Tietz Textbook of

CLINICAL CHEMISTRY *and* MOLECULAR DIAGNOSTICS

Tietz Textbook of CLINICAL CHEMISTRY *and* MOLECULAR DIAGNOSTICS

Carl A. Burtis, Ph.D.
Health Services Division
Oak Ridge National Laboratory
Oak Ridge, Tennessee
Clinical Professor of Pathology
University of Utah School of Medicine
Salt Lake City, Utah

Edward R. Ashwood, M.D.
Professor of Pathology
University of Utah School of Medicine
President and CEO
ARUP Laboratories
Salt Lake City, Utah

David E. Bruns, M.D.
Professor of Pathology
University of Virginia School of Medicine
Director of Clinical Chemistry and Associate Director of Molecular Diagnostics
University of Virginia Health System
Charlottesville, Virginia

FIFTH EDITION

With 909 illustrations

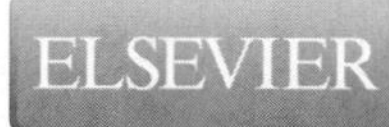

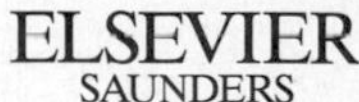

SAUNDERS

3251 Riverport Lane
St. Louis, Missouri 63043

TIETZ TEXTBOOK OF CLINICAL CHEMISTRY AND MOLECULAR DIAGNOSTICS ISBN: 978-1-4160-6164-9

Notices

Knowledge and best practice in this field are constantly changing. As new research and experience broaden our understanding, changes in research methods, professional practices, or medical treatment may become necessary.

Practitioners and researchers must always rely on their own experience and knowledge in evaluating and using any information, methods, compounds, or experiments described herein. In using such information or methods they should be mindful of their own safety and the safety of others, including parties for whom they have a professional responsibility.

With respect to any drug or pharmaceutical products identified, readers are advised to check the most current information provided (i) on procedures featured or (ii) by the manufacturer of each product to be administered, to verify the recommended dose or formula, the method and duration of administration, and contraindications. It is the responsibility of practitioners, relying on their own experience and knowledge of their patients, to make diagnoses, to determine dosages and the best treatment for each individual patient, and to take all appropriate safety precautions.

To the fullest extent of the law, neither the Publisher nor the authors, contributors, or editors assume any liability for any injury and/or damage to persons or property as a matter of product liability, negligence or otherwise, or from any use or operation of any methods, products, instructions, or ideas contained in the material herein.

Library of Congress Cataloging-in-Publication Data

Tietz textbook of clinical chemistry and molecular diagnostics / [edited by] Carl A. Burtis, Edward R. Ashwood, David E. Bruns.—5th ed.
p.; cm.
Textbook of clinical chemistry and molecular diagnostics
Clinical chemistry and molecular diagnostics
Includes bibliographical references and index.
ISBN 978-1-4160-6164-9 (hardcover : alk. paper)
I. Burtis, Carl A. II. Ashwood, Edward R., 1953- III. Bruns, David E., 1941- IV. Tietz, Norbert W., 1926- V. Title: Textbook of clinical chemistry and molecular diagnostics. VI. Title: Clinical chemistry and molecular diagnostics.
[DNLM: 1. Chemistry, Clinical—methods. 2. Molecular Diagnostic Techniques. QY 90]
LC classification not assigned
616.07′56—dc23

2011030889

Publishing Director: Andrew Allen
Managing Editor: Ellen Wurm-Cutter
Publishing Services Manager: Catherine Jackson
Senior Project Manager: Rachel E. McMullen
Senior Designer: Paula Catalano

Printed in the United States of America

Last digit is the print number: 9 8 7 6 5 4 3 2 1

To William L. Roberts, M.D., Ph.D.

A trusted friend and respected colleague

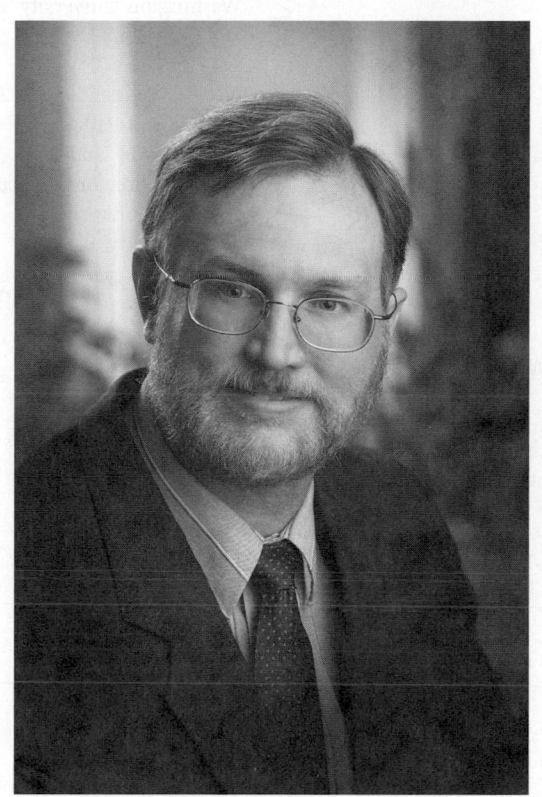

Associate Editors

Ann. M. Gronowski, Ph.D.
Professor, Pathology & Immunology and Obstetrics & Gynecology
Washington University School of Medicine
St. Louis, Missouri

W. Greg Miller, Ph.D.
Professor of Pathology
Director of Clinical Chemistry
Director of Pathology Information Systems
Virginia Commonwealth University Medical Center
Richmond, Virginia

Michael Oellerich, M.D., F.F.Path.(R.C.P.I), F.R.C.Path.
Director, Department of Clinical Chemistry
George-August-University
University Medical Center Göttingen
Göttingen, Germany

François Rousseau, M.D., M.Sc., F.R.C.P.C.
FRSQ/MSSS/CHUQ Research Chair in Technology Assessment and Evidence-Based Laboratory Medicine
Head, Department of Medical Biology
Centre Hospitalier Universitaire de Québec
Titular Professor, Department of Molecular Biology, Medical Biochemistry, & Pathology
Faculty of Medicine, Université Laval
Québec City, Québec, Canada

Mitchell G. Scott, Ph.D.
Professor of Pathology and Immunology
Co-Medical Director, Clinical Chemistry
Division of Laboratory and Genomic Medicine
Washington University School of Medicine
St. Louis, Missouri

Karl V. Voelkerding, M.D.
Professor of Pathology
University of Utah
Medical Director for Genomics and Bioinformatics
ARUP Laboratories
Salt Lake City, Utah

Reviewers

Dave Armbruster, Ph.D., D.A.B.C.C., F.A.C.B.
Scientific Affairs Manager
Global Scientific Affairs
Abbott Diagnostics
Abbott Park, Illinois

Charles Eby, M.D.
Department of Pathology & Immunology
Washington University School of Medicine
St. Louis, Missouri

Doris M. Haverstick, Ph.D.
Department of Pathology
University of Virginia
Charlottesville, Virginia

Marisa A. Needham, Ph.D.
Department of Pathology
University of Virginia
Charlottesville, Virginia

Kristi J. Smock, M.D.
ARUP Laboratories
University of Utah
Salt Lake City, Utah

Contributors

Thomas M. Annesley, Ph.D.
Professor of Clinical Chemistry
University of Michigan Health Center
Ann Arbor, Michigan
Mass Spectrometry

Fred S. Apple, Ph.D.
Medical Director, Clinical Laboratories
Hennepin County Medical Center
Professor of Laboratory Medicine and Pathology
University of Minnesota School of Medicine
Minneapolis, Minnesota
Cardiac Function

Edward R. Ashwood, M.D.
Professor of Pathology
University of Utah School of Medicine
President and CEO
ARUP Laboratories
Salt Lake City, Utah
Introduction to Laboratory Medicine; Clinical Evaluation of Methods; Pregnancy and Its Disorders

Michael N. Badminton, M.B., Ch.B., Ph.D., F.R.C.Path.
Clinical Senior Lecturer
Department of Infection, Immunity, & Biochemistry
School of Medicine
Cardiff University
Cardiff, United Kingdom
The Porphyrias and Other Disorders of Porphyrin Metabolism

Renze Bais, Ph.D., A.R.C.P.A.
Senior Clinical Associate
Department of Medicine
University of Sydney
Chief Operating Officer
Pacific Laboratory Medicine Services, Pathology North
Royal North Shore Hospital
Sydney, NSW, Australia
Enzyme and Rate Analyses; Serum Enzymes

James C. Barton, M.D.
Medical Director, Southern Iron Disorders Center
Clinical Professor of Medicine
University of Alabama at Birmingham
Birmingham, Alabama
Hemoglobin, Iron, and Bilirubin

Howard J. Baum, Ph.D.
Director, Office of Forensic Sciences
New Jersey State Police
Hamilton, New Jersey
Identity Assessment

Lindsay A. L. Bazydlo, Ph.D.
Co-Medical Director, Clinical Chemistry
Assistant Clinical Professor
Department of Pathology, Immunology, & Laboratory Medicine
University of Florida
Gainesville, Florida
Microfabrication and Microfluidics and Their Application to Clinical Diagnostics

Laura Bechtel, Ph.D., D.A.B.C.C.
Director of Clinical Pharmacology
Assistant Attending
Clinical Chemistry Service
Department of Laboratory Medicine
Memorial Sloan-Kettering Cancer Center
New York City, New York
Clinical Toxicology

Roger L. Bertholf, Ph.D.
Director of Clinical Chemistry, Toxicology, and Point-of-Care Testing
University of Florida Health Science Center/Jacksonville
Professor of Pathology
University of Florida College of Medicine
Jacksonville, Florida
Pituitary Function and Pathophysiology; The Adrenal Cortex; The Thyroid: Pathophysiology and Thyroid Function Testing

Aaron D. Bossler, M.D., Ph.D.
Assistant Professor
Department of Pathology
Carver College of Medicine
University of Iowa
Director, Molecular Pathology Laboratory
Director, Molecular Infectious Diseases
University of Iowa Hospitals and Clinics
Iowa City, Iowa
Molecular Methods in Diagnosis and Monitoring of Infectious Diseases

Patrick M. M. Bossuyt, Ph.D.
Professor of Clinical Epidemiology
Department of Clinical Epidemiology, Biostatistics, & Bioinformatics
Academic Medical Center
University of Amsterdam
The Netherlands
Evidence Based Laboratory Medicine

James C. Boyd, M.D.
Associate Professor of Pathology
Director of Core Laboratory Automation
Director of Systems Engineering
Associate Director of Clinical Chemistry and Toxicology
University of Virginia Health System
Charlottesville, Virginia
Selection and Analytical Evaluation of Methods—With Statistical Techniques; Automation in the Clinical Laboratory

David E. Bruns, M.D.
Professor of Pathology
University of Virginia School of Medicine
Director of Clinical Chemistry and Associate Director of Molecular Diagnostics
University of Virginia Health System
Charlottesville, Virginia
Introduction to Laboratory Medicine; Clinical Evaluation of Methods; Evidence Based Laboratory Medicine; Reference Information for the Clinical Laboratory

Carl A. Burtis, Ph.D.
Health Services Division
Oak Ridge National Laboratory
Oak Ridge, Tennessee
Clinical Professor of Pathology
University of Utah School of Medicine
Salt Lake City, Utah
Introduction to Laboratory Medicine; Reference Information for the Clinical Laboratory

Angela M. Caliendo, M.D., Ph.D.
Professor and Vice Chair
Pathology and Laboratory Medicine
Emory University School of Medicine
Director, Emory Medical Laboratories
Emory University Hospital
Atlanta, Georgia
Molecular Methods in Diagnosis and Monitoring of Infectious Diseases

Daniel W. Chan, Ph.D., D.A.B.C.C., F.A.C.B.
Professor of Pathology, Oncology, Radiology, and Urology
Director, Clinical Chemistry Division & Center for Biomarker Discovery and Translation
Co-Director, Pathology Core Laboratories
Department of Pathology
Johns Hopkins Medical Institutions
Baltimore, Maryland
Tumor Markers

Rossa W. K. Chiu, M.B.B.S., Ph.D., F.H.K.A.M. (Pathology), F.R.C.P.A.
Professor
Department of Chemical Pathology
The Chinese University of Hong Kong
Specialist in Chemical Pathology
Honorary Consultant
Prince of Wales Hospital
Hong Kong SAR, China
Principles of Molecular Biology; Nucleic Acid Isolation; Plasma Nucleic Acids

Allan C. Deacon, Ph.D., F.R.C.Path.
Consultant Clinical Scientist (Retired)
Clinical Biochemistry Department
Bedford Hospital
Bedford, United Kingdom
The Porphyrias and Other Disorders of Porphyrin Metabolism

Michael P. Delaney, B.Sc., M.D., F.R.C.P.
Consultant Nephrologist
East Kent Hospitals University NHS Foundation Trust
Kent and Canterbury Hospital
Canterbury, Kent, United Kingdom
Kidney Disease

Paul D'Orazio, Ph.D.
Director, Critical Care Analytical Research and Development
Instrumentation Laboratory
Bedford, Massachusetts
Electrochemistry and Chemical Sensors

Basil T. Doumas, Ph.D.
Professor Emeritus
Department of Pathology
Medical College of Wisconsin
Milwaukee, Wisconsin
Hemoglobin, Iron, and Bilirubin

D. Robert Dufour, M.D., F.C.A.P., F.A.C.B.
Consultant, Pathology and Hepatology
Veterans Affairs Medical Center
Emeritus Professor of Pathology
George Washington University Medical Center
Washington, DC
Liver Disease

John H. Eckfeldt, M.D., Ph.D.
Ellis Benson Professor and Vice Chair for Clinical Affairs
Department of Laboratory Medicine & Pathology
University of Minnesota
Minneapolis, Minnesota
Hemoglobin, Iron, and Bilirubin

Graeme Eisenhofer, Ph.D.
Professor
Department of Medicine III
Institute of Clinical Chemistry and Laboratory Medicine
Chief, Division of Clinical Neurochemistry
University Hospital Carl Gustav Carus Dresden at the Dresden University of Technology
Dresden, Germany
Catecholamines and Serotonin

George H. Elder, M.D., F.R.C.P., F.R.C.Path.
Emeritus Professor
Department of Infection, Immunity, & Biochemistry
School of Medicine
Cardiff University
Cardiff, United Kingdom
The Porphyrias and Other Disorders of Porphyrin Metabolism

Kojo S. J. Elenitoba-Johnson, M.D.
Professor of Pathology
University of Michigan Medical School
University of Michigan Hospital
Ann Arbor, Michigan
Hematopoietic Malignancies

Jens Peter Goetze, M.D., D.M.Sc.
Chief Physician
Department of Clinical Biochemistry
Rigshospitalet
Associate Professor
University of Copenhagen
Copenhagen, Denmark
Cardiac Function

Bruce A. Goldberger, Ph.D.
Professor and Director of Toxicology
Departments of Pathology and Psychiatry
University of Florida College of Medicine
Gainesville, Florida
Chromatography and Extraction

David G. Grenache, Ph.D., M.T.(A.S.C.P.), D.A.B.C.C., F.A.C.B.
Associate Professor of Pathology
University of Utah School of Medicine
Medical Director, Special Chemistry
ARUP Laboratories
Salt Lake City, Utah
Pregnancy and Its Disorders

Ann M. Gronowski, Ph.D.
Professor, Department of Pathology & Immunology
Professor, Department of Obstetrics & Gynecology
Washington University School of Medicine
St. Louis, Missouri
Reproductive Endocrinology and Related Disorders

Amy R. Groszbach, M.ED., M.L.T., M.B.(A.S.C.P.)[C.M.]
Education Specialist II
Molecular Genetics Laboratory, Mayo Clinic
Program Director, Molecular Genetics Technology Internship Program
Mayo School of Health Science, Mayo Clinic
Rochester, Minnesota
Specimen Collection and Processing

Doris M. Haverstick, Ph.D., D.A.B.C.C.
Associate Professor of Pathology
University of Virginia
Charlottesville, Virginia
Specimen Collection and Processing

Charles D. Hawker, Ph.D., M.B.A., F.A.C.B.
Professor (Adjunct) of Pathology
University of Utah School of Medicine
Scientific Director, Automation & Special Projects
ARUP Laboratories
Salt Lake City, Utah
Automation in the Clinical Laboratory

Russell A. Higgins, M.D.
Assistant Professor
Director, Hematology Laboratory
University of Texas Health Science Center San Antonio
San Antonio, Texas
Hemostasis

Trefor Higgins, M.Sc.
Director of Clinical Chemistry
DynaLIFE$_{Dx}$
Clinical Professor
Department of Laboratory Medicine & Pathology
Faculty of Medicine
University of Alberta
Edmonton, Alberta
Hemoglobin, Iron, and Bilirubin

Peter G. Hill, B.Sc., Ph.D., F.R.C.Path, Dip.Hlth.Mgt.
Emeritus Consultant Clinical Biochemist
Royal Derby Hospital
Derby, United Kingdom
Gastric, Pancreatic, and Intestinal Function

Christopher P. Holstege, M.D.
Chief, Division of Medical Toxicology
Associate Professor, Departments of Emergency Medicine and Pediatrics
University of Virginia School of Medicine
Medical Director, Blue Ridge Poison Center
University of Virginia Health System
Charlottesville, Virginia
Clinical Toxicology

Joshua L. Hood, M.D., Ph.D.
Research Instructor
Consortium for Translational Research in Advanced Imaging and Nanomedicine (C-TRAIN)
Washington University
St. Louis, Missouri
Electrolytes and Blood Gases; Physiology and Disorders of Water, Electrolyte, and Acid-Base Metabolism

Gary L. Horowitz, M.D.
Associate Professor of Pathology
Harvard Medical School
Director of Clinical Chemistry
Beth Israel Deaconess Medical Center
Boston, Massachusetts
Establishment and Use of Reference Values

Glen L. Hortin, M.D., Ph.D.
Medical Director
Cincinnati Business Unit
Quest Diagnostics
Cincinnati, Ohio
Chromatography and Extraction; Amino Acids, Peptides, and Proteins

T. Scott Isbell, Ph.D.
Clinical Chemistry Fellow
Department of Pathology & Immunology
Division of Laboratory & Genomic Medicine
Washington University School of Medicine
St. Louis, Missouri
Reproductive Endocrinology and Related Disorders

Allan S. Jaffe, M.D.
Consultant in Cardiology and Laboratory Medicine
Professor of Medicine
Chair, CCLS Division of Laboratory Medicine & Pathology
Mayo Clinic and Medical School
Rochester, Minnesota
Cardiac Function

Ishwarlal Jialal, M.D., Ph.D., F.R.C.Path(London), D.A.B.C.C.
Robert E. Stowell Endowed Chair in Experimental Pathology
Director of the Laboratory for Atherosclerosis and Metabolic Research
Professor of Internal Medicine (Endocrinology, Diabetes, and Metabolism)
University of California Davis Medical Center
Sacramento, California
Pituitary Function and Pathophysiology; The Adrenal Cortex

Emily S. Jungheim, M.D.
Instructor
Washington University
Endocrinologist
Barnes Jewish Hospital
St. Louis, Missouri
Reproductive Endocrinology and Related Disorders

Raymond E. Karcher, Ph.D.
Adjunct Associate Professor
Oakland University
Rochester, Michigan
Clinical Chemist
William Beaumont Hospital
Royal Oak, Michigan
Electrophoresis

Malek Kaumon, M.D., Ph.D.
Professor of Pathology and Laboratory Medicine
University of Pennsylvania School of Medicine
Director, Clinical Immunology & Histocompatibility Laboratory
Hospital of the University of Pennsylvania
Philadelphia, Pennsylvania
Identity Assessment

Steve Kitchen, Ph.D.
Lead Scientist
Department of Coagulation
Sheffield Teaching Hospitals
Sheffield, United Kingdom
Hemostasis

George G. Klee, M.D., Ph.D.
Professor of Laboratory Medicine & Pathology
College of Medicine
Staff Consultant
Department of Laboratory Medicine & Pathology
Mayo Clinic
Rochester, Minnesota
Quality Management

Michael Kleerekoper, M.D., F.A.C.B., F.A.C.P., M.A.C.E.
Clinical Professor of Medicine/Endocrinology
Wayne State University
Detroit, Michigan
Hormones; Bone and Mineral Metabolism

Larry J. Kricka, D.Phil., F.A.C.B., C.Chem., F.R.S.C., F.R.C.Path.
Professor
University of Pennsylvania
Director of General Chemistry
Hospital of the University of Pennsylvania
Philadelphia, Pennsylvania
Optical Techniques; Principles of Immunochemical Techniques

Noriko Kusukawa, Ph.D.
Director, New Technology Assessment & Licensing
ARUP Laboratories
Adjunct Associate Professor of Pathology
University of Utah School of Medicine
Salt Lake City, Utah
Nucleic Acid Techniques; Genomes and Nucleic Acid Alterations

Edmund J. Lamb, Ph.D., F.R.C.Path.
Head, Clinical Biochemistry
East Kent Hospitals University NHS Foundation Trust
Canterbury, Kent, United Kingdom
Kidney Function Tests; Kidney Disease

Geralyn Lambert-Messerlian, Ph.D.
Associate Professor
Department of Pathology & Laboratory Medicine
Alpert Medical School of Brown University
Associate Director
Division of Prenatal & Special Testing
Women and Infants Hospital of Rhode Island
Providence, Rhode Island
Pregnancy and Its Disorders

James P. Landers, Ph.D.
Professor of Chemistry
Professor of Mechanical Engineering
University of Virginia
Associate Professor of Pathology
Member-UVA Cancer Center
University of Virginia School of Medicine
Charlottesville, Virginia
Electrophoresis; Microfabrication and Microfluidics and Their Application to Clinical Diagnostics

Loralie Langman, Ph.D., F.C.A.C.B., D.A.B.C.C. (C.C., M.B., T.C.), D.A.B.F.T.
Director, Toxicology and Drug Monitoring Laboratory
Department of Laboratory Medicine & Pathology
Mayo Clinic
Associate Professor of Laboratory Medicine and Pathology
Mayo Clinic College of Medicine
Rochester, Minnesota
Clinical Toxicology

Vicky A. LeGrys, Ph.D., Dr.A., M.T.(A.S.C.P), C.L.S.(N.C.A.)
Professor
Division of Clinical Laboratory Science
School of Medicine
University of North Carolina at Chapel Hill
Chapel Hill, North Carolina
Electrolytes and Blood Gases

Kristian Linnet, M.D., Ph.D.
Professor, Chief, Section of Forensic Chemistry
Department of Forensic Medicine, Faculty of Health Sciences
University of Copenhagen
Copenhagen, Denmark
Selection and Analytical Evaluation of Methods—With Statistical Techniques

Y. M. Dennis Lo, M.A., D.M., D.Phil., F.R.C.P. (Lond. & Edin.), F.R.C.Path., F.R.S.
Li Ka Shing Professor of Medicine and Professor of Chemical Pathology
Department of Chemical Pathology
The Chinese University of Hong Kong
Honorary Chief of Service
Prince of Wales Hospital
Hong Kong SAR, China
Principles of Molecular Biology; Nucleic Acid Isolation; Plasma Nucleic Acids

Stanley F. Lo, Ph.D., D.A.B.C.C., F.A.C.B
Associate Professor of Pathology
Medical College of Wisconsin
Associate Director, Clinical Laboratories
Children's Hospital of Wisconsin
Milwaukee, Wisconsin
Principles of Basic Techniques and Laboratory Safety

Nicola Longo, M.D., Ph.D.
Professor of Pediatrics and Pathology
Chief, Division of Medical Genetics
Department of Pediatrics
Medical Co-Director, ARUP Biochemical Genetics Laboratory
University of Utah
Salt Lake City, Utah
Newborn Screening and Inborn Errors of Metabolism

Gwendolyn A. McMillin, Ph.D., D.A.B.C.C. (C.C., T.C.)
Clinical Associate Professor of Pathology
University of Utah School of Medicine
Medical Director, Clinical Drug Abuse Testing, Trace Elements
Co-Medical Director, Pharmacogenomics
ARUP Laboratories
Salt Lake City, Utah
Therapeutic Drugs and Their Management; Pharmacogenetics; Reference Information for the Clinical Laboratory

Mark E. Meyerhoff, Ph.D.
Philip J. Elving Professor of Chemistry
The University of Michigan
Department of Chemistry
Ann Arbor, Michigan
Electrochemistry and Chemical Sensors

Thomas P. Moyer, Ph.D.
Professor of Laboratory Medicine
Mayo College of Medicine
Mayo Clinic
Rochester, Minnesota
Therapeutic Drugs and Their Management; Toxic Metals

John D. Olson, M.D., Ph.D.
Professor and Vice Chair for Clinical Affairs
Department of Pathology
University of Texas Health Science Center
Director of Clinical Laboratories
University Health System
San Antonio, Texas
Hemostasis

Mauro Panteghini, M.D.
Professor of Clinical Biochemistry and Clinical Molecular Biology
Department of Clinical Sciences
University of Milan Medical School
Director, Clinical Biochemistry Laboratory
Ospedale "Luigi Sacco"
Milan, Italy
Enzyme and Rate Analyses; Serum Enzymes

Jason Y. Park, M.D., Ph.D., F.A.C.P.
Assistant Professor
Department of Pathology
University of Texas Southwestern Medical Center
Associate Director
Advanced Diagnostics Laboratory
Children's Medical Center
Dallas, Texas
Optical Techniques; Principles of Immunochemical Techniques

Marzia Pasquali, Ph.D., F.A.C.M.G.
Professor of Pathology
University of Utah School of Medicine
Medical Director, Biochemical Genetics & Supplemental Newborn Screening
ARUP Laboratories
Salt Lake City, Utah
Newborn Screening and Inborn Errors of Metabolism

Christopher P. Price, Ph.D., F.R.S.C., F.R.C.Path.
Visiting Professor in Clinical Biochemistry
Department of Primary Care Health Sciences
University of Oxford
Oxford, United Kingdom
Evidence Based Laboratory Medicine; Point-of-Care Testing; Kidney Function Tests; Kidney Disease

Alex J. Rai, Ph.D., D.A.B.C.C., F.A.C.B.
Director, Special Chemistry Laboratory
New York Presbyterian Hospital
Assistant Professor of Pathology
Chief Scientific Officer
Center for Advanced Laboratory Medicine
Department of Pathology & Cell Biology
Columbia University Medical Center
New York, New York
Tumor Markers

Alan T. Remaley, M.D., Ph.D.
Department of Laboratory Medicine
National Institutes of Health
Bethesda, Maryland
Lipids, Lipoproteins, Apolipoproteins, and Other Cardiovascular Risk Factors

Nader Rifai, Ph.D.
Director, Clinical Chemistry
Department of Laboratory Medicine
Children's Hospital Boston
Professor
Harvard Medical School
Boston, Massachusetts
Editor-in-Chief, *Clinical Chemistry*
Washington, D.C.
Lipids, Lipoproteins, Apolipoproteins, and Other Cardiovascular Risk Factors

Juha Risteli, M.D., Ph.D., F.E.B.M.B.
Professor of Clinical Chemistry
Department of Clinical Chemistry
Institute of Diagnostics
University of Oulu
Chief Physician (Part-Time)
Laboratory
Oulu University Hospital
Oulu, Finland
Bone and Mineral Metabolism

Leila Risteli, M.D., Ph.D., M.A., F.E.B.M.B.
Chief Physician
Laboratory
Oulu University Hospital
Adjunct Professor of Medical Biochemistry
University of Oulu
Oulu, Finland
Adjunct Professor of Clinical Chemistry
University of Tampere
Tampere, Finland
Bone and Mineral Metabolism

Norman B. Roberts, M.Sc., Ph.D., C.Chem.
Consultant Clinical Scientist
Department of Clinical Biochemistry
The Royal Liverpool and Broadgreen University Hospitals
Honorary Reader
Clinical Chemistry
The University of Liverpool
Liverpool, United Kingdom
Vitamins and Trace Elements

William L. Roberts, M.D., Ph.D.
Professor of Pathology
University of Utah School of Medicine
Medical Director, Automated Core Laboratory
ARUP Laboratories
Salt Lake City, Utah
Reference Information for the Clinical Laboratory

Alan L. Rockwood, Ph.D., D.A.B.C.C.
Scientific Director for Mass Spectrometry
ARUP Laboratories
Associate Professor (Clinical) of Pathology
University of Utah School of Medicine
Salt Lake City, Utah
Mass Spectrometry

Thomas G. Rosano, Ph.D., D.A.B.C.C., D.A.B.F.T.
Head of Clinical Laboratory Services
Director of Clinical Chemistry & Forensic Toxicology
Professor of Pathology and Laboratory Medicine
Albany Medical Center Hospital & College
Albany, New York
Catecholamines and Serotonin

David B. Sacks, M.B., Ch.B., F.R.C.Path.
Senior Investigator
Chief, Clinical Chemistry
National Institutes of Health
Bethesda, Maryland
Carbohydrates; Diabetes Mellitus

Desmond Schatz, M.D.
Professor and Associate Chairman
Department of Pediatrics
Division of Endocrinology
Medical Director, Diabetes Center
University of Florida
Gainesville, Florida
The Thyroid: Pathophysiology and Thyroid Function Testing

Mitchell G. Scott, Ph.D.
Professor of Pathology and Immunology
Co-Medical Director, Clinical Chemistry
Division of Laboratory & Genomic Medicine
Washington University School of Medicine
St. Louis, Missouri
Electrolytes and Blood Gases; Physiology and Disorders of Water, Electrolyte, and Acid-Base Metabolism

Alan Shenkin, Ph.D.
Professor
Unit of Clinical Chemistry
School of Clinical Sciences
University of Liverpool
Liverpool, England
Vitamins and Trace Elements

Nicholas E. Sherman, Ph.D.
Research Associate Professor
Director of Mass Spectrometry
University of Virginia
Charlottesville, Virginia
Mass Spectrometry

Christine L. H. Snozek, Ph.D.
Assistant Professor
Mayo Clinic College of Medicine
Associate Director, Toxicology and Drug Monitoring Laboratory
Department of Laboratory Medicine & Pathology
Mayo Clinic
Rochester, Minnesota
Therapeutic Drugs and Their Management

Lori J. Sokoll, Ph.D., F.A.C.B.
Associate Professor of Pathology, Oncology, and Urology
Associate Director, Clinical Chemistry Division
Department of Pathology
Johns Hopkins Medical Institutions
Baltimore, Maryland
Tumor Markers

Andrew St. John, Ph.D., M.A.A.C.B.
Consultant
ARC Consulting
Perth, W. Australia
Point-of-Care Testing

Wouter W. van Solinge, Ph.D.
Head of Department and Medical Director, Division Laboratories & Pharmacy
Professor of Clinical Chemistry and Laboratory Medicine
Department of Clinical Chemistry & Haematology
University Medical Center Utrecht
Utrecht University, Faculty of Science
Utrecht Institute for Pharmaceutical Sciences
Division Pharmacoepidemiology & Clinical Pharmacology
Utrecht, The Netherlands
Enzymes of the Red Blood Cell

Richard van Wijk, Ph.D.
Assistant Professor
Laboratory for Red Blood Cell Research
Department of Clinical Chemistry & Haematology
University Medical Center Utrecht
Utrecht, The Netherlands
Enzymes of the Red Blood Cell

Mary Lee Vance, M.D.
University of Virginia School of Medicine Charlottesville, VA
Professor of Medicine and Neurosurgery
Pituitary Function and Pathophysiology; The Adrenal Cortex

Cindy L. Vnencak-Jones, Ph.D., F.A.C.M.G.
Director, Molecular Diagnostics Laboratory
Vanderbilt University Medical Center
Professor, Department of Pathology, Microbiology, & Immunology and Department of Pediatrics
Vanderbilt University School of Medicine
Nashville, Tennessee
Inherited Diseases

G. Russell Warnick, M.S., M.B.A.
Executive Director
Foundation for Health Information and Technology
Chief Science Officer
Health Diagnostic Laboratory
Richmond, Virginia
Lipids, Lipoproteins, Apolipoproteins, and Other Cardiovascular Risk Factors

Victor W. Weedn, M.D., J.D.
Assistant Medical Examiner
Office of the Chief Medical Examiner
Baltimore, Maryland
Identity Assessment

James O. Westgard, Ph.D.
Professor Emeritus
University of Wisconsin Medical School
Madison, Wisconsin
Quality Management

Sharon D. Whatley, Ph.D.
Clinical Biochemist
Department of Medical Biochemistry & Immunology
University Hospital of Wales
Cardiff, United Kingdom
The Porphyrias and Other Disorders of Porphyrin Metabolism

Ronald J. Whitley, Ph.D., D.A.B.C.C., F.A.C.B.
Professor
Department of Pathology & Laboratory Medicine
University of Kentucky
Director of Clinical Chemistry, Toxicology and Core Laboratories
University of Kentucky Medical Center College of Medicine
Lexington, Kentucky
Catecholamines and Serotonin

Thomas M. Williams, M.D.
Professor and Chair of Pathology
University of New Mexico
TriCore Reference Laboratories
Albuquerque, New Mexico
Identity Assessment

William E. Winter, M.D.
Professor, Departments of Pathology, Immunology & Laboratory Medicine, Pediatrics, and Molecular Genetics & Microbiology
Principle Investigator, Type 1 Diabetes TrialNet ICA Core Laboratory
Director, UF Pathology Laboratories, Endocrine Autoantibody Laboratory
Pathology Course Director
University of Florida
Department of Pathology, Immunology, & Laboratory Medicine
Gainesville, Florida
Bone and Mineral Metabolism; Pituitary Function and Pathophysiology; The Adrenal Cortex; The Thyroid: Pathophysiology and Thyroid Function Testing

Carl T. Wittwer, M.D., Ph.D.
Professor of Pathology
University of Utah School of Medicine
Salt Lake City, Utah
Nucleic Acid Techniques; Genomes and Nucleic Acid Alterations

Donald S. Young, M.B., Ph.D.
Professor of Pathology and Laboratory Medicine
University of Pennsylvania Medical School
Philadelphia, Pennsylvania
Preanalytical Variables and Biological Variation

Foreword

Laboratory medicine is at the center of the multidisciplinary healthcare team. Laboratory medicine specialists have a responsibility to convert data into evidence-based knowledge and added value that is then applied to clinical situations in the interests of improved patient outcomes and experiences. To reach this advanced level of knowledge and practice, the laboratory medicine specialist needs support. In the clinical chemistry specialty, that support is available through the *Tietz Textbook of Clinical Chemistry and Molecular Diagnostics*.

The 4th edition of the *Tietz Textbook of Clinical Chemistry and Molecular Diagnostics* published in 2005 enhanced the status of the *Tietz Textbook* as the definitive reference work in the field. In common with so many areas of medicine, clinical chemistry and molecular diagnostics is advancing at a considerable rate, and so this 5th edition is both welcome and important. It brings new knowledge, fresh insights, and a growing appreciation of the central role of laboratory medicine in healthcare.

The 60 chapters in the 5th edition span the full range of clinical chemistry and molecular diagnostics from principles through to pathophysiology and clinical use. Each chapter has been written by international experts, and so the textbook benefits from their many contributions. Their knowledge and expertise have been skillfully blended by the established editorial team of Dr. Carl A. Burtis, Dr. Edward R. Ashwood, and Dr. David E. Bruns, ably assisted by a strong international team of Associate Editors. The result is a text that is comprehensive but easy to read and understand. Whether the reader is a student studying clinical chemistry and molecular diagnostics, an established professional who wants to update knowledge and understanding, or a clinician who wishes to find a specific piece of information, the *Tietz Textbook* will deliver.

This is an important time for clinical chemistry and molecular diagnostics with parallel developments in technology and clinical practice, including the following:

- The advent of a variety of point-of-care testing devices that are sophisticated in design but simple to use, and that bring laboratory medicine to the doctor's office, to the workplace, and to the home
- The impact of automation and robotics in enhancing analytical capacity and throughput in the clinical laboratory
- The impact of DNA sequencing and other genomic technologies that have the potential to rapidly obtain and analyze comprehensive genetic information that will help unravel the mystery of disease causation and will direct targeted therapies
- The appreciation that knowledge acquired from clinical chemistry and other laboratory medicine investigations may be used in evidence-based algorithms and clinical guidelines as part of an integrated approach to healthcare
- The development of personalized medicine, which recognizes that we are all different and uses genetic and other information to predict, prevent, and optimize therapy for the individual person
- The promise of regenerative medicine and living cell–based therapies, which have the potential to repair damaged pathways, rejuvenate the immune system, and restore health to many who now live with chronic disease and tissue damage
- The accessibility of advanced technologies in routine laboratory practice, enabling analysis of the end products of cellular processes and expanding metabolic profiling techniques to the investigation of cancer and metabolic regulatory disorders
- The globalization of healthcare, which facilitates harmonization of practice and assists the rapid development of laboratory medicine services in emerging nations
- The recognition that high quality in the preanalytical, analytical, and postanalytical phases, coupled with demonstrable value for money, is integral to the future of laboratory medicine

These developments all represent subspecialties in their own right, but they are also topics that should be fixed in the mind of every laboratory medicine specialist. True to its reputation and status as the world's leading text, the 5th edition of *Tietz Textbook of Clinical Chemistry and Molecular Diagnostics* addresses all of these issues, in addition to providing the essential foundations from which our discipline has evolved.

Dr. Graham H. Beastall
President of the International Federation of Clinical Chemistry and Laboratory Medicine
University of Glasgow
Mayfield, Birdston, United Kingdom

Dr. Susan A. Evans
Corporate Strategic Planning
Beckman Coulter, Inc.
Brea, California

Preface

The intertwined disciplines of Clinical Chemistry and Molecular Diagnostics continue to expand in depth and breadth, a process that has blurred traditional boundaries between them and other disciplines of laboratory medicine. As a result of this dynamic and relentless explosion of technical and medical advances, clinical laboratories have entered an era of rapid test growth and menu expansion. The knowledge base that defines the field has expanded exponentially, thus placing additional burdens on laboratory professionals to maintain their technical expertise and consultative skills.

To provide an authoritative textbook that contains a current and comprehensive overview of this knowledge base is a challenging and daunting task that threatened to overwhelm our ability to cover all relevant topics. Consequently, to assist us in the endeavor of producing this 5th edition of the *Tietz Textbook of Clinical Chemistry and Molecular Diagnostics,* we organized and recruited a board of associate editors comprising senior and experienced laboratorians. These subject matter experts were asked to edit chapters that contained information most familiar to them. Authorities composing this committee were Drs. Ann Gronowski, W. Greg Miller, Michael Oellerich, Francois Rousseau, Mitchell Scott, and Karl Voelkerding. The three of us thank these associate editors for their hard work and dedication. We are confident that readers of the new edition will discover and benefit from their expertise and superb editing skills and the resultant strengthening of chapters in this new edition. In addition to these associate editors, who edited multiple chapters, we asked colleagues to review single chapters, and we wish to thank Drs. Dave Armbruster, Charles Eby, Doris M. Haverstick, and Kristi J. Smock for their help as reviewers.

Another challenge we faced was the mandate from the publisher that the 5th edition be produced in a single volume. Consequently, we spent many hours reviewing and revising the table of contents. This required some cutting and condensing of chapters and topics, but we were able to retain the chapters on molecular diagnostics, which appeared for the first time in the last edition. Also, because we received multiple requests from readers of previous editions for a chapter on coagulation, we added a chapter on that topic and are grateful to Drs. John Olson, Steve Kitchen, and Russell Higgins for producing a comprehensive and readable chapter on hemostasis and thrombosis.

Many new authors have joined our team of core veterans from previous editions. In fact, 40 of the 99 authors represented in the 5th edition are new to the effort. We believe that these knowledgeable and enthusiastic new authors and our expert core of veteran authors, associate editors, and reviewers of specific chapters have produced chapters that are timely and reflect the state of the art of topics addressed. The international flavor of the book and the global nature of the field are more evident than ever before in the list of countries represented by this outstanding group of colleagues.

Information technology continued to have a significant role in the preparation and production of the 5th edition. As with the last edition, each chapter was submitted electronically. A new tool that was utilized in the 5th edition was Elsevier's Electronic Manuscript Submission System (EMSS). With it, each chapter including figures was uploaded into the book's template. Editors accessed and edited chapters as they became available and then uploaded their revised drafts. Once all 60 chapters were submitted and the editing process completed, the entire book was sent to our project manager at Elsevier, and the production process started. As with previous editions of the *Textbook,* many of the figures, especially those that included chemical structures, were drawn or revised by one of us (E.R.A.) using ChemWindows software (http://www.softshell.com; accessed August 26, 2011). This resulted in a uniform representation of chemical structures and facilitated the integration of figures with text while reducing errors.

We greatly appreciate the opportunity provided to us by Elsevier to participate in the preparation of the 5th edition of this textbook. It has been an exciting, challenging, and educational experience. We have endeavored to ensure that this edition will live up to the reputation and success of its distinguished predecessors. We have benefited from and enjoyed working with the Elsevier staff in St. Louis, especially Managing Editor Ellen Wurm-Cutter and Senior Project Manager Rachel McMullen. Their patience, warm cooperation, sound advice, and professional dedication are gratefully acknowledged.

We would be amiss if we didn't thank the individuals who made all of this possible: our readers. Over the years, we have appreciated and enjoyed having many of you approach us to say how much you enjoyed our books and the significant role they have played in your lives and careers. We have heard from a diverse spectrum of laboratory professionals, including practicing clinical chemists and pathologists; medical, graduate, and medical technology students; clinical chemistry fellows; pathology residents; molecular genetics and pathology fellows; recently board-certified clinical chemists, pathologists, and molecular geneticists; medical librarians; medical researchers; and students who are studying for their Boards. In short, nothing makes us happier than hearing that our book has been helpful and useful!

Regarding the image on the front cover: this visualization depicts the flow of ions and DNA through a single-walled carbon nanotube. Photo courtesy Hao Liu, Arizona State University.

Carl A. Burtis
Edward R. Ashwood
David E. Bruns

Contents

SECTION I

Principles of Laboratory Medicine

CHAPTER 1

Clinical Chemistry, Molecular Diagnostics, and Laboratory Medicine

David E. Bruns, M.D., Edward R. Ashwood, M.D., and Carl A. Burtis, Ph.D.

Clinical chemists, clinical biochemists, chemical pathologists, medical technologists, molecular biologists, and other clinical laboratory scientists are laboratory professionals who play an important role in the global delivery of quality healthcare and public health.[3]

In this chapter, we begin with a general discussion introducing the field of laboratory medicine and the disciplines of clinical chemistry (or clinical biochemistry) and molecular diagnostics. This will include a discussion of the meaning of the term *laboratory medicine* and the relationships among clinical chemistry, molecular diagnostics, laboratory medicine, and evidence-based laboratory medicine. The concepts introduced in this chapter are developed in the remaining chapters of this book.

We end the chapter with a discussion on the ethical issues that clinical chemists/biochemists face in the practice of their profession and issues they will face in the future.

LABORATORY MEDICINE

The term *laboratory medicine* refers to the discipline involved in the selection, provision, and interpretation of diagnostic testing that uses samples from patients. Those active in the field participate in (1) analytical testing, (2) research, (3) administration, (4) teaching activities, and (5) clinical service to varying degrees.

Testing has many uses in laboratory medicine (Box 1-1). In a hospital setting, its use is vital to establish and monitor the severity of a physiologic disturbance. In hospitalized patients, the latter constitutes the largest volume of testing.

Historically, the clinical laboratory as an entity in providing healthcare services began with the manual measurement of a variety of analytes (now termed *measurands*),[10] including (1) metabolites, (2) proteins, (3) lipids, (4) carbohydrates, (5) enzymes, and (6) drugs. The first laboratory attached to a hospital was established in 1886 in Munich, Germany, by Hugo Wilhelm von Ziemssen.[5,8] In the United States, the first clinical laboratory was The William Pepper Laboratory of Clinical Medicine, established in 1895 at the University of Pennsylvania in Philadelphia (http://hss.sas.upenn.edu/microbio/insts2.html). As the demand for these analytical services increased, analytical processes were mechanized and ultimately automated.[9] Technical and scientific advances and the growing understanding of disease at the biochemical and genetic levels have expanded the need for the clinical laboratory to provide analytical services in a broad and diverse spectrum of disciplines (Box 1-2), with clinical chemistry and molecular diagnostics being particularly dynamic as they have developed and expanded alongside the growing understanding of disease at the biochemical and genetic levels. Most individuals entering these two disciplines have backgrounds in biochemistry, molecular biology, physiology, or another biochemistry-related field, and some have backgrounds in areas such as analytical chemistry.[14] Principles of measurement science and metrology, often adapted from the field of analytical chemistry by clinical chemists, have never been more important than they are now, as quantitative molecular methods such as viral load assays and measurement of the numbers of DNA triplet repeats are replacing numerous qualitative techniques throughout medicine.

CLINICAL CHEMISTRY AND LABORATORY MEDICINE

The ties between clinical chemistry and other areas of laboratory medicine have deep roots. Individuals working primarily in the area of clinical chemistry/biochemistry have developed tools and methods that have become part of the fabric of laboratory medicine beyond the clinical chemistry laboratory. Examples include the (1) theory and practice of reference intervals (see Chapter 5), (2) use of both (internal) quality control and proficiency testing (see Chapter 8), (3) introduction of automation into the clinical laboratory (see Chapter 19), and (4) concepts of diagnostic testing (see

BOX 1-1 Uses of Testing in the Clinical Laboratory

- *Confirming* a clinical suspicion (which could include *making* a diagnosis)
- *Excluding* a diagnosis
- Assisting in the *selection, optimization, and monitoring* of treatment
- Providing a *prognosis*
- *Screening* for disease in the absence of clinical signs or symptoms
- Establishing and monitoring the *severity* of a physiologic disturbance

BOX 1-2 Disciplines of the Modern-Day Clinical Laboratory

- Biochemical Genetics
- Blood Banking (Transfusion Medicine)
- Cancer Diagnostics
- Clinical Chemistry/Biochemistry
- Clinical Hematology
- Clinical Immunology
- Cytogenetics
- Drug Monitoring
- Endocrinology Testing
- Hemostasis/Thrombosis (Coagulation) Testing
- Identity Testing
- Infectious Disease Testing
- Information Technology
- Laboratory Management
- Microbiology
- Molecular Cytogenetics
- Molecular Diagnostics
- Nutrition
- Organ Transplantation
- Organ Function Testing
- Pharmacogenetics
- Proteomics
- Quality Management
- Toxicology
- Trace Elements

Chapters 3 and 4). From the physician's and the patient's perspective, no distinction is evident between these specialties, and invariably the repertoire of more than one specialty will be called upon when a clinical decision is made. Examples of clinical scenarios that require tests from multiple laboratory areas include the diagnosis and management of many diseases and the management of patients in intensive care (see Chapters 46 through 59 ["Pathophysiology" section of this text]).

Boundaries between and among the parts of the clinical laboratory have become more blurred with increasing emphasis on the use of chemical and "molecular" (nucleic acid) testing. Molecular diagnostic testing has evolved beyond human genetic testing, an area in which clinical chemists have long been active. Now, clinical chemists in "molecular" laboratories contribute their expertise in laboratory medicine to infectious disease testing, cancer diagnostics, and identity testing, activities that formerly were associated primarily or solely with, respectively, clinical microbiology, hematology, and blood bank laboratories. Successful contribution by clinical chemists to these areas requires an understanding of the principles of laboratory medicine and close collaboration with clinical microbiologists, hematologists, and others who have specialized expertise in those areas of laboratory medicine.

The relationship between the clinical chemist and laboratory medicine has evolved further with the advent of "core" laboratories. These laboratories provide all of the high-volume and emergency testing in many hospitals. Their efficient and reliable operation depends on automation (see Chapter 19), computers, and high levels of quality control and quality management (see Chapter 8). Clinical chemists, who have long been active in these areas, have assumed increasing responsibility in core laboratories and thus have become more involved in areas such as hematology, coagulation, urinalysis, and even microbiology. Thus a new type of "clinical chemist" has emerged, and again the functions require a broader knowledge of laboratory medicine and greater collaboration with other specialists.

A virtual merger of clinical chemistry and laboratory medicine has been suggested in many ways. For example, journals in the field of clinical chemistry publish papers in all of the areas of laboratory medicine. The current logo of the American Association for Clinical Chemistry reads, "AACC—Improving Healthcare through Laboratory Medicine." Moreover, the international association of clinical chemistry societies is now called the International Federation of Clinical Chemistry and Laboratory Medicine. To be active in the field of laboratory medicine today requires, more often than not, familiarity with core concepts in several if not all of the subdisciplines of the field.

During the past two decades, the field of clinical chemistry has been profoundly influenced by new activities in the fields of clinical epidemiology and evidence-based medicine (EBM). Clinical epidemiologists have developed study designs to quantify the diagnostic accuracy (as opposed to analytical accuracy) of the tests developed in laboratory medicine (see Chapter 3). Moreover, they have introduced methods to evaluate the effects and value of laboratory testing in healthcare (see Chapter 2). These developments are expected to play an increasing role in the selection and interpretation of tests. Thus the fourth chapter of this book is devoted to evidence-based laboratory medicine.

ETHICAL ISSUES IN LABORATORY MEDICINE

As in other branches of medicine, practitioners in laboratory medicine are faced with ethical issues, often on a daily basis; examples are listed in Box 1-3.

Specific issues that challenge laboratory professionals include (1) confidentiality of genetic information and patient

BOX 1-3 Ethical Issues in Clinical Chemistry and Molecular Diagnostics

- Confidentiality of genetic information
- Confidentiality of patient medical information
- Allocation of resources
- Codes of conduct
- Publishing issues
- Conflicts of interest

medical information, (2) allocation of healthcare resources, (3) codes of conduct, (4) publishing issues, and (5) conflict of interest.

Confidentiality of Genetic Information

Prominent in the news in the first and second decades of this millennium has been the issue of confidentiality of genetic information. Legislation was considered necessary to prevent denial of health insurance or employment to people found by DNA testing to be at risk of disease. Less appreciated is the fact that the issue of confidentiality of clinical laboratory data predated DNA testing. In fact, many non-DNA tests, old and new, also carry information about risks of illness and death. Clinical laboratorians have long been responsible for maintaining the confidentiality of all laboratory results, a situation made even more critical with the advent of increasingly powerful genetic testing.

Confidentiality of Patient Medical Information

Because new medical tests are constantly needed, laboratory physicians and scientists spend a great deal of time and effort developing new diagnostic tests or evaluating them for use in a specific setting. This process requires use of patient samples and may involve use of patient medical information.[4] Ethical judgments are required regarding the type of informed consent that is needed from patients for use of their samples and clinical information. Clinical laboratory physicians and scientists often serve on institutional review boards that examine proposed research on human subjects. In these discussions, ethical concepts such as equipoise and confidentiality are central to decisions.

Allocation of Resources

Because resources are finite, clinical laboratorians must make ethically responsible decisions about allocation of resources. When a trade-off exists between cost and quality, ethical issues may need to be considered: What is best for patients generally? How can the most good be done with the available resources? For laboratorians in business, the newly appreciated area of business ethics comes into play. One example, recently epitomized by scandals associated with names such as Madoff and Enron, involves the area of accounting, a human endeavor that in the public mind had not been much associated with concerns about ethics.

Codes of Conduct

Most professional organizations publish a Code of Conduct that requires adherence by their members. For example, the American Association for Clinical Chemistry (AACC) has published Ethical Guidelines (http://www.aacc.org/about/ethics/Pages/default.aspx) that require AACC members to endorse principles of ethical conduct in their professional activities, including (1) selection and performance of clinical procedures, (2) research and development, (3) teaching, (4) management, (5) administration, and (6) other forms of professional service.

Publishing Issues

Publication of documents having high scientific integrity depends on authors, editors, and reviewers all working in concert in an environment governed by high ethical standards.[2]

Authors are responsible for honest and complete reporting of original data produced in ethically conducted research studies. Practices such as fraud, plagiarism, and falsification or fabrication of data are unacceptable! The International Committee of Medical Journal Editors (ICMJE)[12] and the Committee on Publication Ethics (COPE)[7] have published policies that address such behavior. Other practices to be avoided include (1) duplicate publication, (2) redundant publication, and (3) inappropriate authorship credit; in addition, ethical policies require that factors that might influence the interpretation of a study must be revealed.

Most journals now have conflict-of-interest policies for both authors and journal editors. For example, *Clinical Chemistry* requires that authors complete a full disclosure form upon manuscript submission. Annually, the Editor and Associate Editors also are required to provide such a form (http://www.clinchem.org).

Conflict of Interest

Concern has been raised over the interrelationships between practitioners in the medical field and commercial suppliers of drugs, devices, equipment, etc., to the medical profession.[13] These concerns led the National Institutes of Health (NIH) in 1995 to require official institutional review of financial disclosure by researchers and management of situations in which disclosure indicates potential conflicts of interest and/or conflicts of effort in research (http://ethics.od.nih.gov/Topics/finance.htm). In 2009, the Institute of Medicine (IOM) issued a report[11] that questioned inappropriate relationships between pharmaceutical and device companies and physicians and other healthcare professionals.[13] Similarly, the relationships between clinical laboratorians and manufacturers and providers of diagnostic equipment and supplies have been scrutinized.

As a consequence of these concerns and as a result of the enactment of various laws designed to prevent fraud, abuse, and waste in Medicare, Medicaid, and other federal programs, professional organizations that represent manufacturers of in vitro diagnostics (IVD) and other device and healthcare companies have published Codes of Ethics. For example, the

Advanced Medical Technology Association (AdvaMed) has revised and published its Code of Ethics that became effective July 1, 2009.[1] Topics discussed in this revised Code include (1) gifts and entertainment, (2) consulting arrangements and royalties, (3) reimbursement for testing, and (4) education. Similarly, the European Diagnostic Manufacturers Association (EDMA) has published its Code of Ethics.[6] In Part A of this document, topics discussed include (1) member-sponsored product training and education, (2) supporting third party educational conferences, (3) sales and promotional meetings, (4) arrangements and consultants, (5) gifts, (6) provision of reimbursements and other economic information, and (7) donations for charitable and philanthropic purposes. Both documents address demands from regulators while nurturing the unique role that laboratorians and other healthcare professionals play in *developing and refining new technology.*[13]

THE FUTURE

Practitioners of clinical chemistry, molecular diagnostics, and laboratory medicine have before them a future full of promise and challenge. New insight into disease and its treatment is exploding, and these insights are based in sciences that are at the heart of the clinical laboratory. The clinical laboratory is the place of translation of these insights into effective healthcare. We honor the important role of ethical laboratory professionals in these efforts and have endeavored to provide in this book chapters prepared by expert authors that help to define the evidence base and knowledge base of the profession.

REFERENCES

1. Advanced Medical Technology Association (AdvaMed). Code of Ethics on interactions with health care professionals. Effective July 1, 2009. Available at: http://www.advamed.org/NR/rdonlyres/FA437A5F-4C75-43B2-A900-C9470BA8DFA7/0/coe_with_faqs_41505.pdf (accessed on 22 February 2011).
2. Annesley TM, Boyd JC, Rifai N. Publication ethics: *Clinical Chemistry* editorial standards. Clin Chem 2009;55:1-4.
3. Centers for Disease Control and Prevention. Laboratory medicine best practices: developing an evidence-based review and evaluation process. Final technical report 2007: phase I. Atlanta, Ga: U.S. Department of Health and Human Services, 2008.
4. Council of Europe. Additional protocol to the convention for the protection of human rights and dignity of the human being with regard to the application of biology and medicine on biomedical research. Law Hum Genome Rev 2004;21:201-14.
5. Dati F. The past, present and future of medical sciences and the evolution of the clinical laboratory (personal communication).
6. European Diagnostic Manufacturers Association (EDMA). Part A: interaction with health care professionals. Available at: http://www.edma-ivd.be (accessed on 22 February 2011).
7. Graf C, Wager E, Bowman A, Fiack S, Scott-Lichter D, Robinson A. Best practice guidelines on publication ethics: a publisher's perspective. Int J Clin Pract Suppl 2007;61:1-26.
8. Guder WG, Büttner J. Clinical chemistry in laboratory medicine in Europe—past, present and future challenges. Eur J Clin Chem Clin Biochem 1997;35:487-94.
9. Griffiths J. Automation and other recent developments in clinical chemistry. Am J Clin Pathol 1992;98(4 Suppl 1):S31-4.
10. International Organization for Standardization (ISO). Guide to the expression of uncertainty in measurement (GUM). ISO/IEC guide 98-1. Geneva, Switzerland: ISO, 2009.
11. Institute of Medicine. Conflict of interest in medical research, education, and practice. Available at: http://www.iom.edu (accessed April 2009).
12. International Committee of Medical Journal Editors. Uniform requirements for manuscripts submitted to biomedical journals: writing and editing for biomedical publication. Available at: http://www.icmje.org/ (accessed October 2008).
13. Malone B. Ethics code changes for diagnostics manufacturers. Clin Lab News 2009;35(6).
14. Scott MG, Dunne WM, Gronowski AM. Education of the PhD in laboratory medicine. Clin Lab Med 2007;27:435-46.

CHAPTER 2

Selection and Analytical Evaluation of Methods—With Statistical Techniques

Kristian Linnet, M.D., Ph.D., and James C. Boyd, M.D.

The introduction of new or revised methods is a common occurrence in the clinical laboratory. Method selection and evaluation are key steps in the process of implementing new methods (Figure 2-1). A new or revised method must be selected carefully and its performance evaluated thoroughly in the laboratory before it is adopted for routine use. Establishment of a new method may also involve evaluation of the features of the automated analyzer on which the method will be implemented.

When a new method is to be introduced to the routine clinical laboratory, a series of evaluations are commonly conducted. Assay imprecision is estimated and comparison of the new assay versus an existing method or versus an external comparative method is undertaken. The allowable measurement range is assessed with estimation of the lower and upper limits of quantification. Interferences and carryover are evaluated when relevant. Depending on the situation, a limited verification of manufacturer claims may be all that is necessary, or, in the case of a newly developed method in a research context, a full validation must be carried out. Subsequent subsections provide details for these procedures. With regard to evaluation of reference intervals or medical decision limits, please see Chapter 5.

Method evaluation in the clinical laboratory is influenced strongly by guidelines.[26,105,106] The Clinical and Laboratory Standards Institute [CLSI, formerly National Committee for Clinical Laboratory Standards (NCCLS)] has published a series of consensus protocols[11-19] for clinical chemistry laboratories and manufacturers to follow when evaluating methods (see the CLSI website at http://www.clsi.org). The International Organization for Standardization (ISO) has also developed several documents related to method evaluation.[43-50] In addition, meeting laboratory accreditation requirements has become an important aspect in the method selection and/or evaluation process with accrediting agencies placing increased focus on the importance of total quality management and assessment of trueness and precision of laboratory measurements. An accompanying trend has been the emergence of an international nomenclature to standardize the terminology used for characterizing method performance. This chapter presents an overview of considerations in the method selection process, followed by sections on method evaluation and method comparison. The latter two sections focus on graphical and statistical tools that are used to aid in the method evaluation process; examples of the application of these tools are provided, and current terminology within the area is summarized.

METHOD SELECTION

Optimal method selection involves consideration of medical need, analytical performance, and practical criteria.

Medical Need and Quality Goals

The selection of appropriate methods for clinical laboratory assays is a vital part of rendering optimal patient care, and advances in patient care are frequently based on the use of new or improved laboratory tests. Ascertainment of what is necessary clinically from a laboratory test is the first step in selecting a candidate method. Key parameters, such as desired turnaround time and necessary clinical utility for an assay, are often derived by discussions between laboratorians and clinicians. When new diagnostic assays are introduced, reliable estimates of clinical sensitivity and specificity must be obtained from the literature or by conducting a clinical outcome study (see Chapter 4). With established analytes, a common scenario is the replacement of an older, labor-intensive method with a new, automated assay that is more economical in daily use. In these situations, consideration must be given to whether the candidate method has sufficient precision, accuracy, analytical measurement range, and freedom from interference to provide clinically useful results (see Figure 2-1).

Analytical Performance Criteria

In evaluation of the performance characteristics of a candidate method, (1) precision, (2) accuracy (trueness),

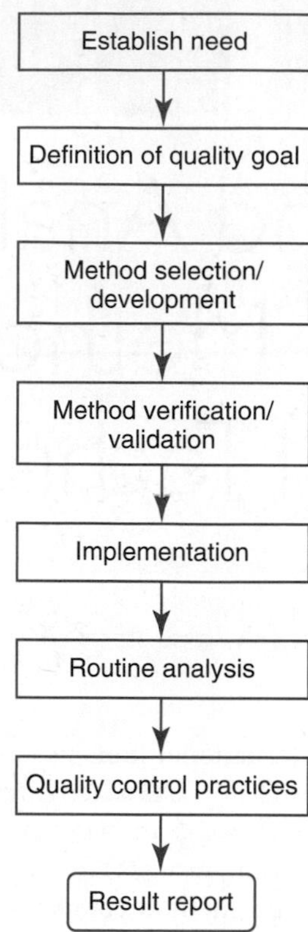

Figure 2-1 A flow diagram that illustrates the process of introducing a new method into routine use.

(3) analytical range, (4) detection limit, and (5) analytical specificity are of prime importance. The sections in this chapter on method evaluation and comparison contain detailed outlines of these concepts and their assessment. Estimated performance parameters for a method are then related to quality goals that ensure acceptable medical use of the test results (see section on "Analytical Goals"). From a practical point of view, the "ruggedness" of the method in routine use is of importance and reliable performance when used by different operators and with different batches of reagents over long time periods is essential.

When a new clinical analyzer is included in the overall evaluation process, various instrumental parameters require evaluation, including (1) pipetting, (2) specimen-to-specimen carryover, (3) reagent lot-to-lot variation, (4) detector imprecision, (5) time to first reportable result, (6) onboard reagent stability, (7) overall throughput, (8) mean time between instrument failures, and (9) mean time to repair. Information on most of these parameters should be available from the instrument manufacturer; the manufacturer should also be able to furnish information on what user studies should be conducted in estimating these parameters for an individual analyzer. Assessment of reagent lot-to-lot variation is especially difficult for a user, and the manufacturer should provide this information.

Other Criteria

Various categories of candidate methods may be considered. New methods described in the scientific literature may require "in-house" development. [Note: Such a test is also referred to as a Laboratory-Developed Test(LDT).] Commercial kit methods, on the other hand, are ready for implementation in the laboratory, often in a "closed" analytical system on a dedicated instrument. When prospective methods are reviewed, attention should be given to the following:

1. Principle of the assay, with original references.
2. Detailed protocol for performing the test.
3. Composition of reagents and reference materials, the quantities provided, and their storage requirements (e.g., space, temperature, light, humidity restrictions) applicable both before and after the original containers are opened.
4. Stability of reagents and reference materials (e.g., their shelf life).
5. Technologist time and required skills.
6. Possible hazards and appropriate safety precautions according to relevant guidelines and legislation.
7. Type, quantity, and disposal of waste generated.
8. Specimen requirements (e.g., conditions for collection and transportation, specimen volume requirements, the necessity for anticoagulants and preservatives, necessary storage conditions).
9. Reference interval of the method, including information on how it was derived, typical values obtained in health and disease, and the necessity of determining a reference interval for one's own institution (see Chapter 5 for details on how to generate a reference interval).
10. Instrumental requirements and limitations.
11. Cost-effectiveness.
12. Computer platforms and interfacing with the laboratory information system.
13. Availability of technical support, supplies, and service.

Other questions concerning placement of the method in the laboratory should be taken into account. They include:

1. Does the laboratory possess the necessary measuring equipment? If not, is there sufficient space for a new instrument?
2. Does the projected workload match with the capacity of a new instrument?
3. Is the test repertoire of a new instrument sufficient?
4. What is the method and frequency of calibration?
5. Is staffing of the laboratory sufficient for the new technology?
6. If training the entire staff in a new technique is required, is such training worth the possible benefits?
7. How frequently will quality control samples be run?
8. What materials will be used to ensure quality control?
9. What approach will be used with the method for proficiency testing?
10. What is the estimated cost of performing an assay using the proposed method, including the costs of calibrators, quality control specimens, and technologists' time?

Questions applicable to implementation of new instrumentation in a particular laboratory may also be relevant. Does the instrument on which the method is implemented satisfy local electrical safety guidelines? What are the power, water, drainage, and air conditioning requirements of the instrument? If the instrument is large, does the floor have sufficient load-bearing capacity?

A qualitative assessment of these factors is often completed, but it is possible to use a value scale to assign points to the various features of a method weighted according to their relative importance; the latter approach allows a more quantitative selection process. Decisions are then made regarding the analytical methods that best fit the laboratory's requirements, and that have the potential for achieving the necessary analytical quality.

BASIC STATISTICS

In this section, fundamental statistical concepts and techniques are introduced in the context of typical analytical investigations. The basic concepts of (1) populations, (2) samples, (3) parameters, (4) statistics, and (5) probability distributions are defined and illustrated. Two important probability distributions—Gaussian and Student *t*—are introduced and discussed.

Frequency Distribution

A graphical device for displaying a large set of data is the *frequency distribution,* also called a *histogram.* Figure 2-2 shows a frequency distribution displaying the results of serum gamma-glutamyltransferase (GGT) measurements of 100 apparently healthy 20- to 29-year-old men. The frequency distribution is constructed by dividing the measurement scale into cells of equal width, counting the number, n_i, of values that fall within each cell, and drawing a rectangle above each cell whose area (and height, because the cell widths are all equal) is proportional to n_i. In this example, the selected cells were 5 to 9, 10 to 14, 15 to 19, 20 to 24, 25 to 29, and so on, with 60 to 64 being the last cell. The ordinate axis of the frequency distribution gives the number of values falling within each cell. When this number is divided by the total number of values in the data set, the relative frequency in each cell is obtained.

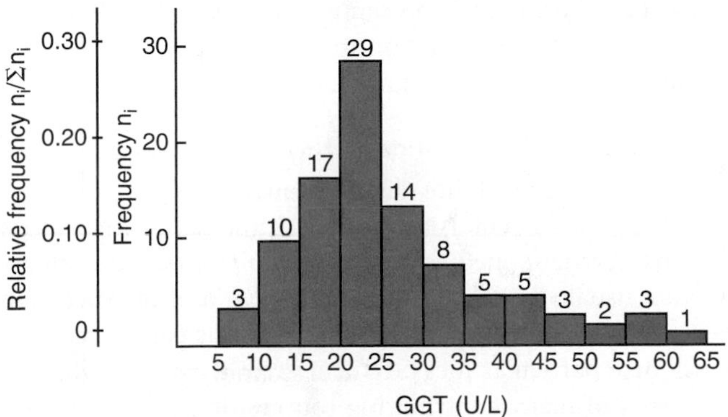

Figure 2-2 Frequency distribution of 100 gamma-glutamyltransferase (GGT) values.

Often, the position of the value for an individual within a distribution of values is useful medically. The *nonparametric* approach can be used to determine directly the *percentile* of a given subject. Having ranked *N* subjects according to their values, the *n*-percentile, $Perc_n$, may be estimated as the value of the $[N(n/100) + 0.5]$ ordered observation.[23] In the case of a noninteger value, interpolation is carried out between neighbor values. The 50-percentile is the median of the distribution.

Population and Sample

The purpose of analytical work is to obtain information and draw conclusions about characteristics of one or more populations of values. In the GGT example, interest is focused on the location and spread of the population of GGT values for 20- to 29-year-old healthy men. Thus, a working definition of a *population* is the complete set of all observations that might occur as a result of performing a particular procedure according to specified conditions.

Most populations of interest in clinical chemistry are infinite in size and so are impossible to study in their entirety. Usually a subgroup of observations is taken from the population as a basis for forming conclusions about population characteristics. The group of observations that has actually been selected from the population is called a *sample.* For example, the 100 GGT values make up a sample from a respective population. However, a sample is used to study the characteristics of a population only if it has been properly selected. For instance, if the analyst is interested in the population of GGT values over various lots of materials and some time period, the sample must be selected to be representative of these factors, as well as of age, sex, and health factors. Consequently, exact specification of the population(s) of interest is necessary before a plan for obtaining the sample(s) can be designed. In the present chapter, a sample is also used as a specimen, depending on the context.

Probability and Probability Distributions

Consider again the frequency distribution in Figure 2-2. In addition to the general location and spread of the GGT determinations, other useful information can be easily extracted from this frequency distribution. For instance, 96% (96 of 100) of the determinations are less than 55 U/L, and 91% (91 of 100) are greater than or equal to 10 but less than 50 U/L. Because the cell interval is 5 U/L in this example, statements such as these can be made only to the nearest 5 U/L. A larger sample would allow a smaller cell interval and more refined statements. For a sufficiently large sample, the cell interval can be made so small that the frequency distribution can be approximated by a continuous, smooth curve, similar to that shown in Figure 2-3. In fact, if the sample is large enough, we can consider this a close representation of the true *population frequency distribution.* In general, the functional form of the population frequency distribution curve of a variable *x* is denoted by $f(x)$.

The population frequency distribution allows us to make probability statements about the GGT of a randomly selected

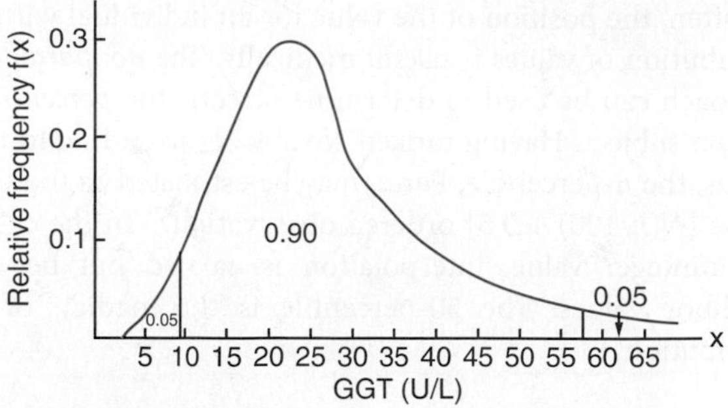

Figure 2-3 Population frequency distribution of gamma-glutamyltransferase (GGT) values.

member of the population of healthy 20- to 29-year-old men. For example, the probability $\Pr(x > x_a)$ that the GGT value x of a randomly selected 20- to 29-year-old healthy man is greater than some particular value x_a is equal to the area under the population frequency distribution to the right of x_a. If $x_a = 58$, then from Figure 2-3, $\Pr(x > 58) = 0.05$. Similarly, the probability $\Pr(x_a < x < x_b)$ that x is greater than x_a but less than x_b is equal to the area under the population frequency distribution between x_a and x_b. For example, if $x_a = 9$ and $x_b = 58$, then from Figure 2-3, $\Pr(9 < x < 58) = 0.90$. Because the population frequency distribution provides all information related to probabilities of a randomly selected member of the population, it is called the probability distribution of the population. Although the true probability distribution is never exactly known in practice, it can be approximated with a large sample of observations.

Parameters: Descriptive Measures of a Population

Any population of values can be described by measures of its characteristics. A *parameter* is a constant that describes some particular characteristic of a population. Although most populations of interest in analytical work are infinite in size, for the following definitions we shall consider the population to be of finite size N, where N is very large.

One important characteristic of a population is its *central location.* The parameter most commonly used to describe the central location of a population of N values is the *population mean* (μ):

$$\mu = \frac{\sum x_i}{N}$$

An alternative parameter that indicates the central tendency of a population is the *median,* which is defined as the 50-percentile, Perc_{50}.

Another important characteristic of a population is the *dispersion* of values about the population mean. A parameter very useful in describing this dispersion of a population of N values is the *population variance* σ^2 (sigma squared):

$$\sigma^2 = \frac{\sum (x_i - \mu)^2}{N}$$

The *population standard deviation* σ, the positive square root of the population variance, is a parameter frequently used to describe the population dispersion in the same units (e.g., mg/dL) as the population values.

Statistics: Descriptive Measures of the Sample

As noted earlier, the clinical chemist usually has at hand only a sample of observations from the population of interest. A *statistic* is a value calculated from the observations in a sample to describe a particular characteristic of that sample. As introduced above, the sample mean x_m is the arithmetical average of a sample, which is an estimate of μ. Likewise, the sample SD is an estimate of σ, and the coefficient of variation (CV) is the ratio of the SD to the mean multiplied by 100%. The equations used to calculate x_m, SD, and CV, respectively, are as follows:

$$x_m = \frac{\sum x_i}{N}$$

$$SD = \sqrt{\frac{\sum (x_i - x_m)^2}{N-1}} = \sqrt{\frac{\sum x_i^2 - \frac{(\sum x_i)^2}{N}}{N-1}}$$

$$CV = \frac{SD}{x_m} \times 100\%$$

where x_i is an individual measurement and N is the number of sample measurements.

Random Sampling

A random selection from a population is one in which each member of the population has an equal chance of being selected. A *random sample* is one in which each member of the sample can be considered to be a random selection from the population of interest. Although much of statistical analysis and interpretation depends on the assumption of a random sample from some fixed population, actual data collection often does not satisfy this assumption. In particular, for sequentially generated data, it is often true that observations adjacent to each other tend to be more alike than observations separated in time. A sample of such observations cannot be considered a sample of random selections from a fixed population. Fortunately, precautions can usually be taken in the design of an investigation to validate approximately the random sampling assumption.

The Gaussian Probability Distribution

The *Gaussian* probability distribution, illustrated in Figure 2-4, is of fundamental importance in statistics for several reasons. As mentioned earlier, a particular analytical value x will not usually be equal to the true value μ of the specimen being measured. Rather, associated with this particular value x will be a particular measurement error $\varepsilon = x - \mu$, which is the result of many contributing sources of error. Pure measurement errors tend to follow a probability distribution similar to that shown in Figure 2-4, where the errors are

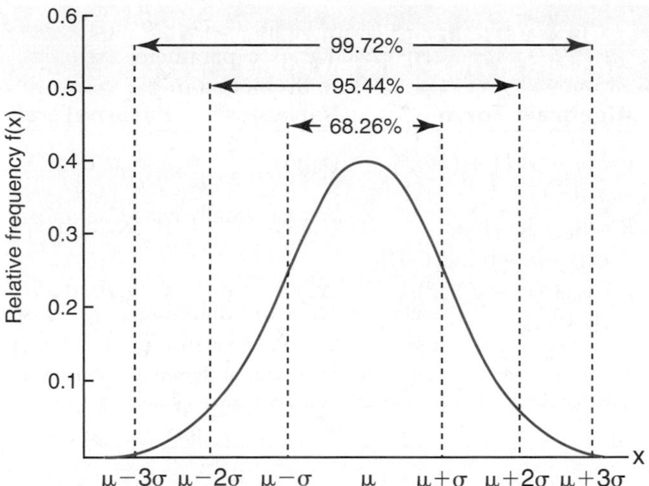

Figure 2-4 The Gaussian probability distribution.

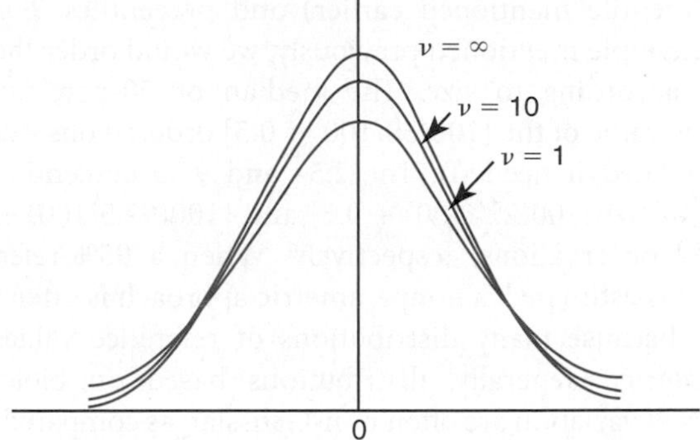

Figure 2-5 The t distribution for v = 1, 10, and ∞.

symmetrically distributed, with smaller errors occurring more frequently than larger ones, and with an expected value of 0. This important fact is known as the central limit effect for distribution of errors: if a measurement error ε is the sum of many independent sources of error, such as $\varepsilon_1, \varepsilon_2, \ldots, \varepsilon_k$, several of which are major contributors, the probability distribution of the measurement error ε will tend to be Gaussian as the number of sources of error becomes large.

Another reason for the importance of the Gaussian probability distribution is that many statistical procedures are based on the assumption of a Gaussian distribution of values; this approach is commonly referred to as *parametric.* Furthermore, these procedures usually are not seriously invalidated by departures from this assumption. Finally, the magnitude of the uncertainty associated with sample statistics can be ascertained based on the fact that many sample statistics computed from large samples have a Gaussian probability distribution.

The Gaussian probability distribution is completely characterized by its mean μ and its variance σ^2. The notation $N(\mu, \sigma^2)$ is often used for the distribution of a variable that is Gaussian with mean μ and variance σ^2. Probability statements about a variable x that follows an $N(\mu, \sigma^2)$ distribution are usually made by considering the variable z,

$$z = \frac{x - \mu}{\sigma}$$

which is called the *standard Gaussian variable.* The variable z has a Gaussian probability distribution with $\mu = 0$ and $\sigma^2 = 1$, that is, z is $N(0, 1)$. The probably that x is within 2 σ of μ [i.e., $\Pr(|x - \mu|<2\sigma)$ =] is 0.9544. Most computer spreadsheet programs can calculate probabilities for all values of z.

Student *t* Probability Distribution

To determine probabilities associated with a Gaussian distribution, it is necessary to know the population standard deviation σ. In actual practice, σ is often unknown, so we cannot calculate z. However, if a random sample can be taken from the Gaussian population, we can calculate the sample standard deviation (SD), substitute SD for σ, and compute the value t:

$$t = \frac{x - \mu}{SD}$$

Under these conditions, the variable t has a probability distribution called the *Student* t *distribution.* The t distribution is really a family of distributions depending on the degrees of freedom ν (= $N - 1$) for the sample SD. Several t distributions from this family are shown in Figure 2-5. When the size of the sample and the degrees of freedom for SD are infinite, there is no uncertainty in SD, and so the t distribution is identical to the standard Gaussian distribution. However, when the sample size is small, the uncertainty in SD causes the t distribution to have greater dispersion and heavier tails than the standard Gaussian distribution, as illustrated in Figure 2-5. Most computer spreadsheet programs can calculate probabilities for all values of t, given the degrees of freedom for SD.

Suppose that the distribution of fasting serum glucose values in healthy men is known to be Gaussian and have a mean of 90 mg/dL. Suppose also that σ is unknown, and that a random sample of size 20 from the healthy men yielded a sample SD = 10.0 mg/dL. Then, to find the probability $\Pr(x > 105)$, we proceed as follows:

1. $t_a = (x_a - x_m)/SD = (105 - 90)/10 = 1.5$.
2. $\Pr(t > t_a) = \Pr(t > 1.5) = 0.08$, approximately, from a t distribution with 19 degrees of freedom.
3. $\Pr(x > 105) = 0.08$.

The Student t distribution is commonly used in significance tests, such as comparison of sample means, or in testing conducted if a regression slope differs significantly from 1. Descriptions of these tests can be found in statistics textbooks[98] and in *Tietz Textbook of Clinical Chemistry,* 3rd edition, 2006, pages 274-287.

Nonparametric Statistics

Distribution-free statistics, often called nonparametric statistics, provides an alternative to parametric statistical procedures that assume data to have Gaussian distributions. Nonparametric descriptive statistics is based on the median

(50-percentile mentioned earlier) and percentiles. For the GGT example mentioned previously, we would order the 100 values according to size. The median or 50-percentile is then the value of the [100(50/100) + 0.5] ordered observation (interpolated if needed). The 2.5- and 97.5-percentiles are values of the [100(2.5/100) + 0.5] and [100(97.5/100) + 0.5] ordered observations, respectively. When a 95%-reference interval is estimated, a nonparametric approach is often preferable, because many distributions of reference values are asymmetric. Generally, distributions based on biological sources of variation are often non-Gaussian as compared with distributions of pure measurement errors that usually are Gaussian.

When the significance of a difference between two estimated mean values is tested, the parametric approach is to use the *t*-test as described in standard textbooks and included in most computer statistical programs. Although the *t*-test assumes Gaussian distributions of values in the two groups to be compared, it is generally robust toward deviations from the Gaussian distribution. The *t*-test occurs in two versions: a paired comparison, where two values are measured for each case; and a nonpaired version, where values of two separate groups are compared. The nonparametric counterpart to the paired *t*-test is the Wilcoxon test, for which paired differences are ordered and tested; for the two-group case, the Mann-Whitney test can be substituted for the *t*-test. The Mann-Whitney test provides a significance test for the difference between median values of the two groups to be compared.[98]

TABLE 2-1 The Four-Parameter Logistic Model Expressed in Three Different Forms

Algebraic Form	Variables*	Parameters†
$y = (a - d)/[1 + (x/c)^{b}] + d$	(x, y)	a, b, c, d
$R = R_0 + K_c/[1 + \exp(-\{a + b \log[C]\})]$	(C, R)	R_0, K_c, a, b
$y = y_0 + (y_{¥} - y_0)(x^{d})/(b + x^{d})$	(x, y)	y_0, $y_{¥}$, b, d

*Concentration and instrument response variables shown in parentheses.
†Equivalent letters do not necessarily denote equivalent parameters.

BASIC CONCEPTS IN RELATION TO ANALYTICAL METHODS

This section defines the basic concepts used in this chapter: (1) calibration, (2) accuracy, (3) precision, (4) linearity, (5) limit of detection, (6) limit of quantification, (7) specificity, and (8) others.

Calibration

The calibration function is the relation between instrument signal *(y)* and concentration of analyte *(x)*, that is,

$$y = f(x)$$

The inverse of this function, also called the measuring function, yields the concentration from response:

$$x = f^{-1}(y)$$

This relationship is established by measurement of samples with known quantities of analyte (calibrators).[22] One may distinguish between solutions of pure chemical standards and samples with known quantities of analyte present in the typical matrix that is to be measured (e.g., human serum). The first situation applies typically to a reference measurement procedure that is not influenced by matrix effects; the second case corresponds typically to a routine method that often is influenced by matrix components, and so preferably is calibrated using the relevant matrix.[90] Calibration functions may be linear or curved and, in the case of immunoassays, may often take a special form (e.g., modeled by the four-parameter logistic curve).[92] This model (logistic in log *x*) has been used for immunoassay techniques and is written in several forms (Table 2-1). An alternative, model-free approach is to estimate a smoothed spline curve, which often is performed for immunoassays; however, a disadvantage of the spline curve approach is that it is insensitive to aberrant calibration values, fitting these just as well as the correct values. If the assumed calibration function does not correctly reflect the true relationship between instrument response and analyte concentration, a systematic error or bias is likely to be associated with the analytical method. A common problem with some immunoassays is the "hook effect" which is a deviation from the expected calibration algorithm in the high concentration range. (The hook effect is discussed in more detail in Chapter 16).

The precision of the analytical method depends on the stability of the instrument response for a given quantity of analyte. In principle, a random dispersion of instrument signal (vertical direction) at a given true concentration transforms into dispersion on the measurement scale (horizontal direction), as is shown schematically (Figure 2-6). The detailed statistical aspects of calibration are complex,[96,98] but in the following sections, some approximate relations are outlined. If the calibration function is linear and the imprecision of the signal response is the same over the analytical measurement range, the analytical standard deviation (SD_A) of the method tends to be constant over the analytical measurement range (see Figure 2-6). If the imprecision increases proportionally to the signal response, the analytical SD of the method tends to increase proportionally to the concentration *(x)*, which means that the *relative* imprecision [coefficient of variation (CV) = SD/*x*] may be constant over the analytical measurement range if it is assumed that the intercept of the calibration line is zero.

With modern, automated clinical chemistry instruments, the relation between analyte concentration and signal is often very stable, so that calibration is necessary only infrequently (e.g., at intervals of several months).[89] Built-in process control mechanisms may help ensure that the relationship remains

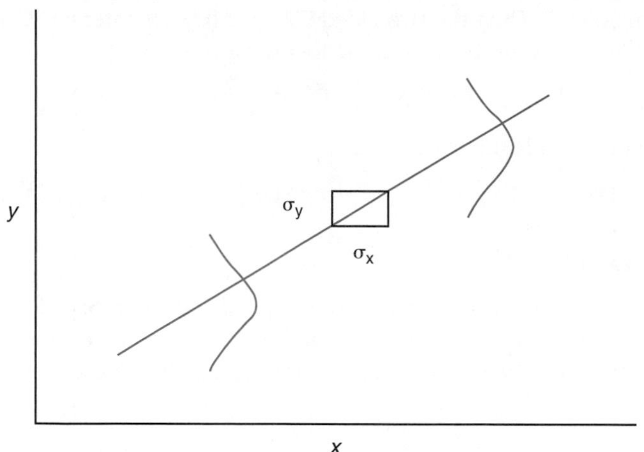

Figure 2-6 Relation between concentration *(x)* and signal response *(y)* for a linear calibration function. The dispersion in signal response (σ_y) is projected onto the *x*-axis and is called assay imprecision [σ_x (=σ_A)].

TABLE 2-2 An Overview of Qualitative Terms and Quantitative Measures Related to Method Performance

Qualitative Concept	Quantitative Measure
Trueness Closeness of agreement of mean value with "true value"	*Bias* A measure of the systematic error
Precision Repeatability (within run) Intermediate precision (long term) Reproducibility (interlaboratory)	*Imprecision (SD)* A measure of the dispersion of random errors
Accuracy Closeness of agreement of a single measurement with "true value"	*Error of measurement* Comprises both random and systematic influences

stable and may indicate when recalibration is necessary. In traditional chromatographic analysis [e.g., high-performance liquid chromatography (HPLC)], on the other hand, it is customary to calibrate each analytical series (run), which means that calibration is carried out daily. Aronsson and associates[1] established a detailed simulation model of the various factors influencing method performance with focus on the calibration function.

Trueness and Accuracy

Trueness of measurements is defined as closeness of agreement between the average value obtained from a large series of results of measurements and the true value.[43] The difference between the average value (strictly, the mathematical expectation) and the true value is the *bias,* which is expressed numerically and so is inversely related to the trueness. Trueness in itself is a qualitative term that can be expressed, for example, as low, medium, or high. From a theoretical point of view, the exact true value for a clinical sample is not available; instead, an "accepted reference value" is used, which is the "true" value that can be determined in practice.[29] Trueness can be evaluated by comparison of measurements by a given routine method and a reference measurement procedure. Such an evaluation may be carried out through parallel measurements of a set of patient samples. The ISO has introduced the trueness expression as a replacement for the term *accuracy,* which now has gained a slightly different meaning. *Accuracy* is the closeness of agreement between the result of a measurement and a true concentration of the analyte.[50] Accuracy thus is influenced by both bias and imprecision and in this way reflects the total error. Accuracy, which in itself is a qualitative term, is inversely related to the "uncertainty" of measurement, which can be quantified as described later (Table 2-2).

In relation to trueness, the concepts *recovery, drift,* and *carryover* may also be considered. *Recovery* is the fraction or percentage increase in concentration that is measured in relation to the amount added. Recovery experiments are typically carried out in the field of drug analysis. One may distinguish between *extraction recovery,* which often is interpreted as the fraction of compound that is carried through an extraction process, and the recovery measured by the entire analytical procedure, in which the addition of an internal standard compensates for losses in the extraction procedure. A recovery close to 100% is a prerequisite for a high degree of trueness, but it does not ensure unbiased results, because possible nonspecificity against matrix components (e.g., an interfering substance) is not detected in a recovery experiment. *Drift* is caused by instrument instability over time, so that calibration becomes biased. Assay *carryover* also must be close to zero to ensure unbiased results. Drift or carryover or both may be conveniently estimated by multifactorial evaluation protocols[58] (see CLSI guideline EP10-A3, "Preliminary Evaluation of Quantitative Clinical Laboratory Measurement Procedures").[14]

Precision

Precision has been defined as the closeness of agreement between independent results of measurements obtained under stipulated conditions.[29] The degree of precision is usually expressed on the basis of statistical measures of imprecision, such as SD or CV ($CV = SD/x$, where x is the measurement concentration), which is inversely related to precision. Imprecision of measurements is solely related to the random error of measurements and has no relation to the trueness of measurements.

Precision is specified as follows[29,44]:

Repeatability: closeness of agreement between results of successive measurements carried out under the same conditions (i.e., corresponding to within-run precision).

Reproducibility: closeness of agreement between results of measurements performed under changed conditions of measurements (e.g., time, operators, calibrators, reagent lots). Two specifications of reproducibility are often used: total or between-run precision in the laboratory, often termed *intermediate precision,* and interlaboratory precision [e.g., as observed in external quality assessment schemes (EQAS)] (see Table 2-2).

The total SD (σ_T) may be divided into within-run and between-run components using the principle of analysis of variance of components (variance is the squared SD)[98]:

$$\sigma^2_T = \sigma^2_{Within\text{-}run} + \sigma^2_{Between\text{-}run}$$

It is not always clear in clinical chemistry publications what is meant by "between-run" variation. Some authors use the term to refer to the total variation of an assay, whereas others apply the term *between-run variance component* as defined earlier. The distinction between these definitions is important but is not always explicitly stated.

In laboratory studies of analytical variation, it is *estimates* of imprecision that are obtained. The more observations, the more certain are the estimates. Commonly the number 20 is given as a reasonable number of observations (e.g., suggested in the CLSI guideline on the topic).[12] To estimate both the within-run imprecision and the total imprecision, a common approach is to measure duplicate control samples in a series of runs. Suppose, for example, that a control is measured in duplicate for 20 runs, in which case 20 observations are present with respect to both components. The dispersion of the means (x_m) of the duplicates is given as follows:

$$\sigma^2_{xm} = \sigma^2_{Within\text{-}run}/2 + \sigma^2_{Between\text{-}run}$$

From the 20 sets of duplicates, we may derive the within-run SD using the following formula:

$$SD_{Within\text{-}run} = [\Sigma d_i^2/(2\times 20)]^{0.5}$$

where d_i refers to the difference between the *i*th set of duplicates. When SDs are estimated, the concept degrees of freedom (df) is used. In a simple situation, the number of degrees of freedom equals $N-1$. For N duplicates, the number of degrees of freedom is $N(2-1) = N$. Thus, both variance components are derived in this way. The advantage of this approach is that the within-run estimate is based on several runs, so that an average estimate is obtained rather than only an estimate for one particular run if all 20 observations had been obtained in the same run. The described approach is a simple example of a *variance component analysis.* The principle can be extended to more components of variation. For example, in the CLSI EP5-A2 guideline, a procedure is outlined that is based on the assumption of two analytical runs per day, in which case within-run, between-run, and between-day components of variance are estimated by a *nested* component of variance analysis approach.[12]

Nothing definitive can be stated about the selected number of 20. Generally, the estimate of the imprecision improves as more observations become available. Exact confidence limits for the SD can be derived from the χ^2 distribution. Estimates of the variance, SD^2, are distributed according to the χ^2 distribution (tabulated in most statistics textbooks) as follows: $(N-1)\ SD^2/\sigma^2 \approx \chi^2_{(N-1)}$, where $(N-1)$ is the degrees of freedom.[98] Then the two-sided 95%-confidence interval (CI) (95%-CI) is derived from the following relation:

$$\Pr[\chi^2_{97.5\%(N-1)} < (N-1)\ SD^2/\sigma^2 < \chi^2_{2.5\%(N-1)}] = 0.95$$

which yields this 95%-CI expression:

$$SD\times[(N-1)/\chi^2_{2.5\%(N-1)}]^{0.5} < \sigma < SD\times[(N-1)/\chi^2_{97.5\%(N-1)}]^{0.5}$$

Example

Suppose we have estimated the imprecision as an SD of 5.0 on the basis of $N = 20$ observations. From a table of the χ^2 distribution, we obtain the following 2.5- and 97.5-percentiles:

$$\chi^2_{2.5\%(19)} = 32.9 \text{ and } \chi^2_{97.5\%(19)} = 8.91$$

where 19 within the parentheses refers to the number of degrees of freedom. Substituting in the equation, we get

$$5.0\times(19/32.9)^{0.5} < \sigma < 5.0\times(19/8.91)^{0.5}$$

or

$$3.8 < \sigma < 7.3$$

For reasonable values of N, approximate limits can be derived from the Gaussian approximation[52,53] that the distribution of the SD is based on expression of the standard error of σ equal to $[\sigma^2/(2\{N-1\})]^{0.5}$. Using the Gaussian approximation, the interval equals $5 \pm t_{19}\ [5^2/(2\{20-1\})]^{0.5}$, which corresponds to $5 \pm 2.093 \times 0.81 = 3.30 - 6.7$. Thus at the sample size of 20, the approximation is not so good because of the asymmetric distribution of the SD. For a sample size of 50, the approximate interval can be calculated to 4.0 to 6.0, which is a somewhat better approximation of the exact interval of 4.2 to 6.25. Generally, it is observed that the uncertainty of the estimated SD is considerable at moderate sample sizes. In Table 2-3, factors corresponding to the 95%-CI are given

TABLE 2-3 Factors Corresponding to 95%-Confidence Interval (CI) Limits for a Standard Deviation

	95%-CI	
N	**Lower**	**Upper**
20	0.760	1.460
30	0.797	1.346
40	0.819	1.283
50	0.835	1.243
60	0.848	1.217
70	0.857	1.198
80	0.865	1.183
90	0.872	1.171
100	0.878	1.161
150	0.898	1.128
200	0.911	1.109
250	0.919	1.096
300	0.926	1.087

as a function of sample size for simple SD estimation according to the χ^2 distribution. These factors provide guidance on the validity of estimated SDs for precision. For individual variance components, the relations are more complicated.

Precision Profile

Precision often depends on the concentration of analyte being considered. A presentation of precision as a function of analyte concentration is the precision profile, which usually is plotted in terms of the SD or the CV as a function of analyte concentration (Figure 2-7, *A-C)*. Some typical examples may be considered. First, the SD may be constant (i.e., independent of the concentration), as it often is for analytes with a limited range of values (e.g., electrolytes). When the SD is constant, the CV varies inversely with the concentration (i.e., it is high in the lower part of the range and low in the high range). For analytes with extended ranges (e.g., hormones), the SD frequently increases as the analyte concentration increases. If a proportional relationship exists, the CV is constant. This may often apply approximately over a large part of the analytical measurement range. Actually, this relationship is anticipated for measurement error that arises because of imprecise volume dispensing. Often a more complex relationship exists. Not infrequently, the SD is relatively constant in the low range, so that the CV increases in the area approaching the lower limit of quantification. At intermediate concentrations, the CV may be relatively constant and perhaps may decline somewhat at increasing concentrations. A square root relationship can be used to model the relationship in some situations as an intermediate form of relation between the constant and the proportional case. A constant SD in the low range can be modeled by truncating the assumed proportional or square root relationship at higher concentrations. The relationship between the SD and the concentration is of importance (1) when method specifications over the analytical measurement range are considered, (2) when limits of quantification are determined, and (3) in the context of selecting appropriate statistical methods for method comparison (e.g., whether a difference or a relative difference plot should be applied, whether a simple or a weighted regression analysis procedure should be used) (see "Relative Distribution of Differences Plot" and "Regression Analysis" sections).

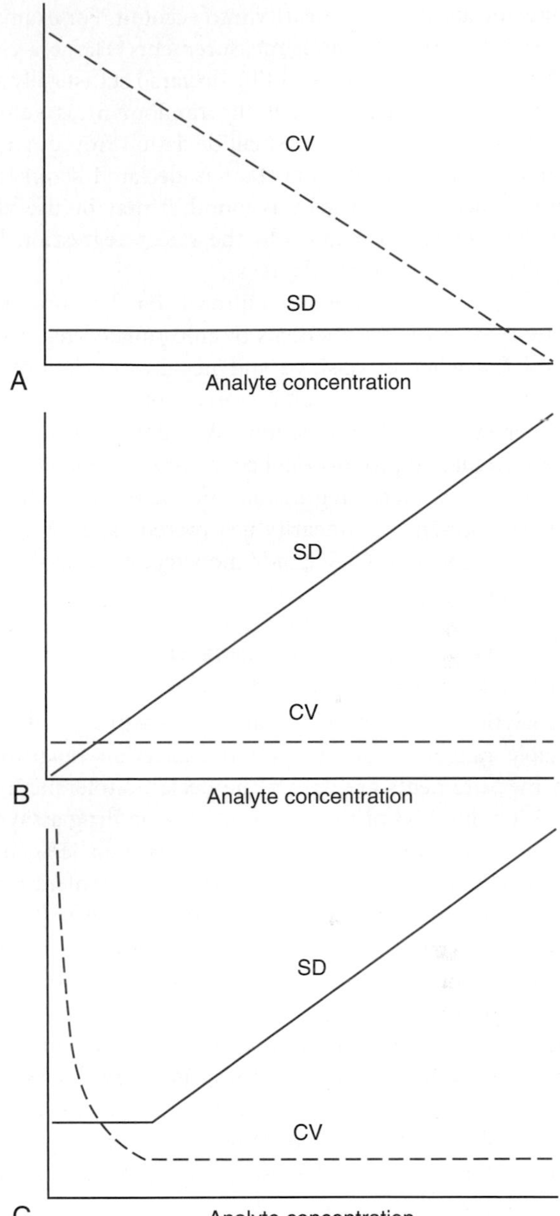

Figure 2-7 Relations between analyte concentration and standard deviation (SD)/coefficient of variation (CV). A, The SD is constant, so that the CV varies inversely with the analyte concentration. B, The CV is constant because of a proportional relationship between concentration and SD. C, A mixed situation with constant SD in the low range and a proportional relationship in the rest of the analytical measurement range.

Linearity

Linearity refers to the relationship between measured and expected values over the analytical measurement range. Linearity may be considered in relation to actual or relative analyte concentrations. In the latter case, a dilution series of a sample may be examined. This dilution series examines whether the measured concentration changes as expected according to the proportional relationship between samples introduced by the dilution factor. Dilution is usually carried out with an appropriate sample matrix [e.g., human serum (individual or pooled serum)].

Evaluation of linearity may be conducted in various ways. A simple, but subjective, approach is to visually assess whether the relationship between measured and expected concentrations is linear. A more formal evaluation may be carried out on the basis of statistical tests. Various principles may be applied here. When repeated measurements are available at each concentration, the random variation between measurements and the variation around an estimated regression line may be evaluated statistically (by an *F*-test).[39] This approach has been criticized because it relates only the magnitudes of random and systematic error without taking the

absolute deviations from linearity into account. For example, if the random variation among measurements is large, a given deviation from linearity may not be declared statistically significant. On the other hand, if the random measurement variation is small, even a very small deviation from linearity that may be clinically unimportant is declared significant. When significant nonlinearity is found, it may be useful to explore nonlinear alternatives to the linear regression line (i.e., polynomials of higher degrees).[32]

Another commonly applied approach for detecting nonlinearity is to assess the residuals of an estimated regression line and test whether positive and negative deviations are randomly distributed. This can be carried out by a runs test[28] (see "Regression Analysis" section). An additional consideration for evaluating proportional concentration relationships is whether an estimated regression line passes through zero or not. The presence of linearity is a prerequisite for a high degree of trueness. A CLSI guideline suggests procedure(s) for assessment of linearity.[11]

Analytical Measurement Range and Limits of Quantification

The analytical measurement range (measuring interval, reportable range) is the analyte concentration range over which measurements are within the declared tolerances for imprecision and bias of the method.[29] Taking drug assays as an example, requirements of a CV% of less than 15% and a bias of less than 15% are common.[95] The measurement range then extends from the lowest concentration [lower limit of quantification (LloQ)] to the highest concentration [upper limit of quantification (UloQ)] for which these performance specifications are fulfilled.

The LloQ is medically important for many analytes. Thyroid-stimulating hormone (TSH) is a good example. As assay methods improved, lowering the LloQ, low TSH results could be distinguished from the lower limit of the reference interval, making the test useful for the diagnosis of hyperthyroidism.

The limit of detection (LoD) is another characteristic of an assay. The LoD may be defined as the lowest value that significantly exceeds the measurements of a blank sample. Thus the limit has been estimated on the basis of repeated measurements of a blank sample and has been *reported* as the mean plus 2 or 3 SDs of the blank measurements. In the interval from LoD up to LloQ, one should report a result as "detected" but not provide a quantitative result. More complicated approaches for estimation of the LoD have been suggested.[18,75,76]

Analytical Sensitivity

The LloQ of a method should not be confused with analytical sensitivity. That is defined as ability of an analytical method to assess small differences in the concentration of analyte.[22] The smaller the random variation of the instrument response and the steeper the slope of the calibration function at a given point, the better is the ability to distinguish small differences in analyte concentrations. In reality, analytical sensitivity depends on the precision of the method. The smallest difference that will be statistically significant equals $2\sqrt{2}\ SD_A$ at a 5% significance level. Historically, the meaning of the term *analytical sensitivity* has been the subject of much discussion.

Analytical Specificity and Interference

Analytical specificity is the ability of an assay procedure to determine the concentration of the target analyte without influence from potentially interfering substances or factors in the sample matrix (e.g., hyperlipemia, hemolysis, bilirubin, antibodies, other metabolic molecules, degradation products of the analyte, exogenous substances, anticoagulants). Interferences from hyperlipemia, hemolysis, and bilirubin are generally concentration dependent and can be quantified as a function of the concentration of the interfering compound.[37] In the context of a drug assay, specificity in relation to drug metabolites is relevant, and in some cases it is desirable to measure the parent drug, as well as metabolites. A detailed protocol for evaluation of interference has been published by the CLSI.[13]

With regard to peptides and proteins, antibodies in different immunoassays may be directed toward different epitopes. Often protein hormones exist in various molecular forms, and differences in specificity of antibodies may give rise to discrepant results. This has been considered for human chorionic gonadotropin (hCG) for which the clinical implications of such molecular variations can be important.[101] Rotmensch and Cole[94] described 12 patients in whom a diagnosis of postgestational choriocarcinoma was made on the basis of false-positive test results for hCG. Most of these patients were subjected to unnecessary surgery or chemotherapy. In each case, the false-positive result was traced to the presence of heterophilic antibodies that interfered with the immunoassay for hCG. Additionally, interference from endogenous antibodies should be recognized. Ismail and colleagues[51] found in a survey comprising more than 5000 TSH results that interference occurred in 0.5% of the samples, leading to incorrect results that in a majority of cases could have changed the treatment. Marks[79] found that almost 10% of immunoassay results from patients with autoimmune disease were erroneous. In many cases, the addition of heterophilic antibody blocking reagent or the study of dilution curves, or both, may help clarify suspected false-positive immunoassay results. Such limitations in the results of immunoassays should be directly communicated to clinicians.

ANALYTICAL GOALS

Setting goals for analytical quality can be based on various principles and a hierarchy has been suggested on the basis of a consensus conference on the subject[85] (Table 2-4). The top level of the hierarchy specifies goals on the basis of clinical outcomes in specific clinical settings, which is a logical principle. For example, one may consider the impact of analytical quality on the error rates of diagnostic or risk classifications.[54,83] A supplementary approach is to study the impact of

TABLE 2-4 Hierarchy of Procedures for Setting Analytical Quality Specifications for Laboratory Methods

I	Evaluation of the effects of analytical performance on clinical outcomes in specific clinical settings
II	Evaluation of the effects of analytical performance on clinical decisions in general:
	A. Data based on components of biological variation
	B. Data based on analysis of clinicians' opinions
III	Published professional recommendations
	A. From national and international expert bodies
	B. From expert local groups or individuals
IV	Performance goals set by
	A. Regulatory bodies
	B. Organizers of EQA schemes
V	Goals based on the current state of the art
	A. Data from EQA/proficiency testing scheme
	B. Data from current publications on methods

EQA, External quality assessment.

imprecision and bias on clinical outcome on the basis of a simulation model, as described by Boyd and Bruns.[6] For a given analyte, a series of specific clinical settings may then be evaluated, and in principle, the most demanding specification then becomes the goal, at least for a general laboratory serving various clinical applications.

Analytical goals related to biological variation have attracted considerable interest.[93] Originally, the focus was on imprecision, and Cotlove and coworkers[21] suggested that the analytical SD (σ_A) should be less than half the within-person biological variation, $\sigma_{Within\text{-}B}$. The rationale for this relation is the principle of adding variances. If a subject is undergoing monitoring of an analyte, the random variation from measurement to measurement consists of both analytical and biological components of variation. The total SD for the random variation during monitoring then is determined by the following relation:

$$\sigma_T^2 = \sigma_{Within\text{-}B}^2 + \sigma_A^2$$

where the biological component includes the preanalytical variation. If σ_A is equal to or less than half the $\sigma_{Within\text{-}B}$ value, σ_T exceeds $\sigma_{Within\text{-}B}$ only by less than 12%. Thus if this relation holds true, analytical imprecision adds limited random noise in a monitoring situation, and the relationship may be called a *desirable* relation. Alternatively, Fraser and associates[35] considered grading of the relationship with additional specifications corresponding to an *optimum* relation (σ_A = 0.25 $\sigma_{Within\text{-}B}$), yielding only 3% additional noise and a *minimum* relation corresponding to 25% additional variation (σ_A = 0.75 $\sigma_{Within\text{-}B}$).[35,36]

In addition to imprecision, goals for bias should be considered. Gowans and colleagues[38] related the allowable bias to the width of the reference interval, which is determined by the combined within- and between-person biological variation, in addition to the analytical variation. On the basis of considerations concerning the included percentage in an interval in the presence of analytical bias, it was suggested that

$$\text{Bias} < 0.25\ (\sigma_{Within\text{-}B}^2 + \sigma_{Between\text{-}B}^2)^{0.5}$$

where $\sigma_{Between\text{-}B}$ is the between-person biological SD component.

Thus the bias should *desirably* be less than one fourth of the combined biological SD. One may further extend the suggested relationships to comprise an optimum relation corresponding to a factor 0.125 and a minimum relation with a factor 0.375. Given a Gaussian distribution of reference values, the desirable relationship corresponds to maximum deviations for proportions outside the interval from the expected 2.5% at each side to 1.4% and 4.4%. This gives an overall deviation of 0.8% from the expected total of 5%, corresponding to a relative deviation of 16%, which may be considered acceptable.[36]

Another principle that has been used is to relate assay goals to the limits set by professional bodies[8] [e.g., the bias goal of 3% for serum cholesterol (originally 5%) set by the National Cholesterol Education Program].[80] Ricos and colleagues[91] have published a comprehensive listing of data on biological variation with a database that is available on the Internet [Ricos et al. Biological variation database. Available at: www.westgard.com/guest17.htm (accessed March 04 2011)].

Qualitative Methods

Qualitative methods, which currently are gaining increased use in the form of point-of-care testing (POCT), are designed to distinguish between results below and above a predefined cutoff value. Note that the cutoff point should not be confused with the detection limit. These tests are assessed primarily on the basis of their ability to correctly classify results in relation to the cutoff value.

Performance Measures

The probability of classifying a result as positive (exceeding the cutoff) when the true value indeed exceeds the cutoff is called *clinical sensitivity.* The probability of classifying a result as negative (below the cutoff) when the true value indeed is below the cutoff is termed *clinical specificity.* Determination of clinical sensitivity and specificity is based on comparison of test results with a gold standard. The gold standard may be an independent test that measures the same analyte, but it may also be a clinical diagnosis determined by definitive clinical methods (e.g., radiographic testing, follow-up, outcomes analysis). Determination of these performance measures is covered in Chapter 3. Clinical sensitivity and specificity may be given as a fraction or as a percentage after multiplication by 100. Standard errors of estimates are derived from the

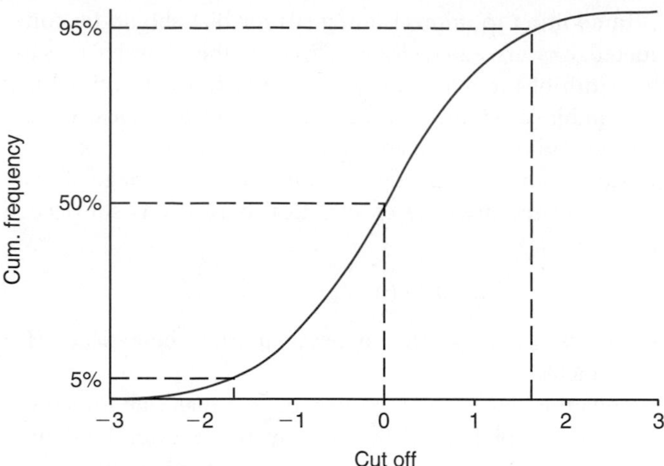

Figure 2-8 Cumulative frequency distribution of positive results. The *x*-axis indicates concentrations standardized to zero at the cutoff point (50% positive results) with unit standard deviation (SD).

binomial distribution.[98] The performance of two qualitative tests applied in the same groups of nondiseased and diseased subjects can be compared using the McNemar test.[64]

One approach for determining the recorded performance of a test in terms of clinical sensitivity and specificity is to determine the true concentration of analyte using an independent reference method. The closer the concentration is to the cutoff point, the larger the error frequencies are expected to be. Actually the cutoff point is defined in such a way that for samples having a true concentration exactly equal to the cutoff point, 50% of results will be positive and 50% will be negative.[33] Concentrations above and below the cutoff point at which repeated results are 95% positive or 95% negative, respectively, have been called the "95% interval" for the cutoff point for that method[33] (note that this is not a CI; Figure 2-8). A CLSI guideline discusses this topic.[15]

Agreement Between Qualitative Tests

As outlined previously, if the outcome of a qualitative test can be related to a true analyte concentration or a definitive clinical diagnosis, it is relatively straightforward to express the performance in terms of clinical specificity and sensitivity. In the absence of a definitive reference or "gold standard," one should be cautious with regard to judgments on performance. In this situation, it is primarily *agreement* with another test that can be assessed. When replacement of an old or expensive routine method with a new or less expensive method is considered, it is of interest to know whether similar test results are likely to be obtained. If both methods are imperfect, however, it is not possible to judge which test has the better performance, unless additional testing by a reference procedure is carried out.

In a comparison study, the same individuals are tested by both methods to prevent bias associated with selection of patients. Basically, the outcome of the comparison study should be presented in the form of a 2 × 2 table, from which

TABLE 2-5 2 × 2 Table for Assessing Agreement Between Two Qualitative Tests

		Test 1	
		+	−
Test 2	+	a	b
	−	c	d
Total		a + c	b + d

various measures of agreement may be derived (Table 2-5). An obvious measure of agreement is the overall fraction or percentage of subjects tested who have the same test result (i.e., both results negative or positive):

$$\text{Overall percent agreement} = (a+d)/(a+b+c+d) \times 100\%$$

If agreement differs with respect to diseased and healthy individuals, the overall percent agreement measure becomes dependent on disease prevalence in the studied group of subjects. This is a common situation; accordingly, it may be desirable to separate this overall agreement measure into agreement concerning negative and positive results:

$$\text{Percent agreement given test 1 positive: } a/(a+c)$$
$$\text{Percent agreement given test 1 negative: } b/(b+d)$$

For example, if there is a close agreement with regard to positive results, overall agreement will be high when the fraction of diseased subjects is high; however, in a screening situation with very low disease prevalence, overall agreement will mainly depend on agreement with regard to negative results. Standard errors of the estimates can be derived from the binomial distribution.[66,98]

A problem with the simple agreement measures is that they do not take agreement by chance into account. Given independence, expected proportions observed in fields of the 2 × 2 table are obtained by multiplication of the fraction's negative and positive results for each test. Concerning agreement, it is excess agreement beyond chance that is of interest. More sophisticated measures have been introduced to account for this aspect. The most well-known measure is kappa, which is defined generally as the ratio of observed excess agreement beyond chance to maximum possible excess agreement beyond chance.[34] We have the following:

$$\text{Kappa} = (I_o - I_e)/(1 - I_e)$$

where I_o is the observed index of agreement and I_e is the expected agreement from chance. Given complete agreement, kappa equals +1. If observed agreement is greater than or equal to chance agreement, kappa is larger than or equal to zero. Observed agreement less than chance yields a negative kappa value.

Example

Table 2-6 shows a hypothetical example of observed numbers in a 2 × 2 table. The proportion of positive results for test 1

TABLE 2-6 2 × 2 Table With Example of Agreement of Data for Two Qualitative Tests

		Test 1		
		+	−	Total
Test 2	+	60	20	80
	−	15	40	55
Total		75	60	135

is 75/(75 + 60) = 0.555, and for test 2, it is 80/(80 + 55) = 0.593. Thus by chance, we expect the ++ pattern in 0.555 × 0.593 × 135 = 44.44 cases. Analogously, the — pattern is expected in (1 – 0.555) × (1 – 0.593) × 135 = 24.45 cases. The expected overall agreement percent by chance I_e is (44.44 + 24.45)/135 = 0.51. The observed overall percent agreement is I_o = (60 + 40)/135 = 0.74. Thus we have

$$\text{Kappa} = (0.74-0.51)/(1-0.51) = 0.47$$

Generally, kappa values greater than 0.75 are taken to indicate excellent agreement beyond chance, values from 0.40 to 0.75 are regarded as showing fair to good agreement beyond chance, and finally, values below 0.40 indicate poor agreement beyond chance. A standard error for the kappa estimate can be computed.[34] Kappa is related to the intraclass correlation coefficient, which is a widely used measure of interrater reliability for quantitative measurements.[34] The considered agreement measures, percent agreement, and kappa can also be applied to assess the reproducibility of a qualitative test when the test is applied twice in a given context.

Various methodological problems are encountered in studies on qualitative tests. An obvious mistake is to let the result of the test being evaluated contribute to the diagnostic classification of subjects being tested (circular argument). Another problem is partial as opposed to complete verification. When a new test is compared with an existing, imperfect test, a partial verification is sometimes undertaken, in which only discrepant results are subjected to further testing by a perfect test procedure. On this basis, sensitivity and specificity are reported for the new test. This procedure (called *discrepant resolution*) leads to biased estimates and should not be accepted.[77] The problem is that for cases with agreement, both the existing (imperfect) test and the new test may be wrong. Thus only a measure of agreement should be reported, not specificity and sensitivity values. In the biostatistical literature, various procedures have been suggested to correct for bias caused by imperfect reference tests, but unrealistic assumptions concerning the independence of test results are usually put forward.

METHOD COMPARISON

Comparison of measurements by two methods is a frequent task in the laboratory. Preferably, parallel measurements of a set of patient samples should be undertaken. To prevent artificial matrix-induced differences, fresh patient samples are the optimal material. A nearly even distribution of values over the analytical measurement range is also preferable. In an ordinary laboratory, comparison of two routine methods will be the most frequently occurring situation. Less commonly, comparison of a routine method with a reference method is undertaken. When two routine methods are compared, the focus is on observed differences. In this situation, it is not possible to establish that one set of measurements is the correct one, and thereby know by how much measurements deviate from the presumed correct concentrations. Rather, the question is whether the new method can replace the existing one without a systematic change in result values. To address this question, the dispersion of observed differences between paired measurements may be evaluated by these methods. To carry out a formal, objective analysis of the data, a statistical procedure with graphics display should be applied. Various approaches may be used: (1) a frequency plot or histogram of the distribution of differences with measures of central tendency and dispersion [distribution of differences (DoD) plot]; (2) a difference (bias) plot, which shows differences as a function of the average concentration of measurements (Bland-Altman plot); or (3) a regression analysis. In the following, a general error model is presented and some typical measurement relationships are considered. Each of the statistical approaches mentioned will be presented in detail, along with a discussion of their advantages and disadvantages.

Basic Error Model

The occurrence of measurement errors is related to the performance characteristics of the assay. It is important to distinguish between pure, random measurement errors, which are present in all measurement procedures, and errors related to incorrect calibration and nonspecificity of the assay. A reference measurement procedure is associated only with pure, random error, whereas a routine method, additionally, is likely to have some bias related to errors in calibration and limitations with regard to specificity. An erroneous calibration function gives rise to a systematic error, whereas nonspecificity gives an error that typically varies from sample to sample. The error related to nonspecificity thus has a random character, but in contrast to the pure measurement error, it cannot be reduced by repeated measurements of a sample. Although errors related to nonspecificity for a group of samples look like random errors, for the individual sample, this type of error is a bias. Because this bias varies from sample to sample, it has been called a *sample-related random bias*.[55,59,60,62] In the following section, the various error components are incorporated into a formal error model.

Measured Value, Target Value, Modified Target Value, and True Value

Upon taking into account that an analytical method measures analyte concentrations with some random measurement error, one has to distinguish between the actual, measured value and the average result we would obtain if the given sample was measured an infinite number of times. If the method is a reference method without bias and nonspecificity, we have the following, simple relationship:

$$x_i = X_{\text{True}i} + \varepsilon_i$$

where x_i represents the measured value, $X_{\text{True}i}$ is the average value for an infinite number of measurements, and ε_i is the deviation of the measured value from the average value. If we were to undertake repeated measurements, the average of ε_i would be zero and the SD would equal the analytical SD (σ_A) of the reference measurement procedure. Pure, random, measurement error will usually be Gaussian distributed.

In the case of a routine method, the relationship between the measured value for a sample and the true value becomes more complicated:

$$x_i = X_{\text{True}i} + \text{Cal-Bias} + \text{Random-Bias}_i + \varepsilon_i$$

The *Cal-Bias* term (calibration bias) is a systematic error related to the calibration of the method. This systematic error may be a constant for all measurements corresponding to an offset error, or it may be a function of the analyte concentration (e.g., corresponding to a slope deviation in the case of a linear calibration function). The *Random-Bias*$_i$ term is a bias that is specific for a given sample related to nonspecificity of the method. It may arise because of codetermination of substances that vary in concentration from sample to sample. For example, a chromogenic creatinine method codetermines some other components with creatinine in serum.[48] Finally, we have the random measurement error term ε_i.

If we performed an infinite number of measurements of a specific sample by the routine method, the random measurement error term ε_i would be zero. The cal-bias and the random-bias$_i$, however, would be unchanged. Thus, the average value of an infinite number of measurements would equal the sum of the true value and these bias terms. This average value may be regarded as the target value ($X_{\text{Target}i}$) of the given sample for the routine method. We have

$$X_{\text{Target}i} = X_{\text{True}i} + \text{Cal-Bias} + \text{Random-Bias}_i$$

As mentioned, the calibration bias represents a systematic error component in relation to the true values measured by a reference measurement procedure. In the context of regression analysis, this systematic error corresponds to the intercept and the slope deviation from unity when a routine method is compared with a reference measurement procedure (outlined in detail later). It is convenient to introduce a modified target value expression ($X'_{\text{Target}i}$) for the routine method to delineate this systematic calibration bias, so that

$$X'_{\text{Target}i} = X_{\text{True}i} + \text{Cal-Bias}$$

Thus, for a set of samples measured by a routine method, the $X_{\text{Target}i}$ values are distributed around the respective $X'_{\text{Target}i}$ values with an SD, which is called σ_{RB}.

If the method is a reference method without bias and nonspecificity, the target value and the modified target value equal the true value, that is,

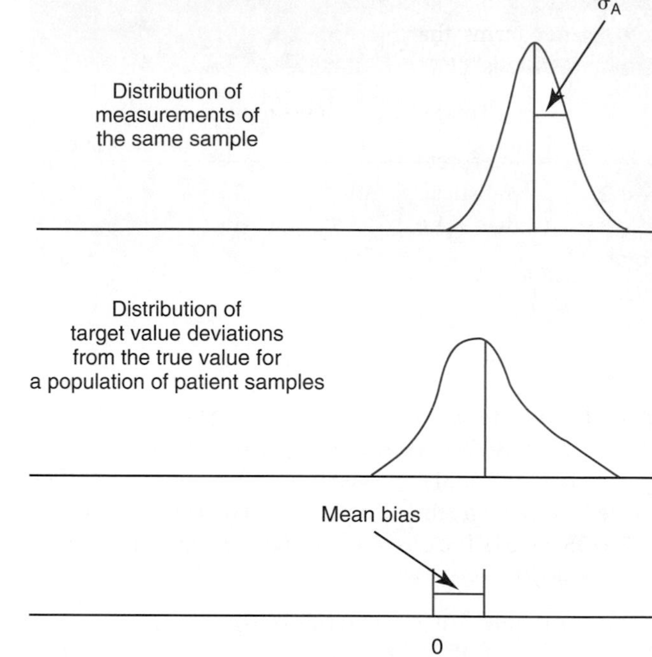

Figure 2-9 Outline of basic error model for measurements by a routine method. *Upper part,* The distribution of repeated measurements of the *same* sample, representing a normal distribution around the target value ($X_{\text{Target}i}$) *(vertical line)* of the sample with a dispersion corresponding to the analytical standard deviation, σ_A. *Middle part,* Schematic outline of the dispersion of target value deviations from the respective true values for a population of patient samples. A distribution of an arbitrary form is displayed. The standard deviation equals σ_{RB}. The vertical line indicates the mean of the distribution. *Lower part,* The distance from zero to the mean of the target value deviations from the true values represents the calibration bias (Mean bias = CAL-Bias) of the method.

$$X_{\text{Target}i} = X'_{\text{Target}i} = X_{\text{True}i}$$

The error model is outlined in Figure 2-9.

Calibration Bias and Random Bias

For an individual measurement, the total error is the deviation of x_i from the true value, that is,

$$\text{Total error of } x_i = \text{Cal-Bias} + \text{Random-Bias}_i + \varepsilon_i$$

Estimation of the bias terms requires parallel measurements between the method in question and a reference method as outlined in detail later. With regard to calibration bias, one should be aware of the possibility of lot-to-lot variation in analytical kit sets. The manufacturer should provide documentation on this lot-to-lot variation, because often it will not be possible for the individual laboratory to investigate a sufficient number of lots to assess this variation. Lot-to-lot variation will show up as a calibration bias that changes from lot to lot.

The previous exposition defines the total error in somewhat broader terms than is often seen. A traditional total error expression is[108]

$$\text{Total error} = \text{Bias} + 2\ \text{SD}_A$$

which often is interpreted as the calibration bias plus 2 SD_A. If a one-sided statistical perspective is taken, the expression is modified to Bias + 1.65 SD_A, indicating that 5% of results are located outside the limit. If a lower percentage is desired, the multiplication factor is increased accordingly, supposing a normal distribution. Interpreting the bias as identical with the calibration bias may lead to an underestimation of the total error.

Random bias related to sample-specific interferences may take several forms. It may be a regularly occurring additional random error component, perhaps of the same order of magnitude as the analytical error. In this context, it is natural to quantify the error in the form of an SD or coefficient of variation. The most straightforward procedure is to carry out a method comparison study based on a set of patient samples in which one of the methods is a reference method, as outlined later. Krouwer[59] formally quantified sample-related random interferences in a comparison experiment of two cholesterol methods and found that the CV of the sample-related random interference component exceeded the analytical CV. Kringle and Bogavich[55] considered random bias of a Jaffe creatinine method by components of variance analysis and found random bias to be a pronounced random error component, constituting 80% of the total random error. This relatively high amount should be interpreted in light of the limited specificity of the Jaffe creatinine measurement principle.

Another form of sample-related random interference is more rarely occurring gross errors, which typically are seen in the context of immunoassays and are related to unexpected antibody interactions (see "Interference" section).[51,79,94] Such an error usually will show up as an outlier in method comparison studies. A well-known source is the occurrence of heterophilic antibodies. Outliers should not just be discarded from the data analysis procedure. Outliers must be investigated to identify their cause, which may be an important limitation in using a given method. Supplementary studies may help clarify such random sample-related interferences and may provide specifications for the assay that limit its application in certain contexts (e.g., with regard to samples from certain patient categories).

Blunders or Clerical Errors

Another reason for outliers in method comparison studies and in daily practice is *blunders* or *clerical errors*. In the past, this type of error usually arose in relation to manual transfer of results. Today, this type of error typically is related to computer error originating at interfaces between computer systems or to instrument failure not detected by the on-analyzer error detection system. Plebani[87] focused on laboratory errors associated with the preanalytical and postanalytical phases. Errors on test order forms and errors related to handling of order forms appear to occur relatively frequently (1 to 5% of recorded cases). In the postanalytical phase, inappropriate interpretation may take place (e.g., in relation to erroneous reference intervals).

Method Comparison Data Model

We here consider the error model described earlier in relation to the method comparison situation. For a given sample measured by two analytical methods, 1 and 2, we have

$$x1_i = X1_{\text{Target}i} + \varepsilon 1_i = X_{\text{True}i} + \text{Cal-Bias1} + \text{Random-Bias1}_i + \varepsilon 1_i$$
$$x2_i = X2_{\text{Target}i} + \varepsilon 2_i$$
$$= X_{\text{True}i} + \text{Cal-Bias2} + \text{Random-Bias2}_i + \varepsilon 2_i$$

From this general model, we may study some typical situations. First, comparison of a routine method with a reference measurement procedure will be treated. Second, comparison of two routine methods is considered.

Comparison of a Routine Method With a Reference Measurement Procedure

Assuming that method 1 is a reference method, the bias components disappear by definition, and we have the following situation:

$$x1_i = X1_{\text{Target}i} + \varepsilon 1_i = X_{\text{True}i} + \varepsilon 1_i$$
$$x2_i = X2_{\text{Target}i} + \varepsilon 2_i$$
$$= X_{\text{True}i} + \text{Cal-Bias2} + \text{Random-Bias2}_i + \varepsilon 2_i$$

The paired differences become

$$(x2_i - x1_i) = \text{Cal-Bias2} + \text{Random-Bias2}_i + (\varepsilon 2_i - \varepsilon 1_i)$$

We thus have an expression consisting of a systematic error term (calibration bias of method 2) and two random terms. The Random-Bias2 term is distributed around Cal-Bias2 according to an undefined distribution. $(\varepsilon 2_i - \varepsilon 1_i)$ is a difference between two random measurement errors that are independent and, commonly, Gaussian distributed. However, we remind the reader that the SD for analytical methods often depends on the concentration, as mentioned earlier. For analytes with a wide analytical measurement range (e.g., some hormones), both sample-related random interferences and analytical SDs are likely to depend on the measurement concentration, often in a roughly proportional manner. It may then be more useful to evaluate the *relative* differences—$(x2_i - x1_i)/[(x2_i + x1_i)/2]$—and accordingly express mean and random bias and analytical error as proportions. An alternative is to partition the total analytical measurement range into segments (e.g., three parts) and consider calibration bias, random bias, and analytical error separately for each of these segments. The segments may be divided preferably in relation to important decision concentrations (e.g., in relation to reference interval limits and/or treatment decision concentrations).

Comparison of Two Routine Methods

In the comparison of two routine methods, the paired differences become

$$(x2_i - x1_i) = (\text{Cal-Bias2} - \text{Cal-Bias1}) + (\text{Random-Bias2}_i - \text{Random-Bias1}_i) + (\varepsilon 2_i - \varepsilon 1_i)$$

The expression again consists of a constant term, the difference between the two calibration biases, and two random terms. The first random term is a difference between two random-bias components that may or may not be independent. If the two field methods are based on the same measurement principle, the random bias terms are likely to be correlated. For example, two chromogenic methods for creatinine are likely to be subject to interference from the same chromogenic compounds present in a given serum sample. On the other hand, a chromogenic method and an enzymatic creatinine method are subject to different types of interfering compounds, and the random bias terms may be relatively independent. In the $\varepsilon 2_i - \varepsilon 1_i$ term, the same relationships as described previously are likely to apply. One may note that the general form of the expressed differences is the same in the two situations. Thus the same general statistical principles actually apply. In the following sections, we will consider the distribution of differences under various circumstances, as well as the measurement relations between methods 1 and 2 on the basis of regression analysis.

Preliminary Practical Work in Relation to a Method Comparison Study

When a method comparison study is to be conducted, the analytical methods to be examined first should be established in the laboratory according to written protocols and should be stable in routine performance. Reagents are commonly supplied as ready-made analytical kits, perhaps implemented on a dedicated analytical instrument (open or closed system). Technologists performing the study should be trained in the procedures and associated instrumentation. Further, it is important that a quality control system is in place to ensure that the methods being compared are running in an in-control state.

Planning a Method Comparison Study

In the planning phase of a method comparison study, several points require attention, including the (1) number of samples necessary, (2) distribution of analyte concentrations (preferably uniform over the analytical measurement range), and (3) representativeness of the samples. To address the latter point, samples from relevant patient categories should be included, so that possible interference phenomena can be discovered. Practical aspects related to storage and treatment of samples (e.g., container) and possible artifacts induced by storage (e.g., freezing of samples) and addition of anticoagulants should be considered. Comparison of measurements should preferably be undertaken over several days (e.g., at least 5 days), so that the comparison of methods does not become dependent on the performance of the methods in one particular analytical run. Finally, ethical aspects (e.g., informed consent from patients whose samples will be used) should be considered in relation to existing legislation.

When the comparison protocol is considered, various guidelines may be consulted. The CLSI Evaluation Protocol (EP) guidelines give advice on various aspects. For example, the CLSI guideline EP-9A2 "Method Comparison and Bias Estimation Using Patient Samples" suggests measurement of 40 samples in duplicate by each method when a new method is introduced in the laboratory as a substitute for an established one.[10] Additionally, it is proposed that a vendor of an analytical test system should have made a comparison study based on at least 100 samples measured in duplicate by each method. The principle of a more demanding requirement for vendors appears reasonable. This initial validation should be comprehensive to disclose the performance of the assay system in detail. Then the requirement for the ordinary user may be more modest. The EP15 guideline "User Verification of Manufacturer's Claims" suggests a more condensed approach based on a bias or difference plot, which does not involve regression analysis and can be carried out using 20 samples.[17] Although these general guidelines on sample size are useful, additional aspects are important. The probability of detecting rarely occurring interferences showing up as outliers should be taken into account when the necessary sample size is considered. Finally, in relation to evaluation of automated methods, special consideration should be given to the sample sequence to evaluate drift, carryover, and nonlinearity (e.g., by a multifactorial design).[58]

Distribution of Differences Plot (DoD plot)

From the end-user viewpoint, it is the differences per se that matter. Thus with regard to the outcome of replacing an established routine method with a new one that perhaps is less expensive or more practical, it is important to focus on the distribution of differences between paired measurements by the old and the new method. A graphic display with assessment of the central tendency and dispersion of differences in the form of an ordinary histogram or frequency polygon plot is useful. The differences may or may not be Gaussian distributed. Because both analytical error components and sample-related random interferences may contribute to the differences, the distribution may be irregular and outliers may occur. Further, the random dispersion elements may be dependent on analyte concentration. Therefore, a nonparametric approach for interpreting the distribution of differences may generally be preferable as a starting point.

Nonparametric Approach

Both the central tendency (median) and extreme percentiles are of interest when the nonparametric approach to the distribution of differences is used. With a traditional 95% level, 2.5- and 97.5-percentiles are considered. A 99% or higher extreme level may be selected, and the related percentiles (0.5- and 99.5-, or more extreme ones) may then be applied for a description of method differences. Nonparametric estimation of the 2.5- and 97.5-percentiles requires 2.5 times as many observations as the parametric approach to obtain the same uncertainty, which implies that sample sizes cannot be too small.[74] Estimating confidence limits of the percentiles

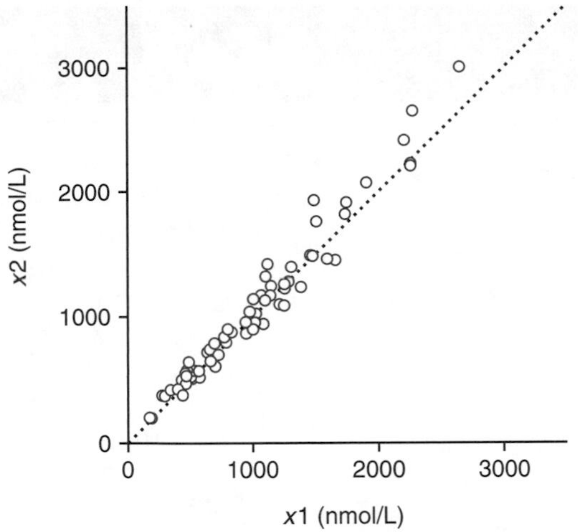

Figure 2-10 A scatter plot of $N = 65$ ($x1$, $x2$) data points for comparison of two drug assays. The *dashed line* is the line of identity.

can give an indication of their imprecision. The CIs can be estimated from the ordered observations as described in Chapter 5 in the section on nonparametric estimation of the 95%-reference interval. Alternatively, a bootstrap procedure can be applied as described.[74] The advantage of the bootstrap procedure is that standard errors can be derived using smaller sample sizes than are used with the simple nonparametric approach.[19]

A method comparison example from the laboratory of one of the authors (K.L.) is considered. Two drug assays developed in-house for serum concentrations of the antipsychotic drug clozapine are compared. The established assay (method 1) is an HPLC method based on manual liquid-liquid extraction. The new method (method 2) is an HPLC method with an automated on-column extraction step. An initial impression of the relation between $x1$ and $x2$ measurements can be obtained from a scatter plot of the 65 measurement sets ($x1$, $x2$) with the identity line outlined (Figure 2-10). The $x1$ measurements range from 177 to 2650 nmol/L, and the range of $x2$ values is from 200 to 3004 nmol/L (i.e., we have a relatively wide analytical measurement range in the present example). A histogram of the difference ($x2 - x1$) is shown in Figure 2-11. Applying a nonparametric data description, we order the observed differences according to size and derive the median difference as the value of the $(0.5N + 0.5)^{\text{th}}$ ordered observation, here 26 nmol/L. In case the order is a noninteger, interpolation between neighbor-ordered values is carried out. A paired nonparametric test, the Wilcoxon test,[98] shows that the median difference was significantly different from zero ($P < 0.02$). The 2.5- and 97.5-percentiles correspond to the values of the $(0.025N + 0.5)^{\text{th}}$ and $(0.975N + 0.5)^{\text{th}}$ ordered observations, respectively, as displayed in Table 2-7.[23,74] For a sample size smaller than 120, it is not possible to derive CIs for the percentiles by the simple nonparametric procedure. Therefore, we also applied the bootstrap procedure to estimate nonparametric percentiles with 90%-CIs[30,74] (see Table 2-7). The bootstrap procedure, which is based on computerized random resampling of the observations, provides slightly different percentile estimates, as shown in Table 2-7. In this way, we obtain an estimation of the size of negative and positive differences with uncertainties. The present example shows a considerable range of differences, with the 2.5-percentile being −169 nmol/L (90%-CI: −214 to −123) and the 97.5-percentile being 356 nmol/L (90% CI: 255 to 457). These relatively large differences should be related to the considerable analytical measurement range for the analyte, and an evaluation of *relative* differences may be more relevant for the present example (see later in this chapter).

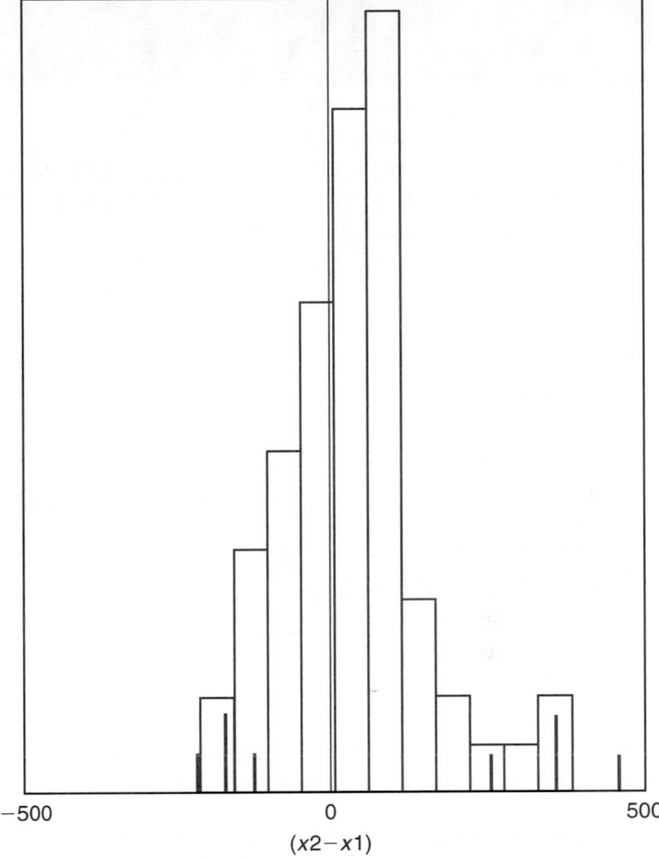

Figure 2-11 Distribution of differences (DoD) plot for comparison of two drug assays: nonparametric analysis. A histogram shows the relative frequency of $N = 65$ differences with demarcated 2.5- and 97.5-percentiles determined nonparametrically. The 90%-confidence intervals (CIs) of the percentiles are shown. These were derived by the bootstrap technique.

In the presented examples, no evident outliers were present. However, outliers deserve special attention.[23] Unless they are related to obvious method or apparatus malfunction, discarding of outliers should be considered with caution. Outliers may indicate the presence of large sample-related random interferences, which may be of major clinical importance (e.g., interference by antibodies or degradation products that occur only rarely). Thus a special investigation of

TABLE 2-7 Analysis of Distribution of Differences for the Comparison of Drug Assays Example. $N = 65$ Single ($x1$, $x2$ Measurements). The Unit is nmol/L

Total range of $x1$ measurements	177 to 2650		
Total range of $x2$ measurements	200 to 3004		
Total range of differences ($x2 - x1$)	−210.00 to 437.00		
Test for normality of differences (Anderson-Darling test)	$P < 0.01$		
Statistical analysis of differences	Simple nonparametric	Bootstrap	Parametric
Median	26.00 ($P < 0.02$)		
Mean			42.00 ($P < 0.01$)
SD			124.42
Coefficient of skewness			+0.83
Coefficient of kurtosis			+1.27
Outlier test (4 SD)			ns
2.5-percentile	−166.00	−169.11	−201.86
97.5-percentile	372.38	355.90	285.86
90%-CI for 2.5-percentile		−214.73 to −123.50	−245.24 to −158.47
90%-CI for 97.5-percentile		255.03 to 456.77	242.47 to 329.24

CI, Confidence interval; *ns*, not significant; *SD*, standard deviation.

outlying results with reanalysis and exploration of the reasons for the outlying observations should be considered.

Parametric Approach

If application of a goodness-of-fit test does not disprove that the distribution of differences is Gaussian distributed, a parametric statistical approach may be undertaken. In the example presented, a significant deviation from normality was present, as assessed by the Anderson-Darling test[65] ($P < 0.01$); therefore, a parametric analysis in principle should not be carried out. However, to demonstrate the procedure, the parametric approach is also carried out (Figure 2-12 and Table 2-7). The mean and SD (SD_{Dif}) of the paired differences ($x2 - x1$) are estimated according to standard procedures. A paired t-test is used to determine whether the mean difference is significantly different from zero ($P < .01$ in this case). The 2.5- and 97.5-percentiles for the differences are estimated as the mean $\pm t_{0.025(N-1)}$ SD_{Dif}. A standard error for the percentiles (SE_{perc}) may be computed and the 90%-CI limits are then derived as ± 1.65 SE_{perc} around the percentiles (see Figure 2-12 and Table 2-7). The parametrically derived 2.5- and 97.5-percentiles (−202 and 286 nmol/L) differ somewhat from the non-parametrically derived percentiles, which in the present context with proven non-normality may be regarded as the most reliable estimates.

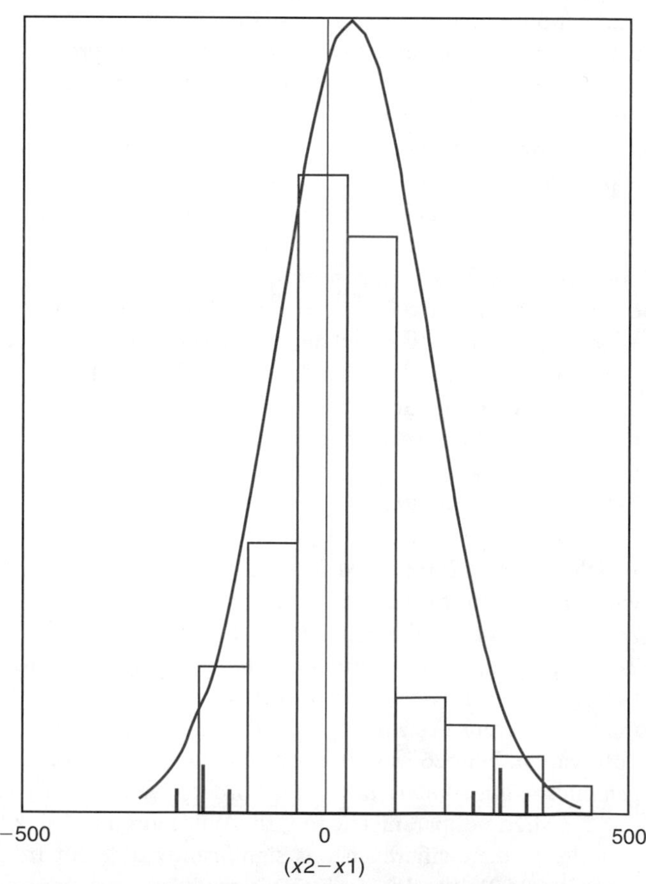

Figure 2-12 Distribution of differences (DoD) plot for comparison of two drug assays: parametric analysis. A histogram shows the relative frequency of $N = 65$ differences with the estimated Gaussian density distribution. Parametrically estimated 2.5- and 97.5-percentiles are shown with 90%-confidence intervals (CIs).

Relative Distribution of Differences Plot (Rel DoD plot)

In some cases in which a wide analytical measurement range (i.e., corresponding to 1 or several decades) is used, the random error components depend on the concentration, as previously mentioned. Analytical SDs may be approximately proportional to the concentration over the major part of the analytical measurement range. In the present example, the

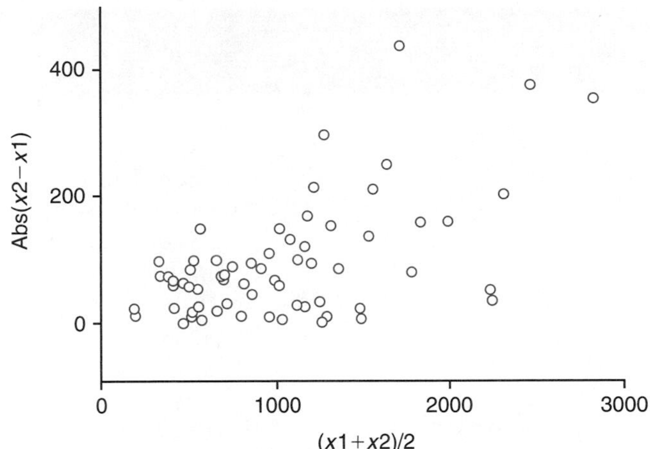

Figure 2-13 Plot of absolute differences (ordinate) against average concentration (abscissa) for the comparison of drug assays example. The scatter increases with the average concentration (r = +0.57).

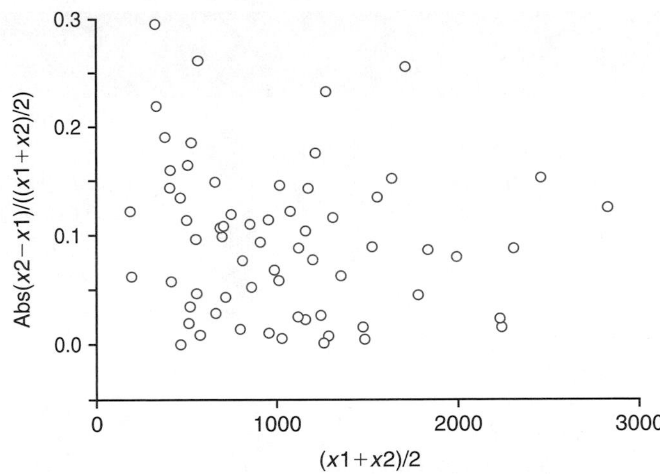

Figure 2-14 Plot of absolute *relative* differences (ordinate) against average concentration (abscissa) for the comparison of drug assays example. The scatter is not significantly correlated with the average concentration (r = −0.15, not significant).

initial scatter plot of ($x1$, $x2$) values suggests that the random error of the differences increases with the concentration (see Figure 2-10). A formal test for this possible relation is to compute the correlation coefficient between the average concentration and the *absolute* value of the differences. This correlation coefficient, r, is +0.57, which is significantly different from zero ($P < 0.001$), and it confirms the relationship of scatter increasing with concentration, which also can be visualized in a scatter plot of the absolute differences against the average concentration (Figure 2-13). A natural next step is to assess the *relative* differences in relation to the average concentration. The correlation coefficient between the absolute values of the relative differences [$|x2 - x1|/(\{x1 + x2\}/2)$] and the average concentration [$(x1 + x2)/2$] was not significantly different ($P > 0.05$) from zero ($r = -0.15$); a scatter plot also suggests a more homogeneous dispersion (Figure 2-14). In this situation, it is more reasonable to deal with *relative* differences or percentage differences [$(\{x2 - x1\}/\{x1 + x2\}/2) \times 100\%$]. The same nonparametric descriptive measures as used earlier may be applied for the central tendency and the dispersion (Figure 2-15). The median relative difference amounts to 0.042, or 4.2%, which is significantly higher than zero ($P < 0.01$) (Wilcoxon test) (Table 2-8). The 2.5- and 97.5-percentiles are −0.15 and 0.26, respectively. The 90%-CIs derived by the bootstrap procedure were −0.16 to −0.14 and 0.21 to 0.30, respectively. Thus from this analysis, we may conclude that the 95% interval for percentage differences ranges from about −15 to +26%.

Finally, we may consider a parametric analysis of the relative differences (Figure 2-16 and Table 2-8). A goodness-of-fit test (Anderson-Darling test; $P > .05$) showed that the relative differences did not depart significantly from a normal distribution, which in this case supports the parametric approach (Figure 2-17). The parametric 2.5- and 97.5-percentiles were

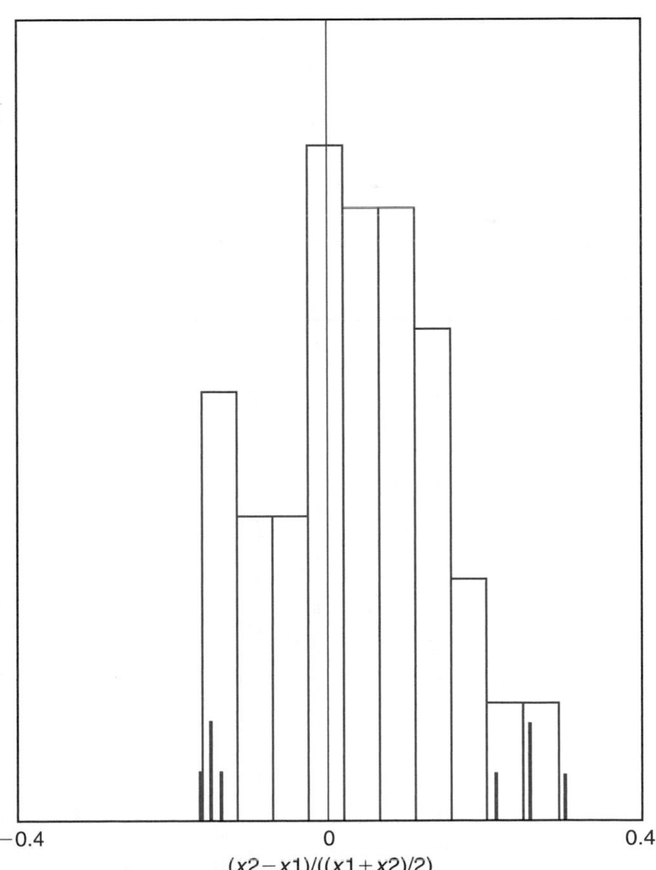

Figure 2-15 Relative distribution of differences (Rel DoD) plot for comparison of two drug assays: nonparametric analysis. A histogram shows the relative frequency of relative differences with demarcated 2.5- and 97.5-percentiles determined nonparametrically. The 90%-confidence intervals (CIs) (bootstrap) of the percentiles are shown.

TABLE 2-8 Analysis of Distribution of *Relative* Differences for the Comparison of Drug Assays Example. $N = 65$

Total range of relative differences	−0.1598 to 0.2953		
Test for normality (Anderson-Darling test)	ns		
Statistical analysis	Simple nonparametric	Bootstrap	Parametric
Median	0.0467 ($P < 0.01$)		
Mean			0.0418 ($P < 0.01$)
SD			0.1109
Coefficient of skewness			+0.05
Coefficient of kurtosis			−0.60
Outlier test			ns
2.5-percentile	−0.1487	−0.1492	−0.1754
97.5-percentile	0.2607	0.2570	0.2591
90%-CI for 2.5-percentile		−0.1627 to −0.1357	−0.2141 to −0.1368
90%-CI for 97.5-percentile		0.2135 to 0.3005	0.2204 to 0.2978

CI, Confidence interval; *ns,* not significant; *SD,* standard deviation.

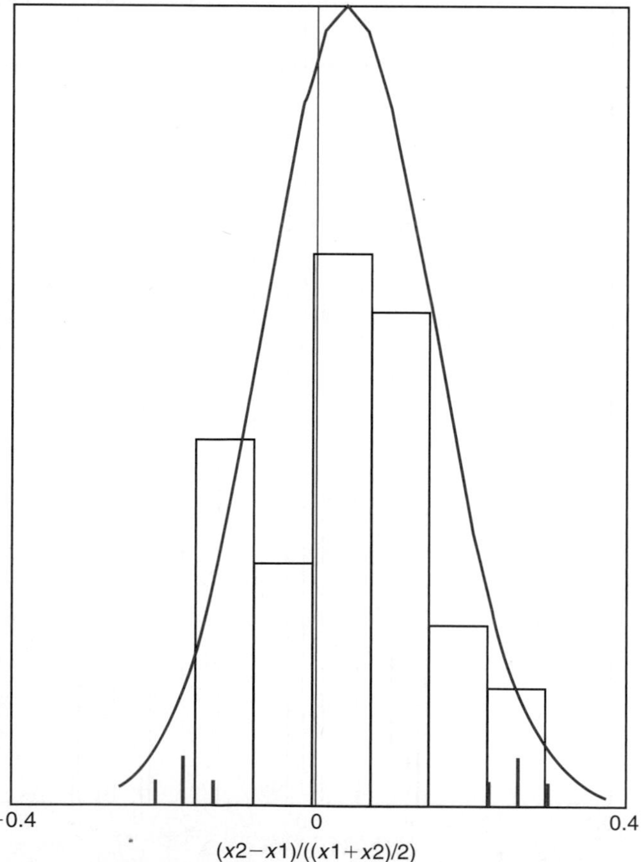

Figure 2-16 Distribution of *relative* differences plot for comparison of two drug assays: parametric analysis. A histogram shows the relative frequency of relative differences with the estimated Gaussian density distribution. Parametrically estimated 2.5- and 97.5-percentiles are shown with 90%-confidence intervals (CIs).

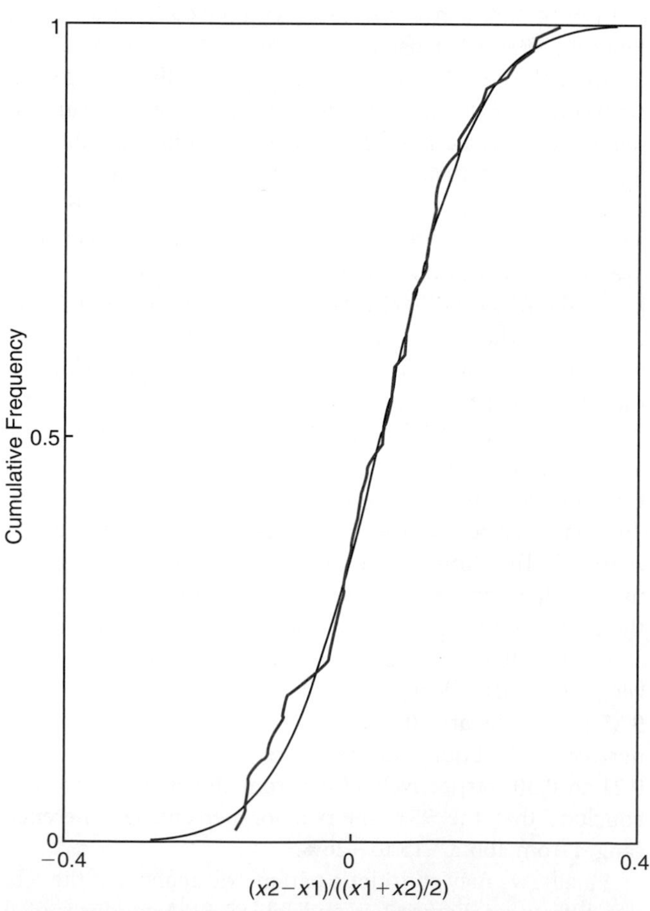

Figure 2-17 Cumulative frequency distribution of relative differences for the comparison of drug assays example. The lighter curve indicates the Gaussian cumulative frequency distribution curve. In accordance with the test for normality, good agreement is observed.

−0.18 and 0.26, respectively. The mean was 0.042, and the SD of the relative differences was 0.11. Thus we may conclude that there is an average bias of about 4%, which might rely on a calibration difference [an estimate of (Cal-Bias2 − Cal-Bias1)], and a random error corresponding to a CV of 11%. The random error CV of 11% is an estimate of the combined dispersion of [(Random-Bias2_i − Random-Bias1_i) + ($\varepsilon 2_i$ − $\varepsilon 1_i$)]. If we ascribe the random variation equally to the two assays, it corresponds to a random error level of $11\%/\sqrt{2}$ = 7.8% for each assay. In the present example, the average bias of 4% and the estimated random variation of differences between the two assays were considered acceptable in relation to the clinical use of the assay, and it was decided to replace the manual assay with the new, automated assay.

Verification of Distribution of Differences in Relation to Specified Limits

In situations in which a field method is being considered for implementation, it may be desired primarily to *verify* whether the differences in relation to the existing method are located within given specified limits, rather than *estimating* the distribution of differences. For example, one may set limits corresponding to ±15% as clinically acceptable and may desire that a majority (e.g., 95% of differences) are located within this interval.

By counting, it may be determined whether the expected proportion of results is within the limits (i.e., 95%). One may accept percentages that do not deviate significantly from the supposed percentage at the given sample size derived from the binomial distribution (Table 2-9). For example, if 50 paired measurements have been performed in a method comparison study, and if it is observed that 46 of these results (92%) are within specified limits (e.g., ±15%), the study supports that the achieved goal has been reached, because the lower boundry for acceptance is 90%. It is clear that a reasonable number of observations should be obtained for the assessment to have acceptable power. If very few observations are available, the risk is high of falsely concluding that at least 95% of the observations are within specified limits, in case it is not true (i.e., committing a type II error).

TABLE 2-9 Lower Bounds (One-Sided 95%-CI) of Observed Proportions (%) of Results Being Located Within Specified Limits for Paired Differences That Are in Accordance With the Hypothesis of at Least 95% of Differences Being Within the Limits

N	Observed Proportions
20	85
30	87
40	90
50	90
60	90
70	90
80	91
90	91
100	91
150	92
200	93
250	93
300	93
400	93
500	93
1000	94

CI, Confidence interval.

Difference (Bland-Altman) Plot

The difference plot suggested by Bland and Altman is widely used for evaluating method comparison data.[3,4] The procedure was originally introduced for comparison of measurements in clinical medicine, but it has also been adopted in clinical chemistry.[69,84,88] The Bland-Altman plot is usually understood as a plot of the differences against the average results of the methods. Thus the difference plot in this version provides information on the relation between differences and concentration, which is useful in evaluating whether problems exist at certain ranges (e.g., in the high range) caused by nonlinearity of one of the methods. It may also be of interest to observe whether differences tend to increase proportionally with the concentration, or whether they are independent of concentration. In some situations, particular interest may be directed toward the low-concentration region. Information on the relation between differences and concentration is useful in the context of how to adjust for an irregularity (e.g., by changing the method to correct for nonlinearity, by restricting the analytical measurement range).

The basic version of the difference plot requires plotting of the differences against the average of the measurements. Figure 2-18 shows the plot for the drug assay comparison

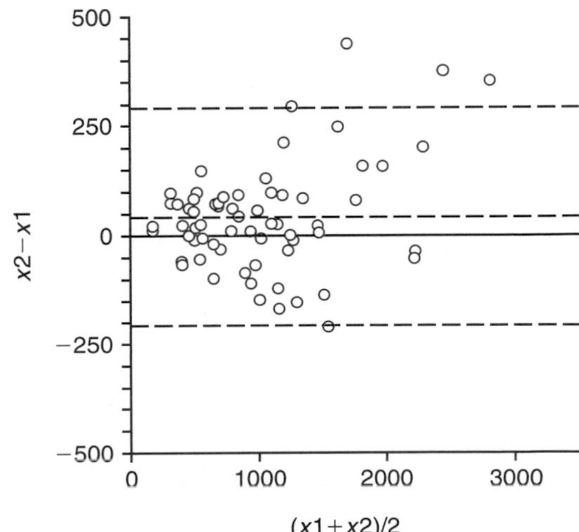

Figure 2-18 Bland-Altman plot of differences for the drug comparison example. The differences are plotted against the average concentration. The mean difference (42 nmol/L) with ±2 standard deviation (SD) of differences is shown *(dashed lines).*

data. The interval ±2 SD of the differences is often delineated around the mean difference (i.e., corresponding to the mean and the 2.5- and 97.5-percentiles considered in the parametric DoD plot).[4]

Nonparametric limits may also be considered. The distribution of the differences as measured on the *y*-axis of the coordinate system corresponds to the relations outlined for the DoD plot, which represents a projection of the differences on the *y*-axis. A constant bias over the analytical measurement range changes the average concentration away from zero. The presence of sample-related random interferences increases the width of the distribution. If the calibration bias depends on the concentration, if the dispersion varies with the concentration, or if both occur, the relations become more complex, and the interval mean ±2 SD of the differences may not fit very well as a 95% interval throughout the analytical measurement range.

The displayed Bland-Altman plot for the drug assay comparison data (see Figure 2-18) shows a tendency toward increasing scatter with increasing concentration, which is a reflection of increasing random error with concentration, as considered in detail in previous paragraphs. Thus a plot of the relative differences against the average concentration is of relevance (Figure 2-19). This plot has a more homogeneous dispersion of values, agreeing with the estimated limits for the dispersion, that is, the relative mean difference $\pm t_{0.025(N-1)}$ SD_{RelDif} equal to $0.042 \pm 1.998 \times 0.11$ corresponding to −0.18 and 0.26, analogous to the situation with the relative DoD plot considered earlier.

Use of *relative* differences in situations with a proportional random error relationship prevents very large differences in the high concentration range from dominating the analysis and making a balanced interpretation difficult. In the low range, the proportional relationship may not necessarily hold

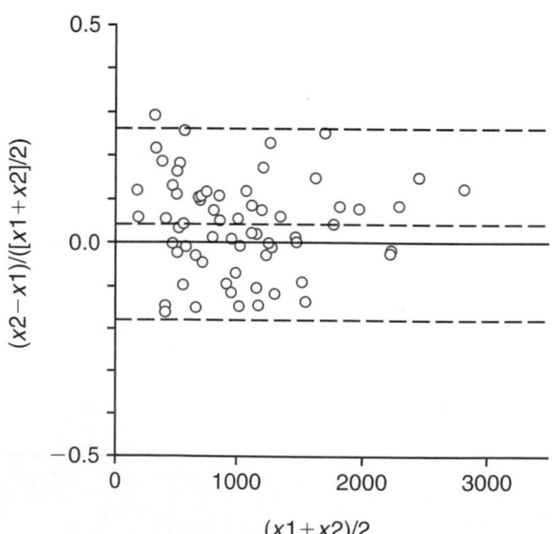

Figure 2-19 Bland-Altman plot of *relative* differences for the drug comparison example. The differences are plotted against the average concentration. The mean relative difference (0.042) with ±2 standard deviation (SD) of relative differences is shown *(dashed lines).*

true, and sometimes the relative difference plot overcompensates for lack of proportionality in this region. It is then possible to truncate the proportional relationship at some lower limit and assume a constant SD for differences below this limit[70] (i.e., corresponding to the relationship in Figure 2-3, *C*). In the actual drug example (see Figure 2-19) with a slightly negative correlation coefficient between relative differences and average concentration, a tendency toward this pattern is seen. An alternative to the relative difference plot is to plot the logarithm of the differences against the average concentration, but this type of plot is more difficult to interpret, because the scale is changed.

Although it is customary to display the *estimated* limits for the differences (often, mean $\pm$ 2 SD_{dif}), one may, as an alternative, display specification limits considered reasonable, as mentioned for the DoD plot.[84] It may then be assessed whether the observed differences conform to these limits, as discussed earlier (see Table 2-9). Application of the difference plot in various specific contexts has been considered.[9,99] It has also been suggested to estimate a regression line for the differences as a function of the average measurement concentration.[103]

A Caution Against Incorrect Interpretation of Paired *t*-Tests in Method Comparison Studies

In association with the difference plot, the paired *t*-test is usually applied as described earlier[3] but one should be careful with regard to the interpretation. For example, consider the case shown below, in which method 2 (*x*2) measurements tend to exceed method 1 (*x*1) measurements in the low range and vice versa at high concentrations (Figure 2-20, *A*). This corresponds to a positive calibration bias in the low range, changing to a negative calibration bias in the high range. In this situation, the overall averages of both sets of measurements are nearly equal, and the paired *t*-test yields a nonsignificant result, because the average paired difference (i.e., the overall bias) is close to zero (Table 2-10). This does not mean that the measurements are equivalent. Subjecting the data to Deming regression analysis (see the next section) clearly discloses the relation[72] (Figure 2-20, *B*). Results of the regression analysis confirm the existence of both a systematic constant error (intercept different from zero) and a systematic proportional error (slope different from 1). Therefore, as pointed out previously, the statistical significance revealed by the paired *t*-test cannot be used to indicate whether measurements are equivalent. The paired *t*-test is just a test for the average bias; it does not say anything about the equivalency of measurements throughout the analytical measurement range.

Regression Analysis

Regression analysis is commonly applied in comparing the results of analytical method comparisons. Typically, an experiment is carried out in which a series of paired values is collected when a new method is compared with an established method. This series of paired observations ($x1_i$, $x2_i$) is then used to establish the nature and strength of the relationship between the tests. This discussion outlines various regression

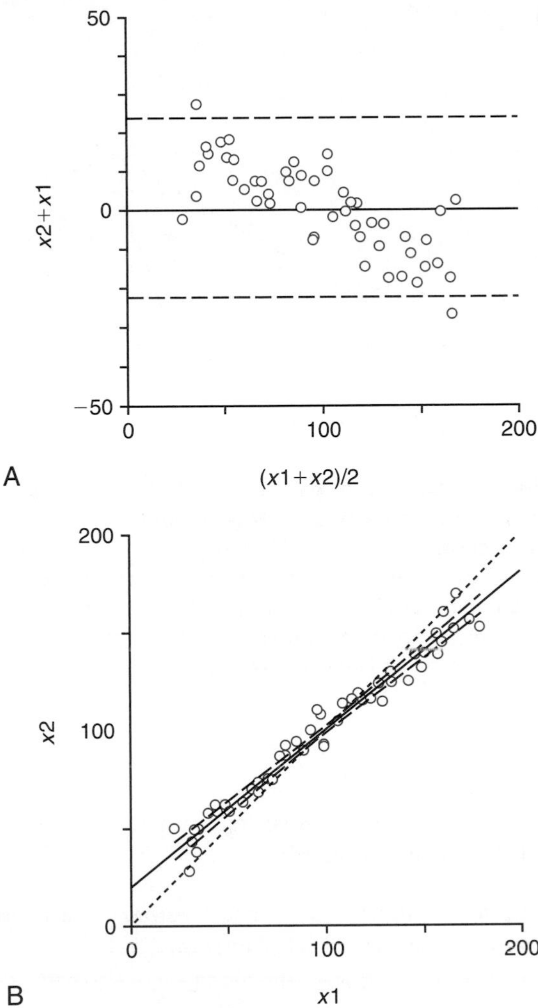

Figure 2-20 Simulated example with positive and negative differences in the low and high ranges, respectively. A, Bland-Altman plot. B, *x-y* plot with diagonal *(dotted straight line)* and estimated Deming regression line *(solid line)* with 95%-confidence curves *(dashed lines).*

models that may be used, gives criteria for when each should be used, and provides guidelines for interpreting the results.

Regression analysis has the advantage that it allows the relation between the target values for the two compared methods to be studied over the full analytical measurement range. If the systematic difference between target values (i.e., the calibration bias between the two methods, or the systematic error) is related to the analyte concentration, such a relationship may not be clearly shown when the previously mentioned types of difference plots are used. Although nonlinear regression analysis may be applied, the focus is usually on linear regression analysis. In linear regression analysis, it is assumed that the systematic difference between target values can be modeled as a constant systematic difference (intercept deviation from zero) combined with a proportional systematic difference (slope deviation from unity), usually related to a discrepancy with regard to calibration of the

TABLE 2-10 Comparison of Paired *t*-Test Results and Deming Regression Results for a Simulated Method Comparison Example With Positive Intercept (a_0 = 20) and Slope Below Unity (b = 0.80). N = 50 ($x1$, $x2$) Measurements

	Paired t-Test	Regression Analysis (Deming)
Mean difference (SEM)	0.78 (1.63)	
t = Mean difference/ SEM	0.78/1.63 = 0.48 (ns)	
Slope (b) [SE(b)]		0.80 (0.027)
$t = (b - 1)/\text{SE}(b)$		−7.4 ($P < 0.001$)
Intercept (a_0) [SE(a_0)]		20.3 (2.82)
$t = (a_0 - 0)/\text{SE}(a_0)$		7.2 ($P < 0.001$)

ns, Not significant; *SEM,* standard error of the mean.

methods. In situations where random errors have a constant SD, unweighted regression procedures are used (e.g., Deming regression analysis). For cases with SDs that are proportional to the concentration, the weighted Deming regression procedure is preferred.

Error Models in Regression Analysis

As outlined previously, we distinguish between the measured value (x_i) and the target value ($X_{\text{Target}i}$) of a sample subjected to analysis by a given method. In linear regression analysis, we assume a linear relationship between values devoid of random error of any kind. In statistical terminology, a so-called structural relationship is assumed.[68,78] Thus, to operate with a linear relationship between values without random measurement error and sample-related random bias, we have to introduce modified target values:

$$X1_{\text{Target}i} = X1'_{\text{Target}i} + \text{Random-Bias1}_i$$
$$X2_{\text{Target}i} = X2'_{\text{Target}i} + \text{Random-Bias2}_i$$

where we now assume a linear relationship between these modified target values:

$$X2'_{\text{Target}i} = \alpha_0 + \beta X1'_{\text{Target}i}$$

In this model, α_0 corresponds to a constant difference with regard to calibration, and ($\beta - 1$) is a proportional deviation. Thus, the systematic error or calibration difference between the measurements corresponds to

$$X2'_{\text{Target}i} - X1'_{\text{Target}i} = \alpha_0 + (\beta - 1)X1'_{\text{Target}i}$$

Because of sample-related random interferences and measurement imprecision (of the type that can be described by a Gaussian distribution, e.g., caused by pipetting variability, signal variability), individually measured pairs of values ($x1_i$, $x2_i$) will be scattered around the line expressing the relationship between $X1'_{\text{Target}i}$ and $X2'_{\text{Target}i}$. Figure 2-21 outlines schematically how the random distribution of $x1$ and $x2$ values occurs around the regression line. We have

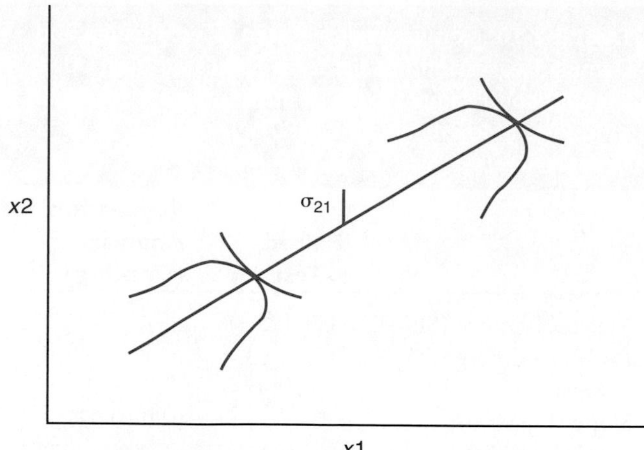

Figure 2-21 Outline of the relation between $x1$ and $x2$ values measured by two methods subject to random errors with constant standard deviations (SDs) over the analytical measurement range. A linear relationship between the modified target values ($X1'_{Targeti}$, $X2'_{Targeti}$) is presumed. The $x1_i$ and $x2_i$ values are Gaussian distributed around $X1'_{Targeti}$ and $X2'_{Targeti}$, respectively, as schematically shown. σ_{21} (σ_{yx}) is demarcated.

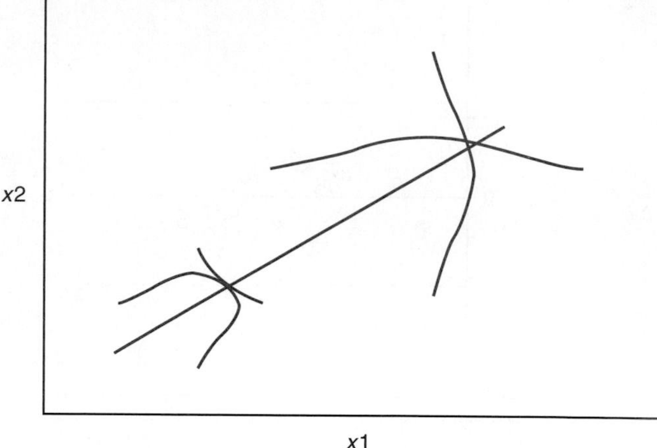

Figure 2-22 Outline of the relation between $x1$ and $x2$ values measured by two methods subject to proportional random errors. A linear relationship between the modified target values is assumed. The $x1_i$ and $x2_i$ values are Gaussian distributed around $X1'_{Targeti}$ and $X2'_{Targeti}$, respectively, with increasing scatter at higher concentrations, as is shown schematically.

$$x1_i = X1_{Targeti} + \varepsilon1_i = X1'_{Targeti} + \text{Random-Bias}1_i + \varepsilon1_i$$
$$x2_i = X2_{Targeti} + \varepsilon2_i = X2'_{Targeti} + \text{Random-Bias}2_i + \varepsilon2_i$$

The random error components may be expressed as SDs, and generally we can assume that sample-related random bias (SD σ_{RB}) and analytical imprecision (SD σ_A) are independent for each analyte, yielding the relations

$$\sigma^2_{ex1} = \sigma^2_{RB1} + \sigma^2_{A1}$$
$$\sigma^2_{ex2} = \sigma^2_{RB2} + \sigma^2_{A2}$$

σ_{ex1} and σ_{ex2} are the total SDs of the distributions of $x1_i$ and $x2_i$ around their respective modified target values, $X1'_{Targeti}$ and $X2'_{Targeti}$. The sample-related random bias components for methods 1 and 2 may not necessarily be independent. They also may not be Gaussian distributed, contrary to the analytical components. Thus when a regression procedure is applied, the explicit assumptions to take into account should be considered. In situations without random bias components of any significance, the relationships simplify to

$$\sigma^2_{ex1} = \sigma^2_{A1}$$
$$\sigma^2_{ex2} = \sigma^2_{A2}$$

In this situation, it usually can be assumed that the error distributions are Gaussian, and estimates of the analytical SDs may be available from quality control data.

Another methodologic problem concerns the question of whether the dispersion of sample-related random bias and the analytical imprecision are constant or change with the analyte concentration, as considered previously in the difference plot sections. In cases with a considerable range (i.e., a decade or longer), this phenomenon should also be taken into account when a regression analysis is applied. Figure 2-22 schematically shows how dispersions may increase proportionally with concentration.

Deming Regression Analysis and Ordinary Least-Squares Regression Analysis (OLR) (Constant SDs)

To reliably estimate the relationship between modified target values (i.e., a_0 for α_0 and b for β), a regression procedure taking into account errors in both $x1$ and $x2$ is preferable (i.e., Deming approach) (see Figure 2-21).[22] Although the OLR procedure is commonly used in method comparison studies, it does not take errors in $x1$ into account but is based on the assumption that only the $x2$ measurements are subject to random errors (Figure 2-23). In the Deming procedure, the sum of squared distances from measured sets of values ($x1_i$, $x2_i$) to the regression line is minimized at an angle determined by the ratio between SDs for the random variations of $x1$ and $x2$. It can be proven theoretically that, given Gaussian *error* distributions, this estimation procedure is optimal. It should here be noted that it is the *error* distributions that should be Gaussian, not the dispersion of values over the measurement range. This is often misunderstood. In Figure 2-24, the symmetric case is illustrated with a regression slope of 1 and equal SDs for the random variations of $x1$ and $x2$, in which case the sum of squared distances is minimized orthogonally in relation to the line.

OLR is not recommended except in special situations. In OLR, the sum of squared distances is minimized in the vertical direction to the line (see Figure 2-24). It can be proven theoretically that neglect of the random error in $x1$ induces a downward biased slope estimate

$$\beta' = \beta[\sigma^2_{X1'target}/(\sigma^2_{X1'target} + \sigma^2_{ex1})] = \beta/[1 + (\sigma_{ex1}/\sigma_{X1'target})^2]$$

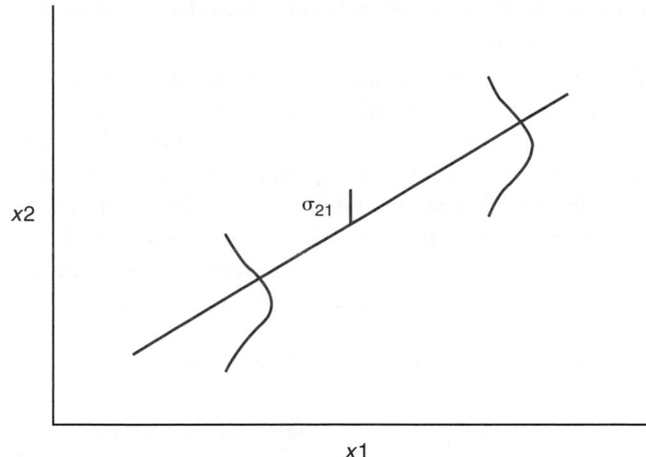

Figure 2-23 The model assumed in ordinary least-squares regression (OLR). The *x*2 values are Gaussian distributed around the line with constant standard deviation (SD) over the analytical measurement range. The *x*1 values are assumed to be without random error. σ_{21} (σ_{yx}) is shown.

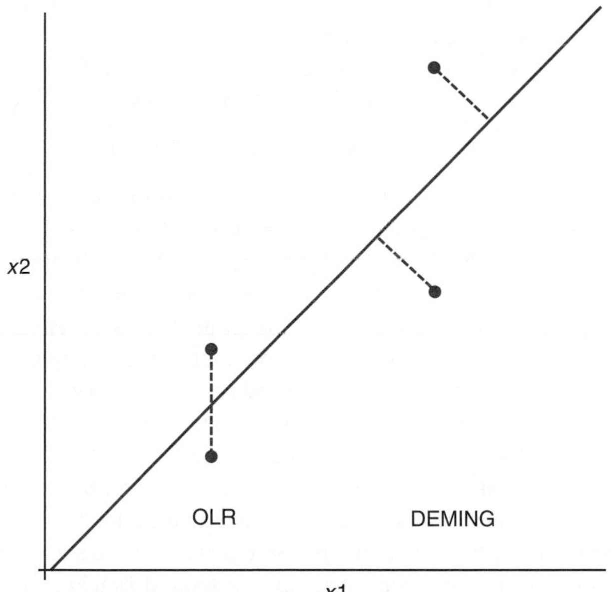

Figure 2-24 In ordinary least-squares regression (OLR), the sum of squared deviations from the line is minimized in the vertical direction. In Deming regression analysis, the sum of squared deviations is minimized at an angle to the line, depending on the random error ratio. Here the symmetric case is displayed with orthogonal deviations. [*Reproduced with permission from* Reference 71 *(Figure 1)*.]

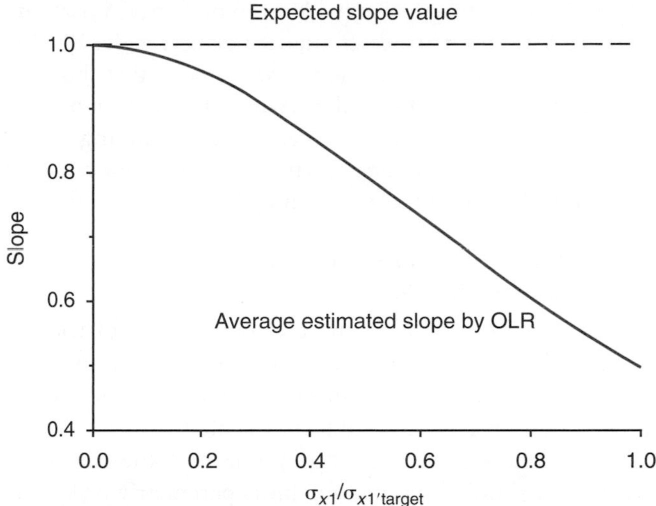

Figure 2-25 Relations between the true (expected) slope value and the average estimated slope by ordinary least-squares regression (OLR). The bias of the OLR slope estimate increases negatively for increasing ratios of the standard deviation (SD) random error in *x*1 to the SD of the *X*1 target value distribution.

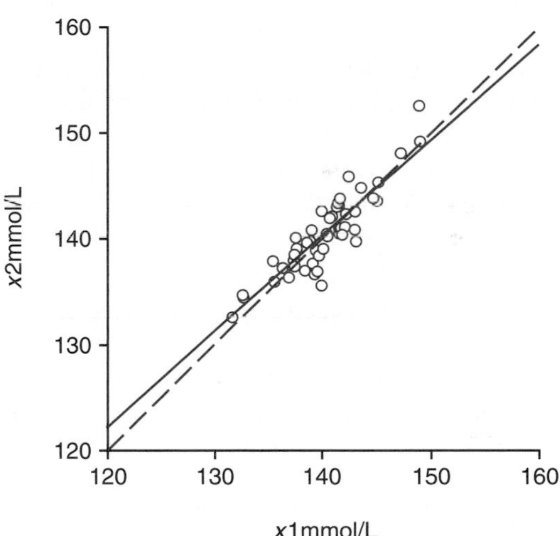

Figure 2-26 Simulated comparison of two sodium methods. The *solid line* indicates the average estimated ordinary least-squares regression (OLR) line, and the *dotted line* is the identity line. Even though no systematic difference is evident between the two methods, the average OLR line deviates from the identity line corresponding to a downward slope bias of about 10%.

where $\sigma_{X1'target}$ is the SD of $X1'$ target values.[98] The magnitude of the bias depends on the ratio between the SD for the random error in $x1$ and the SD of the $X1'$ target values. Figure 2-25 shows the bias as a function of the ratio of the random error SD to the SD of the $X1'$ target value dispersion. For a ratio up to 0.1, the bias is less than 1%. At a ratio of 0.33, the bias amounts to 10%; it increases further for increasing ratios. In a given case, one can take the analytical SD (e.g., from quality control data) and divide by the SD of the measured $x1$ values, which approximately equals the SD of $X1'$ target values. As an example, a typical comparison study for two serum sodium methods may be associated with a downward directed slope bias of about 10% (Figure 2-26).

In the example presented previously, the ratio of the analytical SD to the SD of the target value distribution is large because of the tight physiologic regulation of electrolyte concentrations, which means that the biological variation is limited. Most other types of analytes exhibit wider distributions, and the ratio of error to target value distribution is smaller. For example, for analytes with a distribution of longer than 1 decade and an analytical error corresponding to a CV of 5% at the middle of the analytical measurement range, the OLR slope bias amounts to about −1%.

Computation Procedures for OLR and Deming Regression

Assuming no errors in $x1$ and a Gaussian error distribution of $x2$ with constant SD throughout the analytical measurement range, OLR is the optimal estimation procedure, as proved by Gauss in the eighteenth century. Given errors in both $x1$ and $x2$, the Deming approach is the method of choice.[20] It should be noted for these parametric procedures that only the *error* distributions must be Gaussian or normal. The least-squares principle does not require normality to be applied, but it is optimal under normality conditions, and the nominal type I errors for associated statistical tests for slope and intercept hold true under this assumption. The procedures are generally robust toward deviations from normality, but they are sensitive to outliers because of the squaring principle. Finally, the distribution of the $x1$ and $x2$ values over the measurement range does not have to be normal. A uniform distribution over the analytical measurement range is generally of advantage, but the distribution in principle may take any form. For both procedures, we may evaluate the SD of the dispersion in the *vertical* direction around the line (commonly denoted $SD_{y \cdot x}$ and here given as SD_{21}). We have

$$SD_{21} = [\Sigma(x2_i - X2'_{\text{Targetesti}})^2/(N-2)]^{0.5}$$

Further discussion regarding the interpretation of SD_{21} will be given later.

To compute the slope in Deming regression analysis, the ratio between the SDs of the random errors of $x1$ and $x2$ is necessary, that is,

$$\lambda = (\sigma^2_{RB1} + \sigma^2_{A1})/(\sigma^2_{RB2} + \sigma^2_{A2})$$

SD_As can be estimated from duplicate sets of measurements as

$$SD^2_{A1} = (1/2N]\Sigma[x1_{2i} - x1_{1i})^2$$
$$SD^2_{A2} = (1/2N]\Sigma[x2_{2i} - x2_{1i})^2$$

or they may be available from quality control data. The latter is a practical approach that avoids the need for duplicate measurements by each measurement procedure.

If a specific value for λ is not available and the two routine methods that are compared are likely to be associated with random errors of the same order of magnitude, λ can be set to 1. The Deming procedure is generally relatively insensitive to a misspecification of the λ value.[71]

Formulas for computing slope (β), intercept (α_0), and their standard errors are available from other sources[20,70,98] and will not be provided here. Commonly available software packages for performing regression analysis by both methods will be mentioned later.

Evaluation of the Random Error Around an Estimated Regression Line

The estimated slope and intercept provide an estimate of the systematic difference or calibration bias between two methods over the analytical measurement range. Additionally, an estimate of the random error is important. It is commonplace to consider the dispersion around the line in the vertical direction, which is quantified as $SD_{y \cdot x}$ (here denoted SD_{21}). SD_{21} was originally introduced in the context of OLR, but it also can be considered in relation to Deming regression analysis.

Interpreting $SD_{y \cdot x}$ (SD_{21}) With Random Errors in Both $x1$ and $x2$

With regard to σ_{21}, we have here without sample-related random interferences

$$\sigma^2_{21} = \beta^2\sigma^2_{A1} + \sigma^2_{A2}$$

Thus, σ_{21} reflects the random error both in $x1$ (with a rescaling) and in $x2$. Often β is close to unity, and in this case σ^2_{21} becomes approximately the sum of the individual squared SDs. This relation holds true for both Deming and OLR analyses. Frequently, OLR is applied in situations associated with random measurement error in both $x1$ and $x2$, and in these situations σ_{21} reflects the errors in both.

The presence of sample-related random interferences in both $x1$ and $x2$ gives the following expression:

$$\sigma^2_{21} = (\beta^2\sigma^2_{A1} + \sigma^2_{A2}) + (\beta^2\sigma^2_{RB1} + \sigma^2_{RB2})$$

Thus, the σ_{21} value is influenced by the slope value and the analytical error components σ_{A1} and σ_{A2} (grouped in the first bracket) and σ_{RB1} and σ_{RB2} (grouped in the second bracket). In many cases, the slope is close to unity, in which case we have simple addition of the components. As mentioned earlier, the sample-related random interferences may not be independent. In this case, simple addition of the components is not correct, because a covariance term should be included. However, in a real case, we can estimate the combined effect corresponding to the bracket term. Information on the analytical components is usually available from duplicate sets of measurements or from quality control data. On this basis, the combined random bias term in the second bracket can be derived by subtracting the analytical components from σ_{21}. Overall, it can be judged whether the total random error is acceptable or not. The systematic difference can be adjusted for relatively easily by rescaling one of the sets of measurements. However, if the random error term is very large, such a rescaling does not ensure equivalency of measurements with regard to individual samples. Thus it is important to assess both the systematic difference and the random error when deciding whether a new routine method can replace an existing one.

Assessment of Outliers

The principle of minimizing the sum of squared distances from the line makes the described regression procedures sensitive to outliers, and an assessment of the occurrence of outliers should be carried out routinely. The distance from a suspected outlier to the line is recorded in SD units, and the outlier is rejected if the distance exceeds a predetermined limit (e.g., 3 or 4 SD units). In the case of OLR, the SD unit equals SD_{21}, and the vertical distance is considered. For Deming regression analysis, the unit is the SD of the deviation of the points from the line at an angle determined by the error variance ratio λ. A plot of these deviations, a so-called residuals plot, conveniently illustrates the occurrence of outliers.[68] Figure 2-27, *A*, illustrates an example of Deming regression analysis with occurrence of an outlier and the associated residuals plot *(B)*, which clearly shows the outlier pattern. In this example, the residuals plot was standardized to unit SD. Use of an outlier limit of 4 SD units in this example led to rejection of the outlier, and a reanalysis was undertaken. In this example, rejection of the outlier changed the slope from 1.14 to 1.03. With regard to outliers, these measurements should not be rejected automatically; the reason for their presence should be investigated as a method limitation (e.g., possibly a nonspecificity for the analyte).

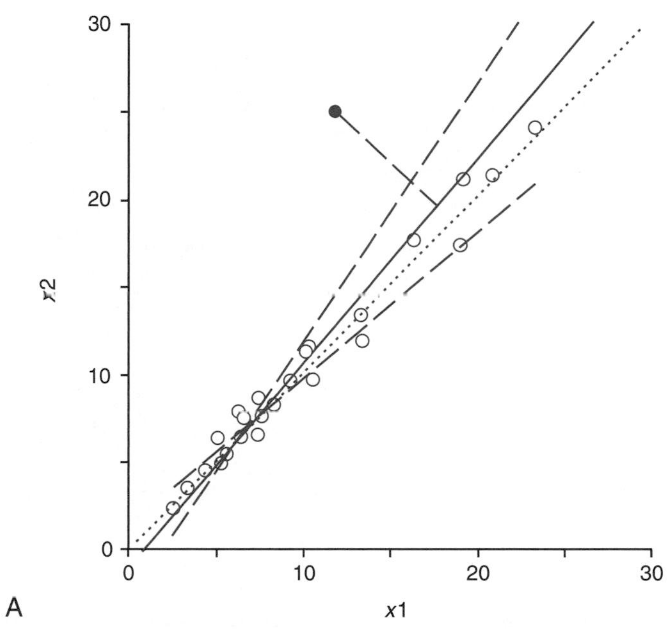

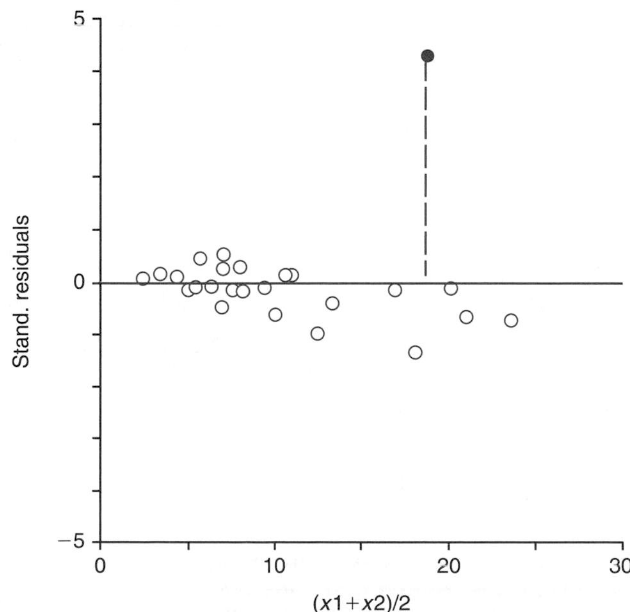

Figure 2-27 A, A scatter plot with the Deming regression line *(solid line)* with an outlier *(filled point)*. The *dotted straight line* is the diagonal, and the *curved dashed lines* demarcate the 95%-confidence region. B, Standardized residuals plot with indication of the outlier.

The Correlation Coefficient

Now that the random error components related to regression analysis have been outlined, some comments on the correlation coefficient may be appropriate. The ordinary correlation coefficient, ρ, also called the Pearson product moment correlation coefficient, is estimated as *r* from sums of squared deviations for *x*1 and *x*2 values as follows:

$$r = p/(uq)^{0.5}$$

where

$$p = \Sigma(x1_i - x1_m)(x2_i - x2_m)$$
$$u = \Sigma(x1_i - x1_m)^2 q = \Sigma(x2_i - x2_m)^2$$

and

$$> x1_m = \Sigma x1_i / N \qquad x2_m = \Sigma x2_i / N$$

A look at the theoretical model reveals that ρ is related to the ratio between the SDs of the distributions of target values ($\sigma_{X1'\text{target}}$ and $\sigma_{X2'\text{target}}$) and the associated independent total random error components (σ_{ex1} and σ_{ex2})[5]:

$$\rho = \sigma_{X1'\text{target}}\sigma_{X2'\text{target}} / [(\sigma^2_{X1'\text{target}} + \sigma^2_{ex1})(\sigma^2_{X2'\text{target}} + \sigma^2_{ex2})]^{0.5}$$

The total random error components comprise both imprecision error and sample-related random interferences (i.e., $\sigma^2_{ex1} = \sigma^2_{A1} + \sigma^2_{RB1}$ and $\sigma^2_{ex2} = \sigma^2_{A2} + \sigma^2_{RB2}$). Thus ρ is a *relative* indicator of the amount of dispersion around the regression line. If the numeric interval of values is short, ρ tends to be low and vice versa for a long range of values. For example, consider simulated examples, where the random errors of *x*1 and *x*2 are the same, but the width of the distributions of measured values differs (Figure 2-28, *A* and *B*). In *(A)*, the target values are uniformly distributed over the range 1 to 3, and in *(B)*, the range is 1 to 6. The random error SD is presumed constant, and it is set to 0.15 for both *x*1 and *x*2, corresponding to a CV of 5% at the value 3. Given sets of 50 paired measurements, the correlation coefficient is 0.93 in case *(A)* and 0.99 in case *(B)*. Further, a single point located outside the range of the rest of the observations exerts a strong influence (Figure 2-28, *C*). In *(C)*, 49 of the observations are distributed within the range 1 to 3, with a single point located apart from the others around the value 6, other factors being equal. The correlation coefficient here takes an intermediate value, 0.97. Thus a single point located away from the rest has a strong influence (a so-called influential point). Note that it is not an outlying point, just an aberrant point with regard to the range.

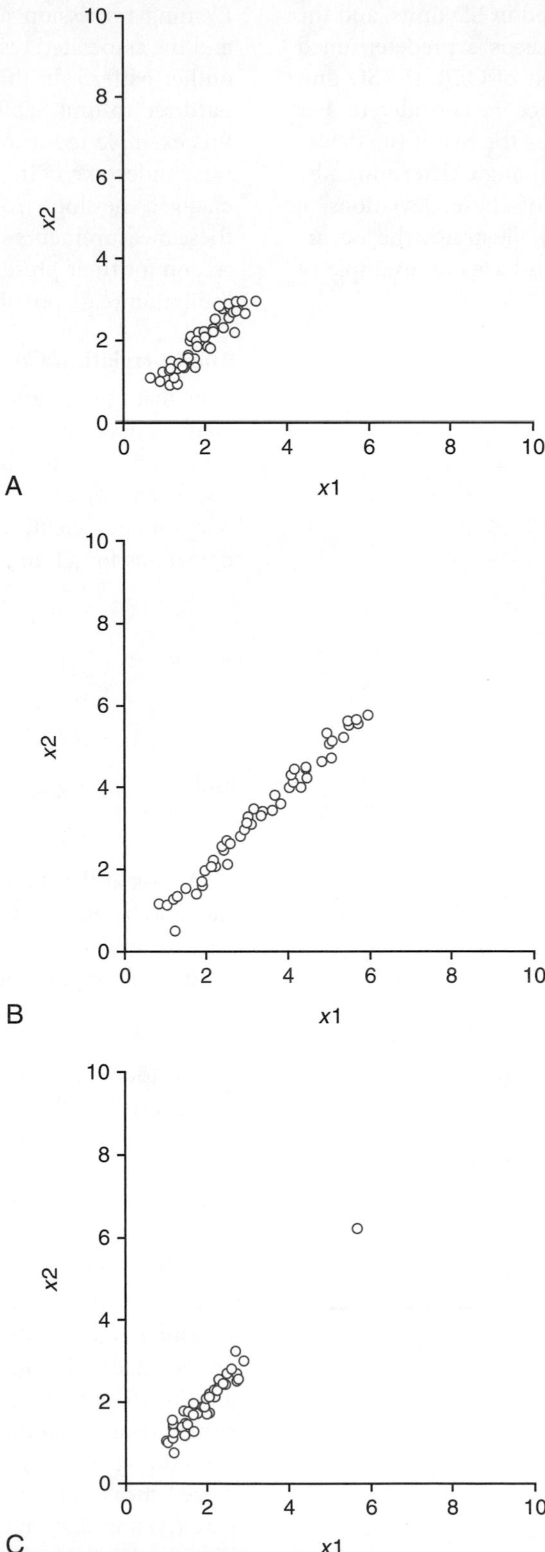

Figure 2-28 Scatter plots illustrating the effect of the range on the value of the correlation coefficient ρ. A, Target values are uniformly distributed over the range 1 to 3 with random errors of both *x*1 and *x*2 corresponding to a standard deviation (SD) of 5% of the target value at 3 (constant error SDs). B, The range is extended to 1 to 6 with the same random error levels. The correlation coefficient equals 0.93 in A and 0.99 in B. C, The effect of a single aberrant point is shown. Forty-nine of the target values are distributed over the range 1 to 3, with a single point at 6. The correlation coefficient is 0.97.

Although σ_{21} is the relevant measure for random error in method comparison studies, ρ is still incorrectly used as a supposed measure of agreement between two methods. It should be noted that a systematic difference due to a difference with regard to calibration is not expressed through ρ but solely in the form of an intercept (α_0) deviation from zero and/or a slope (β) deviation from unity. Thus even though the correlation coefficient is very high, a considerable calibration bias may be noted between the measurements of two methods.

Regression Analysis in Cases of Proportional Random Error

As discussed in relation to the precision profile, for analytes with extended ranges (e.g., 1 or several decades), the SD_A is seldom constant. Rather, a proportional relationship may apply. This may also be true for the random bias components. In this situation, the regression procedures described previously may still be used, but they are not optimal because the standard errors of slope and intercept become larger than is the case when a weighted form of regression analysis is applied. The optimal approaches are weighted forms of regression analysis that take into account the relationship between random error and analyte concentration.[68,70] Given a proportional relationship, a weighted procedure assigns larger weights to observations in the low range; low-range observations are more precise than measurements at higher concentrations that are subject to larger random errors. More specifically, weights are applied in the computations that are inversely proportional to the squared SDs (variances) that express the random error. In the weighted modification of the Deming procedure, distances from ($x1_i$, $x2_i$) to the line are inversely weighted according to the squared SDs at a given concentration (Figure 2-29). The regression procedures are most conveniently performed using dedicated software.

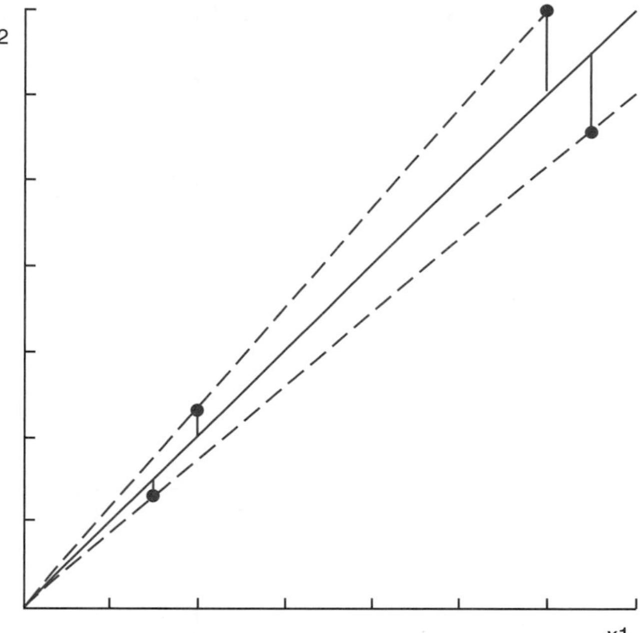

Figure 2-29 Distances from data points to the line in weighted Deming regression assuming proportional random errors in *x*1 and *x*2. The symmetric case is illustrated with equal random errors and a slope of unity yielding orthogonal projections onto the line. *(From Linnet K. Necessary sample size for method comparison studies based on regression analysis. Clin Chem 1999;45:882-94.)*

Testing for Linearity

Splitting of the systematic error into a constant and a proportional component depends on the assumption of linearity, which should be tested. A convenient test is a runs test, which in principle assesses whether negative and positive deviations from the points to the line are randomly distributed over the analytical measurement range. The term *run* here relates to a sequence of deviations with the same sign. Consider for example the situation with a downward trend of $x2$ values at the upper end of the analytical measurement range (Figure 2-30, *A*). The SDs from the line (i.e., the residuals) will tend to be negative in this area instead of being randomly distributed above and below the line[28] (Figure 2-30, *B*). Given a sufficient number of points, such a sequence will turn out to be statistically significant in a runs test.

Nonparametric Regression Analysis (Passing-Bablok)

The slope and the intercept may be estimated by a nonparametric procedure, which is robust to outliers and requires no assumptions of Gaussian error distributions.[81,82] Note, however, that the parametric regression procedures do not presume Gaussian distributions of $x1$ and $x2$ values over the measurement range, but only of the *error* distributions. Thus the main advantage of the nonparametric procedure is its robust performance in the presence of outliers. The method takes measurement errors for both $x1$ and $x2$ into account, but it presumes that the ratio between random errors is related to the slope in a fixed manner:

$$\lambda = (SD^2_{RB1} + SD^2_{A1})/(SD^2_{RB2} + SD^2_{A2}) = 1/\beta^2$$

Otherwise, a biased slope estimate is obtained.[70,82] The procedure may be applied both in situations with random errors with constant SDs and in cases with proportional SDs. The method is not as efficient as the corresponding parametric procedures (i.e., Deming and weighted Deming procedures).[70] Slope and intercept with CIs are provided, together with Spearman's rank correlation coefficient. A software program is required for the procedure.

Interpretation of Systematic Differences Between Methods Obtained on the Basis of Regression Analysis

A systematic difference between two methods is identified if the estimated intercept differs significantly from zero, or if the slope deviates significantly from 1. This is decided on the basis of *t*-tests:

$$t = (a_0 - 0)/SE(a_0)$$
$$t = (b - 1)/SE(b)$$

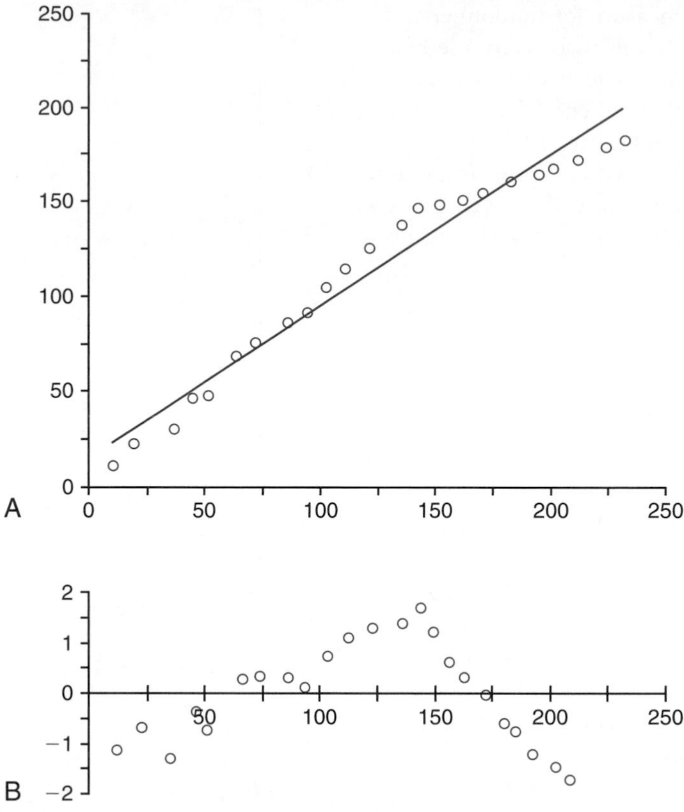

Figure 2-30 ***A,*** **Scatter plot showing an example of nonlinearity in the form of downward deviating** ***x*****2 values at the upper part of the range.** ***B,*** **Plot of residuals showing the effects of nonlinearity. At the upper end of the analytical measurement range, a sequence (run) of negative residuals is present.**

SE(a_0) and SE(b) are the standard errors of the estimated intercept a_0 and the slope b, respectively. Standard errors can be derived by a computerized resampling principle called *the jackknife procedure,* which in practice can be carried out using appropriate software[73] (see section on software). Having estimated a_0 and b, we have the estimate of the systematic difference between the methods, D_c, at a selected concentration, $X1'_{\text{Targetc}}$:

$$D_c = X2'_{\text{Targetestc}} - X1'_{\text{Targetc}} = a_0 + (b-1)X1'_{\text{Targetc}}$$

$X2'_{\text{Targetestc}}$ is the estimated $X2'$ target value at $X1'_c$. Note that D_c refers to the *systematic* difference (i.e., the difference between modified target values corresponding to a calibration difference). The standard error of D_c can be derived by the jackknife procedure using a software program. By evaluating the standard error throughout the analytical measurement range, a confidence region for the estimated line can be displayed. If method comparison is performed to assess the calibration to a reference measurement procedure, correction of a significant systematic difference $Delta_c$ will often be performed by recalibration [$x2_{rec} = (x1 - a_0)/b$]. The associated standard uncertainty is the standard error of $Delta_c$. Even though the intercept and the slope are not significantly different from zero and 1, respectively, the combined expression $Delta_c$ may be significantly different from zero.

Example of Application of Regression Analysis (Weighted Deming Analysis)

Application of weighted Deming regression analysis may be illustrated by the comparison of drug assays example [$N = 65$ ($x1$, $x2$) single measurements]. As outlined in the section on the Bland-Altman plot (see Figure 2-14), in this example the random error of the differences increases with the concentration, suggesting that the weighted form of Deming regression analysis is appropriate. Figure 2-31 shows *(A)* the estimated regression line with 95%-confidence bands and *(B)* a plot of normalized residuals. The nearly homogeneous scatter in the residuals plot supports the assumed proportional random error model and the assumption of linearity. The slope estimate (1.014) is not significantly different from 1 (95%-CI: 0.97 to 1.06), and the intercept is not significantly different from zero (95%-CI: −6.7 to 47.4) (Table 2-11). A runs test for linearity does not contradict the assumption of linearity. The amount of random error is quantified in the form of the SD_{21} proportionality factor equal to 0.11, or 11%. In the present example, with a slope close to unity and two routine methods with assumed random errors of about the same magnitude, we divide the random error by the square root of 2 and get $CV_{x1} = CV_{x2} = 7.8\%$. Quality control data in the laboratory have provided CV_As of 6.1% and 7.2% for methods 1 and 2, respectively. Thus in this example, the random error may be

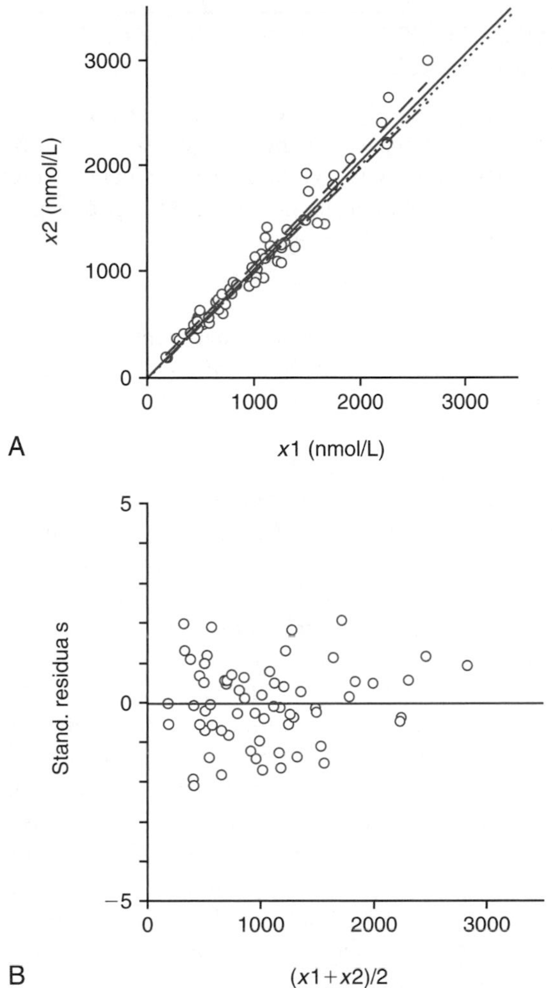

Figure 2-31 An example of weighted Deming regression analysis for the comparison of drug assays. A, The *solid line* is the estimated weighted Deming regression line, the *dashed curves* indicate the 95%-confidence region, and the *dotted line* is the line of identity. B, A plot of residuals standardized to unit standard deviation (SD). The homogeneous scatter supports the assumed proportional error model and the assumption of linearity.

TABLE 2-11 Results of Weighted Deming Regression Analysis for the Comparison of Drug Assays Example, $N = 65$ Single ($x1$, $x2$) Measurements

	Estimate	SE	95%-CI
Slope (b)	1.014	0.022	0.97 to 1.06
Intercept (a_0)	20.3	13.5	−6.7 to 47.4
Weighted correlation coefficient	0.98		
SD_{21} proportionality factor	0.11		
Runs test for linearity	ns		
$Delta_c = X_2 - X_1$ at $X_c = 300$	24.6	9.5	5.72 to 43.6
$Delta_c = X_2 - X_1$ at $X_c = 2000$	48.9	34.2	−19.3 to 117

CI, Confidence interval; *ns,* not significant; *SD,* standard deviation; *SE,* standard error.

attributed largely to analytical error. The assay principle for both methods is HPLC, which generally is a rather specific measurement principle; considerable random bias effects are not expected in this case.

In the table, estimated systematic differences at the limits of the therapeutic interval (300 and 2000 nmol/L) are displayed (24.6 and 48.9 nmol/L, respectively). This corresponds to percentage values of 8.2% and 2.4%, respectively. Estimated standard errors by the jackknife procedure yield the 95%-CIs as shown in the table. At the low concentration, the difference is significant (95%-CI: 5.7 to 44 nmol/L, does not include zero), which is not the case at the high level (95%-CI: −19 to 117 nmol/L). Even though the intercept and slope estimates separately are not significantly different from the null hypothesis values of zero and 1, respectively, the combined difference $Delta_c$ is significant at low concentrations in this example. If the difference is considered of medical importance and both methods are to be used simultaneously in the laboratory, recalibration of one of the methods might be considered.

Discussion of Application of Regression Analysis

Generally, it is recommended that Deming or weighted Deming regression analysis should be used to operate with a type of regression analysis that is based on a correct error model. Most published method evaluations are based on unweighted regression analysis; here the use of unweighted analysis is considered in the setting of proportional random errors.

Basically, the Deming procedure provides unbiased estimates of slope and intercept when the SDs vary, provided that their ratio is constant throughout the analytical measurement range. This aspect is important and means that generally the estimates of slope and intercept are reliable in this frequently encountered situation. However, application of the unweighted Deming analysis in cases of proportional SD_As is less efficient than applying the weighted approach. For uniform distributions of values with range ratios from 2 to 100, 1.2 to 3.7 times as many samples are necessary to obtain the same uncertainty of the slope estimated by the unweighted compared with the weighted approach.[73] Thus the larger the range ratio, the more inefficient is the unweighted method.

MONITORING SERIAL RESULTS

An important aspect of clinical chemistry is monitoring of disease or treatment (e.g., tumor markers in cases of cancer, drug concentrations in cases of therapeutic drug monitoring). To assess changes in a rational way, various imprecision components have to be taken into account. Biological within-subject variation ($SD_{within\text{-}B}$) and preanalytical (SD_{PA}) and analytical variation (SD_A) all have to be recognized. We assume in the following discussion that preanalytical variation is already included in the estimated within-subject variation SD, which often is the case. On this basis, using the principle of adding squared SDs (variances), a total SD (SD_T) can be estimated as follows:

$$SD_T^2 = SD_{Within\ B}^2 + SD_A^2$$

The limit for statistically significant changes then is $k\sqrt{2}\ SD_T$, where k depends on the desired probability level. Considering a two-sided 5% level, k is 1.96. The corresponding one-sided factor is 1.65. If a higher probability level is desired, k should be increased.

Limits for statistically significant changes ($Delta_{stat}$) may be related to changes that are considered of medical importance by clinicians [i.e., action limits ($Delta_{med}$)].[97] Here we will consider a one-sided situation in which an increase is of importance and a 5% significance level is selected (i.e., $Delta_{stat} = 1.65\sqrt{2}\ SD_T = 1.65\ SD_{delta}$). Suppose as a starting point that the true change ($Delta_{true}$) for a patient is zero (Figure 2-32, *A*). If $Delta_{stat}$ is less than $Delta_{med}$, the frequency of false-positive alarms will be less than 5%. If, on the other hand, $Delta_{stat}$ exceeds $Delta_{med}$, the frequency of false-positive alarms will exceed 5% (i.e., medical action will be taken too frequently). Figure 2-32, *A,* illustrates the situation with $Delta_{stat}$ equal to $Delta_{med}$. We now consider the situation with a true change equal to the medically important change (i.e., $Delta_{true} = Delta_{med}$) (Figure 2-32, *B*), where exactly 50% of observed changes exceed the medically important limit. If $Delta_{stat}$ is less than or equal to $Delta_{med}$, less than 5% of patients will exhibit an observed delta value in the opposite direction of the true change (an obviously misleading trend). If the condition is not met, more than 5% will have a misleading change. Finally, in the case where the true change equals the sum of $Delta_{med}$ and $Delta_{stat}$ (Figure 2-32, *C*), more than 95% of observed changes exceed the medically important change, and appropriate action will be taken for most patients.

The outline presented previously illustrates that in the monitoring situation, not only the requirement for statistical significance (i.e., the type I error problem concerning false alarms), but also the type II error problem or the risk of overlooking changes, should be addressed; the latter is an aspect that often is overlooked.[67] Provided that $Delta_{stat}$ is small relative to $Delta_{med}$, both type I and type II errors can be kept small. On the other hand, if $Delta_{stat}$ equals or exceeds $Delta_{med}$, the relative importance of type I and type II errors may be weighed against each other. If the consequences of overlooking a medically important change are serious, one should keep the type II error small and accept a relatively large type I error (i.e., accept the occurrence of false alarms). On the contrary, if overlooking changes only gives rise to minor or transient problems, the priority may be to keep the type I error small. In addition to simple evaluation of a shift between two measurements, as considered here, sequential results may be analyzed using more refined time-series models.[40]

TRACEABILITY AND MEASUREMENT UNCERTAINTY

As outlined previously in the error model sections, laboratory results are likely to be influenced by systematic and random errors of various types. Obtaining agreement of measurements between laboratories or agreement over time in a given laboratory often can be problematic.

Traceability

To ensure reasonable agreement between measurements of routine methods, the concept of traceability comes into focus (See Chapter 8). *Traceability* is based on an unbroken chain of comparisons of measurements leading to a known reference value (Figure 2-33). A hierarchical approach for tracing the values of routine clinical chemistry measurements to reference measurement procedures was proposed by Tietz[105] and has been adapted by the ISO. For well-established analytes, a hierarchy of methods exists with *a reference measurement procedure* at the top, *selected measurement procedures* at an intermediate level, and finally *routine measurement procedures* at the bottom.[8,50,105] A reference measurement procedure is a fully understood procedure of highest analytical quality containing with a complete uncertainty budget given in SI units.[29,46] Reference procedures are used to measure the analyte concentration in *secondary reference materials,* which typically have the same matrix as samples that are to be measured by routine procedures (e.g., human serum). Secondary reference materials are usually of high analytical quality, and certified secondary reference materials must be validated for commutability with clinical samples if they are intended for use as trueness controls for routine methods.[110,111] Otherwise, their use is restricted to those selected measurement procedures for which they are intended. The certificate of analysis should state the methods for which the secondary reference materials have been validated to be commutable with clinical samples. When no information is given for commutability, it must be assumed that the reference material is not commutable with clinical samples, and the user has the responsibility to validate commutability for the methods of interest.[16] Uncertainty of the measurement procedure results in increases from the top level to the bottom. ISO guidelines (15193 and 15194) address requirements for reference methods and reference materials.[46,47]

Using cortisol as an example, the primary reference material is crystalline cortisol with a chemical analysis for impurities [NIST SRM 921, cortisol (hydrocortisone)]. A primary calibrator is then a cortisol preparation with a stated mass fraction (purity) (e.g., 0.998 and a 95% CI of ±0.001). The reference measurement procedure is an isotope-dilution gas chromatography–mass spectrometry method that is calibrated with the primary calibrator. A panel of individual frozen serum samples that have values assigned by the primary reference measurement procedure is available from the Institute for Reference Materials and Measurements (IRMM) as secondary reference materials (ERM-DA451/IFCC).[42] A manufacturer's *selected measurement* procedure is

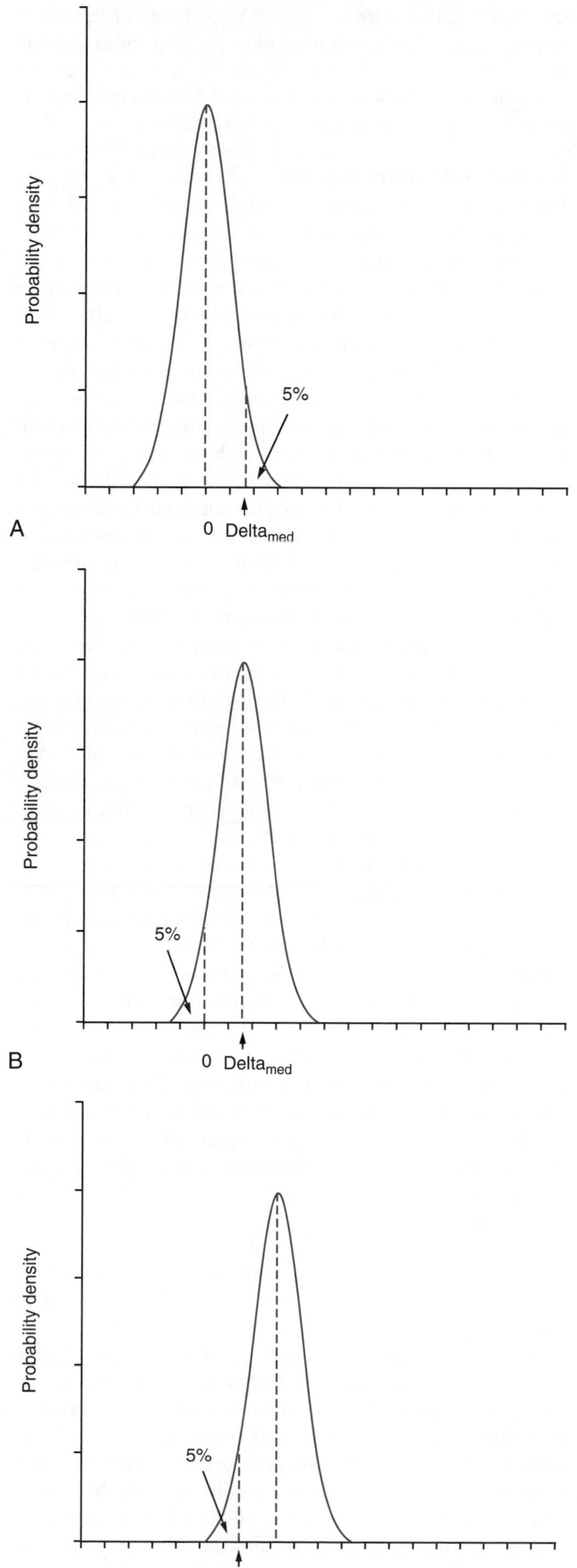

Figure 2-32 The monitoring situation. A, Distribution of observed changes given a true change of zero. B, A true change equal to Delta_{med}. C, A true change of (Delta_{med} + 1.65 SD_{delta}). Delta_{stat} (=1.65 SD_{delta}) equals Delta_{med} in these examples.

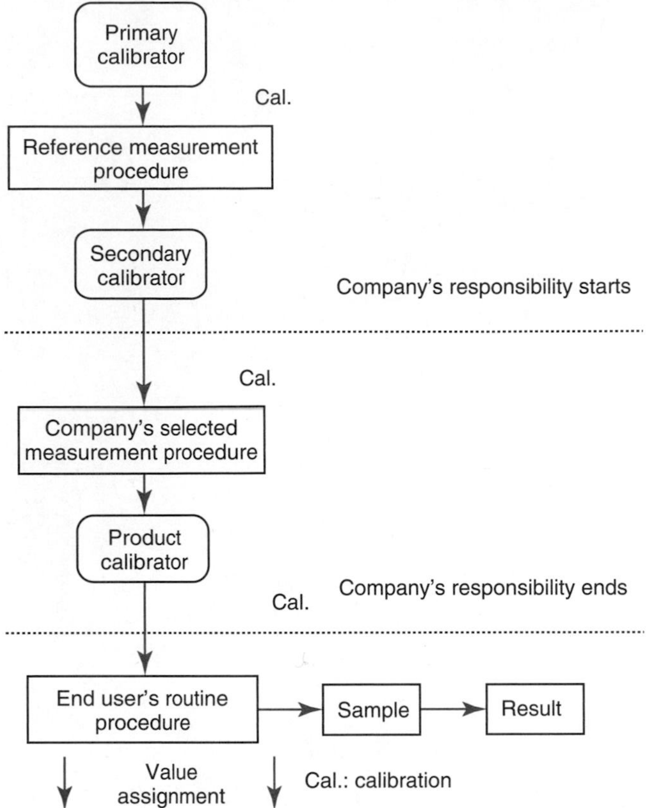

Figure 2-33 The calibration hierarchy from a reference measurement procedure to a routine method. The uncertainty increases from top to bottom.

calibrated with the secondary reference materials and is used for measurement of the quantity in the manufacturer's *product calibrator,* which is the calibrator used for the routine method in clinical laboratories.

Only 25 to 30 of clinical chemistry analytes currently are traceable to SI units, such as electrolytes, some metabolites (glucose, creatinine, and uric acid), steroids, and some thyroid hormones).[104] For plasma proteins, a human reference serum material is available with certified mass concentrations of 12 serum proteins (ERM-DA470k/IFCC) from IRMM. With protein hormones, the existence of heterogeneity or microheterogeneity complicates the problem of traceability.[101,104]

The Uncertainty Concept

To assess in a systematic way, errors associated with laboratory results, the *uncertainty* concept has been introduced into laboratory medicine.[31,45] According to the ISO "Guide to the Expression of Uncertainty in Measurement" (GUM), *uncertainty* is formally defined as "a parameter associated with the result of a measurement that characterizes the dispersion of the values that could reasonably be attributed to the measurand."[45] In practice, this means that the uncertainty is given as an interval around a reported laboratory result that specifies the location of the true value with a given probability (e.g., 95%). In general, the uncertainty of a result, which is traceable to a particular reference, is the uncertainty of that reference together with the overall uncertainty of the traceability chain.[31] Updated information on traceability aspects is available on the website of the Joint Committee on Traceability in Laboratory Medicine (www.bipm.org/en/committees/jc/jctlm/; accessed March 08 2011).

The Standard Uncertainty (u_{st})

The uncertainty concept is directed toward the end user (clinician) of the result, who is concerned about the total error possible, and who is not particularly interested in the question of whether the errors are systematic or random. In the outline of the uncertainty concept, it is assumed that any known systematic error components of a measurement method have been corrected, and the specified uncertainty includes uncertainty associated with correction of the systematic error(s).[45] Although this appears logical, one problem may be that some routine methods have systematic errors dependent on the patient category from which the sample originates. For example, kinetic Jaffe methods for creatinine are subject to positive interference by 2-OXO compounds and to negative interference by bilirubin and its metabolites, which means that the direction of systematic error will be patient dependent and not generally predictable.

In the theory on uncertainty, a distinction between type A and B uncertainties is made. Type A uncertainties are frequency-based estimates of SDs (e.g., an SD of the imprecision). Type B uncertainties are uncertainty components for which frequency-based SDs are not available. Instead, uncertainty is estimated by other approaches or by the opinion of experts. Finally, the total uncertainty is derived from a combination of all sources of uncertainty. In this context, it is practical to operate with *standard uncertainties* (u_{st}), which are equivalent to SDs. By multiplication of a standard uncertainty with a *coverage factor (k),* the uncertainty corresponding to a specified probability level is derived. For example, multiplication with a coverage factor of 2 yields a probability level of ≈95%, given a Gaussian distribution. When the total uncertainty of an analytical result obtained by a routine method is considered, preanalytical variation, method imprecision, sample-related random interferences, and uncertainty related to calibration and bias corrections (traceability) should be taken into account. In expressing the uncertainty components as standard uncertainties, we have the following general relation:

$$u_{st} = [u^2_{PAst} + u^2_{Ast} + u^2_{RBst} + u^2_{Tracst}]$$

where the individual components refer to preanalytical, analytical, sample-related random bias and traceability uncertainty.

Uncertainty can be assessed in various ways; often a combination of procedures is necessary. In principle, uncertainty can be judged *directly* from measurement comparisons or *indirectly* from an analysis of individual error sources according to the law of error propagation ("error budget"). Measurement comparison may consist of a method comparison study with a reference method based on patient samples according to the principles outlined previously or by measurement of commutable certified matrix reference materials (CRMs).

Example of Direct Assessment of Uncertainty on the Basis of Measurements of a Commutable Certified Reference Material

Suppose a CRM is available that was validated to be *commutable* with patient samples for a given routine method with a specified value 10.0 mmol/L and a standard uncertainty of 0.2 mmol/L. Ten repeated measurements in independent runs give a mean value of 10.3 mmol/L with SD 0.5 mmol/L. The standard error of the mean is then $0.5/\sqrt{10} = 0.16$ mmol/L. The mean is not significantly different from the assigned value [$t = (10.3 - 10.0)/(0.2^2 + 0.16^2)^{0.5} = 1.17$]. The total standard uncertainty with regard to traceability is then $u_{\text{Trac st}} = (0.16^2 + 0.2^2)^{0.5} = 0.26$ mmol/L. If the bias had been significant, one might have considered making a correction to the method, and the standard uncertainty would then be the same at the given concentration. Thus measurements of the CRM provide an estimate of the uncertainty related to traceability, *given the assumption of commutability with patient samples*. The other components have to be estimated separately. Concerning method imprecision, long-term imprecision (e.g., observed from quality control measurements) should be used rather than the short-term SD observed for CRM material. Here we suppose that the long-term SD_A is 0.8 mmol/L. Data on preanalytical variation can be obtained by sampling in duplicates from a series of patients or can be a matter of judgment (type B uncertainty) based on literature data or data on similar analytes. We here suppose that SD_{PA} equals half the analytical SD (i.e., 0.4 mmol/L). Finally, we lack data on a possible sample-related random bias component, which we may choose to ignore in the present example. The standard uncertainty of the results then becomes

$$\begin{aligned} u_{st} &= [u_{PAst}^2 + u_{Ast}^2 + u_{RBst}^2 + u_{Tracst}^2]^{0.5} \\ &= (0.4^2 + 0.8^2 + 0.26^2)^{0.5} \\ &= 0.93\ (\text{mmol/L}) \end{aligned}$$

In this case, the major uncertainty component is the long-term imprecision in the laboratory.

Example of Direct Assessment of Uncertainty on the Basis of a Method Comparison Study With a Reference Measurement Procedure Using Patient Samples

Suppose a set of patient samples have been measured by a routine method ($X2$) in parallel with a reference measurement procedure ($X1$), and that a linear relationship exists between measurements. We want to assess a possible calibration bias and evaluate the standard uncertainty of results of the routine method on the basis of regression analysis results and information on standard uncertainty related to the traceability of reference method results. The imprecision of the reference method is 2.5% or, as a fraction (used in the following), 0.025 ($= CV_{A1}$), and the component related to the uncertainty of the traceability chain for the reference method is 0.020 ($= u_{\text{trac st}}$). Proportional measurement errors are assumed for both methods, and a weighted form of Deming regression analysis is applied. The error variance ratio λ is not known exactly, but the reference method is devoid of sample-related random bias, so it is assumed that the random error is about half that of the routine method (i.e., λ is set to $1/2^2 = 1/4$). At a decision point ($X1'_{\text{Targetc}}$) (e.g., corresponding to the upper limit of the 95% reference interval), the systematic difference between methods [$D_c = a_0 + (b - 1)\,X1'_{\text{Targetc}}$] is estimated with standard error (see section on regression):

$$D_c = X2'_{\text{Targetc}} - X1'_{\text{Targetc}} = 20 \text{ mg/L with SE}(D_c) = 1.0 \text{ mg/L}$$

corresponding to a relative SE(D_c) of 0.050 [= (1.0 mg/L)/(20 mg/L)]. For the Deming procedures, the standard error can be conveniently computed by the jackknife procedure. We observe that the difference is highly significant and decide to recalibrate the routine method in relation to the reference method using the estimated slope and intercept [i.e., the recalibrated $x2$ values equals $(x2 - a_0)/b$]. Having done this, the routine method is assumed to have no systematic error in relation to the reference method, but when the uncertainty of the results is considered, we have to add the standard uncertainty of the bias correction. The uncertainty related to traceability for the routine method is now obtained as the uncertainty inherent to the reference method and the comparison step, that is,

$$u_{\text{Tracst}} = (0.020^2 + 0.050^2)^{0.5} = 0.054$$

We are now further interested in deriving estimates of random error components for the routine method from regression analysis results. Both analytical error [e.g., estimated from quality control (QC) data] and sample-related random bias should be assessed, and it should be recognized that the observed total random error is the result of contributions from both measurement methods. Suppose that CV_{21} of the regression analysis has been calculated to be 0.10 (CV_{21} is analogous to SD_{21} or SD_{yx}), given constant measurement errors over the analytical measurement range (i.e., an expression for the random error in the vertical direction in the x-y plot). From the regression section, we have

$$CV_{21}^2 = [CV_{A1}^2 + CV_{A2}^2] + [CV_{RB1}^2 + CV_{RB2}^2]$$

By substituting $CV_{A1} = 0.025$, $CV_{RB1} = 0$, and $CV_{21} = 0.10$, we derive

$$CV_{A1}^2 + CV_{A2}^2 = 0.009375$$

and get

$$CV_{A2}^2 + CV_{RB2}^2 = 0.009372\,[CV_{A2}^2 + CV_{RB2}^2]^{0.5} = 0.0968$$

Thus the total random error of the routine method corresponds to a CV of 0.097. If we had measured samples in duplicate in the method comparison experiment or had available QC data, we could split the total random error into its components. CV_{A2} was here determined to be 0.035 from QC data, which gives 0.090 corresponding to CV_{RB2}. We may here note that the assumed error ratio λ of $(\frac{1}{2})^2$ is not quite correct. According to our results, λ should be $(0.025/0.0968)^2$

Although the Deming regression principle is rather robust toward misspecified λ values, we could choose to carry out a reanalysis with the more correct λ value—a process that could be iterated. Finally, assuming a value of 0.03 for the preanalytical coefficient of variation, we derive a total standard uncertainty estimate of

$$u_{st} = [u^2_{PAst} + u^2_{Ast} + u^2_{RBst} + u^2_{Tracst}]^{0.5}$$
$$(0.03^2 + 0.0968^2 + 0.054^2)^{0.5} = 0.115$$

At the given decision level of 20 mg/L and with a coverage factor of 2, we obtain the 95% uncertainty interval of a single routine measurement as

$$20\ \text{mg/L} \pm (2 \times 0.115 \times 20)\ \text{mg/L} = 15.4 - 24.6\ \text{mg/L}$$

Having estimated the uncertainty as outlined, additional uncertainty sources should be considered. If the comparison was undertaken within a short time period, one might consider adding an additional long-term imprecision component as a variance component to the standard uncertainty expression.

When the two approaches briefly outlined are compared, the latter is the more informative. Using a series of patient samples instead of a pooled sample, individual random bias components are included in the uncertainty estimation, assuming that the patient samples are representative. Also, natural patient samples are preferable to a stabilized pool that perhaps is distributed in freeze-dried form, which may introduce artifactual errors into some analytical systems. Using a commutable CRM, on the other hand, is more practical and in many situations is the only realistic alternative.

With regard to uncertainty estimation from a comparison study of patient samples as outlined previously, one should be careful concerning the uncertainty estimation. First, it is important to estimate correctly the standard error of the difference at selected decision points or at points covering the analytical measurement range (i.e., at the lower limit, in the middle part, and at the upper limit). From the expression of the estimated difference $[D_c = a_0 + (b - 1)\, X1'_{\text{Targetc}}]$, one might at a first glance estimate the standard error (standard uncertainty) by adding (squared) the standard errors of the intercept and the slope. However, simple squared addition of standard errors is correct only when the independence of estimates is given (see later). Estimates of intercept and slope in regression analysis are negatively correlated, which implies that simple squared addition of standard errors leads to an overestimation of the total standard uncertainty.[24] Rather, a direct estimation procedure for the standard error should be applied, as mentioned earlier.

A method comparison study based on genuine patient samples represents as mentioned a real assessment of traceability. In Figure 2-33, the focus is on the calibration aspect intended to *mediate* traceability. One should recognize that the matrix of product calibrators for practical reasons often is artificial (e.g., the matrix of a calibrator may be bovine albumin instead of human serum). Many routine methods are matrix sensitive, which implies that calibrators and patient samples are not commutable. To ensure traceability in this situation, the assigned concentration of a calibrator has to be different from the real concentration.

Indirect Evaluation of Uncertainty by Quantification of Individual Error Source Components

On the basis of a detailed quantitative model of the analytical procedure, the standard approach is to assess the standard uncertainties associated with individual input parameters and combine them according to the law of propagation of uncertainties.[31] The relationship between the combined standard uncertainty $u_c(y)$ of a value y and the uncertainty of the *independent* parameters $x_1, x_2, \ldots x_n$, on which it depends, is

$$u_c[y(x_1, x_2, \ldots)] = [\Sigma c_i^2 u(x_1)^2]^{0.5}$$

where c_i is a sensitivity coefficient (the partial differential of y with respect to x_i). These sensitivity coefficients indicate how the value of y varies with changes in the input parameter x_i. If the variables are not independent, the relationship becomes

$$u_c[y(x_1, x_2, \ldots)] = [\Sigma c_i^2 u(x_1)^2 + \Sigma c_i c_k u(x_i, x_k)^2]^{0.5}$$

where $u(x_i, x_k)$ is the covariance between x_i and x_k, and c_i and c_k are the sensitivity coefficients. The covariance is related to the correlation coefficient ρ_{ik} by

$$u(x_i, x_k) = u(x_i)u(x_k)\rho_{ik}$$

This is a complex relationship that usually will be difficult to evaluate in practice. In many situations, however, the contributing factors are independent, thus simplifying the picture. Below, some simple examples of combined expressions are shown. The rules are presented in the form of combining SDs or CVs given *independent* input components.

$$q = x + y \qquad \text{SD}(q) = [SD(x)^2 + SD(y)^2]^{0.5}$$
$$q = x - y \qquad \text{SD}(q) = [\text{SD}(x)^2 + \text{SD}(y)^2]^{0.5}$$
$$q = ax \qquad \text{SD}(q) = a\text{SD}(x) \text{ and } \text{CV}(q) = \text{CV}(x)$$
$$q = x^p \qquad \text{CV}(q) = p^{0.5}\text{CV}(x)$$
$$q = xy \qquad \text{CV}(q) = [\text{CV}(x)^2 + \text{CV}(y)^2]^{0.5}$$
$$q = x/y \qquad \text{CV}(q) = [\text{CV}(x)^2 + \text{CV}(y)^2]^{0.5}$$

The formulas shown may be used (e.g., to calculate the combined uncertainty of a calibrator solution from the uncertainties of the reference compound, the weighting, and dilution steps) (see later).

Some relations between the SD and non-Gaussian distributions may also be of relevance for uncertainty calculations (type B uncertainties) (Table 2-12). For example, if the uncertainty of a CRM value is given with some percentage, it may be understood as referring to a rectangular probability distribution. In relation to calibration of flasks, the triangular distribution is often assumed.

Example

Briefly, computation of the standard uncertainty of a calibrator solution will be outlined. The concentration C equals the mass M divided by the volume $V(C = M/V)$. We will here express the standard uncertainties as relative values and will

TABLE 2-12 Relations Between Standard Deviation and Range for Various Types of Distributions

Normal Distribution	Rectangular Distribution	Triangular Distribution
SD = Half width of 95%-interval/ $t_{0.975}(\nu)$ ≈ Half width of 95%-interval/2	SD = Half width/√3	SD = Half width/√6

derive the approximate total standard uncertainty by squared addition of the individual contributions. Starting with the mass, the purity is stated on the certificate as 99.4 ± 0.4%. Assuming a rectangular distribution, the relative SD becomes 0.004/√3 = 0.0023. The uncertainty of the weighing process is known in the laboratory to have a CV of 0.1%, or 0.0010. Thus the relative standard uncertainty of the mass becomes

$$u_{M\,st} = (0.0023^2 + 0.0010^2)^{0.5} = 0.0025$$

The certificate of the flask (50 mL at 20 °C) indicates ±0.1 mL as uncertainty. Assuming here a triangular distribution, we derive the standard uncertainty as 0.10 mL/√6 = 0.0408 mL, which is converted to a relative value of 0.000816. The temperature expansion coefficient is given as 0.020 mL per degree change of temperature. Assuming a variability of 20 ± 4 °C, this contribution amounts to ±0.080 mL. Assuming here a rectangular distribution, we get an SD of 0.080/√3 mL, or 0.00092 as a relative SD. The repeatability of the volume dispensing process in the laboratory has been assessed to 0.020 mL expressed as an SD, which corresponds to a relative value of 0.00040. The total standard uncertainty of the volume dispensing process becomes

$$u_{V\,st} = (0.000816^2 + 0.00092^2 + 0.00040^2)^{0.5} = 0.0013$$

The total standard uncertainty of the calibrator solution is

$$\begin{aligned} u_{Cal\,st} &= (u_{M\,st}^2 + u_{v\,st}^2)^{0.5} \\ &= (0.0025^2 + 0.0013^2)^{0.5} \\ &= 0.0028, \text{ or } 0.28\% \end{aligned}$$

Generally, when squared CVs are added, minor contributions in practice can be ignored (e.g., CVs less than a third or a quarter of the other components).[31]

The indirect procedure is mainly of relevance for relatively simple procedures. In some situations, a simulation model of a complex analytical method may be established to estimate the combined uncertainty of the method on the basis of input uncertainties.[1] For closed, automated clinical chemistry procedures, it often will not be possible to discern the individual error elements. Further, the correlation aspect is difficult to take into account in practice. In these cases, the direct procedure of measurement comparison is preferable. However, the indirect procedure has been applied in clinical chemistry.[41,63]

Uncertainty in Relation to Traditional Systematic and Random Error Classifications

As mentioned previously, systematic errors are not included in the uncertainty expression, because it is assumed that they have been corrected. Therefore, it is the uncertainty of the correction procedure that should be taken into account. Otherwise, systematic errors have been added linearly or squared in error propagation models.[86,102] One may further consider that the distinction between systematic effects and random effects may be a matter of the reference frame. For example, a systematic error over time may turn into a random error, because a bias may change over time. Lot-to-lot reagent effects may be interpreted as systematic or random errors. When a laboratory changes from an old to a new lot, a shift in measurement values may occur. Initially this will be considered a systematic change. However, over a long time period involving several lots of reagents, the recorded shifts typically will be up and down and will be regarded as a long-term random error component. Additionally, a bias in a particular laboratory may be viewed as a random error component when dealing with a whole group of laboratories, because individual laboratory biases appear randomly distributed and are quantified as the interlaboratory SD. Thus there are arguments for using the uncertainty concept as outlined earlier to end up with one overall uncertainty expression directed toward the end user of the laboratory result. Still, as mentioned previously, systematic errors linked to samples from specific patient subcategories may constitute a problem because a general correction is not possible. A way to quantify this error contribution is to include samples from all patient subgroups in a balanced way in a method comparison study, so that this error type is incorporated into the uncertainty component related to traceability. Another problem with systematic errors is that they often depend on the analyte concentration. Thus if a commutable CRM is measured at a particular concentration, one should consider whether a bias correction is valid only at the given concentration or generally over the analytical measurement range. Further, the occurrence of outliers caused by rarely occurring interference (e.g., heterophilic antibodies in relation to immunoassays) constitutes a problem.[61] If the uncertainty estimation is based on parametric statistics (standard uncertainty expanded by a coverage factor), inclusion of gross outliers may increase the standard uncertainty considerably and make the uncertainty specification useless. A solution might here be to omit the outliers in the first hand, compute the 95% uncertainty interval, and then finally add a special note with regard to the probability of occurrence of outliers in the uncertainty specification.

Although it may appear complicated to specify the uncertainty in a detailed manner, a rough estimate may be obtained by adding the squares of CVs corresponding to essential uncertainty elements (e.g., grouped as factors outside the laboratory) (derived from the traceability chain), the analytical factors inside the laboratory (intermediate precision), and the preanalytical elements.[56] In estimating uncertainty, it is important to include relevant elements, but one must be careful to avoid counting the same elements twice.

Application of the uncertainty concept in the field of clinical chemistry is subject to some discussion.[57,61]

SOFTWARE PACKAGES

In practice, statistical analyses usually are conducted in spreadsheets or by statistical programs. Concerning the latter, large, general program packages or smaller programs more or less specialized toward the field of clinical chemistry are available. In addition, large, general packages are on the market [e.g., Statistical Package for the Social Sciences (SPSS), SAS, Stata, Systat, StatGraphics]. Among programs of intermediate size, GraphPad (www.graphpad.com) and SigmaStat are worthy of note. Excel (Microsoft) contains various statistical routines. The general programs may lack procedures of interest to clinical chemists (e.g., Deming and Passing-Bablok

BOX 2-1 Abbreviations and Vocabulary

Abbreviations

CI	Confidence interval
CV	Coefficient of variation (= SD/x, where x is the concentration)
CV%	= CV × 100%
CV_A	Analytical coefficient of variation
CV_{RB}	Sample-related random bias coefficient of variation
DoD	Distribution of differences (plot)
ISO	International Organization for Standardization
IUPAC	International Union of Pure and Applied Chemistry
OLR	Ordinary least-squares regression analysis
SD	Standard deviation
SEM	Standard error of the mean (= SD/√N)
SD_A	Analytical standard deviation
SD_{RB}	Sample-related random bias standard deviation
x_m	Mean
x_{mv}	Weighted mean
WLR	Weighted least-squares regression analysis

Vocabulary*

Analyte Compound that is measured.

Bias Difference between the average (strictly the expectation) of the test results and an accepted reference value (ISO 3534-1). Bias is a measure of trueness.[44]

Certified reference material (CRM) is a reference material, one or more of whose property values are certified by a technically valid procedure, accompanied by or traceable to a certificate or other documentation that is issued by a certifying body.

Commutability Ability of a material to yield the same results of measurement by a given set of measurement procedures.

Limit of detection The lowest amount of analyte in a sample that can be detected but not quantified as an exact value. Also called lower limit of detection, minimum detectable concentration (or dose or value).[18]

Lower limit of quantification (LloQ) The lowest concentration at which the measurement procedure fulfills specifications for imprecision and bias (corresponds to the *lower limit of determination* mentioned under *Measuring interval*).

Matrix All components of a material system, except the analyte.

Measurand The "quantity" that is actually measured (e.g., the concentration of the analyte). For example, if the analyte is glucose, the measurand is the concentration of glucose. For an enzyme, the measurand may be the enzyme *activity* or the *mass concentration* of enzyme.

Measuring interval Closed interval of possible values allowed by a measurement procedure and delimited by the *lower limit of determination* and the *higher limit of determination.* For this interval, the total error of the measurements is within specified limits for the method. Also called the *analytical measurement range.*

Primary measurement standard Standard that is designated or widely acknowledged as having the highest metrologic qualities and whose value is accepted without reference to other standards of the same quantity.[47]

Quantity The amount of substance (e.g., the concentration of substance).

Reference material (RM) A material or substance, one or more properties of which are sufficiently well established to be used for the calibration of a method, or for assigning values to materials.

Random error Arises from unpredictable variations in influence quantities. These random effects give rise to variations in repeated observations of the measurand.

Reference measurement procedure Thoroughly investigated measurement procedure shown to yield values having an uncertainty of measurement commensurate with its intended use, especially in assessing the trueness of other measurement procedures for the same quantity and in characterizing reference materials.

Selectivity and/or Specificity Degree to which a method responds uniquely to the required analyte.

Systematic error A component of error that, in the course of a number of analyses of the same measurand, remains constant or varies in a predictable way.

Traceability "The property of the result of a measurement or the value of a standard whereby it can be related to stated references, usually national or international standards, through an unbroken chain of comparisons all having stated uncertainties."[43] This is achieved by establishing a chain of calibrations leading to primary national or international standards, ideally (for long-term consistency) the Système Internationale (SI) units of measurement.

Uncertainty A parameter associated with the result of a measurement that characterizes the dispersion of values that could reasonably be attributed to the measurand, or, more briefly, *uncertainty* is a parameter characterizing the range of values within which the value of the quantity being measured is expected to lie.

Upper limit of quantification (UloQ) The highest concentration at which the measurement procedure fulfills specifications for imprecision and bias (corresponds to the *upper limit of determination* mentioned under *Measuring interval*).

*A listing of terms of relevance in relation to analytical methods is displayed. Many of the definitions originate from Dybkær[29] with statement of original source where relevant (e.g., ISO document number). Others are derived from the Eurachem/Citac guideline on uncertainty.[31] In some cases, slight modifications have been performed for the sake of simplicity.

procedures). Other programs that are specialized for clinical chemistry include Analyze-it (www.analyze-it.com), MedCalc (www.medcalc.be), EP-Evaluator (D. Rhoads Associates, www.dgrhoads.com), and a program distributed by one of the authors (K.L.) called CBstat (www.cbstat.com).

REFERENCES

1. Aronsson T, deVerdier C, Groth T. Factors influencing the quality of analytical methods: a systems analysis, with computer simulation. Clin Chem 1974;20:738-48.
2. Barnett RN. Medical significance of laboratory results. Am J Clin Pathol 1968;50:671-6.
3. Bland JM, Altman DG. Statistical methods for assessing agreement between two methods of clinical measurement. Lancet 1986;i:307-10.
4. Bland JM, Altman DG. Comparing methods of measurement: why plotting difference against standard method is misleading. Lancet 1995;346:1085-7.
5. Bookbinder MJ, Panosian KJ. Using the coefficient of correlation in method-comparison studies. Clin Chem 1987;33:1170-6.
6. Boyd JC, Bruns DE. Quality specifications for glucose meters: assessment by simulation modeling of errors in insulin dose. Clin Chem 2001;47:209-14.
7. Burnett RW, Westgard JO. Selection of measurement and control procedures to satisfy the Health Care Financing Administration requirements and provide cost-effective operation. Arch Pathol Lab Med 1992;116:777-80.
8. Büttner J. Reference materials and reference methods in laboratory medicine: a challenge to international cooperation. Eur J Clin Chem Clin Biochem 1994;32:571-7.
9. Clarke WL, Cox D, Gonder-Frederick LA, Carter W, Pohl SL. Evaluating clinical accuracy of systems for self-monitoring of blood glucose. Diabetes Care 1987;10:622-8.
10. CLSI. Method comparison and bias estimation using patient samples; approved guideline, 2nd edition. CLSI document EP09-A2IR. Wayne, Pa: Clinical and Laboratory Standards Institute, 2010.
11. CLSI. Evaluation of the linearity of quantitative measurement procedures: a statistical approach; approved guideline. CLSI document EP06-A. Wayne, Pa: Clinical and Laboratory Standards Institute, 2003.
12. CLSI. Evaluation of precision performance of quantitative measurement methods; approved guideline, 2nd edition. CLSI document EP05-A2. Wayne, Pa: Clinical and Laboratory Standards Institute, 2004.
13. CLSI. Interference testing in clinical chemistry; approved guideline, 2nd edition. CLSI document EP07-A2. Wayne, Pa: Clinical and Laboratory Standards Institute, 2005.
14. CLSI. Preliminary evaluation of quantitative clinical laboratory measurement procedures; approved guideline, 2nd edition. CLSI document EP10-A3. Wayne, Pa: Clinical and Laboratory Standards Institute, 2006.
15. CLSI. User protocol for evaluation of qualitative test performance; approved guideline, 2nd edition. CLSI document EP12-A2. Wayne, Pa: Clinical and Laboratory Standards Institute, 2008.
16. CLSI. Characterization and qualification of commutable reference materials for laboratory medicine; proposed guideline. CLSI document C53-A. Wayne, Pa: Clinical and Laboratory Standards Institute, 2010.
17. CLSI. User verification of performance for precision and trueness; approved guideline, 2nd edition. CLSI document EP15-A2. Wayne, Pa: Clinical and Laboratory Standards Institute, 2006.
18. CLSI. Protocols for determination of limits of detection and limits of quantitation; approved guideline. CLSI document EP17-A. Wayne, Pa: Clinical and Laboratory Standards Institute, 2004.
19. CLSI. Defining, establishing, and verifying reference intervals in the clinical laboratory; approved guideline, 3rd edition. CLSI document C28-A3c. Wayne, Pa: Clinical and Laboratory Standards Institute, 2010.
20. Cornbleet PJ, Gochman N. Incorrect least-squares regression coefficients in method-comparison analysis. Clin Chem 1979;25:432-8.
21. Cotlove E, Harris EK, Williams GZ. Biological and analytic components of variation in long-term studies of serum constituents in normal subjects. III. Physiological and medical implications. Clin Chem 1970;16:1028-32.
22. Currie LA. Nomenclature in evaluation of analytical methods including detection and quantification capabilities (IUPAC recommendations 1995). Pure Appl Chem 1995;67:1699-1723.
23. David HA. Order statistics. New York: Wiley, 1981:80-2.
24. Davis RB, Thompson JE, Pardue HL. Characteristics of statistical parameters used to interpret least-squares results. Clin Chem 1978;24:611-20.
25. Deming WE. Statistical adjustment of data. New York: Wiley, 1943:184.
26. Directive 98/79/EC of the European Parliament and of the Council of 27 October on in vitro diagnostic medical devices. Off J Eur Comm 1998(Dec 7);L331:1-37.
27. Dixon WJ. Processing data for outliers. Biometrics 1953;9:74-89.
28. Draper NR, Smith H. Applied regression analysis, 3rd edition. New York: Wiley, 1998:192-8.
29. Dybkær R. Vocabulary for use in measurement procedures and description of reference materials in laboratory medicine. Eur J Clin Chem Clin Biochem 1997;35:141-73.
30. Efron B. An introduction to the bootstrap. London: Chapman and Hall, 1993.
31. Ellison SLR, Rosslein M, Williams A, eds. Eurachem/Citac guide: quantifying uncertainty in analytical measurement, 2nd edition. Berlin: Eurachem, 2000:4, 5, 9, 17.
32. Emancipator K, Kroll MH. A quantitative measure of nonlinearity. Clin Chem 1993;39:766-772.
33. European Committee for Clinical Laboratory Standards. Guidelines for the evaluation of diagnostic kits. Part 2. General principles and outline procedures for the evaluation of kits for qualitative tests. Lund, Sweden: ECCLS, 1990.
34. Fleiss JL. Statistical methods for rates and proportions, 2nd edition. New York: Wiley, 1981:Chapter 13.
35. Fraser CG, Petersen PH, Libeer JC, Ricos C. Proposals for setting generally applicable quality goals solely based on biology. Ann Clin Biochem 1997;34:8-12.
36. Fraser CG. Biological variation: from principles to practice. Washington, DC: AACC Press, 2001:50-4, 133-41.
37. Glick MR, Ryder KW. Analytical systems ranked by freedom from interferences. Clin Chem 1987;33:1453-8.
38. Gowans EMS, Petersen PH, Blaabjerg O, Hørder M. Analytical goals for the acceptance of common reference intervals for laboratories throughout a geographical area. Scand J Clin Lab Invest 1988; 48:757-64.
39. Hald A. Statistical theory with engineering applications. New York: Wiley, 1952:534-5, 551-7.
40. Harris EK, Boyd J. Statistical bases of reference values in laboratory medicine. New York: Marcel Dekker, 1995:238-50.
41. Inal BB, Koldas M, Inal H, Coskun C, Gumus A, Doventas Y. Evaluation of measurement uncertainty of glucose in clinical chemistry. Ann N Y Acad Sci 2007;1100:223-6.
42. International Federation of Clinical Chemistry. Approved recommendation (1987) on the theory of reference values. Part 5. Statistical treatment of collected reference values. Determination of reference limits. J Clin Chem Clin Biochem 1987;25:645-56.
43. International Organization for Standardization (ISO). International vocabulary of metrology: basic and general concepts and associated terms (VIM). Geneva: ISO, 2007.
44. International Organization for Standardization (ISO). Statistics: vocabulary and symbols. Part 1. General statistical terms and terms used in probability. ISO 3534-1. Geneva: ISO, 2006.
45. International Organization for Standardization (ISO). Guide 98-1. Uncertainty of measurement. Part 1. Introduction to the expression of uncertainty in measurement. Geneva: ISO, 2009.

46. International Organization for Standardization (ISO). In vitro diagnostic medical devices. Measurement of quantities in samples of biological origin. Requirements for content and presentation of reference measurement procedures (15193). Geneva: ISO, 2009.
47. International Organization for Standardization (ISO). In vitro diagnostic medical devices. Measurement of quantities in samples of biological origin. Requirements for certified reference materials and the content of supporting documentation (15194). Geneva: ISO, 2009.
48. International Organization for Standardization (ISO). Capability of detection. Part 2. Methodology in the linear calibration case (11843-2). Geneva: ISO, 2000.
49. International Organization for Standardization (ISO). Medical laboratories. Particular requirements for quality and competence (15189). Geneva: ISO, 2007.
50. International Organization for Standardization (ISO). In vitro diagnostic medical devices. Measurement of quantities in biological samples. Metrological traceability of values assigned to calibrators and control materials (17511). Geneva: ISO, 2003.
51. Ismail AAA, Walker PL, Barth JH, Lewandowski KC, Jones R, Burr WA. Wrong biochemistry results: two case reports and observational study in 5310 patients on potentially misleading thyroid-stimulating hormone and gonadotropin immunoassay results. Clin Chem 2002;48:2023-9.
52. Kendall MG, Stuart A. The advanced theory of statistics, 4th edition, vol 1. London: C. Griffin & Co., 1977:258, 352.
53. Kendall MG, Stuart A. The advanced theory of statistics, 3rd edition, vol 2. London: C. Griffin & Co., 1973:391-408.
54. Klee G. A conceptual model for establishing tolerance limits for analytical bias and imprecision based on variations in population test distributions. Clin Chim Acta 1997;260:175-88.
55. Kringle RO, Bogavich M. Statistical procedures. In: Burtis CA, Ashwood ER, eds. Tietz textbook of clinical chemistry, 3rd edition. Philadelphia: WB Saunders, 1999:265-309.
56. Kristiansen J. Description of a generally applicable model for the evaluation of uncertainty of measurement in clinical chemistry. Clin Chem Lab Med 2001;39:920-31.
57. Kristiansen J. The guide to expression of uncertainty in measurement approach for estimating uncertainty: an appraisal. Clin Chem 2003;49:1822-9.
58. Krouwer JS. Multifactor protocol designs IV: how multifactor designs estimate the total error by accounting for protocol-specific biases. Clin Chem 1991;37:26-9.
59. Krouwer JS. Estimating total analytical error and its sources. Arch Pathol Lab Med 1992;116:726-31.
60. Krouwer JS. Setting performance goals and evaluating total analytical error for diagnostic assays. Clin Chem 2002;48:919-27.
61. Krouwer JS. Critique of the guide to the expression of uncertainty in measurement methods of estimating and reporting uncertainty in diagnostic assays. Clin Chem 2003;49:1818-21.
62. Lawton WH, Sylvester EA, Young-Ferraro BJ. Statistical comparison of multiple analytic procedures: application to clinical chemistry. Technometrics 1979;21:397-409.
63. Linko S, Örnemark U, Kessel R, Taylor PDP. Evaluation of uncertainty of measurement in routine clinical chemistry: application to determination of the substance concentration of calcium and glucose in serum. Clin Chem Lab Med 2002;40:391-8.
64. Linnet K. Assessing diagnostic tests once an optimal cutoff point has been selected. Clin Chem 1986;32:1341-6.
65. Linnet K. Two-stage transformation systems for normalization of reference distributions evaluated. Clin Chem 1987;33:381-6.
66. Linnet K. A review on the methodology for assessing diagnostic tests. Clin Chem 1988;34:1379-86.
67. Linnet K. Choosing quality control systems to detect maximum medically allowable analytical errors. Clin Chem 1989;35:284-8.
68. Linnet K. Estimation of the linear relationship between the measurements of two methods with proportional errors. Stat Med 1990;9:1463-73.
69. Linnet K, Bruunshuus I. HPLC with enzymatic detection as a candidate reference method for serum creatinine. Clin Chem 1991;37:1669-75.
70. Linnet K. Evaluation of regression procedures for methods comparison studies. Clin Chem 1993;39:424-32.
71. Linnet K. The performance of Deming regression analysis in case of a misspecified analytical error ratio. Clin Chem 1998;44:1024-31.
72. Linnet K. Limitations of the paired t-test for evaluation of method comparison data. Clin Chem 1999;45:314-5.
73. Linnet K. Necessary sample size for method comparison studies based on regression analysis. Clin Chem 1999;45:882-94.
74. Linnet K. Nonparametric estimation of reference intervals by simple and bootstrap-based procedures. Clin Chem 2000;46:867-9.
75. Linnet K, Kondratovich M. Partly nonparametric approach for determining the limit of detection. Clin Chem 2004;50:732-740.
76. Linnet K. Estimation of the limit of detection with a bootstrap-derived standard error by a partly non-parametric approach: application to HPLC drug assays. Clin Chem Lab Med 2005;43: 394-9.
77. Lipman HB, Astles JR. Quantifying the bias associated with use of discrepant analysis. Clin Chem 1998;44:108-15.
78. Mandel J. The statistical analysis of experimental data. New York: Wiley, 1964:290-1.
79. Marks V. False-positive immunoassay results: a multicenter survey of erroneous immunoassay results from assays of 74 analytes in 10 donors from 66 laboratories in seven countries. Clin Chem 2002;48:2008-16.
80. National Cholesterol Education Program. Current status of blood cholesterol measurements in clinical laboratories in the United States: a report from the laboratory Standardization Panel of the National Cholesterol Education Program. Clin Chem 1988;34:193-201.
81. Passing H, Bablok W. A new biometrical procedure for testing the equality of measurements from two different analytical methods. J Clin Chem Clin Biochem 1983;21:709-20.
82. Passing H, Bablok W. Comparison of several regression procedures for method comparison studies and determination of sample sizes. J Clin Chem Clin Biochem 1984;22:431-45.
83. Petersen PH, de Verdier C-H, Groth T, Fraser CG, Blaabjerg O, Hørder M. The influence of analytical bias on diagnostic misclassifications. Clin Chim Acta 1997;260:189-206.
84. Petersen PH, Stöckl D, Blaabjerg O, Pedersen B, Birkemose E, Thienpont L, et al. Graphical interpretation of analytical data from comparison of a field method with a reference method by use of difference plots. Clin Chem 1997;43:2039-46.
85. Petersen PH, Fraser CG, Kallner A, Kenny D, eds. Strategies to set global analytical quality specifications in laboratory medicine. Scand J Clin Lab Invest 1999;59:475-585.
86. Petersen PH, Stöckl D, Westgard JO, Sandberg S, Linnet K, Thienpont L. Models for combining random and systematic errors: assumptions and consequences for different models. Clin Chem Lab Med 2001;39:589-95.
87. Plebani M. Exploring the iceberg of errors in laboratory medicine. Clin Chim Acta 2009;404:16-23.
88. Pollock MA, Jefferson SG, Kane JW, Lomax K, MacKinnon G, Winnard CB. Method comparison: a different approach. Ann Clin Biochem 1992;29:556-60.
89. Powers DM. Establishing and maintaining performance claims. Arch Pathol Lab Med 1992;116:718-25.
90. Prichard FE, Day JA, Hardcastle WA, Holcombe DG, Treble RD. Quality in the analytical chemistry laboratory. Chichester, United Kingdom: Wiley, 1995:136-143, 169.
91. Ricos C, Alvarez V, Cava F, Garcia-Lario JV, Hernandez A, Jimenez CV, et al. Current databases on biological variation: pros, cons and progress. Scand J Clin Lab Invest 1999;59:491-500.
92. Rodbard D, McClean SW. Automated computer analysis for enzyme-multiplied immunological techniques. Clin Chem 1977;23:112-5.

93. Ross JW, Lawson NS. Analytical goals, concentration relationships, and the state of the art for clinical laboratory precision. Arch Pathol Lab Med 1995;119:495-513.
94. Rotmensch S, Cole LA. False diagnosis and needles therapy of presumed malignant disease in women with false-positive human chorionic gonadotropin concentrations. Lancet 2000;355:712-5.
95. Shah VP, Midha KK, Findlay JWA, et al. Bioanalytical method validation: a revisit with a decade of progress. Pharm Res 2000;17:1551-7.
96. Shukla GK. On the problem of calibration. Technometrics 1972;14:547-53.
97. Skendzel LP, Barnett RN, Platt R. Medically useful criteria for analytic performance of laboratory tests. Am J Clin Pathol 1985;83:200-205.
98. Snedecor GW, Cochran WG. Statistical methods, 8th edition. Ames, Iowa: Iowa State University Press, 1989:75, 121, 140-2, 170-4, 177, 237-8, 279.
99. Stöckl D. Beyond the myths of difference plots. [Letter] Ann Clin Biochem 1996;36:575-7.
100. Strike PW. Measurement in laboratory medicine. Oxford: Butterworth-Heinemann, 1996, 162-3.
101. Sturgeon CM, Berger P, Bidart J-M, Birken S, Burns C, Norman RJ, et al. Differences in recognition of the 1st WHO international reference reagents for hCG-related isoforms by diagnostic immunoassays for human chorionic gonadotropin. Clin Chem 2009;55:1484-91.
102. Taylor JR. An introduction to error analysis. Oxford: Oxford University Press, 1982.
103. Thienpont LM, Van Nuwenborg JE, Stöckl D. Intrinsic and routine quality of serum total potassium measurement as investigated by split-sample measurement with an ion chromatography candidate reference method. Clin Chem 1998;44:849-57.
104. Thienpont L, Van Uytfanghe K, De Leenheer AP. Reference measurement systems in clinical chemistry. Clin Chim Acta 2002;323:73-87.
105. Tietz NW. A model for a comprehensive measurement system in clinical chemistry. Clin Chem 1979;25:833-9.
106. U.S. Department of Health and Human Services. Medicare, Medicaid, and CLIA programs: regulations implementing the Clinical Laboratory Improvement Amendments of 1988 (CLIA). Final rule. Fed Register 1992;57:7002-186.
107. U.S. Department of Health and Human Services. Medicare, Medicaid, and CLIA programs: laboratory requirements relating to quality systems and certain personnel qualifications. Final rule. Fed Register 2003;68:3640-714. Available as CMS-2226-F.pdf at: http://wwwn.cdc.gov/clia/chronol.aspx (accessed June 2009).
108. Westgard JO, Hunt MR. Use and interpretation of common statistical tests in method-comparison studies. Clin Chem 1973;19:49-57.
109. Wu CFJ. Jackknife, bootstrap and other resampling methods in regression analysis (with discussion). Ann Stat 1986;14:1261-95.
110. Vesper HW, Miller WG, Myers GL. Reference materials and commutability. Clin Biochem Rev 2007;28:139-47.
111. Vesper HW, Thienpont LM. Traceability in laboratory medicine. Clin Chem 2009;55:1067-75.

CHAPTER 3

Clinical Utility of Laboratory Tests

*Edward R. Ashwood, M.D., and David E. Bruns, M.D.**

A vast majority of medical decisions rely on laboratory testing. Clinicians often ask which test or sequence of tests (1) provides the best information in a specific setting, (2) is the most cost-effective, and (3) offers the most efficient route to diagnosis or considered medical action. In addition, it is often asked, "How does one combine a testing result or testing information with previously obtained information?" In addressing these questions, this chapter focuses on how to use the diagnostic information obtained from a test or a group of tests, and how to compare test results with those of other tests. Designing studies to assess diagnostic accuracy is addressed in Chapter 4, Evidence-Based Laboratory Medicine.

The analytical performance of the methods used for many clinical tests has improved dramatically. However, a test that has high analytical accuracy and precision may provide less useful clinical information than a test that performs worse analytically. For example, a test for free ionized calcium is often more accurate and precise than one for parathyroid hormone (PTH), yet knowledge of ionized calcium is of less value in the assessment of hyperparathyroidism. Pertinent questions include: (1) How does one evaluate the information content of a test? And (2) What procedure should one use to decide among different tests based on their disease discrimination ability? This chapter discusses these and other nonanalytical aspects of test performance that affect a test's overall medical usefulness. Although the techniques described in this chapter have been recommended to clinicians for nearly two decades, few physicians avail themselves of their use. Laboratorians need to take a more active role in promoting these techniques.[5]

DIAGNOSTIC ACCURACY OF TESTS

Whenever a clinician uses a laboratory test, he or she needs to have a clear understanding of the clinical performance characteristics of that test. The extent of agreement of test results with accurate patient diagnosis is represented in several ways, including (1) sensitivity and specificity, (2) predictive values, (3) receiver operating characteristic (ROC) curves, and (4) likelihood ratios.

Sensitivity and Specificity

The *sensitivity* of a test reflects the fraction of those with a specified disease that the test correctly predicts. The *specificity* is the fraction of those without the disease that the test correctly predicts. Table 3-1 shows the classification of unaffected and diseased individuals by test result. *True positives (TP)* are those diseased individuals who are correctly classified by the test. *False positives (FP)* are nondiseased individuals misclassified by the test. *False negatives (FN)* are those diseased patients misclassified by the test. *True negatives (TN)* are nondiseased patients correctly classified by the test.

$$\text{Sensitivity} = \frac{\text{TP}}{\text{TP} + \text{FN}}$$

$$\text{Specificity} = \frac{\text{TN}}{\text{TN} + \text{FP}}$$

Both high sensitivity (few FN) and high specificity (few FP) are desirable characteristics for a test, but one is typically preferred over the other, depending on the clinical situation.

By design, some tests have only positive or negative results and provide qualitative results. These tests, which are termed *dichotomous,* have a single sensitivity and specificity pair for a designated assay cutoff. If a cutoff value is selected to produce high sensitivity, the specificity often will be compromised. Likewise, cutoffs that maximize specificity lower sensitivity.

An example of a dichotomous test is the human immunodeficiency virus (HIV) screening test. This test detects HIV antibodies, producing results that may be nonreactive (negative) or reactive (positive). False positives occur owing to technical errors such as mislabeling or contamination and the

**The authors gratefully acknowledge the original contributions of Edward K. Shultz, Constantin Aliferis, and Dominik Aronsky, upon which portions of this chapter are based, as well as helpful discussions of the revision provided by James C. Boyd.*

TABLE 3-1 Classifications of a Test Result Applied to Unaffected and Diseased Populations

	No. of Patients With Positive Test Result	No. of Patients With Negative Test Result
No. of patients with disease	TP	FN
No. of patients without disease	FP	TN

FN, False negatives (number of diseased patients misclassified by the test); *FP,* false positives (number of nondiseased patients misclassified by the test); *TN,* true negatives (number of nondiseased patients correctly classified by the test); *TP,* true positives (number of diseased patients correctly classified by the test).

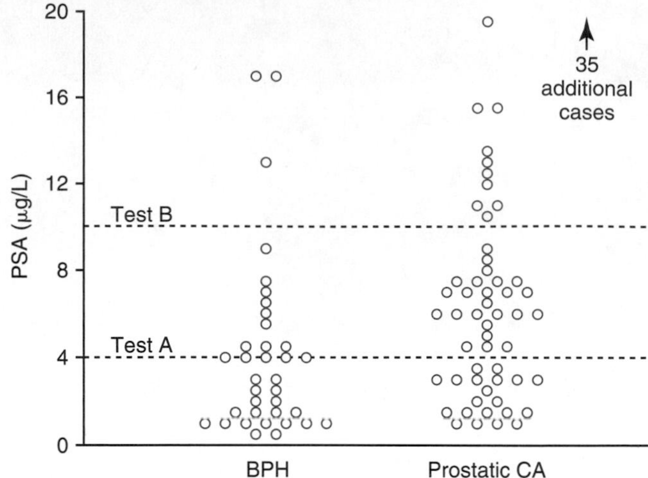

Figure 3-1 Prostate-specific antigen (PSA) concentrations for patients with benign prostatic hyperplasia (BPH) and known prostatic carcinoma (CA) are shown with two decision-level cutoffs.

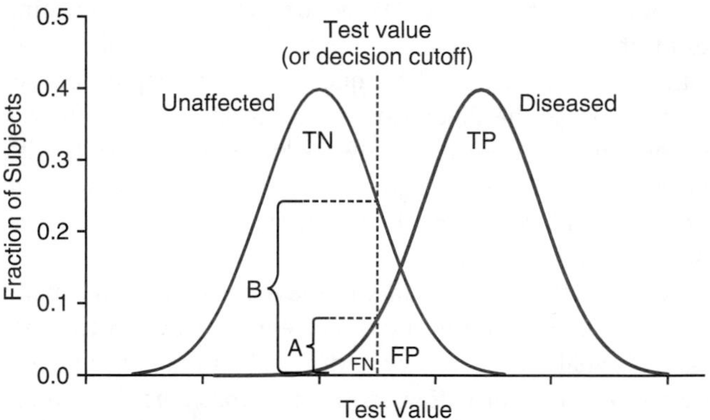

Figure 3-2 Simulated distributions of unaffected and diseased populations. Note that the ratio of diseased patients to healthy patients, A to B, is less than 1 and is very different at the point of decision (the likelihood ratio) from the ratio of TP to FP, which is much greater than 1. *FN,* False negatives; *FP,* false positives; *TN,* true negatives; *TP,* true positives.

presence of cross-reacting antibodies found in individuals such as multiparous women and multiply transfused patients.[28] False negatives occur because of technical errors such as mispipetting and sampling determinants such as testing in early infection (3 to 4 weeks) prior to antibody production. Reported sensitivities and specificities for the HIV screening test vary widely,[16] but reasonable estimates are 96% and 99.8%, respectively. Thus, 4 of 100 HIV-infected subjects will test negative. Only 2 of 1000 noninfected subjects will test positive. The clinical usefulness of an HIV test result from an unknown subject will be explained later in the "Probabilistic Reasoning" section.

As opposed to dichotomous tests, *continuous* tests are those that produce quantitative results. Continuous tests have an infinite number of sensitivity and specificity pairs, as the cutoff varies from lowest to highest decision value.

Figure 3-1 is a dot plot of the performance of a continuous assay for prostatic-specific antigen (PSA) in patients with benign prostatic hyperplasia (BPH) and in those with established carcinoma of the prostate (stages A through D).[8] Often continuous tests are used in a dichotomous fashion by choosing one or more decision cutoffs. Note the two dashed lines crossing the graphs that represent two diagnostic cutoffs. Both tests A and B are PSA tests, but they have different decision cutoffs, namely, 4 µg/L and 10 µg/L. When test A is compared with test B, the decision cutoff of 4 µg/L for test A produces increased sensitivity but at the cost of a decrease in specificity. Thus increased true-positive detection has been traded for an increase in the number of false-positive results. This tradeoff occurs in every test performed in medicine. Not only does it affect the interpretation of quantitative laboratory results, it also affects the opinions of surgical pathologists and radiologists and of the care provider who performs a physical examination.

Figure 3-2 illustrates a hypothetical test that shows higher results in patients who have a disease compared with those who are unaffected. As the decision cutoff is increased, FP decrease and FN increase. At extremely low and extremely high cutoffs, sensitivity and specificity are 100%.

Receiver Operating Characteristic Curves[48]

The dot plot (see Figure 3-1) displays quantitative performance in a limited fashion. For example, one cannot easily estimate sensitivity and specificity for various decision cutoffs using the dot plot. A graphical technique for displaying the same information, called a *receiver operating characteristic (ROC)* curve, began to be used during World War II to examine the sensitivity and specificity associated with radar detection of enemy aircraft. An ROC curve is generated by plotting sensitivity (y-axis) versus 1 − specificity (x-axis).[10a]

Figure 3-3 shows the ROC curve for the data in Figure 3-1. The x-axis plots the fraction of nondiseased patients who

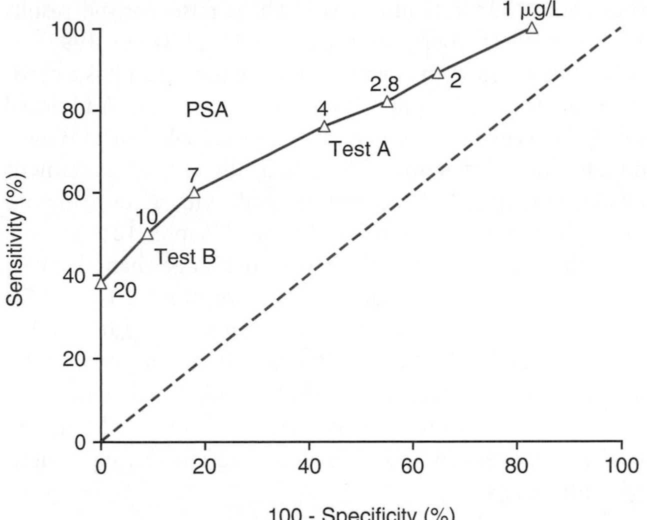

Figure 3-3 Receiver operating characteristic curve of prostate-specific antigen (PSA). Each point on the curve represents a different decision level. The sensitivity and 1 − specificity can be read for tests *A* and *B*, having 4 and 10 μg/L as decision thresholds, respectively.

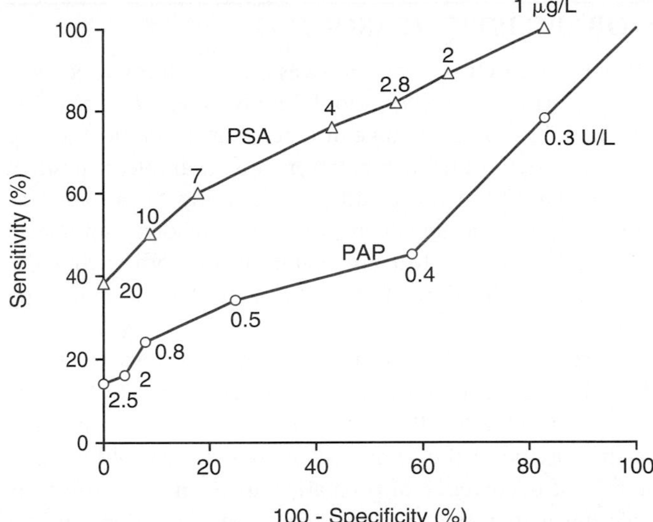

Figure 3-4 Receiver operating characteristic curves of prostatic acid phosphatase (PAP) and prostate-specific antigen (PSA) assays for patients with benign prostatic hyperplasia and prostatic carcinoma. Because the PSA assay curve is above the PAP assay curve at all points, the PSA assay is the better assay for the patients tested.

were erroneously categorized as positive for a specific decision threshold. This "false-positive rate" is mathematically the same as 1 − specificity. The *y*-axis plots the "true-positive rate" (the sensitivity). A "hidden" third axis is contained within the curve itself: the curve is drawn through points that represent different decision cutoff values. Those decision cutoffs are listed as labels on the curve.[18] The entire curve is a graphical display of the performance of the test.

Tests A and B from Figure 3-3 are displayed as two decision points on the ROC curve. The dotted line extending from the lower left to the upper right represents a test with no discrimination and is designated the random guess line. A curve that is "above" the diagonal line describes performance that is better than random guessing. A curve that extends from the lower left to the upper left and then to the upper right is a perfect test. The area under the curve describes the test's overall performance, although usually one is interested only in its performance in a specific region of the curve.[1] One strength of the ROC graph lies in its provision of a meaningful comparison of the diagnostic performance of different tests. In the medical literature, the use of 2 × 2 tables to present the sensitivity and specificity of a test has led to the common logical misconception that a quantitative test has a single sensitivity and specificity. When the initial publication of an assay recommends a cutoff for analysis purposes, the assay is often categorized as sensitive or specific based on this cutoff. Yet, as seen in the ROC curve, every assay can be as sensitive as desired at some cutoff, and as specific as desired at another.

When two procedures are compared, confusion is avoided by using ROC curves instead of accepting statements such as, "Test A is more sensitive, but test B is more specific." For example, the usefulness of the prostatic acid phosphatase assay had been compared for years with that of the PSA assay for diagnostic and follow-up purposes. Various claims were made regarding the relative sensitivity and specificity of the two assays.[12,35]

Figure 3-4 compares the performance of an acid phosphatase assay with that of the PSA assay for discrimination between BPH and prostatic carcinoma in the same cohort of patients. Although each test has been claimed to be "more sensitive but less specific" than the other by various authors, it is clear from the ROC curves that the authors were choosing different points on the two curves. No matter what level of sensitivity is chosen, the PSA assay offers greater specificity than the acid phosphatase assay at the same level of sensitivity. This does not mean that one should conclude that the PSA assay is always superior. It does indicate that for the cohort of patients used to compare the assays, the PSA assay offers superior performance compared with the prostatic acid phosphatase assay. However, the acid phosphatase assay may provide superior diagnostic information to that provided by the PSA assay in subpopulations of the cohort.

The area under the ROC curve is a relative measure of a test's performance. A Wilcoxon statistic (or equivalently, the Mann-Whitney *U*-test) statistically determines which ROC curve has more area under it. These methods are particularly helpful when the curves do not intersect. When the ROC curves of two laboratory tests assessing for the same disease intersect, the tests may exhibit different diagnostic performances, even though the areas under the curve are identical. Test performance depends on the region of the curve (i.e., high sensitivity vs. high specificity) chosen. Details on how individual points on two curves can be compared statistically have been provided elsewhere.[1]

PROBABILISTIC REASONING

Although the ROC curve improves our capability to judge a test's performance, a result should not be interpreted in isolation. The clinician must take into account the clinical setting before rendering an interpretation. For example, a positive HIV screening test has a different meaning for an adult as compared with a newborn. In the newborn, antibodies detected by an HIV test are maternal antibodies; thus the result is an indication of the HIV status of the newborn's mother.

Interpretation of almost all laboratory test results is affected by the probability of the disorder prior to testing. For example, an elevated PSA concentration in a 35-year-old is not interpreted in the same way as in a 70-year-old because the rate of occurrence of prostatic cancer in 35-year-olds is much lower than that in older men.[29] Interpretation must be tempered by knowledge of the prevalence of the disease.

Prevalence

Prevalence is defined as the frequency of disease in the population examined.[44] For example, with step sectioning of prostate tissue from a random sample of men older than 50 years of age, at least a 25% probability of histologic carcinoma is expected (most of the carcinomas identified will never become clinically important, but they are carcinomas nevertheless).[17,34] Several useful techniques have been applied to combine the prevalence with information previously obtained in the results of testing.

Predictive Values

The results of dichotomous tests (and continuous tests used in a dichotomous manner) can be interpreted using predictive values. The *predictive value of a positive test* (PV^+) is the fraction of subjects with a positive test who have the disease. The *predictive value of a negative test* (PV^-) is the fraction of subjects with a negative test who do not have the disease. The predictive value equations are as follows:

$$PV^+ = \frac{TP}{TP + FP}$$

$$PV^- = \frac{TN}{TN + FN}$$

Predictive values are a function of sensitivity, specificity, and prevalence. It is regrettable that clinicians often confuse sensitivity with PV^+. For example, suppose that 1,000,000 U.S. residents were randomly chosen and tested for HIV infection using the HIV screening test. The Centers for Disease Control and Prevention estimates that the prevalence of HIV infection in the United States is 330.4 per 100,000 population.[7] On the basis of this prevalence, about 3304 infected individuals would be expected in a population of 1 million. Because the sensitivity of the HIV test is 96%, about 3172 infected individuals would have a positive test result (i.e., TP = 3172). Similarly, because the specificity of the HIV test is 99.8%, about 2 false positives per 1000 subjects would be expected. Thus about 1993 individuals would have false-positive results (i.e., FP = 1993). Therefore, the PV^+ is 3172/(3172 + 1993), or 61%. Thus an individual with a positive test result has a moderate chance of having a false-positive result. Additional testing is necessary to separate TP individuals from FP individuals. Most laboratories automatically test all specimens having a positive HIV screening result with a confirmatory test such as the HIV Western blot (see Chapter 12).

In this example, the PV^- is much higher than the PV^+. Calculations reveal 132 false-negative results (3304 − 3172) and about 994,703 true negatives [99.8% × (1,000,000 − 3304)]. Thus, the PV^- is 99.987%. Note that many of the false negatives could reflect these infected individuals with early HIV infection prior to antibody development. The limitation of false negatives can be overcome by frequent testing of high-risk individuals.

Odds Ratio

The *odds ratio* (OR) is defined as the probability of the presence of a specific disease divided by the probability of its absence. The odds ratio reflects the prevalence of the disease in a population. For example, the probability of occurrence of a 1.3-cm^3 carcinoma in a 75-year-old man is about 8%. The odds ratio of finding histologic carcinoma measuring greater than 1.3 cm^3 after the prostate is sectioned from the autopsy specimen of a man older than 70 years is thus 0.08/(1 − 0.08), or 1 to 11.5. Findings from a digital rectal examination, from transrectal ultrasonography, or from both consist of other data that affect the previous probability of the presence of prostatic disease.

$$\text{Odds Ratio} = \frac{\text{probability of event}}{1 - \text{probability of event}}$$

Likelihood Ratio

The *likelihood ratio* (LR) is the probability of occurrence of a specific test value given that the disease is present divided by the probability of the same test value if the disease was absent. Many sources (e.g., Henry[20]) indicate that the slope of the ROC curve is equal to the LR for a given test value. Assertions such as these oversimplify the concept of LR. Choi[10] describes three different slopes of the ROC curve, which represent LR in different settings (as illustrated in Figure 3-5):

1. The tangent slope, which is equal to the LR of a *continuous* test at a given test value.
2. The slope from the origin to a test value equal to a decision cutoff, the LR^+ for a positive result of a *dichotomous* test; this slope has a companion slope (which is the slope from the cutoff value to the upper right hand corner of the ROC plot), which represents the LR^- for a negative result of a *dichotomous* test.
3. A slope between any two test values (not illustrated in Figure 3-5), which is termed the *interval LR* and represents the LR of a result that lies between the values; the interval LR is useful for continuous tests that have results grouped into intervals.

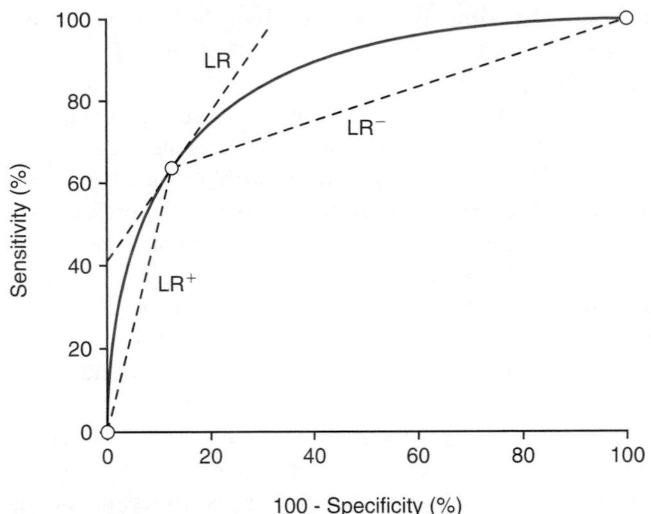

Figure 3-5 Receiver operating characteristic curve illustrating the slopes that define the likelihood ratio (LR) for a continuous test at a specific test result (the gray point), and the positive likelihood ratio (LR^+) and the negative likelihood ratio (LR^-) of a dichotomous test.[10]

For qualitative tests, the *positive likelihood ratio* (LR^+) is equal to the sensitivity/(1 – specificity). Conversely, the *negative likelihood ratio* (LR^-) is the probability of occurrence of a specific test value given that the disease is absent divided by the probability of the same test value if the disease were present. Thus for qualitative tests, the LR^- is specificity/(1 – sensitivity).

For quantitative tests, the LR is the tangent slope of the ROC curve, which equals the ratio of the heights A and B of the two curves at the test value in Figure 3-2. Note that the areas under each curve in Figure 3-2 are the same. The likelihood ratio does not take disease prevalence or any other prior information into account. To arrive at a final probability, one must adjust for the best estimate of the probability of disease before obtaining the test result.

Bayes' Theorem

Bayes' theorem provides a method to calculate the probability of a disease after new information is added to previously obtained information. The basic theorem is usually written as follows:

$$P(D|R) = \frac{P(R|D) \times P(D)}{P(R)}$$

where D is disease and R is a positive result. Thus the above equation is "the probability of disease given a particular result is equal to the probability of that result given the disease (i.e., sensitivity) times the probability of disease (i.e., prevalence) divided by the overall probability of having that result." For a dichotomous test, the probability of a positive result is equal to the numerator of the equation plus $P(R|\text{not } D) \times P(\text{not } D)$, or (1 – specificity) × (1 – prevalence). Thus, Bayes' theorem can be rewritten to express the probability of disease given a positive test result as follows:

$$P(D|R) = \frac{\text{Sensitivity} \times \text{Prevalence}}{\text{Sensitivity} \times \text{Prevalence} + (1 - \text{Specificity}) \times (1 - \text{Prevalence})}$$

Most formulas for Bayes' theorem require computer assistance for rapid solutions. One method, which is performed without a computer, involves using the likelihood version of Bayes' theorem. The odds ratio of the occurrence of a disease is calculated before the test result is known; this information is then combined with the LR. The final result is again in the form of an odds ratio, which can be converted into a probability, if desired. The advantages of this method are that it is relatively easily memorized, and it requires little mathematical calculation. Thus:

$$\text{Odds ratio after testing} = \text{Odds ratio before testing} \times \text{Likelihood ratio of a given test result}$$

Consider interpretation of a slightly elevated PSA (4.0 to 10.0 µg/L) in a patient with BPH. A urologist follows with a transrectal ultrasound examination, which he interprets as giving a positive result for cancer. The urologist has performed biopsies on numerous patients similar to this patient and has had many results that he interprets as negative for cancer. The urologist finds the high number of negative biopsies perplexing, because both screening tests produced positive results. He or she then requests an estimate of the probability of cancer in this patient.

1. *Calculate the odds ratio that carcinoma is present before performing the ultrasound.* Given a PSA of 4.0 to 10.0 µg/L, there is an estimated probability of 12% with biopsy-verifiable carcinoma in a BPH population; thus the probability of no disease is (1 – 0.12) = 0.88. Therefore, the odds ratio for the presence of carcinoma before transrectal ultrasound is performed is 0.12/0.88 = 0.14, or about 1 to 7.3.
2. *Calculate the likelihood ratio of the new information (findings of the transrectal ultrasound).* Screening studies on urology patients report sensitivities for cancer of approximately 92% and specificities that average about 50% for transrectal ultrasound.[6,11,30] The LR^+ is the sensitivity divided by (1 – specificity), or 0.92/0.50 = 1.8.
3. *Calculate the odds ratio after incorporation of the new information.* The revised odds ratio estimate (the product of Steps 1 and 2) is 0.14 × 1.8 = 0.25, or about 1 to 4.
4. *Convert the odds ratio back into probabilities.* The probability equals the odds ratio divided by (1 + odds ratio), or 0.25/1.25 = 0.2.

Although both the PSA and transrectal ultrasound were positive, the probability of a biopsy result positive for carcinoma is only 20%. The urologist had been anticipating a much higher probability because of confusion between sensitivity and predictive value of the PSA and transrectal ultrasound tests.

If the ultrasound findings had been negative, we would use the inverse of the odds ratio coupled with the negative likelihood ratio. The odds ratio of no disease after the PSA assay, (0.88/0.12) = 7.3, multiplied by the negative likelihood ratio

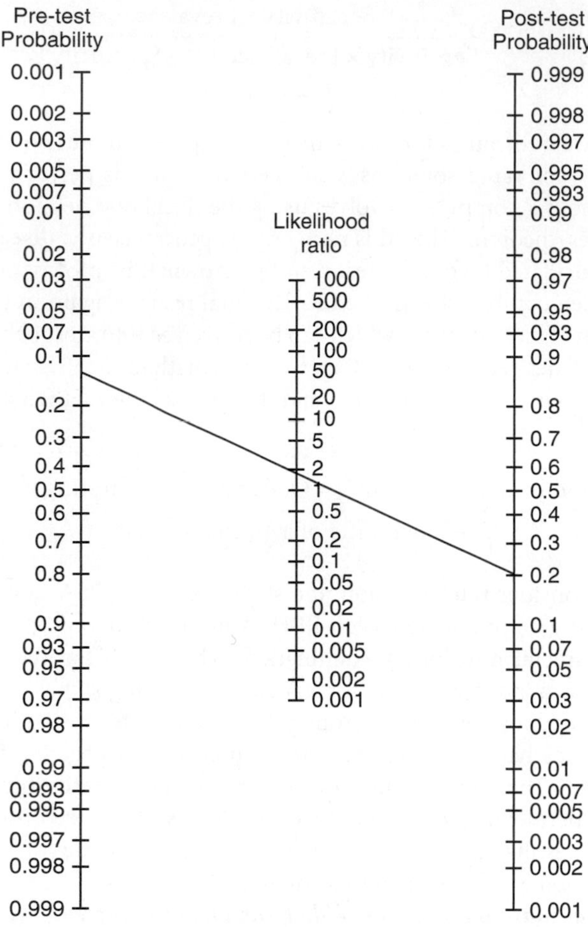

Figure 3-6 Nomogram estimating the post-test probability of a condition given the pretest probability and the likelihood ratio. *(Modified from Boyd JC. Statistical analysis and presentation of data. In: Price CP, Christenson RH, eds. Evidence-based laboratory medicine principles, practice and outcomes, 2nd edition. Washington, DC: AACC Press, 2007:113-40.)*

[specificity/(1 – sensitivity) = 0.5/0.08 = 6.25], is 43. Converting to probabilities yields 43/(43 + 1) = 98% probability of no disease.

The calculation of the post-test probability has also been solved using a convenient nomogram[4] (Figure 3-6). Knowing the pretest probability and the LR, one constructs a line between those two points and extrapolates the line onto the post-test scale.

Limitations of Bayes' Theorem

Although Bayes' theorem is widely recommended as an aid to refine the probabilistic estimates of disease, it rests on the assumption of *test independence,* which often is not present. As an extreme example of the possible errors that can occur when nonindependent tests are used, consider testing the PSA concentration of a BPH patient on three consecutive days. Each day, the PSA value is approximately 10 μg/L. The LR for this result can be estimated from the tangent of the slope at 10 μg/L in Figure 3-2. This slope is approximately 1.2. Using the likelihood form of Bayes' theorem, next multiply the prior odds ratio (assume 10 to 90) by the LR to obtain the odds ratio after 0.13, or a probability of 12% after the first test. The odds ratio is 1.2 × 0.13 = 0.16 after the second test, and finally 0.19 after the third test. This gives a 16% probability of disease. Very little new information has been provided by the second and third tests, yet the probability of disease has apparently increased from 10 to 16%. A less obvious and less extreme example would result from the combination of the prostatic acid phosphatase results with the PSA results. Although this combination does provide some new information, an acid phosphatase result is related to the amount of prostatic tissue, much as a PSA result is. In contrast, the ultrasound examination is a different approach to the diagnosis, and the information it yields should be more independent of the PSA assay than information yielded by the acid phosphatase results. The lack of test independence is also a problem when computerized diagnostic programs that employ a Bayesian approach are used. The amount of independence among different tests for various diseases often must be estimated and tried using a set of test cases.

Judging independence is difficult without collecting a large set of clinical data and examining them mathematically. A useful approach is to think about the incorrect results given by each test. If both tests tend to yield incorrect results for the same patients, then the tests are not independent, and thus Bayes' theorem cannot be applied to the combination of their results to correctly estimate the probability of disease. For example, the presence of prostatitis or BPH will result in a large number of false-positive results for both PSA and prostatic acid phosphatase assays. Although these tests are not measuring the same analyte and do provide some independent information, combining their results using Bayes' theorem is not appropriate. Alternatively, if the tests seem intuitively to be independent, then the errors made by assuming independence are likely to be small.

Combination Testing

Panels of tests are commonly used to increase sensitivity and specificity or are used sequentially to decrease costs. For the practicing laboratorian, the value of panels is limited by sparse literature on the performance of combinations of tests. The same issue of test independence addressed in the previous section makes it difficult to calculate the performance of panels of tests. In addition, the use of multiple tests can increase the probability of the occurrence of false-positive or false-negative results, depending on how the tests are combined. The often used maternal serum screening panel described in Chapter 57 uses four tests, but combines the results using a log normal covariate distribution model, which adjusts for lack of independence among the tests.[41]

Because most reference intervals exclude a fraction of those patients without disease, there is an expected false-positive rate. As multiple tests are added to panels, the probability of false-positive results increases. Efforts to establish multivariate reference intervals that correct for multiple tests and their interrelationships have been made, but the concept has not found widespread acceptance. Although this concept

TABLE 3-2 Performance of Different Test Combinations in Prediction of Prostatic Carcinoma

Test Combination	Sensitivity, %	Specificity, %
PSA > 4 μg/L	78	58
PAP > 0.6 U/L	77	25
PSA > 4 μg/L or PAP > 0.6 U/L	92	19
PSA > 1.5 μg/L	91	36

PAP, Prostatic acid phosphatase; *PSA,* prostate-specific antigen.

is mathematically reasonable, those who have investigated the utility of multivariate reference intervals believe that more work is needed before they will prove useful.

The gain in test performance to be achieved by combining test results may be illusory. As demonstrated by the dot plot in Figure 3-1, and by the ROC curve in Figure 3-3, it is possible to increase sensitivity at the expense of decreased specificity. This does not guarantee that the individual test, if the decision threshold were modified to improve sensitivity, would not have comparable performance. For example, consider the data of Chan and associates[8,9,14,15] for PSA and prostatic acid phosphatase values in patients with BPH and in those with prostatic disease, shown in Table 3-2 (and also in Figure 3-4). Although combining the two individual tests does improve sensitivity, specificity is decreased. Note that using a lower decision threshold for the PSA assay gives comparable sensitivity with improved specificity over the combination.

Two observations are important. First, tables can be as misleading for combinations of tests as they can be for single tests. For example, if only the first three rows of Table 3-2 were published, one might conclude that the combination of the two tests offered superior sensitivity. Second, although in this case the two tests do not offer performance that is comparable with that of the single test, in many cases they do. Although it might be assumed that using a single test is to be preferred given equal performance, it is not always the most cost-effective approach. In this example, the prostatic acid phosphatase assay costs less than the PSA assay. If the combination in row three of Table 3-2 offered performance comparable with that of the PSA assay alone, then using the acid phosphatase assay to exclude some patients and subsequently performing PSA assays on patients with higher PSA values may well be the more economical approach.

A widely held belief[43] is that one should test first with a sensitive test and then follow up the occurrence of positive results with a specific test for best performance. The logic is that if the first test determines which patients are to undergo a second test, then the first test should be the more sensitive of the two, to ensure that the disease has not been missed. It is surprising that even when the first test determines which patients will undergo a second test, the order in which the

TABLE 3-3 Combination Test Performance Maximizing Specificity*

	Sensitivity, %	Specificity, %	Cost
Test A	80	99	$100
Test B	99	80	$100
A followed by B	79.2	99.8	
Prevalence = 0.2			$117
Prevalence = 0.8			$164
B followed by A	79.2	99.8	
Prevalence = 0.2			$136
Prevalence = 0.8			$183

*Results of test A *and* test B must be positive to make a positive diagnosis.

tests are performed does not affect the combination of sensitivity and specificity. However, it does affect the overall cost. In the following examples, two hypothetical tests that are independent are used sequentially. It is assumed that fixed decision limits are used for the two tests, and that the two tests cost the same. Although these tests are hypothetical, the principles are generally applicable to other sequential testing situations.

Example 1. Often care is optimized if it can be confirmed that a disease is not present. In this case, if screening test A yields a positive result, it will be followed by test B; otherwise, testing stops. If test B yields a positive result, then the overall interpretation is a positive result. Because tests A *and* B are necessary for the diagnosis, specificity is improved; however, sensitivity decreases compared with the use of test A alone. As shown in Table 3-3, the average cost of the combination varies with disease prevalence; however, note that performance of the more *specific* test first results in lower expected costs. This lower cost would be accentuated if the second test were to cost more than the first.

The net effect of the use of the test combination compared with the use of test A alone has been to decrease our false-positive rate fivefold while decreasing the true-positive rate by 0.8%. Whether this tradeoff is desirable depends on the implications of missing a diagnosis versus generating false-positive results.

Example 2. Diagnosing a curable disease that has a low-cost therapy often increases the relative worth of sensitivity over specificity. If the first test result is negative, the second test might still be performed to maximize sensitivity. When either of two tests yields a positive result, this would be interpreted as a positive finding overall. This is more typically seen when tests are done simultaneously, but it

TABLE 3-4 Combination Test Performance Maximizing Sensitivity*

	Sensitivity, %	Specificity, %	Cost
Test A	80	99	$100
Test B	99	80	$100
A followed by B	99.8	79.2	
Prevalence = 0.2			$183
Prevalence = 0.8			$136
B followed by A	99.8	79.2	
Prevalence = 0.2			$164
Prevalence = 0.8			$117

*Results of test A *or* test B must be positive to make a positive diagnosis.

also occurs in sequential testing. In Table 3-4, a negative result on the first test is followed by performance of the second test; otherwise, testing stops. If the result of the second test is negative, then the overall interpretation is negative. The cost of performing tests sequentially with this rule varies with prevalence, as seen in Table 3-4.

Using this rule, the combination sensitivity increases as the specificity decreases. Note that the strategy of first using the test with *lower* specificity results in lower average cost.

Following the strategy outlined in Table 3-3, the first test's specificity determines the cost of sequential testing. When the strategy is to confirm all negative results of the first test (see Table 3-4), the first test should be the more sensitive, so as to minimize costs. As demonstrated in the two examples presented earlier, the decision rule used preferentially trades off sensitivity at the expense of specificity, or vice versa. Although independent tests have been used in these examples, the conclusions are the same for dependent tests. It should be remembered that it is the interpretive rule and the two tests that determine the overall panel performance and costs; the order of testing does not affect performance but can dramatically affect costs.

METHODS FOR ASSESSING DIAGNOSTIC ACCURACY

Most studies of diagnostic accuracy are cross-sectional as opposed to longitudinal, attempting to determine the utility of a test at a single point in time. The results of a new test (often referred to as the *index test,* the test of interest) are compared with those from a "gold standard test" using the same subjects, which is more formally called a *reference standard* (the best current practice for establishing the presence of a disorder). The reference standard can include many methods for establishing a subject's health status, such as (1) additional laboratory tests, (2) imaging tests, (3) medical history, (4) physical examination, and (5) clinical changes over time.

Around 1980, some investigators realized that most diagnostic accuracy studies contained serious flaws, introducing biases into reported performance characteristics. The work of advocates for improved study design and reporting led to the development of many important assessment tools.[14] Of note are QUADAS (Quality Assessment of Diagnostic Accuracy Studies)[45] and STARD (Standards for Reporting of Diagnostic Accuracy).[2,3] Both QUADAS and STARD are described in detail in Chapter 4.

Well-designed studies minimize several sources of bias and variation, including those that affect the selection of study subjects (both patients and controls), verification using the reference standard, observer/technician bias, missing or incomplete patient data, and analysis techniques that affect estimates of diagnostic accuracy. A 2006 meta-analysis concluded that most reported studies have shortcomings that variably affect estimates of diagnostic accuracy.[31] Often, an incomplete study description prevents full assessment of potential sources of bias and variation.

Study Subject Ascertainment

Selection of study subjects is a major source of variation in diagnostic accuracy studies. Study subjects can be selected prospectively or retrospectively, consecutively or nonconsecutively, from a variety of medical settings. *Spectrum* describes the breadth of the medical characteristics of subjects involved in the test evaluation. Important aspects include (1) the duration and severity of the disease state, (2) its specific pathologic categorization, and (3) the existence of conditions that may affect test performance. The severity of disease among studied patients with the target condition (varying from mild to life-threatening) and the range of other conditions in the other patients (controls) can affect the apparent diagnostic accuracy of a test. Patient groups can also have variable simultaneously existing medical (comorbid) conditions or alternative diagnoses. Three factors can introduce spectrum variation during the selection of study subjects: (1) study design, (2) method of selection, and (3) consecutive/nonconsecutive series.

Study Design

The best study is one of cohort design, where the index test is performed before it is known whether subjects have the target condition.[31] The alternative design is case-control, in which patients known to have the target condition are selected.[32] Then similar patients are enrolled to form a control group. The discovery that maternal serum inhibin was higher in Down syndrome pregnancies than in unaffected pregnancies used a case-control design.[40] Case-control studies are often used to assess test potential before a prospective cohort study is undertaken. This approach is cost-effective, especially for target conditions with low prevalence. For example, the first report of combining four analyte results into a "quadruple" test for predicting fetal Down syndrome risk used a case-control design,[41] and the follow-up study used a series of patients in a cohort design.[42]

A poorly designed case-control study could include subjects with severe disease and healthy controls (e.g., medical students).[24] Distorted subject selection such as this will uniformly overestimate sensitivity[46] and sometimes will overestimate specificity.[46] Alternatively, selection could be designed to exclude the extreme ends of the spectrum, thereby leading to underestimates of sensitivity and specificity.[32]

Method of Selection

The best method of study subject selection is based on symptoms or signs of the target condition only.[22] For a screening test designed to be used on the general population, study subjects should have no symptoms or signs of the target condition. If a test that is designed to detect early cancer is evaluated in patients with clinically apparent cancer, the test is likely to perform better than when used for persons who do not yet show signs of the condition. This design flaw is called *spectrum variation* (although some authors call this flaw *spectrum bias*).[46] Similarly, if a test were developed to distinguish patients with the target condition from patients with a similar condition, it would be misleading to use healthy subjects as controls when evaluating the diagnostic accuracy of the test. Likewise, demographic features (e.g., sex) should be similar between study subjects and the group to be clinically tested. Cardiovascular studies that enroll only men generally may not be applicable to women.

Consecutive/Nonconsecutive Series

A best design is one that considers a consecutive series of patients, all suspected of having the target condition. Each consenting patient is enrolled, and all study subjects undergo both the index test and then the clinical reference standard. The design must avoid any form of selection bias. All subjects meeting the a priori definition for inclusion are asked to enroll. When other methods are used for subject selection, variation is likely to occur. For example, choosing nonconsecutive patients with very advanced disease is likely to produce an overestimation of sensitivity because the disease severity will be greater (and therefore the index test more abnormal) than observed when the test is used clinically, and many patients have only mild disease.

Test Protocol

Diagnostic accuracy studies should describe the index text well enough to reveal sources of variation between similar tests.

Test technology can evolve over time, improving the diagnostic accuracy of a test. For example, the glycated hemoglobin A_{1c} (HbA_{1c}) methods used in 1993 produced strikingly different results and the National Glycohemoglobin Standardization Program was established to better harmonize methods, and dramatic improvements followed under its leadership.[25] For example, by 2008, harmonization between methods was so successful that HbA_{1c} was recommended for diagnosis.[33]

Verification Procedure

How should the presence or absence of the target condition be established? This question introduces the concept of *verification bias.* The ideal verification of study subjects would rely on a single, instant, 100% accurate reference standard that is independent of the index text.[46] Unfortunately, finding an ideal medical reference standard is rare.

Improper Reference Standard

Often, alternative candidates for gold standards exist, and this confounds simple interpretation. For example, Cooner and associates[11] assumed that patients who had negative ultrasound and digital examination results had no prostatic disease. Based on this assumption, they derived estimates of the performance of the PSA assay in detecting disease. Their standard for the establishment of disease absence was the assessment of biopsy and other test results. This type of reference standard underestimates disease burden cases. When step sections of prostates obtained at autopsy or from patients undergoing radical cystectomy were examined, prostatic carcinoma was found at a rate more than 10 times higher than Cooner and associates had estimated.[13,17,21,26,34] The silent fraction of nonsymptomatic control subjects who were called "normal" in Cooner's study clearly were not free of carcinoma. This resulted in a higher estimate of the disease detection capability (sensitivity) of PSA at a specific decision threshold.

A more subtle issue here is the designation of a true-positive result. Medical professionals have been both frustrated and protected in the past owing to their inability to detect early-stage limited disease; they have been frustrated because earlier detection often would have offered the opportunity to treat disease at a time when a cure is possible, and protected because the temptation to overtreat incidental, clinically insignificant disease did not come into play because of detection limits. This protection is diminishing as the sensitivity and specificity of diagnostic tools increase. The desire to detect early disease now must often be tempered by reflection on what is clinically relevant disease.

It would appear that examination of step sections of patient prostates, although more difficult, might at first seem to be as near an absolute gold standard as possible. However, a great majority of prostatic carcinomas (>99%) are clinically indolent and do not decrease life span or increase morbidity.[15,37] A more reasonable true-positive result should reflect identification of those carcinomas that will progress to cause increased morbidity or mortality if neglected.

In the case of prostatic carcinoma, it has been argued that the size of the carcinoma is the best predictor of morbidity and mortality.[15,37] Minimum tumor sizes from 0.2 to 3 cm^3 have been suggested as worth detecting.[15,37] The Hybritech PSA assay uses 4 µg/L as its cutoff. This can be shown to correspond to an average prostatic carcinoma volume, if present, of approximately 1.3 cm^3.[8,39] A tumor of this size would serve as a reasonable cutoff for a gold standard,[47] but it is difficult to size a tumor before complete prostate removal. Using the biopsy as a gold standard is also problematic. Biopsy will detect clinically insignificant disease by chance, but will miss large tumors owing to sampling error. Yet, by its nature, the sampling error of the biopsy is weighted in favor of ignoring small tumors and detecting large ones.

A subtle example that involves both spectrum variation and improper verification can be seen in the well-known study by Light and coworkers[23] of the utility of the ratio of activity of serum lactate dehydrogenase to that of pleural fluid lactate dehydrogenase. Results appear to document excellent differentiation between effusions and transudates. Unfortunately, when a clinical diagnosis could not be made using the remainder of the clinical information available, the case was excluded from the analysis. For remaining cases, the test offered excellent discrimination. One would expect that small malignancies, which would be less obvious clinically, would have a more indeterminate ratio. The lack of a gold standard resulted in an overly optimistic appraisal of the test's ability to discriminate between effusions and transudates. Similarly, assumptions have been made about the existence of prostatic disease in nonsymptomatic patients, because it has been impractical to take biopsy specimens from these individuals.

Independence

The index test should not be incorporated as part of the reference standard. Some studies have used elevated PSA as a criterion for determining which patients should undergo biopsy. When the test in question is used to determine which patients will have the gold standard test and which ones will be included in the diagnostic set, *test referral bias* occurs. Test referral bias can be shown to erroneously increase the true-positive rate in a study population compared with the clinically relevant population.[36]

Partial Verification

Partial verification occurs when a subset of subjects are evaluated with the reference standard. In a systematic review, Mol and colleagues[27] reported on the effects of partial verification in studies evaluating the usefulness of nuchal translucency for detecting Down syndrome. Ten of the 25 studies suffered from partial verification and reported higher sensitivities than were reported by nonbiased studies.

COST-EFFECTIVENESS AND OUTCOMES RESEARCH

Optimal use of the laboratory requires examination of both the cost of obtaining the result and the value or quality of the information obtained. Determining the quality of various procedures in medicine has been a subject of increasing interest. Key aspects of value received include the amount of improvement noted in healthcare, the extent to which testing is consistent with the wishes and expectations of patients, and the degree to which testing addresses social concerns as embodied in laws and regulations.

The Clinical Laboratory Improvement Act of 1967 (CLIA '67) and the Clinical Laboratory Improvement Amendments of 1988 (CLIA '88) mandate quality control and external quality assurance programs in large part as an effort to address social concerns regarding the quality of testing results. The U.S. Congress appropriated $1.1 billion for Comparative Effectiveness Research (CER) as part of the 2009 American Recovery and Reinvestment Act.[19]

Only indirect measures of the quality of testing in terms of individual or population health benefit are available. The most valuable instruments for measuring the quality of a healthcare intervention, including laboratory testing, assess healthcare outcomes. Outcomes are defined and discussed in Chapter 4. By connecting specific analytical procedures and performance to patient outcomes, it may be possible to directly trade off the increase in cost associated with achieving enhanced performance for actual patient benefit. New tests are often heralded into medical practice enthusiasm. Some are used for years before mounting evidence of their lack of utility becomes available.

An example of the issues involved is seen in the outcomes analysis of screening for prostate cancer. Prostate screening programs are increasing each year, partially accounting for a 600% increase in radical prostatectomies between 1984 and 1990.[29] For each man who dies each year from prostate cancer, prostate cancer progresses slowly in a much larger number, never causing any morbidity. Screening is expensive, and the iatrogenic side effects of surgical treatment for prostate cancer are significant. As a result of these observations, studies have called into question the overall cost-effectiveness of prostate screening. In 2004, Stamey and colleagues concluded that PSA was no longer useful for prostate cancer screening.[38] Their 20-year study showed that in recent years, PSA was related to prostate size, not to the presence of prostate cancer. They concluded that new tests should be sought.

REFERENCES

1. Beck JR, Shultz EK. The use of relative operating characteristic (ROC) curves in test performance evaluation. Arch Pathol Lab Med 1986;110:13-20.
2. Bossuyt PM, Reitsma JB, Bruns DE, Gatsonis CA, Glasziou PP, Irwig LM, et al. Towards complete and accurate reporting of studies of diagnostic accuracy: the STARD initiative. Standards for Reporting of Diagnostic Accuracy. Clin Chem 2003;49:1-6.
3. Bossuyt PM, Reitsma JB, Bruns DE, Gatsonis CA, Glasziou PP, Irwig LM, et al. The STARD statement for reporting studies of diagnostic accuracy: explanation and elaboration. Clin Chem 2003;49:7-18.
4. Boyd JC. Statistical analysis and presentation of data. In: Price CP, Christenson RH, eds. Evidence-based laboratory medicine principles, practice and outcomes, 2nd edition. Washington DC: AACC Press, 2007:113-40.
5. Brook RH. Continuing medical education: let the guessing begin. JAMA 2010;303:359-60.
6. Catalona WJ, Smith DS, Ratliff TL, Dodds KM, Coplen DE, Yuan JJ, et al. Measurement of prostate-specific antigen in serum as a screening test for prostate cancer. N Engl J Med 1991;324:1156-61.
7. Centers for Disease Control and Prevention. Cases of HIV infection and AIDS in the United States and dependent areas, by race/ethnicity, 2003-2007. HIV/AIDS Surveillance Supplemental Report 2009; 14:1-43.

8. Chan DW. PSA as a marker for prostatic cancer. Lab Magmt 1988;26:35-9.
9. Chan DW, Bruzek DJ, Oesterling JE, Rock RC, Walsh PC. Prostate-specific antigen as a marker for prostatic cancer: a monoclonal and a polyclonal immunoassay compared. Clin Chem 1987;33:1916-20.
10. Choi BC. Slopes of a receiver operating characteristic curve and likelihood ratios for a diagnostic test. Am J Epidemiol 1998; 148:1127-32.
10A. Clinical Laboratory Standards Institute. Assessment of the clinical accuracy of laboratory tests using receiver operating characteristic (ROC) plots: approved guideline. CLSI document GP10-A. Wayne, Pa: CLSI, 1995 (reaffirmed 2011).
11. Cooner WH, Mosley BR, Rutherford CL Jr, Beard JH, Pond HS, Bass RB Jr, et al. Clinical application of transrectal ultrasonography and prostate specific antigen in the search for prostate cancer. J Urol 1988;139:758-61.
12. Drago JR, Badalament RA, Wientjes MG, Smith JJ, Nesbitt JA, York JP, et al. Relative value of prostate-specific antigen and prostatic acid phosphatase in diagnosis and management of adenocarcinoma of prostate. Ohio State University experience. Urology 1989;34:187-92.
13. Franks LM. Latent carcinoma of the prostate. J Pathol Bacteriol 1954;68:603-16.
14. Furukawa TA, Guyatt GH. Sources of bias in diagnostic accuracy studies and the diagnostic process. CMAJ 2006;174:481-2.
15. George NJ. Natural history of localised prostatic cancer managed by conservative therapy alone. Lancet 1988;1:494-7.
16. Guy R, Gold J, Calleja JM, Kim AA, Parekh B, Busch M, et al. Accuracy of serological assays for detection of recent infection with HIV and estimation of population incidence: a systematic review. Lancet Infect Dis 2009;9:747-59.
17. Halpert B, Sheehan EE, Schmalhorst WR, Scott R Jr. Carcinoma of the prostate: a survey of 5,000 autopsies. Cancer 1963;16:737-42.
18. Henderson AR, Bhayana V. A modest proposal for the consistent presentation of ROC plots in *Clinical Chemistry*. Clin Chem 1995;41:1205-6.
19. Institute of Medicine. Initial national priorities for comparative effectiveness research. Washington, DC: National Academies Press, 2009.
20. John R, Lifshitz MS, Jhang J, Fink D. Post-analysis: medical decision-making. In: McPherson RA, Pincus MR, eds. Henry's clinical diagnosis and management by laboratory methods, vol 21. St Louis: Saunders Elsevier, 2007:68-75.
21. Kabalin JN, McNeal JE, Price HM, Freiha FS, Stamey TA. Unsuspected adenocarcinoma of the prostate in patients undergoing cystoprostatectomy for other causes: incidence, histology and morphometric observations. J Urol 1989;141:1091-4; discussion 3-4.
22. Knottnerus JA, Muris JW. Assessment of the accuracy of diagnostic tests: the cross-sectional study. J Clin Epidemiol 2003;56:1118-28.
23. Light RW, Macgregor MI, Luchsinger PC, Ball WC Jr. Pleural effusions: the diagnostic separation of transudates and exudates. Ann Intern Med 1972;77:507-13.
24. Lijmer JG, Mol BW, Heisterkamp S, Bonsel GJ, Prins MH, van der Meulen JH, et al. Empirical evidence of design-related bias in studies of diagnostic tests. JAMA 1999;282:1061-6.
25. Little RR, Rohlfing CL, Sacks DB. Status of hemoglobin A_{1c} measurement and goals for improvement: from chaos to order for improving diabetes care. Clin Chem 2011;57:205-14.
26. McNeal JE, Bostwick DG, Kindrachuk RA, Redwine EA, Freiha FS, Stamey TA. Patterns of progression in prostate cancer. Lancet 1986;1:60-3.
27. Mol BW, Lijmer JG, van der Meulen J, Pajkrt E, Bilardo CM, Bossuyt PM. Effect of study design on the association between nuchal translucency measurement and Down syndrome. Obstet Gynecol 1999;94:864-9.
28. Nuwayhid NF. Laboratory tests for detection of human immunodeficiency virus type 1 infection. Clin Diagn Lab Immunol 1995;2:637-45.
29. Parker SL, Tong T, Bolden S, Wingo PA. Cancer statistics, 1996. CA Cancer J Clin 1996;46:5-27.
30. Ragde H, Bagley CM, Aldape HC, Blasko JC. Screening for prostatic cancer with high-resolution ultrasound. J Endourol 1989;3:115-23.
31. Rutjes AW, Reitsma JB, Di Nisio M, Smidt N, van Rijn JC, Bossuyt PM. Evidence of bias and variation in diagnostic accuracy studies. CMAJ 2006;174:469-76.
32. Rutjes AW, Reitsma JB, Vandenbroucke JP, Glas AS, Bossuyt PM. Case-control and two-gate designs in diagnostic accuracy studies. Clin Chem 2005;51:1335-41.
33. Saudek CD, Herman WH, Sacks DB, Bergenstal RM, Edelman D, Davidson MB. A new look at screening and diagnosing diabetes mellitus. J Clin Endocrinol Metab 2008;93:2447-53.
34. Scott R Jr, Mutchnik DL, Laskowski TZ, Schmalhorst WR. Carcinoma of the prostate in elderly men: incidence, growth characteristics and clinical significance. J Urol 1969;101:602-7.
35. Seamonds B, Yang N, Anderson K, Whitaker B, Shaw LM, Bollinger JR. Evaluation of prostate-specific antigen and prostatic acid phosphatase as prostate cancer markers. Urology 1986;28:472-9.
36. Sox HC, Blatt MA, Higgins MC, Marton KI. Medical decision making. Stoneham, Mass: Butterworths, 1988.
37. Stamey TA. Cancer of the prostate: an analysis of some important contributions and dilemmas. Monographs in Urology 1983;3:68-92.
38. Stamey TA, Caldwell M, McNeal JE, Nolley R, Hemenez M, Downs J. The prostate specific antigen era in the United States is over for prostate cancer: what happened in the last 20 years? J Urol 2004; 172:1297-1301.
39. Stamey TA, Yang N, Hay AR, McNeal JE, Freiha FS, Redwine E. Prostate-specific antigen as a serum marker for adenocarcinoma of the prostate. N Engl J Med 1987;317:909-16.
40. Van Lith JM, Pratt JJ, Beekhuis JR, Mantingh A. Second-trimester maternal serum immunoreactive inhibin as a marker for fetal Down's syndrome. Prenat Diagn 1992;12:801-6.
41. Wald NJ, Densem JW, George L, Muttukrishna S, Knight PG. Prenatal screening for Down's syndrome using inhibin-A as a serum marker. Prenat Diagn 1996;16:143-53.
42. Wald NJ, Huttly WJ, Hackshaw AK. Antenatal screening for Down's syndrome with the quadruple test. Lancet 2003;361:835-6.
43. Watts NB. Medical relevance of laboratory tests: a clinical perspective. Arch Pathol Lab Med 1988;112:379-82.
44. Weinstein MC, Fineberg HV. Clinical decision analysis. Philadelphia: WB Saunders, 1980.
45. Whiting P, Rutjes AW, Reitsma JB, Bossuyt PM, Kleijnen J. The development of QUADAS: a tool for the quality assessment of studies of diagnostic accuracy included in systematic reviews. BMC Med Res Methodol 2003;3:25.
46. Whiting P, Rutjes AW, Reitsma JB, Glas AS, Bossuyt PM, Kleijnen J. Sources of variation and bias in studies of diagnostic accuracy: a systematic review. Ann Intern Med 2004;140:189-202.
47. Whitmore WF Jr. Natural history of low-stage prostatic cancer and the impact of early detection. Urol Clin North Am 1990;17:689-97.
48. Zweig MH, Campbell G. Receiver-operating characteristic (ROC) plots: a fundamental evaluation tool in clinical medicine. Clin Chem 1993;39:561-77.

CHAPTER 4

Evidence-Based Laboratory Medicine

Christopher P. Price, Ph.D., F.R.S.C., F.R.C.Path., Patrick M. M. Bossuyt, Ph.D., and David E. Bruns, M.D.

This chapter expands upon the "Principles of Laboratory Medicine." We begin with consideration of the meaning of the term *laboratory medicine* and then go on to describe the role that laboratory medicine plays in an individual's well-being and in patient care. We describe the concepts of evidence-based medicine (EBM) and evidence-based practice (EBP), and illustrate how these are equally applicable to the practice of laboratory medicine. The remainder of the chapter focuses on key concepts of evidence-based laboratory medicine (EBLM). It is hoped that the reader will see these principles as defining one of the key tools operating at the interface between the basic science of medicine and the analytical science applied to diagnostic testing, leading to an emphasis on improving health outcomes. Key chapter topics include diagnostic accuracy of tests, prognostic accuracy of tests, health outcome studies, economic evaluation of diagnostic tests, systematic reviews of diagnostic tests, clinical practice guidelines, and clinical audit. The principles provide a foundation for the rational and appropriate use of diagnostic tests.

CONCEPTS, DEFINITIONS, AND RELATIONSHIPS

In this section, laboratory medicine and its major disciplines are defined, and consideration is given to the roles that they play in the provision of healthcare and well-being.

What Is Laboratory Medicine?

As described in Chapter 1, the term *laboratory medicine* refers to the discipline involved in the selection, provision, and interpretation of diagnostic testing, together with the associated decision making, which uses primarily samples of biological fluids provided by patients. The field of laboratory medicine comprises a number of disciplines, including clinical chemistry (also known as clinical biochemistry), hematology, blood banking (transfusion medicine), clinical immunology, microbiology, and virology. Within this structure there may be a range of subdisciplines, such as toxicology and drug monitoring, endocrinology, hemostasis, genetics, parasitology, and mycology. In some parts of the world, laboratory medicine also encompasses cytology and anatomic pathology (histopathology). However, from the perspective of the patient and the clinical user, these are artificial delineations, as they see the laboratory as a single key diagnostic resource that plays a critical role in clinical decision making. Molecular techniques have come into routine use in recent years, often being developed from an initial academic interest in one particular part of laboratory medicine (e.g., biochemical genetics, identity testing, bacterial subtyping). However, these techniques are being used more widely across the spectrum of laboratory medicine; thus although the analytical element of the service may be consolidated, the emphasis now is on the integration of information to address the clinician's or the patient's needs. Indeed, with the advent of more complex automation, integrating a wider range of analytical methods onto a single platform, aligned with high throughput capability, the boundaries between disciplines are becoming blurred (e.g., with the advent of "blood sciences" laboratories). This notwithstanding, the analytical components of these specialties are delivered from central laboratories or through a more distributed type of service involving smaller satellite laboratories and point-of-care testing (POCT), or both.

Although the core of the practice of laboratory medicine is based on the preanalytical, analytical, and postanalytical elements of routine service, it is underpinned by research and education (with respect to users of the service, as well as those delivering the service), with the whole delivered efficiently through strong clinical leadership and business management. In many cases, the laboratory medicine service also encompasses clinical service, involving direct patient care. The preanalytical service is concerned with ensuring that the *right* patient gets the *right* test at the *right* time, while the analytical service is concerned with getting the *right* result. The postanalytical service works to ensure the *right* interpretation of the result, that the *right* decision is made, and that the *right* action is taken—with the overall objective of obtaining the *best outcome* for the patient. Quality management of the whole process is an important feature of both leadership and management of the service, including service accreditation and clinical governance embracing data management, quality control and proficiency testing, clinical audit, and benchmarking. Some of the concepts of good laboratory practice are discussed in greater detail in other chapters, including automation (see Chapter 19), quality control and quality management (see Chapter 8), and the theory and practice of reference values (see Chapter 5), as well as the broader concept of the use of diagnostic tests (which are illustrated in several of the ensuing chapters). However, it is worth pointing out at this early stage that the term *diagnostic test* is a bit of a misnomer, as the test result is not always used to make a diagnosis; this will be discussed in greater detail when we discuss the underlying concepts of EBM and EBLM.

The use of the laboratory medicine service will vary according to the perspective of the customer, or user. Thus the patient may be interested in one specific question, as might the clinician at the time that he/she sees the patient. They and others may take a longer term view, looking at the way the service can help in longer term management of the patient. The purchaser or commissioner of the service, as well as a policymaker, may take a more holistic view, embracing the full care pathway, or patient journey—a journey in which the laboratory may play different important roles at different stages. Furthermore, different stakeholders may have different expectations.[98] It can be helpful in understanding this to consider the care pathway and the points at which testing may be relevant in a hypothetical pathway, as illustrated in Figure 4-1. Thus testing in laboratory medicine may be directed at (1) *screening* an asymptomatic individual for early evidence of the presence of disease, (2) *confirming* a clinical suspicion (which could include *making* a diagnosis), (3) *excluding* a diagnosis, (4) assisting in the *selection* and *optimization* of treatment, (5) *monitoring* compliance with a treatment protocol, and (6) providing a *prognosis*. Within this framework, test results can be used to establish and monitor the severity of a pathologic disturbance.

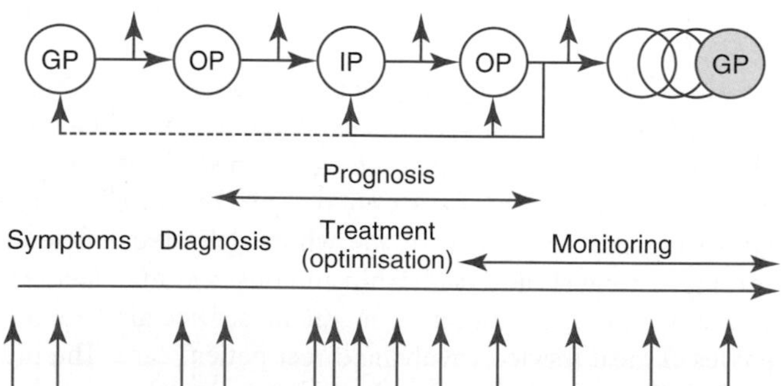

Figure 4-1 A hypothetical patient pathway, different types of clinical questions, and the point at which a diagnostic test might be used. At the point where a diagnosis might be made, it might be a rule-in or a rule-out decision and might include a question about prognosis. *GP*, General practitioner or primary care physician; *IP*, inpatient episode; *OP*, outpatient visit; ↑, point at which a diagnostic test might be required.

WHAT IS EVIDENCE-BASED MEDICINE?

In this brief section, EBM is defined, and its concepts and objectives are outlined; this is followed by a discussion of how these concepts are applied in laboratory medicine.

Definitions, Concepts, and Objectives of Evidence-Based Medicine

EBM has been defined as "the conscientious, judicious, and explicit use of the best evidence in making decisions about the care of individual patients."[121] It has been described in terms of "the integration of best research evidence with clinical expertise and patient values."[51] A key objective of EBM is "to incorporate the best evidence from clinical research into clinical decisions."[51] The words and phrases of these succinct definitions and descriptions of EBM warrant further examination and thought, as they reflect many of the reasons for the development of these concepts, as well as some of the challenges we face in laboratory medicine.

EBM has also been described as "trying to improve the quality of the information on which decisions are based" and in terms of "thinking not about mechanisms but about outcomes."[44] This comment indicates that the importance of EBM lies not in focusing on the science of the condition, or the pathology of the disease, but on how the intervention (test or treatment) can improve the health outcome. The first comment by Glasziou speaks[44] of "the quality of the information" akin to the "best evidence," referred to in the definition by Sackett and associates,[121] both groups emphasizing the use of such information in making decisions. This is why the concepts of EBM are applicable to laboratory medicine, as laboratory medicine is one of the fundamental tools used in making decisions about the care of patients in the practice of medicine.

The concepts of EBM and EBP were derived from initial discussions among a group of epidemiologists at McMaster University preparing a series of articles advising clinicians on how to read clinical journals. Out of these discussions came the term *critical appraisal;* later, the idea of bringing "critical appraisal to the bedside" was born. Implicit in this thinking was the need for good quality evidence and the ability to appraise that evidence and to determine whether it was applicable to the problem at hand and the decision(s) to be made. The initial group grew and evolved into the Evidence-Based Medicine Working Group under the leadership of Gordon Guyatt. The term *evidence-based medicine* first appeared in an editorial by Gordon Guyatt in 1991,[48] and the Working Group subsequently went on to produce a portfolio of papers under the title, *Users' Guides to the Medical Literature.*[51] Many books have now been written on the concepts, teaching, and practice of EBM which illustrate its origins in clinical epidemiology, as well as the challenges faced in adopting this approach to the practice of medicine and to healthcare management and policymaking.[44,93,119,138] Today many thousands of papers and many textbooks address the application of EBM and EBP in all branches of medicine.

The justifications for an evidence-based approach to medicine are founded on the constant requirement for information,[103] the constant addition of new information,[92] the poor quality of access to good information,[1] the decline in up-to-date knowledge or expertise or both with advancing years of an individual clinician's practice,[24] the limited time available to spend with the patient, let alone read the literature,[122] and the variability in individual patients' values and preferences. To this one might add, particularly in relation to laboratory medicine, (1) the lack of awareness of the clinical questions being asked by clinicians, with a consequent lack of focus on patient benefit, (2) the limited number and poor quality of studies linking test results to patient benefit,[85] (3) the poor perception of the value of diagnostic tests, (4) the ever-increasing demand for tests, and (5) the disconnected approach to resource allocation (reimbursement) in laboratory medicine—*silo budgeting*—which addresses only laboratory costs without consideration of benefit outside the laboratory, thus forcing decisions to save expense in the laboratory with insufficient attention to the needs of patients, their caregivers, and payers.

The Practice of EBM

Guyatt and colleagues[49] summarized the practice of EBM as follows: "An evidence-based practitioner must understand the patient's circumstances or predicament; identify knowledge gaps and frame questions to fill those gaps; conduct an efficient literature search; critically appraise the research evidence; and apply that evidence to patient care."

Efficient, and effective, practice of EBM requires the following:

- Knowledge of the *clinical process* and the ability to convert the clinical problem into an answerable question
- Facility to generate focused clinical questions
- Facility to generate evidence [i.e., information (through primary research or searching of the literature)]
- The ability to critically appraise information to generate knowledge
- A critically appraised knowledge resource
- The ability to use the knowledge resource
- A means of accessing and delivering the knowledge resource
- The ability to apply the knowledge appropriately to the clinical problem
- The ability to integrate the knowledge with previous experience in the context of the problem at hand
- A framework of clinical and economic accountability
- A framework of quality management, namely, proper clinical and financial governance

The identification of a clinical problem is both the starting point and the foundation of the service provided by the healthcare professional. Doctors and other healthcare professionals are constantly asking questions, and these can be divided into background questions and foreground questions. *Background questions,* to date more commonly observed being asked by newly qualified professionals by virtue of the way they have been taught, typically deal with knowledge (or underlying science) of the condition (e.g., Why is the circulating level of troponin I increased in a patient suffering with an acute coronary syndrome?). *Foreground questions* are related specifically to the application of knowledge, of experience in treating the condition and using tests (e.g., Will a troponin I measurement help me determine whether this patient is suffering from an acute coronary syndrome?). Clinicians tend to ask more foreground (and fewer background) questions as their experience develops. This may change in coming years as a more evidence and outcomes–based approach to teaching medical students, and training doctors, evolves. Richardson and coworkers[115] argued that all clinical problems could be expressed in the form of a question, and went on to describe a framework for formulating an answerable question: the PICO framework. This will be described in detail later, when the practice of EBLM is discussed. In the area of laboratory medicine, as described later in this chapter, the goal can be expressed in terms of answering a clinical question; appropriate laboratory investigations help to answer the question.[108,109,112] Knowledge of the characteristics of these investigations is needed to decide which test to use, when to use it, and how to interpret the results.

Finding and appraising knowledge that is relevant to the question requires awareness of available information resources, ready access to them, an ability to search the resources effectively, and an ability to critically appraise the relevance of available data. If no evidence is available, then consideration should be given to undertaking a piece of research; in this case, a correctly formulated question becomes the core of the research question. This is called *primary research;* searching for and critically appraising existing peer-reviewed research literature is called *secondary research.*

A knowledge resource in the form of a systematic review (see later in this chapter) should provide critically reviewed evidence of the efficacy, benefits, limitations, and risks of using a test, intervention, or device. Access classically has been gained through scientific journals and textbooks; electronic communications of various sorts (including textbooks and journals) are making access faster and more up-to-date. Professional bodies are now beginning to move away from narrative review to the generation of practice guidelines, their synthesis being based on the discipline of critical appraisal and the process of systematic review. Indeed many health purchasing and commissioning organizations are looking to agencies [e.g., the Agency for Health Research and Quality (AHRQ), www.ahrq.gov, accessed on February 12, 2009] and the National Institute for Health and Clinical Excellence (NICE) (www.nice.org.uk accessed on February 12, 2009) to develop practice guidelines through identification of the best evidence available, generated through both primary and secondary research.

Knowledge on the use of a test or intervention ultimately has to be placed in the context of a framework for clinical and economic accountability, ensuring the highest quality and lowest risk to patients within the resources available. One of the biggest challenges lies in the implementation of new practices and of required changes in existing practices. Many anecdotes tell of a new test being introduced to replace an old test, with the old test remaining on the repertoire of the laboratory! A major part of the implementation process is the education of those involved in using the new test or treatment. Clinical audit, a key element of meeting this objective, underpins the process of clinical governance.

EVIDENCE-BASED MEDICINE AND LABORATORY MEDICINE

When a doctor first sees a patient, that doctor will go through a routine of questioning and observing to identify the signs and symptoms that may be associated with the current health problem; from this process, he/she seeks to establish hypotheses about their etiology. Competing hypotheses may need to be resolved; this may be done in a number of ways, leading to a working diagnosis. Signs and symptoms alone may lead to a diagnosis, or the doctor may want to perform a number of diagnostic tests, including those offered by laboratory medicine. In some cases, the definitive diagnosis may become clear only over time as the nature of the condition evolves, or when a treatment is given (e.g., in the case of prescribing antibiotics in certain situations). In rare instances, a diagnosis is made only following death, with the aid of an autopsy. After a diagnosis, or working diagnosis, has been made, decisions can be made about the process of providing further care (e.g., to treat or not to treat). At this time, in some instances, the nature and severity of the condition will also be assessed to provide a prognosis. Each of these steps, as will be described later, represents a clinical problem (or clinical question) requiring a decision to be made—and action taken. The services of laboratory medicine are included among the tools at the disposal of the clinician to answer questions posed along this pathway, from initial hypothesis generation through to decision making.[119]

The tools of laboratory medicine are called *diagnostic* tests, but—as was mentioned earlier—these tests are used far more broadly than in making a diagnosis. As mentioned earlier and discussed later, they are also used in making a prognosis, excluding a diagnosis, monitoring a treatment or disease process, screening for disease, selecting therapy, evaluating the effects of therapy, and looking for side effects. The process of using a diagnostic test can be described as two processes: one at a macro level, and the other at a micro level. These are illustrated in Figures 4-1 and 4-2.

What Is Evidence-Based Laboratory Medicine?

EBLM is simply the application of principles and techniques of EBM to laboratory medicine. A clinician requesting an investigation has a question and needs to make a decision. The clinician hopes that the test result will help to answer the question and will assist in making the decision. Thus a definition of evidence-based laboratory medicine could be "the conscientious, judicious, and explicit use of best evidence in the use of laboratory medicine investigations for assisting in decision making about the care of individual patients." It might also be expressed more directly in terms of health outcomes as "ensuring that the best evidence on testing is made available, and the clinician is assisted in using the best evidence to ensure that the best decisions are made about the care of the individual patient, and that the probability of improved health outcomes increases." As discussed later, clearly the primary focus is on improving clinical outcomes, but in the delivery of the routine laboratory service, it is also important to consider the operational and economic impact of laboratory investigations.[107,109,112]

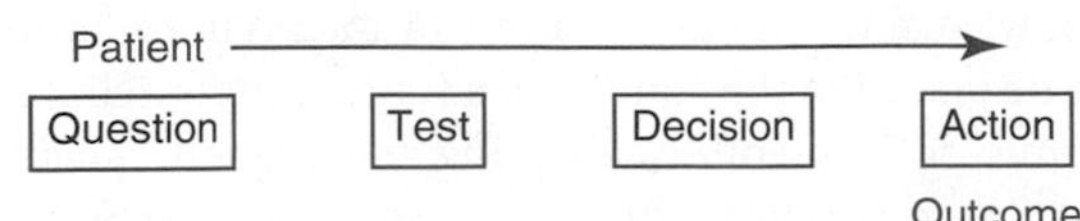

Figure 4-2 A summary of the process from a question leading to a test request, through to action leading to outcome.

The Practice of Evidence-Based Laboratory Medicine

The practice of EBLM employs the skills that have been identified in the practice of EBM, and it is important to acknowledge that the context in which EBLM is practiced is exactly the same as for EBM, focusing on the patient and overall improvement of health outcomes. Three key questions need to be answered:

- Is it a good test?
- If the test is used properly, will it improve patient outcomes?
- Is it worth investing in the test?

A good test is one that reliably answers the question being asked. To do this, the test has to meet three criteria, as will be described in other chapters of this book: (1) analytically the test has to meet accuracy and precision criteria (see Chapter 2), (2) the biological variability and other preanalytical criteria must be understood, and (3) given that the first two criteria are met, the test result must provide an answer to the question being asked; this is called *diagnostic accuracy* (see Chapter 3).

However, having a good test is not sufficient. It has to be used properly, as part of an integrated pathway of care. This is often summarized as "ensuring the *right* patient, gets the *right* test, at the *right* time, that the *right* result is generated, the *right* decision is made, and the *right* action taken, in order that the *right* outcome can be delivered."[112] This is about ensuring that the use of a test leads to a better outcome.

It is also important to be aware of the cost of care, and so it is important to be aware of the value of a test—looking at the value of the test in the immediate context of the care pathway, and more broadly the patient journey, and society as a whole—rather than limiting understanding to the cost of providing the test.

The basic tools required to practice EBLM can be summarized in the A5 cycle for EBLM (Figure 4-3). This EBLM cycle embraces five areas of activity related to the clinical problem[112]:

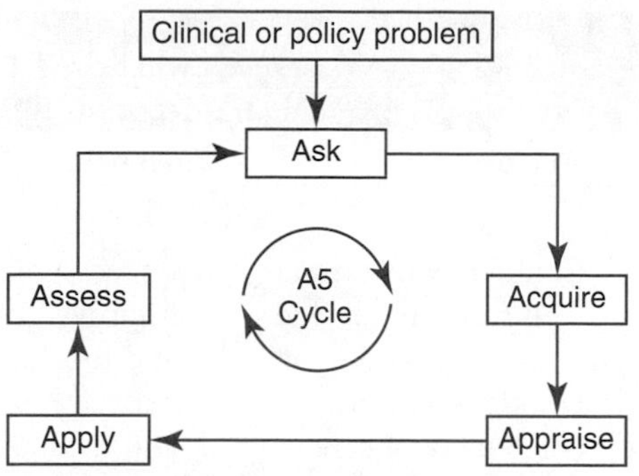

Figure 4-3 The A5 evidence-based laboratory medicine (EBLM) cycle. *(Adapted from Price CP, Lozar Glenn J, Christenson RH. Applying evidence-based laboratory medicine: a step-by-step guide. Washington, DC: AACC Press, 2009.)*

- Asking or formulating the question that describes the problem
- Acquiring the evidence that addresses the question
- Appraising the evidence for relevance and quality
- Applying the knowledge gained from the evidence in resolving the problem
- Assessing or auditing the application to test the process of application, as well as the robustness of the knowledge

However, this may not be enough, and it is helpful to know where and when these skills may be required (i.e., the context).[112] Some examples of the scenarios in which EBLM skills have been applied are given in Table 4-1, and it is evident that a question is being asked in each of these scenarios—from patient through to policymaker.

Types of Questions Addressed in Laboratory Medicine

Referring back to the hypothetical patient, or care, pathway illustrated in Figure 4-1, a number of questions are being asked during the course of this journey. Obviously a patient does not necessarily progress down the whole pathway, as the problem may be resolved by a simple intervention at an early stage. The key clinical questions can be summarized as follows:

- Does this patient have any evidence of the condition? A screening question
- Does this patient have condition X? A "rule-in" diagnostic question
- Can I rule out the patient having condition X? A "rule-out" question
- What is this patient's prognosis? A prognosis question
- Will this treatment work for this patient? A treatment selection question
- Have I got the dose right? A treatment optimization question
- Is this treatment working for this patient? A treatment effectiveness question
- Is the patient following the treatment protocol correctly? A treatment adherence question

Clearly not every question applies in all situations. However, this is not the only perspective that should be considered in the commitment to delivering the highest quality of healthcare. Donabedian[28] advocated an approach to assessing the quality of care based on *structure, process,* and *outcome.* So although the above may represent the main clinical questions, which for these purposes might be grouped under the heading of "Structure," we have also to consider the questions surrounding process and outcomes, and how laboratory medicine services have an impact on these elements of healthcare delivery. We will return to these considerations later.

In the first case, the question relates to the use of a test to screen for early signs of a condition, and in individuals with no evidence of the condition (asymptomatic individuals). Thus an example would be the use of the urine albumin : creatinine ratio to screen for early indications of renal dysfunction in a patient with diabetes. A second example would be the use of fecal occult blood measurement for the early detection of colon cancer in people over the age of 50 years. In both instances, the tests identified are *first-line tests,* and further testing would be undertaken to make or refute the putative diagnosis. Well-accepted criteria for the use of a screening test are often used when population screening is established, as in the second example. These criteria include the diagnostic performance of the test, as well as the existence of an effective treatment and demonstration of improved outcomes for those detected and treated in such a program. So, we are already seeing the close link between the diagnostic test and the intervention when looking at the outcome.

In the second and third cases, the doctor has a clinical suspicion, presumably based on signs and symptoms, and has developed a diagnostic hypothesis, that is, a diagnosis is being sought (rule-in) or rejected (rule-out). A positive diagnostic conclusion would lead to a decision on some form of action, which often involves an intervention. The intention would always be that the cascade from diagnostic question through result, decision, and action should lead to an improved outcome. An example of this scenario in which a test has been used to rule-in a diagnosis would be when a test for acetaminophen indicates that an excessive amount of drug has been ingested, and administration of *N*-acetylcysteine reduces the risk of a fatal outcome. Measurement of acetaminophen in this scenario is referred to as a *rule-in test.* In the scenario for a *rule-out test,* the actions resulting from excluding a diagnosis will invariably involve the evaluation or creation of another hypothesis, and possibly consideration of additional tests. Thus, as an example, when a patient is admitted with atypical chest pain and acute myocardial infarction is suspected, the measurement of troponin may be used to rule-out (or rule-in) acute myocardial necrosis.

At the time that a diagnosis is made, an investigation of prognosis is often undertaken, which may be considered as the assessment of risk. For example, measurement of human immunodeficiency virus (HIV) RNA plasma concentration following initial diagnosis of HIV infection can be used to predict the time interval before immune collapse if the condition is not treated.

Once a diagnosis has been made, consideration moves on to patient management, and it is in this sphere of care that

TABLE 4-1 Examples of Clinical Questions for Which a Laboratory Assessment May Be of Value, and the Associated Action and Potential Outcome (Benefit)

Test	Question	Result	Action	Outcome
Rule-in				
B-type natriuretic peptide (BNP)	Is this breathless patient suffering from heart failure?	450 ng/L	Confirm with cardiac ultrasound, decide to admit and treat	Reduced symptoms, improved morbidity and mortality
Troponin I (TnI)	Has this patient had a myocardial infarction?	7.2 µg/L	Decide to admit, intensity of care required, and treat	Improved morbidity and mortality
Thyroid-stimulating hormone (TSH)	Does this child have hypothyroidism?	12.2 mIU/L	Treat with thyroxine	Improved morbidity and mortality
Urine leukocyte esterase (LE) and nitrite	Does this patient have a urinary tract infection?	Positive LE, positive nitrite, or both	Send urine to laboratory for microscopy, culture and sensitivity, and treat if positive	Appropriate use of antibiotics, improved morbidity
Rule-out				
BNP	Is this breathless patient suffering from heart failure?	56 ng/L	Seek alternative diagnosis	Avoid incorrect diagnosis and treatment
TnI	Has this patient had a myocardial infarction?	<0.1 µg/L	Consider other possible diagnoses and early discharge	Less worry for patient, reduce unnecessary admissions to cardiac care unit
TSH	Does this patient have hypothyroidism?	2.1 mIU/L	No further action	Any parent disquiet allayed
Urine LE and nitrite	Does this patient have a urinary tract infection?	Normal dipstick result	Do not send urine to laboratory, look for alternative causes of symptoms	Inappropriate antibiotic treatment avoided, unnecessary laboratory work avoided
Monitoring				
BNP	Is this patient taking the correct dosage of β-blocker?	No change	Review dosage and patient compliance	No change in symptoms, risk of cardiac event, more clinic visits
BNP	Is this patient taking the correct dosage of β-blocker?	Fallen from 500 to 160 ng/L	No change to dosage, encourage patient	Reduced symptoms and risk of cardiac event
HbA_{1c}	Is this patient complying with treatment protocol?	10.6% (no change in a year)	Consider changing treatment, closer monitoring of compliance, clinic visits, and consultations with diabetes nurse	Increased risk of complications
HbA_{1c}	Is this patient complying with treatment protocol?	5.8%	Congratulate patient, maintain treatment regime	Reduced risk of complications

TABLE 4-1 Examples of Clinical Questions for Which a Laboratory Assessment May Be of Value, and the Associated Action and Potential Outcome (Benefit)—cont'd

Test	Question	Result	Action	Outcome
Prognosis				
BNP	Is this patient's heart failure deteriorating?	Increase from 450 to 2400 ng/L in last year	Advise on palliative care	Poor prognosis
TnI	What is this patient's risk of a further cardiac event?	0.9 μg/L	Consider intervention (e.g., stent)	Increased risk without intervention
Her-2/*neu*	What is this patient's prognosis?	3+ by immunohistochemical staining at primary diagnosis	Consider Herceptin treatment	Poor prognosis

laboratory investigations provide the greatest level of support, certainly as measured by the volume of investigations performed. It is also the most complex area, with tests being used to answer a range of questions, including (1) whether a particular drug is likely to be effective, (2) whether the patient is at risk of suffering an adverse reaction, (3) how to guide the dosing of a drug, (4) how to check for the occurrence of adverse reactions, and (5) in a patient with a chronic disease, how to check for compliance with, and effectiveness of, therapy. In women with metastatic breast cancer, the HER-2/*neu* status is used to assess the potential usefulness of Herceptin therapy. In patients with inflammatory bowel disease prescribed azathioprine, the thiopurine methyltransferase activity status is assessed to warn of the risk of myelosuppression in those with a deficiency of the enzyme. In patients treated with methotrexate, hepatic and kidney function tests are performed at regular intervals to check for evidence of hepatic and renal toxicity. In patients with heart failure, brain natriuretic peptide measurement has been used to guide, or optimize, therapy. Finally, in a person with diabetes, HbA_{1c} measurements are used to assess glycemic control and thus the effectiveness of therapy.

These scenarios illustrate the importance of identifying the triad of *question, decision,* and *action*. Identifying these three components proves to be critical in designing studies of utility or outcomes of testing, as well in the critical appraisal of evidence. They are also important in audit (see later) of the use of investigations from the perspective of both clinical governance (clinical accountability) and financial governance (controlling the test demand in the context of economic governance). Recognition of this triad has led to the definition of an *appropriate test request* as one in which there is a clear clinical question for which the result will provide an answer, enabling the clinician to make a decision and initiate some form of action leading to a health benefit for the patient.[108] In light of the earlier comment, this benefit could be extended to the health provider and to society as a whole to encompass more directly the potential for economic benefit.

BOX 4-1 Examples of Questions That Can Be Asked in Different Settings

- Clinicians inquire about what test to use
- Clinicians inquire how to use a test
- Clinicians and patients inquire about the meaning of a specific test result
- Clinicians inquire about what decision to make upon receipt of a test result
- Clinicians and patients request the introduction of a new test
- Managers request a business case for the introduction of a new test
- National health policymakers want to introduce a screening program
- Laboratory director requires evidence of method performance and the impact on outcome
- Managers want to change the mode of delivery of care (e.g., to a community setting)
- Managers request an audit of utilization of a test
- Laboratory director wishes to stop the use of a test

Examples of questions that specify the detail required to accurately qualify the use of a test result are given in Box 4-1. In practice, the clinical episode involves a series of diagnostic questions with binary responses.[20]

Formulating an Answerable Question in Laboratory Medicine

Reference was made earlier to the PICO framework for the formulation of an answerable question; in its general form, PICO comprises four elements, as illustrated in Box 4-2.

A number of variants of this framework have been described. Given the patient pathway described in Figure 4-1 and the different stages at which a test might be used, the addition of "S" for *setting* has been suggested, giving PICOS or PSICO. The alternative is to qualify the "P" for population or patient according to setting, so that only data appropriate

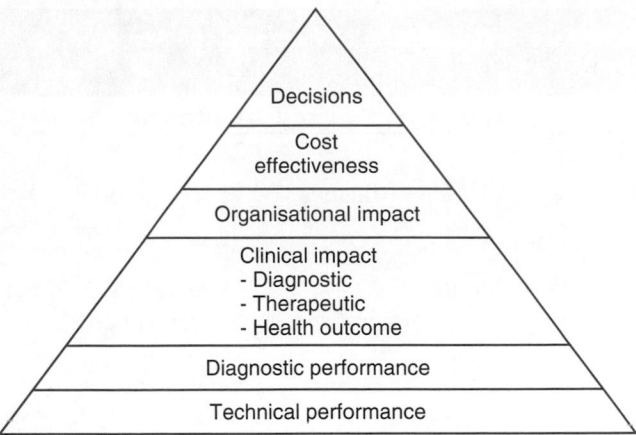

Figure 4-4 A hierarchy of evidence for decision making from technical performance through to impact on health outcomes. *(Adapted from Price CP. Evidence-based laboratory medicine: supporting decision-making. Clin Chem 2000;46:1041-50.)*

BOX 4-2 The PICO Framework: The Core of Structured Question Formulation for Diagnostic Tests

Population, patient, or problem of interest
Intervention, which in laboratory medicine could be the test of interest—the index test
Comparator or control, against which the intervention will be compared
Outcome, which may vary according to the question or the type of study

to that setting are considered. Clinicians who use probabilistic reasoning and likelihood ratios may wish to know the probability associated with the use of earlier tests or observations, and in this case "P" for *prior test* has been suggested, giving PPICO. Finally, time is an important consideration when tests are used (e.g., when looking at the prognostic accuracy of a test and the time over which a patient is observed after the laboratory test has been performed). The time at which samples are taken may also be important (e.g., when the effectiveness of digoxin therapy is monitored). This has led to the use of PICOT.[112]

From Evidence to Outcomes

Fryback and Thornbury[40] developed a hierarchy of evidence in support of their thesis that patient outcome data are the sine qua non of efficacy from the individual patient's perspective. This has been applied to laboratory medicine and is illustrated in Figure 4-4.[107] Surveys of the literature, as well as many systematic reviews, have shown that many of the papers concerned with laboratory medicine, to date, have been concerned with technical (namely, analytical accuracy and precision) and diagnostic (namely, diagnostic accuracy) performance.

Sackett and Haynes[120] described an "architecture for diagnostic research," which was based on four questions:

- Do test results in affected patients differ from those in normal individuals?
- Are patients with certain test results more likely to have the target disorder?
- Do test results distinguish patients with and without the target disorder among those in whom it is clinically sensible to suspect the disorder?
- Do patients undergoing the diagnostic test fare better than similar untested patients?

The first of these questions deals with the basic diagnostic accuracy question, basic because it does not take into consideration the setting in which the question is being asked—which is covered in the third question. The fourth question is the outcome-related question.

CHARACTERIZATION OF THE DIAGNOSTIC ACCURACY OF TESTS

When a new test is developed or an old test is applied to a new clinical question, users need information about the extent of agreement of the test's results with the correct diagnoses of patients. For this purpose, researchers design studies in which results from the new test are compared with results obtained with the clinical reference standard on the same patients. Results of the comparison can be expressed in a number of ways, including clinical sensitivity and specificity, predictive values, likelihood ratios, diagnostic odds ratios, and areas under receiver operating characteristic (ROC) curves (see Chapter 3). We refer to such studies as diagnostic accuracy studies.

Study Design

The following discussion is applicable to the design of a primary research study, in critical appraisal in secondary research, and in the application of information gained from research.

In studies of diagnostic accuracy, the results of one test (often referred to as the index test, the test of interest—I in the PICO framework) are compared with those from the clinical reference standard (sometimes referred to as the reference test). A test can be any method of obtaining additional information on a patient's health status, including not only laboratory tests, imaging tests, and function tests, but also data from the history and physical examination, and genetic data.

The *clinical reference standard* is the best available method for establishing the presence or absence of the target disease or, more generally, the target condition, that is, the suspected condition or disease for which the test is to be applied. The reference standard can be a single test, or a combination of methods and techniques, including clinical follow-up of tested patients. When there is no clear reference procedure, it has been suggested that the best way to assess a new test is by analyzing the consequences when there is disagreement between the new tests and the test in current use.[45] Finally, in some instances, the reference standard may consist of information obtained from an autopsy.

Several potential threats to the internal and external validity of a study of diagnostic accuracy are known, of which only the major ones will be addressed in this section. Poor *internal validity* will produce bias, or systematic error, because the estimates do not correspond to what one would have obtained using optimal methods, whereas poor *external validity* limits the generalizability of the findings, in that the results of the study, even if unbiased, do not correspond to settings encountered by the decision maker. For example, the results of a study of patients in a tertiary care medical center may not be generalizable to patients seen in a general practice, and studies done exclusively in older men may not be applicable to women or children. This shows the importance of the P element in the PICO framework, as well as the S variant.

The ideal study examines a consecutive series of patients, enrolling all consenting patients suspected of the target condition within a specific period. All of these patients then undergo the index test, and then the reference standard. The term *consecutive* refers to total absence of any form of selection, beyond the a priori definition of criteria for inclusion and exclusion, and requires explicit efforts to identify and enroll patients qualifying for inclusion.

Alternative designs are possible; Mol and associates have reviewed the characteristics of good studies of diagnostic tests.[91] Some studies first select patients known to have the target condition, and then contrast the results from these patients with those from a control group. This approach has been used to characterize the performance of tests in settings in which the condition of interest is uncommon, as in maternal serum screening testing for detecting Down syndrome in the fetus. It is also used in preliminary studies to assess the potential of a test before prospective studies of a series of patients are undertaken. With this design, selection of the control group is critical. If the control group consists of healthy individuals only, the diagnostic accuracy of the test will tend to be overestimated, as has been shown in an analysis that compared the results of such studies with results of studies of consecutive series of patients.[83] (See Chapter 3 for further discussion.)

In the ideal study, the results of all patients tested with the test under evaluation are contrasted with the results of a single reference standard. If fewer than all patients are verified with the reference standard, then *partial verification* exists, and verification bias may occur if the selection of subjects for reference testing is not purely random. For example, if selection is associated with the outcome of the index test, or the strength of prior suspicion, or both, then verification bias is certain. In a typical case, some patients with negative test results (test negatives) are not verified by the reference standard if this involves a costly or invasive procedure, and these patients are not included in the analysis. This may result in an underestimation of the number of false-negative results.

A different form of verification bias can happen if more than one reference standard is used and the two reference standards correspond to different manifestations of disease. The use of multiple standards can produce *differential verification bias.* Suppose test-positive patients are verified with further testing, and test-negative patients are verified by clinical follow-up. An example is the verification of suspected appendicitis, with histopathology of the appendix versus natural history as the two forms of the reference standard. A patient is classified as having a false-positive test result if the additional test does not confirm the presence of disease after a positive index test result. Alternatively, a patient is classified as false-negative if an event compatible with appendicitis is observed during follow-up after a negative test result. Yet these are different definitions of disease because not all patients who have positive pathology results would have experienced an event during follow-up if they had been left untreated. The use of two reference standards, one pathologic and the other based on clinical prognosis, can affect the assessment of diagnostic accuracy. It is likely to artificially inflate the estimates of accuracy, compared with the use of a single reference standard in all patients. For additional discussion, see Chapter 3.

A long-standing debate continues on whether or not clinical data should be provided to those performing or reading the index test, especially when that test has a subjective component. Withholding this information is known as *blinding* or *masking.* Often, some clinical information is routinely known by the reader of the test, such as when radiologists see the patients on whom they are performing a test, or a pathologist is told the site from which a biopsy is obtained. Attempts to withhold such information in the context of a study of diagnostic accuracy may create an artificial scenario that has no counterpart in patient care. Thoughtful attention to this question is important in the early phases of designing a study. For most study questions, masking is preferable, because knowledge of the results will tend to increase agreement of the results of the studied (index) test with those of the reference standard (test).

Severity of disease among studied patients with the target condition and the range of other conditions in those without the target condition can affect the apparent diagnostic accuracy of a test. For example, if a test that is designed to detect early cancer is evaluated in patients with clinically apparent cancer, the test is likely to perform better than when used for persons who do not yet show signs of the condition. This problem has been called *spectrum bias* and *spectrum variation* (see Chapter 3). Similarly, if a test is developed to distinguish diseased patients from those with similar complaints but without the target disease, then it may be misleading to use healthy subjects as controls when the diagnostic accuracy of the test is evaluated.

Reporting of Studies of Diagnostic Accuracy: The Role of the STARD Initiative

Complete and accurate reporting of studies of diagnostic accuracy should allow the reader to detect the potential for bias in the study and to assess its ability to generalize the results and their applicability to an individual patient or group. Reid, Lachs, and Feinstein[114] documented that most studies of diagnostic accuracy published in leading general medical journals had poor adherence to standards of clinical epidemiologic research or failed to provide information about adherence to those standards.[7] Similar observations have continued to be made with a number of categories of tests.[86] These reports led to efforts at the journal *Clinical Chemistry* in 1997 to produce a checklist for reporting of studies of diagnostic accuracy.[15] The quality of reporting in that journal increased after introduction of this checklist,[84] although not to an ideal level.[11]

The work of Lijmer and colleagues[83] showed that poor study design and poor reporting are associated with overestimation of the diagnostic accuracy of evaluated tests, indicating the necessity to improve the reporting of studies of diagnostic accuracy for all types of tests, not only those in clinical chemistry. An initiative on Standards for Reporting of Diagnostic Accuracy (STARD) was begun at the 1999 meeting of the Cochrane Diagnostic and Screening Test Methods Working Group. This initiative aimed to improve the quality of reporting of diagnostic accuracy studies by following the model of the successful Consolidated Standards of Reporting Trials (CONSORT) initiative for reporting of trials of therapies (see discussion of outcomes studies later in this chapter).[9]

Key components of the STARD document include a checklist of items to be included in reports of studies of diagnostic accuracy and a flow diagram to document the flow of participants in the study.[9] The checklist was developed from an extensive literature search that identified 75 potential items. The list was pared to 25 items (Figure 4-5) in a consensus meeting of researchers, editors, methodologists, and representatives of professional organizations. The flow diagram (Figure 4-6) has the potential to clearly communicate vital information about the *design* of a study—including the method of recruitment and the order of test execution—and about the *flow* of participants.

The final, single-page checklist (see Figure 4-5) has been endorsed by numerous journals [such as *Journal of the American Medical Association (JAMA)* and *Annals of Internal Medicine*] and published in many of them, including all the major journals of clinical chemistry and other leading journals such as *Radiology*, *British Medical Journal (BMJ)*, and *Lancet*. A separate document explaining the meaning and rationale of each item and briefly summarizing the available evidence was published in *Annals of Internal Medicine* and *Clinical Chemistry*.[10] The STARD group will prepare updates of the STARD document when new evidence on sources of bias or variability becomes available. In the experience of one of the authors of this chapter (D.B.), use of the checklist has enhanced the information content of all manuscripts to which it has been applied at *Clinical Chemistry,* and use of the flow diagram has led to correction of errors in many manuscripts.

Use of the STARD initiative is recommended for all reports on studies of diagnostic accuracy. Most, if not all, of the content of STARD also applies to studies of tests used for prognosis, monitoring, or screening. It is interesting to note that Simel and coworkers recently reported on use of the STARD approach for reporting of diagnostic accuracy of the history and physical examination[133]; this is important in that laboratorians need to be aware of the role that these play in the diagnostic armamentarium of the practicing physician.[141] Smidt and associates[136] found a small improvement in reporting, specifically, in reproducibility of the index test, in assessment of the severity of the condition and other diagnoses, and in estimates of variability of diagnostic accuracy between subgroups. On the other hand, Wilczynski found no improvement to date.[151]

Using the Test Result

In the area of laboratory medicine, the objective can be described in terms of answering a clinical question; appropriate laboratory investigations help to answer the question.[108] Knowledge of the characteristics of these investigations is needed to decide which test to use, when to use it, and how to interpret the results.

The value of test results depends on consideration of a range of preanalytical, analytical, and postanalytical characteristics. Thus, evidence from a study may be unreliable when differences exist in age, sex, ethnic origin, lifestyle, prevalence of the disease in the population, or prevalence of comorbidities. Transferability of study results may be affected by analytical variables, such as patient preparation (effects of fasting, posture, exercise, and biological variation) and method performance (accuracy and precision).

Analytical performance of the test may also have an impact on the outcome of the use of that test, although this is not a factor that is commonly studied. Some information has come from modeling studies, as for example in the case where the impact of the accuracy and precision of blood glucose tests on insulin dosage has been calculated.[13] The impact of the accuracy and precision of total prostate-specific antigen (PSA) methods on the number of cancers detected and of biopsies required has also been modeled.[118] Differences in analytical performance can have an impact on outcomes through differences in the decisions that are made.

At the postanalytical stage, if a result is not received or accessed, then clearly it cannot contribute to an improved outcome. In a systematic study, Kilpatrick and Holding[72] found that when they introduced electronic transmission of data to the emergency department and admissions unit, a notable number of results were never accessed. In another study of POCT for HbA_{1c}, Khunti and colleagues after consultation merely replaced the phlebotomy service with the POCT, with no apparent immediate discussion of the result,[71] thus omitting the key objective for introducing the POCT.[18]

OUTCOME STUDIES

Medical and public health interventions are intended to improve the well-being of patients, the population at large, or population segments, as stated by Fryback and Thornbury[40] and Sackett and Haynes.[120] For therapeutic interventions, patients are interested, for example, not only in whether a drug decreases serum cholesterol or blood pressure (risk factors), but more importantly, whether it decreases the risks of heart attack, stroke, and cardiovascular death. Similarly, on

Section and Topic	Item #		On page #
TITLE/ABSTRACT/ KEYWORDS	1	Identify the article as a study of diagnostic accuracy (recommend MeSH heading sensitivity and specificity).	
INTRODUCTION	2	State the research questions or study aims, such as estimating diagnostic accuracy or comparing accuracy between tests or across participant groups.	
METHODS		Describe	
Participants	3	The study population: The inclusion and exclusion criteria, setting, and locations where the data were collected.	
	4	Participant recruitment: Was recruitment based on presenting symptoms, results from previous tests, or the fact that the participants had received the index tests or the reference standard?	
	5	Participant sampling: Was the study population a consecutive series of participants defined by the selection criteria in items 3 and 4? If not, specify how participants were further selected.	
	6	Data collection: Was data collection planned before the index test and reference standard were performed (prospective study) or after (retrospective study)?	
Test methods	7	The reference standard and its rationale.	
	8	Technical specifications of material and methods involved, including how and when measurements were taken, and/or cite references for index tests and reference standard.	
	9	Definition of and rationale for the units, cutoffs, and/or categories of the results of the index tests and the reference standard.	
	10	The number, training, and expertise of the persons executing and reading the index tests and the reference standard.	
	11	Whether or not the readers of the index tests and reference standard were blind (masked) to the results of the other test and describe any other clinical information available to the readers.	
Statistical methods	12	Methods for calculating or comparing measures of diagnostic accuracy, and the statistical methods used to quantify uncertainty (e.g., 95% confidence intervals).	
	13	Methods for calculating test reproducibility, if done.	
RESULTS		Report	
Participants	14	When study was done, including beginning and ending dates of recruitment.	
	15	Clinical and demographic characteristics of the study population (e.g., age, sex, spectrum of presenting symptoms, comorbidity, current treatments, recruitment centers).	
	16	The number of participants satisfying the criteria for inclusion that did or did not undergo the index tests and/or the reference standard; describe why participants failed to receive either test (a flow diagram is strongly recommended).	
Test results	17	Time interval from the index tests to the reference standard, and any treatment administered between.	
	18	Distribution of severity of disease (define criteria) in those with the target condition; other diagnoses in participants without the target condition.	
	19	A cross tabulation of the results of the index tests (including indeterminate and missing results) by the results of the reference standard; for continuous results, the distribution of the test results by the results of the reference standard.	
	20	Any adverse events from performing the index tests or the reference standard.	
Estimates	21	Estimates of diagnostic accuracy and measures of statistical uncertainty (e.g., 95% confidence intervals).	
	22	How indeterminate results, missing responses, and outliers of the index tests were handled.	
	23	Estimates of variability of diagnostic accuracy between subgroups of participants, readers, or centers, if done.	
	24	Estimates of test reproducibility, if done.	
DISCUSSION	25	Discuss the clinical applicability of the study findings.	

Figure 4-5 The Standards for Reporting of Diagnostic Accuracy (STARD) checklist.

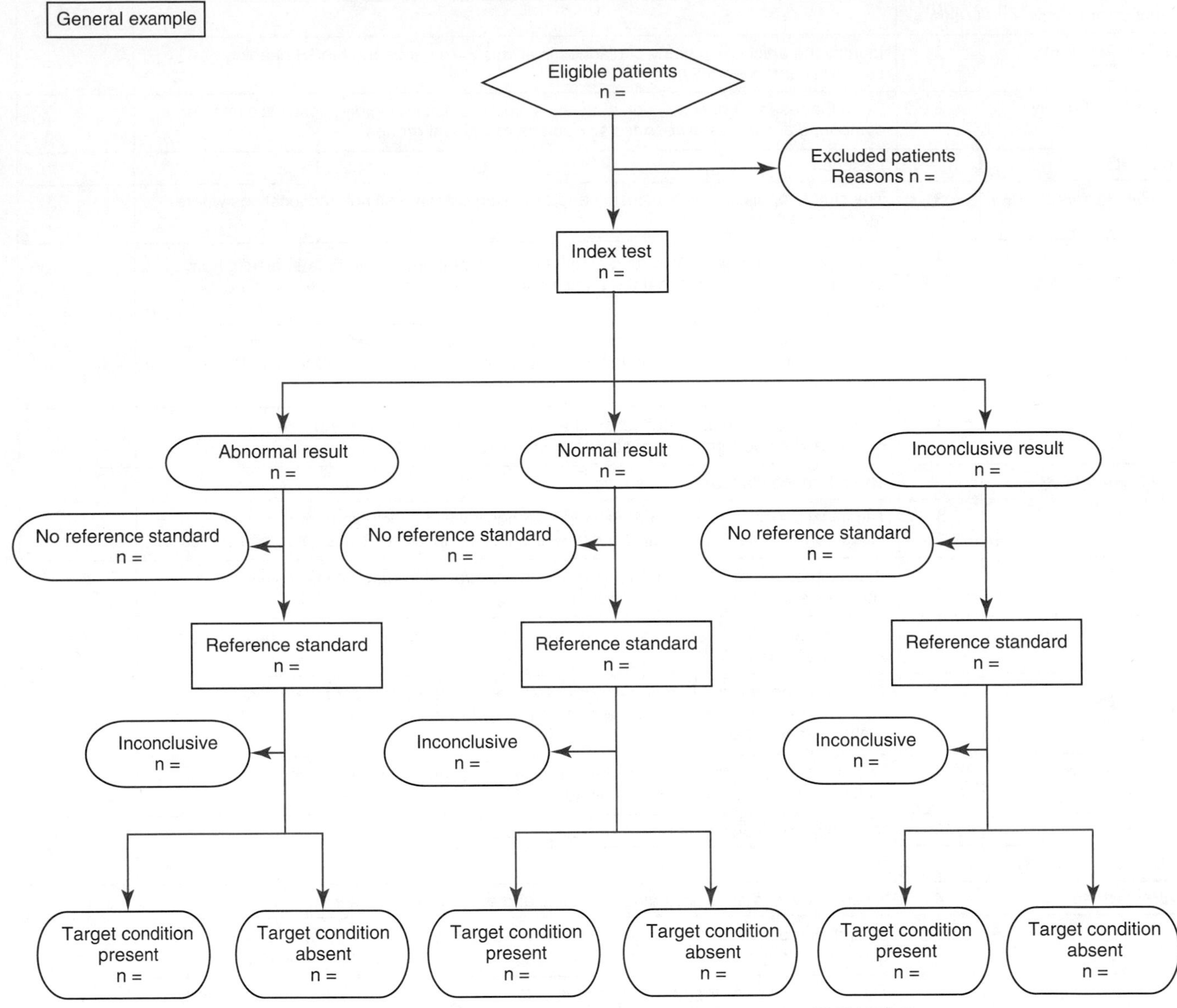

Figure 4-6 The Standards for Reporting of Diagnostic Accuracy (STARD) flow diagram.

the diagnostic side of medicine, patients have little interest in knowing the numeric value of their serum cholesterol concentration or blood pressure unless that knowledge will lead to actions that in some way will improve their quality or quantity of life. For example, a test result may identify the need for a life-saving therapeutic intervention for an existing disease, or it may lead to a change in lifestyle that will decrease the risk of developing a disease. At other times, the test result itself can provide valuable reassurance, as when a genetic test indicates that a family member does not carry a mutation that is present in the family. In still other cases, a laboratory test may provide prognostic information that allows the patient to better plan for the future despite a bad prognosis, or it may provide reassurance that symptoms are not signs of serious disease, thus allowing him or her to better manage the symptoms without fear. Test-related outcomes in these examples range from preventing imminent death to being better able to plan for death.

Who Is Interested in Health Outcomes?

Outcomes studies have taken on considerable importance in medicine. On the therapeutic side of medicine, few drugs can be approved by modern government agencies (or paid for by healthcare organizations or health insurers) without undergoing randomized, controlled trials of their safety and effectiveness. Increasingly, diagnostic testing is entering a similar environment in which physicians, governments, purchasers, commissioners of healthcare (e.g., commercial health insurers), and patients demand evidence of effectiveness of diagnostic procedures. To appreciate this, one need only recall the enormous interest in controversies about the value of mammography and the effectiveness of measuring PSA in serum.

These issues (and many others) hinge on demonstration of improved outcomes.

In the United States, the important Joint Commission defines *quality* as increased probability of desired outcomes and decreased probability of undesired outcomes. The Institute of Medicine defines quality as "the degree to which health services for individuals and populations increase the likelihood of desired health outcomes and are consistent with current professional knowledge."[127]

Up until this point, the focus has been on the patient and his or her interaction with the doctor as the primary caregiver; these individuals may be considered as the two primary stakeholders. Yet we know that healthcare is the product of many healthcare professionals, sometimes referred to as the *clinical team*. The complexity of interactions in this group has to be extended, when the broader issues of healthcare delivery are considered, to include the roles of service provider managers, service purchasers or commissioners, and policymakers. This has been brought more sharply into focus with increased pressure to improve the quality of care and to make more efficient and effective use of resources.[61,62,98] So in the case of laboratory medicine, the identity of stakeholders should be extended to include all of those who have an interest in how the laboratory service can be, and is, used.

Test Results Alone Do Not Generate Improved Health Outcomes

In many clinical scenarios, the first criterion for a useful test is that the result must lead to a change in the probability of the presence of the target condition. Boyd and Deeks,[14] for example, showed that the (pretest) probability of pulmonary embolism fell from about 0.28 to a post-test probability of 0.041 when the D-dimer test result was less than 500 μg/L. The change in probability does not, in itself, make the decision. The clinician must use this information along with other findings and clinical judgment to make decisions or recommendations about care. So, even the knowledge that a test has good diagnostic accuracy is of no value unless it is used correctly, and results are integrated with other observations and the expertise of the clinician.[140]

In most cases, testing is followed by an appropriate intervention to produce a desired outcome, particularly when the outcome is defined as improved morbidity or mortality. A test result alone may provide reassurance or an understanding of the origin of one's complaint, but usually improved outcomes require an intervention in the form of an explanation of the result in the context of the patient's symptoms. Most laboratory medicine research encompasses only test characteristics, including diagnostic accuracy. If these characteristics are not linked to clear consequences for downstream decisions and interventions, such research leads to poor understanding and appreciation of the contribution that the test result makes to improved outcomes. In relation to certain scenarios, it is possible to find valid study data, most particularly when the test result is being used to exclude a diagnosis. Thus in a randomized study of a rapid chest pain evaluation protocol, cardiac markers had a high negative predictive value in the evaluation of patients with chest pain. Testing led to fewer admissions to the coronary care unit, without adverse effects on morbidity and mortality.[99] Reducing the turnaround time for certain tests may improve triage time in the emergency room[82] unless other evaluations (such as other laboratory tests or radiologic investigations) are rate limiting.[69] Reduced length of stay appeared to occur primarily because normal results with the POCT approach enabled some patients to be discharged more quickly (i.e., a rule-out decision).[95] These examples are process outcomes.

What Are Outcomes Studies?

Outcomes may be defined as results of medical interventions in terms of health; evaluation of economic outcomes is discussed later. *Patient outcomes* are results that are perceptible to the patient[5] and are also of importance to caregivers, service provider organizations, and purchasers and commissioners. Outcomes that have been studied commonly include mortality, physiologic measures, clinical events, symptoms, function measures, and patients' experiences with care complication rates (such as the nosocomial infection rate). In studying and comparing diagnostic tests, an improved ability to make a correct diagnosis of a treatable condition may lead to an improvement in one or more of these outcomes. Test results themselves are not widely considered to be outcomes, but an argument can be made that they should be considered as proxy measures of outcome when it is certain that real outcomes will change for the better with a superior test. Some tests are increasingly being used as surrogate outcome measures in intervention studies when a strong relationship has been documented between test results and morbidity or mortality; examples include the use of HbA_{1c} and the urine albumin:creatinine ratio in studies on the management of diabetes mellitus.

Outcomes studies must be distinguished from studies of prognosis. Studies of the prognostic value of a test ask the question, "Can the test be used to predict the future course of disease, in terms of patient outcome?" By contrast, outcomes studies ask questions such as, "Does use of the test improve outcomes?" For example, a study of the former type asks the question, "Does the concentration of a cardiac troponin in serum correlate with the mortality rate after myocardial infarction?" An outcomes study might ask, "Is the mortality rate of patients with suspected myocardial infarction decreased when physicians use troponin testing to guide therapy?" Recent outcomes studies have asked questions such as the following: "Is availability of POCT in the emergency room, compared with testing performed in the hospital laboratory, associated with a decreased length of stay for patients in the emergency department?"[69,82,95,104] and "Does routine testing of elderly patients before cataract surgery decrease postoperative complication rates?"[125]

Design of Clinical Outcomes Studies

The randomized controlled trial (RCT) is the de facto standard for studies of the health effects of medical interventions. In these studies, patients are randomized to receive either a therapy to be tested or an alternative (a placebo or a conventional treatment), and outcomes are measured. RCTs have been used to evaluate therapeutic interventions, including drugs, radiation therapy, and surgical interventions, among others. Measured outcomes vary from hard evidence, such as mortality and morbidity, to softer evidence, such as patient-reported satisfaction and surrogate end points typified by markers of disease activity (e.g., HbA_{1c}, urine albumin: creatinine ratio as mentioned earlier).

The high impact of RCTs of therapeutic interventions has led to scrutiny of their conduct and reporting. An interdisciplinary group (largely clinical epidemiologists and editors of medical journals) developed a guideline known as CONSORT[90] for the conduct of these studies. Although initially designed for trials of therapies, CONSORT provides useful reminders when outcomes studies of tests in laboratory medicine are designed or appraised. Key features of the guideline include a checklist (Figure 4-7) of items to include in the report and a flow diagram (Figure 4-8) of patients in the study, which are similar to those used for STARD.

The optimal design of an RCT of a diagnostic test is not always obvious. A classical design is to randomize patients to receive or not receive a test, and then to modify therapy from conventional therapy to a different therapy based on test results among tested patients. This approach leads to interpretive problems.[8] For example, if the new therapy is always effective, the tested group will always fare better even if the test is a coin toss, because only the tested group had access to the new therapy. The conclusion that the testing was valuable would thus be wrong. A similar problem occurs if the tested group had merely an increased access to the therapy. (A

Checklist of items to include when reporting a randomized trial

PAPER SECTION and topic	Item	Description	Reported on page #
TITLE & ABSTRACT	1	How participants were allocated to interventions (*e.g.*, "random allocation," "randomized," or "randomly assigned").	
INTRODUCTION Background	2	Scientific background and explanation of rationale.	
METHODS Participants	3	Eligibility criteria for participants and the settings and locations where the data were collected.	
Interventions	4	Precise details of the interventions intended for each group and how and when they were actually administered.	
Objectives	5	Specific objectives and hypotheses.	
Outcomes	6	Clearly defined primary and secondary outcome measures and, when applicable, any methods used to enhance the quality of measurements (*e.g.*, multiple observations, training of assessors).	
Sample size	7	How sample size was determined and, when applicable, explanation of any interim analyses and stopping rules.	
Randomization—Sequence generation	8	Method used to generate the random allocation sequence, including details of any restriction (*e.g.*, blocking, stratification).	
Randomization—Allocation concealment	9	Method used to implement the random allocation sequence (*e.g.*, numbered containers or central telephone), clarifying whether the sequence was concealed until interventions were assigned.	
Randomization—Implementation	10	Who generated the allocation sequence, who enrolled participants, and who assigned participants to their groups.	
Blinding (masking)	11	Whether or not participants, those administering the interventions, and those assessing the outcomes were blinded to group assignment. When relevant, how the success of blinding was evaluated.	

Figure 4-7 The Consolidated Standards of Reporting Trials (CONSORT) checklist.

Statistical methods	12	Statistical methods used to compare groups for primary outcome(s); methods for additional analyses, such as subgroup analyses and adjusted analyses.	
RESULTS Participant flow	13	Flow of participants through each stage (a diagram is strongly recommended). Specifically, for each group report the numbers of participants randomly assigned, receiving intended treatment, completing the study protocol, and analyzed for the primary outcome. Describe protocol deviations from study as planned, together with reasons.	
Recruitment	14	Dates defining the periods of recruitment and follow-up.	
Baseline data	15	Baseline demographics and clinical characteristics of each group.	
Numbers analyzed	16	Number of participants (denominator) in each group included in each analysis and whether the analysis was by "intention-to-treat." State the results in absolute numbers when feasible (*e.g.*, 10/20, not 50%).	
Outcomes and estimation	17	For each primary and secondary outcome, a summary of results for each group, and the estimated effect size and its precision (*e.g.*, 95% confidence interval).	
Ancillary analyses	18	Address multiplicity by reporting any other analyses performed, including subgroup analyses and adjusted analyses, indicating those pre-specified and those exploratory.	
Adverse events	19	All important adverse events or side effects in each intervention group.	
DISCUSSION Interpretation	20	Interpretation of the results, taking into account study hypotheses, sources of potential bias or imprecision, and the dangers associated with multiplicity of analyses and outcomes.	
Generalizability	21	Generalizability (external validity) of the trial findings.	
Overall evidence	22	General interpretation of the results in the context of current evidence.	

Figure 4-7, cont'd

possible example is the apparent benefit of fecal occult blood testing in decreasing the incidence of colon cancer when the tested group is more likely to undergo colonoscopy and removal of premalignant lesions in the colon. Even a random selection of patients for colonoscopy might achieve results similar to those obtained for the group tested for fecal occult blood.) This problem will lead to the erroneous conclusion that the test itself is useful. By contrast, if the new therapy is always worse than the conventional treatment, patients in the tested group will do worse and the test will be judged worse than useless, no matter how accurate it is. Similarly, if the two treatments are equally effective, the outcomes will be the same with or without testing; this scenario will lead to the conclusion that the test is not good, no matter how diagnostically accurate it is. When a truly better therapy becomes available, the test may prove to be valuable, so it is important to not discount the test's potential based on a study with a new therapy that offers no advantage over the old therapy.

Bossuyt and colleagues[8] described a study design to determine whether ultrasound testing of the fetus can be used to identify those women with growth-restricted fetuses who can be safely managed at home rather than in the hospital. In a common study design, women with fetuses showing intrauterine growth restriction (IUGR) are randomized to receive Doppler ultrasound. Women with positive test results would be kept in the hospital, and those with negative test results would go home. Women in the control arm would stay in the hospital—the usual approach. One can see here that if some women benefit from home care, whereas all other women do equally well with either of the two treatments, home care patients will do better regardless of the intrinsic value of the ultrasound test. Thus patients in the tested arm will fare

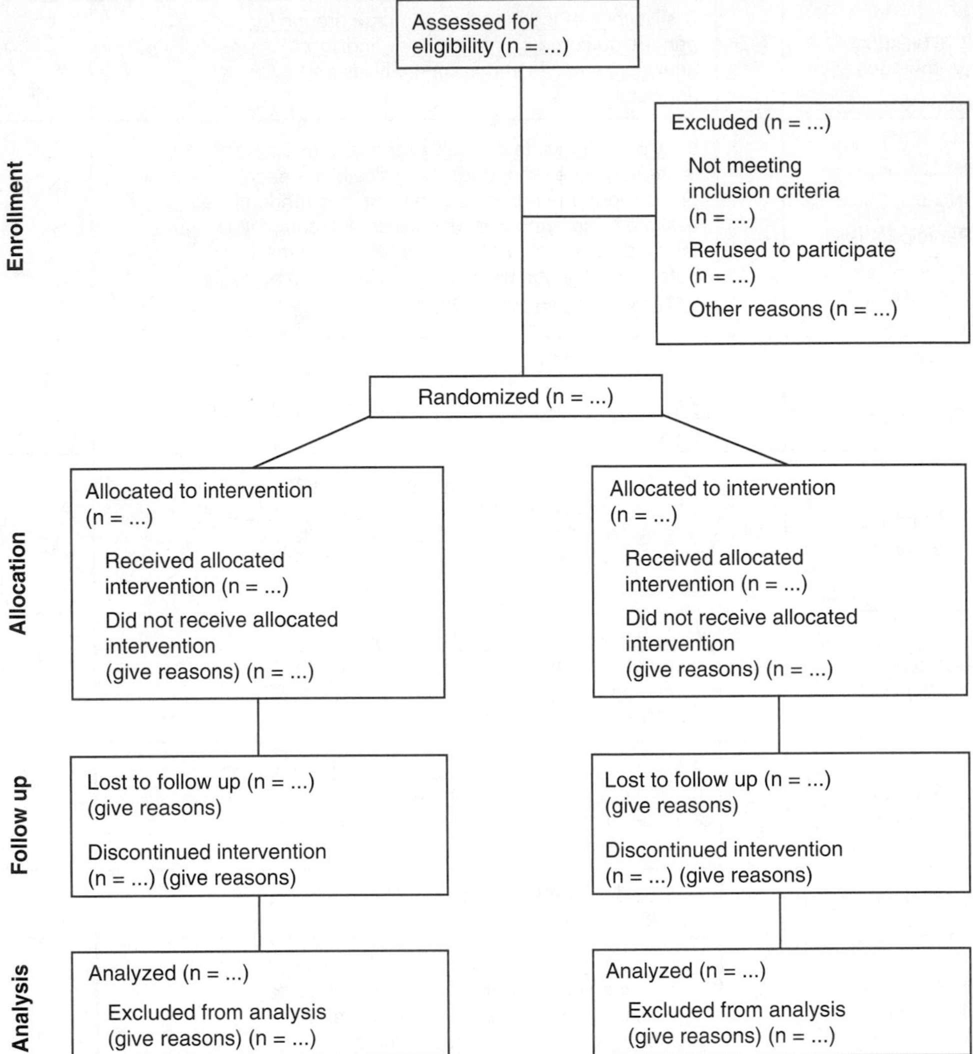

Figure 4-8 The Consolidated Standards of Reporting Trials (CONSORT) flow diagram for patients in a randomized controlled trial (RCT).

better, and the testing itself will erroneously be declared a success. By contrast, a proper interpretation would be that the strategy worked well, and a testable hypothesis might be generated from the study that all patients can be sent home without testing.

Alternative designs have been described to address the question of use of ultrasound in women with IUGR.[8] In one design, all patients undergo the new test, but the results are hidden during the trial. Patients are randomized to receive or not receive the new therapy. In this design, the new test should be adopted only if there is an improvement in patient outcome caused by switching to the new therapy, and if that improvement in outcome is associated with the test outcome. For example, the improvement may be larger in the subgroup that had positive test results on ultrasound compared with the subgroup that had negative test results.

An RCT is not always feasible. Alternatives to the RCT include studies that use historical or contemporaneous control patients in whom the intervention was not undertaken. Other studies include patients with and patients without the outcome of interest. These studies are called case-control studies. Uncertainty about the comparability of the controls and the patients in such designs is a threat to the validity of these studies. One approach that has been proposed for the study of diagnostic tests is the *before-and-after study,* in which patients are cared for using one test or testing strategy for a given period of time (the "before" period), and then the testing strategy is changed (e.g., to the new test) for another (equal) period (the "after" period) and the outcome measures collected and compared between the two periods. A number of concerns have been raised about the validity of this approach, including the size of the patient cohorts required to ensure homogeneity and other effects that may occur during the two periods (e.g., differences between summer and winter). It has been suggested that this approach is valid when an *add-on test* is considered.[77]

Researchers have turned to other methods of exploring the outcomes of testing strategies. To address the multitude of options when several tests are available, decision analysis has been proposed. These studies rely on a model that links data on diagnostic accuracy with data on health outcomes. Patients with true-positive test results receive the benefits of treatment for the target condition, in contrast with patients who have true-negative test results. On the other hand, those with false-positive test results undergo the risk of the side effects associated with treatment, without the benefits. For an example, see Perrier and associates.[106]

Comparative Effectiveness

In 2008, the U.S. Senate introduced legislation under the Comparative Effectiveness Research Act "to improve the quality of healthcare that Americans receive, by creating national priorities for, and conducting and distributing research findings of, the effectiveness of different health care treatments." Although this legislation stalled in committee, it was reintroduced as part of the 2009 American Recovery and Reinvestment Act, which appropriated $1.1 billion to establish the Health Care Comparative Effectiveness Research Institute. This institute will "review evidence and produce new information on how diseases, disorders, and other health conditions can be treated to achieve the best clinical outcome for patients. The Congressional Budget Office has signalled that national healthcare spending could be reduced if physicians and patients had more unbiased data on the effectiveness of the treatments available to them."

On comparative effectiveness, the Institute of Medicine has said that "within the overall umbrella of clinical effectiveness research, the most practical need is for studies of comparative effectiveness, the comparison of one diagnostic or treatment option to one or more others. In this respect, primary comparative effectiveness research involves the direct generation of clinical information on the relative merits or outcomes of one intervention in comparison to one or more others. Secondary comparative effectiveness research involves the synthesis of primary studies (usually multiple) to allow conclusions to be drawn. Secondary comparisons of the relative merits of different diagnostic or treatment interventions can be done through collective analysis of the results of multiple head-to-head studies, or indirectly, in which the treatment options have not been directly compared to each other in a clinical evaluation but reside in larger databases. Conclusions utilize inferential adjustments based on the relative effect of each intervention to a specific comparison, often a placebo."[63]

In a briefing to the Center for Medical Technology Policy, Tunis observed that comparative effectiveness comprised "a set of analytic tools that allow for the comparison of one treatment—drug, device, or procedure—to another treatment on the basis of risks, benefits, and potentially, cost." Tools include systematic reviews of evidence; modeling; retrospective analyses of databases [either electronic health records (EHRs) or administrative data used to process claims]; and prospective, but nonrandomized controlled trials research (e.g., adaptive trials, practical trials). The research setting is real-world healthcare interactions, rather than randomized and controlled trials. Thus it includes key methods associated with the practice of EBLM, as well as other initiatives in the field of EBP, including health technology assessment and outcomes research.[55,146,149]

CRITICAL APPRAISAL AND SYSTEMATIC REVIEWS OF DIAGNOSTIC TESTS

Critical appraisal of data is an important part of determining whether they provide robust information in both primary (experimental) and secondary (literature) research. Information from a number of studies can then be brought together and summarized in systematic reviews, and this can increase the certainty or strength of the information. Systematic reviews are recent additions to the medical literature. In contrast to traditional narrative reviews, these reviews aim to answer a precisely defined clinical question (hence the value of the PICO framework), and to do so in a way that is transparent and is designed to minimize bias. The defining features of systematic reviews include (1) a clear definition of the clinical question to be addressed, (2) an extensive and explicit strategy to find all studies (published or unpublished) that may be eligible for inclusion in the review, (3) criteria by which studies are included and excluded, (4) a mechanism to assess the quality of each study, and, in some cases, (5) synthesis of results with the use of statistical techniques of meta-analysis. By contrast, traditional reviews are subjective, are rarely well focused on a clinical question, lack explicit criteria for selection of studies to be reviewed, do not indicate criteria by which to assess the quality of included studies, and rarely use meta-analysis.

The explicit method of systematic reviews suggests that persons skilled in the art of systematic reviewing should be able to reproduce the data of a systematic review, just as researchers in chemistry or biochemistry expect to be able to reproduce published primary studies in their fields. This concept strengthens the credibility of systematic reviews, and workers in the field of EBM generally consider well-conducted systematic reviews of high-quality primary studies to constitute the highest level of evidence on a medical question.

Why Systematic Reviews?

The explosion of research and the vastness of the medical literature are such that no one can read, much less digest, all relevant work. The massive amount of new technology, the poor quality of narrative reviews,[94] and the necessity to provide an accurate digest for practicing clinicians[42] constitute the background to the call for a more systematic review of literature. Reference has already been made, earlier in this chapter, to the poor quality of reporting of studies, as well as the poor design of studies, and so although critical appraisal skills are essential to reading individual reports of studies, they are also essential to the process of undertaking a systematic review. Systematic reviewing is essentially secondary research and combines the second and third elements of the

A5 EBLM cycle (see Figure 4-3); both will be described in the next section.

Systematic reviews can achieve multiple objectives. They can identify the number, scope, and quality of primary studies by using an extensive search strategy; provide a summary of the diagnostic accuracy of a test; compare the diagnostic accuracies of tests; determine the dependence of reported diagnostic accuracies on quality of study design; identify the dependence of diagnostic accuracy on characteristics of the patients or method for the test; and identify areas that require further research and recognize questions that are well answered and for which further study may not be necessary.

Conducting a Systematic Review

Systematic reviewing is time consuming and requires multiple skills. Usually a team is required, and the team should include persons with searching skills, statistical skills, and experience in performing such a review. A crucial starting point is that the team must agree on the clinical problem (the question) to be tackled and on the scope of the review. This can be achieved with the help of the PICO framework.

It is also helpful at the outset to identify whether a similar review has been undertaken recently. Such a search will help to focus the review and will indicate whether, indeed, the planned review is required, or if the answer to the question has already been found. The Cochrane Collaboration serves as an excellent source of reviews, but unfortunately few are reviews of diagnostic tests (accessed at www.cochrane.org on March 21, 2011).[57] The Cochrane Collaboration has established a working group on Diagnostic Test Accuracy whose mission is to ensure the preparation and publication of quality systematic reviews (accessed at http://srdta.cochrane.org March 22, 2011). The Database of Abstracts of Reviews of Effectiveness (DARE) (accessed at www.york.ac.uk/inst/crd/ on March 21, 2011), which is run by the Centre for Reviews and Dissemination at the University of York in the United Kingdom, contains reviews of some diagnostic tests. Other resources include electronic databases, such as PubMed and Embase, and recent clinical practice guidelines, which are likely to cite systematic reviews that were available at the time of the guideline's development (see section on guidelines later in this chapter). Horvath and colleagues[58] and Price and coworkers[112] list additional resources.

The review team must develop a protocol for the project. A protocol should include the following,[4,58,70,105] in addition to a title, background information, composition of the review group, and a timetable:

- The clinical question(s) to be addressed in the review
- Search strategy
- Inclusion and exclusion criteria for selection of studies
- Method of and checklists for critical appraisal of studies
- Method of data extraction and data extraction forms
- Method of study synthesis and summary measures to be used

Description of all of the details is beyond the scope of this chapter, and only some highlights will be discussed. Review of the references cited here is recommended before embarking on a systematic review. Leeflang and associates have reviewed the method for conducting a systematic review of diagnostic test accuracy; this article illustrated the limitations of some of the approaches that have been taken.[80] A step-by-step guide published in 2009 can be consulted to take the reader through each of the steps of question formulation, searching strategy, and critical appraisal, together with worked examples.[112]

The Clinical Question and Criteria for Selection of Studies

Among the steps in conducting a systematic review of a diagnostic test (Box 4-3), the most important is identification of the clinical question for which the test result is required to give an answer, and thus formulation of the question that forms the basis of the review. The PICO framework is used to formulate the question. A wide range of questions can be addressed in a systematic review in diagnostic medicine, including (1) the diagnostic accuracy of the test, (2) the prognostic accuracy of the test, (3) the clinical value of using the test, and (4) the operational or economic value of using the test. Questions that arise are similar in structure but require different approaches.

Examples of structured questions, with PICO annotation, are given below:

Diagnostic accuracy of a test: In patients coming to the emergency department with shortness of breath (P), can the measurement of B-type natriuretic peptide (BNP) or N-terminal pro-BNP (I) predict (identify the presence of) heart failure (O) as assessed by the cardiac ejection fraction measured by echocardiography (C)? Note in this case that echocardiography is the control or current procedure rather than the reference standard, which is now regarded as the independent opinion of two experienced cardiologists.

Prognostic accuracy of a test: In patients with chronic kidney disease (P), can the measurement of BNP or N-terminal pro-BNP (I) predict the likelihood of death (O)? Note that in this type of study, there is no comparator (or control) term.

BOX 4-3 Key Steps in Conducting a Systematic Review of a Diagnostic Test

Identify the clinical question.
Define the inclusion and exclusion criteria.
Search the literature.
Identify the relevant studies.
Select studies against explicit quality criteria.
Extract data and assess quality.
Analyze and interpret data.
Present and summarize findings.

Clinical value of a test in improving patient outcomes (called a phase 4 evaluation of a test by Sackett and Haynes[120]*):* In patients attending the hospital for treatment of heart failure (P), can the measurement of BNP or N-terminal pro-BNP (I) help as a guide to therapy or improve the ability to treat heart failure as assessed by the rate of subsequent readmission for heart failure (O), compared with the current practice, which does not involve the use of a biochemical test (C)? Note that in this example, the rate of readmission for heart failure is a surrogate measure of the quality of management of the heart failure.

Operational value of a test improving the economic outcome in managing a patient: In patients with shortness of breath (P), can the measurement of BNP or N-terminal pro-BNP using POCT in a primary care setting (I) rule out the presence of heart failure (O) as assessed by the cardiac ejection fraction measured by echocardiography (C)? In this case, the economic benefit would be a reduction in the need to refer for echocardiography every breathless patient with suspicion of heart failure.

Note that each question employs the PICO framework. More complex questions often arise. Thus a question may involve comparing the diagnostic accuracies of two or more tests, or it may address improvement in diagnostic accuracy derived by adding results of a new test to results of an existing test or tests. A complex outcome question may involve the utility of therapeutic drug testing at the time of a clinic visit to reduce clinic visits by helping to establish optimum drug dosages; this is an operational question, but it could also be considered as a clinical question, such as "Has the new protocol reduced the number of adverse events (e.g., rejection episodes) or has it improved patient satisfaction?" Similarly when looking at POCT for a monitoring test (e.g., HbA_{1c}), it is possible to consider the clinical benefits (reduction in HbA_{1c} level, or delay in the onset of complications), as well as the economic benefits (reduction in the number of clinic visits or in the need for hospitalization associated with onset of complications).

The clinical question leads to inclusion and exclusion criteria for studies to be included in the review. These criteria include the patient cohort and the setting in which the test is to be used, as well as the outcome measures to be considered. These are all important, as both the patient setting and the nature of the question affect the diagnostic performance of a test.[108]

When the questions to be addressed are defined, the review group must agree on the scope of the review. Irwig and colleagues[64] summarized two main approaches to defining the scope of a systematic review of studies of diagnostic accuracy:

- Restrict the review to studies of high quality directly applicable to the problem of immediate interest to the reviewer.
- Explore the effects of variability in study quality and other characteristics (e.g., setting, type of population, disease spectrum) on estimates of accuracy, using subgroup analysis or modeling.

The second approach is more complex but allows estimates of such things as the applicability of estimates of diagnostic accuracy to different settings and the effects of study design and inherent patient characteristics (e.g., age, sex, symptoms) on estimates of a test's diagnostic accuracy.

Search Strategy

Searching of the primary literature is usually carried out in three ways: (1) an electronic search of literature databases, (2) hand searching of key journals, and (3) review of the references of key review articles. It is usual to search both Medline and Embase, as the overlap between the two can be as low as 35%.[137] Searching of databases is a detailed exercise, and the help of a librarian or information scientist is recommended. An incorrectly structured search can generate a large number of irrelevant references and can miss crucial references.[76] Guidance that is tailored to searching for studies of diagnostic accuracy in the published literature is available in Irwig and associates.[61] A step-by-step guide through a search is given by Price and coworkers.[112]

Additional studies may be found in the "gray" literature that is not indexed by the major databases. These sources include theses, conference proceedings, technical reports, and monographs. Consultation with individuals active in the field may uncover studies in these sources and studies that are being prepared for publication.

Data Extraction and Critical Appraisal of Studies

Depending on the number of papers identified in the search, an initial review of the abstract may be undertaken to check for relevance, in an attempt to reduce the number of papers that need to be read. Identified papers should be read independently by two persons and data extracted according to a template. A checklist of items to extract from primary studies in preparing a systematic review on test diagnostic accuracy [**Qu**ality **A**ssessment of **D**iagnostic **A**ccuracy in **S**ystematic Reviews (QUADAS)] is available online (http://www.ncbi.nlm.nih.gov/pmc/articles/PMC305345/, accessed on March 23, 2011).[152] The STARD checklist can be used as an additional guide in designing the template.[9] Similarly, a checklist of items to extract from primary studies in preparing a systematic review on test prognostic accuracy is available online from the Critical Appraisal Skills Programme for a cohort study appropriate for evaluating a prognostic study (http://www.sph.nhs.uk/what-we-do/public-health-workforce/resources, accessed on March 23, 2011), adapted from Reference 50, as well as in a step-by-step guide to critical appraisal.[50,112] A checklist for an outcome study has also been adapted for use with a diagnostic test.[112]

The quality of studies must be assessed as part of the systematic review. Rating schemes for the quality of primary studies have been concerned mostly with studies of therapeutic interventions. These schemes have focused on the type of study design, with large RCTs routinely considered to have the highest level of quality and other designs given lower ratings. Glasziou and associates[43] have pointed out, however, that different types of clinical questions (such as questions related to diagnostic approaches) often require different types of study design. Thus, a randomized trial, although ideal for studies of the effects of interventions, is not the most appropriate design for studying whether (their examples) computerized or human reading of cervical smears is better (or to study the natural history of a disease or the cause of a disease). Moreover, a study may use a good design but suffer from serious drawbacks in other dimensions, such as (1) study of a small cohort, (2) the number of patients lost to follow-up, and (3) the characteristics of patients recruited. Thus adequate grading of the quality of studies must go beyond the categorization of study design.[43,80]

Summarizing the Data

Characteristics and data from critically appraised studies should be presented in tables. Data should include sensitivities, specificities, and likelihood ratios wherever possible. These can then be summarized in plots that provide an indication of the variation among studies; Whiting and associates have discussed the graphical presentation of diagnostic information.[153] The summary should also include an assessment of the quality of each study, using an explicit scoring system. A review should present critical analysis of the data highlighted in the review.

Meta-Analysis

It may be possible to undertake a meta-analysis if data are available from a number of similar studies (i.e., asking the same question in the same type of patient and in the same or similar clinical settings). Meta-analyses can explore sources of variability in the results of clinical studies, increase confidence in the data and conclusions, and signal when no additional studies are necessary. However, the conclusions will depend on the papers chosen for analysis; in the case of self-monitoring of blood glucose in patients with type 2 diabetes, a number of systematic reviews have been published in recent years, with the papers chosen for meta-analysis varying between reviews—notwithstanding the fact that later reviews will have included more recent studies.[22,88,89,124,139,145,150] For guidelines on conduct of meta-analyses of RCTs, see the Preferred Reporting Items for Systematic Reviews and Meta-Analyses (PRISMA) statement at www.prisma-statement.org (accessed March 23, 2011).

Although meta-analyses are hampered in diagnostic research by the paucity of high-quality primary studies,[64] the quality of these studies is improving.[84] For descriptions of meta-analytic techniques in diagnostic research, including the summary ROC curve, see papers by Irwig and colleagues[65,66] and Deeks[25] and book chapters by Boyd[12] and Perera and Heneghen.[105] Deeks has argued that likelihood ratios provide the most transparent expression of the utility of a test, because they enable the clinician to calculate the post-test probability if the pretest probability is known (see examples in Chapter 3).[25]

ECONOMIC EVALUATION OF DIAGNOSTIC TESTS

Healthcare costs worldwide have surged in recent decades. For example, in 2009, the United States spent $2.5 trillion dollars, or 17.2% of its gross domestic product, on healthcare (see www.cms.hhs.gov/NationalHealthExpendData, accessed March 23, 2011); this is expected to rise to $4.5 trillion dollars and 19.6% of gross domestic product by 2019. Although direct laboratory costs are small in comparison, evidence from individual studies shows that test results have a profound influence on medical decision making and therefore on the total cost of healthcare.

Who Uses Economic Evaluations of Diagnostic Test?

The perspective from which an economic evaluation is performed affects the design, conduct, and results of the evaluation. For example, the perspective may be that of a patient, a service provider, a payer (government health agency or health insurance company), or society. The perspective may be long term or short term. The perspective is a practical consideration when one is attempting to assess the benefit of a particular test or device as part of a more complex clinical protocol. Perspective is also important in relation to many of the routine decisions made about a diagnostic test. The questions below illustrate the importance of perspective:

- What is the cost of the test result produced on analyzer A compared with analyzer B?
- What is the cost of the test result produced by laboratory A compared with laboratory B?
- What is the cost of the test result produced by POCT compared with the laboratory?
- Will provision of rapid testing for the emergency department reduce the length of patient stay in the department and thus decrease cost for the hospital?
- Will HbA_{1c} testing in a clinic save time for *patients* by providing results at the time of the clinic visit? Will it save money for the patients' *employers* by reducing employees' time away from work for physician appointments? Will it save time for the physician and thus money for the *clinic?* Will it improve care of diabetes (perhaps by facilitating counseling at the time of the clinic visit) for the *patient* as indicated by independent measures of glycemic control? Will it save money for the *health system* by improving glycemic control and thus decreasing hospitalizations? Will it provide benefit for *society* by decreasing society's healthcare costs (for hospitalizations) and enhancing patients' quality of life and contributions to society?

The first scenario is the type of evaluation made in making a deal for new equipment; this is part of a simple procurement exercise. The outcome is the same: the provision of a given test result, to a given standard of accuracy and precision, within a given time; this is part of the procurement specification. The second question might appear to be the same, but it is not, and undoubtedly, it will have to take into account other issues, namely, the logistical issues associated with sample transport or the level of communication support provided by the laboratories; again it is part of a procurement exercise. To make a relevant evaluation concerning the value of POCT, it is important to take into account implications outside of the laboratory that may result from a delay in sending the sample to another laboratory, as well as cost implications outside of the laboratory.

Most economic evaluations of diagnostic tests will have a perspective beyond the bounds of the laboratory if the value of the test is to be appreciated and understood. Unfortunately, many of the early economic data on POCT looked solely at the costs of producing the test result.[81] These studies overlooked the potential value of the key objective of producing the result more quickly, namely, that a decision can be made immediately and a treatment instituted or changed. When a test is proposed to reduce the use of other resources within the hospital (e.g., use of drugs or blood products or other expensive diagnostic technology), the expectation is that the clinical outcome will be unchanged or improved (e.g., the patient is not put at risk by using less blood or less expensive technology). When provision of a test result may have a longer-term impact, as in management of chronic disease, use of intermediate measures of outcome may be especially important.

Quality of Evidence in Economic Evaluations

A hierarchy of evidence regarding clinical tests[40,107] (see Figure 4-4) begins with assessment of the test's technical performance and proceeds through study of the test's diagnostic performance to identification of potential benefits and thus to economic evaluation. The hierarchy has also been expressed as moving up from the efficacy of a test through efficiency to effectiveness of a test.[87] This hierarchy of evidence can also be seen in the context of the data required to make decisions about the implementation of a test.[107] It therefore lies at the heart of the process of policymaking and service management.[93] Economic evaluation provides a means of evaluating the comparative costs of alternative care strategies, as well as health outcomes at the highest level in terms of life-years gained and social benefit.[34,134]

Design of Economic Evaluation Studies

Health economics is concerned with the *costs* and *consequences* of decisions made about the care of patients. It therefore involves identification, measurement, and valuation of both the costs and the consequences. This process is complex and is an inexact science.[96] Approaches to economic evaluation include (1) cost minimization, (2) cost benefit, (3) cost-effectiveness, and (4) cost utility analysis (Table 4-2).

Cost minimization can be considered as the simplest approach and provides the least information; it is an evaluation of the costs of alternative approaches that produce the same outcome. In the area of diagnostic testing, it is applicable only to the costs of alternative suppliers of the same test, device, or instrument. Therefore, it is a technique that is limited to the procurement process, where the specifications of the service are already established and the outcomes clearly defined. It might be considered as providing the "cost per test," an often quoted parameter that is not, however, a true economic evaluation because it does not identify an outcome except the provision of a test result.

Cost-benefit analysis determines whether the cost of the benefit exceeds the cost of the intervention, and therefore whether the intervention is worthwhile. The value of the consequence or benefit is assessed in monetary terms; this can be challenging, because it may require the analyst to equate a year of life to a monetary amount. A number of methods may be used, including the *human capital approach,* which assesses the individual's productivity (in terms of earnings), and the *willingness to pay approach,* which is more of a modeling approach based on determination by questionnaire of what individuals are prepared to pay. Cost-benefit evaluation is not widely used, but it might have some value in comparisons of different testing modalities. An example is the economic evaluation of the use of BNP measurement in the diagnosis of heart failure and the appropriate use of echocardiography, which used decision tree modeling and showed that a test could be justified for ruling-out a diagnosis of heart failure on both clinical and economic grounds.[128]

Cost-effectiveness analysis looks at the most efficient way of spending a fixed budget; the effects are measured in terms of a natural unit. The ultimate natural unit is the life-year, but

TABLE 4-2 Approaches to Economic Evaluation

Type of Evaluation	Test Evaluated	Effect or Outcome	Decision Criteria
Cost-minimization	Alternative tests or delivery options	Identical outcomes	Least expensive alternative
Cost-benefit	Alternative tests or delivery options	Improved effect or outcome	Effect evaluated purely in monetary terms
Cost-effectiveness	Alternative tests or delivery options	Common unit of effect but differential effect	Cost per unit of effect (e.g., dollars per life-years gained)
Cost-utility	Alternative tests or delivery options	Improved effect or outcome	Outcome expressed in terms of survival and quality of life

more practical measures include reduction in the frequency of hypoglycemic episodes and the number of strokes prevented. Surrogate measures with clear relationships to morbidity and mortality have also been used (e.g., change in blood pressure). When an intervention is assessed, the number of cases of disease prevented may be used as a measure of benefit, as in the case of alternative approaches to the management of patients with suspected peptic ulcer.[36] In this study, investigative and treatment strategies were compared for outcome measures of cost per ulcer cured and cost per patient treated. The serologic testing strategy was found to be more effective than endoscopy by both measures.

Cost-utility analysis includes the quality and the quantity of the health outcome, most often looking at the quality of the life-years gained. The cost of the intervention is assessed in monetary terms, but the outcomes are expressed in quality-adjusted life years (QALYs). Approaches that assess quality of life include Quality of Wellbeing,[67] Health Utilities Index,[144] and EuroQol.[73] Cost-utility analysis has seen little use in the study of diagnostic tests, probably because of the complexity of the clinical process involving both diagnostic test and treatment necessary to produce a measurable clinical outcome. However, it has been used to assess the utility of some screening programs.

The inclusion of a quality of life component can affect choices among alternatives. In the Centers for Disease Control and Prevention Diabetes Cost-Effectiveness Study, the lifetime costs and benefits of opportunistic screening for diabetes were compared with those of current practice,[19] with primary outcome measures of life-years saved and QALYs. The incremental cost effectiveness was found to be $35,768 per life year gained and $13,376 per QALY, showing that adjustment for quality of life has a major impact on cost-effectiveness. This suggests that in addition to extension of life through screening, a gain in quality of life increases the attractiveness of the benefits accruing from screening.

The addition of new technology often increases both cost and benefit. A cost-effectiveness study of screening for colorectal cancer (vs. no screening) showed that the least expensive strategy was a single sigmoidoscopy at 55 years of age, with an incremental cost-effectiveness ratio of $1200 per life-year saved.[39] Alternative strategies gave incremental cost-effectiveness ratios of $21,200, $51,200, and $92,900 with the addition of increasingly complex and frequent screening for fecal occult blood.

When tests increase both cost and benefit, decisions about their use will depend on factors such as willingness to pay and other political and individual pressures. An amount of $50,000 per QALY has been used in the United States as a reference point, the amount deriving from a decision by the U.S. Congress to approve dialysis treatment for end-stage renal failure.[78] Although they provide useful comparative data, concerns have arisen about the use of tables of cost per QALY.[29]

The underlying goal of economic evaluation is to compare the costs that will be incurred with an estimate of the gain; for this, there are four possible findings and three possible decisions:

- Testing more costly but providing greater benefit—possibly introduce depending on overall gain
- Testing more costly but providing less benefit—do not introduce test
- Testing less costly but providing greater benefit—introduce test
- Testing less costly but providing less benefit—possibly introduce test depending on the size of the loss in benefit and the magnitude of savings (which may be able to produce a demonstrably greater benefit if spent on a different intervention or test).

These options have been expressed graphically in a two-dimensional plot called the *cost-effectiveness plane,*[6,101] with cost on the horizontal axis and benefit on the perpendicular axis.

In exactly the same way as for studies on diagnostic performance and for outcomes studies, a minimal set of criteria is used to evaluate an economic study of a diagnostic test. A suggested list of criteria includes the following[31]:

- Clear definition of economic question, including perspective of the evaluation [e.g., patient, society, employer, health insurance company, hospital (provider) administrator] and whether it is a long-term versus a short-term perspective
- Description of competing alternatives
- Evidence of effectiveness of the intervention
- Clear identification and quantification of costs and consequences, including incremental analysis
- Appropriate consideration of effects of differential timing of costs and benefits
- Performance of sensitivity analysis, that is, how sensitive are results to changes in assumptions or in input (e.g., cost of drugs, expected benefit in life-years)?
- Inclusion of summary measure of efficiency, ensuring that all issues are addressed

Two reviews of economic evaluations of diagnostic tests have shown poor adherence to the criteria outlined previously, with only about half of evaluated papers meeting the criteria.[30,129]

Choice of Outcome Measures

Tests are not always evaluated in terms of life-years gained. Even for cost-effectiveness and cost-utility studies, surrogate clinical measures and surrogate economic measures may have a place.[26] Use of surrogate measures of clinical outcomes requires the existence of a clear, demonstrated relationship between the measure and morbidity and mortality. Even if such a relationship is demonstrated, however, changes in the surrogate do not reliably lead to changes in the associated patient-important outcome.[17] This limits the strength of inferences from such studies.

Many of the questions listed above address issues within the clinical episode (i.e., the part of the episode of care that directly involves use of the test), but evaluation of the longer-term value or benefit of a diagnostic test is more complex. Long-term costs and benefits, as in management of a chronic condition such as diabetes, may be influenced by other (confounding) factors. Complexity depends on the relationship between test and treatment, and also on the compliance of both patient and clinician in use of the test and the treatment. Thus in the case of diabetes, measurement of blood glucose and HbA_{1c} is an integral part of management. Although short-term studies have been done,[47] rigorous economic evaluations of the long-term use of these tests are rare. Economic modeling of both the Diabetes Control and Complications Trial (DCCT) and the United Kingdom Prospective Diabetes Study (UKPDS) demonstrated the economic benefits of intensive glycemic control[27,46] but did not indicate the value of the testing component. An observational study of the implementation of an intensive glycemic control program demonstrated long-term savings from improved clinical outcomes that reduced clinic visits and hospital admissions and their attendant costs.[148]

Modeling has been used in a number of cases to assess the potential impact of using a test, albeit it has not involved complex pathways. The introduction of screening for *Chlamydia* using a molecular technique was modeled on early experience of the technology in a smaller clinical study.[59,60] Modeling has also been used to determine the potential value of screening for type 2 diabetes using blood glucose testing.[113]

Clinical Outcomes and Economic Evaluation in Decision Making and Changing Practice

The stream of new tests in laboratory medicine requires frequent decisions about whether or not to implement them. Examples of outcomes discussed illustrate that they can be characterized into *clinical* and *economic* outcomes. An alternative approach is to look at these in terms of *clinical* and *process* outcomes,[26] although it can also be helpful to consider economic outcomes in terms of *operational* and *economic/cost* outcomes.[112] Recognition of operational outcomes can be helpful when issues of change in practice and the design of an implementation plan for a new intervention are considered. This can be particularly helpful in the use of POCT.[111] Economic evaluations can help in making these decisions. The finite resources for healthcare require use of an objective means of determining how resources are allocated, and how the efficiency and effectiveness of service delivery can be improved.

Use of economic evaluations faces several challenges. First, the laboratory medicine budget is usually controlled independently of the other costs of healthcare. This is often referred to as *silo budgeting.* In practical terms, the budget for testing is established independently of the budgets for all other services, including budgets for which the contemplated diagnostic test might be able to provide savings. Second, achievement of a favorable outcome (e.g., from a reduction in length of stay or a decrease in admissions to the coronary care unit) is of use from a management standpoint only if the potential savings can be turned into real money (leveraged). Third, the introduction of a new test or testing modality (e.g., POCT) will undoubtedly lead to a change in practice, and so benefits can be achieved only if the change in practice can be implemented. Finally, even if the desired cost savings is achieved, silo budgeting means that the savings are seen in a budget different from that of the laboratory, while the laboratory budget shows only an increased burden of cost. Fortunately, the drawbacks of silo budgeting are being recognized, and a broader view of health economics seems to be developing in some healthcare settings. With the advent of *pay-for-performance,* thought has to be given as to how the incentives can be extended to laboratory medicine.[110]

Regardless of any problems involved in introducing them, economic evaluations can provide an objective measure of what can be achieved and the standard against which the change in practice can be audited after implementation.

CLINICAL PRACTICE GUIDELINES AND CARE PATHWAYS

Patient-centered goals of EBLM cannot be reached by primary studies and systematic reviews alone. The results of these investigations must be turned into action; it has been recognized for many years that translation of research findings into clinical practice takes many years, and furthermore that there is considerable variation in practice once a technology has been disseminated. Increasingly, health systems and professional groups in medicine have turned to the use of clinical practice guidelines as one tool to facilitate implementation of lessons from primary studies and systematic reviews. So, some of the important motivations for development of guidelines have been to decrease variability in practice, to improve the use of best practice, and to make this available to all.

Although most guidelines have been developed primarily for use by clinicians, publication of guidelines on the Internet and descriptions of them in articles in the popular press have led to their use by patients and their families.[16] The development of such guidelines is a challenging new area about which some things are becoming clearer, including the absence of tested guidelines for the development of laboratory-related guidelines. The principles underlying the development of guidelines in laboratory medicine have been described[102]; however, the paucity of outcomes data for laboratory medicine investigations means that the inclusion of laboratory medicine investigations in care pathway guidelines is still limited. This has led to the use of consensus guidelines as an interim measure, while offering the benefit of professional consensus as a means of reducing variability in practice.[135]

What Is a Clinical Guideline?

Clinical practice guidelines have been described as "systematically developed statements to assist practitioner and patient decisions about appropriate healthcare for specific clinical circumstances."[37] This definition appears broad enough to accommodate the laboratory-related guidelines that are appearing in the literature and on the Internet. Guidelines of various sorts have long addressed issues of concern to laboratorians, such as requirements or goals for accuracy, precision, and turnaround time of tests and considerations about the frequency of repeat tests in the monitoring of patients. In contrast to many earlier pronouncements on such issues, the focus of modern clinical practice guidelines, such as recent ones on laboratory testing in diabetes[123] and liver disease,[32,33] is the patient in the "specific clinical circumstances" referred to in the definition of clinical practice guidelines. The new ingredient in development of these guidelines is the tool kit of EBM and clinical epidemiology, which allow the guidelines to grow in a more transparent way from well-conducted studies and systematic reviews.

What Is a Care Pathway?

Care pathways have been described as "defining the expected course of events in the care of a patient, with a particular condition, within a set timescale."[74,93] They follow from the clinical guideline in that they define not only the expected flow or sequence of care, but also the times at which care might be expected to be available, and then the expected outcomes. As is implied in the definition of care pathways, this is intended to lead to a more standardized approach to the care of patients with the same condition, which itself has led to the development of the concept of *managed care*.[68]

The Process of Developing Clinical Guidelines

When guidelines are developed by a professional group (such as specialist physicians or laboratory-based practitioners), the recommendations (e.g., to perform a diagnostic procedure in a given setting) may be suspected of promoting the welfare of the professional group. In contrast, when guidelines are prepared under the auspices of payers for healthcare (e.g., governments, insurance companies), the recommendations may be seen as cost-control measures. In this setting, a key danger is that the absence of evidence of benefit from a medical intervention may be interpreted as evidence of absence of benefit. It is therefore helpful to have a transparent process for the development of guidelines.

Steps in the Development of Guidelines

The development of guidelines is best undertaken with a step-by-step plan. One such scheme is shown in Figure 4-9, only selected issues of which will be discussed here. For a more detailed discussion, see Bruns and Oosterhuis[16] or Oosterhuis and coworkers.[102]

Selection and Refinement of a Topic

The critical importance of this first step is analogous to the importance of the corresponding step in development of a systematic review. The scope must not exceed the capabilities (in time, funding, and expertise) of the group, the topic must not be without evidence (or the guideline will lack credibility), and the area must be one requiring attention (or the guideline will have little value and will attract no attention).

Guidelines can address clinical conditions (such as diabetes and liver disease), symptoms (chest pain), signs (abnormal bleeding), or interventions, whether therapeutic (coronary angioplasty and aspirin) or diagnostic (cardiac markers). The priority for a guideline should be as follows: Is there variation in practice that suggests uncertainty? Is the issue of public health importance, such as the increasing problem of diabetes and obesity? Is there a perceived necessity for cost reduction?

The critical issues to be addressed must be identified and distinguished from those that may be considered peripheral or simply beyond the scope that can reasonably be included. Ideally, this process involves a multidisciplinary group, consisting of clinicians, laboratory experts, patients, and likely users of the guidelines. The scope will be affected by the staff (if any) and by financial support available to the guideline group. The cost is usually underestimated.

Determination of Target Group and Establishment of a Multidisciplinary Guideline Development Team

The intended audience must be identified: Is it nurses, general practice physicians, clinical specialty physicians, laboratory specialists, or patients? The Guideline Development team should include representatives of all key groups involved in management of the target condition. In development of guidelines in laboratory medicine, teams ideally include relevant medical specialists, laboratory experts, methodologists (for expertise in statistics, literature search, critical appraisal, and guideline development), and those who deliver services [such as nurse practitioners and patients (for guidelines on home monitoring of glucose), laboratory technicians, and laboratory managers (for a guideline that addresses turnaround times for cardiac markers)].

Because the composition of the guideline development group affects recommendations, with those who perform procedures more likely to recommend their use,[79] potential conflicts of interest of all members must be noted. The role, if any, of sponsors (commercial or nonprofit) in the guideline development process must be agreed upon and reported. Ideally, staff support is available for arranging meetings and conference calls and assisting with publication and other forms of dissemination (e.g., audioconferences).

A minimum group size of six has been recommended.[131] Making the team larger than 12 to 15 persons can inhibit the airing of each person's views. A recommended tool is the use of subgroups to focus on specific questions, with a steering committee responsible for coordination and production of the final guideline. Other ways of using subgroups can be envisioned.

Identifying and Assessing the Evidence

When available, well-performed systematic reviews form the most important part of the evidence base for guidelines. Systematic reviews are necessary when variation between studies is expected, which sometimes is attributable to effects too small to be measured. When no systematic reviews exist, the group effectively must undertake to produce one. The level of evidence supporting each conclusion in the review will affect the recommendations made in the guidelines.

Translating Evidence Into a Guideline and Grading the Strength of Recommendations

The process of reaching recommendations within an expert group is poorly understood. For clinical practice guidelines,

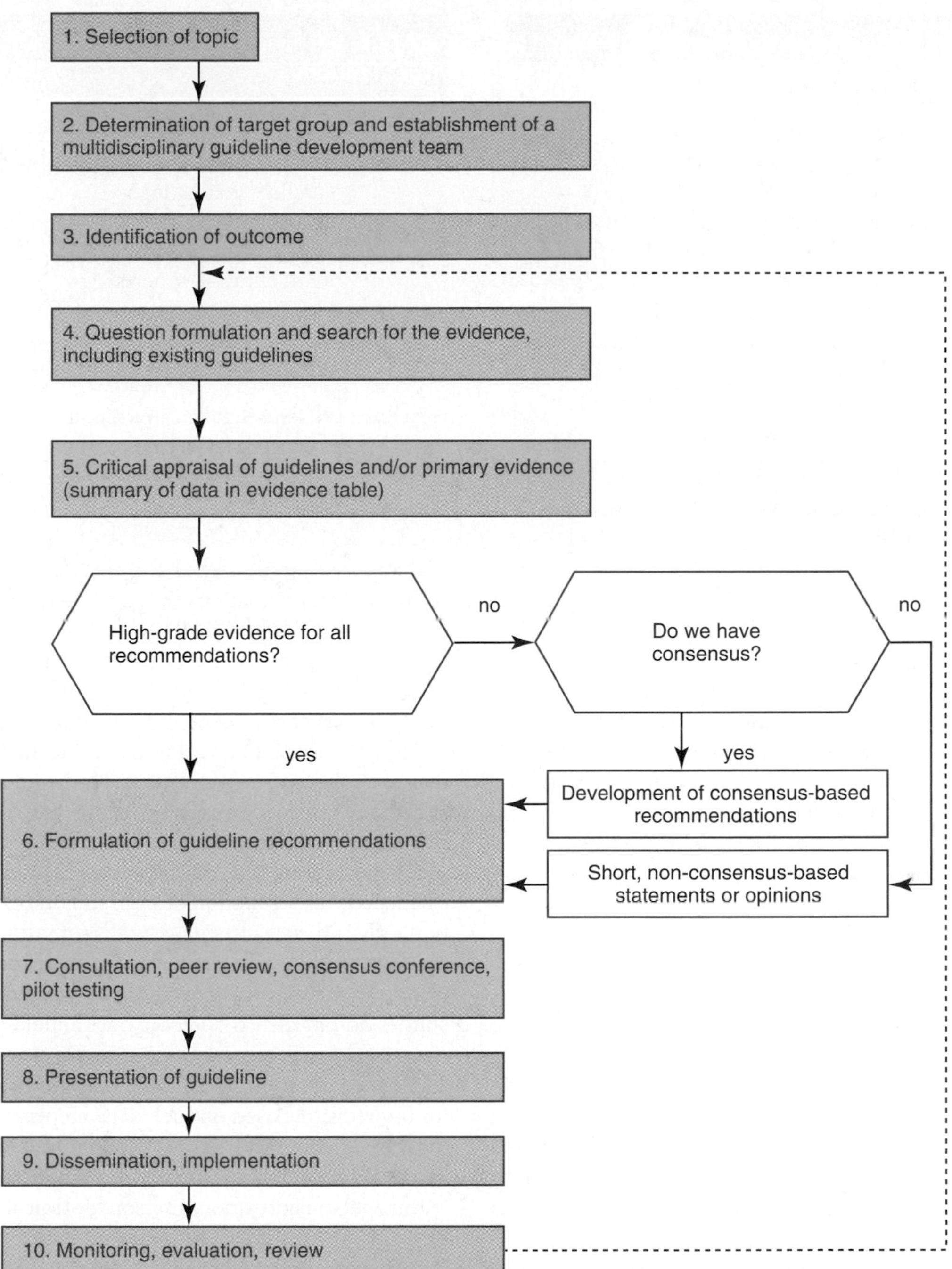

Figure 4-9 Steps in the development of a clinical practice guideline. *(Modified from Oosterhuis WP, Bruns DE, Watine J, Sandberg S, Horvath AR. Evidence-based guidelines in laboratory medicine: principles and methods. Clin Chem 2004;50:806-18.)*

the process may involve balancing of costs and benefits after values are assigned and the strength of evidence is assessed. Conclusive evidence for recommendations is only rarely available. Authors of guidelines thus have an ethical responsibility to make very clear the level of evidence that supports each recommendation.

Various schemes are available for grading the level of evidence, and one of them should be adopted and used explicitly.[16,102] Reservations have been expressed about many of the grading systems, as well as the way in which they are used.[43] In 2000, a group of researchers—the Grading of Recommendations Assessment, Development, and Evaluation (GRADE) Working Group—began to look at the issues surrounding grading the levels of evidence (accessed www.gradeworkinggroup.org/index.htm on February 16, 2009). This group proposed a scheme for grading of evidence that has overcome some of the limitations of other schemes; at its core, it has four levels of evidence, as shown in Table 4-3.[53] The approach developed judges the evidence in relation to the study design, study quality, consistency, and directness for

TABLE 4-3 A System to Rate the Strength of Evidence

Rating	Qualification
High	Further research is very unlikely to change our confidence in the estimate of effect.
Moderate	Further research is likely to have an important impact on our confidence in the estimate of effect and may change the estimate.
Low	Further research is very likely to have an important impact on our confidence in the estimate of effect and is likely to change the estimate.
Very low	Any estimate of effect is very uncertain.

Abstracted from Guyatt GH, Oxman AD, Vist GE, Kunz R, Falck-Ytter Y, Alonso-Coello P, et al; GRADE Working Group. GRADE: an emerging consensus on rating quality of evidence and strength of recommendations. BMJ 2008;336:924-6.

TABLE 4-4 Hierarchy of Criteria for Quality Specifications

Level	Basis
1A	Medical decision making: use of test in specific clinical situations
1B	Medical decision making: use of test in medicine generally
2	Guidelines—"experts"
3	Regulators or organizers of external quality assurance schemes
4	Published data on state of the art

From Fraser CG, Petersen PH. Analytical performance characteristics should be judged against objective quality specifications. Clin Chem 1999;45:321-3.

each outcome identified[2,52,126] and has been demonstrated in a pilot study.[3] A new grading scheme focused on guidelines for diagnostic testing has been developed in conjunction with the 2011 NACB guidelines on diabetes testing that were in press at the time of writing of this chapter.

The level of evidence does not always predict the strength of a recommendation, as recommendations may follow directly from clinical studies or may be extrapolated from study results. The GRADE Working Group identified four factors that could influence the strength of recommendations: (1) the balance between desirable and undesirable effects (e.g., adverse events, adverse impact on mortality and morbidity), (2) the quality of evidence, (3) the values and preferences of stakeholders, and (4) cost. Specifically, in the context of the use of a diagnostic test, the situation may arise wherein the diagnostic accuracy is excellent, but no effective treatment is available. The GRADE Working Group proposed a binary system for grading the strength of recommendations: strong and weak.[54]

The highest level of evidence (A in some systems) is rare in guidelines on the use of diagnostic tests. Recommendations made in the National Academy of Clinical Biochemistry (NACB) guidelines on laboratory testing in diabetes[123] were graded by the scheme of the American Diabetes Association. A vast majority of the recommendations were graded only as level E (expert opinion) by the authors of the guidelines, and only three were graded as level A. The high proportion of recommendations in the NACB document supported only by expert opinion is far from unique or peculiar to that document or to guidelines for diagnostic tests. A similar experience was found with the NACB practice guidelines for POCT.[100]

For analytical goal setting or quality specifications for analytical methods in guidelines, randomized controlled clinical trials (outcomes studies) are rarely available. As discussed by Bruns and Oosterhuis,[16] a different hierarchy of evidence (Table 4-4) may be useful for grading of such laboratory-related recommendations.[38] The highest level of evidence is evidence related to patient outcomes. It is conceivable that even statistical modeling of specific clinical decisions could be considered as a subtype of evidence related to medical needs. For example, Klee and coworkers[75] have shown rates of misclassification of cardiac risk as a function of analytical bias of cholesterol assays, and Roddam and associates[118] have shown the impact of imprecision and inaccuracy of total PSA methods on the numbers of cancers detected and biopsies performed. Similarly, error rates in insulin dosing can be calculated[13] as a function of imprecision (or bias or both) of home glucose measurements, with increasing imprecision (or bias) of the glucose assay leading to increasingly frequent errors in the administered dose of insulin. Although such studies do not directly demonstrate an effect on patient outcomes, they may represent a distinct advance over anecdotes, and an expert group can make reasoned recommendations for imprecision based on such data and mathematical modeling when the clinical action follows a well-defined rule.

Level 1B in Table 4-4 refers primarily to the concepts of within-person and among-person biological variation. Levels of optimum, desirable, and minimum performance for both imprecision and bias have been defined on the basis of these concepts.[38] When a test is to be used for monitoring, use of this type of quality specification for imprecision appears appropriate in guidelines. Failure to use this approach is difficult to justify, because data on within-person and among-person biological variation are available for virtually all commonly used tests.[117] The quality specifications relate directly to the ability to use assays for monitoring and the ability to use common reference intervals within a population. These may be considered patient-centered objectives in a broad sense, if not in a narrow one.

Obtaining External Review and Updating the Guidelines

Three types of external examiners can evaluate the guideline[131]:

- Experts in the clinical content area—to assess completeness of the literature review and the reasonableness of recommendations
- Experts on systematic reviewing and guideline development—to review the process of guideline development
- Potential users of the guidelines

In addition, journals, sponsoring organizations, and other potential endorsers of the guidelines may undertake formal reviews. Each of these reviews can add value. An approach has been proposed for the evaluation of guidelines, referred to as the AGREE instrument [developed by AGREE (Appraisal of Guidelines, Research, and Evaluation for Europe)] at www.agreecollaboration.org (accessed on March 23, 2011). This instrument has been used for review of guidelines in the management of diabetes, with particular reference to laboratory medicine testing.[97] Participants found that guidelines produced by agencies with clear procedures for guideline development were of a higher quality, and that agencies producing guidelines for laboratory practice tended to have more preanalytical and analytical guidance then those that encompassed both analytical and therapeutic interventions. Horvath[56] has pointed out that there is considerable variation in the approaches used to grade the quality of evidence and the strength of recommendations. A key feature of this variation is the quality of evidence considered acceptable, which, in the case of clinicians, the ultimate users of clinical guidelines, is provided by the RCT. Clinicians make decisions based on a range of indicators, including test results, and the utility of tests is often evaluated in isolation; it is not always possible to perform an RCT in which the diagnostic test is the only variable between experimental and control arms of the study. As Horvath points out, the GRADE group has suggested that if robust data from an RCT are not available, then guidance should be based on studies of diagnostic accuracy, with inferences made about the likely impact on patient outcomes.[126] However, Horvath's conclusion is surely right, that is, that there should be international agreement on the whole process of formulating and reporting guidelines, with transparency of process as the key.

As part of the guideline development process, a plan for updating should be developed. The importance of this step is underscored by the finding that one of the most common reasons for nonadherence to guidelines is that the guidelines are outdated.[147] Consistent with this finding, a study of clinical practice guidelines of the Agency for Healthcare Research and Quality showed that about half the guidelines were outdated in 5.8 years [95%-confidence interval (CI): 5.0 to 6.6 years].[132] No more than 90% of conclusions were still valid after 3.6 years (95%-CI: 2.6 to 4.6 years). These findings suggest that the time interval between completion and review of a guideline should be short.

APPLYING EVIDENCE AND CLINICAL AUDIT

Applying the evidence and auditing the process are the final steps in the EBLM A5 cycle; in themselves, these steps are part of a cycle (Figure 4-10). The term *audit* is associated with a particular connotation in healthcare, namely, clinical audit, and refers to the review of case histories of patients against the benchmark of current best practice.[130] The clinical audit was proposed as a tool to improve clinical practice, and a 2002 study indicates that it can do so, although the effects are modest.[143] A more general role for audit, however, is that it can be used as part of the wider management exercise of benchmarking performance with the use of relevant performance indicators against the performance of peers, as well as for the introduction of new tests and the deletion of redundant tests.[112]

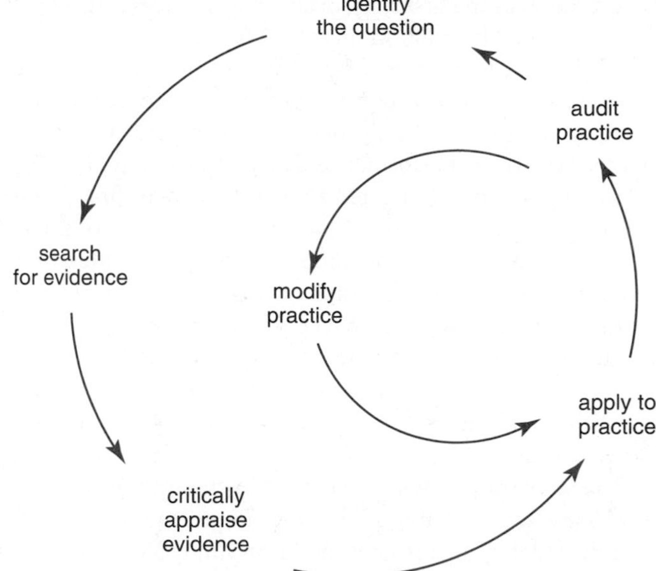

Figure 4-10 The audit cycle. *(From Price CP. Evidence-based laboratory medicine: supporting decision-making. Clin Chem 2000; 46:1041-50.)*

Five distinct activities can be considered under the broad umbrella of an audit: (1) solving problems associated with the process or outcome, (2) monitoring workload in the context of controlling demand, (3) monitoring the introduction of a new test and/or changes in practice, (4) deleting a redundant test, and (5) monitoring compliance with best practices (e.g., with guidelines).

The components of the audit cycle are depicted in Figure 4-10. All audit activities embrace the principles of EBLM, namely, that there is a clinical question for which the test result should provide an answer, and that the answer will lead to a decision made and an action taken, followed by an improved health outcome. Evidence should be available to support the use of the test in the setting for which it is being developed.

Audit to Help Solve Problems

All audits involve the collection of observational data and comparison against a standard or specification. In many cases, a standard does not exist, and maybe not even a specification. In those cases, it is important to establish a specification as the first stage of auditing a process. This specification should be built on the PICO framework (i.e., a properly structured question). Such a specification may then generate observations, which can lead to the creation of a standard. At the outset, it provides the comparative measure against which the performance data collected can be judged.

Solving a problem related to a process may first involve collecting data on aspects of the process that are considered to have an influence on outcome, with the goal of identifying rate-limiting steps. For example, a study of test result turnaround times might collect data on phlebotomy waiting time, quality of patient identification, transport time, sample registration time, quality of sample identification, sample preparation time, analysis time, test result validation time, and result delivery time.

The study of process may extend to the way in which the results are accessed and used. For example, the use of POCT in an emergency department (not in an audit) did not decrease the length of stay, despite the fact that delivery time for the results was much shorter than when results were provided by the laboratory.[69] The authors concluded that the test result generation was not the rate-limiting step.[69] Murray, in a similar study,[95] did find a reduction in the length of stay and identified a subset of patients in whom the POCT results could be used to rule-out diagnoses, allowing a faster discharge. Investigators noted that in other cases, the triage decision was delayed by the need for results from the laboratory. Lee-Lewandrowski and colleagues,[82] when looking at how to reduce turnaround times and length of stay in the emergency department, began their study by identifying which tests might be contributing to triage delays (i.e., they identified the clinical need and formulated the appropriate question before commencing their study).

Monitoring Workload and Demand

The true demand for a test will depend on the number of patients and the spectrum of disease in each case for which the test is appropriate. The appropriateness of the test request is a valuable arbiter in situations in which workload or demand for tests is questioned. A portfolio of evidence helps to define the basis for the appropriate use of tests. When an audit of workload for a test is conducted, it is possible to ask a number of questions, usually by questionnaire, that are directly related to the original generation of evidence upon which use of the test should be based (guidelines). These include the following:

- What clinical question is being asked?
- What decision will be aided by the results of the test?
- What action will be taken following the decision?
- What risks are associated with not receiving the result?
- What are the expected outcomes?
- Is there evidence to support the use of the test in this setting?
- And, for tests ordered urgently, why was this test result required urgently?

This approach is likely to identify unnecessary use of tests, misunderstandings about the use of tests, and instances of use of the wrong test. With the advent of electronic requesting and the electronic patient record, it is possible to build this approach into a routine practice.

After receipt of results from the questionnaire, a number of actions may be taken, depending on the findings of the survey. They are likely to include (1) feedback of results to users; (2) reeducation of users; (3) identification of unmet needs and research to satisfy, for example, a need for advice on alternative tests; (4) creation of an algorithm or guideline on use of the test; and (5) reaudit in 6 months' time to review for changes in practice. Any algorithm may be embedded in the electronic requesting package to provide an automatic bar to inappropriate requesting (e.g., to prevent liver function tests from being requested every day).

Monitoring the Introduction of a New Test

In this situation, the main objectives of the audit are to ensure (1) that the change in practice that is often consequent upon the introduction of a new test has been made, and (2) that the outcomes originally predicted are being delivered. The development of any new test should lead to evidence that identifies the following ways in which the test is going to be used:

- Identification of the clinical question(s), patient cohort, clinical setting, etc.
- Identification of preanalytical and analytical requirements for the test
- Identification of any decision support algorithm into which the test might have to be inserted (e.g., use in conjunction with other tests, signs, or symptoms)
- Identification of the decision(s) that is (are) likely to be made on receipt of the result
- Identification of the action(s) likely to be taken on receipt of the result
- Identification of the likely outcome(s)
- Identification of any risks associated with introduction of a new test
- Evidence (and strength of that evidence) that supports the use of the test and the outcomes to be expected
- Identification of any changes in practice (e.g., deletion of another test from the repertoire, move to POCT, reduction in laboratory workload)

This summary of use with portfolio of evidence forms the basis of the *standard operating procedure* for clinical use of the test, the core of the educational material for users of the service, and the basis for conducting the audit.

Before auditing the introduction of a new test, it is obviously important to have ensured that a full program of education of users has been completed, and that any changes in practice have been accommodated in the clinic and/or ward routines. Thus if a test is moving to the point-of-care, then the necessary training and certification of operators must have been completed.

Deleting a Redundant Test

This may be one of the most challenging aspects of demand management, as it involves a change in practice. However, when an evidence base exists to underpin the use of a new test, the replacement an older test can be of immense value, particularly because it can help to frame the education program that is made available to all users of the laboratory as part of the introduction of the test. This is also where evidence from comparative effectiveness research can be of value. Audit can play an important part at several stages in deleting a redundant test, from demonstrating that the old test does not deliver the required outcomes, through to introduction through a pilot study and auditing of full implementation.

Monitoring Adherence to Best Practice

This is the scenario that probably best reflects the way in which the clinical audit was first envisaged and practiced. Typically, it is based on a review of randomly selected cases from a clinical team with the review undertaken by an independent clinician. This approach is the most likely to identify when a test has not been performed and to identify unnecessary testing. The audit is best performed against some form of benchmark, which may be a local, regional, or national guideline; a guideline appropriately written (see earlier) will have taken into account the best evidence available, and in so doing will take away any bias that may exist between clinical teams.

In recent years, registers have been established to track the performance of health institutions and organizations. Typically, such registers are disease specific and will measure outputs at a high level (e.g., morbidity, mortality).[23,35,41] In some cases (e.g., the U.K. Renal Registry), the data collected are extensive and include laboratory information.[142] This depth of data is extremely helpful to the laboratory specialist because it begins to provide a basis for looking at issues, such as the impact of the analytical performance of certain tests on clinical outcomes.

APPLYING THE PRINCIPLES OF EVIDENCE-BASED LABORATORY MEDICINE IN ROUTINE PRACTICE

It is worth reflecting back on a few of the statements highlighted at the outset of this chapter as they apply to the practice of laboratory medicine:

- EB(L)M is about the explicit use of best evidence in the care of individual patients.
- EB(L)M is about integrating evidence with clinical expertise and patient preferences and values.
- EB(L)M is not about mechanisms, but about outcomes.
- EB(L)M is about improving knowledge on which decisions are made.

The concepts of EBLM provide the logic on which all of the elements of practice are founded. The tools of EBLM provide the means of delivering the highest quality of service in meeting the needs of all stakeholders involved in healthcare—from patient through to policymaker. However, it should be realized that the application of EBP appears more challenging in the specific case of laboratory medicine, especially in the case of the generation of evidence of benefit, compared with, for example, the generation of evidence for pharmaceutical interventions. Yet this may be a myth born solely out of an excessive focus on the basic science of disease and the pursuit of analytical excellence—at the expense of an emphasis on outcomes. In addition, a preponderance of studies on diagnostic tests have employed retrospective sampling; in themselves these investigations are unable to test whether the availability of a diagnostic test result can have any impact on decision making—which has to be one of the key requirements for improving outcomes.

The ways in which the test is used, once its efficacy has been demonstrated, will be embodied in the laboratory handbook, which, increasingly, will be electronic, fully searchable in real time, and built into clinical protocols and care pathways. Such a handbook can then be supported by an information resource, again searchable, which will inform the clinician (and the patient) of the strength of evidence to support use of the test in a specific situation. Use of these resources is practical, as shown by Richardson and Burdette, who observed that information resources could be accessed during patient consultations, with each access completed in 4 to 5 seconds.[116]

Demonstration of improved outcomes provides validation of the test and provides the data on which some form of economic analysis can be undertaken. As indicated earlier, this will show where the benefits are generated and what the costs and savings will be—costs to the laboratory medicine budget and savings elsewhere in the health economy. This information will enable a business case to be produced, supporting a reimbursement strategy, the style of which will depend on the type of healthcare system. The real challenge, however, comes in identifying the changes in practice that undoubtedly will have to be implemented should the test be introduced (e.g., to leverage benefits derived from reduction in length of stay, faster optimization of therapy, earlier discharge, and rule-out decisions in primary care).[112]

The evidence base then underpins the activities that ensure maintenance of a high quality of service: (1) provision of a knowledge resource that summarizes the evidence and its application, (2) use of this resource in education and training of health professionals, and (3) audit to ensure correct implementation and maintenance of good practice.

EBM expects clinicians to use primary studies of diagnostic performance and outcomes to guide decision making. However, as has been observed during the course of this chapter, few such studies are available for diagnostic tests and devices. Furthermore, in the case of many tests, it will be difficult to undertake such studies, in that use of established markers has become embedded in routine practice and consensus guidelines. In these cases, it will be necessary to depend on a more audit style of evaluation to attempt to validate the use of a test.[21] Although this may appear as a limitation, it still embodies many of the principles of EBP in laboratory medicine—crucially, recognition of the question for which the test result is seeking to provide an answer.

Furthermore, the focus on outcomes will certainly help to demonstrate the value of the laboratory medicine service.

REFERENCES

1. Antman EM, Lau J, Kupelnick B, Mosteller F, Chalmers TC. A comparison of results of meta-analyses of randomized control trials and recommendations of clinical experts: treatments for myocardial infarction. JAMA 1992;268:240-8.
2. Atkins D, Best D, Briss PA, Eccles M, Falck-Ytter Y, Flottorp S, et al. Grading quality of evidence and strength of recommendations. BMJ 2004;328:1490.
3. Atkins D, Briss PA, Eccles M, Flottorp S, Guyatt GH, Harbour RT, et al. Systems for grading the quality of evidence and the strength of recommendations II: pilot study of a new system. BMC Health Serv Res 2005;5:25.
4. Battaglia M, Bucher H, Egger M, et al (writing committee). The Bayes Library of Diagnostic Studies and Reviews, 2nd edition. Basel: Division of Clinical Epidemiology and Biostatistics, Institute of Social and Preventive Medicine, University of Berne and Basel Institute for Clinical Epidemiology, University of Basel, Switzerland; 2002:1-60. Available at: www.ispm.unibe.ch (accessed on February 16, 2009).
5. Bissell MG. Laboratory related measures of patient outcomes: an introduction. Washington, DC: AACC Press, 2000.
6. Black WC. The CE plane: a graphic representation of cost-effectiveness. Med Decis Making 1990;10:212-4.
7. Bogardus ST Jr, Concato J, Feinstein AR. Clinical epidemiological quality in molecular genetic research: the need for methodological standards. JAMA 1999;281:1919-26.
8. Bossuyt PM, Lijmer JG, Mol BW. Randomised comparisons of medical tests: sometimes invalid, not always efficient. Lancet 2000;356:1844-7.
9. Bossuyt PM, Reitsma JB, Bruns DE, Gatsonis CA, Glasziou PP, Irwig LM, et al. Towards complete and accurate reporting of studies of diagnostic accuracy: the STARD initiative. Standards for Reporting of Diagnostic Accuracy. Clin Chem 2003;49:1-6.
10. Bossuyt PM, Reitsma JB, Bruns DE, Gatsonis CA, Glasziou PP, Irwig LM, et al. The STARD statement for reporting studies of diagnostic accuracy: explanation and elaboration. Clin Chem 2003;49:7-18.
11. Bossuyt PM. The quality of reporting in diagnostic test research: getting better, still not optimal. Clin Chem 2004;50:458-66.
12. Boyd JC. Statistical analysis and presentation of data. In: Price CP, Christenson RH, eds. Evidence-based laboratory medicine: principles, practice and outcomes, 2nd edition. Washington, DC: AACC Press, 2007:113-40.
13. Boyd JC, Bruns DE. Quality specifications for glucose meters: assessment by simulation modeling of errors in insulin dose. Clin Chem 2001;47:209-14.
14. Boyd JC, Deeks JJ. Analysis and presentation of data. In: Price CP, Christenson RH, eds. Evidence-based laboratory medicine: from principles to outcomes. Washington, DC: AACC Press, 2003:115-36.
15. Bruns DE, Huth EJ, Magid E, Young DS. Toward a checklist for reporting of studies of diagnostic accuracy of medical tests. Clin Chem 2000;46:893-5.
16. Bruns DE, Oosterhuis WP. From evidence to guidelines. In: Price CP, Christenson RH, eds. Evidence-based laboratory medicine: from principles to outcomes. Washington, DC: AACC Press, 2003:187-208.
17. Bucher H, Guyatt G, Cook D, Holbrook A, McAlister F. Surrogate outcomes. In: Guyatt G, Rennie D, eds. The users' guides to the medical literature: a manual for evidence-based clinical practice. JAMA and Archive Journals. Chicago: American Medical Association, 2002:393-413.
18. Cagliero E, Levina E, Nathan D. Immediate feedback of HbA1c levels improves glycemic control in type 1 and insulin-treated type 2 diabetic patients. Diabetes Care 1999;22:1785-9.
19. CDC Diabetes Cost-Effectiveness Study Group, Centers for Disease. The cost-effectiveness of screening for type 2 diabetes. JAMA 1998;280:1757-63.
20. Christenson RH, Duh S-H, Price CP. Identifying the question: the laboratory's role in testing provisional assumptions aimed at improving patient outcomes. In: Price CP, Christenson RH, eds. Evidence-based laboratory medicine: from principles to outcomes. Washington, DC: AACC Press, 2003:21-37.
21. Collinson PO. The role of audit in laboratory medicine. In: Price CP, Christenson RH, eds. Evidence-based laboratory medicine: principles, practice and outcomes, 2nd edition. Washington, DC: AACC Press, 2007:347-73.
22. Coster S, Gulliford MC, Seed PT, Powrie JK, Swaminathan R. Monitoring blood glucose control in diabetes mellitus: a systematic review. Health Technol Assess 2000;4:1-93.
23. Cystic Fibrosis Registry of Australia. Available at: www.cysticfibrosisaustralia.org/dataregistry.shtml (accessed on February 16, 2009).
24. Davis DA, Thomson MA, Oxman AD, Haynes RB. Changing physician performance: a systematic review of the effect of continuing medical education strategies. JAMA 1995;274:700-5.
25. Deeks JJ. Systematic reviews in health care: systematic reviews of evaluations of diagnostic and screening tests. BMJ 2001;323:157-62.
26. Deeks J. Assessing outcome following tests. In: Price CP, Christenson RH, eds. Evidence-based laboratory medicine: principles, practice and outcomes, 2nd edition. Washington, DC: AACC Press, 2007: 95-111.
27. Diabetes Control and Complications Trial Research Group. Lifetime benefits and costs of intensive therapy as practiced in the Diabetes Control and Complications Trial. JAMA 1996;276:1409-15.
28. Donabedian A. An introduction to quality assurance in health care. Oxford: Oxford University Press, 2003.
29. Drummond MF, Torrance GW, Mason J. Cost-effectiveness league tables: more harm than good? Soc Sci Med 1993;37:33-40.
30. Drummond MF, Jefferson TO. Guidelines for authors and peer reviewers of economic submissions to the BMJ. The BMJ Economic Evaluation Working Party. BMJ 1996;313:275-83.
31. Drummond MF, O'Brien BJ, Stoddart GL, Torrance GW. Methods for the valuation of health care programs, 2nd edition. Toronto: Oxford University Press, 1997.
32. Dufour DR, Lott JA, Nolte FS, Gretch DR, Koff RS, Seeff LB. Diagnosis and monitoring of hepatic injury. I. Performance characteristics of laboratory tests. Clin Chem 2000;46:2027-49.
33. Dufour DR, Lott JA, Nolte FS, Gretch DR, Koff RS, Seeff LB. Diagnosis and monitoring of hepatic injury. II. Recommendations for use of laboratory tests in screening, diagnosis, and monitoring. Clin Chem 2000;46:2050-68.
34. Eisenberg JM. Clinical economics: a guide to the economic analysis of clinical practices. JAMA 1989;262:2879-86.
35. European Network of Cancer Registries. Available at: www.encr.com.fr (accessed on February 16, 2009).
36. Fendrick AM, Chernew ME, Hirth RA, Bloom BS. Alternative management strategies for patients with suspected peptic ulcer disease. Ann Intern Med 1995;123:260-8.
37. Field MJ, Lohr KN, eds. Clinical practice guidelines: directions for a new program. Washington, DC: National Academy Press; 1990:38.
38. Fraser CG, Petersen PH. Analytical performance characteristics should be judged against objective quality specifications. Clin Chem 1999;45:321-3.
39. Frazier AL, Colditz GA, Fuchs CS, Kuntz KM. Cost-effectiveness of screening for colorectal cancer in the general population. JAMA 2000;284:1954-61.
40. Fryback DG, Thornbury JR. The efficacy of diagnostic imaging. Med Decis Making 1991;11:88-94.
41. Gaucher Registry. Available at: www.gaucherregistry.com (accessed on February 16, 2009).
42. Glasziou P, Irwig L, Bain C, Colditz G. Systematic reviews in health care: a practical guide. Cambridge, United Kingdom: Cambridge University Press, 2001.
43. Glasziou P, Vandenbroucke JP, Chalmers I. Assessing the quality of research. BMJ 2004;328:39-41.

44. Glasziou P, Del Mar C, Salisbury J. Evidence based practice workbook, 2nd edition. Oxford: Blackwell Publishing, 2007.
45. Glasziou P, Irwig L, Deeks JJ. When should a new test become the current reference standard? Ann Intern Med 2008;149:816-22.
46. Gray A, Raikou R, McGuire A, et al. Cost effectiveness of an intensive blood glucose control policy in patients with type 2 diabetes: economic analysis alongside randomised controlled trail (UKPDS 41). BMJ 2000;320:1373-8.
47. Grieve R, Beech R, Vincent J, Mazurkiewicz J. Near patient testing in diabetes clinics: appraising the costs and outcomes. Health Technol Ass 1999;3:1-74.
48. Guyatt GH. Evidence-based medicine. ACP Journal Club 1991;114: A-16.
49. Guyatt GH, Haynes RB, Jaeschke RZ, Cook DJ, Green L, Naylor CD, et al. Users' guides to the medical literature: XXV. Evidence-based medicine: principles for applying the users' guides to patient care. Evidence-Based Medicine Working Group. JAMA 2000;284:1290-6.
50. Guyatt GH, Meade MO, Jaeschke RZ, et al. Practitioners of evidence based care: not all clinicians need to appraise evidence from scratch but all need some skills. BMJ 2000;320:954-5.
51. Guyatt G, Rennie D, eds. User's guide to the medical literature: a manual for evidence-based clinical practice. JAMA and Archive Journals. Chicago: American Medical Association, 2002:3-12.
52. Guyatt GH, Oxman AD, Kunz R, Vist GE, Falck-Ytter Y, Schünemann HJ; GRADE Working Group. What is "quality of evidence" and why is it important to clinicians? BMJ 2008;336:995-8.
53. Guyatt GH, Oxman AD, Vist GE, Kunz R, Falck-Ytter Y, Alonso-Coello P, et al; GRADE Working Group. GRADE: an emerging consensus on rating quality of evidence and strength of recommendations. BMJ 2008;336:924-6.
54. Guyatt GH, Oxman AD, Kunz R, Falck-Ytter Y, Vist GE, Liberat A, et al; GRADE Working Group. Going from evidence to recommendations. BMJ 2008;336:1049-51.
55. Hanney S, Buxton M, Green C, Coulson D, Raftery J. An assessment of the impact of the NHS Health Technology Assessment Programme. Health Technol Assess 2007;11:iii-iv, ix-xi, 1-180.
56. Horvath AR. Grading quality of evidence and strength of recommendations for diagnostic tests and strategies. Clin Chem 2009;55:853-5.
57. Horvath AR, Pewsner D, Egger M. Systematic reviews in laboratory medicine: potentials, principles and pitfalls. In: Price CP, Christenson RH, eds. Evidence-based laboratory medicine: from principles to outcomes. Washington, DC: AACC Press, 2003:137-58.
58. Horvath AR, Pewsner D. Systematic reviews in laboratory medicine: principles, processes and practical considerations. Clin Chim Acta 2004;342:23-39
59. Howell MR, Quinn TC, Gaydos CA. Screening for *Chlamydia trachomatis* in asymptomatic women attending family planning clinics: a cost effectiveness analysis of three strategies. Ann Intern Med 1998;128:277-84.
60. Hu D, Hook EW 3rd, Goldie SJ. Screening for *Chlamydia trachomatis* in women 15 to 29 years of age: a cost-effectiveness analysis. Ann Intern Med 2004;141:501-13.
61. Institute of Medicine. To err is human: building a safer health system. Washington, DC: National Academy Press, 2000.
62. Institute of Medicine. Bridging the quality chasm: a new health system for the 21st century. Washington, DC: National Academy Press, 2001.
63. Institute of Medicine Roundtable on Evidence Based Medicine. Earning what works best: the nation's needs for evidence on comparative effectiveness in health care, 2007. Available at: www.iom.edu/Object.File/Master/43/390/Comparative%20 Effectiveness%20White%20Paper%20(F).pdf (assessed on February 15, 2009).
64. Irwig L, Glasziou P. Cochrane Methods Group on Systematic Review of Screening and Diagnostic Tests: recommended methods, Updated 6 June 1996. Available at: http://www.cochrane.org/cochrane/sadtdoc1.htm (accessed on March 15, 2003).
65. Irwig L, Macaskill P, Glasziou P, Fahey M. Meta-analytic methods for diagnostic test accuracy. J Clin Epidemiol 1995;48:119-30.
66. Irwig L, Tosteson ANA, Gatsonis C, Lau J, Colditz G, Chalmers TC, et al. Guidelines for meta-analyses evaluating diagnostic tests. Ann Intern Med 1994;120:667-76.
67. Kaplan RM, Anderson JP. A general health policy model: update and applications. Health Serv Res 1988;23:203-35.
68. Kassirer JP. Managed care and the morality of the marketplace. N Engl J Med 1995;333:50-2.
69. Kendall J, Reeves B, Clancy M. Point of care testing: randomised, controlled trial of clinical outcome. BMJ 1998;316:1052-7.
70. Khan KS, ter Riet G, Glanville J, Sowden AJ, Kleijnen J, eds. Undertaking systematic reviews of research on effectiveness: CRD's guidance for those carrying out or commissioning reviews. CRD Report No. 4, 2nd edition. York, United Kingdom: NHS Centre for Reviews and Dissemination, University of York, York Publishing Services Ltd, March 2001.
71. Khunti K, Stone MA, Burden AC, Turner D, Raymond NT, Burden M, et al. Randomised controlled trial of near-patient testing for glycated haemoglobin in people with type 2 diabetes mellitus. Br J Gen Pract 2006;56:511-7.
72. Kilpatrick ES, Holding S. Use of computer terminals on wards to access emergency test results: a retrospective audit. BMJ 2001;322: 1101-3.
73. Kind P. The EuroQol instrument: an index of health-related quality of life. Quality of Life and Pharmacoeconomics in Clinical Trials. Philadelphia: Lippincott-Raven, 1996:191-201.
74. Kitchiner D, Davidson C, Bundred P. Integrated care pathways: effective tools for continuous evaluation of clinical practice. J Eval Clin Pract 1996;2:65-9.
75. Klee GG, Schryver PG, Kisabeth RM. Analytic bias specifications based on the analysis of effects on performance of medical guidelines. Scand J Clin Lab Invest 1999;59:509-12.
76. Klovning A, Sandberg S. Searching the literature. In: Price CP, Christenson RH, eds. Evidence-based laboratory medicine: from principles to outcomes, 2nd edition. Washington, DC: AACC Press, 2007:189-212.
77. Knottnerus JA, Buntinx F, eds. The evidence base of clinical diagnosis, 2nd edition. London, United Kingdom: Wiley-Blackwell BMJ Books, 2008.
78. Laupacis A, Feeny D, Detsky AS, Tugwell PX. How attractive does a new technology have to be to warrant adoption and utilization? Tentative guidelines for using clinical and economic evaluations. CMAJ 1992;146:473-81.
79. Leape LL, Park RE, Kahan JP, Brook RH. Group judgments of appropriateness: the effect of panel composition. Qual Assur Health Care 1992;4:151-9.
80. Leeflang MM, Deeks JJ, Gatsonis C, Bossuyt PM; Cochrane Diagnostic Test Accuracy Working Group. Systematic reviews of diagnostic test accuracy. Ann Intern Med 2008;149:889-97.
81. Lee-Lewandrowski E, Laposata M, Eschenbach K, Camooso C, Nathan DM, Godine JE, et al. Utilization and cost analysis of bedside capillary glucose testing in a large teaching hospital: implications for managing point of care testing. Am J Med 1994;97:222-30.
82. Lee-Lewandrowski E, Corboy D, Lewandrowski K, Sinclair J, McDermot S, Benzer TI. Implementation of a point-of-care satellite laboratory in the emergency department of an academic medical center: impact on test turnaround time and patient emergency department length of stay. Arch Pathol Lab Med 2003;127:456-60.
83. Lijmer JG, Mol BW, Heisterkamp S, Bonsel GJ, Prins MH, van der Meulen JH, et al. Empirical evidence of design-related bias in studies of diagnostic tests. JAMA 1999;282:1061-6.
84. Lumbreras-Lacarra B, Ramos-Rincón JM, Hernández-Aguado I. Methodology in diagnostic laboratory test research in *Clinical Chemistry* and *Clinical Chemistry and Laboratory Medicine*. Clin Chem 2004;50:530-6.

85. Lundberg GD. The need for an outcomes research agenda for clinical laboratory testing. JAMA 1998;280:565-6.
86. Mallett S, Deeks JJ, Halligan S, Hopewell S, Cornelius V, Altman DG. Systematic reviews of diagnostic tests in cancer: review of methods and reporting. BMJ 2006;333:413-9.
87. Marshall DA, O'Brien BJ. Economic evaluation of diagnostic tests. In: Price CP, Christenson RH, eds. Evidence-based laboratory medicine: from principles to outcomes, 2nd edition. Washington, DC: AACC Press, 2003:159-86.
88. McAndrew L, Schneider SH, Burns E, Leventhal H. Does patient blood glucose monitoring improve diabetes control? A systematic review of the literature. The Diabetes Educator 2007;33:991-1011.
89. McGeoch G, Derry S, Moore RA. Self-monitoring of blood glucose in type-2 diabetes: what is the evidence? Diabetes Metab Res Rev 2007;23:423-40.
90. Moher D, Schulz KF, Altman DG, for the CONSORT Group. The CONSORT statement: revised recommendations for improving the quality of reports of parallel group randomized trials 2001. JAMA 2001;285:1987-91. Available at: http://www.consort-statement.org/revisedstatement.htm (accessed on February 16, 2009).
91. Mol BW, Lijmer JG, Evers JL, Bossuyt PM. Characteristics of good diagnostic studies. Semin Reprod Med 2003;21:17-25.
92. Moore RA. Evidence-based clinical biochemistry. Ann Clin Biochem 1997;34:3-7.
93. Muir Gray JA. Evidence-based healthcare: how to make health policy and management decisions, 2nd edition. Edinburgh: Churchill Livingstone, 2001.
94. Mulrow CD. The medical review article: state of the science. Ann Intern Med 1987;106:485-8.
95. Murray RP, Leroux M, Sabga E, Palatnick W, Ludwig L. Effect of point of care testing on length of stay in an adult emergency department. J Emerg Med 1999;17:811-4.
96. Mushlin AI, Ruchlin HS, Callahan MA. Cost effectiveness of diagnostic tests. Lancet 2001;358:1353-5.
97. Nagy E, Watine J, Bunting PS, Onody R, Oosterhuis WP, Rogic D, et al; IFCC Task Force on the Global Campaign for Diabetes Mellitus. Do guidelines for the diagnosis and monitoring of diabetes mellitus fulfill the criteria of evidence-based guideline development? Clin Chem 2008;54:1872-82.
98. National Academy of Engineering and Institute of Medicine. Building a better delivery system: a new engineering/health care partnership. Washington, DC: The National Academies Press, 2005.
99. Ng SM, Krishnaswamy P, Morissey R, Clopton P, Fitzgerald R, Maisel AS. Ninety-minute accelerated critical pathway for chest pain evaluation. Am J Cardiol 2001;88:611-7.
100. Nichols JH, Christenson RH, Clarke W, Gronowski A, Hammett-Stabler CA, Jacobs E, et al. Executive summary: the National Academy of Clinical Biochemistry Laboratory Medicine practice guideline: evidence-based practice for point-of-care testing. Clin Chim Acta 2007;379:14-28; discussion 29-30.
101. O'Brien BJ, Heyland D, Richardson WS, Levine M, Drummond MF. Users' guide to the medical literature. XIII. How to use an article on economic analysis of clinical practice. B. What are the results and will they help me in caring for my patients? Evidence-Based Medicine Working Group. JAMA 1997;277:1802-6.
102. Oosterhuis WP, Bruns DE, Watine J, Sandberg S, Horvath AR. Evidence-based guidelines in laboratory medicine: principles and methods. Clin Chem 2004;50:806-18.
103. Osheroff JA, Forsythe DE, Buchanan BG, Bankowitz RA, Blumenfeld BH, Miller RA. Physicians' information needs: analysis of questions posed during clinical teaching. Ann Intern Med 1991;114:576-81.
104. Parvin CA, Lo SF, Deuser SM, Weaver LG, Lewis LM, Scott MG. Impact of point-of-care testing on patients' length of stay in a large emergency department. Clin Chem 1996;42:711-7.
105. Perera R, Heneghen C. Systematic review and metaanalysis. In: Price CP, Christenson RH, eds. Evidence-based laboratory medicine: principles, practice and outcomes, 2nd edition. Washington, DC: AACC Press, 2007:245-74.
106. Perrier A, Nendaz MR, Sarasin FP, Howarth N, Bounameaux H. Cost-effectiveness analysis of diagnostic strategies for suspected pulmonary embolism including helical computed tomography. Am J Respir Crit Care Med 2003;167:39-44.
107. Price CP. Evidence-based laboratory medicine: supporting decision-making. Clin Chem 2000;46:1041-50.
108. Price CP. Applications of the principles of evidence-based medicine to laboratory medicine. Clin Chim Acta 2003;333:147-54.
109. Price CP, Christenson RH, eds. Evidence-based laboratory medicine: principles, practice and outcomes, 2nd edition. Washington, DC: AACC Press, 2007.
110. Price CP, Christenson RH. Evaluating new diagnostic technologies: perspectives in the UK and US. Clin Chem 2008;54:1421-3.
111. Price CP, St John A. Point-of-care testing for managers and policymakers: from rapid testing to better outcomes. Washington, DC: AACC Press, 2006.
112. Price CP, Lozar Glenn J, Christenson RH. Applying evidence-based laboratory medicine: a step-by-step guide. Washington, DC: AACC Press, 2009.
113. Raikou M, McGuire A. The economics of screening and treatment in type 2 diabetes. Pharmacoeconomics 2003;21:543-64.
114. Reid MC, Lachs MS, Feinstein AR. Use of methodological standards in diagnostic test research: getting better but still not good. JAMA 1995;274:645-51.
115. Richardson WS, Wilson MC, Nishikawa J, Hayward RSA. The well-built clinical question: a key to evidence-based decisions. ACP J Club 1995;123:A12-A13.
116. Richardson WS, Burdette SD. Practice corner: taking evidence in hand. Evidence-based medicine. ACP J Club 2003;8:4-5.
117. Ricos C, Alvarez V, Cava F, Garcia-Lario JV, Hernandez A, Jimenez CV, et al. Desirable specifications for total error, imprecision, and bias, derived from biological variation. Available at: http://www.westgard.com/biodatabase1.htm (accessed on February 16, 2009).
118. Roddam AW, Price CP, Allen NE, Ward AW. Assessing the clinical impact of prostate-specific antigen assay variability and nonequimolarity: a simulation study based on the population of the United Kingdom. Clin Chem 2004;50:1012-6.
119. Sackett DL, Haynes RB, Guyatt GH, Tugwell P. Clinical epidemiology: a basic science for clinical medicine, 2nd edition. Boston: Little, Brown, 1991:3-4.
120. Sackett DL, Haynes RB. The architecture of diagnostic research. BMJ 2002;324:539-41.
121. Sackett DL, Rosenberg WMC, Muir Gray JA, Haynes RB, Richardson WS. Evidence-based medicine: what it is and what it isn't. BMJ 1996;312:71-2.
122. Sackett DL, Straus SE. Finding and applying evidence during clinical rounds: the "evidence cart." JAMA 1998;280:1336-8.
123. Sacks DB, Bruns DE, Goldstein DE, Maclaren NK, McDonald JM, Parrott M. Guidelines and recommendations for laboratory analysis in the diagnosis and management of diabetes mellitus. Clin Chem 2002;48:436-72.
124. Sarol JN, Nicodemus NA, Tan KM, Grava MB. Self-monitoring of blood glucose as part of a multi-component therapy among non-insulin requiring type 2 diabetes patients: a meta-analysis (1966-2004). Curr Med Res Opin 2005;21:173-84.
125. Schein OD, Katz J, Bass EB, Tielsch JM, Lubomski LH, Feldman MA, et al. The value of routine preoperative medical testing before cataract surgery: study of medical testing for cataract surgery. N Engl J Med 2000;342:168-75.
126. Schünemann HJ, Oxman AD, Brozek J, Glasziou P, Jaeschke R, Vist GE, et al; GRADE Working Group. Grading quality of evidence and strength of recommendations for diagnostic tests and strategies. BMJ 2008;336:1106-10.
127. Schuster MA, McGlynn EA, Pham CB, Spar MD, Brook RH. The quality of health care in the United States: a review of articles since 1987. In: Committee on Quality of Health Care in America, eds. Bridging the quality chasm: a new health system for the 21st century. Washington, DC: National Academy Press, 2001:231-49.

128. Scott MA, Price CP, Cowie MR, Buxton MJ. Cost-consequences analysis of natriuretic peptide assays to refute symptomatic heart failure in primary care. Br J Cardiol 2008;15:199-204.
129. Severens JL, van der Wilt GJ. Economic evaluation of diagnostic tests: a review of published studies. Int J Technol Assess Health Care 1999;15:480-96.
130. Shaw CD. Measuring against clinical standards. Clin Chim Acta 2003;333:115-24.
131. Shekelle PG, Woolf SH, Eccles M, Grimshaw J. Clinical guidelines: developing guidelines. BMJ 1999;318:593-6.
132. Shekelle PG, Ortiz E, Rhodes S, Morton SC, Eccles MP, Grimshaw JM, et al. Validity of the Agency for Healthcare Research and Quality clinical practice guidelines: how quickly do guidelines become outdated? JAMA 2001;286:1461-7.
133. Simel DL, Rennie D, Bossuyt PM. The STARD statement for reporting diagnostic accuracy studies: application to the history and physical examination. J Gen Intern Med 2008;23:768-74.
134. Sloan FA. Valuing health care. Cambridge, United Kingdom: Cambridge University Press, 1995:1-273.
135. Smellie WS, Finnigan DI, Wilson D, Freedman D, McNulty CA, Clark G. Methodology for constructing guidance. J Clin Pathol 2005;58:249-53.
136. Smidt N, Rutjes AW, van der Windt DA, Ostelo RW, Bossuyt PM, Reitsma JB, et al. The quality of diagnostic accuracy studies since the STARD statement: has it improved? Neurology 2006;67:792-7.
137. Smith BJ, Darzins PJ, Quinn M, Heller RF. Modern methods of searching the medical literature. Med J Aust 1992;157:603-11.
138. Strauss SE, Richardson WS, Glasziou P, Haynes RB. Evidence-based medicine: how to teach and practice EBM, 3rd edition. Edinburgh: Elsevier Churchill Livingstone, 2005.
139. St John A, Davis WA, Price CP, Davis TM. The value of self-monitoring of blood glucose: a review of recent evidence. J Diabetes Complications 2010;24:129-41.
140. Summerton N. Diagnostic testing: the importance of context. Br J Gen Pract 2007;57:678-9.
141. Summerton N. The medical history as a diagnostic technology. Br J Gen Pract 2008;58:273-6.
142. The Renal Association. Available at: www.renalreg.com (accessed on February 16, 2009).
143. Thompson O'Brien MA, Oxman AD, David DA, Haynes RB, Freemantle N, Harvey EL. Audit and feedback: effects on professional practice and health care outcomes (Cochrane Review). In: The Cochrane Library, issue 4. Oxford: Update Software, 2002.
144. Torrance GW, Furlong W, Feeny D, Boyle M. Multi-attribute preference functions: health utilities index. Pharmacoeconomics 1995;7:503-20.
145. Towfigh A, Romanova M, Weinreb JE, Munjas B, Suttorp MJ, Zhou A, et al. Self-monitoring of blood glucose levels in patients with type 2 diabetes mellitus not taking insulin: a meta-analysis. Am J Manag Care 2008;14:468-75.
146. Tunis SR. Comparative effectiveness: basic terms and concepts. Available at: http://www.allhealth.org/briefingmaterials/Tunis4-27-07-699.pdf (accessed on February 15, 2009).
147. van Wijk MA, van der Lei J, Mosseveld M, Bohnen AM, van Bemmel JH. Compliance of general practitioners with a guideline-based decision support system for ordering blood tests. Clin Chem 2002;48:55-60.
148. Wagner EH, Sandhu N, Newton KM, McCulloch DK, Ramsey SD, Grothaus LC. Effect of improved glycemic control on health care costs and utilization. JAMA 2001;285:182-9.
149. Walley T. Evaluating laboratory diagnostic tests: international collaboration to set standards and methods is urgently needed. BMJ 2008;336:569-70.
150. Welschen LM, Bloemendal E, Nijpels G, Dekker JM, Heine RJ, Stalman WA, et al. Self-monitoring of blood glucose in patients with type 2 diabetes who are not using insulin: a systematic review. Diabetes Care 2005;28:1510-17.
151. Wilczynski NL. Quality of reporting of diagnostic accuracy studies: no change since STARD statement publication—before-and-after study. Radiology 2008;248:817-23.
152. Whiting P, Rutjes AWS, Reitsma JB, Bossuyt PMM, Kleijnen J. The development of QUADAS: a tool for the quality assessment of studies of diagnostic accuracy included in systematic reviews. BMC Med Res Methodol 2003;3:25.
153. Whiting PF, Sterne JA, Westwood ME, Bachmann LM, Harbord R, Egger M, et al. Graphical presentation of diagnostic information. BMC Med Res Methodol 2008;8:20.

CHAPTER 5

Establishment and Use of Reference Values

*Gary L. Horowitz, M.D.**

Medicine is an art and a science in the service of fellow human beings. To improve the health of their patients, physicians (1) collect empirical data, (2) interpret these data using scientific knowledge and professional experience, (3) make decisions concerning diagnoses, (4) recommend preventive measures, and (5) execute therapeutic actions.

THE CONCEPT OF REFERENCE VALUES

Health is necessarily a relative concept.[27] However, to say that health is *relative* implies that the condition of individuals must be related to something.

Interpretation by Comparison

Data collected during the medical interview, clinical examination, and supplementary investigations must be interpreted by *comparison* with reference data. The physician does this when making a diagnosis. If the condition of the patient resembles what is considered typical of a particular disease, the physician may base the diagnosis on this observation (positive diagnosis). This diagnosis is made more likely if observed symptoms and signs do not fit the patterns characterizing a set of alternative diseases (diagnosis by exclusion). Such disease patterns are examples of reference data necessary for the medical interpretation. Also, the different degrees of health have their sets of characteristics that serve as reference sources for judging the health of an individual.

The process of medical interpretation by comparison may be more or less formalized. Some diagnoses are recognized by an intuitive assessment based on clinical experience. Others are based on reasoning using advanced knowledge of normal and pathologic anatomy, physiology, and biochemistry and of other relevant areas of medical science. Sometimes, the evaluation is of a qualitative nature; in other cases, it may be quantitative. The decision making may even be computer assisted, using rules based on the laws of probability and statistical techniques or on formalized medical knowledge (expert systems, artificial intelligence).

The interpretation of medical laboratory data is an example of decision making by comparison. Therefore, *reference values* are needed for all tests performed in the clinical laboratory, not only from healthy individuals but from patients with relevant diseases.

Ideally, an observed value *in an individual* should be related to *relevant* collections of reference values, such as values from healthy persons, from the undifferentiated hospital population, from persons with typical diseases, and from ambulatory individuals, along with previous values from the same subject.[78] A patient's laboratory result simply is not medically useful if appropriate data for comparison are lacking.

Normal Values—An Obsolete Term

Historically, the term *normal values* was frequently used to refer to medical data used for purposes of comparison. However, use of the term often leads to confusion because the word "normal" has several different connotations.[59] For example, three medically important but very different meanings of "normal" are given in the following:

1. *Statistical sense:* Values are often qualified as "normal" if their observed distribution seems to follow closely the theoretical *normal distribution* of statistics—the Gaussian probability distribution. This use of "normal" has sometimes misled people to believe that the distribution of biological data is symmetric and bell shaped, like the Gaussian distribution. But on closer examination, this usually is not correct. To exorcize the "ghost of Gauss," Elveback and colleagues recommend not using the term *normal limits.*[20] For a similar reason, the term *normal distribution* should be avoided and replaced by the term *Gaussian distribution.*
2. *Epidemiologic sense:* Another meaning of "normal" is illustrated by the following statement: It is "normal" to find that the activity of gamma-glutamyltransferase

**The author gratefully acknowledges the original contribution by Helge Eric Solberg, on which major portions of this chapter are based.*

(GGT) in serum is between 7 and 47 IU/L, whereas it is considered "abnormal" to have a serum GGT value outside these limits. Here a more exact statement would read as follows: Approximately 95% of the values obtained, when the activity of GGT in sera collected from individuals considered to be healthy is measured, are included in the interval 7 to 47 IU/L. The obsolete concept of *normal values* in part carried this meaning. Alternative terms for "normal" in this sense are *common, frequent, habitual, usual,* and *typical.*

3. *Clinical sense:* The term "normal" also is often used to indicate that values show the absence of certain diseases or the absence of risks for the development of diseases. In this sense, a *normal value* is considered as a sign of health. Better descriptive terms for such values are *healthy,* nonpathologic, and *harmless.*

Because of confusion resulting from the different meanings of normal, the term *normal values* is obsolete and should not be used.

To prevent the ambiguities inherent in the term *normal values,* the concept of *reference values* was introduced and implemented in the 1980s.[28,78] This was an important event in establishing a scientific basis for clinical interpretation of laboratory data.[84]

Terminology

The International Federation of Clinical Chemistry and Laboratory Medicine (IFCC) recommends the term *reference values* and related terms, such as *reference individual, reference limit, reference interval,* and *observed values.*[42] The definitions given below and the presentation in the following sections of this chapter are in accordance with IFCC recommendations.*

The definition of *reference values* is based on that of the reference individual[42]:

> Reference individual: *An individual selected for comparison using defined criteria.*

As mentioned previously, for the interpretation of values obtained from an individual under clinical investigation, appropriate comparison values are needed. To provide such values, suitable individuals must be selected. The characteristics of the individuals in each group chosen for comparison should be clearly defined. Their age and gender must be specified, along with the conditions for the specimen collection, and whether they should be healthy or have a certain disease. The definition of a reference individual also covers cases in which the individual under clinical investigation is his or her own reference, as discussed in a later section on subject-based reference values.

*A note on the literature: The Expert Panel on Theory of Reference Values of the IFCC has Produced a series of the six recommendations on the establishment and use of reference values.[42] A 1989 review by Solberg and Gräsbeck[78] gives in-depth information on this topic.

A reference value may then be defined as follows[42]:

> Reference value: *A value obtained by observation or measurement of a particular type of quantity on a reference individual.*

If, for example, the activity of GGT is measured in sera collected from a group of reference individuals selected for comparison according to a sufficiently exact set of criteria, the GGT results are considered reference values.

The observed value is defined as follows[42]:

> Observed value: *A value of a particular type of quantity obtained by observation or measurement and produced to make a medical decision. Observed values can be compared with reference values, reference distributions, reference limits, or reference intervals.*

Or, rephrased: an observed value is the laboratory result obtained by analysis of a specimen collected from an individual under clinical investigation. Some call such values "test values," but the word "test" in this term is ambiguous (a laboratory test? a statistical test?), and it should be avoided.

The IFCC also defines other terms related to the concept of reference values: reference population, reference sample group, reference distribution, reference limit, and reference interval.[42] Some of these terms are introduced in later sections of this chapter.

The term *reference range* is sometimes used for the IFCC-recommended term *reference interval.* This use is incorrect, as the statistical term *range* denotes the difference (a single value!) between maximum and minimum values in a distribution.[45]

Clinical Decision Limits

The terms *reference limits* and *clinical decision limits* should not be confused.[63,84] *Reference limits* is descriptive of the reference distribution; they tell us something about the observed variation of values in the selected subset of reference individuals. Comparison of new values with these limits conveys information about similarity to the given reference values. In contrast, *clinical decision limits* provide optimum separation among clinical categories. The latter limits may be based on analysis of reference values from several groups of individuals (healthy persons and patients with relevant diseases) and are used for the purpose of differential diagnosis.[28,63,81] Alternatively, such values are established scientifically on the basis of outcome studies and are used as clinical guidelines for treatment. Examples of current decision limits include the National Cholesterol Education Program guidelines for cholesterol,[21] the American Diabetes Association recommendations for glycated hemoglobin,[60] and the American Academy of Pediatrics guidelines on neonatal bilirubin[5]; each assumes that measurements of the involved analytes are accurate.

In this context, it is critical to point out another difference between reference limits and clinical decision limits. For most analytes, a laboratory should establish (or verify) its own reference limits. This is especially true for new analytes. But for other analytes, in particular those with clinical decision limits, physicians tend to use the national (or international) guidelines. In the 2010 Clinical and Laboratory Standards Institute (CLSI) guidelines,[15] this point is given much-deserved emphasis. Laboratory efforts that once would have been dedicated to establishing or verifying reference intervals should, for these analytes, be redirected toward establishing accuracy. It does little good to establish one's own reference limits if physicians will (and should) use national guidelines. Methods to establish the accuracy of one's method are discussed in Chapters 2 and 8.

Types of Reference Values

In practice it is often necessary or convenient to give a short description associated with the term *reference values,* such as *health-associated reference values* (close to what was understood by the obsolete term *normal values*). Other examples of such qualifying words are *diabetic, hospitalized diabetic,* and *ambulatory diabetic.* These short descriptions prevent the common misunderstanding that reference values are associated only with health.

Subject-Based and Population-Based Reference Values

Subject-based reference values are previous values from the same individual, obtained when he or she was in a known state of health. *Population-based* reference values are those obtained from a group of well-defined reference individuals and are usually the types of values referred to when the term *reference values* is used with no qualifying words. This chapter deals primarily with population-based values. It should be noted, however, that for some tests, intraindividual variation may be small relative to interindividual differences. In such cases (e.g., creatinine,[25] immunoglobulins[80]), population-based reference intervals may actually mask clinically significant intraindividual changes, as noted later in this chapter.

It is also important to note that this chapter focuses on population-based *univariate reference values* and quantities derived from them. For example, if separate reference values for cholesterol and triglycerides in serum are used, two sets of univariate reference values are produced. The term *multivariate reference values* denotes that results of two or more analytes obtained from the same set of reference individuals are treated in combination. Serum cholesterol and triglyceride values may be used, for example, to define a bivariate reference region. This subject is addressed briefly in a later section.

Requirements

Certain conditions apply for a valid comparison between a patient's laboratory results and reference values[19]:

1. All groups of reference individuals should be clearly defined.
2. The patient examined should sufficiently resemble the reference individuals (in all groups selected for comparison) in all respects other than those under investigation.
3. The conditions under which the specimens were obtained and processed for analysis should be known.
4. All quantities compared should be of the same type.
5. All laboratory results should be produced using adequately standardized methods under sufficient analytical quality control (see Chapters 3 and 8).

To these general requirements one may add others that become necessary when more advanced techniques for decision making are applied.[84]

6. Stages in the pathogenesis of diseases that are the objectives for diagnosis should be demarcated. For example, although some overlap occurs, the clinical grades of congestive heart failure (CHF) are distinguished by progressive increases in levels of N-terminal (NT)-proBNP.[65]
7. Clinical diagnostic sensitivity and specificity, prevalence, and clinical costs of misclassification should be known for all laboratory tests used. For example, in some instances, one might want to know whether a given BNP (or NT-proBNP) value is "healthy," in which case one would want to use reference values for age- and gender-matched individuals with no evidence of CHF. In contrast, faced with a patient complaining of shortness of breath in the emergency room, one might want instead to know, not so much whether any degree of CHF is present, but whether the patient's CHF is sufficiently advanced to be the cause of the shortness of breath.[49,54]

SELECTION OF REFERENCE INDIVIDUALS

A set of *selection criteria* determines which individuals should be included in the group of reference individuals.[42,78] Such selection criteria include statements describing the source population and specifications of criteria for health or for the disease of interest.

Often, separate reference values for each sex and for different age groups,[8A] as well as other criteria, are necessary. Our group of reference individuals therefore may have to be divided into more homogeneous subgroups. For this purpose, specific rules for the division, called *stratification* or *partitioning criteria,* are needed.

It is important to distinguish between selection and partitioning criteria. First, selection criteria are applied to obtain a group of reference individuals. Thereafter, this group is divided into subgroups using partitioning criteria. Whether a specific criterion (e.g., gender) is a selection or a partitioning criterion depends on the purpose of the actual project. For example, gender is a selection criterion if reference values only from female subjects are necessary.

Concept of Health in Relation to Reference Values

There is an obvious requirement for health-associated reference values for quantities measured in the clinical laboratory. But the concept of health[27] is problematic; much confusion may arise if the selection criteria for health are not clearly stated for a specific project.

The World Health Organization has defined health as "a state of complete physical, mental and social well-being and not merely the absence of disease or infirmity." This is an attempt to define *absolute health,* but as such, absolute health is never attained.

Thus in the context of reference values, a more modest concept of health is needed. Past experience has taught that health is a *relative concept.* It is possible to be ill in one respect and healthy in another. For example, what is considered healthy in a developing country may be judged to be rather unhealthy in Western Europe and North America.

Furthermore, the diagnosis of health should not be based solely on excluding pathology. This fact, which has been named the *privative concept of health,* may cause difficulties. If no signs of disease are demonstrated, uncertainty remains, because such signs might be detected on closer examination. The "feeling" of health is not a reliable criterion because of its subjectivity. In addition, an individual may try to conceal an illness for various reasons (e.g., to qualify for life insurance).

When reference values are produced, the following questions are asked: (1) Why are these values needed? (2) How are they going to be used? (3) To what extent does the intended purpose of the project determine how health is identified? In short, a *goal-oriented concept of health* is needed.

Gräsbeck suggested the following general definition of health, which summarizes the relative, privative, and goal-oriented aspects discussed previously[27]: *Health is characterized by a minimum of subjective feelings and objective signs of disease, assessed in relation to the social situation of the subject and the purpose of the medical activity, and it is in the absolute sense an unattainable ideal state.*

Strategies for Selection of Reference Individuals

Several methods have been suggested for the selection of reference individuals. Table 5-1 shows a variety of concepts that may be used to describe a sampling scheme. The concepts of each pair are mutually exclusive. For example, the sampling may be direct or indirect. One may, however, combine one concept from several pairs to obtain a more exact description. For example, the selection may be direct, a priori or a posteriori, and nonrandom.

The merits and disadvantages of these strategies are described in the following sections. It is not possible to recommend one sampling scheme that is superior in all respects and applicable to all situations. One must choose the optimal approach for a given project and state clearly what has been done.

Direct or Indirect Sampling?

Direct selection of reference individuals (see Table 5-1) concurs with the concept of reference values as recommended by the IFCC,[42] and it is the basis for the presentation in this chapter. Its only disadvantages are the problems and costs of obtaining a representative group of reference individuals.

These practical problems have led to the search for simpler and less expensive approaches such as the *indirect* method.[6,28] This method is based on the observation that most analysis results produced in the clinical laboratory seem to be "normal." An example of an indirect method is shown in Figure 5-1. As seen, the values of serum sodium

TABLE 5-1 Strategies for Selection of Reference Individuals

Direct	Individuals are selected from a parent population using defined criteria.
Indirect	Individuals are not considered, but certain statistical methods are applied to analytical values in a laboratory database to obtain estimates with specified characteristic.
A priori*	Direct method (see above) in which individuals are selected for specimen collection and analysis if they fulfill defined inclusion criteria.
A posteriori	Direct method using an already existing database containing both analysis results and information on a large number of individuals. Values of individuals fulfilling defined inclusion criteria are selected.
Random	Process of selection giving each item (individual or test result) an equal chance of being chosen.
Nonrandom	Process of selection giving each item an unequal chance of being chosen.

*Note: The terms a priori and a posteriori signify in this context "before" and "after" and refer to when inclusion criteria are applied.

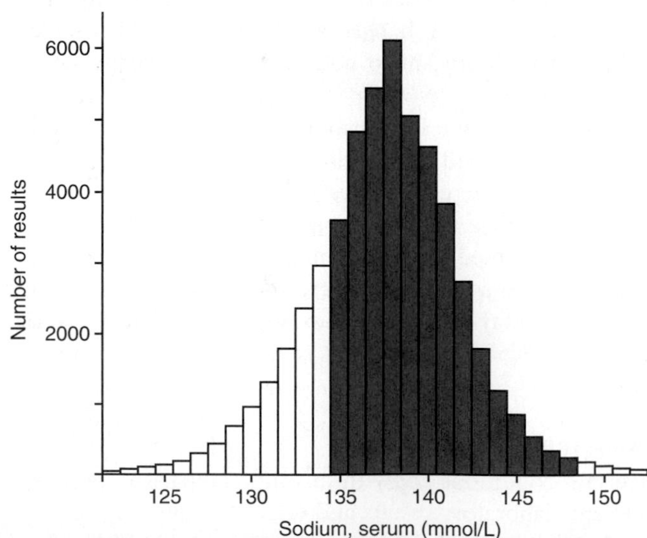

Figure 5-1 Distribution of sodium concentrations in serum obtained in a routine laboratory. The histogram shows the distribution of 53,128 serum sodium concentrations measured in consecutive clinical specimens during a 6-month period in 1982 at Rikshospitalet, Oslo, Norway. The shaded area is within health-associated reference limits (135 to 148 mmol/L), as determined by a direct method (193 healthy adults of both sexes).

concentrations from hospitalized patients have a distribution with a preponderant central peak and a shape similar to a Gaussian distribution. The underlying assumption of the indirect method is that this peak is composed mainly of *normal values.* Advocates of the method therefore claim that it is possible to estimate the *normal interval* if the distribution of *normal values* from this distribution is extracted. However, as shown in Figure 5-1, *normal limits* determined by the indirect method on the basis of this distribution would be seriously biased compared with the health-associated reference limits. Note, for example, the substantial proportion of values below 135 mmol/L—the true, health-associated, lower reference limit. (The term "normal" is used here intentionally to distinguish between the concepts of *normal values* and *reference values.*)

Several mathematical methods have been used to extract the distribution of *normal values* from routine laboratory data.[6,28]

The indirect method, however, has at least two major deficiencies:

1. Estimates of the lower and upper *normal limits* depend heavily on the particular mathematical method used and on its underlying assumptions.
2. The indirect method destroys the scientific basis for obtaining and comparing reference values. The results for each hospital would depend on the characteristics of the hospital's patient group at that particular time. These results would vary not only across hospitals but for the same hospital at different times. The outcome would be a compilation of unstable values for each analyte.

Hospital databases may, however, be used for the establishment of reference values that are fully concordant with IFCC recommendations.[46,76] The requirement is that laboratory data should be *combined with information stored in clinical databases* (i.e., to apply a direct sampling strategy instead of the distribution-based indirect method). Laboratory results are to be used as reference values only if stated clinical criteria are fulfilled. One may define criteria for selecting individuals who have a specified state of health or the disease for which reference data are necessary. Usually certain constraints are imposed on the use of their laboratory results, such as allowing only one result of each analyte under study from each selected individual. Such reference values have a potential advantage over those based on direct sampling from other types of populations: hospital-based reference values are ideal for interpretation of results from hospitalized patients because they are produced under similar conditions.

A Priori or A Posteriori Sampling?

When carefully performed, both a priori and a posteriori sampling (see Table 5-1) may result in reliable reference values. The choice is often a question of practicality. Both require the same set of successive steps, but the order of some of these operations differs depending on the mode of selection: a priori or a posteriori.[28]

The first step in the process of producing reference values for a laboratory test should always be the collection of quantitative information about sources of biological variation for the analyte studied. A search through relevant literature may yield the required information (see Chapter 6).[71,85] If relevant information cannot be found in the literature, pilot studies may be necessary before the selection of reference individuals is planned in detail.

Serum sodium is an example of a biological analyte that is affected by only a few sources of biological variation. However, the list of factors may be rather long for other analytes, such as serum enzymes, proteins, and hormones.

It is important to distinguish between controllable and noncontrollable sources of biological variation. Some factors may be controlled by standardization of the procedure for preparation of reference individuals and specimen collection (see a later section of this chapter). Other factors, such as age and gender, may be relevant partitioning criteria. Remaining sources of variation should be considered when criteria for the selection of reference individuals are defined.

The a priori strategy is best suited for smaller studies. Possible reference individuals from the parent population are interviewed and examined clinically and by selected laboratory methods to decide whether they fulfill the defined inclusion criteria. If the decision is positive, specimens for analysis are collected by a standardized procedure (including the necessary preparation of individuals before the collection).

The a posteriori method is based on the availability of a large collection of data on medically examined individuals and measured quantities. Studies thoroughly planned by centers for health screening or preventive medicine may provide such data. It is important that data be collected by a strictly standardized and comprehensive protocol concerning (1) sampling from the parent population, (2) registration of demographic and clinical data on participating individuals, (3) preparation for and execution of specimen collection, and (4) handling and analysis of the specimens. If these requirements are met, values may be selected after application of the defined inclusion criteria to individuals found in the database. The selection of individuals from large hospital databases (see earlier discussion) is another example of the application of an a posteriori method. In this case, however, the quality of data may be lower than in well-planned population studies.

A study performed in Kristianstad, Sweden,[8] highlights a practical problem often met when reference individuals are selected: the number of subjects fulfilling the inclusion criteria may be too small. In this study, only 17% of participants were accepted into the study, according to the criteria used, leaving an insufficient reference sample group. The frequency of exclusion was higher among women and in older age groups.

This problem has two possible solutions:

1. The exclusion criteria may be relaxed. As already discussed, the set of relevant sources of biological variation differs among different analytes. One may define a minimum set of exclusion criteria for a given laboratory test. In the Kristianstad study, the complete group of individuals could probably be used for establishment of

reference values for serum sodium, and most of the individuals would be acceptable for the determination of reference values for several other analytes.[8]

2. Another design of the sampling procedure could reduce the practical problems and costs of obtaining a sufficiently large group of reference individuals. The Kristianstad study showed that 75% of excluded subjects could have been identified using only a simple questionnaire.[8] In the upper age group, this percentage was even higher. Therefore, preliminary screening of a large number of individuals from the parent population, using a carefully designed autoanamnestic questionnaire (i.e., of or related to the current or previous medical history of a patient), would result in a much smaller sample of individuals for examination clinically and by laboratory methods. If 3000 individuals had been prescreened in Kristianstad, and if only the individuals remaining in the reduced sample were subjected to a closer examination, a group of 240 reference individuals would have been obtained.

The two modifications of the protocol may also be combined.

Random or Nonrandom Sampling?

Ideally, the group of reference individuals should be a random sample of all individuals fulfilling the inclusion criteria defined in the parent population. Statistical estimation of distribution parameters (and their confidence intervals) and statistical hypothesis testing require this assumption.

For several reasons, most collections of reference values are, in fact, obtained by a nonrandom process.[33] This means that all possible reference individuals in the entire population under study do not have an equal chance of being chosen for inclusion in the usually much smaller sample of individuals studied. A strictly random sampling scheme in most cases is impossible for practical reasons. It would imply the examination of and application of inclusion criteria to the entire population (thousands or millions of persons), and then the random selection of a subset of individuals from among those accepted.

It is important to realize that a random sample is not obtained, in the strict sense, if individuals are randomly selected from the entire population, and then inclusion criteria are applied to sort out the subset of individuals fulfilling these criteria, even though this may be the best approximation to be obtained. Usually the situation is less satisfactory. A sample of reference individuals obtained by selecting among (1) blood donors, (2) persons working in a factory, or (3) hospital staff, or by (4) selection from hospital databases definitely is not the result of random sampling of possible reference individuals in the general population.

The conclusions are obvious: (1) the best reference sample obtainable must be used with all practical considerations taken into account, and (2) the data should be used and interpreted with due caution, with awareness of the possible bias introduced by the nonrandomness of the sample selection process.

Selection Criteria and Evaluation of Subjects

The selection of reference individuals consists essentially of applying defined criteria to a group of examined candidate persons.[42] The required characteristics of the reference values determine which criteria should be used in the selection process. Box 5-1 lists some important criteria to consider when production of health-associated reference values is the aim.

In practice, consideration of which *diseases* and *risk factors* to exclude is difficult (see the discussion on the concept of health earlier in this chapter). The answer lies in part in the intended purpose of establishing reference values; the project must be goal oriented.

For example, even the definition of *obesity* is problematic. It might be based on a known or assumed contribution to the risk for development of a specified disease. However, scientific data of this type are seldom available for the studied population. Another possibility for establishing obesity is to use upper limits based on weight measurements in different age, gender, and height groups of the general population, using, for example, the national age-, gender-, and height-specific mean weight + 20% as the upper limit. However, national differences are great. Tables of optimum or ideal weights have been published by life insurance companies; they may be more appropriate for delineation of obesity than this formula.

Similar problems affect the definition of *hypertension* in relation to the establishment of health-associated reference values and exclusion criteria based on *laboratory examinations*. It has been argued that a circular process might happen when laboratory tests are used to assess the health of subjects

BOX 5-1 Examples of Exclusion Criteria for Health-Associated Reference Values*

Diseases
Risk Factors
Obesity
Hypertension
Risks from occupation or environment
Genetically determined risks

Intake of Pharmacologically Active Agents[46,86]
Drug treatment for disease or suffering
Oral contraceptives
Drug abuse
Alcohol
Tobacco

Specific Physiologic States
Pregnancy
Stress
Excessive exercise

*The box lists only some major classes of criteria. It should be supplemented with other relevant criteria based on known sources of biological variation (see Chapter 6).[71,85]

who are subsequently used as healthy control subjects for laboratory tests. But actually there is no difference, in this context, between measuring height, weight, and blood pressure and performing selected laboratory tests, provided that these laboratory tests are neither those for which reference values are produced nor tests that are significantly correlated with them.[27]

It is particularly difficult to define selection criteria when establishing reference values for a geriatric population.[22] In higher age groups, it is "normal" to have minor or major diseases and to take drugs. One solution is to collect values at one time and to use the values of survivors after a defined number of years.[27,61]

Usually the clinical evaluation of candidate individuals is based on (1) an anamnestic interview or questionnaire (i.e., the complete history recalled and recounted by a patient), (2) a physical examination, and (3) supplementary investigations. Anamnestic and examination forms tailored to the requirements of the actual project facilitate the evaluation and document the decisions made.

Partitioning of the Reference Group

It may also be necessary to define *partitioning criteria* for the subclassification of the set of selected reference individuals into more homogeneous groups (Box 5-2).[42] (The question of determining when stratification of the reference sample group is necessary and justified is discussed in later sections.) In practice, the number of partitioning criteria should usually be kept as small as possible to ensure sufficient sample sizes to derive valid estimates.

Age and *gender* are the most frequently used criteria for subgrouping, because several analytes vary notably among different age and gender groups (see Chapter 6).[22,71,85] Age may be categorized by equal intervals (e.g., by decades) or by intervals that are narrower in the periods of life where greater variation is observed. In some cases, it is more convenient to use qualitative age groups, such as (1) postnatal, (2) infancy, (3) childhood, (4) prepubertal, (5) pubertal, (6) adult, (7) premenopausal, (8) menopausal, and (9) geriatric. Height and weight also have been used as criteria for categorizing children.

Additional factors are discussed in Chapter 6.[71,85]

BOX 5-2 Examples of Partitioning Criteria for Possible Subgrouping of the Reference Group

- Age (not necessarily categorized by equal intervals)
- Gender
- Genetic factors
  - Ethnic origin
  - Blood groups (ABO)
  - Histocompatibility antigens (HLA)
  - Genes
- Physiologic factors
  - Stage in menstrual cycle
  - Stage in pregnancy
  - Physical condition
- Other factors
  - Socioeconomic
  - Environmental
  - Chronobiological

HLA, Human leukocyte antigen.

SPECIMEN COLLECTION

Several preanalytical factors influence the values of biological quantities, such as the concentrations of components in blood and in other specimens and the amount excreted in feces, urine, or sweat. This topic is covered elsewhere (see Chapter 6).* In this discussion, only aspects of special relevance to the generation of reliable reference values are highlighted.[4,42]

Preanalytical standardization of the (1) preparation of individuals before specimen collection, (2) procedure of specimen collection itself, and (3) handling of the specimen before analysis may eliminate or minimize bias or variation from these factors. This reduces biological "noise" that might otherwise conceal important biological "signals" of disease, risk, or treatment effect.

Preanalytical Standardization

Preanalytical procedures used before routine analysis of patient specimens and when reference values are established should be as similar as possible. In general, it is much easier to standardize routines for studies of reference values than those used in the daily clinical setting, especially when specimens are collected in emergency or other unplanned situations. Thus two approaches have been suggested:

1. Only such factors that may be relatively easily controlled in the clinical setting should be part of the standardization when reference values are produced.
2. The rules for preanalytical standardization when reference values are produced (Table 5-2) should also be used for the clinical situation. For example, it has been shown that it is possible to apply these rules rather closely in the clinical setting for both hospitalized and ambulatory patients.[78] The same philosophy forms the basis for recommendations concerning routine blood specimen collection.†

However, either philosophy is concordant with the concept of reference values, provided that the conditions under which reference values are produced are clearly stated.

Analyte-Specific Considerations

The magnitudes of preanalytical sources of variation clearly are not equal for different analytes (see Chapter 6).‡ In fact, some believe that only those factors that cause unwanted variation in the biological quantities for which reference values are being generated should be considered. For example,

*References 23, 28, 29, 71, 78, 85, and 92.
†References 3, 4, 13, 14, 42, 50, and 57.
‡References 23, 28, 29, 71, 78, 85, and 92.

TABLE 5-2 Standardization of Preanalytical Factors in the Establishment of Reference Values for Adult Individuals

The Day Before Specimen Collection	
Food	Ordinary intake; last meal before 2200 hours
Alcohol	Maximum of one small bottle of beer (or equivalent of other beverage) taken with a meal
Abstinence	No solid food or tobacco and maximum of one glass of water after 2200 hours
Subjects Lying in Bed; Collection in the Morning	
Rest	Bed rest from 2200 hours until collection; a short visit to the toilet allowed, but minimum of 1 hour before collection
Collection	Between 0700 and 0900 hours (record time); supine position with the arm approximately in the horizontal plane
Ambulatory Subjects; Collection in the Morning	
Rise	1 to 3 hours before collection (record time)
Transport	Public or car transport for maximum of 45 minutes; walking a maximum of 500 meters (<550 yd) at moderate speed
Rest	Sitting for at least 15 minutes; arm muscle work not allowed
Collection	Between 0800 and 1000 hours (record time); sitting position with the arm approximately 45° below the horizontal position
Ambulatory Subjects; Collection in the Afternoon	
Breakfast	A light meal in the morning (approximately 310 kcal, 1300 kJ) composed of milk, coffee, or tea (maximum two cups); two open sandwiches with butter, slices of lunch meat/cheese, or marmalade
Activity	No exercise or heavy work
Rest	Sitting at least 15 minutes; arm muscle work not allowed
Collection	Between 1300 and 1500 hours (record time); minimum of 4 hours after breakfast; otherwise as above
Collection and Handling of Specimen*	
Venipuncture	In the cubital fold; no tourniquet; finger pressure proximal to the site allowed
Difficulties	A new attempt on opposite arm after 15 minutes' rest

*Consult Chapter 7 for a discussion of other requirements for the collection and handling of specimens.
Based on Scandinavian recommendations.[4,28]

body posture during specimen collection is highly relevant for the establishment of reference values for nondiffusible analytes, such as albumin in serum, but irrelevant for establishment of serum sodium values.[23]

Alternatively, several constituents are analyzed routinely in the same clinical specimen. Therefore, it would be impractical to devise special systems for every single type of quantity.[78] Consequently, three standardized procedures for blood specimen collection by venipuncture have been recommended[4,28]: (1) collection in the morning from hospitalized patients, (2) collection in the morning from ambulatory patients, and (3) collection in the afternoon from ambulatory patients. Table 5-2 summarizes these procedures. However, such schemes have to be modified depending on local conditions and necessities and on the intended use of the reference values produced. Published checklists[42,78] may be helpful in the design of a scheme.

A special problem is caused by drugs taken by individuals before specimen collection,[44,86,93] and it may be necessary to distinguish between indispensable and dispensable medications. If possible, dispensable medication should always be avoided for at least 48 hours. The use of indispensable drugs, such as contraceptive pills or essential medication, may be a criterion for exclusion or partitioning.

In emergency or other unplanned clinical situations, even a partial application of the standardized procedure for collection has been shown to be of great value.[28]

The Necessity for Additional Information

The clinical situation often is different from a controlled research situation; specimens have to be taken (1) during operations, (2) in emergency situations, and (3) when patients are unwilling or unable to follow instructions. Therefore the clinician needs additional information for interpretation of a patient's values in relation to reference values obtained under fairly standardized conditions.

An *empirical approach*[78] is to produce other sets of reference values, such as postprandial values, postexercise values, or postpartum values.[28] Such a method, however, is very expensive and does not cover all situations that could possibly arise.

Another, more general solution to the problem is called the *predictive approach*.[78] Starting from a set of ordinary reference values and using quantitative information on the effects of various factors, such as (1) intake of food, alcohol, and drugs; (2) exercise; (3) stress; or (4) posture, expected reference values that fit the actual clinical setting (see Chapter 6) could be estimated.[71,85]

More studies of such effects are needed, especially for the combined effect of two or more sources of variation. For example, is the combined effect of alcohol and contraceptive drugs on GGT activity in serum less than, equal to, or greater than the sum of their individual effects?

ANALYTICAL PROCEDURES AND QUALITY CONTROL

Essential components of the required definition of a set of reference values are specifications concerning (1) the analysis method (including information on equipment, reagents, calibrators, type of raw data, and calculation method), (2) quality control (see Chapter 8), and (3) reliability criteria (see Chapter 2).[28,42]

Specifications should be so carefully described that another investigator will be able to reproduce the study, and the user of reference values will then be able to evaluate their comparability with values obtained by methods used for producing the patient's values in a routine laboratory. To ensure comparability between reference values and observed values, the same analytical method should be used.

It is often claimed that analytical quality should be better when reference values rather than routine values are produced. This may be true for accuracy; all measures should be taken to eliminate bias. The question of imprecision is more difficult because it depends in part on the intended use of the reference values. Increases in analytical random variation result in widening of the reference interval.[28] For some special uses of reference values, the narrower reference interval obtained by a more precise analytical method may be appropriate. However, this usually is not true for routine clinical use of reference values. Interpretation is simplest if a patient's values and reference values are comparable with regard to analytical imprecision. For the same reason, it is advisable to analyze specimens from reference individuals in several runs to include between-run components of variation. A safe way to obtain comparability is to include these specimens in routine runs together with real patient specimens.

STATISTICAL TREATMENT OF REFERENCE VALUES

This section deals with two main topics: the partitioning of reference values into more homogeneous classes, and the determination of reference limits and intervals.[42A] The subject matter is presented in the order in which data often are treated. Figure 5-2 gives an outline and refers to corresponding sections in the text. Before the presentation of methods, some statistical concepts used are briefly discussed (see also Chapter 2). A textbook by Harris and Boyd gives an excellent survey of the statistical bases of reference values in laboratory medicine.[34]

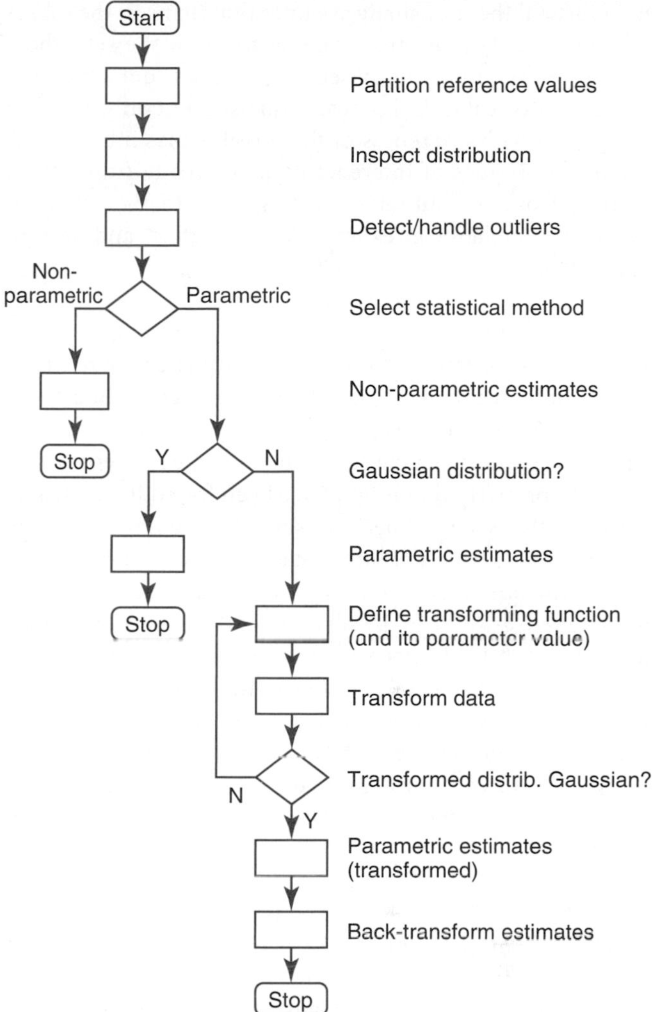

Figure 5-2 The statistical treatment of reference values. The boxes in the flow chart refer to sections in the text. Note: The order of the three first actions (partitioning, inspection, and detection and/or handling of outliers) may vary, depending on the distribution and the statistical methods applied. *N*, No; *Y*, yes.

Basic Statistical Concepts

Sample

The first step in the establishment of reference values is the selection of a group of reference individuals. In practice, it usually is not feasible to gather observations on all possible reference individuals of a certain category of the general population. Therefore, a smaller group (sometimes called the reference *sample* group) is examined. This *subset* is so chosen that it is expected to give the desired information about the characteristics of the complete *set* of individuals (the reference *population*).[42]

The reference *population* is often considered to be *hypothetical* because its characteristics are not observed directly; neither the number (the set size) nor the properties of all of its individuals are known. An obvious requirement is that individuals in the subset are typical of those in the complete set. Statistical theory usually assumes that items in the subset are selected at *random* from among those in the set; otherwise, the subset may be biased. If items are not randomly selected, statistical techniques are still used, but only with due caution and with awareness of the possible bias introduced.

Two main types of inferences may be made from values obtained from the subset (sample group) to the set (total reference population): estimating properties and testing hypotheses.

Estimating Properties

In practice, properties of the set are estimated. A *reference limit* (a percentile) of a biological quantity, such as the activity of serum GGT, based on subset reference values, is an example of a *point estimate* (a single value). It is considered representative of the property that might have been found if all possible values in the set had been observed. If many randomly selected subsets from the same set are examined, several estimates with some variation around the "true" value of the set are obtained. Also, it is possible to produce an *interval estimate* bounded by limits within which the "true" value is located with a specified confidence: the *confidence interval.* The parameter is expressed as a number in the interval 0 to 1, indicating the degree on the scale between "never" and "always." A reference limit for serum GGT can thus be associated by a confidence interval showing its region of uncertainty.

Testing Hypotheses

Also, the hypotheses about the distribution can be tested. For example, the hypothesis that the distribution of values for serum GGT activities is of the Gaussian type (the *null* hypothesis) can be stated. If true, this will enable determination of the reference limits with relatively few points. If deviations of subset values from the Gaussian distribution are small, they can be ascribed to variation caused by chance alone. In that case, it is possible to use statistical methods based on the Gaussian distribution. However, the hypothesis must be rejected if it is unlikely that observed deviations from the Gaussian distribution are caused by chance alone. *Statistical tests* provide quantitative approaches to these types of decisions: the null hypothesis is rejected if the statistical test shows that the probability of the hypothesis being true is less than a stated *significance level.* The *probability* (*P*) is a number in the interval of 0 to 1, indicating the degree on the scale between "unlikely" and "certain." If a significance level of 0.05 is stated, the Gaussian hypothesis is tested for the distribution of serum GGT activities; it should be rejected if the probability obtained by the test is, for example, $P = 0.01$. Then the alternative hypothesis that the distribution is non-Gaussian is accepted. The *power* of a statistical test is the probability of rejection when the null hypothesis is false.

Describing the Distribution

In the following sections, the term *reference distribution*[42] is used for the distribution of reference values (x). The two statistics *arithmetic mean* $\bar{x}$ and *standard deviation* (s_x) are measures of its location and the dispersion of values in it, respectively. They are defined as follows:

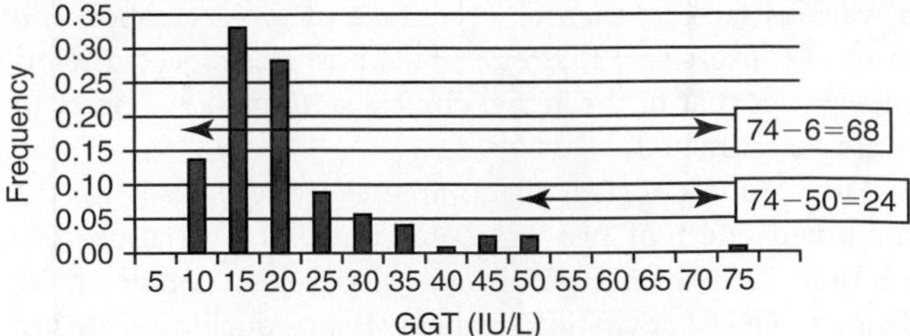

Figure 5-3 Observed distribution of 124 gamma-glutamyltransferase (GGT) values in serum (IU/L). The *upper arrow* indicates the range of observed values (highest – lowest, or 74 – 6 = 68); the *lower arrow* indicates the difference between the highest value and the next highest value (74 – 50 = 24). Because the quotient (24/68 = 0.35) exceeds 0.33, Dixon's range test indicates that the highest value is an outlier and therefore is omitted from all further analyses.

$$\bar{x} = \frac{\sum x}{n}$$

$$s_x = \sqrt{\frac{\sum (x-\bar{x})^2}{n-1}} = \sqrt{\frac{\sum x^2 - \frac{\left(\sum x\right)^2}{n}}{n-1}}$$

where $\boldsymbol{x}$ represents each of the n reference values in the subset (or a subclass of it).

An observed distribution may be presented as a table or graph (histogram) showing the number of observations in small intervals (Figure 5-3). The number of observations in an interval divided by the total number of observations in the distribution (its size) is an estimator of the probability of finding a value in the corresponding interval of the hypothetical *probability distribution* of the population (assuming random sampling). By consecutive summing of all these ratios, starting with the leftmost interval of the observed distribution, an estimate is obtained of the hypothetical *cumulative probability distribution,* shown plotted on Gaussian probability paper in Figure 5-4, *B*.

Reference Limits: Interpercentile Interval

As mentioned previously, reference values provide a basis for interpretation of laboratory data. In clinical practice, one usually compares a patient's result with the corresponding *reference interval,* which is bounded by a pair of *reference limits.*[42] This interval, which may be defined in different ways, is a useful condensation of the information carried by the total set of reference values.

Types of reference intervals that have been used include (1) tolerance, (2) prediction, and (3) interpercentile intervals.[42,78] Selection from among these types of intervals may be important for certain well-defined statistical problems, but their numeric differences are negligible when based on at least 100 reference values.

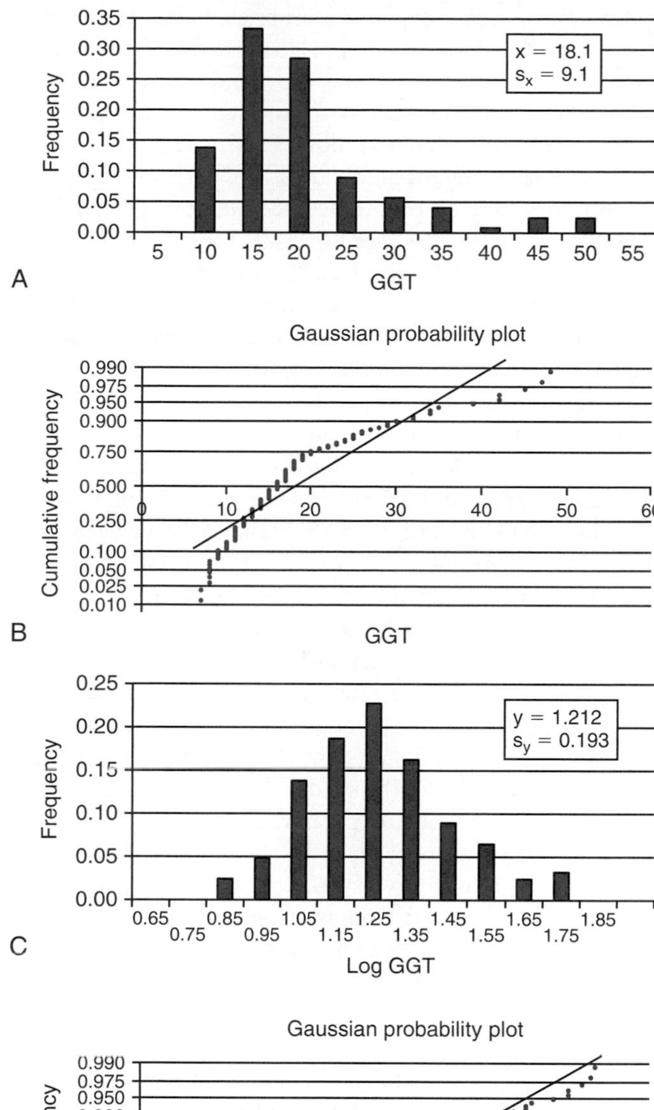

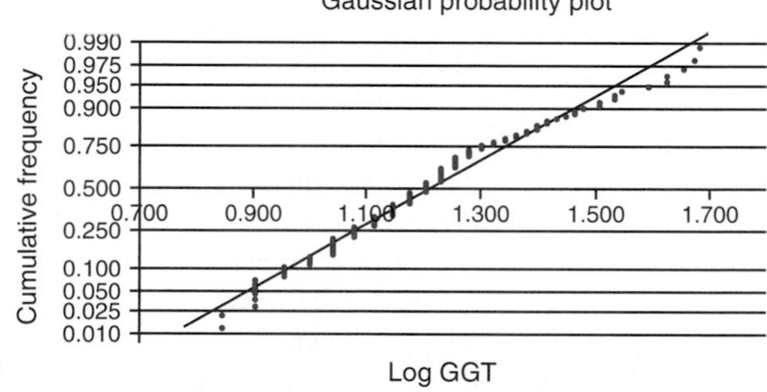

Figure 5-4 Distribution of 123 remaining gamma-glutamyltransferase (GGT) values from reference subjects. A, A histogram of the original, untransformed data. B, Shows the cumulative frequency of the data from A, plotted on Gaussian probability paper. C, A histogram of the logarithmic transformed data. D, The cumulative frequency of the data from C plotted on Gaussian probability paper.

This discussion will be confined to the *interpercentile interval,* which is (1) simple to estimate, (2) more commonly used, and (3) recommended by the IFCC.[42] It is defined as an interval bounded by two percentiles of the reference distribution. A *percentile* denotes a value that divides the reference distribution such that specified percentages of its values have magnitudes less than or equal to the limiting value. For example, if 47 IU/L is the 97.5-percentile of serum GGT values, then 97.5% of the values are equal to or below this value.

It is an arbitrary but common convention to define the reference interval as the *central 95%-interval* bounded by the 2.5- and 97.5-percentiles.[42] Another size or an asymmetric location of the reference interval may be more appropriate in particular cases. To prevent ambiguity, the definition of the interval should always be stated. The estimation of percentiles presented in the following sections is based on the conventional central 95% interval, but the techniques are easily adapted to other locations of the limits.

The percentiles are point estimates of population parameters. Accordingly, they are unbiased estimates only if the subset of values was selected randomly from the population. But, as was discussed earlier, random sampling is often difficult to achieve. The interpercentile interval may always be used, however, as a summary or description of the subset reference distribution.

The precision of a percentile as an estimate of a population value depends on the size of the subset; it is less precise when few observations are reported. If the assumption of random sampling is fulfilled, the *confidence interval* of the percentile (i.e., the limits within which the true percentile is located with a specified degree of confidence) can be determined. The 0.90 confidence interval of the 2.5-percentile (lower reference limit) for serum GGT values may, for example, be 6 to 8 IU/L. Finding the true percentile in this interval with a confidence of 0.90 could be expected if all serum GGT values in the total reference population were measured.

Methods Used To Determine Interpercentile Intervals

The interpercentile interval is typically determined using a parametric or a nonparametric method.[34,42]

The *parametric method* for determination of percentiles and their confidence intervals assumes a certain type of distribution, and it is based on estimates of population parameters, such as the mean and the standard deviation. For example, a parametric method is used if it is thought that the true distribution is Gaussian and the reference limits (percentiles) are determined as the values located 2 standard deviations below and above the mean. In fact, most of the parametric methods are based on the Gaussian distribution. If the reference distribution does not appear to be Gaussian, mathematical functions may be used that transform data to a distribution that approximates a Gaussian shape. Some positively skewed distributions (Figure 5-5, *A*) may, for example, be made symmetric by using logarithms of the data values.

In contrast, the *nonparametric method* makes no assumptions concerning the type of distribution and does not use estimates of distribution parameters. Percentiles are determined simply by cutting off the required percentage of values in each tail of the subset reference distribution (typically 2.5%).

The simple nonparametric method for determination of percentiles is recommended by IFCC[42] and CLSI.[15] The more

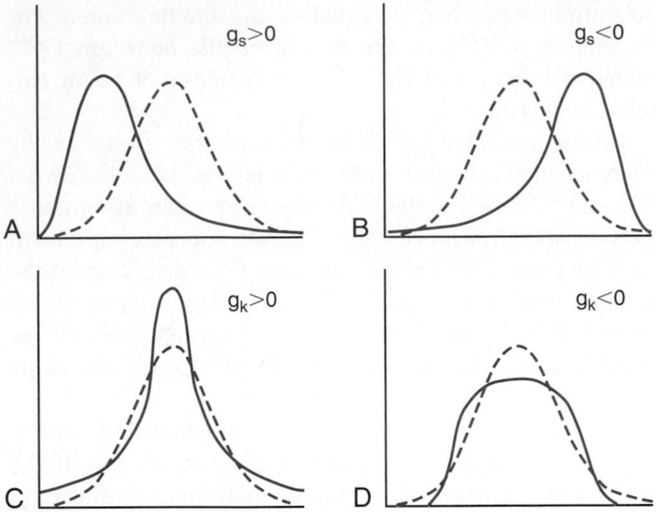

Figure 5-5 Skewness and kurtosis. The two *upper figures* show asymmetric distributions (A, positive skewness; B, negative skewness). The two *lower figures* show distributions with non-Gaussian peakedness (C, positive kurtosis; D, negative kurtosis). The Gaussian distribution *(dashed curve)* is shown in all graphs for comparison. Values of the coefficients of skewness (g_s) and kurtosis (g_k) are also shown.

complex parametric method is seldom necessary, but it will be presented here owing to its popularity and frequent misapplication. Other methods will be mentioned later in this chapter, but they require the use of computer techniques. When results obtained using proper application of any of these methods are compared, it is usually found that estimates of the percentiles are very similar. Detailed descriptions of nonparametric and parametric methods are given later in this chapter.

Sample Size

In general, the theoretical lower limit of the sample size required for estimation of the 100α and $100(1 - \alpha)$ percentiles is equal to $1/\alpha$. Thus, estimation of the 2.5-percentile requires at least $1/0.025 = 40$ observations (per partition). For the nonparametric approach in particular, a sample size of at least 120 reference values has been recommended; otherwise, one cannot determine confidence intervals for the reference limits.[34,42]

It should be noted that for any method (parametric or nonparametric), the precision of the percentiles increases as the number of observations increases, as is shown by narrowing of their confidence intervals. Also, the more highly skewed a distribution is, the larger is the number of reference values needed to obtain reasonable confidence intervals.[51]

Partitioning of Reference Values

The best order of the first three actions outlined in Figure 5-2 (1—partitioning of reference values, 2—inspection of the distribution, and detection and/or 3—elimination of outliers) may in some cases be different from that shown in the figure. For example, it might be more appropriate to eliminate outliers before testing for partitioning. No strict rules for the order of these actions can be given as it depends on data and the statistical methods applied. With this caution in mind, the presentation in this chapter follows Figure 5-2.

The subset of reference individuals and corresponding reference values may be partitioned according to gender, age, and other characteristics (see Box 5-2). The process of partitioning is also called (1) stratification, (2) categorization, and (3) subgrouping, and its results are called (1) partitions, (2) strata, (3) categories, (4) classes, and (5) subgroups. In this chapter, the terms *partitioning* (for the process) and *(sub) classes* (for its result) are used.

The aim of partitioning is to provide a better basis for comparison of clinical laboratory results: *class-specific* reference intervals (e.g., age- and gender-specific reference intervals).

Various statistical criteria for partitioning have been suggested.[34,47] For example, an intuitive criterion states that partitioning is necessary if differences between classes are statistically significant (rejection of the "null" hypothesis of equal distributions). The distribution of reference values in the classes may show different locations (mean values vary) or different intraclass variations (standard deviations vary). These differences may be tested by statistical methods, which are not described here. The reader is referred to Chapter 2 and to standard textbooks of parametric[68,72] and nonparametric statistics.[12]

Differences in location or variation, however, may be statistically significant and still may be too small to justify replacing a single total reference interval with several class-specific intervals. Alternatively, statistically nonsignificant differences can lead to situations in which the proportions of each subclass above the upper or below the lower reference limits (without partitioning) are much different from the desired 2.5% on each side. Harris and Boyd[34] therefore suggested criteria based on the ratio between subclass standard deviations, a normal deviate test of means, and calculation of critical decision values dependent on the sample size.

Lahti and coworkers[47,48] focused on distances between reference limits instead of distances between means, and suggested new distance and proportion criteria for partitioning. Their model makes it possible to account for unequal subclass prevalences and is applicable to distributions of various types.

Partitioning requires large samples of reference values. If these are not used, subclass sizes may be too small for reliable estimates of reference intervals.

To solve the subclass size problem, it has been suggested to estimate regression-based reference intervals. Instead of dividing, for example, the total material into several age classes, one may construct continuous age-dependent reference limits and their confidence regions. Simulation studies have shown that this method produces reliable estimates with small sample sizes.[88]

When the intended purpose of the reference interval is to detect individual changes in biochemical status, subject-based reference values may be more appropriate than class-specific reference intervals for interpretation.[31,32,34]

In the following sections, a homogeneous reference distribution and either the complete distribution (if partitioning has been shown to be unnecessary) or a subclass distribution (after partitioning) are assumed.

Inspection of Distribution

It is always advisable to display the reference distribution graphically and to inspect it. A *histogram,* as shown in Figure 5-3, is easily prepared and is the type of data display best suited for visual inspection. Examination of the histogram serves as a safeguard against misapplication or misinterpretation of statistical methods, and it may reveal valuable information about the data. Data should be evaluated for the following characteristics of the distribution:

1. Highly deviating values *(outliers)* may represent erroneous values.
2. *Bimodal* or *polymodal* distributions have more than one peak and may indicate that the distribution is nonhomogeneous because of mixing of two or more distributions. If so, the criteria used to select reference individuals should be reevaluated, or partitioning of the values according to age, gender, or other relevant factors should be attempted.
3. The shape of the distribution should be noticed. It may be asymmetrical, or it may be more or less peaked than the symmetrical and bell-shaped Gaussian distribution (see Figure 5-5). The asymmetry most frequently observed with clinical chemistry data is positive *skewness* (see Figure 5-5, *A*). A symmetric distribution with positive *kurtosis** has a high and slim peak and a greater number of values in both tails than the Gaussian type of distribution (see Figure 5-5, *C*). Conversely, negative kurtosis indicates that the distribution has a broad and flat top with relatively few observations in the tails (see Figure 5-5, *D*). Asymmetry and non-Gaussian peakedness may be combined.
4. The visual inspection may also provide initial estimates of the location of reference limits that are useful as checks on the validity of computations.

Identification and Handling of Erroneous Values

An *erroneous value* can be traced to a gross deviation from the prescribed procedure for establishment of reference values.[33] Such values may deviate significantly from proper reference values *(outliers)* or may be hidden in the reference distribution. Only a strict experimental protocol, with adequate controls at each step, can eliminate the latter type of erroneous values.

Visual inspection of a histogram is a reliable method for identification of possible outliers. It is important to keep in mind, however, that values far out in the long tail of a skewed distribution may easily be misinterpreted as outliers. If the distribution is positively skewed, inspection of a histogram displaying logarithms of the values may aid in the visual identification of outliers.

Some outliers may also be identified by *statistical tests* (see Chapter 2), but no single method is capable of detecting outliers in every situation that may occur. The number of techniques suggested or recommended is, for this reason, very large.[7,34,37] The two main problems encountered can be described as follows:

1. Many tests assume that the type of the true distribution is known before the test is used. Some of these specifically require that the distribution be Gaussian. However, biological distributions very often are non-Gaussian, and their types are seldom known in advance. Furthermore, statistical tests of types of distribution are unreliable in the presence of outliers. This unreliability poses a difficult dilemma: some tests for outliers assume that the type of distribution is known, but tests for determining the type of distribution require that outliers be absent! As a consequence, it may be difficult to transform the distribution to Gaussian form before outliers are identified by statistical tests. Some tests are relatively insensitive to departures from a Gaussian distribution. This is the case with Dixon's *range test,* in which a value is identified as an extreme outlier if the difference between the two highest (or lowest) values in the distribution exceeds one third of the range of all values (see Figure 5-3).[34,42,64]
2. Several tests for outliers assume that a data set contains only a single outlier. The limitation of these tests is obvious. Some tests may detect a specified number of outliers, or they may be run several times, discarding one outlier in each pass of data. The range test, however, usually fails in the presence of several outliers. It is possible to estimate the standard deviation using data remaining after *trimming* of both tails of the distribution by a specified percentage of observations.[34,38] Outliers could be identified by this method as the values lying 3 or 4 standard deviations from the arithmetic mean. This method assumes, however, that the true distribution is Gaussian.

Horn and coworkers[40] have published a novel method in two stages for outlier detection that seems to provide a promising solution to both of the problems just mentioned. With this method, one executes the following:

1. Mathematically transform the data to approximate a Gaussian distribution. Horn used the Box-Cox transformation,[10] but other transformations that correct for skewness (see later) probably would also work. As mentioned earlier, it is impossible to achieve exact symmetry by transformation in the presence of outliers, but this does not seem to be critical with Horn's method.
2. Identify (or eliminate) outliers using a criterion based on the central 50% of the distribution, thus reducing the masking effect of several outliers. Compute the interquartile range (IQR) between the lower and upper

*Kurtosis is a measure of the "peakedness" of the probability distribution of a real-valued random variable. A high kurtosis distribution has a sharper *peak* and longer, fatter *tails;* a low kurtosis distribution has a more rounded peak and shorter thinner tails.

quartiles of the distribution (Q_1 and Q_3, respectively): $IQR = Q_3 - Q_1$. Then identify as outliers data lying outside the two fences

$$Q_1 - 1.5 * IQR \text{ and } Q_3 + 1.5 * IQR$$

Deviating values identified as possible outliers cannot always be discarded automatically. Values should be included or excluded on a rational basis. For example, records of the dubious values should be checked and errors corrected. In some cases, deviating values should be rejected because non-correctable causes have been found, such as in previously unrecognized conditions that qualify individuals for exclusion from the group of reference individuals.

Methods for Determining Reference Values

Nonparametric, parametric, bootstrap, and robust methods are used to determine reference intervals.

Nonparametric Method

This method consists essentially of cutting off a specified percentage of the values from each tail of the reference distribution. Three techniques may be used:

1. The percentiles may be determined *graphically* by plotting the cumulative distribution on Gaussian probability paper (see Figure 5-4, *B* and *D*).
2. A *mathematical function* may be fitted to the reference distribution.[34,66,70] The percentiles are then determined using the fitted function.
3. Very simple and reliable methods are based on *rank numbers*.[42,53,64] They also allow nonparametric estimation of the confidence intervals of the percentiles.[64] This method can easily be applied manually or with a spreadsheet program.

The rank-based method as recommended by the IFCC[42] and CLSI[15] requires the following steps:

1. First, the *n* reference values are sorted in ascending order of magnitude.
2. Next, the individual values are ranked. For example, the minimum value has rank number 1, the next value has rank number 2, and so on, until the maximum value, which has rank number *n*. Consecutive rank numbers should be given to two or more values that are equal ("ties").
3. The rank numbers of the 100α and $100(1 - \alpha)$ percentiles are computed as $\alpha(n + 1)$ and $(1 - \alpha)(n + 1)$, respectively. Thus the limits of the conventional 95%-reference interval have rank numbers equal to $0.025(n + 1)$ and $0.975(n + 1)$.
4. The percentiles are determined by finding the original reference values that correspond to the computed rank numbers, provided that the rank numbers are integers. Otherwise, one should interpolate between the two limiting values.
5. Finally, the confidence interval of each percentile is determined by using the binomial distribution.[64] Table 5-3 provides data for the 0.90-confidence interval of the 2.5- and 97.5-percentiles. For the relevant sample size *n*, rank numbers for the lower and upper limits should be found for the 2.5-percentile; those same values are subtracted from (n + 1) to find the rank numbers for the 97.5-percentile.

TABLE 5-3 Nonparametric Confidence Intervals of Reference Limits*

	Rank Numbers	
Sample Size	**Lower**	**Upper**
119-132	1	7
133-160	1	8
161-187	1	9
188-189	2	9
190-218	2	10
219-248	2	11
249-249	2	12
250-279	3	12
280-307	3	13
308-309	4	13
310-340	4	14
341-363	4	15
364-372	5	15
373-403	5	16
404-417	5	17
418-435	6	17
436-468	6	18
469-470	6	19
471-500	7	19

*The table shows the rank numbers of the 0.90-confidence interval of the 2.5-percentile for samples with 119 to 500 values. To obtain the corresponding rank numbers of the 97.5-percentile, subtract the rank numbers in the table from ($n = 1$), where *n* is the sample size.
From IFCC.[42]

Table 5-4 provides a detailed example of the nonparametric determination of 95%-reference limits using the serum GGT reference values first shown in Figure 5-3.

Parametric Method

The parametric method is much more complicated than the simple nonparametric method and requires computer software to process the data. The method is presented here under separate headings for testing of type of distribution, transformation of data, and estimation of percentiles and their confidence intervals.

It should be noted that commonly used statistical computer program packages[9,69,79] aid in the estimation of reference limits, but these packages may lack some of the techniques described in this chapter. The RefVal,[77] CBstat,[52] and Medcalc (http://www.medcalc.be/manual/referenceinterval.php) programs implement these methods.

Testing Fit to Gaussian Distribution

The parametric method for estimating percentiles assumes that the true distribution is Gaussian. This fact was frequently ignored in the past and caused Elveback[20] to warn against "the

TABLE 5-4 Nonparametric Determination of Reference Interval*

Calculation of Rank Numbers of Percentiles

Lower:	0.025(123 + 1) = 3.1 (i.e., Rank #3)
Upper:	0.975(123 + 1) = 120.9 (i.e., Rank #121)

Original Values Corresponding to These Rank Numbers

Lower limit (2.5-percentile):	7 IU/L
Upper limit (97.5-percentile):	47 IU/L

Rank Numbers and Values of the 0.90-Confidence Limits

Lower Reference Limits

Rank numbers (see Table 5-3):	#1 and #7
Values:	6 and 8 IU/L

Upper Reference Limits

Rank numbers (see Table 5-3):	(123+1) – 7 = #117 and (123 + 1) – 1 = #123
Values:	39 and 50 IU/L

Summary

Lower reference limit:	7(6 to 8) IU/L
Upper reference limit:	47(39 to 50) IU/L

GGT Value	Frequency	Rank Order
6	1	1
7	2	2, 3
8	6	4-9
9	4	10-13
10	4	14-17
11	9	18-26
12	7	27-33
13	7	34-40
14	9	41-49
15	9	50-58
16	8	59-66
17	11	67-77
18	8	78-85
19	5	86-90
20	3	91-93
21	2	94, 95
22	2	96, 97
23	2	98, 99
24	2	100, 101
25	3	101-104
26	2	105, 106
27	1	107
28	1	108
29	2	109, 110
30	1	111
32	2	112, 113
34	2	114, 115
35	1	116
39	1	117
42	2	118, 119
45	1	120
47	1	121
48	1	122
50	1	123

*This table shows an example using the 123 serum gamma-glutamyltransferase (GGT) values displayed in Figure 5-4, *A*. See text for a description of the nonparametric method.

TABLE 5-5 Summary of GGT Reference Interval Determination by Three Methods

Method	Lower Limit (Confidence Interval)	Upper Limit (Confidence Interval)	Values Below Lower Limit	Values Above Upper Limit
Nonparametric	7 (6 to 8)	47 (39 to 50)	1	2
Parametric—untransformed data	0 (–2 to 2)	36 (34 to 38)	0	7
Parametric—transformed data	7 (6 to 8)	40 (35 to 44)	1	6

The table summarizes the 95%-reference intervals and associated 90%-confidence limits generated by each of three methods for the same data set. The numbers of observed values deemed lower and higher than the corresponding interval for each method are given in the last two columns. Because the original data are positively skewed, note that the parametric techniques generate intervals that are biased low. Note too that the parametric technique on untransformed data has a lower confidence interval, which is actually less than 0.

ghost of Gauss." Negligence often results in seriously biased estimates of reference limits. After elimination of the outlier from the GGT reference values in Figure 5-3, the mean and standard deviation of the remaining 123 serum GGT reference values are 18.1 and 9.1 (see Figure 5-4, *A*), from which the reference interval is calculated as 0 ± 1.960 S_x, or 0 to 36 IU/L (vs. the nonparametric values of 7 and 47 IU/L; Table 5-5). More highly positively skewed distributions may even result in negative values for the lower reference limit.

Therefore, a critical phase in the parametric method is testing the goodness-of-fit of the reference distribution to a hypothetical Gaussian distribution. If the Gaussian hypothesis must be rejected at a specified significance level, one is left with two alternatives (see Figure 5-2): either the nonparametric method can be used, or a mathematical transformation of data can be applied to approximate the Gaussian distribution. Only when the Gaussian hypothesis is not rejected by the test can one pass directly to parametric estimation of percentiles and their confidence intervals (see Figure 5-2).

Goodness-of-fit tests have been reviewed by Mardia.[56] These tests can be broadly classified as (1) graphical procedures, (2) coefficient-based tests, and (3) tests that are based on shape differences between observed and theoretical distributions.

1. *The graphical procedure* consists of plotting the cumulative distribution on probability paper, which has a nonlinear vertical axis based on the Gaussian distribution (see Figure 5-4, *B* and *D*). The plot should be close to a straight line if the distribution is Gaussian.
2. *Coefficient-based tests* use statistical measures of skewness and kurtosis (see Figure 5-5). Formulas for calculating these parameters are available elsewhere.[17,42,72,75,78] For Gaussian (and other symmetric distributions), the *coefficient of skewness* is zero; the sign of a nonzero coefficient indicates the type of skewness present in the data (see Figure 5-5, *A* and *B*). The *coefficient of kurtosis* is approximately zero for the Gaussian distribution. The sign of a nonzero coefficient indicates the type of kurtosis present in the data (see Figure 5-5, *C* and *D*). The statistical significance of these two coefficients may be found by referring to tables for testing skewness and kurtosis.[72]
3. Tests of *shape differences* that have been used to evaluate goodness-of-fit include the (1) Kolmogorov-Smirnov, (2) Cramer-von Mises, and (3) Anderson-Darling tests.[42,56,75,78,82] The Anderson-Darling test is recommended by the IFCC.[42] Computer programs for all three tests are available.[77]

Transformation of Data: Simple Method

In the previous section, it was shown that $0 \pm 1.960\ S_x$ of the serum GGT data in Figure 5-4, *A*, resulted in biased reference limits (too low values), as was to be expected with this positively skewed distribution. However, it is often possible to transform data mathematically to obtain a distribution of transformed values that approximates a Gaussian distribution. With these new values, the 2.5- and 97.5-percentiles are localized at 2 standard deviations on both sides of the mean. The estimates may then be transformed back to the original measurement scale by using the inverse mathematical function.

It is frequently observed that *logarithmically transformed* values, $y = \log(x)$, of a positively skewed distribution fit the Gaussian distribution rather closely. In other cases, *square roots* of the values, $y = \sqrt{x}$, result in a better approximation to the Gaussian distribution. This is the basis for the common use of logarithmic and square root transformations when reference limits are estimated. The method is applicable only to positively skewed distributions and is easily performed with a spreadsheet program. The procedure is as follows:

1. Test the fit of the distribution of original data to the Gaussian distribution. If the distribution has approximately Gaussian shape, the 2.5- and 97.5-percentiles are calculated directly as $0 \pm 1.960\ S_x$. Otherwise, continue with the following steps.
2. Transform data by the logarithmic function $y = log\ (x)$ or by the square root function $y = \sqrt{x}$, then test the fit to the Gaussian distribution. If the transformed distribution is significantly different from Gaussian shape, try another transformation or estimate the percentiles by the nonparametric method (see earlier in this chapter). Continue with the next step if the transformation resulted in a Gaussian distribution.
3. Compute the mean y and the standard deviation s_y of transformed data. Then estimate the 2.5- and 97.5-percentiles in the transformed data scale as

$$\overline{y} \pm 1.960\ S_y$$

4. The final step is reconversion of these percentiles to the original data scale. The inverse functions of the two transformations described here are as follows:

$$\text{Inverse of logarithmic function: } x = 10^y$$
$$\text{Inverse of square root function: } x = y^2$$

It is also possible to estimate the confidence limits of percentiles determined by the parametric method. This method is presented in a later section.

Example: As noted earlier, the original GGT data reference distribution is not Gaussian but is, similar to many biological distributions, skewed to the right (see Figure 5-4, *A*). However, by using the logarithm of the serum GGT values, a distribution very close to Gaussian shape (see Figure 5-4, *C*) is obtained. This observation is confirmed in Figure 5-4, *B* and *D*, where the cumulative probabilities are shown graphed on Gaussian probability paper; the original data are not linear, but the transformed data form a reasonably good line. As shown, the mean and standard deviation of the transformed data are $\overline{y} = 1.212$ and $s_y = 0.193$, respectively, that is, the mean value is 1.212 (corresponding to $10^{1.212}$, or 16 in the original scale). The transformed 2.5-percentile is then $1.212 - (1.960 \times 0.193) = 0.835$. On reconversion to the original data scale, a value of $10^{0.835} = 6.84$ is obtained. The lower reference limit of serum GGT is thus 7 IU/L. Similarly, it is found that the upper reference limit is 39 IU/L. These values are in closer agreement with those found by the nonparametric method: 7 and 47 IU/L (see Tables 5-4 and 5-5).

Transformation of Data: Two-Stage Method

Because simple logarithmic and square root transformations often fail to produce the desired Gaussian shape of the distribution, Harris and DeMets[36] introduced the two-stage method: first, use a function that transforms the distribution to symmetry (zero coefficient of skewness), and then apply another function that removes any remaining non-Gaussian kurtosis. Several mathematical functions may serve the purpose.[34,78] The IFCC recommends[42] the two-stage procedure based on the exponential function[55] and the modulus function[43]; the procedure is implemented in the RefVal computer program.[77] Successive approximations to symmetry and to Gaussian kurtosis (i.e., the iterative determination of the function parameters) are monitored by the coefficient-based tests, whereas the final evaluation has to be done by an independent test (e.g., the Anderson-Darling test, as mentioned earlier in this chapter).

Parametric Estimates of Percentiles and Their Confidence Intervals

General estimates for the 100α and 100(1 − α) percentiles and their 0.90-confidence intervals can be determined by the following method, provided that data (original or transformed) fit the Gaussian distribution[42]:

As noted earlier, the 100α and 100(1 − α) *percentiles* are calculated as follows:

$$(\text{mean}) \pm (\text{c}) * (\text{standard deviation})$$

where *c* is the (1 − α) standard Gaussian deviate, as can be found in statistical tables. For the 2.5-and 97.5-percentiles, the (1 − 0.025) = 0.975 standard Gaussian deviate, c, has a value of 1.960.

The 0.90-*confidence intervals* of these percentiles are then determined as follows[42,78]:

$$percentile = \pm 2.81 \frac{S_y}{\sqrt{n}}$$

where s_y is the standard deviation of the reference values (original or transformed) and *n* is the number of values. This formula is a special case of a general formula that can be used for confidence intervals of other sizes or for other percentiles.[42,78]

Example: The parametric estimate of the 2.5-percentile of serum GGT was determined previously by the logarithmic transformation as $10^{0.835} = 6.8$. The 0.90-confidence limits of the lower percentile are then

$$0.835 - 2.81 * (0.193/\sqrt{123}) = 0.786 \qquad 10^{0.786} = 6.1$$
$$0.835 + 2.81 * (0.193/\sqrt{123}) = 0.884 \qquad 10^{0.884} = 7.7$$

Thus the complete estimate of the 2.5-percentile (and its 0.90-confidence interval) is 7 (6 to 8) IU/L. The 97.5-percentile is, by the same method, found to be 39 (35 to 43) IU/L. Table 5-5 summarizes data from the three methods used to determine reference intervals from GGT data.

Other Methods for Calculating Reference Limits

Other methods have been recommended for calculating reference limits including the so-called bootstrap and robust methods. Neither of these methods makes assumptions about the underlying distribution; it need not be Gaussian. Both require the use of computer software, as they involve numerous iterations and somewhat complicated calculations.

Bootstrap Method

Bootstrap-based methods are reliable for estimating reference intervals.[34,53,70] The following version uses the rank-based nonparametric method; it is simple and reliable:

1. First, random samples, each of size *m*, are selected, with replacement, from the original set of *n* reference values. One selects "with replacement" if each value randomly selected from the original set remains available, so that it may be selected again in the random selection of the next value. In other words, even if there is only one occurrence of a specific value in the original set of n values, it may appear more than once in one, or more, random samples of size m.The number of resamples should be high (500 is a reasonable number of iterations).
2. For each resample, the upper and lower reference limits (percentiles) are next estimated by the rank-based nonparametric procedure described previously. These estimates from each iteration are saved.
3. Upon completion of all iterations, the final lower reference limit is calculated as the mean of the estimates of the lower reference limit; similarly, the final upper reference limit is calculated as the mean of the estimates of the upper reference limit.
4. Finally, the 0.90-confidence interval of each reference limit is calculated from the distribution of the percentile estimates, that is, with 500 iterations, the 25th rank order value represents the 5th percentile, and the 475th rank order value represents the 95th percentile.

Among available methods for estimating reference limits and their confidence intervals, the bootstrap method may be among the most reliable.[34,53] The location of estimated percentiles is always dependent on the characteristics of the particular subset of reference values. Only two methods may be used to obtain percentile estimates that approach population values: using a very large sample, or performing repeated sampling from the same parent population. Both methods are obviously expensive. In practice, the bootstrap method is a good alternative: (1) it is economical because it is based upon resampling from a single subset of reference values (but a minimum of 100 values is needed)[53]; (2) it provides robust percentile estimates (with the mentioned single-sample limitation); and (3) the widths of the confidence intervals approach asymptotically those that would have been obtained by repeated sampling from the parent population.[18] However, computer processing software is needed to run the large number of bootstrap iterations.

The reader should note that the bootstrap version described here uses rank-based nonparametric percentile estimates. However, the bootstrap principle may be employed with any kind of estimation, parametric or nonparametric.

Robust Method

The robust method has the form of the parametric method described earlier, but instead of using the mean and the standard deviation of the sample, it uses robust measures of location and spread. For example, instead of using the mean, it uses the median: in a series of 10 values, if the highest value is doubled, the mean changes appreciably, but the median does not change at all and thus is considered robust. Briefly, the steps involved are as follows:

1. Symmetry of the data is ensured, using transformations if necessary (e.g., Box-Cox transformation[10]).
2. Initial robust measures of location (median) and spread (median absolute deviation) are found.
3. Using a *biweight estimation* technique, in which more weight is given to observations closer to the center and progressively less to values farther from the center, new estimates of location and spread are found until successive results are satisfactorily close.

4. With final robust values of location and spread, the upper and lower limits are calculated, in a manner analogous to that described for the parametric technique.
5. Confidence intervals are then estimated using the bootstrapping technique described in the previous section.

Similar to the bootstrap method, this method does not require a Gaussian distribution. It is resistant to outliers and may be applied to very small numbers of observations. Details on the method are available.[41]

TRANSFERABILITY OF REFERENCE VALUES

Determination of reliable reference values for each test in the laboratory's repertoire is a major task that is often far beyond the capabilities of the individual laboratory. Therefore, it would be convenient if reference values generated in another laboratory could be used. This is especially important when ethical considerations limit the number of available individuals (e.g., when pediatric reference values are produced). Then, cooperative establishment of reference values may be necessary.

A major prerequisite for transfer of reference values is that the populations must be comparable (i.e., no major ethnic, social, or environmental differences should be noted between them). If they are not, a separate reference interval study must be done.

Analytical Issues

In practice, even if the populations are comparable, the problem of analytical transferability remains. The optimal, but usually very unrealistic, situation assumes that analytical methods, including their calibration and quality assurance, are identical in the laboratories. A more pragmatic approach involves (1) standardization of analytical protocols, (2) common calibration, (3) design of a sufficiently efficient external quality control scheme, and (4) the use of mathematical transfer functions if results still are not directly comparable.

The parameters of transfer functions may be estimated from results obtained by analysis of a sufficient number of patient specimens spanning the relevant range of concentrations in all participating laboratories.[15] Sometimes, functions obtained by simple linear regression suffice: using $y = a_0 + a_1{*}x$, the constant term a_0 compensates for systematic shifts among methods, whereas the coefficient term a_1 adjusts for proportional differences. In other cases, a more elaborate system for transfer of laboratory data is necessary.[83] It should be noted that the mentioned transfer functions account only for analytical bias; however, adjustments for differences in imprecision may also be designed.

Multicenter Trials

Another way to assist individual laboratories in generating reference values is to pool data from multiple sites to obtain the requisite minimum 120 samples (per partition). *Multicenter production of reference values* is gaining acceptance, both as a theoretical concept and as a practical approach. A Spanish study[24] introduced a cooperative model, simulating a virtual laboratory for 15 biochemical quantities. A project in the Nordic countries (NORIP) has produced common reference intervals for 25 analytes.[62,67]

On a less rigorous but more pragmatic level is the so-called Reference Range Service of the College of American Pathologists (CAP).[16] Each participating laboratory submits data for each analyte under consideration from 20 reference individuals, including each individual's gender, age, and race/ethnic background. In addition, each laboratory indicates the specific analytical method it uses (e.g., instrument, reagents). CAP pools the data for each specific method and then applies the nonparametric technique described previously to generate reference intervals for that method. With sufficient numbers of participating laboratories, it becomes possible to generate reasonable 95%-reference intervals, with 90%-confidence limits, for multiple partitions. As more laboratories, with more diverse reference individuals, participate, it becomes possible to generate more information. In addition, as methods become more standardized, pooling data from different methods may become possible, thereby increasing even further CAP's ability to partition the data. The main advantage of the service is that each laboratory is required to submit data on just 20 samples.

Verification of Transfer

Whether a laboratory adopts reference values from (1) a package insert, (2) another laboratory, or (3) a multicenter trial, it is important that the laboratory verifies the appropriateness of those values for its own use.[34] This verification is the final check that the laboratory has implemented the analytical method correctly, and that the laboratory's own population is comparable with that used for the original reference value study.

Comparison of a locally produced, small subset of values with the large set produced elsewhere using traditional statistical tests often is not appropriate, because the underlying statistical assumptions are not fulfilled and the sample sizes are unbalanced. Relatively sophisticated methods using nonparametric tests[87] or Monte Carlo sampling[39] have been described. Notwithstanding these caveats, a reasonably practical alternative has been recommended by CLSI: with a sample size of 20 reference values, one verifies the appropriateness of a proposed reference interval so long as no more than two values are outside the proposed limits.[15] One obvious deficiency of this test is that it does not detect the situation where the reference interval of the local group is narrower than that of the study group. Nonetheless, it does provide reasonable reassurance that a proposed reference interval is used.

PRESENTATION OF AN OBSERVED VALUE IN RELATION TO REFERENCE VALUES

An observed value (patient's value) may be compared with reference values. This comparison is often similar to hypothesis testing, but it is seldom statistical testing in the strict sense. Ideally, the patient and the reference individuals should match [i.e., the hypothesis is stated that they were all picked from the same set (population)]. Often, however, this is not the case. Thus it is advisable to consider the reference values as the yardstick for a less formal assessment than hypothesis testing.

The clinician should always be supplied with as much information about the reference values as is needed for their interpretation. Reference intervals for all laboratory tests may be presented to clinicians in a booklet, together with information about (1) analysis methods, (2) their imprecision, and (3) descriptions of the reference values. The goal is to present enough information to clinicians for rational clinical judgments.

In addition, a convenient presentation of an observed value in relation to reference values may be a great help for the busy clinician.[19,28,42,74]

Presentation of the observed value, together with a *listing of all reference values* for the corresponding test, is a feasible procedure only when few reference values are available. When there are many reference values, it is more convenient to present the *reference distribution* in a table, graphically in the form of a histogram (see Figure 5-4, *A* and *C*), or by a plot of the cumulative distribution (see Figure 5-4, *B* and *D*). A very informative presentation of the observed value involves showing its location on a graph. A more condensed technique is to present the observed value and the *reference interval* on the same report sheet. The reference intervals may be preprinted on report forms, or the computer system may select the appropriate age- and gender-specific reference interval from a file and print it next to the test result. This type of presentation is often graphical.[28]

It is also possible to compute various *mathematical indices* or to *flag* the results on reports using convenient symbols. When such presentation methods are used, the original observed value should also be reported to allow comparison with results of other laboratory tests and metabolic calculations.

An observed value may be classified as low, usual, or high (three classes), depending on its *location in relation to the reference interval.* On reports, it is convenient to flag unusual results (e.g., by using "L" and "H" for "low" and "high," respectively).[28]

A more detailed division of the value scale has also been advocated.[19] Regions outside the reference interval may be subdivided to indicate how unusual the observed value is. The reference interval may also be subclassified. The advantages are doubtful, however, because the shape of the reference distribution is not taken into account.

Another popular method is to express the observed value by a *statistical distance measure.* All such distances are ratios of the following type:

$$\frac{\text{observed value} - \text{measure of location}}{\text{measure of dispersion}}$$

The *SD unit,* or normal equivalent deviate, is such a measure. It is calculated as the difference between the observed value and the mean of the reference values divided by their standard deviation.[30] Several similar ratios have been suggested[22]; all produce very confusing values if the reference distribution is very skewed. An observed value (e.g., with an SD unit of 2.2) would be above the 97.5-percentile if the reference distribution had a Gaussian shape, but it might be well below the upper reference limit of a positively skewed distribution. If this occurs, mathematical transformation of the reference distribution to the Gaussian shape may be used to resolve this problem.[73]

Reporting the observed value as a *percentile* of the reference distribution provides a very accurate measure of the relation.[19,66] An observed serum GGT value of 48 IU/L may, for example, be reported as 48 IU/L (99th percentile). Alternatively, the probability of finding a value closer to the mean than the observed value, the *index of atypicality,* can be estimated.[2,74]

When observed values of several analytes are reported simultaneously, it is possible to use multivariate analogs of the SD unit and the index of atypicality (see later).[1,2]

ADDITIONAL TOPICS

Multivariate, Population-Based Reference Regions

The topic of previous sections of this chapter has been univariate population-based reference values and quantities derived from them. However, such values do not fit the common clinical situation in which observed values of several different laboratory tests are available for interpretation and decision making. For example, the average number of individual clinical chemistry tests requested on each specimen received in the author's laboratory is roughly six; in many laboratories, this number is even larger. Two models are used for interpretation by comparison in this situation. Each observed value can be compared with the corresponding reference values or interval (i.e., a *multiple, univariate comparison is performed*); or the set of observed values can be considered as a single multivariate observation and can be interpreted as such by a *multivariate comparison.* In this section, the relative merits of these two approaches are discussed, and methods for the latter type of comparison are presented.

The Multivariate Concept

A univariate observation, such as a single laboratory result, may be represented graphically as a point on a line—the axis. Results obtained by two different laboratory tests performed on the same specimen (a bivariate observation) are then displayed as a point in a plane defined by two perpendicular axes. With three results, a trivariate observation and a point in a space are defined by three perpendicular axes, and so forth. The possibility of visualization of a multivariate observation is lost when there are more than three dimensions. Still, one can consider the multivariate observation as a point in a multidimensional hyperspace with as many mutually perpendicular axes as there are results of different tests. The prefix *hyper-* signifies, in this context, "more than three dimensions." Such multivariate observations are also called *patterns* or *profiles.* A multivariate distribution thus is represented by a cluster of points on a plane, in a space, or in a hyperspace, depending on the dimensionality of the observation.[1,7,73,89] Several statistical methods are based on multivariate methods, some of which are straightforward extensions of well-known univariate methods.[58]

The Multiple, Univariate Reference Region

The univariate reference interval is bounded by two reference limits (lower and upper) on the result axis. Figure 5-6 shows the univariate reference intervals for two laboratory tests: one depicted on the *x*-axis, and the other, on the *y*-axis. Together, they describe a square in the plane of the two axes. Similarly, three or more univariate reference intervals define boxes or hyperboxes in the (hyper)space. By multiple, univariate comparison, it can be decided whether a multivariate observation point lies inside or outside this square, box, or hyperbox. However, this method has two very serious deficiencies[91]: an observation may lie outside the limits of the region without being unusual (see Figure 5-6, point *a*), or it may be found on the inside and still be an atypical observation (see Figure 5-6, point *b*). If the central 95%-interval is used, 5% of the values by definition are expected to be located in the two tails of the univariate reference distribution. However, more than 5% of the values would be located outside the square or (hyper)box created by several 95%-intervals. To be exact, $100(1 - 0.95^m)$ percent of multivariate reference values would be excluded by the method of multiple, univariate comparison (*m* being the number of different tests, or the dimensionality). For example, one would expect to find $100(1 - 0.95^{10}) =$ 40% of false positives when 10 laboratory tests are used. This discouraging result has been verified in several multiphasic screening programs. Therefore, a better method is needed.

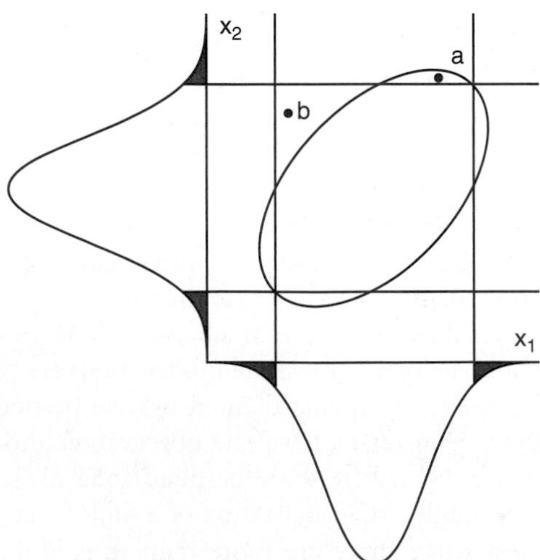

Figure 5-6 Bivariate reference region *(ellipse)* compared with the region defined by the two univariate reference intervals *(box).*

The Multivariate Reference Region

It is possible to define a common multivariate reference region[1,2,11,34,89,91] on the basis of joint distribution of reference values for two or more laboratory tests. This multivariate region is not a right-angled area, or hyperbox, but is more like an ellipse in the plane (see Figure 5-6) or an ellipsoid hyperbody in hyperspace. This region may be a straightforward extension of the univariate 95% interval to the multivariate situation; it may be set to enclose 95% of central multivariate reference data points. In this case, one would expect to find only 5% false positives.

The use of multivariate reference regions usually requires the assistance of a computer program, which takes a set of results obtained by several laboratory tests on the same clinical specimen and calculates an index. Interpretation of a multivariate observation in relation to reference values is then the task of comparing the index with a threshold value estimated from the reference values. Obviously, this is much simpler than comparing each result with its proper reference interval.

This index is essentially a distance measure and is known as *Mahalanobis' squared distance* (D^2). It is analogous to the square of the standard deviation for single reference values. It expresses the multivariate distance between the observation point and the common mean of the reference values, taking into account the dispersion and the correlation of the variables.[1,2,11,34,89,91] More interpretational guidance may be obtained from this distance by expressing it as a percentile analogous to the percentile presentation of univariate observed values.[11] Also, the index of atypicality has a multivariate counterpart.[1,2]

Although the theory of multivariate reference regions has been known for a while, surprisingly few applications of it have been reported in the literature. An important report reviews the topic and presents the results of a very careful study on the multivariate 95% region for a 20-test chemistry profile.[11] Some of the most important findings can be summarized as follows:

1. Sixty-eight percent of subjects had at least one test result outside univariate reference intervals, which was close to what was theoretically expected: $100(1 - 0.95^{20}) =$ 64%.
2. By contrast, only 5% of patterns were outside the multivariate reference region (as expected).
3. Transformation to approximately Gaussian shape of the univariate distributions was necessary.
4. A test profile may be distinctly unusual in the multivariate sense even though each individual result is within its proper reference interval (e.g., see point *b* in Figure 5-6).
5. The multivariate reference region could detect minor deviations of multiple analytes.
6. Conversely, it could also be insensitive to highly deviating results for a single analyte.
7. Sensitivity could be increased by defining multivariate reference regions for subsets of physiologically related tests.

Subject-Based Reference Values

Figure 5-7 depicts the inherent problem associated with population-based reference values. It shows two hypothetical reference distributions. One represents the common reference distribution based on single specimens obtained from a group of different reference individuals. It has a true (hypothetical) mean μ and a standard deviation σ. The other distribution is based on several specimens collected over time in a single individual, the *i*th individual. Its hypothetical mean is μ_i and its standard deviation σ_i.

If an observed value is located outside the subject's 2.5- and 97.5-percentiles, the personal or *subject-based reference interval,* the cause may be a change in biochemical status, suggesting the presence of disease. Figure 5-7 shows that such an observed value may still be within the population-based reference interval. The sensitivity of the latter interval to changes in a subject's biochemical status depends accordingly on the location of the individual's mean μ_i relative to the common mean μ and to the relative magnitudes of the corresponding standard deviations σ_i and σ. A mean μ_i close to μ and a small σ_i relative to σ may conceal the individual's changes entirely within the population-based reference interval.

Harris[31,32] analyzed this topic and found that the ratio R of intraindividual (personal) variation over interindividual (among subjects) variation provides a criterion for the usefulness of the population-based reference interval. The population-based reference interval has less than the desired sensitivity to changes in biochemical status if the ratio value is $R \leq 0.6$. This interval is a more trustworthy reference if $R > 1.4$, at least for the individual whose standard deviation σ_i is close to the average value. Published data[31,90] usually show that homeostatically tightly controlled quantities, such as serum electrolytes, have high ratio values. Population-based reference intervals of such analytes suffice for clinical use. In contrast, serum proteins and enzymes have very low ratios because they are not under the same degree of metabolic control. Here, subject-based reference intervals seem more appropriate.

Two specific examples mentioned earlier may help to clarify this concept further. Figure 5-8 depicts immunoglobulin (Ig)M values from several healthy individuals over the course of several days. As illustrated, the intraindividual differences are small as compared with interindividual differences. Even though the population-based reference interval might extend from 200 to 1600 mg/dL, it would be most unusual (abnormal) for any patient's IgM value to change by more than 200 mg/dL, even if the value remained within the population-based reference interval. Similarly, it is well known that any given patient's serum creatinine value is reasonably constant,[25] which is related both to glomerular filtration rate (GFR) and to lean muscle mass. If the latter is constant, then changes in GFR are inversely proportional to the serum creatinine (see Chapters 25 and 48). That is, even though a typical (population-based) reference interval for serum creatinine might extend from 62 to 106 μmol/L (0.7 to 1.2 mg/dL), a change from 65 to 105 μmol/L in a given patient would be distinctly abnormal, representing the loss of almost half of the GFR.

Two solutions can be proposed to the problem of the clinical insensitivity of population-based reference intervals:

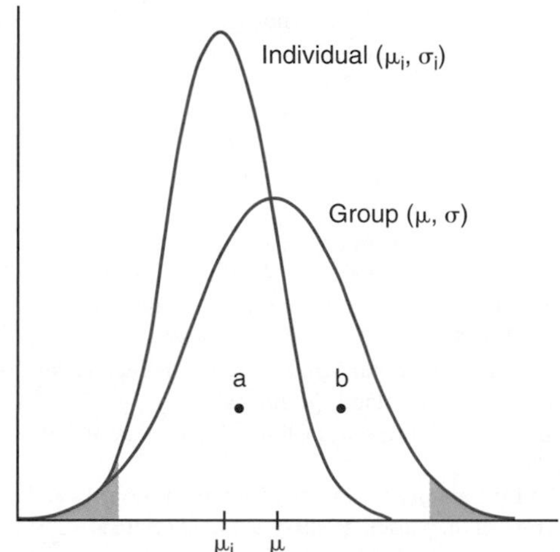

Figure 5-7 Relationship between population-based and subject-based reference distributions and reference intervals. The example is hypothetical, and the two distributions are, for simplicity, Gaussian. Note that points *a* and *b* are within the population-based reference interval, but only point *a* would be "normal" for this particular subject. *(Modified from Harris EK. Effects of intraindividual and interindividual variation on the appropriate use of normal ranges. Clin Chem 1974;20:1536.)*

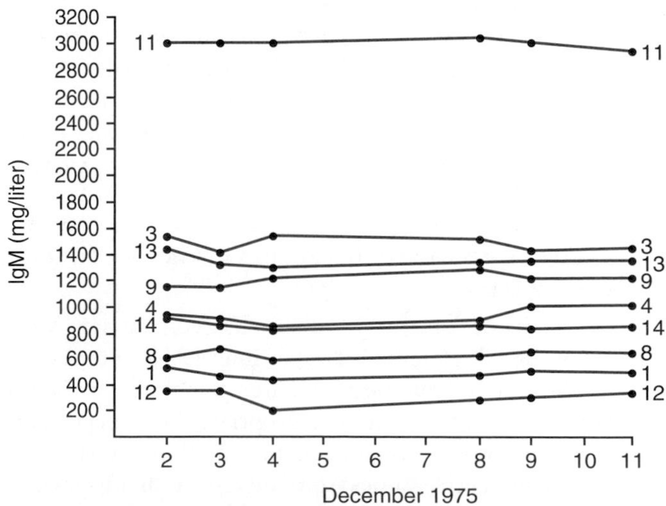

Figure 5-8 Serial immunoglobulin (Ig)M values over several days from reference individuals. Note that intraindividual variability is very small compared with interindividual variability. *(From Statland BE, Winkel P, Killingsworth LM. Factors contributing to intra-individual variation of serum constituents: 6. Physiological day-to-day variation in concentrations of 10 specific proteins in sera. Clin Chem 1976;22:1635-6.)*

1. One can try to reduce variation in reference values by *partitioning* into more homogeneous subclasses, as was discussed in a previous section. However, increasing the ratio, R, for example, from 0.6 to 1.4 by partitioning requires that one can obtain the rather dramatic reduction of 37% in standard deviation.[31] This often is difficult to attain in practice.
2. The other possibility is to use the patient's previous values, obtained when the patient was in a defined state of health, as the reference for any future value. Application of *subject-based reference values* becomes more feasible as health screening by laboratory tests and computer storage of results become available to large segments of the general population.

Two not completely separated classes of models may be used for construction of subject-based reference intervals: statistical and physiologic models.[34]

1. Harris has developed several models based on statistical *time series analysis.*[31-35] At one extreme, a stationary or *homeostatic model* is suitable for analytes showing relatively fast, random fluctuations around a constant mean (set point). The set point is estimated from past values that are given equal weights. Another model, the nonstationary *random-walk model,* allows a changing set point over time in healthy subjects. Then, more recent values are given heavier weights during estimation of the current set point. Intermediate and more or less complex models exist. Some of these data-following methods are suitable for adaptive forecasting in situations in which the time intervals are short (e.g., during hospitalization).[33] They might thus be implemented on a computer as part of a laboratory cumulative reporting system. The reader is referred to papers by Harris for details on statistical time series models.[31-35]
2. It is also possible to construct *physiologic models* that use known physiologic and biochemical time-dependent relationships. Winkel has developed a time series model for monitoring plasma progesterone in pregnancy using the assumption of a simple exponential growth curve for the size of the placenta.[90]

Dynamic versus Static Interpretation of Clinical Chemistry Data

Interpretation of observed values by comparison with population-based reference values or intervals is not the only way that clinical data may be used. Often, dynamic approaches to data interpretation are more appropriate. Time-dependent variation may provide important information. Time series analysis of consecutive values from the same individual is one example. Other examples include dynamic analysis of kinetic processes in the organism, such as intermediary metabolism and the exchange of substances between metabolic pools. For example, it is possible to design a model for urea turnover in the body.[26] The model defines (1) rates of urea input from various sources to the extracellular fluid, (2) exchange of urea across cell membranes, (3) urea degradation in the gut, (4) handling of urea by the kidneys, and so forth. Such a model may facilitate interpretation of serum urea values with the purpose of detecting hemorrhage or necrosis after major surgery and evaluating the magnitude of these complications. Biochemical model building, estimation of model parameters from observed values, and computer simulation of the models may add greatly to our understanding.

REFERENCES

1. Albert A, Harris EK. Multivariate interpretation of clinical laboratory data. New York: Marcel Dekker, 1987.
2. Albert A, Heusghem C. Relating observed values to reference values: the multivariate approach. In: Gräsbeck R, Alström T, eds. Reference values in laboratory medicine. Chichester, United Kingdom: John Wiley, 1981:289-96.
3. Alström T, Dahl M, Gräsbeck R, Hagenfeldt L, Hertz H, Hjelm M, et al. Recommendation for collection of skin puncture blood from children with special reference to production of reference values. Scand J Clin Lab Invest 1987;47:199-205.
4. Alström T, Gräsbeck R, Lindblad B, Solberg HE, Winkel P, Vinikka L. Establishing reference values from adults: recommendation on procedures for the preparation of individuals, collection of blood, and handling and storage of specimens. Scand J Clin Lab Invest 1993;53: 649-52.
5. American Academy of Pediatrics Subcommittee on Hyperbilirubinemia. Management of hyperbilirubinemia in the newborn infant 35 or more weeks of gestation. Pediatrics 2004;114:297-316.
6. Baadenhuijsen H, Smit JC. Indirect estimation of clinical chemical reference intervals from total hospital patient data: application of a modified *Bhattacharya* procedure. J Clin Chem Clin Biochem 1985;23:5829-39.
7. Barnett V, Lewis T. Outliers in statistical data. Chichester, United Kingdom: John Wiley, 1994.
8. Berg B, Nilsson JE, Solberg HE, Tryding N. Practical experience in the selection and preparation of reference individuals: empirical testing of the provisional Scandinavian recommendations. In: Gräsbeck R, Alström T, eds. Reference values in laboratory medicine. Chichester, United Kingdom: John Wiley, 1981:55-64.

8A. Bjerner J. Age-dependent biochemical quantities: an approach for calculating reference intervals. Scand J Clin Lab Invest 2007;67: 707-22.

9. BMDP. Cork, Ireland: Statistical Solutions. Available at: http://www.statsol.ie/ (accessed June 2009).
10. Box GEP, Cox DR. Analysis of transformations. J R Stat Soc 1964;B26:211-52.
11. Boyd JC, Lacher DA. The multivariate reference range: an alternative interpretation of multi-test profiles. Clin Chem 1982;28:259-65.
12. Bradley JV. Distribution-free statistical tests. Englewood Cliffs, NJ: Prentice-Hall, 1968.
13. Clinical and Laboratory Standards Institute. Procedures for the collection of diagnostic blood specimens by venipuncture. CLSI Document H03-A6. Wayne, Pa: Clinical Laboratory and Standards Institute, 2007.
14. Clinical and Laboratory Standards Institute. Procedures and devices for the collection of diagnostic capillary blood specimens. CLSI Document H04-A6. Wayne, Pa: Clinical and Laboratory Standards Institute, 2008.
15. Clinical and Laboratory Standards Institute. Defining, establishing, and verifying reference intervals in the clinical laboratory. CLSI Document C28-A3c. Wayne, Pa: Clinical and Laboratory Standards Institute, 2010.
16. College of American Pathologists. 2009 surveys catalogue. Available at: http://www.cap.org/apps/docs/proficiency_testing/surveys_catalog/2009_surveys_catalog.pdf (accessed March 2011).
17. Cramer H. Mathematical methods of statistics. Princeton, NJ: Princeton University Press, 1999.
18. Davison AC, Hinkley DV. Bootstrap methods and their application. Cambridge, United Kingdom: Cambridge University Press, 1997:46-52.

19. Dybkær R. Observed value related to reference values. In: Gräsbeck R, Alström T, eds. Reference values in laboratory medicine. Chichester, United Kingdom: John Wiley, 1981:263-78.
20. Elveback LR, Guillier CL, Keating FR. Health normality and the ghost of Gauss. JAMA 1970;211:69-75.
21. Expert Panel on Detection, Evaluation, and Treatment of High Blood Cholesterol in Adults. Executive summary of the Third Report of the National Cholesterol Education Program (NCEP) Expert Panel on Detection, Evaluation, and Treatment of High Blood Cholesterol in Adults (Adult Treatment Panel III). JAMA 2001;285:2486-97.
22. Faulkner WR, Meites S, eds. Geriatric clinical chemistry: reference values. Washington, DC: AACC Press, 1997.
23. Felding P, Tryding N, Hyltoft Petersen P, Hørder M. Effects of posture on concentrations of blood constituents in healthy adults: practical application of blood specimen collection procedures recommended by the Scandinavian Committee on Reference Values. Scand J Clin Lab Invest 1980;40:615-21.
24. Ferré-Masferrer M, Fuentes-Arderiu X, Alvarez-Funes V, et al. Multicentric reference values: shared reference limits. Eur J Clin Chem Clin Biochem 1997;35:715-8.
25. Fraser CG. Biological variation: from principles to practice. Washington, DC: AACC Press, 2001:15-17.
26. Groth T, de Verdier CH. The potential use of biochemical-physiological simulation models in clinical chemistry. Scand J Clin Lab Invest 1979;39:103-10.
27. Gräsbeck R. Health as seen from the laboratory. In: Gräsbeck R, Alström T, eds. Reference values in laboratory medicine. Chichester, United Kingdom: John Wiley, 1981:17-24.
28. Gräsbeck R, Alström T, eds. Reference values in laboratory medicine: the current state of the art. Chichester, United Kingdom: John Wiley, 1981.
29. Guder WG, Narayanan S, Wisser H, Zawta B. Samples: from the patient to the laboratory: the impact of preanalytical variables on the quality of laboratory results, 2nd edition. Darmstadt, Germany: GIT Verlag, 2001.
30. Gullick HD, Schauble MK. SD unit system for standardized reporting and interpretation of laboratory data. Am J Clin Pathol 1972;57:517-25.
31. Harris EK. Effects of intra- and interindividual variation on the appropriate use of normal ranges. Clin Chem 1974;20:1535-42.
32. Harris EK. Some theory of reference values. I. Stratified (categorized) normal ranges and a method for following an individual's clinical laboratory values. Clin Chem 1975;21:1457-64.
33. Harris EK. Statistical aspects of reference values in clinical pathology. In: Stefanini M, Benson ES, eds. Progress in clinical pathology, volume 7. New York: Grune & Stratton, 1981:45-66.
34. Harris EK, Boyd JC. Statistical bases of reference values in laboratory medicine. New York: Marcel Dekker, 1995.
35. Harris EK, Cooil BK, Shakarji G, et al. On the use of statistical models of within-person variation in long-term studies of healthy individuals. Clin Chem 1980;26:383-91.
36. Harris EK, DeMets DL. Estimation of normal ranges and cumulative proportions by transforming observed distributions to Gaussian form. Clin Chem 1972;18:605-12.
37. Hawkins DM. Identification of outliers. London: Chapman and Hall, 1980.
38. Healy MJR. Outliers in clinical chemistry quality-control schemes. Clin Chem 1979;25:675-7.
39. Holmes EW, Kahn SE Molnar PA, Bermes EW Jr. Verification of reference ranges by using a Monte Carlo sampling technique. Clin Chem 1994;40:2216-22.
40. Horn PS, Feng L, Li Y, Pesce AJ. Effect of outliers and nonhealthy individuals on reference interval estimation. Clin Chem 2001;47: 2137-45.
41. Horn PS, Pesce AJ. Reference intervals: a user's guide. Washington, DC: AACC Press, 2005.
42. International Federation of Clinical Chemistry, Expert Panel on Theory of Reference Values. Approved recommendation on the theory of reference values. Part 1. The concept of reference values. J Clin Chem Clin Biochem 1987;25:337-42; Part 2. Selection of individuals for the production of reference values. J Clin Chem Clin Biochem 1987;25:639-44; Part 3. Preparation of individuals and collection of specimens for the production of reference values. J Clin Chem Clin Biochem 1988;26:593-8; Part 4. Control of analytical variation in the production transfer and application of reference values. Eur J Clin Chem Clin Biochem 1991;29:531-5; Part 5. Statistical treatment of collected reference values: determination of reference limits. J Clin Chem Clin Biochem 1987;25:645-56; Part 6. Presentation of observed values related to reference values. J Clin Chem Clin Biochem 1987;25:657-62.
42A. Ichihara K, Boyd JC; IFCC Committee on Reference Intervals and Decision Limits (C-RIDL) An appraisal of statistical procedures used in derivation of reference intervals. Clin Chem Lab Med. 2010;48:1537-51.43. John JA, Draper NR. An alternative family of transformations. Appl Statistics 1980;29:190-7.
43. John JA, Draper NR. An alternative family of transformations. Appl Statistics 1980;29:190-7.
44. Kallner A, Tryding N. IFCC guidelines to the evaluation of drug effects in clinical chemistry: based on the IFCC recommendations of the Expert Panel on Drug Effects in Clinical Chemistry. Scand J Clin Lab Invest 1989;49(Suppl 195):1-29.
45. Kendall MG, Buckland WR. A dictionary of statistical terms, 5th edition. London: Longman, 1990.
46. Kouri T, Kairisto V, Virtanen A, et al. Reference intervals developed from data for hospitalized patients: computerized method based on combination of laboratory and diagnostic data. Clin Chem 1994;40:2209-15.
47. Lahti A, Petersen PH, Boyd JC, et al. Objective criteria for partitioning Gaussian-distributed reference values into subgroups. Clin Chem 2002;48:338-52.
48. Lahti A, Petersen PH, Boyd JC, Rustad P, Laake P, Helge Erik Solberg HE. Partitioning of nongaussian-distributed biochemical reference data into subgroups. Clin Chem 2004;50:891-900.
49. Lainchbury JG, Campbell E, Frampton CM, Yandle TG, Nicholls MG, Richards AM. Brain natriuretic peptide and N-terminal brain natriuretic peptide in the diagnosis of heart failure in patients with acute shortness of breath. J Am Coll Cardiol 2003;42:728-35.
50. Lindblad B, Alström T, Bo Hansen A, Gräsbeck R, Hertz H, Holmberg C, et al. Recommendation for collection of venous blood from children with special reference to production of reference values. Scand J Clin Lab Invest 1990;50:99-104.
51. Linnet K. Two-stage transformation systems for normalization of reference distributions evaluated. Clin Chem 1987;33:381-6.
52. Linnet K. CBstat: a program for statistical analysis in clinical biochemistry: reference manual. Risskov, Denmark: K Linnet, 1999:1-53.
53. Linnet K. Nonparametric estimation of reference intervals by simple and bootstrap-based procedures. Clin Chem 2000;46:867-9.
54. Maisel AS, Krishnaswamy P, Nowak RM, McCord J, Hollander JE, Duc P, et al. Rapid measurement of B-type natriuretic peptide in the emergency diagnosis of heart failure. N Engl J Med 2002;347:161-7.
55. Manly BFJ. Exponential data transformations. The Statistician 1976;25:37-42.
56. Mardia KV. Tests of univariate and multivariate normality. In: Krishnaiah PR, ed. Handbook of statistics, volume 1. Analysis of variance. Amsterdam: North-Holland Publishing, 1980:279-320.
57. Meites S, Levitt MJ. Skin-puncture and blood-collecting techniques for infants. Clin Chem 1979;25:183-9.
58. Morrison DF. Multivariate statistical methods, 3rd edition. New York: McGraw-Hill, 1990.
59. Murphy EA. The normal and the perils of the sylleptic argument. Perspect Biol Med 1972;15:566-82.
60. Nathan DM, Buse JB, Davidson MB, Heine RJ, Holman RR, Sherwin R, et al. Management of hyperglycemia in type 2 diabetes: a consensus algorithm for the initiation and adjustment of therapy. A consensus statement from the American Diabetes Association and the European Association for the Study of Diabetes. Diabetes Care 2006;29:1963-72.

61. Nilsson SE, Evrin PE, Tryding N, et al. Biochemical values in persons older than 82 years of age: report from a population-based study of twins. Scand J Clin Lab Invest 2003;63:1-14.
62. Rustad P, Felding P, eds. Transnational biological reference intervals: procedures and examples from the Nordic Reference Interval Project 2000. Scand J Clin Lab Invest 2004;64:265-441.
63. Pincus MR. Interpreting laboratory results: reference values and decision making. In: Henry JB, ed. Clinical diagnosis and management by laboratory methods, 19th edition. Philadelphia: WB Saunders, 1996:74-91.
64. Reed AH, Henry RJ, Mason WB. Influence of statistical method used on the resulting estimate of normal range. Clin Chem 1971;17:275-84.
65. Roche Diagnostics proBNP II package insert. Available at: https://www.mylabonline.com/extranet/psupport/elecdoc/elecsys/04988540001v2.pdf (accessed June 2009).
66. Rossing RG, Hatcher WE. A computer program for estimation of reference percentile values in laboratory data. Comput Progr Biomed 1979;9:69-74.
67. Rustad P, Felding P. Transnational biological reference intervals: procedures and examples from the Nordic Reference Interval Project 2000. Scand J Clin Lab Invest 2004;64:265-441.
68. Sachs L. Applied statistics: a handbook of techniques. New York: Springer-Verlag, 1982.
69. SAS System. Cary, NC: SAS Institute, 2009. Available at: http://www.sas.com/ (accessed June 2009).
70. Shultz EK, Willard KE, Rich SS, Connelly DP, Critchfield GC. Improved reference-interval estimation. Clin Chem 1985;31:1974-8.
71. Siest G, Henny J, Schiele F, Young DS, eds. Interpretation of clinical laboratory tests: reference values and their biological variation. Foster City, Calif: Biomedical Publications, 1985.
72. Snedecor GW, Cochran WG. Statistical methods, 8th edition. Ames, Iowa: Iowa State University Press, 1989.
73. Solberg HE. Discriminant analysis. Crit Rev Clin Lab Sci 1978;9:209-42.
74. Solberg HE. Presentation of observed values in relation to reference values. Bull Mol Biol Med 1983;8:21-6.
75. Solberg HE. Statistical treatment of reference values in laboratory medicine: testing the goodness-of-fit of an observed distribution to the Gaussian distribution. Scand J Clin Lab Invest 1986;46(Suppl 184):125-32.
76. Solberg HE. Using a hospitalized population to establish reference intervals: pros and cons [Editorial]. Clin Chem 1994;40:2205-6.
77. Solberg HE. RefVal: a program implementing the recommendations of the International Federation of Clinical Chemistry on the statistical treatment of reference values. Comput Meth Progr Biomed 1995;48:247-56. (Also see Clin Chem Acta 1993;222:19-21.)
78. Solberg HE, Gräsbeck R. Reference values. Adv Clin Chem 1989;27:1-79.
79. SPSS. Chicago, Ill: SPSS Inc, 2009. Available at: http://www.spss.com/ (accessed June 2009).
80. Statland BE, Winkel P, Killingsworth LM. Factors contributing to intra-individual variation of serum constituents: 6. Physiological day-to-day variation in concentrations of 10 specific proteins in sera. Clin Chem 1976;22:1635-8.
81. Statland BE. Clinical decision levels for lab tests. Oradell, NJ: Medical Economics Books, 1987.
82. Stephens MA. EDF statistics for goodness of fit and some comparisons. J Am Stat Assoc 1974;69:730-7.
83. Strike PW, Michaeloudis A, Green AJ. Standardizing clinical laboratory data for the development of transferable computer-based diagnostic programs. Clin Chem 1986;32:22-9.
84. Sunderman FW. Current concepts of "normal values," "reference values," and "discrimination values" in clinical chemistry [Editorial]. Clin Chem 1975;21:1873-7.
85. Tietz NW, ed. Clinical guide to laboratory tests, 3rd edition. Philadelphia: WB Saunders, 1995.
86. Tryding N, Tufvesson C, Sonntag O, eds. Drug effects in clinical chemistry, 7th edition. Stockholm: Apoteksbolaget, 1996. [The references are found in a separate book: Tryding N, Tufvesson C, eds. References to drug effects in clinical chemistry. Stockholm: Apoteksbolaget, 1996.]
87. Van Der Meulen EA, Boogard PJ, Van Sittert NJ. Use of small-sample-based reference limits on a group basis. Clin Chem 1994;40:1698-702.
88. Virtanen A, Kairisto V, Uusipaikka E. Regression-based reference limits: determination of sufficient sample size. Clin Chem 1998;44:2353-8.
89. Winkel P. Patterns and clusters: multivariate approach for interpreting clinical chemistry results. Clin Chem 1973;19:1329-38.
90. Winkel P. The use of the subject as his own referent. In: Gräsbeck R, Alström T, eds. Reference values in laboratory medicine. Chichester, United Kingdom: John Wiley, 1981:65-78.
91. Winkel P, Lyngbye J, Jorgensen K. The normal region: a multivariate problem. Scand J Clin Lab Invest 1972;30:339-44.
92. Young DS. Effects of preanalytical variables on clinical laboratory tests, 3rd edition. Washington, DC: AACC Press, 2007.
93. Young DS. Effects of drugs on clinical laboratory tests, 5th edition. Washington, DC: AACC Press, 2000.

CHAPTER 6

Preanalytical Variables and Biological Variation

Donald S. Young, M.B., Ph.D.

The human body is composed of many different compounds and elements; the concentration or activity of these analytes in body fluids may reflect an individual's health or pathophysiological state. Many factors other than disease may affect the concentration or activity of these analytes.[31,49]

PREANALYTICAL VARIABLES

Preanalytical variables fall under two categories: those that are controllable and those that are not. Those that can be controlled have short-lived effects. Duration of the other factors is much longer. Standardization of specimen collection practices minimizes the variables that cause changes in test values within 1 day or from one day to another, thereby reducing the difficulty in interpretation of values. However, in clinical practice, standardization is rarely possible. Thus one must understand the influences of controllable and uncontrollable variables on the composition of body fluids.

Controllable Variables

Controlling variations begins with specimen collection. Collecting appropriate blood specimens involves both proper preparation of the individual and attention to the details of the technique of specimen collection. Controllable variables include physiologic variables such as posture, prolonged bed rest, exercise, physical fitness and training, circadian variation, and travel. Diet, life-style, stimulants, drugs, herbal preparations, and recreational drug ingestion are additional examples of variables that can be controlled. A few of the more important influences are discussed in this chapter.

In clinical practice, it is rarely possible to standardize specimen collection conditions to the extent that is ideal for proper interpretation of results. However, certain actions should be taken in an attempt to ensure proper specimens for testing. An essential element is proper identification of the patient and his/her specimen. At least two permanent identifiers [i.e., patient names (last and first), date of birth, medical record number] need to be used, with the same information contained on the test requisition form and on the specimen label. If specimens are collected for medicolegal purposes, a chain of custody system must be established to ensure that all persons handling or processing the specimen are identified. To protect both the patient and the phlebotomists when blood specimens are collected, the phlebotomist should wear gloves and protective impervious clothing. To draw specimens from infectious patients, the phlebotomist should also wear a facemask and goggles.

If pertinent for the requested tests, the phlebotomist should verify that the patient is fasting. Ideally, a patient should have remained in the same position for 30 minutes before a specimen is collected, and in the same position as likely to be appropriate for the next specimen to be collected (e.g., supine if an inpatient, sitting if an outpatient). A tourniquet should be used to facilitate location of a vein for venipuncture, but application for longer than 1 minute begins to induce hemoconcentration. An appropriately sized needle should be used to lessen the possibility of hemolysis. Other precautions must also be taken to prevent hemolysis—no shaking of tubes or vigorous mixing of blood or puncturing of skin before the alcohol used to clean the skin has evaporated.[105] Hemolysis may lead to false results through leakage of analytes from erythrocytes or through interference with certain photometric methods.[104] The extent of the interference is typically related to the degree of hemolysis. Use of an evacuated blood tube system to collect blood is preferred to use of a syringe to minimize hemolysis, and blood collected into one type of tube should never be transferred into another tube. Each laboratory must define which types of specimens are appropriate for the analytical methods that it uses. Generally, plasma allows more rapid processing of specimens for chemistry tests, but anticoagulants may interfere with some analytical methods.[104] However, serum concentrations of potassium and phosphate may be as much as 8.4% and 7.0% higher, respectively, than in plasma, and other analytes may be affected to a lesser extent.[58] The composition of blood from different vascular locations (e.g., capillary, artery, vein) may be slightly different, so consistent use of the same source of blood is desirable.[105]

Although testing of urine is common, the types of specimens needed for different tests can be quite different. For example, the first morning specimen is usually the most concentrated and is most appropriate for microscopic examination, whereas specimens collected over 24 hours are most appropriate for quantitative measurements. The appropriate preservative for urine specimens depends on the analytes to be measured (e.g., alkalinized specimens are most appropriate for porphyrins and uric acid, whereas no preservative or acidification is more appropriate for other analytes). Cerebrospinal fluid and abnormal fluids such as pleural or ascitic fluid must be collected under sterile conditions because microbiological testing is frequently required at the same time as chemistry tests. In such situations, chemistry tests should be performed on the specimen in the first tube, and the second tube should be used for culture to eliminate contamination from tissue debris or skin bacteria.

Once specimens have been collected, they should be transported rapidly to a laboratory for testing. If a blood collection site is distant from a laboratory, specimens should be collected into evacuated blood tubes containing a thixotropic polymer gel and should be centrifuged on site. The gel forms an effective barrier between the separated serum or plasma and cells, so no leakage of cellular constituents occurs into the plasma or serum above the gel. Centrifugation of specimens should be done within 2 hours of blood collection, and within the laboratory, if specimens cannot be tested in a timely manner, they must be held under appropriate storage conditions—at room temperature, refrigerated, or frozen, depending on the analyte—until testing takes place.[105]

Physiologic Variables

Physiologic variables that are controllable that affect analytical results include (1) posture, (2) prolonged bed rest, (3) exercise, (4) physical training, (5) circadian variation, and (6) travel.

Posture

In an adult, a change from a lying to an upright position results in a reduction of the person's blood volume of about 10% (≈600 to 700 mL). Because only protein-free fluid passes through the capillaries to the tissue, this change in posture results in a reduction of the plasma volume of the blood and an increase (≈8 to 10%) in the plasma protein concentration. Normally, the decrease with the change from lying to standing is complete in 10 minutes. However, an interval of 30 minutes is required for the reverse change to occur when one goes from standing to lying.

The typical pressure at the arterial end of a capillary is 24 mm Hg (3.2 kPa), and at the venous end 10 mm Hg (1.3 kPa), although this varies with the distance of the capillary from the heart.[74] Transfer of fluid and solute across a capillary wall depends on a complex interaction of hydrostatic and osmotic pressures of capillary and interstitial fluids. Fluid moves into the interstitial space at the arteriolar end of the capillary and returns to the capillary at the venular end. A greater volume of fluid leaves the capillary at the arteriolar end than is returned to the venous end. Excess fluid drains into the lymphatic system. When an individual lies down, fluid return to the capillaries is increased, because capillary pressure is reduced. The volume of fluid returning to capillaries progressively declines when an individual is recumbent for a long time. Heart rate and systolic and diastolic blood pressures are greater in the upright than in the recumbent individual. Change in posture from lying to standing increases the secretion of catecholamines, aldosterone, angiotensin II, renin, and antidiuretic hormone (vasopressin). Epinephrine and norepinephrine concentrations in plasma may double within 10 minutes, but no change in their urinary excretion is noted. The increase in plasma aldosterone and plasma renin activity is slower, but their concentrations may still double within 1 hour. Concentrations of other hormones may also increase as a result of the relative hemoconcentration induced by standing. Typically, a 5 to 15% increase in the concentrations of most cellular elements and protein-bound molecules is also noted with a change from lying to an erect position.

Substantial changes also take place with a change from lying to a sitting position, or from standing to a supine or sitting position.[16] Reduction of the extracellular fluid volume with standing reduces the renal blood flow and causes a reduction in the glomerular filtration rate (GFR) and in urine production. Changes are apparent in 1 hour. Within 2 hours of becoming recumbent, an individual's hemoglobin and hematocrit may decrease by as much as 6.5% as the result of hypervolemia. This is associated with a reduction in the concentration of plasma protein on the order of 8% and of protein-bound constituents.[38] Although postural changes affect urinary sodium excretion, its plasma concentration is only slightly affected. Urinary excretion of sodium and lithium (used to treat some forms of schizophrenia) is reduced in response to increased aldosterone secretion, but the normal diurnal variation persists.[41] When an individual stands, his urinary pH decreases and excretion of bicarbonate is reduced as hydrogen ions are exchanged for sodium. Excretion of protein is reduced in most individuals with reduction of the glomerular filtration rate that occurs with standing. Orthostatic proteinuria is a condition in which protein is present when individuals are standing but is essentially absent when they are recumbent. This phenomenon may be caused by increased glomerular permeability from increased venous pressure. The incidence of orthostatic proteinuria is probably less than 5%.

Changes in concentration of proteins and protein-bound constituents in serum with postural changes are greater in hypertensive patients than in normotensive patients, in individuals with a low plasma protein concentration than in those with a normal concentration, and in the elderly compared with the young.[25,26] Most of the plasma oncotic pressure is attributable to albumin because of its high concentration, so that protein malnutrition—with its associated reduction in plasma albumin concentration—reduces the retention of fluid within the capillaries. Conversely, the impact of postural changes is less in individuals with abnormally high concentrations of protein, such as those with a monoclonal gammopathy (multiple myeloma). In general, the concentrations of freely diffusible constituents with molecular weights of less

TABLE 6-1 Change in Concentration of Serum Constituents With Change from Lying to Standing

Constituent	Average Increase, %
Alanine aminotransferase	7
Albumin	9
Alkaline phosphatase	7
Amylase	6
Aspartate aminotransferase	5
Calcium	3
Cholesterol	7
Immunoglobulin (Ig)A	7
IgG	7
IgM	5
Thyroxine	11
Triglycerides	6

From Felding P, Tryding N, Hyltoft Petersen P, Hørder M. Effects of posture on concentrations of blood constituents in healthy adults: practical application of blood specimen collection procedures recommended by the Scandinavian Committee on Reference Values. Scand J Clin Lab Invest 1980;40:615-21.

than 5000 Da are unaffected by postural changes. However, a significant increase in potassium (≈0.2 to 0.3 mmol/L) occurs after an individual stands for 30 minutes.[27] This increase in K^+ has been attributed to the release of intracellular potassium from muscle. Changes in the concentration of some major serum constituents with changes in posture are listed in Table 6-1.

Application of a tourniquet at the time of blood collection mimics the effect of a change from a lying to a standing position, raising the plasma concentrations of proteins and protein-bound constituents, the activities of enzymes and the counts of blood cells, and the blood hematocrit and hemoglobin concentrations.

Prolonged Bed Rest

Plasma and extracellular fluid volumes decrease within a few days of the start of bed rest. Consequently, the blood hematocrit may increase by as much as 10% within 4 days. Usually a slight reduction in total body water is noted, but with 2 weeks' bed rest the plasma volume reverts to its pre-bed rest value.[38]

Concentrations of protein-bound constituents are also reduced, although mobilization of calcium from bones with an increased free ionized fraction compensates for the reduced protein-bound calcium, so serum total calcium is less affected. Indeed, a paradoxical increase in the total plasma calcium concentration may occur. Plasma 1,25-dihydroxyvitamin D and 25-hydroxyvitamin D concentrations may decrease by as much as 20%. Plasma aspartate aminotransferase activity is usually slightly less in individuals confined to bed than in those undertaking normal physical activity. Initially and paradoxically, CK activity is increased as a result of its release from skeletal muscles, but ultimately, CK activity may be less than in active, healthy individuals. Serum potassium may be reduced by up to 0.5 mmol/L over 3 weeks in association with a reduction in skeletal muscle mass.

Prolonged bed rest is associated with increased urinary nitrogen excretion, which increases by up to 15% after 2 weeks. Calcium excretion steadily increases up to 7 weeks of rest, increasing by a maximum of about 60%. Excretion of sodium, potassium, phosphate, and sulfate is also increased but to a much smaller extent; hydrogen ion excretion is reduced, and this is presumably caused by decreased metabolism of skeletal muscle.[22] The amplitude of circadian variation of plasma cortisol is reduced by prolonged immobilization, and urinary excretion of catecholamines may be reduced to one third of the concentration in an active individual. Vanillylmandelic acid (VMA) excretion is reduced by one fourth after 2 to 3 weeks of bed rest.

When an individual becomes active after a period of bed rest, longer than 3 weeks is required before calcium excretion reverts to normal, and another 3 weeks before positive calcium balance is achieved. A period of several weeks is required before positive nitrogen balance is restored.

Exercise

In considering the effects of exercise, the nature and extent of the exercise should be taken into account.[86] Static or isometric exercise, usually of short duration but of high intensity, uses previously stored ATP and creatine phosphate, whereas more prolonged exercise must use ATP generated by normal metabolic pathways. Changes in concentrations of analytes that result from exercise are largely due to shifts of fluid between intravascular and interstitial compartments and changes in hormone concentrations stimulated by the change in activity and by the loss of fluid due to sweating. Plasma concentrations of β-endorphin and catecholamines may more than double within a minute of initiation of strenuous exercise. Hemoconcentration, affecting high molecular weight constituents, follows strenuous exercise. The physical fitness of an individual may also affect the extent of change in the concentration of a constituent; the length of time after exercise when a specimen was collected also influences the concentrations of measured analytes. Such factors account for sometimes conflicting reports in the literature.

With *moderate exercise,* the provoked stress response causes an increase in blood glucose, which stimulates insulin secretion. The arteriovenous difference in glucose concentration is increased more than 5-fold from about 14 mg/dL (0.8 mmol/L) at rest, depending on the duration and intensity of exercise in association with greater tissue demand for glucose.[97] Plasma pyruvate and lactate are increased by increased metabolic activity of skeletal muscle. Even mild exercise may increase the plasma lactate twofold. Arterial pH and PCO_2 are reduced by exercise. Reduced renal blood flow causes a slight increase in the serum creatinine concentration. Competition for renal excretion between urate, lactate, and products of increased tissue catabolism causes the plasma urate concentration to increase. Exercise causes a reduction in cellular ATP, which increases cellular permeability. Increased permeability causes slight increases in the serum activities of enzymes originating from skeletal muscle, such as AST, LD, CK, and aldolase.[94] The increase in CK is largely attributable to its CK-MM isoform, although small increases in CK-MB may also be observed. The increase in enzyme activity tends to be greater in unfit than in fit individuals. Performing normal daily activities over 4 hours may increase serum CK activity by as much as 50% in some healthy individuals.[48] Mild exercise produces a slight decrease in serum cholesterol and triglyceride concentrations that may persist for several days. Those who walk for about 4 hours each week have an average cholesterol concentration 5% lower and HDL concentration 3.4% higher than inactive individuals.

In general, the effects of *strenuous exercise* are exaggerations of those occurring with mild exercise. Thus hypoglycemia and increased glucose tolerance may occur. Plasma lactate may be increased tenfold during exercise but soon returns to normal in fit individuals. Severe exercise increases the concentration of plasma proteins owing to an influx of protein from interstitial spaces, which occurs after an initial loss of both fluid and protein through the capillaries. Plasma concentrations of total proteins increase by about 9% and renal glomerular permeability increases, leading to increased proteinuria.[75] Plasma fibrinolytic activity is also increased. Strenuous exercise may more than double CK activity, but the activity of enzymes with primarily liver or kidney origin is little changed, although hepatic and renal blood flow is reduced.

Strenuous exercise for 10 minutes increases plasma renin activity by 400%. Cortisol secretion is stimulated, and the normal diurnal variation may be abolished.[21] Urinary free cortisol excretion and plasma concentrations of cortisol, aldosterone, growth hormone (somatotropin), and prolactin are also increased by exercise. Plasma insulin concentration is decreased by exercise. Strenuous exercise increases both plasma and urinary concentrations of catecholamines. Changes in concentrations of cortisol and other stress-stimulated increased hormone concentrations are presumed to release leukocytes, primarily neutrophils, from the bone marrow into the peripheral circulation. Following strenuous exercise, the leukocyte count has been observed to increase to about 25,000 cells/μL.[41]

Blood pH, oxygen saturation, and venous bicarbonate concentrations are decreased by strenuous exercise. The concentration of triglycerides is reduced briefly by exercise, but the free fatty acid concentration is greatly increased; serum creatinine and urea nitrogen concentrations are also increased. Although the creatinine concentration returns rapidly to normal on cessation of exercise, the increased urea nitrogen concentration persists for some time. Reversible, benign hematuria and proteinuria with increased excretion of leukocytes and erythrocytes occur commonly with exercise and worsen in proportion to the extent of exercise. These may persist for 3 days following strenuous sports, but this does not warrant investigation. Urinary steroid excretion increases in response to the stress of exercise.

Some representative changes in concentration or activity of serum constituents induced by exercise are listed in Table 6-2.

Physical Training

Athletes generally have a higher serum activity of enzymes of skeletal muscular origin at rest than do nonathletes. However, the response of these enzymes to exercise is less in athletes than in other individuals. Reduced release of enzymes from skeletal muscle in well-trained individuals has been attributed to an increase in the number and size of mitochondria, allowing the muscle to better metabolize glucose, fatty acids, and ketone bodies. The proportion of CK that is CK-MB is much greater in trained than in untrained individuals.[14] Serum concentrations of urea, urate, creatinine, and thyroxine are higher in athletes than in comparable untrained individuals. Urinary excretion of creatinine is also increased. These changes are probably related to increased muscle mass and greater turnover of muscle mass in athletes.

TABLE 6-2 Effects of Strenuous Exercise on Selected Serum Constituents*

Constituent Value	% Increase	Constituent Value	% Decrease
Acid phosphatase	11	Albumin	4
Alanine aminotransferase	41	Bilirubin	4
Alkaline phosphatase	3	Iron	11
Aspartate aminotransferase	31	Lactate dehydrogenase	1
Calcium	1	Potassium	8
Chloride	1	Sodium	1
Cholesterol	3	Total lipids	12
Creatinine	17		
Phosphate	12		
Total protein	3		
Urea nitrogen	3		
Uric acid	4		

From Statland BE, Winkel P, Bokelund H. Factors contributing to variation of serum constituents in healthy subjects. In: Siest G, ed. Organisation des laboratoires: biologie perspective. Paris: L'Expansion Scientifique Francaise, 1975:717-50.

*Changes were determined 15 minutes after conclusion of 20 minutes of exercise.

Body fat is reduced by physical training. This is associated with increased HDL-cholesterol and decreased LDL-cholesterol and triglyceride concentrations, the extent of which varies with the intensity and duration of training.

Circadian Variation

Many constituents of body fluids exhibit cyclical variation throughout the day.[95,100] Factors contributing to such variation include posture, activity, food ingestion, stress, daylight or darkness, and sleep or wakefulness. The cyclical pattern tends to be similar among individuals who work during the day and sleep at night, although it is different in night workers. These cyclical variations may be quite large; therefore the timing of specimen collection must be strictly controlled. For example, the concentration of serum iron may increase by as much as 50% from 0800 to 1400, and that of cortisol by a similar amount between 0800 and 1600. Serum potassium has been reported to decline from 5.4 mmol/L at 0800 to 4.3 mmol/L at 1400.[88,89] The typical total variation in several commonly measured serum constituents over 6 hours is illustrated in Table 6-3. Total variation is contrasted with analytical error.

Hormones are secreted in bursts, and this, together with the cyclical variation to which most hormones are subject, may make it very difficult to interpret their plasma concentrations properly.[99] Corticotropin secretion is influenced by cortisol-like steroids, but it is also affected by posture and by light, darkness, and stress. Its secretion is increased threefold to fivefold from its minimum between afternoon and midnight to its maximum around waking. Growth hormone and epinephrine concentrations exhibit similar change throughout the day. Cortisol concentrations are greatest around 0600 to 0800 hours, and one study reported mean minima and maxima of 15.8 μg/dL and 111 μg/dL, respectively, at different times during the day.[52]

Maximum renin activity normally occurs early in the morning during sleep; its minimum occurs late in the afternoon. The plasma aldosterone concentration shows a similar pattern. GFR varies inversely with the secretion of renin, probably through constriction of renal efferent arterioles.[42] GFR is least at the time of maximum renin secretion and is 20% greater in the afternoon, when renin activity is at a minimum. Excretion of 17-ketosteroids and 17-hydroxycorticosteroids is low at night and reaches a maximum about midafternoon.

No circadian variation in plasma concentrations of FSH and LH is noted in men, but a 20 to 40% increase in plasma testosterone occurs during the night. Prolactin is secreted, similar to other hormones such as LH and FSH, in multiple bursts; prolactin concentration is greatest during sleep.[99] The pituitary gland regulates hormone secretion primarily through negative feedback generated by increased circulating concentrations of circulating hormones. To perform a precise assessment of the concentration of a hormone, several measurements may be required.

Serum TSH is at a maximum between 0200 and 0400, and is at a minimum between 1800 and 2200. The variation is on the order of 50 to 206%.[52] Variations in serum thyroxine concentrations also occur, but these appear to be related to changes in the concentration of binding protein brought about by changes in posture. These variations are maximal at

TABLE 6-3 Total and Analytical Variation for Serum Tests on Specimens Obtained at 0800 and 1400*

Constituent	Mean	Total Variation, %	Analytical Variation, %
Sodium, mmol/L	141	1.9	1.8
Potassium, mmol/L	4.4	7.1	2.8
Calcium, mg/dL	10.8	3.2	2.7
Chloride, mmol/L	102	3.8	3.4
Phosphate, mg/dL	3.8	10.7	2.4
Urea nitrogen, mg/dL	14	22.5	2.5
Creatinine, mg/dL	1.0	14.5	6.3
Uric acid, mg/dL	5.6	11.5	2.6
Iron, μg/dL	116	36.6	3.4
Cholesterol, mg/dL	193	14.8	5.7
Albumin, g/dL	4.5	5.5	3.9
Total protein, g/dL	7.3	4.8	1.7
Total lipids, g/L	5.3	25.0	3.6
Aspartate aminotransferase, U/L	9	25	6
Alanine aminotransferase, U/L	6	56	17
Acid phosphatase, U/L	3	15	8
Alkaline phosphatase, U/L	63	20	3
Lactate dehydrogenase, U/L	195	16	12

*11 male subjects, age 21 to 27 years, studied at 0800, 1100, and 1400.

From Winkel P, Statland BE, Bokelund H. The effects of time of venipuncture on variation of serum constituents. Am J Clin Pathol 1975;64:433-47.

between 1000 and 1400. Total protein concentration may vary by as much as 10% over 24 hours, but variation in individual proteins may be even greater.

Growth hormone secretion is greatest shortly after sleep commences. Conversely, basal plasma insulin is higher in the morning than later in the day, and its response to glucose is also greatest in the morning and least at about midnight. When a glucose tolerance test is given in the afternoon, higher glucose values occur than when the test is given early in the day. Higher plasma glucose occurs in spite of a greater insulin response, which is nevertheless delayed and less effective.

Urinary excretion of catecholamines and their metabolites is less at night than during the day. The effect is related to activity, because in night workers, excretion is less during the day.

Peak urinary excretion of sodium and potassium occurs about noon, whereas excretion of calcium and magnesium is greatest during the night. Urinary phosphate excretion is low at night, with the result that serum phosphate is as much as 30% higher at night than during the morning. Urinary volume and creatinine excretion are low during the night. Creatinine clearance may be reduced by up to 10% during the night. Night urine contains excess ammonia, and its titratable acidity is high.[90]

Blood cell concentrations are affected by circadian rhythms, with neutrophil and lymphocyte counts increasing by 61% and 67%, respectively, at their peaks from their nadir concentrations.[52]

Travel

Travel across several time zones affects the normal circadian rhythm. Five days is required to establish a new stable diurnal rhythm after travel across 10 time zones. Changes in laboratory test results are attributable to altered pituitary and adrenal function. Urinary excretion of catecholamines is usually increased for 2 days, and serum cortisol is reduced. During a 20-hour flight, serum glucose and triglyceride concentrations increase, while glucocorticoid secretion is stimulated. During such a prolonged flight, fluid and sodium retention occurs, but urinary excretion returns to normal after 2 days.[11]

Space travel is associated with a decrease in blood and plasma volumes and is further associated with increases in plasma antidiuretic hormone, atrial natriuretic peptide, growth hormone, cortisol, and corticotropin concentrations.[60] In contrast, the plasma renin activity may be decreased by as much as 50%. Plasma aldosterone may also decrease but to a lesser extent. In spite of the stress of space travel, plasma concentrations of catecholamines are usually unaffected. Space travel leads to bone demineralization and a negative calcium and phosphate balance, primarily caused by increased excretion of these minerals. However, concentrations of commonly measured analytes generally do not exceed the reference range when astronauts adapt to space travel.[102]

Diet

Diet has considerable influence on the composition of plasma. Studies with synthetic diets have shown that day-to-day changes in the amount of protein are reflected within a few days in the composition of nitrogenous components of plasma and in the excretion of end products of protein metabolism.

Four days after the change from a normal diet to a high-protein diet, doubling of the plasma urea concentration occurs, along with an increase in its urinary excretion.[9] Serum cholesterol, phosphate, urate, and ammonia concentrations are also increased. High protein intake increases both serum and urinary urea and urate. A high-fat diet, in contrast, depletes the nitrogen pool because of the requirement for excretion of ammonium ions to maintain acid-base homeostasis. A high-fat diet increases the serum concentration of triglycerides but reduces serum urate. Reduction of fat intake reduces serum lactate dehydrogenase activity. Ingestion of very different amounts of cholesterol has little effect on its serum concentration; an increase in intake of 50% may affect the serum concentration by only 5 to 10 mg/dL (0.13 to 0.26 mmol/L).[54] Ingestion of monounsaturated fat instead of saturated fat reduces cholesterol and LDL-cholesterol concentrations. When polyunsaturated fat is substituted for saturated fat, the concentrations of triglycerides and HDL-cholesterol are reduced. Notwithstanding the conclusions of previous studies, a 2009 report suggests that different types of diets have a similar influence on the plasma concentrations of lipids, and that total caloric ingestion is the primary influence on an individual's body mass and blood lipid concentrations, with total and LDL-cholesterol and triglyceride concentrations decreasing and HDL-cholesterol increasing similarly when volunteers were fed different weight-loss diets.[81]

When dietary carbohydrates consist mainly of starch or sucrose rather than other sugars, the serum activities of ALP and LD are increased. AST and ALT activities are also influenced by the type of sugar ingested, being higher with a sugar diet than with a starch-based diet.[51] Plasma triglyceride concentration is reduced when sucrose intake is decreased. Peak glucose concentration tends to be less during a glucose tolerance test in individuals habitually ingesting a bread diet than when a high-sucrose diet is ingested. A high-carbohydrate diet decreases the serum concentrations of LDL-cholesterol, triglycerides, cholesterol, and protein. Individuals who eat many small meals throughout the day tend to have total LDL- and HDL-cholesterol concentrations that are lower than when food of the same type and amount is eaten in three meals.[2]

In addition to the types of foods and drinks ingested, specific food-related situations influence plasma composition. These include vegetarianism, obesity, malnutrition, fasting, and starvation.

Food Ingestion

The concentration of certain plasma constituents is affected by the ingestion of a meal, with the time between ingestion of a meal and collection of blood affecting the plasma concentrations of many analytes. For example, fasting overnight for 10 to 14 hours before blood collection noticeably decreases the variability in concentration of many analytes and is seen as the optimal time for fasting around which to standardize blood collections.[24] The biggest increases in serum concentration that occur after a meal are noted for glucose and triglycerides.[13] The increase in ALP (mainly intestinal isoenzyme) is greater when a fatty meal is ingested and is influenced by the blood group of the individual and the substrate used for the enzyme assay. Activities of alanine and aspartate aminotransferases may increase by 10 to 20% following a meal.[49] In addition, lipemia following a meal may affect some analytical methods used to measure serum constituents. Ultracentrifugation or the use of serum blanks can reduce the adverse analytical effects of lipemia.

The effects of a meal may be long lasting. Thus ingestion of a protein-rich meal in the evening may cause increases in concentration of serum urea nitrogen, phosphorus, and urate that are still apparent 12 hours later.[1] Nevertheless, these changes may be less than the typical intraindividual variability. Large protein meals at lunch or in the evening increase serum cholesterol and growth hormone concentrations for at least 1 hour after a meal. The effect of carbohydrate meals on blood composition is less than that of protein meals. No change in the cortisol concentration is noted when breakfast is taken, probably because cortisol completely occupies all cortisol binding sites on its binding protein in the early morning. Glucagon and insulin secretions are stimulated by a protein meal, and insulin is also stimulated by carbohydrate meals.

In response to a meal, the stomach secretes hydrochloric acid, causing a reduction in the plasma chloride concentration. Venous blood from the stomach contains an increased amount of bicarbonate. This condition reflects a mild metabolic alkalosis ("alkaline tide") and increased PCO_2. The metabolic alkalosis is sufficient to reduce serum-free ionized calcium by 0.2 mg/dL (0.05 mmol/L). After ingestion of a meal, the liver becomes the prime site for metabolism of ingested substances. Ingestion of therapeutic drugs with meals may have considerable influence on the characteristic absorption and metabolism of each drug.

The effects of ingestion of a 700-kcal (2.93-MJ) meal on some commonly measured blood constituents are illustrated in Table 6-4. These effects differ with different meals. Thus the glucose increase is often greater and phosphate is usually decreased after a carbohydrate meal.[90]

Ingestion of one glass of water leads to statistically, but not clinically, significant alterations in the concentration of several commonly measured test constituents. When 75 g glucose is ingested with water, as in a glucose tolerance test, the concentration of glucose is increased. This stimulates the secretion of insulin. Insulin causes the release of sodium from cells and stimulates the transport of potassium into cells.

TABLE 6-4 Influence of a Standard 700-kcal Meal on Serum Constituents*

Constituent	Before Meal	2 h After† Meal
Alanine aminotransferase, U/L	31	33
Albumin, g/dL	4.5	4.6
Alkaline phosphatase, U/L	46	46
Aspartate aminotransferase, U/L	22	28
Bilirubin, total, mg/dL	0.7	0.8
Calcium, mg/dL	9.9	10.0
Cholesterol, mg/dL	220.0	220.0
Glucose, mg/dL	71	82*
Lactate dehydrogenase, U/L	198	198
Phosphate, mg/dL	3.1	3.6*
Potassium, mmol/L	3.8	4.0*
Sodium, mmol/L	140	141
Protein, total, g/dL	7.8	7.9
Urea nitrogen, mg/dL	16	16
Uric acid, mg/dL	6.0	6.2

*Results are mean values in 200 healthy individuals.
†Note that other studies have reported different changes based on different content and amounts of food.
From Steinmetz J, Panek E, Sourieau F, Siest G. Influence of food intake on biological parameters. In: Siest G (ed). Reference values in human chemistry. Basel: Karger, 1973:193-200; Cohn JS, McNamara JR, Cohn SD, et al. Postprandial plasma lipoprotein changes in human subjects of different ages. J Lipid Res 1988;29:469-79. (These investigators have reported increases in plasma triglyceride concentrations greater than 150% after a high-fat meal.)

Ingestion of Specific Foods and Beverages

Constituents of food and drink affect the composition of plasma. Bran, serotonin, and caffeine are examples of such constituents.

Bran. Habitual ingestion of bran, which is widely promoted to improve the concentration of lipids, impedes absorption of certain compounds, including calcium, cholesterol, and triglycerides, from the gastrointestinal tract. The concentration of calcium may be reduced by as much as 0.3 mg/dL (0.08 mmol/L) and that of triglycerides by 20 mg/dL (0.23 mmol/L), especially if triglycerides were high initially.[46] Pectin and dietary fibers reduce serum apolipoprotein B and cholesterol concentrations.

Food Constituents. The composition of common foods is often overlooked. Many fruits, such as bananas, and vegetables that contain 5-hydroxytryptamine (serotonin) cause increased excretion of 5-HIAA. Avocados impair glucose tolerance by affecting insulin secretion. Onions reduce plasma glucose and the insulin response to glucose. Garlic ingestion may reduce serum cholesterol concentrations by about 9%.[104]

Caffeine. Caffeine is contained in many beverages, including coffee, tea, and colas, and has a considerable effect on the concentration of blood constituents. Caffeine stimulates the adrenal medulla, causing increased secretion of epinephrine, reflected in a two- to threefold increase in the plasma epinephrine concentration. Excretion of the catecholamines and their metabolites is increased and a slight increase in plasma glucose concentration occurs as a result of increased gluconeogenesis with concomitant impairment of glucose tolerance.[5] The adrenal cortex is also affected; plasma cortisol is increased, and this is accompanied by increased excretion of free cortisol, 11-hydroxycorticoids, and 5-HIAA. The effect of caffeine may be so great that the normal diurnal variation of plasma cortisol may be suppressed. Plasma renin activity may also be increased following caffeine ingestion. Caffeinated, but not decaffeinated, coffee causes diuresis with a transient increase in excretion of sodium and potassium. It does this by inhibiting the reabsorption of electrolytes in the ascending loop of Henle of the renal nephrons.[66]

Caffeine has a marked effect on lipid metabolism. Ingestion of two cups of coffee may increase the plasma free fatty acid concentration by as much as 30% and those of glycerol, total lipids, and lipoproteins to a lesser extent. Activation of triglyceride lipase causes an increase in nonesterified fatty acid concentration. Prolonged ingestion of caffeine (e.g., over several weeks) causes a slight reduction in the serum cholesterol concentration but an increase in the serum triglyceride concentration. Because the effect on plasma LDL-cholesterol and apolipoprotein B is greater in individuals drinking decaffeinated coffee than in those drinking regular coffee, the effects may be unrelated to caffeine.[92]

Caffeine is also a potent stimulant of the secretion of gastric juice, hydrochloric acid, and pepsin. The serum gastrin concentration may be increased by as much as five times after three cups of coffee are ingested. Coffee has a diuretic effect, and it increases the excretion of erythrocytes and renal tubular cells in the urine. Caffeine increases the absolute amounts of sodium, potassium, calcium, and magnesium in urine—an effect that is not observed with decaffeinated coffee.

Vegetarianism

In long-standing vegetarians, the concentration of VLDL-cholesterol is reduced, typically by 12%, compared with nonvegetarians. Total lipid and phospholipid concentrations are reduced, and concentrations of cholesterol and triglycerides may be only two thirds of those in individuals on a mixed diet. Both HDL- and LDL-cholesterol concentrations are affected. In strict vegetarians, the LDL-cholesterol concentration may be 37% less and the HDL-cholesterol concentration 12% less than in nonvegetarians. The cholesterol : HDL-cholesterol ratio is decreased. Effects are less notable in individuals who have been on a vegetarian diet for only a short time. Lipid concentrations are also less in individuals who eat only a vegetable diet than in those who consume eggs and milk as well. Little difference is seen in the concentration of protein or the activities of enzymes in the serum of long-standing vegetarians and individuals on a mixed diet. A vegetarian diet does not appear to affect liver function in that liver function tests are similar in vegans and nonvegans.[37] The serum creatinine concentration may be slightly reduced in vegetarians because of reduced ingestion of protein, but urinary excretion of creatinine and its clearance may be almost 40% less than in meat-eaters.[61] Plasma concentrations of trace elements tend to be reduced in vegans. For example, serum copper may be reduced by 20%, selenium by 10%, and zinc by more than 10% after individuals have consumed a lactovegetarian diet for 3 months.[87] Although the plasma concentration of many vitamins is increased, that of vitamin B_{12} may be reduced in vegetarians to a concentration approaching that observed in deficiency. An explanation for the low vitamin B_{12} and the high bilirubin still has to be established. Differences in the composition of serum of vegetarians and nonvegetarians are shown in Table 6-5. Urinary pH is usually higher in vegetarians than in meat-eaters as the result of reduced intake of precursors of acid metabolites.

TABLE 6-5 Comparison of Blood Constituents Between Vegetarians and Nonvegetarians

Constituent	Vegetarians	Nonvegetarians
S-Albumin, g/dL	4.2	4.3
P-Calcium, mg/dL	9.4	9.7
P-Cholesterol, mg/dL	213	252
P-HDL cholesterol, mg/dL	66	66
B-Glucose, mg/dL	90	101
B-Hemoglobin, g/dL	13.9	14.3
P-Triglycerides, mg/dL	106	124
B-Urea nitrogen, mg/dL	14	16
P-Uric acid, mg/dL	5.3	5.8

B, Whole blood; *P*, plasma; *S*, serum.
From Gear JS, Mann JI, Thorogood M, Carter R, Jelfs R. Biochemical and haematological variables in vegetarians. Br Med J 1980;280:1415.

Malnutrition

In malnutrition, the plasma concentrations of most proteins, including total protein, albumin, prealbumin, and β-globulin, are reduced. The frequently increased concentration of γ-globulin does not fully compensate for the decrease in other proteins. Concentrations of complement C3, retinol-binding globulin, transferrin, and prealbumin decrease rapidly with the onset of malnutrition and are measured to define the severity of the condition.[72] Plasma concentrations of lipoproteins are reduced, and serum cholesterol and triglycerides may be only 50% of the concentrations in healthy individuals. In spite of severe malnutrition, glucose concentration is maintained close to that in healthy individuals. However, the concentrations of serum urea nitrogen and creatinine are greatly reduced as a result of decreased skeletal mass, and creatinine clearance is decreased.

The plasma cortisol concentration is increased, largely as the result of an increase in the free cortisol moiety, but also possibly because of decreased metabolic clearance. Plasma concentrations of total T_3 and T_4 are considerably reduced, with the thyroxine concentration being most affected. This is due in part to reduced concentrations of TBG and prealbumin.

Erythrocyte and plasma folate concentrations are reduced in protein-calorie malnutrition, but the serum vitamin B_{12}

concentration is unaffected or may even be slightly increased.[55] Plasma concentrations of vitamins A and E are reduced, but the extent depends on the cause and duration of the malnutrition (e.g., dietary or iatrogenic, such as bariatric surgery). The blood hemoglobin concentration is reduced, but the serum iron concentration initially is little affected by malnutrition, although decreased plasma transferrin concentrations ultimately lead to reduced iron concentrations.

The activity of most of the commonly measured enzymes is reduced but increases with restoration of good nutrition.

Long-Term Fasting and Starvation

Withdrawal of most caloric intake has been used to treat certain cases of obesity. Such withdrawal provokes many metabolic responses. The body attempts to conserve protein at the expense of other sources of energy, such as fat. The blood glucose concentration decreases by as much as 18 mg/dL (1 mmol/L) within 3 days of the start of a fast, in spite of the body's attempts to maintain glucose production.[67] Insulin secretion is greatly reduced, whereas glucagon secretion may double in an attempt to maintain normal glucose concentration. Lipolysis and hepatic ketogenesis are stimulated. Amino acids are released from skeletal muscle, and the plasma concentration of branched-chain amino acids may increase by as much as 100% with 1 day of fasting, but the urea concentration decreases. Ketoacids and fatty acids become the principal sources of energy for muscle. This results in an accumulation of organic acids that leads to a metabolic acidosis with reduction of blood pH, PCO_2, and plasma bicarbonate concentrations. In addition, the concentrations of ketone bodies (acetoacetic acid, β-hydroxybutyric acid, and acetone), fatty acids, and glycerol in serum rise considerably. When individuals are fasted for 60 hours compared with the usual 12 hours typically used in clinical practice to obtain baseline laboratory values, plasma insulin concentrations are reduced by half and those of C-peptide by more than one third. In contrast, concentrations of glucagon, epinephrine, and norepinephrine are doubled, and that of growth hormone is increased fivefold.[10]

The breakdown of fat leads to a transient increase in body water. Typically, however, an osmotic diuresis soon reduces the blood volume. Fasting for 6 days increases plasma concentrations of cholesterol and triglycerides but causes a decrease in HDL-cholesterol concentration.[82] After individuals lived for 4 weeks on a 400-kcal diet, the concentrations of urea and triglycerides and the activity of gamma-glutamyltransferase decreased by 20 to 50%, whereas concentrations of urate, derived from nucleoprotein, and creatinine and the activity of AST increased by 20 to 40%.[96] Reduced GFR and competition for excretion from lactate and ketoacids contribute to the increased urate concentration.

Hepatic blood supply may be reduced with starvation. BSP retention is increased, and serum bilirubin rises; unconjugated bilirubin more than doubles within 48 hours.[3] Slight increases in the serum activities of aspartate and alanine aminotransferase and of lactate dehydrogenase are observed within 2 weeks of the start of a fast, but return to baseline within 4 to 6 weeks.[34] Enzyme changes may be linked more to focal necrosis of the liver than to general circulatory impairment.

In spite of the catabolism of tissue induced by starvation, the serum protein concentration is little affected initially; ultimately, a reduction occurs. With the onset of starvation, aldosterone secretion increases, leading to increased urinary excretion and decreased plasma concentration of potassium. Magnesium, calcium, and phosphate are affected similarly, although the urinary excretion of phosphate gradually declines. Although the plasma urea concentration is not significantly affected by 10 days of starvation, the absolute urinary excretion of urea, total nitrogen, and creatinine is increased over the first few days of starvation.[15]

Plasma growth hormone concentration may rise by as much as 15 times at the start of a fast but may return to normal after 3 days. Reduced energy expenditure is associated with decreased concentrations of thyroid hormones. Free and total triiodothyronine is decreased by up to 50% within 3 days of the start of a fast. Free thyroxine concentration is also affected, but to a lesser extent; total thyroxine is little changed. Urinary free cortisol is decreased by fasting, and the plasma cortisol concentration (free and total) shows a slight increase, together with loss of the normal diurnal variation.

Early in refeeding, sodium retention occurs as a result of decreased sodium and chloride excretion in the urine.[77] The reduction in potassium excretion takes longer. These events are associated with an even greater secretion of aldosterone than occurs during the period of fasting. Abnormal concentrations of most constituents rapidly revert to normal with refeeding. Nitrogen balance soon becomes positive, especially if the nonprotein calories are derived mainly from carbohydrate.

Life-Style

Life-style factors that affect the concentrations of commonly measured analytes include smoking and alcohol ingestion.

Smoking

Smoking, through the action of nicotine, may affect several laboratory tests. The extent of the effect is related to the number of cigarettes smoked and to the amount of smoke inhaled.

Through stimulation of the adrenal medulla, nicotine increases the concentration of epinephrine in the plasma and the urinary excretion of catecholamines and their metabolites.[18] Glucose concentration may be increased by 10 mg/dL (0.56 mmol/L) within 10 minutes of smoking a cigarette. The increase may persist for 1 hour. Plasma lactate is increased by about 0.3 μmol/L and because the pyruvate concentration is reduced by about 20 μmol/L the lactate:pyruvate ratio increases significantly within 10 minutes. Plasma insulin concentration shows a delayed response to the increase in blood glucose, rising about 1 hour after a cigarette is smoked. Typically, the plasma glucose concentration is higher in smokers than in nonsmokers, and glucose tolerance is mildly impaired

TABLE 6-6 Reported Increased Concentrations in Serum in Smokers

Constituent	% Change
Albumin	3
Cholesterol	3-4
Glucose	10
LDL-cholesterol	2
Phospholipids	5
Triglycerides	9-20
Urea nitrogen	10
VLDL-cholesterol	10

From Siest G, Henny J, Schiele F, (eds). Interpretation des examens de laboratoire. Basel: Karger, 1981; Craig W, Palomaki GE, Haddow JE. Cigarette smoking and serum lipid and lipoprotein concentrations: an analysis of published data. Br Med J 1989;298:784-8.

in smokers. The plasma growth hormone concentration is particularly sensitive to smoking. It may increase 10-fold within 30 minutes after an individual has smoked a cigarette.[64]

Plasma cholesterol, triglyceride, and LDL-cholesterol concentrations are higher (by about 3%, 9%, and 2%, respectively) in smokers than in nonsmokers. In contrast, serum apolipoprotein A-I and HDL-cholesterol concentrations are lower in smokers than in nonsmokers, by 8.9% and 5.7%, respectively.[17] Free fatty acid concentration tends to be variable, but inhalation during smoking produces an immediate increase in free fatty acids of about 30%. Serum C-reactive protein concentrations in current smokers may be almost twice as high as in nonsmokers (2.53 mg/L vs. 1.35 mg/L).[98] Some of the effects of smoking on serum constituents are listed in Table 6-6.

Smoking also affects the adrenal cortex; plasma 11-hydroxycorticosteroids may be increased by 75% with heavy smoking. In addition, the plasma cortisol concentration may increase by as much as 40% within 5 minutes of the start of smoking, although the normal diurnal rhythmicity of cortisol is unaffected. Smokers excrete more 5-hydroxyindoleacetic acid than do nonsmokers.

The blood erythrocyte count is increased in smokers. The amount of carboxyhemoglobin may exceed 10% of the total hemoglobin in heavy smokers, and the increased number of cells compensates for impaired ability of the red cells to transport oxygen. The blood PO_2 of the habitual smoker is usually about 5 mm Hg (0.7 kPa) less than in the nonsmoker, whereas the PCO_2 is unaffected. The blood leukocyte concentration is increased by as much as 30% in smokers, but the leukocyte concentration of ascorbic acid is greatly reduced. The lymphocyte count is increased as a proportion of the total leukocyte count.

Fluid retention caused by nicotine causes a mild decrease in the plasma protein concentration but without demonstrable effect on the calcium concentration or on the activity of serum enzymes. The plasma urate concentration is less in smokers than in nonsmokers, probably as a result of lessened intake of food by smokers. Both the serum urea and creatinine concentrations tend to be less in smokers than in nonsmokers.

Nicotine is a potent stimulant of the secretion of gastric juice. Volume and acid secretion are increased within 1 hour of smoking several cigarettes. In contrast, the bicarbonate concentration and the volume of pancreatic juice are reduced.

Smoking affects the body's immune response. For example, serum immunoglobulin (Ig)A, IgG, and IgM concentrations are generally lower in smokers than in nonsmokers, whereas the IgE concentration is higher. Smokers, more often than nonsmokers, may show the presence of antinuclear antibodies. The concentration of carcinoembryonic antigen has been reported to be as much as 70% higher in habitual smokers than in nonsmokers. The serum vitamin B_{12} concentration is often notably reduced in smokers, and the decrease is in inverse proportion to the serum concentration of thiocyanate.

The sperm count of male smokers is often reduced compared with that in nonsmokers: the number of abnormal forms is greater, and sperm motility is less.

Although an individual may have smoked previously, some residual influences may continue to be observed. Thus the erythrocyte folate concentration, on average, may be as much as almost 10% less compared with the concentration in nonsmokers. The reduction in serum concentration may be even greater. Plasma fibrinogen concentrations are increased by smoking, but it takes longer than 5 years after individuals stop smoking before fibrinogen concentrations revert to those in life-long nonsmokers.[65] Although the hematocrit reverts to nonsmoker levels within 5 years of cessation, it may take as long as 20 years before the leukocyte count becomes the same as in nonsmokers.[98]

Alcohol Ingestion

A single moderate dose of alcohol has few effects on laboratory tests. Ingestion of enough alcohol to produce mild inebriation may increase the blood glucose concentration by 20 to 50%. The increase may be even higher in persons with diabetes. More commonly, inhibition of gluconeogenesis occurs and becomes apparent as hypoglycemia and ketonemia as ethanol is metabolized to acetaldehyde and to acetate. Hypoglycemia is most common in children, alcoholics, and the malnourished. Lactate and acetate accumulate and compete with urate for excretion in the kidneys, so that the serum urate is also increased. Marked hypertriglyceridemia after alcohol ingestion is due to a combination of increased triglyceride formation in the liver and impaired removal of chylomicrons and VLDL from the circulation. The effect is most noticeable when alcohol is ingested with a fatty meal and may persist for longer than 12 hours. When moderate amounts of alcohol are ingested for 1 week, the serum triglyceride concentration is increased by more than 20 mg/dL (0.23 mmol/L). The plasma concentration of aldosterone may be increased by as much as 150% and that of prolactin by 40 to 50% within 2 to 4 hours of alcohol ingestion. Acute alcohol ingestion has been reported to increase the activity of several serum enzymes, including GGT, isocitrate dehydrogenase, and ornithine carbamoyltransferase.[33] A single acute ingestion of alcohol (1 g/kg body weight) has been shown to be enough to increase the serum activity of GGT by almost 10% 4 hours later, and by about 100% 24 hours later—a manifestation of hepatic microsomal enzyme induction.[71]

Prolonged moderate ingestion of alcohol may increase the HDL-cholesterol concentration, which is associated with reduced plasma concentration of cholesterol ester transfer protein (CETP). Phenols in wine with potent antioxidant activity are probably responsible for reducing the oxidation of LDL-cholesterol.

Intoxicating amounts of alcohol stimulate the release of cortisol, although the effect is related more to the intoxication than to the alcohol per se. Sympatheticomedullary activity is increased by acute alcohol ingestion but without detectable effect on the plasma epinephrine concentration and with only a mild effect on norepinephrine. With intoxication, plasma concentrations of catecholamines are substantially increased. Acute ingestion of alcohol leads to a sharp reduction in plasma testosterone in men, with an increase in the plasma luteinizing hormone concentration. Acute ethanol ingestion also leads to a mild diuresis by inhibiting antidiuretic hormone secretion.[80]

Chronic alcohol ingestion affects the activity of many serum enzymes. GGT activity has been extensively studied, and increased activity of the enzyme is used as a marker of persistent drinking. The increase may be as much as 1000-fold. Chronic alcoholism is associated with many characteristic biochemical abnormalities, including abnormal pituitary, adrenal cortical, and medullary function. AST and ALT activities may be increased by 250% and 60%, respectively, in habitual alcohol users. Alcohol ingestion also has considerable influence on serum HDL-cholesterol and total cholesterol concentration.[104] Measurement of carbohydrate-deficient transferrin is becoming increasingly popular as a means of identifying habitual alcohol ingestion. Desialylation of proteins occurs because of inhibition of enzymatic glycosylation in the liver by alcohol. Increased mean cell volume (MCV) has also been used as a marker of habitual alcohol use and may be related to folic acid deficiency or a direct toxic effect of alcohol on red blood cell precursors.

Drug Administration

It is rare for a patient to be hospitalized without receiving medication. For certain medical conditions, more than 10 drugs may be administered at one time. Even many healthy individuals take several drugs regularly, such as vitamins, oral contraceptives, or sleeping tablets. Individuals with chronic diseases often ingest drugs on a continuing basis. The effects of drugs on laboratory tests may be manifest through their therapeutic intent, but also through side effects and patient idiosyncratic responses to their administration. Effects on the composition of body fluids are likely to be more apparent when large doses of a drug are administered for a long time than when administration of a single dose occurs on an isolated occasion. Coadministration of certain drugs may influence the metabolism of one or the other to alter their plasma concentrations and pharmacologic effects.[70] Drugs may also have in vitro effects on laboratory tests, often through spectral interferences with colorimetric methods. A comprehensive listing of the effects of drugs on laboratory tests is available.[103] Only a few representative effects are discussed here.

Many drugs, when administered intramuscularly, cause sufficient muscle irritation to increase amounts of enzyme released into the serum. Activities of CK, aldolase, and the skeletal muscle component of lactate dehydrogenase are increased in the serum. The increased activities may persist for several days after a single injection, and consistently high values may be observed during a course of treatment. *Penicillin* derivatives given intramuscularly are particularly likely to increase the activity of these enzymes, although any drug given intramuscularly appears capable of increasing enzyme activity.

Opiates, such as morphine or meperidine, can cause spasm of the sphincter of Oddi. The spasm transmits pressure back to the liver, causing release of liver and pancreatic enzymes into the serum.

Oral contraceptives affect many different constituents measured in the clinical laboratory. Tests are affected by both progestin and estrogen components. The overall effect depends on the proportion and amount of the two components. Many of the effects are related to estrogen-induced synthesis of hormone-binding proteins in the liver. This leads to increased plasma concentrations of thyroid hormones, glucocorticoids, and sex steroids, although concentrations of the free hormones are unaffected. Contraceptives containing only progestin may be associated with reduced plasma HDL-concentrations and increased LDL-cholesterol concentrations. With modern low-dose contraceptives, effects on lipid metabolism may be clinically insignificant, although the ethinyl estradiol component may increase the concentration of some coagulation factors.[62]

Diuretic drugs often cause a mild reduction of the plasma potassium concentration; hyponatremia may be observed. Hypercalcemia may occur with hemoconcentration, but occasionally the free ionized and protein-bound fraction is increased. Thiazides may cause hypokalemia, which is often associated with hyperglycemia and reduced glucose tolerance, especially in those with diabetes. Thiazides may cause prerenal azotemia with hyperuricemia as a result of decreased renal blood flow and GFR as a result of reduced blood volume. Thiazides, similar to other diuretics, by causing hemoconcentration increase the plasma concentration of lipids. Many thiazides induce microsomal enzymes and thus affect lipoprotein concentrations with increased concentrations of LDL-cholesterol and total cholesterol and triglycerides, the extent being dependent on the type, dose, and frequency of use of the diuretic.

The broad variety of possible effects of a single drug on clinical laboratory tests is exemplified by phenytoin, which is used to treat some cases of epilepsy. With long-term treatment, many patients have reduced serum calcium and phosphate concentrations and increased ALP activity. Phenytoin induces the synthesis of bilirubin-conjugating enzymes in the liver. Consequently, the serum total bilirubin concentration is reduced, serum GGT activity is increased, and urinary glucaric acid excretion is augmented. A few cases of increased serum aminotransferase activity have been reported, together with prolongation of the prothrombin time. Occasionally, cholestatic, cytotoxic, or mixed hepatic injury may occur. The overall incidence of slight alteration of liver function is about 25%.

Phenytoin may cause hyperglycemia and glycosuria by inhibiting insulin secretion.[62] It decreases the urinary excretion of some steroids by stimulating the conversion of cortisol to 6-β-hydroxycortisol; it also diminishes serum FSH and the sperm count in semen, and thereby reduces fertility. Phenytoin also lowers the serum thyroxine concentration, probably by competitive displacement of thyroxine from its protein-binding sites; free thyroxine also tends to be low. Serum triiodothyronine is low, probably as a result of stimulated metabolism in the liver, but the concentration of TSH is unaffected by the altered thyroxine metabolism. Phenytoin administration may lead to osteomalacia with reduced plasma calcium concentration and increased serum alkaline phosphatase activity. This is probably attributable to the combined effects on vitamin D metabolism and reduced absorption of calcium. Concurrent administration of drugs that are metabolized by the P450 cytochrome system may decrease the rate of metabolism of phenytoin and increase its plasma concentration. Phenytoin may reduce the concentration of other drugs.[70] Barbiturates also induce the hepatic cytochrome enzyme system and may affect the concentrations of coadministered drugs.

Some drugs interfere with analytical methods.[103] Many studies have been done at supraphysiologic concentrations so the reported effects can be discounted, but at physiologic concentrations, spironolactone may appear to increase the concentration of analytes measured by fluorometric methods. Fluorescein, used topically for the diagnosis of various ocular disorders, may be present at a sufficiently high concentration in the plasma to cause a positive interference with analytical methods using fluorescence, particularly fluorescent polarization immunoassays. Icodextrin and mannitol, used with hemodialysis, may cause positive interference with point-of-care glucose testing devices that use coupled glucose-6-phosphate dehydrogenase methods.

Radiographic contrast agents not only may cause renal damage in some patients, but some, such as gadodiamide, which is used to enhance magnetic resonance images and is a powerful chelating agent, may interfere with the measurement of calcium, iron, and magnesium when blood specimens are collected shortly after administration of the dye.[76]

Ingestion of ascorbic acid can raise its plasma concentration to 30 mmol/L. With ascorbic acid ingestion, the vitamin may be present in sufficiently high amounts in urine and feces to render negative positive dipstick tests for hemoglobin in urine and for occult blood in feces.

Herbal Preparations

Herbal preparations are now commonly ingested in by many Americans. Lack of regulatory standardization means that the composition of mixtures with the same name may vary markedly and the purity of individual components cannot be assured. Thus observed effects may vary considerably from one preparation to another. The major concern with ingestion of herbs is their effect on the metabolism of therapeutic drugs.[56] St. John's Wort *(Hypericum perforatum)* acts primarily by increasing the expression of the cytochrome P450-3A *(CYP3A)* gene in the liver, which accelerates the breakdown of many drugs, reducing their plasma concentrations and effectiveness. When coadministered with cyclosporine or tacrolimus, their circulating concentrations have been reported to be reduced by more than 50%. St. John Wort decreases the circulating concentration of digoxin, the norethindrone component of many oral contraceptives, the antifungal drug vericonazole, the antiviral agent indinavir, and a variety of other drugs. Several studies have recorded marked reductions in the half-life and plasma concentration of warfarin (Coumadin) when it is coadministered. Ginseng ingestion may also reduce the plasma prothrombin time and international normalized ratio (INR) in patients who are taking warfarin. Ginseng also reduces the plasma glucose concentration in persons with type 2 diabetes. Grapefruit juice may be ingested and contains inhibitors of intestinal cytochrome P450-3A4, thereby increasing the bioavailability of drugs such as methadone, amiodarone, and simvastatin.

Garlic ingestion may cause an approximate 10% reduction in serum cholesterol concentration; it also significantly reduces the plasma concentration of the HIV protease inhibitor saquinavir. Both ginkgo biloba and ginseng have been reported to lessen hyperglycemia in patients with type 2 diabetes mellitus. Aloe vera, senna, and cascara sagrada have a laxative effect through anthraquinone derivatives that they contain, but their prolonged use may lead to hypokalemia, provoking hyperaldosteronism. Abuse of other laxatives may cause the same problems.

Many herbal preparations affect liver function. Germander has been reported to cause liver cell necrosis, and bishop's weed infrequently causes cholestatic jaundice. Tonka beans can cause reversible liver damage. Comfrey has been associated with at least one death from liver failure. Liver damage may be caused by impure constituents of herbal mixtures, and physicians should always question patients who present with apparent liver damage about their use of herbal preparations.

Noncontrollable Variables

Examples of noncontrollable preanalytical variables include those related to biological, environmental, and long-term cyclical influences and those related to underlying medical conditions.

Biological Influences

Better agreement has been noted between the serum concentrations or activities of several constituents in monozygotic twins than in dizygotic twins.[104] Evidence underscores the importance of genetics in determining the concentration of blood constituents. An influence of heredity on the plasma concentrations of cholesterol, glucose, urea nitrogen, urate, and bilirubin has been substantiated.

An association of blood type with concentration of certain constituents (uric acid, α_1-antitrypsin, cholesterol, and ALP) has been established. In women with blood group O, the blood hemoglobin concentration is generally less than in women with other blood groups. Histocompatibility antigens have an underlying genetic basis but can be markedly influenced by prior blood transfusions.

The age, sex, and race of the patient influence the results of individual laboratory tests.[73,84] They are discussed individually in various chapters of this book, and reference intervals for various analytes as a function of some of these biological influences are listed in Chapter 60.

Age

Age has a notable effect on reference intervals; typical changes in serum composition that occur with age are listed in Table 6-7, although the degree of change differs in various reports. In general, individuals are considered as belonging to one of four groups: the newborn, the older child to puberty, the sexually mature adult, and the elderly adult.

Newborn. The body fluids of the newborn infant reflect both the trauma of birth and changes related to the infant's adaptation to an independent existence. The composition of the blood is affected by the maturity of the infant at birth. The erythrocyte count and the hemoglobin concentration in the neonate at birth are much higher than those of the adult, but within a few days of birth erythrocytes degrade in response to the higher oxygen concentration than that to which the fetus was exposed in utero. In the mature infant, most of the hemoglobin is present in the adult form, hemoglobin A, whereas in the immature infant, much of the hemoglobin may be found in the fetal form, hemoglobin F. In both mature and immature infants, the arterial blood oxygen saturation is very low initially. A metabolic acidosis develops in newborns as the result of accumulation of organic acids, especially lactic acid. The acid-base status, however, reverts to normal within 24 hours.

Within a few minutes of an infant's birth, fluid passes from the blood vessels into the extravascular spaces. This fluid is similar to plasma, except that fluid lost from the intravascular space contains no protein. Consequently, the plasma protein concentration increases. The serum activities of several enzymes, including CK, AST, and LD, are high after birth, with CK activity being almost three times higher than cord blood activity 12 hours after birth, and with AST activity doubling and LD activity increasing by more than 50%.[57]

In infants, even in the absence of disease, the concentration of bilirubin rises after birth because of enhanced erythrocyte destruction. Its concentration peaks about the third to fifth day of life. Conjugation of bilirubin is relatively poor in the neonate as a result of immature liver function. The physiologic jaundice of the newborn rarely produces serum bilirubin values greater than 5 mg/dL (85 μmol/L). Distinguishing this naturally occurring phenomenon from other conditions that produce neonatal hyperbilirubinemia may be difficult, and the chronological course of hyperbilirubinemia is important.

The blood glucose concentration is low in newborns because of their small glycogen reserves, although some attribute the low glucose to adrenal immaturity. Blood lipid concentrations are low but reach 80% of adult values after 2 weeks. The plasma sodium concentration in an infant at birth is slightly higher than in an adult; at 12 hours, it decreases to below the adult value before rising to a value slightly greater than in the adult. The chloride concentration changes similarly, and these changes are largely related to fluid transfer in

TABLE 6-7 Influence of Age on Mean Concentration of Serum Constituents in Males

		CHANGE COMPARED WITH <29-YEAR VALUE			
	Measured Value <30 y	**30-39 y**	**40-49 y**	**50-59 y**	**60-69 y**
Albumin, g/dL	4.6	−0.2	−0.3	−0.4	−0.6
Alkaline phosphatase, U/L	51	−3	−1	1	4
Aspartate aminotransferase, U/L	41	3	3	1	1
Bilirubin, mg/dL	0.4	0.1	0	0	0
Calcium, mg/dL	9.8	−0.1	−0.2	−0.2	−0.3
Cholesterol, mg/dL	211	29	43	48	36
Creatinine, mg/dL	11	0	0.1	0.1	0
Glucose, mg/dL	108	1	6	2	9
Phosphorus, mg/dL	4.0	−0.1	−0.3	−0.2	−0.2
Total protein, g/dL	7.6	−0.1	−0.2	−0.2	−0.2
Urea nitrogen, mg/dL	15	1	1	2	3
Uric acid, mg/dL	5.9	0	0.2	−0.1	−0.2

From Leonard PJ. The effect of age and sex on biochemical parameters in blood of healthy human subjects. In: Siest G, ed. Reference values in human chemistry. Basel: Karger, 1973:134-40.

and out of the blood capillaries. The plasma potassium concentration may be as high as 7 mmol/L at birth, but it falls rapidly thereafter. Plasma calcium is also high initially but falls by as much as 1.4 mg/dL (0.35 mmol/L) during the first day of life.

The plasma urea nitrogen concentration decreases after birth as the infant synthesizes new protein, and the concentration does not begin to rise until tissue catabolism becomes prominent. The plasma amino acid concentration is low as a result of synthesis of tissue protein, although urinary excretion of amino acids may be high because of immaturity of the tubular reabsorptive mechanisms. The plasma urate concentration is high at birth, but the high clearance of urate soon reduces the plasma concentration to below the adult value.

The serum thyroxine concentration of the healthy newborn, similar to that in the pregnant woman, is considerably higher than in the nonpregnant adult. After birth, an infant secretes TSH, which causes a further increase in the serum thyroxine concentration. The physiologic hyperthyroidism gradually declines over the first year of life.

It should be noted that the maturity of a baby at birth may have a marked effect on the concentration of some of his or her blood constituents. For example, plasma aldosterone may be as much as five times higher in premature infants as in mature babies for up to 7 days after birth.

Childhood to Puberty. Many changes in the composition of body fluids take place between infancy and puberty. Most of these changes are gradual, and abrupt changes to adult concentrations rarely occur.

The plasma protein concentrations increase after infancy, and adult concentration values are attained by the age of 10 years. Serum IgG increases slightly out of proportion to the increase in concentration of α_2-globulin. The serum activity of most enzymes decreases during childhood to adult values by puberty or earlier, although the activity of ALT may continue to rise, at least in men, until middle age. Serum ALP activity is high in infancy but decreases during childhood and rises again with growth before puberty. Indeed, during puberty GGT values can be fourfold higher than in adults. The activity of the enzyme is better correlated with skeletal growth and sexual maturity than with chronological age; it is greatest at the time of maximum osteoblastic activity occurring with bone growth. Activity decreases rapidly after puberty, especially in girls. Total and LDL-cholesterol concentrations also increase during the rapid growth spurt.

The serum creatinine concentration increases steadily from infancy to puberty, parallel to the development of skeletal muscle; until puberty, little difference in the concentration is noted between sexes. The serum urate concentration decreases from its high at birth until age 7 to 10 years, at which time it begins to increase, especially in boys, until about age 16 years.

The Adult. Adult values are usually taken as the reference for comparison with those of the young and the elderly. Concentrations of most test constituents remain constant between puberty and menopause in women, and between puberty and middle age in men.

During the midlife years, serum total protein and albumin concentrations decrease slightly. A slight decrease in serum calcium concentration may be noted in both sexes. In men, serum phosphate decreases greatly after age 20 years; in women, phosphate also decreases until menopause, when a sharp increase takes place. Serum urate concentrations peak in men in their twenties and in women during middle age. Urea concentration increases in both sexes in middle age. Age does not affect the serum creatinine concentration in men but does increase the concentration in women. Serum total cholesterol and triglyceride concentrations increase in both men and women at a rate of 2 mg/dL (0.02 mmol/L) per year to a maximum between ages 50 and 60 years. The activity of most enzymes in serum is greater during adolescence than during adult life. This enhanced enzyme activity presumably reflects the greater physical activity of the adolescent.

The Elderly Adult. The plasma concentrations of many constituents are increased in women after menopause (Table 6-8).[101]

Renal concentrating ability is reduced in the elderly adult, so that creatinine clearance may decline by as much as 50% between the third and ninth decades. This decreased clearance is caused more by a decrease in urinary creatinine excretion as a result of decreased lean body mass than by altered renal function. The proximal tubular maximum capacity for glucose reabsorption declines steadily from about 360 mg/min/1.73 m^2 at age 20 to 29 years to 230 mg/min/1.73 m^2 at age 80 to 89 years.[28] The plasma urea concentration rises with age, as does the urinary excretion of protein. Serum median IgG and IgM concentrations are reduced in the elderly, although serum IgA concentrations in men are increased slightly in the elderly. Serum ALP begins to rise in women at menopause, so that in elderly women activity of this enzyme may actually be higher than in men. The concentration of glucose in plasma 1 hour after a loading dose rises by 8 mg/dL (0.44 mmol/L) per decade.

TABLE 6-8 Changes in Composition of Serum with Menopause

Constituent	% Increase
Alanine aminotransferase	12
Albumin	2
Alkaline phosphatase	25
Apolipoprotein A-1	4
Aspartate aminotransferase	11
Cholesterol	10
Glucose	2
Phosphate	10
Phospholipids	8
Sodium	1.5
Total protein	0.7
Uric acid	10

From Wilding P, Rollason JG, Robinson D. Pattern of change for various biochemical constituents detected in well population screening. Clin Chim Acta 1972;41:375-87.

Hormone concentrations are also affected by aging. However, changes in concentration are much less pronounced than an endocrine organ's response to stimuli. Triiodothyronine concentration decreases by up to 40% in persons older than 40 years of age. Although thyroxine secretion is reduced, the thyroxine concentration is not changed, because its degradation is also reduced, with a mean of almost 90 μg/d thyroxine iodine at about age 20 years and 45 μg/d at about age 45 years.[40] The plasma parathyroid hormone concentration does decrease with age. Cortisol secretion is reduced, although the serum concentration may not be affected. Reduced secretion leads to a reduction in the urinary excretion of 17-hydroxycorticosteroids. 17-Ketosteroid excretion in the elderly adult is about half that in the younger adult. The secretion and metabolic clearance of aldosterone are decreased, with a reduction of 50% in the plasma concentration. The aldosterone response to sodium restriction is diminished. Basal insulin concentration is unaffected by aging, but its response to glucose is reduced. In men, the secretion rate and concentration of testosterone are reduced after age 50 years. In women, the concentrations of FSH and LH are increased in the blood and urine, with concentrations increasing progressively with increasing age.[83]

Estrogen secretion in women begins to decrease before menopause and continues at a greater rate after menopause, whereas gonadotropins show a feedback-mediated reciprocal rise. Serum concentrations of estrogens decrease by 70% or more, and urinary excretion of estrogens is decreased comparably. The decreased estrogen secretion may be responsible for the increase in serum cholesterol that occurs up to age 60 years in women. Estrogen secretion in men also declines with age.[59]

Sex

Until puberty, few differences in laboratory data are noted between boys and girls. After puberty, characteristic changes in the concentrations of sex hormones, including prolactin in women, become apparent. After puberty, the serum activities of ALP, ALT, AST, CK, and aldolase are greater in men than in women (see Chapter 60). The higher activity of enzymes originating from skeletal muscle in men is related to their greater muscle mass. After menopause, the activity of ALP increases in women until it is higher than in men. Although total LD activity is similar in men and women, the activities of the LD-1 and LD-3 isoenzymes are higher, and LD-2 is less in young women than in men. These differences disappear after the menopause.

The blood hemoglobin concentration is lower in women; thus, serum bilirubin concentrations are also slightly lower. Increased turnover of erythrocytes in women leads to their having a higher reticulocyte count than men. Serum iron is low during a woman's fertile years, and her plasma ferritin may be only one third of the concentration in men. The reduced iron concentration in women is attributable to menstrual blood loss. In contrast, the serum copper concentration tends to be higher in women than in men. Total cholesterol and LDL-cholesterol concentrations are typically higher in men than in women, whereas the α-lipoprotein, apolipoprotein A-1, and HDL-cholesterol concentrations are less. Plasma concentrations of creatinine, urea, and urate are higher in men than in women, and urinary excretion of amino acids is greater.[103] Creatinine clearance is greater in men than in women. The effect of age on the difference in concentration of some serum constituents between men and women is illustrated in Table 6-9.

Race

Differentiation of the effects of race from those of socioeconomic conditions is often difficult. Nevertheless, the total serum protein concentration is known to be higher in blacks than in whites. This is largely attributable to a much higher γ-globulin, although concentrations of α_1- and β-globulins

TABLE 6-9 Influence of Sex on Composition of Serum at Different Ages*

		CHANGE COMPARED WITH <29-YEAR VALUE			
	Measured Value <30 y	30-39 y	40-49 y	50-59 y	60-69 y
Albumin, g/dL	0.1	0.1	0	0	−0.1
Alkaline phosphatase, U/L	14	12	−8	2	−1
Aspartate aminotransferase, U/L	5	8	8	1	−1
Bilirubin, mg/dL	0.1	0.1	0.1	0.1	0.1
Calcium, mg/dL	0.1	0.1	0.1	−0.1	−0.2
Cholesterol, mg/dL	−14	2	6	−16	−34
Creatinine, mg/dL	0.2	0.2	0.2	0.2	0.1
Glucose, mg/dL	5	3	6	0	6
Phosphorus, mg/dL	0.1	0.1	0.0	−0.1	−0.2
Total protein, g/dL	−0.1	−0.1	−0.1	−0.1	−0.2
Urea nitrogen, mg/dL	3	3	3	2	0
Uric acid, mg/dL	1.5	1.7	1.7	1.0	0.5

*Male values are higher than female values, except where indicated by a minus sign.
From Leonard PJ. The effect of age and sex on biochemical parameters in blood of healthy human subjects. In: Siest G. Reference values in human chemistry. Basel: Karger, 1973:134-40.

usually are also increased. Serum albumin is typically less in blacks than in whites. In black men, serum IgG is often 40% higher and serum IgA may be as much as 20% higher than in white men.[11]

The activity of CK and LD is usually much higher in both black men and women than in whites. This effect presumably is related to the amount of skeletal muscle, which tends to be greater in blacks than in whites. Because of their greater skeletal development, black children usually have a higher serum ALP at puberty than do white children. γ-Glutamyltransferase activity may be as much as twice as high in black men and women than in whites.[63] Amylase activity also tends to be higher in blacks than in whites.[79]

Carbohydrate and lipid metabolism differs in blacks and whites.[6] Glucose tolerance is less in blacks, Polynesians, Native Americans, and Inuits than in comparable age- and sex-matched whites. This is substantiated by a plasma glucose 1 hour after glucose challenge that may be as much as 15 to 25 mg/dL (0.8 to 1.4 mmol/L) higher in blacks than in whites. After age 40 years, serum cholesterol and triglyceride concentrations are consistently higher in both white men and women than in blacks. The lipoprotein (Lp) (a) concentration in blacks may be twice as high as in whites. These may be dietary rather than racial factors, because the concentration of plasma lipids has been shown to be different for the same racial group in different parts of the world. Black Americans of both sexes have lower leukocyte counts than white Americans, largely caused by a lower number of granulocytes, but their monocyte count is also less. Some indigenous groups of the Pacific (e.g., Maoris of New Zealand) have notably higher mean serum urate concentrations than white populations.

Environmental Factors

Environmental factors that affect laboratory results include altitude, ambient temperature, and place of residence.

Altitude

In individuals living at a high *altitude,* blood hemoglobin and hematocrit are greatly increased because of reduced atmospheric PO_2.[23] Erythrocyte 2,3-diphosphoglycerate is also increased, and the oxygen dissociation curve is shifted to the right. Increased erythrocyte concentration leads to increased turnover of nucleoproteins and excretion of urate. The fasting, basal concentration of growth hormone is high in individuals living at a high altitude, but concentrations of renin and aldosterone are decreased in healthy individuals. Different studies have reported no change in plasma sodium and potassium concentrations by high altitude, although others have reported increased concentrations and osmolality with a change from a mean of 290 mosmol/kg (mmol/kg) at sea level to 302 mosmol/kg (mmol/kg) at 6300 m.[7] Serum concentrations of C-reactive protein, transferrin, and β_2-globulin are notably increased with transition to a high altitude. Urinary creatinine concentration and clearance are decreased at high altitudes. Plasma and urine concentrations of catecholamine are increased with increased altitude. The increase is on the order of twofold, largely caused by norepinephrine.[19] Complete adaptation to a high altitude takes many weeks, whereas adjustment to lower altitudes takes less time.

Ambient Temperature

Ambient temperature affects the composition of body fluids. Acute exposure to heat causes the plasma volume to expand by an influx of interstitial fluid into the intravascular space, and by reduction of glomerular filtration. The plasma protein concentration may decrease by up to 10%. Sweating may cause salt and water loss, but usually no changes are seen in the plasma sodium and chloride concentrations. Plasma potassium concentration may decrease by as much as 10% as potassium is taken up by the cells. If sweating is extensive, hemoconcentration rather than hemodilution may occur.

Place of Residence

The geographic location where individuals live may affect the composition of their body fluids. Thus a significant increase in serum concentrations of cholesterol, triglycerides, and magnesium has been observed in people living in areas with hard water. Trace element concentrations are also affected by locale, for example, in areas where much ore smelting occurs, serum concentrations of the trace elements involved may be increased. Carboxyhemoglobin concentrations are higher in areas where there is much heavier automobile traffic than in rural areas (as was true for blood lead in the 1970s in the United States). Individuals who are exposed to ultraviolet light from sunshine typically have higher concentrations of 25-hydroxyvitamin D than those with minimal exposure, but concentrations are also affected by dietary vitamin D, season, age, and gender.[93]

Long-Term Cyclical Changes

Long-term cyclical changes affect laboratory results. Seasonal influences and the menstrual cycle are examples of such changes.

Seasonal Influences

Seasonal influences on the composition of body fluids are small compared with those related to changes in posture or misuse of a tourniquet. Probable factors are dietary changes as different foods come into season, and altered physical activity as more or different forms of exercise become feasible. Evaluation of seasonal variations is difficult because they depend on the definition of a season and on the magnitude of temperature change from one season to another. Day-to-day variability in the composition of body fluids is greater in summer than in winter.

In summer in the Northern hemisphere, the blood volume increases in association with the higher temperature. In winter, the plasma protein increases by as much as 10%. Serum urate concentrations appear to be 5 to 7% higher in summer than in winter. Urea concentrations are affected similarly. Serum triglyceride concentrations are up to 10% higher in summer, whereas the serum cholesterol has been reported to be higher in winter than in summer and has been negatively correlated with ambient temperature. The increased winter cholesterol concentration has been attributed to less physical exercise, greater food intake, and lesser amounts of sunshine. However, similar changes in animals suggest that humoral factors may also be involved. Activities of serum enzymes arising from skeletal muscle are higher in summer than in winter, presumably as a result of increased physical activity. The increase in serum lactate dehydrogenase activity may be as much as 20%.

Calcium metabolism is affected by an individual's exposure to sunlight. Dehydrocholecalciferol in the skin is converted by ultraviolet irradiation to cholecalciferol, which is further metabolized in the liver and kidney to 1,25-dihydroxycholecalciferol. The calcium concentration in serum is decreased in summer to a mean of 10.0 mg/dL (2.5 mmol/L) from a mean of 10.7 mg/dL (2.7 mmol/L) in winter.[50] Calcium elimination in urine may be increased by as much as 30% from winter to summer.[39] Seasonal changes appear to affect other endocrine systems as well. A lower plasma glucose concentration may be observed and glucose tolerance is improved during summer. Serum concentrations of thyroid hormones are generally unaffected, but the serum concentration of triiodothyronine is decreased by 20% in summer, and its urinary excretion is increased. The TSH response to thyroid-releasing hormone is increased during summer. Excretion of metabolites of adrenal hormones usually is greater in summer than in winter. This could be attributable to greater physical activity.

Exposure to sunshine for as little as one weekend during summer may cause enough photodegradation of bilirubin to reduce the serum concentration by 20%. Protracted exposure to sun during the summer leads to a consistently lower bilirubin concentration than during the winter. Some seasonal effects on the composition of body fluids are listed in Table 6-10.

Influence of Menstrual Cycle

The plasma concentrations of many female sex hormones and other hormones are affected by the menstrual cycle (see also Chapters 53 through 56).[104] Thus the plasma corticosterone concentration is as much as 50% higher in the luteal phase than in the follicular phase. The urinary excretion of 17-hydroxycorticosteroids reaches a peak at midcycle. Plasma androstenedione concentration and plasma aldosterone concentration increase from the follicular phase to the luteal phase of the menstrual cycle. On the preovulatory day, the aldosterone concentration may actually be twice that of the early part of the follicular phase. The change in renin activity is almost as great. These changes are usually more pronounced in women who retain fluid before menstruation. Urinary catecholamine excretion increases at midcycle and remains high throughout the luteal phase. These changes within the menstrual cycle make it essential to do repetitive measurements on women at the same time during the cycle.

Plasma cholesterol and triglyceride concentrations tend to be highest at midcycle, corresponding to the time of maximum estrogen secretion. The cyclical variation in cholesterol is not observed with anovulatory cycles. The plasma albumin concentration decreases significantly in the luteal phase of the menstrual cycle compared with the concentration at the time of menstruation (by about 0.6 g/L).[53] The plasma fibrinogen concentration decreases greatly at menstruation. The serum calcium correlates with changes in albumin. The plasma parathyroid hormone concentration is significantly higher during the follicular phase than the luteal phase.[36] Creatinine and urate concentrations are highest at the time of menstruation and are lowest toward the end of the intermenstrual period.

The plasma iron concentration may be very low with the onset of menstruation; the magnesium concentration is least at this point of the cycle. Plasma sodium and chloride concentrations increase up to the onset of menstruation but may fall by 2 mmol/L with the postmenstrual diuresis.

The plasma ascorbic acid concentration is low at the time of ovulation, whereas that of folate is unaffected by the menstrual cycle. Serum CK activity may be slightly reduced at the time of ovulation, but the activities of other enzymes appear to be unaffected by the menstrual cycle.

TABLE 6-10 Seasonal Effects on Composition of Serum

	Concentration		
Constituent	**Highest**	**Lowest**	**% Difference Between High and Low**
Alanine aminotransferase	Winter	Spring, summer	5.0
Albumin	Fall	Summer	1.2
Aspartate aminotransferase	Spring	Fall	11.7
Calcium	Fall	Winter	1.0
Creatinine	Summer	Winter	4.7
Glucose	Fall	Spring	1.5
Lactate dehydrogenase	Summer	Winter	1.8
Triglycerides	Spring	Fall	5.4
Urea nitrogen	Fall	Spring, summer	3.2
Uric acid	Summer	Winter	4.3

Reprinted by permission of Elsevier Science from Letellier G, Desjarlais F. Study of seasonal variations for eighteen biochemical parameters over a four-year period. Clin Biochem 1982;15:206-10. Copyright © by Canadian Society of Clinical Chemists.

Underlying Medical Conditions

Some general clinical conditions have an effect per se on the composition of body fluids. These conditions may exist in addition to the primary complaint that prompted a patient's admission to the hospital. For example, obesity, blindness, fever, shock and trauma, and transfusions and infusions all affect one or more laboratory results.

Obesity

Serum concentrations of cholesterol, triglycerides, and β-lipoproteins are positively correlated with obesity.[41] One study in twins has shown that for an average increase of 7.3% in body mass index, increases of 2.5% in total cholesterol concentration, 3% in LDL-cholesterol concentration, and 18.2% in triglyceride concentration were observed.[16] The increase in the concentration of cholesterol is attributable to LDL-cholesterol because HDL-cholesterol is typically reduced. The serum urate concentration is also correlated with body weight, especially in individuals weighing more than 80 kg.[69] Serum LD activity and glucose concentration are increased in both sexes with increasing body weight.[85] In men, serum AST, creatinine, total protein, and blood hemoglobin concentration increase with increasing body weight. In women, serum calcium increases with increasing body weight. In both sexes, serum phosphate decreases with increased body mass.

Cortisol production is increased in obese individuals. However, increased metabolism maintains the serum concentration unchanged so that urinary excretion of 17-hydroxycorticosteroids and 17-ketosteroids is increased. Because the growth hormone concentration is reduced in obese individuals, it responds poorly to normal stimulation challenges such as glucose, arginine, or acute glucocorticoid administration. Plasma insulin concentration is increased, but glucose tolerance is impaired in the obese (see Chapter 26). Plasma glucose concentrations are increased. Although the serum thyroxine concentration is unaffected by obesity, serum triiodothyronine correlates significantly with body weight and increases further with overeating. In obese men, the plasma testosterone concentration is reduced.

Plasma concentrations of acute-phase reactants tend to be higher in obese than in lean individuals. Fasting concentrations of pyruvate, lactate, citrate, and unesterified fatty acids are higher in obese individuals than in those of normal body weight. Serum iron and transferrin concentrations are low. Plasma adiponectin and ghrelin concentrations are significantly reduced in obese individuals compared with those in lean individuals, whereas concentrations of leptin, especially free leptin, soluble leptin receptor, resistin, C-peptide and estrogens tend to be increased (see Chapter 46).

Blindness

With blindness, normal stimulation of the hypothalamic-pituitary axis is reduced. Consequently, certain features of hypopituitarism and hypoadrenalism may be observed.[8] In some blind individuals, the normal diurnal variation of cortisol may persist; in others it does not. Generally, plasma cortisol concentrations are reduced in blind people. Urinary excretion of 17-ketosteroids and 17-hydroxycorticosteroids is reduced. Plasma sodium and chloride are often low in blind individuals, probably as a result of reduced aldosterone secretion. Plasma glucose may be reduced in blind people, and insulin sensitivity is often decreased. The excretion of urate is reduced. Renal function may be slightly impaired, as evidenced by slight increases in serum creatinine and urea nitrogen.

Negative nitrogen balance may occur in blind people, and the serum protein concentration may be reduced. The serum cholesterol is frequently increased, and the bilirubin concentration may exceed the upper limit of normal. The diurnal variation of serum iron is often lost.

Pregnancy

Many changes in the concentrations of analytes occur during pregnancy, and proper interpretation of test results is dependent on knowledge of the duration of pregnancy (see Chapter 57).

Substantial hormonal changes occur during pregnancy, including several not normally associated with reproduction. Many of these changes are related to the great increase in blood volume that occurs during pregnancy, from about 2600 mL early in pregnancy to 3500 mL at about 35 weeks. This hemodilution reduces the concentration of plasma proteins. The total protein concentration is most reduced by the decrease in albumin concentration. However, the concentration of some transport proteins, including ceruloplasmin and thyroxine-binding globulin, is increased as a consequence of estrogen-stimulated hepatic synthesis. This results in increased concentrations of copper, cortisol, and thyroxine, for example. The concentrations of cholesterol and triglycerides are notably increased in association with increased concentrations of apolipoprotein A and B. In contrast, pregnancy creates a relative deficiency of iron and ferritin.

Urine volume increases during pregnancy, so that it is typically 25% greater in the third trimester than in the nonpregnant woman. The glomerular filtration rate increases by 50% during the third trimester. This results in increased urinary excretion of hydroxyproline and increased creatinine clearance.

Pregnancy triggers many physiologic stress reactions and is associated with increased concentrations of acute-phase reactant proteins. The erythrocyte sedimentation rate increases fivefold during pregnancy, largely as a result of an increase in the fibrinogen concentration.

Stress

Physical and mental stress influences the concentrations of many plasma constituents. Anxiety stimulates increased secretion of aldosterone, angiotensin, catecholamines, cortisol, prolactin, renin, growth hormone, TSH, and antidiuretic hormone. Plasma concentrations of albumin are decreased by up to 5%, and cholesterol may be increased to a greater extent, but fibrinogen, glucose, insulin, and lactate concentrations may increase to a much greater degree. The magnitude of the changes is dependent on the nature and duration of the stress.

Fever

Fever provokes many hormonal responses.[78] Hyperglycemia occurs early and stimulates the secretion of insulin, which improves glucose tolerance; however, insulin secretion does not necessarily reduce the blood glucose concentration because increased secretion of growth hormone and glucagon also occurs. Fever appears to reduce the secretion of thyroxine, as do acute illnesses even without fever. In response to increased corticotropin secretion, the plasma cortisol concentration is increased, and its normal diurnal variation may be abolished. Urinary excretion of free cortisol and other steroids is increased. As acute fever subsides, or if it lessens but still persists for a prolonged period, hormone responses diminish.

Glycogenolysis and a negative nitrogen balance occur with the onset of fever. These are prompted by the typically decreased food intake and wasting of skeletal muscle that may accompany fever. Although an increase in blood volume is usually noted with fever, the serum concentrations of creatinine and urate are usually increased. Aldosterone secretion is increased with retention of sodium and chloride. Secretion of antidiuretic hormone also contributes to retention of water by the kidneys. Increased synthesis of protein occurs in the liver, and the plasma concentrations of acute-phase reactants and glycoproteins are increased. Plasma concentrations of cytokines may be substantially increased.

Fever accelerates lipid metabolism. Serum concentrations of cholesterol, nonesterified fatty acids, and the other lipids may decrease initially, but within a few days the free fatty acid concentration may increase. Fever is often associated with a respiratory alkalosis caused by hyperventilation. This pH increase causes a reduction in the plasma phosphate concentration, with increased excretion of phosphate and other electrolytes.[4] Serum iron and zinc concentrations decline with accumulation of both elements in the liver. The copper concentration increases because of increased production of ceruloplasmin by the liver. Some representative changes in serum composition induced by fever are listed in Table 6-11.

TABLE 6-11 Effects of Fever on Composition of Serum

Constituent	Baseline Value	Concentration After Induction of Fever: 18 h	48 h	72 h	96 h
Sodium, mmol/L	141	130	130	132	135
Chloride, mmol/L	99	91	89	92	94
Potassium, mmol/L	3.6	3.5	3.0	3.4	3.6
Calcium, mg/dL	9.7	8.4	8.5	9.0	9.1
Phosphate, mg/dL	3.3	2.3	3.2	3.2	3.7
Magnesium, mg/dL	1.85	1.62	1.73	1.78	1.70
Creatinine, mg/dL	1.10	1.03	1.04	1.00	1.09
Urea nitrogen, mg/dL	13.4	14.0	15.2	18.5	17.4
Uric acid, mg/dL	5.0	5.5	5.7	6.2	6.2

From Beisel WR, Goldman RF, Joy RJT. Metabolic balance studies during induced hyperthermia in man. J Appl Physiol 1968;24:1-10.

Shock and Trauma

Regardless of the cause of shock or trauma, certain characteristic biochemical changes may result.[20] For example, corticotropin secretion is stimulated to produce a three- to fivefold increase in the serum cortisol concentration. 17-Hydroxycorticosteroid excretion is greatly increased, although excretion of 17-ketosteroids and metabolites of adrenal androgens may be unaffected. Aldosterone secretion is stimulated. Plasma renin activity is increased, as are secretions of growth hormone, glucagon, and insulin. Anxiety and stress increase the excretion of catecholamines. The stress of surgery has been shown to reduce serum triiodothyronine by 50% in patients without thyroid disease.

The general metabolic response to shock includes the normal response to stress with mobilization of lipids, although the serum triglyceride concentration is not usually affected. Following acute myocardial infarction and other cardiac events, notable decreases tend to occur in LDL- and HDL-cholesterols and in apolipoprotein B and A-I concentrations, with an increase in the triglyceride concentration. Surgical procedures and intercurrent illnesses produce similar effects. Thus, it is not recommended to assess serum lipids for future cardiac risk during the acute phase of such events. Even minor illnesses, such as colds, can affect lipid concentrations. The concentrations of lipids revert to normal within 1 month of the event. Plasma glucose concentration is increased in response to stress, and glucose tolerance is reduced.

Immediately after an injury, fluid is lost to extravascular tissue, with a resulting decrease in plasma volume. If the decrease is enough to impair circulation, glomerular filtration is diminished. Diminished renal function leads to the accumulation of urea and other end products of protein metabolism in the circulation. In burned patients, serum total protein concentration falls by as much as 0.8 g/dL because of both loss to extravascular spaces and catabolism of protein. Serum α_1-, α_2-, and γ-globulin concentrations are increased, but not enough to compensate for the reduced albumin concentration. The plasma fibrinogen concentration responds dramatically to trauma and may double within 2 to 8 days after surgery. The concentration of C-reactive protein rises at the same time.

TABLE 6-12 Incidence of Increased Activity of Serum Enzymes and Isoenzymes After Surgery

Enzyme	%
CK	76
CK-2 isoenzyme	6
Aspartate aminotransferase	50
α-Hydroxybutyrate dehydrogenase	28
LD-1 isoenzyme	18
LD-1 > LD-2	10
LD-5 isoenzyme	20

From Krafft J, Fink R, Rosalki SB. Serum enzymes and isoenzymes after surgery. Ann Clin Biochem 1977;14:294-6.

The muscle damage associated with the trauma of surgery increases the serum activity of enzymes originating in skeletal muscle, and this increased activity may persist for several days. Typical alterations in activity of serum enzymes following surgery are illustrated in Table 6-12. Increased tissue catabolism requires increased oxygen consumption and also leads to the production of acid metabolites. Thus blood lactate may increase two- to threefold. With tissue anoxia and impairment of renal and respiratory function, a metabolic acidosis develops. With tissue destruction, urinary excretion of the major biochemical components of skeletal muscle is increased.

Transfusion and Infusions

The protein-rich fluid lost from the intravascular space after trauma is replaced with protein-poor fluid from the interstitial spaces. Subsequently, this is replaced by a fluid similar in composition to plasma. Transfusion of whole blood or plasma raises the plasma protein concentration; the extent of this increase depends on the amount of blood administered. Serum LD activity, primarily LD-1 and LD-2 isoenzymes, is increased by the breakdown of transfused erythrocytes. Transfusions to replace blood lost because of injury reduce sodium, chloride, and water retention precipitated by the injury. Serum iron and transferrin concentrations are reduced immediately after an injury, but extensive blood transfusions can lead to siderosis and an increased serum iron concentration. Serum potassium may increase with transfusion of stored blood.

Infusions of glucose solutions usually result in a reduction in both plasma phosphate and potassium concentrations because these compounds are taken up by erythrocytes. Infusions of solutions of albumin may increase plasma ALP activity if the albumin has been prepared from placenta. Because of the possible influence of infused components on the concentration of circulating constituents, it is inadvisable to collect blood for analysis less than 8 hours after infusion of a fat emulsion or 1 hour after infusion of carbohydrates, amino acids, and protein hydrolysates or electrolytes.

BIOLOGICAL VARIABILITY*

Data from studies of biological variation may be used to assess the importance of changes in test values within an individual from one occasion to another, determining the appropriateness of reference intervals and, in conjunction with data from analytical variation, establishing laboratory analytical goals.[29-31] Application by clinicians of information on biological variability could enhance their ability to precisely identify important changes in test results in their patients. Properly determined reference intervals are used most appropriately in outpatient practice to provide a rough guide as to whether an individual is healthy with respect to an individual analyte. Other concepts, outlined in the following sections, have greater application for hospital inpatient practice, where day-to-day changes in laboratory test values are important for monitoring a patient's response to treatment.

Overview

Categories of biological variation include (1) within an individual and (2) between individuals. The change in laboratory data around a hemostatic set point from one occasion to another within one person is called within-subject or intraindividual variation (Table 6-13). The difference between set points of different individuals is called interindividual variation. Average intraindividual variability varies greatly for different analytes, even within the same biochemical class of compounds (e.g., 6.1% for total cholesterol, 7.4% for HDL-cholesterol, 9.5% for LDL-cholesterol, 22.6% for triglycerides). Major factors influencing reported intraindividual and interindividual variability primarily include the number of individuals in a study, the standardization (or lack thereof) of patient preparation and specimen collection conditions, the number of measurements per individual, and the homogeneity of the studied population.

Often, biological variability influences clinical decisions. For example, Mogadam and associates showed that intraindividual variability in LDL concentrations led to 10% of subjects moving from high risk for cardiovascular events status to normal, or vice versa.[68] Where clinicians rely inappropriately on the upper and lower limits of the reference interval as finite decision points for treatment, this will result in some patients receiving unnecessary treatment, and others, who should be candidates for treatment, going untreated and potentially lost to follow-up because their test values suggested that they were healthy. Emphasis on target values for lipid concentrations, for example, in effect only establishes different decision points than those historically inferred from reference intervals.

Test values in a healthy population used to derive a conventional reference interval are subject to a variety of

*Note: The author has based much of the discussion of biological variability on C.G. Fraser's book, entitled *Biological Variation: From Principles to Practice* (Washington, DC: AACC Press, 2001:1-151). This source should be consulted for further details.

TABLE 6-13 Comparison of Intraindividual and Interindividual Variations and Indices of Individuality

Analyte	Intraindividual Variation, %	Interindividual Variation, %	Index of Individuality
Alanine aminotransferase	24.3	41.6	0.58
Albumin	3.1	4.2	0.74
Alkaline phosphatase	32.6	39.0	0.84
Bilirubin	25.6	30.5	0.85
Calcium	1.9	2.8	0.68
Chloride	1.2	1.5	0.80
Creatine kinase	22.8	40.0	0.57
Creatinine	4.3	12.9	0.33
Lactate dehydrogenase	6.6	14.7	0.45
Magnesium	3.6	6.4	0.56
Phosphate	8.5	9.4	0.90
Potassium	13.6	13.4	1.02
Protein	2.7	4.0	0.68
Sodium	0.7	1.0	0.70
Urea nitrogen	12.3	18.3	0.67
Uric acid	8.6	17.2	0.50

From Fraser CG. Biological variation: from principles to practice. Washington, DC: AACC Press, 2001. Reprinted with permission of AACC Press.

influences, including endogenous, exogenous, genetic or ethnic, and laboratory factors. The statistical approach used to calculate the interval also has considerable influence on the derived reference interval (see Chapter 5). No individual has test results that would span the entire reference interval. Indeed all results within a healthy individual typically encompass only a small part of most reference intervals. Stratification into more appropriate intervals for subpopulations is sometimes required. The most typical stratifications are based on sex and age. Stinton and colleagues[91] have advocated that separate reference intervals are justified when the difference between the means of potentially different populations (e.g., men and women, blacks and whites) is greater than 25% of the 95%-reference interval of the entire population. An alternative approach to defining whether stratification is appropriate is that of Harris and Boyd, which involves calculation of the standard deviations of all results from each of the potentially different populations; if the standard deviation of 1 is more than 1.5 times another, stratification is justified.[44]

Inherent in any reported laboratory test results on patients are influences of (1) biological variation, (2) analytical variation or error, (3) preanalytical and postanalytical sources of variation, and (4) possible pathophysiologic alterations. When repeated measurements are made over time in one individual, even under standardized conditions, considerable variability in the test results is noted. Variability within the individual is attributable to both analytical and intraindividual factors, but intraindividual (within-subject) variability is typically less than the variability seen among a group of individuals. This means that when analytical variability is constant, a statistically significant change in the test results in one individual might occur, yet all results still could lie within the reference interval established by the results obtained from many individuals. Many studies have demonstrated remarkable constancy over the years in terms of intraindividual variability. For those analytes that are influenced by the endocrine system, variation tends to be even less than for those that have no hormonal regulation, especially those that are affected by dietary factors. In general, biological variability is only slightly affected by age or by diseases that do not directly cause abnormal concentrations of a specific analyte.[32]

Calculating Total Variation

To determine what confidence should be placed in a test result, it is useful to evaluate the variability of test values. Factors influencing a test value are preanalytical, analytical, and within an individual. Because sources of variation (squares of the standard deviations) are additive, the total variation (SD_T^2) for any one laboratory result is

$$SD_T^2 = SD_P^2 + SD_A^2 + SD_I^2$$

where

SD_P = Standard deviation of preanalytical variation
SD_A = Standard deviation of analytical variation
SD_I = Standard deviation of within-individual biological variation

It is possible to substitute the coefficient of variation for the standard deviation in the above equation. If the conditions of patient preparation, sample collection, and sample handling are standardized, preanalytical variation is minimized and total variation is then determined by the combined influence of analytical and intraindividual variations, thus:

$$CV_T = (CV_A^2 + CV_I^2)^{1/2}$$

Reference Change Values

To determine whether the difference between consecutive results for a single analyte in a patient might have clinical significance, Harris and Yasaka developed the concept of *reference change values*.[45] An *RCV,* also known as *critical difference,* is the value that must be exceeded before a change in consecutive test results is statistically significant at a predetermined probability. The concept introduces a scientific approach to an area where clinicians have largely relied on their intuition and experience. Historically, clinicians' impressions of clinically significant differences between results have varied markedly. Fraser and coworkers showed that systematically calculated critical differences for many analytes tend to be less than physicians' assumptions of clinically significant differences.[32]

RCV takes into account both analytical and within-individual variations discussed earlier. It is calculated using the following equation:

$$RCV = 2^{1/2} \times Z \times (CV_A^2 + CV_I^2)^{1/2}$$

where Z = Z-score (also called *standard normal deviate*). Z-scores vary with the desired probability for the change. The Z-scores for different probabilities may be derived from statistical tables. For the widely used probability of 95% for clinical laboratory decisions, the Z-score is 1.96. When inserted in the formula above, the formula becomes

$$RCV = 2.77 \times (CV_A^2 + CV_I^2)^{1/2}$$

In practice, a Z-score of 1.96 for a 95% probability is used to identify a significant RCV. A Z-score of 2.58 is used for a 99% probability to ensure an even more significant RCV. The higher the probability used in the calculation, the greater is the likelihood that all identified changes will be true changes. Yet greater certainty with the higher probability may make some physicians believe that the change is obvious, and that such large RCVs may mask trends in test values. The CV_A used for the calculation should be appropriate for the range of test values, as low analytical variability enhances the likelihood that calculated changes will be statistically significant. The probability of change is then largely influenced by intraindividual variation, CV_I. To enhance the utility of the RCV, intraindividual variability should also be minimized, with standardization of patient preparation and specimen collection and processing practices. Standardization is more readily achieved in hospital practice, where uniform timing of collections by trained phlebotomists is often possible, than in outpatient practices.

The change in values between successive measurements in a hospitalized patient is generally greater than the change in values reported in the literature as derived from studies of healthy individuals, because of the change in the patient's medical condition and its response to treatment. RCVs are not constant, and a significant change is likely to be smaller over the short term than over a longer time span. Thus application of RCVs derived from healthy individuals over a short time will identify an inappropriately large number of apparently significant changes in hospitalized patients. CV_I varies between individuals, so that calculations using the mean CV_I flag a disproportionately large number of significant changes. Table 6-14 shows the effects of using different probabilities of significant changes.

Index of Individuality

Although it would be preferable if the range of values in an individual when healthy could be used as the reference for the same individual when he or she is ill, this is largely impractical. The less specific reference interval derived from many individuals must be used as a guide to determine whether a specific result is abnormal. The *index of individuality* (II) allows a comparison of total within-subject (intraindividual) variation to between-subject (interindividual) variation. It is calculated as the ratio of total intraindividual variation to interindividual biological variation as follows:

$$II = \frac{[CV_A^2 + CV_I^2]^{1/2}}{CV_G}$$

where CV_A is the analytical variability, CV_I the intraindividual variability, and CV_G the interindividual variability. In clinical

TABLE 6-14 Significance of Changes in Serial Results: Probability That Changes Between Successive Values Are Significant, %

		Probability					
Analyte	**Units**	**60**	**70**	**80**	**90**	**95**	**99**
Alanine aminotransferase	U/L	3	5	8	13	16	23
Albumin	g/L	<1	1	2	3	4	5
Alkaline phosphatase	U/L	4	9	13	20	26	36
Amylase	U/L	2	5	8	13	16	23
Bilirubin	mmol/L	<1	1	2	3	4	6
Calcium	mmol/L	0.02	0.04	0.06	0.09	0.12	0.17
Chloride	mmol/L	1	2	3	4	5	7
Cholesterol	mmol/L	0.2	0.3	0.5	0.8	1.1	1.5

From Fraser CG. Biological variation: from principles to practice. Washington, DC: AACC Press, 2001. Reprinted with permission of AACC Press.

practice for most analytes, CV_A is small in comparison with CV_I or CV_G and can be ignored; the formula for II is thus simplified to

$$II = \frac{CV_I}{CV_G}$$

A low index of individuality indicates that an analyte has marked individuality, and a high index indicates that an analyte has little individuality. Harris has demonstrated that it is appropriate to use the reference interval for an analyte to make clinical decisions only when CV_I:CV_G is greater than 1.4.[43] When II is less than 0.6, conventional population reference values are of little value and may be misleading. Little variation in test values for an analyte within one person (i.e., a high index of individuality) means that an individual could have considerable changes in laboratory data that might have clinical significance for him or her, yet all these values could fall within the population reference interval. In theory, such analytes are of little use for the diagnosis of disease unless the changes are markedly abnormal.

Index of Heterogeneity

The *index of heterogeneity* (IH) provides a means of determining whether individuals within a population have similar within-individual variation for a given analyte. It is defined as the ratio of CV of $(SD^2_A + SD^2_I)^{1/2}$ to $[2/(n - 1)]^{1/2}$, where A and I are the analytical and within-subject variations, and n is the number of specimens per subject. The higher the index of heterogeneity, the greater is the intraindividual variation.

Reliability Coefficient

The *reliability coefficient* (R) is the ratio of between-subject variation to total variation. This is another measure of individuality. It is calculated as the between-individual variance divided by the total variation.

$$R = \frac{CV_G^2}{CV_A^2 + CV_I^2 + CV_G^2}$$

The reliability coefficient will always be between 0 and 1. If it approaches 1, this means that there is very little variation in results over time within one individual, indicating that great confidence can be placed in a single result, and that repeated measurements are unnecessary.

Quality Specifications for Total Error Allowable

Analytical variations may increase the number of results in a healthy population outside a previously established reference interval. A positive analytical bias increases the number of high values, and a negative bias decreases the number to below the lower reference limit. It is possible to link the maximum tolerable analytical bias to biological variability.[32] The relationship below is derived on the assumption that the maximum acceptable bias is less than one quarter of the sum of intraindividual and interindividual variations within a population.

$$\text{Analytical bias} = < 0.25 \times (CV_I^2 + CV_G^2)^{1/2}$$

By substituting different factors in the above formula, different targeted analytical biases can be identified. If less analytical bias is deemed to be appropriate (e.g., one fifth of the total biological variation instead of one quarter), 0.20 would be substituted for 0.25. It has been suggested that analytical precision should be less than one half of the mean intraindividual variation ($CV_A = 0.50\ CV_I$). Total error is derived from the sum of imprecision and bias. From the formula above,

$$\text{Total allowable analytical error} < 1.65 \times 0.50 \times CV_I + 0.25 \times (CV_I^2 + CV_G^2)^{1/2}$$

The factor 1.65 is derived from 90% of the distribution of results excluding the highest and lowest 5% of values. Again, substituting different values for 0.50 and 0.25 above allows different goals to be established.

Other formulas have been used to determine quality specifications for bias. Generally, analytical bias should be less than one quarter of interindividual biological variation:

$$B_A < 0.250 \times (CV_I^2 + CV_G^2)^{1/2}$$

But optimum performance is also defined by substituting 0.125 for 0.250 in the above formula, and minimum performance is defined by substituting 0.375 for 0.250. When the factor 0.125 is used, 1.8% of values are outside one reference limit and 3.3% outside the other. When 0.375 is used, 1.0% of values are outside one reference limit and 5.7% are outside the other.[31] Fraser has stated that the lower number should be used when desirable performance standards are easily attained, and 0.375 should be used when performance goals are not readily attainable with current procedures.[32] Most of the literature has reported total error in terms of the sum of bias plus 1.65 times the precision (TE_A = Bias + 1.65 SD or CV of interindividual variation).

Biological variation has been included in a goal to determine analytical interference.[35] This goal specifies that

$$\text{Interference (\%)} < CV_I - (1.96CV_A + SE)$$

where SE represents the percentage systematic error (inaccuracy).

Assessment of Mode of Reporting Test Results

The RCV concept is used to determine the most appropriate mode to report several analytes where several possibilities exist. For example, the amount of an analyte in urine could be reported in terms of concentration, absolute amount per unit of time, or amount relative to that of creatinine. The mode with the smallest relative change value is the most informative. Data on analytical and intraindividual variation together with RCV can pinpoint the most appropriate type of specimen for certain analyses. Howey and associates[47] studied random, early morning, and 24-hour urine specimens to determine the most appropriate means to monitor microalbuminuria. The first morning specimen became the preferred specimen because of its smallest within-individual variation, smallest heterogeneity in intraindividual variances, and smallest RCV between consecutive measurements.

Data on biological variability are used to assist in selection of the most appropriate test in a given situation. For example, creatinine clearance and urine creatinine have less intraindividual variation than serum creatinine, so that creatinine clearance is a better choice than serum creatinine for initial assessment of renal function in an individual, but the lower RCV for serum creatinine makes this test better for monitoring individuals. However, the need for urine collection reduces the practicality of using clearance in the initial assessment of renal function. Findings of studies to determine whether the GFR calculated from the serum creatinine concentration might enhance the utility of the serum measurement still have to be thoroughly assessed.

REFERENCES

1. Addis T, Barrett E, Poo LJ, Yuen DW. The relation between the serum urea concentration and the protein consumption of normal individuals. J Clin Invest 1947;26:869-74.
2. Arnold LM, Ball MJ, Duncan AW, Mann J. Effect of isoenergetic intake of three or nine meals on plasma lipoproteins and glucose metabolism. Am J Clin Nutr 1993;57:446-51.
3. Barrett JV. Hyperbilirubinemia of fasting. JAMA 1971;217:1349-53.
4. Beisel WR, Goldman RF, Joy RJT. Metabolic balance studies during induced hyperthermia in man. J Appl Physiol 1968;24:1-10.
5. Bellet S, Roman, L, DeCastro O, Kim KE, Kershbaum A. Effect of coffee ingestion on catecholamine release. Metabolism 1969;18:288-91.
6. Benedek TG, Sunder JH. Comparison of serum lipid and uric acid content in white and Negro men. Am J Med Sci 1970;260:331-40.
7. Blume FD, Boyer SJ, Braverman LE, Cohen A, Dirkse J, Mordes JP. Impaired osmoregulation at high altitude. JAMA 1984;252:524-6.
8. Bodenheimer S, Winter JSD, Faiman C. Diurnal rhythms of serum gonadotropins, testosterone, estradiol and cortisol in blind men. J Clin Endocrinol Metab 1973;37:472-5.
9. Brohult J. Effects of high protein and low protein diets on ornithine carbamoyl transferase activity in human serum (S-OCT). Acta Med Scand 1969;185:357-62.
10. Carlson MG, Snead WL, Campbell PJ. Fuel and energy metabolism in fasting humans. Am J Clin Nutr 1994;60:29-36.
11. Carruthers M, Arguelles AE, Mosovich A. Man in transit: biochemical and physiological changes during intercontinental flights. Lancet 1976;1:977-81.
12. Chobianian AV, Lille RD, Tercyak A, Blevins P. The metabolic and hemodynamic effects of prolonged bed rest in normal subjects. Circulation 1974;49:551-9.
13. Cohn JS, McNanmara JR, Cohn SD, Ordovas JM, Schaefer EJ. Postprandial plasma lipoprotein change in human subjects of different ages. J Lipid Res 1988;29:469-79.
14. Collinson PO, Chandler HA, Stubbs PJ, Moseley DS, Lewis D, Simmons MD. Measurement of serum troponin T, creatine kinase MB isoenzyme, and total creatine kinase following arduous physical training. Ann Clin Biochem 1995;32:450-3.
15. Consolazio CF, Matoush LO, Johnson HL, Nelson RA, Krzywicki HJ. Metabolic aspects of acute starvation in normal humans (10 days). Am J Clin Nutr 1967;20:672-83.
16. Cooper GR, Smith SJ, Myers GL, Sampson EJ, Magid E. Biological variation in the concentration of serum lipids: sources, meta-analysis, estimation and minimization by relative range measurements. J Int Fed Clin Chem 1995;7:23-8.
17. Craig W, Palomaki GE, Haddow JE. Cigarette smoking and serum lipid and lipoprotein concentrations: an analysis of published data. Br Med J 1989;298:784-8.
18. Cryer PE, Haymond MW, Santiago JV, Shah SD. Norepinephrine and epinephrine release and adrenergic mediation of smoking-associated hemodynamic and metabolic events. N Engl J Med 1976;295:573-7.
19. Cunningham WL, Becker EJ, Kreuzer F. Catecholamines in plasma and urine at high altitude. J Appl Physiol 1965;20:607-10.
20. Cuthbertson DP, Tilstone WJ. Metabolism during the post-injury period. Adv Clin Chem 1969;12:1-55.
21. Davies CTM, Few JD. Effects of exercise on adrenocortical function. J Appl Physiol 1972;35:887-91.
22. Deitrick JE, Whedon GD, Shorr E. Effects of immobilization upon various metabolic and physiologic functions of normal men. Am J Med 1948;4:3-36.
23. Eaton JW, Brewer GJ, Grover RG. Role of red cell 2,3-diphosphoglycerate in the adaptation of man to altitude. J Lab Clin Med 1969;73:603-9.
24. Einer G, Zawta B. Praanalytikfibel, 2nd edition. Heidelberg, Leipzig: Barth-Verlag, 1991.
25. Eisenberg S, Wolf PC. Plasma volume after posture changes in hypertensive subjects. Arch Intern Med 1965;115:17-22.
26. Felding P, Tryding N, Hyltoft Petersen P, Hørder M. Effects of posture on concentrations of blood constituents in healthy adults: practical application of blood specimen collection procedures recommended by the Scandinavian Committee on Reference Values. Scand J Clin Lab Invest 1980;40:615-21.
27. Fogh-Andersen N, Altura BM, Altura BT, Siggaard-Andersen O. Composition of interstitial fluid. Clin Chem 1995;41:1522-5.
28. Falzone JA Jr, Shock NW. Physiological limitations and age. Public Health Rep 1956;71:1185-93.
29. Fraser CG. Desirable performance standards for clinical chemistry tests. Adv Clin Chem 1983;23:299-339.
30. Fraser CG. Data on biological variation: essential prerequisites for introducing new procedures? Clin Chem 1994;40:1671-3.
31. Fraser CG. Biological variation: from principles to practice. Washington, DC: AACC Press, 2001.
32. Fraser CG, Cummings ST, Wilkinson SP, Neville RG, Knox JDE, Ho O, et al. Biological variability of 26 clinical chemistry analytes in elderly people. Clin Chem 1989;5:783-6.
33. Freer DE, Statland BE. The effects of ethanol (0.75g/kg body weight) on the activities of selected enzymes in sera of healthy adults: 1. Intermediate-term effects. Clin Chem 1977;23:830-4.
34. Friis R, Vaziri ND, Akbarpour F, Afrsiabi A. Effect of rapid weight loss with supplemented fasting on liver tests. J Clin Gastroenterol 1987;9:204-7.
35. Fuentes-Arderiu X, Fraser CG. Analytical goals for interference. Ann Clin Biochem 1991;28:393-5.
36. Gorai I, Taguchi Y, Chaki O, Kikuchi R, Nakayama M, Yang BC, et al. Serum soluble interleukin-6 receptor and biochemical markers of bone metabolism show significant variations during the menstrual cycle. J Clin Endocrinol Metab 1998;83:326-32.
37. Gear JS, Mann JI, Thorogood M, Carter R, Jelfs R. Biochemical and haematological variables in vegetarians. Br Med J 1980;280:1415.
38. Greenleaf JE. Physiological responses to prolonged bed rest and fluid immersion in humans. J Appl Physiol Respir Environ Exerc Physiol 1984;57:619-33.
39. Green AG. Circannual excretory patterns in man. J Clin Pathol 1974;27:932.
40. Gregerman RI, Gaffney GW, Shock NW. Thyroxine turnover in euthyroid man with special reference to changes with age. J Clin Invest 1962;41:2065-74.
41. Guder WG, Narayanan S, Wisser H, Zawta B. Diagnostic samples: from the patient to the laboratory, 4th edition. Weinheim, Germany: Wiley-Blackwell, 2009.
42. Hall JE, Guyton AC, Jackson TE, Coleman TG, Lohmeier TE, Trippodo NC. Control of glomerular filtration rate by renin-angiotensin system. Am J Physiol 1977;233:F366-F72.
43. Harris EK. Statistical aspects of reference values in clinical pathology. Prog Clin Pathol 1981;8:45-66.

44. Harris EK, Boyd JC. On dividing reference data into sub-groups to produce separate reference ranges. Clin Chem 1990;36:265-70.
45. Harris EK, Yasaka T. On the calculation of a "reference change" for comparing two consecutive measurements. Clin Chem 1983;29:25-30.
46. Heaton KW, Pomare EW. Effect of bran on blood lipids and calcium. Lancet 1974;303:49-50.
47. Howey JE, Browning MCK, Fraser CG. Selecting the optimum specimen for assessing slight albuminuria and a strategy for clinical investigation: novel uses of data on biological variation. Clin Chem 1987;33:2034-8.
48. Hudgson P, Gardner-Medwin D, Pennington RJT, Walton JN. Studies of the carrier state in the Duchenne type of muscular dystrophy. Part I. Effect of exercise on serum creatine kinase activity. J Neurol Neurosurg Psychiatr 1967;30:416-8.
49. Irjala KM, Gronroos PE. Preanalytical and analytical factors affecting laboratory results. Ann Med 1998;30:267-72.
50. Iwanami M, Osiba S, Yamada T, Yoshimura H. Seasonal variations in serum inorganic phosphate and calcium with special reference to parathyroid activity. J Physiol 1959;149:23-33.
51. Irwin MI, Staton AJ. Dietary wheat and starch: effect on levels of five enzymes in blood serum of young adults. Am J Clin Nutr 1969;22:701-9.
52. Kanabrocki EL, Sothern RB, Scheving LE, Vesely DL, Tsai TH, Shelstad J, et al. Reference values for circadian rhythms of 98 variables in clinically healthy men in the fifth decade of life. Chronobiol Int 1990;7:445-61.
53. Kim I, Yetley EA, Calvo MS. Variations in iron-status measures during the menstrual cycle. Am J Clin Nutr 1993;58:705-9.
54. Keys A, Anderson JT, Mickelsen O, Adelson SF, Fidanza F. Diet and serum cholesterol in men: lack of effect of dietary cholesterol. J Nutr 1956;59:39-56.
55. Khalil M, Tanios A, Moghazy M, Aref MK, Mahmoud S, el-Lozy M. Serum and red cell folates, and serum vitamin B12 in protein calorie malnutrition. Arch Dis Child 1973;48:366-8.
56. Klinger C, Pond D. PDR: guide to drug interactions, side effects, and indications, 63rd edition. Montvale, NJ: Physicians' Desk Reference, 2008.
57. Lackmann GD. Reference values for selected enzyme activities in serum from healthy neonates. Clin Biochem 1996;29:599-602.
58. Ladenson JH, Tsai L-MB, Michael JM, Kessler G, Joist JH. Serum versus heparinized plasma for eighteen common chemistry tests. Am J Clin Pathol 1974;62:545-52.
59. Lamberts SWJ, van den Beld AW, van der Lely A-J. The endocrinology of aging. Science 1997;278:419-24.
60. Leach CS, Cintron NM, Krauhs JM. Metabolic changes observed in astronauts. J Clin Pharmacol 1991;31:921-7.
61. Lew SQ, Bosch JP. Effect of diet on creatinine clearance and excretion in young and elderly healthy subjects and in patients with renal disease. J Am Soc Nephrol 1991;2:856-65.
62. Loose DS, Stancel GM. Estrogens and progestins. In: Brunton LL, Lazo JS, Parker KL, eds. Goodman and Gilman's the pharmacological basis of therapeutics, 11th edition. New York: McGraw-Hill, 2006.
63. Manollo TA, Burke GL, Savage PJ, Jacobs DR Jr, Sidney S, Wagenknecht LE, et al. Sex- and race-related differences in liver-associated serum chemistry tests in young adults in the CARDIA study. Clin Chem 1992;38:1853-9.
64. Marchesi C, Chiodera P, Volpi R, Dassò L, Menozzi P, Coiro V. Blunted GH response to nicotine from cigarette smoking in 4 week abstinent alcoholics. Neuroendocrinol Lett 1991;13:349-54.
65. Meade TW, Imeson J, Stirling Y. Effect of changes in smoking and other characteristics on clotting factors and the risk of ischaemic heart disease. Lancet 1987;2:966-7.
66. Mendyka BE. Fluid and electrolyte disorders caused by diuretic therapy. AACN Clin Issues Crit Care Nurs 1992;3:672-80.
67. Merimee TJ, Fineberg ES. Homeostasis during fasting: II. Hormone substrate differences between men and women. J Clin Endocrinol Metab 1982;37:698-702.
68. Mogadam M, Ahmed SW, Mensch AH, Godwin ID. Within-person fluctuations of serum cholesterol and lipoproteins. Arch Intern Med 1998;150:1645-8.
69. Munan L, Kelly A, PetitClerc C. Association with body weight of selected chemical constituents in blood. Clin Chem 1978;24:772-7.
70. Narayanan S, Young DS. Effects of herbs and natural products on clinical laboratory tests. Washington, DC: AACC Press, 2007.
71. Nemesanszky E, Lott JA, Arato M. Changes in serum enzymes in moderate drinkers after an alcohol challenge. Clin Chem 1988;34:525-7.
72. Olusi SO, McFarlane H, Osunkoya BO, Adesina H. Specific protein assays in protein calorie malnutrition. Clin Chim Acta 1975;62: 107-16.
73. Pelsers MM, Chapelle JP, Knapen M, Vermeer C, Muijtjens AM, Hermens WT, et al. Influence of age and sex and day-to-day and within-day biological variation on plasma concentrations of fatty acid-binding protein and myoglobin in healthy subjects. Clin Chem 1999;45:441-3.
74. Pitts RF. Physiology of the kidney and body fluids, 3rd edition. Chicago, Ill: Year Book Medical Publishers, 1974.
75. Poortmans JR, Haralambie G. Biochemical changes in a 100 km run: proteins in serum and urine. Eur J Appl Physiol 1979;40:245-54.
76. Proctor KAS, Rao LV, Roberts WL. Gadolinium magnetic resonance contrast agents produce analytic interference in multiple serum assays. Am J Clin Pathol 2004;121:282-92.
77. Rapport A, From GLA, Husdan H. Metabolic studies in prolonged fasting: I. Inorganic metabolism and kidney function. Metabolism 1965;14:31-46.
78. Rayfield EJ, Curnow RT, George DT, Beisel WR. Impaired carbohydrate metabolism during a mild viral illness. N Engl J Med 1973;289:618-21.
79. Rosalki SB. Genetic influences on diagnostic enzymes in plasma. Enzyme 1988;39:95-109.
80. Rubini ME, Kleeman CR, Lamdin E. Studies on alcohol diuresis. I. The effect of ethyl alcohol ingestion on water, electrolyte and acid-base metabolism. J Clin Invest 1955;34:439-47.
81. Sacks FM, Bray GA, Carey VJ, Smith SR, Ryan DH, Anton SD, et al. Comparison of weight-loss diets with different compositions of fat, protein, and carbohydrates. N Engl J Med 2009;360:859-73.
82. Savendahl L, Underwood LE. Fasting increases serum total cholesterol, LDL cholesterol and apolipoprotein B in healthy, nonobese humans. J Nutr 1999;129:2005-8.
83. Scaglia H, Medina M, Pinto-Ferreira AL, Vázques G, Gual C, Pérez-Palacios G. Pituitary LH and FSH secretion and responsiveness in women of old age. Acta Endocrinol 1976;81:673-9.
84. Sebastian-Gambaro MA, Liron-Hernandez FJ, Fuentes-Arderiu X. Intra- and inter-individual biological variability data bank. Eur J Clin Chem Clin Biochem 1997;35:845-52.
85. Siest G, Henny J, Schiele F, eds. Interpretation des examens de laboratoire. Basel: Karger, 1981.
86. Slentz CA, Houmard JA, Johnson JL, Bateman LA, Tanner CJ, McCartney JS, et al. Inactivity, exercise training and detraining, and plasma lipoproteins. STRRIDE: a randomized, controlled study of exercise intensity and amount. J Appl Physiol 2007;103:432-42.
87. Srikumar TS, Johansson GK, Ockerman PA, Gustafsson JA, Akesson B. Trace element status in healthy subjects switching from a mixed to a lactovegetarian diet for 12 mo. Am J Clin Nutr 1992;55:885-90.
88. Statland BE, Winkel P. Selected pre-analytical sources of variation. In: Gräsbeck R, Alström T (eds). Reference values in laboratory medicine. New York: Wiley, 1981:127-37.
89. Statland BE, Winkel P, Bokelund H. Factors contributing to intraindividual variation of serum constituents: 1. Within-day variation of serum constituents in healthy subjects. Clin. Chem 1973;19:1374-9.
90. Steinmetz J, Panek E, Sourieau F, Siest G. Influence of food intake on biological parameters. In: Siest G (ed). Reference values in human chemistry. Basel: Karger, 1973:193-200.

91. Stinton TJ, Crowley D, Bryant SJ. Reference values of calcium, phosphate, and alkaline phosphatase as derived on the basis of multi-analyzer profiles. Clin Chem 1986;32:76-8.
92. Superko HR, Bortz W Jr, Williams PT, Albers JJ, Wood PD. Caffeinated and decaffeinated coffee effects on plasma lipoprotein cholesterol, apolipoproteins, and lipase activity: a controlled, randomized trial. Am J Clin Nutr 1991;54:599-605.
93. Thomas MK, Lloyd-Jones DM, Thadani RI, Shaw AC, Deraska DJ, Kitch BT, et al. Hypovitaminosis D in medical inpatients. N Engl J Med 1998;338:777-83.
94. Thomson WHS, Sweetin JC, Hamilton IJD. ATP and muscle enzyme efflux after physical exertion. Clin Chim Acta 1975;59: 241-5.
95. Touitou Y, Haus E (eds). Biologic rhythms in clinical and laboratory medicine. Berlin: Springer, 1992.
96. Vermeulan A. Effects of a short term (4 weeks) protein-sparing modified fast on plasma lipids and lipoproteins in obese women. Ann Nutr Metab 1990;34:133-42.
97. Wahren J, Felig P, Ahlborg G, Jorfeldt L. Glucose metabolism during leg exercise in man. J Clin Invest 1971;50:2715-25.
98. Wannamethee SG, Lowe GD, Shaper AG, Rumley A, Lennon L, Whincup PH. Associations between cigarette smoking, pipe/cigar smoking, and smoking cessation, and haemostatic and inflammatory markers for cardiovascular disease. Eur Heart J 2005;26:1765-73.
99. Weitzman ED. Circadian rhythms and episodic hormone secretion. Ann Rev Med 1976;27:225-43.
100. Wesson LG Jr. Electrolyte excretion in relation to diurnal cycles of renal function. Medicine 1964;43:547-92.
101. Wilding P, Rollason JG, Robinson D. Pattern of change for various biochemical constituents detected in well population screening. Clin Chim Acta 1975;41:375-87.
102. Wu AHB, Taylor GR, Graham GA, McKinley BA. The clinical chemistry and immunology of long-duration space missions. Clin Chem 1993;39:22-36.
103. Young DS. Effects of drugs on clinical laboratory tests, 5th edition. Washington, DC: AACC Press, 2000.
104. Young DS. Effects of preanalytical variables on clinical laboratory tests, 3rd edition. Washington, DC: AACC Press, 2007.
105. Young DS, Bermes EW Jr, Haverstick DM. Specimen collection and processing. In: Burtis CA, Ashwood ER, Bruns DE (eds). Tietz textbook of clinical chemistry and molecular diagnostics, 4th edition. Philadelphia: Elsevier, 2006.

ADDITIONAL READING

Fraser CG. Biological variation: from principles to practice. Washington, DC: AACC Press, 2001.

Guder WG, Narayanan S, Wisser H, Zawta B. Diagnostic samples: from the patient to the laboratory, 4th edition. Weinheim, Germany: Wiley-Blackwell, 2009.

Narayanan S, Young DS. Effects of herbs and natural products on clinical laboratory tests, Washington, DC: AACC Press, 2007.

Soldin SJ, Brugnara C, Wong EC. Pediatric reference intervals, 6th edition. Washington, DC: AACC Press, 2007.

Wu AHB: Tietz clinical guide to laboratory tests, 4th edition. Philadelphia: WB Saunders, 2006.

CHAPTER 7

Specimen Collection and Processing

*Doris M. Haverstick, Ph.D., D.A.B.C.C., and Amy R. Groszbach, M.E.D., M.L.T., M.B.(A.S.C.P.)[C.M.]**

Proper collection, identification, processing, storage, and transport of common sample types associated with requests for diagnostic testing are critical to the provision of quality test results. Many errors can occur during these steps. Minimizing these errors through careful adherence to the concepts discussed here and to individual institutional policies will result in more reliable information for use by healthcare professionals in providing quality patient care.

This chapter provides a review and discussion of common types of specimens and samples used for diagnostic testing.

TYPES OF SPECIMENS

Types of biological specimens that are analyzed in clinical laboratories include (1) whole blood; (2) serum; (3) plasma; (4) urine; (5) feces; (6) saliva; (7) spinal, synovial, amniotic, pleural, pericardial, and ascitic fluids; and (8) various types of solid tissue. The Clinical and Laboratory Standards Institute (CLSI) has published several procedures for collecting many of these specimens under standardized conditions.[4-16]

Blood

Blood for analysis may be obtained from veins, arteries, or capillaries. Venous blood is usually the specimen of choice, and venipuncture is the method for obtaining this specimen. Arterial puncture is used mainly for blood gas analyses. In young children and for many point-of-care tests, skin puncture is frequently used to obtain what is mostly capillary blood. The process of collecting blood is known as phlebotomy (from *phleb,* which means vein, and *tome,* to cut or incise) and should always be performed by a trained phlebotomist.

Venipuncture

In the clinical laboratory, venipuncture is defined as all of the steps involved in obtaining an appropriate and identified blood specimen from a patient's vein.[12]

Preliminary Steps

Before any specimen is collected, the phlebotomist must confirm the identity of the patient.[4] Two or three items of identification should be used (e.g., [1] name, [2] medical record number, [3] date of birth, [4] address if the patient is an outpatient). In specialized situations, such as paternity testing or other tests of medico-legal importance, establishment of a chain of custody for the specimen may require additional patient identification, such as a photograph, provided as part of the identification process or taken to confirm the identity of the patient.

Identification must be an active process. Where possible, the patient should state his or her name, and the phlebotomist should verify information on the patient's wrist band if the patient is hospitalized. If the patient is an outpatient, the phlebotomist should ask the patient to state his or her name and should confirm the information on the test requisition form with identifying information provided by the patient. In the case of pediatric patients, the parent or guardian should be present and should provide active identification of the child. In many institutions at this point in the process, the patient should be asked about latex allergies. If latex allergy is present and if latex gloves or a latex tourniquet may be used, the phlebotomist should secure an alternative tourniquet and put on gloves that are latex free. Finally, for some tests for genetic diseases, the performing laboratory may request a signed consent form from the patient; this should be completed at this time if it was not provided by the requesting physician.

Before collection of a specimen, a phlebotomist should dress in personal protective equipment (PPE), such as an impervious gown and gloves applied immediately before approaching the patient, to adhere to standard precautions against potentially infectious material and to limit the spread of infectious disease from one patient to another.[14] If the phlebotomist is to collect a specimen from a patient in isolation in a hospital, the phlebotomist must put on a clean gown and

**The authors gratefully acknowledge the original contributions by Drs. Donald S. Young and Edward W. Bermes, on which portions of this chapter are based.*

gloves and a face mask and goggles before entering the patient's room. The face mask limits the spread of potentially infectious droplets, and the goggles limit the possible entry of infectious material into the eye. The extent of the precautions required will vary with the nature of the patient's illness and the institution's policies and bloodborne pathogen plan, to which a phlebotomist must adhere. If airborne precautions are indicated, the phlebotomist must wear an N95 TB respirator.

If appropriate, the phlebotomist should verify that the patient is fasting, what medications are being taken or have been discontinued as required, and so forth. The patient should be comfortable, seated or supine (if sitting is not feasible), and should have been in this position for as long as possible before the specimen is drawn. For an outpatient, it is generally recommended that patients be seated before completion of the identification process to maximize their relaxation. At no time should venipuncture be performed on a standing patient. Either of the patient's arms should be extended in a straight line from the shoulder to the wrist. An arm with an inserted intravenous line should be avoided, as should an arm with extensive scarring or a hematoma at the intended collection site. If a woman has had a mastectomy, arm veins on that side of the body should not be used, because the surgery may have caused lymphostasis (blockade of normal lymph node drainage), affecting the blood composition. If a woman has had double mastectomies, blood should be drawn from the arm of the side on which the first procedure was performed. If the surgery was done within 6 months on both sides, a vein on the back of the hand or at the ankle should be used.

Before performing a venipuncture, the phlebotomist should estimate the volume of blood to be drawn and should select the appropriate number and types of tubes for the blood, plasma, or serum tests requested. In many settings, this will be facilitated by computer-generated collection recommendations and should be designed to collect the minimum amount necessary for testing. The sections below on "Order of Draw for Multiple Collections" and "Collection With Evacuated Blood Tubes" discuss in greater detail the recommended order of draw for multiple specimens and types of tubes. In addition to tubes, an appropriate needle must be selected. The most commonly used sizes are 19 to 22 gauge. (The larger the gauge number, the smaller the bore.) The usual choice for an adult with normal veins is 20 gauge; if veins tend to collapse easily, a size 21 is preferred. For volumes of blood from 30 to 50 mL, an 18-gauge needle may be required to ensure adequate blood flow. A needle is typically 1.5 inches (3.7 cm) long, but 1-inch (2.5-cm) needles, usually attached to a winged or butterfly collection set, are also used. All needles must be sterile, sharp, and without barbs. If blood is drawn for trace element measurements, the needle should be stainless steel and should be known to be free from contamination.

Location

The median cubital vein in the antecubital fossa, or crook of the elbow, is the preferred site for collecting venous blood in adults because the vein is large and is close to the surface of the skin.[12,20] Veins on the back of the hand or at the ankle may be used, although these are less desirable and should be avoided in people with diabetes and other individuals with poor circulation. In the inpatient setting, it is appropriate to collect blood through a cannula that is inserted for long-term fluid infusions at the time of first insertion to avoid the need for a second stick. For severely ill individuals and those requiring many intravenous injections, an alternative blood-drawing site should be chosen. Selection of a vein for puncture is facilitated by palpation. An arm containing a cannula or an arteriovenous fistula should not be used without consent of the patient's physician. If fluid is being infused intravenously into a limb, the fluid should be shut off for 3 minutes before a specimen is obtained and a suitable note made in the patient's chart and on the result report form. Specimens obtained from the opposite arm are preferred.[12] Specimens below the infusion site in the same arm may be satisfactory for most tests, except for those analytes that are contained in the infused solution (e.g., glucose, electrolytes).

Preparation of Site

The area around the intended puncture site should be cleaned with whatever cleanser is approved for use by the institution. Three commonly used materials are a prepackaged alcohol swab, a gauze pad saturated with 70% isopropanol, and a benzalkonium chloride solution (Zephiran chloride solution, 1:750). Cleaning of the puncture site should be done with a circular motion and from the site outward. The skin should be allowed to dry in the air. No alcohol or cleanser should remain on the skin because traces may cause hemolysis and invalidate test results. Once the skin has been cleaned, it should not be touched until after the venipuncture has been completed.

Timing

The time at which a specimen is obtained is important for those blood constituents that undergo marked diurnal variation (e.g., corticosteroids, iron) and for those used to monitor drug therapy (see Chapter 34). For most current molecular diagnostic tests, the time of day is unlikely to contribute to altered or invalid test results. Furthermore, timing is important in relation to specimens for alcohol or drug measurements in association with medico-legal considerations.

Venous Occlusion

After the skin is cleaned, a blood pressure cuff or a tourniquet is applied 4 to 6 inches (10 to 15 cm) above the intended puncture site (distance for adults). This obstructs the return of venous blood to the heart and distends the veins (venous occlusion). When a blood pressure cuff is used as a tourniquet, it is usually inflated to approximately 60 mm Hg (8.0 kPa). Tourniquets typically are made from precut soft rubber strips or from Velcro. It is rarely necessary to leave a tourniquet in place for longer than 1 minute, but even within this short time the composition of blood changes. Although the changes that occur in 1 minute are slight, marked changes

TABLE 7-1 Changes in Composition of Serum When Venous Occlusion Is Prolonged from 1 Minute to 3 Minutes*†

Increase	%	Decrease	%
Total protein	4.9	Potassium	6.2
Iron	6.7		
Total lipids	4.7		
Cholesterol	5.1		
Aspartate aminotransferase	9.3		
Bilirubin	8.4		

*To estimate the probable effect of a factor on results, relate percent increase or decrease shown (or intimated) in table to analytical variation (±% CV) routinely found for analytes.
†Mean values obtained from 11 healthy individuals.
From Statland BE, Bokelund H, Winkel P. Factors contributing to intraindividual variation of serum constituents: effects of posture and tourniquet application on variation of serum constituents in healthy subjects. Clin Chem 1974;20:1513-9.

have been observed after 3 minutes for many chemistry analytes (Table 7-1). No known changes affect molecular diagnostics.

The composition of blood drawn first—that is, the blood closest to the tourniquet—is most representative of the composition of circulating blood. The first-drawn specimen should therefore be used for those analytes such as calcium that are pertinent to critical medical decisions.[25] Blood drawn later shows a greater effect from venous stasis. Thus the first tube may show a 5% increase in protein, whereas the third tube may show a 10% change.[22] The concentration of protein-bound constituents is also influenced by stasis. Prolonged stasis may increase the concentration of protein or protein-bound constituents by as much as 15%. A uniform procedure for the order of draw for tests should therefore be established (see later). If it is possible to collect only a small volume of blood, the priority of which tests to perform should be established.

The increase in activity of creatine kinase and aspartate aminotransferase in serum seen after venipuncture may be caused by hemoconcentration, by slight trauma to tissue as the needle pierces the skin, and by stasis of blood in the tissue.

Pumping of the fist before venipuncture should be avoided because it causes an increase in plasma potassium, phosphate, and lactate concentrations. Lowering of blood pH by accumulation of lactate causes the plasma ionized calcium concentration to increase.[24] The ionized calcium concentration reverts to normal 10 minutes after the tourniquet is released.

Stress associated with blood collection can have effects on patients at any age. As a consequence, plasma concentrations of cortisol and growth hormone may increase. Stress occurs particularly in young children who are frightened, struggling, and held in physical restraint. Collection under these conditions may cause adrenal stimulation leading to an increased plasma glucose concentration or may create increases in the serum activities of enzymes that originate in skeletal muscle.

TABLE 7-2 Recommended Order of Draw for Multiple Specimen Collection

Stopper Color	Contents	Inversions
Yellow	Sterile media for blood culture	8
Royal blue	No additive	0
Clear	Nonadditive; discard tube if no royal blue used	0
Light blue	Sodium citrate	3-4
Gold/red	Serum separator tube	5
Red/red, orange/yellow, royal blue	Serum tube, with or without clot activator, with or without gel	5
Green	Heparin tube with or without gel	8
Tan (glass)	Sodium heparin	8
Royal blue	Sodium heparin, sodium EDTA	8
Lavender, pearl white, pink/pink, tan (plastic)	EDTA tubes, with or without gel	8
Gray	Glycolytic inhibitor	8
Yellow (glass)	ACD for molecular studies and cell culture	8

Modified from information in CLSI. Tubes and additives for venous blood specimen collection: CLSI-approved standard H1-A6, 6th edition. Wayne, Pa: Clinical and Laboratory Standards Institute, 2010; Kiechle FL, ed. So you're going to collect a blood specimen: an introduction to phlebotomy, 11th edition. Northfield, Ill: College of American Pathologists, 2005.

Order of Draw for Multiple Blood Specimens

In a few patients, backflow from blood tubes into veins occurs owing to a decrease in venous pressure. The dangerous consequences of this occurrence may be prevented if only sterile tubes are used for collection of blood. Backflow is minimized if the arm is held downward and blood is kept from contact with the stopper during the collection procedure. To minimize problems if backflow should occur, and to optimize the quality of specimens—especially to prevent cross-contamination with anticoagulants—blood should be collected into tubes in the order outlined in Table 7-2. This table also provides the recommended number of inversions for each tube type because it is critical that complete mixing of any additive with the blood collected be accomplished as quickly as possible.

Collection With Evacuated Blood Tubes

Evacuated blood tubes are usually considered to be less expensive and are more convenient and easier to use than syringes, and thus are the collection device of choice in many institutions. Evacuated blood tubes may be made of soda-lime or borosilicate glass or plastic (polyethylene terephthalate). Because of the decreased likelihood of breakage and subsequent exposure to infectious materials, many laboratories have converted from glass tubes to plastic tubes. Several types of evacuated tubes may be used for venipuncture collection.[12] They vary by the type of additive added and the volume of the tube. The different types of additives are identified by the color of the stopper used (Table 7-3). Serum or plasma separator tubes are available that contain an inert, thixotropic, polymer gel material with a specific gravity of approximately 1.04. Aspiration of blood into the tube and subsequent centrifugation displace the gel, which settles like a disk between cells and supernatant when the tube is centrifuged. A minimum relative centrifugal force (RCF) of 1100 ×g is required for gel release and barrier formation in most tubes. Release of intracellular components into the supernatant is prevented by the barrier for several hours or, in some cases, for a few days. These separator tubes may be used as primary containers from which serum or plasma can be directly aspirated by a number of analytical instruments. Additional tubes, not listed, are sold for special applications,

TABLE 7-3 Coding of Stopper Color to Indicate Additive in Evacuated Blood Tube

Tube Type	Additive	Stopper Color	Alternative
Gel separation tubes	Polymer gel/silica activator	Red/black	Gold
	Polymer gel/silica activator/lithium heparin	Green/gray	Light gray
Serum tubes (nonadditive)	Silicone-coated interior	Red	Red
	Uncoated interior	Red	Pink
Serum tubes (with additives)	Thrombin (dry additive)	Gray/yellow	Orange
	Particulate clot activator	Yellow/red	Red
	Thrombin (dry additive)	Light blue	Light blue
Whole blood/plasma tubes	K_2 EDTA (dry additive)	Lavender	Lavender
	K_3 EDTA (liquid additive)	Lavender	Lavender
	Na_2 EDTA (dry additive)	Lavender	Lavender
	Citrate, trisodium (coagulation)	Light blue	Light blue
	Citrate, trisodium (erythrocyte sedimentation rate)	Black	Black
	Sodium fluoride (antiglycolic agent)	Gray	Light/gray
	Heparin, lithium (dry or liquid additive)	Green	Green
	Potassium oxalate/sodium fluoride	Light gray	Light gray
	Lithium heparin/iodoacetate	Light gray	Light gray
Specialty Tubes (Microbiology)			
Blood culture	Sodium polyanethol sulfonate (SPS)	Light yellow	Light yellow
Specialty Tubes (Chemistry)			
Lead	Heparin, potassium (liquid additive)	Tan	Tan
	Heparin, sodium (dry additive)	Royal blue	Royal blue
Trace elements	Silicone-coated interior (serum tube)	Royal blue	Royal blue
Stat chemistry	Thrombin	Gray/yellow	Orange
Specialty Tubes (Molecular Diagnostics)			
Plasma	K_2 EDTA (dry additive)/polymer gel/silica activator	Opalescent white	Opalescent white
	ACD solution A (Na_3 citrate, 22.0 g/L; citric acid, 8.0 g/L; dextrose, 24.5 g/L)	Bright yellow	Bright yellow
	ACD solution B (Na_3 citrate, 13.2 g/L; citric acid, 4.8 g/L; dextrose, 14.7 g/L)	Bright yellow	Bright yellow
Mononuclear cell preparation tube	Sodium citrate with density gradient polymer fluid	Blue/black	Blue/black
	Sodium heparin with density gradient polymer fluid	Green/red	Green/red

Modified from information in CLSI. Tubes and additives for venous blood specimen collection: CLSI-approved standard H1-A6, 6th edition. Wayne, Pa: Clinical and Laboratory Standards Institute, 2010; Becton Dickinson Web page (http:/www.bd.com/).

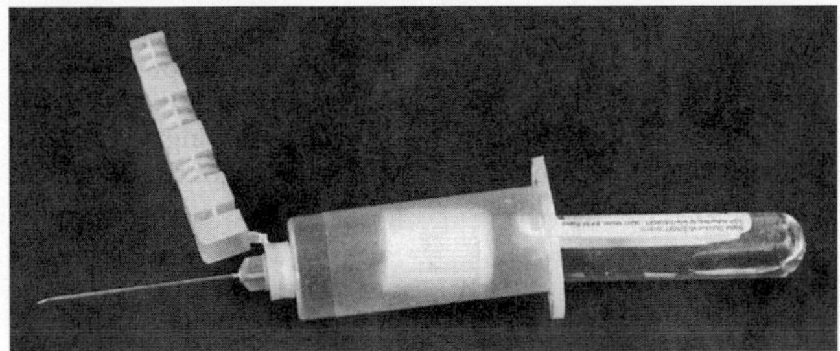

Figure 7-1 Assembled venipuncture set. *(From Flynn JC. Procedures in phlebotomy, 3rd edition. St Louis: Saunders, 2005.)*

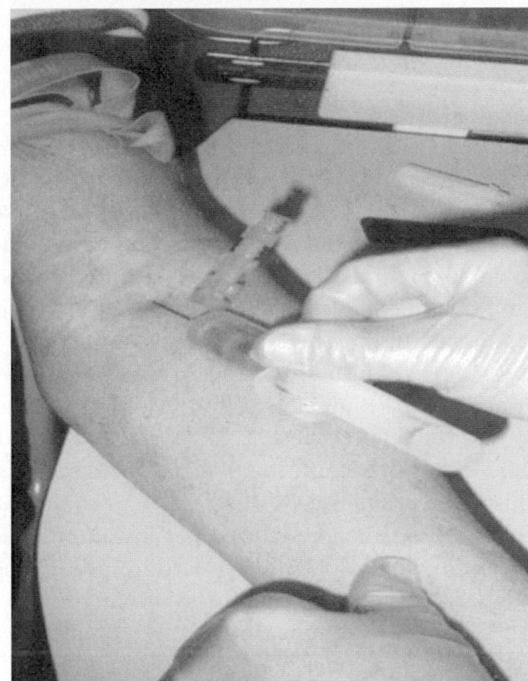

Figure 7-2 Venipuncture. *(Courtesy Ruth M. Jacobsen, Mayo Clinic, Rochester, Minn.)*

such as RNA isolation. These less common tubes must be validated by each laboratory before use if not approved by the manufacturer for the specific analysis to be conducted.

Stoppers may contain zinc, invalidating the use of evacuated blood tubes for zinc measurement, and TBEP [tris(2-butoxyethyl) phosphate], a constituent of rubber, which may interfere with the measurement of certain drugs. With time, the vacuum in evacuated tubes is lost and their effective draw diminishes. The silicone coating also decays with age. Therefore the stock of these tubes should be rotated and careful attention paid to the expiration date. Blood collected into a tube containing one additive should never be transferred into other tubes, because the first additive may interfere with tests for which a different additive is specified. Additionally, transfer of the additive from one tube to another should be minimized (or adverse effects reduced) through strict adherence to recommendations for order of tube use (see Table 7-2).

A typical system for collecting blood in evacuated tubes is shown in Figure 7-1.[17] This is an example of a commonly used single-use device that incorporates a cover that is designed to be placed over the needle when collection of the blood is complete, thereby reducing the risk of puncture of the phlebotomist by the now contaminated needle. A needle or winged (butterfly) set is screwed into the collection tube holder, and the tube is then gently inserted into this holder. The tube should be gently tapped to dislodge any additive from the stopper before the needle is inserted into a vein; this prevents aspiration of the additive into the patient's vein.

After the skin has been cleaned, the needle should be guided gently into the patient's vein (Figure 7-2); once the needle is in place, the tube should be pressed forward into the holder to puncture the stopper and release the vacuum. **As soon as** blood begins to flow into the tube, the tourniquet should be released without moving the needle (see earlier discussion on venous occlusion). The tube is filled until the vacuum is exhausted. It is critically important that the evacuated tube be filled completely. Many additives are provided in the tube based on a "full" collection; deviation or short draws can be a source of preanalytical error because they can significantly affect test results.[7] Once the tube is filled completely, it should be withdrawn from the holder, mixed gently by inversion, and replaced by another tube, if this is necessary. Other tubes may be filled using the same technique with the holder in place. When several tubes are required from a single blood collection, a shut-off valve—consisting of rubber tubing that slides over the needle opening—is used to prevent spillage of blood during exchange of tubes.

Blood Collection With Syringe

Syringes are customarily used for patients with difficult veins. If a syringe is used, the needle is placed firmly over the nozzle of the syringe, and the cover of the needle is removed. If the syringe has an eccentric nozzle, the needle should be arranged with the nozzle downward but the bevel of the needle upward. The syringe and the needle should be aligned with the vein to be entered and the needle pushed into the vein at an angle to the skin of approximately 15 degrees. When the initial resistance of the vein wall is overcome as it is pierced, forward pressure on the syringe is eased, and the blood is withdrawn by gently pulling back the plunger of the syringe. Should a second syringe be necessary, a gauze pad may be placed under the hub of the needle to absorb the spill; the first syringe is then quickly disconnected, and the second put in place to continue the blood draw. Using the same needle or a new needle, the cap of the evacuated tube should be punctured and the evacuated tube allowed to fill passively. Uncapping the evacuated tube is not recommended. Vigorous withdrawal of blood into a syringe during collection or forceful transfer from the syringe to the receiving vessel may cause hemolysis of blood. Hemolysis is usually less when blood is drawn through a small-bore needle than when a larger-bore needle is used.

Completion of Collection

When blood collection is complete and the needle withdrawn, the patient should be instructed to hold a dry gauze pad over the puncture site, with the arm raised to lessen the likelihood of leakage of blood. The pad may then be held in place by a bandage or by a nonadhesive strap (which avoids pulling hairs on the arm when it is removed); these are removed after 15 minutes. With a collection device, such as that shown in Figure 7-1, the needle is covered, and the needle and the tube holder are immediately discarded into a sharps container. In the event that a winged (butterfly) set is used, the wings are pushed forward to cover the needle, or with newer available equipment, a button is pressed, releasing a spring that retracts the needle. If a syringe was used, the needle and syringe (still attached) should be discarded in a hazardous waste receptacle.

All tubes should then be labeled per institutional policy. Most institutions have a written procedure prohibiting the advance labeling of tubes because this is seen as providing the potential for mislabeling, one of the most common sources of preanalytical error. Some institutions recommend showing the labeled tube to the patient to further confirm correct identification. Gloves should be discarded in a hazardous waste receptacle if visibly contaminated, or in noncontaminated trash if not visibly contaminated. Before applying new gloves and proceeding to the next patient, and depending on institutional policy, clinicians should use an alcohol-based cleanser or soap and water to wash their hands.

Venipuncture in Children

The techniques for venipuncture in children and adults are similar. However, children are likely to make unexpected movements, and assistance in holding them still is often desirable. A syringe or an evacuated blood tube system may be used to collect specimens. A syringe should be the tuberculin type or should have a 3-mL capacity, except when a large volume of blood is required for analysis. A 21- to 23-gauge needle or a 20- to 23-gauge butterfly needle with attached tubing is appropriate to collect specimens. In general, in the pediatric population, alternative collection through skin puncture is often used.

Skin Puncture

Skin puncture is an open collection technique in which the skin is punctured by a lancet and a small volume of blood is collected into a microdevice. Skin puncture blood is more like arterial blood than venous blood. In practice, it is used in situations in which (1) sample volume is limited (e.g., pediatric applications), (2) repeated venipunctures have resulted in severe vein damage, or (3) patients have been burned or bandaged and veins therefore are unavailable for venipuncture. This technique is also commonly used when the sample is to be applied directly to a testing device in a point-of-care testing situation or to filter paper. It is most often performed on (1) the tip of a finger, (2) an earlobe, and (3) the heel or big toe of infants. For example, in an infant younger than 1 year, the lateral or medial plantar surface of the foot should be used for skin puncture; suitable areas are illustrated in Figure 7-3.[1] In older children, the plantar surface of the big toe may also be used, although blood collection from anywhere on the foot should be avoided on ambulatory patients. The complete procedure for collecting blood from infants using skin puncture is described in a CLSI document.[10]

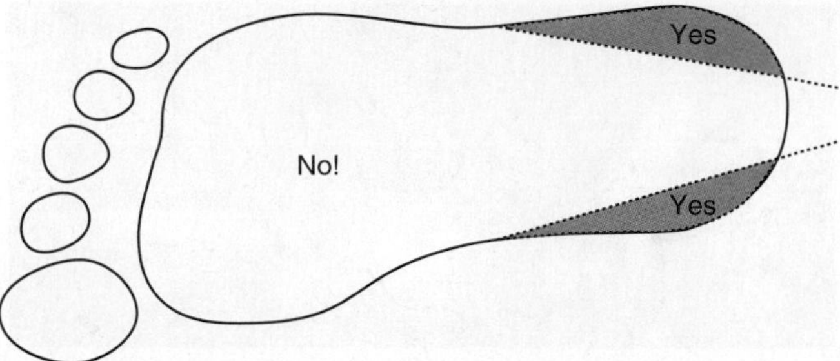

Figure 7-3 Acceptable sites for skin puncture to collect blood from an infant's foot. *(Modified from Blumenfeld TA, Turi GK, Blanc WA. Recommended site and depth of newborn heel punctures based on anatomical measurements and histopathology. Lancet 1979;1:230-3. Reprinted with permission from Elsevier.)*

To collect a blood specimen by skin puncture, the phlebotomist first thoroughly cleans the skin with a gauze pad saturated with an approved cleaning solution, as outlined earlier for venipuncture. If an alcohol swab is used, the alcohol must be allowed to evaporate from the skin so that hemolysis does not occur. When the skin is dry, it is quickly punctured by a sharp stab with a lancet. The depth of the incision should be less than 2.5 mm to prevent contact with bone. To minimize the possibility of infection, a different site should be selected for each puncture. The finger should be held in such a way that gravity assists collection of blood at the fingertip and the lancet held to make the incision as close to perpendicular to the fingernail as possible.[20] Massage of the finger to stimulate blood flow should be avoided because it causes the outflow of debris and tissue fluid, which does not have the same composition as plasma. To improve circulation of the blood, the finger (or the heel in the case of heelsticks) may be warmed by application of a warm, wet washcloth or a specialized device, such as a heel warmer, for 3 minutes before the lancet is applied. The first drop of blood is wiped off, and subsequent drops are transferred to the appropriate collection tube by gentle contact. Filling should be done rapidly to prevent clotting, and introduction of air bubbles should be prevented.

As the name suggests, blood is collected into capillary blood tubes by capillary action. A variety of collection tubes are commercially available (Figure 7-4). Containers are commercially available that contain different anticoagulants, such as sodium and ammonium heparin, and some are available in brown glass for collection of light-sensitive analytes, such as bilirubin (see later section on anticoagulants). As with evacuated blood tubes, to prevent the possibility of breakage and the spread of infection, capillary devices frequently are

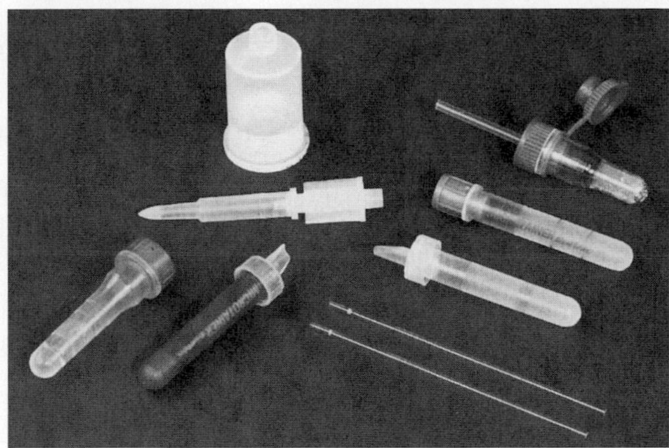

Figure 7-4 Microcollection tubes. *(From Flynn JC. Procedures in phlebotomy, 3rd edition. St Louis: Saunders, 2005.)*

plastic or coated with plastic. A disadvantage of some of the collection devices shown in Figure 7-4 is that blood tends to pool in the mouth of the tube and must be flicked down the tube, creating a risk of hemolysis. Drop-by-drop collection should be avoided because it increases hemolysis. The correct order of filling of these devices is the same as for evacuated blood tubes (see Table 7-2).

For collection of blood specimens on filter paper for molecular genetic testing and neonatal screening,[5] the skin is cleaned and punctured as described previously. The first drop of blood should be wiped away. Then the filter paper is gently touched against a large drop of blood that is allowed to soak into the paper to fill the marked circle. Only a single application per circle should be made to prevent nonuniform analyte concentration.[5] The paper is examined to verify that there has been complete penetration of the paper. The procedure is repeated to fill all the circles. Avoid milking or squeezing the finger or foot because this procedure contributes tissue fluids. The filter papers should be air-dried (generally for 2 to 3 hours to prevent mold or bacterial overgrowth) before storage in a properly labeled paper envelope. Blood should never be transferred onto filter paper after it has been collected in capillary tubes because partial clotting may have occurred, compromising the quality of the specimen. However, blood collected into an evacuated tube containing an anticoagulant may be applied directly to the filter paper. This is a convenient way to store a sample for possible future molecular testing (with patient consent). These blood spots are handled in the same manner as neonatal screening specimens, with air drying and storage in a dry protected environment.

Arterial Puncture

Arterial puncture requires considerable skill and is usually performed only by physicians or specially trained technicians or nurses. Preferred sites of arterial puncture are, in order, the (1) radial artery at the wrist, (2) brachial artery in the elbow, and (3) femoral artery in the groin. Because leakage of blood from the femoral artery tends to be greater, especially in the elderly, sites in the arm are used most often. The proper technique for arterial puncture is described in a CLSI document.[11]

In the neonate, an indwelling catheter in the umbilical artery is best to obtain specimens for blood gas analysis. In the older child or adult in whom it is impossible to perform an arterial puncture, a capillary puncture may be performed to obtain arterialized capillary blood. Such a specimen yields acceptable values for pH and PCO_2, but not always for PO_2. In the older child or adult, the preferred puncture site is the earlobe; in the young child or infant, it is the heel. Capillary blood specimens are particularly inappropriate when blood circulation is poor and thus should be avoided when a patient has reduced cardiac output, hypotension, or vasoconstriction. For each capillary puncture, the skin should be warmed first with a hot, moist towel to improve the circulation. The puncture itself should be performed as described previously; a free flow of blood is essential. Heparinized capillary tubes containing a small metal bar are used to collect the blood. Tubes should be sealed quickly and the contents mixed well by using a magnet to move the metal bar up and down in the tube so that a uniform specimen is available for analysis.

Anticoagulants and Preservatives for Blood

Serum is defined as the watery portion of blood that remains after coagulation has occurred and is the specimen of choice for many analyses, including viral screening and protein electrophoresis. Samples are collected into tubes with no additive or with a clotactivator and must be allowed to complete the coagulation process before further processing. Plasma is defined as the noncellular component of anticoagulated whole blood and is increasingly being used for routine chemistry testing to decrease turnaround time. Sometimes considerable differences may be observed between the concentrations of analytes in serum and in plasma, as shown in Table 7-4. For molecular diagnostics, anticoagulated whole blood or plasma is more likely to be the specimen of choice. A number of anticoagulants are available, including heparin, ethylenediaminetetraacetic acid (EDTA), sodium fluoride, citrate, acid citrate dextrose (ACD, oxalate, and iodoacetate.

Heparin

Heparin is the most widely used anticoagulant for chemistry and hematology testing. It is a mucoitin polysulfuric acid and is available as sodium, potassium, lithium, and ammonium salts, all of which adequately prevent coagulation. This anticoagulant accelerates the action of antithrombin III, which neutralizes thrombin and thus prevents the formation of fibrin from fibrinogen. Most blood tubes are prepared with approximately 0.2 mg heparin for each milliliter of blood (1000 units/mL) to be collected. The heparin is usually present as a dry powder that is hygroscopic and dissolves rapidly. Heparin has the disadvantages of high cost and a more temporary action of anticoagulation than is attained by chemical means, such as those discussed below. It produces a blue background in blood smears that are stained with Wright's stain. In addition, heparin is said to inhibit acid phosphatase

TABLE 7-4 Differences in Composition Between Plasma and Serum*

Plasma Value > Serum Value, %		No Difference Between Serum and Plasma Values	Plasma Value < Serum Value, %	
Calcium	0.9	Bilirubin	Albumin	1.3
Chloride	0.2	Cholesterol	Alkaline phosphatase	1.6
Lactate dehydrogenase	2.7	Creatinine	Aspartate aminotransferase	0.9
Total protein	4.0		Bicarbonate	1.8
			Creatine kinase	2.1
			Glucose	5.1
			Phosphorus	7.0
			Potassium	8.4
			Sodium	0.1
			Urea	0.6
			Uric acid	0.2

From Ladenson JH, Tsai L-MB, Michael JM, Kessler G, Joist JH. Serum versus heparinized plasma for eighteen common chemistry tests. Am J Clin Pathol 1974;62:545-52. Copyright 1974 by the American Society of Clinical Pathologists. Reprinted with permission.

*To estimate the probable effect of a factor on results, relate percent increase or decrease shown (or intimated) in table to analytical variation (±% CV) routinely found for analytes.

activity and to interfere with the binding of calcium to EDTA in analytical methods for calcium involving complexing with EDTA.

It should be noted that heparin is unacceptable for most tests performed using the polymerase chain reaction (PCR) because of inhibition of the polymerase enzyme by this large molecule. In some special circumstances, a heparin tube can be shared with a molecular diagnostic laboratory if a non-heparinized tube is not available. DNA can be extracted from heparinized samples, but amplification may be reduced.

Ethylenediaminetetraacetic Acid

EDTA is a chelating agent of divalent cations such as Ca^{2+} and Mg^{2+} that is particularly useful for (1) hematologic examinations, (2) isolation of genomic DNA, and (3) qualitative and quantitative virus determinations by molecular techniques, because it preserves the cellular components of blood. It is used as the disodium, dipotassium, or tripotassium salt, the last two being more soluble. It is effective at a final concentration of 1 to 2 g/L of blood. Higher concentrations hypertonically shrink the red cells. EDTA prevents coagulation by binding calcium, which is essential for the clotting mechanism. Newer advances using EDTA include the inclusion of a gel barrier to separate plasma from cells (white tubes; see Table 7-3). In blue/black tubes (see Table 7-3), incorporation of a density gradient allows recovery of nucleated cells after centrifugation, thus increasing the yield of DNA.

EDTA, probably by chelation of metallic cofactors, inhibits alkaline phosphatase, creatine kinase, and leucine aminopeptidase activities. Because it chelates calcium and iron, EDTA is unsuitable for specimens for calcium and iron analyses using photometric or titrimetric techniques. As an anticoagulant, it has little effect on other clinical tests, although the concentration of cholesterol has been reported to be decreased by 3 to 5%.

Sodium Fluoride

Sodium fluoride is a weak anticoagulant that is often added as a preservative for blood glucose. As a preservative, together with another anticoagulant such as potassium oxalate, it is effective at a concentration of approximately 2 g/L blood. It exerts its preservative action by inhibiting the enzyme systems involved in glycolysis, although such inhibition is not immediate[23] and a certain amount of degradation occurs during the first hour after collection. Most specimens are then preserved at 25 °C for 24 hours or at 4 °C for 48 hours. Without an antiglycolytic agent, the blood glucose concentration decreases approximately 100 mg/L (0.56 mmol/L) per hour at 25 °C. The rate of decrease is faster in newborns because of the increased metabolic activity of their erythrocytes and in leukemic patients because of the high metabolic activity of the white cells. Sodium fluoride is poorly soluble, and blood must be well mixed before effective antiglycolysis occurs.

If sodium fluoride is used alone for anticoagulation, three to five times greater concentrations than the usual 2 g/L are required. This high concentration and inhibition of the glycolytic cycle are likely to cause fluid shifts and a change in the concentration of some analytes. Fluoride is also a potent inhibitor of many serum enzymes and in high concentrations also affects urease, used to measure urea nitrogen in many analytical systems.

Citrate

Sodium citrate solution, at a concentration of 34 to 38 g/L in a ratio of 1 part to 9 parts of blood, is widely used for coagulation studies,[7] although the correct ratio of blood to anticoagulant is critical because the effect is easily reversible by addition of standard amounts of Ca^{2+} that are based on a proper collection volume. Because citrate chelates calcium, it is unsuitable as an anticoagulant for specimens for measurement of this element. It also inhibits aminotransferases and alkaline phosphatase but stimulates acid phosphatase when phenylphosphate is used as a substrate. Because citrate complexes molybdate, it decreases the color yield in phosphate measurements that involve molybdate ions and produces low results.

Acid Citrate Dextrose

As indicated previously, the collection of specimens into EDTA is often used for isolation of genomic DNA from the patient. However, additional and complementary diagnostic tests, such as cytogenetic testing, may be requested at the same time. For this reason, samples for molecular diagnostics are often collected into ACD anticoagulant, so as to preserve both the form and the function of the cellular components. There are two ACD tube designations: ACD A and ACD B. These differ only by the concentrations of the additives (see Table 7-3). Both enhance the vitality and recovery of white blood cells for several days after collection of the specimen, thus they are suitable for both molecular diagnostic testing and cytogenetic testing.

Solution A is used for an 8.5-mL blood draw (10 mL total volume), whereas solution B is used for a 3-mL or a 6-mL blood draw (7 mL total volume). The specific test(s) requested will determine the size of tube necessary for specimen collection.

Oxalates

Sodium, potassium, ammonium, and lithium oxalates inhibit blood coagulation by forming rather insoluble complexes with calcium ions. Potassium oxalate ($K_2C_2O_4 \bullet H_2O$), at a concentration of approximately 1 to 2 g/L of blood, is the most widely used oxalate. At concentrations of greater than 3 g oxalate per liter, hemolysis is likely to occur.

Combined ammonium and/or potassium oxalate does not cause shrinkage of erythrocytes. However, other oxalates have been known to cause shrinkage by drawing water into the plasma. Reduction in hematocrit may be as much as 10%, causing a reduction in the concentration of plasma constituents of 5%. As fluid is lost from the cells, an exchange of electrolytes and other constituents across the cell membrane occurs. Oxalate inhibits several enzymes, including acid and alkaline phosphatases, amylase, and lactate dehydrogenase, and may cause precipitation of calcium as the oxalate salt.

Iodoacetate

Sodium iodoacetate at a concentration of 2 g/L is an effective antiglycolytic agent (with the caveats mentioned earlier) and a substitute for sodium fluoride. Because it has no effect on urease, it is often used when glucose and urea tests are performed on a single specimen. It inhibits creatine kinase but appears to have no notable effects on other clinical tests.

Influence of Site of Collection on Blood Composition

Blood obtained from different sites differs in composition. Skin puncture blood is more like arterial blood than venous blood. Thus there are no clinically significant differences between freely flowing capillary blood and arterial blood in pH, PCO_2, PO_2, and oxygen saturation. The PCO_2 of venous blood is up to 6 to 7 mm Hg (0.8 to 0.9 kPa) higher. Venous blood glucose is as much as 70 mg/L (0.39 mmol/L) less than capillary blood glucose.

TABLE 7-5 Difference in Composition of Capillary and Venous Serum*

Capillary Value Greater Than Venous Value, %		No Difference Between Capillary and Venous Values	Capillary Value Less Than Venous Value, %	
Glucose	1.4	Phosphate	Bilirubin	5.0
Potassium	0.9	Urea	Calcium	4.6
			Chloride	1.8
			Sodium	2.3
			Total protein	3.3

*To estimate the probable effect of a factor on results, relate percent increase or decrease shown (or intimated) in table to analytical variation (±% CV) routinely found for analytes.

From Kupke IR, Kather B, Zeugner S. On the composition of capillary and venous blood serum. Clin Chim Acta 1981;112:177-85.

Blood obtained by skin puncture is contaminated to some extent with interstitial and intracellular fluids. The major differences between venous serum and capillary serum are illustrated in Table 7-5.

Collection of Blood from Intravenous or Arterial Lines

When blood is collected from a central venous catheter or arterial line, it is necessary to ensure that the composition of the specimen is not affected by the fluid that is infused into the patient. The fluid is shut off using the stopcock on the catheter, and 10 mL of blood is aspirated through the stopcock and discarded before the specimen for analysis is withdrawn. This is particularly important for molecular diagnostics because the stopcock is often heavily saturated with heparin to prevent clotting. Blood properly collected from a central venous catheter and compared with blood drawn from a peripheral vein at the same time shows notable differences in composition. A comparison of arterial blood with central and peripheral venous blood is illustrated in Table 7-6.

In theory, blood may be collected from the veins of an arm below an intravenous line without interference from the fluid being infused, because retrograde blood flow does not occur in the veins, and the fluid that is infused must first circulate through the heart and return to the tissue before it reaches the sampling site. However, as stated previously, collection from the arm without the intravenous line is recommended.[12]

Hemolysis

Hemolysis is defined as the disruption of the red cell membrane resulting in the release of hemoglobin and may be the consequence of intravascular events (in vivo hemolysis) or

TABLE 7-6 Influence of Collection Site on Composition of Plasma*

	Arterial	Central Venous	Peripheral Venous
Alanine aminotransferase, U/L	62	61	81
Albumin, g/L	36	37	39
Alkaline phosphatase, U/L	114	113	107
Amylase, U/L	149	148	177
Aspartate aminotransferase, U/L	20	20	21
Calcium, mg/L	81	82	83
Chloride, mmol/L	99	97	101
Creatine kinase, U/L	82	73	91
Creatinine, mg/L	14	13	12
γ-Glutamyltransferase, U/L	13	14	14
Potassium, mmol/L	4.0	3.9	3.8
Sodium, mmol/L	144	145	144
Total protein, g/L	66	68	77
Urea nitrogen, mg/L	320	310	250
Uric acid, mg/L	81	81	79

From Rommel K, Koch C-D, Spilker D. Einfluss der Materialgewinnung auf klinisch-chemische Parameter in Blut, Plasma und Serum bei Patienten mit stabilem und zentralisiertem Kreislauf. J Clin Chem Clin Biochem 1978;16:373-80.
*To estimate the probable effect of a factor on results, relate percent increase or decrease shown (or intimated) in table to analytical variation (±% CV) routinely found for analytes.

may occur subsequent to or during blood collection (in vitro hemolysis). Serum and plasma show visual evidence of hemolysis when the hemoglobin concentration exceeds 50 mg/dL. Once the level exceeds 150 to 200 mg/dL, the plasma will appear bright red to most observers. Slight hemolysis has little effect on most test values. However, a notable effect may be observed on those constituents that are present at a higher concentration in erythrocytes than in plasma. Thus plasma activities or concentrations of aldolase, total acid phosphatase, lactate dehydrogenase, isocitrate dehydrogenase, potassium, magnesium, and phosphate are particularly increased by hemolysis. The inorganic phosphate in serum increases rapidly as the organic esters in the cells are hydrolyzed. An additional band caused by hemoglobin may be observed on serum protein electrophoresis. Most manufacturers now provide data on the effects of hemolysis on the analytical performance of individual tests, and this should be evaluated in the selection of individual methods.

Although the amount of free hemoglobin could be measured and a calculation made to correct test values affected by hemoglobin, this practice is undesirable because factors other than hemoglobin could contribute to the altered test values, and it would be impossible to assess their impact. Hemolysis may affect many unblanked or inadequately blanked analytical methods.[27]

In molecular diagnostic testing, hemoglobin may interfere with the amplification reaction, particularly when reverse transcriptase (RT)-PCR is the first step in the analysis of RNA. In some situations, the isolation of nucleic acid is sufficiently selective that free hemoglobin from the ruptured cells is removed and will not cause a problem. However, with hemolyzed blood, alternative or additional extraction methods are usually needed to ensure that RNA is fully and accurately transcribed, and that the greatest amplification of DNA is achieved.

URINE

The type of urine specimen to be collected is dictated by the tests to be performed. Untimed or random specimens are suitable for only a few chemical tests; usually, urine specimens must be collected over a predetermined interval of time, such as 4, 12, or 24 hours. A clean, early morning, fasting specimen is usually the most concentrated specimen, and thus is preferred for microscopic examinations and for the detection of abnormal amounts of constituents, such as proteins, or of unusual compounds, such as chorionic gonadotropin. The clean timed specimen is one obtained at specific times of the day or during certain phases of the act of micturition. Bacterial examination of the first 10 mL of urine voided is most appropriate to detect urethritis, whereas the midstream specimen is best for investigating bladder disorders. The double-voided specimen is the urine excreted during a timed period after complete emptying of the bladder; it is used, for example, to assess glucose excretion during a glucose tolerance test. Its collection must be timed in relation to the ingestion of glucose. Similarly, in some metabolic disorders, urine must be collected during or immediately after symptoms of the disease appear (see Chapter 33 on porphyrins).

When they are to be tested for their alcohol and drugs of abuse content, urine specimens are collected under rigorous conditions requiring chain of custody documentation. (See Chapter 35 for details of such a collection.)

Catheter specimens are used for microbiological examination in critically ill patients or in those with urinary tract obstruction, but should not normally be obtained just for examination of chemical constituents. The suprapubic tap specimen is a useful alternative, because the tap is unlikely to cause infection. After appropriate cleaning of the skin over the full bladder, a 22-gauge spinal needle is passed through a small wheal made by a local anesthetic. The bladder is penetrated and the urine withdrawn into the syringe.

Even though tests in the clinical laboratory are not usually affected by lack of sterile collection procedures, the patient's genitalia should be cleaned before each voiding to minimize the transfer of surface bacteria to the urine. Cleansing is essential if the true concentration of white cells is to be obtained.

Currently, urine is an uncommon specimen type in the molecular diagnostic laboratory for genomic testing, although some laboratories use urine samples for bladder cancer screening and monitoring of therapy for bladder cancer. However, urine is frequently used for molecular testing for infectious agents, such as *Chlamydia,* a common sexually transmitted organism, or BK virus, associated with potential rejection and/or failure of transplanted kidneys. Because most requests involve a specific organism, an untimed or random urine specimen collected into a sterile container with no preservative is usually acceptable.

Timed Urine Specimens

The collection period for timed specimens should be long enough to minimize the influence of short-term biological variations. When specimens are to be collected over a specified period of time, the patient's close adherence to instructions is important. The bladder must be emptied at the time the collection is to begin and this urine discarded. Thereafter all urine must be collected until the end of the scheduled time. If a patient has a bowel movement during the collection period, precautions should be taken to prevent fecal contamination of the urine. If a collection has to be made over several hours, urine should be passed into a separate container at each voiding and then emptied into a larger container for the complete specimen. This two-step procedure prevents the danger of patients splashing themselves with a preservative, such as acid. The large container should be stored at 4 °C during the entire collection period.

Before beginning a timed collection, a patient should be given written instructions with regard to diet or drug ingestion, if appropriate, to avoid interference of ingested compounds with analytical procedures. Thus instructions for collection of specimens for 5-hydroxyindoleacetic acid measurements should specify avoidance of avocados, bananas, plums, walnuts, pineapples, eggplant, acetaminophen, and cough syrups containing glyceryl guaiacolate (guaifenesin). These dietary components are sources of 5-hydroxytryptamine and should be avoided for this reason; the other compounds interfere with certain analytical procedures but may not interfere with highly specific analytical methods. Each laboratory should determine its own requirements. See also specimen information for specific analytes in the respective chapters.

For 2-hour specimens, a prelabeled 1-L bottle is generally adequate. For a 12-hour collection, a 2-L bottle usually suffices; for a 24-hour collection, a 3- or 4-L bottle is appropriate for most patients. A single bottle allows adequate mixing of the specimen and prevents possible loss of some of the specimen if a second container does not reach the laboratory. Urine should not be collected at the same time for two or more tests requiring different preservatives. Aliquots for an analysis such as a microscopic examination should not be removed while a 24-hour collection is in process. Removal of aliquots is not permissible even when the volume removed is measured and corrected, because excretion of most compounds varies throughout the day, and test results will be affected. Appropriate information regarding the collection, including warnings with respect to handling of the specimen, should appear on the bottle label.

When a timed collection is complete, the specimen should be delivered without delay to the clinical laboratory, where the volume should be measured. This may be done by using graduated cylinders or by weighing the container and the urine when preweighed or uniform containers are used. The mass in grams may be reported as if it were the volume in milliliters. There is rarely a need to measure the specific gravity of a weighed specimen because errors in analysis usually exceed the error arising from failure to correct the volume of urine for its mass.

Before a specimen is transferred into small containers for each of the ordered tests, it must be thoroughly mixed to ensure homogeneity, because the specific gravity, volume, and composition of the urine all may vary throughout the collection period. The small container into which an aliquot is transferred should not be a plastic bottle if toluene or another organic compound has been used as a preservative; metal-free containers must be used for trace metal analyses.

Collection of Urine from Children

Collection of a timed specimen from an infant is difficult, but fortunately such specimens are rarely required. The scrotal or perineal area is cleaned and dried first, and any natural or applied skin oils are removed. For an untimed specimen, a plastic bag (U-Bag, Hollister Inc, Chicago Ill; or Tink-Col, C.R. Bard Inc, Murray Hill, NJ) is placed around the infant's genitalia and is left in place until urine has been voided.

A metabolic bed is used to collect timed specimens from infants. The infant lies on a fine screen above a funnel-shaped base containing a drain, under which a container is placed to receive urine. The fine screen retains fecal material. Nevertheless, the urine is likely to be contaminated, to some extent, by such material.

To obtain a sterile urine specimen for culture from an infant, a suprapubic tap is performed. The collection of specimens from older children is done as in adults, using assistance from a parent when this is necessary.

Urine Preservatives

The most common preservatives and the tests for which preservatives are required are listed in Table 7-7. Preservatives have different roles but usually are added to reduce bacterial action or chemical decomposition, or to solubilize

TABLE 7-7 Commonly Used Urine Preservatives

Preservative	Concentrations/Volumes
HCl	6 mol/L; 30 mL per 24 hour collection
Acetic acid	50%; 25 mL per 24 hour collection
Na_2CO_3	5 g per 24 hour collection
HNO_3	6 mol/L; 15 mL per 24 hour collection
Boric acid	10 g per 24 hour collection
Toluene	30 mL per 24 hour collection
Thymol	10% in isopropanol; 10 mL per 24 hour collection

Adapted from information provided in CLSI. Routine urinalysis and collection, transportation, and preservation of urine specimens: CLSI-approved guideline GP16-A3. Wayne, Pa: Clinical and Laboratory Standards Institute, 2009.

constituents that otherwise might precipitate out of solution. Another application is to decrease atmospheric oxidation of unstable compounds. Some specimens should not have *any* preservatives added because of the possibility of interference with analytical methods.

One of the most acceptable forms of preservation of urine specimens is refrigeration immediately after collection; it is even more successful when combined with chemical preservation. Urinary preservative tablets that contain a mixture of chemicals, such as potassium acid phosphate, sodium benzoate, benzoic acid, hexamethylene tetramine, sodium bicarbonate, and mercuric oxide [Starplex Scientific Inc (www.starplexscientific.com)], have been used for chemical and microscopic examination. Because these tablets contain sodium and potassium salts among others, they should not be used for analysis of these analytes. The preservative tablets act mainly by lowering the pH of the urine and by releasing formaldehyde. Formalin has also been used for preserving specimens, but in large amounts it precipitates urea and inhibits certain reactions (e.g., the dipstick esterase test for leukocytes). Acidification to below pH 3 is widely used to preserve 24-hour specimens and is particularly useful for specimens for determination of calcium, steroids, and vanillylmandelic acid (VMA). However, precipitation of urates will occur, thereby rendering a specimen unsuitable for measurement of uric acid.

Sulfamic acid (10 g/L urine) has also been used to reduce pH. Boric acid (5 mg/30 mL) has been used, but it too causes precipitation of urates. Although thymol and chloroform were widely used in the past to preserve specimens for chemical and microscopic urinalysis, it is now recognized that specimens for these tests should be analyzed immediately, and that the addition of preservatives is both largely ineffective and a source of interference with several analytical methods. Toluene is the only organic solvent that is still used as a preservative. When present in a large enough amount, it acts as a barrier between the air and the surface of the specimen. Toluene, however, does not prevent the growth of anaerobic microorganisms and, because of its flammable nature, is a safety hazard. A mild base, such as sodium bicarbonate or a small amount of sodium hydroxide, is used to preserve porphyrins, urobilinogen, and uric acid. A sufficient quantity should be added to adjust the pH to between 8 and 9.

Feces

Small aliquots of feces are frequently analyzed to detect the presence of "hidden" blood—also known as "occult" blood. Detecting this blood is considered an effective means to discover "the presence of a bleeding ulcer or malignant disease in the gastrointestinal tract. The utility of screening for occult blood is that it is included as part of many periodic health examinations. Tests for occult blood should be done on aliquots of excreted stools rather than on material obtained on the glove of a physician doing a rectal examination, because this procedure may cause enough bleeding to produce a positive result. In other instances, the small amount of stool present on the glove may not be representative of the whole, so that bleeding may not be recognized.

In the newborn, the first specimen from the bowel (meconium) may be used for detection of maternal drug use during the gestational period, which requires specific attention to the details of collection and identification (see Chapter 35). Feces from infants and children may be screened for tryptic activity to detect cystic fibrosis. In the infant, fecal material for these tests is usually recovered from the child's diaper. See Chapter 21 for a discussion of the measurement of trypsin in feces.

In adults, measurement of fecal nitrogen and fat in 72-hour specimens is used to assess the severity of malabsorption; measurement of fecal porphyrins is occasionally required to characterize the type of porphyria (see Chapter 33). Usually, no preservative is added to the feces, but the container should be kept refrigerated throughout the collection period, and care should be taken to prevent contamination from urine. When the collection is complete, the container and feces are weighed, and the mass of excreted feces is calculated. The specimen is homogenized and aliquoted so that the amount of fat or nitrogen excreted per day and the proportion of dietary intake excreted can be calculated.

For metabolic balance studies, collections of stool are usually made over a 72-hour period. Many balance studies are carried out in conjunction with research on the metabolism of such elements as calcium. It is important for such studies that a patient be on a controlled diet for a sufficiently long time before commencement of the study, so that a steady state has been attained.

Testing of patient DNA in stool is uncommon, but DNA isolated from fecal samples is representative of the genetic composition of the colonic mucosa at the time of stool collection. The differential and quantitative analysis of stool DNA integrity has been proposed as a sensitive and specific biomarker useful for the detection of colorectal cancer.[2]

Cerebrospinal Fluid

Cerebrospinal fluid (CSF) is normally obtained from the lumbar region, although a physician may occasionally request analysis of fluid obtained during surgery from the cervical region or from a cistern or ventricle of the brain. CSF is examined when there is a question as to the presence of (1) a cerebrovascular accident, (2) meningitis, (3) demyelinating disease, or (4) meningeal involvement in malignant disease. Lumbar punctures should always be performed by a physician. The physician thoroughly cleans the skin of the lumbar region below the termination of the spinal cord where the cauda equina goes through the spinal canal. The physician then makes a small bleb in the skin over the space between the third and fourth or fourth and fifth lumbar vertebrae with 2% procaine and introduces a spinal needle [22-gauge, 3.5 inches (9 cm) long] through the bleb into the spinal canal. The pressure is then measured with a manometer and 3 to 4 mL of fluid allowed to drip into plain tubes. The tubes should be sterile, especially if microbiological tests are required. Because the initial specimen may be contaminated by tissue debris or skin bacteria, the first tube should be used for chemical or serological tests, the second for microbiological tests, and the third for microscopic and cytologic examination. The same procedure is used for infants and children, but the volume of fluid withdrawn should be the minimum for the requested tests.

Up to 20 mL of spinal fluid can be safely removed from an adult, although this amount is not usually required. Antiglycolytic agents usually are not added to the tube for glucose measurement; rapid processing of specimens, a clinical requirement for tests on spinal fluid, ensures that little metabolism of glucose occurs even in the presence of many bacteria. To allow proper interpretation of spinal fluid glucose values, a simultaneous blood specimen should be obtained. The most common use of spinal fluid in molecular diagnostics is for the rapid identification of an infectious agent and for T- and B-cell gene rearrangements associated with hematologic malignancies.

Synovial Fluid

Synovial fluid is a clear thixotropic fluid that serves as a lubricant in a joint, tendon sheath, or bursa. The technique used to obtain it for examination is called *arthrocentesis*. Synovial fluid is withdrawn from joints to aid characterization of the type of arthritis and to differentiate noninflammatory effusions from inflammatory fluids. Normally, only a very small amount of fluid is present in any joint, but this volume is usually very much increased in the presence of inflammatory conditions. Arthrocentesis should be performed by a physician using sterile procedures, and the technique must be modified from joint to joint depending on the anatomic location and the size of the joint. The skin over the joint is cleaned with an antiseptic, such as iodine, and then is anesthetized with an agent like ethyl chloride. A needle of appropriate size is introduced into the joint, and the required amount of fluid is aspirated into the syringe. The physician should establish priorities for the tests to be performed in case the available volume is insufficient for all tests. Sterile plain tubes should be used for culture and for glucose and protein measurements; an EDTA tube is necessary for total leukocyte, differential, and erythrocyte counts. Microscopic slides are prepared for staining with Gram's or other stains indicated, and for visual inspection.

The most common use of synovial (joint) fluid in molecular diagnostics is to assess the presence of infectious microorganisms that lead to complications of great severity. Examples of organisms that the laboratory may test for include (1) *Borrelia burgdorferi,* the causative agent in Lyme disease; (2) *Staphylococcus aureus* for the presence of a staph infection; and (3) aerobic gram-negative bacilli for the presence of *Salmonella, Pasteurella,* or *Pseudomonas,* which can lead to loss of limbs if left untreated.

Amniotic Fluid

Collection of amniotic fluid is a technique known as amniocentesis. It is performed by a physician (1) for prenatal diagnosis of congenital disorders, (2) to assess fetal maturity, or (3) to look for Rh isoimmunization or intrauterine infection. Virtually any molecular diagnostic assay can be applied to the DNA from an amniotic fluid specimen. Some of the more common molecular diagnostic assays include tests for cystic fibrosis, sickle cell anemia, Tay-Sachs disease, and thalassemia.

Gestational timing for sample collection is dependent upon the clinical question. Although ultrasound is not essential, amniocentesis is best performed with its assistance to aid localization of the placenta and to determine the presentation of the fetus. The best sites for obtaining amniotic fluid are behind the neck of the fetus or below its head, or may include other unoccupied areas of the amniotic cavity.

The skin is cleaned and anesthetized as for other similar procedures, and 10 mL of fluid is aspirated into a syringe connected to the spinal needle that is typically used. Sterile containers, such as polypropylene test tubes or urine cups, are used to transport the fluid to the laboratory. Few complications result from amniocentesis. Occasionally a bloody tap is made, but normally the fluid is clear and yellow. The blood may come from the uterine wall, the placenta, or even the fetus. Determination of fetal hemoglobin can be used to help ascertain the source, if it is important to do so.

For prenatal determination of genetic disorders, the cellular content of the amniocentesis sample may not provide sufficient nucleic acid for analysis. To perform cytogenetic studies and to obtain more DNA, the fluid is usually cultured under highly specialized conditions to expand the number of cells. Nine to 12 days of culturing is used to obtain a sufficient number of cells for DNA extraction. The cells are gently removed from the surface of the flask through the use of the enzyme trypsin, mixed, and placed into a collection tube. The sample is then ready for DNA extraction.

Chorionic Villus Sampling

Chorionic villus sampling (CVS) allows for earlier diagnosis of inherited genetic disorders than is possible with amniotic fluid analysis. With CVS, testing can be performed at a gestation period of 10 to 12 weeks, whereas with amniotic fluid, testing generally is not performed until week 15 to 20 of gestation. CVS is the technique of inserting a catheter or needle into the placenta and removing some of the chorionic villi, or vascular projections, from the chorion. This tissue has the same chromosomal and genetic makeup as the fetus and can be used to test for disorders that may be present in the fetus. When chorionic villus is sampled, ultrasound is performed to assess the placenta and determine its position. The sample of the placenta is obtained through the vagina or through the abdomen, depending on the location of the placenta. The specimen is examined under a microscope by a physician at the time of collection to determine the quality, quantity, and integrity of the chorionic villi. Once it is received by the laboratory, the quality of the specimen is further assessed by examination for branching, budding, and veining. The specimen is then placed in culture medium and is allowed to grow for up to 3 weeks. Once the cells are fully confluent, they are treated in the way that cells from amniotic fluid (earlier) are treated for DNA extraction.

Maternal cell contamination testing is used to definitively identify the source of isolated cells in an amniotic fluid sample and in CVS. Such confirmation of the source of the sample is strongly recommended for any prenatal diagnostic testing and may be required as a quality monitor in some laboratories.

Pleural, Pericardial, and Ascitic Fluids

The pleural, pericardial, and peritoneal cavities normally contain a small amount of serous fluid, which lubricates the opposing parietal and visceral membrane surfaces. Inflammation or infection affecting the cavities causes fluid to accumulate. The fluid may be removed to determine whether it is an effusion or an exudate—a distinction made possible by protein or enzyme analysis. The fluid may also be examined for cellular elements.[6] The primary uses of these fluids in the molecular diagnostic laboratory are for infectious agent identification and possibly for the detection of cancer cells.[24]

The collection procedure is called *paracentesis.* When specifically applied to the pleural cavity, the procedure is a *thoracentesis;* if applied to the pericardial cavity, a *pericardiocentesis.* Paracentesis should be performed only by skilled and experienced physicians. Pericardiocentesis has now been largely supplanted by echocardiography.

The skin over the intended puncture site should be cleaned with 70% isopropanol and then allowed to dry in the air. A spinal needle is inserted into the body cavity through a small bleb in the skin raised by injection of a local anesthetic. Fluid is then withdrawn by a syringe and is transferred to appropriate tubes for analysis. Paracentesis is rarely associated with complications. Occasionally, blood-stained fluid is obtained through puncture of a small blood vessel. If adhesions are present between the intestine and the abdominal wall, a part of the intestine could be perforated by a peritoneal tap. With thoracentesis, pneumothorax and bronchopleural fistulas are potential complications.

Saliva

Although measurement of the concentrations of certain analytes in saliva has been advocated,[3] clinical application of methods that use saliva has been limited. Exceptions include measurement of blood group substances to determine secretor status and genotype. Measurement of a drug in saliva has been suggested to estimate the free, pharmacologically active concentration of the drug in serum. There is, however, a considerable difference in pH between saliva and serum, and ratios of bound-to-free drug may not be the same. Fortunately, ultrafiltration techniques are now available that facilitate the processing of serum for free drug analysis.

Several slightly different techniques have been devised for the collection of saliva. Usually an individual is asked to rinse out his or her mouth with water and then chew an inert material, such as a piece of rubber or paraffin wax, from 30 seconds to several minutes. The first mouthful of saliva is discarded; thereafter the saliva is collected into a small glass bottle. Newer devices require the patient to put a small amount of table sugar in the palm of the hand and then touch the table sugar with the tongue. Table sugar promotes the production of saliva. Depending on the collection tube, saliva can be used as a source of DNA or RNA.

Buccal Cells

Collection of buccal cells (cells of the oral cavity of epithelial origin) has been identified as providing an excellent source of genomic DNA. Collection of buccal cells is often viewed as less invasive than collection of blood. It is particularly useful for collecting cells with the patient's genomic DNA when the patient has had blood transfusions and thus has blood with another person's (or persons') DNA. Similarly, it is useful after bone marrow transplantation when the circulating blood cells are derived wholly or partially from the donor of the bone marrow. Two methods are used commonly to collect buccal cells: rinsing with mouthwash and using swabs or cytobrushes.

Rinsing of the oral cavity generally provides a higher yield of cells than can be obtained by using swabs. For these collections, the patient is provided with a small amount of mouthwash and is instructed to rinse well for a minimum of 60 seconds, then return the mouthwash to a collection tube. There is no harm in doing this longer than 60 seconds, but shortening the time may decrease the yield of buccal cells. Mouthwash solutions high in phenol and ethanol are destructive to recovered cells and should be avoided. It is necessary for each laboratory to validate a list of acceptable solutions.

Swabs or cytobrushes have also been used to collect buccal cells for molecular genetics testing. For swabs, a sterile Dacron or rayon swab with a plastic shaft is preferred because calcium alginate swabs or swabs with wooden sticks may contain substances that inhibit PCR-based testing. After collection, the swab or cytobrush should be stored in an air-tight plastic container or immersed in liquid, such as phosphate-buffered saline (PBS) or viral transport medium. In general, the yield of cells and nucleic acid is lower with physical scraping using swabs or cytobrushes than with rinsing.

Solid Tissue

Traditionally, the solid tissue most often analyzed in the clinical laboratory was malignant tissue from the breast for estrogen and progesterone receptors. During surgery, at least 0.5 to 1 g of tissue is removed and trimmed of fat and nontumor material. This tissue is quickly frozen, within 20 minutes, preferably in liquid nitrogen or in a mixture of dry ice and alcohol. A histologic section should always be examined at the time of analysis of the specimen to confirm that the specimen is indeed malignant tissue.

The same procedure may be used to obtain and prepare solid tissue for toxicologic analysis; however, when trace element determinations are to be made, all materials used in the collection or handling of the tissue should be made of plastic or materials known to be free of contaminating trace elements (see also Chapter 31).

Somatic gene analyses, such as T-cell receptor rearrangement and clonal expansion, are now providing important information for clinicians. Additionally, mutations in malignant tissues may be used to direct therapy (see Chapter 43). For these studies, the molecular diagnostic laboratory often receives tissue that has been formalin-fixed and paraffin-embedded (FFPE). In general, neutral buffered formalin, containing no heavy metals, will not interfere with amplification reactions. However, recovery of nucleic acids is greatly decreased if the tissue has been overfixed. DNA can still be extracted from tissue embedded in paraffin, but the DNA will be degraded to low molecular weight fragments. In most cases, segments of DNA will amplify in a PCR reaction, but Southern blot methods will be problematic, as most require high molecular weight DNA.

Tissue structure can be retained without permanent fixation by freezing specimens in an optimal cutting temperature compound (OCT). OCT is a mixture of polyvinyl alcohol and polyethylene glycol that surrounds but does not infiltrate the tissue. The sample is then frozen at ≈–80 °C, and sections are prepared for review by a pathologist. OCT is fully water soluble and should be completely removed from a tissue specimen before it is used as a source of DNA. In general, DNA of higher molecular weight can be extracted from OCT-fixed tissues compared with that extracted from FFPE samples.

Hair and Nails

Currently, the use of hair or nail in molecular diagnostics is limited to forensic analysis (genomic DNA identification). Hair and fingernails or toenails have been used for trace metal and drug analyses. However, collection procedures have been poorly standardized, and quantitative measurements are better obtained from blood or urine.

HANDLING OF SPECIMENS FOR ANALYSIS

Steps that are important for obtaining a valid specimen for analysis include (1) identification, (2) preservation, (3) separation and storage, and (4) transport.

Maintenance of Specimen Identification

Proper identification of the specimen must be maintained at each step of the testing process.[4] The minimum information on a label should include a patient's name, location, and identifying number, and the date and time of collection. All labels should conform to the laboratory's stated requirements to facilitate proper processing of specimens. No specific labeling should be attached to specimens from patients with infectious diseases to suggest that these specimens should be handled with special care. All specimens should be treated as if they are potentially infectious.[14]

In practice, every specimen container must be adequately labeled even if the specimen must be placed in ice, or if the container is so small that a label cannot be placed along the tube, as might happen with a capillary blood tube. Direct labeling of a capillary blood tube by folding the label like a flag around the tube is preferred. For small volumes of urine submitted in a screw-cap urine cup and any specimen submitted in a screw-cap test tube or cup, the label should be placed on the cup or tube directly, not on the cap.

Preservation of Specimens

The practitioner must ensure that specimens are collected into the correct container and are properly labeled; in addition, specimens must be properly treated both during transport to the laboratory and from the time the serum, plasma, or cells have been separated until analysis. For some tests, specimens must be kept at 4 °C from the time the blood is drawn until the specimens are analyzed, or until the serum or plasma is separated from the cells. Examples are specimens for ammonia and blood gas determinations, such as PCO_2, PO_2, and blood pH (see Chapter 28). Transfer of these specimens to the laboratory must be done by placing the specimen container in ice water. Specimens for acid phosphatase, lactate and pyruvate, and certain hormone tests (e.g., gastrin and renin activity) should be treated the same way. A notable decrease in pyruvate and increase in lactate concentration occurs within a few minutes at ambient temperature (see Chapter 28).

For all test constituents that are thermally labile, serum and plasma should be separated from cells in a refrigerated centrifuge. Specimens for bilirubin or carotene and for some drugs, such as methotrexate, must be protected from both daylight and fluorescent light to prevent photodegradation.

Hemolysis may occur in pneumatic tube systems unless the tubes are completely filled and movement of the blood tubes inside the specimen carrier is prevented.[26] The pneumatic tube system should be designed to eliminate sharp curves and sudden stops of specimen carriers, because these factors are responsible for much of the hemolysis that may occur. With many systems, however, the plasma hemoglobin concentration may be increased, and the serum activity of red cell enzymes, such as lactate dehydrogenase, may also be increased. Nonetheless, the amount of hemolysis is usually so small that it can be ignored. In special cases, such as a patient's undergoing chemotherapy whose cells are fragile, samples should be centrifuged before they are placed in the pneumatic tube system or identified as "messenger delivery only."

For the molecular diagnostic laboratory, it's challenging to recover RNA from transported specimens. Depending on the tissue source, RNA yields will vary, primarily because of the amount of RNA present at the time of collection. Specimens from liver, spleen, or heart have large amounts of RNA, but specimens from skin, muscle, and bone have lower RNA content. Increasingly, creative solutions to this issue continue to be produced (e.g., see www.dnagenotek.com) with collection kits that contain stabilizers and even the first reagents required for extraction, all of which have the effect of maximizing the recoverable nucleic acid. Tissue samples should be frozen immediately. Alternatively, a blood specimen should never be frozen before separation of the cellular elements because of hemolysis and released heme that may interfere with subsequent amplification processes. For tissue samples, it is critical to choose the disruption method best suited for the specific type of tissue. Thorough cellular disruption is critical for high RNA quality and yield. RNA that is trapped in intact cells is often removed with cellular debris by centrifugation.[18]

For specimens that are collected in a remote facility with infrequent transportation by courier to a central laboratory, proper specimen processing must be done in the remote facility so that appropriately separated and preserved plasma or serum is delivered to the laboratory. This necessitates that the remote facility has ready access to all commonly used preservatives and wet ice.

Separation and Storage of Specimens

Plasma or serum should be separated from cells as soon as possible and certainly within 2 hours.[21] Premature separation of serum, however, may permit continued formation of fibrin, which can clog sampling devices in testing equipment. If it is impossible to centrifuge a blood specimen within 2 hours, the specimen should be held at room temperature rather than at 4 °C to decrease hemolysis. For most plasma samples used for molecular diagnostics, the plasma should be removed from the primary tube promptly after centrifugation and held at −20 °C in a freezer capable of maintaining this temperature. Frost-free freezers should be avoided because they have a wide temperature swing during the freeze-thaw cycle. Note, however, that 4 °C or −20 °C is not the optimum storage temperature for all tests; some lactate dehydrogenase isoenzymes, for instance, are more stable at room temperature than at 4 °C. Although changes in concentration of test constituents have been observed when serum or plasma is stored in a gel separator tube in a refrigerator for 24 hours, these changes do not appear to be large enough to be of clinical significance.

Specimen tubes should be centrifuged with stoppers in place. Closure reduces evaporation, which occurs rapidly in a warm centrifuge with the air currents set up by centrifugation. Stoppers also prevent aerosolization of infectious particles. Specimen tubes containing volatiles, such as ethanol, *must* be stoppered while they are spun. Centrifuging specimens with the stopper in place maintains anaerobic conditions, which are important in the measurement of carbon dioxide and ionized calcium. Removal of the stopper before centrifugation allows loss of carbon dioxide and an increase in blood pH. Control of pH is especially important for the enzymatic measurement of acid phosphatase, which is labile under alkaline conditions engendered by CO_2 loss.

Cryopreservation of white blood cells and DNA is one method to store and maintain samples for extended periods of time. Whole blood specimens can be centrifuged, and white cells removed and cryopreserved at −20 °C until these cells are required for DNA extraction. For even longer periods of storage, isolated DNA can be stored at −70 °C. The extracted DNA should not be exposed to repetitive cycles of freezing and thawing because this can lead to shearing of the DNA. After these extracted DNA samples have completely thawed, it is important to fully mix the sample to ensure a homogeneous specimen.

Transport of Specimens

Although the remaining discussion uses the specific example of referral laboratory testing by another laboratory, many of the issues discussed, such as regulations related to shipping,[13] are also relevant to a laboratory that receives specimens from outlying clinics via a (laboratory-owned and/or operated) courier service. This may involve validating specific transport/storage conditions that are in conflict with existing CLSI recommendations.[9,19]

Before a referral laboratory is used for any tests, the quality of its work should be verified by the referring laboratory. Guidelines for selection and evaluation of a referral laboratory have been published.[15] For laboratories accredited by the College of American Pathologists (CAP), it is a requirement that the referring laboratory validate that the referral laboratory is CLIA certified by obtaining a copy of the CLIA certificate before specimens are shipped. For molecular diagnostic testing, this is of particular importance, because often the latest genetic test being requested by a physician has not yet been moved from research interest status to patient care status and may not be available in a CLIA-certified laboratory.

Specimen type and quantity and specimen handling requirements of the referral laboratory must be observed, and in laboratories operating under CLIA '88 regulations, test results reported by a referral laboratory must be identified as such when they are filed in a patient's chart. The director of a referring laboratory has the responsibility to ensure that specimens will be adequately transported to the referral laboratory. Also, the director should determine the benefits of different services and should keep in mind that the fastest service is usually the most expensive. The director should also know that specimens should not be sent to a referral laboratory at the end of the week, because more delays in transit occur during weekends than during the working week, and deterioration of specimens is more likely.

It should be assumed that transport from a referring laboratory to a referral laboratory may take as long as 72 hours. Under optimal conditions, a referring laboratory should retain enough specimen for retesting should an unanticipated problem arise during shipment. The tube used for holding a specimen (primary container) should be so constructed that the contents do not escape if the container is exposed to extremes of heat, cold, or sunlight. Reduced pressure of 0.50 atmosphere (50 kPa) may be encountered during air transport, together with vibration, and specimens should be protected from these adverse conditions by a suitable container. Variability in temperature is a significant factor causing instability of test constituents.

Polypropylene and polyethylene containers are usually suitable for specimen transport. Glass should be avoided. Polystyrene is unsuitable because it may crack when frozen. Containers must be leakproof and should have a Teflon-lined screw cap that does not loosen under the variety of temperatures to which the container may be exposed. The materials of both stopper and container must be inert and must not have any effect on the concentration of the analyte.

In situations in which sample delivery for molecular analysis will be delayed, extracted nucleic acid, usually DNA only, can be transported in a buffer solution or water, or it can be dried down and shipped as a loose powder. With either method, DNA should be transported at ambient temperatures and should not be exposed to extremely high temperatures for an extended period of time because it will begin to degrade, and testing may be compromised.

The shipping or secondary container used to hold one or more specimen tubes or bottles must be constructed to prevent the tubes from banging against each other. Corrugated, fiberboard, or Styrofoam boxes designed to fit around a single specimen tube are commonly used. A padded shipping envelope provides adequate protection for shipping single specimens. When specimens are shipped as drops of blood on filter paper (e.g., for neonatal screening), the paper should be enclosed in a paper envelope to ensure that the sample remains dry. The initial paper envelope can be placed in a shipping envelope and transported to the testing facility; rapid shipping is rarely required for dried blood on paper.

For transport of frozen or refrigerated specimens, a Styrofoam container should be used. The container walls should be 1 inch (2.5 cm) thick to provide effective insulation. The container should be vented to prevent buildup of carbon dioxide under pressure and a possible explosion. Solid carbon dioxide (dry ice) is the most convenient refrigerant material for keeping specimens frozen, and temperatures as low as −70 °C can be achieved. The amount of dry ice required in a container depends on the size of the container, the efficiency of its insulation, and the length of time for which the specimens must be kept frozen. One piece of solid dry ice (about 3 inches × 4 inches × 1 inch) in a container with 1-inch Styrofoam walls and a volume of 125 cubic inches (2000 cm^3) will maintain a single specimen frozen for 48 hours.

Various laws and regulations apply to the shipment of biological specimens.[4,8,14] Although they theoretically apply only to etiologic agents (known infectious agents), all specimens should be transported as if the same regulations applied. Airlines have rigid regulations covering the transport of specimens. Airlines deem dry ice a hazardous material; therefore the transport of most clinical laboratory specimens is affected by the regulations, and those who package the specimens should be trained in the appropriate regulations, such as those put forth by the U.S. Air International Transport Association (IATA).

The various modes of transport of specimens influence the shipping time and cost, and each laboratory will need to make its own assessment as to adequate service. The objective is to ensure that the properly collected, processed, and identified specimen arrives at the testing facility in time and under the correct storage conditions so that the analytical phase can then proceed.

REFERENCES

1. Blumenfeld TA, Turi GK, Blanc WA. Recommended site and depth of newborn heel skin punctures based on anatomic measurements and histopathology. Lancet 1979;1:230-3.
2. Boynton KA, Summerhayes IC, Ahlquist DA, Shuber AP. DNA integrity as a potential marker for stool-based detection of colorectal cancer. Clin Chem 2003;49:2112-3.
3. Carroll T, Raff H, Findling JW. Late-night salivary cortisol for the diagnosis of Cushing's syndrome: a meta-analysis. Endocr Pract 2009; 6:1-17.
4. CLSI. Accuracy in patient and sample identification: proposed guideline. CLSI Document GP33-A. Wayne, Pa: Clinical and Laboratory Standards Institute, 2010.
5. CLSI. Blood collection on filter paper for newborn screening programs: approved standard, 5th edition. CLSI Document LA04-A5. Wayne, Pa: Clinical and Laboratory Standards Institute, 2007.
6. CLSI. Body fluid analysis for cellular composition: approved guideline. CLSI Document H56-A. Wayne, Pa: Clinical and Laboratory Standards Institute, 2006.
7. CLSI. Collection, transport, and processing of blood specimens for testing plasma-based coagulation assays and molecular hemostasis assay: approved guideline, 5th edition. CLSI Document H21-A5. Wayne, Pa: Clinical and Laboratory Standards Institute, 2008.
8. CLSI. Collection, transport, preparation, and storage of specimens for molecular methods: approved guideline. CLSI Document MM13-A. Wayne, Pa: Clinical and Laboratory Standards Institute, 2006.
9. CLSI. Ionized calcium determinations: precollection variables, specimen choice, collection, and handling: approved guideline, 2nd edition. CLSI Document C31-A2. Wayne, Pa: Clinical and Laboratory Standards Institute, 2001.
10. CLSI. Procedures and devices for the collection of diagnostic capillary blood specimens: approved standard, 6th edition. CLSI Document H04-A6. Wayne, Pa: Clinical and Laboratory Standards Institute, 2008.
11. CLSI. Procedures for the collection of arterial blood specimens: approved standard, 4th edition. CLSI Document H11-A4. Wayne, Pa: Clinical and Laboratory Standards Institute, 2004.
12. CLSI. Procedures for the collection of diagnostic blood specimens by venipuncture: approved standard, 6th edition. CLSI Document H3-A6. Wayne, Pa: Clinical and Laboratory Standards Institute, 2007.
13. CLSI. Procedures for the handling and transport of diagnostic specimens and etiologic agents: approved standard, 3rd edition. CLSI Document H5-A3. Wayne, Pa: Clinical and Laboratory Standards Institute, 1994.
14. CLSI. Protection of laboratory workers from occupationally acquired infections: approved standard, 3rd edition. CLSI Document M29-A3. Wayne, Pa: Clinical and Laboratory Standards Institute, 2005.
15. CLSI. Selecting and evaluating a referral laboratory: approved standard. CLSI Document GP9-A. Wayne, Pa: Clinical and Laboratory Standards Institute, 1998.
16. CLSI. Sweat testing: sample collection and quantitative chloride analysis: approved guideline, 3rd edition. CLSI Document C34-A3. Wayne, Pa: Clinical and Laboratory Standards Institute, 2009.
17. Flynn JC. Procedures in phlebotomy, 3rd edition. St Louis: Saunders, 2005.
18. Groszbach A. Nucleic acid preparation. Presented at: 4th Annual University of Connecticut Molecular Review Symposium, 26th Annual

Meeting of the Association of Genetic Technologists, May 30, 2001, Minneapolis, Minn.

19. Haverstick DM, Brill LB, Scott MG, Bruns DE. Preanalytical variables in measurement of free (ionized) calcium in lithium heparin-containing blood collection tubes. Clin Chim Acta 2009;403:102-4.
20. Kiechle FL, ed. So you're going to collect a blood specimen: an introduction to phlebotomy, 11th edition. Northfield, Ill: College of American Pathologists, 2005.
21. Laessig RH, Indriksons AA, Hassemer DJ, et al. Changes in serum chemical values as a result of prolonged contact with the clot. Am J Clin Pathol 1976;66:598-604.
22. McNair P, Nielsen SL, Christiansen C, Axelsson C. Gross errors made by routine blood sampling from two sites using a tourniquet applied at different positions. Clin Chim Acta 1979;98:113-8.
23. Mikesh LM, Bruns DE. Stabilization of glucose in blood specimens: mechanism of delay in fluoride inhibition of glycolysis. Clin Chem 2008;54:930-2.
24. Natsugoe S, Tokuda K, Matsumoto M. Molecular detection of free cancer cells in pleural lavage fluid from esophageal cancer patients. Int J Mol Med 2003;12:771-5.
25. Renoe BW, McDonald JM, Ladenson JH. The effects of stasis with and without exercise on free calcium, various cations, and related parameters. Clin Chim Acta 1980;103:91-100.
26. Steige H, Jone JD. Evaluation of pneumatic tube system for delivery of blood specimens. Clin Chem 1971;17:1160-4.
27. Young DS. Effects of preanalytical variable on clinical laboratory tests, 3rd edition. Washington, DC: AACC Press, 2007.

CHAPTER 8

Quality Management

George G. Klee, M.D., Ph.D.,
and James O. Westgard, Ph.D.

The principles of quality management, assurance, and control have become the foundation by which clinical laboratories are managed and operated. This chapter begins with a discussion of the fundamentals of total quality management followed by discussions of (1) total quality management of the clinical laboratory, (2) laboratory error and the Six Sigma process, (3) elements of a quality assurance program, (4) control of preanalytical variables, (5) control of analytical variables, (6) control of analytical quality using stable control materials, (7) control of analytical quality using patient data, (8) external quality assessment and proficiency testing programs, and (9) identification of sources of analytical errors. We conclude the chapter with a discussion on quality initiatives, including the ISO 9000 certification process.

FUNDAMENTALS OF TOTAL QUALITY MANAGEMENT[127]

Public and private pressures to contain healthcare costs are accompanied by pressures to improve quality. Seemingly contradictory pressures for both cost reduction and quality improvement (QI) require that healthcare organizations adopt new systems for managing quality. When faced with these same pressures, other industries implemented *total quality management,* or TQM.[116] TQM may also be referred to as (1) total quality control (QC), (2) total quality leadership, (3) continuous quality improvement, (4) quality management science, or, more generally, (5) industrial quality management. TQM provides both a management *philosophy* for organizational development and a management *process* for improving the quality of all aspects of work. Many healthcare organizations have adopted the concepts and principles of TQM.[12,101]

Fundamental Concepts

In this chapter, *quality* is defined as conformance with the requirements of users or customers. More directly, *quality* refers to satisfaction of the needs and expectations of users or customers. The focus on users and customers is important, particularly in service industries such as healthcare. Users of healthcare laboratories are often nurses and physicians; their customers are patients and other parties who pay the bills.

Cost must be understood in the context of quality. If *quality* means conformance with requirements, then *quality costs* must be understood in terms of "costs of conformance" and "costs of nonconformance," as illustrated in Figure 8-1. In industrial terms, costs of conformance are divided into prevention costs and appraisal costs. Costs of nonconformance consist of internal and external failure costs. For a laboratory testing process, calibration is a good example of a cost incurred to prevent problems. Likewise, quality control is a cost for appraising performance, a repeat run is an internal failure cost for poor analytical performance, and repeat requests for tests because of poor analytical quality are an external failure cost.

This understanding of quality and cost leads to a new perspective on the relationship between them. Improvements in quality can lead to reductions in cost. For example, with better analytical quality, a laboratory would be able to reduce waste; this, in turn, would reduce cost. The father of this fundamental concept was the late W. Edwards Deming, who developed and internationally promulgated the idea that quality improvement reduces waste and leads to improved productivity, which, in turn, reduces costs and provides a competitive advantage.[42] As a result, the organization stays in business and is able to continue providing jobs for its employees.

Fundamental Principles

Quality improvement occurs when problems are eliminated permanently. Industrial experience has shown that 85% of all problems are process problems that are solvable only by managers; the remaining 15% are problems that require the action and improvement in performance of individual workers. Thus quality problems are primarily management problems because only management has the power to change work processes.

This emphasis on processes leads to a new view of the organization as a system of processes (Figure 8-2). For example, physicians might view a healthcare organization as a provider of processes for patient examination (A), patient testing (B), patient diagnosis (C), and patient treatment (D). Healthcare administrators might view the activities in terms of processes for admitting patients (A), tracking patient services (B), discharging patients (C), and billing for costs of

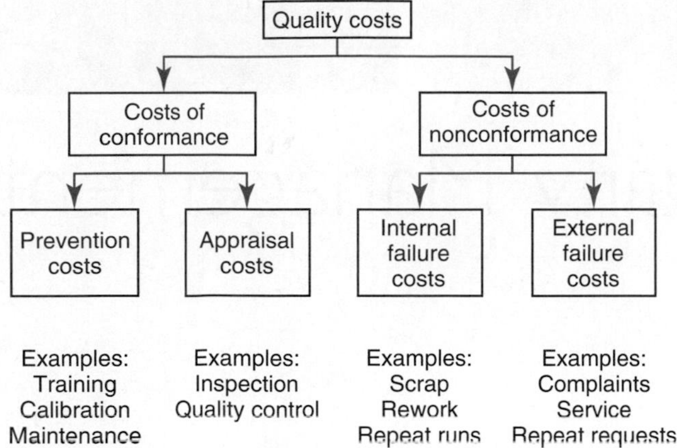

Figure 8-1 The cost of quality in terms of the costs of conformance and the costs of nonconformance with customer requirements. *(From Westgard JO, Barry PL. Cost-effective quality control: managing the quality and productivity of analytical processes. Washington, DC: AACC Press, 1986.)*

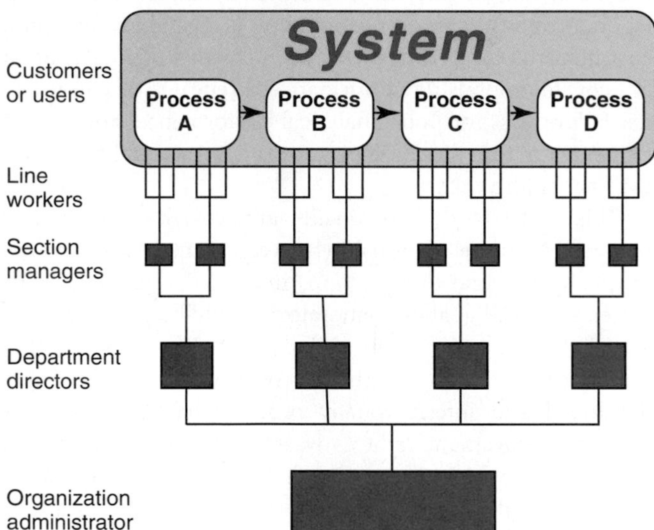

Figure 8-2 Total quality management (TQM) view of an organization as a system of processes.

service (D). Laboratory directors might understand their responsibilities in terms of processes for acquisition of specimens (A), processing of specimens (B), analysis of samples (C), and reporting of test results (D). Laboratory analysts might view their work as processes for acquiring samples (A), analyzing samples (B), performing quality control (C), and releasing patient test results (D). The total system for a healthcare organization involves the interaction of all of these processes and many others. Given the primary importance of these processes for accomplishing the work of the organization, TQM views the organization as a support structure rather than as a command structure. As a support structure, the most immediate processes required for delivery of services are those of frontline employees. The role of upper management is to support the frontline employees and to *empower* them to identify and solve problems in their own work processes.

The importance of empowerment is easily understood if a problem involves processes from two different departments. For example, if a problem occurs that involves the link between process A and process B in Figure 8-2, the traditional management structure requires that the problem be passed up from the line workers to a section manager or supervisor, a department director, and an organization administrator. The administrator then works back through an equal number of intermediaries in the other department. Direct involvement of line workers and their managers should provide more immediate resolution of the problem.

However, such problem solving requires a carefully structured process to ensure that root causes are identified and proposed solutions verified. Juran's "project-by-project" quality improvement process[53] provides detailed guidelines that have been widely adopted and integrated into current team problem-solving methods.[11,12,97] These methods outline distinct steps for (1) carefully defining the problem, (2) establishing baseline measures of process performance, (3) identifying root causes of the problem, (4) identifying a remedy for the problem, (5) verifying that the remedy actually works, (6) "standardizing" or generalizing the solution for routine implementation of an improved process, and (7) establishing ongoing measures for monitoring and controlling the process.

The quality improvement project team provides a new flexible organization unit. A *project team* is a group of employees appointed by management to solve a specific problem that has been identified by management or staff. The team comprises members from any department and from any level of the organization and includes anyone whose presence is necessary to understand the problem and identify the solution. Management initiates the project, and the team is empowered and supported to identify the root cause and verify a solution; management then becomes involved in replanning the process (i.e., planning the implementation of changes in a laboratory process, defining and standardizing the improved process, and establishing appropriate measures for ongoing evaluation and control of the process).[129]

TOTAL QUALITY MANAGEMENT OF THE CLINICAL LABORATORY

The principles and concepts of TQM have been formalized into a quality management process (Figure 8-3). The traditional framework for managing quality in a healthcare laboratory has emphasized the establishment of quality laboratory processes (QLPs), QC, and quality assessment (QA). A QLP includes analytical processes and the general policies, practices, and procedures that define how work is done. QC emphasizes statistical control procedures but also includes nonstatistical check procedures, such as linearity checks, reagent and standard checks, and temperature monitors. QA, as currently applied, is primarily concerned with broader measures and monitors of laboratory performance, such as (1) turnaround time, (2) specimen identification, (3) patient

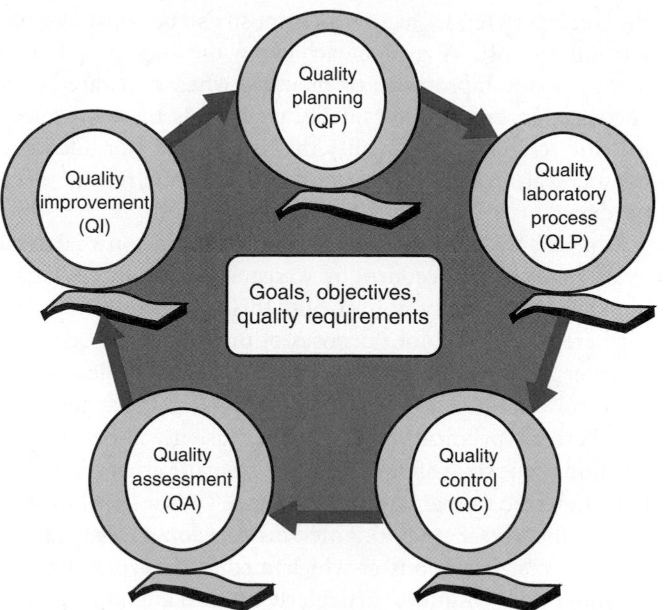

Figure 8-3 Total quality management (TQM) framework for managing quality in a healthcare laboratory. *(From Westgard JO, Burnett RW, Bowers GN. Quality management science in clinical chemistry: a dynamic framework for continuous improvement of quality. Clin Chem 1990;36:1712-6.)*

identification, and (4) test utility. Quality "assessment" is the proper name for these activities rather than quality "assurance." Measuring performance does not by itself improve performance and often does not detect problems in time to prevent negative outcomes. Quality assurance requires that causes of problems be identified through QI and eliminated through quality planning (QP), or that QC be able to detect problems early enough to prevent their consequences.

To provide a fully developed system and framework for managing quality, the QI and QP components must be established.[37,80,127] QI provides a structured problem-solving process for identifying the root cause of a problem and for identifying a remedy for the problem. QP is necessary to (1) standardize the remedy, (2) establish measures for monitoring performance, (3) ensure that the performance achieved satisfies quality requirements, and (4) document the new QLP. The new process is then implemented through QLP, measured and monitored through QC and QA, improved through QI, and replanned through QP. These five components, working together in a feedback loop, illustrate how continuous QI is accomplished and how quality assurance is built into laboratory processes.

The "five-Q" framework also defines how quality is able to be managed objectively using the "scientific method" or the *PDCA cycle* (**p**lan, **d**o, **c**heck, **a**ct). QP provides the planning step, QLP establishes standard processes for doing things, QC and QA provide measures for checking how well things are done, and QI provides a mechanism for acting on those measures. The method that we naturally apply in scientific experiments should also serve as the basis for objective management decisions.

ESTABLISHING QUALITY GOALS AND ANALYTICAL PERFORMANCE LIMITS

Fundamental requirements for all objective quality control systems are clearly defined quality goals. Laboratories must define their service goals and establish clinical and analytical quality requirements for testing processes. Without such quality goals, there is no objective way to determine whether acceptable quality is being achieved, or to identify processes that have to be improved, or to design new processes that ensure that a specified level of quality will be attained.

The establishment of medically relevant analytical performance limits is not an easy task. Each assay and each clinical application of each assay logically should have its own optimal and its own acceptable performance limits. Systematic and random errors generally affect applications differently; therefore independent assessment of the quality goals for these two types of errors may be most practical. Systematic errors have the most profound effect on medical diagnostic decisions, especially those involving specific diagnostic limits. Medical guidelines may specify numeric decision limits such as 200 mg/dL of cholesterol in the National Cholesterol Education Program (NCEP) guideline.[4,8] Analytical tolerance limits for systematic errors may be very tight near the decision limit and less stringent for measurements farther from the decision values. Performance limits for random errors can be bounded by biological variations as follows.

$$SD_{total} = \sqrt{SD^2_{analytical} + SD^2_{biological}}$$

If analytical imprecision is less than 25% of the biological variation [measured as standard deviation (SD) or coefficient of variation (CV)], then the total combined analytical and biological SD or CV will be increased by less than 3% compared with the biological variation [e.g., $\sqrt{(0.25)^2 + (1.00)^2} = \leq 1.03$]. If an assay is used to monitor test changes within an individual over time, the within person biological variation would be the appropriate bonding limit. Values for biological variation were published in a 1999 paper by C. Ricos.[90] Updated values are available at the website www.westgard.com (assessed March 22, 2011).[122]

The establishment of analytical performance goals may represent a compromise between what would be optimal for best medical practice and what is realistically achievable by current technology, given healthcare cost constraints. The optimal systematic error generally is zero, particularly around the decision levels. Consequences of systematic error depend on the uncertainties associated with the other decision variables and the degree of redundancy incorporated into the decision algorithms. When medical decisions are based on multiple independent measurements, the adverse effects of errors in any one measurement are less than when a critical decision is based on only one measurement.

Two types of system analysis are used to determine what analytical performance is achieved with a particular laboratory system. The first is called a *bottom-up analysis,* and the second is a *top-down analysis.*[6,7] In the bottom-up analysis, the system is divided into multiple components. The uncertainties of all components are defined and statistically combined to obtain the total uncertainty of the complete system. The systematic errors add linearly, whereas the random errors add by the square root of the sum of squares.

Total systematic error (SE) and total random error (if independent) are defined as follows:

$$\text{Total Systematic Error (SE)} = \text{Systematic Error}_1 + \text{Systematic Error}_2 + \text{Systematic Error}_N$$

$$\text{Total Random Error} = \sqrt{(\text{Random Error}_1)^2 + (\text{Random Error}_2)^2 + \ldots\ldots (\text{Random Error}_N)^2}$$

(Note: If the component errors are not statistically independent, covariances must be accounted for when adding the random errors.)

Error limits for each of these components are obtained from (1) the manufacturers, (2) published literature, or (3) in-house validation studies.

The top-down analysis generally utilizes quality control measurements and/or proficiency testing results. In-house quality control measurements may underestimate the total errors, particularly if the target values for the controls are not independently assigned, or if the data are collected only over a short period of time. Potential differences across multiple calibrators and differences across multiple reagent lots should be accounted for in estimating total analytical variations. On the other hand, between-laboratory proficiency testing data may overestimate the analytical variation within an individual laboratory.

The performance characteristics obtained from assessment of laboratory processes have been used to back-calculate the system performance that a laboratory is able to realistically achieve. Maximum tolerance ranges utilized in QC programs (the specifications promised to clinicians) must be wider than the limits measured by bottom-up or top-down assessments to provide adequate statistical power to ensure that the laboratory consistently meets performance expectations. For example, if the analytical performance assessment of a laboratory process shows a CV of 5%, the maximum tolerance range for the QC may be set at ±30%, and clinicians should be advised that analytical variation will not exceed ±30% (based on ±6 sigma tolerance specifications). Even if only 4 sigma confidence limits are used, clinicians should be advised that variation may be up to ±20%. The concepts of Six Sigma reliability and the metrics for establishing effective operating QC limits are further explained later in this chapter. Therefore, if the medical utility of the assay can tolerate these wider limits, system integrity would be much better in maintaining this level of performance.

It should be noted that quality goals cannot be set on an absolute basis because they vary from laboratory to laboratory, depending on the medical missions of the healthcare facilities and the professional interests of the physicians using the laboratory tests. Quality goals must also be considered in relation to cost. A goal of achieving the highest possible quality is not appropriate or practical when costs are being curtailed. In establishing quality goals, it is therefore more realistic to specify the quality that is necessary or adequate for medical applications of the laboratory test results to be produced.

The balance of this chapter focuses primarily on analytical quality and the procedures by which it is monitored. Goals for analytical quality are established in the same way that they are established for purposes of method evaluation (see Chapter 2). The philosophy is to define an "allowable analytical error" based on "medical usefulness" requirements. A "total error" specification is useful because it will permit calculation of the sizes of random and systematic errors that have to be detected to maintain performance within the allowable error limit (see Chapter 2).[85] Medical decision concentrations (i.e., the concentrations at which medical interpretation of laboratory test results is particularly critical) are important in establishing the analytical concentrations at which analytical performance has to be most carefully monitored. Thus analytical goals are established by specifying the allowable analytical error and the critical medical decision concentration. Method evaluation is only the first step in validating that analytical performance satisfies those goals. Quality control procedures should provide for continuing verification that those goals are being achieved during routine service.

LABORATORY ERROR AND THE SIX SIGMA PROCESS

A study by the Institute of Medicine found that more than 1 million preventable injuries and 44,000 to 98,000 preventable deaths occur annually in the United States.[60,64] Additional publications have offered suggestions for minimizing medical errors in general.[13,40,64-66,94] The magnitude of laboratory errors and the use of the Six Sigma process in controlling them are discussed in the following sections.

Number of Errors Made in the Clinical Laboratory

A study of 363 incidents captured by a laboratory's quality assurance program in a hospital enumerated the sources and impact of errors.[92] Incidents included those in which (1) physicians' orders for laboratory tests were missed or incorrectly interpreted; (2) patients were not properly prepared for testing or were incorrectly identified; (3) specimens were collected in the wrong containers or were mislabeled or mishandled; (4) the analysis was incorrect; (5) data were entered improperly; or (6) results were delayed, not available, or incomplete, or they conflicted with clinical expectations. Upon evaluating the data, the authors found no effect on patient care for 233 patients; 78 patients were not harmed but were subjected to an unnecessary procedure not associated with increased patient risk; and 25 patients were not harmed but were subjected to an additional risk of inappropriate care. Of the total number, preanalytical mistakes accounted for 218

(45.5%), analytical for 35 (7.3%), and postanalytical for 226 (47.2%). Nonlaboratory personnel were responsible for 28.6% of the mistakes. An average of 37.5 patients per 100,000 treated were placed at increased risk because of mistakes in the testing process.

Witte and colleagues investigated rates of error within the analytical component and found that widely discrepant values were rare, occurring in only 98 of 219,353 analyses.[145] When these results were converted into a standard metric of errors per million episodes, an error rate of 447 ppm was calculated.[13] In another study, Plebani and Carraro identified 189 mistakes from a total of 40,490 analyses, with a relative frequency of 0.47% (4667 ppm). The distribution of mistakes was 68.2% preanalytical (3183 ppm), 13.3% analytical (620 ppm), and 18.5% postanalytical (863 ppm).[86] Most laboratory mistakes did not affect patients' outcomes, but in 37 patients, laboratory mistakes were associated with additional inappropriate investigations, thus resulting in an unjustifiable increase in costs. In addition, laboratory mistakes were associated with inappropriate care or inappropriate modification of therapy in 12 patients. The authors concluded that "promotion of quality control and continuous improvement of the total testing process, including pre-analytical and post-analytical phases, seems to be a prerequisite for an effective laboratory service."[86]

In a study of common immunoassays, Ismail and colleagues found only 28 false results from 5310 patients (5273 ppm).[51] However, as a result of incorrect immunoassay results attributable to interference, 1 patient had 15 consultations, 77 laboratory tests, and an unnecessary pituitary computed tomography scan. The authors stress (1) the necessity for good communication between clinician and laboratory personnel, (2) the importance of the clinical context, and (3) the necessity for use of multiple methods of identifying erroneous test results—a necessity for a rigorous and robust quality system. Heterophilic antibody blocking studies were most effective in identifying interference, but in 21% of patients with false results, dilution studies or alternative assays were necessary to identify the problem. In a similar study, Marks enlisted participation from 74 laboratories from a broad international spectrum of settings and found that 6% of analyses gave false-positive results and, as in the Ismail study, found that use of a heterophilic blocking reagent corrected approximately one third of these.[72] Further evaluation of the data showed no consistent pattern for false results: errors were distributed across donors, laboratories, and systems of analysis. In reviewing the data from these last two studies, Leape suggested setting up a system that would ensure that every result was given a rigorous review before being reported.[64]

Bonini et al conducted several MEDLINE studies of laboratory medical errors and found large heterogeneity in study design and quality and lack of a shared definition of *laboratory error.*[17] However, even with these limitations, they concluded that most such errors occur in the preanalytical phase and suggested that these could be reduced by the implementation of a more rigorous method for error detection and classification and the adoption of proper technologies for error reduction. Thus current QA programs that monitor only the analytical phase of the total process have to be expanded to include both preanalytical (see Chapter 6) and postanalytical phases (www.westgard.com/essay34/assessed March 22, 2011). Through expanded monitoring, the total process would then be managed so as to reduce or eliminate all defects within the process.[86]

Six Sigma Principles and Metrics

Six Sigma,[41A,46A,48] is an evolution in quality management that is being widely implemented in business and industry in the new millennium.[89] Six Sigma metrics are being adopted as the universal measure of quality to be applied to their processes and the processes of their suppliers. The principles of Six Sigma go back to Motorola's approach to TQM in the early 1990s and the performance goal that "6 sigma's or 6 standard deviations of process variation should fit within the tolerance limits for the process," hence, the name Six Sigma (http://mu.motorola.com/accessed March 22, 2011). For this development, Motorola won the Malcolm Baldridge Quality Award in 1988.

Six Sigma provides a more quantitative framework for evaluating process performance and more objective evidence for process improvement. The goal for process performance is illustrated in Figure 8-4, which shows the tolerance specifications or quality requirements for that measurement set at −6S and +6S. Any process can be evaluated in terms of a sigma metric that describes how many sigma's fit within the tolerance limits. The power of the sigma metric comes from its role as a universal measure of process performance that facilitates benchmarking across industries.

Two methods can be used to assess process performance in terms of a sigma metric (Figure 8-5). One approach is to measure outcomes by inspection. The other approach is to measure variation and predict process performance. For processes in which poor outcomes can be counted as errors or defects, the defects are expressed as defects per million (DPM), then are converted to a sigma metric using a standard table available in any Six Sigma text.[48] This conversion from defects per million to sigma levels is an

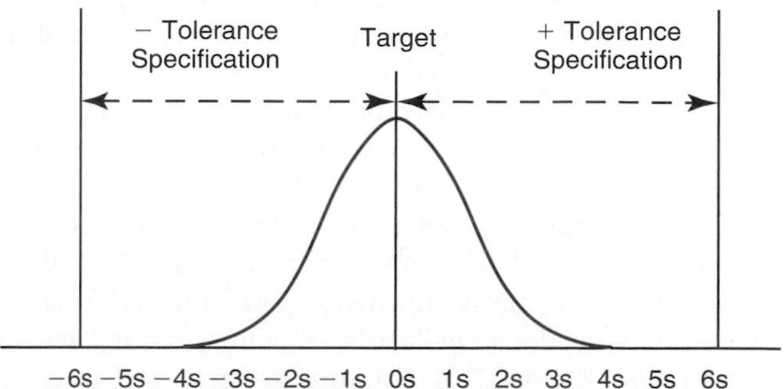

Figure 8-4 Six Sigma goal for process performance "tolerance specification" represents the quality requirement.

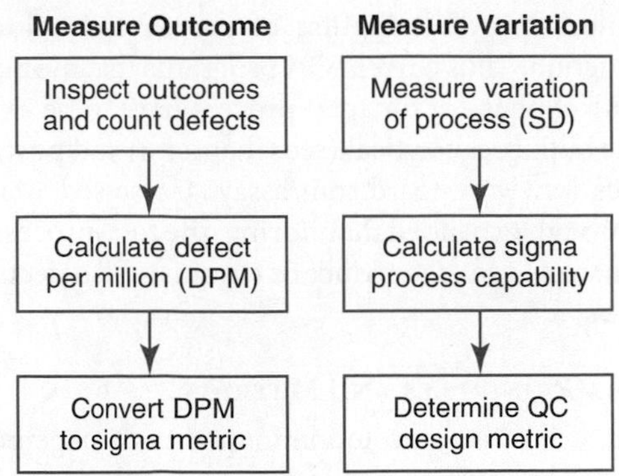

Figure 8-5 Six Sigma methods for measuring process performance. The method of measuring process variation is applicable to analytical testing processes.

enumeration of the area under the error curve plus or minus the tolerance limits (±2 S = 308,500 DPM; ±3 S = 66,800 DPM; ±4 S = 4350 DPM; ±5 S = 230 DPM; ±6 S = 3.4 DPM). In practice, Six Sigma provides a general method by which to describe process outcomes on the sigma scale.

To illustrate this assessment, consider the rates of malfunction for cardiac pacemakers. Analysis of approved annual reports submitted by manufacturers to the Food and Drug Administration (FDA) between 1990 and 2002 revealed that 2.25 million pacemakers were implanted in the United States. Overall, 17,323 devices were explanted because of confirmed malfunction.[70] The defect rate then is estimated at 7699 DPM (17,323/2,250,000), or 0.77%, which corresponds to a sigma of 3.92 using a DPM-to-sigma conversion calculator (http:www.isixsigma.com/sixsigma/six_sigma_calculator.asp?m=basic/accessed March 22, 2011). For comparison or benchmarking purposes, airline baggage handling has been described as 4.15 sigma performance, and airline safety (0.43 deaths per million passenger miles) as better than Six Sigma performance. A defect rate of 0.033% would be considered excellent in any healthcare organization, where error rates from 1 to 5% are often considered acceptable.[13] A 5.0% error rate corresponds to a 3.15 sigma performance, and a 1.0% error rate corresponds to 3.85 sigma. Six Sigma shows that the goal should be error rates of 0.1% (4.6 sigma) to 0.01% (5.2 sigma) and ultimately 0.001% (5.8 sigma).

The first application describing sigma metrics in a healthcare laboratory was published by Nevalainen et al[79] in the year 2000. This application focused on preanalytical and postanalytical processes. Order accuracy, for example, was observed to have an error rate of 1.8%, or 18,000 DPM, which corresponds to 3.6 sigma performance. Hematology specimen acceptability showed a 0.38% error rate, or 3800 DPM, which is a 4.15 sigma performance. The best performance observed was for the error rate in laboratory reports, which was only 0.0477%, or 477 DPM, or 4.80 sigma performance. The worst performance was therapeutic drug monitoring timing errors of 24.4%, or 244,000 DPM, which is 2.20 sigma performance.

Of the studies discussed in the previous section, it is possible to convert the error rates computed in DPM to sigma metrics. For example, for the Ross-Boone study,[92] the computed DPM corresponds to a 3.3 sigma long-term performance. For the Plebani et al study[86] a DPM of 620 DPM corresponds to a 3.2 sigma long-term performance. In the Ismail et al study,[51] a DPM of 5273 corresponds to a 2.6 sigma long-term performance. On average, this indicates about 3.0 sigma long-term performance.

The application of sigma metrics for assessing analytical performance depends on measuring process variation and determining *process capability* in sigma units.[95,110,126] This approach makes use of the information on precision and accuracy that laboratories acquire initially during method validation studies and have available on a continuing basis from internal and external quality control. An important aspect of this method is that the capability, or predictive performance, of the process must be ensured by proper quality control; therefore the ease of assessment comes with the responsibility to design and implement QC procedures that will detect medically important errors.

To apply this method, the tolerance limits are taken from performance criteria for external quality assessment programs or regulatory requirements [such as the U.S. Clinical Laboratory Improvement Amendment (CLIA) criteria for acceptable performance in proficiency testing]; process variation and bias can be estimated from method validation experiments, peer-comparison data, proficiency testing results, and routine QC data. For laboratory measurements, it is straightforward to calculate the sigma performance of a method from the imprecision: SD or CV and inaccuracy (bias) observed for a method and the quality requirement (allowable total error, TE_a) for the test [Sigma = $(TE_a - \text{bias})/SD$]. For a cholesterol test with an NCEP total error of 9%, method bias of 1.0%, and method CV of 2.0%, the sigma metric is 4.0 [(9.0 − 1.0)/2]. If the method had a CV of 3.0% and a bias of 3.0% (the maximum allowable figures according to NCEP guidelines), the sigma metric is 2.0. Sigma metrics from 6.0 to 3.0 represent the range from "best case" to "worst case." Methods with Six Sigma performance are considered "world class"; methods with sigma performance less than 3 are not considered acceptable for production.

Those conclusions can be readily understood by considering the amount of quality control that is necessary for measurement processes having different performance metrics. Figure 8-6 shows a *power function graph* that describes the probability of rejecting an analytical run on the *y*-axis versus the size of the systematic error that has to be detected on the *x*-axis. The bold vertical lines correspond to methods having 3, 4, and 5 sigma performance (left to right). The different lines or power curves correspond to the control rules and the number of control measurements given in the key at the right (top to bottom). These different QC procedures have different sensitivities or capabilities for detecting analytical errors. Practical goals are to achieve a probability of error detection of 0.90 (i.e., a 90% chance of detecting the critically sized systematic error), while keeping the probability of false

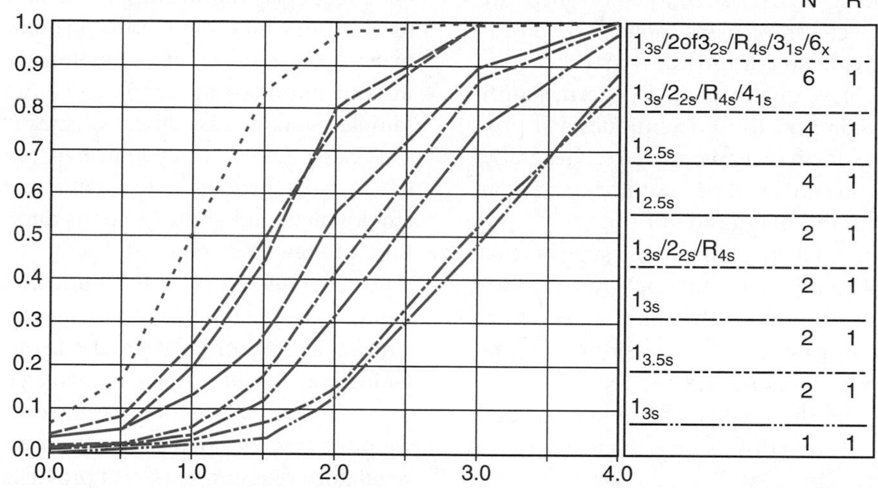

Figure 8-6 The probability for rejection is shown on the *y*-axis versus the size of the systematic error on the *x*-axis *(bottom scale)* or the sigma-metric of the measurement procedure *(top scale)*. The *vertical lines* represent measurement procedures having 3-sigma, 4-sigma, and 5-sigma performance. The key at the right identifies quality control (QC) procedures. The curves in the graph, top to bottom, match the list in the key, top to bottom. *N*, Total number of control measurements; *Pfr*, probability for false rejection; *R*, number of runs to which the QC procedure is applied.

rejection at 0.05 or less (i.e., 5% or lower chance of false alarms). This is easy to accomplish for processes with 5 to 6 sigma performance; it requires more careful selection and increased QC efforts for processes from 4 to 5 sigma, and it becomes very difficult and expensive for processes less than 4 sigma.

As demonstrated previously, the application of Six Sigma principles and metrics is very valuable for all phases of the laboratory testing process.[41A,46B] Because the core business of the laboratory is to produce accurate test results, it makes sense to first apply Six Sigma to the analytical processes. This also is the easiest application because there are tolerance limits in the form of acceptability criteria from peer-comparison and proficiency-testing programs, QC data available for estimating method precision, and peer data available for estimating method bias. Laboratories should next expand their efforts to the preanalytical and postanalytical processes, knowing that their core processes are producing the necessary analytical quality.

Effect of Analytical Bias on Clinical Decisions

Changes in analytical bias directly shift the distribution of patient test values. If the elevated values on a test are associated with specific clinical actions, then the shifts in analytical bias can notably alter the number of patients having test values that exceed the action limit.[56] For example, for a serum calcium assay with an action limit of 10.1 mg/dL, an upward bias of 0.2 mg/dL changes the number of patients subjected to further investigation from 6.5 to 15.0%. Similarly, analytical shifts in other critical analytes can cause notable clinical problems, such as false elevations of prostate-specific antigen values, triggering prostate ultrasound examinations and biopsies, and false elevation of thyroid-stimulating hormone (TSH), triggering additional thyroid examinations. These small analytical shifts can have major downstream effects on healthcare costs.

LEAN PRODUCTION

Lean production is a quality process that is focused on creating more value by eliminating activities that are considered waste. For example, any inefficient activity or process that consumes resources or adds cost or time without creating value is revised or eliminated. In practice, it focuses on *system level* improvements (as opposed to *point improvements*). Because of its success in enhancing efficiency environments,[10] the lean approach has proven useful wherever a defined set of activities is working to produce a product or service. For example, a "lean team" at Saint Mary's Hospital, a Mayo Clinic hospital in Rochester, Minnesota, used lean production to improve the efficiency of its paper ordering system for laboratory work in its intensive care unit.[69] Because the goal of lean production is to enhance efficiency and the Six Sigma Process to improve quality, they have been combined and integrated into the management of several organizations, including healthcare facilities[84,115,144] and clinical[99,106] and molecular diagnostic[28] laboratories.[46]

ELEMENTS OF A QUALITY ASSURANCE PROGRAM

Attainment of quality goals in a clinical laboratory requires a comprehensive quality assurance program. *Quality assurance* is used here to represent practices that are generally recommended for ensuring that desired quality goals are achieved. It is a broad spectrum of plans, policies, and procedures that together provide an administrative structure for a laboratory's efforts to achieve quality goals. The term *quality control* is often used to represent those techniques and procedures that monitor performance parameters. Generally, these are quantitative techniques that monitor particular sources of errors, estimate the magnitude of the errors, and alert laboratory personnel when indications suggest that quality has deteriorated. A quality assurance program involves virtually everything and everybody in the clinical laboratory. An error in any one step during the (1) acquisition, (2) processing, (3) analysis of a specimen, and (4) reporting of a laboratory test result affects the quality of the analysis and causes the laboratory to fall short of its quality goals.

Commitment

Dedication to quality service must be central and reflect a team effort. Otherwise, quality goals are not likely to be achieved. Quality must be a major consideration in all management decisions because any single decision may compromise other plans and practices for attaining quality goals. A true commitment is required by laboratory directors, managers, and supervisors if the efforts of other laboratory personnel are to be successful.

Facilities and Resources

Laboratories must have the administrative support necessary to provide the quality of services desired. This means having (1) adequate space, (2) equipment, (3) materials, (4) supplies, (5) staffing, (6) supervision, and (7) budgetary resources. These resources provide the basis upon which quality services are developed and maintained.

Personnel Competency and Training*

People are critical components of a total quality system, and training and education are vital to the performance of personnel. A key factor in successful training and assessment of laboratory staff is the planning and implementation of targeted education programs. Given the shortage of clinical laboratorians in many countries, laboratories are providing in-depth training for both new and existing staff and are assessing their competency on an ongoing basis. In the United States, CLIA requires competency assessment as part of the laboratory quality system. In other countries, ISO 15189 requires competency assessment as part of the technical requirements for medical laboratories.

CLIA identifies the following six elements as required components of a laboratory competency assessment program: (1) direct observation of routine patient test performance; (2) monitoring of the recording and reporting of test results; (3) review of intermediate test results, QC records, proficiency testing results, and preventive maintenance records; (4) direct observation and performance of instrument maintenance and function checks; (5) assessment of test performance through testing previously analyzed specimens, internal blind testing samples, or external proficiency testing samples; and (6) assessment of problem-solving skills.[87]

Assessment of competence in job tasks as required by CLIA must be conducted semiannually the first year of employment and annually thereafter, and upon implementation of new test methods before patient test results are reported. Guidelines to assist in the development and documentation of competency assessment are available from the Clinical and Laboratory Standards Institute (CLSI). The CLSI Guideline, *Training and Competence Assessment,* gives detailed instructions on how to develop and implement a training and competency assessment program that meets regulatory requirements, and provides examples of forms for documentation and record keeping.[38]

Design of an in-service training program based on instructional systems design includes the following elements: (1) analysis, (2) design, (3) implementation, and (4) evaluation. It begins with a needs assessment or gap analysis to determine employee performance requirements, to identify deficiencies, and to evaluate existing education and training resources. It requires the development of measurable instructional objectives that are based on the specific skills and competencies required of the employee to perform the job or task, and selection of an appropriate teaching strategy. The in-service training program also considers how an instructional program will be delivered and a range of organizational factors that may impact the successful delivery of the instruction. These include (1) employee participation, (2) scheduling, (3) availability of subject matter experts to teach, (4) budget constraints, and (5) assessment of learning outcomes. It provides evaluation of the effectiveness of the instructional program.[39]

A workforce deficiency sometimes found with laboratory personnel is lack of academic education in basic quality control practices and statistical methods of analysis. Without formal training in statistical quality control for the clinical laboratory, employees are often taught what to do, but may not understand the "why," which can impact their ability to troubleshoot and problem-solve. This background understanding is difficult to teach in short, "in-service" laboratory sessions and generally is better provided in a more structured program. Implementing an in-house education program in basic quality control practices that is dependent on the availability of subject matter experts to provide the instruction may not be feasible. A cost-effective, alternative approach is to access experts through existing Web-based training programs and complement this with local problem-oriented examples.

In the face of increased pressures to reduce operating costs, including expenses associated with attendance at and travel to conferences, Internet education programs provide an effective, cost-efficient way to implement in-service training. Web-based training programs in quality control concepts are available through both professional organizations and private

*This information was provided by Susan M. Lehman, Director, Clinical Laboratory Science Program, Mayo Clinic, Rochester, MN.

companies. As an example, the Mayo Clinic identified that a gap in academic education in basic quality control concepts existed based on the diversity of its workforce and the varying academic backgrounds required for its highly specialized laboratories. To provide the desired level of academic education to its employees in a way that could be readily accomplished, employees were enrolled in the course *Basic QC Practices* available on the Web through Westgard QC Inc. The e-learning content of the curriculum includes the following modules: (1) statistical quality control, (2) construction and interpretation of Levey-Jennings control charts, (3) electronic checks and sources of error, (4) CLIA '88 regulations for QC, (5) control materials and limitations of QC, (6) multirule and multilevel interpretation of QC data, (7) false rejection and error detection, (8) troubleshooting, (9) regulatory guidelines, (10) QC documentation and record keeping, and (11) external quality assessment programs. In addition, the online curriculum was customized to employees' specific needs by adding staff lectures, six 2-hour laboratory sessions, assignments tailored to the clinical laboratory practice at Mayo, and pretesting and post-testing to assess competency.

Implementation of this in-house training program in basic quality control by the Mayo Clinic followed the educational model designed for the Clinical Laboratory Science Program. The didactic component is provided in an e-learning platform and is underscored by transactional distance theory,[76] whereby the three modalities of learner interaction with content, instructor, and fellow learners were integrated into the online module. Each lesson plan also includes a supplemental laboratory module taught by traditional methods of interaction between instructor and learner, which is closely anchored in the context of the work performed. Finally, the curricular model implements the *reverse lecture-homework paradigm,* whereby learners complete the Web-supported didactic modules asynchronously as "homework" assignments (Figure 8-7, *A*) and complete the laboratory lessons in the classroom (work setting) under the guidance and direction of the instructor/supervisor (Figure 8-7, *B*).

The in-service training program in quality control concepts follows the CLSI academic curricular model and applies the reverse lecture-homework paradigm (see Figure 8-7). To implement the program, employees complete 14 online lessons asynchronously, as "homework," and participate in 6 scheduled laboratory sessions taught in the traditional format, over a period of 3 weeks. The electronic curriculum includes employee interaction with the written quality control course content ("learner-content"), threaded discussions ("learner-learner"), and email ("learner-instructor"). The online material is applied directly during "hands-on" instructor-facilitated laboratory sessions that are problem-based and consist of a combination of case studies, laboratory activities, and discussions.

Implementing an e-learning platform allows the curricular model to expand the number of students over time toward an improved economy of scale. For academic programs, this approach allows for a potential increase in class size with minimal additional expenses. For in-service training, an electronic curriculum provides the opportunity to share training across different physical sites in a healthcare delivery system. This sharing will eliminate the costs associated with duplication of effort, reduce the operating cost to cover additional employees, and decrease the startup costs for new academic and in-service programs at additional sites.

Technical Procedures

Technical procedures necessary for laboratory services include the following:

1. Control of preanalytical conditions or variables, such as test requests, patient preparation, patient identification, specimen acquisition, specimen transport, specimen processing, specimen distribution, preparation of work lists and logs, and maintenance of records (see Chapters 6 and 9).[149]

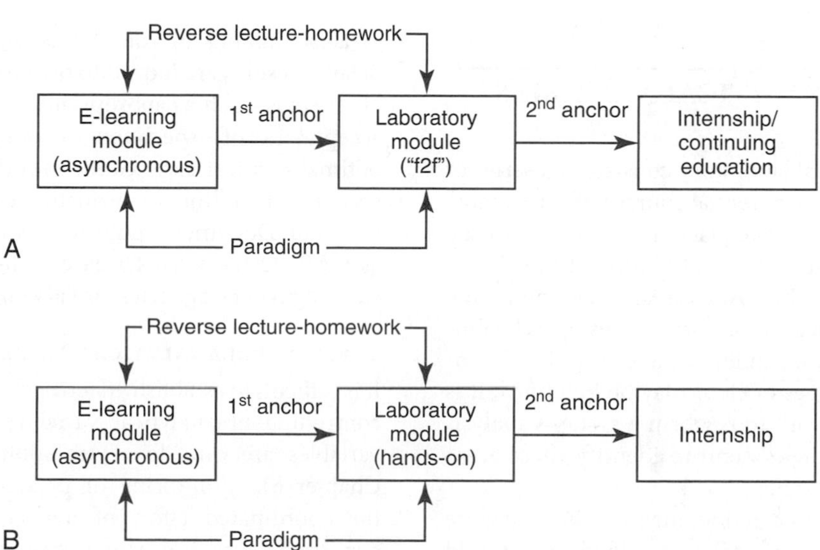

Figure 8-7 Examples of reverse lecture-homework paradigms.

2. Control of analytical variables, which include analytical methods, standardization and calibration procedures, documentation of analytical protocols and procedures, and monitoring of critical equipment and materials.
3. Monitoring of analytical quality through the use of statistical methods and control charts.
4. Control of postanalytical conditions or variables.

Problem-Solving Mechanism

Although it is a particularly critical element in a quality assurance program, the necessity for a mechanism for problem solving is often underemphasized. Such a mechanism provides the link between identification of a problem and implementation of a solution to the problem. It is a *feedback loop* that responds to an error signal by making adjustments to reduce the size of the error or to prevent its recurrence. For problems limited to individual methods or instrument systems, delegation of responsibility for the systems may provide the corrective mechanism. Specialized troubleshooting skills need to be developed and improved and preventive maintenance programs instituted. For problems that occur more generally, the in-service training program can be an important part of the mechanism but often requires additional input from a QC specialist or supervisor to initiate the use of this mechanism and to help define its objectives. A different approach to problem solving is the use of quality teams that meet regularly to analyze problems and identify solutions.[97] By involving personnel, quality teams heighten interest and commitment to quality and provide a creative feedback mechanism.

The comprehensive nature of quality assurance programs and their missions, goals, and activities have been discussed in greater detail by Eilers.[44] Detailed outlines of the elements of cost management for quality assurance are available,[45,54] as are detailed recommendations by professional organizations, such as the College of American Pathologists (CAP),[1] the CLSI,[33,35-37] and the International Federation of Clinical Chemistry,[22-27] and books devoted to quality assurance practices in clinical laboratories.[29,120]

TABLE 8-1 Laboratory Testing Processes and Their Potential Errors

Process	Potential Errors
Test ordering	Inappropriate test
	Handwriting not legible
	Wrong patient identification
	Special requirements not specified
	Cost or delayed order
Specimen acquisition	Incorrect tube or container
	Incorrect patient identification
	Inadequate volume
	Invalid specimen (e.g., hemolyzed, too dilute)
	Collected at wrong time
	Improper transport conditions
Analytical measurement	Instrument not calibrated correctly
	Specimen mixup
	Incorrect volume of specimen
	Interfering substance present
	Instrument precision problem
Test reporting	Wrong patient identification
	Report not posted in chart
	Report not legible
	Report delayed
	Transcription error
Test interpretation	Interfering substances not recognized
	Specificity of test not understood
	Precision limitations not recognized
	Analytical sensitivity not appropriate
	Previous values not available for comparison

CONTROL OF PREANALYTICAL VARIABLES

Systems Analysis

The operation of the clinical laboratory consists of a series of processes, each of which has potential sources of error. Table 8-1 shows the processes that take place from the time of the physician's initial request for a test to the time of final interpretation of the test result. This *systems analysis* identifies the critical processes for a typical laboratory; however, each laboratory situation is somewhat different, and additional processes and additional sources of error may be identified. It is important for each laboratory to perform a systems analysis of its own laboratory testing system to identify those areas where errors are likely to occur.

Once the processes have been documented, those that are most susceptible to error should be identified and should receive the most attention. Often, processes that lead to the greatest number of complaints, such as lost specimens or delayed results, are judged to be most important, even though other steps, such as appropriateness of test selection and the acceptability of a specimen, may be of greater importance for optimal medical care. Guidelines describing procedures for specimen handling are available from organizations such as the CLSI. Documents put forth by accrediting agencies, such as CAP,[1] Centers for Disease Control and Prevention, and state regulatory agencies, are also helpful in this regard.

Types of Preanalytical Variables

It is difficult to establish effective methods for monitoring and controlling preanalytical variables because many of these variables are outside of traditional laboratory areas (see Chapter 6). Monitoring of preanalytical variables requires the coordinated effort of many individuals and hospital departments, each of which must recognize the importance of these efforts in maintaining a high quality of service.

Accomplishing such monitoring may require support from outside the laboratory, particularly from the institution's clinical practice committee or some similar authority. Variables to consider are discussed in the following section.

Test Usage and Practice Guidelines

Traditionally, laboratory test utilization has been monitored or controlled to some degree, but current emphasis on the cost of medical care and government regulation of medical care has increased their importance. For example, clinical practice committees may decide that only certain tests are necessary for emergency care and therefore limit their availability. Peer review audits may lead to the development of other guidelines concerning the appropriate use of diagnostic tests in different clinical situations. Numerous patient care strategies and guidelines are being developed that directly impact laboratory usage.[55] For example, implementation guidelines for the use of bleeding times at the University of Massachusetts Medical Center resulted in a substantial reduction in test requests.[78] Careful monitoring of test requests and their appropriateness is likely to increase in importance, and the laboratory will likely have a role in identifying situations in which test utilization can be optimized and in providing in-service education to effect changes in ordering patterns.

Patient Identification

Correct identification of patients and specimens is a major concern for laboratories. The highest frequency of error occurs with the use of handwritten labels and request forms. One method for checking identification is to compare identifiers such as the patient's name and his or her unique hospital number. The identification on the specimen label should also correspond with the identification supplied with the test requisition. The use of plastic embossed patient identification cards to imprint the patient's name on test request forms and on blood collection labels can eliminate transcription and identification errors but does not guarantee that the patient name on the labels correctly identifies the donor of the specimen. Integration of bar code technology into the analytical systems used by clinical laboratories has significantly reduced within laboratory specimen identification problems (see Chapter 19).

Turnaround Time

Delayed and lost test requisitions, specimens, and reports have been major problems for laboratories. An essential feature in monitoring the cause of delays is the recording of actual times of specimen collection, receipt in the laboratory, and reporting of test results. This has been done manually by placing time stamps in key locations such as blood-drawing centers, specimen-processing stations, result-reporting areas, and wards or chart-posting areas. It also has been done more effectively by programming computer systems to automatically document the times of test requests, specimen acquisition, processing, analysis, and reporting.[91] Turnaround time has been monitored like any other QC variable, and limits established to flag "out-of-range" specimens. Lists of delayed specimens also provide a powerful mechanism for detecting lost specimens or reports. Resolution of problems in this area is aided by a systems analysis of laboratory operations, which helps to identify those steps and areas that cause delays and disruptions in service. A good system for monitoring patient, specimen, and information flow may be obtained through integration of the light wand and/or bar code or optical character identification system with a computer that could automatically track each specimen at each of the steps from test request to result posting.

Transcription Errors

In laboratories where electronic identification and tracking have not been implemented, a substantial risk of transcription error exists is associated with manual entry of data, even with double checking of results. Computerization will reduce this type of transcription error, as such systems often have error detection routines programmed into the terminal entry functions, such as check digits, limit checks, test correlation checks, and verification checks with master hospital files. Implementation of electronic data exchanges eliminates many of these transcription errors.

Patient Preparation

Laboratory tests are affected by many factors such as recent intake of food, alcohol, or drugs, and by smoking, exercise, stress, sleep, posture during specimen collection, and other variables (see Chapter 6). Proper patient preparation is essential for test results to be meaningful. Although responsibility for this usually resides with personnel outside the laboratory, the laboratory must define the instructions and procedures for patient preparation and specimen acquisition. These procedures should be included in hospital procedure manuals and should be transmitted to patients in both oral and written instructions. Compliance with these instructions is monitored directly when the laboratory employs its own phlebotomists. Specific inquiry should be made regarding patient preparation before specimens are collected, and efforts should be made to correct noncompliance. For tests in which standardization of the collection is very important (such as for plasma catecholamines), specimens should be collected in a controlled environment with appropriate supervision.

Specimen Collection

The techniques used to acquire a specimen affect many laboratory tests (see Chapter 7).[104] For example, prolonged tourniquet application causes local anoxia to cells and excessive venous back pressure. The anoxia causes small solutes (such as potassium) to leak from cells, and the venous pressure concentrates cells, proteins, and substances bound to proteins (such as calcium). Blood collected from an arm into which an intravenous infusion is running can be diluted or contaminated. Collection of blood through an indwelling catheter should be avoided because it is a major source of contamination. Hemolysis during and after collection alters the concentration of any analyte that has a red blood cell/plasma concentration differential. Improper containers and incorrect preservatives greatly affect test results and make them inappropriate. One way to monitor and control this aspect of laboratory processing is to have a specially trained laboratory team assigned to specimen collection. All members of the team should be given explicit instruction in the proper methods of specimen collection. The identification of the person collecting a specimen should be maintained. Individuals who process the specimens should be trained to look for and document collection problems. Physicians should be encouraged to report clinically inconsistent results. Similarly, errors detected by limit checks, delta checks (differences between consecutive results on individual patients), or other algorithms should be recorded. Any collection problems should be reviewed with the individuals collecting the specimens. Pride of workmanship should be encouraged, and quality performance should be rewarded.

Specimen Transport

The stability of specimens during transport from the patient to the laboratory is seldom monitored; however, this aspect may be critical for some tests when performed locally and for most tests when sent to regional centers and commercial laboratories.[33] Most laboratories have recommendations for specimen storage and transport, but many of these are empirical and lack adequate scientific documentation. Even the definition of *stability* is not well agreed upon; some investigators accept changes less than 10%,[61,143] and others relate stability to medically significant changes[93] or a percentage of established analytical variability.[112]

In controlling specimen transport, the essential feature is the authority to reject specimens that arrive in the laboratory in an obviously unsatisfactory condition (such as a thawed specimen that should have remained frozen). As with other QC procedures, a small number of problems are expected, but if the error rate gets too large, systems analysis of transport procedures with resulting modifications may be necessary. In tests in which stability is a major problem, the design of specific control procedures appropriate for those tests may be necessary. Potential procedures would include the use of devices to record minimum and maximum temperatures and the use of refrigerated packs in shipping containers.

Accessioning and Documentation

When the serum aliquot tubes arrive in the laboratory, various logging and monitoring systems are necessary. In laboratories without computerized reporting, a request and/or report form generally accompanies the specimens. The specimen should be inspected to confirm adequacy of volume and freedom from problems that would interfere with the assay, such as lipemia or hemolysis. The specimens are then stored appropriately, and identification information and arrival time are recorded in a master log. If analyses are performed in batches, specimen identification generally is recorded in specific locations on the worksheets using the information on the tube labels. After analysis, results are recorded on the worksheet, and if both the assay and the individual test results pass the QC criteria, the test results are transferred to the result forms for reporting. However, before the results are reported, a second technologist should verify the adequacy of the QC and should check for transcription errors by comparing results on the report forms with those on the master log. Specimens that require further analysis because of dilution or assay problems should be indicated on the master log or on a delayed report log.

Specimen Separation and Aliquoting

Separating and aliquoting blood specimens are directly under the control of the laboratory. The main variables are the centrifuges, the containers used, and the personnel.

Centrifuge Performance

Centrifuges are discussed in Chapter 9. For QC purposes, centrifuges should be monitored by checking the speed, timer, and temperature.

Container Monitoring

Evaporation can substantially alter test results; therefore all containers should be sealed or the surface area of the liquids contained in them protected. Collection tubes, pipettes, stoppers, and aliquot tubes are sources of calcium and trace metal contamination. Also, glass beads and other materials added to blood specimens to aid in the separation of serum from cells may cause contamination. Manufacturers should provide reassurance that materials used are tested for contamination by calcium and possibly other elements. Cork stoppers should not be used on specimens intended for calcium determinations because false elevations of 10 to 50% may occur. Some of the plasticizers used in making plastic containers interfere with drug analyses. Also, some plastic materials adsorb trace amounts of some analytes and should not be used for substances in low concentration, such as parathyroid hormone.[52] Also, the effects of evaporation are important matters of concern during processing, storage, and analysis. Because of the intricate relationship between specimen processing and analytical testing, supplies and processing procedures should not be changed without consulting the personnel responsible for analytical testing (see also Chapter 7).

Clerical Errors

An elegant system for monitoring manual clerical functions was developed to detect errors in blood banking records.[109] In this system, known errors are discretely introduced into the system using fictitious patients. The types of errors introduced are chosen to represent errors likely to occur or errors that cause major problems. The fictitious reports are routed to dummy locations and eventually are returned to the QC technologist. One can calculate the efficiency of the laboratory error detection program by comparing the number of fictitious errors discovered versus the number introduced. This efficiency factor is then used to estimate the actual laboratory error rate based on the number of true errors discovered in the laboratory. Implementation of this scheme requires the cooperation of laboratory personnel and the involvement of a QC specialist. Through a combination of paranoia and pride of workmanship, most personnel are more conscientious when they know they are being monitored. A substantial increase in the rate of error detection was observed shortly after this plan was implemented in the blood bank. Public display of individual error rates encourages pride in workmanship.

CONTROL OF ANALYTICAL VARIABLES

Reliable analytical methods are obtained by a careful process of selection, evaluation, implementation, maintenance, and control (see Chapter 2).

Certain variables—water quality, calibration of analytical balances, calibration of volumetric glassware and pipettes, stability of electrical power, and the temperature of heating baths, refrigerators, freezers, and centrifuges—should be monitored on a laboratory-wide basis because they will affect many of the methods used in the laboratory (see Chapter 9). In addition, certain variables will relate more directly to individual analytical methods, and these require that procedures be developed to deal specifically with the characteristics of those methods.

Choice of Analytical Method

Selection and evaluation of analytical methods are discussed in Chapter 2. It is important to recognize, however, that the initial evaluation of a method often takes place in a setting somewhat more idealized than the production setting. Therefore, it is desirable to have a startup period in the service laboratory before test results are to be reported. This period allows time to (1) discover any additional problems, (2) develop maintenance programs that alleviate those problems, and (3) train a sufficient number of analysts to support the routine service operation.

Reference Materials and Methods

Reference materials and methods used are major factors in determining the quality and reliability of the analytical values produced by a clinical laboratory. Uriano[113] and Tietz[111] have defined a hierarchy of analytical methods and reference materials that shows the relationship between them. For example, *definitive methods* are those of highest quality that are used to validate reference methods and primary reference materials. *Primary reference materials* are those of the highest quality that are used in the (1) development and validation of reference methods, (2) calibration of definitive and reference methods, and (3) production of secondary reference materials. *Reference methods* are used to validate field methods. *Secondary reference materials* are used to provide working calibrators for field methods and to assign values to control materials. *Control materials* are used only to monitor field methods.

Definitions of Relevance to Analytical Quality

Many organizations have developed definitions for terms of analytical relevance to the clinical laboratory. Depending on the organization that developed them and the circumstances and culture under which they were developed, definitions for the same term are often slightly different. As part of its global harmonization effort, the CLSI has developed the Harmonized Terminology Database, which is a compilation of internationally accepted terminology (http://www.clsi.org/Content/NavigationMenu/Resources/HarmonizedTerminologyDatabase/Harmonized_Terminolo.htm/accessed March 22, 2011). To use it, one clicks on the Website and then simply enters the term of interest, and definitions for that term are listed. Standard, internationally preferred terms and definitions are highlighted in **blue.** Terms and definitions in black are acceptable; but *only if* the standard internationally preferred terms and definitions are unacceptable for a certain context. Terms highlighted in **red** *are not* acceptable in the international standards community.

In general, the international standards community uses the definitions listed in the *Vocabulary of Basic and General Terms in Metrology* (VIM) document produced by the International Organization for Standardization (ISO). Several of these definitions that are of particular interest to clinical laboratorians are listed in Table 8-2.

ANALYTICAL TRACEABILITY

Considerable effort has been spent in developing a traceable accuracy base for measurands of clinical interest (Figure 8-8).[3,9,41,111,114] The driver to develop such a base was the European Directive 98/79/EC, which requires that "the traceability of values assigned to calibrators and/or control materials must be assured through available reference measurement procedures and/or available reference materials of a higher order" (www.ce-mark.com/ivd.pdf/accessed March 22, 2011). It became effective on December 7, 2003.

In 2002, the Joint Committee for Traceability in Laboratory Medicine (JCTLM) was created to provide a worldwide platform to promote and give guidance on internationally recognized and accepted equivalence of measurements in laboratory medicine and traceability to appropriate measurement standards (http://www.bipm.org/en/committees/jc/jctlm/accessed March 22, 2011), and to review and list reference methods, materials, and laboratories that provide higher order measurement methods. The original three principal participants in JCTLM were the International Bureau of Weights and Measures (BIPM), the International Federation for Clinical Chemistry and Laboratory Medicine (IFCC), and the International Laboratory Accreditation Cooperation. Other key participants include producers of certified reference materials [e.g., National Institute for Standards and Technology (NIST), the Institute for Reference Materials and Measurements (IRMM)]. In vitro diagnostic (IVD) manufacturers are represented by the Advanced Medical Technology Association (AdvaMed) and the European Diagnostic Manufacturers Association (EDMA); external quality assessment and proficiency testing organizations; standards organizations (e.g., CLSI, ISO/Technical Committee 212); and regulatory bodies [e.g., FDA, European Union (EU) authorities, European Commission].

TABLE 8-2 ISO/VIM Definitions of Relevance to the Clinical Laboratory

ISO ID	Term	Definition
2.1	Measurement	Process of experimentally obtaining one or more quantity values that can reasonably be attributed to a quantity
2.2	Metrology	Science of measurement and its application
2.3	Measurand	Quantity intended to be measured
2.4	Measurement principle	Phenomenon serving as the basis of a measurement
2.5	Measurement method	Generic description of a logical organization of operations used in a measurement
2.6	Measurement procedure	Detailed description of a measurement according to one or more measurement principles and to a given measurement method, based on a measurement model and including any calculation to obtain a measurement result
2.7	Reference measurement procedure	Measurement procedure accepted as providing measurement results fit for their intended use in assessing measurement trueness of measured quantity values obtained from other measurement procedures for quantities of the same type, in calibration, or in characterizing reference materials
2.8	Primary reference procedure	Reference measurement procedure used to obtain a measurement result without relation to a measurement standard for a quantity of the same type
2.9	Measurement result	Set of quantity values being attributed to a measurand, together with any other available relevant information
2.13	Measurement accuracy	Closeness of agreement between a measured quantity value and a true quantity value of a measurand
2.14	Measurement trueness	Closeness of agreement between the average of an infinite number of replicate measured quantity values and a reference quantity value
2.15	Measurement precision	Closeness of agreement between indications or measured quantity values obtained by replicate measurements on the same or similar objects under specified conditions
2.17	Systematic measurement error	Systematic error component of measurement error that in replicate measurements remains constant or varies in a predictable manner
2.18	Measurement bias	Estimate of a systematic measurement error
2.19	Random measurement error	Random error component of measurement error that in replicate measurements varies in an unpredictable manner
2.20	Repeatability condition of measurement	Out of a set of conditions that includes the same measurement procedure, same operators, same measuring system, same operating conditions, and same location, and replicate measurements on the same or similar objects over a short period of time
2.21	Measurement repeatability	Measurement precision under a set of repeatability
2.39	Calibration	Operation that, under specified conditions, in a first step, establishes a relation between quantity values with measurement uncertainties provided by measurement standards and corresponding indications with associated measurement uncertainties and, in a second step, uses this information to establish a relation for obtaining a measurement result from an indication
2.40	Calibration hierarchy	Sequence of calibrations from a reference to the final measuring system, where the outcome of each calibration depends on the outcome of the previous calibration
2.41	Metrological traceability	Property of a measurement result whereby the result can be related to a reference through a documented unbroken chain of calibrations, each contributing to measurement uncertainty
2.46	Metrological comparability	Comparability of measurement results, for quantities of a given type, that are metrologically traceable to the same reference
2.42	Metrological traceability chain	A sequence of measurement standards and calibrations that is used to relate a measurement result to a reference

ISO, International Organization for Standardization; *VIM,* Vocabulary of Basic and General Terms in Metrology.
From International vocabulary of basic and general terms in metrology (VIM). Geneva, Switzerland: International Organization for Standardization, 2008. (Note: A Corrigendum or correction of this document was published by the BIPM in 2010.)

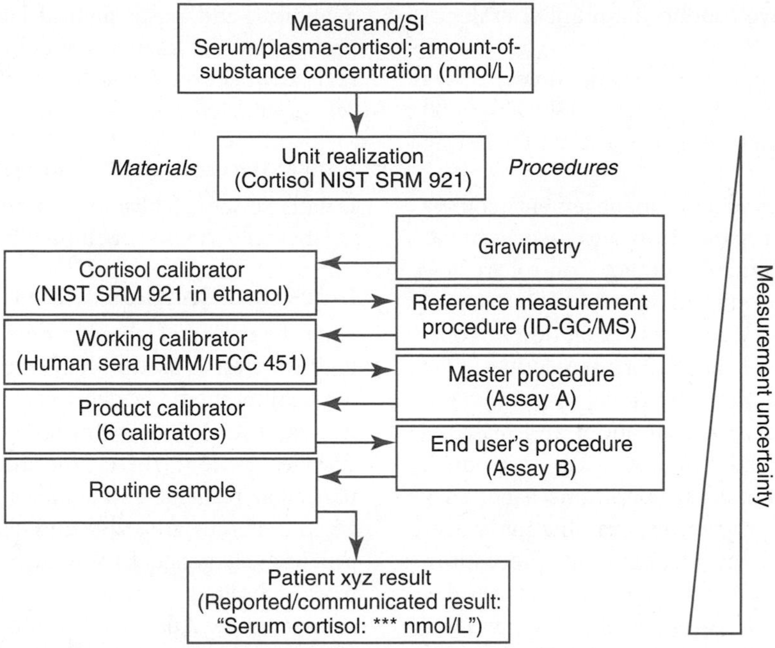

Figure 8-8 Example of traceability chain developed for serum cortisol measurements. Arrows pointing to the left indicate value assignment activity using the procedure; arrows pointing to the right indicate calibration activity using the material. *(Reproduced from Vesper HW, Thienpont LM. Traceability in laboratory medicine. Clin Chem 2009;55:1067-75. With permission from The American Association for Clinical Chemistry. Publishing for Clinical Chemistry Journal.)*

The JCTLM has created two working groups: (1) JCTLM WG-I, Reference Materials and Reference Procedures, and (2) JCTLM WG-II, Reference Laboratory Networks. They are responsible for providing practical support to the worldwide IVD industry in establishing metrological traceability for values assigned to calibrators and/or control materials as required by the European Directive on in vitro diagnostics and by comparable regulations in other countries. Also, the JCTLM is considering forming two additional working groups—one dealing with publications (WR-III), and one with master comparisons (WG-IV).

Role of International Organization for Standardization (ISO)

ISO is a worldwide federation of national standards bodies from more than 150 countries (http://www.iso.ch) accessed March 22, 2011. The work of the ISO results in international agreements, which are published as international standards. The ISO 9000 standards are examples of such standards, and they have been applied on a worldwide basis. The ISO has several technical committees that address quality issues of interest to clinical laboratorians.

ISO 9000

ISO 9000 is a set of standards for ensuring quality management and quality assurance in manufacturing and service industries. They were first published in 1987 and are used worldwide, with more than 80 countries adopting them as national standards. ISO 9000 certification is a tangible expression of an organization's commitment to quality that is recognized internationally. Many major diagnostic companies and healthcare facilities have received ISO 9000 certification.

The ISO 9000 standards include the following:

ISO 9000:2005: Quality management systems—Fundamentals and vocabulary

ISO 9001:2008: Quality management systems—Requirements

ISO 9004:2009: Managing for the sustained success of an organization—A quality management approach

ISO Technical Advisory Groups for Laboratory Standards

The ISO has a number of technical committees that relate to quality activities in the clinical laboratory. For example, in response to a CLSI [then National Committee for Clinical Laboratory Standards (NCCLS)] proposal, the ISO organized in 1995 a Technical Advisory Group (TC 212—Clinical Laboratory Testing and In Vitro Diagnostic Testing Systems). The ISO has delegated responsibility for managing TC 212 to the American National Standards Institute (ANSI), which, in turn, has delegated this responsibility to CLSI. Creation of this technical committee provides a focus for coordination of international standardization in the field of laboratory medicine and in vitro diagnostic test systems. Four working groups for TC 212 have been organized:

- WG 1—Quality management in the clinical laboratory
- WG 2—Reference systems
- WG 3—In vitro diagnostic products
- WG-4—Antimicrobial susceptibility testing

These working groups have produced a number of documents (Table 8-3).

ISO 15189:2007 is an example of an ISO document; it was published by the ISO in 2007 and is based on ISO 9001:2000 and ISO 17025:2005, the latter being a standard for testing and calibration laboratories.

ISO 15189:2007 identifies specific management requirements, such as laboratory organization and management, a quality management system, document control, review of contracts, evaluation by referral laboratories, external services and supplies, advisory services, resolution of complaints, identification and control of nonconformities, corrective action, preventive action, continual improvement, quality and technical records, internal audit, and management review. Technical requirements cover personnel, accommodation and environmental conditions, laboratory equipment, preexamination procedures, examination procedures, assurance of quality of examination procedures, postexamination procedures, and reporting of results. Annexes provide tables that correlate the requirements between ISO 9001:2000 and ISO/IEC 17025:2005. In addition, there are annexes with recommendations for protection of laboratory information systems, ethics in laboratory medicine, and point-of-care testing (POCT).

Other ISO technical committees that relate to quality in healthcare include (1) TC 48—Laboratory Glassware and Related Apparatus; (2) TC 76—Transfusion, Infusion, and Injection Equipment for Medical Use; (3) TC 176—Quality Management and Quality Assurance; (4) TC 210—Quality Management and Corresponding General Aspects for Medical Devices; and TC 215—Health Informatics. ISO/TC 76 is particularly concerned with development of standards for glass containers for blood transfusions, plastic containers for blood collection and transfusion, and blood specimen containers for hematology and biochemistry.

Preparing for ISO Accreditation

In 2002, Burnett compared ISO standards and synthesized an "ideal standard" that became a practical guide for laboratories preparing for ISO accreditation.[21] In his comparison, he supplements the original ISO standards and illustrates their application and provides many examples of specific forms and policies that would be appropriate for a laboratory. He also provides additional technical information about the quality required for the "intended use" of laboratory tests, which is important if the goal of uniform quality is to be achieved for a patient who moves from place to place and from country to country.

Documentation of Analytical Protocols

Step-by-step procedures for performing analytical determinations are critical if the methods are to provide the same results when used by different analysts over a long period of time. Maintaining such consistency requires written protocols or methods and procedure manuals. Examples of process and procedure documents are available in a CLSI document,[35] which includes template documents for preanalytical, analytical, and postanalytical laboratory activities. Method procedures and manuals should be reviewed annually and revised whenever changes occur. It is also a good practice to retain outdated procedures in an archival file.

Establishment of Reference Intervals

Details for the establishment of reference values are presented in Chapter 5. A CLSI document is also available on the topic.[34]

Inventory Control of Materials

Stable operation of laboratory methods is critically dependent on the materials used with the methods. Storage temperatures for stability should be defined and monitored. Procedures are necessary to inventory materials and initiate orders when supplies are low. These procedures must be tailored to the particular reagents and supplies that are in use. In general, when materials are stable and changes in lot numbers cause problems, large stocks should be maintained, although this may be limited by economic considerations, shelf life, and storage space. Adequate inventory should be maintained to allow time for additional shipment and testing of additional supplies should the current shipment be unsatisfactory. Formal inventory control procedures will help minimize required storage by initiating orders when stock reaches a certain predetermined level. Many companies will ship reagents on a standing order once usage rates are established. In fact, with the arrival of rapid transportation and delivery capabilities, a laboratory is now able to order reagents and supplies and receive them in a very short period of time—a "just-in-time" approach to inventory control.

Input Control of Materials

Along with inventory management, the quality of materials should be monitored when they are received. Interruptions in service can be prevented by testing the adequacy of materials before their introduction for routine use. It is particularly important that patient results from new lots of reagents and calibrators be compared with those obtained with previous lots. It also is important to measure QC materials and reassign target values if they change with new lots of reagents. New lots of blood-drawing tubes, processing tubes, and the like should undergo some parallel or comparison testing before their routine use. In establishing pretesting procedures for monitoring incoming materials, it should be recognized that this kind of testing is costly, in terms of both time and money.

Another part of input control is the proper labeling of reagents and materials. Proper identification should include the name, lot number (particular manufacturing batch) and concentration, date received, date prepared, date opened, date of expiration, and recommended storage conditions. In practice, such information is provided by manufacturers via a human-readable bar code.

Monitoring Method Changes

An essential tool for solving analytical problems is a record or log of all changes and problems occurring with a method.

TABLE 8-3 ISO Standards Relevant to Clinical Laboratories

Number	Title
Published Standards	
ISO 15190:2003	Medical Laboratories—Requirements for Safety
ISO 15193:2009	In Vitro Diagnostic Medical Devices—Measurement of Quantities in Samples of Biological Origin—Presentation of Reference Measurement Procedures
ISO 15194:2009	In Vitro Diagnostic Medical Devices—Measurement of Quantities in Samples of Biological Origin—Description of Reference Materials
ISO 15195:2003	Laboratory Medicine—Requirements for Reference Measurement Laboratories
ISO/AWI 15197	In Vitro Diagnostic Test Systems—Requirements for Blood-Glucose Monitoring Systems for Self-testing in Managing Diabetes Mellitus
ISO 15198:2004	Clinical Laboratory Medicine—In Vitro Diagnostic Medical Devices—Validation of User Quality Control Procedures by the Manufacturer
ISO 17511:2003	In Vitro Diagnostic Medical Devices—Measurement of Quantities in Biological Samples—Metrological Traceability of Values Assigned to Calibrators and Control Materials
ISO 17593:2007	Clinical Laboratory Testing and In Vitro Medical Devices—Requirements for In Vitro Monitoring Systems for Self-testing of Oral Anticoagulant Therapy
ISO/TR 18112:2006	Clinical Laboratory Testing and In Vitro Diagnostic Test Systems—In Vitro Diagnostic Medical Devices for Professional Use—Summary of Regulatory Requirements for Information Supplied by the Manufacturer
ISO 18113-1:2009	In Vitro Diagnostic Medical Devices—Information Supplied by the Manufacturer (Labeling)—Part 1: Terms, Definitions, and General Requirements
ISO 18113-2:2009	In Vitro Diagnostic Medical Devices—Information Supplied by the Manufacturer (Labeling)—Part 2: In Vitro Diagnostic Reagents for Professional Use
ISO 18113-3:2009	In Vitro Diagnostic Medical Devices—Information Supplied by the Manufacturer (Labeling)—Part 3: In Vitro Diagnostic Instruments for Professional Use
ISO 18113-4:2009	In Vitro Diagnostic Medical Devices—Information Supplied by the Manufacturer (Labeling)—Part 4: In Vitro Diagnostic Reagents for Self-testing
IISO 18113-5:2009	In Vitro Diagnostic Medical Devices—Information Supplied by the Manufacturer (Labeling)—Part 5: In Vitro Diagnostic Instruments for Self-testing
ISO 18153:2003	In vitro Diagnostic Medical Devices—Measurement of Quantities in Biological Samples—Metrologic Traceability of Values for Catalytic Concentration of Enzymes Assigned Calibrators and Control Materials
ISO 19001:2002	In Vitro Diagnostic Medical Devices—Information Supplied by the Manufacturer With In Vitro Diagnostic Reagents for Staining in Biology
ISO 20776-1:2006	Clinical Laboratory Testing and In Vitro Diagnostic Test Systems—Susceptibility Testing of Infectious Agents and Evaluation of Performance of Antimicrobial Susceptibility Test Devices—Part 1: Reference Method for Testing the In Vitro Activity of Antimicrobial Agents Against Rapidly Growing Aerobic Bacteria Involved in Infectious Diseases
ISO 20776-2:2006	Clinical Laboratory Testing and In Vitro Diagnostic Test Systems—Susceptibility Testing of Infectious Agents and Evaluation of Performance of Antimicrobial Susceptibility Test Devices—Part 2: Evaluation of Performance of Antimicrobial Susceptibility Test Devices
ISO/TS 22367:2008	Medical Laboratories—Reduction of Error Through Risk Management and Continual Improvement
ISO/TS 22367:2008	Medical Laboratories—Reduction of Error Through Risk Management and Continual Improvement Cor 1:2009
IISO/TR 22869:2005	Medical Laboratories—Guidance on Laboratory Implementation of ISO 15189:2003
IISO 22870:2006	Point-of-Care Testing (POCT)—Requirements for Quality and Competence
Standards Under Development	
ISO/WD 11764	Clinical Laboratory Testing—Susceptibility Testing of Fungi
ISO 15189:2007	Medical Laboratories—Particular Requirements for Quality and Competence
ISO 15197:2003	In Vitro Diagnostic Test Systems—Requirements for Blood Glucose Monitoring Systems for Self-testing in Managing Diabetes Mellitus
ISO/DIS 23640	In Vitro Diagnostic Medical Devices—Stability Determination and/or Verification of In Vitro Diagnostic Reagents
ISO/CD TS 25680	Medical Laboratories—Calculation and Expression of Measurement Uncertainty

This should include the date, time, analyst, and any changes in lots of reagents, materials, or calibrators. All instrument maintenance should be recorded, including all work performed by service personnel from outside the laboratory. The occurrence of control problems should be indicated, along with actions taken to resolve the problems. Periodic review of these logs should lead to implementation of preventive maintenance programs, based on the frequency of occurrence of particular problems.

CONTROL OF ANALYTICAL QUALITY USING STABLE CONTROL MATERIALS AND CONTROL CHARTS

In the routine operation of clinical laboratories worldwide, the performance of analytical methods is routinely monitored by analyzing specimens whose concentrations or activities are known, followed by comparing observed values with known values. Known values are usually represented by an interval of acceptable values, or upper and lower limits for control (control limits). When observed values fall within the control limits, the analyst is assured that the analytical method is functioning properly. When observed values fall outside the control limits, the analyst should be alerted to the possibility of problems in the analytical determination. A number of books are available that discuss the application of QC in the operation of the clinical laboratory.[19,29,118,119,130] CLSI document C24 is a good consensus guideline for statistical QC.

Control Materials

Specimens that are analyzed for QC purposes are called *control materials.* They are required to be (1) stable, (2) available in aliquots or vials, and (3) amenable to analysis periodically over a long time. Little vial-to-vial variation should occur, so that differences between repeated measurements are attributed to the analytical method alone. The control material preferably should have the same matrix as the test specimens of interest (e.g., a protein matrix may be best when serum is the test material to be analyzed by the analytical method).[73] Materials from human sources have generally been preferred, but because there is some risk of hepatitis infection, bovine and synthetic materials offer a certain advantage in safety. The concentration of analyte should be in normal and abnormal intervals, corresponding to concentrations that are critical in the medical interpretation of test results.

In practice, clinical laboratories are able to purchase materials from one of several companies that manufacture control sera or "control products." These are generally supplied as liquid, frozen, or lyophilized materials that are reconstituted by adding water or a specific diluent solution. Also available are materials that have matrices representing urine, spinal fluid, and whole blood. Liquid control materials have the potential advantage of eliminating errors caused by reconstitution. However, the matrices of these control materials may contain other materials that are a potential source of error with some analytical methods and instruments.

When commercial control materials are selected, several other elements, in addition to the matrix of the product, should be considered. Stability is critical because it is often desirable to purchase a year's supply of one manufacturing lot or batch. Different batches (or lot numbers) of the same material will have different concentrations, which require new estimates of the mean and standard deviation. The size of the aliquots or vials should be convenient for analytical methods to be monitored. Larger vials are generally less expensive (on a per milliliter basis), but unused materials may eliminate any savings. Two or three different materials should be selected to provide concentrations that monitor performance at different medical decision levels. There may be some advantage in selecting materials from different manufacturers to minimize possible problems with a given manufacturing process. Alternatively, a series of materials designed by one manufacturer to have a certain relationship between concentrations can be used to gain additional information regarding linearity and accuracy.

Control products are purchased as assayed or unassayed materials. Assayed materials come with a list of values for the concentrations that are expected for that material. This list often includes both the mean and the standard deviation for several of the common analytical methods and preferably for a reference method used to measure a particular analyte. Because of the work required to determine these values, assayed materials in general are more expensive. Although the stated assay values are useful in selecting the desired materials, it is advisable to determine the mean and the standard deviation in the user's laboratory, because this process improves the performance characteristics of statistical control procedures.

General Principles of Control Charts

The most common method of comparing the values observed for control materials with their known values is the use of control charts. Control charts are simple graphical displays in which the observed values are plotted versus the time when the observations were made.* The known values are represented by an acceptable range of values, as indicated on the chart by lines for upper and lower control limits. When plotted points fall within control limits, this is generally interpreted to mean that the method is performing properly. When points fall outside the control limits, this may signify a problem with the analytical system or with the controls.

Control limits are usually calculated from the mean ($\bar{x}$) and standard deviation(s) obtained from repeated measurements on known specimens by the particular analytical method that is to be controlled. The mean ($\bar{x}$) and standard deviation(s) are calculated from the following equations:

*Although the discussions in this chapter imply that plots are manually prepared, in actual practice, a wide variety of computer software packages are available for statistically calculating and plotting QA data.

$$\bar{x} = \frac{\sum x_i}{n}$$

$$s = \sqrt{\frac{n\sum_{i=1}^{n} x_i^2 - \sum_{i=1}^{n} (x_i)^2}{n(n-1)}}$$

where x_i is an individual control observation and n is the number of observations in the time period being monitored (see Chapter 2). The initial estimate should be based on measurements obtained over a period of at least 20 days when the method is working properly. These conditions are necessary because the measurements are used to characterize the distribution of values that is expected during stable routine operation of the analytical method.

Also, not all sources of variability may be encountered during this 20-day interval. For example, some sources of variability, such as reagent lot changes, changes with different matrix-related biases for the QC materials, calibrator lot changes with small shifts in results, maintenance cycles, etc, occur at periodic intervals. These sources of variability explain why the cumulative estimate of SD is more reliable as a measure of expected variability, because it includes more sources of variability. The initial estimate may not be entirely reliable owing to the low number of data points and possible outliers in the data. The estimates are revised when more data have been accumulated by recording n and the summations of x_i and x_i2, then using the cumulative totals in the previous equations to obtain cumulative means and standard deviations. The effects of outliers can be minimized by eliminating values exceeding the mean by more than ±3.1 to ±3.8 s (where the exact factor depends on the total number of data points: 3.14 for $n = 30$; 3.22, $n = 40$; 3.33, $n = 60$; 3.41, $n = 80$; 3.47, $n = 100$; 3.66, $n = 200$; 3.83, $n = 400$).

It is assumed that the error distribution of the analytical method is Gaussian (see Chapter 2). The control limits are set to include most of the control values, usually 95 to 99.7%, which correspond to the mean ±2 or 3 SDs. Because it should be a relatively rare occurrence to observe a value in the tails of the distribution (only 1 out of 20 times for 2 s limits and 3 out of 1000 for 3 s limits), such an observation is suspect and suggests that something has happened to the analytical method. Such an occurrence could have caused a shift in the mean (an accuracy problem), which would result in a higher probability of exceeding the limits, or it could have caused an increase in the SD (a precision problem), which would widen the distribution and also result in a higher probability of exceeding the limits.

Figure 8-9, *A*, illustrates how the distributions of control values will appear for three different situations: (1) stable performance where only an occasional observation exceeds the control limits, (2) occurrence of a systematic error that shifts the mean of the distribution and causes a much higher expectation or probability of observing control values outside one of the control limits, and (3) occurrence of an increase in random error or imprecision, which widens the distribution and causes a much higher probability of observing a control value outside either of the control limits.

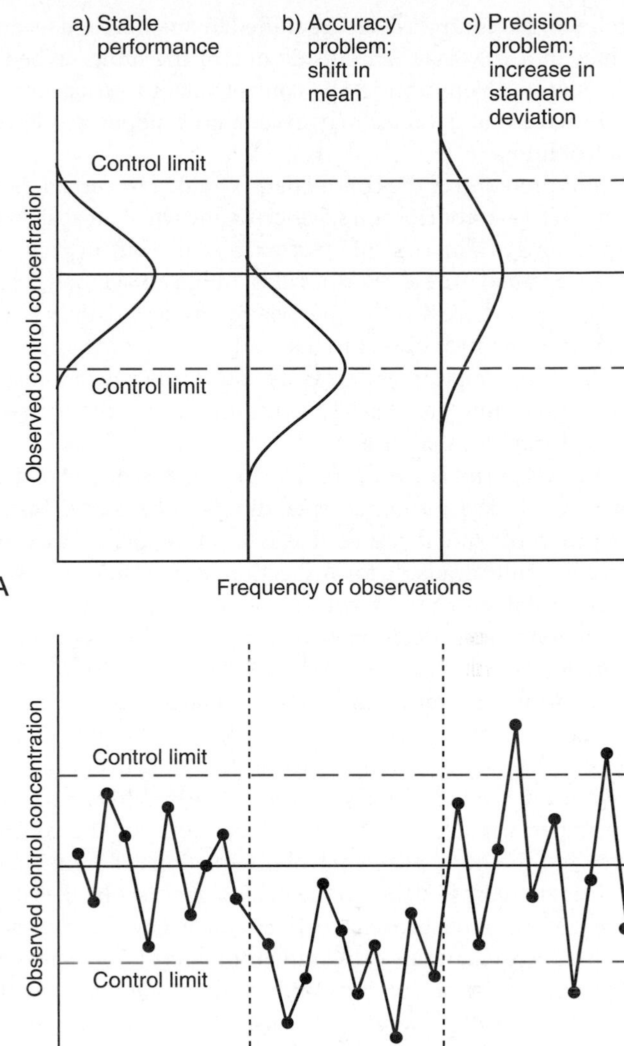

Figure 8-9 Conceptual basis of control charts. A, Frequency distributions of control observations for different error conditions. B, Display of control values representing those distributions when concentration is plotted versus time on a control chart.

Control charts are used to compare observed control values with control limits and to provide a visual display that can be quickly inspected and reviewed. These charts have the concentration or observed value plotted on the *y*-axis versus time of observation on the *x*-axis. It is common practice to plot 1 month's data on a chart—usually only one or two points a day—but the time axis should be chosen to be appropriate for the method being monitored. An example of a control chart is shown in Figure 8-9, *B*, where the control values represent the three situations in Figure 8-9, *A*, with 10 values per situation for a total of 30 values. When the analytical method is operating properly, the control values fall predominantly within the control limits. When there is an accuracy problem, the control values are shifted to one side, and several values in a row may fall outside one of the limits. When a precision problem occurs, the control values fluctuate much more widely, and values may exceed both upper and lower control limits.

Interpretation of the control data is guided by certain decision criteria or control rules, which define when an analytical run is judged "in control" (acceptable) or "out of control" (unacceptable). These control rules are given symbols, such as A_L, or n_L, where A is the abbreviation for a statistic, n is the number of control observations, and L refers to the control limits. For example, 1_{3s} refers to a control rule where 1 observation exceeding the mean ±3 s control limits is the criterion for rejecting the analytical run.

Analytical run is used here to refer to that segment of data for which a decision on acceptability is to be made. This is the group of patient results that is to be reported based on control results available for inspection at that time.

The total number of control observations available for inspection when a decision is to be made on the acceptability of an analytical run is designated as "N." For example, when one control observation precedes and one follows a group of 10 patient samples whose results are to be reported, two control observations are included in this analytical run.

The different control procedures discussed here have different performance capabilities, depending on the control rules and the number of control observations chosen. These choices should be related to the quality goals set by the laboratory. Many of the procedures in use today have been chosen not for best performance, but rather for ease of use in manual implementation or rule availability in the QC software of instruments and laboratory information systems. Tetrault and Steindel contend that the best set of control rules will vary from method to method.[109] Knowledge of the performance characteristics of control procedures is necessary to select control rules and n's that will detect relevant laboratory problems without causing too many "false alarms" (rejections when there are no analytical problems). Experienced analysts often employ a series of informal rules or judgments to reduce the number of false alarms without knowing their effects on the detection of real problems, or true alarms. There should be some quantitative assessment of these two characteristics—false alarms and true alarms—whenever capabilities of new control procedures are assessed or established control procedures are reviewed.

Performance Characteristics of a Control Procedure

The performance of a control procedure is described by its probability for rejection.[137] *Probability* refers to the likelihood that an event will occur; in this case, the event is the rejection of an analytical run. Ideally, there should be no rejections of analytical runs when the analytical method is performing properly. Alternatively, when analytical errors occur, the control procedure should provide a rejection signal. This corresponds to having a probability of 0.00 in the first situation and a probability of 1.00 in the second.

The term *probability for false rejection* (p_{fr}) is used to describe the first situation, in which no analytical errors are present except for the inherent imprecision or inherent random error of the analytical method. (Some random error is always associated with an analytical method, even when it is working properly. This is the random error that is estimated by the replication experiment during method evaluation studies.) When only this inherent random error is present, without any additional errors, the probability for false rejection should be zero. The frequency of false rejection is critical, because false rejections are like false alarms. Too many false alarms cause the analyst to disregard the alarm system, even when the alarm is occurring as a result of real errors that should be corrected.

Probability for error detection (p_{ed}) is the term used to describe the second case, in which there is an analytical error, in addition to the inherent or background random error. The probability for error detection should be high (near 1.00) when these errors are large enough to invalidate the quality goals for the analytical method. Unfortunately, this is difficult to achieve because the control procedure is attempting to detect a signal (additional error) in the presence of noise (inherent random error).

These critical performance characteristics—probability for false rejection and probability for error detection—are summarized by graphs of probability for rejection (y-axis) versus the size of analytical error (x-axis). Graphs such as that shown in Figure 8-10 are called *power functions* because they describe the statistical power of the control procedure.[135] The different lines on the graph represent different numbers of control observations (e.g., n = 1, 2, and 4 for the three lines on this graph). The probability for false rejection is given by the

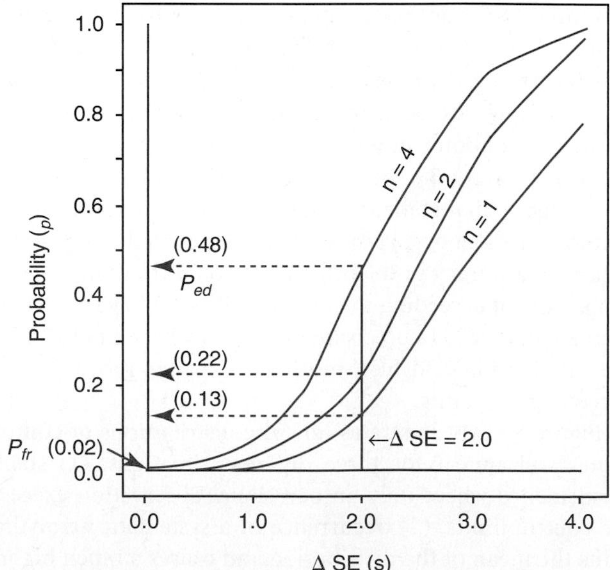

Figure 8-10 Power function graph presenting probability for rejection on the *y*-axis versus size of the error on the *x*-axis. The different lines represent numbers of control observations, in this case, *n* = 1, 2, and 4.

y-intercept, the point where each line intersects the *y*-axis. For this control procedure with *n* from 1 to 4, p_{fr} is 0.01 to 0.02, or 1 to 2%. The probability for error detection can be determined for an error of any size by locating the size of the error on the *x*-axis, drawing a line up to intersect the power function curve, drawing a horizontal line from the point of intersection to the *y*-axis, and reading the probability for rejection from the scale on the *y*-axis. For this control procedure, p_{ed} is 0.13 for $n = 1$, 0.22 for $n = 2$, and 0.48 for $n = 4$. Thus there is a 13 to 48% chance of detecting an error of this size with this control procedure, depending on the number of control observations used.

Two power function graphs are necessary: one to describe the performance for random error (RE) and the other for the performance for systematic error (SE). For RE, as shown in Figure 8-11, *A*, the *x*-axis is labeled ΔRE. A value of 1.0 is consistent with the standard deviation of the analytical method; when the system is working properly, a value of 2.0 corresponds to a doubling of the initial standard deviation, 3.0 to a tripling, and so forth. For systematic error, the *x*-axis is labeled ΔSE (Figure 8-11, *B*). A value of 1.0 s corresponds to a systematic shift equivalent to the size of the standard deviation, a value of 2.0 s to a shift equivalent to two times s, and so forth.

Power functions are determined by mathematical calculations or by computer simulation studies, the latter having been used in clinical laboratories to characterize many of the commonly used control procedures.[47,135] Power functions are useful for evaluating the performance capabilities of individual control procedures, for comparing the performance of different control procedures, and for designing new procedures with improved performance characteristics. The best control procedure is the one with the lowest probability for false rejection and the highest probability for detecting those errors that are large enough to invalidate the analytical quality goals for the method.

The sizes of the analytical errors that must be detected if the control procedure is to maintain a specified quality can be determined from a general analytical model for translating quality requirements into laboratory process specifications.[142]

$$TE_a = bias_{meas} + \Delta SE_{cont} s_{meas} + z\Delta RE_{cont} s_{meas}$$

TE_a is the analytical quality requirement expressed as an allowable total error. Minimum total error requirements for between laboratory proficiency testing evaluations are defined by the CLIA proficiency testing criteria for acceptable performance (see later section). $Bias_{meas}$ is the analytical measurement bias (stable inaccuracy), s_{meas} is the analytical measurement standard deviation (stable imprecision), ΔSE_{cont} is the change in systematic error (unstable inaccuracy) to be detected by the control procedure, ΔRE_{cont} is the change in random error (unstable imprecision) to be detected by the control procedure, and *z* is related to the chance of exceeding the quality requirement. When *z* is 1.65, a maximum defect rate of 5% may occur before an analytical run is rejected.

This analytical model is solved for ΔSE_{cont} (by setting ΔRE_{cont} to 1.0) or for ΔRE_{cont} (by setting ΔSE_{cont} to 0.0) to determine the critical sizes of errors that must be detected to maintain performance within the specified quality:

$$\Delta SE_{crit} = [(TE_a - |bias_{meas}|)/s_{meas}] - 1.65$$
$$\Delta RE_{crit} = (TE_a - |bias_{meas}|)/1.65\, s_{meas}$$

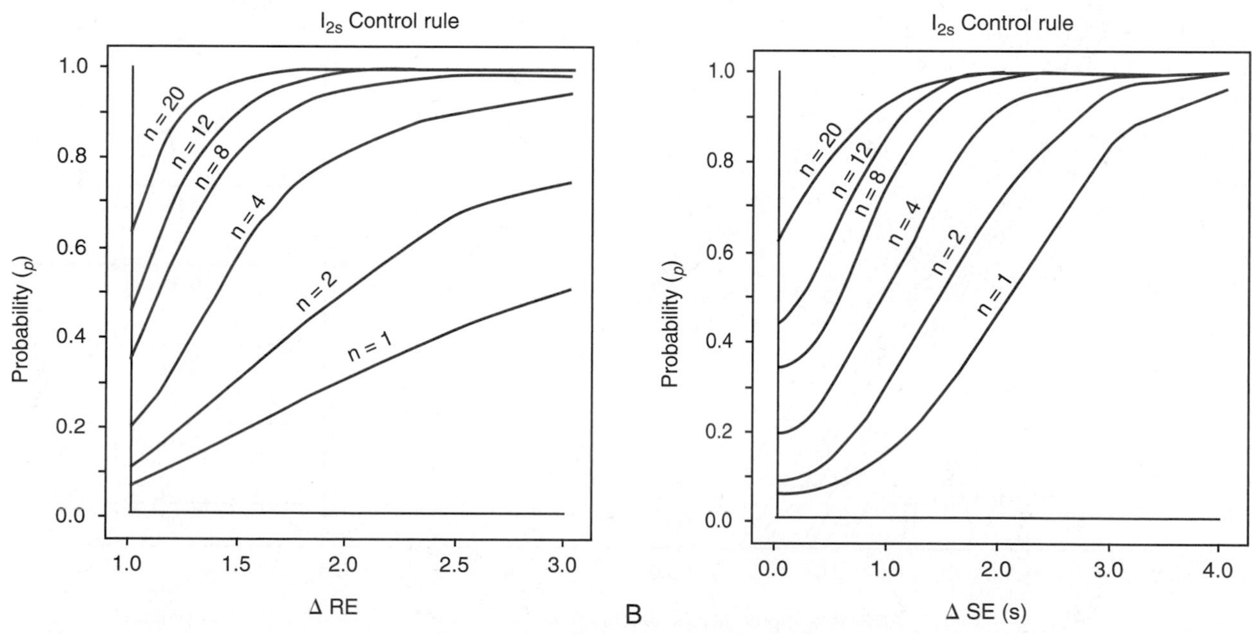

Figure 8-11 Power functions for 12s control rule. A, Random error. B, Systematic error. *(From Westgard JO, Groth T. Power functions for statistical control rules. Clin Chem 1979;25:863-9.)*

ΔSE_{crit} is the critical systematic error that would shift the distribution enough to cause 5% of the test results to exceed TE_a; ΔRE_{crit} is the critical increase in random error that would widen the distribution enough to cause 5% of the test results to exceed TE_a ($z = 1.65$ for 5% on one side; $z = 1.96$ for 2.5% on each side).

For example, if TE_a were specified as 10 mg/dL at a concentration of 120 mg/dL, and s_{meas} were estimated as 2.0 mg/dL and $bias_{meas}$ as 0.0 mg/dL, ΔSE_{crit} would be 3.35, and ΔRE_{crit} would be 3.03. This indicates that the control procedure has to be able to detect a systematic shift equivalent to 6.7 mg/dL (3.35 s) and a random error equivalent to a standard deviation of 6.1 mg/dL (3.03 s).

With knowledge of these values for critical errors and the power functions for a control procedure, it is possible to make a critical assessment of the performance achievable by different statistical control procedures. The quality of the control procedures themselves can be evaluated and related to the quality goals defined for the laboratory.

The relationship between the quality requirement for a test, the imprecision and inaccuracy that are allowable, and the QC that is necessary is shown graphically by a chart of operating specifications (OPSpecs chart).[117,121] Figure 8-12 shows such a chart that has been prepared for a TE_a of 10%, single rules and multirules with *n*'s that are commonly used in laboratories, and a p_{ed} of 0.90 or 90% error detection for systematic errors. This OPSpecs chart is derived from the analytical quality planning model shown earlier, setting ΔRE to 1.0, then rearranging as follows:

$$bias_{meas} = TE_a - (\Delta SE_{cont} + 1.65)s_{meas}$$

Notice that this equation has the form of a straight line ($Y = a + bX$), where the *y*-intercept *(a)* is TE_a and the slope *(b)* depends on the sensitivity of the QC procedure. The value for ΔSE_{cont} is obtained from power curves for the control rules and *n*'s of interest and for specified probabilities, such as 90% and 50%.[117] A plot of $bias_{meas}$ versus s_{meas} will describe the allowable limits of imprecision and inaccuracy for different control rules and different numbers of control measurements. A QC procedure can be selected by plotting the observed inaccuracy and imprecision as the method's operating point, then identifying the control rules and *n*'s of the lines above the operating point.

For this example, where the observed imprecision is 2.0% and the observed inaccuracy is 1.0%, the four lines above the operating point correspond to the top four QC procedures listed in the key on the right. All four will provide at least 90% detection of critical systematic errors, but their false rejection rates will vary from 0.03 to 0.18, or 3 to 18%. Appropriate choices would be the $1_{2.5s}$ single rule with $n = 4$, or the $1_{3s}/2_{2s}/R_{4s}/4_{1s}$ multirule with $n = 4$, to keep false rejections low.

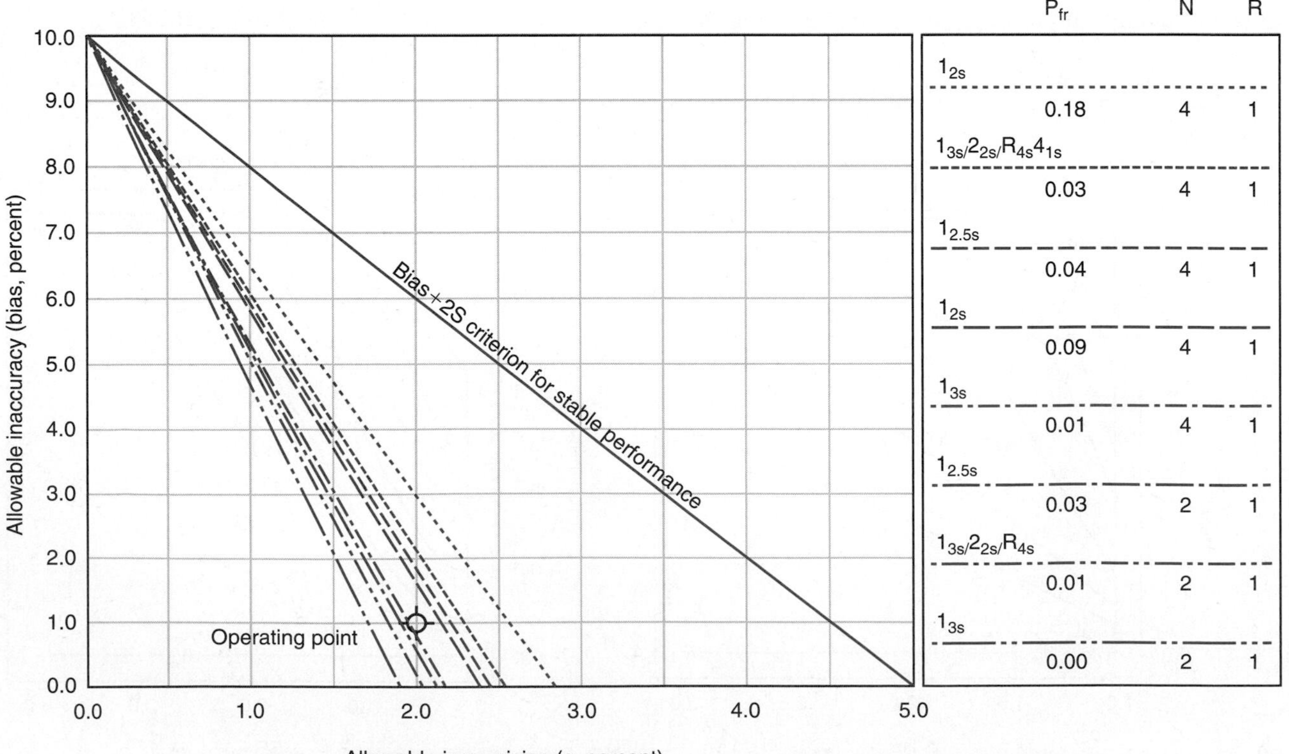

Figure 8-12 Operating specifications chart for an analytical quality requirement of 10% (*Te$_a$*) and an analytical quality assurance for systematic error of 90%. Allowable inaccuracy is plotted on the *y*-axis versus allowable imprecision on the *x*-axis.

Step-by-Step Process for Selecting QC Procedures

Laboratories should establish a systematic process for selecting appropriate QC procedures. The necessity for this is illustrated by the statement in the U.S. CLIA regulations[101] that "the laboratory must evaluate instrument and reagent stability and operator variance in determining the number, type, and frequency of testing calibration or control materials and establish criteria for acceptability used to monitor test performance during a run of patient specimens." Given that most laboratories must also satisfy certain national proficiency testing requirements, analytical requirements for quality have been defined by regulatory or professional groups for many of the common tests.

1. Define the analytical quality requirement in the form of an allowable total error (TE_a). Ideally, these goals should be based on the impact of analytical uncertainty on medical decisions. However, in the absence of evidence-based clinical criteria, proficiency testing criteria provide a surrogate starting point for defining the minimum quality that must be achieved.
2. Evaluate method performance to obtain estimates of imprecision and inaccuracy. Obtain initial estimates from replication and comparison of methods experiments. Obtain ongoing estimates from routine QC and proficiency testing surveys.
3. Obtain power function graphs for the control rules and *n*'s of interest, or OPSpecs charts for the defined TE_a. Power function graphs and OPSpecs charts for commonly used QC procedures with *n*'s of 2, 3, 4, and 6 are available in the scientific literature,[134,135] in workbook format,[125] and also from computer programs (EZ Rules and QC Validator 2.0, Westgard QC Inc., Madison, Wis.; http://www.westgard.com/accessed March 22, 2011).
4. Calculate the critical systematic error and draw a vertical line showing its location on the power function graph, or plot the observed imprecision and inaccuracy of your method on the OPSpecs chart for the TE_a of interest.
5. Assess the probabilities for error detection and false rejection.
6. Select control rules and *n*'s that provide 90% detection of the critical systematic error and less than 5% false rejections. For less critical assays with stable methods, consider 50% error detection if necessary to keep the numbers of control measurements and false rejections low.
7. Select a total QC strategy to provide an appropriate balance between statistical and nonstatistical process improvement and preventive maintenance QC procedures. With 90% error detection, depend on the statistical QC component and perform the minimal preventive maintenance, instrument function checks, and method validation tests required by good laboratory practice, manufacturers' instructions, and regulatory and accreditation guidelines.

   With 50 to 90% error detection, balance the efforts between statistical and nonstatistical QC procedures; improve method performance by reducing the bias and reducing imprecision, especially with laboratory-developed procedures. With less than 50% error detection, increase the efforts for nonstatistical QC to prevent problems from occurring and improve method performance, or consider replacing the method to achieve better imprecision and inaccuracy and more cost-effective operation of the testing process.
8. Reassess for changes in method performance as necessary. Cost-effective QC depends on doing the right QC to ensure that the desired quality is achieved at minimum cost.[130] If method performance improves, less QC will be necessary; if method performance deteriorates, more QC will be necessary. Adjust the QC design as necessary for any changes in method performance.

Detailed applications based on calculated critical systematic errors have been presented for a multitest chemistry analyzer[57,139]; detailed applications using OPSpecs charts have been presented for automated immunoassays[77]; and illustrative examples using OPSpecs charts have also been provided for a variety of tests in chemistry, hematology, coagulation, endocrinology, toxicology, and immunology.[125] Manual application of this QC planning process is performed in just a minute using a workbook of OPSpecs charts that cover the range of analytical quality requirements from 1 to 50% and common single and multirules with *n*'s from 2 to 6.[125] Computer support is necessary to use clinical quality requirements stated in the form of a medically important change or a decision interval for test interpretation; clinical requirements are more complicated and require an expanded quality planning model that accounts for additional preanalytical factors, such as within run biological variation.[140]

With manual or computer-supported QC planning, laboratories are able to identify appropriate control rules and the minimum number of control measurements that will ensure that the desired quality is achieved at the minimum cost. These control rules and *n*'s are usually implemented by setting up a Levey-Jennings control chart or a Westgard multirule chart, and less often by a cumulative sum chart or mean and range charts.

Levey-Jennings Control Chart

Control charts were first introduced into the clinical chemistry laboratory by Levey and Jennings in 1950.[67] They demonstrated how the industrial control procedures developed by Shewhart[102] could be used with the mean and range of duplicate measurements from clinical chemical methods. In an alternate chart, single control values are plotted directly. This "single-value" chart was adopted by most laboratories because data calculations were not required before the control results were plotted. Today, this single-value chart is commonly known as a *Levey-Jennings chart,* even though Levey and Jennings recommended plotting the mean and range of replicate measurements. To use a Levey-Jennings control chart, follow these steps:

1. Analyze samples of the control material by the analytical method to be controlled on at least 20 different days during stable method performance. Calculate the mean and standard deviation for those results.

2. Construct a control chart manually on graph paper or electronically using graphical software. Label the y-axis "control value" and set the range of concentrations to include the mean ±4 s. Draw horizontal lines for the mean and the upper and lower control limits. Set the control limits as the mean ±3 s when the number of control observations, n, is 2 or greater. When n is 1, control limits may be set as the mean ±2 s. (See the following discussion of performance characteristics.) Label the x-axis in terms of time, using day, run number, control observation number, or whatever is most appropriate for recording the relative time of the control observations.
3. Introduce control specimens into each analytical run, record the values, and plot each value on the control chart.
4. When the control values fall within the control limits, interpret the run as being "in control" and report the patient results. When a single control value exceeds control limits, stop the method; *do not* report patient results. Inspect the method to determine the cause for the errors. Resolve the problem, then repeat the entire run—specimens and control samples. Determine control status for the new run in the same manner.

An example of a Levey-Jennings chart is shown in Figure 8-13, where control limits have been set as the mean ±3 s. Power functions for a Levey-Jennings chart having 3 s control limits, or a 1_{3s} control rule, are shown in Figure 8-14. The probability for false rejection is seen to be less than 0.05 or 5% even when n is very large. The probability for error detection increases as n increases, but for an n of 2 to 4, the procedure is not very sensitive for random or systematic errors. Figure 8-11 shows the power functions for a Levey-Jennings chart having 2 s control limits, or the 1_{2s} control rule. Observe that the y-intercept increases rapidly as n increases. The probabilities for false rejection are as follows: $n = 1$, 0.05; $n = 2$, 0.09; $n = 4$, 0.18; $n = 8$, 0.33; $n = 12$, 0.46; and $n = 20$, 0.64. Because probabilities for false rejection greater than 0.05 or 5% are not desirable, use of the 1_{2s} rule is limited to the case where $n = 1$. In practice, the 1_{2s} rule has been widely used with a higher n. However, such use causes a false rejection problem that may compromise the usefulness of the control procedure. There is no easy way to tell whether the rejection signal is due to the background random error (false

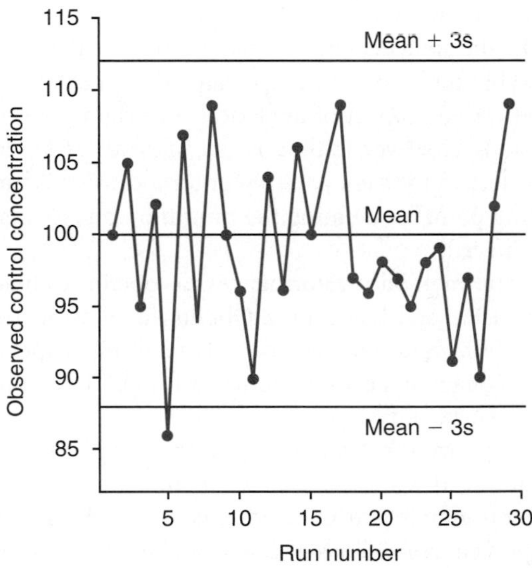

Figure 8-13 Levey-Jennings control chart having control limits set as the mean ±3 s. Concentration is plotted on the y-axis versus time (run number) on the x-axis.

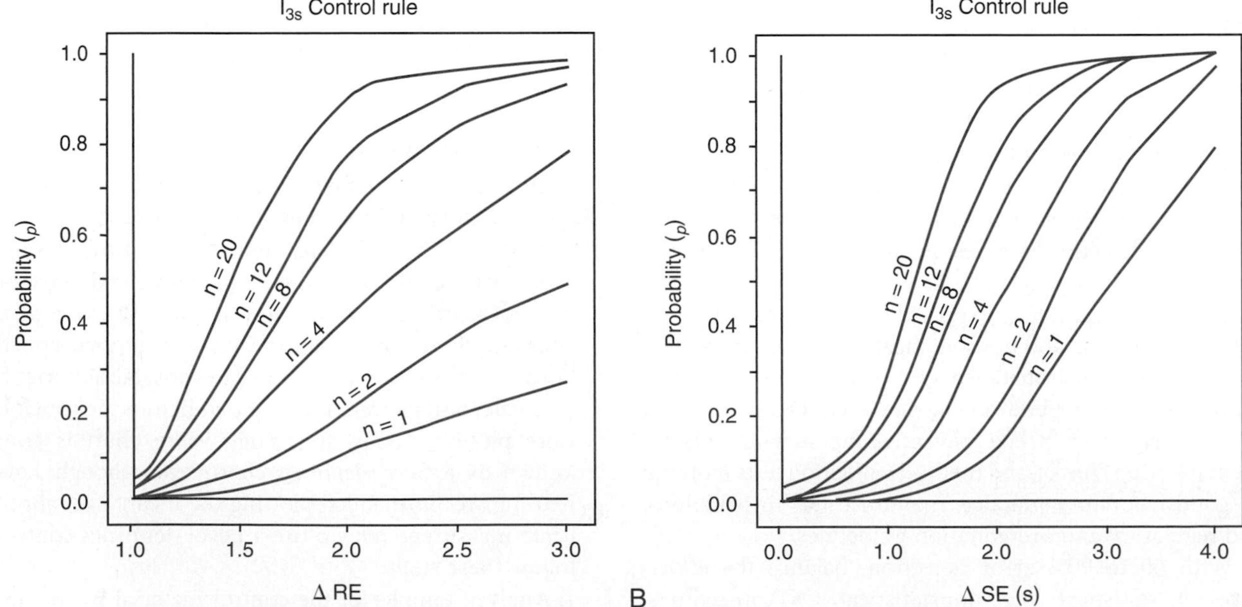

Figure 8-14 Power functions for the 13s control rule. A, Random error. B, Systematic error. *(From Westgard JO, Groth T. Power functions for statistical control rules. Clin Chem 1979;25:863-9.)*

rejection), or whether an additional error has occurred (true rejection). This difficulty has led to a more qualitative interpretation of the control results and often to routine repetition of the control measurements (and sometimes patient sampling) whenever a control value exceeds a 2 s limit. When the second or repeated control value is observed to be outside the 2 s control limits, this provides evidence for a true rejection, and problem-solving procedures should be started. A similar false rejection problem arises when multichannel instrument systems are controlled using the 1_{2s} rule on each of several channels. For one control material being analyzed by 4, 8, 12, and 20 channels, the chances that the control value on at least one channel exceeds its 2 s limits are 18%, 33%, 46%, and 64%, respectively. Such a high rate of values exceeding control limits may cause the same percentage of work to be routinely repeated, obviously compromising the efficiency of the laboratory and increasing its costs. It is important to recognize the seriousness of the false rejection problem and its relationship to the control limits chosen for the Levey-Jennings chart. These false rejections are in effect an inherent property of the control procedure. They occur because of the control limits that have been selected—not because of any problems with the analytical method. Therefore the use of 2 s control limits cannot be generally recommended. With the use of 3 s control limits, the false rejection problem is eliminated, but unfortunately error detection is also reduced.

Westgard Multirule Chart

The *multirule* procedure developed by Westgard and associates[128] uses a series of control rules for interpreting control data. The probability of false rejections is kept low by selecting only those rules whose individual probabilities for false rejection are very low (0.01 or less). The probability for error detection is improved by selecting those rules that are particularly sensitive to random and systematic errors. The procedure requires a chart having lines for control limits drawn at the mean ± 1 s, 2 s, and 3 s, and is adapted to existing Levey-Jennings charts by the addition of one or two sets of control limits.

The following control rules are used.

Rule	Description
1_{2s}	One control observation exceeding the mean ± 2 s is used only as a "warning" rule that initiates testing of the control data by the other control rules.
1_{3s}	One control observation exceeding the mean ± 3 s is a rejection rule that is primarily sensitive to random error.
2_{2s}	Two consecutive control observations exceeding the same mean plus 2 s or mean minus 2 s limit is a rejection rule that is sensitive to systematic error.
R_{4s}	One observation exceeding the mean plus 2 s and another exceeding the mean minus 2 s is a rejection rule that is sensitive to random error.
4_{1s}	Four consecutive observations exceeding the mean plus 1 s or the mean minus 1 s is a rejection rule that is sensitive to systematic error.
10_0	Ten consecutive control observations falling on one side of the mean (above or below, with no other requirement on size of the deviations) is a rejection rule that is sensitive to systematic error.

Use of the multirule procedure is similar to use of a Levey-Jennings chart, but the data interpretation is more structured. To use the multirule procedure, follow these steps:

1. Analyze samples of the control material by the analytical method to be controlled on at least 20 different days during stable method performance. Two different materials having appropriate concentrations are recommended, but a single material can be used. Calculate the mean and standard deviation for the results for each control material being used.
2. Manually or electronically construct a control chart for each of the control materials being used. The observed concentration or control value should be plotted on the *y*-axis, setting the range of concentrations to include the mean ± 4 s. Draw horizontal lines for the mean, the mean ± 1 s, the mean ± 2 s, and the mean ± 3 s. It may be desirable to use different colors for these lines, perhaps green, yellow, and red for the 1 s, 2 s, and 3 s limits, respectively. The *x*-axis should be scaled for time, day, or run number, and labeled accordingly.
3. Introduce two control specimens into each analytical run, one for each of the two concentrations when two different materials have been selected. Record the control values and plot each on its respective control chart.
4. When both control observations fall within the 2 s limits, accept the analytical run and report the patient results. When one of the control observations exceeds a 2 s limit, this is a warning condition that warrants further investigation. Inspect the control data using the 1_{3s}, 2_{2s}, R_{4s}, and 10_0 rules. When any one of these rules indicates that the run is out of control, reject the analytical run and do not report the patient results. When all of these rules indicate that the run is in control, accept the analytical run and report the patient results.
5. When a run is out of control, determine the type of error occurring based on the control rule that has been violated. Look for sources of that type of error. Correct the problem, then reanalyze the entire run, including both control and patient samples.

An example application of the multirule procedure is shown in Figure 8-15, where the top chart is for a high-concentration control material and the bottom chart is for a low-concentration material. Table 8-4 summarizes the interpretation of the charted data, providing the run number, the accept and/or reject decision, control rules violated, and the type of error suspected based on the rule violations. It is important to note that the R_{4s} rule is applied only within a run, so that between run systematic errors are not wrongly interpreted as random errors. However, the rule may be applied "across" materials, meaning that one of the observations can be on the low material and the other on the high material, as long as they are within the same run. On the other hand, note that the 2_{2s}, 4_{1s}, and 10_0 rules can be applied across runs and materials. This effectively increases *n* and improves the error detection capabilities of the procedure.

Power functions for the multirule procedure are shown in Figure 8-16 for *n* from 2 to 6. The probability for false rejection will be much lower at these *n*'s than for the Levey-Jennings chart having 2 s control limits. However, the false rejections do increase as *n* increases, limiting *n* to a maximum of 4 to 6. For larger *n*'s, it would be necessary to modify the procedure by eliminating the R_{4s} rule, or by replacing this approximate range rule with an exact range rule (see discussion of Shewhart range procedure later in this chapter).

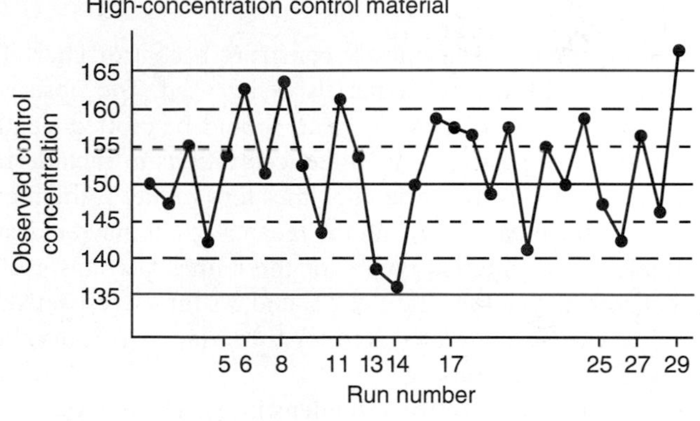

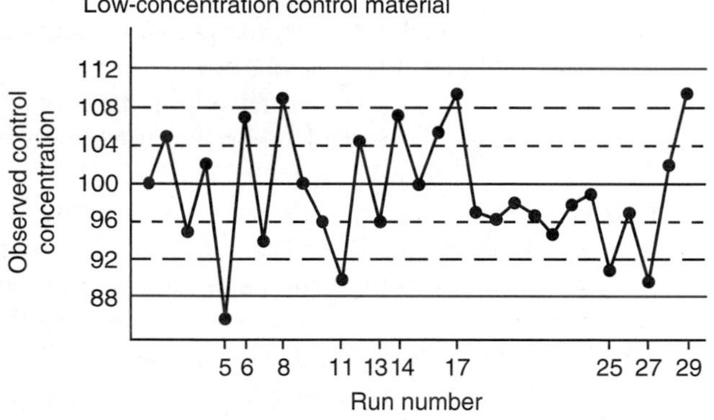

Figure 8-15 Westgard multirule control chart having control limits drawn at the mean ± 1 s, 2 s, and 3 s. Concentration is plotted on the y-axis versus time (run number) on the x-axis. A, Chart for high-concentration control material. B, Chart for low-concentration control material. *(From Westgard JO, Barry PL, Hunt MR, Groth T. A multi-rule Shewhart chart for quality control in clinical chemistry. Clin Chem 1981;27:493-501.)*

Comparison of the probability for error detection between the multirule procedure and the Levey-Jennings chart having 3 s limits shows improved error detection for the multirule procedure. The R_{4s} rule improves the detection of random error, and the 2_{2s}, 4_{1s}, and 10_0 rules improve the detection of systematic error. Elimination of the 10_0 rule does not cause much loss in error detection but does considerably reduce the quantity of control data that must be inspected; thus the simplification may make the multirule procedure easier to use.

Cumulative Sum (Cusum) Control Chart

The single-value control charts discussed in the previous sections provide a display of the differences between observed values and the expected mean. Control rules, such as 2_{2s}, 4_{1s}, and 10_0, provide one way of determining when these successive differences no longer appear to be random (too many in a row on one side of a limit). A more exact and quantitative method is the cumulative sum control procedure or cusum chart. To set up a cusum chart, follow these steps:

1. Analyze the control material by the analytical method to be controlled on at least 20 different days, and calculate the mean and standard deviation of those results. (This is the same as the initial step required for a Levey-Jennings chart or for a multirule chart.)
2. Manually or electronically construct a control chart. Label the *y*-axis "cusum." Draw a horizontal line at the midpoint of the *y*-axis to represent a cusum of zero. Set the range of values above and below to be about 10 times the standard deviation. Label the *x*-axis in terms of time, using day, run number, control observation number, or whatever is most appropriate for recording the relative time of the control observation.
3. Introduce control specimens into each analytical run and record the value obtained.
4. Calculate the difference between the value and the expected mean. Obtain the cusum by adding this difference to the cumulative sum of the previous differences. Plot the cusum on the control chart and inspect the plot.
5. Interpret the charted data by evaluating the slope of the cusum line. A steep slope suggests that a systematic error is present and that the run is out of control.

TABLE 8-4 Interpretation of Example Control Data Using the Westgard Multirule Procedure

Run Number	Decision on Run		Control Rule Violated					Type of Error	
	Accept	Reject	1_{3s}	2_{2s}	R_{4s}	4_{1s}	10_0	RE	SE
5		X	X				X		
6	X								
8		X		X				X	
11		X			X		X		
13	X								
14		X		X				X	
17		X				X		X	
25	X		X				X		X
29		X	X	X				X	

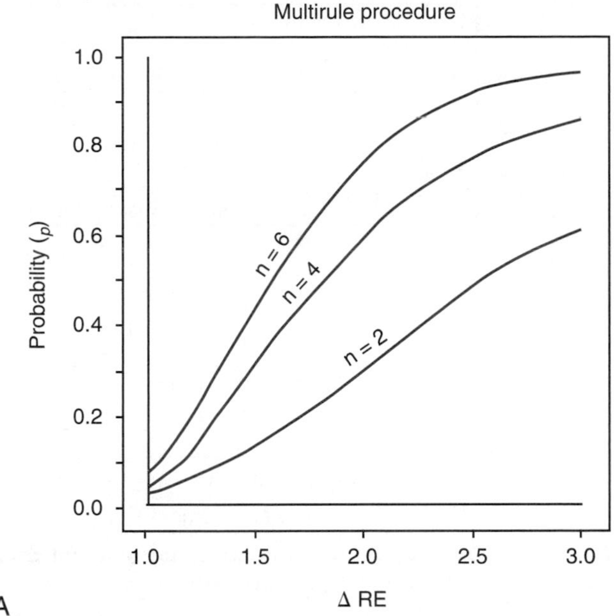

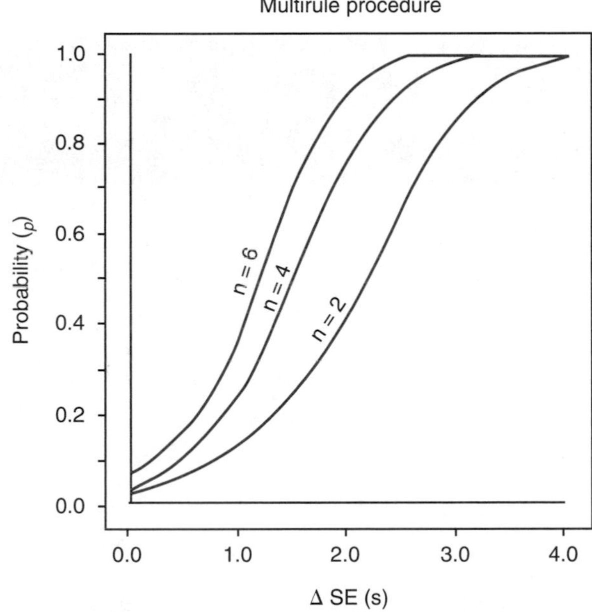

Figure 8-16 Power functions for Westgard multirule control procedure. A, Random error. B, Systematic error. *(From Westgard JO, Barry PL, Hunt MR, Groth T. A multi-rule Shewhart chart for quality control in clinical chemistry. Clin Chem 1981;27:493-501.)*

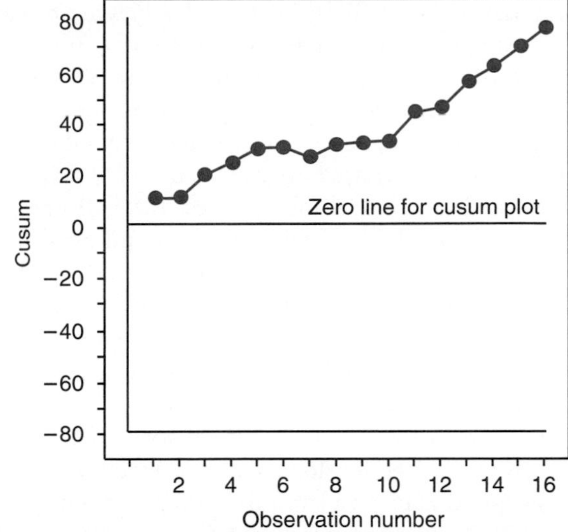

Figure 8-17 V-mask cumulative sum control chart (e.g., data in Table 19-4). The cumulative sum of the differences from the mean is plotted on the y-axis versus time (control observation number) on the x-axis.

TABLE 8-5 Example Cusum Calculations and Tabular Record for V-Mask Cusum Chart (for Control Material With $\bar{x}$ *(x bar) = 100,* s = 5.0)

Control Observation Number	Control Value	D_i	C_{si}
1	110	+10	+10
2	100	0	+10
3	108	+8	+18
4	105	+5	+23
5	105	+5	+28
6	101	+1	+29
7	96	−4	+25
8	105	+5	+30
9	101	+1	+31
10	101	+1	+32
11	111	+11	+43
12	102	+2	+45
13	110	+10	+55
14	107	+7	+62
15	107	+7	+69
16	107	+7	+76

Example calculations are shown in Table 8-5. These cusum values are plotted versus observation numbers in Figure 8-17. When control values scatter on both sides of the mean, giving both positive and negative differences, the cusum will alternate in sign, and the plotted values will wander back and forth across the zero line on the control chart. When the control values fall mostly on one side of the mean so that most of the differences have the same sign, the cusum value increases in magnitude, and the plotted values will move away from the zero line of the control chart.

It is more difficult to judge the control status from cusum charts than from Levey-Jennings or multirule charts. The approach that has been used most extensively is to make the judgment based on the slope of the cusum line. In industry, this has often been done by constructing templates having a V-shaped section removed from a rectangular sheet of clear plastic. This V-shaped cutout establishes the angle that is the control limit and gives the technique its name of V-*mask cusum.* The apex of the V-mask is positioned on the control chart at a specified distance in front of the most recent cusum observation. If all of the plotted values are contained within the angle of the V-mask, the method is judged to be in control. If any of the plotted values fall outside the angle of the V-mask, the method is judged to be out of control. Although this technique for interpreting cusum data is very objective, V-mask overlays have not been very widely used or recommended for clinical laboratories. Instead, interpretation has been based on visual inspection and on judgment of the angle of the cusum line, sometimes aided by the use of special graph paper having an underlying pattern of 45-degree angles (∠∠∠∠∠∠∠.) across the chart. When this special graph paper is used, the convention has been to scale the graph so that a change of 2 s on the *y*-axis is the same distance between two points on the *x*-axis. The 45-degree angle then represents the slope expected when the observed mean is approximately 2 s from the expected mean.

An alternative way of interpreting cusum data is to use a numerical limit for the cusum value itself, a technique known as *decision limit cusum*. Particular decision limit schemes are characterized by two parameters: *k*, a factor for calculating the threshold, and *h*, a factor for calculating the decision limit or control limit. The cusum calculations do not start until a control value exceeds a certain threshold above (k_u) or below (k_l), the expected mean (0). Once exceeded, the differences from the threshold are calculated and summed for successive observations to provide the cusum. This process continues until the cusum exceeds the upper and lower control limits (h_u and h_l) and the method is judged out of control, or until the cusum changes sign, in which case the cusum calculation is stopped and the method is judged to be in control. An example of the cusum calculations for the decision limit technique is given in Table 8-6.

These example data are plotted in Figure 8-18. One advantage of the decision limit cusum chart is that it has horizontal lines for control limits, permitting the cusum chart to be interpreted in a manner similar to a Levey-Jennings chart. This form of interpretation requires less experience and judgment, thus making possible more consistent interpretation when many analysts use the control procedure. Another advantage of the decision limit technique is that it can be implemented using only tabular operations (without charting), thus making it very easy to program for computerized handling of control data.

Although interpretation is easier and more objective, selecting the threshold and control limits is somewhat difficult. This selection is done with the aid of nomograms, which are complicated to understand and use; therefore it is initially perhaps best to use one of the decision limit schemes recommended in the clinical chemistry literature.[136] For manual implementation, set the threshold at the $x \pm 1.0$ s and the control limits at 2.7 s. For computer implementation, set the threshold at the $x \pm 0.5$ s and the control limits at 5.1 s. This latter procedure will be sensitive to smaller errors because of the choice of the lower threshold. However, the charting is not as convenient when performed manually, particularly when the cusum is used in combination with the 1_{3s} control rule to provide better detection of random errors.[136]

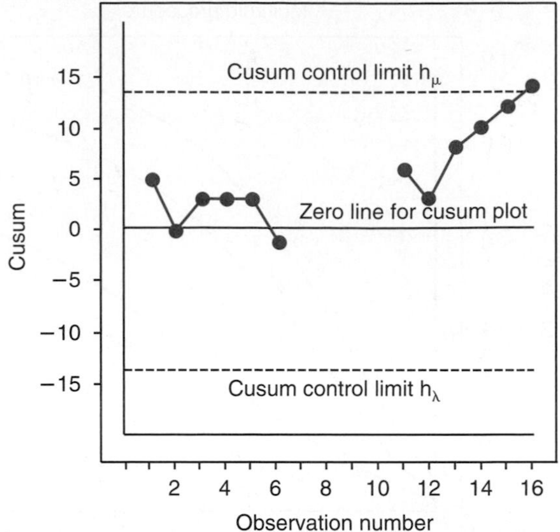

Figure 8-18 Decision limit cumulative sum control chart (e.g., data in Table 19-5). The cumulative sum of the differences from the threshold is plotted on the *y*-axis versus time (control observation number) on the *x*-axis.

TABLE 8-6 Example Cusum Calculations and Tabular Record for Decision Limit Cusum (for Control Material With $\bar{x}$ *(x bar)* = *100*, s = 5.0; for Control Chart With k_u = 105, k_l = 95, h_u = 13.5, h_l = 13.5)

Control Observation Number	Control Value	d_i	Cs_i	Comment
1	110	+5	+5	Start cusum calculation
2	100	−5	0	
3	108	+3	+3	
4	105	0	+3	
5	105	0	+3	
6	101	−4	−1	End cusum calculation
7				
8	105			
9	101			
10	101			
11	111	+6	+6	Start cusum calculation
12	102	−3	+3	
13	110	+5	+8	
14	107	+2	+10	
15	107	+2	+12	
16	107	+2	+14	

When compared with the Levey-Jennings chart with 3 s limits, the cusum procedure provides better detection of systematic errors but less sensitivity for random errors. Because of the low sensitivity to random errors, cusum should not be used alone, but rather should be included with a

Levey-Jennings procedure on a combined chart[136] or used as a separate chart along with a Levey-Jennings chart. Performance is similar to the multirule procedure for low *n*'s, at least as far as detecting systematic errors. However, the multirule procedure is more sensitive to random errors because of the added R_{4s} rule.

Alternative Calculations and Applications

Moving averages and moving standard deviations are used in industry and sometimes in clinical laboratories. With these procedures, *n* is chosen, measurements are collected until *n* is attained, and then the mean and the standard deviation are calculated. With each additional measurement, the oldest measurement is dropped, the newest is added, and new estimates of the mean and the standard deviation are obtained after each new control measurement, rather than waiting for new groups of *n* measurements. Parvin[82] has proposed the use of a multimean rule that combines the means of control values observed in consecutive runs. Similar updated means and standard deviations are obtained from exponential smoothing, a calculation procedure that provides an average that weighs recent observations more heavily than older observations.[134] The *smoothed mean* is sensitive to trends that are just beginning to develop, and therefore it is often referred to as a *trend analysis procedure.* The calculations are too complicated to be implemented manually, but the availability of computer software makes these calculations feasible in clinical laboratories.

Power functions for mean (or Z-test), range, and χ^2 (or standard deviation) control procedures, when compared with those for previous control procedures, show higher probabilities for error detection, particularly at larger *n*'s. The probability for false rejection can be set at a suitably low level by proper choice of control limits. Thus these control procedures appear to offer better performance characteristics than single-value control charts because they have higher error detection and lower false rejection as *n* increases.

The use of mean and standard deviation control procedures (or related procedures) to monitor accuracy and precision is a direct extension of the practices of method evaluation, the mean being used to monitor systematic error and the standard deviation to monitor random error. This relationship helps explain why control procedures having *n*'s from 1 to 4 have relatively low power or error detection capability. It is no surprise that it is more difficult to estimate precision and accuracy using quality control procedures with *n*'s of 1 to 4 than with method evaluation procedures using *n*'s of 20 to 40. For low *n*'s, all control procedures have relatively low power. As *n* increases, power will increase, particularly for procedures using mean, range, S-charts, Z-tests, and χ^2-tests, moving averages and moving standard deviations, and trend analysis. Future practices in statistical quality control in clinical laboratories will undoubtedly make greater use of these procedures.

The integration of powerful computer hardware and software into analytical systems has made it practical to use complicated control procedures on a routine basis in clinical laboratories. Calculations on control data, once properly programmed, are performed quickly and without mistakes. Graphical displays can be generated, with color added to aid the interpretation of control data. Specific control rules are programmed to provide "accept" and "reject" signals or printouts. Records are maintained to document instrument changes, preventive maintenance, and control problems. Monthly summary statistics and quality control reports are generated. Many of these features, along with many of the statistical control procedures that have been described, are found in quality control software programs that are commercially available today.

CONTROL OF ANALYTICAL QUALITY USING PATIENT DATA

QC mechanisms based on patient data provide additional information useful in monitoring the quality of laboratory analyses. These procedures are often time consuming and generally are not sensitive enough to serve as the only means of QC. However, many of the control problems detected with these techniques may not be evident with conventional QC systems. A quality assurance program should make appropriate use of "patient data procedures," and both individual and multiple patient results have been used for QC purposes.

Individual Patient Results

Patient test results are the final product of most laboratory procedures, and monitoring of these results is the most direct form of QC. Unfortunately, procedures for monitoring results are not very sensitive and have low probabilities for error detection. The most effective procedure is the clinical correlation of test results with other information related to the patient, especially surgical findings, response to therapy, and autopsy data. Less sensitive but easier to implement are comparisons with previous test values and correlation with related test results. The easiest procedure is the comparison of test results with physiologic or probabilistic limits.

Clinical Correlation

Operationally, it is impractical for high-volume, core laboratories to correlate all test results with the clinical status of the patient. In general, the clinician ordering the tests is in a better position to evaluate the appropriateness of test results. However, clinicians often order a test because they are uncertain of the exact clinical status of their patient and base their diagnoses heavily on the laboratory test results. In such cases, it is circular reasoning to correlate clinical diagnoses with laboratory test results. Clinical correlation studies are best done retrospectively when laboratory test results are directly related to other evidence, such as surgical findings. Unfortunately, most laboratory tests do not correlate perfectly with disease states, and one must evaluate multiple cases before determining the diagnostic efficiency of a given test (as discussed further in Chapter 3). In an individual patient, clinical correlation can identify impossible or highly unlikely test results that cannot be flagged in the laboratory, such as a normal serum bilirubin concentration in a highly jaundiced patient. Clinicians should be encouraged to report these discrepancies to the laboratory, and a mechanism should be available to follow up with these problems. Also, after using a test for a period of time, many clinicians can detect alterations in test results, and although this is not reliable for documenting problems, informal discussions with clinicians frequently using the test can aid in identifying aspects of laboratory tests that should be further investigated.

A focus on linking laboratory tests with patient care outcomes (see Chapter 4) requires an integrated healthcare system in which all processes are operating properly.[49,146] This integrated system includes (1) correct assessment of the patient's problem, (2) ordering of the correct tests, (3) accurate and timely analytical performance, (4) correct interpretation of the test results, and (5) implementation of appropriate clinical actions that produce the expected response in the patients.

Correlation With Other Laboratory Tests

As in clinical correlation, a single test result can be judged to be implausible in a limited number of situations, but the combination of several test results is impossible or very unlikely. If the tests involved in these comparisons are performed at the same time, it is often possible to identify errors and correct problems before reporting the test results to the clinicians. Even though very few tests have exact clinical relationships, and one often must consider statistical percentages rather than the results of a single patient to identify malfunctions, several relationships provide some possibilities for monitoring an individual patient's results, at least for purposes of initiating further review:

1. *Blood typing.* There is a close association between the ABO blood antigens on erythrocytes and isoantibodies found in plasma. Exceptions are found in patients recently transfused with whole blood.
2. *Anion gap.* To maintain electrical neutrality, the sum of the charges of anions in a blood sample must equal the sum of the charges of cations when expressed in molar concentrations. With all units in mmol/L, an anion gap (AG) can be calculated as follows:

$$AG = (Na^+ + K^+) - (Cl^- + HCO_3^-)$$

   Values less than approximately 3 mmol/L or greater than about 21 mmol/L may indicate error. Elevated values may be found in patients with renal failure, diabetic acidosis, cardiac failure, anoxia, and other conditions (see Chapter 49). Low values occur in hypoproteinemia and with intravenous hydration. The capabilities of AG control procedures were studied by Cembrowski and coworkers,[32] who recommend that the average AG of groups of eight or more patients be used to provide a more sensitive statistical control.
3. *Acid-base balance.* The Henderson-Hasselbalch equation is also used to calculate theoretical bicarbonate and total CO_2 concentrations when pH and PCO_2 are measured. Theoretical and measured results generally agree within 2.0 mmol/L.
4. *Thyroxine-TSH.* Normally, thyroxine sends negative feedback to the pituitary and reduces the secretion of TSH. Patients with serum thyroxine concentrations above 8.0 μg/dL seldom have elevated concentrations of TSH. Exceptions occur in secondary and tertiary hyperthyroidism.

Intralaboratory Duplicates

In practice, samples often are divided into two aliquots and analyzed, and the duplicates used for control purposes. This is a simple quality control procedure that does not require stable control materials; therefore it is used when stable materials are not available, or as a supplemental procedure when stable control materials are available. The differences between duplicates are plotted on a range type of control chart that has limits calculated from the standard deviation of the differences.[130] When duplicates are obtained from the same method, this range chart monitors only random error and thus is not adequate for ensuring the accuracy of the analytical method. When duplicates are obtained from two different laboratory methods, then the range chart actually monitors both random and systematic errors but cannot separate the two types of errors. Such a procedure is very effective in identifying biases between methods that may indicate the need to recalibrate a method or instrument. Interpretation becomes more difficult, particularly when there are stable systematic differences or biases between the two analytical methods. Multiplicative factors may be necessary to deal with proportional differences, and additive factors may be necessary to allow for constant differences. Interpretation of observed differences becomes more qualitative; nevertheless, this procedure still provides a useful way of monitoring the consistency of data being generated by the laboratory.

Delta Checks With Previous Test Results

Certain errors, particularly errors in specimen identification, have been detected by comparing laboratory test results with values obtained on previous specimens from the same patient. The expected variability of test results depends on both the analyte and the time interval between determinations. Ladenson has defined delta check limits based on a 3-day interval in terms of a percentage change from the initial value.[62] His check limits for some common tests are shown in Table 8-7.

In identifying specimen-related errors, it is helpful to examine multiple test parameters, including hematologic tests, because differences in a profile of test results often are more obvious and more statistically significant than are changes in individual tests. For example, in a 1979 study, the performance of several delta check methods was evaluated, including two discriminant functions, for detecting mislabeled specimens; a false-positive rate of 5% and an error detection of about 50% for mislabeled specimens were observed.[138]

Limit Checks

A patient's test results should be reviewed to check that they are within the physiologic ranges compatible with life. These

TABLE 8-7 Recommended Limits for Delta Checks

Test	Delta Check Limit, %
Albumin	20
Bilirubin, total	50
Calcium, total	15
Creatine kinase	99
Creatinine	50
Phosphorus	20
Potassium	20
Protein, total	20
Sodium	5
Thyroxine	25
Urea nitrogen	50
Uric acid	40

From Ladenson JH. Patients as their own controls: use of the computer to identify "laboratory error." Clin Chem 1975;21:1648-53.

TABLE 8-8 Recommended Reference Values for Limit Checks

Test	Low Warning	High Warning
Albumin, g/dL	1.5	6
Alkaline phosphatase,* U/L	5	300
Amylase,* U/L	20	1000
Bilirubin, mg/dL	0.2	10.0
Calcium, mg/dL	6.5	13.0
Creatine kinase, U/L	5	1500
Creatinine, mg/dL	0.3	7.5
Phosphorus, mg/dL	1.0	8.0
Potassium, mmol/L	3.0	6.0
Sodium, mmol/L	120	150
Urea nitrogen, mg/dL	3	50
Uric acid, mg/dL	1.0	12.0

*Values are method dependent.
From Whitehurst P, DiSilvio TV, Boyadjian G. Evaluation of discrepancies in patients' results: an aspect of computer-assisted quality control. Clin Chem 1975;21:87-92.

limit checks are helpful for detecting clerical errors, such as transposed digits or misplaced decimal points. This checking can be combined with warning limit checks for detecting and verifying possible, but infrequently occurring, test results. These warning limits are dependent on the test methodology and on characteristics of the patient population being tested. Table 8-8 shows limits for some common tests. Many automated chemistry instruments have monitors that allow autorelease of test results within defined limits, which are wider than some of the values listed in this table. For example, the Roche Diagnostics Module and Cobas Systems have auto release limits of 23 to 1050 U/L for alkaline phosphatase and 0.1 to 30.0 mg/dL for total bilirubin.

Multiple Patients

Test Distribution Statistics

Statistics based on distributions of test results from large numbers of patients are useful for detecting systematic errors (shifts and drifts) but are of no value for detecting random errors (increased variability or scatter). They are useful adjuncts to the fundamental control procedures, which use stable control materials, but should not be substituted for them. Patient values include numerous sources of variation—demographic, biological, pathologic, and preanalytical (see Chapter 6)[149]—in addition to the analytical variation caused by the analytical method. As a result, individual test values have too much variability to have any utility for QC; however, the mean of multiple test values or groups of patients is more stable and therefore may be useful for control purposes.

Changes in the means of patient populations may be caused by multiple variables (see Chapters 3 and 5). Changes in the demographic and clinical characteristics of patients, such as the ratio of males to females, the ratio of hospitalized patients to outpatients, or the presence of many specimens from a specialty clinic, can alter the mean value. Similarly, changes in preanalytical conditions[149] such as tourniquet time and specimen storage alter patient population means and therefore can be monitored by the use of patient means. These variables are not monitored by those control procedures employing stable materials; thus *patient mean procedures* provide additional capabilities and should be used in conjunction with other control procedures. Population statistics are most useful when patients are segmented into groups such as different clinics, different phlebotomists, and so forth. These subgroups generally have smaller within group variations, which helps improve the detection of systemic changes. The smaller the within group variance, the better the ability to detect an analytical or preanalytical assay change.

Statistical Methods for Monitoring Patient Means

The *mean of normals* or *average of normals* (AON) approach calls for establishing limits, usually the limits for reference values, for "trimming" patient data.[141] Values outside these limits are eliminated from the calculations, thus reducing the response to outliers and subpopulations and also to real errors. An alternative approach has been to use the median as the control statistic; this may be a more sensitive indicator of change than the mean. More complicated estimates have been recommended to account for hospitalized patients having slightly different test values from those of ambulatory patients. A weighted mean based on the percentage of patients in each category has greater sensitivity for error detection, particularly for measurements of the serum concentrations of total protein, albumin, and calcium.

Bull's algorithm has been widely employed for online monitoring of automated hematologic cell counters.[108] Bull and colleagues[20] evaluated six statistics for monitoring erythrocyte indices: the sample mean, two moving average means, the mean of a truncated sample, John's mean, and the median. They assessed the usefulness of these different statistics by mathematically introducing both abrupt bias changes and cyclic time changes. The moving average statistics were found to have superior error detection. The batch size used in calculating the moving average regulates smoothing of the data. Large batch sizes not only smooth out undesired individual patient effects, but also increase the number of specimens (and time) necessary to detect instrument malfunction. A weighted moving average based on a batch size of 20 specimens was recommended. Cembrowski has developed power function graphs to provide quantitative information on both single-rule and multirule variations of Bull's algorithm.[31,68]

Control statistics based on patient data have been readily implemented in computerized laboratories.[54] However, several authors have shown that these control procedures are not as sensitive as procedures using stable control material. All of these statistics are designed to detect systematic errors and have virtually no power for detecting random error. The relative sensitivity of these statistics for detection of systematic errors, as compared with stable control materials, is dependent on three factors: (1) variation in patient test values (and the test statistics derived from them), (2) analytical variation, and (3) the number of specimens relative to the number of controls. Low patient variability, high analytical variability, and a high ratio of specimens to controls favor patient-based QC procedures. Patient test result variability depends not only on the analyte measured, but also on the population being tested. Populations consisting mainly of healthy individuals generally have lower test variability than populations of inpatients and medical specialty clinics. Results from several quantitative studies of these variables and their effects on the statistical power of procedures using patient means have been reported by a number of investigators. Cembrowski and associates, Ye and colleagues,[30,54,147] and Smith and Kroft[103,104] have further evaluated the performance and relationship of AON and Bull's algorithms and have proposed an exponentially adjusted moving mean whose performance can be optimized for individual applications.

Combined Use of Liquid Controls and Moving Averages of Patient Values for Quality Control Monitoring

Distributions of measured test values have been used to supplement traditional liquid controls for monitoring analytical bias. These patient specimen measurements generally have much larger variances than liquid controls because they contain biological, pathophysiologic, and preanalytical sources of variation, in addition to the analytical variation. However, if some of these sources of variation are controlled, averaging techniques often are used to generate tracking parameters, which have variations of the same order of magnitude as liquid controls. Demographic information about specific patients such as age, sex, and medical provider service area have been used to adjust test values, resulting in smaller variances of group means for the monitoring parameters. The larger the number of patient results included in a mandatory group, the smaller the variations between averages of these groups; however, the use of larger groups delays the time to detection of changes. Variations of the group mean decrease approximately proportionately to the square root of the number of patient values included in the group. Various statistical techniques have been used to calculate a QC statistic from patient values, such as the exponentially adjusted moving mean proposed by Smith and Kroft.[103,104] In general, there is a trade-off between decreased variance versus increased time for error detection when larger numbers of patient values are used in these QC statistics. For most chemistry tests, 50 to 100 patient test values often are necessary.[54,57,147] An advantage of test value distributions over liquid controls is the inclusion of preanalytical variation caused by specimen collection, transport, and storage. This allows patient value–derived QC parameters to detect changes in these variables, in addition to changes in the analytical testing.

Figure 8-19 illustrates an algorithm for combining liquid controls with a patient value–derived parameter. The same multirule evaluation systems used for liquid controls have been used for tracking the patient value–derived QC statistic. Set points and threshold values are assigned to this derived parameter to optimize the power for error detection for systematic error. Note that the averaging algorithms used to generate these derived parameters average out random errors, so these derived parameters are not useful for detecting random errors. As illustrated in the figure, this combined control protocol is most accurate when both the liquid control and the patient-derived control move in the same direction (both high, or both low). When the controls move discordantly, further investigation is necessary to define whether the problem is related to instability of liquid controls, changes in patient characteristics (such as many sick patients seen at one time), preanalytical test changes, or other causes.

EXTERNAL QUALITY ASSESSMENT AND PROFICIENCY TESTING PROGRAMS

All of the control procedures described earlier in the chapter have focused on monitoring a single laboratory. These procedures constitute what is called *internal quality control*[124] to distinguish them from procedures used to compare the performance of different laboratories, the latter being known as *external quality assessment*. The two are complementary activities, internal QC being necessary for the daily monitoring of the precision and accuracy of the analytical method, and external quality assessment being important for maintaining long-term accuracy of the analytical methods.[22,23]

In practice, internal QC procedures detect changes in performance only between the present operation and the "stable" operation that was characteristic during the baseline period, when the analytical method was thought to be operating properly. Although the procedures detect systematic and random errors, the only systematic errors detected are those changes from the original baseline. If the method actually had some undetected systematic errors during the baseline period, those systematic errors would be included in the mean that was used to calculate control limits for the procedure. Thus only systematic changes from this original mean will be detected by internal QC procedures.

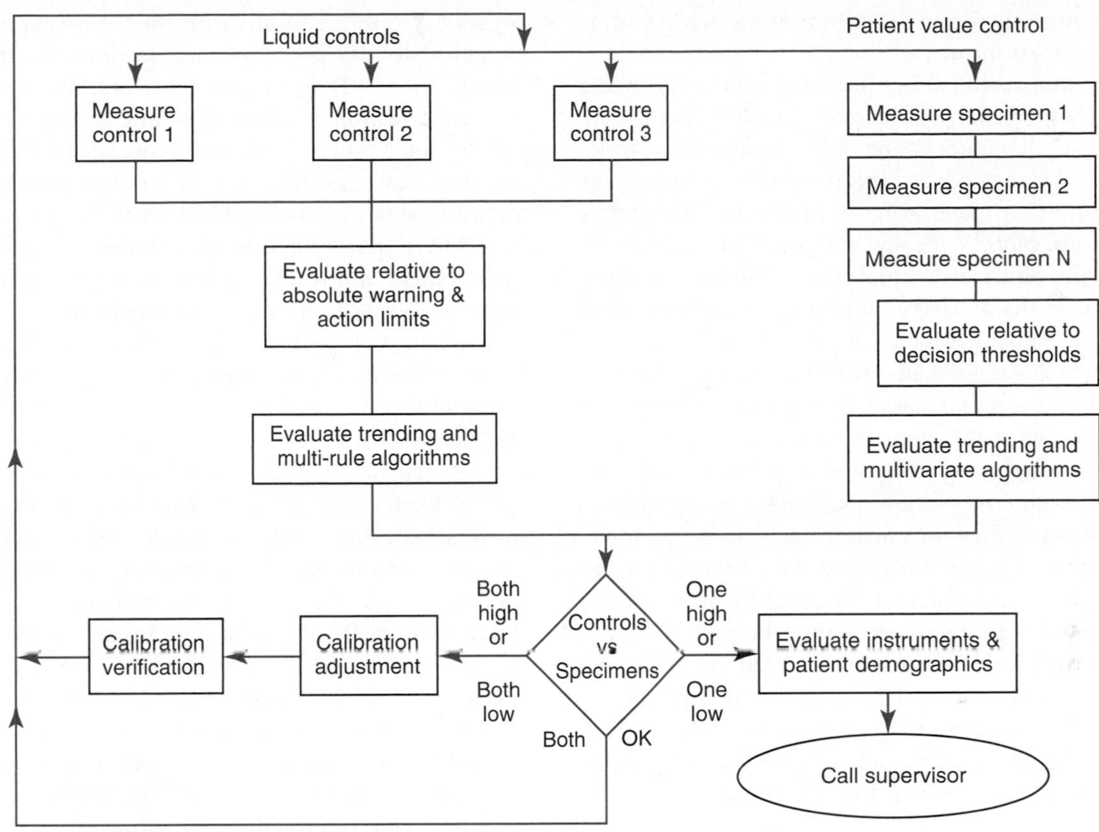

Figure 8-19 Protocol for combining liquid controls and a patient value–derived control.

Initial method evaluation studies are essential to ensure that systematic errors are not present before the baseline period and the determination of mean and control limits. The accuracy of the method should be initially established by comparison with other analytical methods (and recovery and interference studies) and should continue to be monitored by comparison with other analytical methods. Ongoing comparison-of-methods studies are desirable to ensure that systematic errors do not slowly increase and go undetected by internal QC procedures. These ongoing comparison studies are provided by external QA programs, which in turn form the basis for proficiency testing programs.

Quality Control Comparison Programs

Several external QA programs are available to laboratories, some sponsored by professional societies and others offered by manufacturers of control materials. The basic operation of these programs involves having all participating laboratories analyze the same lot of control material, usually daily as part of the internal QC activities. Results are sent to the sponsoring group for the data analysis. Summary reports are prepared by the program sponsor and are distributed to all participating laboratories. This reporting takes time for processing of all data from a large number of laboratories; thus the data analysis is not available in real time and is useful only for monthly reviews and periodic problem-solving activities. However, with advances in telecommunications and the arrival of the World Wide Web, real-time external QC is a possibility.

Reports often include extensive data analysis, statistical summaries, and plots. The mean of all results or the mean of results from peer laboratories (those performing the test with similar methods) is taken as the target value and is used for comparison with the individual laboratory's result. Different programs do this in different ways. For example, the statistical significance of any difference between an individual laboratory's observed result and the group mean can be tested by use of the *t*-test. When the difference is significant, the laboratory is alerted that its results are biased compared with the results of most of the other laboratories. Another approach is to divide the difference by the overall standard deviation of the group, and then to express the difference in terms of the number of standard deviations as follows:

$$\text{SDI} = \frac{\text{Laboratory Result} - \text{Group Mean}}{\text{Group SD}}$$

where *SDI* is the abbreviation for standard deviation interval or index, and *Group SD* is the standard deviation for the group or a selected subset of the group. Differences greater than 2 or 3 indicate that a laboratory is not in agreement with the rest of the laboratories in the program. These calculations reduce all test results to the same values, which makes it possible to interpret the data without reference to the exact mean and *s* for each analytical method. For example, a value of +2.0

has the same meaning for any test, indicating that the value is 2 s above its target mean.

Additional information about the nature of the systematic error is obtained when two different control materials are analyzed by each laboratory. For example, the laboratory's observed mean for material A is plotted on the y-axis versus its observed mean for material B on the x-axis; these graphs are called *Youden plots.*[148] Ideally, the point for a laboratory should fall at the center of the plot. Points falling away from the center but on the 45-degree line suggest a proportional analytical error. Points falling away from the center but not on the 45-degree line suggest an error that is constant for both materials or an error that occurs with just one material.

The operation of quality control comparison programs is greatly improved by using a PC and appropriate software. Operationally, comparisons are performed more quickly using the PC as a terminal for transmitting data via the Internet to the central computer. Processing of the data to compare the results from many different laboratories is then performed, and reports are returned to the laboratory. Because individual control observations are entered into the PC, control data are then immediately tested by internal control procedures to determine control status. Thus in practice, the PC integrates the internal QC and the external comparison procedures into a more efficient program for QA.

Proficiency Testing and Laboratory Accreditation

Proficiency testing (PT) programs are a type of external quality assessment in which simulated patient specimens made from a common pool are analyzed by the laboratories enrolled in the program. Results are returned to a central facility and are evaluated to determine the "quality" of each laboratory's performance. Government and licensing agencies are increasingly using PT as an objective method for accrediting laboratories, thereby giving them official authorization to operate.[96]

An example of using PT for such a purpose is the U.S. Government's mandate that clinical laboratories be accredited and licensed. Historically, this developed after a series of newspaper articles were published that focused on laboratory quality problems and led to a determined effort by the U.S. government to protect patients' interests and the public welfare.[15,16] In 1988, the U.S. Congress subsequently revised the Clinical Laboratory Improvement Act of 1967 (CLIA '67) and passed the Clinical Laboratory Improvement Amendment (CLIA '88); it mandates PT as a major part of the laboratory accreditation process.[2,101] The implementation rules for this legislation have been evolving, with the final legislative rule being published on January 24, 2006.[100] Additional interpretative guidelines were published by the Centers for Medicare and Medicaid Services (CMS) in January 2004 in the form of the *State Operations Manual.* Appendix C of that document refers specifically to guidelines for laboratories and laboratory testing services.[5]

The initial CLIA '88 regulations focused primarily on the analytical process. However, it was later stressed that the quality of the "total testing process" must be monitored, in addition to the precision and accuracy of the analytical phase.[83,86,92,145] Thus as mentioned earlier in this chapter, current QA programs that monitor only the analytical phase of the total process have to be expanded to include both preanalytical (see Chapter 6) and postanalytical phases (www.westgard.com/essay34/accessed March 22, 2011).

CLIA requires all U.S. laboratories to register with the government and to identify the tests they perform. Certain tests are "waived," meaning that any laboratory can perform those tests as long as they follow the manufacturers' directions. There are no other requirements for quality management of those tests. Laboratories that perform "nonwaived" tests are subject to the complete CLIA regulations and must be inspected periodically by the government or by certain professional organizations that are deemed to have standards at least as stringent as the CLIA requirements. Two such organizations are the College of American Pathologists (CAP) and the Joint Commission on Accreditation of Healthcare Organizations (JCAHO). The CLIA implementation rules and interpretative guidelines outline the criteria for acceptable performance in laboratory inspection and accreditation.

CLIA requirements cover several broad classes: (1) Subpart J. Facility Administration; (2) Subpart K. Quality Systems; (3) Subpart M. Personnel; and (4) Subpart Q. Inspection. The final rule dealt mainly with changes to the subpart on Quality Systems, with particular attention to preanalytical, analytical, and postanalytical systems. It places increased emphasis on having quality systems to monitor preanalytical and postanalytical processes, yet the biggest impact of the final rule is on analytical quality assessment and analytical quality systems.[131]

In general, the performance characteristics of PT programs for detecting bias and imprecision are evaluated using methods similar to those listed for assessing internal QC.[63] A commonly used evaluation criterion has been the comparison of PT test results with those of peer groups, considering all values that exceed 3 SD to be "unacceptable." This rule fails to detect many of the laboratories that have poor performance, especially those that have precision problems.[43] The initial CLIA '88 proposal called for the PT of two specimens four times per year, but the final rule expanded this to the study of five samples three times per year, so as to improve the capability of detecting "unacceptable" performance.

CLIA '88 criteria grouped laboratory tests into "specialty" and "subspecialty" categories, and specifically representative tests to be monitored in each category.[101] To be totally "successful" in a given category, a laboratory must produce correct results on four out of five specimens for each of the analytes in that category and must have an overall score of at least 80% for three consecutive challenges. If there are more than two incorrect results for any analyte, the laboratory is considered "on probation." If a laboratory has two or more incorrect results for any analyte or has an overall score less than 80% on two of three consecutive surveys, it is classified as "suspended" and must cease testing all analytes in that specialty category until its status is reinstated.

The CLIA regulations have established fixed limits (percentages or absolute values from target) for evaluating PT performance. These test categories and limits are shown in Table 8-9. Target values for these analytes will be established by the agencies implementing PT programs under the federal guideline[101] that states, "Target value means either the mean of all responses after removal of outliers (those responses greater than 3 standard deviations from the original mean) or the mean established by definitive or reference methods acceptable for use in the National Reference System (NRS) for the Clinical Laboratory by the CLSI. In instances in which definitive or reference methods are not available, a comparative method may be used. If the method group is less than 20 participants, 'target value' means the overall mean after outlier removal (as defined above) unless acceptable scientific reasons are available to indicate that such an evaluation is not appropriate."

Accepted reference methods do not exist for many of these *controlled analytes,* and even when they do exist, the values obtained for PT specimens with some analytical systems may not match those obtained with the reference method owing to differences in matrices and analyte form.[110]

CLIA '88 regulations specify that PT specimens should be treated in the same manner as patient specimens and require that personnel performing the tests sign a statement attesting that they have complied with the regulations. In reality, PT specimens must be treated differently than those from patients, because many are lyophilized or sealed in containers, and reporting of their results requires different forms and generally is not computerized.

A new requirement of the final CLIA regulations is that laboratories must perform method validation studies on all new tests introduced after April 24, 2003. Before this, laboratories that implemented new methods and analytical systems that had been cleared by the FDA could simply follow manufacturers' directions for operation and assume that the manufacturers' performance claims were valid. With issuance of the final rule, the performance of all new tests must be validated in each laboratory to document the reportable range, precision, accuracy, and reference intervals. For some methods, it may also be necessary to determine the detection limit and to test for possible interferences.

Another major change in the final rule was the elimination of an earlier provision that would have required the FDA to review a manufacturer's QC instructions. This was a key provision for allowing laboratories to simply follow a manufacturer's directions. However, with elimination of that provision, laboratories now have greater responsibility for establishing effective QC systems that will monitor the complete analytical process, take into account the performance specifications of the method, detect immediate errors, and monitor long-term precision and accuracy.

The most controversial change in the final rule is the introduction of *equivalent QC procedures.* CLIA sets a minimum level of QC that must be performed by all laboratories. Typically, this requires two levels of controls to be analyzed every 24 hours, or for some tests, one level of control to be analyzed every 8 hours. The new guidelines for equivalent QC may allow laboratories to reduce daily QC to weekly or even monthly QC for analytical systems that have built-in procedural controls. The provision is obviously targeted for POCT or near-patient testing (NPT), where personnel lack the skills to perform QC and instead rely on instrument checks, most notably electronic checks or electronic QC. In spite of arguments about the inadequacy of electronic QC,[123] it has become widely accepted in POCT and NPT applications. Although at least one example of an analytical system with improved QC technology requires little or no operator initiation of QC,[133] most analytical systems have yet to demonstrate the performance that would justify a reduction of daily QC to only weekly or monthly QC.

In the United States, as a result of personnel standards of the CLIA and current staffing shortages, many laboratories have been left without the technical and analytical skills to manage quality effectively. Consequently, in the authors' opinion, the use of statistical QC is declining in many laboratories (www.westgard.com/essay34/accessed March 22, 2011). Thus QC has come to mean *quality compliance* rather than quality control. The consequences of a regulatory approach to quality have to be carefully assessed relative to other initiatives. Regulation does not appear to be an adequate substitute for professional responsibility for quality.

To summarize this section, PT programs are far from ideal monitors of laboratory performance. In a study of PT survey problems at the Mayo Clinic, more than half of the errors on surveys were directly related to deficiencies in the surveys (such as invalid specimens and inappropriate evaluation criteria), and only 28% could be linked to specific analytical problems.[58] A PT program piloted by the New York State Department of Health involves obtaining aliquots of patient specimens that are routinely processed by the laboratory at the time of its annual inspection.[88] These specimens are reanalyzed in the state's laboratories using reference methods, and the results are compared with those obtained during inspection. This prevents problems such as the presence of unnatural specimens and laboratory clerical errors related to reporting of PT results. Other specimen stability problems, methodologic interferences, and potential clerical errors at the reference laboratories probably continue to occur.

IDENTIFYING THE SOURCES OF ANALYTICAL ERRORS

The control procedures discussed in the previous sections provide a means of alerting the analyst to problems that may cause the quality of analytical performance to fall short of the goals set by the laboratory. However, these control procedures do not identify the sources of the analytical errors to solve the control problems. The following additional procedures are often necessary to identify these sources.

Physical Inspection

When alerted to a control problem, the first step should be to carefully inspect the analytical method, equipment,

TABLE 8-9 HCFA/CLIA Proficiency Testing Criteria for Acceptable Performance

Analyte or Test	Acceptable Performance
Routine Chemistry	
Alanine aminotransferase	Target value ±20%
Albumin	Target value ±10%
Alkaline phosphatase	Target value ±30%
Amylase	Target value ±30%
Aspartate aminotransferase	Target value ±20%
Bilirubin, total	Target value ±0.4 mg/dL or ±0% (greater)
Blood gas PCO_2	Target value ±55 mm Hg or ±8% (greater)
Blood gas pH	Target value ±0.04
Blood gas PO_2	Target value ±3 standard deviations (SD)
Calcium, total	Target value ±1.0 mg/dL
Chloride	Target value ±5%
Cholesterol, high-density lipoprotein	Target value ±30%
Cholesterol, total	Target value ±10%
Creatine kinase	Target value ±30%
Creatine kinase isoenzymes	MB elevated (presence or absence) or target value ±3 SD
Creatinine	Target value ±0.3 mg/dL or ±15% (greater)
Glucose	Target value ±6 mg/dL or ±10% (greater)
Iron, total	Target value ±20%
Lactate dehydrogenase (LD)	Target value ±20%
LD isoenzymes	LD 1/LD 2 positive or negative or target value ±30%
Magnesium	Target value ±25%
Potassium	Target value ±0.5 mmol/L
Sodium	Target value ±4 mmol/L
Total protein	Target value ±10%
Triglycerides	Target value ±25%
Urea nitrogen	Target value ±2 mg/dL or ±9% (greater)
Uric acid	Target value ±17%
Endocrinology	
Cortisol	Target value ±25%
Free thyroxine	Target value ±3 SD
Human chorionic gonadotropin	Target value ±3 SD or positive or negative
T_3 uptake	Target value ±3 SD
Triiodothyronine	Target value ±3 SD
Thyroid-stimulating hormone	Target value ±3 SD
Thyroxine	Target value ±20% or 1.0 μg/dL (greater)
Toxicology	
Alcohol, blood	Target value ±25%
Blood lead	Target value ±10% or ±4 μg/dL (greater)
Carbamazepine	Target value ±25%
Digoxin	Target value ±20% or 0.2 ng/mL (greater)
Ethosuximide	Target value ±20%
Gentamicin	Target value ±25%
Lithium	Target value ±0.3 mmol/L or ±0% (greater)
Phenobarbital	Target value ±20%
Phenytoin	Target value ±25%
Primidone	Target value ±25%
Procainamide (and metabolite)	Target value ±25%
Quinidine	Target value ±25%
Theophylline	Target value ±25%
Tobramycin	Target value ±25%
Valproic acid	Target value ±25%

TABLE 8-9 HCFA/CLIA Proficiency Testing Criteria for Acceptable Performance—cont'd

Analyte or Test	Acceptable Performance
Hematology	
Cell identification	90% or greater consensus on identification
White cell differentiation	Target ±3 SD based on percentage of different types of white cells
Erythrocyte count	Target ±6%
Hematocrit	Target ±6%
Hemoglobin	Target ±7%
Leukocyte count	Target ±15%
Platelet count	Target ±25%
Fibrinogen	Target ±20%
Partial thromboplastin time	Target ±15%
Prothrombin time	Target ±15%
General Immunology	
α_1-antitrypsin	Target value ±3 SD
α-fetoprotein	Target value ±3 SD
Antinuclear antibody	Target value ±2 dilution or positive or negative
Antistreptolysin O	Target value ±2 dilution or positive or negative
Anti–human immunodeficiency virus	Reactive or nonreactive
Complement C3	Target value ±3 SD
Complement C4	Target value ±3 SD
Hepatitis (HbsAg, anti-HBc, HbeAg)	Reactive (positive) or nonreactive (negative)
Immunoglobulin (Ig)A	Target value ±3 SD
IgE	Target value ±3 SD
IgG	Target value ±25%
IgM	Target value ±3 SD
Infectious mononucleosis	Target value ±2 dilution or positive or negative
Rheumatoid factor	Target value ±2 dilution or positive or negative
Rubella	Target value ±2 dilution or positive or negative

From the U.S. Department of Health and Human Services. Clinical Laboratory Improvement Amendments of 1988. Final rules and notice. 42 CFR Part 493. Federal Register 1992;57:7188-288.

reagents, and specimens. Does everything look, feel, smell, and sound correct? An inspection may seem to be a very qualitative and subjective technique, but it can be exceedingly useful when performed with checklists developed for specific analytical methods. This inspection should include a review of records documenting changes that have occurred with the instrument and reagents. Brief instrument function checks are often performed to verify proper system performance and to separate chemical and instrumental sources of error. An experienced analyst can often spot the problem by making this kind of inspection, whereas inexperienced analysts will be aided by formal checklists.

Relationship of Type and Source of Error

The type of error itself provides a clue about the source of the error. For example, systematic errors are often related to calibration problems (impure calibration materials, improper preparation of calibrating solutions, erroneous set point and assigned values, unstable calibrating solutions, contaminated solutions, inadequate calibration techniques, nonlinear or unstable calibration functions, unstable reagent blanks, and inadequate sample blanks). Random errors are more likely caused by lack of reproducibility in the pipetting of samples and reagents, by the dissolving of reagent tablets and the mixing of sample and reagents, and by lack of stability of temperature baths, timing regulation, and photometric and other sensors. Individual analytical methods may not be subject to all of these possible sources of error; rather, there may be only a few plausible sources for a particular type of error. Experienced analysts often know what these common sources are for their particular analytical methods and quickly identify the sources once the type of error is known.

Some information about the type of error occurring is obtained by knowing to which errors the control procedures respond. As discussed earlier in this chapter, different control rules have different sensitivities to detect random and systematic errors. However, in practice, it is often possible to make a good judgment as to the type of error occurring based on the control procedure that provides the alert. Control procedures that employ patient samples rather than stable control materials can help identify preanalytical sources of error, such as sample handling and processing.* External quality assessment procedures that employ frozen patient samples[14,59,74,75,81,98,107] may provide more extensive information about errors than what is available from internal procedures. Information from all of these procedures is complementary and, when used in combination, provides a more complete assessment of the types of errors occurring and their possible sources.

Method Evaluation Experiments

When the type of error cannot be easily identified and quantified from available control data, it may be necessary to use the experiments employed in method evaluation studies (see Chapter 3). A *comparison-of-methods experiment* may be used to estimate systematic errors when another routine method is available for measuring the analyte of interest. Interpretation of the results must consider that observed differences between the two methods could be caused by either method and therefore cannot be assigned to the method under investigation unless the quality of the "comparison" method is well documented. Recovery, interference, and linearity experiments may be more specific in estimating systematic errors, including the constant or proportional nature of systematic errors.

To identify sources of random error, a *replication experiment* is designed to estimate the contributions from several different components. For example, when duplicates are analyzed within a run for several different runs, the data are used to determine the components of within run and between run variations. This process isolates the errors that occur in different time periods, which in turn may help reveal the sources of the random error. Replication experiments of this type, using analysis of variance statistical techniques, are tailored to particular analytical systems to identify the major factors that contribute to the random error of those analytical methods. Performance of control procedures also depends on the different components of variance, and it is particularly important that the between run component be kept as small as possible.[132]

Although the discussions in this chapter imply that plots are manually prepared, in actual practice, a wide variety of computer software packages are available for statistically calculating and plotting QA data.

Optimization Techniques

More complicated experimental techniques, such as factorial experiments, *simplex optimization,* and *response surface optimization,* have been used to solve complex control problems. These techniques generally are used by laboratorians only for laboratory development of tests because only manufacturers typically have access to this information for FDA-approved assays.[18,50,71,105] Youden[148] described the use of a series of experiments in which several factors could be varied simultaneously, thus reducing the total number of experiments necessary to determine how these factors affect the performance of the analytical method. These "factorial" experiments have been used for testing the "ruggedness" of an analytical method (i.e., its responsiveness to any disturbance in chosen experimental conditions). A properly optimized method should be rugged—this means that small changes in the analytical conditions should not greatly affect analytical performance. Formal optimization strategies have been employed to decide on those analytical conditions. These techniques provide systematic approaches for selecting the analytical conditions that minimize errors and reduce control problems.

*References 39, 41, 67, 69, 77-90, 104, 110, and 117.

REFERENCES

1. Anonymous. CAP standards for accreditation of medical laboratories. Available at: www.cap.org (accessed on March 21, 2011).
2. Anonymous. Clinical Laboratory Improvement Amendments of 1988. Stat 42 USC 201. HR 5471. Vol. Public Law, 1988:100-578.
3. Anonymous. Establishing calibration traceability for quantitative assays—CD. Washington, DC: AACC Press, 2002.
4. Anonymous. Executive summary of the third report of the National Cholesterol Education Program (NCEP) Expert Panel on Detection, Evaluation, and Treatment of High Blood Cholesterol in Adults (Adult Treatment Panel III). JAMA 2001;285:2486-97.
5. Anonymous. Interpretive guidelines for laboratories. Available at: https://www.cms.gov/CLIA/03_Interpretive_Guidelines_for_Laboratories.asp (accessed on March 21, 2011).
6. Anonymous. Quantifying uncertainty in analytical measurement. Available at: http://www.measurementuncertainty.org/ (accessed in March 21, 2011).
7. Anonymous. Statistical methods of uncertainty analysis: ISO 7C69/SC6/WG7 draft 2. Available at: http://www.itl.nist.gov/div898/carroll/u.htm (accessed in March 21, 2011).
8. Ardern CI, Katzmarzyk PT, Janssen I, Church TS, Blair SN. Revised Adult Treatment Panel III guidelines and cardiovascular disease mortality in men attending a preventive medical clinic. Circulation 2005;112:1478-85.
9. Armbruster D, Miller RR. The Joint Committee for Traceability in Laboratory Medicine (JCTLM): a global approach to promote the standardisation of clinical laboratory test results. Clin Biochem Rev 2007;28:105-14.
10. Bauer JC. Performance improvement—lean times ahead. J Healthc Inf Manag 2009;23:4-5.
11. Berry TH. Managing the total quality transformation. St Louis: McGraw-Hill Book Co, 1991.
12. Berwick DM, Godfrey AB, Roessner J. Curing health care: new strategies for quality improvement. San Francisco: Jossey-Bass Publishers, 1990.
13. Blumenthal D. The errors of our ways. Clin Chem 1997;43:1305.
14. Bock JL, Endres DB, Elin RJ, Wang E, Rosenzweig B, Klee GG. Comparison of fresh frozen serum to traditional proficiency testing material in a College of American Pathologists survey for ferritin, folate, and vitamin B12. Arch Pathol Lab Med 2005;129:323-7.
15. Bogdanich W. False negative: medical labs, trusted and largely error-free, are far from infallible-haste, misuse of equipment, specimen mix-ups afflict even best labs at times-regulation: weak and spotty. The Wall Street Journal, February 2, 1987.
16. Bogdanich W. Inaccuracy in testing cholesterol hampers war on heart disease: some diagnoses are skewed by glitches such as use of ill-calibrated lab gear: missing the mark by 100 percent. The Wall Street Journal, February 3, 1987.
17. Bonini P, Plebani M, Ceriotti F, Rubboli F. Errors in laboratory medicine. Clin Chem 2002;48:691-8.

18. Bota A, Gella FJ, Canalias F. Optimization of adenosine deaminase assay by response surface methodology. Clin Chim Acta 2000;290:145-57.
19. Brooks ZC, Plaut D. Quality control from "data" to "decisions": basic concepts. Washington, DC: AACC Press, 2002.
20. Bull BS, Elashoff RM, Heilbron DC, Couperus J. A study of various estimators for the derivation of quality control procedures from patient erythrocyte indices. Am J Clin Pathol 1974;61:473-81.
21. Burnett D. A practical guideline to accreditation in laboratory medicine. London: Association of Clinical Biochemists, 2002.
22. Buttner J, Borth R, Broughton PM, Bowyer RC. Approved recommendation (1983) on quality control in clinical chemistry. Part 4. Internal quality control. J Clin Chem Clin Biochem 1983;21:877-84.
23. Buttner J, Borth R, Boutwell JH. International Federation of Clinical Chemistry approved recommendation (1983) on quality control in clinical chemistry: V. External quality control. J Clin Chem Clin Biochem 1983;21:885-92.
24. Buttner J, Borth R, Boutwell JH. International Federation of Clinical Chemistry provisional recommendation on quality control in clinical chemistry: I. General principles and terminology. Clin Chem 1976;22:532-9.
25. Buttner J, Borth R, Boutwell JH. International Federation of Clinical Chemistry provisional recommendation on quality control in clinical chemistry: II. Assessment of analytical methods for routine use. Clin Chem 1976;22:1922-32.
26. Buttner J, Borth R, Boutwell JH. International Federation of Clinical Chemistry provisional recommendation on quality control in clinical chemistry: III. Calibration and control materials. Clin Chem 1977;23:1784-90.
27. Buttner J, Borth R, Boutwell JH. International Federation of Clinical Chemistry provisional recommendation on quality control in clinical chemistry: VI. Quality requirements from the point of view of health care. Clin Chim Acta 1977;74:F1-9.
28. Cankovic M, Varney RC, Whiteley L, Brown R, D'Angelo R, Chitale D, et al. The Henry Ford production system: LEAN process redesign improves service in the molecular diagnostic laboratory: a paper from the 2008 William Beaumont hospital symposium on molecular pathology. J Mol Diagn 2009;11:390-9.
29. Cembrowski GS, Carey RN. Laboratory quality management: QC and QA. Chicago: ASCP Press, 1989.
30. Cembrowski GS, Chandler EP, Westgard JO. Assessment of "average of normals" quality control procedures and guidelines for implementation. Am J Clin Pathol 1984;81:492-9.
31. Cembrowski GS, Westgard JO. Quality control of multichannel hematology analyzers: evaluation of Bull's algorithm. Am J Clin Pathol 1985;83:337-45.
32. Cembrowski GS, Westgard JO, Kurtycz DF. Use of anion gap for the quality control of electrolyte analyzers. Am J Clin Pathol 1983;79:688-96.
33. CLSI. Collection, transport, and processing of blood specimens for testing plasma-based coagulation assays and molecular hemostasis assays: approved guideline, 5th edition. CLSI Document H21-A5. Wayne, Pa: Clinical and Laboratory Standards Institute, 2008.
34. CLSI. Defining, establishing, and verifying reference intervals in the clinical laboratory: approved guideline, 3rd edition. CLSI Document C28-A3c. Wayne, Pa: Clinical and Laboratory Standards Institute, 2010.
35. CLSI. Laboratory Documents: Development and control: approved guideline, 5th edition. CLSI Document GP02-A5. Wayne, Pa: Clinical and Laboratory Standards Institute, 2006.
36. CLSI. Nomenclature and definitions for use in the NRSCL and other NCCLS documents: proposed standard. CLSI Document NRSCl 08-A. Wayne, Pa: Clinical and Laboratory Standards Institute, 1998.
37. CLSI. A quality management system model for health care: approved guideline, 2nd edition. CLSI Document HS01-A2. Wayne, Pa: Clinical and Laboratory Standards Institute, 2004.
38. CLSI. Training and competence assessment: approved guideline, 3rd edition. CLSI Document GP21-A3. Wayne, Pa: Clinical and Laboratory Standards Institute, 2009.
39. Coldeway DO. Instructional systems design. Madison, Wis: University of Wisconsin Madison, 2005.
40. Davies HT. Exploring the pathology of quality failings: measuring quality is not the problem—changing it is. J Eval Clin Pract 2001;7:243-51.
41. De Bievre P. The 2007 International Vocabulary of Metrology (VIM), JCGM 200:2008 (ISO/IEC Guide 99): meeting the need for intercontinentally understood concepts and their associated intercontinentally agreed terms. Clin Biochem 2009;42:246-8.
41A. DelliFraine JL, Langabeer JR 2nd, Nembhard IM. Assessing the evidence of Six Sigma and Lean in the health care industry. Qual Manag Health Care. 2010;19:211-25.
42. Deming WE. Out of the crisis. Cambridge, Mass: Massachusetts Institute of Technology Center for Advanced Study, 1987.
43. Ehrmeyer SS, Laessig RH. Ability of the 1(2)s rule to detect substandard performance in interlaboratory proficiency testing. Clin Chem 1987;33:788-91.
44. Eilers RJ. Quality assurance in health care: missions, goals, activities. Clin Chem 1975;21:1357-67.
45. Elin RJ. Notes on standards: elements of cost management for quality assurance. Pathologist 1980;34:182-3, 194.
46. George M. Lean six sigma: combining six sigma quality with lean production. New York: McGraw-Hill, 2002.
46A. Glasgow JM, Scott-Caziewell JR, Kaboli PJ. Guiding inpatient quality improvement: a systematic review of Lean and Six Sigma. Jt Comm J Qual Patient Saf. 2010;36:533-40.
46B. Gras JM, Philippe M. Application of the Six Sigma concept in clinical laboratories: a review. Clin Chem Lab Med. 2007;45:789-96.
47. Groth T, Falk H, Westgard JO. An interactive computer simulation program for the design of statistical control procedures in clinical chemistry. Comput Programs Biomed 1981;13:73-86.
48. Harry SR. Six sigma: the breakthrough management strategy revolutionizing the world's top corporations. New York: Currency, 2000.
49. Hay ID, Klee GG. Linking medical needs and performance goals: clinical and laboratory perspectives on thyroid disease. Clin Chem 1993;39:1519-24.
50. Horstkotte B, Tovar Sanchez A, Duarte CM, Cerda V. Sequential injection analysis for automation of the Winkler methodology, with real-time SIMPLEX optimization and shipboard application. Anal Chim Acta 2010;658:147-55.
51. Ismail AA, Walker PL, Barth JH, Lewandowski KC, Jones R, Burr WA. Wrong biochemistry results: two case reports and observational study in 5310 patients on potentially misleading thyroid-stimulating hormone and gonadotropin immunoassay results. Clin Chem 2002;48:2023-9.
52. Juppner H, Mohr H, Hesch RD. Adsorption of parathyrin: pitfall for solid phase assays using radiolabelled antibodies? J Clin Chem Clin Biochem 1980;18:585-90.
53. Juran JM. Quality improvement for services. Wilton, Conn: Juran Institute Inc, 1986.
54. Kazmierczak SC. Laboratory quality control: using patient data to assess analytical performance. Clin Chem Lab Med 2003;41: 617-27.
55. Kelly JT. Role of clinical practice guidelines and clinical profiling in facilitating optimal laboratory use. Clin Chem 1995;41:1234-6.
56. Klee GG. Tolerance limits for short-term analytical bias and analytical imprecision derived from clinical assay specificity. Clin Chem 1993;39:1514-8.
57. Klee GG. Use of patient test values to enhance the quality control of PSA assays. Clin Chem 2003;49:A94.
58. Klee GG, Forsman RW. A user's classification of problems identified by proficiency testing surveys. Arch Pathol Lab Med 1988;112:371-3.
59. Knight GJ, Palomaki GE, Klee GG, Schreiber WE, Cole LA. A comparison of human chorionic gonadotropin- related components in fresh frozen serum with the proficiency testing material used by the College of American Pathologists. Arch Pathol Lab Med 2005;129: 328-30.

60. Kohn KT, Donaldson MS. To err is human: building a safer health system. Washington, DC: National Academy Press, 1993.
61. Kubasik NP, Ricotta M, Hunter T, Sine HE. Effect of duration and temperature of storage on serum analyte stability: examination of 14 selected radioimmunoassay procedures. Clin Chem 1982;28:164-5.
62. Ladenson JH. Patients as their own controls: use of the computer to identify "laboratory error." Clin Chem 1975;21:1648-53.
63. Laessig RH, Ehrmeyer SS. Use of computer modeling to predict the magnitude of intralaboratory error tolerated by proposed CDC interlaboratory proficiency testing performance criteria. Clin Chem 1988;34:1849-53.
64. Leape LL. Striving for perfection. Clin Chem 2002;48:1871-2.
65. Leape LL, Berwick DM, Bates DW. What practices will most improve safety? Evidence-based medicine meets patient safety. JAMA 2002;288:501-7.
66. Leape LL. Robert E. Gross lecture. Making health care safe: are we up to it? J Pediatr Surg 2004;39:258-66.
67. Levey S, Jennings ER. The use of control charts in the clinical laboratory. Am J Clin Pathol 1950;20:1059-66.
68. Lunetzky ES, Cembrowski GS. Performance characteristics of Bull's multirule algorithm for the quality control of multichannel hematology analyzers. Am J Clin Pathol 1987;88:634-8.
69. Lusky K. Trimming the fat from lab processes. CAP Today May, 2006. (http://www.cap.org, assessed March 22, 2011)
70. Maisel WH, Moynahan M, Zuckerman BD, Gross TP, Tovar OH, Tillman DB, et al. Pacemaker and ICD generator malfunctions: analysis of Food and Drug Administration annual reports. JAMA 2006;295:1901-6.
71. Maneeboon T, Vanichsriratana W, Pomchaitaward C, Kitpreechavanich V. Optimization of lactic acid production by pellet-form *Rhizopus oryzae* in 3-L airlift bioreactor using response surface methodology. Appl Biochem Biotechnol 2010;161:137-46.
72. Marks V. False-positive immunoassay results: a multicenter survey of erroneous immunoassay results from assays of 74 analytes in 10 donors from 66 laboratories in seven countries. Clin Chem 2002;48:2008-16.
73. Miller WG. Specimen materials, target values and commutability for external quality assessment (proficiency testing) schemes. Clin Chim Acta 2003;327:25-37.
74. Miller WG, Myers GL, Ashwood ER, Killeen AA, Wang E, Ehlers GW, et al. State of the art in trueness and interlaboratory harmonization for 10 analytes in general clinical chemistry. Arch Pathol Lab Med 2008;132:838-46.
75. Miller WG, Myers GL, Ashwood ER, Killeen AA, Wang E, Thienpont LM, et al. Creatinine measurement: state of the art in accuracy and interlaboratory harmonization. Arch Pathol Lab Med 2005;129:297-304.
76. Moore MG. On a theory of independent study. London: Croon Helm, 1983.
77. Mugan K, Westgard JO. Planning QC procedures for immunoassays. J Clin Immunoassay 1994;17:216-22.
78. Nardella A, Farrell M, Pechet L, Snyder LM. Continuous improvement, quality control, and cost containment in clinical laboratory testing: enhancement of physicians' laboratory-ordering practices. Arch Pathol Lab Med 1994;118:965-8.
79. Nevalainen D, Berte L, Kraft C, Leigh E, Picaso L, Morgan T. Evaluating laboratory performance on quality indicators with the six sigma scale. Arch Pathol Lab Med 2000;124:516-9.
80. Nevalainen DE. The quality systems approach. Arch Pathol Lab Med 1999;123:566-8.
81. Palmer-Toy DE, Wang E, Winter WE, Soldin SJ, Klee GG, Howanitz JH, et al. Comparison of pooled fresh frozen serum to proficiency testing material in College of American Pathologists surveys: cortisol and immunoglobulin E. Arch Pathol Lab Med 2005;129:305-9.
82. Parvin CA. Comparing the power of quality-control rules to detect persistent systematic error. Clin Chem 1992;38:358-63.
83. Peddecord KM, Hammond HC. Clinical laboratory regulation under the Clinical Laboratory Improvement Amendments of 1988: can it be done? Clin Chem 1990;36:2027-35.
84. Persoon TJ, Zaleski S, Frerichs J. Improving preanalytic processes using the principles of lean production (Toyota Production System). Am J Clin Pathol 2006;125:16-25.
85. Petersen PH, Stockl D, Westgard JO, Sandberg S, Linnet K, Thienpont L. Models for combining random and systematic errors. Assumptions and consequences for different models. Clin Chem Lab Med 2001;39:589-95.
86. Plebani M, Carraro P. Mistakes in a stat laboratory: types and frequency. Clin Chem 1997;43:1348-51.
87. Prevention CfDCa. Code of Federal Regulations: 42CFR493.1451. Standard: technical supervisor responsibilities. Available at: http://www.cdc.gov/clia/regs/toc.aspx (accessed on August 25, 2009).
88. Rej R, Norton C. External assessment of laboratory cholesterol measurements using patient specimens. Clin Chem 1989;35:1069.
89. Revere L, Black K. Integrating Six Sigma with total quality management: a case example for measuring medication errors. J Healthc Manage 2003;48:377-91; discussion 392.
90. Ricos C, Alvarez V, Cava F, Garcia-Lario JV, Hernandez A, Jimenez CV, et al. Current databases on biological variation: pros, cons and progress. Scand J Clin Lab Invest 1999;59:491-500.
91. Rollo JL, Fauser BA. Computers in total quality management: statistical process control to expedite stats. Arch Pathol Lab Med 1993;117:900-5.
92. Ross JW. Assessing the effect of mistakes in the total testing process on the quality of patient care. Minneapolis, Minn: DuPont Press, 1991.
93. Rossing RG, Foster DM. The stability of clinical chemistry specimens during refrigerated storage for 24 hours. Am J Clin Pathol 1980;73:91-5.
94. Samore MH, Evans RS, Lassen A, Gould P, Lloyd J, Gardner RM, et al. Surveillance of medical device-related hazards and adverse events in hospitalized patients. JAMA 2004;291:325-34.
95. Sarewitz SJ. Evaluating laboratory performance with the six sigma scale. Arch Pathol Lab Med 2000;124:1748.
96. Savage RA. Proficiency testing and laboratory quality: lessons from the Ontario program. Arch Pathol Lab Med 1989;113:983-4.
97. Scholtes PR. The team handbook. Madison, Wis: Joiner Associates Inc, 1988.
98. Schreiber WE, Endres DB, McDowell GA, Palomaki GE, Elin RJ, Klee GG, et al. Comparison of fresh frozen serum to proficiency testing material in College of American Pathologists surveys: alpha-fetoprotein, carcinoembryonic antigen, human chorionic gonadotropin, and prostate-specific antigen. Arch Pathol Lab Med 2005;129:331-7.
99. Schweikhart SA, Dembe AE. The applicability of Lean and Six Sigma techniques to clinical and translational research. J Investig Med 2009;57:748-55.
100. Services for. Medicare, Medicaid, and CLIA programs: laboratory requirements relating to quality systems and certain personnel qualifications. Final rule. Federal Register 2006:3640-714.
101. Services for Clinical Laboratory Improvement Amendments of 1988. Final rules and notice. 42 CFR Part 493. Federal Register 1992:7188-288.
102. Shewhart WA. Economic control of quality of the manufactured product. New York: Van Nostrand, 1931.
103. Smith FA, Kroft SH. Exponentially adjusted moving mean procedure for quality control: an optimized patient sample control procedure. Am J Clin Pathol 1996;105:44-51.
104. Smith FA, Kroft SH. Optimal procedures for detecting analytic bias using patient samples. Am J Clin Pathol 1997;108:254-68.
105. Soylak M, Narin I, Bezerra MA, Ferreira SL. Factorial design in the optimization of preconcentration procedure for lead determination by FAAS. Talanta 2005;65:895-9.
106. Stankovic AK, DiLauri E. Quality improvements in the preanalytical phase: focus on urine specimen workflow. Clin Lab Med 2008;28:339-50, viii.
107. Steele BW, Wang E, Klee GG, Thienpont LM, Soldin SJ, Sokoll LJ, et al. Analytic bias of thyroid function tests: analysis of a College of

American Pathologists fresh frozen serum pool by 3900 clinical laboratories. Arch Pathol Lab Med 2005;129:310-7.
108. Taswell HF, Smith AM, Sweatt MA, Pfaff KJ. Quality control in the blood bank—a new approach. Am J Clin Pathol 1974;62:491-5.
109. Tetrault GA. Daily quality control exception practices. Chicago, Ill: College of American Pathologists, 1994.
110. Thienpont LM, Van Uytfanghe K, De Leenheer AP. Reference measurement systems in clinical chemistry. Clin Chim Acta 2002;323:73-87.
111. Tietz NW. A model for a comprehensive measurement system in clinical chemistry. Clin Chem 1979;25:833-9.
112. Trisolini MG. Applying business management models in health care. Int J Health Plann Manage 2002;17:295-314.
113. Uriano GA. Role of reference materials and reference methods in the measurement process. In: Validation of the measurement process. Washington, DC: American Chemical Society, 1977:140.
114. Vesper HW, Thienpont LM. Traceability in laboratory medicine. Clin Chem 2009;55:1067-75.
115. Vest JR, Gamm LD. A critical review of the research literature on Six Sigma, Lean and StuderGroup's Hardwiring Excellence in the United States: the need to demonstrate and communicate the effectiveness of transformation strategies in healthcare. Implement Sci 2009;4:35.
116. Warwood S, Antony J. A simple, semi-prescriptive self-assessment model for TQM. Qual Assur 2003;10:67-81.
117. Westgard JO. Assuring analytical quality through process planning and quality control. Arch Pathol Lab Med 1992;116:765-9.
118. Westgard JO. Basic method validation, 2nd edition. Washington, DC: AACC Press, 2003.
119. Westgard JO. Basic planning for quality. Washington, DC: AACC Press, 2000.
120. Westgard JO. Basic QC practices, 2nd edition. Madison, Wis: Westgard, QC Inc, 2002.
121. Westgard JO. Charts of operational process specifications ("OPSpecs charts") for assessing the precision, accuracy, and quality control needed to satisfy proficiency testing performance criteria. Clin Chem 1992;38:1226-33; discussion 1245-50.
122. Westgard JO. Desirable specifications for total error, imprecision, and bias, derived from intra- and inter-individual biologic variation. Available at: http://www.westgard.com/guest32/index.php?option=com_content&view=article&id=238:biodatabase1&catid=37:quality-requirements&Itemid=66 (accessed on March 22, 2011).
123. Westgard JO. Electronic quality control, the total testing process, and the total quality control system. Clin Chim Acta 2001;307:45-8.
124. Westgard JO. Internal quality control: planning and implementation strategies. Ann Clin Biochem 2003;40:593-611.
125. Westgard JO. OPSpecs manual, expanded edition. Operating specifications for imprecision, inaccuracy, and quality control. Ogunquit, Maine: Westgard QC, 1996.
126. Westgard JO. Six sigma quality design and control: desirable precision and requisite QC for laboratory testing processes. Madison, Wis: Westgard QC, 2001.
127. Westgard JO, Barry PL. Total quality control: evolution of quality management systems. Lab Med 1989;20:377-84.
128. Westgard JO, Barry PL, Hunt MR, Groth T. A multi-rule Shewhart chart for quality control in clinical chemistry. Clin Chem 1981;27:493-501.
129. Westgard JO, Barry PL, Tomar RH. Implementing total quality management (TQM) in health-care laboratories. Clin Lab Manage Rev 1991;5:353-5, 358-9, 362-6.
130. Westgard JO, Barry PL. Cost-effective quality control: managing the quality and productivity of analytical processes. Washington, DC: AACC Press, 1986.
131. Westgard JO, Ehrmeyer SS, Darcy TP. CLIA final rules for quality systems: quality assessment issues and answers. Madison, Wis: Westgard QC, 2004.
132. Westgard JO, Falk H, Groth T. Influence of a between-run component of variation, choice of control limits, and shape of error distribution on the performance characteristics of rules for internal quality control. Clin Chem 1979;25:394-400.
133. Westgard JO, Fallon KD, Mansouri S. Validation of iQM active process control technology. Point of Care 2003;2:1-7.
134. Westgard JO, Groth T. Design and evaluation of statistical control procedures: applications of a computer "quality control simulator" program. Clin Chem 1981;27:1536-45.
135. Westgard JO, Groth T. Power functions for statistical control rules. Clin Chem 1979;25:863-9.
136. Westgard JO, Groth T, Aronsson T, de Verdier CH. Combined Shewhart-Cusum control chart for improved quality control in clinical chemistry. Clin Chem 1977;23:1881-7.
137. Westgard JO, Groth T, Aronsson T, Falk H, de Verdier CH. Performance characteristics of rules for internal quality control: probabilities for false rejection and error detection. Clin Chem 1977;23:1857-67.
138. Westgard JO, Klee GG. Quality management, 3rd edition. Philadelphia: WB Saunders, 1999:404.
139. Westgard JO, Oryall JJ, Koch DD. Predicting effects of quality-control practices on the cost-effective operation of a stable, multitest analytical system. Clin Chem 1990;36:1760-4.
140. Westgard JO, Petersen PH, Wiebe DA. Laboratory process specifications for assuring quality in the U.S. National Cholesterol Education Program. Clin Chem 1991;37:656-61.
141. Westgard JO, Smith FA, Mountain PJ, Boss S. Design and assessment of average of normals (AON) patient data algorithms to maximize run lengths for automatic process control. Clin Chem 1996;42:1683-8.
142. Westgard JO, Wiebe DA. Cholesterol operational process specifications for assuring the quality required by CLIA proficiency testing. Clin Chem 1991;37:1938-44.
143. Wilding P, Zilva JF, Wilde CE. Transport of specimens for clinical chemistry analysis. Ann Clin Biochem 1977;14:301-6.
144. Winch S, Henderson AJ. Making cars and making health care: a critical review. Med J Aust 2009;191:28-9.
145. Witte DL, VanNess SA, Angstadt DS, Pennell BJ. Errors, mistakes, blunders, outliers, or unacceptable results: how many? Clin Chem 1997;43:1352-6.
146. Wong ET. Improving laboratory testing: can we get physicians to focus on outcome? Clin Chem 1995;41:1241-7.
147. Ye JJ, Ingels SC, Parvin CA. Performance evaluation and planning for patient-based quality control procedures. Am J Clin Pathol 2000;113:240-8.
148. Youden WJ. Statistical techniques for collaborative tests. Washington, DC: Association of Official Analytical Chemists, 1969.
149. Young DS. Effects of preanalytical variables on clinical laboratory tests, 3rd edition. Washington, DC: AACC Press, 2007.

SECTION II

Analytical Techniques and Instrumentation

CHAPTER 9

Principles of Basic Techniques and Laboratory Safety

*Stanley F. Lo, Ph.D., D.A.B.C.C., F.A.C.B.**

To reliably perform qualitative and quantitative analyses on body fluids and tissue, the clinical laboratorian must understand the basic *principles and techniques* of analytical chemistry. Valcárcel has generically defined analytical chemistry as "a metrological science that develops, optimizes, and applies measuring processes intended to derive quality analytical information in order to solve the measuring problems posed."[25] Factors that affect the analytical process and operation of the clinical laboratory include knowledge of (1) the concept of solute and solvent; (2) units of measurement; (3) chemicals; (4) reference materials; (5) basic techniques, such as volumetric sampling and dispensing, centrifugation, measurement of radioactivity, gravimetry, thermometry, buffer solution, and processing of solutions; and (6) safety.

CONCEPT OF SOLUTE AND SOLVENT

Many analyses in the clinical laboratory are concerned with determination of the presence or measurement of the concentration of substances in solutions, the solutions most often being blood, serum, urine, spinal fluid, or other body fluids (see Chapter 7).

A *solution* is a homogeneous mixture of one or more *solutes* dispersed molecularly in a sufficient quantity of a dissolving *solvent.* In laboratory practice, solutes are typically measured and are frequently referred to as analytes or measurands. A solution may be gaseous, liquid, or solid. A clinical laboratorian is concerned primarily with the measurement of gases or solids in liquids, where there is always a relatively large amount of solvent in comparison with the amount of solute.

Expressing Concentrations of Solutions

The following equations define the expression of concentrations:

$$\text{Mole} = \frac{\text{mass (g)}}{\text{gram molecular weight (g)}}$$

$$\text{Molarity of a solution} = \frac{\text{number of moles of solute}}{\text{number of liters of solution}}$$

$$\text{Molality of a solution} = \frac{\text{number of moles of solute}}{\text{number of kilograms of solvent}}$$

$$\text{Normality of a solution} = \frac{\text{number of gram equivalents of solute}}{\text{number of liters of solution}}$$

$$\begin{array}{c}\text{Gram equivalent weight}\\ \text{(as oxidatant or reductant)}\end{array} = \frac{\text{formula weight (g)}}{\text{difference in oxidation state}}$$

In the past, milliequivalent (mEq) was used to express the concentration of electrolytes in plasma. Now, the recommended unit for expressing the concentration of an electrolyte in plasma is millimoles per liter (mmol/L). For example, if a sample contains 322 mg of Na per deciliter then the serum contains 3220 mg/L. The molar concentration of Na is

$$\text{mmol/L} = \frac{\text{mg/L}}{\text{mg molecular mass}} = \frac{322 \times 10 \times 1}{23} = 140 \text{ mmol/L}$$

In clinical laboratory practice, a *titer* is thought of as the lowest dilution at which a particular reaction takes place. Titer is customarily expressed as a ratio, for example, 1:10 or 1 to 10.

Regarding gases in solution, Henry's law states that the solubility of a gas in a liquid is directly proportional to the pressure of the gas above the liquid at equilibrium. Thus as the pressure of a gas is doubled, its solubility is also doubled. The relationship between pressure and solubility varies with the nature of the gas. When several gases are dissolved at the same time in a single solvent, the solubility of each gas is

The author gratefully acknowledges the original contributions of Drs. Edward W. Bermes, Stephen E. Kahn, Donald S. Young, Edward R. Powsner, and John C. Widman, on which portions of this chapter are based.

proportional to its partial pressure in the mixture. The solubility of most gases in liquids decreases with an increase in temperature, and indeed boiling a liquid frequently drives out all dissolved gases. Traditionally, the unit used to describe the concentration of gases in liquids has been percent by volume (vol/vol). Using the SI, gas concentrations are expressed in moles per cubic meter (mol/m^3).

UNITS OF MEASUREMENT

A meaningful measurement is expressed with both a number and a unit. The unit identifies the dimension—mass, volume, or concentration—of a measured property. The number indicates how many units are contained in the property.

Traditionally, measurements in the clinical laboratory have been made in metric units. In the early development of the *metric system,* units were referenced to length, mass, and time. The first absolute systems were based on the centimeter, gram, and second (CGS), and then the meter, kilogram, and second (MKS). The Système Internationale d'Unités (SI) is a different system that was accepted internationally in 1960. The *units of the system* are called SI units.

International System of Units

Base, derived, and supplemental units are the three classes of SI units.[20] The eight fundamental base units are listed in Table 9-1. A *derived unit* is derived mathematically from two or more base units (Table 9-2). A *supplemental unit* is a unit that conforms to the SI but has not been classified as either base or derived. At present, only the radian (for plane angles) and the steradian (for solid angles) are classified this way.

The Conférence Générale des Poids et Mésures (CGPM) recognizes that some units outside the SI continue to be important and useful in particular applications. An example is the liter as the reference volume in clinical analyses. Liter is the name of the submultiple (cubic decimeter) of the SI unit of volume, the cubic meter. Considering that 1 cubic meter represents some 200 times the blood volume of an adult human, the SI unit of volume is neither a convenient nor a reasonable reference volume in a clinical context. Nevertheless, the CGPM recommends that such exceptional units as the liter should not be combined with SI units and preferably should be replaced with SI units whenever possible.

The minute, hour, and day have had such long-standing use in everyday life that it is unlikely that new SI units derived from the second could supplant them. Some other non-SI units are still accepted, although they are rarely used by most individuals in their daily lives but have been very important in some specialized fields. Details of the SI system are found in an expanded version of this chapter.[2]

In practical application of units, certain values are too large or too small to be expressed conveniently. Numeric values are brought to convenient size when the unit is appropriately modified by official prefixes (Table 9-3).

Standardized Reporting of Test Results

To describe test results properly, it is important that all necessary information be included in the test description. Systems developed for expressing results produced by the clinical laboratory include the Laboratory Logical Observation Identifiers, Names, and Codes (Lab LOINC),[15-17] and the Nomenclature, Properties, and Units (NPU) developed by the

TABLE 9-1 SI Base Units

Quantity	Name	Symbol
Length	meter	m
Mass	kilogram	kg
Time	second	S
Electrical current	ampere	A
Thermodynamic temperature	kelvin	K
Amount of substance	mole	mol
Luminous intensity	candela	cd
Catalytic amount	katal	kat

TABLE 9-2 Examples of SI-Derived Units Important in Clinical Medicine, Expressed in Terms of Base Units

Quantity	Name	SI Symbol	Expression in Terms of SI Base Units	Expression in Terms of Other SI Units
Volume	cubic meter	m^3	m^3	
Mass density	kilogram per cubic meter	kg/m^3	kg/m^3	
Concentration of amount of substance	mole per cubic meter	mol/m^3	mol/m^3	
Frequency	hertz	Hz	s^{-1}	
Force	newton	N	$m\bullet kg\bullet s^{-2}$	
Pressure	pascal	Pa	$m^{-1}\bullet kg\bullet s^{-2}$	N/m^2
Energy, work, quantity of heat	joule	J	$m^2\bullet kg\bullet s^{-2}$	N•m
Power	watt	W	$m^2\bullet kg\bullet ^{s-3}$	J/s
Electric potential, potential difference, electromotive force	volt	V	$m^2\bullet kg\bullet s^{-3}\bullet A^{-1}$	$W\bullet A^{-1}$

TABLE 9-3 Metric Prefixes of SI Units*

Factor	Prefix	Symbol
10^{24}	yotta	Y
10^{21}	zetta	Z
10^{18}	exa	E
10^{15}	peta	P
10^{12}	tera	T
10^{9}	giga	G
10^{6}	mega	M
10^{3}	kilo	k
10^{2}	hecto	h
10^{1}	deka†	da
10^{-1}	deci	d
10^{-2}	centi	c
10^{-3}	milli	m
10^{-6}	micro	µ
10^{-9}	nano	n
10^{-12}	pico	p
10^{-15}	femto	f
10^{-18}	atto	a
10^{-21}	zepto	z
10^{-24}	yocto	y

*The Eleventh Conférence Générale des Poids et Mésures (CGPM) (1960, Resolution 12) adopted a first series of prefixes and symbols of prefixes to form the names and symbols of the decimal multiples and submultiples of SI units. Prefixes for 10^{-15} and 10^{-18} were added by the 12th CGPM (1964, Resolution 8) and those for 10^{15} and 10^{18} by the 15th CGPM (1975, Resolution 10), and those for 10^{21}, 10^{24}, and 10^{-24} were proposed by the Comité International des Poids et Mésures (CIPM) (1990) for approval by the 19th CGPM (1991).

†Outside the United States, the spelling "deca" is used extensively.

From The International System of Units (SI). Washington, DC: National Institute of Standards and Technology, 1991.

International Federation of Clinical Chemistry/International Union of Pure and Applied Chemistry (IFCC/IUPAC).

Lab LOINC System

The Lab LOINC system is a universal coding system for reporting laboratory and other clinical observations to facilitate electronic transmission of laboratory data within and between institutions (http://www.loinc.org). It has several thousand observations in its database. For each observation, there is a code, a long formal name, a short 30-character name, and synonyms. A mapping program termed "Regenstrief LOINC Mapping Assistant" (RELMA) is available to map local test codes to LOINC codes and to facilitate searching of the Lab LOINC database. Both Lab LOINC and RELMA are available at no cost from http://loinc.org/relma (accessed March 16, 2011).

NPU

The NPU system recommends that the following items be included with each test result:

1. The name of the system or its abbreviation
2. A dash (two hyphens)
3. The name of the analyte (never abbreviated) with an initial capital letter
4. A comma
5. The quantity name or its abbreviation
6. An equal sign
7. The numeric value and the unit or its abbreviation

Applications

The Lab LOINC and NPU coding systems are used in context with existing standards, such as the Systematized Nomenclature of Medicine, Clinical Terms (SNOMED CT). Other such coding systems are the ASTM E1238 (American Society for Testing and Materials), HL7 version 2.2 (Health Level Seven; http://www.hl7.org; accessed March 16, 2011), and CEN ENV 1613—a standard developed by the European Committee for Standardization of the Comité Européen de Normalisation (CEN) Technical Committee 251 (http://www.cen.eu/ accessed March 16, 2011).

SNOMED CT is a comprehensive clinical terminology, originally created by the College of American Pathologists (CAP) and, as of April 2007, owned, maintained, and distributed by the International Health Terminology Standards Development Organisation (IHTSDO) in Denmark (http://www.ihtsdo.org; accessed March 16, 2011). IHTSDO is a not-for-profit association that develops and promotes use of SNOMED CT to support safe and effective health information exchange. In practice, the CAP continues to support SNOMED CT operations under contract to the IHTSDO and provides SNOMED-related products and services as a licensee of the terminology.

On April 1, 2009, the owners of LOINC, NPU, and SNOMED CT began an operational trial of prospective divisions of labor in the generation of laboratory test terminology content. This trial will provide practical experience and important information on opportunities to decrease duplication of effort in the development of laboratory test terminology and to ensure that SNOMED CT works effectively in combination with LOINC or NPU.

CHEMICALS

The quality of the analytical results produced by the laboratory is a direct indication of the purity of the chemicals used as analytical reagents. The availability and quality of the reference materials used to calibrate assays and to monitor their analytical performance also are important.

Laboratory chemicals are available in a variety of grades. The solutes and solvents used in analytical work are *reagent grade chemicals,* among which water is a solvent of primary importance.

Reagent Grade Water

Preparation of many reagents and solutions used in the clinical laboratory requires "pure" water. Single-distilled water fails to meet the specifications for Clinical Laboratory Reagent Water (CLRW) established by the Clinical Laboratory and Standards Institute (CLSI).[10] Because the terms *deionized*

TABLE 9-4 Clinical Laboratory and Standards Institute (CLSI) Specifications for Reagent Water

	CLRW
Microbiological content,* colony-forming units per mL, cfu/mL (maximum)	10
pH	Not applicable
Resistivity,† MΩ per centimeter (MΩcm), 25 °C	≥10 (in line)
Silicate, mg SiO_2/L (maximum)	0.05
Particulate matter‡	Water passed through 0.2-μm filter
Organics	Water passed through activated carbon

*Microbiological content. The microbiological content of viable organisms, as determined by total colony count after incubation at 36 ± 1 °C for 14 hours, followed by 48 hours at 25 ± 1 °C, and reported as colony-forming units per mL (cfu/mL).
†Specific resistance or resistivity. The electrical resistance in ohms measured between opposite faces of a 1-cm cube of an aqueous solution at a specified temperature. For these specifications, the resistivity will be corrected for 25 °C and reported in MΩ/cm. The higher the quantity of ionizable materials, the lower will be the resistivity and the higher the conductivity.
‡Particulate matter. When water is passed through a membrane filter with a mean pore size of 0.2 μm, it is considered to be free of particulate matter; when water is passed through a bed of activated carbon, it is considered to contain minimum organic material.
From CLSI. Preparation and testing of reagent water in the clinical laboratory, 4th edition. CLSI Document C3-A4. Wayne, Pa: CLSI, 2006.

water and *distilled water* describe preparation techniques, they should be replaced by reagent grade water, followed by the designation of CLRW, which better defines the specifications of the water and is independent of the method of preparation (Table 9-4).

Preparation of Reagent Grade Water

Distillation, ion exchange, reverse osmosis, and ultraviolet oxidation are processes used to prepare reagent grade water. In practice, water is filtered before any of these processes are used.

Distillation

Distillation is the process of vaporizing and condensing a liquid to purify or concentrate a substance or to separate a volatile substance from less volatile substances. It is the oldest method of water purification. Problems with distillation for preparing reagent water include the carryover of volatile impurities and entrapped water droplets that may contain impurities into the purified water. This will result in contamination of the distillate with volatiles, sodium, potassium, manganese, carbonates, and sulfates. As a result, water treated by distillation alone does not meet the specific conductivity requirement of type I water.

Ion Exchange

Ion exchange is a process that removes ions to produce mineral-free *deionized water.* Such water is most conveniently prepared using commercial equipment, which ranges in size from small, disposable cartridges to large, resin-containing tanks. Deionization is accomplished by passing feed water through columns containing insoluble resin polymers that exchange H^+ and OH^- ions for the impurities present in ionized form in the water. The columns may contain cation exchangers, anion exchangers, or a *mixed-bed resin exchanger,* which is a mixture of cation- and anion-exchange resins in the same container.

A single-bed deionizer generally is capable of producing water that has a specific resistance in excess of 1 MΩ/cm. When connected in series, mixed-bed deionizers usually produce water with a specific resistance that exceeds 10 MΩ/cm.

Reverse Osmosis

Reverse osmosis is a process by which water is forced through a semipermeable membrane that acts as a molecular filter. The membrane removes 95 to 99% of organic compounds, bacteria, and other particulate matter and 90 to 97% of all ionized and dissolved minerals, but fewer of the gaseous impurities. Although this process is inadequate for producing reagent grade water for the laboratory, it may be used as a preliminary purification method.

Ultraviolet Oxidation

Ultraviolet oxidation is another method that works well as part of a total system. The use of ultraviolet radiation at the biocidal wavelength of 254 nanometers eliminates many bacteria and cleaves many ionizing organics that are then removed by deionization.

Quality, Use, and Storage of Reagent Grade Water

Type III water may be used for glassware washing. (Final rinsing, however, should be done with the water grade suitable for the intended glassware use.) It may also be used for certain qualitative procedures, such as those used in general urinalysis.

Type II water is used for general laboratory testing not requiring type I water. Storage should be kept to a minimum; storage and delivery systems should be constructed to ensure a minimum of chemical or bacterial contamination.

Type I water should be used in test methods requiring minimal interference and maximal precision and accuracy. Such procedures include trace metal, enzyme, and electrolyte measurements, and preparation of all calibrators and solutions of reference materials. This water should be used immediately after production. No specifications for storage systems for type I water are given because it is not possible to maintain high resistivity while drawing off water and storing it.

Testing for Water Purity

At a minimum, water should be tested for microbiological content, pH, resistivity, and soluble silica,[10] and the maximum interval in the testing cycle for purity of reagent water should be 1 week. It should be noted that measurements taken at the time of production may differ from those taken at the time and place of use. For example, if the water is piped a long distance, consideration must be given to deterioration en route to the site of use. To meet the specifications for high-performance liquid chromatography (HPLC), in some instances it may be necessary to add a final 0.1-μm membrane filter. The water can be tested by HPLC using a gradient program and monitoring with an ultraviolet (UV) detector. No peaks exceeding the analytical noise of the system should be found.

Reagent Grade or Analytical Reagent Grade (AR) Chemicals

Chemicals that meet specifications of the American Chemical Society (ACS) are described as reagent or analytical reagent grade. These specifications have also become the de facto standards for chemicals used in many high-purity applications. These are available in two forms: (1) lot-analyzed reagents, in which each individual lot is analyzed and the actual amount of impurity reported, and (2) maximum impurities reagents, for which maximum impurities are listed. The Committee on Analytical Reagents of the ACS periodically publishes "Reagent Chemicals" listing specifications (http://pubs.acs.org/reagents/index.html; accessed March 16, 2011). These reagent grade chemicals are of very high purity and are recommended for quantitative or qualitative analyses.

Ultrapure Reagents

Many analytical techniques require reagents whose purity exceeds the specifications of those described previously. Manufacturers offer selected chemicals that have been especially purified to meet specific requirements. There is no uniform designation for these chemicals and organic solvents. Terms such as *spectrograde, nanograde,* and *HPLC pure* have been used. Data of interest to the user (e.g., absorbance at a specific UV wavelength) are supplied with the reagent.

Other designations of chemical purity include chemically pure (CP), USP and NF grade [chemicals produced to meet specifications set down in the U.S. Pharmacopeia (USP) or the National Formulary (NF)]. Chemicals labeled *purified, practical, technical,* or *commercial grade* should not be used in clinical chemical analysis without prior purification.

REFERENCE MATERIALS

A *reference material* is a material or substance with one or more physical or chemical properties that is sufficiently well established to be used for (1) calibrating instruments, (2) validating methods, (3) assigning values to materials, and (4) evaluating the comparability of results. Reference materials are of prime importance in establishing *metrologic transferability* (http://www.bipm.org; accessed March 16, 2011),[1,26] a term defined as "the property of a measurement result whereby the result can be related to a reference through a documented unbroken chain of calibrations, each contributing to the measurement uncertainty."[13]

Primary, secondary, standard, and certified are types of reference materials.

Primary Reference Materials

Primary reference materials are highly purified chemicals that are directly weighed or measured to produce a solution whose concentration is exactly known. The IUPAC has proposed a degree of 99.98% purity for primary reference materials. These highly purified chemicals may be weighed out directly for the preparation of solutions of selected concentration or for the calibration of solutions of unknown strength. They are supplied with a certificate of analysis for each lot.

Secondary Reference Materials

Secondary reference materials are solutions whose concentrations cannot be prepared by weighing the solute and dissolving a known amount into a volume of solution. The concentration of secondary reference materials is usually determined by analysis of an aliquot of the solution by an acceptable reference method, using a primary reference material to calibrate the method.

Standard Reference Materials (SRMs)

Standard reference materials (SRMs) for clinical and molecular laboratories are available from the National Institute of Standards and Technology (NIST; http://ts.nist.gov; accessed March 16, 2011). Cholesterol, the first SRM developed by the NIST, was issued in 1967. It should be noted that not all SRMs have the properties and the degree of purity specified for a primary standard, but each has been well characterized for certain chemical or physical properties and is issued with a certificate that gives results of the characterization. These may then be used to characterize other materials.

Examples of SRMs that are available from the NIST for use in clinical and molecular diagnostics laboratories include (1) pure crystalline standards (Table 9-5), (2) human-based standards (Table 9-6), (3) animal blood standards (Table 9-7), (4) standards containing drugs of abuse in urine and human hair (Table 9-8), and (5) SRMs used for DNA profiling/crime scene investigations (Table 9-9).

Certified Reference Materials (CRMs)

Certified reference materials (CRMs) are available for clinical and molecular laboratories from the Institute for Reference Materials and Measurements (IRMM) in Geel, Belgium (http://www.irmm.jrc.be; accessed March 16, 2011). The IRMM is one of the seven institutes of the Joint Research Centre (JRC), a Directorate-General of the European Commission (EC). Other acronyms used to label IRMM reference materials include ERM (European Reference Materials), BCR (Community Bureau of Reference of the Commission of the European Communities), and the IFCC (International Federation of Clinical Chemistry).

Examples of available IRMM standards are listed in Tables 9-10 and 9-11. Reference materials also are available from the World Health Organization (WHO; http://www.who.int/biologicals; accessed March 16, 2011).

TABLE 9-5 Standard Reference Materials (SRMs)—Pure Crystalline Standards

SRM Number	Analyte
998	Angiotensin I (human)
916a	Bilirubin
915b	Calcium Carbonate
911c	Cholesterol
921	Cortisol (hydroxycortisone)
914a	Creatinine
917b	D-Glucose (dextrose)
920	D-Mannitol
937	Iron Metal (clinical)
928	Lead Nitrate
924a	Lithium Carbonate
929a	Magnesium Gluconate Dihydrate
918b	Potassium Chloride
919b	Sodium Chloride
1595	Tripalmitin
912a	Urea
913a	Uric Acid
925	VMA (4-Hydroxy-3-Methoxy-DL-Mandelic Acid)
8327	Peptide Reference Materials (For Molecular Mass and Purity Measurements)

Available from the National Institute of Standards and Technology (www.nist.gov; accessed March 16 2011).

TABLE 9-6 Standard Reference Materials (SRMs)—Human Serum Based

SRM Number	Description
909b	Human Serum (Contains 12 Analytes)
1951b	Lipids in Frozen Human Serum
956b	Electrolytes in Frozen Human Serum
965a	Glucose in Frozen Human Serum
967	Creatinine in Frozen Human Serum
970	Ascorbic Acid in Frozen Human Serum
1952a	Cholesterol in Frozen Human Serum
968c	Fat-Soluble Vitamins in Human Serum
1589a	PCBs, Pesticides, and Dioxins/Furans in Human Serum
1599	Anticonvulsant Drug Level Assay (Valproic Acid and Carbamazepine)
900	Antiepilepsy Drug Level Assay
1955	Homocysteine and Folate in Human Serum

PCBs, Polychlorinated biphenyls.
Available from the National Institute of Standards and Technology (www.nist.gov; accessed March 16, 2011).

TABLE 9-7 Standard Reference Materials (SRMs)—Miscellaneous

SRM Number	Description
955c	Lead in Caprine (Goat) Blood
966	Toxic Elements in Bovine Blood
1598	Inorganic Constituents in Bovine Serum
927d	Bovine Serum Albumin
2921	Cardiac Troponin Complex
2389	Amino Acids in HCl
1400	Bone Ash
1486	Bone Ash

Available from the National Institute of Standards and Technology (www.nist.gov; accessed March 16, 2011).

TABLE 9-8 Standard Reference Materials (SRMs) for Drugs of Abuse in Urine and Human Hair

SRM	Description
1508 a	Cocaine Metabolite in Urine
RM 8444	Cotinine in Urine
1507b	Marijuana Metabolite in Urine
2381	Morphine and Codeine in Urine
2382	Morphine Glucuronide in Urine
1511	Multi Drugs of Abuse in Urine
2379	Drugs of Abuse in Human Hair I
2379	Drugs of Abuse in Human Hair I

Available from the National Institute of Standards and Technology (www.nist.gov; accessed March 16, 2011).

TABLE 9-9 Standard Reference Materials (SRMs) for Use in DA Profiling/Crime Scene Investigations

SRM	Description
2372	Human DNA Quantitation Standard
2390	DNA Profiling Standard—RFLP
2391b	PCR-Based DNA Profiling Standard
2392	Human Mitochondrial DNA Sequencing (3 Components)
2392-1	Human Mitochondrial DNA Sequencing (1 Component)
2394	Heteroplasmic Mitochondrial DNA Mutation Detection Standard
2395	Human Y-Chromosome DNA Profiling Standard
2396	Oxidative DNA Damage Mass Spectrometry Standard
2399	Fragile X Human DNA Triplet Repeat Standard

PCR, Polymerase chain reaction; *RFLP,* restriction fragment length polymorphism.
Available from the National Institute of Standards and Technology (www.nist.gov accessed March 16, 2011).

TABLE 9-10 Reference Materials Available from the Institute for Reference Materials and Measurements (www.irmm.jrc.be; accessed March 16, 2011)

Number	Description
BCR-304	Lyophilized Human Serum
BCR-573; 574; and 575	Creatinine in Human Serum
IRMM-468 and 469	Thyroxine (T_4) and Triiodothyronine (T_3), Two Levels Each
ERM-DA451/IFCC	Cortisol Reference Panel of Fresh Frozen Human Serum
ERM-DA192 and 193	Cortisol in Human Serum
BCR-348R and BCR-DA347	Progesterone in Human Serum
BCR-576; 577; and 578	17-β-Estradiol in Human Serum
ERM-CE-194; 195; and 196	Pb and Cd in Lyophilized Bovine Blood
BCR-634; 635; and 636	Pb and Cd in Lyophilized Human Blood
BCR-637; 638; and 639	Al, Se, and Zn in Human Serum
BCR-393	Lyophilized APO A1 from Human Serum
BCR-457	Human Thyroglobin (Tg)
BCR-486	Purified Alpha Fetoprotein (AFP)
BCR-613	Prostate Specific Antigen (PSA) in the Reconstituted Material
BCR-405	Glycated Hemoglobin (HbA1c) in Human Hemolysate
ERM-DA470k	Human Serum Proteins
ERM-DA472/IFCC	C-Reactive Protein (CRP)
BCR-522	Hemiglobincyanide (HCN) in Bovine Blood Lysate
IRMM/IFCC-466 and 467	Hemoglobin Isolated from Whole Blood
BCR-410	Prostatic Acid Phosphatase from Human Prostate
BCR-647	Human Adenosine Deaminase (ADA1) from Human Erythrocytes
BCR-693	Human Pancreatic Lipase from Pancreatic Juice
BCR-6974	Human Pancreatic Lipase (Recombinant)
ERM-AD452/IFCC	γ-Glutamyltransferase from Pig Kidney
ERM-AD453/IFCC	Human Lactate Dehydrogenase Isoenzyme 1
ERM-AD454/IFCC	Alanine Aminotransferase from Pig Heart
ERM-AD455/IFCC	Creatine Kinase (CK-MB) from Human Heart
IRMM/IFCC-456	Human Pancreatic α-Amylase
ERM-AD457/IFCC	Aspartate Transaminase (AST)

TABLE 9-11 Standards Certified for DNA Sequence Available from the Institute for Reference Materials and Measurements (www.irmm.jrc.be; accessed March 16, 2011)*

Number	Plasmid DNA
IRMM/IFCC-490	Sequence of 609 bp DNA Fragment from Human Prothrombin Gene (G20210 Wildtype Sequence)
IRMM/IFCC-491	Sequence of 609 bp DNA Fragment from Human Prothrombin Gene (Point Mutation G20210A)
IRMM/IFCC-492	Sequence of 609 bp DNA Fragment from Human Prothrombin Gene (G20210 Wildtype and Point Mutation G20210A Sequences)

*Availability: Each polypropylene vial contains approximately 1 ng plasmid DNA in a volume of 50 μL of a tris/EDTA solution.
bp, Base pairs.

BASIC TECHNIQUES AND PROCEDURES

Basic practices used in clinical and molecular diagnostic laboratories include (1) optical, (2) chromatographic, (3) electrochemical, (4) electrophoretic, (5) mass spectrometric, (6) enzymatic, and (7) immunoassay techniques. These techniques are discussed in detail in Chapters 10 through 16. Here we discuss the basic techniques of volumetric sampling and dispensing, centrifugation, measurement of radioactivity, gravimetry, thermometry, controlling hydrogen ion concentration, and processing solutions.

Volumetric Sampling and Dispensing

Clinical chemistry procedures require accurate volumetric measurements to ensure accurate results. For accurate work, only Class A glassware should be used. Class A glassware is certified to conform to the specifications outlined in NIST circular C-602.

Pipettes

Pipettes are used for the transfer of a volume of liquid from one container to another. They are designed either (1) to contain (TC) a specific volume of liquid or (2) to deliver (TD) a specified volume. Pipettes used in clinical, molecular diagnostic, and analytical laboratories include (1) manual transfer and measuring pipettes, (2) micropipettes, and (3) electronic and mechanical pipetting devices. Developments in improved design of pipetting systems include robotic automation, the capability to provide electronic and personal computer (PC) control of pipetting devices, and careful attention to advanced ergonomic design features. Automatic photometric pipette calibration systems are also available that reduce the time needed to periodically check pipettes and potentially allow more efficient use of personnel.

Transfer and Measuring Pipettes

A transfer pipette is designed to transfer a known volume of liquid. Measuring and serologic pipettes are scored in units such that any volume up to a maximum capacity is delivered.

Transfer Pipettes. *Transfer pipettes* include both volumetric and Ostwald-Folin pipettes (Figure 9-1). They consist of a cylindrical bulb joined at both ends to narrower glass tubing. A calibration mark is etched around the upper suction tube, and the lower delivery tube is drawn out to a gradual taper. The bore of the delivery orifice should be sufficiently narrow to allow rapid outflow of liquid and incomplete drainage cannot cause measurement errors beyond tolerances specified.

A volumetric transfer pipette (Figure 9-1, *A*) is calibrated to deliver accurately a fixed volume of a dilute aqueous solution. The reliability of the calibration of the volumetric pipette decreases with decreased size, and therefore special micropipettes have been developed.

Ostwald-Folin pipettes (Figure 9-1, *B*) are similar to volumetric pipettes but have the bulb closer to the delivery tip and are used for accurate measurement of viscous fluids, such as blood or serum. In contrast to a volumetric pipette, an Ostwald-Folin pipette has an etched ring near the mouthpiece, indicating that it is a blow-out pipette. With the use of a pipetting bulb, the liquid is blown out of the pipette only after the blood or serum has drained to the last drop in the delivery tip. When filled with opaque fluids, such as blood, the top of the meniscus must be read. Controlled slow drainage is required with all viscous solutions so that no residual film is left on the walls of the pipette.

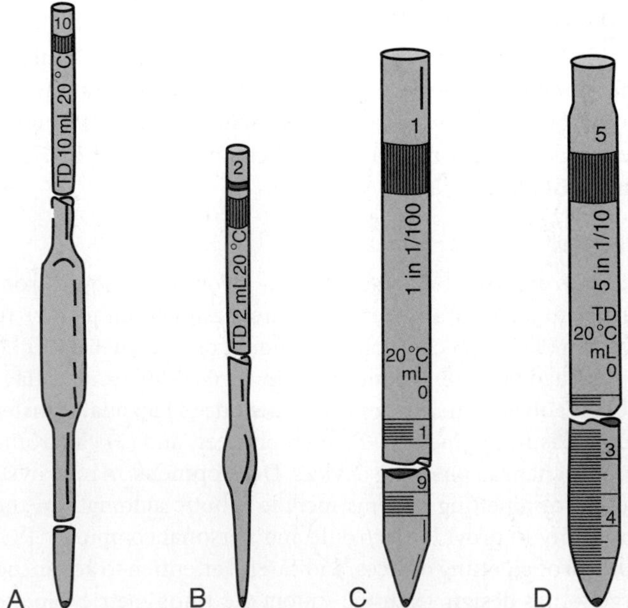

Figure 9-1 Pipettes. A, Volumetric (transfer). B, Ostwald-Folin (transfer). C, Mohr (measuring). D, Serologic (graduated to the tip).

Measuring Pipettes. The second principal type of pipette is the *graduated* or *measuring pipette* (Figure 9-1, *C*). This is a piece of glass tubing that is drawn out to a tip and graduated uniformly along its length. Two types are available. The Mohr pipette is calibrated between two marks on the stem, whereas the serologic pipette has graduated marks down to the tip. The serologic pipette (Figure 9-1, *D*) must be blown out to deliver the entire volume of the pipette and has an etched ring (or pair of rings) near the bulb end of the pipette signifying that it is a blow-out pipette. Mohr pipettes require controlled delivery of the solution between the calibration marks. Serologic pipettes have a larger orifice than do Mohr pipettes and thus drain faster. In practice, measuring pipettes are used principally for measurement of reagents and generally are not considered sufficiently accurate for measuring samples and calibrators.

Pipetting Technique

There are general pipetting techniques that apply to the pipettes described previously. For example, pipetting bulbs should always be used, and pipettes must be held in a vertical position when the liquid level is adjusted to the calibration line and during delivery. The lowest part of the meniscus, when it is sighted at eye level, should be level with the calibration line on the pipette. The flow of liquid should be unrestricted when volumetric pipettes are used, and the tips should be touched to the inclined surface of the receiving container for 2 seconds after the liquid has ceased to flow.

With graduated pipettes, the flow of liquid may have to be slowed during delivery. Serologic pipettes are calibrated to the tip, and the etched glass ring on top of the pipette signifies that it is to be blown out. First, the pipette is allowed to drain, and then the remaining liquid is blown out.

Micropipettes

Micropipettes are pipettes used for the measurement of microliter volumes. With such devices, the remaining volume that coats the inner wall of a pipette causes notable error. For this reason, most micropipettes are calibrated to contain (TC) the stated volume rather than to deliver it (TD). Proper use requires rinsing the pipette with the final solution after the contents are delivered into the diluent. Volumes are expressed in microliters (μL); the older term *lambda* is no longer recommended. Micropipettes generally are available in small sizes, ranging from 1 to 500 μL. Also, they are available for volumes as low as 0.2 μL.

Semiautomatic and Automatic Pipettes and Dispensers. Figure 9-2, *A* and *B*, illustrates two types of adjustable micropipetting devices that demonstrate unique ergonomic design features. These devices are programmable and are used for simultaneously dispensing aliquots of liquid into multiple wells. In practice, with the use of disposable plastic tips, they allow simultaneous aspiration and delivery of solutions to multiple sample micro wells. Each channel is piston driven to allow the user to pipette with as few or as many tips as necessary. Aliquots of liquid as small as 0.2 μL are dispensed at three different aspiration or dispense rates.

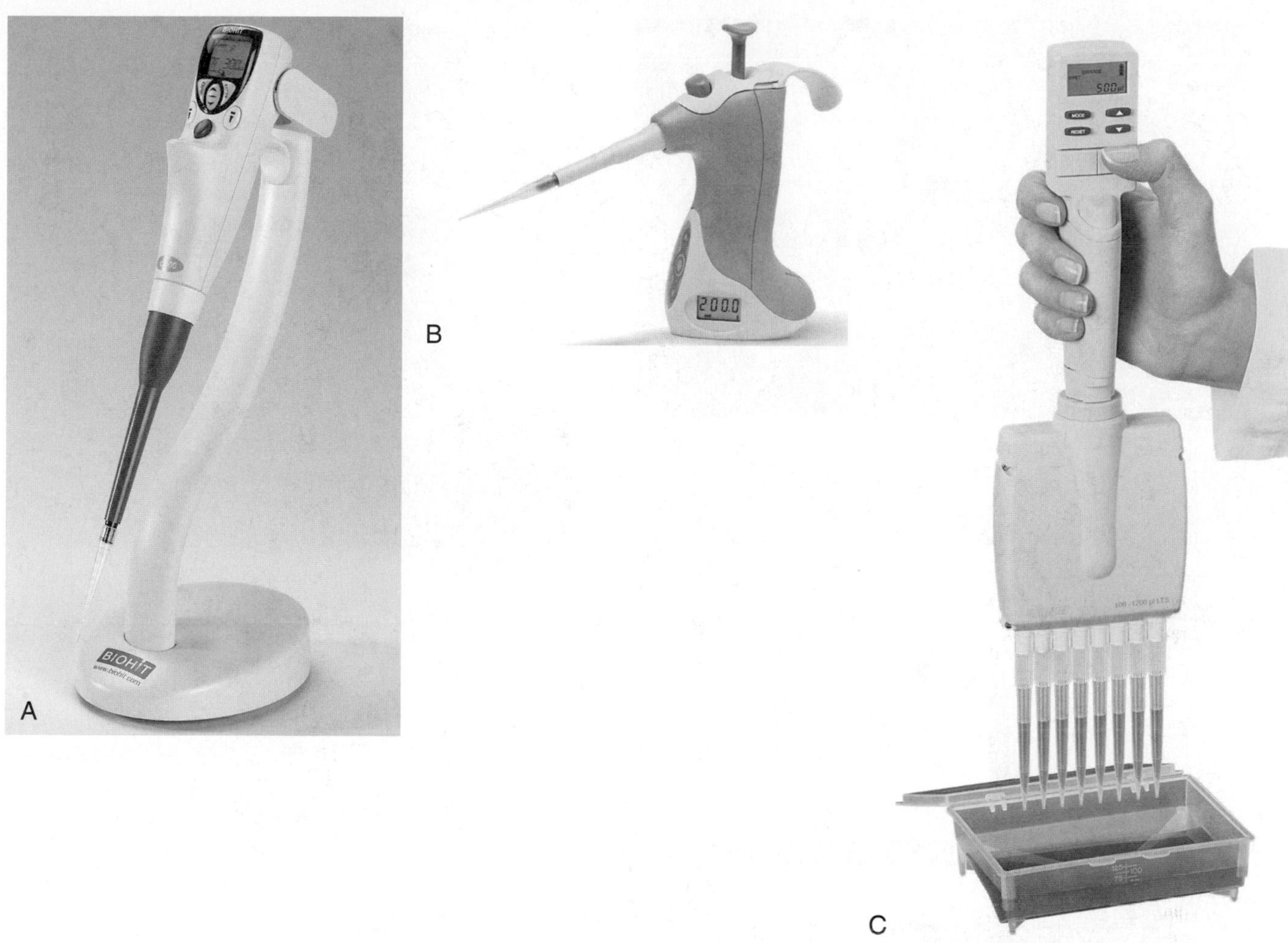

Figure 9-2 A, Adjustable volume micropipetting device with ergonomic design. B, Adjustable volume electronic micropipetting device with ergonomic design. C, Electronic programmable multichannel pipette. *(A, Courtesy Biohit Plc. **B,** Courtesy VistaLab Technologies, Inc. **C,** Courtesy Rainin Instrument LLC.)*

Semiautomatic manual and electronic versions of pipettes and dispensers are available in sizes ranging from 0.5 μL to 10 mL. Figure 9-2, *C,* illustrates an electronically operated, positive-displacement multichannel pipettor. This device aspirates and dispenses its predefined volumes (from 0.5 to 200 μL) when its plunger is moved through a complete cycle. Its disposable, fluid containment tips are made of a plastic material that tends to retain less inner surface film than does glass. Such pipettes (1) avoid the risk of cross-contamination among samples, (2) eliminate the necessity for washing between samples, and (3) improve the precision of measurements. Models that allow for digital adjustment of the volume aspirated and dispensed are available.

Figure 9-3, *A,* shows an automatic dispensing apparatus that aspirates and dispenses preset volumes of two different liquids by means of two motor-driven syringes, one for metering a volume of the sample and one for metering a volume of the diluent. It is possible to adjust this device to aspirate as little as 1 μL of one liquid and to deliver it with as much as 999 μL of the other. This type of device, available as a dilutor or dispenser, is obtainable as a manual, electronic, or computer-controlled device. The device is microprocessor controlled and is easily programmed. Twenty-one dispensing programs are stored in memory and retrieved. This type of liquid dispensing device is also obtainable as a computer-controlled system.

A more versatile piece of equipment is the robotic liquid handling workstation shown in Figure 9-3, *B.* This automated pipetting station is used with individual reaction tubes and also with 96- and 384-well microtiter plates. Depending on the design of the system, a single probe or multiple probes may be used to rapidly transfer programmed volumes of solution from one container to microtiter plates (e.g., so that the transfer to all 96 wells is complete in 1 minute). In some systems, liquid sensing is incorporated into the sample probes to minimize contact with sample and reagents even though automatic washing of the probes is performed between specimens. Two-dimensional (X-Y) movement of probes and tubes or microtiter plates is built into the pipetting stations to minimize the necessity for operator intervention. This

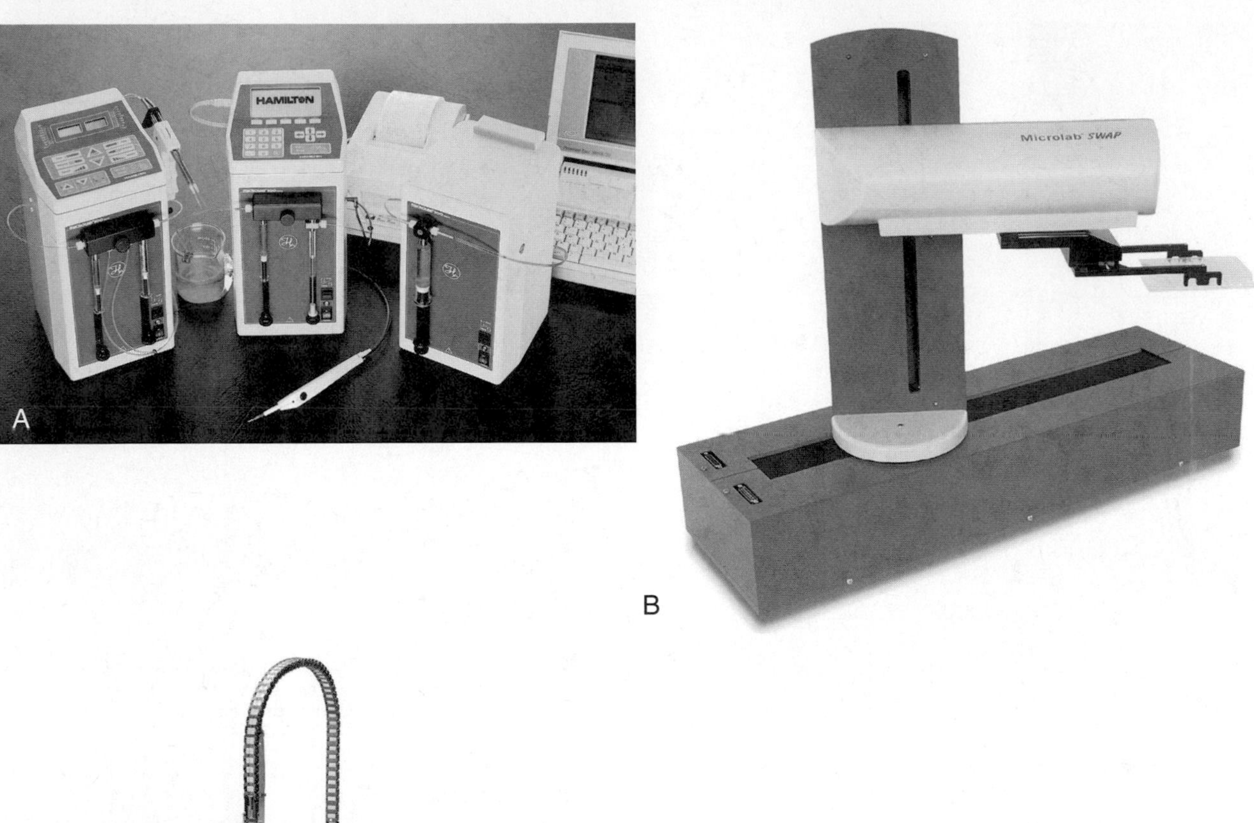

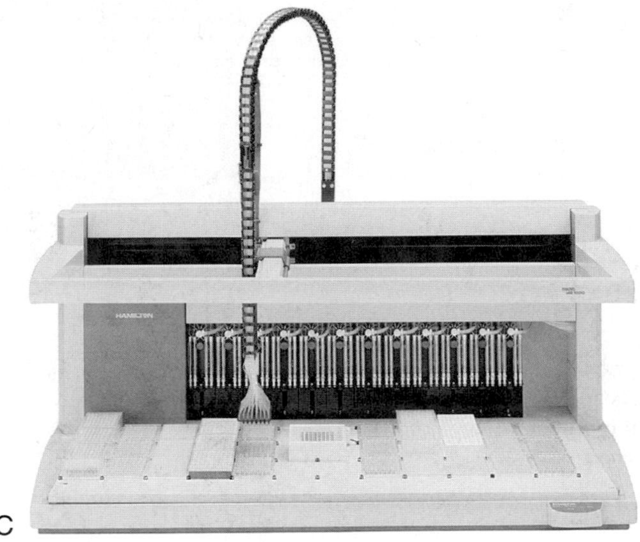

Figure 9-3 A, Personal computer (PC)-controlled diluting and/or dispensing apparatus that aspirates and dispenses preset volumes of one or two different liquids, such as a diluent and sample, by means of motor-driven syringes. B and C, Robotic liquid handling workstations. *(A and B, Courtesy Hamilton Co.)*

device dispenses programmed volumes from 0.5 to 1000 μL in serial dilutions from 4 to 16 channels employing an auto-loaded system with barcodes for positive identification.

Volumetric Flasks

Volumetric flasks (Figure 9-4) are used to measure exact volumes; they are commonly found in sizes varying from 1 to 4000 mL. In practice, they are used primarily in preparing solutions of known concentration, and they are available in various grades. The most accurate are certified as meeting standards set forth by the NIST.

An important factor in the use of a volumetric apparatus is the requirement for an accurate adjustment of the meniscus. A small piece of card that is half black and half white is most useful. The card is placed 1 cm behind the apparatus with the white half uppermost and the top of the black area about 1 mm below the meniscus. The meniscus then appears as a clearly defined, thin black line. This device also is useful in reading the meniscus of a burette.

Volumetric equipment should be used with solutions equilibrated to room temperature. Solutions diluted in volumetric flasks should be repeatedly mixed during dilution so that the contents are homogeneous before the solution is made up to final volume. Errors caused by expansion or contraction of liquids on mixing are thereby minimized.

Volumetric flasks should be thoroughly cleaned and dried before calibration. The flask is then weighed and filled with carbon dioxide–free deionized water until just above the

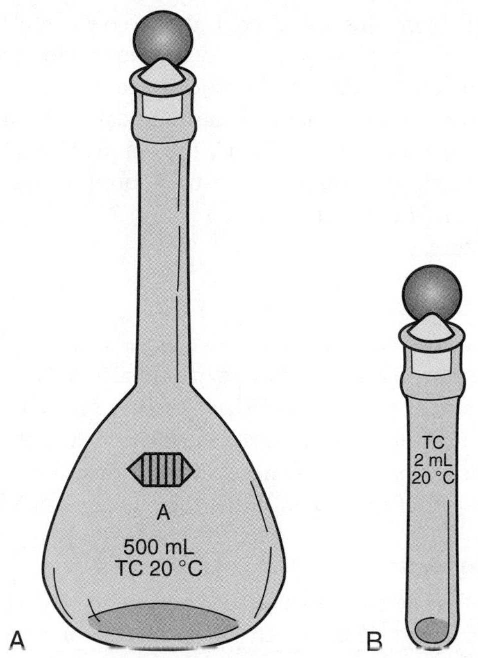

Figure 9-4 Volumetric flasks. A, Macro. B, Micro.

graduation mark. The neck of the flask just above the water level should be kept free of water. The meniscus mark is set at the graduation line by removing excess water, and the flask is reweighed. The final weight is corrected for the equilibrated water and air temperature to obtain the volume of the flask. Flasks also may be calibrated by the spectrophotometric technique described in the next section.

CENTRIFUGATION

Centrifugation is the process of using centrifugal force to separate the lighter portions of a solution, mixture, or suspension from the heavier portions. A *centrifuge* is a device by which centrifugation is effected.

In the clinical laboratory, centrifugation is used to

1. Remove cellular elements from blood to provide cell-free plasma or serum for analysis (see Chapter 7).
2. Concentrate cellular elements and other components of biological fluids for microscopic examination or chemical analysis.
3. Remove chemically precipitated protein from an analytical specimen.
4. Separate protein-bound or antibody-bound ligand from free ligand in immunochemical and other assays (see Chapter 16).
5. Extract solutes in biological fluids from aqueous to organic solvents.
6. Separate lipid components such as chylomicrons from other components of plasma or serum, and lipoproteins from one another (see Chapter 27).

Types of Centrifuges

Several types of centrifuges are used in the clinical laboratory including (1) horizontal-head, (2) swinging-bucket, (3) fixed-angle head, (4) angle-head, (5) ultracentrifuge, and (6) axial units. In addition, the development of automatic balancing centrifuges has enabled centrifugation to be incorporated as an integral step in the total automation of laboratory testing (see Chapter 19).

Principles of Centrifugation

The correct term to describe the force required to separate two phases in a centrifuge is *relative centrifugal force (RCF)*. Units are expressed as number of times greater than gravity (e.g., 500 ×g).

RCF is calculated as follows:

$$RCF = 1.118 \times 10^{-5} \times r \times rpm^2$$

where

1.118×10^{-5} is an empirical factor

r = radius in centimeters from the center of rotation to the bottom of the tube in the rotor cavity or bucket during centrifugation

rpm = the speed of rotation of the rotor in revolutions per minute

The RCF of a centrifuge may also be determined from a nomogram distributed by manufacturers of centrifuges. RCF is derived from the distance from the rotor center to the bottom of the tube, whether the tube is horizontal to, or at an angle to, the rotor center.

The time required to sediment particles depends on the (1) rotor speed, (2) radius of the rotor, and (3) effective path length traveled by the sedimented particles, that is, the depth of the liquid in the tube. Duplication of conditions of centrifugation is often desirable. The following is a useful formula for calculating the speed required of a rotor whose radius differs from the radius with which a prescribed RCF was originally defined:

$$\text{rpm (alternate rotor)} = 1000 \times \sqrt{\frac{RCF,\ original\ rotor}{11.18 \times r(cm),\ alternate\ rotor}}$$

The length of time for centrifugation is calculated so that running with an alternate rotor of a different size is equivalent to running with the original rotor:

$$\text{time (alternate rotor)} = \frac{\text{time} \times RCF\ \text{(original rotor)}}{\text{RCF (alternate rotor)}}$$

Note, however, that it may not be possible to reproduce conditions exactly when a different centrifuge is used. Descriptions of times of centrifugation include the time for the rotor to reach operating speed (which may vary from instrument to instrument) and do not include deceleration time, during which sedimentation is still occurring but less efficiently. Even with maximal braking, deceleration may take as long as 3 minutes in some centrifuges.

Operation of the Centrifuge

For proper operation of a centrifuge, only those tubes recommended by their manufacturer should be used. The material used for the tube must withstand the RCF to which the tube is likely to be subjected. Polypropylene tubes generally are capable of withstanding RCFs of up to 5000 ×g. The tubes should have a tapered bottom, particularly if a supernatant is to be removed, and should be of a size to fit securely into the rack to be centrifuged. The top of the tube should not protrude so far above the bucket that the swing into a horizontal position is impeded by the rotor.

For smooth operation of the centrifuge, the rotor must be properly balanced. The weight of racks, tubes, and their contents on opposite sides of a rotor should not differ by more than 1% or by an acceptable limit established by the manufacturer. Centrifuges that automatically balance their rotors are now available.

Tubes of collected blood should be centrifuged before they are unstoppered to reduce the probability of an aerosol being produced when the tube is opened. The practice of using a wooden applicator to release a clot stuck to the top of the tube or to its stopper should be avoided; it is a potential cause of hemolysis. Centrifugation at an appropriate RCF usually ensures that the clot is released from the tube wall and is drawn to the bottom of the tube.

Despite years of experience with centrifuges, just a few specific recommendations can be made for RCF or time for centrifugation of blood specimens. For example, CLSI standard H18-A4[5] proposes an RCF of 1000 to 1200 ×g for 10 ± 5 minutes. Standards have not been established for centrifugation of other specimens, such as serum to which a protein precipitant has been added.

Operating Practice

Cleanliness of a centrifuge is important in minimizing the possible spread of infectious agents, such as hepatitis viruses. With proper operation of a centrifuge, few tubes break. In case of breakage, the racks and chamber of the centrifuge must be carefully cleaned. Any spillage should be considered a possible bloodborne pathogen hazard. Gray dust arising from sandblasting of the chamber by fragments of glass indicates tube breakage and possible contamination, necessitating cleaning of the chamber. Broken glass embedded in cushions of tube holders may be a continuing cause of breakage if cushions are not inspected and replaced as part of the cleanup procedure.

The speed of a centrifuge should be checked at least once every 3 months. The measured speed should not differ by more than 5% from the rated speed under specified conditions. All the speeds at which the centrifuge is commonly operated should be checked. The centrifuge timer should be checked weekly against a reference timer (such as a stopwatch) and should not be more than 10% in error. Commutators and brushes should be checked at least every 3 months. Brushes (where used) should be replaced when they show considerable wear. However, in many modern induction-driven motors, brushes have been eliminated, thus removing a source of dust that causes motor failure.

Because centrifuges generate heat, the temperature in the chamber in many centrifuge models may increase by as much as 5 °C after a single run. When the material to be centrifuged has a labile temperature, a refrigerated centrifuge should be used. In the simplest form, a refrigerator unit is mounted beside the centrifuge, and cold air is blown into the rotor chamber. This approach is usually inadequate to stabilize the low temperature. In more sophisticated centrifuges, refrigeration coils around the chamber make it possible to maintain a preset temperature within ±1 °C. The temperature of a refrigerated centrifuge should be measured monthly under reproducible conditions and should be within 2 °C of the expected temperature.

Measurement of Radioactivity

The rapid acceptance and extensive use of nonisotopic immunoassays by the clinical laboratory have resulted in decreased use of radioimmunoassays (RIAs) and ultimately a decreased requirement for their use in measuring radioactivity. Because of this deemphasis on the necessity of measuring radioactivity, only a brief discussion of the topic is presented here.

Basic Concepts

An *atom* is the smallest unit of an element having the properties of that element. An individual atom consists of a positively charged nucleus around which revolve negatively charged electrons. The *nucleus* is composed of positively charged protons and neutral neutrons. The *atomic number* (Z) of an element is the number of protons in its nucleus; the total number of nucleons and protons plus neutrons is its *mass number* (A). A *nuclide* is an atomic species with a given atomic number and a given mass number. *Isotopes* are nuclides with the same atomic number but different mass numbers. These represent various nuclear species of the same element. Radionuclides of clinical interest are listed in Table 9-12.

Radioactive Decay

Radioactive decay is a property of the atomic nucleus that provides evidence of nuclear instability. The rate of decay is unaffected by temperature, pressure, concentration, or any other chemical or physical condition, but is a characteristic of each individual radionuclide.

Alpha Decay. To achieve stable configurations, heavy elements, particularly those with atomic numbers above 70, may shed some of their nuclear mass by emitting a two-proton, two-neutron fragment identifiable after emission as a helium nucleus. Because nuclear radiations were observed before their identity was known, this fragment was called an *alpha* (α-) *particle,* and its emission is termed α-*decay.* Alpha particles are relatively large in mass and interact strongly with matter but are absorbed by as little as a sheet of paper. However, because they are so heavy, even with low velocity, their momentum is high. Consequently, they do not travel far, but when they collide with other molecules, they do a lot of damage; therefore α-emitters are considered to be very hazardous.

Beta Decay. For some heavy nuclides and for almost all those with atomic numbers below 60, stability is achieved by a rearrangement of the nucleus in which the total number of nucleons is unchanged. In terms of the neutron-proton model of the nucleus, this rearrangement is the conversion of a neutron to a proton or vice versa. During such conversions,

TABLE 9-12 Radiation Properties of Some Radionuclides Used in the Clinical Laboratory

			Maximum Energy of Radiation (MeV)†	
Nuclides	**Half-life**	**Decay Type***	**Beta**	**Gamma**
^{3}H	12.3 y	β^-	0.186	None
^{14}C	5730 y	β^-	0.155	None
^{32}P	14.3 d	β^-	1.71	None
^{35}S	87 d	β^-	0.167	None
^{51}Cr	27.7 d	EC	None	0.320
^{57}Co	272 d	EC	None	0.122, 0.136, 0.014
^{58}Co	71 d	EC, β^-	0.474	0.811, annihilation photons only
^{59}Fe	45 d	β^-	0.475, 0.273	1.10, 1.29
^{99}Mo	66 h	β^-	1.21, 0.450	0.740, 0.181, 0.778
^{99m}Tc	6.0 h	IT	None	0.141
^{125}I	60 d	EC	None	0.035
^{131}I	8.04 d	β^-	0.607, 0.336	0.364, 0.637, 0.284

*β^-, β^+, EC, and IT refer to β-decay, positron decay, electron capture, and isomeric transition, respectively. Where nuclides are known to have more than one mode of decay, they are listed in the order of their prevalence.

†Energies are given only for the more prevalent β- and γ-radiations and are in approximate order of prevalence. Electron capture (EC) decay also yields the characteristic x-rays of the daughter; the energies of the x-rays are not included in this listing. As noted in the gamma column, positron decay (β^+) is accompanied by annihilation radiation, which consists principally of a pair of 0.511 MeV photons.

the nucleus emits either a negative electron or its positive equivalent, a *positron.* Emission of the negative electron, named the *beta* (β-) *particle,* is what is usually meant by the term *β-decay.*

Emission of a negative β-particle leaves the nucleus with one additional positive charge, a neutron is converted to a proton, and the nucleus assumes the next higher atomic number. Negative β-emission is characteristic of a nucleus that has more neutrons than required by its protons for stability. For example, tritium (^{3}H) is an unstable isotope of hydrogen, consisting of a proton, an electron, and two neutrons. When an atom of tritium decays, one of the neutrons is converted to a proton, one β-particle and one neutrino are released, and a helium isotope (^{3}He) remains. Tritium is called a "soft" β-emitter because its β-particles have relatively low velocities. A hard β-emitter, such as *phosphorus* 32 (^{32}P), is more hazardous because its β-particles carry more kinetic energy; however, it is easier to detect.

Other examples of nuclides that decay by negative β-emission are carbon-14 (^{14}C), iron-59 (^{59}Fe), and iodine-131 (^{131}I). Negatively charged β-particles are smaller in mass and interact less with matter than β-particles and easily penetrate paper and cardboard, but they are absorbed by metal sheets.

Electron Capture. An alternative decay process to the emission of positive β-particles is the capture of an electron. In this process, an orbital electron is "absorbed" by the nucleus. The end effect on nuclear structure is the same; a proton appears to have changed into a neutron, the atomic number decreases by one, and the atomic mass remains the same. For example, ^{125}I decays exclusively by electron capture to tellurium-125.

Gamma Radiation and Internal Conversion. Gamma radiation is high-energy electromagnetic radiation that resembles x-rays. An example of a γ-emitter is ^{131}I. Because γ-rays are high-energy photons, their penetrating power is very high and more difficult to shield.

Activity and Half-life

The rate of decay of a radioactive source is called its *activity* and is simply the rate at which radioactive parent atoms decay to more stable daughter atoms. In practice, it is often convenient to describe the rate of decay in terms of *half-life* ($t_{1/2}$), the time required for a nuclide's activity to decrease to half its initial value:

$$t_{1/2} = \frac{\ln 2}{\lambda} = \frac{0.693}{\lambda}$$

where λ is the decay constant characteristic of a given nuclide.

This equation is useful in planning experiments and in disposing of radioactive waste. For disposal, a rule of thumb is that a decay time of seven half-lives reduces the activity to less than 1% of its original value ($2^{-7} = 1/128 = 0.78\%$), and after 10 half-lives, to less than 0.1%.

Units of Radioactivity

The *becquerel* (Bq) is the SI unit of radioactivity and is defined as one decay per second (dps). Because 1 Bq is a very small amount of activity, the activity of typical chemistry samples is often expressed in kilobecquerels (kBq). The *curie* (Ci) is the older, *conventional unit;* it is defined as 3.7×10^{10} dps. One curie equals 37 gigabecquerels (GBq). Because the becquerel is inconveniently small and the curie very large, they are typically used as their multiples or submultiples, for example, megabecquerels (MBq) and millicuries (mCi). One mCi equals 37 MBq.

Specific Activity

The term *specific activity* has several meanings. It may refer to (1) radioactivity per unit mass of an element, (2) radioactivity per mass of labeled compound, or (3) radioactivity per unit volume of a solution. The denominator of reference must be specified. In terms of radioactivity per unit mass, the maximum specific activity attainable for each radionuclide is that for the pure radionuclide. For example, pure ^{14}C has a specific activity of 62 Ci/mol or 4400 Ci/kg. As usually available, ^{14}C is a tracer for compounds in which it represents only a small fraction of the total carbon, most of which is the naturally occurring mixture of stable ^{12}C and stable ^{13}C. If no stable element is present, the radionuclide is said to be *carrier free*.

Detection and Measurement of Radioactivity

Autoradiography, gas ionization, and fluorescent scintillation serve as the basis for techniques used to detect and measure radioactivity in the clinical laboratory.

Autoradiography

In *autoradiography*, a photographic emulsion is used to visualize molecules labeled with a radioactive element. For example, this technique is used to visualize nucleic acids and fragments that have been hybridized with nucleic acid probes labeled with ^{32}P (see Chapter 17). With such techniques, nucleic acid probes labeled with radioactive ^{32}P are incubated with target nucleic acid. After hybridization, hydrolysis, and separation of fragments by gel electrophoresis, a photographic film is applied to the covered gel and is allowed to incubate. Alternatively, the nucleic acid fragments are transferred to a nylon membrane, and the photographic film is applied to the membrane. With either approach, the film is developed with the resulting image reflecting the radioactivity of the target nucleic acid fragments.

Gas-Filled Detectors

Detectors filled with certain gases or gas mixtures are designed to capture and measure ions produced by radiation within the detector. Gas-filled detectors used to measure radioactivity include the (1) ionization chamber, (2) proportional counter, and (3) Geiger counter. In the clinical chemistry laboratory, the Geiger counter is used as a portable radiation monitor.

Scintillation Counting

In the scintillation process, absorption of radiation produces a flash of light. The principal types of scintillation detectors found in the clinical chemistry laboratory are the sodium iodide *crystal scintillation detector* and the *organic liquid scintillation detector*. Because of the crystal detector's relative ease of operation and economy of sample preparation, most clinical laboratory procedures have been developed to measure nuclides, such as ^{125}I, which is counted efficiently in a crystal detector. A liquid scintillation detector is used to measure pure β-emitters, such as tritium or ^{14}C.

Crystal Scintillation Detector. The *well detector* (often referred to as a γ-counter) is a common type of crystal scintillation detector and has a hole drilled in the end or side of the cylindrical crystal to accept a test tube. Because it is hygroscopic, the crystal is hermetically sealed in an aluminum can with a transparent quartz window at one end through which blue-violet (420 nm) scintillations are detected. The photons of gamma emitters, such as ^{51}Cr, ^{57}Co, ^{59}Fe, ^{125}I, and ^{131}I (see Table 9-8) in the sample, easily penetrate the specimen tube and the thin, low-density can, and enter the crystal where they are likely to be absorbed in the thick, high-density sodium iodide. A well counter is not suitable for measuring β-radiation because such radiation does not penetrate the sample container and the aluminum lining of the wall.

Liquid Scintillation Detector. This detector measures radioactivity by recording scintillations occurring within a transparent vial that contains the unknown sample and liquid scintillator. Because the radionuclide is intimately mixed with, or actually dissolved in, the liquid scintillator, the technique is ideal for the pure β-emitters, such as ^{3}H, ^{14}C, and ^{32}P. Typical efficiencies for liquid scintillation counting in the absence of significant quenching are 60% for tritium and 90% for ^{14}C.

The liquid scintillator is known as the *scintillation cocktail* and contains at least two components (the primary solvent and the primary scintillator). The *primary solvent* is usually one of the aromatic hydrocarbons such as toluene, xylene, or pseudocumene (1,2,4-trimethyl benzene). The *primary scintillator* absorbs energy from the primary solvent and converts it into light. The usual material is 2,5-diphenyloxazole (PPO) used in a concentration of 3 to 6 g/L. PPO emits ultraviolet light of 380 nm. In addition, other components added to the liquid scintillator include (1) a *secondary solvent* to improve the solubility of aqueous samples; (2) a surfactant to stabilize or emulsify the sample; (3) a *secondary scintillator*, sometimes referred to as a wavelength shifter, to absorb the ultraviolet photons of the primary scintillator and reemit the energy at a longer wavelength, which facilitates the response of some photomultiplier tubes; and (4) one or more *adjuvants*, such as suspension agents, solubilizers for biological tissue, and antifreezes, to prevent freezing and separation of water at low temperatures.

Description of other components of a scintillation counter and discussion of relevant topics are found in an earlier edition of this textbook.[23]

GRAVIMETRY

Mass is an invariant property of matter. Gravimetry is the process used to measure the mass of a substance. Weight is a function of mass under the influence of gravity, a relationship expressed by the relationship

$$\text{Weight} = \text{Mass} \times \text{Gravity}$$

Two substances of equal weight and subject to the same gravitational force have equal mass. Mass is determined using a balance to compare the mass of an unknown with that of a known mass. This comparison is called *weighing,* and the absolute standards with which masses are compared are called *weights.* In practice, the terms *mass* and *weight* are used synonymously.

The classic form of a *balance* is a beam poised on an agate knife-edge fulcrum, with a pan hanging from each end of the beam and a rigid pointer hanging from the beam at the poised point. With the object to be weighed on one pan and weights of equal mass on the other pan, the pointer comes to rest at an equilibrium or balance point between the extremes of the path of excursion. The weight required to achieve the equilibrium is therefore equal to the weight of the substance being weighed.

Principles of Weighing

In practice, one of two modes of weighing is used: (1) analytical weights are added to equal the weight of the object being weighed, or (2) the material to be weighed is added to a balance pan to achieve equilibrium with a preset weight. This second mode is used more commonly in clinical laboratories, where the major necessity is to weigh a fixed quantity of chemical so that a calibrator or reagent solution of known concentration may be prepared. Before a sample of the chemical is weighed, the weight of the container must be determined to subsequently allow for deducting the weight of the container from the gross weight of the container plus sample to obtain the net weight of the sample. This is called "taring." When taring is impractical, the weight of the empty container must be subtracted from the combined weight of the container and the material to obtain the weight of the material alone.

Types of Balances

Double- and single-pan and electronic balances are frequently used in the clinical laboratory.

Double-Pan Balance

A double-pan balance conforms to the classic design, consisting of a single beam with arms of equal length. Standard weights are usually added by hand to the right-side pan to counterbalance the weight of the object on the other, but in some models, a dial or vernier with chain is used to make fine adjustments to the mass associated with the right-side pan. In *single-pan* balances, the arms are of unequal length. The object to be weighed is placed on the pan attached to the shorter arm. A restoring force is applied mechanically or electronically to the other arm to return the beam to its null position. Double- and triple-beam balances are forms of the unequal-arm balance.

Single-Pan Balance

The single-pan balance is a commonly used balance in the clinical laboratory. It is most often electronically operated and self-balancing. Such a balance may be coupled directly to a computer or recording device. In the electronic single-pan balance, a load on the pan causes the beam to tilt downward. A null detector senses the position of the beam and indicates when the beam has deviated from the equilibrium point.

Electronic Balance

In an electronic balance, an electromagnetic force is applied to return the balance beam to its null position. This force is proportional to the weight on the pan. Most electronic balances have a built-in provision for taring so that the mass of the container is subtracted easily from the total mass measured. In addition, in many modern balances, a built-in computer compensates for changes in temperature and provides both automatic zero tracking and calibration.

Analytical Weights

Analytical weights are used to counterbalance the weight of objects weighed on two-pan balances and to verify the performance of both single- and two-pan balances. The NIST recognizes five classes of analytical weights. Class S weights are used for calibrating balances. In the clinical laboratory, balances should be calibrated at least monthly and before very accurate analytical work is conducted. These weights are typically made from brass or stainless steel and are lacquered or plated for protection. The fractional weights of a set of class S standards are usually made of platinum or aluminum. Tolerances of the different weights have been defined by the NIST. For class S weights from 1 to 5 g, the tolerance is ±0.054 mg, from 100 to 500 mg it is ±0.025 mg, and from 1 to 50 mg it is ±0.014 mg.

Thermometry

In the clinical chemistry laboratory, measurements of temperature are made primarily to verify that devices measure within their prescribed temperature limits. Water baths and heated cells where reactions take place are examples of such devices, as are refrigerators, whose temperatures must be measured and recorded daily to meet laboratory regulatory requirements.

The two most popular types of thermometers in the chemistry laboratory are liquid-in-glass thermometers and thermistor probes.

All thermometers must be verified against a certified thermometer before they are placed into use. For example, the NIST SRM 934 is a mercury-in-glass thermometer with calibration points at 0 °C, 25 °C, 30 °C, and 37 °C. Some manufacturers supply liquid-in-glass thermometers that have ranges greater than the SRM thermometer and are verified to have been calibrated against the NIST thermometers. Details of verification of the calibration of a thermometer have been described.[9] The NIST also supplies several materials that melt at a known temperature, including gallium (SRM 1968), which melts at 29.7723 °C, and rubidium (SRM 1969), which melts at 39.3 °C.

Controlling Hydrogen Ion Concentration

In the laboratory, hydrogen ion concentration is controlled with buffers. *Buffers* are defined as substances that resist changes in the pH of a system. All weak acids or bases, in the presence of their salts, form buffer systems. The actions of buffers and their role in maintaining the pH of a solution are explained with the aid of the Henderson-Hasselbalch equation, which is derived as follows.

Chemically, the ionization of a weak acid, HA, and of a salt of that acid, BA, is represented as follows:

$$HA \rightleftarrows H^+ + A^-$$

$$BA \rightleftarrows B^+ + A^-$$

The dissociation constant for a weak acid (K_a) may be calculated from the following equation:

$$K_a = \frac{[H^+][A^-]}{[HA]}$$

Thus

$$[H^+] = K_a \times \frac{[HA]}{[A^-]}$$

or

$$\log[H^+] = \log K_a + \log\frac{[HA]}{[A^-]}$$

where brackets indicate the concentration of the compound contained within. Now multiplying throughout by −1, we obtain

$$-\log[H^+] = -\log K_a - \log\frac{[HA]}{[A^-]}$$

By definition, pH = −log[H] and $pK_a = -\log K_a$, therefore

$$pH = pK_a + \log\frac{[A^-]}{[HA]}$$

This equation is known as the Henderson-Hasselbalch equation. Because A^- is derived principally from the salt, the equation is also written as

$$pH = pK_a + \log\frac{[salt]}{[undissociated\ acid]}$$

or simply as

$$pH = pK_a + \log\frac{[salt]}{[acid]}$$

where [salt] = $[A^{-1}]$ = concentration of dissociated salt and [acid] = [HA] = concentration of undissociated acid.

This derivation demonstrates that the pH of the system is determined by the pK_a of the acid and the ratio of $[A^{-1}]$ to [HA]. The buffer has its greatest buffer capacity at its pK_a [the pH at which the (A^{-1}) = (HA)].

The capacity of the buffer decreases as the ratio deviates from 1. In general, buffers should not be used at a pH greater than 1 unit from their pK_a. If the ratio is beyond 50/1 or 1/50, the system is considered to have lost its buffering capacity. This point is approximately 1.7 pH units to either side of the pK_a of the acid

$$pH = pK_a \pm 1.7$$

Procedures for Processing Solutions

Several procedures are used routinely to process solutions in the clinical laboratory, including those used for diluting, concentrating, and filtering solutions.

Dilution

Dilution is the process by which the concentration or activity of a given solution is decreased by the addition of solvent. In laboratory practice, most dilutions are made by transferring an exact volume of a concentrated solution into an appropriate flask and then adding water or other diluent to the required volume, with appropriate mixing to ensure homogeneity. A serial dilution is a sequential set of dilutions in mathematical sequence. A given dilution is expressed as the amount, either volume or weight, of a solute (analyte) in a specified volume. For example, a 1:5 volume-to-volume (vol/vol) dilution contains one volume in a total of five volumes (one volume plus four volumes).

To prevent errors that arise when two liquids of very different composition are mixed, the technique of diluting to volume is used. Instead of adding 90 mL of water to 10 mL of concentrated solution, the 10 mL of concentrated solution should be pipetted into a 100-mL volumetric flask. Water is added to bring the volume to the 100-mL mark on the neck of the flask.

When a dilution is performed, the following equation is used to determine the volume (V_2) necessary to dilute a given volume (V_1) of solution of a known concentration (C_1) to the desired lesser concentration (C_2):

$$C_1 \times V_1 = C_2 \times V_2$$

or

$$V_2 = \frac{C_1 \times V_1}{C_2}$$

Likewise, the equation is also used to calculate the concentration of the diluted solution when a given volume is added to the starting solution.

Evaporation

Evaporation is a process used to convert a liquid or a volatile solid into vapor. It is used in the clinical laboratory to remove liquid from a sample, thereby increasing the concentrations of analyte(s) left behind.

Lyophilization

Lyophilization (also known as "freeze drying") is used in laboratory medicine for the preparation of (1) calibrators, (2) control materials, (3) reagents, and (4) individual specimens for analysis. Lyophilization entails first freezing a material at −40 °C or less and then subjecting it to a high vacuum. Very low temperatures cause the ice to sublimate to a vapor state. The solid nonsublimable material remains behind in a dried state.

Filtration

Filtration is defined as the passage of a liquid through a filter and is accomplished by gravity, pressure, or vacuum. *Filtrate* is the liquid that has passed through the filter. The purpose of filtration is to remove particulate matter from the liquid. Many filtrations in the clinical laboratory are carried out with *filter paper* and with plastic *membranes* of controlled pore size.

Membrane filters are used (1) under vacuum, (2) with positive pressure, or (3) with gravity. Filters have been incorporated into certain disposable tips for use with semiautomatic pipettes. These filters minimize the exchange of aerosol droplets between the tips and the pipette. This is of particular importance for DNA amplification and microbiological procedures. Other membrane filters are designed for ultrafiltration and are available with a variety of pore sizes for selective filtration. *Ultrafiltration* is a technique for removing dissolved particles using an extremely fine filter. It is used to concentrate macromolecules, such as proteins, because smaller dissolved molecules pass through the filter.

SAFETY

In the United States, the Federal Occupational Safety and Health Act of 1970 marked the beginning of formal regulatory oversight of employee safety. Since 1970, the Occupational Safety and Health Administration (OSHA) and the Centers for Disease Control and Prevention (CDC) have published numerous safety standards that apply to clinical laboratories. Each year, as The Joint Commission (JC) and the College of American Pathologists (CAP) revise their guidelines, more attention is devoted to safety. Consideration for the health and responsibility for the safety of employees are now accepted as obligations of all employers and laboratory directors. In May of 1988, OSHA expanded the Hazard Communication Standard to apply to hospital workers. Part of this standard is frequently referred to as the "Lab Right to Know Standard."

There are many aspects to the safe operation of a clinical laboratory. Key elements for safety in the clinical laboratory include

1. A formal safety program.
2. Documented policies and effective use of mandated plans and/or programs in the areas of chemical hygiene, control of exposure to bloodborne pathogens, tuberculosis control, and ergonomics.
3. Identification of significant occupational hazards, such as biological, chemical, fire, and electrical hazards, and clear identification and documentation of policies for employees to deal with each type of hazard (e.g., packaging and shipping of diagnostic specimens and infectious substances).
4. Recognition that there are additional important and relevant safety areas of concern. These areas include effective waste management and bioterrorism and chemical terrorism response plans in the event of potential threats or casualties involving these types of agents.

Safety Program

Every clinical laboratory must have and implement a comprehensive formal safety program. Regardless of the size of the clinical laboratory, a specific individual should be designated as the "Safety Officer" or "Chair of the Safety Committee" and given the responsibility to implement and maintain a safety program. Safety is each employee's responsibility, but responsibility for the entire program begins with the laboratory leadership (directors, administrative directors, supervisors, managers, etc.) and is delegated through the leadership to the safety officer or safety committee. This individual or committee then has the duties of providing guidance to laboratory leadership on matters related to the provision of a safe workplace for all employees. Although a small institution may have one individual who deals with all safety-related matters for all departments, including the laboratory, OSHA mandates that the laboratory specifically have a chemical hygiene officer, who is designated on the basis of training or experience to provide technical guidance in the development of the *chemical hygiene plan (CHP)* discussed later.

An integral part of the laboratory safety program is the education and motivation of all laboratory employees in all matters related to safety. All new employees should be given a copy of the general laboratory safety manual as part of their orientation. The continuing education program of the laboratory should include periodic talks on safety. Safety information is available from a variety of sources to support the continuing education element of the safety program.[6,7,11]

Another important part of the laboratory safety program relates to ensuring that the laboratory environment meets accepted safety standards. This would include, but would not be limited to, attention to such items as (1) proper labeling of chemicals, (2) types and locations of fire extinguishers, (3) hoods that are in good working order, (4) proper grounding of electrical equipment, (5) ergonomic issues (which include equipment, such as pipetting devices, laboratory furniture, and prevention of musculoskeletal disorders),[19] and (6) providing means for the proper handling and disposal of biohazardous materials, including all patient specimens.[7]

Safety Equipment

OSHA requires that institutions provide employees with all necessary personal protective equipment (PPE). Key important safety items are (1) clothing (such as laboratory coats, gowns, and/or scrubs), (2) gloves, and (3) eye protection. These safety items should be used in areas where they are appropriate. Eye washers or face washers should be available in every chemistry laboratory. Many types are available, and some simply connect to existing plumbing. A handheld eye and/or face safety spray is a requisite safety device and is typically placed in a position next to each sink using only a few inches of space. Safety showers, strategically located in the laboratory, must be available and should be tested on a regular schedule.

Heat-resistant (nonasbestos) gloves should be available for handling hot glassware and dry ice. Safety goggles, glasses, and visors, including some that fit conveniently over regular eyeglasses, are available in many sizes and shapes. Personnel wearing contact lenses should be aware of the danger of irritants getting under a lens, making it difficult to irrigate the eye properly. Shatterproof safety shields should be used in front of systems posing a potential danger because of implosion (vacuum collapse) or pressure explosions. *Desiccator* guards should be used with vacuum desiccators. Hot beakers should be handled with tongs. Inexpensive polyethylene pumps are available to pump acids from large bottles. Spill kits for acids, caustic materials, or flammable solvents come in various sizes. Such kits and the other appropriate safety materials should be located in convenient and appropriate sites in the laboratory.

A chemical fume hood is a necessity for every clinical chemistry laboratory. In practice, it is used for (1) opening any container of a material that gives off harmful vapors, (2) preparing reagents that produce fumes, and (3) heating flammable solvents. In the event of an explosion or a fire in the hood, closing its window contains the fire.

Safety Inspections

It is good laboratory practice to organize a safety inspection team from the laboratory staff. This team is responsible for conducting periodic and scheduled safety inspections of the laboratory.[8]

In the United States, several regulatory, private accreditation, state, and federal organizations may conduct a safety inspection of the laboratory. Some of these safety inspections may occur unannounced. From an external perspective, OSHA inspectors have the authority to enter a clinical laboratory unannounced and, on presentation of credentials, inspect it. The inspection may be regular or may occur as the result of a complaint. In addition, the Commission on Inspection and Accreditation of the CAP inspects clinical laboratories and uses various safety checklists (available to the laboratory before inspection) when evaluating a laboratory for accreditation. Although the The Joint Commission (JC) will accept CAP accreditation of a laboratory, it still may conduct a safety inspection of the laboratory when it inspects the hospital. The CAP and JC conduct their accreditation inspections, which may include a full laboratory or laboratory safety component, unannounced.

Depending on the group designated as responsible for accrediting a particular laboratory, selected laboratories may be subject to inspections for the purposes of accreditation and/or safety only by state agencies or local Centers for Medicare and Medicaid Services (CMS) groups. Inspections may be made on a regular basis by state or local health departments or by local fire departments to determine conformance with their particular safety requirements. Currently a laboratory that meets federal or state OSHA requirements is likely to satisfy the standards of any other inspecting agency.

Plans for the Clinical Laboratory

In 1991, OSHA mandated that all clinical laboratories in the United States must have a CHP and an exposure control plan. OSHA has since updated their requirements for the exposure control plan to provide new examples of engineering controls and to place significantly greater responsibility on employers to minimize and manage employee occupational exposure to bloodborne pathogens.[21] The CAP and other groups require that an accredited laboratory must have a documented tuberculosis exposure control plan that conforms with biosafety guidelines published by the CDC.[3] Elements of the plan must include regularly defined intervals for employee exposure, as well as process controls, to minimize exposure to aerosolization of *Mycobacterium tuberculosis.*

In addition, it is now recognized that the workplace setting of a clinical laboratory exposes employees to the occupational risk of developing various musculoskeletal disorders. As a result, the focus of OSHA on laboratories that have an effective ergonomics program has led to federal, state, and private accreditation groups addressing this area of occupational safety. However, considerable controversy on this issue is ongoing, with a final ergonomics rule published and then withdrawn in 2001.[14]

Chemical Hygiene Plan

Major elements of a CHP include listing of responsibilities for employers, employees, and a chemical hygiene officer. Also, every laboratory must have a complete chemical inventory that is updated annually. A copy of the *Material Safety Data Sheet (MSDS),* which defines each chemical as toxic, carcinogenic, or dangerous, must be on file and readily accessible and available to all employees 24 hours a day, 7 days a week. The MSDS contains important information for the benefit of laboratory employees. The chemical manufacturer's information as supplied on the MSDS is used to ascertain whether a certain chemical is hazardous. Each MSDS must give the product's identity as it appears on the container label and the chemical and common names of its hazardous components. The MSDS also provides physical data on the product, such as boiling point, vapor pressure, and specific gravity. Easily recognized characteristics of the chemical are also listed on the line for "appearance and odor." Information about hazardous properties is given in detail on the MSDS; this includes fire and explosion hazard data and health-related data, including the threshold limit value (TLV), exposure limits, and toxicity values. The TLV is the exposure allowable for an employee during one 8-hour day. It also notes effects of overexposure and details first-aid procedures. Each MSDS also provides information on spill and disposal procedures and protective personal gear and equipment requirements.

Exposure Control Plan

OSHA regulations require that each laboratory develop, implement, adhere to, and maintain a plan that ensures the protection of laboratory workers against potential exposure to bloodborne pathogens,[6,8] and that ensures that medical wastes produced by the laboratory are managed and handled in a safe and effective manner.[7,8] OSHA regulations also place responsibility on employers to implement new developments in exposure control technology; to solicit the input of employees directly involved in patient care in the identification, evaluation, and selection of these work practice controls; and in certain instances to maintain a log for employee percutaneous injuries from sharp devices, such as syringe needles.[21] Organizationally, the plan should include sections on (1) purpose, (2) scope, (3) applicable references, (4) applicable definitions, (5) definition of responsibilities, and (6) detailed procedural steps.

When implementing the plan, each laboratory employee must be placed into one of the following three groups.

Group I: A job classification in which all employees have occupational exposure to blood or other potentially infectious materials.

Group II: A job classification in which some employees have occupational exposure to blood or other potentially infectious materials.

Group III: A job classification in which employees do not have any occupational exposure to blood or other potentially infectious materials.

Tuberculosis Control Plan

The purpose of the tuberculosis control plan is to prevent the transmission of tuberculosis (TB), which occurs when an individual inhales a droplet that contains *Mycobacterium tuberculosis. M. tuberculosis* is aerosolized when an infected individual sneezes, speaks, or coughs (http://www.cdc.gov/tb/publications/guidelines/control_elim.htm/accessed April 26, 2011). Transmission of TB and exposure to TB are greatly diminished with (1) early identification and isolation of patients at risk, (2) environmental controls, (3) appropriate use of respiratory protection equipment, (4) education of laboratory employees, and (5) early initiation of therapy.

An effective tuberculosis control plan will include determination of exposure at regular intervals for all employees who are at occupational risk. Engineering and work practice controls are particularly important in laboratory areas, such as surgical pathology and microbiology. But there is clearly a risk of exposure from specimens of patients with suspected or confirmed tuberculosis in every section of the laboratory, including chemistry.

Pandemic Plan

A *pandemic* is an epidemic of infectious disease that spreads through populations across a large region or even worldwide. An influenza pandemic is a worldwide outbreak or epidemic caused by an influenza virus. For example, the influenza pandemic of 1918-1919 killed between 20 and 40 million people with more than 500,000 deaths reported in the United States alone (http://1918.pandemicflu.gov; accessed March 16, 2011).

Influenza viruses capable of causing a pandemic (1) must cause human disease, (2) have novel surface antigens, and (3) must be able to be spread effectively from person to person. Beginning in 1997, an outbreak of avian influenza (strain H5N1) affected birds in several countries in Asia, Africa, and Europe. This strain has been shown to cause lethal disease among humans and created concern that it might evolve into a strain of virus capable of causing a pandemic. Subsequently, many states in the United States developed pandemic influenza control or response plans (http://www.pandemicflu.gov; accessed March 16, 2011).[24]

A novel influenza A (H1N1) of swine origin was first detected in April of 2009.[22] This virus was found to be highly infectious, easily spreading from person to person, and led to an outbreak of illness in the United States and internationally as well (http://www.cdc.gov/h1n1flu; accessed March 16, 2011). A global pandemic was declared by the World Health Organization in June of 2009.

Because of the potential for exposure of individuals working in healthcare settings, the CDC has published recommendations for establishing infection control.[4] These recommendations provide guidance for all individuals who may be processing or performing diagnostic testing on clinical specimens from patients with suspected novel influenza A (H1N1) virus infection, or performing viral isolation.

Ergonomics Program

Several areas of occupational risk for development of musculoskeletal disorders have been identified in the clinical laboratory. These include (1) routine laboratory activity, (2) functionality of the workspace (including laboratory floor matting, bright lighting, and noise generation), and (3) equipment design (computer keyboards and displays, workstations, and chairs). One particular laboratory function, pipetting and related pipette design, has received considerable attention. As depicted in Figure 9-2, pipettes are being designed with the goal of reducing an employee's risk of developing cumulative stress disorders caused by awkward posture, repetitive motion, and repeated use of force.

The CAP requires accredited laboratories to have a comprehensive and defined ergonomics program that is designed to prevent work-related musculoskeletal disorders through prevention and engineering controls. The documented ergonomics plan should include elements of employee training regarding the areas of risk, engineering controls to minimize or eliminate risks, and an assessment process to identify problematic issues for documentation and remediation.

Hazards in the Laboratory

Various types of hazards are encountered in the operation of a clinical laboratory. These hazards must be identified and labeled, and work practices developed for dealing with them. The major categories of hazards encountered include (1) biological, (2) chemical, (3) electrical, and (4) fire hazards.

Identification of Hazards

Clinical laboratories deal with each of the nine classes of hazardous materials. These are classified by the United Nations (UN) as (1) explosives, (2) compressed gases, (3) flammable liquids, (4) flammable solids, (5) oxidizer materials, (6) toxic materials, (7) radioactive materials, (8) corrosive materials, and (9) miscellaneous materials not elsewhere classified. Shipping and handling of class 6 toxic materials, specifically biological and potentially infectious materials, has received considerable attention. In 2002, the U.S. Department of Transportation (DOT) released a revised rule with standards for infectious substance hazardous material handling.[12] Warning labels aid in the identification of chemical hazards during shipment. Under regulations of the DOT, chemicals that are transported in the United States must carry labels based on the UN classification. DOT placards or labels are diamond shaped with a digit imprinted on the bottom corner that identifies the UN hazard class (1 to 9). The hazard is identified more specifically in printed words placed along the horizontal axis of the diamond. Color coding and a pictorial art description of the hazard supplement the identification of hazardous material on the label; the artwork appears in the top corner of the diamond (Figure 9-5, *A*).

The system is used by the DOT for shipping hazardous materials; however, when the hazardous material reaches its destination and is removed from the shipping container, this identification is lost. The laboratory must then label each individual container. Usually the information necessary to classify the contents of the container appropriately is contained on the shipping label and should be noted. Important first aid information is usually provided on this label.

Even though OSHA at present prescribes the use of labels or other appropriate warnings, no single uniform labeling system for hazardous chemicals exists for use by clinical laboratories. Appropriate hazard warnings include any words, pictures, symbols, or combinations that convey the health or physical hazards of the container's contents and must be specific as to the effect of the chemical and the specific target organs involved. The National Fire Protection Association (NFPA) has developed the 704-M Identification System, which classifies hazardous material from 0 to 4 (most hazardous) according to flammability and reactivity (instability). This system uses diamond-shaped labels (Figure 9-5, *B*), which are available from most companies that sell laboratory safety equipment. The labels are color coded and are divided into quadrants. Three of the quadrants have a characteristic color and represent a type of hazard. A number in the quadrant indicates the degree of hazard. The fourth (lower) quadrant contains information of special interest to firemen.

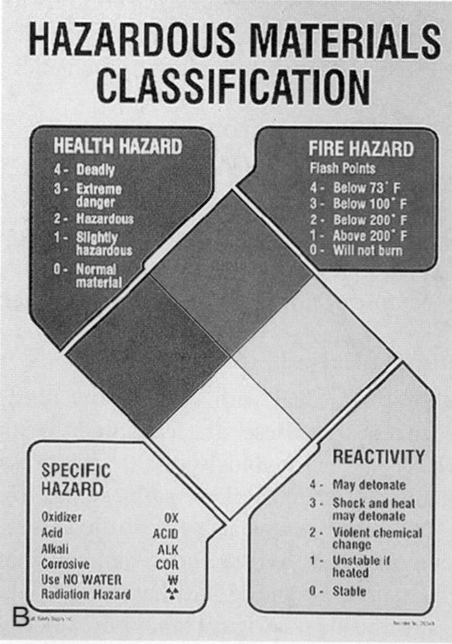

Figure 9-5 A, Department of Transportation label for corrosives. B, Labeling identification system of the National Fire Protection Association. *(Courtesy Lab Safety Supply Inc., Janesville, Wis.)*

Biological Hazards

It is essential to minimize the exposure of laboratory workers to infectious agents, such as the hepatitis viruses, human immunodeficiency virus (HIV), and flu viruses. Exposure to infectious agents results from (1) accidental puncture with needles, (2) spraying of infectious materials by a syringe or spilling and splattering of these materials on bench tops or floors, (3) centrifuge accidents, and (4) cuts or scratches from contaminated vessels. Any unfixed tissue, including blood slides, must also be treated as potentially infectious material.

OSHA has mandated that all U.S. laboratories have an exposure control plan. In addition, the National Institute for Occupational Safety and Health (NIOSH), a functional unit of the CDC, has prepared and widely distributed a document entitled *Universal Precautions* that specifies how U.S. clinical laboratories should handle infectious agents.[18] In general, it mandates that clinical laboratories treat all human blood and other potentially infectious materials as if they were known to contain infectious agents, such as hepatitis B virus (HBV), HIV, and other bloodborne pathogens. These requirements apply to all specimens of (1) blood, (2) serum, (3) plasma, (4) blood products, (5) vaginal secretions, (6) semen, (7) cerebrospinal fluid, (8) synovial fluid, and (9) concentrated HBV or HIV viruses. In addition, any specimen of any type that contains visible traces of blood should be handled using these universal precautions.

Universal precautions also specify that barrier protection must be used by laboratory workers to prevent skin and mucous membrane contamination from specimens. These barriers, also known as PPE, include (1) gloves, (2) gowns, (3) laboratory coats, (4) face shields or mask and eye protection, (5) mouthpieces, (6) resuscitation bags, (7) pocket masks, and (8) other ventilator devices. For some individuals, latex allergy is a problem when latex gloves are used for barrier protection. For such individuals, medical grade non-latex gloves made of materials such as vinyl, nitrile, neoprene, or thermoplastic elastomer are available. If latex gloves are to be used, they should be made of powder-free, low-allergen latex.

New products for increasing employee protection against needlesticks include an array of novel containers for sharps (e.g., needles, scalpels, glass) and biological safety disposal bags and needle sheaths that may be closed following venipuncture without physically touching the needle or the sheath. Although additional studies on their efficacy and effects on laboratory test results are required, microlaser devices are now available for piercing a patient's skin to collect a capillary blood specimen.

The CLSI has published a similar set of recommendations,[6,8] several of which are specified as requirements in the OSHA exposure control plan. They include the following:

"1. Never perform mouth pipetting and never blow out pipettes that contain potentially infectious material.
2. Do not mix potentially infectious material by bubbling air through the liquid.
3. Barrier protection, such as gloves, masks, and protective eye wear and gowns, must be available and used when drawing blood from a patient and when handling all patient specimens. This includes the removal of stoppers from tubes. Gloves must be disposable, nonsterile latex or of other material to provide adequate barrier protection. Phlebotomists must change gloves and adequately dispose of them between drawing blood from different patients.
4. Wash hands whenever gloves are changed.
5. Facial barrier protection should be used if there is a significant potential for the spattering of blood or body fluids.
6. Avoid using syringes whenever possible and dispose of needles in rigid containers (Figure 9-6, *A*) without handling them (Figure 9-6, *B*).
7. Dispose of all sharps appropriately.
8. Wear protective clothing, which serves as an effective barrier against potentially infective materials. When leaving the laboratory, the protective clothing should be removed.
9. Strive to prevent accidental injuries.
10. Encourage frequent hand washing in the laboratory; employees must wash their hands whenever they leave the laboratory.
11. Make a habit of keeping your hands away from your mouth, nose, eyes, and any other mucous membranes. This reduces the possibility of self-inoculation.
12. Minimize spills and spatters.
13. Decontaminate all surfaces and reusable devices after use with appropriate U.S. Environmental Protection Agency (EPA)-registered hospital disinfectants. Sterilization, disinfection, and decontamination are discussed in detail in CLSI publication M29-A3.[6]
14. No warning labels are to be used on patient specimens since all should be treated as potentially hazardous.
15. Biosafety level 2 procedures should be used whenever appropriate.

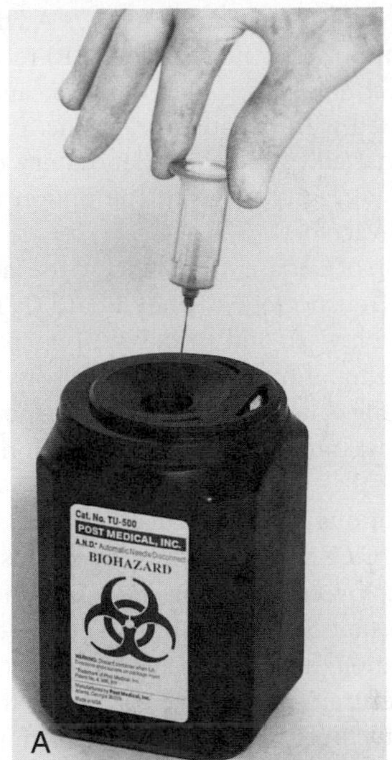

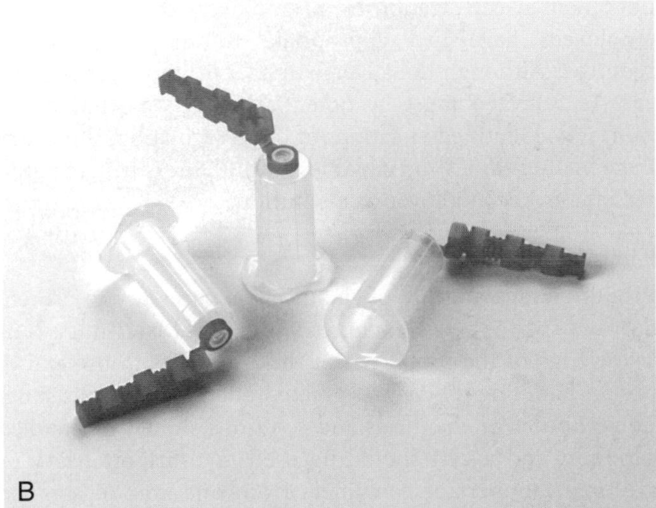

Figure 9-6 A, Convenient needle disposal system for sharps. B, Needle sheathing devices for prevention of body contact with needle. *(B, Courtesy MarketLab Inc.)*

16. Before centrifuging tubes, inspect them for cracks. Inspect the inside of the trunnion cup for signs of erosion or adhering matter. Be sure that rubber cushions are free from all bits of glass.
17. Use biohazard disposal techniques (e.g., 'Red Bag').
18. Never leave a discarded tube or infected material unattended or unlabeled.
19. Periodically, clean out freezer and dry-ice chests to remove broken ampoules and tubes of biological specimens. Use rubber gloves and respiratory protection during this cleaning.
20. OSHA requires that hepatitis B vaccine be offered to all employees at risk of potential exposure as a regular or

occasional part of their duties. CDC's Advisory Committee on Immunization Practices (ACIP) recommends that medical technologists, phlebotomists, and pathologists be vaccinated with hepatitis B vaccine. It is a regulatory mandate that all of the above laboratory employees at a minimum [at least] be given the option to receive free hepatitis B vaccine."

Investigation of tragic air accidents in the late 1990s by the U.S. National Transportation Safety Board (NTSB) led to the development of revised and strict requirements for the shipping and handling of hazardous materials by DOT, in cooperation with the International Air Transport Association (IATA) and the International Civil Aviation Organization (ICAO).[12]

These regulations place particular emphasis on the hazardous material (HAZMAT) training that must be given to laboratory employees regarding shipping and handling of infectious substances. Elements include general awareness and familiarization, function-specific information, and safety training. Proper training, particularly in the areas of package labeling and documentation (including a shipper's declaration of contents for dangerous goods), is mandatory, and documented certification from employers that the relevant employees have had appropriate training programs is required. Although the adverse impact of improper training can be reflected most by potential human morbidity and mortality, identified violations of these regulations also carry large financial fines and penalties for both the infringing individual and the employer or institution.

Chemical Hazards

Proper storage and use of chemicals is necessary to prevent dangers, such as burns, explosions, fires, and toxic fumes. Thus knowledge of the properties of the chemicals in use and of proper handling procedures greatly reduces dangerous situations. Bottles of chemicals and solutions should be handled carefully, and a cart should be used to transport heavy or multiple numbers of containers from one area to another. Glass containers with chemicals should be transported in rubber or plastic containers that protect them from breakage and, in the event of breakage, contain the spill. Appropriate spill kits should be available in strategic locations.

Spattering from acids, caustic materials, and strong oxidizing agents is a hazard to clothing and eyes and is a potential source of chemical burns. A bottle should never be held by its neck but instead firmly around its body with one or both hands, depending on the size of the bottle. Acids must be diluted by slowly adding them to water while mixing; water should never be added to concentrated acid. When working with acid or alkali solutions, safety glasses should be worn. Acids, caustic materials, and strong oxidizing agents should be mixed in the sink. This provides water for cooling and for confinement of the reagent in the event that the flask or bottle breaks.

All bottles containing reagents must be properly labeled. It is good practice to label the container before adding the reagent, thus preventing the possibility of having an unlabeled reagent. The label should bear the (1) name and concentration of the reagent, (2) initials of the person who made up the reagent, and (3) date on which the reagent was prepared. When appropriate, the expiration date should also be included. The labels should be color coded or an additional label added to designate specific storage instructions, such as the requirement for refrigeration or special storage related to a potential hazard. All reagents found in unlabeled bottles should be disposed of using appropriate procedures and precautions.

Strong acids, caustic materials, and strong oxidizing agents should be dispensed by a commercially available automatic dispensing device. Under no circumstances is mouth pipetting permitted.

In some instances, all waste materials are not collected in the same container. With certain pieces of equipment, strong acids or other hazardous materials are pumped directly into the drain. This should always be accompanied by a steady flow of water from the faucet. Safety glasses should be used by instrument operators when acids are pumped under pressure.

Perchloric acid, because it is potentially explosive in contact with organic materials, requires careful handling. Perchloric acid should not be used on wooden bench tops, and bottles of this acid should be stored on a glass tray. Disposal may be accomplished by adding the acid dropwise (using a splatter shield) to at least 100 volumes of cold water and pouring the diluted acid down the drain with large amounts of additional cold water. Special perchloric acid hoods, with special wash-down facilities, should be installed if large amounts of this acid are used.

Special care is necessary when dealing with mercury. Even small drops of mercury on bench tops and floors may poison the atmosphere in a poorly ventilated room. The element's ability to amalgamate with a number of metals is well known. After an accidental spillage of mercury, the spill area should be cleaned carefully until no droplets are remaining. All containers of mercury should be kept well stoppered. Because it is highly hazardous, most recommend that no mercury be used in the laboratory.

The EPA controls the disposal of nonradioactive hazardous wastes. The Resource Conservation and Recovery Act of 1976 (RCRA) states that disposal of materials classifiable within any of the nine UN hazardous materials classes is enforced in such a way that health and safety professionals involved in the disposal of such materials are personally liable for each individual violation.

A CLSI publication[7] covers hazardous waste disposal; however, many municipalities and states have their own regulations. These agencies should be contacted by the laboratory for specifics.

Volatile chemicals and compressed gases pose specific hazards.

Hazards from Volatiles

The use of organic solvents in a clinical laboratory represents a potential fire hazard and hazards to health from inhalation of toxic vapors or skin contact. These solvents should be used in a fume hood. Storage of organic solvents is regulated by rules set down by OSHA. However, some local fire department rules are more stringent. Solvents should be stored in an OSHA-approved metal storage cabinet that is properly vented. The maximum working volume of flammable solvents allowed outside storage cabinets is 5 gallons per room. No more than 60 gallons of type I and II solvents may be stored in a single cabinet. No more than three cabinets may be located in each 5000 sq ft of laboratory space.

Vaporization is a major problem in the ignition and spread of fires. Vapors from flammable and combustible liquids and solids form a flammable mixture with air. They are characterized by their flash point, where the flash point is defined as the lowest temperature at which a solvent gives off flammable vapors in the close vicinity of its surface. The mixture at its flash point ignites when exposed to a source of ignition. At temperatures below the flash point, the vapor given off is considered too lean for ignition.

Disposal of flammable solvents in storm sewers or sanitary sewers generally is not allowed. Exceptions are small amounts of those materials that are miscible with water, but even disposal of these should be followed by large amounts of cold water. Other solvents should be collected in safety cans. Separate cans should be used for ether and for chlorinated solvents; all other solvents may be combined in a third can. The cans should be stored, in keeping with storage quantity rules, in a safety cabinet until pickup by a waste disposal firm. A more economical approach is to transfer the solvents to larger cans or drums in an outside storage facility, so that pickup can be less frequent. Some large institutions have their own in-house disposal facilities.

Hazards from Compressed Gases

DOT regulations cover the labeling of cylinders of compressed gases that are transported by interstate carriers. The diamond-shaped labels described previously are used on all large cylinders and on any boxes containing small cylinders. Some general rules for handling large cylinders of compressed gas are as follows:

1. Always transport cylinders using a hand truck to which the cylinder is secured.
2. Leave the valve cap on a cylinder until the cylinder is ready for use, at which time the cylinder should have been secured by a support around the upper one third of its body. Disconnect the hose or regulator, shut off the valve, and replace the cap before the cylinder is completely empty to prevent the possibility of development of a negative pressure. Place an "empty" sign or label on the cylinder.
3. Chain or secure cylinders at all times even when empty.
4. Always check cylinders for the composition of their contents before connection.
5. Never force threads; if a regulator does not thread readily, something is wrong.

The precautions cited for large, refillable gas cylinders also apply to small cylinders that are not refillable. Propane cylinders and cylinders of calibrating gases for blood gas equipment are examples of disposable cylinders. Cylinders in floor-standing base supports require the additional security of a chain or strap attached to a wall or fixed piece of furniture. Local fire department regulations (which vary considerably from place to place) govern the disposal of exhausted cylinders.

Electrical Hazards

Electrical wires or connections are potential shock or fire hazards. Worn wires on all electrical equipment should be replaced immediately, and all equipment should be grounded using three-prong plugs. OSHA regulations stipulate that the requirements for grounding of electrical equipment of the National Electrical Code (published by NFPA) be met. If grounded receptacles are not available, a licensed electrician should be consulted for proper alternative grounding techniques. Some local codes are more stringent than OSHA requirements and do not allow for two-pole mating receptacles with adapters for a three-pole plug.

Use of extension cords is prohibited. This standard is more stringent than any other existing regulation. In some instances, an extension cord may have to be used temporarily. In such cases, the cord should (1) be less than 12 feet in length, (2) include at least 16 American Wire Gauge (AWG) wire, (3) be approved by the Underwriters Laboratory (UL), and (4) have only one outlet at the end. If several outlets are necessary in a single area, a power strip with its own fuse or circuit breaker may be installed at least 3 inches above bench top level. Several manufacturers now sell devices to check for high resistance in neutral or ground wiring or excess voltage in neutral wiring.

Electrical equipment and connections should not be handled with wet hands, nor should electrical equipment be used after liquid has been spilled on it. The equipment must be turned off immediately and dried thoroughly. In case of a wet or malfunctioning electrical instrument that is used by several people, the plug should be pulled and a note cautioning coworkers against use should be left on the instrument.

Fire Hazards

NFPA and OSHA publish standards covering subjects from emergency exits (including means of egress) to safety and firefighting equipment. NFPA also publishes the National Fire Codes. Many state and local agencies have adopted these codes (some of which are more stringent than OSHA requirements), thus making them legally enforceable.

Every laboratory should have the necessary equipment to extinguish or confine a fire in the laboratory and to extinguish a fire on the clothing of an individual. Easy access to safety showers is essential. A safety shower should have a pull chain attached to the wall at a convenient height or hanging down from the shower head; the chain should have a large ring attached so that the shower may be easily activated, even with eyes closed. Fire blankets for smothering fire on clothing should be available in an easily accessible wall-mounted case. The blanket is unrolled from the case and is rolled around the

TABLE 9-13 Classification of Fires and Fire Extinguisher Requirements

Type of Hazard	Class of Fire	Recommended Extinguisher Agents
Ordinary combustibles: wood, cloth, paper	A	Water, dry chemical foam, loaded steam
Flammable liquids and gases: solvents and greases, natural or manufactured gases	B	Dry chemical, carbon dioxide, loaded steam, Halon 1211 or 1301 foam
Electrical equipment: any energized electrical equipment. If electricity is turned off at source, this reverts to a class A or B.	C	Dry chemical, carbon dioxide, Halon 1211 or 1301 foam
Combinations of ordinary combustibles and flammable liquids and gases	A and B	Dry chemical, loaded steam, foam
Combinations of ordinary combustibles and electrical equipment	A and C	Dry chemical
Combinations of flammable liquids and gases and electrical equipment	B and C	Dry chemical, carbon dioxide, Halon 1211 or 1301 foam
Combinations of ordinary combustibles, flammable liquids and gases, and electrical equipment	A, B, and C	Triplex dry chemical

body by taking hold of the rope that is attached to the blanket and turning the body around. The location of this equipment and the locations of fire alarms and maps of evacuation routes are dictated by the local fire marshal.

Various types of fire extinguishers are available. The type to use depends on the type of fire. Because it is impractical to have several types of fire extinguishers present in every area, dry chemical fire extinguishers are among the best all-purpose extinguishers for laboratory areas. An extinguisher should be provided near every laboratory door and, in a large laboratory, at the end of the room opposite the door. Everyone in the laboratory should be instructed in the use of these extinguishers and any other available firefighting equipment. All fire extinguishers should be tested by qualified personnel at intervals specified by the manufacturer. The three classes of fires and the type of fire extinguisher to be used for each are listed in Table 9-13. Every fire extinguisher is labeled as to the type of fire it should be used to extinguish.

Two additional types of fires, designated "D" and "E," should be handled only by trained personnel. Type D fires include those involving powdered metal materials (e.g., magnesium). A special powder is used to fight this hazard. A type E fire is one that cannot be put out or is liable to result in a detonation (such as an arsenal fire). A type E fire is usually allowed to burn out while nearby materials are appropriately protected.

Many clinical laboratories now have a computer that is housed in a temperature- and humidity-controlled room. The most popular automatic fire control system used for these rooms is Halon 1301 (bromotrifluoromethane). Although this is the least toxic of the halons, NFPA regulations require a warning sign at the entrance to the room and availability of self-contained breathing equipment.

REFERENCES

1. Armbruster D, Miller RR. The Joint Committee for Traceability in Laboratory Medicine (JCTLM): a global approach to promote the standardisation of clinical laboratory test results. Clin Biochem Rev 2007;28:105-14.
2. Bermes EW Jr, Kahn SE, Young DS. General laboratory techniques and procedures. In: Burtis CA, Ashwood ER, Bruns DE, eds. Tietz textbook of clinical chemistry and molecular diagnostics, 4th edition. Philadelphia: WB Saunders, 2006:3-40.
3. Biosafety in microbiological and biomedical laboratories, 4th edition. Washington, DC: Department of Health and Human Services, Centers for Disease Control and Prevention, National Institutes of Health. Washington, DC: U.S. Government Printing Office, May 1999.
4. Centers for Disease Control and Prevention. H1N1 influenza virus biosafety guidelines for laboratory workers. Available at: http://www.cdc.gov/h1n1flu/guidelines_labworkers.htm (accessed May 5, 2009).
5. CLSI. Procedures for the handling and processing of blood specimens: approved guideline, 3rd edition. CLSI Document H18-A4. Wayne, Pa: Clinical and Laboratory Standards Institute, 2010.
6. CLSI. Protection of laboratory workers from occupationally acquired infections: approved guideline, 3rd edition. CLSI Document M29-A3. Wayne, Pa: Clinical and Laboratory Standards Institute, 2005.
7. CLSI. Clinical laboratory waste Management: approved Guideline, 2nd edition. CLSI Document GP5-A3. Wayne, Pa: Clinical and Laboratory Standards Institute, 2011.
8. CLSI. Clinical laboratory safety, 2nd edition. CLSI Document GP17-A2. Wayne, Pa: Clinical and Laboratory Standards Institute, 2004.
9. CLSI. Temperature calibration of water baths, instruments, and temperature sensors: approved guideline, 2nd edition. CLSI Document I09-A2. Wayne, Pa: Clinical and Laboratory Standards Institute, 1990.
10. CLSI. Preparation and testing of reagent water in the clinical laboratory: approved guideline, 4th edition. CLSI Document C03-A4. Wayne, Pa: Clinical and Laboratory Standards Institute, 2006.
11. Davis DL. Laboratory safety. Washington, DC: AACC Press, 2008.
12. Department of Transportation. 49 CFR, Part 171. Hazardous materials: revisions to standards for infectious substances. Final rule. Federal Register 67, No 157, Wednesday, August 14, 2002.
13. De Bièvre P. The 2007 International Vocabulary of Metrology (VIM), JCGM 200:2008 (ISO/IEC Guide 99): meeting the need for intercontinentally understood concepts and their associated intercontinentally agreed terms. Clin Biochem 2009;42:246-8.
14. Ergonomics program. Final rule: removal. Occupational Safety and Health Administration (OSHA). Federal Register 2001;666:20403.
15. McDonald CJ, Huff SM, Suico JG, Hill G, Leavelle D, Aller R, et al. LOINC, a universal standard for identifying laboratory observations: a 5-year update. Clin Chem 2003;49:624-33.

16. McDonald CJ, Huff SM, White TM, et al. LOINC update extended clinical observation, performance measures, attachments, mapping and translations (Spanish and simplified Chinese). Presented at: American Medical Informatics Association (AMIA) Symposium, January 20-23, 2005, Key West, Fla.
17. McDonald CJ, Huff SM, White T, Banning P. New developments in the LOINC coding world. Presented at: American Medical Informatics Association (AMIA) Symposium, November 11-15, 2006, Washington, DC. (http://loinc.org; accessed March 16, 2011).
18. National Institute for Occupational Safety and Health. Updated U.S. Public Health Service guidelines for the management of occupational exposures to HBV, HCV, and HIV and recommendations for postexposure prophylaxis. MMWR 2001;50:1-50.
19. National Institute for Occupational Safety and Health (NIOSH). Musculoskeletal disorders and workplace factors: a critical review of epidemiologic evidence for work-related musculoskeletal disorders of the neck, upper extremities, and low back. Centers for Disease Control (NIOSH) Publication No. 97-141. Atlanta, Ga: Centers for Disease Control, July 1997.
20. National Institute of Standards and Technology. The international system of units (SI). NIST Special Publication 811. Gaithersburg, Md: National Institute of Standards and Technology (http://www.nist.gov), 1994.
21. Occupational exposure to bloodborne pathogens: needlesticks and other sharps injuries. Final rule. Occupational Safety and Health Administration (OSHA). Federal Register 2001;66:5318-25.
22. Poon LL, Chan KH, Smith GJ, Leung CS, Guan Y, Yuen KY, et al. Molecular detection of a novel human influenza (H1N1) of pandemic potential by conventional and real-time quantitative RT-PCR assays. Clin Chem 2009:55:1555-58.
23. Powsner ER, Widman JC. Basic principles of radioactivity and its measurement. In: Burtis CA, Ashwood ER, eds. Tietz textbook of clinical chemistry, 3rd edition. Philadelphia: WB Saunders, 1999:113-32.
24. State Pandemic Plans. Pandemicflu.gov Available at: http://www.pandemicflu.gov (accessed March 16, 2011).
25. Valcárcel M. A modern definition of analytical chemistry. Trends Anal Chem 1997;16:124-31.
26. Vesper HW, Thienpont LM. Traceability in laboratory medicine. Clin Chem 2009;55:1067-75.

CHAPTER 10

Optical Techniques

*Larry J. Kricka, D.Phil., F.A.C.B., C.Chem., F.R.S.C., F.R.C.Path., and Jason Y. Park, M.D., Ph.D., F.C.A.P.**

Many determinations made in the clinical laboratory are based on measurements of radiant energy emitted, transmitted, absorbed, scattered, or reflected under controlled conditions. The principles involved in such measurements are considered in this chapter.

NATURE OF LIGHT

Electromagnetic radiation includes radiant energy that extends from cosmic rays with wavelengths as short as 10 nm up to radio waves longer than 1000 km. However, in this chapter, the term *light* is used to describe radiant energy from the ultraviolet and visible portions of the spectrum (180 to 800 nm).

The wavelength of light is defined as the distance between two peaks as the light travels in a wavelike manner. This distance is expressed in nanometers (nm) for wavelengths commonly used in photometry. Other units include

$$1\ \text{nm} = 1\ \text{millimicron}\ (\text{m}\mu) = 10\ \text{Angstroms}\ (\text{Å}) = 10^{-9}\ \text{m}$$

In addition to possessing wavelength characteristics, light has properties that indicate that it is composed of discrete energy packets called *photons*. The relationship between the energy of photons and their frequency is given by the equation

$$E = h\nu \qquad (1)$$

where E = energy in ergs, ν = frequency of light in cycles per second, and h = Planck's constant (6.62×10^{27} erg seconds). The frequency of light (ν) is related to the wavelength by an equation

$$\nu = \frac{c}{\lambda} \qquad (2)$$

where c = speed of light in a vacuum (3×10^{10} cm/s), and λ = wavelength in centimeters. Combining equations (1) and (2) results in

$$E = \frac{hc}{\lambda} \qquad (3)$$

This equation shows that the energy of light is inversely proportional to the wavelength. For example, ultraviolet (UV) radiation at 200 nm possesses greater energy than infrared (IR) radiation at 750 nm.

The human eye is able to detect radiant energy with wavelengths between about 380 and 750 nm, but modern instrumentation permits measurements at both shorter wavelength (UV) and longer wavelength (IR) portions of the spectrum. Sunlight, or light emitted from a tungsten filament, is a mixture of wavelengths or a spectrum of radiant energy of different wavelengths that the eye recognizes as "white." Table 10-1 shows approximate relationships between wavelengths and color characteristics for the UV, visible, and short IR portions of the spectrum. Thus a solution will appear green when viewed against white light if it transmits light maximally between 500 and 580 nm but absorbs light at other wavelengths. Similarly, a solid object appears green if it reflects light in this region (500 to 580 nm) but absorbs light at other portions of the spectrum. In general, if we compare the intensity of light transmitted by a colored solution versus that of a reference solution over the entire spectrum, we obtain a typical spectral transmittance curve characteristic for that spectrum. Such curves are shown in Figure 10-1 for solutions of nickel sulfate *(a)* and potassium permanganate *(b)*. Inspection of the curves should lead us to predict that the color of solution *a* is green because light is transmitted maximally near the green portion of the spectrum. Curve *b*, on the other hand, illustrates the spectrum of a solution that transmits light maximally in the blue, violet, and red portions of the spectrum. The eye recognizes this mixture of colors as purple.

SPECTROPHOTOMETRY

Photometry is defined as the measurement of light; *spectrophotometry* is defined as the measurement of the intensity of light at selected wavelengths. Spectrophotometric analysis is a widely used method of quantitative and qualitative analysis in the chemical and biological sciences. The method depends on the light-absorbing properties of the substance or a

**The authors gratefully acknowledge the original contributions by Dr. Merle A. Evenson and Dr. Thomas O. Tiffany, upon which portions of this chapter are based.*

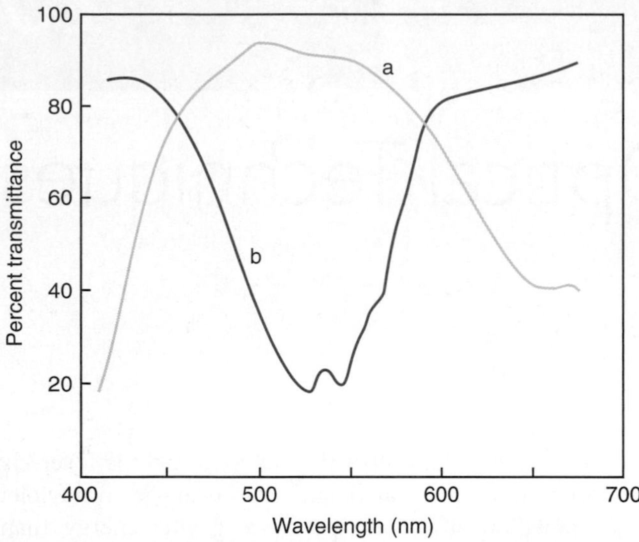

Figure 10-1 Spectral transmittance curves of nickel sulfate *(a)* and potassium permanganate *(b)*. Arbitrary concentrations read versus water as a blank (Beckman DB-G spectrophotometer).

TABLE 10-1 Ultraviolet, Visible, and Short Infrared Spectrum Characteristics

Wavelength, nm	Region Name	Color Observed*
<380	Ultraviolet†	Invisible
380-440	Visible	Violet
440-500	Visible	Blue
500-580	Visible	Green
580-600	Visible	Yellow
600-620	Visible	Orange
620-750	Visible	Red
800-2500	Near infrared	Not visible
2500-15,000	Mid infrared	Not visible
15,000-1,000,000	Far infrared	Not visible

*Owing to the subjective nature of color, the wavelength intervals shown are only approximations.

†The ultraviolet (UV) portion of the spectrum is sometimes further divided into "near" UV (200-380 nm) and "far" UV (<220 nm). This arbitrary distinction has a practical basis, because silica used to make cuvets transmits light effectively at wavelengths ≥220 nm.

derivative of the substance being analyzed. The intensity of transmitted light passing through a solution containing an absorbing substance (chromogen) is decreased by the absorbed fraction. This fraction is detected, measured, and used to relate the light transmitted or absorbed to the concentration of the analyte in question.

Basic Concepts

Consider an incident light beam with intensity I_0 passing through a square cell containing a solution of a compound that absorbs light of a certain wavelength, λ. Given that the intensity of the transmitted light beam is I_S, then transmittance *(T)* of light is defined as

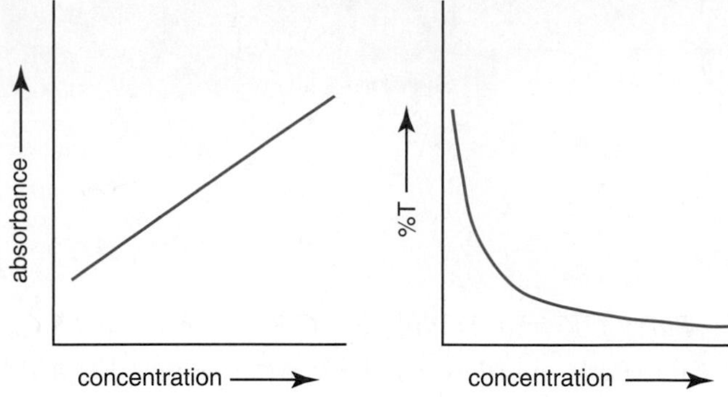

Figure 10-2 Absorbance and %*T* relationship.

$$T = \frac{I_S}{I_0} \tag{4}$$

A portion of the incident light, however, may be reflected by the surface of the cell or may be absorbed by the cell wall or solvent. To focus attention on the compound of interest, elimination of these factors is necessary. This is achieved using a reference cell identical to the sample cell, except that the compound of interest is omitted from the solvent in the reference cell. The transmittance *(T)* through this reference cell is I_R divided by I_O; the transmittance for the compound in solution then is defined as *I* divided by I_R. In practice, the light beam is blocked and the detector signal set to zero transmittance, then a reference cell is inserted and the detector signal adjusted to an arbitrary scale reading of 100 (corresponding to 100% transmittance), followed by the cell containing the sample to be measured, and the percent transmittance reading is made on the sample. As we increase the concentration of the compound in solution, we find that transmittance varies inversely and logarithmically with concentration (Figure 10-2). Consequently, it is more convenient to define a new term, absorbance *(A)*, which will be directly proportional to the concentration. Thus the amount of light absorbed *(A)* as the incident light passes through the sample is equivalent to

$$A = -\log\frac{I_S}{I_R} = -\log T \tag{5}$$

Analytically, the amount of light absorbed or transmitted is related mathematically to the concentration of the analyte in question by Beer's law.

Beer's Law—Relationship Between Transmittance, Absorbance, and Concentration

Beer's law (also known as the Beer-Lambert law) states that the concentration of a substance is directly proportional to the amount of light absorbed or inversely proportional to the logarithm of the transmitted light (see Figure 10-2). Mathematically, Beer's law is expressed as

$$A = abc \tag{6}$$

TABLE 10-2 Spectrophotometry Nomenclature

Name	Symbol	Definition
Absorbance	A	$\log T$ or $\log I_0/I$
Absorptivity	a	A/bc (c in g/L)
Molar absorptivity	ε	A/bc (c in mol/L)
Path length	b	Internal cell or sample length, in cm
Transmittance	T	I/I_0*
Wavelength unit	nm	10^{-9} m
Absorption maximum	λmax	Wavelength at which maximum absorption occurs

*I/I_0 is the ratio of the intensity of transmitted light to incident light.

where

A = Absorbance

a = Proportionality constant defined as absorptivity

b = Light path in centimeters

c = Concentration of the absorbing compound, usually expressed in moles per liter

This equation forms the basis of quantitative analysis by absorption photometry. When b is 1 cm and c is expressed in moles per liter, the constant a is called the molar absorptivity. The value for a is a constant for a given compound at a given wavelength under prescribed conditions of solvent, temperature, pH, and so forth. The nomenclature of spectrophotometry is summarized in Table 10-2. Values for a are useful for characterizing compounds, establishing their purity, and comparing the sensitivity of measurements obtained on derivatives. Pure bilirubin, for example, when dissolved in chloroform at 25 °C, has a molar absorptivity of 60,700 ± 1600 at 453 nm. The molecular weight of bilirubin is 584. Hence a solution containing 5 mg/L (0.005 g/L) should have an absorbance of

$$A = (60{,}700) \times \left(= -\frac{0.005}{584}\right) = 0.520 \qquad (7)$$

The molar absorptivity of the complex between ferrous iron and *s*-tripyridyltriazine is 22,600, whereas that with 1,10-phenanthroline is 11,000. Thus for a given concentration of iron, *s*-tripyridyltriazine produces a complex with an absorbance about twice that of the complex with 1,10-phenanthroline. Consequently, *s*-tripyridyltriazine is a more sensitive reagent to use in the measurement of iron.

Application of Beer's Law

In practice, a calibration relationship between absorbance and concentration is established experimentally for a given instrument under specified conditions using a series of reference solutions that contain increasing concentrations of analyte. Frequently, a linear relationship exists up to a certain concentration or absorbance. When this linear relationship exists, the solution is said to obey Beer's law up to this point. Within this limitation, a calibration constant *(K)* may be derived and used to calculate the concentration of an unknown solution by comparison with a calibrating solution.

Certain precautions must be observed with the use of such calibration constants. For example, under no circumstances should the calibration constants be used when the calibrator or unknown readings exceed the linear portion of the calibration relationship. In other words, calibration constants are used only when the curve obeys Beer's law. At least two and preferably more calibrators should be included in each series of determinations to permit direct comparison of unknown readings with calibrators or to calculate the calibration constant. These multiple calibrators are necessary because variations in reagents, working conditions, and cell diameters and deterioration or changes in instruments may result in day-to-day changes in the absorbance value for the calibrator. A nonlinear calibration curve may be used if a sufficient number of calibrators of varying concentrations are included to cover the entire range encountered for readings on unknowns.

In some cases, a pure reference material may not be readily available, and constants may be provided that were obtained on pure materials and reported in the literature. In general, published constants should be used only if the method is followed in detail and readings are made on a spectrophotometer capable of providing light of high spectral purity at a verified wavelength. Use of broader-band light sources usually leads to some decrease in absorbance. For example, the absorbance of nicotinamide adenine dinucleotide (NADH) at 340 nm is frequently used as a reference for determination of enzyme activity, based on a molar absorptivity of 6.22×10^3 (see Chapter 15). This value is acceptable only under the carefully controlled conditions previously described and should not be used unless these conditions are met. Published values for molar absorptivities and absorption coefficients should be used only as guidelines until they are verified by readings on pure reference materials for a given instrument. In addition, Beer's law is followed only if the following conditions are met:

- Incident radiation on the substance of interest is monochromatic.
- The solvent absorption is insignificant compared with the solute absorbance.
- The solute concentration is within given limits.
- An optical interferant is not present.
- A chemical reaction does not occur between the molecule of interest and another solute or solvent molecule.

Instrumentation

Modern instruments isolate a narrow wavelength range of the spectrum for measurements. Those that use filters for this purpose are referred to as *filter photometers;* those that use prisms or gratings are called *spectrophotometers*. Spectrophotometers are classified as single or double beam.

The major components of a *single-beam spectrophotometer* are shown schematically in Figure 10-3. In such an instrument, a beam of light is passed through a monochromator that isolates the desired region of the spectrum to be used

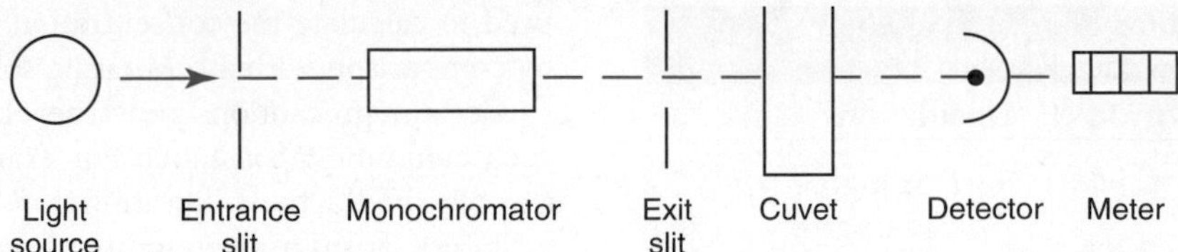

Figure 10-3 Major components of a single-beam spectrophotometer.

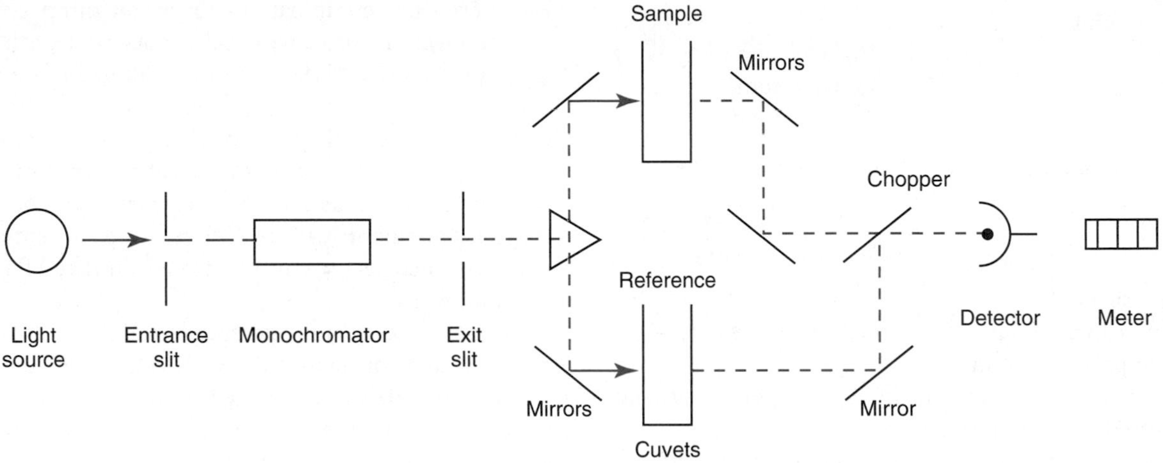

Figure 10-4 Double-beam spectrophotometer.

for measurements. The light next passes through an absorption cell (cuvet), where a portion of the radiant energy is absorbed, depending on the nature and concentration of the substance in the solution. Any light not absorbed is transmitted to a detector, which converts light energy to electrical energy that is registered on a meter or recorder or digitally displayed.

In operation, an opaque block is substituted for the cuvet, so that no light reaches the photocell, and the meter is adjusted to read 0% *T*. Next, a cuvet containing a reagent blank is inserted, and the meter is adjusted to read 100% *T* (zero absorbance). The composition of the reagent blank should be identical to that of calibrating or unknown solutions except for the substance to be measured. Calibrating solutions containing various known concentrations of the substance are inserted, and readings are recorded. Finally, a reading is made of the unknown solution, and its concentration is determined by comparison with readings obtained on the calibrators. In most spectrophotometers, digital hardware and software are integral components and perform these functions automatically.

Figure 10-4 illustrates schematically a typical double-beam instrument that uses a light-beam chopper (a rotating wheel with alternate silvered sections and cutout sections) inserted after the exit slit. A system of mirrors passes portions of the light reflected off the chopper alternately through the sample and a reference cuvet onto a common detector. The chopped-beam approach, using one detector, compensates for light source variation and for sensitivity changes in the detector.

Components

The basic components of a spectrophotometer include (1) a light source, (2) a device to isolate light of a desired wavelength, (3) a cuvet, (4) a photodetector, (5) a readout device, and (6) a data system.

Light Sources

Types of light sources used in spectrophotometers include incandescent lamps, xenon discharge lamps, light-emitting diodes, and lasers.

Incandescent, Arc, and Cathode Lamps. The light source for measurements in the visible portion of the spectrum is usually a tungsten light bulb. The lifetime of a tungsten filament is greatly increased by the presence of a low pressure of iodine or bromine vapor within the lamp. An example is the *quartz-halogen* lamp, which has a fused-silica envelope and which provides high-intensity light over a wide spectrum for extended operating periods (2000 to 5000 hours) before replacement is necessary.

However, a tungsten light source does not supply sufficient radiant energy for measurements in the UV region (below 320 nm). In the UV region of the spectrum, hydrogen and deuterium lamps, as well as high-pressure mercury and xenon arc lamps, provide sources of continuous spectra in the UV region with some sharp emission lines. These sources are more commonly used in UV absorption measurements. Low-pressure mercury vapor lamps also provide spectra in the UV region and are useful for calibration purposes, but they are not very practical for absorbance measurements, because of their limited wavelengths.

Mercury arc lamps emit an intense 254-nm resonance line and are widely used as detectors in high-performance liquid chromatography (HPLC) (see Chapter 13). Alternatively, some HPLCs employ a miniature hollow cathode lamp as a very-narrow-wavelength intense source. For example, a zinc hollow cathode lamp emits a line at 214 nm that is close to the maximum wavelength of peptide bond absorption (206 nm); this emission property permits the usage of such lamps to measure peptides and proteins. Details on the hollow cathode lamp are found in the section on "Atomic Absorption Spectrophotometry." The hollow cathode lamp also has a long, useful lifetime if a lower-current, nonpulsed power supply is used.

Laser Sources. A laser (light amplification by stimulated emission of radiation) is a device that controls the way that energized atoms release photons; lasers are used as light sources in spectrophotometers because they provide intense light of a narrow wavelength. Through selection of different materials, different wavelength(s) of light are emitted by different types of lasers (Table 10-3).

Three properties of laser sources distinguish them from "conventional" sources: (1) spatial coherence is a property of lasers that allows beam diameters in the range of several microns; (2) lasers produce monochromatic light; and (3) lasers have pulse widths that vary from microseconds (flash lamp–pulsed lasers) to nanoseconds (nitrogen lasers) to picoseconds or less (mode-locked lasers) in duration. Air-cooled argon ion lasers produce about 25 mW of energy output at 488 nm and have plasma tube lifetimes of 6000 hours or longer. Continuous-wave dye lasers typically use an argon ion laser with an output of 1 W or less as an energy pump and use different fluorescent dyes to achieve excitation wavelength ranges of 400 to 800 nm. Helium-neon and helium-cadmium lasers are useful because of their low cost and ease of operation, and because they emit a number of excitation wavelengths; however, the power output of helium-neon lasers has been limited to about 2 mW at 594 nm.

Infrared diode lasers are used in compact disc players and laser printers, and in bar code readers (see Chapter 19). They are solid-state devices, typically constructed of gallium arsenide, and energy is pumped into them at a low potential of −1.5 V. Depending on its construction, the wavelength output of the laser ranges from 550 to 1810 nm. Development of inexpensive near-IR lasers has led to interest in using reflective techniques in the near-IR region of the spectrum (0.8 to 2.5 μm wavelength). Reflectance spectrophotometry is now used clinically for the transcutaneous measurement of bilirubin in neonates.[14] Another application of reflectance spectrophotometry is measurement of blood oxygen saturation in near-IR and IR regions.

TABLE 10-3 Various Types of Lasers and the Wavelengths at Which They Operate

Laser	Wavelengths, nm
Argon fluoride	193
Argon fluoride	248
Helium-cadmium	325 or 442
Nitrogen	337
Argon (blue)	488
Argon (green)	514
Helium-neon (green)	543
Light-emitting diode—GaP	550 or 700
Rhodamine 6G dye (tunable)	570-650
Laser diode (AlGaInP, GaAlAs)	633-1660
Helium-neon (red)	633
Ruby ($CrAlO_3$) (red)	694
Light-emitting diode—GaAs	880
Light-emitting diode—Si	1100
Neodymium-YAG (yttrium aluminum garnet)	1064
Carbon dioxide	9300, 9600, 10,300, or 10,600

Spectral Isolation

Radiant energy of a desired wavelength can be isolated and that of other wavelengths excluded in various ways, including the use of (1) filters (interference or dichroic filters), (2) prisms, and (3) diffraction gratings. Combinations of lenses and slits may be inserted before or after the monochromatic device to render light rays parallel or to isolate narrow portions of the light beam. Variable slits may be used to permit adjustments in total radiant energy to reach the photocell.

Filters. The simplest type of filter is a thin layer of colored glass. Certain metal complexes or salts, dissolved or suspended in glass, produce colors corresponding to the predominant wavelengths transmitted. The spectral purity of a filter or other monochromator is usually described in terms of its *spectral bandwidth.* This is defined as the width, in nanometers, of the spectral transmittance curve at a point equal to one half the peak transmittance. Because glass filters have spectral bandwidths of approximately 50 nm, they are referred to as *wide-bandpass filters.*

Other glass filters include narrow-bandpass and sharp-cutoff types. Operationally, a cutoff filter typically shows a sharp rise in transmittance over a narrow portion of the spectrum and is used to eliminate light below a given wavelength. Historically, narrow-bandpass filters were constructed by combining two or more sharp-cutoff filters or regular filters. Currently, however, the availability of high-intensity light sources now favors the use of narrow-bandpass interference filters.

A narrow-bandpass interference or dichroic filter uses a dielectric material of controlled thickness sandwiched between two thinly silvered pieces of glass. The thickness of the layer determines the wavelength of energy transmitted after constructive and destructive wavelength interference caused by reflections between the glass surfaces separated by the dielectric spacing. These filters have narrow spectral bandwidths, usually from 5 to 15 nm. Because they also transmit harmonics, or multiples, of the desired wavelength, accessory glass filters are required to eliminate undesired wavelengths. Thus an interference filter designed for 620 nm will also transmit some radiation at 310 and 1240 nm unless accessory cutoff filters are provided to absorb this undesired stray light.

Prisms and Gratings. Prisms and diffraction gratings are widely used as monochromators. A *prism* separates white light into a continuous spectrum because shorter wavelengths are bent, or refracted, more than longer wavelengths as they pass through the prism. A *diffraction grating* is prepared by depositing a thin layer of aluminum-copper alloy on the surface of a flat glass plate, then ruling many small parallel grooves into the metal coating. Better gratings contain 1000 to 2000 lines/mm and must be made with great care. These are then used as molds to prepare less expensive replicas for general use in instruments.

Modern holographic gratings are made using a laser in a "high-precision machining" mode. The focused beam of the laser is accurately scanned over a photosensitive material termed a *photoresist.* After multiple lines have been scribed on the photoresist, chemicals are used to dissolve and elute the exposed photoresist to create channels that become the lines of the grating. A layer of a highly reflective material is then sputtered onto the surface of the laser-etched channels, and the grating is ready for use. A flat photoresistive surface or a concave surface can be used to make this type of grating. These types of gratings are extremely accurate, have low light scatter, and are widely used in the spectrophotometers found in clinical chemistry instruments. For example, most UV-visible spectrophotometers and virtually all IR spectrophotometers use reflective gratings. In addition, HPLC detectors frequently use a concave holographic reflective grating in their optical system.

Each line ruled on the grating, when illuminated, reflects light and gives rise to a tiny spectrum. An array of parallel wave fronts are formed that reinforce those wavelengths in phase and cancel those not in phase. The net result is a uniform linear spectrum. Some instruments contain diffraction gratings that produce spectral bandwidths of 20 nm or more; higher-priced instruments may have a resolution of 0.5 nm or less.

The flat surface grating discussed previously is called a plane *transmission grating.* Lines are engraved on the surface of a mirror, which may be a polished metal slab or a glass plate on which a thin, metallic film has been deposited. A grating may also be ruled at a specified angle, so that a maximum fraction of the radiant energy is directed into wavelengths diffracted at a selected angle. This type of grating is called an *echelette* and is said to have been given a *blaze* at a particular angle or to have been blazed at a certain wavelength (e.g., 250 nm).

Selection of a Wavelength Isolation Device. The type of monochromator chosen depends on the analytical purpose for which it is to be used. For example, narrow spectral bandwidths are required in spectrophotometers for resolving and identifying sharp absorption peaks that are closely adjacent. Lack of agreement with Beer's law will occur when a part of the spectral energy transmitted by the monochromator is not absorbed by the substance being measured. This is more commonly observed with wide-bandpass instruments. In practice, an increase in absorbance and improved linearity with concentration are usually observed with instruments that operate at narrower bandwidths of light. This is especially true for substances that exhibit a sharp peak of absorption.

The *natural bandwidth* of an absorbing substance is defined as "the bandwidth of the spectral absorbance curve at a point equal to one half of the maximum absorbance." As a general rule, for peak absorbance readings to be within 99.5% of true values, the spectral bandwidth should not exceed 10% of the natural bandwidth. For example, many chemistry procedures used in the clinical laboratory produce an absorbing species for which the natural bandwidth ranges from 40 to over 200 nm. The natural bandwidth of NADH is 58 nm (λmax = 339 nm). Therefore, for accurate measurements of this compound, a spectral bandwidth of 6 nm or less should be used.

In practice, the wavelength selected is usually at the peak of maximum absorbance to attain the maximum measurement; however, it may be desirable to choose another wavelength to minimize interfering substances. For example, turbidity readings on a spectrophotometer are greater in the blue region than in the red region of the spectrum, but the latter region is chosen for turbidity measurements to avoid absorption of light by bilirubin (460 nm) or hemoglobin (417 and 575 nm). The absorbing species developed in the alkaline picrate procedure for creatinine produces a relatively flat peak in the visible region of the spectrum at approximately 480 nm, but the reagent blank itself absorbs light strongly below 500 nm. A compromise is made by selecting a wavelength at 520 nm to minimize the contribution of the blank. Blank readings should, of course, be kept to a minimum. A small difference between two large numbers is subject to greater uncertainty; hence minimizing absorbance of the blank improves precision and accuracy. The linear working range of a method can be expanded by not measuring at the peak absorbance. However, measurements should not be taken on the steep slope of an absorption curve, because a slight error in wavelength adjustment would introduce a significant error in absorbance readings.

Cuvets

A cuvet (also often termed a cuvette) is a small vessel used to hold a liquid sample to be analyzed in the light path of a spectrometer. Cuvets may be round, square, or rectangular and are constructed from glass, silica (quartz), or plastic. Square or rectangular cuvets have plane-parallel optical surfaces and a constant light path. The most popular have a 1.0-cm light path, held to close tolerances. Ordinary borosilicate glass or plastic cuvets are suitable for measurements in the visible portion of the spectrum. For readings below 340 nm, however, quartz cells are usually required. Some plastic cells have good clarity in both the visible and UV range but can present problems related to tolerances, cleaning, etching by solvents, and temperature deformations. Many of the plastic cuvets are designed for disposable, single-use applications. However, in many clinical analyzers, cuvets are cleaned and reused many times before optical degradation requires them to be replaced.

Cuvets must be clean and optically clear, because etching or deposits on the surface affect absorbance values. Cuvets used in the visible range are cleaned by copious rinsing with tap water and distilled water. Alkaline solutions should not be left standing in cuvets for prolonged periods, because alkali slowly dissolves glass and produces etching. Cuvets may be cleaned in mild detergent or soaked in a mixture of concentrated HCl: water: ethanol (1:3:4). Cuvets should never be soaked in dichromate cleaning solution, because the solution is hazardous and tends to adsorb onto and discolor the glass.

Cuvets used for measurements in the UV region should be handled with special care. Invisible scratches, fingerprints, or residual traces of previously measured substances may be present and may absorb significantly. A good practice is to fill all such cuvets with distilled water and measure the absorbance for each against a reference blank over the wavelengths to be used. This value should be essentially zero.

Photodetectors

A *photodetector* is a device that converts light into an electric signal that is proportional to the number of photons striking its photosensitive surface. The photomultiplier tube is a commonly used photodetector for measuring light intensity in the UV and visible regions of the spectrum. Alternatively, photodiodes are solid-state devices that are also used in modern instruments. In older instruments, barrier layer cells (also known as *photovoltaic cells*) were used as photodetectors, because they were rugged and less expensive.

Photomultiplier Tubes. A photomultiplier tube (PMT) contains (1) a cathode, (2) a light-sensitive metal, and (3) a series of dynodes, all of which are enclosed in an evacuated glass enclosure. As many as 10 to 15 stages or dynodes are present in common photomultipliers. Photons that strike the photoemissive cathode emit electrons that are accelerated toward the dynodes. Additional electrons are generated at each dynode. Depending on the number of dynodes and the accelerating voltage, the cascading effect creates 10^5 to 10^7 electrons for each photon hitting the first cathode. This amplified signal is finally collected at the anode, where it can be measured.

When such a tube is operated, voltage is applied between the photocathode and each successive stage. The normal incremental increase in voltage at each photomultiplier stage is from 50 to 100 V larger than that of the previous stage (Figure 10-5). Typically, a conventional PMT tube has approximately 1500 V applied to it.

PMTs have (1) extremely rapid response times, (2) are very sensitive, and (3) are slow to fatigue. Because these tubes are very sensitive and have a rapid response, they must be carefully shielded from all stray light. A PMT with the voltage applied should never be exposed to room light because it will

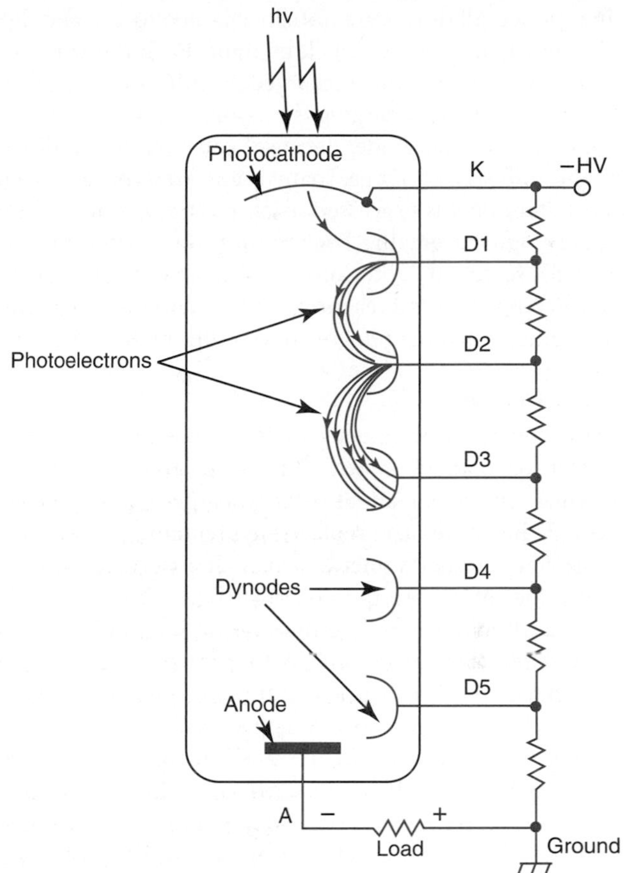

Figure 10-5 Schematic diagrams of a glass photomultiplier tube.

burn out. The rapid response times of PMTs are needed when a spectrophotometer is being used to determine an absorption spectrum of a compound. Also, PMTs are sensitive over a wide range of wavelengths.

When voltage is applied to a PMT in the absence of any incident light, some current is usually produced. This current is called *dark current*. It is desirable to have the dark current of a PMT at its lowest level because this current appears as background noise.

Photodiodes. Photodiodes are solid-state photodetectors that are fabricated from photosensitive semiconductor materials such as (1) silicon, (2) gallium arsenide, (3) indium antimonide, (4) indium arsenide, (5) lead selenide, and (6) lead sulfide. These materials absorb light over a characteristic wavelength range (e.g., 250 nm to 1100 nm for silicon). Their development and use as detectors in spectrophotometers have resulted in instruments capable of measuring light at a multitude of wavelengths. When a photodetector consists of two-dimensional arrays of diodes, it is known as a photodiode array. Each photodetector within the array responds to a specific wavelength. For example, photodiode arrays have been designed to have a 2-nm resolution per diode from 200 to 340 nm, and a 1-nm resolution per diode from 340 to 800 nm.

In practice, all diodes are initially charged to 5 V, and they discharge when they are struck by light. Each diode then is sequentially scanned and recharged to 5 V. The amount of energy required for recharging is proportional to the quantity of light striking that diode. Because scan time for all diodes is in the millisecond range, many scans are typically taken. The resultant data is processed using a variety of algorithms, including signal averaging, background subtraction, and correction for scattered light. Consequently, an optical spectrum of an ongoing chemical reaction can be monitored as a function of time with a high degree of resolution and accuracy.

Readout Devices

Electrical energy from a detector is displayed on some type of meter or readout system. In the past, analog devices were widely used as readout devices in spectrophotometers. However, they have been replaced by digital readout devices that provide a visual numeric display of absorbance or converted values of concentrations. Spectrophotometers may be equipped with recorders in addition to or instead of a digital display. These are synchronized to provide line traces of transmittance or absorbance as a function of time or wavelength. When a continuous tracing of absorbance versus wavelength is recorded, the resultant display is called an *absorption spectrum.* If a substance absorbs light, distinct peaks of absorbance will be observed (see Figure 10-1). Measuring the absorption spectra of an unknown sample and comparing them with spectra from known compounds is very useful for qualitative purposes. For example, this type of procedure is especially useful for identification of drugs that absorb in the UV region.

Performance Parameters

In most spectrophotometric analytical procedures, the absorbance of an unknown is compared directly with that of a calibrator or a series of calibrators. Under these circumstances, minor errors in wavelength calibration, variation in spectral bandwidths, and the presence of stray light are compensated for and usually do not contribute serious errors. Use of a series of calibrators covering a wide range of concentrations also provides a measure of linearity (i.e., agreement with Beer's law for a given procedure and instrument). When calculations are based on published or previously determined values for molar absorptivities or absorption coefficients, however, the spectrophotometer must be checked more rigorously. Performance verification of spectrophotometers on a periodic basis also improves reliability of routine comparative analyses.

To verify that a spectrophotometer is performing satisfactorily, the device must be shown to be able to operate within the specifications provided for it. Parameters to be tested include (1) wavelength accuracy, (2) spectral bandwidth, (3) stray light, (4) linearity, and (5) photometric accuracy.

The National Institute of Standards and Technology (NIST) provides several standard reference materials (SRMs) for spectrophotometry that are useful in the calibration or verification of the performance of photometers or spectrophotometers (e.g., SRM 930e is for the verification and calibration of the transmittance and absorbance scales of visible absorption spectrometers) (http://www.nist.gov, accessed March 23, 2011).

The Institute for Reference Materials and Measurements (IRMM) belongs to the European Commission and provides reference materials for verification of the performance of photometers or spectrophotometers. These materials are listed in the IRMM ERM Reference Materials Catalogue (http://www.irmm.jrc.be, accessed March 23, 2011).

Wavelength Calibration

With narrow-spectral-bandwidth instruments, a *holmium oxide glass* may be scanned over the range of 280 to 650 nm. This material shows very sharp absorbance peaks at defined wavelengths, and the operator may compare the wavelength scale readings that produce maximum absorbance with established values. If compared values do not coincide, a calibration correction table can be constructed to relate scale readings to true wavelengths. A typical spectral transmittance curve for holmium oxide glass is shown in Figure 10-6. Selected absorption peaks for this filter, which are suitable for calibration purposes, occur at the following wavelengths: 279.3, 418.5, 287.6, 536.4, 333.8, 637.5, and 360.8 nm. Solutions of holmium oxide in dilute perchloric acid have also been recommended and may be used with any spectrophotometer.

With broader-bandpass instruments, a didymium filter may be used to verify wavelength settings. This filter should show a minimum percent transmittance at 530 nm against an air blank (Figure 10-7). Because didymium has several absorption peaks, the setting should be verified grossly by visual examination of transmitted light. This light should appear green at 530 nm.

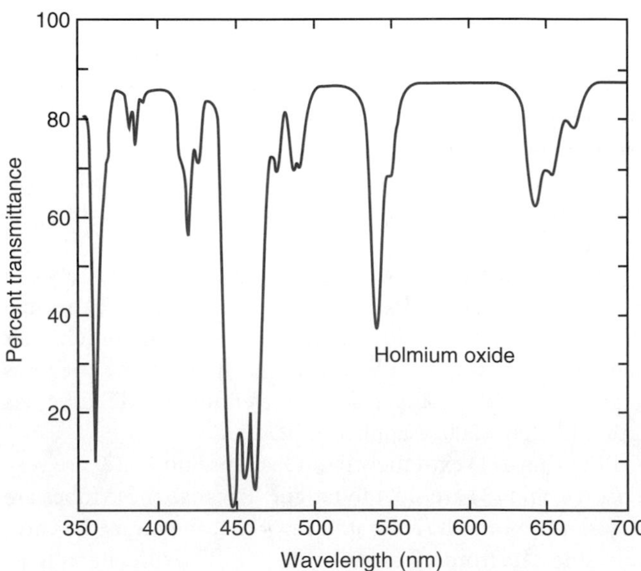

Figure 10-6 Spectral transmittance curve of holmium oxide filter.

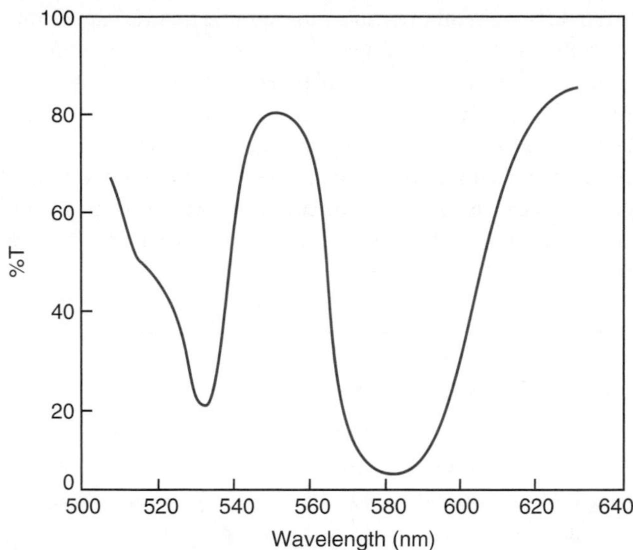

Figure 10-7 Spectral transmittance curve of a didymium filter (Perkin-Elmer Model 35 spectrophotometer, 8-nm nominal spectral bandwidth).

Spectral Bandwidth

The apparent width of an emission band at half-peak height is taken to be the spectral bandwidth of the instrument. The spectral bandwidth may also be calculated from the manufacturer's specifications. Interference filters with spectral bandwidths of 1 to 2 nm are available and may be used to check those instruments with a nominal spectral bandwidth of 8 nm or more.

Stray Light

Stray light, in general terms, is radiation of wavelengths outside the narrow band nominally transmitted by the monochromator that hits the detector. A perfect monochromator would transmit light only within its bandpass. In practice, scattering and diffraction inside the monochromator introduce light of other wavelengths into the exit beam. This light is further modified by other components of the spectrophotometer and by the sample itself. Stray light is usually defined as a ratio or percent to the total detected light.

Other sources of unwanted light include light leaks and fluorescence of the sample. Light leaks should be excluded by covering the cell compartments. Light arising from fluorescence can increase the signal to the detector and cause an apparent decrease in absorbance. These sources of light are not included in the usual definition of stray light.

The major effect of stray light on the performance of a spectrophotometer is an absorbance error, especially in the upper end of the absorbance range of the instrument. Most spectrophotometers are equipped with one or more stray-light filters. Thus a blue filter is used with a tungsten lamp for wavelength settings below about 400 nm. When the spectrophotometer is set to 350 nm, for example, most of the stray light is of wavelengths in the visible range. The blue filter absorbs most of the visible light but transmits well in this UV portion of the spectrum. By analogy, a red filter is used for wavelengths in the range of 650 to 800 nm.

Cutoff filters are satisfactory for the detection of stray light. These may be of glass, similar to the stray-light filters discussed previously, and produce a sharp cut in the spectrum with almost complete absorption on one side and high transmittance on the other. Liquid cutoff filters are satisfactory and convenient in the UV range, where stray light is usually more of a problem. A 50-g/L aqueous solution of sodium nitrite should show essentially 0% *T* when read against water over the range of 300 to 385 nm. Acetone, read against water, should show 0% *T* over the range of 250 to 320 nm.

TABLE 10-4 Absorbance Values for Acidic Potassium Dichromate Solutions on a Calibrated Spectrophotometer

	Absorbance	
Wavelength, nm	**Solution A**	**Solution B**
235 (min)	0.626 ± 0.009	1.251 ± 0.019
257 (max)	0.727 ± 0.007	1.454 ± 0.015
313 (min)	0.244 ± 0.004	0.488 ± 0.007
350 (max)	0.536 ± 0.005	1.071 ± 0.011

Photometric Accuracy

Neutral density filters (SRM 1930) available from the NIST are used to check an instrument's photometric accuracy. In addition, solutions of potassium dichromate ($K_2Cr_2O_7$) may be used for overall checks on photometric accuracy. In practice, analytical reagent grade $K_2Cr_2O_7$ is dried at 110 °C for 1 hour, and then the following solutions in 0.005 mol/L sulfuric acid are prepared:

Solution A: 0.0500 g/L for the absorbance range from 0.2 to 0.7

Solution B: 0.1000 g/L for the absorbance range from 0.4 to 1.4

Measurements should be made in 10-mm cells with the temperature controlled in the range of 15 to 25 °C, using 0.005 mol/L sulfuric acid as the reference. Table 10-4 gives the expected values for the two absorbance maxima and minima of the solutions based on literature values. Because the natural bandwidth of solution A at 350 nm is approximately 63 nm, the values shown apply strictly to spectrophotometers with a spectral bandwidth of 6 nm or less.

Multiple-Wavelength Readings

Background interference due to interfering chromogens can often be eliminated or minimized by inclusion of blanks or by reading absorbance at two or three wavelengths. In one approach, termed *bichromatic,* absorbance is measured at two wavelengths—one corresponding to peak absorbance and another at a point near the base of the peak to serve as a baseline. The difference in absorbance at the two wavelengths is related to concentration.

Before the correction is used, knowledge of the shape of the absorption curve for the substance of interest and of the interference is required. The linearity of the baseline shift should be verified by measuring the absorption spectrum of commonly encountered interferences. Care should be exercised in the use of the correction because if it is not properly used, it may introduce larger errors than would be observed without correction. For example, such a situation may occur if the background reading is not linear over the region measured.

REFLECTANCE PHOTOMETRY

In *reflectance photometry,* diffuse reflected light is measured. The reaction mixture in a carrier is illuminated with diffused light, and the intensity of the reflected light from the chromogen is compared with the intensity of light reflected from a reference surface. Because the intensity of reflected light is nonlinear in relation to the concentration of the analyte, the Kubelka-Munk equation or the Clapper-Williams transformation is commonly used to convert the data into a linear format (see Chapter 19). The electro-optical components used in reflectance photometry are essentially the same as those required for absorbance photometry, except that the geometry of the system is modified so that the light source and the detector are located next to each other on one side of the sample, as opposed to on opposite sides of the sample cuvet as in absorption photometry. Reflectance photometry is used as the measurement method with dry-film chemistry systems.

FLAME EMISSION AND INDUCTIVELY COUPLED PLASMA SPECTROPHOTOMETRY

Flame emission spectrophotometry is based on the characteristic emission of light by atoms of many metallic elements when given sufficient energy, such as that supplied by a hot flame. The wavelength to be used for the measurement of an element depends on the selection of a line of sufficient intensity to provide adequate sensitivity and freedom from other interfering lines at or near the selected wavelength. For example, lithium produces a red, sodium a yellow, potassium a violet, rubidium a red, and magnesium a blue color in a flame. These colors are characteristic of the metal atoms that are present as cations in solution. Under constant and controlled conditions, the light intensity of the characteristic wavelength produced by each of the atoms is directly proportional to the number of atoms that are emitting energy, which in turn is directly proportional to the concentration of the substance of interest in the sample. Although this technique once was used widely for analysis of sodium, potassium, and lithium in body fluids, it now has been replaced largely by electrochemical techniques.

Inductively coupled plasma (ICP) atomic emission spectroscopy is a technique for elemental analysis (e.g., trace metals) that uses an inductively coupled plasma to produce excited species that emit light at wavelengths characteristic of a particular element present in the sample. An ICP spectrometer consists of an optical spectrometer and an ICP torch. The torch produces an argon gas plasma (10,000°K) by means of radiofrequency induction coil and an electric spark. A nebulized sample is injected into the argon gas plasma, and elements in the sample become excited and the electrons emit energy at a characteristic wavelength as they return to ground state. The emitted light is then measured by optical spectrometry.

ATOMIC ABSORPTION SPECTROPHOTOMETRY

Atomic absorption (AA) spectrophotometry is used widely in clinical laboratories to measure elements such as aluminum, calcium, copper, lead, lithium, magnesium, zinc, and other metals.

Basic Concepts

Atomic absorption is an absorption spectrophotometric technique in which a metallic atom in the sample absorbs light of a specific wavelength. However, the element is not appreciably excited in the flame, but is merely dissociated from its chemical bonds (atomized) and placed in an unexcited or ground state (neutral atom). Thus, the ground state atom absorbs radiation at a very narrow bandwidth corresponding to its own line spectrum. A hollow cathode lamp with the cathode made of the material to be analyzed is used to produce a wavelength of light specific for the atom. Thus, if the cathode were made of sodium, sodium light at predominantly 589 nm would be emitted by the lamp. When the light from the hollow cathode lamp enters the flame, some of it is absorbed by the ground-state atoms in the flame, resulting in a net decrease in the intensity of the beam from the lamp. This process is referred to as *atomic absorption.*

A specific hollow cathode lamp serves as the light source, and the sample heated in the flame is the sample in the cuvet. The path length of the flame is the light path through the cuvet. Hence, most of the atoms are in the ground state and are able to absorb light emitted by the cathode lamp. In general, AA methods are approximately 100 times more sensitive than flame emission methods. In addition, owing to the unique specificity of the wavelength from the hollow cathode lamp, these methods are highly specific for the element being measured.

Instrumentation

Figure 10-8 shows the basic components of an AA spectrophotometer. The hollow cathode lamp is made of the metal of the substance to be analyzed and is different for each metal analysis. In some cases, an alloy is used to make the cathode, resulting in a multielement lamp. The hollow cathode lamp usually contains argon or neon gas at a pressure of a few millimeters of mercury. An argon-filled lamp produces a blue-to-purple glow during operation, and the neon produces a reddish-orange glow inside the hollow cathode lamp. Quartz, or special glass that allows transmission of the proper

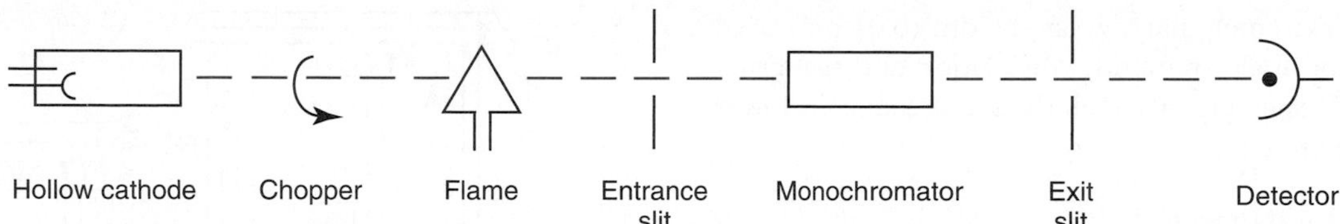

Figure 10-8 Basic components of an atomic absorption spectrophotometer.

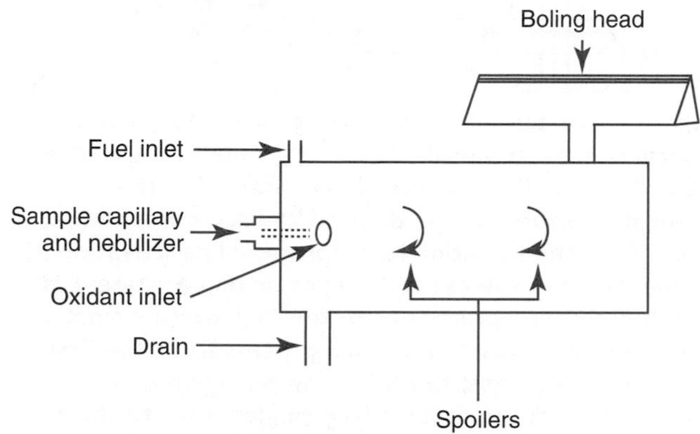

Figure 10-9 Laminar flow burner.

wavelength, is used as a window. A current is applied between the two electrodes inside the hollow cathode lamp, and metal is sputtered from the cathode into the gases inside the glass envelope. When the metal atoms collide with the neon or argon gases, they lose energy and emit their characteristic radiation. Calcium has a sharp, intense, analytical emission line at 422.7 nm, which is used most frequently for calcium analysis. In an ideal interference-free system, only calcium atoms absorb the calcium light from the hollow cathode as it passes through the flame.

A pulsed hollow cathode lamp and a tuned amplifier are incorporated into most AA instruments. Operationally, the power to the hollow cathode lamp is pulsed, so that light is emitted by the lamp at a certain number of pulses per second. On the other hand, all of the light originating from the flame is continuous. When light leaves the flame, it is composed of pulsed, unabsorbed light from the lamp and a small amount of nonpulsed flame spectrum and sample emission light. The detector senses all light, but the amplifier is electrically tuned to the pulsed signals and can subtract the background light measured when the lamp is off and the total light that includes both lamp and flame background light. In this way, the electronics, in conjunction with the monochromator, discriminates between the flame background emission and the sample atomic absorption.

Figure 10-9 shows a laminar flow premix burner and illustrates how the sample is aspirated, volatilized, and burned to form atoms of the metal in the gas phase. Note that the gases are mixed and the sample is atomized before it is burned. An advantage of this system is that the larger droplets go to waste while the fine mist enters the flame, thus producing a less noisy signal.

In *flameless AA* techniques (carbon rod or "graphite furnace"), the sample is placed in a depression on a carbon rod in an enclosed chamber. Strips of tantalum or platinum metal may also be used as sample cups. In successive steps, the temperature of the rod is raised to dry, char, and finally atomize the sample into the gas phase in the chamber. The atomized element then absorbs energy from the corresponding hollow cathode lamp. This approach is more sensitive than conventional flame methods and permits determination of trace metals in small samples of blood or tissue.

With flameless AA, a novel approach used to correct for background absorption is called the *Zeeman correction.*[16] In Zeeman background correction, the light source or the atomizer is placed in a strong magnetic field. In practice, because Zeeman correction requires special lamps, the analyte is placed in the magnetic field. The intense magnetic field splits the degenerate (i.e., of equal energy) atomic energy levels into two components that are polarized parallel and perpendicular to the magnetic field, respectively. The parallel component is at the resonance line of the source, whereas the two perpendicular components are shifted to different wavelengths. The two components interact differently with polarized light. A polarizer is placed between the source and the atomizer, and two absorption measurements are taken at different polarizer settings. One measures both analyte and background absorptions, A_t, the other only the background absorption, A_{bc}. The difference between the two absorption readings is the corrected absorbance.

The major advantage of the Zeeman correction method is that the same light source at the same wavelength is used to measure the total and the background absorption. The implementation is complex and expensive, and the strength of the magnetic field needs to be optimized for every element, but the method gives more accurate results at higher background levels than are attained with the other correction techniques.

Interferences in Atomic Absorption Spectrophotometry

Interferences in AA spectroscopy are divided into spectral and nonspectral interferences.

Spectral Interferences

Spectral interferences include absorption by other closely absorbing atomic species, absorption by molecular species, scattering by nonvolatile salt particles or oxides, and background emission (which can be electronically filtered). Absorption by other atomic species usually is not a problem because of the extremely narrow bandwidth (0.01 nm) used in the absorption measurements. Absorption and scattering by molecular species are particularly problematic in lower atomizing temperatures.

Nonspectral Interferences

Nonspectral interferences may be nonspecific or specific. *Nonspecific interferences* affect nebulization by altering the viscosity, surface tension, or density of the analyte solution, and consequently the sample flow rate. Certain contaminants also decrease desolvation and atomization efficiency by lowering the atomizer temperature. *Specific interferences* are also called *chemical interferences* because they are more analyte dependent. *Solute volatilization interference* refers to the situation in which the contaminant forms nonvolatile species with the analyte. An example is phosphate interference in the determination of calcium that is caused by the formation of calcium–phosphate complexes. The phosphate interference is overcome by adding a cation, usually lanthanum or strontium; the cation competes with calcium for the phosphate. Enhancement effects are also observed, in which the addition of contaminants increases the volatilization efficiency. Such is the case with aluminum, which normally forms nonvolatile oxides but in the presence of hydrofluoric acid forms more volatile aluminum fluoride. *Dissociation interferences* affect the degree of dissociation of the analyte. Analytes that form oxides or hydroxides are especially susceptible to dissociation interferences. *Ionization interference* occurs when the presence of an easily ionized element, such as K, affects the degree of ionization of the analyte, which leads to changes in the analyte signal. Ionization interference is controlled by adding a relatively high concentration of an element that is easily ionized to maintain a more consistent concentration of ions in the flame and to suppress ionization of the analyte. In the case of *excitation interference,* the analyte atoms are excited in the atomizer, with subsequent emission at the absorption wavelength. This type of interference is more pronounced at higher temperatures.

FLUOROMETRY

Fluorescence refers to the condition when a molecule absorbs light at one wavelength and reemits light at a longer wavelength. An atom or molecule that fluoresces is termed a *fluorophore. Fluorometry* is defined as the measurement of emitted fluorescent light. Fluorometric analysis is a widely used method of quantitative analysis in the chemical and biological sciences; it is a very accurate and sensitive technique.

Basic Concepts

Figure 10-10 illustrates the relationship between absorption, fluorescence, and phosphorescence. As indicated, each molecule contains a series of closely spaced energy levels. Absorption of a quantum of light energy by a molecule causes the transition of an electron from the singlet ground state to one of a number of possible vibrational levels of its first singlet state. The actual number of molecules in the excited state under typical reaction conditions and excited with a typical 150-W light source is very small and is estimated to be about 10^{-13} mole per mole of fluorophore. Once the molecule is in an excited state, it returns to its original energy state in several ways. These include (1) radiation-less vibrational equilibration, (2) the fluorescence process from the excited singlet state, (3) quenching of the excited singlet state, (4) radiation-less crossover to a triplet state, (5) quenching of the first triplet state, and (6) the phosphorescence process of light emission from the triplet state.

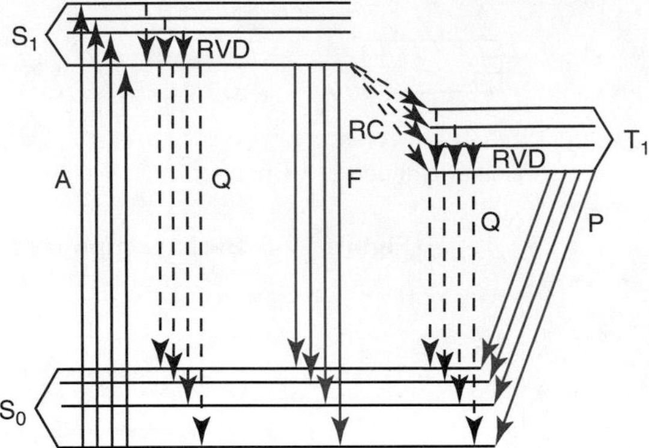

Figure 10-10 Luminescence energy-level diagram of typical organic molecule. S_0 is the ground-level singlet state; S_1 is the first excited singlet state; *A* is the absorption process; T_1 is the first excited triplet state; and *RVD* is the radiation-less vibrational deactivation. *Q* is quenching of the excited singlet or triplet state; *F* is the fluorescence process from the first excited singlet state; *P* is the phosphorescence process from the first excited triplet state; and *RC* is the radiation-less crossover from the first excited singlet state to the first excited triplet state.

As shown in Figure 10-10, vibrational equilibration before fluorescence results in some loss of the excitation energy. The emitted fluorescence light is therefore of less energy or has a longer wavelength than the excitation light. The difference between the maximum wavelength of the excitation light and the maximum wavelength of the emitted fluorescence light is a constant referred to as the *Stokes shift.* This constant is a measure of energy lost during the lifetime of the excited state (radiation-less vibrational deactivation) before returning to the ground singlet level (fluorescence emission).

Time Relationships of Fluorescence Emission

The time required for a molecule to absorb radiant energy and to be promoted to an excited state is approximately 10^{-15} s. The length of time for vibrational equilibration to occur to the lowest excited state is of the order of 10^{-14} to 10^{-12} s. The length of time required for fluorescence emission to occur is of the order of 10^{-8} to 10^{-7} s. Relatively speaking, there is a considerable time delay between the (1) absorption of light energy, (2) return to the lowest excited state, and (3) emission of fluorescence light. This time relationship is shown in Figure 10-11. In this figure, phase I represents the

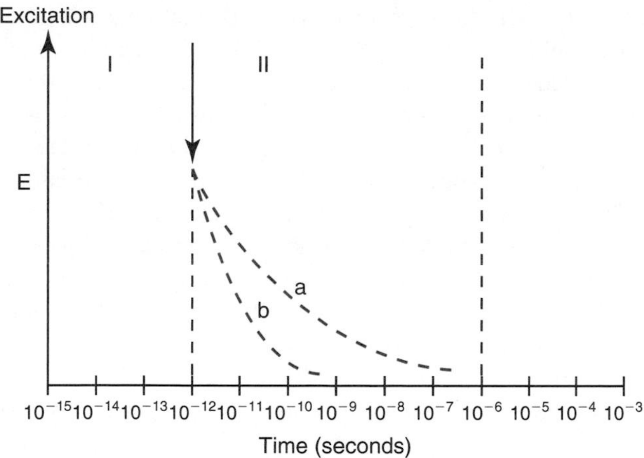

Figure 10-11 Fluorescence decay process. *E* is the absorption of energy; *I* is the vibrational deactivation time phase; *II* is the fluorescence emission time phase; *a* is long fluorescence decay time; and *b* is short fluorescence decay time.

time period between absorbance of light energy and radiationless loss of energy during vibrational rearrangement to the lowest excited energy state. This time period is represented by the up and down arrows in the diagram. Phase II shows the emission and decay of a short-lived *(b)* and a longer-lived *(a)* fluorophore. If the fluorescence emission is measured over time following a pulse of light from an excitation source, such as a xenon lamp or laser, the intensity of the emitted light decays as a first-order process similar to radioactive decay (i.e., phase II of Figure 10-11). The time required for the emitted light to reach 1/e of its initial intensity, where *e* is the Naperian base 2.718, is called the average lifetime of the excited state of the molecule, or the fluorescence decay time.

The time delay between absorption of quanta of energy and fluorescence is used in fluorescence instrumentation called *time-resolved fluorometers.*[8] Advantages of a time-resolved fluorometer include the elimination of background light scattering due to Rayleigh and Raman signals and a short-lived fluorescence background with a consequent dramatic increase in signal-to-noise and detection sensitivity.

Time-resolved fluorometry[3] falls into one of two categories, depending on how the fluorescence emission response is measured: (1) pulse fluorometry, in which the sample is illuminated with an intense brief pulse of light and the intensity of the resulting fluorescence emission is measured as a function of time with a fast detector system, or (2) phase fluorometry, in which a continuous-wave laser illuminates the sample, and the fluorescence emission response is monitored for impulse and frequency response.[8]

Relationship of Concentration and Fluorescence Intensity

The relationship of concentration to the intensity of fluorescence emission is derived from the Beer-Lambert law. By expansion through a Taylor series, rearrangement, logarithm base conversion, and basic assumptions about dilute solutions, the following equation is obtained:

$$F = ø[I_o(2.3 - abc)] \quad (8)$$

where

F = relative fluorescence intensity
ø = fluorescence efficiency (i.e., the ratio between quanta of light emitted and quanta of light absorbed)
I_0 = initial excitation intensity
a = molar absorptivity
b = volume element defined by geometry of the excitation and emission slits
c = the concentration in mol/L

Equation (8) indicates that fluorescence intensity is directly proportional to the concentration of the fluorophore and the excitation intensity. This relationship holds only for dilute solutions, in which absorbance is less than 2% of the exciting radiation; the fluorescence intensity becomes nonlinear as the absorbance of the solution increases to above 2% of the exciting radiation. This phenomenon, called the *inner filter effect,* is discussed in more detail in a later section. Other factors influencing the measurement of fluorescence intensity include the sensitivity of the detector and the degree of background light scatter seen by the detector.

Fluorescence intensity measurements are more sensitive than absorbance measurements. The magnitude of absorbance of a chromophore in solution is determined by its concentration and the path length of the cuvet. The magnitude of fluorescence intensity of a fluorophore is determined by its concentration, the path length, and the intensity of the light source. The sensitivity of fluorescence measurements can be 100 to 1000 times greater than the sensitivity of absorbance measurements through the use of more intense light sources, digital signal filtering techniques, and sensitive emission photometers. All of these are incorporated into conventional spectrofluorometric instrumentation, described later in this chapter.

Frequently, fluorescence measurements are expressed in relative intensity units. The word *relative* is used because the intensity measured is not an absolute quantity. It is a small part of the total fluorescence emission, and its magnitude is defined by the instrument slit width, detector sensitivity, monochromator efficiency, and excitation intensity. Because these are instrument-related variables, establishing an absolute intensity unit for a given concentration of a fluorophore that is valid from instrument to instrument is difficult, if not impossible.

Fluorescence Polarization

Light is composed of electrical and magnetic waves at right angles to each other. Light waves produced by standard excitation sources have their electrical vectors oriented randomly. Light waves, passed through certain crystalline materials (polarizers), have their electrical vectors oriented in a single plane and are said to be plane-polarized. Fluorophores absorb light most efficiently in the plane of their electronic energy levels. If their rotational relaxation (Brownian movement) is slower than their fluorescence decay time, as is the case for large fluorescent-labeled molecules, the emitted fluorescence light will be polarized. Because small molecules have rotational relaxation times that are much shorter than their fluorescence decay time, their emitted fluorescence light is depolarized. However, if the small fluorescent molecule is attached to a macromolecule, or if it is placed in a viscous solution, the small molecule will emit polarized light. Fluorescence polarization, *P*, is defined by the following equation:

$$P = \frac{(I_v - I_h)}{(I_v + I_h)} \quad \textbf{(9)}$$

where

I_v = intensity of the emitted fluorescence light in the vertical plane

I_h = intensity of the emitted fluorescence light in the horizontal plane

As indicated, *P* is the difference between the two observed intensities divided by their sum. Fluorescence polarization is measured by placing a mechanically or electrically driven polarizer between the sample cuvet and the detector. A diagram of a fluorescence polarization measurement system is shown in Figure 10-12. In the normal instrumentation mode, the sample is excited with polarized light to obtain maximum sensitivity. First, the polarization analyzer is positioned to measure the intensity of the emitted fluorescence light in the vertical plane (I_v); then the polarization analyzer is rotated 90° to measure the emitted fluorescence light intensity in the horizontal plane (I_h). *P* is then calculated manually or automatically by using equation (9).

Fluorescence polarization is used to quantitate analytes by using the change in fluorescence depolarization following immunologic reactions (see Chapter 16). Quantitation is accomplished by adding a known quantity of fluorescent-labeled analyte molecules to a reaction solution containing an antibody specific to the analyte. The labeled analyte binds to the antibody and causes a change in its rotational relaxation time, resulting in fluorescence polarization. The addition of a nonlabeled analyte, such as an unknown quantity of a therapeutic drug in a serum specimen, will result in competition for binding to the antibody with the fluorescent-labeled analyte. This change in binding of the fluorophore-labeled analyte causes a change in fluorescence polarization that is inversely proportional to the amount of analyte contained in a given sample. Because the change in fluorescence polarization is a direct response to the reaction mixture, the bound fluorophore need not be separated from free fluorophore. Thus fluorescence polarization is applicable to homogeneous assays of low molecular weight analytes, such as therapeutic drugs.[10]

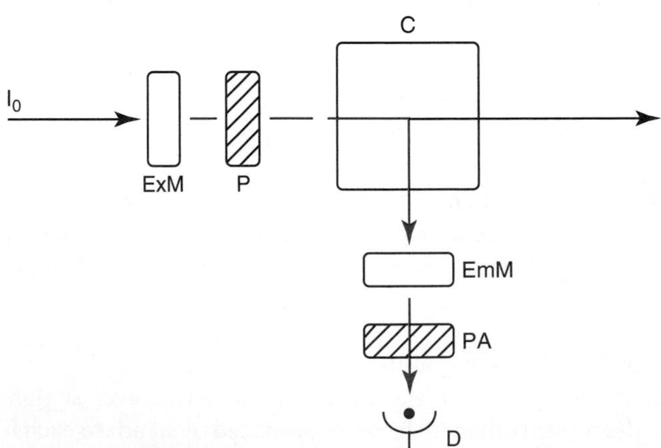

Figure 10-12 Schematic diagram of a fluorescence polarization analyzer. *P* is the polarizer used to provide polarized excitation light; *PA* is the polarizer analyzer, which is rotated to provide measurements of parallel and perpendicular polarized fluorescence emission intensity. *ExM* is the excitation monochromator; *EmM* is the emission monochromator; *D* is the detector; and *C* is the reaction cell or cuvet.

Instrumentation

Fluorometers and spectrofluorometers are used to measure fluorescence. Operationally, a fluorometer uses interference filters, glass filters, gratings, or prisms to produce monochromatic light for sample excitation and for isolation of fluorescence emission.

Components

Basic components of fluorometers and spectrofluorometers include (1) an excitation source, (2) an excitation monochromator, (3) a cuvet, (4) an emission monochromator, and (5) a detector.

Excitation Source

The absorption spectra of most fluorescent compounds of interest are in the spectral region of 300 to 700 nm. The fluorescence emission intensity is proportional to the initial excitation intensity and to concentration and size of the volume element being measured in the sample cell. Therefore, an intense lamp capable of emitting radiant energy over a large spectral region is desirable. Excitation sources used in fluorometers and spectrophotometers include xenon, quartz halogen, and mercury arc lamps and lasers. Some provide high-intensity spectra at one or more wavelengths; others provide a continuum over the spectral range of interest.

Xenon Lamp. The xenon lamp is a popular excitation source, as it provides a continuum of relatively high-intensity radiant energy over the spectral region of 250 to 800 nm. It is widely used for certain fluorescence applications because of its high energy output, stability of lamp flashes, and higher ultraviolet and visible spectral output. These flash lamps can be pulsed at rates up to 2500 pulses per second. Light output is typically in the 0.01- to 0.1-J interval, with a spectral distribution ranging from 250 to 800 nm. The life of flash lamps varies from 10^6 to 10^9 flashes, with spectral stability maintained throughout the life of the flash lamp. A limitation of xenon lamps for analytical use is arc wandering or flicker. However, the use of current-stabilized power supplies has minimized this problem and improved the performance of fluorescence instrumentation using xenon lamps.

Lasers. Laser sources (discussed earlier in the "Spectrophotometry" section) are widely used in fluorescence applications in which highly intense, well-focused, and essentially monochromatic light is required. Examples of these applications include time-resolved fluorometry, flow cytometry, pulsed laser confocal microscopy, laser-induced fluorometry, and light scattering measurements for particle size and shape. Several different types of lasers are available as an excitation source for fluorescence measurements (see Table 10-3).

Excitation and Emission Monochromator

Monochromators used in fluorescence instrumentation include interference filters, colored glass filters, gratings, and prisms. Most modern analytical instruments using interference filters use the all-dielectric multicavity filter or a hybrid Fabry-Perot coupled-dielectric-layer filter (a filter with metal reflective layers). Either type of filter is combined with appropriate sharp cutoff glass filters to form a single filter package, which removes undesired transmission of higher orders and provides narrow bandwidth, higher peak wavelength transmission, and increased band slope. The increased slope of the spectral band makes the transition from peak transmission to nontransmission more abrupt, which is very important for the spectral separation of excitation and emission bands with a small Stokes shift.

Colored glass filters selectively absorb certain wavelengths of light. These filters have been used for both excitation and emission wavelength selection, but they are more susceptible to transmitting stray light and unwanted fluorescence.

Grating monochromators are devices that isolate regions of the spectrum. The spectral resolution of the light at the slit is a function of slit width and resolution of the grating. Spectrofluorometers generally use larger slit widths than absorbance spectrophotometers to obtain higher excitation intensities. An advantage of the grating monochromator is that it provides selectivity of the excitation and emission wavelengths required when working with new fluorophores with absorbance and emission maxima for which specially fabricated interference filters may not exist. The rotation of the grating is digitally controlled when spectral scans of fluorescence excitation and emission are automated. In the conventional operation of a spectrofluorometer, the excitation wavelength or the emission wavelength is held constant, and the other is scanned. With more automated instrumentation, both excitation and emission monochromators are synchronized and scanned together at programmed rates. This provides a change in emission intensity as a function of change in excitation and emission wavelength and gives an additional dimension of specificity to fluorescence measurements. Because of their high degree of monochromaticity, lasers are used as both the excitation light source and the monochromator. When a laser is used as a combination excitation source and monochromator, a narrow-band interference filter is usually placed before the detector to eliminate additional orders of emission.

Cuvet

As with spectrophotometers, cuvets are used in fluorometers and spectrofluorometers to hold the liquid sample to be analyzed. For fluorescence instruments, the cuvets used are typically square or rectangular and are constructed from a material that allows the excitation and the emitting light to pass (glass or plastic for visible light; quartz for ultraviolet light). However, some plastic cuvets contain ultraviolet absorbers that fluoresce, causing unwanted background signal and loss of sensitivity.

With fluorometers and spectrofluorometers, placement of the cuvet and excitation beam relative to the photodetector is critical in establishing the optical geometry for fluorescence measurements. Because fluorescence light is emitted in all directions from a molecule, several excitation/emission geometries are used to measure fluorescence (Figure 10-13). Although the end-on approach allows the adaptation of a fluorescence detector to existing 180° absorption instruments, it is not widely used, because its sensitivity is limited by the quality of the excitation and/or emission interference filter pair, the excitation and/or emission spectral band overlap, and the inner filter effect. In practice, most commercial spectrofluorometers and fluorometers use the right angle–detector approach, because it minimizes the background signal that limits analytical sensitivity. The front

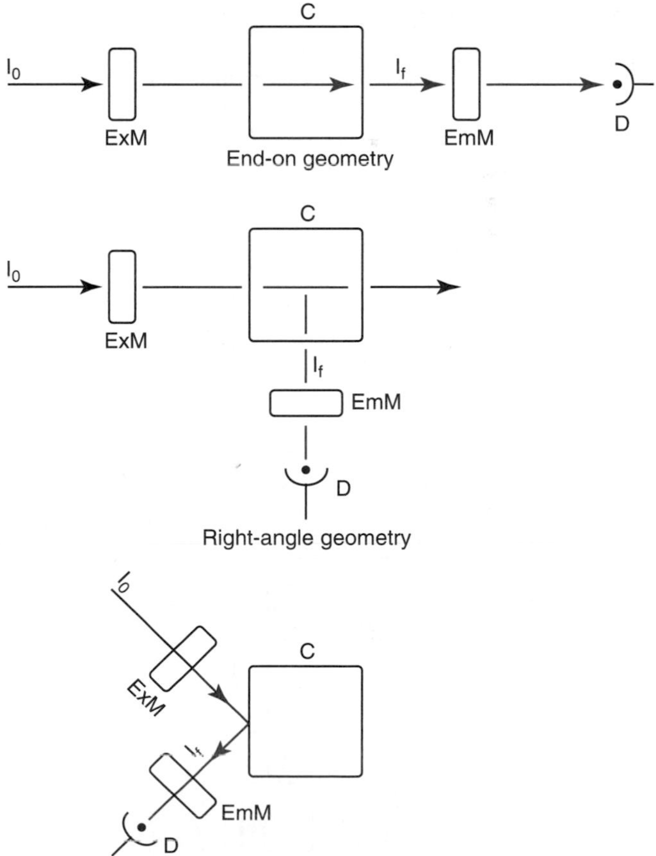

Figure 10-13 Fluorescence excitation/emission geometries: I_0 is the initial excitation energy; *ExM* is the excitation monochromator; *C* is the sample cuvet; I_f is the fluorescence intensity; *EmM* is the emission monochromator; and *D* is the detector.

surface approach provides the greatest linearity over a broad range of concentration because it minimizes the inner filter effect. The front surface approach shows similar sensitivity to the right-angle detectors but is more susceptible to background light scatter. Front surface fluorometry has been widely applied to heterogeneous solid phase fluorescence immunoassay systems.

To accommodate these different geometries, the sample cell is oriented at different angles in relation to the excitation source and the detector. Major concerns related to the geometry of the sample cell include light scattering, the inner filter effect, and the sample volume element seen by the detector. Figure 10-14, *A*, shows the sample cell and slit arrangement for a conventional fluorescence spectrophotometer with the excitation and emission slits oriented at a right angle. S_1 and S_2 designate the excitation and emission slits, respectively. The position of the emission slit and the width of the slit are important. If the emission slit is located near the front edge of the sample cell, as shown in Figure 10-14, *B*, the inner filter effect is minimized. If the emission slit width is increased, sensitivity will increase, but specificity may decrease.

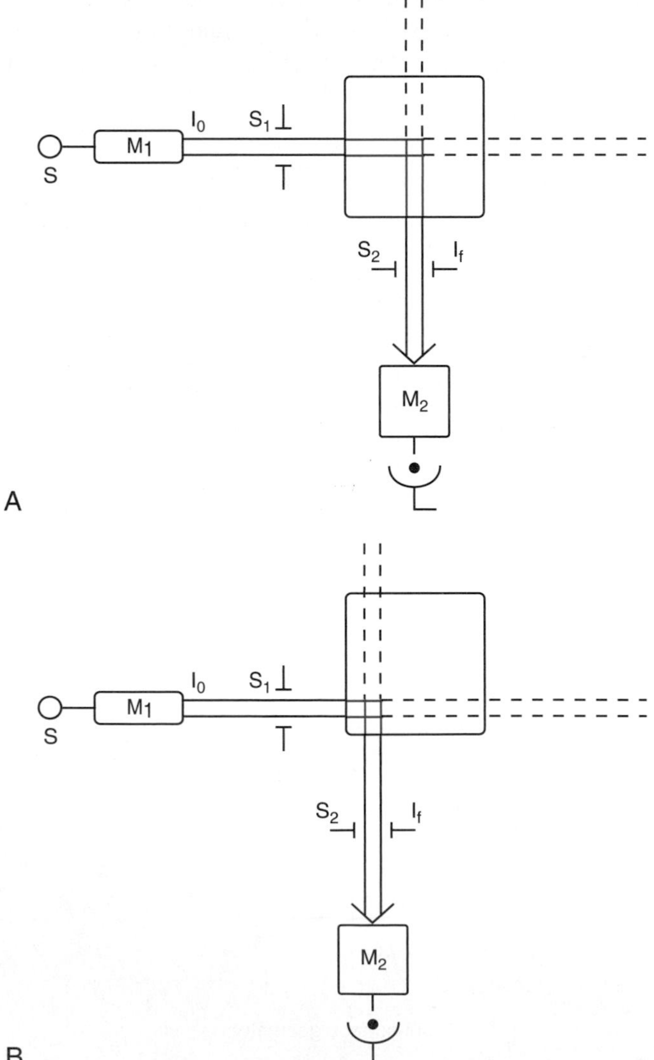

Figure 10-14 Two right-angle fluorescence sample cuvet positions. A shows the standard 90° configuration. B shows the offset positioning of the cuvet to minimize the inner filter effect.

Photodetectors

As with spectrophotometric instruments, a number of devices are used as photodetectors in fluorometric instruments, including the photomultiplier tube (PMT) and the charge-coupled detector (CCD). In addition, visual observation is used for some applications.

Visual Observation. Because the human eye is a very sensitive detector with a wide range of spectral recognition, qualitative fluorescent thin-layer chromatographic methods in the clinical laboratory use short- and long-wavelength ultraviolet lamp sources coupled with visual observation.

Photomultiplier Tube. For quantitative assays, the most commonly used detector in fluorometers and spectrofluorometers is the PMT. Important features of the PMT for fluorescence measurements consist of (1) a wide choice of spectral responses, (2) nanosecond photon response time, and (3) sensitivity. Sensitivity is due to the possible gain of 10^6 electrons at the anode of the PMT for each incident photon hitting the photo cathode.

Depending on the light level (photon flux) striking the PMT cathode and the desired sensitivity, measurement of electron flow at the PMT anode is accomplished in different ways. At high light intensities, analog techniques for measurement of PMT current are used. The analog signal is converted to a digital signal for computer use or for panel digital display. At low light levels, spikes or pulses generated at the cathode of the PMT are counted. The number of pulses that occur per unit of time is directly proportional to the intensity of emitted fluorescence light striking the PMT. This method is called *photon counting.* The use of photon counting increases the signal-to-noise ratio and decreases the lower limit of detection of the measurement of fluorophores at very low concentrations.

Charge-Coupled Detector. CCDs are multichannel devices with a dynamic range and a signal-to-noise ratio that are superior to those of PMTs.[4,21] These solid-state devices are composed of a large number of photo-detecting shift registers that are read horizontally and vertically. CCDs were first used for astronomy applications and in ground-based optical telescopes, in which sensitive low-light measurements are required. Because of their ability to detect very low levels of light, they have been used for molecular fluorescence measurement of very low concentrations of fluorescent molecules[21] and as quantitative electronic imagers for quantitative confocal microscopy.[11] A data-reading technique called *binning* has been developed that allows multielement devices to have functional elements linked together, much like rectangular slit widths.

Performance Verification

As with spectrophotometers, NIST provides a number of SRMs for use in calibration or verification of the performance of fluorometers or fluorospectrophotometers. These include SRM 936a (quinine sulfate dihydrate) for calibrating such instruments and SRM 1932 (fluorescein) for establishing a reference scale for fluorescence measurements (http://www.nist.gov/accessed April 26, 2011).

Types of Fluorometers and Spectrofluorometers

Fluorometers and fluorescence spectrophotometers that offer a variety of features are available. These features include ratio referencing, microprocessor-controlled excitation and emission monochromators, pulsed xenon light sources, photon counting, rhodamine cells for corrected spectra, polarizers, flow cells, front-surface viewing adapters, multiple cell holders, and microprocessor-based data reduction systems.

In addition to the basic spectrofluorometer discussed earlier, other types of fluorometric instruments include a ratio-referencing spectrofluorometer, a time-resolved fluorometer, a flow cytometer, and a hematofluorometer.

Ratio-Referencing Spectrofluorometer

A typical ratio-referencing spectrofluorometer is illustrated in Figure 10-15. Basically, this is a simple right-angle instrument that uses two monochromators (M1 and M2), two photomultiplier tube detectors (D1 and D2, the reference and sample PMTs), and a xenon lamp source. The light from the exciter monochromator (M1) is split, and a small portion (10%) is directed to the reference PMT (D1) for ratio-referencing purposes. The remaining excitation light is focused into the sample cuvet (C). Emission optics are positioned at a right angle to the excitation optics. An emission monochromator (M2) is used to select or scan the desired portion of the emission spectra, which is directed to the sample PMT (D2) for measurement of emission intensity. Output signals from the reference and sample PMTs are amplified (A1 and A2), and the ratio of the sample to the reference signal is provided by a digital display or a chart recorder. The operational mode of a ratio fluorometer is similar to that of a spectrofluorometer; however, only discrete excitation and emission wavelengths are available, and use of this type of instrument is precluded from scanning fluorophores to obtain emission and excitation spectra. The ratio filter fluorometer is most useful for obtaining concentration measurements at defined excitation and emission wavelengths.

The ratio-referencing spectrofluorometer is operated at fixed excitation and emission wavelength settings for concentration measurements; alternatively, it is used to measure the excitation or emission spectrum of a given compound. Measurement of the concentration of a specimen is accomplished in a similar manner as with a single-beam fluorometer. A blank and a calibrating solution are measured first; then the unknown specimens are measured. The ratio-referencing spectrofluorometer in Figure 10-15 offers two advantages over single-beam spectrofluorometers. First, it eliminates short- and long-term xenon lamp energy fluctuations (i.e., arc flicker and lamp decay) and thus minimizes the need for frequent calibration of the instrument during analysis. Second, it provides "essentially" corrected excitation spectra by compensating for wavelength-dependent energy fluctuations.

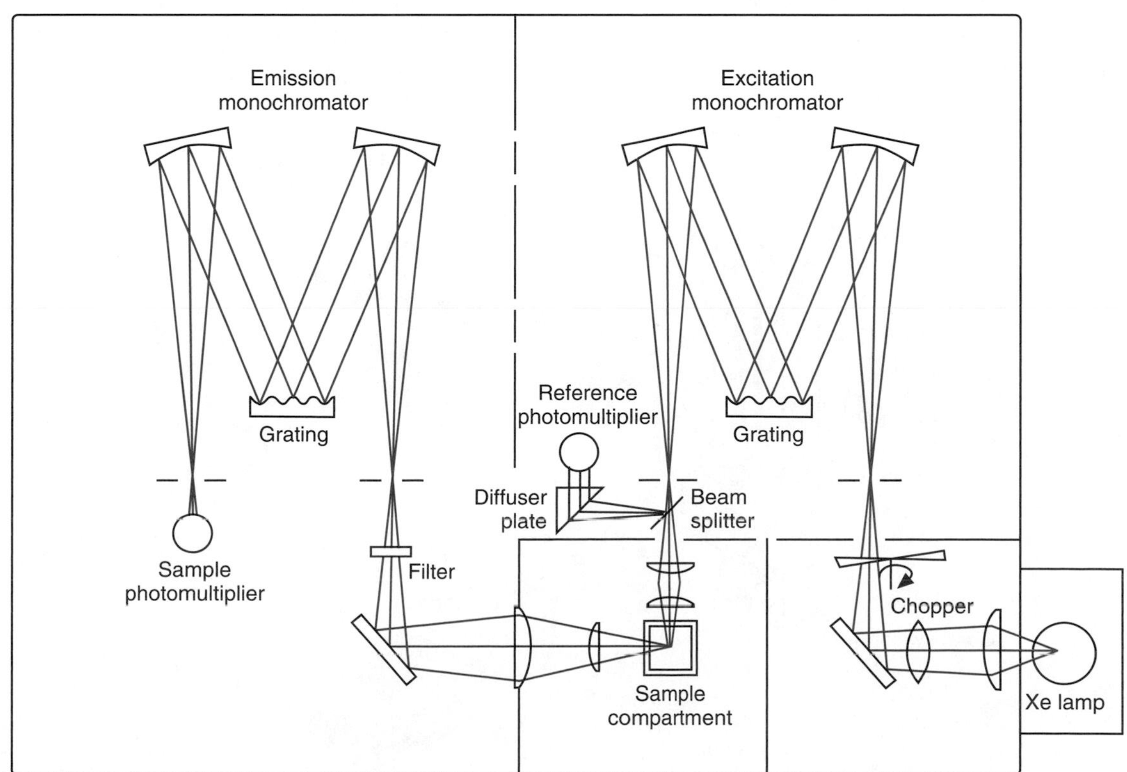

Figure 10-15 Diagram of a typical ratio-referencing spectrofluorometer.

Time-Resolved Fluorometer

The time-resolved fluorometer was introduced in the mid-1970s, when Weider developed a pulsed nitrogen laser fluorometer in conjunction with a lanthanide-based immunoassay system to measure the fluorescence decay of lanthanide chelates as a means of eliminating background interferences from light scatter and short decay time fluorescence compounds. The time-resolved fluorometer[3,17] is similar to the ratio-referencing fluorometer, with the exceptions that the light source is pulsed and the detector monitors, in a fast photon-counting mode, the exponential decay of the fluorescence signal after excitation. Time-resolved fluorometry requires the use of long-lived fluorophores, such as the lanthanide (rare earth) metal ions europium (Eu^{3+}) and samarium (Sm^{3+}). Whereas most fluorescence compounds have decay times of 5 to 100 ns, europium chelates decay in 0.6 to 100 s. Thus time-resolved fluorescence assays take advantage of the difference in lifetimes of fluorophore and background fluorescence by measuring the decaying fluorescence signal. This eliminates background interferences and at the same time averages the signal to improve the precision of measurement. Detection limits of approximately 10^{-13} mol/L can be achieved with time-resolved fluorometry; this is an improvement of about four orders of magnitude compared with conventional fluorometric measurements. For example, Eu^{3+}-labeled nanoparticles in combination with time-resolved fluorometry have been used to develop a highly sensitive immunoassay for free and total prostate-specific antigen having a functional sensitivity of 0.5 ng/L.[7,18,19]

Flow Cytometer

Cytometry refers to the measurement of physical and/or chemical characteristics of cells or, by extension, of other biological particles. Flow cytometry is a process in which such measurements are made while cells or particles pass, preferably in single file, through the measuring apparatus in a fluid stream. Flow sorting extends flow cytometry by using electrical or mechanical means to divert and collect cells with one or more measured characteristics that fall within a range or ranges of values set by the user.[13-16]

Operationally, flow cytometry combines laser-induced fluorometry with particle light scattering analysis that allows different populations of molecules, cells, or particles to be differentiated by size and shape using low-light and right-angle light scattering. The use of a laser is ideally suited for low-angle light scattering. These cells, molecules, or particles are labeled with specific fluorescent labels, such as β-phycoerythrin, fluorescein isothiocyanate, rhodamine-6G, and other dye-labeled antibodies. As they move in a fluid stream through the flow cell, simultaneous fluorescence and light scattering measurements are automatically performed by the flow cytometer. Most flow cytometers incorporate two or more fluorescence emission detection systems, so that multiple fluorescent labels can be used. In this manner, molecules, cells, or particles can be classified by size, shape, and type according to their light scattering and fluorescent properties. A schematic diagram of a flow cytometer is shown in Figure 10-16. An optical stop is placed in the 180° beam after the flow capillary to block the main laser beam and permit low-angle forward light scattering measurements. The 90° emission signal is split and directed to two PMTs to determine right-angle light scattering and detect at least two separate fluorescence emission signals. Two narrow-bandpass interference filters (530 nm and 596 nm) are placed in front of the two 90° fluorescence emission PMTs. A computer with substantial resident software is employed to reduce the

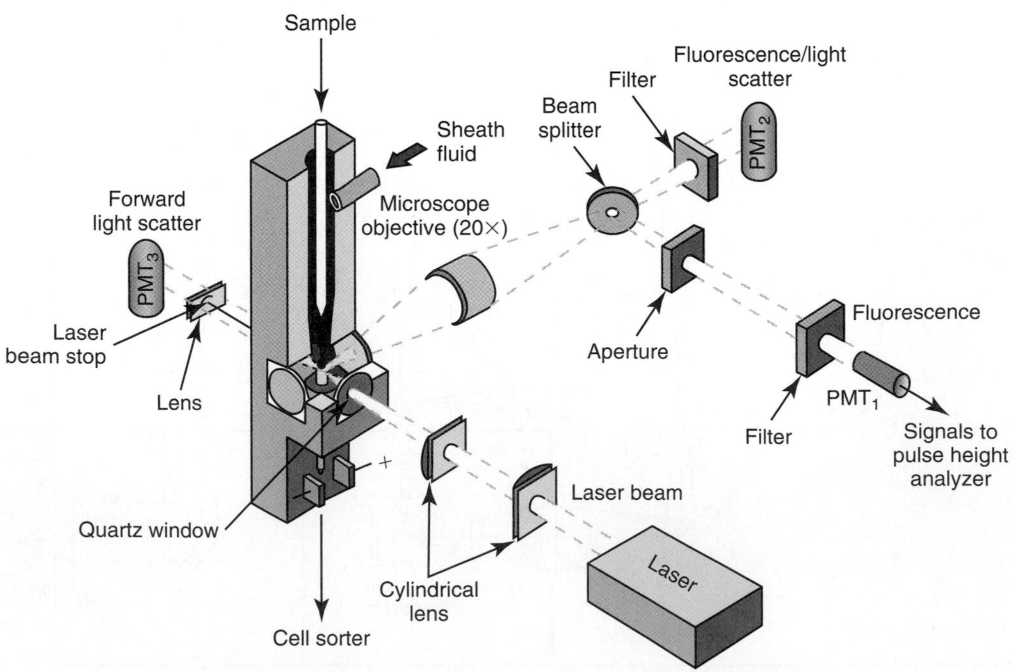

Figure 10-16 Schematic diagram of a flow cytometer.

acquired data to appropriate histograms for final result reporting. Cell-sorting electrodes are shown in the schematic drawing. Most commercial flow cytometers use one or more laser light sources. For example, the LSR II (BD Biosciences, Rockville, MD) can be equipped with seven lasers [355 nm (UV), 405 nm (violet), 488 nm (blue), 532 nm (green), 594 nm (yellow), 638 nm (red), and 785 nm (IR)], which are used to simultaneously measure 18 emission spectra.

Flow cytometers are able to measure multiple parameters, including (1) cell size (forward scatter), (2) granularity (90° scatter), (3) DNA content, (4) RNA content, (5) DNA (A + T)/(G + C) nucleotide ratios, (6) chromatin structure, (7) antigens, (8) total protein content, (9) cell receptors, (10) membrane potential, and (11) calcium ion concentration as a function of pH. These parameters are used in hematology, immunology (e.g., in T-cell subsets, tissue typing, lymphocyte stimulation, and antigen-antibody reactions), oncology (e.g., in diagnosis, prognosis, and treatment monitoring), microbiology (e.g., in bacterial identification and antibiotic sensitivity), virology, genetics (e.g., in karyotyping and carrier state detection), parasitology, and reproduction and fertility studies, and may have application in cervical cytology. Flow cytometry also has potential applications for the development of sensitive laser-induced fluoroimmunoassays. Phycoerythrin is a large phycobiliprotein molecule [molecular weight (MW) = 250,000 Da] with the fluorescence emission equivalent of 25 rhodamine-6G molecules, a quantum yield of 0.98, a broad emission spectrum of 530 to 630 nm, and low photodecomposition. It is an excellent label for cells and possibly for use in new fluoroimmunoassays.

Of particular note have been the development and use of particle-based flow cytometric assays. With this technology, a flow cytometer is combined with microspheres that are used as the solid support for conventional immunoassay, affinity assay, or DNA hybridization assay.[22] The resultant system is very flexible, and its use has led to the development of multiplexed assays that simultaneously measure many different analytes in a small sample volume.

Hematofluorometer

The *hematofluorometer* is a single-channel front-surface photofluorometer dedicated to the analysis of zinc protoporphyrin in whole blood (see Chapter 33). A typical hematofluorometer uses a quartz-tungsten lamp, a narrow-bandpass excitation filter (420 nm), front-surface optics, a narrow-bandpass filter (594 nm), and a PMT. A drop of whole blood is placed on a small rectangular glass slide that serves as a cuvet.

Limitations of Fluorescence Measurements

Factors that influence fluorescence measurements include concentration effects (e.g., inner filter effects, concentration quenching), background effects (due to Rayleigh and Raman scattering), solvent effects (e.g., interfering nonspecific fluorescence, quenching from the solvent), sample effects (e.g., light scattering, interfering fluorescence, sample adsorption), temperature effects, and photodecomposition (bleaching) of the sample.

Inner Filter Effects

The linear relationship between concentration and fluorescence emission [equation (8)] is valid when solutions that absorb less than 2% of the exciting light are used. As the absorbance of the solution increases above this amount, the relationship becomes nonlinear, a phenomenon known as the *inner filter effect.* It is caused by loss of excitation intensity across the cuvet path length as excitation light is absorbed by the fluorophore. Thus as the fluorophore becomes more concentrated, absorbance of the excitation intensity increases, and loss of the excitation light as it travels through the cuvet increases. This effect is most often encountered with a right-angle fluorescence instrument, in which the emission slits are set to monitor the center of the sample cell, where absorbance of excitation light is greater than at the front surface of the cuvet. Therefore it is less problematic if a front-surface fluorescence instrument is used. However, most fluorescence measurements are made on very dilute solutions, and the inner filter effect therefore is not a problem.

Concentration Quenching

Another related phenomenon that results in a lower quantum yield than expected is called *concentration quenching.* This can occur when a macromolecule, such as an antibody, is heavily labeled with a fluorophore, such as fluorescein isothiocyanate. When this compound is excited, the fluorescence labels are in such close proximity that radiation-less energy transfer occurs. Thus, the resulting fluorescence is much lower than expected for the concentration of the label. This is a common problem in flow cytometry and laser-induced fluorescence when attempts are made to enhance detection sensitivity by increasing the density of the fluorescing label.

Light Scattering

Light scattering—Rayleigh and Raman—limits the use of fluorescence measurements. Rayleigh scattering occurs with no change in wavelength. For fluorophores with small Stokes shifts, the excitation and emission spectra overlap and are particularly susceptible to loss of sensitivity because of background light scatter. Rayleigh-type light scatter is controlled by the use of well-defined emission and excitation interference filters, or by appropriate monochromator settings and the use of polarizers.

Raman scattering occurs with lengthening of a wavelength. This type of light scattering is independent of excitation wavelength and is a property of the solvent. Because Raman light scattering appears at longer wavelengths than the exciting radiation, it is a difficult interference to eliminate when working at very low fluorophore concentrations. As an example, the wavelength shift in water is ≈50 nm at an excitation wavelength of 365 nm, and ≈75 nm at an excitation wavelength of 436 nm. This shift would represent a problem if the excitation maximum of a fluorophore was 365 nm and the emission maximum was 415 nm. Raman light scattering is controlled by setting the excitation and emission wavelengths far enough apart to prevent the Raman scatter. It is also controlled by narrowing the slit width on the excitation monochromator. However, both options tend to decrease sensitivity.

Cuvet Material and Solvent Effects

Certain quartz glass and plastic materials that contain ultraviolet absorbers will fluoresce. Some solvents, such as ethanol, are also known to cause appreciable fluorescence. It is therefore important when developing a fluorescence assay to assess the background fluorescence of all components of the reaction mixture. Solvents and cuvets with minimal fluorescence emission are commercially available; these reagents minimize background fluorescence problems.

Quenching by the solvent can be a problem and should be investigated when a new fluorometric method is established. Quenching is related to the interaction of the fluorophore with the solvent or with a solute dissolved in the solvent. Such interaction results in loss of fluorescence owing to energy transfer or other mechanisms, but no effect on the absorbance spectrum of the fluorophore is noted. An example of quenching is the loss of fluorescence when halides are added to quinine in dilute sulfuric acid. Quenching can be a useful tool for studying molecular structure, because fluorescence emission is sensitive to and specific for changes in atomic and molecular structure.

Sample Matrix Effects

A serum or urine sample contains many compounds that fluoresce. Thus the sample matrix is a potential source of unwanted background fluorescence and must be examined when new methods are developed. The most serious contributors to unwanted fluorescence are proteins and bilirubin. However, because protein excitation maxima are in the spectral region of 260 to 290 nm, their contribution to overall background fluorescence is minor when excitation above 300 nm occurs.

Light scattering of proteins and other macromolecules in the sample matrix has been known to cause unwanted background signal. Lipemic samples, for example, are noted for their intense light scattering, and the relative contributions of lipids to the background signal of a fluorescence measurement should be investigated when setting up a new method.

In addition to background interferences, dilute solutions of some fluorophores in the concentration range of 10^{-9} mol/L and below will adsorb to the walls of glass cuvets and other reaction vessels. Also, dilute solutions of fluorophores, when excited over long periods of time, are susceptible to photodecomposition by intense excitation light. Operationally, these problems are avoided by selecting proper reaction vessels, adding wetting agents, and minimizing the length of time a sample is exposed to the excitation light.

Temperature Effects

The fluorescence quantum efficiency of many compounds is sensitive to temperature fluctuations. Therefore, the temperature of the reaction must be regulated to within ±0.1 °C. In general, fluorescence intensity decreases with increasing temperature by approximately 1 to 5% per degree Celsius. Furthermore, collisional quenching decreases with increasing viscosity, thus reducing quenching of fluorescence. Operationally, fluorescence intensity is therefore enhanced by increasing reaction viscosity or lowering solvent temperature. Temperature effects are minimized by controlling reaction temperature and warming samples or reagents, or both, if they have been refrigerated.

Photodecomposition

In conventional fluorometry, excitation of weakly fluorescing or dilute solutions with intense light sources will cause photochemical decomposition of the analyte (photobleaching).

The following steps help to minimize photodecomposition effects:

1. Always use the longest feasible wavelength for excitation that does not introduce light scattering effects.
2. Decrease the duration of excitation of the sample by measuring the fluorescence intensity immediately after excitation.
3. Protect unstable solutions from ambient light by storing them in dark bottles.
4. Remove dissolved oxygen from the solution.

In addition, highly intense laser light sources with an energy output greater than 5 to 10 mW are used for flow cytometry, fluorescence microscopy, and laser-induced fluorescence measurements. These intense light sources rapidly photodecompose some fluorescence analytes. This decomposition introduces nonlinear response curves and loss of the majority of the sample fluorescence. Fluorescence-based assays for analytes at ultralow concentrations require optimization of laser intensity and use of a sensitive detector.

PHOSPHORESCENCE

Phosphorescence is the luminescence produced by certain substances (e.g., zinc sulfide) after radiant energy or other types of energy are absorbed. Phosphorescence is distinguished from fluorescence in that light emission results from the relaxation of molecules in an excited triplet electronic state, as opposed to an excited singlet electronic state in fluorescence emission. The decay time of emission of phosphorescence light is usually longer (10^{-4} to 10^{2} s) than the decay time of fluorescence emission because of the longer lifetime of molecules in an excited triplet state. Phosphorescence shows a larger shift in emitted light wavelength than is seen with fluorescence.

CHEMILUMINESCENCE, BIOLUMINESCENCE, AND ELECTROCHEMILUMINESCENCE

Chemiluminescence, bioluminescence, and *electrochemiluminescence* are types of luminescence in which the excitation event is caused by a (1) chemical,[14A] (2) biochemical, or (3) electrochemical reaction, and not by photoillumination.

Basic Concepts

The physical event of light emission in chemiluminescence, bioluminescence, and electrochemiluminescence is similar to fluorescence in that it occurs from an excited singlet state, and light is emitted when the electron returns to the ground state.

Chemiluminescence and Bioluminescence

Chemiluminescence is the emission of light when an electron returns from an excited or higher energy level to a lower energy level. The excitation event is caused by a chemical reaction and involves the oxidation of an organic compound, such as luminol, isoluminol, acridinium esters, or luciferin, by an oxidant (e.g., hydrogen peroxide, hypochlorite, oxygen); light is emitted from the excited product formed in the oxidation reaction. These reactions occur in the presence of catalysts, such as enzymes (e.g., alkaline phosphatase, horseradish peroxidase, microperoxidase), metal ions, or metal complexes (e.g., Cu^{2+} and Fe^{3+} phthalocyanine complex), and hemin.[2,5,6,12,23]

Bioluminescence is a special form of chemiluminescence found in biological systems. In bioluminescence, an enzyme or a photoprotein increases the efficiency of the luminescence reaction. Luciferase and aequorin are two examples of these biological catalysts. The quantum yield (e.g., total photons emitted per total molecules reacting) is approximately 0.1 to 10% for chemiluminescence, and 10 to 30% for bioluminescence.

Chemiluminescence assays are ultrasensitive (attomole to zeptomole detection limits) and have wide dynamic ranges. They are now widely used in automated immunoassay and DNA probe assay systems [e.g., acridinium ester and acridinium sulfonamide labels, 1,2-dioxetane substrates for alkaline phosphatase labels, enhanced-luminol reaction for horseradish peroxidase labels (see Chapter 16)].

Electrochemiluminescence

Electrochemiluminescence differs from chemiluminescence in that the reactive species that produce the chemiluminescent reaction are electrochemically generated from stable precursors at the surface of an electrode.[1] A ruthenium (Ru^{2+}), tris(bipyridyl) chelate is the most commonly used electrochemiluminescence label, and electrochemiluminescence is generated at an electrode via an oxidation-reduction–type reaction with tripropylamine. This chelate is very stable and relatively small and has been used to label haptens or large molecules (e.g., proteins, oligonucleotides). The electrochemiluminescence process has been used in both immunoassays and nucleic acid assays. Advantages of this process include (1) improved reagent stability, (2) simple reagent preparation, and (3) enhanced sensitivity. With its use, detection limits of 200 fmol/L and a dynamic range extending over six orders of magnitude can be obtained.

Instrumentation

Luminometers are instruments used to measure chemiluminescence and electrochemiluminescence.[2] Basic components are (1) the sample cell housed in a light-tight chamber, (2) the injection system used to add reagents to the sample cell, and (3) the detector. The detector is usually a PMT. However, CCD, x-ray film, or photographic film has been used to image chemiluminescence reactions on a membrane or in the wells of a microplate. For electrochemiluminescence, the reaction vessel incorporates an electrode, at which electrochemiluminescence is generated.

Limitations of Chemiluminescence and Electrochemiluminescence Measurements

Light leaks, light piping, and high background luminescence from assay reagents and reaction vessels (e.g., plastic tubes exposed to light) are common factors that degrade analytical performance. The extreme sensitivity of chemiluminescence assays requires stringent controls on the purity of reagents and the solvents (e.g., water) used to prepare reagent solutions. Efficient capture of light emission from reactions that produce a flash of light requires an efficient injector that provides adequate mixing when the triggering reagent is added to the reaction vessel. Chemiluminescent and electrochemiluminescent assays have a wide linear range, usually several orders of magnitude, but very high-intensity light emission can lead to pulse pile-up in PMTs, and this can lead to a serious underestimation of true light emission intensity.

NEPHELOMETRY AND TURBIDIMETRY

Light scattering is a physical phenomenon that results from the interaction of light with particles in solution. Nephelometry and turbidimetry are analytical techniques used to measure scattered light. Light scattering measurements have been applied to immunoassays of specific proteins and haptens.

Basic Concepts

Light scattering occurs when radiant energy passing through a solution encounters a molecule in an elastic collision, which results in scattering of the light in all directions. Unlike fluorescence emission, the scattered light is of the same frequency as the incident light.

Factors that influence light scattering include effects of particle size, wavelength dependence, distance of observation, effects of polarization of incident light, concentration of the particles, and molecular weight of the particles.

Particle Size

The Rayleigh scattering equation (see next section) applies to the scattering of light from small particles with much smaller dimensions than the wavelength of incident light (e.g., particle size $<\lambda/10$). When the dimensions of the particles are much smaller than the wavelength of the incident light, each particle is subjected to the same electric field strength at the same time. Reradiated or scattered light waves from the small particle are in phase and reinforce each other. As the particles become larger than the incident light wave, radiated light waves are no longer all in phase. Reinforcement of radiation occurs in some directions, and destructive interference occurs in others. Scattering patterns from these large particles are characteristic of the size and shape of the particle.

Wavelength Dependence of Light Scattering

In 1871, Lord Rayleigh derived the following equation, which demonstrates the relationship of the intensity (I_S) of scattered light to the intensity (I_0) of incident light:

$$\frac{I_S}{I_0} = \frac{16\pi^2 a \sin^2 \phi}{\lambda^4 r^2} \quad \textbf{(10)}$$

where

I_s = intensity of scattered light
I_0 = intensity of the excitation light
a = polarizability of the small particle
θ = angle of observation
λ = wavelength of incident light
r = distance from light scattering to the detector

As indicated, the intensity of light scattering is inversely proportional to the wavelength of the incident light. Another useful observation from equation (10) is the fact that scattered light intensity is also inversely proportional to the distance r from the light scattering particles to the detector. Thus, the detector should be located close to the analytical cell by the juxtaposition of the cell to the detector or by the use of good collection optics.

Concentration and Molecular Weight Factors in Light Scattering

The direct relationship of light scattering to the concentration of particles and to the molecular weight of particles is derived from equation (10), showing that

$$\frac{I_S}{I_0} = \frac{4\pi^2 \left(\frac{dn}{dc}\right)^2 Mc \sin^2 \phi}{N_a \lambda^4 r^2} \quad \textbf{(11)}$$

where

I_s = intensity of scattered light from small particles excited by polarized light
I_0 = incident intensity
dn/dc = change in refractive index of the solvent with respect to change in solute concentration
M = molecular weight (g/mol)
c = concentration (g/mL) of the particles
θ = angle of observation
N_a = Avogadro's number
λ = wavelength of the incident light
r = distance from light scattering to the detector

The important observation to be made from equation (11) is the direct relationship of light scattering to the concentration and the molecular weight of particles.

Effects of Polarized Light on Light Scattering

Equations (10) and (11) are different forms of the Rayleigh expression for light scattering from small particles if excited by polarized light. Figure 10-17, *A*, shows the effects of polarized and nonpolarized light on light scattering intensity from small particles as a function of scattering angle. Curve 2 shows a spherically symmetric intensity diagram as predicted by equation (10). Curve 3 is the resultant intensity diagram when curves 1 and 2 are summed and is the scattering angular intensity diagram obtained when light scatters from small particles excited with nonpolarized light. Curves 1 and 2 represent intensity diagrams from vertically and horizontally polarized light components that are considered to comprise nonpolarized light. The Rayleigh light scattering expression for small particles excited by nonpolarized light is given by equation (12):

$$\frac{I_S}{I_0} = \frac{2\pi^2 \left(\frac{dn}{dc}\right)^2 Mc\,(1+\cos\phi)}{N_a \lambda^4 r^2} \quad \textbf{(12)}$$

Two important observations can be made from equation (12) and Figure 10-17, *A*. First, the total light scattered by small particles is less when excited by polarized light than by nonpolarized light, and reduction of background signal from light scattering in fluorescence measurements is achieved if an appropriately oriented polarizer is used in front of the emission detector. Second, light scattering intensity from small particles excited by nonpolarized light shows symmetric angular dependence of light scattering about the 90° axis (refer to Figure 10-17, *A*, curve 3).

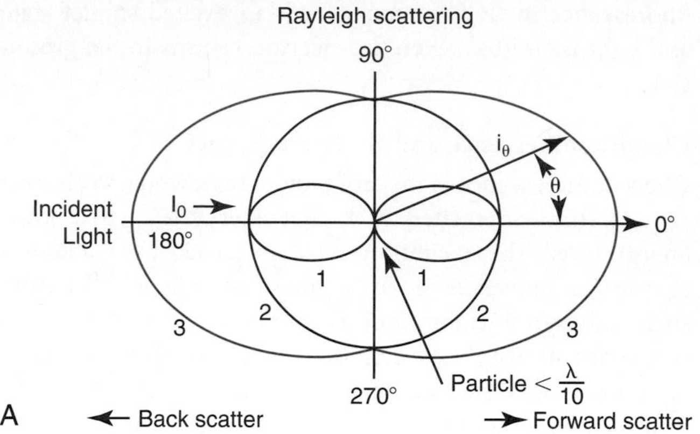

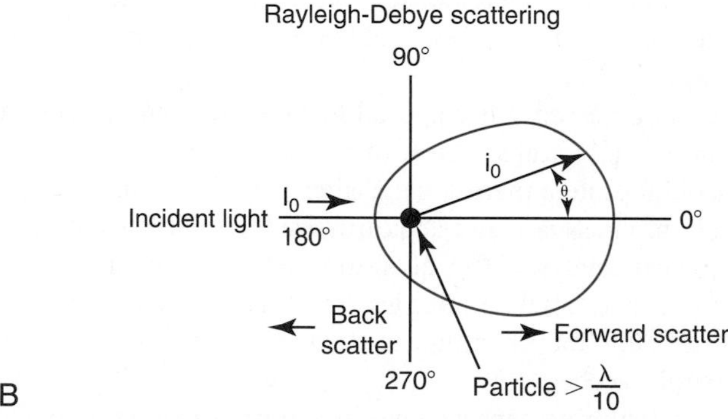

Figure 10-17 Intensity of scatter in different directions under different particle size conditions relative to the wavelength of light. Panel A shows the angular dependence of light scattering intensity with nonpolarized and polarized incident light for small particles (1, 2, and 3). Panel B shows the angular dependence of light scattering with nonpolarized light for larger particles.

Angular Dependence of Light Scattering

The angular dependence of light scattering from small particles (i.e., less than λ/10), as indicated in the previous section, is represented by Figure 10-17, *A*. Examination of Figure 10-17, *A* (curve 3), shows that light scatter intensity values for forward scatter and back scatter (I_0 at 0° and 180°) from small particles excited by nonpolarized light are equal. However, light scatter intensity at 90° is much less. As particles become larger (e.g., >λ/10), the angular dependence of light scatter takes on the dissymmetric relationship shown in Figure 10-17, *B*. In this situation, light-scattering intensities at forward and back angles are not equal; forward scatter intensity is much larger. Also, light scattering intensity at 90° is much less than intensity at the forward (0°) angle. As particles become even larger, this dissymmetry increases even further. This dissymmetry and the change in angular dependence of light scattering with change in the size of particles are very useful for characterization and differentiation of various classes of macromolecules and cells. As was previously mentioned, this property of light scattering is being used in the design of flow cytometers. These instruments measure near forward light scattering and right-angle light scattering from cellular particles flowing through an optical cell and excited by a high-intensity laser. The ratio of near forward light scattering intensity to right-angle light intensity is used in these instruments to distinguish among cell sizes.

Light Scattering and Plasma Proteins

The expression for light scattering given in equation (10) holds true in dilute solution for small particles if the largest dimension is less than one tenth the wavelength of the incident light. Thus the upper limit on the size of particles exhibiting Rayleigh scattering is about 40 nm when visible light is used at 400 nm. Many of the plasma proteins—such as immunoglobulins, β-lipoproteins, and albumin—are below this limit. For larger particles (≈40 to 400 nm), the angular dependence of the scattered light loses symmetry around the 90° axis, as seen in Figure 10-17, and shows an increase in forward scattering. Some plasma proteins of the immunoglobulin M class, chylomicrons, and aggregating immunoglobulin–antigen complexes fall into this size category. Scattering from particles in this size range is known as Rayleigh-Debye scattering, and the equation for this type of scattering becomes more complex. Particles such as red blood cells and bacteria are larger yet (i.e., 7000 to 40,000 nm). These particles show a complex angular dependence of light scattering, and this type of scattering from very large particles is called Mie scattering. These large particles produce a predominance of scattered light in a narrow angular region in the forward direction.

Measurement of Scattered Light

Turbidimetry and nephelometry are methods used to measure scattered light. Such measurement has proven useful for the quantitation of serum proteins (see Chapters 15 and 22).

Turbidimetry

Turbidity decreases the intensity of the incident beam of light as it passes through a solution of particles. Measurement of this decrease in intensity is called *turbidimetry*. Analogous to absorption spectroscopy, turbidity is defined as follows:

$$I = I_0 e^{-bt} \tag{13}$$

or

$$t = \frac{1}{b} \ln \frac{I_0}{I} \tag{14}$$

where

t = turbidity

b = path length of incident light through the solution of light scattering particles

I = intensity of transmitted light

I_0 = intensity of incident light

Turbidity is measured at 180° from the incident beam or, more simply, in the same manner as absorbance measurements are made in a spectrophotometer. Turbidity can be measured on most spectrophotometers and automated clinical chemistry analyzers. The stability and resolution of modern microprocessor-driven spectrophotometers and photometers have greatly improved their ability to measure turbidity with accuracy and precision.

Nephelometry

Nephelometry is defined as the detection of light energy scattered or reflected toward a detector that is not in the direct path of the transmitted light.[9] Common nephelometers measure scattered light at right angles to the incident light. The ideal nephelometric instrument would be free of stray light, and neither light scatter nor any other signal would be seen by the detector when the solution in front of the detector is free from particles. However, because of stray light-generating components in the optical system and in the sample cuvet or the sample itself, a truly dark field situation is difficult to obtain when making nephelometric measurements. Some nephelometers are designed to measure scattered light at an angle other than 90° to take advantage of the increased forward scatter intensity caused by light scattering from larger particles (e.g., immune complexes).

Selection of Method

The choice between turbidimetry and nephelometry depends on the application and the available instrumentation. Nephelometry, however, still offers some advantage in terms of sensitivity when low-level antigen-antibody reactions are measured.[10]

Instrumentation

Turbidimeters and nephelometers are used to measure the intensity of light scattering.

Turbidimeter

Turbidimetric measurements are easily performed on photometers or spectrophotometers and require little optimization.

The principal concern of turbidimetric measurements is signal-to-noise ratio. Photometric systems with electro-optical noise in the range of ±0.0002 absorbance unit or less are useful for turbidity measurements.

Nephelometer

Although light scattering can be measured with standard analytical fluorometers or photometers, the angular dependence of light scattering intensity has resulted in the design of special nephelometers. These devices place the PMT detector at appropriate angles to the excitation light beam. The design principle of a nephelometer is similar to the design principle applied in fluorescence measurement. The major operational difference between the fluorometer and the nephelometer is that the excitation and detection wavelengths will be set to the same value when operating a nephelometer. The principal concerns of light scatter instrumentation include excitation intensity, wavelength, distance of the detector from the sample cuvet, and minimization of external stray light. As shown in Figure 10-18, the basic components of a nephelometer include (1) a light source, (2) collimating optics, (3) a sample cell, and (4) collection optics, which include light scattering optics, a detector optical filter, and a detector. The schematic diagram also shows the different angles from the incident light beam where the detector, filter, and optics are placed to measure light scattering. Figure 10-18, *A*, shows the straight-through arrangement for turbidimetry, whereas Figure 10-18, *B* and *C*, shows arrangements frequently found in nephelometers. The detector arrangement shown in Figure 10-18, *B*, is used for measurement of forward scatter at 30°—the optical arrangement used with some commercial nephelometers.

Operationally, the optical components used in turbidimeters and nephelometers are similar to those used in fluorometers and photometers. For example, the light sources commonly used are quartz-halogen lamps, xenon lamps, and lasers. He-Ne lasers, which operate at 633 nm, typically have been used for light scattering applications, such as nephelometric immunoassays and particle size and shape determinations. The laser beam is used specifically in some nephelometers because of its high intensity; in addition, the coherent nature of laser light makes it ideally suited for nephelometric applications.

In addition, ratio-referencing fluorometers are well suited for nephelometric measurements.

Limitations of Light Scattering Measurements

Antigen excess and matrix effects are limitations encountered in the use of turbidimeters and nephelometers for measurement of analytes of clinical interest.

Antigen Excess

Antigen-antibody reactions are complex and appear to result in a mixture of aggregate sizes. As turbidity increases during addition of antigen to antibodies, the signal increases to a maximum value and then decreases. The point at which the decrease begins marks the beginning of the phase of antigen excess; this phenomenon is explained in Chapter 16. Consequently, light scattering methods for quantitation of antigen-antibody reactions must provide a method for detecting

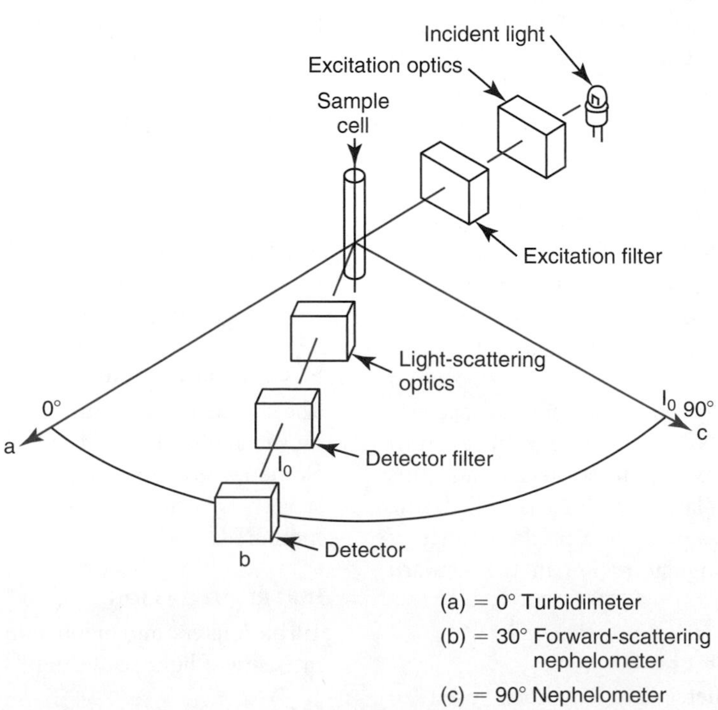

Figure 10-18 Schematic diagram of light scattering instrumentation showing (A) the optics position for a turbidimeter; (B) the optics position for a forward scattering nephelometer; and (C) the optics position for a right-angle nephelometer.

antigen excess. The kinetics of immune complex formation measured by nephelometry or turbidimetry is sufficiently different in each of the three phases—antibody excess, equivalence, and antigen excess—that computer algorithms have been developed to flag antigen excess automatically.[9,20]

Matrix Effects

Particles, solvent, and all serum macromolecules scatter light. Lipoproteins and chylomicrons in lipemic serum provide the highest background turbidity or nephelometric intensity. With appropriate dilutions, the relative intensity of light scattering from a lipemic sample is less than that of the antiserum blank. However, as the concentration of the antigen in serum decreases and correspondingly less dilute samples are used, background interference from lipemic samples becomes greater. An effective method for minimizing this background interference is the use of rate measurements, in which the initial sample blank is eliminated. Large particles, such as suspended dust, also cause significant background interference. This background interference is controlled by filtering all buffers and diluted antisera before analysis is attempted.

REFERENCES

1. Blackburn GF, Shah HP, Kenten JH, Leland J, Kamin RA, Link J, et al. Electrochemiluminescence detection for development of immunoassays and DNA probe assays for clinical diagnostics. Clin Chem 1991;37:1534-9.
2. DeLuca M, McElroy WD. Bioluminescence and chemiluminescence, part B. In: Methods in enzymology, volume 133. San Diego: Academic Press, 1986.
3. Diamandis E, Christopoulos TK. Europium chelate labels in time-resolved fluorescence immunoassays and DNA hybridization assays. Anal Chem 1990;62:1149A-57A.
4. Epperson PM, Sweedler JV, Billhorn RB, Sims GR, Denton MB. Applications of charge transfer devices in spectroscopy. Anal Chem 1988;60:327A-35A.
5. Fletcher P, Andrew KN, Calokerinos AC, Forbes S, Worsfold PJ. Analytical applications of flow injection with chemiluminescence detection—a review. Luminescence 2001;16:1-23.
6. Galban J, Andreu Y, Sierra JF, de Marcos S, Castillo JR. Intrinsic fluorescence of enzymes and fluorescence of chemically modified enzymes for analytical purposes: a review. Luminescence 2001;16:199-210.
7. Harma H, Soukka T, Lovgren T. Europium nanoparticles and time-resolved fluorescence for ultrasensitive detection of prostate-specific antigen. Clin Chem 2001;47:561-8.
8. Heiftje GM, Vogelstein EE. A linear response theory approach to time-resolved fluorometry. In: Wehry EL, ed. Modern fluorescence spectroscopy, volume 4. New York: Plenum Press, 1981:25-50.
9. Hills LP, Tiffany TO. Comparison of turbidimetric and light scattering measurements of immunoglobulins by use of a centrifugal analyzer with absorbance and fluorescence light scattering optics. Clin Chem 1980;26:1459-66.
10. Jolley ME, Stroupe SD, Schwenzer KS, Wang CJ, Lu-Steffes M, Hill HD, et al. Fluorescence polarization immunoassay. III. An automated system for therapeutic drug determination. Clin Chem 1981;27:1575-9.
11. Masters BR, Kino GS. Charge coupled devices for quantitative Nipkow Disk real-time scanning confocal microscopy. In: Shotton D, ed. Electron light microscopy: the principles and practice of video-enhanced contrast, digital intensified fluorescence, and confocal scanning light microscopy. New York: Wiley-Liss, 1993.
12. Mestre YF, Zamora LL, Calatayud JM. Flow-chemiluminescence: a growing modality of pharmaceutical analysis. Luminescence 2001;16:213-35.
13. Patrick CW. Clinical flow cytometry: milestones along the pathway of progress. MLO Med Lab Obs 2002;34:0-16.
14. Petersen JR, Okorodudu AO, Mohammad AA, Fernando A, Shattuck KE. Association of transcutaneous bilirubin testing in hospital with decreased readmission rate for hyperbilirubinemia. Clin Chem 2005;51:540-4.

14A. Rodríguez-Orozco AR, Ruiz-Reyes H, Medina-Serriteño N. Recent applications of chemiluminescence assays in clinical immunology. Mini Rev Med Chem 2010;10(14):1393-400.

15. Shapiro HM. Practical flow cytometry, 4th edition. Hoboken, NJ: John Wiley & Sons, 2003.
16. Slavin W. Atomic absorption spectroscopy: the present and future. Anal Chem 1982;54:685A-94A.
17. Soini E, Kojola H. Time-resolved fluorometer for lanthanide chelates: a new generation of nonisotopic immunoassays. Clin Chem 1983;29:65-8.
18. Soukka T, Paukkunen J, Harma H, Lonnberg S, Lindroos H, Lovgren T. Supersensitive time-resolved immunofluorometric assay of free prostate-specific antigen with nanoparticle label technology. Clin Chem 2001;47:1269-78.
19. Soukka T, Antonen K, Harma H, Pelkkikangas AM, Huhtinen P, Lovgren T. Highly sensitive immunoassay of free prostate-specific antigen in serum using europium(III) nanoparticle label technology. Clin Chim Acta 2003;328:45-58.
20. Sternberg J. A rate nephelometer for measuring specific proteins by immunoprecipitin reactions. Clin Chem 1977;25:1456-64.
21. Sweedler JV, Billhorn RB, Epperson PM, Sims GR, Denton MB. High performance charge transfer devices. Anal Chem 1988;60:282A-91A.
22. Vignali DA. Multiplexed particle-based flow cytometric assays. J Immunol Methods 2000;243:243-55.
23. Ziegler MM, Baldwin TO, eds. Bioluminescence and chemiluminescence, part C. In: Methods in enzymology, volume 305. San Diego: Academic Press, 2000.

CHAPTER 11

Electrochemistry and Chemical Sensors

*Paul D'Orazio, Ph.D., and Mark E. Meyerhoff, Ph.D.**

Electrochemical and optical sensors (and associated biosensors) are firmly established in clinical analysis systems. Sensors for measurement of blood gases, electrolytes, and metabolites are particularly well suited for incorporation into automated, point-of-care, and critical-care analyzers (see Chapters 19, 20, and 28, respectively), because of their ease of use, low maintenance, and ability to measure clinically important analytes in undiluted blood.[62] When integrated into chromatographic systems (see Chapter 13), electrochemical detectors provide a highly sensitive and selective means of detecting a variety of other analytes, such as therapeutic drugs, neurotransmitters, glutathione, and homocysteine. Also, electrochemical detection has been applied successfully for monitoring coagulation reactions, detecting toxic lead in blood samples, and developing novel ultrasensitive immunoassays. When bioelements are integrated with electrodes, the resultant biosensors further expand the analytical capabilities of such devices. In addition, the development and application of *optodes,* based on some of the same selective chemistries used in electrochemical devices, have resulted in another analytical tool for measuring blood gases and electrolytes.

In this chapter, the fundamental electrochemical principles of (1) potentiometry, (2) voltammetry/ amperometry, (3) conductance, and (4) coulometry will be summarized and clinical applications presented. Next, optodes and biosensors will be discussed. The chapter concludes with a discussion of in vivo and minimally invasive sensors.

POTENTIOMETRY AND ION-SELECTIVE ELECTRODES

Potentiometry is widely used clinically for the measurement of pH, PCO_2, and electrolytes (Na^+, K^+, Cl^-, Ca^{2+}, Mg^{2+}, Li^+) in whole blood, serum, plasma, and urine, and as the basis for some biosensors for metabolites of clinical interest.

Basic Concepts

Potentiometry is the measurement of an electrical potential difference between two electrodes (half-cells) in an electrochemical cell (Figure 11-1) when the cell current is zero (galvanic cell). Such a cell consists of two electrodes (electron and metallic conductors) that are connected by an electrolyte solution (ion conductor). An *electrode,* or *half-cell,* consists of a single metallic conductor that is in contact with an electrolyte solution. Ion conductors have been composed of one or more phases that are either in direct contact with each other or separated by membranes permeable only to specific cations or anions (see Figure 11-1). One of the electrolyte solutions is the unknown or test solution; this solution may be replaced by an appropriate reference solution for calibration purposes. By convention, the cell notation is shown so that the left electrode (M_L) is the reference electrode, and the right electrode (M_R) is the *indicator (measuring) electrode* [see later equation (3)].[11]

The *electromotive force* (E or EMF) is defined as the maximum difference in potential between the two electrodes (right minus left) obtained when the cell current is zero. The cell potential is measured using a *potentiometer,* of which the common pH meter is a special type. The *direct-reading potentiometer* is a voltmeter that measures the potential across the cell (between the two electrodes); however, to obtain an accurate potential measurement, it is necessary that no current flow through the cell. This is accomplished by incorporating high resistance within the voltmeter (input impedance $>10^{12}\ \Omega$). Modern direct-reading potentiometers are accurate and can be modified to provide direct digital displays or printouts.

Within any one conductive phase, the potential is constant as long as the current flow is zero. However, a potential difference arises between two different phases in contact with each other. The overall potential of an electrochemical cell is the sum of all potential gradients that exist between different

The authors gratefully acknowledge the original contributions of Drs. Richard A. Durst and Ole Siggard-Andersen on which portions of this chapter are based.

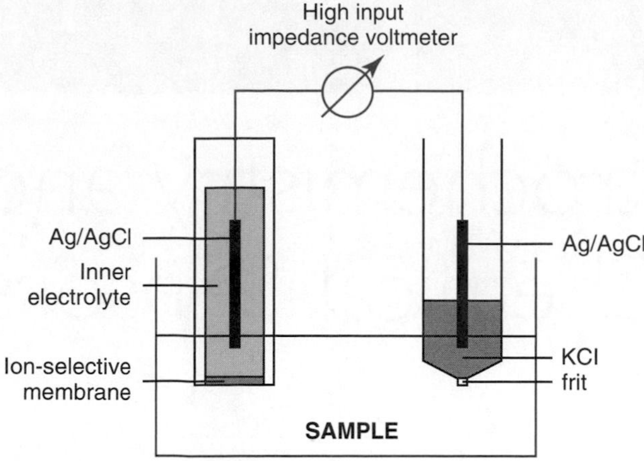

Figure 11-1 Schematic of ion-selective membrane electrode–based potentiometric cell.

phases of the cell. The potential of a single electrode with respect to the surrounding electrolyte and the absolute magnitude of the individual potential gradients between phases are unknown and cannot be measured. Only *potential differences* between two electrodes (half-cells) can be measured. Potential gradients can be classified as (1) redox potentials, (2) membrane potentials, or (3) diffusion potentials. Generally, it is possible to devise a cell in such a manner that all potential gradients except one are constant. This potential then can be related to the activity of a specific ion of interest (e.g., H^+, Na^+).

Types of Electrodes

Many different types of electrodes are used for potentiometric applications. They include redox, ion-selective membrane (glass and polymer), and PCO_2 electrodes.

Redox Electrodes

Redox potentials are the result of chemical equilibria involving electron transfer reactions:

$$\text{Oxidized form (Ox)} + ne^- \longleftrightarrow \text{Reduced form (Red)} \quad \textbf{(1)}$$

where n represents the number of electrons involved in the reaction. Any substance that accepts electrons is an *oxidant* (Ox), and any substance that donates electrons is a *reductant* (Red). The two forms, Ox and Red, represent a redox couple (conjugate redox pair). Usually, homogeneous redox processes take place only between two redox couples. In such cases, electrons are transferred from a reductant (Red_1) to an oxidant (Ox_2). In this process, Red_1 is oxidized to its conjugate Ox_1, whereas Ox_2 is reduced to Red_2:

$$Red_1 + Ox_2 \longleftrightarrow Ox_1 + Red_2 \quad (2)$$

In an electrochemical cell, electrons may be accepted from or donated to an inert metallic conductor (e.g., platinum). A reduction process tends to charge the electrode positively (remove electrons), and an oxidation process tends to charge the electrode negatively (add electrons). By convention, a heterogeneous redox equilibrium [equation (2)] is represented by the cell

$$M_L|Red_1 - Ox_1 \vdots\vdots Ox_2 - Red_2|M_R \quad (3)$$

A positive potential ($E > 0$) for this cell signifies that the cell reaction proceeds spontaneously from left to right; $E < 0$ signifies that the reaction proceeds from right to left; and $E = 0$ indicates that the two redox couples are at mutual equilibrium.

The *electrode potential* (reduction potential) for a redox couple is defined as the couple's potential measured with respect to the standard hydrogen electrode, which is set equal to zero (see later discussion of hydrogen electrode). This potential, by convention, is the electromotive force of a cell, where the standard hydrogen electrode is the reference electrode (left electrode) and the given half-cell is the indicator electrode (right electrode). The reduction potential for a given redox couple is shown by the Nernst equation:

$$E = E^0 - \frac{N}{n} \times \log\frac{aRed}{aOx} = E^0 - \frac{0.0592V}{n} \times \log\frac{aRed}{aOx} \quad (4)$$

where

E = electrode potential of the half-cell
E^0 = standard electrode potential when $a_{Red}/a_{Ox} = 1$
n = number of electrons involved in the reduction reaction
$N = (R \times T \times \ln 10)/F$ (the Nernst factor if $n = 1$)
$N = 0.0592$ V if $T = 298.15$ K (25 °C)
$N = 0.0615$ V if $T = 310.15$ K (37 °C)
R = gas constant (= 8.31431 Joules × K^{-1} × mol^{-1})
T = absolute temperature (unit: K, kelvin)
F = Faraday constant (= 96,487 Coulombs × mol^{-1})
ln 10 = natural logarithm of 10 = 2.303
a = activity
$aRed/aOx$ = product of mass action for the reduction reaction

Redox electrodes currently in use include (1) inert metal electrodes immersed in solutions containing redox couples and (2) metal electrodes whose metal functions as a member of the redox couple.

Inert Metal Electrodes

Platinum and *gold* are examples of inert metals used to record the redox potential of a redox couple dissolved in an electrolyte solution. The *hydrogen electrode* is a special redox electrode for pH measurement. It consists of a platinum or gold electrode that is electrolytically coated (platinized) with highly porous platinum (platinum black) to catalyze the electrode reaction:

$$H^+ + e^- \longleftrightarrow \frac{1}{2}H_2 \quad (5)$$

The electrode potential is given by

$$E = E^0 - N \times \log\frac{(fH_2)^{1/2}}{aH^+} \quad (6)$$

or

$$E = E^0 - N \times [\log(fH_2)^{1/2} - \log aH^+] \qquad (7)$$

where

$E^0 = 0$ at all temperatures (by convention)

f_{H2} = fugacity of hydrogen gas

a_{H+} = activity of hydrogen ions

$-\log a_{H+}$ = negative log of H^+ activity (pa_{H+} or pH)

When the partial pressure of hydrogen (PH_2) in the solution (and hence f_{H2}) is maintained constant by bubbling hydrogen through the solution, the potential is a linear function of log a_{H+} (= −pH). In the *standard hydrogen electrode (SHE),* the electrolyte consists of an aqueous solution of hydrogen chloride with a_{HCl} equal to 1.000 (or c_{HCl} = 1.2 mol/L) in equilibrium with a gas phase, and with f_{H2} equal to 1.000 (or PH_2 = 101.3 kPa = 1 atm). The SHE is also used as a reference electrode.

Metal Electrodes Participating in Redox Reactions

The silver-silver chloride electrode is an example of a metal electrode that participates as a member of a redox couple. The silver-silver chloride electrode consists of a silver wire or rod coated with $AgCl_{(s)}$ that is immersed in a chloride solution of constant activity; this sets the half-cell potential. The Ag/AgCl electrode is itself considered a potentiometric electrode, as its phase boundary potential is governed by an oxidation-reduction electron transfer equilibrium reaction that occurs at the surface of the silver:

$$AgCl_{(solid)} + e^- \longleftrightarrow Ag^{\circ}_{(solid)} + Cl^- \qquad (8)$$

The Nernst equation for the reference half-cell potential of an Ag/AgCl reference electrode is written as follows:

$$E_{Ag/AgCl} = E^0_{Ag/AgCl} + \frac{RT}{nF} \times \ln \frac{a_{AgCl}}{a_{Ag} a_{Cl-}} \qquad (9)$$

Because AgCl and Ag are both solids, their activities are equal to unity ($a_{AgCl} = a^0_{Ag} = 1$). Therefore, from equation (9), the half-cell potential is controlled by the activity of chloride ion in solution (a_{Cl-}) contacting the electrode.

The Ag/AgCl electrode is used both as an internal reference element in potentiometric ion-selective electrodes (ISEs) and as an external reference electrode half-cell of constant potential, required to complete a potentiometric cell (see Figure 11-1). In both cases, the Ag/AgCl electrode must be in equilibrium with a solution of constant chloride ion activity.

The Ag/AgCl element of the external reference electrode half-cell is in contact with a high-concentration solution of a soluble chloride salt. Saturated potassium chloride is commonly used. A porous membrane or frit is frequently employed to separate the concentrated KCl from the sample solution. The frit serves both as a mechanical barrier to hold the concentrated electrolyte within the electrode and as a diffusional barrier to prevent proteins and other species in the sample from coming into contact with the internal Ag/AgCl element, which could poison and alter its potential. The interface between two dissimilar electrolytes (concentrated KCl/calibrator or sample) occurs within the frit and develops the liquid-liquid junction potential (E_j), a source of error in potentiometric measurements. The difference in liquid-liquid junction potential between calibrator and sample (residual liquid junction potential) is responsible for this error and can be minimized and usually neglected in practice if the compositions of the calibrating solutions are matched as closely as possible to the sample with respect to ionic content and ionic strength. An equitransferant electrolyte at high concentration as the reference electrolyte further helps to minimize the residual liquid junction potential. Potassium chloride at a concentration ≥2 mol/L is preferred. Differences of approximately −2% in the measurement of sodium by ISEs have been demonstrated when the KCl concentration in the reference electrolyte is lowered from 3 to 0.5 mol/L.[28] The magnitude of the residual liquid junction potential may also be estimated by the Henderson equation[106] with sufficient knowledge of ionic activities, ionic charges, and ionic mobilities for each electrolyte on both sides of the junction and the temperature. Using this estimate, a correction to the overall cell potential may be applied.

The presence of erythrocytes in the sample may affect the magnitude of the residual liquid junction potential in a less predictable manner. For example, erythrocytes in blood of normal hematocrit are estimated to produce approximately 1.8 mmol/L positive error in the measurement of sodium by ISEs when an open, unrestricted liquid-liquid junction is used.[13] This bias may be minimized if a restrictive membrane or frit is used to modify the liquid-liquid junction.

The *calomel electrode* consists of mercury covered by a layer of calomel (Hg_2Cl_2), which is in contact with an electrolyte solution containing Cl^-. Calomel electrodes are frequently used as reference electrodes for pH measurements using glass pH electrodes.

Ion-Selective Electrodes

Membrane potentials are caused by the permeability of certain types of membranes to selected anions or cations. Such membranes are used to fabricate ISEs that selectively interact with a single ionic species. The potential produced at the membrane-sample solution interface is proportional to the logarithm of the ionic activity or concentration of the ion in question. Measurements with ISEs are simple, often rapid, nondestructive, and applicable to a wide range of concentrations.

The ion-selective membrane is the "heart" of an ISE, as it controls the selectivity of the electrode. Ion-selective membranes are typically composed of glass, crystalline, or polymeric materials. The chemical composition of the membrane is designed to achieve an optimal permselectivity toward the ion of interest. In practice, other ions exhibit finite interaction with membrane sites and will display some degree of interference for determination of an analyte ion. In clinical practice, if the interference exceeds an acceptable quantity, a correction is required.

The Nicolsky-Eisenman equation describes the selectivity of an ISE for the ion of interest over interfering ions:

$$E = E^0 + \left[\frac{2.303\ RT}{z_i F}\right] \log\left(a_i + \sum K_{i/j} a_j^{z_i/x_j}\right) \qquad (10)$$

where

a_i = activity of the ion of interest

a_j = activity of the interfering ion

$K_{i/j}$ = selectivity coefficient for the primary ion over the interfering ion. Low values indicate good selectivity for the analyte *i* over the interfering ion *j*

z_i = charge of primary ion

z_j = charge of interfering ion

All other terms are identical to those in the Nernst equation [equation (4)].

Various approaches may be used to determine the selectivity of an ISE for a primary ion over an interfering ion.[7,14] A straightforward approach is the *separate solution method,* whereby the potential of an ISE is determined in solutions of the primary and interfering ions separately, but at equal ionic activities. The selectivity coefficient is then calculated as follows:

$$\log K_{ij} = \frac{\dfrac{E_j - E_i}{2.303\,RT}}{nF} + \left(1 - \frac{z_i}{z_j}\right)\log a_i \tag{11}$$

Most ISEs used in clinical practice have sufficient selectivity and do not require correction for interfering ions. Oesch and associates have published required ISE selectivity coefficients for ions commonly measured in clinical chemistry over other ions found in blood.[88] Table 11-1 shows required selectivity coefficients for the measurement of cations of interest in clinical chemistry over potentially interfering cations, assuming an acceptable maximum interference of 1% for the ion of interest.

Glass membrane and polymer membrane electrodes are two types of ISEs that are commonly used in clinical chemistry applications.

The Glass Electrode

Glass membrane electrodes are employed to measure pH and Na^+, and as an internal transducer for PCO_2 sensors. The H^+ response of thin glass membranes was first demonstrated in 1906 by Cremer.[26] In the 1930s, practical application of this phenomenon for measurement of acidity in lemon juice was made possible by the invention of the pH meter by Arnold Beckman.[11] Glass electrode membranes are formulated from melts of silicon and/or aluminum oxide mixed with oxides of alkaline earth or alkali metal cations. By varying the glass composition, electrodes with selectivity for H^+, Na^+, K^+, Li^+, Rb^+, Cs^+, Ag^+, Tl^+, and NH_4^+ have been demonstrated.[33] However, glass electrodes for H^+ and Na^+ are today the only types with sufficient selectivity over interfering ions to allow practical application in clinical chemistry. A typical formulation for H^+ selective glass is 72% SiO_2; 22% Na_2O; 6% CaO, which has a selectivity order of $H^+ >>> Na^+ > K^+$. This glass membrane has sufficient selectivity for H^+ over Na^+ to allow error-free measurements of pH in the range of 7.0 to 8.0 [$[H^+] = 10^{-7}$ to 10^{-8} mol/L] in the presence of >0.1 mol/L Na^+. Glass pH electrodes with selectivity coefficients ($K_{H/Na}$) over Na^+ of 10^{-7} and better have been realized. By altering slightly the formulation of the glass membrane to 71% SiO_2; 11% Na_2O; 18% Al_2O_3, its selectivity order becomes $H^+ > Na^+ > K^+$. Thus, the preference of the glass membrane for H^+ over Na^+ is greatly reduced, resulting in a practical sensor for Na^+ at pH values typically found in blood.[32]

TABLE 11-1 Required Selectivities for Cation-Selective Ion-Selective Electrodes for Whole Blood, Plasma, and Serum Measurements

Primary Ion (i)	Required Selectivity Coefficient ($\log K_{i/j}$) for Interfering Cation (J)					
	H^+	Li^+	Na^+	K^+	Mg^{2+}	Ca^{2+}
H^+	—	−6.5	−8.5	−7.0	−7.7	−7.7
Li^+*	2.1	—	−4.3	−2.8	−3.5	−3.6
Na^+	4.4	−0.1	—	−0.6	−1.2	−1.3
K^+	2.8	−1.7	−3.6	—	−2.8	−2.9
Mg^{2+}	8.9	0.1	−3.9	−0.9	—	−2.4
Ca^{2+}	9.3	0.4	−3.6	−0.6	−1.9	—

*Assumes a therapeutic range for Li^+ between 0.7 and 1.5 mmol/L.

Polymer Membrane Electrodes

Polymer membrane ISEs are employed for monitoring pH and for measuring electrolytes, including K^+, Na^+, Cl^-, Ca^{2+}, Li^+, Mg^{2+}, and CO_3^{2-} (for total CO_2 measurements). They are the predominant class of potentiometric electrodes used in modern clinical analysis instruments.

Mechanisms of response of these ISEs fall into three categories: (1) charged, dissociated ion exchanger; (2) charged associated carrier; and (3) neutral ion carrier (ionophore).[6,15] An early charged-associated ion-exchanger type ISE for Ca^{2+} was developed and commercialized for clinical application in the 1960s based on the Ca^{2+}-selective ion-exchange/complexation properties of 2-ethylhexyl phosphoric acid dissolved in dioctyl phenyl phosphonate.[37] A porous membrane was impregnated with this cocktail and mounted at the end of an electrode body. This type of sensor was referred to as the "liquid membrane" ISE. Later, a method was devised whereby these ingredients could be cast into a plasticized poly(vinyl chloride) (PVC) membrane that was more rugged and convenient to use. This same approach is still used today to formulate PVC-based ISEs for clinical use.[84]

A major breakthrough in the development and routine application of PVC-type ISEs was the discovery by Simon and coworkers that the neutral antibiotic valinomycin could be incorporated into organic liquid membranes (and later plasticized PVC membranes), resulting in a sensor with high selectivity for K^+ over Na^+ ($K_{K/Na} = 2.5 \times 10^{-4}$).[97] The K^+ ISE based on valinomycin was the first example of a neutral carrier ISE and is used extensively today for the routine measurement of K^+ in blood. Figure 11-2 shows the response of the valinomycin-based K^+ ISE in the presence of physiologic concentrations of Na^+, Ca^{2+}, and Mg^{2+}. The wide linear range of this ISE over three orders of magnitude makes it suitable for the measurement of K^+ in blood and urine. The K^+ range

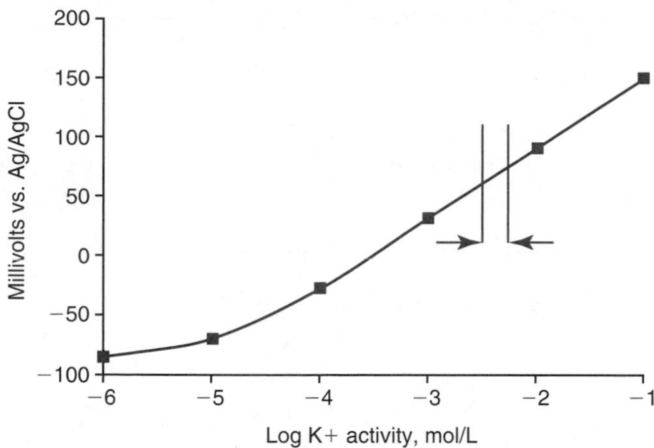

Figure 11-2 Typical electromotive force (EMF) response of potassium selective membrane electrode to changes in activity of potassium in the sample solution. Bracketed interval represents the normal reference interval of potassium concentration in blood. *(From D'Orazio P. In: Lewendrowski K, ed. Clinical chemistry: laboratory management and clinical correlations. Philadelphia: Lippincott, Williams and Wilkins, 2002:455.)*

in blood is only a small portion of the electrode linear range and is spanned by a total ΔEMF of about 9 mV. Interference from other cations, seen as deviation from linearity, is not apparent at K^+ activities $>10^{-4}$ mol/L. Other, less selective polymer-based ISEs (e.g., for the measurement of Mg^{2+} and Li^+) are subject to interference from Ca^{2+}/Na^+ and Na^+, respectively, requiring simultaneous determination and correction for the presence of significant concentrations of interfering ions.[81,99]

Studies regarding the relationship between molecular structure and ionic selectivity have resulted in the development of polymer-based ISEs using a number of naturally occurring and synthetic ionophores, with sufficient selectivity for application in clinical analysis. The chemical structures of several of these neutral ionophores are illustrated in Figure 11-3.

Dissociated anion exchanger-based electrodes employing lipophilic quaternary ammonium salts as active membrane components are still used commercially for the determination of Cl^- in whole blood, serum, and plasma despite some limitations.[68] Selectivity for this type of ISE is controlled by extraction of the ion into the organic membrane phase and is a function of the lipophilic character of the ion (because, unlike with the carriers described earlier, no direct binding interaction occurs between the exchanger site and the anion in the membrane phase). Thus, the selectivity order for Cl^- ISE based on an anion exchanger is fixed as $R^- > ClO_4^- > I^- > NO_3^- > Br^- > Cl^- > F^-$. Application of the Cl^- ion-exchange electrode therefore is limited to samples without significant concentrations of anions more lipophilic than Cl^-. Blood samples containing salicylate or thiocyanate, for example, will produce positive interference for the measurement of Cl^-. Repeated exposure of the electrode to the anticoagulant heparin will lead to loss of electrode sensitivity toward Cl^- because of extraction of negatively charged heparin into the membrane. Indeed, this extraction process has been used successfully to devise a method to detect heparin concentrations in blood by potentiometry,[75] as well as to develop a simple potentiometric technique to screen for the presence of toxic, high charge density polyanion contaminants (e.g., oversulfated chondroitin sulfate) in biomedical grade heparin preparations.[127]

High selectivity for carbonate anion can be achieved using a neutral carrier ionophore possessing trifluoroacetophenone groups doped within a polymeric membrane.[65,107] Such ionophores form negatively charged adducts with carbonate anions, and the resulting electrodes have proven useful in commercial instruments for determination of total carbon dioxide in serum/plasma, after dilution of the blood to a pH value in the range of 8.5 to 9.0, where a significant fraction of total carbon dioxide will exist as carbonate anions.

A typical formulation of a PVC membrane ISE used in clinical instrumentation consists of the following:

1 to 3 wt% ionophore
≈64 wt% plasticizer
≈30 wt% PVC
<1 wt% additives

The plasticizer is crucial in controlling the polarity of the membrane and thus, along with the ionophore, plays a pivotal role in determining the selectivity of the membrane toward the ion of interest. A large lipophilic anion (e.g., tetraphenylborate derivative) is often included as an additive for preparation of cation-selective ISE membranes. This anion serves as a counteranion for the cation of interest as it is extracted into the membrane phase, forming a positively charged complex with the neutral ionophore. However, it is the ratio of bound to unbound ionophore sites at the membrane surface that determines the magnitude of the phase boundary potential generated by the ISE membrane.[3] Thus, the selective response to the activity of the ion of interest is an interfacial property of the given ISE membrane.

Studies have demonstrated that the ultimate detection limits of polymer membrane–type ISEs are controlled in part by the leakage of analyte ions from the internal solution to the outer surface of the membrane, and into the sample phase in close contact with the membrane.[78] Hence, lower limits of detection can be achieved by decreasing the concentration of the primary analyte ion within the internal solution of the electrode. Further, this leakage of analyte ions, coupled with an ion-exchange process at the membrane sample interface when the selectivity of the membrane over other ions is assessed, can often yield a measured potentiometric selectivity coefficient that underestimates the true selectivity of the membrane. To determine "unbiased" selectivity coefficients by the separate solution method, the membrane should not be exposed to the analyte ion for extended periods of time, and the concentration of analyte ion in the internal solution should be low.[8] To avoid leakage of primary ions from the inner solution of conventional polymer membrane ISEs, new more stable designs for solid-state ion sensors have been suggested, in which the ionophore-doped polymer

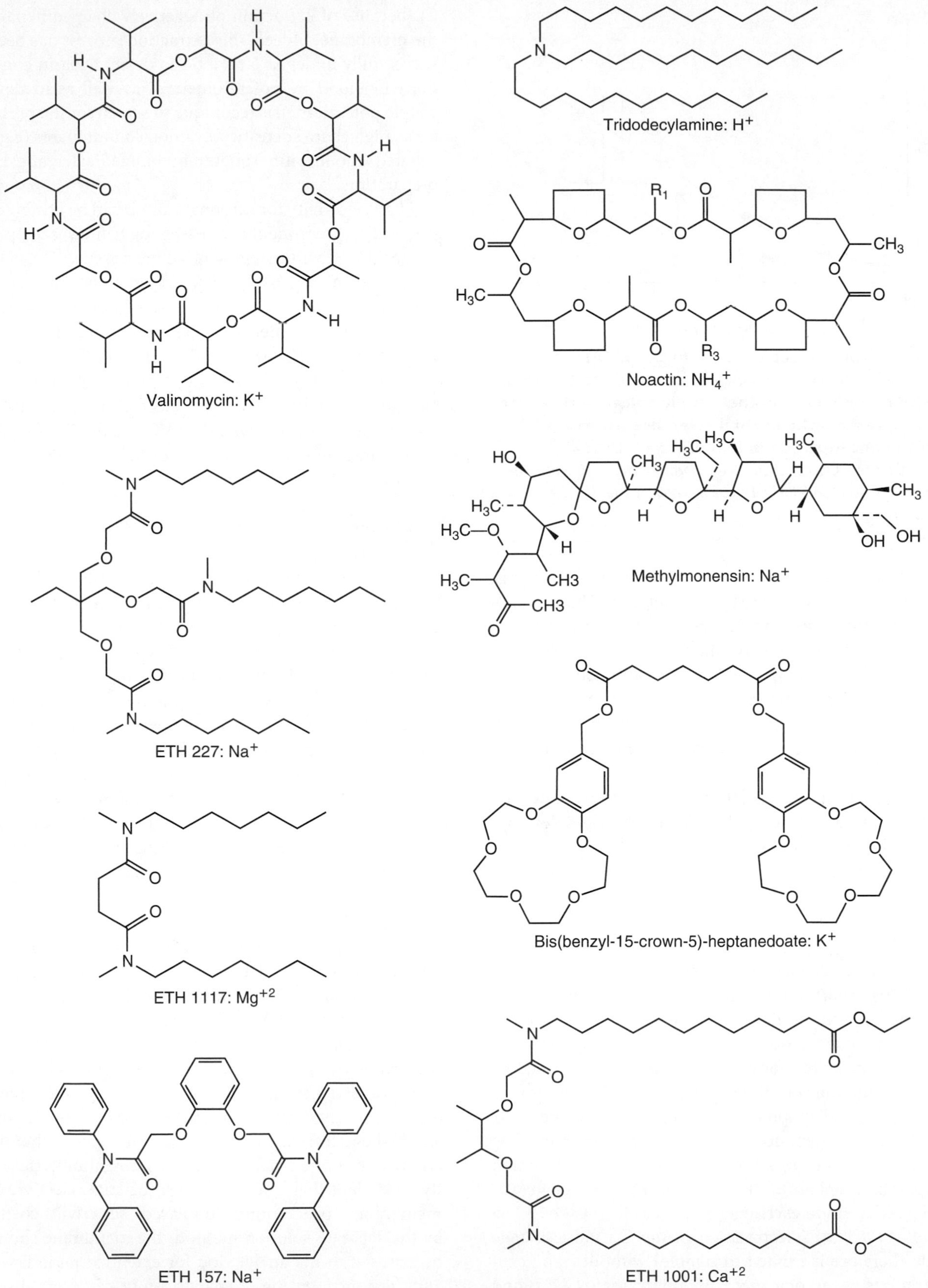

Valinomycin: K^+

Tridodecylamine: H^+

Noactin: NH_4^+

Methylmonensin: Na^+

ETH 227: Na^+

Bis(benzyl-15-crown-5)-heptanedoate: K^+

ETH 1117: Mg^{+2}

ETH 157: Na^+

ETH 1001: Ca^{+2}

Figure 11-3 Structures of common ionophores used to fabricate polymer membrane–type ion-selective electrodes (ISEs) for clinical analysis.

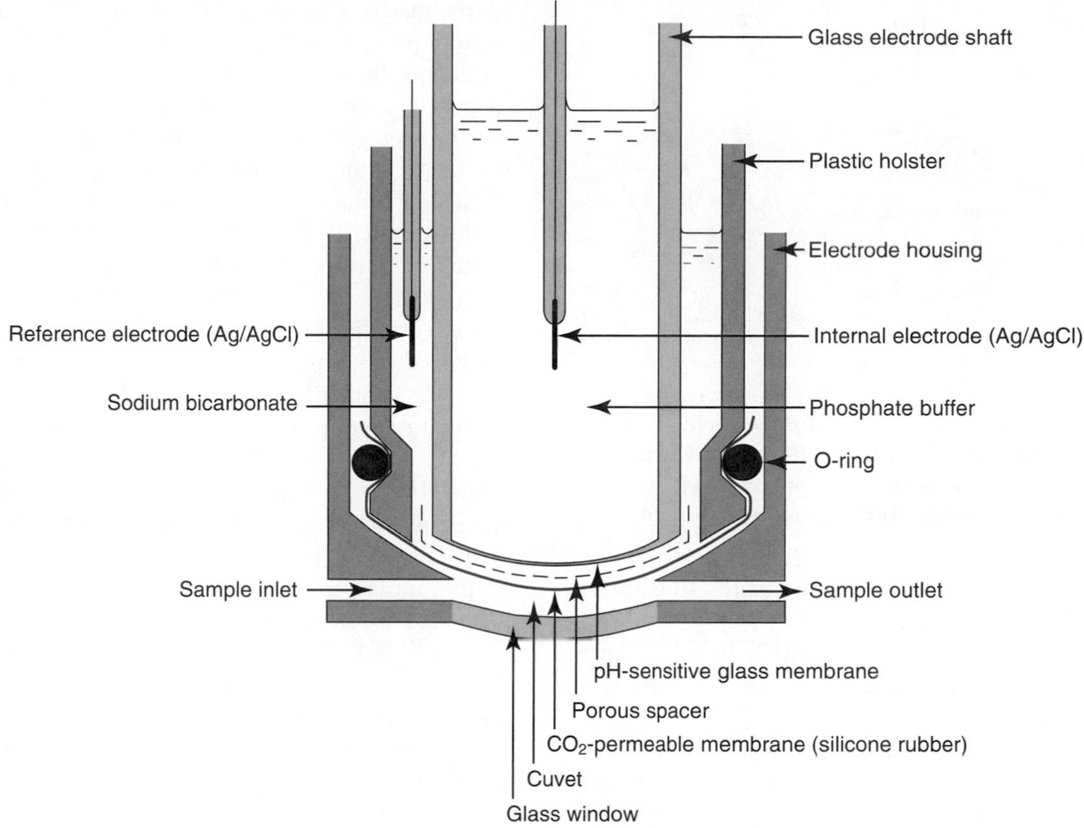

Figure 11-4 Schematic of Severinghaus-style PCO_2 sensor used to monitor CO_2 concentrations in blood samples. *(From Siggard-Andersen O. The acid-base status of the blood, 4th edition. Baltimore: Williams & Wilkins, 1974:172.)*

ion-sensing membrane [based on more water repellent poly(methylmethacrylate)/poly(decylmethacrylate copolymer)] is coated onto a conductive poly(3-octylethiophene 2,5-diyl) (POT) polymer layer on the surface of an underlying gold electrode.[121]

An interesting application of sodium selective polymer (or glass) membrane electrodes is seen in the determination of whole blood hematrocrit.[58] Because intracellular sodium concentrations are much lower than those in the plasma phase, the change in sodium concentration (dilution) measured potentiometrically before and after erythrocyte lysis can be used to assess the hematocrit of the blood sample. This approach can be coupled with simultaneous measurement of changes in potassium ion concentration as determined with a valinomycin-based polymer membrane ISE to quantify the concentration of potassium ions within red blood cells.[96]

Electrodes for PCO_2

Electrodes have been developed to measure PCO_2 in body fluids. The first PCO_2 electrode, developed in the 1950s by Stow and Severinghaus, used a glass pH electrode as the internal element in a potentiometric cell for measurement of the partial pressure of carbon dioxide.[4] This important development paved the way for commercial availability of the three-channel blood analyzer (pH, PCO_2, PO_2) to give the complete picture of the oxygenation and acid-base status of blood.

Figure 11-4 shows a diagram of a typical Severinghaus-style electrode for PCO_2. A thin membrane (≈20 μm), permeable only to gases and water vapor, is in contact with the sample. Membranes of silicone rubber, Teflon, and other polymeric materials are suitable for this purpose. On the opposite side of the membrane is a thin electrolyte layer consisting of a weak bicarbonate salt (about 5 mmol/L) and a chloride salt. A pH electrode and an Ag/AgCl reference electrode are in contact with this solution. The PCO_2 electrode is a self-contained potentiometric cell. Carbon dioxide gas from the sample or calibration matrix diffuses through the membrane and dissolves in the internal electrolyte layer. Carbonic acid is formed and dissociates, shifting the pH of the bicarbonate solution in the internal layer as follows:

$$CO_2 + H_2O \rightleftarrows H_2CO_3 \leftrightarrow H^+ + HCO_3^- \quad \textbf{(12)}$$

and

$$\Delta \log PCO_{2(\text{sample})} \approx \Delta pH_{(\text{internal layer})} \quad \textbf{(13)}$$

The relationship between the sample PCO_2 and the signal generated by the internal pH electrode is logarithmic and is governed by the Nernst equation. The electrode may be calibrated using precision gas mixtures or using solutions with stable PCO_2 concentrations. Although Severinghaus-style electrodes for PCO_2 have gained widespread use in modern blood gas analyzers, the format in which such sensors may be

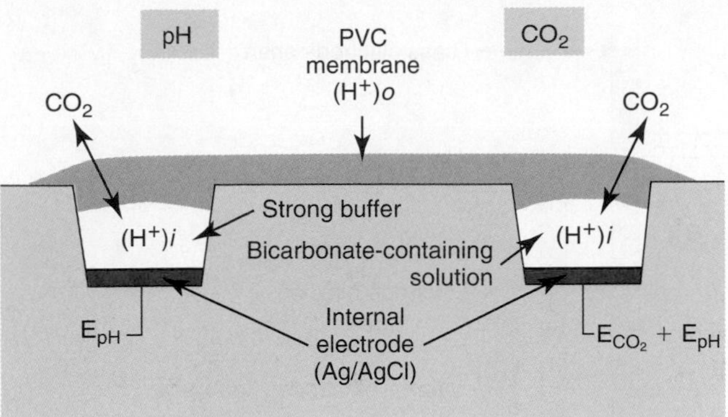

Figure 11-5 Differential planar PCO_2 potentiometric sensor design, based on two identical polymeric membrane pH electrodes, but with different internal reference electrolyte solutions. Both pH sensing membranes are prepared with H^+-selective ionophore.

constructed is limited by size, shape, and ability to fabricate the internal pH sensitive element.

A slightly different potentiometric cell for PCO_2 is shown in Figure 11-5. This cell arrangement uses two PVC-type pH-selective electrodes in a differential mode. The electrode membranes contain a lipophilic amine-type neutral ionophore that exhibits very high selectivity for H^+ (see Figure 11-3). One electrode has an internal layer that is buffered, and the other is unbuffered, consisting of a low concentration of bicarbonate salt. Carbon dioxide gas from the sample or calibration matrix diffuses across the outer H^+-selective PVC membranes of both sensors. On the unbuffered side, CO_2 diffusion produces a potential shift at the internal interface of the pH-responsive membrane proportional to sample PCO_2 concentration. The signal at the electrode with the buffered internal layer is unaffected by CO_2 that diffuses across the membrane. Consequently, one half of the sensor responds to pH alone, and the other half responds to both pH and PCO_2. The signal difference between the two electrodes cancels any contribution of sample pH to the overall measured cell potential. The differential signal is proportional only to PCO_2. Unlike the traditional Severinghaus-style electrode, this differential potentiometric cell PCO_2 sensor has been commercialized in a planar format and is more easily adaptable to mass production in sensor arrays.[16]

Direct Potentiometry by ISE—Units of Measure and Reporting for Clinical Applications

Older analytical methods such as flame photometry for the measurement of electrolytes provide the total *concentration (c)* of a given ion in the sample, usually expressed in units of millimoles of ion per liter of sample (mmol/L). *Molality (m)* is a measure of the moles of ion per mass of water (mmol/kg) in the sample. Using the sodium ion as an example, the relationship between concentration and molality is given by

$$c_{Na^+} = m_{Na^+} \times \rho H_2O \quad \textbf{(14)}$$

where ρH_2O is the mass concentration of water in kg/L. For normal blood plasma, the mass concentration of water is approximately 0.93 kg/L, but in specimens with elevated lipids or protein, the value may be as low as 0.8 kg/L. In these specimens, the difference between concentration and molality may be as great as 20%. A significant advantage of direct potentiometry by ISE for the measurement of electrolytes is that the technique is sensitive to molality and therefore is not affected by variations in the concentration of protein or lipids in the sample. Techniques such as flame photometry, ISE methods requiring sample dilution (also called *indirect potentiometry*), and other photometric methods requiring sample dilution are affected by the presence of protein and lipids. In these methods, only the water phase of the sample is diluted, producing results lower than molality as a function of the concentration of protein and lipids in the sample. Thus there is a risk for errors, such as a falsely low Na^+ concentration (pseudohyponatremia), in cases of extremely elevated protein and lipid concentrations (see also Chapter 28).[2]

In addition to the difference between molality and concentration, measurement of ions by direct potentiometry provides yet another unit of measurement known as *activity (a)*, the concentration of free, unbound ion in solution. Unlike methods sensitive to ion concentration, ISEs do not sense the presence of complexed or electrostatically "hindered" ions in the sample. The relationship between activity and concentration using, again, sodium ion as an example, is expressed as

$$a_{Na^+} = \gamma_{Na^+} \times c_{Na^+} \quad \textbf{(15)}$$

where γ is a dimensionless quantity known as the activity coefficient. The activity coefficient is primarily dependent on ionic strength of the sample as described by the Debye-Huckel equation:

$$\log\gamma = \frac{(A \times z^2 \times I^{0.5})}{1 + B \times a \times I^{0.5}} \quad \textbf{(16)}$$

where A and B are temperature-dependent constants (A = 0.5213 and B = 3.305 in water at 37 °C), a is the ion size parameter for a specific ion, and I is the ionic strength ($I = 0.5\ \Sigma m \times z^2$, where z is the charge number of the ions). Equation (16) shows that a decrease in the activity coefficient occurs with an increase in ionic strength. This effect is more pronounced when the charge *(z)* of the ion is high. Activity coefficients for ions in biological fluids, such as blood and serum, are difficult to calculate with accuracy because of the uncertain contribution of macromolecular ions, such as proteins, to the overall ionic strength. However, assuming that the normal ionic strength of blood plasma is 0.160 mol/kg, estimates of activity coefficients at 37 °C are as follows: Na^+ = 0.75, K^+ = 0.74, and Ca^{2+} = 0.31. Referring to equation (15), activity and concentration will differ greatly in samples of physiologic ionic strength, especially for divalent ions.

Physiologically, ionic activity is assumed to be more relevant than concentration when chemical equilibria or biological processes are considered. Practically, however, *ionic concentration* is the more familiar term in clinical practice, forming the basis of reference intervals and medical decision

TABLE 11-2 Examples of Two-Value Calibrating Solutions for Measurement of pH and Electrolytes by Direct Potentiometry*

Analyte	Calibration Point, mmol/L	Slope Point, mmol/L	Expected Signal Δ, millivolts
Na^+	140	110	6.6
K^+	4.0	8.0	18
Ca^{2+}	1.25	2.50	9
Cl^-	100	80	6
pH	7.38 (pH units)	6.84 (pH units)	32.4

*Ionic strength adjusted to 160 mmol/kg with buffer salts and inert electrolytes.

concentrations for electrolytes. Early in the evolution of ISEs as practical tools in clinical chemistry, it was decided that changing clinical reference intervals to a system based on activity instead of concentration was impractical and carried the risk for clinical misinterpretation. A pragmatic approach for using ISEs in modern analyzers without changing established concentration-based reference intervals is to formulate calibration solutions with ionic strengths and ionic compositions as close as possible to those of blood plasma. In this way, the activity coefficient of each ion in the calibrating solutions approximates that in the sample matrix, allowing calibration and measurement of electrolytes in units of concentration instead of activity.[90]

A typical set of solutions for multi-ISE calibration in an analyzer is shown in Table 11-2. Two points are used to calibrate each ISE. The difference in the cell potential generated by these two solutions (ΔE) is used to calculate the response slope of the cell (slope = ΔE/Δlog c), where *c* is the concentration of ion in each calibrating solution, substituted for activity. The standard electrode potential, E^0, is calculated as the *y*-intercept. Determination of ion concentration in an unknown sample is then a straightforward solution of the Nickolsky-Eisenman equation [equation (10)], after the cell potential generated by the sample is measured.

Calibration of the cell is done in units of concentration; however, as mentioned earlier, direct potentiometry is sensitive to the molality of the ion, which is related to concentration by the water content of the sample [equation (14)]. The water content of aqueous calibrating solutions shown in Table 11-2 is approximately 0.99 kg/L. The water content of normal blood plasma is ≈0.93 kg/L. Molality is 7% greater than concentration in this normal plasma specimen. The direct potentiometric cell will report results approximately 6% greater than the concentration in normal specimens because of this difference in water content between sample and calibrator (0.99/0.93 = 1.06). Direct potentiometry presents an advantage in that the technique is not affected by the presence of protein and lipids in the sample; however, the application of clinical reference intervals based on concentration again poses a risk for confusion and clinical misinterpretation. Most manufacturers of electrolyte measurement systems have overcome this problem in a practical way by following Clinical and Laboratory Standards Institute (CLSI) guidelines recommending the use of correlation factors to standardize ISE measurements to units of concentration. These factors may be obtained by standardizing the ISE measurement to certified reference materials based on human serum, with electrolyte values assigned in units of concentration.[21,22,49] Appropriate correlation factors are then applied to sample calculations using algorithms resident in the instrument software.

VOLTAMMETRY/AMPEROMETRY

Voltammetric and amperometric techniques are among the most sensitive and widely applicable of all electroanalytical methods.

Basic Concepts

In contrast to potentiometry, voltammetric and amperometric methods are based on electrolytic electrochemical cells in which an external voltage is applied to a polarizable working electrode (measured vs. a suitable reference electrode: $E_{appl} = E_{work} = E_{ref}$), and the resulting cathodic (for analytical reductions) or anodic (for analytical oxidations) current of the cell is monitored and is proportional to the concentration of analyte present in the test sample. Current flows only if E_{appl} is greater than a certain voltage (decomposition voltage), determined by the thermodynamics for a given redox reaction of interest [$Ox + ne^- \rightleftharpoons Red$; defined by the E^0 value for that reaction (standard reduction potential)] and the kinetics for heterogeneous electron transfer at the interface of the working electrode. Often, slow kinetics of electron transfer for the redox reaction on a given inert working electrode (Pt, carbon, gold, etc.) mandates use of a much more negative (for reductions) or positive (for oxidations) E_{appl} than predicted based merely on the E^0 for a given redox reaction. This is called an *overpotential* (η). Regardless of whether an overpotential for electron transfer exists, a specific oxidation or reduction reaction occurs at the surface of the working electrode in voltammetry/amperometry, and it is the charge transfer at this interface (current flow) that provides the analytical information.

For electrolytic cells that form the basis of voltammetric and amperometric methods.

$$E_{appl} = E_{cell} + \eta - iR_{cell} \tag{17}$$

where E_{cell} is the thermodynamic potential between the working and reference electrodes in the absence of an applied external voltage. When the external voltage is greater or less than this equilibrium potential, plus or minus any overpotential (η), then current will flow because of an oxidation or reduction reaction at the working electrode. A voltammogram is simply the plot of observed current, *i*, versus E_{appl} (Figure 11-6). In amperometry (see later), a fixed voltage is applied and the resulting current is monitored. The amount of current is inversely related to the resistance of the

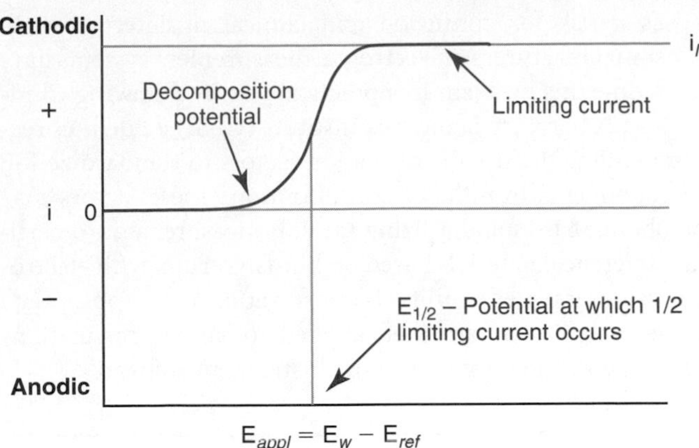

Figure 11-6 Illustration of the current versus voltage curve (voltammogram) obtained for oxidized species (Ox) reduced (Red) at the surface of the working electrode, as the E_{appl} is scanned more negatively and the solution is stirred to yield a steady-state response.

electrolyte solution and to any "apparent" resistance that develops because of mass transfer of the analyte species to the surface of the working electrode. Because electrochemical reactions are heterogeneous, occurring only at the surface of the working electrode, the amount of current observed is also highly dependent on the surface area (A) of the working electrode.

When a potential is applied to a working electrode that will oxidize or reduce a species in the solution phase contacting the electrode, the electrochemical reaction causes the concentration of electroactive species to decrease at the surface of the electrode (Figure 11-7), a process termed *concentration polarization.* This in turn causes a concentration gradient of analyte species between the bulk sample solution and the surface of the electrode.[35] When the bulk solution is stirred, the diffusion layer of analyte grows out from the surface of the electrode very quickly to a fixed distance controlled by how vigorously the solution is stirred. This diffusion layer is termed the *Nernst layer* and has a finite thickness (δ) after a relatively short time period (see Figure 11-7) when the solution is moving (convection). Voltammetry carried out in the presence of convection (by stirring the solution, rotating the electrode, flowing solution by electrode, etc.) is called *steady-state voltammetry.* When the solution is not moving, the diffusion layer grows further and further with time (i.e., not constant), creating larger and larger δ values over time. This is termed *non–steady-state voltammetry* and often results in peak currents in i versus E_{appl} plots for electrolytic cells.

In steady-state voltammetry, when the potential of the working electrode is scanned past a value that will cause an electrochemical reaction, the current will rise rapidly and then will plateau, even as E_{appl} changes further. Figure 11-6 illustrates such a wave for a hypothetical reduction of an oxidized species (Ox) via an n electron reduction to a reduced species (Red). When the applied potential is much more negative than required, the current reaches a limiting value (termed the limiting current, i_l). This limiting current is

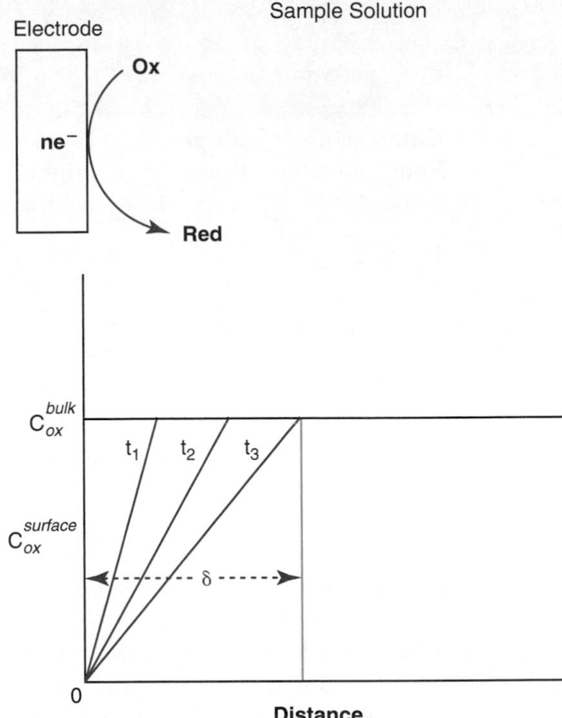

Figure 11-7 Concept of electrochemical reaction increasing diffusion layer thickness (concentration polarization) of analytes via reduction (or oxidation) at the surface of the working electrode. As time (t) increases, the diffusion layer thickness grows quickly to a value determined by degree of convection in the sample solution.

proportional to the concentration of the electroactive species (Ox in this case) as expressed by the following equation:

$$i_l = nFA\left(\frac{D}{\delta}\right)C_{ox} \qquad (18)$$

where i is the measured current in amperes, n equals the number of electrons in the electrochemical reaction (reduction in this case), F is Faraday's constant (96,487 coulombs/mol), A is the electrochemical surface area of the working electrode (in cm^2) (assuming a planar electrode geometry), D is the diffusion coefficient (in cm^2/sec) of the electroactive species (Ox in this case), δ is the diffusion layer thickness (in cm), and C is the concentration of the analyte species in mol/cm^3. The D/δ term is often denoted as m_o, the mass transfer coefficient of the Ox species to the surface of the working electrode. Note that equation (18) indicates a linear relationship for limiting current and concentration. The exact same equation applies for detecting reduced species by an oxidation reaction at the working electrode. In this case, by convention, the resulting anodic current is considered a negative current. As shown in Figure 11-6, the potential of the working electrode that corresponds to a current that is exactly one half the limiting current is termed the $E_{1/2}$ value. This value is not dependent on analyte concentration. The $E_{1/2}$ is determined by the thermodynamics (E^0) of the given redox reaction, the solution conditions (e.g., if protons are involved in reaction, then the pH will influence the $E_{1/2}$ value), and any overpotential caused by slow electron transfer, etc., at a particular working electrode surface. The $E_{1/2}$ values are indicative of a given species undergoing an electrochemical reaction under specified conditions; hence, the $E_{1/2}$ values enable one to distinguish one electroactive species from another in the same sample. If the $E_{1/2}$ values for various species differ significantly (e.g., >120 mV), then measurements of several limiting currents in a given voltammogram can yield quantitative results for several different species simultaneously.

Electrochemical cells employed to carry out voltammetric or amperometric measurements can involve a two- or three-electrode configuration. In the two-electrode mode, external voltage is applied between the working electrode and a reference electrode, and the current monitored. Because the current must also pass through the reference electrode, such current flow can potentially alter the surface concentration of electroactive species that poises the actual half-cell potential of the reference electrode, changing its value by a concentration polarization process. For example, if an Ag/AgCl reference electrode were used in a cell in which a reduction reaction for the analyte occurs at the working electrode, then an oxidation reaction would take place at the surface of the reference electrode:

$$Ag^0 + Cl^- \rightarrow AgCl_{(s)} + 1\,e^- \tag{19}$$

Hence, the activity/concentration of chloride ions near the surface of the electrode would decrease, which would make the potential of the reference electrode more positive than its true equilibrium value based on the actual activity of chloride ion in the reference half-cell, because the Nernst equation for this half-cell is

$$E_{Ag/AgCl} = E^0_{Ag/AgCl} - 0.059\log(a^{surface}_{Cl^-}) \tag{20}$$

Such concentration polarization of the reference electrode is prevented by keeping the current density (J; amperes/cm^2) very low at the reference electrode. This is achieved in practice by making sure that the area of the working electrode in the electrochemical cell is much smaller than the surface area of the reference electrode; hence the total current flow will be limited by this much smaller area, and J values for the reference will be very small, as desired, to prevent concentration polarization.

To completely eliminate changes in reference electrode half-cell potentials, a three-electrode potentiostat is often employed. In simple terms, the potentiostat applies a voltage to the working electrode, which is measured versus a reference electrode via a zero current potentiometric-type measurement, but the current flow is between the working electrode and a third electrode, called the *counter electrode.* Thus if reduction takes place at the working electrode, oxidation would occur at the counter electrode; but no net reaction would take place at the surface of the reference electrode, because no current flows through this electrode. A potentiostat circuit is relatively simple to construct using modern operational amplifiers.

In voltammetric methods, the E_{appl} is varying via some waveform to alter the working electrode potential as a function of time and the resulting current measured. The current change occurs at the decomposition potential range, which is best when specific for a given analyte. However, the location of the current response as a function of E_{appl} provides information on the nature of the species present (e.g., $E_{1/2}$), along with a concentration-dependent signal. This scan of E_{appl} can be linear (linear sweep voltammetry) or it can have more complex shapes that enable greatly enhanced sensitivity to be achieved for monitoring the concentration of a given electroactive species (e.g., normal pulsed voltammetry, differential pulse voltammetry, square wave voltammetry).[91] When a dropping mercury electrode (DME) is used, such voltammetric methods are considered polarographic methods of analysis.

Amperometric methods differ from voltammetry in that E_{appl} is fixed, generally at a potential value that occurs in the limiting current plateau region of the voltammogram and simply monitors the resulting current, which will be proportional to concentration. Amperometry can be more sensitive than common voltammetric methods because background charging currents, which arise from changing the E_{appl} as a function of time in voltammetry, do not exist. Hence, when selectivity can be assured at a given E_{appl} value, amperometry may be preferred to voltammetric methods for more sensitive quantitative measurements.

Applications

Molecular oxygen is capable of undergoing several reduction reactions, all with a significant overpotential at solid electrodes, such as Pt, Au, or Ag. For example, the following reaction,

$$O_2 + 2H_2O + 4e^- \rightarrow 4OH^- \quad (E^0 = +0.179 \text{ vs Ag/AgCl; 1 M Cl}^-) \tag{21}$$

exhibits an $E_{1/2}$ at around −0.500 V on a Pt electrode (vs. a Ag/AgCl reference electrode), with a limiting current plateau beginning at approximately −0.600 V. This reaction is used to monitor the PO_2 in blood, which is the basis of the widely used Clark-style amperometric oxygen sensor (Figure 11-8). This device employs a small area planar platinum electrode as a working electrode (encased in insulating glass or other material) and an Ag/AgCl reference electrode, typically with a cylindrical design (see Figure 11-8). This two-electrode electrolytic cell is placed within a sensor housing, on which a gas-permeable membrane (e.g., polypropylene, silicone rubber, Teflon) is held at the distal end. The inner working platinum electrode is pressed tightly against the gas-permeable membrane to create a thin film of internal electrolyte solution (usually buffer with KCl added). Oxygen in the sample can permeate across the membrane and can be reduced in accordance with the above electrochemical reaction. An E_{appl} of −0.650 or −0.700 V versus Ag/AgCl (within the limiting current regime) to the Pt working electrode will result in an observed current that is proportional to the PO_2 present in

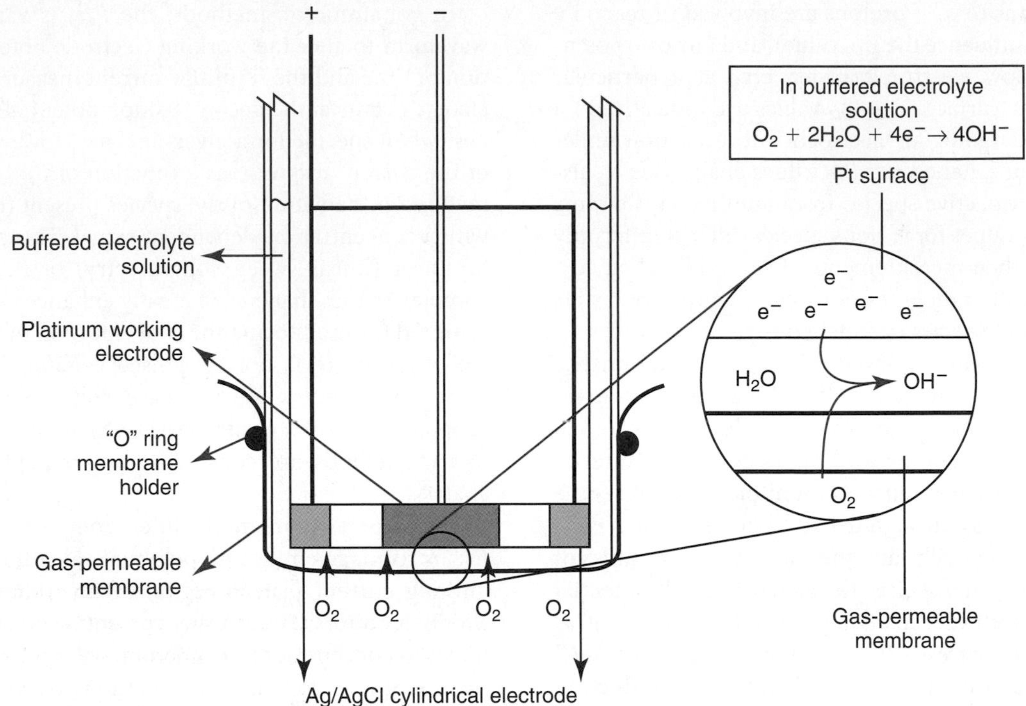

Figure 11-8 Design of Clark-style amperometric oxygen sensor used to monitor PO_2 in blood.

the sample (including whole blood). In the absence of any oxygen, the current at this applied voltage under amperometric conditions will be very near zero.

The outer gas-permeable membrane enables the Clark electrode to detect oxygen with very high selectivity over other easily reduced species that might be present in a given sample (e.g., metal ions, cystine). Indeed, only other gas species or highly lipophilic organic species can partition into and pass through such gas-permeable membranes. One type of interference in clinical samples can be caused by certain anesthesia gases, such as nitrous oxide, halothane, and isoflurane. These species can also diffuse through the outer membrane of the sensor, can be electrochemically reduced at the platinum electrode, and can yield a false-positive value for the measurement of PO_2.[30] However, optimized gas-permeable membrane materials and appropriate control of the applied potential to the cathode of the sensor have greatly reduced this problem in modern instruments. The outer gas-permeable membranes also help restrict the diffusion of analyte to the inner working electrode; hence the membrane can control the mass transport of analyte [D/δ term in equation (18)] such that in the presence or absence of sample convection, mass transport of oxygen to the surface of the platinum working electrode is essentially the same.

The basic design of the Clark amperometric PO_2 sensor can be used to detect other gas species by altering applied voltage to the working electrode. For example, it is possible to detect nitric oxide (NO) with high selectivity using a similar gas electrode design in which the platinum is polarized at +0.900 versus Ag/AgCl to oxidize diffusing NO to nitrate at the platinum anode.[12] Such NO sensors can be used for a variety of biomedically important studies to deduce the amount of NO locally at or near the surface of various NO-producing cells.

Beyond amperometric devices, one specialized method of detecting trace concentrations of toxic metal ions in clinical samples is anodic stripping voltammetry (ASV). In ASV, a carbon working electrode is used (sometimes further coated with an Hg film), and the E_{appl} is first fixed at a very negative E_{appl} voltage, so that all metal ions in the solution will be reduced to elemental metals (M^0) within the mercury film and/or on the surface of the carbon. Then the E_{appl} is scanned more positively, and reduced metals deposited in and/or on the surface of the working electrode are reoxidized, giving a large anodic current peak proportional to the concentration of metal ions in the original sample. The potential at which these peaks are observed indicates which metal is present, and the height of stripping peak current is directly proportional to the concentration of the metal ion in the original sample. Such ASV techniques can be used to detect the total concentration of Pb in whole blood samples, providing a rapid screening method for lead exposure and poisoning.[36]

Another biomedical example of modern voltammetry is a rapid scan cyclic voltammetric technique that has been used to quantify dopamine in brain tissue of freely moving animals.[101] In this application, oxidation of dopamine to a quinone species at an implanted microcarbon electrode (at approximately +0.600 V vs. Ag/AgCl) yields peak currents proportional to dopamine concentrations. The electrode can be used to measure this neurotransmitter in different regions of the brain or in a fixed location. Often, pharmacologic or electrical stimulation can be employed to measure the change

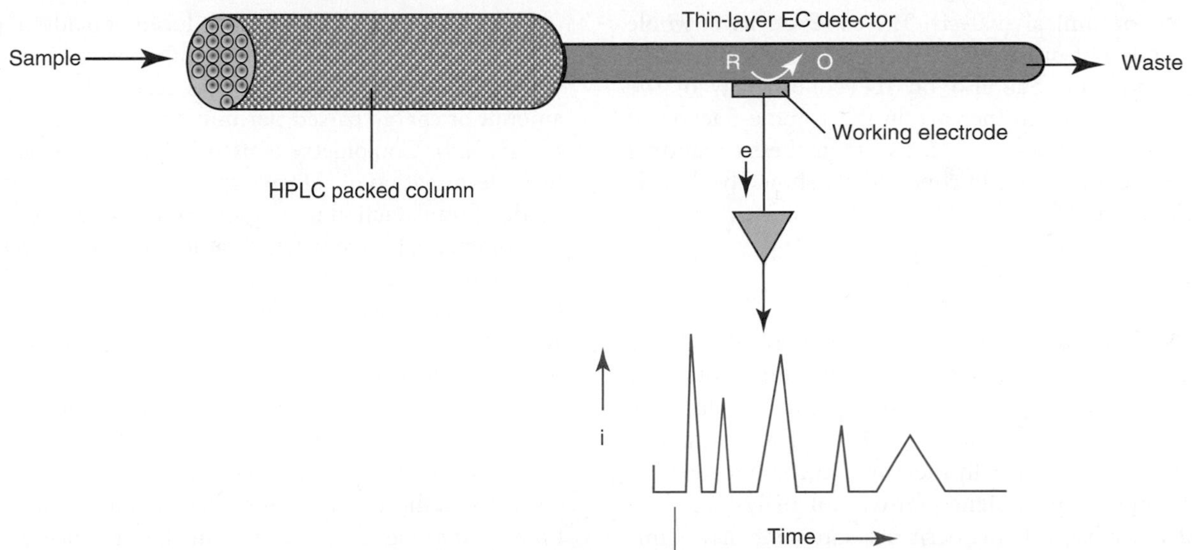

Figure 11-9 Schematic of liquid chromatography with electrochemical detection (LC-EC) system, with electrochemical detector monitoring elution of analytes from a high-performance liquid chromatography (HPLC) column by their oxidation or reduction (shown here as example) at a suitable thin-layer working electrode.

in local dopamine concentrations due to such stimulation techniques.

Although voltammetric/amperometric techniques can be applied to detect a wide range of species, the selectivity offered for measurements in complex clinical samples—where many species can be electroactive—is rather limited. For example, as stated in the previous discussion relevant to the Clark oxygen sensor, in the absence of the gas-permeable membrane, other species that can be reduced at or near the same E_{appl} as oxygen would cause significant interference.

To expand the range of analytes that can be detected with voltammetric/amperometric methods, electrochemical techniques can be used as highly sensitive detectors for modern high-performance liquid chromatography (HPLC) systems (see Chapter 13). In liquid chromatography with electrochemical detection (LC-EC), eluting solutes are detected by flow-through electrodes (usually carbon or mercury) designed to have extremely low dead volumes (Figure 11-9). The electrodes can be operated in amperometric or voltammetric modes (with high scan speeds), and several electrodes can be operated simultaneously in series or in parallel flow arrangements to gain additional selectivity.[57] For example, homocysteine can be measured with (1) the addition of reducing agents to a serum sample to generate free homocysteine, (2) precipitation of proteins in the sample (with trichloroacetic acid), and (3) separation of the serum components on a reversed-phase octadecylsilane HPLC column. The eluting homocysteine is detected and measured with online electrochemical detection via homocysteine oxidation to the corresponding mercuric dithiolate complex:

$$2RSH + Hg \rightarrow Hg(RS)_2 + 2H^+ + 2e^- \quad \textbf{(22)}$$

using a thin-layer Hg/Au amalgam electrode poised at +0.150 V versus Ag/AgCl.[105] Integration of the eluting band for homocysteine provides quantitative results, with very high selectivity. Similarly, catechols and catecholamines can be readily detected in serum by a similar LC-EC method, with eluted catechols oxidized to quinones at a flow-through carbon working electrode poised at potentials typically >0.200 V versus Ag/AgCl. Further, a host of therapeutic drugs can also be quantitated in serum or urine via LC-EC methods.

CONDUCTOMETRY

Conductometry is an electrochemical technique used to determine the quantity of an analyte present in a mixture by measurement of its effects on the electrical conductivity of the mixture. It is the measure of the ability of ions in solution to carry current under the influence of a potential difference. In a conductometric cell, potential is applied between two inert metal electrodes. An alternating potential with a frequency between 100 and 3000 Hz is used to prevent polarization of the electrodes. A decrease in solution resistance results in an increase in conductance, and more current is passed between the electrodes. The resulting current flow is also alternating. The current is directly proportional to solution conductance. Conductance is considered the inverse of resistance and may be expressed in units of ohm^{-1} (siemens). In clinical analysis, conductometry is frequently used for measurement of the volume fraction of erythrocytes in whole blood (hematocrit) and as the transduction mechanism for some biosensors.

Erythrocytes act as electrical insulators because of their lipid-based membrane composition. This phenomenon was used first in the 1940s to measure the volume fraction of erythrocytes in whole blood (hematocrit) by conductivity[103] and is used today to measure hematocrit on multianalyte instruments for clinical analysis. The conductivity of whole blood depends not only on the volume fraction and shape of the erythrocytes, but also on the conductivity of the surrounding plasma. An increase in the volume fraction of erythrocytes that are less conductive than the surrounding plasma leads to a decrease in conductivity shown by the following relationship[124]:

$$G_b = \frac{a}{1} + \frac{H}{100 - H} \times c \qquad (23)$$

where G_b is the conductivity of whole blood, a is the plasma conductivity, H is the percent of hematocrit, and c is a factor for erythrocyte orientation. In practice, plasma conductivity also contains correction factors for Na^+ and K^+ concentrations. These cations are usually measured in conjunction with hematocrit on systems designed for clinical analysis.

Conductivity-based hematocrit measurements have limitations.[112] Abnormal protein concentrations will change plasma conductivity and interfere with measurement. Low protein concentrations resulting from dilution of blood with protein-free electrolyte solutions during cardiopulmonary bypass surgery will result in erroneously low hematocrit values by conductivity. Preanalytical variables, such as insufficient mixing of the sample, will also lead to errors.[133] Hemoglobin is the preferred analyte to monitor blood loss and the need for transfusion during trauma and surgery. However, electrochemical measurement of hematocrit in conjunction with blood gases and electrolytes remains in use mainly because of simplicity and convenience, despite some limitations.

Another clinical application of conductance is for electronic counting of blood cells in suspension. Termed the *Coulter principle,* it relies on the fact that the conductivity of blood cells is lower than that of a salt solution used as a suspension medium.[25] The cell suspension is forced to flow through a tiny orifice. Two electrodes are placed on either side of the orifice, and a constant current is established between the electrodes. Each time a cell passes through the orifice, resistance increases; this causes a spike in the electrical potential difference between the electrodes. The pulses are then amplified and counted.

COULOMETRY

Coulometry measures the electrical charge passing between two electrodes in an electrochemical cell. The amount of charge passing between the electrodes is directly proportional to oxidation or reduction of an electroactive substance at one of the electrodes. The number of coulombs transferred in this process is related to the absolute amount of electroactive substance by Faraday's law:

$$Q = n \times N \times F \qquad (24)$$

where

Q = is the amount of charge passing through the cell (unit: C = coulomb = ampere × second)

n = the number of electrons transferred in the oxidation or reduction reaction

N = the amount of substance reduced or oxidized in moles

F = Faraday constant (96,487 coulombs/mol)

The measurement of current is related to charge as the amount of charge passed per unit time (ampere = coulomb per second). Coulometry is used in clinical applications for the determination of chloride in serum or plasma and as the mode of transduction in certain types of biosensors.

Commercial coulometric titrators have been developed for determination of chloride. A constant current is applied between a silver wire (anode) and a platinum wire (cathode). At the anode, Ag is oxidized to Ag^+. At the cathode, H^+ is reduced to hydrogen gas. At a constant applied current, the number of coulombs passed between the anode and the cathode is directly proportional to time (coulombs = amperes × seconds). Therefore, the absolute number of silver ions produced at the anode may be calculated from the amount of time current passes through it. In the presence of Cl^-, Ag^+ ions formed are precipitated as $AgCl_{(s)}$, and the amount of free Ag^+ in solution is low. When all Cl^- ions have been complexed, a sudden increase in the concentration of Ag^+ in solution is noted. Excess Ag^+ is sensed amperometrically at a second Ag electrode, polarized at negative potential. The excess Ag^+ is reduced to Ag, producing a current. When this current exceeds a certain value, the titration is stopped. The absolute number of Cl^- ions present in the sample is calculated from the time during which titration with Ag^+ was in progress. Given the volumetric amount of serum or plasma sample originally used, it is possible to calculate the concentration of Cl^- in the sample. Coulometric titration is one of the most accurate electrochemical techniques because the method measures the absolute quantity of electroactive substance in the sample. Coulometry is considered the gold standard for determination of chloride in serum or plasma. However, the method is subject to interference from anions in the sample with affinity for Ag^+ greater than chloride, such as bromide,[129] and is not commonly used in today's clinical laboratories.

OPTICAL CHEMICAL SENSORS

An *optode* is an optical sensor used in analytical instruments to measure blood gases and electrolytes. Optodes have certain advantages over electrodes, including (1) ease of miniaturization, (2) less noise (no transduction wires), (3) potential long-term stability using ratiometric-type measurements at multiple wavelengths,[108] and (4) do not require a separate reference electrode. These advantages initially promoted the development of optical sensor technology for design of intravascular blood gas sensors (see in vivo sensor section later). However, the same basic sensing principles can be used in clinical chemistry instrumentation designed for more classical in vitro measurements on discrete samples. In such systems, light can be brought to and from the sensing site by optical fibers or simply by appropriate positioning of light sources [light-emitting diodes (LEDs)], filters, and photodetectors to monitor absorbance (by reflectance), fluorescence, or phosphorescence (Figure 11-10).

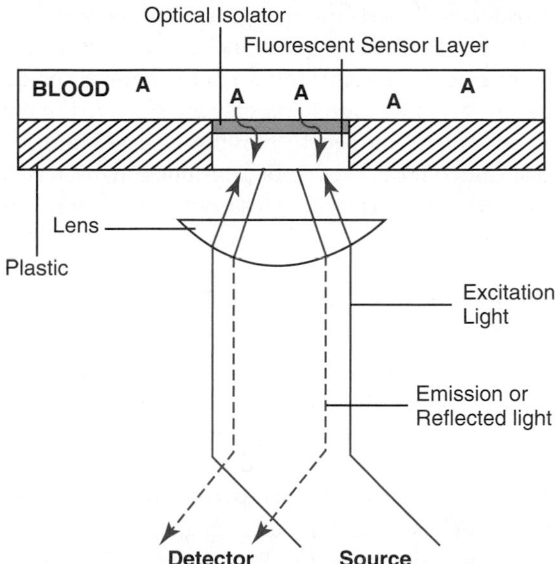

Figure 11-10 General design for in vitro optical sensor designed to detect given analyte in blood sample. Polymer film contains dye that changes spectral properties in proportion to the amount of analyte in the sample phase. Example shown is for sensing film that changes luminescence (fluorescence or phosphorescence).

Basic Concepts

Optical sensors devised for PO_2 measurements are typically based on immobilization of certain organic dyes (e.g., pyrene, diphenylphenanthrene, phenanthrene, fluoranthene) or metal ligand complexes [e.g., ruthenium(II) tris(dipyridine), Pt and Pd metalloporphyrins] within hydrophobic polymer films (e.g., silicone rubber) in which oxygen is very soluble.[29] The fluorescence or phosphorescence of such species at a given wavelength is often quenched in the presence of paramagnetic species, including molecular oxygen. In the case of embedded fluorescent dyes, the intensity of the emitted fluorescence of such films will decrease in proportion to the partial pressure of the oxygen (PO_2) in the sample in contact with the polymer film, in accordance with the Stern-Volmer equation for quenching:

$$\frac{I_0}{I_{PO_2}} = 1 + kPO_2 \quad (25)$$

where

I_0 = fluorescence intensity in the absence of any oxygen
I_{PO_2} = fluorescence intensity at a given partial pressure of oxygen (PO_2)
k = quenching constant for the particular fluorophore used

Hence a linear relationship exists between the ratio I_0/I_{PO2} and the PO_2 in the sample phase. The larger the Stern-Volmer constant, the greater is the degree of quenching for the given fluorophore. However, it is important that the quenching constant is in a range that will yield linear Stern-Volmer behavior over the physiologically relevant range of PO_2 in blood. For example, if k is too large, then maximum quenching possible will occur over a range of PO_2 that is less than physiologic.

Phosphorescence intensity or phosphorescence lifetime measurements of immobilized metal ligand complexes can also be employed (i.e., binding of oxygen decreases excited state lifetimes). Sensors based on changes in luminescent lifetime have the inherent advantage of being insensitive to perturbations in the optical path length and the amount of active dye present in the sensing layer.

Optical pH sensors require immobilization of appropriate pH indicators [e.g., fluorescein, 8-hydroxy-1,2,6-pyrene trisulfonate (HPTS), phenol red] within thin layers of hydrophilic polymers (e.g., hydrogels), because equilibrium access of protons to the indicator is essential. The absorbance or fluorescence of the protonated or deprotonated form of the species can be used for sensing purposes.[108] One issue with respect to using immobilized indicators for accurate physiologic pH measurements is the effect of ionic strength on the pKa of the indicator. Because optical sensors measure the concentration of protonated or deprotonated dye as an indirect measure of hydrogen ion activity, variations in ionic strength of the physiologic sample can influence the accuracy of the pH measurement.

Applications

Optical sensors suitable for the determination of PCO_2 employ optical pH transducers (with immobilized indicators) as inner transducers in an arrangement similar to the classical Severinghaus-style electrochemical sensor design (see Figure 11-4). The addition of bicarbonate salt within the pH sensing hydrogel layer creates the required electrolyte film layer, which varies in pH depending on the partial pressure of carbon dioxide (PCO_2) in equilibrium with the film. The optical pH sensor is covered by an outer gas-permeable hydrophobic film (e.g., silicone rubber) to prevent proton access, yet it allows CO_2 equilibration with the pH sensing layer. As the partial pressure of the CO_2 in the sample increases, the pH of the bicarbonate layer decreases, and the corresponding decrease in the deprotonated form of the indicator (or increase in the protonated form) is sensed optically.

Two approaches have been used to sense electrolyte ions optically in physiologic samples. One method employs many of the same lipophilic ionophores developed for polymer membrane–type ISEs (see Figure 11-3).[6,15] These species are doped into very thin hydrophobic polymeric films along with a lipophilic pH indicator. In the case of cation ionophores (e.g., valinomycin for sensing potassium), when cations from the sample are extracted by the ionophore into the thin film, the pH indicator (RH) loses a proton to the sample phase to maintain charge neutrality within the organic film (yielding R^-). This results in a change in the optical absorption or fluorescence spectrum of the polymer layer. If the thickness of the films is kept at $<10\ \mu m$, equilibrium response times on the order of <1 min have been achieved. The main limitation of this design is that the pH of the sample phase also influences the overall extraction equilibrium for ions into the film.

Thus simultaneous and independent measurement of sample pH is required, or buffered dilution and/or pH control of the sample phase is necessary to obtain accurate measurements of electrolytes.

A second technique used to sense electrolyte ions is immobilization of a cation and/or anion recognition agent within a hydrogel matrix, similar to the pH sensors described earlier. The recognition agent in this case is not usually lipophilic; therefore it must be covalently anchored to the hydrogel, so that it does not leach into the sample phase. The agent is designed so that selective cation or anion binding alters the absorbance or fluorescence spectrum of the species within the hydrogel. Typically, this is achieved by linking ion recognition and chromophoric properties within a single organic molecule. Such ion sensors have been used successfully in at least one commercial blood gas-electrolyte analyzer using an array of sensors of the generic design similar to that illustrated in Figure 11-10.

BIOSENSORS

A biosensor is a specific type of chemical sensor consisting of a biological recognition element and a physicochemical transducer, often an electrochemical[52,117] or an optical device. The biological element is capable of recognizing the presence and activity and/or concentration of a specific analyte in solution. The recognition may be a *biocatalytic reaction (enzyme-based biosensor)* or a *binding process (affinity-based biosensor)* when the recognition element is, for example, an antibody, DNA segment, or cell receptor. Interaction of the recognition element with a target analyte results in a measurable change in a solution property locally at the surface of the device, such as formation of a product or consumption of a reactant. The transducer converts the change in solution property into a quantifiable electrical signal. The mode of transduction may be one of several, including electrochemical or optical measurement and measurement of mass or heat. The present discussion will be limited to biosensors based on electrochemical and optical modes of transduction because they constitute the majority of biosensors used for clinical applications.

Enzyme-Based Biosensors With Amperometric Detection

Enzyme-based biosensors based on electrochemical transducers, specifically amperometric electrodes, are the most commonly used for clinical analyses and the most frequently cited in the literature.[51] Clark and Lyons developed the first amperometric biosensor; it was used to measure glucose in blood and was based on immobilizing glucose oxidase on the surface of an amperometric PO_2 sensor.[20] A solution of glucose oxidase was physically entrapped between the gas-permeable membrane of the PO_2 electrode and an outer semipermeable membrane (Figure 11-11, see general design). The outer membrane was of a low molecular weight cutoff to allow substrate (glucose) and oxygen from the sample to pass, but not proteins and other macromolecules. In this way, enzymes could be concentrated at the sensor's surface. Oxidation of glucose, catalyzed by glucose oxidase as follows,

$$\text{Glucose} + O_2 \xrightarrow{\text{glucose oxidase}} \text{gluconic acid} + H_2O_2 \quad \textbf{(26)}$$

consumes oxygen near the surface of the sensor. The rate of decrease in PO_2 is a function of the glucose concentration and is monitored by the PO_2 electrode. A steady-state reduced partial pressure of oxygen can be achieved at the surface in a short period of time, yielding a steady-state current value that

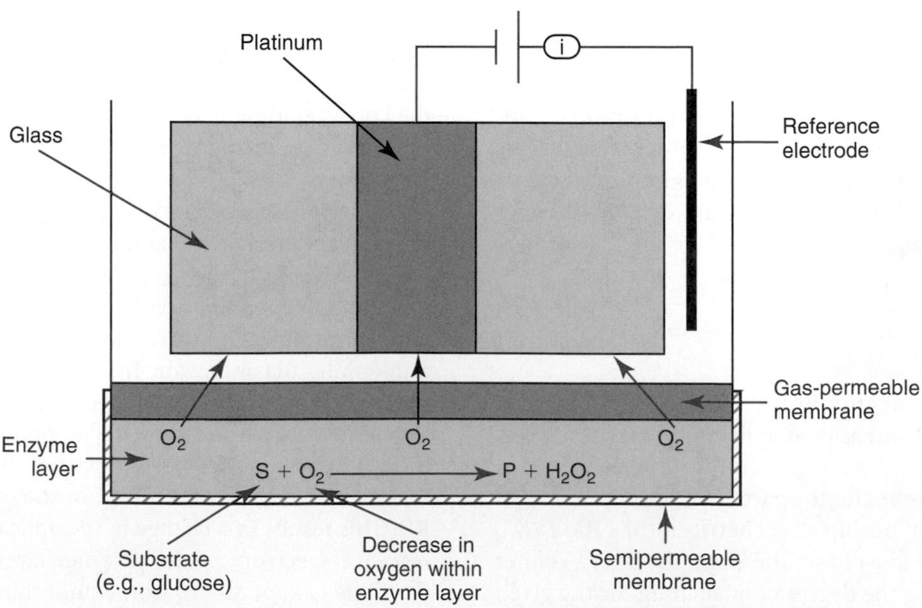

Figure 11-11 Illustration of enzyme electrode prepared using oxidase enzyme immobilized at the surface of amperometric PO_2 sensor. Increase in substrate concentration *S* reduces the amount of oxygen present at the surface of the sensor.

decreases as a function of glucose concentration in the sample.

If the polarizing voltage of the PO_2 electrode is reversed, making the platinum electrode positive (anode) relative to the Ag/AgCl reference electrode, and if the gas-permeable membrane is replaced with a hydrophilic membrane containing the immobilized enzyme, it is possible to oxidize the H_2O_2 produced by the glucose oxidase as follows:

$$H_2O_2 \rightarrow 2H^+ + O_2 + 2e^- \quad (27)$$

The steady-state current produced is now directly proportional to the concentration of glucose in the sample.

In practice, a sufficiently high voltage (overpotential) must be applied to the platinum anode to drive the oxidation of the hydrogen peroxide. An applied voltage of +0.7 volts or greater (relative to Ag/AgCl) is typically used. Figure 11-12 illustrates this basic hydrogen peroxide detection design, which is suitable for use in devising clinically useful sensors for glucose, but also for a host of other substrates for which suitable oxidase enzymes generate hydrogen peroxide.

Immobilization of enzymes in the early biosensors was a simple entrapment method behind a membrane of low molecular weight cutoff; this approach is still used in some commercial applications. Many other schemes for enzyme immobilization for biosensor development have been suggested.[48] Most common are cross-linking of the enzyme with an inert protein, such as bovine serum albumin (BSA), using glutaraldehyde, simple adsorption of enzyme to electrode surfaces, and covalent binding of enzymes to insoluble carriers, such as nylon or glass. Another immobilization technique involves bulk modification of an electrode material, mixing enzymes with carbon paste, which serves as both the enzyme immobilization matrix and the electroactive surface.[45]

One of the first biosensor-based systems for the measurement of glucose in blood was commercialized by Yellow Springs Instruments, Inc. (YSI), Yellow Springs, Ohio, in 1975, and used the amperometric detection of H_2O_2 as the measurement principle (see Figure 11-12). Dependence of the measured glucose value on oxygen concentration in the sample was a problem because significantly less than the

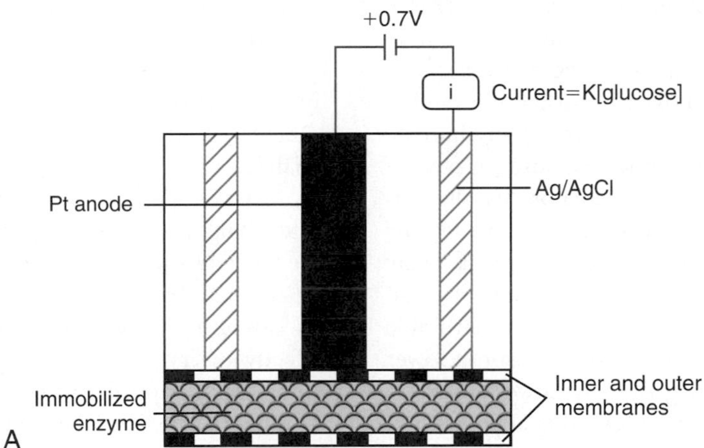

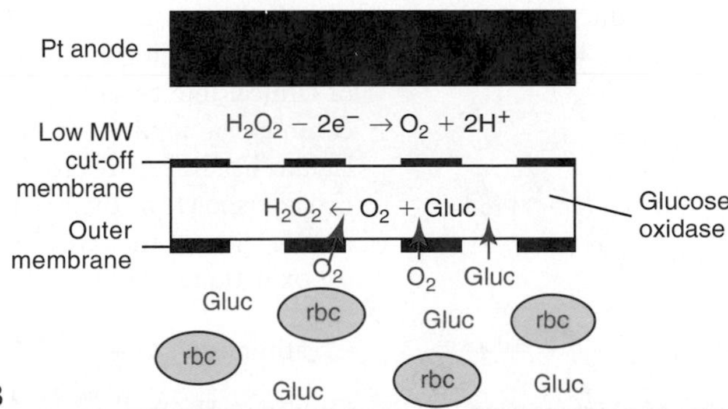

Figure 11-12 A, Design of amperometric enzyme electrode based on anodic detection of hydrogen peroxide generated from oxidase enzymatic reaction (e.g., glucose oxidase). B, Expanded view of the sensing surface shows the different membranes and electrochemical processes that yield the anodic current proportional to the substrate concentration in the sample. *(From Meyerhoff M. New in vitro analytical approaches for clinical chemistry measurements in critical care. Clin Chem 1990;36:1570.)*

stoichiometric amount of dissolved oxygen is present in blood to support the glucose oxidase reaction and produce a linear relationship of signal with glucose concentration. This is especially true at high concentrations of glucose found in samples from diabetic patients (>500 mg/dL). In the case of the YSI system, sample and calibration solutions are diluted at least 1 : 10 in buffer (depends on model), which is in equilibrium with atmospheric PO_2, fixing the oxygen concentration in the calibrator and sample at a constant value.

The problem of oxygen limitations of biosensors based on oxidase enzymes has been addressed by designing semipermeable membranes that restrict diffusion of the primary analyte (substrate) to the enzyme layer, avoiding saturation of the enzyme and keeping the ratio of oxygen to analyte always in excess of 1. This extends the linearity of response to analyte concentrations substantially higher than the K_m of the enzyme, and reduces the signal dependence on oxygen. Outer track-etched polycarbonate membranes are commonly used,[98] as are membranes of poly(vinyl chloride), polyurethanes, and silicone emulsions.[77] Another approach has been to use an oxygen-rich electrode material as a reservoir of oxygen to support the bioreaction. A fluorocarbon (Kel-F Oil) has been used to formulate a carbon paste electrode to act as a source of oxygen and as the working electrode.[126]

Electron acceptors other than oxygen can serve as mediators in the glucose oxidase reaction and completely eliminate any dependence of the amperometric response on oxygen concentration of the sample. The mediator, usually co-immobilized with the enzyme, transports electrons to the anode surface, where it is reoxidized, resulting in a cyclic reaction mechanism (Figure 11-13). Mediators with electron transfer kinetics (little or no overpotential) more favorable than that of oxygen allow operation of the sensor at lower applied potentials (+0.2 V vs. Ag/AgCl or lower) than are typically used for the oxidation of H_2O_2. This approach not only eliminates dependency of the reaction rate on oxygen, it also serves to reduce the contribution from oxidizable interfering substances (e.g., uric acid, ascorbic acid, acetaminophen) to the sensor response. Examples of mediators that have been used include quinones and conductive organic salts, such as tetrathiafulvalene-tetracyanoquinodimethane (TTF-TCNQ).[38,93] Ferricyanide and ferrocene derivatives have also been employed,[17] including commercial application in a first-generation device for home blood glucose monitoring. Dimethylferrocene is impregnated into a graphite electrode to which glucose oxidase has been immobilized. Reduced glucose oxidase from the enzymatic reaction is reoxidized by electrochemically generated ferricinium ion. Current produced during this cycling mechanism is proportional to the concentration of glucose in the blood sample.

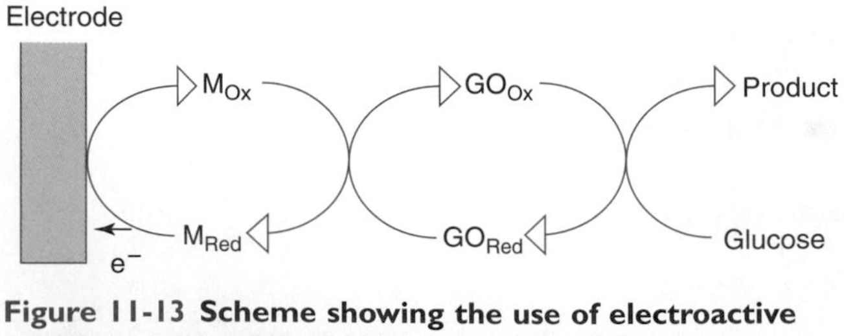

Figure 11-13 Scheme showing the use of electroactive mediator in the design of an amperometric enzyme electrode. The mediator accepts electrons directly from the enzyme and is oxidized at the surface of the working electrode, creating a more oxidized mediator to continue this process. *(From D'Orazio P. In: Lewendrowski K, ed. Clinical chemistry: laboratory management and clinical correlations. Philadelphia: Lippincott, Williams & Wilkins, 2002:464.)*

Another technique used to decrease interferences from easily oxidized species in a blood sample when traditional H_2O_2 electrochemical detection is used is to employ selectively permeable membranes in proximity to the electrode surface that allow transport of H_2O_2 to the electrode surface, but reject the interfering substances based on size exclusion (see Figure 11-12, *B*). An example is as simple as a low molecular weight cutoff membrane, such as cellulose acetate, used in many commercial amperometric biosensors.[61] Also used are electropolymerized films, such as poly(phenylenediamine) formed in situ, to reject interfering substances based on size.[34] Another approach employed in a commercial application involves using a second correcting electrode, identical to the working electrode, but without enzyme, sensitive only to the presence of oxidizable interfering substances. The resulting differential signal is proportional to the concentration of analyte.

A novel approach used for elimination of electroactive interfering substances in a commercially available glucose sensor is to directly "wire" the redox center of the enzyme glucose oxidase to a metallic, amperometric electrode using an osmium (III/IV)-based redox hydrogel.[89] Osmium sites effectively serve as mediators and can accept electrons directly from the entrapped enzyme, without the need for oxygen. This approach allows the operating potential of the electrode to be dramatically lowered to +0.2 V versus the saturated calomel reference electrode (SCE), where currents resulting from electro-oxidation of ascorbate, urate, acetaminophen, and L-cysteine are negligible.

Substitution of other oxoreductase enzymes for glucose oxidase allows amperometric biosensors for other substrates of clinical interest to be constructed. Practical sensors with commercial application in critical care analyzers for blood lactate have been realized.[1] By using the multiple enzyme cascade shown in the reactions discussed here, an amperometric biosensor for creatinine is also possible. Electrochemical oxidation of H_2O_2 is the detection mechanism.

$$\text{Creatinine} + H_2O \xrightarrow{\text{creatinine amidohydrolase}} \text{Creatine} \tag{28}$$

$$\text{Creatine} + H_2O \xrightarrow{\text{creatine amidinohyrdrolase}} \text{Sarcosine} + \text{Urea} \tag{29}$$

$$\text{Sarcosine} + H_2O + O_2 \xrightarrow{\text{sar cos ine oxidase}} \text{Glycine} + \text{formaldehyde} + H_2O_2 \tag{30}$$

This three-enzyme scheme suffers interference from endogenous creatine in the sample, requiring correction. Low concentrations of creatinine found in blood (≤100 µmol/L) must be measured in the presence of oxidizable interfering substances, sometimes present at higher concentrations than the analyte.[56] Special electroactive layers within the biosensor have been proposed to remove redox-active interfering substances.[109] Because the useful life of the creatinine biosensor based on these reactions requires three enzymes to retain activity, reusable commercial biosensors for creatinine based on this measurement principle typically have suffered from a short (few days) useful life, but improvements in enzyme immobilization methods and/or use of stabilizers/activators within calibrating reagents may yield creatinine sensor devices with much longer lifetimes. The importance of developing creatinine sensors and progress to date in this field have recently been summarized in detail by Lad and colleagues.[64]

Enzyme-Based Biosensors With Potentiometric and Conductometric Detection

Ion-selective electrodes can be used as transducers in potentiometric biosensors. An example is a biosensor for urea [blood urea nitrogen (BUN)] based on a polymer membrane ISE (vinyl chloride) for ammonium ion (Figure 11-14).[63] The enzyme urease is immobilized at the surface of the ammonium-selective ISE based on the antibiotic nonactin (see structure of ionophore in Figure 11-3) and catalyzes the hydrolysis of urea to NH_3 and CO_2.

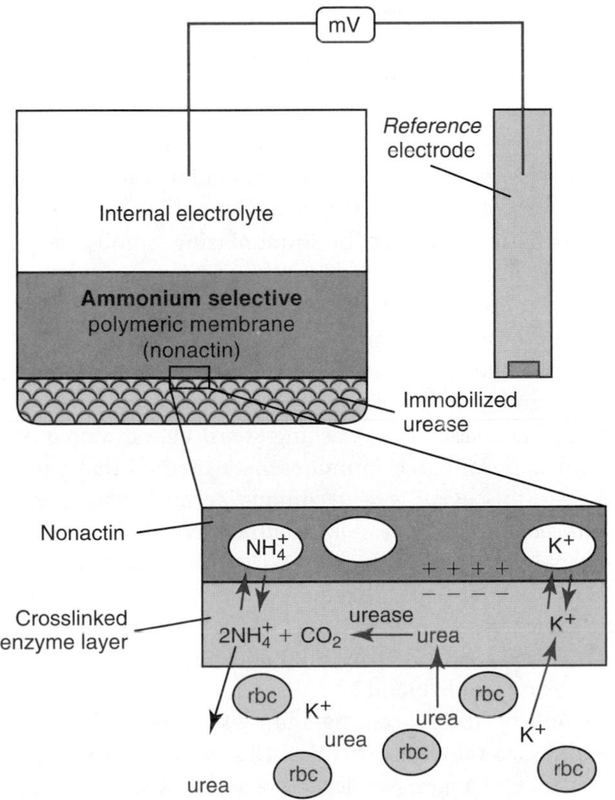

Figure 11-14 Potentiometric enzyme electrode for determination of blood urea, based on urease enzyme immobilized on the surface of an ammonium ion–selective polymeric membrane electrode.

$$\text{Urea} \xrightarrow{\text{urease}} 2NH_3 + CO_2 \quad (31)$$

The ammonia produced forms NH_4^+, which is sensed by the ISE. The signal generated by the NH_4^+ produced is proportional to the logarithm of the concentration of urea in the sample. The response may be steady state or transient. Typically, correction for background potassium is required, because the nonactin ionophore has limited selectivity for ammonium over potassium ($K_{NH4/K} = 0.1$). Potassium is measured simultaneously with urea and is used to correct the output of the urea sensor using the Nicolsky-Eisenman equation [equation (10)].

The approach already described for measurement of urea using an enzyme-based potentiometric biosensor assumes that the turnover of urea to ammonium at steady state provides a constant ratio of ammonium ions to urea, independent of concentration. This is rarely the case, especially at higher substrate concentrations, resulting in a nonlinear sensor response. The linearity of the sensor is also limited by the fact that hydrolysis of urea produces a local alkaline pH in the vicinity of the ammonium-sensing membrane, partially converting NH_4^+ to NH_3 (pKa = 9.3). Ammonia (NH_3) is not sensed by the ISE. The degree of nonlinearity may be reduced by placement of a semipermeable membrane between enzyme and sample to restrict diffusion of urea to the immobilized enzyme layer.

A change in solution conductivity has also been used as a transduction mechanism in enzyme-based biosensors. Examples include the measurement of glucose, creatinine, and acetaminophen using interdigitated electrodes.[27] Practical applications of conductometric biosensors are few because of the variable ionic background of clinical samples and the requirement to measure small conductivity changes in media of high ionic strength. A commercial system for the measurement of urea in serum, plasma, and urine is a BUN analyzer (Beckman-Coulter, Brea, Calif) based on the enzyme urease.[31] Dissolution of products to NH_4^+ and HCO_3^- produces a change in sample conductivity. The initial rate of change in conductivity is measured to compensate for the background conductivity of the sample. This approach is limited to the measurement of analytes at relatively high concentrations because of small changes in conductivity produced by low concentrations of analyte.

Enzyme-Based Biosensors With Optical Detection

Optical sensors with immobilized enzymes and indicator dyes have been developed for the measurement of glucose and other substrates of clinical interest.[66] These biosensors are based on optical detection chemistries for pH and oxygen, described earlier in this chapter, and rely on absorbance/reflectance, fluorescence, and luminescence as modes of detection. Enzyme immobilization methods resemble those used to construct electrochemical biosensors, including physical entrapment or encapsulation in a gel matrix, physical adsorption onto substrates, and covalent binding or absorption on an insoluble support. Using an example based on an optode for PO_2, a sensitive indicator is co-immobilized with an oxidase enzyme at the end of a fiber optic probe. The probe is used to monitor fluorescence of the indicator. Quenching of fluorescence of the indicator by O_2 is followed. A decrease in PO_2 resulting from a reaction catalyzed by the enzyme will result in less quenching of the indicator and a fluorescent signal directly proportional to the concentration of substrate. In an example of an optical biosensor probe for glucose, an oxygen-sensitive cationic dye, $Ru(phen)_3^{2+}$, is immobilized along with glucose oxidase on the surface of an optical fiber.[85] A decrease in PO_2 arising from the enzyme-catalyzed oxidation of glucose results in an increase in luminescence intensity of the ruthenium tris(phenanthrene).

Similar optical biosensors have been prepared for many other analytes. For example, a cholesterol optical biosensor has been devised based on fluorescence quenching of an oxygen-sensitive dye that is coupled to consumption of oxygen resulting from the enzyme-catalyzed oxidation of cholesterol by the enzyme cholesterol oxidase.[120] Serum bilirubin has been detected using bilirubin oxidase, co-immobilized with a ruthenium dye, on an optical fiber.[69] The bilirubin sensor was reported to exhibit a lower detection limit of 10 μmol/L, a linear range up to 30 mmol/L, and a typical reproducibility of 3% (CV), certainly adequate for clinical application.

The pH change resulting from enzyme-catalyzed reactions has also been measured optically. The indicator dye fluorescein is often used as a pH-sensitive indicator to construct such sensors. The protonated form of fluorescein does not fluoresce, but the conjugate base strongly fluoresces at 530 nm, when excited at 490 nm. Using glucose oxidase as the enzyme, a pH optode has been used to follow the formation of gluconic acid.[119] A disadvantage of optical sensors based on pH changes is that they are strongly dependent on the pH and buffer capacity of the sample. Moreover, the working range of the sensor is determined by the pKa of the indicator, 6.8 to 7.2 for fluorescein, depending on ionic strength of the sample matrix. A pH-sensitive indicator may also be used to follow enzymatic reactions that produce ammonia (e.g., urease action on urea).

Affinity Sensors

Affinity sensors are a special class of biosensors in which the immobilized biological recognition element is a binding protein, antibody (immunosensors), or oligonucleotide (e.g., DNA, aptamers) with high binding affinity and high specificity toward a clinically important analyte/partner. Such sensors are being developed as alternatives to conventional binding assays to enhance the speed and convenience of a wide range of assays that normally would be run on large, sophisticated instruments in a central laboratory. Affinity sensors may be more easily adapted than traditional assays to systems developed for point-of-care testing for infectious disease, cardiac markers, or other cases where speed and ease of use are required. Ideally, direct binding of the immobilized species with its target in a clinical sample should yield a sensor signal proportional to the concentration of the analyte. However, direct sensing (without use of exogenous labels/tracers) of the binding events at analyte concentrations that would cover the full range for clinical applications is very difficult to achieve. Further, high affinity of such binding reactions, required to achieve optimal sensitivity, also limits the reversibility of such devices (slow reverse rate constant). Indeed, unlike ISEs, oxygen sensors, and many of the enzyme-based biosensors described previously, affinity sensors based on electrochemical, optical, or other transduction modes are typically single-use devices. For repeated multiuse applications, some type of regeneration step (pH change, temperature change, etc.) to dissociate the tight binding between the recognition element and the target is required. A thermally reversible immunosensor, demonstrated to retain activity and specificity for up to 30 assays, has recently been described.[72] The sensor consists of an antibody conjugated to a polymer, which undergoes a reversible phase transition in response to temperature. Altering temperature produces a change in orientation of the conjugated polymer and affinity between the conjugate and a target antigen, resulting in a reversible antigen-antibody binding reaction.

Most affinity-type sensors that function well for real clinical measurements are based on labeled reagents such as enzymes, fluorophores, and electrochemical tags, and hence function more like traditional binding/immunoassays, except that one recognition element is immobilized on the surface of a suitable electrode or another type of transducer.[74,79,111] For example, electrochemical oxygen sensors have been used to carry out heterogeneous enzyme immunoassays (sandwich or competitive type), using catalase as a labeling enzyme (catalyzes $H_2O_2 \rightarrow 2H^+$ and O_2) and immobilizing capture antibodies on the outer surface of the gas-permeable membrane. After binding equilibration and washing steps, the amount of bound enzyme is detected by adding the substrate and following the increase in current generation caused by local production of oxygen near the surface of the sensor.

The basic advantage of immobilizing affinity reagents on the surfaces of electrodes and optical sensing devices is somewhat diminished when separate washing steps are required to remove unbound label species. Indeed, true biosensors should yield analytically useful responses in the presence of undiluted physiologic samples, without the need for discrete incubation and washing steps. One example of an electrochemical-based immunosensor method that partially achieves this goal is a technique termed *nonseparation electrochemical enzyme immunoassay (NEEIA)*.[82] The basic concept is illustrated in Figure 11-15. As indicated, no separation or washing steps are required. This method was used to detect prostate-specific antigen (PSA) and human chorionic gonadotropin (hCG) at ng/mL concentrations in undiluted plasma and whole blood.[82]

A host of "direct" sensing affinity sensors have been proposed, based on electrochemical (including capacitance and impedance changes), optical, thermal, mass, and acoustic detection methods.[54,74,79,111,125] Direct affinity sensors eliminate the need for labeled reagents because the binding reaction results in a change in a property that may be monitored directly. Of these, few have adequate specificity to be used in

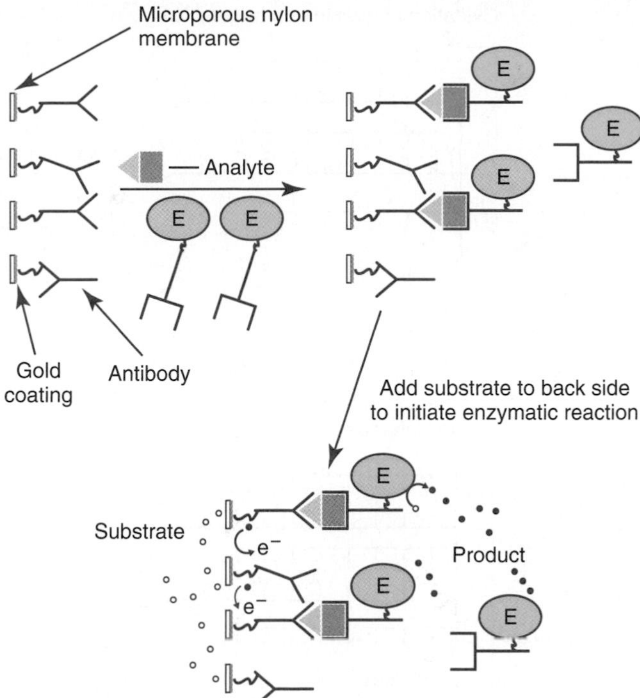

Figure 11-15 Principle of nonseparation electrochemical enzyme immunoassay (NEEIA) concept, configured in sandwich immunoassay mode to detect a given protein analyte. Enzyme label on reporter antibody generates an electroactive product that is detected at the surface of the porous gold electrode when substrate for enzyme is added to the back side of the membrane.

complex clinical samples, owing to significant signals arising from nonspecific binding. One report, however, suggests that alpha fetoprotein can be detected reliably in serum samples via a quartz crystal microbalance mass detector, possessing immobilized anti–alpha fetoprotein antibodies on the surface of the quartz crystal transducer.[19] Increasing concentrations of analyte in the sample yield increased binding to the surface, changing the mass loaded because of the immunologic reaction. Incubation times as low as 20 minutes are required to achieve results that compare favorably with those of a conventional radioimmunoassay method for serum samples. Direct immunosensors for sensitive assays of tumor markers have been reported. Examples include an electrochemical immunosensor for PSA with an enhanced lower limit of detection, based on an alternating current (AC)-impedance measurement,[10] and assay for carcinoma antigen 125 using a quartz crystal microbalance.[113] The former uses a control sensor with immobilized immunoglobulin (Ig)G antibody instead of anti-PSA to subtract out effects from nonspecific binding to achieve a limit of detection of 1 pg/mL toward PSA.

Some success for direct sensing affinity sensors has also been achieved in the area of DNA sensors.[54] Generally, with such devices, a segment of DNA complementary to the target strand is immobilized on a suitable transducer. DNA sensors show particular promise as the basis of point-of-care test devices, for example, for rapid detection of bacterial pathogens.[55,70] Methods for immobilizing DNA segments on electrode surfaces are similar to protein immobilization methods used for other biosensors. Electrically conducting polymers such as polypyrrole, polyaniline, and polythiophene are possible matrices for immobilization of a DNA segment using physical entrapment, covalent attachment, and affinity interactions as methods of immobilization.[95] The conducting polymer not only serves as an immobilization matrix but also plays an active role in the transduction mechanism, providing communication between the DNA binding event and an underlying metallic electrode. Electrochemical DNA sensors can operate in direct (based on electrochemical oxidation of guanine in target DNA) (see Figure 11-15, *A*) or indirect (with exogenous electrochemical markers/labels) (see later and Figure 11-16, *B*) transduction modes. For example, Ozkan and coworkers demonstrated a relatively simple label-free electrochemical *genosensor* to detect the presence of factor V Leiden mutations, using capture probes with inosine substituted for guanosine nucleic acids.[92] Probes were developed to bind wild-type and mutant DNA, based on known base sequences in regions of wild and mutant DNA species. These probes were immobilized on the surface of carbon paste working electrodes. After polymerase chain reaction (PCR) amplification of the sample DNA, a small volume of such samples (10 μL) is incubated for 6 minutes with the probe-modified electrode. Then, after a quick washing step, the presence of the target amplicon bound to the surface can be observed by differential pulse voltammetry using an anodic scan. The presence of a guanine oxidation peak, occurring at +1.00 V versus the Ag/AgCl reference, indicates the presence of the target DNA in the original sample. Another example of a direct DNA sensor uses a field effect transistor coated with an organic semiconducting polymer, poly(3-hexylthiophene).[131] Single-stranded DNA was immobilized at the source/drain electrodes. Single- and double-stranded DNA could be differentiated based on differences in the drain current caused by differences in resistance produced by the two types of DNA.

Weng and associates[128] have suggested an impedance-based detection scheme to monitor DNA hybridization using a boron-doped diamond electrode as the underlying transducer. Using single-stranded oligo sequences immobilized on the diamond electrode, a large decrease in AC impedance was detected when the surface was exposed to complementary single-stranded DNA sequences. Remarkable detection limits of 10^{-19} g/mL were reported using this approach.

DNA detection using electrochemical-labeled oligonucleotides or electrochemical probes that selectively intercalate into hybridized DNA duplexes represents a growing area of investigation, with several "gene" sensor arrays of this type poised to become commercial products (see Chapter 17). As illustrated in Figure 11-16, *B*, when the intrinsic electroactivity of guanine [that requires use of electrode-immobilized capture oligo probes with inosine replacing guanosine (see above)] is not used, detection of hybridization of a target DNA sequence is achieved in either of two ways. In one case, after the immobilized capture oligo anchored to the electrode

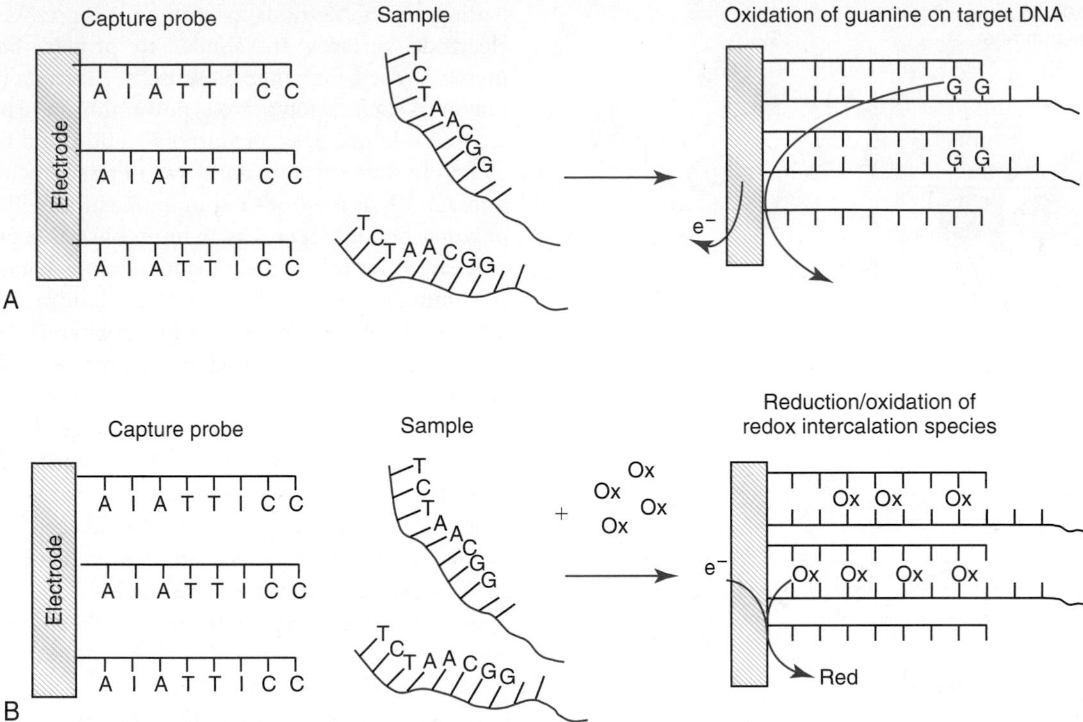

Figure 11-16 Examples of DNA biosensor configurations. A, Direct electro-oxidation detection of guanosine bases in target DNA after hybridization with immobilized capture probe on electrode surface. B, Electrochemical detection of hybridization using exogenous redox species that intercalates into hybridized complex between immobilized capture DNA probe and target DNA.

surface is allowed to bind the target sequence, hybridization is detected by exposing the surface of the electrode to an exogenous electroactive species [Co(III)tris-phenanthroline, ruthenium complexes, etc.] that can interact (intercalate) with the duplex but not single-stranded DNA. After unbound electroactive species are washed away, the presence of hybridization can be readily detected by voltammetry, scanning the potential of the underlying electrode to oxidize or reduce any intercalated electroactive species, with the current detected being proportional to the number of duplex DNA species on the surface of the electrode. Another route involves the detection of target DNA via a sandwich-type binding assay, using an electrochemical-labeled oligonucleotide [oligo labeled with ferrocene, osmium(III) trisbipyridine, etc.] to bind to another sequence of targeted DNA different from the capture oligo on the surface of the electrode. Sequential exposure of the electrode to the sample of DNA (usually after amplification via PCR), excessive labeled reporter oligo (a wash solution), and electrochemical detection of surface-bound label yields the analytical signal. Again, the amount of current monitored is proportional to the number of target DNA species present in the original sample.

A variant of the sandwich-type DNA assay scheme just discussed involves using proximity-dependent surface hybridization of a ferrocene-labeled reporter oligo nucleic acid sequence.[134] In this approach, a thiolated capture oligo probe is immobilized on a gold electrode. When the complementary target DNA was introduced, it was complementary to the region of the capture probe that is farther from the surface of the gold. The reporter oligo with the ferrocene label was prepared to be complementary to one end of the target and to the sequence of the surface immobilized capture probe closest to the gold electrode. Hence, in the presence of the target, the ferrocene tracer ends up being positioned extremely close to the surface of the gold, making it more easily observed electrochemically via a simple differential pulse voltammetric scan, allowing femtomolar detection of the target DNA.

Affinity sensors based on synthetic oligonucleotides, known as *aptamers,* have been explored as recognition elements for a variety of biosensing applications, including small molecules, proteins, and cells. In practice, aptamers are generated and selected in vitro to bind targets for which antibodies and other protein receptors are not easily obtained. Aptamers have been demonstrated to function in biosensors using various transduction methods, including optical sensing (using fluorescently labeled aptamers)[87] and acoustic, mass (cantilever-based), and electrochemical sensing, using, for example, aptamer probes labeled with a redox species such as ferrocene.[86,73] Practical applications for aptamer-based affinity sensors in clinical chemistry are still emerging. Model analytes such as adenosine triphosphate (ATP) and thrombin have been used to demonstrate proof of concept for sensing schemes aimed at producing reversible sensors.[73] The method by which aptamers are selected against their targets makes them inherently suited to displacement assays because of greatly reduced affinity for the labeled form of the target. Thrombin-binding aptamer was shown to have an order of magnitude less affinity for thrombin labeled with horseradish peroxidase than native thrombin. A rapid (10 minute) displacement assay for thrombin was demonstrated with sensitive detection limits of 4.5 and <1 nanomolar using optical and electrochemical detection, respectively.[9]

CHEMICAL SENSORS BASED ON NANOTECHNOLOGY

Nanotechnology is defined as the study of the synthesis, properties, and application of structures and materials having at least one critical dimension on the scale of approximately 100 nm.[94] Structures such as nanowires, nanoparticles, and carbon nanotubes offer unique electrical, optical, and magnetic properties that can be exploited for chemical sensing. The large surface area available on nanostructures for immobilization of labels and biological recognition elements offers the potential for high signal amplification. Developments in the field of DNA nanodevices have resulted in complex molecular detection and amplification schemes, which may outperform PCR in terms of sensitivity and ease of use.[110]

The flexibility and the unique shape of carbon nanotubes and the presence of reactive groups on their surface has led to their being used as biocatalytic and affinity biosensors.[100,122] Direct electron transfer between immobilized glucose oxidase and carbon nanotubes allows construction of glucose biosensors without mediators. In addition, enhanced electron transfer between proteins and carbon nanotubes results in lower overpotentials and higher peak currents observed for the voltammetric response of several molecules at electrodes modified with carbon nanotubes.[100] For DNA sensors, using carbon nanotubes in a detector for the hybridization event provides an efficient way to amplify the label-free electrochemical detection of DNA hybridization and to enhance charge transfer between surface-anchored DNA sequences and carbon nanotubes.[114,125]

Nanomaterial labels, including gold, silver, and semiconductor nanoparticles, have been shown to result in large signal enhancements and to lower limits of detection in electrochemical immunosensors for disease-related protein biomarkers, and for detection of DNA hybridization events.[71] Gold nanoparticles have been used as both immobilization platforms and labels for electrochemical immunosensors.[80] Electrodes with layers of densely packed 5-nm gold nanoparticles were used as a matrix for immobilization of horseradish peroxidase in a sandwich immunoassay for PSA with a detection limit of 0.5 pg/mL.[104] In an optical assay, oligonucleotide targets labeled with gold nanoparticles instead of fluorophore probes have been shown to enhance sensitivity toward the oligonucleotide target by up to two orders of magnitude.[115] A commercial system using gold nanoparticle probes is the Verigene System (Nanosphere, Northbrook, Ill), which is capable of detecting single-nucleotide polymorphisms related to some common genetic disorders, such as thrombophilia, alterations of folate metabolism, cystic fibrosis, and hemochromatosis.

Other examples of nanotechnology applied to chemical sensing are emerging. For example, nanopores down to 1.4 nm in diameter have been created in lipid bilayers through the action of the protein α-hemolysin. A pore with nanometer-scale dimensions has a size comparable with that of a single large molecule (protein, single-stranded DNA). The molecule must be charged to be driven through the pore by an electric field. The contribution of the large molecule to the passage of electric (ionic) current through the pore is small compared with that of mobile small ions, allowing detection of the target analyte down to a single molecule.[67] Microfabricated cantilevers made of silicon or silicon nitride have been used as transducers in affinity biosensors for monitoring (1) DNA hybridization, (2) antigen-antibody interactions, or (3) absorption of bacteria. Mechanical bending of the cantilever on the order of nanometers, in response to affinity reactions, is monitored. Although the sensitivity of cantilever biosensors is limited by nonspecific binding, the technology is equivalent in sensitivity to that of other label-free methods, for example, in the picomolar range for detection of oligonucleotides, and in the ng/mL range for measurement of antigens.[39]

IN VIVO AND MINIMALLY INVASIVE SENSORS

Progress has been made in the development of miniaturized, implantable electrochemical/optical sensors that can be used for in vivo, real-time monitoring of clinically important species. Unfortunately, the biological response toward such sensors (e.g., clotting) can have a dramatic impact on the analytical accuracy of such indwelling probes[5,41,50,76,83] and has prevented their widespread use in clinical practice. However, progress is being made toward improving the reliability of in vivo measurements, and some commercial products for subcutaneous glucose monitoring are already on the market (see later).

Analytical sensors that can be implanted within human blood vessels or subcutaneously mandate that such sensing devices have an outside diameter of <0.6 mm. Both electrochemical and optical sensor technologies have been employed to create devices of the required size. These are basically miniaturized versions of the electrochemical and optical sensor devices described previously. However, in addition to their small size, such devices must exhibit very stable output signals, because reliable calibration of the probes with calibrating solutions is not possible once the probes are inserted. Although so-called in situ calibration is possible (periodically removing an in vitro blood sample to obtain current values of analytes and updating in vivo sensor output to this value), if the frequency of such in situ calibrations is high, the true advantage of having an in vivo probe is greatly diminished.

Continuous in vivo measurement of oxygen saturation (SaO_2) has been achieved by placing small optical fibers into the bloodstream via a catheter and then measuring the reflective absorbance of the blood at two or three appropriately selected wavelengths based on the absorbance spectra of oxy- and deoxy-Hb.[23] In addition, implantable analytical sensors that provide continuous readings of blood gases (pH/PCO_2/PO_2), when inserted within the radial artery, especially for critically ill patients already fitted with an arterial line, have been developed.[102] Such sensors are usually based on the classical Clark-style design, in which oxygen is reduced at a microplatinum, silver, or gold working electrode confined (along with Ag/AgCl reference) within a narrow-diameter gas-permeable catheter tube made of a given polymer (Figure 11-17, *A*), with the resulting current being proportional to the partial pressure of oxygen in the medium surrounding the catheter. Indwelling electrochemical pH and PCO_2 sensors are typically potentiometric devices, based on polymer membrane pH electrode technology or the use of solid-state metal oxide–based pH sensors. Incorporation of lipophilic proton ionophores (e.g., tridodecylamine; see Figure 11-3) within the walls of plastic tubing provides a convenient means of preparing a novel dual-lumen pH/PCO_2 sensing design that has been demonstrated in animal experiments to provide accurate in vivo results.[116]

Miniaturization of electrode designs that enable several sensors to be bundled into a single implantable device, however, remains a significant engineering challenge. Consequently, many efforts aimed at developing commercially viable intravascular blood gas sensors for simultaneously monitoring pH, PCO_2, and PO_2 have employed modern optical fiber–based technology alone or in combination with

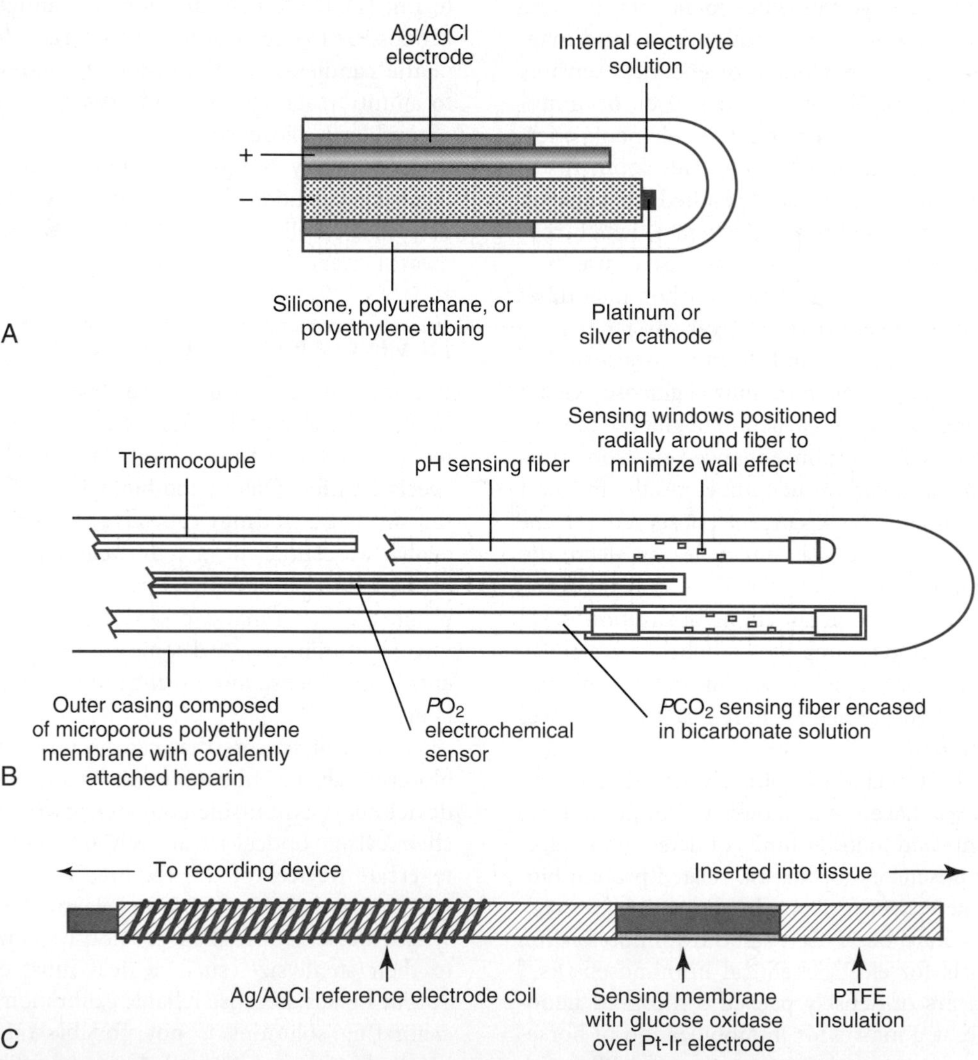

Figure 11-17 Schematics of various implantable electrochemical/optical sensors useful for continuous in vivo monitoring. A, Catheter-style amperometric oxygen sensor. B, Design of Paratrend intravascular combined PO_2, PCO_2, and pH sensor (hybrid electrochemical/optical design). C, Needle-type electrochemical glucose sensor useful for monitoring glucose subcutaneously to track blood glucose concentrations continuously.

a single electrochemical device. Because the outer diameter of available fibers continues to decrease, it is now possible to bundle three or more separate chemically sensitive fibers within a single catheter with an outer diameter <600 μm for implantation within human radial arteries, without dampening the pressure waveform detected by a microelectronic pressure transducer within the arterial line. Absorbance-, fluorescence-, and phosphorescence-based chemistries have been investigated in the design of sensors with suitable selectivity and calibration stability.[83] Appropriate indicators are usually immobilized on the distal ends of the fibers, although alternate configurations/locations have also been proposed. Most optical oxygen measurements are made with indicators whose luminescence is quenched in the presence of oxygen, whereas pH sensors are prepared by immobilizing pH indicators (e.g., phenol red) in hydrogel type films.[108] Optical sensors for PCO_2 can be easily prepared from the same pH sensors by incorporating bicarbonate salt in the hydrogel layer and then covering this layer with a gas-permeable polymeric film (usually silicone rubber material), as described previously in the section on optical sensors.

Despite significant efforts by a number of large biomedical companies in the 1980s/1990s, only the Paratrend probe was commercially available for a period of time for the intravascular measurement of blood gases. As shown in Figure 11-17, *B*, this indwelling sensor consisted of a novel hybrid design, in which oxygen is sensed electrochemically (catheter form of Clark sensor), while pH and PCO_2 are determined via fiber-based optical fluorescence sensors.[123] Although acceptable clinical performance of the Paratrend was reported, frequent in situ recalibrations have been suggested.[24] A later version of this product replaced the electrochemical oxygen sensor with an optical fiber design. However, continued problems with in vivo performance and concomitant costs of using the device have prevented widespread use, and the product is no longer available.

Another class of in vivo chemical sensor that is now available consists of glucose sensors designed to help manage diabetic patients, with the ultimate goal of attaining fully automated feedback control of subcutaneous insulin delivery via newly devised, highly portable insulin pumps. Because such sensors need to function within patients outside the hospital setting and for extended time periods (days, weeks), placement of such devices subcutaneously, rather than intravascularly, is desirable.[60] In addition, sensors are being developed that could be implanted within the vena cava for periods of 1 year. In the case of subcutaneous devices, several studies have shown that concentrations of glucose in interstitial fluid track blood concentrations closely, although some time delay has been noted in achieving identical values in the two sample environments.[12]

Implantable glucose (and lactate) sensors have been based, almost exclusively, on electrochemical transducers. For example, one such sensor is based on using dual oxygen sensors in a single catheter design for indwelling blood glucose and lactate measurements.[46] One oxygen sensor with immobilized glucose or lactate oxidase provides response to glucose concentrations (decreasing surface oxygen in response to increased glucose or lactate), while the second matched oxygen sensor, without enzyme, is able to correct for unknown and varying amounts of endogenous PO_2. Others have focused on the design of probes with amperometric detection of the hydrogen peroxide (via oxidation) at an underlying iridium/platinum anode similar in operation to those used in vitro in commercial instruments.[132] With such designs, the use of outer polymer films to restrict glucose (or lactate) diffusion relative to oxygen is critical to achieve a linear electrochemical response to glucose from normal (90 mg/dL) to elevated concentrations found in diabetic patients (>500 mg/dL). Figure 11-17, *C*, illustrates a design in which the needle-type probe is constructed by multiple membrane coatings and electrodeposition of the glucose oxidase layer.[18] Designs similar to this are among the currently Food and Drug Administration (FDA)-approved sensors available for subcutaneous monitoring of glucose.[44,47,59] In one instance, the sensor is actually fabricated on a very narrow planar substrate, rather than on a cylindrical wire–based system. Relatively frequent calibration of all such sensors is still required via periodic in vitro blood tests, especially in the early stages after subcutaneous implantation.[44]

Instead of implanting glucose sensors intravascularly or subcutaneously, an alternative approach employs electrochemical glucose sensors to monitor glucose concentrations in interstitial fluid brought to the surface of the sensors via an iontophoresis process.[44,118] Electrical current is passed through the skin to move fluid in a given direction toward the surface of the electrochemical glucose sensors that are based on peroxide detection (see Chapter 26 for additional discussion of this device).

Current research and development efforts have focused on the use of more biocompatible coatings to reduce the biological response of intravascular and subcutaneous devices. These efforts are based on the expectation that such developments will be critical to ultimate success in developing implanted sensors that yield continuous analytical results that match closely those attained by conventional in vitro test methods. One new approach in this direction employs novel NO release/generating polymers to coat the surface of intravascular sensors.[40,41,130] The potent antiplatelet activity of NO has been shown to greatly reduce the formation of thrombus on the surface of implantable electrochemical oxygen sensing catheters, and to yield much more accurate continuous PO_2 values in animal experiments. Further, NO has been shown to decrease the inflammatory response that occurs for glucose sensors implanted subcutaneously.[43,53]

REFERENCES

1. Aduen J, Bernstein WK, Khastigir T, Miller J, Kerzner R, Bhatiani A, et al. The use and clinical importance of a substrate specific electrode for rapid determination of blood lactate concentrations. JAMA 1994;272:1678-85.
2. Apple FS, Koch DD, Graves S, Ladenson JH. Relationship between direct potentiometric and flame photometric measurement of sodium in blood. Clin Chem 1982;28:1931-5.

3. Armstrong RD, Lockhart JC, Todd M. The mechanism of transfer of K^+ between aqueous solutions and PVC membranes containing valinomycin. Electrochim Acta 1986;31:591-4.
4. Astrup P, Severinghaus JW. The history of blood gases, acids and bases. Copenhagen: Munksgaard, 1986.
5. Baker DA, Gough DA. Dynamic delay and maximal dynamic error in continuous biosensors. Anal Chem 1996;68:1292-7.
6. Bakker E, Bühlmann P, Pretsch E. Carrier-based ion-selective electrodes and bulk optodes. 1. General characteristics. Chem Rev 1997;97:3083-132.
7. Bakker E, Pretsch E, Bühlmann P. Selectivity of potentiometric ion sensors. Anal Chem 2000;72:1127-33.
8. Bakker E. Determination of improved selectivity coefficients of polymer membrane ion-selective electrodes by conditioning with a discriminated ion. J Electrochem Soc 1996;143:L83-5.
9. Baldrich E, Acero JL, Reekmans G, Laureyn W, O'Sullivan CK. Displacement enzyme linked aptamer assay. Anal Chem 2005;77:4774-84.
10. Barton AC, Davis F, Higson SPJ. Labeless immunosensor assay for prostate specific antigen with picogram per milliliter limits of detection based upon an AC impedance protocol. Anal Chem 2008;80:6198-205.
11. Bates RG. Determination of pH: theory and practice. New York: John Wiley & Sons, 1973.
12. Bedioui F, Villeneuve N. Electrochemical nitric oxide sensors for biological samples—principle, selected examples and applications. Electroanalysis 2003;15:5-18.
13. Bijster P Vader HL, Vink CLJ. Influence of erythrocytes on direct potentiometric determination of sodium and potassium. Ann Clin Biochem 1983;20:116-20.
14. Buck RP, Lindner E. Recommendations for nomenclature of ion-selective electrodes. Pure Appl Chem 1994;66:2527-36.
15. Bühlmann P, Pretsch E, Bakker E. Carrier-based ion-selective electrodes and bulk optodes. 2. Ionophores for potentiometric and optical sensors. Chem Rev 1998;98:1593-687.
16. Burgess B, Martin G. Combined pH and dissolved carbon dioxide gas sensor. U.S. Patent 4,818,361. Washington, DC: U.S. Patent Office, April 4, 1989.
17. Cass AEG, Davis G, Francis GD, Hill HAO, Aston WJ, Higgins IJ. Ferrocene mediated enzyme electrode for amperometric determination of glucose. Anal Chem 1984;56:667-71.
18. Chen X, Matsumoto N, Hu Y, Wilson GS. Electrochemically mediated electrodeposition/electropolymerization to yield a glucose microbiosensor with improved characteristics. Anal Chem 2002;74:368-72.
19. Chou SF, Hsu WL, Hwang JM, Chen CY. Determination of alpha-fetoprotein in human serum by a quartz crystal microbalance-based immunosensor. Clin Chem 2002;48:913-8.
20. Clark LC Jr, Lyons C. Electrode systems for continuous monitoring in cardiovascular surgery. Ann N Y Acad Sci 1962;102:29-45.
21. Clinical and Laboratory Standards Institute. A designated comparison method for the measurement of ionized calcium in serum: approved standard. CLSI Document C39-A. Wayne, Pa: CLSI, 2000.
22. Clinical and Laboratory Standards Institute. Standardization of sodium and potassium ion selective electrode systems to the flame photometric reference method: approved standard, 2nd edition. CLSI Document C29-A2. Wayne, Pa: CLSI, 2000.
23. Collison ME, Meyerhoff ME. Chemical sensors for bedside monitoring of critically ill patients. Anal Chem 1990;62:425A-37A.
24. Coule LW, Truemper EJ, Steinhart CM, Lutin WA. Accuracy and utility of a continuous intra-arterial blood gas monitoring system in pediatric patients. Crit Care Med 2001;29:420-6.
25. Coulter WH. Means for counting particles suspended in a fluid. U.S. Patent 2,656,508. Washington, DC: U.S. Patent Office, October 20, 1953.
26. Cremer M. Uber die Ursahce der Elektromotorishcen eigneschaften der Gewebe, Zugliech ein beitrag zur lehre von den Polyphasichen Elektrolytketten. Z Biol 1906;47:562-608.
27. Cullen D, Sethi R, Lowe C. A multi-analyte miniature conductance biosensor. Anal Chim Acta 1990;231:33-40.
28. Czaban JD, Cormier AD, Legg KD. Establishing the direct potentiometric normal range for Na/K: residual liquid junction potential and activity coefficient effects. Clin Chem 1982;28:1936-45.
29. Demas JN, DeGraff BA, Coleman PB. Oxygen sensors based on luminescence quenching. Anal Chem 1999;71:793A-800A.
30. Eberhard P, Mindt W. Interferences of anesthetic gases at oxygen sensors. In: Birth defects: original article series 1979;XV:65-74.
31. Eckfeldt J, Levine AS, Greiner C, Kershaw M. Urinary urea: are currently available methods adequate for revival of an almost abandoned test? Clin Chem 1982;28:1500-2.
32. Eisenman G, Rudin DO, Casby JU. Glass electrode for measuring sodium ion. Science 1957;126:831-4.
33. Eisenman G. Theory of membrane electrode potentials: an examination of the parameters determining the selectivity of solid and liquid ion exchangers and of neutral ion sequestering molecules. In: Durst RA, ed. Ion-selective electrodes. NBS Special Publication 314. Washington, DC: U.S. Government Printing Office, 1969:1-56.
34. Emr S, Yacynych A. Use of polymer films in amperometric biosensors. Electroanalysis 1995;7:913-23.
35. Faulkner LR. Understanding electrochemistry: some distinctive concepts. J Chem Ed 1983;60:262-4.
36. Feldman BJ, Oserioh JD, Hata BH, D'Alessandro A. Determination of lead in blood by square wave anodic stripping voltammetry at a carbon disk ultramicroelectrode. Anal Chem 1994;66:1983-7.
37. Frant MS. Where did ion selective electrodes come from? The story of their development and commercialization. J Chem Ed 1997;74:159-66.
38. Frew J, Hill HA. Electrochemical biosensors. Anal Chem 1987;59:933A-44A.
39. Fritz J. Cantilever biosensors. Analyst 2008;133:855-63.
40. Frost MC, Rudich SM, Zhang H, Marashio MA, Meyerhoff ME. In vivo biocompatibility and analytical performance of intravascular oxygen sensors prepared with improved nitric oxide-releasing silicone rubber coating. Anal Chem 2002;74:5942-7.
41. Frost M, Meyerhoff ME. In-vivo chemical sensors: tackling biocompatibility. Anal Chem 2006;78:7370-7.
42. Gerritsen M, Jansen JA, Lutterman JA. Performance of subcutaneously implanted sensors for continuous monitoring. Netherlands J Med 1999;54:167-79.
43. Gifford R, Batchelor MM, Lee Y, Gokulrangan G, Meyerhoff ME, Wilson GS. Mediation of in-vivo glucose sensor inflammatory response via nitric oxide release. J Biomed Mater Res 2005;75A:755-66.
44. Girardin CM, Hout C, Gonthier M, Delvin E. Continuous glucose monitoring: a review of biochemical perspectives and use in type 1 diabetes. Clin Biochem 2009;49:136-42.
45. Gorton L. Carbon paste electrodes modified with enzymes, tissues and cells. Electroanalysis 1995;7:23-45.
46. Gough DA, Lucisano JW, Pius HST. Two dimensional enzyme electrode sensor for glucose. Anal Chem 1985;57:2351-7.
47. Gross TM, Bode BW, Einhorn D, Kayne DM, Reed JH, White NH, et al. Performance evaluation of the MiniMed Continuous Glucose Monitoring System during patient home use. Diabetes Technol Ther 2000;2:49-56.
48. Guilbault GG. Handbook of immobilized enzymes. New York: Marcel-Dekker, 1984.
49. Gunaratna PC, Koch WF, Paule RC, Cormier AD, D'Orazio P, Greenberg N, et al. Frozen human serum reference material for standardization of sodium and potassium measurements in serum or plasma by ion selective electrode. Clin Chem 1992;38:1459-65.
50. Halbert SA. Intravascular monitoring: problems and promise. Clin Chem 1990;36:1581-4.
51. Heller A. Amperometric biosensors. Curr Opin Biotechnol 1996;7:50-4.
52. Henning TP, Cunningham DD. Biosensors for personal diabetes management. In: Ramsay G, ed. Commercial biosensors: application

to clinical, bioprocess, and environmental samples. New York: John Wiley & Sons, 1998:3-46.
53. Hetrick EM, Prichard HL, Klitzman B, Schoenfisch MH. Reduced foreign body response at nitric oxide-releasing subcutaneous implants. Biomaterials 2007;28:4571-80.
54. Homs MC. DNA sensors. Anal Letters 2002;35:1875-94.
55. Kalogianni DP, Litos IK, Christopoulos TK, Ioannou PC. Dipstick-type biosensor for visual detection of DNA with oligonucleotide-decorated colored polystyrene microspheres as reporters. Biosens Bioelectron 2009;24:1811-5.
56. Killard AJ, Smyth MR. Creatinine biosensors: principles and design. Trends Biotechnol 2000;18:433-7.
57. Kissinger P. LCEC: the combination of liquid chromatography and electrochemistry. J Chem Ed 1983;60:308-11.
58. Kobos RK, Abbott SD, Levin HW, Kilkson H, Peterson DR, Dickson JW. Electrochemical determination of hemoglobin, hematocrit and hemolysis. Clin Chem 1987;33:153-8.
59. Kondepati VR, Heise HM. Recent progress in analytical instrumentation for glycemic control in diabetic and critically ill patients. Anal Bioanal Chem 2007;388:545-63.
60. Koschchinsky T, Heinemann L. Sensors for glucose monitoring: technical and clinical aspects. Diabetes Metab Res Rev 2001;17:113-23.
61. Kost GJ, Nguyen TH, Tang Z. Whole blood glucose and lactate: trilayer biosensors, drug interference, metabolism and practice guidelines. Arch Pathol Lab Med 2000;124:1128-34.
62. Kost GJ. New whole blood analyzers and their impact on cardiac and critical care. Crit Rev Clin Lab Sci 1993;30:153-202.
63. Kuan SS, Guilbault GG. Ion selective electrodes and biosensors based on ISEs. In: Turner APF, Karube I, Wilson GS, eds. Biosensors, fundamentals and applications. Oxford: Oxford University Press, 1987.
64. Lad U, Khokhar S, Kale GM. Electrochemical creatinine biosensors. Anal Chem 2008;80:7910-7.
65. Lee HJ, Yoon IJ, Yoo CL, Pyun HJ, Cha GS, Nam H. Potentiometric evaluation of solvent polymeric carbonate-selective membranes based on molecular tweezer-type neutral carriers. Anal Chem 2000;72:4694-9.
66. Leiner MJP. Luminescence chemical sensors for biomedical applications: scope and limitations. Anal Chim Acta 1991;255:209-22.
67. Lemay SG. Nanopore-based biosensors: the interface between ionics and electronics. ACS Nano 2009;3:775-9.
68. Lewandowski R, Sokalski T, Hulanicki A. Influence of aspirin on in vitro direct potentiometry of chloride in serum. Clin Chem 1989;35:2146.
69. Li X, Rosenweig Z. A fiber-optic sensor for rapid analysis of bilirubin in serum. Anal Chim Acta 1997;353:263-73.
70. Liao JC, Mastali M, Li Y, Gau V, Suchard MA, Babbitt J, et al. Development of an electrochemical DNA biosensor for bacterial pathogen detection. J Mol Diagn 2007;9:158-68.
71. Liu G, Lin Y. Nanomaterial labels in electrochemical immunosensors and immunoassays. Talanta 2007;74:308-17.
72. Liu Y, Meng S, Mu L, Jin G, Zhong W, Kong J. Novel renewable immunosensors based on temperature-sensitive PNIPAAm bioconjugates. Biosens Bioelectron 2008;24:710-5.
73. Lu Y, Li X, Zhang L, Yu P, Su L, Mao L. Aptamer-based electrochemical sensors with aptamer-complementary DNA oligonucleotides as probe. Anal Chem 2008;80:1883-90.
74. Luppa PB, Sokoll LJ, Chan DW. Immunosensors—principles and applications to clinical chemistry. Clin Chim Acta 2001;314:1-26.
75. Ma SC, Meyerhoff ME, Yang V. Heparin-responsive electrochemical sensor: a preliminary report. Anal Chem 1992;64:694-7.
76. Mahutte CK. On-line arterial blood gas analysis with optodes: current status. Clin Biochem 1998;31:119-30.
77. Maines A, Ashworth D, Vadgama P. Diffusion restricting outer membranes for greatly extending linearity measurements with glucose oxidase enzyme electrodes. Anal Chim Acta 1996;333: 223-31.
78. Mathison S, Bakker E. Effect of transmembrane electrolyte diffusion on the detection limit of carrier-based potentiometric ion sensors. Anal Chem 1998;70:303-9.
79. Medyantseva EP, Khaldeeva EV, Budnikov GK. Immunosensors in biology and medicine: analytical capabilities, problems, and prospects. J Anal Chem 2001;56:886-900.
80. Merkoci A. Electrochemical biosensing with nanoparticles. FEBS J 2007;274:310-6.
81. Metzger E, Aeschimann R, Egli M, Suter G, Dohner R, Ammann D, et al. 3,7-Dioxa-azela-amides as ionophores for lithium ion selective liquid membrane electrodes. Helvetica Chim Acta 1986;69:1821-8.
82. Meyerhoff ME, Duan C, Meusel M. Novel nonseparation sandwich-type electrochemical enzyme immunoassay system for detecting marker proteins in undilute blood. Clin Chem 1995;41:1378-84.
83. Meyerhoff ME. In vivo blood-gas and electrolyte sensors: progress and challenges. Trends Anal Chem 1993;12:257-66.
84. Moody GJ, Thomas JDR. Selective ion sensitive electrodes. Watford, United Kingdom: Merrow, 1971.
85. Moreno-Bondi MC, Wolfbeis OS, Leiner MJP, Schaffar BPH. Oxygen optrode for use in a fiber-optic glucose biosensor. Anal Chem 1990;62:2377-80.
86. Navani NK, Li Y. Nucleic acid aptamers and enzymes as sensors. Curr Opin Chem Biol 2006;10:272-81.
87. Nutiu R, Li Y. Aptamers with fluorescence-signaling properties. Methods 2005;37:16-25.
88. Oesch U, Ammann D, Simon W. Ion-selective membrane electrodes for clinical use. Clin Chem 1986;32:1448-59.
89. Ohara TJ, Rajagopalan R, Heller A. "Wired" enzyme electrodes for amperometric determination of glucose or lactate in the presence of interfering substances. Anal Chem 1994;66:2451-7.
90. Osswald HF, Wuhrmann HR. Calibration standards for multi ion analysis in whole blood samples. In: Lubbers DW, Acker H, Buck RP, Eisenman G, Kessler M, Simon W, eds. Progress in enzyme and ion-selective electrodes. Berlin: Springer-Verlag, 1981:74-8.
91. Osteryoung J. Pulse voltammetry. J Chem Ed 1983;60:296-8.
92. Ozkan D, Erdem A, Kara P, Kerman K, Meric B, Hassmann J, et al. Allele-specific genotype detection of factor V Leiden mutation from polymerase chain reaction amplicons based on label-free electrochemical genosensor. Anal Chem 2002:74:5931-6.
93. Pandey PC, Upadhyay S, Upadhyay B. Peroxide biosensors and mediated electrochemical regeneration of redox enzymes. Anal Biochem 1997;252:136-42.
94. Patolsky F, Zheng G, Lieber CM. Nanowire sensors for medicine and the life sciences. Nanomedicine 2006;1:51-65.
95. Peng H, Zhang L, Soeller C, Travas-Sejdic J. Conducting polymers for electrochemical DNA sensing. Biomaterials 2009;30:2132-48.
96. Pietrzak M, Meyerhoff ME. Determination of potassium in red blood cells using unmeasured volumes of whole blood samples and combined sodium/potassium selective membrane electrode measurements. Anal Chem 2009;81:596-605.
97. Pioda LA, Simon W, Bosshard HR, Curtius CH. Determination of potassium ion concentration in serum using a highly selective liquid-membrane electrode. Clin Chim Acta 1970;29:289-93.
98. Reddy SM, Vadgama PM. Membranes to improve amperometric sensor characteristics. In: Kress-Rogers E, ed. Handbook of biosensors and electronic noses. New York: CRC Press, 1997:111-35.
99. Rehak N, Cecco SA, Niemela JE, Hristova EN, Elin RJ. Linearity and stability of the AVL and Nova magnesium and calcium ion selective electrodes. Clin Chem 1996;42:880-7.
100. Rivas GA, Rubianes MD, Rodriguez MC, Ferreyra NF, Luque GL, Pedano ML, et al. Carbon nanotubes for electrochemical sensing. Talanta 2007;74:291-307.
101. Robinson DL, Venton BJ, Helen MLAV, Wightman RM. Detecting sub-second dopamine release with fast-scan voltammetry in freely moving rats. Clin Chem 2003;49:1763-73.
102. Rolfe P. In vivo chemical sensors for intensive-care monitoring. Med Biol Eng Comput 1990;28:B34-B47.

103. Rosenthal RL, Tobias CW. Measurement of the electrical resistance of human blood: use in coagulation studies and cell volume determinations. J Lab Clin Med 1948;33:1110-22.
104. Rusling JF, Sotzing G, Papadimitrakopoulosa F. Designing nanomaterial-enhanced electrochemical immunosensors for cancer biomarker proteins. Bioelectrochemistry 2009;76:189-94.
105. Rubenstein D, Yahashita GT. Determination of homocysteine, penicillamine and their symmetrical and mix disulfides by liquid chromatography with electrochemical detection. Anal Biochem 1989;180:259-63.
106. Salling N, Siggaard-Andersen O. Liquid junction potentials between plasma or erythrolysate and KCl solutions. Scand J Clin Lab Invest 1971;28:33-40.
107. Scott WJ, Chapoteau E, Kumar A. Ion-selective membrane electrode for rapid automated determinations of total carbon dioxide. Clin Chem 1986;312:137-41.
108. Seitz WR. Chemical sensors based on fiber optics. Anal Chem 1984;56:16A-34A.
109. Shin JH, Choi YS, Lee HJ, Choi SH, Ha J, Yoon IJ, et al. A planar amperometric creatinine biosensor employing an insoluble oxidizing agent for removing redox-active interferences. Anal Chem 2001;73: 5965-71.
110. Simmel FC. Toward biomedical applications for nucleic acid nanodevices. Nanomedicine 2007;2:817-30.
111. Stefan RI, van Staden JF, Aboul-Enein HY. Immunosensors in clinical analysis. Fresenius J Anal Chem 2000;366:659-68.
112. Stott RAW, Hortin GL, Wilhite TR, Miller SB, Smith CH, Landt M. Analytical artifacts in hematocrit measurements by whole blood chemistry analyzers. Clin Chem 1995;41:306-11.
113. Tang D, Yuan R, Chai Y. Quartz crystal microbalance immunoassay for carcinoma antigen 125 based on gold nanowire-functionalized biomimetic interface. Analyst 2008;133:933-8.
114. Tang X, Bansaruntip S, Nakayama N, Yenilmez E, Chang YI, Wang Q. Carbon nanotube DNA sensor and sensing mechanism. Nano Lett 2006;6:1632-6.
115. Taton TA, Mirkin CA, Letsinger RL. Scanometric DNA array detection with nanoparticle probes. Science 2000;289:1757-60.
116. Telting-Diaz M, Collison ME, Meyerhoff ME. Simplified dual lumen catheter design for simultaneous potentiometric monitoring of carbon dioxide and pH. Anal Chem 1994;66:576-83.
117. Thevenot DR, Toth K, Durst RA, Wilson GS. Electrochemical biosensors: recommended definitions and classifications. Biosens Bioelectron 2001;16:121-31.
118. Tierney MJ, Tamada JA, Potts RO, Jovanovic L, Garg S. Clinical evaluation of the GlucoWatch biographer: a continual, noninvasive glucose monitor for patients with diabetes. Biosens Bioelectron 2001;16:621-9.
119. Trettnak W, Leiner MJP, Wolfbeis OS. Fiber optic glucose sensor with a pH optrode as the transducer. Biosensors 1988;4:15-26.
120. Trettnak W, Wolfbeis OS. A fiber-optic cholesterol biosensor with an oxygen optrode as the transducer. Anal Biochem 1990;184:124-7.
121. Veder JP, DeMarco R, Clarke G, Chester R, Nelson A, Prince K. Elimination of undesirable water layers in solid-contact polymeric ion-selective electrodes. Anal Chem 2008;80:6731-40.
122. Veetil JV, Ye K. Development of immunosensors using carbon nanotubes. Biotechnol Prog 2007;23:517-31.
123. Venkatesh B, Clutton-Brock TH, Hendry SP. Continuous measurement of blood gases using a combined electrochemical and spectrophotometric sensor. J Med Eng Technol 1995;18:165-8.
124. Visser KR. Electrical conductivity of stationary and flowing blood at low frequencies. Med Biol Eng Comput 1992;30:636-40.
125. Wang J, Kawde AN, Musameh M. Carbon-nanotube-modified glassy carbon electrodes for amplified label-free electrochemical detection of DNA hybridization. Analyst 2003;128:912-6.
126. Wang J, Lu F. Oxygen rich oxidase enzyme electrodes for operation in oxygen-free solutions. J Am Chem Soc 1998;120:1048-50.
127. Wang L, Buchanan S, Meyerhoff ME. Rapid detection of high charge density polyanion contaminants in biomedical heparin preparations using potentiometric polyanion sensors. Anal Chem 2008;80:9845-7.
128. Weng J, Zhang J, Li H, Sun L, Lin C, Zhang Q. Label-free DNA sensor by boron-doped diamond electrode using an AC impedimetric approach. Anal Chem 2008;80:7075-83.
129. Wenk RE, Lustgarten JA, Pappas NJ, Levy RI, Jackson R. Serum chloride analysis, bromide detection, and the diagnosis of bromism. Am J Clin Pathol 1976;64:49-57.
130. Wu Y, Meyerhoff ME. Nitric oxide releasing/generating polymers for development of implantable chemical sensors with improved biocompatibility. Talanta 2008;75:642-50.
131. Yan F, Mok SM, Yu J, Chan HLW, Yang M. Label-free DNA sensor based on organic thin film transistors. Biosens Bioelectron 2009;24:1241-5.
132. Yang Q, Atanasov P, Wilkins E. A needle-type sensor for monitoring glucose in whole blood. Biomed Instrum Technol 1997;31:54-62.
133. Zaloga GP, Hill TP, Strickland RA, Kennedy D, Visser M, Ford K, et al. Bedside blood gas and electrolyte monitoring in critically ill patients. Crit Care Med 1989;17:920-5.
134. Zhang Y, Wang Y, Wang H, Jiang JH, Shen GL, Yu RQ, Li J. Electrochemical DNA biosensor based on the proximity-dependent surface hybridization assay. Anal Chem 2009;81:1982-7.

CHAPTER 12

Electrophoresis

Raymond E. Karcher, Ph.D.,
and James P. Landers, Ph.D.*

Developments in *deoxyribonucleic acid (DNA)* testing, improvements in ease of performance through automation, and advantages of speed and miniaturization afforded by the technique of *capillary electrophoresis (CE)* have led to a renaissance and growth of *electrophoresis* as an analytical tool that is widely used in clinical laboratories. These developments and improvements have enabled clinical laboratories to keep pace with higher volumes of testing and to introduce more sophisticated technology to meet the demands of modern clinical practice. This chapter will review the principles and practice of the technique and will separately discuss conventional, capillary, and microchip electrophoresis. Particular attention is given to newer methods and their promise in fields such as *genomics* and *proteomics.*

BASIC CONCEPTS AND DEFINITIONS

Electrophoresis is a comprehensive term that refers to the migration of charged solutes or particles of any size in a liquid medium under the influence of an electrical field. *Iontophoresis* and *isotachophoresis (ITP)* are similar terms but refer specifically to the migration of small ions. The first electrophoresis method used to study proteins was the free solution or moving boundary method devised by Tiselius in 1937. This technique was used in research to measure electrophoretic mobility and to study protein-protein interaction. It was able to resolve the serum proteins into only four component mixtures, with the α_1 fraction incompletely separated from albumin.

Zone electrophoresis refers to the migration of charged molecules of proteins, usually in a porous supporting medium like agarose gel film, such that each protein zone is sharply separated from neighboring zones by a protein-free area. Zones are visualized by staining with a protein-specific stain to produce an *electropherogram* that is then scanned and quantified using a densitometer. The support medium can also be handled after drying and kept as a permanent record. It is a most commonly applied technique in clinical chemistry and is used to separate proteins in serum, urine, cerebrospinal fluid (CSF), other physiologic fluids, erythrocytes and tissue, and nucleic acids in various tissue cells.

Although electrophoretic separation of biologically relevant macromolecules in gels (or paper) has been the workhorse of modern biomedical research, the advent of *capillary electrophoresis (CE)* has revolutionized separations. Intense interest in carrying out electrophoretic separation in capillaries with inner diameters ranging from 20 to 75 μm has resulted from its unprecedented resolving power, separation speed, and small sample analysis capabilities. However, the true significance of CE to the separations community is seen in its ability to apply these separation principles in a multimodal approach to a variety of analytes that obviously included proteins and polynucleic acids, but also peptides, small drug-like molecules, and even ions.

THEORY OF ELECTROPHORESIS

Depending on the charge they carry, ionized solutes move toward either the cathode (negative electrode) or the anode (positive electrode) in an electrophoresis system. For example, positive ions (cations) migrate to the cathode, and negative ions (anions) to the anode. An ampholyte (a molecule that is either positively or negatively charged, formerly called a *zwitterion*) becomes positively charged in a solution that is more acidic than its isoelectric point (pI)* and migrates toward the cathode. In a more alkaline solution, the ampholyte becomes negatively charged and migrates toward the anode. Because proteins contain many ionizable amino (—NH_2) and carboxyl (—COOH) groups, and because the bases in nucleic acids may also be positively or negatively charged, they both behave as ampholytes in solution.

The rate of migration of ions in an electrical field depends on the factors listed in Box 12-1. The equation expressing the driving force in such a system is given by

$$F = (X)(Q) = \frac{(EMF)\ (Q)}{d} \quad (1)$$

where

F = the force exerted on an ion

*The isoelectric point of a molecule is the pH at which it has no net charge and will not move in an electrical field.

*The authors gratefully acknowledge the original contributions of Drs. Emmanuel Epstein and Kern L. Nuttall, on which portions of this chapter are based.

BOX 12-1 Factors Affecting the Motility of Ions in an Electrophoretic System

Net charge of the molecules
Size and shape of the molecules
Strength of the electrical field
Support medium properties
Ionic strength of the buffer
Temperature

X = the current field strength (V/cm) (i.e., voltage drop per unit length of medium)
Q = the net charge on the ion
EMF = the electromotive force [voltage (V) applied]
d = the length of the electrophoretic medium (cm)

Steady acceleration of the migrating ion is counteracted by a resisting force characteristic of the solution in which migration occurs. This force, expressed by Stokes' law, is

$$F' = 6\pi r\eta v \quad (2)$$

where
F' = the counter force
π = 3.1416
r = the ionic radius of the solute
η = the viscosity of the buffer solution in which migration is occurring
v = the rate of migration of the solute = velocity, length (l) traveled per unit of time (cm/s)

The force F' counteracts the acceleration that would be produced by F if no counter force were present, and the result of the two forces is a constant velocity. Therefore, when

$$F = F' \quad (3)$$

then

$$6\pi r\eta v = (X)(Q) \quad (4)$$

or

$$\frac{v}{X} = \frac{1 \times d}{t \times E} = \frac{Q}{6\pi r\eta} = \mu \quad (5)$$

where v/X is the rate of migration (cm/s) per unit field strength (E/cm), defined as the electrophoretic mobility. It is expressed by the symbol μ and has the units $cm^2/(V)(s)$.

Electrophoretic mobility is directly proportional to the net charge and inversely proportional to the size of the molecule and the viscosity of the electrophoresis medium. In practice, the equation $\mu = m^2/(V)(s)$ is used to calculate electrophoretic mobility. For example, if albumin travels 3 cm (l) on a 10-cm (d)-long agarose gel and does so in 75 minutes (or 75 × 60 s) at a voltage of 250 V, then

$$\mu = \frac{(3)(10)}{(75)(60)(250)} = 2.7 \times 10^{-5}\ cm^2/(V)(s)$$

Because 1 mobility unit is defined as 10^{-5} $cm^2/(V)(s)$, this result is converted to 2.7 mobility units. Mobility may be positive or negative, depending on whether a protein migrates in the same or the opposite direction as the electrophoretic field (defined as extending from the anode to the cathode). In the example just given, electrophoresis was performed at pH 8.6, where proteins have a negative charge; therefore migration occurred from the cathode to the anode, and the mobility would be −2.7 mobility units.

In addition to the factors listed in Box 12-1, other factors that affect electrophoretic mobility include electroendosmosis (endosmosis) and wick flow. Electroendosmosis affects mobility by causing uneven movement of water through the support medium. An electrophoretic support medium, such as a gel in contact with water, takes on a negative charge caused by adsorption of hydroxyl ions. These ions are fixed to the surface and are immobile. Positive ions in solution cluster about the fixed negative charge sites, forming an ionic cloud of mostly positive ions. The number of negative ions in the solution increases with increasing distance from the fixed negative charge sites until eventually positive and negative ions are present in equal concentrations (Figure 12-1).

When current is applied to such a system, charges attached to the immobile support remain fixed, but the cloud of ions in solution moves to the electrode of opposite polarity.

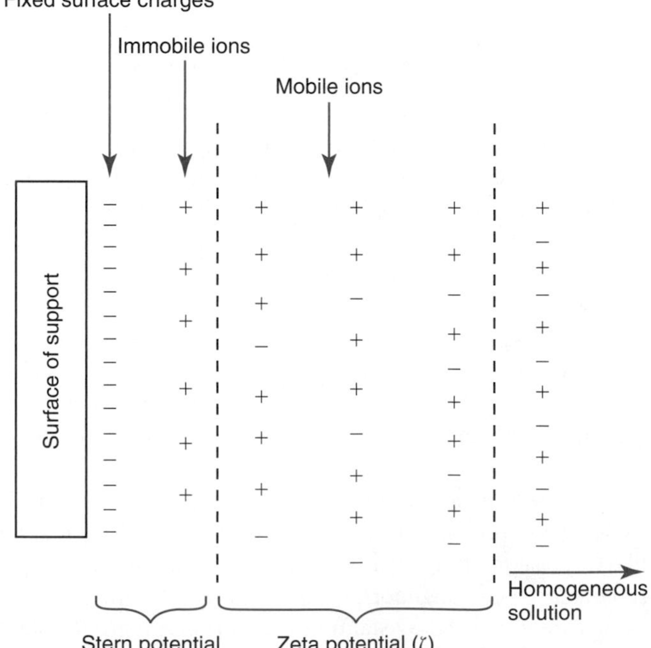

Figure 12-1 Distribution of + and − ions around the surface of an electrophoretic support. Fixed on the surface of the solid is a layer of − ions. (These may be + ions under suitable conditions.) A second layer of + ions is attracted to the surface. These two layers compose the Stern potential. The large, diffuse layer containing mostly + ions is the electrokinetic or zeta potential. Extending farther from the surface of the solid is homogeneous solution. The Stern potential plus the zeta potential equals the electrochemical potential, or epsilon potential.

Because ions in solution are highly hydrated, this results in movement of the solvent as well. Movement of solvent and its solutes relative to the fixed support is referred to as *endosmosis* and causes preferential movement of water in one direction. Macromolecules in solution that move in the direction opposite this flow may remain immobile or may even be swept back toward the opposite pole if they are insufficiently charged. In media in which endosmosis is strong, such as conventional cellulose acetate and unpurified agarose gel, γ-globulins are swept back from the application point. Because the inner surface of a glass capillary contains many such charged groups, endosmosis is very strong and is actually the primary driving force for migration in CE systems. In practice, the endosmosis in CE is manipulated, however, to modify the magnitude of the endosmotic effect. In electrophoretic media in which surface charges are minimal (starch gel, purified agarose gel, or polyacrylamide gel), endosmosis is minimal.

Wick flow results from the movement of buffer into the support medium. During electrophoresis, heat evolved because of the passage of current through a resistive medium can cause evaporation of solvent from the electrophoretic support. This drying effect draws buffer into the support, and, if significant, the flow of buffer can affect protein migration and hence the calculated mobility.

CONVENTIONAL ELECTROPHORESIS

In this section, (1) instrumentation, (2) general electrophoretic operations, (3) technical and practical considerations, and (4) types of conventional electrophoresis are discussed.

INSTRUMENTATION

Although modern electrophoresis equipment and systems vary considerably in form and degree of automation, the essential components common to all systems (Figure 12-2) include two reservoirs *(1)*, which contain the buffer used in the process, a means of delivering current from a power supply via platinum or carbon electrodes *(2)*, which contact the buffer, and a support medium *(3)* in which separation takes place connecting the two reservoirs. In some systems, wicks *(4)* may connect the medium to the buffer solution or directly to the electrodes. The entire apparatus is enclosed *(5)* to minimize evaporation and protect both the system and the operator. The direct current power supply sets the polarity of the electrodes and delivers current to the medium.

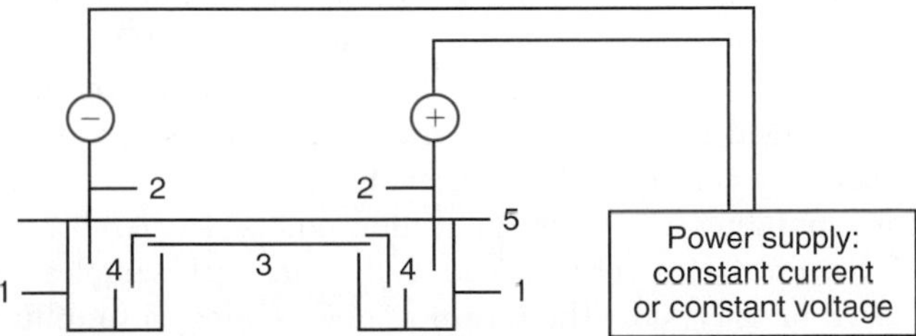

Figure 12-2 A schematic diagram of a typical electrophoresis apparatus showing two buffer boxes with baffle plates *(1)*, electrodes *(2)*, electrophoretic support *(3)*, wicks *(4)*, cover *(5)*, and power supply.

Power Supplies

The power supply drives the movement of ionic species in the medium and allows adjustment and control of the current or the voltage. With more sophisticated units, the power may be controlled as well, and conditions may be programmed to change during electrophoresis. Capillary systems use power supplies capable of providing voltages in the kilovolt range.

Current flowing through a medium that has resistance produces heat:

$$Heat = (E)(I)(t) \quad (6)$$

where

E = EMF in volts (V)
I = current in amperes (A)
T = time in seconds (s)

This heat is released into the medium and increases the thermal agitation of all dissolved ions, and therefore the conductance of the system (decreases resistance). With constant-voltage power supplies, the resultant rise in current increases both protein migration and evaporation of water from the medium. Any water loss increases the ion concentration and further decreases the resistance *(R)*. Under these circumstances, the current and therefore the migration rate will progressively increase. To minimize these effects, it is best to use a constant-current power supply. According to Ohm's law,

$$E = (I)(R) \quad (7)$$

Therefore if R decreases, the applied EMF also decreases, keeping the current constant. This in turn decreases the heat effect and stabilizes the migration rate.

For *isoelectric focusing (IEF)* (see later section), a power supply that provides constant power is advisable. During electrophoresis, current drops significantly because of lower conductivity as carrier ampholytes focus at their isoelectric points, and because of creation of zones of pure water. If a constant voltage supply is used, frequent voltage adjustments may be necessary. As a result, constant current power supplies are not customarily used in IEF. *Pulsed-power* or *pulsed-field* techniques (see later section) require a power supply that can periodically change the orientation of the applied field relative to the direction of migration.

Buffers

Buffer ions have a twofold purpose in electrophoresis: they carry the applied current, and they set the pH at which electrophoresis is carried out. Thus they determine (1) the type of electrical charge on the solute, (2) the extent of ionization of the solute, and therefore (3) the electrode toward which the solute will migrate. The buffer's ionic strength determines the thickness of the ionic cloud (buffer and nonbuffer ions) surrounding a charged molecule, the rate of its migration, and the sharpness of the electrophoretic zones. With increasing concentration of ions, the ionic cloud increases in size, and the molecule becomes more hindered in its movement. For the separation of serum proteins, the barbital or tris-boric acid ethylenediaminetetraacetic acid (EDTA) buffers remain the most popular.

According to Joule's law, power produced when current flows through a resistive medium is dissipated as heat. This heat increases in direct proportion to the resistance, but also in proportion to the square of the current. The reduction in resistance caused by a high ionic strength buffer therefore leads to increased current and excessive heat. These buffers yield sharper band separations, but the benefits of sharper resolution are diminished by the Joule (heat) effect that leads to denaturation of heat-labile proteins or degradation of other components.

Ionic strength (also denoted by the symbol μ) is computed according to the following:

$$\mu = 0.5\sum c_i z_i^2 \quad \textbf{(8)}$$

where

c_i = ion concentration in mol/L

z_i = the charge on the ion

The ionic strength μ of an electrolyte (buffer) composed of monovalent ions is equal to its molarity (mol/L). The ionic strength of a 1-mol/L electrolyte solution with one monovalent and one divalent ion is 3 mol/L, and for a doubly divalent electrolyte, it is 4 mol/L.

A relatively high ionic strength buffer used in *high-resolution electrophoresis* improves the separation of serum proteins into as many as 13 bands, with two or more bands in the α_1, α_2, and β-globulin regions and one or more additional bands seen in various pathologic conditions. Because of higher conductivity and the associated heat produced, it is necessary to reduce the temperature of the system to 10 to 14 °C. "Submarine" techniques, in which gels are submersed in circulating buffer cooled by an external cooling device or are supported on an electrophoresis chamber cooled by circulating water or an integral Peltier plate,[41] provide exact temperature control. Effective cooling with less precise temperature control may also be achieved using chambers designed with a sealed compartment of cooled ethylene glycol, which is in contact with the gel during running.

Because buffers used in electrophoresis are good culture media for the growth of microorganisms, they should be refrigerated when not in use. Moreover, a cold buffer is preferred in an electrophoretic run, because it improves resolution and decreases evaporation from the electrophoretic support. Buffer used in a small-volume apparatus should be discarded after each run because of pH changes resulting from the electrolysis of water that accompany electrophoresis. If volumes used are larger than 100 mL, buffer from both reservoirs may be combined, mixed, and reused up to four times.

Support Media

The support medium provides the matrix in which protein separation takes place. Various types of support media have been used in electrophoresis and range from pure buffer solutions in a capillary to insoluble gels (e.g., sheets, slabs, or columns of starch, agarose, or polyacrylamide) or membranes of cellulose acetate. Gels are cast in a solution of the same buffer to be used in the procedure and may be used in a horizontal or vertical direction. In either case, maximum resolution is achieved if the sample is applied in a very fine starting zone. Separation is based on differences in charge-to-mass ratio of the proteins and, depending on the pore size of the medium, possibly molecular size.

Starch Gel

Starch gel was the first gel medium to be used for electrophoresis (SGE) and is only of historical interest. It separated proteins by both charge-to-mass ratio and molecular size, and because proteins compacted on the surface of the gel before migrating into it, they formed narrow bands with improved resolution.

Cellulose Acetate

Cellulose acetate, a thermoplastic resin made by treating cellulose with acetic anhydride to acetylate the hydroxyl groups, also is primarily of historical interest. When dry, the membranes contain about 80% air space within the interlocking cellulose acetate fibers and are opaque, brittle films. As the film is soaked in buffer, the air spaces fill with liquid, and it becomes pliable. Samples were applied with a twin-wire applicator or the edge of a glass slide. Because of their opacity, stained membranes needed to be made transparent (cleared) for densitometry by soaking in 95:5 methanol:glacial acetic acid. Cleared membranes were strong and could be stored as a permanent record, but because of the necessity for presoaking and clearing, cellulose acetate has largely been replaced by agarose gel in most clinical applications.

Agarose

Agarose is a linear polymer containing alternating D-galactose and 3,6-anhydro-L-galactose monomers. It is the purified, essentially neutral fraction of agar obtained by separating agarose from agaropectin, a more highly charged fraction containing acidic sulfate and carboxylic side groups. Because the pore size in agarose gel is large enough for all proteins to pass through unimpeded, separation is based only on the charge-to-mass ratio of the protein. Advantages of agarose gel include its lower affinity for proteins and its native clarity after drying, which permits excellent densitometry. It is essentially free of ionizable groups and so exhibits little endosmosis.

Most routine procedures for agarose electrophoresis (AGE) are now performed using commercially produced, prepackaged microzone gels, and the sample is applied by means of a comb or a thin plastic template, with small slots corresponding to sample application points. The template is placed on the agarose surface, and 5- to 7-μL samples are placed on each slot. The serum sample is allowed to diffuse into the agarose for 5 minutes, excess sample is removed by blotting, and the template is removed. AGE separation for most routine serum applications requires an electrophoresis time of 20 to 30 minutes.

Polyacrylamide Gel

Polyacrylamide is a polymeric matrix consisting of linear chains of acrylamide cross-linked with bis-acrylamide. It is thermostable, transparent, strong, and relatively chemically inert, and—depending on concentration—can be made in a wide range of pore sizes. Its average pore size in a typical 7.5% gel is about 5 nm (50 Å)—large enough to allow most serum proteins to migrate unimpeded. However, proteins with a molecular radius and/or length that exceeds critical limits will be impeded in their migration. Some of these proteins are (1) fibrinogen, (2) β-lipoprotein, (3) α_2-macroglobulin, and (4) γ-globulins. Thus separation is based on both charge-to-mass ratio and molecular size (a phenomenon referred to as *molecular sieving*), and serum proteins can be resolved into more individual fractions than with agarose gel. Furthermore, these gels are uncharged, thus eliminating electroendosmosis. Precast minigels are available in a variety of concentrations and acrylamide-to-bis-acrylamide ratios suitable for most protein or nucleic acid separations. Because of the potential carcinogenicity of acrylamide, however, appropriate caution must be exercised when handling this material if gels are prepared by hand.

Attempts to improve the hydrophilic nature of polyacrylamide have led to the development of mono- and di-substituted monomers, one of which is *N*-acryloyl-tris(hydroxymethyl) aminomethane, or poly NAT™.[5] This material is more hydrophilic than polyacrylamide, and its matrix has larger pores, thereby presenting less resistance to the passage of large molecules. It is ideally suited to the separation of DNA fragments up to 20 kilobases (kb) in size using a homogeneous (nonpulsed) electric field. Fragments that differ in size by as little as 2% can be resolved. Gels are submersed in buffer during use, allowing temperatures to be tightly controlled at values between 50 and 60 °C. Use of elevated temperatures results in shorter run times and more reproducible band migration.

Automated Systems

Because of increased volume of testing, primarily for serum proteins, many laboratories are converting to automated systems for electrophoresis. Such a system is the Helena SPIFE 4000 (Helena Laboratories, Beaumont, Tex), an automated electrophoresis system providing automated reagent application and a variety of gel sizes that permit analysis of 10 to 100 samples simultaneously. It also features (1) in-line sample application, (2) automated electrophoretic separation and staining of analytes, (3) multiple staining capability, and (4) positive sample identification. The Interlab Microgel system (Interlab Srl, Rome, Italy) also fully automates the process and integrates (1) sample application, (2) temperature-controlled electrophoresis, (3) staining, and (4) densitometry into a single unit with the capability of managing four gels simultaneously. Other systems that have partially automated the procedure or incorporated the ability to process sequentially multiple gels of different compositions include the (1) Phast System (Pharmacia LKB, Gaithersburg, Md), (2) HITE Fractoscan (Olympus, Invicon, München, Germany), (3) Hydragel-Hydrasys (Sebia Inc., Durham, NC), and (4) High-Performance Gel Electrophoresis (HPGE)-1000 system (LabIntelligence Inc., Belmont, Calif). Most CE systems (see "Capillary Electrophoresis" section) have autosampling capability for sequentially processing specimens, but the Sebia Capillarys permits simultaneous processing of seven samples by using multiple capillaries. Newer microchip-based analyzers like the Agilent 2100 Bioanalyzer (Agilent Technologies Inc., Santa Clara, Calif) significantly miniaturize and increase the speed of the process for separating proteins, nucleic acids, or even entire cells. These advances substantially reduce the labor component associated with this technique.

General Operations

General operations performed in conventional electrophoresis include (1) separation, (2) detection, (3) quantification, and (4) a number of "blotting" techniques.

Electrophoretic Separation

When electrophoresis is performed on precast microzone agarose gels, the following steps are typical: (1) excess buffer is removed from the support surface by blotting, taking care that bubbles are not present; (2) 5 to 7 μL of sample is applied using a comb or a plastic template and is allowed to diffuse into the gel; it is then blotted to remove the excess; (3) the gel is placed into the electrode chamber; (4) electrophoresis is performed at specified current, voltage, or power; (5) the gel is rinsed, fixed, and then dried; (6) the gel is stained and redried; and (7) the gel is scanned in a densitometer. If isoenzymes are to be determined, substrate dye solution is incubated on the gel to stain zones before fixing and drying. Alternative procedures would be required if the more sophisticated methods described later are used.

Detection and Quantification

Once separated, proteins may be detected by staining followed by quantification using a densitometer, or by direct measurement using an optical detection system set at 210 nm.

Staining

If staining is used to visualize separated proteins, the proteins usually are fixed first by precipitating them in the gel with a chemical agent such as acetic acid or methanol. This prevents diffusion of proteins out of the gel when submersed in the stain solution. The amount of dye taken up by the sample is affected by many factors, such as the type of protein and the degree of denaturation of the proteins by fixing agents.

Table 12-1 lists dyes commonly used in electrophoresis, along with suggested wavelengths for quantification by densitometry. Most commercial methods for serum protein electrophoresis use Amido Black B or members of the Coomassie Brilliant Blue series of dyes for staining. Isoenzymes are typically visualized by incubating the gel in contact with a solution of substrate, which is linked structurally or chemically to a dye before fixing. Silver nitrate and silver diammine stain proteins and polypeptides with sensitivity 10- to 100-fold greater than that of conventional dyes.[52] Selective fixing and

TABLE 12-1 Suggested Wavelengths for Quantitation of Protein Zones by Direct Densitometry After Staining

Separation Type	Stain	Nominal Wavelength, nm
Serum proteins in general	Amido Black (Naphthol Blue Black)	640
	Coomassie Brilliant Blue G–250 (Brilliant Blue G)	595
	Coomassie Brilliant Blue R–250 (Brilliant Blue R)	560
	Ponceau S	520
Isoenzymes	Nitrotetrazolium Blue	570
Lipoprotein zones	Fat Red 7B (Sudan Red 7B)	540
	Oil Red O	520
	Sudan Black B	600
DNA fragments	Ethidium bromide (fluorescent)	254 (Ex) 590 (Em)
CSF proteins	Silver nitrate	—

CSF, Cerebrospinal fluid.

staining of protein subclasses also can be achieved by combining a stain molecule with an antiglobulin, as is done in immunofixation.

Improvements in conducting sensitive measurements have been achieved by linking an enzyme such as alkaline phosphatase or peroxidase to a single or double antibody specific for particular proteins such as oligoclonal immunoglobulin (Ig)G,[53] or by spraying separated proteins with luminal and peroxide to develop chemiluminescence, which, in turn, exposes x-ray film to form a permanent image.[64] Chemiluminescence has been used in this way to quantify IgE (Lumi-Phos 530, Lumigen, Inc., Southfield, Mich),[67] and DNA fragments have been detected by linking with a fluorescent dye label.[35]

In practice, a typical stain solution may be used several times before it is replaced. A good rule of thumb is that a stain solution of 100 mL may be used for a combined total of 387 cm^2 (60 in^2) of agarose film. The stain solution may be considered faulty if leaching of stained protein zones occurs in the 5% acetic acid wash solution. Whenever protein zones appear too lightly stained, the stain or substrate reagent—in the case of isoenzymes—should always be suspected. Stain solution must be stored tightly covered to prevent evaporation.

Quantification

A *densitometer* is used to quantify stained zones. This instrument measures the absorbance of each fraction as the gel (or other medium) is moved past a photometric optical system and displays an *electropherogram* on a recorder chart or computer display. Microprocessor-containing units automatically integrate the area under each peak and report each as a percent of total or as absolute concentration or activity computed from the total protein or activity of enzyme in the sample.

Reliable densitometric quantitation requires (1) light of an appropriate wavelength, (2) linear response from the instrument, and (3) a transparent background in the medium being scanned. Linearity may be tested with a neutral density filter designed with separated or adjacent areas of linearly increasing density. The densities are permanent and have expected absorbance values. The very small sample sizes used and the transparency of agarose gels satisfy the requirement for a clear background. Nevertheless, problems occur with densitometry because of differences in the quantity of stain taken up by individual proteins and differences in protein zone sizes.

Essential features of a densitometer include (1) the ability to scan gels 25 to 100 mm in length; (2) electronic adjustment of the most intense peak to full scale; (3) automatic background zeroing (peaks are not lost or "cut off"); (4) variable wavelength control over the range of 400 to 700 nm; (5) variable slits to allow adjustment of the beam size; (6) an integrating device with both automatic and manual selection of cut points between peaks; and (7) automatic indexing, a feature that advances the electrophoresis strip from one sample channel to the next.

Desirable features of a densitometer include computerized integration and printout, built-in diagnostics for instrument troubleshooting, choice of one of several scanning speeds, and ability to measure in the reflectance mode. Models with a separate computer for data processing permit storage and reformatting of data, if desired, and reprinting or delayed transmission to a host computer.

DNA analysis requires the ability to scan larger gels, which may contain several dozen bands of DNA fragments of different length. Modern automated electrophoresis systems also use larger gels containing 30 or more samples, which are scanned on a new generation of densitometers referred to as *flat bed scanners* or *digital image analyzers.* These instruments are capable of scanning and storing digitized light intensity readings from large areas and use ultrasensitive charge-coupled device (CCD) detectors having a resolution of up to 1200 dots per inch (21 μm). Sophisticated data processing software permits manipulation of stored image information to produce conventional scans and computations or more complex outputs, such as overlaying and subtraction of patterns from two different samples.

Blotting Techniques

In 1975, Edward Southern developed a technique that is widely used to detect fragments of DNA. This technique, known as *Southern blotting,*[24] first requires electrophoretic separation of DNA or DNA fragments by AGE. Next, a strip of nitrocellulose or a nylon membrane is laid over the agarose gel, and the DNA or DNA fragments are transferred or "blotted" onto it by capillary, electro-, or vacuum blotting. They are then detected and identified by hybridization with a labeled, complementary nucleic acid probe. This technique is widely used in (1) molecular biology for identifying a particular DNA sequence; (2) determining the presence, position, and number of copies of a gene in a genome; and (3) typing DNA (see Chapters 17, 38, and 39 for further details).

Northern and *Western* blotting techniques,[24] named by analogy to Southern blotting, were subsequently developed to separate and detect ribonucleic acids (RNAs) and proteins, respectively. Northern blotting is carried out identically to Southern blotting except that a labeled RNA probe is used for hybridization. Western blotting is used to separate, detect, and identify one or more proteins in a complex mixture. It involves first separating the individual proteins by polyacrylamide gel and then transferring or "blotting" onto an overlying strip of nitrocellulose or a nylon membrane by electro-blotting. The strip or membrane is then reacted with a reagent that contains an antibody raised against the protein of interest.

Technical and Practical Considerations

In performing electrophoretic separations, a number of technical and practical aspects need to be considered, as they affect the process.

Sampling

To achieve a proper balance between sensitive measurements and resolution, the amount of serum protein applied to an electrophoretic support must be optimum. Albumin is about 10 times more concentrated in serum than the smallest fraction, the α_1-globulins. Therefore, the amount of serum applied should prevent overloading with albumin, but should still be adequate to quantify α_1-globulin. For separation of serum proteins using polyacrylamide gel electrophoresis (PAGE), 3 μL of serum containing approximately 210 μg of total protein is applied. For alkaline phosphatase isoenzymes, up to 25 μL of a normal serum may be applied (less may be used if activity is greatly increased). Urine specimens require 50- to 100-fold concentration or extended application time for adequate sensitivity, and CSF may or may not require concentration, depending on the staining approach used.

Discontinuities in Sample Application

Discontinuities in sample application may be caused by (1) dirty applicators, (2) uneven absorption by sample combs, or (3) inclusion of an air bubble if sample is pipetted onto the gel. The pipette tip should be checked for air bubbles before sample is applied to the agarose gel template.

Unequal Migration Rates

Unequal migration of samples across the width of the gel may be caused by dirty electrodes, which may cause uneven application of the electric field, or by uneven wetting of the gel. If wicks are used to connect the gel to a power supply, uneven wetting of the wicks could cause unequal migration or bowing of sample lanes at the gel edges. Gels must be kept horizontal during storage to avoid sagging and uneven thickness. Finally, gels that may have been stored too close to heat sources (e.g., in a cabinet over a light fixture) could have partially and unevenly dried areas, contributing to similar problems.

Distorted, Unusual, or Atypical Bands

Distorted protein zones may be caused by bent applicators, incorporation of an air bubble during sample application, overapplication, or inadequate blotting of the sample. Distorted zones may also be caused by excessive drying of the electrophoretic support before or during electrophoresis. Irregularities (other than broken zones) in the sample application probably are due to excessively wet agarose gels. Portions of applied samples may look washed out.

In most cases, unusual bands are artifacts that may be easily recognized. Hemolyzed samples are frequent causes of increased β-globulin (where free hemoglobin migrates) or an unusual band between the α_2- and β-globulins, the result of a hemoglobin–haptoglobin complex. A band occurring at the starting point of an electropherogram may be fibrinogen. The sample should be verified as being serum before this band is reported as an abnormal protein. The α- and β-lipoproteins may migrate ahead of their normal positions in some samples. Occasionally, a split albumin zone is observed in the rare, benign, genetically related condition of bis-albuminemia. However, a grossly widened albumin zone could be due to albumin-bound medication and not to faulty practice of electrophoresis.

Atypical bands in an isoenzyme pattern may be the result of binding by an immunoglobulin (a macroenzyme), causing abnormal migration of one or more of the normal isoenzymes. Occasionally, an irregular but sharp protein zone is seen at the starting point. Unlike fibrinogen or other proteins that may be seen at about the same point, the artifact lacks the regular, somewhat diffuse appearance that proteins normally show; it is actually denatured protein resulting from deteriorated serum. When faced with an unusual band anywhere in a serum protein pattern, the possibility that it is a true paraprotein must always be considered. Finally, it is good laboratory practice to include a control serum with each electrophoretic run to evaluate its quality and that of the densitometer.

Types of Electrophoresis

With different media in different physical formats and a variety of instrumental configurations, several different types of electrophoretic techniques are used for the separation of a diverse range of analytes.

Slab Gel Electrophoresis

Traditional methods, using a rectangular gel regardless of thickness, are referred to collectively by the term *slab gel electrophoresis*. Its main advantage is its ability to simultaneously separate several samples in one run. Starch, agarose, and polyacrylamide media have all been used in this format. It is the primary method used in clinical chemistry laboratories for separation of various classes of serum or CSF proteins and DNA and RNA fragments. Gels (usually agarose) may be cast on a sheet of plastic backing or completely encased within a plastic-walled cell, which allows horizontal or vertical electrophoresis and submersion for cooling, if necessary.

Slab gels may be cast with additives such as (1) ampholytes, which create a pH gradient (see "Isoelectric Focusing Electrophoresis"), or (2) sodium dodecyl sulfate (SDS), which denatures proteins [see "Two-Dimensional (2D) Electrophoresis"]. In some applications, a gradient of concentration or denaturant is created in the gel to improve separation.[14] Very thin gradient or nongradient gels have been used to improve the efficiency and speed of separation of DNA fragments.[63] In addition to conventional serum proteins, applications include separation of isoenzymes, lipoproteins, hemoglobins, and fragments of DNA and RNA. One-dimensional separations of the last two often involve the addition of a mixture of known fragment size markers, referred to as a *ladder,* in one lane to enable size identification of sample fragments.

Disc Electrophoresis

Protein electrophoresis using agarose gel yields only five zones, namely, (1) albumin, and (2) α_1-, (3) α_2-, (4) β-, and (5) γ-globulins, although some subfractionation of the α_2- and β-globulins is possible with high-resolution gels. *Disc electrophoresis* was developed by Davis and Ornstein to improve this situation and derived its name from *discontinuities* in the electrophoretic matrix caused by layers of polyacrylamide or starch gel that differ in composition and pore size. These gels may yield 20 or more fractions and were widely used to study individual proteins in serum, especially genetic variants and isoenzymes.

With this technique, samples are separated in a three-gel system prepared in situ. Such a system is constructed of a small-pore *separation gel,* followed by a thin segment of large-pore *spacer gel,* then another thin layer of large-pore monomer solution containing a small amount of serum—about 3 μL—was polymerized in open-ended glass tubes. When electrophoresis begins, all protein ions stack up on the separation gel in a very thin zone. This process improves resolution and concentrated protein components so that preconcentration of specimens with low protein content (e.g., CSF) may not be necessary. A schematic representation of serum protein electrophoresis is shown in Figure 12-3.

Isoelectric Focusing Electrophoresis

IEF separates amphoteric compounds, such as proteins, with increased resolution in a medium possessing a stable pH gradient. The protein becomes "focused" at a point on the gel as it migrates to a zone where the pH of the gel matches the protein's isoelectric point (pI). At this point, the charge of the protein becomes zero, and its migration ceases. Figure 12-4 illustrates the procedure and shows the electrophoretic conditions before and after current is applied. The protein zones are very sharp, because the region associated with a given pH is very narrow. Ordinary diffusion is also counteracted by the acquisition of a charge, as a protein varies from its pI position and subsequently migrates back because of electrophoretic forces (Figure 12-5). Proteins that differ in their pI values by only 0.02 pH unit have been separated by IEF.

The pH gradient is created with *carrier ampholytes,* a group of amphoteric polyaminocarboxylic acids that have slight differences in pKa value and molecular weights of 300 to 1000. Mixtures of 50 to 100 different compounds are added to the medium and create a "natural pH gradient" when individual ampholytes reach their pI values during electrophoresis. They establish narrow buffered zones, with stable but slightly different pHs, through which the slower-moving proteins migrate and stop at their individual pIs.

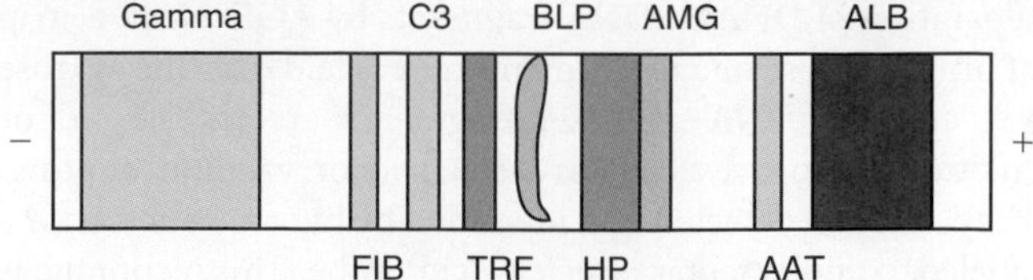

Figure 12-3 **A simplified schematic drawing of a protein pattern from the serum of a subject with haptoglobin type 2-1 [separation by polyacrylamide gel electrophoresis (PAGE)]. Some zones contain more than the one protein shown, as demonstrated by immunologic techniques. *AAT,* α_1-Antitrypsin; *ALB,* albumin; *AMG,* α_2-macroglobulin; *BLP,* β-lipoprotein; *C3,* complement 3; *FIB,* fibrinogen; *gamma,* γ-globulin; *HP,* haptoglobin; *TRF,* transferrin.**

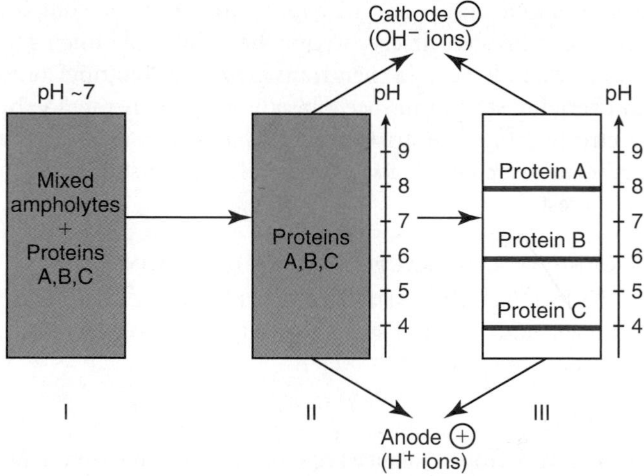

Figure 12-4 **Schematic of an isoelectric focusing (IEF) procedure. *I,* A homogeneous mixture of carrier ampholytes, pH range 3 to 10, to which *proteins A, B,* and *C,* with isoelectric point (pI) of 8, 6, and 4, respectively, were added. *II,* Current is applied and carrier ampholytes rapidly migrate to pH zones where the net charge is zero (the pI value). *III, Proteins A, B,* and *C* migrate more slowly to their respective pI zones, where migration ceases. The high buffering capacity of the carrier ampholyte creates stable pH zones in which each protein may reach its pI.**

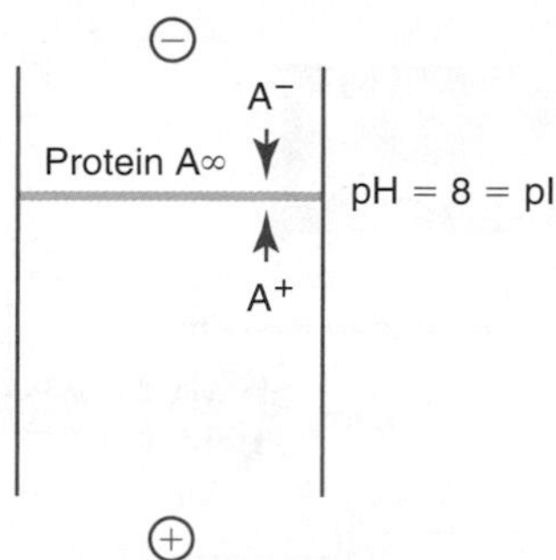

Figure 12-5 After the pH where protein A has a net charge of zero (Å) is attained, diffusion toward the cathode bestows a negative charge on A (A^-), and migration in the electric field forces A^- back to Å. Diffusion toward the anode causes A to take on the opposite charge A^+, and migration is toward the cathode and toward the point where Å exists. Isoelectric focusing processes of this type cause focus of proteins and formation of sharp zones.

As Figure 12-4 illustrates, the anode is surrounded by a dilute acid solution, and the cathode by a dilute alkaline solution. After focusing, the most negatively charged carrier ampholytes and proteins will be found at the anodal end, and the most positively charged near the cathodal end of the electrophoretic matrix. The other carrier ampholytes and proteins focus at intermediate points according to their isoelectric points. Because carrier ampholytes are generally used in relatively high concentrations, a high-voltage power source (up to 2000 V) is necessary (power is in the vicinity of 2 to 50 W, depending on experimental conditions). As a result, the electrophoretic matrix must be cooled. A modification of this technique (IPG-IEF), in which an immobilized pH gradient (IPG) is produced in the gel before the sample is applied, is reported to improve resolution and reproducibility.[13]

PAGE-IEF is widely used in analytical work, as it is essentially free of electroendosmosis. The polyacrylamide gel must have a large enough pore size, however, that protein migration will not be impeded by molecular sieving effects. In actual practice, impeded migration of some proteins, such as IgM, cannot be prevented. AGE-IEF has the advantages that operating conditions are simple, and that large pore sizes make it unlikely that any proteins will be excluded on the basis of molecular size. IEF has been applied to the separation of alkaline phosphatase isoenzymes and is widely used in neonatal screening programs to test for variant hemoglobins (see Chapter 32). Off-gel techniques carry out the separation in free solution with sample containing ampholytes loaded into each of a linear series of wells separated by semipermeable membranes and in contact with a pH gradient strip. Electrophoresis separates sample proteins into different wells depending on their pI values. Separated fractions are further resolved in a second similar focusing step or taken directly to further separation by 2D electrophoresis (see later section) or liquid chromatography-mass spectrometry (LC-MS/MS; see Chapter 14).[17,73] This technique has been useful in the study of the human proteome.

Isotachophoresis

ITP completely separates smaller ionic substances into adjacent zones that contact one another with no overlap, and all migrate at the same rate. In this technique, background electrolyte (buffer) is not mixed with the sample, so current flow is carried entirely by charged sample ions. An aliquot of a sample is typically placed in a capillary between a leading electrolyte solution that contains faster-migrating ions than any in the sample and a trailing solution containing slower-migrating ions than any in the sample. Once a faster-moving component separates completely from a slower-moving one, any further separation creates a region of depleted charge and increases the resistance and therefore the local voltage in that region. Increased voltage causes the slower component to migrate faster and close the gap, thereby concentrating it and increasing the conductivity of its zone until it matches that of the faster ion. Ultimately, all ions migrate at the rate of the fastest ion in zones that differ in size depending on their original concentrations. Zone size is determined by measuring ultraviolet (UV) absorbance, temperature difference, or conductivity as the sample passes a detector. Applications include the separation of small anions and cations, organic and amino acids, and peptides, nucleotides, nucleosides, and proteins.

Pulsed-Field Electrophoresis

In pulsed-field electrophoresis, power is alternately applied to different pairs of electrodes or electrode arrays, so the electrophoretic field is cycled between two directions. The directions can differ spatially by 105° to 180°, and molecules must reorient themselves to the new field direction during each cycle before migration can continue. Because reorientation time depends on molecular size, net migration becomes a function of the frequency of field alteration. This permits separation of very large molecules, such as DNA fragments greater than 50 kb, which cannot be resolved by the relatively small pores in agarose or polyacrylamide gels.[46] Fragments of 50 to 400 kb can be resolved using 10-s pulse times, whereas larger fragments up to 7 megabases in size or intact chromosomes require pulse times of several hours for complete resolution. This technique has been applied to typing various strains of bacterial DNA for research or epidemiologic studies.[10,19,54,56]

Two-Dimensional (2D) Electrophoresis

Two-dimensional (2D) electrophoresis is extensively used in the field of proteomics to study families of proteins and search for genetic- or disease-based differences, or to study the protein content of cells of various types.[37] It has also been applied to the study of human gene mutations[68] and the DNA of various bacteria and tumor cells as a means to earlier diagnosis.[14,51] By combining charge-dependent IEF in the first dimension with molecular weight–dependent electrophoresis in the second, the technique is able to resolve up to 1100 separate protein spots using autoradiographic detection, and up to 400 using Coomassie dyes. The first-dimension separation is carried out in a large-pore medium, such as agarose gel or large-pore polyacrylamide gel. The second dimension is often polyacrylamide in a linear or gradient format.

Conventional 2D electrophoresis uses PAGE-IEF in 130 × 2.5-mm (internal diameter) tubes for the first dimension and covers a pH range of 3 to 10 units. After electrophoresis is complete, the gel is extruded from the tube and is placed in contact with a thin, polyacrylamide gradient gel slab that incorporates SDS. At the end of the process, the polypeptides are detected by one of several different methods. SDS is commonly used in the second dimension, because it denatures proteins to polypeptides by reducing disulfide bonds and depolymerizing proteins. When native proteins, such as enzymes, are desired for further study, nondenaturing sample preparation and electrophoresis conditions must be used.

Separated proteins are detected by the use of Coomassie dyes, silver staining, radiography (exposure of photographic film to emissions of isotopically labeled polypeptides or chemiluminescence), or fluorographic analysis (x-ray film exposed to tritium-labeled polypeptides in the presence of a scintillator). The latter two methods represent the most sensitive methods and are 100 to 1000 times more sensitive than staining with Coomassie dyes. Difference gel electrophoresis (DIGE) permits two samples to be compared on the same 2D gel by labeling each with a different fluorophor. Although each separated spot contains protein from both samples, selective excitation and scanning software allow differences in expression to be qualitatively identified.[47,59]

Newer developments in this area combine analytical techniques to achieve 2D separation by linking, for example, liquid IEF with nonporous silica reverse-phase high-performance liquid chromatography (HPLC; see Chapter 13) and detecting intact proteins by electrospray ionization, time of flight, and mass spectrometry[65,66,71] (see Chapter 14).

CAPILLARY ELECTROPHORESIS

With CE, the classic techniques of (1) zone electrophoresis, (2) ITP, (3) IEF, and (4) gel electrophoresis are carried out in a small-bore (10- to 100-μm internal diameter) fused silica capillary tube, 20 to 200 cm in length.[44]

Two distinct advantages of the capillary format include the (1) ability to apply much higher voltages than in traditional electrophoresis and (2) ease of automation. Applications are also more extensive and include separation of low molecular weight ions, in addition to proteins and other macromolecules. Even uncharged molecules can be separated using CE in the micellar electrokinetic chromatography (MEKC) mode discussed later in this section. CE has also proved useful for separation of (1) inorganic ions, (2) amino acids, (3) organic acids, (4) drugs, (5) vitamins, (6) porphyrins, (7) carbohydrates, (8) oligonucleotides, (9) proteins, and (10) DNA fragments.[9,26,62,74]

Instrumentation

A schematic diagram of a typical instrumental configuration for CE is shown in Figure 12-6. As indicated, the capillary serves as an electrophoretic chamber, analogous to a lane on

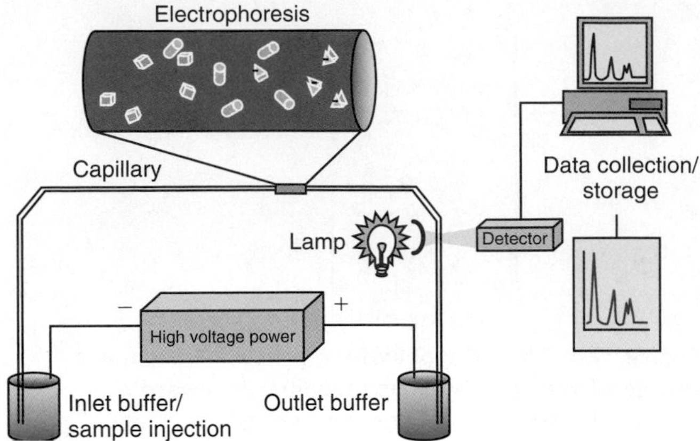

Figure 12-6 A schematic for capillary electrophoresis (CE) instrumentation.

a gel, that is connected to buffer reservoirs at either end, which, in turn, are connected to a high-voltage power supply. It is important to note that at some point along the length of the capillary (typically close to the end), a detector is interfaced for online detection. Improved heat dissipation from the capillary (as opposed to a slab gel) permits the application of voltages in the range of 10 to 30 kV, which enhances separation efficiency and reduces separation time, in some cases to less than 1 minute. Only a few microliters of the sample are required, with injected volumes in the nanoliter range. The small sample plug volume minimizes distortions in the applied field caused by the presence of analytes or other sample species.

In contrast to the cumbersome and time-consuming tasks of conventional electrophoresis, CE is easily automated. Analogous to HPLC technology, samples typically are stored in a temperature-controlled environment and are automatically injected into the capillary, with a variety of detector types available; the resulting electropherograms are analyzed and manipulated in much the same manner as chromatograms.

The Capillary Format

The capillaries used as separation columns in CE are most commonly made from fused silica (pure glass) coated with a thin exterior covering of polyimide to provide strength and flexibility. Although capillaries have been made from other materials, such as polyethylene or Teflon, such capillaries have seen limited use. The polyimide coating is usually removed from a small portion of the capillary close to the terminal end, creating a window for online optical detection. The outer diameter of the capillary tubing typically varies from 180 to 375 μm, the inner diameter from 20 to 180 μm, and the total length from 20 cm up to several meters. Noncylindrical capillary tubing suitable for CE is now available from some commercial providers. For example, rectangular capillaries (Polymicro Technologies, Phoenix, Ariz) provide a flat surface that is more amenable to optical detection than that of their curved counterparts.

Sample Injection

In CE, sample volumes of 1 to 50 nL are loaded into the capillary by (1) *hydrodynamic injection* or (2) *electrokinetic (EK) injection.* With hydrodynamic injection, an aliquot of a sample is introduced by applying positive pressure at the inlet vial or vacuum at the outlet vial. The volume of sample loaded is governed by a number of parameters, including (but not limited to) (1) the inner diameter of the capillary, (2) buffer viscosity, (3) applied pressure, (4) temperature, and (5) time. With some earlier commercial or homemade systems, gravity was used as the source of pressure by raising the inlet vial (or lowering the outlet vial), thus allowing "siphoning" to occur for a timed interval. With EK injection, an aliquot of a sample is introduced by applying a voltage for a timed interval. The magnitude of the voltage is dependent on the analyte and buffer system used but typically involves field strength three to five times lower than that used for separation. It is important to note that although hydrodynamic methods introduce a sample representative of the bulk specimen, EK injection favors the preferential movement of more electrokinetically mobile analytes into the capillary.

In practice, to maintain high separation efficiency, the sample plug length is usually less than 2% of the total capillary length.

Direct Detection

With CE, separated analytes are detected and measured as they migrate past a point on the capillary that is optically interrogated. Optical detection is based on classical methods, such as (1) photometric absorbance, (2) refractive index, and (3) fluorescence (see Chapter 10). As with HPLC, ultraviolet-visible photometers are widely used as detectors to monitor CE separations.[49] To interface such online detectors with the capillary, a *detection window* is created toward the outlet end of the capillary. This "window," which serves as an inline cuvet, typically is formed by burning off the polyimide with a small flame and cleaning the window with ethanol. This configuration allows high-efficiency separation, with the inner diameter of the capillary tube defining the optical path length (OPL) of the inline cuvet. Because absorbance is directly proportional to the length of the cuvet (OPL) used in an optical system, the 20- to 100-μm inner diameter of the capillary limits UV-visible absorbance detection limits to concentrations of 10^{-8} to 10^{-6} mol/L.

Improving Limits of Detection

Several approaches have been devised to improve the limit of detection of online CE detectors. These include (1) increasing the diameter of the OPL, (2) using more sensitive optical techniques, and (3) preconcentrating the sample.

Increased OPL. Capillary tubes modified at the detector window with a "bubble" cell (a glass-blown expansion of the internal diameter of the capillary tube) can increase the detection capability of the OPL by almost an order of magnitude, with concomitant lowering of the system's limit of detection. Alternatively, a "Z" geometry has been developed that increases the OPL via detection down the core of the capillary, with possible lengths up to 1 mm.

Sensitive Optical Detectors. Sensitive optical techniques that have been used with CE include (1) fluorescence, (2) refractive index, (3) chemiluminescence, (4) Raman spectrophotometry, and (5) circular dichroism.[62] The most sensitive optical detection method used in CE is laser-induced fluorescence (LIF), which is capable of detection limits in the 10^{-18} to 10^{-21} mol/L (or lower) range. This detection mode is easily accomplished with analytes that may be easily labeled with a fluorescent substrate (e.g., intercalators for double-stranded DNA) or may be naturally fluorescent (e.g., proteins or peptides containing tryptophan). CE systems have also been interfaced with mass spectrometers,[58] and electrochemical detection methods[15] have been developed, although such detectors must be isolated electrically from the electrophoretic voltages.

Online Sample Concentration. Another technique used in CE systems to enhance their limit of detection is preconcentration of the sample. One of the simplest methods for sample preconcentration is to induce a "stacking" effect with the sample components, which is accomplished by exploiting the ionic strength differences between the sample matrix and the separation buffer.[6] This results from the fact that sample ions have decreased electrophoretic mobility in a higher conductivity environment. When voltage is applied to the system, sample ions in the sample plug instantaneously accelerate toward the adjacent separation buffer zone. Upon crossing the boundary, the higher conductivity environment induces a decrease in electrophoretic velocity and subsequent "stacking" of the sample components into a smaller buffer zone than the original sample plug. Within a short time, the ionic strength gradient dissipates and the charged analyte molecules begin to move from the "stacked" sample zone toward the cathode. Stacking has been used with hydrostatic or EK injection and typically yields a tenfold enhancement in sample concentration, resulting in a lower limit of detection.

An alternative approach to stacking is "focusing" a technique that is based on pH differences between the sample plug and the separation buffer. This has been shown to be very useful for analysis of peptides, mainly because of their relative stability over a wide pH range.[1] By increasing the pH of the sample to above that of the net pI of the analytes of interest and flanking the sample plug with low pH separation buffer zones (i.e., an equivalent volume of low pH separation buffer following introduction of the sample plug), negatively charged peptides are electrophoretically driven toward the anode. Upon entering the lower pH separation buffer, a pH-induced change in their charge state causes a reversal in their electrophoretic mobility, resulting in "focusing" of the peptides at the interface of the sample (high pH) and low pH buffer plugs (similar to those in isoelectric focusing). After the pH gradient dissipates, the peptides, again positively charged, migrate toward the cathode as a sharp zone. This approach has been applied to a variety of analytes but is limited to those that are able to withstand inherent changes in pH without substantial denaturation, and may yield as much as a fivefold enhancement of a system's limit of detection.[61]

Other types of sample concentration enhancement approaches applicable to CE include ITP[69] and those involving concentration of an online solid phase.[50] This latter method shows much promise for both small and large molecules and is discussed in detail in the review by Wettstein and Strausbauch.[70]

Indirect Detection

When strong chromophores are lacking in the analyte of interest, absorbance and fluorescence detection have been used in an indirect mode.[11,34,42] With the absorbance technique, a strongly absorbing ion is added to the running electrolyte and is monitored at a wavelength that gives a constant, high background absorbance. As solute ions move into their discrete zones during the electrophoretic process, they displace the indirect detection agent through mutual repulsion, and this produces a decrease in background absorbance as the zone passes through the detector. Reagents with appropriate fluorescence properties have been employed in a similar manner. Indirect detection of amino acids by CE has been demonstrated, with the potential for use in diagnosis of aminoacidurias.[38] Investigators have demonstrated the direct extrapolation of this technique to microchip detection when UV detection is difficult, if not impossible.

Technical Considerations

Temperature and surface effects influence the separation capabilities of CE. Artifacts also have been known to arise with CE.

Temperature Effects

In most slab or tube platforms for electrophoresis, moderate electric fields (up to 1000 volts) are used, because the Joule heating that accompanies the use of higher field strengths causes (1) nonuniform temperature gradients, (2) local changes in viscosity, and (3) subsequent zone broadening. CE is distinguished from other forms of electrophoresis by the fact that extraordinarily high fields (30,000 volts) are used to obtain rapid, high-efficiency separations. The problems encountered with noncapillary platforms are prevented by effective dissipation of Joule heat by forced air convection or liquid cooling of the capillary, both of which are possible because of the narrow bore of the capillary. The Joule heat produced is a function of (1) buffer type, (2) concentration, (3) voltage applied, (4) capillary inner diameter, and (5) length, and can be determined for any given system by generating an *Ohm's law plot,* which allows easy determination of the maximum voltage that can be used effectively.[40] Reducing the inner diameter of the capillary, the ionic strength of the running buffer, or the applied voltage will reduce the heat produced by the electrophoretic process. It should be noted that reducing the inner diameter will compromise the detection limit of UV measurements (smaller OPL); reducing the applied field is less desirable in that resolution is directly proportional to the applied field. Consequently, attempts should be made to alter other parameters before reducing inner diameter or the applied field.

Surface Effects

As in electrophoresis in general, the flow of fluid [electroosmotic or electroendosmotic flow (EOF)] in CE is a consequence of surface charge on the solid support. In CE, EOF is a significant factor in the separation process. The charge on the inner surface of a fused silica capillary is determined by the ionization state of the silanol groups (SiOH) that populate it. Interaction of positively charged buffer species with bound surface anions generates a layer of mobile cations that move toward the cathode when voltage is applied. This induces a very strong EOF that mobilizes all analytes in the same direction, regardless of their charge. Separation is consequently achieved because of differences in the electrophoretic migration rates of analytes superimposed on this EOF.

Because the driving force of the flow is distributed along the wall of the capillary, the flow profile is nearly flat or plug-like, contrasting with the laminar or parabolic flow generated by a pressure-driven system caused by shear forces at the wall. A flat flow profile is beneficial because it does not contribute to the dispersion of solute zones. The magnitude and direction of the EOF are influenced by several parameters, including (1) type of electrolyte used, (2) pH, (3) ionic strength, (4) use of additives (e.g., surfactants, organic solvents), and (5) polarity and magnitude of the applied electric field.

Although advantageous for dissipation of Joule heat, the large surface area-to-volume ratio of the inner capillary space increases the likelihood of analyte adsorption onto the surface of its inner wall. This causes phenomena such as peak tailing and even total and irreversible adsorption of the analyte. Adsorption is typically noted between cationic solutes and the negatively charged inner wall of the capillary, primarily through ionic interactions (with deprotonated silanols), but also involves hydrophobic interactions (with siloxanes). Because of the numerous charges and hydrophobic regions, significant adsorptive effects have been noted, especially for highly cationic proteins. In practice, adsorption of substances, whether from the sample or from the buffer, to the inner surface of the capillary will alter migration times and other separation characteristics; unaddressed, the capillary eventually may become "fouled." Buffer components and/or additives, such as surfactants, can often render permanent changes to the inner surface of the capillary (through adsorption) and may warrant dedication of specific capillaries for use with particular surfactants.

To minimize these inner wall effects, capillaries are conditioned by chemical treatment, most commonly with base, to remove adsorbates and rejuvenate the surface. A typical wash method includes flushing the chamber with 10 to 20 capillary volumes of 0.1 to 1.0 mol/L NaOH, followed by flushing with "run" buffer. To prevent exposing the capillary surface to drastic fluctuations in pH, conditioning procedures for separations at low pH may be better served by using strong acids (e.g., HNO_3), surfactants (e.g., SDS), or organic solvents, such as acetonitrile or methanol.

Modes of Operation

Modes in which CE systems are operated include (1) capillary zone electrophoresis (CZE), (2) MEKC, (3) capillary gel electrophoresis (CGE), (4) capillary IEF, and (5) capillary ITP.

Capillary Zone Electrophoresis

CZE, also called *open-tube* or *free-solution* CE, is the simplest form of CE. It includes *capillary ion electrophoresis,* which refers to the analysis of inorganic ions by CZE, often utilizing indirect detection. The power of the CZE mode is its ability to electrophoretically resolve charged species without a sieving matrix; this applies to a broad spectrum of analytes ranging from proteins, peptides, and amino acids to small molecules (e.g., drugs) and ions.

Serum Protein Analysis

Compared with AGE and CAE, CZE is more advantageous for serum protein analysis.[22,23,45] Figure 12-7 shows a comparison of the separation of serum proteins by (1) cellulose acetate (CAE), (2) agarose (AGE), and (3) CE. The presence of the classical zones with CE is apparent, albeit in reversed order, as is the identification of serum protein abnormalities in gamma regions. Retrospective studies have shown CE to be effective for detecting monoclonal proteins, which could then be immunotyped by conventional techniques.[45] Moreover, one study demonstrated the utility of CE in performing both serum protein electrophoresis and immunotyping for more than 1500 serum samples.[23] These and other studies put forth the same conclusion: that CE is more sensitive than AGE in identifying abnormalities. Other studies have shown the value of CZE in serum protein analysis. For example, in 2005, Luraschi and associates[31] described the use of CZE coupled with immunosubtraction to detect and characterize low concentrations of free γ-heavy chains in serum. In this study, they showed that a patient with γ-heavy chain disease could be detected by serum protein analysis in CZE in tandem with immunosubtraction. However, although studies have proven the clear utility of CZE for serum protein analysis, Bossuyt and coworkers[33] point to the fact that CZE is not flawless, describing a case where CZE failed to detect μ-heavy chain disease in a 90-year-old woman. This is countered by Maisnar and colleagues,[32] who submit that the laboratory diagnosis of patients with μ-heavy chain disease is typically challenging, and that detection of the monoclonal protein by standard electrophoretic approaches may fail in up to 75% of cases of μ-heavy chain disease. They describe a patient with multiple malignancies for whom CZE with immunotyping allowed the detection and characterization of monoclonal μ-heavy chains.

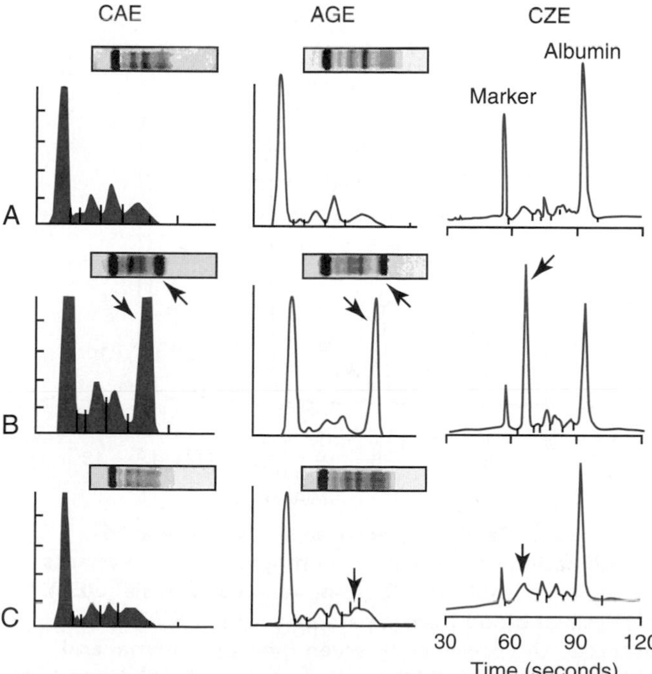

Figure 12-7 Rapid protein electrophoresis of serum protein; comparison with scanning densitometry profiles obtained from cellulose acetate (CAE) and agarose (AGE) electrophoresis. Panel A, Normal serum. Panel B, Patient serum containing a large M-protein. Panel C, Patient serum containing a small monoclonal protein. ***Arrows*** **indicate the position of the monoclonal proteins.**

Finally, CZE for serum protein analysis is evolving in a high-throughput format that has leveraged the success of multiplexed CE systems developed for DNA analysis. Two commercial systems have evolved: the Beckman Paragon 2000 (Beckman Analytical, Milan, Italy) and Sebia CAPILLARYS (Sebia, Durham, NC). Although several studies have illustrated the potential of these systems for serum paraprotein characterization (essentially supplanting AGE and IFE),[2,12,20] studies have not yet settled the issue of paraprotein detection sensitivity and specificity for the clinical community.[3,28,29] For example, Yang and associates[75] compared the CAPILLARYS 2 system versus standard serum protein AGE for the detection and identification of monoclonal proteins in patient serum samples. After defining sensitivity for both, they concluded that AGE and CZE had the same specificity for detection of monoclonal proteins, but that CZE/immunosubtraction was slightly less sensitive than standard immunofixation in the detection of IgM and light chains.

Artifacts in Serum Protein Analysis

With CE utilizing online optical detection, artifacts can occur in the form of "system peaks." These often originate from the sample or from the interfaces between the sample and the separation buffer, because any species that absorbs at the detection wavelength will generate a response. This differs from protein slab gel electrophoresis, wherein detection specificity is governed by a protein-specific stain. It is not uncommon, for example, for buffer species present in the sample but not in the separation buffer to generate system peaks. However, clinical serum protein electrophoresis provides one example whereby artifacts are eliminated by CE.

One problem associated with conventional electrophoresis of serum proteins is its proclivity for point-of-application artifacts. These are bands that result from the fact that electrophoretic mobility (e.g., with AGE) is bidirectional from the point of application. Consequently, the point of application remains part of the scanned area of interest. These bands must be immunotyped to distinguish real monoclonal proteins from artifacts—a process that is costly and time-consuming. CE prevents point-of-application artifacts in two ways. First, net mobility in CE results from the vectorial addition of both protein electrophoretic mobility and EOF. As a result of this unidirectional movement (toward the detector), the point of application is not scanned by detector. Second, unlike AGE, where precipitates cannot exit the loading well and enter the gel (thus appearing as a band in the scanned region of the gel), no gel matrix is present in CZE to impede electrophoretic migration, because analysis occurs in free solution. This was demonstrated by Clark and colleagues, who evaluated a small subset of serum samples containing monoclonal proteins that remained at the point of application on agarose gels (and cellulose acetate) but were handled by CZE with ease.[7] These precipitates may be euglobulin or cryoprecipitates and may or may not contain a monoclonal protein; only immunoelectrophoresis or immunofixation can identify the presence of monoclonal proteins.

Micellar Electrokinetic Chromatography (MEKC)

MEKC is a hybrid of electrophoresis and chromatography. MEKC, a mode that is separate and distinct from capillary electrokinetic chromatography (CEC), is an effective electrophoretic technique, because it can be used for the separation of neutral and charged solutes. The separation of neutral species is accomplished by exploiting micelles formed in the running buffer when the concentration of surfactant exceeds the critical micelle concentration (e.g., 8 to 9 mmol/L for SDS). During electrophoresis, neutral micelles can interact with analytes in a chromatographic manner through hydrophobic interactions in which analytes are micellized based on their degree of hydrophobicity. Under these conditions, partitioning into the micelle is the driving force for separation. With charged micelles (e.g., SDS), analytes can also interact through electrostatic interactions via the charge on the surface of the micelle.

Capillary Gel Electrophoresis

CGE is directly comparable with traditional slab or tube gel electrophoresis because the separation mechanisms are identical. Size separation is achieved with a suitable polymer, which acts as a molecular sieve or sizing mechanism. As charged analytes migrate through the polymer network, they become hindered to a degree that is governed by their size (larger molecules are hindered more than smaller ones). Macromolecules, such as DNA and SDS-saturated proteins, cannot be separated without a gel or some other separation mechanism, because they have a mass-to-charge ratio that is size independent. The term *gel* in CGE is a misnomer, primarily because cross-linked "gels," as we know them in slab format, are not routinely used in CE. A more suitable term is a *sieving matrix* or *soluble polymer network*, a linear polymeric structure that is soluble, has reasonably low viscosity, and is capable of self-entangling in a manner that forms pores through which sieving can occur. A variety of polymeric matrices have been defined for DNA (e.g., polyacrylamide, cellulosic materials) and protein analysis (e.g., dextran-base matrices), provided that pores can be formed inherently that have diameters in the range of tens to hundreds of nanometers. One of the requirements that often accompany this type of analysis is reduction of electro-osmotic flow. This is accomplished by covalently, adsorptively, or dynamically coating the surface. Cross-linked polyacrylamide was the main polymer of choice for this but recently has been supplanted by a host of polymeric matrices that not only provide effective molecular sieving but also adsorptively coat the capillary surface.[27,65] An example of CGE separation of DNA is provided in a later section.

Capillary Isoelectric Focusing Electrophoresis

Capillary isoelectric focusing electrophoresis (cIEF) is comparable with tube IEF and is governed by the same principles and procedures. It differs from conventional IEF in that it can be carried out using a free solution of ampholytes or a precast gel. As expected with a CE mode, and unlike conventional IEF, the focused zones migrate past the online detector during the focusing process or following it. Figure 12-8 shows an example of this, where separation by cIEF is completed in ≈15 minutes, circumventing conventional IEF protocols and/or the necessity for other electrophoretic methods (e.g., CAE), both of which are much less time efficient.[18]

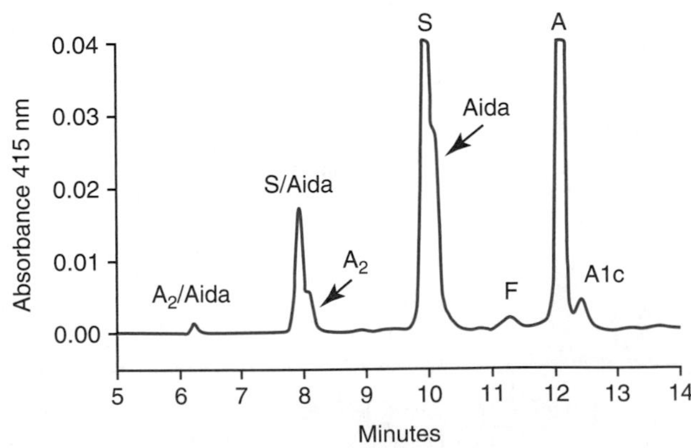

Figure 12-8 Capillary electrophoresis (CE)-based identification of uncommon hemoglobin (Hb) variants by capillary isoelectric focusing electrophoresis (cIEF).[18] Analysis of blood from a patient with Hb S/Aida trait detected the presence of seven different normal and abnormal structural Hb variants, some of which are not detectable by conventional electrophoresis because of lack of sensitivity or inadequate resolution. The four abnormal variants include Hb S, Aida, S/Aida hybrid, and A_2/Aida. Identifying ∀-variants of Hb A_2 by cIEF helps discriminate between α- and β-globin gene mutations in samples containing unknown Hb variants. Glycated Hb A (HbA_{1c}) is also apparent in the electropherogram.

Capillary Isotachophoresis

Capillary ITP has essentially the same features as ITP in other formats, except that conditions of pure ITP usually are not achieved but is not commonly used as a bonafide CE mode. Instead, it is more typically used for online sample preconcentration (as described earlier). Also, it functions as a preconcentrating step in a mixed mode with CZE, MEKC, or CGE. However, ITP may be undergoing a renaissance. Work done by groups such as the Santiago Group at Stanford is beginning to show that rigorous modeling of the process may begin to tease new capabilities and applications out of a technique that has been largely unheralded over the decades since Eaverarts first revealed it as a sample preparation technique for liquid chromatography.[57]

MICROCHIP ELECTROPHORESIS

Over the past decade, microchip electrophoresis has undergone substantial development, including (1) integrated microchip designs, (2) advanced detection systems, and (3) new applications.[8,16,30,36] In the arena of clinical diagnosis, the main analytes of interest for extrapolation to the microchip platform are proteins and DNA.[27,66A]

Among the attributes of microchip electrophoresis separation, the most notable is high speed—normally fourfold to tenfold faster than conventional CE, and at least an order of magnitude faster than the slab gel format. Other advantages of microchips include (1) simplicity, (2) capability for chip integration of multiple functions, and (3) certainly the potential for automation.

Instrumentation

Although similar in principle, instrumentally, the microchip system differs from its CE counterpart. For example, with the microchip approach, (1) separation channels, (2) sample injection channels, (3) reservoirs, and (4) sample preparation and/or (5) precolumn or postcolumn reactors are all fabricated onto the surface of a microchip, using photolithographic processes defined by the microelectronics industry (see Chapter 18 for additional details on the manufacturing of such devices). Thus creation of a truly multifunctional, "integrated" analytical device embedded in a single monolithic substrate is possible. The classic "cross-T" design of a single-channel microchip involves a short (injection) channel that intersects a longer (separation) channel and includes a reservoir at the end of each of these, as shown in Figure 12-9. The setup for LIF detection on a single-channel microchip is shown in Figure 12-10.

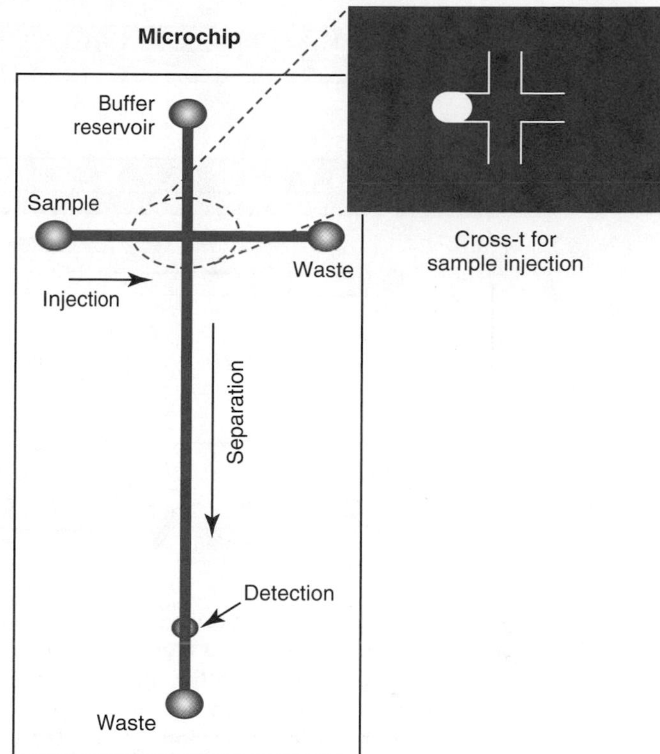

Figure 12-9 Simple cross-T microstructure design on chips used for electrophoretic separation.

When solution volumes required to fill the architecture are compared, it is seen that the volume of the separation channel on a microchip is roughly an order of magnitude smaller (low nanoliters) than conventional capillary systems. With their decreased volume requirements (nanoliter and even picoliter range), pressure injection is more challenging (but not impossible), and the electrokinetic sample injection mode is used primarily. In practice, an injection voltage of several hundred volts is applied across the sample and sample waste reservoirs to migrate the sample to the injection cross, which typically represents an injection volume of 50 to 100 pL. A separation voltage (1 to 4 kV) is then applied to the separation channel; this induces separation of the analyte zones before they reach the detection window downstream. It is important to note that, although the sample volume injected is ≈100 to 500 pL, the actual sample volume necessary (for handling) is still ≈2 to 4 μL, depending on the reservoir size.

Detection with a microchip occurs primarily through LIF, because this is easily implemented with the planar configuration of the microchip (see Figure 12-10). Limits of detection for fluorescein-like fluors have been easily demonstrated at 10^{-11} mole and even as low as 10^{-13} moles—a mass detection limit of a few hundred molecules.[43] This allows for detection, for example, of polymerase chain reaction (PCR)-amplified DNA fragments at a quantity that competes with ^{32}P-autoradiography from Southern blots.[48] Typical microchip separation times are around 50 to 200 seconds.

Fabrication of Microchips

Standard cross-T configuration microchips are commercially available from several small vendors, but chips of more complex architecture tend to be fabricated in the laboratories that use them. They are constructed from substrates such as (1) glass (Pyrex-like or soda lime), (2) silicon (as per microelectronic chips), or (3) a variety of polymeric materials (plastics), or (4) they may be cast from silicone-like materials (polydimethylsiloxane).[25] The first two of these

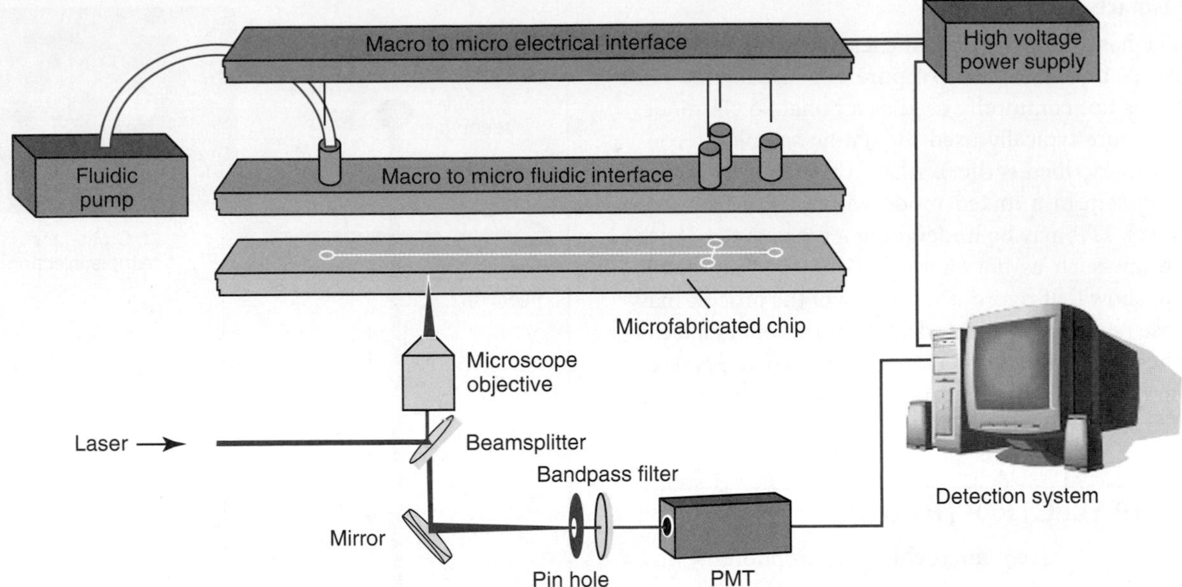

Figure 12-10 Detection system for laser-induced fluorescence (LIF) detection on microchips. Fluidic and electrical interfaces are indirectly fundamental to the detection system. The fluidic interface drives the preparation and flushing of the chip before separation and after separation, and the electrical interface drives the electrophoretic separation and controls the flow of fluid through the chip architecture via electrokinetic valving.

types constitute the vast majority of electrophoretic devices described in the literature.

A buffered solution of hydrofluoric acid is used to etch the desired structures into a glass wafer, thereby producing a series of U-shaped troughs [typically 70 μm (w) × 20 μm (d)] that interconnect appropriately. Smooth walls are typically achieved, but channels are U-shaped because of downward and lateral etching by the etch solution. Consequently, features are often designed to be smaller than they have to be to allow for this type of spreading. Following successful etching, the etched wafer is bonded to a second piece of glass, into which reservoirs have been drilled, to enclose chambers and channels of the device.

Molecular Diagnostics Using Microchips

As a result of the ease with which double-stranded (ds)DNA will fluoresce via high-affinity dsDNA fluorescent intercalators, and the excellent detection sensitivity that results from LIF, DNA separations on microchips have developed more rapidly than protein separations. Consequently, capillary and microchip types of electrophoresis have emerged as alternatives to traditional slab gel electrophoresis for DNA analysis; this is signified by sequencing of the human genome by Celera using primarily CE-based separation. A variety of polymers have been defined as *sieving matrices,* effective for molecular sieving and size-based microchip DNA separations, many of which had been used previously in CE.

As described in the CE section, the chemical nature of the microchannel surface is equally important in DNA separation, where electro-osmotic flow has to be minimized or eliminated. For microchip-based electrophoretic DNA analysis, the chip surface must be passivated to reduce EOF. This is accomplished through covalent modification with polymers such as polyacrylamide (PA)[21]; however, PCR samples must be desalted to achieve optimal resolution and acceptable longevity.[4,60] More attractive alternatives developed for CE involve polymers that have dual functionality, in that they both coat the microchannel surface and act as effective sieving polymers. Polydimethylacrylamide (PDMA) and the cellulosic polymers, hydroxyethyl cellulose and hydroxypropyl cellulose, have been shown to be very effective in this respect.[55]

In practice, microchip electrophoresis has been extensively utilized for the molecular diagnosis of disease based on PCR amplification of DNA (see Chapter 18).[27] For example, rudimentary microchip designs have been used to demonstrate the application of this platform in the most simplistic form, that is, detecting the presence of a PCR product of diagnostic significance. This has been demonstrated with a number of applications, including detection of (1) herpes simplex viral DNA in CSF for diagnosis of encephalitis, (2) gene rearrangements correlative with lymphoproliferative disorders, (3) polymorphisms in the methylenetetrahydrofolate reductase (MTHFR) gene, (4) tetranucleotide repeats associated with hypercholesterolemia, and the (5) diagnosis of fragile X syndrome and (6) muscular dystrophy. More complicated DNA assays have been accomplished on electrophoretic microchips, including single-stranded conformation polymorphism (SSCP) and heteroduplex analysis for the detection of common mutations in the breast cancer susceptibility genes, *BRCA1* and *BRCA2.*[27]

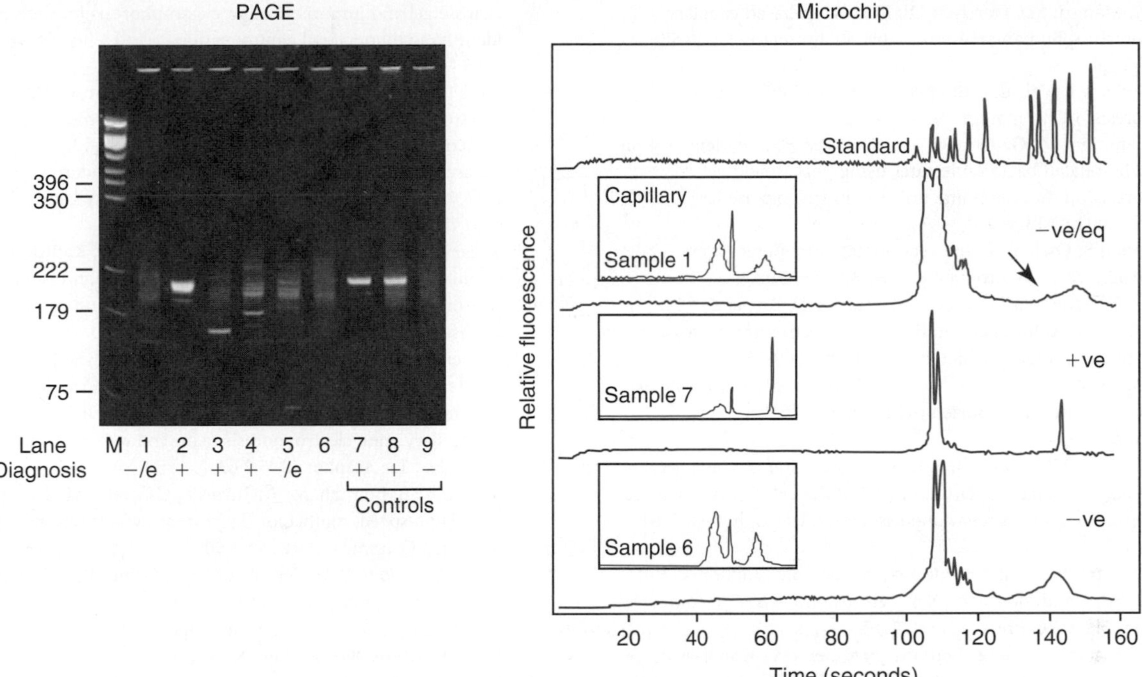

Figure 12-11 Electrophoretic detection of T-cell receptor γ-gene rearrangement products. Left, Slab gel electrophoresis of amplified products resulting from polymerase chain reaction (PCR) of nine patient samples. Right, Capillary *(inset)* and microchip separations of select samples analyzed by gel electrophoresis on the left. The top profile results from separation of a DNA sizing standard. Sample 6 was consistent with a negative diagnosis for gene rearrangement; sample 7 was positive, as indicated by the dominant peak signifying clonality (peak at 142 seconds); sample 1 was deemed negative and/or equivocal based on the suspicious peak indicated by the *arrow*. Separation in both systems used hydroxyethylcellulose (HEC) as a polymeric sieving matrix and applied fields of 300 volts/cm and 275 volts/cm, respectively, for the capillary and microchip systems.[39]

An example of microchip DNA separation applied to the diagnosis of lymphoproliferative disorders is shown in Figure 12-11.[39] The high-resolution (8%) acrylamide slab gel used for conventional analysis is given on the left for comparison. Because of the short separation length of the electrophoretic chamber (≈4 cm) and the use of applied electrical fields comparable with those used in CE, separation on the microchip is complete in 160 seconds (in comparison with 8 hours for the slab gel). Other examples are seen in chip-based methods for DNA extraction from sample, PCR amplification of purified DNA, and a method to inject this material with a DNA ladder for electrophoretic interrogation, with all processes interfaced on a single chip. Using whole blood from a mouse infected with *Bacillus anthracis,* analysis of less than 1 μL of blood allowed the detection of an *anthracis*-specific PCR product in less than 30 minutes, demonstrating the power of integrated microchip-based analysis.

More complicated microchip systems have been developed to address the high-throughput requirements of molecular diagnostics laboratories (see Chapters 17 and 39). For example, high-throughput genetic typing has been performed on a 96-channel radial capillary array electrophoresis microplate with an unprecedented sample throughput of ≈0.6 samples/s.[36,60] This has been extrapolated to a variety of other applications, including genotyping of the marker gene for diagnosis of hereditary hemochromatosis.[72]

REFERENCES

1. Abersold R, Morrison HD. Analysis of dilute peptide samples by capillary zone electrophoresis. J Chromatogr 1990;516:79-88.
2. Bossuyt X, Bogaerts A, Schiettekatte G, Blanckaert N. Detection and classification of paraproteins by capillary immunofixation/subtraction. Clin Chem 1998;44:760-4.
3. Bossuyt X, Lissoir B, Mariën G, Maisin D, Vunckx J, Blanckaert N, et al. Automated serum protein electrophoresis by Capillarys. Clin Chem Lab Med 2003;41:704-10.
4. Carrilho E. DNA sequencing by capillary array electrophoresis and microfabricated array systems. Electrophoresis 2000;21:55-65.
5. Chiari M, Micheletti C, Nesi M, Fazio M, Righetti PG. Towards new formulations for polyacrylamide matrices: *N*-acryloylaminoethoxyethanol, a novel monomer combining high hydrophilicity with extreme hydrolytic stability. Electrophoresis 1994;15:177-86.
6. Chien R-L, Burgi DS. Field amplified sample injection in high-performance capillary electrophoresis. J Chromatogr 1991;559:141-52.
7. Clark R, Katzmann JA, Kyle R, Fleisher M, Landers JP. Differential diagnosis of gammopathies by automated capillary electrophoresis: analysis of serum samples problematic by agarose gel electrophoresis. Electrophoresis 1998;19:2479-84.

8. Colyer CL, Mangru SD, Harrison DJ. Microchip-based capillary electrophoresis of human serum proteins. J Chromatogr A 1997; 781:271-76.
9. Deyl Z, Tagliaro F, Miksik I. Biomedical applications of capillary electrophoresis. J Chromatogr 1994;656:3-27.
10. Drinka P, Stemper M, Gauerke C, Miller J, Reed K. The identification of genetically related bacterial isolates using pulsed field gel electrophoresis on nursing home units: a clinical experience. J Am Geriatr Soc 2004;52:1373-7.
11. Foret F, Fanali S, Ossicini L. Indirect photometric detection in capillary zone electrophoresis. J Chromatogr 1989;470:299-308.
12. Gay-Bellile C, Bengoufa D, Houze P, Le Carrer D, Benlakehal M, Bousquet B, et al. Automated multicapillary electrophoresis for analysis of human serum proteins. Clin Chem 2003;49:1909-15.
13. Gorg A, Postel W, Gunther S. The current state of two-dimensional electrophoresis with immobilized pH gradients. Electrophoresis 1988;9:531-46.
14. Gurtler V, Barrie HD, Mayall BC. Use of denaturing gradient gel electrophoresis to detect mutation in VS2 of the 16S-23SrDNA spacer amplified from *Staphylococcus aureus* isolates. Electrophoresis 2001; 22:1920-4.
15. Haber C. Electrochemical detection in capillary electrophoresis. In: Landers JP, ed. Handbook of capillary electrophoresis, 2nd edition. Boca Raton, Fla: CRC Press, 1997:425-47.
16. Harrison DJ, Manz A, Fan Z, Leudi H, Widmer HM. Capillary electrophoresis and sample injection systems integrated on a planar glass chip. Anal Chem 1992;64:1926-32.
17. Heller M, Michel P, Morier P, Crettaz D, Wenz C, Tissot J, et al. Two-stage off-gel isoelectric focusing: protein followed by peptide fractionation and application to proteome analysis of human plasma. Electrophoresis 2005;26:1174-88.
18. Hempe JM, Vargas A, Craver RD. Clinical analysis of structural hemoglobin variants and Hb A1c by capillary isoelectric focusing. In: Petersen JR, Mohammad AA, eds. Clinical and forensic applications of capillary electrophoresis. Totowa, NJ: Humana Press, 2001:145-63.
19. Hennekine JA, Kerouanton A, Brisabois A, DeBuyser ML. Discrimination of *Staphylococcus aureus* biotypes by pulsed-field gel electrophoresis of DNA macro-restriction fragments. J Appl Microbiol 2003;94:321-9.
20. Henskens Y, de Winter J, Pekelharing M, Ponjee G. Detection and identification of monoclonal gammopathies by capillary electrophoresis. Clin Chem 1998;44:1184-90.
21. Hjerten S. High-performance electrophoresis—elimination of electroendosmosis and solute adsorption. J Chromatogr 1985;347:191-8.
22. Katzmann JA, Clark R, Namyst-Goldberg C, Sanders L, Kyle RA, Landers JP. Identification of monoclonal proteins by capillary electrophoresis: quantitative comparison with acetate and agarose electrophoresis. Electrophoresis 1997;18:1775-80.
23. Katzmann JA, Clark R, Sanders E, Landers JP, Kyle RA. Prospective study of serum protein capillary zone electrophoresis and immunotyping of monoclonal proteins by immunosubtraction. Am J Clin Pathol 1998;110:503-9.
24. Kendrew J, ed. The encyclopedia of molecular biology. Oxford: Blackwell Science, 1994.
25. Lacher NS, de Rooij NF, Verpoorte E, Lunte SM. Comparison of the performance characteristics of poly(dimethylsiloxane) and Pyrex microchip electrophoresis devices for peptide separations. J Chromatogr A 2003;1004:225-35.
26. Landers JP. Clinical capillary electrophoresis. Clin Chem 1995;41:495-509.
27. Landers JP. Molecular diagnostic analyses using electrophoretic microchips. Anal Chem 2003;75:2919-27.
28. Lissoir B, Wallemacq P, Maisin D. Serum protein electrophoresis: comparison of capillary zone electrophoresis Capillarys (Sebia) and agarose gel electrophoresis Hydrasys (Sebia). Ann Biol Clin (Paris) 2003;61:557-62.
29. Litwin CM, Anderson SK, Philipps G, Martins TB, Jaskowski TD, Hill HR. Comparison of capillary zone and immunosubtraction with agarose gel and immunofixation electrophoresis for detecting and identifying monoclonal gammopathies. Am J Clin Pathol 1999;112:411-7.
30. Liu YJ, Foote RS, Jabobson SC, Ramsey RS, Ramsey JM. Electrophoretic separation of proteins on a microchip with noncovalent postcolumn labeling. Anal Chem 2000;72:4606-13.
31. Luraschi P, Infusino I, Zorzoli I, Merlini G, Fundaro C, Franzini C. Heavy chain disease can be detected by capillary zone electrophoresis. Clin Chem 2005;51:247-9.
32. Maisnar V, Tichy M, Stulik J, Urban P, Adam Z, Kadlckova E, et al. Capillary immunotyping electrophoresis and high resolution two-dimensional electrophoresis for the detection of μ-heavy chain disease. Clin Chim Acta 2008;389:171-3.
33. Marien G, Verhoef G, Bossuyt X. Detection of heavy chain disease by capillary zone electrophoresis. Clin Chem 2005;51:1302-3.
34. Marsh DB, Nuttall KL. Methylmalonic acid in clinical urine specimens by capillary zone electrophoresis using indirect photometric detection. J Capillary Electrophor 1995;2:63-7.
35. McGrath SB, Bounpheng M, Torres L, Calavetta M, Scott CB, Rines D, et al. High speed, multicolor fluorescent two-dimensional gene scanning. Genomics 2001;78:83-90.
36. Medintz I, Wong WW, Sensabaugh G, Mathies RA. High speed single nucleotide polymorphism typing of a hereditary haemochromatosis mutation with capillary array electrophoresis microplates. Electrophoresis 2000;21:2352-8.
37. Molloy MP. Two-dimensional electrophoresis of membrane proteins using immobilized pH gradients. Anal Biochem 2000;280:1-10. Review.
38. Munro NJ, Finegold DN, Landers JP. Indirect fluorescence detection of amino acids on electrophoretic microchips. Anal Chem 2000;72: 2765-73.
39. Munro NJ, Snow K, Kant J, Landers JP. Molecular diagnostics on microfabricated electrophoretic devices: translating slab gel-based T- and B-cell lymphoproliferative disorder assays from the capillary to the microchip. Clin Chem 1999;45:1906-17.
40. Nelson RJ, Burgi DS. Temperature control in capillary electrophoresis. In: Landers JP, ed. Handbook of capillary electrophoresis. Boca Raton, Fla: CRC Press, 1994:549-62.
41. Nelson RJ, Paulus A, Cohen AS, Guttman A, Krager BL. Use of Peltier thermoelectric devices to control column temperature in high-performance capillary electrophoresis. J Chromatogr 1989; 80:111-27.
42. Nielen MW. Quantitative aspects of indirect UV detection in capillary zone electrophoresis. J Chromatogr 1991;588:321-6.
43. Ocvirk G, Tang T, Harrison DJ. Optimization of confocal epifluorescence microscopy for microchip-based miniaturized total analysis systems. The Analyst 1998;123:1429-34.
44. Oda RP, Bush VJ, Landers JP. Clinical applications of capillary electrophoresis. In: Landers JP, ed. Handbook of capillary electrophoresis, 2nd edition. Boca Raton, Fla: CRC Press, 1997:639-73.
45. Oda RP, Clark RJ, Katzmann JA, Landers JP. Capillary electrophoresis as a clinical tool for the analysis of protein in serum and other body fluids. Electrophoresis 1997;18:1715-23.
46. O'Reilly MJ, Kinnon C. The technique of pulsed field gel electrophoresis and its impact on molecular immunology. J Immunol Methods 1990;131:1-31.
47. O'Riordan E, Goligorsky M. Emerging studies of the urinary proteome: the end of the beginning? Review. Curr Opin Nephrol Hypertens 2005;14:579-85.
48. Pancholi P, Oda RP, Mitchell PS, Persing DA, Landers JP. Clinical diagnostic detection of hepatitis C and herpes simplex viral PCR amplification products by capillary electrophoresis with laser-induced fluorescence. Mol Diagn 1997;2:27-38.
49. Pentoney SL Jr, Sweedler JV. Optical detection techniques for capillary electrophoresis. In: Landers JP, ed. Handbook of capillary electrophoresis, 2nd edition. Boca Raton, Fla: CRC Press, 1997:379-423.
50. Peri-Okonny UL, Kenndler E, Stubbs RJ, Guzman NA. Characterization of pharmaceutical drugs by a modified nonaqueous

capillary electrophoresis—mass spectrometry method. Electrophoresis 2003;24:139-50.

51. Pohlod-Miller S, Fanning J, Gu P, Crist KA, You M. Detection of genomic alterations in human endometrial cancer by two-dimensional gel electrophoresis. Am J Obstet Gynecol 2002;186:855-7.
52. Rabilloud T. A comparison between low background silver diammine and silver nitrate protein stains. Electrophoresis 1992;13:429-39.
53. Sadaba M, Porque P, Masjuan J, Alvarez-Cermeno J, Bootello A, Villar L. An ultrasensitive method for the detection of oligoclonal IgG bands. J Immunol Methods 2004;284:141-5.
54. Saeedi B, Hallgren A, Jonasson J, Nilsson LE, Hanberger H, Isaksson B. Modified pulsed-field gel electrophoresis protocol for typing of enterococci. APMIS 2002;110:869-74.
55. Sanders JC, Breadmore MC, Kwok YC, Horsman KM, Landers JP. Hydroxypropyl cellulose as an adsorptive coating sieving matrix for DNA separations: artificial neural network optimization of polymer and electrolyte conditions for microchip analysis. Anal Chem 2003;75:986-94.
56. Sandt C, Krouse D, Cook C, Hackman A, Chmielecki W, Warren N. The key role of pulsed-field gel electrophoresis in investigation of a large multiserotype and multistate food-borne outbreak of salmonella infections centered in Pennsylvania. J Clin Microbiol 2006;44:3208-12.
57. Schoots AC, Everaerts FM. Isotachophoresis as a preseparation technique for liquid chromatography. J Chromatogr 1983;277:328-32.
58. Severs JC, Smith RD. Capillary electrophoresis-mass spectrometry. In: Landers JP, ed. Handbook of capillary electrophoresis, 2nd edition. Boca Raton, Fla: CRC Press, 1997:791-826.
59. Sharma K, Lee S, Han S, Lee S, Francos B, McCue P, et al. Two-dimensional fluorescence difference gel electrophoresis analysis of the urine proteome in human diabetic nephropathy. Proteomics 2005;5:2648-55.
60. Shi Y, Simpson PC, Scherer JR, Wexler D, Skibola C, Smith MT, et al. Radial capillary array electrophoresis microplate and scanner for high-performance nucleic acid analysis. Anal Chem 1999;71:5354-61.
61. Shihabi ZK. Effects of sample matrix on capillary electrophoretic analysis. In: Landers JP, ed. Handbook of capillary electrophoresis, 2nd edition. Boca Raton, Fla: CRC Press, 1997:457-77.
62. St. Claire RL. Capillary electrophoresis. Anal Chem 1996;68:569R-86R.
63. Szoke M, Sasvari-Szelely M, Guttman A. Ultra-thin-layer agarose gel electrophoresis. I. Effect of the gel concentration and temperature on the separation of DNA fragments. J Chromatogr A 1999;830:465-71.
64. Tao Q, Wang Z, Zhao H, Baeyens W, Delanghe J, Huang L, et al. Direct chemiluminescent imaging detection of human serum proteins in two-dimensional polyacrylamide gel electrophoresis. Proteomics 2007;7:3481-90.
65. Tian H, Brody LB, Mao D, Landers JP. Effective capillary electrophoresis-based heteroduplex analysis through surface coatings and polymers. Anal Chem 2000;72:5483-92.
66. Tian R, Wei L, Qin R, Li Y, Du Z, Xia W, et al. Proteome analysis of human pancreatic ductal adenocarcinoma tissue using two-dimensional gel electrophoresis and tandem mass spectrometry for identification of disease-related proteins. Dig Dis Sci 2008;53:65-72.
66A. Tran NT, Ayed I, Pallandre A, Taverna M. Recent innovations in protein separation on microchips by electrophoretic methods: an update. Electrophoresis. 2010 Jan;31(1):147-73.
67. Vesterberg O, Acevedo F, Bayard C. Sensitive quantification of proteins by electrophoresis in gels by use of chemiluminescence. Electrophoresis 1995;16:1390-3.
68. Vijg J, van Orsouw NJ. Two-dimensional gene scanning: exploring human genetic variability. Electrophoresis 1999;20:1239-49.
69. Wainright A, Williams SJ, Ciambrone G, Xue Q, Wei J, Harris D. Sample pre-concentration by isotachophoresis in microfluidic devices. J Chromatogr A 2002;979:69-80.
70. Wettstein PJ, Strausbauch MA. Fraction collection in micro-preparative capillary electrophoresis. In: Landers JP, ed. Handbook of capillary electrophoresis, 2nd edition. Boca Raton, Fla: CRC Press, 1997:841-64.
71. Wittmann-Liebold B, Graack H, Pohl T. Two-dimensional gel electrophoresis as a tool for proteomics studies in combination with protein identification by mass spectrometry. Review. Proteomics 2006;6:4688-703.
72. Woolley AT, Sensabaugh GF, Mathies RA. High-speed DNA genotyping using microfabricated capillary array electrophoresis chips. Anal Chem 1997;9:2181-6.
73. Xiao Z, Conrads T, Lucas D, Janini G, Schaefer C, Buetow K, et al. Direct ampholyte-free liquid-phase isoelectric peptide focusing: application to the human serum proteome. Electrophoresis 2004;25:128-33.
74. Xu Y. Capillary electrophoresis. Anal Chem 1995;67:463R-73R.
75. Yang Z, Harrison K, Park YA, Chaffin C, Thigpen B, Easley P, et al. Performance of the Sebia CAPILLARYS 2 for detection and immunotyping of serum monoclonal paraproteins. Am J Clin Pathol 2007;128:293-9.

CHAPTER 13

Chromatography and Extraction

Glen L. Hortin, M.D., Ph.D., and
*Bruce A. Goldberger, Ph.D.**

Biological fluids are complex mixtures, and clinical tests for specific components contained in these fluids often entail one or more sequential separation steps to isolate or enrich the component of interest. Common methods for achieving separation include (1) chromatography, (2) extraction, (3) differential precipitation, and (4) electrophoresis (see Chapter 12). This chapter describes basic concepts and principles of chromatographic and extraction techniques that are used as analytical techniques or as methods to prepare specimens for analysis.

CHOMATOGRAPHY

Chromatography is a process in which components of a mixture are separated by differential distribution between a mobile phase and a stationary phase.[12,48,66] Components with greater distribution into the stationary phase are retained and move through the system more slowly. The initial description of this technique by Mikhail Tswett in 1903 entailed the separation of plant pigments into separate colored bands on a column of calcium carbonate.[13] He originated the term *chromatography,* derived from chroma and graphein (Greek for "color" and "to write"), and this term has continued to be used even though most separations do not involve colored components.

Planar and column are the two basic forms of chromatography (Figure 13-1). In planar chromatography, the stationary phase is coated on a sheet of paper (paper chromatography) or is bound to a solid surface [thin-layer chromatography (TLC)]. For paper chromatography, the stationary phase is a layer of water or a polar solvent coated onto paper fibers. In TLC, a thin layer of particles of a material such as silica gel is spread uniformly on a glass plate or a plastic or aluminum sheet. When the thin layer consists of particles with small diameters (4.5 μm), the technique is known as *high-performance, thin-layer chromatography* (HPTLC).

In column chromatography, the stationary phase may be a pure silica or polymer, or it may be coated onto, or chemically bonded to, support particles.[6] The stationary phase may be "packed" into a tube, or it may be coated onto the inner surface of the tube. Column chromatography includes both gas chromatography (GC)[47] and liquid chromatography (LC)[62]; with classification dependent on whether the mobile phase is a gas or a liquid. Operationally, the instrument used to perform a GC or LC separation is known as a *gas* or *liquid chromatograph.* When the stationary phase in LC consists of small-diameter particles, the technique is known as high-performance liquid chromatography (HPLC). When a gas or liquid chromatograph is connected to a mass spectrometer, the combined or "hyphenated" techniques are gas chromatography–mass spectrometry (GC-MS) and liquid chromatography–mass spectrometry (LC-MS).[23]

In analytical GC and LC, the mobile phase, or eluent, exits from the column and passes through a detector that produces an electronic signal that is plotted as a function of (1) time, (2) distance, or (3) volume. The resulting graphical display is a chromatogram (Figure 13-2).

Retention time or volume is the interval or volume required for a solute to pass from the injector, through the column, and to the detector. Data represented by the chromatogram are used to help identify and quantify the solute(s). Because eluting solutes are displayed graphically as a series of peaks, they are frequently referred to as chromatographic peaks. These peaks are described in terms of peak (1) width, (2) height, and (3) area. In planar chromatography, the separated zones are detected by their natural colors or are visualized through chemical modification that produces colored "spots" or "bands," which are used to qualitatively identify various analytes, or to quantify them.

Separation Mechanisms

Chromatographic separations are classified by the chemical or physical mechanisms used to separate the solutes (Figure

*The authors gratefully acknowledge the contributions of Drs. M. David Ullman, Carl A. Burtis, and Larry D. Bowers to this chapter in previous editions.

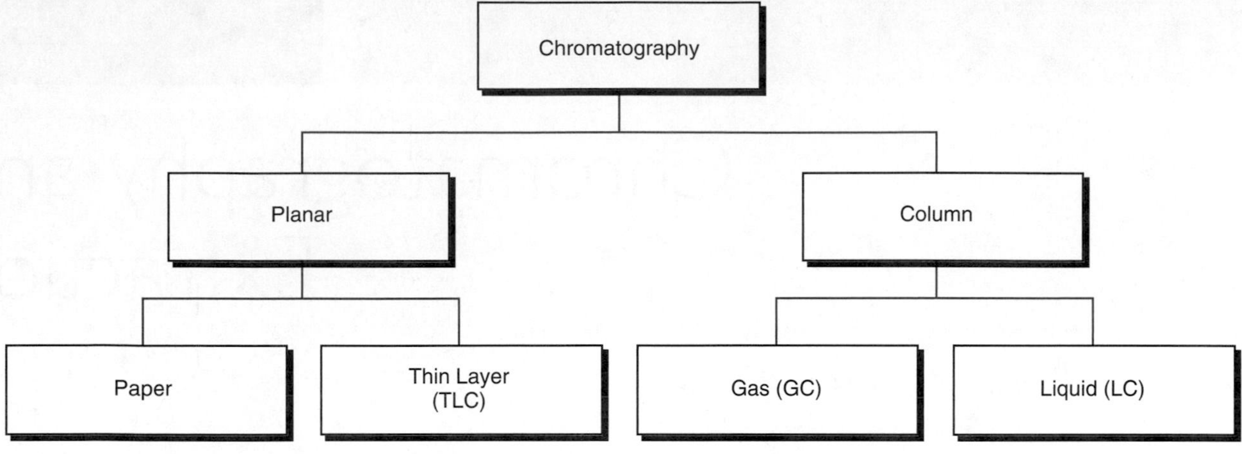

Figure 13-1 Forms of chromatography.

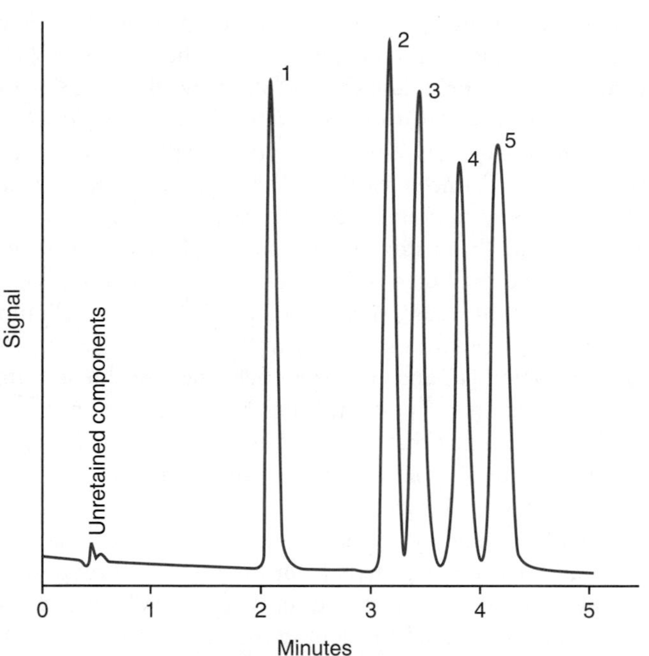

Figure 13-2 Chromatogram from an HPLC reversed-phase separation of tricyclic antidepressants with the use of a UV photometer detector set at 215 nm. Signal is displayed at 0.1 AUFS. ***AUFS,*** **Absorbance units full scale;** ***HPLC,*** **high-performance liquid chromatography;** ***UV,*** **ultraviolet.** *(Courtesy Vydac/The Separations Group, Hesperia, Calif.)*

13-3). These include (1) ion-exchange, (2) adsorption, (3) partition, (4) affinity, and (5) size-exclusion mechanisms. Predominantly, clinical applications use chromatographic separations based on ion-exchange and partition mechanisms.

Ion-Exchange

Ion-exchange chromatography relies on the exchange of ions between charged groups bound to a stationary phase and ions of opposite charge in the mobile phase (see Figure 13-3). Depending on the charge of the stationary phase, components binding to the column may be cations (positively charged) or anions (negatively charged). Cation-exchange solid phases contain covalently bound, negatively charged functional groups. Examples include strongly acidic groups, such as sulfonate ions, or weakly acidic groups, such as carboxyl or carboxymethyl. Anion-exchange solid phases have strongly basic quaternary amines, such as triethylaminoethyl groups, or weakly basic groups, such as aminoethyl (AE) and diethylaminoethyl (DEAE) groups. Separations are performed under conditions where analytes are charged and bind to the ion-exchange stationary phase. Solutes are eluted with a solution containing competing counterions, such as sodium for cation exchange and chloride for anion exchange, and, in some cases, by adjustment of pH to decrease the charge of bound ions or the ion-exchange surface. Important factors in performance of ion-exchange chromatography include (1) type of stationary phase ionic group, (2) charge density, (3) stationary phase matrix, (4) type and concentration of ions in the mobile phase, and (5) mobile phase pH. Many stationary phases exhibit mixed mode retention by a combination of ion exchange and adsorptive binding. As an example, ion-exchange resins used for amino acid analysis are able to separate amino acids with virtually the same charge because of variable adsorptive interactions of different amino acids with the stationary phase. Some solid-phase extraction media are designed to have mixed hydrophobic–ion-exchange retention, offering improved selectivity versus extraction

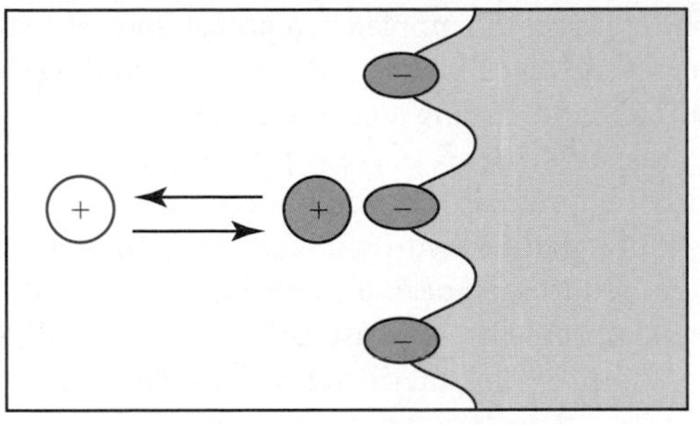

Ion-exchange chromatography

Separation is based on exchange of ions between surface and eluents.

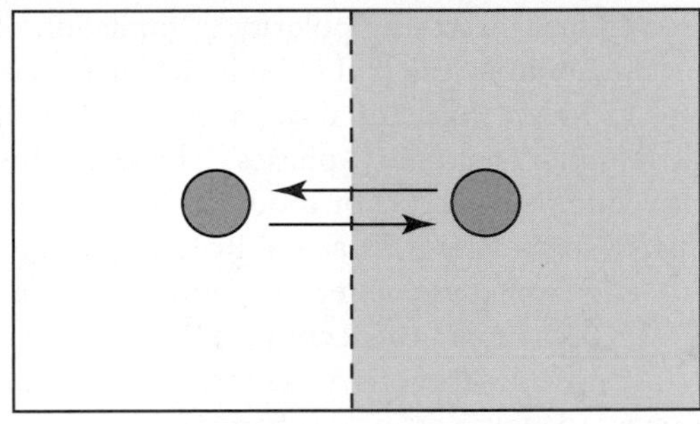

Partition chromatography

Separation is based on solute partitioning between two liquid phases.

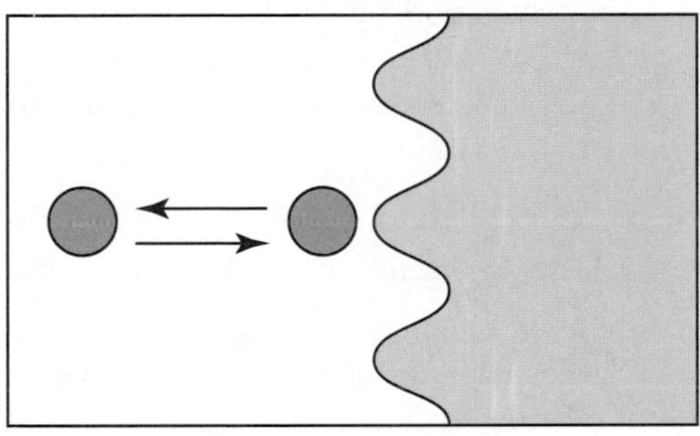

Adsorption chromatography

Separation is due to a series of adsorption/desorption steps.

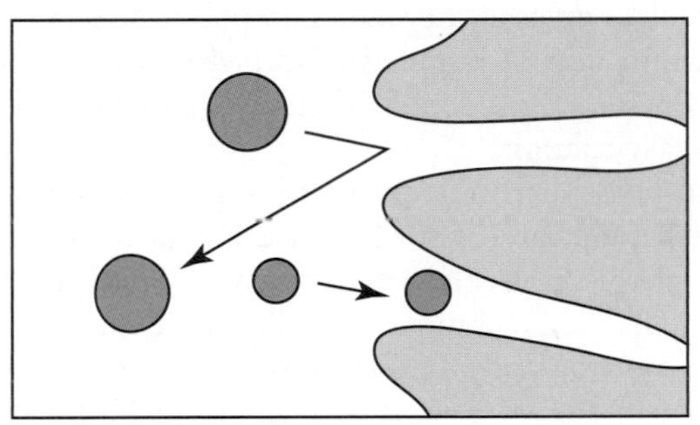

Size-exclusion chromatography

Separation is based on molecular size.

Figure 13-3 Examples of separation mechanisms used in chromatography. *(Courtesy James K. Hardy, Akron, Ohio [http://ull.chemistry.uakron.edu].)*

media designed predominantly for hydrophobic or ion-exchange extractions.

Ion-exchange chromatography has a number of clinical applications, including analyses of amino acids and hemoglobins. It is also used to analyze small inorganic and organic ions with conductivity detection, a technique termed *ion chromatography.* Water purification is an important preparative application of ion-exchange chromatography consists of using mixed-bed resins with both cation and anion exchangers. Ions are removed by exchange of hydrogen ions for other cations and hydroxyl ions for other anions. The hydrogen ions and hydroxyl ions displaced by salt ions form water.

Adsorption

The basis of separation by adsorption chromatography is the difference between adsorption and desorption of solutes at the surface of a solid particle (see Figure 13-3). Electrostatic, hydrogen-bonding, and dispersive (van der Waals) interactions are the physical forces that control this type of chromatography.[17,28] As solvent molecules compete for binding to the stationary phase, the strength of binding to the stationary phase depends on the properties of the stationary phase and of the mobile phase. In general, for a polar stationary phase, elution tracks the polarity of the components in a mixture: less polar ones elute first, followed by those of increasing polarity.[7]

In GC, this mode is used to separate low molecular weight compounds such as methyl, ethyl, isopropyl alcohols from compounds that are normally gases at room temperature. It uses particles of support, such as "molecular sieves," alumina, and styrene-divinylbenzene copolymers. In LC, three types of adsorbents are generally used: (1) nonpolar, (2) acid polar, and (3) basic polar. Nonpolar adsorbents include charcoal and polystyrene-divinylbenzene. The main acidic polar adsorbent is silica gel, the surface silanol (SiOH) groups of which adsorb basic substances. Alumina is the main basic adsorbent for retaining acidic substances. Florisil has also been used as a basic adsorbent when catalytic decomposition of the analyte is observed with alumina.

Hydrophilic interaction liquid chromatography (HILIC) is a type of adsorption chromatography that is used to separate highly polar compounds that form hydrogen bonds with a stationary phase having a relatively polar surface.[8,26,41] Examples of stationary phases used for HILIC include (1) unmodified silica, (2) silica with bonded zwitterionic groups, (3) hydroxyl-rich compounds, and (4) amide-rich compounds. Initial binding of solutes to the stationary phase is performed in relatively hydrophobic solvent, and elution is attained with solvents of increasing polarity. A limitation of HILIC for clinical laboratory use is that biological fluids are highly polar and include a substantial quantity of salts that also interact with polar stationary phases. Therefore, the specimen may need to be extracted or modified by the addition of a less polar solvent such as acetonitrile to promote binding to the stationary phase. Interest is growing in the application of HILIC as a separation technique linked to mass spectrometry, but most separations in clinical laboratories have relied on reversed-phase or ion-exchange separations.

Partition Chromatography

The differential distribution of solutes between two immiscible liquids is the basis for separation by partition chromatography (see Figure 13-3).[46,55,56] Operationally, one of the immiscible liquids serves as the stationary phase. To prepare this phase, a thin film of liquid is adsorbed or chemically bonded onto the surface of support particles or onto the inner wall of a capillary column.

In reversed-phase, partition chromatography, the (1) stationary phase is nonpolar, (2) mobile phase is relatively polar, and (3) hydrophobic molecules are preferentially retained. It is the most widely used technique for solid-phase extraction and liquid chromatography in the clinical laboratory. An example of separation of several antidepressant drugs by reversed-phase chromatography is shown in Figure 13-2. Examples of stationary phases for reversed-phase adsorption include silica with bonded hydrophobic groups such as octadecyl (C18), octyl (C8), phenyl, or butyl (C4) and polystyrene-divinylbenzene. For solid-phase extractions, similar materials are used including copolymers of styrene with more hydrophilic monomers that form stationary phases with balanced hydrophobic-hydrophilic character or with charged groups that offer mixed-mode extraction with both hydrophobic and ion-exchange retention.[6,20,55] The retention characteristics of silica-based stationary phases depend on (1) the nature of bonded phases, (2) the amount of bonded phase (often expressed as % carbon load), (3) the surface area of the particles, (4) the pore size of the particles, and (5) the quantity of accessible silanol groups on silica particles that depend on surface treatments such as "end-capping," where such groups are replaced by trimethylsilyl groups. For reversed-phase separations, solutions are applied in relatively polar solvent such as water or water with a low concentration of organic solvent such as methanol or acetonitrile. Reversed-phase separations are often used with aqueous specimens such as blood and urine, because most of the solvent (water) and inorganic salts pass through the column with minimal retention. The partitioning of solutes in reversed-phase separations usually is favored by adjustment of pH to minimize the charge of solutes, such as decreasing the pH so that organic acids are in uncharged forms, or adding ion-pairing agents that yield less polar ion pairs. Prior to the introduction of a sample, hydrophobic stationary phases may require conditioning or "wetting" with a solvent such as methanol before equilibrating with a more polar solvent. Some stationary phases, such as C18-silica, may undergo "phase collapse" of the bonded phase if run in completely aqueous solvent, which probably represents the aliphatic bonded phase folding down onto the surface and having decreased access to solvent. During a solid-phase extraction, drawing air into the column can similarly require reapplication of organic solvent to wet surfaces. Use of balanced hydrophobic-hydrophilic phases for extractions reduces the need for wetting of the stationary phase and avoids problems of phase collapse with loading of aqueous solutions.[19,55] Polymeric stationary phases usually have higher capacity than bonded silica stationary phases, because the entire particle serves as the stationary phase.

Elution of compounds in reversed-phase separations relies on competition of molecules in the mobile phase with molecules bound to the stationary phase. Elution is hastened by changing the solvent strength with a linear or stepwise gradient, or by changing the pH to increase the polarity of solutes. The strength of solvents, sometimes referred to as the *eluotropic series,* for reversed-phase separations generally follows this order:

Pentane > Cyclohexane > Toluene > Dichloromethane >
Ethylacetate > Acetonitrile > Ethanol > Methanol > Water

More hydrophobic solvents generally are stronger eluents for reversed-phase separations. For normal-phase chromatography (polar stationary phase, nonpolar mobile phase), the eluotropic series is reversed. In practice, it is also possible to change the solvent strength by using mixtures of solvents and gradients of changing proportions of solvents during an analysis (Figure 13-4).[9] It is also possible to modify the

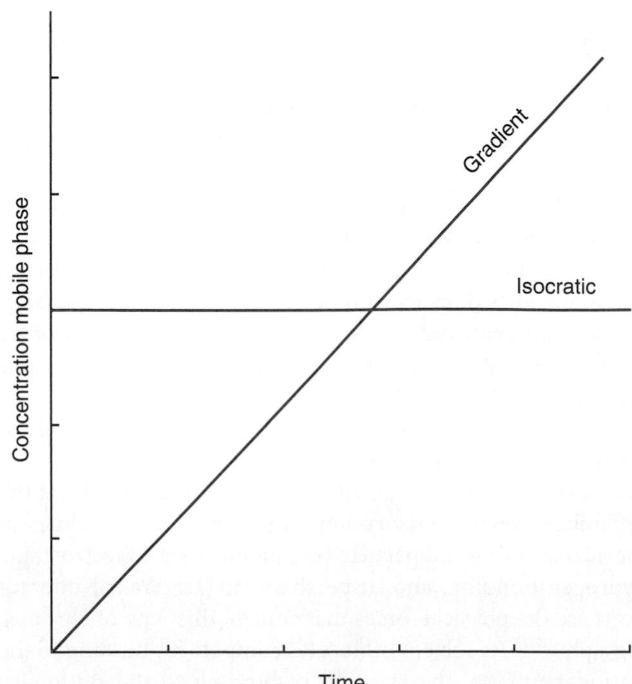

Figure 13-4 Examples of isocratic (constant composition) and gradient elution (varying composition) in LC. *LC,* Liquid chromatography.

polarity of aqueous solutions by changing the salt concentration. This characteristic is employed in a variation of reversed-phase chromatography termed *hydrophobic interaction chromatography,* which has been applied mainly for separation of proteins. Binding to a weakly hydrophobic stationary phase containing interaction groups such as phenyl or butyl groups is promoted by loading specimens in a high-salt concentration, and elution is achieved by lowering the salt concentration rather than by adding an organic solvent.

A wide range of solid phases for reversed-phase separations have slightly different specificities, and some have mixed modes of separation.[6,16,39] Some solid phases such as porous graphite or fluorinated hydrocarbons or hydrophobic stationary phases with embedded polar groups offer different selectivities than traditional C18-silica. Stationary phases bonded on silica have weak cation-exchange and normal-phase properties, depending on the quantity of accessible hydroxyl groups on the silica. Basic compounds may exhibit peak tailing caused by ion exchange with the silica. Ion-exchange properties of silica are minimized by chemically modifying the surface to block hydroxyls and by operating at low pH. Silica tends to dissolve slowly at pH > 7, so that silica particles usually require separations below pH 8, unless the silica is stabilized by surface treatment.[5] Other types of stationary phases such as polystyrene or porous graphite are stable at high pH and allow separations over a broader pH range.

Because of its wide diversity of stationary phases with differing selectivities and varying ability to change solvent conditions and ion-pairing agents, reversed-phase chromatography is a very versatile technique, and separations often achieve high efficiency and , sharp peaks. Compounds representing the greatest challenge for reversed-phase separations are small ions and highly polar compounds such as sugars or amino acids, which tend to be weakly retained by reversed-phase media, and basic compounds, which may exhibit peak tailing as the result of interactions with silica. Derivatization of some compounds such as amino acids has been employed to improve reversed-phase retention and to add chromophores or fluorophores to improve detection.[48] Separation of large peptides or proteins requires stationary phases with larger pore sizes than are routinely used for separation of small molecules.[3,32,63]

Chiral Separations

Many biological molecules occur as specific stereoisomeric forms, such as L-amino acids, and in some cases, only a particular stereoisomer of a therapeutic drug may be active. In general, the two mirror-image forms of a compound or enantiomers have very similar physical properties and do not separate in most chromatographic analyses. Separation of enantiomers generally requires use of a stationary phase that has an enantiomeric component that will interact with molecules in a stereospecific manner. For example, chiral stationary phases (CSPs) that contain groups such as derivatized L-amino acids or stereospecific carbohydrates have been used to separate enantiomers.[52,62A,72]

Size Exclusion Chromatography

Size exclusion chromatography, also known as (1) gel filtration, (2) gel permeation, (3) steric exclusion, (4) molecular exclusion, or (5) molecular sieve chromatography, is a technique that separates molecules or other particles based on size (Figure 13-5). In this technique, the stationary phase consists of porous particles with an inert surface designed to have minimal adsorption of components. Materials used for stationary phases include cross-linked dextran, polyacrylamide, agarose, polystyrene, and porous glass with an inert surface coating. Beads of these materials are porous and have pore sizes that allow small molecules to enter. Molecules too large to enter the pores remain entirely in the mobile phase and are rapidly eluted from the column. Molecules that are intermediate in size have access to various fractions of the pore volume and elute between large and small molecules according to the following relation:

$$V_r = V_0 + KV_i$$

where V_r is the retention volume, V_0 is the void volume between particles, K is the fraction of the pore volume accessible to the molecule, and V_i is the volume within the support particles.

By calibrating a size-exclusion column with molecules of known size, it is possible to estimate the molecular size of proteins or other molecules.[64] However, this is a relatively low-resolution technique, and separation of components requires substantial proportional differences in molecular weight. The diameter of globular proteins changes only in proportion to the cube root of molecular weight, so that an eightfold difference in molecular weight is required to yield a twofold change

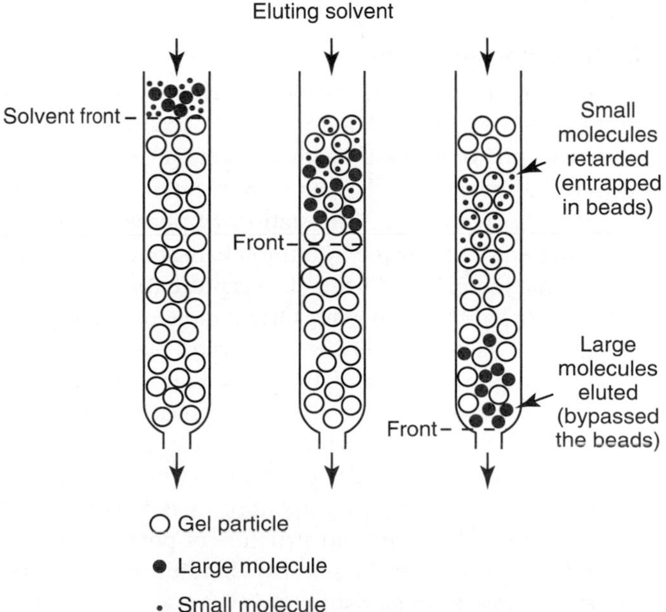

Figure 13-5 Schematic representation of gel filtration column chromatography. *(Modified from Bennett TP. Graphic biochemistry, vol 1: chemistry of biological molecules. New York: Macmillan, 1968.)*

in diameter.[64] Linear polymers, such as DNA, and proteins denatured with sodium dodecylsulfate or guanidine hydrochloride have a much larger diameter for the same molecular weight, and diameter changes approximately in proportion to the square root of molecular weight, allowing better resolution of linear molecules relative to molecular weight than of globular molecules. Therefore, analysis of molecules under denaturing conditions provides the ability to resolve molecules with smaller differences in molecular weight.

Size exclusion chromatography allows the separation of molecules under physiologic salt conditions; this is useful for identifying intact complexes of molecules such as lipoproteins, antibody-antigen complexes, and other binding proteins and their ligands under mild nondenaturing conditions. Also, it is used as a rapid preparative technique for salt exchange or to remove small molecules from large molecules using small centrifuge or gravity flow columns.

Other Size Exclusion Separations

Separations by size exclusion also are performed with ultrafiltration membranes or particles with defined pore sizes. Ultrafiltration is employed in the clinical laboratory as a preparative technique to separate small molecules such as amino acids or drugs, which pass through the membrane in the ultrafiltrate, from proteins, which remain in the retentate fraction. Ultrafiltration and equilibrium dialysis serve as means of separating free from protein-bound components, such as for measurement of free phenytoin or thyroxine concentrations. Ultrafiltration also is used as a technique for concentrating proteins in dilute solutions, such as urine, for analysis by electrophoresis or other techniques. Ultrafiltration is useful mainly for separating molecules or particles that have large differences in size, typically more than a 10-fold difference in molecular weight.

Affinity Chromatography

Specific molecular interactions are used as the basis for affinity chromatography (Figure 13-6).[25,57] Examples include (1) interactions of antibody with antigen, (2) enzyme with substrate, (3) aptamer with ligand, (4) receptor with ligand, and (5) lectin with sugar. The stationary phase for affinity chromatography is prepared by immobilizing one component of an interaction pair and using it to capture the other component of the interaction pair. Orientation of the capture molecule and its accessibility are important elements in the function of capture molecules. Using a spacer to provide distance from the surface of the stationary phase may improve access and function of the capture molecule. An alternative approach to developing affinity matrices without immobilized ligands is to form molecularly imprinted surfaces on the capture phase.[38] The shape and structure of pores formed by molecular imprinting yield selective binding of molecules that have a complementary structure.

To perform affinity chromatography, a solution is applied to the stationary phase under conditions that allow specific binding to the capture molecule, and nonbound components are removed by extensive washing of the stationary phase.

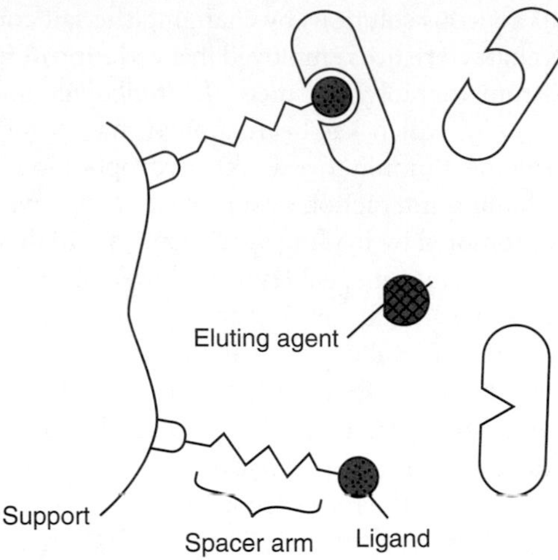

Figure 13-6 Principle of affinity chromatography. The analyte (enzyme, antibody, antigen, tissue receptor, etc.) binds to the support-bound ligand. Subsequently, it is eluted with a general eluent (such as a chaotropic agent), a pH change, or a biospecific eluent (such as an inhibitor or substrate).

Specifically bound components are eluted by adding competing ligand or changing conditions such as pH or ionic strength, so as to eliminate binding to the stationary phase. Affinity separations may be performed batchwise with sedimentation of the stationary phase, or by column chromatography. Chromatographic elution often is seen with stepwise change of solvent to allow elution of desired components in a single fraction.

The power of affinity chromatography lies in its selectivity. Affinity chromatography is widely applied to purifying antibodies and other proteins used in clinical assays. Lectin affinity chromatography offers a means of assessing changes in the oligosaccharide structures bound to glycoproteins. Immobilized phenylboronic acid has been used to separate glycated hemoglobin from unmodified hemoglobin. Most heterogenous assays in the clinical laboratory are based on the selective extraction or capture of a specific target molecule onto a solid phase with elution of all other molecules (see Chapter 16). Immunodepletion or immunopartitioning of high-abundance proteins has been used as a means of preparing biological specimens for proteomic analysis to assist in the detection of lower-abundance components.[53]

Resolution

Resolution (R_s) is a measure of the separation between two components (Figure 13-7). Improved resolution may result from sharper peaks (higher chromatographic efficiency) or from a greater separation between peaks (higher selectivity), as described in Figure 13-8. It is expressed mathematically as follows:

$$R_s = \frac{t_r(B) - t_r(A)}{\left[\dfrac{w(A) - w(B)}{2}\right]}$$

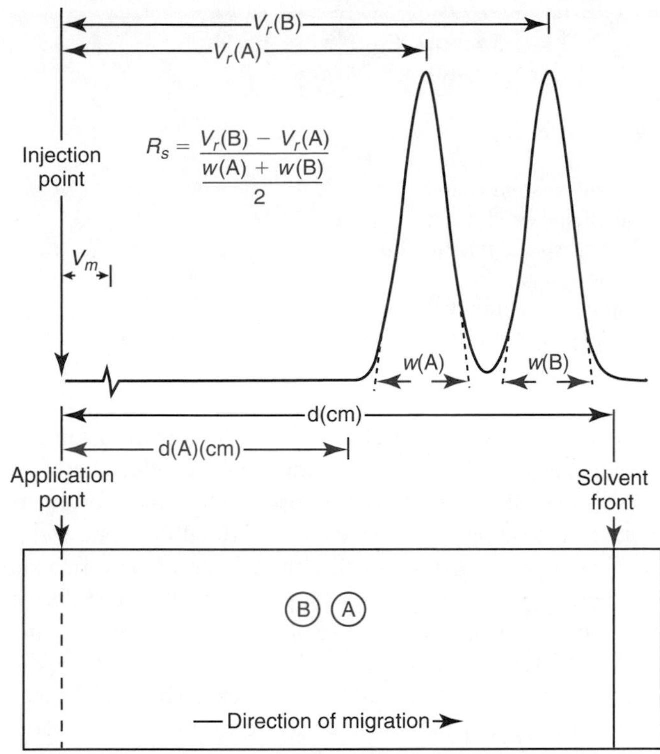

Figure 13-7 Schematic diagram of chromatograms obtained from a column and a planar chromatograph. In planar chromatography *(bottom)*, strongly retained compound *B* migrates less than weakly retained compound *A*. In column chromatography *(top)*, compound *B* is eluted later than compound *A*. *d(A)* and *d(B)*, Distance traveled by solutes *A* and *B*; R_s, resolution; V_m, volume between injector and detector; $V_r(A)$ and $V_r(B)$, retention volumes for solutes *A* and *B*; *w(A)* and *w(B)*, peak widths at base for solutes *A* and *B*.

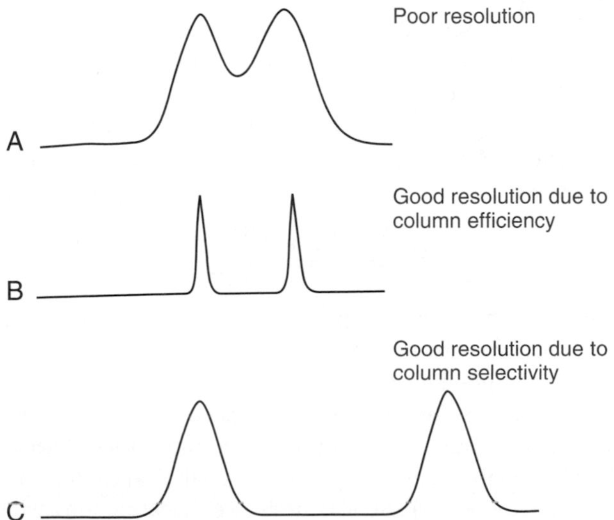

Figure 13-8 Effects of selectivity and efficiency on chromatographic resolution. A, Poor resolution. B, Good resolution because of high column efficiency. C, Good resolution because of column selectivity. *(From Johnson EL, Stevenson R. Basic liquid chromatography. Palo Alto, Calif: Varian Associates, 1978.)*

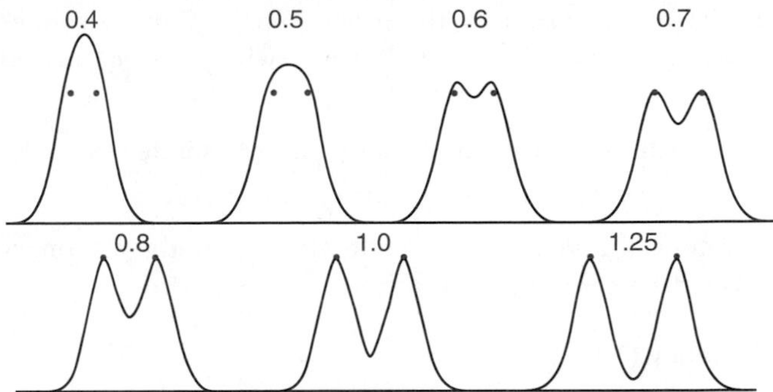

Figure 13-9 Separation of chromatographic peaks present in a 1 : 1 ratio as a function of resolution (R_s). *(From Snyder LR. A rapid approach to selecting the best experimental conditions for high-speed liquid column chromatography. Part I. Estimating initial sample resolution required by a given problem. J Chrom Sci 1972;10:202.)*

where

$t_r(A)$ = retention time for solute A
$t_r(B)$ = retention time for solute B
$w(A)$ = peak width (units of time) measured at base for solute A
$w(B)$ = peak width (units of time) measured at base for solute B

Retention may be expressed in units of time (previous equation) or volume (see Figure 13-7). A resolution of 1.25 or greater reflects baseline separation of peaks; lower resolution represents increasing degrees of overlap between peaks, as described in Figure 13-9. Resolution is improved by enhancing efficiency (achieving narrower peaks) or by improving selectivity to increase the separation between the two components. Two ways to increase resolution are by using a longer column and by selecting a column with higher efficiency. Either of these measures increases N, the number of theoretical plates. Resolution increases proportionally with the square root of N, so that doubling of column length (doubling of N) will increase resolution by a factor of 1.41.

Retention Factor

The retention factor k′ is a measure of the time a solute resides in the stationary phase relative to the time it resides in the mobile phase. Mathematically, it is the ratio of the adjusted retention volume(v_r) or retention time (t_r) to the void volume (v_0) or hold-up time (t_0) (the time for unretained components to elute from the column).

$$k' = \frac{v_r - v_0}{v_0} = \frac{t_r - t_0}{t_0}$$

A k′ of 0 indicates no binding between a solute and the stationary phase. Greater partitioning into the stationary phase results in longer retention times and increased k′. In practice, it is desirable to have a k′ between 1 and 10 for optimal separations that do not take an excessive length of time.

In planar chromatography, such as paper and thin-layer chromatography, all separation of solutes must occur within the distance traveled by the mobile phase. Thus, a solute's migration is expressed by its R_f value, which is calculated as follows:

$$R_f = \frac{\text{distance from application point to solute center}}{\text{distance from application point to solvent front}}$$

Therefore, the greater the solute affinity for the stationary phase, the smaller the R_f value.

Efficiency (N)

Ideally, a component moving through a chromatographic column migrates as a very narrow band. However, nonuniformity of flow, diffusion, and mass transfer effects between particles and the mobile phase produce band broadening. Chromatographic efficiency is considered to be highest when band broadening is minimized. Column efficiency is commonly expressed as N, the number of theoretical plates. For a peak forming a Gaussian curve, $N = (\frac{t_r}{\sigma})^2$, where t_r is retention time and σ is the standard deviation of the curve measured as time. A practical way to calculate N is based on the measurement of peak width ($w_{1/2}$) at half the maximal peak height; $w_{1/2}$ represents 2.354 σ. Therefore,

$$N = 5.55\left[\frac{t_r}{w_{1/2}}\right]^2 = \left[\frac{t_r}{\sigma}\right]^2$$

An increase in N represents improved chromatographic efficiency and sharper peaks. Efficiency is often expressed as the number of theoretical plates per column length (N/L). The efficiency and the number of theoretical plates for a column are directly related to the column length, but usually a tradeoff of longer analysis times for longer columns occurs. Column efficiency also is expressed as the height equivalent of a theoretical plate (HETP):

$$HETP = \frac{L}{N}$$

In theory, a theoretical plate is equivalent to the length of a column necessary to allow one equilibration of the solute to occur between stationary and mobile phases. To increase the efficiency of a column, the number of theoretical plates is increased. In practice, this typically is accomplished by increasing the length of the column.

The flow rate has a major effect on chromatographic efficiency as described by the van Deemter equation:

$$HETP = A + \frac{B}{v} + Cv$$

where

A = a constant related to *eddy-diffusion*
B = a constant related to longitudinal diffusion
C = a constant related to kinetics of mass transfer between mobile and stationary phases
v = the mobile phase velocity

Decreasing values for HETP represent improved efficiency, in that the number of theoretical plates for a particular column length is increased. The van Deemter equation predicts that optimization of flow rates involves a balance between peak broadening at low flow rates from diffusion and at high flow rates from increased mass transfer effects between mobile and stationary phases. It also predicts that, for a particular chromatographic system, an optimal flow rate yields the best efficiency. Empirically, the effects of flow rate on efficiency are tested by measuring peak widths at different flow rates. In practice, there usually is no interest in defining the complete van Deemter curve, but rather in identifying the highest flow rate that does not result in excessive peak broadening. The usual goal is to identify conditions for the most rapid analysis time that still yields adequate separations.

Factors that affect chromatographic efficiency are listed in Box 13-1. In practice, efficiency is improved by using (1) smaller particles, (2) nonporous particles, or (3) a coated capillary surface as the stationary phase to minimize mass transfer effects (the C constant in the van Deemter equation). This allows the use of higher mobile phase flow rates without peak broadening, resulting in faster separations. The limiting factor in reducing particle size is the increased resistance to flow and the need to operate at higher pressures.

BOX 13-1 Factors That Affect Chromatographic Efficiency

Column length
Flow rate
Initial injection volume
Mobile-phase viscosity
Particle size of stationary phase
Temperature
Uniformity of the stationary phase
Volume of connecting tubing

Selectivity

Selectivity of a separation of two components reflects variable partitioning of different components between the two phases of an extraction or between the stationary and mobile phases of a chromatographic system. The *selectivity factor* (α) for two components A and B is the ratio of retention factors for two components:

$$\alpha = \frac{k'(B)}{k'(A)} = \frac{[t_r(B) - t_0]}{[t_r(A) - t_0]}$$

with the later eluting component B in the numerator. If two components have the same retention times, then $\alpha = 1$. Separations of components generally seek to identify conditions in which there are moderate differences in retention times of components. This is achieved through appropriate selection of mobile phase, stationary phase, and analytical conditions. A large selectivity coefficient is desirable in extractions where analysts seek to selectively extract one component. However, a large selectivity component in chromatography may result in the need to change the mobile phase or temperature during an analysis to achieve elution of both components within a practical length of time. An α of 1.1 or greater for two components usually represents adequate chromatographic separation.

Peak Capacity

Peak capacity is the theoretical maximum of the number of components that are able to be separated in a single chromatographic analysis[20,51,54]; it assumes a continuous distribution of peaks separated by four standard deviations. In practice, the number of components that are resolved will be lower than expected, because retention times of components are not evenly distributed. The peak capacity, therefore, serves as an upper limit for the number of components that are able to be resolved and as a performance measure for a chromatographic method. The peak capacity of high-performance liquid chromatographic (HPLC) separation usually is limited to several hundred peaks. Some gains in peak capacity are achieved by (1) increasing column length, (2) elution with solvent gradients, (3) extended run times, or (4) increasing chromatographic efficiency. However, the greatest gain in peak capacity is achieved by using two-dimensional or multidimensional chromatography, where the different dimensions usually are performed sequentially (with the second dimension representing analyses of fractions collected from the first dimension).[20,58] Peak capacities of greater than 10,000 have been achieved for two-dimensional HPLC separations, but this requires prolonged analysis time for each sample to perform multiple runs in the second dimension. Linking of chromatographic methods to other analytical methods or detectors, such as mass spectrometers, with the capacity to resolve or detect multiple components serves as an alternative approach to overcome the fundamental limitation of chromatographic peak capacity without extending analysis time. This enables the practical analysis of up to thousands of components in a single specimen, such as for metabolomic[22] or proteomic analysis.[42]

Planar Chromatography

Paper chromatography and thin-layer chromatography (TLC) are classified as planar techniques.[59] TLC uses a thin layer of sorbent, such as silica gel, microparticulate cellulose, or alumina, spread uniformly on a glass plate, plastic sheet, or aluminum foil. The sample is added as a small spot or band on the plate, which is placed in a closed container with the lower edge within, and the sample band just above, the mobile phase (Figure 13-10). After the mobile phase travels a desired distance by capillary action, the plate is removed from the tank and dried. Separated components are located and identified by procedures such as (1) ultraviolet (UV) illumination (fluorescence); (2) spraying with specific, color-generating reagents; or (3) autoradiography. Paper chromatography and TLC tend to be used primarily for qualitative analysis. They allow two-dimensional separations using a different solvent in a second direction or the parallel analysis of multiple specimens. Applications of these techniques include analysis of amniotic fluid for lecithin-to-sphingomyelin ratios and screening of urine samples for drugs or metabolites such as amino acids that accumulate in hereditary disorders. These techniques (1) are relatively simple, (2) do not require much equipment, and (3) allow parallel analysis of multiple specimens for one-dimensional separations. However, application in clinical laboratories has been decreasing because of lack of automation and limited ability to perform precise quantification.

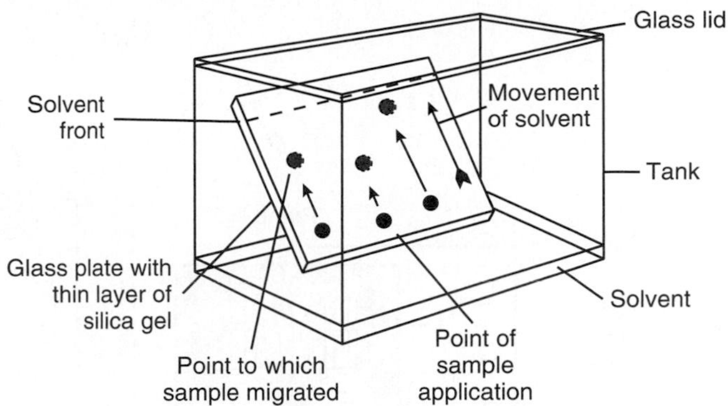

Figure 13-10 Illustration of thin-layer chromatography (TLC). The solvent moves up the thin layer of adsorbent by capillary action. *(Modified from Bennett TP. Graphic biochemistry, vol 1: chemistry of biological molecules. New York: Macmillan, 1968.)*

Liquid Chromatography

Separation by LC is based on the distribution of the solutes between a liquid mobile phase and a stationary phase.[62] In HPLC, particles of small diameter are used as the stationary-phase support. Because pressure drop is related to the square of the particle diameter, relatively high pressures are required to pump liquids through efficient HPLC columns. Consequently, the technique has also been referred to as *high-pressure liquid chromatography.* In the clinical laboratory, HPLC is the most widely used form of LC. It is an extremely versatile technique because of the wide variety of separation mechanisms, stationary phases, solvents, and detectors that have been employed.

Instrumentation

The components of a liquid chromatograph are illustrated in Figure 13-11.[36]

Solvent Reservoir

Solvents used as the mobile phase are contained in solvent reservoirs. In their simplest forms, the reservoirs are glass bottles or flasks into which "feed lines" to the pump are inserted. To remove particles from solvents, inline filters are placed on the inlets of the feed lines. Most also have a means of sparging solutions with a gas such as helium to remove dissolved oxygen that will interfere with the response of some detectors. Removal of gas bubbles and oxygen or "degassing" has also been achieved by applying a vacuum to the reservoir or to gas exchange devices placed in the flow path from reservoirs.

Solvent Delivery System

The solvent delivery system includes (1) valves, (2) a gradient mixing chamber, (3) pressure sensors, (4) pulse dampers, and

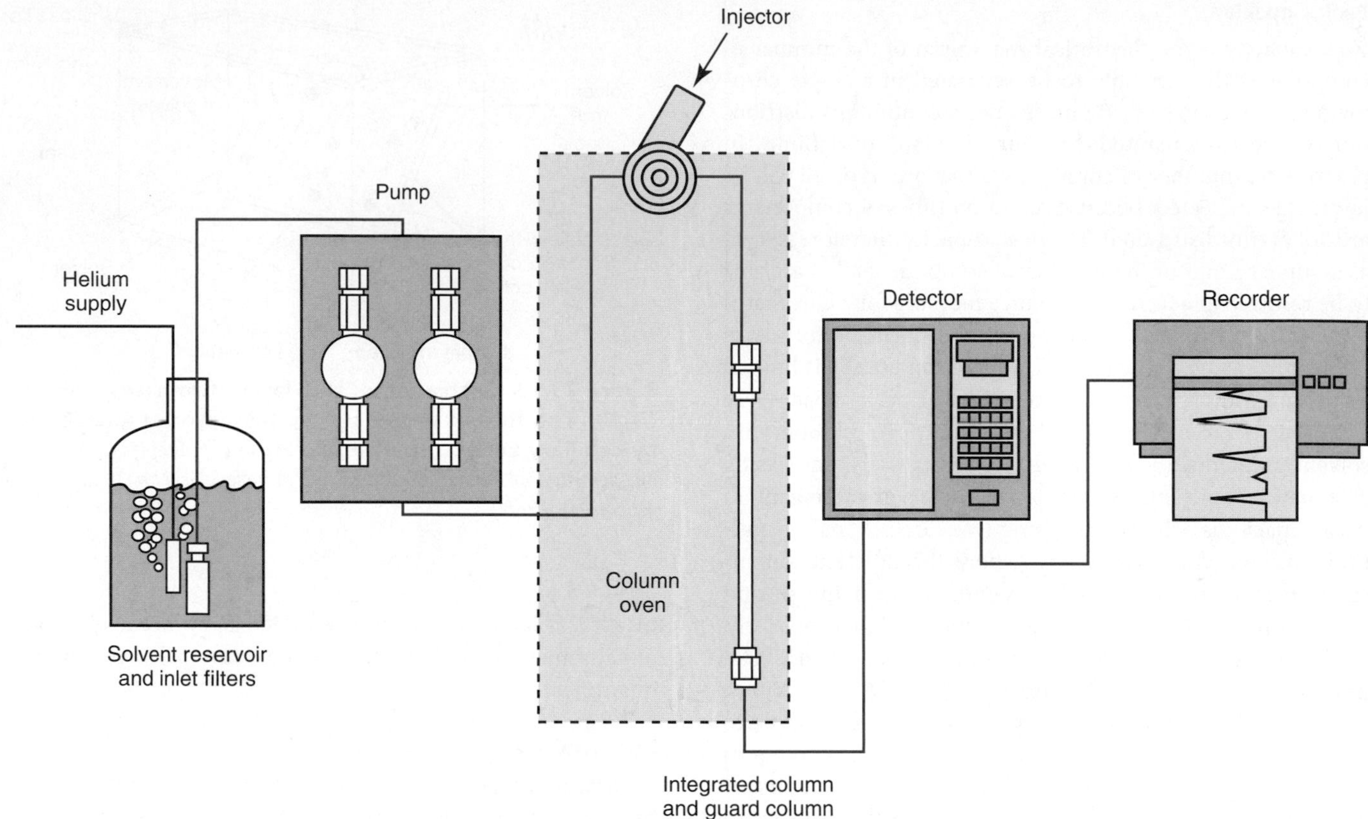

Figure 13-11 Diagram of a liquid chromatograph. HPLC components and types of columns. *(Courtesy Restek Corporation, Bellefonte, Pa.)*

(5) pumps to provide controlled flow and delivery of the correct solvent mixture. Several types of pumps have been used in liquid chromatography. For example, peristaltic and diaphragm-type pumps have been used, but they are suitable only for low-pressure chromatography. Piston-type or syringe-type pumps are used to achieve higher pressures. Reciprocating piston pumps are commonly used for HPLC, and the reciprocating action of the pump generates pulsation that is minimized by electronic pump control and pulse dampers in the flow path. Pulsation in flow is undesirable because of increases in baseline noise of many detectors.

Until recently, the upper pressure limit of most HPLC applications was about 400 bar (6000 psi), but some newer systems are designed for operation up to as high as 1000 bar (15,000 psi).[15,21,32A,67A,73] Such systems are termed UHPLC (for ultra-high performance or ultra-high pressure liquid chromatography). Operation at higher pressure limits not only requires appropriately designed pumps but also places some constraints on tubing, connections, and columns.

Systems for HPLC have pressure sensors to detect any obstruction to flow and usually shut down the system above defined pressure limits to prevent damage to components. At very high pressures, some solvents become slightly compressible and some compensation for solvent compression needs to be made to achieve constant flow rates.[21] Another extreme of operation is seen at very low flow rates for very small-bore microfluidic and capillary columns. Adaptation to low flow rates ($<\cong$10 μL/min) may require specially designed pumping systems or flow splitting of the output from a standard pumping system. Use of flow rates in the nL/min range has been referred to as nanoflow chromatography and has been coupled to mass spectrometry by nanospray interfaces, which offer very high ionization efficiency.

A variety of techniques have been used to vary solvent composition, including the use of switching valves that change to different solvents at prescribed times, or the mixing of two or more solvents to form a solvent gradient. Gradients may be generated by a proportioning valve linked to two or more solvent reservoirs before the inlet to a single pump, or by two or more pumps linked to different solvents. The output of two pumps passes into a mixing chamber to thoroughly mix the solvents, and the composition is adjusted by varying the flow rates of the two pumps. Static mixers rely on flow-generated turbulence, whereas dynamic mixers use magnetic stirrers. Solvent miscibility and viscosity affect mixing characteristics; inadequate mixing may result in poorer chromatographic performance.

Sample Injector

The first step of an LC separation is the introduction of an aliquot of sample into the column via an injector. The most widely used type of injector is the fixed-loop injector that is switched into or out of the flow path by manual or automated injection. In the inject mode, the loop is switched into the flow path, and the sample is carried downstream and into the column. The loop continues as part of the flow path until it is switched back to the fill position. Important characteristics of injection systems are their (1) reproducibility, (2) amount of carryover, and (3) range of injected volumes. Some automated injectors have the capability of injecting multiple aliquots or of mixing a sample and a reagent for derivatization reactions prior to injection. Refrigeration of specimens may be an important characteristic needed for analysis of specimens with limited stability, particularly when large batches of specimens will be analyzed.

Column Heaters/Chillers

Control of column temperature is a factor in the reproducibility and efficiency of LC separations. However, unlike GC separations, where temperature gradients are employed, in LC separations, a constant column temperature is maintained. It is achieved using a variety of techniques such as (1) column chambers, (2) water jackets, (3) temperature-controlled blankets, or (4) heating/cooling blocks. In addition, operation at high flow rates might require a heater/exchanger, usually a coil of tubing with good heat exchange properties, placed before the column inlet.

In operation, a stable column temperature is required to generate reproducible retention times. In addition, an increased column temperature (1) lowers solvent viscosity, (2) increases the rate of mass transfer between mobile and stationary phases, and (3) allows the use of higher flow rates and hence shortened analysis time. The thermal stability of the sample, however, imposes an upper limit on temperature. Also, in some instances, sample stability may require separations to be performed at reduced temperatures. Preparative work for proteins sometimes is performed in cold rooms or refrigerated cabinets to decrease the rates of denaturation and proteolytic degradation. Some systems for temperature control have the ability to operate at temperatures below room temperature through the action of Peltier coolers or other refrigeration systems. Important characteristics of column heater/chillers include temperature range, constancy of temperature, and number and length of columns that they accommodate.

Columns

The wide selection of columns available for liquid chromatography is based on combinations of packing materials and tubing of different diameters and lengths. Columns often include an inlet filter to remove particulate matter; a short guard column with the same packing material may be used to protect the more expensive separation column. The relatively inexpensive guard columns are replaced periodically and extend the usable life of the column.

The size of the column used depends on its application. The size of open or low-pressure columns, used for applications such as desalting or for affinity or ion-exchange purification, usually is related to the capacity needed for the separation. Gel-filtration columns, such as small centrifuge columns used for desalting, can accommodate specimens up to about 10% of column volume. The size of affinity columns depends on the amount of compound that needs to be separated and the capacity of the packing material.

TABLE 13-1 Size of Columns Commonly Used in Analytical HPLC

Column Terminology	Column ID, mm	Optimum Flow Rate
Standard	4.6	1.25 mL/min
	4.0	1.0 mL/min
Narrow bore	3.0	0.6 mL/min
	2.0	200 μL/min
Microbore/capillary	1.0	50 μL/min
	0.5	12 μL/min
	0.3	4 μL/min

HPLC, High-performance liquid chromatography; *ID,* internal diameter.

Column Dimensions. Modern column technology has produced columns in different dimensions with the tendency toward smaller internal volumes prevailing for analytical, especially hyphenated, techniques (see Chapter 14). For use in the clinical laboratory, most analytical HPLC columns are fabricated from tubes made of 316 stainless steel that have internal diameters (IDs) ranging from 0.3 mm to 5 mm and lengths from 50 mm to 250 mm (Table 13-1). Column end fittings, which have zero dead volume and frits to retain the support particles, are used to connect the column to the injector on the inlet end and the detector on the outlet end. Generally, lower detection limits are achieved with columns having smaller IDs. These smaller ID columns are manufactured from narrow-bore (approximately 2.1 mm ID) and microbore (approximately 1.0 mm ID) tubes.[2,34] In addition to providing improved efficiency, columns with smaller IDs use decreased volumes of mobile phase. For example, a 2-mm-ID column requires much less solvent than a 4.6-mm-ID column (see Table 13-1).

Capillary columns used in LC are constructed by coating the inner wall of a fused silica tube with a thin film of liquid phase. These columns vary from 0.1 to 0.5 mm in ID and from 10 to 50 cm in length.

Column Stationary Phase. The type of stationary phase in the column is the major determinant of selectivity and resolution of separations. The typical physical form of the stationary phase usually is a packed bed of small particles or a monolithic porous rod.[6,33,67,68]

Particulate Column Packings. Great variety is seen in the particles used to form packed beds, with particle diameters varying from 1.8 to 10 μm. As mentioned previously, the backpressure generated by packed beds varies approximately inversely with the square of the particle diameter. Thus, a twofold reduction in particle size results in about a fourfold increase in backpressure. Low-pressure separations, with packing materials such as cross-linked dextrans and agarose, commonly use particles of 50 to 200 μm in diameter.

Historically, separations by HPLC in clinical laboratories commonly used particles of about 5 μm in diameter, but there is a trend toward the use of progressively smaller particles extending to diameters <2 μm.[73] Smaller particles offer higher separation efficiency with the tradeoff of higher resistance to solvent flow and the need to operate at higher pressures. The use of columns with small-diameter particles has led to a new generation of HPLC systems with pressure limits of up to about 1000 bar (15,000 psi), which is about twofold to threefold higher than most previous HPLC systems.[73] High pressures may introduce some other changes related to compressibility of solvent, compression heating, and altered retention times.[15,21]

Types of particulate packings include (1) bonded, (2) polymeric, (3) chiral, and (4) restricted access materials.[5,6,16,39,67,68]

Bonded Phase Packings. In this type of packing, the stationary phase is bonded chemically to the surface of silica particles through a silica ester or silicone polymeric linkage. Bonded phase packings (1) are mechanically and chemically stable, (2) have long lifetimes, and (3) provide excellent chromatographic performance. They are available for ion-exchange and both normal-phase and reversed-phase chromatography. In normal-phase HPLC, the functional groups of the stationary phase are polar relative to those of the mobile phase, which usually consists of nonpolar solvents, such as hexane. Examples of polar functional groups for normal-phase HPLC packings are silanol, amino, and nitrile groups. Reversed-phase HPLC requires a nonpolar stationary phase. The most popular reversed-phase packing is the C18 type, in which octadecylsilane molecules are bonded to silica particles. A column with octadecyl packing is often called an *ODS column* [octadecyl silica (ODS)]. Reversed-phase column retention and selectivity characteristics are altered via attachment of other groups, such as octyl, phenyl, or cyanopropyl, to the silica.

Polymeric Packings. Graphitized carbon or mixed copolymers are used as polymeric packing (e.g., polystyrene-divinylbenzene) or are further derivatized with ion-exchange or C4, C8, or C18 functional groups. The performance of columns filled with these packings is comparable with that of silica-based columns and is stable from pH 2 to 13.

Chiral Packings. Chiral packings are used to separate enantiomers, which are mirror-image forms of the same compound. In the clinical laboratory, this type of packing is used to separate and quantify drug enantiomers.

Restricted Access Packings. With this type of packing, the outer surfaces of the support particles are protected by a hydrophilic network. Smaller solutes, such as drugs, pass through the network into the pores, which are coated with hydrophobic stationary phase. Large protein molecules are denied access to the inner core and pass through the column. Columns filled with restricted access packing allow the direct injection of biological samples with high protein concentrations; this bypasses sample preparation and improves analytical accuracy.

Monolithic Columns. As opposed to columns packed with discrete particles, monolithic columns are cylinders of silica- or polymer-based monolithic rods. Such columns have bimodal pore structures with large pores (approximately 2-μm diameter) that create high pore density, and smaller ones (approximately 13-nm diameter) that create a large internal surface area. They have been found to be capable of efficient fast separations, as they allow higher flow rates than particulate columns at reasonable backpressures. In addition, they are capable of fast mass transfer and have high binding capacity. The lower back pressure provides highly reproducible column characteristics because many of the factors that degrade particulate columns are eliminated (e.g., packing down and channeling). The monolithic rods are encased in inert polytetrafluoroethylene (PTFE) tubing and housed in stainless steel tubes. The inert tubing eliminates void volumes at the stainless steel tube/monolithic rod interface, thus improving resolution. Two additional advantages of these columns are that they can be used with mobile phase flow gradients (e.g., increasing flow rate at the end of a separation), and several columns can be coupled in a series to improve resolution with little increase in flow backpressure. Capillary monolithic columns also are available.

Of clinical interest, monolithic columns are being used to perform reversed-phase separations of peptides and proteins.[3,32,63,74]

Detectors

Many different types of detectors have been used as monitors in liquid chromatographs (Table 13-2). A key and integral component of such detectors is the flow cell through which the eluate from the chromatographic column passes. Dissolved analytes are detected and an electronic signal generated.

Operationally, detectors are used individually or are linked in series. In addition, postcolumn reactors have been interposed between the column and the detector to perform a chemical reaction such as the reaction of ninhydrin with amino acids to generate products with a stronger and more specific signal.

Photometers and Spectrophotometers. UV and visible photometers measure the radiant energy absorbed by compounds as they elute from the chromatographic column (see Chapter 10). These detectors operate in the radiant energy regions of 190 to 400 nm and 400 to 700 nm, respectively. The devices are versatile and detect many solutes because most aromatic compounds are detected in the ultraviolet region from 250 to 300 nm, and many other compounds are detectable in the ultraviolet region from 190 to 220 nm, where amide, carboxylic acids, and many other groups have substantial absorbance.

Photometers may operate as fixed-wavelength or variable-wavelength detectors. Most fixed-wavelength UV photometers use the intense 254-nm resonance line produced by a mercury arc lamp. This type of detector is extremely sensitive and is capable of operation at 0.005 absorbance unit full scale (AUFS). To provide fixed-wavelength detectors with greater flexibility, other less intense resonance lines of the mercury lamp are used. Alternatively, a phosphor is placed between

TABLE 13-2 Examples of Detectors Used in High-Performance Liquid Chromatography

Type of Detector	Principle of Operation	Range of Application	Detection Limit	Comments
Spectrophotometer	Measures absorbance of light at a single wavelength	Diverse	<1 ng	Analyte must absorb UV or visible light or must be derivatized
Spectrophotometer (diode array)	Measures absorbance of light at many wavelengths	Diverse	<1 ng	Detector provides complete spectra qualitative and quantitative information
Fluorometer	Measures fluorescence	Very selective	pg to ng	Analyte must fluoresce or be derivatized
Electrochemical	Electrochemically measures oxidized/reduced analyte	Selective	pg to ng	Detector is useful for catecholamines
Mass spectrometer	Detects ions after separation by mass-to-charge ratio	Diverse	fg to ng	Analytes must be converted to ionized form
Conductivity	Measures conductivity by ions	Selective	1 ng	Detection of ions used in ion chromatography
Refractometer	Measures change in refractive index	Universal	1 μg	Detection of most compounds but relatively low sensitivity
Evaporative light scattering	Light scattering by solutes after solvent evaporation	Nonvolatile compounds	1 ng	Detection of all nonvolatile compounds
Charged aerosol detector	Charged particle detection compounds	Nonvolatile	<1 ng	Detection of all nonvolatile compounds

the lamp and the flow cell, and the emitted fluorescence resulting from the 254-nm excitation is used as the light source. This latter approach is used in the dual-wavelength photometers that operate at two fixed wavelengths (e.g., 254 nm and 280 nm). The intense 214-nm or 229-nm resonance lines of a zinc or cadmium arc lamp, respectively, may be used for detection at lower wavelengths, where more compounds have strong absorbance.

The second type of photometer is the variable-wavelength detector. It operates at a wavelength selected from a given wavelength range. Thus the detector is "tuned" to operate at the absorbance maximum for a given analyte or set of analytes; this greatly enhances the applicability and selectivity of the detector. Another advantage of this detector is its ability to operate at lower wavelengths (e.g., 190 nm). Because more compounds (e.g., cholesterol) absorb at lower wavelengths, this capability enhances the versatility of the detector. At lower wavelengths, however, many solvents absorb UV light and cannot be used as mobile phases. Fortunately, acetonitrile and methanol, two widely used solvents in reversed-phase chromatography, have low UV absorptions at 200 nm.

Diode arrays also are used as HPLC detectors because they rapidly yield spectral data over the entire wavelength range of 190 to 600 nm in about 10 ms.[37] During operation, the diode array detector passes polychromatic light through the detector flow cell. The transmitted light is dispersed by a diffraction grating and then is directed to a photodiode array, where the intensity of light at multiple wavelengths in the spectrum is measured. Such detectors have been helpful in the identification of drugs in urine and serum.

In practice, it is necessary to use solvents, ion pairing agents, and buffers with low absorbance at wavelengths of interest to maintain a low background signal. Water, acetonitrile, methanol, isopropanol, and hexane are solvents that allow ultraviolet detection down to wavelengths of 200 nm, as are phosphate buffers. Many other solvents and buffers have substantial absorbance in the ultraviolet region that may limit ultraviolet detection. Also, flow cells of low volume are used in HPLC to avoid band broadening.

A problem with the operation of photometric detectors is the outgassing that occurs in the solvent as it exits from the high pressure of the column and into the low-pressure flow cell of the detector. Because these detectors are very sensitive, they detect these bubbles as noise that degrades the signal-to-noise ratio of the detector. Effective degassing of solvents and maintenance of some backpressure across the detector helps to minimize bubble formation.

Fluorometers. As discussed in Chapter 10, fluorescence occurs when a molecule absorbs light at one wavelength and reemits light at a longer wavelength. Online fluorometers are used in liquid chromatographs to detect fluorescing compounds as they elute from the column. Fluorescence detectors are generally more sensitive than photometric ones. In addition, precolumn or postcolumn reactors have been used to chemically tag a compound with a fluorescent label for subsequent detection. For example, amino acids and other primary amines often are labeled with a dansyl or fluorescamine tag, followed by HPLC separation and fluorometric detection. Most fluorometers used with liquid chromatographs are relatively simple in design and are extremely selective and sensitive for compounds fluorescing within the detector's operating wavelength range. Deuterium or xenon arc lamps or lasers have been used as light sources in such detectors.

Electrochemical Detectors. In amperometric electrochemical detectors (see Chapters 11 and 30), an electroactive analyte enters the flow cell, where it may be oxidized or reduced at an electrode surface under a constant potential.[70] Use of multiple electrodes and cyclic changes in voltage allow detection of multiple components at different potentials and cyclic cleaning of the electrode. Electroactive compounds of clinical interest conveniently analyzed by HPLC with electrochemical detection include the urinary catecholamines (see Chapter 30), thiol-containing compounds such as homocysteine, and ascorbic acid. In addition, electrochemically active tags (e.g., bromine) are added to compounds such as unsaturated fatty acids or prostaglandins.

Coulometric detectors are also used. When placed in a series, such detectors are used to detect and quantify coeluting compounds that differ in their half-wave potentials (the potential at half-signal maximum) by at least 60 mV. These detectors are extremely selective and sensitive, with reasonably wide linear response ranges. They are used in the clinical laboratory for analysis of metanephrines, vanillylmandelic acid, homovanillic acid, and 5-hydroxyindole acetic acid in human urine without extensive sample preparation.

Low-sensitivity conductivity detectors also have been used to monitor gradients of varying salt composition in ion-exchange chromatography. The other application of conductivity detectors is their use in ion chromatography.[24] Elution of ions separated by anion- or cation-exchange chromatography can be detected with high sensitivity. Conductivity from a specific ion is related to its concentration, charge, and mobility. This technique is best suited for analysis of small inorganic and organic ions that have high mobility. It has been applied to measure components such as sulfate in biological fluids, but primary applications of this technique have been nonclinical.

Refractive Index Detectors. These detectors sense a change in the refraction of light as solutes pass through its flow cell. They offer a means of detecting substances, such as alcohols, polyethylene glycol, salts, and sugars that have low absorbance at wavelengths commonly used for spectrophotometric detection.[35,60]

Mass Spectrometry. As mentioned earlier, when a gas or liquid chromatograph is connected to a mass spectrometer (see Chapter 14), the combined or "hyphenated" techniques are referred to as gas chromatography–mass spectrometry (GC-MS) and liquid chromatography–mass spectrometry (LC-MS).[23,59A,69,69A] These very sensitive and specific techniques have increasing application in clinical and research laboratories and in the emerging field of proteomics.[4,18,27,43-45] For many applications, the high specificity of tandem mass spectrometers allows very short HPLC runs to be used, because most compounds do not need to be completely separated.

A critical element in linking a GC or an HPLC to a mass spectrometer is the interface between them. For example, the interface between the liquid chromatograph and the mass spectrometer has the challenging task of removing solvent molecules and transferring components from a liquid solution into a charged form in vacuum for analysis by the mass spectrometer. Therefore, all buffers used for chromatography need to be volatile to avoid overloading and contaminating the interface. For the same reason, a switching valve often is used to divert salts and other unretained components eluting early in the HPLC separation to waste. The switching valve then directs later parts of the HPLC run to the mass spectrometer. Several different ionization techniques, including electrospray, chemical ionization, and photoionization, are discussed in greater detail in Chapter 14.

Other Detectors. A number of other types of detectors have been used with liquid chromatographs, but primarily for research applications. Dynamic light scattering detectors measure light scattering related to molecular size and have been found useful in characterizing the size of large molecules and complexes.[49] Nuclear magnetic resonance has been performed on specimens passing through flow cells and may be useful for applications such as lipoprotein analysis, metabolomics, and characterization of metabolites of drugs. There has been an interest in detectors that are more sensitive than refractive index detectors for compounds with low spectrophotometric absorbance.

New types of detectors also have been developed that provide nearly universal detection of compounds that are nonvolatile.[35,60] For example, with the evaporative light scattering detector, solvent is evaporated by nebulizing the chromatographic effluent with a stream of gas. Nonvolatile solutes remain as particles in the gas stream, and particles are detected by measuring light scattering at an angle from incident light. Light scattering is proportional to the mass of nonvolatile substances. Detection limits of about 1 ng for compounds such as glucose have been achieved. Potential applications include analysis of lipids, sugars, and other compounds difficult to detect photometrically. A second type of evaporative detector, the charged aerosol detector, ionizes solutes with a corona discharge and measures ion currents rather than light scattering. This approach is very sensitive for most compounds. A disadvantage of such evaporative detectors is that they destroy the specimen so that components cannot be collected for further analysis or coupled for subsequent analysis by another detector.

System Controller and Data System

By using the simplest form of instrumentation for a liquid chromatograph, it is possible to perform injections and pump adjustments manually and to record results on a strip chart recorder. This may be suitable for infrequent preparative separations, but for high-volume applications in the clinical laboratory, there usually is an interest in automating the injections and chromatographic runs with hardware and software for system control. The system controller manages (1) sample injections; (2) solvent delivery; (3) temperature control; (4) and detectors; and (5) it provides an auditable record of analyst, method, calibration, controls, and specimens. Data systems take the thousands of data points from an individual run and identify a set of peaks with parameters such as retention times, peak areas, peak heights, and peak widths. Comparison of these parameters with those generated from reference materials yields identification of peaks and quantitative values. Software for data analysis becomes more critical as data streams become larger, such as from diode array and mass spectrometric detection, and multiple components are analyzed in a single run; libraries of spectra or other databases are searched for identification of compounds, peptides, or nucleic acid sequences.

Safety

Normal laboratory precautions must be exercised during HPLC operation. Most organic solvents are flammable. The column effluent should be collected in a suitable container and stored appropriately before disposal. The explosive release of pressure in an HPLC system is not a major hazard; liquids compress only slightly and therefore accumulate little energy.

Supercritical Fluid Chromatography (SFC)

Under pressure, carbon dioxide occurs as a liquid that has some favorable properties as a solvent for chromatography.[1,40] It has low viscosity and high diffusion coefficients and dissolves many hydrophobic compounds. Consequently, SFC has performance characteristics somewhat intermediate between liquid and gas chromatography.[65] A variety of organic modifiers have been mixed with carbon dioxide to serve as the solvent. Columns are packed with a variety of stationary phases similar to those used for liquid chromatography. This technique has been used for analysis of lipids and other hydrophobic components that are soluble in liquid carbon dioxide. SFC has been applied to pharmaceutical research and analysis of natural products but, because of the need for specialized equipment, it has found limited use in clinical laboratories.

Gas Chromatography

GC was first developed by James and Martin in 1952 to separate fatty acids.[30] With this technique, a gaseous mobile phase is used to pass a mixture of volatile solutes through a column containing the stationary phase.[47] The mobile phase is typically an inert gas, such as nitrogen, helium, hydrogen, or argon, referred to as the *carrier gas*. Solute separation is based on relative differences in the solutes' vapor pressures and interaction with the stationary phase. Thus a more volatile solute elutes from the column before a less volatile one. In addition, a solute that selectively interacts with the stationary phase elutes from the column after one with a lesser degree of interaction. The column effluent carries the separated solutes to the detector in the order of their elution. Solutes are identified qualitatively by their similar retention times.[14] Furthermore, peak size (area or height) is proportional to the amount of solute detected and is used to quantify it.

Gas-solid chromatography (GSC) and gas-liquid partition chromatography (GLC) are variations of GC. In GSC, separations occur primarily through differences in absorption at the solid phase surface. In GLC, a nonvolatile liquid is coated or chemically bonded onto particles of column packing or directly onto the wall of a capillary column. Separation occurs primarily through differences in solute partitioning between the gaseous mobile phase and the liquid stationary phase.

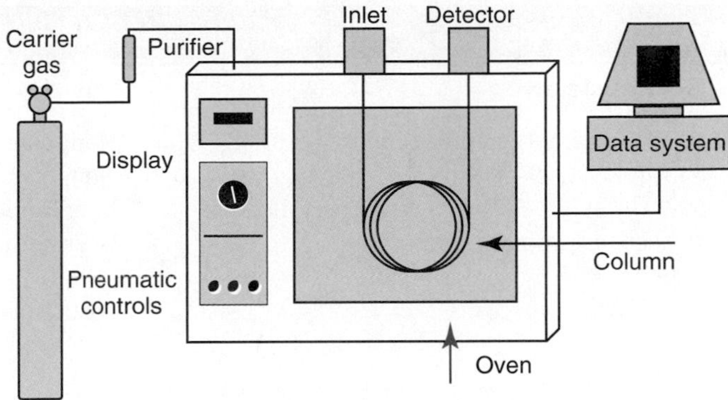

Figure 13-12 Diagram of a gas chromatograph. *(Courtesy Restek Corporation, Bellefonte, Pa.)*

Instrumentation

The components of a gas chromatograph are illustrated in Figure 13-12.

Columns

Both packed and capillary columns are used in gas chromatographs. Packed columns are filled with support particles that are used uncoated (GSC) or have been coated or chemically bonded with the stationary phase (GLC). Such columns vary from 1 to 4 mm in ID and from 1 m or more in length, and are fabricated from tubes of glass or stainless steel. Although narrow columns are more efficient, wider columns have increased sample capacities. For example, fast GC is a type of GC in which high-speed separations are achieved with short lengths of narrow-bore capillary columns in conjunction with rapid oven temperature ramp rates and increased linear velocity of the carrier gas.

Types of capillary columns include (1) porous layer open tubular (PCOT), (2) support coated open tubular (SCOT), and (3) wall-coated open tubular (WCOT) columns. In PCOT columns there is a porous layer on the inner wall. Porosity is achieved by either chemical means (e.g., etching) or by the deposition of porous particles on the wall from a suspension. The porous layer serves as a support for a liquid stationary phase or as the stationary phase itself (http://goldbook.iupac.org/P04763.html/accessed April 6, 2011). PLOT columns primarily are utilized for gas analysis and the separation of low molecular weight hydrocarbons.

The SCOT columns have their inner wall lined with a thin layer of support material onto which the stationary phase is adsorbed. Wall-coated open tubular columns consist of a capillary tube whose inner wall is coated with a liquid stationary phase. They are the most popular of the three types of capillary columns and are fabricated by coating the inner wall of a fused silica tube whose ID and length varies from 0.1 to

TABLE 13-3 Stationary Phases Commonly Used in Gas Chromatography for Clinical Separations

Composition	Polarity	Similar Phases	Applications
100% dimethyl-polysiloxane	Nonpolar	OV-1, SE-30	Drugs, amino acid derivatives
5% diphenyl–95% dimethyl-polysiloxane	Nonpolar	OV-101, SP-2100	Drugs
50% diphenyl–50% dimethyl-polysiloxane	Intermediate	OV-17	Drugs, steroids, glycols
50% cyanopropylmethyl–50% phenylmethyl-polysiloxane	Intermediate	OV-225	Fatty acid methyl esters, carbohydrate derivatives
Polyethylene glycol	Polar	Carbowax 20M	Acids, alcohols, glycols, ketones

0.5 mm and from 10 to 150 m, respectively. The ultrapure fused silica capillary tubing used in their manufacture is very fragile and to physically strengthen the tubing, a thin outside coating of polyimide or aluminum is added, which improves column durability. These modified capillary columns have the structural strength and flexibility necessary to withstand coiling and placement in ovens.

In addition to the packed and capillary columns, progress has been made in the development of micro GC columns on silicon chips.[1A] These microdevices have great potential for high-speed GC, a miniature GC, and eventually even a pocket GC.[10]

A variety of compounds have been used as the stationary phase in GLC. These include (1) methyl silicone polymers, (2) substituted silicone polymers, and (3) silicone polyesters (Table 13-3). These materials are coated or are chemically bonded onto the surface of the support particles or onto the walls of the column. Although they are more expensive, bonded materials are preferred because of their stability.

Carrier Gas Supply and Flow Control

The function of the carrier gas supply and flow control is to provide carrier gas to the chromatographic column and to regulate its flow through the system. Operationally, a constant flow of carrier gas is required for column efficiency and reproducible elution times. Systems that provide constant flow rates vary from simple mechanical devices to sophisticated electronic ones. More demanding temperature-programmed operation (discussed later) requires a more sophisticated differential flow controller, such as an electronic pressure control system programmed to regulate the carrier gas flow rate and pressure during a chromatographic run. Such a controller may be operated in a constant-flow or a constant-pressure mode. In the constant-flow mode, the pressure required to maintain a constant flow independent of carrier gas viscosity is calculated. A pressure transducer then measures and maintains the inlet pressure required for the constant flow.

The magnitude of the carrier gas flow rate depends on the type of column. For example, packed columns require a flow rate from 10 to 60 mL/min. Flow rates for capillary columns are much lower (1 to 2 mL/min), and maintenance of a constant flow rate is even more critical for the efficient operation of these columns. Microprocessor controls with specialized valves are currently used to control flow rates.

A number of gases are used as carrier gases, depending on the column and the detector. Hydrogen and helium are the carrier gases of choice with capillary columns. Only high-purity hydrogen and helium should be used because carrier gas impurities (1) harm the column, (2) negatively influence the performance of some detectors, and (3) adversely affect quantification in trace analysis. For packed columns, the most frequently used carrier gas is nitrogen, which is used with flame ionization (FID), electron capture (ECD), or thermal conductivity (TCD) detectors. Helium is used with FIDs and TCDs, and nitrogen-argon-methane gas mixtures are used with the ECD. Carrier gases must be dry, and the tubing used to connect the gas source to the GC must be uncontaminated. Molecular sieve beds and specialized inline traps are commonly used to remove the moisture, hydrocarbon, and/or oxygen content of the carrier gas.[11]

Injector

The injection of an aliquot of the sample to be analyzed into the column begins the chromatographic process and has to be done with minimal disruption of the gas flow into the column. In most clinical GC methods, samples are dissolved in nonaqueous liquids introduced into the column via an automated, highly precise, and rapid inline injector. With packed columns, a glass microsyringe is used to inject a 1- to 10-μL aliquot of the dissolved sample through a septum, which serves as the interface between the injector and the chromatographic system. In practice, the syringe needle is inserted through the injector septum and into a heating region. The volatile analytes and the solvent are then "flash-vaporized" and swept into the column by the carrier gas. To ensure rapid and complete solute volatilization, the temperature of the injector is typically maintained at least 30 to 50 °C higher than the column temperature.

Common problems with GC analysis include septum leaks and adsorption of components from the sample onto the septum during injection. In addition, because the septum is heated, decomposition products often form and "bleed" into the column. This results in spurious peaks, termed *ghost* peaks, which appear in the chromatogram. Septum bleed is greater at higher injection port temperatures. To minimize this problem, a Teflon-coated, low-bleed septum is used. The inner surface of the septum is purged continuously with the carrier gas that is vented before it passes into the column. This approach is especially effective, and most commercial injectors are equipped with continuous-purge capabilities. The septum is a consumable component of the gas chromatograph and should be replaced at least once every 100 injections.

Because of the low sample capacities and carrier gas flow rates used with capillary columns, split and splitless injection techniques are used to introduce samples into the columns. In the split mode, only a small portion of the vaporized sample enters the column, whereas in the splitless mode, most of the sample enters the column.[66] Operationally, the split flow mode is used for samples that contain relatively high concentrations of the target analyte(s); the splitless mode is used for samples that contain relatively low concentrations of the target analyte(s).

Temperature-programmable injection ports are available and may be used in the split or splitless mode. The sample is injected at a temperature slightly higher than the boiling point of the solvent. Most of the sample components condense on glass or fused silica wool in the injector insert, while the solvent is removed. The injector is then rapidly heated at rates of up to 100 °C/min. The rapid heating vaporizes the analytes, which then move into the column. Very rapid heating is advantageous in that thermally labile compounds are exposed to high temperatures for only a short time. Separation of solvent removal and analyte vaporization allows injection of sample volumes up to hundreds of microliters. This obviously improves analyte detection when the sample matrix is not the limiting factor.

Temperature Control

Operationally, both packed and capillary GC columns require careful control of the column, injector, and detector temperatures. Control of the column temperature is achieved when the column is placed in an oven, or when the column is heated directly by resistive heating.[31] Injector and detector temperatures usually are controlled by electrical resistance heating. Depending on the application, the column temperature is maintained at a constant preset value (isothermal operation) during the chromatographic run or is varied as a function of time (temperature-programmed or temperature-gradient operation).

In practice, temperature-programmed column heating is used for most clinical applications. With temperature programming, the solutes having the lower boiling points elute first, followed by those having higher boiling points. Consequently, a complex mixture of solutes with a wide range of boiling points is separated into sharp, distinct chromatographic peaks in less time than with isothermal operation. The temperature is programmed and controlled by a computer and its resident software.

In capillary gas chromatographs, accurate and precise control of column and injector temperatures is required to obtain optimal performance and reliable results. Temperature control of the column is especially important, particularly in qualitative applications in which the retention times or volumes of eluting peaks are compared with those of authentic standards for compound identification. A change of only 1 °C causes a 5% change in retention time. In addition, instability of the column temperature adversely affects retention time or volume comparability among instruments or among values in the literature. Temperature gradients in the oven and rapid temperature programming rates also causes variable analyte retention.

The thermal stability of the stationary phase is also important. Because each stationary phase has a range of thermal stability, it is important to control column temperature within the specified operating range. For the nonpolar phases, the temperature limit is determined by the stability of the polyimide coating. The introduction of aluminum clad columns notably broadens the usable temperature range. Oxidation at higher temperatures limits the operating temperature of intermediate to polar phases.

Before any column is used, it must be "thermally conditioned" by heating the column at various temperatures for different lengths of time. This removes volatile contaminants, including residual monomers, in the polymeric stationary phase. In addition, thermal conditioning of used columns removes accumulated nonvolatile contaminants that cause unstable baselines. To condition a column thermally, it is disconnected from the detector and purged for at least 5 minutes with pure carrier gas. It is then heated to above 50 °C. The column temperature is cycled through a normal temperature program three or four times. Alternatively, the column can be maintained at the maximum operating temperature for 12 to 24 hours. Thermal conditioning of columns at lower temperatures prolongs the life of the column, but longer conditioning times are required to achieve baseline stability. Preconditioned capillary columns are also available.

Detectors

A variety of sensitive detectors are used with gas chromatographs (Table 13-4). These include universal units that detect most analytes and extremely selective devices that detect only specific ones. Examples include (1) FID, (2) thermionic selective (TSD), (3) ECD, (4) photoionization (PID), (5) TCD, and (6) mass spetrometers. Many other devices have been used as GC detectors, and it has become common practice to place two or more detectors in a series to enhance analytical specificity and sensitivity. Different types of mass spectrometers are also used as detectors for gas chromatographs (see Chapter 14).

Flame Ionization Detector. The FID is a commonly used detector in clinical laboratories. A common application is the analysis of ethanol and other volatiles in blood and other aqueous specimens. Chromatograms of volatiles analyzed by headspace gas chromatography with FID detection is shown in Figure 13-13. Its advantages include simplicity, reliability, versatility, and ease of operation. During operation, the column effluent is mixed with hydrogen and air, and the eluting compounds are burned by a flame. About one molecule in 10,000 produces an organic cation and releases an electron, which is detected by a collector electrode positioned above the flame. The magnitude of the generated current is related to the mass of carbon material delivered to the

TABLE 13-4 Examples of Detectors Used in Gas Chromatographs

Type of Detector	Principle of Operation	Selectivity	Limit of Detection	Comments
Thermal conductance (TCD)	Measures thermal conductivity change in carrier gas on elution of compounds	Universal	<400 pg propane/mL He	
Flame ionization (FID)	CHNO + heat → $CHNO^+$ + e^-; electrons collected for detection	Hydrocarbon	10-100 pg CHO	
Thermionic selective (TSD; NPD)	Alkali bead selectively ionizes N- or P-containing compounds	N, P	0.4-10 pg N 0.1-1.0 pg P	
Electron capture (ECD)	$e^- + R + N_2 \rightarrow Re^- + N_2 + e^-$; excess electrons collected; concentration inversely related	Electronegative groups	0.05-1.0 pg Cl^--containing compounds	
Mass spectrometer (MS)	$e^- + ABC \rightarrow A^+ BC$; monitor mass-to-charge ratio by scanning or single-ion monitoring (SIM)	Universal (tunable)	1 ng scan 10 pg SIM	Provides structural confirmation; ion ratios constant in SIM
Photoionization (PID)	CHNO + photon → $CHNO^+$ + e^-; detect electron	Hydrocarbon	1-10 pg CHO	May be improvement on FID
Electrolytic conductivity (Hall)	Postcolumn reaction detector for selective detection of halogen-, S-, or N-containing compounds	Halogen-, S-, and N-containing compounds	0.1-1.0 pg Cl 2.0 pg S 4.0 pg N	
Flame photometric (FPD)	P- and S-containing hydrocarbons emit light when burned in FID-type flame; emitted light detected	P- and S-containing compounds	0.9 pg CHP 20 pg CHS	
Fourier transform infrared (FTIR)	Infrared wavelength light absorbed by the compound of interest	Universal (tunable)	1 ng strong infrared absorber	Scanned for structural information or absorbance—measured for quantitation

CHNO, Carbon, hydrogen, nitrogen, oxygen containing compound; *CHO,* carbon, hydrogen, oxygen containing compound; *CHP* carbon, hydrogen, phosphorous containing compound; *CHS,* carbon, hydrogen, sulfur containing compound.

detector; after measurement, it is used for detection and quantification of the eluting solutes.

Thermionic Selective Detector. The TSD, also known as the *nitrogen-phosphorus detector (NPD),* is a modification of the FID in which an alkali bead is heated electrically in the area directly above the jet. In the presence of alkali atoms in the flame, nitrogen-containing compounds produce a 15 times greater, and phosphorus-containing compounds a 300 times greater, response. The TSD is frequently used in analytical laboratories for the detection of organic bases and acids.

Electron Capture Detector. The operating principle of the ECD is based on the reaction between electronegative compounds and thermal electrons. Electrons are normally provided from a radioactive source, such as ^{63}Ni or ^{3}H housed in the detector. A collector electrode is pulsed to collect "excess" electrons. This is called the *standing current.* If electronegative species are not present in the detector cell, the nitrogen or argon/methane (95/5) sweep gas removes most of the electrons from the cell. When a compound capable of capturing an electron passes through the cell, some electrons are removed and a decrease in the standing current is observed. The use of nitrogen or argon/methane is important, because these gases reduce the energy of the electrons via collisions and thus improve the ability of the compounds to "capture" them. It is also important that the gases are very pure and dry, because oxygen and water can foul the detector. In some detector designs, the collection pulse rate is varied to maintain a constant amount of current. Then the pulses are counted, and this number is used to determine the concentration of electronegative species passing through the cell. The

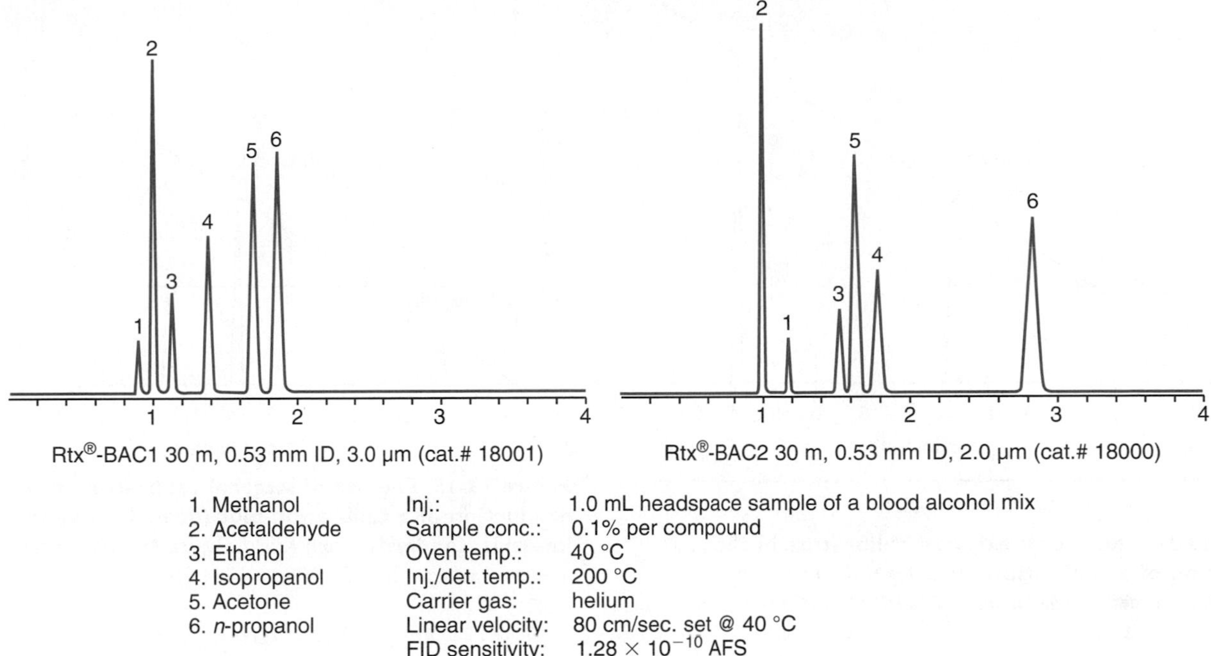

Figure 13-13 Chromatograms of volatiles analyzed by headspace gas chromatography. *(Courtesy Restek Corporation, Bellefonte, Pa.)*

ECD is a concentration-dependent detector. The presence of electronegative constituents, such as fluorine, chlorine, bromine, and iodine, enhances the response of the ECD. Because not all compounds contain these functional groups, derivatization with reagents containing polychlorinated or polyfluorinated groups to increase detector response is a common practice.

Photoionization Detector. The PID is a variant of the FID. With the PID, however, energy for ionization is provided by an intense UV lamp rather than by a flame.

Thermal Conductivity Detector. The TCD is based on the principle that addition of a compound to a gas alters the thermal conductance of the gas.

Mass Spectrometry. Mass spectrometers are also used as detectors for gas chromatographs (see HPLC section earlier or Chapter 14).

Computer/Controller

As with most modern analytical instruments, an automated GC is computer controlled with the computer functioning as both a process controller and a data processor. For example, as a process controller, the computer regulates various para meters, such as (1) carrier gas composition and flow rate; (2) column backpressure; (3) column and detector temperatures; (4) sample injection, detector selection and operation; and (5) the various timing steps that command the operation of the system. For data processing, the computer monitors signals generated by the system's detectors and commands the acquisition and storage of data at specified time intervals. The area, or height, of each chromatographic peak is determined from the stored data, and this information is used to compute the analyte concentration represented by each peak. Available algorithms for this computation include those based on calibration curves or conversion factors from internal or external calibration. If desired, a complete report can be prepared and printed for each chromatographic run. Alternatively, data are stored to be recalled and reprocessed, with different integration parameters.

Qualitative and Quantitative Analyses

Chromatography is used to qualitatively identify and quantify the analyte(s) of interest.

Analyte Identification

The retention time or volume at which an unknown solute elutes from a column, or the distance traveled on a plate, is often compared and matched with that of a reference compound. The appearance of a solute peak, band, or spot at the same time, volume, or distance as that of a reference compound is consistent with the two compounds being the same. This simultaneous appearance does not prove identity, however, because other compounds can have the same retention time or volume or can travel the same distance as the reference compound.

In planar chromatography, reference compounds are chromatographed with the unknown sample. Tentative identification is made by comparison of migration distances and detection characteristics of the reference compounds with those of the unknown analytes. If the R_f of the unknown analyte and the R_f of the reference compound do not match, the compounds are judged to be different. If they match, the compounds are presumed to be identical. However, because

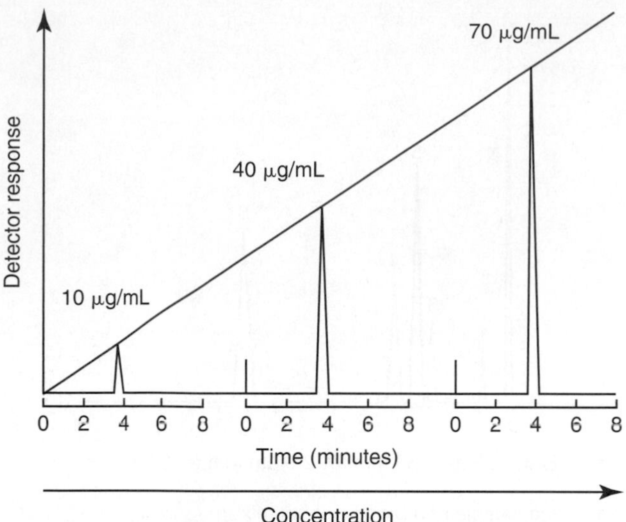

Figure 13-14 The use of external calibrators in the production of a calibration plot. *(From Krull I, Swartz M. Quantitation in method validation. LC-GC 1998;16:1084-90.)*

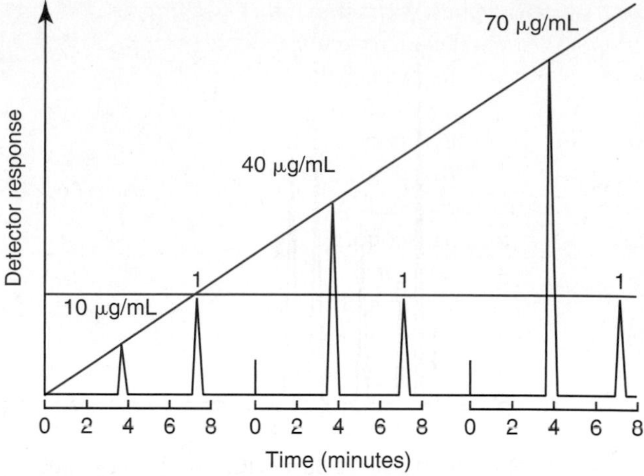

Figure 13-15 The use of internal calibrators in the production of a calibration plot (peak 1 being the internal standard). *(From Krull I, Swartz M. Quantitation in method validation. LC-GC 1998;16:1084-90.)*

more than one compound can have the same R_f in a particular chromatographic system, the presumptive identification should be confirmed by the use of specific spray reagents, antibody complexation, or isolation of the compound followed by chemical and/or instrumental analysis. Software is now available for compound identification by library searching of UV spectra based on corrected R_f values.

With capillary GC and LC columns, it is possible to simultaneously introduce the components of a single injection into two columns made of dissimilar stationary phases. These columns are connected to separate detectors of the same or a different type. Matching the retention properties of a single analyte with a reference compound on two columns of dissimilar phases enhances the chance for correct identification of the analyte. The most reliable analyte identification, however, is provided by a detector that features structural information, such as a mass spectrometer (see Chapter 14).

Analyte Quantification

Electronic signals from the detector(s) are also used to produce quantitative information. Both external and internal calibrating techniques have been used. With external calibration, reference solutions containing known quantities of analytes are processed in a manner identical to samples containing the analyte (Figure 13-14). A calibration curve of (1) peak height, (2) peak area, or (3) spot density versus calibrator concentration is constructed and used to calculate the concentration of the analyte in the samples. With internal calibration, also called *internal standardization,* reference solutions of known analyte concentrations are prepared, and a constant amount of a different compound, the internal standard, is added to each reference solution and each sample (Figure 13-15). By plotting the ratio of the peak height (or area) or spot density of the analyte to the peak height (or area) or spot density of the internal standard versus the concentration of the analyte, a calibration curve that corrects for systematic losses is constructed. This curve is then used to compute the analyte concentration in the samples by interpolation.

EXTRACTION AND DIFFERENTIAL PRECIPITATION

Extraction and differential precipitation refer to the separation of components into discrete fractions, often two separate liquid fractions or a liquid and a solid fraction that may be separated by centrifugation or filtration. A simple example of extraction is the separation of components into two immiscible solvents in a separatory funnel. Different components are partitioned differentially into two phases, which then are physically separated. Extraction or differential precipitation is often used to simplify specimens and to remove components such as proteins that may interfere with subsequent chromatographic or analytical methods. Extraction may also be used as a method to concentrate specimens; extraction by volatile organic solvents is often followed by evaporation, yielding an extract with a higher concentration than the original specimen. Differential precipitation uses conditions whereby some components are soluble, while others are precipitated. Precipitation of proteins in biological fluids with acid or organic solvent is often used to separate them differentially from drugs or other small molecules that remain in solution. Other examples include differential precipitation of albumin and globulins with salt solutions and lipoprotein fractions by selective precipitating agents.

Use of solid-phase extraction has been increasing for many applications,[61] and solid phases are packed in a variety of formats, including small open columns, cartridges, 96-well plates, and pipet tips.[19,55] The use of particles with pore sizes smaller than 10 nm (100 Å) results in exclusion of most proteins from pores, leading to removal of proteins from the retentate. Solid-phase extraction can be performed on many specimens in parallel on a vacuum manifold or on extraction plates in 96-well formats. Solid-phase extraction generally yields more selective extraction than does liquid-liquid extraction, because it is possible to perform washing steps before elution of the desired components with solvents of defined composition. Solid-phase extraction may be amenable to automation with robots in a separate process from later chromatography steps, or the use of online extraction as an initial separation step in a chromatographic process.[50,71] Use of online extraction linked to liquid chromatographic separations improves the automation and reproducibility of sample handling, [29]

REFERENCES

1. Bamba T. Application of supercritical fluid chromatography to the analysis of hydrophobic metabolites. J Sep Science 2008;31:1274-8.

1A. Breadmore MC, Dawod M, Quirino JP. Recent advances in enhancing the sensitivity of electrophoresis and electrochromatography in capillaries and microchips (2008-2010). Electrophoresis. 2011 Jan;32(1):127-48

2. Brennan RA, Yin H, Killeen KP. Microfluidic gradient formation for nanoflow chip LC. Anal Chem 2007;79:9302-9.
3. Causon TJ, Nordborg A, Shellie RA, Hilder EF. High temperature liquid chromatography of intact proteins using organic polymer monoliths and alternative solvent systems. J Chromatogr A 2010;1217:3519-24.
4. Chen G, Pramanik BN. Application of LC/MS to proteomics studies: current status and future prospects. Drug Discov Today 2009;14:465-71.
5. Claessens HA, van Straten MA. Review on the chemical and thermal stability of stationary phases for reversed-phase liquid chromatography. J Chromatogr A 2004;1060:23-41.
6. Cserháti T. Carbon-based sorbents in chromatography: new achievements. Biomed Chromatogr 2009;23:111-8.
7. Cooper WT. Normal-phase liquid chromatography. In: Myers RA, ed. Encyclopedia of analytical chemistry. New York: John Wiley & Sons, 2000:11428-42.
8. Dejaegher B, Mangelings D, Vander Heyden Y. Method development for HILIC assays. J Sep Sci 2008;31:1438-48.
9. Dolan JW, Snyder LR. Gradient elution chromatography. In: Meyers RA, ed. Encyclopedia of analytical chemistry. Chichester: John Wiley & Sons, 2000:11342-60.
10. Eiceman GA. Instrumentation of gas chromatography in clinical chemistry. In: Meyers RA, ed. Encyclopedia of analytical chemistry. Chichester: John Wiley & Sons, 2000:10671-9.
11. Eiceman GA, Gardea-Torresdey J, Overton E, Carney K, Dorman F. Gas chromatography. Anal Chem 2002;74:22771-80.
12. Ettre LS: Nomenclature for chromatography: IUPAC recommendations 1993. Pure Appl Chem 1993;65:819-72.
13. Ettre LS. Tswett and the invention of chromatography. LC/GC North Am 2003;21:458-67.
14. Etxebarria N, Zuloaga O, Olivares M, Bartolomé LJ, Navarro P. Retention-time locked methods in gas chromatography. J Chromatogr A 2009;1216:1624-9.
15. Fallas MM, Neue UD, Hadley MR, McCalley DV. Investigation of the effect of pressure on retention of small molecules using reversed-phase ultra-high pressure liquid chromatography. J Chromatogr A 2008;1209:195-205.
16. Forgacs E. Retention characteristics and practical applications of carbon sorbents. J Chromatogr A 2002;975:229-43.
17. Fornstedt T. Characterization of adsorption processes in analytical liquid-solid chromatography. J Chromatogr A 2010;1217:792-812.
18. Gergov M, Nokua P, Vuori E, Ojanperä I. Simultaneous screening and quantification of 25 opioid drugs in post-mortem blood and urine by liquid chromatography-tandem mass spectrometry. Forensic Sci Int 2009;186:36-43.
19. Gilar M, Bouvier ESP, Compton BJ. Advances in sample preparation in electromigration, chromatographic and mass spectrometric separation methods. J Chromatogr A 2001;909:111-35.
20. Gilar M, Daly AE, Kele M, Neue UD, Gebler JC. Implications of column peak capacity on the separation of complex peptide mixtures in single- and two-dimensional high-performance chromatography. J Chromatogr A 2004;1061:183-192.
21. Gilpin RK, Zhou W. Ultrahigh-pressure liquid chromatography: fundamental aspects of compression and decompression heating. J Chromatogr Sci 2008;46:248-53.
22. Gowda GA, Zhang S, Gu H, Asiago V, Shanaiah N, Raftery D. Metabolomics-based methods for early disease diagnostics. Expert Rev Mol Diagn 2008;8:617-33.
23. Gross ML, Caprioli RM, Niessen W. The encyclopedia of mass spectrometry, vol 8: hyphenated methods. Amsterdam: Elsevier, 2006:1-1068.
24. Haddad PR, Nesterenko PN, Buchberger W. Recent developments and emerging directions in ion chromatography. J Chromatogr A 2008; 1184:456-73.
25. Hage DS. Affinity chromatography: a review of clinical applications. Clin Chem 1999;45:593-615.
26. Hao Z, Xiao B, Weng N. Impact of column temperature and mobile phase components on selectivity of hydrophilic interaction chromatography (HILIC). J Sep Sci 2008;31:1449-64.
27. Hoofnagle AN. Quantitative clinical proteomics by liquid chromatography–tandem mass spectrometry: assessing the platform. Clin Chem 2010;56:161-4.
28. Hurtubise RJ. Adsorption chromatography. In: Cazes J, ed. Encyclopedia of chromatography, 2nd edition, vol 2. Boca Raton: Taylor & Francis, 2005:21-4.
29. Hyötyläinen T. Critical evaluation of sample pretreatment techniques. Anal Bioanal Chem 2009;394:743-58.
30. James AT, Martin AJP. Separation and identification of methyl esters of saturated and unsaturated fatty acids from n-pentanoic to n-octadecanoic acids. Analyst 1952;77:915.
31. Jain V, Phillips JB. Fast temperature programming on fused-silica open-tubular capillary columns by direct resistive heating. J Chromatogr Sci 1995;33:55-9.
32. Jandera P, Urban J, Skeríková V, Langmaier P, Kubícková R, Planeta J. Polymethacrylate monolithic and hybrid particle-monolithic columns for reversed-phase and hydrophilic interaction capillary liquid chromatography. J Chromatogr A 2010;1217:22-33.

32A. Jorgenson JW. Capillary liquid chromatography at ultrahigh pressures. Annu Rev Anal Chem. 2010;3:129-50.

33. Kobayashi H, Ikegami T, Kimura H, Hara T, Tokuda D, Tanaka N. Properties of monolithic silica columns for HPLC. Anal Sci 2006;22:491-501.
34. Koster S, Verpoorte E. A decade of microfluidic analysis coupled with electrospray mass spectrometry: an overview. Lab Chip 2007; 7:1394-412.
35. Kou D, Manius G, Zhan S, Choksi HP. Size exclusion chromatography with corona charged aerosol detector for the analysis of polyethylene glycol polymer. J Chromatogr A 2009;1216:5424-8.
36. LaCourse WR. Column liquid chromatography: equipment and instrumentation. Anal Chem 2002;74:2813-32.
37. Lambert WE, Van Bocxlaer JF, De Leenheer AP. Potential of high-performance liquid chromatography with photodiode array detection in forensic toxicology. J Chromatogr B Biomed Sci Appl 1997;689:45-53.
38. Lee WC, Cheng CH, Pan HH, Chung TH, Hwang CC. Chromatographic characterization of molecularly imprinted polymers. Anal Bioanal Chem 2008;390:1101-9.
39. Lesellier E, West C. Description and comparison of chromatographic tests and chemometric methods for packed column classification. J Chromatogr A 2007;1158:329-60.
40. Li F, Hsieh Y. Supercritical fluid chromatography–mass spectrometry for chemical analysis. J Sep Sci 2008;31:1231-7.

41. Lienqueo ME, Mahn A, Salgado JC, Asenjo JA. Current insights on protein behavior in hydrophobic interaction chromatography. J Chromatogr B 2007;849:53-68.
42. Lu B, Xu T, Park SK, Yates JR. Shotgun protein identification and quantification by mass spectrometry. Methods Mol Biol 2009; 564:261-88.
43. Makawita S, Diamandis EP. The bottleneck in the cancer biomarker pipeline and protein quantification through mass spectrometry–based approaches: current strategies for candidate verification. Clin Chem 2010;56:212-22.
44. Maurer HH. Current role of liquid chromatography–mass spectrometry in clinical and forensic toxicology. Anal Bioanal Chem 2007;388: 1315-25.
45. Maurer HH. Perspectives of liquid chromatography coupled to low- and high-resolution mass spectrometry for screening, identification, and quantification of drugs in clinical and forensic toxicology. Ther Drug Monit 2010;32:324-7.
46. Martin AJP, Synge RLM. A new form of chromatography employing two liquid phases. I. A theory of chromatography. II. Applications to the microdetermination of the higher monoamino acids in proteins. Biochem J 1941;35:1358.
47. McNair HM, Miller JM. Basic gas chromatography, 2nd edition. Malden, Mass: Wiley Interscience, 2009.
48. Miller JM. Chromatography: concepts and contrasts, 2nd edition. Malden, Mass: Wiley Interscience, 2009.
49. Mogridge J. Using light scattering to determine the stoichiometry of protein complexes. Methods Mol Biol 2004;261:113-8.
50. Mullett WM. Determination of drugs in biological fluids by direct injection of samples for liquid-chromatographic analysis. J Biochem Biophys Methods 2007;70:263-73.
51. Neue UD. Theory of peak capacity in gradient elution. J Chromatogr A 2005;1079:153-61.
52. Okamoto Y, Ikai T. Chiral HPLC for efficient resolution of enantiomers. Chem Soc Rev 2008;37:2593-608.
53. Pernemalm M, Lewensohn R, Lehtio J. Affinity prefractionation for MS-based plasma proteomics. Proteomics 2009;9:1420-7.
54. Petersson P, Heaton FA, Euerby MR. Maximizing peak capacity and separation speed in liquid chromatography. J Sep Sci 2008;31:2346-57.
55. Poole CF. New trends in solid-phase extraction. Trends Anal Chem 2003;22:362-73.
56. Poole CF, Poole SK. Foundations of retention in partition chromatography. J Chromatograph A 2009;1216:1530-50.
57. Roque AC, Lowe CR. Affinity chromatography: history, perspectives, limitations and prospects. Methods Mol Biol 2008;421:1-21.
58. Shalliker RA, Gray MJ. Concepts and practice of multidimensional high-performance liquid chromatography. Adv Chromatogr 2006;44:177-236.
59. Sherma J. Planar chromatography. Anal Chem 2008;80:4235-57.
59A. Shushan B. A review of clinical diagnostic applications of liquid chromatography-tandem mass spectrometry. Mass Spectrom Rev. 2010 Nov-Dec;29(6):930-44.
60. Sinclair I, Charles I. Applications of the charged aerosol detector in compound management. J Biomol Screen 2009;14:531-7.
61. Snow NH. Sample preparation for gas chromatography using solid-phase microextraction with derivatization. Adv Chromatogr 2010;48:373-88.
62. Snyder LR,Lloyd R. Snyder (Author) > Visit Amazon's Lloyd R. Snyder Page Find all the books, read about the author, and more. See search results for this author Are you an author? Learn about Author Central Kirkland JJ, Dolan JW. Introduction to modern liquid chromatography, 3rd edition. New York: Wiley, 2009.
62A. Stalcup AM. Chiral separations. Annu Rev Anal Chem (Palo Alto Calif). 2010;3:341-63.
63. Tang J, Gao M, Deng C, Zhang X. Recent development of multi-dimensional chromatography strategies in proteome research. J Chromatogr B Analyt Technol Biomed Life Sci 2008;866:123-32.
64. Tarvers RC, Church FC. Use of high-performance size-exclusion chromatography to measure protein molecular weight and hydrodynamic radius. Int J Peptide Protein Res 1985;26:539-49.
65. Taylor LT. Supercritical fluid chromatography. Anal Chem 2008;80:4285-94.
66. Ullman MD, Burtis CA. Chromatography. In: Burtis CA, Ashwood ER, Bruns DE, eds. Tietz textbook of clinical chemistry, 4th edition. Philadelphia: WB Saunders, 2006:141-63.
67. Unger KK, Skudas R, Schulte MM. Particle packed columns and monolithic columns in high-performance liquid chromatography—comparison and critical appraisal. J Chromatogr A 2008;1184:393-415.
67A. Varma D, Jansen SA, Ganti S. Chromatography with higher pressure, smaller particles and higher temperature: a bioanalytical perspective. Bioanalysis 2010 Dec;2(12):2019-34.
68. Vlakh EG, Tennikova TB. Applications of polymethacrylate-based monoliths in high-performance liquid chromatography. J Chromatogr A 2009;1216:2637-50.
69. Vogeser M, Seger C. A decade of HPLC-MS/MS in the routine clinical laboratory—goals for further developments. Clin Biochem 2008;41: 649-62.
69A. Vogeser M, Seger C. Pitfalls associated with the use of liquid chromatography-tandem mass spectrometry in the clinical laboratory. Clin Chem 2010 Aug;56(8):1234-44.
70. Wang C, Xu J, Zhou G, Qu Q, Yang G, Hu X. Electrochemical detection coupled with high-performance liquid chromatography in pharmaceutical and biomedical analysis: a mini review. Comb Chem High Throughput Screen 2007;10:547-54.
71. Wang S, Miller A. A rapid liquid chromatography–tandem mass spectrometry analysis of whole blood sirolimus using turbulent flow technology for online extraction. Clin Chem Lab Med 2008;46:1631-4.
72. Ward TJ. Chiral separations. Anal Chem 2008;80:4363-72.
73. Wu N, Clausen AM. Fundamental and practical aspects of ultrahigh pressure liquid chromatography for fast separations. J Sep Sci 2007; 30:1167-82.
74. Zacharis CK. Accelerating the quality control of pharmaceuticals using monolithic stationary phases: a review of recent HPLC applications. J Chromatogr Sci 2009;47:443-51.

CHAPTER 14

Mass Spectrometry

Alan L. Rockwood, Ph.D., D.A.B.C.C.,
Thomas M. Annesley, Ph.D.,
*and Nicholas E. Sherman, Ph.D.**

Mass spectrometry (MS) is a powerful qualitative and quantitative analytical technique that is used to measure a wide range of clinically relevant analytes. When MS is coupled with gas or liquid chromatographs, the resultant analyzers have expanded analytical capabilities with widespread clinical applications. In addition, because of its ability to identify and quantify proteins, MS is a key analytical tool that is used in the emerging field of proteomics.

We begin this chapter with a discussion of the basic concepts and definitions of MS followed by discussions of MS instrumentation and clinical applications, and we end the chapter with a discussion of logistic/operational/quality issues. In this chapter, it is impossible to cover all concepts in a field as vast as mass spectrometry, even if one limits one's focus to clinical mass spectrometry. The Clinical and Laboratory Standards Institute (CLSI) has published recommendations on clinical mass spectrometry that can serve as a good next step for study of this topic and another gateway into the extensive literature on this topic.[27]

BASIC CONCEPTS AND DEFINITIONS

MS is the branch of science that deals with all aspects of mass spectrometers and the results obtained with them. *Molecular mass* (sometimes referred to as *molecular weight*) is measured in units of *unified atomic mass unit* (u), also known as the *dalton* (Da). The mass of a carbon atom in its lowest energy state is defined as 12 Da. Although the term *atomic mass unit (amu)* has been regarded as equivalent to the Da, it is only approximately equal to the Da and now is considered an obsolete unit; its use to refer to the Da is strongly discouraged. A *mass spectrometer* is an analytical instrument that first ionizes a target molecule and then separates and measures the mass of a molecule or its fragments. *Mass analysis* is the process by which one or more ionic species are identified according to the *mass-to-charge ratio (m/z)*.[117] The analysis is qualitative, quantitative, and extremely useful for determining the elemental composition and structure of both inorganic and organic compounds.

All MS techniques require an *ionization* step in which an ion is produced from a neutral atom or molecule. In fact, the development of versatile ionization techniques caused MS to become the excellent analytical tool it is today. In 2002, John Fenn and Koichi Tanaka shared the Nobel Prize for their development of electrospray[43,44] and laser desorption[72,92,115] ionization, respectively.

Ions may undergo *fragmentation* in a mass spectrometer. An unfragmented ion of the original molecule is called the *molecular ion.* If the ionization source is *soft,* meaning that it produces little fragmentation, the most abundant peak in the mass spectrum (the *base* peak) may be the molecular ion. Ions that are formed by fragmentation of a molecular ion in the ion source are known as *fragment ions.* If the ion source is *hard,* meaning that it produces extensive fragmentation, the base peak may be one of the fragment ions. By convention, the base peak in a mass spectrum is assigned a relative abundance value of 100%.

Fragment ions that are formed in a separate dissociation cell in a *tandem mass spectrometer* are known as *product ions.* A tandem mass spectrometer consists of two mass spectrometers operated in sequence, or a single mass spectrometer capable of sequential measurement of ions. Generally, ions are dissociated into product ions between the two stages of m/z analysis.

A *mass spectrum* is represented by the relative abundance of each ion plotted as a function of its m/z ratio (Figure 14-1). Usually, each ion has a single charge ($z = 1$); thus the m/z ratio is equal to the mass. However, in some cases, the charge may be represented by some other integer number, in which case the m/z ratio is not equal to the mass, but rather is some fraction of the mass.

Monitoring ions with higher mass usually results in lower limits of detection because fewer background ions are present. A peak in a mass spectrum can be characterized by its *resolution,* $[(m/z)/(\Delta m/z)]$, where $\Delta m/z$ is the width of the mass

The authors gratefully acknowledge the original contributions by Larry D. Bowers on which portions of this chapter are based. We also wish to acknowledge technical assistance by Jacquelyn McCowen-Rose and helpful suggestions from N. Leigh Anderson, Julianne C. Botelho, Pierre Chaurand, David K. Crockett, Ulrich Eigner, Steven A. Hofstadler, Andrew N. Hoofnagle, Gary H. Kruppa, Mark M. Kushnir, Donald Mason, Michael Morris, Maria M. Ospina, and Hubert W. Vesper.

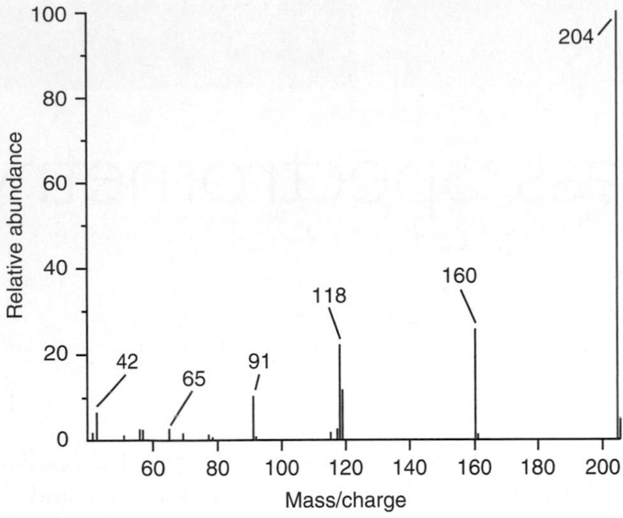

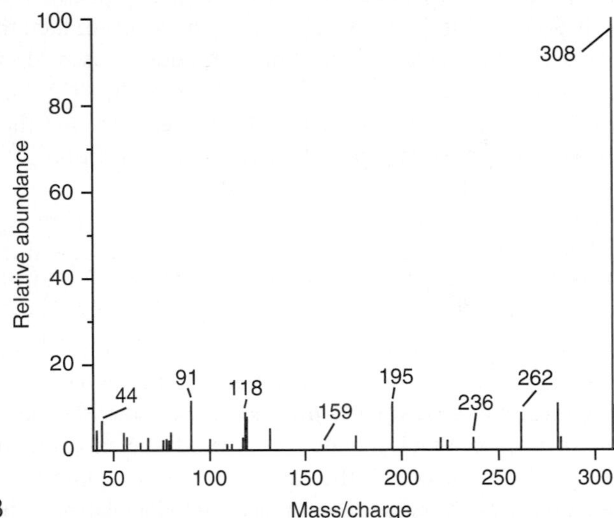

Figure 14-1 Mass spectrum of the pentafluoropropionyl (A) and carbethoxyhexafluorobutyryl (B) derivatives of D-methamphetamine.

spectral peak. This parameter characterizes the ability of a mass spectrometer to separate nearby masses from each other.

By setting the relative abundance of the base peak to 100% and therefore using the relative, rather than absolute, abundance of each ion fragment, instrument-dependent variability is minimized, and the mass spectrum can be compared with spectra obtained on other instruments. Because fragmentation at specific bonds depends on their chemical nature, the mass spectrum can be interpreted in terms of the molecular structure of the analyte. In some cases, the chemical structure of the analyte can be deduced, or at least reconciled with features found in the mass spectrum. Computer-based libraries of spectra are also available to assist in identification of the analyte(s). In some applications, the mass spectrum of an analyte may be matched against mass spectra in a database, thereby identifying the analyte by its mass spectral *fingerprint.*

When interfaced to a liquid or gas chromatograph, the mass spectrometer functions as a powerful detector, providing structural information in real time on individual analytes as they elute from a chromatographic column. Depending on the operating characteristics of the mass spectrometer and the chromatographic peak width, several mass spectral scans can be acquired across the peak. The sum of all ions produced is displayed as a function of time to yield a *total ion chromatogram.*

The mass spectrometer is considered to be a "universal detector" because all compounds have mass. The data system can also be programmed to display chromatograms of only preselected ions acquired during data acquisition. The resultant display is called an *extracted ion chromatogram,* sometimes referred to as an *extracted ion profile.* Both of these displays have the appearance of a chromatogram with signal intensity plotted as a function of time. Retention times can be measured and peak heights or peak areas can be integrated for use in quantitative analysis.

Sample preparation is critical to successful mass spectrometry, particularly when one is dealing with complex matrices, such as are commonly encountered in clinical chemistry. This typically involves one or more of the following steps: (1) protein precipitation, (2) solid-phase extraction, (3) liquid-liquid extraction, or (4) *derivatization.* Derivatization is the process of chemically modifying the target compound(s) to be more favorably analyzed by mass spectrometry. Derivatization usually involves the addition of some well-defined functional group. The goals of derivatization vary, depending on the application, but typically include one or more of the following: (1) increased volatility, (2) greater thermal stability, (3) modified chromatographic properties, (4) greater ionization efficiency, or (5) favorable fragmentation properties.

When only a few analytes are of interest for quantitative analysis and their mass spectrum is known, the mass spectrometer is programmed to monitor only those ions of interest. This selective detection technique is known as *selected ion monitoring* (SIM). Because SIM focuses on a limited number of ions, more ion signal is collected for each selected *m/z.* This increases the signal-to-noise ratio of the analyte and improves the lower limit of detection. In general, an unknown is considered identified if the relative abundances of three or four ions agree within ±20% of those from a reference compound.

A chemical element may be composed of a single *isotope* or multiple isotopes. Each isotope of an element has the same number of protons in its nucleus but different numbers of neutrons. For example, naturally occurring carbon is composed primarily of two isotopes: ^{12}C, whose nuclei contain six protons and six neutrons, and ^{13}C, whose nuclei contain six protons and seven neutrons. Some elements, such as arsenic, have only a single isotope in the naturally occurring state.

A distinct advantage of the mass spectrometer is that it can simultaneously differentiate and quantify a compound with a normal abundance of isotope from an analog enriched with a stable isotope [e.g., (1) ^{2}H relative to ^{1}H, (2) ^{13}C relative to ^{12}C, (3) ^{15}N relative to ^{14}N, (4) ^{18}O relative to ^{16}O]. A compound labeled with a stable isotope is used as an *internal*

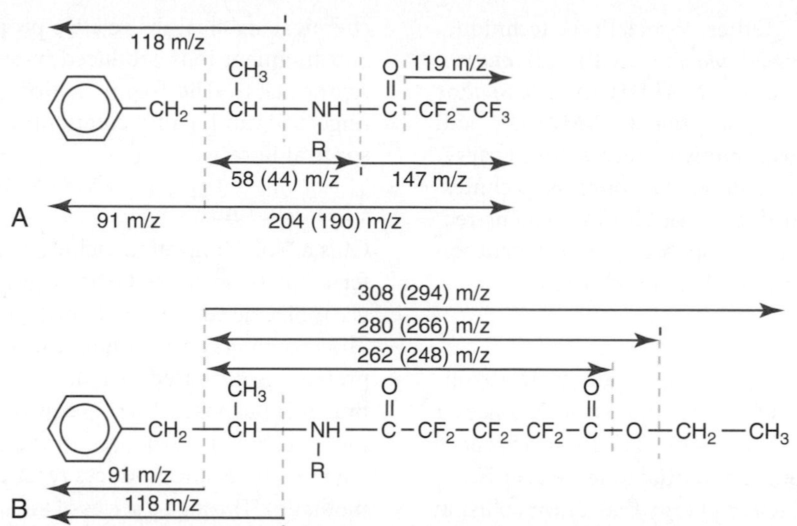

Figure 14-2 Fragmentation patterns for the pentafluoropropionyl (A) and carbethoxyhexafluorobutyryl (B) derivatives of methamphetamine (R = CH_3) and amphetamine (R = H; *masses in parentheses*). Compare the predicted masses with the spectrum shown in Figure 14-1. Note that for the pentafluoropropionyl derivative, only one ion (204, 190 *m/z*) is characteristic of the aliphatic portion of the molecule.

standard because it behaves nearly identically to the native compound during sample preparation and chromatographic analysis. The internal standard must have a sufficient amount of heavy isotope so that no naturally occurring isotope (such as ^{2}H or ^{13}C) contributes significantly to the ion current. For the methamphetamine derivatives shown in Figure 14-2, an internal standard with at least three ^{2}H or ^{13}C atoms is preferred, because at this point the natural abundance of these isotopes is ≈0.1% at 3 mass units above the molecular ion $[(M+3)^+]$. Placement of the stable isotope atoms in the structure is also important. For example, the *m/z* 204 ion for methamphetamine represents the aliphatic portion of the molecule (loss of the aromatic ring). If five deuterium atoms were present on the aromatic ring of methamphetamine, the pentafluoropropionyl derivatives of both native and isotope-labeled drug would yield the *m/z* 204 ion. Similarly, the stable isotope must be located so that it will not exchange with solvent molecules. The ability to quantify a compound relative to an isotopic species of known or fixed concentration is known as *isotope dilution analysis,* and the specific mass spectrometric technique is known as isotope dilution mass spectrometry (IDMS). The IDMS technique has been used to develop definitive methods for a number of clinically relevant analytes including drugs of abuse.

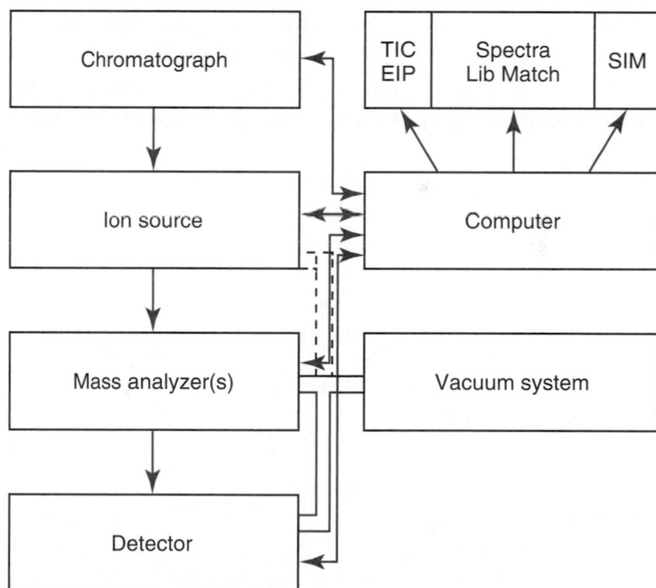

Figure 14-3 Block diagram of the components of a chromatograph–mass spectrometer system. The mass analyzer and the detector are always under vacuum. The ion source may be under vacuum or under near-atmospheric pressure conditions, depending on the ionization mode. The computer system is an integral part of data acquisition and output.

INSTRUMENTATION

A mass spectrometer consists of (1) an ion source, (2) a vacuum system, (3) a mass analyzer, (4) a detector, and (5) a computer (Figure 14-3).

Ion Source

Many approaches have been used to form ions in both high-vacuum and near-atmospheric pressure conditions. *Electron ionization* (EI) and *chemical ionization* (CI) are ionization techniques used when gas-phase molecules are introduced directly into the analyzer from a gas chromatograph. In other analyses, such as high-performance liquid chromatography-mass spectrometry (HPLC-MS), *electrospray ionization* (ESI), *atmospheric pressure chemical ionization* (APCI), and *atmospheric pressure photoionization* (APPI) interfaces are used as ionization sources.[19,41,50,60] Other ionization techniques include (1) *inductively coupled plasma* (ICP), (2) *matrix-assisted laser desorption ionization* (MALDI), (3) *atmospheric pressure matrix-assisted laser desorption* (AP-MALDI), and (4) a number of other less well-known sources. This chapter will limit its discussion to ion sources of interest to clinical chemical analysis. The CLSI document C-50A contains recommendations for matching the capabilities of different ion source technologies to various application classes.[27]

Electron Ionization

In EI, gas-phase molecules are bombarded by electrons emitted from a heated filament and attracted to a collector electrode (Figure 14-4). This process must occur in a vacuum to prevent filament oxidation. A potential difference of 70 eV generates electrons with sufficient energy that a near collision with most organic molecules produces a *radical* cation that is both an ion and a radical.[117] The radical ion then often undergoes unimolecular rearrangement and dissociation to produce a cation and a radical:

$$AB^{+\bullet} \longrightarrow A^{+} + B^{\bullet}$$

Positive ions are repelled or drawn out of the ionization chamber by an electrical field. The cations are then electrostatically focused and introduced into the mass analyzer. EI is primarily used as an ion source in gas chromatography–mass spectrometry (GC-MS). As determined by their chemical stability, the relative proportions of molecular ions and fragment ions produced in an EI source are reasonably reproducible. The fragmentation pattern is often used as a fingerprint to identify compounds by comparison with mass spectral libraries.

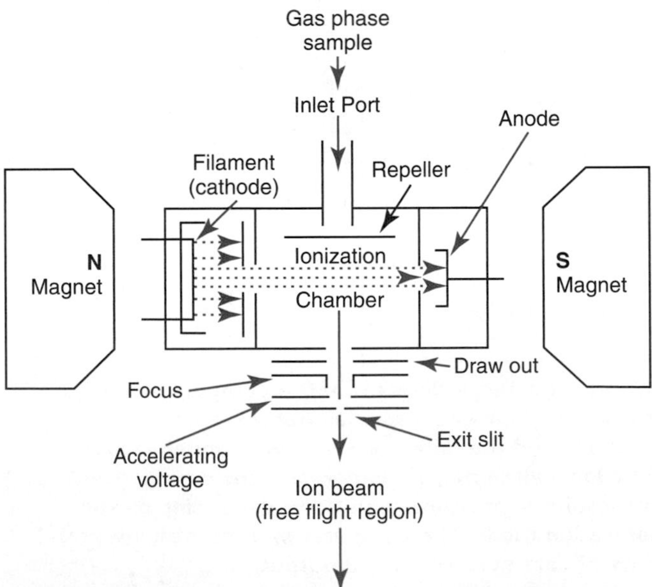

Figure 14-4 Electron impact ion source. The small magnets are used to collimate a dense electron beam, which is drawn from a heated filament placed at a negative potential. The electron beam is positioned in front of a repeller, which is at a slightly positive potential compared with the ion source. The repeller sends any positively charged fragment ions toward the opening at the front of the ion source. The accelerating plates strongly attract the positively charged fragment ions.

Chemical Ionization

CI is a "soft" ionization technique in which a proton is transferred to, or abstracted from, a gas-phase analyte by a reagent gas molecule such as methane, ammonia, isobutane, or water. The reagent gas is bled into a special CI source so the source pressure is increased to about 0.1 torr. (Note: For virtually all practical purposes "torr" is equivalent to "mm Hg" and is the more customary term used in the field of mass spectrometry.) An electron beam produces reactive species (such as CH_5^+ for methane). Through a series of ion-molecule reactions, analyte ions become charged, usually via attachment of a proton. In most cases, relatively little fragmentation occurs. Negative ion electron capture CI is also possible and has become popular for quantification of drugs such as benzodiazepines. Negative ion formation occurs when thermalized electrons are captured by an electronegative substituent, such as chlorine or fluorine on the analyte. When applicable, negative ion CI has very low limits of detection. CI also is used as an ion source in GC-MS.

Electrospray Ionization

ESI is a soft ionization technique in which a sample is ionized at atmospheric pressure before introduction into the mass analyzer.[121,126] The sample, typically an HPLC effluent, is passed through a narrow metal or fused silica capillary to which a 3- to 5-kV voltage has been applied (Figure 14-5, *A*). The partial charge separation between the liquid and the capillary results in instability in the liquid that in turn results in expulsion of a series of charged droplets from a Taylor cone, which forms at the tip of the capillary. A coaxial nebulizing gas, which is used in several types of ESI sources, helps direct the charged droplets toward a counter-electrode. The droplets evaporate as they migrate through the atmospheric pressure region, expelling smaller droplets as the charge-to-volume ratio exceeds the Raleigh instability limit. The proton- or ammonium-adduct of the molecule, which may be associated with solvent molecules, is "desolvated" to form "bare" ions and is typically formed in the ionization process. However, other ionization products are sometimes observed, such as metal ion adducts with analyte molecules, or ions formed by redox processes. Ions then pass through a sampling cone and one or more extraction cones (skimmers) before entering the high-vacuum region of the mass analyzer.

One unusual feature of ESI is the production of multiple charged ions, particularly from peptides and proteins. It is common to observe approximately one charge for every 10 amino acid residues in a protein. For example, because a molecule of mass 20,000 can yield 20 charges, it can be detected at *m/z* 1000 (20,000/20) on a lower resolution and with a less expensive analyzer. This greatly extends the accessible mass range of such an instrument. In these cases, one

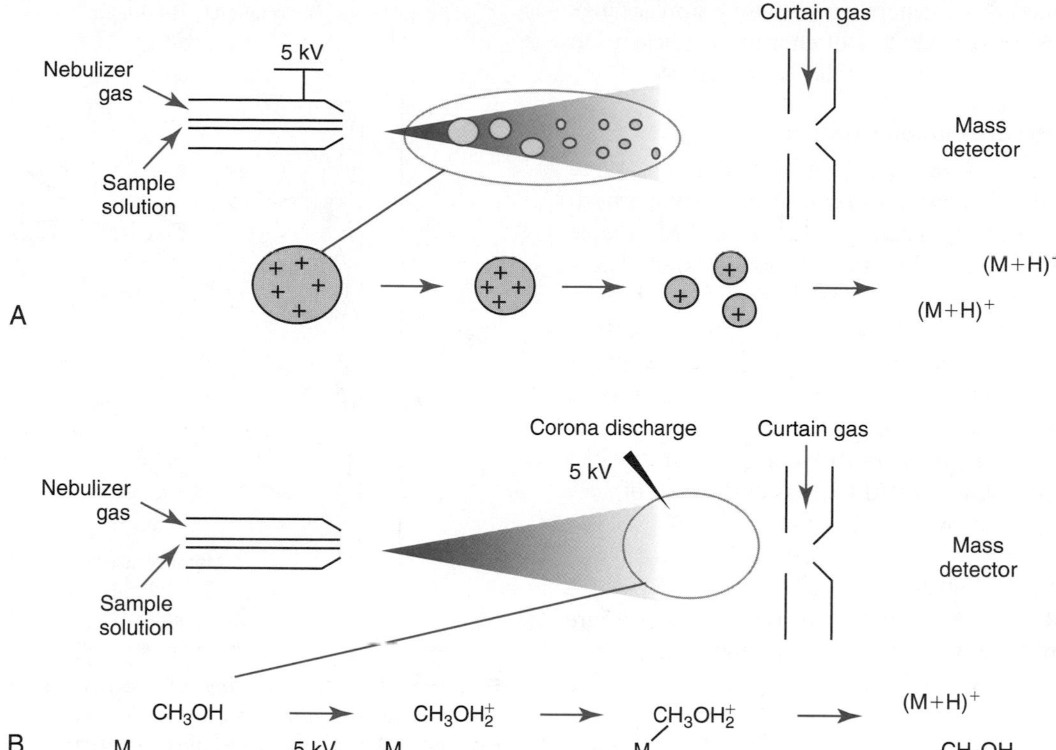

Figure 14-5 Schematics of (A) electrospray and (B) atmospheric pressure chemical ionization sources. Note the different points where ionization occurs, as described in the text.

usually observes a series of peaks, with each peak corresponding to a different number of charges. Nucleic acid polymers can also produce a series of multiply charged ions, particularly when ESI mass spectra are acquired in negative ion mode.

It should be noted that Figure 14-5 is a simplified illustration of the probe being directed toward the sampling cone of the mass detector. To enhance performance and minimize contamination of the mass detector, many modern hardware configurations have offset the probe and/or the mass detector relative to the sampling cone.

ESI tends to be an efficient ion source for polar compounds or for compounds that are ionized in solution, which include a high percentage of medically interesting compounds. ESI, along with APCI, allows an effective interface between a liquid chromatograph and a mass spectrometer. These have become the most widely used ion sources in clinical mass spectrometry.

Atmospheric Pressure Chemical Ionization

APCI is similar to ESI in the sense that ionization takes place at atmospheric pressure, involves nebulization and desolvation, and uses the same sample and extraction cones as ESI. The major difference lies in the mode of ionization. In APCI, no voltage is applied to the inlet capillary. Instead, a separate corona discharge needle[17] is used to generate a corona discharge. Somewhat analogously to the processes occurring in a CI source, ions generated by the corona discharge undergo ion-molecule reactions such as the following:

$$CH_3OH + H^+ \longrightarrow CH_3OH_2^+$$
$$A(\text{analyte}) + CH_3OH_2^+ \longrightarrow AH^+ + CH_3OH$$

or

$$H_2O + H^+ \longrightarrow H_3O^+$$
$$A(\text{analyte}) + H_3O^+ \longrightarrow AH^+ + H_2O$$

Because eluent solvent molecules (e.g., water, methanol) are present in excess relative to analytes in the sample, they are predominantly ionized early in the ion molecule cascade and then act as a reagent gas that reacts secondarily to ionize analyte molecules (Figure 14-5, *B*). Because the products of these secondary reactions may contain clusters of solvent and analyte molecules, a heated transfer tube or a countercurrent flow of a curtain gas, such as nitrogen, is used to decluster the ions. As with ESI, APCI is a soft ionization technique that produces relatively little fragmentation. Thus, compared with EI, the mass spectrum produced by APCI and other soft ionization techniques is less useful for analyte identification by mass spectral fingerprinting. However, because the ion current is concentrated into a single mass spectral peak (or relatively few mass spectral peaks if isotope peaks are considered), APCI and other soft ion sources are well matched to the requirements of tandem mass spectrometry (discussed later) and the combination of the two used for quantitative analysis. APCI and ESI are generally useful for a similar range of compounds. However, APCI is often a more efficient ion source than ESI for relatively nonpolar compounds.

Atmospheric Pressure Photoionization

APPI is a relatively new and less frequently used ion source in clinical chemistry that provides a complementary approach to ESI or APCI. The physical configuration of an APPI source is similar to that for APCI, but an ultraviolet photon flux is used instead of a corona discharge needle to generate ions in the gas phase.[100,111,112] In APPI, an ionizable dopant, such as toluene or acetone, is often infused coaxially to the nebulizer to provide a source of ions that provide charge or proton transfer to analytes, thus increasing the efficiency of analyte ionization. APPI has a similar range of application to APCI but is often more useful than APCI for compounds of very low polarity, such as many steroids.

Inductively Coupled Plasma

As with ESI, APCI, and APPI, ICP is an atmospheric pressure ionization method. However, unlike most atmospheric pressure ionization methods, which are "soft" (i.e., producing little fragmentation), ICP is the ultimate in "hard" ionization, typically leading to complete atomization of the sample during ionization. Consequently, its primary use is for elemental analysis. In the clinical laboratory, it is particularly useful for trace metal and heavy metal analysis in tissue or body fluids. ICP is extremely sensitive (e.g., parts per trillion) and is capable of extremely high dynamic ranges.

Following sample preparation, which generally includes the addition of an internal standard such as yttrium and sometimes includes an acid digestion step, the sample is introduced into the ion source via a nebulizer fed by a peristaltic pump. The nebulized sample is transmitted into hot plasma generated at atmospheric pressure by inductively coupling power into the plasma using a high-powered, radiofrequency (RF) generator. A small orifice samples the plasma, and ions are transmitted to the mass analyzer through a series of differential pumping stages. The atmospheric sampling apparatus is conceptually similar to that of other atmospheric pressure ion sources, such as electrospray, except that the device must withstand the extremely high temperatures generated by the plasma.

ICP-MS is comparatively free from most interference. However, some interfering species can be extremely troublesome. Most interfering species are small polyatomic ions formed in the torch via ion-molecule reactions. For example, ArO^+ interferes with iron at *m/z* 56. One solution to this problem is to use a reaction cell, which consists of a moderate-pressure gas placed before the *m/z* analyzer.[12] A reactant gas, such as NH_3, is bled into the reaction cell. The reactant gas reacts with polyatomic interferences and removes them before introduction into the *m/z* analyzer. Another approach to removing interferences of the same nominal mass is to use a high-resolution mass spectrometer, which is capable of resolving species with similar nominal mass.[12] For example, the masses of ArO^+ and $^{56}Fe^+$ differ by 0.022 Da—a difference that is easily resolved using a high-resolution mass spectrometer.

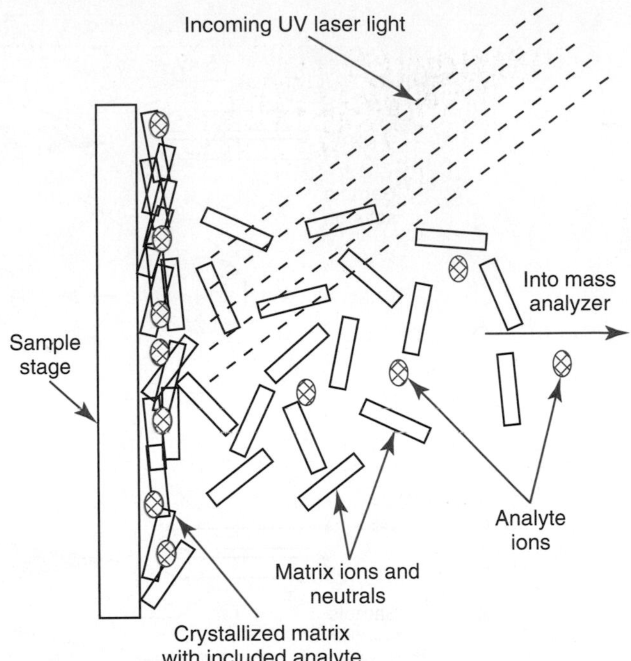

Figure 14-6 A generic view of the process of matrix-assisted laser desorption ionization. Cocrystallized matrix and analyte molecules are irradiated with an ultraviolet (UV) laser. The laser vaporizes the matrix, producing a plume of matrix ions, analyte ions, and neutrals. Gas-phase ions are directed into a mass analyzer.

Matrix-Assisted Laser Desorption/Ionization

MALDI and related techniques rely on energy transfer processes from a pulsed laser beam to the sample for ion generation. In most cases, the analyte is dissolved in a solution of matrix, a small molecular weight UV-absorbing compound, and this solution is placed on a target that is introduced into the mass spectrometer. A UV laser vaporizes small amounts of matrix and analyte into a plume of ions that is directed into a mass analyzer (Figure 14-6). MALDI is another of the "soft" ionization methods. Related techniques include atmospheric pressure matrix-assisted laser desorption/ionization, in which the MALDI process occurs at atmospheric pressure rather than reduced pressure, and surface-enhanced laser desorption ionization (SELDI), which uses a MALDI target surface modified with some type of affinity capture property [hydrophobic, ionic, immobilized metal affinity chromatography (IMAC), DNA, antibody, etc].

Ionization Methods of Potential Interest

Sonic spray ionization is one of the lesser used ionization methods with potential utility for clinical mass spectrometry.[53,54] It is as yet uncertain whether this technology has sufficient advantages over ESI and APCI to find frequent application, although it may find application for the analysis of thermally labile compounds. Desorption electrospray ionization (DESI)[114] and direct analysis in real time (DART)[28] are two relatively new ionization methods that exemplify the generation of ions from surfaces at atmospheric pressure. Most applications of DESI and DART to date have been directed toward minimal sample preparation.

Ionization Methods of Historical Interest

The older literature includes several ionization methods or sample introduction methods that, although promising, or even widely used at one time, hold little interest for current practice in clinical chemistry. These include (1) *fast atom bombardment* (FAB), (2) *thermospray* (TSI), (3) *direct liquid introduction* (DLI), (4) *plasma desorption*, (5) *field ionization* (FI), (6) *field desorption* (FD), (7) *surface ionization mass spectrometry* (SIMS), (8) *laser desorption* (LD), and others. ESI and APCI ion sources have largely rendered these techniques obsolete.

Vacuum System

With the exception of certain ion trap mass spectrometers, ion separation in any of the mass analyzers requires that the ions do not collide with any other molecules during their interaction with magnetic or electric fields. This requires the use of a vacuum from 10^{-3} to 10^{-9} torr, depending on mass analyzer type. The length of the ion path in the analyzer must be less than the mean free path length, unless collisions play a role in mass analysis. Fourier transform ion cyclotron resonance (FT-ICR) requires the lowest pressure (10^{-9} torr). The quadrupole ion trap (QIT) tolerates the highest pressure (10^{-3} torr), a pressure range in which some collisions occur between ions and background gas. Routine quality assurance checks for vacuum leaks should include evaluation of air and water in the mass analyzer.

Efficient high-vacuum pumps generally do not operate well near atmospheric pressure. Thus the vacuum system must have a mechanical vacuum pump to evacuate the system to a pressure at which the high-vacuum pumps are effective. Mechanical pumps require routine maintenance, such as ballasting and replacing the pump oil. The diffusion pump is the least expensive and most reliable high-vacuum pump. Turbomolecular pumps and cryopumps are also used on mass analyzers, having largely replaced diffusion pumps. These high-vacuum pumps also require routine maintenance for optimal operation. A key consideration in construction of the vacuum system is pumping speed. The ability of the pump to maintain the vacuum by removing any gas (or solvent vapor) that enters the system determines the flow rate of gas or liquid that is introduced into the mass spectrometer. In general, higher pump capacities are associated with lower detection limits because noise arising from the gas background is reduced.

Mass Analyzers, Tandem Mass Spectrometers, and Ion Detectors

The term *mass spectrometry* is somewhat a misnomer because mass spectrometers do not measure molecular mass, but rather they measure mass-to-charge ratio. This fact is fundamental to the physical operating principles of mass spectrometers and consequently affects all aspects of instrumentation design and operation and interpretation of results. The symbol m/z is used to denote mass-to-charge ratio and conventionally has been defined as a dimensionless quantity.[97] However, a "dimensionless" mass-to-charge ratio is not consistent with equations of ion motion in the presence of electric and magnetic fields, which require units of mass divided by charge. Furthermore, the m/z scale sometimes is loosely discussed in terms of daltons (Da, also known as unified atomic mass units, u), although strictly speaking, Da is a unit of mass, not mass-to-charge ratio. Despite these nomenclature issues, the present chapter often follows conventional practices by discussing m/z in terms of mass and Da.

To help avoid some of the confusion surrounding the use of m/z, it has been proposed that it should be defined explicitly as quantity having units of mass-to-charge ratio, with mass specified in daltons and charge specified in elementary charges, and that this unit should be called the *Thomson* (Th) in honor of one of the pioneers of MS.[29,36] This terminology is sometimes seen in the literature but has not yet been widely adopted.

General Classes of Mass Spectrometers

Mass spectrometers are broadly classified into two groups: beam-type instruments and trapping-type instruments. In a beam-type instrument, the ions make one pass through the instrument and then strike the detector, where they are destructively detected. The entire process, from the time an ion enters the analyzer until the time it is detected, generally takes microseconds to milliseconds.

In a trapping-type analyzer, ions are held in a spatially confined region of space through a combination of magnetic and/or electrostatic and/or RF electrical fields. The trapping fields are manipulated in ways that allow m/z measurements to be performed. Trapping times may range from a fraction of a second to minutes, although most clinical applications are at the low end of this range. Detection of the ions in a trapping-type instrument may be destructive or nondestructive, depending on the specific type of mass spectrometer used. In this context, "destructive" means that ions are destroyed in the detection process. Additional discussions of mass analyzers, tandem mass spectrometers, and ion detectors are available,[35,107] and the CLSI document C-50A contains recommendations for matching the capabilities of different m/z analyzers to various application classes.[27]

Beam-Type Designs

The main beam-type mass spectrometer designs are (1) quadrupole, (2) magnetic sector, and (3) time-of-flight (TOF). It is convenient to categorize beam-type instruments into two broad categories, those that produce a mass spectrum by scanning the m/z range over a period of time (quadrupole and magnetic sectors) and those that acquire successive instantaneous snapshots of the mass spectrum (TOF). This categorization is not hard and fast. Certain instrument

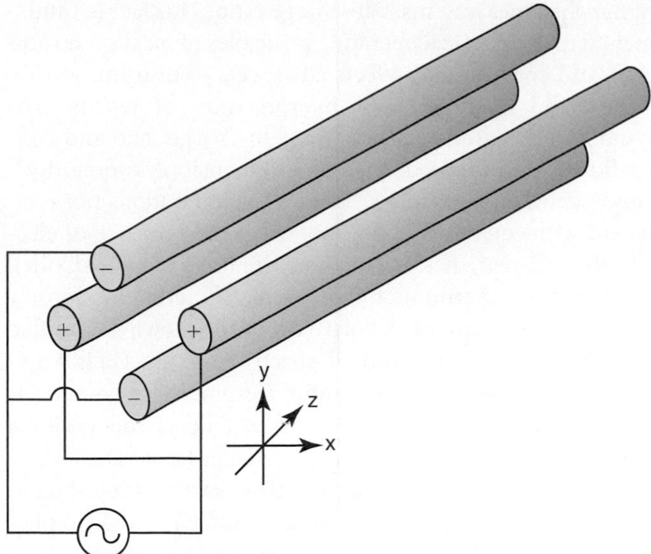

Figure 14-7 Diagram of quadrupole mass filter, including the radiofrequency (RF) part of voltages applied to the quadrupole rods.

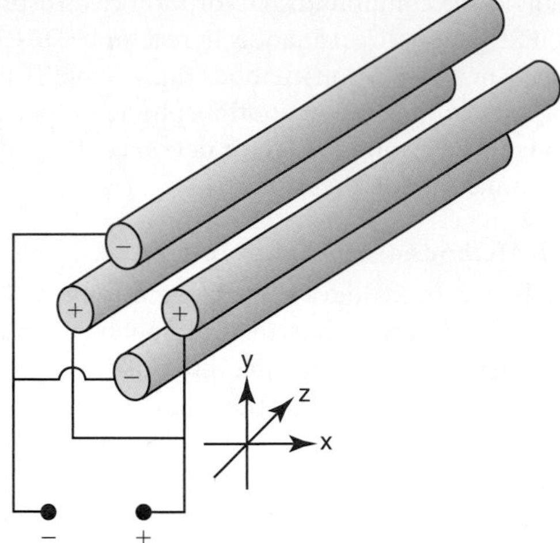

Figure 14-8 Direct current (DC) voltages applied to quadrupole rod assembly.

designs have been adapted to scanning or nonscanning operations. Nevertheless, the categorization is a useful one because it covers the majority of instruments currently available, and because scanning and nonscanning instruments are adapted for different optimal usages.

Quadrupole. Quadrupole mass spectrometers, sometimes known as quadrupole mass filters (QMFs), are currently the most widely used mass spectrometers, having displaced magnetic sector mass spectrometers as the standard instrument. Although these instruments lag behind magnetic sector instruments in terms of (1) sensitivity, (2) upper mass range, (3) resolution, and (4) mass accuracy, they offer an attractive and practical mix of features that accounts for their popularity, including (1) ease of use, (2) flexibility, (3) adequate performance for most applications, (4) relatively low cost, (5) noncritical site requirements, and (6) highly developed software systems.

A quadrupole mass spectrometer consists of four parallel electrically conductive rods arranged in a square array (Figure 14-7). The four rods form a long channel through which the ion beam passes. The beam enters near the axis at one end of the array, passes through the array in a direction generally parallel to the axis, and exits at the far end of the array. The ion beam entering the quadrupole array may contain a mixture of ions of various m/z values, but only ions of a very narrow m/z range (typically $\Delta m/z<1$) are successfully transported through the device to reach the detector. Ions outside this narrow range are ejected radially. The $\Delta m/z$ range represents a pass band, analogous to the pass band of an interference filter in optics (see Chapter 10), which is why quadrupole mass spectrometers are often referred to as *mass filters* rather than *mass spectrometers.*

Quadrupole mass spectrometers rely on a superposition of RF and constant direct current, or DC potentials applied to the quadrupole rods. DC voltages are applied to the electrodes in a quadrupolar pattern. For example, a positive DC potential is applied to electrodes 1 and 3, as indicated in Figure 14-8, and an equivalent negative DC potential is applied to electrodes 2 and 4. The DC potentials are relatively small, on the order of a few volts. Superimposed on the DC potentials are RF potentials, also applied in a quadrupolar fashion. RF potentials range up to the kilovolt range, and frequency is on the order of 1 MHz. The frequency is typically fixed and highly stable, although variable frequency operation is possible in principle.

The physical principles underlying the operation of a quadrupole mass spectrometer are rigorously described by solutions of a complicated differential equation, the Mathieu equation.[33] When an ion is subjected to a quadrupolar RF field, its trajectory is described qualitatively as a combination of fast and slow oscillatory motions. For descriptive purposes, the fast component will be ignored here. The slow component oscillates about the quadrupolar axis; this resembles the motion of a particle in a fictitious harmonic *pseudopotential.* The frequency of this oscillation is sometimes called the *secular frequency.*

The *effective force* associated with the pseudopotential is directed inward toward the quadrupolar axis and is proportional to the distance from the axis. It therefore acts as a confining force, preventing ions from being ejected radially from the quadrupolar assembly. Figure 14-9, *A,* shows an example of an ion confined by an RF-only quadrupole. Below a certain m/z cutoff frequency (which depends on the frequency and amplitude of the RF field), ions are ejected rather than confined. Figure 14-9, *B,* shows an example of an ion ejected by an RF-only quadrupolar field. This establishes the low mass cutoff for the m/z pass band. The effective confining force is strongest just above the low m/z cutoff, and then decreases asymptotically toward zero at high m/z.

The DC part of the quadrupolar potential is independent of m/z. Positive ions are attracted toward the negative poles.

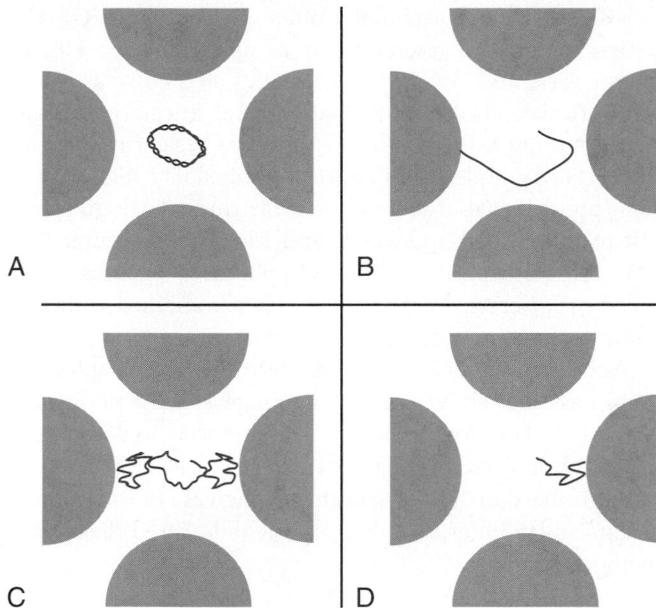

Figure 14-9 Ion trajectories showing confinement and ejection in quadrupole mass filters. A, Ion confinement by radiofrequency (RF)-only field. B, Ion ejection by RF-only field. C, Ion confinement with a combination of RF and direct current (DC) fields. D, Ion ejection with a combination of RF and DC fields. All trajectories were simulated using Simion software (Scientific Instrument Services, Inc., Ringoes, NJ).

Negative ions are attracted toward the positive poles. Attraction increases as the distance from the quadrupolar axis increases. Because a quadrupolar DC potential always has both negative and positive poles, the quadrupolar DC potential always contributes to ejection in at least one direction. Whether ejection of an ion of a particular *m/z* actually occurs depends on whether the ejecting force caused by the quadrupolar DC potential overcomes the effective confining force caused by the pseudopotential generated by the RF field. Above a certain *m/z* value, the DC part dominates, and ions are ejected radially from the device. This establishes an upper *m/z* limit for ion transmission. Figures 14-9, *C* and *D,* shows examples of ion trajectories under the influence of combined RF-DC fields, one being confined and the other being ejected. Trajectories in Figure 14-9 were calculated using the Simion ion optics computer program.[31]

A rigorous description of low- and high-mass cutoffs is found in so-called stability diagrams, which graphically describe the lower and upper *m/z* cutoffs of a quadrupole mass spectrometer in terms of parameters related to voltages, frequencies, and *m/z*. The third edition of this book presents an example of a stability diagram. However, to fully understand the meaning of the stability diagram, one must delve more deeply into a mathematical description than can be done here.

The combination of lower and upper *m/z* limits establishes a pass band ($\Delta m/z$), and ultimately a resolution $[(m/z)/(\Delta m/z)]$. With relatively few exceptions, quadrupole instruments are limited to a resolution of several thousand, which is sufficient to achieve isotopic resolution for singly charged ions of *m/z* as high as several thousand.

A quadrupole MS may be operated in an SIM mode or a scanning mode. In SIM mode, both DC and RF voltages are fixed. Consequently, both the center of the pass band and the width of the pass band are fixed. For example, the mass spectrometer may be set to pass ions of *m/z* 363 ± 0.5. Both the center *m/z* and the $\Delta m/z$ are adjusted by the appropriate choice of DC and RF.

In the scanning mode of operation, the RF and/or DC voltages are continuously varied to scan a range of *m/z* values. As with the SIM mode, the $\Delta m/z$ is determined by the RF and DC voltages. Usually the scan function is designed to maintain a constant $\Delta m/z$ across the full *m/z* range. Thus the resolution increases as *m/z* increases. The value of $\Delta m/z$ is frequently chosen in the range 0.5 to 0.7 to resolve isotopic peaks across the full *m/z* range.

Magnetic Sectors. Because magnetic sector mass spectrometers are rarely used in the clinical laboratory they will not be described in detail here. For an introduction to magnetic sector technology, refer to the third edition of this book. It should be noted, however, that these classic mass spectrometers are easy to understand (given a basic understanding of physics); are versatile, reliable, and highly sensitive; and in their "double focusing" variation are capable of very high *m/z* resolution and mass accuracy. However, they are typically expensive, large, and heavy. In addition, they have the reputation of being difficult to use. Consequently, other instruments have largely displaced magnetic sector mass spectrometers.

Time-of-Flight. TOF mass spectrometry (TOF-MS) is a nonscanning technique whereby a full mass spectrum is acquired as a snapshot rather than by sweeping through a sequential series of *m/z* values while sampling the sample. TOF mass spectrometers have several advantages, including (1) a nearly unlimited *m/z* range, (2) high acquisition speed, (3) high mass accuracy, (4) moderately high resolution, (5) high sensitivity, and (6) reasonable cost. They are also well adapted to pulsed ionization sources, which is an advantage in some applications, particularly with MALDI and related techniques.[14]

A major advantage of modern TOF mass spectrometers is that some of them produce so-called accurate mass measurements, sometimes loosely referred to as *exact mass,* which is typically accurate to a few parts per million (ppm). This allows TOF measurements to confirm the molecular formula of a compound. Unlike magnetic sector instruments, which are also capable of accurate mass measurements. TOF mass spectrometers are conceptually simple to understand because they are based on the fact that a lighter ion travels faster than a heavier ion, provided that both have the same kinetic energy. Figure 14-10 presents a simplified conceptual diagram of a TOF mass spectrometer. It resembles a long pipe. Ions are created or injected at the source end of the device and are then accelerated by a potential of several kilovolts. They travel down the flight tube and strike the detector at the far end of

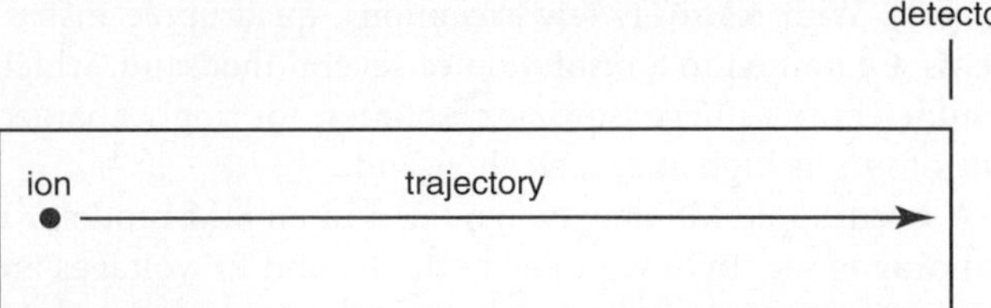

Figure 14-10 Diagram of simplified time-of-flight mass spectrometer.

the flight tube. The time it takes to traverse the tube is known as the flight time; this is related to the mass-to-charge ratio of the ion.

The flight time for an ion of mass m and kinetic energy E to travel a distance L in a region free of electric fields is given by

$$t = L\left(\frac{m}{2E}\right)^{1/2}$$

A sample calculation for an ion of molecular weight 200 Da (3.32×10^{-25} kg) with a kinetic energy of 10 keV (1.60×10^{-15} J), traveling through a distance of 1 m, yields a flight time of 10.18 ms, and an ion of molecular weight 201 takes just 25 ns longer. To accurately capture such fleeting signals, the data recording system must operate on a $\approx$1 ns or shorter time scale. Advances in signal processing electronics have made this practical at relatively modest cost, and this has been a major factor in the rise in popularity of TOF-MS.

TOF is inherently a pulsed technique; it couples readily to pulsed ionization methods, with MALDI being the most common example, although it is also possible to couple TOF with continuous ion sources such as EI, ESI, and APCI. However, the continuous nature of these sources causes a natural mismatch between continuous ion sources and TOF-MS, which is a pulsed technique. This mismatch is overcome by using a technique known as orthogonal acceleration TOF-MS (OA-TOF-MS), in which the ion beam is injected orthogonal to the axis of the TOF-MS.[32,78,106] During the injection period, the acceleration voltage is turned off. Once the injection region is filled with the traversing beam, the acceleration voltage is quickly turned on, and the TOF timing cycle starts. The process is cycled repeatedly. The overall duty cycle for this method can be more than 10%; this represents a vast improvement over the traditional method of gating the ion beam. For full spectrum capability with continuous ion sources, orthogonal injection TOF mass spectrometers are generally considered to have the lowest detection limits of all mass spectrometers. However, for the monitoring of a single m/z rather than a full mass spectrum, the use of SIM mode with a quadrupole MS provides superior limits of detection.

Improved resolution is an additional benefit conferred by orthogonal acceleration as applied to TOF-MS. Although a complete explanation is beyond the scope of this book, in brief, orthogonal acceleration reduces the resolution degrading effects that would normally accompany the kinetic energy variations of individual ions in the ion beam. Use of an ion mirror is a second technique often employed in TOF-MS design to improve resolution by compensating for kinetic energy variations.[82,101] Such instruments are known as *reflectrons.* To date, TOF-MS has had a lesser impact in clinical chemistry, but it seems read to take on a greater role in the future. For example, the full-spectrum capability, high resolution (up to 40,000 in some current instruments), high speed (10 to 100 stored spectra/s), and high mass accuracy of TOF-MS seem ideally suited to applications such as high-speed drug screens in toxicology when combined with fast chromatographic sample introduction.

Another area where TOF-MS provides an advantage is high-mass analysis, where its mass range is nearly unlimited. In MALDI-TOF, for example, it is not unusual to detect proteins with molecular weights exceeding 100,000. The ability for high-mass analysis is expected to increase in importance as clinical laboratories embrace proteomic-based diagnostic methods.

Trapping Mass Spectrometers

In contrast to beam-type designs, these mass spectrometers are based on the trapping of ions to capture and hold ions for an extended length of time in a small region of space. Trapping times vary from a fraction of a second to minutes. Compared with beam-type instruments, the division between scanning and nonscanning instruments has less meaning for ion-trapping instruments. The main practical difference between scanning and nonscanning instruments is related to distortions in chromatographic mass spectral data arising from the finite scan time of the mass spectrometer in relation to the chromatographic peak width of the chromatographic sample introduction scheme (peak skew). In terms of producing skewed spectra, trapping devices are more similar to nonscanning instruments, such as TOF (no skew), than to scanning instruments. This is because the sample is captured in an instant and then is analyzed at leisure. Because the sample is captured in an instant, no skewing of the spectra occurs, regardless of whether the m/z analysis is performed by a scanning procedure or a nonscanning procedure.

Traditionally, ion traps have been classified as (1) a quadrupole ion trap (QIT), which relies on RF fields to provide ion trapping; (2) a linear ion trap, which is closely related to the QIT in its operating principles; and (3) an ion cyclotron resonance (ICR) mass spectrometer, which relies on a combination of magnetic fields and electrostatic fields for trapping. A fourth, the orbitrap, is a more recent introduction into the field of ion trap mass spectrometry.[81A]

Quadrupole Ion Trap. QITs are relatively compact, inexpensive, and versatile instruments that are excellent for (1) exploratory studies, (2) structural characterization, and (3) sample identification. They are also used for quantitative analysis, although quantitative analysis is not the best use for these devices when compared with quadrupole-based instruments.

Operation of the QIT is based on the same physical principle as the quadrupole mass spectrometer described earlier. Both devices make use of the ability of RF fields to confine

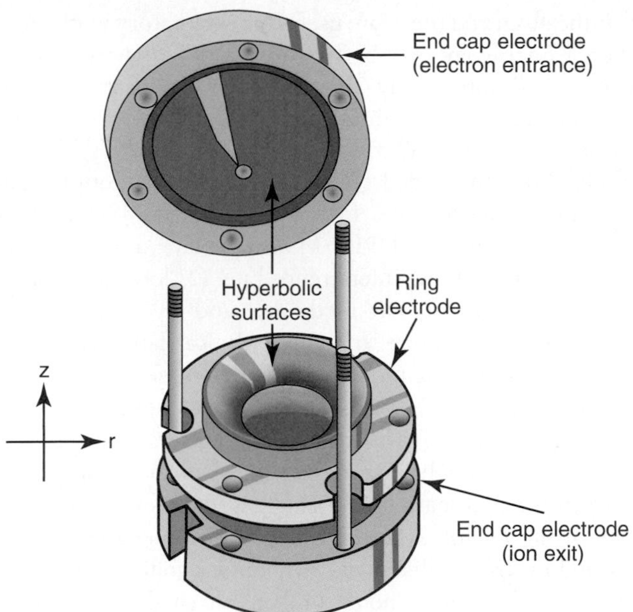

Figure 14-11 Diagram of quadrupole ion trap.

ions. However, the RF field of an ion trap is designed to trap ions in three dimensions rather than to allow the ions to pass through as in a QMF, which confines ions in only two dimensions. This difference has a large impact on the operation and limitations of the QIT.

The physical arrangement of a QIT is different from that of a QMF. If an imaginary axis is drawn through the y-axis of the quadrupole rods, and the rods are rotated around the axis, a solid ring with a hyperbolic inner surface results from the x-axis pair of rods. The two y-axis rods form two solid end caps. A diagram of an ion trap is given in Figure 14-11. The description of the fields within the electrodes must now include a radial component and an axial (between the end caps) component. This slightly changes the precise conditions required for ion confinement when compared with a QMF, although the qualitative description of ion confinement discussed previously is still valid.

A discussion of the several ways of scanning a QIT is beyond the scope of this chapter, except to mention that ions may be ejected from the trap in an m/z-dependent fashion for detection using an external electron multiplier.

QITs are among the most versatile of mass spectrometers, rivaled only in this respect by the ICR mass spectrometer. Notably, QITs are especially well adapted for performing multiple stages of tandem mass spectrometry (MS^n). The QIT also shares some advantages with TOF-MS. In particular, ion trap mass spectrometry is known for high sensitivity. Furthermore, sampling is decoupled from scanning, so no mass spectral peak skewing is seen in GC-MS and HPLC-MS. However, owing to ion-ion repulsion effects, which can reduce dynamic range and produce mass misassignments at high signal levels, QITs do not seem ideal for quantitative analysis applications that dominate clinical chemistry at the present time.

Linear Ion Trap. This is an RF ion trap that is based on a modified linear QMF. Rather than being a pass-through device, as in a normal linear QMF, electrostatic fields are applied to the ends to prevent ions from exiting out the ends of the device. When trapped in this manner, ions can be manipulated in many of the same ways as in a QIT. An advantage of the linear quadrupole trap is that the trapping field can be turned off at will and the device operated as a normal QMF. Thus a single device combines most of the features of a QIT and QMF and is extremely versatile. Commercial triple quadrupole mass spectrometers are being offered in which the third quadrupole is modified to function as a linear trap. Exploration of the capabilities of the linear ion trap is a very active field of research, and one can expect many new capabilities to be discovered in the next few years.

Ion Cyclotron Resonance. The ICR-MS excels in high-resolution and high-mass accuracy measurements.[84] Measurements at resolution exceeding 1 million are not unusual. ICR is a trapping technique that shares many of the advantages of RF ion traps. However, there are even more ways to manipulate ions in an ICR-MS than in QIT, and MS^n (multiple stages of MS/MS) measurements are easily done with an ICR-MS. Sensitivity of an ICR-MS is generally high. Furthermore, sampling is decoupled from spectral acquisition, so no peak skewing is seen in chromatographic experiments—a feature that ICR shares with TOF and QIT.

An ICR-MS is based on the principle that ions immersed in a magnetic field undergo circular motion (cyclotron motion). A typical ICR-MS uses a high-field (3 to 12 tesla) superconducting magnet. Within this field and within a high vacuum is mounted a "cell" typically composed of six metal electrodes, arranged as the faces of a cube. Ions are suspended inside the cell and undergo cyclotron motion, which keeps ions from being lost radially (the radial direction being defined as perpendicular to the magnetic field lines). A low (~1 V) potential is applied to the end caps to keep ions from leaving the trap axially. Thus the combination of electric and magnetic fields keeps ions confined within the cell.

Each m/z is associated with a specific cyclotron frequency. Ions circulating in the ICR cell induce an electrical current in detection electrodes, and after certain mathematical operations are performed on the signal (principally a Fourier transform), a mass spectrum is recovered. Each m/z value present in the sample produces a peak in the transformed signal. Because of the frequent use of FT in ICR, the technique is often referred to as FT-ICR, or FTMS.

Although this technique has many advantages, including (1) high mass accuracy, (2) ultrahigh resolution, and (3) the ability to perform MS^n, ICR-MS has several disadvantages, including (1) instrument costs are high; (2) site requirements, both in terms of space and in terms of access restrictions, are very demanding; (3) it uses a high-field superconducting magnet; and (4) its magnetic field introduces safety concerns, such as flying iron objects. Practical problems with this instrument include (1) the erasing of credit cards and other magnetically encoded strips; (2) costs of operation, care, and maintenance are high because the instruments consume liquid helium, and they must never be allowed to go dry; and (3) a highly skilled individual is necessary to operate it.

Orbitrap. The suitability of a new type of mass analyzer, the orbitrap, for clinical analysis has yet to be evaluated. However, the high resolution and mass accuracy of the orbitrap demand that its potential for clinical analysis be considered in the future. The orbitrap mass analyzer has similar resolution and mass accuracy to the ICR but does not require a magnetic field. This innovation minimizes many of the ICR disadvantages listed previously, although cost is still high. The analyzer is based on an early ion storage device—the Kingdon trap.[67] After many variations over the years, Makarov and associates produced a modified version that eventually was marketed in 2006.[79-81A] The commercial instrument can easily achieve resolutions up to 100,000 with sub-ppm mass accuracy, has a four orders of magnitude dynamic range, and has sampling decoupled from spectral acquisition (as in the ICR).

An orbitrap-MS is based on trapping within electrostatic fields.[96] The actual device is a rodlike central electrode surrounded by a barrel-like outer electrode.[59] When ions are introduced perpendicular to the central electrode and a radial potential is applied between electrodes, the ions spiral (orbit) around the central electrode and are effectively trapped in a radial direction. Trapping in the axial direction is an indirect result of the shape of the electrodes, together with the potentials that are applied to the electrodes. Ion trapping therefore involves both orbital motion around the central electrode and axial oscillations.

The trapping potential in the axial direction is of the form of a harmonic oscillator, and because the frequency of a harmonic oscillator is independent of oscillation amplitude, this frequency is very stable and well behaved. The *m/z* can be calculated from the frequency of axial oscillation

$$\omega = \left(kz/m\right)^{0.5}$$

where *m* and *z* are the mass and charge, and *k* is the constant determined by trap geometry, dimensions, and applied potential. The image current made in the outer electrode by this motion is acquired in the time domain and can be Fourier-transformed to produce a frequency spectrum, which is then converted to *m/z* by the previous equation. With its ability to perform accurate mass measurements, especially when combined with a linear ion trap to form a hybrid tandem mass spectrometer, the orbitrap has excellent potential for proteomics research. However, the capabilities, advantages, and disadvantages of this new type of instrument are still an active area of research. For example, one recent publication noted anomalous isotope ratios observed under high-resolution operating conditions.[42] It is a curious point that the anomalies are compound dependent, and a theoretical explanation for them has yet to appear in the literature.

Tandem Mass Spectrometers

Tandem mass spectrometry, or mass spectrometry/mass spectrometry (MS/MS), has become a mainstay in clinical laboratories, where it has found extensive application in the quantitative analysis of routine samples.[20] However, it is also excellent for structural characterization and compound identification, and therefore useful for exploratory work, even when a final assay may be based on a different technology such as an immunoassay. The most important feature of this technique is its very high selectivity together with its ability to measure very low concentrations of analyte(s). When coupled with the added selectivity of a gas or liquid chromatograph, interferences in a well-designed MS/MS assay (and particularly an HPLC-MS/MS assay) are very low. Because of its (1) low interference rate, (2) low consumable cost (as with most MS methods), and (3) high sample throughput rates, more and more clinical laboratories are purchasing and using tandem mass spectrometers.

The physical principle of tandem mass spectrometry is based on the use of two mass spectrometers (mass filters) arranged sequentially in tandem, with a "collision cell" placed between the two mass filters. The first filter is used to select a *precursor ion* of a particular *m/z.* The precursor ion is directed into the collision cell, where ions collide with background gas molecules and are broken into smaller ions. These product ions of the dissociation process are referred to as *product ions* because they are products derived from the precursor ion. The second mass filter acquires the mass spectrum of the product ions. In the older literature, precursor and product ions are often referred to as parent and daughter ions, respectively.

A variety of scan functions are possible with tandem mass spectrometers. In practice, a product ion scan involves setting the first mass spectrometer or mass filter, MF1, to select a given *m/z,* and scanning through the full mass spectrum of product ions using the second mass spectrometer or mass filter, MF2. This scan function is often used for structural characterization.

A precursor ion scan reverses this relationship, with the second mass filter, MF2, set to select a specific product ion, and MF1 is scanned through the spectrum of precursor ions. The scan tells us which precursor ions produce a specific product ion—a capability that is often used to analyze for specific classes of compounds. For example, acylcarnitines are often analyzed by searching for the precursors to the *m/z* 85 product ion.

In a constant neutral loss scan, the two mass filters are scanned synchronously, with a constant *m/z* offset between precursor and product ion. This scan indicates which ions lose a particular neutral fragment. For example, an offset of 18 *m/z* units would select for ions losing H_2O in the dissociation process.

Another scan function is multiple reaction monitoring, or MRM. This is not actually a scan function but consists of a series of precursor/product ion pairs, with the mass spectrometer set to jump through the table of parent/product ion pairs in a cyclic fashion. This is primarily used for quantitative analysis of a few selected target compounds and is a close analog to SIM monitoring as used in GC-MS. MRM is also performed in a *static mode,* where the two mass filters are set to monitor just one precursor and one product ion. This is especially good for quantitative mass spectrometry.

The key to the high selectivity of MS/MS is that it characterizes a compound by two physical properties—precursor ion mass and product ion mass—rather than by a single property. If combined with chromatographic separation, retention time is added to the characterization, and the analytes are characterized by three physical properties. This imparts a very high degree of selectivity to the analysis and eliminates the vast majority of potential interferences.

As with single-stage mass spectrometers, tandem mass spectrometers are roughly categorized as beam-type instruments and trapping instruments. The most popular beam-type instrument is the triple quadrupole. In this instrument, the first quadrupole (Q1) functions as MF1, and the third quadrupole (Q3) functions as MF2. Between these two quadrupoles is another quadrupole, Q2, which functions as the collision cell. The pressure is raised in Q2 (e.g., greater than 10^{-3} torr) to the point that ions traversing Q2 undergo several collisions, leading to dissociation of precursor ions. The Q2 is operated as an "RF-only" quadrupole, ideally passing all ions regardless of *m/z,* although in reality the pass band may cover a ≈10 : 1 *m/z* range.

Two magnetic sector instruments have also been operated in tandem, with a collision cell placed between the two instruments. These instruments permit high-resolution selection of both precursor and product ions. However, they are now rarely used because they are expensive and cumbersome to operate. A single (as opposed to a pair in tandem) double-focusing mass spectrometer has also been used as a tandem mass spectrometer by a technique known as *linked scanning.* A product ion scan by linked scanning involves low resolution for the first *m/z* selection and high resolution for the second *m/z* selection.

So-called hybrid mass spectrometers include a combination of two different types of mass spectrometers in a tandem arrangement. The combination of a magnetic sector mass spectrometer with a quadrupole mass spectrometer was an early instrument of this type. More popular today is the combination of a quadrupole for the first stage of *m/z* selection and a TOF for the second *m/z* analyzer. Subsequently, a linear ion trap has been combined with an orbitrap. Hybrid instruments are presently used mainly for proteomics research. These instruments also have a problem in performing true precursor ion scans or constant neutral loss scans, though it is possible to mimic these functions by post-processing data, provided the full precursor-product ion map was generated in the experiment.

QIT, linear ion trap, and ICR mass spectrometers can also be used as tandem mass spectrometers. Unlike beam-type instruments, which are referred to as "tandem in space," trapping mass spectrometers are "tandem in time," meaning that ions are held in one region of space while the parent ion is selected and dissociated and the daughter ion analyzed sequentially in time. The ability to perform tandem mass spectrometry is inherent in the design of most trapping mass spectrometers. Generally, little or no additional hardware is required, and tandem capability is supplied via a software change. An exception is the orbitrap, which does not seem to be amenable to tandem mass spectrometry when used alone. However, when incorporated into a hybrid instrument, with a different type of mass spectrometer supplying the first stage of mass spectrometry (such as a linear ion trap), and with the orbitrap supplying the final stage of MS, tandem mass spectrometry is possible in an orbitrap-containing instrument. Most trap-based instruments are capable of multiple stages of mass spectrometry. Thus, product ions may be further dissociated to produce another generation of product ions (MS/MS/MS, or MS^3). In principle, any number of dissociation stages may be performed. This capability finds its greatest use in structural characterization, such as in the sequencing of peptides, and is less useful for quantitative analysis. Trapping designs are extremely versatile, but unlike triple quadrupoles, these instruments are unable to perform true precursor ion scans or constant neutral loss scans.

Detectors

With the exception of ICR-MS, orbitrap, and some ICP-MS instruments, most modern mass spectrometers use electron multipliers for ion detection. The main classes of electron multipliers used as MS detectors include the (1) discrete dynode multipliers; (2) continuous dynode electron multipliers (CDEMs), also known as channel electron multipliers (CEMs); and (3) microchannel plate (MCP) electron multipliers, also known as multichannel plate electron multipliers. Although different in detail, all three work on the same physical principle. Additional detectors used in mass spectrometers are the Faraday cup and image current detection.

Figure 14-12 presents a conceptual diagram of the operation of a discrete dynode electron multiplier. When an ion strikes the first dynode, it causes the ejection of one or more electrons ("secondary electrons") from the dynode surface. The electron is accelerated toward the second dynode by a voltage difference of ≈100 V. Upon striking the second dynode, this electron causes the ejection of additional electrons, typically 2 or 3 in number. The second group of electrons is then accelerated toward the third dynode and, upon striking the third dynode, causes the ejection of several more

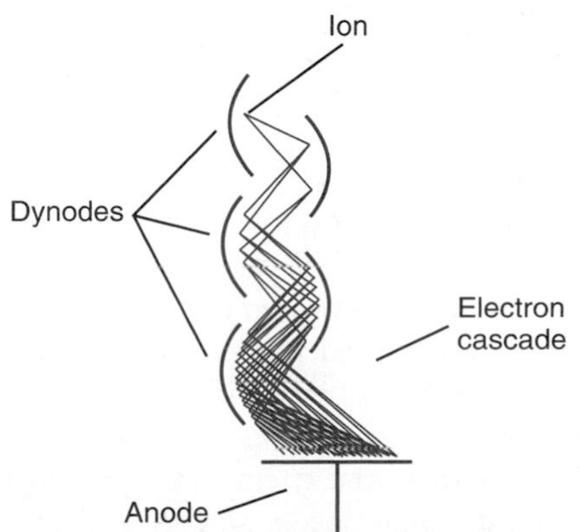

Figure 14-12 Discrete dynode electron multiplier showing dynode structure and generation of electron cascade.

electrons. This process is repeated through a chain of dynodes, numbering between 12 and 24 for most designs. The cascade process typically produces a gain of 10^4 to 10^8, meaning that the generation of one electron at the first dynode produces a pulse of 10^4 to 10^8 electrons at the end of the cascade. The duration of the pulse is very short, typically less than 10 ns.

Continuous dynode electron multipliers work on the same principle as discrete dynode electron multipliers but differ in their physical construction. The set of dynodes of a discrete dynode electron multiplier is replaced by a single continuous resistive surface that acts both as a (continuous) voltage divider to establish the potential gradient and as the secondary electron-generating surface. A microchannel plate electron multiplier is essentially a monolithic array of miniaturized CDEMs fabricated in a single wafer or disk of glass. Sometimes these are stacked into a "chevron" configuration for added gain.

The Faraday cup is not an electron-multiplying device, but rather a simple electrode that intercepts the ion beam directly. This current is amplified using electronic amplifiers. Because the Faraday cup measures signal intensity directly, rather than indirectly (as in saturation-prone electron multipliers), it provides an absolute measure of ion current and is useful when signal levels are too high for electron multiplier–based detection. Some instruments use both electron multiplier— and Faraday cup–based detection to provide for extended dynamic range—a capability that is especially useful for elemental analysis of trace metals in samples.

Detection in ICR occurs via image current detection. This is closely related to the Faraday detection cup in the sense that the ion current is detected directly. However, ions are not destroyed in the process of image current detection and are available for remeasurement. This feature is one of the keys to the versatility of ICR mass spectrometers. Image current detection is also used in the orbitrap.

Closely linked to the detection system is the electronic and signal processing system. In instruments that use electron multiplier detection (the vast majority of mass spectrometers), the raw signal from the detector is processed in one of two ways: (1) individual pulses (corresponding to individual ions) may be counted, as in so-called ion counting systems, or (2) the signal may be converted to a digital representation of the analog signal using an analog-to-digital converter, as in so-called analog detection.

Computer and Software

Because of their (1) mass resolution capabilities, (2) scanning functions, and (3) ability to automatically switch from positive to negative ionization modes, and (4) speed with which multiple *m/z* signals are acquired, modern MS instruments generate enormous quantities of raw data. In addition, the use of MS in such areas as (1) proteomics,[1A] (2) biomarker discovery, (3) synthetic combinatorial chemistry, (4) high-throughput drug discovery, (5) pharmacogenomics, (6) toxicology, and (7) therapeutic drug monitoring requires that MS manufacturers provide sophisticated computers and software programs.

In toxicology laboratories, one important function of the data system is library searching to assist in compound identification. Several commercial libraries, including the Wiley Registry of Mass Spectral Data (http://player.accuradio.com/player/slipstream/accuclassical/?channel=classical&sub=SubCrossover/accessed April 08, 2011), the NIST Mass Spectral Database (http://chemdata.nist.gov/accessed April 08, 2011), and the Pfleger, Maurer, and Weber drug libraries (http://www.sisweb.com/software/ms/wiley.htm/accessed April 08, 2011), are available. In addition, many laboratories generate their own libraries. The quality and quantity of available spectra, the search algorithm, and whether condensed or full spectra are searched are all important factors in spectral matching.

In proteomics and biomarker discovery, complex mass spectra from single proteins, protein mixtures, or protein digests are obtained. Data systems aid in characterization of spectral data to identify such properties as intact protein mass, amino acid subsequences, and post-translational modifications. Fragmentation information can also be compared with peptide databases to identify structural mutations that may be present.

The most important function of software in MS systems containing a chromatographic component is the generation and data processing of chromatograms from SIM or MRM data. Chromatographic peaks are integrated using automatic integration programs (with manual integration over-ride), and integrated peak intensities serve as the basis for quantitative analysis. Calibration curves are generated by the data processing programs, and quantitative results from individual samples are generated from the calibration curves created by the data system. Data systems also contain report generation capabilities, although in current MS instruments, the data reporting functions generally are not interfaced directly to laboratory information management systems.

Software programs are also available to locate and identify components in complex chromatographic separations. Deconvolution protocols have been developed that identify and characterize the mass spectra of coeluting compounds. In addition to proprietary deconvolution protocols embedded in the data systems of mass spectrometers supplied by some vendors, a popular deconvolution software program known as AMDIS (Association of Medical Directors of Information Systems, Lake Almanor, CA/ http://www.amdis.org/accessed April 08,2011) is available as a free download on the Internet.[1] In some cases, two separate sets of chromatographic data can be compared to evaluate similarities or unique differences (e.g., controls vs. disease state).

CLINICAL APPLICATIONS

Mass spectrometers coupled with gas or liquid chromatographs (GC-MS or LC-MS) serve as versatile analytical instruments that combine the resolving power of a chromatograph with the exquisite specificity and detection limits of a mass spectrometer. [102A] Such instruments are powerful analytical tools that are used by clinical laboratories to identify and quantify organic analytes. They provide structural and quantitative information in real time on individual analytes as they elute from a chromatographic column. These coupled techniques require only nanogram or picogram quantities of an analyte for analysis. Specific applications of these coupled instruments are found in Chapters 34 and 35.

MALDI-TOF mass spectrometers and ICP ionization techniques have also enhanced the analytical capabilities of mass spectrometers. In addition, an important application of MS is its use as the primary analytical tool in the rapidly developing and expanding fields of proteomics and metabolomics.

Gas Chromatography–Mass Spectrometry

GC-MS has been used for the analysis of biological compounds for several decades. This technique is used by the U.S. National Institute of Standards and Technology for the development of definitive methods to qualify standard reference materials and to assign certified values to many clinical analytes, including cholesterol, glucose, creatinine, and urea nitrogen (see Chapter 9). One of the most common applications of GC-MS is drug testing for clinical or forensic purposes (see Chapter 35). Many drugs have relatively small molecular weights and nonpolar and/or volatile properties, making these compounds particularly suitable for analysis by GC. Electron impact ionization with full-scan mass detection is the most widely used approach for comprehensive drug screening. Unknown compounds can be identified by comparison of their full mass spectrum with a mass spectral library or database. In addition, vendors have recently reintroduced GC tandem quadrupole (GC-MS/MS) mass spectrometers, which should expand the capability of GC-MS to perform improved targeted analysis, thus enhancing existing screening and mass spectral identification properties of GC-MS.

GC-MS has many applications beyond drug testing. Numerous xenobiotic compounds are readily analyzed by GC-MS. Applications for anabolic steroids, pesticides, pollutants, and inborn errors of metabolism have been described.[64,90,109]

One important limitation to GC-MS is the requirement that compounds be sufficiently volatile to allow transfer from the solid phase to the mobile carrier gas and thus to elute from the analytical column to the detector. Although many biological compounds are amenable to chromatographic separation with GC, numerous compounds are too polar or too large to be analyzed with this technique. In many cases, chemical derivatization is necessary to create sufficiently volatile forms of compounds. Knapp's classic work on derivatization may be consulted for more information.[68]

Despite its limitations, GC-MS has several positive attributes. Fast and effective separations have been achieved with numerous commercial nonpolar columns. This technique has excellent limits of quantification and reproducibility. Last, some analytes, such as organic acids, are better suited to GC-MS because less interference may be present compared with atmospheric pressure ionization LC-MS.

Liquid Chromatography–Mass Spectrometry

As has been discussed earlier, several interface techniques have been developed for coupling a liquid chromatograph to a mass spectrometer, notably ESI and APCI, which have allowed LC-MS and LC-MS/MS to be successfully applied to a wide range of compounds. In theory, as long as a compound can be dissolved in a liquid, it can be introduced into an LC-MS system. Thus, in addition to low molecular weight polar and nonpolar analytes, large molecular weight compounds such as proteins can be analyzed using this technique.

LC-MS/MS has gained momentum in the arena of toxicology screening and confirmation.[38,88,89] Because a scan mode for MF1 looks for such a large range of potentially unnecessary precursor ions, many data acquisition protocols employ preselected sets of time-dependent targeted MRM precursor/product pairs that cover the drugs that are most often used by patients (Figure 14-13, *A*). For example, within the chromatographic time window of 1.5 to 2.0 minutes, the MRM transitions for selected sympathomimetic amines might be monitored (136→119 for amphetamine, 166→148 for pseudoephedrine, 220→84 for Ritalin). During the next defined time window, a new set of MRM transitions are monitored, and so on for the rest of the chromatographic run. A related approach is the use of targeted MRM, in which recognition of a chromatographic peak containing a preselected MRM transition triggers a product ion scan in a process called *information-dependent acquisition,* also known as *data-dependent acquisition.*

Although not presently widely applied to toxicology screening, coupling of TOF mass spectrometers to GC or LC provides a new approach to the identification of drugs. Because TOF is capable of achieving high mass resolution and has the ability of accurately measuring low quantities, the need for compound fragmentation may be minimized, allowing compound identification based on retention time and exact mass.[2]

The number of quantitative LC-MS/MS assays introduced for the measurement of clinically important compounds has markedly increased. For example, compounds that have been of special interest include (1) immunosuppressant drugs,[127] (2) biogenic amines,[37] (3) 25(OH)-vitamin D,[69] (4) antiretroviral drugs,[70,98] (5) psychoactive drugs,[34,110,124] (6) methylmalonic acid,[74,77] (7) thyroid hormones,[128] and (8) steroids.[75,108] When quantification of a specific compound is desired, the most effective approach is MRM analysis, as diagrammed in Figure 14-13, *B*. Both mass filters MF1 and MF2 are set in a static mode, whereby only a single precursor ion specific for the compound being measured is passed through MF1. This preselected precursor ion is then fragmented in the collision cell, and a specific product fragment ion derived from the compound of interest is passed by MF2 to the detector. Because only one ion is monitored in MF1 and one ion in MF2, as opposed to scanning for multiple ions, the MRM approach allows much greater specificity as well as lower limits of quantification.

Another area where MS/MS is used clinically is screening and confirmation of genetic disorders and inborn errors of

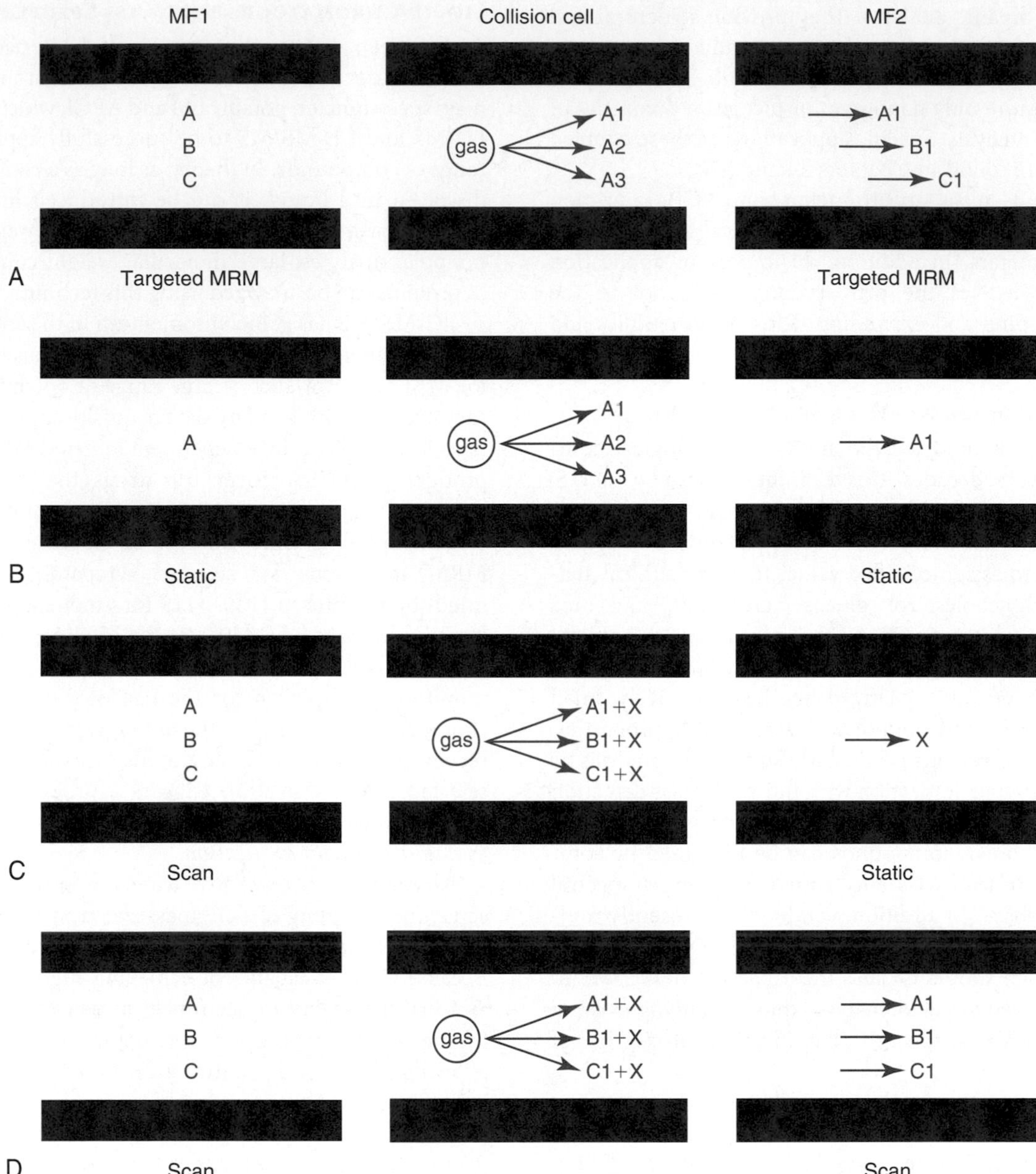

Figure 14-13 Scan modes in mass spectrometry/mass spectrometry (MS/MS). A, Multiple reaction monitoring (MRM), where *A, B, C, A1, B1,* and *C1* are ions. Monitoring of MS/MS transitions *A* → *A1*, *B* → *B1*, and *B* → *C1* is multiplexed. For simplicity, only the dissociation of *A* is shown in a collision cell in the figure. B, MRM of a single compound, where only one MS/MS transition is monitored. C, Precursor ion scan, where *A, B, C,* and *X* are all ions. The second mass filter (MF2) is fixed to monitor the mass-to-charge ratio (*m/z*) corresponding to ionic species *X*, and the first mass filter (MF1) is scanned through a range of *m/z* values. D, Constant neutral loss scan, where *X* is uncharged and *A, B, C, A1, B1,* and *C1* are ions. The two mass filters are scanned with a constant *m/z* offset between the two corresponding to the mass of *X*.

metabolism (see Chapter 58).[23,24] The ability to analyze multiple compounds in a single analytical run makes this technique an efficient tool for screening purposes. Often MS/MS is of sufficient selectivity to eliminate the need to incorporate LC separation, a simplification that can lead to considerable improvement in sample throughput. Electrospray-MS/MS has become the recognized reference method for carnitine and acylcarnitine analysis to identify organic acidemias and fatty acid oxidation defects.[22,51] In the case of acylcarnitine and amino acid analysis, these compounds vary widely in their polarity, which creates problems with consistency of response factors. To address this, most procedures employ a butyl ester derivatization of the carboxyl group to force cationic character upon the amino acids and thus yield similar ionization efficiencies for these compounds.[18] Acylcarnitines can be analyzed without derivatization[25] but most often are monitored as butyl esters, where their identification is based on a data acquisition mode known as a *precursor ion scan* (see Figure 14-13, *C*).[21,99] This data acquisition mode makes use of the fact that acylcarnitines have a common collision-induced *m/z* 85 product ion (represented by *X* in Figure 14-13, *C*) that is selectively monitored in MF2. MF1 is set to full scan for any precursor *m/z* that fragmented to yield this product ion, thus identifying acylcarnitines present in the sample (see Figure 14-13, *C*).

Analysis of amino acids by LC-MS/MS has typically been performed using a data acquisition mode known as *constant neutral loss* (see Figure 14-13, *D*).[23] Alpha-amino acids share a common neutral product, butylformate, which has a mass of 102 Da (represented by *X* in Figure 14-13, *D*). By scanning for both product (MF2) and precursor (MF1) ions, and by keeping a constant offset between the two mass *m/z* analyzers (e.g., a difference of 102 *m/z* units), any *m/z* differences that equal 102 Da can be used to identify the presence of an amino acid.

One advantage of LC-MS/MS relative to GC-MS is that in many cases it is unnecessary to derivatize the target compounds. The example of butyl ester derivatization was discussed previously. In this example, the derivative has more favorable fragmentation properties than the underivatized compounds. Similarly, the dibutyl ester of methylmalonic acid, when run in positive ion mode ESI, has more favorable MS/MS spectra than the underivatized compound run in negative ion mode ESI; in addition, the dibutyl esters of dicarboxylic acids are more efficiently ionized in positive ion mode ESI than the underivatized compound run in positive ion mode ESI.[74] The most frequent reason for using derivatization in LC-MS and LC-MS/MS is to achieve improved ionization efficiency. Gao and colleagues have emphasized this issue in an extensive discussion of derivatization in ESI and APCI mass spectrometry.[48]

Not illustrated in Figure 14-13 is a product ion scan mode. In this scan mode, the first mass filter is fixed to pass a specific *m/z*, and the second mass filter is scanned over a range of *m/z* values. This scan mode is very useful for structural studies of targeted ions, such as in peptide sequencing applications by MS/MS, but is less useful for routine screening applications or quantitative analysis.

MALDI Mass Spectrometry

MALDI (usually coupled with a TOF analyzer) has been used to analyze many different classes of compounds. Notably, it has been widely applied in discovery applications for the detection and identification of proteins and peptides. Primary limitations include high background signal and a higher coefficient of variation that seems inherent in the MALDI ionization process. In addition, MALDI is essentially a batch-type process that does not interface naturally with online separation processes such as HPLC.

MALDI-TOF is often used to determine the identity of proteins through peptide mass fingerprinting (PMF). This technique has been used to identify a large number of two-dimensional (2D) gel spots for the bacterial pathogen *Pseudomonas aeruginosa*.[105] The procedure generally involves in-gel tryptic digestion followed by accurate mass measurement of the peptides. The generated mass list is then compared with theoretical tryptic masses for proteins in a database (Figure 14-14 and Table 14-1). This procedure, which works best for organisms with complete and annotated genomes, is very rapid (<2 min per sample) because 100 or more samples may be automatically processed and deposited on a single MALDI target plate. In the previous example,[105] the group rapidly identified a large number of proteins that were expressed differently between laboratory and pathogenic bacteria. In addition, it was found that some proteins were listed as "hypothetical," meaning they were previously undescribed or confirmed to be expressed, and that theoretical molecular weights and/or isoelectric points (pIs) in some cases were extremely different from those measured in the gel, indicating possible terminal clipping and/or post-translational modification. These observations are extremely useful in targeting areas of focus, given the large quantity of data generated by this technique.

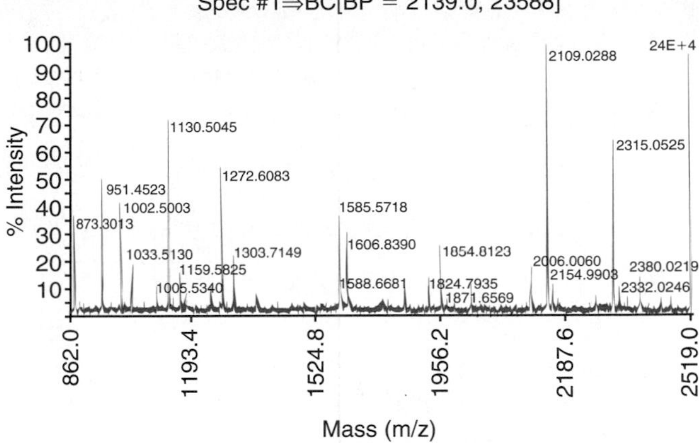

Figure 14-14 An example of a matrix-assisted laser desorption ionization (MALDI)–time-of-flight (TOF) spectrum showing peptides generated in a tryptic digest of a spot cored from a two-dimensional (2D) sodium dodecyl sulfate polyacrylamide gel electrophoresis (SDS-PAGE). The 16 most abundant *m/z* values were submitted to the MS-Fit database for searching against the nonredundant database. The results for this search are shown in Table 14-1.

An interesting emerging clinical application of MALDI-TOF involves identification of organisms, such as bacteria. A method has been described that attempts to identify bacteria by fingerprinting proteins that were extracted using gentle conditions.[120] The basis of this technique is that different bacteria should express unique proteins in the 2- to 20-kDa mass range, allowing classification according to the protein mass fingerprint. Problems[120] include lack of actual protein mass information for various bacteria and lack of investigation into different strains of the same bacteria. The

TABLE 14-1 Example of Printout of Bacterial Identification Through PMF Using MALDI-TOF*

Rank	MOWSE Score	# (%) Masses Matched	Protein MW (Da)/pI	Species	NCBInr.81602 Accession #	Protein Name
1	1.07e+008	14/16 (87%)	101754.9/9.15	*Saccharomyces cerevisiae*	6321275	(Z72685) ORF YGL163c

1. 14/16 matches (87%). 101754.9 Da, pI = 9.15. Acc. #6321275. *Saccharomyces cerevisiae.* (Z72685) ORF YGL163c.

m/z Submitted	MH$^+$ Matched	Delta ppm	Start	End	Peptide Sequence (Click for Fragment Ions)	Modifications
870.4746	870.4797	−5.8732	598	606	(K) GVGGSQPLR(A)	
873.3981	873.3929	5.9793	774	779	(K) DCFIYR(F)	
951.4901	951.4900	0.1050	814	821	(R) LFSSDNLR(Q)	
1002.5385	1002.5373	1.2224	515	522	(K) NFENPILR(G)	
1033.5513	1033.5543	−2.8793	46	55	(K) NTHIPPAAGR(I)	
1130.6349	1130.6322	2.4037	120	128	(R) LSHIQYTLR(R)	
1130.6349	1130.6322	2.4037	514	522	(R) KNFENPILR(G)	
1159.6039	1159.6071	−2.7957	56	67	(R) IATGSDNIVGGR(S)	
1272.6508	1272.6483	1.9865	734	746	(K) AGGCGINLIGANR(L)	
1303.7573	1303.7599	−1.9457	270	280	(K) ILRPHQVEGVR(F)	
1585.7190	1585.7215	−1.5602	446	459	(K) NCNVGLMLADEGHR(L)	
1606.8861	1606.9029	−10.4650	22	35	(R) LVPRPINVQDSVNR(L)	
2138.0756	2138.0704	2.4250	747	765	(R) LILMDPDWNPAADQQALAR(V)	
2315.1093	2315.0951	6.1321	401	423	(K) SSMGGGNTTVSQAIHAWAQAQGR(N)	
2388.0671	2388.0731	−2.5004	293	313	(K) DYLEAEAFNTSSEDPLKSDEK(A)	

*A generated mass list is compared with theoretical tryptic masses for proteins in a database. Match quality is used for pathogen identification. *MALDI-TOF,* Matrix-assisted laser desorption ionization–time-of-flight; *MOWSE,* MOlecular Weight SEarch method; *MW,* molecular weight; *m/z,* mass-to-charge ratio; *PMF,* peptide mass fingerprinting; MH+, ion formed by attachment of a proton to molecule M.

protein mass fingerprints must be catalogued for each bacterium and determined to be completely reproducible for a given extraction method.

Some of these drawbacks were addressed in a MALDI technique that targets ribosomal proteins.[40] This technique was evaluated using 1116 isolates collected in a routine clinical microbiology laboratory and was described as being fast, reliable, and easy to use. More than 95% of clinical isolates were correctly identified, and most of the incorrectly identified isolates were placed in the correct genus or a closely related genus.

MALDI mass spectrometry has the reputation of being a nonquantitative technique. However, some progress has been made toward its use as a quantitative technique.[113] If this application becomes routine, it could have major benefits for clinical mass spectrometry because the time to acquire a mass spectrum by MALDI is only a few seconds. This could dramatically improve throughput. However, it seems likely that this application would require off-line separation prior to loading of the MALDI target, to obtain sufficient selectivity for clinical applications.

ICP Mass Spectrometry

ICP-MS is used for the determination of trace and toxic elements in many types of samples (see Chapters 31 and 36).[9,10] and references 9 and 10). However, it is known that the toxicity of an element may depend on the organic or inorganic state in which the element is present. In these cases, it is more important to ascertain the concentrations of toxic species rather than the total concentration of the element. To extend the usefulness of this technique, GC and HPLC systems have been coupled to ICP-MS to separate individual elemental species before ICP-MS analysis.[83]

Proteomics, Genomics, and Metabolomics

The past 20 years have seen tremendous progress in genomics, with hundreds of genomes completed or near completion and many now parsed and annotated. However, this information has often failed to provide vast new understanding into cellular function, mainly because of the myriad changes that occur to proteins produced from the genome throughout the life cycle of a cell.[1A] In the mid 1990s, MS came to the forefront of analytical techniques used to study proteins, and the term *proteomics* was coined. Although the definition of proteomics is still debated, for the present discussion it is taken to encompass knowledge of the structure, function, and expression of all proteins in the biochemical or biological contexts of all organism.[65] In a more basic and practical sense, proteomics refers to the identification and quantification of proteins and their post-translational modifications in a given system or systems. This is a challenging task in that a given gene may have many distinct chemical protein isoforms. In addition, many other molecules (metals, lipids, etc.) interact with proteins in a noncovalent fashion. Therefore in a genome, such as the human genome, a repertoire of more than a million "proteins" may require identification and quantification. Proteome analysis is a powerful tool for investigating (1) biomarkers of disease, (2) antigens of pathogens, (3) drug target proteins, and (4) post-translational modifications, as well as for other investigations.

Two foundations are necessary to begin this daunting challenge. The first is the basic sequence expected for each possible protein in a cell (i.e., a completed genome). The second is instrumentation, which currently consists of advanced mass spectrometers that identify and quantify protein isoforms in an automated fashion at very low limits of detection. Both foundations are now essentially in place, and the field of proteomics has leapt forward over the past several years. However, the goal previously stated is far from being met, and considerable advances will have to be made before we truly examine all the proteins in a cell.

Currently, MS is routinely used to accomplish many tasks in proteomics. The most basic task is protein identification. The typical approach is known as the *bottom-up* method, whereby proteins are separated—by gel electrophoresis or by solution-based methods—and then digested. The resulting enzymatic fragments are analyzed and used to identify the protein(s) present. This process is time consuming and has many pitfalls. Increasingly, much research has been devoted to analysis of mixtures of proteins. These mixtures are derived from cellular compartments, tissue, or immunoprecipitation. Although it solves many problems associated with analysis of proteins isolated by gels, this technique suffers one major drawback: complexity. Currently, both instrumentation and analysis software are not sufficiently advanced to allow easy identification of all the proteins in truly complex mixtures. As a result, much emphasis has been placed on separation methods for proteins and/or peptides. Many groups have introduced methods to begin handling this level of complexity. The most popular approaches include subcellular fractionation, multidimensional chromatography, and affinity labeling and/or purification. By combining these approaches, several thousand protein species can be identified routinely. Obviously these numbers are better than those obtained through bottom-up methods from gels, but they still fall far short of those necessary for complete proteomics.

Two additional areas that have to be addressed are quantification and de novo sequencing and/or post-translational modification. First, most identified proteins must be quantified in relation to changes in cell state or cell type. Quanti fication in MS for these purposes is relative comparing a standard condition to a perturbed one. Current techniques in this area involve labeling a subset of peptides (isotope-coded affinity tagging) or all peptides (metabolic labeling). Although some problems exist with the labeling, the g reatest—as with identification—involves the sheer complexity of the sample to be analyzed. Label-free approaches for LC-MS/MS quantitative proteomics have also appeared in the literature.[103] The second problem is both separate and related. Post-translational modifications clearly are the major control mechanisms in cells.[94,95] For example, in the field of phosphoproteomics, mass spectrometry has become a powerful technology for the analysis of in vivo phosphorylation in signaling pathways.[94,95] Mass spectrometry is unique as a technique because it will both identify and exactly locate a modification. However, the software needed to automate this process lags far behind the ability to collect data. What is lacking is software for de novo sequencing that will reliably interpret a mass spectrum with little or no user intervention, especially in the area of post-translational modification. Currently, highly skilled mass spectrometrists manually interpret most modified spectra, adding days or even weeks of analysis time per sample. These two problems, in addition to sample complexity, will have to be solved before proteomics evolves into a mature field.

The term *proteomics* is often used in the context of biomarker discovery. To date, very few markers discovered using proteomics methods have migrated to the clinical laboratory. Some of the reasons for the dearth of new protein biomarkers have recently been discussed.[16] From a broader view, however, proteomics may also include the application of mass spectrometry for the analysis of previously recognized proteins and peptides. For example, mass spectrometric methods for the analysis of carbohydrate-deficient transferrin have been developed, including a reference method[93] and a method for routine patient testing. Additional areas of application of mass spectrometry include analysis of the proteome of the pathogenic mold *Aspergillus fumigatus* with the aim of identifying vaccine candidates and new allergens.[6]

A method of analysis of thyroglobulin, a well-known tumor marker, has been described.[56] Although the limit of quantification of this thyroglobulin method still needs to be improved before it is suitable for routine clinical application, it represents substantial progress in the application of mass spectrometry for practical analysis of proteins.

Promising proof-of-principle research has been performed on the characterization of hemoglobinopathies by mass spectrometry.[8,122,123] Most hemoglobin methods using mass spectrometry do not detect the intact tetramer but rather detect separate hemoglobin chains or peptides products from enzymatic digests of hemoglobin. However, as shown by Rockwood and coworkers,[102] and shortly thereafter by Ganem and associates,[46,47] the retention of higher order structure, such as noncovalent complexes, is possible when ions are transferred from solution to gas phase, and hemoglobin tetramers have been observed by mass spectrometry.[5] Another hemoglobin application, a reference method for hemoglobin A_{1c} using mass spectrometry, has been approved by the International Federation of Clinical Chemistry and Laboratory Medicine (IFCC).[62] A method used for hepcidin, a recently discovered peptide hormone believed to be a master regulator of iron status, has been published.[71]

Genetic applications for clinical mass spectrometry are beginning to emerge. For example, MALDI-TOF has been used for mutation detection in myeloproliferative disorders,[45] DNA methylation analysis,[61,119] and gene expression analysis.[7]

A very promising genomic approach for pathogen identification uses polymerase chain reaction amplification of selected regions of a pathogen genome, followed by accurate mass measurement using ESI-TOF-MS. From the accurate mass information, a DNA base composition is computed, and the results are matched to pathogen DNA base compositions in a database.[39,55]

A burgeoning area where MS plays a role is the emerging field of *metabolomics*. This scientific area involves the investigation and characterization of small molecules, including byproducts, present in biological fluids under different conditions that include (1) normal homeostasis, (2) disease states, (3) stress, (4) dietary modification, (5) treatment protocols, (6) aging, and (7) others. In a fashion similar to a mass spectrum providing a fingerprint signature for a specific molecule, it has been speculated that compounds identified and evaluated in metabolomic studies may provide a fingerprint signature for a current physiologic state.

In practice, metabolites are identified through comparison with (1) known reference materials if available, (2) commercial or in-house developed mass spectral libraries or metabolite databases, (3) interpretation of mass spectra, or (4) ancillary techniques such as nuclear magnetic resonance (NMR). As with other applications of MS, both GC-MS and LC-MS have a place in such studies. GC-MS has some potential advantages that were described earlier. To use GC-MS, however, the metabolites in the sample must be volatile, or a separate derivatization step is needed to observe additional compounds. Furthermore, the molecular ion, reflecting the mass of a compound, may not be observed.

LC-MS has its own usefulness in metabolomics because it has potentially wider applicability to polar and nonpolar compounds. LC-MS allows observation of the pseudomolecular ion. However, because reference materials or isotope-labeled internal reference materials do not exist for validating ionization efficiencies or recoveries for newly identified unknown compounds, the effects of ion suppression (discussed later) remain a potential confounding factor. Compared with proteomic research, metabolomic research faces the added difficulties that the MS/MS spectra are more difficult to interpret, no "sequence information" is found in the MS/MS spectra, and DNA and protein sequence databases are of no use in interpreting the results.

Mass spectral imaging of tissue sections is another emerging technology intended for clinical applications that holds great promise. The most common approach is to apply MALDI mass spectrometry to image tissue sections.[26,30] A mass spectrum is acquired at each spot on a regularly spaced array on the sample. From these data, an image is constructed for each m/z. The images provide a spatial map of chemical composition (primarily peptides) from the sample. Another approach uses laser ablation, followed by ICP-MS, to provide a spatial map of the inorganic elemental composition of the sample.[11] This technique can be extended to immunohistochemical imaging by using metal-labeled antibodies.[104] With this scheme, it is possible to use different labels on different antibodies to do multiplexed imaging of several different targets on the same sample.

Practical Aspects of Mass Spectrometry—Logistics, Operations, and Quality

In many respects, the logistics, operations, and quality processes for clinical mass spectrometry laboratories follow well-established clinical laboratory standards and processes. However, mass spectrometers are complex instruments and most manufacturers of instrumentation are still learning how to best support their clients in the clinical laboratory. Consequently, the adoption of mass spectrometry, and especially the more complex technologies such as LC-MS/MS, places added demands on training, competency, and service beyond those of more familiar and well-established technologies used in clinical laboratories.

In contrast to techniques such as optical spectrophotometry, mass spectrometers tend to require more frequent tuning, calibration, and optimization, and the laboratory inspection checklist of the College of American Pathologists specifies that mass spectrometers be tuned daily.[15] In addition, the frequency of calibrations and optimizations needed to maintain instruments in fit-for-purpose condition will vary, depending on the requirements of the assays being performed, the instrumentation used, and other factors.

The term *calibration* is used in at least two distinct ways in mass spectrometry. The first is calibration of the m/z scale of the instrument, usually referred to as *mass calibration*. The other is calibration for quantitative analysis.

Schedules for mass calibration vary between laboratories, types of instruments used, and types of assays being run. For example, if accurate mass measurements are an important part of a method, as with many assays that employ TOF mass spectrometry, then very frequent mass calibration is typically required. In some cases, internal mass reference materials are included within each run, or even within each sample. For applications that are less dependent on mass accuracy, such as most quantitative methods that rely on a quadruple mass filter, mass calibration may be performed less frequently. For example, mass calibration may be performed every few weeks, with verification of mass calibration performed more frequently—as often as daily in some laboratories.

Based on validation results obtained in individual laboratories, schedules for calibration for quantitative analysis may vary. For example, some laboratories calibrate an assay daily, while others calibrate every run.

One advantage of mass spectrometry is that most methods in the mass spectrometry laboratory avoid the use of highly specialized reagents such as antibodies. Consumables are mostly generic items, such as solvents, chromatography columns, and sample vials or 96-well plates. This tends to buffer the laboratory from supply disruptions of specialized reagents, and in some cases can decrease consumable costs as well. However, consumables must be carefully selected and monitored for quality, and some laboratories have experienced intermittent cases of contaminated supplies. Solvent quality is of particular concern. For example, one study documented wide variations in methanol quality from different suppliers, which can lead to large differences in ionization efficiency in ESI sources.[4]

Whenever possible, a quantitative method should use isotopically labeled internal reference materials of the same chemical composition (except for the isotope labels) for each target analyte. However, it is not always possible to obtain isotopically labeled versions of each target analyte, in which case one should select a closely related chemical analog as an internal standard.

Mass spectrometry provides several opportunities for enhancing analytical quality, and therefore improving patient care. The high degree of selectivity of mass spectrometry, particularly when included as a part of hyphenated techniques (GC-MS, LC-MS, LC-MS/MS, etc.) reduces the likelihood of interference compared with immunoassays or simple separation-based techniques (GC or LC), particularly for small molecule analysis, where cross-reactivity is a concern.[57] Perhaps as important as a high degree of selectivity, mass spectrometry provides a means to detect the presence of interferences when they occur. With methods that produce fragmentation, in the ion source (as in EI) or in a collision cell (as in MS/MS), fragment ions are produced in reproducible intensity ratios. By monitoring one or more ion ratios, and by comparing these ratios to ratios obtained from authentic reference materials measured in the same run, it is possible to detect many occurrences of interfering compounds on a sample-by-sample basis.[76]

In addition, accurate mass measurements are useful for detecting interferences if one is using an instrument capable of such measurements, such as a TOF mass spectrometer. To illustrate, the accurate mass of protonated cortisol ($C_{21}H_{31}O_5^+$) is 363.2166 Da, whereas the accurate mass of one of the isotope peaks of protonated fenofibrate ($C_{20}H_{22}ClO_4^+$) is 363.1180 Da—a difference of 270 ppm. Therefore, an interference of even a few percent by fenofibrate in a cortisol analysis would be detectable as a shift in mass of the cortisol peak on an instrument capable of low single-digit ppm mass accuracy.

Obviously, detection of interferences by mass measurement alone becomes more difficult as the mass of the interfering compound approaches that of the target compound, but given the ability to detect interferences at a ≈20% level or better, and assuming a mass spectrometer of ≈3 ppm mass accuracy, a reasonable estimate is that one could detect interferences for all compounds with $|\Delta m/z|$ >30 ppm relative to the target compound. Given the cortisol example discussed earlier, 22 chemical formulas for ions are within 30 ppm of the mass of protonated cortisol, provided we limit our list to the composition constraints listed earlier. Interferences from these would be difficult or impossible to detect by mass measurement alone, but for the other 131 chemical formulas discussed that are outside of the 30 ppm window interference, detection by mass measurement alone is feasible. Thus, accurate mass would likely detect the majority of possible interferences, but a non-negligible minority of potentially interfering compounds would be difficult or impossible to detect.

In developing methods using MS/MS, it is important to carefully assess which MS/MS transitions are to be used. Not all are created equal, particularly with regard to selectivity. In preliminary studies in method development, it is useful to first develop a list of possible MS/MS transitions, based on product ion spectra of pure reference materials . It is generally advisable at this point to strike those transitions from the list that are likely to be nonspecific. Water loss peaks are prime candidates for exclusion, although exclusion of water loss peaks is not always a feasible option if no other high-abundance peaks are available. In the case of methods that rely on derivatization, it is usually best to remove those ions from the list that are products of the derivatization reagent rather than the original target molecule, as these often lack specificity. More transitions can be struck from the list by running a series of patient samples. Those MS/MS transitions that show high background or other interferences are best eliminated from consideration. If pure reference materials of related compounds show similar MS/MS transitions, they may also be candidates to be struck from the list, although if the method is an LC-MS/MS method and the related compounds have different retention times from the target compounds, they may be acceptable. It is also often useful to optimize the collision energy during method development to minimize the likelihood of interferences.

Ion suppression is another quality issue that should be evaluated during method validation.[3] First described in 1993,[63,116] ion suppression is a matrix effect that results from the presence of coeluting nonvolatile or less volatile compounds that change the efficiency of spray droplet formation, ionic properties, and evaporation. These nonvolatile materials, which include salts, ion-pairing agents, endogenous compounds, drugs, and/or metabolites, compete with analyte ions for access to the droplet surface or transfer to the gas phase, which, in turn, affects the amount of charged ion in the gas phase that ultimately reaches the detector.[66] Anions, such as phosphate or borate in buffers, can also neutralize the effective ionization of an analyte. Phospholipids present in blood have been demonstrated to be a major contributor to ion suppression.[125] Impurities in solvents can result in ion suppression.[4]

The presence of ion suppression, or other deleterious matrix effects, can be evaluated via several experimental protocols.[27] One involves comparison of (1) the instrument response for reference materials (including any internal standards) injected directly in the mobile phase, and (2) the same amount of compound spiked into preextracted samples.[86] Data for the standard in the mobile phase provide a relative 100% response value. Data for the same amount of compound spiked into preextracted samples show the effects of sample matrix on MS response (ion suppression).

A second protocol involves postcolumn continuous infusion of compound into the MS detector.[13,58,91] The

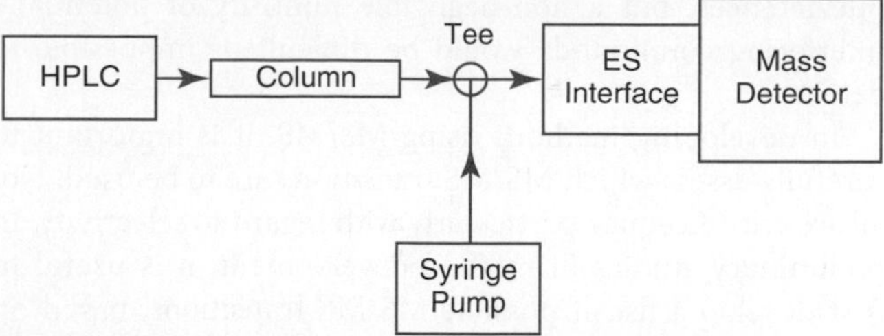

Figure 14-15 Postcolumn infusion system. Mobile phase or specimen extracts are injected into the high-performance liquid chromatography (HPLC) system. The analyte being evaluated is continuously infused, post column, and is mixed with the column effluent through a tee before entering the electrospray interface.

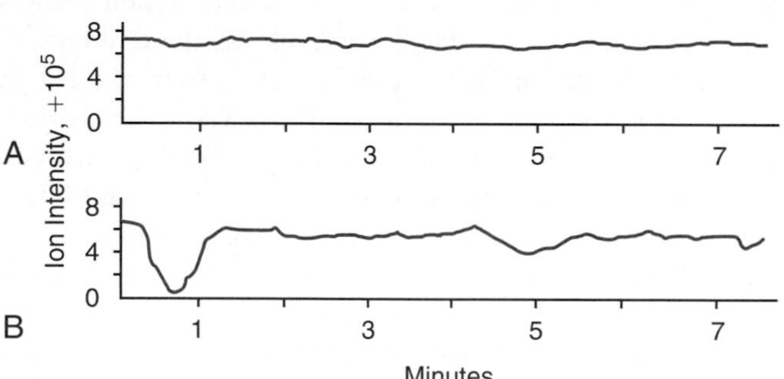

Figure 14-16 Infusion chromatograms for hypothetical analytes. A, Mobile-phase injection. B, Serum liquid-liquid extract injection. These profiles illustrate that ion suppression can be greater than 90%, that a recovery time may exist, and that suppression is not limited to the solvent front region. For a comprehensive presentation of these types of effects, the reader is referred to References 13, 58, and 91.

instrumental setup includes a syringe pump connected via a tee to the column effluent (Figure 14-15). Because the compound being tested is introduced into the mass detector at a constant rate, a constant electrospray ionization response should ideally be observed (Figure 14-16, *A*) if no ionization interferences occur when an extract from a biological specimen, such as serum, is injected into the HPLC portion of the instrument. In actuality, it is common to see suppression of the signal at the time point that corresponds to the void volume of the column (see Figure 14-16, *B*). The degree of ion suppression and the recovery time to full response can vary from compound to compound[13] and from sample to sample and can be dependent on the sample preparation method. Because endogenous compounds from the specimen matrix can continue to elute at any time during the chromatographic run, ion suppression is not limited to the column void. The observed degree of ion suppression can also be dependent on the injection volume and the concentration of the analyte being monitored,[118] which is related to the matrix-to-analyte ratio.[52] It should be noted that the degree of the matrix effect might differ even between different samples of the same biological material, as has been amply shown by Matuszewski et al.[85,87]

Ion suppression is not limited to HPLC-MS or ESI interfaces. For MALDI analysis, arginine-containing peptides have been reported to dominate the peptide pattern for protein digests,[73] the extent of which depends on the matrix used. The presence of ionic detergents, such as Triton X-100 and Tween 20, has been shown to cause signal suppression in MALDI experiments, which can be countered by modifications to the matrix.[49]

REFERENCES

1. Anonymous. Available at: http://chemdata.nist.gov/mass-spc/amdis/ (accessed 2010).

1A. Anderson Nl. Counting the proteins in plasma. Clin Chem 56.1775-6, 2010.

2. Annesley T, Majzoub J, Hsing A, Wu A, Rockwood A, Mason D. Mass spectrometry in the clinical laboratory: how have we done, and where do we need to be? Clin Chem 2009;55:1236-9.
3. Annesley TM. Ion suppression in mass spectrometry. Clin Chem 2003;49:1041-4.
4. Annesley TM. Methanol-associated matrix effects in electrospray ionization tandem mass spectrometry. Clin Chem 2007;53:1827-34.
5. Apostol I. Assessing the relative stabilities of engineered hemoglobins using electrospray mass spectrometry. Anal Biochem 1999;272:8-18.
6. Asif AR, Oellerich M, Amstrong VW, Riemenschneider B, Monod M, Reichard U. Proteome of conidial surface associated proteins of *Aspergillus fumigatus* reflecting potential vaccine candidates and allergens. J Proteome Res 2006;5:954-62.
7. Au WY, Lam V, Pang A, Lee WM, Chan JL, Song YQ, et al. Glucose-6-phosphate dehydrogenase deficiency in female octogenarians, nanogenarians, and centenarians. J Gerontol A Biol Sci Med Sci 2006;61:1086-9.
8. Bateman RH, Green BN, Morris M. Electrospray ionization mass spectrometric analysis of the globin chains in hemoglobin heterozygotes can detect the variants HbC, D, and E. Clin Chem 2008;54:1256-7.
9. Batista BL, Grotto D, Rodrigues JL, Souza VC, Barbosa F Jr. Determination of trace elements in biological samples by inductively coupled plasma mass spectrometry with tetramethylammonium hydroxide solubilization at room temperature. Anal Chim Acta 2009;646:23-9.
10. Beauchemin D. Inductively coupled plasma mass spectrometry. Anal Chem 2002;74:2873-93.
11. Becker JS. Inorganic mass spectrometry. Chichester, England: John Wiley & Sons, 2007:366-75.
12. Becker JS. Inorganic mass spectrometry. Chichester, England: John Wiley & Sons, 2007:181-87.
13. Bonfiglio R, King RC, Olah TV, Merkle K. The effects of sample preparation methods on the variability of the electrospray ionization response for model drug compounds. Rapid Commun Mass Spectrom 1999;13:1175-85.
14. Bucknall M, Fung KYC, Duncan JW. Practical quantitative biomedical applications of MALDI-TOF mass spectrometry. J Am Soc Mass Spectrom 2002;13:1015-27.
15. CAP (College of American Pathologists). Accreditation checklists. CHM 18600, 2009.
16. Carr SA, Anderson L. Protein quantitation through targeted mass spectrometry: the way out of biomarker purgatory? Clin Chem 2008;54:1749-52.
17. Carroll DI, Dizdic I, Stillwell RN, Haegele KD, Horning EC. Atmospheric pressure ionization mass spectrometry: corona discharge ion source for use in liquid chromatograph-mass spectrometer-computer analytical system. Anal Chem 1975;47:2369-73.
18. Casetta B, Tagliacozzi D, Shushan B. Development of a method for rapid quantitation of amino acids by liquid chromatography-tandem mass spectrometry (LC-MSMS) in plasma. Clin Chem Lab Med 2000;38:391-401.

19. Cech NB, Enke CG. Practical implications of some recent studies in electrospray ionization fundamentals. Mass Spectrom Rev 2001; 20:362-87.
20. Chace DH. Mass spectrometry-based diagnostics: the upcoming revolution in disease detection has already arrived. Clin Chem 2003;49:1227-8; author reply 28-9.
21. Chace DH. Mass spectrometry in newborn and metabolic screening: historical perspective and future directions. J Mass Spectrom 2008;42:163-70.
22. Chace DH, DiPerna JC, Mitchell BL, Sgroi B, Hofman LF, Naylor EW. Electrospray tandem mass spectrometry for analysis of acylcarnitines in dried postmortem blood specimens collected at autopsy from infants with unexplained cause of death. Clin Chem 2001;47:1166-82.
23. Chace DH, Kalas TA. A biochemical perspective on the use of tandem mass spectrometry for newborn screening and clinical testing. Clin Biochem 2005;38:296-309.
24. Chace DH, Kalas TA, Naylor EW. Use of tandem mass spectrometry for multianalyte screening of dried blood specimens from newborns. Clin Chem 2003;49:1797-817.
25. Chalcraft KR, Britz-McKibbin P. Newborn screening of inborn errors of metabolism by capillary electrophoresis-electrospray ionization-mass spectrometry: a second-tier method with improved specificity and sensitivity. Anal Chem 2009;81:307-14.
26. Chaurand P, Sanders ME, Jensen RA, Caprioli RM. Proteomics in diagnostic pathology: profiling and imaging proteins directly in tissue sections. Am J Pathol 2004;165:1057-68.
27. CLSI. Mass spectrometry in the clinical laboratory. General principles and practice: approved guideline, vol C-50A, 1st ed. Wayne, Pa: Clinical Laboratory Standards Institute, 2007.
28. Cody RB, Laramee JA, Durst HD. Versatile new ion source for the analysis of materials in open air under ambient conditions. Anal Chem 2005;77:2297-302.
29. Cooks RG, Rockwood AL. The "Thomson": a suggested unit for mass spectroscopists. Rapid Commun Mass Spectrom 1991;5:93.
30. Cornett DS, Reyzer ML, Chaurand P, Caprioli RM. MALDI imaging mass spectrometry: molecular snapshots of biochemical systems. Nat Methods 2007;4:828-33.
31. Dahl D. Simion 6.0 ion optics computer program.
32. Dawson JHJ, Gilhaus M. Orthogonal-acceleration time-of-flight mass spectrometer. Rapid Commun Mass Spectrom 1989;3:155-59.
33. Dawson PH. Quadrupole mass spectometry and its applications, 65-78. New York: Elsevier Scientific Publishing, 1976.
34. de Castro A, Concheiro M, Quintela O, Cruz A, Lopez-Rivadulla M. LC-MS/MS method for the determination of nine antidepressants and some of their main metabolites in oral fluid and plasma: study of correlation between venlafaxine concentrations in both matrices. J Pharm Biomed Anal 2008;48:183-93.
35. de Hoffman E, Stroobant V. Mass spectrometry principles and applications, 63-122, 132-155, 2nd edition. New York: John Wiley & Sons, 2001.
36. de Hoffman E, Stroobant V. Mass spectrometry principles and applications: appendix 1, 361, 2nd edition. New York: John Wiley & Sons, 2001.
37. de Jong WH, Graham KS, van der Molen JC, Links TP, Morris MR, Ross HA, et al. Plasma free metanephrine measurement using automated online solid-phase extraction HPLC tandem mass spectrometry. Clin Chem 2007;53:1684-93.
38. Drees JC, Stone JA, Olson KR, Meier KH, Gelb AM, Wu AH. Clinical utility of an LC-MS/MS seizure panel for common drugs involved in drug-induced seizures. Clin Chem 2009;55:126-33.
39. Ecker DJ, Sampath R, Massire C, Blyn LB, Hall TA, Eshoo MW, Hofstadler SA. Ibis T5000: a universal biosensor approach for microbiology. Nat Rev Microbiol 2008;6:553-8.
40. Eigner U, Holfelder M, Overdorfer K, Betz-Wild U, Bertsch D, Fahr A-M. Performance of a matrix-assisted laser deorption ionization-time-of-flight mass spectrometry system for the identification of bacterial isolates in the clinical routine laboratory. Clin Lab 2009;55:289-96.
41. Ermer J, Vogel M. Applications of hyphenated LC-MS techniques in pharmaceutical analysis. Biomed Chromatogr 2000;14:373-83.
42. Erve JC, Gu M, Wang Y, DeMaio W, Talaat RE. Spectral accuracy of molecular ions in an LTQ/Orbitrap mass spectrometer and implications for elemental composition determination. J Am Soc Mass Spectrom 2009;20:2058-69.
43. Fenn JB. Electrospray wings for molecular elephants (Nobel Lecture). Angew Chem Int Ed Engl 2003;42:3871-94.
44. Fenn JB, Mann M, Meng CK, Wong SF, Whitehouse CM. Electrospray ionization for mass spectrometry of large biomolecules. Science 1989;6:64-71.
45. Fu JF, Shi JY, Zhao WL, Li G, Pan Q, Li JM, et al. MassARRAY assay: a more accurate method for JAK2V617F mutation detection in Chinese patients with myeloproliferative disorders. Leukemia 2008;22:660-3.
46. Ganem B, Li YT, Henion JD. Detection of noncovalent receptor-ligand complexes by mass spectrometry. J Am Chem Soc 1991;113:6294-96.
47. Ganem B, Li YT, Henion JD. Observation of noncovalent enzyme substrate and enzyme product complexes by ion spray mass spectrometry. J Am Chem Soc 1991;113:7818-19.
48. Gao S, Zhang ZP, Karnes HT. Sensitivity enhancement in liquid chromatography/atmospheric pressure ionization mass spectrometry using derivatization and mobile phase additives. J Chromatogr B Analyt Technol Biomed Life Sci 2005;825:98-110.
49. Gharahdaghi F, Kirchner M, Fernandez J, Mische SM. Peptide-mass profiles of polyvinylidene difluoride-bound proteins by matrix-assisted laser desorption/ionization time-of-flight mass spectrometry in the presence of nonionic detergents. Anal Biochem 1996;233:94-9.
50. Glish GL, Vachet RW. The basics of mass spectrometry in the twenty-first century. Nat Rev Drug Discov 2003;2:140-50.
51. Hardy DT, Preece MA, Green A. Determination of plasma free carnitine by electrospray tandem mass spectrometry. Ann Clin Biochem 2001;38:665-70.
52. Heller DN. Ruggedness testing of quantitative atmospheric pressure ionization mass spectrometry methods: the effect of co-injected matrix on matrix effects. Rapid Commun Mass Spectrom 2007; 21:644-52.
53. Hirabayashi A, de la Mora JF. Charged droplet formation in sonic spray. Int J Mass Spectrometr Ion Processes 1998;175:277-82.
54. Hirabayashi A, Sakairi M, Koizumi H. Sonic spray mass spectrometry. Anal Chem 1995;67:2878-82.
55. Hofstadler SA, Sampatha R, Blyna LB, Eshooa MW, Halla TA, Jianga Y, et al. TIGER: the universal biosensor. Int J Mass Spectrometrom 2005;242:23-41.
56. Hoofnagle AN, Becker JO, Wener MH, Heinecke JW. Quantification of thyroglobulin, a low-abundance serum protein, by immunoaffinity peptide enrichment and tandem mass spectrometry. Clin Chem 2008;54:1796-804.
57. Hoofnagle AN, Wener MH. The fundamental flaws of immunoassays and potential solutions using tandem mass spectrometry. J Immunol Methods 2009;347:3-11.
58. Hsieh Y, Chintala M, Mei H, Agans J, Brisson JM, Ng K, Korfmacher WA. Quantitative screening and matrix effect studies of drug discovery compounds in monkey plasma using fast-gradient liquid chromatography/tandem mass spectrometry. Rapid Commun Mass Spectrom 2001;15:2481-7.
59. Hu Q, Noll RJ, Li H, Makarov A, Hardman M, Graham Cooks R. The Orbitrap: a new mass spectrometer. J Mass Spectrom 2005;40: 430-43.
60. Huang C, Wachs T, Conboy JJ, Henion JD. Atmospheric pressure ionization mass spectrometry. Anal Chem 1990;62:713A-25A.
61. Igarashi J, Muroi S, Kawashima H, Wang X, Shinojima Y, Kitamura E, et al. Quantitative analysis of human tissue-specific differences in methylation. Biochem Biophys Res Commun 2008;376:658-64.
62. Jeppsson JO, Kobold U, Barr J, Finke A, Hoelzel W, Hoshino T, et al. Approved IFCC reference method for the measurement of HbA1c in human blood. Clin Chem Lab Med 2002;40:78-89.

63. Kebarle P, Tang L. From ions to solution in the gas phase: the mechanism of electrospray mass spectrometry. Anal Chem 1993;65:972A-86A.
64. Kelley RJ. Diagnosis of Smith-Lemli-Opitz syndrome by gas chromatography/mass spectrometry of 7-dehydrocholesterol in plasma, amniotic fluid, and cultured skin fibroblasts. Clin Chem Acta 1995;236:45-58.
65. Kenyon GL, DeMarini DM, Fuchs E, Galas DJ, Kirsch JF, Leyh TS, et al. Defining the mandate of proteomics in the post-genomics era: workshop report. Mol Cell Proteomics 2002;1:763-80.
66. King R, Bonfiglio R, Fernandez-Metzler C, Miller-Stein C, Olah T. Mechanistic investigation of ionization suppression in electrospray ionization. J Am Soc Mass Spectrom 2000;11:942-50.
67. Kingdon KH. A method for the neutralization of electron space charge by positive ionization at very low gas pressures. Phys Rev 1923;21:408-18.
68. Knapp DR. Handbook of analytical derivatization reactions. New York: John Wiley & Sons, 1979.
69. Knox S, Harris J, Calton L, Wallace AM. A simple automated solid-phase extraction procedure for measurement of 25-hydroxyvitamin D3 and D2 by liquid chromatography-tandem mass spectrometry. Ann Clin Biochem 2009;46:226-30.
70. Koal T, Burhenne H, Romling R, Svoboda M, Resch K, Kaever V. Quantification of antiretroviral drugs in dried blood spot samples by means of liquid chromatography/tandem mass spectrometry. Rapid Commun Mass Spectrom 2005;19:2995-3001.
71. Kobold U, Dulffer T, Dangl M, Escherich A, Kubbies M, Roddiger R, Wright JA. Quantification of hepcidin-25 in human serum by isotope dilution micro-HPLC-tandem mass spectrometry. Clin Chem 2008;54:1584-6.
72. Koy C, Mikkat S, Raptakis E, Sutton C, Resch M, Tanaka K, Glocker MO. Matrix-assisted laser desorption/ionization- quadrupole ion trap-time of flight mass spectrometry sequencing resolves structures of unidentified peptides obtained by in-gel tryptic digestion of haptoglobin derivatives from human plasma proteomes. Proteomics 2003;3:851-8.
73. Krause E, Wenschuh H, Jungblut PR. The dominance of arginine-containing peptides in MALDI-derived tryptic mass fingerprints of proteins. Anal Chem 1999;71:4160-5.
74. Kushnir MM, Komaromy-Hiller G, Shushan B, Urry FM, Roberts WL. Analysis of dicarboxylic acids by tandem mass spectrometry: high-throughput quantitative measurement of methylmalonic acid in serum, plasma, and urine. Clin Chem 2001;47:1993-2002.
75. Kushnir MM, Rockwood AL, Bergquist J. Liquid chromatography-tandem mass spectrometry applications in endocrinology. Mass Spectrom Rev 2010;29:480-502.
76. Kushnir MM, Rockwood AL, Nelson GJ, Yue B, Urry FM. Assessing analytical specificity in quantitative analysis using tandem mass spectrometry. Clin Biochem 2005;38:319-27.
77. Lakso HA, Appelblad P, Schneede J. Quantification of methylmalonic acid in human plasma with hydrophilic interaction liquid chromatography separation and mass spectrometric detection. Clin Chem 2008;54:2028-35.
78. Lazar IM, Lee ED, Rockwood AL, Lee ML. General considerations for optimizing a capillary electrophoresis-electrospray time-of-flight mass spectrometry system. J Chromatogr A 1998;829:279-88.
79. Makarov A. Electrostatic axially harmonic orbital trapping: a high-performance technique of mass analysis. Anal Chem 2000;72:1156-62.
80. Makarov A, Denisov E, Kholomeev A, Balschun W, Lange O, Strupat K, Horning S. Performance evaluation of a hybrid linear ion trap/orbitrap mass spectrometer. Anal Chem 2006;78:2113-20.
81. Makarov A, Denisov E, Lange O, Horning S. Dynamic range of mass accuracy in LTQ orbitrap hybrid mass spectrometry. J Am Soc Mass Spectrom 2006;17:977-82.
81A. Makarov A, Scigelova M. Coupling liquid chromatography to Orbitrap mass spectrometry. J Chromatogr A. 2010 Jun 18;1217(25): 3938-45.
82. Mamyrin BA, Karataev VI, Shmikk DV, Zagulin VA. Mass reflectron: new non-magnetic time-of-flight high-resolution mass spectrometer. Zh Eksp Teor Fiz 1973;64:82-9.
83. Mandal BK, Ogra Y, Suzuki KT. Speciation of arsenic in human nail and hair from arsenic-affected area by HPLC-inductively coupled argon plasma mass spectrometry. Toxicol Appl Pharmacol 2003; 189:73-83.
84. Marshall AG, Hendrickson CL, Jackson GS. Fourier transform ion cyclotron resonance mass spectrometry: a primer. Mass Spectrom Rev 1998;17:1-35.
85. Matuszewski BK. Standard line slopes as a measure of a relative matrix effect in quantitative HPLC-MS bioanalysis. J Chromatogr B Analyt Technol Biomed Life Sci 2006;830:293-300.
86. Matuszewski BK, Constanzer ML, Chavez-Eng CM. Matrix effect in quantitative LC/MS/MS analyses of biological fluids: a method for determination of finasteride in human plasma at picogram per milliliter concentrations. Anal Chem 1998;70:882-9.
87. Matuszewski BK, Constanzer ML, Chavez-Eng CM. Strategies for the assessment of matrix effect in quantitative bioanalytical methods based on HPLC-MS/MS. Anal Chem 2003;75:3019-30.
88. Maurer HH. Current role of liquid chromatography-mass spectrometry in clinical and forensic toxicology. Anal Bioanal Chem 2007;388:1315-25.
89. Maurer HH. Mass spectrometric approaches in impaired driving toxicology. Anal Bioanal Chem 2009;393:97-107.
90. Maurer HH. Role of gas chromatography-mass spectrometry with negative ion chemical ionization in clinical and forensic toxicology, doping control, and biomonitoring. Ther Drug Monit 2002;24:247-54.
91. Muller C, Schafer P, Stortzel M, Vogt S, Weinmann W. Ion suppression effects in liquid chromatography-electrospray-ionisation transport-region collision induced dissociation mass spectrometry with different serum extraction methods for systematic toxicological analysis with mass spectra libraries. J Chromatogr B Analyt Technol Biomed Life Sci 2002;773:47-52.
92. Nakanishi T, Okamoto N, Tanaka K, Shimizu A. Laser desorption time-of-flight mass spectrometric analysis of transferrin precipitated with antiserum: a unique simple method to identify molecular weight variants. Biol Mass Spectrom 1994;23:230-33.
93. Oberrauch W, Bergman AC, Helander A. HPLC and mass spectrometric characterization of a candidate reference material for the alcohol biomarker carbohydrate-deficient transferrin (CDT). Clin Chim Acta 2008;395:142-5.
94. Oellerich T, Gronborg M, Neumann K, Hsiao HH, Urlaub H, Wienands J. SLP-65 phosphorylation dynamics reveals a functional basis for signal integration by receptor-proximal adaptor proteins. Mol Cell Proteomics 2009;8:1738-50.
95. Olsen JV, Blagoev B, Gnad F, Macek B, Kumar C, Mortensen P, Mann M. Global, in vivo, and site-specific phosphorylation dynamics in signaling networks. Cell 2006;127:635-48.
96. Perry RH, Cooks RG, Noll RJ. Orbitrap mass spectrometry: instrumentation, ion motion and applications. Mass Spectrom Rev 2008;27:661-99.
97. Price P. Standard definition of terms relating to mass spectrometry. J Am Soc Mass Spectrom 1991;2:336-48.
98. Remmel RP, Kawle SP, Weller D, Fletcher CV. Simultaneous HPLC assay for quantification of indinavir, nelfinavir, ritonavir, and saquinavir in human plasma. Clin Chem 2000;46:73-81.
99. Rinaldo P, Cowan TM, Matern D. Acylcarnitine profile analysis. Genet Med 2008;10:151-6.
100. Robb DB, Covey TR, Bruins AP. Atmospheric pressure photoionization: an ionization method for liquid chromatography-mass spectrometry. Anal Chem 2000;72:3653-9.
101. Rockwood AL. An improved time of flight mass spectrometer. Cincinnati, Ohio: 34th Annual American Society for Mass Spectrometry, 1986:173-4.
102. Rockwood AL, Busman M, Smith RD. Coulombic effects in the dissociation of large highly charged ions. Int Natl J Mass Spectrom Ion Processing 1991;111:103-29.

102A. Rodriguez H, Tezak Z, Mesri M, Carr SA, Liebler DC, Fisher SJ, et al. Analytical validation of protein-based multiplex assays: a workshop report by the NCI-FDA interagency oncology task force on molecular diagnostics. Clin Chem 2010 Feb;56(2):237-43.
103. Schwarz E, Levin Y, Wang L, Leweke FM, Bahn S. Peptide correlation: a means to identify high quality quantitative information in large-scale proteomic studies. J Sep Sci 2007;30:2190-7.
104. Seuma J, Bunch J, Cox A, McLeod C, Bell J, Murray C. Combination of immunohistochemistry and laser ablation ICP mass spectrometry for imaging of cancer biomarkers. Proteomics 2008;8:3775-84.
105. Sherman NE, Stefansson B, Fox JW, Goldberg JB. *Pseudomonas aeruginosa* and a proteomic approach to bacterial pathogenesis. Dis Markers 2001;17:285-93.
106. Sin CH, Lee ED, Lee ML. Atmospheric pressure ionization time-of-flight mass spectrometry. Anal Chem 1991;63:2897-900.
107. Siuzdak G. Mass analyzers and ion detectors. In: Siuzdak G, ed. Mass spectrometry for biotechnology. San Diego: Academic Press, 1996: 32-55.
108. Soldin SJ, Soldin OP. Steroid hormone analysis by tandem mass spectrometry. Clin Chem 2009;55:1061-6.
109. Stelland F, ten Brink HJ, Kok RM, Jacobs C. Stable isotope dilution analysis of very long chain fatty acids in plasma, urine, and amniotic fluid by electron capture negative ion mass fragmentography. Clin Chem Acta 1990;192:133-44.
110. Subramanian M, Birnbaum AK, Remmel RP. High-speed simultaneous determination of nine antiepileptic drugs using liquid chromatography-mass spectrometry. Ther Drug Monit 2008;30: 347-56.
111. Syage JA, Evans MD, Hanold KA. Photoionization mass spectrometry. Am Lab 2000;12:24-9.
112. Syage JA, Hanning-Lee MA, Hanold KA. A man-portable, photoionization time-of-flight mass spectrometer. Field Anal Chem Toxicol 2000;4:204-15.
113. Szajli E, Feher T, Medzihradszky KF. Investigating the quantitative nature of MALDI-TOF MS. Mol Cell Proteomics 2008;7:2410-8.
114. Takats Z, Wiseman JM, Gologan B, Cooks RG. Mass spectrometry sampling under ambient conditions with desorption electrospray ionization Science 2004;306:471-3.
115. Tanaka K. The origin of macromolecule ionization by laser irradiation (Nobel Lecture). Angew Chem Int Ed Engl 2003;42:3860-70.
116. Tang L, Kebarle P. Dependence of ion intensity in electrospray mass spectrometry on the concentration of the analytes in the electrosprayed solution. Anal Chem 1993;65:3654-68.
117. Todd JFT. Recommendations for nomenclature and symbolism for mass spectrometry. IUPAC recommendations. Pure Appl Chem 1991;63:1541-66.
118. van Hout MWJ, Hoffland CM, Niederlander HAG, de Jong GJ. On-line coupling of solid-phase extraction with mass spectrometry for the analysis of biological samples. II. Determination of clenbuterol in urine using multiple-stage mass spectrometry in an ion-trap spectrometer. Rapid Commun Mass Spectrom 2000;14:2103-11.
119. Wang SC, Oelze B, Schumacher A. Age-specific epigenetic drift in late-onset Alzheimer's disease. PLoS One 2008;3:e2698.
120. Wang Z, Dunlop K, Long SR, Li L. Mass spectrometric methods for generation of protein mass database used for bacterial identification. Anal Chem 2002;74:3174-82.
121. Whitehouse CM, Dreyer RN, Yamashita M, Fenn JB. Electropray interface for liquid chromatographs and mass spectrometers. Anal Chem 1985;57:675-9.
122. Wild BJ, Green BN, Cooper EK, Lalloz MR, Erten S, Stephens AD, Layton DM. Rapid identification of hemoglobin variants by electrospray ionization mass spectrometry. Blood Cell Mol Dis 2001;27:691-704.
123. Wild BJ, Green BN, Stephens AD. The potential of electrospray ionization mass spectrometry for the diagnosis of hemoglobin variants found in newborn screening. Blood Cell Mol Dis 2004;33:308-17.
124. Wohlfarth A, Weinmann W, Dresen S. LC-MS/MS screening method for designer amphetamines, tryptamines, and piperazines in serum. Anal Bioanal Chem 2010;396:2403-14.
125. Xia YQ, Jemal M. Phospholipids in liquid chromatography/mass spectrometry bioanalysis: comparison of three tandem mass spectrometric techniques for monitoring plasma phospholipids, the effect of mobile phase composition on phospholipids elution and the association of phospholipids with matrix effects. Rapid Commun Mass Spectrom 2009;23:2125-38.
126. Yamashita M, Fenn JB. Electrospray ion source: another variation on the free-jet theme. J Phys Chem A 1984;88:4451-9.
127. Yang Z, Wang S. Recent development in application of high performance liquid chromatography-tandem mass spectrometry in therapeutic drug monitoring of immunosuppressants. J Immunol Methods 2008;336:98-103.
128. Yue B, Rockwood AL, Sandrock T, La'ulu SL, Kushnir MM, Meikle AW. Free thyroid hormones in serum by direct equilibrium dialysis and online solid-phase extraction—liquid chromatography/tandem mass spectrometry. Clin Chem 2008;54:642-51.

CHAPTER 15

Enzyme and Rate Analyses

*Renze Bais, Ph.D., A.R.C.P.A., and Mauro Panteghini, M.D.**

Enzymes are proteins with catalytic properties; *clinical enzymology* is the application of the science of enzymes to the diagnosis and treatment of disease. The principles of clinical enzymology will be introduced and discussed in this chapter, as will information on how enzymes are measured and how they are used as analytical reagents in various types of rate analysis. Individual topics include basic principles, enzyme kinetics and analytical enzymology, and rate analyses.

BASIC PRINCIPLES

This section begins with a presentation of enzyme nomenclature, which is followed by a discussion of enzymes as proteins and catalysts.

Enzyme Nomenclature

Historically, individual enzymes were identified using the name of the substrate or group upon which they act and then adding the suffix *-ase*. For example, the enzyme hydrolyzing urea was ure*ase*. Later, the type of reaction involved was also identified, as in carbonic anhydrase, D-amino acid oxidase, and succinate dehydrogenase. In addition, some enzymes had been given empirical names such as trypsin, diastase, ptyalin, pepsin, and emulsin.

Because this combination of trivial common names and semisystematic names was found to be inadequate, in 1955 the International Union of Biochemistry (IUB) appointed an Enzyme Commission (EC) to study the problem of enzyme nomenclature. Its subsequent recommendations, with periodic updating, provide a rational and practical basis for identifying all enzymes now known and enzymes that will be discovered in the future (http://www.chem.qmw.ac.uk/iubmb/enzyme/accessed May 6, 2011).[11]

With the IUB system, a systematic and trivial name is provided for each enzyme. The systematic name describes the nature of the reaction catalyzed and is associated with a unique numeric code. The trivial or practical name, which may be identical to the systematic name but is often a simplification of it, is suitable for everyday use. The unique numeric designation for each enzyme consists of four numbers, separated by periods (e.g., 2.2.8.11), and is prefixed by the letters *EC*, denoting *Enzyme Commission*. The first number defines the class to which the enzyme belongs. All enzymes are assigned to one of six classes, characterized by the type of reaction they catalyze: (1) oxidoreductases, (2) transferases, (3) hydrolases, (4) lyases, (5) isomerases, and (6) ligases. The next two numbers indicate the subclass and the sub-subclass to which the enzyme is assigned. For example, these may differentiate the amino-transferring subclass from the phosphate-transferring category, or the ethanol acceptor sub-subclass from that accepting acyl groups. The last number is the specific serial number given to each enzyme within its sub-subclass.

To illustrate how this system is used to name an enzyme, consider the enzyme creatine kinase, which catalyzes the following reaction:

$$\text{ATP} + \text{creatine} \rightleftarrows \text{ADP} + \text{creatine phosphate}$$

Its system number is

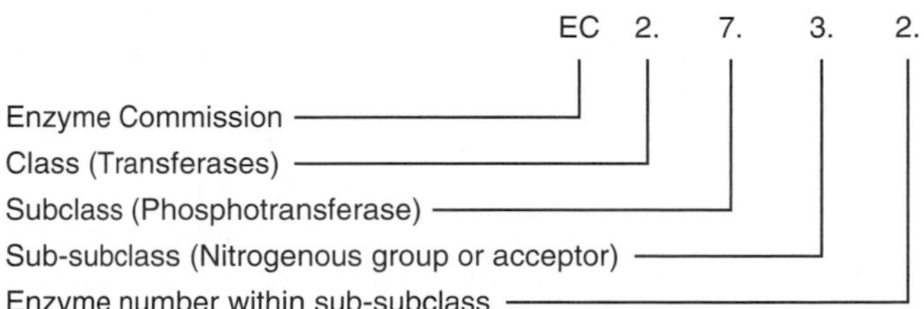

Table 15-1 lists some selected enzymes of clinical interest, identified by trivial, abbreviated, and systematic names and by their code numbers.

Although it is not recommended by the EC, it is a common and convenient practice to use capital letter abbreviations for the names of certain enzymes, such as ALT (formerly GPT) for alanine aminotransferase. Other examples are AST for aspartate aminotransferase, LD for lactate dehydrogenase, and CK for creatine kinase (see Table 15-1).

Enzymes as Proteins

All enzyme molecules possess the primary, secondary, and tertiary structural characteristics of proteins (see Chapter 21).

**The authors gratefully acknowledge the original contributions by Drs. A. Ralph Henderson and Donald W. Moss upon which portions of this chapter are based.*

TABLE 15-1 Enzyme Commission (EC) Numbers, Systematic and Trivial Names, Together With Frequently Adopted Abbreviations of Enzymes of Major Clinical Importance

EC Number	Systematic Name	Trivial Name	Abbreviation
1.1.1.27	L-Lactate: NAD^+ oxidoreductase	Lactate dehydrogenase	LD
1.4.1.3	L-Glutamate: $NAD(P)^+$ oxidoreductase (deaminating)	Glutamate dehydrogenase	GLD
2.3.2.2	(γ-Glutamyl)-peptide: amino acid γ-glutamyltransferase	γ-Glutamyltransferase	GGT
2.6.1.1	L-Aspartate: 2-oxoglutarate aminotransferase	Aspartate aminotransferase (transaminase)	AST
2.6.1.2	L-Alanine: 2-oxoglutarate aminotransferase	Alanine aminotransferase (transaminase)	ALT
2.7.3.2	ATP: creatine *N*-phosphotransferase	Creatine kinase	CK
3.1.1.3	Triacylglycerol acylhydrolase	Lipase	LPS
3.1.1.7	Acetylcholine acetylhydrolase	Acetylcholinesterase, true cholinesterase, choline esterase I	—
3.1.1.8	Acylcholine acylhydrolase	Pseudocholinesterase, butyryl cholinesterase, choline esterase II (serum cholinesterase)	CHE
3.1.3.1	Orthophosphoric-monoester phosphohydrolase (alkaline optimum)	Alkaline phosphatase	ALP
3.1.3.2	Orthophosphoric-monoester phosphohydrolase (acid optimum)	Acid phosphatase	ACP
3.1.3.5	5′-Ribonucleotide phosphohydrolase	5′-Nucleotidase	NTP
3.2.1.1	1,4-α-D-Glucan glucanohydrolase	Amylase	AMY
3.4.21.4		Trypsin	TRY
4.1.2.13	D-Fructose-1,6-bisphosphate D-glyceraldehyde-3-phosphate-lyase	Aldolase	ALD

In addition, most enzymes exhibit quaternary structure. The *primary* structure, the linear sequence of amino acids linked through their α-carboxyl and α-amino groups by peptide bonds, is specific for each type of enzyme molecule. Each polypeptide chain is coiled up into three-dimensional secondary and tertiary structure. *Secondary* structure refers to the conformation of limited segments of the polypeptide chain, namely α-helices, β-pleated sheets, random coils, and β-turns. The arrangement of secondary structural elements and amino acid side chain interactions that define the three-dimensional structure of the folded protein is referred to as its *tertiary* structure. In many cases, biological activity, such as the catalytic activity of enzymes, requires two or more folded polypeptide chains (subunits) to associate to form a functional molecule. The arrangement of these subunits defines the *quaternary* structure. The subunits may be copies of the same polypeptide chain (e.g., the MM isoenzyme of creatine kinase, the H_4 isoenzyme of lactate dehydrogenase), or they may represent distinct polypeptides.

The application of physical methods, such as x-ray crystallography and multidimensional nuclear magnetic resonance (NMR), has provided structural insights upon which enzyme mechanisms have been built. Furthermore, the tools of molecular biology, such as molecular cloning, have enabled the purification and characterization of enzymes that previously were available only in minute amounts. Molecular biology also enables the manipulation of the amino acid sequence of enzymes, and site-directed mutagenesis (substituting one amino acid residue for another) and deletion mutagenesis (eliminating sections of the primary structure) have enabled the identification of chemical groups that participate in ligand binding and in specific chemical steps during catalysis.

In general, no feature of primary structures, such as repetition of particular amino acid sequences, is common to all enzyme molecules. However, considerable homologies of sequence are found between enzymes that appear to share a common evolutionary origin, such as the proteases, trypsin and chymotrypsin, and similarities of sequence are even more marked among the members of a family of isoenzymes. The amino acid sequence in the immediate neighborhood of the active center of the enzyme (discussed later) is often closely similar in enzymes of related function (e.g., the *serine proteases* are so called because they all have this amino acid in the active center).

Enzyme molecules differ in the proportion of secondary structures—such as α-helices—they contain, although no enzyme molecule so far studied approaches the large proportion of α-helices found in myoglobin and hemoglobin. The tertiary structures of different types of enzyme molecules are as individually characteristic as their primary structures;

nevertheless, some common features exist. Enzyme molecules are roughly globular in overall shape, with a preponderance of polar amino acid side chains on the outside of the molecule and nonpolar side chains in the interior. The ionizable residues in contact with the surrounding medium are responsible for many of the properties of the enzyme molecules in solution, such as their migration in an electric field and their solubility. Covalent disulfide bridges may link different parts of the polypeptide chains in some enzyme molecules, but the three-dimensional structure is mainly stabilized by the large number of hydrophobic interactions that are formed between the nonpolar side chains in the interior of the molecule.

The biological activity of a protein molecule depends generally on the integrity of its structure, and any disruption of its structure is accompanied by loss of activity, a process known as *denaturation*. If the process of denaturation is minimal, it may be reversed with the recovery of enzyme activity upon removal of the denaturing agent. However, prolonged or severe denaturing conditions result in an irreversible loss of activity. Denaturing conditions include elevated temperatures, extremes of pH, and chemical addition. Heat inactivation of most enzymes takes place at an appreciable rate at room temperature and in most cases becomes almost instantaneous above 60 °C. The polymerases are an exception and retain activity at temperatures as high as 90 °C—a property that has been made use of in the polymerase chain reaction (see Chapter 17). Low temperatures are used to preserve enzyme activity, especially in aqueous solutions, such as serum (see Chapter 22). Extremes of pH also cause unfolding of enzyme molecular structures and, except for a few exceptions, should be avoided when enzyme samples are preserved. Addition of chemicals, such as urea and detergents, disrupts hydrogen bonds and hydrophobic interactions so that exposure of enzymes to strong solutions of these reagents results in inactivation.

Specificity and the Active Center

With the exception of enzymes such as proteases, nucleases, and amylases, which act on macromolecular substrates, enzyme molecules are considerably larger than the molecules of their substrates. Consideration of the structure of an enzyme's active site and its relationship to the structures of the enzyme's substrate(s) in its ground and transition states is necessary to understand the rate enhancement and specificity of the chemical reactions performed by the enzyme. The active site of an enzyme will vary between enzymes but in general,[5]

1. The active site of an enzyme is relatively small compared with the total volume of the enzyme molecule because its structure may involve less than 5% of the total amino acids in the molecule.
2. The active sites of enzymes are three-dimensional structures that are formed as a result of the overall tertiary structure of the protein. This results when the amino acids and cofactors in the active site of an enzyme are spatially structured in an exact, three-dimensional relationship with respect to one another and the structure of the substrate molecule.
3. Typically, the attraction between the molecules of the enzyme and its substrate molecules is noncovalent binding. Physical forces used in this type of binding include hydrogen bonding, electrostatic and hydrophobic interactions, and van der Waals forces.
4. Active sites of enzymes typically occur in clefts and crevices in the protein. This excludes bulk solvent and reduces the catalytic activity of the enzyme.
5. The specificity of substrate binding is a function of the exact special arrangement of atoms in the enzyme active site that complements the structure of the substrate molecule.

Isoenzymes and Other Multiple Forms of Enzymes

An *isoenzyme* is defined as "one of a group of related enzymes catalyzing the same reaction but having different molecular structures and characterized by varying physical, biochemical, and immunologic properties." However, the IUB recommends that use of the term *isoenzyme* be restricted to forms that originate at the level of the genes that encode the structures of the enzyme proteins in question.[4]

Isoenzymes may occur within a single organ or even within a single type of cell. The forms can be distinguished on the basis of differences in various physical properties, such as electrophoretic mobility and resistance to chemical or thermal inactivation. They often have significant quantifiable differences in catalytic properties, but all forms of a particular enzyme retain the ability to catalyze its characteristic reaction.

The existence of multiple forms of enzymes in human tissue has important implications in the study of human disease. The presence in different organs of isoenzymes with distinctive properties helps in our understanding of organ-specific patterns of metabolism, but genetically determined variations in enzyme structure between individuals account for such characteristics as differences in sensitivity to drugs and differences in metabolism, which manifest themselves as hereditary metabolic diseases. For diagnostic enzymology, the existence of multiple forms of enzymes, whether due to genetic or nongenetic causes, provides opportunities to increase the diagnostic specificity and sensitivity of enzyme assays in body fluid samples.

Similar to other proteins, enzymes usually elicit the production of antibodies when they are injected into animals of a species other than those in which they originate. Even small structural differences between closely similar molecules, such as the members of a family of isoenzymes, are often sufficient to render them antigenically distinct, allowing antibodies to be produced specific to a single type of molecule. The availability of enzyme-specific antisera opens up a wide range of methods in enzyme analysis, some of which—such as immunoassay—do not depend on the catalytic activity of the enzyme molecules. The availability of immunochemical methods has been particularly important in the analysis of isoenzyme mixtures. Many commercial immunoassays now use monoclonal antibodies to increase specificity.

Genetic Origins of Enzyme Variants

True isoenzymes result from the existence of more than one gene locus coding for the structure of the enzyme protein. Many human enzymes (perhaps more than one third) are known to be determined by more than one structural gene locus. Genes at the different loci have undergone differential modifications during the course of evolution, so that the enzyme proteins coded by them no longer have identical structures, although they are recognizably similar; in other words, they are isoenzymes.

The multiple genes that determine a particular group of isoenzymes are not necessarily closely linked on one chromosome. For example, the structural genes that code for human salivary and pancreatic amylases both are located on chromosome 1, whereas the genes that code for cytoplasmic and mitochondrial malate dehydrogenase are carried on chromosomes 2 and 7, respectively. Among the enzymes of clinical importance that exist as isoenzymes because of the presence of multiple-gene loci are lactate dehydrogenase, creatine kinase, α-amylase, and some forms of alkaline phosphatase.

An enzyme can exist in molecular forms that differ from one individual to another because of the existence of alternative alleles that are inherited according to mendelian laws. These give rise to gene products with the same function, and isoenzymes that result from the existence of allelic genes are termed *allozymes.* The proportion of human gene loci subject to allelic variation is considerable, and the probability that individual human beings will differ to some degree in their isoenzyme patterns is correspondingly high.

The number of allelic variants and the frequency with which particular variants occur within the population vary considerably from one enzyme to another. For example, mutations at either of the two principal loci that determine human lactate dehydrogenase are extremely rare, but a high incidence of mutant alleles occurs at the single locus that determines the structure of placental alkaline phosphatase. More than 400 mutations in the glucose-6-phosphate dehydrogenase gene have now been identified on the X chromosome [up-to-date genetic information on this and other enzymes can be obtained from the Online Mendelian Inheritance in Man (OMIM) database at http://www.ncbi.nlm.nih.gov/Omim/searchomim.html/accessed May 6, 2011]. Some of these alleles are extremely rare, whereas others occur with appreciable frequency in particular populations or geographical locations. When isoenzymes, because of variation at a single locus, occur with appreciable frequency in a human population, the population is said to be *polymorphic* with respect to the isoenzymes in question.

Another category of multiple molecular forms can arise when enzymes are oligomeric and consist of molecules made up of subunits. The association of different types of subunits in various combinations gives rise to a range of active enzyme molecules. When the subunits are derived from different structural genes—multiple loci or multiple alleles—the hybrid molecules so formed are called *hybrid isoenzymes.* The ability to form hybrid isoenzymes is evidence of considerable structural similarities between the different subunits. Hybrid isoenzymes can be formed in vitro, but they are also formed in vivo in cells in which different types of constituent subunits are present in the same subcellular compartment.

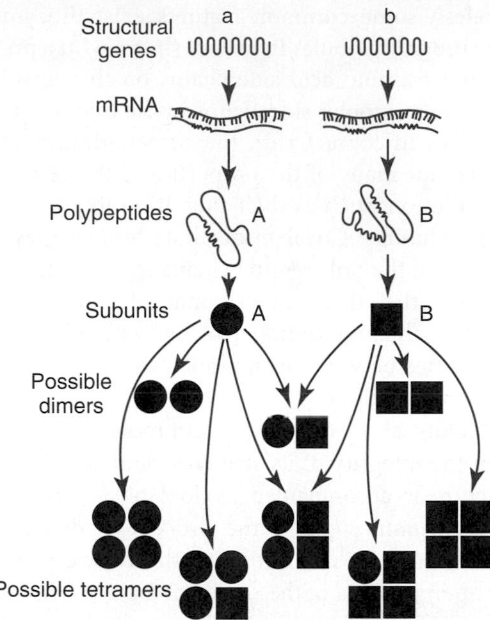

Figure 15-1 Diagram showing the origin of isoenzymes, assuming the existence of two distinct gene loci. When the active enzymes are polymers containing more than one subunit, hybrid isoenzymes consisting of mixtures of different subunits may be formed. One such isoenzyme can be formed in the case of a dimeric enzyme, such as creatine kinase, and three if the enzyme is a tetramer (e.g., lactate dehydrogenase). In both cases, two homopolymeric isoenzymes can also exist. *(From Moss DW. Isoenzyme analysis. London: The Chemical Society, 1979. Reprinted by permission of The Royal Society of Chemistry. Reproduced by permission of The Royal Society of Chemistry.)*

The number of different hybrid isoenzymes that can be formed from two nonidentical protomers depends on the number of subunits in the complete enzyme molecule. For a dimeric enzyme, one mixed dimer (hybrid isoenzyme) can be formed. If the enzyme is a tetramer, three heteropolymeric isoenzymes may be formed (Figure 15-1). Examples of hybrid isoenzymes include the mixed MB dimer of creatine kinase and the three hybrid isoenzymes—LD-2, LD-3, and LD-4—of lactate dehydrogenase.

Nongenetic Causes of Multiple Forms of Enzymes

Post-translational modifications of enzyme molecules give rise to multiple forms known as *isoforms* (Figure 15-2).

Modifications of residues in the polypeptide chains of enzyme molecules takes place in living cells to yield multiple forms. For example, removal of amide groups accounts for some of the heterogeneity of amylase and carbonic anhydrase (each of these enzymes also exists as a true isoenzyme). Modification can also take place as a result of extraction

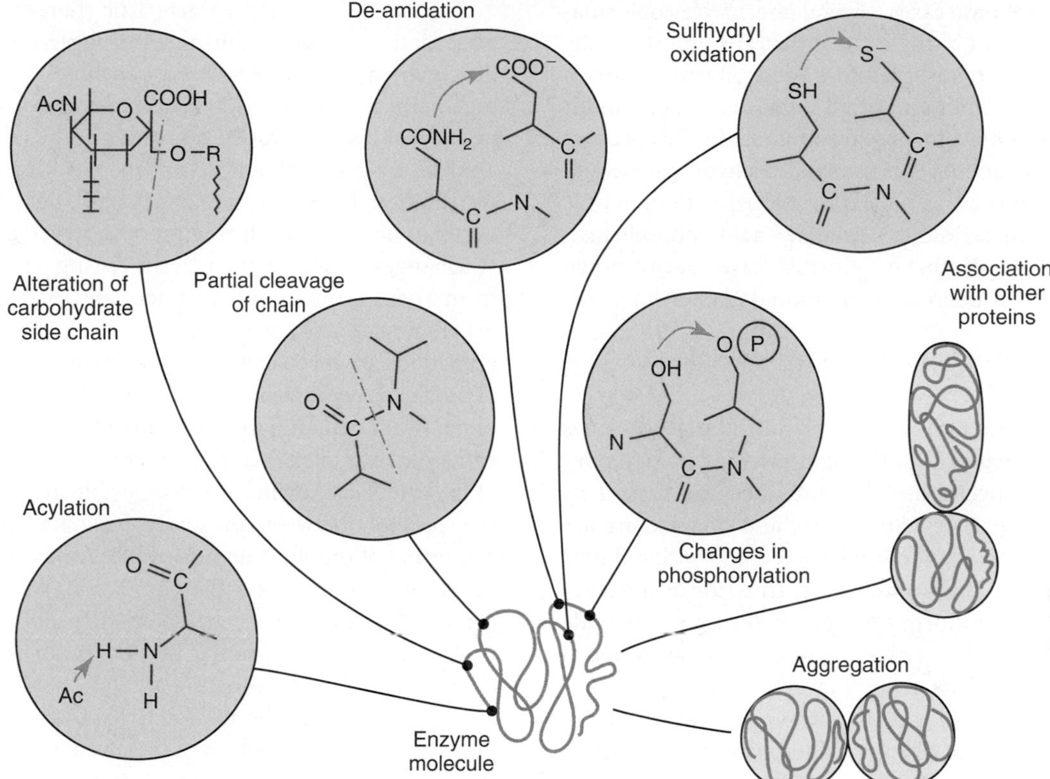

Figure 15-2 Nongenetic modifications that may give rise to multiple forms of enzymes. *(From Moss DW. Isoenzymes. London: Chapman & Hall, 1982.)*

procedures. Many erythrocyte enzymes, including adenosine deaminase, acid phosphatase, and some forms of phosphoglucomutase, contain sulfhydryl groups that are susceptible to oxidation. In hemolysates, oxidation may be brought about by the action of oxidized glutathione, although in intact cells, this compound is present in its reduced form. Thus, variant enzyme molecules with altered molecular charge may be generated.

Serum isoforms of creatine kinase are formed as part of the normal clearance process of the cell. Human myocardial and skeletal muscle tissues have the CK-MM and CK-MB isoenzymes, which are modified upon release into the circulation. This modification is due to sequential removal of the C-terminal amino acid, lysine, by the action of carboxypeptidase (see Chapter 22 for additional details).

Modifications affecting nonprotein components of enzyme molecules may also lead to molecular heterogeneity. Many enzymes are glycoproteins, and variations in carbohydrate side chains are a common cause of nonhomogeneity of preparations of these enzymes. Some carbohydrate moieties, notably *N*-acetylneuraminic acid (sialic acid), are strongly ionized and consequently have a profound effect on some properties of enzyme molecules.[1] For example, removal of terminal sialic acid groups from human liver and/or bone alkaline phosphatase with neuraminidase greatly reduces the electrophoretic heterogeneity of the enzyme.

Aggregation of enzyme molecules with each other or with nonenzymatic proteins may give rise to multiple forms that can be separated by techniques that depend on differences in molecular size. For example, four catalytically active cholinesterase components with molecular weights ranging from about 80,000 to 340,000 are found in most sera, with the heaviest component, C_4, contributing most of the enzyme activity. Other enzyme forms are also occasionally present, but it appears that the principal serum cholinesterase fractions can be attributed to different states of aggregation of a single monomer.

A specific form of interaction between enzymatic and nonenzymatic proteins is the cause of unusual enzyme components noted when some samples of human plasma are fractionated by electrophoresis or chromatography. These components are the result of the combination of apparently normal enzyme or isoenzyme molecules with plasma immunoglobulins. The enzyme–protein complexes *(macrocomplexes)* thus formed may themselves be heterogeneous. Since the identification of *macroamylase,* the first such enzyme–immunoglobulin complex to be identified, similar complexes have been observed involving lactate dehydrogenase, creatine kinase, alkaline phosphatase, and other enzymes.

A single polypeptide chain in theory exists in an infinite number of different conformations. However, one specific conformation generally appears to be the most stable for any given sequence of amino acids, and this conformation is assumed by the chain as it is synthesized within the cell. Thus, the primary structure of the polypeptide chain also determines its three-dimensional secondary and tertiary structures. It is conceivable that in some cases, several alternative conformations ("conformers") of a single chain that are almost equally stablel may be present, and therefore these alternative forms may coexist. This possibility was first suggested to account for the heterogeneity noted in preparations of the cytoplasmic and mitochondrial isoenzymes of malate dehydrogenase and has also been proposed as an explanation for the multiple electrophoretic zones of erythrocyte acid phosphatase. However, no multiple-enzyme forms have been shown unequivocally to be due to conformational isomerism.

Distribution of Isoenzymes and Other Multiple Forms of Enzymes

The existence of multiple-gene loci and the isoenzymes derived from them has presumably conferred an evolutionary advantage on the species and has thus become part of its normal metabolic pattern. Some of these adaptations are related to the division of function between and within different types of specialized cells and tissues. Thus, the distribution of isoenzymes is not uniform throughout the body, and wide variations in the activities of different isoenzymes are found at the organ, cellular, and subcellular levels. Tissue-specific differences are also found in the distributions of some multiple forms of enzymes that are not due to the existence of multiple-gene loci. The tissue-specific distribution of isoenzymes and other multiple forms of enzymes provides the basis for organ-specific diagnosis through isoenzyme measurements.

Certain gene loci may be expressed almost exclusively in a single tissue, perhaps at a particular stage in development. In addition to the two gene loci that determine the two most common subunits of lactate dehydrogenase, a third locus is active only in mature testes. It determines the structure of a third type of subunit, X or C, which makes up a specific isoenzyme, LD-X or LD_C, found only in testes. The isoenzyme of ALP that occurs in the human placenta is the product of a single structural gene locus, which is distinct from the loci that specify the structures of other forms of ALP, and the product of the placental phosphatase locus is normally detectable only in the placenta.

A particularly striking example of the local expression of multiple-gene loci is provided by distinct isoenzymes that occur exclusively in specific subcellular organelles. Differences between mitochondrial isoenzymes and their functionally analogous counterparts in the cytoplasm have been demonstrated in several cases (e.g., for aspartate aminotransferase and malate dehydrogenase).

Changes in Isoenzyme Distribution During Development and Disease

The patterns of several sets of isoenzymes change during normal development in tissues from many species. For example, during the embryonic development of skeletal muscle, the proportions of the electrophoretically more cathodal isoenzymes—both LD and CK—progressively increase in this tissue until approximately the sixth month of intrauterine life, when the pattern resembles that of differentiated muscle.

The liver also shows characteristic changes in the patterns of several isoenzymes during embryogenesis. In early fetal development, three aldolase isoenzymes—A, B, and C—together with various hybrid tetramers, can be detected in extracts of liver. However, at birth as in the adult liver, aldolase B is the predominant isoenzyme. Striking changes in the distribution of isoenzymes of alcohol dehydrogenase also occur in human liver during prenatal development.

Changes in isoenzyme patterns during development result from changes in the relative activities of gene loci within developing cells of a particular type (e.g., muscle cells). Other alterations in the balance of isoenzymes within the whole organism may derive from changes in the number or activity of cells that contain large amounts of a characteristic isoenzyme. An example of this is the increased number and activity of the osteoblasts, which are responsible for mineralization of the skeleton between the early postnatal period and the beginning of the third decade of life. An excess of ALP from active osteoblasts enters the circulation, where its presence can be recognized by its characteristic properties, and where it elevates the total serum ALP activity of young people to above that of skeletally mature adults. An ALP from the liver also contributes to the total activity of this enzyme in the plasma of healthy people, and the amount of this isoenzyme in plasma shows a small, progressive increase with age. The reason for the latter age-dependent change is not known, but it may result from increased synthesis of the isoenzyme by hepatocytes in response to continuing exposure to inducing factors.

Certain diseases, such as the progressive muscular dystrophies, appear to involve failure of the affected tissues to mature normally or to maintain a normal state. Cancer cells show progressive loss of the structure and metabolism of the healthy cells from which they arise. Therefore, the pattern of isoenzymes of mature, differentiated tissue may be lost or modified if normal differentiation is arrested or reversed, and many examples of isoenzyme changes accompanying such processes have been reported.

The distributions of isoenzymes of aldolase, LD, and CK in the muscles of patients with progressive muscular dystrophy have been found to be similar to those in the earlier stages of development of fetal muscle. Isoenzyme abnormalities in dystrophic muscle have been interpreted as failure to reach or maintain a normal degree of differentiation. Isoenzyme patterns seen in regenerating tissues may also show some tendency to approach fetal distributions. This tendency may result from relaxation or modification of control systems in rapidly dividing cells and may account for some of the isoenzyme changes noted (e.g., in muscle in acute polymyositis).

Reemergence of fetal patterns of isoenzyme distribution is a feature of malignant transformation in many tissues. This phenomenon was first studied extensively in the case of lactate dehydrogenase isoenzymes. Malignant tumors in general show a significant shift in the balance of isoenzymes toward electrophoretically more cathodal forms such as LD-4 and LD-5. The decline in activity of the LD-1 and LD-2 isoenzymes results in patterns that are reminiscent of those occurring in embryonic tissues. Tumors of prostate, cervix, breast, brain, stomach, colon, rectum, bronchus, and lymph nodes are among those that show this transformation. In contrast, comparatively benign gliomas show a relative increase in anionic isoenzymes. A relative increase in the proportion of cathodal isoenzymes of LD has also been observed in tissue adjacent to malignant tumors (e.g., the colon), although the cells in these regions are morphologically normal.

Differences in Properties Between Multiple Forms of Enzymes

Structural differences between the multiple forms of an enzyme give rise to greater or lesser differences in physicochemical properties, such as electrophoretic mobility, resistance to inactivation, and solubility, or in catalytic characteristics, such as the ratio of reaction with substrate analogs or response to inhibitors. Methods of isoenzyme analysis have therefore been designed to investigate a wide range of catalytic and structural properties of enzyme molecules.[9] However, it is usually possible to make only limited deductions about the nature of the underlying structural differences between isoenzymes that are responsible for the dissimilar properties. Equally, the changes in catalytic and other properties that may result from specific structural alterations in enzyme molecules are difficult to predict from current theoretical knowledge of the relationship between structure and function of proteins.[22]

Techniques of molecular biology, such as gene cloning and sequencing, have revolutionized the investigation of the primary structures of isoenzymes. Differences in primary structures between isoenzymes, whether derived from multiple-gene loci or from different alleles, are now known to exist in a growing number of cases. Furthermore, many questions have been answered about whether multiple-enzyme forms represented true (genetically determined) isoenzymes or arose from post-translational modification.

Isoenzymes caused by the existence of multiple-gene loci usually differ quantitatively in catalytic properties. These differences may be manifested in such characteristics as molecular activity, K_m values for substrate(s), sensitivity to various inhibitors, and relative rates of activity with substrate analogs (when the specificity of the isoenzymes allows the substrate to be varied), underscoring the biological importance of isoenzymatic variation. In contrast, multiple-enzyme forms that arise by such post-translational modifications as aggregation usually have similar catalytic properties.

Multilocus isoenzymes also usually differ in terms of antigenic specificity, although these differences may be less pronounced among isoenzymes that have emerged relatively recently in evolutionary history and are closely related in structure. Immunological cross-reaction is not uncommon among multilocus isoenzymes. Multiple-enzyme forms caused by postsynthetic modification frequently have common antigenic determinants. Isoenzymes derived from allelic genes (allozymes) are often antigenically similar, even to the extent that they may cross-react with antisera to the common isoenzyme even when a mutation has abolished enzyme activity altogether. The capacity for detecting differences between antigenically similar isoenzyme molecules depends on the extent of monoclonal antibody specificity.

Differences in resistance to denaturation (e.g., by heat, concentrated urea solutions, detergents) are commonly found between true isoenzymes, whether these are the products of multiple loci or multiple alleles. Other multiple forms of enzymes often do not differ or differ only slightly in this respect. The most commonly exploited difference between isoenzymes is the difference in net molecular charge that results from the altered amino acid compositions of the molecules; this forms the basis of separation by zone electrophoresis, ion-exchange chromatography, or isoelectric focusing. Separation methods that depend on differences in molecular size, such as gel filtration, do not distinguish between the small size differences that often exist between true isoenzyme molecules but are important in the detection of multiple forms that involve aggregation or association of enzyme molecules with other proteins.

Enzymes as Catalysts

A *catalyst* is a substance that modifies and increases the rate of a particular chemical reaction without being consumed or permanently altered; enzymes are *protein catalysts* of biological origin. *Metabolism* is a coordinated series of chemical reactions that occur within a living cell to provide energy and accomplish biosynthesis. The process can be regarded as an integrated series of enzymatic reactions, and some diseases as a derangement of the normal pattern of metabolism. Apart from these fundamental considerations, it is the remarkable properties of enzymes that make them such sensitive indicators of pathologic change.

Because of their remarkable catalytic activity, a given number of enzyme molecules convert an enormous number of substrate molecules to products within a short time. This property is used to measure increased amounts of enzymes in the bloodstream, although the amount of enzyme protein released from damaged cells is small compared with the total quantity of nonenzymatic proteins in blood. Thus a change in the quantity of a particular enzyme is recognized by its characteristic effect on a given chemical reaction.

Units for Expressing Enzyme Activity

When enzymes are measured by their catalytic activities, the results of such determinations are expressed in terms of the concentration of the number of activity units present in a convenient volume or mass of specimen. The unit of activity is the measure of the rate at which the reaction proceeds (e.g., the quantity of substrate consumed or product formed in a chosen unit of time). In clinical enzymology, the activity of an enzyme is generally reported in terms of unit of volume, such as activity per 100 mL or per liter of serum or per 1.0 mL of packed erythrocytes. Because the rate of the reaction depends on experimental parameters, such as pH, type of buffer, temperature, nature of substrate, ionic strength, concentration of activators, and other variables, these parameters must be specified in the definition of the unit.

To standardize how enzyme activities are expressed, the EC proposed that the unit of enzyme activity should be defined as the quantity of enzyme that catalyzes the reaction of 1 μmol of substrate per minute, and that this unit should be termed the *international unit* (U). Catalytic concentration is to be expressed in terms of U/L or kU/L, whichever gives the more convenient numeric value. In this chapter, the symbol U is used to denote the international unit. In those instances in which there is some uncertainty about the exact nature of the substrate, or when difficulty is encountered in calculating the number of micromoles reacting (as with macromolecules such as starch, protein, and complex lipids), the unit is to be expressed in terms of the chemical group or residue measured in the following reaction (e.g., glucose units, amino acid units formed).

The International System of Units (SI)-derived unit for catalytic activity (see Chapter 9) is the *katal,* defined as moles converted per second. The name *katal* had been used for this unit for decades but did not become an official SI-derived unit until 1999 with Resolution 12 of the 21st French Conférence Général des Poids et Mesures (CGPM), on the recommendation of the International Federation of Clinical Chemistry and Laboratory Medicine (IFCC). Both the International Union of Pure and Applied Chemistry (IUPAC) and the IUB now recommend that enzyme activity be expressed in moles per second, and that the enzyme concentration be expressed in terms of katals per liter (kat/L).[8] Thus, 1 U = 10^{-6} mol/60 s = 16.7×10^{-9} mol/s, or 1.0 nkat/L = 0.06 U/L.

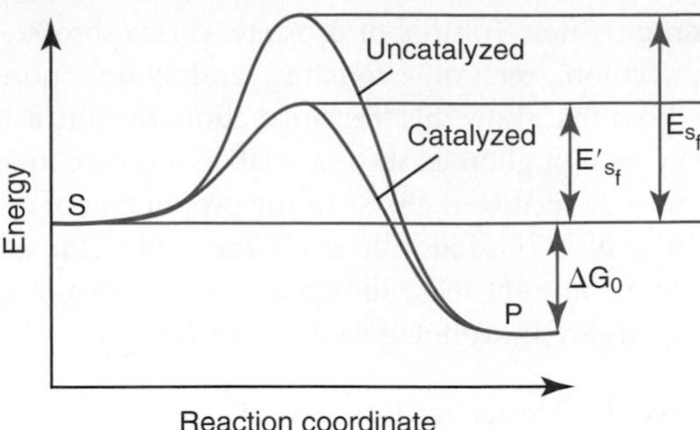

Figure 15-3 Activation energy barrier and reaction course, with and without enzyme catalysis. E_{Sf} is the activation energy for the forward reaction (S → P) in the absence of a catalyst, and E'_{Sf} is the activation energy in the presence of a catalyst. ΔG_0 is the change in free energy for the reaction.

ENZYME KINETICS

The Enzyme–Substrate Complex

Enzymes act through the formation of an enzyme–substrate (*ES*) complex, in which a molecule of substrate is bound to the *active center* of the enzyme molecule. The binding process transforms the substrate molecule to its activated state. The energy required for this transformation is provided by the free energy of binding of *S* to *E.* Therefore, activation takes place without the addition of external energy, so that the energy barrier to the reaction is lowered and the breakdown to products is accelerated (Figure 15-3). The ES complex breaks down to give the reaction products *(P)* and free enzyme *(E)*:

$$E + S \rightleftharpoons ES \longrightarrow P + E \tag{1}$$

All reactions catalyzed by enzymes are in theory reversible. However, in practice, the reaction is usually found to be more rapid in one direction than in the other, so that an equilibrium is reached in which the product of the forward or the backward reaction predominates, sometimes so markedly that the reaction is virtually irreversible.

If the product of the reaction in one direction is removed as it is formed (e.g., because it is the substrate of a second enzyme present in the reaction mixture), the equilibrium of the first enzymatic process will be displaced so that the reaction will proceed to completion in that direction. Reaction sequences in which the product of one enzyme-catalyzed reaction becomes the substrate of the next enzyme and so on, often through many stages, are characteristic of biological processes. In the laboratory also, several enzymatic reactions may be linked together to provide a means of measuring the activity of the first enzyme or the concentration of the initial substrate in the chain. For example, the activity of CK is usually measured by a series of linked reactions, and the concentration of glucose is determined by consecutive reactions catalyzed by hexokinase and glucose-6-phosphate dehydrogenase.

When a secondary enzyme-catalyzed reaction, known as an *indicator reaction,* is used to determine the activity of a different enzyme, the primary reaction catalyzed by the enzyme to be determined must be the rate-limiting step. Conditions are chosen to ensure that the rate of reaction catalyzed by the indicator enzyme is directly proportional to the rate of product formation in the first reaction.

Factors Governing the Rate of Enzyme-Catalyzed Reactions

Factors that affect the rate of enzyme-catalyzed reactions include enzyme and substrate concentration, pH, temperature, and the presence of inhibitors, activators, coenzymes, and prosthetic groups.

Enzyme Concentration

The simplest enzymatically catalyzed reaction for converting substrate S into product P with the intermediate formation of an ES complex is as follows:

$$E_f + S \underset{k_{-1}}{\overset{k_1}{\rightleftharpoons}} ES \xrightarrow{k_2} E_f + P \tag{2}$$

where

E_f = free enzyme
k_1 = rate constant for the association of the complex
k_1 = rate constant for the dissociation of the complex
ES = enzyme–substrate complex
k_2 = rate constant for breakdown of ES to E_f and P
P = product

Michaelis and Menten assumed that equilibrium is attained rapidly among E, S, and ES, with the effect of product formation (ES → P) on the concentration of ES being negligible. In addition, the formation of product is written as an irreversible process because there is no product in the solution under initial conditions. Therefore the overall rate of the reaction under otherwise constant conditions is proportional to the concentration of the ES complex.

Provided that an excess of free substrate molecules is present, addition of more enzyme molecules to the reaction system increases the concentration of the ES complex and thus the overall rate of reaction. This accounts for the observation that the rate of reaction is generally proportional to the concentration of enzyme present in the system and is the basis for the quantitative determination of enzymes by measurement of reaction rates. Reaction conditions are selected to ensure that the observed reaction rate is proportional to enzyme concentration over as wide a range as possible.

Substrate Concentration

In addition to explaining the dependence of reaction rate on enzyme concentration under conditions in which excess substrate is present, the formation of an ES complex accounts for the hyperbolic relationship between reaction velocity and substrate concentration (Figure 15-4). In this section, single-substrate, two-substrate, and consecutive enzyme reactions will be discussed.

Single-Substrate Reactions

If the enzyme concentration is fixed and the substrate concentration is varied, the rate of reaction is first order with respect to substrate concentration and proportional to substrate concentration at low values of the latter. Under these conditions, only a fraction of the enzyme is associated with substrate, and the rate observed reflects the low concentration of the ES complex. At high substrate concentrations, variation in substrate concentration has no effect on rate, and the reaction is zero order with respect to substrate concentration. Under these conditions, all the enzyme is bound to the substrate, and a much higher rate of reaction is obtained. Moreover, because all the enzyme is now present in the form of the complex, no further increase in complex concentration and no further increment in reaction rate are possible. The maximum possible velocity for the reaction has been reached. The significance of substrate-rate curves was first emphasized by Michaelis and Menten, and such curves are referred to as *Michaelis-Menten plots.*

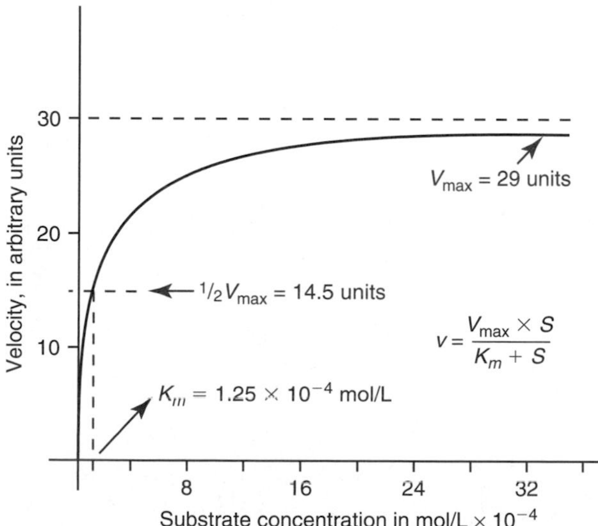

Figure 15-4 Michaelis-Menten curve relating velocity (rate) of an enzyme-catalyzed reaction to substrate concentration. The value of K_m is given by the substrate concentration at which one half of the maximum velocity is obtained.

Referring again to equation (2), the overall rate of the reaction (v) is determined by the rate at which product is formed:

$$v = \frac{d[P]}{dt} = k_2[ES] \tag{3}$$

The formation of ES will depend on the rate constant k_1 and the availability of enzyme and substrate. If it its assumed the system is in a steady state with the ES complex being formed and broken down at the same rate so that overall $[ES]$ is constant, then the steady-state equation is

$$k_1[E][S] = k_{-1}[ES] + k_2[ES] \tag{4}$$

This equation can be rearranged to

$$[ES] = \frac{k_1[E][S]}{k_{-1} + k_2} \tag{5}$$

when these rate constants are combined into a single term; writing the Michaelis constant (K_m) as

$$K_m = \frac{k_{-1} + k_2}{k_1} \tag{6}$$

and then substituting this into equation (5) gives

$$[ES] = \frac{[E][S]}{K_m} \tag{7}$$

Because the total amount of enzyme in the system does not change,

$$[E_t] = [ES] + [E] \tag{8}$$

and upon substituting equation (3) into equation (7) and eliminating (ES) using equation (8),

$$v = k_2 \times \frac{[E_t] \times [S]}{K_m + [S]} \tag{9}$$

For a given amount of enzyme, the maximum reaction velocity (V_{max}) is reached when all of the enzyme is saturated with substrate (i.e., $[ES]$ = $[Et]$), and therefore, $V_{max} = k_2 \times [Et]$. Substituting this in equation (9) gives

$$v = \frac{V_{max}[S]}{K_m + [S]} \tag{10}$$

A plot of v against $[S]$ gives a section of a rectangular hyperbola (see Figure 15-4), and this is the shape of the curve that is found experimentally for most enzymes. When $[S] = K_m$, it can be shown with manipulation of equation (10) that K_m is the substrate concentration at which the reaction proceeds at one half of its maximum velocity. In practice, it is now customary to restrict K_m to the experimentally determined substrate concentration at which $v = 0.5V_{max}$ and to use the symbol K_s to represent the true ES association constant, where this is known.

Although it is simple to set up an experiment to determine the variation of v with $[S]$, the exact value of V_{max} is not easily determined from hyperbolic curves. Furthermore, many enzymes deviate from ideal behavior at high substrate concentrations and indeed may be inhibited by excess substrate, so the calculated value of V_{max} cannot be achieved in practice. In the past, it was common practice to transform the Michaelis-Menten equation (10) into one of several reciprocal forms [equations (11) and (12)], and either $1/v$ was plotted against $1/[S]$, or $[S]/v$ was plotted against $[S]$.

$$\frac{1}{v} = \left(\frac{K_m}{V_{max}} \times \frac{1}{[S]}\right) + \frac{1}{V_{max}} \quad (11)$$

$$\frac{[S]}{v} = \left(\frac{1}{V_{max}} \times [S]\right) + \frac{K_m}{V_{max}} \quad (12)$$

Equation (11), for example, when plotted, results in a *Lineweaver-Burk* plot that gives a straight line with intercepts at $1/V_{max}$ on the ordinate and $-1/K_m$ on the abscissa. For illustrative purposes, the data for Figure 15-4 are replotted in Lineweaver-Burk form in Figure 15-5.

It is now routine practice to determine kinetic constants such as K_m and V_{max} using a software package. A large number of such packages are available; these vary from specialized routines for kinetic simulations or for data fitting to general mathematical, statistical, or graphical packages (http://med.umich.edu/biochem/enzresources/software.ttm/ accessed March 30, 2011). These packages are free (public domain, shareware, or free license) or are commercially available. An example of the former is the ENCORA 1.2 freeware package available from R.J.W. Slats and colleagues at the Delft University of Technology (http://www.bt.tudelft.nl/ http://med.umich.edu/biochem/enzresources/software.ttm/ accessed March 30, 2011), which was developed for an enzymatic kinetic parameter fitting using progressive curve analysis. DynaFit is an example of a commercially available routine (http://www.biokin.com/dynafit/accessed March 30, 2011) that performs nonlinear least-squares regression of chemical kinetic, enzyme kinetic, or ligand receptor binding data. The data can be initial reaction velocities for different concentrations of varied species (e.g., inhibitor concentration vs. velocity), or reaction progress curves (e.g., time vs. absorbance). SigmaPlot 11 is another example of commercially available software that will compute and plot enzyme kinetic data (http://www.sigmaplot.com/products/sigmaplot/enzyme-mod.php/accessed March 30, 2011).

The value of K_s has been used to compare the binding of homologous or related substrates to the same enzyme. Also, if measured against the same substrate under defined conditions, the K_m value can be used to compare the properties of similar enzymes from different sources. Isoenzymes

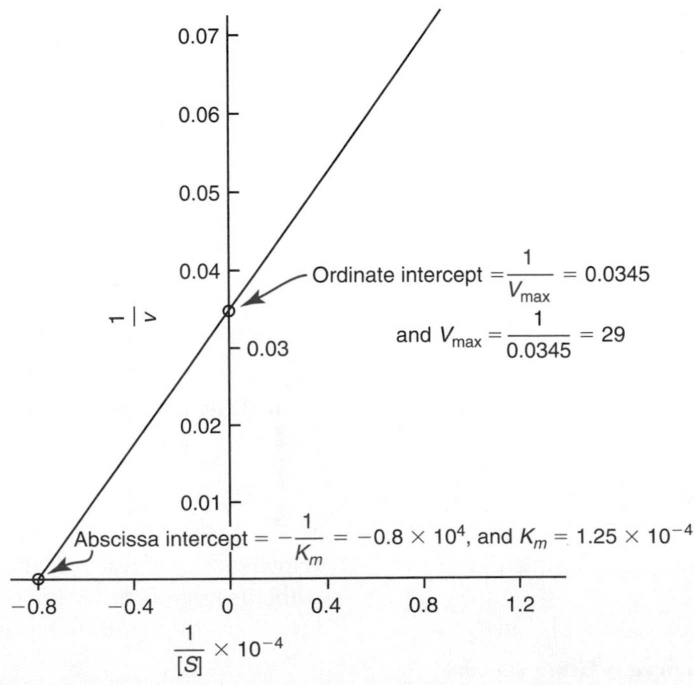

Figure 15-5 Lineweaver-Burk transformation of the curve in Figure 15-4, with $1/v$ plotted on the ordinate (y-axis), and $1/[S]$ on the abscissa (x-axis). The indicated intercepts permit calculation of V_{max} and K_m. The units of v and $[S]$ are those given in Figure 15-4.

determined by distinct genetic loci typically differ in their K_m (e.g., for the isoenzymes of lactate dehydrogenase).

When setting up methods of enzyme assay, it is necessary to (1) explore the relationship between reaction velocity and substrate concentration over a wide range, (2) determine K_m, and (3) detect any inhibition at high substrate concentrations. Zero-order kinetics is maintained if the substrate is present in large excess (i.e., concentrations at least 10 and preferably 100 times that of the value of K_m). When $[S] = 10 \times K_m$, v is approximately 91% of the theoretical V_{max}. The K_m values for the majority of enzymes are on the order of 10^{-5} to 10^{-3} mol/L; therefore substrate concentrations are usually chosen to be in the range of 0.001 to 0.10 mol/L. On occasion, the optimal concentrations of substrate cannot be used (e.g., when the substrate has limited solubility, or when the concentration of a given substrate inhibits the activity of another enzyme needed in a coupled reaction system).

Two-Substrate Reactions

Most enzymes catalyze reactions with two or more interacting substrates symbolized by the following equation:

$$\underset{S_1}{Substrate\ 1} + \underset{S_2}{Substrate\ 2} \overset{E}{\rightleftharpoons} \underset{P_1}{Product\ 1} + \underset{P_2}{Product\ 2} \quad \textbf{(13)}$$

When one of the substrates is water (i.e., when the process is one of hydrolysis), with the reaction taking place in aqueous solution, only a fraction of the total number of water molecules present participates in the reaction. The small change in the concentration of water has no effect on the rate of reaction and these pseudo-one substrate reactions are described by one-substrate kinetics. More generally, the concentrations of both substrates may be variable, and both may affect the rate of reaction. Among the bisubstrate reactions important in clinical enzymology are the reactions catalyzed by dehydrogenases, in which the second substrate is a specific coenzyme, such as the oxidized or reduced forms of nicotinamide adenine dinucleotide (NADH), or nicotinamide adenine dinucleotide phosphate (NADPH), and the amino-group transfers catalyzed by the aminotransferases.

If a bisubstrate reaction proceeds by way of intermediate ES complexes, so that

$$E + S_1 \rightleftharpoons ES_1 \quad \textbf{(14)}$$

followed by

$$ES_1 + S_2 \rightleftharpoons ES_1S_2 \longrightarrow P_1 + P_2 + E \quad \textbf{(15)}$$

and if S_1 and S_2 combine with separate sites on the enzyme molecule, the rate of reaction is given by

$$v = \frac{V_{max} \times [S_1][S_2]}{[S_1][S_2] + [S_2]K_m^1 + [S_1]K_m^2 + K_S^1 K_m^2} \quad \textbf{(16)}$$

K^1_m and K^2_m are the K_m values for the two substrates, and $[S_1]$ and $[S_2]$ are their concentrations. K^1_s is the equilibrium constant for the reversible reaction between the enzyme and S_1. If the equation is rearranged into the double reciprocal form

$$\frac{1}{v} = \frac{1}{[S_1]}\left(\frac{K_m^1}{V_{max}} + \frac{K_m^2 K_S^1}{[S_2]V_{max}}\right) + \frac{1}{V_{max}}\left(1 + \frac{K_m^2}{[S_2]}\right) \quad \textbf{(17)}$$

a plot of $1/v$ against $1/[S_1]$ gives a straight line, but both the slope of the line and its intercept on the ordinate are dependent on $[S_2]$, the concentration of the second substrate (Figure 15-6, *A*). Similarly, a plot of $1/v$ against $1/[S_2]$ is rectilinear but with the slope and intercept dependent on $[S_1]$.

Values of K_m and V_{max} for each substrate are derived from experiments in which the concentration of the first substrate is held constant at saturating quantities while the concentration of the second substrate is varied, and vice versa. There is no reason why the K_m values for the two substrates should be the same or even similar (e.g., pyruvate and NADH, the two-substrate pair in the reaction catalyzed by lactate dehydrogenase of beef heart, have K_m values of 2×10^{-5} mol/L and 3×10^{-6} mol/L, respectively).

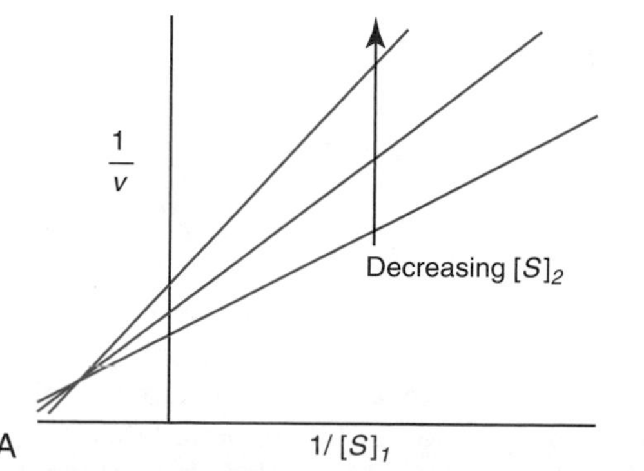

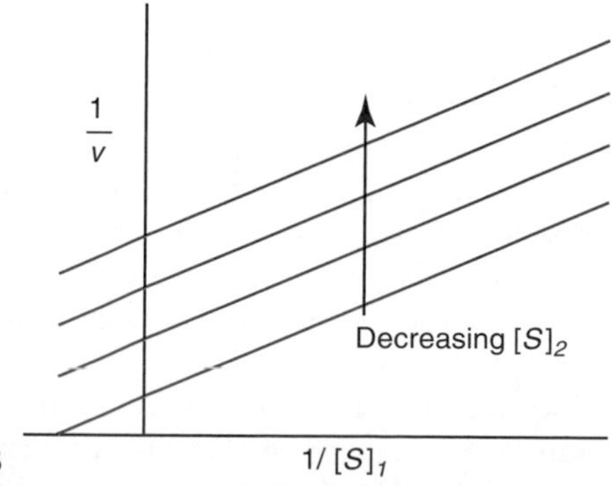

Figure 15-6 Double-reciprocal plots of 1/v against 1/[S₁] for two-substrate reactions, showing the effect of falling concentration of the second substrate, [S₂]. A, In a dehydrogenase reaction in which a ternary complex is formed. B, In a *ping-pong bi-bi* reaction mechanism (e.g., aminotransferase) in which no ternary complex is formed. *(From Moss DW. Measurement of enzymes. In: Hearse DJ, de Leiris J, eds. Enzymes in cardiology: diagnosis and research. New York: John Wiley & Sons Inc, 1979. Reprinted by permission of John Wiley & Sons, Inc.)*

In some bisubstrate reactions, no ternary complex ES_1S_2 is formed, because the binding of the first substrate is followed by release of the first product before the second substrate is bound and the second product is released. This sequence is described as a *ping-pong bi-bi* type of reaction. It occurs in reactions catalyzed by aminotransferases.

The relationship between reaction velocity and the concentrations of the two substrates in *ping-pong bi-bi* reactions reduces to the form

$$v = \frac{V_{max} \times [S_1][S_2]}{[S_1][S_2] + [S_2]K_m^1 + [S_1]K_m^2} \quad \textbf{(18)}$$

The reciprocals of v and $[S_1]$ are related by the equation

$$\frac{1}{v} = \frac{1}{[S_1]} \times \frac{K_m^1}{V_{max}} + \frac{1}{V_{max}}\left(1 + \frac{K_m^2}{[S_2]}\right) \quad \textbf{(19)}$$

so that a plot of $1/v$ against $1/[S_1]$ is unchanged in slope by variation in $[S_2]$, but the intercept on the ordinate and therefore the value of V_{max} changes as $[S_2]$ is varied (see Figure 15-6, *B*). Similar equations describe the variation of V_{max} with $[S_1]$ when $1/v$ is plotted as a function of $1/[S_2]$.

The selection of reaction conditions for the measurement of enzymatic activity involving two substrates is approached empirically by varying the concentration of the first substrate and keeping the concentration of the second substrate constant until maximum activity is reached. The process is then repeated with the concentration of the first substrate held at the value thus determined, while the concentration of the second substrate is varied.

In practice, the choice of substrate concentrations is limited by such considerations as the solubility of the substrates, the viscosity and initial absorbance of concentrated solutions, and the relative costs of the reagents. Furthermore, the selection of appropriate substrate concentrations is only one of the factors to be considered in formulating an optimal assay system for the measurement of a specific enzyme activity. Critical choices must also be made with respect to other, frequently interdependent factors that affect reaction rate, such as the concentrations of activators and the nature and pH of the buffer system.

Consecutive Enzymatic Reactions

As discussed previously, an enzymatic reaction is usually found to be more rapid in one direction than the other, so that the reaction is essentially irreversible. If the product of the reaction in one direction is removed as it is formed (i.e., because it is the substrate of a second enzyme present in the reaction mixture), the equilibrium of the first enzymatic process is displaced so that the reaction may continue to completion in that direction. Reaction sequences in which the product of one enzyme-catalyzed reaction becomes the substrate of another enzyme, often through many stages, are characteristic of metabolic processes. Analytically, as indicated earlier, several enzymatic reactions also may be linked together to provide a means of measuring the activity of the first enzyme or the concentration of the initial substrate in the chain.

When a linked enzyme assay, known as an *indicator reaction,* is used to determine the activity of a different enzyme, it is essential that the primary reaction be the rate-limiting step. For example, in the determination of aspartate aminotransferase activity, the indicator reaction is the reduction of the 2-oxoglutarate formed in the aminotransferase reaction to malate by malate dehydrogenase and NADH. The activity of the indicator enzyme must be sufficient to ensure the virtually instantaneous removal of the product of the first reaction so as to prevent significant reversal of the first reaction. The measured enzyme typically is acting under conditions of saturation with respect to its substrate; however, the concentration of the substrate of the indicator enzyme (i.e., the product of the first reaction) remains in the region of the Michaelis-Menten curve in which v is directly proportional to $[S]$. Therefore the rate of reaction catalyzed by the indicator enzyme is directly proportional to the rate of product formation in the first reaction.

During a lag period that occurs after the start of the first reaction, the concentration of its product reaches a steady state. Because the rate of the second reaction depends on the activity of the indicator enzyme and on the concentration of its substrate (the product of the primary reaction), the duration of the lag period is reduced by increasing the concentration of the indicator enzyme, thus lowering the steady-state concentration of the product of the primary reaction.

The rate of the indicator reaction, v_i, is related to substrate concentration and therefore to the product concentration $[P]$ by the Michaelis-Menten equation

$$v_i = \frac{V_{max}^i \times [P]}{[P] + K_m^i} \quad \textbf{(20)}$$

in which V^i_{max} and K^i_m are the maximum velocity and K_m of the indicator enzyme, respectively. For the rate of the indicator reaction not to be the rate limiting factor, v_i must at least equal the limiting velocity of the primary reaction, v_t, which the assay system is expected to measure. Therefore, the minimum activity of indicator enzyme needed is given by

$$v_t = \frac{V_{max}^i \times [P]}{[P] + K_m^i} \quad \textbf{(21)}$$

or is rearranged as

$$V_{max}^i = v_t\left(1 + \frac{K_m^i}{[P]}\right) \quad \textbf{(22)}$$

The ratio of activities of the indicator and primary enzymes varies from one assay method to another, depending on (1) the range of activity measured, (2) the K_m of the indicator enzyme, and (3) the lag period that is considered acceptable. Nevertheless the catalytic concentration of the indicator enzyme in the reaction mixture must always be much greater than that of the enzyme being determined.

Effect of pH

The rate of enzyme-catalyzed reactions typically shows a marked dependence on pH (Figure 15-7). Many of the

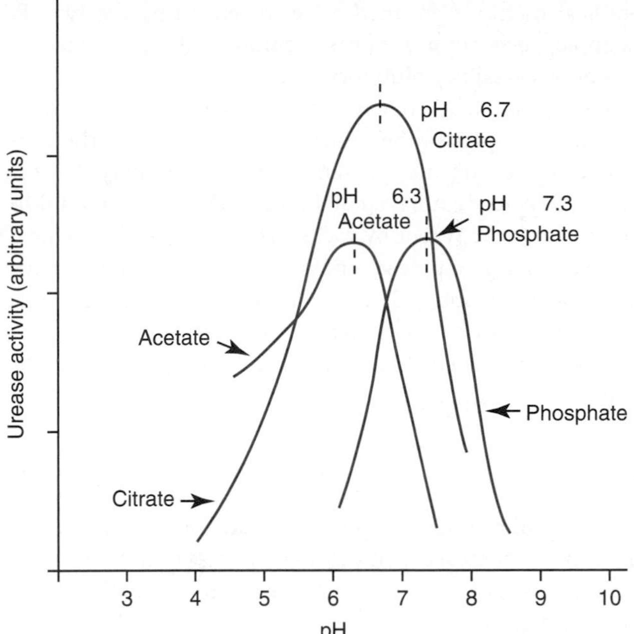

Figure 15-7 The pH activity curves for urease show the effects of buffer species on pH optimum. *(Modified from Howell SF, Sumner JB. The specific effects of buffers upon urease activity. J Biol Chem 1934;104:619.)*

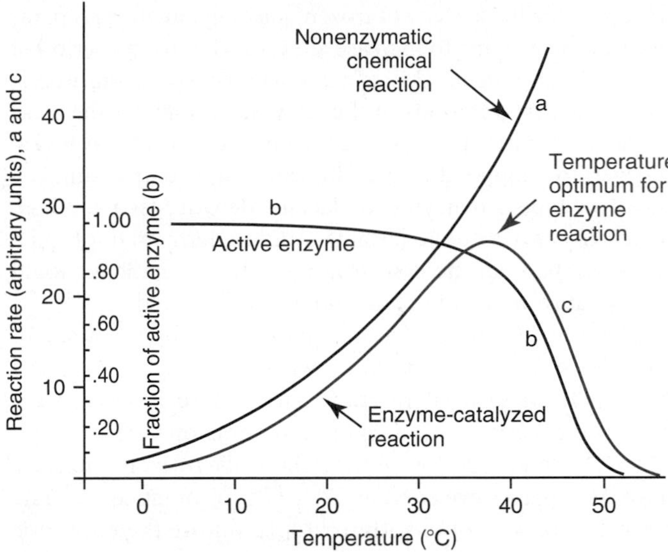

Figure 15-8 Schematic diagram showing effects of temperature on the rate of non–enzyme-catalyzed and enzyme-catalyzed reactions.

enzymes in blood plasma show maximum activity in vitro in the pH range from 7 to 8. However, activity has been observed at pH values as low as 1.5 (pepsin) and as high as 10.5 (ALP). The optimal pH for a given forward reaction may be different from the optimal pH found for the corresponding reverse reaction. The form of the pH-dependence curve is the result of a number of separate effects, including ionization of the substrate and the extent of dissociation of certain key amino acid side chains in the protein molecule, both at the active center and elsewhere in the molecule. Both pH and ionic environment will also have an effect on the three-dimensional conformation of the protein and therefore on enzyme activity to such an extent that enzymes may be irreversibly denatured at extreme values of pH.

The pronounced effects of pH on enzyme reactions emphasize the need to control this variable by means of adequate buffer solutions. Enzyme assays should be carried out at the pH of optimal activity, because the pH-activity curve has its minimum slope near this pH, and a small variation in pH will cause a minimal change in enzyme activity. The buffer system must be capable of counteracting the effect of adding the specimen (e.g., serum itself is a powerful buffer) to the assay system, as well as the effects of acids or bases formed during the reaction (e.g., formation of fatty acids by the action of lipase). Because buffers have their maximum buffering capacity close to their pK_a values, whenever possible a buffer system should be chosen with a pK_a value within 1 pH unit of the desired pH of the assay (see Chapter 11). Interaction between buffer ions and other components of the assay system (e.g., activating metal ions) may eliminate certain buffers from consideration.

Temperature

The rate of an enzymatic reaction is proportional to its reaction temperature. For most enzymatic reactions, values of Q_{10} (the relative reaction rates at two temperatures differing by 10 °C) vary from 1.7 to 2.5. However, an increase in the rate of the catalyzed reaction is not the only effect of increasing temperature on an enzymatic reaction. In theory, the initial rate of reaction measured instantaneously will increase with a rising temperature. In practice, however, a finite time is needed to allow the components of the reaction mixture, including the enzyme solution, to reach temperature equilibrium and to permit the formation of a measurable amount of the product. During this period, the enzyme is undergoing thermal inactivation and denaturation, a process that has a very large temperature coefficient for most enzymes and thus becomes virtually instantaneous at temperatures of 60 to 70 °C. The counteracting effects of the increased rate of the catalyzed reaction and more rapid enzyme inactivation as the temperature increases account for the existence of an apparent *optimal temperature* for enzyme activity (Figure 15-8).

As stated earlier, at some critical temperature, an enzyme will undergo thermal inactivation influenced by a number of factors. These include the presence of substrate and its concentration, the pH, and the nature and ionic strength of the buffer. The presence of other proteins, as in serum samples, may help to stabilize enzymes. Storage of serum samples at low temperatures is necessary to minimize loss of enzyme activity while awaiting analysis, although repeated freezing and thawing should be avoided. However, individual enzymes vary in their stability characteristics, and appropriate storage conditions vary correspondingly. Amylase, for example, is stable at room temperature (22 to 25 °C) for 24 hours, whereas acid phosphatase is exceedingly unstable, even when refrigerated, unless kept at a pH below 6.0. ALP exhibits an unusual property: the tendency for the activity of frozen, partially purified preparations of the enzyme to increase after thawing over a period of 24 hours or longer. This effect is shared by reconstituted, lyophilized preparations of the enzyme and affects their use for quality control purposes. A few enzymes are inactivated at refrigerator temperatures; a clinically important example is the liver-type isoenzyme of lactate dehydrogenase, LD-5, which appears to be less stable at lower temperatures. As a result, sera for lactate dehydrogenase determinations should be kept at room temperature and not refrigerated.

Historically, the choice of temperature for the assay of enzymes of clinical importance was the subject of extensive debate. The choice of reaction temperature has become a nonissue because most analytical systems operate at 37 °C. Reference methods for several clinically relevant enzymes have now been developed at 37 °C.[14-21] In practice, accurate temperature control to within ±0.1 °C during the enzymatic reaction is essential.

Inhibitors and Activators

The rates of enzymatic reactions are often affected by substances other than the enzyme or substrate. These modifiers may be inhibitors because their presence reduces the reaction rate, or activators because they increase the rate of reaction. Activators and inhibitors are usually small molecules (compared with the enzyme itself) or even ions. They vary in specificity from modifiers that exert similar effects on a wide range of different enzymatic reactions at one extreme, to substances that affect only a single reaction. Reagents, such as strong acids or multivalent anions and cations that denature or precipitate proteins, destroy enzyme activity and thus may be regarded as extreme examples of nonspecific enzyme inhibitors. These effects usually are not included in discussions of enzyme inhibition, although they have obvious practical implications in the treatment and storage of specimens in which enzyme activity is to be measured. The activity of some enzymes depends on the presence of particular chemical groups, such as reduced sulfhydryl (–SH) groups, in the active center. Reagents that alter these groups (e.g., oxidants of SH groups) therefore act as general inhibitors of such enzymes.

Some phenomena of enzyme activation or inhibition are caused by interactions between the modifier and a nonenzymatic component of the reaction system, such as the substrate (e.g., Mg^{2+} combining with ATP to form MgATP, the required substrate for the creatine kinase reaction). In most cases, however, the modifier combines with the enzyme itself in a manner analogous to the combination of enzyme and substrate.

Inhibition of Enzyme Activity

Inhibitors are classified as reversible or irreversible. *Reversible inhibition* implies that the activity of the enzyme is fully restored when the inhibitor is removed from the system in which the enzyme acts by some physical separative process, such as dialysis, gel filtration, or chromatography. An *irreversible inhibitor* combines covalently with the enzyme so that physical methods are ineffective in separating the two. For example, organophosphorous compounds are extremely potent irreversible inhibitors of esterases, including acetylcholinesterase. The enzyme breaks one of the bonds in the inhibitor, but part of the molecule is left bound to the active center of the enzyme, preventing further activity. In some cases, enzymes that have combined with irreversible inhibitors can be reactivated by a chemical reaction that removes the blocking group (e.g., the phosphoryl enzymes formed with organophosphorous compounds sometimes can be reactivated by treatment with oximes or hydroxamic acids).

Reversible Inhibition. Reversible inhibition is characterized by the existence of equilibrium between enzyme, *E*, and inhibitor, *I*:

$$E + I \rightleftharpoons EI \tag{23}$$

The equilibrium constant of the reaction, K_i (the *inhibitor constant*), is a measure of the affinity of the inhibitor for the enzyme, just as K_m generally reflects the affinity of the enzyme for its substrate.

A *competitive* inhibitor is usually a structural analog of the substrate that can combine with the free enzyme in such a way that it competes with the normal substrate for binding at the active site. The actual rate of the reaction is strictly dependent on the relative concentrations of substrate and inhibitor. Two equilibriums are therefore possible:

$$E + S \rightleftharpoons ES \longrightarrow E + Products \tag{24}$$

and

$$E + I \rightleftharpoons EI \tag{25}$$

The equation that relates the observed reaction velocity to the concentrations of substrate, [*S*], and inhibitor, [*I*], is as follows:

$$v = \frac{V_{max}[S]}{[S] + K_m\left(1 + \frac{[I]}{K_i}\right)} \tag{26}$$

This is the Michaelis-Menten equation, but with K_m modified by a term including the inhibitor concentration and the inhibitor constant, V_{max} is unaltered. Therefore, curves of v against [*S*] in the presence and absence of inhibitor reach the same limiting value at high substrate concentrations, but when the inhibitor is present, K_m is apparently greater. Plots of $1/v$ against $1/[S]$ with and without inhibitor intersect the ordinate at the same point but have different slopes and intercepts on the abscissa (Figure 15-9).

Competitive inhibition is responsible for the inhibition of some enzymes by excess substrate because of competition between substrate molecules for a single binding site. In two-substrate reactions, high concentrations of the second substrate may compete with binding of the first substrate. For example, aspartate aminotransferase is inhibited by excess concentrations of the substrate 2-oxoglutarate, and this inhibition is competitive with respect to L-aspartate. Therefore, to maintain a given velocity at high 2-oxoglutarate concentrations, the concentration of L-aspartate has to be

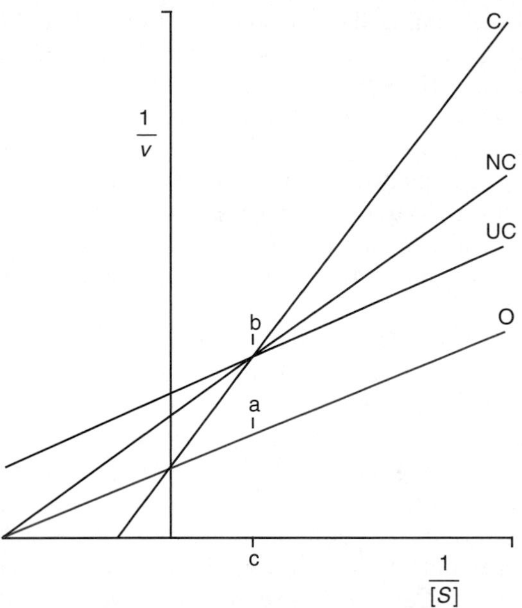

Figure 15-9 Effects of different types of inhibitors on the double-reciprocal plot of 1/v against 1/[S]. Each of the inhibitors has been assumed to reduce the activity of the enzyme by the same amount, represented by the change in 1/v from *a* to *b* at a substrate concentration of *c*. Line O is the plot for enzyme without inhibitor, C with a competitive inhibitor, NC with a noncompetitive inhibitor, and UC with an uncompetitive inhibitor. *(From Moss DW. Measurement of enzymes. In: Hearse DJ, de Leiris J, eds. Enzymes in cardiology: diagnosis and research. New York: John Wiley & Sons Inc., 1979. Reprinted by permission of John Wiley & Sons, Inc.)*

increased above the value needed at lower concentrations of 2-oxoglutarate.

Competitive inhibition also contributes to the reduction in the rate of an enzymatic reaction over time. For example, a rate reduction can occur because increasing concentrations of reaction products tend to drive the reaction backward, if it is freely reversible. A product may itself be an inhibitor of the forward reaction, so even if the reaction is not readily reversible, it proceeds against a rising concentration of inhibitor. A familiar example of *product inhibition* is the release of the competitive inhibitor, inorganic phosphate, by the action of ALP on its substrates. In this case, both organic phosphates and inorganic phosphates bind to the active center of the enzyme with similar affinities (i.e., K_m and K_i are of the same order of magnitude).

Product inhibition is a cause of nonlinearity of reaction progress curves during fixed-time methods of enzyme assay. For example, oxaloacetate produced by the action of aspartate aminotransferase inhibits the enzyme, particularly the mitochondrial isoenzyme. The inhibitory product may be removed as it is formed by a coupled enzymatic reaction: malate dehydrogenase converts the oxaloacetate to malate and at the same time oxidizes NADH to NAD^+.

Competitive inhibition by metal ions occurs when two metal ions compete for the same binding site on the enzyme. Sodium and lithium are potent inhibitors of pyruvate kinase, for which potassium is an obligatory activator.

A *noncompetitive* inhibitor is usually structurally different from the substrate. It is assumed to bind at a site on the enzyme molecule that is different from the substrate-binding site; thus, there is no competition between inhibitor and substrate, and a ternary enzyme–substrate–inhibitor (ESI) complex is formed. Attachment of the inhibitor to the enzyme does not alter the affinity of the enzyme for its substrate (i.e., K_m is unaltered), but the ESI complex does not break down to give products. Because the substrate does not compete with the inhibitor for binding sites on the enzyme molecule, increasing the substrate concentration does not overcome the effect of a noncompetitive inhibitor. Thus, V_{max} is reduced in the presence of such an inhibitor, whereas K_m is not altered, as the Lineweaver-Burk plot shows (see Figure 15-9).

Uncompetitive inhibition is produced by a combination of the inhibitor with the ES complex. It is more common in two-substrate reactions, in which a ternary ESI complex forms after the first substrate has combined with the enzyme. In uncompetitive inhibition, parallel lines are obtained when plots of $1/v$ against $1/[S]$ with and without the inhibitor are compared (see Figure 15-9), that is, both K_m and V_{max} are decreased.

Irreversible Inhibition. Irreversible inhibitors render the enzyme molecule inactive by covalently and permanently modifying a functional group required for catalysis. An irreversible inhibitor is not in equilibrium with the enzyme. Its effect is progressive with time, becoming complete if the amount of inhibitor present exceeds the total amount of enzyme. The rate of the reaction between enzyme and inhibitor is expressed as the fraction of the enzyme activity that is inhibited in a fixed time by a given concentration of inhibitor. The velocity constant of the reaction of the inhibitor with the enzyme is a measure of the effectiveness of the inhibitor.

When the inhibitor is added to the enzyme in the presence of its substrate, the reaction between the enzyme and the inhibitor may be delayed because some of the enzyme molecules are combined with the substrate and are therefore protected from reacting with the inhibitor. However, as the substrate molecules react chemically, the active centers become available, and inhibition eventually will become complete, even though an excess of substrate may have been present initially. Furthermore, the addition of more substrate is ineffective in reversing the inhibition in contrast to its effect on reversible competitive inhibition.

Irreversible inhibitors have been useful in mapping active sites by covalently modifying different types of functional groups in the enzyme molecule to establish whether such groups are necessary for catalytic activity.

A physiologically important category of irreversible enzyme inhibition is exemplified by various trypsin inhibitors. These are proteins that bind to trypsin irreversibly, nullifying its proteolytic activity. One such inhibitor is present in the α_1-globulin fraction of serum proteins; others are found in soybeans and lima beans. Similar proteolysis inhibitors present in plasma prevent the accumulation of excess thrombin and other coagulation enzymes, thus keeping the coagulation process under control.

Inhibition by Antibodies. The combination of enzyme molecules with specific antibodies often has no effect on catalytic activity, which is retained by the enzyme–antibody complex.[2] However, in some cases, the reaction of the enzyme and antibody reduces or even abolishes enzymatic activity. The most probable explanation for this type of inhibition is that the antibody molecule restricts access of the substrate molecules to the active center by steric hindrance or, in extreme cases, completely masks the substrate-binding site. However, it appears that some examples of enzyme inhibition by combination with antibodies are caused by a conformational change induced in the enzyme molecule.

Inhibition of the activity of an enzyme molecule labeled with a hapten (e.g., morphine) as a result of combination with a specific antibody forms the basis for a homogeneous enzyme immunoassay (EMIT, Siemens Healthcare Diagnostics, Deerfield, Ill; http://www.medical.siemens.com/accessed March 30, 2011). See Chapter 16 for additional details.

Enzyme Activation

Activators increase the rates of enzyme-catalyzed reactions by promoting formation of the most active state of the enzyme itself or of other reactants, such as the substrate. This generalization covers a wide variety of mechanisms of activation.

Many enzymes contain metal ions as an integral part of their structures (e.g., zinc in ALP and carboxypeptidase A). The function of the metal may be to stabilize tertiary and quaternary protein structures. Removal of divalent metal ions by treatment with an appropriate quantity of ethylenediaminetetraacetic acid (EDTA) solution is accompanied by conformational changes and inactivation of the enzyme. The enzyme often can be reactivated by dialysis against a solution of the appropriate metal ion or simply by addition of the ion to the reaction mixture. Reactivation may take some time, because rearrangement of polypeptide chains into the active conformation is not instantaneous.

When the activator ion is an essential part of the functional enzyme molecule, whether as a purely structural element or with an additional catalytic role, it is usually incorporated quite firmly into the enzyme molecule. Therefore it is not usually necessary to add the activator to reaction mixtures, and an excess of the ion may even have an inhibitory effect. However, in some cases, the activating ion is attached only weakly or transiently to the enzyme (or its substrate) during catalysis. Enzyme samples therefore may be deficient in the ion, so that addition of the ion increases the reaction rate or indeed may be essential for the reaction to take place. For example, all phosphate transfer enzymes (kinases), such as creatine kinase, require the essential presence of Mg^{2+} ions. Other common activating cations are Mn^{2+}, Fe^{2+}, Ca^{2+}, Zn^{2+}, and K^+. More rarely, anions may act as activators. Amylase functions at its maximal rate only if Cl^- or other monovalent anions, such as Br^- or NO_3^-, are present. Addition of 5 mmol/L of chloride increases amylase activity almost threefold, at the same time shifting the pH optimum from 6.5 to 7.0. The chloride ion may combine with a positively charged group in the enzyme, changing the ionization constant of a group important in catalysis. However, other anions—such as bromide—are less effective activators of amylase, so some degree of specificity is involved in the process of activation. Some enzymes require the obligate presence of two activating ions. K^+ and Mg^{2+} are essential for the activity of pyruvate kinase, and both Mg^{2+} and Zn^{2+} are required for ALP activity.

The velocity of the reaction depends on the concentration of a reversible activator in a fashion similar to its dependence on substrate concentration, and an activator constant, K_a, analogous to K_m, can be determined from data relating enzyme activity to increasing activator concentration in the presence of excess substrate. The simplest interpretation of K_a is that it is the dissociation constant of the equilibrium between E and the activator, A. However, this is true only when the combination of enzyme and activator is independent of the reaction between E and S, and the same value for K_a is obtained at all concentrations of the substrate. If the free enzyme and the enzyme–substrate complex have different affinities for the activator, the value for K_a varies with $[S]$.

Apparent activation of an enzyme may be observed whenever a substance that can counteract the presence of some inhibiting agent is added.

Coenzymes and Prosthetic Groups

Coenzymes are usually more complex molecules than activators, although they are smaller molecules than the enzyme proteins themselves. Some compounds, such as the dinucleotides NAD and NADP, are classified as coenzymes and are specific substrates in two-substrate reactions. Their effects on the rate of reaction follow the Michaelis-Menten pattern of dependence on substrate concentration. The structures of these two coenzymes are identical except for the presence of an additional phosphate group in NADP; nevertheless, individual dehydrogenases, for which these coenzymes are substrates, are predominantly or even absolutely specific for one or the other form.

Coenzymes such as NAD and NADP are bound only momentarily to the enzyme during the course of the reaction, as is the case for substrates in general. Therefore no reaction takes place unless the appropriate coenzyme is present in solution (e.g., by adding it to the reaction mixture in the assay of dehydrogenase activity). In contrast to these entirely soluble coenzymes, some coenzymes are more or less permanently bound to the enzyme molecules, where they form part of the active center and undergo cycles of chemical change during the reaction. When bound, the coenzyme is known as a prosthetic group.

The active *holoenzyme* results from the combination of the inactive *apoenzyme* with the *prosthetic group.* An example of a prosthetic group is pyridoxal-5′-phosphate (P-5′-P), a component of AST and ALT. The P-5′-P prosthetic group undergoes a cycle of conversion of the pyridoxal moiety to pyridoxamine and back again during the transfer of an amino group from an amino acid to an oxo-acid. Prosthetic groups, such as activators with a structural role, do not usually have to be added to elicit full catalytic activity of the enzyme unless previous treatment has caused the prosthetic group to be lost from some enzyme molecules. However, both normal and pathologic serum samples contain appreciable quantities of apo-aminotransferases, which are converted to active holoenzymes through a suitable period of incubation with P-5′-P.

A study of the formulas of coenzyme and prosthetic groups shows that many contain structures derived from the vitamins (see Chapter 31). Thus, the nicotinamide portion of NAD and NADP derives from the vitamin niacin, whereas the P-5′-P prosthetic group of the aminotransferases is a derivative of pyridoxine, vitamin B_6. Other derivatives of the B-group vitamins participate in enzymatic reactions.

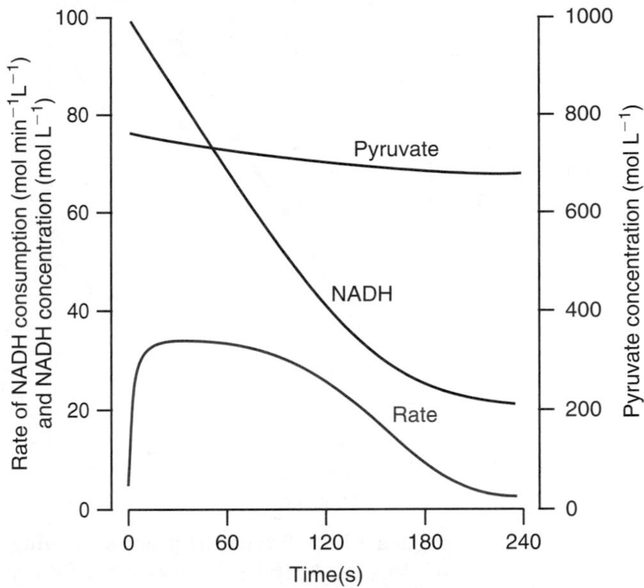

Figure 15-10 Changes in substrate concentrations and rates of reaction during an assay of lactate dehydrogenase activity at 37 °C in phosphate buffer, with pyruvate and nicotinamide adenine dinucleotide (NADH) as substrates. The reaction is followed by observing the fall in absorbance at 340 nm as NADH is oxidized to NAD^+. The rate of reaction rises rapidly to a maximum value, from which it declines only slightly until about half the NADH has been used up. During this phase of the reaction, the rate is essentially zero order with respect to substrate concentration. At the point at which the rate falls below about 90% of its maximum value, NADH concentration is approximately 10 × K_m. The K_m for NADH is on the order of 5 × 10^{-6} mol/L, whereas for pyruvate it is 9 × 10^{-5} mol/L. Thus an initial pyruvate concentration approximately 10 times that of NADH is used. (Concentrations are per liter of reaction mixture.) *(From Moss DW. Measurement of enzymes. In: Hearse DJ, de Leiris J, eds. Enzymes in cardiology: diagnosis and research. New York: John Wiley & Sons Inc., 1979. Reprinted by permission of John Wiley & Sons, Inc.)*

ANALYTICAL ENZYMOLOGY

Analytically, the clinical laboratorian is concerned with measuring the activity or mass in serum or plasma of enzymes that are predominantly intracellular and that are physiologically present in the serum in low concentrations only. By measuring changes in the concentrations of these enzymes in disease, it is possible to infer the location and nature of pathologic changes in the tissues of the body.

Measurement of Reaction Rates

The rate of an enzyme-catalyzed reaction is directly proportional to the amount of active enzyme present in the system. Consequently, determination of the rate of reaction under defined and controlled conditions provides a measurement of the amount of enzyme in a sample such as serum.

Determination of reaction rate involves the kinetic measurement of the amount of change produced within a defined time interval.[6,23A] Both *fixed-time* and *continuous-monitoring* methods are used to measure reaction rates. In the fixed-time method, the amount of change produced by the enzyme is measured after the reaction is stopped at the end of a fixed-time interval. In the continuous-monitoring method, the progress of the reaction is monitored continuously. These two methods have different advantages and limitations. To appreciate them, it is necessary to consider the way in which the rate of an enzymatic reaction varies with time.

The progress of conversion of the substrate into products in the presence of an enzyme is monitored by measuring the decreasing concentration of the substrate or the increasing concentration of the products. Measurement of product formation is preferable, as determination of the increase in concentration of a substance above an initially zero or low concentration is analytically more reliable than measurement of a decline from an initially high concentration.

At the moment when the enzyme and the substrate are mixed, the rate of the reaction is zero. The rate then typically rises rapidly to a maximum value, which remains constant for a period of time (Figure 15-10). During the period of constant reaction rate, the rate depends only on enzyme concentration and is completely independent of substrate concentration. The reaction is said to follow zero-order kinetics, because its rate is proportional to the zero power of the substrate concentration. Ultimately, however, as more substrate is consumed, the reaction rate declines and enters a phase of first-order dependence on substrate concentration. Other factors that contribute to the decline in reaction rate include accumulation of products that may be inhibitory, the growing importance of the reverse reaction, and even enzyme denaturation. Although it is possible to compare the rates of reaction produced by different amounts of an enzyme under first-order conditions, it is obviously easier to standardize such comparisons when the enzyme concentration is the only variable that influences the reaction rate. Therefore, enzyme assays are usually made under conditions that are initially saturating with respect to substrate concentration. The rate of reaction during the zero-order phase is determined by

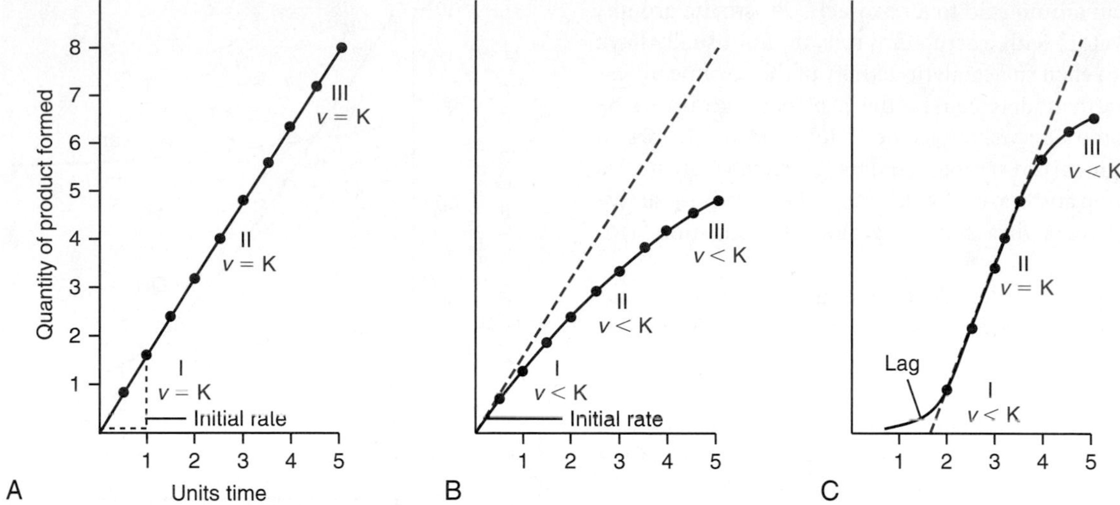

Figure 15-11 Forms of graphs showing change in enzyme reaction rate as a function of time. In A, the rate is constant during the entire run, and rates calculated as *I, II,* and *III* will be identical to the initial rate. In B, the rate falls off continuously; rates calculated at *I, II,* and *III* will be different and less than the true initial rate. In C, a measurement at *II* will be representative of the maximum rate, but at *I* (lag period) and *III* (substrate depletion), it will be less than at *II*.

measuring the product formed during a fixed period of incubation where the rate remains constant. This is illustrated in Figure 15-11. Measurement of reaction rates at any portion of curve A gives results that are identical to the true *initial rate.* However, curve B deviates from linearity over its entire course, and rates fall off with time. From curve C, correct results are obtained only if the rate is measured along segment II. Incorrect results are obtained if the rate is measured during the lag phase (I) or during phase III.

Careful selection of reaction conditions, such as the concentrations of substrates and cofactors, improves the reaction progress curves, eliminating lag phases and prolonging the period of linearity, so that fixed-time methods of analysis become feasible. Improvements in optical techniques, leading to more reliable and sensitive measurement of product formation, have also allowed the duration of incubation to be shortened compared with older assays. This has resulted in a corresponding increase in the interval over which enzyme activity is measured. Nevertheless, an upper limit of activity exists in all fixed-time methods, above which progress curves will no longer be linear. In this case, the amount of change measured over the fixed-time interval no longer represents true zero-order rate conditions.

The upper limit of activity acceptable in the unmodified method must be chosen so that samples with activities below it are presumed with a high degree of certainty to give linear progress curves; alternatively, if the limit is set too low, many samples will be reanalyzed unnecessarily. Samples that are above the limit should ideally be reassayed by shortening the incubation period until a constant reaction rate is obtained. However, this is difficult or impossible in some automated methods, in which the duration of incubation is fixed by the configuration of the apparatus. It then becomes necessary to dilute the specimen; however, dilution may not always result in a proportional change in activity.

The initial rate of reaction theoretically increases without limit as enzyme concentration increases, as long as no other factor, such as substrate concentration, becomes limiting. In practice, the reaction rate becomes so rapid at high enzyme activities that it is impossible to measure the initial rate of reaction, even with continuous-monitoring methods. Therefore, an upper limit of activity that is measurable without modification of the assay procedure exists even in continuous-monitoring methods, but this limit is usually much higher than that applicable in corresponding fixed-time methods. Fewer samples therefore require special treatment. Furthermore, continuous monitoring allows identification of the appropriate zero-order portion of the progress curve for each sample and identification of samples that require special treatment. Continuous-monitoring methods therefore provide a decisive advantage in enzyme assay and should be used whenever possible.

Measurement of Substrates

The amount of substrate transformed into products during an enzyme-catalyzed reaction can be measured with any appropriate analytical method, such as spectrophotometry, fluorometry, or chemiluminescence.[8A] For example, if an enzyme reaction is accompanied by a change in the absorbance characteristics of some component of the assay system, in the visible or ultraviolet spectrum, it can be photometrically observed while it is proceeding. *Self-indicating* reactions of this type are particularly valuable, as they allow continuous monitoring. Important examples of self-indicating reactions are determination of dehydrogenase activity by monitoring the change in absorbance at 339 (340) nm of the coenzyme NADH or NADPH during oxidation or reduction, and measurement of ALP activity by the generation of the yellow *p*-nitrophenolate ion from the substrate *p*-nitrophenyl phosphate in alkaline solution. These indicator reactions are so versatile that coupled reactions are frequently used to provide an observable optical change accompanying a primary reaction in which such a change is not present.

The introduction of prism or diffraction-grating spectrophotometers capable of isolating a narrow beam of monochromatic light in the ultraviolet or visible spectrum and with stable and sensitive photomultipliers as detectors has greatly improved the reproducibility of photometric measurements (see Chapter 10). Consequently, it is customary to make use of the known molar absorptivity of well-defined reaction products (such as NADH) when calculating changes in their concentrations based on measurements made with spectrophotometers. However, the absorbance and wavelength accuracy of the spectrophotometer should be checked regularly. (See Chapter 10 for details on validating the performance of a spectrophotometer.)

Optimization, Standardization, and Quality Control

To measure enzyme activity reliably, all factors that affect the reaction rate—other than the concentration of active enzyme—need to be optimized and rigidly controlled. Furthermore, because the reaction velocity is at or near its maximum under optimal conditions, a larger analytical signal is obtained that can be more accurately and precisely measured than a smaller signal obtained under suboptimal conditions. Much effort therefore has been devoted to determining optimal conditions for measuring the activities of enzymes of clinical importance.

Optimization

Optimization of reaction conditions for enzyme assays traditionally has been carried out by varying a single factor and studying its effect on the reaction rate, then repeating the experiment with a second factor and so on, until effects of all the variables have been tested. An optimal combination of variables is selected on the basis of these experiments, and the validity of the chosen conditions is verified. Not only is this approach labor intensive, it also is difficult to adapt in situations in which the effects of different variables are interdependent, as is frequently the case in enzyme analysis. This traditional empirical approach to optimization has been replaced by newer techniques of simplex co-optimization and response-surface methodology.[13]

Standardization

Despite considerable effort, the goal of a single universally used procedure to measure the catalytic activity of a given enzyme has not been achieved. Consequently, current enzyme standardization efforts are focused on the development of a system that allows comparability of test results, independent of the measurement method. To achieve this, a "reference system" based on the concepts of metrologic traceability and on the hierarchy of analytical methods has been proposed.[7,12,24] A reference procedure and certified reference materials form the basis of the metrological traceability chain (Figure 15-12).[1,3] As part of this hierarchy, reference procedures at 37 °C for the most common enzymes have been developed, and a group of reference laboratories are being selected to perform enzyme measurements at an appropriately high metrologic level.[14-21]

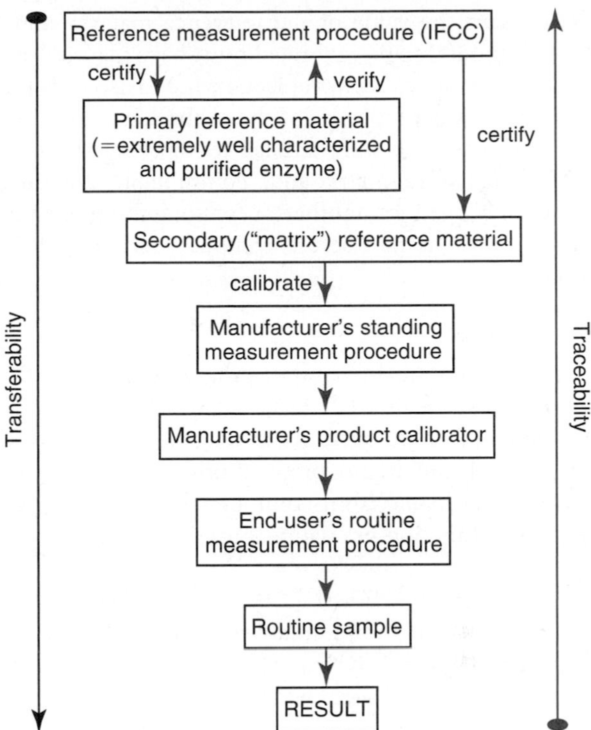

Figure 15-12 The proposed reference system for enzyme measurement showing the traceability of the laboratory result to the reference measurement procedure. *(From Panteghini M, Ceriotti F, Schumann G, Siekmann L. Establishing a reference system in clinical enzymology. Clin Chem Lab Med 2001;39:795-800. Reprinted with permission of Walter de Gruyter.)*

Reference procedures set standards of precision and accuracy against which the relative performance of methods intended for routine use are judged. The reference procedure is used to assign a certified value to the reference material. This certified material is then used by the manufacturers to assign values to commercial calibrators, resulting in traceability of the value obtained in the laboratory.

Several studies have demonstrated that enzyme preparations with reproducible properties and purity and having assured stability can be made. These may be derived from animal sources in which the enzymes closely resemble their human counterparts, although new possibilities have been created by gene-transfer and recombinant techniques.

For a reference system to be capable of standardizing the results of different assays of a given enzyme activity, some conditions must be satisfied.[10] First, the reference procedure used to assign the value of the reference material and the routine method(s) to be calibrated must have identical specificities for the analyte enzyme isoenzyme or isoform under study. Second, the properties of the calibrator material must be the same as or closely similar to those of the analyte enzyme in its natural matrix and, "commutable" and capable of being exchanged for another or for something else that is equivalent with human serum samples for that particular method.

Quality Control

The application of quality control programs is as essential in enzyme analysis as in other forms of clinical analysis if the results obtained are to be useful in diagnosis and treatment.

Lyophilized and liquid preparations containing various enzymes are available from commercial sources, and these have a useful function in quality control.

Measurement of Enzyme Mass Concentration

Many immunoassays for human enzymes and isoenzymes measuring protein mass instead of catalytic activity have been described. To develop such assays, purified enzyme protein has to be prepared to (1) act as a calibrator, (2) be labeled, and (3) be used to raise the enzyme-specific antibody. These methods identify all molecules with the antigenic determinants necessary for recognition by the antibody, so that inactive enzyme molecules that are immunologically unaltered are measured along with active molecules. This has been found to be significant in the determination of some digestive enzymes, such as trypsin, when inactive precursors and inhibitors of catalytic activity are present in plasma. In the majority of cases, however, no degradation or changes in the active enzyme occur in blood so that the clinical equivalence of the different measurement approaches (i.e., estimation of catalytic activity and mass concentration) is obtained.

Immunoassays typically are not used for determination of total activities for the more important diagnostic enzymes, as these assays generally cannot compete in terms of speed, precision, and cost with automated measurements of catalytic activity. Furthermore, several enzyme activities in serum are due to mixtures of immunologically distinct forms, so an assay using a single type of antibody usually determines only one of the enzyme forms. However, this disadvantage in the determination of total enzyme activity becomes a marked advantage in the measurement of specific isoenzymes and isoforms, and immunologic methods have assumed great importance in isoenzyme analysis for diagnostic purposes.

Enzymes as Analytical Reagents

Enzymes are used as analytical reagents for the measurement of several metabolites and substrates and in immunoassays to detect and quantify immunologic reactions.

Measurement of Metabolites

The use of enzymes as analytical reagents to measure metabolites frequently offers the advantage of great specificity for the substance being determined. This high specificity typically removes the need for preliminary separation or purification stages, so the analysis can be carried out directly on complex mixtures such as serum. Uricase (urate oxidase), urease, and glucose oxidase are examples of highly specific enzymes used in clinically important assays, such as the measurement of uric acid, urea, and glucose in biological fluids. However, high specificity cannot always be achieved in practice, and knowledge of the substrate specificities of reagent enzymes is therefore essential to allow possible interferences with the assay to be anticipated and corrected. Coupled reactions are often used to construct an enzymatic analytical system for determining a particular compound. An example of this is the determination of glucose by the hexokinase reaction. Hexokinase converts sugars other than glucose to their 6-phosphate esters. However, the indicator reaction used to monitor this change is catalyzed by glucose-6-phosphate dehydrogenase, an enzyme that is highly specific for its substrate; so the overall process is highly specific for glucose.

In practice, both equilibrium and kinetic (rate) methods have been developed that use enzymes as reagents.[23]

Equilibrium Methods

Most assays used to determine the amount of a substance enzymatically are allowed to continue to completion, so that all substrate has been converted into a measurable product. These methods are called *end point* or, more correctly, *equilibrium* methods, because the reaction ceases when equilibrium is reached. Reactions in which the equilibrium point corresponds virtually to complete conversion of the substrate are obviously preferable for this type of analysis. However, an unfavorable equilibrium can often be displaced in the desired direction by additional enzymatic or nonenzymatic reactions that convert or "trap" a product of the first reaction (e.g., in measuring lactate with lactate dehydrogenase, the pyruvate formed can be trapped by the addition of hydrazine, with which it forms an irreversible hydrazone).

Theoretically, the time required to transform a fixed quantity, Q, of substrate into products is inversely proportional to the amount of enzyme, $[E]$, present:

$$Q = k_1 + [E] \times t \qquad \textbf{(27)}$$

and

$$[E] = \frac{Q}{k_1} \times \frac{1}{t} \qquad \textbf{(28)}$$

where k_1 is the rate constant and t is the elapsed time. Equilibrium methods therefore may require the use of appreciable amounts of enzyme for each sample, to avoid inconveniently long incubation periods. As the substrate concentration falls to low quantities toward the end of the reaction, the K_m of the enzyme becomes important in determining the reaction rate. Enzymes with high affinities for their substrates (low K_m values) therefore are most suitable for equilibrium analysis. Equilibrium methods are largely insensitive to minor changes in reaction conditions. It is not necessary to have exactly the same amount of enzyme in each reaction mixture or to maintain the pH or temperature absolutely constant, provided that the variations are not so great that the reaction is not completed within the fixed time allowed.

Kinetic Methods

First-order or pseudo–first-order reactions are the most important reactions for the kinetic determination of substrate concentration. For any first-order reaction, the substrate concentration $[S]$ at a given time t after the start of the reaction is given by

$$[S]=[S_0]\times e^{-kt} \tag{29}$$

where $[S_0]$ is the initial substrate concentration, e is the base of the natural log, and k is the rate constant.

The change in substrate concentration $\Delta[S]$ over a fixed-time interval, t_1 to t_2, is related to $[S_0]$ by the equation

$$[S_0]=\frac{-\Delta[S]}{e^{-kt_1}-e^{kt_2}} \tag{30}$$

As this equation indicates, the change in substrate concentration over a fixed-time interval is directly proportional to its initial concentration. This is a general property of first-order reactions.

For an enzymatic reaction, first-order kinetics is followed when $[S]$ is small compared with K_m. Thus,

$$v=\frac{V_{\max}}{K_m}\times[S] \tag{31}$$

or

$$v=k[S] \tag{32}$$

Therefore, the first-order rate constant, k, is equal to $\frac{V_{\max}}{K_m}$.

Methods in which some property related to substrate concentration (such as absorbance, fluorescence, chemiluminescence, etc.) is measured at two fixed times during the course of the reaction are known as *two-point* kinetic methods. Theoretically, they are most accurate for the enzymatic determination of substrates. However, these methods are technically more demanding than equilibrium methods, and all factors that affect reaction rate, such as pH, temperature, and amount of enzyme, must be kept constant from one assay to the next, as must the timing of the two measurements. These conditions can readily be achieved in automatic analyzers. A reference solution of the analyte (substrate) must be used for calibration. To ensure first-order reaction conditions, the substrate concentration must be low compared with the K_m (i.e., on the order of less than $0.2 \times K_m$). Enzymes with high K_m values therefore are preferred for kinetic analysis to obtain a wider usable range of substrate concentrations.

Immunoassay

In enzyme immunoassay, enzyme-labeled antibodies or antigens first are allowed to react with ligand; then an enzyme substrate is added. Enzymes such as (1) ALP, (2) horseradish peroxidase, (3) glucose-6-phosphate dehydrogenase, and (4) β-galactosidase all have been used as enzyme labels. A modification of this methodology is the enzyme-linked immunoabsorbent assay (ELISA), in which one of the reaction components is bound to a solid-phase surface. In this technique, an aliquot of sample is allowed to interact with the solid-phase antibody. After washing, a second antibody labeled with enzyme is added to form an Ab–Ag–Ab–enzyme complex. Excess free enzyme–labeled antibody then is washed away, and the substrate is added; the conversion of substrate is proportional to the quantity of antigen. In immunoassays, it is not the specificity of labeled enzymes that is important, but their sensitivity.

Analytical Applications of Immobilized Enzymes

For some types of enzymatic analyses, enzyme consumption is reduced by the use of immobilized enzymes that are reused for several analyses. Immobilized enzymes have been chemically bonded to adsorbents, such as (1) microcrystalline cellulose,(2) diethylaminoethyl (DEAE) cellulose, (3) carboxymethyl cellulose, and (4) agarose. Diazo, triazine, and azide groups are used to join the enzyme protein to the insoluble matrix, forming particles in contact with the substrate solution or a surface in contact with substrate solution, such as a membrane or a coating on the inner surface of a vessel holding the substrate solution. Among enzymes available in such immobilized form are (1) urease, (2) hexokinase, (3) α-amylase, (4) glucose oxidase, (5) trypsin, and (6) leucine aminopeptidase. Stability to heat and other forms of inactivation is considerably increased compared with enzymes in solution. Immobilized proteolytic enzymes are not subject to autodigestion. However, some properties of the enzyme, such as its K_m or its pH optimum, may be altered.

Electrochemical techniques such as (1) potentiometry, (2) polarography, and (3) microcalorimetry have been chosen in exploiting the benefits of immobilized enzymes (see Chapter 11). Enzymes incorporated into membranes form part of enzyme electrodes. The surface of an ion-sensitive electrode is coated with a layer of porous gel in which an enzyme has been polymerized. When the electrode is immersed in a solution of the appropriate substrate, the action of the enzyme produces ions to which the electrode is sensitive. For example, an oxygen electrode coated with a layer containing glucose oxidase has been used to determine glucose from the amount of oxygen consumed in the reaction. Urea has been estimated by the combination of a selective ammonium ion–sensitive electrode and a urease membrane.

Measurement of Isoenzymes and Isoforms

A number of analytical techniques have been used to measure isoenzymes or isoforms. They include (1) electrophoresis (see Chapter 12), (2) chromatography (see Chapter 13), (3) chemical inactivation, and (4) differences in catalytic properties, but the most widely used methods are now based on immunochemical methods.

Electrophoresis

Various forms of electrophoresis have been used to separate isoenzymes, but generally they are not used routinely because they are time-consuming, difficult to quantify, and relatively expensive. Isoelectric focusing (see Chapter 12) has been used successfully to separate isoforms that differ in the amount of covalently bound sugar residues, such as sialic acid.

Chromatography

Ion-exchange chromatography makes use of differences in net molecular charge at a given pH to separate isoenzymes. A typical ion-exchange material is DEAE cellulose, in which ionizable DEAE groups are attached to an inert cellulose matrix. Ion-exchange chromatography is not in general as highly resolving of closely similar proteins as is zone electrophoresis, but relatively large quantities of proteins can be separated with good recovery of enzymatic activity, so the method is of great value in enzyme purification.

Other forms of chromatography that have been applied to fractionation of isoenzyme mixtures include high-performance liquid chromatography (HPLC) and affinity chromatography. The latter makes use of differences between isoenzymes in their affinities for a specific ligand that is attached to an inert insoluble support used as the stationary phase in a chromatography column or in a batch technique.

Chemical Inactivation and Differences in Catalytic Properties

Selective inactivation under controlled conditions has been used in isoenzyme characterization. The method is based on differences in stability that result from small changes in the structure of protein molecules. Elevated temperatures or concentrated solutions of urea or other reagents were used to denature the enzyme. Rates of enzyme inactivation by these agents are critically dependent on the conditions of the experiment, which therefore must be strictly controlled if reliable comparisons between samples are to be made.

Differences in catalytic properties, such as (1) differences in K_m, relative rates of reaction with substrate analogs (when the specificity of the enzyme allows for variation in the structure of the substrate), (2) pH optima, and (3) response to inhibitors, typically exist between isoenzymes that are the products of multiple-gene loci. These differences can serve as the basis of methods of identification and measurement of particular isoenzymes.

These techniques generally are not used routinely, as they have been largely superseded by other, more convenient methods such as immunoassay methods.

Immunochemical Assays

Immunochemical methods of isoenzyme analysis are particularly applicable to isoenzymes derived from multiple-gene loci, because these are usually most clearly antigenically distinct. However, the greater discriminating power of monoclonal antibodies has potentially brought all multiple forms of an enzyme within the scope of immunochemical analysis. Some of these methods make use of catalytic activity of the isoenzymes. For example, residual activity may be measured after reaction with antiserum. Radioimmunoassays in which isoenzyme labeled with a radioactive tracer competes with unlabeled isoenzyme for antibody-binding sites have also been applied to isoenzyme measurement. These methods do not depend on the catalytic activity of the isoenzyme being determined. However, with the development of automated immunoassay systems, the most common routine methods for measuring isoenzymes, such as CK-MB, are solid-phase ELISAs.

The choice and application of various methods of isoenzyme analysis in clinical enzymology in relation to specific isoenzyme systems are discussed in Chapter 22.

REFERENCES

1. Armbruster D, Miller RR, The Joint Committee for Traceability in Laboratory Medicine (JCTLM). A global approach to promote the standardisation of clinical laboratory test results. Clin Biochem Rev 2007; 28:105-14.
2. Bais R, Huxtable A, Edwards JB. Human prostatic acid phosphatase: properties of the native enzyme, and the enzyme-antibody complex. Ann Clin Biochem 1983;20:374-80.
3. Canalias F, Camprubí S, Sánchez M, Gella FJ. Metrological traceability of values for catalytic concentration of enzymes assigned to a calibration material. Clin Chem Lab Med 2006;44:333-9.
4. Commission on Biochemical Nomenclature. I. Nomenclature of multiple forms of enzymes. J Biol Chem 1977;252:5939-41.
5. Copeland RA. Enzymes: a practical introduction to structure, mechanism, and data analysis. Basel: VCH Publishers, 1996.
6. Harris TK, Keshwani MM. Measurement of enzyme activity. Methods Enzymol 2009;463:57-71.
7. Infusino I, Schumann G, Ceriotti F, Panteghini M. Standardization in clinical enzymology: a challenge for the theory of metrological traceability. Clin Chem Lab Med 2010;48:301-7.
8. IUPAC Commission on Quantities and Units and IFCC Expert Panel on Quantities and Units. Approved recommendations (1978): quantities and units in clinical chemistry. Clin Chim Acta 1979;96:157F-83F.

8A. Marquette CA, Blum LJ. Chemiluminescent enzyme immunoassays: a review of bioanalytical applications. Bioanalysis 2009 Oct;1(7): 1259-69.

9. Moss DW. Isoenzyme analysis. London: The Chemical Society, 1979.
10. Moss DW. Enzyme reference materials: their place in diagnostic enzymology. Ann Biol Clin 1994;52:143-6.
11. Nomenclature Committee, I.E. Recommendations of the Nomenclature Committee of IUB on the nomenclature and classification of enzymes (1978). New York: Academic Press, 1979.
12. Panteghini M, Ceriotti F, Schumann G, Siekmann L. Establishing a reference system in clinical enzymology. Clin Chem Lab Med 2001;39:795-800.
13. Rautela GS, Snee RD, Miller WK. Response-surface co-optimization of reaction conditions in clinical chemical methods. Clin Chem 1979; 25:1954-64.
14. Schumann G, Aoki R, Ferrero CA, Ehlers G, Férard G, Gella FJ, et al. IFCC primary reference procedures for the measurement of catalytic activity concentrations of enzymes at 37°C. Part 8: reference procedure for the measurement of catalytic concentration of α-amylase. Clin Chem Lab Med 2006;44:1146-55.
15. Schumann G, Bonora R, Ceriotti F, Clerc-Renaud P, Ferrero CA, Férard G, et al. IFCC primary reference procedures for the measurement of catalytic activity concentrations of enzymes at 37°C. Part 2: reference procedure for the measurement of catalytic concentration of creatine kinase. Clin Chem Lab Med 2002;40:635-42.
16. Schumann G, Bonora R, Ceriotti F, Clerc-Renaud P, Ferrero CA, Férard G, et al. IFCC primary reference procedures for the measurement of catalytic activity concentrations of enzymes at 37°C. Part 3: reference procedure for the measurement of catalytic concentration of lactate dehydrogenase. Clin Chem Lab Med 2002;40:643-8.

17. Schumann G, Bonora R, Ceriotti F, Ferard G, Ferrero CA, Franck PFH, et al. IFCC primary reference procedures for the measurement of catalytic activity concentrations of enzymes at 37°C. International Federation of Clinical Chemistry and Laboratory Medicine. Part 4: reference procedure for the measurement of catalytic concentration of alanine aminotransferase. Clin Chem Lab Med 2002;40:718-24.
18. Schumann G, Bonora R, Ceriotti F, Ferard G, Ferrero CA, Franck PFH, et al. IFCC primary reference procedures for the measurement of catalytic activity concentrations of enzymes at 37°C. International Federation of Clinical Chemistry and Laboratory Medicine. Part 5: reference procedure for the measurement of catalytic concentration of aspartate aminotransferase. Clin Chem Lab Med 2002;40:725-33.
19. Schumann G, Bonora R, Ceriotti F, Clerc-Renaud P, Ferard G, Ferrero CA, et al. IFCC primary reference procedures for the measurement of catalytic activity concentrations of enzymes at 37°C. International Federation of Clinical Chemistry and Laboratory Medicine. Part 6: reference procedure for the measurement of catalytic concentration of γ-glutamyltransferase. Clin Chem Lab Med 2002;40:734-8.
20. Siekmann L, Bonora R, Burtis CA, Ceriotti F, Clerc-Renaud P, Férard G. IFCC primary reference procedures for the measurement of catalytic activity concentrations of enzymes at 37°C. Part 1: the concept of reference procedures for the measurement of catalytic activity concentrations of enzymes. Clin Chem Lab Med 2002;40:631-4.
21 Siekmann L, Bonora R, Burtis CA, Ceriotti F, Clerc-Renaud P, Férard G, et al. IFCC primary reference procedures for the measurement of catalytic activity concentrations of enzymes at 37°C. International Federation of Clinical Chemistry and Laboratory Medicine. Part 7: certification of four reference materials for the determination of enzymatic activity of gamma-glutamyltransferase, lactate dehydrogenase, alanine aminotransferase and creatine kinase accord. Clin Chem Lab Med 2002;40:739-45.
22. Stein M, Gabdoulline RR, Wade RC. Calculating enzyme kinetic parameters from protein structures. Biochem Soc Trans 2008;36:51-4.
23. Tiffany TO, Jansen JM, Burtis CA, Overton JB, Scott CD. Enzymatic kinetic rate and end-point analyses of substrate using a GeMSAEC Fast Analyzer. Clin Chem 1972;18:829-40.
23A. Uttamchandani M, Moochhala S.Microarray-based enzyme profiling: recent advances and applications (Review). Biointerphases. 2010 Sep; 5(3):FA24-31.
24. Wu AH. Standardization of assays for clinically important enzymes that have high biologic variation: what is all the fuss about? Clin Chem Lab Med. 2010;48:299-300.

CHAPTER 16

Principles of Immunochemical Techniques

*Larry J. Kricka, D.Phil., F.A.C.B., C.Chem., F.R.S.C., F.R.C.Path., and Jason Y. Park, M.D., Ph.D., F.A.C.P.**

Immunochemical reactions form the basis of a diverse range of sensitive and specific clinical assays. In a typical immunochemical analysis, an antibody is used as a reagent to detect an antigen of interest. The exquisite specificity and the high affinity of antibodies for their antigens, coupled with the ability of antibodies to cross-link antigens, allow the identification and quantitation of specific substances by a variety of methods. The principles of the methods most commonly used in the clinical laboratory are discussed in this chapter. This introduction is intended to acquaint the reader with the structure and function of antibodies (immunoglobulins) in relation to their use as reagents in immunoanalyses.

BASIC CONCEPTS

The binding of antibodies and their complementary antigens forms the basis of all immunochemical techniques.

Antibodies

Antibodies are immunoglobulins that are capable of binding specifically to a wide array of natural and synthetic antigens, including proteins, carbohydrates, nucleic acids, lipids, and other molecules. Immunoglobulins consist of five general classes designated as immunoglobulin (Ig)G, IgA, IgM, IgD, and IgE. IgG is used most commonly in immunochemical reagents. A schematic diagram of the IgG molecule is shown in Figure 16-1. IgG is a glycoprotein [molecular weight (MW), 158,000 Da] composed of two heavy (γ) and two light (κ or λ) chains joined by disulfide bonds. Each chain (H or L) is the product of three (L) or four (H) distinct gene segments. These are the constant (C), joining (J), diversity (D), and variable (V) genes that undergo combinatorial joining during B-cell development. Several hundred germline V genes, 5 to 10 J genes, 15 D genes (H chain only), and a single C gene have been identified for each heavy or light chain class. During B-cell development, the V, D, and J (H chain) or V and J (L chain) undergo random rearrangement and splicing, and this recombined product then is spliced to the constant region gene. This combinatorial diversity, along with somatic mutations that occur at the splicing sites, generates a tremendous diversity of antibody specificities. When a B-cell clone expressing a particular antibody specificity on its surface is "selected" by an antigen, it expands and differentiates into a plasma cell that secretes the specific antibody. For more information on immunoglobulins, see Chapter 21.

The variable amino acid sequence at the amino terminal end (≈105 amino acids) of each chain determines the antigenic specificity of the particular antibody. Each unique variable region is a product of a single plasma cell line or clone. A complex antigen is capable of eliciting a multiplicity of antibodies with different specificities that are derived from different cell lines. Antibodies derived in this manner are termed *polyclonal* and exhibit diverse specificities in their reactivity with the immunogen. Each unique region of the antigen molecule that will bind a complementary antibody is termed an *epitope* (antigenic determinant).

Immunogens

An *immunogen* is a protein or a substance coupled to a carrier that when introduced into a foreign host is capable of inducing the formation of an antibody in the host. The antibody produced may be circulating *(humoral)* or tissue bound *(cellular)*.

A *hapten* is a small, chemically defined determinant that when conjugated to an immunogenic carrier stimulates the synthesis of antibody specific for the hapten. It is capable of binding an antibody but cannot by itself stimulate an immune response.

**The author gratefully acknowledges the original contribution by Dr. Gregory Buffone, upon which portions of this chapter are based.*

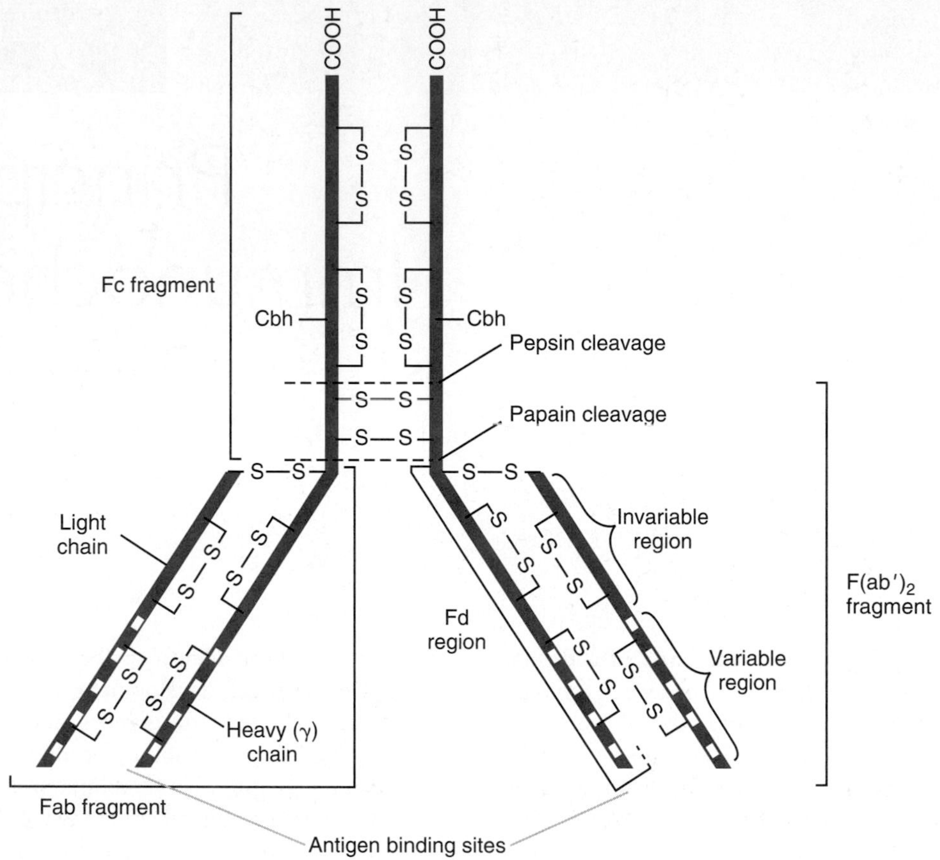

Figure 16-1 Schematic diagram of immunoglobulin (Ig)G antibody molecule showing carbohydrate (Cbh), disulfide bonds (—S—S—), and major fragments produced by proteolytic enzyme treatment (F[ab′]$_2$, Fc, Fab, Fd).

Continued stimulation by an immunogen results in increased production of immunoglobulins of different types and of high-affinity binding characteristics for antigens. After the first exposure to an immunogen, a latent period (induction) occurs during which no antibody is present in serum; this period may last from 5 to 10 days.

The strength or energy of interaction between the antibody and the antigen is described by two terms. *Affinity* refers to the thermodynamic quantity defining the energy of interaction of a single antibody-combining site and its corresponding epitope on the antigen. *Avidity* refers to the overall strength of binding of an antibody and its antigen and includes the sum of the binding affinities of all the individual combining sites on the antibody. For example, IgG has two antigen-binding sites, whereas IgM has 10 antigen-binding sites per antibody molecule. Thus affinity is a property of the substance bound (antigen), and avidity is a property of the binder (antibody). For polyclonal antibodies, avidity is difficult to determine primarily because of the diversity of the antibody population.

Polyclonal antiserum is raised in a normal animal host in response to immunogen administration. In contrast, *monoclonal antibodies* are produced in a very different manner and represent the product of a single clone or plasma cell line, rather than a heterogeneous mixture of antibodies produced by many plasma cell clones in response to immunization. Monoclonal antibodies are now widely used as reagents in immunoassay techniques.[44,59] The usual method of production of monoclonal antibodies involves fusing antibody-producing plasma cells from the spleens or lymph nodes of mice that have been immunized several times over a 2- to 4-week period with a murine myeloma cell line from tissue culture in the presence of polyethylene glycol (PEG)(PEG promotes membrane and thus cell fusion through an unknown mechanism). The murine myeloma cell line is an immortalized plasma cell line. The murine myeloma cell lines most commonly used are deficient in the enzyme hypoxanthine guanine phosphoribosyl transferase (HGPRT) and therefore cannot synthesize purine bases from thymidine and hypoxanthine in the presence of aminopterin. Following fusion, the cells are placed into a selection medium containing hypoxanthine, aminopterin, and thymidine (HAT medium) to grow *fused hybrid cell* lines selectively. The fused hybrid cells can survive in a HAT medium, because these cells combine the immortality of the myeloma cell with the genetic material of the splenic plasma cell necessary for synthesis of thymidine in the presence of aminopterin. The unfused myeloma cells are killed by the HAT medium because they do not have the HGPRT gene, and the unfused spleen cells cannot be maintained in the culture. Colonies arising from the fused cells are then screened for antibody production, and cell lines secreting antibody of the desired specificity are cloned in subcultures. In this way, a single clonal line can be isolated that produces an antibody with a selected specificity and affinity for a single antigen.

Because of the unique ability of a monoclonal antibody to react with a single epitope on a multivalent antigen, the majority of monoclonal antibodies will not cross-link and precipitate macromolecular antigens. Consequently, monoclonal antibodies have not found broad applicability in traditional precipitin methods. A practical advantage of using monoclonal antibodies is that two different antibody specificities can be used in a single incubation step. A solid phase antibody specific for a unique epitope and another labeled antibody specific for a different epitope can react with an antigen in a single step. This eliminates the incubating and washing steps that usually would be required for polyclonal antibodies.

Phage display technology provides a new in vitro approach for producing antibodies (single chain Fv fragments, Fab fragments, and whole antibody molecules) that mimic the immune system but do not require B-cell immortalization.[15,89] V genes coding for the heavy and light chain variable domains of immunoglobulin isolated from lymphocytes are amplified by the polymerase chain reaction and ligated into a filamentous bacteriophage vector to form combinatorial libraries of V_H and V_L genes. Individual bacteriophages display copies of a specific antibody on their surface, and the phage library can be screened for the antibody of a defined specificity using immobilized antigen ("panning"). Large libraries displaying antibodies formed from more than 10^{12} different V_H and V_L combinations can be constructed; this provides a rich source of antibodies with binding constants of 10^8 to 10^9 L/mol. Soluble antibody from selected bacteriophages can be secreted from infected bacteria (e.g., *Escherichia coli*) in yields greater than 500 mg/L.

ANTIGEN-ANTIBODY BINDING

Binding Forces

The strength of the binding of an antigen to an antibody depends on several forces acting cooperatively. These include van der Waals-London dipole-dipole interaction, hydrophobic interaction, and ionic coulombic bonding.[42]

Van der Waals-London Dipole-Dipole Interactions

Van der Waals-London binding is caused by the attraction between atoms when they are brought together in close proximity. These interactions are basically electrostatic in nature and are applicable to polarizable, noncharged molecules, whose structure allows the electron cloud around the molecule to be distorted by outside forces in such a way that a transient dipole is produced. Such polarization results in the formation of an instantaneous dipole moment, which in turn induces a dipole moment in adjacent molecules. The induced dipole moment is oriented in an antiparallel fashion with respect to the original dipole moment, such that a net attractive force is produced. These forces operate over short distances (4 to 6 nm) and are more significant for larger molecules. Because polarizability varies inversely with temperature, the attractive force is inversely proportional to the temperature.

Hydrophobic Interaction

Hydrophobic interactions result because the association of nonpolar groups is energetically favored in aqueous or other polar solutions. In proteins, hydrophobic interactions serve to bend and fold a molecule in a way that brings nonpolar R groups inside to the less polar interior; polar R groups are oriented outside toward the more polar aqueous environment. Thus hydrophobic bonding forms an interior, hydrophobic protein core, where most hydrophobic side chains can closely associate and weakly bind. Hydrophobic interaction enhances or stabilizes antigen-antibody binding but is not necessarily the major force in such binding.[76]

Coulombic Bonds

Coulombic bonding results from the attraction between charged groups on the antigen and the antibody, primarily COO^- and NH_4^+. The attraction between the charged groups is greatest in a medium with a low dielectric constant caused by reduced interaction of the solvent or other solute (salts) with the macromolecular ions. In a medium of high dielectric constant (aqueous solutions containing added salt), a diffuse double layer of charged particles will tend to shield the attraction of the charged species in the reactive sites of the antigen and antibody. This inhibition under certain circumstances can considerably reduce the binding constant for many antigen-antibody systems.

Given these forces, one would predict that changing pH, temperature, and ionic strength of the reaction medium should influence the binding of antigen and antibody. However, given a lower and upper limit of pH of 6 and 8 and an incubation temperature between 25 °C and 35 °C, these variables have only minimal effect on the rate of association and immune complex formation.[58,78] In fact, extremes in pH (less than 4.0 and greater than 8.0) can cause inhibition of binding or dissociation of already formed antigen-antibody complexes. Changes in ionic strength will produce a significant effect on the rate of binding of antigen and antibody. This concept is studied further in the following sections.

Reaction Mechanism

The binding of antigen to antibody is not static but is an equilibrium reaction that proceeds in three phases. The initial reaction (phase 1) of a multivalent antigen (Ag_n) and a bivalent antibody (Ab) occurs very rapidly in comparison with subsequent growth of the complexes (phase 2) and is depicted by the following equation:

$$Ag_n + Ab \underset{k_{-1}}{\overset{k_1}{\rightleftharpoons}} Ag_nAb \underset{k_{-2}}{\overset{k_2}{\rightleftharpoons}} Ag_aAb_b \qquad (1)$$

where $k_1 >>> k_2$, n is the number of epitopes per molecule, and a and b are the numbers of antigen and antibody molecules per complex. Phase 3 of the reaction involves precipitation of the complex after a critical size is reached. The speed of these reactions depends on electrolyte concentration, pH, and temperature, and on antigen structure and antibody class and the binding affinity of the antibody. The concentration of NaCl is important, and in most cases saline (NaCl, 0.15 mol/L) is used. Higher concentrations of NaCl can lead to smaller amounts of precipitate; this is due not to increased solubility of the antigen-antibody complex, but to an equilibrium shift causing a given amount of antigen to combine with smaller amounts of antibody. Decreasing the NaCl concentration can lead to increased precipitation of other proteins.

It is best to use dilute Ab and Ag solutions for determining the influence of such factors as (1) ionic species, (2) ionic strength, and (3) pH. Use of dilute solutions slows the growth of antigen-antibody complexes, and a more stable and more homogeneous population of complexes results.

Factors Influencing Binding

Factors that influence the strength of binding between an antigen and an antibody include ion species, ionic strength, and polymers used in the solution.

Ion Species and Ionic Strength Effects

Cationic salts produce an inhibition of the binding of antibody with a cationic hapten.[30] The order of inhibition by various cations is $Cs^+ > Rb^+ > NH_4^+ > K^+ > Na^+ > Li^+$. This order corresponds to the decreasing ionic radius and the increasing radius of hydration. Similar results were found for anionic haptens and anionic salts. For example, the order of inhibition of binding for anionic salts is $CNS^- > NO^-3 > I^- > Br^- > Cl^- > F^-$, which again is in the order of decreasing ionic radius and increasing radius of hydration. If the competition theory as suggested by these experiments is correct, one would expect the degree of inhibition to be a concentration-dependent phenomenon, and indeed the rate of formation of immune complexes is slower in normal saline (NaCl, 0.15 mol/L) than the same reaction carried out in deionized water. Given the previous observation, F^- should be the anion of choice for immunochemical reaction buffers. In fact, F^- does provide a modest improvement over Cl^-, but the advantage is so small that laboratories rarely substitute toxic fluoride ion for innocuous chloride ion in buffer solutions. A small but measurable difference in the initial rate of combination of antigen and antibody can be seen for phosphate as compared with tris buffer. In general, the most notable differences in reaction rates for the various anionic species evaluated are seen when t is less than 5 minutes. When reactions are evaluated at longer times (i.e., t greater than 5 minutes), the difference in the rate of Ag-Ab complex formation is relatively small for different anionic species.[58]

Polymer Effect[54]

In general, the solubility of a protein in the presence of different linear polymers is inversely proportional to the molecular weight of the polymer (i.e., the higher the molecular weight of the polymer, the lower is the solubility of the protein). For example, in the presence of Dextran 500, the solubility of α-crystalline < fibrinogen < γ-globulin < albumin <<< tyrosine.[52,53] Laurent thus proposed a steric exclusion mechanism to explain the effects of polymers on protein solubility.[53] Assuming a fixed total volume (V_T) of solvent being occupied by both polymer and protein and defining the volume occupied by polymer as V_E (excluded volume, i.e., volume not accessible to proteins) and the volume occupied by protein as V', then the relation

$$V_T = V' + V_E \qquad (2)$$

implies that any increase in V_E caused by an increase in number or size of polymer molecules forces a decrease in V' and an effective increase in the concentration of protein molecules. Hence, as V_E is increased, the *effective* protein concentration is increased, the probability of collision and self-association of protein molecules is increased, and large insoluble aggregates are formed.

BOX 16-1 Linear Polymers Used to Enhance Antigen-Antibody Reactions

Polyethylene glycol (Carbowax)
Polypropylene glycol
Dextran
Polyvinyl alcohol
Modified cellulose
Polyvinyl pyrrolidone

Studies by Hellsing[34,35] have provided support for the steric exclusion model and have demonstrated that (1) the *composition* of the immune complex formed is not affected by the presence of a polymer; (2) no complex is formed between the polymer and the antigen, antibody, or immune complex; (3) the polymer effect is dependent on the molecular weight of both antigen and polymer; and (4) the use of polymer in a reaction mixture can increase the precipitation of an immune complex with low-avidity antibody. Addition of polymer to a mixture of antigen and antibody causes a notable increase in the rate of immune complex growth, especially during the early phase of the reaction. Numerous polymer species have been tested (Box 16-1) for applications in immunochemical methods. The most desirable characteristics of the polymer are high molecular weight, a high degree of linearity (minimal branching), and high aqueous solubility. Most investigators have found PEG 6000 in concentrations of 3 to 5 g/dL to be most useful.

Types of Reactions

Types of antigen-antibody reactions that are of analytical importance include the precipitin reaction and those noted at a solid-liquid interface.

The Precipitin Reaction

If the number of antibody-combining sites is notably greater than the antigen-epitope sites ([Ab] >>> [Ag]), then antigen-binding sites are quickly saturated by antibodies before

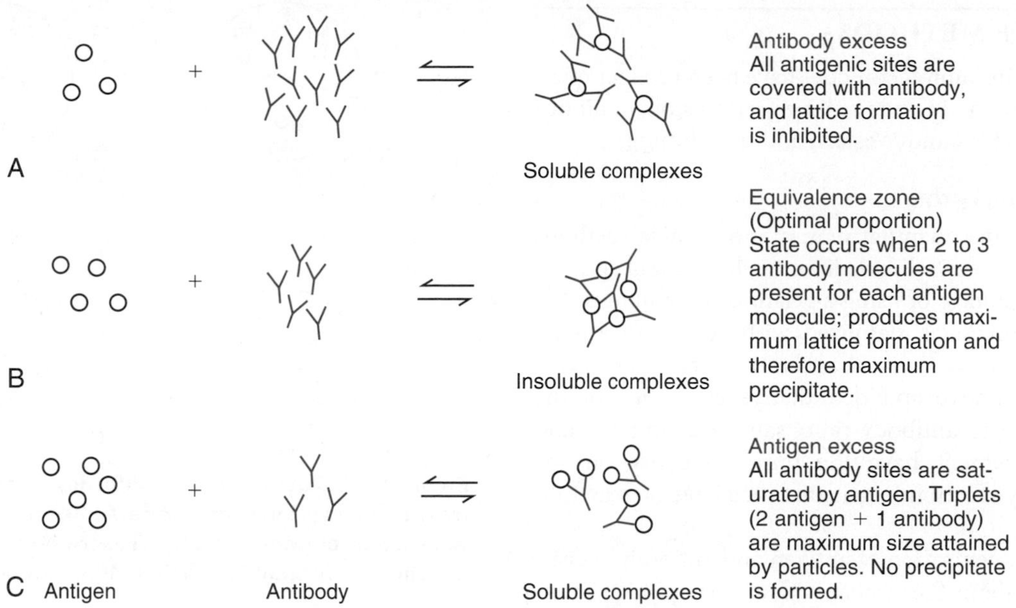

A

Soluble complexes

Antibody excess
All antigenic sites are covered with antibody, and lattice formation is inhibited.

B

Insoluble complexes

Equivalence zone
(Optimal proportion)
State occurs when 2 to 3 antibody molecules are present for each antigen molecule; produces maximum lattice formation and therefore maximum precipitate.

C Antigen Antibody Soluble complexes

Antigen excess
All antibody sites are saturated by antigen. Triplets (2 antigen + 1 antibody) are maximum size attained by particles. No precipitate is formed.

Figure 16-2 Schematic diagram for precipitin reaction.

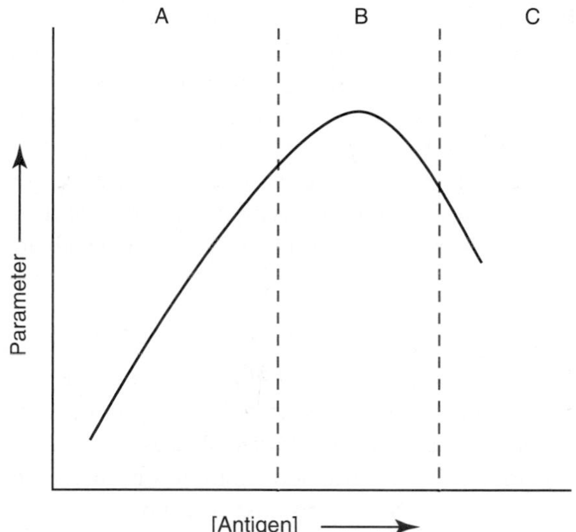

Figure 16-3 Schematic diagram of precipitin curve illustrating zones of antibody excess *(A)*, equivalence *(B)*, and antigen excess *(C)*. The parameter measured may be the quantity of protein precipitated, light scattering, or another measurable parameter. Antibody concentration is held constant in this example.

cross-linking can occur, along with the formation of small insoluble antigen-antibody complexes (Figure 16-2, *A*). When an antibody is in moderate excess (i.e., [Ab] > [Ag]), the probability of cross-linking of Ag by Ab is more likely, and hence large insoluble complex formation is favored (Figure 16-2, *B*). When [Ag] is in great excess, large complexes would be less probable (Figure 16-2, *C*). This model describes the results observed when antigens and antibodies are mixed in various concentration ratios. The curve shown in Figure 16-3 is a schematic diagram of the classical precipitin curve. Although the concentration of total antibody is constant, the concentration of free antibody $[Ab]_f$ (i.e., not bound to antigen) and free antigen $[Ag]_f$ varies throughout the range for any given Ag/Ab ratio. A low Ag/Ab ratio exists in *A* of Figure 16-3 (zone of antibody excess). Under these conditions, $[Ab]_f$ exists in solution, but $[Ag]_f$ does not. As total antigen increases, the size of the immune complexes increases up to equivalence (Figure 16-3, *B*), where little or no $[Ab]_f$ or $[Ag]_f$ exists. This is the zone of maximum immune complex size. This equivalence zone does not represent a ratio of exact molar equivalence of reactants but is the optimal combining ratio for cross-linking in the particular system under evaluation. As Ag/Ab increases (Figure 16-3, *C*), the immune complex size will decrease and $[Ag]_f$ will increase (zone of antigen excess). No $[Ab]_f$ should exist in this area of the curve. However, for a given Ag/Ab ratio, the population of immune complexes formed at equilibrium will be heterogeneous with respect to size and composition.

Reactions at a Solid-Liquid Interface

If the antigen or antibody of interest is bound to a solid phase such as a synthetic particle (polystyrene or cellulose), the protein will exist in a microenvironment that is different from that of a protein in free solution. Water surrounding the protein is more highly ordered near the surface of the solid phase, and the condition that results is more favorable for van der Waals-London dipole-dipole interaction and coulombic bonding. This situation favors the formation of both low- and high-avidity antigen-antibody complexes, and hence can provide lower detection limits for analytical applications.

Because of the exquisite specificity and the high affinity of antibodies for specific antigens, thousands of immunoassays have been developed to detect and measure a wide variety of biological analytes. In the next two sections, qualitative and quantitative immunotechniques are discussed.

QUALITATIVE METHODS

Various types of immunotechniques have been used for qualitative purposes; these include passive gel diffusion, immunoelectrophoresis (IEP), and Western and dot blotting.

Passive Gel Diffusion

Many qualitative and quantitative immunochemical methods are performed in a semisolid medium, such as agar or agarose. The primary advantage of using a gelatinous medium is that the diffusion process is stabilized with regard to mixing caused by vibration, and visualization of precipitin bands is allowed for qualitative and quantitative evaluation of the reaction. Antigen-to-antibody ratio, salt concentration, and polymer enhancement have the same influence on the antigen-antibody reaction in gels that they have on reactions in solution.

The initial concentration of antigen and antibody is critical. Each molecule in the system will achieve a unique concentration gradient with time. When the leading fronts of antigen and antibody diffusion overlap, the reaction will begin, but formation of a precipitin line will not occur until moderate antibody excess is achieved. A precipitin band may form and be dissolved many times by an incoming antigen before equilibrium is established, and the position of the precipitin band becomes stable. Because heavier molecules diffuse more slowly, the position of the precipitin band is in part a function of the molecular masses of both antigen and antibody. The precipitin band acts as a specific barrier; neither specific antigen nor antibody can penetrate without being precipitated by the other, but unrelated molecules can cross the band of precipitation freely. Basic approaches to passive diffusion include simple diffusion and double diffusion. With simple diffusion, a concentration gradient is established for only a single reactant. *Single immunodiffusion* usually depends on diffusion of an antigen into agar impregnated with antibody. A quantitative technique based on this principle is radial immunodiffusion (RID), which is discussed later. The second approach is double diffusion, in which a concentration gradient is established for both reactants (antigen and antibody).

Double immunodiffusion in two dimensions is a historical immunotechnique known as the Ouchterlony method. It allows direct comparison of two or more test materials and provides a simple method for determining whether the antigens in the test specimens are identical, cross-reactive, or nonidentical.

The simplest method uses an agar dish or slide with holes cut as shown in Figure 16-4. When the same antigen is in adjacent wells, the lines of precipitation fuse and are continuous—this is a reaction of identity (Figure 16-4, *A*). When the precipitin bands cross each other, this is a reaction of nonidentity (Figure 16-4, *B*); if the two antigens are related but are not identical, a reaction of partial identity is observed (Figure 16-4, *C*). Here the cardinal point is that the precipitate serves as a barrier that does not block unrelated diffusing reactants. As shown in Figure 16-4, *D*, when two related antigens, Ag and Ag_1, are in separate wells, and the respective antibodies, Ab and Ab_1, are in the third well, an AgAb precipitate forms on one side and blocks further diffusion of Ab from the antibody well. However, on the other side, the Ag_1Ab_1 precipitate does not stop Ab from migrating further and forming an AgAb spur.

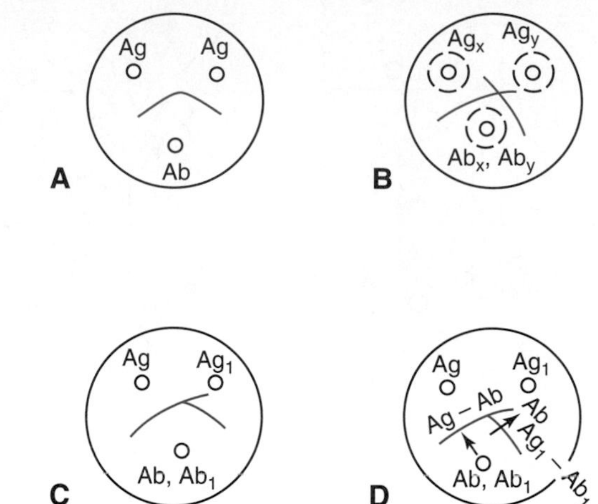

Figure 16-4 Double immunodiffusion in two dimensions by the Ouchterlony technique. A, Reaction of identity; B, reaction of nonidentity; C, reaction of partial identity; D, scheme for spur formation. *Ab,* Antibody; *Ag,* antigen.

Note that a negative reaction does not necessarily imply absence of antibody or antigen. A negative reaction can result from using amounts of material too small for the detection limit of the method, or the antibody may be nonprecipitating.

Immunoelectrophoresis (IEP)

If several antigens of interest exist in a solution (e.g., spinal fluid or serum), the various protein species can be separated and identified by IEP. This technique has been used extensively for the study of antigen mixtures and for evaluation of the specificity of antiserum.[43]

The procedure is performed using an agarose gel medium poured onto a thin plastic sheet. The sample to be analyzed is placed in a reservoir in the gel, and an electrical field is applied across the gel surface. During electrophoresis, the proteins in the serum are separated according to their electrophoretic mobilities (Figure 16-5). Following electrophoresis, an antiserum against the protein of interest is placed in a trough parallel and adjacent to the electrophoresed sample. Simultaneous diffusion of the antigen from the separated sample and the antibody from the trough leads to the formation of precipitin arcs, whose shape and position are characteristic of individual separated proteins within the specimen. By comparison with a known control separated on the same plate, individual proteins can be tentatively identified.

Crossed Immunoelectrophoresis (CRIE)

This technique, also known as two-dimensional IEP, is a variation of IEP wherein electrophoresis is also used in the second

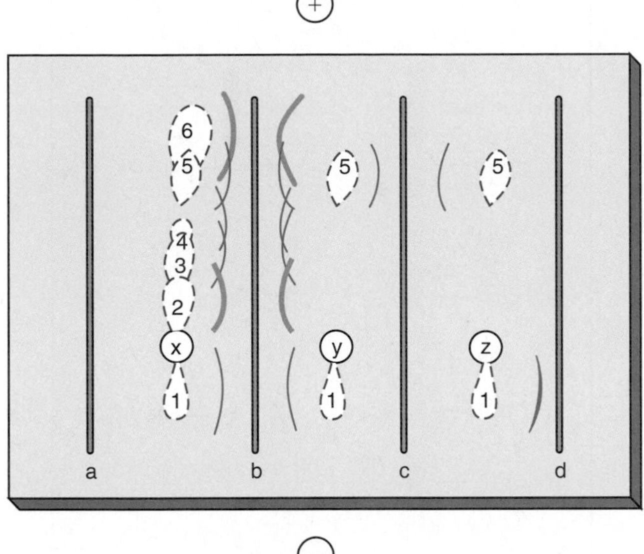

Figure 16-5 Configuration for immunoelectrophoresis. Sample wells are punched in the agar and/or agarose, sample is applied, and electrophoresis is carried out to separate the proteins in the sample. Antiserum is loaded into the troughs and the gel incubated in a moist chamber at 4 °C for 24 to 72 hours. Track *x* represents the shape of the protein zones after electrophoresis; tracks y and z show the reactions of proteins 5 and 1 with their specific antisera in troughs *c* and *d*. Antiserum against protein *1-6* is present in trough *b*.

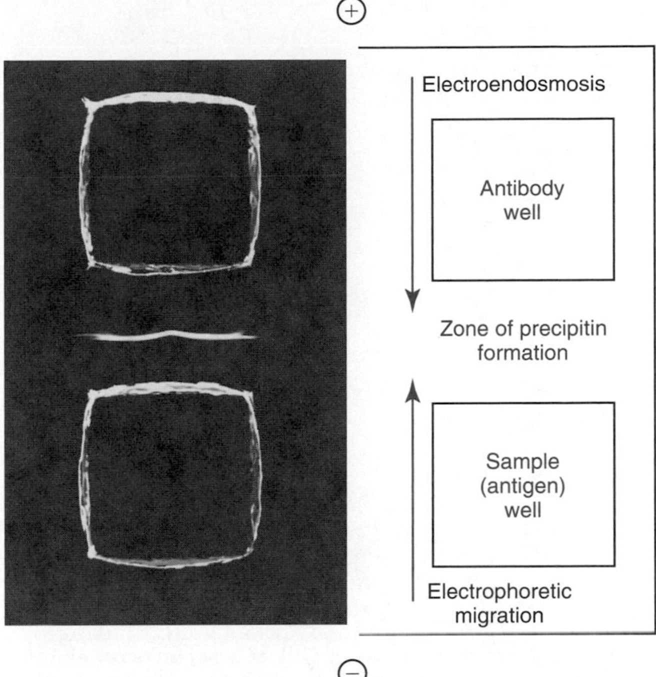

Figure 16-6 Counterimmunoelectrophoresis (CIE) showing positive reaction between anti–*Haemophilus influenzae* B *(upper well)* and a cerebrospinal fluid (CSF) sample containing *H. influenzae* B *(lower well).*

dimension to drive the antigen into a gel containing antibodies specific for the antigens of interest.[50] This technique is more sensitive and produces higher resolution than IEP. For more information on CRIE, see the previous edition of this textbook.

Counterimmunoelectrophoresis (CIE)

With CIE, two parallel lines of wells are punched in the agar. One row is filled with antigen solution, and the opposing row is filled with antibody solution (Figure 16-6). If the solutions were allowed to passively diffuse, a precipitin line would form between the opposing wells in 18 to 24 hours. With CIE, this process is accelerated by applying a voltage across the gel so that the antigen and the antibody move toward each other. Qualitative information (i.e., identification of antigen) is provided within 1 to 2 hours. Historically, this method has found application in the detection of bacterial antigens in blood, urine, and cerebrospinal fluid.

Immunofixation (IF)

This technique has gained widespread acceptance as an immunochemical method for identifying proteins.[3] As in IEP and CRIE, a first-dimension electrophoresis is performed in agarose gel to separate proteins in the sample. Subsequently, antiserum spread directly on the gel causes the protein(s) of interest to precipitate. The immune precipitate is trapped within the gel matrix, and all other nonprecipitated proteins are removed by washing the gel. The gel may then be stained for identification of the proteins. IF is technically more efficient than IEP or CRIE, and it produces patterns that are interpreted more easily. The usefulness of IF, which is now widely used for the evaluation of myeloma proteins, is illustrated in Figure 16-7.

Western Blotting

The techniques discussed previously use direct evaluation of the immunoprecipitation of the protein(s) in a gel. However, certain media, such as polyacrylamide, do not lend themselves to direct immunoprecipitation, nor is there always sufficient antigen concentration to produce an immunoprecipitate that will be retained in the gel during subsequent processing. Under these circumstances, a technique termed *Western blotting* can be used (see Chapter 12).[11,26] This technique involves an electrophoresis step followed by transfer of separated proteins onto an overlying strip of nitrocellulose or a nylon membrane by a process called *electro-blotting.* Once the proteins are in the membrane, they can be detected using antibodies labeled with probes, such as radioactive isotopes or enzymes. When such probes are used, the limits of detection can be 10 to 100 times lower than when direct immunoprecipitation and staining of proteins are conducted. This technique is analogous to *Southern blotting* (electrophoresed DNA blotted onto a membrane), and *Northern blotting* (electrophoresed RNA blotted onto a membrane).

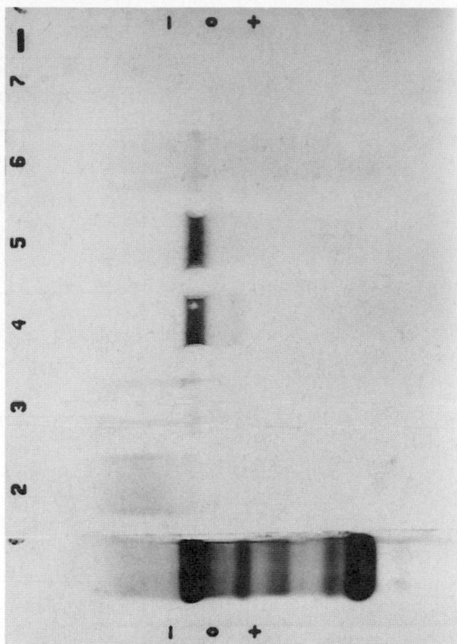

Figure 16-7 Immunofixation (IF) of a serum containing an immunoglobulin (Ig)M kappa paraprotein. ***Lane 1,*** **Serum electrophoresis stained for protein;** ***lane 2,*** **anti-IgG, Fc piece specific;** ***lane 3,*** **anti-IgA, α-chain specific;** ***lane 4,*** **anti-IgM, μ-chain specific;** ***lane 5,*** **anti-κ light chain;** ***lane 6,*** **anti-λ light chain.** *(Courtesy Katherine Bayer, Protein Laboratory, Hospital of the University of Pennsylvania, Philadelphia, Pa.)*

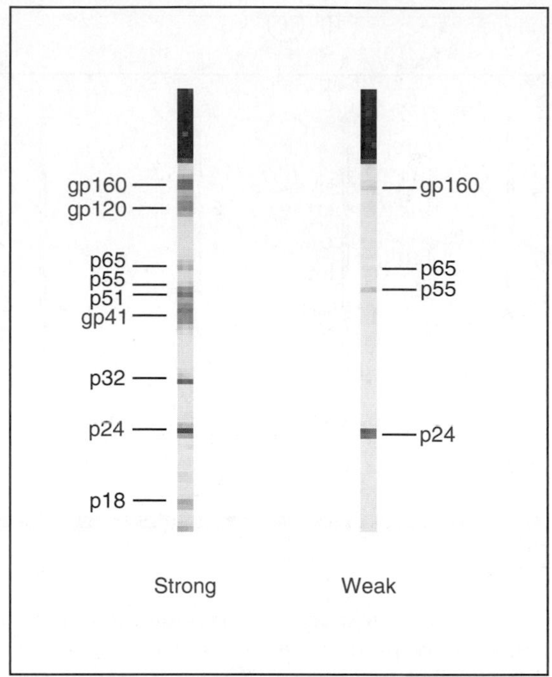

Figure 16-8 Western blot analysis of serum samples strongly positive and weakly positive for human immunodeficiency virus type 1 (HIV-1) antibody. Core proteins (GAG, group-specific antigens) p18, p24, and p55; polymerase (POL) p32, p51, and p65; envelope proteins (ENV) gp41, gp120, and gp160. *(Courtesy Bio-Rad Laboratories Diagnostics Group, Irvine, Calif.)*

An example of this technique applied to the detection of human immunodeficiency virus type 1 (HIV-1) antibodies is shown in Figure 16-8. HIV-1 antigens are separated according to molecular weight by gel electrophoresis and then are transferred to a nitrocellulose membrane by electro-blotting. A serum sample is then incubated with a strip of the membrane. HIV-1 antibodies in the sample bind to the viral antigens transferred to the strip as discrete bands. After washing, the strip is incubated with an alkaline phosphatase antihuman immunoglobulin conjugate. After a further washing step, the nitrocellulose strip is incubated with an alkaline phosphatase substrate solution (5-bromo-4-chloro-3-indolyl phosphate and nitroblue tetrazolium) to reveal where anti–HIV-1 antibody is bound to specific viral antigens fixed in the membrane.

Protein transfer and immobilization following separation by electrophoresis, isoelectric focusing, sodium dodecyl sulfate polyacrylamide electrophoresis (see Chapter 12 for further discussion of these techniques), or other methods provide a powerful tool for the analytical study of proteins present in low concentrations in cell culture or body fluids. When applied to antigen assays, concentrations of antigen as low as 500 ng/mL or 2.5 ng/band in the gel can be detected by this method. The detection limit of the technique can be lowered to approximately 100 pg by using chemiluminescence labels on the antibody.[10,47]

Dot Blotting

A similar technique that bypasses the electrophoretic separation step is known as *dot blotting.* A protein sample to be analyzed is applied to a membrane surface as a small "dot" and is dried. The membrane is then exposed to a labeled antibody specific for the test antigen contained in the dotted protein mixture. After washing, bound labeled antibody is detected with a photometric or chemiluminescent detection system.

QUANTITATIVE METHODS

Several immunochemical techniques have been used to quantify analytes of clinical interest. They include radial immunodiffusion (RID) and electroimmunoassays, turbidimetric and nephelometric assays, and labeled immunochemical antibody assays.

Radial Immunodiffusion and Electroimmunoassay

Typically, the two most commonly encountered gel-based methods for quantitative immunochemical studies are RID immunoassay and electroimmunoassay ("rocket" technique).

Radial Immunodiffusion Immunoassay

With this technique, a concentration gradient is established for a single reactant, usually the antigen. The antibody is uniformly dispersed in the gel matrix. Antigen is allowed to passively diffuse from a well into the gel, and immune precipitation occurs until antibody excess exists. The antigen-antibody interaction is manifested by a defined ring of precipitation around the antigen well, and ring diameter will increase with increased antigen concentration. Calibrators are run at the same time as the sample, and a calibration curve of ring diameter versus concentration is plotted. Under equilibrium conditions, a linear relationship exists between antigen concentration and the square of the precipitin ring diameter.[57] In addition, the precision of the measurement of the ring diameter is better when equilibrium is established. However, quantitative data can also be derived by reading the ring diameter before equilibrium is established.[23] This approach, although less precise, is often more practical for a clinical laboratory if time is at a premium. Antigen concentrations are calculated in both the preequilibrium and equilibrium methods[23,57] by plotting the square of the precipitin ring diameter against calibrating antigen concentrations. RID can be made more sensitive by using PEG to enhance precipitin line formation or by using ^{125}I- or enzyme-labeled reagents.[33,61,69]

Electroimmunoassay

In *electroimmunoassay,* as in RID, a single concentration gradient is established for the antigen, but in this case, an applied voltage is used to drive the antigen from the application well into a homogeneous suspension of antibody in the gel (Figure 16-9).[51] Unlike RID, this produces a unidirectional migration of antigen and results in a lower limit of detection for electroimmunoassay methods. The height of the resulting rocket-shaped precipitin line is proportional to the antigen concentration. Quantitation is affected by using calibrators on the same plate and estimating the concentrations of unknowns from the heights of the "rockets" obtained. The calibration curve is linear only over a narrow concentration range, so samples may have to be diluted or concentrated as necessary. Electroimmunoassay methods produce the best results, with antigens having a strong anodic mobility and intermediate to low molecular weight. Proteins such as transferrin, C3, or IgG, with low anodal mobility or virtually no net charge at pH 8.6 (the most common pH used for the method), can be modified by carbamylation or can be run at a lower pH to make their measurements by electroimmunoassay feasible. Other modifications, such as use of an intermediate gel that causes precipitation of C3, allow measurement of C3d in human serum and illustrate the exceptional versatility of this method.[9]

Turbidimetric and Nephelometric Assays

Turbidimetry and nephelometry are convenient techniques for measuring the rate of formation of immune complexes in vitro. Instrumental principles for these methods are described in Chapter 10. It has been found that the reaction between antigen and antibody begins within milliseconds and continues for hours.[30] Both turbidimetric and nephelometric immunochemical methods using rate and pseudoequilibrium protocols have been described for proteins, antigens, and haptens. In rate assays, measurements are usually made within the first few minutes of the reaction, when the largest change *(dIs/dt)* in intensity of scattered light *(Is)* with respect to time occurs. For so-called equilibrium assays, it is necessary to wait 30 to 60 minutes. For the purpose of this discussion, such conditions are referred to as *pseudoequilibrium,* because true equilibrium is not reached within the time allowed for these assays. Measurement of the *rate* of immune complex formation can also be used for quantitative immunochemical studies. Either *dIs/dt* or the time required to reach peak rate can be related to antigen concentration in a manner analogous to any other rate methodology. Rate nephelometric assays have the advantage that blank correction is not required, and that several samples can be assayed in a few minutes instead of the 30 to 60 minutes required for pseudoequilibrium methods.[6,14,37] The analytical performance of nephelometric or turbidimetric assays can be significantly improved by increasing the reaction rate by adding water-soluble linear polymers. This allows the use of much lower reactant concentrations and results in more stable immune complexes.[13]

Nephelometric methods in general are more sensitive than turbidimetric assays and have an average lower limit of detection of 0.1 to 10 mg/L for a serum protein. Lower detection limits are obtained in cerebrospinal fluid and urine because of their lower lipid and protein concentrations, resulting in a better signal-to-noise ratio. In addition, for low molecular weight proteins [e.g., myoglobin (MW, 17,800 Da)], assay

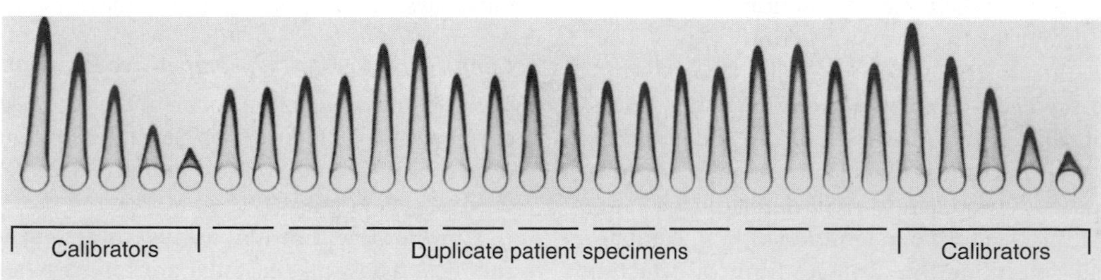

Figure 16-9 Rocket immunoelectrophoresis of human serum albumin. Patient samples were applied in duplicate. Standards were placed at opposite ends of the plate.

detection limits can be lowered using a latex-enhanced procedure based on antibody-coated latex beads.[29]

Nephelometric and turbidimetric assays have also been applied to the measurement of drugs (haptens) using *inhibition techniques.* The reagent is made by attaching the drug of interest to a carrier molecule, such as bovine serum albumin. The hapten-bound albumin then competes with free hapten (drug introduced in sample) for the antihapten antibody. In the presence of free hapten, immune complex formation is decreased, because more antibody sites are saturated; thus light scattering is decreased. This decrease in light scattering is related to the concentration of free hapten. Both kinetic and pseudoequilibrium methods have been described.[25]

Particle-enhanced turbidimetric inhibition immunoassay (PETINIA) is another type of agglutination immunoassay that measures decreasing agglutination in the presence of increasing concentrations of analyte. The reagents comprise an antibody to the analyte of interest and a reagent analyte of interest linked to a latex bead. In the absence of analyte in a specimen, reagent antibody binds to the reagent analyte linked to the latex bead, resulting in increased turbidity. When a specimen with high analyte levels is added to the reagents, the reagent antibody is bound by the analyte in the specimen and not to the reagent analyte linked to the latex bead. Thus, the presence of specimen analyte results in less turbidity.

Labeled Immunochemical Assays

The previously discussed methods rely on immune complex formation as an index of antigen-antibody reaction. As demonstrated previously in equation (1), the overall reaction occurs in sequential phases, and only the final phase is the formation of the immune complex. However, the initial binding of the antibody and antigen has been demonstrated to be very useful analytically and has been used with labeled antigens and antibodies to develop many sensitive and specific immunochemical assays. The reaction describing this initial binding and the kinetic constant for the overall reaction are shown in equations (3a) and (3b), respectively:

$$\mathrm{Ab} + \mathrm{Ag} \underset{k_{-1}}{\overset{k_1}{\rightleftharpoons}} \mathrm{AbAg} \quad \textbf{(3a)}$$

$$K = \frac{[\mathrm{AbAg}]}{[\mathrm{Ab}][\mathrm{Ag}]} \quad \textbf{(3b)}$$

where

k_1 = the rate constant for the forward reaction

k_{-1} = the rate constant for the reverse reaction

K = the equilibrium constant for the overall reaction

As would be predicted from the law of mass action, the concentration of Ab, Ag, and AbAg will be dependent on the magnitude of k_1 and k_{-1}. For polyclonal antiserum, the average avidity of the antibody populations will determine K (typically 10^8 to 10^{10} L/mol), and the magnitude of k_1 in comparison with k_{-1} will determine the ultimate limit of detection attainable with a given antibody population.

The original assays used radioactive labels, but concerns about safe handling and disposal of radioactive reagents and waste have led to the development of alternative nonisotopic labels (Table 16-1).[47,66] In this section, the methodologic principles on which these assays are based and the factors that affect their analytical sensitivity are discussed. In addition, specific examples of these assays and the types of labels that are used in them are evaluated. Commercial versions and applications of these assays are discussed in other chapters (see Chapters 10 and 19).

TABLE 16-1 Labels Used for Nonisotopic Immunoassay

Chemiluminescent	Acridinium ester, sulfonyl acridinium ester, isoluminol
Cofactor	Adenosine triphosphate, flavin adenine dinucleotide
Enzyme	Alkaline phosphatase, marine bacterial luciferase, β-galactosidase, firefly luciferase, glucose oxidase, glucose-6-phosphate dehydrogenase, horseradish peroxidase, lysozyme, malate dehydrogenase, microperoxidase, urease, xanthine oxidase
Fluorophore	Europium chelate, fluorescein, phycoerythrin, terbium chelate
Free radical	Nitroxide
Inhibitor	Methotrexate
Metal	Gold sol, selenium sol, silver sol
Particle	Bacteriophage, erythrocyte, latex bead, liposome, quantum dot
Phosphor	Upconverting lanthanide-containing nanoparticle
Polynucleotide	DNA
Substrate	Galactosyl-umbelliferone

Methodologic Principles

To exploit the exquisite specificity and the enhanced sensitivity that are possible with immunochemical assays, various methodological principles have been applied in their development. These include competitive and noncompetitive reaction formats and different processing schemes for performing the assays.

Competitive versus Noncompetitive Reaction Formats

The two major reaction formats that are used in immunochemical assays (Figure 16-10) are termed *competitive* (limited reagent assays) and *noncompetitive* (excess reagent, two-site, or sandwich assays).

Competitive Immunoassays. In a *competitive* immunochemical assay, all reactants are mixed together *simultaneously* or *sequentially.* In the simultaneous approach, the labeled antigen (Ag*) and the unlabeled antigen (Ag) compete for binding to the antibody. In such a system, the avidity of

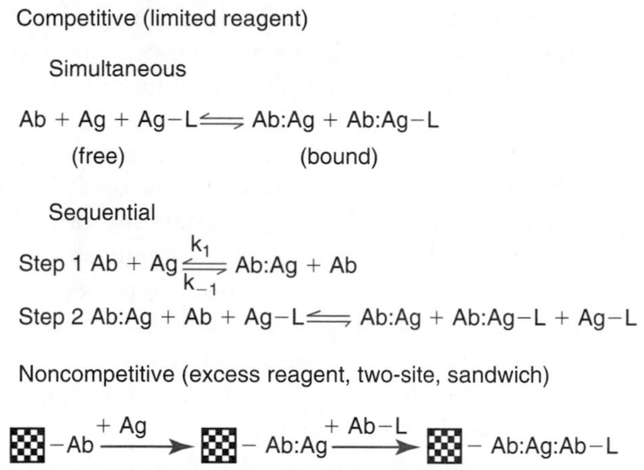

Competitive (limited reagent)

Simultaneous

$$\text{Ab} + \text{Ag} + \text{Ag–L} \rightleftharpoons \text{Ab:Ag} + \text{Ab:Ag–L}$$

(free) (bound)

Sequential

$$\text{Step 1 } \text{Ab} + \text{Ag} \underset{k_{-1}}{\overset{k_1}{\rightleftharpoons}} \text{Ab:Ag} + \text{Ab}$$

$$\text{Step 2 } \text{Ab:Ag} + \text{Ab} + \text{Ag–L} \rightleftharpoons \text{Ab:Ag} + \text{Ab:Ag–L} + \text{Ag–L}$$

Noncompetitive (excess reagent, two-site, sandwich)

▩–Ab —(+ Ag)→ ▩– Ab:Ag —(+ Ab–L)→ ▩– Ab:Ag:Ab–L

Figure 16-10 Immunoassay designs. *L*, Label.

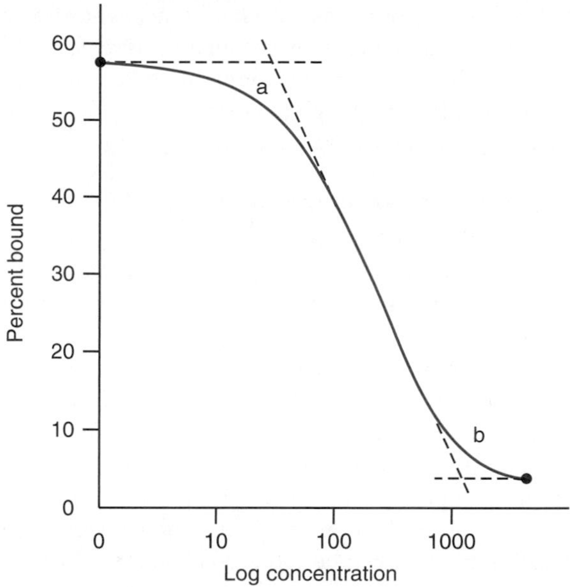

Figure 16-11 A schematic diagram of the dose-response curve for a typical competitive immunoassay. The analytically useful portion of the curve is bracketed by points *a* and *b*.

the antibody for both labeled and unlabeled antigen must be the same. Under these conditions, the probability of the antibody binding the labeled antigen is inversely proportional to the concentration of unlabeled antigen; hence, bound label is inversely proportional to unlabeled antigen concentration.

In a *sequential* competitive assay, unlabeled antigen is first mixed with excess antibody, and binding is allowed to reach equilibrium (see Figure 16-10, step 1). Labeled antigen is then sequentially added (step 2) and is allowed to equilibrate. After separation, the bound labeled antigen is determined and is used to calculate the unlabeled antigen concentration. Using this two-step method, a larger fraction of the unlabeled antigen is bound by the antibody than in the simultaneous assay, especially at low antigen concentrations. Consequently, this strategy provides a twofold to fourfold improvement in the detection limit of provided $k_1 >> k_{-1}$. This improvement in detection limit results from an increase in AgAb binding (and thus a decrease in Ag* binding), which is favored by the sequential addition of Ag and Ag*. If $k_1 >> k_{-1}$, dissociation of AgAb becomes more likely, resulting in increased competition between Ag* and Ag. A typical competitive immunochemical assay binding curve is shown in Figure 16-11.

Noncompetitive Immunoassays. In a *noncompetitive immunochemical assay*, a capture antibody first is passively adsorbed or covalently bound to the surface of a solid phase. Various approaches for attaching the capture antibody are shown in Box 16-2. The simplest involves direct attachment to the solid phase. However, this can lead to some loss of antibody-binding capacity because of steric factors or attachment of the antibody via its Fab region. To protect the binding properties of the antibody, more complex sequences have been devised. For example, the solid support is coated with an antispecies antibody, and then the antispecies antibody used to immobilize the capture antibody via an antigen-antibody reaction.

In the first stage of the assay, the antigen from the sample is allowed to react with the solid phase, capture antibody; other proteins are washed away, and a labeled antibody (conjugate) is added that reacts with the bound antigen through a second and distinct epitope. After washing again, the bound label is determined, and its concentration or activity is directly proportional to the concentration of the antigen.

BOX 16-2 Immobilization Schemes for Preparation of Solid Phase Antibodies for Use in Immunoassay

- AB
- Anchor protein-reptavidin:biotin-AB
- Antispecies Ab:AB

AB, Capture antibody.

In noncompetitive assays, the capture and labeled antibody are polyclonal or monoclonal. If monoclonal antibodies having specificity for distinct epitopes are used, it is possible to incubate the sample and conjugate simultaneously with the capture antibody, thus simplifying the assay protocol.

Noncompetitive immunoassays are performed in a simultaneous (one-step) or sequential (two-step) mode. However, in the simultaneous mode, a situation can occur in which a high concentration of analyte can saturate both capture and labeled antibodies. When this occurs, the calibration curve of the assay exhibits a "hook effect," in which the assay response drops off at high analyte concentrations. Under these conditions, the analyte is present in such high concentrations that it reacts simultaneously with the capture antibody and the labeled antibody. This reduces the number of complexes formed and produces a falsely low result. Assays for analytes for which the normal pathologic concentration range is very wide (e.g., tumor markers) are particularly prone to this problem. Dilutions of a sample are usually reanalyzed to check for this type of analytical interference. The hook effect can be eliminated by adopting a sequential assay format[64] and by ensuring that the concentrations of capture and labeled antibody are sufficiently high to cover analyte concentrations over the entire analytical range of the assay.

Heterogeneous versus Homogeneous Immunochemical Assays

Immunochemical assays that require separation of free from bound labels are termed *heterogeneous;* those that do not are called *homogeneous.*

Heterogeneous Assays. Heterogeneous assays implicitly assume that $k_1 >> k_{-1}$ and that a variety of physical separation techniques are used to separate the free-label (Ag*) from the bound-label antigen (Ag*Ab). The most widely used of these techniques are precipitation and solid phase adsorption.

Precipitation of the bound-labeled antigen (Ag*Ab) from the reaction mixture can be achieved chemically by the addition of a protein-precipitating chemical, such as $(NH_4)_2SO_4$, or immunologically by the addition of a second, "precipitating" antibody. In the latter approach, if the primary antibody was obtained from rabbit antiserum, the precipitating antibody would be contained in a goat or sheep antiserum raised against rabbit globulin. This approach has the advantage that it can be used for practically any assay; however, it has the disadvantage that it usually requires longer assay times and additional processing steps.

Solid phase adsorption is the separation technique that currently is the most popular and widely used in both manual and automated immunoassays (see Chapter 19). In this technique, the binding and competition of labeled and unlabeled antigens for the binding sites of the antibody occur on the surface of a solid support onto which the capture antibody has been attached by physical adsorption or covalent bonding. Several different types of solid support have been used, including the inner surface of plastic tubes or wells of microtiter plates and the outer surface of insoluble materials, such as cellulose or magnetic latex beads or particles. With the tubes and microtiter plates, the solid surface containing the attached antibody and the bound antigen is washed "in place," and indicator reagents are subsequently added to complete the assay. When beads or particles are used, they are added directly to the reaction mixture and after incubation are removed by centrifugation or magnetic separation. After the supernatant has been removed by siphoning or decanting, the beads or particles are washed and indicator reagents subsequently added to complete the assay.

Homogeneous Assays. The development of homogeneous assays that do not require separation of bound- and free-labeled antibody or antigen was a major advance in the field of immunochemical analysis. In this type of assay, the activity of the label attached to the antigen is directly modulated by antibody binding, with the magnitude of the modulation being proportional to the concentration of the antigen or antibody being measured. Consequently, in practice it is necessary to incubate only the sample containing the analyte antigen with the labeled antigen and antibody and then to directly measure the activity of the label "in place," thus making these assays technically easier and faster. The original homogeneous immunoassay was developed for drug analysis and used a nitroxide spin label; this was termed a *free radical immunoassay technique.*[55] The electron spin resonance spectrum of this label was modulated when the nitroxide-labeled drug was bound by a drug-specific antibody. This procedure was quickly superseded by homogeneous immunoassays that used enzyme labels and could be performed on spectrophotometric analyzers [see subsequent descriptions of enzyme multiplied immunoassay technique (EMIT) and cloned enzyme donor immunoassay (CEDIA)].[36,70] A homogeneous sandwich format chemiluminescent immunoassay has also been developed that expands the scope of homogeneous assays to large molecules [see subsequent description of luminescent oxygen channeling immunoassay (LOCI)].[80]

Analytical Detection Limits

The analytical detection limits of competitive and noncompetitive immunoassays are determined principally by the affinity of the antibody and the detection limit of the label used, respectively.[21,39,40,67] Calculations have indicated that a lower limit of detection of 10 fmol/L (i.e., 600,000 molecules of analyte in a typical sample volume of 100 μL) is possible in a competitive assay using an antibody with an affinity of 10^{12} L/mol. Table 16-2 illustrates theoretical detection limits for isotopic and nonisotopic labels. A radioactive label, such as ^{125}I, has low specific activity (7.5 million labels necessary for detection of 1 disintegration/s) compared with enzyme labels and chemiluminescent and fluorescent labels. Enzyme labels provide an amplification (each enzyme label produces many detectable product molecules), and the detection limit for an enzyme can be improved by replacing the conventional photometric detection reaction by a chemiluminescent or bioluminescent reaction. The combination of amplification and an ultrasensitive detection reaction makes noncompetitive chemiluminescent immunoassays among the most sensitive types of immunoassay. Fluorescent labels also have high specific activity, and a single high-quantum yield fluorophor can produce 100 million photons/s. In practice, several factors degrade the detection limit of an immunoassay; these include background signal from the detector, assay reagents, and nonspecific binding of the labeled reagent.

Secondary labels, such as biotin, can be used to introduce amplification into an immunoassay. The binding constant of the biotin-avidin complex is extremely high (10^{15} L/mol); capitalizing on this system allows immunoassay systems to be devised that are even more sensitive than simple antibody systems. A biotin-avidin system uses a biotin-labeled soluble antibody. Biotin can be attached to the antibody in relatively high proportion without loss of immunoreactivity.[5,31] When an avidin-conjugated label is added, a complex of Ag:Ab-biotin:avidin label is formed. Further amplification can be achieved by a biotin:avidin:biotin linkage, because the binding ratio of biotin : avidin is 4 : 1. If the label is an enzyme, then large numbers of enzyme molecules in the complete complex provide a large increase in enzymatic activity coupled with

TABLE 16-2 Detection Limits for Isotopic and Nonisotopic Immunoassay Labels

Label	Detection Limit in Zeptomoles* (10^{-21} moles)	Method
Alkaline phosphatase	50,000	Photometry
	300	Time-resolved fluorescence
	100	Fluorescence
	10	Enzyme cascade
	1	Chemiluminescence
β-D-Galactosidase	5000	Chemiluminescence
	1000	Fluorescence
Europium chelate	10,000	Time-resolved fluorescence
Glucose-6-phosphate dehydrogenase	1000	Chemiluminescence
Horseradish peroxidase	2,000,000	Photometry
	1	Chemiluminescence
^{125}I	1000	Scintillation
Ruthenium (II) tris(bipyridyl)	20†	Electrochemiluminescence

*One zeptomole = 10^{-3} attomoles or 10^{-6} femtomoles.
†Personal communication.

the small amount of antigen being determined, and the assay is correspondingly more sensitive.

Examples of Labeled Immunoassays

In the decade following the pioneering developments of Yalow and Berson,[93] all competitive and noncompetitive immunoassays used a radioactive label in a competitive assay format. Since the introduction of enzyme immunochemical assays in the 1970s,[55,70] a vast array of sophisticated immunochemical assays have evolved. Specific examples of several of these assays follow; others are briefly described in Box 16-3.

Radioimmunoassay

Radioimmunoassays (RIAs) were developed in the 1960s and used radioactive isotopes of iodine (^{125}I, ^{131}I) and tritium (^{3}H) as labels.[20,93] Radiolabeling of antigen with an isotope can cause changes in reactivity with the antibody. Therefore labeled and unlabeled antigens always need to be evaluated when a competitive assay is used to ensure that the antibody reacts equally with each form. Labeled antibody noncompetitive assays (immunoradiometric or "sandwich" assay) have the advantage of not requiring a quantity of purified antigen because the antigen does not have to be labeled. This also obviates potential problems that may be caused by iodination of labile antigens. Antibodies are relatively stable proteins that are less difficult to label without damaging the function of the protein. Combinations of labels (e.g., ^{57}Co and ^{125}I) have been used for simultaneous assays of lutropin and follitropin,[87] and thyrotropin and free thyroxine.

Enzyme Immunoassay (EIA)

Enzyme immunoassays use the catalytic properties of enzymes to detect and quantify immunologic reactions. In practice, enzyme-labeled antibodies or antigens (i.e., conjugates) are first allowed to react with ligands. Bound label is then separated and enzyme substrates are subsequently added. Measurement of the resultant decrease in substrate concentration or increase in product concentration is used to detect or quantify the antigen-antibody reaction. Alkaline phosphatase, horseradish peroxidase, glucose-6-phosphate dehydrogenase, and β-galactosidase enzyme labels predominate in EIA.[27,28] Enzyme-labeled antibody and antigen conjugates are prepared by covalent coupling procedures using bifunctional reagents [e.g., glutaraldehyde, *N*-succinimidyl-3-(pyridyl) propionate].[4]

Various detection systems have been used to monitor and quantify EIAs. Assays that produce compounds that can be monitored photometrically are very popular, because compact, high-performance photometers are available. However, EIAs that use fluorescent- or chemiluminescent-labeled substrates or products are often preferred to photometry-based assays owing to the inherent sensitivity of fluorescent and chemiluminescent measurements (see Chapter 10 and Table 16-2). Immunoassays that incorporate horseradish peroxidase as a label can be assayed by chemiluminescence using a mixture of (1) luminol, (2) peroxide, and an (3) enhancer such as *p*-iodophenol, or by using an acridan derivative.[2] Umbelliferone phosphate is a nonfluorescent substrate that is converted to the highly fluorescent umbelliferone by alkaline phosphatase.[24] A very sensitive assay for alkaline phosphatase labels uses a chemiluminescent adamantyl 1,2-dioxetane aryl phosphate substrate.[10] The enzyme dephosphorylates the substrate, which decomposes with a concomitant long-lived glow of light [detection limit for alkaline phosphatase using this assay is ≈1 zeptomole (10^{-21} moles)]. Enzyme cascade reactions have also been applied to the detection of enzyme labels in EIA; the principle of a cascade assay for alkaline phosphatase is illustrated in Figure 16-12. The advantage of such an assay is that it combines the amplification properties of two enzymes—the alkaline phosphatase label and the alcohol dehydrogenase in the assay reagent—thus producing a very sensitive assay (see Table 16-2).

BOX 16-3 Examples of Other Nonisotopic Immunoassays

Bioluminescent Immunoassays[66]
Native or recombinant apoaequorin (from the bioluminescent jellyfish *Aequorea*) is used as the label. It is activated by reaction with coelenterazine, and light emission at 469 nm is triggered by reaction with calcium ions (calcium chloride).

Erenna Immunoassay[72,74,79,91]
The Erenna Immunoassay System utilizes a modified microparticle-based sandwich immunoassay and single-molecule counting technology. It integrates capillary flow, laser-induced fluorescence, a highly sensitive detection optics module, and a 384-well plate format for sample analysis.

Fluorescence Excitation Transfer Immunoassay[81]
Homogeneous competitive assay in which a fluorophore (donor)-labeled antigen competes with an antigen in the sample for binding sites on an antibody labeled with a fluorescent dye (acceptor). The fluorescence of the donor is quenched when it is bound to the acceptor-labeled antibody.

Immuno-PCR[71]
Heterogeneous immunoassay in which a piece of single- or double-stranded DNA is used as a label for an antibody in a sandwich assay. Bound DNA label is amplified using the polymerase chain reaction (PCR). The amplified DNA product is separated by gel electrophoresis and quantitated by densitometric scanning of an ethidium-stained gel.

Nanotechnology-Based Assays[6,17,18,49,92-95]
A variety of immunoassays that employ nanoparticles, spheres, or tubes as solid phases.

Phosphor Immunoassay[60,96]
Heterogeneous immunoassay in which an upconverting phosphor nanoparticle is used as a label. The nanoparticle (200- to 400-nm diameter) is a crystalline lanthanide oxysulfide. It absorbs two or more photons of infrared light (980 nm) and produces light emission at a shorter wavelength (anti-Stokes shift). The phosphorescence is not influenced by reaction conditions (e.g., temperature, buffer), and no upconverted signal is received from biological components in the sample (low background). Multiplexing is possible because different types of particles produce different wavelengths of phosphorescence [e.g., yttrium/erbium oxysulfides are green (550 nm), yttrium/thulium oxysulfide particles are blue (475 nm)].

Quantum Dot Immunoassay[16,32,68]
Heterogeneous immunoassay in which a nanometer-sized (less than 10 nm) semiconductor quantum dot is used as a label. A quantum dot is a highly fluorescent nanocrystal composed of CdSe, CdS, ZnSe, InP, or InAs or a layer of ZnS or CdS on, for example, a CdSe core. Multiplexing is possible with these labels because the emission properties can be modulated by changing the size and composition of the nanocrystal (e.g., CdS emits blue light, InP emits red light).

Solid Phase, Light-Scattering Immunoassay[65]
Indium spheres are coated on glass to measure an antibody binding to an antigen. Binding of antibodies to antigens increases dielectric layer thickness, which produces a greater degree of scatter than in areas where only an antigen is bound. Quantitation is achieved by densitometry.

Surface Effect Immunoassay[75]
An antibody is immobilized on the surface of a waveguide (a quartz, glass, or plastic slide, or a gold- or silver-coated prism), and binding of an antigen is measured directly by total internal reflection fluorescence, surface plasmon resonance, or attenuated total reflection.

Types of enzyme-linked immunoassay include (1) enzyme-linked immunosorbent assay (ELISA), (2) EMIT, and (3) CEDIA.

Enzyme-Linked Immunosorbent Assay. ELISA is a heterogeneous EIA technique that is widely used in clinical analyses.[22,83] In this type of assay, one of the reaction components is nonspecifically adsorbed or covalently bound to the surface of a solid phase, such as a microtiter well, a magnetic particle, or a plastic bead. This attachment facilitates separation of bound- and free-labeled reactants. In the most common approach to using the ELISA technique, an aliquot of sample or calibrator containing the antigen to be quantitated is added to and allowed to bind with a solid phase antibody. After washing, enzyme-labeled antibody is added and forms a "sandwich complex" of solid phase Ab-Ag-Ab enzyme. Unbound antibody is then washed away, and enzyme substrate is added. The amount of product generated is proportional to the quantity of antigen in the sample. Specific antibodies in a sample can also be quantified using an ELISA procedure, in which antigen instead of antibody is bound to a solid phase and the second reagent is an enzyme-labeled antibody specific for the analyte antibody. Also, ELISA assays have been used extensively for detection of antibodies to viruses and autoantigens in serum or whole blood.[84] In addition, enzyme conjugates coupled with substrates that produce visible products have been used to develop ELISA-type assays with results that can be interpreted visually. Such assays have been found to be very useful in screening, point-of-care, and home testing applications.

Enzyme Multiplied Immunoassay Technique. EMIT is a homogeneous EIA that is very widely used in clinical analyses, an illustration of which is shown in Figure 16-13. Because EMIT does not require a separation step, it is simple to perform and has been used to develop a wide variety of drug, hormone, and metabolite assays.[70] Because of their operational simplicity, EMIT-type assays are easily automated and are included in the repertoire of many automated clinical and immunoassay analyzers (see Chapter 19). In this technique, antibody against the analyte drug, hormone, or metabolite is added together with substrate to the patient's sample. Binding

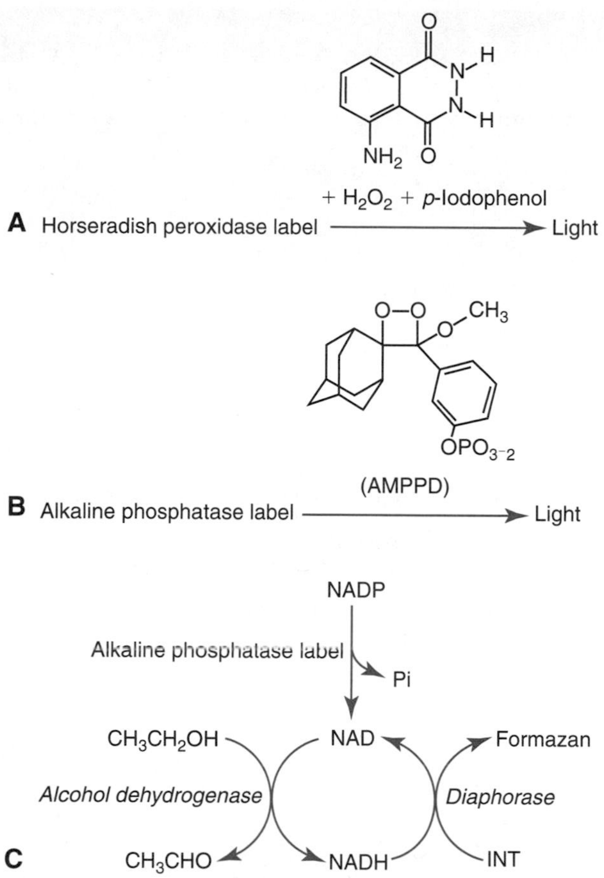

Figure 16-12 Ultrasensitive assays for horseradish peroxidase and alkaline phosphatase labels. A, Chemiluminescent assay for horseradish peroxidase label using luminol. B, Chemiluminescent assay for an alkaline phosphatase label using AMPPD. C, Photometric assay for an alkaline phosphatase label using a cascade detection reaction. *INT,* *p*-Iodonitrotetrazolium violet.

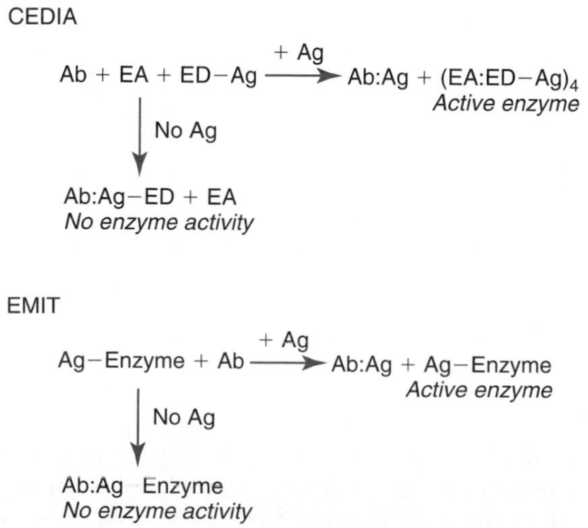

Figure 16-13 Cloned enzyme donor immunoassay (CEDIA) and enzyme multiplied immunoassay technique (EMIT) homogeneous immunoassays. *EA,* Enzyme acceptor; *ED,* enzyme donor.

of the antibody and analyte occurs. An aliquot of the enzyme conjugate of the analyte is then added as a second reagent; the enzyme hapten (analyte) conjugate binds with the excess analyte antibody, forming an antigen-antibody complex. This binding of the analyte antibody with the enzyme analyte conjugate affects enzyme activity by physically blocking access of the substrate to the active site of the enzyme, or by changing the conformation of the enzyme molecule and thus altering its activity. To complete the assay, the resultant enzyme activity is measured. The relative change in enzyme activity resulting from the formation of the antigen-antibody complex is proportional to the hapten concentration in the patient's sample. Concentration of the analyte is calculated from a calibration curve prepared by analyzing calibrators that contain known quantities of the analyte in question.

Cloned Enzyme Donor Immunoassay. As shown in Figure 16-13, CEDIA is a homogeneous EIA; it was the first EIA designed and developed using genetic engineering techniques.[36] Inactive fragments (the enzyme donor and acceptor) of β-galactosidase are prepared by manipulation of the Z gene of the *lac* operon of *E. coli.* These two fragments spontaneously reassemble to form active enzyme even if the enzyme donor is attached to an antigen. However, binding of antibody to the enzyme donor antigen conjugate inhibits reassembly, and no active enzyme is formed. Thus competition between the antigen and the enzyme donor antigen conjugate for a fixed amount of antibody in the presence of the enzyme acceptor modulates the measured enzyme activity (high concentrations of the analyte antigen produce the least inhibition of enzyme activity; low concentrations produce the greatest inhibition).

Fluoroimmunoassay

Examples of fluorophores that are used as labels in *fluoroimmunoassay* and their properties are listed in Table 16-3.[90] Initially, background fluorescence from drugs, drug metabolites, and protein-bound substances, such as bilirubin, limited the usefulness of this technique. However, this problem has largely been overcome by the use of rare earth (lanthanide) chelates and background rejection (time-resolved) procedures (see Chapters 10 and 19).[19,73] Fluorescent emissions from lanthanide chelates (e.g., europium, terbium, samarium) are long lived (greater than 1 μs) compared with the typical background fluorescence encountered in biological specimens. In a time-resolved fluoroimmunoassay, a europium chelate label is excited by a pulse of excitation light (0.5 μs), and the long-lived fluorescence emission from the label is measured after a delay (400 to 800 μs). By this time, any short-lived background signal has decayed.

Fluorescent polarization immunoassay is a type of homogeneous fluoroimmunoassay that is widely used to measure drugs and other small molecules (Figure 16-14).[41,63] The polarization of the fluorescence from a fluorescein-antigen conjugate is determined by its rate of rotation during the lifetime of the excited state in solution. A small, rapidly rotating fluorescein antigen conjugate has a low degree of polarization; however, binding to a large antibody molecule slows

TABLE 16-3 Properties of Fluorescent Labels

Fluorophore	Excitation, nm	Emission, nm	Fluorescence Quantum Yield*	Lifetime, ns
Fluorescein isothiocyanate	492	520	0.0-0.85	4.5
Europium (β-naphthoyl trifluoroacetone)	340	590, 613	–	500,000
Phycobiliprotein	550-620	580-660	0.5-0.98	–
Rhodamine B isothiocyanate	550	585	0.0-0.7	3.0
Umbelliferone	380	450	–	–

*Fluorescence quantum yield: fraction of molecules that emit a photon.

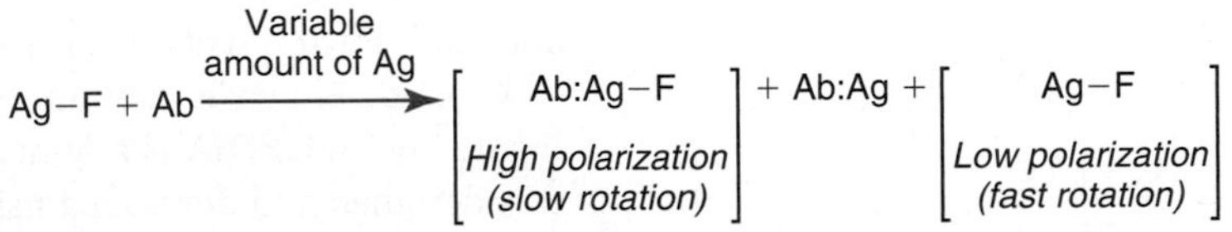

$$\text{Ag-F} + \text{Ab} \xrightarrow{\text{Variable amount of Ag}} \left[\begin{matrix}\text{Ab:Ag-F} \\ \textit{High polarization} \\ \textit{(slow rotation)}\end{matrix}\right] + \text{Ab:Ag} + \left[\begin{matrix}\text{Ag-F} \\ \textit{Low polarization} \\ \textit{(fast rotation)}\end{matrix}\right]$$

Figure 16-14 Homogeneous polarization fluoroimmunoassay. *F*, Fluorescein.

down the rate of rotation and increases the degree of polarization. Thus binding to antibody modulates polarization, and a homogeneous assay is possible.[42,56] As listed in Box 16-3, other types of homogeneous fluoroimmunoassays have been described in the literature.[28,46,64,81]

Chemiluminescence Immunoassay

Chemiluminescence is the name given to light emission produced during a chemical reaction (see Chapter 10). Isoluminol and acridinium esters are important examples of chemiluminescent labels used in *chemiluminescent immunoassay.* Oxidation of isoluminol by hydrogen peroxide in the presence of a catalyst, such as microperoxidase, produces a relatively long-lived light emission at 425 nm, and oxidation of an acridinium ester by alkaline hydrogen peroxide in the presence of a detergent (e.g., Triton X-100) produces a rapid flash of light at 429 nm. Acridinium and sulfonyl acridinium esters are high specific activity labels (detection limit for the label is 800 zeptomoles) that can be used to label both antibodies and haptens (Figure 16-15, *A*).[1,86]

Luminescent oxygen channeling immunoassay (LOCI) is a particularly important type of chemiluminescent immunoassay (Figure 16-16). It is one of the few homogeneous immunoassays that operate in a noncompetitive ("sandwich") format and can be used to assay large molecules. LOCI utilizes two reagent particles (sensitizer and chemiluminescer particles) that form a complex with the analyte of interest.[81] The presence of analyte links the two reagent latex particles in close proximity. The first particle contains a photosensitizer (e.g., phthalocyanine) and in the presence of light converts oxygen to singlet oxygen. The second chemiluminescer particle contains a chemiluminescent agent (e.g., olefin) that reacts with singlet oxygen to form a dioxetane that decomposes and emits light. This reaction occurs only if the two particles are in close proximity and the singlet oxygen can

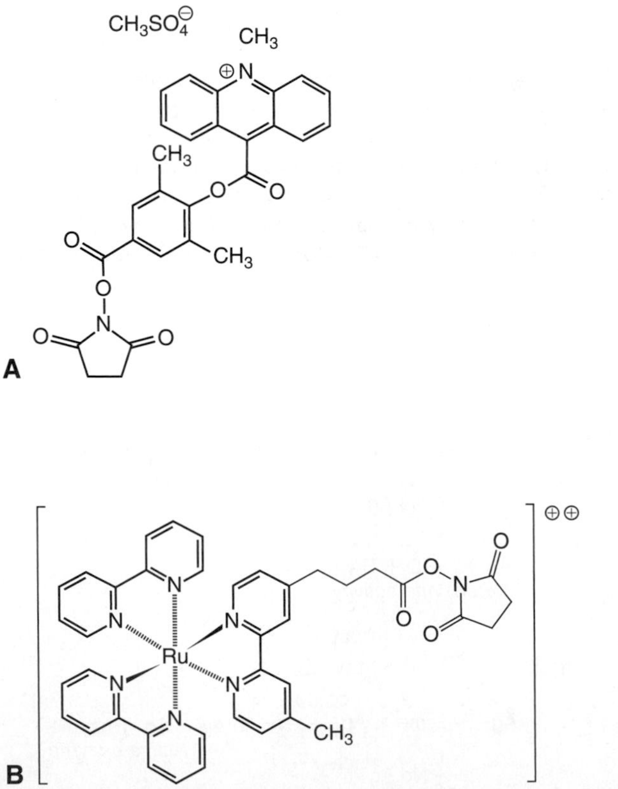

Figure 16-15 Luminescent labels. A, Chemiluminescent acridinium ester label. B, Electrochemiluminescent ruthenium (II) tris(bipyridyl) NHS ester label. *(From Law S-J, Miller T, Piran U, Klukas C, Chang S, Unger J. Novel poly-substituted aryl acridinium esters and their use in immunoassay. J Biolumin Chemilumin 1989;4:88-98. Reprinted by permission of John Wiley & Sons Ltd.)*

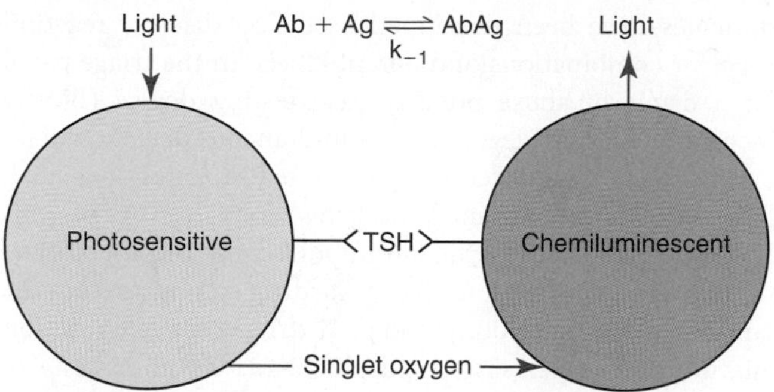

Figure 16-16 Example of a luminescent oxygen channeling immunoassay (LOCI). Note that thyroid-stimulating hormone (TSH)-linked microbeads are energized by light, which results in singlet oxygen activating the chemiluminescent bead to emit light of a specific wavelength.

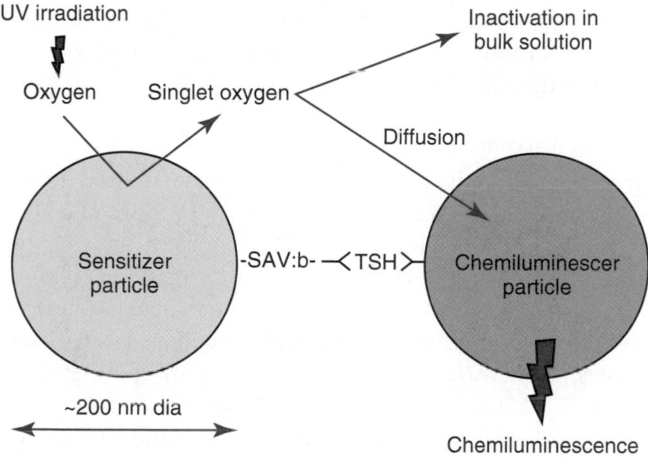

Figure 16-17 Example of luminescent oxygen channeling immunoassay (LOCI) for thyroid-stimulating hormone (TSH). In this assay, TSH links two latex microbeads—one containing a photosensitive reagent, and the other, a precursor of a chemiluminescent reagent.

diffuse efficiently from the sensitizer particle to the chemiluminescer particle. Singlet oxygen does not react with unbound chemiluminescer particles because of the short lifetime of this transient species in an aqueous environment.

An example of a sandwich immunoassay for thyroid-stimulating hormone (TSH) is illustrated in Figure 16-17. TSH binds to a biotinylated anti-TSH antibody, and this complex links the streptavidin-coated sensitizer particle to the anti-TSH antibody–coated chemiluminescer particle. Exposure of light results in emission of singlet oxygen from the photosensitive particle. The singlet oxygen activates the chemiluminescent particle to emit light that is then measured.[81]

Electrochemiluminescence Immunoassay

Ruthenium (II) tris(bipyridyl) (see Figure 16-15, *B*) undergoes an electrochemiluminescent reaction (620 nm) with tripropylamine at an electrode surface, and this chelate is now

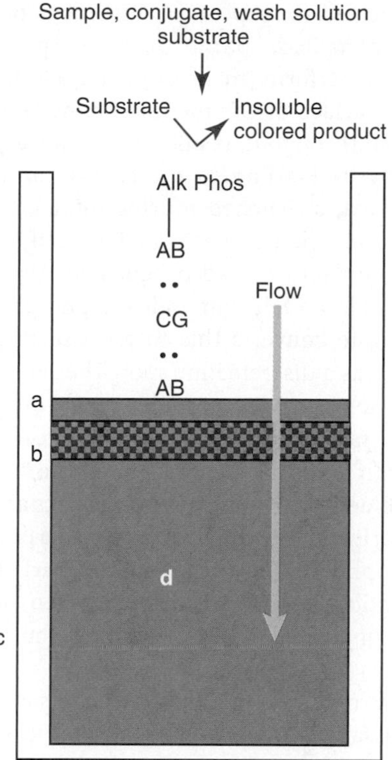

Figure 16-18 ICON immunoassay device (*a*, immobilized antibody membrane; *b*, separating membrane; *c*, container; *d*, adsorbent pad). *AB*, Monoclonal antibody to hCG; *hCG*, human chorionic gonadotropin.

used as a label in competitive and sandwich *electrochemiluminescence immunoassays*. Using this label, various assays have been developed in a flow cell using magnetic beads as the solid phase. Beads are captured at the electrode surface, and an unbound label is washed out of the cell by a wash buffer. Label bound to the bead undergoes an electrochemiluminescent reaction, and the light emission is measured by an adjacent photomultiplier tube.[7,38]

Simplified Immunoassays

Integration of the technical advances made in molecular immunology with those made in the material and processing sciences has resulted in the development of a number of "simplified" immunoassays for use in physicians' offices or the home (i.e., the so-called point-of-care market). Early efforts were directed toward pregnancy and fertility testing and were based on agglutination and inhibition of agglutination using labeled red blood cells or latex particles in a slide format. Subsequently, sandwich immunoassays have been adapted for similar applications. For example, as listed in the package insert, the ICON II pregnancy test (Beckman Coulter, Fullerton, Calif) is an operationally simple and sensitive assay for human chorionic gonadotropin (hCG) that detects hCG down to 10 mIU/mL for serum and 20 mIU/mL for urine. As shown in Figure 16-18, the ICON II test is a sandwich EIA device that uses a murine monoclonal antibody, which is immobilized onto the surface of a microporous nylon membrane located on top of an adsorbent pad.[82] The pad functions as a capillary pump to draw liquid through the membrane. To perform an analysis, an aliquot of urine is added to the surface of the membrane; hCG is removed as liquid is drawn through it, resulting in removal of hCG from the sample by its binding to the capture antibody on the membrane. Next, a matched murine monoclonal anti-hCG antibody alkaline phosphatase conjugate is added and is allowed to drain into the adsorbent pad. Wash solution is then added, followed by an indoxyl phosphate substrate. Bound conjugate converts this to an insoluble indigo dye, which appears as a discrete blue spot. The second generation of the ICON test includes two additional control zones. An immobilized anti–alkaline phosphatase zone acts as a procedural control; it binds the alkaline phosphatase conjugate and appears as a blue spot. Another zone contains an immobilized irrelevant murine monoclonal antibody; this detects the presence of heterophile antibodies in samples, particularly human antimouse antibodies.[8] These mimic antigen and bridge the capture and conjugated mouse antibodies, thus yielding what appears to be a positive result.

Newer tests require only the addition of sample, thus simplifying the assay protocol and minimizing possible malfunction resulting from operator error. Numerous one-step pregnancy tests are now available.[62] One uses a colloidal selenium particle (160-nm diameter) labeled with monoclonal anti–α-hCG antibody, which is red and easily visible. Sample (urine) is applied to the sample well and soaks into a glass fiber pad containing the conjugate. Any hCG in the urine sample combines with the selenium-labeled antibody, and the mixture migrates along a nitrocellulose track to a region where a line of polyclonal anti-hCG antibody and an orthogonal line of anti–α-hCG:hCG complex has been immobilized. The complex captures unreacted selenium-labeled anti–α-hCG to form a minus sign visible in the viewing window. If hCG is present in the urine sample, then the selenium-labeled anti–α-hCG:hCG complexes bind to the immobilized polyclonal anti-hCG, and a plus sign is formed, denoting a positive result. The remainder of the reaction mixture migrates to the end of the track and reacts with a Quinaldine Red pH indicator in an "end-of-assay" window to signal that the flow in the device has functioned correctly.

Another test device uses an absorbent strip that contains blue beads attached to an anti-hCG monoclonal antibody. As urine moves by capillary action through the strip, labeled antibodies are mobilized and move up the test strip, which contains regions of immobilized antibodies loaded with a blue dye. Each strip has separate windows for the positive, negative, and procedural controls. If hCG is present at a level of 25 mIU/mL or greater, a blue line becomes visible in the test region window. This region remains clear if the test is negative. A blue line appears in the reference region of the result window to show the test is complete and has worked correctly.

Simultaneous multianalyte immunoassays in which two or more analytes are detected in a single assay represent a further means of work simplification in immunoassay. Two different strategies have been developed based on discrete reaction zones or combinations of different labels. In the triage panel for a drugs of abuse point-of-care testing device (Biosite Incorporated, San Diego, Calif), simultaneous detection of up to nine drugs is achieved using discrete test zones on a small piece of nylon membrane.[12] Each test zone consists of antibodies for a specific drug immobilized on the membrane surface. This zone captures free gold-drug conjugate from the sample, antidrug antibody, and gold-drug conjugate reaction mixture and appears as a purple band. Combinations of distinguishable labels, such as europium (613 nm; emission lifetime, 730 μs) and samarium (643 nm; emission lifetime 50 μs) chelates, provide the basis of quantitative simultaneous immunoassays. These two chelates have different fluorescence emission maxima and different fluorescence decay times and thus can be easily distinguished by making measurements at 613 nm, delay time 0.4 ms (europium), and 643 nm, delay time 0.05 ms (samarium). An assay for free and bound prostate-specific antigen and an assay for myoglobin and carbonic anhydrase III are examples of tests combined in this simultaneous assay format.[54,85]

Protein Microarrays

Arrays of hundreds or thousands of micrometer-sized dots of antigens or antibodies immobilized on the surface of a glass or plastic chip are emerging as an important tool in proteomic studies and in assessing protein-protein interactions. This format facilitates simultaneous multianalyte immunoassays using, for example, enzyme or fluorophore-labeled conjugates. The arrays are made by printing or spotting 1-nL drops of protein solutions onto a flat surface, such as a glass microscope slide. In a typical sandwich assay, the array on the surface of the slide is incubated with sample and then with conjugate. Bound conjugate is detected with chemiluminescence or fluorescein using a scanning device. The pattern of the signal provides information on the presence and amount of individual analytes in the sample or the reactivity of a single analyte with the range of proteins arrayed on the surface of the slide.[77] (Such devices are discussed in greater detail in Chapter 10.)

Interferences in Immunoassays

Immunological assays are prone to interferences, in spite of the use of highly specific antibodies for molecular recognition of the analyte. Falsely low results can occur because of the hook effect at high antigen concentrations (see earlier discussion). False-negative or false-positive results are encountered if the sample contains anti–animal immunoglobulin antibodies. For example, in a two-site sandwich assay for hCG based on mouse antibodies, any human antimouse antibodies (HAMA) present in the specimen will recognize the immobilized mouse capture and mouse conjugate antibodies and will form a complex that is indistinguishable from an immobilized capture antibody:hCG:conjugate complex. This leads to a false-positive result. A false-negative result will be obtained if the HAMA react with the capture antibody or the conjugate to such an extent that specific antibody binding to hCG is prevented. Many different types of circulating anti–animal immunoglobulin antibodies have been detected (e.g., human antigoat, human antibovine antibodies) and shown to interfere in immunoassays. In practice, this type of interference is minimized by including additives in the immunoassay reagents such as nonimmune serum or IgG from the species used to raise the antibodies used in the assay.[8,45,48]

CELL AND TISSUE-BASED IMMUNOCHEMICAL TECHNIQUES

Other analytical methods of clinical interest that employ antibodies include immunohistochemistry and agglutination assays.

Immunohistochemistry

The use of labeled antibody reagents as specific probes for protein and peptide antigens allows the researcher and the pathologist to evaluate single cells or pieces of tissue for their synthetic capability and/or phenotypic identity. Immunohistochemistry has been rapidly expanded by immunoenzymatic methods, especially with regard to the use of horseradish peroxidase–labeled (immunoperoxidase) assays. Using enzyme labels provides several advantages over fluorescent labels. They permit the use of fixed tissue embedded in paraffin, which provides excellent preservation of cell morphology and eliminates the problem of autofluorescence from tissue. In addition, immunoperoxidase stains are permanent, and only a standard light microscope is necessary to identify labeled features. The immunoperoxidase methods are also applicable to electron microscopy. Several approaches for immunoenzymatic assays have been used, including direct, indirect, peroxidase-antiperoxidase, and enzyme bridge methods.

Agglutination Assays

Agglutination assays have been used for many years for the qualitative and quantitative measurement of antigens and antibodies. In an agglutination method, the visible clumping of particulates, such as cells and latex particles, is used as an indicator of the primary reaction of antigen and antibody. Agglutination methods require stable and uniform particulates, pure antigen, and specific antibody. IgM antibodies are more likely to produce complete agglutination than are IgG antibodies because of the size and valence of the IgM molecule. Therefore, when only IgG antibodies are involved, it may be necessary to use chemical enhancement or an antiglobulin agglutination method. As with all immunochemical reactions in which aggregation is the measured end point, the ratio of antigen to antibody is critical. Extremes in antigen or antibody concentration will result in inhibition of aggregation.

An incomplete agglutination reaction is one in which the primary reaction occurs, but no or only minimal aggregation of the particles occurs. Many particles, such as erythrocytes and bacteria in solution, have a net negative charge (zeta potential), which causes mutual repulsion.[88] For successful agglutination, the antigen-antibody reaction must overcome this normal resistance. In the case of a weak antigen-antibody reaction, or one in which only IgG is involved, this mutual repulsion may be sufficient to inhibit agglutination completely or partially. In systems in which incomplete agglutination results, enhancement may be achieved by lowering the ionic strength or by introducing polymeric molecules, such as polymerized albumin (5% to 30%), dextran, polybrene, polyvinylpyrrolidone, or PEG.[88]

Hemagglutination refers to agglutination reactions in which the antigen is located on an erythrocyte. Erythrocytes not only are good passive carriers of antigen, they also are easily coated with foreign proteins and can be easily obtained and stored.

Direct testing of erythrocytes for blood group, Rh, and other antigenic types is used widely in blood banks; specific antisera, such as anti-A, anti-C, and anti-Kell, are used to detect such antigens on the erythrocyte surface.

In *indirect* or *passive* hemagglutination, the erythrocytes are used as a particulate carrier of foreign antigen (and in some tests of antibodies); this technique has wide applications. Other materials available in the form of fine particles, such as bentonite and latex, also have been used as antigen carriers, but they are more difficult to coat, standardize, and store. In a related variation of this technique, known as *hemagglutination inhibition,* the ability of antigens, haptens, or other substances to specifically inhibit hemagglutination of sensitized (coated) cells by antibody is determined.

In general, agglutination methods are sensitive but are not as quantitative as other immunochemical methods discussed thus far. Nonisotopic immunoassays, especially EIAs, are as convenient as agglutination reactions and therefore are replacing agglutination methods in many laboratories.

REFERENCES

1. Adamczyk M, Chen YY, Fishpaugh JR, Mattingly PG, Pan Y, Shreder K, et al. Linker-mediated modulation of the chemiluminescent signal from *N*(10)-(3-sulfopropyl)-*N*-sulfonylacridinium-9-carboxamide tracers. Bioconj Chem 2000;11:714-24.
2. Akhavan-Tafti H, Sugioka K, Arghavani Z, Desilva R, Handley RS, Sugioka Y, et al. Lumigen™ PS: Chemiluminescent detection of horseradish peroxidase by enzymatic generation of acridinium esters. Clin Chem 1995;41:1368-9.
3. Alper CA, Johnson AM. Immunofixation electrophoresis: a technique for the study of protein polymorphism. Vox Sang 1969;17:445-52.
4. Avrameas S, Ternynck T, Guesdon JL. Coupling of enzymes to antibodies and antigens. Scand J Immunol 1978;8(Suppl 7):7-23.
5. Bayer EA, Wilcheck M. The use of the avidin-biotin complex as a tool in molecular biology. Methods Biochem Anal 1980;26:2-42.
6. Bi S, Zhou H, Zhang S. Multilayers enzyme-coated carbon nanotubes as biolabel for ultrasensitive chemiluminescence immunoassay of cancer biomarker. Biosens Bioelectron 2009;24:2961-6.
7. Blackburn GF, Shah HP, Kenten JH, Leland J, Kamin RA, Link J, et al. Electrochemiluminescence detection for development of immunoassays and DNA probe assays for clinical diagnostics. Clin Chem 1991;37:1534-9.
8. Boscato LM, Stuart MC. Heterophilic antibodies: a problem for all immunoassays. Clin Chem 1988;34:27-33.
9. Brandshund I, Siersted SE, Teisner B. Double-decker rocket immunoelectrophoresis for direct quantitation of complement split products with C3d specificities in plasma. J Immunol Methods 1981;44:63-71.

10. Bronstein I, Edwards B, Voyta JC. 1,2-Dioxetanes: novel chemiluminescent enzyme substrates: applications to immunoassays. J Biolumin Chemilumin 1989;4:99-111.
11. Brunette WN. Western blotting: electrophoretic transfer of proteins from sodium dodecyl sulfate-polyacrylamide gels to unmodified nitrocellulose and radiographic detection with antibody and radioiodinated protein A. Anal Biochem 1981;112:195-203.
12. Buechler KF, Moi S, Noar B, McGrath D, Villela J, Clancy M, et al. Simultaneous detection of seven drugs of abuse by the Triage™ panel for drugs of abuse. Clin Chem 1992;38:1678-4.
13. Buffone GJ, Lewis SA. Advantages of small angle light scattering measurements in immunonephelometry. In: Peeters H, Wright PH, eds. Plasma protein pathology. New York: Pergamon Press, 1979:55-61.
14. Buffone GJ, Savory J, Cross RE, Hammond JE. Evaluation of kinetic light scattering as an approach to the measurement of specific proteins with the centrifugal analyzer. I. Methodology. Clin Chem 1975;21: 1731-4.
15. Burton DR, Barbas CF III. Human antibodies from combinatorial libraries. Adv Immunol 1994;57:191-280.
16. Chan WC, Maxwell DJ, Gao X, Bailey RE, Han M, Nie S. Luminescent quantum dots for multiplexed biological detection and imaging. Curr Opin Biotechnol 2002;13:40-6.
17. Chen J, Wang C, Irudayaraj J. Ultrasensitive protein detection in blood serum using gold nanoparticle probes by single molecule spectroscopy. J Biomed Opt 2009;14:040501.
18. Cui D, Pan B, Zhang H, Gao F, Wu R, Wang J, et al. Self-assembly of quantum dots and carbon nanotubes for ultrasensitive DNA and antigen detection. Anal Chem 2008;80:7996-8001.
19. Diamandis EP. Multiple labeling and time-resolvable fluorophores. Clin Chem 1991;37:1486-91.
20. Ekins RP. The estimation of thyroxine in human plasma by an electrophoretic technique. Clin Chim Acta 1960;5:453-9.
21. Ekins RP. Current concepts and future developments. In: Collins WP, ed. Alternative immunoassays. New York: John Wiley & Sons Inc, 1985:219-37.
22. Engvall E, Perlmann P. Enzyme-linked immunosorbent assay (ELISA): quantitative assay of immunoglobulin G. Immunochemistry 1971;8: 871-4.
23. Fahey JL, McKelvey EM. Quantitative determination of serum immunoglobulins in antibody agar plates. J Immunol 1965;94:84-90.
24. Fiore M, Mitchell J, Doan T, Nelson R, Winter G, Grandone C, et al. The Abbott IMx™ automated benchtop immunochemistry analyzer system. Clin Chem 1988;34:1726-32.
25. Gauldie J, Bienenstock J. Automated nephelometric analysis of haptens. In: Ritchie R, ed. Automated immunoanalysis, vol 7, part 1. New York: Marcel Dekker Inc, 1978:321-33.
26. Gershoni JM, Palade GE. Electrophoretic transfer of proteins from sodium dodecyl-sulfate-polyacrylamide gels to a positively charged membrane filter. Anal Biochem 1982;124:396-405.
27. Giegel JL, Brotherton MM, Cronin P, D'Aquino M, Evans H, Heller ZH, et al. Radial partition immunoassay. Clin Chem 1982;28:1894-98.
28. Gosling JP. A decade of development in immunoassay methodology. Clin Chem 1990;36:1408-27.
29. Grange J, Roch AM, Quash GA. Nephelometric assay of antigens and antibodies with latex particles. J Immunol Methods 1977;18:365-75.
30. Grossberg AL, Chen CC, Rendina L, Pressman D. Specific cation effects with antibody to a hapten with a positive charge. J Immunol 1962;88:600-3.
31. Guesdon JL, Ternynck T, Avrameas S. The use of avidin-biotin interaction in immunoenzymatic techniques. J Histochem Cytochem 1979;27:1131-9.
32. Han M, Gao X, Su JZ, Nie S. Quantum-dot-tagged microbeads for multiplexed optical coding of biomolecules. Nat Biotechnol 2001;19:631-5.
33. Harrington JL, Fenton JW, Pert H. Polymer-induced precipitation of antigen-antibody complexes: "precipiplex reactions." Immunochemistry 1971;8:413-21.
34. Hellsing K. Immune reactions in polysaccharide media: polysaccharide-enhanced precipitation reactions with antigens of various sizes. Biochem J 1969;114:145-9.
35. Hellsing K. Immune reactions in polysaccharide media. I. The effect of dextran on the reaction between ^{125}I-labeled human serum albumin and gamma-G-globulin from rabbit. Acta Chem Scand 1966;20: 1251-62.
36. Henderson DR, Friedman SB, Harris JB, Manning WB, Zoccoli MA. CEDIA, a new homogeneous immunoassay system. Clin Chem 1986;32:1637-41.
37. Hills LP, Tiffany TO. Comparison of turbidimetric and light-scattering measurements of immunoglobulins by use of a centrifugal analyzer with absorbance and fluorescence-light-scattering optics. Clin Chem 1980;26:1459-66.
38. Hoyle NR. The application of electrochemiluminescence to immunoassay-based analyte detection. In: Campbell AK, Kricka LJ, Stanley PE, eds. Bioluminescence and chemiluminescence: fundamentals and applied aspects. Chichester: Wiley, 1994:28-31.
39. Jackson TM, Ekins RP. Theoretical limitations on immunoassay. Methods Enzymol 1986;74:28-60.
40. Jackson TM, Ekins RP. Theoretical limitations of immunoassay sensitivity: current practice and potential advantages of fluorescent Eu^{3+} chelates as non-radioisotopic tracers. J Immunol Methods 1986; 87:13-20.
41. Jolley ME, Stroupe SD, Wang CJ. Fluorescence polarization immunoassay. I. Monitoring aminoglycoside antibiotics in serum and plasma. Clin Chem 1981;27:1190-7.
42. Kabat EA. Structural concepts in immunology and immunochemistry, 2nd edition. New York: Holt, Rinehart & Winston Inc, 1976.
43. Keren DF. High resolution electrophoresis and immunofixation techniques. Boston: Butterworth-Heineman, 1994.
44. Kohler G, Milstein C. Continuous cultures of fused cells secreting antibody of predefined specificity. Nature 1975;256:495-7.
45. Kohse KP, Wisser H. Antibodies as a source of analytical errors. J Clin Chem Clin Biochem 1990;28:881-92.
46. Kricka LJ. Ligand-binder assays. New York: Marcel Dekker Inc, 1985.
47. Kricka LJ. Chemiluminescent and bioluminescent techniques. Clin Chem 1991;37:1472-81.
48. Kricka LJ. Human anti-animal antibody interferences in immunological assays. Clin Chem 1999;45:942-56.
49. Lai G, Yan F, Ju H. Dual signal amplification of glucose oxidase—functionalized nanocomposites as a trace label for ultrasensitive simultaneous multiplexed electrochemical detection of tumor markers. Anal Chem 2009;81:9730-6.
50. Laurell CB. Antigen-antibody crossed electrophoresis. Anal Biochem 1965;10:358-61.
51. Laurell CB. Electroimmunoassay. Scand J Clin Lab Invest 1972; 29(Suppl 124):21-37.
52. Laurent TC. In: Quintarelei G, ed. The chemical physiology of mucopolysaccharides. Boston: Little, Brown & Co Inc, 1968:153.
53. Laurent TC. The interaction between polysaccharides and other macromolecules. 5. The solubility of proteins in the presence of dextran. Biochem J 1963;89:253-7.
54. Leinonen J, Lovgren T, Vornanen T, Stenman U-H. Double-label time-resolved immunofluorometric assay of prostate-specific antigen and its complex with alpha1-antichymotrypsin. Clin Chem 1993; 39:2098-103.
55. Leute RK, Ullman EF, Goldstein A, Herzenberg LA. Spin immunoassay technique for determination of morphine. Nature 1972;236:93-4.
56. Li TM, Benovic JL, Burd JF. Serum theophylline determination by fluorescence polarization immunoassay utilizing an umbelliferone derivative as a fluorescent label. Anal Biochem 1981;118:102-7.
57. Mancini G, Carbonara AO, Heremans JF. Immunochemical quantitation of antigens by single radial immunodiffusion. Immunochemistry 1965;2:235-54.
58. Marrack JR, Richards CB. Light scattering studies of the formation of aggregates in mixtures of antigen and antibody. Immunology 1970; 20:1019-40.

59. McCormack RT, Ludwig JR, Wolfert RL. Advances in design, generation, and manipulation of monoclonal antibodies. In: Nakamura RM, Kasahara Y, Rechnitz GA, eds. Immunochemical assays and biosensor technology for the 1990s. Washington DC: American Association for Microbiology, 1992:57-82.
60. Niedbala RS, Feindt H, Kardos K, Vail T, Burton J, Bielska B, et al. Detection of analytes by immunoassay using up-converting phosphor technology. Anal Biochem 2001;293:22-30.
61. Nygren H, Stenberg M. Diffusion-in-gel enzyme-linked immunosorbent assay (DIG-ELISA): quantification of antigen by diffusion over an antibody-coated surface. Scand J Clin Lab Invest 1982;42:355-9.
62. Osikowicz G, Beggs M, Brookhart P, Caplan D, Ching S, Eck P, et al. One step chromatographic immunoassay for qualitative determination of choriogonadotrophin in urine. Clin Chem 1990;36:1586.
63. Popelka SR, Miller DM, Holen JT, Kelso DM. Fluorescence polarization immunoassay. II. Analyzer for rapid, precise measurement of fluorescence polarization with use of disposable cuvettes. Clin Chem 1981;27:1198-201.
64. Price CP, Newman DJ, eds. Principles and practice of immunoassay, 2nd edition. New York: Stockton Press, 1996.
65. Rej R, Keese CR, Giaever I. Direct immunochemical determination of aspartate aminotransferase isoenzymes. Clin Chem 1981;27:1597-601.
66. Rigl CT, Patel MT, Rivera HN, Stults NL, Smith DF. A bioluminescent immunoassay based on the recombinant photoprotein. In: Campbell AK, Kricka LJ, Stanley PE, eds. Bioluminescence and chemiluminescence: fundamentals and applied aspects. Chichester: Wiley, 1994:345-8.
67. Rodbard D. Data processing for radioimmunoassays: an overview. In: Natelson S, Pesce AJ, Mietz AA, eds. Clinical immunochemistry, vol 3. Washington DC: American Association for Clinical Chemistry, 1978: 477-94.
68. Rosenthal SJ. Bar-coding biomolecules with fluorescent nanocrystals. Nat Biotechnol 2001;19:621-2.
69. Rowe DS. Radioactive single radial diffusion: a method for increasing the sensitivity of immunochemical quantitation of proteins in agar gel. Bull WHO 1969;40:613-16.
70. Rubenstein KE, Schneider RS, Ullman EF. "Homogeneous" enzyme immunoassay: new immunochemical technique. Biochem Biophys Res Commun 1972;47:846-51.
71. Sano T, Smith CL, Cantor CR. Immuno-PCR: very sensitive antigen detection by means of specific antibody-DNA conjugates. Science 1992;258:120-2.
72. Schultze AE, Konrad RJ, Credille KM, Lu QA, Todd J. Ultrasensitive cross-species measurement of cardiac troponin-I using the Erenna immunoassay system. Toxicol Pathol 2008;36:777-82.
73. Soini E, Kojola J. Time-resolved fluorometer for lanthanide chelates: a new generation of non-isotopic immunoassays. Clin Chem 1983;29: 65-8.
74. St Ledger K, Agee SJ, Kasaian MT, Forlow SB, Durn BL, Minyard J, et al. Analytical validation of a highly sensitive microparticle-based immunoassay for the quantitation of IL-13 in human serum using the Erenna immunoassay system. J Immunol Methods 2009;350:161-70.
75. Sutherland R, Simpson B, Allman B. Surface effect immunoassay. In: Price CP, Newman DJ, eds. Principles and practice of immunoassay. New York: Stockton Press, 1991:515-42.
76. Tanford C. The hydrophobic effect: formation of micelles and biological membranes. New York: John Wiley & Sons Inc, 1980.
77. Templin MF, Stoll D, Schrenk M, Traub PC, Vohringer CF, Joos TO. Protein microarray technology. Trends Biotechnol 2002;20:160-6.
78. Tengerdy RP. Reaction kinetic studies of the antigen antibody reaction. J Immunol 1967;99:126-32.
79. Todd J, Freese B, Lu A, Held D, Morey J, Livingston R, et al. Ultrasensitive flow-based immunoassays using single-molecule counting. Clin Chem 2007;53:1990-5.
80. Ullman EF, Kirakossian H, Switchenko AC, Ishkanian J, Ericson M, Wartchow CA, et al. Luminescent oxygen channeling assay (LOCI): sensitive, broadly applicable homogeneous immunoassay method. Clin Chem 1996;42:1518-26.
81. Ullman EF, Khana PL. Fluorescence excitation transfer immunoassay (FETI). Methods Enzymol 1981;74: 28-60.
82. Valkirs GE, Barton R. ImmunoConcentration™: a new format for solid-phase immunoassays. Clin Chem 1985;31:1427-31.
83. Van Weeman BK, Schuurs AH. Immunoassay using antigen-enzyme conjugates. FEBS Letts 1971;15:232-6.
84. Voller A, Bartlett A, Bidwell DE. Enzyme immunoassays with special reference to ELISA techniques. J Clin Pathol 1978;31:507-19.
85. Vuori J, Rasi S, Takala T, Vaananen K. Dual-label time-resolved fluoroimmunoassay for simultaneous detection of myoglobin and carbonic anhydrase III. Clin Chem 1991;37:2087-92.
86. Weeks I, Campbell AK, Woodhead JS. Two-site immunochemiluminometric assay for human alpha-1 fetoprotein. Clin Chem 1983;29:1480-3.
87. Wians FH Jr, Dev J, Powell MM, Heald JI. Evaluation of simultaneous measurements of lutropin and follitropin with the SimulTropin™ radioimmunoassay kit. Clin Chem 1986;32:887-90.
88. Williams CA, Chase MM, eds. Methods in immunology and immunochemistry, vol 3. New York: Academic Press Inc, 1970: 1-125.
89. Winter G, Griffiths AD, Hawkins RE, Hoogenboom HR. Making antibodies by phage display technology. Ann Rev Immunol 1994; 12:433-55.
90. Wood P. Heterogeneous fluoroimmunoassay. In: Price CP, Newman DJ, eds. Principles and practice of immunoassay. New York: Stockton Press, 1991:365-92.
91. Wu AH, Shea E, Lu QT, Minyard J, Bui K, Hsu JC, et al. Short- and long-term cardiac troponin I analyte stability in plasma and serum from healthy volunteers by use of an ultrasensitive, single-molecule counting assay. Clin Chem 2009;55:2057-9.
92. Xie C, Xu F, Huang X, Dong C, Ren J. Single gold nanoparticles counter: an ultrasensitive detection platform for one-step homogeneous immunoassays and DNA hybridization assays. J Am Chem Soc 2009;131:12763-70.
93. Yalow RS, Berson SA. Assay of plasma insulin in human subjects by immunological methods. Nature 1959;184:1648-69.
94. Yang XY, Guo YS, Bi S, Zhang SS. Ultrasensitive enhanced chemiluminescence enzyme immunoassay for the determination of alpha-fetoprotein amplified by double-codified gold nanoparticles labels. Biosens Bioelectron 2009;24:2707-11.
95. Yin Z, Cui R, Liu Y, Jiang L, Zhu JJ. Ultrasensitive electrochemical immunoassay based on cadmium ion-functionalized PSA-PAA nanospheres. Biosens Bioelectron 2010;25:1319-24.
96. Zijlmans HJ, Bonnet J, Burton J, Kardos K, Vail T, Niedbala RS, et al. Detection of cell and tissue surface antigens using up-converting phosphors: a new reporter technology. Anal Biochem 1999;267: 30-6.

CHAPTER 17

Nucleic Acid Techniques

Carl T. Wittwer, M.D., Ph.D.,
and Noriko Kusukawa, Ph.D.

Molecular diagnostics requires techniques to detect extremely low concentrations of nucleic acids in a background of complex genomic structure. This chapter begins by considering the enzymes that allow us to process nucleic acids into forms suitable for analytical interrogation. We briefly touch on chemical and other processes that aid us in handling nucleic acids (nucleic acid isolation is discussed in detail in Chapter 39). We then discuss amplification techniques that are often necessary to observe or quantify nucleic acid sequences of interest. The tools used to detect or visualize nucleic acids are discussed. Finally, specific methods are described that allow identification, quantification, and/or segregation of individual nucleic acid species.

Molecular diagnostics is a highly competitive field, both in academics and in industry. Those using particular techniques, instruments, or probe designs may defend their choices with a commitment that approaches religious fervor. In this chapter, cute trade names and commercial references are avoided. To misquote the Bard's fool, "if you think our presentation less familiar, please accept that our intent was not to offend, perhaps inspection of the references will mend."

ENZYMES THAT ACT ON NUCLEIC ACIDS

Nucleic acid enzymes are critical tools for the techniques used in molecular diagnostics. Common enzymes that act on nucleic acids include those that synthesize nucleic acid polymers and those that process them into shorter fragments. These enzymes are critical for DNA replication and RNA transcription and must be present in all cells that replicate. In addition, a variety of unique enzymes found in bacteria and viruses act on specific nucleic acid sequences. Many of these enzymes have been purified and synthesized in vitro, sometimes "engineered" with alterations that improve their performance or stability. Our ability to manipulate nucleic acids in vitro with these enzymes has made modern molecular biology possible. Enzymes are used extensively in nucleic acid diagnostics, including sample preparation, probe labeling, signal generation, and amplification of targets and probes.

Nucleases are enzymes that hydrolyze one or more phosphodiester bonds in nucleic acid polymers.[67] Nucleases may require a free hydroxyl end *(exonucleases),* with specificity for the 3′ or 5′ end, or may act only on internal bonds *(endonucleases).* Nucleases can be DNA or RNA specific and may act only on double- or single-stranded polymers. For example, DNAse I digests double-stranded DNA (dsDNA), and S1 nuclease acts only on single-stranded DNA (ssDNA). DNase I can be used to specifically degrade DNA in nucleic acid mixtures when only RNA is of interest. RNAses are very stable enzymes that are common laboratory contaminants.

DNA glycosylases are enzymes that remove damaged nitrogenous bases while leaving the sugar-phosphate backbone of DNA intact. Uracil *N*-glycosylase (UNG) from the bacterium *Escherichia coli* is commonly used in molecular diagnostics to prevent carryover contamination of DNA from previous amplification reactions (see Contamination Control to Avoid False-Positive Results later in this chapter for details).

Restriction endonucleases are found in bacteria; these enzymes prevent replication of foreign DNA.[99] Their action is sequence specific, requiring recognition sequences of usually 4 to 10 nucleotides on a dsDNA molecule. Often, these recognition sequences are palindromic (meaning that the same sequence occurs on both of the complementary DNA strands). At each location where these sequences are found, the enzyme cuts both strands in a reproducible manner, resulting in staggered or blunt-end cuts. For example, *Eco*RI is a restriction enzyme from *E. coli* that recognizes the six-base sequence GAATTC and cuts between the G and the A on both strands, producing a staggered cut:

5′ … G/AATTC … 3′
3′ … CTTAA/G … 5′

Note that "blunt-end" cuts would be produced if an enzyme hydrolyzed the bond between A and T. Some restriction enzymes recognize nonpalindromic asymmetric sequences and cut outside of the recognition sequence. An example is *Fok*I, which recognizes the sequence 5′GGATG, and then cuts the two DNA strands 9 and 13 bases downstream of the recognition sequence, generating a four-base 5′ overhang.

Restriction enzymes are used for digesting large strands of DNA into smaller fragments and for preparing DNA from different sources to be joined together in cloning procedures. *Nicking enzymes* are restriction enzymes that cut only one strand of double-stranded nucleic acid. *Methylation-sensitive enzymes* are restriction enzymes that distinguish between cytosine and 5-methylcytosine in the recognition sequence. In humans, methylation of cytosine is a common epigenetic modification of DNA and is important because it affects gene expression.

Ligases catalyze the formation of phosphodiester linkages between two nucleic acid chains.[48] DNA ligases are not sequence specific but require the presence of a complementary template. In contrast, RNA ligases used in mRNA processing do not require a template but are sensitive to sequence.

Polymerases catalyze the synthesis of complementary nucleic acid polymers using a parent strand as a template.[48] In vitro, these enzymes can extend an oligonucleotide primer that is annealed to a template strand. Extension requires that the 3′-OH of the extending end is free, and that nucleotide triphosphates (NTPs) are present in the reaction mixture. Extension stops if you run out of template or NTPs, or if no 3′-OH groups are available at the extending end. DNA polymerases generate DNA strands from a DNA template, whereas RNA polymerases generate RNA strands from a DNA template. Thermostable polymerases, such as *Thermus aquaticus (Taq)* DNA polymerase, are essential reagents for the automation of many nucleic acid amplification procedures because of their stability at the high temperatures used in these procedures. Some DNA polymerases also have exonuclease activity that can be 3′ to 5′, 5′ to 3′, or both. A polymerase with 3′ to 5′ exonuclease activity can correct mismatched base pairs at the 3′-end of the extending chain. Such *proofreading activity* increases polymerase *fidelity* by decreasing the number of errors or misincorporated bases. A polymerase with 5′ to 3′ exonuclease activity can increase polymerase *processivity* by cleaving any blocking probes or secondary structures, thereby increasing the number of bases incorporated for each extension.

Reverse transcriptase is found in retroviruses and catalyzes the synthesis of DNA from an RNA (or DNA) template.[2] Retroviruses have RNA genomes, and reverse transcriptase activity is required as part of their replication. Reverse transcriptases do not have proofreading activity and therefore are error prone compared with polymerases. This, however, allows viruses to mutate quickly and develop drug resistance. In vitro, reverse transcriptase is used to make complementary DNA (cDNA) copies of RNA in samples and may be used for cloning, probe preparation, and nucleic acid assays.

NUCLEIC ACID TREATMENTS THAT DO NOT USE ENZYMES

Sometimes nonenzymatic methods are used to process nucleic acids before amplification and/or analysis. This is not an exhaustive list, and others are discussed during various parts of the remainder of this chapter.

Sonication, shearing, or *chemical cleavage* can be used to cut DNA or RNA into smaller fragments so as to make the analytical processes that follow more efficient. Sonication generates nucleic acid fragments of 100 to 1000 bases in length, depending on the conditions used. Shearing can be performed by a compressed air device known as a *nebulizer.* For chemical cleavage, several metal-ion–catalyzed chemistries can cleave single-stranded and double-stranded nucleic acids. Some alkylating compounds can cleave and label nucleic acids at the same time. One example is 5-(bromomethyl)-fluorescein, which is catalyzed by metal ions to fragment RNA or DNA, and then labels those fragments with fluorescein.[10] This can be used in nucleic acid preparation for microarray analysis.

Bisulfite treatment of DNA is used to analyze the methylation status of cytosine (C) residues in DNA. Sodium bisulfite ($NaHSO_3$),[36] optionally used together with ammonium bisulfite,[97] converts C into uracil (U), but does not affect 5-methylcytosine. The chemical process of bisulfite treatment is shown in Figure 17-1. The process works effectively only on single-stranded DNA, and so the sample needs to be denatured by heat, alkali, or chaotropic agents such as urea or formamide. Analysis of the bisulfite-treated DNA is usually performed after nucleic acid amplification. DNA polymerases used for amplification will treat 5-methylcytosine as C (no change in sequence), but they will treat unmethylated C that is converted to U as a T (thus a sequence change of C to T). Many methods can be used to detect and quantify the altered sequences that result from bisulfite treatment of methylated DNA, including preferential amplification, detection with probes, melting techniques, and sequencing.[49] One limitation of bisulfite treatment is that it significantly degrades DNA.

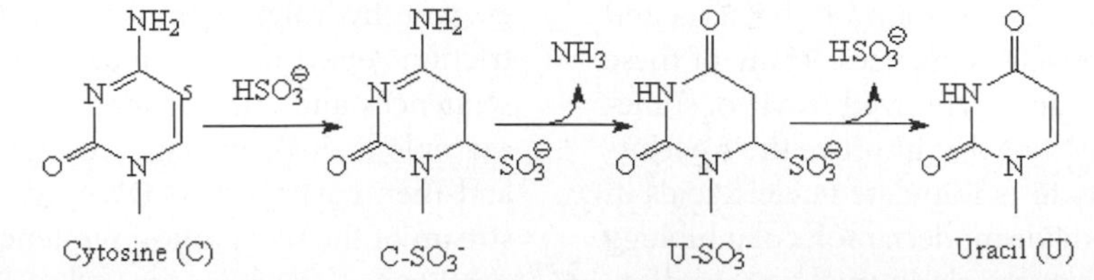

Cytosine (C) — HSO_3^- → $C\text{-}SO_3^-$ → (NH_3) $U\text{-}SO_3^-$ → (HSO_3^-) Uracil (U)

Figure 17-1 Bisulfite-mediated conversion of cytosine (C) to uracil (U) occurs in three steps. The first step is the addition of bisulfite to C. This reaction occurs at acid pH. The second step is the deamination of cytidine-bisulfite ($C\text{-}SO_3^-$) to produce uracil-bisulfite ($U\text{-}SO_3^-$), which is optimal at pH 5 to 6. Prior to analysis, $U\text{-}SO_3^-$ is converted to U by adjusting the pH to alkali. The majority of methylation on the C residue in mammalian cells occurs at the carbon 5 position (shown in the structure of C), resulting in 5-methylcytosine, which is resistant to bisulfite-mediated conversion.

Depending on the protocol, as much as 90% of the DNA can be lost.

Affinity enrichment of methylated DNA is an alternative to bisulfite treatment that may provide higher yields. One example is to enrich methylated DNA by immunoprecipitation with an antibody raised against DNA containing 5-methylcytosine.[117] Up to 90-fold enrichment in methylated DNA can be achieved by immunoprecipitation. Another method is to use methylated DNA binding protein to capture double-stranded methylated DNA on an affinity column or other solid support.[83]

Reversal of formalin (formaldehyde) cross-linking is required before DNA or RNA can be analyzed from tissues prepared in formalin-fixed paraffin-embedded (FFPE) blocks. Formalin modifies nucleic acids with monomethylol groups, which cause nucleic acids to cross-link by forming methylene bridges to amino groups.[63] These cross-links interfere with many processes, including reverse transcription and polymerase reactions. Heating the DNA or RNA reverses cross-linking, and most protocols use alkali (pH 9 to 12) conditions to reverse formalin cross-linking in DNA and acid (pH 3 to 6) conditions for RNA. Depending on the age of the FFPE specimen, nucleic acid can be degraded into short fragments.

AMPLIFICATION TECHNIQUES

Achieving adequate detection limits is a central concern for clinical applications of nucleic acid analysis. Techniques that increase the amount of the nucleic acid target, the detection signal, or the probe are referred to as *amplification methods*. Examples of amplification methods are listed in Table 17-1. In *target amplification*, a well-defined segment of the nucleic acid region of interest (the target sequence) is copied many times by in vitro methods. Areas outside the target are not amplified. In *signal amplification*, the amount of target stays the same, but the signal is increased by one of several methods, including sequential hybridization of branching nucleic acid structures and continuous enzyme action on substrate that may be recycled. Finally, in *probe amplification*, the probe (or a product of the probe) is amplified only in the presence of the target. Amplification techniques often can achieve more than a million-fold amplification in less than an hour.

Polymerase Chain Reaction (PCR)—Target Amplification

When the amount of target nucleic acid is increased by synthetic in vitro methods, target amplification occurs. PCR[90] is the best known and most widely applied of the target amplification methods. Because of the commercial availability of thermostable DNA polymerases, kits, and instrumentation, this method has been widely adopted in research and is routinely used in the clinical laboratory.

Details of the PCR Process

PCR requires a thermostable DNA polymerase, (deoxy) nucleotides of each base (collectively referred to as *dNTPs*), the target sequence, and a pair of oligonucleotides (referred to as *primers*) complementary to opposite strands flanking the sequence to be amplified (the target sequence). In the first step, target duplexes are denatured into single strands by heat (Figure 17-2). When the mixture is cooled, primers provided in great excess (usually over a million times the concentration of the initial target) specifically anneal to complementary sequences on the target. Once the primers are annealed, the action of the polymerase synthesizes two new DNA strands by extending each of the two primers at their 3′ end. The primers are designed to recognize sequences of the target that

TABLE 17-1 Common Amplification Techniques

Techniques	Amplifies	Enzymes Used	Thermal Cycling
Polymerase chain reaction (PCR)[90]	Target	DNA polymerase (thermostable)	Yes
Transcription-mediated amplification (TMA)[46] Self-sustained sequence replication (3SR)[32] Nucleic acid sequence–based amplification (NASBA)[15]	Target	Reverse transcriptase; RNA polymerase; RNase H	No
Strand displacement amplification (SDA)[114]	Target	*Hinc*II; DNA polymerase I (exonuclease deficient)	No
Loop-mediated amplification (LAMP)[75]	Target	DNA polymerase	No
Whole genome amplification (WGA) or multiple displacement amplification (MDA)[19]	Target	Φ29 DNA polymerase	No
Ligase chain reaction (LCR)[120]	Target	DNA ligase (thermostable)	Yes
Antisense RNA amplification (aRNA)[80]	Target	T4 DNA polymerase; Klenow; S1 nuclease; T7 polymerase	No
Branched DNA (bDNA)[14]	Signal	Alkaline phosphatase	No
Serial invasive signal amplification[35]	Signal	Cleavase	No
Rolling circle amplification (RCA)[3,60] Ramification amplification (RAM)[131]	Probe	T4 gene 32 protein; Φ29 DNA polymerase; DNA ligase (RAM)	No

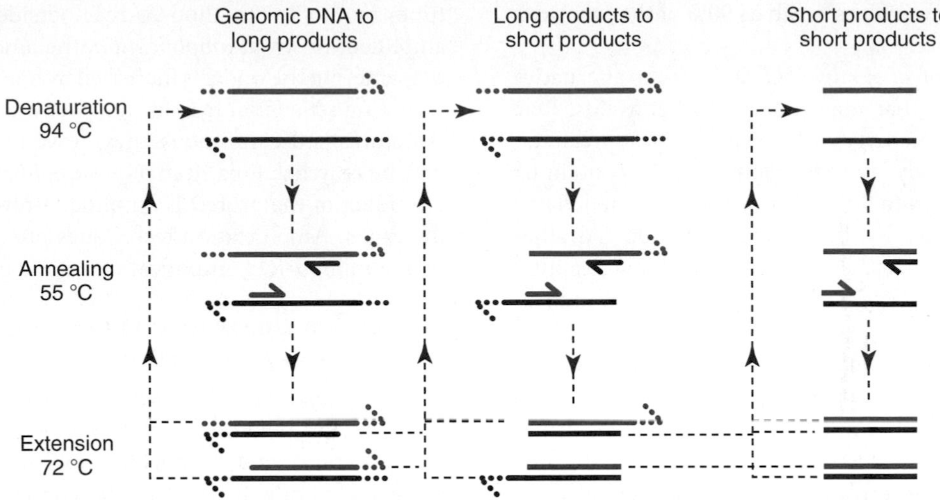

Figure 17-2 Schematic diagram of the polymerase chain reaction (PCR). Repetitive cycles of denaturation, annealing, and extension are paced by temperature cycling of the reaction. Two primers (indicated as short segments) anneal to opposite template strands *(long red and black lines)* to define the region to be amplified. Extension occurs from the 3′-ends *(indicated with half arrowheads)*. In each cycle, genomic DNA is denatured and annealed to primers that extend in opposite directions across the same region, producing long products of undefined length. Long products generated by extension of one of the primers anneal to the other primer during the next cycle, producing short products of defined length. Any short products present produce more short products. After n cycles, 2^n new copies of the amplified region (n long products + [2^n – n] short products) are generated from each original genomic copy. A similar approach can be used to amplify RNA targets by initial reverse transcription of the RNA template to produce the DNA template.

are close enough together that the polymerase extends each strand far enough to include the priming site of the other primer. Usually, the optimal temperature for polymerization (or DNA synthesis) is an intermediate temperature between the annealing temperature (at which primer hybridizes to its target) and the denaturation temperature (at which the newly generated DNA strand dissociates from its template). The second cycle also begins with denaturation, but now twice as many strands (the original genomic DNA and the extension products from the first cycle) are available for primer annealing and subsequent extension. Temperature cycling (typically) employs three temperatures: a high temperature sufficient to denature the target sequence, a low temperature that allows annealing of the primers to the target, and a third temperature optimal for polymerase extension. The instrument that takes samples through the multiple steps of changing temperature is known as a *thermocycler.*

Repetitive thermocycling results in the exponential accumulation of the short product (consisting of primers and all intervening sequences). If the efficiency of each cycle is optimal, the number of target sequences doubles each cycle (the efficiency is 100% or 1.0). PCR efficiency depends on the primers and the temperature-cycling conditions, along with the presence or absence of polymerase inhibitors. Amplified products accumulate exponentially in the beginning cycles of PCR. At some point, however, the efficiency of amplification falls and eventually the amount of product plateaus (Figure 17-3) as the result of exhaustion of components or competition between primer and product annealing (i.e., the single strands of product are at such high concentrations that they anneal to each other rather than to the primers). The S-curve shape is similar to the logistical model for population growth. In a typical PCR reaction using 0.5 μmol/L of each primer, the maximum DNA concentration achievable is about 100 billion copies/μL.

With the addition of an initial reverse transcriptase step to form cDNA from RNA in the sample, RNA targets can be successfully amplified into DNA copies. Reverse transcription and DNA amplification steps usually are catalyzed by two different polymerases, but some thermostable enzymes (such as the *Tth* polymerase) have both DNA polymerase and reverse transcription activities, so that both steps can be performed in the same tube with the same enzyme.

After amplification, the products can be detected by various methods. Gel electrophoresis with ethidium bromide staining is a classical qualitative method that may suffice for many applications. When greater accuracy is required, one of the primers can be fluorescently labeled so that after PCR, the fragments can be sized on a *DNA sequencing* device. Alternatively, some form of hybridization assay can be used to verify or analyze the amplified product. Automated methods are always attractive, and closed-tube methods are particularly advantageous in the clinical laboratory. Adding a fluorescent dye or probe before amplification allows thermocyclers

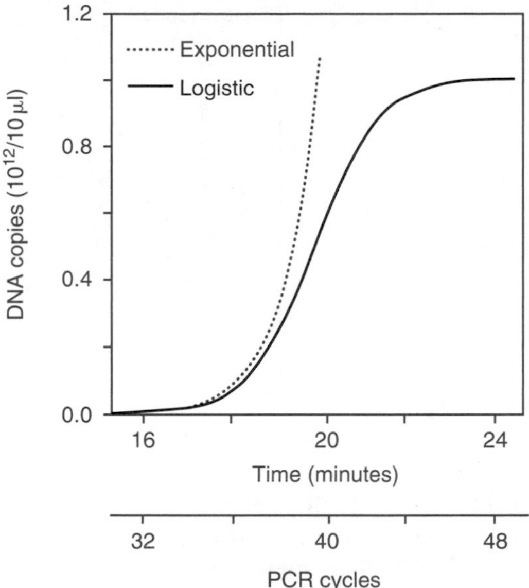

Figure 17-3 Exponential and logistic curves for DNA amplified by polymerase chain reaction (PCR). A doubling time of 30 seconds is assumed for PCR, that is, given the equation $N_t = N_0e^{rt}$, in which N_t is the amount of DNA at time t and N_0 is the initial amount of DNA, r is 1.386 min^{-1} for PCR. A carrying capacity of 100 billion copies of PCR product per µL was used, assuming that the reaction is primer limited at one-third the primer concentration (initially at 0.5 µmol/L, or 300 billion primer pairs per µL). Starting with only one target copy, it takes 23 minutes (46 cycles) to amplify the target to saturation. *(Modified with permission of the publisher from Wittwer CT, Kusukawa N. Real-time PCR. In: Persing DH, Tenover FC, Versalovic J, eds. Molecular microbiology: diagnostic principles and practice. Washington, DC: ASM Press, 2004:71-84. © 2004 ASM Press.)*

equipped with optical detection to analyze the reaction as it progresses (real-time PCR) or after the reaction is complete (end point melting) without the need to process the sample for a separate analysis step.

PCR Kinetics and Rapid Cycling

It is natural to think about PCR in terms of three events—denaturation of double-stranded target, annealing of primers to their targets, and extension of the DNA strand from the primer—that occur at three temperatures, each requiring a certain amount of time. Indeed, it is common to perform PCR by holding the reaction mixture at three different temperatures (e.g., denaturation at 94 °C, annealing at 55 °C, and extension at 72 °C). Standard thermocycling instruments that use conical tubes focus on accurate temperature control of the heating block at equilibrium, not on the dynamic control of the sample temperature. As a result, sample temperatures are not well defined during transitions, and long cycle times have become standard to ensure that samples reach target temperatures. Reproducibility between instruments and manufacturers is poor, and PCR may require hours to complete 30 cycles of amplification.

The kinetics of PCR suggests that *rapid transitions* between temperatures with minimal or no pauses (temperature plateaus) provide a better paradigm of PCR amplification (Figure 17-4). Denaturation, annealing, and extension are very rapid reactions as shown by experiments in capillaries.[125] The use of temperature "spikes" at denaturation and annealing, instead of extended temperature plateaus, allows for rapid cycling with the appropriate instrumentation.[129] The actual time required for PCR depends on the size of the product, but when it is less than 500 base pairs (bp), 30 cycles are easily completed in 15 minutes. Furthermore, rapid amplification improves specificity. Figure 17-5 shows PCR amplification of the same product amplified at different cycling speeds. With conventional slow cycling, many nonspecific products are generated (cycling profile A). These products disappear as the cycling time is decreased (profiles B, C, and D). In fact, amplification yield and product specificity are optimal when denaturation and annealing times are minimal.

Requirements for denaturation, annealing, and extension in PCR have been reviewed.[128] Initial denaturation of genomic DNA may be required before PCR cycling, depending on how the DNA sample was prepared. Boiling of the sample or an initial denaturation step of 5 to 10 seconds before PCR cycling may be necessary. During PCR, however, denaturation occurs very rapidly. Even for long PCR products, denaturation is complete in less than 1 second after the denaturation temperature is reached. Anything greater than a denaturation time of "0" serves only to degrade the polymerase. If longer denaturation times are required, either the sample is not reaching temperature or heat-activated polymerases are being used. Product specificity is optimal when annealing times are less than 1 second. Longer annealing times may be required if the primer concentrations are low. The required extension time for each cycle depends on the length of the PCR product. Extension is not instantaneous, although it is much faster than common practice would suggest. Extension rates of *Taq* polymerase under optimal conditions are 50 to 100 bases per second. Despite its common use, a 5 to 10 minute final extension is not necessary to complete extension. Products can be as small as 40 bp to about 40 kilobases (kb). To amplify products longer than 2 kb, mixtures of polymerases that include some 3′-exonuclease activity to edit mismatched nucleotides are usually used. Instead of separate annealing and extension temperatures, both processes can be carried out at the same temperature, resulting in two-temperature, instead of three-temperature, cycling. Although this simplifies the demand on instrumentation and programming, it limits the choice of primers and requires a longer extension time at suboptimal temperatures.

PCR Optimization and Primer Design

In addition to the temperature-cycling conditions, the specificity of PCR depends on the choice of primers and the Mg^{2+} concentration. The choice of primers often dictates the quality and success of the amplification reaction. To select primers, the sequence of the target must be known. Some guidelines for primer selection are intuitive and helpful:

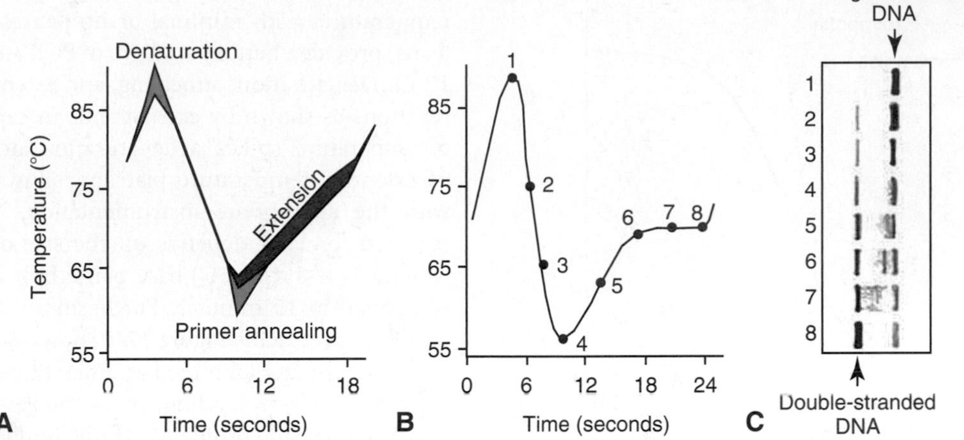

Figure 17-4 A visual demonstration of polymerase chain reaction (PCR) kinetics. The three phases of PCR (denaturation, annealing, and extension) occur as the temperature is continuously changing (A). Toward the end of PCR temperature cycling, the reaction contains single- and double-stranded PCR products. When different points of the cycle are sampled (by snap-cooling the mixture in ice water, (B) and analyzed, the transition from denatured single-stranded DNA to double-stranded DNA is revealed as a continuum (C). Progression of the extension reaction can be followed by additional bands appearing between the single- and double-stranded DNA (time points 5 to 7). *(Modified with permission from Wittwer CT, Herrmann MG. Rapid thermal cycling and PCR kinetics. In: Innis M, Gelfand D, Sninsky J, eds. PCR applications. San Diego: Academic Press, 1999:211-29. © 1999 Academic Press.)*

1. Avoid primers that anneal to themselves or to other primers. Particularly avoid complementation at the 3′-end of primers, and especially do not use a primer that has reciprocal 3′-end complementation.
2. Choose primers that are specific to the target. Avoid simple sequence repeats and common repeated sequences, such as *Alu* repeats. If your target has close relatives, design your primers so that they will anneal only to your intended target. Targets that need to be avoided include pseudogenes (for genomic DNA) and related bacterial or viral strains (for microorganisms).
3. One should avoid primers that have sequence complementary to internal sequences of the intended product, especially at the 3′-ends of the primers.
4. Primers should have between 18 and 25 bases that are matched in melting temperature (Tm) to each other. A primer greater than 17 bases long has a good chance of being unique in the human genome.
5. Unless there is a reason to amplify longer targets, product length should be less than 500 bps. Even shorter products (<200 bps) amplify with the highest efficiency.
6. It is important to search for sequences similar to the candidate primers that are present in the background DNA likely to be present in your assay (http://www.ncbi.nlm.nihgov/BLAST/). Many primer selection programs are available commercially and others can be freely obtained over the Internet. However, very few if any of the selection rules have been empirically tested.

For exponential PCR, priming sites must be oriented appropriately within a close distance. The desired target can be favored by choosing a small product size and rapid cycling.

Detection Limits of PCR

When PCR is performed under optimal conditions, a single copy of the target can be detected. In practice, however, the statistical probability of distributing at least a single copy from a dilute template solution into the PCR must be considered. The Poisson distribution indicates that if, on average, one target copy is present per tube, 37% of the tubes will have no target, 37% will have one target, and the remainder will have more than one target. About three copies on average are necessary for 95% of the tubes to include at least one copy. Therefore, the limit of detection (95% probability) of any single PCR cannot be lower than three copies per reaction. This limitation of low copy analysis holds true for any amplification technique.

3′-End of PCR Products

Taq DNA polymerase and other polymerases have a terminal transferase activity that may add a single unpaired nucleotide on the 3′-end of PCR product strands. In the presence of all four dNTPs, dATP is preferentially added. This means that some percentage of the double-stranded products generated by PCR will have a protruding A at one or both ends. Although this does not influence most detection protocols, it can complicate some systems with high size resolution. On the other

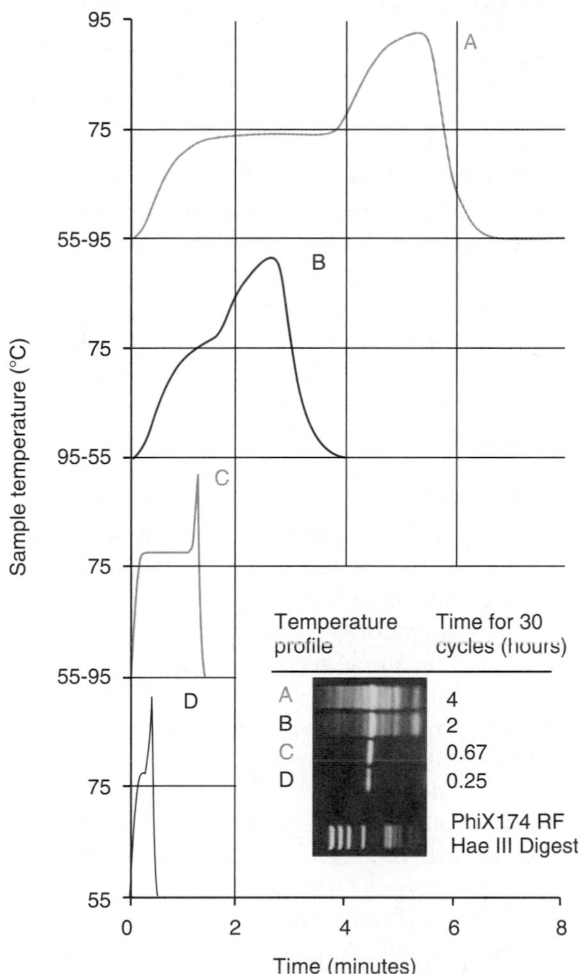

Figure 17-5 Rapid polymerase chain reaction (PCR) improves product specificity. Human genomic DNA samples were cycled 30 times through temperature profiles *A, B, C,* and *D.* Increased specificity of amplification of the 536 bp β-globin fragment is seen with faster cycling (*C* and *D*). *(Reprinted by permission of the publisher from Wittwer CT, Garling DJ. Rapid cycle DNA amplification: time and temperature optimization. BioTechniques 1991;10:76-83. © 1991 Eaton Publishing.)*

hand, this feature is useful for high-efficiency cloning and ligation of PCR products.[134]

Contamination Control to Avoid False-Positive Results

Because PCR can detect a single molecule of target sequence, a small amount of contamination in a sample can easily produce a false-positive result. The greatest potential for contamination comes from the product of the amplification reaction, referred to as the *amplicon* (used interchangeably with *PCR product*). After amplification, each reaction mixture may contain as many as one trillion copies of the amplicon. Thus, minute aerosol droplets contain more than enough target for robust amplification. Amplicon can contaminate reagents, pipettes, and glassware. It is easy to turn a laboratory into a Dr. Seuss fiasco.[95] Experience has dictated the use of laboratory procedures that minimize contamination by amplicons.[52] These include physically separated areas for preamplification and postamplification steps, positive-displacement or filter barrier pipettes to minimize aerosol contamination, and the use of prealiquoted reagents. The most effective way of all is to not let the product out of the tube. Methods that perform amplification, detection, and characterization in a closed tube virtually eliminate the risk of product contamination. Even with these precautions, a negative control or blank (all reactants minus target DNA) is one of the most important controls for PCR.

In combination with the precautions listed previously, chemical modifications can be made to the amplicon so it becomes an unsuitable template for further amplification. One of the commonly practiced chemical modifications is to substitute deoxyuridine 5′-triphosphate (dUTP) for deoxythymidine 5′-triphosphate (dTTP) in amplification reactions, which results in incorporation of U in place of T in the amplified product. A bacterial enzyme, UNG, degrades DNA that contains U. Because U is not normally found in DNA, only amplicons will be susceptible to degradation by UNG treatment, and a new target DNA will not be affected. During a brief incubation step before amplification, uracil-containing DNA strands that are carried over from previous amplifications are enzymatically degraded such that they cannot serve as substrates for further amplification. UNG is then inactivated during the first denaturation cycle, so newly formed amplicon can accumulate normally during the reaction. However, UNG may regain activity, even after multiple cycles of amplification, if the temperature of the reaction mixture drops to below 55 °C. Residual UNG activity may also affect the detection limit (and the sensitivity of quantitative PCR assays) if amplified products are held at room temperature before detection. Often, PCR is carried out with dUTP but not with UNG until amplicon contamination is suspected.

An inexpensive method for reducing contamination in PCR consists of exposing the amplicon to ultraviolet (UV) light (such as a transilluminator) for a certain amount of time (usually 15 minutes) immediately after the amplification procedure. UV light creates unamplifiable pyrimidine dimers in the amplicon molecules. However, this procedure may not be compatible with all detection methods.

Inhibition Control to Avoid False-Negative Results

PCR is a resilient process that does not require highly purified nucleic acid. In practice, however, clinical samples may contain impurities that can inhibit polymerase activity. To ensure reliable amplification, some form of nucleic acid purification is often used. The idiosyncratic nature of PCR inhibitors contained in clinical specimens requires demonstration that the sample (or preparation of nucleic acid purified from it) will allow amplification. A control nucleic acid sequence, usually different from the target, can be added to the sample (or to the extract from the sample). Failure to amplify this control indicates that further purification of the sample is required to remove inhibitors of PCR.

Hot Start Techniques

PCR sensitivity and specificity can be compromised by the formation of unintended low molecular weight artifacts. This process is initiated before PCR, when the primers, template, and polymerase are all together at temperatures below the annealing temperature of PCR. Even at low temperatures, if a primer momentarily anneals to another primer or to an undesired target region, *Taq* DNA polymerase may extend the complex. If the extension product, in turn, is primed and extended, then unintended, double-stranded products can be formed (e.g., primer-dimers) that serve as amplification templates throughout the reaction. Primer-dimers can be distinguished from the intended target by their molecular weight or melting temperature, but they also influence the efficiency of the intended amplification and decrease the sensitivity of the assay.

The formation of primer-dimers can be minimized in several ways. All limit the activity of polymerase until the temperature is increased (thus the strategy is often collectively called *hot start*). One method of hot start involves the use of antibody (or an aptamer) to bind and inactivate the polymerase at room temperature. The binding agent is released upon heating, allowing polymerase activation. Another method uses wax or paraffin to create a physical barrier between the essential components in the reaction. This barrier may be created by putting some of the reaction components into the bottom of the tube and overlaying them with molten wax. Cooling solidifies the wax, and the missing components (usually the polymerase, or magnesium, which is essential for polymerase activity) can be placed on top. The wax melts when the temperature reaches 60 to 80 °C, and all components are mixed together by convection while the molten wax floats on top and prevents evaporation of the sample. Various commercial wax beads encasing one or more critical components are available. Finally the polymerase, primers, or dNTPs can be chemically blocked so that extension cannot occur until activation by heat, usually requiring an extended initial denaturation period of 10 to 20 minutes.

Asymmetric PCR and Allele-Specific PCR

Conventional PCR uses primers that are present in equal amounts, thereby ensuring that most of the products are double-stranded amplicons. *Asymmetric PCR* uses different concentrations of the two primers to generate more of one strand than of the other. For instance, the use of primer A at 0.5 μmol/L and primer B at 0.005 μmol/L produces mostly single-stranded DNA extended off the more abundant primer. This is useful for sequencing or making single-stranded probes. Yield of the product, however, may be low. With less extreme ratios (e.g., primer A at 0.5 μmol/L and primer B at 0.2 μmol/L), the yield is mostly preserved, with one strand produced in enough excess to make it more available for probe hybridization.

Another variant method called *allele-specific PCR* enables preferential amplification of one genetic allele over another. The 3′-end of one primer is placed at the polymorphic site and is extended readily only if it is completely complementary to the target. This strategy is used for distinguishing a gene from its pseudogenes and for genotyping of single-nucleotide polymorphisms (SNPs). Allele-specific PCR can also be used to determine haplotypes.[66]

Single-Molecule PCR or Digital PCR

Conventional PCR averages the amplification results of the many individual template molecules in a reaction. Because of this averaging, certain questions are difficult to answer. For example, quantification of copy number variants and minor allele fractions in the background of wild-type DNA, although possible, is difficult by bulk PCR. It is also difficult to determine whether multiple variants are on the same or different chromosomes. Single-molecule PCR (sometimes also called *digital PCR*) is a technique that uses a dilute solution of template that is distributed across many reaction compartments such that each of those compartments will have no template or a single molecule of template. Instead of conventional tubes, these compartments may be minute aqueous droplets in a water-in-oil emulsion *(emulsion PCR),*[102] PCR colonies *(polonies)* on a thin film of acrylamide gel,[68] or clusters on the surface of a planar flowcell generated by bridge amplification,[4] or they may be found on beads with clonally amplified template attached to their surface.[62,96] When amplification is observed in one of the massively parallel reactions, this means that clonal amplification occurred from a single template molecule. By analyzing each of these clonal reactions, it is possible (1) to determine whether multiple sequence variants are carried on one chromosome or split among two chromosomes, (2) to detect hemizygous gene or exon level deletions, and (3) to count minority events such as a mutation in a gene that is present in a very small fraction of cells in the specimen. Single-molecule PCR is used as the first step for many of the high-throughput sequencing methods reviewed later in this chapter.

Other Forms of Target Amplification

Several other methods for target amplification have been developed and are described briefly here.

Transcription-Based Amplification Methods

Transcription-based amplification methods are modeled after the replication of retroviruses. These methods are known by various names, including transcription-mediated amplification (TMA),[30,43] nucleic acid sequence–based amplification (NASBA),[15] and self-sustained sequence replication (3SR) assays.[32] They amplify their target without temperature cycling (isothermally) and use the collective activities of reverse transcriptase, RNase H, and RNA polymerase. The most widely used is TMA, illustrated in Figure 17-6. Two primers, a reverse transcriptase, and an RNA polymerase are used. The primer complementary to the RNA target has a 5′-tail that includes a promoter sequence for RNA polymerase. This primer anneals to the target RNA and is extended by the reverse transcriptase, creating an RNA/DNA duplex. The RNA strand is degraded by the RNAse H activity of the reverse transcriptase, allowing the second primer to anneal.

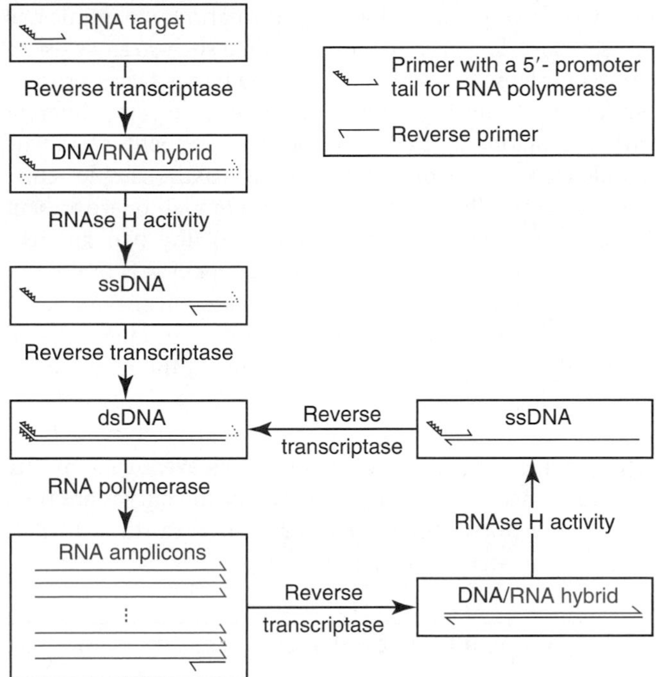

Figure 17-6 Schematic diagram of transcription-mediated amplification (TMA). Starting with a single-stranded RNA target, a primer with an RNA polymerase promoter on its 5′-end is extended by reverse transcriptase to form a DNA/RNA hybrid. The reverse transcriptase also has RNAse H activity that subsequently degrades the RNA strand to leave single-stranded DNA (ssDNA). A second primer then binds to the ssDNA, and extension forms double-stranded DNA (dsDNA) with the attached RNA polymerase promoter. RNA polymerase then makes 100 to 1000 copies of RNA, some of which are again primed by the second primer. Repeated cycles of reverse transcription, DNA/RNA hybrid degradation by RNAse H activity, dsDNA formation by reverse transcriptase, and further transcription by RNA polymerase exponentially produce ssRNA amplicons. Single-stranded targets are amplified isothermally, while double-stranded targets are first denatured to single strands.

The reverse transcriptase then extends the second primer to create double-stranded DNA that includes the promoter. RNA polymerase recognizes the promoter and initiates transcription, producing 100 to 1000 copies of RNA. Each strand of RNA then binds and extends the second primer, forming a RNA/DNA hybrid; the RNA in the hybrid is degraded, the promoter primer binds and extends to produce double-stranded DNA that can be transcribed, and the cycle repeats. As in PCR, all reagents are included and amplification is exponential with completion in less than an hour. Unlike PCR, these methods do not require temperature cycling (except for an initial heat denaturation if a DNA template is used). They are particularly advantageous when the target is RNA (e.g., human immunodeficiency virus [HIV] and hepatitis C virus [HCV] in blood bank nucleic acid testing).

Strand Displacement Amplification

Another isothermal amplification technique is strand displacement amplification (SDA).[114] After heat denaturation of DNA in the presence of four primers—dCTP, dGTP, dUTP, and a modified deoxynucleotide (dATPαS)—two enzymes are added: an exonuclease-deficient polymerase and a restriction enzyme. The two flanking primers that enter into exponential amplification have a restriction site added to their 5′-end and get nicked by the restriction enzyme, allowing displacement of strands that in turn can be primed, extended, and nicked. Deoxy-ATPαS is used so that restriction sites include a hemiphosphorothioate linkage to allow single-strand nicking, instead of cutting through the double strands.

Loop-Mediated Amplification Methods

The target amplification methods presented so far produce a defined length of RNA or DNA according to primer placement. In contrast, loop-mediated methods produce a wide range of different length concatemers of the target sequence. Primer design includes tails at the 5′-end of some of the primers that are complementary to the target sequence. After replication of complementary strands, these ends become free 3′-ends capable of extension. By forming a loop, these 3′-ends prime and extend the hairpin (self-priming) initiating concatemer formation. After initial DNA denaturation, the process can be isothermal if strand displacement primers are included. In the basic version, two strand displacement primers and two loop-forming primers recognize six segments in the target.[75] In another version, allele-specific amplification with five primers and one competitive probe recognizes seven segments in the target.[1] In both versions, a variety of product concatemers are formed, and the reactions can be completed in less than 1 hour.

Whole Genome and Whole Transcriptome Amplification

Instead of specific amplification of one target to improve sensitivity, methods that amplify all genomic DNA or mRNAs are useful when the target is in short supply. For example, *multiple-displacement amplification* uses exonuclease-resistant random hexamers and a highly processive polymerase to amplify DNA nonspecifically.[19] Initial DNA denaturation is not necessary, and the reaction proceeds isothermally. Similarly, messenger RNA can be generically amplified with a poly(T) primer modified with an RNA polymerase promoter.[80] After reverse transcription, second-strand DNA synthesis, and transcription, antisense RNA is produced. Both whole genome and antisense RNA amplification are also useful as nucleic acid purification methods before amplification or detection.

Other Approaches to Amplification

It is not always necessary to amplify the target DNA or cDNA sequence. Instead of target amplification, signal amplification or probe amplification can be used.

Branched-Chain DNA: Signal Amplification

Instead of increasing the concentration of target, signal amplification techniques use nucleic acids to magnify the detection signal. The branched-chain DNA (bDNA) method is one of these techniques in common use. The bDNA approach hybridizes the target nucleic acid to multiple capture probes affixed to a microtiter well.[108] This is followed by hybridization to a series of "extender," "preamplifier," and amplifier probes. The final, highly branched amplifier probe includes multiple copies of signal-generating enzymes that act on a chemiluminescent substrate to produce light. Nucleotide analogs isoC and isoG (isomers of C and G that are complementary to each other but not to other nucleotides) are often used to increase the specificity of the signaling cascade.

Serial Invasive Amplification: Signal Amplification

When two probes overlap on one target, an "invasive" cleavage reaction can be catalyzed by certain structure-specific nucleases. The cleaved fragment, in turn, can cause invasive cleavage of a secondary probe in the shape of a hairpin. The hairpin probe can be designed as a fluorogenic indicator by using a reporter/quencher pair of dyes that are separated by cleavage. This serial sequence of events (primary invasion and cleavage, followed by secondary invasion and cleavage of an indicator probe) is known as the serial invasive signal amplification reaction.[35] After DNA denaturation, cooling, and the addition of enzymes, the reaction is run at a temperature at which both the primary and secondary reactions recycle.

Rolling Circle Amplification: Probe Amplification

If a primer is annealed to a closed circle of DNA in the presence of a processive, displacing polymerase, the complement of the circle will be synthesized over and over again with displacement of the tandem repeats.[60] If two primers are used in opposite orientation, progressively more complex branches will be formed in an exponential reaction. The rolling circle can be formed by ligation of the two ends of a linear probe on template DNA. Ligation may happen directly, after polymerization through a gap, or after annealing of an additional, allele-specific oligonucleotide.

End Point Quantification in Amplification Assays

Molecular diagnostic assays may be qualitative (presence/absence of a target or genotype identification) or quantitative (the original concentration of a target sequence in the sample). When amplification is part of the assay, many variables need to be carefully controlled for accurate and precise quantification. Variation in extraction efficiency, the presence of enzyme inhibitors, lot-to-lot variation in enzyme and reagent performance, and day-to-day variation in reaction and detection conditions need to be addressed by methods that attempt quantification.

Quantitative analysis at the end point of amplification is usually carried out with the use of calibrators with known amounts of target or a target mimic. Sample nucleic acid may be quantified by comparison with an *internal standard* of known amount that is added at the time of sample processing to control for efficiency of nucleic acid purification. These internal standards can be DNA fragments, plasmids, or RNA packaged into synthetic phage or virus particles to mimic real viruses (so-called *armored RNA*[115]). One such strategy uses a *competitor* template, which is amplified by the target primers but generates an amplicon with sequence or size different from that of the expected amplicon. This competitor template is added in varying amounts to replicates of the sample before amplification. When the target and the competitor are present in equal concentrations, the amounts of the two different products will also be the same. The competitor is present in the same tube as the sample, so any variation in enzyme activity affects both products identically. This method is not used frequently in clinical applications because of the requirement for multiple assays on each patient sample.

Real-time (continuous) analysis is simpler and more powerful for quantification than end point assays. Reactions are monitored over time, and the profiles of the curves are used to calculate initial target concentrations. Real-time PCR is described in later sections of this chapter.

DETECTION TECHNIQUES

Molecular diagnostics uses both generic and specific methods of nucleic acid detection. Nucleic acids can be quantified in bulk by optical techniques, and specific methods of detection and quantification use sequence-specific primers and/or probes.

Generic Measurement and Visualization of Nucleic Acids

To measure or visualize nucleic acids generically, two approaches are commonly used: UV absorbance and fluorescent dyes.

UV Absorbance

Nucleic acid molecules absorb ultraviolet light maximally at 260 nm owing almost entirely to the constituent bases. This property can be used to measure the nucleic acid content of a solution. DNA double helices have lower UV absorbance than an equivalent number of nucleotide monomers, and when DNA is denatured into single strands (ssDNA) (e.g., by heat or pH), UV absorbance increases.[6] If a double-stranded DNA preparation is pure, a 50 mg/L solution has an absorbance of 1.0 at 260 nm. RNA has a greater absorbance, so only about 30 mg/L gives an absorbance of 1.0. More precise estimates for oligonucleotides are based on dinucleotide contributions.[8] It is common to assess the purity of a nucleic acid preparation by its ratio of absorbances at 260 nm and 280 nm *(260 : 280 ratio)*. In contrast to nucleic acids, proteins absorb maximally at 280 nm. A pure preparation of nucleic acid should have a 260 : 280 ratio between 1.7 and 2.0 that depends on base content. Lower values suggest significant protein contamination.

Fluorescent Staining of Nucleic Acids

Although absorbance measurements are simple and precise, they are not sensitive. Fluorescent stains that bind to nucleic acid are 1000 to 10,000 times more sensitive than absorbance measurements. The best known example of a nucleic acid dye is ethidium bromide, a positively charged, intercalating dye for double-stranded DNA and to a lesser extent, single-stranded DNA and RNA. Cyanine dyes are also popular stains for nucleic acids; they do not fluoresce unless they are bound to nucleic acids, thus providing very low background. With the appropriate optics, single molecules of DNA can be visualized with cyanine-based nucleic acid stains.[79] Nucleic acid dyes can detect DNA and RNA in gels or in solution (such as in real-time PCR).

Reporter Molecules and Labeled Probes

Ultraviolet absorbance and fluorescent dyes in themselves do not discriminate between different nucleic acid sequences (i.e., they are not sequence specific). Specificity in nucleic acid assays almost always comes from the hybridization of two complementary nucleic acid strands. Many reporter molecules can be covalently attached or incorporated into nucleic acid probes. Use of these probes can reveal the physical presence or location of sequences complementary to the nucleic acid portion of the probe.

Radioactivity

The first probes used in nucleic acid detection were radioactively labeled. Radioactive labels are still favored in some research settings because of the sensitivity attained with probes of high specific activity. The most frequently used isotopic labels are ^{32}P and ^{33}P, which are incorporated into the probe by enzymatic reactions. *Nick translation* is a classical method of labeling double-stranded DNA fragments. Nicks are introduced randomly into each strand of DNA by DNase I, and the resulting 3′-OH groups form priming sites for DNA polymerase. Labeled nucleotides are incorporated as the polymerase extends the strand by digesting and removing the unlabeled strand. Another method of labeling double-stranded DNA is *random priming*, in which the nucleic acid is denatured and is allowed to anneal with short oligonucleotides of random sequence. The 3′-end of an annealed primer forms an initiation site for the DNA polymerase, which incorporates labeled nucleotides using single-stranded regions of the DNA as the template. Labeled nucleic acid can also be synthesized by PCR, or if a labeled RNA is desired, it can be prepared with the use of a double-stranded DNA fragment containing a promoter sequence for RNA polymerase and incorporating radiolabeled ribonucleotides by transcription.

Additional enzymatic reactions are useful for labeling oligonucleotides. T4 polynucleotide kinase may be used to label the 5′-end of an oligonucleotide. Alternatively, terminal deoxynucleotidyl transferase (TdT) can add labeled nucleotides onto the 3′-end in a *tailing* reaction. No template is required, and the number and type of nucleotides can be controlled by the reaction conditions. A somewhat longer probe than the original oligonucleotide is obtained with additional labeled bases at the 3′-end. The sensitivity that is achieved with radioactive nucleic acid probes is determined by the radioactivity of the label, its extent of incorporation, and the detection time. Radioactively labeled probes have a short shelf life limited by isotopic decay and radiolysis of the nucleic acid. This inherent instability, along with concerns of radioisotope safety and disposal, restricts the use of radioactive probes in the clinical laboratory.

Indirect Probe Detection

The first practical example of nonradioactive probes used a biotin-labeled analog of dUTP.[53] Despite the altered steric configuration, this nucleotide is incorporated by both DNA polymerase and terminal transferase. Other functional groups, such as digoxigenin, may also be used as affinity labels through chemical linkage to a dUTP and incorporation into polynucleotides. Alternatively, oligonucleotide probes can be labeled during synthesis with biotin or amino linkers for subsequent attachment to indicator molecules. Labels at the 5′- or 3′-end of the molecule are usually preferred because central modifications may interfere with hybridization.

Biotin and other affinity labels do not generate detectable signals on their own. However, they can initiate signal amplification mediated by high-affinity binding with antibodies, or in the case of biotin, with avidin or streptavidin. These binding molecules can be linked to enzymes—such as alkaline phosphatase, peroxidase, or luciferase—connecting a single target to a single enzyme. Enzyme activity is monitored by detecting catalytic turnover of enzyme substrates that result in colorimetric, fluorescent, or chemiluminescent signals.

Affinity labels can be used to capture and localize targets to an area of a solid support. For example, biotinylated probes can be affixed to a streptavidin-coated surface. After incubation with the target nucleic acid, a second probe is added, which may be directly labeled with fluorescence or conjugated through another affinity label to an enzyme. Any background or nonspecific localization of reagents results in amplification of an undesired signal along with the desired signal, and these methods usually require multiple separation and washing steps to decrease the background.

Electronic detection of nucleic acids is attractive for its simplicity. Hybridization events can be detected by redox indicators that recognize the DNA duplex, or by other hybridization-induced changes in electrochemical parameters, such as conductivity or capacitance.[78,107] However, it is difficult to make electronic methods sensitive and specific enough that nucleic acid amplification is not required.

Fluorescent Labels

Advances in oligonucleotide synthesis and fluorescence detection have made fluorescently labeled probes the preferred reporter for nucleic acid analysis. Many fluorescent labels are now available, allowing color multiplexing for applications such as DNA sequencing, fragment length analysis, DNA arrays, and real-time PCR as reviewed later in this chapter. Techniques such as fluorescence polarization, fluorescence resonance energy transfer (FRET), and fluorescence quenching can provide additional detection specificity. Fluorescence polarization can be used to distinguish free from bound label, if the molecular rotation of the probe changes upon binding.[51] Molecular rotation primarily depends on the size of the molecule, so binding of a small probe onto a large target results in a polarization increase that can be measured. FRET techniques depend on the distance between two spectrally distinct fluorescent labels. Two labeled probes may be brought closer together by adjacent hybridization. Alternatively, two labels on the same probe may end up farther apart by hydrolysis or hybridization. Fluorescence quenching or augmentation does not always require FRET. For example, fluorescence may change merely by hybridization of a fluorescent oligonucleotide to its target. The effect depends on the dye and on inherent quenching from G residues in the target and/or probe.[16,72] Alternatively, quenching moieties can be purposely incorporated into probes.[55,106]

DISCRIMINATION TECHNIQUES

Nucleic acid discrimination techniques are divided into three categories:

1. Electrophoretic methods that physically separate nucleic acids based on molecular size and/or shape.
2. Alternatives to electrophoresis that determine the size, base content, and/or sequence of nucleic acids without electrophoresis. Examples include high-performance liquid chromatography (HPLC), mass spectrometry, and high-throughput sequencing.
3. Hybridization assays that identify specific nucleic acids by annealing or melting of complementary nucleic acids.

Some techniques use both electrophoresis and hybridization.

Electrophoresis

Electrophoresis is the most commonly used method for DNA and RNA analysis. Both DNA and RNA are negatively charged and will migrate toward the positively charged electrode when an electrical field is present within an appropriately buffered solution. Separation of different nucleic acids occurs when mixtures are allowed to travel through a neutral sieving polymer under the electrical field. Separation is based primarily on molecular size, with smaller molecules traveling faster through the polymer than larger ones (Figure 17-7). When very large molecules (≥50 kb) have to be separated, pulsed electrical fields are used to help move these molecules through the polymer matrix.[64] Separation also occurs based on the physical conformation, or shape, of the molecule. For instance, (1) single-stranded molecules may fold into secondary structures or they may stay as flexible linear structures; (2) linear double-stranded molecules may form heteroduplexes with mismatched bases or they may stay in their original homoduplex forms; and (3) circular double-stranded nucleic acids may be nicked and take a relaxed open-circular structure or they can be in a more compact superhelical structure. Under nondenaturing conditions, each of these shapes may influence the way nucleic acid molecules travel through the electrophoretic matrix. Separation based on shape can provide useful information, but it can also confuse size-based analysis. Electrophoresis of DNA is performed under nondenaturing or denaturing conditions depending on the application.

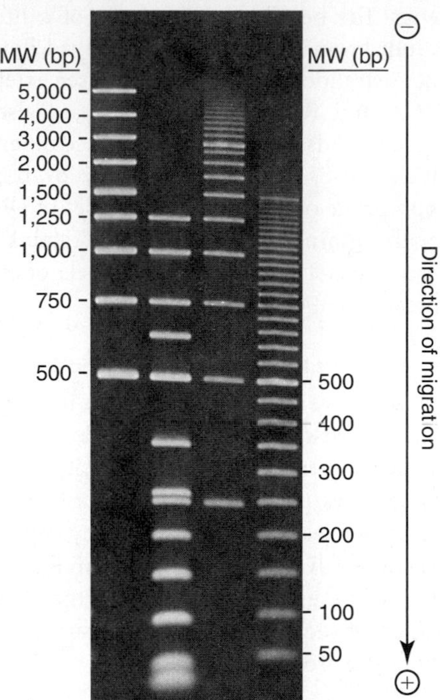

Figure 17-7 A photograph of multiple DNA fragments after agarose gel electrophoresis (1% w/v, SeaKem LE agarose gel) showing the separation of double-stranded DNA molecules by size. *(Photograph courtesy of Lonza Rockland Inc, Rockland, Maine.)*

RNA electrophoresis is commonly performed as a quality control check before transcript quantification or microarray expression analysis. RNA can be degraded easily by tissue or environmental RNAses, so it is important to assess the quality of the RNA used in these methods. Because RNA often has secondary structure, electrophoresis is usually performed under denaturing conditions to abolish these structures. Microfluidic chips with integrated microelectrophoresis are commercially available to rapidly assess RNA integrity by inspection of ribosomal RNA peaks (Figure 17-8). Although specific transcripts are not detected by this method, only small amounts of starting RNA are needed.

Agarose and *polyacrylamide* are the two types of polymers commonly used in electrophoresis. Several chemical variants of the polymers are commercially available and are tailored for different separation ranges and applications. The choice of polymer and polymer concentration (usually expressed as % w/v) is dictated by (1) the size of nucleic acid to be separated, (2) the resolution that is required, and (3) how the result will be visualized and analyzed. Using various concentrations, an agarose gel can separate nucleic acid fragments as small as 20 bp to over 10 Mb (10,000 kb), including chromosomes of yeast, fungi, and parasites. However, the resolution of agarose is limited, usually to a size difference of 2 to 5%. Agarose polymers are cast in trays (sometimes commercially supplied as precast gels) and submerged in buffer. The

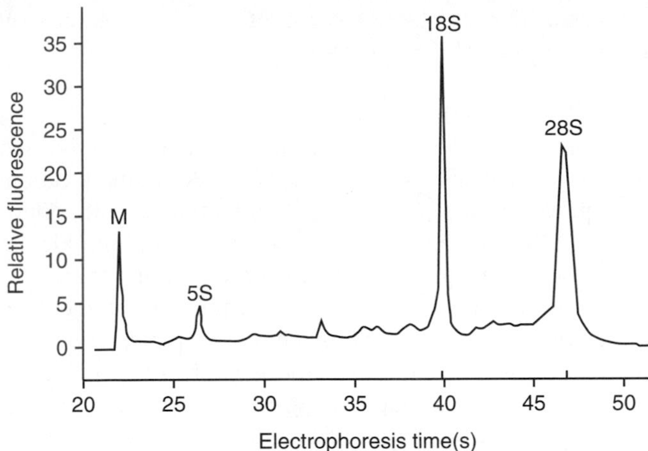

Figure 17-8 Microelectrophoresis of human white blood cell RNA. After isolation of white blood cells and extraction of total RNA, samples were denatured, stained with a fluorescent dye, and applied to a commercial microelectrophoresis platform for assessment of RNA quality. Prominent 18S and 28S bands of ribosomal RNA suggest the RNA is largely intact. Also indicated are a reference marker (M) and the 5S ribosomal band. Note that electrophoresis was performed in less than 1 minute.

gels are permeable to fluorescent nucleic acid–binding dyes, and results may be recorded as a photographic image of the stained gel under ultraviolet illumination.

Polyacrylamide polymers are suited for high-resolution separation (down to about 0.1% size differences) of short molecules (up to about 2 kb) and are the primary polymer for single-stranded nucleic acid separation, such as dideoxy-termination sequencing. Polyacrylamide may be used as a linear polymer solution, which is filled in capillaries *(capillary electrophoresis),* or as cross-linked gels, which are cast between two plastic or glass plates *(slab gel electrophoresis).* Polyacrylamide gels are permeable to fluorescent stains, and nucleic acids can also be silver stained. In addition, the optical clarity of polyacrylamide polymers makes them ideal for visualizing emission signals from fluorescently labeled fragments using laser-induced fluorescence detection.

Table 17-2 lists common electrophoresis-based techniques described further in this section.

TABLE 17-2 Commonly Used Electrophoresis-Based Techniques

Techniques Using Electrophoresis	Abbreviation	Primary Application
PCR/Restriction fragment length polymorphism	RFLP	Detection
PCR (RT-PCR) fragment analysis		Detection
Southern blotting		Detection
Northern blotting		Detection
Dideoxy-termination sequencing		Detection
Single-nucleotide extension assay	SNE	Detection
Oligo ligation assay	OLA	Detection
Multiplex ligation-dependent probe amplification	MLPA	Quantification
Heteroduplex migration assay	CSGE	Scanning
Single-strand conformation polymorphism analysis	SSCP, SSCA	Scanning
Denaturing gradient gel electrophoresis	DGGE	Scanning
Temperature-gradient electrophoresis	TGGE, TGCE	Scanning

CSGE, Conformation-sensitive gel electrophoresis; *PCR*, polymerase chain reaction; *RT-PCR*, reverse-transcriptase PCR.

Restriction Fragment Length Polymorphism

DNA extracted from a cell is extremely long and is usually cut into shorter fragments before electrophoresis to enhance mobility. Restriction endonucleases cut double-stranded DNA into fragments of reproducible size; the same enzyme produces the same fragments in different specimens if they contain the same DNA sequence. If an alteration in the DNA abolishes or creates a cleavage site recognized by the enzyme (or changes the spacing between two cleavage sites), then different sized fragments will be produced. These changes in fragment lengths (or polymorphisms) that result from restriction digestion are called *restriction fragment length polymorphisms* (RFLPs). However, restriction digestion produces thousands of fragments. To be useful, specific fragments need to be visualized.

Southern and Northern Blotting

Southern blot analysis (Figure 17-9) separates restriction fragments by agarose gel electrophoresis and transfers (blots) them to a membrane for easier manipulation in the following steps and for selective visualization by labeled probes. It reveals polymorphisms in the DNA sequence based on the RFLP profile. After electrophoresis, acid treatment fragments the DNA to make it easier to blot, and base treatment denatures the DNA to single strands for better binding to the membrane and probe hybridization. After neutralization, the DNA is transferred to a nitrocellulose or nylon membrane and immobilized. The membrane is then incubated with one or more probes that hybridize to the fragments of interest. The hybridized probes then are visualized by autoradiography or chemiluminescence. Southern blotting detects RFLPs, including large structural alterations such as deletions, duplications, insertions, and rearrangements. The procedure was named after its inventor, E. M. Southern,[100] and was the first

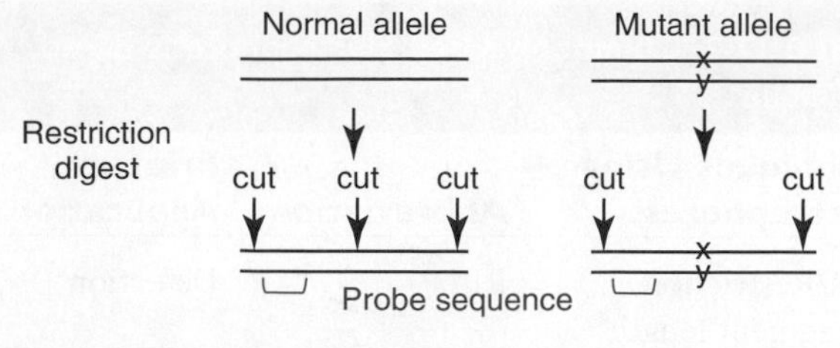

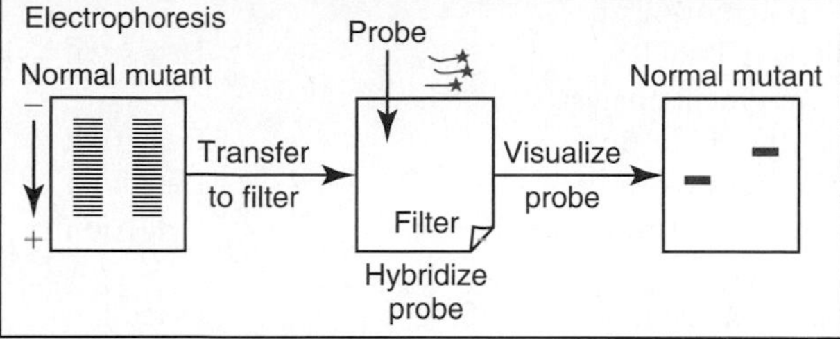

Figure 17-9 Schematic of Southern blotting. Genomic DNA is isolated from a normal specimen and from a mutant specimen that carries the polymorphic allele (*x,y*). The normal specimen has a site in the middle that is recognized by a restriction enzyme, while the mutant allele disrupts this site. After restriction enzyme digestion of genomic DNA, both samples are separated by agarose electrophoresis. At this point, no discrete bands are visible over the background of many fragments that are generated by the enzyme. DNA is transferred to a filter and is hybridized with a short DNA probe that is labeled. This probe hybridizes to the genomic sequence on one side of the polymorphic site. After visualization of the probe on film, a larger fragment is seen in the specimen with the mutant allele compared with the smaller digested fragment seen in the normal specimen.

discrimination method with adequate sensitivity and specificity for DNA analysis of single-copy genes in complex genomes. However, it requires large amounts of DNA (10 to 50 μg/lane) and is very labor intensive and time consuming. Today, it has largely been replaced by PCR.

Northern blotting was named not for its inventor but as a companion technique that uses RNA rather than DNA as the test nucleic acid. After electrophoresis, RNA is transferred from the gel onto a membrane followed by hybridization with a specific labeled probe. Because RNA molecules have defined lengths and are much shorter than genomic DNA, it is not necessary to cleave RNA before electrophoresis. However, because of the secondary structure of RNA, it is necessary to perform electrophoresis under denaturing conditions, usually formaldehyde/formamide buffers in agarose gels. RNA extracted from cells consists primarily of ribosomal and transfer RNA. Messenger RNA makes up only 1 to 2% of total cellular RNA. After electrophoresis and staining, intact RNA reveals two clearly visible bands of ribosomal RNA. Electrophoresis of about 10 μg of RNA is usually sufficient to allow visualization of the mRNA of interest after hybridization with a probe. Northern blotting provides information about the size of mRNA transcripts. Although only partly quantitative, the relative concentration of a particular transcript can be estimated by reference to a constitutively expressed control transcript, such as β-actin mRNA.

PCR Product Length

PCR product analysis by electrophoresis is frequently used to query the quality and specificity of PCR amplification. PCR products are visualized by staining the gel with a fluorescent DNA-binding dye, such as ethidium bromide. In some cases, the presence of an amplification product is directly diagnostic (e.g., detection of sequences found only in a bacterium, virus, or fungus in a human sample). The specificity of the amplification reaction is verified by the known size of the fragment. Internal negative and positive controls are used to control for potential contamination and to establish detection sensitivity.

Small insertions, deletions, rearrangements, and changes in the number of repeated sequences can also be detected by monitoring PCR product length on gels. Length differences may be large and easily picked up with agarose gel electrophoresis, or they may be small enough to require a denaturing polyacrylamide matrix. Fluorescent primers may be incorporated into the product during PCR to simplify detection of fragment lengths. These techniques are commonly used in the diagnosis of inherited diseases and in identity assessment.

PCR/RFLP

Many sequence alterations (e.g., single base substitutions) do not change the length of DNA. However, they can be amplified easily by PCR and usually are detected as RFLPs after treatment with restriction enzymes. After PCR, the products are digested with one or more enzymes and analyzed by electrophoresis. For example, if a sample has a mutation that disrupts an enzyme recognition site, this can be distinguished from a sample that does not have the mutation. Such an assay will produce one uncut PCR fragment when the mutation is present and two shorter fragments when the mutation is absent (Figure 17-10). If the mutation is present as a heterozygote (one normal and one mutant copy of DNA), then one long and two shorter fragments will be observed. Usually it is possible to design the assay so that the fragments can be easily resolved by agarose electrophoresis. One variant of this method uses reverse-transcribed mRNA, which lacks the introns that would be present in the DNA. In this way, multiple exons can be analyzed in a single PCR reaction.

Heteroduplex Migration

Heteroduplex migration analysis [also called *conformation-sensitive gel electrophoresis (CSGE)*] reveals the presence of sequence variants by the altered electrophoretic mobility of a double-stranded DNA fragment that contains one or more mismatched bases (a heteroduplex) versus one that is perfectly matched (a homoduplex). Originally described as a PCR artifact,[71] heteroduplex migration analysis has become a popular mutation-scanning technique, primarily because of its technical simplicity. With this technique, dsDNA generated by PCR is denatured, is allowed to re-anneal, and then is separated by electrophoresis under slightly denaturing

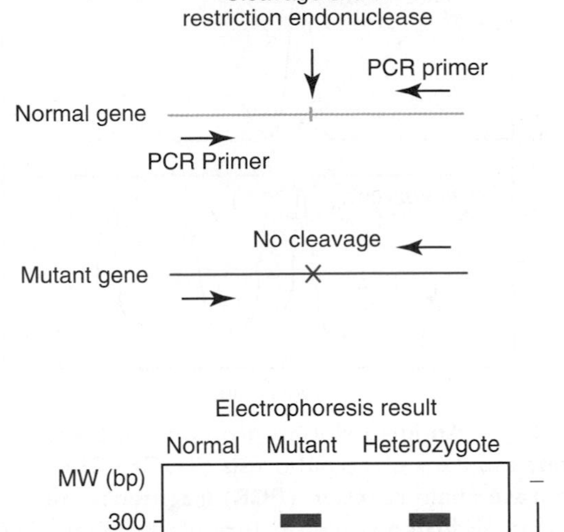

Figure 17-10 An example of polymerase chain reaction–restriction fragment length polymorphism (PCR-RFLP). A DNA fragment amplified by PCR carries a site (a unique sequence of generally four or more bases) that is recognized and cleaved by a restriction endonuclease. If a mutation is present, this site is altered and is no longer recognized by the enzyme. Electrophoresis reveals that the fragment from a normal specimen was indeed cut by the enzyme, generating two fragments shorter than the original length, while the fragment from a homozygous mutant was not cut, and the original length of the amplicon is preserved. In a heterozygous mutant, both the original fragment and the shorter fragments are visible.

conditions (e.g., 15% urea, 40 °C) on polyacrylamide gels. Detection is performed by silver staining of the gel or by fluorescence detection if one of the PCR primers is labeled. Heteroduplexes usually migrate more slowly than homoduplexes during electrophoresis (Figure 17-11). Although mutant alleles are often present as heterozygotes in a clinical specimen, homozygous mutations require mixing with wild-type DNA for mutations to be detected.

Heteroduplex migration detects single-nucleotide polymorphisms in fragments as large as 600 bp. The principal factor influencing sensitivity is the combination of the mismatched bases. Greater mobility differences (relative to the homoduplex) occur in the order of G:G/C:C > A:C/T:G = A:G/T:C > A:A/T:T.[39] This technique and other variant-scanning methods are useful when a wide variety of sequence alterations might be present. Particularly when most of the samples tested are wild-type ("normal"), it is more economical to scan for the presence of variants before performing specific genotyping or DNA sequencing.

Single-Strand Conformation Polymorphism

Single-strand conformation polymorphism analysis (SSCP or SSCA) is another electrophoresis technique used to scan for unknown variants in nucleic acid sequence. Similar to heteroduplex migration, it first requires PCR amplification. The amplicon is diluted and is denatured with heat and formamide; the resulting single-stranded DNA is separated by nondenaturing polyacrylamide electrophoresis (usually run at 4 °C). During electrophoresis, the single-stranded molecules fold into three-dimensional structures according to their primary sequence. Electrophoretic mobility then becomes a function of size and shape of the folded single-stranded molecules. If the sequence of a reference sample

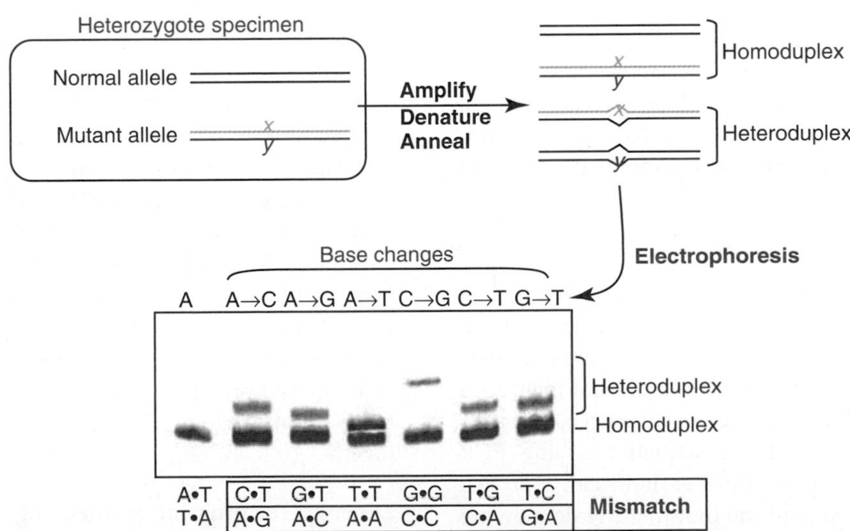

Figure 17-11 A schematic of heteroduplex migration analysis. When amplified DNA from a heterozygous specimen is denatured and cooled, the fragments re-anneal in four combinations. Electrophoresis on a specialized polyacrylamide gel reveals the presence of heteroduplexes by extra band(s) appearing above the homoduplex band.

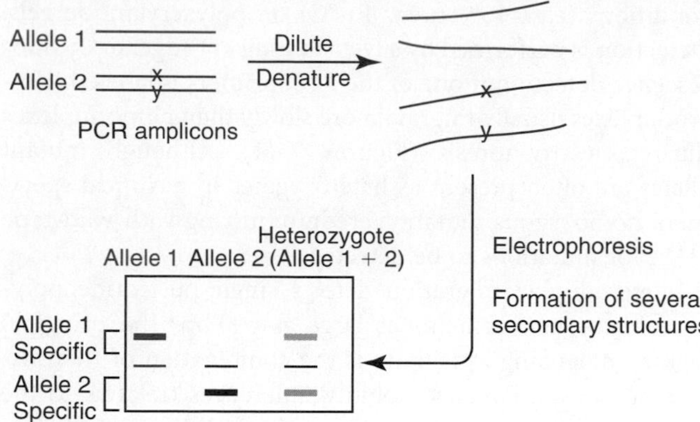

Figure 17-12 A schematic of single-strand conformation polymorphism analysis (SSCP). Polymerase chain reaction (PCR) amplicons carrying the polymorphic site *(shown as x and y)* are diluted and then denatured to form single-stranded fragments. During electrophoresis, they assume secondary structures. When conditions are right, polymorphisms are detected by differential band patterns compared with a known sample.

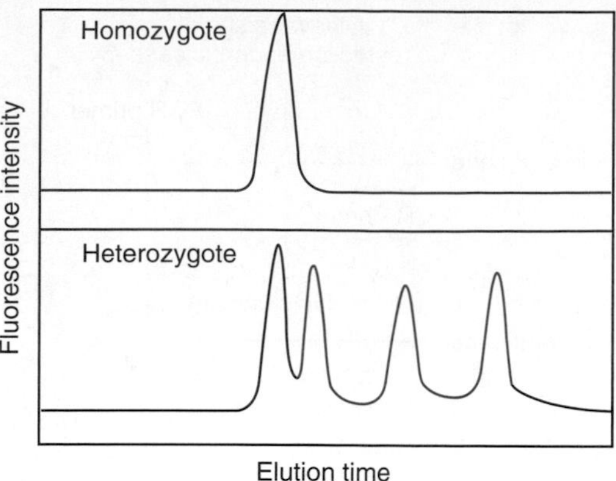

Figure 17-13 An ideal elution profile from temperature-gradient capillary electrophoresis (TGCE). The polymerase chain reaction (PCR) fragments are denatured and then cooled before electrophoresis (see diagram in Figure 17-11). Only one peak is visible for the PCR product of a normal homozygous specimen, whereas all four possible duplexes are visible and are separated from each other in a heterozygous mutant specimen. The shape of the elution profile (rather than the elution time) is used to compare unknowns with control samples.

differs from that of the fragment being tested, even by only a single nucleotide, often at least one of the strands, if not both, will adopt different conformations and exhibit a unique banding pattern (Figure 17-12). Since its introduction in 1989,[76] SSCP has emerged as a popular strategy used to detect sequence variants. Results can be visualized by silver staining of the gel or by fluorescent detection using labeled PCR primers. Unlike heteroduplex migration, there is no need to mix reference materials to detect the presence of homozygous variants. The sensitivity of SSCP depends on the GC content of the fragment and the assay conditions.[40] GC content is the amount of guanine and cytosine in a polynucleic acid usually expressed as percentage of total bases. Different conditions may be required to detect all mutations, sometimes making multiple runs necessary for a single target sequence. Furthermore, the results of SSCP are difficult to interpret when one sequence gives rise to multiple single-stranded conformations, some of which may be difficult to see, depending on amplification and electrophoresis conditions. It is also difficult to establish reliable protocols for fragments greater than ≈200 bp.

Denaturing Gradient Gel Electrophoresis

Denaturing gradient gel electrophoresis (DGGE) is yet another technique used to scan for unknown variants in nucleic acid sequence. Separation of PCR products is performed at a constant temperature within a gel that includes a concentration gradient of denaturants, such as urea, along the direction of electrophoresis. If the sequence of the PCR product is known, the detection rate of variants can approach 100%. However, only variants in the first melting domain are detected, so it may be necessary to limit the length of the PCR product and/or attach an artificial GC-rich sequence *(GC clamp)* to one end of the fragment to provide adequate separation.[12]

Temperature Gradient Electrophoresis

Temperature gradient gel electrophoresis (TGGE) is similar to DGGE. However, instead of using chemical denaturants, a temporal or spatial temperature gradient is used to provide the denaturing effect. For example, if the electrophoresis gel is in contact with a metal plate, a linear temperature gradient can be established perpendicular or parallel to the direction of electrophoresis.[86] Separation occurs according to size, shape, and thermal stability of the nucleic acids. If the temperature gradient is perpendicular to the direction of electrophoresis, intramolecular conformational changes show up as continuous transition curves, while strand separation leads to discontinuous transitions. Heteroduplexes are detected by a shift of the transition curves to lower temperatures.

Temperature gradients over time have been applied during capillary electrophoresis.[56] The temperature of the capillary array is increased by 0.5 to 0.7 °C/min and nucleic acid migration monitored by fluorescence in the presence of an intercalating dye. Heteroduplexes are detected by a change in the peak profile, which, under ideal conditions, may show all four possible duplexes as peaks[27] (Figure 17-13). Multiple samples can be run at the same time. However, as with heteroduplex techniques, homozygous variants are difficult to discriminate from a homozygous normal sample without mixing the two together to form heteroduplexes.

Dideoxy-Termination Sequencing

DNA sequencing[26] is routinely performed in the clinical laboratory. RNA is sequenced by first converting RNA to DNA by reverse transcriptase. Nucleic acid sequence is determined and compared with a reference sequence with an error rate

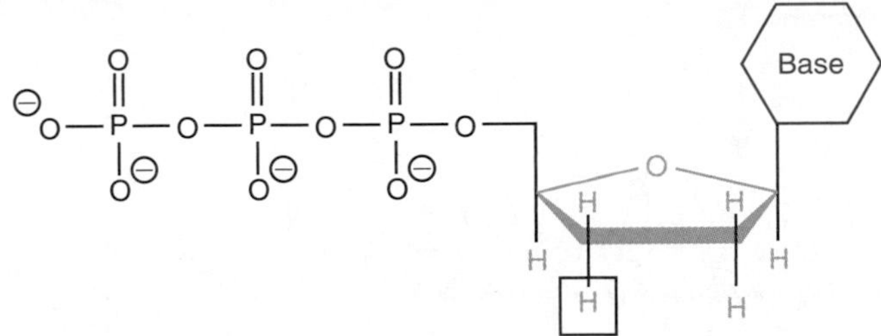

Figure 17-14 A dideoxynucleotide. Notice the absence of the 3′-OH that is usually present in standard deoxynucleotides. This lack of a 3′-OH prevents polymerase extension because no phosphoester bond can form. Incorporation of a dideoxynucleotide forces termination of polymerase extension.

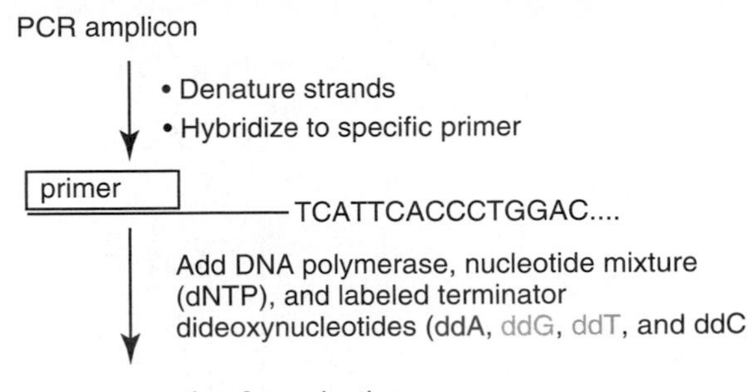

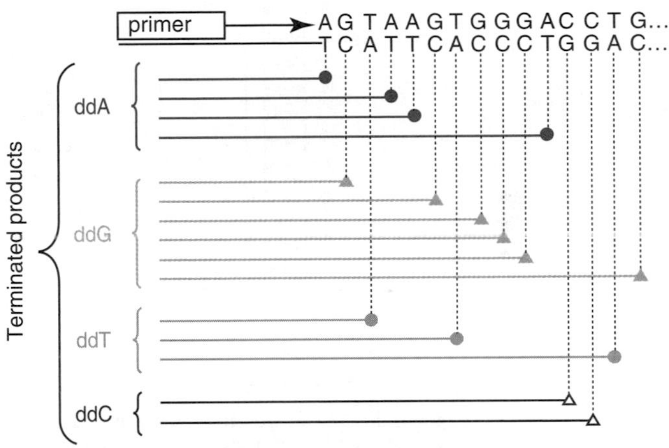

Figure 17-15 The dideoxy-termination reaction for sequencing. A polymerase chain reaction (PCR) amplicon is denatured and then hybridized to a specific oligonucleotide primer. As the DNA polymerase extends the primer by incorporating bases [(deoxy)nucleotides (dNTPs)] complementary to the template, it occasionally incorporates a terminator base analog (ddA, ddG, ddT, or ddC) that stops further extension. The result is a mixture of extended products of varying lengths. Each terminator base may be labeled with one of four different fluorescent tags (shown as different symbols in the diagram). Alternatively, the primer can carry four different fluorescent tags in individual chain-termination reactions [containing only one dideoxy-nucleoside triphosphate (ddNTP)] performed in separate tubes. The original procedure incorporated a radioactive dNTP during extension, allowing monochromatic detection of the truncated fragments in four electrophoresis lanes.

of 0.1% (one misidentified base in 1000). Often the sequence is analyzed on both strands (sense and antisense) for even greater accuracy. Any deviation from the reference sequence is identified by using computer programs to match the sequences. Base changes resulting in an altered amino acid code, stop codons, deletions, or insertions can be identified. The most common sequencing strategy uses PCR in the first step to amplify the region of interest, followed by a variable chain-termination reaction developed by F. Sanger in the late 1970s.[91] This reaction (also referred to as *Sanger sequencing*) generates fragments that are terminated at various lengths by incorporation of one of the four dideoxynucleotide base analogs (Figure 17-14) during extension from a sequencing primer (Figure 17-15). Dideoxynucleotides lack both 3′- and 2′-hydroxyl groups on the pentose ring. Because DNA chain growth requires the addition of deoxynucleotides to the 3′OH group, incorporation of dideoxynucleotides terminates chain growth. The most common method for generating these terminated fragments is *cycle sequencing,* repeating the steps of annealing, chain extension-termination, and denaturation by temperature cycling, similar to PCR. The fragments generated are tagged with a fluorescent dye (with the use of labeled primers or labeled terminator dideoxynucleotides), are separated by electrophoresis, and are detected by fluorescence as the fragments travel past a detector (Figure 17-16). When fluorescently labeled primers are used, four tubes are needed, each with one of the four dideoxy-terminators. If four colors are used, then the termination reactions can be combined before electrophoresis, and only one capillary is necessary. Alternatively, the use of four terminators of different colors makes it possible to streamline the process down to one tube for the termination reactions and one capillary. After PCR and cycle sequencing, about 600 bases can be resolved in less than 2 hours by capillary electrophoresis, and 96 of 384 samples can be run in parallel. DNA sequencing in the clinical laboratory is commonly used in viral genotyping such as HIV for drug resistance and HCV to establish prognosis and appropriate therapy. Sequencing is also used for bacterial speciation by analysis of ribosomal DNA and to identify mutations in many genetic diseases.

New technology now allows high-throughput sequencing of entire organisms in one operation. Massively parallel amplification in microscopic reactions (such as emulsion droplets) is followed by extension or ligation reactions that are observed with fluorescence (see next section). However, complete sequencing of only one gene (exons and splice sites) in the clinical laboratory for the detection of disease-causing mutations is still an expensive proposition by targeted dideoxy-termination sequencing. This is especially true for population screening (in which most samples will not have a

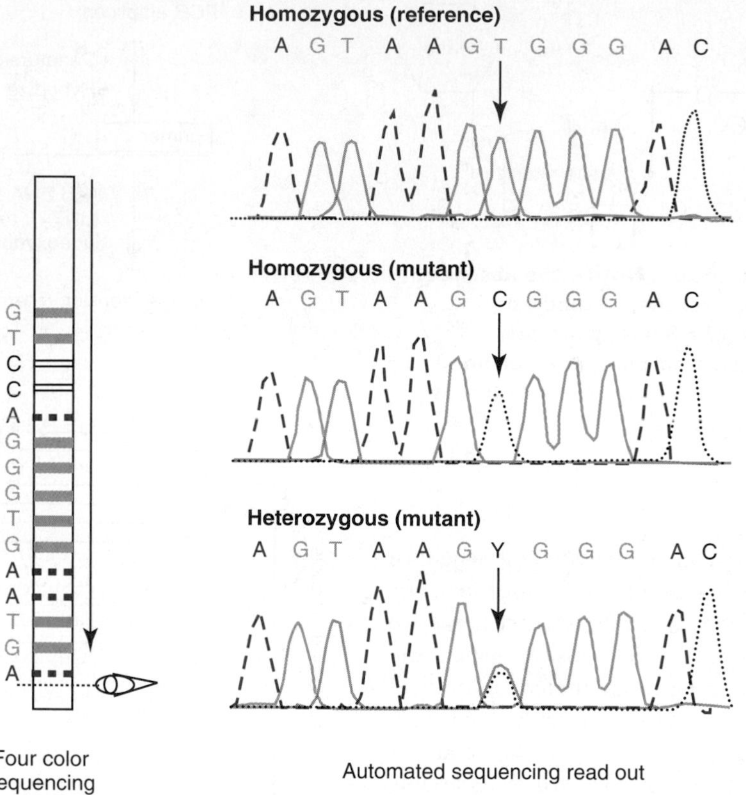

Figure 17-16 Schematic of DNA sequencing. Extension products (see Figure 17-15) are labeled with different color dyes for each of the four terminator reactions and are separated by electrophoresis. The four-color strategy allows automated end point fluorescence detection *(shown by the eye icon)*. The direction of fragment migration is from top to bottom. The sequence is read from left to right in the electropherogram generated by the sequencer. Examples of a reference sample (homozygous T at the polymorphic site), a mutant sample (homozygous C), and a heterozygous mutant sample (T and C, reported as Y) are shown.

mutation), but also for patients with symptoms of the disease. Therefore, in genetic testing, DNA sequencing is often performed after a negative result is obtained from targeted analysis of common mutations, or after a *mutation scanning assay* has determined the exons that need to be sequenced or otherwise genotyped.

Single Nucleotide Extension (SNE)

Also known as *single-base primer extension* or *minisequencing,* single nucleotide extension (SNE) assays involve the annealing of an oligonucleotide primer to a single-stranded PCR amplicon at a location that is immediately adjacent to, but does not include, the site of the single base variant, followed by enzymatic extension of the primer in the presence of polymerase and dideoxynucleotide terminators. For example, each of the four terminators can be labeled with a unique fluorescent label so that it is possible to detect which base was incorporated. SNE assays can be multiplexed on capillary electrophoresis instruments by varying the lengths of the primers so that each SNP is resolved by size in one electrophoresis run. Many SNE detection methods are available other than electrophoresis, including (1) photometric detection on microtiter plates, (2) product capture detection systems on DNA microarrays, (3) bead hybridization assays detected by flow cytometry, (4) solution-based fluorescence polarization detection systems, and (5) mass spectrometry. SNE assays are particularly useful when the target of interest contains 5 to 50 disease-causing single base variants. SNE assays do not work well if polymorphisms are present in the primer-binding site. Nor are they usually designed to detect polymorphisms at a position other than immediately adjacent to the 3′-end of the primer.

Oligo Ligation

Another assay format frequently used for SNP detection is the oligo ligation assay (OLA). Two oligonucleotide probes are hybridized to adjacent sequences of amplified target DNA, with the variation site positioned at the end of one probe (Figure 17-17). DNA ligase covalently joins the two probes only if both probes are perfectly hybridized to the target, including the polymorphic base. A probe matching the normal base and another probe matching the variant base are usually prepared. These two can be discriminated through differential electrophoretic mobility by varying the length of

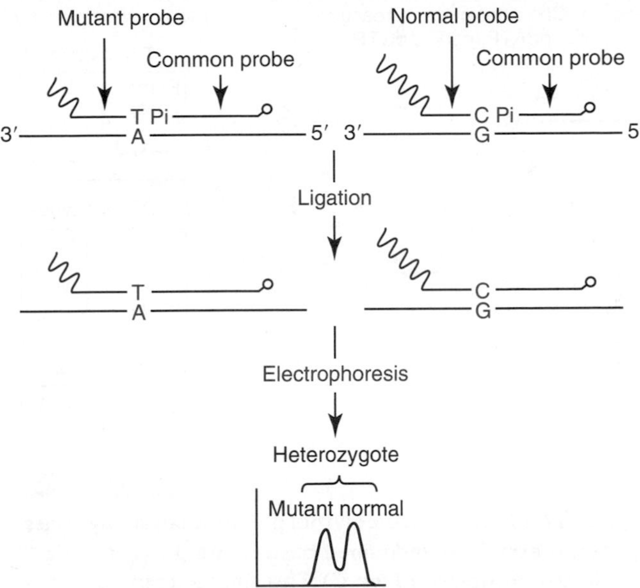

Figure 17-17 Oligo ligation assay of a heterozygous single-nucleotide polymorphism (SNP). A mutant probe with a 3′-T *(upper left)* hybridizes to the mutant DNA with an opposing *A*, while a normal probe with a 3′-C *(upper right)* hybridizes to the normal DNA with an opposing *G*. The probes are also attached to mobility modifying tails of different lengths *(wavy lines)*. Hybridized next to these probes is the common probe with a 5′-phosphate (Pi) and a 3′-fluorescent tag. In the presence of ligase, adjacent probes are covalently joined to generate longer probes, each with a fluorescent tag and a mobility-modifying tail. Probes that are mismatched to the target at their 3′-ends may hybridize, but they are not ligated. Electrophoresis and end point, laser-induced detection of ligated probes reveal the different alleles by their different mobility. Multiple SNP sites can be analyzed in one electrophoresis assay by varying tail lengths and/or by using multicolor fluorescence tags.

their 5′-tails. These tails can be noncomplementary poly A or poly C tails or pentaethylene oxide (PEO) units. The probe hybridizing to both alleles (the *common probe*) provides the reporter molecule, usually a fluorescent label. Multiplexing of SNP detection is achieved by attaching different fluorescent labels to the common probes and by varying the length of the tails on the allele-specific probes. Following ligation, probes for multiple SNP sites are separated by denaturing capillary electrophoresis.

Multiplex Ligation-Dependent Probe Amplification

Muliplex ligation-dependent probe amplification (MPLA)[7] is a convenient method for relative quantification of up to 10 to 50 targets. This method is particularly useful in screening for deletions or duplications of multiple exons within a gene. For each target, two probes are designed that hybridize adjacent to each other so that they can be ligated. The two probes have unique tails that do not hybridize to the target and that are the same between targets. After hybridization and ligation, the probes are amplified by PCR with a common primer pair (complementary to the tails). One of the primers is fluorescently labeled at its 5′-end. Because probes of different lengths are used, multiple PCR products of different sizes are produced and separated on a sequencing gel. Relative peaks heights or areas are compared for relative quantification.

Alternatives to Electrophoresis

Electrophoresis is not required to determine the size, base content, and/or sequence of nucleic acids. Some of these alternatives to electrophoresis are attractive in the clinical laboratory because of compatibility with automation and capacity for high throughput. Some examples include pyrosequencing, mass spectrometry, HPLC, and high-throughput sequencing.

Pyrosequencing

Pyrosequencing[89] is a sequencing-by-synthesis method that does not require dideoxy-termination or electrophoresis. A sequencing primer is hybridized to a single-stranded template generated by PCR. Four enzymes, a DNA polymerase, ATP sulfurylase, luciferase and apyrase, and two substrates—adenosine 5′-phosphosulfate and luciferin—are included in the reaction mixture (Figure 17-18). One of the four dNTPs is added to the reaction, with dATPαS substituted for dATP because it is incorporated by the polymerase but is not a luciferase substrate. If the base is complementary to the template strand, DNA polymerase catalyzes its incorporation. Each incorporation event is accompanied by release of a pyrophosphate (PPi) so that the quantity of PPi produced is equimolar to the amount of incorporated nucleotide. The release of PPi is monitored by conversion of PPi and adenosine 5′-phosphosulfate into adenosine triphosphate (ATP) by ATP sulfurylase, and ATP in turn drives conversion of luciferin into oxyluciferin, which generates visible light. The light produced is proportional to the number of nucleotides incorporated. Apyrase, which is a nucleotide-degrading enzyme, continuously degrades ATP and unincorporated dNTP. This switches off the light in preparation for the next dNTP addition. As the process is repeated by adding one dNTP at a time, the complementary DNA strand is built and the nucleotide sequence is determined. Because the technique can be automated, it is useful when the sequences of a large number of short segments need to be determined.

Mass Spectrometry

Matrix-assisted laser-desorption ionization time-of-flight (MALDI-TOF) mass spectrometry can be used to genotype sequence polymorphisms.[9,82] With mass spectrometry, no label is necessary because the alleles differ in mass. After isolation of genomic DNA, a specific DNA fragment including the polymorphic site is amplified by PCR. Heat-labile alkaline phosphatase is added to the reaction to dephosphorylate any residual nucleotides, preventing future incorporation and interference with the primer extension assay. Samples are then heated to inactivate the alkaline phosphatase. An extension primer is hybridized directly or closely

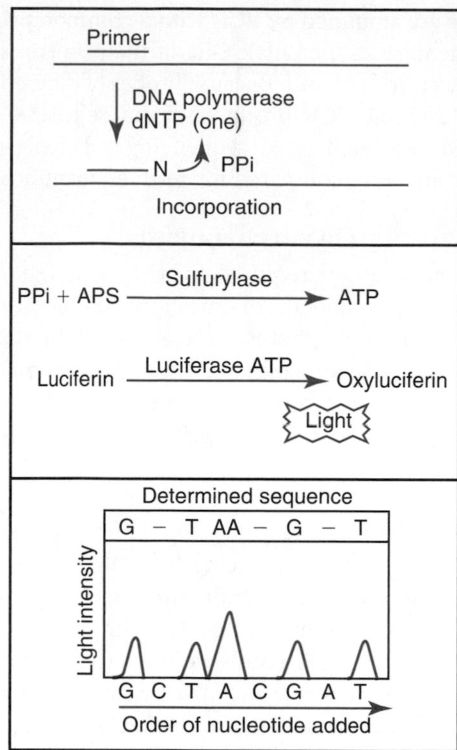

Figure 17-18 Schematic of pyrosequencing. Individual (deoxy)nucleotides (dNTPs) are added one by one to the single-stranded template, a primer, and a polymerase. Pyrophosphate is generated if the dNTP is complementary to the next base on the template *(top)*. Any pyrophosphate produced reacts with adenosine-5′-phosphosulfate (APS) to produce adenosine triphosphate (ATP), which in turn generates light in the presence of luciferase *(middle)*. The sequence can be determined from the order of dTNP addition and from the intensity of light produced *(bottom)*.

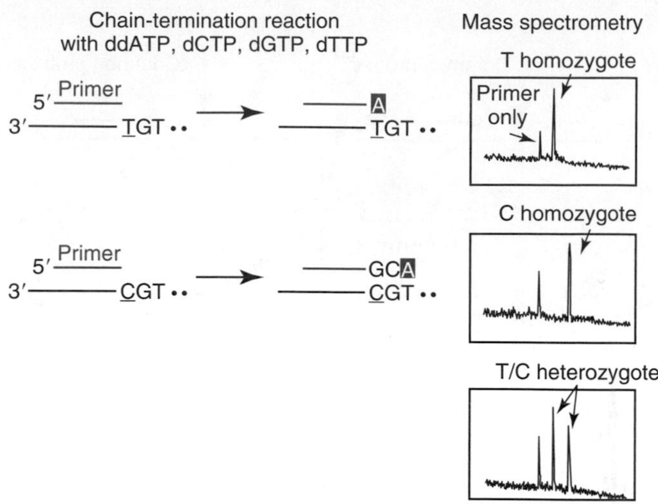

Figure 17-19 Sequence polymorphism analysis by mass spectrometry. The *underlined* base is the polymorphic site in the template (T or C). The single-stranded template is primed and extended in the presence of three (deoxy)nucleotides (dNTPs) and one dideoxy-nucleoside triphosphate (ddNTP), producing fragments of different mass depending on the sequence. The boxed "A" in this example indicates the incorporated terminator adenine base. The mass of terminated products is precisely measured by matrix-assisted laser-desorption ionization time-of-flight (MALDI-TOF) mass spectrometric data (relative intensity vs. m/z).

adjacent to the polymorphic site. Unlabeled deoxynucleotides are incorporated and terminated with a dideoxynucleotide, generating allele-specific diagnostic products of different mass. Salt is removed from the sample, and ≈10 nL of it is spotted onto an array coated with 3-hydroxypicolinic acid. This is placed into the MALDI-TOF, which measures the mass of the extension products. Once the mass is measured, the genotype is determined (Figure 17-19). Despite the complexity, automated systems processing 384 to 1536 samples at once are available.

High-Performance Liquid Chromatography (HPLC)

HPLC is commonly used for separating and purifying oligonucleotides. Separation usually is based on ion-pair, reversed-phase chromatography and is particularly useful for purifying fluorescently labeled probes guided by absorbance and fluorescent elution profiles.

A variant of this technology is denaturing HPLC (dHPLC). Denaturing HPLC is run at a single elevated temperature to partially denature double-stranded DNA. Similar to gel-based heteroduplex detection, dHPLC reveals the presence of heteroduplexes as additional peaks that are shifted in retention compared with homoduplexes.[130] Retention of double-stranded DNA is governed by electrostatic interactions and an acetonitrile gradient. DNA detection is most often performed by UV absorbance, although fluorescence or mass spectroscopy can also be used. Limitations of dHPLC include sequential (one at a time) analysis and the need to analyze some samples at multiple temperatures when more than one melting domain is present.

High-Throughput Sequencing

The need to understand the full extent of genome-wide human variation has led to the development of new high-throughput sequencing techniques.[111] Compared with dideoxy-termination sequencing (Sanger sequencing), these techniques generate between several hundred thousand and several hundred million times more sequence data in one operation, at fifty times to tens of thousands times lower cost per base. The techniques, none of which uses electrophoresis, are still evolving such that throughput and cost continue to improve. Much of the progress that has been made in this technology is dependent on progress in optical data processing, bioinformatics, and overall computer power. As the cost and turnaround time of these methods continues to decrease, they will be increasingly used in the clinical laboratory.

Most high-throughput sequencing techniques start by randomly fragmenting DNA into small pieces, usually less than 1 kb, and many between 100 and 500 bases. Short *adapter* sequences are attached to each fragment by the use of ligase or other enzymes such as terminal transferase. The primary role of these adapters is to provide priming sites for each fragment to initiate massively parallel sequencing reactions. Adapters also facilitate initial capture of DNA fragments onto solid surfaces and spatially restrict clonal amplification products generated from the fragments onto beads or spots on an array surface. Clonal amplification is performed by one of several methods, including the following:

- *Emulsion PCR,* in which one strand of the template fragment is captured on one bead and is clonally amplified inside a water-in-oil droplet, generating a bead tethered by single-stranded amplicons (Figure 17-20). The beads are then deposited onto a glass slide[96] or into discrete wells on a fiberoptic slide.[62]
- *Bridge amplification,* which generates clusters of single-stranded amplicons tethered to the surface of a planar flowcell in which the clusters are spatially separated (Figure 17-21).[4]
- *Rolling circle amplification,* which generates concatemers of templates that self-assemble into DNA balls in solution and are deposited onto ordered spots on a silicon array.[21]

Sequence determination of nucleic acids is performed on these clonally amplified templates in a massively parallel fashion using sequencing by ligation or sequencing by synthesis, which includes *pyrosequencing* and iterative single-base extension using cleavable four-color nucleotide terminators that are removed each step after fluorescent interrogation.[4]

Sequencing by Ligation

Sequencing by ligation is used in a number of high-throughput sequencing techniques, as it is suited for parallel operations even though the read length produced by each reaction is very short. Instead of using dideoxy-termination or electrophoresis, sequencing by ligation uses an immobilized template to which two types of ligatable oligonucleotides (anchor and probe) are hybridized repetitively. First, an anchor oligonucleotide is hybridized to a known portion of the immobilized template. Then, a mixture of probes about eight bases long compete for ligation to the anchor. Each of the competing probes has one position with a defined base (A, T, G, or C) indicated by the color of a fluorescent label at the far end of the probe. The remaining bases of the probe may be degenerate (meaning that all four bases are used in the synthesis, creating a combination of 4^m different probes, where m is the number of degenerate base positions), or they may be universal bases (nucleotide analogs that pair with any of the four bases). The terminal fluorescent label blocks further concatenation of probes. At a stringent temperature, only the ligated anchor-probe complex remains hybridized to the template, and the defined base position is decoded by the color of the fluorescent label. The next cycle begins by stripping away the anchor-probe complex from the template and repeating the process, but offset by one base by using a different anchor. Eventually, a short string of bases immediately adjacent to the anchoring site is determined. A variant of the technique uses two defined bases on each labeled probe and extends the read

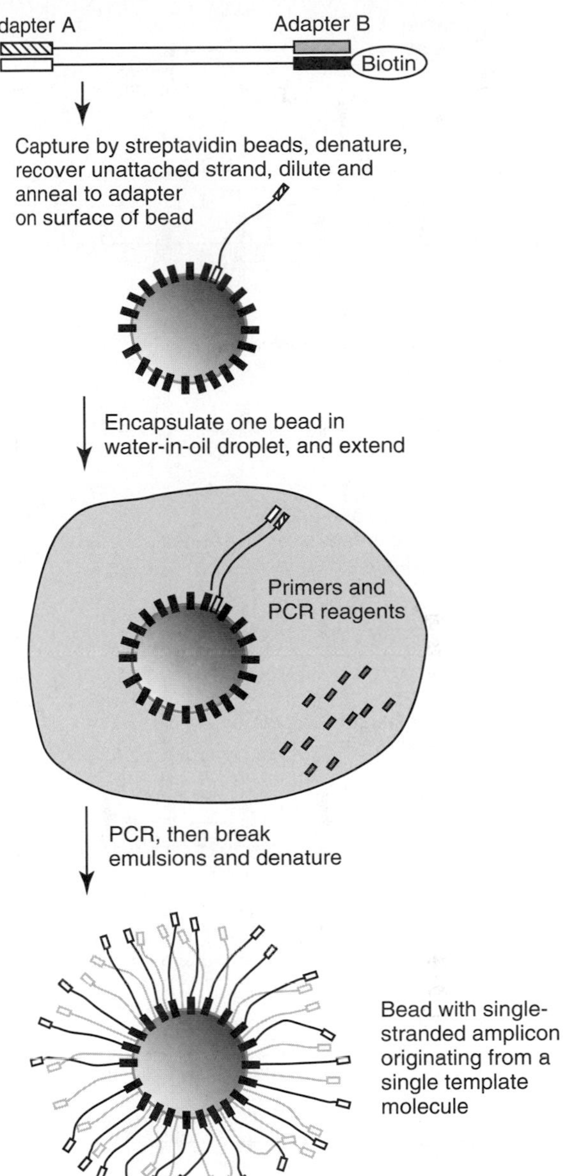

Figure 17-20 Emulsion polymerase chain reaction (PCR). Two adapters (*adapters A* and *B*) are randomly ligated to DNA fragments. *Adapter B* has a biotin on its 5′ end. Fragments with *adapter B* on one or both ends are captured by streptavidin beads, while fragments with only *adapter A* are washed away *(not shown)*. Then fragments are denatured, and the free strand with *adapter A* and *adapter B* at each end is collected (fragments with *adapter B* on both ends will not be released from the streptavidin bead). One molecule of the single-stranded template is then captured on a bead coated with adapter and is encapsulated inside a water-in-oil droplet that contains PCR reagents and primers. After PCR, the emulsion is broken and the DNA is denatured. This generates a bead with a large number of clonal single strands tethered to it. The bead is then deposited into one of many wells on a fiberoptic slide, or onto a glass slide for sequence analysis *(not shown)*.

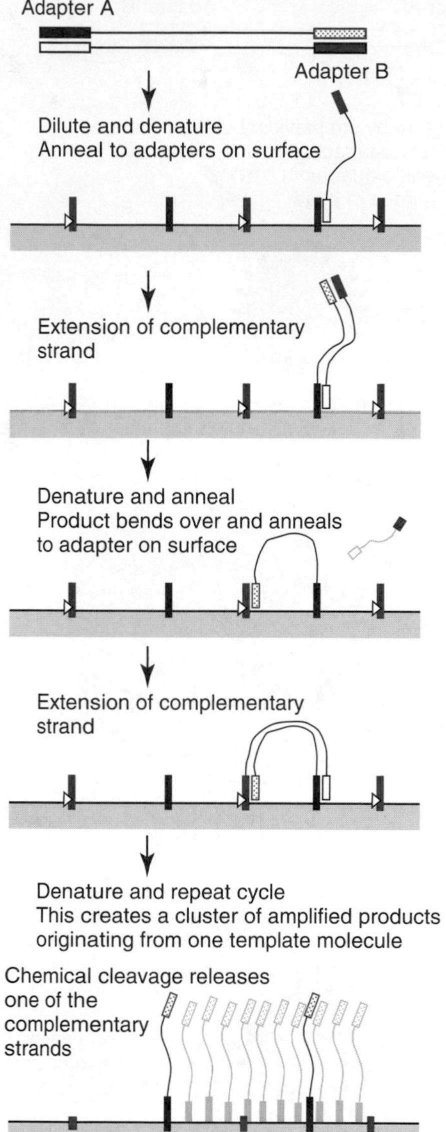

Figure 17-21 Bridge amplification. Two adapters (*A* and *B*) are ligated to a DNA template. Once diluted and denatured into single strands, the template is captured onto a flowcell surface by annealing to one of the two surface-bound primers that share sequences with *adapter A* or *B*. The polymerase reagent introduced into the flowcell extends the primer and generates the complementary strand of the template. The denaturant (usually sodium hydroxide) is introduced to the flowcell to release the original template strand. The free end of the newly synthesized strand anneals to a nearby primer by bending over, and a second round of reagent addition catalyzes the synthesis of another complementary strand. By repeating many of these cycles, a clonal cluster that consists of about 1000 copies of single-stranded template tethered to the surface is generated. This cluster is still a mixture of both complementary strands. One of the strands is selectively eliminated by treatment with periodic acid that cleaves the diol linkage present in one of the surface-bound primers *(open triangle on red primer)*. The cluster now contains only one of the template strands and is ready for sequence analysis.

length by cleaving part of the probe after recording the label (Figure 17-22).

High-Throughput Sequencing Without Amplification

Some high-throughput sequencing methods do not require template amplification. Sensitive optical techniques are used to observe incorporation of fluorescent nucleotides during strand synthesis on single template molecules. One such method observes real-time DNA synthesis by a single polymerase molecule immobilized inside a nanostructure array. The method uses four-color dNTPs whose label cleaves off as nucleotides are incorporated into the newly synthesized DNA strand. Each addition of a base is observed as a short pulse of one of the colors representing one of four bases. Long contiguous reads are possible.[23] If high accuracy can be achieved, this method has advantages for efficient sequence assembly, analyses of repetitive sequences and de novo sequencing. In contrast, many of the other high-throughput sequencing methods generate short sequence reads (30 to 70 bases long) that have to be aligned and analyzed to derive a consensus, then stitched together, and compared with reference genome sequences. Accurate assembly of sequence data relies on sufficient coverage or redundancy across the sequenced region (at least 15-fold redundancy is thought to be required for accurate resequencing[98]), and informatics tools for this process are still evolving.

Hybridization Assays: Principles

All hybridization assays are based on the ability of single-stranded nucleic acids to form specific double-stranded hybrids. The process requires (1) that probe and target nucleic acids are mixed under conditions that allow specific complementary base pairing, and (2) that a method is available to detect any resulting double-stranded nucleic acids. A *probe* indicates a nucleic acid whose identity is known, and the *target* or *sample* is a nucleic acid whose identity or abundance is revealed by hybridization. In some of the methods discussed here, hybridization occurs between a target in solution and a probe that is tethered to a solid surface. In *homogeneous* or *real-time* techniques, both the probes and the targets are in solution, and hybridization and detection occur without washing steps. Some of the homogeneous methods also monitor the dissociation of hybridized duplexes under controlled heating, revealing the identities of the hybridized duplexes by *melting curve* signatures.

As with any assay, both positive and negative controls are necessary. Positive controls contain sequences complementary to the probe, assess assay sensitivity, and ensure that the probe will hybridize to the target under the assay conditions. Negative controls without target sequence assess assay specificity and detect positive contamination if present.

Hybridization Thermodynamics

The favored structure of DNA under physiologic conditions is an ordered double-stranded helix held together by noncovalent interactions. The duplex structure is most stable when all opposing bases are complementary, allowing for maximal

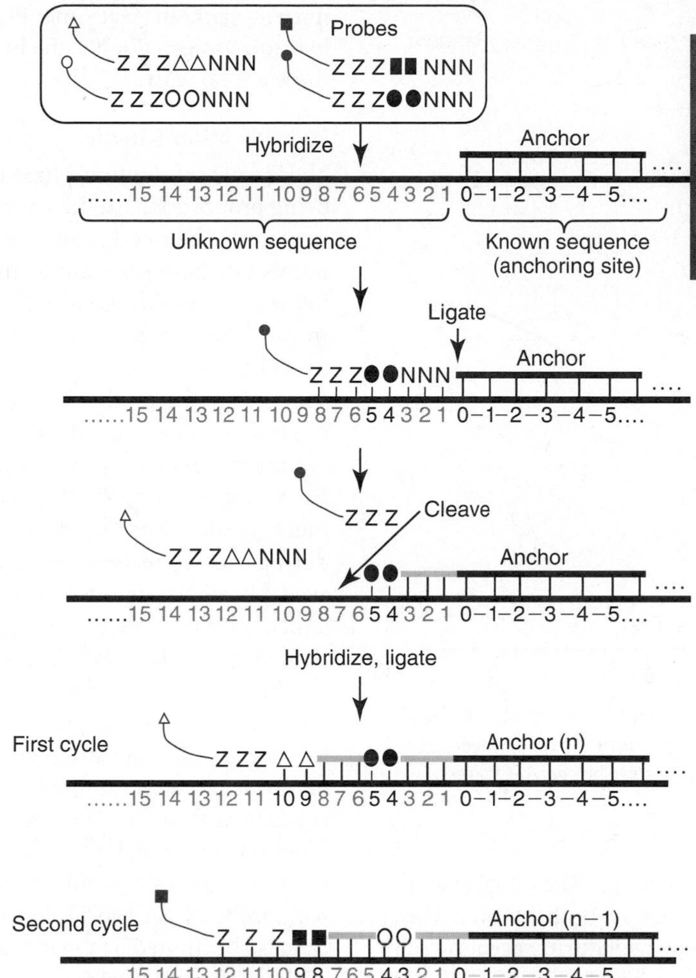

Figure 17-22 Sequencing by ligation (two-base encoding method). An anchor oligonucleotide is hybridized to known sequences of the template (anchoring site). Structures of octamer (8-mer) probes are shown. *N* represents a degenerate base (A, T, C, or G), *Z* represents a universal base that pairs with any base, and the defined bases (●, ○, ■, △) occupy the fourth and fifth base positions. The probes are color-coded by one of four labels *(shown in red),* with each color representing a set of four two-base combinations (e.g., color 1 is AT, TA, CG, or GC; color 2 is AC, CA, TG, or GT; color 3 is TC, CT, AG, or GA; and color 4 is AA, TT, GG, or CC). Once a probe hybridizes to the sequence adjacent to the anchoring site, ligase will connect the probe to the anchor. After the color is recorded, part of the probe is cleaved, and the label is removed together with some of the probe bases. This makes it possible for another probe to ligate to the extending complex. In fact, many rounds of ligation/cleavage can be performed, each time elongating the anchor-probe complex and providing additional two-base possibilities. After a few rounds of probe ligation/cleavage, the anchor-probe complex is stripped, and the next cycle, which is offset by one base, repeats the process. Cycles are repeated until one of the defined bases on the probe pairs with a known base on the anchoring site, allowing decoding of all of the two-base combinations. For example, in the first cycle, two-base possibilities for positions 4, 5, 9, and 10 are determined. In the second cycle, which is offset by one base (n-1), possibilities for positions 3, 4, 8, and 9 are determined. This process is repeated until the defined base on the probe pairs with the first base on the anchoring site (position 0). Because the identity of that base is known, the 0/1 base combination is decoded, which in turn decodes base position 2 and so on, until all of the two-base combinations are decoded.

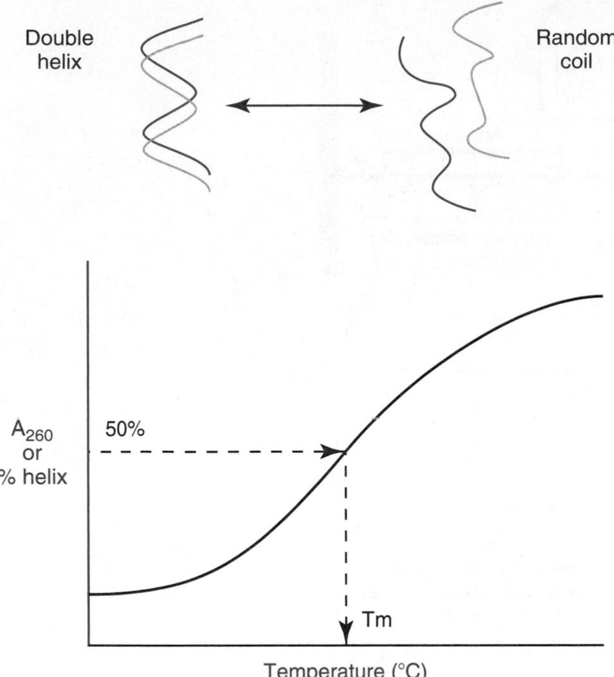

Figure 17-23 Absorbance melting curve of double-helical nucleic acid. *(Modified with permission from Piper MA, Unger ER. Nucleic acid probes: a primer for pathologists. Chicago: ASCP Press, 1989.)*

hydrogen bonding and base stacking. The noncovalent binding between two DNA strands is both specific (i.e., sequence dependent) and reversible. Denaturing agents (such as high temperature, formamide, or extremes of pH) favor dissociation of the double-stranded molecule into two separate random coils (Figure 17-23). On removal of the denaturant, single strands attempt to re-form duplexes, strongly favoring interactions that maximize complementary base pairing. Because temperature is the denaturant most easily manipulated, double- to single-strand transformation is referred to as *melting,* and the temperature at which one half of the DNA is melted is referred to as the *melting temperature,* or *Tm,* of the duplex. Duplexes with mismatched base pairs are less stable than those with a perfect sequence match and thus melt at a lower temperature. The reverse process, in which two complementary strands recombine to form a stable duplex molecule, is referred to as *annealing* or *hybridization.* Hybridization can occur between DNA strands, RNA strands, and strands of nucleic acid analogs (such as peptide nucleic acids[74]), in all combinations.

The hybridization environment defines the degree of base pair mismatch that can be tolerated in a duplex structure. Conditions of high *stringency* (low salt concentration, high formamide concentration, and high temperature) require exact base pairing. As the stringency is lowered by increasing the salt concentration, lowering the formamide concentration, or lowering temperature, more base pair mismatches can be tolerated in a duplex structure. The stringency of a hybridization reaction is determined by hybridization conditions and any washing steps designed to remove nonspecific nucleic acid. In real-time PCR and melting analysis, the hybridization solution is the buffer in which PCR occurs, and there are no washing steps.

Hybridization Kinetics

The kinetics of solution-phase hybridizations is second order, being proportional to the concentrations of both hybridizing strands.[118] The rate-limiting step is nucleation, where a small number of base pairs are formed in the correct orientation, followed by rapid "zippering" of complementary sequences. In the case of a probe present in great excess to the target, hybridization proceeds as a pseudo-first order reaction, depending only on the concentration of the target. However, the time required to hybridize the probe to a given fraction of the target remains proportional to the probe concentration. For example, during PCR, the concentration of primers is much greater than that of the target, and the reaction rate during each annealing step depends on the concentration of available single-stranded product, but the time required to anneal primers to a certain fraction of the target is proportional to the primer concentration.

The availability of nucleic acids for hybridization can also be an issue. In PCR, primer annealing competes with the formation of double-stranded product. As the concentration of product increases during PCR, some double-stranded product is formed before primer annealing can occur (see Figure 17-4). Similarly, when double-stranded probes are used at high concentrations, probe self-annealing interferes with probe-target hybridization. Available hybridization sites can also be limited by the intramolecular secondary structure of the probe or target (e.g., as seen in SSCP).

In addition to probe concentration and availability, the length of the probe and the nucleic acid complexity affect hybridization rates. Rates are directly proportional to the square root of the probe length and inversely proportional to complexity, defined as the total number of base pairs present in nonrepeating sequences. Mismatches up to about 10% have little effect on hybridization rates.

Hybridization rates are also influenced by many factors in the reaction environment, most notably temperature and ionic strength. Above the Tm, no stable hybrids are present, although transient complexes may form. As the temperature is lowered below the Tm, hybridization rates increase until a broad maximum occurs about 20 to 25 °C below the Tm. Hybridization rates also increase with ionic strength. Divalent cations such as Mg^{2+} have a much stronger effect than monovalent cations such as Na^+ or K^+.

When the nucleic acid target or probe is immobilized on a solid support, the kinetics of hybridization is even more complex. Many of the preceding observations still hold true, but the rate and extent of solid-phase hybridization are lower than with solution-phase hybridization. Depending on the concentrations of the reactants, solid-phase hybridization can be nucleation limited or diffusion limited. Optimal efficiency of solid-phase hybridization is achieved under conditions that facilitate diffusion of the probe to the support and that favor hybridization over strand reassociation if double-stranded probes are used. This usually means a small volume of hybridization solution and relatively low probe concentrations. In practice, solid-phase hybridization assays are empirically designed. Time of hybridization and probe concentration are the two variables most frequently adjusted in the assay. Conditions that tend to maximize the extent of hybridization and minimize the background or nonspecific attachment of the probe are selected.

Probes

Similar to antibodies in immunoassays, probes in nucleic acid hybridization assays can be unlabeled or labeled with one of a variety of reporter molecules, depending on the technique used to detect hybridization. Probes may be cloned (recombinant), generated by PCR, or synthesized (oligonucleotides). They may be DNA, RNA, or nucleic acid analogs, and single-stranded or double-stranded. Selection, purification, and labeling of probes are crucial to the success of hybridization assays.

Cloned Probes

Cloned probes consist of a known segment of DNA inserted into a plasmid vector that is propagated by growth in a bacterium. Many different plasmid vectors are now available; pBR322 was one of the first in common use.[7] Some plasmids, such as the F plasmid of *E. coli,* can be used to carry insert sizes that are very long (several hundred kb) and are called *bacterial artificial chromosomes,* or BACs. The entire plasmid DNA (insert plus vector sequences) may be used as a probe, or the insert may be purified first from the vector sequences. The latter method is obviously more cumbersome but may result in reduced background. The resulting probe is a double-stranded DNA probe, and it must be denatured before use.

Some vectors contain RNA promoter regions adjacent to the inserted DNA sequence. These regions permit generation of RNA transcripts from the DNA insert. Because only one strand is copied during RNA synthesis, single-stranded RNA probes are generated. Controlling the orientation of the insert in relation to the promoter region allows the production of transcripts in the "sense" direction (i.e., same as mRNA) or the "antisense" direction (i.e., complementary to mRNA).

PCR-Generated Probes

PCR-generated probes are simple to prepare.[45] During amplification, the PCR product typically is labeled with nucleotides that are radioactive or fluorescent, or have attached affinity labels. If desired, single-stranded probes can be obtained by amplifying with a biotin-labeled primer, followed by solid-phase separation with streptavidin.

Oligonucleotide Probes

Oligonucleotide probes are even easier to obtain than PCR-generated probes. These probes are usually 15 to 45 bases of single-stranded nucleic acid that are chemically synthesized to a specified base sequence. Most commonly, they are DNA, but RNA or nucleic acid analogs can be used. Automated, efficient, and accurate methods of synthesis continue to lower the cost of production. Sequence information is now routinely available in public databases [e.g., the National Institutes of Health (NIH) genetic sequence database, GenBank], and a similarity check for probe sequences can be performed using public algorithms (e.g., BLAST). Probe sequences must be carefully chosen to minimize cross-hybridization with pseudogenes (eukaryotes) or related species (bacteria and viruses). The melting temperature of the probe should allow both favorable hybrid stability and discrimination between related sequences under the stringency of the assay. Oligonucleotide probes are often prepared with covalent attachment of a reporter molecule (such as fluorescent dyes) or affinity labels that allow them to be attached to solid supports. Probes used in homogeneous (real-time) PCR are usually oligonucleotides with a fluorescent label.

Estimating Tms of Oligonucleotide Probes

Probe Tm prediction based on nearest neighbor thermodynamic parameters has improved with compilation of a unified database.[93] Consideration of all possible single-base mismatches and dangling ends further extends the usefulness of these estimates.[92] However, prediction parameters are typically determined using 1 M NaCl, far from typical assay conditions, so it is not surprising that predicted Tms are often at variance from observation. Empirical correction factors[77,112] that may include the concentrations of various cations, dNTPs, the target, and common additives may enhance prediction accuracy and are often used in software programs and Internet sites for in silico Tm estimation. Most fluorescent dyes also stabilize duplexes,[69,123] but this increase in Tm is seldom incorporated into predictions. For these reasons, absolute Tm predictions are seldom accurate in common laboratory and PCR buffers. However, relative Tms (i.e., the difference in Tm between two related probes, such as a probe that is matched and one that is mismatched to a single base variant) are considerably more accurate.[61]

Purity of Labeled Oligonucleotide Probes

The purity of labeled oligonucleotide probes is important for hybridization assays and critical in real-time PCR. Commercial oligonucleotides with a fluorescent label are of variable quality, and their concentration and purity should be assessed before use. Mass spectroscopy and/or coelution of absorbance (A_{260}) and fluorescence peaks on reversed-phase HPLC can indicate probe purity. Quantitative estimates of probe purity can also be obtained by simple absorbance measurements. The extinction coefficient of the oligonucleotide at 260 nm [$e_{260(oligo)}$] is first calculated from its sequence by tabulated values.[8] Some software programs and commercial suppliers provide the related value, nmol per absorbance unit at 260 nm, or nmol/$A_{260(oligo)}$, which is related to the extinction coefficient by the formula $e_{260(oligo)} = 10^6/[\text{nmol}/A_{260(oligo)}]$. Next the concentration of the fluorescent label (C_{fluor}) is calculated from its molar absorptivity[126]:

$$C_{fluor} = A_{\lambda max\ of\ fluor} / e_{\lambda max\ of\ fluor} \tag{1}$$

The concentration of the fluorescently labeled oligonucleotide is then calculated as

$$C_{oligo} = [A_{260} - (A_{\lambda max\ of\ fluor} \times e_{260(fluor)} / e_{\lambda max\ of\ fluor})] / e_{260(oligo)} \quad (2)$$

The equation takes into account the A_{260} contribution from the fluorophore. Similar equations for more than one label can be derived. The concentrations of fluorophore and oligonucleotide should be nearly equal (i.e., the ratio of fluorophore to oligonucleotide should be near 1). Acceptable ratios are between 0.8 and 1.2. Ratios less than 0.8 suggest incomplete labeling or destruction of the attached dye. Ratios greater than 1.2 suggest the presence of free dye or degraded labeled oligonucleotides. A ratio near 1 is a necessary but not a sufficient criterion of a pure probe.

Hybridization Assays: Examples

Hybridization reactions can be divided into two broad categories: *solid-phase,* in which either probe or target is tethered to a solid support while the other is in solution, and *solution-phase,* in which both are in solution (Table 17-3). It is somewhat surprising to note that nucleic acids bound on a solid matrix can still bind complementary nucleic acids. Solid-phase assays are useful because multiple samples can be processed together, facilitating control, washing, and separation procedures. However, hybridization on a solid support is less efficient than solution hybridization, and the kinetics is slower and more difficult to predict. Both solid-phase and liquid-phase assays are used routinely in the clinical laboratory. Solid-phase assays include dot blots, line probes, arrays, in situ hybridization, and Southern and Northern blotting.

Several classical methods first hybridize in solution and then separate the bound from the unbound labeled probe. Exclusion chromatography, and binding by hydroxyapatite, magnetic particles, or other affinity capture methods allow selective measurement of the labeled probe-target hybrid. For example, *hybrid capture* methods use an immobilized antibody that is specific for RNA-DNA hybrids that are formed during solution-phase hybridization of a DNA sample and an unlabeled RNA probe. The assay can be adapted to microtiter plate format for automation of washing and detection.

Solution hybridization has now been combined with amplification, detection, and quantification—all in the same tube. Such closed-tube, real-time assays do not require any addition, washing, or separation steps.

TABLE 17-3 Hybridization Assays

Solid phase Hybridization	Dot-blot and line-probe assays
	Arrays (microarrays and medium-density arrays)
	Microbead assays
	In situ hybridization
	Southern and Northern blotting
Solution phase Hybridization	Real-time (or homogeneous) PCR
	PCR melting analysis
	Single-molecule visualization
	Other classical techniques

PCR, Polymerase chain reaction.

Dot-Blot and Line-Probe Assays

Conventional hybridization assays on membranes are known as dot blots or line probes, depending on the geometry of the individual spots. Nucleic acids are applied with suction, using a commercially available manifold that results in a shape that may be round (dot) or elongated (line or slot). After immobilization, the membrane is incubated with complementary nucleic acid at a constant temperature, followed by one or more washes to discriminate matched from mismatched nucleic acid. This method allows multiple probe-target hybridizations to be carried out simultaneously under identical conditions.

Two general formats are used for these assays: multiple samples may be affixed to the solid support and interrogated by a small number of probes ("sample-down"), or multiple probes may be attached to the support and a small number of samples used ("probe-down") (Figure 17-24). In the sample-down format, purified nucleic acid or amplified fragments from multiple samples are immobilized on the support.

In the probe-down format, unlabeled probes bound to the filter are allowed to interact directly with a specimen that carries the label (a technique also known as *reverse dot blot*). Alternatively, instead of having to label the sample, a set of secondary probes can be used for signal generation. Signal probes are attached to the filter only through sample-mediated hybridization; the sample nucleic acid forms a sandwich between the immobilized probe and the signal-generating probe. Results of a dot-blot or line-probe assay are usually qualitative: if hybridization has occurred, a signal is generated at the specified spot and a simple yes/no interpretation is given. Similar assays have been developed substituting microtiter plate wells for filters. This requires chemical modification of the plastic wells to bind short DNA probes at one end, allowing the bound probes to hybridize to sample, but this approach is more amenable to automation of washing and detection.

Medium-Density Arrays

Dot-blot and line-probe assays have largely been replaced by medium-density arrays that typically analyze 20 to 500 spots. Medium-density arrays are emerging in the clinical laboratory for testing multiple mutations in specimens for genetic disease, oncology, and pharmacogenetics. Many companies are involved in the supply of arrays, and the industry is moving swiftly.[37,44] These arrays do not need to be attached to a two-dimensional surface as long as their "address" can be decoded. For example, microspheres can be coded by fluorescence intensity in two different channels, while

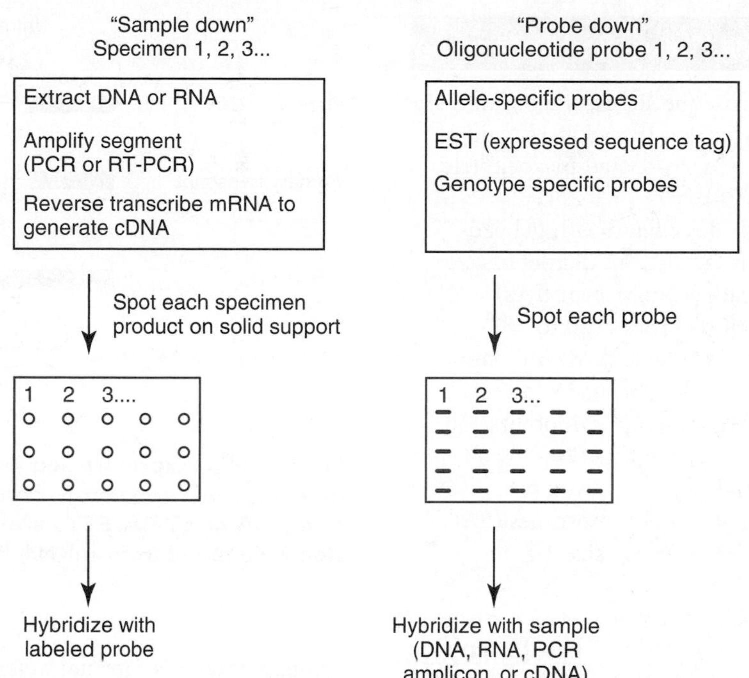

Figure 17-24 Two modes of dot-blot and line-probe assays. In the "sample-down" mode, DNA, cDNA, RNA, or amplified products are attached to the solid support and hybridized to labeled probes in solution. Alternatively, different probes are spotted onto the support ("probe-down"), and the sample is in solution.

fluorescence in a third channel monitors hybridization. All channels can be read simultaneously using a flow cytometer.[47] Some characteristics of arrays are listed in Table 17-4.

Microarrays

Extending further the density of hybridization assays, microarrays (also called *DNA arrays* or *DNA chips*) were introduced in the mid 1990s.[94] Compared with medium-density arrays, spot sizes in microarrays are decreased (typically to less than 200 microns in diameter) such that one array contains thousands to millions of spots. This dimensional change requires specialized detection equipment, software, and informatics to analyze the data. Microarrays are fabricated on solid surfaces (generally on glass, but sometimes on other supports, such as gel pads or coated gold surfaces) by synthesis of oligonucleotides on these surfaces or by physical spotting of probes with the aid of robotic arraying equipment or electronic addressing. The promise of microarrays is accompanied by challenges, including the need for strict requirements for controls and good experimental design. Because of their massively parallel capacity, microarrays have attracted tremendous interest among researchers who wish to monitor the whole genome for (1) single-nucleotide polymorphisms, (2) gene expression, and (3) copy number variants.

Single-Nucleotide Polymorphism (SNP) Arrays

Because SNPs represent the most common genetic difference between individuals, much effort has focused on correlating SNP alleles to phenotype and disease association. Microarrays that analyze human SNPs ("SNP chips") provide the technology to genotype most known human SNPs in one experiment. Nearby SNP alleles tend to cluster together as haplotypes, so disease association by haplotype simplifies the analysis. Although some valuable markers have been found by these genome-wide association studies,[31] the yield of useful disease markers obtained by these methods has been disappointing and many difficulties remain, such as identifying adequate control populations.[88] SNP arrays are also used to assess copy number variation and to genotype SNPs of known association with disease.

Gene Expression Arrays

Early gene expression arrays often used expressed-sequence-tag (EST) libraries. ESTs are short sequences that are expressed in certain cells, tissues, or organs at different developmental stages (Figure 17-25). An example of a two-color comparative EST microarray for gene expression studies is shown in Figure 17-26. Because the human genome is now completely sequenced, mRNA probes are usually directly synthesized on microarrays today. Modern gene expression arrays can measure the mRNA transcribed from all human genes in one experiment. They have been applied to almost every conceivable human condition, including neoplastic, inflammatory, and psychiatric. The promise consists of better diagnosis, molecular staging, prognosis, and therapy through understanding of disease pathogenesis. In oncology, arrays have led

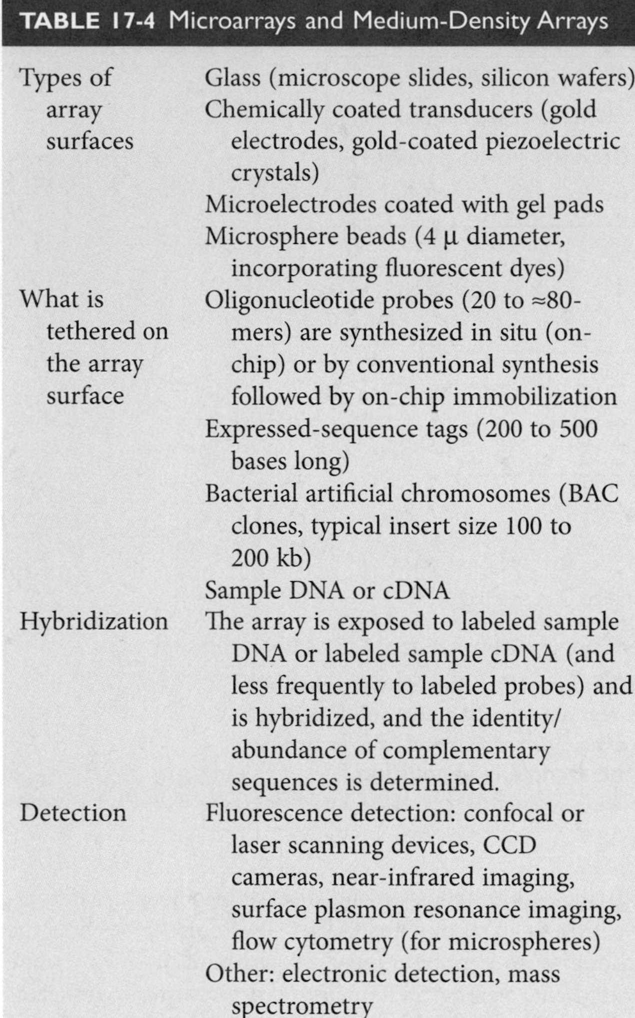

TABLE 17-4 Microarrays and Medium-Density Arrays

Types of array surfaces	Glass (microscope slides, silicon wafers) Chemically coated transducers (gold electrodes, gold-coated piezoelectric crystals) Microelectrodes coated with gel pads Microsphere beads (4 μ diameter, incorporating fluorescent dyes)
What is tethered on the array surface	Oligonucleotide probes (20 to ≈80-mers) are synthesized in situ (on-chip) or by conventional synthesis followed by on-chip immobilization Expressed-sequence tags (200 to 500 bases long) Bacterial artificial chromosomes (BAC clones, typical insert size 100 to 200 kb) Sample DNA or cDNA
Hybridization	The array is exposed to labeled sample DNA or labeled sample cDNA (and less frequently to labeled probes) and is hybridized, and the identity/abundance of complementary sequences is determined.
Detection	Fluorescence detection: confocal or laser scanning devices, CCD cameras, near-infrared imaging, surface plasmon resonance imaging, flow cytometry (for microspheres) Other: electronic detection, mass spectrometry

CCD, Charge-coupled device.

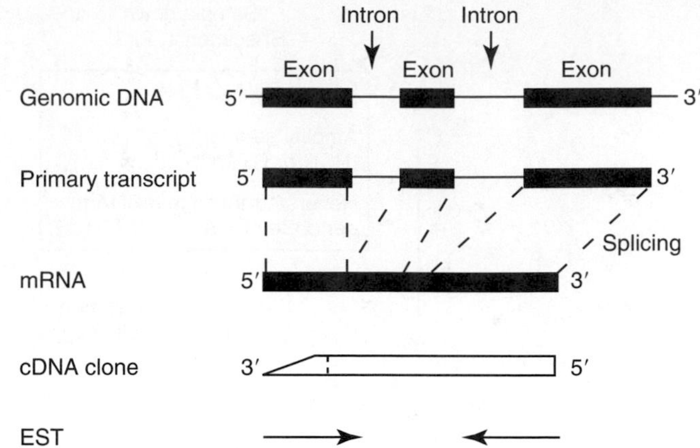

Figure 17-25 Expressed sequence tags (ESTs) can be used as probes to identify expressed genes by hybridizing to mRNA or cDNA. ESTs are generated from cDNA clones obtained from mRNA libraries.

to new diagnostic and prognostic markers in breast cancer,[109] bladder cancer,[110] leukemia,[34] and sarcoma,[17] among others. In the clinical laboratory, expression arrays are used directly in only a limited number of diagnostic or prognostic tests. Most arrays are used in marker discovery projects and for selection of a smaller panel of expression targets that are then analyzed by other quantitative methods such as real-time PCR that provide greater precision and dynamic range.

Copy Number Variant Arrays

One important clinical application of microarrays is the genome-wide analysis of deletions and duplications, also referred to as analysis of copy number variants, or CNVs. CNV analyses using microarrays are steadily augmenting, and in some cases replacing, traditional cytogenetic chromosome analysis (karyotyping) and fluorescence in situ hybridization (FISH) analysis (see next section) through higher resolution of microarray data. Similar to gene expression arrays, many of the CNV arrays use two-color comparative hybridization to determine the gene dosage in a specimen compared with a normal reference genome (comparative genomic hybridization, or CGH). Arrays for CGH may use BACs carrying large fragments of the genome as probes, or oligonucleotide probes for even higher resolution and data density. An example of CNV analysis using an oligonucleotide CGH array is shown in Figure 17-27. SNP arrays can also detect copy number changes by loss of heterozygosity (this method is sometimes referred to as *virtual karyotyping*). Unlike CGH, SNP arrays have the advantage of analyzing the specimen without the need to mix the reference genome with the specimen. SNP arrays can also detect copy number neutral changes caused by uniparental disomy that are not detected by CGH methods. Chromosomal abnormalities identified by CNV arrays in a clinical setting are usually confirmed by FISH or other methods.

In Situ Hybridization

In situ hybridization is a specialized type of solid support assay in which morphologically intact tissues, cells, or chromosomes affixed to a glass microscope slide provide the matrix for hybridization. The process is analogous to immunohistochemistry, except that nucleic acids instead of antibodies are used as probes. The strength of the method lies in linking morphologic evaluation with detection of specific nucleic acid sequences. When fluorescent probes are applied to metaphase chromosome spreads or interphase nuclei, the technique is referred to as fluorescent in situ hybridization, or *FISH.* Numeric aberrations or translocations of chromosomes can be detected rapidly. FISH can also be combined with immunohistochemistry so that information on both the amount of protein expression and the gene dosage can be found on the same slide. In situ hybridization is appropriate when localization of a target in tissue is important. However, experience in histology is necessary for accurate interpretation. In situ hybridization can provide information on the level of mRNA expression, but not on the size or structure of the mRNA. As might be expected, hybridization within a

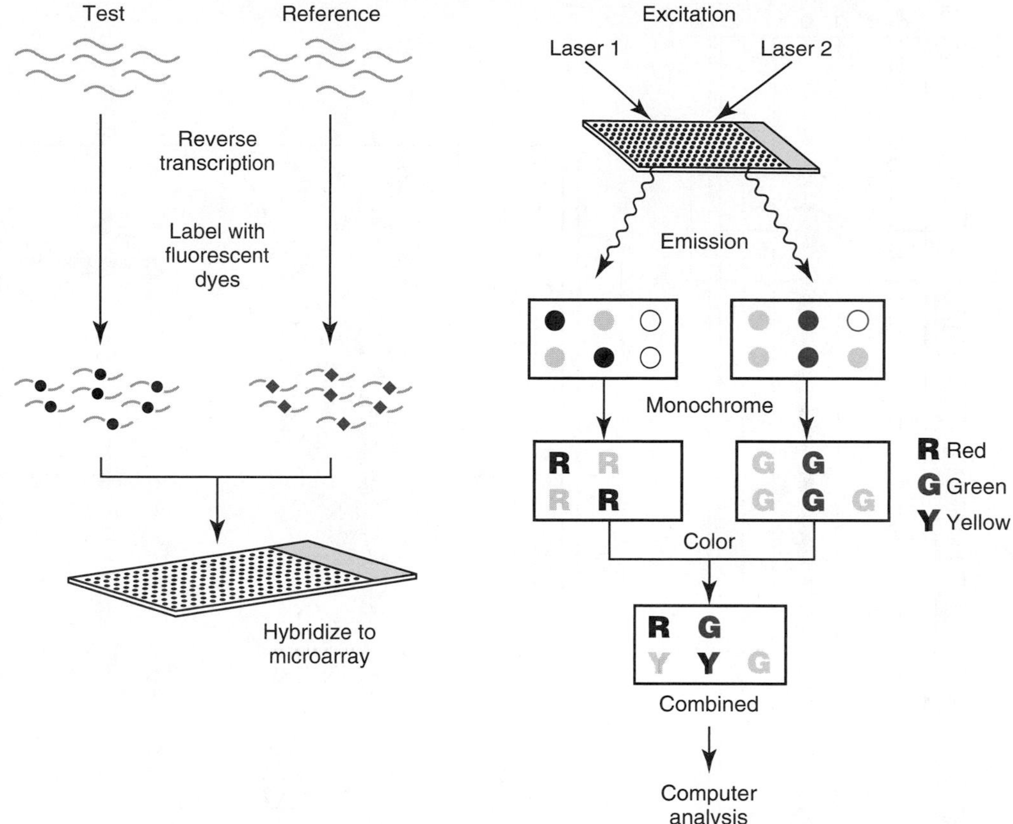

Figure 17-26 A two-color microarray experiment. An array of DNA clones representing expressed-sequence tags (ESTs) is affixed to a glass slide. Messenger RNAs in the test and reference specimen are converted into differentially labeled cDNA by reverse transcription and incorporation of two different fluorescent dyes. The two samples are hybridized together onto the array. The array is washed, and the image is captured twice, each time with a laser of a wavelength that excites one of the dyes but not the other. The monochromatic images are then converted to two colors [green for the test sample (G), and red for the reference (R)], and the images are combined. If the abundance of cDNA is the same in each of the two samples, then the composite spot will be shown as yellow (Y). If one is in greater abundance, then that color will be preserved. Upregulation and downregulation of gene expression are then analyzed by software.

tissue matrix is more variable than in solution or on well-characterized chemical surfaces.

Single-Copy Visualization

If a nucleic acid probe is labeled with many fluorescent molecules, it is possible to optically visualize a single copy of the nucleic acid target by fluorescent microscopy. One technique uses reporter probes that are labeled with a long string of multicolored fluorescent labels.[28] Several tandem color segments on the reporter probe each consist of about a hundred fluorophores, and the combination of different color segments uniquely identifies the target. The target nucleic acid is hybridized in solution with the reporter probe together with a capture probe and is washed, immobilized, stretched, and oriented on the surface of an optical slide. Each captured target is then identified by the color code of the reporter and is counted (Figure 17-28). Unfortunately, much of the target is lost during the washing step; therefore, the sensitivity of this technique is not as high as that of real-time PCR (see next section). A minimum of about 2000 target copies is currently required for quantification above background. However, the ability of the method to multiplex more than 150 reporter probes in one reaction tube and to count individual molecules is attractive. One application of this technique is direct measurement of mRNA expression in tissue specimens prepared from formalin-fixed paraffin blocks without the need for cDNA preparation or PCR.

Real-Time PCR

In real-time PCR, data are collected during nucleic acid amplification rather than at a single end point. The technique uses fluorescent reporter molecules and instrumentation that records fluorescence during thermal cycling. Data obtained provide information on the identity, quantity, and sequence

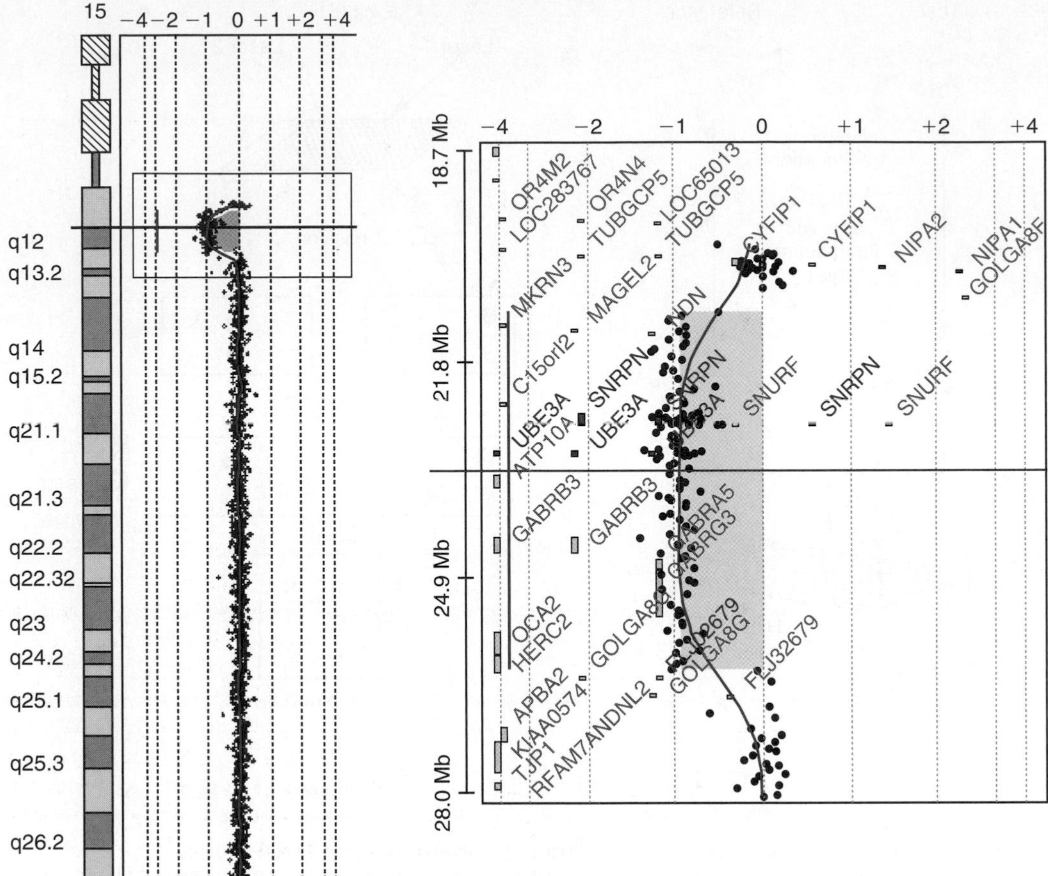

Figure 17-27 Copy number variation identified with a comparative genomic hybridization array made from oligonucleotides. DNA from a subject is fragmented, labeled with Cy5, and hybridized onto a microarray, together with Cy3-labeled reference DNA. On the array are nearly 44,000 oligonucleotide probes, each about 60 bases long and tiled across the whole genome at an average spacing of 75 kb. Shown on the left panel are results of probes on chromosome 15 (all other chromosomes are analyzed in this assay but are not shown). Each dot represents a specific probe to which the subject's DNA hybridizes. Their positions (0, −1, +1, etc.) reflect the dosage of the subject's DNA relative to the reference DNA. A majority of the probes line up on "0," indicating no quantitative difference compared with the reference DNA. Probes in the 15q11 to 15q13 region, however, are on the "−1" line, indicating that the subject has a deletion of that region in one of the chromosomes. A closer view of that region *(right panel)* shows that among the deleted genes are *UBE3A*, which causes Angelman syndrome, and *SNRPN*, which causes Prader-Willi syndrome. Because the method does not distinguish the methylation status of the deleted alleles, this result alone cannot determine which of the two disorders the subject has. *(Courtesy Sarah South, Ph.D., ARUP Laboratories.)*

of the nucleic acid sample. Fluorescent dyes or probes capable of signaling the relative quantity of DNA are added to the PCR mixture before amplification. The same reaction tube is used for amplification and fluorescence monitoring, and there are no sample transfers, reagent additions, binding or washing steps, thereby eliminating the risk of product contamination in subsequent reactions. Because the process is simple and fast, real-time PCR is replacing many conventional techniques in the clinical laboratory.

Real-time PCR was first described using ethidium bromide to monitor the accumulation of a double-stranded PCR product with the fluorescence signal recorded once each cycle.[41,42] If target DNA is present, fluorescence increases. How early during PCR one begins to see a signal depends on the initial amount of target DNA, and this provides a systematic method of quantification. Further, when fluorescence is continuously monitored as the temperature is raised, a melting curve can be generated. Often the first derivative of this melting curve is plotted to visually aid a person in determining the position of the melting temperature. Melting analysis can be used to verify the identity of the amplified product and to detect sequence variants down to a single base

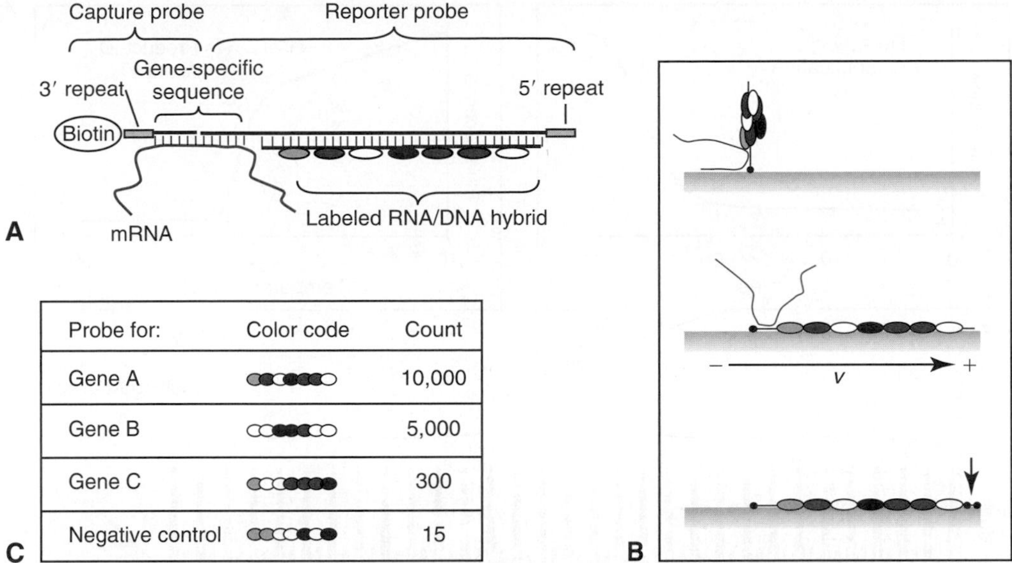

Figure 17-28 Single-copy visualization. A pair of probes (capture probe and reporter probe) hybridize to the mRNA target in solution through gene-specific probe sequences (A). The reporter probe has seven color segments, each segment made of ≈900 RNA bases that are labeled with about a hundred fluorophores of one color. The labeled portion of the probe is a DNA/RNA hybrid that can be observed as a ≈3 nm fluorescent spot. Excess probes and unbound DNA are removed and the target complex is immobilized on a streptavidin-coated slide through the biotin on the capture probe (B, top). An electrical current is applied, and the complex is stretched (B, middle). The reporter probe is immobilized in extended form by biotin-labeled oligonucleotides complementary to its 5′ repeat sequence (B, bottom). The color code of the probe is read by an epi-fluorescent microscope, and each unique probe is counted (C). Normally, a number of negative control probes are present in the hybridization solution to establish nonspecific background counts.

(Figure 17-29). Real-time PCR and melting analysis can be considered as "dynamic" hybridization assays in which formation and dissociation of the probe-target duplex (or product duplex) are monitored in real time.

Dyes and Probe Formats for Real-Time PCR

Many different fluorescent reporter systems are used in real-time PCR, and some of the more common ones are shown in Figure 17-30. Many methods use probes with sequences complementary to the target. Others rely on double-stranded DNA binding dyes and the specificity afforded by PCR primers. Some have the additional option of melting analysis to verify the melting temperature of the probe or product.

Double-Stranded DNA Binding Dyes

Although ethidium bromide was the first dye used in real-time PCR, cyanine dyes are more widely used today. Several cyanine dyes have fluorescent properties similar to those of fluorescein, allowing the use of commonly available real-time optics.[22,127] The fluorescence increases as double-stranded DNA is produced during PCR (Figure 17-30, *row one*). Double-stranded DNA binding dyes are commonly used for real-time quantification, particularly in the research setting when the specificity of a probe is not needed and the cost of probes is prohibitive.

One disadvantage of some cyanine dyes is that they inhibit amplification at dye concentrations that are needed to saturate the amount of DNA produced by PCR. As a result, there is not enough dye to go around, and low Tm products are poorly detected in multiplex amplifications. However, alternative "saturating" DNA dyes that do not inhibit PCR have been developed. These dyes also detect heteroduplexes and enable very simple solutions for genotyping and mutation scanning.[84,123]

Fluorescently Labeled Primers

Labeled primers can also be used to monitor PCR. In one system, a primer with a 5′-hairpin is labeled with a fluorophore and a quencher so that fluorescence is quenched in the hairpin conformation. When the primer straightens out during PCR, fluorescence increases[73] (Figure 17-30, *row six*). If the sequence of the primer is carefully considered, the quencher moiety is not necessary.[72] Nonhairpin primers with a single label can also be used for detection and genotyping because of changes in fluorescence that occur with hybridization.[33]

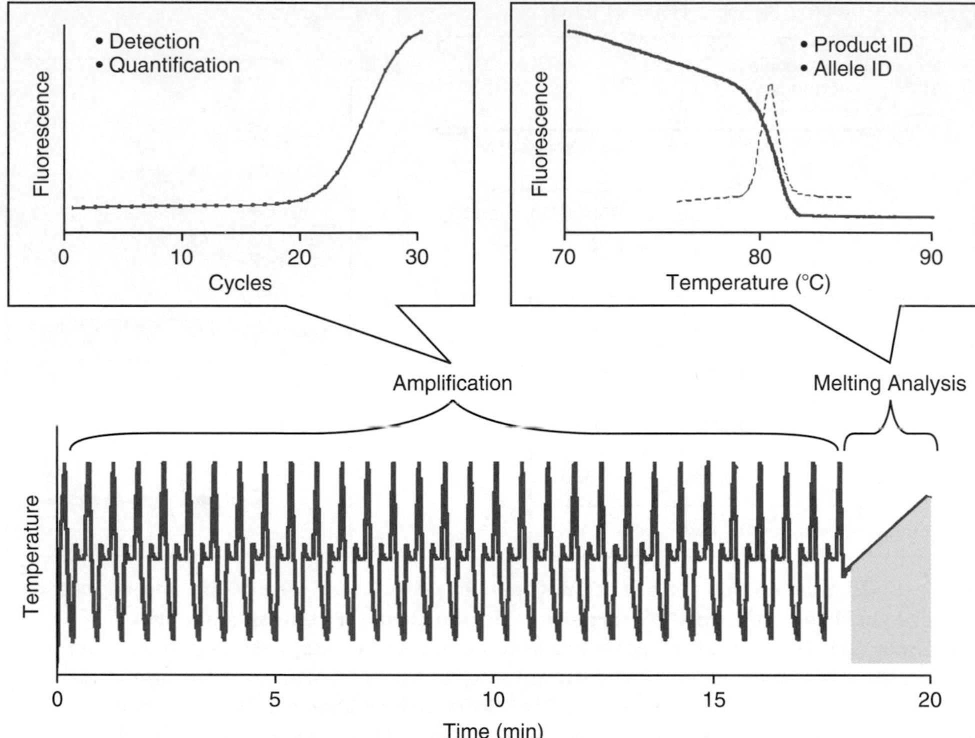

Figure 17-29 Real-time monitoring during amplification and melting analysis. The *bottom panel* shows a typical rapid-cycle temperature profile that is followed by a temperature ramp for melting analysis. When fluorescence is monitored during amplification once each cycle *(dotted lines),* information is provided on the presence or absence of specific target sequences and allows quantification of the target. When fluorescence is monitored continuously through the melting phase *(shaded area),* information can be provided that verifies target identification or establishes genotype. *(Modifed with permission of the publisher from Wittwer CT, Kusukawa N. Real-time PCR. In: Persing DH, Tenover FC, Versalovic J, et al, eds. Molecular microbiology: diagnostic principles and practice. Washington, DC: ASM Press, 2004:71-84.)*

One advantage of fluorescently labeled primers over dsDNA dyes is that multiplexing is possible. However, with both dsDNA dyes and labeled primers, reaction specificity depends on the primers. Any double-stranded product that is formed will be detected, including primer-dimers. Therefore, hot start techniques to increase specificity and melting curve analysis to confirm the desired product are useful.

Probe-Specific Detection

The use of fluorescent probes in PCR adds another level of specificity to the process. Fluorescent probes that hybridize to PCR products during amplification change fluorescence by two possible mechanisms: (1) a covalent bond between two dyes is broken by hydrolysis or is made through ligation, or (2) the fluorescence change follows reversible hybridization of the probe to the target. Following this distinction, when an irreversible covalent bond is involved, the probes are called *hydrolysis probes.* When probes reversibly change fluorescence on duplex formation, they are called *hybridization probes.* One major difference between the two probe types is that melting analysis is possible with hybridization probes, but not with probes that have been hydrolyzed.

Hybridization Probes. These probes change fluorescence upon hybridization, usually by fluorescence resonance energy transfer.[54,127] Two interacting fluorophores may be placed on adjacent probes (Figure 17-30, *row two*), or one may be placed on a primer and the other on a probe (Figure 17-30, *row three*). Only one probe with one fluorophore may be necessary if fluorescence is quenched by deoxyguanosine residues.[16] Another single-labeled probe design uses thiazole orange attached to a peptide nucleic acid.[101] In each of these designs, the fluorescence change that occurs with hybridization is reversible with melting.

Hydrolysis Probes. A fluorophore-labeled probe can be synthesized with a quencher located in a position that allows it to quench fluorescence from the fluorophore. If the probe is hydrolyzed between the fluorophore and the quencher during PCR, fluorescence will increase. The most common implementation uses the 5′-exonuclease activity of some DNA polymerases to hydrolyze the probe and dissociate the labels (Figure 17-30, *row four*). This method has been simplified by putting the fluorophores on opposite ends of the probe.[59] Hybrid-stabilizing agents, such as a minor groove binder, can be added to the probe to make the system more robust.[50]

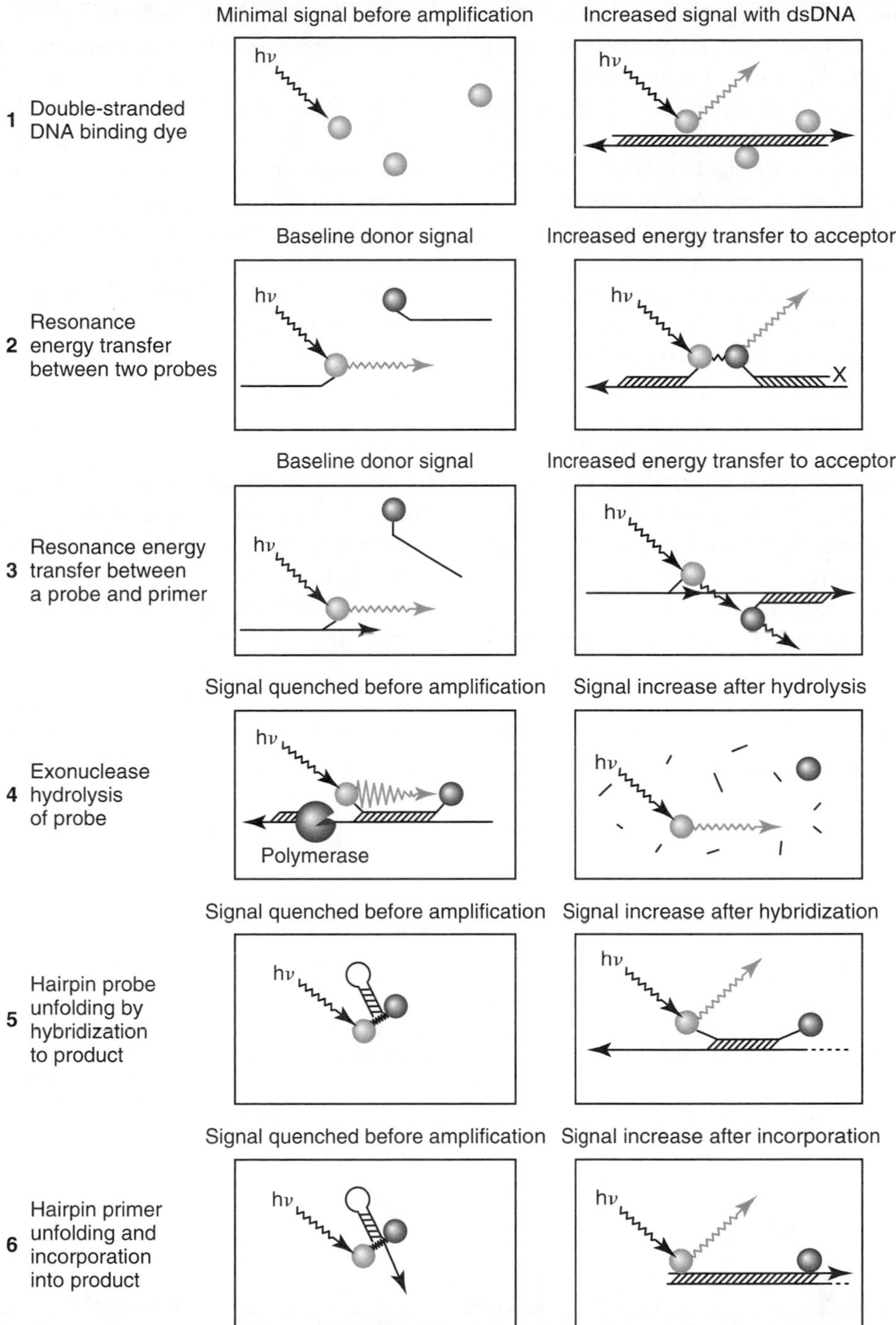

Figure 17-30 Common probes and dyes for real-time polymerase chain reaction (PCR). ***(1)*** **Double-stranded DNA dyes show a significant increase in fluorescence when bound to DNA (*hv* = excitation light).** ***(2)*** **Adjacent hybridization probes. Fluorescence resonance energy transfer (FRET) is illustrated between a donor and acceptor fluorophore. The "*x*" indicates termination of the 3′-end of the probe to prevent polymerase extension.** ***(3)*** **FRET between a labeled primer and a single hybridization probe.** ***(4)*** **Hydrolysis probes are cleaved between a fluorescent reporter and a quencher, resulting in increased fluorescence.** ***(5)*** **Hairpin probes are quenched in the native conformation, but increase in fluorescence when hybridized.** ***(6)*** **Hairpin primers retain their native, quenched conformation until they are incorporated into a double-stranded product.** *(Modified with permission of the publisher from Pritham GH, Wittwer CT. Continuous fluorescent monitoring of PCR. J Clin Lig Assay 1998;21:404-12. © 1998 Clinical Ligand Assay Society Inc.)*

Dual-labeled probes can also be cleaved using a DNAzyme (a DNA molecule that acts as a catalyst) generated during PCR.[104] Finally, irreversible ligation can be used for homogeneous genotyping with a fluorescent readout.[13] Hydrolysis probes generate fluorescence through changes in covalent bonds. The change in fluorescence signal is irreversible, and melting analysis of the hydrolyzed probe is not useful.

Mixed Mechanism Probes. Several probe systems appear to function by both hydrolysis and hybridization mechanisms. These include hairpin probes, self-probing amplicon primers, and displacement probes. A hairpin probe functions similarly to a hairpin primer in that it is designed to increase in fluorescence when the distance between the quencher and the reporter increases upon target hybridization (Figure 17-30, *row five*). Similarly, primers that result in self-probing amplicons have a hairpin that separates quencher from reporter when hybridized.[119] Competitive displacement probes separate quencher and reporter by competitive hybridization.[57] However, in all three cases, polymerases with exonuclease activity usually are used, and the labeled probes are potential substrates for exonuclease cleavage. Indeed, their amplification growth curves often resemble irreversible hydrolysis rather than reversible hybridization (Figure 17-31). Conversely, many exonuclease probes, especially probes labeled on each end, show significant hybridization signals.[59]

Detection and Quantification in Real-Time PCR

When fluorescence is monitored once each cycle in the presence of a dye, the data closely follow the expected logistic shape discussed earlier (see Figures 17-3 and 17-31, *top left*). However, with hydrolysis probes, fluorescence is cumulative and continues to increase even after the amount of product reaches a plateau (Figure 17-31, *top middle*). In contrast, reactions monitored with hybridization probes may show a decrease in fluorescence at high cycle number[124] (Figure 17-31, *top right*). Despite differences in the curve shape, all real-time systems follow the amount of product being produced during PCR, and this information is used for detection and quantification.

Detection

A fluorescent signal that increases during PCR and follows one of the expected curve shapes suggests that the specific target is present and was amplified. In contrast, a signal that stays at background even after 40 PCR cycles suggests that the target is absent and that no amplification occurred. Algorithms that analyze the entire curve may be more robust than simple threshold methods.[122] Positive controls (to rule out inhibitory factors) and negative controls (to rule out product contamination and nonspecific signal generation) are necessary. Melting analysis can be used to verify the expected Tm

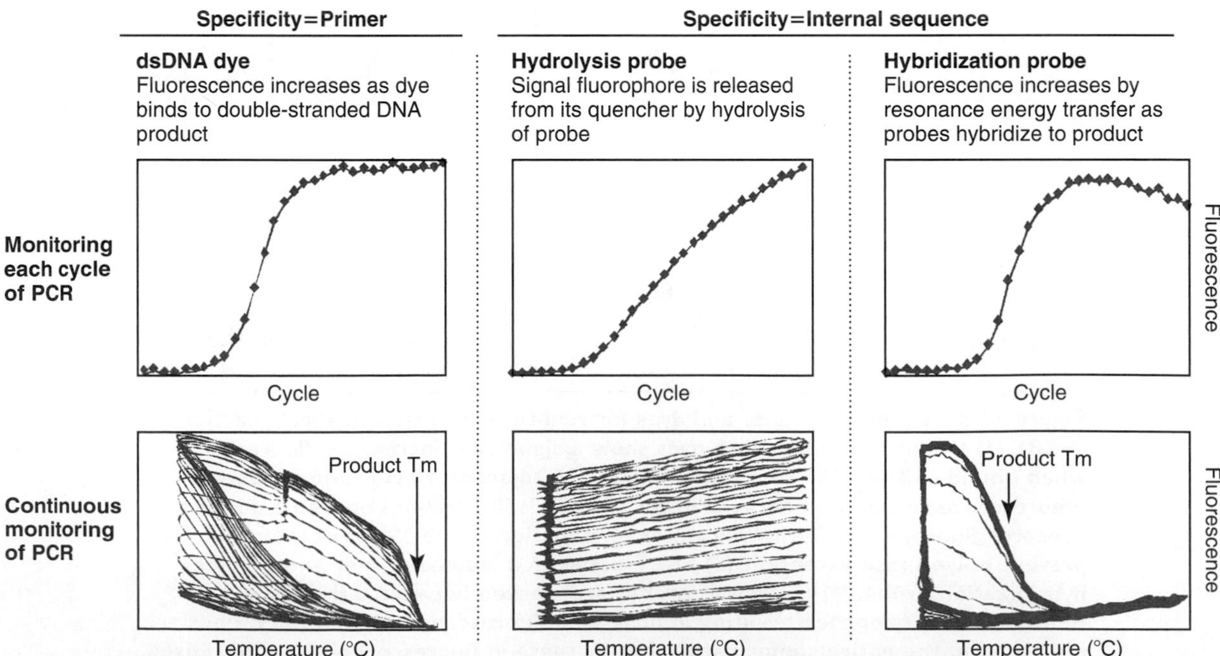

Figure 17-31 Monitoring in real time. The *top row* shows data collected once each polymerase chain reaction (PCR) cycle, and the *bottom row* shows data collected continuously (5 times per second) during all PCR cycles. Three different reporter systems are shown. *(Modified with permission of the publisher from Wittwer CT, Kusukawa N. Real-time PCR. In: Persing DH, Tenover FC, Versalovic J, et al, eds. Molecular microbiology: diagnostic principles and practice. Washington, DC: ASM Press, 2004:71-84.)*

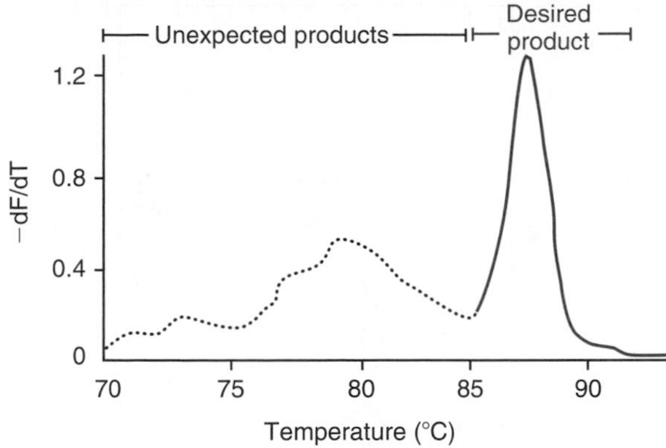

Figure 17-32 First-derivative melting curve showing the target (at high Tm, *solid line*) and nonspecific polymerase chain reaction (PCR) products (at lower Tms, *dotted line*). *(Modified by permission of the publisher from Morrison TB, Weiss JJ, Wittwer CT. Quantification of low-copy transcripts by continuous SYBR Green I monitoring during amplification. Biotechniques 1998;24:954-63. © 1998 Eaton Publishing.)*

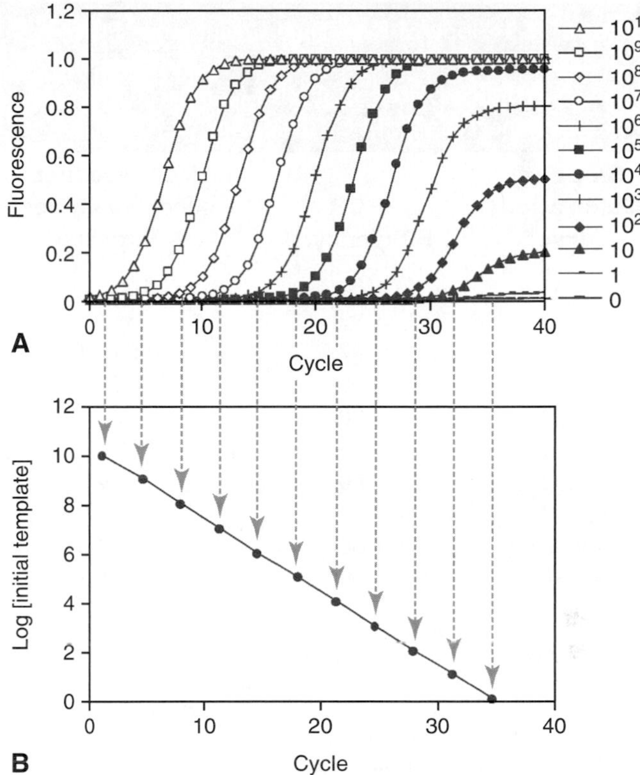

Figure 17-33 Quantification by real-time polymerase chain reaction (PCR). Shown are typical real-time curves for amplification reactions of varying initial target concentrations (A), and the log of the initial concentration plotted against the quantification cycle (B) as calculated by the second derivative maximum (see Figure 17-35). *(Modified with permission of the publisher from Wittwer CT, Kusukawa N. Real-time PCR. In: Persing DH, Tenover FC, Versalovic J, et al, eds. Molecular microbiology: diagnostic principles and practice. Washington, DC: ASM Press, 2004:71-84.)*

of the probe or product if the fluorescence generated is reversible with hybridization.

When assay specificity depends on the primers (e.g., with DNA dyes or labeled primers), the possibility of amplifying undesired targets or primer-dimers is a concern. One way to eliminate or decrease the detection of unexpected targets is to acquire fluorescence during each cycle at a temperature just below the melting transition of the expected target. To illustrate the concept, Figure 17-32 shows a first-derivative melting curve of products at the end of a PCR that shows unexpected products along with the desired product. The signal was generated with a dye that detects all double-stranded DNA. The plot reveals both lower Tm species that are unexpected products and a single Gaussian-shaped peak that is centered on the target's predicted Tm. If fluorescence is acquired during each cycle at (in this case) 85 °C, the unexpected products will be denatured and will not contribute to the signal.[70]

Multiplex detection is possible with probes that are labeled with different colors or with probes or amplicons that have different melting temperatures. Examples in the clinical laboratory include probe multiplexing to detect the presence of more than one infectious organism, or to discriminate an internal control template from the target.

Quantification

Real-time PCR offers a convenient and systematic approach to quantification by monitoring the amount of product each cycle. Perhaps the most popular clinical use of real-time PCR is in the assessment of viral load, particularly for HIV and HCV. The clinical need for quantification is well established, and real-time methods give rapid and precise answers. However, other amplification systems, particularly transcription-based and branched DNA methods, are also used in this highly competitive field. Additional quantitative applications of real-time PCR include quantification of mRNAs (after reverse transcription) in gene expression studies and assessment of gene dosage in genetics and oncology.

One of the advantages of real-time PCR is its large dynamic range. Figure 17-33, *A*, shows an extended range of quantification standards in a typical real-time PCR. As the initial template concentration increases, the curves shift to earlier cycles. The extent of this shift depends on the PCR efficiency (Table 17-5). The cycle at which fluorescence rises correlates inversely with the log of the initial template concentration and is the quantification cycle or Cq (Figure 17-33, *B*). This "cycle" is actually a *virtual* cycle that includes a fractional component determined by interpolation, which can be calculated by several methods. One method uses the maximum of the *second derivative* of the curve to determine Cq (Figure 17-34). The second derivative of the amplification curve is estimated numerically with Savitzky-Golay polynomials.[81] The second derivative is derived from the shape of the curve,

TABLE 17-5 Slope of Real-Time Quantitative PCR Standard Curve, PCR Efficiency, and the Amount of PCR Product Produced After 30 Cycles Compared With the Amount Expected With PCR Efficiency of 100%

Slope of Calibration Curve*	PCR Efficiency, %	PCR Product After 30 Cycles, % Expected
−3.32	100	100
−3.35	99	86
−3.38	97.5	69
−3.45	95	47
−3.59	90	22
−3.74	85	10
−3.92	80	4
−4.34	70	1
−4.90	60	0.1
−5.68	50	0.02

*Assuming the log (initial template) is plotted on the *x*-axis as the independent variable, and the quantification cycle is plotted on the *y*-axis as the dependent variable, the slope of the calibration curve is as follows: Slope = ΔCycle/Δlog (initial template). Percent PCR efficiency is calculated as $(10^{-1/\text{Slope}} - 1) \times 100$.
PCR, Polymerase chain reaction.

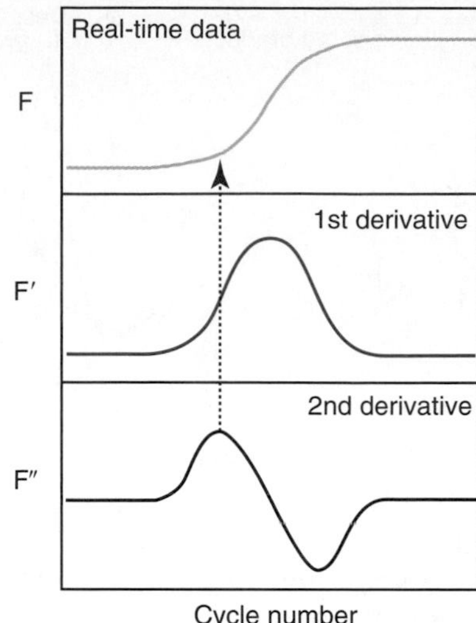

Figure 17-34 Finding the fraction cycle number for quantification. Real-time fluorescence data *(F)* from the amplification reaction are shown with the first *(F′)* and second *(F″)* derivatives. The maximum of the second derivative provides one way to determine the quantification cycle, Cq. *(Modified with permission of the publisher from Wittwer CT, Kusukawa N. Real-time PCR. In: Persing DH, Tenover FC, Versalovic J, et al, eds. Molecular microbiology: diagnostic principles and practice. Washington, DC: ASM Press, 2004:71-84.)*

and there is no need to adjust baselines or worry about normalizing the fluorescence values. Alternatively, in *threshold analysis,* a fluorescence level is selected that intersects with the amplification curves, and fractional cycle numbers are found by interpolation. However, when the sample fluorescence does not reach the threshold (as may happen with low copy samples), quantification is not possible.

Accuracy and Precision

The accuracy of real-time PCR quantification depends not only on the method chosen to analyze the curves, but also on the quality of the quantification standards used. Purified PCR products quantified by spectrophotometry are easily obtained. When serially diluted, these calibrators can accurately quantify the amount of target in human genomic DNA.[81] Synthesized oligonucleotides, purified plasmids, and genomic DNA can also be used as calibrators. *Limiting dilution* analysis can also be used to determine the amount of "amplifiable" DNA.[70] Sometimes absolute quantification is not needed, and quantification relative to one or more reference genes is performed. In this case, selection of the reference genes and PCR efficiency are critical. The precision of quantitative real-time PCR depends on the initial number of template copies in the reaction. When the initial target concentration is low, imprecision is high. Part of the variance comes from stochastic limitations as defined by the Poisson distribution described earlier. In addition, PCR efficiency is more variable at low copy numbers. Technical guidelines for performing quantitative PCR experiments have been published.[11]

Melting Analysis

Not only can amplification, detection, and quantification be performed by homogeneous hybridization, but detailed genotyping information can also be obtained. Genotyping is best performed in the same tube by monitoring the melting of hybridized duplexes during controlled heating, producing a melting curve signature for the duplex. Such a signature monitors melting over of a range of temperatures in contrast to the single-temperature analysis of conventional hybridization techniques, such as dot blots or microarrays. The advantages of complete melting curves also apply when different homogeneous techniques are compared. For example, methods that rely on hydrolysis for signal generation and/or those that acquire data only at one temperature are more susceptible to genotyping errors.[103] Real-time amplification and melting analysis make up a powerful combination of techniques that require only temperature control and sampling of fluorescence. Many other genotyping techniques require complex separation and/or detection equipment after PCR. Real-time PCR with melting curve analysis allows detection, quantification, and genotyping in less than 30 minutes (see Figure 17-29) without ancillary processing or additional equipment. A book series has been published on methods and applications of rapid-cycle, real-time PCR.[20,65,85,121]

When fluorescence is monitored continuously within each cycle of PCR, the hybridization characteristics of PCR products and probes can be observed.[128] Continuous spirals of fluorescence versus temperature are produced (see Figure

17-31, *bottom panels*).[127] With dyes, the melting characteristics of the amplified DNA identify the product.[87] No hybridization information is revealed with hydrolysis probes, whereas the melting of hybridization probes is readily apparent. Probe melting occurs at a characteristic temperature that can be exploited to confirm target identity and to analyze sequence alterations under the probe.

For routine testing in the clinical laboratory, a single melting curve is usually performed at the end of PCR instead of monitoring hybridization throughout the entire PCR process (see Figure 17-29). Immediately after the last PCR cycle, samples are momentarily denatured (94 °C), cooled to about 10 °C below the lowest temperature of interest, and heated at a rate of 0.1 to 0.3 °C/s, while fluorescence is continuously monitored. When hybridization probes are used, rapid cooling maximizes formation of probe-target duplexes while minimizing formation of the duplex PCR product. Primer asymmetry and use of 5′-exonuclease–deficient polymerases often augment the probe signal.

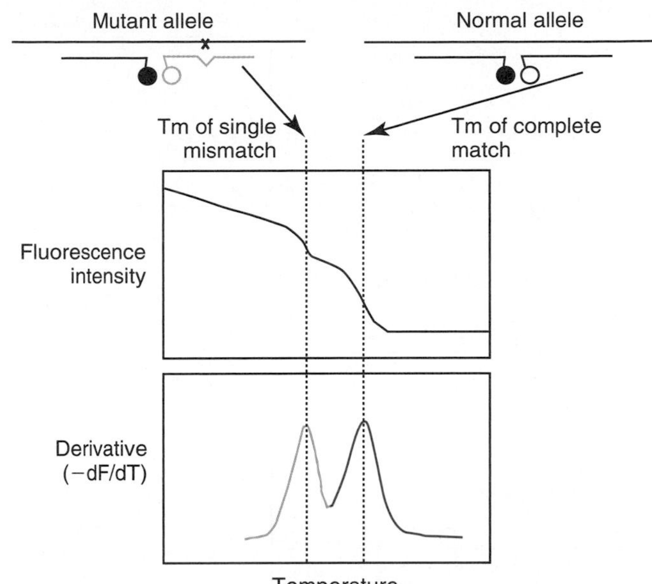

Figure 17-35 Melting curve single-nucleotide polymorphism (SNP) genotyping. A heterozygous specimen with an SNP under the probe is amplified and melted. Two temperature transitions are visible: one from the mutant allele that is mismatched with the probe and melts at a lower temperature, and one from the normal allele that is completely matched with the probe and melts at a higher temperature. The derivative plot shows the melting temperatures of both the mutant-probe and the normal-probe duplexes as peaks. *(Modified with permission of the publisher from Bernard PS, Pritham GH, Wittwer CT. Color multiplexing hybridization probes using the apolipoprotein E locus as a model system for genotyping. Anal Biochem 1999;273:221-228. © 1999 Academic Press.)*

SNP Genotyping

A hybridization probe pair placed over a heterozygous polymorphism is shown in Figure 17-35. The reporter probe is complementary to the normal allele. As the temperature is increased, the mismatched mutant hybrid melts first, giving the first transition, followed by the matched normal hybrid. The melting temperatures of both hybrids are easily seen in the derivative plots.[81] A well-optimized probe design will provide a Tm difference of 4 to 10 °C for a single base mismatch under the probe.

SNP genotyping by melting curve analysis can be achieved with a variety of probe and dye methods. Figure 17-36, *A* shows the design of the traditional hybridization probe pair[5] and the results of homozygous wild-type, mutant, and heterozygous samples that are well discriminated from each other. Virtually the same result can be achieved by using a single hybridization probe in which the fluorescent signal is quenched on the free probe, but is dequenched as it forms a hybrid with the target (Fig. 17-36, *B*).[16] The third row shows genotyping with an *unlabeled probe* and a saturating DNA binding dye.[132] Both probe and amplicon melting transitions are present. The fourth row shows similar results using a *snapback primer*,[133] an unlabeled probe attached as a 5′-tail to one of the primers. The advantage of these last two methods is that they do not require fluorescently labeled probes. Finally, SNP genotyping is possible by amplicon melting alone if a saturating DNA binding dye is used (Fig. 17-36, *E*).[58] However, the temperature difference between genotypes is small, and high-resolution melting is required for accurate genotyping.

High-Resolution Melting Analysis

In earlier sections of this chapter, heteroduplex detection (by electrophoresis or by HPLC) was discussed as a means to scan stretches of DNA in which the presence of variation is suspected. Melting analysis with saturating dyes can detect heteroduplexes with better sensitivity than these methods and does not require any processing or separation.[84] Although conventional fluorescent melting analysis could distinguish PCR products that differed by only about 1 to 2 °C,[87] high-resolution melting instruments now provide precision and resolution improvement of at least 10-fold[123] and require only a few minutes.[38] Typically, melting data are normalized between 0% and 100% fluorescence, and different homozygotes are distinguished by Tm. Heterozygotes are best detected when comparing the melting curve shapes by shifting the curves along the temperature axis until they overlap. An example of heteroduplex detection and SNP genotyping by melting curve analysis is shown in Figure 17-37. Major applications of high-resolution melting include genotyping, mutation scanning, and sequence matching. High-resolution melting analysis has been reviewed.[24,25,113]

Comparison of Closed-Tube SNP Genotyping Methods

Many methods are available for SNP genotyping, and the method of choice depends on several factors, including turnaround time, batch size, and throughput requirements. The necessities of high-volume genomic research are different

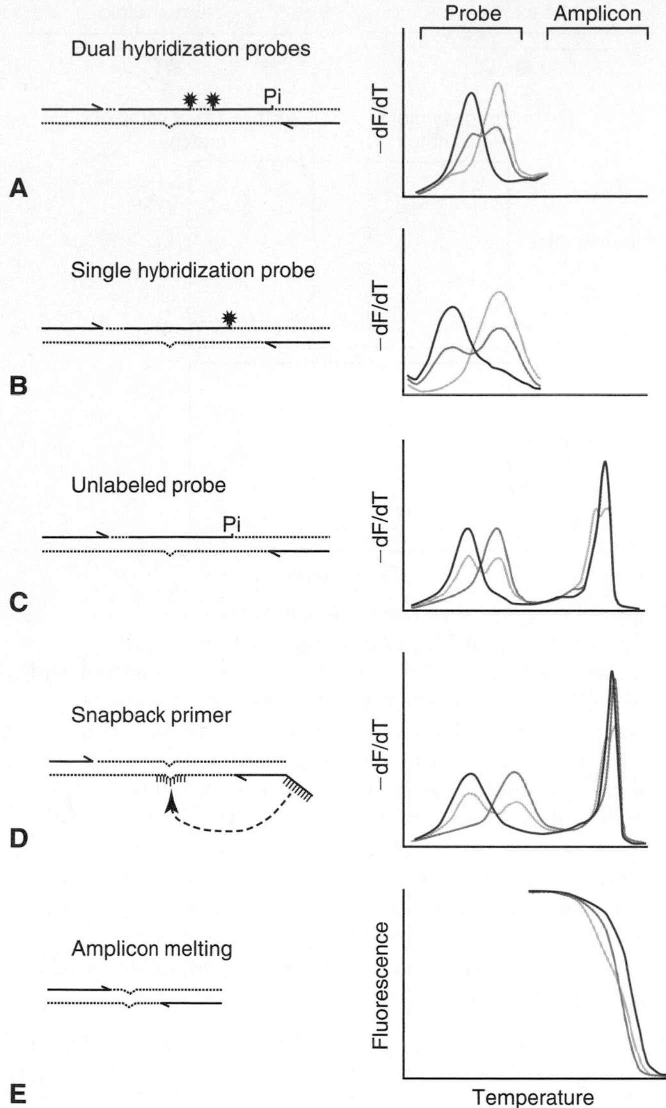

Figure 17-36 Five designs for single-nucleotide polymorphism (SNP) genotyping and corresponding melting curve results. The traditional dual hybridization probe design (A) uses a pair of probes: one labeled with an acceptor fluorophore and the other with a donor fluorophore. The single hybridization probe design (B) lacks the second probe. The unlabeled probe design (C) does not require a covalently attached fluorescent label, using instead a saturating DNA binding dye in solution. Snapback primers (D) are similar to unlabeled probes, with the probe attached to one primer as a 5′-tail. Finally, amplicon melting (E) uses only two regular polymerase chain reaction (PCR) primers, relying on high-resolution melting analysis to distinguish the small differences between genotypes. The two homozygotes are differentiated by melting temperature (Tm), and the heterozygote differs in shape from the contribution of heteroduplexes. Pi indicates a 3′-phosphate or other blocker that prevents polymerase extension.

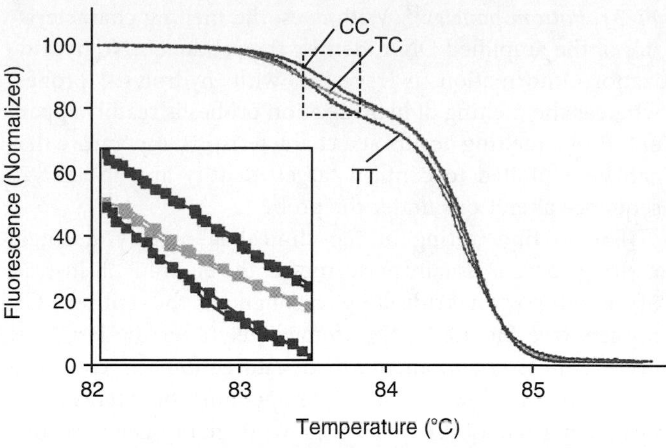

Figure 17-37 A single base change in a 544 bp fragment detected by melting analysis. Shown are high-resolution melting curves of polymerase chain reaction (PCR) amplicons from the gene *HTR2A* carrying a single-nucleotide polymorphism (SNP). Results are shown for six individuals, two different individuals for each of the three genotypes: wild-type homozygote (TT), mutant homozygote (CC), and heterozygote (TC). Two melting domains are present because of differing GC content. The SNP was present in the lower melting domain. The inset magnifies a portion of the data, showing that all three genotypes can be discriminated. *(Modified by permission of the publisher from Wittwer CT, Reed GH, Gundry CN, et al. High-resolution genotyping by amplicon melting analysis using LC Green. Clin Chem 2003;49:853-60. © AACC.)*

from those of a clinical reference laboratory, a medical clinic, or the STAT laboratories of the future.

Methods for homogeneous SNP analysis in a closed system differ greatly in their level of complexity (Table 17-6). The number of oligonucleotides required varies from 2 to 5. The simpler techniques do not require probes at all, although some of the more complex methods require up to three labels or modifications on each probe. All of these methods use fluorescence and solution hybridization. Some of the methods that use melting analysis will detect more than two alleles if present; those based on allele-specific amplification or end point analysis are limited to two.

The five simplest homogeneous SNP typing methods do not use fluorescently labeled probes. Amplicon melting requires only two primers and a heteroduplex-detecting DNA dye (see Figure 17-36, *E*).[58] The snapback primer system also requires only two primers—one with a self-probing 5′-tail (see Figure 17-36, *D*).[133] Unlabeled probe genotyping requires two primers and one 3′-blocked probe (see Figure 17-36, *C*).[132] Allele-specific PCR requires three primers and is based on a preference by the polymerase to extend only a perfectly matched primer. Genotyping can be obtained in two wells by monitoring fluorescence at each cycle,[29] or in one well by incorporating GC-clamp(s) so that alleles can be differentiated at the end of PCR by their melting temperatures.[116] Intermediate in complexity are hybridization probe

TABLE 17-6 Comparison of Homogeneous (Closed-Tube) SNP Genotyping Methods (In Order of Increasing Complexity)

Method	Oligonucleotides	Modifications	Comments
Amplicon melting[58]	2	0	Simplest and least expensive
Snapback primers[133]	2	1	Self-complementary 5′-tail
Allele-specific PCR (real-time)[29]	3	0	Requires one well for each allele
Unlabeled probes[132]	3	1	3′-phosphate on probe
Allele-specific PCR (melting)[116]	3	1-2	GC clamps
Single hybridization probe[16]	3	1-2	3′-phosphate if 5′-fluorophore
Dual hybridization probes[5]	4	2-3	3′-phosphate if 5′-fluorophore
Hydrolysis probes[55]	4	4	
Dual-labeled hairpin probes[105]	4	4	
Self-probing amplicon[119]	3-4	6	
Minor groove binder hydrolysis probe[18]	4	6	
Serial invasive signal amplification[35]	5	4	

GC, Short 5′-oligonucleotide tail of G and C bases used to modify allele Tm; *PCR*, polymerase chain reaction; *SNP*, single-nucleotide polymorphism.

melting assays. Designs with single[16] or dual hybridization[5] probes are shown in Figure 17-36, *A, B*.

The more complex closed-tube methods for SNP genotyping are end point assays. Allele-specific hydrolysis[55] and hairpin probes[105] are commonly used. Self-probing amplicons[119] and minor groove binder hydrolysis probes[18] both require three modifications on two probes for SNP typing. Finally, serial invasive signal amplification is a method of homogeneous genotyping that does not require PCR.[35]

CONCLUSION

Molecular diagnostics remains a developing field in laboratory medicine. Current progress in nucleic acid techniques is extraordinary, driven by the promise of great return. Can drug therapy be tailored to each individual by appropriate molecular tests? Can diagnostic biochips parallel the microelectronics revolution, continuing to provide more information at less expense? Will complete genome sequencing for individual predisposition testing become a reality? Although we are still years away from immediate, comprehensive testing, the time for personalized diagnostics will come. In the end, the rate-limiting factors seldom involve technology, but rather our ability to correlate test results with disease. Nevertheless, simple, powerful, and cost-effective techniques will aid this quest.

Molecular analysis often requires multiple steps, including sample preparation, amplification, and analysis. As a result, successful automation is critical for routine adoption in the clinical laboratory. However, to corruptly paraphrase Henry David Thoreau in Civil Disobedience: "I heartily adhere to the motto: The best automation is not needing to automate." The simplest techniques are often the best. As with immunoassays, methods that require separation and washing steps are being replaced by rapid, homogeneous methods. How to maintain this simplicity while handling the increased data density provided by current technology is a central challenge for molecular diagnostics today.

REFERENCES

1. Aomori T, Yamamoto K, Oguchi-Katayama A, Kawai Y, Ishidao T, Mitani Y, et al. Rapid single-nucleotide polymorphism detection of cytochrome P450 (CYP2C9) and vitamin K epoxide reductase (VKORC1) genes for the warfarin dose adjustment by the SMart-amplification process version 2. Clin Chem 2009;55:804-12.
2. Baltimore D. Viral RNA-dependent DNA polymerase. Biotechnology 1992;24:3-5.
3. Baner J, Nilsson M, Mendel-Hartvig M, Landegren U. Signal amplification of padlock probes by rolling circle replication. Nucleic Acids Res 1998;26:5073-8.
4. Bentley DR, Balasubramanian S, Swerdlow HP, Smith GP, Milton J, Brown CG, et al. Accurate whole human genome sequencing using reversible terminator chemistry. Nature 2008;456:53-9.
5. Bernard PS, Ajioka RS, Kushner JP, Wittwer CT. Homogeneous multiplex genotyping of hemochromatosis mutations with fluorescent hybridization probes. Am J Pathol 1998;153:1055-61.
6. Blackburn GM, Gait MJ, eds. Nucleic acids in chemistry and biology. New York: IRL Press at Oxford University Press, 1990.
7. Bolivar F, Rodriguez RL, Greene PJ, Betlach MC, Heynker HL, Boyer HW, et al. Construction and characterization of new cloning vehicles. II. A multipurpose cloning system. Biotechnology 1992;24:153-71.
8. Borer P. Handbook of biochemistry and molecular biology. In: Fasman GD, ed. Boca Raton, Fla: CRC Press, 1975:589.
9. Braun A, Little DP, Koster H. Detecting CFTR gene mutations by using primer oligo base extension and mass spectrometry. Clin Chem 1997;43:1151-8.
10. Browne KA. Metal ion-catalyzed nucleic acid alkylation and fragmentation. J Am Chem Soc 2002;124:7950-62.
11. Bustin SA, Benes V, Garson JA, Hellemans J, Huggett J, Kubista M, et al. The MIQE guidelines: minimum information for publication of quantitative real-time PCR experiments. Clin Chem 2009;55:611-22.
12. Cariello NF, Scott JK, Kat AG, Thilly WG, Keohavong P. Resolution of a missense mutant in human genomic DNA by denaturing gradient gel electrophoresis and direct sequencing using in vitro DNA amplification: HPRT Munich. Am J Hum Genet 1988;42:726-34.
13. Chen X, Livak KJ, Kwok PY. A homogeneous, ligase-mediated DNA diagnostic test. Genome Res 1998;8:549-56.
14. Collins ML, Irvine B, Tyner D, Fine E, Zayati C, Chang C, et al. A branched DNA signal amplification assay for quantification of nucleic acid targets below 100 molecules/ml. Nucleic Acids Res 1997;25:2979-84.
15. Compton J. Nucleic acid sequence-based amplification. Nature 1991;350:91-2.

16. Crockett AO, Wittwer CT. Fluorescein-labeled oligonucleotides for real-time PCR: using the inherent quenching of deoxyguanosine nucleotides. Anal Biochem 2001;290:89-97.
17. Davicioni E, Wai DH, Anderson MJ. Diagnostic and prognostic sarcoma signatures. Mol Diagn Ther 2008;12:359-74.
18. de Kok JB, Wiegerinck ET, Giesendorf BA, Swinkels DW. Rapid genotyping of single nucleotide polymorphisms using novel minor groove binding DNA oligonucleotides (MGB probes). Hum Mutat 2002;19:554-9.
19. Dean FB, Hosono S, Fang L, Wu X, Faruqi AF, Bray-Ward P, et al. Comprehensive human genome amplification using multiple displacement amplification. Proc Natl Acad Sci U S A 2002;99:5261-6.
20. Dietmaier C, Wittwer CT, Sivasubrananian N. Rapid cycle real-time PCR methods and applications: genetics and oncology. Berlin: Springer, 2002.
21. Drmanac RT, Callow M, Drmanac S. High throughput genome sequencing on DNA arrays. U.S. Patent Application 20090155781, Complete Genomics Inc, June 18, 2009.
22. Dujols VE, Kusukawa N, McKinney JT, Dobrowolski SF, Wittwer CT. High-resolution melting analysis for scanning and genotyping. In: Dorak MT, ed. Real-time PCR. New York: Garland Science, 2006:157-71.
23. Eid J, Fehr A, Gray J, Luong K, Lyle J, Otto G, et al. Real-time DNA sequencing from single polymerase molecules. Science 2009;323: 133-8.
24. Erali M, Voelkerding KV, Wittwer CT. High resolution melting applications for clinical laboratory medicine. Exp Mol Pathol 2008;85:50-8.
25. Farrar JS, Reed GH, Wittwer CT. High resolution melting curve analysis for molecular diagnostics. In: Patrinos GP, Ansorge WJ, eds. Molecular diagnostics, 2nd edition. London: Elsevier, 2010, 229-45.
26. Franca LT, Carrilho E, Kist TB. A review of DNA sequencing techniques. Q Rev Biophys 2002;35:169-200.
27. Gao Q, Yeung ES. High-throughput detection of unknown mutations by using multiplexed capillary electrophoresis with poly(vinylpyrrolidone) solution. Anal Chem 2000;72:2499-506.
28. Geiss GK, Bumgarner RE, Birditt B, Dahl T, Dowidar N, Dunaway DL, et al. Direct multiplexed measurement of gene expression with color-coded probe pairs. Nat Biotechnol 2008;26:317-25.
29. Germer S, Higuchi R. Single-tube genotyping without oligonucleotide probes. Genome Res 1999;9:72-8.
30. Giachetti C, Linnen JM, Kolk DP, Dockter J, Gillotte-Taylor K, Park M, et al. Highly sensitive multiplex assay for detection of human immunodeficiency virus type 1 and hepatitis C virus RNA. J Clin Microbiol 2002;40:2408-19.
31. Grant SF, Hakonarson H. Microarray technology and applications in the arena of genome-wide association. Clin Chem 2008;54:1116-24.
32. Guatelli JC, Whitfield KM, Kwoh DY, Barringer KJ, Richman DD, Gingeras TR. Isothermal, in vitro amplification of nucleic acids by a multienzyme reaction modeled after retroviral replication. Proc Natl Acad Sci U S A 1990;87:1874-8.
33. Gundry CN, Vandersteen JG, Reed GH, Pryor RJ, Chen J, Wittwer CT. Amplicon melting analysis with labeled primers: a closed-tube method for differentiating homozygotes and heterozygotes. Clin Chem 2003;49:396-406.
34. Haferlach T, Bacher U, Kohlmann A, Haferlach C. Discussion of the applicability of microarrays: profiling of leukemias. Methods Mol Biol 2009;509:15-33.
35. Hall JG, Eis PS, Law SM, Reynaldo LP, Prudent JR, Marshall DJ, et al. Sensitive detection of DNA polymorphisms by the serial invasive signal amplification reaction. Proc Natl Acad Sci U S A 2000;97:8272-7.
36. Hayatsu H, Wataya Y, Kai K, Iida S. Reaction of sodium bisulfite with uracil, cytosine, and their derivatives. Biochemistry 1970;9:2858-65.
37. Heller MJ. DNA microarray technology: devices, systems, and applications. Annu Rev Biomed Eng 2002;4:129-53.
38. Herrmann MG, Durtschi JD, Bromley LK, Wittwer CT, Voelkerding KV. Amplicon DNA melting analysis for mutation scanning and genotyping: cross-platform comparison of instruments and dyes. Clin Chem 2006;52:494-503.
39. Highsmith WE, Jr, Jin Q, Nataraj AJ, O'Connor JM, Burland VD, Baubonis WR, et al. Use of a DNA toolbox for the characterization of mutation scanning methods. I: construction of the toolbox and evaluation of heteroduplex analysis. Electrophoresis 1999;20:1186-94.
40. Highsmith WE, Jr, Nataraj AJ, Jin Q, O'Connor JM, El-Nabi SH, Kusukawa N, Garner MM. Use of DNA toolbox for the characterization of mutation scanning methods. II. Evaluation of single-strand conformation polymorphism analysis. Electrophoresis 1999;20:1195-203.
41. Higuchi R, Fockler C, Dollinger G, Watson R. Kinetic PCR analysis: real-time monitoring of DNA amplification reactions. Biotechnology (N Y) 1993;11:1026-30.
42. Higuchi R, Dollinger G, Walsh PS, Griffith R. Simultaneous amplification and detection of specific DNA sequences. Biotechnology (N Y) 1992;10:413-17.
43. Hill CS. Molecular diagnostic testing for infectious diseases using TMA technology. Expert Rev Mol Diagn 2001;1:445-55.
44. Holloway AJ, van Laar RK, Tothill RW, Bowtell DD. Options available—from start to finish—for obtaining data from DNA microarrays II. Nat Genet 2002;32(Suppl):481-9.
45. Hopfenbeck JA, Holden JA, Wittwer CT, Kjeldsberg CR. Digoxigenin-labeled probes amplified from genomic DNA detect T-cell gene rearrangements. Am J Clin Pathol 1992;97:638-44.
46. Jonas V, Alden MJ, Curry JI, Kamisango K, Knott CA, Lankford R, et al. Detection and identification of *Mycobacterium tuberculosis* directly from sputum sediments by amplification of rRNA. J Clin Microbiol 1993;31:2410-6.
47. Kellar KL, Iannone MA. Multiplexed microsphere-based flow cytometric assays. Exp Hematol 2002;30:1227-37.
48. Kornberg A, Baker T. DNA replication, 2nd edition, New York: WH Freeman and Company, 1992:101-273, 307-22.
49. Kristensen LS, Hansen LL. PCR-based methods for detecting single-locus DNA methylation biomarkers in cancer diagnostics, prognostics, and response to treatment. Clin Chem 2009;55:1471-83.
50. Kutyavin IV, Afonina IA, Mills A, Gorn VV, Lukhtanov EA, Belousov ES, et al. 3′-Minor groove binder-DNA probes increase sequence specificity at PCR extension temperatures. Nucleic Acids Res 2000;28:655-61.
51. Kwok PY. SNP genotyping with fluorescence polarization detection. Hum Mutat 2002;19:315-23.
52. Kwok S, Higuchi R. Avoiding false positives with PCR. Nature 1989;339:237-8.
53. Langer PR, Waldrop AA, Ward DC. Enzymatic synthesis of biotin-labeled polynucleotides: novel nucleic acid affinity probes. Proc Natl Acad Sci U S A 1981;78:6633-7.
54. Lay MJ, Wittwer CT. Real-time fluorescence genotyping of factor V Leiden during rapid-cycle PCR. Clin Chem 1997;43:2262-7.
55. Lee LG, Connell CR, Bloch W. Allelic discrimination by nick-translation PCR with fluorogenic probes. Nucleic Acids Res 1993;21:3761-6.
56. Li Q, Liu Z, Monroe H, Culiat CT. Integrated platform for detection of DNA sequence variants using capillary array electrophoresis. Electrophoresis 2002;23:1499-511.
57. Li Q, Luan G, Guo Q, Liang J. A new class of homogeneous nucleic acid probes based on specific displacement hybridization. Nucleic Acids Res 2002;30:E5.
58. Liew M, Pryor R, Palais R, Meadows C, Erali M, Lyon E, Wittwer C. Genotyping of single-nucleotide polymorphisms by high-resolution melting of small amplicons. Clin Chem 2004;50:1156-64.
59. Livak KJ, Flood SJ, Marmaro J, Giusti W, Deetz K. Oligonucleotides with fluorescent dyes at opposite ends provide a quenched probe system useful for detecting PCR product and nucleic acid hybridization. PCR Methods Appl 1995;4:357-62.
60. Lizardi PM, Huang X, Zhu Z, Bray-Ward P, Thomas DC, Ward DC. Mutation detection and single-molecule counting using isothermal rolling-circle amplification. Nat Genet 1998;19:225-32.

61. Lyon E. Discovering rare variants by use of melting temperature shifts seen in melting curve analysis. Clin Chem 2005;51:1331-2.
62. Margulies M, Egholm M, Altman WE, Attiya S, Bader JS, Bemben LA, et al. Genome sequencing in microfabricated high-density picolitre reactors. Nature 2005;437:376-80.
63. Masuda N, Ohnishi T, Kawamoto S, Monden M, Okubo K. Analysis of chemical modification of RNA from formalin-fixed samples and optimization of molecular biology applications for such samples. Nucleic Acids Res 1999;27:4436-43.
64. Maule J. Pulsed-field gel electrophoresis. Mol Biotechnol 1998;9:107-26.
65. Meuer S, Wittwer CT, Nakaguawara K. Rapid cycle real-time PCR: methods and applications. Berlin: Springer, 2001.
66. Michalatos-Beloin S, Tishkoff SA, Bentley KL, Kidd KK, Ruano G. Molecular haplotyping of genetic markers 10 kb apart by allele-specific long-range PCR. Nucleic Acids Res 1996;24:4841-3.
67. Mishra NC, ed. Nucleases: molecular biology and applications. Hoboken: Wiley, 2002:344.
68. Mitra RD, Butty VL, Shendure J, Williams BR, Housman DE, Church GM. Digital genotyping and haplotyping with polymerase colonies. Proc Natl Acad Sci U S A 2003;100:5926-31.
69. Moreira BG, You Y, Behlke MA, Owczarzy R. Effects of fluorescent dyes, quenchers, and dangling ends on DNA duplex stability. Biochem Biophys Res Commun 2005;327:473-84.
70. Morrison TB, Weis JJ, Wittwer CT. Quantification of low-copy transcripts by continuous SYBR Green I monitoring during amplification. Biotechniques 1998;24:954-8, 960, 962.
71. Nagamine CM, Chan K, Lau YF. A PCR artifact: generation of heteroduplexes. Am J Hum Genet 1989;45:337-9.
72. Nazarenko I, Pires R, Lowe B, Obaidy M, Rashtchian A. Effect of primary and secondary structure of oligodeoxyribonucleotides on the fluorescent properties of conjugated dyes. Nucleic Acids Res 2002;30:2089-195.
73. Nazarenko IA, Bhatnagar SK, Hohman RJ. A closed tube format for amplification and detection of DNA based on energy transfer. Nucleic Acids Res 1997;25:2516-21.
74. Nielsen PE. PNA technology. Mol Biotechnol 2004;26:233-48.
75. Notomi T, Okayama H, Masubuchi H, Yonekawa T, Watanabe K, Amino N, Hase T. Loop-mediated isothermal amplification of DNA. Nucleic Acids Res 2000;28:E63.
76. Orita M, Iwahana H, Kanazawa H, Hayashi K, Sekiya T. Detection of polymorphisms of human DNA by gel electrophoresis as single-strand conformation polymorphisms. Proc Natl Acad Sci U S A 1989;86: 2766-70.
77. Owczarzy R, Moreira BG, You Y, Behlke MA, Walder JA. Predicting stability of DNA duplexes in solutions containing magnesium and monovalent cations. Biochemistry 2008;47:5336-53.
78. Park SJ, Taton TA, Mirkin CA. Array-based electrical detection of DNA with nanoparticle probes. Science 2002;295:1503-6.
79. Perkins TT, Quake SR, Smith DE, Chu S. Relaxation of a single DNA molecule observed by optical microscopy. Science 1994;264:822-6.
80. Phillips J, Eberwine JH. Antisense RNA amplification: a linear amplification method for analyzing the mRNA population from single living cells. Methods 1996;10:283-8.
81. Press W, Teukolsky S, Vetterling W, Flannery B. Salvitsky-Golay smoothing filters. In: Numerical recipes in C: the art of scientific computing. New York: Cambridge University Press, 1992:650-5.
82. Pusch W, Wurmbach JH, Thiele H, Kostrzewa M. MALDI-TOF mass spectrometry-based SNP genotyping. Pharmacogenomics 2002;3:537-48.
83. Rauch T, Pfeifer GP. Methylated-CpG island recovery assay: a new technique for the rapid detection of methylated-CpG islands in cancer. Lab Invest 2005;85:1172-80.
84. Reed GH, Wittwer CT. Sensitivity and specificity of single-nucleotide polymorphism scanning by high-resolution melting analysis. Clin Chem 2004;50:1748-54.
85. Reischl U, Wittwer CT, Cockerill F. Rapid cycle real-time PCR: methods and applications: microbiology and food analysis. Berlin: Springer, 2002.
86. Riesner D, Steger G, Zimmat R, Owens RA, Wagenhofer M, Hillen W, et al. Temperature-gradient gel electrophoresis of nucleic acids: analysis of conformational transitions, sequence variations, and protein-nucleic acid interactions. Electrophoresis 1989;10:377-89.
87. Ririe KM, Rasmussen RP, Wittwer CT. Product differentiation by analysis of DNA melting curves during the polymerase chain reaction. Anal Biochem 1997;245:154-60.
88. Roeder K, Luca D. Searching for disease susceptibility variants in structured populations. Genomics 2009;93:1-4.
89. Ronaghi M, Uhlen M, Nyren P. A sequencing method based on real-time pyrophosphate. Science 1998;281:363-5.
90. Saiki RK, Gelfand DH, Stoffel S, Scharf SJ, Higuchi R, Horn GT, et al. Primer-directed enzymatic amplification of DNA with a thermostable DNA polymerase. Science 1988;239:487-91.
91. Sanger F, Nicklen S, Coulson AR. DNA sequencing with chain-terminating inhibitors. Proc Natl Acad Sci U S A 1977;74:5463-7.
92. SantaLucia J Jr, Hicks D. The thermodynamics of DNA structural motifs. Annu Rev Biophys Biomol Struct 2004;33:415-40.
93. SantaLucia J Jr. A unified view of polymer, dumbbell, and oligonucleotide DNA nearest-neighbor thermodynamics. Proc Natl Acad Sci U S A 1998;95:1460-5.
94. Schena M, Shalon D, Davis RW, Brown PO. Quantitative monitoring of gene expression patterns with a complementary DNA microarray. Science 1995;270:467-70.
95. Seuss D. The cat in the hat comes back! New York: Random House, 1958.
96. Shendure J, Porreca GJ, Reppas NB, Lin X, McCutcheon JP, Rosenbaum AM, et al. Accurate multiplex polony sequencing of an evolved bacterial genome. Science 2005;309:1728-32.
97. Shiraishi M, Hayatsu H. High-speed conversion of cytosine to uracil in bisulfite genomic sequencing analysis of DNA methylation. DNA Res 2004;11:409-15.
98. Smith DR, Quinlan AR, Peckham HE, Makowsky K, Tao W, Woolf B, et al. Rapid whole-genome mutational profiling using next-generation sequencing technologies. Genome Res 2008;18:1638-42.
99. Smith HO. Nucleotide sequence specificity of restriction endonucleases. Science 1979;205:455-62.
100. Southern EM. Detection of specific sequences among DNA fragments separated by gel electrophoresis. J Mol Biol 1975;98:503-17.
101. Svanvik N, Stahlberg A, Sehlstedt U, Sjoback R, Kubista M. Detection of PCR products in real time using light-up probes. Anal Biochem 2000;287:179-82.
102. Tawfik DS, Griffiths AD. Man-made cell-like compartments for molecular evolution. Nat Biotechnol 1998;16:652-6.
103. Teupser D, Rupprecht W, Lohse P, Thiery J. Fluorescence-based detection of the CETP TaqIB polymorphism: false positives with the TaqMan-based exonuclease assay attributable to a previously unknown gene variant. Clin Chem 2001;47:852-7.
104. Todd AV, Fuery CJ, Impey HL, Applegate TL, Haughton MA. DzyNA-PCR: use of DNAzymes to detect and quantify nucleic acid sequences in a real-time fluorescent format. Clin Chem 2000;46:625-30.
105. Tyagi S, Bratu DP, Kramer FR. Multicolor molecular beacons for allele discrimination. Nat Biotechnol 1998;16:49-53.
106. Tyagi S, Kramer FR. Molecular beacons: probes that fluoresce upon hybridization. Nat Biotechnol 1996;14:303-8.
107. Umek RM, Lin SW, Vielmetter J, Terbrueggen RH, Irvine B, Yu CJ, et al. Electronic detection of nucleic acids: a versatile platform for molecular diagnostics. J Mol Diagn 2001;3:74-84.
108. Urdea MS, Horn T, Fultz TJ, Anderson M, Running JA, Hamren S, et al. Branched DNA amplification multimers for the sensitive, direct detection of human hepatitis viruses. Nucleic Acids Symp Ser 1991: 197-200.
109. van't Veer LJ, Dai H, van de Vijver MJ, He YD, Hart AA, Mao M, et al. Gene expression profiling predicts clinical outcome of breast cancer. Nature 2002;415:530-6.
110. van der Kwast TH, Bapat B. Predicting favourable prognosis of urothelial carcinoma: gene expression and genome profiling. Curr Opin Urol 2009;19:516-21.

111. Voelkerding KV, Dames SA, Durtschi JD. Next-generation sequencing: from basic research to diagnostics. Clin Chem 2009;55:641-58.
112. von Ahsen N, Wittwer CT, Schutz E. Oligonucleotide melting temperatures under PCR conditions: nearest-neighbor corrections for Mg(2+), deoxynucleotide triphosphate, and dimethyl sulfoxide concentrations with comparison to alternative empirical formulas. Clin Chem 2001;47:1956-61.
113. Vossen RH, Aten E, Roos A, den Dunnen JT. High-resolution melting analysis (HRMA): more than just sequence variant screening. Hum Mutat 2009;30:860-6.
114. Walker GT, Linn CP, Nadeau JG. DNA detection by strand displacement amplification and fluorescence polarization with signal enhancement using a DNA binding protein. Nucleic Acids Res 1996;24:348-53.
115. WalkerPeach CR, Winkler M, DuBois DB, Pasloske BL. Ribonuclease-resistant RNA controls (armored RNA) for reverse transcription PCR, branched DNA, and genotyping assays for hepatitis C virus. Clin Chem 1999;45:2079-85.
116. Wang J, Chuang K, Ahluwalia M, Patel S, Umblas N, Mirel D, et al. High-throughput SNP genotyping by single-tube PCR with Tm-shift primers. Biotechniques 2005;39:885-93.
117. Weber M, Davies JJ, Wittig D, Oakeley EJ, Haase M, Lam WL, Schubeler D. Chromosome-wide and promoter-specific analyses identify sites of differential DNA methylation in normal and transformed human cells. Nat Genet 2005;37:853-62.
118. Wetmur JG. DNA probes: applications of the principles of nucleic acid hybridization. Crit Rev Biochem Mol Biol 1991;26:227-59.
119. Whitcombe D, Theaker J, Guy SP, Brown T, Little S. Detection of PCR products using self-probing amplicons and fluorescence. Nat Biotechnol 1999;17:804-7.
120. Wiedmann M, Wilson WJ, Czajka J, Luo J, Barany F, Batt CA. Ligase chain reaction (LCR): overview and applications. PCR Methods Appl 1994;3:S51-64.
121. Wittwer C, Hahn M, Kaul K. Rapid cycle real-time PCR: methods and applications: quantification. Berlin: Springer, 2004.
122. Wittwer C, Kusukawa N. Real-time PCR. In: Persing DH, Tenover FC, Relman DA, White TJ, Tang YW, Versalovic J, Unger ER, eds. Diagnostic molecular microbiology: principles and applications. Washington: ASM Press, 2004:71-84.
123. Wittwer CT, Reed GH, Gundry CN, Vandersteen JG, Pryor RJ. High-resolution genotyping by amplicon melting analysis using LC Green. Clin Chem 2003;49:853-60.
124. Wittwer CT, Ririe KM, Andrew RV, David DA, Gundry RA, Balis UJ. The LightCycler: a microvolume multisample fluorimeter with rapid temperature control. Biotechniques 1997;22:176-81.
125. Wittwer CT, Garling DJ. Rapid cycle DNA amplification: time and temperature optimization. Biotechniques 1991;10:76-83.
126. Wittwer CT, Herrmann MG, Gundry CN, Elenitoba-Johnson KS. Real-time multiplex PCR assays. Methods 2001;25:430-42.
127. Wittwer CT, Herrmann MG, Moss AA, Rasmussen RP. Continuous fluorescence monitoring of rapid cycle DNA amplification. Biotechniques 1997;22:130-1, 4-8.
128. Wittwer CT, Rasmussen RP, Ririe KM. Rapid PCR and melting analysis. In: Bustin SA, ed. The PCR revolution: impact on basic and clinical science. New York: Cambridge University Press, 2010, 48-69.
129. Wittwer CT, Herrmann MG. Rapid thermal cycling and PCR kinetics. In: Innis M, Gelfand D, Sninsky J, eds. PCR methods manual. San Diego: Academic Press, 1999:211-29.
130. Xiao W, Oefner PJ. Denaturing high-performance liquid chromatography: a review. Hum Mutat 2001;17:439-74.
131. Zhang DY, Zhang W, Li X, Konomi Y. Detection of rare DNA targets by isothermal ramification amplification. Gene 2001;274:209-16.
132. Zhou L, Myers AN, Vandersteen JG, Wang L, Wittwer CT. Closed-tube genotyping with unlabeled oligonucleotide probes and a saturating DNA dye. Clin Chem 2004;50:1328-35.
133. Zhou L, Errigo RJ, Lu H, Poritz MA, Seipp MT, Wittwer CT. Snapback primer genotyping with saturating DNA dye and melting analysis. Clin Chem 2008;54:1648-56.
134. Zhou MY, Gomez-Sanchez CE. Universal TA cloning. Curr Issues Mol Biol 2000;2:1-7.

CHAPTER 18

Microfabrication and Microfluidics and Their Application to Clinical Diagnostics

Lindsay A. L. Bazydlo, Ph.D., and James P. Landers, Ph.D.

BACKGROUND

The first miniaturized analytical device with some degree of functionality was reported in 1979, when the separation of a simple mixture of low molecular weight compounds was achieved in only a few seconds in a microdevice fabricated in silicon.[156] The significance of this development can be appreciated only by a relativistic view of state of the art separation techniques common to the laboratories of that time. The 1970s saw most chemical separations carried out using open-column, paper, and thin-layer chromatographic processes, while gas chromatography (GC), having experienced several decades of development, was only beginning to mature into a bona fide technology for small molecule analysis. Pressure liquid chromatography began to evolve into a method that would bring faster analysis times with higher resolution, and the late 1970s saw new chemistries amenable to reverse-phase liquid chromatographic separations for improved resolution of similar compounds. Electrophoresis was the workhorse for large biomolecule separations, with Laemmli having established denaturing separations of proteins in acrylamide gels[81] and O'Farrell having just defined the power of two-dimensional (2D) gel separations for proteins[119]; the advent of sequencing gels[137] and the use of agarose gels for nucleic acid separations followed later that decade.

On that backdrop, envision the stark contrast of a paper that described a gas chromatographic analyzer fabricated out of silicon (Figure 18-1) using the tools under development for a microelectronics industry that was still in its infancy. The work of Terry and associates[156] provided the first evidence that microfabrication could be used to create micro-miniaturized devices for analytical separations. Despite that, the scientific community did not immediately recognize the significance of this achievement nor see this as a glimpse into a future that would be seeded, in no uncertain terms, by Widmer's group at CIBA in Basel, Switzerland, roughly a decade later. Although several papers followed this initial work, it was not until the concept of a total analysis system (TAS), first proposed by Manz and colleagues in 1990,[104] that the idea of miniaturization had a significant impact. The TAS concept was originally motivated by a lack of adequate sensors for detection of specific species from a complex mixture. It was hypothesized in the seminal Manz paper[104] that, by improving the sample treatment steps and thereby increasing the selectivity of the sensor, an ultrasensitive sensor would not be required if interfering chemical compounds were removed. A TAS, as proposed, entailed initial sampling, transport of the sample, sample pretreatment steps, and final detection of the analyte. Miniaturization of all of the processes required for total analysis, a micro–total analysis system (µTAS), would allow development of a TAS that performs these functions at the site of measurement. Additional benefits are derived from decreasing the size of a TAS, such as decreased volumes of sample and reagent and the potential for drastically reduced analysis times.

MICRODEVICE FABRICATION

Since the inception of the µTAS concept, the field has expanded to exploit multiple different substrates for microchip fabrication. Initial work in this field involved silicon or glass as the microchip substrate and has been extended to polymers such as polydimethylsiloxane and polymethylmethacrylate. This section highlights the traditional processes used for fabricating glass and silicon devices, namely, photolithography and etching, and then discusses polymeric microchip fabrication broadly while highlighting two popular plastic substrate choices.

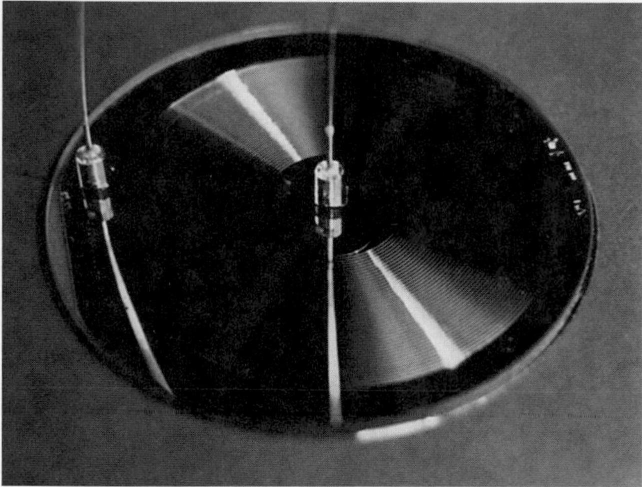

Figure 18-1 First microfabricated analytical device—integrated gas chromatograph (GC) microfabricated into silicon substrate.[118]

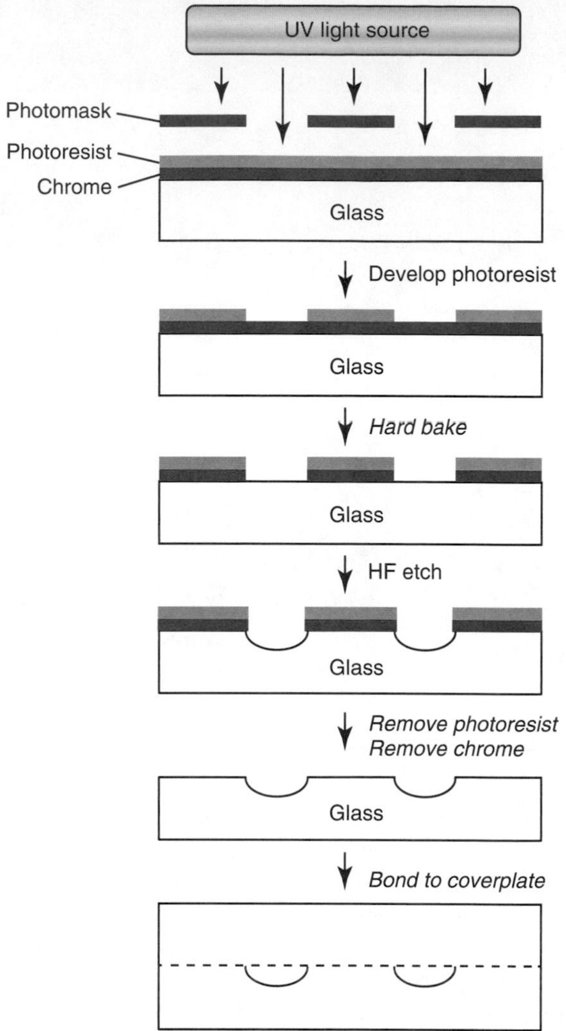

Figure 18-2 Glass microchip fabrication method. A diagram illustrating the processes involved in microchip fabrication using standard photolithography and wet chemical etching methods.

Photolithography and Glass Etching Techniques

In standard photolithography practices, glass is obtained with a photoresist and metal layer deposited onto the wafer (see Figure 18-2 for a schematic of the process). The function of these films is twofold: to allow for channel design and for glass protection during the chemical etching step. A chrome metal layer is first deposited onto the glass because of its tight bonding with both glass and silicon. This layer provides extra protection from hydrofluoric acid (HF) during wet chemical etching. On top of the metal is a layer of photoresist that allows for channel patterning. The traditional mode of application is to spin-coat the photoresist on top of the metal layer, although there are alternatives to this approach, such as the constant-volume injection method.[92] Because such fine precision can be attained using photolithography, application of the photoresist is performed under cleanroom conditions using specialized instrumentation. In most cases, glass can be purchased with both the photoresist and metals already applied.

Transfer of the channel pattern to the photoresist involves using a photomask containing the design. The photomask can be a film mask or a metal mask. For either mask, the microfluidic design is created using software (Adobe Illustrator, AutoCAD, etc). A film mask can be printed by a high-resolution printer, allowing for microfluidic channels on the order of 40 to 200 μm, while metal masks allow fabrication of structures of higher resolution (<20 μm). A photomask containing the pattern is placed on top of the photoresist, and the "sandwich" is exposed to ultraviolet (UV) light. The glass is then placed in a developer solution and the photoresist removed. The exposed chrome is then removed, exposing the glass only in the places where channels are to be etched.

Glass channels are achieved by wet chemical etching using a solution of HF. The etching rate of the solution depends on the concentration of HF in the etching solution—the higher the concentration of HF, the faster the etch rate. An etch rate of 10 μm/min can be achieved with a 49% HF etch solution[87] in borosilicate glass. The use of wet chemical etching results in an isotropically etched channel, where the glass is etched equally in all directions. This type of etching results in a channel architecture that has a semihemisphere shape (see Figure 18-2). Once the channels have been etched to their desired width/depth, access holes are drilled and the devices bonded. For glass-glass bonding, thermal bonding is widely used. With this technique, both glass wafers to be bonded are thoroughly cleaned, aligned, and brought into intimate contact. The bonding process takes place at a temperature of 620 to 690 °C over 6 to 8 hours and can be achieved using a programmable furnace. Multiple bonding cycles are typically required to get a fully bonded device, which is one of the biggest drawbacks to thermal bonding. Other approaches have been developed, such as room temperature bonding techniques,[17,57,67,128] UV-curable adhesives,[59,141] and silicate solutions.[63,78,139]

Alternatives to Traditional Photolithography and Wet Chemical Etching

Application of a photoresist requires a spin-coater and clean-room conditions, which can be fairly expensive. Alternatives to the use of a photoresist have been developed, where patterned polydimethylsiloxane (PDMS) was affixed to the glass wafer to be etched and HF flowed through the PDMS channels.[134] Enzyme nanolithography has achieved nanometer-sized depressions in a protein surface. Scanning probe microscopy was used to control a nanopipet, which delivered proteases to a dried bovine serum albumin film.[61,62] Although wet chemical etching does not require expensive instrumentation, the desire for high aspect ratio structures or for more control over the dimensions of the channel can lead to other types of etching techniques. For example, high aspect ratio structures were obtained in glass and fused silica wafers by using powder blasting,[7] fast atom beam etching[54] and deep reactive ion etching (DRIE).[16] All of these methods involve bombarding the wafer surface with particles; however, DRIE uses chemically reactive ions, typically fluoride, to collide and remove surface atoms while fast atom beam etching uses neutral particles.

POLYMERIC MATERIALS

Because of the expense involved in the fabrication of glass microchips, interest is increasing in the idea of using plastic materials as microfluidic substrates. Some of the key factors to consider when choosing a polymeric material for microchips include surface chemistry, optical clarity, chemical compatibility, temperature stability, and desired application. Glass microfluidic devices make an excellent platform for electrophoretic separations that utilize electro-osmotic flow (EOF), because of the abundance of silanol groups on the surface. This same surface can be difficult in applications such as polymerase chain reaction (PCR), because the glass surface can react with necessary components, thereby inhibiting the reaction. Polyimide is a thermoplastic polymer with a neutral surface charge that provides an excellent vessel for PCR,[37] yet it has less than optimal visible light transmittance, making optical detection difficult with this material. Another driving force for finding alternatives to glass for microfluidics involves generally easier fabrication methods.

As the list of possible substrates for microfluidic devices grows, ways of making fabrication easier and more streamlined with these materials are becoming more innovative. Polyester-toner microdevices have been made on overhead transparencies using laser printers.[20,21,26] The channel geometry is simply printed onto the transparency (where the absence of toner dictates the channels) and placed together with another piece of blank transparency containing only access holes. The sandwich is bonded by lamination, and the toner printing results in channels that are approximately 6 μm deep. These microchips have been used for electrophoretic separations using a number of different detection methods. SU-8 is a negative photoresist that has been used as a substrate for microfluidic devices. Fabrication of these devices takes advantage of the photoresist properties of SU-8 and allows the device to build in a number of layers.[162] The first layer is homogeneously spun onto silicon; this is followed by complete cross-linking with UV exposure. A second layer is spun onto the first layer and covered with a photomask during UV exposure, which allows the channel pattern transfer. The third layer is separately spun onto a piece of glass, completely cross-linked through UV exposure, and then placed onto the second layer. A low-temperature baking step, UV exposure of the whole device, and removal of the glass and silicon pieces complete the device. Thermoset polyester (TPE) is an unsaturated polyester in which cross-linking occurs upon addition of a catalyst; TPE can be fabricated using many of the same techniques as are used with PDMS (see section later).[166] Poly(cyclolefin), the same material used in making compact discs, has also been used in microfluidic devices.[73] Hot embossing is used to make these chips, and a silicon master allows for channel dictation. A cover plate is bonded to enclose the device, using heat and pressure to generate a complete seal.

Polydimethylsiloxane (PDMS)

Polydimethylsiloxane (PDMS) is one of the most popular polymeric materials used as substrates. Fabrication is fairly easy involving the combination of elastomeric base and curing agent. The PDMS surface has methyl groups on the surface, imparting a hydrophobic nature, and is flexible and optically transparent. The flexibility of PDMS allows it to be a highly chosen substrate for valving, and it can be both reversibly and irreversibly[5,6,73] sealed to a variety of surfaces. Several different PDMS fabrication methods have been reported (see Sun[151] for a review), with replica molding[73] and rapid prototyping being two processes that are readily used. Rapid prototyping involves the use of a master, which, once made, allows for fast and easy replication of that design. The master is made by using a negative photoresist, such as SU-8, spun onto a silicon or glass wafer. The microfluidic channel design is imparted onto the photoresist using photolithography and the wafer subsequently developed. Because SU-8 is a negative photoresist, only where the light is incident is where the photoresist is rendered insoluble, while the remaining photoresist remains soluble in the developer solution. This leaves photoresist only where the channels are, exposing the glass everywhere else. Etching of the glass results in the reverse architecture of the glass microfluidic layer, where the channels are raised instead of imprinted. The height of the photoresist over the glass dictates the depth of the PDMS channels. Although photolithography is still used in fabrication of the master, once made, multiple devices can be made easily.

PDMS is produced when an elastomeric base and a curing agent are mixed in the appropriate ratios. Once mixed, they are poured over the master and are allowed to cure; this can happen at room temperature overnight, although heating quickens the process. The cured PDMS can then be peeled from the master and bonded with the substrate of choice. The bonding method will depend on the substrate used for the coverplate; PDMS/PDMS devices can be reversibly bonded by putting the two pieces into contact with one another. Irreversible bonding of PDMS/PDMS can be achieved through a number of different methods, one being activation of the surface by plasma oxidation.[6,73] Liu and coworkers reported another method, in which they altered the elastomer base to curing agent ratios, using 20 : 1 for the fluidic layer and 5 : 1 for the cover plate. The device was assembled and placed in an oven, at which point the two layers fused as the result of the distribution of excess reagents between the two layers.[5]

Plexiglas (PMMA)

Poly(methylmethacrylate) (PMMA) has become a popular substrate choice for microfluidic devices. PMMA is considered a thermoset polymer that softens into a viscous liquid when heated above its glass transition temperature. Multiple methods of fabrication are available, and the channel surface is easily modified to adapt to a particular application; see references 6 and 151 for reviews of polymer fabrication techniques. Hot embossing[80,131] is a technique that can be used with a variety of substrates; it consists of heating the polymer above the glass transition temperature and stamping the substrate with the desired microfluidic pattern. To make PMMA devices using this technique, a metal or silicon stamp is brought into contact with the PMMA and is embossed using a constant force and elevated temperatures to partially melt the substrate. The embossing process can be completed in less than 10 minutes, and once the apparatus has cooled, the stamp and the substrate can be carefully separated. This same process can also be done at room temperature using PMMA as a substrate; this yields channel dimensions that vary by less than 2%.[184] Injection molding, another fabrication technique used to make PMMA devices,[29] incorporates the use of a metal or silicon stamp. This involves heating the PMMA at high temperatures, which results in the formation of a viscous liquid. The PMMA is then pushed into the mold by applying high pressure and is allowed to cool; it is then removed from the mold. Both of these methods result in devices with micron-sized channels and are useful for mass production of devices with the same microfluidic pattern.

Certain applications require the use of sub-micron-sized features; x-ray lithography is capable of making these small channels and intricate structures. Figure 18-3 shows an example of post structures that can function as a solid phase for DNA chromatography. Solid phases for DNA extraction traditionally are created with silica beads, sol-gels, or silica bead/sol-gel hybrids (see section on DNA extraction). However, phases can also be microfabricated during the microchip fabrication process. This can be done by using a direct write process or a mask, typically fabricated in a thick gold layer because it can absorb the x-rays. Where the x-rays are incident upon the PMMA, the polymer degrades. The

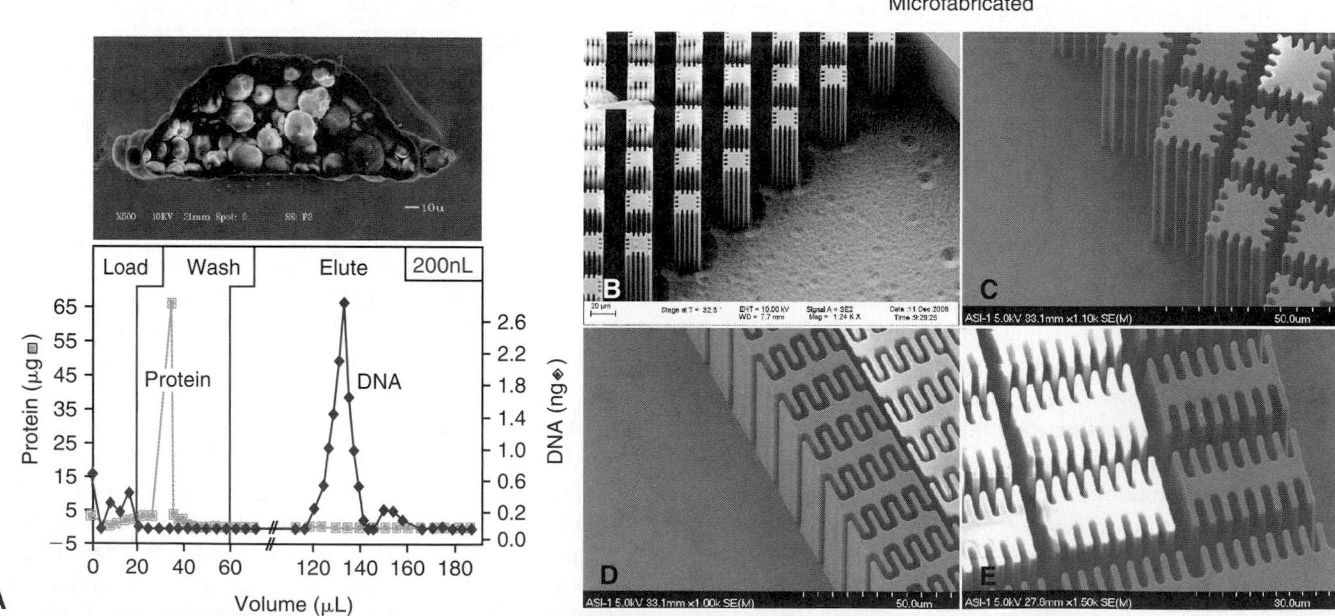

Figure 18-3 Solid phase for on-chip DNA purification/chromatography. A, Microchromatogram *(lower)* showing the separation of protein and nucleic acid components from 200 nL of human whole blood on a sol gel–immobilized silica solid phase *(upper)*. B through E, Two designs for microfabricated solid phases use a LIGA process to generate polymethylmethacrylate (PMMA) (PlexiGlas) posts for the chromatographic process. The dimensions are as follows: B, 14 μm square posts with ≈3 μm extensions with 17 μm distance between posts. C, 14 μm square posts with ≈3 μm extensions with 4 μm distance between posts. D, 6 μm × 30 μm posts with 5 μm extensions. E, 6 μm × 30 μm posts with 8 μm extensions.

device is placed into a developer solution which removes degradation products by solubilization. The length of exposure along with the energy used dictates the depth of the channels. Laser ablation is also used to make submicron features in PMMA devices. This involves bombarding the surface with a pulsed UV source to damage the polymer structure.[149] With both of these last two techniques, high aspect ratio features can be accomplished; however, neither of these methods is ideal for situations involving mass production of the same design.

SEPARATION AND DETECTION OF CLINICALLY RELEVANT ANALYTES

Miniaturized electrophoresis was the first and most dominant embodiment of a µTAS, with the driving force for the miniaturization related to an enhancement in its analytical performance, rather than a simple reduction in size.[104] Because separation efficiency is a function of the applied voltage, microfluidic devices use shorter separation lengths, along with application of high voltages typical of capillary separation, resulting in fast, efficient separations.

A core component in the development of microfluidic technology has been the use of microchips as an analytical platform for electrophoretic separation.[46] Components required for microchip-based electrophoresis (ME) include a detection system, a power supply, and a computer with programmable software for controlling application of voltage, for data collection, and for conditioning of raw data. A number of different detection systems can be used with microchips; however, a fluorescence detection system, essentially a homemade fluorescence microscope, is the most widely used.[46] In terms of selection of the components, power supply selection is critical, because a required number of voltage outputs are needed for electrokinetic injection of the sample and application of the desired electric field. For chip-based separations, the cross-t design originally proposed by Verheggen and associates[165] for electrokinetic injection of sample is the most popular. With this design, a minimum of four voltage outputs are required to control the sample injection and separation. As the complexity of the chip design increases, more outputs may be necessary, particularly if electrokinetic pumping of reagents and buffers is involved. The user is cautioned, however, that effective electrokinetic mobilization of solutions through the microchip architecture is limited to reagents that are low in conductivity and not high in organic solvent concentration; this results in obvious limitations with many clinical samples and, thus, may necessitate the implementation of pressure-driven fluidic control.

For injection, both pressure-driven and electric field–driven injection modes are used, as they are in capillary electrophoresis (CE). The pressure-driven injection mode commonly used in CE, which avoids bias associated with analytes that have a wide range of electrophoretic mobilities, is less popular with chip-based injection. That said, Karlinsey and colleagues[77] demonstrated that integrated diaphragm pumps on a hybrid PDMS-glass microchip could perform pressure sample injection for subsequent electrophoretic separations. The same type of electrokinetic bias associated with CE could be avoided on-chip with pressure injection, and pressure injection could be achieved with sample volumes as low as 500 nL while sample composition was maintained. This was later used by Easley and colleagues[32] for integrated microchip detection of infectious pathogens in blood. However, the injection mode that dominates for most applications in microchip electrophoresis is electrokinetic injection (driven by electrophoretic mobility and/or electroosmotic effects).

The more popular electrokinetic sample injection is dominated by two types—pinched and gated—that are used in standard cross-t design chips. With the pinched injection, a small sample plug is electrokinetically mobilized into the injection cross-t via a voltage applied between the sample and the sample waste reservoir and orthogonal to the separation channel.[65] Once the cross-t is adequately populated with sample, sample injection is accomplished by reconfiguring the primary electric field between the inlet buffer and the outlet buffer reservoirs. Injection "bleed" of sample into the separation channel is minimized by applying a small voltage to the sample and the sample waste. A gated injection allows the sample to electrokinetically migrate through the cross-t toward the sample waste reservoir and then is directed into the separation column by temporarily terminating the potential at the buffer reservoir via a high-voltage relay and allowing the sample to migrate into the separation channel electrokinetically.[66] Unlike a pinched injection, the injected plug volume is dependent on the amount of time the buffer reservoir potential is off. Additionally, this type of injection is susceptible to bias based on differences in analyte electrophoretic mobility.

Electrophoretic Separations

When chip-based separations are performed, the separation channel in a cross-t design provides the counterpart of the capillary in CE, although with a substantially truncated separation length (Figure 18-4). Many of the parameters governing electrophoretic separation in capillaries apply to chip-based separations. For example, like capillaries, one of the benefits of glass-based devices is their inherent ability to dissipate the Joule heat generated from use of the high electric fields needed to facilitate rapid separation. However, the same type of Ohm's law plot (applied voltage vs. current) that would be used to test buffer compatibility with high electric field application should be carried out here as well.[83] Using the appropriate buffer for the separation of interest, the channel surface must be conditioned in a manner not dissimilar to those processes used with capillary systems. If separations requiring EOF are performed, the rigorous cleaning method suggested for fused silica capillaries is required to ensure proper surface regeneration, but attention must be paid to hydration of the glass. The entire cross-t channel architecture of the device is filled, including the reservoirs, to ensure good electrical contact between the platinum electrodes and the solution. The holes drilled into the

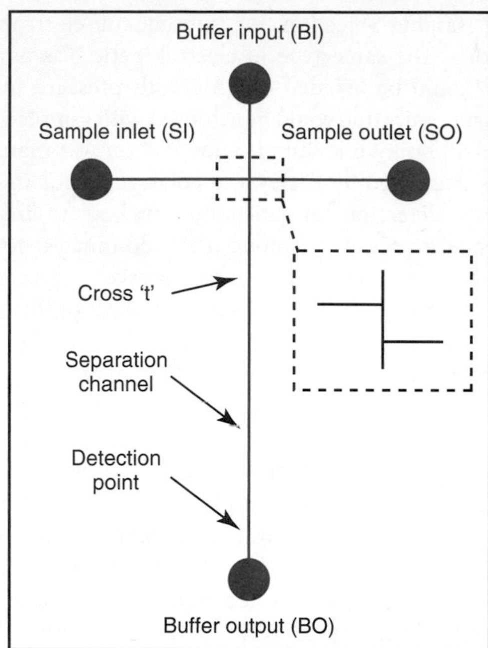

Figure 18-4 Schematic of microchip electrophoresis device design. The reservoirs are labeled as follows: *SI* is the sample inlet, *SO* is the sample outlet, *BI* is the buffer inlet, and *BO* is the buffer outlet. A closer view of the cross-t can be seen in the *dotted box*.

microfluidic device to function as reservoirs (i.e., buffer/sample microvials) may not be large enough to hold a sufficient volume of buffer to avoid buffer depletion. The user must remain cognizant of this and, even with expanded reservoirs generated by commercial "nanoports," or homemade trimmed pipette tips, replenishment of the buffer may be needed.

For sample injection, separation, and detection in a chip of simple design (see Figure 18-4), the sample is placed in the reservoir (SI) and a voltage is applied between SI to SO to inject the sample into the separation channel in a manner consistent with the injection mode chosen. Separation is initiated by application of voltage to BO and BI where electrophoresis of the sample analytes down the separation channel ensues. A point along the separation channel, most commonly at a location close to BO, is used for detection. The detection mode most commonly used is optical detection, and laser-induced fluorescence is popular because of its sensitivity. The detector system [e.g., a laser and photomultiplier tube (PMT)] is positioned at a point in the separation channel commensurate with providing the necessary effective separation length (L_{eff}) for the separation; sample analytes passing that detection point are excited, and the resultant fluorescence is collected. Although the electric fields (E; volts/cm) applied in microchip electrophoresis approach (but do not exceed) those used in capillaries, reduction of the L_{eff} is more easily achieved in microchips. The reservoirs and electrodes required to apply voltage to capillaries limit the minimal L_{eff} to tens of centimeters; microchips, in contrast, can easily allow for separation distances of a few centimeters. It is interesting to note that the U-shaped channel in microchips has little effect on the resolution of separations under high electric fields. The plug profile typically associated with capillaries and known to play a role in yielding high-efficiency (number of theoretical plates) separations does not seem to be adversely affected by the semihemispherically shaped channels.

Detection on Microchips

A detection system is required to measure the number and quantity of analytes electrophoretically separated in the channel as they pass the detection point. With increasing popularity of microchips for separation, a variety of different detection options have evolved that include optical detection methods that are, for the most part, similar to those employed in CE. However, electrochemical, conductivity, and mass spectrometric approaches have also been developed. For optical detection, the most prevalent method in CE and high-performance liquid chromatography (HPLC)—ultraviolet-visible spectroscopy (UV-VIS) detection—is not as common with chip-based electrophoresis, primarily because of challenges with the short optical path length (channel depth) in miniaturized systems and the difficulties involved in coupling light into and out of these channels.[167] That said, a number of reports have detailed progress with UV-VIS detection in analytical microsystems.[10,28,41,91,102,108,183] However, no universally successful method akin to that on CE has been devised. A number of other optical detection schemes for microchips have evolved with varied success and applicability, including infrared,[126] nuclear magnetic resonance (NMR),[175] surface plasmon resonance,[74] thermal lens microscopy,[161] and chemiluminescence/electrochemiluminescence.[55]

The most prevalent detection system used for chip-based separation is laser-induced fluorescence (LIF).[71] It not only is an extremely sensitive method for detection in chemical separations (subzeptomole detection limits), it also is well suited to detection in small volumes, hence, its widespread popularity in capillary electrophoresis separations. A number of reviews have detailed the components required for LIF, have provided a guide to alignment of the optical system, and have described the keystone elements (analyte velocity, probe volume, optimized signal-to-noise ratio as a function of excitation intensity) necessary to achieve sensitive detection.[71,75] Components of an LIF system consist of a light detection module, such as a photomultiplier tube or a charge-coupled detector (CCD) camera, a laser source, optics for alignment of the excitation/emission, an excitation source, and a computer for data collection. LabVIEW software (National Instruments, Austin, Tex), which is commonly used as the interface, allows easy application–specific computer programming to provide software interfaces that permit collection of data and control the detection system.[71,75] A typical method for performing LIF detection on a microchip is to bring the excitation light from a laser of light-emitting diode into the microchannel orthogonal to the device plane, which is relatively simple to align, and to then focus the beam into the channel using a microscope objective or some combination of achromatic lenses. LIF emission is collected with a separate objective or lens combination, spatially and spectrally filtered, and recorded on a photodetector. Confocal detection systems were popular in the capillary electrophoresis literature early on,[51] when focusing and collection optics were one and the same, and the excitation and emission wavelengths were separated with a dichroic beam splitter. Variations in LIF detection setup exist, however, and He and colleagues presented a detailed illustration of their laser-induced detection system, in which excitation is brought into the microchannel from an angle.[50] Two relatively recent reviews provide detailed descriptions of the fundamentals and practice of LIF detection in microanalytical systems.[71,75]

Chip-based detection systems can involve multipoint detection in a single channel or the multichannel detection that is key to high-throughput analysis. For multipoint detection, waveguides can be incorporated into the microchip design for detection at multiple points along the same channel[109] and applied to microchip isoelectric focusing (IEF).[42] Yao and coworkers[186] carried out whole channel imaging during the IEF separation of proteins using a CCD array, ironically using organic LEDs as the excitation source. Alternatively, Raisi and coworkers used a scanning fluorescence detector and a single PMT to scan the entire separation channel.[132] In terms of multichannel scanning, Huang and associates used an acousto-optic deflector (AOD) to change the diffraction angle of an incident laser beam to address an eight-channel device designed for parallel DNA separations.[58] However, the most significant advances have involved the multichannel microdevices designed by Mathies and coworkers for high-throughput analysis. Paegal and colleagues multiplexed 96 channels on a radial capillary electrophoresis microchannel plate,[125] demonstrating that the microchip platform could compete with the 96 capillary arrays that had evolved for CE. Radial microdevices of this ilk for DNA analysis containing as many as 384 channels[34] have been demonstrated as possible.[143] More recently, this group reviewed the types of applications possible with these high-throughput chip-based systems.[95]

Multicolor LIF detection is not essential for all applications but certainly for some involving key genetic analysis techniques. Expanding the number of photodetectors needed to sample at multiple emission wavelengths is the simple approach that has been used for multicolor DNA sequencing[98] and genotyping[142] on microchips; however, Backhouse and associates used a diffraction grating to disperse the LIF emission onto a CCD array for four-color sequencing,[2] and Simpson and colleagues used a transmission imaging spectrograph with a wide imaging area to disperse LIF emission from a two-color genotyping experiment run in 48 parallel channels onto a CCD array.[144] More recently, a system was developed to complement the microchip platform by featuring a single acousto-optic tunable filter (AOTF) and a single PMT.[76] The filter behaves similarly to the previously described AOD, except that when an acoustic wave traveling through the crystal at a specific frequency interacts with the light, only select wavelength bands are diffracted by the crystal and collected by the PMT.[75]

Exemplary Separations

Separation of Nucleic Acids

Although small molecules were the target analytes in early chip-based separations (fluorescein and calcein),[47,105] the separation of amino acids[46] (Figure 18-5) changed the landscape to one that could involve biomolecules of interest and eventually led to a literature dominated by the separation of DNA fragments using laser-induced fluorescence as the detection method. The significance of the early studies showing electrophoretic separation of analytes in a planar glass system was less about faster analysis times and more about the drastic reduction in reagent consumption. It was this unprecedented analytical potential that paved the way for DNA separations in microdevices, shoring up the threat that CE was bringing to large, unwieldy slab gels that were slow to run, cumbersome to manipulate, and labor intensive to use in high-throughput mode. Early work from Mathies and coworkers laid the groundwork for successful separation in 120 seconds of ΦX174 Hae III restriction fragments ranging from 70 to 1000 bp.[180] This technology was advanced by this group, which accomplished high-resolution separations and DNA sequencing using multicolor fluorescence detection.[97,179]

Although Karlinsey and associates showed that using an AOTF for multicolor detection could be applied to short tandem repeat (STR) profiling for human identification, the microchip-based separation of amplified gene products for STRs of clinical significance has also been demonstrated. For example, fragile X syndrome has been correlated with a CGG repeat expansion seen in the 5′-untranslated region of the familial MR type I *(FMR1)* gene. Individuals with the

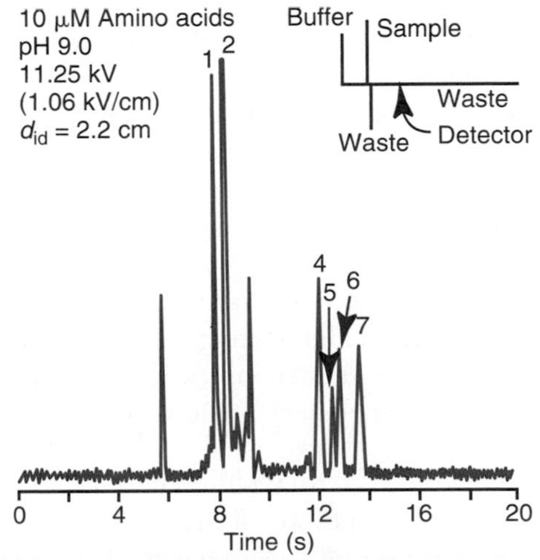

Figure 18-5 Rapid microchip electrophoresis of amino acids. Electropherogram of the resultant separation of six fluorescein isothiocyanate (FITC)-labeled amino acids. The numbered peaks are as follows: *1*, Arg; *2*, FITC hydrolysis product; *3*, Gln; *4*, Phe; *5*, Asn; *6*, Ser; and *7*, Gly. The *inset* shows the microchip diagram of the device used in this separation. *(Reprinted from Harrison DJ, Fluri K, Seiler K, Fan ZH, Effenhauser CS, Manz A. Micromachining a miniaturized capillary electrophoresis-based chemical-analysis system on a chip. Science 1993;261:895-7.)*

premutation show an unstable number of $(CGG)_n$ repeats and generally are asymptomatic; however, identifying the number of trinucleotide repeats is critical for genetic counseling. Sung and colleagues[152] used microchip separations that were completed in less than 1 minute to identify these trinucleotide repeats using a polymethyl(methacrylate) (Plexiglas) microchip; this represented a roughly 100-fold reduction in analysis time when compared with the 70 minutes consumed by the conventional slab gel approach. Similarly, Cantafora and colleagues[14] used microchip electrophoresis to detect the D19S394 tetranucleotide repeat $(AAAG)_n$. This repeat is highly polymorphic (with the number of repeats typically ranging from 1 to 17) and is a short recombination distance from the low-density lipoprotein (LDL) receptor gene, making it suitable for the study of familial hypercholesterolemia (FH). Analysis was performed using the commercial microchip electrophoresis system, with instrument control by dedicated software for completely automated sample injection, fluid manipulation, and data collection. This system is designed to analyze 25 to 500 base pair (bp) double-stranded (ds)DNA fragments with 5 bp resolution. Using this, 70 carriers of two LDL receptor mutations common in Northern Italy were compared with 100 healthy controls, and the microchip-based technique was successfully used for the sizing of D19S394 needed for a simple cosegregation analysis.

Nemoda and coworkers[117] used a microchip with 96 robotically loaded electrophoretic lanes for analysis of 20 bp repetitive sequence elements within the 5′-regulatory region of the serotonin transporter gene *(5-HTT)*. Two amplified products, one for each of two common alleles (a short 14-repeat and a long 16-repeat sequence), that were shown to have an impact on transcription of this key synaptic transporter, could be separated and detected in about 4 minutes. The reduction in analysis time for the 334 samples that were genotyped for variable repeats was dramatic in comparison with that required for conventional slab gel electrophoresis. This technology was applied in a similar way to the detection of variable repeat alleles of the dopamine receptor *(DR)* gene using PCR and microchip electrophoresis.[4] Following PCR amplification of a variable number of repeats of a 48 bp sequence, chip electrophoresis allowed separation and detection of the products in 90 seconds, highlighting the potential of pharmacogenetic analysis for mutations shown to correlate with effective doses of methylphenidate in school children.[43]

Mutation Detection via Microchip Analysis

An early diagnostic application of electrophoretic microchips involved the detection of T-cell receptor (TCR) gene rearrangement, where normal samples yield amplified PCR fragments representative of a polyclonal lymphocyte population, while lymphoma patients display a monoclonal population. Munro and coworkers[113] were able to separate B- and T-cell gene rearrangement PCR products on microchips, providing diagnostic information in an assay where the electrophoresis consumed only 160 seconds (Figure 18-6). This marked a 60-fold decrease in analysis time compared with conventional slab gel methods, with no loss in diagnostic capacity. More recently, Legendre and associates[85] demonstrated a microchip separation method for analyzing post-PCR products from patients' samples that were both positive and negative for T-cell lymphoma. They showed the resultant electropherograms, where negative samples show three broad peaks, characteristic of a range of different sized PCR products generated, and positive samples show the presence of one or two strong peaks, caused by the presence of a clonal cell population. These separations required less than 5 minutes on a microdevice—a more than 8-fold reduction in time when compared with commercial capillary electrophoresis.

With heteroduplex analysis (HDA), a common method for mutation detection, denaturation of the sample DNA followed by controlled re-annealing generates homoduplexes or heteroduplexes, depending on whether wild-type or mutant DNA is present. The relative presence of these can be parsed out via differences in the electrophoretic mobilities of the duplexes stemming from the degree of sequence mismatch. Tian and colleagues[158] used HDA-based electrophoresis to target *BRCA1* and *BRCA2* germline mutations. Using microchip HDA analysis, they demonstrated the detection of six different deletion, insertion, and point *BRCA* mutations in separations that were complete in 130 seconds, proving the microchip platform to be a powerful and efficient mutation screening. Similarly, Footz and coworkers[36] compared a microchip-based HDA technique versus denaturing HPLC (dHPLC) using glass microchips and a commercial self-coating sieving polymer. They showed that eight sequence variants of *BRCA1* and *BRCA2* genes could be detected, even without optimization of PCR amplification or of chip HDA conditions, demonstrating that the microfluidic technique could provide sensitivity similar to that of an extensively optimized dHPLC system.

An alternative mode of mutation detection, allele-specific PCR (AS-PCR), is commonly used for the rapid detection of known single-base DNA polymorphisms. AS-PCR was used by Medintz and associates[107] on a capillary array electrophoretic microplate for high-speed single-nucleotide polymorphism (SNP) analysis of the *HFE* gene, which is associated with hereditary hemochromatosis (HH). The HH disorder is an autosomal recessive disease of iron metabolism, affecting roughly 1 of every 300 people of Native American descent. The disease has been linked to an S65D (193A>T) substitution. In this analysis, two different fluorescently labeled primers were designed to detect the HH-associated substitution mutation [S65C (193 A>T)], with the A- and T-specific amplicons identified by both size and color. Using microchip electrophoresis on a radial 96-channel array, analysis of 96 samples could be completed in an unprecedented 10 minutes. This work was later extended by Emrich and colleagues[34] into a 384-lane microfabricated capillary array electrophoresis device for massively parallel genetic analysis, demonstrating the high-throughput SNP genotyping made possible by microchip-based microchannel arrays.

The AS-PCR was also exploited by Tian and coworkers,[157] in conjunction with HDA analysis of *BRCA* mutations. The wild-type homozygotes and heterozygotes were distinguished

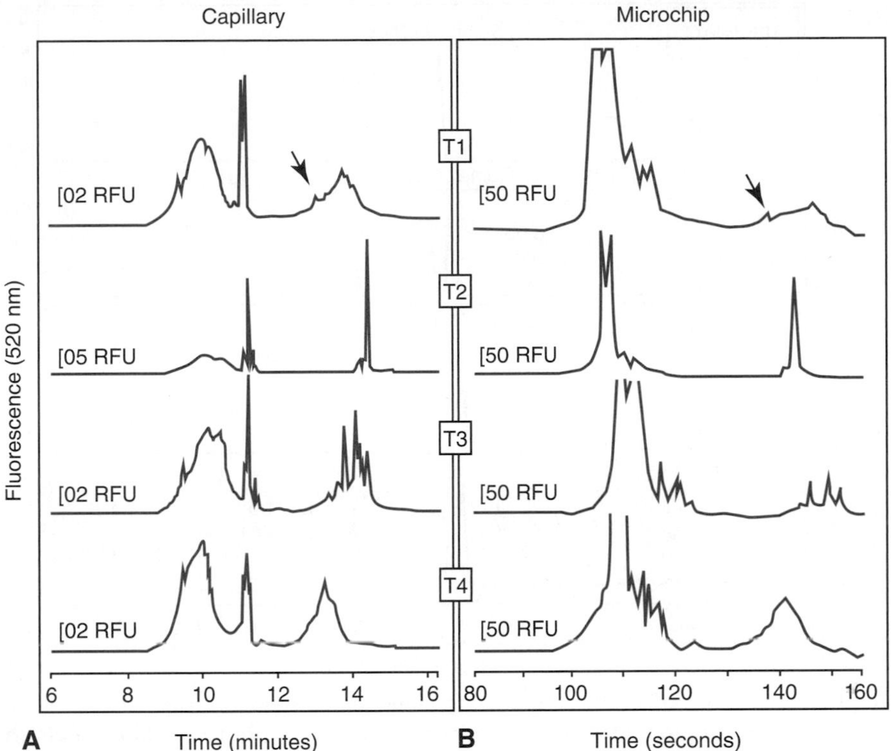

Figure 18-6 Microchip electrophoretic detection of T-cell receptor gene rearrangements. Electropherograms of T-cell receptor gene rearrangement products performed in (A) capillary or (B) microchip. Samples T2 and T3 are both positive samples, sample T4 is a negative sample, and sample T1 shows a sample interpreted as negative/equivocal. *(Modified from Munro NJ, Snow K, Kant JA, Landers JP. Molecular diagnostics on microfabricated electrophoretic devices: from slab gel- to capillary- to microchip-based assays for T- and B-cell lymphoproliferative disorders. Clin Chem 1999;45:1906-17.)*

on the basis of the number of peaks observed after chip-based electrophoretic separation (Figure 18-7). Alleles were identified in less than 180 seconds by microchip electrophoresis, for a total analysis time (including a 10-minute DNA purification and a 1.2- to 2-hour PCR amplification) of less than 2.5 hours. The method was simple and rapid, and because no enzymatic digestion was used, post-PCR processing was not required.

Chowdhury and associates[18] used microchip analysis to probe gene variants within the thiopurine-*S*-methyltransferase *(TPMT)* gene using AS-PCR and restriction fragment length polymorphism (RFLP)-PCR followed by chip-based electrophoresis with multicolor LIF. With both AS-PCR and microchip electrophoresis integrated into a single microchip that accepted off-chip purified DNA, this chip enabled PCR-RFLP-μCE analysis to be performed in 3 hours, compared with 9 hours for conventional methods,[18] and over 24 hours with an oligonucleotide array microdevice.[116] Excluding prepurification, the costs of the polymeric microchip and reagents used by these authors for a single analysis totaled only $10, demonstrating the potential of microfluidics to provide disposable chips for both reduced sample handling and contamination risk, as well as cost-effective decentralized point-of-care testing.

Single-stranded conformational polymorphism (SSCP), developed by Orita and colleagues[124] in the late 1980s, involves thermal denaturation of the sample post PCR amplification, followed by rapid cooling ("snap-cooling"), allowing single-stranded oligonucleotides to take on a self-annealed three-dimensional (3D) conformation. The discriminating aspect of this mutation detection method is the fact that the 3D conformation depends on the intrastrand base pair sequence, with different alleles forming differing conformations that can be resolved electrophoretically. For smaller PCR products (<200 bp), SSCP can resolve single base pair mutations with greater than 90% accuracy—this can approach 100% accuracy when coupled with heteroduplex analysis.[1,36] Following on their work with HDA, Tian and coworkers[160] were the first to implement SSCP on an electrophoretic microchip to detect mutations in two breast cancer genes, *BRCA1* and *BRCA2*. Following multiplex PCR amplification using fluorescently labeled primers and snap-cooling on ice to induce intrastrand secondary structures and separation of the products by microchip electrophoresis, resolution of the fluorescently tagged amplicons was possible in 130 seconds or less, representing analysis speed that was orders of magnitude faster than with slab gel analysis and even capillary electrophoresis.

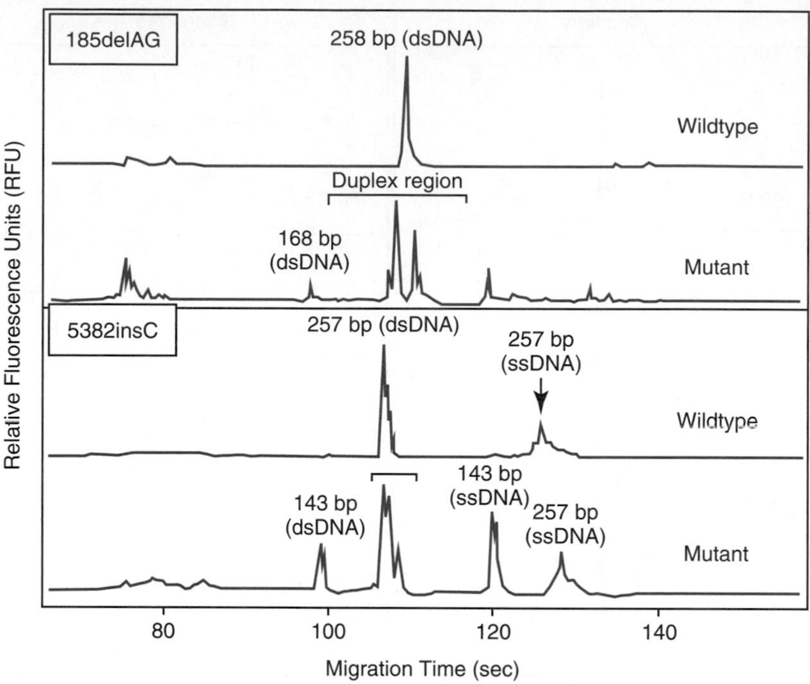

Figure 18-7 Fast mutation detection using allele-specific polymerase chain reaction (PCR) and heteroduplex analysis on a microfluidic electrophoretic chip. Panels show AS-PCR heteroduplex analysis results for wild-type and heterozygous mutants associated with a deletion (185delAG) and insertion (5382insC) mutation. The separation was in a chip containing a poly(vinylpyrrolidone) (PVP)-coated microchannel with an effective length of 55 mm filled with tris-borate-EDTA (TBE) buffer containing hydroxyethyl cellulose and glycerol; detection was laser-induced fluorescence. *(Modified from Tian H, Brody LC, Fan S, Huang Z, Landers JP. Capillary and microchip electrophoresis for rapid detection of known mutations by combining allele-specific DNA amplification with heteroduplex analysis. Clin Chem 2001;47:173-85.)*

Vahedi and associates[164] followed this work with fusion of HA and SSCP on a single electrophoretic microchip. Using the manual addition of formamide to the PCR amplicons from *BRCA1* exon 20, and *HFE* exon 2, they were able to electrokinetically inject into a traditional cross-t microchip, with subsequent separation yielding heteroduplex data. Although the ability to do sequential HA and SSCP on the same microchip with the same sample is advantageous, it is important to recognize that the manual addition of formamide to the sample reservoir removes the ability to repeat the HA analysis. An additional discriminator involves real-time labeling of the heteroduplex and SSCP products with intercalating dyes (as opposed to using fluorescently labeled primers). Shortly after, the same group[103] demonstrated that detection of all three major *HFE* mutations could be accomplished using similar HA/SSCP technology, but again, using the cumbersome manual addition of formamide. Barron's group addressed the issue of optimization of HA and SSCP on a microchip using PCR amplicons of p53 exons 5 through 9.[53] PCR-amplified products were subjected to HA and SSCP via heat denaturation followed by snap-cooling on ice. By evaluating a variety of sieving mediums and channel coatings synthesized and characterized by this group, and by using a high-pressure loading device to accommodate loading of the highly viscous polymers into microchip channels, they identified a polymer (600 kDa linear polyacrylamide) and a hydrophobic wall coating (poly-*N*-hydroxyethylacrylamide) that seemed to provide optimal resolution of DNA conformational variants by microchip electrophoresis.

Other Mutation Detection Schemes

Zhou and colleagues[191] exploited the fact that aberrant methylation of the *p16* suppressor gene is recognized as an early event in many forms of cancer, especially of the lungs, making methylation detection a potential biomarker for early detection. They compared a modified, seminested methylation-specific PCR on a plastic (PMMA) electrophoresis microchip versus conventional slab gel electrophoresis for the detection of tumor-associated *p16* gene hypermethylation in plasma and tissue DNA. In a blinded approach, they analyzed 153 specimens by microchip electrophoresis (94 cancer patients, 30 positive, and 30 negative controls). Not only were they able to identify all positive and negative controls, they also correctly identified the cancerous samples both faster and at a rate 26.6% higher than that attainable by conventional slab gel electrophoresis.

Jabasini and coworkers[64] presented a multiplexed PCR assay to probe nonobstructive spermatogenic failure based on interstitial deletions on the Y chromosome. Their method specifically targeted the amplification of three DNA sequence-tagged sites on the human Y chromosome, which were subsequently separated on a 12-lane microchip electrophoresis system. With this separation system, 36 DNA markers (3 per separation × 12 lanes) were analyzed in less than 180 seconds, with acceptable resolution despite the only 11 bp difference between them. This type of rapid interrogation of specific deletion events commonly associated as a genetic cause of male infertility greatly enhances the potential for diagnostic testing for infertility, supplanting a conventional method that is cumbersome and time consuming. Yung and associates[188] sought a microfluidic solution for detecting two common epidermal growth factor receptor *(EGFR)* mutations in the plasma/tumor tissues of patients suffering from non–small cell lung cancers. Using a digital PCR-based approach, they were able to quantitatively probe mutations at two exons that account for more than 85% of clinically important *EGFR* mutations associated with responsiveness to tyrosine kinase inhibitors. The digital PCR system allowed 9180 PCR amplifications to be carried out simultaneously in nanoliter reaction volumes. With sensitivity at the single-molecule level, mutations in clinical specimens could be detected at low levels, and quantities of mutant and wild-type sequences were determined in a manner that predicted treatment response. Knowing that microsatellite instability (MSI) is associated with ≈15% of colorectal (as well as gastric and endometrial) carcinomas, and that this impacts clinical prognosis, Odenthal and colleagues[122] interrogated the five microsatellite loci (Bat25, Bat26, D2S123, D5S346, and D17S250) using an electrophoretic microchip with 40 patient samples having known MSI status (Figure 18-8). Results obtained from microfluidic chip analysis of the PCR products in all cases resulted in genetic profiles for the five microsatellite loci that correlated well with data derived from more conventional technology.

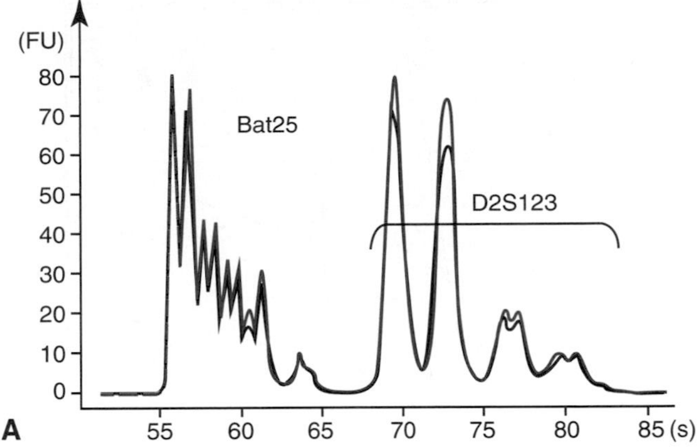

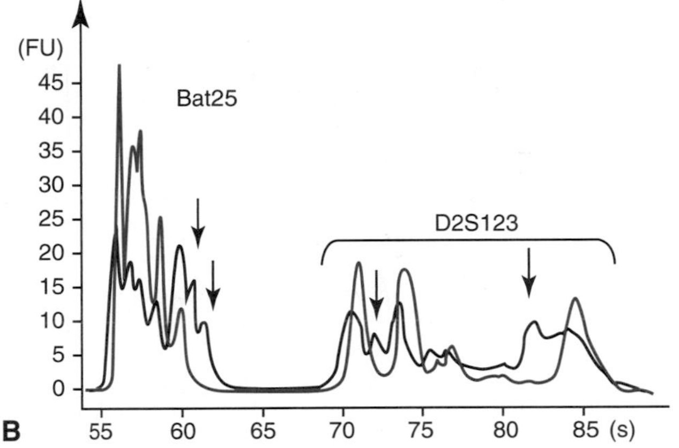

Figure 18-8 Microchip electropherograms of microsatellite markers in colorectal cancer. The separations are from polymerase chain reaction (PCR) products of both normal *(red)* and tumor *(blue)* tissue. A, The resultant electropherogram from stable microsatellites, as seen by the matching profiles from both samples. B, Indicative of instable microsatellites, as shown by deviations in the electrophoretic pattern. The tissues used were taken from cases with a known microsatellite instability status. *(Reprinted from Odenthal M, Barta N, Lohfink D, et al. Analysis of microsatellite instability in colorectal carcinoma by microfluidic-based chip electrophoresis. J Clin Pathol 2009;62:850-2.)*

Separation of Proteins

Although the literature is ripe with methods used for capillary electrophoretic separation of proteins, a vast majority of these involve nondenaturing separation in the absence of sodium dodecyl sulfate (SDS). Although this simple (no sieving matrix) and powerful (resolution) method can be used for protein analysis, sizing information is lost, and this is often an important component of protein-based clinical assays. In addition, the most common mode for the detection of proteins by CE is UV absorbance (200, 214, or 280 nm), and this has been difficult to translate to the microchip. Although LIF can easily be used (via massive development effort for DNA separations), it typically requires fluorescent labeling of the proteins, which has its own inherent limitations. Bousse and coworkers adapted SDS–polyacrylamide gel electrophoresis (PAGE) to a microdevice for the high-speed separation of proteins[11] with fluorescence detection that must use an on-chip, noncovalent labeling process; this technology has been commercialized in a glass microdevice with associated instrumentation (Agilent's Bioanalyzer, Agilent Technologies, Santa Clara, Calif). Giordano and associates[70] described a similar method for circumventing the covalent labeling of proteins with a "dynamic," on-chip approach that used commercially available fluorescent dyes in the separation medium to allow size-based protein analysis in a glass microchip. In a subsequent report,[38] they optimized conditions for dynamic interaction of the dye with protein, yielding a rapid, sensitive method for protein sizing and quantitation on microchips with a limit of detection (LoD) of 500 ng/mL for bovine serum albumin (BSA). On-chip analysis of patient serum samples allowed abnormalities in the levels of γ-globulins to be determined. Figure 18-9 shows partially purified human plasma separated on a glass microchip in comparison with that done in an 11% acrylamide SDS-PAGE gel, and clearly shows that the use of dynamic labeling enhances sensitivity without loss of resolution.

Nonglass substrates have been shown effective for protein separation as well. Liu and colleagues[94] showed that PMMA

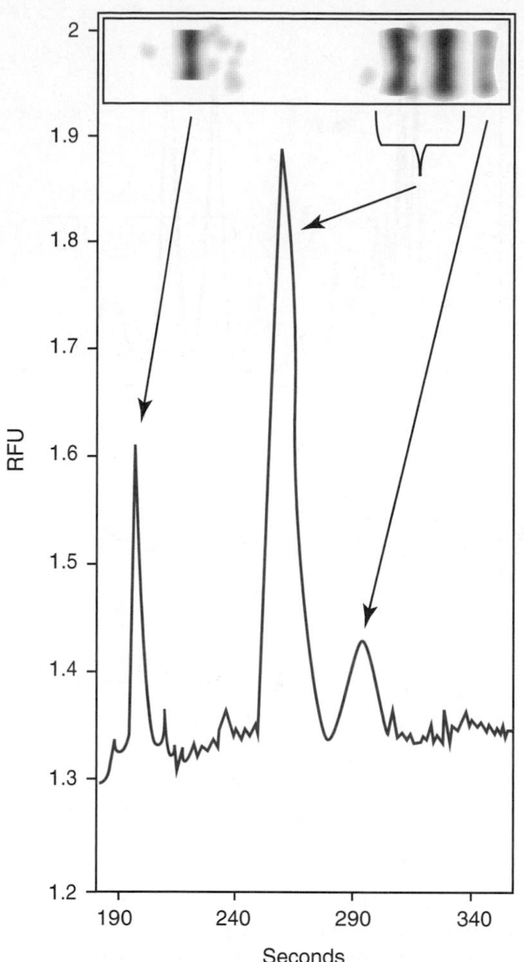

Figure 18-9 Comparison of 11% acrylamide sodium dodecyl sulfate-polyacrylamide gel electrophoresis (SDS-PAGE) gel separation of partially purified human plasma versus microchip-based capillary electrophoresis-SDS (CE-SDS) analysis. Separation conditions include 25 mM/L Tris-CHES, 1 mM DTT, 0.1% SDS, 370 V/cm field strength, electrokinetic injection, and 0.2% (v/v) NanoOrange (excitation 488 nm, emission 590 nm). *(Reprinted from Giordano BC, Jin LJ, Couch AJ, Ferrance JP, Landers JP. Microchip laser-induced fluorescence detection of proteins at submicrogram per milliliter levels mediated by dynamic labeling under pseudonative conditions. Anal Chem 2004;76:4705-14.)*

microchips containing microchannels that had been passivated with polyethylene glycol could provide adequate resolution of the components of BSA; Roman and coworkers[135] used micellar-electrokinetic chromatography in a PDMS microdevice to perform high-resolution separations of standard protein using SDS-coated surfaces. The second most common mode of conventional protein separation in cross-linked gels, isoelectric focusing, has also been translated to the microchip platform using a variety of detection modes such as LIF, UV detection, and whole-column detection.[44,90,154] Guillo and coworkers circumvented the standard CE-type methods to mobilize focused zones past the detector (EOF or chemical mobilization) by using on-chip pumping generated by diaphragm pumps in a three-layer device containing deformable membranes. They illustrated success with this approach by defining the separation of L-lysine and L-histidine and by defining the dependence of resolution on mobilization flow rates.[42] Moreover, they analyzed low (<10 kDa) and high (>10 kDa) molecular weight fractions from patient urine when peaks in the former were assumed to represent a combination of metabolites and amino acids containing primary amino groups, such as creatine, methionine, phenyalanine, histidine, peptides, and small proteins, while the latter reflected larger proteins often present in urine at much lower concentrations. More recently, Xian and associates[182] used a microfluidic chip to evaluate the serum from 38 patients with type 2 diabetes, with focus on alterations in high-density lipoprotein (HDL) subfractions. Their results showed meaningful clinical correlations for total HDL and HDL2b and its ratio with triglycerides, suggesting that the microchip-based method may have predictive value when applied clinically.

Separation of Small Molecules and Ions

The vast majority of the microfluidic chip literature is focused on the separation of nucleic acids or proteins; however, other clinically relevant biological species have been shown to be measurable on microchips. Small molecule metabolites represent a significant portion of the assays carried out in clinical chemistry laboratories; therefore, development of microfluidic platforms that could address the detection and quantitation of metabolites, potentially in multiplexed form, would be powerful.

Wang and Chatrathi[171] showed that a glass microchip could be used to electrophoretically separate and detect glucose, uric acid, and ascorbic acid. These oxidizable species were detected by a downstream amperometric detector, with glucose detected in <100 seconds and all three detected within a few hundred seconds. Munro and colleagues[112] used glass microchips and indirect fluorescence detection (detection without fluorescent labeling) to separate 19 amino acids for urinanalysis (Figure 18-10, *A*). They reported on the detection of amino acids in a normal urine sample (Figure 18-10, *B*) and two abnormal urine specimens. The first abnormal urine sample was taken from a patient suspected of having nephropathic cystinosis with onset of Fanconi syndrome, for whom microchip analysis detected a generalized hyperaminoaciduria (Figure 18-10, *C*). The second abnormal sample was taken from a patient who exhibited symptomatic indicators for amino acid metabolic disorders in which glycine, serine, threonine, and histidine determined to be elevated via HPLC could be identified by microchip electrophoretic analysis (Figure 18-10, *D*). Deng and coworkers[23] used a microfluidic electrophoretic system interfaced with mass spectrometry as the detector to quantitate carnitine and select acylcarnitines in urine; Lunte and associates[127] used chip-based electrophoresis with electrochemical detection for the quantitation of homocysteine and glutathione in plasma samples at levels as high as 50 μmol/L, exceeding the reference interval (5 to 15 μmol/L) for healthy individuals. Henry and colleagues[35] measured uric acid concentrations in urine using a silicone (PDMS)/glass microchip with on-board

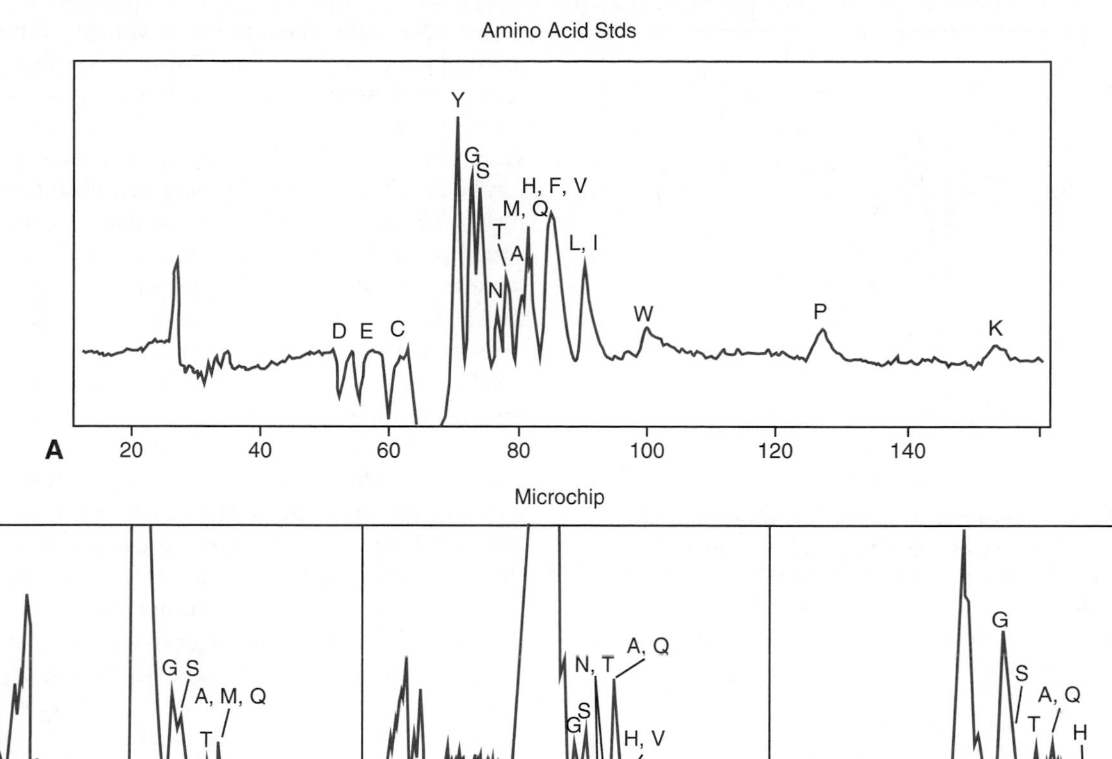

Figure 18-10 Indirect detection of the 19 amino acids by microchip electrophoresis. Electropherograms from (A) a sample containing amino acid standards, (B) a normal urine sample, (C) abnormal urine sample 1, and (D) abnormal urine sample 2. *A*, Alanine; *C*, cysteine; *D*, aspartic acid; *E*, glutamic acid; *F*, phenylalanine; *G*, glycine; *H*, histidine; *I*, isoleucine; *K*, lysine *L*, leucine; *M*, methionine; *N*, asparagine; *P*, proline; *Q*, glutamine; *S*, serine; *T*, threonine; *tau*, taurine; *V*, valine; *W*, tryptophan; *Y*, tyrosine. *(Modified from Munro NJ, Huang Z, Finegold DN, Landers JP. Indirect fluorescence detection of amino acids on electrophoretic microchips. Anal Chem 2000;72:2765-73.)*

amperometric detection. Similarly, Wang and Chatrathi[170] showed that markers of renal function—creatine, creatinine, *p*-aminohippuric acid, and uric acid—could be measured electrochemically in urine in roughly 5 minutes. Detector response was linear over the range of 15 to 110 µM, and analysis time was rapid (<30 seconds). Van den Berg and coworkers[169] developed an integrated glass microchip system that carried out sample cleanup followed by ion separation and detection for quantitation of lithium ion with conductivity detection. Using a simple sample collector requiring less than <10 µL of test fluid and an integrated filter membrane that prevented transport of blood cells into the microchip, they were able to separate sodium/calcium from lithium and magnesium within 20 seconds with a detection limit for lithium of 0.150 mmol/L (Figure 18-11). Investigators validated the device against routine lithium testing of five patients, demonstrating that the microchip-based system provided rapid analysis and comparable results and, hence, had the potential for point-of-care testing of electrolytes in serum and whole blood.

Using a simple, low-cost, PDMS-based microfluidic system, Songjaroen and associates[147] demonstrated that a chip-based two-point alkaline picrate kinetic reaction for determination of urinary creatinine was possible. Knowing that the reaction of creatinine with picric acid under alkaline conditions could be monitored photometrically using a miniature fiberoptic spectrometer (at 510 nm) interfaced with the PDMS chip, they showed linearity in detection from 0 to 40 mg/L creatinine, with a concentration detection limit of 3.3 mg/L (with a signal-to-noise ratio S/N = 3). Investigators concluded that the method was highly correlated with conventional spectrophotometric results obtained from urine samples.

Using a more generic metabolite detection approach, Do and colleagues[25] described a microfluidic chip system for the measurement of oxygen, glucose, and lactate in whole blood.

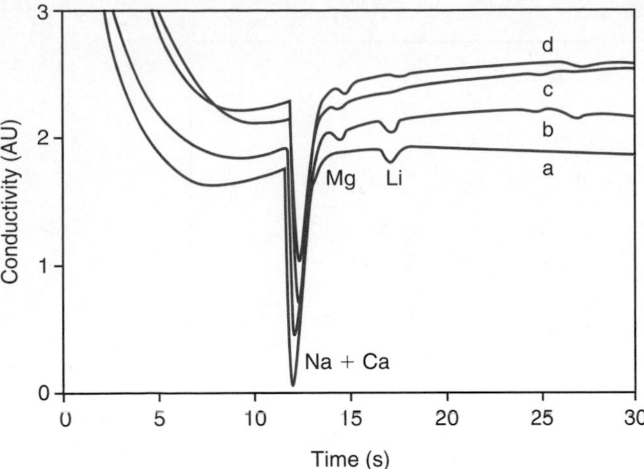

Figure 18-11 Microchip-based detection of lithium in blood samples. Electropherogram of *(a)* an aqueous calibration mixture containing 140 mmol/L sodium and 2 mmol/L lithium, *(b)* citrated whole blood enriched with 2 mmol/L lithium, *(c)* whole blood without anticoagulant, and *(d)* heparinized plasma from a patient on lithium therapy containing 0.62 mmol/L lithium. *(Reprinted from Vrouwe EX, Luttge R, Vermes I, van den Berg A. Microchip capillary electrophoresis for point-of-care analysis of lithium. Clin Chem 2007;53:117-23.)*

A reasonably compact portable analyzer was described that had multianalyte detection capabilities with a disposable microchip that accepted as little as 3.5 μL of blood. With total analysis times on the order of a few hundred seconds (sampling and sensing included), lactate and glucose could be detected in the ranges of 1 to 7 mmol/dL and 50 to 350 mg/dL, respectively, and dissolved oxygen in the range of 50 to 350 mg/dL could be measured.

MICROFLUIDIC VALVING

Volumes used in microfluidic devices can range from picoliters to microliters, with typical total solution volumes in the nanoliter range. A hurdle to the development of true "lab-on-a-chip" devices was absence of a method that could be used to reliably control these small volumes of fluid using practical fabrication methods. This capability was provided by the Quake[163] and Mathies groups,[40] which developed robust valves that were simple to fabricate. Key to these valving approaches was the use of a flexible PDMS membrane that could be pneumatically actuated to produce on-chip valves or fluidic switches. Although elastomeric membranes are not the only material amenable to such use, they represent the only substrate that has been used extensively thus far in the microfluidics field. Use of PDMS in microfluidics was, in fact, pioneered by Whiteside's group,[27,106] which developed the soft lithography techniques used by Quake and colleagues[163] to fabricate their valves.

The type of valve implemented in a microfluidic device typically can be categorized as "normally open" or "normally closed." Normally open, pressure-actuated valves are fabricated in the push-down[163] or push-up[150] configuration. A key feature of these types of valves is the essentially zero dead volume valving critical to effective fluid control on microdevices, but also having the inherent advantage that the valves can be arranged into high-density architectures (≥30 valves/mm^{-2}).[3] Moreover, with at least three valves coupled in series, peristaltic pumps can be created,[163] allowing precise metering of solutions within the device at flow rates up to 2.35 nL/s.

Normally closed, negative pressure–actuated valves developed by the Mathies group[40] are opened by vacuum, with the option of applying positive pressure to promote closing. Rather than patterning PDMS by soft lithography, these valves are defined by patterned glass layers (chemically etched) that sandwich a PDMS membrane. This provides a distinction from valves fashioned using soft lithography, in that most of the channel architecture can be made from glass; this can be advantageous when microchips are needed that are more rigid in structure (glass substrate) and that have enhanced chemical resistivity, while valving capabilities are maintained. The disadvantage of these valves is that the dead volume is not negligible; this is related to lower achievable valve density compared with the Quake valves, although the valves can be designed for <10 nL dead volume[40] and have been shown to be useful for injection of samples that are submicroliter in volume.[30,39] Either type of valve—normally closed or normally open—can be arranged into a diaphragm pumping configuration (at least three valves) with reported flow rates up to 25 μL/min.[40] It is notable that glass-based, normally closed valves are capable of pumping at rates approximately two orders of magnitude greater than their normally open counterparts. These types of devices have been used for amino acid detection,[145,146] DNA computing,[39] pressure injection for electrophoresis microchips,[32] and DNA sequencing,[9] and as fully integrated genetic analysis devices.[31]

Quake's group defined normally open valving systems on PDMS-glass hybrid chips.[150,163] These normally open, pressure-actuated valves are primarily fabricated as push-down valves and are typically restricted to a depth of less than ≈20 μm. A key feature of this type of valve is that it is essentially zero dead volume and can be arranged into high-density architectures (≥30 valves/mm^{-2}).[3] Valves coupled in series can perform as peristaltic pumps, thus providing on-board valving and pumping for precise metering of solutions within the device at flow rates up to 2.35 nL/s^{-1}. These valves have proved functional through implementation in a wide variety of applications such as protein crystallization,[45] nucleic acid processing,[56] multistep radiolabel synthesis,[84] and, more recently, sequencing of the human genome.[130]

APPLICATIONS

Nucleic Acids

DNA Extraction

Analytical techniques for nucleic acid (NA) extraction have been transferred in an effort to lessen sample handling, reduce potential contamination, and expedite analysis time.[31,68,123] Several different approaches have been used for NA purification and preconcentration; the most widely used involves the use of silica-based solid supports. With the use of chemistries similar to commercially available silica-based NA extraction kits, the sample is lysed in a high–ionic strength, chaotropic-containing buffer. NA is loaded onto the silica support in this lysis buffer, and the high-salt environment drives NA onto the solid phase. An alcohol, typically ethanol or isopropanol, is rinsed over the phase to remove cellular debris, and the NA eluted from the phase using a low salt buffer, typically a Tris solution that is compatible with PCR. The silica solid support can exist in many different forms and has been demonstrated as a bead-packed column,[159] as micropillars fabricated into the channel,[19,176,177,185] as sol-gel,[140,173,174,181] and as immobilized silica particles.[8,12,86,178] Other methods used for microchip NA purification involve similar microfluidic strategies but with the use of different extraction chemistries. For example, pH-induced NA capture and release systems have been reported for NA extraction to avoid the harsh solutions used in silica-based extractions.[15,115] A microchannel was coated with a chitosan polymer, which has a pKa of 6.3, allowing for a loading step in pH 5 buffer and elution at pH 9 in a totally aqueous environment.[15,115] Even though the surface area-to-volume ratio of a microchannel is not optimal for performing NA extraction, Wu and associates were able to show 75% extraction efficiencies of DNA from 1.5 μL whole blood.

Polymerase Chain Reaction

Conventional means of performing PCR involve the reaction in a tube, placed in a stationary heating block that thermocycles through desired temperatures. Microfluidic PCR has greatly enhanced this process of conventional PCR by reducing volumes, introducing innovative thermocycling techniques, and allowing for amplification reactions that are limited only by the kinetics of the polymerase. One of the greatest advantages of microchip PCR is the decreased thermocycling times when compared with thermal block. Multiple different approaches have been developed, including infrared-mediated heating,[37,60,121,136] where a lamp is used to selectively heat the solution, and strategies by which thermocycling components are fabricated directly into the microchip, such as titanium/platinum heaters[82,93,190] and Peltier elements.[78] Another approach to thermocycling involves flow through a PCR device that exploits discrete temperature zones in the microdevice, when the PCR master mix solution is fluidically mobilized through different zones to change the temperature of the solution.[48,79,120] Using this strategy, Hashimoto and colleagues[48] were able to amplify 500-bp and 997-bp fragments in 1.7 and 3.2 minutes, respectively; investigators attribute this to the kinetic limit of nucleotide incorporation by *Taq* polymerase.

Integration

One of the long-standing goals in the microfluidic field has been to create a fully integrated device for which all components needed to perform an analysis are included in the microchip. The benefits of a device capable of this are many, ranging from faster analysis times to use of a completely closed system, leading to a decrease in potential sources of contamination. An example of this type of integrated device is the microgenetic analysis (MGA) device described by Easley and coworkers in 2006.[31] In this work, the authors were able to start with a sample—lysed blood or a human nasal aspirate—and perform DNA extraction, amplification, and electrophoretic separation for pathogen identification. Analysis time required for identification of *Bacillus anthracis* was just 24 minutes, and the sample remained completely enclosed in the microfluidic device throughout the entire process. Figure 18-12, *A*, illustrates all three processes: DNA extraction, PCR amplification, and three replicates of electrophoretic separation. Figure 18-12, *B*, shows a zoomed-in image of the electropherogram, illustrating reproducibility of the separation with the desired PCR product highlighted in red and surrounded by a DNA marker for sizing of the fragment. Figure 18-12, *C*, shows the glass microfluidic device encased in the PMMA macrointerface to microinterface; the actual size of the encompassed device is roughly equivalent to a deck of cards. In 2007, another report emerged that could identify bird flu (the H5N1 strain) in a droplet.[129] The authors were able to manipulate the 100-nL droplet through the use of magnetic beads and to isolate viral RNA, followed by ultrafast real-time RT-PCR, with the whole process requiring 28 minutes. This report states that compared with commercially available tests, their assay shows comparable sensitivity and is 440% faster and 2000 to 5000% cheaper.

Integrated microchips capable of genetic analysis have also been developed, with a focus on human genotyping and DNA sequencing. In 2006, Blazej and colleagues reported a bioprocessor microfabricated from glass and PDMS that integrates the three Sanger sequencing steps: amplification, post-PCR sample purification, and electrophoresis, all in one device.[9] They were able to read up to 556 continuous bases with 99% accuracy from only 1 fmol of DNA. The same group also developed a portable microsystem capable of rapid forensic short tandem repeat (STR) typing.[96] In this work, the authors designed both the microchip and a portable instrument capable of PCR thermal cycling, electrophoretic separation, four-color laser excited fluorescence, and fluidic control through the use of pneumatic valves. They showed STR typing of amelogenin (sex-determining marker) and 3 Y chromosome STR loci within 1.5 hours using their microsystem. They reported a limit of detection of 20 copies of male standard DNA in the reactor.

Hybridization Arrays

DNA hybridization arrays are powerful tools that allow for the interrogation of many genes in a single sample. Microarrays consist of slides, typically made from glass or plastic, that have multiple, different short DNA oligonucleotide probes affixed to the surface. The sample can be applied to the array, and through a predetermined detection scheme,

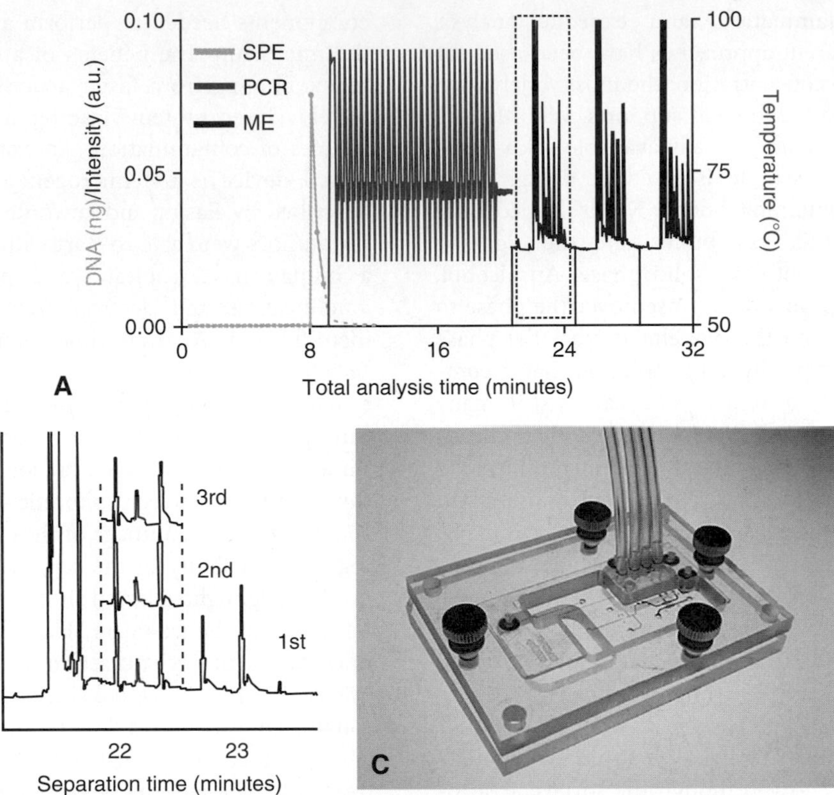

Figure 18-12 Integrated analysis for the detection of *Bacillus anthracis* from blood samples. A, A schematic representing DNA extraction [solid phase extraction (SPE)], polymerase chain reaction (PCR), and microchip electrophoresis (ME), all graphed with respect to time. ME shows three repetitive injections and separations. B, A magnified view of the ME from (A), where the PCR product is highlighted in red and is flanked by a DNA marker for sizing. All three injections and separations are shown. C, A photograph of the glass device enclosed in the polymethylmethacrylate (PMMA) manifold for microinterfacing to macrointerfacing. *(Modified from Easley CJ, Karlinsey JM, Bienvenue JM, Legendre LA, Roper MG, Feldman SH, et al. A fully integrated microfluidic genetic analysis system with sample-in-answer-out capability. Proc Natl Acad Sci U S A 2006;103:19272-7.)*

data can be obtained based on the hybridization of DNA sequences from the sample with those patterned on the slide. This is a very provocative technique that yields a lot of information from just a single sample. To fully understand the potential of this method, please see Chapter 17 by Wittwer for a more in-depth discussion.

PROTEINS

Immunoassays

Protein immunoassays are key to many biochemical analyses, in the clinical arena and in research, and these assays have also been adapted to a microfluidic format. The basic elements of a microfluidic-based immunoassay are the same when compared with a conventional assay, involving a mode for solution transport, a reaction solid phase, and a detection mechanism. One of the biggest differences between the two formats is the size, with conventional assays done in volumes on the order of 50 µL, where microfluidic assays are generally done in volumes less than 1 µL; this leads to a large difference in diffusion rates, which is one of the time-limiting factors in immunoassays. A comparison was performed to evaluate the effects of microtiter and microfluidic formats on diffusion.[138] Figure 18-13 shows a comparative schematic of the two different formats. The authors reported that it required nearly 15 hours for immunoreactions to occur in the microtiter format (Figure 18-13, *A*), while the signal intensity became constant after only 10 minutes in the 100 µm deep microchannel (Figure 18-13, *B*) packed with beads. They credit the decrease in reaction time to a reduction in diffusion distance due to the increased surface area-to-volume ratio. The longest distance that needs to be covered in a microtiter plate is 1.5 mm, whereas that distance is estimated to be less than 20 µm in a bead-packed microchannel. Because diffusion time is equal to the square of the diffusion distance, the time required for the same molecule to diffuse in the bead-packed microchannel is more than 5600 times shorter than in a microtiter plate.

Several microfluidic immunoassays have been used for clinical applications reported in the literature. Herr and

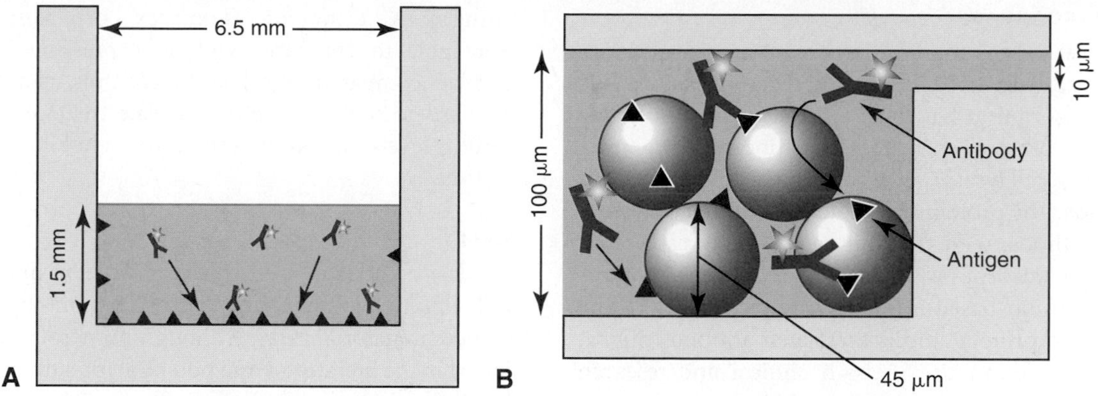

Figure 18-13 Illustration of antigen-antibody interactions in (A) microtiter and (B) microchip formats. *(Reprinted with permission from Sato K, Tokeshi M, Odake T, et al. Integration of an immunosorbent assay system: analysis of secretory human immunoglobulin A on polystyrene beads in a microchip. Anal Chem 2000;72:1144-7.)*

associates[52] demonstrated the use of a microchip-based point-of-care diagnostic immunoassay for the measurement of proteinaceous disease biomarkers in saliva. They evaluated saliva samples from both healthy subjects and those with moderate to severe periodontitis and looked for the detection of matrix metalloproteinase-8 (MMP-8). They performed sample loading, sample enrichment, and rapid diffusive mixing of sample and primary antibody, as well as electrophoretic separations of antibody-sample complexes from the unbound primary antibody—all integrated on the device; the electropherograms from these samples are shown in Figure 18-14, *A*. A linear regression analysis, shown in Figure 18-14, *B*, compares the microchip system versus the commercially available enzyme-linked immunosorbent assay (ELISA). Measurement of MMP-8 was accomplished within 10 minutes, requiring only 20 μL of saliva. Another group developed a microdevice for the immunofluorescent detection of viruses[99] using antibody-coated microbeads for analyte capture and quantum dots for detection. When they compared their device with a conventional ELISA method for detecting the presence of Singapore grouper iridovirus (SGIV), a marine iridovirus, the microfluidic format improved detection sensitivity from 360 ng/mL to 22 ng/mL, decreased detection time to less than 30 minutes, and reduced the quantity of antibodies required by a factor of 14.3. A PMMA device was developed for the detection of biomarkers in serum.[100] In this report, the authors demonstrated the detection of alpha fetoprotein (AFP) in healthy human serum. The microchip consisted of a channel coated with poly(ethyleneimine), containing abundant NH_2 groups to assist in capture of the monoclonal antibody to the channel surface. The sample was flowed through the channel, followed by a horseradish peroxidase–conjugated AFP antibody, and detection was achieved using a three-electrode electrochemical detection system. Investigators reported a detection limit of 1 pg/mL of AFP and a detectable linear concentration range of 1 to 500 pg/mL using their method.

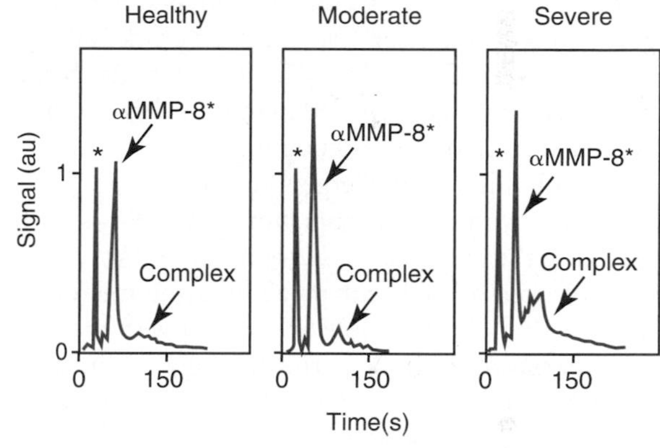

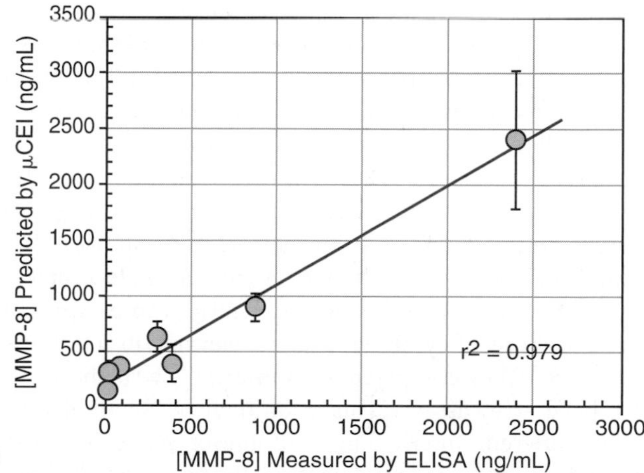

Figure 18-14 Measurement of matrix metalloproteinase (MMP)-8 in saliva. A, μCEI (microchip electrophoretic immunoassay) measurements of MMP-8 from a healthy patient and from patients who have been diagnosed with moderate or severe periodontitis. B, Linear regression analysis comparing the μCEI method versus a commercial enzyme-linked immunosorbent assay (ELISA) for the detection of MMP-8 ($y = 0.91 \times +181.7$, $r^2 = 0.979$). *(Reprinted from Herr AE, Hatch AV, Throckmorton DJ, et al. Microfluidic immunoassays as rapid saliva-based clinical diagnostics. Proc Natl Acad Sci U S A 2007;104:5268-73.)*

Protein Microarrays

In their simplest form, protein microarrays consist of planar substrates affixed with proteins for sample interrogation. This rudimentary description has been expanded over the years, where the term "protein" encompasses antibodies, cytokines, tissue, and whole cell lysates, and "substrate" can include glass and microbeads. The proteins are attached through a number of different methods, with the four most widely used techniques involving adsorption, covalent binding, affinity interaction, and diffusion-based immobilizing techniques.[148] The most widely used protein chip is the planar antibody microarray, which has found use in both clinical and research applications. This involves the immobilization of a few hundred antibodies to capture proteins of interest from a more complex sample. In a report searching for alterations in cell signaling in colon cancer, the authors used a protein microarray with 224 antibodies affixed to the surface to identify altered proteins.[101] They screened soluble protein extracts from tumor biopsies of 11 different patients, all with varying stages of colorectal cancer. Using this experimental approach, the authors were able to identify new potential biomarkers that are preferentially expressed in this cancer. Another group enhanced the microarray by coupling it with microfluidics for immunoglobulin (Ig)E allergen testing.[22] They used glass slides coated with a novel copolymer that allows for immobilization of the allergens in their native conformation. Their fully automated assay is enhanced by using microfluidics to achieve mixing of the sample and serum with the surface of the microarray and can be performed in 25 minutes.

Microbeads provide another format that is used to probe protein and nucleic acid interactions. In this format, the protein is attached to microbeads, such as polystyrene microspheres, and detection can be accomplished through the use of laser-induced fluorescence or color coding of the beads, for example. Microbead-based arrays also allow for multiplexing, where one sample can be probed for multiple analytes, and this is followed by analysis via flow cytometry. When flow cytometry is used for detection, the beads can be discriminated by size using side scatter, or by fluorescence, where each capture protein has a different fluorochrome attached.[111] The ability to analyze multiple analytes from a single sample was demonstrated by Tarnok and colleagues, who evaluated the concentrations of cytokines that are elevated in infections in children.[155] They compared a commercially available fluorescent bead array assay versus traditional ELISA for detection of six different interleukins and tumor necrosis factor-α. Using flow cytometry for detection, the bead array had a calibration range that was 10 times wider when compared with ELISA results, and the authors were able to decrease the amount of blood used by more than 80% for three of the analytes. The authors showed that the bead array performed comparatively with ELISA and offered additional benefits, such as decreased operating time and the ability to multiplex the detection of multiple analytes in one sample. In another example of the usefulness of bead-based arrays, the authors analyzed up to 100 different serum cytokines in a single well in melanoma patients with interferon alpha2b treatment.[189] Using xMAP technology (Luminex Corp, Austin, Tex), they were able to compare cytokine expression in melanoma patients compared with healthy controls using fluorescence as the detection scheme to correlate treatment with altered serum levels of proinflammatory cytokines and growth factors.

Cells

The last decade has seen efforts to develop microchip-based cell culture platforms for performing multiplex culturing and combinatorial assay. Although numerous reports can be found in the literature,[33] the potential for culturing and assaying in the same microdevice offers numerous benefits. For example, Yu and coworkers[187] demonstrated the ability to culture NIH 3T3 fibroblast, B16 melanoma, and HeLa cells and, in a parallel manner, to assay for drug-induced apoptotic responses and demonstrate "on-chip" transfection of a reporter gene, followed by live-cell imaging of transcriptional activation of cyclooxygenase-2 expression. Perhaps more pertinent to this chapter is the ability to use microdevices for the capture of circulating tumor cells (CTCs).

Although this is still open to question, CTCs are emerging as a potential alternative to invasive biopsies as a source of tumor tissue for the detection, characterization, and monitoring of nonhematologic cancers.[110] The number of CTCs is a proven independent predictor of survival in patients with breast, prostate, lung, and colon cancers, and the importance of CTC analysis will continue to grow. The ability to identify, isolate, propagate, and molecularly characterize CTC subpopulations could further the discovery of cancer stem cell biomarkers and expand our understanding of the biology of metastasis. Although it is currently unclear how treatment decisions will be influenced by CTC analysis, or whether patient outcomes will be improved by decisions based on CTC data, the future of CTC analysis appears promising.

The only commercially available technique that is Food and Drug Administration (FDA) approved for CTC isolation is the CellSearch assay (Veridex LLC, Raritan, NJ). This automated, highly reproducible technique has been in use for several years. It utilizes ferrofluid nanoparticles coated with streptavidin and epithelial cell adhesion molecule (EpCAM) antibodies to isolate CTCs and can reliably detect CTCs in approximately 36% of patients with metastatic cancer.[1a] However, microfluidic assays for CTC isolation have begun to emerge from several research groups with the promise that this approach will be more sensitive. Nagrath and associates[114] showed that viable CTCs (i.e., tumor-derived epithelial cells) could be isolated from the whole blood of cancer patients. In this work, the authors flowed samples through an array of microposts coated with anti-EpCAM antibodies. Device characterization experiments determined a calculated capture efficiency of 65% using non–small cell lung carcinoma cells spiked into phosphate buffered saline (PBS). Peripheral blood samples from 116 patients with metastatic lung, prostate, pancreatic, breast, and colon cancers were analyzed, and CTCs were identified in 115 (99%) samples. More recently, Tan and colleagues[153] presented a label-free microdevice capable of isolating cancer cells from whole blood based on physical properties (size and deformability) that are discriminators. The authors fabricated crescent-shaped isolation wells to act as a sieve, capturing the larger tumor cells (approximately 17 μm) in contrast to erythrocytes and leukocytes, whose cell diameters can range from 8 to 25 μm, yet their deformable nature lets them traverse capillaries that are 2 to 5 μm in diameter. Using breast and colon cancer cells, they showed an isolation efficiency of ≈80%. Soper and colleagues[1b] used plastic (PMMA) microdevices to isolate a small number of CTCs also using antibodies against EpCAM. They sampled milliliter input volumes of whole blood in less than 40 minutes and showed the capture of CTCs in small volumes (several hundred nanoliters) that could be detected with an integrated conductivity sensor following release from the capture surface. The highly quantitative (>97%) recovery of CTCs directly from whole blood by capture channels points to microfluidic devices as the next generation of devices to supplant CellSearch-type assays.

In a completely orthogonal approach with a different application, Lenshof and coworkers[88] reported the use of an acoustophoresis-based separation microchip to prepare plasma from whole blood for clinical applications. This work derived from earlier work from this group, in which they had used acoustic energy transduced to the microchannel from a piezo interfaced with the chip in a microfluidic system to cleanse blood of fat microglobules contaminating filtrate during open thorax surgery.[72] In that application, investigators exploited ultrasounds to set up standing acoustic waves (Figure 18-15, *B*) in the microfluidic channel, which augmented the

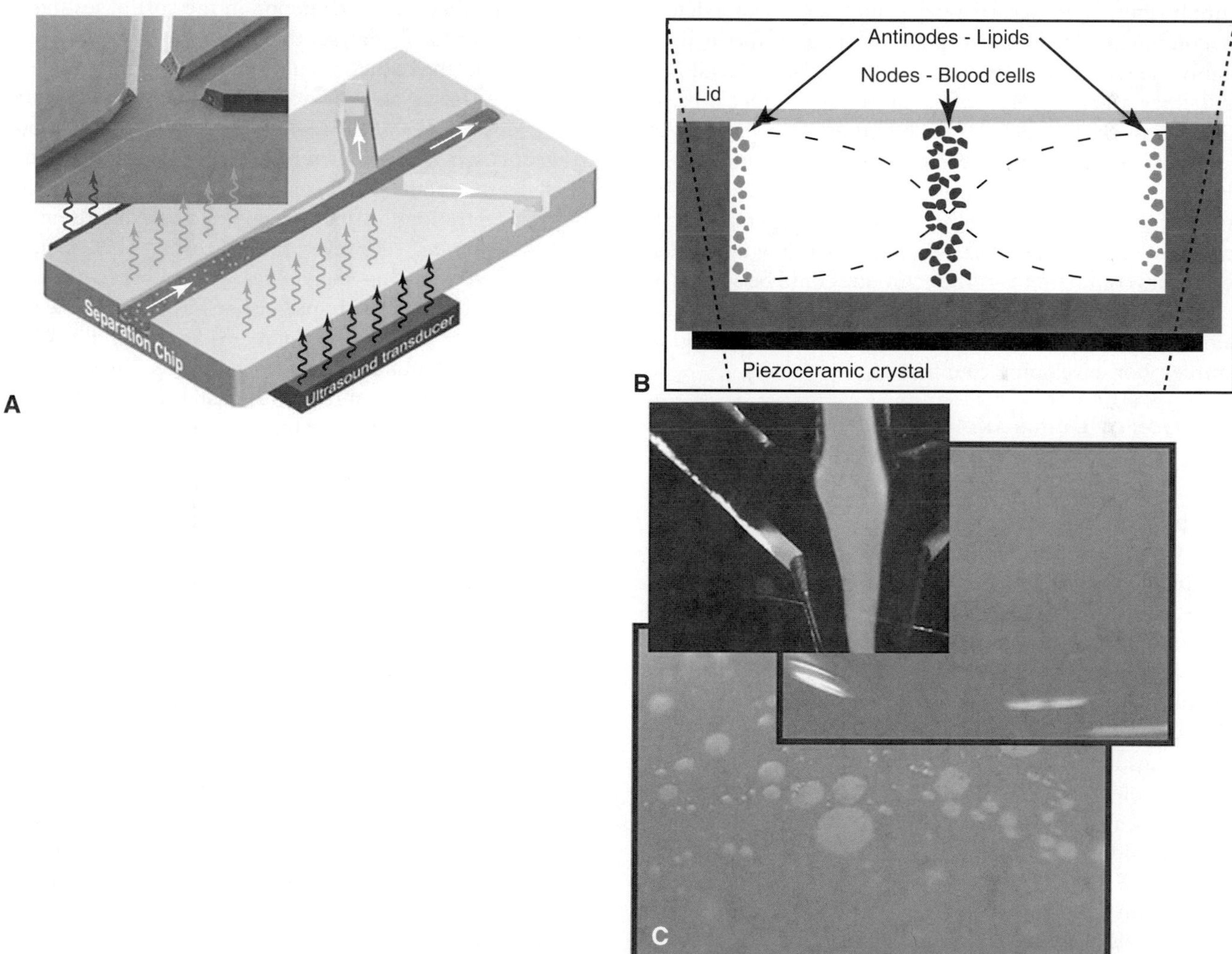

Figure 18-15 Cell-particle separation using standing acoustic waves. A, An illustration of the device, showing the flow of erythrocytes. B, A schematic of the acoustic standing wave, where the less compressible particles with higher density (erythrocytes) migrate to the nodes, and the lipid emboli move to the antinodes. C, The three panels show still images of the blood before *(bottom image)* and after *(middle image)* processing by the device. The lipid particles that are evident before *(bottom image)* are not visible after *(middle image)* the microfluidic separation. The *top image* shows an image of the chip during the separation, where the erythrocytes can be seen in the middle of the channel and the lipid particles are seen as white patch on the side of the channel. *(Reprinted from Jonsson H, Holm C, Nilsson A, Petersson F, Johnsson P, Laurell T. Particle separation using ultrasound can radically reduce embolic load to brain after cardiac surgery. Ann Thorac Surg 2004;78:1572-7.)*

flow of particles in a size-dependent way (also affected by density and compressibility). In a manner amenable to handling hundreds of milliliters per hour of pericardial blood during surgery, they showed that lipid particles purported to be associated with microembolisms could be cleansed from the blood (Figure 18-15, *C*). The Lenshof group[88] sought to remove cells in a single flow-through step process to yield high-quality plasma of low cellular content, in contrast to purifying them through a multistep process. They not only demonstrated that the plasma generated by the method meets European standard requirements for plasma in terms of the number of erythrocytes per liter ($<6.0 \times 10^{-9}$), they also successfully linked the plasmapheresis microchip to an antibody microarray chip for prostate-specific antigen (PSA) detection.

Wang and coworkers[172] used a PDMS chip to count CD4+ T lymphocytes in a microchannel. Using fluorescence detection combined with resistive pulse sensing mediated by a metal oxide semiconductor field effect transistor (MOSFET) signal, they were able to define the total number of cells passing through the channel, while fluorescence was used to detect cells tagged with a specific fluorophore. The CD4+ T cells counted and the percentage of total lymphocytes determined by the chip-based method showed comparable accuracy with data obtained with a commercial flow cytometer. The authors comment that this technique could be applied to the diagnosis of human immunodeficiency virus (HIV) and could greatly reduce the cost, making it more accessible to resource-poor developing countries.

Detection of Drugs and Drug Metabolites

The advent of rapid and simple analytical systems in the early 1990s set the stage for what point-of-care-testing platforms would bring to clinical diagnostics. In 1992, Biosite Inc (San Diego, Calif) released the Triage Drugs of Abuse Panel for the rapid detection of amphetamines/methamphetamines, cocaine, opiates, phencyclidine, and tetrahydrocannabinol.[13] This event preceded release of a similar kit in which acetaminophen, barbiturates, benzodiazepines, methadone, propoxyphene, and tricyclic antidepressants were detected via the Triage TOX Drug Screen (Biosite Inc). Assays for therapeutic drugs or drugs of abuse that employ chemistries that are deployable on-site are simple to use from raw sample (e.g., urine), are single-use and disposable, and highlight the need for microfluidic systems capable of rapid, information-rich analysis.

Thormann and coworkers[168] were the first to demonstrate the use of electrophoretic microdevices for drug analysis, showing that serum theophylline could be measured using micellar electrokinetic chromatography to carry out an immunoassay on microchip. Henion's group,[24] having pioneered effective microfabricated interfaces between microchip and mass spectrometer, demonstrated that imipramine and desipramine could be quantitated in human plasma. Similarly, Locascio and associates[69] used plastic microdevices (both copolyester and PDMS) for drug screening and residue analysis of barbiturates and phenobarbital, exploiting an on-board affinity preconcentration step. The problem with these assays is that no device has yet been produced that meets the requirements of "user friendliness" for the busy clinical laboratory or the rigid specifications demanded for recording quality assurance data.

LIMITATIONS OF MICROFLUIDIC SYSTEMS

Challenges in developing mass-producible microfluidic devices that can enhance productivity in the clinical chemistry laboratory are ongoing. First and foremost, integrated microfluidic systems with *sample-in-answer-out* capabilities are required to avoid generating devices that only incrementally improve part of the overall analytical process; these devices need to be not only robust in performance but turnkey in operation. Second, small volumes that lie at the heart of microfluidics offer a reduction in the cost of testing over more conventional analyses that use larger reagent volumes. For example, the reduction in master mix volume needed for PCR in an integrated microfluidic system (reduced from 25 μL down to 500 nL) represents a 50-fold reduction in reagent costs.[31] A report from the Yager Laboratory demonstrated a microfluidic T-mixer capable of measuring phenytoin concentrations in blood samples using less than 1 μL within 1 minute.[49] However, the microscale also extends to small sample volume capabilities, typically in the tens of microliters. Although this may be fine for some clinical applications, others require the microdevices to handle volumes ranging from hundreds of microliters to as much as several milliliters (testing for minimal residual disease), while forensic applications may require the concentration and detection of hundreds of milliliters of sample (e.g., food safety). It is in this respect that *large-volume reduction strategies* will be needed to concentrate the analytes of interest from large-volume samples into volumes that can be processed by the chip. The acoustic-based approaches described are ideal for cell and particle concentrations from larger volumes,[72] and chip-based methods for extracting nucleic acids from milliliter volume samples are being developed.[133] Third, new approaches to *fluidic control* on microdevices need to be devised. Although developments since 2000 have revolutionized microfluidic systems, allowing very different chemistries on the device to be chemically isolated yet fluidically connected via mechanical valves,[40,163] novel, compact valving strategies that minimize external hardware are needed. Leslie and associates[89] have shown that passive fluidic control elements may present the possibility of flow control without valve actuation, relying solely on frequency-specific pumping for control of flow. Fourth, although microfabrication of devices in glass once dominated the analytical microchip landscape, other chip substrates need to be explored. Polymeric substrates (e.g., PDMS, PMMA) are becoming increasingly popular and likely represent the future. The ability to hot emboss microfluidic structures in plastic substrates presents a direct path to the inexpensive, single-use, disposable microdevices that will be a must for adoption in clinical testing. Fifth, and finally, engineering of the hardware, firmware, and software needs serious engagement in a collaborative effort with analytical chemists (who develop the "chemware") to define benchtop instrumentation amenable to turn-key operation by unskilled operators. Only then will rugged and "portable" instrumentation be developed with robust performance capabilities, and this will lay the groundwork for miniaturization of the instrument to hand-held, personal digital assistant (PDA)-like devices that will perform total biochemical analysis.

FUTURE OF MICROFLUIDICS IN CLINICAL DIAGNOSTICS

The barrier to implementing new technology in the clinical diagnostics sector is palpable, not because of lack of "need," but because competition is fierce, the sector is dominated by a handful of behemoth multinationals, and the profit margins are small. Although "need" should drive the development of new technologies, such as microfluidics, other driving forces often factor in. It is interesting when one views this retrospectively and outside the realm of "sector needs." A precedent has been established for national security applications to provide a large, powerful driving force for technology development. This is supported by historical recapitulation of the development of microelectronics, which was driven largely by the race-to-space and by military/civil needs. World War II drove the development of electronic circuits that were substantially smaller in size, weight, and power consumption, especially for implementation in aircraft. Layered on top of this was the need for NASA to have smaller, lightweight, more powerful circuits for the space-limited spacecraft that were evolving. Similarly, computer science and computer engineering were shaped by military funding of the early stages of digital computing, during which most of the basic technologies for digital computing were developed through a program focused on the development of an automated radar shield. It is not beyond the realm of possibility that the clinical sector will be the recipient of analytical microfluidic technology as a result of the development of *biowarfare detection* systems. This area saw serious capital investment come into play with the advent of 9/11 and can experience a fast track to market because it circumnavigates the FDA 510(k) approval process.

In addition, the focus on *personalized medicine* appears to be ever increasing—something that may be inevitable as we witness the aging of an educated population (i.e., baby boomers). The shift away from the passive role that the patient has traditionally played in the management of his or her health care to one that is more preemptive or active, even proactive, at some point will present new markets of opportunity to the diagnostic testing community. Microfluidic platforms may well play a significant role in making clinical testing more personalized. It is not unreasonable to envision the availability of self-test molecular diagnostic kits that allow a patient to do a rapid (and affordable) screen for the current flu season virus before incurring the costs associated with a weekend visit to the Emergency Room. Certainly, multiple technical challenges will have to be addressed before such visions can ever become a reality. Thorough validation and FDA approval will be required; although lengthy and arduous, these processes should not be insurmountable. A number of major bona fide issues are tethered to the technology, but the demonstrated advantages made possible by the field of microfluidics make it one likely vehicle to take us into an era where the term *personalized medicine* is not nebulous but, in fact, is commonplace. All that remains to be seen is whether the ethical, personal, societal, and political issues are adequately addressed.

REFERENCES

1. Atha DH, Wenz H-M, Morehead H, Tian J, O'Connell CD. Detection of p53 point mutations by single strand conformation polymorphism: analysis by capillary electrophoresis. Electrophoresis 1998;19:172-9.

1a. Adams AA, Okagbare PI, Feng J, Hupert ML, Patterson D, Göttert J, et al. Highly efficient circulating tumor cell isolation from whole blood and label-free enumeration using polymer-based microfluidics with an integrated conductivity sensor. J Am Chem Soc 2008;130:8633-41.

1b. Allard WJ, Matera J, Miller MC, Repollet M, Connelly MC, Rao C, et al. Tumor cells circulate in the peripheral blood of all major carcinomas but not in healthy subjects or patients with nonmalignant diseases. Clin Cancer Res 2004;10:6897-904.

2. Backhouse C, Caamano M, Oaks F, Nordman E, Carrillo A, Johnson B, et al. DNA sequencing in a monolithic microchannel device. Electrophoresis 2000;21:150-6.
3. Balagadde FK, You L, Hansen CL, Arnold FH, Quake SR. Long-term monitoring of bacteria undergoing programmed population control in a microchemostat. Science 2005;309:137-40.
4. Barta C, Ronai Z, Nemoda Z, Szekely A, Kovacs E, Sasvari-Szekely M, et al. Analysis of dopamine D4 receptor gene polymorphism using microchip electrophoresis. J Chromatogr A 2001;924:285-90.
5. Becker H, Gartner C. Polymer microfabrication methods for microfluidic analytical applications. Electrophoresis 2000;21:12-26.
6. Becker H, Locascio LE. Polymer microfluidic devices. Talanta 2002;56:267-87.
7. Belloy E, Pawlowski AG, Sayah A, Gijs MAM. Microfabrication of high-aspect ratio and complex monolithic structures in glass. J Microelectromech S 2002;11:521-7.
8. Bienvenue JM, Duncalf N, Marchiarullo D, Ferrance JP, Landers JP. Microchip-based cell lysis and DNA extraction from sperm cells for application to forensic analysis. J Forensic Sci 2006;51:266-73.
9. Blazej RG, Kumaresan P, Mathies RA. Microfabricated bioprocessor for integrated nanoliter-scale Sanger DNA sequencing. Proc Natl Acad Sci U S A 2006;103:7240-5.
10. Blom MT, Chmela E, Oosterbroek RE, Tijssen R, van den Berg A. On-chip hydrodynamic chromatography separation and detection of nanoparticles and biomolecules. Anal Chem 2003;75:6761-8.
11. Bousse L, Mouradian S, Minalla A, Yee H, Williams K, Dubrow R. Protein sizing on a microchip. Anal Chem 2001;73:1207-12.
12. Breadmore MC, Wolfe KA, Arcibal IG, Leung WK, Dickson D, Giordano BC, et al. Microchip-based purification of DNA from biological samples. Anal Chem 2003;75:1880-6.
13. Buechler KF, Moi S, Noar B, McGrath D, Villela J, Clancy M, et al. Simultaneous detection of seven drugs of abuse by the Triage panel for drugs of abuse. Clin Chem 1992;38:1678-84.
14. Cantàfora A, Blotta I, Bruzzese N, Calandra S, Bertolini S. Rapid sizing of microsatellite alleles by gel electrophoresis on microfabricated channels: application to the D19S394 tetranucleotide repeat for cosegregation study of familial hypercholesterolemia. Electrophoresis 2001;22:4012-5.
15. Cao W, Easley CJ, Ferrance JP, Landers JP. Chitosan as a polymer for pH-induced DNA capture in a totally aqueous system. Anal Chem 2006;78:7222-8.

16. Ceriotti L, Weible K, de Rooij NF, Verpoorte E. Rectangular channels for lab-on-a-chip applications. Microelectron Eng 2003;67:865-71.
17. Chiem N, Lockyear-Shultz L, Andersson P, Skinner C, Harrison DJ. Room temperature bonding of micromachined glass devices for capillary electrophoresis. Sensor Actuat B Chem 2000;63:147-52.
18. Chowdhury J, Kagiala GV, Pushpakom S, Lauzon J, Makin A, Atrazhev A, et al. Microfluidic platform for single nucleotide polymorphism genotyping of the thiopurine S-methyltransferase gene to evaluate risk for adverse drug events. J Mol Diagn 2007;9:521-9.
19. Christel LA, Petersen K, McMillan W, Northrup MA. Rapid, automated nucleic acid probe assays using silicon microstructures for nucleic acid concentration. J Biomech Eng 1999;121:22-7.
20. Coltro WK, da Silva JA, da Silva HD, Richter EM, Furlan R, Angnes L, et al. Electrophoresis microchip fabricated by a direct-printing process with end-channel amperometric detection. Electrophoresis 2004;25:3832-9.
21. Coltro WK, Lunte SM, Carrilho E. Comparison of the analytical performance of electrophoresis microchannels fabricated in PDMS, glass, and polyester-toner. Electrophoresis 2008;29:4928-37.
22. Cretich M, Di Carlo G, Giudici C, Pokoj S, Lauer I, Scheurer S, et al. Detection of allergen specific immunoglobulins by microarrays coupled to microfluidics. Proteomics 2009;9:2098-107.
23. Deng Y, Henion J, Li J, Thibault P, Wang C, Harrison DJ. Chip-based capillary electrophoresis/mass spectrometry determination of carnitines in human urine. Anal Chem 2001;73:639-46.
24. Deng Y, Zhang H, Henion J. Chip-based quantitative capillary electrophoresis/mass spectrometry determination of drugs in human plasma. Anal Chem 2001;73:1432-9.
25. Do J, Lee S, Han J, Kai J, Hong CC, Gao C, et al. Development of functional lab-on-a-chip on polymer for point-of-care testing of metabolic parameters. Lab Chip 2008;8:2113-20.
26. do Lago CL, da Silva HD, Neves CA, Brito-Neto JG, da Silva JA. A dry process for production of microfluidic devices based on the lamination of laser-printed polyester films. Anal Chem 2003;75:3853-8.
27. Duffy DC, McDonald JC, Schueller OJA, Whitesides GM. Rapid prototyping of microfluidic systems in poly(dimethylsiloxane). Anal Chem 1998;70:4974-84.
28. Duggan MP, McCreedy T, Aylott JW. A non-invasive analysis method for on-chip spectrophotometric detection using liquid-core waveguiding within a 3D architecture. Analyst 2003;128:1336-40.
29. Dumitrescu OR, Baker DC, Foster GM, Evans KE. Near infrared spectroscopy for in-line monitoring during injection moulding. Polymer Testing 2005;24:367-75.
30. Easley CJ. Development and application of microfluidic genetic analysis systems. Charlottesville: University of Virginia, 2006.
31. Easley CJ, Karlinsey JM, Bienvenue JM, Legendre LA, Roper MG, Feldman SH, et al. A fully integrated microfluidic genetic analysis system with sample-in-answer-out capability. Proc Natl Acad Sci U S A 2006;103:19272-7.
32. Easley CJ, Karlinsey JM, Landers JP. On-chip pressure injection for integration of infrared-mediated DNA amplification with electrophoretic separation. Lab Chip 2006;6:601-10.
33. El-Ali J, Sorger PK, Jensen KF. Cells on chips. Nature 2006;442:403-11.
34. Emrich CA, Tian H, Medintz IL, Mathies RA. Microfabricated 384-lane capillary array electrophoresis bioanalyzer for ultrahigh-throughput genetic analysis. Anal Chem 2002;74:5076-83.
35. Fanguy JC, Henry CS. The analysis of uric acid in urine using microchip capillary electrophoresis with electrochemical detection. Electrophoresis 2002;23:767-73.
36. Footz T, Somerville MJ, Tomaszewski R, Sprysak KA, Backhouse CJ. Heteroduplex-based genotyping with microchip electrophoresis and dHPLC. Genetic Testing 2003;7:283-93.
37. Giordano BC, Ferrance J, Swedberg S, Huhmer AF, Landers JP. Polymerase chain reaction in polymeric microchips: DNA amplification in less than 240 seconds. Anal Biochem 2001;291:124-32.
38. Giordano BC, Jin LJ, Couch AJ, Ferrance JP, Landers JP. Microchip laser-induced fluorescence detection of proteins at submicrogram per milliliter levels mediated by dynamic labeling under pseudonative conditions. Anal Chem 2004;76:4705-14.
39. Grover WH, Mathies RA. An integrated microfluidic processor for single nucleotide polymorphism-based DNA computing. Lab Chip 2005;5:1033-40.
40. Grover WH, Skelley AM, Liu CN, Lagally ET, Mathies RA. Monolithic membrane valves and diaphragm pumps for practical large-scale integration into glass microfluidic devices. Sensor Actuat B Chem 2003;89:315-23.
41. Guihen E, Glennon JD. Rapid separation of antimicrobial metabolites by microchip electrophoresis with UV linear imaging detection. J Chromatogr A 2005;1071:223-8.
42. Guillo C, Karlinsey JM, Landers JP. On-chip pumping for pressure mobilization of the focused zones following microchip isoelectric focusing. Lab Chip 2007;7:112-8.
43. Hamarman S, Fossella J, Ulger C, Brimacombe M, Dermody J. Dopamine receptor 4 (DRD4) 7-repeat allele predicts methylphenidate dose response in children with attention deficit hyperactivity disorder: a pharmacogenetic study. J Child Adolesc Psychopharmacol 2004;14:564-74.
44. Han J, Singh AK. Rapid protein separations in ultra-short microchannels: microchip sodium dodecyl sulfate-polyacrylamide gel electrophoresis and isoelectric focusing. J Chromatogr A 2004;1049:205-9.
45. Hansen CL, Skordalakes E, Berger JM, Quake SR. A robust and scalable microfluidic metering method that allows protein crystal growth by free interface diffusion. Proc Natl Acad Sci U S A 2002;99:16531-6.
46. Harrison DJ, Fluri K, Seiler K, Fan ZH, Effenhauser CS, Manz A. Micromachining a miniaturized capillary electrophoresis-based chemical-analysis system on a chip. Science 1993;261:895-7.
47. Harrison DJ, Manz A, Fan ZH, Ludi H, Widmer HM. Capillary electrophoresis and sample injection systems integrated on a planar glass chip. Anal Chem 1992;64:1926-32.
48. Hashimoto M, Chen PC, Mitchell MW, Nikitopoulos DE, Soper SA, Murphy MC. Rapid PCR in a continuous flow device. Lab Chip 2004;4:638-45.
49. Hatch A, Kamholz AE, Hawkins KR, Munson MS, Schilling EA, Weigl BH, et al. A rapid diffusion immunoassay in a T-sensor. Nat Biotechnol 2001;19:461-5.
50. He B, Tait N, Regnier F. Fabrication of nanocolumns for liquid chromatography. Anal Chem 1998;70:3790-7.
51. Hernandez L, Escalona J, Joshi N, Guzman N. Laser-induced fluorescence and fluorescence microscopy for capillary electrophoresis zone detection. J Chromatogr 1991;559:183-96.
52. Herr AE, Hatch AV, Throckmorton DJ, Tran HM, Brennan JS, Giannobile WV, et al. Microfluidic immunoassays as rapid saliva-based clinical diagnostics. Proc Natl Acad Sci U S A 2007;104:5268-73.
53. Hestekin CN, Jakupciak JP, Chiesl TN, Kan CW, O'Connell CD, Barron AE. An optimized microchip electrophoresis system for mutation detection by tandem SSCP and heteroduplex analysis for p53 gene exons 5-9. Electrophoresis 2006;27:3823-35.
54. Hibara A, Saito T, Kim HB, Tokeshi M, Ooi T, Nakao M, et al. Nanochannels on a fused-silica microchip and liquid properties investigation by time-resolved fluorescence measurements. Anal Chem 2002;74:6170-6.
55. Hofmann O, Miller P, Sullivan P, Jones TS, deMello JC, Bradley DDC, et al. Thin-film organic photodiodes as integrated detectors for microscale chemiluminescence assays. Sensor Actuat B Chem 2005;106:878-84.
56. Hong JW, Studer V, Hang G, Anderson WF, Quake SR. A nanoliter-scale nucleic acid processor with parallel architecture. Nat Biotechnol 2004;22:435-9.
57. Howlader MMR, Suehara S, Suga T. Room temperature wafer level glass/glass bonding. Sensor Actuat A Phys 2006;127:31-6.

58. Huang Z, Munro N, Huhmer AF, Landers JP. Acousto-optical deflection-based laser beam scanning for fluorescence detection on multichannel electrophoretic microchips. Anal Chem 1999;71:5309-14.
59. Huang ZL, Sanders JC, Dunsmor C, Ahmadzadeh H, Landers JP. A method for UV-bonding in the fabrication of glass electrophoretic microchips. Electrophoresis 2001;22:3924-9.
60. Huhmer AF, Landers JP. Noncontact infrared-mediated thermocycling for effective polymerase chain reaction amplification of DNA in nanoliter volumes. Anal Chem 2000;72:5507-12.
61. Ionescu RE, Marks RS, Gheber LA. Manufacturing of nanochannels with controlled dimensions using protease nanolithography. Nano Lett 2005;5:821-7.
62. Ionescu RE, Marks RS, Gheber LA. Nanolithography using protease etching of protein surfaces. Nano Lett 2003;3:1639-42.
63. Ito T, Sobue K, Ohya S. Water glass bonding for micro-total analysis system. Sensor Actuat B Chem 2002;81:187-95.
64. Jabasini M, Ewis AA, Fouad M, Dang F, Ping G, Shinka T, et al. Rapid multiplexing and simultaneous detection of human spermatogenetic failure with a 12 lane microchip electrophoresis system. Biol Pharm Bull 2006;29:1487-9.
65. Jacobson SC, Hergenroder R, Koutny LB, Warmack RJ, Ramsey JM. Effects of injection schemes and column geometry on the performance of microchip electrophoresis devices. Anal Chem 1994;66:1107-13.
66. Jacobson SC, Koutny LB, Hergenroder R, Moore AW, Ramsey JM. Microchip capillary electrophoresis with an integrated postcolumn reactor. Anal Chem 1994;66:3472-6.
67. Jia ZJ, Fang Q, Fang ZL. Bonding of glass microfluidic chips at room temperatures. Anal Chem 2004;76:5597-602.
68. Jiang G, Harrison DJ. mRNA isolation in a microfluidic device for eventual integration of cDNA library construction. Analyst 2000; 125:2176-9.
69. Jiang Y, Wang PC, Locascio LE, Lee CS. Integrated plastic microfluidic devices with ESI-MS for drug screening and residue analysis. Anal Chem 2001;73:2048-53.
70. Jin LJ, Giordano BC, Landers JP. Dynamic labeling during capillary or microchip electrophoresis for laser-induced fluorescence detection of protein-SDS complexes without pre- or postcolumn labeling. Anal Chem 2001;73:4994-9.
71. Johnson ME, Landers JP. Fundamentals and practice for ultrasensitive laser-induced fluorescence detection in microanalytical systems. Electrophoresis 2004;25:3513-27.
72. Jonsson H, Holm C, Nilsson A, Petersson F, Johnsson P, Laurell T. Particle separation using ultrasound can radically reduce embolic load to brain after cardiac surgery. Ann Thorac Surg 2004;78:1572-7.
73. Kameoka J, Craighead HG, Zhang H, Henion J. A polymeric microfluidic chip for CE/MS determination of small molecules. Anal Chem 2001;73:1935-41.
74. Kanda V, Kariuki JK, Harrison DJ, McDermott MT. Label-free reading of microarray-based immunoassays with surface plasmon resonance imaging. Anal Chem 2004;76:7257-62.
75. Karlinsey JM, Landers JP. AOTF-based multicolor fluorescence detection for short tandem repeat (STR) analysis in an electrophoretic microdevice. Lab Chip 2008;8:1285-91.
76. Karlinsey JM, Landers JP. Multicolor fluorescence detection on an electrophoretic microdevice using an acoustooptic tunable filter. Anal Chem 2006;78:5590-6.
77. Karlinsey JM, Monahan J, Marchiarullo DJ, Ferrance JP, Landers JP. Pressure injection on a valved microdevice for electrophoretic analysis of submicroliter samples. Anal Chem 2005;77:3637-43.
78. Khandurina J, McKnight TE, Jacobson SC, Waters LC, Foote RS, Ramsey JM. Integrated system for rapid PCR-based DNA analysis in microfluidic devices. Anal Chem 2000;72:2995-3000.
79. Kopp MU, Mello AJ, Manz A. Chemical amplification: continuous-flow PCR on a chip. Science 1998;280:1046-8.
80. Kricka LJ, Fortina P, Panaro NJ, Wilding P, Alonso-Amigo G, Becker H. Fabrication of plastic microchips by hot embossing. Lab Chip 2002;2:1-4.
81. Laemmli UK. Cleavage of structural proteins during the assembly of the head of bacteriophage T4. Nature 1970;227:680-5.
82. Lagally ET, Scherer JR, Blazej RG, Toriello NM, Diep BA, Ramchandani M, et al. Integrated portable genetic analysis microsystem for pathogen/infectious disease detection. Anal Chem 2004;76:3162-70.
83. Landers JP. Introduction to capillary electrophoresis. In: Landers JP, ed. Handbook of capillary and microchip electrophoresis and associated microtechniques, 3rd edition. Boca Raton, Fla: CRC Press, 2008:3-74.
84. Lee CC, Sui G, Elizarov A, Shu CJ, Shin YS, Dooley AN, et al. Multistep synthesis of a radiolabeled imaging probe using integrated microfluidics. Science 2005;310:1793-6.
85. Legendre L, Leslie D, Morris C, Barron AE, McClure R, Landers JP. A fully integrated microfluidic genetic analysis device for the detection of blood cancers. Paris: MicroTas, 2007.
86. Legendre LA, Bienvenue JM, Roper MG, Ferrance JP, Landers JP. A simple, valveless microfluidic sample preparation device for extraction and amplification of DNA from nanoliter-volume samples. Anal Chem 2006;78:1444-51.
87. Legendre LA, Ferrance JP, Landers JP. Microfluidic devices for electrophoretic separations: fabrication and use. In: Landers JP, ed. The handbook of capillary and microchip electrophoresis and associated microtechniques, 3rd edition. Boca Raton, Fla: CRC Press, 2008:335-58.
88. Lenshof A, Ahmad-Tajudin A, Jaras K, Sward-Nilsson AM, Aberg L, Marko-Varga G, et al. Acoustic whole blood plasmapheresis chip for prostate specific antigen microarray diagnostics. Anal Chem 2009;81:6030-7.
89. Leslie DC, Easley CJ, Seker E, Karlinsey JM, Utz M, Begley MR, et al. Frequency-specific flow control in microfluidic circuits with passive elastomeric features. Nature Physics 2009;5:231-5.
90. Li Y, DeVoe DL, Lee CS. Dynamic analyte introduction and focusing in plastic microfluidic devices for proteomic analysis. Electrophoresis 2003;24:193-9.
91. Liang Z, Chiem N, Ocvirk G, Tang T, Fluri K, Harrison DJ. Microfabrication of a planar absorbance and fluorescence cell for integrated capillary electrophoresis devices. Anal Chem 1996;68: 1040-6.
92. Lin CH, Lee GB, Chang BW, Chang GL. A new fabrication process for ultra-thick microfluidic microstructures utilizing SU-8 photoresist. J Micromech Microeng 2002;12:590-7.
93. Liu CN, Toriello NM, Mathies RA. Multichannel PCR-CE microdevice for genetic analysis. Anal Chem 2006;78:5474-9.
94. Liu J, Enzelberger M, Quake S. A nanoliter rotary device for polymerase chain reaction. Electrophoresis 2002;23:1531-6.
95. Liu P, Mathies RA. Integrated microfluidic systems for high-performance genetic analysis. Trends Biotechnol 2009;27: 572-81.
96. Liu P, Seo TS, Beyor N, Shin KJ, Scherer JR, Mathies RA. Integrated portable polymerase chain reaction-capillary electrophoresis microsystem for rapid forensic short tandem repeat typing. Anal Chem 2007;79:1881-9.
97. Liu SR, Ren HJ, Gao QF, Roach DJ, Loder RT, Armstrong TM, et al. Automated parallel DNA sequencing on multiple channel microchips. Proc Natl Acad Sci U S A 2000;97:5369-74.
98. Liu SR, Shi YN, Ja WW, Mathies RA. Optimization of high-speed DNA sequencing on microfabricated capillary electrophoresis channels. Anal Chem 1999;71:566-73.
99. Liu WT, Zhu L, Qin QW, Zhang Q, Feng H, Ang S. Microfluidic device as a new platform for immunofluorescent detection of viruses. Lab Chip 2005;5:1327-30.
100. Liu Y, Wang H, Huang J, Yang J, Liu B, Yang P. Microchip-based ELISA strategy for the detection of low-level disease biomarker in serum. Anal Chim Acta 2009;650:77-82.
101. Madoz-Gurpide J, Canamero M, Sanchez L, Solano J, Alfonso P, Casal JI. A proteomics analysis of cell signaling alterations in colorectal cancer. Mol Cell Proteomics 2007;6:2150-64.

102. Malcik N, Ferrance JP, Landers JP, Caglar P. The performance of a microchip-based fiber optic detection technique for the determination of Ca2+ ions in urine. Sensor Actuat B Chem 2005;107:24-31.
103. Manage D, Zheng Y, Somerville M, Backhouse C. On-chip HA/SSCP for the detection of hereditary haemochromatosis. Microfluidics and Nanofluidics 2005;1:364-72.
104. Manz A, Graber N, Widmer HM. Miniaturized total chemical analysis systems: a novel concept for chemical sensing. Sensor Actuat B Chem 1990;1:244-8.
105. Manz A, Harrison DJ, Verpoorte EM, Fettinger JC, Paulus A, Ludi H, et al. Planar chips technology for miniaturization and integration of separation techniques into monitoring systems: capillary electrophoresis on a chip. J Chromatogr 1992;593:253-8.
106. McDonald JC, Duffy DC, Anderson JR, Chiu DT, Wu H, Schueller OJ, et al. Fabrication of microfluidic systems in poly(dimethylsiloxane). Electrophoresis 2000;21:27-40.
107. Medintz I, Wong WW, Sensabaugh G, Mathies RA. High speed single nucleotide polymorphism typing of a hereditary haemochromatosis mutation with capillary array electrophoresis microplates. Electrophoresis 2000;21:2352-8.
108. Mogensen KB, Eriksson F, Gustafsson O, Nikolajsen RP, Kutter JP. Pure-silica optical waveguides, fiber couplers, and high-aspect ratio submicrometer channels for electrokinetic separation devices. Electrophoresis 2004;25:3788-95.
109. Mogensen KB, Kwok YC, Eijkel JCT, Petersen NJ, Manz A, Kutter JP. A Microfluidic device with an integrated waveguide beam splitter for velocity measurements of flowing particles by Fourier transformation. Anal Chem 2003;75:4931-6.
110. Molnar B, Sipos F, Galamb O, Tulassay Z. Molecular detection of circulating cancer cells: role in diagnosis, prognosis and follow-up of colon cancer patients. Dig Dis 2003;21:320-5.
111. Morgan E, Varro R, Sepulveda H, Ember JA, Apgar J, Wilson J, et al. Cytometric bead array: a multiplexed assay platform with applications in various areas of biology. Clin Immunol 2004;110:252-66.
112. Munro NJ, Huang Z, Finegold DN, Landers JP. Indirect fluorescence detection of amino acids on electrophoretic microchips. Anal Chem 2000;72:2765-73.
113. Munro NJ, Snow K, Kant JA, Landers JP. Molecular diagnostics on microfabricated electrophoretic devices: from slab gel- to capillary- to microchip-based assays for T- and B-cell lymphoproliferative disorders. Clin Chem 1999;45:1906-17.
114. Nagrath S, Sequist LV, Maheswaran S, Bell DW, Irimia D, Ulkus L, et al. Isolation of rare circulating tumour cells in cancer patients by microchip technology. Nature 2007;450:1235-9.
115. Nakagawa T, Tanaka T, Niwa D, Osaka T, Takeyama H, Matsunaga T. Fabrication of amino silane-coated microchip for DNA extraction from whole blood. J Biotechnol 2005;116:105-11.
116. Nasedkina TV, Fedorova OE, Glotov AS, Chupova NV, Samochatova EV, Maiorova OA, et al. Rapid genotyping of common deficient thiopurine S-methyltransferase alleles using the DNA-microchip technique. Eur J Hum Genet 2006;14:991-8.
117. Nemoda Z, Ronai Z, Szekely A, Kovacs E, Shandrick S, Guttman A, et al. High-throughput genotyping of repeat polymorphism in the regulatory region of serotonin transporter gene by gel microchip electrophoresis. Electrophoresis 2001;22:4008-11.
118. Nieradko L, Malecki K. Silicon components for gas chromatograph. Available at: http://www.cs.cmu.edu/~sensing-sensors/readings/silicon_gas_chromatogaph.pdf (accessed May 24, 2011).
119. O'Farrell PH. High resolution two-dimensional electrophoresis of proteins. J Biol Chem 1975;250:4007-21.
120. Obeid PJ, Christopoulos TK, Crabtree HJ, Backhouse CJ. Microfabricated device for DNA and RNA amplification by continuous-flow polymerase chain reaction and reverse transcription-polymerase chain reaction with cycle number selection. Anal Chem 2003;75:288-95.
121. Oda RP, Strausbauch MA, Huhmer AF, Borson N, Jurrens SR, Craighead J, et al. Infrared-mediated thermocycling for ultrafast polymerase chain reaction amplification of DNA. Anal Chem 1998;70:4361-8.
122. Odenthal M, Barta N, Lohfink D, Drebber U, Schulze F, Dienes HP, et al. Analysis of microsatellite instability in colorectal carcinoma by microfluidic-based chip electrophoresis. J Clin Pathol 2009;62: 850-2.
123. Oleschuk RD, Shultz-Lockyear LL, Ning Y, Harrison DJ. Trapping of bead-based reagents within microfluidic systems: on-chip solid-phase extraction and electrochromatography. Anal Chem 2000;72:585-90.
124. Orita M, Iwahana H, Kanazawa H, Hayashi K, Sekiya T. Detection of polymorphisms of human DNA by gel electrophoresis as single-strand conformation polymorphisms. Proc Natl Acad Sci U S A 1989;86: 2766-70.
125. Paegel BM, Emrich CA, Weyemayer GJ, Scherer JR, Mathies RA. High throughput DNA sequencing with a microfabricated 96-lane capillary array electrophoresis bioprocessor. Proc Natl Acad Sci U S A 2002;99:574-9.
126. Pan T, Kelly RT, Asplund MC, Woolley AT. Fabrication of calcium fluoride capillary electrophoresis microdevices for on-chip infrared detection. J Chromatogr A 2004;1027:231-5.
127. Pasas SA, Lacher NA, Davies MI, Lunte SM. Detection of homocysteine by conventional and microchip capillary electrophoresis/electrochemistry. Electrophoresis 2002;23:759-66.
128. Pigeon F, Biasse B, Zussy M. Low-temperature Pyrex glass wafer direct bonding. Electron Lett 1995;31:792-3.
129. Pipper J, Inoue M, Ng LF, Neuzil P, Zhang Y, Novak L. Catching bird flu in a droplet. Nat Med 2007;13:1259-63.
130. Pushkarev D, Neff NF, Quake SR. Single-molecule sequencing of an individual human genome. Nat Biotechnol 2009;27:847-52.
131. Qi S, Liu X, Ford S, Barrows J, Thomas G, Kelly K, et al. Microfluidic devices fabricated in poly(methyl methacrylate) using hot-embossing with integrated sampling capillary and fiber optics for fluorescence detection. Lab Chip 2002;2:88-95.
132. Raisi F, Belgrader P, Borkholder DA, Herr AE, Kintz GJ, Pourhamadi F, et al. Microchip isoelectric focusing using a miniature scanning detection system. Electrophoresis 2001;22:2291-5.
133. Reedy CR, Bienvenue JM, Coletta L, Strachan BC, Bhatri N, Greenspoon SA, et al. Volume reduction solid phase extraction of DNA from dilute, large volume biological samples. Forensic Sci Int Genet 2010;4:206-12.
134. Rodriguez I, Spicar-Mihalic P, Kuyper CL, Fiorini GS, Chiu DT. Rapid prototyping of glass microchannels. Anal Chim Acta 2003; 496:205-15.
135. Roman GT, Carroll S, McDaniel K, Culbertson CT. Micellar electrokinetic chromatography of fluorescently labeled proteins on poly(dimethylsiloxane)-based microchips. Electrophoresis 2006;27:2933-9.
136. Roper MG, Easley CJ, Legendre LA, Humphrey JA, Landers JP. Infrared temperature control system for a completely noncontact polymerase chain reaction in microfluidic chips. Anal Chem 2007;79:1294-300.
137. Sanger F, Coulson AR. Use of thin acrylamide gels for DNA sequencing. FEBS Lett 1978;87:107-10.
138. Sato K, Tokeshi M, Odake T, Kimura H, Ooi T, Nakao M, et al. Integration of an immunosorbent assay system: analysis of secretory human immunoglobulin A on polystyrene beads in a microchip. Anal Chem 2000;72:1144-7.
139. Satoh A. Water glass bonding. Sensor Actuat A Phys 1999;72:160-8.
140. Satterfield BC, Stern S, Caplan MR, Hukari KW, West JA. Microfluidic purification and preconcentration of mRNA by flow-through polymeric monolith. Anal Chem 2007;79:6230-5.
141. Satyanarayana S, Karnik RN, Majumdar A. Stamp-and-stick room-temperature bonding technique for microdevices. J Microelectromech S 2005;14:392-9.
142. Schmalzing D, Koutny L, Chisholm D, Adourian A, Matsudaira P, Ehrlich D. Two-color multiplexed analysis of eight short tandem repeat loci with an electrophoretic microdevice. Anal Biochem 1999;270:148-52.

143. Shi Y, Simpson PC, Scherer JR, Wexler D, Skibola C, Smith MT, et al. Radial capillary array electrophoresis microplate and scanner for high-performance nucleic acid analysis. Anal Chem 1999;71: 5354-61.
144. Simpson JW, Ruiz-Martinez MC, Mulhern GT, Berka J, Latimer DR, Ball JA, et al. A transmission imaging spectrograph and microfabricated channel system for DNA analysis. Electrophoresis 2000;21:135-49.
145. Skelley AM, Cleaves HJ, Jayarajah CN, Bada JL, Mathies RA. Application of the Mars Organic Analyzer to nucleobase and amine biomarker detection. Astrobiology 2006;6:824-37.
146. Skelley AM, Scherer JR, Aubrey AD, Grover WH, Ivester RH, Ehrenfreund P, et al. Development and evaluation of a microdevice for amino acid biomarker detection and analysis on Mars. Proc Natl Acad Sci U S A 2005;102:1041-6.
147. Songjaroen T, Maturos T, Sappat A, Tuantranont A, Laiwattanapaisal W. Portable microfluidic system for determination of urinary creatinine. Anal Chim Acta 2009;647:78-83.
148. Spisak S, Guttman A. Biomedical applications of protein microarrays. Curr Med Chem 2009;16:2806-15.
149. Srinivasan R. Controlled degradation and ablation of polymer surfaces by ultraviolet-laser radiation. Polymer Degradation and Stability 1987;17:193-203.
150. Studer V, Hang G, Pandolfi A, Ortiz M, Anderson WF, Quake SR. Scaling properties of a low-actuation pressure microfluidic valve. J Appl Phys 2004;95:393-8.
151. Sun Y, Kwok YC. Polymeric microfluidic system for DNA analysis. Anal Chim Acta 2006;556:80-96.
152. Sung W-C, Lee G-B, Tzeng C-C, Chen S-H. Plastic microchip electrophoresis for genetic screening: the analysis of polymerase chain reactions products of fragile X (CGG)n alleles. Electrophoresis 2001;22:1188-93.
153. Tan SJ, Yobas L, Lee GY, Ong CN, Lim CT. Microdevice for the isolation and enumeration of cancer cells from blood. Biomed Microdevices 2009;11:883-92.
154. Tan W, Fan ZH, Qiu CX, Ricco AJ, Gibbons I. Miniaturized capillary isoelectric focusing in plastic microfluidic devices. Electrophoresis 2002;23:3638-45.
155. Tarnok A, Hambsch J, Chen R, Varro R. Cytometric bead array to measure six cytokines in twenty-five microliters of serum. Clin Chem 2003;49:1000-2.
156. Terry SC, Herman JH, Angel JB. A gas chromatographic air analyzer fabricated on a silicon wafer. IEEE Trans Elec Dev 1979;26:1880.
157. Tian H, Brody LC, Fan S, Huang Z, Landers JP. Capillary and microchip electrophoresis for rapid detection of known mutations by combining allele-specific DNA amplification with heteroduplex analysis. Clin Chem 2001;47:173-85.
158. Tian H, Brody LC, Landers JP. Rapid detection of deletion, insertion, and substitution mutations via heteroduplex analysis using capillary- and microchip-based electrophoresis. Genome Res 2000;10:1403-13.
159. Tian H, Huhmer AF, Landers JP. Evaluation of silica resins for direct and efficient extraction of DNA from complex biological matrices in a miniaturized format. Anal Biochem 2000;283:175-91.
160. Tian HJ, Jaquins-Gerstl A, Munro N, Trucco M, Brody LC, Landers JP. Single-strand conformation polymorphism analysis by capillary and microchip electrophoresis: a fast, simple method for detection of common mutations in *BRCA1* and *BRCA2*. Genomics 2000;63:25-34.
161. Tokeshi M, Yamaguchi J, Hattori A, Kitamori T. Thermal lens micro optical systems. Anal Chem 2005;77:626-30.
162. Tuomikoski S, Franssila S. Free-standing SU-8 microfluidic chips by adhesive bonding and release etching. Sensor Actuat A Phys 2005; 120:408-15.
163. Unger MA, Chou HP, Thorsen T, Scherer A, Quake SR. Monolithic microfabricated valves and pumps by multilayer soft lithography. Science 2000;288:113-6.
164. Vahedi G, Kaler K, Backhouse CJ. An integrated method for mutation detection using on-chip sample preparation, single-stranded conformation polymorphism, and heteroduplex analysis. Electrophoresis 2004;25:2346-56.
165. Verheggen TP, Beckers JL, Everaerts FM. Simple sampling device for capillary isotachophoresis and capillary zone electrophoresis. J Chromatogr 1988;452:615-22.
166. Vickers JA, Dressen BM, Weston MC, Boonsong K, Chailapakul O, Cropek DM, et al. Thermoset polyester as an alternative material for microchip electrophoresis/electrochemistry. Electrophoresis 2007;28:1123-9.
167. Viskari PJ, Landers JP. Unconventional detection methods for microfluidic devices. Electrophoresis 2006;27:1797-810.
168. von Heeren F, Verpoorte E, Manz A, Thormann W. Micellar electrokinetic chromatography separations and analyses of biological samples on a cyclic planar microstructure. Anal Chem 1996;68:2044-53.
169. Vrouwe EX, Luttge R, Vermes I, van den Berg A. Microchip capillary electrophoresis for point-of-care analysis of lithium. Clin Chem 2007;53:117-23.
170. Wang J, Chatrathi MP. Microfabricated electrophoresis chip for bioassay of renal markers. Anal Chem 2003;75:525-9.
171. Wang J, Chatrathi MP, Tian B, Polsky R. Microfabricated electrophoresis chips for simultaneous bioassays of glucose, uric acid, ascorbic acid, and acetaminophen. Anal Chem 2000;72:2514-8.
172. Wang YN, Kang Y, Xu D, Chon CH, Barnett L, Kalams SA, Li D. On-chip counting the number and the percentage of CD4+ T lymphocytes. Lab Chip 2008;8:309-15.
173. Wen J, Guillo C, Ferrance JP, Landers JP. DNA extraction using a tetramethyl orthosilicate-grafted photopolymerized monolithic solid phase. Anal Chem 2006;78:1673-81.
174. Wen J, Guillo C, Ferrance JP, Landers JP. Microfluidic-based DNA purification in a two-stage, dual-phase microchip containing a reversed-phase and a photopolymerized monolith. Anal Chem 2007;79:6135-42.
175. Wensink H, Benito-Lopez F, Hermes DC, Verboom W, Gardeniers HJ, Reinhoudt DN, et al. Measuring reaction kinetics in a lab-on-a-chip by microcoil NMR. Lab Chip 2005;5:280-4.
176. Witek MA, Hupert ML, Park DS, Fears K, Murphy MC, Soper SA. 96-well polycarbonate-based microfluidic titer plate for high-throughput purification of DNA and RNA. Anal Chem 2008;80:3483-91.
177. Witek MA, Llopis SD, Wheatley A, McCarley RL, Soper SA. Purification and preconcentration of genomic DNA from whole cell lysates using photoactivated polycarbonate (PPC) microfluidic chips. Nucleic Acids Res 2006;34:e74.
178. Wolfe KA, Breadmore MC, Ferrance JP, Power ME, Conroy JF, Norris PM, Landers JP. Toward a microchip-based solid-phase extraction method for isolation of nucleic acids. Electrophoresis 2002;23: 727-33.
179. Woolley AT, Mathies RA. Ultra-high-speed DNA sequencing using capillary electrophoresis chips. Anal Chem 1995;67:3676-80.
180. Woolley AT, Mathies RA. Ultra-high-speed DNA fragment separations using microfabricated capillary array electrophoresis chips. Proc Natl Acad Sci U S A 1994;91:11348-52.
181. Wu Q, Bienvenue JM, Hassan BJ, Kwok YC, Giordano BC, Norris PM, et al. Microchip-based macroporous silica sol-gel monolith for efficient isolation of DNA from clinical samples. Anal Chem 2006;78:5704-10.
182. Xian X, Ma Y, Uang DD, Huang W, Wang Y, Mueller O, et al. Reduced high-density lipoprotein 2b in non-obese type 2 diabetic patients analysed by a microfluidic chip method in a case-control study. Biomarkers 2009;14:619-23.
183. Xu F, Jabasini M, Zhu B, Ying L, Cui X, Arai A, et al. Single-step quantitation of DNA in microchip electrophoresis with linear imaging UV detection and fluorescence detection through comigration with a digest. J Chromatogr A 2004;1051:147-53.
184. Xu J, Locascio L, Gaitan M, Lee CS. Room-temperature imprinting method for plastic microchannel fabrication. Anal Chem 2000;72:1930-3.

185. Xu Y, Vaidya B, Patel AB, Ford SM, McCarley RL, Soper SA. Solid-phase reversible immobilization in microfluidic chips for the purification of dye-labeled DNA sequencing fragments. Anal Chem 2003;75:2975-84.
186. Yao B, Yang H, Liang Q, Luo G, Wang L, Ren K, et al. High-speed, whole-column fluorescence imaging detection for isoelectric focusing on a microchip using an organic light emitting diode as light source. Anal Chem 2006;78:5845-50.
187. Yu ZT, Kamei K, Takahashi H, Shu CJ, Wang X, He GW, et al. Integrated microfluidic devices for combinatorial cell-based assays. Biomed Microdevices 2009;11:547-55.
188. Yung TK, Chan KC, Mok TS, Tong J, To KF, Lo YM. Single-molecule detection of epidermal growth factor receptor mutations in plasma by microfluidics digital PCR in non-small cell lung cancer patients. Clin Cancer Res 2009;15:2076-84.
189. Yurkovetsky ZR, Kirkwood JM, Edington HD, Marrangoni AM, Velikokhatnaya L, Winans MT, et al. Multiplex analysis of serum cytokines in melanoma patients treated with interferon-alpha2b. Clin Cancer Res 2007;13:2422-8.
190. Zhong R, Pan X, Jiang L, Dai Z, Qin J, Lin B. Simply and reliably integrating micro heaters/sensors in a monolithic PCR-CE microfluidic genetic analysis system. Electrophoresis 2009;30:1297-305.
191. Zhou XM, Shao SJ, Xu GD, Zhong RT, Liu DY, Tang JW, et al. Highly sensitive determination of the methylated p16 gene in cancer patients by microchip electrophoresis. J Chromatogr B Analyt Technol Biomed Life Sci 2005;816:145-51.

CHAPTER 19

Automation in the Clinical Laboratory

James C. Boyd, M.D., and Charles D. Hawker, Ph.D., M.B.A., F.A.C.B.

The term *automation* has been applied in clinical chemistry to describe the process whereby an analytical instrument performs many tests with only minimal involvement of an analyst. The availability of automated instruments enables laboratories to process much larger workloads without comparable increases in staff. The evolution of automation in the clinical laboratory has paralleled that in the manufacturing industry, progressing from fixed automation, whereby an instrument performs a repetitive task by itself, to programmable automation, which allows the instrument to perform a variety of different tasks. Intelligent automation also has been introduced into some individual instruments or systems to allow them to self-monitor and respond appropriately to changing conditions.

One benefit of automation is a reduction in the variability of results and errors of analysis through the elimination of tasks that are repetitive and monotonous for most individuals. The improved reproducibility gained by automation has led to a significant improvement in the quality of laboratory tests.

Many small laboratories now have consolidated into larger, more efficient entities in response to market trends involving cost reduction. The drive to automate these mega-laboratories has led to new avenues in laboratory automation. No longer is automation simply being used to assist the laboratory technologist in test performance; it now includes (1) processing and transport of specimens, (2) loading of specimens into automated analyzers, (3) assessment of the results of the tests performed, and (4) storage of specimens. We believe that automating these additional functions is crucial to the future prosperity of the clinical laboratory.[1,2]

This chapter discusses the principles that apply to automation of the individual steps of the analytical process—both in individual analyzers and in the integration of automation throughout the clinical laboratory.

BASIC CONCEPTS

Automated analyzers generally incorporate mechanized versions of basic manual laboratory techniques and procedures. However, modern instrumentation is packaged in a wide variety of configurations. The most common configuration is the random-access analyzer. In *random-access analysis*, analyses are performed sequentially on a collection of specimens, with each specimen analyzed for a different selection of tests. Tests performed in random-access analysis are selected through the use of different vials of reagents stored on board the analyzer. This approach permits measurement of a variable number and variety of analytes in each specimen. Profiles or groups of tests are defined for a specimen at the time the tests to be performed are entered into the analyzer (1) via a keyboard, (2) by instruction from a laboratory information system in conjunction with bar coding on the specimen tube, or (3) by operator selection of appropriate reagent packs.

Historically, other *analyzer configurations* used include continuous-flow and centrifugal analyzers. Continuous-flow analyzers were the first automated analyzers used in clinical laboratories. Initially, these analyzers were used in a *single-channel analysis* configuration and carried out a *sequential analysis* of each specimen. Subsequently, *multiple-channel analysis* versions were developed, in which analysis of each specimen was performed on every channel in parallel. Results from nonrequested tests in the test profile were discarded as necessary after the analysis was complete. Inflexibility in the menu of tests that could be performed on these analyzers eventually led to their replacement in the marketplace by more versatile configurations.

Centrifugal analyzers used discrete pipetting to load *aliquots* of specimens and reagents sequentially into the discrete chambers in a rotor, and the specimens subsequently were analyzed in parallel *(parallel analysis)* by spinning the rotor to exert centrifugal force to mix the specimens and reagent and to drive the mixtures into cuvettes located on the periphery of the rotor. Such analyzers could be operated in a multiple-specimen/single-chemistry or a single-specimen/multiple-chemistry mode. Although such technology was developed as part of the space program and is suitable for application in a zero gravity environment, it was not sufficiently versatile to compete with other random-access

BOX 19-1 Unit Operations in an Analytical Process

Specimen identification
Specimen delivery
Specimen processing
Sample introduction and internal transport
Sample loading and aspiration
Reagent handling and storage
Reagent delivery
Chemical reaction phase
Measurement approaches
Signal processing, data handling, and process control

BOX 19-2 Technologies Used for Automatic Identification and Data Collection

Bar coding
Optical character recognition
Magnetic stripe and magnetic ink character recognition
Voice identification
Radiofrequency identification (RFID)
Touch screens
Light pens
Hand print tablets
Optical mark readers
Smart cards

analyzers and has largely been abandoned for use in the routine laboratory.

AUTOMATION OF THE ANALYTICAL PROCESSES

The following individual steps required to complete an analysis often are referred to collectively as *unit operations* (Box 19-1). These operations are described individually in this section, and examples demonstrate how they have been automated in terms of operational and analytical performance. In most automated systems, these steps usually are performed sequentially, but with some instruments, they may occur in parallel.

Specimen Identification

Typically, the identifying link (identifier) between patient and specimen is noted at the patient's bedside, and maintenance of this connection throughout (1) transport of the specimen to the laboratory, (2) subsequent specimen analysis, and (3) preparation of a report is essential. Several technologies are available for automatic identification and data collection purposes (Box 19-2). In practice, automatic identification includes only those technologies that electronically detect a unique characteristic or unique data string associated with a physical object. For example, identifiers such as (1) serial number, (2) part number, (3) color, (4) manufacturer, (5) patient name, and (6) medical record number have been used to identify an object or patient through the use of electronic data processing. In the clinical laboratory, labeling with a bar code has become the technology of choice for purposes of automatic identification.

Labeling

In many laboratory information systems, electronic entry of a test order in the laboratory or at a nursing station for a uniquely identified patient generates a specimen label bearing a unique laboratory accession number. A record is established that remains incomplete until a result (or a set of results) is entered into the computer against the accession number. The unique label is affixed to the specimen collection container when the specimen is obtained. Proper alignment of the label on a specimen tube is critical for subsequent specimen processing when bar-coded labels are used. Arrival of the specimen in the laboratory is recorded by a manual or computerized log-in procedure. In other systems, the specimen is labeled at the patient's bedside, and patient identification and collection information is provided; then the labeled specimen is submitted to the laboratory with a requisition form. There it is assigned an accession number as part of the log-in procedure, which is usually a computerized process.

After accessioning, specimens undergo the technical handling processes. For those processes requiring physical removal of serum or plasma from the original tube, secondary labels bearing essential information from the original label must be affixed to any secondary tubes created. Some automated analyzers sample directly from the original collection tube while simultaneously reading the accession number from the bar code label on the tube. Secondary bar code labels, if necessary, may be generated at the time of accessioning, or in some analyzers by a built-in printer that is activated when the analyzer is programmed.

Many methods are used to achieve secondary labeling when bar code labels are not available. A number may be handwritten on the specimen cup, or a coded label may be affixed to the original tube or to a specimen cup. The label numbers require correlation with a manual or computer-generated work or load list. The load list usually records accession numbers in sequence with the physical positions of cups or tubes in the loading zone of the analyzer. This loading zone may be (1) a revolving tray or turntable, (2) a mechanical belt, or (3) a rack or set of racks by which specimens are delivered in a predetermined order to the sample aspiration station of the analyzer.

In those analyzers that do not automatically link specimen identity and sample aspiration, the sequence of results produced must be linked manually with the sequence of entry of specimens. Some analyzers print out or transmit to a host computer each result or set of results from a specimen through the position of the specimen in the loading zone or the accession number programmed to that position.

Bar Coding

A major advance in the automation of specimen identification in the clinical laboratory is the incorporation of bar coding technology into analytical systems. A bar coding system consists of a bar code printer and a bar code reader, or scanner. One- and two-dimensional bar coding systems are available. A one-dimensional bar code is an array of rectangular bars and spaces arranged in a predetermined pattern according to unambiguous rules to represent elements of data referred to as *characters*. A bar code is transferred and affixed to an object by a *bar code label* that carries the bar code and, optionally, other noncoded readable information. *Symbology* is the term used to describe the rules specifying the way data are encoded into the bars and spaces. The width of the bars and spaces, as well as the number of each, is determined by a specification for that symbology. Different combinations of bars and spaces represent different characters. When a bar code scanner is passed over the bar code, the light beam from the scanner is absorbed by the dark bars and is not reflected; the beam is reflected by the light spaces. A photocell detector in the scanner receives the reflected light and converts that light into an electrical signal that then is digitized. A one-dimensional bar code is "vertically redundant" in that the same information is repeated vertically—the heights of the bars can be truncated without any loss of information. In practice, vertical redundancy allows a symbol with printing defects, such as spots or voids, to be read.

In practice, a bar code label (often generated by the laboratory information system and bearing the sample accession number) is placed onto the specimen container and is subsequently "read" by one or more bar code readers placed at key positions in the analytical sequence. The resultant identifying and ancillary information then is transferred to and processed by the system software. Initiating bar code identification at a patient's bedside ensures greater integrity of the specimen's identity in an analyzer. Systems to transfer information concerning a patient's identity to blood tubes at the patient's bedside have been introduced in many hospitals, and several companies are now offering these systems.

Unequivocal positive identification of each specimen is achieved in analyzers with bar code readers. Advantages of the use of bar code labels include the following:

1. Elimination of work lists for the system
2. Avoidance of mistakes made in the placement of tubes in the analyzer or during sampling
3. Avoidance of the need for analysis of specimens in a defined sequence
4. Decrease in identification errors.

Examples of types of bar codes that are used in chemistry analyzers are illustrated in Figure 19-1.

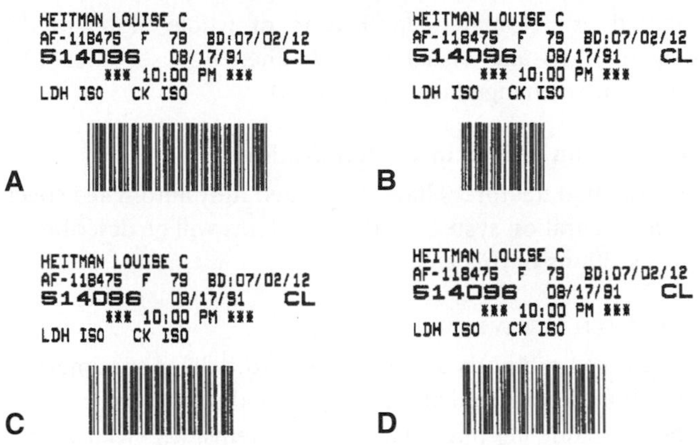

Figure 19-1 Examples of bar codes used in chemistry analyzers containing the same information. A, Code 39. B, Code I 2/5. C, Code 128B. D, Codabar. *(Courtesy Computer Transceiver Systems, Inc.)*

Identification Errors

Many opportunities arise for the mismatch of specimens and results. The risks begin at the bedside and are compounded with each processing step a specimen undergoes between collection from the patient and analysis by the instrument. The risks are particularly great when hand transcription is invoked for accessioning, labeling and relabeling, and creation of load lists. An incorrect accession number, one in which the digits are transposed, or a load list with transposed accession numbers may cause test results to be attributed to the wrong patient. An additional hazard exists when specimens must be inserted into certain positions in the loading zone defined by a load list. Human misreading of the specimen label or the loading list may cause misplacement of specimens, calibrators, or controls. Automatic reading of bar code labels reduces the error rate from 1 in 300 characters (for human entry) to about 1 in 1 million characters barring (1) minor imperfections in printed bar codes, (2) improper bar code scanner resolution, or (3) skewed orientation of bar code labels on containers, all of which can result in read errors.

Specimen Preparation

The clotting of blood in specimen collection tubes, their subsequent centrifugation, and the transfer of serum to secondary tubes require a finite time to complete. If performed manually, the process results in a delay in the preparation of a specimen for analysis. To eliminate the problems associated with specimen preparation, systems are being developed to automate this process.

Use of Whole Blood for Analysis

When whole blood is used in an assay system, specimen preparation time is essentially eliminated. Automated or semiautomated ion-selective electrodes, which measure ion activity in whole blood rather than ion concentration, have been incorporated into automated systems to provide certain test results within minutes of the drawing of a specimen. This approach now is used commonly for assays of electrolytes and some other common analytes. Another approach involves manual or automated application of whole blood to dry reagent films and visual or instrumental observation of a quantitative change (see Chapter 20).

Automation of Specimen Preparation

Several manufacturers have developed fully automated specimen preparation systems. (These systems will be described in later sections of this chapter.)

Specimen Delivery

Automated methods are often used to deliver specimens to the laboratory instead of the historic method (courier service). These include (1) pneumatic tube systems, (2) electric track vehicles, and (3) mobile robots.

Pneumatic Tube Systems

Pneumatic tube systems provide rapid specimen transportation and are reliable when installed as point-to-point services. However, when switching mechanisms are introduced to allow carriers (the bullet-shaped containers used to hold specimens) to be sent to various locations, mechanical problems may occur and may cause misrouting of carriers. In addition, close attention to the design of the pneumatic tube system is necessary to prevent hemolysis of the specimen. Avoidance of sudden accelerations and decelerations and the use of proper packing material inside the carriers will minimize hemolysis.

Electric Track Vehicles

Electric track vehicles have a larger carrying capacity than pneumatic tube systems and do not have problems with damaging specimens by acceleration and/or deceleration forces. Some systems maintain the carrier in an upright position with the use of a gimbal (a device that permits a body to incline freely in any direction or suspends it so it will remain level when its support is tipped), enabling the carrier to move both vertically and horizontally on an installed electric track. The containers can hold dry ice or refrigerated gel packs with specimens if desired. They are especially useful in quickly transporting specimens between floors or between laboratory locations that are some distance from each other, by making use of the space in the ceiling plenum above the laboratory. A primary disadvantage is the cost of moving the track and loading/unloading stations if the laboratory is expanding or moving; in addition, the stations may be larger than the pneumatic tube stations. If the station is not located directly in the central laboratory (centralized testing; core laboratory), additional staff may be necessary to unload the carts and transport the specimens to their final destination, and the electric track system may not achieve its desired goal of rapid specimen transport.

Mobile Robots

Automated guided vehicles (AGVs), also called mobile robots, have been used successfully to transport laboratory specimens both within the laboratory and outside the central laboratory.[13] They are easily adapted to carry various sizes and shapes of specimen containers and are reprogrammable with changes in laboratory geometry. In addition, in a busy laboratory setting, delivery of specimens to laboratory benches by a mobile robot can be more frequent than human pickup and has been shown to be cost-effective. Inexpensive models follow a line on the floor, whereas others have more sophisticated guidance systems. Their limitations include the need to batch specimens for greater efficiency and, in most cases, the requirement for laboratory personnel to place specimens onto or remove specimens from the mobile robot at each stopping place. Some mobile robots have been integrated with robotic systems that automate loading and unloading of specimens; others initiate an audible or visual signal of their arrival at a specified station so that employees are able to load or unload the specimens being transported. Box 19-3 lists several vendors that provide mobile robot systems for clinical laboratories.

BOX 19-3 Vendors of Mobile Robot Systems

Aethon TUG
www.aethon.com
Cardinal Health HELPMATE
www.cardinalhealth.com
CCRI ROBOCART
www.robocart.com
Egemin PACKMOBILE
www.egeminusa.com
FMC Technologies
www.fmcsgvs.com
Frog MEDIMOVER
www.frogusa.com
Mobile Robots, Inc. MOTIVITY
www.mobilerobots.com

Specimen Loading and Aspiration

In most situations, the specimen for automatic analysis is serum or plasma. Many analyzers directly sample serum from primary collection tubes of various sizes. With such analyzers, the collection tubes most frequently used contain separator material that forms a barrier between serum or plasma and cells (see Chapter 7).

Many analyzers also sample from cups or tubes filled with serum transferred from the original specimen tubes. Often the design of the sampling cup is unique for a particular analyzer. Each cup should be designed to minimize dead volume, that is, the excess serum that must be present in a cup to permit aspiration of the full volume required for testing. Cups must be made of inert material so they do not interact with the analytes being measured. Specimen cups also should be disposable to minimize cost and contamination, and their shape should, even without a cap, minimize evaporation by minimizing the surface area of sample exposed to the air.

Specimens may undergo other forms of degradation in addition to evaporation. For example, specimens that contain thermolabile constituents may undergo degradation of such analytes if held at ambient temperatures. Other constituents, such as bilirubin, are photolabile. Thermolability is minimized when both specimens and calibrators are held in a refrigerated loading zone. Photodegradation is reduced by the use of semiopaque cups and placement of smoke- or orange-colored plastic covers over the specimen cups.

The loading zone of an analyzer is the area in which specimens are held in the instrument before they are analyzed. The holding area may be a circular tray, a rack or series of racks built into a cassette, or a serpentine chain of containers into which individual tubes are inserted. When specimens are not identified automatically, they must be presented to the sampling device in the correct sequence, as specified by a loading list. The sampling mechanism determines the exact volume of sample removed from the specimen.

For most analyzers, specimens for a subsequent run may be prepared on a separate tray while one run is already in progress. This process permits machine operation and human actions to proceed in parallel for optimal efficiency. In some analyzers, specimens may be added continuously by the operator as they become available. A desirable feature of any automated analyzer is the ability to insert new specimens ahead of specimens already in place in the loading zone. This feature allows the timely analysis of a specimen with a high medical priority. When specimen identification is machine-read, it is possible for the operator to easily reposition specimens in the loading zone. When specimen identification is tied to a loading list, however, insertion or repositioning of specimens must be accompanied by revision of the loading list.

Transmission of infectious diseases by automated equipment is a concern in clinical laboratories. The method of transmission by equipment is primarily through splatter of serum or blood during the acquisition of samples from rapidly moving specimen probes. The use of level sensors, which restrict the penetration of sample probes into specimens, and provision of software for smoother motion control greatly reduce splatter.

Because the potential for contamination exists when the stoppers of primary containers are opened or "popped" to decant serum into specimen cups, several firms have developed closed-container sampling systems for use in their automated hematology and chemistry analyzers. In these systems, the specimen probe passes through a hollow needle that initially penetrates the primary container's rubber stopper. This configuration prevents damage or plugging of the specimen probe while allowing the level sensor (used to reduce carryover and to detect short samples) to remain active. After the specimen probe is withdrawn, the outer hollow needle also is withdrawn, so the stopper reseals and no specimen escapes. Closed-container sampling is used widely in hematology analyzers.

Sample Pretreatment

Automation of analytical procedures requires the capability to remove proteins and other interferents from some specimens to ensure the specificity of an analytical method. Dialysis, column chromatography, and filtration have been used for this purpose.

Sample Introduction and Internal Transport

The method used to introduce the sample into the analyzer and its subsequent transport within the analyzer is the major difference between continuous-flow and discrete systems. In continuous-flow systems, the sample is aspirated through the sample probe into a stream of flowing liquid, whereby it is transported to analytical stations in the instrument. In *discrete analysis*, the sample is aspirated into the sample probe and then is delivered, often with reagent, through the same orifice into a reaction cup or other container. Carryover is a potential problem with both types of systems.

Technicon Instruments Corporation pioneered the use of peristaltic pumps and plastic tubing to advance the sample and reagents in continuous-flow analysis. Peristaltic pumps trap a "slug" of fluid between two rollers that occlude the tubing. As the rollers travel over the tubing, the trapped fluid is pushed forward and, as the leading roller lifts from the tubing, is added to the fluid beyond it. The peristaltic pump still is used in some hematology analyzers and analyzers with ion-selective electrodes, as well as for wash systems.

Discrete Processing Systems

Positive–liquid displacement pipettes are used for sampling in most discrete automated systems in which specimens, calibrators, and controls are delivered by a single pipette to the next stage in the analytical process.

A positive-displacement pipette may be designed for one of two operational modes: (1) to dispense only aspirated sample into the reaction receptacle, or (2) to flush out sample together with diluent. Both systems use a plastic or glass syringe with a plunger, the tip of which usually is made of Teflon.

Pipettes may be categorized as (1) fixed-, (2) variable-, or (3) selectable-volume (see Chapter 9). Selectable-volume pipettes allow the selection of a limited number of predetermined volumes. Pipettes with unlimited or selectable volumes are used in systems that allow many different applications, whereas fixed-volume pipettes usually are used for samples and reagents in instruments dedicated to the performance of only a small variety of tests.

Carryover

Carryover is defined as the transfer of a quantity of analyte or reagent from one specimen reaction into a subsequent one. Because it erroneously affects analytical results from the subsequent reaction, carryover should be minimized or eliminated. In discrete systems with disposable reaction vessels and measuring cuvets, carryover is caused by the pipetting system. In instruments with reusable cuvets or flowcells, carryover may also arise from incomplete cleaning of the cuvettes or flowcells between assays.

Most manufacturers of discrete systems reduce sample-to-sample carryover by using disposable pipette tips or by incorporating wash stations for the sample probe that flush the internal and external surfaces of the probe with copious amounts of diluent. An adequate ratio of flush and rinse to specimen volume controls carryover in many cases to acceptable values. Appropriate choice of sample probe material, geometry, and surface conditions also influences carryover. Some systems wipe the outside of the sample probe to prevent transfer of a portion of the previous specimen into the next specimen cup. Use of disposable sample probe tips allows complete elimination of contamination of one sample by another inside the probe, as well as the carryover of one specimen into the specimen in the next cup, because a new pipette tip is used for each pipetting.

In practice, the reduction of sample-to-sample carryover is a more stringent requirement for automated analyzers that perform immunoassays in which some analytes (e.g., human chorionic gonadotropin) have a wide range of concentrations. Some systems use extra steps, such as additional washes, or an additional washing device to reduce carryover for selected tests to acceptable limits. Because extra steps reduce overall throughput, additional rinsing functions are initiated (by computer operator selection) only for assays with a large analytical measurement range.

Sample-to-sample carryover can be detected by the preparation of two sample pools—one having a very high analyte concentration (H), the other having a low concentration (L). By running sequences of tests such as HHHLLLHHLL-HHLL, if sample-to-sample carryover is present, higher results will be noted in the low-concentration sample analyses that immediately follow a high-concentration sample analysis.

Reagent-to-reagent carryover also can occur on discrete systems that use a common reagent probe for pipetting all reagents; its minimization or elimination requires use of the same approaches just described for sample-to-sample carryover. Detection of reagent-to-reagent carryover can be difficult for end-users and usually requires the involvement of the instrument vendor. Users should be aware that the introduction of third party reagents in "open" channels on otherwise closed systems may introduce problems with reagent-to-reagent carryover. Consultation with the system manufacturer is advised to determine how to test for and minimize such carryover.

Reagent Handling and Storage

Many automated systems use liquid reagents stored in plastic or glass containers. For those analyzers in which a working inventory is maintained in the system, the volumes of reagents stored depend on the number of tests to be performed without operator intervention.

For many analyzers in which specimens are not processed continuously, reagents are stored in laboratory refrigerators and are introduced into the instruments as required. In larger systems, sections of the reagent storage compartments are maintained at 4 to 10 °C.

Some systems use reagents or antibodies that have been immobilized in a reaction coil or chamber to allow their repetitive use in a chemical reaction. Other systems use enzymes immobilized on membranes coupled to sensing electrodes. The reaction products then are measured by the sensing device. Only a buffer is required as a diluent and a wash solution; thus the membrane has an extended life, which lowers the cost of each test.

Reagent Identification

Labels on reagent containers include information such as (1) reagent identification, (2) volume of the contents or the number of tests for which the contents of the containers are to be used, (3) expiration date, and (4) lot number. Many reagent containers now carry bar codes that contain some or all of this information, and the manufacturer is able to retrieve any pertinent information when necessary.

Other advantages of using reagent bar codes include (1) facilitation of inventory management, (2) ability to insert reagent containers in random sequence, and (3) ability to automatically dispense a particular volume of liquid reagent. Furthermore, when a bar code reader is coupled with a level-sensing system on the reagent probe, it alerts the operator as to whether a sufficient quantity of reagent exists to complete a workload.

A bar code on a reagent container may also contain information about (multiple) calibrators, such as the definition of a calibration curve algorithm and values of curve constants defined at the time of reagent manufacture. Accompanying calibrator materials provided in their own bar code tubes at the time of manufacture ensure that calibration functions are integrated properly into the analysis.

Open versus Closed Systems

Automated analyzers are classified as "open" or "closed." In an open analyzer, the operator is able to change the parameters related to an analysis and to prepare "in-house" reagents or use reagents from a variety of suppliers. Such analyzers usually have considerable flexibility and adapt readily to new methods and analytes.

A closed-system analyzer is one in which reagents and calibrators are provided only by the manufacturer and other reagents or methods cannot be used.

Reagent Delivery

Liquid reagents are acquired and delivered to mixing and reaction chambers by pumps (through tubes) or by positive-displacement syringe devices. In those analyzers in which more than one reagent is acquired and dispensed by the same syringe, washing or flushing of the probe is essential to prevent reagent carryover.

Chemical Reaction Phase

Sample and reagents react in the chemical reaction phase. Factors that are important in this phase include (1) vessel in which the reaction occurs; (2) cuvet in which the reaction is monitored; (3) timing of the reaction(s); (4) mixing and transport of reactants; (5) thermal conditioning of fluids; and (6) for some immunoassay systems, separation of bound and unbound fractions.

Type of Reaction Vessel and Cuvet

In continuous-flow systems, each specimen passes through the same continuous stream and is subjected to the same analytical reactions as every other specimen and at the same rate. In such systems, the reaction occurs in the flow-through component.

In discrete systems, each specimen in a batch has its own physical and chemical space, separate from every other specimen. Discrete analyzers use individual (disposable or reusable) reaction vessels transported through the system after sample and reagent have been dispensed, or they use a stationary reaction chamber.

Reaction vessels are reused in many instruments. The time before reusable cuvet/reaction vessels must be replaced depends on their composition and the washing mechanisms used. Some manufacturers have computer algorithms that automatically control when individual cuvet/reaction vessels are discarded, depending on how many assays and what types of assays have been performed in a given cuvet.

Mixing of Reactants

Various techniques are used to mix reactants. In a discrete system, these include (1) forceful dispensing; (2) magnetic stirring; (3) vigorous lateral displacement; (4) physical stirring; and (5) vigorous lateral displacement. Dry reagent systems obviate the need for mixing because the serum completely interacts with the dry chemicals as it flows through the matrix of the reaction unit. However, regardless of the technique used, mixing is a difficult process to automate and one that can contribute to reaction-to-reaction carryover among reused components.

Thermal Regulation

Thermal regulation requires the establishment of a controlled-temperature environment in close contact with the reaction container and efficient heat transfer from the environment to the reaction mixture. Various technologies have been used for temperature regulation, including air baths, water baths, and piezoelectric devices.

Separation in Immunoassay Systems

Automation of immunoassay procedures requires the separation of free and bound fractions of heterogeneous immunoassays. Several approaches have been used. For example, several automated immunoassay analyzers use bound antibodies or proteins in a solid-phase format. With this approach, the binding of antigens and antibodies occurs on a solid surface to which the antibodies or other reactive proteins have been adsorbed or chemically bonded. Different types of solid phases are used, including (1) beads, (2) coated tubes, (3) microtiter plates, (4) magnetic and nonmagnetic microparticles, and (5) fiber matrices. Additional details on automated systems that use various solid phases are found in books by Wild,[17] and Price and Newman.[12]

Measurement Approaches

Automated chemistry analyzers traditionally have relied on photometers and spectrophotometers to measure the absorbance of the reaction produced in the chemical reaction phase. Alternative approaches now being incorporated into analyzers include reflectance photometers, fluorometers, and luminometers. Immunoassay systems have used reaction schemes that produce fluorescence, chemiluminescence, and electrochemiluminescence to enhance sensitivity. Ion-selective electrodes and other electrochemical techniques also are used widely.

Photometry/Spectrophotometry

Measurement of absorbance requires the following three basic components (see Chapter 10): (1); an optical source; (2) a means of spectral isolation; and (3) a detector.

Optical Source

Radiant energy sources used in automated systems include (1) tungsten, (2) quartz-halogen, (3) deuterium, (4) mercury, (5) xenon lamps, and (6) lasers. In the quartz-halogen lamp, low-pressure halogen vapor (e.g., iodine, bromine) is enclosed in a fused silica envelope in which a tungsten filament serves as an incandescent light source. The spectrum produced includes wavelengths from approximately 300 to 700 nm.

Spectral Isolation

In automated systems, spectral isolation commonly is achieved with interference filters. Typical interference filters have peak transmissions of 30% to 80% and bandwidths of 5 to 15 nm (see Chapter 10). In several multitest analyzers, filters are mounted in a filter wheel, and the appropriate filter is moved into place under command of the system's computer. Monochromators with movable gratings and slits provide a continuous choice of wavelengths. They offer great flexibility and are suited especially for the development of new assays. However, because relatively few wavelengths are required for analyses in routine analyzers, many manufacturers use a stationary, holographically ruled grating, coupled with a stationary photodiode array, to isolate the spectrum. These two elements also are coupled with fiber optic light guides to transfer the passage of light energy through cuvets at locations convenient for mechanization. Use of these passive elements enhances the reliability of a system because no moving parts are required for spectral isolation (Figure 19-2).

Photometric Detectors

Photodiodes are used as detectors in many automated systems, either as individual components or in multiples as an array. Photomultiplier tubes are required in many immunoassay systems to provide a high signal-to-noise ratio and fast detector response times for fluorescent and chemiluminescent measurements.

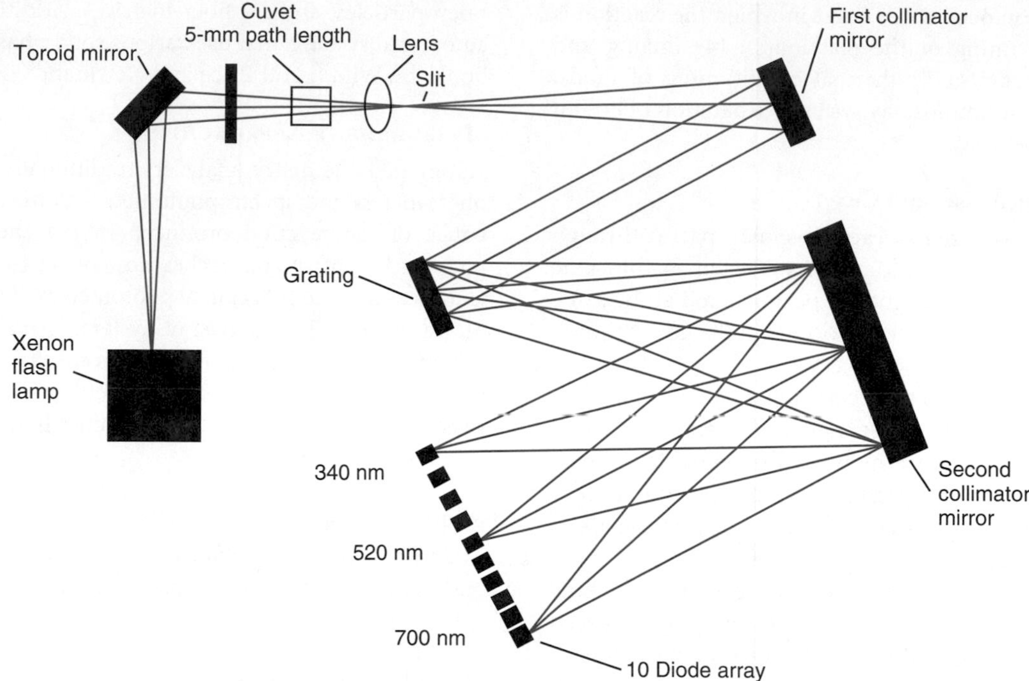

Figure 19-2 Use of a diode array in the SYNCHRON CX7 monochromator reduces requirements for moving parts. For simplicity, ray traces for only three wavelengths are shown. *(Courtesy Beckman Coulter, Inc.; www.beckmancoulter.com.)*

Proper alignment of cuvets with the light path(s) is important in both automated and manual analyzers. In addition, stray energy and internal reflections must be kept to acceptable levels. If the light path is not perpendicular to the cuvet, inaccuracy and imprecision may occur, particularly in rate analyses.

Reflectance Photometry

In reflectance photometry, diffuse reflected light is measured. The reflected light results from illumination, with diffused light, of a reaction mixture in a carrier or from the diffusion of light by a reaction mixture in an illuminated carrier. The intensity of the reflected light from the reagent carrier is compared with that reflected from a reference surface. Because the intensity of reflected light is nonlinear with concentration of the analyte, mathematical algorithms commonly are used to linearize the relation of reflectance to concentration.[16]

Fluorometry

Fluorescence is the emission of electromagnetic radiation by a species that has absorbed exciting radiation from an outside source. Intensity of emitted (fluorescent) light is directly proportional to concentration of the excited species (see Chapter 10).

Fluorometry is used widely for automated immunoassay. It is approximately 1000 times more sensitive than comparable absorbance spectrophotometry, but background interference due to fluorescence of native serum is a major problem. This interference is minimized by (1) careful design of the filters used for spectral isolation, (2) selection of a fluorophor with an emission spectrum distinct from those of interfering compounds, or (3) use of time- or phase-resolved fluorometry (see Chapter 10).

Different optical configurations are represented in different manufacturers' equipment. Right-angle fluorescence measurement is one of the common approaches used, with emitted light passing through the emission interference filter to a photomultiplier tube. In fluorescence polarization, the light source is in the form of polarized light. Measurement then is made of the change in the degree of polarized light emitted by a fluorescent molecule (see Chapters 10 and 16).

Turbidimetry and Nephelometry

Turbidimetry and nephelometry are optical techniques that are applicable particularly to methods measuring precipitate formation in antigen-antibody reactions (see Chapter 16). These techniques are used to measure plasma proteins and for therapeutic drug monitoring.

Chemiluminescence and Bioluminescence

Chemiluminescence and bioluminescence differ from fluorometry in that the excitation event is caused by a chemical or electrochemical reaction and not by photoluminescence (see Chapter 10). The applications of chemiluminescence and bioluminescence have increased significantly with the development of automated instrumentation and new reagent systems. Because of their attamole-to-zeptomole detection limits, chemiluminescence and bioluminescence reactions have been used widely as direct and indicator labels in the development of immunoassays.

Electrochemical

A variety of electrochemical methods have been incorporated into automated systems. The most widely used electrochemical approach involves ion-selective electrodes. These electrodes have replaced flame photometry in the determination of sodium and potassium. Electrochemical detectors also have been used for the measurement of other electrolytes and for indirect application in the analysis of several other serum constituents (see Chapter 11). The relationship between ion activity and the concentrations of ions in the specimens must be established with calibrating solutions, and such electrodes need to be recalibrated frequently to compensate for alterations in electrode response.

Peristaltic pumps are used to move the sample into chambers containing fixed sample and reference electrodes. The electrodes must remain in contact with the specimen from 7 to 45 seconds to reach steady-state conditions. The most common arrangement is to provide electrodes to assay three analytes, typically, sodium, potassium, and chloride. Because specimens and calibrators usually flow past a group of electrodes, results for all analytes are reported for most systems. Ion-selective electrode capability also has been incorporated into medium-sized and large automated analyzers as integrated three- and four-parameter modules; this incorporation has increased significantly these systems' throughputs because several results are produced in parallel.

Signal Processing, Data Handling, and Process Control

The interfacing and integration of computers into automated analyzers and analytical systems has had a major impact on the acquisition and processing of analytical data. Analog signals from detectors are converted to digital signals. Computer software then processes the digital data into useful and meaningful output. Data processing has allowed automation of complex calibration relationships. Computer workstations provide a central point of communication with the user regarding (1) instrument status, (2) order entry, (3) result display, (4) quality control functions, (5) instrument troubleshooting, and (6) autoverification of results. Several functions performed by computers in automated analyzers are listed in Box 19-4.

Test Autoverification

Autoverification is the process whereby patient results generated from interfaced instruments are compared by computer software against laboratory-defined acceptance parameters. If results fall within these defined parameters, the results are automatically released for reporting with no additional laboratory staff intervention. Any data that fall outside the defined parameters are reviewed by laboratory staff prior to reporting. Autoverification has been implemented in various ways, such as by using the laboratory information system to compare results against acceptance parameters, or, alternatively, by performing this function in separate computers that are interposed between the laboratory analyzer and the laboratory information system (termed *middleware* by some

BOX 19-4 Signal and Data Processing Functions Performed by Computers of Automated Analyzers

Data Acquisition and Calculation

Acquisition of response signal and signal averaging
Subtraction of blank response
Correction of response of sample for interferences (e.g., multiwavelength spectrophotometric corrections)
Linear regression for determining slope
($\Delta A/\Delta t$) of rate reactions; ($\Delta A/\Delta C$) of absorbance/concentration relation; ($\Delta R/\Delta C$) of any response parameter to concentration
Statistics (mean, Standard Deviation, Coefficient of Variation) on patient or control values
Mathematical transformation of nonlinear relations to linear counterpart
Mathematical transformation of results to alternative reporting units

Monitoring

Test for fit of data to criteria for calibration or rate reactions
Test of patient result against reference interval criteria
Test of control result against criteria of a quality control standard of performance
Test of moving average of patient results against quality criteria for detecting assay drift

Display

Display of specimens currently being analyzed, tests ordered on each specimen, and expected times of completion
Accumulation of sets of patient results
Collation of results for patient-oriented printout
Warning messages provided to alert operator to instrument malfunction, need for maintenance, or unusual clinical situation
Quality control charts provided for operator review
Troubleshooting flowcharts provided to assist operator

Control, Data Storage, Communications

Control of electromechanical operation of the analyzer
Ensurance that all functions are performed uniformly in the correct sequence
Acquisition, assessment, processing, and storage of operational data from the analyzers
Serial RS-232c or Ethernet interfaces provided with laboratory information systems

Workstation Functions

Point of interaction with the instrument operator provided
Test orders accepted
Monitoring of the testing process
Assistance with analysis of process quality
Facilities for review and verification of test results provided
Assistance with the review of completed test results
Assistance with rule-based autoverification

observers). Most autoverification systems use rule-based decision logic. The rules applied in such systems require careful development and validation by laboratories before and after they are implemented. Guidance for implementation, validation, and monitoring of autoverification systems is provided in a recent document from the Clinical and Laboratory Standards Institute.[6]

INTEGRATED AUTOMATION FOR THE CLINICAL LABORATORY

Significant progress has been made in automating preanalytical and postanalytical activities and integrating these operations with analytical systems. Several versions of stand-alone pre-analytical or "front-end" automation systems, which have largely automated various specimen processing steps, have become available. More options are also available as modules for total laboratory automation systems, and many vendors have increased the number of different analyzers that can be interfaced to their automation.

Large-scale automation of the laboratory usually includes an automated specimen processing area where specimens are (1) identified, (2) labeled, (3) scheduled for analysis, (4) centrifuged, and (5) sorted. After specimens are processed, automated specimen conveyor devices transport specimens to appropriate workstations in the laboratory, where they are analyzed without human intervention. Rules-based expert system software (1) assists with the review of laboratory results by automatically releasing results that have no associated problems, and (2) identifies any problematic results to bring to the attention of trained medical technologists. All specimens are catalogued after analysis and stored in a central storage facility, which may include automated storage and retrieval functions. As previously discussed, particularly important aspects of large-scale automation projects are the approaches used to process and transport specimens and the overall integration of automated components into a smoothly functioning whole.

WORKSTATIONS

The task of integrating laboratory automation begins with the laboratory workstation. In general, a clinical laboratory workstation is usually dedicated to a defined task and contains appropriate laboratory instrumentation to carry out that task. Frequently, the workstation in the modern laboratory is defined in terms of the automated analyzer that is being used. Current laboratory instruments and systems are highly developed for stand-alone operation and fit into the workstation concept. Movement of specimens into and out of the workstation is accomplished by manual transport, and instrument operator activities are largely independent of those at other workstations. On a typical instrument, the operator follows a manufacturer-recommended sequence of calibration, quality control, and daily maintenance activities, and uses the instrument's front-panel functions to introduce specimens for analysis. If the analyzer has a bidirectional interface with a laboratory information system (LIS) and bar code reading capabilities, information regarding what assays to run on each specimen is downloaded from the LIS, and the operator simply loads bar code–labeled specimens into the specimen input area. The built-in diagnostics supplied in most modern analyzers provide sufficient "intelligence" in the analyzer that the operator is able to "walk away" from the instrument for short periods, confident of its reliable operation. Nevertheless, the operator needs to attend periodically to (1) instrument operation, (2) replenishing of reagents or other disposables, (3) evaluation of instrument diagnostic messages, and (4) introduction of new specimens into the specimen input tray.

INSTRUMENT CLUSTERS

To reduce labor costs, instrument manufacturers are developing approaches that will allow a single technologist to simultaneously control and monitor the functions of several instruments. Initially, such workstations were configured with *clusters* of identical instruments, such as chemistry, immunochemistry, or hematology analyzers. More advanced instrument clusters may incorporate both chemistry and immunoassay analyzers from the same vendor; a possible extension of this concept is the development of clusters of unlike instruments that cross traditional laboratory disciplines. An example might be a cluster of chemistry and hematology analyzers.

A cluster of analyzers has its own central computer control module with software designed to assist the operator in monitoring the functions of each analyzer and to aid in the review of laboratory results generated by the cluster. Access to the many front-panel functions of each analyzer is provided by the interface between the analyzer and the central control module. Thus, the technologist loads specimens onto each instrument in the cluster and then monitors subsequent instrument operation and reviews the results at the central workstation. By incorporating the activities of what would be *several* workstations in most current laboratories into a *single* integrated workstation, this approach shows promise in saving laboratory manpower.

WORK CELLS

Another extension of the instrument cluster concept is the addition of robotic specimen handling and preparation. A robotic system is used to carry out various specimen preparation steps, such as checks of specimen adequacy, centrifugation, aliquot preparation and labeling, transport, and storage of specimens. The robotic system is then responsible for introducing specimens into the appropriate analyzer, allowing the technologist to assume a primarily monitoring role that also includes reagent replenishment, calibration, control operations, and instrument maintenance. An interface between the central control module and the robot controller (or combining these functions on a single computer) allows the activities of the robotic cluster to be fully coordinated.

Automated Specimen Processing

Although the manual operations carried out in a specimen processing area look simple, considerable complexity underlies them. Consequently, specimen processing has been one of the most difficult areas of the clinical laboratory to automate. This has been approached in various ways using both integrated and modular approaches, which are discussed in the following sections. Each specimen passing through a specimen processing area has to undergo a series of operations, including (1) receiving the specimen, (2) inspecting it for appropriateness (labeling, container type, temperature, and quantity of specimen), (3) logging onto the LIS, (4) labeling the specimen with an accession number, and (5) separating urgent and stat specimens from routine specimens. Also, specimens have to be sorted for centrifugation and aliquoted or otherwise prepared for the appropriate laboratory station.

Stand-Alone Specimen Processing Systems

An example of a stand-alone specimen processing system is shown in Figure 19-3. Similar systems place processed specimens into racks that must be transported manually to the testing areas, with some exceptions. Some of these are about the size of a large automated analyzer, and others may be a little larger. They may be a good choice for laboratories (1) with daily workloads of 500 to 2000 specimens, (2) with space limitations, or (3) that desire an upgrade path and ease of use with different analyzers from different vendors. Some laboratories may choose to use multiples of a stand-alone specimen processing system to automate archiving and preanalytical specimen processing.

These systems will (1) receive incoming specimens, (2) sort, (3) decap, (4) aliquot, and (5) label aliquot specimen containers with bar codes. All are interfaced to the laboratory's LIS. Some systems include automated centrifugation. Several of the systems sort into instrument-specific racks for analyzers from a number of different vendors. In addition, some users apply these systems to aliquot and sort reference or "send-out" testing, saving considerable time in locating the original specimens after testing in their own laboratory.

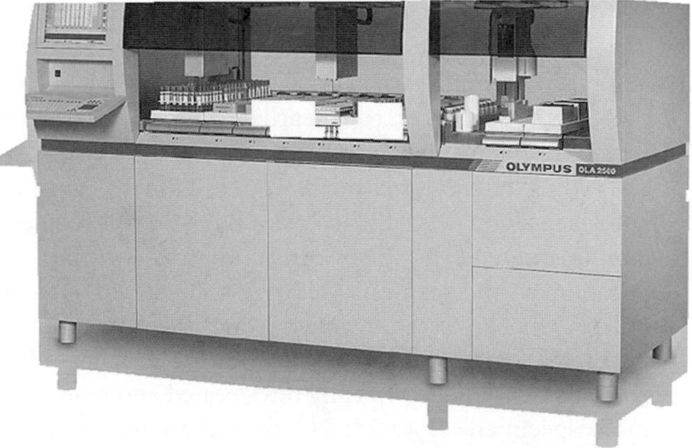

Figure 19-3 The Beckman Coulter Auto-Mate 2500 Lab Automation System is a work cell that performs presorting, specimen volume inspection, decapping, aliquoting, and destination sorting into racks specific to different analyzers with a throughput of up to 650 tubes per hour aliquoted and 800 per hour sorted. *(Courtesy Beckman Coulter, www.beckmancoulter.com.)*

Integrated and Modular Automation Systems

Several manufacturers offer integrated or modular automation systems for specimen processing that include additional functionality. A listing of automation vendors and their Websites can be found in Box 19-5. In addition to the functions described in the preceding section, these systems typically add (1) conveyor transport, (2) interfacing to automated analyzers, (3) more sophisticated process control, and, in some cases, (4) a specimen storage and retrieval system. All systems are of modular design, allowing the customer to choose the modules/features that should be included. Some systems use an open design, which permits interfaces to analyzers from a variety of vendors, whereas other systems are of a closed design and are interfaced only to the vendor's own or a limited number of analyzers. It should be noted that closed systems typically do not have process control software that is independent of the instruments or system, but rather the automation process control is integrated to work with the vendor's analyzers.

BOX 19-5 Vendors of Clinical Laboratory Automation Systems

Abbott Diagnostics
www.abbottdiagnostics.com/accessed April 18, 2011
Aim Lab (formerly Ai Scientific)
www.aimlab.com/accessed April 18, 2011
Beckman Coulter
www.beckmancoulter.com/accessed April 18, 2011
Integrated Laboratory Automation Solutions
www.lab-ilas.com/accessed April 18, 2011
Labotix Automation
www.labotix.com/accessed April 18, 2011
m-u-t America
www.mut-group.com/accessed April 18, 2011
Ortho-Clinical Diagnostics
www.orthoclinical.com/accessed April 18, 2011
PVT LabSystems
www.pvtlabsystems.com/accessed April 18, 2011
Roche Diagnostics
us.labsystems.roche.com/accessed April 18, 2011
Sarstedt
www.sarstedt.com/accessed April 18, 2011
Siemens Healthcare Diagnostics
www.siemens.com/diagnostics/accessed April 18, 2011
Sysmex America
www.sysmex.com/usa/accessed April 18, 2011
Yaskawa America, Motoman Robotics Division
www.motoman.com/labauto//accessed April 18, 2011

To achieve maximum effectiveness of an automation system, process control software should be able to read the specimen's identification (ID) bar code and obtain information from the laboratory's LIS about specimen type and ordered tests. This process control software is usually referred to as the Laboratory Automation System (LAS), not to be confused with the actual hardware of a laboratory automation system. The reader is referred to the Clinical Laboratory and Standards Institute (CLSI) standard on automation communications[5] for further information on LAS. It should then determine the processes the specimen requires and the exact route or course of action for each specimen. It should be able to (1) calculate the number of aliquots and the proper volume for each depending on the tests requested, (2) route the specimens to analyzers, (3) recap the specimens, and (4) retain the specimens for automatic recall. The software should be able to monitor analyzers for in-control production status and automatically make decisions if a test is not available. Specimen integrity checking should be automatic; rules-based decisions should monitor specimen quality and make these decisions. Finally, most process control software should include (1) "autoverification," which is validation of analyzer results by making rules-based decisions that flag exceptions for technologist review, and (2) "autoretrieval" of specimens for repeat, reflex, and dilution testing.

Although most of these systems are restricted to handling specific types of specimen containers, they are capable of processing much of the daily workload of a large clinical laboratory. A few laboratories with daily workloads as low as 600 to 800 specimen tubes have justified these systems because of a shortage of technical help, but typically these systems are designed for laboratories with workloads of 1000 to 10,000 specimens per day. In addition to process control software and the ability to be interfaced to the laboratory's LIS, each of these systems incorporates some or all of the following components:

1. *Specimen input area:* A holding area where bar code–labeled specimens are introduced into the system.
2. *Bar code reading stations:* Multiple bar code readers are placed at critical locations in the processing system to track specimens and provide information for their proper routing to various stations in the processing system.
3. *Transport system:* Segments of a conveyor belt line that move specimens to the appropriate location.
4. A *high-level device to sort or route specimens:* A device that separates specimens by type (such as by tube height) or by order code and passes them to the transport system or to a system using racks. A high-level sorter is often used to separate specimens that require centrifugation, or other processing steps, from specimens that do not, or to route specimens into completely different pathways within the total automation system.[8]
5. *Automated centrifuge:* An area of the specimen processor in which specimens requiring centrifugation are removed from the conveyor belt, introduced into a centrifuge that is automatically balanced, centrifuged (refrigerated or at room temperature), and then removed from the centrifuge and placed back on the transport system.
6. *Level detection and evaluation of specimen adequacy (specimen integrity):* An area in which sensors are used to evaluate the volume of specimen in each specimen container and to look for the presence of hemolysis, lipemia, or icterus.
7. *Decapper station:* An area or device in the automated system in which specimen caps or stoppers are automatically removed and discarded into a waste container.
8. *Recapper station:* An area or device in the automated system in which specimen tubes are automatically recapped with new stoppers or covered with an air-tight closure.
9. *Aliquoter:* A machine that aspirates appropriately sized aliquots from each original specimen container and places them into bar coded secondary specimen containers for sorting and transport to multiple analytical workstations. The LAS generally instructs the aliquoter as to how many aliquots of what volumes are required, based on the bar code ID of the specimen.
10. *Interface to automated analyzer:* A direct physical connection to an automated analyzer that permits the analyzer's sampling probe to aspirate directly from an open specimen container while the container is still on the conveyor, or that may robotically lift the container from the conveyor and place it in the analyzer. Some automation systems interface only to their own brand of analyzers or to a limited number of systems, whereas other automation systems use a so-called open design that complies with CLSI standards and permits interfaces to a variety of automated analyzers.
11. *Sorter:* An automated sorter to sort specimens not going to a conveyor-interfaced analyzer or workstation. Such a sorter typically sorts into 30 to 100 different sort groups in racks or carriers. In some systems, the racks are specific to certain analyzers for convenience.
12. *Take-out stations:* Temporary storage areas for specimens before or after analysis. The take-out station may be the same as the sorter described earlier, where specimens are sorted for manual delivery. However, it may also serve as a holding area (stockyard) for specimens awaiting autoverification of results in case a repeat test is required.
13. *Storage and retrieval system:* This unit may serve the same function as the take-out station or stockyard—that of holding specimens after analysis in case a specimen is necessary for a repeat test—but it has one major difference. These units are typically refrigerated and hold many more specimens (3 to 15,000) than the typical take-out station or stockyard. Depending on daily workloads, the laboratory may be able to retain up to 1 week's worth of specimens for possible repeat or additional tests. Specimen containers are loaded and retrieved with a robot.

Conveyor Belts

The main feature of integrated or so-called total laboratory automation systems is the use of conveyor belts. Ordinary industrial conveyor belts have been used successfully when only transportation is required. However, in the past, when conveyors were integrated with other robotic systems to automate preanalytical and/or postanalytical functions, this technology had difficulty in handling the large variety of specimen containers found in the clinical laboratory. To increase the variety of types of specimen containers that are carried on a conveyor belt system, specimens are placed into specially designed carriers that fit on the conveyor belt line. Sometimes known as "pucks" or "racks" (depending on whether they carry individual specimens or groups of specimens), the carriers have receptacles for variously sized tubes, generally ranging from 13 × 75 mm to 16 × 100 mm—sizes that are consistent with the CLSI Standard AUTO01-A.[3] The industrial, motor-driven conveyor belts used in typical laboratory automation systems have transport rates of a few hundred pucks per hour up to 2000 per hour. In addition, linear synchronous motors (LSMs) and magnetic pucks are now being used for clinical laboratory automation (www.magnemotion.com/accessed April 18, 2011). This technology, which is an order of magnitude faster than present conveyors and has virtually no moving parts, may become the next generation of specimen transport for clinical laboratory automation systems.

Two types of conveyor belt systems are typically used as illustrated in Figure 19-4. Figure 19-4, *A*, depicts a loop conveyor that has a single module for both input of new specimens and removal of completed specimens, and the flow around the loop goes past the processing and analytical modules. Specimens may be sampled directly by the analytical instrument while on the conveyor, or a robot attached to the workstation may remove selected specimens from the conveyor for analysis. Figure 19-4, *B*, depicts a unidirectional conveyor in which specimens are input at one end of the belt, flow past various processing and analytical modules, and arrive at the opposite end, where they are removed. Analyzers access specimens in the same way as the loop conveyor. Depending on the vendor, both of these conveyor types can have bypass lanes that enable specimens not stopping at some modules to bypass them and proceed to other modules. This approach has the advantage that it does not require that specimens be aliquoted because specimens pass by all workstations at which tests are performed. It should also be noted that if specimens are robotically removed from their carriers on the

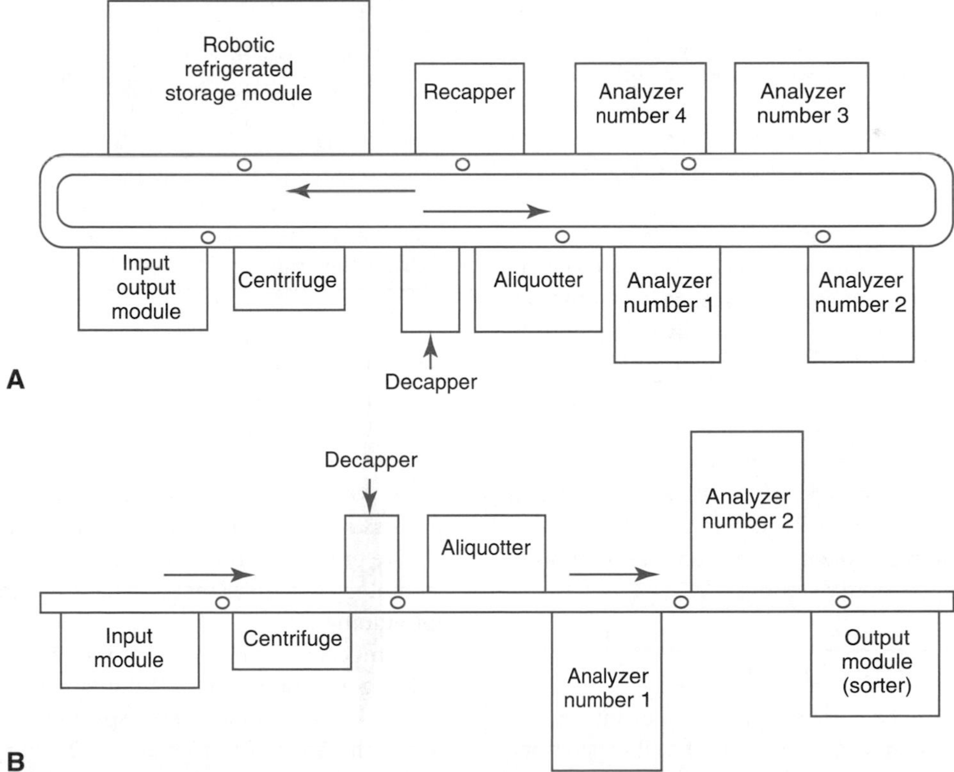

Figure 19-4 A, A depiction of a laboratory automation system employing a continuous loop–type conveyor. In this concept, a single module is used for loading of new specimens and unloading of completed specimens. Depending on the needs of the laboratory, all other modules illustrated are options that can be included or not. B, A depiction of a laboratory automation system employing a unidirectional conveyor. In this concept, separate modules are required for loading of new specimens and unloading of completed specimens. The output module may also perform sorting of specimens for other testing. Other modules can be included, depending on the laboratory's needs.

line for testing, systems for queuing empty carriers to return the tubes to the conveyor and to identify which specimen is in each carrier would be required.

Transfer of specimens from the conveyor belt to the laboratory workstation has been implemented in various ways. For example, some manufacturers have equipped their laboratory instruments with devices to move specimen containers from conveyor belt systems onto the analyzers, while others have installed the ability for the analyzer to sample directly from specimen containers remaining on the conveyor. In practice, the automation system requires a device that stops the tube in the exact location required by the analyzer for sample transfer and verifies and transfers the tube's bar code identification to the analyzer. The CLSI Standard AUTO05-A[4] specifies a common "point in space" that is this exact location for all analyzers and automation conveyor systems.

Depending on the particular automation system, specimens for "stat" testing may or may not be processed and analyzed at speeds that are faster than if manually handled. Laboratories that are purchasing laboratory automation systems are advised to learn how each system handles stat specimens.

Automated Specimen Sorting

In addition to the sorting described previously for stand-alone specimen processing systems and integrated automation systems, stand-alone sorting systems are available, most of which sort into racks for transfer to particular laboratory sections or analyzers. In some cases, the racks may be specific for a specific analyzer, eliminating additional handling of tubes.

Automated Specimen Storage and Retrieval

Automated capability to store and retrieve specimens on demand and with readily known exact storage locations is an important aspect of automated specimen delivery systems. In addition to those automated storage and retrieval options in some of the integrated systems described earlier, several automated or semiautomated options for storage and retrieval, as well as LIS modules and PC-based software systems, permit laboratories to track trays or racks of specimens in their own freezers or refrigerators. Some large reference laboratories have adapted large storage systems commonly used in other industries into their laboratory settings.

PRACTICAL CONSIDERATIONS

In this section, the practical considerations that influence a laboratory's decision to automate part or all of its operations are discussed. A 2007 review[9] outlined how a large hospital laboratory evaluated its needs for automation; the selection and decision processes used by that hospital may provide a useful supplement to this discussion.

Evaluation of Requirements

Any consideration of total or modular laboratory automation should start with an evaluation of requirements.[7] Such an evaluation begins with mapping of the current laboratory work-flow from the arrival of patient specimens through completion of testing and reporting of results. Box 19-6 lists potential work-flow steps that should be mapped. Mapping of material (specimen) flows and data flows is directly related to process flow and will assist the laboratory in determining process steps that (1) are bottlenecks, (2) waste labor, and (3) are prone to error.[10] Work flow mapping thus enables the laboratory to better identify what steps should be considered for automation.

Some laboratorians use 80% as a "rule of thumb" in guiding decisions about automation. Clinical laboratories have many exceptional tests, specimen containers, and handling situations. Nevertheless, if 80% of specimen containers and handling situations can be standardized and automated, the laboratory will achieve a dramatic reduction in its labor usage and costs, which should be sufficient to justify the investment in automation and the planning and evaluation time involved.

Once the laboratory's work-flow has been mapped and its requirements have been identified, alternative solutions are considered. Vendors are invited to make presentations and to host visits of the laboratory management team to other

BOX 19-6 Clinical Laboratory Steps for Work Flow Mapping

Unpacking from transport containers
Presorting
Temperature preservation
Order entry
Document management (requisitions, etc.)
Labeling
Sorting
Centrifugation
Labeling of aliquot tubes
Decapping
Pouring of aliquots
More sorting
Delivery to laboratory sections
More sorting
Preparing work lists
Labeling analyzer-specific tubes for specimens
Pouring or pipetting analyzer-specific specimens
Loading tubes on analyzers
Performing tests (steps such as extraction, centrifugation, precipitation, dilution, etc., are not specifically listed)
Unloading analyzers
Recapping
Data manipulations (calculations)
Results review and verification
Reporting of results
Delivery of specimens to archival storage system
Archival storage of specimens
Reflexive testing
Repeat testing, diluting, if necessary
Additional physician-ordered testing
Specimen retrieval for additional or repeat testing
Disposal of expired specimens

laboratories where vendors have successful installations. It is important at this stage to focus on the requirements identified by work flow mapping and to not allow the vendor to try to sell equipment that may not be necessary.

Problems of Integration

Building a highly integrated laboratory generates many potential problems. Most vendors of clinical laboratory automation systems prefer customer settings in which the integrated analyzers are their own brand. However, many laboratories may prefer to use analyzers from a vendor that is different from their automation system vendor, making integration of instruments and robotic devices from different manufacturers necessary. Decisions must be made concerning which device will be the master controller and which vendor will develop the software that provides overall control of the automation scheme. In addition, individuals or firms that will be responsible for configuration of the automation to the geometry and production schedule of the laboratory must be recruited and trained. Over the past decade, automation vendors have gained considerable experience implementing integrated systems. Although some clinical laboratories have had unsatisfactory experiences, integrated systems are becoming more commonplace.

The reader is referred to the CLSI standard AUTO03-A2 and, in particular, to the Functional Control Model (Section 4.2), which describes the relationships between the LIS, LAS, and various devices.[5] In this model, and throughout the series of CLSI automation standards, the term *LAS* represents the computer system that controls the automation system, not the actual automation hardware. Most often, it is the LAS that has the requisite process control software to support automation. The functional control model, which is depicted in Figure 19-5, supports analytical instruments that may be physically attached to the automation system and analyzers that may not be attached but are still interfaced to the LIS. The model does not give dominance to the LIS or the LAS, but rather allows for essential information flow in either direction to make the most efficient use of the strengths of each system. Although not specified in the AUTO03-A2 standard, some vendors have implemented redundant clustered computers as their LAS to protect customers from downtime associated with failure of a single computer.

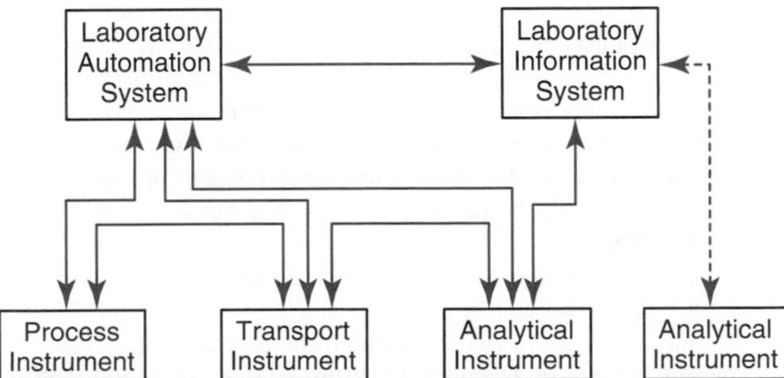

Figure 19-5 Functional control model of the CLSI AUTO3-A2 standard. The *solid lines and arrows* depict logical information flows supported by the standard. The *dotted line and arrows* show logical information flows permitted, but not supported, by the standard. *(Clinical and Laboratory Standards Institute. Laboratory automation: communications with automated clinical laboratory systems, instruments, devices, and information systems. CLSI Approved Standard AUTO3-A2. Wayne, Pa: Clinical and Laboratory Standards Institute, 2009. Figure reproduced with permission of CLSI.)*

Device Integration

One objective in developing an integrated laboratory is to link laboratory instruments and devices into an automated system to maximize the number of functions automated. Automatic specimen introduction requires the development of mechanical interfaces between each laboratory analyzer and devices such as conveyor belts, mobile robots, or robot arms. Some systems have added enhancements such as electronic interfaces for laboratory instruments to allow remote computer control of front-panel functions, notification of instrument status information, and coordination of the distribution of specimens between instruments. In the ideal integrated clinical laboratory automation system, the LAS may be a process controller that would integrate, automate, and monitor many of the decision-making tasks that occur in the daily activity of a laboratory. For example, the LAS would notify an operator that a particular analyzer (even if it is from a different vendor) may be running low on a reagent or may have a fault condition. The LAS (process controller) would control and schedule nonanalytical modules such as automated centrifuges, aliquoters, decappers, and so forth. Most existing LIS systems have no process control capability, and their interfaces with laboratory analyzers provide only the ability to download accession numbers and the tests requested on each specimen, and to upload results generated by the analyzer. The distribution of tasks must be carefully specified in developing such a communications network.

OTHER AREAS OF AUTOMATION

In addition to the automated devices described previously, a variety of other instruments and processes have been automated and used in the clinical laboratory. They include (1) urine analyzers, (2) cell counters, (3) nucleic acid analyzers, (4) microtiter plate systems, (5) automated pipetting stations, and (6) point-of-care testing analyzers.

Urine Analyzers

Many of the same analytical principles are used for the quantification of serum and urine constituents. It is more difficult, however, to automate testing of urine than serum because of the broad range of concentrations of many urine constituents. This requires a low limit of detection to measure low concentrations and expanded linearity to permit measurements of high concentrations without dilution. This requirement, together with the relatively low demand for urine tests compared with that for serum tests, slowed the development of analyzers designed specifically for urine constituents. However, with the deployment of new-generation analyzers, automation of urinalysis is gaining acceptance in many laboratories.[14]

Cell Counters

Analyzers that perform a complete blood count (CBC) have been automated through the use of (1) the "Coulter principle," which is based on cell conductivity, (2) light scatter, and (3) flow cytometry. Individual blood cells are analyzed by application of one or more of these techniques. The Coulter principle is based on changes in electrical impedance produced by nonconductive particles suspended in an electrolyte as they pass through a small aperture between electrodes. In the sensing zone of the aperture, the volume of electrolyte displaced by the particle (cell) is measured as a change in voltage that is proportional to the volume of the particle. By carefully controlling the quantity of electrolyte drawn through the aperture, several thousand particles per second are counted and sized individually. Red blood cells, white blood cells, and platelets are identified by their sizes. Alternating current in the radiofrequency range short-circuits the bipolar lipid layer of the cell membrane, allowing energy to penetrate the cell. Information about intracellular structure, including chemical composition and nuclear volume, is collected with this technique.

Flow cytometry typically uses cells stained with a supravital or fluorescent dye that travel in suspension one by one past a laser light source. (Unstained cells also are measured.) Scattered light and emitted light are collected in front of the light source and at right angles, respectively. Information derived through measurement of light scatter when a cell is struck by the laser beam is then used to estimate (1) cell shape, (2) cell size, (3) cellular granularity, (4) nuclear lobularity, and (5) cell surface structure. Some cell counters classify white cells using the Coulter principle, cell conductivity, and light scattering of unstained cells to differentiate cell types, whereas other cell counters use multiple flow cytometry channels or a combination of flow cytometry, cell conductivity, and light scattering.

Nucleic Acid Analyzers

Automation of the analysis of nucleic acids developed rapidly as an outgrowth of the Human Genome Project.[18] Several manufacturers have developed automation to assist with the isolation of nucleic acids and with analysis of nucleic acids using several amplification schemes and nucleic acid sequencing. Many of these techniques have been miniaturized using chip technology (see Chapter 18).[11,15] Microfluidic chip-based approaches hold promise for reducing analysis time and reagent consumption, and for reducing the costs associated with robotics and laboratory apparatus needed for the macroscale approaches.

Microtiter Plate Systems

Microtiter plate systems are commonly used in immunoassays and nucleic acid analyses. As used for enzyme-linked immunosorbent assays (ELISAs), microtiter plates usually are made of polystyrene and have 48 or 96 wells coated with antibody specific for the antigen of interest. After incubation of serum in the microtiter plate well, the well is washed to remove unbound antigen, and a second antibody with conjugated indicator enzyme is added. After a second incubation period, the well is washed to remove the unbound conjugate. A color-producing product is developed by the addition of enzyme substrate, and the reaction is terminated at a specific time. With the development of automated pipetting stations, the liquid handling steps required for microtiter plate assays have been fully automated to make microtiter plate assays a viable technology for carrying out large numbers of immunoassays. Automated pipetting stations have a cartesian robot with a pipette fixed to the end of a probe that moves about a rectangular space. The probe is capable of moving in the *x*-, *y*-, and *z*-axes. Liquids may be aspirated and dispensed in any location within the rectangular space. Measurement of absorbance and data processing are also automated in such automated instruments.

Automated Pipetting Stations

Pipetting stations may be used to automate an analytical procedure for which an automated analyzer does not exist or cannot be cost justified. Most pipetting robots (1) are relatively easy to program, (2) rarely malfunction, and (3) are capable of delivering aliquots of liquids with extreme precision and accuracy. Multiple-channel pipetting robots allow parallel processing of specimens with 8- or 12-channel probes to handle microtiter plates.

REFERENCES

1. Boyd J. Tech sight. Robotic laboratory automation. Science 2002;295:517-8.
2. Boyd JC, Felder RA. Preanalytical automation in the clinical laboratory. In: Ward-Cook KM, Lehmann CA, Schoeff LE, Williams RH, eds. Clinical diagnostic technology: the total testing process, volume 1. The preanalytical phase. Washington, DC: AACC Press, 2002:107-29.
3. Clinical and Laboratory Standards Institute. Laboratory automation: specimen container/specimen carrier. CLSI Approved Standard AUTO01-A. Wayne, Pa: Clinical and Laboratory Standards Institute, 2000.
4. Clinical and Laboratory Standards Institute. Laboratory automation: electromechanical interfaces. CLSI Approved Standard AUTO05-A. Wayne, Pa: Clinical and Laboratory Standards Institute, 2001.
5. Clinical and Laboratory Standards Institute. Laboratory automation: communications with automated clinical laboratory systems, instruments, devices, and information systems. CLSI Approved Standard AUTO03-A2. Wayne, Pa: Clinical and Laboratory Standards Institute, 2009.
6. Clinical and Laboratory Standards Institute. Autoverification of clinical laboratory test results. CLSI Approved Standard AUTO10-A. Wayne, Pa: Clinical and Laboratory Standards Institute, 2006.
7. Hawker CD, Garr SB, Hamilton LT, Penrose JR, Ashwood ER, Weiss RL. Automated transport and sorting system in a large reference laboratory. Part 1: Evaluation of needs and alternatives and development of a plan. Clin Chem 2002;48:1751-60.
8. Hawker CD, Roberts WL, Garr SB, Hamilton LT, Penrose JR, Ashwood ER, et al. Automated transport and sorting system in a large reference laboratory. Part 2: Implementation of the system and performance measures over three years. Clin Chem 2002;48:1761-67.
9. Melanson SEF, Lindeman NI, Jarolim P. Selecting automation for the clinical chemistry laboratory. Arch Pathol Lab Med 2007;131:1063-9.
10. Middleton S, Mountain P. Process control and on-line optimization. In: Kost GJ, ed. Handbook of clinical automation,

robotics, and optimization. New York: John Wiley & Sons, 1996: 515-40.
11. Paegel BM, Blazej RG, Mathies RA. Microfluidic devices for DNA sequencing: sample preparation and electrophoretic analysis. Curr Opin Biotechnol 2003;14:42-50.
12. Price CP, Newman DJ, eds. Principles and practice of immunoassay, 2nd edition. New York: Stockton Press, 1997.
13. Sasaki M, Kageoka T, Ogura K, Kataoka H, Ueta T, Sugihara S. Total laboratory automation in Japan: past, present, and the future. Clin Chim Acta 1998;278:217-27.
14. Shayanfar N, Tobler U, von Eckardstein A, Bestmann L. Automated urinalysis: first experiences and a comparison between the Iris iQ200 urine microscopy system, the Sysmex UF-100 flow cytometer and manual microscopic particle counting. Clin Chem Lab Med 2007;45:1251-6.
15. Shen Y, Wu BL. Microarray-based genomic DNA profiling technologies in clinical molecular diagnostics. Clin Chem 2009;55:659-69.
16. Walter B: Dry reagent chemistries in clinical analysis. Anal Chem 1983;55:498A-514B.
17. Wild D, ed. The immunoassay handbook, 3rd edition. San Diego, Calif: Elsevier, 2005.
18. Voelkerding KV, Dames SA, Durtschi JD. Next-generation sequencing: from basic research to diagnostics. Clin Chem 2009;55:641-58.

CHAPTER 20

Point-of-Care Testing

Christopher P. Price, Ph.D., F.R.S.C., F.R.C.Path., and Andrew St. John, Ph.D., M.A.A.C.B.

Advances in a range of analytical and fabrication technologies, such as (1) thin film sensors, (2) semiconductor engineering, (3) plastic molding, (4) microfluidics, (5) nanotechnology, and (6) consumer electronics, have made it possible to adapt most of the methods used in the laboratory to the point-of-care setting.[78] This prompts the question as to whether there is the beginning of a general movement of testing away from the central laboratory to the point of care.[112,113,120] Christensen and associates believe that point-of-care testing (POCT) is one of the key enablers required to deliver changes in healthcare provision through disruptive innovation, namely, radically changing the way that healthcare is delivered.[23]

Although early POCT technologies were very much associated with acute clinical needs (e.g., medical emergencies), it is more appropriate to define POCT as "when a test is performed at the time at which the test result enables a decision to be made and an action taken that leads to an improved health outcome." Other terms used to describe POCT have included (1) "bed side,"[97] (2) "near patient,"[32] (3) "physician's office,"[87] (4) "extralaboratory,"[108] (5) "decentralized,"[6] (6) "off site," (7) "satellite," (8) "kiosk," (9) "ancillary," and (10) "alternative site" testing[50]; many of the latter descriptors identify a specific location where the test is intended to be performed, while others clearly describe the adjunctive nature of the testing site to the central laboratory. "Self-testing" should be added to these descriptions to reflect that there is an increasing repertoire of tests that are, performed by patients themselves.

In the hospital setting, POCT has been described in (1) coronary care units,[31] (2) intensive care units,[46] (3) surgical wards,[36] (4) emergency rooms,[41,81] and (5) pediatric units,[42,119] and for monitoring patients with acute[49,54] and chronic conditions.[1] More testing is now being performed using POCT in primary care, both to help in rapid diagnosis and to determine the appropriateness of triage to secondary care, as well as to manage patients with chronic conditions. The "wish list" for the capability to perform POCT in primary care is extensive![92] However a systematic review conducted in 1997 provided little high quality evidence to support this utility.[57]

Although POCT can be viewed as a means to deliver results rapidly to where they are needed (clinical need), it can also be seen as a means of reducing the complexity of the process associated with obtaining a test result (process need). Clinical needs met by POCT can include clinical urgency and improving the interaction between the patient and the clinician/carer to achieve greater patient empowerment and the potential to improve the clinical outcome. Similarly, process needs met by POCT can improve the immediate patient/clinician/carer interaction as alluded to previously, as well as the longer process of the whole patient journey and the patient experience.

Improving clinical and process outcomes has the potential to reduce errors and wastage of resources while also reducing the cost of care and increasing societal gain. This argument can be applied simply to the testing process (Figure 20-1) or to the wider aspects of the whole patient journey. Thus, such a radical change in the provision of healthcare can be seen to have several potential advantages, while exposing stakeholders to different risks, and hence disadvantages (Box 20-1).

Thus an important feature of POCT is identification of healthcare needs and performance requirements associated with meeting those needs, which must be complemented by the quality management and reimbursement strategies required to ensure "fitness for purpose."

The following sections of this chapter describes the technology available for POCT and the organizational factors that are important when POCT is implemented in a healthcare setting. The chapter concludes with a short discussion of the future of POCT.

ANALYTICAL AND TECHNOLOGICAL SOLUTIONS

The commercial POCT market is reported to make up nearly 30% of the total in vitro diagnostics (IVD) market and is worth in excess of $13 billion (U.S.).[68] Within this market are a wide variety of devices that are difficult to classify succinctly but that can be divided into smaller, single-use, hand-held devices and larger benchtop devices that may be single- or multiple-use items (Table 20-1). An additional group, is the wearable devices, an example of which was the GlucoWatch G2 Biographer.[124]

Although all manufacturers of diagnostic medical devices aim to make their devices simple to use and to reduce the risk of error, these goals assume a greater imperative for POCT devices because they are likely to be used by personnel who have not received laboratory training and who lack the skills required to detect when devices may not be working correctly and are giving incorrect results. Thus much of the ingenuity and engineering that have gone into producing the myriad of POCT devices that exist today have been directed toward achieving these goals. The novel mechanical design and engineering solutions are matched in importance by software that makes the device operate in a way that minimizes the risks of mechanical failure and operator error.

This section focuses on some of the key technologies that are used in hand-held and benchtop devices, including specific design features that are aimed at preventing misuse or errors, and refers to some commercial examples. Box 20-2 provides a summary of the ideal requirements for a POCT device against which new technologies and devices are assessed. Readers requiring additional information are referred to more comprehensive texts[75,109] or to vendors of POCT devices.

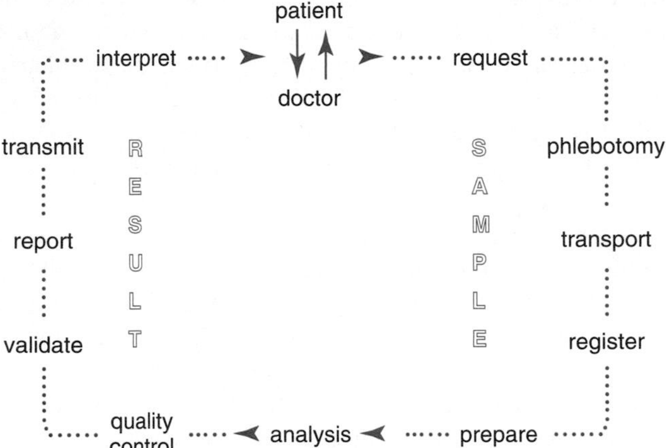

Figure 20-1 Schematic representation of the key steps in requesting, delivering, and using a diagnostic test result.

Hand-Held, Single-Use Devices

No hard and fast definition of a hand-held device as compared with a benchtop instrument is available, but one typical definition used by Kricka and Thorpe is that hand-held

BOX 20-1 Potential Advantages and Disadvantages of Point-of-Care Testing

Advantages

- Reduced turnaround time for test results
- Improved patient management; improved interaction between patient and carer
- Improved patient morbidity and mortality
- Reduction in the administrative work associated with test requesting and reporting
- Reduced risk of errors
- Reduction in clinic visits
- Reduction in hospital admissions
- Improved cost of care

Disadvantages

- Increase in administrative work associated with training and certification of operators
- Caregiver required to perform test
- Increased risk of error if tests are performed by untrained operators

TABLE 20-1 Classification of Types of Point-of-Care Testing Instruments or Devices

Type of Technology	Analytical Principle	Analytes
Single-use, qualitative or semiquantitative cartridge/strip tests	Reflectance	Urine and blood chemistry
	Lateral flow or flow-through immunoassays	Infectious disease agents, cardiac markers, hCG
Single-use quantitative cartridge/strip tests with a reader device	Reflectance	Glucose
	Electrochemistry	Glucose
	Reflectance	Blood chemistry
	Light scattering/optical motion	Coagulation
	Lateral flow, flow-through, or solid phase immunoassays	Cardiac markers, drugs, CRP, allergy, fertility tests
	Microfluidics, PCR	*Chlamydia*
	Immunoturbidimetry	HbA_{1c}, urine albumin
	Spectrophotometry	Blood chemistry
	Electrochemistry	pH, blood gases, electrolytes, metabolites
Multiple-use quantitative cartridge/benchtop devices	Electrochemistry	pH, blood gases, electrolytes, metabolites
	Fluorescence	pH, blood gases, electrolytes, metabolites
	Multiwavelength spectrophotometry	Hemoglobin species, bilirubin
	Time-resolved fluorescence	Cardiac markers, drugs, CRP
	Electrical impedance	Complete blood count

PCR, Polymerase chain reaction.

BOX 20-2 Ideal Requirements for a Point-of-Care Testing System

First results in a minute or less
Portable instruments with consumable reagent cartridges
Single-step operating protocol
Capability of performing direct specimen analysis on whole blood, CSF, urine, and stool specimens (nonprocessed samples)
Simple operating procedures that do not require a laboratory-trained operator
Flexible test menus
Results that meet the analytical specifications that are "fit-for-purpose," and with accuracy and precision comparable with those of the central laboratory, if necessary
Built-in/integrated calibration and quality control
Ambient temperature storage for reagents
Results provided as hard copy, stored, and available for transmission
Low instrument cost
Service by exchange
Built-in regulatory record keeping

devices are up to about the size of the electronic book readers that are now gaining popularity.[79] Hand-held devices first appeared in the form of paper strips many centuries ago for the testing of urine. Test strips as we know them today were introduced in the 1940s and 1950s through companies such as Ames and Roche, while the first disposable immunochemical test could be deemed to be the relatively rapid (2 hours) pregnancy test presented by Wampole in 1970.

To provide some insight into the wealth of different designs that make up disposable hand-held devices, four categories of devices will be reviewed in some detail (1) urine or blood dipsticks; (2) glucose and coagulation strips together with accompanying meters; (3) lateral flow devices including immunosensors; and (4) cartridge or cassette devices. A key attribute of all these devices is that they are used only once and therefore are referred to as single-use devices. Test strips were originally designed to be read by the operator, and with some devices this is still the case, but many strips are now used in conjunction with meters or reading devices. Advances in meter design have been greatly influenced by advances in consumer electronics, and the ability of POCT devices to meet the goals mentioned previously is a consequence of both the design of the strip or analytical system and the meter with which the strip or device is used. Control and communication systems are a major component of all POCT devices other than qualitative or semiquantitative strip tests that do not require a reader or measurement device. In even the smallest device, a control subsystem coordinates all the other systems and ensures that all required processes for an analysis take place in the correct order. Operations that require control include (1) insertion or removal of the strip, cartridge, or cassette; (2) temperature control; (3) sample injection or aspiration; (4) sample detection; (5) mixing; timing of incubation and detection processes (such as absorbance measurement); and (6) waste removal. Fluid movement often is accomplished by mechanical means through pumps or centrifugation, and by fluidic properties, such as surface tension; the latter can be a critical element in the design of simple strip tests and in microfabricated systems.[72]

Urine and Blood Dipsticks

Dipsticks are relatively simple in construction and are composed of a pad of porous material, such as cellulose, that is impregnated with reagent and then dried.[134] The reaction is indicated by a visible color reaction that is compared with a chart. More complex pads are composed of several layers, the uppermost of which is a semipermeable membrane that prevents red cells from entering the matrix. Despite their simplicity, critical operator factors can affect the result, and manufacturers have tried to overcome some of these problems through innovative designs. Thus not all strips now require that the whole pad be covered with the sample to obtain a reliable result. Although reactions in dipsticks do not always proceed to completion, the time between placement of the sample on the pad and comparison of the resulting color with a color chart is less critical for some strips than for others.

However, the need for reproducible timing has driven the need to use small meters to complete the measurement process. This also has the added benefit of reducing operator variability in assessing the color change. For blood tests, it may be necessary to remove all blood before placing the sample in the reflectance meter, but some manufacturers have overcome this problem by reading the color from the underside of the strip.

Further progress with these single-stick devices has included the use of multiple pads for measurement of (1) different concentrations of the same analyte, such as hemoglobin and glucose[134]; (2) both albumin and creatinine (semiquantitative) to obtain an albumin-to-creatinine ratio[114]; and (3) up to 10 different urine analytes; as well as the use of a reflectance meter to quantitate the color change.[85] Table 20-2 lists some of the tests performed by single or multipad dipsticks and the chemistry used for analysis.

Glucose Strips and Meters

Point-of-care glucose testing using disposable strips represents a market that was worth nearly $10 billion (U.S.) in 2008.[68] The size of the market has driven considerable innovation in strip and meter design in an effort to produce devices produce results comparable with those obtained through laboratory methods. Significant improvement has been noted in attributes such as ease of use; however, limitations of this technology are particularly important when testing is conducted in hospitals.

Glucose strips are biosensors in that they all use an enzyme as the recognition agent; glucose oxidase (GO), hexokinase (HK), or glucose dehydrogenase (GDH) with photometric (reflectance) or, more commonly, electrochemical detection may be used.[98] Each strip comprises several layers, each having a specific function. When blood is added, both water

TABLE 20-2 Examples of Single or Multipad Stick Tests

Test	Sample	Chemistry
Acetaminophen	Whole blood	Acyl dehydrogenase
Alanine aminotransferase	Whole blood	Alanine/glutamate
Albumin	Whole blood, urine	Dye binding
Cholesterol	Whole blood	Cholesterol oxidase
Creatinine	Whole blood, urine	Copper complexation
Glucose	Whole blood	Glucose oxidase
Lactate	Whole blood	Lactate dehydrogenase
Uric acid	Whole blood	Uricase
Alcohol	Urine	Alcohol dehydrogenase
Bilirubin	Urine	2,4-Dichloroaniline
Hemoglobin	Urine	Peroxidase activity
Leukocyte esterase	Urine	Pyrrole amino ester hydrolysis
Ketones	Urine	Sodium nitroprusside reaction
Nitrite	Urine	*p*-Arsanilic acid reaction
pH	Urine	Double indicator principle
Protein	Urine	Protein error of indicators
Specific gravity	Urine	Polyacid pH change
Urobilinogen	Urine	Ehrlich's reaction

and glucose must pass into the film or analytical layer; for photometric systems, erythrocytes must be excluded. These processes are achieved by what is called the separating layer that contains various components, including glass fiber fleeces, membranes, and special latex formulations. In photometric systems, a spreading layer is important for fast homogeneous distribution of the sample, whereas electrochemical strips use capillary fill systems. The support layer is usually a thin plastic material that in the case of reflectance-based strips may have reflective properties. Additional reflectance properties have been achieved through the inclusion of substances such as titanium oxide, barium sulfate, and zinc oxide.

The use of different chemistries and detection systems is driven by a number of requirements, including (1) accurate and precise results with freedom from common interferences, (2) rapid response of detection, (3) ease of use, and (4) low cost. The relative importance of these goals differs somewhat between meters used in the hospital, where there can be significant problems due to interferences, and those used by patients for self-monitoring, when ease of use and low cost are priorities.

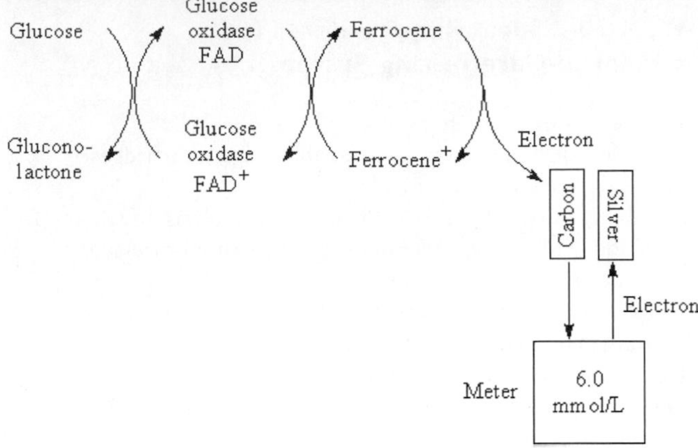

Figure 20-2 Schematic diagram of the reactions taking place in a MediSense electrochemical glucose strip. *(Modified from Henning TP, Cunningham TP. Biosensors for personal diabetes management. In: Ramsay G, ed. Commercial biosensors. New York: John Wiley & Sons, 1998:3-46.)*

A major advance in the development process was the use of ferrocene and its derivatives as immobilized mediators in the construction of electrochemical glucose strips.[33] The strip is composed of an Ag-AgCl reference electrode and a carbon-based active electrode, both manufactured using screen printing technology with the ferrocene or its derivatives contained in the printing ink. The sample is placed in the sample observation window, and the hydrophilic layer serves to direct the sample over the reagent layer. Conversion of glucose is accompanied by the reduction of ferrocene and the release of electrons (Figure 20-2).[33] Another significant advance has been the use of techniques such as capillary filling to ensure that the right amount of sample is in place.

In practice, glucose strips are produced in large batches; after extensive quality assurance procedures, each batch is given a code that is stored in a magnetic strip on the underside of each test strip. This code describes the performance of the batch, including the calibrating relationship between the photometric or electrochemical signal and the concentration of glucose. For many years, it was necessary to provide a means for recalibrating a meter (e.g., providing the algorithm on a bar coded strip that could be read by the meter) when a new batch of strips was employed, which led to errors when patients forgot to perform the recalibration.[115] However, strips now can be manufactured with sufficient consistency such that recalibration between different lots is no longer required.[8]

Parallel with advances in strip technology has been the evolution of the consumer electronics industry, in particular the miniaturization of electronics.[95] The latter, together with the use of amperometric methods, has enabled the production of smaller meters, nonwipe strips, sample volumes

<1 μL, less need to clean instrument optics, and results obtained within 5 seconds. Some meters also include substantial information technology (IT) capability, including the ability to lock users out if they have not completed required procedures such as quality control (QC) and the capacity to store and download patient results. In conjunction with docking stations and data managers is the capability to institute the type of informatics procedures that are required of central laboratory testing, such as identification and possible lockout of operators, together with transmission of results to the laboratory information system (LIS), along with accompanying patient information.

Thus the capability of glucose meters has advanced significantly over the years and is such that appropriately trained and motivated patients with diabetes can monitor their own glucose with a reasonable degree of assurance and tailor their insulin therapy accordingly. The use of glucose meters in sick or hospitalized patients has been more problematic. For example, a major problem with glucose oxidase methods was their susceptibility to the ambient tension of oxygen in blood, which may vary substantially in critically ill patients. This interference was essentially removed by using glucose dehydrogenase as the enzyme, but several reports and at least one death have been the result of maltose interference in glucose dehydrogenase strips that use the pyrroloquinolinequenone form of the enzyme (GDH-PQQ), the maltose being given as part of the patient's therapy.[43] Subsequently, improved strips such as the StatStrip by Nova BioMedical (Waltham, Mass) appear to overcome this problem.[58]

In addition, evaluation reports indicate that this newer design is not affected by hematocrit, unlike most other glucose strips. Hematocrit can vary substantially in young infants and in critically ill adults with the glucose concentration being inversely related to the hematocrit; those who look after the critically ill need to be aware of this phenomenon. Many interferent issues and the resulting performance gap between glucose meters and laboratory results have been brought into sharp focus with the adoption of procedures such as tight glycemic control (TGC) in intensive care unit (ICU) patients.[132] Although meter performance has undoubtedly improved over the years, reports show that the analytical performance of most current meters is not good enough for them to be used in TGC protocols.[14] An International Organization for Standardization (ISO) document reviews the performance goals required for meters in hospitals, in physician and practitioner offices, and for patients performing self-monitoring.[62]

Coagulation Strips and Meters

The clinical need to monitor anticoagulant therapy in both acute and chronic medical settings has been well defined, and the value of POCT devices has been demonstrated in several studies.[36,53] The number of patients requiring long-term anticoagulant therapy is growing, and coagulation monitoring is one of the largest sectors of the POCT market after glucose monitoring and pregnancy testing. General features of a typical coagulation meter include a design that utilizes fingerstick samples in the case of home or clinic monitoring, with minimal demands on the user in terms of sample application. The reaction usually takes place in a cassette or test strip that is maintained at a temperature above 37 °C to maximize reaction kinetics and minimize changes in outside temperature. The latest generation of portable meters generally used in hospital locations is much easier to use, compared with earlier systems, and requires smaller specimen volumes.

Manufacturers have used a variety of systems to detect the clotting event in coagulation meters, but newer detection technologies that are classified broadly as electrochemical are used in HemoSense and Roche CoaguChek XS instruments. With the HemoSense InRatio2 coagulation meter (HemoSense Inc., Inverness Medical Innovations, Waltham, Mass) for measurement of prothrombin time (PT), clotting is detected by impedance rather than by current.[64] Because this device is likely to be used by patients, it has various features designed to make QC automatic or to require minimal involvement of the patient. These include a test strip that has three channels—one for the patient test and two for different concentrations of internal QC reference materials; all three channels operate simultaneously when a patient sample is applied to the strip (Figure 20-3). Similar features of integrated on-board QC operate in other smaller meters or devices likely to be used by patients, such as the ITC ProTime Microcoagulation System (ITC, Edison, NJ). Several studies have shown that the ProTime device can be used satisfactorily by patients for self-testing purposes.[99,100] Many meters have QC lockout features that prevent operation of the device when QC results are not within prescribed limits, as well as software to detect common errors such as expired reagents

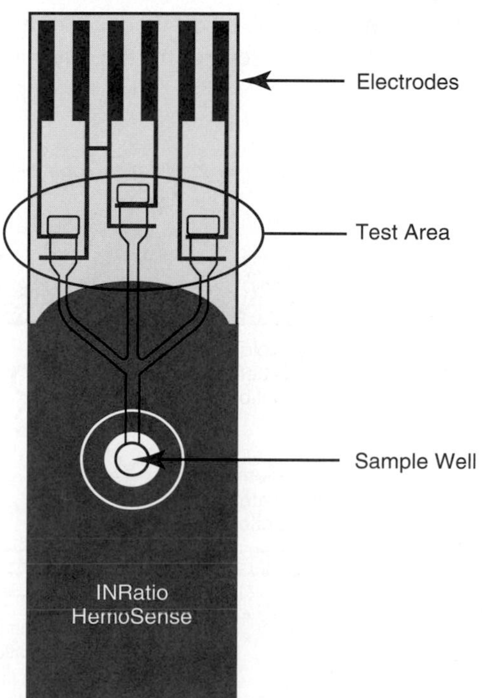

Figure 20-3 Schematic diagram of the HemoSense PT strip. *(Courtesy Hemesense.)*

and incorrect specimen placement or volume. The Roche CoaguChek XS (Roche Diagnostics, Mannheim, Germany) uses a similar amperometric detection principle. Thrombin-activated cleavage of thromboplastin in the strip leads to generation of electrochemically active phenylenediamine, and when the current generated by this species reaches a certain value, the PT can be determined.[105] Environmental changes in the strip that might occur as the result of incorrect handling are detected by an integrated QC system in the strip, which, under the Clinical Laboratory Improvement Amendments (CLIA) of the United States, means there is no need to run liquid quality controls on the strip.

One persistent problem that remains for point-of-care coagulation testing is the poor correlation between POCT devices and coagulation analyzers in the central laboratory. This is a particular problem for activated clotting time (ACT), for which a so-called gold standard for comparison does not exist.[106] Reports in the literature indicate that despite improvements and progress with standardization, lack of agreement can still be a problem.[69,125]

Lateral Flow Strips

Many POC tests use lateral flow strips, usually for immunoassays; the original application that was filed as a patent in 1979 was called an *immunochromatograph.*[48,111] These devices are biological sensors in which the recognition agent is usually an antibody that binds to the analyte. Detection of the binding event or signal transducer usually occurs via an optical mechanism—reflectance or fluorescence spectrophotometry—for quantification. A typical sandwich immunoassay format in a lateral flow is the Roche Troponin T test shown in Figure 20-4.[3,30] Two antibodies are present in the strip: one labeled with gold particles, and the other conjugated to biotin. When whole blood is added to the test well, it flows through the fleece, separating the plasma, and the troponin binds to the two antibodies. The antibody-troponin complex flows along the cellulose nitrate strip and reaches the capture zone, which contains streptavidin. The latter binds to the biotin in the troponin complex, immobilizing it and appearing as a purple band due to the presence of gold particles on one of the antibodies. Unreacted gold-labeled antibody is able to move down the strip, where it is captured by a synthetic peptide that contains the epitope of human cardiac troponin T, which is visualized as a separate second band. This band indicates that the sample has flowed along the strip and the device has worked correctly, which represents a form of built-in control.

A growing application of lateral flow strip immunoassay is for infectious disease testing and the rapid detection of various infectious antigens and antibodies, including (1) *Chlamydia trachomatis,*[65] (2) group A streptococci,[21] (3) *Helicobacter pylori,*[51] (4) infectious mononucleosis,[40] and (5) human immunodeficiency virus.[67]

Although many lateral flow strips rely on visual reading by the operator, an increasing number are used in conjunction with meters or reading devices. An integral part of many of these instruments is a charge-coupled device (CCD) camera that is a multichannel light detector, similar to a photomultiplier tube in a spectrophotometer, but with a higher signal-to-noise ratio so it detects much lower signals at low quantities of light. For example, the Roche Cardiac Reader contains a CCD that will quantitate separate lateral flow immunoassay strips for measurement of troponin T, myoglobin, and D-dimer.

Several immunosensor-based devices have been developed that are capable of measuring a panel of analytes, such as cardiac markers,[4] drugs of abuse tests,[17] and fertility tests.[12] With these devices, a mixture of antibodies is placed at the origin, and complementary antibodies for various analytes are located at varying positions along the porous strip. In the

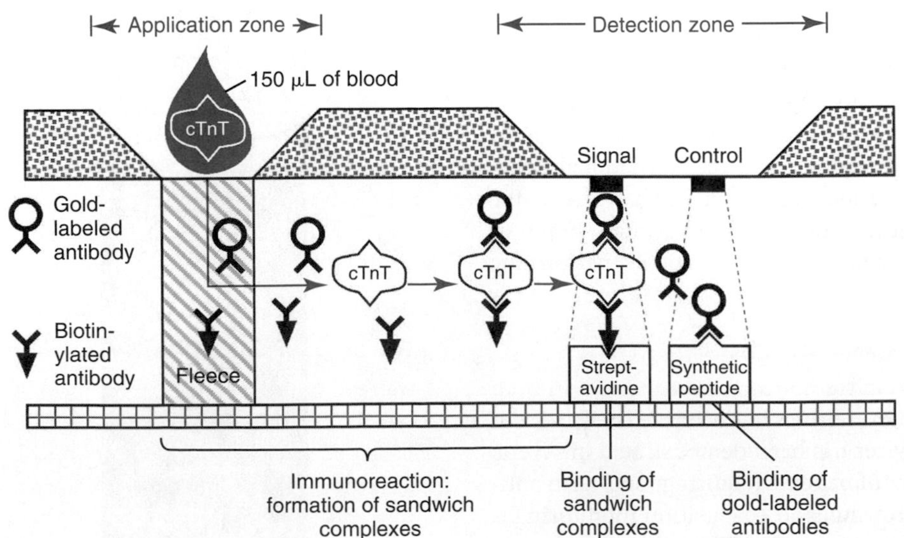

Figure 20-4 Schematic diagram of a lateral flow immunoassay strip for troponin T. *(Courtesy Roche Diagnostics.)*

case of drugs of abuse, devices are designed such that positive responses are obtained only if the concentration is above a precalibrated cutoff value.[17]

Although lateral flow devices are the most common form of POCT immunosensor, other formats include a flow-through design.[130] Alternative detection mechanisms to reflectance or absorbance are also being investigated; these include (1) surface plasmon resonance, (2) evanescent wave, (3) fixed-polarized ellipsometry, and (4) diffraction.

Cartridge or Cassette Devices

Another major category of single-use devices consists of integrated cartridges or cassettes that operate in conjunction with a hand-held meter. The most common example is the i-Stat Analyzer (Abbott Laboratories, Chicago, Ill), which when introduced some 2 decades ago, measured only blood gases, electrolytes, and glucose but now has a menu that includes creatinine, certain coagulation parameters, and troponin.[11,39] To achieve the full menu requires different combinations of cartridges. Each of these contains sensors or electrodes as wafer structures constructed with thin metal oxide films using microfabrication techniques directly comparable with those used in the computer industry.[35] Another important component of the cartridge is the microfluidic network, which directs and controls the movement of calibration liquids and blood sample to each of the sensors.[72] This device was one of the first to introduce the concept of electronic QC, a procedure that checks the status of the cartridge prior to analysis of a patient sample. Although this is a valuable procedure, it is agreed by most laboratory professionals that it cannot substitute for conventional QC procedures.[135] The size of the device allows it to be used directly at the bedside and via the use of a docking station or cradle connected to the LIS or hospital information system (HIS); patient results can be captured and retained in the patient record. Some hospitals use these systems for all critical care testing; others retain them as a backup or use them in locations where testing is done relatively infrequently.

The need for clean air fabrication means that the cost of I-stat–type devices is relatively high, which has driven research into alternative and less costly ways to manufacture such complex cartridges. One example is the Epoc system (Epocal Inc., Ottawa, Ontario, Canada), which uses technology from the smart-card industry by manufacturing blood gas, electrolyte, and immunoassay devices as credit card–sized items on 35-mm tape-on-reel format.[80] Similar to the I-Stat system, the cards are used in conjunction with a hand-held meter, but this type of technology has significant advantages in terms of manufacturing cost.

In a similar vein, microfluidic cards are now being developed as an alternative to more conventional cassettes for a number of applications, including polymerase chain reaction (PCR)-based tests for infectious agents. In one approach under development by Atlas Genetics (Bristol, United Kingdom; www.atlasgenetics.com/accessed April 14, 2011), the disposable card (Figure 20-5) has many functions, which use a common architecture to ensure a simple, low-cost device that combines sample preparation, PCR amplification, and electrochemical detection. The lower molding contains fluidic channels through which reagents are moved using a series of bellows and valves created by the flexible rubber layer. This enables an instrument to remain isolated from the fluids in the card by simply applying pressure to the card to run the assay. The foil on the bottom of the card has excellent barrier properties for long-term storage of wet reagents, while providing a low-resistance path for rapid thermocycling.[55]

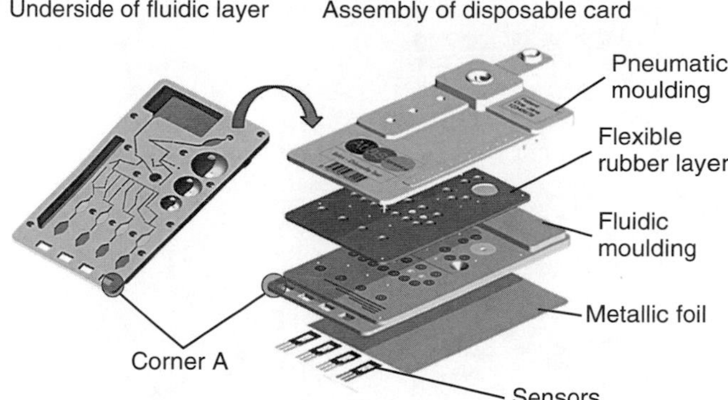

Figure 20-5 Schematic diagram of a microfluidic card employing a molecular test for *Chlamydia trachomatis*. *(Courtesy Atlas Genetics, Bristol, United Kingdom.)*

Multiple-Use Cartridges and Benchtop Systems

A significant proportion of multiple-use systems are used for critical care testing in locations such as the ICU, the surgical suite, and the emergency room. The technology for measuring blood gases and associated parameters has existed for many years, but the menus of so-called blood gas instruments have recently been extended to include biosensors for parameters such as glucose, lactate, and urea. Although they use similar technology to that described previously, they differ in that the sensors are designed to be reusable.[34] To improve convenience for non–laboratory trained users such as nurses and doctors, the sensors have been incorporated with reagents and calibrators into a single cartridge or pack that is placed in the body of a small to medium-sized, portable critical care analyzer (Figure 20-6). Each pack will measure a certain number of samples during a particular time period, after which replacement is a relatively simple procedure. This type of technology is available as the (1) Instrumentation Laboratory GEM Premier 3000 and 4000 (Instrumentation Laboratory GEM, Bedford, Mass),[9,10] (2) Radiometer ABL800 (Radiometer ApS, Copenhagen, Denmark),[84] and (3) Siemens Healthcare Diagnostics Rapidpoint 400 (Deerfield, Ill).[86]

Other key developments for critical care devices include liquid calibration systems that use a combination of aqueous base solutions and conductance measurements to calibrate the pH and PCO_2 electrodes, with oxygen being calibrated with an oxygen-free solution and room air.[90] This dispenses with the need for gas bottles. Another important innovation is the integration of automated QC packages into these analyzers, which ensure that QC samples are analyzed at regular

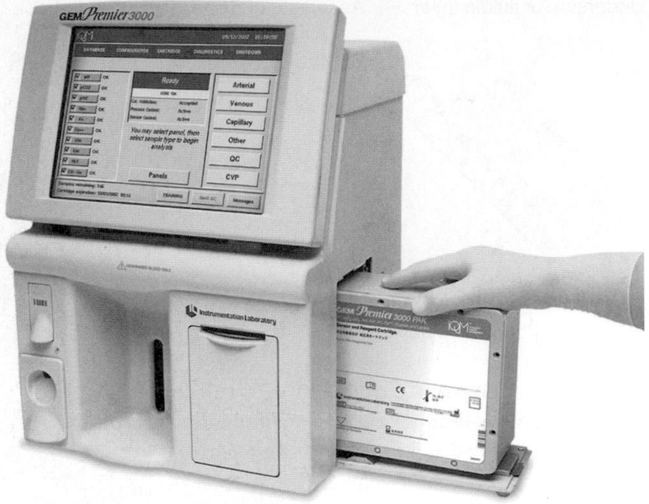

Figure 20-6 The GEM Premier 3000 critical care analyzer. *(Courtesy Instrumentation Laboratory, Lexington, Mass.)*

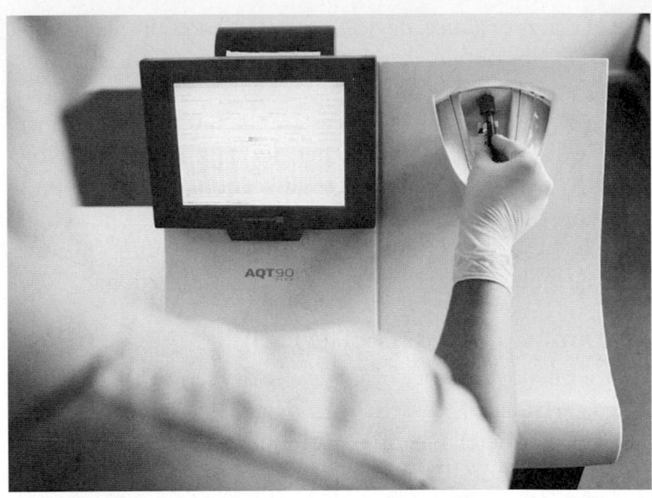

Figure 20-7 Touchscreen of the Radiometer AQT Flex analyzer. *(Courtesy Radiometer, Copenhagen, Denmark.)*

intervals. These comprise packs or bottles of QC material that are contained within the instrument and are sampled at predetermined intervals with onboard software interpreting the results and generating alerts, if necessary. Such devices can even be remotely monitored and programmed to respond to problems with instruments located long distances from the central laboratory.[56]

Critical care POCT instruments are also available for measuring various hemoglobin species and performing CO-oximetry determinations. The latter relies upon multiwavelength spectrophotometry where light absorption by hemolyzed blood is measured at up to 60 or more wavelengths to determine the concentration of the five hemoglobin species.[16] Manufacturers have extended the capability of multiwavelength spectrophotometry to measure bilirubin directly in whole blood.[13,117]

The menu of critical care tests is also being extended to parameters that can be measured only by immunoassay. Two particularly important parameters required for acute care are troponin and beta–**chorionic gonadotropin** (CG). As has been described, both can be measured using hand-held devices, usually using lateral flow or similar technology, but the precision and accuracy of such techniques are occasionally not fit for the purpose for which they are intended. Thus manufacturers have devised larger instruments for immunoassay measurement that are capable of comparable analytical quality to laboratory instruments, but they use whole blood, thus facilitating their use close to patient care. The Radiometer AQT90 Flex uses an all-in-one dry-reagent concept and the well-established technique of time-resolved fluorescence used in laboratory-based instruments. Whole blood or plasma samples are used, and the instrument includes an automated sample aspiration module, thus minimizing the time that operators have to interact with the instrument and reducing the risk of preanalytical error (Figure 20-7). The sample is added automatically to the cup containing assay-specific reagents, and in the case of troponin, the assay is a one-step immunofluorometric assay using two biotinylated antibodies for capture and one europium-labeled antibody for detection. Whole blood results are corrected for hematocrit using conductance measurement and are available in less than 20 minutes.[52]

The case for performing acute care testing close to the patient is obvious and well established. In recent years, healthcare providers have seen the need to improve the process for managing patients with chronic conditions such as diabetes. Part of this improvement includes the provision of laboratory testing at the time of the actual consultation; in the case of diabetes care, this has created the need for point-of-care devices that can measure key analytes such as glycated hemoglobin ($HbA1_C$), lipids, and urinary albumin.

Several small devices exist for measurement of HbA_{1c}, but as indicated in a study performed with nurses in a diabetes clinic, only one was considered capable of meeting the required analytical specifications for the monitoring of HbA_{1c}.[121] The DCA 2000 uses an established analytical method of light scattering immunoassay for glycated hemoglobin, but the measurement has been incorporated into a single-use cartridge (Figure 20-8) that is placed in a small benchtop instrument and requires minimal interaction with the operator.[102,107] The Axis-Shield Affionion AS100 (Axis-Shield plc, Dundee, Scotland) is a newer, not dissimilar, cartridge-based analyzer that measures C-Reactive Protein (CRP) as well as HbA_{1c} with analytical performance adequate for the monitoring of HbA_{1c} in patients with diabetes.[5]

Other developments in POCT benchtop technologies have included small instruments for measuring cellular components of blood. Thus the Chempaq analyzer and associated cassettes (Figure 20-9) employ an impedance sensor to count blood cells, which can differentiate between cell types and subgroups by measuring their size, expressed as a change in electrical impedance, when the cells pass the sensor. The

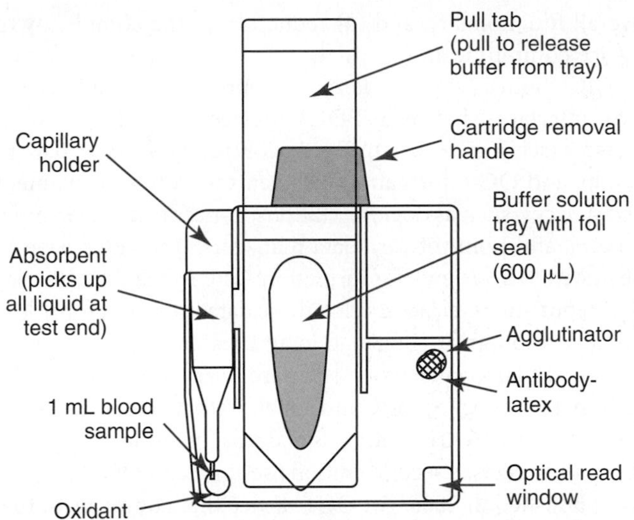

Figure 20-8 Schematic diagram of the Bayer DCA 2000 HbA_{1c} immunoassay cartridge. *(Courtesy Seimens Medical Diagnostics.)*

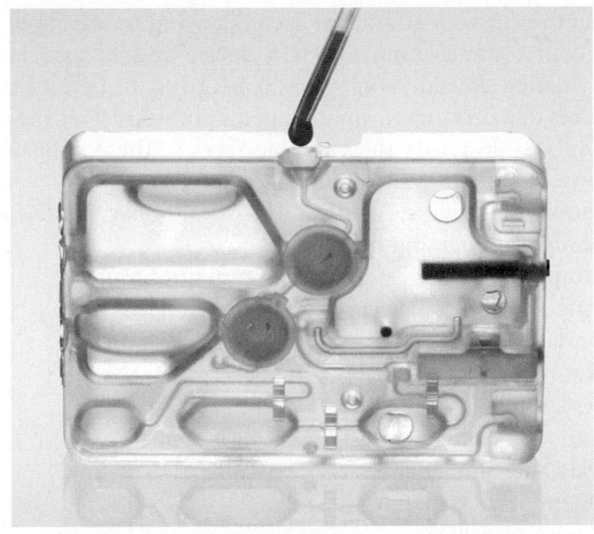

Figure 20-9 Schematic diagram of the Chempaq CBC Analyzer. *(Courtesy Chempaq A/S, Farum, Denmark.)*

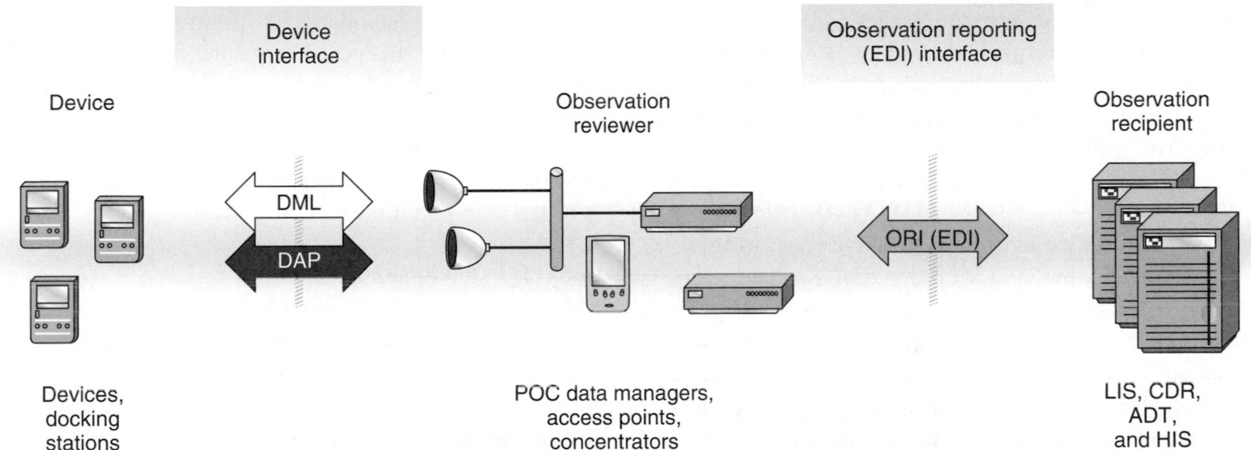

Figure 20-10 Schematic diagram of the interfaces between point-of-care testing (POCT) devices and information systems. *(Clinical Laboratory Standards Institute. Point-of-care connectivity: approved standard, 2nd edition. CLSI Document POCT01-A2. Wayne, Pa: CLSI, 2006.)*

disposable unit (termed the PAQ) contains two chemical reagents. The first reagent is an isotonic solution, which dilutes the blood and enables quantitation of red blood cells (Mean Cell Volume) and platelets (PLT). The second reagent is used to lyse the red blood cells (RBC)s, thereby enabling quantitation of white blood cells, a three-part differential, and hemoglobin.The reagent used to measure hemoglobin lyses the red blood cell membrane, releasing hemoglobin and further causing chemical reformulation of released hemoglobin to form a stable methemoglobin complex. The amount of hemoglobin is measured using spectrophotometry at two different wavelengths.[116] A white cell counter (HemoCue WBC Analyzer, HemoCue, Cypress, Calif) has been described that uses a digital photomicroscope and specially designed software with image analysis algorithms to detect white cells following staining of the nuclei with methylene blue dye.[101]

INFORMATICS AND POCT

POCT devices require the same variety of informatic functions required by conventional laboratory analyzers. Primarily, these functions are associated with electronic transfer of data from analyzers to the LIS and ultimately into a patient's electronic medical record. This provides healthcare professionals with quick, accurate, and appropriate access to the patient's medical history and information. In reality, it is rare for POCT devices to be directly connected to the LIS, and they are usually connected via some sort of docking station and/or data management system (DM), which, in turn, is connected to the LIS (Figure 20-10).

Informatic Requirements in POCT Devices

With advances in software and hardware capabilities, it is possible to considerably enhance the value and quality of the patient result with additional accompanying information. In the course of selecting a POCT device and its associated informatics, consideration should be given to devices that ensures that certain information items always accompany the patient result across the two interfaces.[26] These obligatory information items include the following:

- Patient identifiers: medical record number (MRN) or similar number and name
- Sample identifiers or accession number (AN)
- Date and time of specimen collection
- Type of specimen
- Test requested
- Test result
- Units to be attributed to the result if applicable
- Date and time of analysis
- Operator identifier
- Device identifier
- Error messages and action messages

Other optional information items that operators may wish to transfer from the device to the DM and possibly to the LIS include (1) reference interval, if not generated by the LIS; (2) specific comments (e.g., error messages); (3) consumable material details (e.g., lot number and expiry date); (4) calibration information, including expiration date; (5) QC parameters; and (6) date and time of system alerts, such as "low battery" and "calibration due."

Development of POCT Connectivity Standards

Although the importance of linking POCT devices to information systems and enhancing the value of the patient result is clear, problems have been associated with achieving this goal, primarily because of interfacing difficulties. These difficulties arose because specific vendor instruments and accompanying DM systems came with proprietary interfaces that rarely allowed devices from other vendors to be linked without significant cost. Because it is common for laboratories to use POCT devices from multiple vendors, this lack of ability to connect different devices through a single DM led to many devices not being linked to any sort of information system. Consequently, patient results often did not get entered into the patient record, thus running the risk of duplicate testing, or they were entered manually with risk of transcription error.[66,122]

At the time, it was thought that the development of a set of common universal "plug and play" interfacing standards for incorporation into all POCT devices would address this problem. Such standards would ensure that POCT devices meet critical user requirements, such as (1) bidirectionality; (2) device connection commonality; (3) commercial software intraoperability, security; and (4) QC and/or regulatory compliance. Accordingly, the Connectivity Industry Consortium (CIC) of more than 30 companies involved in the POCT industry designed a set of connectivity standards that incorporated the following features: (1) use of a proven architecture and notation, (2) use of existing standards and architectural patterns wherever possible, (3) focus on services that would enable software intraoperability and add value to overall functionality, and (4) reduction in the complexity of device communications.

CIC connectivity standards are represented simply as the two interfaces between POCT devices and information systems (see Figure 20-10). The device interface passes patient results and QC information between the POCT instrument and devices, such as docking stations, concentrators, terminal servers, and point-of-care data managers. The latter have to be linked to a variety of information systems via the observation reporting interface or electronic data interface, for transmission of ordering information and patient results.

The initial connectivity standard was approved by the National Committee for Clinical Laboratory Standards [now the Clinical and Laboratory Standards Institute (CLSI)] in 2001, and a revised second edition (designated POCT01-A2)[25] was published in 2006. A POCT device that conforms to this standard should be able to communicate with DM and LIS systems, allowing exchange of data and information in a standardized format, irrespective of vendor or location.

Unfortunately, the uptake of POCT01-A2 has not been as rapid as was anticipated, and not all POCT device companies have adopted the standard. To promote awareness of the potential benefits that could be gained from a universal connectivity standard, CLSI published POCT02-A, "An Implementation Guide of POCT01 for Healthcare Providers," a document that provides in relatively nontechnical terms an explanation of connectivity and what users should look for in POCT01-compliant devices.[26]

Benefits of Connectivity and Future Developments

One of the most important benefits of connectivity is to facilitate the transfer and capture of patient POCT and quality-related data into permanent medical records.[22] Other destinations for point-of-care data include the bedside monitors and clinical information systems that reside in critical care units. These systems integrate data from various sources, including vital signs and diagnostic results. In conjunction with clinical guidelines and expert systems, they can produce critical care maps used in the management of the critically ill patient.[49] Integration of POCT data with other laboratory and clinical information is now commonly seen in disease management systems supporting the care of patients with chronic diseases, such as diabetes mellitus and hyperlipidemia. In the case of diabetes mellitus, the DM serves to maintain a record of blood glucose results and any other observations that the patient wishes to record, to bring to the attention of the clinician at the next clinic visit. This record is then used to help patients in the management of their own disease. In the case of hyperlipidemia, data may be fed into an algorithm together with other observations to calculate a risk score that is used by the patient and his or her clinician to identify life-style, dietary, and therapy changes, together with expected outcomes (e.g., reduced risk of cardiovascular disease). Linking POCT with decision support tools and associated treatment algorithms is seen as the future in a number of situations, including glycemic control in intensive care,[132] management of diabetes,[47] management of heart failure,[82] and assistance with self-dosing for patients on anticoagulants.[53]

Improvements in the quality management of POCT are also assisted by an ability to easily link devices to networks and to those who are ultimately responsible for the device. Most manufacturers of POCT devices now provide software to allow central laboratories to monitor their instruments in remote locations. In conjunction with network technology, remote control software not only allows monitoring of the performance of the device, it also enables those responsible for the instrument to carry out some service procedures or even to shut the instrument down completely if required. Such software can manage a large number of devices that may be geographically dispersed, and, by reducing the necessity to physically visit each device, its use can result in significant staff savings.[56]

Informatic-related features for the future include greater adoption of the POCT01-A2 standard. Although one can appreciate that some device vendors may prefer to always retain their proprietary interfaces rather than open their systems to competitor devices, there remains a call by users for more universal connectivity.[83] A randomized controlled trial of POCT in general practice in Australia was groundbreaking in many respects, but it did not include the use of any form of comprehensive data management or informatics, partly because the devices used were obtained from multiple vendors, and it was impossible to easily interface them to a single data management system.[15] A second important demand for the future is wireless connectivity, which would provide many management benefits, particularly for those devices used in conjunction with docking stations.[93]

IMPLEMENTATION AND MANAGEMENT CONSIDERATIONS

Implementation, management, and maintenance of a high-quality POCT service require proper organization, training, and management. Consequently, several factors must be considered, including (1) establishing need, performance specifications, risks, and change management challenges; (2) organizing and implementing a POCT Coordinating Committee; (3) establishing a POCT testing policy and accountability; (4) procuring equipment and its evaluation; (5) training and certification of operators, and establishing a QC, quality assurance, and audit policy; (6) ensuring documentation; (7) establishing a policy for accreditation and regulation of POCT, which, in certain situations (e.g., a hospital setting), may require conformance to accreditation and regulatory requirements applicable to the local laboratory.

Several published guidelines on POCT are based on the ISO standard 22870 ["Point-of-Care Testing (POCT): Requirements for Quality and Competence"].[59] Separate ISO standards have been put forth for self-testing of blood glucose[60] and for monitoring for oral anticoagulation therapy.[61] The CLSI has published a second edition of its guidelines for POCT,[27] as have a number of organizations in other countries.[2,7,89] The following paragraphs summarize some of the main features of these guidelines.

ESTABLISHMENT OF NEED, RISKS, AND CHANGE MANAGEMENT CHALLENGES

As with laboratory testing in general, the decision to implement a POCT service requires definition of (1) the healthcare need; (2) the clinical, operational, and economic benefits; (3) the performance requirements; (4) the clinical risks; and (5) the costs involved.

Box 20-3 lists typical questions that should be asked when one is establishing the requirement for a POCT service. Analytical performance specifications are an important part of these considerations. Reference has already been made to the fact that the performance should be "fit for purpose," and although this is often considered equivalent to laboratory performance, in many cases, little formal evidence is available to support this conjecture. Thus one situation where laboratory quality method precision has been shown to be important is in the measurement of blood glucose to support tight glycemic control of patients in the intensive care unit. On the other hand, a semiquantitative POCT method for measurement of the urine albumin-to-creatinine ratio may be acceptable for the rule-out of albuminuria in a primary care setting. Fitness for purpose therefore is based on the combination of need, performance, and outcome.

Responses to the questions should help the clinician to identify what benefits are likely to accrue to the patient, the caregiver and/or the healthcare provider organization by introducing a more rapid service. An economic assessment of the costs of delivering the current service and the costs associated with the POCT service should be conducted. The

BOX 20-3 Assessing the Need for a Point-of-Care Testing Service

Which tests are required?
What is the turnaround time required?
What clinical question is being asked when requesting this test?
What clinical decision is likely to be made upon receipt of the result?
What action is likely to be taken upon receipt of the result?
What outcome should be expected from the action taken?
Why isn't the laboratory able to deliver the required service?
Will POCT provide the required accuracy and precision of the result?
Is staff available to perform the test?
Are facilities adequate to perform the test and store the equipment and reagents?
Will you abide by the organization's POCT policy?
Are there operational benefits to this POCT strategy?
Are there economic benefits to this POCT strategy?
Will a change in practice be required to deliver these benefits?
Is it feasible to make the changes in practice that might be required?

benefits must be identified and accounted for in a way similar to that involved in identifying the cost of other elements of the health service. The total cost of the current service and that of a revised service based on POCT should be determined. Total cost will include all resources used to deliver the service, including personnel and process management functions. In addition, potential cost savings due to decreased length of stay or substitution of physician time for another care provider's time must be considered, as reducing costs may be the key objective in using POCT.

A risk assessment should also be conducted that will focus primarily on procedures and processes that have to be put in place to ensure the maintenance of a high quality of service.[74] Issues of concern include (1) robustness of the POCT device; (2) quality of the results produced, including changes in accuracy and/or precision and/or specificity of POCT results compared with central laboratory results, and how such changes will influence interpretation of results and clinical action based on those results; (3) competence of the operator of the device; (4) effectiveness of the process for transmission of results to the caregiver; (5) competence of the caregiver to interpret the results provided; (6) procedures in place to ensure that an accurate record of the results is kept; (7) identification of what practice changes may have to be made to deliver the benefits that have been identified; (8) how the staff will be retrained if appropriate; and (9) how changes in practice will be implemented.[70,94,110,118]

ORGANIZATION AND IMPLEMENTATION OF A COORDINATING COMMITTEE

It is important to consult with all parties involved in delivering, and receiving, a POCT service. This is best achieved by establishing a POCT Coordinating Committee. Such a committee is charged with managing the whole process of delivering a high-quality POCT service. Committee members should include representatives of those who use the service and those who deliver the service, together with a representative of the organization's management team. The users will include physicians, nurses, other healthcare providers, and maybe even a patient. The providers should include at least one representative from the laboratory and of those involved in the use of other diagnostic and therapy equipment close to the patient (e.g., respiratory measurement technologists, nurses). Typically, a laboratory professional will chair such a committee because it is the laboratory that will provide the necessary backup if a service failure occurs; furthermore, the laboratory professional will have had training and will have gained expertise regarding the analytical issues that are likely to arise. For many reasons, the committee should report to the medical director of the provider organization. The committee should then designate members who will take responsibility for overseeing the training and certification of all POCT operators, and also for QC and quality assurance. The work of the committee should be governed by the organization's policy on POCT.

BOX 20-4 Elements of a Point-of-Care Testing (POCT) Policy

Catalog information—review time
- Approved by
- Original distribution
- Related policies
- Further information
- Policy replaces

Introduction—background
- Definition
- Accreditation of services
- Audit of services

Laboratory services in the organization—location
- Logistics
- Policy on diagnostic testing

Management of POCT—committee and accountability
- Officers
- Committee members
- Terms of reference
- Responsibilities
- Meetings

Equipment and consumable procurement—criteria for procurement
- Process of procurement

Standard operating procedures
- Training and certification of staff—training
- Certification
- Recertification

Quality control and quality assurance—procedures
- Documentation and review

Health and safety procedures

Bibliography

POCT POLICY AND ACCOUNTABILITY

Implementation of a POCT service requires a POCT policy that establishes all of the procedures required to ensure delivery of high-quality service, together with the responsibility and accountability of all staff associated with the POCT. This may be (1) part of the organization's total quality management system,[63] (2) part of its clinical governance policy,[44] and (3) required for accreditation purposes.[19,20] The elements of a POCT policy are listed in Box 20-4.

EQUIPMENT PROCUREMENT AND EVALUATION

Equipment procurement and evaluation involve first identifying candidate POCT equipment having the prerequisite analytical and operational capabilities to meet the clinical requirements of a POCT service. Performance requirements should then be established and compared with the performance characteristics of these devices (obtained from the manufacturer or assessed as part of the procurement exercise). These characteristics include parameters such as accuracy, precision, specificity for the analyte, turnaround time (TAT), calibration frequency, potential interferents, calibrator and reagent stability, lot-to-lot variation for reagents and calibrators, and QC requirements. In addition, operational requirements have to be identified, and the potential for operator error (e.g., effects of delayed addition of the sample and use of an incorrect sample volume) determined. Independent validation of these analytical and operational characteristics can be obtained from (1) published evaluations performed by agencies such as the Medicine and Healthcare Products Regulatory Agency (MHRA) in the United Kingdom; (2) Norwegian Quality Improvement of Primary Care Laboratories[96]; and (3) reports in the peer-reviewed literature. When performance data are reviewed, particular attention should be paid to the precision and accuracy of measurement, including concordance between results from the POCT device and the routine laboratory method, because patients are likely to be managed using both analytical systems. Evaluation of analytical performance is discussed in a CLSI guideline on selection criteria for POCT equipment.[28]

An economic assessment of the equipment, including the costs of consumables and servicing, should also be completed. Any comparison of costs with the laboratory service will highlight only the cost per test, which, as stated earlier, will not give an accurate assessment of the cost-effectiveness of using the system. However, it is helpful at this point to obtain a good assessment of the relative staff costs associated with different systems, because these are likely to be key features in the decision-making process.

After comparison data have been obtained, tabulated, and interpreted, a POCT device is selected if the assessment has indicated value in using such an approach. It is recommended that the laboratory professional should then conduct a short evaluation of the equipment to gain familiarization with the system. This evaluation will help to determine the content of the training program that will be used, as well as a troubleshooting protocol. Such an evaluation should document the concordance between results generated with the device and those provided by the laboratory. All of this information should then be recorded in a logbook associated with the equipment. In addition, the organization may wish to undertake some form of safety check, give the device some form of local code, and enter the code into the local equipment register.

TRAINING AND CERTIFICATION OF OPERATORS

The confidence of the clinician, the healthcare provider, and the patient in results generated by a POCT device depends heavily on the robustness of the instrument and the competence of the operator, assuming that it has already been shown to meet the analytical requirements of the clinical setting. Many of the agencies involved in the regulation of healthcare delivery now require that all personnel associated with the delivery of diagnostic results demonstrate their competence through a process of regulation, and this applies equally to POCT personnel.

BOX 20-5 Main Elements of a Point-of-Care Testing Training Program

Understanding the context of the test—pathophysiologic context
- Clinical requirement for the test
- Action taken on basis of result
- Nature of test and method used

Patient preparation required—relevance of diurnal variation
- Relevance of drug therapy

Sample requirement and specimen collection
Preparation of analytical device—machine and/or consumables
Performance of test
Performance of quality control
Documentation of test result and quality control result
Reporting of test result to appropriate personnel
Interpretation of result and sources of advice
Health and safety issues (e.g., disposal of sample and test device, cleaning of machine and test area)

The elements of a training program are listed in Box 20-5. In practice, such a program is tailored to suit the needs of the individual and the organization.[123] These may include formal presentation to groups, or on a one-to-one basis, self-directed learning using agreed documentation, or computer-aided learning. For example, several of the current models of blood gas and electrolyte analyzers have onboard computer-aided training modules. Whatever the training strategy employed, it is important to document satisfactory completion of training, and that the individual has been tested and found competent with a combination of questions concerned with understanding and practical demonstration of the skills gained. The latter can be achieved by performing tests on a series of QC materials and repeat testing of samples that have been analyzed recently (parallel testing). Finally, the operator should be observed on a minimum of three occasions throughout the procedure involved in the POCT.

Competence on a long-term basis is maintained through regular practice of skills and continuing education; it is important to build these features into any education and training program. Regular review of performance in QC and quality assurance programs will provide a means of overseeing the competence of operators. However, this is not always sufficient, particularly when operators are employed on irregular shifts or may not always be called upon to perform POCT. In this latter situation, it may be necessary to create specific arrangements for individuals to undertake tests on QC material. The error log may highlight when problems are arising. However, the most important thing is to encourage an open approach to the assessment of competence, so that operators themselves can seek help if they believe that problems are occurring. Such an open approach should be supported with audit and performance review meetings where problems are aired and developments discussed. Regular assessment of competence should be built into a formal program for recertification that will be a requirement of most accreditation programs.

QUALITY CONTROL, QUALITY ASSURANCE, AND AUDIT

Quality control and quality assurance programs provide a formal means of monitoring the quality of a service (see Chapter 8). The within-organization QC program offers a relatively short-term view of performance and typically compares current performance with acceptance criteria for the measurement device. External quality assurance (proficiency testing) on the other hand takes a longer-term view and in some respects addresses other issues surrounding the quality of the result. Thus external quality assurance method compares the testing performance at different sites and/or with different pieces of equipment or methods.[18,131] An audit is a more retrospective form of analysis of performance and, furthermore, it can provide a more holistic view of the whole process. However, the foundation to ensuring good quality remains a successful training and certification scheme.

Classically, quantitative within-laboratory (or within-organization) QC involves analysis of a sample for which the analyte concentration is known, either because the material has been analyzed on many occasions and the distribution of results documented, or because it has been analyzed independently and the mean and interval range of results have been quoted for the method used. The essence of using within-laboratory QC material is to establish the interval of results that is acceptable; the current analytical result is compared with the interval of results deemed acceptable (see Chapter 8). The QC result must then be documented, usually graphically, because it shows the conformity of results to pre-established acceptance criteria and any trends in results that may be occurring. The major aim is to use a means of documentation that ensures that comparative performance is assessed.

Several challenges have been put forth regarding the classical approach with POCT. The first concerns the frequency of testing—should a QC sample be analyzed every time that (1) a sample is analyzed, (2) a new operator uses the system, (3) a new lot number of reagents is used, or (4) the system is recalibrated? No consistent agreement on the correct approach has been reached, and one probably has to be guided by the reproducibility and overall analytical performance of the system and local circumstances, such as the (1) number and competence of the operators, (2) frequency with which the system is used, and (3) risk to the patient of an erroneous result not being detected. For a benchtop and/or multitest analyzer, the frequency of measuring QC samples conforms to regulatory requirements applicable to the measurement setting. It can be argued that with the frequent turnover of staff in larger institutions, frequency should be a minimum of once per shift—three times a day. Many critical care analyzers can be programmed to perform a QC check at intervals set by those responsible for the device.

For single-use POCT disposable devices, the previous strategy does not completely monitor the quality of the test system.[103,135] For example, when conventional QC material is analyzed on a unit-use or single-test POCT system, only that testing unit is monitored. Thus it is impossible to test every unit with control material because by definition they are single-test systems. Under these circumstances, greater dependence is placed on the manufacturing reproducibility of devices, to ensure a good quality service.[24]

Some users may wish to continue with a QC testing strategy that is similar to that applied for multiuse devices. If testing is infrequent, another approach that can be used would be to analyze a QC sample whenever a change to the testing system occurs, such as with a different batch of testing materials or a different operator.[27] However, it is important to follow the manufacturer's recommendations. Other QC approaches may be used, but many do not test the whole process. For example, the use of a plastic surrogate reflectance pad as a QC sample will test only the performance of the reflectance meter and not processes such as sample addition, reagent stability, reagent calibration, or performance of the test. Similarly, other forms of electronic QC checks only verify the functionality of the electronic systems.[135]

External quality assurance or proficiency testing is a systematic approach to QC monitoring in which standardized samples are analyzed by one or more laboratories to determine the capability of each participant. With this approach, the operator has no knowledge of the analyte concentration. Results are transmitted to a central authority, which then prepares a report and returns a copy to each participating laboratory. The report will identify the results obtained for the complete group of participants and may be classified according to the different methods used by participants in the scheme. The scheme may encompass both laboratory and POCT users, which gives an opportunity to compare results with laboratory-based methods. In practice, external quality assurance or proficiency testing is used in POCT to determine and document long-term performance and concordance of results among users of the same POCT devices, and, when commutable samples are used, between the POCT service and an organization's central laboratory. It is also possible to operate an external quality assurance scheme within a hospital or organizational setting; such a scheme typically would be run by qualified laboratory personnel. If authentic patient samples are used for a scheme within a hospital or organizational setting, the results reported by the laboratory and by other POCT sites within the same organization can be compared. This can be important when patients are managed in several departments, or when devices are not available and samples are taken to other sites for testing. When deteriorating or poor performance is identified in one of these schemes, it is important to document the problem and then to provide and document a solution. It may be necessary as part of this exercise to review some of the patient's notes to ensure that incorrect results have not been reported and inappropriate clinical actions taken. In addition, if the solution highlights a vulnerable feature of the process overall or for one particular operator, process improvement or retraining must be instituted.

An example of data from an external quality assurance scheme for POCT is shown in Figure 20-11. Such schemes are run on national and international bases, and some Website schemes are listed in the references.[29,126,133]

MAINTENANCE AND INVENTORY CONTROL

Implementation and maintenance of a POCT service require that a supply of devices (both instrumentation and consumables) be maintained at all times, and that this is supported by a formal program. This approach may be taken for larger benchtop systems within a large organization; however, similar arrangements (e.g., rapid replacement of faulty units) can be achieved for smaller organizations (e.g., a physician's office laboratory) through an appropriate arrangement with the supplier. In the case of consumables, the key points in this process are to (1) adhere to recommended storage conditions for reagents, calibrators, and controls, (2) be aware of the stated shelf life of consumables, and (3) ensure that stocks are released in time for any preanalytical preparation to be accommodated (e.g., thawing). When multiple sites are using the same materials, a central purchasing, supply, and inventory control system should be put in place—not only to gain benefit from bulk purchasing, but also to ensure that individual systems are not supplied unknowingly with different batches of consumables.

Complexity in the maintenance of reusable devices will vary from system to system, but clear guidelines will be available from the manufacturer and should be adhered to rigorously. Issues that usually require particular vigilance include expiration dates, biocontamination, electrical safety, maintenance of optics, and inadvertent use of inappropriate consumables.

DOCUMENTATION

Documentation of all aspects of a POCT service has been a major issue for many years, compounded by the fact that the storage of data in laboratory and hospital information systems has often been limited and inconsistent. Thus it is critically important to keep an accurate record of the test request, the result, and the action taken—as an absolute minimum. Although the last point may be seen as beyond the scope of the laboratory, the incidence of errors in laboratory medicine that have been attributed to preanalytical and postanalytical phases suggests that the laboratory should play a more integrated role in the whole care process. Some of the issues concerning documentation are now being resolved with the advent of the electronic patient record, electronic requesting, and better connectivity of POCT instrumentation to information systems (see earlier discussion). Documentation should extend from the standard operating procedure(s) for the POCT systems to records of training and certification of

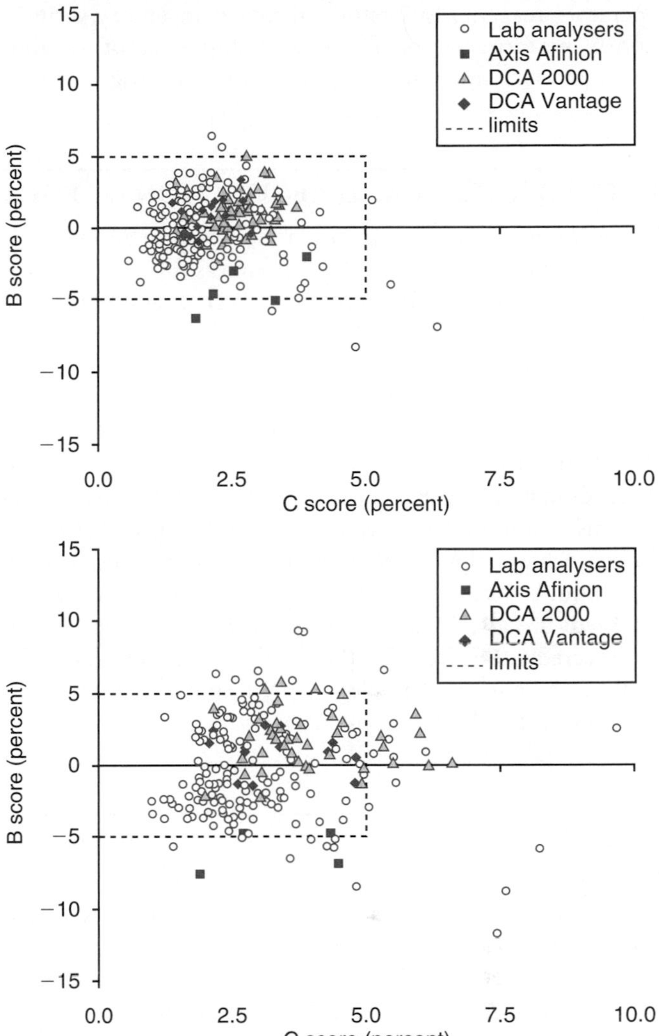

Figure 20-11 Extract of data from a recent distribution of the U.K. NEQAS Glycated Hemoglobin scheme. The "*B score*" is the average of % biases of all samples distributed within the six-distribution rolling time window. In the HbA_{1c} scheme, three samples are sent out per month, so this will be 18 samples. Data are trimmed by 10% at either end of the ranked data set, so that the middle 14 results are used to calculate average % bias and hence the *B score*. The "*C score*" is the standard deviation of the *B score*, adjusted by the method of Healy to correct for the amount of trimming performed. The *B score* therefore is a smoothed, robust indicator of average bias, and the *C score* is an estimator of the variability of this bias for different samples with different analyte concentrations in the scoring time window. A high *C score* may have components of within-run imprecision, between-run reproducibility, batch-to batch reagent variability, and concentration-dependent bias. The limits of B and *C scores* shown by *dotted lines* on the plots are those agreed to by the National Quality Assurance Advisory Panel for Chemical Pathology, outside of which laboratories are deemed to have unacceptable performance. Laboratories with scores persistently outside these limits may be contacted by the Panel, and ultimately intervention may be required. *(Courtesy Dr. J. Middle, U.K. NEQAS.)*

operators, reagents, calibrator and control inventory, verification of performance of devices and shipments of consumables, and QC and external quality assurance, together with error logs and any corrective action taken.

ACCREDITATION AND REGULATION OF POCT

The features of the organization and management of POCT described previously should be the same as those for accreditation of any diagnostic services.[19,20] Accreditation of POCT should be part of the overall accreditation of laboratory medicine services, or indeed should be part of the accreditation of the full clinical service, as has been the case for several years in many countries, including the United States and the United Kingdom. Thus the Clinical Laboratory Improvement Amendments of 1988 (CLIA) and the final rule on quality systems requirements as specified in 2003 legislation in the United States stipulate that all POCT must meet certain minimum standards.[127-129] In the United States, the Centers for Medicare and Medicaid Services, the Joint Commission on Accreditation of Healthcare Organizations, and the College of American Pathologists are responsible for inspecting sites, and each is committed to ensuring compliance with testing regulations for POCT.[38]

FUTURE OF POCT

In the previous edition of this chapter, we suggested that the three key drivers for expansion of POCT services in the future will be (1) changes in the way healthcare is provided, (2) patients' needs and expectations, and (3) technological innovations. We also observed that trends in the way that clinical care is being delivered are completely opposite to those in which diagnostic testing services are moving. Observations on healthcare provision in the United States as put forth by the Institute of Medicine[73] have been reiterated in many other countries,[113] with similar conclusions such as recommending more patient-centered care, improved access, and better choices for patients. Christensen and coworkers[23] suggested that POCT and information technologies (namely, connectivity, the electronic patient record, and decision support systems) provide some of the key technologies to enable a disruptive solution to the provision of healthcare, namely, offering solutions to the problems that many health systems face today by radically changing the way that care is organized and delivered.

Patient expectations are increasing and will drive the trend toward a more patient-focused style of care, with fewer clinic visits, shorter waiting times, and an expectation of better care. POCT has been shown to be capable of shorter "lengths of stay" and, in many cases, improved health outcomes. As health service decision makers (both purchasers and providers) realize that it is possible to achieve lower "costs per patient episode" with the use of POCT, more effort will be put into this testing modality. So what will facilitate this revolution? The answer lies in new technology—in terms of the development of new delivery platforms and the discovery of new markers—with the use of new business models and value networks.[23,109]

Considerable efforts are being made to develop and manufacture miniaturized analytical devices (see Chapter 18) that will enable faster analytical times to be achieved, with smaller sample requirements. Several examples in the field of microfabricated devices have been shown to meet these aspirations.[76-78,109] In the future, continued technological advances will result in even smaller devices that can be tailored for a large number of analytes and that are very simple to operate.

Noninvasive testing remains the "holy grail" for POCT, and over the past two decades, evidence has suggested some success in this area. Most work has been performed on a range of imaging techniques that seek a signature of the molecule of interest (e.g., glucose) from among the many signatures of the extracellular and tissue matrices.[71,88,91,104] Alternative approaches have sought to access the extracellular fluid space or to sample extracellular fluid directly, as with the Glucowatch[124] and other developments.[109]

Areas of testing that are showing significant progress include (1) testing for infectious agents using molecular-based techniques, (2) testing for predisposition to disease, and (3) assessing an individual's response profile toward a new drug. In all three scenarios, the key to having a POCT is the need for early decision making to implement therapy (or life-style change), together with the need for patient counseling. The technology is clearly available to detect any form of biological entity at the point-of-care, including very rapid analysis of deoxyribonucleic acid (DNA) from saliva samples.[45,109] However, many ethical issues surround analysis for genetic predisposition and tests for certain infectious diseases (see Chapter 1). These developments notwithstanding, evidence also indicates that POCT is being used increasingly in the management of long-term conditions—probably the area where the greatest volume of testing is focused.

If one accepts that patient empowerment is a key development in healthcare for the future, self-testing is likely to increase. This is an area that is well established for blood glucose and is increasingly used in the management of oral anticoagulation therapy. As emphasis slowly moves toward health promotion and wellness monitoring, issues of access to testing will become significant drivers of the use of diagnostic tests. Perhaps the most interesting aspect of patient empowerment, however, is the fact that it changes the relationship between the patient and the health professional. It could be argued that in the not too distant future, the patient will not be expected to make an appointment or to travel to see the health professional, but rather will expect better access and convenience. This vision requires a totally new way of assessing "clinical need" and a better understanding of all of the processes of care, as well as stakeholder needs, as advocated by Donabedian,[37] who investigated system redesign in search of improved quality of care.[109] This may lead to a totally different perspective on the repertoire (and combinations) of tests required for POCT, as well as on the way in which care is delivered.

REFERENCES

1. Aarsand AK, Alter D, Frost SJ, Kaplanis R, Klovning A, Price CP, et al. Diagnosis and management of diabetes mellitus. In: Nichols JH, ed. The National Academy of Clinical Biochemistry: laboratory medicine practice guidelines. Evidence-based practice for point-of-care testing, 2007, p 187. Available at: http://www.aacc.org/AACC/members/nacb/LMPG/OnlineGuide/PublishedGuidelines/poct/default.htm (accessed on April 14, 2011).
2. Academy of Medical Laboratory Science, Association of Clinical Biochemists in Ireland, Irish Medicines Board and RCPI Faculty of Pathology. Guidelines for safe and effective management and use of point of care testing. Available at: http://www.amls.ie/images/forms/poct%20guide.pdf (accessed on April 14, 2011).
3. Antmann EM, Grudzien C, Sachs DB. Evaluation of a rapid bedside assay for detection of serum cardiac troponin T. JAMA 1995;273:1279-82.
4. Apple FS, Christenson RH, Valdes R, Wu AHB, Andriak AJ, Duh SH, et al. Simultaneous rapid measurement of whole blood myoglobin, creatine kinase MB, and cardiac troponin I by the Triage Cardiac Panel for detection of myocardial infarction. Clin Chem 1999;273:1279-82.
5. Arabadjief M, Nichols JH. Evaluation of the Afinion AS100 point-of-care analyzer for hemoglobin A1c. Point of Care 2009;8:11-5.
6. Ashby JP, ed. The patient and decentralised testing. Lancaster, UK: MTP Press Ltd, 1988.
7. Australasian Association of Clinical Biochemists. Point of care testing implementation guide. Available at: http://www.aacb.asn.au/admin/?getfile=1442 (accessed on April 14, 2011).
8. Baum JM, Monhaut NM, Parker DR, Price CP. Improving the quality of self-monitoring blood glucose measurement: a study in reducing calibration errors. Diabetes Technol Ther 2006;8:347-57.
9. Beneteau-Burnat B, Bocque MC, Lorin A, Martin C, Vaubourdolle M. Evaluation of the blood gas analyzer Gem PREMIER 3000. Clin Chem Lab Med 2004;42: 96-101.
10. Beneteau-Burnat B, Pernet P, Pilon A, Latour D, Goujon S, Feuillu A, et al. Evaluation of the GEM Premier 4000: a compact blood gas CO-oximeter and electrolyte analyzer for point-of-care and laboratory testing. Clin Chem Lab Med 2008;46:271-9.
11. Bingham D, Kendall J, Clancy M. The portable laboratory: an evaluation of the accuracy and reproducibility of I-STAT. Ann Clin Biochem 1999;36:66-71.
12. Bonnar J, Flynn A, Freundl G, Kirkman R, Royston R, Snowden R. Personal hormone monitoring for contraception. Brit J Fam Planning 1999;24:128-34.
13. Borgard JP, Szymanowicz A, Pellae I, Szmidt-Adjidé V, Rota M. Determination of total bilirubin in whole blood from neonates: results from a French multicenter study. Clin Chem Lab Med 2006;44:1103-10.
14. Boyd JC, Bruns DE. Quality specifications for glucose meters: assessment by simulation modeling of errors in insulin dose. Clin Chem 2001;47:209-14.
15. Bubner TK, Lawrence CO, Gialamas A, Yelland LN, Ryan P, Wilson KJ, et al. Effectiveness of point-of-care testing for therapeutic control of chronic conditions: results from the PoCT in General Practice Trial. Med J Aust 2009;190:624-6.
16. Brunelle JA, Degtiarov AM, Moran RF, Race LA. Simultaneous measurement of total hemoglobin and its derivatives in blood using CO-oximeters: analytical principles; their application in selecting analytical wavelengths and reference methods; a comparison of the results and the choices made. Scand J Clin Lab Invest 1996;56(Suppl 224):47-69.
17. Buechler KF, Moi S, Noar B, McGrath D, Villela J, Clancy M, et al. Simultaneous detection of seven drugs of abuse by the triage panel for drugs of abuse. Clin Chem 1992;38:1678-84.
18. Bullock DG. Quality control and quality assurance. In: Price CP, St John A, Hicks JH, eds. Point-of-care testing. Washington DC: AACC Press, 2004:137-45.
19. Burnett D. Accreditation and point-of-care testing. Ann Clin Biochem 2000;37:241-3.
20. Burnett D. A practical guide to accreditation in laboratory medicine. London: ACB Venture Publications, 2002:1-314.
21. Chapin KC, Blake P, Wilson CD. Performance characteristics and utilization of rapid antigen test, DNA probe, and culture for detection of group A streptococci in an acute care clinic. J Clin Microbiol 2002;40:4207-10.
22. Chin HL, Krall MA. Successful implementation of a comprehensive computer-based patient record system in Kaiser Permanente Northwest: strategy and experience. Eff Clin Pract 1998;1:51-60.
23. Christensen CM, Grossman JH, Hwang J. The innovator's prescription: a disruptive solution to health care. New York: McGraw Hill, 2009:1-441.
24. Clinical Laboratory Standards Institute. Quality management for unit-use testing: approved guideline. CLSI Document EP18-A. Volume 22 Number 28 Wayne, Pa: CLSI, 2002.
25. Clinical Laboratory Standards Institute. Point-of-care connectivity: approved standard, 2nd edition. CLSI Document POCT01-A2. Wayne, Pa: CLSI, 2006.
26. Clinical Laboratory Standards Institute. Implementation guide of POCT01 for healthcare providers: approved guideline. CLSI Document POCT02-A. Wayne, Pa: CLSI, 2008.
27. Clinical Laboratory Standards Institute. Point-of-care in vitro diagnostic (IVD) testing: approved guidelines, 2nd edition. CLSI Document POCT4-A2. Wayne, Pa: CLSI, 2006.
28. Clinical Laboratory Standards Institute. Selection criteria for point of care testing devices. CLSI Document POCT09-A. Wayne, Pa: CLSI, 2010.
29. College of American Pathologists. Information (e.g., drugs of abuse testing program). Available at: www.cap.org (accessed on April 14, 2011).
30. Collinson PO, Gerhardt W, Katus HA, Muller-Bardoff M, Braun S, Schricke U, et al. Multicenter evaluation of an immunological rapid test for the detection of troponin T in whole blood samples. Eur J Clin Chem Clin Biochem 1996;34:591-8.
31. Collinson PO, John C, Lynch S, Rao A, Canepa-Anson R, Carson E, et al. A prospective randomized controlled trial of point-of-care testing on the coronary care unit. Ann Clin Biochem 2004;41:397-404.
32. Crook M. Handbook of near-patient testing. London: Greenwich Medical Media Limited, 1999:1-116.
33. D'Costa EJ, Higgins IJ, Turner AP. Quinoprotein glucose dehydrogenase and its application in an amperometric glucose sensor. Biosensors 1986;2:71-87.
34. D'Orazio P. Biosensors in clinical chemistry. Clin Chim Acta 2003;334:41-69.
35. Davis G. Microfabricated sensors and the commercial development of the i-Stat® point-of-care system. In: Ramsay G, ed. Commercial biosensors. New York: John Wiley & Sons, 1998:47-76.
36. Dickinson KJ, Troxler M, Homer-Vanniasinkam S. The surgical application of point-of-care haemostasis and platelet function testing. Br J Surg 2008;95:1317-30.
37. Donabedian A. An introduction to quality assurance in health care. Oxford: Oxford University Press, 2003:1-200.
38. Ehrmeyer SS, Laessig RH. Regulation, accreditation and education for point-of-care testing. In: Kost G, ed. Principles and practice of point-of-care testing. Philadelphia: Lippincott Williams and Wilkins, 2002:434-43.
39. Erickson KA, Wilding P. Evaluation of a novel point-of-care system: the i-Stat portable clinical analyzer. Clin Chem 1993;39:283-7.
40. Farhat SE, Finn S, Chua R, Smith B, Simor AE, George P, et al. Rapid detection of infectious mononucleosis-associated heterophile antibodies by a novel immunochromatographic assay and a latex agglutination test. J Clin Microbiol 1993;31:1597-600.
41. Fermann GJ, Suyama J. Point of care testing in the emergency department. J Emerg Med 2002;22:393-404.

42. Fiallos MR, Hanhan UA, Orlowski JP. Point-of-care testing. Pediatr Clin North Am 2001;48:589-99.
43. Flore KM, Delanghe R. Analytical interferences in point-of-care testing glucometers by icodextrin and its metabolites: an overview. Perit Dial Int 2009;4:377-83.
44. Freedman DB. Clinical governance: implications for point-of-care testing. Ann Clin Biochem 2002;39:421-3.
45. French DJ, Archard CL, Andersen MT, McDowell DG. Ultra-rapid DNA analysis using HyBeacon probes and direct PCR amplification from saliva. Mol Cell Probes 2002;16:319-26.
46. Giuliano KK, Perkins S. Implementing a point-of-care testing program in the critical care setting. Clin Leadersh Manag Rev 2002;16:139-47.
47. Gomez EJ, Hernando Pérez ME, Vering T, Rigla Cros M, Bott O, García-Sáez G, et al. The INCA system: a further step towards a telemedical artificial pancreas. IEEE Trans Inf Technol Biomed 2008;12:470-9.
48. Grubb AO, Glad UC Inventors. Immunoassay with test strip having antibodies bound thereto. U.S. Patent 4,168,146; September 18, 1979.
49. Halpern MT, Palmer CS, Simpson KN, Chesley FD, Luce BR, Suyderhoud JP, et al. The economic and clinical efficiency of point-of-care testing for critically ill patients: a decision-analysis model. Am J Med Qual 1998;13:3-12.
50. Handorf CR. College of American Pathologists Conference XXVIII on alternate site testing: introduction. Arch Pathol Lab Med 1995;119: 867-71.
51. Harrison JR, Bevan J, Furth EE, Metz DC. AccuStat whole blood fingerstick test for *Helicobacter pylori* infection: a reliable screening method. J Clin Gastroenterol 1998;27:50-3.
52. Hedberg P, Wennecke G. A preliminary evaluation of the AQT90 FLEX Tnl immunoassay. Clin Chem Lab Med 2009;47:376-8.
53. Heneghan C, Alonso-Coello P, Garcia-Alamino JM, Perera R, Meats E, Glasziou P. Self-monitoring of oral anticoagulation: a systematic review and meta-analysis. Lancet 2006;367:404-11.
54. Heslop L, Howard A, Fernando J, Rothfield A, Wallace L. Wireless communications in acute health-care. J Telemed Telecare 2003;9:187-93.
55. Hillier SC, Flower SE, Frost CG, Jenkins ATA, Keay R, Braven H, et al. An electrochemical gene detection assay utilising T7 exonuclease activity on complementary probe–target oligonucleotide sequences. Electrochem Comm 2004;6:1227-32.
56. Hirst D, St. John A. Keeping the spotlight on quality from a distance. Accred Qual Assur 2000;5;9-13.
57. Hobbs FD, Delaney BC, Fitzmaurice DA, Wilson S, Hyde CJ, Thorpe GH, et al. A review of near patient testing in primary care. Health Technol Assess 1997;1:1-230.
58. Holtzinger C, Szelag E, DuBois JA, Shirey TL, Presti S. Evaluation of a new POCT bedside glucose meter and strip with hematocrit and interference corrections. Point of Care 2008;7:1-6.
59. International Organization for Standardization. ISO 22870:2006. Point-of-care testing (POCT): requirements for quality and competence. Available at: http://www.iso.org/iso/catalogue_detail.htm?csnumber=35173 (accessed on April 14, 2011).
60. International Organization for Standardization. ISO 15197:2003. In vitro diagnostic test systems: requirements for blood-glucose monitoring systems for self-testing in managing diabetes mellitus. Available at: http://www.iso.org/iso/search.htm?qt=self+testing+for+blood+glucose&searchSubmit=Search&sort=rel&type=simple&published=on (April 14, 2011).
61. International Organization for Standardization. ISO 17593:2007. Clinical laboratory testing and in vitro medical devices: requirements for in vitro monitoring systems for self-testing of oral anticoagulant therapy. Available at: http://www.iso.org/iso/search.htm?qt=oral+anticoagulation+therapy&searchSubmit=Search&sort=rel&type=simple&published=on (accessed on April 14, 2011).
62. International Organization for Standardization. N283 position paper clinical for ISO 15197. Performance goals for glucose meters: clinical perspective. Geneva: ISO, 2003.
63. Jacobs E, Hinson KA, Tolnai J, Simson E. Implementation, management and continuous quality improvement of point-of-care testing in an academic health care setting. Clin Chim Acta 2001;307:49-59.
64. Jina A. A novel point-of-care prothrombin time monitoring system. Chest 2000;118(Suppl):2835.
65. Johnson RE, Newhall WJ, Papp JR, Knapp JS, Black CM, Gift TL, et al. Screening tests to detect *Chlamydia trachomatis* and *Neisseria gonorrhoeae* infections—2002. MMWR Recomm Rep 2002;51:1-38; quiz CE1-4.
66. Jones R, St. John A. Informatics in point-of-care testing. In: Price CP, St. John A, Hicks JM, eds. Point-of-care testing. Washington, DC: AACC Press, 2004:197-208.
67. Jurgens R, Elliott R. Rapid HIV screening at the point of care: legal and ethical issues. Can HIV AIDS Policy Law Newsl 2000;5:28-33.
68. Kalorama Information Worldwide Point of Care Diagnostics, 2009. Available at: http:www.KaloramaInformation.com (accessed on April 14, 2011).
69. Karon BS, McBane RD, Chaudhry R, Beyer LK, Santrach PJ. Accuracy of capillary whole blood international normalized ratio on the CoaguChek S, CoaguChek XS, and i-STAT 1 point-of-care analyzers. Am J Clin Pathol 2008;130:88-92.
70. Kendall J, Reeves B, Clancy M. Point of care testing: randomised, controlled trial of clinical outcome. BMJ 1998;316:1052-7.
71. Khalil OS. Spectroscopic and clinical aspects of noninvasive glucose measurements. Clin Chem 1999;45:165-75.
72. Khandurina J, Guttman A. Bioanalysis in microfluidic devices. J Chromatogr A 2002;943:159-83.
73. Kohn LT, Corrigan JM, Donaldson MS, eds. To err is human: building a safer health system. Institute of Medicine. Washington, DC: National Academies Press, 2000:1-287.
74. Kost GJ. Preventing medical errors in point-of-care testing: security, validation, safeguards, and connectivity. Arch Pathol Lab Med 2001;125:1307-15.
75. Kost GJ, ed. Principles and practice of point-of-care testing. Philadelphia: Lippincott Williams & Wilkins, 2002:1-654.
76. Kricka LJ. Microchips, microarrays, biochips, and nanochips: personal laboratories for the 21st century. Clin Chim Acta 2001;307:219-23.
77. Kricka LJ. Microchips: the hitchhiker's guide to analytical microchips. Washington: AACC Press, 2002:1-94.
78. Kricka LJ. Point-of-care technologies for the future: technological innovations and hurdles to implementation. Point of Care 2009;8:42-5.
79. Kricka LJ, Thorpe GHG. Technology of handheld devices for point-of-care testing. In: Price CP, St. John A, Kricka LJ, eds. Point-of-care testing, 3rd edition. Washington, DC: AACC Press, 2010:27-42
80. Lauks IR, inventor. Point-of-care in-vitro blood analysis system. U.S. Patent 6,845,327; January 18, 2005.
81. Lee-Lewandrowski E, Corboy D, Lewandrowski K, Sinclair J, McDermott S, Benzer TI. Implementation of a point-of-care satellite laboratory in the emergency department of an academic medical center: impact on test turnaround time and patient emergency department length of stay. Arch Pathol Lab Med 2003;127:456-60.
82. Lehmann CA, Mintz N, Giacini JM. Impact of telehealth on heathcare utilization by congestive heart failure patients. Dis Manage Health Outcomes 2006;14:163-9.
83. Lewandrowski K. Three wishes for POCT testing: a compendium of unmet needs from the perspective of practitioners in the field. Point of Care 2008;7:86-88.
84. Lindemans J, Hoefkens P, van Kessel AL, Bonnay M, Kulpmann WR, van Suijlen JD. Portable blood gas and electrolyte analyzer evaluated in a multiinstitutional study. Clin Chem 1999;45:111-17.
85. Lott JA, Johnson WR, Luke KE. Evaluation of an automated urine chemistry reagent-strip analyzer. J Clin Lab Anal 1995;9:212-17.
86. Magny E, Renard MF, Launay JM. Analytical evaluation of Rapidpoint 400 blood gas analyzer. Ann Biol Clin (Paris) 2001;59:622-8.
87. Mass D. Consulting to physician office laboratories. In: Snyder JR, Wilkinson DS, eds. Management in laboratory medicine, 3rd edition. New York: Lippincott, 1998:443-50.

88. MacKenzie HA, Ashton HS, Spiers S, Shen Y, Freeborn SS, Hannigan J, et al. Advances in photoacoustic noninvasive glucose testing. Clin Chem 1999;45:1587-95.
89. Medicines and Healthcare Products Regulatory Agency. DB 2002(03). Management and use of IVD point of care test devices. Available at: http://www.mhra.gov.uk/Publications/Safetyguidance/DeviceBulletins/CON007333 (accessed on April 14, 2011).
90. Mollard J-F. Single phase calibration for blood gas and electrolyte analysis. In D'Orazio P, ed. Preparing for critical care analyses in the 21st century. Proceedings of the 16th International Symposium. Washington: AACC Press, 1996.
91. Nadeau RG, Groner W. The role of a new noninvasive imaging technology in the diagnosis of anemia. J Nutr 2001;131:1610S-4S.
92. National Institute of Biomedical Imaging and Bioengineering/National Heart, Lung, and Blood Institute/National Science Foundation Workshop Faculty; Price CP, Kricka LJ. Improving healthcare accessibility through point-of-care technologies. Clin Chem 2007;53:1665-75.
93. Nichols JH. The future of point-of-care testing. Point of Care 2008;7:271-73.
94. Nichols JH, Kickler TS, Dyer KL, Humbertson SK, Cooper PC, Maughan WL, et al. Clinical outcomes of point-of-care testing in the interventional radiology and invasive cardiology setting. Clin Chem 2000;46:543-50.
95. Niewenhaus JH, van Kasteel M. The role of consumer electronics in point-of-care testing. In: Price CP, St. John A, Kricka LJ, eds. Point-of-care testing, 3rd edition. Washington, DC: AACC Press, 2010:97-106.
96. Norwegian Quality Improvement of Primary Care Laboratories. Available at: www.noklus.no (accessed on April 14, 2011).
97. Oliver G. On bedside testing. London: HK Lewis, 1884:1-128.
98. Oliver NS, Toumazou C, Cass AE, Johnston DG. Glucose sensors: a review of current and emerging technology. Diabet Med 2009;26:197-210.
99. Oral Anticoagulation Monitoring Study Group. Point-of-care prothrombin time measurement for professional and patient self-testing use: a multicenter clinical experience. Am J Clin Pathol 2001;115:288-96.
100. Oral Anticoagulation Monitoring Study Group. Prothrombin measurement using a patient self-testing system. Am J Clin Pathol 2001;115:280-7.
101. Osei-Bimpong A, Jury C, McLean R, Lewis SM. Point-of-care method for total white cell count: an evaluation of the HemoCue WBC device. Int J Lab Hematol 2009;31:657-64.
102. Parsons MP, Newman DJ, Newall RG, Price CP. Validation of a point-of-care assay for the urinary albumin:creatinine ratio. Clin Chem 1999;45:414-17.
103. Phillips DL. Quality systems for unit-use testing devices. Clin Chem 1997;43:893-6.
104. Pickup J, Rolinski O, Birch D. In vivo glucose sensing for diabetes management: progress towards non-invasive monitoring. BMJ 1999;319:1289-92.
105. Plesch W, Wolf T, Breitenbeck N, Dikkeschei LD, Cervero A, Perez PL, et al. Results of the performance verification of the CoaguChek XS system. Thromb Res 2008;123:381-9.
106. Prisco D, Paniccia R. Point-of-care testing of hemostasis in cardiac surgery. Thromb J 2003;1:1-10.
107. Pope RM, Apps JM, Page MD, Allen K, Bodansky HJ. A novel device for the rapid in-clinic measurement of haemoglobin A1c. Diabet Med 1993;3:260-3.
108. Price CP. Quality assurance of extra-laboratory analyses. In: Marks V, Alberti KG, eds. Clinical biochemistry nearer the patient II. London: Bailliere Tindall, 1987:166-78.
109. Price CP, St. John A, Kricka LJ, eds. Point-of-care testing: needs, opportunity and innovation, 3rd edition. Washington, DC: AACC Press, 2010:1-582.
110. Price CP, St. John A. Point-of-care testing for managers and policymakers. Washington, DC: AACC Press, 2006:1-120.
111. Price CP, Thorpe GH. Disposable analytical devices for point-of-care testing. In: Price CP, Hicks JM, eds. Point-of-care testing. Washington, DC: AACC Press, 1999:19-40.
112. Price CP. Point-of-care testing. BMJ 2001;322:1285-8.
113. Price CP. Point of care testing: potential for tracking disease management outcomes. Dis Manage Health Outcomes 2002;10:749-61.
114. Pugia MJ, Lott JA, Clark LW, Parker DR, Wallace JF, Willis TW. Comparisons of urine dipsticks with quantitative methods for microalbuminuria. Eur J Clin Chem Clin Biochem 1997;35:693-700.
115. Raine CH. Self-monitored blood glucose: a common pitfall. Endo Pract 2003;9:137-9.
116. Rao LV, Ekberg BA, Connor D, Jakubiak F, Vallaro GM, Snyder M. Evaluation of a new point of care automated complete blood count (CBC) analyzer in various clinical settings. Clin Chim Acta 2008;389:120-5.
117. Rolinski B, Kuster H, Ugele B, Gruber R, Horn K. Total bilirubin measurement by photometry on a blood gas analyzer: potential for use in neonatal testing at the point of care. Clin Chem 2001;47:1845-7.
118. Scott MG. Faster is better—it's rarely that simple! Clin Chem 2000;46:441-2.
119. Sirkin A, Jalloh T, Lee L. Selecting an accurate point-of-care testing system: clinical and technical issues and implications in neonatal blood glucose monitoring. J Spec Pediatr Nurs 2002;7:104-12.
120. St. Louis P. Status of point-of-care testing: promise, realities, and possibilities. Clin Biochem 2000;33:427-40.
121. St John A, Davis TM, Goodall I, Townsend MA, Price CP. Nurse-based evaluation of assays for glycated hemoglobin. Clin Chim Acta 2005;365:257-263.
122. Stephens EJ. Developing open standards for point-of-care connectivity. IVD Technol 1999;10:22-5.
123. Storto Poe S, Case-Cromer DL. Nursing strategies for point-of-care testing. In: Kost G, ed. Principles and practice in point-of-care testing. Philadelphia: Lippincott Williams and Wilkins, 2002:214-35.
124. Tamada JA, Garg S, Jovanovic L, Pitzer KR, Fermi S, Potts RO. Noninvasive glucose monitoring: comprehensive clinical results. Cygnus Research Team. JAMA 1999;282:1839-44.
125. Tripodi A, Chantarangkul V, Mannucci P. Near-patient testing devices to monitor oral anticoagulant therapy. Br J Haematol 2001;113:847-52.
126. United Kingdom National External Quality Assessment Scheme. Information (e.g., cholesterol testing programme). Available at: www.ukneqas.org.uk (accessed on April 14, 2011).
127. U.S. Department of Health and Human Services. Medicare, Medicaid and CLIA Programs. Regulations implementing the Clinical Laboratory Improvement Amendments of 1988 (CLIA): final rule. Federal Register 1992;57:7002-186.
128. U.S. Department of Health and Human Services. Medicare, Medicaid and CLIA Programs. Regulations implementing the Clinical Laboratory Improvement Amendments of 1988 (CLIA) and Clinical Laboratory Act program fee collection. Federal Register 1993;58:5215-37.
129. U.S. Department of Health and Human Services. Medicare, Medicaid and CLIA Programs. Laboratory requirements relating to quality systems and certain personnel qualifications: final rule. Federal Register 2003;68:3639-3714.
130. Valkirs GE, Barton R. Immunoconcentration™: a new format for solid-phase immunoassays. Clin Chem 1985;31:1427-31.
131. van den Besselaar AM. Accuracy, precision, and quality control for point-of-care testing of oral anticoagulation. J Thromb Thrombolysis 2001;12:35-40.
132. Van Herpe T, De Moor B, Van den Berghe G. Towards closed-loop glycaemic control. Best Pract Res Clin Anaesthesiol 2009;23:69-80.
133. Wales External Quality Assessment Scheme. Information (e.g., urinalysis program). Available at: www.weqas.co.uk (accessed on 14 April, 2011).
134. Walter B. Dry reagent chemistries. Anal Chem 1983;55:A498-514.
135. Westgard JO. Electronic quality control, the total testing process, and the total quality system. Clin Chim Acta 2001;307:45-8.

SECTION III

Analytes

CHAPTER 21

Amino Acids, Peptides, and Proteins

Glen L. Hortin, M.D., Ph.D*

Amino acids, peptides, and proteins are crucial for virtually all biological processes. Amino acids have diverse roles in metabolism, neurotransmission, and intercellular signaling, as well as serving as structural subunits of peptides and proteins. Peptides include many hormones, signaling molecules, and protein fragments that are of physiologic and diagnostic significance. Nucleic acids provide the information or software program, and proteins serve as the hardware that performs most cellular functions. Proteins are multifunctional and constitute the machinery of life. Biologically, they (1) form many important intracellular and extracellular structures; (2) generate energy through catalysis and electron transfer; (3) produce motility through contractile elements; (4) assemble molecules; (5) serve as ion channels and pumps; (6) act as carriers; (7) perform immune defense; (8) serve as receptors, hormones, and cytokines for intercellular regulation; and (9) constitute signaling networks for intracellular regulation.

In humans, more than 20,000 genes encode proteins. Completion of the sequence of the human genome defines much of the sequence information for proteins and facilitates the identification of protein and peptide sequences. The number of proteins is greater than the number of genes, however, because of variable splicing of messenger RNA (mRNA), somatic recombination and mutation, proteolytic processing, and numerous post-translational modifications of proteins. The Human Antibody Initiative has developed specific antibodies for thousands of human proteins, and these antibodies have been used to assemble a Human Protein Atlas that uses immunohistochemistry to define the expression of more than 5000 proteins in different tissues of the body (http://www.proteinatlas.org/accessed April 19, 2011).[124] These efforts serve as major resources for identification of tissue sources of proteins and potential assay reagents. Many proteins are secreted or leak out of cells in response to cellular injury or turnover, allowing their analysis in biological fluids such as blood and urine. The *proteome* represents the complete set of proteins in an organism or subcompartment of an organism such as the plasma space.[3] Initial efforts of the Human Proteome Organization's (HUPO's) Plasma Proteome Project tentatively identified sequences of about 3000 gene products in plasma, and many structural variants of these gene products may exist.[114,117] Several databases include extensive information about the sequence and post-translational modification of proteins. The U.S. National Library of Medicine and the Swiss Institute of Bioinformatics maintain gene and protein databases and sequence analysis tools that are available via the Internet [http://www.ncbi.nlm.nih.gov/accessed April 19, 2011 and http://ca.expasy.org/accessed April 19, 2011; The HIP2 Database (Healthy Human Individual's Integrated Plasma Proteome); http://bio.informatics.iupui.edu/HIP2/accessed April 19, 2011/] and include data on more than 12,000 protein entries].[134] The Human Protein Reference Database and Human Proteinpedia are additional resource (http://www.hprd.org/accessed April 19, 2011).[101] Most databases are designed mainly to assist with peptide and protein identification, and more data are needed related to the abundance of components in healthy and diseased populations, which is the usual basis for diagnostic applications.[2,3,60]

This chapter begins with a discussion of the properties and metabolism of amino acids. Inherited disorders of amino acid metabolism are discussed in Chapter 58. A general description of protein structure is followed by information on several high-abundance proteins in plasma and several other fluids including cerebrospinal fluid. This chapter provides limited discussion of urinary proteins, which are covered in Chapters 25 and 48. Virtually all tissues contribute proteins to plasma via secretion or cell injury. The resulting diversity of plasma proteins leads to high informational content and broad clinical utility of the analysis of proteins in plasma or serum. Other proteins are discussed in the chapters on enzymes (see Chapter

The author gratefully acknowledges the previous contributions of A. Myron Johnson, Robert H. Christenson, Hassan M.E. Azzazy, Lawrence M. Silverman, and Elizabeth M. Rohlfs, on which portions of this chapter are based.

22), tumor markers (see Chapter 24), lipoproteins (see Chapter 27), hormones (see Chapter 29), and specific disease processes. Chapter 32 describes analysis of hemoglobins, which are the major protein component of whole blood and are major plasma components when red blood cell lysis occurs.

AMINO ACIDS

Amino acids are major metabolic intermediates and the basic structural units of proteins. Their measurement in physiological fluids assists with fundamental studies of metabolism and the diagnosis of pathologic processes and inherited conditions.

Basic Biochemistry

Amino acids are organic compounds containing both an amino group (—NH_2) and a carboxyl group (—COOH) or another acidic group such as sulfonic acid (—SO_3). Technically, proline, hydroxyproline, and sarcosine are imino acids (—NH—), but they usually are grouped together with amino acids. Those occurring in proteins are α-amino acids, with amino groups linked to the α-carbon, as diagrammed here:

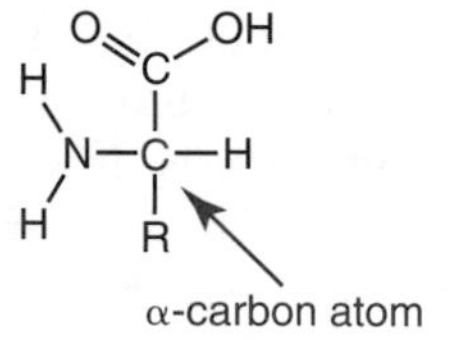

α-carbon atom

R represents a variety of different sidechains as listed in Table 21-1. Amino acids in physiologic fluids also include β-amino acids such as β-alanine and taurine, and γ-amino acids such as γ-aminobutyric acid (GABA).

With the exception of glycine, all α-amino acids are asymmetric about the α-carbon, with four different groups linked to this carbon. Most α-amino acids in humans, including all of the amino acids incorporated into protein, have the L-configuration. Small quantities of D-amino acids occur in physiological fluids. In most cases, these are not known to have specific functions. An exception is D-serine, which represents 5 to 20% of total serine in cerebrospinal fluid; D-serine may serve as a neurotransmitter.[41] Amino acids with the D-configuration occur in some bacterial products, foods, and pharmaceuticals. D-Amino acid oxidases in liver and kidney convert D-amino acids to ketoacids, which can be metabolized. L-Amino acids in proteins undergo slow racemization to a mixture of L- and D-amino acids over many years. Aspartic acid undergoes the most rapid racemization and can be used to estimate the time of synthesis of proteins undergoing very slow turnover, such as lens proteins in the eye or collagens in intervertebral disks, where half-lives may exceed 50 years.[145] Two amino acids—threonine and isoleucine—have a second asymmetric carbon, and the stereoisomers are referred to as *allothreonine* and *alloisoleucine.* Table 21-1 diagrams the structures of the 21 amino acids that are encoded by codons in messenger RNA and incorporated into proteins. Twenty amino acids are incorporated into most proteins. Selenocysteine is a special case of an amino acid synthesized on a specific transfer RNA and incorporated into a few sites in only about 25 proteins.[92] Many additional amino acids are generated by post-translational modification of proteins or by metabolism.

Acid-Base Properties of Amino Acids

Acid-base properties of amino acids depend on the amino and carboxyl groups attached to the α-carbon and on the basic or acidic groups occurring on some sidechains (R). In the physiologic pH range of plasma near pH 7.4, the carboxyl group is dissociated, and the amino group is protonated to give the following structure:

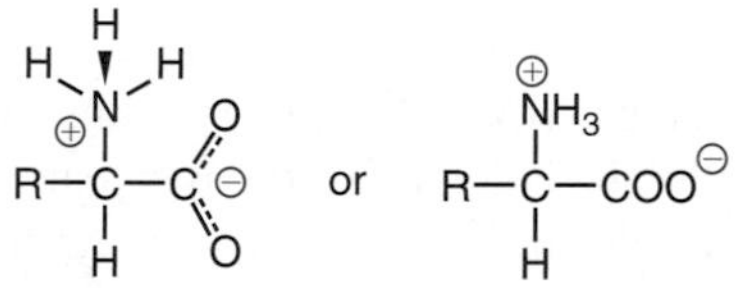

$$R-CH(NH_3^{+})-COO^{-}$$

Thus, at neutral pH, amino acids have both positively and negatively charged groups and occur as zwitterions.

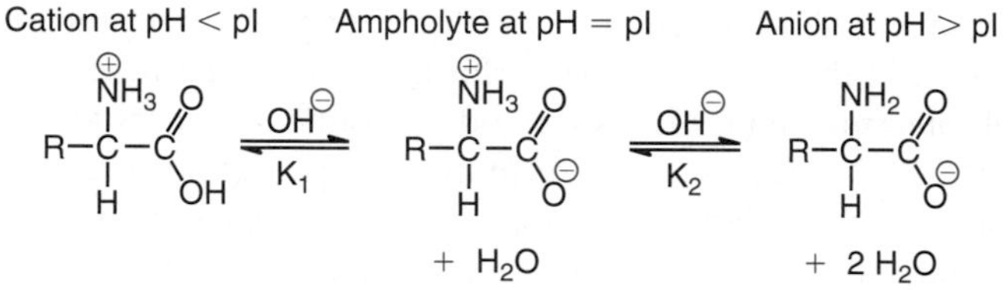

Cation at pH < pI ⇌ (OH^-, K_1) Ampholyte at pH = pI ⇌ (OH^-, K_2) Anion at pH > pI

$$R-CH(NH_3^{+})-COOH \underset{K_1}{\overset{OH^-}{\rightleftharpoons}} R-CH(NH_3^{+})-COO^{-} + H_2O \underset{K_2}{\overset{OH^-}{\rightleftharpoons}} R-CH(NH_2)-COO^{-} + 2\,H_2O$$

The pH at which an ionizable group, such as an amino or carboxyl group, occurs equally in charged and uncharged forms is referred to as the pK for that group. Amino acids have two or more pKs, including one for the carboxyl, one for the amino group, and an additional pK if an ionizable sidechain is present. The isoelectric point (pI) is the pH where an amino acid or other molecule has a net charge of 0. For a typical neutral amino acid such as glycine, the pI of 5.97 is midway between the pK_1 of 2.34 for the carboxylic acid and the pK_2 of 9.60 for the amino group. Ionization constants for amino acids are given in Table 21-2. The pKs of amino acid sidechains in proteins vary somewhat because of the influence of neighboring amino acids.

The buffering capacity of ionizable groups is primarily in a pH range within ±1 of the pK for the respective groups. Amino acids and proteins therefore have a limited buffering capacity near physiologic pH, mainly caused by the contribution of imidazole sidechains of histidine. Amino acids serve as buffers at pHs near the pKs of their ionizable groups; glycine, for example, sometimes is used as a buffer near pH 2.5 or 9.5.

Hydrophobicity, Solubility, and Stability of Amino Acids

Sidechains produce variation in the properties of different amino acids. Table 21-1 shows the structures of amino acids, molecular weights, and the Kyte and Doolittle index of the hydrophobicity of their sidechains.[83] Amino acids with longer

TABLE 21-1 Amino Acids Incorporated into Protein, Their Properties and Structures

Name and Abbreviation	HI	MW*	Structure at pH 6-7	Comments
I. Neutral Amino Acids				
Alanine Ala, A	1.8	89.09	$H_3C-CH(NH_3^{\oplus})-COO^{\ominus}$	Important metabolic substrate in alanine cycle; substrate for ALT
Leucine Leu, L	3.8	131.17	$(H_3C)_2CH-CH_2-CH(NH_3^{\oplus})-COO^{\ominus}$	Essential; branched-chain R group; ketogenic; metabolism is faulty in maple syrup urine disease
Isoleucine Ile, I	4.5	131.17	$H_3C-CH_2-CH(CH_3)-CH(NH_3^{\oplus})-COO^{\ominus}$	Essential; partly ketogenic; see leucine above
Valine Val, V	4.2	117.17	$(H_3C)_2CH-CH(NH_3^{\oplus})-COO^{\ominus}$	Essential; partly ketogenic; see leucine above
Proline Pro, P	1.6	115.13	pyrrolidine ring ($NH_2^{\oplus}$) $-COO^{\ominus}$	Has α-imino rather than α-amino; high content in collagens and can be hydroxylated to hydroxyproline; destabilizes α-helical structures
Methionine Met, M	1.9	149.21	$H_3C-S-CH_2-CH_2-CH(NH_3^{\oplus})-COO^{\ominus}$	Essential; important as donor of methyl groups; provides sulfur for other sulfur-containing compounds
Phenylalanine Phe, F	2.8	165.19	$C_6H_5-CH_2-CH(NH_3^{\oplus})-COO^{\ominus}$	Essential; elevated concentrations in phenylketonuria as conversion to Tyr is impaired.
Tryptophan Trp, W	–0.9	204.22	indole (N) $-CH_2-CH(NH_3^{\oplus})-COO^{\ominus}$	Essential; metabolites in carcinoid disease; contains indole ring; precursor of serotonin, melatonin
Glycine Gly, G	–0.4	75.07	$H-CH(NH_3^{\oplus})-COO^{\ominus}$	No stereoisomer; used in biosynthesis of purines and porphyrins; transfer to bile acids, hippurates, and other conjugates
Serine Ser, S	–0.8	105.09	$HO-CH_2-CH(NH_3^{\oplus})-COO^{\ominus}$	Source of one-carbon groups for folates; can undergo post-translational addition of phosphate, sugars
Threonine Thr, T	–0.7	119.12	$HO(H_3C)CH-CH(NH_3^{\oplus})-COO^{\ominus}$	Essential; can undergo post-translational addition of phosphate or sugars
Cysteine Cys, C	2.5	121.16	$HS-CH_2-CH(NH_3^{\oplus})-COO^{\ominus}$	Sulfhydryl group in active sites of some enzymes; forms disulfides; homocysteine is homolog with sidechain one carbon longer
Selenocysteine Sec, U		168.05	$HSe-CH_2-CH(NH_3^{\oplus})-COO^{\ominus}$	Active form of selenium; found in some enzymes involved in oxidation-reduction reactions; formed on a specific transfer RNA

Continued

TABLE 21-1 Amino Acids Incorporated into Protein, Their Properties and Structures—cont'd

Name and Abbreviation	HI	MW*	Structure at pH 6-7	Comments
Tyrosine Tyr, Y	−1.3	181.19	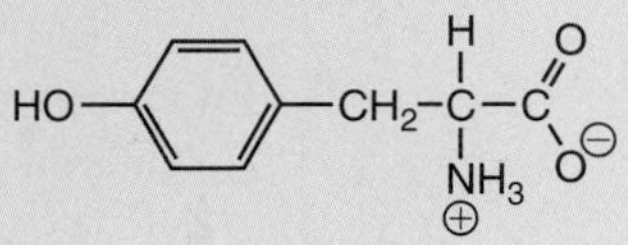 $HO-C_6H_4-CH_2-CH(NH_3^{\oplus})-COO^{\ominus}$	Usually nonessential; intermediate in synthesis of catecholamines, thyroxine, and melanin; functional phenolic group
Glutamine Gln, Q	−3.5	146.15	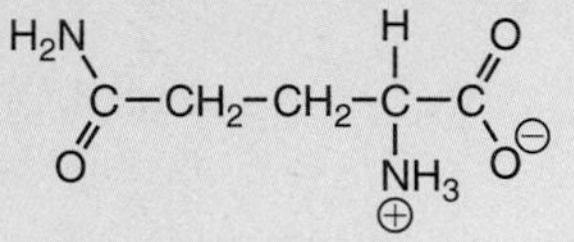 $H_2N-C(=O)-CH_2-CH_2-CH(NH_3^{\oplus})-COO^{\ominus}$	Transport form of ammonia; supplies nitrogen atoms used in purine and pyrimidine biosynthesis
Asparagine Asn, N	−3.5	132.12	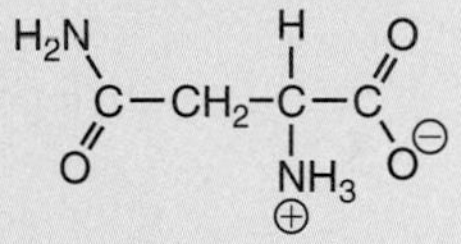 $H_2N-C(=O)-CH_2-CH(NH_3^{\oplus})-COO^{\ominus}$	Attachment site of oligosaccharides in Asn-Xxx-(Ser or Thr) sequences
Acidic Amino Acids				
Aspartic acid Asp, D	−3.5	133.10	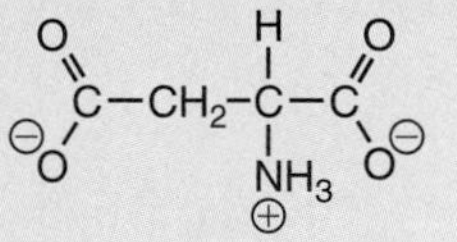 $^{\ominus}OOC-CH_2-CH(NH_3^{\oplus})-COO^{\ominus}$	Precursor for pyrimidine and purine biosynthesis; a substrate in urea cycle
Glutamic acid Glu, E	−3.5	147.13	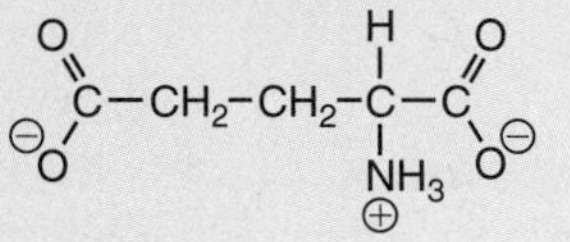 $^{\ominus}OOC-CH_2-CH_2-CH(NH_3^{\oplus})-COO^{\ominus}$	Transport form of ammonia γ-glutamyl transfer from glutathione; a neurotransmitter
Basic Amino Acids				
Lysine Lys, K	−3.9	146.19	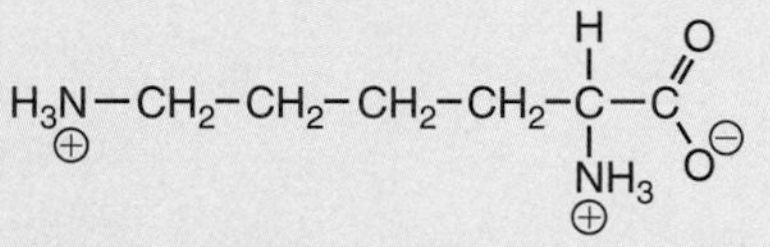 $H_3N^{\oplus}-CH_2-CH_2-CH_2-CH_2-CH(NH_3^{\oplus})-COO^{\ominus}$	Essential; sidechain has an additional amino group
Arginine Arg, R	−4.5	174.20	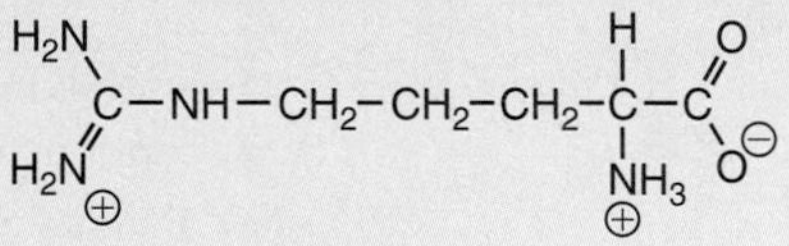 $(H_2N)(H_2N^{\oplus}=)C-NH-CH_2-CH_2-CH_2-CH(NH_3^{\oplus})-COO^{\ominus}$	Involved in urea synthesis; sidechain has a guanidinium group
Histidine His, H	−3.2	155.16	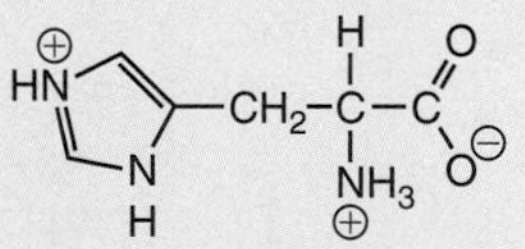 imidazolium ($^{\oplus}HN$, N–H) $-CH_2-CH(NH_3^{\oplus})-COO^{\ominus}$	The imidazole group has a pK near physiologic pH, so charge can vary with physiologic pH change

*A higher value for hydropathy index (HI)[83] indicates greater hydrophobicity of amino acid sidechains.

aliphatic or aromatic sidechains such as isoleucine, leucine, and phenylalanine have greater hydrophobicity than shorter sidechains such as alanine, indicating lower water solubility. Neutral amino acids having polar groups such as hydroxyl or amide groups in their sidechains are more hydrophilic. Acidic amino acids have sidechains with carboxylic acids, and basic amino acids have sidechains with amino, guanidine, or imidazole groups. Acidic and basic sidechains generally represent highly polar and water-soluble sidechains. The structural diversity of sidechains contributes to the participation of amino acids in many metabolic pathways and the ability to form proteins with wide variation in structure and physical properties. The occurrence of an imino rather than an amino group in proline results in some differences in physical properties and reactivity of proline and in the geometry of peptides containing proline.

Amino acids generally occur freely in solution in plasma and other physiologic fluids, with a few exceptions. The thiol group of cysteine and homocysteine and small peptides such as cysteinylglycine and glutathione oxidize easily and become linked to other molecules via disulfides in the extracellular space, which is an oxidizing environment. This contrasts with the cytoplasm, which is predominantly a reducing environment maintained by a high concentration of glutathione in reduced form.[127] In plasma, cysteine occurs as cystine (dimeric cysteine linked via a disulfide) or as a mixed disulfide with

TABLE 21-2 Ionization Constants of Ionizable Groups in Free Amino Acids and in Proteins*

Ionizing Group		Range of pK Values: Free Amino Acids	Range of pK Values: Proteins
Principal carboxyl = pK_1	$-C(=O)O^{\ominus}$	1.7-2.6	3.0-3.2
α-Amino = pK_2	$-NH_3^{\oplus}$	9.0-10.8	7.6-8.4
Second carboxyls of Glu and Asp	$-C(=O)O^{\ominus}$	3.8-4.3	3.0-4.5
Imidazole nitrogen of His	$=NH^{\oplus}-$	6.0	6.0-7.0
Sulfhydryl of Cys	$-SH$	8.3	9.1-10.8
Phenolic hydroxyl of Tyr	$-OH$	10.1	9.2-9.8
ε-Amino of Lys	$-NH_3^{\oplus}$	10.5	9.4-10.6
Guanidinium group of Arg	$-NH-C(NH_2)=NH_2^{\oplus}$	12.5	11.5-12.6

*The pK value for the primary carboxyl varies from 1.71 for Cys to 2.63 for Thr. The pK for the α-amino group varies from 8.95 for Lys to 10.78 for Cys. In protein chains, the local environment modifies the pK for any given ionizable group. The amino acid symbols are listed in Table 21-1.

albumin or other proteins. About half of cysteine is covalently bound to protein and can be released by the addition of reducing agents. Analysis of amino acids without reduction detects only the cystine component. Homocysteine, cysteinylglycine, and glutathione are similarly distributed as mixed disulfides with cysteine or protein.[157] During storage of plasma specimens, some change in the distribution of homocysteine occurs, and the proportion bound to protein increases.[59,157] Tryptophan is another amino acid that occurs approximately 50% bound to albumin, although in this case the binding is noncovalent.

Most amino acids are water soluble and stable in plasma specimens, again with a few exceptions. Solubility of cystine and a few of the more hydrophobic amino acids can be limiting in some disorders of transport or metabolism. Crystals of cystine, leucine, or tyrosine may deposit when concentrations become elevated in urine in cystinuria or tyrosinemia or within intracellular compartments in cystinosis. Glutamine degrades in solution as the result of intramolecular cyclization to pyroglutamic acid (also termed *5-oxoproline*) with release of ammonia. Quantification of glutamine therefore requires rapid processing of specimens and frozen storage, similar to requirements for ammonia analysis. Homocysteine (usually measured as total homocysteine after reduction) is stable in plasma but requires rapid processing of blood specimens to avoid elevation resulting from continuing release from cells.[128] Arginine can be degraded in specimens with increased arginase concentrations; some arginase is present in erythrocytes and may be increased by hemolysis.[112]

Amino Acid Metabolism

Amino acids participate in many metabolic pathways, in addition to serving as a substrate for protein synthesis.[31] In the healthy state, women require ≈46 g/d and men ≈56 g/d of dietary protein (0.8 g/kg body weight), and substantial increases in demand occur during growth and in many disease states.[118] Dietary protein is digested by proteases in the stomach and small intestine to yield amino acids. Endogenous protein turnover serves as another source of free amino acids. Dietary sources and endogenous turnover, therefore, serve as dual sources of amino acids for protein synthesis. Eight amino acids used for protein synthesis—(1) isoleucine, (2) leucine, (3) lysine, (4) methionine, (5) phenylalanine, (6) threonine, (7) tryptophan, and (8) valine—are not synthesized by humans and therefore are considered "essential" constituents of the diet. Meat, milk, eggs, and fish contain a full range of essential amino acids. Gelatin is deficient in tryptophan, and individual plant sources of protein may be deficient in lysine, methionine, or tryptophan. Diets based on a single source of plant protein may be deficient in some amino acids. When liver function is compromised,[162] cysteine and tyrosine become essential because they are not converted from their usual precursors methionine and phenylalanine. Arginine may be conditionally essential.[112] Essential amino acids usually have been defined for the entire body, but additional amino acids may be essential for specific tissues or for some human cells in culture. As an example, administration of asparaginase to deplete asparagine is useful therapy for acute lymphoblastic leukemia, because the lymphoblasts are not able to synthesize asparagine. Glutamine is considered to be an important metabolic substrate for immune cells and enterocytes.[132] Supplementation of glutamine and arginine may be beneficial in critically ill patients.[162]

Requirements for dietary protein to maintain nitrogen balance increase per unit body weight during infancy and childhood when there are demands for protein for growth, and in pregnancy, lactation, and states of protein loss or catabolic states.[24,80] Daily requirements increase by up to 3.5 to 4 g protein/kg body weight for premature infants.[50] A diet severely deficient in protein and consisting primarily of high-starch foods can lead to kwashiorkor, with decreased serum albumin, immune deficiency, edema, ascites, growth failure, apathy, and many other symptoms.[67] Marasmus results when protein and energy sources such as carbohydrates are deficient; protein-calorie starvation causes generalized wasting of muscles and subcutaneous tissues and lesser edema. Inadequate nutrition is frequently a problem in surgical, burn, or trauma patients in a catabolic state and with decreased food intake.[69] Negative nitrogen balance can contribute to delayed wound healing and impaired immunity. Measurements of plasma markers such as albumin or prealbumin are indicators of adequacy of the amino acid supply. Protein intake is related to urinary urea and acid excretion in the form of sulfate. A high-protein diet promotes excretion of acidic urine, and a vegetarian diet of a neutral urine. In kidney disease, high protein intake appears to be harmful, and protein restriction has been used as a therapeutic intervention to slow the progress of kidney disease.[89]

Amino acids normally are released from dietary protein by degradation with pepsin in the acidic environment of the stomach and with pancreatic hydrolases added in the duodenum.[31] Digestion of protein may be impaired by gastric or pancreatic disorders. Uptake by intestinal and other cells occurs by active transport with several separate transport systems that handle neutral amino acids, acidic amino acids, basic amino acids, and cystine, glycine, and proline. Amino acids are actively transported by γ-glutamyltransferases that transport amino acids by linking them to glutamic acid transferred from glutathione. Active transport maintains higher concentrations of amino acids inside cells than outside in the extracellular space and, in renal tubules, reclaims most amino acids that undergo glomerular filtration.[70]

Amino acids are critical intermediates in many metabolic pathways, including the urea cycle for converting ammonia to urea and the alanine cycle for transferring nitrogen and fuel sources from muscle to liver, both described later. Other major pathways include ammonia generation in the kidney from glutamine and glutamic acid, glutathione formation and reduction to maintain a reducing environment intracellularly, and the glutathione cycle for cellular uptake of molecules.[127] Amino acids are precursors for many hormones and signaling molecules such as thyroid hormones, catecholamines, serotonin, melatonin, nitric oxide, and hydrogen sulfide. Activated pathways for metabolism of tryptophan and cysteine are effector pathways for interferon action.[139] Serine is a major source of one-carbon units transferred by tetrahydrofolic acid for purine synthesis, methylation of deoxyuridylic acid to thymidylic acid, and conversion of homocysteine to methionine. Glycine, aspartic acid, glutamine, and serine contribute atoms to purine and pyrimidine synthesis. Glycine and arginine are precursors for creatine synthesis. Methionine serves as a methyl donor after activation as S-adenosylmethione for a wide range of methylation reactions, including creatine synthesis, protein methylation, and choline synthesis, and yields homocysteine as a byproduct. Several amino acids participate in conjugation reactions that serve as excretory pathways and generate products such as glycine or taurine conjugates with bile acids. Cysteine and glutathione form mercapturates with reactive compounds as a protective mechanism. Metabolism of the sulfur-containing amino acids generates sulfate, which is excreted in urine in increased amounts with consumption of high-protein diets.

The alanine cycle is a metabolic pathway that allows muscle cells to use amino acids as a fuel source and to export excess nitrogen in the form of alanine, which then is metabolized in the liver as diagrammed in Figure 21-1. In muscle cells, ammonia is transferred from amino acids to pyruvate by aminotransferases to form alanine. Alanine is excreted from muscle cells and is taken up by the liver, where aminotransferases transfer ammonia from alanine to 2-oxoglutarate, forming pyruvate and glutamic acid. Pyruvate can serve as a substrate for gluconeogenesis or for energy, and glutamate serves as a donor for urea synthesis. This pathway explains the need for high aminotransferase catalytic amounts in liver and muscle.

The urea cycle converts ammonia to urea in the liver (see Chapter 50). Ammonia, bicarbonate, and ATP join in formation of carbamoylphosphate, which is transferred to ornithine to form citrulline. Aspartic acid and citrulline are condensed to form arginosuccinic acid, which, in turn, is cleaved to arginine and fumaric acid. Arginase hydrolyzes arginine to urea and ornithine to allow the cycle to repeat. Net changes from the cycle include input of ammonia, bicarbonate, aspartic acid, and energy in the form of ATP and output of urea and fumaric acid. Urea usually is viewed simply as a waste product, with urea production related to protein intake. However, one beneficial action of urea is its contribution to the ability of kidneys to concentrate urine. Urea is the main component accounting for high osmolality in the renal medulla, and maximal urinary concentrating ability decreases when protein intake is low and urea production is decreased.

Amino Acid Concentrations

Plasma amino acid concentrations are high during the first days of life, especially in premature neonates, but they tend to be low in infants with low birth weight for gestational age because of placental insufficiency. *Plasma* amino acid concentrations vary by about 30% during the day; therefore, blood specimens should be collected at the same time each day. Values are highest in midafternoon and lowest in early morning. This diurnal variation affects detection of heterozygous defects in metabolism.[70]

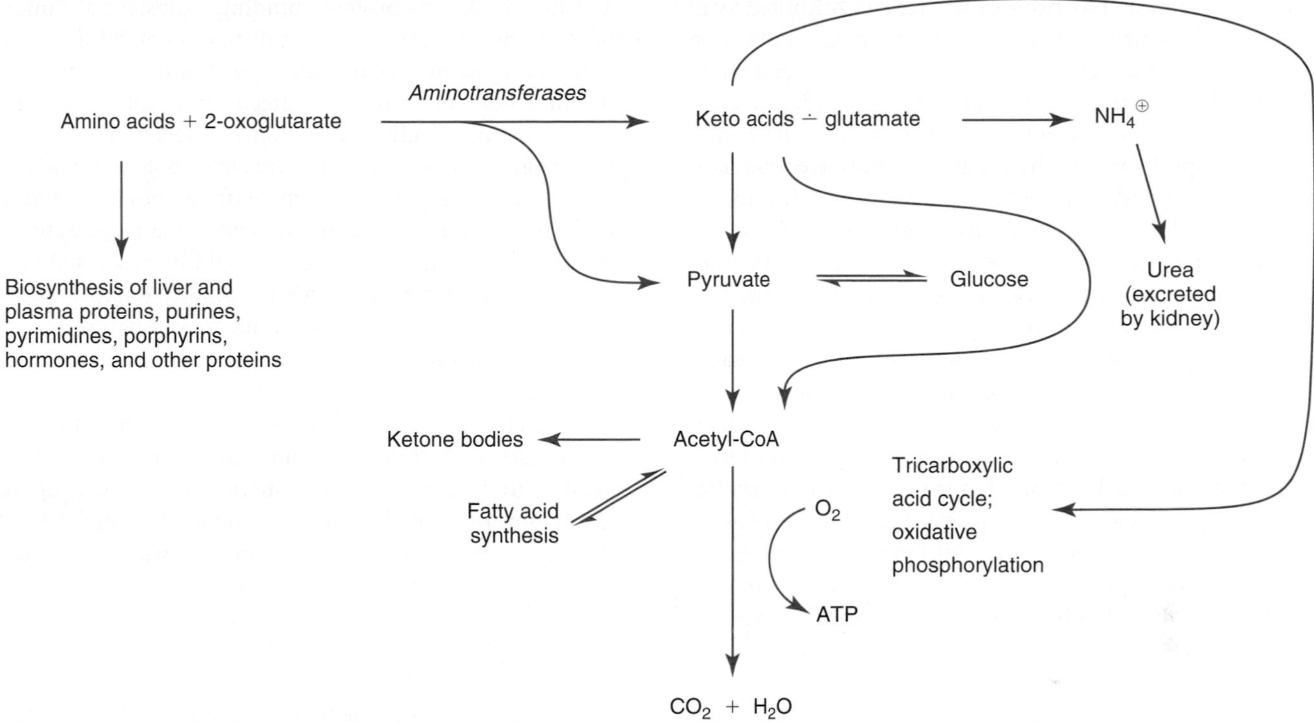

Figure 21-1 A generalized scheme of amino acid metabolism in the liver. Alanine represents one of the major metabolic substrates.

Most amino acids in blood undergo efficient glomerular filtration but are reabsorbed in proximal renal tubules by saturable transport systems (see Chapter 48). Increased renal excretion of amino acids *(aminoaciduria)* results from overload from increased plasma concentrations or from tubular impairment related to hereditary disorders or tubular injury. Amino acid excretion in urine varies with renal tubular maturation. Premature infants, especially during the first week, have a generalized aminoaciduria; even at full term, amino acid excretion is greater than in normal adults. In the urine of normal adults, glycine is the most abundant amino acid, followed by histidine, taurine, glutamine, serine, and alanine. Amounts of 1-methylhistidine may be high, depending on meat intake.

For adults, CSF concentrations of most amino acids, except for glutamine, are several-fold lower than in plasma. Glutamine is the main component, with usual concentrations of 0.4 to 1.0 mmol/L that are slightly higher than in plasma. Most amino acids other than alanine, serine, and threonine have CSF concentrations <0.03 mmol/L. Newborns have a smaller gradient of amino acid concentrations versus plasma than do adults.

Cells generally have intracellular amino acid concentrations higher than plasma concentrations. Intracellular concentrations of glutathione are in the mmol/L range. Many cells maintain high concentrations of taurine, which may serve as an antioxidant and as a component for regulation of intracellular osmolality. Regulation of intracellular amino acid concentrations may be one mechanism for controlling intracellular osmolality, particularly in tissues such as the renal medulla and brain.[5]

Clinical Implications of Amino Acid Concentrations

Historically, clinical laboratory assessments of plasma and urinary amino acids have been used primarily to detect or monitor inborn errors of metabolism, as detailed in Chapter 58. Measurement of plasma homocysteine is of clinical interest, as increased homocysteine is an indicator of deficiency of folic acid or vitamin B_{12} and is correlated with risk of cardiovascular disease.[71,128] Fasting concentrations of plasma homocysteine are relatively constant within individuals and are correlated with risk for cardiovascular disease and thrombosis. Many hypotheses have been advanced for how homocysteine might be a cause of cardiovascular disease or thrombosis, but these hypotheses have been undermined by some recent intervention trials that have not observed decreased cardiovascular disease in response to lowering of homocysteine by increased intake of folic acid and vitamin B_{12}.[71] However, even if homocysteine does not cause cardiovascular disease, it could still serve as a measurable risk factor.

Measurement of amino acids has not been extensively used in clinical practice for monitoring of patients with nutritional, metabolic, infectious, or psychiatric disorders. In part, this is because plasma amino acid concentrations do not always reflect severe deficiencies in malnutrition states; most amino acid metabolism and function are intracellular. Also amino acid analysis has been expensive, with limited availability and slow turnaround time. Metabolomic studies may provide increased insight into metabolic pathways and potential clinical applications of measurement of amino acids. Several amino acid concentrations are of potential clinical interest. Drops in tryptophan concentration are associated with depression and other psychiatric disease.[107] Tryptophan degradation along the kynurenine pathway and cysteine metabolism by cysteine dioxygenase are stimulated by interferon, so that quantification of tryptophan, cysteine, and their metabolites is an indicator of immune activation.[139] Concentrations of arginine and citrulline are indicators of activation of the nitric oxide synthase pathway and adequacy of the substrate arginine for nitric oxide synthesis. This pathway may be important for pathogenesis of vascular disorders in sickle cell disease, asthma, and other disorders and may be a pharmacologic target.[43,111] Increased concentrations of asymmetric dimethylarginine, which inhibits nitric oxide synthase, may be physiologically significant in the development of cardiovascular and kidney disease.[75] Glutamine concentration may be monitored to assess the nutritional adequacy of postsurgical patients and those with other conditions.[132,162] Measurements of intracellular concentrations of glutathione or ratios of reduced and oxidized glutathione may serve as measures of oxidative stress, nutritional depletion in cancer or other states, or overdose with toxic compounds such as acetaminophen. Advances in the ability to measure amino acids rapidly and efficiently may expand clinical application of amino acid measurements.

Analysis of Amino Acids

Methods used to measure amino acids in biological samples are detailed in Chapter 58. The standard method for many years was the cation-exchange chromatography with spectrophotometric detection after postcolumn reaction with ninhydrin, as developed by Stein and Moore in the 1950s. This method quantifies 30 to 40 components in plasma and urine. However, newborn screening programs usually apply tandem mass spectrometry, and an increasing range of chromatographic and mass spectrometric methods are being applied to amino acid analysis. Analytical procedures usually involve deproteinization prior to analysis by precipitation with acids or organic acid or by ultrafiltration. This yields good recovery of most amino acids, except recovery of tryptophan may vary as the result of protein binding; substantial amounts of cysteine, homocysteine, and thiol-containing peptides such as cysteinylglycine and glutathione are linked via disulfide bonds to proteins.[157] Recovery of total cysteine and homocysteine requires reduction of specimens before precipitation steps. Most amino acids are stable in blood specimens, except for glutamine, which undergoes intramolecular cyclization to form pyroglutamic acid (5-oxoproline) with the release of ammonia. Specimens should be processed rapidly and stored frozen to preserve glutamine. Rapid processing of specimens is needed for accurate determination of homocysteine to avoid effects of homocysteine excretion from blood cells.[128]

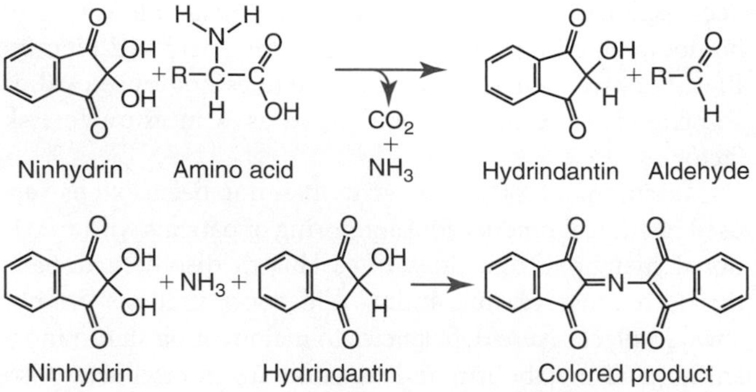

Ninhydrin + Amino acid → CO_2 + NH_3 + Hydrindantin + Aldehyde

Ninhydrin + NH_3 + Hydrindantin → Colored product

Several methods are available for measurement of total homocysteine, including immunoassay after enzymatic conversion to S-adenosylhomocysteine, enzyme cycling reactions, chromatographic or electrophoretic methods after derivatization, chromatographic analysis with electrochemical detection, and tandem mass spectrometry.

PEPTIDES AND PROTEINS

This section describes the basic biochemistry of peptides and proteins, and provides details on several high-abundance plasma proteins and selected methods for protein analysis used in the clinical laboratory.

Peptide and Protein Structure

A *peptide bond* is the amide bond formed between the amino group of one amino acid and the carboxyl group of a second amino acid. An example of a peptide bond joining two amino acids is diagrammed with the peptide bond enclosed by a box:

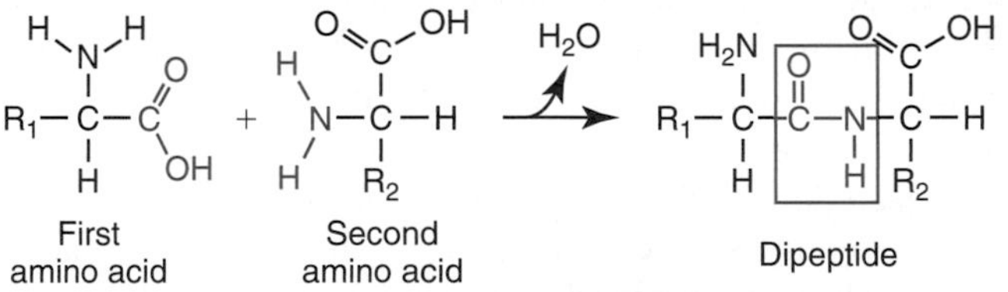

First amino acid + Second amino acid → (H_2O) Dipeptide

Isopeptide bonds refer to amide bonds linking amino acids via amino acid sidechains; an example is glutathione, in which the γ-carboxyl of glutamic acid is linked to the amino group of cysteine. Polymers of several amino acids are termed *peptides,* and amino acid sequences are described from the amino- or N-terminus, the amino acid with a free α-amino group. The final amino acid in the chain is the carboxy- or C-terminus. Peptide bonds, similar to all amide bonds, are planar structures that fix the geometry about the bonds, so that the major conformational flexibility of the peptide backbone results from rotation about the axes of the two bonds to the α-carbon. Short peptides are identified by the number of constituent amino acids, such as dipeptide, tripeptide, tetrapeptide, or pentapeptide. When peptides reach sufficient length to have a defined globular structure—about 50 or more residues—polypeptides begin to be referred to as *proteins.*

The terms *proteose* and *peptone* refer to partial digestion products of proteins, sometimes used as a source of amino acids for bacterial culture or other purposes.

The structures of peptides and proteins consist of five elements:

1. *Primary structure* is the sequence of amino acids in a peptide or protein. Post-translational modifications of amino acids contribute to increased diversity.
2. *Secondary structure* is the restriction of the peptide backbone by hydrogen bonds between different peptide bonds. Elements of secondary structure include α-helix, β-sheet, and β-turn. An α-helix has about 3.6 residues per turn, and hydrogen bonds are between amide oxygens and amide hydrogens 4 residues later. A β-sheet involves hydrogen bonds between the peptide bonds of adjacent peptide chains arranged in parallel or antiparallel configurations. *Random coils* refer to segments of peptide that lack defined secondary structure. Turns are commonly located on the surface of proteins and represent frequent sites of mutation because fewer constraints are imposed on sidechain packing than on interior regions of a protein.
3. *Tertiary structure* refers to folding of the polypeptide chain and elements of secondary structure into a compact three-dimensional shape. Folding is a complex process driven by energy minimization of intramolecular and solvent interactions. Hydrophobic groups tend to fold into the interior with less exposure to solvent, and charged and polar sidechains tend to be located on the surface, where sidechains are exposed to solvent. The three-dimensional structure is stabilized by intramolecular hydrogen bonds, van der Waals forces, and hydrophobic interactions. Disulfide bonds between cysteine residues stabilize three-dimensional structure. High stability of a structure is reflected by maintenance of structures up to high temperatures. *Denaturation of protein* refers to unfolding that occurs with temperature change or in the presence of organic solvents, detergents, or reagents that disrupt hydrogen bonds. Limited denaturation can be reversible, but extensive unfolding and denaturation of proteins often lead to aggregation and precipitation, which is difficult to reverse.
4. *Quaternary structure* refers to the incorporation of two or more polypeptide chains or subunits into a larger unit. Examples are creatine kinase with two subunits and lactate dehydrogenase and hemoglobin with four subunits.
5. Ligands and prosthetic groups provide additional functional and structural elements, such as metals in metalloenzymes, heme in hemoglobin and cytochromes, and lipids in lipoproteins. Proteins without their associated ligands are often referred to as apoproteins (e.g., apotransferrin without iron, apolipoproteins without lipid).

Many proteins are organized with subassemblies of smaller structural units or domains somewhat analogous to a string of beads. Similar domains may occur in different proteins, but diversity in structure is possible through assembly of domains in different combinations and three-dimensional configurations. This is exemplified by a number of proteins of the coagulation and complement systems that are formed from different combinations of small globular domains. Many gene products have arisen from duplication of common ancestral genes. Homologous genes not only commonly have sequence homology but fold into similar three-dimensional structures. The serpin (originally from serine proteinase inhibitor) superfamily consists of more than 1000 related proteins in different organisms that have been subdivided into 16 clades (lettered A through P).[88] Humans have 36 serpins, of which 29 are protease inhibitors and 7 lack protease inhibitor function.[88] Serpins that act as protease inhibitors in plasma include α_1-antitrypsin, α_1-antichymotrypsin, α_2-antiplasmin, antithrombin III, C1 inhibitor, heparin cofactor II, protein C inhibitor, and plasminogen activator inhibitor-1. Some serpins without known protease inhibitor function are cortisol-binding globulin, thyroxine-binding globulin, angiotensinogen, intracellular proteins, heat shock protein 47, and the tumor suppressor maspin. Serpins illustrate how a common structure is adapted to multiple functions. Extensive information about structures of serpins provides insight into disorders of protein conformation and folding discussed later. Other examples of families of plasma proteins are the albumin and lipocalin families. The albumin family includes albumin, α-fetoprotein, and afamin.[121] The lipocalin family includes several plasma proteins such as α_1-acid glycoprotein, retinol-binding protein, apolipoprotein D, α_1-microglobulin, prostaglandin D synthase (β-trace), β-lactoglobulin, neutrophil gelatinase-associated lipocalin (NGAL), inter-α-trypsin inhibitor, and C8 γ-chain.[171] Lipocalins generally have a barrel-shaped structure that is well suited to serve as a carrier for small molecules.

Disorders of Protein Folding

Protein folding is an error-prone process, and many molecular chaperones work to refold, prevent aggregation of misfolded proteins, or degrade misfolded proteins.[28,44] Several heat shock proteins that increase in response to a variety of stresses are molecular chaperones. When cells detect increased accumulation of misfolded proteins, an adaptive mechanism—the unfolded protein response—is activated.[135] This response increases production of chaperones and slows general protein synthesis to allow more time to fold new proteins. Despite these protective mechanisms, several families of age-related, genetic, and infectious diseases appear connected to disorders of protein folding and protein aggregation. Prion diseases are infectious diseases in which the transmissible agent may be protein that catalyzes misfolding of endogenous proteins. In Alzheimer's disease, accumulation of deposits of amyloid may contribute to pathogenesis. Polyglutamine diseases result from genetic expansion of repeat units encoding glutamine and are associated with Huntington's disease or other neurodegenerative disorders; polyglutamine sequences aggregate as β-sheets.[169] TDP 43 proteinopathies are neurodegenerative disorders, including amyotrophic lateral sclerosis, resulting from aggregation of transactive response DNA-binding protein.[81] Several inherited disorders related to mutations in specific proteins probably result from problems in protein folding. In α_1-antitrypsin deficiency, hepatic injury results from aggregation and accumulation of misfolded protein.[14,144] In cystic fibrosis, the cystic fibrosis transmembrane conductance regulator (CFTR) protein has a one–amino acid deletion that may influence interactions with chaperones and the stability of the protein. Accumulation of misfolded proteins has been suggested as a pathogenic mechanism contributing to vascular, cardiac, and beta cell failure in diabetes.[44,135]

Protein Synthesis and Processing

Proteins are synthesized by ribosomes reading from the 5′-end of mRNA. Triplet codons in mRNA are matched with complementary sequence in transfer RNA carrying specific amino acids. Protein synthesis begins with an AUG codon encoding methionine, and the polypeptide chain is synthesized from the N-terminus. As originally outlined by Blobel in the signal hypothesis, proteins that are secreted, located in vesicular compartments, or oriented on the external surface of cell membranes usually contain an N-terminal signal peptide about 15 to 30 amino acids in length. Signal peptides interact with signal recognition particles and attach ribosomes to the endoplasmic reticulum (ER). Nascent peptide chains are inserted through the membrane of the ER as the protein is synthesized. Signal peptides of most secretory proteins are removed even before synthesis of the entire protein chain is completed. Some post-translational modifications such as asparagine-linked, also termed N-linked, glycosylation occur in the ER.[100] This modification entails assembly on a dolichol carrier of a branched oligosaccharide ending with multiple mannose subunits, and the oligosaccharide is transferred en bloc to asparagine residues that are in the sequence Asn-Xxx-(Ser or Thr), where Xxx can be any amino acid but proline. Within the cisternal compartments of the ER and Golgi apparatus, many biosynthetic processing steps occur. The structures of N-linked oligosaccharides are modified into a complex set of structures that usually end in sialic acids; a variety of O-linked oligosaccharides are attached, primarily to Ser and Thr, and many modifications of sidechains occur, such as phosphorylation, sulfation, hydroxylation of Pro, Lys and Asp, and carboxylation of Glu at selected sites in proteins. Oligosaccharide processing may change in different physiologic states and may serve as a marker for disease.[45] Numerous molecular chaperones assist with folding and disulfide bond formation of proteins, including peptidylprolyl isomerases and disulfide isomerases.[28]

Many proteins and peptides are synthesized as larger precursors. Proinsulin, discovered as the precursor for insulin by Steiner in the 1960s, served as the prototype of a peptide precursor. Proinsulin is a single polypeptide chain that sequentially contains the B-chain of insulin, connecting or C-peptide, and the A-chain of insulin. The C-peptide is excised by proteases and insulin is produced, with A- and B-chains linked by two disulfides. Synthesis of insulin as a precursor assists in appropriate formation of disulfide bonds. Most small bioactive peptides (e.g., gastrin, ACTH, angiotensin, bradykinin, vasopressin, thyrotropin-releasing hormone) are synthesized as precursors, and peptides are released by proteolysis prior to release or extracellularly. Many larger proteins are synthesized as precursors as well, including albumin, haptoglobin, and C3 and C4. Synthesis as precursors aids in appropriate folding and assembly of disulfides for proteins such as haptoglobin, C3, and C4, which are cleaved into multiple peptide chains.

Different sets of post-translational modifications occur on intracellular proteins. N- and O-linked glycosylation typical of extracellular proteins does not occur; instead, reversible addition of N-acetylglucosamine to Ser and Thr is noted.[49] Reversible phosphorylation of proteins by signaling cascades of kinases and phosphatase serve as important regulatory systems. Many other biosynthetic modifications influence protein function and intracellular localization. Modification of histones and nuclear proteins by acetylation and methylation affects transcription. Coupling of the small protein ubiquitin is a mechanism for targeting proteins for degradation into peptides by proteasomes. This is an important process for degrading misfolded or damaged proteins, for protein turnover, and for generating peptides that are presented for immune surveillance and activation.[53]

In addition to biosynthetic modifications, proteins undergo chemical modification by free radicals and other reactants. As an example, glucose reacts with amine groups to generate reversible Schiff's bases; some of the reaction products rearrange to more stable glucose conjugates, and the products are referred to as glycated proteins. Amounts of hemoglobin A_{1c} and glycated plasma protein measured as fructosamine serve as measures of exposure to glucose. Side-chain carbonyls serve as an indicator of free radical generation. Nitrotyrosine can be assessed as a measure of exposure to reactants. Oxidants can modify a number of amino acid sidechains, including oxidation of methionine to methionine sulfoxide and sulfone and cysteine to cysteic acid. Albumin serves as a model for many chemical modifications of plasma proteins.[105,121]

Physical Properties of Proteins

Variable amino acid sequences and three-dimensional structures of different proteins result in variation in physical properties. Tyrosine and tryptophan residues absorb light at 280 nm, and the abundance of these amino acids determines the strength of absorbance of a peptide or protein. Absorption at 280 nm, therefore, is used to quantify a purified protein. Tryptophan residues are intrinsic fluorescent groups with variable fluorescence efficiency and lifetimes, depending on their local environment. Some proteins, such as hemoglobin, contain heme or other chromophores that can be assessed at visible wavelengths. Peptide bonds have strong absorbance at wavelengths below 220 nm, so that spectrophotometric detection in this range detects all peptides and proteins, and absorbance is much greater than at 280 nm. Ionizable groups in proteins exert a strong effect on physical properties and changes in structure that occur in response to changes in pH. Common ranges of pKs are shown in Table 21-2, although the ionization of individual amino acids may be influenced strongly by neighboring amino acids. Differing physical properties serve as the basis of methods to separate proteins (see also Chapter 12). Some important characteristics include the following:

1. *Differential solubility.* The solubility of proteins is affected by pH, ionic strength, temperature, and the dielectric constant (addition of solvents such as ethanol). Changing solvent pH affects the net charges of a protein; at its pI (net charge zero), a protein in polar solvent usually has its lowest solubility. Changing ionic strength affects the hydration and solubility of proteins. "Salting-in" and "salting-out" procedures were early methods for separating and characterizing proteins. Serum was originally divided into albumin, which is soluble in water, and globulins, which require salt to remain in solution. Albumin also stays in solution at high concentrations of salts such as ammonium sulfate that precipitate globulins. Addition of organic solvents and polyethylene glycol has been used for differential precipitation. Fractional precipitation of plasma with ethanol, using protocols developed by Cohn and coworkers, leads to several Cohn fractions that are enriched in immunoglobulins, α- and β-globulins, or albumin (fraction V). Polyethylene glycols induce precipitation by steric exclusion and, therefore, preferentially precipitate large proteins or complexes.
2. *Molecular size.* Separation of small and large molecules can be achieved by dialysis or ultrafiltration. Size exclusion chromatography, ultracentrifugation, and electrophoresis perform size separations under native conditions where proteins and peptides are in native globular states or under denaturing conditions. Addition of reducing agents allows separation of disulfide-linked components. Polyacrylamide gel electrophoresis in the presence of the denaturing detergent sodium dodecylsulfate is a method for estimating the molecular weight of polypeptide chains in proteins.
3. *Molecular mass.* Advances in mass spectrometry allow the determination of masses of peptides and proteins with increasing accuracy. Peptides and proteins can be ionized by matrix-assisted laser desorption/ionization (MALDI) or by electrospray ionization. Highest detection sensitivity and mass accuracy are for peptides, and tandem mass spectrometry can be applied for sequence analysis of peptides. Large proteins with extensive mass heterogeneity due to variable modifications pose challenges related to their high mass and the formation of multiple peaks.
4. *Electrical charge.* Ion-exchange chromatography, isoelectric focusing, and electrophoresis separate peptides and proteins based on charge.
5. *Surface adsorption.* Adsorption of peptides and proteins to particles have been used as the basis for separations. Hydrophobic interaction chromatography and reverse-phase chromatography rely on differential hydrophobic interactions of peptides or proteins.
6. *Affinity chromatography.* Specific ligands, antibodies, or other recognition molecules have been used to separate peptides or proteins selectively.

Plasma Proteins

Plasma is a complex mixture of proteins representing thousands of gene products.[2,57,117] The most abundant products are proteins secreted directly into the circulation primarily by the liver, and immunoglobulins contributed by lymphatic tissue. Classical methods for protein fractionation and purification over several decades led to isolation and characterization of about 100 of the most abundant plasma proteins.[3] The 12 most abundant proteins represent more than 95% of total protein mass, and a progressive decline in abundance of other components has been noted.[2,60] Albumin alone represents more than 50% of the total mass of protein and an even higher proportion of the number of molecules, so that albumin is the main factor in colloid osmotic pressure (oncotic pressure). For some purposes, such as evaluation of contributions to oncotic pressure, inhibitory capacity of proteases, and binding capacity for ions, drugs, or small molecules, it is useful to express abundance of proteins on a molar basis rather than as mass abundance, and a slightly different set of proteins is identified that includes some lower molecular weight proteins that do not represent major components by mass. Lists of the 30 most abundant proteins by mass and molecular abundance are provided in Table 21-3.

It is apparent, for example, that although α_2-macroglobulin (AMG) is the most abundant protease inhibitor by mass abundance, α_1-antitrypsin and several other protease inhibitors have a higher molar concentration and capacity for protease inhibition.

The most appropriate way to express protein abundance depends on the method of analysis. Signal intensities of stained bands in gels and chromatographic separations with photometric detection usually relate to protein mass. Signal responses in immunoassays and mass spectrometry usually correspond to numbers of particles (i.e., the molar abundance of proteins). Components with highest molar abundance in Table 21-3 are easiest to detect by immunoassay (allowing use of less sensitive methods such as immunoturbidimetry and immunonephelometry) and generally will yield tryptic peptides with the highest abundance for mass spectrometric detection.[60] Use of molar abundance allows better comparison of the stoichiometry of molecular forms of proteins and different proteins that differ substantially in molecular weight. Currently, concentration of proteins s are typically expressed in units of mass or molarity. High-abundance proteins most often are reported in units of mass per volume by clinical laboratories in the United States.

The Plasma Proteome and Peptidome

Plasma contains a complex mixture of thousands of proteins and peptides. The complete set of proteins is referred to as the *proteome.* Current efforts to compile a database of components found in plasma include more than 12,000 protein entries.[134] Considerable variation among proteins is related to post-translational and genetic variation.[114] In addition to the diversity of proteins, plasma contains complex mixtures of peptide components—the peptidome—which only recently has been fully appreciated.[122] Although many peptides are

TABLE 21-3 High-Abundance Plasma Proteins Ranked According to Reference Intervals by Mass or Molar Abundance

	Ranked by Mass Abundance (mg/L)		Ranked by Molar Abundance (μmol/L)	
Rank	**Protein**	**Concentration**	**Protein**	**Concentration**
1	Albumin	35,000-52,000	Albumin	500-800
2	Immunoglobulin G	7000-16,000	Immunoglobulin G	40-120
3	Transferrin	2000-3600	Apolipoprotein A-I	30-70
4	Immunoglobulin A	700-4000	Apolipoprotein A-II	30-60
5	α_2-Macroglobulin	1300-3000	Transferrin	25-45
6	Fibrinogen	2000-4000	α_1-Antitrypsin	18-40
7	α_1-Antitrypsin	900-2000	Haptoglobin	6-40
8	Apolipoprotein A-I	910-1940	α_1-Acid glycoprotein	15-30
9	C3	900-1800	α_2HS-glycoprotein	9-30
10	IgM	400-2300	Immunoglobulin A	5-30
11	Haptoglobin	300-2000	Hemopexin	9-20
12	Apolipoprotein B	600-1550	Apolipoprotein C-III	6-20
13	α_1-Acid glycoprotein	500-1200	Fibrinogen	5-18
14	α_2HS-glycoprotein	400-1300	Gc-Globulin	8-14
15	Hemopexin	500-1150	Apolipoprotein C-I	6-12
16	Gc-Globulin (vitamin D-BP)	400-700	C3	5-10
17	Factor H	240-740	α_1-Antichymotrypsin	4-9
18	α_1-Antichymotrypsin	300-600	Apolipoprotein D	2-10
19	Inter-α-trypsin inhibitor	200-700	Prealbumin	4-8
20	Apolipoprotein A-II	260-510	β_2-Glycoprotein I	3-6
21	C4b-binding protein	200-530	Apolipoprotein A-IV	3-6
22	Ceruloplasmin	200-500	Apolipoprotein C-II	2-7
23	Factor B	180-460	Serum amyloid A4	3-6
24	Prealbumin	200-400	Inter-α-trypsin inhibitor	3-5
25	Gelsolin	200-400	Antithrombin III	3-5
26	Fibronectin	300	α_1B-glycoprotein	3-5
27	C1 inhibitor	190-370	Gelsolin	3-5
28	C4	100-400	Ceruloplasmin	2-5
29	Plasminogen	150-350	Factor H	2-5
30	Antithrombin III	170-300	Factor B	2-5

Based on values in Hortin GL, Sviridov D, Anderson L. High-abundance polypeptides of the human plasma proteome comprising the top 4 logs of polypeptide abundance. Clin Chem 2008;54:1608-16.

cleared rapidly by renal clearance and peptidolysis, some peptides accumulate bound to albumin or other carrier proteins.[122] The peptidome is of potential diagnostic interest because of its large diversity and information content, reflection of activity of physiologic proteases, and suitability for direct analysis by mass spectrometry. Many approaches for proteome analysis are known, including (1) two-dimensional electrophoresis and chromatography, (2) microarrays of antibodies or other proteins, and (3) mass spectrometry with electrospray ionization or matrix-assisted laser desorption/ionization.[2,29,56,117,134,149] Analysis of multiple components expands the ability to examine changes in patterns of protein concentration versus traditional analysis of one protein at a time, and high-resolution separation techniques offer the opportunity to identify many structural changes, as well as quantitative changes, in proteins. Sequence analysis can be performed rapidly on small peptides, allowing identification of components. Simultaneous analysis of many peptides or proteins offers opportunities to empirically identify protein markers for disease without knowing beforehand which protein to test for. It has been suggested that mass spectrometric patterns of peptides might serve as signatures of disease that could be interpreted by complex pattern recognition by computers.[122] However, it is not clear how usual standards of laboratory practice, such as calibration, quality control, and verification of accuracy, would be assessed.[55] The U.S. Food and Drug Administration has proposed guidelines for in vitro *diagnostic multivariate index assays* to address special issues raised by this approach. Although untargeted empirical analysis may be a useful discovery approach, most methods for multiplex analysis of peptides and proteins for clinical use are likely to rely on targeted analysis. Substantial advances have been made in the quantitative analysis of proteins by digesting proteins into peptides with the protease trypsin and then quantitating released tryptic peptides by tandem mass spectrometry using isotopically labeled internal standard peptides. It has been proposed that *proteotypic peptides* (peptides that are unique to a single protein) for more than 20,000 proteins should be identified to provide a means of quantifying virtually any human protein.[2] Peptide quantification via tandem mass spectrometry is being applied to measurement even of relatively low-abundance proteins such as thyroglobulin and troponins,[54,79] and it may serve as a valuable method for measuring bioactive peptides. Multiplex immunoassays are coming into routine clinical laboratory use as the result of microparticle or planar arrays.[78,90] Products currently available for clinical use measure several components; highly multiplexed assays still present some challenges with respect to reproducibility and quality control.[32]

Plasma Protein Concentrations

The characteristic of proteins that has been applied most frequently is their plasma concentration, and the range of plasma concentrations of different proteins measured in clinical assays extends well over 10 logs of concentration.[3,60] Relative to the highest abundance protein, albumin, concentrations of plasma proteins decrease progressively over several logs of concentration for proteins released from tissues of smaller cell mass, and the ability of endogenous proteins to enter the circulation generally decreases hierarchically: (1) proteins secreted directly into plasma, (2) cell membrane proteins shed into the circulation, (3) secretory proteins in exocrine secretions, (4) high-abundance cytoplasmic proteins, (5) low-abundance cytoplasmic proteins, (6) transmembrane proteins, and (7) organellar proteins that must traverse more than one membrane to exit cells. Many proteins serve as useful markers of physiology and disease, as these processes alter the production or release of proteins into plasma. Changes in plasma concentrations of secretory proteins usually reflect changes in synthetic rates, secretion, or clearance, and plasma concentrations of cytoplasmic and organellar proteins tend to reflect cellular injury and rates of leakage into plasma. In addition to endogenous sources of proteins, multiple exogenous sources of proteins include infectious organisms, dietary sources, and therapeutic interventions. For diagnostic purposes, clinical laboratories currently assess only a small proportion of the thousands of gene products in the circulation and identify only a small proportion of diversity of post-translational processing. Antibodies and T-cell receptors represent special cases wherein somatic recombination and mutation result in repertoires of millions of sequences and binding specificities. A small portion of this diversity is assessed by serological or functional assay.

Plasma concentrations of proteins depend not only on rates of production and efficiency of entry to the circulation, but also on rates of clearance. Proteins and peptides substantially smaller than albumin are cleared from the circulation by glomerular filtration unless they are bound to larger carriers, such as small apolipoproteins bound to lipoprotein particles or retinol-binding protein bound to prealbumin.[116] Peptides and small proteins not bound to carriers are cleared with half-lives of about 2 hours under conditions of normal kidney function and accumulate to higher concentrations in kidney failure. Examples of proteins and peptides that increase dramatically in renal failure include β_2-microglobulin, cystatin C, immunoglobulin light chains, parathyroid hormone fragments, complement factor D, Clara cell protein (CC16), atrial natriuretic peptide, interleukins, and, to a lesser extent, retinol-binding protein. Accumulation of components in renal failure identifies components with renal clearance[161] as a primary clearance mechanism; hundreds of increased plasma peptide components can be detected by mass spectrometry.[136] Many bioactive peptides in plasma, such as insulin, intact parathyroid hormone, and kinins, have much shorter circulating half-lives of only a few minutes, indicating receptor-mediated uptake or degradation by exopeptidases or endopeptidases.[56] Proteins the size of albumin or larger generally have an upper limit of about 7 days for their circulating half-lives because of pinocytosis and degradation by cells. Two exceptions to this are albumin and immunoglobulin G, which have a receptor-mediated process to recycle these proteins from pinocytotic vesicles. The recycling mechanism extends the half-life of albumin and immunoglobulin severalfold.[131,165] Many proteins are subject to uptake by specific receptors or degradation by proteolysis. Half-lives $<$7 days suggest clearance mechanisms other than bulk pinocytosis.

Major Plasma Proteins

Protein abundance of major components, as listed in Table 21-3, probably reflects the concentrations of proteins needed for major physiologic processes. Transport proteins, protease inhibitors, antibodies, complement factors, and coagulation components are well represented. Many of the proteins in Table 21-3 have been measured for diagnostic purposes. Only a few of the high-abundance proteins represent diagnostic orphans. Clinical laboratory analysis of α_2HS-glycoprotein (fetuin-A) has been limited, and its physiologic significance, possibly related to regulation of mineral deposition in bone, has been unclear.[102] Gelsolin has not been measured frequently, although it may have an important function, together with Gc-globulin (also known as vitamin D–binding protein), in clearing actin and preventing actin filament formation in the circulation.

Historically, major plasma proteins were classified according to electrophoretic mobilities in agarose gels at pH 8.6. Table 21-4 lists several major plasma proteins of diagnostic interest in order of electrophoretic mobility, together with other characteristics. Only about 10 of the most abundant plasma proteins by mass are prominently observed by staining of agarose gels; other, more selective procedures are needed to analyze lesser plasma protein components. Detailed descriptions of several high-abundance proteins are provided in this chapter; other chapters describe other plasma proteins, including enzymes (see Chapter 22), lipoproteins (see Chapter 27), hormones (see Chapter 29), and hemoglobin, fibrinogen, and other coagulation proteins (see Chapters 32 and 59).

Plasma concentrations and molecular forms of major secretory proteins vary in response to nutritional, physiologic,

TABLE 21-4 Properties of Selected Plasma Proteins

Electrophoretic Region	Protein	Half-Life	pI	MW, daltons	Function, Comments
Prealbumin	Retinol-binding protein (RBP)	12 h		21,000	Carrier of retinol (vitamin A) Complexed to prealbumin
Prealbumin	Prealbumin (transthyretin)	48 h	4.7	54,980 (tetramer)	Transports thyroid hormone Binds RBP
Albumin	Albumin	15-19 d	4-5.8	66,438	Maintains oncotic pressure Transports fatty acids, bilirubin, and other organic molecules; binds calcium, drugs
α_1	α_1-Antitrypsin (AAT)	4 d	4.8	51,000	A serine protease inhibitor (serpin); inhibits neutrophil elastase
	α_1-Acid glycoprotein (AAG, orosomucoid)	5 d	2.7-4	40,000	Carrier for steroid hormones Binds cationic drugs, a lipocalin
α_2	Haptoglobin (Hp, HAP)	2 d	≈4.1 (type 1-1)	85,000-840,000	Binds hemoglobin; molecular weight depends on phenotype (1-1, 2-1, or 2-2)
	α_2-Macroglobulin (AMG)	5 d	5.4	720,000 (tetramer)	General proteolytic inhibitor Homologous to C3 and C4
	Ceruloplasmin (CER)	4.5 d	4.4	132,000	Oxidizes iron to Fe^{+3} Blue color from copper ligand
β_1	Transferrin (Tf, siderophilin)	7 d	5.7	79,600	Transports iron, two Fe^{+3} binding sites
	C4, fourth component of complement	X		206,000	Covalently binds to target molecules, releases C4a peptide
β_2	C3, third component of complement	2-3 d		180,000	Covalently binds to target molecules, releases C3a peptide
	β_2-Microglobulin	X		11,800	Component of HLA on cell surfaces
γ	IgG	24 d	6-7.3	150,000	Antibody from secondary responses Four subclasses: IgG1, IgG2, IgG3, IgG4
	IgA	6 d		≈160,000	Major secretory antibody; two subclasses
	IgM	5 d		900,000	Antibody from primary responses
	C-reactive protein (CRP)	18-20 h	6.2	≈115,000 (pentamer)	Nonspecific defense; binds phospholipid

and genetic factors. Development of reference materials and value transfer to routine clinical assays represent a challenge for each protein.[11] The interim consensus reference intervals for 14 plasma proteins are listed in Table 21-5.[22] Molecular forms, in some cases such as haptoglobin and apolipoprotein(a), differ substantially with genetic variation. Many factors affect the concentrations of specific plasma proteins, including age, gender, genetic variation, diet, hormonal variation, inflammatory processes, and many other factors. The example of changes in several proteins in response to

TABLE 21-5 Interim Consensus Reference Intervals for 14 Plasma Proteins in Human Serum Referenced to CRM 470[22]*

Protein	g/L	mg/dL
α_1-Acid glycoprotein	0.5-1.2	50-120
Albumin	35-52	3500-5200
α_1-Antitrypsin	0.9-2.0	90-200
C3*	0.9-1.8*	90-180†
C4	0.1-0.4	10-40
Ceruloplasmin	0.2-0.6	20-60
C-reactive protein	<5	<0.5
Haptoglobin	0.3-2.0	30-200
IgA	0.7-4.0	70-400
IgG	7-16	700-1600
IgM	0.4-2.3	40-230
Prealbumin	0.2-0.4	20-40
α_2-Macroglobulin	1.3-3.0	130-300
Transferrin	2.0-3.6	200-360

*Values are applicable only to adults between 20 and 60 years of age.
†Values are slightly lower in samples assayed <8 hours after draw.
From Dati F, Schumann G, Thomas L, et al. Consensus of a group of professional societies and diagnostic companies on guidelines for interim reference ranges for 14 proteins in serum based on the standardization against the IFCC/BCR/CAP reference material (CRM 470). Eur J Clin Chem Clin Biochem 1996;34:517-20.

TABLE 21-6 Effects of Steroid Hormones on Plasma Protein Concentrations

	Corticoid	Androgen	Estrogen
Prealbumin	+	+	–
Albumin	–	N	–
α_1-Lipoprotein	N	–	++
α_1-Acid glycoprotein	+	+	–
α_1-Antitrypsin	N	+	++
Haptoglobin	+	++	–
Ceruloplasmin	N	N	+++
Transferrin	N	+	+
β-Lipoprotein	++	+	N
IgG	–	N	–

+, Increase; –, decrease; *N*, no change.
Modified from Whicher JT. Abnormalities of plasma proteins. In: Williams DL, Marks V, eds. Biochemistry in clinical practice. London: William Heinemann, 1983:221-50.

steroid hormones shown in Table 21-6 illustrates how physiologic and pharmacologic factors can strongly influence plasma protein concentrations.

The Acute-Phase Response

Systemic inflammation in response to infection, tissue injury, or inflammatory disease triggers changes in hepatic production of multiple plasma proteins, as indicated in Table 21-7.

TABLE 21-7 The Acute Phase Response (APR): Changes in Plasma Protein Concentrations

Positive APR	C-reactive protein (extreme)
	Serum amyloid A (extreme)
	α_1-Acid glycoprotein
	α_1-Antitrypsin
	α_1-Antichymotrypsin
	Antithrombin III
	C3, C4, and C9
	C1 inhibitor
	C4b-binding protein
	Ceruloplasmin
	Factor B
	Ferritin
	Fibrinogen
	Haptoglobin
	Hemopexin
	Lipopolysaccharide-binding protein
	Mannan-binding protein (lectin)
	Plasminogen
	Procalcitonin
Negative APR	Albumin
	Apolipoprotein A-I
	Apolipoprotein B
	α_2-HS glycoprotein
	IGF-I
	Prealbumin
	Retinol-binding protein
	Thyroxine-binding globulin
	Transferrin

Data from Craig WY, Ledue TB, Ritchie RF. Plasma proteins: clinical utility and interpretation. Scarborough, Maine: Foundation for Blood Research, 2001; Gabay C, Kushner I. Acute-phase proteins and other systemic responses to inflammation. N Engl J Med 1999;340:448-54; and Vollmer T, Piper C, Kleesiek K, Dreier J. Lipopolysaccharide-binding protein: a new biomarker for infectious endocarditis? Clin Chem 2009;55:295-302.

This process, mediated by the action of interleukin-6 (IL-6) and other cytokines has been termed the *acute-phase response (APR)*.[42] It is a nonspecific reaction to inflammation, comparable with the increase in temperature or leukocyte count. Studies have suggested that it is possible to therapeutically block the APR with inhibitors of tumor necrosis factor α (TNF-α), which may be beneficial in some cases where products of the APR contribute to inflammation or deposit in tissues as amyloid.[74] In the APR, synthesis of a few proteins, including albumin, transferrin, and prealbumin, is downregulated; such proteins are termed *negative acute-phase reactants.* Albumin concentrations fall faster than expected from decreased synthesis; acute response might also reflect increased capillary permeability and redistribution of albumin to extracellular fluids. Production of a number of proteins, including α_1-antitrypsin (AAT), α_1-acid glycoprotein (AAG), haptoglobin (Hp), ceruloplasmin, C4, C3, and fibrinogen increases several-fold. Production of C-reactive protein (CRP) and serum amyloid A (SAA) increase greatly, and plasma concentrations can increase up to 1000-fold or more in extreme cases. The decrease in apolipoprotein A-I, coupled with increases in serum amyloid A, results in remodeling of high-density lipoproteins (HDLs) from forms with apolipoprotein A-I as the major component to forms with increased amounts of serum amyloid A. These changes in composition of HDL have been related to decreased capacity for reverse cholesterol transport and antioxidant activity, and a general change in function of HDL from anti-inflammatory to proinflammatory.[47]

Procalcitonin is another component measured to assess APRs. Procalcitonin is a polypeptide of 116 amino acids that serves as the precursor for calcitonin in C cells of the thyroid. In response to inflammation, procalcitonin begins to be synthesized by other tissues, such as liver, kidney, and pancreas, where it is not cleaved into smaller peptide components,[137] and plasma concentrations increase more rapidly than other acute-phase reactants from a very low baseline concentration. Plasma concentrations of individual acute-phase proteins rise at different rates—first, procalcitonin, CRP, SAA, and α_1-antichymotrypsin; after the first 12 hours, AAG; after 24 to 48 hours, AAT, Hp, C4, and fibrinogen; and finally, C3 and Cp. All reach maxima within 2 to 5 days following an acute insult and then decrease in the same order as their increase. Measurement of CRP and SAA, which have the greatest change in concentration, can be used to monitor the progress of an inflammatory reaction or its response to treatment. Increased erythrocyte sedimentation rate (ESR) is another indicator of inflammation. Fibrinogen concentrations are considered a major determinant of ESR, so that ESR probably relates to changes in fibrinogen in the acute-phase response. APRs to bacterial infection usually are stronger than those to viral infection, and procalcitonin or other acute-phase reactants sometimes are measured in newborns or in complex adult patients to try to rapidly identify patients with bacterial infection before results from bacterial culture can be obtained.[7,84] Procalcitonin measurements therefore assist in determining whether antibiotic therapy should be used. Concentrations of procalcitonin are low in infants, and a cutoff of 0.12 ng/mL has been recommended to detect bacterial infection in infants presenting with fever.[98] Concentrations below a higher cutoff of 0.5 ng/mL indicate low risk of sepsis in adult patients in intensive care units. Lipopolysaccharide-binding protein is another acute-phase reactant that has been suggested as a useful marker for detecting infection; concentrations of lipopolysaccharide-binding protein are markedly increased in most patients with infectious endocarditis in comparison with noninfectious valvular disease.[163] Qualitative changes in proteins also are seen with the APR, such as altered changes in glycosylation of proteins.[45] Changes in glycosylation of immunoglobulins may have an immunomodulatory effect.[72]

Chronic infection, such as viral hepatitis, yields different changes in the composition of plasma proteins compared with acute infection. Stimulation of lymphocytes to produce antibodies leads initially to increased amounts of IgM and later to increased IgG and IgA antibodies to the infectious agent. Many plasma proteins have been used as indicators of impaired liver function in cirrhotic liver disease, including α_2-macroglobulin, apolipoprotein A-I, haptoglobin, vitronectin, and fibronectin, and measures of some of these components have been included in several different multiparameter indices of hepatic fibrosis.[46]

Differences Between Plasma and Serum Proteins

Plasma refers to the fluid portion of blood after cells are removed by centrifugation. Some type of anticoagulant needs to be added to prevent coagulation of blood due to contact with foreign surfaces in blood collection devices (see Chapter 7). Common anticoagulants include dry heparin or EDTA or solutions containing citrate. Dry additives produce only slight osmotic effects on plasma volume, and citrate solutions introduce some specimen dilution. Variation in platelet concentration is noted, depending on the time of centrifugation and the force applied. Preparation of platelet-poor plasma commonly requires spinning specimens twice to ensure platelet removal and remove their contribution to plasma proteins. Platelets undergo some activation and release of their granules during routine blood collection, and specialized blood collection tubes with additives such as theophylline, adenosine, and dipyridamole that suppress platelet activation are needed to assess plasma concentrations of some components contained in platelets.[66]

Serum is the fluid component of blood after blood is allowed to clot. It differs from plasma in several respects.[56,93,126] An approximate 4% decrease in total protein content is related mainly to removal of fibrinogen during coagulation. This results in serum having a lower viscosity than plasma, because fibrinogen contributes to plasma viscosity. Besides fibrinogen, several other clotting factors are removed in the clot and activation peptides released into serum. An increase in complexes of proteases is seen with inhibitors. Platelets are trapped in the clot, but during coagulation, platelets release their granules, which contain hundreds of proteins, including platelet factor 4 and thromboglobulins.[18,66] Activation of coagulation proteases during clotting may modify a variety of other proteins, and substantial amounts of exopeptidase activity in serum degrade small peptides. Given the complex processes that occur in the conversion of plasma to serum, many protein and peptide components differ substantially in plasma and serum. For proteomic analysis, plasma (usually EDTA) rather than serum generally is recommended, because plasma represents a protein and peptide composition more similar to that seen in in vivo conditions. Serum offers a slight advantage for analysis of some abundant components such as immunoglobulins because the reduced specimen viscosity improves specimen delivery, decreases precipitates formed during freezing and thawing, and decreases the opportunity for fibrin formation in specimens. Most of the high-abundance components described in this chapter are relatively stable globular proteins that are not degraded substantially during clotting of plasma and can be analyzed on serum or plasma specimens. For traditional agarose protein electrophoresis, serum is the preferred specimen, because fibrinogen yields a prominent band near the β-λ border that can be mistaken for or can obscure a paraprotein.

Determination of Total Protein

Plasma normally contains about 6.5 to 8.5 g/dL protein, and serum about 4% less. Determination of total protein in biological fluids in some respects represents a greater challenge than analysis of a specific protein, because variable protein composition of biological fluids leads to variable carbohydrate composition, charge, and physical characteristics of proteins in the mixture. Many methods of protein analysis respond differentially to different proteins and present problems when applied to specimens of varying protein composition. Most methods other than the biuret method have not been thoroughly examined for interactions with small peptide components as well as intact proteins, and this may become a significant issue in renal failure with increased accumulation of peptides and small proteins.[161]

Specific Methods. Many methods have been developed to measure the total protein content of biological fluids. Several are reviewed here.

Kjeldahl Method. This method is rarely used in clinical laboratories but is of historical importance and is sometimes used as a reference method. Protein nitrogen is converted to ammonium ion by heating with sulfuric acid in the presence of a catalyst. Ammonium ion is measured by alkalinization, distillation, and acid titration, or by Nessler's reagent. Protein is estimated to contain 16% nitrogen (multiply N by 6.25). Errors in protein estimation occur if the amino acid composition is unusual, and if nitrogen content differs from 16%. Nonprotein N, such as from urea and amino acids, also is measured, so a protein precipitation step may be required. The Kjeldahl method was one of the first methods used for reproducible total protein measurement, but it is time-consuming and impractical for routine use. This method has been used to assign values to reference materials for the biuret method.[70]

Biuret Method. Under strongly alkaline conditions, Cu^{2+} ions form multivalent complexes with peptide bonds in proteins. Binding shifts the absorption spectrum of Cu^{2+} ions to shorter wavelengths, leading to a color change from blue to violet that has been termed the *biuret reaction.* Binding of Cu^{2+} ions to the organic compound biuret yields a similar color change, hence the name. Absorbance change from protein addition is measured spectrophotometrically at ≈540 nm, and this serves as a relatively simple method for quantifying protein. Absorbance changes at 540 nm also result from binding of Cu^{2+} ions by many compounds that can form chelates with five- or six-member rings, where amino, amide, or hydroxyl groups bind to Cu^{2+} ions.[58] Such compounds include (1) serine, (2) asparagine, (3) ethanolamine, (4) tris(hydroxymethyl)aminomethane, and (5) many others. Small compounds lead to a smaller spectral shift than proteins. Historically, the biuret method was not considered to react with amino acids and dipeptides, but absorbance changes occur with some amino acids, with amino acid amides, and with dipeptides.[58] The biuret action also was considered to react equally according to peptide content with all proteins and peptides longer than two amino acids, but subsequently, peptides containing proline were noted to have reduced reactivity, and some sidechains may contribute.[58] As long as proteins are not extremely proline-rich or do not have a very unusual composition, different proteins probably have similar reactivities with respect to peptide content as long as the biuret reaction is performed in the typical end point manner. Bilirubin, lipemia, and other serum components can introduce slight interference with serum measurement by biuret assays, and calibration with albumin results in a slight bias relative to a Kjeldahl method.[17] Interference has also been noted for immunoglobulin lambda light chains.[155]

Biuret rate assays are also available but should be considered as a separate category from equilibrium assays. Cu^{2+} ions complex with small molecules and accessible sites in proteins almost instantaneously; additional absorbance change over time for the kinetic analysis probably depends on the rate of unfolding of a protein and exposure of additional binding sites for Cu^{2+} ions under strongly alkaline conditions. Different proteins are likely to unfold at different rates.[58] An advantage of the kinetic biuret assay is the decreased effect of low molecular weight compounds; they usually react before the measuring interval occurs.

Direct Optical Methods. Absorbance of UV light at 200 to 225 nm and 270 to 290 nm have been used to measure protein concentrations and is commonly applied to monitor chromatographic separations of peptides and proteins. Absorbance at 280 nm depends primarily on the tryptophan and tyrosine content of a protein. This technique works best for purified proteins with known absorptivity. For complex mixtures, accuracy and specificity suffer from variable content of tryptophan and tyrosine and from absorbance of low molecular weight compounds such as free amino acids, uric acid, and bilirubin. At 200 to 225 nm, peptide bonds are chiefly responsible for UV absorbance (70% at A_{205}); specific absorption by proteins at these shorter wavelengths is 10 to 30 times greater than at 280 nm.[70] Many low molecular weight compounds such as urea also have absorbance at *wavelengths* below 220 nm. Accurate measurement of proteins by this method may require removal of low molecular weight molecules before absorbance measurements are performed. Several other optical methods using infrared or Raman analysis of specimens offer methods for total protein determination based on complex spectral analysis.[63]

Dye-Binding Methods. Dye-binding methods depend on shifts in the absorbance spectra of dyes when they bind to proteins. Variable binding of dyes to different proteins is a limitation. Calibration with a protein mixture may be hard to define consistently. Calibration with a pure protein such as albumin may not simulate binding to the complex mixture of proteins in serum or plasma. Using the dye Coomassie brilliant blue, immunoglobulins often give only 60% of the response of an equivalent concentration of albumin or transferrin.[70] This dye binds to polypeptide chains under acidic conditions, resulting in decreased absorbance at 465 nm and increased absorbance at 595 nm. Dye-binding methods offer good sensitivity, and pyrogallol red has become one of the most commonly used dyes for analysis of fluids with lower protein concentrations such as urine and CSF.

Lowry (Folin-Ciocalteu) Method. The detection limit of the Lowry method is about 100 times lower than that of the biuret method. Specimens are mixed with an alkaline copper solution followed by addition of the Folin-Ciocalteu reagent. Phosphotungstic acid and phosphomolybdic acid are reduced to tungsten blue and molybdenum blue by copper complexed with peptide and by tyrosine and tryptophan residues. Absorbance of products is measured at 650 to 750 nm. Reactivity of proteins varies with the content of tyrosine and tryptophan. Low molecular weight compounds including tryptophan and tyrosine and drugs such as salicylates, chlorpromazine, tetracyclines, and some sulfa drugs also give positive interference. Analysis of a fluid such as urine with high concentrations of phenolic compounds requires removal of low molecular weight substances before protein is measured.[70]

Refractometry. Refractometry is a method used to rapidly estimate protein at high concentrations. Accuracy decreases at protein concentrations <35 g/L, where salts, glucose, and other low molecular weight compounds have a larger proportional effect on refractive index.[70] Refractometry is used more often in clinical laboratories to assess the concentration of solutes in urine specimens than for determining total protein.

Turbidimetric and Nephelometric Methods. Many different reagents have been used to aggregate protein for turbidimetric or nephelometric assays, including (1) trichloroacetic acid, (2) sulfosalicylic acid, (3) sulfosalicylic acid combined with sodium sulfate, and (4) benzethonium chloride or (5) benzalkonium salts under alkaline conditions. Precipitation methods for total protein assay depend on forming a suspension of uniform, insoluble protein particles, which scatter incident light. Albumin and globulins often give different reactivities in precipitation methods.

Calibration of Total Protein Methods. Bovine or human albumin is commonly used to calibrate biuret methods, which react nearly equivalently with the peptide content of most proteins (see section on the biuret method). Protein mixtures with usual albumin-to-globulin ratios often have been recommended for calibration of other methods, with total protein content established by the biuret or Kjeldahl method.

Reference Intervals. The total protein concentration of serum obtained from healthy ambulatory adults is 6.3 to 8.3 g/dL and 6.0 to 7.8 g/dL for adults at bed rest. Plasma usually contains a protein concentration about 0.3 g/dL higher (unless diluted by a volume of anticoagulant such as citrate solution) because of the content of fibrinogen and other proteins removed during clotting to form serum. *Hemoconcentration* and relative *hyperproteinemia,* with increased concentrations of all plasma proteins, occur with inadequate water intake or excessive water loss as in severe vomiting, diarrhea, Addison's disease, or diabetic acidosis. Some hemoconcentration also occurs with standing (reduced intravascular volume) or prolonged tourniquet time during blood collection. *Hemodilution* and relative hypoproteinemia, with decreased concentrations of all plasma proteins, occur with water intoxication or salt retention syndromes, during massive intravenous infusions, and physiologically when a recumbent position is assumed. A recumbent position decreases total protein concentration by 0.3 to 0.5 g/dL and many individual proteins including albumin by up to 10%.[70] This reflects the redistribution of extracellular fluid from the extravascular space to the intravascular space and therefore dilution of a constant amount of plasma protein in a larger volume.

Of the individual serum proteins, albumin is present in such high concentrations that low concentrations of this protein alone may cause *hypoproteinemia.* Hypoalbuminemia is very common and has many causes. Mild *hyperproteinemia* may be caused by an increase in the concentration of specific proteins normally present in relatively low concentration as, for example, in dehydration, with increases in acute-phase reactants, or with increases in polyclonal immunoglobulins as a result of infection. Marked hyperproteinemia may be caused by high concentrations of the *monoclonal immunoglobulins* produced in paraproteinemias.

Prealbumin (Transthyretin) and Retinol-Binding Protein (RBP)

Prealbumin and RBP are nonglycosylated transport proteins. RBP is bound to prealbumin, which was named for its electrophoretic mobility. In 1981, the term *transthyretin* was proposed for prealbumin to reflect its binding and transport of both thyroid hormones and RBP. Both *prealbumin* and *transthyretin* are terms in common use.

Biochemistry and Function. Prealbumin (MW 35 kDa) is composed of four identical, noncovalently bound subunits, forming triiodothyronine (T_3)- and thyroxine (T_4)-binding sites. It binds and transports ≈10% of both hormones. (Thyroxine-binding globulin transports ≈70%, and albumin binds ≈20%.) Because of negative cooperativity of thyroid hormone binding, usually only one prealbumin-binding site is occupied. Prealbumin's synthesis is stimulated by glucocorticosteroid hormones, androgens, and many nonsteroidal anti-inflammatory drugs (NSAIDs), including aspirin. Prealbumin is synthesized in the liver and to a lesser extent in the choroid plexus of the brain.[138] Synthesis in the choroid plexus may account for relatively high concentrations of prealbumin in CSF.

RBP is a 21-kDa transport protein for all-*trans* retinol, the active form of vitamin A. RBP is synthesized in the liver and in adipose tissue.[16] Minor variants that lack one or two C-terminal residues are observed by mass spectrometry.[114] Studies in the metabolism literature sometimes refer to RBP as retinol-binding protein-4.[160] Zinc is required for synthesis, and retinol is required for its transportation by the Golgi apparatus.[70] In plasma, RBP occurs mainly as a 1 : 1 complex with prealbumin, slowing glomerular filtration of RBP. Prealbumin usually has twofold to threefold molar excess over RBP. Uptake of retinol by target cells is followed by dissociation of the prealbumin-RBP complex and clearance of apoRBP (RBP without retinol) from the circulation by the kidneys. RBP has a half-life of only about 12 hours, but it is extended in renal failure.[161]

Clinical Significance of Prealbumin and RBP. If vitamin A intake is adequate and renal function is normal, concentrations of prealbumin and RBP often rise and fall in parallel. Adipocytes appear to be a significant site for synthesis of RBP, and its concentrations may increase with obesity or syndromes of insulin resistance.[160]

Increased Plasma Concentrations. Serum RBP increases in chronic renal disease, including diabetic nephropathy.[161] Concentrations are increased with corticosteroid or NSAID therapy and in Hodgkin's disease. Interest in RBP has been stimulated by recognition that it is synthesized in adipose tissues, and that excretion from adipose tissue may increase in syndromes of insulin resistance, together with other products of adipocytes such as leptin, adiponectin, and resistin.[16,160]

Decreased Plasma Concentrations. Decreased concentrations of prealbumin and RBP are seen primarily in liver disease, protein malnutrition, and the APR. Zinc deficiency results in low serum concentrations of both RBP and vitamin A. Prealbumin concentrations are often used as an indicator of adequacy of protein nutrition because of its relatively short half-life, high proportion of essential amino acids, and small pool size. However, it is a negative APR. Concentrations also fall in cirrhosis of the liver and protein-losing diseases of the gut or kidneys. An acute-phase reactant, such as CRP, should be assayed along with prealbumin if concentrations are to be used to estimate nutritional status. History and physical examination are also important aspects of nutritional assessment.[25]

Genetic Aspects. The gene coding for prealbumin is on chromosome 18q. More than 75 genetic variants have been described, a few affecting T_4 binding. Variants with increased affinity for T_4 are associated with euthyroid *hyper*thyroxinemia, similar to albumin variants with increased T_4 affinity. Changes in T_4 binding affect total T_4 measurements but not other assessments of thyroid function such as thyrotropin or free T_4.

Some prealbumin variants are associated with tissue deposition of amyloid fibrils. These autosomal dominant hereditary amyloidoses include amyloidotic cardiomyopathy, familial amyloidotic polyneuropathy, and senile systemic amyloidosis (see later section in this chapter on amyloidoses). Variants can be detected by mass spectrometry or by genetic analysis.[8,143] The *RBP* gene is on chromosome 10q, and clinically significant variants are not described.

Laboratory Considerations and Reference Intervals. Prealbumin migrates as a minor component anodal to albumin on routine serum electrophoresis and is not routinely observed by most methods. It is a proportionately greater component of CSF. Prealbumin and RBP usually are measured by immunonephelometric or immunoturbidimetric methods. The adult reference interval for RBP is 3.0 to 6.0 mg/dL. The RBP concentration at birth is 1.1 to 3.4 mg/dL and at 6 months increases to 1.8 to 5.0 mg/dL. The adult reference interval for prealbumin, based on the Certified Reference Material (CRM) 470, is 20 to 40 mg/dL (0.2 to 0.4 g/L).[22] Concentrations in healthy neonates are approximately half those found in adults; they increase into puberty, with a larger increase noted in boys than girls, and decrease in both sexes after age 50.[70]

Albumin

The name *albumin* (*L. albus* = white) originated from the white precipitate formed during the boiling of acidic urine from patients with proteinuria. Normally, albumin is the most abundant plasma protein from the fetal period onward, accounting for about half of the plasma protein mass. It is a major component of most body fluids, including interstitial fluid, CSF, urine, and amniotic fluid. More than half of the total pool of albumin is in the extravascular space. The monograph by Peters is a source of extensive information about albumin.[121]

Biochemistry of Albumin. Albumin has a nonglycosylated polypeptide chain of 585 amino acids and a calculated molecular weight of 66,438 Da. It has a heart-shaped three-dimensional structure stabilized by 17 intrachain S-S bonds.[121] It is a relatively stable protein, resisting denaturation up to higher temperatures than most plasma proteins. Albumin has a high abundance of charged amino acids that contribute to high solubility, and it has a net negative charge of about −12 at neutral pH.[37] Albumin therefore contributes about 6 to 10 mmol/L to the anion gap at normal albumin concentrations of 0.5 to 0.8 mmol/L, and lesser amounts at lower albumin concentrations. At a pH of 8.6 for alkaline electrophoresis, albumin has a net charge of about −25, resulting in high mobility toward the anode. One unpaired cysteine at position 34 occurs partially in reduced form and partially in exchangeable disulfide bonds with small compounds such as cysteine and homocysteine. The unpaired cysteine has an unusually low pK of <6 and high rates of disulfide exchange.[121] Consequently, it serves as a major plasma carrier of compounds with free sulfhydryls.

Albumin is synthesized by hepatocytes. The synthetic reserve of the liver is substantial; in nephrotic syndrome, albumin synthesis can increase threefold above normal. The synthetic rate is controlled primarily by colloidal osmotic pressure (COP) and secondarily by protein intake.[121] As noted previously, albumin is a negative acute-phase reactant.[42] Catabolism occurs mainly by pinocytosis by multiple tissues, with lysosomal degradation of protein to amino acids. Normally, only small amounts (10 to 20% of the total catabolized) are lost into the gastrointestinal tract and the glomerular filtrate.[121] Albumin losses by these routes may become substantial, however, in protein-losing enteropathies and glomerular disorders, resulting in nephrotic states. Burn injuries also result in major losses of albumin. The normal plasma half-life of albumin is 15 to 19 days. Albumin and IgG have several-fold longer plasma half-lives than most proteins because of the action of a recycling receptor, the neonatal IgG receptor, that recovers these two proteins from pinocytosed fluids.[131,165]

At high concentrations of albumin, the receptor may be saturated and the half-life of albumin decreased. At low concentrations of albumin, such as in analbuminemia (described later), the half-life of albumin is markedly extended.

Function of Albumin. Albumin is not essential for humans; rare individuals with analbuminemia have been found.[121] However, the large metabolic expenditure for abundant albumin formation, mechanisms of regulation, and specific recycling mechanisms argue for beneficial functions. Albumin may serve as a storage form of amino acids that can be delivered to tissues in catabolic states and as an antioxidant, particularly through the action of its free sulfhydryl group. The two most clearly defined functions of albumin are (1) serving as the major component of colloid osmotic pressure (patients in hypoalbuminemic states, such as nephrotic syndromes, are prone to develop edema; albumin solutions sometimes are administered as a replacement fluid to try to acutely maintain intravascular volume); and (2) serving as a transporter for a diverse range of substances, including fatty acids and other lipids, bilirubin, foreign substances such as drugs, thiol-containing amino acids, tryptophan, calcium, and metals.[121] Some of these substances, such as fatty acids and unconjugated bilirubin, have very low solubility in water in the absence of a carrier molecule; albumin therefore serves as an important carrier for a variety of hydrophobic metabolic substrates and drugs, assisting with transport to the liver or other sites of metabolism. Albumin has up to six binding sites for free fatty acids. The reference interval of 0.28 to 0.89 mmol/L[156] for free fatty acids corresponds to a stoichiometry of about one fatty acid per albumin molecule, and this ratio increases in obesity and other states with increased free fatty acids. Purified albumin usually contains bound fatty acids unless special stripping procedures are used.[121]

Clinical Significance of Albumin

Increased Plasma Concentrations. Increased concentrations of albumin occur with dehydration or artifactually from prolonged tourniquet time or specimen evaporation prior to analysis. High albumin concentrations therefore suggest problems with hydration or specimen handling.

Decreased Plasma Concentrations. Low concentrations of albumin are associated with decreased survival and poorer outcomes in kidney and cardiovascular disease.[1,62] Decreased albumin concentrations can result from decreased synthesis, increased metabolic turnover, increased distribution to extravascular fluids, or losses from glomerular and gastrointestinal disorders, burns, or other wounds. Decreased synthesis occurs with rare genetic variants, acute-phase responses, and liver dysfunction. Hypoalbuminemia leads to decreases in the anion gap. Albumin usually binds half the calcium in the circulation; therefore, decreased albumin concentrations need to be considered in interpretation of total calcium concentrations that may be expressed as values corrected for calcium concentration.[85]

Analbuminemia. Only about 20 families with inherited analbuminemia have been reported.[121] Although affected individuals have plasma albumin concentrations <0.5 g/L (≤1% of normal), symptoms often are absent or consist of mild edema, lipodystrophy, and dyslipidemia. No increased risk for atherosclerosis has been noted. The plasma half-life of infused albumin in affected individuals is prolonged to 50 to 60 days.

Inflammation. Inflammatory disorders lower albumin by (1) increasing capillary permeability, allowing increased distribution of albumin into the extravascular space; (2) decreasing synthesis in response to inflammatory cytokines such as IL-6; (3) responding to increased quantities of positive acute-phase reactants that contribute to oncotic pressure; and (4) increasing the catabolism of albumin by cells.[121]

Hepatic Disease. The liver has synthetic capacity to maintain albumin concentrations until parenchymal damage or loss is severe, with loss of more than 50% of function. Mechanisms other than direct loss of function may lead to lower albumin concentrations. Potential mechanisms include nutritional deficiencies, direct inhibition of synthesis by toxins such as alcohol, and increased distribution of albumin in extravascular spaces.[70]

Urinary Loss/Kidney Disease. Normally, the glomerular filtration barrier efficiently prevents entry into the urinary ultrafiltrate by proteins the size of albumin or larger.[116] Usually, only 1 to 2 g/d of albumin passes through the glomerular barrier, and 99.9% of albumin in the glomerular ultrafiltrate is taken up by proximal tubules of the kidney and degraded. Only about 10 mg/d of albumin is normally excreted in urine. Small increases and urine albumin excretion to >30 mg/d are indicators of early stages of glomerular or tubular injury.[105] This has been termed *microalbuminuria* ("micro" refers to excretion of small amounts, not a smaller form, of albumin). (See Chapter 25 on kidney function tests.) Nonpathologic increases in albumin excretion are observed in some individuals with postural changes, strenuous exercise, and fever. Therefore, urinary albumin should be collected under controlled conditions, and collection repeated if a question arises. First or second voided specimens in the morning may decrease postural effects. Severe glomerular injury and nephrotic syndromes are characterized by excretion of >3.5 g/d. In nephrotic syndrome, the glomerular leakage of proteins is increased but some size selectivity is retained; therefore, very large proteins are still retained. Even though the liver compensates through increased protein synthesis, concentrations of proteins up to about 200 kDa, including albumin, decrease substantially. Concentrations of very large proteins, such as α_2-macroglobulin (AMG), larger isotypes of Hp (genotypes 2-1 and 2-2), cholinesterase, and apolipoprotein B are increased.

Gastrointestinal Loss. Protein-losing enteropathy may result in losses as great as those seen in the nephrotic syndrome. If protein-losing enteropathy occurs secondary to lymphangiectasis, larger proteins—especially the immunoglobulins—may be lost in large quantities. Patients with Ménétrier's disease who have gastric protein losses or inflammatory bowel disease of the intestinal tract, such as Crohn's disease with intestinal losses, can develop hypoalbuminemia.[36]

Protein-Calorie Malnutrition. Albumin concentrations serve as a means of detecting and monitoring protein-calorie malnutrition, because concentrations vary directly with adequacy of intake. However, the response of albumin to increased or decreased protein ingestion is relatively slow, in part because of its relatively long half-life. Also, effects of acute or chronic inflammation may decrease the correlation of albumin concentration with nutrition.[70]

Burn Injury. Patients with burn injury can experience severe losses of albumin from wounds. Severely decreased plasma albumin concentrations probably relate to combined effects of epithelial losses, accelerated catabolism, and stimulation of the acute-phase response.[69]

Edema and Ascites. Edema and ascites rarely are the result of decreased plasma albumin concentrations per se. Usually they occur secondary to increased vascular permeability, which permits the loss of albumin into these spaces. Albumin concentrations in these fluids vary from very low to higher than those in plasma, the latter in particular with certain forms of ascites.[52] Increased volumes of extravascular fluid may be large enough to contain a substantial portion of total body albumin. In patients with edema or ascites associated with low plasma albumin, effects of albumin infusion are transient because of rapid equilibration with extravascular fluid. In acute hypovolemic shock, albumin infusion may help to maintain vascular volume, but rapid infusion may result in symptoms of hypocalcemia due to calcium binding by albumin.

Genetic Aspects of Albumin. The albumin gene is on chromosome 4, linked to homologous genes for α-fetoprotein (AFP) and vitamin D–binding protein (Gc-globulin). Inherited analbuminemia has been reported in a few families. Inheritance is autosomal recessive, with heterozygotes having low normal to moderately reduced concentrations.[121] More than 80 different inherited structural variants of albumin have been described, most with normal concentrations of albumin. All variants have a population frequency of <1 : 1000. Variants may have altered electrophoretic migration, leading to two bands for albumin or *bisalbuminemia* for heterozygotes. Variants with abnormal intramolecular disulfide bonding, such as Alb Hawkes Bay, may form homodimers or heterodimers with other proteins such as α_1-antitrypsin AAT.[121] Electrophoretic variants of albumin and bisalbuminemia may be acquired as effects of bound drugs or metabolites. Most albumin isoforms have normal function; an exception consists of increased or decreased binding affinities for T_4 of certain albumin variants. Variants with increased affinity for T_4 yield familial dysalbuminemic hyperthyroxinemia, where total serum T_4 is elevated, although individuals are euthyroid and have normal thyrotropin concentrations.

Laboratory Considerations for Albumin

Plasma and Serum. Most clinical laboratories assay albumin in plasma or serum samples by dye-binding methods, which rely on a shift in the absorption spectrum of dyes such as bromcresol green (BCG) or purple (BCP) upon albumin binding. The affinity of these dyes is higher for albumin than for other proteins, providing some specificity for albumin. BCP generally is slightly more specific for albumin and yields lower values than BCG, particularly for patients with kidney failure.[85] Heparin in collection tubes is reported to affect some dye-binding methods.[104] Dye-binding assays also tend to be less accurate when the serum or plasma protein composition is abnormal. Dye-binding methods have decreased accuracy for patients with cirrhosis, possibly related to oxidized or other modified forms of albumin.[166] Unfortunately, disorders with abnormal plasma protein compositions, such as kidney and liver disease, often present situations in which accurate analysis is most desired. Albumin concentrations are considered an important indicator of adequate nutrition in patients with kidney failure, and guidelines for monitoring patients with kidney failure recommend correcting total calcium values for albumin concentration.[85] Guidelines also recommend nutritional supplementation of patients with kidney failure to maintain serum albumin concentrations of at least 40 g/L by the BCG method.[1] Low albumin concentrations are a strong predictor of unfavorable outcomes for many clinical disorders, including patients on chronic hemodialysis. Albumin concentrations increasingly are used as a measure of quality of care by physicians or patient care units, so that methods of analysis and accuracy of results are of increasing concern to many medical professionals. Serum albumin also is used as a criterion in the staging of patients with multiple myeloma, with albumin ≥3.5 g/dL necessary for patients to be in stage I with best prognosis.[82] Estimation of albumin concentration by serum protein electrophoresis yields discordant values with immunonephelometry and BCG methods for some patients with high paraprotein concentrations.[147]

Many ligands of albumin, including drugs and metabolites, bind to albumin but usually do not affect dye-binding assays of serum or plasma significantly unless their concentrations are very high. Because of their simplicity and low cost, dye-binding assays are likely to remain the predominant means for assaying albumin in serum and plasma. In assessment of albumin in ascitic fluid, dye-binding methods have been noted to give spuriously high results.[33]

Densitometric scans of electrophoretic patterns can determine the percentage of protein made up of albumin. Along with a measure of total protein concentration, albumin concentration can be calculated. Care is needed in calibrating assays and determining ranges of linear responses of staining or absorbance measurements in capillary electrophoresis. Scanning often offers low precision and linearity, and multiple measurements are combined, generally resulting in albumin measurement with lower accuracy, less precision, and greater potential for interference.[147] Immunoturbidimetry and immunonephelometry offer greater specificity and accuracy of albumin measurement than other methods, along with the higher sensitivity needed for specimens with low albumin concentrations such as urine and CSF.

Reference Intervals of Albumin. Based on the international protein reference CRM 470, the recommended interim reference interval for albumin in serum of adults 20 to 60 years of age is 35 to 52 g/L (3.5 to 5.2 g/dL).[22] Albumin concentrations reach adult concentrations around 20 to 30 weeks' gestation and remain relatively constant until at least 20 years of age. Concentrations then slowly decrease with age in both sexes. Concentrations are lower in individuals living in the subtropics and tropics, probably because of higher immunoglobulin concentrations secondary to infection. Concentrations are posture dependent, increasing by up to 10 to 15% if an individual is standing versus recumbent. This reflects a shift of fluid between intravascular and extravascular spaces; albumin is preferentially retained in the intravascular space. A similar increase in albumin results from prolonged tourniquet time before blood collection.

α_1-Acid Glycoprotein (AAG)

AAG, also known as orosomucoid, was one of the first plasma glycoproteins to be isolated and extensively characterized. AAG is a major constituent of the seromucoid fraction of plasma, which consists of a group of proteins that are "slimy" ("mucoid" is from Greek *myxa* = slime) because of their high carbohydrate content.

Biochemistry of AAG. AAG actually consists of two proteins that are products of homologous genes on chromosome 9. Each of the two gene products has a polypeptide chain of 183 amino acids, but the two differ at about 21 positions. About two thirds of AAG is the product of the *AAG-1* (or *ORM1*) gene. Both have a molecular mass of 35 to 40 kDa, of which ≈45% is carbohydrate (CHO), including ≈12% sialic acid; 5-N-linked oligosaccharides include a variable mixture of biantennary, triantennary, and tetraantennary structures with terminal sialic acids, resulting in heterogeneity of AAG upon isoelectric focusing.[38] Oligosaccharide structures and charge of AAG change with inflammation, as do many proteins.[45,72]

AAG is synthesized mainly by hepatocytes, but granulocytes and monocytes may contribute to plasma concentrations in sepsis. Removal of desialylated AAG by hepatic asialoglycoprotein receptors contributes to catabolism. The plasma half-life of intact AAG is ≈3 days, whereas that of the desialylated protein is only a few minutes.[70]

Function of AAG. AAG is a *lipocalin,* a family of homologous proteins, including RBP, many of which bind lipophilic substances. AAG binds a large number of basic and lipophilic compounds, including progesterone and related steroid hormones. Binding of drugs to AAG increases the total plasma concentration while reducing the proportion of drug that is free and bioactive. Affected drugs include propranolol, quinidine, chlorpromazine, cocaine, imatinib, and benzodiazepines. Because AAG concentrations may change several-fold in acute-phase responses, interpretation of total drug concentrations for some drugs requires measurement of AAG or alternative measurements of free rather than total drug concentrations. Besides its carrier function, AAG has been proposed to serve a variety of functions, including downregulation of the immune response, depression of phagocytosis by neutrophils, inhibition of platelet aggregation, inhibition of mitosis, inhibition of viruses and parasites, and action as a cofactor for lipoprotein lipase; it also acts as a contributor to capillary selectivity.[70]

Clinical Significance of AAG. Various pathologic conditions are associated with increased and decreased concentrations of AAG.

Increased Plasma Concentrations

Acute-Phase Response. Plasma AAG concentrations increase up to fourfold in response to inflammation or tissue necrosis, with peak concentrations noted around 3 to 5 days after the initial insult. As an example, AAG serves as an indicator of the clinical activity of ulcerative colitis.

Hormonal Effects. AAG concentrations are increased by glucocorticoid hormones, either endogenous (e.g., Cushing's syndrome) or exogenous, along with Hp and prealbumin concentrations.

Decreased Plasma Concentrations

Hormonal Effects. Synthesis and plasma AAG concentrations are decreased by estrogens.

Sieving Protein Loss. AAG is slightly smaller than albumin and therefore is lost in the urine in nephrotic syndrome and in gastrointestinal secretions in protein-losing enteropathy.

Laboratory Considerations for AAG. The major applications of AAG measurement are to monitor APRs and to assess effects on drug binding. Measurement of total drug concentrations may require correction for AAG concentration.[70] Hormonal effects and the APR are similar for AAG and haptoglobin, so that measurement of AAG may assist in interpreting whether changes in haptoglobin are due to in vivo hemolysis (which does not affect AAG concentrations). Although AAG is one of the proteins of highest concentration in the α_1-globulin region on routine serum electrophoresis, it does not stain well with protein stains because of its high carbohydrate content. It can be visualized by using periodic acid–Schiff or other carbohydrate stains. AAG usually is quantified by immunoturbidimetry, immunonephelometry, or radial immunodiffusion (RID).

Reference Intervals for AAG. The proposed interim reference interval for white adolescents and adults is 0.5 to 1.2 g/L (50 to 120 mg/dL), based on CRM 470.[22] Concentrations at birth are only 20 to 30% of this, but approximately adult concentrations are reached by 6 to 12 months of age.

α_1-Antitrypsin (AAT)

Schultze described AAT in 1955, recognizing inhibition of trypsin. However, AAT inhibits a variety of serine proteinases, leading to the term α_1-*proteinase inhibitor.* Both names are used currently. *AAT* is the term commonly used by clinicians and clinical laboratorians, but phenotypes are commonly abbreviated as Pi.

Biochemistry of AAT. AAT has a single polypeptide chain of 394 amino acid residues with 3 *N*-linked oligosaccharides, giving a total MW of ≈51 kDa. It is SerpinA1 of the serpin superfamily (where *A* refers to subgroup or clade). It has Met as a reactive site residue at residue 358, helping to define its specificity for inhibition of elastase and its susceptibility to inactivation by oxidation of the methionine sidechain.[14] Serpins are suicide inhibitors of serine proteases, which abortively try to cleave the inhibitor at the reactive site residue but remain covalently linked to the reactive site residue because of a conformational shift of the inhibitor upon cleavage. Serpins usually occur in a "stressed" conformation, and cleavage leads to a dramatic conformational shift to a "relaxed" form. AAT and other serpins serve as important models for conformational change in protein function and aggregation.[14]

Most AAT in plasma is synthesized by the hepatocytes, and AAT genotype changes with liver transplantation. AAT is an acute-phase reactant, with hepatic synthesis and plasma concentrations rising up to several-fold. Catabolism occurs by several routes, in addition to usual bulk pinocytosis of plasma proteins: AAT-protease complexes are removed by serpin-enzyme complex receptors [low-density lipoprotein (LDL)-related receptor],[68] along with several other serpin-enzyme complexes. Proteases complexed with AAT also may be transferred to AMG; AMG-protease complexes are removed even faster by the liver than are AAT-protease complexes. AAT can also be removed by asialoglycoprotein receptors, which bind AAT that loses sialic acid. The normal plasma half-life is 6 to 7 days for the Pi M genotype; Pi S and perhaps other variants have a shorter half-life and secondarily lower plasma concentrations.

Function of AAT. AAT covalently binds to the active sites of serine proteases, thus blocking their enzymatic activity. Other members of the serpin superfamily include the proteinase inhibitors α_1-antichymotrypsin, α_2-antiplasmin, antithrombin III, heparin cofactor II, and C1 inhibitor, plus angiotensinogen, thyroxine-binding globulin, and other proteins with no apparent inhibitory activity.[88] AAT is one of the 10 most abundant plasma proteins and the most abundant protease inhibitor on a molar basis. AAT inhibits many proteases, but physiologically, one of its most critical actions is inhibiting elastase released from neutrophils. As first established by Laurell, deficiency of AAT is associated with emphysema related to elastin degradation in the lung by neutrophil elastase. Smoking serves as a cofactor in this process by stimulating chronic inflammation and neutrophil infiltration in the lungs, and by promoting inactivation of AAT through oxidation of its reactive site Met residue.[14]

Clinical Significance of AAT

Increased Plasma Concentrations. Plasma AAT concentrations are increased in the APR and with estrogens.

Acute-Phase Response. In acute inflammatory processes, serum AAT concentrations begin to rise after approximately 24 hours and peak at 3 to 4 days. Synthesis is stimulated by cytokines, particularly IL-6, and by AAT-elastase complexes taken up via the LDL-related receptor. Cytokines, including IL-6, induce a broader APR. Inflammation of hepatocytes may be associated with increased serum AAT without the other components of the APR.[70]

Estrogens. Synthesis of AAT is stimulated by estrogens; elevated concentrations are seen particularly during late pregnancy and during estrogen therapy.

Decreased Plasma Concentrations. Plasma AAT concentrations are decreased with genetic deficiency, increased turnover, and urinary or gastrointestinal loss.

Genetic Deficiency. More than 75 genetic variants of AAT have been noted, and prevalence of clinical AAT deficiency in the United States is estimated at 1:3000 to 1:5000.[144] About 10% of individuals express genetic variants of AAT, but clinical disorders usually occur only in individuals expressing variants at both alleles. Severe genetic deficiency of AAT (Pi ZZ or Pi Z null genotypes) increases risk for pulmonary emphysema, and onset of disease is relatively early, with changes beginning in the second to fourth decades of life in 90% of Pi ZZ individuals. Progression of emphysema is highly variable, but age at onset and median age at death are, on average, younger in smokers. Patients with Pi SZ genotype have less risk for lung disease than those with Pi ZZ genotype.[144]

AAT deficiency also is associated with liver disease, including neonatal cholestasis or hepatitis, cirrhosis, and hepatocellular carcinoma. About 10% of infants with Pi ZZ or Pi Znull genotype have prolonged obstructive jaundice; 2% progress to liver failure in childhood.[144] Early differentiation of cholestasis from AAT deficiency and biliary atresia can be challenging histologically.[70] Liver disease with AAT variants has a risk for progression to hepatocarcinoma. Hepatic injury in AAT deficiency probably is related to intracellular accumulation of AAT, but many factors may determine disease progression.[144]

Increased Utilization. Low concentrations of AAT are seen in neonatal respiratory distress syndrome, severe neonatal hepatitis, and severe preterminal pancreatic disease. In nonfatal pancreatitis, concentrations increase from the APR, and increased concentrations of complexes with trypsin may indicate diagnosis or prognosis in patients with possible pancreatitis.

Urinary or Gastrointestinal Loss. AAT is similar in size to albumin; therefore, urinary and gastrointestinal losses occur in parallel to those noted with albumin in nephrotic syndromes and protein-losing enteropathies. AAT is normally present in excreted stool, mostly complexed to pancreatic trypsin and elastase. Evaluation of AAT excretion in stool is used as a measure of protein-losing enteropathy (see section on stool protein).[6,152]

Genetic Aspects of AAT. The gene for AAT (*Pi,* for protease inhibitor) is found on chromosome 14. It is a polymorphic gene with more than 75 genetic isotypes of AAT, designated as Pi (pronounced *pee eye*) plus letters from B to Z in order of decreasing electrophoretic mobility, with B being the most anodal.[12] About 30 variants are associated with decreased AAT.[144] The usual or wild type is Pi M. In many populations, 10% or more of individuals are heterozygous for AAT variants. Most clinical disorders occur in individuals with two variant alleles. Numbers or subscripted place names indicate subtypes (e.g., Pi M1 and Pi M_{malton}); null is used for deleted or nonproducing alleles. Several variants are associated with reduced plasma concentrations, with an aggregate population frequency of about 1:3000. AAT concentrations are reduced to about Pi P 25%, Pi S 60%, Pi W 80%, Pi Z 15%, and Pi null 0%. Pi Z is most common among northern Europeans, and Pi S is most common in those in southwestern Europe. Pi Z, clinically the most important deficiency variant, has a lys → glu substitution at position 342, whereas Pi S has a 264 glu → val substitution. Mutations resulting in Pi null are rare. The concentrations and the variants are codominant; therefore an individual with Pi MZ, for example, would have a concentration of ≈58% of the normal Pi MM concentration [(100 + 15)/2]. One variant, Pi $M_{pittsburgh}$, with a Met → Arg substitution at position 358 (the reactive site residue), inhibits elastase poorly but inhibits clotting enzymes, including thrombin and kallikrein. Heterozygotes for this variant have a bleeding disorder because of its anticoagulant effects.[140] This variant demonstrates the importance of reactive site residue in serpin specificity.

Laboratory Considerations for AAT. The Global Initiative for Chronic Obstructive Lung Disease recommends quantitative testing of AAT for patients with chronic obstructive pulmonary disease with family history or onset before age 45.[144] AAT usually is quantified by immunoturbidimetry or immunonephelometry. AAT represents the majority of serum inhibitory activity versus trypsin and elastase and could be assessed by inhibition assays of these enzymes. Leukocyte proteases may be released into serum stored on the clot after blood drawing, and the proteases may complex with AAT, altering both electrophoretic mobility and immunochemical quantification. Bacterial contamination and release of bacterial proteases can have a similar effect. Serum should be removed from the retracted clot and stored aseptically at 4 °C (for up to 3 to 4 days) or at −70 °C (for long-term storage). Phenotyping of AAT usually is performed by isoelectric focusing. For genotyping, the most important types to detect are Z and S, but a large number of other rare alleles are known, and it is important to consider what variants are detected.

AAT usually is the major serum component stained in the α_1-globulin band on agarose gel electrophoresis. Decreases in the α_1-band suggest a quantitative decrease in AAT or variants with altered mobility. Variants forming dimers with albumin have altered electrophoretic mobility but normal concentrations. The two other highest abundance α_1-globulins, AAG and α-lipoprotein, do not stain well with peptide stains because of their high contents of carbohydrate and lipid, respectively. Five to eight AAT bands are found on acid gel electrophoresis or isoelectric focusing (pIs approximately 4.2 to 4.9, depending on the genetic phenotype), as shown in Figure 21-2.

Microheterogeneity within a single genetic variant results primarily from variation in oligosaccharides and, in the case of the two most cathodal bands, absence of the first 5 amino acids of the peptide chain.[70]

Reference Intervals for AAT. For adults, the recommended consensus reference interval, based on CRM 470, is 0.9 to 2.0 g/L (90 to 200 mg/dL) for individuals with the Pi MM phenotype,[22] with a median of approximately 1.3 g/L. Concentrations are slightly higher in women in childbearing years and in elderly individuals. Concentrations are also higher in patients with inflammatory disorders, malignancy, or trauma, and in women who are pregnant, on estrogen

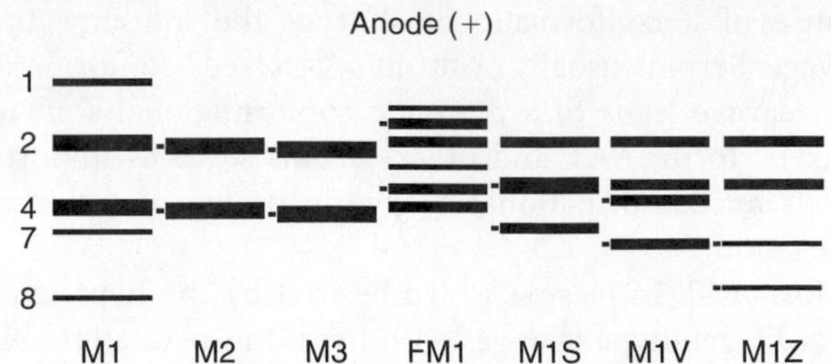

Figure 21-2 Diagram of common variants of α_1-antitrypsin, as demonstrated by isoelectric focusing. The five major bands are shown for M1, but only the 2 and 4 bands are shown for the other variants *(with dots to the left of each)*. Variants F, S, V, and Z are shown in combination with M1 for the sake of clarity. If cysteine is added to the samples before focusing, the F-2 and F-4 bands shift to the locations of the faint bands.

therapy, or taking oral contraceptives. Neonates have higher concentrations, possibly because of maternal estrogen. Individuals with concentrations below 70 mg/dL should be phenotyped or genotyped, especially if they or family members have diseases that may be associated with AAT deficiency. AAT concentrations in Pi ZZ genotypes usually are 0.1 to 0.5 g/L (10 to 50 mg/dL). AAT replacement therapy, with weekly infusions, has been approved by the U.S. Food and Drug Administration for patients with AAT <56 mg/dL (<11 μmol/L).[144]

α_2-Macroglobulin (AMG)

AMG is a large protein with Mr of ≈720 kDa. It is a versatile protease inhibitor with a different mechanism than serpins. AMG is homologous to complement components C3 and C4 and, like those proteins, contains an internal thioester that is activated by proteolytic cleavage and reacts to bind covalently to neighboring molecules.

Biochemistry of AMG. AMG has four identical subunits with MW of 180 kDa, occurring as a pair of dimers. The dimers are disulfide-linked, whereas the pairs are held together by noncovalent bonds. The dimer is the active unit; one molecule of AMG binds up to two protease molecules. Each monomer contains a reactive thioester, which is formed internally between cysteine and glutamine sidechains at positions 949 and 952 in the peptide chain. The thioester is exposed when a "bait" region is cleaved by a protease. The thioester reacts to form covalent bonds with the protease, thus immobilizing it, but the active site of proteases is not blocked and retains activity versus low molecular weight substrates.[61,77] AMG is synthesized primarily by hepatocytes and has a half-life of several days. However, once AMG's thioester is cleaved clearance occurs within minutes via a hepatic receptor. Also, desialylated AMG is removed rapidly by asialoglycoprotein receptors.

Function of AMG. AMG is a versatile inhibitor of many proteases, including enzymes in the kinin, complement, coagulation, and fibrinolytic pathways and classes of proteases not inhibited by serpins. In addition, AMG accepts transfer of proteases complexed to serpins (e.g., elastase-AAT), and AMG-protease complexes are then rapidly removed by receptors. Because of its large size, AMG is restricted primarily to the vascular space. In addition to serving as a protease inhibitor, AMG may serve as a transport molecule for cytokines, growth factors, and zinc. Transport functions may contribute to apparent activity of AMG in modulating immunologic and inflammatory reactions. Oxidation dissociates AMG tetramers into dysfunctional dimers. Thus as is the case for AAT and other serpins, inhibitory activity is reduced or eradicated by increased concentrations of oxidants (such as those from cigarette smoke or from neutrophils).[70]

Clinical Significance of AMG

Increased Plasma Concentrations. Increased plasma concentrations of AMG relate to hormonal effects, age, and the nephrotic syndrome.

Hormonal Effects. Synthesis and plasma concentrations of AMG are increased by estrogens; women of childbearing age have higher concentrations than men of the same age.

Age. Synthesis rates in infants and children are up to three times adult concentrations. High concentrations of AMG may delay clinical signs and symptoms until after puberty in individuals with antithrombin III or C1 inhibitor deficiency.

Nephrotic Syndrome. Hepatic synthesis is increased in the nephrotic syndrome, as is synthesis of most other proteins made by the liver, in attempts to compensate for decreased oncotic pressure. Elevated AMG concentrations may partially compensate physiologically for renal loss of lower molecular weight proteinase inhibitors.[70]

Decreased Plasma Concentrations. Decreased plasma concentrations of AMG result from various genetic conditions, pancreatitis, *and* prostatic carcinoma. AMG does not change markedly in the acute-phase response. AMG has been measured as one component of some multiparameter indices of hepatic fibrosis.[46]

Genetic. See "Genetic Aspects," later in this chapter.

Pancreatitis. In severe attacks of acute pancreatitis, plasma concentrations of antithrombin III and AMG may be markedly decreased; other inhibitors are normal or increased, and protease-antiprotease complexes are increased. In the peritoneal fluid, all major protease inhibitors are decreased or absent.[70]

Prostatic Carcinoma. Plasma concentrations of AMG are decreased before treatment for advanced carcinoma of the prostate and return to normal with successful treatment. AMG binds to prostate-specific antigen (PSA), and concentrations of the complexes are elevated in plasma during active disease, as is the case with PSA-α_1-antichymotrypsin complexes. In vitro, PSA added to serum has a higher affinity for AMG than for α_1-antichymotrypsin. In vivo, the complexes are probably removed very rapidly by the liver, as are other protease complexes with AMG; usually, free PSA and PSA-α_1-antichymotrypsin are the only forms detected.

Genetic Aspects of AMG. The gene for AMG is on chromosome 12, near genes for pregnancy zone protein and for its membrane receptor (LDL-related protein). No individuals with complete genetic deficiency of AMG have been described. Genetic variants are known, however. Two reported heterozygous mutations affected the function of AMG, and one patient with decreased AMG developed chronic lung disease in childhood.

Laboratory Considerations for AMG. AMG and Hp together constitute most of the α_2-globulin zone on routine clinical serum electrophoresis. In the newborn period and with in vivo hemolysis, AMG alone is the major contributor to this zone. Native and cleaved forms of AMG cannot be distinguished on routine electrophoresis. Higher-resolution separations indicate native AMG migrating slightly cathodal to AMG that has split its thioester. Monoclonal antibodies specific for the two forms indicate that normal plasma contains 0.8 to 1.9% of AMG in the complexed form.[70]

Reference Intervals for AMG. The interim recommended reference interval for white adults is 1.3 to 3.0 g/L (130 to 300 mg/dL).[22] Concentrations are approximately twice this in children at a maximum at 2 to 4 years of age; concentrations in women are 20 to 30% higher than in men after age 40.

Ceruloplasmin (Cp)

Cp is an α_2-globulin that contains about 95% of serum copper. Each molecule of Cp contains 6 to 8 copper atoms, most of which are tightly bound. A solution of Cp is blue (*L. caeruleus* = blue), and elevated concentrations of Cp may lend plasma a green tint.

Biochemistry of Cp. Cp has a polypeptide chain with 1046 amino acids and three asparagine-linked oligosaccharides, along with a total carbohydrate content of 8 to 10%. MW of intact Cp is 132 kDa. Size and charge heterogeneity results from variations in glycosylation, the number of copper atoms, peptide chain variations from alternative DNA splicing, and polymerization. Cp is highly susceptible to proteolysis, leading to earlier reports of more than one peptide chain.[70]

Cp is synthesized primarily by hepatic parenchymal cells, with small amounts from macrophages and lymphocytes. The peptide chain is formed first, then copper is added from an intracellular ATPase (absent in Wilson's disease). Copper appears to be essential for the normal folding of Cp and possibly for normal oligosaccharide attachment. Much of apoCp synthesized in the absence of copper or the ATPase is degraded intracellularly; some apoCp reaches the circulation, where it has a shortened half-life of a few hours. Consequently, serum Cp is low in Wilson's disease.[96] The normal half-life of Cp is 4 to 5 days.

Function of Cp. Cp is a catalyst for redox reactions in plasma.[141] Cp oxidizes Fe^{2+} to Fe^{3+} (Figure 21-3), which is important for allowing binding of iron to transferrin. Cp helps control membrane lipid oxidation—probably by direct oxidation of cations—thus preventing their catalysis of lipid peroxidation. In the presence of superoxide, Cp promotes LDL oxidation, which may contribute to atherosclerosis.[39] Neurologic disorders in hereditary Cp deficiency (aceruloplasminemia) may be due to disordered iron transport in the brain.[154] Cp appears to have a limited role in plasma copper transport to tissues. Albumin and transcuprein appear to

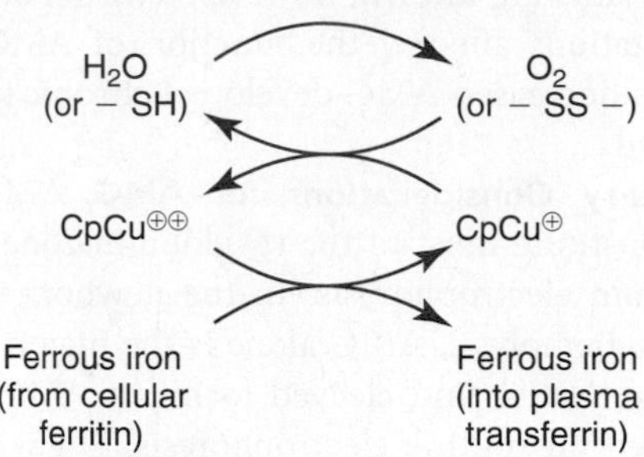

Figure 21-3 Proposed function of ceruloplasmin copper ($CpCu2^+$) as an electron recipient from cellular ferrous iron. The resulting oxidation of Fe2' to the ferric state permits its binding and transport by plasma transferrin. $CpCu^+$ is oxidized (regenerated to $CpCu2^+$) by reaction with oxygen, oxidized thiol groups, or other oxidizing substances. *(Modified from Johnson AM. Ceruloplasmin. In: Ritchie RF, Navolotskaia O, eds. Serum proteins in clinical medicine, volume I, Laboratory section. Scarborough, Maine: Foundation for Blood Research, 1996:13.01-13.03.)*

be the major copper transport proteins, especially following absorption from the intestinal tract.

Clinical Significance of Cp. Cp is most often measured by immunoassays as a screening test for Wilson's disease. Several factors, including diet, hormone concentrations, and other genetic disorders, may influence plasma concentrations. Immunochemical assays may not distinguish between the active, copper-replete holoCp and apoCp, which is released into the circulation in most of the disorders associated with low total Cp concentrations. Functional assays may be helpful to monitor patients on copper-lowering therapy.[96]

Increased Plasma Concentrations. Synthesis of Cp is increased modestly in the APR. This increase occurs relatively slowly, peaking at 4 to 20 days after a single, acute insult. Synthesis is stimulated markedly by estrogens, with moderate increases seen in women taking estrogen-containing medications, and larger increases noted during pregnancy.

Decreased Plasma Concentrations. Cp concentrations are decreased as a result of various primary and secondary deficiencies.

Genetic Deficiency. Inherited aceruloplasminemia has been reported in several families.[154] Neurodegeneration occurs in these patients associated with iron deposition in the brain. This argues strongly that a major role of Cp is to maintain normal iron transport, particularly in the brain.

Secondary Deficiency. Low plasma Cp concentrations caused by lack of incorporation of Cu^{2+} into the molecule during synthesis are much more common than aceruloplasminemia. Cp deficiency may be due to dietary Cu^{2+} insufficiency (including malabsorption), inability to release Cu^{2+} from the gastrointestinal epithelium into the circulation, or inability to insert Cu^{2+} into the developing Cp molecule. In all cases, apoCp (non–copper containing) is still synthesized, but most apoCp is catabolized intracellularly, and plasma apoCp has a much shorter half-life than Cp. Cp concentrations also may be low in blood loss or in gastrointestinal or renal protein-losing syndromes.

Dietary Cp deficiency is due to nutritional copper deficiency and is associated with neutropenia, thrombocytopenia, low serum iron, and hypochromic, normocytic, or macrocytic anemia unresponsive to iron therapy. The deficiency may be due to inadequate dietary intake, long-term parenteral nutrition without copper supplementation, malabsorption, penicillamine therapy, or combinations of these. Therapy includes dietary changes or copper supplementation, plus treatment of the primary cause of malabsorption if known.[95]

Menkes' disease is an X-linked inherited disorder in which dietary copper is absorbed by gastrointestinal cells that lack an ATPase for copper transfer to plasma.[95] Hence, copper is not available to the liver for incorporation into Cp. Affected infants manifest sparse, brittle, and kinky hair, growth restriction, and neurologic degeneration, with death occurring during the first few years of life if untreated. Subcutaneous injections of copper histidine partially reverse the deleterious effects if started early in life; some residual Menkes' ATPase activity (i.e., incomplete deficiency) may be necessary for this response, however. Patients with deficient gastrointestinal *and* blood-brain barrier transport of copper have been described; neurologic symptoms in these patients are not reversed by copper therapy.[70]

Wilson's disease, or hepatolenticular degeneration, differs from dietary deficiency and Menkes' disease in that body copper is markedly increased and is deposited in tissue, including the hepatic parenchymal cells, the brain, and the periphery of the iris (resulting in the characteristic Kayser-Fleischer rings).[96,97] Copper is absorbed and transported to the liver, but the absence of a hepatocellular P type of ATPase encoded on chromosome 13 prevents incorporation of copper into Cp. Symptoms in patients with Wilson's disease usually begin in the second or third decade of life. However, mutations that eliminate gene function may lead to onset of liver disease as early as 3 years of age. The initial clinical presentation may show acute hepatitis or chronic active hepatitis; neurologic signs (e.g., clumsiness, dysarthria, ataxia, tremors); renal indications (e.g., renal tubular acidosis with aminoaciduria); or, less commonly, hemolysis secondary to acute release of free copper from tissue. Treatment aims to decrease tissue copper overload through chelation with agents such as penicillamine or trientene and inhibition of dietary copper intake with supplemental zinc.[96]

Most patients with Wilson's disease have low plasma Cp concentrations. A cutoff of 0.2 g/L often has been used, but slight adjustment may be indicated for different populations and assays; an optimal cutoff of 0.14 g/L is recommended from one recent study.[97] However, inflammatory diseases or pregnancy may bring Cp concentrations of affected individuals to above cutoff values. Cp concentrations are slightly reduced in obligate heterozygotes. Low Cp concentrations are also seen in other disorders, as noted earlier. Clinical diagnosis of Wilson's disease therefore requires the presence of classical signs of the disease, documentation of copper excess, or both. Slit-lamp examination of corneas for Kayser-Fleischer rings, assays of urine copper, and, if these are not diagnostic, liver biopsy for quantitative copper assay may be required for definitive diagnosis. Genetic analysis of the defective ATPase also permits definitive diagnosis in most cases, even in the absence of clinical abnormalities.

Genetic Aspects of Cp. Several variants or isotypes of the Cp gene are found on chromosome 3, but none of these, except for genetic deficiency (aceruloplasminemia), has known clinical significance. The most prevalent isotypes are CpA, CpB, and CpC, which are detectable by electrophoresis followed by immunofixation or functional staining; CpB is the common, or "wild," isotype.[70]

Laboratory Considerations for Cp. Cp usually is measured by immunoturbidimetry or immunonephelometry. It is subject to oxidation and proteolytic degradation during storage that may affect immunoreactivity. This lability may create problems with calibrators, controls, and quality control materials, and with patient samples. Depending on the degree of degradation and the assay method used, apparent concentrations may increase or decrease. Serum or plasma from patient samples should be separated as soon as possible after collection and assayed promptly or stored under proper conditions (up to 3 days at 4 °C; longer storage at −70 °C).[70] Cp also can be assessed for oxidase activity. Activity assay may serve as a better indicator of functional protein when therapy for copper chelation or other potential sources of copper deficiency is provided.[96]

Reference Intervals for Cp. Cp is undetectable before 20 weeks' gestation. Plasma concentrations gradually rise by term to 25 to 40% of normal adult concentrations, and by 6 months of age to nearly adult concentrations (Table 21-8). Serum Cp concentrations reach a maximum at 2 or 3 years of age, then fall slowly until adolescence, when adult concentrations are reached. Concentrations are higher in women during their menstrual years (and longer if estrogen replacement therapy is used). A genetic influence on synthetic rates is apparent; concentrations within families vary less than concentrations among families. Studies have examined the optimal cutoff value for detecting Wilson's disease and suggest a cutoff of 0.14 g/L, but this may require adjustment for local populations.[96] The recommended interim reference interval for all adults of both sexes, based on CRM 470, is 0.2 to 0.6 g/L (20 to 60 mg/dL).[22]

TABLE 21-8 Plasma Ceruloplasmin Reference Intervals*

Age	Reference Interval (mg/L)	
Cord (term)	50-330	
Birth-4 months	150-560	
5-6 months	260-830	
7-36 months	310-900	
4-12 y	250-450	
	Male	**Female**
13-19 y	150-370	220-500
Adults	220-400	250-600 (no OC)
		270-660 (OC; estrogens)
		300-1200 (pregnant†)

*Converted to CRM 470 values from multiple references.
†Second and third trimesters; concentrations increase with increasing gestational age.
OC, Oral contraceptives.

Haptoglobin (Hp)

Hp is an α_2-glycoprotein that binds hemoglobin (*G. haptein* = to bind).

Biochemistry of Hp. Hp is synthesized as a single peptide chain by hepatocytes and is cleaved into α- and β-chains. The α-chain has some homology to kringle 5 of plasminogen; the β-chain, with 245 amino acid residues plus oligosaccharides, is related to serine proteases. The protein is polymorphic, with two types of α-chain—α^1 and α^2—leading to three Hp genotypes—Hp 1-1, 2-1, and 2-2—that respectively are homozygous for α^1, heterozygous for α^1 and α^2, and homozygous for α^2. Variable numbers of α- and β-chains combine and become covalently linked by disulfides to form Hp. Hp 1-1 consists of four peptide chains $\alpha^1{}_2\beta_2$ with a total MW of 85 kDa. Hp 2-2 consists of multiple forms, including $\alpha^1{}_2\beta_2$, $\alpha^1{}_2\alpha^2\beta_3$, $\alpha^1{}_2\alpha^2{}_2\beta_4$, $\alpha^1{}_2\alpha^2{}_3\beta_5$, and higher multimers, with MW ranging from 86 to 300 kDa. Hp 2-2 consists of $\alpha^2{}_3\beta_3$, $\alpha^2{}_4\beta_4$, $\alpha^2{}_5\beta_5$, and higher multimers, ranging from 170 to 900 kDa.[87]

Hp scavenges hemoglobin in the vascular space. Hemoglobin released by hemolysis dissociates into αβ dimers at low concentrations, and these dimers of hemoglobin subunits bind to Hp. Each Hp molecule can bind hemoglobin ab dimers, equivalent in number to Hp b-chain binds in the molecule. Hp 1-1 binds hemoglobin with higher affinity than other phenotypes.[70] Hp-hemoglobin complexes are bound by CD163 receptors and are rapidly removed by reticuloendothelial cells, which degrade proteins and heme and reuse iron and amino acids. This process prevents renal clearance of hemoglobin until Hp-binding capacity is exceeded. Because Hp is degraded after complexing with hemoglobin, its concentration drops severely when intravascular hemolysis occurs.[43] The normal plasma half-life of Hp is about 5.5 days. Hemolysis of specimens after blood collection does not decrease amounts of Hp.

Function of Hp. Hp clears hemoglobin from the circulation, thereby preventing iron loss via renal hemoglobin excretion. Hp may have other functions, including antioxidant activity of Hp-hemoglobin complexes, inhibition of cathepsin B release by phagocytes, and bacteriostatic action. Hp synthesis is stimulated by inflammation but not by hemolysis (and depletion of Hp), suggesting important roles of Hp in inflammatory and immune responses.[70] In chronic hemolytic states, such as sickle cell disease, where haptoglobin is depleted, circulating hemoglobin increases, contributing to vascular disorders such as pulmonary hypertension by binding nitric oxide.[43]

Clinical Significance of Hp. Hp has a capacity to bind only about 1% of the hemoglobin in red cells at usual hematocrits, so intravascular lysis of a small proportion of red cells completely depletes plasma Hp.[87] Once Hp capacity is exceeded, free hemoglobin in the circulation increases. Free hemoglobin can oxidize to methemoglobin, followed by dissociation of metheme from globin. Metheme binds to hemopexin (high affinity) or albumin (low affinity), keeping it in solution. Hemopexin-heme complexes are removed by the reticuloendothelial system (as with Hp-hemoglobin complexes, but more slowly), with subsequent intracellular catabolism of the complex and a decrease in the hemopexin concentration in plasma.[70] Hemopexin synthesis is unaffected by other factors (such as estrogen) that decrease Hp synthesis, so low values usually reflect severe or prolonged hemolysis. Similar to Hp, it is a positive (but weak) APR. Disorders with increased red cell breakdown are associated with chronic depletion of Hp and hemopexin. Methemalbumin may be seen when Hp and hemopexin are depleted. Hp depletion may also allow excess hemoglobin αβ dimers to undergo glomerular filtration. Absorption and catabolism of hemoglobin subunits by the proximal tubules can lead to tubular injury from iron toxicity. If the absorptive capacity of the proximal tubules is exceeded, overflow proteinuria of hemoglobin into urine occurs. Evaluation of hemoglobinuria tries to distinguish prerenal, renal, and postrenal sources of hemoglobin.

Hp depletion is usually a sensitive biochemical indicator of intravascular hemolysis, followed by hemopexin depletion and finally by the presence of methemalbuminemia, hemoglobinuria, or both. Hp, therefore, is part of the assessment of possible transfusion reactions or other causes of hemolysis. However, Hp concentrations must be considered together with potential sources of protein loss or an APR, which increases Hp.

Haptoglobin phenotypes 2-1 and 2-2 are associated with increased risk of cardiovascular disease relative to phenotype 1-1, possibly related to lower average Hp concentrations, hemoglobin affinity, and limited extravascular distribution of those genotypes.[20] The Hp 2-2 phenotype is associated with higher serum iron, ferritin, and transferrin saturation, perhaps because of its preferential uptake by CD163 receptors.[70] Possible clinical associations of the Hp polymorphism have been considered in many studies.[15]

Increased Plasma Concentrations. Increased concentrations of Hp are seen in the APR and in protein-losing syndromes and are associated with corticosteroid effects.

Acute-Phase Response. Hp synthesis is increased in the APR 4 to 6 days after stimulation and takes about 2 weeks to fall to normal after the stimulus is removed.

Protein-Losing Syndromes (in Association With Hp 2-1 or 2-2 Phenotype). Most protein-losing syndromes, such as the nephrotic syndromes, compensate by increasing hepatic protein synthesis, including Hp, although Hp 1-1 is relatively small and losses are similar to albumin. Hp 2-1 and 2-2 phenotypes express large forms of Hp that have lower clearance rates, so they are increased in concentration in some protein-losing states.

Corticosteroid Effects. Glucocorticoids and androgens increase synthesis and plasma concentrations of Hp. Exogenous steroids, such as dexamethasone, may enhance the response to interleukins rather than directly affecting synthesis.

Decreased Plasma Concentrations. Decreased concentrations of Hp are seen with genetic deficiency, hemolytic disease, ineffective erythropoiesis, estrogens, and hepatocellular disease, and in neonates.

Genetic Deficiency. Genetic absence (anhaptoglobinemia, or *Hp0*) and hypohaptoglobinemia are rare. Detection of genetic Hp deficiency is complicated by high rates of hemolytic disease, either genetic (e.g., hemoglobinopathies, glucose-6-phosphatase deficiency) or acquired (e.g., malaria).

Hemolytic Disease and Ineffective Erythropoiesis. As discussed previously, Hp concentrations are a sensitive indicator of in vivo hemolysis. Splenomegaly and ineffective hematopoiesis also decrease Hp concentrations. The latter, with increased hemolysis of red cells and their precursors in bone marrow, is seen in megaloblastic anemias (vitamin B_{12} or folate deficiency) and in many hemoglobinopathies.

Estrogens. Endogenous or exogenous estrogens (e.g., in late pregnancy, in oral contraceptive therapy) decrease Hp synthesis and plasma concentrations.

Hepatocellular Disease. Most forms of acute or chronic hepatocellular disease, including acute viral hepatitis and cirrhosis, are associated with decreased concentrations of Hp, possibly caused in part by altered estrogen metabolism. Biliary obstruction is associated with increased Hp concentrations in the absence of severe hepatocellular disease.

Newborn Period. Hp is absent or present in very low concentration in most newborns as a result of hepatic immaturity. In addition, hemopexin concentrations in newborns are on average one fifth adult concentrations.

Genetic Aspects of Hp. The gene encoding Hp is on chromosome 16. Polymorphism of the α-chain accounts for the commonly recognized Hp isotypes. Additional genotype variation, related to point mutations, can be detected by changes in electrophoretic mobility or isoelectric focusing.[87] The distribution of Hp 1-1, 2-1, and 2-2 genotypes varies markedly in different populations (Figure 21-4). The 1-1 genotype occurs in more than 50% of the population in some African and indigenous South American populations, but in only about 10 to 20% of most European and North American whites and in <10% of most Asian populations.[15,87]

Laboratory Considerations for Hp. Immunoturbidimetry and immunonephelometry usually are employed for clinical assays. RID requires correction for Hp genotype because of the different molecular sizes and the diffusion of different Hp genotypes. Traditionally, Hp was measured by assaying peroxidase activity after mixing serum with an excess of free hemoglobin, the so-called hemoglobin-binding capacity. On average, 1 mg hemoglobin is bound by 1.5 mg Hp, depending on the genotype.[70]

Reference Intervals for Hp. The recommended reference interval for Hp in serum for adults is 0.3 to 2.0 g/L (30 to 200 mg/dL).[22] Concentrations are low to absent in the

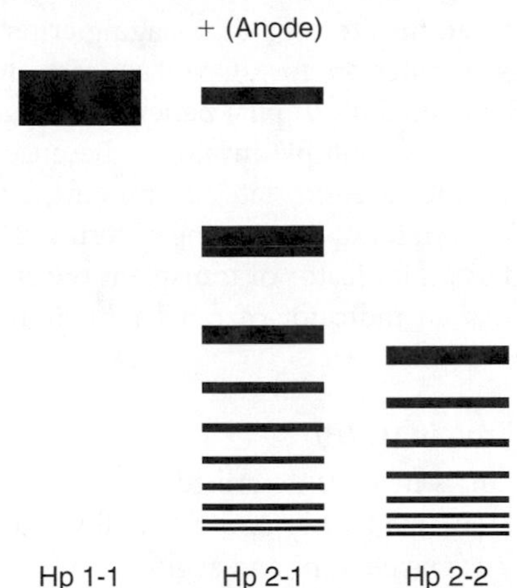

Figure 21-4 Common phenotypes of haptoglobin, as shown by sieving gel electrophoresis of haptoglobin-hemoglobin complexes. *(From Langlois MR, Delanghe JR. Biological and clinical significance of haptoglobin polymorphism in humans. Clin Chem 1996;42:1589-600.)*

neonatal period and low in women who are pregnant or on exogenous estrogen therapy, including oral contraceptives. For children, the reference interval is approximately 0.2 to 1.6 g/L. Concentrations of Hp vary with genotype as follows: 0.57 to 2.27 g/L in Hp 1-1, 0.44 to 1.83 g/L in Hp 2-1, and 0.38 to 1.50 g/L in Hp 2-2.[70,87]

Transferrin (Tf)

Transferrin (originally named *siderophilin*) is the principal plasma transport protein for iron (Fe^{3+}); Chapter 32 describes iron metabolism.

Biochemistry of Tf. Transferrin (Tf) has a molecular weight of 79.6 kDa, including 5.5% carbohydrate. It is a single polypeptide chain, with two *N*-linked oligosaccharides and two homologous domains, each with an Fe^{3+}-binding site. It is synthesized mainly in the liver, with lesser amounts in the choroid plexus of the brain. Plasma concentrations are regulated primarily by iron; in iron deficiency, plasma Tf concentrations rise and on successful treatment with iron return to normal. Tf has a usual half-life of 8 to 10 days. As with albumin, about half of Tf exists in extravascular fluids. Tf reversibly binds two ferric ions and associated anions, usually bicarbonate. The two binding sites for iron have high affinity at physiologic pH, but lower affinity at decreased pH, allowing release of iron in intracellular compartments. Tf has an absorbance maximum at 470 nm related to its iron complex.

Function of Tf. Iron metabolism is discussed in greater detail in Chapter 32. Apotransferrin binds iron absorbed from the intestine or released from catabolism of hemoglobin after oxidation of ferrous (Fe^{2+}) to ferric (Fe^{3+}) ions by Cp. Tf is bound by surface receptors for Tf and is internalized into intracellular compartments where Fe^{3+} is released from Tf. Fe^{3+} is reduced to Fe^{2+} for storage in ferritin or utilization in iron-containing molecules such as hemoglobin and cytochromes. After delivery of iron, apotransferrin is recycled back into the circulation.

Clinical Significance of Tf

Increased Plasma Concentrations. High concentrations of Tf occur in iron deficiency anemia, as well as in pregnancy and during estrogen administration.[70] Plasma Tf concentrations assist in evaluating hypochromic microcytic anemia and in monitoring treatment. In iron deficiency, Tf is increased but iron saturation is decreased. On the other hand, in anemia of chronic disease, Tf concentration may be normal or low, but iron saturation is high. In iron overload (e.g., hereditary hemochromatosis, recurrent red cell transfusion), Tf concentration is normal, but saturation (normally 30 to 38%) exceeds 55% and may be as great as 100%. Interpreting serum iron and iron saturation is complicated by large diurnal variation. Serum iron concentration is highest in morning and decreases markedly in the evening. In cases of iron overload, some iron may circulate bound to other proteins such as albumin. Saturation >100% may be observed for toxic overdoses of iron or with administration of parenteral iron preparations.

Decreased Plasma Concentrations. Transferrin is a negative APR; low concentrations occur in inflammation or malignancy. Decreased synthesis occurs with chronic liver disease (see Chapter 50) and malnutrition. Protein loss, as in the nephrotic syndrome or protein-losing enteropathies, also results in low concentrations. In hereditary atransferrinemia, a very low concentration of Tf is accompanied by iron overload and severe hypochromic anemia resistant to iron therapy.

Carbohydrate-Deficient Transferrin (CDT). Glycosylation of transferrin may be decreased or absent in certain circumstances. Congenital disorders of glycosylation affect glycosylation of many proteins, including Tf, and result in varying multisystem dysfunction, usually with brain involvement. Disorders of glycosylation can be identified by separations of Tf by electrophoresis or isoelectric focusing due to decreased charge from sialic acids.[9,100]

CDT, which migrates in a β_2 rather the usual β_1 position of Tf, occurs in CSF and has been used as in indicator of CSF leakage in fluid from the ear or nasal passages (see later section on CSF proteins). Increased CDT in plasma also has been used as an indicator of alcohol abuse. Transfer of oligosaccharides is deficient, so that none or one oligosaccharide is attached rather than two as in normal Tf. The decreased amount of sialic acid and the negative charge of CDT allow separation from normal Tf by (1) electrophoresis, (2) capillary electrophoresis, (3) ion-exchange chromatography, or (4) isoelectric focusing. Genetic variants of Tf may complicate interpretation of results based on charge separation. Mass spectrometry analyzes Tf after antibody capture and determines the ratio of CDT to total Tf based on peaks separated by mass/charge.[143] An immunoassay for CDT detects an epitope in CDT that is blocked in Tf by glycosylation.[168] CDT usually is a minor component (<2% of total Tf). Determining the best cutoff value for detecting alcohol abuse may require adjustments per method of analysis, gender, and other factors.

Only about 30% of individuals become positive at four drinks per day, but CDT rises with higher alcohol intake.[168]

Genetic Aspects of Tf. The Tf gene is on chromosome 3. At least 22 genetic variants of Tf have been identified, with up to 25% heterozygotes present in some populations. The wild type is Tf C. Tf variants all bind iron and have no recognized significance except for the rare congenital deficiency, atransferrinemia. However, they may be misinterpreted as monoclonal immunoglobulins or as CDT.

Laboratory Considerations for Tf. Transferrin is commonly assayed by immunoturbidimetry and immunonephelometry. It migrates in the β_1 region on routine serum electrophoresis; genetic variants may have altered mobility. Tf can be estimated from total iron-binding capacity (see Chapter 32).

Reference Intervals for Tf. Serum reference intervals based on CRM 470[22] are as follows:

	g/L	mg/dL
Newborn	1.17-2.50	117-250
Adults (20-60 y)	2.0-3.6	200-360
>60 y	1.6-3.4	160-340

β_2-Microglobulin (BMG)

β_2-Microglobulin is a small protein that increases in immune activation and in renal failure, because its major clearance mechanism is glomerular filtration.

Biochemistry of BMG. BMG is a small protein 99 residues in length with MW of 11.8 kDa. It is the noncovalently bound light chain subunit of class I major histocompatibility complex molecules on the surfaces of all nucleated cells. BMG is shed into the blood, particularly by B lymphocytes and some tumor cells. BMG is a nonglycosylated polypeptide chain with one intrachain disulfide bridge. Its small size allows efficient glomerular filtration, resulting in a plasma half-life of ≈110 minutes. Minor variants can arise from proteolysis in plasma during renal failure and in urine.[19]

Clinical Significance of BMG. High plasma concentrations occur in renal failure, inflammation, and neoplasms, especially those associated with B lymphocytes. Patients with renal failure have a large increase in BMG, because glomerular filtration usually is the primary clearance mechanism.[19,161] For example, compared with a reference interval of 0.7 to 1.8 mg/L,[60] plasma or serum BMG concentrations in patients on low-flux renal dialysis are about 40 mg/L. High-flux renal dialysis yields values of about 20 mg/L.[153] BMG concentrations and efficiency of BMG clearance during dialysis are clinically significant in chronic renal failure, because high plasma concentrations of BMG promote deposition of BMG as amyloid, leading to systemic amyloidosis in many patients on long-term dialysis.[19] In patients with chronic lymphocytic leukemia, high BMG concentrations are a prognostic marker for decreased treatment-free survival and overall survival, although some correction should be made for patients with renal failure.[23] In the International Staging System for multiple myeloma, serum or plasma BMG concentrations are used as a staging criterion.[82] BMG <3.5 mg/L is a criterion for stage I disease and a better prognosis. BMG ≥5.5 mg/L puts patients in stage III with a poorer prognosis of multiple myeloma. Because BMG concentrations are increased in states of immune activation and increased turnover, serial monitoring of serum BMG also has been applied as an indicator of transplant rejection. Urinary BMG serves as an indicator of renal tubular function (see Chapter 25).

C-Reactive Protein (CRP)

Tillet and Francis in 1930 described a substance in the sera of acutely ill patients that bound cell wall C-polysaccharide of *Streptococcus pneumoniae* and agglutinated the organisms. In 1941, the substance was shown to be a protein and named C-reactive protein. A long history of using CRP as a marker for inflammation has been documented.[130]

Biochemistry of CRP. CRP consists of five identical, nonglycosylated polypeptide subunits of 23,028 Da noncovalently associated to form a disk-shaped structure with radial symmetry and total mass of ≈115 kDa. Its pentameric structure leads to the family name pentraxin for CRP and related proteins such as serum amyloid P and pentraxin-3 (PTX3).[99] CRP binds not only the polysaccharides present in many bacteria, fungi, and protozoal parasites but—in the presence of free calcium ions—phosphorylcholine; phosphatidylcholines such as lecithin; and polyanions such as nucleic acids. In the absence of calcium ions, CRP also binds polycations such as histones. CRP has a circulating half-life of 18 to 20 hours.[129]

Function of CRP. CRP aids in nonspecific host defense against infectious organisms and breakdown products of cells. CRP complexes activate the classical complement pathway starting at C1q (see next section), resulting in phagocytosis via C3b receptors. However, CRP complexes bind factor H, a complement inhibitory factor, greatly reducing the activation of late components (C5 to C9) and positive feedback via the alternative pathway (see later section on complement). CRP is catabolized when complexes are engulfed by phagocytes. However, whether CRP is catabolized by any other route is not clear. No genetic abnormalities have been reported for circulating CRP.

Clinical Significance of CRP

Acute-Phase Response (APR). CRP is one of the strongest acute-phase reactants, with plasma concentrations rising up to 1000-fold after myocardial infarction, stress, trauma, infection, inflammation, surgery, or neoplastic proliferation.[21,42] Concentrations >5 to 10 mg/L suggest the presence of an infection or inflammatory process. Concentrations are generally higher in bacterial than viral infection, although concentrations >100 mg/L (10 mg/dL) may be seen in uncomplicated influenza and infectious mononucleosis. The increase with inflammation occurs within 6 to 12 hours and peaks at about 48 hours. It is generally proportional to tissue damage. Because the increase is nonspecific, however, it cannot be interpreted without other clinical information. Umbilical cord blood normally has low CRP (0.01 to 0.35 mg/L), but with intrauterine (fetal) bacterial infection, concentrations may be as high as 260 mg/L.[70]

Determination of CRP is clinically useful to screen for organic disease; to assess activity of inflammatory diseases, such as rheumatoid arthritis; to detect intercurrent infections in systemic lupus erythematosus (SLE), in leukemia, or after surgery (secondary rise in plasma concentration); to detect rejection in renal allograft recipients; and to detect neonatal septicemia and meningitis.[70] For unknown reasons, CRP responses vary in some diseases that otherwise are apparently similar. For example, the CRP response in SLE and ulcerative colitis, even when signs and symptoms of inflammation are obvious, is slight in contrast to the strong response in rheumatoid arthritis and Crohn's disease.[70]

Risk of Cardiovascular Disease. Epidemiologic studies demonstrate that increased serum CRP concentrations are associated with risk of cardiovascular disease (see Chapter 27).[110] Increased concentrations may reflect low-grade, chronic intimal inflammation. The use of CRP for these purposes requires assays with detection limits <0.3 mg/L that generally are referred to as high-sensitivity CRP assays.[130] Usually, separate assays are used to assess large increases in CRP with inflammation due to the much higher concentrations that must be measured.

Laboratory Considerations for CRP. CRP is normally present in plasma at a concentration <5 mg/L. High concentrations in inflammatory states are measured with direct immunoturbidimetric or immunonephelometric assays using antibody to CRP. High-sensitivity assays to measure CRP in healthy subjects often require particle-enhanced (also termed *latex-enhanced*) immunoturbidimetric or immunonephelometric assays or sandwich-type assay formats. CRP migrates on agarose gel electrophoresis anywhere from the slow-γ to mid-β regions, depending on the calcium ion content of the buffer. Quantities are too small to yield a visibly stained band except in extreme inflammation.

Reference Interval for CRP. The reference interval for CRP in adults is 0-≤5 mg/L (0.5 mg/dL) using less-sensitive assays applied to detection of inflammatory responses.[22] High-sensitivity assays are needed to measure CRP in healthy individuals and to use CRP as an indicator of cardiovascular risk. A cutoff of 2 mg/L or more was used for increased cardiovascular risk in the JUPITER trial.[110]

Complement Proteins

The complement system consists of more than 20 proteins, synthesized primarily by the liver. Complement deficiencies are associated with a variety of disease processes, but diagnosis is often overlooked.[146] The complement system has been divided into six groups by function:

1. The *classical pathway,* which includes C1, C4, C2, and C3 (in order of activation)
2. The *alternative pathway,* which includes C3, factors B and D, and properdin
3. The lectin pathway
4. The *membrane attack complex,* which includes C5 through C9
5. *Inhibitors* and *inactivators* of the previous pathways, including C1 inhibitor, factors H and I, and C4b-binding protein (C4bp)
6. *Cellular regulators and receptors* for activated or cell-bound complement factors

In the late 1800s, Bordet found that heat-labile and heat-stable fractions of serum contributed to in vitro killing of microorganisms and, therefore, protection of animals against infection. Ehrlich termed the labile fraction *complement;* immunoglobulins made up the stable fraction. Protein fractionation in the 1960s identified the nine "classical" components, and the current numbering of components was adopted by the World Health Organization in 1968. Deficiency of any component in the classical pathway can be identified using assays of hemolytic activity commonly expressed as CH50, the dilution yielding 50% hemolysis.[158]

The classical pathway is activated primarily by antibody-antigen complexes. An antibody-independent or alternative pathway, also termed the *properdin pathway,* was initially identified through activation of hemolytic activity with cobra venom factor. The alternative pathway is activated by the classical pathway (providing amplification), by bacterial lipopolysaccharides, cellular proteases, or cobra venom factor. A third pathway, the lectin pathway, is activated by binding of ficolins or mannan-binding protein (MBP; also referred to as mannose-binding protein or lectin, or mannan-binding lectin) to mannose-rich oligosaccharides that are present in the cell walls of many microorganisms.[113,159,173] The three types of ficolin and MBP work analogous to C1q in activating two associated protease zymogens: mannan-binding protein–associated serine protease-I and -II (MASP-I and MASP-II). MASP-II cleaves C4 and C2 analogous to the action of C1s. Activation of pathways generates cascades of protease activation and cleavage products, as outlined in Figure 21-5.

During activation, many of the complement components are enzymatically cleaved into two fragments. The larger fragments are designated by a lowercase *b,* and the smaller ones by a lowercase *a.* The larger fragments usually contain a binding site for membranes, immune complexes, and protein association, or, in several cases, represent proteases that activate subsequent component(s). Thus the larger cell-bound fragment of C3 is C3b, whereas the small fragment C3a is released to serve as an anaphylatoxic and chemotactic peptide. Inactivated fragments are designated by the letter *i* (e.g., C3bi). C3i represents C3 in which the thioester essential for activity has degraded. The persisting membrane-bound portion of C3b after inactivation is called C3d, and the major fragment after enzymatic cleavage in solution is called C3c. Activated complexes often are indicated by a bar over the components.

Complement activation results in opsonization or lysis of microorganisms, immune complexes, and debris, and immune activation and recruitment of white cells through release of inflammatory mediators. A few of the effector pathways are listed here:

1. Release of bioactive peptides, C3a and C5a in particular, which act as anaphylatoxins and chemotaxins.

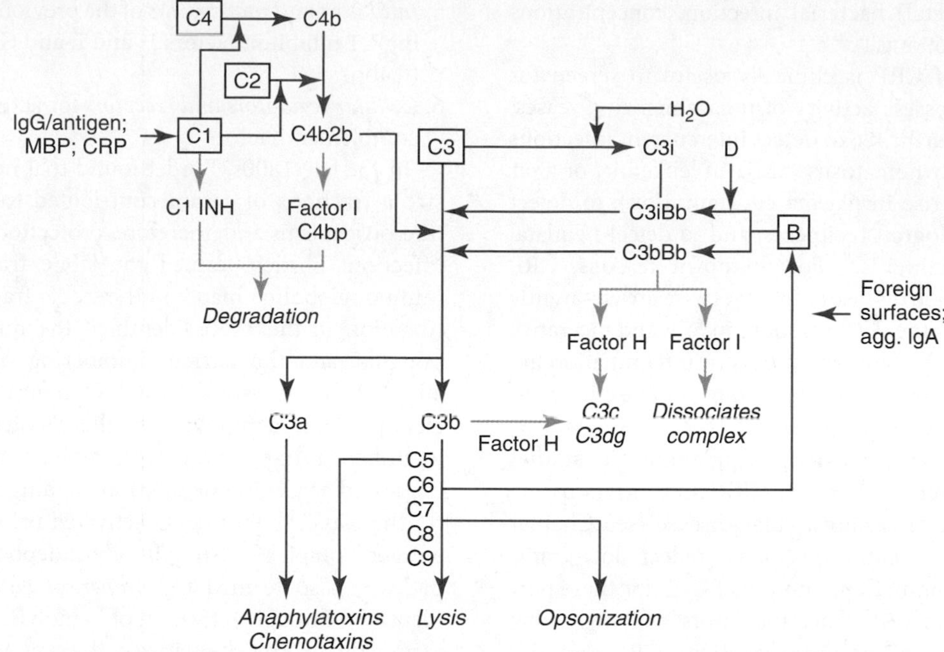

Figure 21-5 The complement cascades. Activation via the classical pathway is shown on the left and via the alternative pathway on the right. Continuous slow hydrolysis of C3 to C3i is shown at the center top. Direct activation of C3 by neutrophil and plasma proteases also may occur. The control mechanisms are shaded. *(Courtesy J.W. Whicher, with modifications.)*

Anaphylatoxins stimulate the release of histamine from mast cells, contraction of smooth muscles, and increased vascular permeability. Chemotaxins attract neutrophils and macrophages into areas of inflammation.

2. Surface-bound C3b and C4b are opsonins, mediating the binding of microbes or immune complexes to complement receptors on phagocytes, which ingest the particles. (*Opsonin* is derived from a Greek word for "preparing food for ingestion.")
3. Activating the membrane-attack complex through C9 is cytolytic by creating holes in cell membranes. This mechanism appears to be important mainly for control of neisserial infections in human beings, as indicated by genetic deficiencies of C6-C9.
4. C4b and C3b solubilize immune complexes by disrupting lattice formation and directing their removal through opsonization.
5. C3d-kallikrein complexes promote the release of neutrophils from bone marrow.
6. Activation of C1s and C2b can activate the clotting, fibrinolytic, and kinin systems and platelets.
7. Interactions of complement complexes with cellular receptors influence antibody responses.

Through these mechanisms, complement factors are major mediators of inflammatory responses to infection or injury. Increased vascular permeability permits the passage of additional antibody, complement, and phagocytes into extravascular spaces, aiding in the killing and removal of infectious agents and immune complexes. Complement activation by the lectin pathway or CRP binding represents innate responses that may be important in early responses to infection, in immunosuppressed patients, and in infancy before high concentrations of antibody are produced versus a pathogen.[159] After antibodies are produced, complement serves as a further effector mechanism. The high incidence of systemic lupus erythematosus and inflammatory disease in patients with complement deficiencies suggests that complement also has roles in suppressing inflammation, possibly through clearance of immune complexes.

The constant slow ongoing activation of complement factors would lead to accumulation of complement factors on cells such as red blood cells and would result in their lysis or clearance if factors were not present on cell surfaces to suppress complement activation and promote removal of C3b and C4b bound to cell surfaces. A few of these factors include decay-accelerating factor (DAF or CD55), protectin (CD59), membrane cofactor protein (MCP), and complement receptor 1. Deficiency of these factors can lead to lysis of red cells or other cells. As an example, in the disorder paroxysmal nocturnal hematuria (PNH), amounts of DAF and CD59 on cell surfaces are decreased by deficiency of enzymes that generate glycosyl-phosphatidylinositol linkages that attach DAF, CD59, and other proteins to cell membranes.[119] Complement regulatory factors on cell surfaces help to prevent destruction of endogenous cells at the same time that foreign cells are destroyed by complement.

The clinical importance of the complement system is demonstrated by the disease associations seen in inherited deficiency of various components, with examples listed in Table 21-9. Deficiencies do not simply increase susceptibility to

TABLE 21-9 Clinical Disorders Associated With Inherited Deficiencies of Complement Components

Component	Frequency of Deficiency	Associated Disorders
Ficolins 1-3	Rare?	Recurrent infection
MBP	5%	Infection in infancy; less effect on adults
MASP	Rare?	Recurrent infection (e.g., pneumococcal); inflammation
C1q*	Relatively rare	SLE; DLE; GN
C1r, C1s	Rare	SLE; DLE; infection
C2	≥0.0003% (homozygous)	Recurrent infection, vasculitis; SLE, DLE (no antinuclear antibody); half of affected individuals are asymptomatic
C3	Rare	Severe and recurrent bacterial infection, especially with encapsulated, pyogenic bacteria
C4A	13% (heterozygous)	SLE, DLE
C4B	13% (heterozygous)	IgA nephropathy; infection
Combined C4	35% one null; 8-10% 2 nulls; ≈1% 3 nulls; <0.1% 4 null alleles	Total deficiency: SLE, GN, DLE (many are anti-dsDNA negative but anti-Ro/SSA positive)
C5-C9	Rare	Severe or recurrent infection with *Neisseria* species
Properdin	Rare	*X*-linked; neisserial infection
Factor D	Rare	Recurrent infection
Factor H or I	Rare	Hypercatabolism of C3; recurrent bacterial infection; hemolytic-uremic syndrome in factor H deficiency
C1 inhibitor	0.002%	Hereditary angioedema (autosomal dominant)
Decay accelerating Factor (DAF, CD 55)	Rare	Paroxysmal nocturnal hematuria (PNH) related to decreased DAF and CD59 on cell surfaces

*Both quantitative and qualitative (functional) deficiencies reported.
DLE, Discoid lupus erythematosus; *GN,* glomerulonephritis; *SLE,* systemic lupus erythematosus (or SLE-like disease).
Modified from Colten HR, Rosen FS. Complement deficiencies. Annu Rev Immunol 1992;10:809-34; and Unsworth DJ. Complement deficiency and disease. J Clin Pathol 2008;61:1013-7.

infectious disease but are also associated with autoimmune disorders such as SLE and Sjögren's syndrome.[158] Despite the redundancy of multiple pathways of complement activation, deficiencies in early components of individual pathways are associated with clinical disorders. As an example, genetic deficiency of just one of the three ficolins is associated with recurrent infection.[113] Deficiency of mannan-binding protein may affect about 5% of many populations and is associated with recurrent infection in childhood, before antibodies reach high concentrations, and in patients with bone marrow transplants.[158,159] Partial deficiency of C4 also is fairly common. Genetic polymorphism is recognized for a number of components. The genetic aspects of C3 and C4 are discussed here.

C3: The Third Component of Complement

C3 is the most abundant complement component and is cleaved by all pathways of complement activation (see Figure 21-5). C3 is homologous to C4, C5, and AMG. A reactive internal thioester in C3 forms covalent bonds to target molecules and surfaces when it is activated.

Biochemistry and Function of C3

C3 is synthesized as a precursor that is cleaved into two disulfide-linked chains, α (110 kDa) and β (75 kDa). An internal thioester forms in the α-chain between sidechains of glutamine and cysteine that are separated by two residues. C3 contains ≈3% carbohydrate. C3 is synthesized mainly by hepatocytes; endotoxin induces synthesis by monocytes and fibroblasts. Activation via any pathway of complement activation results in the cleavage of C3. The small fragment C3a acts as an anaphylatoxin and a chemotactic factor. Upon cleavage of C3, the reactive thioester in the large fragment C3b becomes accessible and rapidly forms covalent bonds with neighboring molecules. C3b anchored to other molecules then participates in the cascade generating the membrane-attack complex. C3b also acts as an opsonin, binding to receptors on phagocytic cells, resulting in the ingestion of bacteria, viruses, and other foreign particles by these cells. C3 has a usual half-life of 2 to 3 days.

Low rates of hydrolysis of the thioester of C3 generate C3i continuously in plasma. C3i can bind factor B, which then is cleaved by factor D. The resulting C3iBb complex is a weak C3 convertase, producing slow activation of C3. Upon activation of the classical pathway, membrane-bound C3b forms similar complexes with factor B; C3bBb is a more active C3 convertase. The resulting positive feedback amplifies the complement activity many-fold. Normal control mechanisms prevent complete activation and depletion of C3. Factor H speeds dissociation of factor Bb from convertases, and factor I cleaves C3b to C3c and C3dg. Hereditary deficiency of factor H or factor I can lead to depletion of C3. Properdin and so-called nephritic factors (autoantibodies) also increase complement activation by stabilizing C3bBb and protecting it from factors H and I.[70]

Clinical Significance

Increased Plasma Concentrations. C3 concentrations increase with the APR, with biliary obstruction, and with focal glomerulosclerosis.[70]

Acute-Phase Response. C3 synthesis is induced by cytokines IL-1, IL-6, and TNF-α. Concentrations rise modestly after trauma or surgery and during inflammatory processes (Table 21-10).

Biliary Obstruction. C3 concentrations increase in biliary obstruction in direct proportion to hyperbilirubinemia.

Focal Glomerulosclerosis. In contrast to nephritic disorders, in which most patients with active disease have low concentrations of C3, about 30% of patients with idiopathic focal glomerulosclerosis have elevated concentrations, which indicate a favorable prognosis.

Decreased Plasma Concentrations. Decreased concentrations of C3 occur with genetic deficiency, increased turnover, and infancy.

Genetic Deficiency. Inherited primary deficiency of C3 is associated with a greatly increased risk for infection, particularly with encapsulated bacteria. Deficiency of the inactivators of C3, including factors H and I, results in secondary deficiency of C3 and a similar clinical disorder.

Acquired Deficiency. Any process increasing activation of C3 in vivo usually is associated with decreased plasma concentrations; examples are lupus nephritis and severe infection. Turnover is increased and extended by the presence of C3 nephritic factor. In addition to increasing consumption of C3, acute poststreptococcal glomerulonephritis can decrease synthesis for several weeks. Sequential concentrations of C3 can monitor recovery from this disorder. Low C3 concentrations in patients with systemic lupus nephritis suggest risk of active nephritis. Fulminant septicemia, in particular with *Neisseria meningitidis,* is associated with hypocomplementemia, whether or not shock develops.

Infancy. Concentrations in neonates are approximately two thirds of adult concentrations, which are reached by ≈1 year of age.

TABLE 21-10 Diseases in Which Estimates of Complement Factors May Be Useful for Diagnosis

Disease	Complement Status
Systemic lupus erythematosus	C4 usually low, C3 sometimes low*
Rheumatoid vasculitis	C3 usually low*
Subacute bacterial endocarditis	Both C3* and C4 low
Shunt nephritis	Both C3* and C4 low
Poststreptococcal glomerulonephritis	C3 low,* usually returns to normal in 3 months
Mesangiocapillary glomerulonephritis	C3 low* (persistent), C4 normal
Polymyalgia rheumatica	C3 conversion products found
Mixed cryoglobulinemia	C3 conversion products found
Gram-negative bacteremic shock (early diagnosis)	C3 low,* C4 normal, factor B low
Gram-positive bacteremia	Both C3* and C4 low
Disseminated cytomegalovirus infection	C4 very low, C3* normal or increased

*C3 conversion products also present

Genetic Aspects of C3

C3 is coded by a gene on chromosome 19. More than 25 known inherited variants are demonstrable by prolonged agarose gel electrophoresis of serum; the most common are C3S and C3F (for "slow" and "fast," respectively). Most are associated with normal concentrations and function; one, C3f, has the same mobility as C3F but is present in approximately 50% of the normal concentration. Genetic deficiency is discussed earlier under "Clinical Significance."[70]

Laboratory Considerations for C3

C3 is usually quantified by immunoturbidimetric or immunonephelometric methods. Because of differences in immunochemical reactivity of C3 and C3c, reference materials should be completely converted to C3c and stabilized, as is the case for the international reference material CRM 470.[167] C3 concentrations measured on fresh samples may be lower than after storage for 8 hours or longer, possibly as the result of conversion of C3 to C3i or C3c. Intact C3 in serum migrates on agarose gel electrophoresis in the β_2-region in the presence of free Ca^{2+}. However, it is a relatively labile protein, with conversion to more anodal forms, C3c and C3dg, on extended storage. Electrophoretic variants, including C3F, may be confused with monoclonal immunoglobulins. Assays for complement activation require plasma samples obtained with precautions to limit activation by plasmin, C1s, and leukocyte proteases. Centrifugation should be performed immediately, and the separated plasma should be frozen at below −40 °C.

Reference Intervals for C3

C3 concentrations are low in newborns, then rise and remain relatively constant after the first year of life. The recommended reference interval for adults, based on CRM 470, is 0.9 to 1.8 g/L (90 to 180 mg/dL).[22] Concentrations are slightly lower in fresh serum (assayed within 8 hours after drawing).

The Fourth Component of Complement: C4

C4 is actually a pair of two highly homologous proteins C4A and C4B from closely linked genes that differ only in a few amino acids (note that these are different from the cleavage products C4A and C4B). C4A and C4B are homologous to C3, C5, and AMG.

Biochemistry and Function of C4

C4 has a molecular mass of 206 kDa, including ≈4% carbohydrate. Most synthesis occurs in hepatocytes; some may occur in monocytes or other tissues. C4 is synthesized as a single chain (proC4) that is cleaved into three chains: α, β, and γ, linked by disulfide bonds. The α-chain has an internal thioester that, on activation, becomes accessible and forms covalent bonds with neighboring molecules, resulting in "fixation" to membranes, viruses, and immune complexes.

C4 participates in the classical pathway. However, most individuals with C4 deficiency do not have increased susceptibility to bacterial infection, suggesting that the alternative pathway can compensate for the lack of classical pathway activation in removal of bacterial agents; C4 may be more critical for clearance of infecting viruses and immune complexes. C4b2b bound to immune complexes prevents their precipitation and promotes immune complex clearance by the CRa receptor. C4A and C4B have differential specificities in their surface reactivities and may have differential effects on immune complex clearance. C4a, the small fragment released on activation of C4, is a weak anaphylatoxin.

Clinical Significance of C4

Increased Plasma Concentrations. C4 concentrations are modestly increased by the APR.

Decreased Plasma Concentrations. C4 concentrations are low in genetic deficiency, increased turnover, and infancy.

Genetic Deficiency. Complete deficiency of C4 is rare and is strongly associated with autoimmune or collagen vascular disease, particularly SLE, and, in a few cases, with susceptibility for infection.[158] Partial deficiency of C4 is much more common. Isolated deficiency of C4A is markedly increased in patients with SLE as well, but it is not clear whether this results from decreased clearance of immune complexes or from linkage to other genes. Approximately 20% of individuals with deficiency of IgA also have homozygous deficiency of C4A, as do some with combined IgA and IgG subclass deficiencies, suggesting that the gene for a B-cell maturation factor is linked to C4A.

Acquired Deficiency. Concentrations of C4 are more commonly depressed because of consumption; most individuals with SLE and low C4 concentrations do not have genetic deficiency. Other disorders associated with consumption and low concentrations include hereditary angioedema (C1 inhibitor deficiency), autoimmune hemolytic anemia, and autoimmune nephritis.

Infancy. C4 concentrations in newborn infants are approximately 50 to 75% of adult concentrations.

Genetic Aspects of C4

C4 is coded by two genes, C4A and C4B, in the major histocompatibility complex region of chromosome 6p, closely linked to the genes for C2, factor B, and HLA-DR. Linkage to immune response genes may account for most disease associations of C4 variants with deficiency. The C4A and C4B proteins differ by only four amino acids near the thioester in the α-chain, and these sequence differences alter reactivity. C4A binds more efficiently with amino groups in proteins and C4B with hydroxyl groups in oligosaccharides. C4d fragments of C4A and C4B bound to erythrocytes are the Rodgers and Chido blood group antigens. Both C4 loci are highly polymorphic, mostly because of substitutions in the α-chain. Either or both loci may be deleted, unexpressed, or duplicated; as a result, a given individual may have zero to four copies of each locus. Both the total C4 concentration and the ratio of C4A to C4B depend on the number of copies of each locus. Most C4A variants have 25 to 35% of the hemolytic activity of the C4B alleles.[70]

Laboratory Considerations for C4

C4 usually is measured by immunoturbidimetric or immunonephelometric methods. Low concentrations alone cannot differentiate between genetic and acquired deficiency; tests for breakdown products (e.g., C4a des-arginine) or neoantigens may assist in detecting increased turnover. C4 has β_1 electrophoretic mobility, similar to that of transferrin, but normally is not visualized because of its low concentration. Phenotyping of C4 proteins can be performed by electrophoresis of neuraminidase-treated EDTA plasma, followed by immunofixation. Hemolytic gel overlay can help identify C4B bands. DNA genotyping can also determine the types in most cases but cannot distinguish between synthesizing and nonsynthesizing genes. If C4 concentrations are to be used to monitor disease activity in patients with SLE, genotyping or phenotyping of C4 may be indicated.[70]

Reference Intervals for C4

As with C3, concentrations are low in neonates but relatively constant after the first year of life. The recommended interim reference interval for adults, based on CRM 470, is 0.1 to 0.4 g/L (10 to 40 mg/dL).[22] The baseline plasma concentration of C4 in individuals with one or more null genes is lower.

IMMUNOGLOBULINS

Immunoglobulins (antibodies) are preferentially generated against foreign immunogens and initiate clearance of the foreign molecule or organism. Failure of regulatory mechanisms sometimes leads to autoantibodies that contribute to autoimmune disease. Immunoglobulins are characterized by tremendous sequence heterogeneity of their antigen-binding sites that allows binding of a diverse range of molecules.

Basic Biochemistry of Immunoglobulins

The major immunoglobulin molecules in humans consist of one or more basic units built of two identical heavy (H) chains and two identical light (L) chains.[70,125] Each of the four chains has one variable and one (L chain) or three to four (H chain) constant domains, with the variable region involved in antigen recognition and binding (see Chapter 16). Extensive diversity in the variable domains is generated by somatic recombination and mutation of the immunoglobulin genes. Individual plasma cells or clonally expanded cells are committed to synthesis of a single variable domain sequence for heavy and light chains. The amino acid sequences of the variable domains at the N-terminal ends of the four chains form two antigen-binding sites with a high degree of variation in binding specificity, allowing diversity in binding specificity. The constant domains are the same for every immunoglobulin molecule of a given subclass and carry sites for binding to complement receptors and activation of complement.

Immunoglobulins are synthesized by plasma cells, the progeny of B-lymphocyte stem cells in bone marrow (Table 21-11). More mature B lymphocytes, found mainly in lymph nodes and in blood, develop receptor immunoglobulins on their surface membranes. Recombination of segments of the variable regions of genes by the recombinases RAG1 and RAG2 helps generate diversity that allows recognition of a wide range of antigens.[115] Upon binding a target antigen, these B lymphocytes proliferate and develop into a clone of plasma cells producing antibody to the target antigen. Somatic mutation of immunoglobulins by activation-induced DNA deaminase leads to further diversity of immunoglobulin variable region and antibody maturation—generally leading to antibodies with higher affinity. B lymphocytes at first have IgM surface receptors and secrete IgM as the first or "primary" response to an antigen. Membrane and secreted forms of the antibody arise from differential splicing of the messenger RNA for heavy chains, which adds a transmembrane segment to the membrane-bound form. Heavy chains of the IgM surface receptor molecules undergo class switching to produce immunoglobulins with γ- or α-heavy chains (IgG or IgA), but the variable regions remain unchanged; as the cells change into plasma cells, second exposure to the same antigen causes a larger secondary or anamnestic response of IgG secretion.

The variable domains contain the antigen-binding regions, and the constant domains of the heavy chains contain sites for complement activation and receptor binding. Cleavage of immunoglobulins with pepsin or papain can yield antigen-binding fragments (Fab) and constant region fragments (Fc). Variations in the constant domains of heavy chains (Fc region) result in the classes and subclasses into which immunoglobulins are grouped: IgM, IgG (four subclasses), IgA (two subclasses), IgD, and IgE, respectively, containing heavy chains μ, γ, α, δ, and ε.[70,125]

Light chains, which are produced independently and in slight excess of heavy chains, are of two types—kappa (κ) and lambda (λ)—defined by constant domains with different structures. The heavy-chain genes are located on chromosome 14; κ-light chains are encoded by a gene on chromosome 2, whereas the λ-chain gene is on chromosome 22. Each plasma cell expresses only one type of light chain, so that each immunoglobulin molecule contains only one type of light chain. The proportions of κ:λ typically are about 2:1 in immunoglobulins. Light chains are usually synthesized in excess and secreted as free light chains, but concentrations usually remain low because of rapid glomerular filtration (see section on free light chains later).

Biochemistry of Individual Immunoglobulins

The individual immunoglobulins IgG, IgA, IgM, IgD, and IgE actually represent families of proteins with different sequences in their variable regions rather than typical proteins with defined sequences.

Immunoglobulin G (IgG)

IgG accounts for 70 to 75% of the total immunoglobulins in plasma. Only 35% is found in the plasma space, and 65% is extravascular. IgG consists of two γ-heavy and two light chains, linked by disulfides (see Chapter 16); its molecular weight is $\approx$150 kDa, usually including one N-linked oligosaccharide on each heavy chain. The oligosaccharide structure may change in inflammatory states and affect interactions with receptors.[72] On agarose gel electrophoresis, IgG migrates broadly in the γ- and slow β-regions as a result of its heterogeneity of charge from sequence variation.

Immunoglobulin G has four subclasses: IgG_1, IgG_2, IgG_3, and IgG_4. The circulating half-life of IgG_1, IgG_2, and IgG_4 is about 22 days—much longer than most plasma proteins—because of recycling from pinocytic vesicles via binding to the neonatal immunoglobulin receptor. IgG_3, which does not bind to the receptor, has a half-life of 7 days.[131,165] IgG_1 and

TABLE 21-11 B-Lymphocyte Lineage and Associated Malignant Neoplasms

		Immunoglobulins		
Stages in Maturation and Proliferation	Principal Site	Surface Receptor	Secreted Into Blood	Associated Malignant Neoplasms
Stem cell ↓	Bone marrow	None	None	Acute lymphoblastic leukemia
Early B lymphocyte antigen → ↓	Lymph nodes	IgM, IgD	None	Lymphoma, chronic lymphocytic leukemia (85%)
Late B-lymphocyte antigen → ↓	Lymph nodes	IgM ↓	IgM	Lymphoma, chronic lymphocytic leukemia (15%), and Waldenström's macroglobulinemia
Plasma cell	Lymphatic tissue, bone marrow	IgG, IgA	IgG, IgA	Multiple myeloma

IgG_3 strongly activate complement via the classical pathway, IgG_2 is weakly complement fixing, and IgG_4 does not activate complement. Clustering of multiple IgG molecules is required to activate complement. Both IgG_1 and IgG_3 bind Fc receptors on phagocytic cells, activate killer monocytes (K cells), and cross the placenta via receptor-mediated active transport. IgG_1 is the principal IgG to cross the placenta, and neonatal concentrations are similar to maternal concentrations. Neonates have low production of IgG as the result of immaturity of their immune systems, and IgG concentrations fall through infancy as maternally acquired antibody is cleared.

Immunoglobulin M (IgM)

IgM is produced at earlier stages of B-cell development. In the immature immune systems of neonates, IgM is the major immunoglobulin synthesized. In adult serum, it is the third most abundant immunoglobulin, usually accounting for 5 to 10% of total circulating immunoglobulins. IgM as a membrane receptor molecule is monomeric, but most of the serum IgM is a pentamer, which contains five monomers similar to IgG linked via disulfides to the small J chain. Plasma cell malignancies may secrete monomeric IgM in addition to, or instead of, pentamers. The high molecular weight of IgM (970 kDa; ≈10% carbohydrate) prevents its ready passage into extravascular spaces. IgM is not transported across the placenta and therefore is not involved in hemolytic disease of neonates. It activates complement even more efficiently than IgG; binding of one IgM molecule may be adequate to activate complement. In rare hyper-IgM syndromes, class switching to IgG and IgA is deficient, shedding light on the process of class switching. Affected patients have deficiency of IgG and IgA and increased susceptibility to infection.[30]

Immunoglobulin A (IgA)

Approximately 10 to 15% of serum immunoglobulin is IgA, which contains about 10% carbohydrate, with both N- and O-linked oligosaccharides, has a molecular weight of 160 kDa, and has a half-life of 6 days. In its monomeric form, its structure is similar to that of IgG, but 10 to 15% of IgA in serum is dimeric, particularly IgA_2, which is more resistant to destruction by pathogenic bacteria than IgA_1. On electrophoresis, IgA migrates in the β-γ region, anodal to most IgG. IgA is an important component of mucosal immunity.[170] *Secretory* IgA is found in tears, sweat, saliva, milk, colostrum, and gastrointestinal and bronchial secretions. Secretory IgA has a molecular weight of 380 kDa and consists of two molecules of IgA: a secretory component (70 kDa) and a J chain (15.6 kDa). It is synthesized mainly by plasma cells in the mucous membranes of the gut and bronchi and in the ductules of the lactating breast. The secretory component assists with transport of secretory IgA across mucosal epithelium and into secretions. Secretory IgA in colostrum and milk is more abundant than IgG and may aid in protection of neonates from intestinal infection. IgA can activate complement by the alternative pathway (see Figure 21-5), but the exact role of IgA in serum is not clear.

Immunoglobulin D (IgD)

IgD accounts for <1% of serum immunoglobulin. It is monomeric, contains about 12% carbohydrate, and has a molecular weight of 184 kDa. Its structure is similar to that of IgG. Similar to IgM, IgD is a surface receptor for antigen on B lymphocytes, but its primary function is unknown.

Immunoglobulin E (IgE)

IgE is so rapidly and firmly bound to specific IgE receptors on mast cells that only trace amounts of it are normally present in serum. IgE contains 15% carbohydrate and has a molecular weight of 188 kDa; its quaternary structure is similar to that of IgG. IgE binds to mast cells via sites on its Fc region. When the antigen (allergen) cross-links two of the attached IgE molecules, the mast cell is stimulated to release histamine and other vasoactive amines that increase vascular permeability and smooth muscle contraction, mediating type 1 hypersensitivity reactions such as hay fever, asthma, urticaria, and eczema. Rare regulatory disorders with hyperproduction of IgE lead to a primary immunodeficiency disorder, Job's syndrome, with eczema, recurrent infection, and markedly increased IgE.[40] IgE molecules specific for particular allergens are analyzed to identify the specificity of allergies. The total serum concentration of IgE may be increased in allergic disorders.

Free Immunoglobulin Light Chains

Light chains are usually synthesized in slight excess versus quantities required for intact immunoglobulins. Consequently, small amounts of free light chain, representing only about 0.1% of total immunoglobulin, usually are present in serum or plasma. Amounts in plasma are kept low by renal clearance. Free κ-light chains (23 kDa) are cleared about three times faster than free λ-light chains (a disulfide-linked dimer of 46 kDa), which have a half-life of 4 to 6 hours. Consequently, even though production of κ-light chains is about twice as great as that of λ-light chains, the plasma concentration of free λ-light chains is usually higher, except in renal failure.[65] Free light chains usually are not functional, but immunoassays specific for free light chains are applied to detect plasma cell disorders.[27]

Clinical Significance

Normally, serum contains a diverse, polyclonal mixture of antibodies with varying amino acid sequences, which represent multiple "idiotypes" (i.e., the products of many different clones of plasma cells, each producing a specific immunoglobulin molecule). Benign or malignant proliferation of one such clone produces a high concentration of a single monoclonal antibody, which may appear as a sharp, narrow band on protein electrophoresis. Unbalanced production of free light chains might also lead to a second band representing free light chains. If a few clones proliferate, several sharp bands may be seen (e.g., the oligoclonal bands seen in electrophoresis of CSF in demyelinating diseases such as multiple sclerosis, or in serum following successful bone marrow transplantation, or early during a response to such organisms as *Streptococcus pneumoniae*). Therefore, disease may be associated with a decrease or an increase in normal polyclonal immunoglobulins or an increase in one or more monoclonal immunoglobulins.

Immunoglobulin Deficiency

Immune defense depends on four complex, interactive systems: cell-mediated immunity; humoral antibodies (immunoglobulins); the phagocytic system; and the complement system. The last two systems are nonspecific in that they have no immunologic memory for the antigen. Immunodeficiency states may be the result of deficiency of a single factor or combinations affecting multiple systems of immune defense. Analysis of serum or plasma proteins allows detection primarily of deficiencies of antibody and complement systems. Several genetic disorders with immunoglobulin deficiency are summarized in Box 21-1. Diagnosis of major deficiencies in immunoglobulin production is clinically important because infants will be at increased risk of infection as their maternally acquired antibodies decline, and replacement therapy with IgG will be needed. The most common primary deficiencies involve only one or two immunoglobulin classes (IgA) or subclasses (IgA or IgG subclasses) or ability to generate antibodies versus polysaccharides; such deficiencies may be associated with increased susceptibility to infection, depending on the degree of reduction of immunoglobulin concentrations.[148] IgA deficiency varies markedly in different populations, occurring in about 1:500 whites, and much less frequently in Asian populations. IgA deficiency usually is not associated with severe infection, but the risk of nonsevere infection with *Giardia* or other organisms may be increased. IgA deficiency may lead to false-negative assays for autoantibodies for celiac disease detection, and affected individuals have some risk of anaphylaxis if they receive blood products containing IgA. Detection of antibodies to IgA serves as an indicator of risk of transfusion reactions.[13] Selective deficiency of IgG subclasses is not rare, but it is unclear whether it is an important risk for infection. Deficiency of IgG2 may be related to poorer responses to polysaccharide antigens and increased risk of infection with encapsulated organisms.[148]

Infants have transient physiologic deficiency of IgG, with a nadir at about 3 months of age; prolonged or severe physiologic deficiency may be associated with increased infection rates, especially with encapsulated bacteria. Concentrations of maternal IgG, transferred across the placenta, rise rapidly in the fetus during the last half of pregnancy but then drop over a few months following birth (Figure 21-6). Two groups of neonates are at risk for clinically significant IgG deficiency: premature infants, who start with less maternal IgG, and infants with delayed initiation of IgG synthesis. Monitoring of IgG concentrations can identify this problem. Rising IgM and normal salivary IgA concentrations at 6 weeks of age suggest a favorable prognosis. Contact of the neonate with environmental antigens normally causes B lymphocytes to begin to multiply and IgM concentrations to start to rise, followed weeks to months later by IgA and IgG.[70]

Polyclonal Hyperimmunoglobulinemia

Polyclonal increases in plasma immunoglobulins are the normal response to infection. IgG response predominates in autoimmune responses; IgA in skin, gut, respiratory, and renal infections; and IgM in primary viral infections and bloodstream parasites such as malaria. Chronic bacterial infection may cause increased concentrations of all immunoglobulins. Selective changes in immunoglobulin concentrations assist in the differential diagnosis of liver disease and of intrauterine infection. In *primary biliary cirrhosis,* the IgM concentration is greatly increased; in *chronic active hepatitis,* IgG and sometimes IgM are increased; and in *portal cirrhosis,* IgA and sometimes IgG are increased. In *intrauterine infection,* production of IgM by the fetus increases, and the IgM concentration in umbilical cord blood is increased. Measurements of total IgE are used in the management of asthma and other allergic conditions, especially in children. Measurements of allergen-specific IgE assist in identifying allergens that trigger hypersensitivity responses.[48]

BOX 21-1 Causes of Immunoglobulin Deficiency

Secondary Causes (Common)

Defective Synthesis (IgM Falls First, Then IgA, Finally IgG)

Multiple myeloma, lymphoma, chronic lymphocytic leukemia
Toxic reaction (e.g., renal failure, diabetes mellitus)
Drugs (e.g., phenytoin, penicillamine)
In neonates: prematurity, transient delay in initiation of synthesis

Abnormal Loss of Proteins

Nephrotic syndrome, burns, protein-losing enteropathy

Primary or Inherited Causes (Rare)

Failure of Antibody Production

Generalized (severe pyogenic infections occur)
Infantile X-linked Bruton's type
Acquired, variable, unclassifiable, occurring at any age
Selective immunoglobulin deficiency of

- IgA: most common (1:700), increased allergic or autoimmune disease
- IgG and IgA (IgM increased): recurrent pyogenic infection
- IgA and IgM: giardiasis common
- IgG: recurrent pyogenic infection
- IgM: susceptibility to autoimmune disease and to septicemia following splenectomy

Combined Failure of Antibody- and Cell-Mediated Immunity

Severe combined immunodeficiency. Swiss and sex-linked types, death in infancy from fungal or viral infection
Associated with thymoma, achondroplasia, or thrombocytopenia and eczema (Wiskott-Aldrich syndrome)

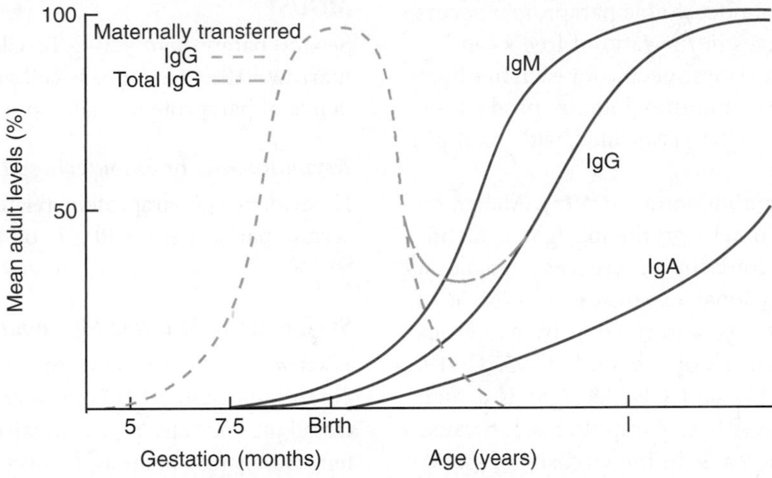

Figure 21-6 Serum immunoglobulin concentrations as percent of mean adult concentrations before birth and for the first year of life.

Monoclonal Immunoglobulins (Paraproteins)

A single clone of plasma cells produces immunoglobulin molecules with a single defined amino acid sequence. If the clone expands greatly, the concentration of its particular protein in the patient's serum may produce a discrete band on electrophoresis, often referred to as an M-spike or M-protein, which stands out from the diffuse background. These monoclonal immunoglobulins, termed *paraproteins,* may be polymers, monomers, individual immunoglobulin chains such as free light chains or heavy chains, or fragments of immunoglobulins. About 60% of paraproteins are associated with plasma cell malignancies (multiple myeloma or solitary plasmacytoma), and approximately 15% are due to overproduction by B lymphocytes, mainly in lymph nodes (lymphomas, chronic lymphocytic leukemia, Waldenström's macroglobulinemia, or heavy-chain disease). Up to 25% of paraproteins are benign and have been termed *monoclonal gammopathy of undetermined significance (MGUS).* The incidence of MGUS increases with age, with 1% incidence for people 50 to 70 years of age and 3% incidence for people older than 70. Occurrence of MGUS is associated with increased risk of progression to multiple myeloma that should be monitored. Multiple myeloma appears to be preceded consistently by MGUS.[86]

The primary clinical interest in identifying paraproteins is to detect or monitor proliferative disorders of B cells. However, from the laboratory standpoint, paraproteins are also significant as a potentially unpredictable source of interference with many assays. Paraproteins may aggregate or precipitate in a variety of photometric reactions and hematology analyzers. Occasionally, specimens with paraproteins form gels that can plug sample probes of and disable automated analyzers (see discussion of cryoglobulins later).

Many patients with paraproteins have nonspecific presentations such as anemia or infection. Identification of paraproteins in serum usually is based on serum protein electrophoresis and immunofixation electrophoresis (described in a later section), and urine protein electrophoresis and urine immunofixation electrophoresis are helpful mainly in identifying patients with free immunoglobulin light chains. Urinary free light chains, as described by Bence-Jones in the 1850s, were the first tumor marker. Free light chains, particularly in urine, are often referred to as *Bence-Jones proteins,* although this term was originally used to refer to a subset of free light chains in urine that precipitated and redissolved upon heating. Introduction of capillary electrophoresis and assays for free light chains in serum has led to a variety of approaches for detecting paraproteins.[82,103] Serum protein electrophoresis together with analysis of free light chains in serum appears to have a diagnostic yield similar to use of immunofixation on serum and urine, except for lower detection of MGUS.[73] Analysis of free light chains tends to detect residual disease or recurrence at lower concentrations than does immunofixation.[73,82]

Malignancies of B cells that commonly express paraproteins are described as follows:

Multiple Myeloma. *Multiple myeloma* is a clonal malignant neoplasm of plasma cells.[70,82] The plasma cells usually proliferate diffusely throughout the bone marrow, but occasionally they form a solitary tumor or *plasmacytoma.* Osteolytic bone lesions are produced and the other bone marrow cells are reduced, so that thrombocytopenia, anemia, and leukopenia develop. Production of normal plasma cells is suppressed; consequently, synthesis of other immunoglobulins is reduced, and recurrent infection may occur. The incidence of multiple myeloma is low in individuals younger than 60 years but increases with age. Patients may present with symptoms of a bone lesion such as pain or fracture, but more often present with nonspecific symptoms such as weight loss, anemia, hemorrhage, recurrent infection, or renal failure. A normal serum alkaline phosphatase concentration may be observed in a patient with destructive bone lesions.[70] Cardinal diagnostic features of the disease include findings of neoplastic plasma cells in bone marrow aspirate, radiologic demonstration of osteolytic lesions, and identification of a paraprotein in serum or urine. All patients who could conceivably have the disease should be screened for paraproteins;

nonsecretory myeloma with undetectable paraprotein occurs but is uncommon.[73,82] Changes in the ratio of free κ- and γ-light chains determined with assays specific for each free light chain also indicate aberrant immunoglobulin production. Table 21-12 lists the paraproteins associated with multiple myeloma.

Waldenström's Macroglobulinemia (WM). Malignant proliferation of plasmacytoid cells producing IgM is distinguished from multiple myeloma by differences in biology, outcome, and treatment.[26] Clonal expansion in WM is of more immature B cells that are characterized by numerous cell surface markers, including surface IgM, CD5, CD19, and CD20, and lacking CD10 and CD23.[82] IgM is a high molecular weight protein, and IgM paraproteins can cause concentration-dependent increases in the viscosity of blood, leading to hyperviscosity syndromes. Serum viscosity measurement helps to assess this problem. Monoclonal IgM also may behave as a cryoglobulin.

Lymphoid Tumors. *Lymphoid tumors,* such as lymphomas or chronic lymphocytic leukemias, arise from less mature stages in B-lymphocyte development; about one in five produce paraproteins, usually of the IgM class.

Classification of Plasma Cell Proliferative Disorders

Analysis of paraproteins and other laboratory studies play an important role in classification and staging of plasma cell proliferative disorders. Evidence of end-organ injury related to paraproteins is provided by hypercalcemia (calcium ≥11.5 g/dL or 2.875 mmol/L), impaired renal function (creatinine >1.95 mg/dL or 172 μmol/L), anemia, and bone lesions. Criteria for diagnosis and classification of plasma cell disorders developed by the International Myeloma Working Group have been summarized.[82]

MGUS

Serum paraprotein <30 g/L. Clonal plasma cells in bone marrow <10%. No other B-cell proliferative disorder. No evidence of paraprotein-related organ injury.

Asymptomatic or Smoldering Multiple Myeloma

No evidence of paraprotein-related organ or tissue injury, but serum paraprotein >30 g/L or bone marrow plasma cells >10%.

Symptomatic Multiple Myeloma

Paraprotein is detected in serum or urine (40% have serum paraprotein <30 g/L); bone marrow or plasmacytoma with clonal plasma cells; organ impairment related to the paraprotein. Rarely (3% of multiple myeloma), nonsecretory multiple myeloma occurs without detectable paraprotein.

Waldenström's Macroglobulinemia (WM)

Monoclonal IgM detected. Bone marrow infiltration with ≥10% small lymphocytes with typical immunophenotype, excluding other lymphoproliferative disorders.

Solitary Plasmacytoma

Solitary localized tumor of bone or soft tissue with clonal plasma cells and normal bone marrow. No other bone lesions or evidence of paraprotein-related organ injury.

Systemic Amyloid Light Chain (AL) Amyloidosis

Four criteria must be met: evidence of organ injury from systemic amyloidosis, positive amyloid staining, evidence of immunoglobulin light chains in amyloid deposits, and paraproteins or other evidence of a monoclonal plasma cell disorder.

TABLE 21-12 Monoclonal Immunoglobulins (Paraproteins) in Multiple Myeloma

Plasma Paraprotein	Incidence,* %	Age of Occurrence,* Mean	Incidence of Free Light Chain in Urine, %	Comments
IgG	50	65	60	Patients more susceptible to infection; paraproteins reach highest concentrations
IgA	25	65	70	Tend to have hypercalcemia and amyloidosis
Free light chain only	20	56	100	Often renal failure; bone lesions; amyloidosis; poor prognosis
IgD	2	57	100	90% λ type; often have extraosseous lesion, amyloidosis, renal failure; poor prognosis
IgM	1	—	100	May or may not have hyperviscosity syndrome
IgE	0.1	—	Most	—
Biclonal	1	—	—	—
None detected	<1	—	0	Usually reduction of normal immunoglobulins

*Approximate.

POEMS Syndrome

POEMS is a syndrome with polyneuropathy, organomegaly, endocrinopathy, monoclonal protein, and skin changes. Three criteria must be met: (1) presence of a monoclonal plasma cell disorder, (2) peripheral neuropathy, and (3) other related features.[82]

A couple of other plasma cell disorders that are not always included with classification lists are light chain deposition disease, in which free light chains are deposited in tissues but lack characteristics of amyloid; and plasma cell leukemia, which is identified by plasma cell counts in peripheral blood >2000/μL and plasma cells >20% of white blood cells.[73]

Heavy-Chain Disease

Heavy-chain disease is a rare disorder in which clonal production of immunoglobulin heavy chains occurs. The heavy chains are shorter than normal and lack a segment that forms disulfide bonds with light chains because of faulty recombination of variable and constant regions of heavy chains during somatic recombination. This explains the failure of heavy chains to form intact immunoglobulins. The most common form is α-chain disease, which may be associated with intestinal infiltration with the clonal population of lymphocytes and problems with malabsorption. Less commonly, heavy-chain disease may result from clonal production of γ-chains or μ-chains.

Staging of Multiple Myeloma and Monitoring of Treatment Responses

The International Staging System has been developed for objective stratification of the risk of rapid progression of multiple myeloma. It does not have a role in staging of other plasma cell disorders. Stage 1 multiple myeloma has β_2-microglobulin <3.5 mg/L and albumin ≥3.5 g/dL. Stage II has BMG ≥3.5 mg/L and <5.5 mg/L or albumin <3.5 g/dL. Stage III has BMG ≥5.5 mg/L.[82] The method of determining albumin has the potential to affect the staging of some patients. For specimens with high paraprotein concentrations, albumin concentrations estimated from serum protein electrophoresis differ from measurements by immunonephelometry or BSG.[147] A more complex staging system, the Durie-Salmon system, has been in use since 1975 and divides patients into three stages based on degree of anemia, hypercalcemia, paraprotein concentration, and number of bone lesions.[82] Recommendations for considering cytogenetic and genetic characteristics as prognostic factors, as well as LDH concentrations and serum free light chain ratios, have been proposed.[82]

Monitoring and classification of treatment responses rely on multiple factors.[82] Detection and quantification of paraproteins are major factors in assessing treatment responses. Increases in serum paraprotein concentration or urine excretion usually indicate disease progression. Decreases in paraprotein usually indicate response to treatment. Negative results from immunofixation electrophoresis for paraprotein detection serve as a major criterion in complete responses.[82] Assessment of the κ:λ ratio of free light chains in serum sometimes serves as a more sensitive indicator of paraproteins than does immunofixation electrophoresis.[73,82]

Cryoglobulinemia and Amyloid Disease

Deposition of monoclonal immunoglobulin light chains or, more rarely, heavy chains in tissues can produce systemic amyloidosis as discussed in a later section of this chapter. Cryoglobulins are serum proteins or protein complexes that precipitate at temperatures lower than normal core body temperature.[142] Precipitation of cryoglobulins in tissues can result in vasculitis and ischemic injury to peripheral tissues at a lower temperature and tissue loss of fingers, toes, nose, and other sites. Patients need to be kept in a warm environment until treatment can lower cryoglobulin concentrations. Type I cryoglobulins consist of monoclonal immunoglobulins, often IgM. Occasionally, specimens with high paraprotein concentrations will gel, and this can present major problems with plugging sample probes of automated analyzers. Most cryoglobulins consist of immunoglobulin mixed with a monoclonal component (type II) or without a monoclonal component (type III cryoglobulin). Mixed cryoglobulins often present with chronic infection, particularly with hepatitis C. Cryoglobulins require transport and processing of specimens at temperatures near body temperature to prevent loss of the cryoglobulin during serum formation and centrifugation. For cryoglobulin analysis, serum usually is stored for 7 days under refrigeration. Cryoglobulins precipitated by centrifugation should redissolve in saline when warmed to 37 °C, whereas cryofibrinogen will not dissolve. Monoclonal immunoglobulins may have unusual solubility characteristics that include not only gelling or precipitating at low temperatures, but also behaving as pyroglobulins (precipitating at 56 °C) or precipitating as a result of pH changes. Unusual solubility or physical characteristics may contribute to unpredictable interferences of paraproteins in a variety of photometric assays due to precipitation and turbidity under assay conditions as described in many reports; a recent example describes interference with the biuret assay.[155] Cryoglobulins also are recognized to interfere with automated hematology analyzers.

Laboratory Considerations

Methodologies

Immunoglobulins are typically quantified by immunoturbidimetry or immunonephelometry (see Chapters 10 and 16). Immunochemical assays of polyclonal immunoglobulins involve determining the concentration of a mixture of protein molecules having similar constant regions but different variable regions (idiotypes). Reagent antisera and reference immunoglobulin calibrators used in most immunochemical assays have been generated against normal human sera containing a mixture of immunoglobulin subclasses and idiotypes. However, a monoclonal immunoglobulin has only a few of the determinants with which the antiserum usually reacts, and antigen excess may be reached at relatively low

IMMUNOGLOBULIN REFERENCE INTERVALS

Body Fluid	IgG, mg/dL	IgA, mg/dL	IgM, mg/dL	IgD, mg/dL	IgE, mg/dL
Serum					
Newborn (4 d)	700-1480	0-2.2	5-30		
20-60 y	700-1600	70-400	40-230	0-8	0-380
>60 y	600-1560	90-410	30-360		
CSF	0-5.5	0-0.6	0-1.3		
Saliva	≈11				

concentrations. If a paraprotein is suspected or previously identified, the assays should be performed at two or more dilutions to check for this; corrected for dilution, the values should agree within ≈10%. Furthermore, if a new batch of antiserum is introduced, the relationship between paraprotein concentration and the calibration curve is likely to change. For these reasons, many laboratories estimate the concentration of paraproteins by electrophoresis and densitometry.

Reference Intervals

Reference intervals for IgG and IgM in various human adult populations differ around the world because of different degrees of antigenic stimulation. IgA concentrations, however, are relatively unaffected by environmental factors. Newborn infants have B lymphocytes with antigen receptors of the IgM type but do not have significant rates of immunoglobulin synthesis. Essentially all of the IgG in neonates has been transferred across the placenta from the mother.

Amyloidosis

Amyloidosis is a pathologic process in which aggregations of proteins as β-sheet structures form deposits in tissues. The aggregates are relatively stable filamentous structures, resistant to proteolysis and normal clearance mechanisms, so they can accumulate over time. *Amyloid* (Greek, "resembling starch") received its name from Virchow because it stained with iodine like starch.

Biochemistry of Amyloid

Amyloid represents primarily an aggregate of misfolded proteins resulting from overproduction of a specific protein or synthesis of fragments or genetic variants of proteins that are more prone to aggregation.[120] At least 26 different proteins are identified as primary components of amyloid. Serum amyloid P, apolipoprotein E, and glycosaminoglycans also are found as minor components of many amyloid deposits. Depending on the site of amyloid deposition, variable injury results to the kidneys, brain, heart, peripheral nerves, or other tissues. In the past, amyloid has often been classified according to the types of tissue injury caused.[70] From a diagnostic standpoint, it may be more useful to classify amyloid according to the protein serving as the primary component of the amyloid deposits, as in Table 21-13. Amyloidosis cannot be diagnosed directly from analysis of plasma proteins, because it is a process occurring in tissues. Diagnosis may be made from analysis of tissues obtained as aspirates of fat, rectal biopsies, or biopsies of affected tissues. The β-sheet structure of amyloid has characteristic staining with Congo red dye. Serum amyloid P (SAP) binds to most types of amyloid deposits, and radiolabeled SAP has been used for nuclear imaging of amyloid deposition, although this technique has been available at only a few centers.[120]

One of the diagnostic challenges that the physician faces after the presence of amyloid is detected is the need to identify the protein that is forming the amyloid deposits.[123] Immunohistochemistry or other analyses of amyloid deposits may assist in identifying the protein. Analysis of plasma proteins may identify monoclonal immunoglobulin light chains or increases in serum amyloid A or β_2-microglobulin that contribute to the deposition of amyloid. Patients with severe inflammatory disorders such as rheumatoid arthritis and with chronic renal failure undergoing dialysis are at high risk of AA and $A\beta_2$ amyloidosis because of the relatively high concentrations of serum amyloid A and β_2-microglobulin. Patients suspected of having heritable forms of amyloidosis require analysis of plasma protein or gene sequencing to identify genetic variants of proteins such as prealbumin (transthyretin). A combined screening strategy using sequential mass spectrometric analysis of prealbumin and genetic analysis has been described.[8] More than 75 amyloidogenic variants of prealbumin are recognized. Hereditary forms of amyloidosis generally are inherited in an autosomal dominant manner. Variants of many proteins have been associated with amyloidosis—apolipoproteins A-I and A-II, fibrinogen α-chain, gelsolin (Finnish-type amyloidosis), cystatin C (localized deposition in cerebral blood vessels), calcitonin (localized in thyroid medullary carcinoma), amylin (deposition in pancreatic islets of patients with type 2 diabetes), prolactin (deposited in the pituitary), atrial natriuretic factor (in cardiac atria), keratin (cutaneous deposits), lysozyme, and other proteins.[120,150] Alzheimer's disease is associated with deposition of Aβ-peptide in brain tissue, although the pathogenic role of amyloid remains controversial. The Aβ-peptide of about 42 amino acid residues in length is released by proteolytic cleavage of a transmembrane protein, the amyloid β precursor protein. Increased concentrations of Ab -peptide in CSF may serve as an indicator of the production of this amyloidogenic peptide.[112A,172]

TABLE 21-13 Classification and Protein Deposition in Selected Amyloidoses

Protein	Type	Causes
Systemic		
Immunoglobulin light chain	AL	Plasma cell dyscrasias, multiple myeloma
Immunoglobulin heavy chain	AH	Rare, plasma cell dyscrasias
Serum amyloid A	AA	Inflammation as in rheumatoid arthritis, tuberculosis
Prealbumin (Transthyretin)	ATTR	Genetic variants of prealbumin
β_2-Microglobulin	$A\beta_2$	Accumulation of β_2-microglobulin in renal failure
Localized		
Amyloid β-protein	Aβ	Cleavage of amyloid β-precursor protein; Alzheimer's disease
Amylin	IAPP	Type 2 diabetes, accumulation in pancreatic islets
Cystatin C	ACys	Genetic variant of cystatin C, deposition in cerebral vessels
Keratin	Aker	Cutaneous deposition of keratin
Gelsolin		Genetic variant of gelsolin, Finish-type amyloidosis
Procalcitonin		Local deposition in thyroid medullary carcinoma

Clinical Significance of Amyloid

AL and AH Amyloidosis

Monoclonal production of free immunoglobulin light chains or, rarely, heavy chains is associated with benign or malignant expansion of clones of plasma cells.[108] The fibrillar proteins consist of homogeneous immunoglobulin light polypeptide chains mainly of the 8 (especially 8_{VI}) type, their amino-terminal variable fragments, or both. AL proteins have a molecular weight of 14 to 22 kDa and an affinity for clotting factor X, which may decrease plasma concentrations of this factor with associated bleeding.[150] Because they always include the variable portion of the immunoglobulin light chain, they differ from one case to another. AL deposits may occur in the tongue, heart, lymph nodes, spleen, joints, peripheral nerves, and skin.

AA Amyloidosis

Serum amyloid A (SAA) synthesis is strongly induced by inflammation; similar to CRP, its concentration can increase up to 1000-fold.[42] Three different genes for SAA are known. SAA-4 is a constitutively expressed protein not induced by the APR; SAA-1 and SAA-2 are gene products induced by inflammation. SAA-1 is a small nonglycosylated protein of 11,683 Da that also occurs in some truncated forms.[34,56] All forms of SAA bind to high-density lipoproteins and appear to supplant apolipoprotein A-I in inflammatory conditions, because apolipoprotein A-I is a negative acute-phase reactant. Fragments of SAA of 5 to 9 kDa are amyloidogenic. AA amyloidosis occurs in rheumatoid arthritis (incidence up to 20%) and other inflammatory joint diseases, and in chronic infections such as tuberculosis and osteomyelitis. Deposits of AA protein are also observed in nonlymphoid tumors such as renal and gastric carcinomas and in Hodgkin's disease. Deposits of AA protein most often are found in the kidneys, liver, and spleen, usually resulting in nephrotic syndrome and hepatosplenomegaly.[70] Studies have shown that blocking inflammatory responses with inhibitors of TNF-α offers one approach to lower SAA concentrations and to decrease renal injury.[74]

ATTR Amyloidosis

Deposition of prealbumin (transthyretin) has been shown to result from more than 75 different genetic variants.[8,120] One common presentation has been termed *senile amyloidosis* or *senile cardiac amyloidosis* related to cardiac failure resulting from amyloid deposition in the heart; amyloid deposits also occur in other tissues. Other presentations may include polyneuropathies and neurologic disorders that may relate to the relatively high abundance of prealbumin in the central nervous system.

Methods for Analyzing Proteins

Analysis of high-abundance proteins in body fluids depends on a variety of methods for total protein analysis, electrophoretic methods, and specific quantitative immunoassays based on turbidimetry, nephelometry, and radial immunodiffusion. Mass spectrometry is used increasingly for qualitative analysis of high-abundance protein components. Analysis of low-abundance components by functional assays and other immunoassay techniques is described in other chapters.

Immunochemical Methods

Nephelometric and turbidimetric methods are performed as equilibrium or rate methods for measuring the amount of light scattering by antigen-antibody complexes. Limits of detection of ≈10 mg/L are attained with routine nephelometric and turbidimetric methods, adding antibodies in solution. Binding antibodies to particles of latex or other materials enhances light scattering and can lower limits of detection by 10- to 100-fold. Such assays may be described as latex-enhanced or as particle-enhanced assays. Radial immunodiffusion methods usually are able to detect down to a minimum of 10 to 20 mg/L. These methods are generally adequate for the high-abundance plasma proteins described in this chapter. Nephelometric and turbidimetric assays commonly offer within-run coefficients of variation (CVs) of <5%, except as limits of detection are approached. RID has higher within-run and run-to-run CVs. Turbidimetric methods can be applied on most chemistry analyzers capable of performing photometric methods. Nephelometry requires instrumentation capable of measuring light scattering at an angle.

Calibration of Immunochemical Methods

Older reference preparations such as WHO 6HSP and USNRP for the measurement of complement, immunoglobulins, and a few other proteins had values assigned in international units (IU). Certified reference material 470 was developed through combined efforts of multiple organizations with concentration values versus USNRP for albumin, AMG, complement factors C3 and C4, Cp, Hp, and IgA, IgG, and IgM. Concentration values were assigned for AAT (α_1-protease inhibitor), α_1-antichymotrypsin, AAG (orosomucoid), and transferrin against highly purified and thoroughly characterized purified proteins, and for C-reactive protein against WHO 85/506, using the factor 1 IU = 1 mg/dL. CRM 470 has been used to standardize manufacturers' controls and calibrators, resulting in decreased variation between assays, and tentative reference values for white adults have been established.[22] Minor differences in assays remain based on different antibody specificities.

Specimen Collection and Storage for Immunoassay

Test specimens should be nonhemolyzed, cell-free serum, urine, or CSF. CSF specimens may require centrifugation if cells are present. Serum and CSF samples may be stored at 2 to 8 °C for up to 3 days or at −20 °C for longer periods. Repeated freezing and thawing of specimens may cause denaturation of some proteins and should be avoided.

Electrophoretic Techniques

Electrophoresis is used to separate proteins by charge and thereby to assess protein variants or the concentrations of specific components in serum or other fluids. Electrophoretic techniques commonly performed in clinical laboratories include nondenaturing electrophoresis on cellulose acetate strips or agarose gels, capillary electrophoresis (CE), immunofixation, and "Western blotting." Protein separation in one or two dimensions with polyacrylamide gel is a powerful separation technique frequently used for research.[3]

Serum Protein Electrophoresis

Generally, serum rather than plasma is used for electrophoresis of proteins on agarose gels to avoid the fibrinogen band at the β-γ interface. The principles of electrophoresis are described in Chapter 12. Figure 21-7 illustrates examples of serum electrophoretic patterns for normal and pathologic specimens. Analysis usually is performed with low–ionic strength buffers (≈0.05) at pH ≈ 8.6. For agarose gels, the usual sample is 3 to 5 µL, applied evenly across a lane. Much smaller volumes are injected for capillary electrophoresis via electrokinetic or hydrostatic injection. Separation times are typically about 1 hour for agarose gels and a few minutes for capillary electrophoresis. A variety of stains are used to visualize proteins in gels, including amido black, Ponceau S, Coomassie brilliant blue, and related dyes. Levels of detection and linearity of protein detection vary with different dyes. Only a few of the most abundant proteins are visualized, and intensities of bands with protein stains usually relate to the mass of peptide; oligosaccharides and lipids may reduce rather than contribute to band intensities. Therefore, glycoproteins with a high proportion of carbohydrate (e.g., AAG) have lower detection responses than a nonglycosylated protein such as albumin. Quantitative analysis relies on densitometry, which provides relative proportions of different components rather than absolute amounts. Quantitation of individual components relies on calculations based on total protein concentration. Lipophilic stains such as Sudan black are needed to visualize lipoproteins such as HDL (α_1-lipoprotein), VLDL (pre-β-region), LDL (β-lipoprotein), or chylomicrons (origin) (see also Chapter 27). Capillary electrophoresis detects proteins passing through a flow cell by their light absorbance at wavelengths below 220 nm. This offers a more unbiased assessment of protein concentration than staining intensity, as absorbance of proteins in the low ultraviolet region is more consistently related to mass. Small molecules at high concentrations, such as metabolites, radiocontrast dyes, or drugs, may also yield absorbance peaks, and this presents problems with analysis of urine specimens.

The major clinical application of serum protein electrophoresis is the detection of monoclonal immunoglobulins (paraproteins) to assist in the diagnosis and monitoring of multiple myeloma and related disorders. Most of the monoclonal immunoglobulins are observed in the β-region or γ-region. Quantitation of monoclonal components serves as a means of monitoring disease progression and response to therapy. Identification of paraproteins requires distinction from a variety of other sources of additional bands or pseudoparaproteins by means such as immunofixation electrophoresis as described later. Incompletely clotted specimens contain fibrinogen. Genetic or post-translational variants of proteins such as transferrin, haptoglobin, and C3 may migrate in different than usual positions. Large increases in CRP may yield a detectable band in the β- or γ-region. Increased lysozyme in monocytic leukemia may produce a band in the post-γ-region. Hemoglobin will yield a band in hemolyzed specimens.

Many other findings of potential clinical significance have been reported:

1. Changes in albumin concentration or migration. Decreases in concentration suggest nutritional deficiency, protein-losing disorders, APR, or advanced liver disease. Changes in mobility or bisalbuminemia may indicate genetic variants or increased binding of fatty acids or drugs; usually this is not of great clinical significance.
2. Changes in the α_1-region relate to changes in AAT, and to a lesser degree in AAG or HDL. Decreases are associated with AAT deficiency or protein-losing disorders. Increases are related to inflammation.
3. Changes in the α_2-region usually relate to changes in HPT and AMG. Migration of HPT varies with genotype. HPT

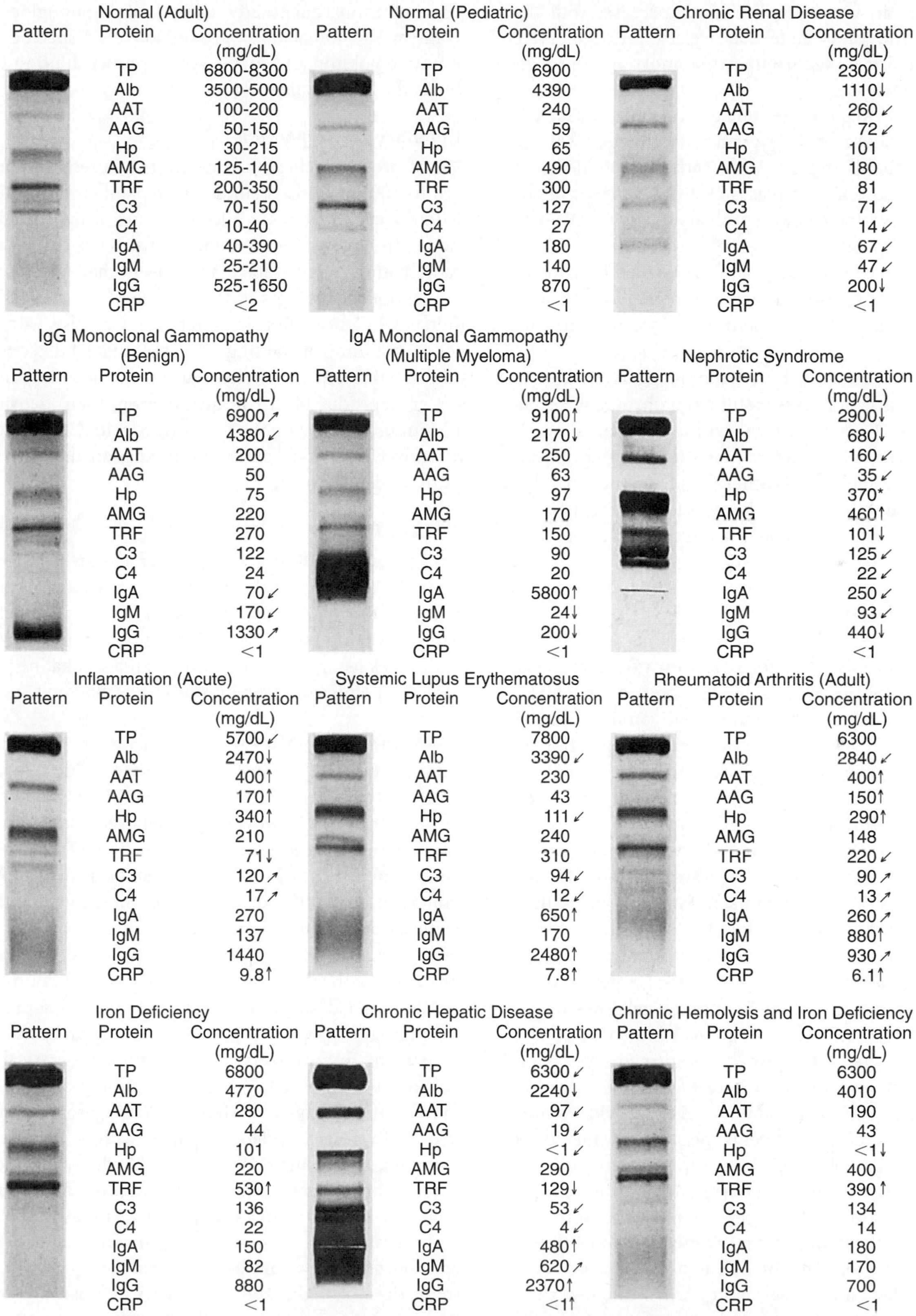

Normal (Adult)

Protein	Concentration (mg/dL)
TP	6800-8300
Alb	3500-5000
AAT	100-200
AAG	50-150
Hp	30-215
AMG	125-140
TRF	200-350
C3	70-150
C4	10-40
IgA	40-390
IgM	25-210
IgG	525-1650
CRP	<2

Normal (Pediatric)

Protein	Concentration (mg/dL)
TP	6900
Alb	4390
AAT	240
AAG	59
Hp	65
AMG	490
TRF	300
C3	127
C4	27
IgA	180
IgM	140
IgG	870
CRP	<1

Chronic Renal Disease

Protein	Concentration (mg/dL)
TP	2300↓
Alb	1110↓
AAT	260↙
AAG	72↙
Hp	101
AMG	180
TRF	81
C3	71↙
C4	14↙
IgA	67↙
IgM	47↙
IgG	200↓
CRP	<1

IgG Monoclonal Gammopathy (Benign)

Protein	Concentration (mg/dL)
TP	6900↗
Alb	4380↙
AAT	200
AAG	50
Hp	75
AMG	220
TRF	270
C3	122
C4	24
IgA	70↙
IgM	170↙
IgG	1330↗
CRP	<1

IgA Monclonal Gammopathy (Multiple Myeloma)

Protein	Concentration (mg/dL)
TP	9100↑
Alb	2170↓
AAT	250
AAG	63
Hp	97
AMG	170
TRF	150
C3	90
C4	20
IgA	5800↑
IgM	24↓
IgG	200↓
CRP	<1

Nephrotic Syndrome

Protein	Concentration (mg/dL)
TP	2900↓
Alb	680↓
AAT	160↙
AAG	35↙
Hp	370*
AMG	460↑
TRF	101↓
C3	125↙
C4	22↙
IgA	250↙
IgM	93↙
IgG	440↓
CRP	<1

Inflammation (Acute)

Protein	Concentration (mg/dL)
TP	5700↙
Alb	2470↓
AAT	400↑
AAG	170↑
Hp	340↑
AMG	210
TRF	71↓
C3	120↗
C4	17↗
IgA	270
IgM	137
IgG	1440
CRP	9.8↑

Systemic Lupus Erythematosus

Protein	Concentration (mg/dL)
TP	7800
Alb	3390↙
AAT	230
AAG	43
Hp	111↙
AMG	240
TRF	310
C3	94↙
C4	12↙
IgA	650↑
IgM	170
IgG	2480↑
CRP	7.8↑

Rheumatoid Arthritis (Adult)

Protein	Concentration (mg/dL)
TP	6300
Alb	2840↙
AAT	400↑
AAG	150↑
Hp	290↑
AMG	148
TRF	220↙
C3	90↗
C4	13↗
IgA	260↗
IgM	880↑
IgG	930↗
CRP	6.1↑

Iron Deficiency

Protein	Concentration (mg/dL)
TP	6800
Alb	4770
AAT	280
AAG	44
Hp	101
AMG	220
TRF	530↑
C3	136
C4	22
IgA	150
IgM	82
IgG	880
CRP	<1

Chronic Hepatic Disease

Protein	Concentration (mg/dL)
TP	6300↙
Alb	2240↓
AAT	97↙
AAG	19↙
Hp	<1↙
AMG	290
TRF	129↓
C3	53↙
C4	4↙
IgA	480↑
IgM	620↗
IgG	2370↑
CRP	<1↑

Chronic Hemolysis and Iron Deficiency

Protein	Concentration (mg/dL)
TP	6300
Alb	4010
AAT	190
AAG	43
Hp	<1↓
AMG	400
TRF	390↑
C3	134
C4	14
IgA	180
IgM	170
IgG	700
CRP	<1

Figure 21-7 Electrophoretic patterns typical of normal conditions and of some pathologic conditions (agarose gel). ***Upward- and downward-pointing arrows*** **indicate increase and decrease from the reference interval, respectively.** ***Right- or left-slanting arrows*** **indicate variation from normal to an increase or from normal to a decrease from the reference interval, respectively. The** ***asterisk*** **indicates Hp 2-2 phenotype.**

decreases with in vivo hemolysis and increases with the APR. AMG and high molecular weight forms of HPT increase in nephrotic syndrome, while most other protein components decrease.

4. Bands in the β-region are related to transferrin, C3, and LDL. Migration of transferrin may change from the β_1-region to the β_2-region with carbohydrate-deficient transferrin. Transferrin decreases and C3 increases in the APR. Transferrin increases in iron deficiency. LDL may increase in dyslipidemias.
5. An increase between β- and γ-bands, so-called bridging of β- and γ-bands, suggests an increase in IgA as seen with cirrhosis, respiratory tract or skin infection, and rheumatoid arthritis.
6. Increases or decreases in the γ-region suggest changes in immunoglobulins. Increases result from chronic infection or paraproteins. Decreases occur with many immunodeficiency states. Multiple myeloma may suppress general production of immunoglobulins other than from the expanded clone. Therefore, a decrease in the γ-region may suggest the need for additional studies such as immunofixation electrophoresis to detect paraproteins.

Immunofixation Electrophoresis

Immunofixation electrophoresis (IFE) has largely replaced immunoelectrophoresis (IEP) for detection of paraproteins. IFE provides easier interpretation. A comparison of IFE and IEP for two patients with monoclonal gammopathies is shown in Figure 21-8. After electrophoretic separation in agarose, IEP relies on antibody diffusion from troughs parallel to lanes, while IFE involves antibody overlaid directly on lanes. To perform IFE, a patient's serum is run in multiple lanes on an agarose gel. One lane is fixed to provide the overall pattern of proteins. Other lanes are overlaid with specific antisera, usually separate antisera versus κ and λ light chains and γ, μ, and α-immunoglobulin heavy chains. Antibody dilutions are adjusted to provide approximate equivalence with immunoglobulins separated in the gel, so as to form immune complexes precipitated in the gel. Proteins not precipitated are washed from the gel to lower background, and precipitated proteins are stained. Paraproteins characteristically yield sharper precipitin bands than the heterogeneous polyclonal immunoglobulins. IFE provides more sensitive detection of paraproteins because of the lower background and signal amplification from immune complex formation, and helps distinguish paraproteins from pseudoparaproteins. Immunofixation helps identify the immunoglobulin type of the paraprotein. Sometimes, more than one clone may be expanded, or free light chain may occur together with intact immunoglobulin. Uncommonly, paraproteins may be of the IgD or IgE class. They should be detected by antisera versus light chains but require δ or ε heavy chain specific antisera to distinguish them from free light chains. High concentrations of paraproteins may yield prozones during immunofixation, requiring specimen dilution for optimal studies. For paraproteins present in high concentrations, quantitative analysis of immunoglobulins can confirm the unbalanced production of a specific class of immunoglobulin and may assist in proper dilution of specimens for immunofixation.

Capillary Electrophoresis

CE of proteins relies on zone electrophoresis in small-bore (10 to 100 μm), fused silica capillary tubes 20 to 200 cm in length (see Chapter 12). Electrokinetic or hydrostatic injection introduces a small amount of protein that is resolved rapidly under high voltage. One of the challenges is to avoid adsorption of proteins to the surface of the capillary. CE is suitable for automation and offers rapid analysis with no need for gel handling or staining. Direct ultraviolet detection offers slightly different specificity than protein staining and offers better reproducibility of quantitation than densitometry. Immunofixation cannot be performed with CE. Immunosubtraction with specific antisera is used as an alternative procedure to identify paraproteins.[103]

Western Blotting

For Western blotting, proteins separated on a gel are transferred by diffusion or electroblotting onto a membrane made of materials such as nitrocellulose or polyvinylidene fluoride. Proteins bound on the membrane are identified with specific antibodies using labels such as peroxidase, alkaline phosphatase, or chemiluminescent probes (see Chapter 12).

Mass Spectrometry (MS)

Multiple types of MS instrumentation provide qualitative or quantitative information about proteins (see Chapter 14). An advantage of MS is the ability to analyze a large number of components in a single analysis, including rapid sequence analysis of peptides. MS, therefore, has been an enabling technology in *proteomics,* defined as the effort to study the complete set of proteins in an organism or in subcompartments of an organism such as plasma.[3,57] Ionization of peptides and proteins has been accomplished by electrospray or matrix-assisted laser desorption/ionization (MALDI) sources. Electrospray sources take a solution containing proteins and form a spray of fine droplets with an applied electrical charge. Solvent is evaporated, generating multiply charged protein ions for mass analysis. In MALDI sources, proteins are deposited on a target surface together with a light-absorbing compound (the matrix) such as dihydroxybenzoic acid.[56] Under a high vacuum, the matrix and proteins are vaporized by pulses of light from a laser; proteins usually are preferentially ionized in a singly charged form. Once proteins are ionized, they can be separated by quadrupoles, ion traps, time-of-flight, and other types of mass analyzers.[29] In general, MS is better suited to analyzing small peptides than proteins, because it provides better resolution, a smaller number of charge states of ions, and better detection sensitivity.[29,56] It is difficult to quantitatively interpret the absolute magnitude of detector responses in MS, but accurate ratios of similar peptides can be determined. Use of stable

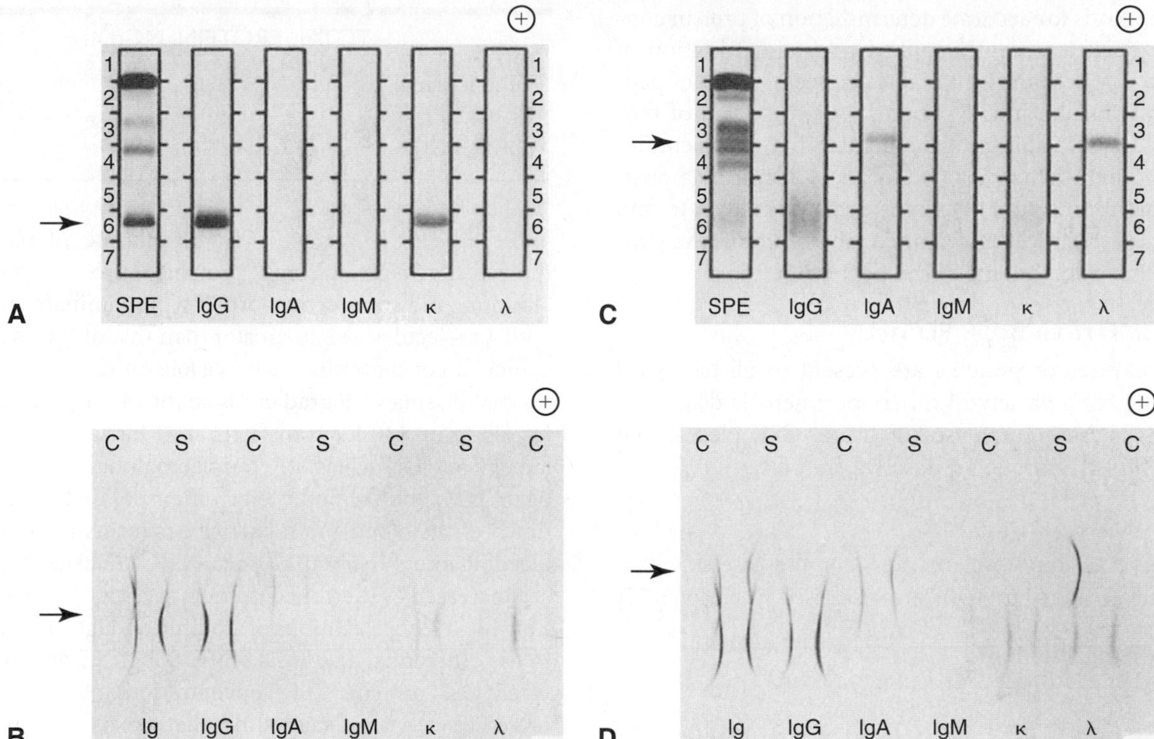

Figure 21-8 Comparison of immunofixation electrophoresis (IFE) and immunoelectrophoresis (IEP) for two patients with monoclonal gammopathies. A, Patient specimen with an IgG (κ) monoclonal protein as identified by IFE. The *arrow* indicates the position of monoclonal protein. After electrophoresis, each track except SPE is reacted with its respective antiserum; then all tracks are stained for visualization of the respective protein bands. (SPE, chemically fixed serum protein electrophoresis; IgG, IgA, IgM, κ, and λ indicate antiserum used on each track.) B, Same specimen as in A, with proteins identified by IEP. The *arrow* indicates the position of monoclonal protein. Normal control (C) and patient sera (S) are alternated. After electrophoresis, antiserum is added to each trough as indicated by the labels Ig (polyvalent Ig antiserum), IgG, IgA, IgM, κ, and λ. The antisera react with separated proteins in the specimens to form precipitates in the shape of arcs. The IgG and κ arcs are shorter and thicker than those in the normal control, showing the presence of the IgG (κ) monoclonal protein. Concentrations of IgA, IgM, and λ-light chains are also reduced. C, Patient specimen with an IgA (λ) monoclonal protein identified by IFE procedure as described in A. D, Same specimen as in C with proteins identified by IEP as described in B. Abnormal IgA and λ-arcs for the patient specimen indicate an elevated concentration of a monoclonal IgA (λ) protein. All separations were performed using the Beckman-Coulter Paragon system.

isotope-labeled internal standards allows the absolute quantitation of peptides or proteins (based on analysis of proteotypic peptides released by proteolysis). Use of tandem MS with an intermediate fragmentation step between two stages of MS separation offers high sensitivity and specificity for the quantitative analysis of peptides, as it does for most small molecules. Quantitative analysis usually uses selected ion monitoring (also referred to as multiple reaction monitoring for multiple components), which selects particular precursor and product ions for analysis. This form of analysis is performed very efficiently by triple quadrupole MS. Qualitative analysis of peptides, identifying their sequences and post-translational modification, often uses mass spectrometers such as ion traps that are well suited for scanning all peptide fragments generated by fragmentation.[29]

Advantages of using MS for quantitative analysis include the ability to analyze components without developing specific antibodies and the ability to multiplex a large number of measurements.[7] MS can provide information about post-translational modifications that is difficult to assess by immunoassays and chromatographic or electrophoretic techniques. Examples of clinical applications include identification of genetic variants of prealbumin and carbohydrate-deficient transferrin.[8] MS techniques are likely to increasingly serve as reference methods for accurate determination of protein concentrations, such as recently applied for standardization of hemoglobin A_{1c} measurement and for concentrations of peptides such as insulin and C-peptide.[106] For analysis of bioactive peptides, the ability to distinguish between peptides differing in length by one or two amino acids or by a post-translational modification often is critical. MS is likely to find increased use for clinical laboratory analysis of bioactive peptides and other components of the peptidome.

Proteins in Other Body Fluids

Complex mixtures of proteins are present in all biological fluids; analysis of a variety of other specimens is diagnostically useful, including analyses of urine, CSF, pleural and peritoneal fluids, amniotic fluid, saliva, and feces.

Urinary Proteins

Proteins serve as important markers for the assessment of kidney injury. Urinary proteins are discussed in Chapter 25.

Proteins in Amniotic Fluid

See Chapter 57.

Proteins in Saliva

Saliva has a very different protein composition compared with plasma, with amylase and small peptide components representing major components; a variety of diagnostic applications of salivary protein analysis are being explored.[64] Protein composition varies with the site and method of sampling of saliva. In Sjögren's syndrome with lymphoid infiltration of salivary glands, β_2-microglobulin concentrations rise in saliva. Saliva is tested for secretory IgA in infantile hypogammaglobulinemia.

Proteins in Cerebrospinal Fluid

CSF is the extracellular fluid around the brain and spinal column. CSF usually has total protein concentrations about 100-fold lower than plasma and a different protein composition, as most proteins have limited passage across the blood-brain barrier. CSF for testing most frequently is obtained by a spinal tap in the lumbar region.[94,164]

Biochemistry of CSF

CSF is secreted by the choroid plexuses, around the cerebral vessels, and along the walls of the ventricles of the brain. It fills the ventricles and cisternae, bathes the spinal cord, and is reabsorbed into the blood through the arachnoid villi. CSF turnover is rapid, exchanging totally about four times daily. More than 80% of CSF protein content originates from plasma by ultrafiltration and pinocytosis; the remainder is derived from intrathecal synthesis. The lowest protein concentration and the smallest proportion of larger protein molecules are in the ventricular fluid; as the CSF passes down to the lumbar spine (where specimens are usually collected), the protein concentration increases. This gradient in concentration at different concentrations of the CNS is illustrated by the following reference intervals[156]:

TOTAL PROTEIN, MG/DL	
Ventricular fluid	5-15
Cisternal fluid	15-25
Lumbar fluid	15-48

Because CSF is mainly an ultrafiltrate of plasma, low molecular weight plasma proteins such as prealbumin, albumin, and transferrin normally predominate. No protein with a molecular weight greater than that of IgG is present in sufficient concentration to be visible on electrophoresis. The normal plasma/CSF gradient is about 14 for prealbumin, 240 for albumin, 140 for transferrin, 800 for IgG, and >1000 for larger proteins such as IgA, α_2-macroglobulin (AMG), fibrinogen, IgM, and β-lipoprotein.[35] If partial or complete breakdown of the blood-brain barrier occurs, as in meningitis or bleeding into the subdural space, AMG concentrations in CSF are increased.[91] The concentration of AMG alone, or its relationship to concentrations of albumin and IgG, may be helpful in the differential diagnosis of neurologic disorders or of elevated CSF protein. CSF concentrations of AMG normally increase with age, suggesting that partial but progressive breakdown of the blood-CSF barrier occurs with aging. Bleeding into the CSF also raises AMG concentrations in this fluid.

The electrophoretic pattern of normal CSF after concentration of the fluid has two striking features—a prealbumin band and two transferrin bands—one at β_2 in addition to the usual β_1 position. The β_2-transferrin has decreased charge because it is carbohydrate deficient. Both β_2-transferrin and another relatively abundant CSF protein, prostaglandin D synthase or β-trace, have been used to determine whether clear fluids from nasal or ear passages represent leakage of CSF, so-called CSF rhinorrhea and otorrhea.[4] Prostaglandin D synthase is a protein of about 30 kDa that is relatively enriched in CSF relative to serum or plasma, where it normally is cleared rapidly by glomerular filtration. Apolipoprotein E serves as one of the major lipid transport proteins because of the relative lack of other lipoproteins such as HDL and LDL to carry lipids.

Clinical Significance

The blood-brain or blood-CSF barrier limits exchange of many compounds, particularly large compounds such as proteins. Analyses of total protein and specific proteins in CSF are used primarily to detect increased permeability of the blood-CSF barrier to plasma proteins or increased production or release of specific proteins, such as immunoglobulins, myelin basic protein, or amyloid beta peptides in the CNS (Table 21-14).

Increased Permeability. The permeability of the blood-CSF barrier to plasma proteins increases with inflammation in bacterial or viral meningitis, encephalitis, or poliomyelitis and with high intracranial pressure resulting from a brain tumor, intracerebral hemorrhage, or traumatic injury. Highest elevations of CSF total protein are seen in bacterial meningitis. Lumbar CSF protein increases when the CSF

TABLE 21-14 Cerebrospinal Fluid Total Protein in Various Diseases

Clinical Condition	Appearance and Cells × 10^6/L	Total Protein, mg/dL
Normal	Clear, colorless; 0-5 lymphocytes	15-45*
Increased Admixture of Proteins From Blood		
Increased capillary permeability:		
• Bacterial meningitis	Turbid, opalescent, purulent, usually >500 polymorphs	80-500
• Cryptococcal meningitis	Clear or turbid; 50-150 polymorphs or lymphocytes	25-200
• Leptospiral meningitis	Clear to slight haze; polymorphs early, then 5-100 lymphocytes	50-100
• Viral meningitis	Clear or slight haze, colorless; usually up to 500 lymphocytes	30-100
• Encephalitis	Clear or slight haze, colorless; usually up to 500 lymphocytes	15-100
• Poliomyelitis	Clear, colorless; up to 500 lymphocytes	10-300
• Brain tumor	Usually clear; 0-80 lymphocytes	15-200 (usually normal)
Mechanical obstruction:		
• Spinal cord tumor†	Clear, colorless, or yellow	100-2000
Hemorrhage		
Cerebral hemorrhage	Colorless, yellow, or bloody; blood cells	30-150
Local immunoglobulin production:		
• Neurosyphilis	Clear, colorless; 10-100 lymphocytes	50-150
• Multiple sclerosis‡	Clear, colorless; 0-10 lymphocytes	25-50
Both increased capillary permeability and local immunoglobulin production:		
• Tuberculous meningitis	Colorless, fibrin clot, or slightly turbid; 50-500 lymphocytes	50-300 (occasionally up to 1000)
• Brain abscess	Clear or slightly turbid	20-120
After myelography (inflammatory reaction)		Slight increase

*Premature infant: up to 400 mg/dL. Children: 30-100 mg/dL. Old age: up to 60 mg/dL.
†Froin's syndrome: lumbar fluid values are much higher than cisternal fluid values.
‡Similar values may occur in certain other chronic inflammatory conditions of the nervous system.

circulation is obstructed above the collection site (as by a spinal cord tumor). Increased permeability results in CSF composition closer to that of plasma.

Intrathecal Synthesis. Increased intrathecal synthesis of immunoglobulins, particularly IgG, occurs in demyelinating diseases of the CNS, especially multiple sclerosis.[164] In multiple sclerosis, patchy demyelination of axons in the CNS interferes with nerve conduction and leads to varying neurologic symptoms. B lymphocytes that infiltrate the lesions release immunoglobulins, primarily IgG, into CSF.

Laboratory Considerations for CSF

Various analytical techniques are used to assess the increased permeability of the blood-CSF barrier to plasma proteins and to detect intrathecal synthesis of immunoglobulins.

Determination of Total Protein in CSF. The total protein concentration in CSF is an indicator of blood-CSF permeability. The protein concentration of CSF usually is more than 100-fold lower than for plasma, and methods with greater sensitivity or increased specimen volume are required for measuring total serum or plasma protein. In practice, methods commonly used by clinical laboratories to measure total CSF protein include (1) pyrogallol red, (2) benzethonium chloride, (3) reverse-biuret, and (4) biuret. The reverse-biuret method measures free copper remaining after formation of biuret complexes by reduction and complexation with a chelating dye. Analyzers often use the same method, possibly with some adjustment of specimen volume, for CSF and urine protein. The usual reference interval for CSF IgG in adults is 0.8 to 4.2 mg/dL; for total protein, 15 to 45 mg/dL. Total protein concentrations are considerably higher in neonates, and in healthy elderly adults. In CSF from premature and full-term neonates, concentrations up to 400 mg/dL for premature and 130 mg/dL for full-term neonates); in healthy elderly adults, concentrations up to 60 mg/dL are considered normal. In newborns, a progressive decline in the reference interval CSF protein is seen over the first few weeks of life, with values approaching adult concentrations at >4 months of age.[10] Use of age-adjusted reference intervals for the first few weeks of life is most important.

Increased Permeability. A more specific measure of the permeability of the blood-CSF barrier involves determination of the ratio of albumin concentration in CSF versus plasma. This ratio, the *CSF/serum albumin index,* usually is calculated for CSF albumin in mg/dL and for serum protein in g/L, effectively multiplying values by 1000.

A CSF/serum albumin index <9 indicates an intact blood-CSF barrier. Values of 9 to 14 represent slight impairment, 14 to 30 moderate impairment, and >30 severe impairment. The index helps correct for variation in serum albumin concentration.

Intrathecal Synthesis. Measurement of the CSF/serum immunoglobulin ratio and assessment of oligoclonal immunoglobulin bands on electrophoretic separations of CSF serve as assays for intrathecal immunoglobulin synthesis. At least 90% of cases of multiple sclerosis give positive findings, but increased immunoglobulins and oligoclonal immunoglobulins may be found in other inflammatory diseases of the CNS, such as infection caused by bacteria, viruses, fungi, or parasites; neurosyphilis; subacute sclerosing panencephalitis; and Guillain-Barré syndrome. Multiple sclerosis is less likely if CSF total protein exceeds 100 mg/dL, or if the CSF leukocyte count is >50/μL. The CSF albumin concentration in 70% of cases of multiple sclerosis is within the reference interval.

Increases in CSF IgG concentration or in the CSF/serum IgG ratio may result from increased permeability of the blood-CSF barrier, increased local production of IgG, or both. To identify intrathecal production specifically, correction for increased permeability is necessary. Corrections use *CSF and serum* albumin and IgG concentrations in one of several ways:

1. Concentrations *in CSF* of IgG and albumin are measured, and the IgG/albumin ratio is calculated. A ratio >0.27 is considered indicative of increased synthesis; in about 70% of cases of multiple sclerosis, the ratio exceeds 0.27.

$$\text{Ratio} = \frac{\text{IgG}_{\text{CSF}}\,(\text{mg/dL})}{\text{Albumin}_{\text{CSF}}\,(\text{mg/dL})}$$

2. Concentrations in *CSF and serum* of IgG and albumin are measured, and the CSF immunoglobulin index is calculated.

$$\text{Index} = \frac{\text{IgG}_{\text{CSF}}\,(\text{mg/dL}) \times \text{Albumin}_{\text{serum}}\,(\text{g/dL})}{\text{Albumin}_{\text{CSF}}\,(\text{mg/dL}) \times \text{IgG}_{\text{serum}}\,(\text{g/dL})}$$

The reference interval for the index is 0.30 to 0.70. Values >0.70 indicate increased IgG synthesis; in more than 80% of cases of multiple sclerosis, this index exceeds 0.70. This CSF immunoglobulin index is now a frequently used index.

3. The rate of intrathecal IgG synthesis can be estimated by the empirically derived Tourtellotte's formula. The rate of synthesis of IgG in milligrams per day is equal to

$$5\ \text{dL/d}\left[\left[\left\{\text{IgG}_{\text{CSF}} - \frac{\text{IgG}_{\text{serum}}}{369}\right\} - \left\{\left(\text{Albumin}_{\text{CSF}} - \frac{\text{Albumin}_{\text{serum}}}{230}\right) \times \frac{0.43\,(\text{IgG}_{\text{serum}})}{\text{Albumin}_{\text{serum}}}\right\}\right]\right]$$

where protein concentrations are in mg/dL. The first bracketed term represents the difference between IgG found in CSF and the IgG expected if the blood-brain barrier is intact. The second bracketed term represents the same for albumin but is corrected by a factor of 0.43, corresponding to the ratio of molecular weights of albumin to IgG, assuming that 1 mole of IgG accompanies every mole of albumin that passes the blood-brain barrier; 369 and 230 originate from the normal serum/CSF ratios for IgG and albumin. The reference interval for the synthesis rate is 0 to 3.3 mg/d. Values exceeding 8 mg/d are found in most cases of multiple sclerosis. This estimator provides no more clinical information than the IgG index; the complex formula merely rearranges the results for serum and CSF IgG and albumin and then factors in several constants.

Determination of Specific Proteins in CSF

Analyses of albumin and immunoglobulins are applied as described previously. CSF concentrations of a protein component of the fatty myelin sheath, *myelin basic protein,* are an indicator of myelin turnover. CSF concentrations of myelin basic protein appear to correlate with exacerbation and remission of multiple sclerosis, but proteolysis may yield different forms of the protein.[94] A number of other proteins such as S100B and neuron-specific enolase are potential markers for traumatic or ischemic brain injury.[76] In acute leukemia and lymphoma with central nervous system involvement, the concentration of β_2-microglobulin BMG is increased in CSF. Concentrations of tau protein y decrease in Alzheimer's disease.[172]

Reference Intervals for CSF Proteins

The reference interval for albumin in lumbar CSF by RID is 17.7 to 25.1 mg/dL. In normal CSF, IgA, IgD, and IgM are <0.2 mg/dL. Reference intervals for IgG are age related; their means increase from 3.5 mg/dL in the 15- to 20-year-old age group to 5.8 mg/dL in adults aged 60 years or older. A usual reference interval for CSF IgG in adults is 0.8 to 4.2 mg/L.[70,156]

Proteins in Peritoneal and Pleural Fluids

Pathologic accumulations of fluid in the peritoneal and pleural cavities or elsewhere vary greatly in protein content. They may be ultrafiltrates with low protein concentrations relative to plasma and scant amounts of large proteins (transudates) or, in response to local inflammation and increased vascular permeability, fluids (exudates) may have protein concentrations approaching those of plasma and significant amounts of large proteins such as immunoglobulins and

AMG. The distinction between transudates and exudates assists in diagnosing the cause of fluid formation. The major cause of pleural transudates is congestive heart failure. Exudates occur with infection, pleuritis, pulmonary embolism, and cancer. Criteria for identifying exudates in pleural fluid were proposed by Light: pleural fluid protein : serum protein >0.5; pleural LDH : serum LDH >0.6; pleural fluid LDH >200 IU/L.[51] Pleural fluid may be turbid from large numbers of white cells, fibrin particles, or chylomicrons. Chylous effusions (containing chylomicrons) result from lymphatic obstruction related to cancer, surgery, trauma, sarcoidosis, or other causes.[109] Lymphatics, particularly the major trunk, the thoracic duct, serve as the major route for chylomicrons from the intestines to the blood circulation. Entry of chylomicrons into the pleural space, therefore, is related in part to dietary fat intake to generate chylomicrons, and fasting lowers the fat content of chylous effusions. Chylomicrons in fluids may be identified by separation of a cream layer upon standing or by triglyceride analysis.

For peritoneal fluid, the serum-ascites albumin gradient (i.e., the difference between serum and peritoneal fluid albumin) helps distinguish transudates (mainly in portal hypertension from cirrhosis) from infection and other causes of ascites. Usually, the serum albumin-ascites albumin gradient is >1.1 g/dL in portal hypertension and is lower than 1.1 g/dL for other causes that generate exudates.[133]

Fecal Proteins

Assay of fecal α_1-antitrypsin is used as an indicator of protein losses into the gastrointestinal tract in protein-losing enteropathies and inflammatory bowel disease. Fecal AAT preferably is determined as clearance on a timed collection to determine an excretion rate ratioed versus the serum AAT concentration.[6] Correction for serum AAT concentration is necessary because of variation in serum AAT from severe enteric losses or from acute-phase responses. AAT is relatively stable in the lower digestive tract but is digested in the stomach at acid pH. Therefore, suppression of acid secretion is necessary to use AAT excretion as a measure of gastric protein-losing enteropathy.[152] An alternative measure of increased gastrointestinal loss of protein has been injection of radiolabeled albumin with monitoring of radioactivity into stool. For inflammatory bowel disease, it may be more useful to have indicators of inflammation rather than leakage of plasma proteins. Fecal content of products secreted by white cells, such as lactoferrin and calprotectin, has been used as a measure of disease activity in inflammatory bowel disease.[151]

REFERENCES

1. Amaral S, Hwang W, Fivush B, Neu A, Frankenfield D, Furth S. Serum albumin concentration and risk of mortality and hospitalization in adolescents on hemodialysis. Clin J Am Soc Nephrol 2008;3:759-67.
2. Anderson NL, Anderson NG, Pearson TW, Borchers CH, Paulovich AG, Patterson SD, et al. A human proteome detection and quantitation project. Mol Cell Proteomics 2009; 8:883-6.
3. Anderson NL, Anderson NG. The human plasma proteome: history, character, and diagnostic prospects. Mol Cell Proteomics 2002;1:845-67.
4. Bachmann-Harildstad G. Diagnostic values of beta-2 transferrin and beta-trace protein as markers for cerebrospinal fluid fistula. Rhinology 2008;46:82-5.
5. Beck FX, Neuhofer W. Response of renal medullary cells to osmotic stress. Contrib Nephrol 2005;148:21-34.
6. Becker K, Frieling T, Haussinger D. Quantification of fecal alpha 1-antitrypsin excretion for assessment of inflammatory bowel diseases. Eur J Med Res 1998;3:65-70.
7. Becker KL, Snider R, Nylen ES. Procalcitonin assay in systemic inflammation, infection, and sepsis: clinical utility and limitations. Crit Care Med 2008;36:941-52.
8. Bergen HR, Zeldenrust SR, Butz ML, Snow DS, Dyck PJ, Dyck JB, et al. Identification of transthyretin variants by sequential proteomic and genomic analysis. Clin Chem 2004;50:1544-52.
9. Biffi S, Tamaro G, Bortot B, Zamberlan S, Severini GM, Carrozzi M. Carbohydrate-deficient transferrin (CDT) as a biochemical tool for the screening of congenital disorders of glycosylation (CDGs). Clin Biochem 2007;40:1431-4.
10. Biou D, Benoist JF, Huong CN, Morel P, Marchand M. Cerebrospinal fluid protein concentrations in children: age-related values in patients without disorders of the central nervous system. Clin Chem 2000;46:399-403.
11. Blirup-Jensen S, Johnson AM, Larsen M. IFCC Committee on Plasma Proteins. Protein standardization. V: value transfer. A practical protocol for the assignment of serum protein values from a reference material to a target material. Clin Chem Lab Med 2008;46:1470-9.
12. Bornhorst JA, Calderon FRO, Procter M, Tang W, Ashwood ER, Mao R. Genotypes and serum concentrations of human alpha-1-antitrypsin "P" protein variants in a clinical population. J Clin Pathol 2007;60:1124-8.
13. Brown R, Nelson M, Aklilu E, Kabani D, Yang S, Blayney B, et al. An evaluation of the DiaMed assays for immunoglobulin A antibodies (anti-IgA) and IgA deficiency. Transfusion 2008;48:2057-9.
14. Carrell RW, Lomas DA. Alpha1-antitrypsin deficiency—a model for conformational diseases. N Engl J Med 2002;346:45-53.
15. Carter K, Worwood M. Haptoglobin: a review of the major allele frequencies worldwide and their association with diseases. Int J Haematol 2007;29:92-110.
16. Chehab FF. Obesity and lipodystrophy—where do the circles intersect? Endocrinology 2008;149:925-34.
17. Chromy V, Svachova B, Novosad L, Jarkovsky J, Sedlak P, Horak P, et al. Albumin-based or albumin-linked calibrators cause a positive bias in serum proteins assayed by the Biuret method. Clin Chem Lab Med 2009;47:91-101.
18. Coppinger JA, Maguire PB. Insights into the platelet releasate. Curr Pharm Des 2007;13:2640-6.
19. Corlin DB, Sen JW, Ladefoged S, Lund GB, Nissen MH, Heegaard NH. Quantification of cleaved beta2-microglobulin in serum from patients undergoing chronic dialysis. Clin Chem 2005;51:1177-84.
20. Costacou T, Ferrell RE, Orchard TJ. Haptoglobin genotype: a determinant of cardiovascular complication risk in type 1 diabetes. Diabetes 2008;57:1702-6.
21. Craig WY, Ledue TB, Ritchie RF. Plasma proteins: clinical utility and interpretation. Scarborough, ME: Foundation for Blood Research, 2001.
22. Dati F, Schumann G, Thomas L, Aguzzi F, Baudner S, Bienvenu J, et al. Consensus of a group of professional societies and diagnostic companies on guidelines for interim reference ranges for 14 proteins in serum based on the standardization against the IFCC/BCR/CAP reference material (CRM 470). Eur J Clin Chem Clin Biochem 1996;34:517-20.
23. Delgado J, Pratt G, Phillips N, Briones J, Fegan C, Nomdedeu J, et al. Beta(2)-microglobulin is a better predictor of treatment-free survival in patients with chronic lymphocytic leukemia if adjusted according to glomerular filtration rate. Br J Haematol 2009;145:801-5.

24. Denne SC, Poindexter BB. Evidence supporting early nutritional support with parenteral amino acid infusion. Semin Perinatol 2007;31:56-60.
25. Devoto G, Gallo F, Marchello C, Racchi O, Garbini R, Bonassi S, et al. Prealbumin concentrations as a useful tool in the assessment of malnutrition in hospitalized patients. Clin Chem 2006;52:2281-5.
26. Dimopoulos MA, Gertz MA, Kastritis E, Garcia-Sanz R, Kimby EK, Leblond V, et al. Update on treatment recommendations from the Fourth International Workshop on Waldenstrom's macroglobulinemia. J Clin Oncol 2009;27:120-6.
27. Dispenzieri A, Kyle R, Merlini G, Miguel JS, Ludwig H, Hajek R, et al. International Myeloma Working Group guidelines for serum free light chain analysis in multiple myeloma and related disorders. Leukemia 2009;23:215-24.
28. Dobson CM. Protein folding and misfolding. Nature 2003;426: 884-90.
29. Domon B, Aebersold R. Mass spectrometry and protein analysis. Science 2006;312:212-7.
30. Durandy A, Peron S, Fischer A. Hyper-IgM syndrome. Curr Opin Rheumatol 2006;18:369-76.
31. Elango R, Ball RO, Pencharz PB. Amino acid requirements in humans: with a special emphasis on the metabolic availability of amino acids. Amino Acids 2009;37:19-27.
32. Ellington AA, Kullo IJ, Bailey KR, Klee GG. Measurement and quality control issues in multiplex protein assays: a case study. Clin Chem 2009;55:1092-9.
33. Engel H, Bac DJ, Brouwer R, Blijenberg BG, Lindemans J. Diagnostic analysis of total protein, albumin, white cell count and differential in ascitic fluid. Eur J Clin Chem Clin Biochem 1995;33:239-42.
34. Erikson N, Benditt EP. Serum amyloid A (ApoSAA) and lipoproteins. Methods Enzymol 1986;128:311-20.
35. Felgenhauer K. Protein size and cerebrospinal fluid composition. Klin Wochenschr 1974;52:1158-64.
36. Ferrante M, Penninckx F, De Hertogh G, Geboes K, D'Hoore A, Noman M, et al. Protein-losing enteropathy in Crohn's disease. Acta Gastroenterol Belg 2006;69:384-9.
37. Fogh-Andersen N, Bjerrum BJ, Siggaard-Andersen O. Ionic binding, net charge, and Donnan effect of human serum albumin as a function of pH. Clin Chem 1993;39:48-52.
38. Fournier T, Medjoubi NN, Porquet D. Alpha-1-acid glycoprotein. Biochim Biophys Acta 2000;1482:157-171.
39. Fox PL, Mazumder B, Ehrenwald E, Mukhopadhyay CK. Ceruloplasmin and cardiovascular disease. Free Radic Biol Med 2000;28:1735-44.
40. Freeman AF, Domingo DL, Holland SM. Hyper IgE (Job's) syndrome: a primary immunodeficiency with oral manifestations. Oral Dis 2009;15:2-7.
41. Fuchs SA, de Sain-van der Velden MG, de Barse MM, Roeconcentrationd MM, Hendriks M, Dorland L, et al. Two mass-spectrometric techniques for quantifying serine enantiomers and glycine in cerebrospinal fluid: potential confounders and age-dependent ranges. Clin Chem 2008;54:1443-50.
42. Gabay C, Kushner I. Acute-phase proteins and other systemic responses to inflammation. N Engl J Med 1999;340:448-54.
43. Gladwin MT, Vichinsky E. Pulmonary complications of sickle cell disease. N Engl J Med 2008;359:2254-65.
44. Glembotski CC. Endoplasmic reticulum stress in the heart. Circ Res 2007;101:975-84.
45. Gornick, O, Lauc G. Glycosylation of serum proteins in inflammatory diseases. Dis Markers 2008;25:267-78.
46. Gressner OA, Weiskirchen R, Gressner AM. Biomarkers of liver fibrosis: clinical translation of molecular pathogenesis or based on liver-dependent malfunction tests. Clin Chim Acta 2007;381:107-13.
47. Hahn BH, Grossman J, Ansell BJ, Skaggs BJ, McMahon M. Altered lipoprotein metabolism in chronic inflammatory states: proinflammatory high-density lipoprotein and accelerated atherosclerosis is systemic lupus erythematosus and rheumatoid arthritis. Arthritis Res Ther 2008;10:213.
48. Hamilton RG, Franklin Adkinson N. In vitro assays for the diagnosis of IgE-mediated disorders. J Allergy Immunol 2004;114:213-25.
49. Hart GW, Housley MP, Slawson C. Cycling of O-linked beta-N-acetylglucosamine on nucleocytoplasmic proteins. Nature 2007;446:1017-22.
50. Hay WW. Strategies for feeding the preterm infant. Neonatology 2008;94:245-54.
51. Heffner JE. Discriminating between transudates and exudates. Clin Chest Med 2006;27:241-52.
52. Henderson JM, Stein SF, Kutner M, Wiles MB, Ansley JD, Rudman D. Analysis of twenty-three plasma proteins in ascites: the depletion of fibrinogen and plasminogen. Ann Surg 1980;192:738-42.
53. Hochstrasser M. Origin and function of ubiquitin-like proteins. Nature 2009;458:422-9.
54. Hoofnagle AN, Becker JO, Wener MH, Heinecke JW. Quantification of thyroglobulin, a low-abundance serum protein, by immunoaffinity peptide enrichment and tandem mass spectrometry. Clin Chem 2008;54:1796-804.
55. Hortin GL. Can mass spectrometric protein profiling meet desired standards of clinical laboratory practice? Clin Chem 2005;51:3-5.
56. Hortin GL. The MALDI-TOF mass spectrometric view of the plasma proteome and peptidome. Clin Chem 2006;52:1223-37.
57. Hortin GL, Jortani SA, Ritchie JC, Valdes R, Chan DW. Proteomics: a new diagnostic frontier. Clin Chem 2006;52:1218-22.
58. Hortin GL, Meilinger B. Cross-reactivity of amino acids and other compounds in the Biuret reaction: interference with urinary peptide measurements. Clin Chem 2005;51:1411-9.
59. Hortin GL, Seam N, Hoehn GT. Bound homocysteine, cysteine, and cysteinylglycine distribution between albumin and globulins. Clin Chem 2006;52:2258-64.
60. Hortin GL, Sviridov D, Anderson L. High-abundance polypeptides of the human plasma proteome comprising the top 4 logs of polypeptide abundance. Clin Chem 2008;54:1608-16.
61. Hortin GL, Warshawsky I, Laude-Sharp M. Macromolecular chromogenic substrates for measuring proteinase activity. Clin Chem 2001;47:215-22.
62. Horwich TB, Kalantar-Zadeh K, MacLellan RW, Fonarow GC. Albumin concentrations predict survival in patients with systolic heart failure. Am Heart J 2008;155:883-9.
63. Hosafci G, Klein O, Oremek G, Mantele W. Clinical chemistry without reagents? An infrared spectroscopic technique for determination of clinically relevant constituents of body fluids. Anal Bioanal Chem 2007;387:1815-22.
64. Hu S, Loo JA, Wong DT. Human saliva proteome analysis and disease biomarker discovery. Expert Rev Proteomics 2007;4:531-8.
65. Hutchison CA, Harding S, Hewins P, Mead GP, Townsend J, Bradwell AR, et al. Quantitative assessment of serum and urinary free light chains in patients with chronic kidney disease. Clin J Am Soc Nephrol 2008;3:1684-90.
66. Ivandic BT, Spanuth E, Haase D, Lestin HG, Katus HA. Increased plasma concentrations of soluble CD40 ligand in acute coronary syndrome depend on in vitro platelet activation. Clin Chem 2007;53:1231-4.
67. Jahoor F, Badaloo A, Reid M, Forrester T. Protein metabolism in severe childhood malnutrition. Ann Trop Paediatr 2008;28:87-101.
68. Jensen JK, Dolmer K, Gettins PG. Specificity of binding of the low density lipoprotein receptor-related protein (LRP) to different conformational states of the clade E serpins PAI-1 and PN1. J Biol Chem 2009;284:17989-97.
69. Jeschke MG, Finnerty CC, Kulp GA, Przkora R, Micak RP, Nerndon DN. Combination of recombinant human growth hormone and propranolol decreases hypermetabolism and inflammation in severely burned children. Pediatr Crit Care Med 2008;9:209-16.
70. Johnson AM. Amino acids, peptides, and proteins. In: Burtis CA, Ashwood ER, Bruns DE, eds. Tietz textbook of clinical chemistry, 4th edition. Philadelphia: WB Saunders, 2006:531-95.
71. Joseph J, Handy DE, Loscalzo J. Quo vadis: whither homocysteine research? Cardiovasc Toxicol 2009;9:53-63.

72. Kaneko Y, Nimmerjahn F, Ravetch JV. Anti-inflammatory activity of immunoglobulin G resulting from Fc sialylation. Science 2006;313:670-3.
73. Katzmann JA, Kyle RA, Benson J, Larson DR, Snyder MR, Lust JA, et al. Screening panels for detection of monoclonal gammopathies. Clin Chem 2009;55:1-6.
74. Keersmaekers T, Claes K, Kuypers DR, de Vlam K, Verschueren P, Westhovens R. Long-term efficacy of infliximab treatment for AA-amyloidosis secondary to chronic inflammatory arthritis. Ann Rheum Dis 2009;68:759-61.
75. Kielstein JT, Zoccali C. Asymmetric dimethylarginine: a novel marker of risk and a potential target for therapy in chronic kidney disease. Curr Opin Nephrol Hypertens 2008;17:609-15.
76. Kochanek PM, Berger RP, Bayir H, Wagner AK, Jenkins LW, Clark RS. Biomarkers of evolving damage in traumatic and ischemic brain injury: diagnosis, prognosis, probing mechanisms, and therapeutic decision making. Curr Opin Crit Care 2008;14:135-41.
77. Kolodziej SJ, Klueppelberg HU, Nolasco N, Ehses W, Strickland DK, Stoops JK. Three-dimensional structure of the human plasmin alpha2-macroglobulin complex. J Struct Biol 1998;123:124-33.
78. Kricka LJ, Master SR, Joos TO, Fortina P. Current perspectives in protein array technology. Ann Clin Biochem 2006;43:457-67.
79. Kuhn E, Addona T, Keshishian H, Burgess M, Mani DR, Lee RT, et al. Developing multiplexed assays for troponin I and interleukin-33 in plasma by peptide immunoaffinity enrichment and targeted mass spectrometry. Clin Chem 2009;55:1108-17.
80. Kurpad AV. The requirements of protein and amino acid during acute and chronic infections. Indian J Med Res 2006;124:129-148.
81. Kwong LK, Uryu K, Trojanowski JQ, Lee VM. TDP-43 proteinopathies: neurodegenerative protein misfolding diseases without amyloidosis. Neurosignals 2008;16:41-51.
82. Kyle RA, Rajkuma SV. Criteria for diagnosis, staging, risk stratification and response assessment of multiple myeloma. Leukemia 2009;23:3-9.
83. Kyte J, Doolittle RF. A simple method for displaying the hydropathic character of a protein. J Mol Biol 1982;157:105-132.
84. Lam HS, Ng PC. Biochemical markers of neonatal sepsis. Pathology 2008;40:141-8.
85. Labriola B, Wallemacq P, Gulbis B, Jadoul M. The impact of the assay for measuring albumin on corrected ("adjusted") calcium concentrations. Nephrol Dial Transplant 2009;24:1834-8.
86. Landgren O, Kyle RA, Pfeiffer RM, Katzmann JA, Caporaso NE, Hayes RB, et al. Monoclonal gammopathy of undetermined significance (MGUS) consistently precedes multiple myeloma: a prospective study. Blood 2009;113:5412-7.
87. Langlois MR, Delanghe JR. Biological and clinical significance of haptoglobin polymorphism in humans. Clin Chem 1996;42:1589-600.
88. Law RH, Zhang Q, McGowan S, Buckle AM, Silverman GA, Wong W, et al. An overview of the serpin superfamily. Genome Biol 2006;7:216.
89. Lentine K, Wrone EM. New insights into protein intake and progression of renal disease. Curr Opin Nephrol Hypertens 2004;13:333-6.
90. Ling MM, Ricks C, Lea P. Multiplexing molecular diagnostics and immunoassays using emerging microarray technologies. Expert Rev Mol Diagn 2007;7:87-98.
91. Livrea P, Trojano M, Simone IL, Zimatore GB, Pisicchio L, Logroscino G, et al. Heterogeneous models for blood-cerebrospinal fluid barrier permeability to serum proteins in normal and abnormal cerebrospinal fluid/serum protein concentration gradients. J Neurol Sci 1984;64:245-58.
92. Lu J, Holmgren A. Selenoproteins. J Biol Chem 2009;284:723-7.
93. Lundblad RL. The evolution from protein chemistry to proteomics: basic science to clinical application. Boca Raton, Fla: CRC Press, 2006.
94. Luque FA, Jaffe SL. Cerebrospinal fluid analysis in multiple sclerosis. Int Rev Neurobiol 2007;79:341-56.
95. Madsden E, Gitlin JD. Copper deficiency. Curr Opin Gastroenterol 2007;23:187-92.
96. Mak CM, Lam CW. Diagnosis of Wilson's disease: a comprehensive review. Crit Rev Clin Lab Sci 2008;45:263-90.
97. Mak CM, Lam WW, Tam S. Diagnostic accuracy of serum ceruloplasmin in Wilson disease: determination of sensitivity and specificity by ROC curve analysis among ATP7B-genotyped subjects. Clin Chem 2008;54:1356-62.
98. Maniaci V, Dauber A, Weiss S, Nylen E, Becker KL, Bachur R. Procalcitonin in young febrile infants for the detection of serious bacterial infections. Pediatrics 2008;122:701-10.
99. Mantovani A, Garlanda C, Doni A, Bottazzi B. Pentraxins in innate immunity: from C-reactive protein to the long pentraxin PTX3. J Clin Immunol 2008;28:1-13.
100. Marklova E, Albahri Z. Screening and diagnosis of congenital disorders of glycosylation. Clin Chim Acta 2007;385:6-20.
101. Mathivanan S, Pandey A. Human proteinpedia as a resource for clinical proteomics. Mol Cell Proteomics 2008;7:2038-47.
102. Matthews ST, Deutsch DD, Iyer G, Hora N, Pati B, Marsh J, et al. Plasma alpha2-HS glycoprotein concentrations in patients with acute myocardial infarction quantified by a modified ELISA. Clin Chim Acta 2002;319:27-34.
103. McCudden CR, Mathews SP, Hainsworth SA, Chapman JF, Hammett-Stabler CA, Willis MS, et al. Performance comparison of capillary and agarose electrophoresis for the identification and characterization of monoclonal immunoglobulins. Am J Clin Pathol 2008;129:451-8.
104. Meng QH, Krahn J. Lithium heparinized blood-collection tubes give falsely low albumin results with an automated bromcresol green method in haemodialysis patients. Clin Chem Lab Med 2008;46:396-400.
105. Miller WG, Bruns DE, Hortin GL, Sandberg S, Aakre KM, McQueen MJ, et al. Current issues in measurement and reporting of urinary albumin excretion. Clin Chem 2009;55:24-38.
106. Miller WG, Thienpont LM, Van Uytfanghe K, Clark PM, Lindstedt P, Nilsson G, et al. Toward standardization of insulin immunoassays. Clin Chem 2009;55:1011-8.
107. Miura H, Ozaki N, Sawada M, Isobe K, Ohta T, Nagatsu T. A link between stress and depression: shifts in the balance between the kynurenine and serotonin pathways of tryptophan metabolism and the etiology and pathophysiology of depression. Stroke 2008;11:198-209.
108. Mizazaki D, Yazaki M, Gono T, Kametani F, Tsuchiya A, Matsuda M, et al. AH amyloidosis associated with an immunoglobulin heavy chain variable region (VH1) fragment: a case report. Amyloid 2008;15:125-8.
109. Moldonado F, Hawkins FJ, Daniels CE, Doerr CH, Decker PA, Ryu JH. Pleural fluid characteristics of chylothorax. Mayo Clin Proc 2009;84:129-133.
110. Mora S, Musunuru K, Blumenthal RS. The clinical utility of high-sensitivity C-reactive protein in cardiovascular disease and the potential implication for JUPITER on current practice guidelines. Clin Chem 2009;55:219-28.
111. Morris CR. Asthma management: reinventing the wheel in sickle cell disease. Am J Hematol 2009;84:234-41.
112. Morris SM. Arginine: beyond protein. Am J Clin Nutr 2006;83:508S-12S.
112A. Mulder C, Verwey NA, van der Flier WM, Bouwman FH, Kok A, van Elk EJ, et al. Amyloid-∃(1-42), total tau, and phosphorylated tau as cerebrospinal fluid biomarkers for the diagnosis of Alzheimer disease. Clin Chem 2010;56:248-53.
113. Munthe-Fog B, Hummelshoj T, Honore C, Madsen HO, Permin H, Garred P. Immunodeficiency associated with FCN3 mutation and ficolin-3 deficiency. N Engl J Med 2009;360:2637-44.
114. Nedelkov D, Kiernan UA, Niederkofler EE, Tubbs KA, Nelson RW. Investigating diversity in human plasma proteins. Proc Natl Acad Sci U S A 2005;102:10852-7.
115. Neuberger MS. Antibody diversification by somatic mutation: from Burnet onwards. Immunol Cell Biol 2008;86:124-32.
116. Norden AGW, Lapsley M, Lee PJ, Pusey CD, Schenman SJ, Tam FWK, et al. Glomerular protein sieving and implications for renal failure in Fanconi syndrome. Kidney Int 2001;60:1885-92.

117. Omenn GS, States DJ, Adamski M, Blackwell TW, Menon R, Hermjakob H, et al. Overview of the HUPO Plasma Proteome Project: results from the pilot phase with 35 collaborating laboratories and multiple analytical groups, generating a core dataset of 3020 proteins and a publicly-available database. Proteomics 2005;5:3226-45.
118. Otten JJ, Hellweg JP, Meyers LD. Dietary reference intakes: the essential guide to nutrient requirements. Washington, DC: National Academy of Sciences Press, 2006.
119. Parker C, Omine M, Richards S, Nishimura J, Bessler M, Ware R, et al. Diagnosis and management of paroxysmal nocturnal hemoglobinuria. Blood 2005;106:3699-709.
120. Pepys MB. Amyloidosis. Annu Rev Med 2006;57:223-41.
121. Peters T Jr. All about albumin: serum albumin—biochemistry, genetics, and medical applications. Washington, DC: AACC Press, 1996.
122. Petricoin EF, Belluco C, Araujo RP, Liotta LA. The blood peptidome: a higher dimension of information content for cancer biomarker discovery. Nat Rev Cancer 2006;6:961-7.
123. Picken MM. New insights into systemic amyloidosis: the importance of diagnosis of specific type. Curr Opin Nephrol Hypertens 2007;16:196-203.
124. Ponten F, Jirstrom K, Uhlen M. The human protein atlas—a tool for pathology. J Pathol 2008;216:387-93.
125. Pumphrey RSH. Structure and function of immunoglobulin. In: Ward AM, Whicher JT, eds. Immunochemistry in clinical laboratory medicine. Lancaster, UK: MTP Press, 1979:85-98.
126. Rai AJ, Vitzthum F. Effects of preanalytical variables on peptide and protein measurements in human serum and plasma: implications for clinical proteomics. Expert Rev Proteomics 2006;3:409-26.
127. Rebrin I, Sohal RS. Pro-oxidant shift in glutathione redox state during aging. Adv Drug Deliv Rev 2008;60:1545-52.
128. Refsum H, Smith AD, Ueland PM, Nexo E, Clarke R, McPartlin J, et al. Facts and recommendations about total homocysteine determinations: an expert opinion. Clin Chem 2004;50:3-32.
129. Ridker PM. Clinical application of C-reactive protein for cardiovascular disease detection and prevention. Circulation 2003;107:363-9.
130. Ridker PM. C-reactive protein: eighty years from discovery to emergence as a major risk marker for cardiovascular disease. Clin Chem 2009;55:209-215.
131. Roopenian DC, Akilesh S. FcRn: the neonatal Fc receptor comes of age. Nat Rev Immunol 2007;7:715-25.
132. Roth E. Nonnutritive effects of glutamine. J Nutr 2008;138:2025S-31S.
133. Runyon BA, Montano AA, Akriviadis EA, Antillon MR, Irving MA, McHutchison JG. The serum-ascites albumin gradient is superior to the exudate-transudate concept in the differential diagnosis of ascites. Ann Intern Med 1992;117:215-20.
134. Saha S, Harrison SH, Shen C, Tang H, Radivojac P, Arnold RJ, et al. HIP2: an online database of human plasma proteins from healthy individuals. BMC Med Genom 2008;1:12.
135. Scheuner D, Kaufman RJ. The unfolded protein response: a pathway that links insulin demand with beta-cell failure and diabetes. Endocr Rev 2008;29:317-33.
136. Schiffer E, Mischak H, Vanholder RC. Exploring the uremic toxins using proteomic technologies. Contrib Nephrol 2008;160:159-71.
137. Schneider HG, Lam QT. Procalcitonin for the clinical laboratory: a review. Pathology 2007;39:383-90.
138. Schreiber G, Aldred AR, Jaworowski A, Nilsson C, Achen MG, Segal MB. Thyroxine transport from blood to brain via transthyretin synthesis in choroid plexus. Am J Physiol 1990;258:R338.
139. Schrockensnadel K, Wirleitner B, Winkler C, Fuchs D. Monitoring tryptophan metabolism in chronic immune activation. Clin Chim Acta 2006;364:82-90.
140. Scott CF, Carrell RW, Glaser CB, Kueppers F, Lewis JH, Colman RW. Alpha-1-antitrypsin Pittsburgh: a potent inhibitor of human plasma factor XIa, kallikrein, and factor XIIf. J Clin Invest 1986;77:631-4.
141. Sharp P. The molecular basis of copper and iron interactions. Proc Nutr Soc 2004;63:563-9.
142. Shihabi ZK. Cryoglobulins: an important but neglected clinical test. Ann Clin Lab Sci 2006;36:395-408.
143. Shimizu A, Nakanishi T, Miyazaki A. Detection and characterization of variant and modified structures of proteins in blood and tissues by mass spectrometry. Mass Spectrom Rev 2006;25:686-712.
144. Silverman EK, Sandhaus RA. Alpha1-antitrypsin deficiency. N Engl J Med 2009;360:2749-57.
145. Sivan SS, Wachtel E, Tsitron E, Sakkee N, van der Ham F, DeGroot J, et al. Collagen turnover in normal and degenerate human intervertebral discs as determined by the racemization of aspartic acid. J Biol Chem 2008;283:8796-801.
146. Sjoholm AG, Jonsson G, Braconier JH, Sturfelt G, Truedsson L. Complement deficiency and disease: an update. Mol Immunol 2006;43:78-85.
147. Snozek CLH, Saenger AK, Greipp PR, Bryant SC, Kyle RA, Rajkumar SV, et al. Comparison of bromcresol green and agarose protein electrophoresis for quantitation of serum albumin in multiple myeloma. Clin Chem 2007;53:1099-103.
148. Stiehm ER. The four most common pediatric immunodeficiencies. J Immunotoxicol 2008;5:227-34.
149. Stoevesandt O, Taussig MJ, He M. Protein microarrays: high-throughput tools for proteomics. Expert Rev Proteomics 2009;6:145-57.
150. Sucker C, Hetzel GR, Grabensee B, Stockschlaeder M, Scharf RE. Amyloidosis and bleeding: pathophysiology, diagnosis, and therapy. Am J Kidney Dis 2006;47:947-55.
151. Sutherland AD, Gearry RB, Frizelle FA. Review of fecal biomarkers in inflammatory bowel disease. Dis Colon Rectum 2008;51:1283-91.
152. Takeda H, Nishise S, Furukawa M, Nagashima R, Shizawa H, Takahashi T. Fecal clearance of alpha 1-antitrypsin with lansoprazole can detect protein-losing gastropathy. Dig Dis Sci 1999;44:2313-8.
153. Tattersall J. Clearance of beta-2-microglobulin and middle molecules in haemodiafiltration. Contrib Nephrol 2007;158:201-9.
154. Texel SJ, Xu X, Harris ZL. Ceruloplasmin in neurodegenerative diseases. Biochem Soc Trans 2008;36:1277-81.
155. Tichy M, Friedecky B, Budina M, Maisner V, Buchler T, Holeckova M, et al. Interference of IgM-lambda paraprotein with biuret-type assay for total serum protein quantification. Clin Chem Lab Med 2009;47:235-6.
156. Tietz NW, ed. Clinical guide to laboratory tests, 3rd edition. Philadelphia: WB Saunders, 1995.
157. Ueland PM. Homocysteine species as components of plasma redox thiol status. Clin Chem 1995;41:340-2.
158. Unsworth DJ. Complement deficiency and disease. J Clin Pathol 2008;61:1013-7.
159. Van Asbeck EC, Hoepelman AIM, Scharringa J, Herpers BL, Verhoef J. Mannose binding lectin plays a crucial role in innate immunity against yeast by enhanced complement activation and enhanced uptake of polymorphonuclear cells. BMC Microbiol 2008;8:229.
160. Von Eynatten M, Humpert PM. Retinol-binding protein-4 in experimental and clinical metabolic disease. Expert Rev Mol Diagn 2008;8:289-99.
161. Vanholder R, De Smet R, Glorieux G, Argiles A, Baurmeister U, Brunet P, et al. Review on uremic toxins: classification, concentration, and interindividual variability. Kidney Int 2003;63:1934-43.
162. Vermeulen MA, van de Poll MC, Ligthart-Melis GC, Dejong CH, van den Tol MP, Boelens PG, et al. Specific amino acids in the critically ill patient—exogenous glutamine/arginine: a common denominator? Crit Care Med 2007;35(9 Suppl):S568-76.
163. Vollmer T, Piper C, Kleesiek K, Dreier J. Lipopolysaccharide-binding protein: a new biomarker for infectious endocarditis? Clin Chem 2009;55:295-302.
164. Walsh MJ, Tourtellotte WW: The cerebrospinal fluid in multiple sclerosis. In: Hallpike JF, Adams CWM, Tourtellotte WW, eds. Multiple sclerosis. London: Chapman & Hall, 1983:275-358.

165. Wani MA, Haynes LC, Kim J, Bronson CL, Chaudhury C, Mohanty S, et al. Familial hypercatabolic hypoproteinemia caused by deficiency of the neonatal Fc receptor, FcRN, due to a mutant beta2-microglobulin gene. PNAS USA 2006;103:5084-9.
166. Watanabe A, Matsuzaki S, Moriwaki H, Suzuki K, Nishiguchi S. Problems in serum albumin measurement and clinical significance of albumin microheterogeneity in cirrhotics. Nutrition 2004;2:351-7.
167. Whicher JT. BCR/IFCC reference material for plasma proteins (CRM 470). Community Bureau of Reference. International Federation of Clinical Chemistry. Clin Biochem 1998;31:459-65.
168. Whitfield JB, Dy V, Madden PA, Heath AC, Martin NG, Montgomery GW. Measuring carbohydrate-deficient transferring by direct immunoassay: factors affecting diagnostic sensitivity for excessive alcohol intake. Clin Chem 2008;54:1158-65.
169. Williams AJ, Paulson HL. Polyglutamine neurodegeneration: protein misfolding revisited. Trends Neurosci 2008;31:521-8.
170. Woof JM, Mestecky J. Mucosal immunoglobulins. Immunol Rev 2005;206:64-82.
171. Xu S, Venge P. Lipocalins as biochemical markers of disease. Biochim Biophys Acta 2000;1482:298-307.
172. Zetterberg H. Update on amyloid-beta homeostasis markers for sporadic Alzheimer's disease. Scand J Clin Lab Invest 2009;69:18-21.
173. Zhang XL, Ali MA. Ficolins: structure, function and associated diseases. Adv Exp Med 2008;632:105-15.

CHAPTER 22

Serum Enzymes

Mauro Panteghini, M.D.,
and Renze Bais, Ph.D., A.R.C.P.A.

Measurements of enzymes are used in medicine in two major ways. Enzymes are measured in serum and other bodily fluids to detect injury to a tissue that makes up the enzyme. Enzymes are also measured, often within a tissue, to identify abnormalities or absence of the enzyme, which may cause disease.

Injury to tissue releases cellular substances that can be used as plasma markers of tissue damage. Many of the clinically useful markers of cellular damage are enzymes. For a substance to serve as a biochemical marker of damage to a specific organ or tissue, it must arise predominantly from the organ or tissue of interest. Highly specific markers have been identified (e.g., cardiac troponin I, which is found only in cardiac myocytes). Some enzymes are found predominantly in specialized tissue (e.g., lipase in the pancreas); others, more widely distributed, have tissue-specific isoenzymes or isoforms (e.g., the pancreatic isoenzyme of α-amylase, the bone isoform of alkaline phosphatase) that can be evaluated to enhance tissue and organ specificity.

The timing of the enzyme's diagnostic window is another important aspect to be considered when these markers are used to evaluate acute injury. According to Noe,[52] the diagnostic window for an injury marker is the interval of time following an episode of injury during which plasma concentrations of the marker are increased, thereby demonstrating the occurrence of injury. Marker substances that rapidly enter the circulation (i.e., early indicators) tend to have diagnostic windows that begin soon after onset of the injury. On the contrary, those biomarkers that are slowly released into the circulation and/or are slowly cleared from the circulation (i.e., late indicators) generally have diagnostic windows that begin later and last long after the time of injury.

DIAGNOSTIC ENZYMOLOGY

In general, clinical laboratorians are principally concerned with changes in activity in the serum or plasma of enzymes that are predominantly intracellular and physiologically present in the blood at low activity concentrations only. Changes in the serum activities of these enzymes are used to infer the location and nature of pathologic changes in tissues of the body. Therefore, an understanding of the factors that affect the rate of release of enzymes from their cells of origin and the rate at which they are cleared from the circulation is necessary to interpret correctly changes in activity that occur with disease.

Factors Affecting Enzyme Concentrations in Plasma or Serum[35,36]

The measured activity of an enzyme in blood is the result not only of the total amount released from its cells of origin, but also of the rate of enzyme catabolism in the circulation, the escape to the extracellular enzyme pool, and the rate at which it is inactivated or removed.

Leakage of Enzymes from Cells

Enzymes are retained within their cells of origin by the plasma membrane surrounding the cell. The plasma membrane is a metabolically active part of the cell, and its integrity depends on the cell's production of ATP. Any process that impairs ATP production by depriving the cell of oxidizable substrates or by reducing the efficiency of energy production by restricting the access of oxygen (ischemia or anoxia) promotes deterioration of the cell membrane. The earliest sign of impaired energy metabolism is the efflux of potassium with influx of sodium; water thus accumulates within the cell, causing it to swell. The next and most serious stage is the entry of Ca^{2+}, which stimulates intracellular enzymes, leading to both cell damage and disruption of the cell membrane. Finally, free radicals formed during these processes may cause further damage. The membrane becomes leaky; if cellular injury becomes irreversible, the cell will die, although enzyme loss may also occur without the occurrence of irreversible injury. Small molecules are the first to leak from damaged or dying cells, followed by larger molecules, such as enzymes and other proteins. Cytosolic proteins appear early on in the plasma, followed much later by mitochondrial and membrane-bound enzymes. It appears that ATP must decline to below a certain level before substantial enzyme release occurs. Ultimately, the complete content of the necrotic cells is discharged.

Because of very high concentrations of enzymes within the cells—thousands or even tens of thousands times greater than concentrations in extracellular fluid—and because extremely small amounts of enzyme can be detected by their catalytic activity, increased enzyme activity in the extracellular fluid or plasma is an extremely sensitive indicator of even minor cellular damage, some causes of which are listed in Table 22-1.

A reduction in the supply of oxygenated blood perfusing any tissue will promote enzyme release, such as occurs in myocardial infarction. Cells of the affected region rapidly begin to deteriorate and die, releasing their protein and enzyme contents to the systemic circulation, which accounts for the rapid rise in serum biomarkers that is characteristic of this condition. The liver is also very sensitive to hypoxia, which results from diminished cardiac output (heart failure). Direct attack on the cell membranes by such agents as viruses or organic chemicals also causes enzyme release, which is particularly important in the case of the liver. Skeletal muscles also contribute enzymes to blood. Again, the cause may be poor perfusion, hypothermia, or direct trauma to the muscles (crush injuries). Infection, inflammation (polymyositis), degenerative changes (dystrophies), drugs, and alcohol (alcoholic myopathy) will cause enzyme leakage from myocytes.

TABLE 22-1 Causes of Cell Damage or Death

Category	Examples
Hypoxia (an extremely common accompaniment of clinical disease)	Loss of blood supply due to narrowing (atheromatous plaques) or blocking (thrombosis) of artery or vein; ischemic-perfusion injury; inadequate oxygenation due to cardiorespiratory failure; loss of oxygen-carrying capacity, CO poisoning, and anemia
Chemicals and drugs	Environmental pollutants—lead, mercury; drugs—use and abuse; alcohol; tobacco
Physical agents	Trauma; extremes of heat and radiation; electrical energy; toxic chemicals
Microbiological agents	Bacteria, viruses, fungi, protozoa, and helminths
Immune mechanisms	Immune disorders can cause tissue damage by a number of mechanisms: 1. Anaphylaxis (causing release of vasoactive amines) 2. Cytotoxicity (causing the target cell to be lysed) 3. Immune complex disease (leading to release of lysosomal enzymes) 4. Cell-mediated hypersensitivity (leading to cytotoxicity)
Genetic defects	Disorders with polygenic inheritance—diabetes mellitus, gout
	Mendelian disorders—X-linked disorders, autosomal dominant and recessive disorders, disorders with variable modes of transmission and inborn errors of metabolism
Nutritional disorders	Protein-calorie malnutrition, vitamin deficiencies, mineral deficiencies; obesity and its consequences

Based on the classification of Robbins and colleagues. In: Basic pathology, 3rd edition. Philadelphia: WB Saunders, 1981.

Efflux of Enzymes from Damaged Cells

Once conditions for leakage of enzymes from cells have become established, the speed and extent to which the process is reflected in enzyme changes in the blood depend on several factors.

The driving force of enzyme release is the steep concentration gradient that exists between the interior and the exterior of the cells. The rate of escape of enzyme molecules is presumably controlled to some extent by diffusion; therefore, smaller enzyme molecules might be expected to appear in the extracellular fluid earlier than larger ones.

The way in which released enzyme molecules are transferred from the interstitial fluid to the blood varies from one tissue to another; they may pass directly through the capillary wall, or lymphatic transfer may occur. Direct transfer occurs to a large extent in the liver, which is a highly vascular tissue with many permeable capillaries, although evidence suggests that liver enzymes may also be subject to lymphatic transfer. On the other hand, the capillaries of skeletal muscle are relatively impermeable, and in this tissue it is probable that released enzymes mainly reach the circulatory system by way of drainage from the lymphatic system. Lymph drainage is also important in transporting enzymes released from damaged intestinal, pancreatic, and myocardial cells to the circulation, although, following myocardial infarction, a minor proportion of myocardial enzymes reaches the circulation by direct capillary transfer.

The intracellular location of the leaking enzymes affects the rates at which they appear in the circulation. As would be expected, the most sensitive indicators of cell damage are the molecules that are present in the soluble fraction of the cell. Release of structurally bound membrane proteins requires both a leaky cell membrane and a dissociation or degradation, which is a slower process.[39] Enzymes associated with subcellular structures, such as mitochondria, are less readily released into the circulation and often indicate irreversible cellular injury. This fact has been used in attempts to distinguish reversible leakage, presumed to reflect damage only to the cell membrane, from necrotic lesions, in which intracellular structures are destroyed.

The relation between tissue injury and the appearance of enzymes in the circulation is most clearly seen in myocardial infarction, in which a relatively short episode of damage is followed by rapid transfer of enzymes to the circulatory system. About 24 hours after a myocardial infarction, the pattern of relative activity of various enzymes in the circulatory system closely resembles that in myocardial tissue. These relationships are less clearly recognized in other conditions, such as chronic liver disease, in which enzyme release is a process that continues over a period of time. The pattern of relative enzyme activities in serum in chronic disease may also become distorted by differential rates of removal of enzymes from the circulation and possibly by differential changes in rates of enzyme synthesis in affected tissue.

Release of enzymes from damaged or dying cells and changes in the rate of enzyme production constitute the most important mechanisms by which changes in enzyme activity in the serum or plasma are produced. However, other possibilities exist and appear to account for some changes of diagnostic importance. For example, much of the γ-glutamyltransferase activity of liver cells is located on their exterior surfaces. It is possible that ectoenzymes such as this may be eluted from the surfaces, especially where detergent action of the blood is increased through accumulation of bile salts. This process does not involve cell damage in the sense of increased membrane permeability, as evidenced by lack of correlation between activities in the serum of γ-glutamyltransferase and the aminotransferases in liver disease of different types.

Altered Enzyme Production

Small amounts of intracellular enzymes physiologically present in the plasma can be assumed to result from wear and tear of cells or leakage of enzyme from healthy cells. This contribution of enzymes to the circulating blood may decrease as the result of a genetic deficiency of enzyme production (e.g., as is the case for alkaline phosphatase in hypophosphatasia or in individuals homozygous for the "silent" gene for serum cholinesterase), or when enzyme production is depressed as a result of disease (e.g., cholinesterase in liver disease). However, cases in which enzyme production is increased are of more general interest in diagnostic enzymology. For example, an increase in the number and activity of alkaline phosphatase–producing osteoblasts of bone is responsible for the increased concentration of alkaline phosphatase in the serum of normally growing children. Increased osteoblastic activity also accounts for increased concentrations of this enzyme in the serum in various types of bone disease.

The process of enzyme induction also increases enzyme production. An example of such induction is the increased activity of γ-glutamyltransferase in serum, which results from administration of drugs such as barbiturates or phenytoin, and from intake of ethanol.

Clearance of Enzymes

Significant evidence is available about the way in which enzymes are cleared from the circulation. Few enzyme molecules are small enough to pass through the glomerulus of the kidney; therefore urinary excretion is not a major route for elimination of enzymes from the circulation. An exception to this is α-amylase; increased concentrations of this enzyme in the blood (e.g., after *acute pancreatitis*) are accompanied by increased excretion in the urine.

Evidence now suggests that many enzymes are not inactivated in the plasma but are rapidly removed, probably by the reticuloendothelial system, such as the bone marrow, spleen, and liver (Kupffer cells), or, to a lesser extent, by nearly all cells in the body. The mechanism appears to consist of receptor-mediated endocytosis (the process of recognition, specific accumulation, and uptake of protein by specific cell surface receptors followed by fusion with lysosomes, digestion of ingested protein, and recycling of the receptor back to the cell membrane). For example, hepatic Kupffer cells have been shown to take up several tissue-derived enzymes—such as creatine kinase, adenylate kinase, cytoplasmic and mitochondrial aspartate aminotransferase, and malate and alcohol dehydrogenases—by receptor-mediated endocytosis, which may have affinity for lysine residues on these enzymes. The adult isoform of intestinal alkaline phosphatase is a galactosyl-terminal glycoprotein that reacts with a galactosyl-specific receptor on the hepatocyte membrane and undergoes subsequent endocytosis. This process is rapid, accounting for the extremely short plasma half-life of this isoform. However, in hepatic cirrhosis, in which considerable reduction in parenchymal cell mass often occurs, the plasma concentration and half-life of the isoform increase. Other alkaline phosphatase isoenzymes and isoforms are sialoglycoproteins that do not react with the galactosyl receptor and therefore are protected from rapid uptake from blood. Indeed, examples are known of excessive sialylation of alkaline phosphatases produced by malignant cells, prolonging their plasma half-lives and facilitating their detection. This example illustrates the importance of understanding the processes by which enzymes are cleared from plasma.

The half-lives of enzymes in plasma vary from a few hours to several days, but in most cases, the average half-life ($t_{1/2}$) is 6 to 48 hours. Rates of decay may also be expressed as k_d values—the fractional disappearance rate—and the relationship to $t_{1/2}$ values is as follows:

$$k_d = 2.303 \log \frac{2}{t_{1/2}} = \frac{0.693}{t_{1/2}}$$

Typical disappearance rates from human blood for several clinically relevant enzymes are shown in Figure 22-1.

Selection of Enzyme Tests

The selection of which enzyme to measure in serum for diagnostic or prognostic purposes depends on a number of factors. An important factor is the distribution of enzymes among the various tissues, shown, for example, for aspartate aminotransferase, alanine aminotransferase, and creatine kinase in Figure 22-2. The main enzymes of established clinical value, together with their tissues of origin and their major clinical applications, are listed in Table 22-2.

The mass of the damaged or malfunctioning organ, together with the enzyme cell/blood gradient, obviously has a profound influence on the resulting elevation of enzyme

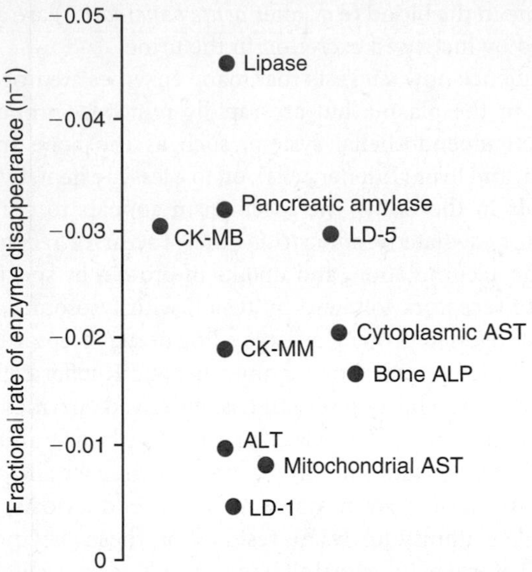

Figure 22-1 Fractional disappearance rates (k_d, in hours^{-1}) from human blood of the most important enzymes.

activity in blood. Thus the gradient of activity of prostatic acid phosphatase between prostate and blood is about $10^3:1$, and the mass of that organ is 20 g. By contrast, the cell and/or blood gradient of alanine aminotransferase in the liver cell is $10^4:1$, and the mass of the liver can exceed 1000 g. Obviously, fewer cells have to be damaged in the liver than in the prostate for the abnormality to be detected by an enzyme elevation in blood. If on the other hand, total organ involvement occurs, then clearly the vast number of affected liver cells will markedly elevate blood concentrations of any liver enzyme. It has been estimated that if only 1 liver cell in every 750 is damaged, elevation in the blood concentration of alanine aminotransferase would be detectable.

Knowledge of the intracellular location of enzymes can assist in determining the nature and severity of a pathologic process if suitable enzymes are assayed in the blood. For instance, a mild, reversible viral inflammation of the liver, such as a mild attack of viral hepatitis, is likely to increase only the permeability of the cell membrane, while allowing cytoplasmic enzymes to leak out into the blood, whereas a

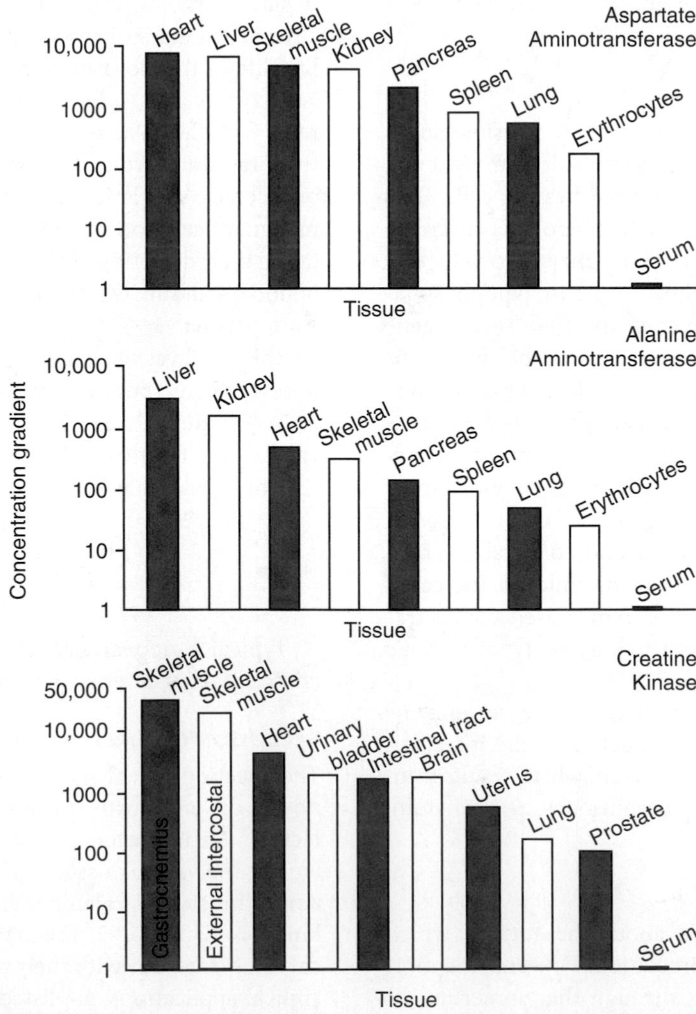

Figure 22-2 The concentration gradients between some human tissues and serum for aspartate transaminase, alanine transaminase, and creatine kinase. The concentration gradient axis is logarithmic.

TABLE 22-2 Distribution of Diagnostically Important Enzymes

Enzyme	Principal Sources of Enzyme in Blood	Principal Clinical Applications
Alanine aminotransferase	Liver	Hepatic parenchymal disease
Alkaline phosphatase	Liver, bone, intestinal mucosa, placenta	Hepatobiliary disease, bone disease
Amylase	Salivary glands, pancreas	Pancreatic disease
Aspartate aminotransferase	Heart, liver, skeletal muscle, erythrocytes	Hepatic parenchymal disease
Creatine kinase	Skeletal muscle, heart	Muscle disease, myocardial infarction
γ-Glutamyltransferase	Liver, pancreas, kidney	Hepatobiliary disease
Lactate dehydrogenase	Heart, erythrocytes, lymph nodes, skeletal muscle, liver	Hemolytic and megaloblastic anemias, leukemia and lymphomas, oncology
Lipase	Pancreas	Pancreatic disease
5′-Nucleotidase	Liver	Hepatobiliary disease

severe attack causing cell necrosis also disrupts the mitochondrial membrane, and both cytoplasmic and mitochondrial enzymes are detected in the blood. Finally, in selecting a suitable enzyme to assay in blood for diagnostic purposes, the clearance way and the rate at which its activity disappears from the blood are of significance. As previously indicated, the most commonly assayed enzymes are those with half-lives in the range of 12 hours or greater.

Several enzymes of diagnostic utility are discussed in this chapter. To better clarify their clinical meaning, the individual enzymes are discussed relative to the organ in which they are clinically most important. Overlap may occur for this classification as the same enzyme may be used for investigating disease in several organs.

MUSCLE ENZYMES

Enzymes in this category include creatine kinase, aldolase, and glycogen phosphorylase.

Creatine Kinase

Creatine kinase (EC 2.7.3.2; adenosine triphosphate : creatine *N*-phosphotransferase; CK) is a dimeric enzyme (82 kDa) that catalyzes the reversible phosphorylation of creatine (Cr) by adenosine triphosphate (ATP).

Creatine + Adenosine triphosphate ⇌ Phosphocreatine (creatine phosphate) + Adenosine diphosphate + $H^{\oplus}$

pH = 9.0 (forward); CK, Mg^{2+}; pH = 6.7 (reverse)

Physiologically, when muscle contracts, ATP is converted to adenosine diphosphate (ADP), and CK catalyzes the rephosphorylation of ADP to ATP using creatine phosphate (CrP) as the phosphorylation reservoir.

Optimal pH values for the forward (Cr + ATP → ADP + CrP) and reverse (CrP + ADP → ATP + Cr) reactions are 9.0 and 6.7, respectively. At neutral pH, the formation of ATP is favored; a pH of 9.0 is optimal for the formation of CrP, another high-energy compound. Mg^{2+} is an obligate activating ion that forms complexes with ATP and ADP. The optimal concentration range for Mg^{2+} is narrow, and excess Mg^{2+} is inhibitory. Many metal ions, such as Mn^{2+}, Ca^{2+}, Zn^{2+}, and Cu^{2+}, inhibit enzyme activity, as do iodoacetate and other sulfhydryl-binding reagents. Activity is inhibited by excess ADP and by citrate, fluoride, nitrate, acetate, iodide, bromide, malonate, and L-thyroxine.[3] Uratc and cystine are potent inhibitors of the enzyme in serum. Even chloride and sulfate ions inhibit activity, and the concentrations of these ions should be kept low in any enzyme assay system based on the CrP + ADP (reverse) reaction. The enzyme in serum is relatively unstable, activity being lost as a result of sulfhydryl group oxidation at the active site of the enzyme. Activity can be partially restored by incubating the enzyme preparation with sulfhydryl compounds, such as *N*-acetylcysteine, dithiothreitol (Cleland reagent), and glutathione. The current agent of choice is *N*-acetylcysteine, which has the advantage of being a very soluble substance used at a final concentration of 20 mmol/L in the assay reagent.

CK activity is greatest in striated muscle and heart tissue, which contain some 2500 and 550 U/g of protein, respectively. Other tissues, such as the brain, the gastrointestinal tract, and the urinary bladder, contain significantly less activity, and the liver and erythrocytes are essentially devoid of activity (Table 22-3).

CK is a dimer composed of two subunits, each with a molecular weight of about 40,000 Da. These subunits (B and M) are the products of loci on chromosomes 14 and 19, respectively. Because the active form of the enzyme is a dimer, only three different pairs of subunits can exist: BB (or CK-1), MB (or CK-2), and MM (or CK-3). The Commission

TABLE 22-3 Approximate Concentrations of Tissue Creatine Kinase (CK) Activity (Expressed as Multiples of CK Activity Concentrations in Serum) and Cytoplasmic Isoenzyme Composition

	Relative CK	Isoenzymes, %		
Tissue	**Activity**	**CK-BB**	**CK-MB**	**CK-MM**
Skeletal muscle (type I, slow twitch, or red fibers)	50,000	<1	3	97
Skeletal muscle (type II, fast twitch, or white fibers)	50,000	<1	1	99
Heart	10,000	<1	22	78
Brain	5000	100	0	0
Smooth Muscle				
Gastrointestinal tract	5000	96	1	3
Urinary bladder	4000	92	6	2

on Biochemical Nomenclature has recommended that isoenzymes be numbered on the basis of their electrophoretic mobility, with the most anodal form receiving the lowest number. Accordingly, the CK isoenzymes are numbered CK-1, CK-2, and CK-3. The distribution of these isoenzymes in the various tissues of humans is shown in Table 22-3. All three of these isoenzyme species are found in the cytosol of the cell or are associated with myofibrillar structures. However, there exists a fourth form that differs from the others both immunologically and by electrophoretic mobility. This isoenzyme (CK-Mt) is located between the inner and outer membranes of mitochondria, and it constitutes, in the heart for example, up to 15% of total CK activity. The gene for CK-Mt is located on chromosome 15.

CK activity may also be found in macromolecular form—the so-called macro-CK. Macro-CK is found, often transiently, in the sera of up to 6% of hospitalized patients, but only a minor proportion of these have increased CK activities in serum. It exists in two forms: types 1 and 2. Type 1 is a complex of CK, typically CK-BB, and an immunoglobulin, often IgG, but other complexes have been described, such as CK-MM with IgA. Macro-CK type 1 is not of pathologic significance, but it can be the cause of elevated CK results, resulting in diagnostic confusion and leading to unnecessary further investigation. Prevalence has been estimated as between 0.8 and 2.3%, but this is dependent on the method used and the population studied.[17] Macro-CK type 2 is oligomeric CK-Mt, with a reported prevalence of between 0.5 and 2.6%. It is found predominantly in adults who are severely ill with malignancy or liver disease, or in children who have notable tissue distress. The appearance of this isoenzyme in serum is usually associated with a poor prognosis. Macro-CK can interfere with the assay of CK-MB by some immunoinhibition methods.

Both M and B subunits have a C-terminal lysine residue, but only the former can be hydrolyzed by the action of carboxypeptidases present in blood. Carboxypeptidases B (EC 3.4.17.2) and N (arginine carboxypeptidase; EC 3.4.17.3) sequentially hydrolyze the lysine residues from CK-MM to produce two CK-MM isoforms: CK-MM_2 (one lysine residue removed) and CK-MM_1 (both lysine residues removed). Loss of the positively charged lysine produces a more negatively charged CK molecule with greater anodic mobility at electrophoresis. Because CK-MB has only one M subunit, the dimer coded by the M and B genes is named CK-MB_2 and the lysine-hydrolyzed dimer is named CK-MB_1. The assay of the CK isoforms requires a special technique, such as high-voltage electrophoresis (with gel cooling), high-performance liquid chromatography (HPLC), or immunoassay.[61]

Clinical Significance

Serum CK is increased in nearly all patients when injury, inflammation, or necrosis of skeletal or heart muscle occurs.

Elevation of serum CK activity may be the only sign of subclinical neuromuscular disorders.[43] In case series, 30 to 44% of asymptomatic subjects with persistent hyperCKemia up to fivefold the upper reference limit (URL) have myopathy. Serum CK activity is greatly elevated in all types of muscular dystrophy. In progressive muscular dystrophy (particularly Duchenne sex-linked muscular dystrophy), enzyme activity in serum is highest in infancy and childhood (7 to 10 years of age) and may be increased long before the disease is clinically apparent. Serum CK activity characteristically falls as patients get older and as the mass of functioning muscle diminishes with progression of the disease. About 50 to 80% of asymptomatic female carriers of Duchenne dystrophy show threefold to sixfold increases in CK activity. High values of CK are noted in viral myositis, polymyositis, and similar muscle diseases. However, in neurogenic muscle diseases, such as myasthenia gravis, multiple sclerosis, poliomyelitis, and parkinsonism, serum enzyme activity is not increased. Very high activity is also encountered in malignant hyperthermia, an inherited life-threatening condition characterized by high fever and brought on by administration of inhalation anesthesia (usually halothane) to the affected individual.

Skeletal muscle that is diseased or damaged (such as by extreme exercise) may contain significant proportions of CK-MB owing to the phenomenon of "fetal reversion," in which fetal patterns of protein synthesis reappear. Thus serum CK-MB isoenzyme may increase in such circumstances. This explanation may also account for the elevated CK-MB values sometimes observed in chronic renal failure (uremic myopathy).

In acute rhabdomyolysis due to crush injury, with severe muscle destruction, serum CK activities exceeding 200 times the URL may be found. If the CK remains below 5000 U/L (about 30 times the URL) during the first 3 days after the insult, the probability of developing acute renal failure appears to be low.[5] Serum CK can also be increased by other direct trauma to muscle, including intramuscular injection and surgical intervention. Finally, a number of drugs when given at pharmacologic doses can increase serum CK activities. The drugs principally responsible are statins, fibrates, antiretrovirals, and angiotensin II receptor antagonists. Varying degrees of myopathy may occur with statin use, ranging from mild myalgic syndrome alone to rhabdomyolysis (0.02%).[86]

Changes in serum CK and its MB isoenzyme following acute myocardial infarction have been the mainstay of diagnosis for many years.[14] However, it is now more advantageous to use more cardiac-specific nonenzymatic markers, such as cardiac troponin I or T. CK-MB determination can still be used with some success to estimate the extent of myocardial necrosis to assist with assessment of infarct prognosis. When peak CK-MB is compared with estimates of infarct size, good correlations can be obtained (Table 22-4). A problem with using CK-MB for this purpose is the requirement for frequent sampling to ensure that peak CK-MB values are correctly identified.

Hypothyroidism is a common cause of endocrine myopathy. About 60% of hypothyroid subjects show an average elevation of CK activity fivefold greater than the URL. The major isoenzyme present is CK-MM, suggesting muscular involvement.

During normal childbirth, a sixfold elevation in maternal total serum CK activity occurs. Surgical intervention during labor further increases the activity of CK in serum. CK-BB may be elevated in neonates, particularly in brain-damaged or very low birth weight newborns. The presence of CK-BB in blood, usually at low concentrations, may however represent a physiologic finding in the first days of life.

Methods for Determination of Creatine Kinase Activity

Numerous photometric, fluorometric, and coupled enzyme methods have been developed for the assay of CK activity, using the forward (Cr → CrP) or the reverse (Cr ← CrP) reaction. Currently, all commercial assays for total CK are based on the reverse reaction, which proceeds about six times faster than the forward reaction.

$$\text{Creatine phosphate} + \text{ADP} \xrightarrow[\text{pH 6.7}]{CK} \text{creatine} + \text{ADP}$$

$$\text{ADP} + \text{glucose} \xrightarrow{HK} \text{glucose-6-phosphate} + \text{ADP}$$

$$\text{Glucose-6-phosphate} + \text{NADP}^{\oplus} \xrightarrow{G6PD} \text{6-phosphogluconate} + \text{NADPH} + \text{H}^{\oplus}$$

CK catalyzes the conversion of CrP to Cr with concomitant phosphorylation of ADP to ATP. The ATP produced is measured by hexokinase (HK)/glucose-6-phosphate dehydrogenase (G6PD) coupled reactions that ultimately convert $NADP^+$ to NADPH, which is monitored spectrophotometrically at 340 nm. Szasz and colleagues optimized the assay by adding *N*-acetylcysteine to activate CK, EDTA to bind Ca^{2+} and to increase the stability of the reaction mixture, and adenosine pentaphosphate (Ap_5A) in addition to AMP to inhibit adenylate kinase (AK).[85] A reference method based on this previous experience was developed by the International Federation of Clinical Chemistry and Laboratory Medicine (IFCC) for the measurement of CK at 37 °C.[76]

Specimens for CK analysis include serum and plasma heparin. Anticoagulants other than heparin should not be used in collection tubes because they inhibit CK activity. CK activity in serum is relatively unstable and is rapidly lost during storage. Average stabilities are less than 8 hours at room temperature, 48 hours at 4 °C, and 1 month at −20 °C. Therefore the serum specimen should be chilled to 4 °C if the serum is not analyzed immediately, and stored at −80 °C if analysis is delayed for longer than 30 days. It is not necessary to add any thiol agent for storage because the optimized assay formulation containing EDTA, 2 mmol/L, and *N*-acetylcysteine, 20 mmol/L, reactivates CK in serum to the extent of 99% after it has been stored for 1 week at 4 °C. A moderate degree of hemolysis is tolerated because erythrocytes contain no CK activity. However, severely hemolyzed specimens are unsatisfactory because enzymes and intermediates (AK, ATP, and G6P) liberated from the erythrocytes may affect the lag phase and side reactions occurring in the assay system.

Reference Intervals

Serum CK activity is subject to a number of physiologic variations. It is influenced by sex, age, race, muscle mass, and physical activity. The distributions of CK activity are notably skewed toward higher values in reference populations. Men have higher values than women, and blacks have higher values than nonblacks. In white subjects, the reference interval was found to be 46 to 171 U/L for males and 34 to 145 U/L for females, when measured with an assay traceable to the IFCC 37 °C reference procedure.[81] Newborns generally have

TABLE 22-4 Decision Limits of CK-MB Mass Peak for Infarct Size Definition

Microscopic myocardial infarction (focal necrosis)	<10 µg/L
Small myocardial infarction (<10% left ventricle)	10-60 µg/L
Medium myocardial infarction (10-30% left ventricle)	60-225 µg/L
Large myocardial infarction (>30% left ventricle)	>225 µg/L

higher CK activity resulting from skeletal muscle trauma during birth. Serum CK in infants decreases to the adult reference interval by 6 to 10 weeks.

CK activity in the serum of healthy people is due almost exclusively to CK-MM activity (although small amounts of CK-MB may be present) and is the result of physiologic turnover of muscle tissue. Exercise and muscle trauma can increase serum CK.[7] Sustained exercise, such as that performed by well-trained long-distance runners, increases the CK-MB content of skeletal muscle, which may produce abnormal serum CK-MB concentrations.

Methods for Separation and Quantification of Creatine Kinase Isoenzymes

Electrophoretic methods are useful for separation of all CK isoenzymes. The isoenzyme bands are visualized by incubating the support (e.g., agarose, cellulose acetate) with a concentrated CK assay mixture using the reverse reaction. NADPH formed in this reaction is then detected by observing the bluish-white fluorescence after excitation by long-wave (360 nm) ultraviolet light. NADPH may be quantified by fluorescent densitometry, which is capable of detecting bands of 2 to 5 U/L. The mobility of CK isoenzymes at pH 8.6 toward the anode is BB > MB > MM, with the MM remaining cathodic to the point of application. The discriminating power of electrophoresis also allows the detection of abnormal bands (Figure 22-3). Disadvantages of electrophoresis include that the turnaround time is relatively long, the procedure is highly labor intensive and is not adaptable to clinical chemistry analyzers, and interpretative skills are required.

Immunochemical methods are applicable to the direct measurement of CK-MB. Immunoinhibition techniques measuring the catalytic activity of the B subunit of CK dimer were first introduced. T

Although a modification was developed to avoid these interferences, interferences from CK-BB, macro-CKs, or CK-Mt led to low specificity of most immunoinhibitin methods. Furthermore, because the CK-B subunit accounts for one half of CK-MB activity, the change in absorbance should be doubled to obtain CK-MB activity. This resulted in a significant decrease in the analytical sensitivity of the method.

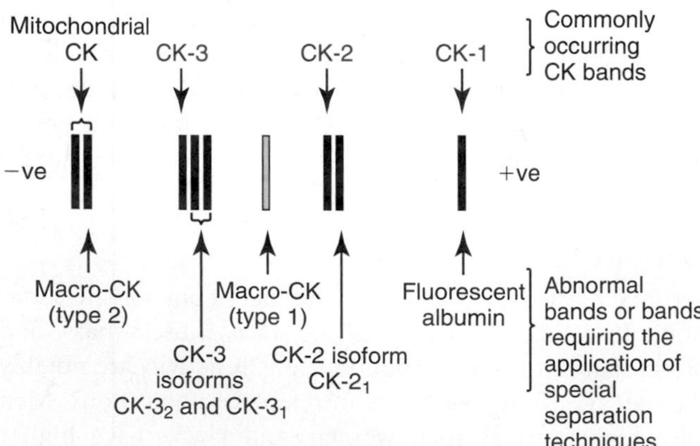

Figure 22-3 A diagrammatic representation of the electrophoretic pattern of CK isoenzymes (some of which are seen, in blood, only in disease) and some of the reported anomalous forms.

Currently, the most common approach is to measure concentrations of the CK-MB protein ("mass") by using immunoassays with monoclonal antibodies.[58] Measurements use the "sandwich" technique, in which one antibody specifically recognizes only the MB dimer. The sandwich technique ensures that only CK-MB is estimated because neither CK-MM nor CK-BB reacts with both antibodies. Mass assays are more sensitive than activity-based methods with a limit of detection for CK-MB usually less than 1 μg/L. Other advantages include sample stability, noninterference with hemolysis, anticoagulants or other catalytic activity inhibitors, full automation, and fast turnaround time. With CM-MB mass assays, the upper reference limit for males is 5.0 μg/L, with values for females being less than male values, although many laboratories use a single reference limit (male).

Aldolase

Aldolase (EC 4.1.2.13; D-fructose-1,6-bisdiphosphate D-glyceraldehyde-3-phosphate-lyase; ALD) catalyzes the splitting of D-fructose-1,6-diphosphate to D-glyceraldehyde-3-phosphate (GLAP) and dihydroxyacetone-phosphate (DAP), an important reaction in the glycolytic breakdown of glucose to lactate.

ALD is a tetramer with subunits determined by three separate gene loci. Only two of these loci, those producing A and B subunits, appear to be active simultaneously in most tissues, so the most common isoenzyme pattern consists of various proportions of the components of a five-member set of isoenzymes, of which two members correspond to the A and B homopolymers. The locus that determines the structure of the C subunit is active in brain tissue, as is the A locus, so this tissue contains ALD A and C, together with the three corresponding heteropolymers.

Clinical Significance

Serum ALD determinations have been of some clinical interest in primary diseases of skeletal muscle. Some researchers believe that increased ALD activity is useful in distinguishing neuromuscular atrophies from myopathies in combination with the CK/AST ratio.[27] In general, however, measurement of ALD activity in the serum of subjects with suspected muscle disease does not add information to that available more readily from measurement of other enzymes, especially CK.[22] At the time of this book's writing, ALD measurement has largely been discontinued within clinical laboratories and is not routinely available.

Methods for Measurement of Aldolase Activity

All assay methods are based on the forward ALD-catalyzed reaction. In the analytical approach on which all commonly used procedures and kits are based, the ALD reaction is coupled with two other enzyme reactions. Triosephosphate isomerase (EC 5.3.1.1) is added to ensure rapid conversion of all GLAP to DAP. Glycerol-3-phosphate dehydrogenase (EC 1.1.1.8) is added to reduce DAP to glycerol-3-phosphate, with NADH acting as hydrogen donor. The decrease in NADH concentration is then measured.

ALD activity in serum is quite stable. Activity is unchanged at ambient temperatures for up to 48 hours and at 4 °C for several days. Hemolyzed specimens should not be used; plasma is preferred over serum because of the possible release of platelet enzyme during the clotting process.

Reference Intervals

The reference interval for the activity of ALD in adults is 2.5 to 10 U/L, measured at 37 °C. However, a definite sex difference has been noted, with men having higher values. Serum ALD activity in the neonate is fourfold that seen in adult, and in children is twice that in the adult. Adult values are attained by the time the child reaches puberty.[91]

Glycogen Phosphorylase

Glycogen phosphorylase (EC 2.4.1.1; α-1,4-D-glucan:orthophosphate D-glucosyltransferase; GP) plays an essential role in the regulation of carbohydrate metabolism by mobilizing glycogen. It catalyzes the first step in glycogenolysis, in which glycogen is converted to glucose-1-phosphate. The physiologic role of muscle GP is to provide fuel for the energy supply required for muscle contraction. GP exists in the myocyte in association with glycogen and the sarcoplasmic reticulum, forming a macromolecular complex. The degree of association of GP with this complex depends on the metabolic state of the muscle. With the onset of tissue hypoxia, when glycogen is broken down and disappears, GP becomes soluble and can move from the peri–sarcoplasmic reticulum compartment directly into the extracellular fluid.

GP exists as a dimer composed of two identical subunits (molecular mass as a monomer of about 97,000 Da). Three GP isoenzymes are found in human tissues: GP-LL, GP-MM, and GP-BB. Adult skeletal muscle contains only GP-MM. GP-LL is the predominant isoenzyme in liver and all other human tissues except for heart, skeletal muscle, and brain. GP-BB is the predominant isoenzyme in the human brain. In the heart, the isoenzymes BB and MM are found, but GP-BB is the predominant isoenzyme in the myocardium as well.

Clinical Significance

In preliminary studies, GP-BB was significantly more sensitive than CK-MB and myoglobin for the diagnosis of acute myocardial infarction within the first 4 hours after onset of chest pain.[2] However, GP-BB is not a heart-specific protein, and its specificity as a marker for myocardial damage is limited.

Methods for Measurement of Glycogen Phosphorylase Isoenzyme BB

Manual ELISA assays are available for measurement of the isoenzyme GP-BB. The calculated upper reference limit is 10 μg/L.

LIVER ENZYMES

Enzymes in this category include alanine and aspartate aminotransferases, glutamate dehydrogenase, alkaline phosphatase, 5′-nucleotidase, γ-glutamyltransferase, and glutathione S-transferase. The aminotransferases, alkaline phosphatase and γ-glutamyltransferase, are widely used and available on automated analyzers. They have long been mistakenly called, as a group, "liver function tests." They are not, of course, but the habit sometimes persists. The others have not been adopted as widely.

The most common alterations in liver enzyme activities encountered in clinical practice is divided into two major pathophysiology subgroups—hepatocellular damage (elevated transaminase and glutamate dehydrogenase activities) and cholestasis (elevated alkaline phosphatase, 5′-nucleotidase, and γ-glutamyltransferase activities)—although certain liver diseases may display a mixed biochemical picture.

Aminotransferases

The aminotransferases constitute a group of enzymes that catalyze the interconversion of amino acids to 2-oxo-acids by transfer of amino groups. Aspartate aminotransferase (EC 2.6.1.1; L-aspartate:2-oxoglutarate aminotransferase; AST) and alanine aminotransferase (EC 2.6.1.2; L-alanine:2-oxoglutarate aminotransferase; ALT) are examples of aminotransferases that are of clinical interest.

The 2-oxoglutarate/L-glutamate couple serves as one amino group acceptor and donor pair in all amino-transfer reactions; the specificity of the individual enzymes derives from the particular amino acid that serves as the other donor of an amino group. Thus AST catalyzes the following reaction:

$$\underset{\text{L-Aspartate}}{^{-}OOC{-}CH_2{-}CH(NH_2){-}COO^{-}} + \underset{\text{2-Oxoglutarate}}{^{-}OOC{-}CH_2{-}CH_2{-}C(=O){-}COO^{-}} \xrightleftharpoons{AST,\ P\text{-}5'\text{-}P} \underset{\text{Oxaloacetate}}{^{-}OOC{-}CH_2{-}C(=O){-}COO^{-}} + \underset{\text{L-Glutamate}}{^{-}OOC{-}CH_2{-}CH_2{-}CH(NH_2){-}COO^{-}}$$

ALT catalyzes the analogous reaction as follows:

$$\underset{\text{L-Alanine}}{CH_3{-}CH(NH_2){-}COO^{-}} + \underset{\text{2-Oxoglutarate}}{^{-}OOC{-}CH_2{-}CH_2{-}C(=O){-}COO^{-}} \xrightleftharpoons{ALT,\ P\text{-}5'\text{-}P} \underset{\text{Pyruvate}}{CH_3{-}C(=O){-}COO^{-}} + \underset{\text{L-Glutamate}}{^{-}OOC{-}CH_2{-}CH_2{-}CH(NH_2){-}COO^{-}}$$

The reactions are reversible, but the equilibria of the AST and ALT reactions favor formation of aspartate and alanine, respectively.

Pyridoxal-5′-phosphate (P-5′-P) and its amino analog, pyridoxamine-5′-phosphate, function as coenzymes in amino-transfer reactions. The P-5′-P is bound to the apoenzyme and serves as a true prosthetic group. P-5′-P bound to the apoenzyme accepts the amino group from the first substrate, aspartate or alanine, to form enzyme-bound pyridoxamine-5′-phosphate and the first reaction product, oxaloacetate or pyruvate, respectively. The coenzyme in amino form then transfers its amino group to the second substrate, 2-oxoglutarate, to form the second product, glutamate. P-5′-P is thus regenerated.

Both coenzyme-deficient apoenzymes and holoenzymes may be present in serum. Therefore, addition of P-5′-P under conditions that allow recombination with the enzymes usually produces an increase in aminotransferase activity. In accordance with the principle that all factors affecting the rate of reaction must be optimized and controlled, the IFCC recommends addition of P-5′-P in aminotransferase methods to ensure that all enzymatic activity is measured.

Transaminases are widely distributed throughout the body. AST is found primarily in the heart, liver, skeletal muscle, and kidney, whereas ALT is found primarily in the liver and kidney, with lesser amounts in heart and skeletal muscle (Table 22-5). ALT is exclusively cytoplasmic; both mitochondrial and cytoplasmic forms of AST are found in cells. These are genetically distinct isoenzymes with a dimeric structure composed of two identical polypeptide subunits of about 400 amino acid residues.

Clinical Significance

Liver disease is the most important cause of increased transaminase activity in serum. In most types of liver disease, ALT activity is higher than that of AST; exceptions may be seen in alcoholic hepatitis, hepatic cirrhosis, and liver neoplasia. In viral hepatitis and other forms of liver disease associated with acute hepatic necrosis, serum AST and ALT activities are elevated even before the clinical signs and symptoms of disease (such as jaundice) appear. Activities for both enzymes may reach values as high as 100 times the upper reference limit, although 10-fold to 40-fold elevations are most frequently encountered. The most efficient aminotransferase threshold for diagnosing acute liver injury lies at seven times the upper reference limit (sensitivity and specificity >95%). Peak values of transaminase activity occur between the 7th and 12th days; activities then gradually decrease, reaching normal levels by the 3rd to 5th week if recovery is uneventful. Peak activities bear no relationship to prognosis and may fall with worsening of the patient's condition.

Persistence of increased ALT for longer than 6 months after an episode of acute hepatitis is used to diagnose chronic hepatitis. Most patients with chronic hepatitis have maximum ALT less than seven times the upper reference limit. ALT may be persistently normal in 15 to 50% of patients with chronic hepatitis C, but the likelihood of continuously normal ALT decreases with an increasing number of measurements. In patients with acute hepatitis C, ALT should be measured periodically over the next 1 to 2 years to determine if it becomes and stays normal.[15]

The picture in toxic hepatitis is different from that in infectious hepatitis. In acetaminophen-induced hepatic injury, the transaminase peak is more than 85 times the upper reference limit in 90% of cases—a value rarely seen with acute viral hepatitis. Furthermore, AST and ALT activities typically peak early and fall rapidly.[15]

Nonalcoholic fatty liver disease (NAFLD) is the most common cause of aminotransferase increases other than viral and alcoholic hepatitis. NAFLD includes a spectrum of liver pathology, from simple steatosis to nonalcoholic steatohepatitis (NASH), in which inflammatory changes and focal necrosis may progress to liver fibrosis, cirrhosis, and hepatic failure. NAFLD is now considered to be an additional feature of the "metabolic syndrome." Indeed, serum aminotransferase elevation in NAFLD is associated with higher body mass index, waist circumference, serum triglycerides, and fasting insulin and lower HDL cholesterol—all features characteristic of this syndrome.

Aminotransferase activities observed in cirrhosis vary with the status of the cirrhotic process and range from the upper reference limit to four to five times higher, with an AST/ALT ratio (AAR) greater than 1. This appears to be attributable to a reduction in ALT production in a damaged liver, associated with reduced clearance of AST in advancing liver fibrosis. An AAR ≥1 has ≈90% positive predictive value for diagnosing the presence of advanced fibrosis in patients with chronic liver disease. Furthermore, the amount of elevation in the AAR can reflect the grade of fibrosis in these patients.

Twofold to fivefold elevations of both enzymes occur in patients with primary or metastatic carcinoma of the liver, with AST usually being higher than ALT, but activities are often normal in the early stages of malignant infiltration of the liver. Slight or moderate elevations of AST and ALT activities have been observed after administration of various medications, such as nonsteroidal anti-inflammatory drugs, antibiotics, antiepileptic drugs, statins, or opiates.

TABLE 22-5 Transaminase Activities in Human Tissues, Relative to Serum as Unity

	AST	ALT
Heart	7800	450
Liver	7100	2850
Skeletal muscle	5000	300
Kidneys	4500	1200
Pancreas	1400	130
Spleen	700	80
Lungs	500	45
Erythrocytes	15	7
Serum	1	1

From King J. Practical clinical enzymology. London: D Van Nostrand Co Ltd, 1965.

Over-the-counter medications and herbal preparations are also implicated. In patients with increased transaminases, negative viral markers, and a negative history for drugs or alcohol ingestion, the work-up should include less common causes of chronic hepatic injury (e.g., hemochromatosis, Wilson's disease, autoimmune hepatitis, primary biliary cirrhosis, sclerosing cholangitis, celiac disease, α_1-antitrypsin deficiency).[67]

Although serum activities of both AST and ALT become elevated whenever disease processes affect liver cell integrity, ALT is the more liver-specific enzyme. Serum elevations of ALT activity are rarely observed in conditions other than parenchymal liver disease.[34] Moreover, elevations of ALT activity persist longer than do those of AST activity. Thus the incremental benefit of determination of AST, in addition to ALT, may be limited.

After acute myocardial infarction, increased AST activity appears in serum, as might be expected from the high AST concentration in heart muscle. AST activity also is increased in progressive muscular dystrophy and dermatomyositis, reaching concentrations up to eight times normal; they are usually normal in other types of muscle disease, especially in those of neurogenic origin. Pulmonary emboli can increase AST to two to three times normal, and slight to moderate elevations are noted in acute pancreatitis, crushed muscle injury, and hemolytic disease.

Generally, mitochondrial AST (m-AST) activity in serum shows a marked increase in patients with extensive liver cell degeneration and necrosis. Of particular interest is the usefulness of the ratio between m-AST and total AST activities for diagnosing alcoholic hepatitis. The ratio seems to identify the liver cell "necrotic type" condition (i.e., slight enzyme increase concomitant with relatively high activities of mitochondrial enzymes) typical of alcoholic hepatitis.[56]

Several authors have described AST linked to immunoglobulins, or macro-AST. Typical findings include a persistent increase in serum AST activity in an asymptomatic subject, with absence of any demonstrable pathology in organs rich in AST. Increased AST activity might reflect decreased clearance of the abnormal complex from plasma. Macro-AST has no known clinical relevance. However, identification is important to avoid unnecessary diagnostic procedures in these subjects. Laboratory procedures for the demonstration of macro-AST include electrophoresis with specific enzyme stain (atypical origin band) and differential precipitation with polyethylene glycol (PEG) 6000 (see "Amylase" section later in this chapter).

Methods for Measurement of Transaminase Activity

The assay system for measuring transaminase activity contains two amino acids and two oxo-acids. Because no convenient method is available for assaying amino acids, formation or consumption of the oxo-acids is measured. Continuous-monitoring methods are commonly used to measure transaminase activity by coupling transaminase reactions to specific dehydrogenase reactions. The oxo-acids formed in the transaminase reaction are measured indirectly by enzymatic reduction to corresponding hydroxy acids, and the accompanying change in NADH concentration is monitored spectrophotometrically. Thus oxaloacetate, formed in the AST reaction, is reduced to malate in the presence of malate dehydrogenase (MD).

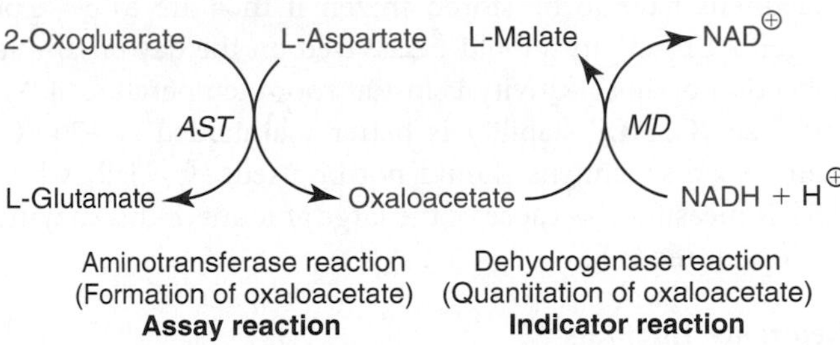

Pyruvate formed in the ALT reaction is reduced to lactate by lactate dehydrogenase (LD). The substrate, NADH, and an auxiliary enzyme, MD or LD, must be present in sufficient quantity so that the reaction rate is limited only by the amounts of AST and ALT, respectively. As the reactions proceed, NADH is oxidized to NAD^+. The disappearance of NADH is followed by measuring the decrease in absorbance at 340 nm for several minutes, either continuously or at frequent intervals. The change in absorbance per minute (ΔA/min) is proportional to the micromoles of NADH oxidized and in turn to micromoles of substrate transformed per minute. A preliminary incubation period is necessary to ensure that NADH-dependent reduction of endogenous oxo-acids in the sample is completed before 2-oxoglutarate is added to start the transaminase reaction. After a brief lag phase, the change in absorbance (ΔA) is monitored. As already mentioned, supplementation with P-5′-P ensures that all transaminase activity of the sample is measured.

Because of the large numbers of AST and ALT activity measurements performed daily in clinical laboratories throughout the world, standardization of transaminase measurements is a priority need for patient care. As discussed in Chapter 8, the reference system approach, based on the concepts of metrologic traceability and the hierarchy of analytical measurement procedures, gives clinical laboratories and the medical community universal means of creating and ensuring the comparability of results. In this system, the IFCC reference measurement procedure forms the highest metrologic level and thereby constitutes the definition of the respective measurable enzyme quantity.[30] Primary IFCC procedures for the measurement of catalytic activity concentrations of AST and ALT at 37 °C have been published.[79,80] Values assigned to the manufacturer's product calibrators and measurement results of lower metrologic levels, including those used in daily routine practice, should be traceable to these top-level reference measurement procedures, thus improving the accuracy and comparability of transaminase results. It should be remembered that the concept of the reference system is valid only if the reference procedure and corresponding routine procedures have identical, or at least very similar, specificities for the measured enzyme. Thus it will not be possible to calibrate procedures for aminotransferases that do not incorporate P-5′-P using a procedure that does, such as the IFCC reference procedure, because the ratio of pre-formed holoenzyme to apoenzyme differs among specimens.

AST activity in serum is stable for up to 48 hours at 4 °C. Specimens have to be stored frozen if they are to be kept longer. ALT activity should be assayed on the day of sample collection because activity is lost at room temperature, 4 °C, and −25 °C. ALT stability is better maintained at −70 °C. Hemolyzed specimens should not be used, especially when AST is measured, because of the large amount of this enzyme present in red cells.

Reference Intervals[25,29]

Using methods traceable to the IFCC reference system, the AST upper reference limit for adults, calculated as the 97.5-percentile of the reference distribution, is 35 U/L, with no significant sex-related differences. Conversely, a clear difference in ALT activities has been noted between adult males and females. Corresponding ALT upper reference limits are 60 U/L and 42 U/L respectively. ALT does not reveal a distinct age dependency during childhood, whereas serum AST activity in neonates and in children younger than 3 years old is twice that in adults. Adult values are attained by the time the child reaches puberty.

Methods for Separation and Quantification of AST Isoenzymes

AST isoenzymes can be separated into anionic (cytoplasmic AST) and cationic bands (m-AST) by electrophoresis. However, the low concentration of m-AST in normal sera is usually below the limit of detection of this method. Immunoprecipitation assays using antibodies directed against both mitochondrial and cytosolic isoenzymes allow instead measurement of low concentrations of the m-AST isoenzyme present in serum. A homogeneous inhibition assay using proteinase K (EC 3.4.21.14) for selective proteolysis of cytosolic AST has been described and made amenable to automation, permitting m-AST to be measured with convenience that approaches that of the total AST assay.[63]

About 5 to 10% of the activity of total AST in serum from healthy individuals is of mitochondrial origin. The upper reference limit for m-AST activity measured at 37 °C is 3.0 U/L.

Glutamate Dehydrogenase

Glutamate dehydrogenase [EC 1.4.1.3; L-glutamate: NAD(P)$^+$ oxidoreductase, deaminating; GLD] is a mitochondrial enzyme found mainly in the liver, heart muscle, and kidneys, but small amounts occur in other tissue, including brain and skeletal muscle tissue, and in leukocytes.

GLD is a zinc-containing enzyme that consists of six polypeptide chains. The smallest active molecule has a molecular weight of about 350,000 Da, but larger polymers are also found. The enzyme catalyzes the removal of hydrogen from L-glutamate to form the corresponding ketimino-acid, which undergoes spontaneous hydrolysis to 2-oxoglutarate.

$$\text{L-Glutamate} + NAD^{+} \underset{\text{Glutamate dehydrogenase}}{\rightleftharpoons} \text{Ketimino-acid} + NADH + H^{+}$$

$$\text{Ketimino-acid} + H_2O \xrightarrow{\text{Spontaneous}} \text{2-Oxoglutarate} + NH_3$$

Although NAD$^+$ is the preferred coenzyme, NADP$^+$ also acts as the hydrogen acceptor. GLD is inhibited by metal ions, such as Ag$^+$ and Hg$^+$, by several chelating agents, and by L-thyroxine.

Clinical Significance[74]

GLD is increased in the serum of patients with hepatocellular damage. Fourfold or fivefold elevations are seen in chronic hepatitis; in cirrhosis, increases are only up to twofold. Very large rises in serum GLD occur in halothane toxicity, and notable increases are seen in response to some other hepatotoxic agents.

GLD potentially offers differential diagnostic potential in the investigation of liver disease, particularly when interpreted in conjunction with other enzyme test results. The key to this differential diagnostic potential is to be found in the intraorgan and intracellular distribution of the enzyme as discussed earlier in this chapter. As an exclusively mitochondrial enzyme, GLD is released from necrotic cells; therefore, when compared with hepatic disorders with extensive necrosis, release is less in diffuse inflammatory processes, and in these conditions, the release of cytoplasmic enzymes, such as ALT, is quantitatively more pronounced. Together with m-AST, GLD is of value in estimating the severity of liver cell damage.

GLD is more concentrated in the central areas of the liver lobules than in the periportal zones. This pattern of distribution is the reverse of that of ALT. Pronounced release of GLD therefore is to be expected in conditions in which centrilobular necrosis occurs (e.g., as a result of ischemia, in halothane toxicity).

Methods for Determination of Glutamate Dehydrogenase Activity

Continuous-monitoring methods have been developed for determination of GLD using both forward and reverse reactions. The equilibrium favors the formation of glutamate, and higher reaction rates are observed when 2-oxoglutarate is used as a substrate. Serum is added to a solution of NADH, an ammonium salt, and ADP in buffer at pH 7.5, and the reaction is initiated by the addition of the substrate, 2-oxoglutarate. The rate of decrease in absorbance at 340 nm is measured. The German Society for Clinical Chemistry has published optimum reaction conditions for 37 °C.[13] Oxamate is incorporated into the reaction mixture because this acid inhibits LD activity, avoiding the critical consumption of NADH by this enzyme in serum.

GLD activity in serum is stable at 4 °C for 48 hours and at −20 °C for several weeks.

Reference Intervals

The GLD upper reference limits are 6 U/L (women) and 8 U/L (men) when a method optimized at 37 °C is used.

Alkaline Phosphatase

Alkaline phosphatase [EC 3.1.3.1; orthophosphoric-monoester phosphohydrolase (alkaline optimum); ALP] catalyzes the alkaline hydrolysis of a large variety of naturally occurring and synthetic substrates.

ALP activity is present in most organs of the body and is especially associated with membranes and cell surfaces located in the mucosa of the small intestine and the proximal convoluted tubules of the kidney, in bone (osteoblasts), liver, and placenta. Although the exact metabolic function of the enzyme is not yet understood, it appears that ALP is associated with lipid transport in the intestine and with the calcification process in bone.

ALP exists in multiple forms, some of which are true isoenzymes, encoded at separate genetic loci (Figure 22-4).[47] Bone, liver, and kidney ALP forms share a common primary structure coded for by the same genetic locus, but they differ in carbohydrate content.[45]

Some divalent ions, such as Mg^{2+}, Co^{2+}, and Mn^{2+}, are activators of the enzyme, and Zn^{2+} is a constituent metal ion. The correct ratio of Mg^{2+}/Zn^{2+} ions is necessary to avoid displacement of Mg^{2+} and to attain optimal activity. Phosphate, borate, oxalate, and cyanide ions are inhibitors of ALP activity. Variations in Mg^{2+} and substrate concentrations change the pH optimum. The type of buffer present (except at low concentrations) affects the rate of enzyme activity. Buffers can be classified as inert (carbonate and barbital), inhibiting (glycine and propylamine), or activating [2-amino-2-methyl-1-propanol (AMP), tris (hydroxymethyl) aminomethane (TRIS), and diethanolamine (DEA)].

The ALP activity present in the sera of healthy adults originates mainly in the liver, with most of the rest coming from the skeleton. The respective contributions of these two forms to the total activity are age dependent. Minimal amounts of intestinal ALP may also be present, particularly in the sera of individuals of blood group B or O (i.e., those who are secretors of blood group substances). Because intestinal ALP activity in serum may increase after a meal, ALP should be measured preferentially in fasting sera.

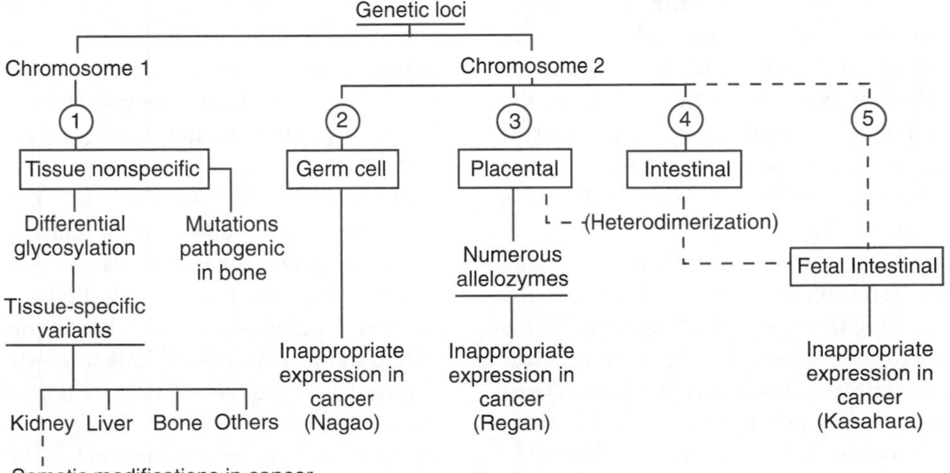

Figure 22-4 Identities, chromosomal assignments, and main physiologic and pathologic expression of genes encoding human alkaline phosphatases. The gene names (and gene symbols) are alkaline phosphatase, liver/bone/kidney (*ALPL*); alkaline phosphatase, intestinal (*ALPI*); alkaline phosphatase, placental (*ALPP*); and alkaline phosphatase, placental-like 2 (*ALPPL2*). *Broken lines* show two alternative proposed origins of the fetal intestinal alkaline phosphatase; the sequence of a cDNA is reportedly identical to that of adult intestinal alkaline phosphatase. All isoenzymes and isoforms are glycoproteins, imposing a further level of microheterogeneity. Different processes of cleavage or preservation of the membrane-anchoring domain can generate additional isoforms. *(Modified from Moss DW. Perspectives in alkaline phosphatase research. Clin Chem 1992;38:2486-92.)*

Clinical Significance

Elevations in serum ALP activity commonly originate from one or both of two sources: liver and bone. Consequently, serum ALP measurements are of particular interest in the investigation of two groups of conditions: hepatobiliary disease and bone disease associated with increased osteoblastic activity (see "Bone Enzymes" section later in this chapter).

Serum ALP was the first enzyme to be used for the investigation of hepatic disease. The response of the liver to any form of biliary tree obstruction induces the synthesis of ALP by hepatocytes. Some of the newly formed enzyme enters the circulation to increase the enzyme activity in serum.[48] Elevation tends to be more notable (greater than threefold) in extrahepatic obstruction (e.g., by stone, by cancer of the head of the pancreas) than in intrahepatic obstruction and is greater the more complete the obstruction. Serum enzyme activities may reach 10 to 12 times the upper reference limit and usually return to normal on surgical removal of the obstruction. A similar increase is seen in patients with advanced primary liver cancer or widespread secondary hepatic metastases. Liver diseases that principally affect parenchymal cells, such as infectious hepatitis, typically show only moderately (less than threefold) increased or even normal serum ALP activities. Increases may also be seen as a consequence of a reaction to drug therapy. Intestinal ALP isoenzyme, an asialoglycoprotein normally cleared by the hepatic asialoglycoprotein receptors, is often elevated in patients with liver cirrhosis.

An increase of up to two to three times normal is observed in women in the third trimester of pregnancy, with the additional enzyme being of placental origin. Reports have also described a benign familial elevation in serum ALP activity due to increased concentrations of intestinal ALP.[57] Transient, benign increases in serum ALP may be observed in infants and children, with changes often more than 10 times the upper reference limit. Increases in both liver and bone forms are seen. These changes seem to reflect a reduction in the removal of ALP from blood caused by transient modifications of enzyme glycosylation.[83]

A result of the application of techniques of isoenzyme analysis to the characterization of ALP in serum was the discovery that forms of the enzyme essentially identical to the normal placental isoenzyme appear in the sera of some patients with malignant disease. These carcinoplacental isoenzymes (e.g., Regan isoenzyme) appear to result from de-repression of the placental ALP gene. As described later, the presence of these isoenzymes can be readily detected in serum by their stability at 65 °C. Tumors have also been found to produce ALPs that appear to be modified forms of nonplacental isoenzymes (Kasahara isoenzyme).

Methods for Determination of Alkaline Phosphatase Activity

Numerous methods have been developed for determining ALP activity. In general, methodologic developments have been directed toward increasing the speed and sensitivity of the assay by selecting readily hydrolyzed substrates and phosphate-accepting buffers, and toward the use of continuous-monitoring methods based on "self-indicating" substrates.

The most popular of the chromogenic or self-indicating substrates for ALP is 4-nitrophenyl phosphate (usually abbreviated 4-NPP, or PNPP from the older name, *p*-nitrophenyl phosphate). This ester is colorless, but the final product is yellow at the pH of the reaction:

4-Nitrophenyl phosphate (colorless) + H_2O —(ALP, Mg^{2+}, pH 10.3)→ 4-Nitrophenoxide (colorless, benzenoid form) + phosphate; 4-Nitrophenoxide (colorless, benzenoid form) ⇌ (Rearranges at alkaline pH) 4-Nitrophenoxide (yellow, quinonoid form)

The enzyme reaction is continuously monitored by observing the rate of formation of the 4-nitrophenoxide ions. With improvement in reaction conditions, this reaction forms the basis of current recommended and standard methods of ALP assay. Other self-indicating substrates include phenolphthalein monophosphate, thymolphthalein phosphate, and α-naphthyl phosphate. With the ALP methods discussed, the liberated phosphate group is transferred to water. The rate of phosphatase action is enhanced, however, if certain amino alcohols are used as phosphate-accepting buffers. Among these activators are compounds such as AMP, DEA, TRIS, ethylaminoethanol (EAE), and *N*-methyl-D-glucamine (MEG). Enzyme activity in the presence of optimal concentrations of these buffers is twofold to sixfold greater than in the presence of a nonactivating buffer, such as carbonate.

ALP catalyzes the hydrolysis of 4-NPP, forming phosphate and free 4-nitrophenol (4-NP, PNP), which in dilute acid solutions is colorless. Under alkaline conditions, 4-NP is converted to the 4-nitrophenoxide ion, which has a very intense yellow color. The rate of formation of 4-NP by the action of the enzyme on 4-NPP at 37 °C is then monitored at 405 nm with a recording spectrophotometer. The (provisional) IFCC-recommended method uses 4-NPP as the substrate and AMP as the phosphate-acceptor buffer. It includes Mg^{2+} and Zn^{2+}, optimal concentrations of which are controlled by the addition of Mg^{2+} and Zn^{2+}, and the chelating agent *N*-hydroxyethylethylenediaminetriacetic acid (HEDTA). Although Zn^{2+} ions are present in a total concentration of 1 mmol/L, most are bound to HEDTA, leaving only a small, experimentally determined optimal concentration of free ions. A similar situation exists for Mg^{2+} ions. Thus HEDTA acts as a metal ion buffer, maintaining optimal concentrations of both ions.[88]

Serum or heparinized plasma, free of hemolysis, should be used. Complexing anticoagulants—such as citrate, oxalate, and EDTA—must be avoided, because they bind cations, such as Mg^{2+} and Zn^{2+}, which are necessary cofactors for ALP activity measurement. Blood transfusion (containing citrate) causes a transient decrease in serum ALP through a similar mechanism. Freshly collected serum samples should be kept at room temperature and assayed as soon as possible but preferably within 4 hours after collection. In sera stored at a refrigerated temperature, ALP activity increases slowly (2%/d). Frozen specimens should be thawed and kept at room temperature for 18 to 24 hours before measurement to achieve full enzyme reactivation.

Reference Intervals[66,90]

ALP activities in serum vary with age. Children show higher ALP activity than healthy adults as a result of the leakage of bone ALP from osteoblasts during bone growth. Using methods traceable to the IFCC procedure at 37 °C, the following reference intervals (central 95-percentiles) have been established:

Sex	Age	Reference Interval
Males/Females	4-15 y	54-369 U/L
Males	20-50 y	53-128 U/L
	≥60 y	56-116 U/L
Females	20-50 y	42-98 U/L
	≥60 y	53-141 U/L

Activities in growing children are highly variable.

Methods for Separation and Quantification of Alkaline Phosphatase Isoenzymes

Assays for ALP isoenzymes are needed when (1) the source of an elevated ALP in serum is not obvious and should be clarified; (2) the main clinical question is concerned with detecting the presence of liver or bone involvement; and (3) it is important to ascertain any modifications in the activity of osteoblasts to monitor disease activity and the effects of appropriate therapies in the case of metabolic bone disorders.

Criteria that have been used to differentiate the isoenzymes and other multiple forms of ALP include (1) electrophoretic mobility; (2) stability to denaturation by heat or chemicals; (3) response to the presence of selected inhibitors; (4) affinity for specific lectins; and (5) immunochemical characteristics.[68]

The same electrophoretic techniques are used for the separation of ALP isoenzymes in serum as for separation of serum proteins. After electrophoresis, ALP zones are made visible by incubating the gel in a solution of buffered substrate (e.g., 1-naphthyl phosphate, to which a chromogenic system, usually represented by a diazonium salt, is added; in the case of electrophoresis on cellulose acetate, the strips are covered with an agar gel layer containing the staining system). The liver ALP typically moves most rapidly toward the anode. Bone ALP, which typically gives a more diffuse zone than the liver form, has slightly reduced anodal mobility, although the two zones usually overlap to some extent. Intestinal ALP migrates more slowly than the bone enzyme, whereas the placental isoenzyme commonly appears as a discrete band overlying the diffuse bone fraction. An additional band, which is frequently present in the serum of patients with various hepatic diseases, contains a high molecular weight form of ALP but is also strongly negatively charged. Therefore it moves slowly in starch gel or may even fail to enter polyacrylamide gel, but it migrates more anodally than the main liver zone on nonsieving media, such as cellulose acetate. Investigations of this form have revealed that it corresponds to the main liver form attached to the membrane moiety *[membrane particle (fragment) ALP]*.[60]

Complexes between ALP and immunoglobulins, or macro-ALP, occur occasionally in serum, giving rise to abnormally migrating bands in the γ-globulin zone; however, they do not provide specific diagnostic information in the present state of knowledge.

Two approaches have been proposed to improve the electrophoretic separation between bone and liver ALPs. Both methods exploit differences in the carbohydrate portions of the two forms of ALP. With one, electrophoresis is carried out in the presence of wheat germ lectin, binding the *N*-acetylglucosamine residues present in different amounts on individual fractions, which retards bone ALP migration more than liver enzyme migration.[72] With the other, serum is treated briefly (i.e., for 15 minutes at 37 °C) with neuraminidase to remove a portion of the terminal sialic acid residues. Because the sialic acid residues of bone ALP are more readily attacked than those of liver ALP, the electrophoretic mobility of the bone form is reduced more than that of liver ALP. The improved separation allows quantitative estimates to be made by densitometric scanning (Figure 22-5).[49] As an alternative to electrophoretic fractionation of ALP, measurement of γ-glutamyltransferase, which is increased in liver disease but not in bone disease, may be a useful rapid tool to distinguish between the two diseases as the explanation for an increased serum ALP.

Overnight incubation of the serum sample with neuraminidase is used to confirm the presence of intestinal ALP. This treatment reduces the anodal mobility of all ALP isoenzymes except that of intestinal origin, which is neuraminidase resistant because terminal sialic acid residues are not present in the molecule. Because placental ALP is heat stable, incubation of the serum sample at a temperature as high as 65 °C for 30 minutes provides a convenient test for the presence of this isoenzyme. Immunologic methods provide the best quantitative measurements of intestinal or placental ALPs. Much more difficult is the production of antibodies that selectively react with different products of the tissue-nonspecific ALP gene, including liver- and bone-derived isoforms, as these antibodies should recognize specific sugar sidechains instead of a particular amino acid sequence. Until now, no monoclonal antibodies have fully discriminated between liver and bone ALPs. Despite lack of complete specificity, commercially available immunoassays of bone ALP

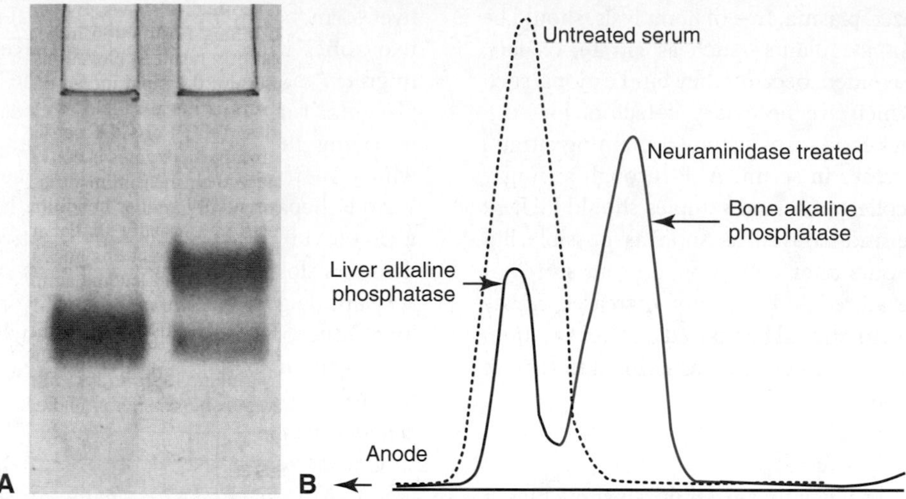

Figure 22-5 A, Polyacrylamide-gel electrophoresis of bone and liver alkaline phosphatases in human serum. *Left,* Mixture of two sera containing, respectively, entirely bone phosphatase and entirely liver phosphatase. *Right,* Mixture of the same two sera after each has been treated with neuraminidase for 10 minutes at 37 °C. The anodal direction is downward. The more anodal zone is liver phosphatase. B, Densitometric scans of electrophoretic patterns shown in A. *Broken line,* Scan of mixture of untreated sera; *solid line,* scan of mixture of sera treated briefly with neuraminidase. *(From Moss DW, Edwards RK. Improved electrophoretic resolution of bone and liver alkaline phosphatases resulting from partial digestion with neuraminidase. Clin Chim Acta 1984;143:177-82.)*

may offer some advantages, but their value has not been convincingly demonstrated, in part because measurements of total ALP provide the required clinical information in many situations.

5′-Nucleotidase

5′-Nucleotidase (EC 3.1.3.5; 5′-ribonucleotide phosphohydrolase; NTP) is a phosphatase that acts only on nucleoside-5′-phosphates, such as adenosine-5′-phosphate (AMP) and adenylic acid, releasing inorganic phosphate.

NH_2 … $CH_2OPO_3^{\ominus\ominus}$ … HO OH

Adenosine-5′-monophosphate (AMP)

H_2O $HOPO_3^{\ominus\ominus}$

Nucleotidase
pH 6.6 to 7.0

NH_2 … CH_2OH … HO OH

Adenosine

NTP is a glycoprotein that is widely distributed throughout the tissues of the body and is principally localized in the cytoplasmic membrane of the cells in which it occurs. Its pH optimum is between 6.6 and 7.0.[84]

Clinical Significance

Despite its ubiquitous distribution, serum NTP activities appear to reflect hepatobiliary disease with considerable specificity. NTP is increased threefold to sixfold in those hepatobiliary diseases in which there is interference with the secretion of bile. This may be due to extrahepatic causes (a stone or tumor occluding the bile duct), or it may arise from intrahepatic conditions, such as cholestasis caused by chlorpromazine, malignant infiltration of the liver, or biliary cirrhosis. When parenchymal cell damage is predominant, as in infectious hepatitis, serum NTP activity is only moderately elevated.

The assay of NTP activity has been considered of value as an addition to measurement of nonspecific total ALP in patients with suspected hepatobiliary disease, and abnormal NTP activity is routinely interpreted as evidence of a hepatic origin of increased ALP activity in serum. However, approximately half of individuals in whom liver ALP activity is increased in serum may simultaneously show a normal NTP. On the other hand, increased NTP in the serum of patients with normal liver ALP is very often associated with the presence of liver disease. Thus the frequent dissociation of the two enzyme activities supports the usefulness of determining both (liver) ALP and NTP to enhance diagnostic efficiency in diseases of the liver.[54]

Methods for Determination of 5′-Nucleotidase Activity

The substrates most generally used in measuring the activity of NTP are AMP and IMP (inosine-5′-phosphate). However, these substrates are organic phosphate esters and thus can be hydrolyzed to an appreciable degree by other nonspecific (alkaline) phosphatases, even at a pH as low as 7.5, which is the pH assumed optimal for NTP activity. Methods for the estimation of NTP in serum therefore must incorporate some means for correcting for the hydrolysis of the substrate by the nonspecific phosphatases.

In a commercially available assay, serum NTP catalyzes the hydrolysis of IMP to yield inosine, which is then converted to hypoxanthine by purine-nucleoside phosphorylase (EC 2.4.2.1). Hypoxanthine is oxidized to urate with xanthine oxidase (EC 1.2.3.2). Two moles of hydrogen peroxide are produced for each mole of hypoxanthine liberated and converted to uric acid. The formation rate of hydrogen peroxide is monitored by a spectrophotometer at 510 nm by the oxidation of a chromogenic system. The effect of ALPs on IMP is inhibited by β-glycerophosphate. This material is substrate for ALP but not for NTP, and by forming substrate complexes with the former enzyme, it reduces the proportion of total ALP activity that is directed to the hydrolysis of the NTP substrate, IMP.[6]

NTP activity in serum or plasma heparin is stable for at least 4 days at 4 °C and 4 months at −20 °C.

Reference Interval

The reference interval for NTP activity at 37 °C is from 3 to 9 U/L, with no sex-related differences.

γ-Glutamyltransferase

Peptidases are enzymes that catalyze the hydrolytic cleavage of peptides to form amino acids or smaller peptides. They constitute a broad group of enzymes of varied specificity, and some individual enzymes act as amino acid transferases and catalyze the transfer of amino acids from one peptide to another amino acid or peptide. γ-Glutamyltransferase (EC 2.3.2.2; γ-glutamyl-peptide : amino acid γ-glutamyltransferase; GGT) catalyzes the transfer of the γ-glutamyl group from peptides and compounds to an acceptor.[21] The γ-glutamyl acceptor is the substrate itself, some amino acid or peptide, or even water, in which case simple hydrolysis takes place. The enzyme acts only on peptides or peptide-like compounds containing a terminal glutamate residue joined to the remainder of the compound through the terminal (-γ-) carboxyl. Glycylglycine is five times more effective as an acceptor than is glycine or the tripeptide (gly-gly-gly), but little is known about the optimal properties of the acceptor cosubstrate. The peptidase transfer reaction is considerably faster than the simple hydrolysis reaction. An example of a reaction catalyzed by the enzyme is shown here:

γ-Glutamyl-*p*-nitroanilide *Substrate (donor)* + Glycylglycine *Acceptor* $\xrightarrow[\text{pH 8.2}]{\gamma\text{-Glutamyltransferase}}$ *p*-Nitroaniline *Donor residue* + *p*-Glutamylglycylglycine *Transfer product*

GGT is present (in decreasing order of abundance) in proximal renal tubule, liver, pancreas, and intestine. The enzyme is present in cytoplasm (microsomes), but the larger fraction is located in the cell membrane and may transport amino acids and peptides into the cell across the cell membrane in the form of γ-glutamyl peptides. GGT is critical for the maintenance of adequate intracellular levels of reduced glutathione, a major antioxidant agent.[93]

GGT activity in serum comes primarily from liver. The enzyme in serum is heterogeneous with respect to both net molecular charge (e.g., shown by electrophoresis) and size. These forms appear to derive from post-translational modifications of a single type of enzyme molecule rather than resulting from the existence of true isoenzymes. For example, high molecular weight forms may represent the release of cell membrane fragments into the circulation. Despite numerous investigations, clear correlations between patterns of multiple forms and particular diseases cannot be discerned.

Clinical Significance

Even though renal tissue has the highest concentration of GGT, the enzyme present in serum appears to originate primarily from the hepatobiliary system. GGT is a sensitive indicator of the presence of hepatobiliary disease, being elevated in most subjects with liver disease regardless of cause, but its usefulness is limited by lack of specificity. Similar to ALP, it is highest in cases of intrahepatic or posthepatic biliary obstruction, reaching activities some 5 to 30 times the upper reference limit. High elevations of GGT are also observed in patients with primary or secondary (metastatic) liver neoplasm. Moderate elevations (two to five times normal) occur in infectious hepatitis. Patients with chronic hepatitis C infection and high pretreatment serum GGT are unlikely to have a sustained virologic response to interferon treatment. Small increases in GGT activity are observed in more than 50% of patients with NAFLD, and similar but transient increases are noted in cases of drug intoxication. In acute and chronic pancreatitis and in some pancreatic malignancies (especially if associated with hepatobiliary obstruction), enzyme activity may be 5 to 15 times the upper reference limit.

Elevated activities of GGT are found in the sera of patients with alcoholic hepatitis and in the majority of sera from people who are heavy drinkers. Increased concentrations of the enzyme are also found in the serum of subjects receiving anticonvulsant drugs such as phenytoin and phenobarbital. Such an increase in GGT activity in serum may reflect induction of new enzyme activity by the action of the alcohol and drugs and/or their toxic effects on microsomal structures in liver cells.

In acute myocardial infarction, GGT activity is usually normal. If there is a rise, it occurs at about the fourth day, reaches a maximum value in another 4 days, and probably implies liver damage secondary to cardiac insufficiency.

Unlike ALP, GGT is not increased in conditions in which osteoblastic activity is increased.

Recent epidemiologic evidence has shown that serum GGT activity possesses an independent prognostic value for cardiovascular morbidity and mortality. Indeed, experimental work has documented that active enzyme is present in atherosclerotic plaques, and this appears related to the ability of GGT to mediate redox/pro-oxidant reactions at a cellular level.[16]

Methods for Determination of γ-Glutamyltransferase Activity

Early GGT assays used L-γ-glutamyl-*p*-nitroanilide (GGPNA) as the substrate, with glycylglycine serving as the γ-glutamyl residue acceptor. However, GGPNA has limited solubility in the reaction mixture, and it is therefore difficult to obtain saturating substrate concentrations. The *p*-nitroaniline produced in the reaction is determined by its yellow color, which is monitored at 405 nm.

Derivatives of GGPNA are also available and have been used in other methods. With these derivatives, various groups have been introduced into the benzene ring to increase solubility in water. The most useful of these substrates is L-γ-glutamyl-3-carboxy-4-nitroanilide, which is readily soluble in water and is split by GGT at a rate comparable with that observed with GGPNA. In the IFCC reference measurement procedure for GGT, L-γ-glutamyl-3-carboxy-4-nitroanilide serves as the substrate, with glycylglycine serving as an acceptor. Buffering is provided by glycylglycine itself. The temperature of the reaction is 37 °C, and the wavelength of measurement of the reaction product, 5-amino-2-nitrobenzoate, is 410 nm.[78]

GGT is a comparatively stable enzyme in vitro. Activity is stable for at least 1 month at 4 °C and for 1 year at −20 °C.

Nonhemolyzed serum is the preferred specimen, but EDTA plasma has also been used. Heparin may produce turbidity in the reaction mixture; citrate, oxalate, and fluoride depress GGT activity by 10 to 15%.

Reference Intervals

In adults, the upper reference limit for GGT activity in serum is 40 U/L for females and 70 U/L for males, when measured with an assay traceable to the IFCC reference procedure.[29] Reference limits are approximately twofold higher in people of African ancestry. In normal full-term neonates, GGT activity at birth is approximately six to seven times the adult reference range. The activity then declines, reaching adult values by the age of 5 to 7 months.[10]

Glutathione S-Transferase

Cytosolic glutathione S-transferases (EC 2.5.1.18; GST) are dimeric enzymes that catalyze the nucleophilic addition of glutathione to the electrophilic centers of a wide variety of chemical structures, accomplishing detoxification reactions. In addition, GSTs exert part of the glutathione peroxidase activity and have an important function in intracellular binding and transport of a wide variety of both endogenous and exogenous compounds. The family of human enzymes is divided into four main classes: α, μ, π, and θ.[23]

α-GST is found at high concentrations in the human liver and is released quickly and in large quantities from damaged hepatocytes into the bloodstream.

Clinical Significance

α-GST is an emerging marker for assessing hepatocellular damage. Unlike aminotransferases, which are found predominantly in the periportal hepatocytes, α-GST is evenly distributed across the liver acinus and therefore is released in all types of hepatocyte injury. In liver transplant recipients, α-GST was found to be more valuable than AST in detecting early rejection episodes postoperatively and less susceptible to the confounding effects of infection.

Methods for Determination of Glutathione S-Transferase

Several problems have been associated with GST activity measurements. First, normal plasma activity is low and difficult to measure. Second, GST binds a number of anions, such as bile salts and bilirubin, that inhibit enzyme activity. Immunoassays have been described that allow the precise and specific measurement of α-GST concentrations. The only methodologic problem relates to the speed of the assays, which take several hours.

Reference Interval

Using a commercially available enzyme immunoassay for α-GST, the upper reference limit was 11.4 μg/L.[71]

PANCREATIC ENZYMES

The most commonly used serum biomarkers for investigation of pancreatic disease, and more specifically acute pancreatitis, are digestive enzymes. Assays of (P-type) amylase, lipase, and trypsin are applied. Pancreatic function and pathology are discussed in Chapter 51.

Amylase

α-Amylase (EC 3.2.1.1; 1,4-α-D glucan glucanohydrolase; AMY) is an enzyme of the hydrolase class that catalyzes the hydrolysis of 1,4-α-glucosidic linkages in polysaccharides. Both straight-chain (linear) polyglucans, such as amylose, and branched polyglucans, such as amylopectin and glycogen, are hydrolyzed, but at different rates. In the case of amylose, the enzyme splits the chains at alternate α-1,4-hemiacetal (–C–O–C–) links, forming maltose and some residual glucose; maltose, glucose, and a residue of limit dextrins are formed if branched-chain polyglucans are used as substrate. The enzyme does not attack the α-1,6-linkages at the branch points. AMYs are calcium metalloenzymes, with the calcium essential for functional integrity. However, full activity is displayed only in the presence of various anions—such as chloride, bromide, nitrate, cholate, or monohydrogen phosphate—with chloride and bromide being the most effective activators. AMY in human serum has a moderately sharp pH optimum at 6.9 to 7.0.

AMYs normally occurring in human plasma are small molecules with molecular weights varying from 54,000 to 62,000 Da. The enzyme is thus small enough to pass through the glomeruli of the kidneys, and AMY is the only plasma enzyme normally found in urine. AMY is present in a number of organs and tissues.[94] The greatest concentration is noted in the salivary glands, which secrete a potent AMY (S-type) to initiate hydrolysis of starches while the food is still in the mouth and esophagus. The action of the S-AMY, once referred to as *ptyalin,* is terminated by acid in the stomach. In the pancreas, the enzyme (P-type) is synthesized by acinar cells and then is secreted into the intestinal tract by way of the pancreatic duct system. In the intestinal tract, effective action of pancreatic and intestinal AMY is favored by mildly alkaline conditions in the duodenum. Intestinal maltase then further hydrolyzes maltose to glucose. AMY activity is also found in extracts from semen, testes, ovaries, fallopian tubes, striated muscle, lungs, and adipose tissue. The enzyme is present in colostrum, tears, and milk. Epithelial tumors of lung and ovary may also contain considerable AMY activity. Ascitic and pleural fluids may contain AMY as a result of the presence of a tumor or pancreatitis.

The enzyme present in normal serum and urine is predominantly of pancreatic (P-AMY) and salivary gland (S-AMY) origin. These isoenzymes are products of two closely linked loci on chromosome 1. AMY isoenzymes also undergo post-translational modification of deamidation, glycosylation, and deglycosylation to form a number of isoforms. Indeed, nonenzymic deamidation appears to be the mechanism for "aging" that occurs when AMY is sequestered (e.g., pancreatic pseudocysts) or subjected to prolonged in vitro storage. Although P-AMY is not glycosylated, S-AMY may exist in both glycosylated and deglycosylated forms; these isoforms can be separated in both serum and urine using isoelectric focusing or electrophoresis. Individuals with isolated P-AMY deficiency, a rare condition, have carbohydrate maldigestion resulting in abdominal distention, flatulence, loose stools, and poor weight gain.

Clinical Significance

Blood AMY activity is physiologically low and constant and greatly increases in acute pancreatitis and salivary gland inflammation. In acute pancreatitis, a rise in serum AMY activity occurs within 5 to 8 hours of symptom onset; activities typically return to normal by the third or fourth day. A fourfold to sixfold elevation in AMY activity above the upper reference limit is usual, with maximal concentrations attained in 12 to 72 hours. The magnitude of the elevation of serum enzyme activity is not related to the severity of pancreatic involvement; however, the greater the rise, the greater the probability of acute pancreatitis. A portion of the clearance of AMY from the circulation occurs via renal excretion into the urine, and increased serum activity is reflected in an increase in urinary AMY activity. As compared with serum AMY, urine AMY reaches higher concentrations and persists for longer periods. The clinical specificity of AMY for the diagnosis of acute pancreatitis is low (20 to 60%, depending on the mix of the patient population studied) because increased values are also found in a number of acute intra-abdominal disorders and in several extrapancreatic conditions (Table 22-6).

Lack of specificity of total AMY measurement has led to interest in the direct measurement of P-AMY instead of total enzyme activity for the differential diagnosis of patients with acute abdominal pain. By applying the best decision limit (an activity equal to threefold the upper reference limit), the clinical specificity of P-AMY for the diagnosis of acute pancreatitis was greater than 90%.[65] Sensitivity in late detection of this condition is also notably improved with P-AMY. P-AMY values remain elevated in 80% of patients with uncomplicated pancreatitis 1 week after onset, when only 30% still show increased total AMY activity. This long-standing increase in P-AMY activity in serum also makes redundant the traditional measurement of total AMY in urine—a test performed to achieve better diagnostic sensitivity in the late phase of pancreatitis.

Biliary tract diseases, such as cholecystitis, cause up to fourfold elevation in serum P-AMY activity as a result of primary or secondary pancreatic involvement. Various intra-abdominal events can lead to a significant increase in serum P-AMY activities up to a fourfold elevation and sometimes beyond. Such increases may be due to leakage of P-AMY from the intestine into the peritoneal cavity and then into the circulation.

In renal insufficiency, serum AMY activity is increased in proportion to the extent of renal impairment (usually, no more than five times the upper reference limit).

TABLE 22-6 Causes of Hyperamylasemia

Pancreatic disease	Pancreatitis, any cause (P-AMY↑)*
	Pancreatic trauma (P-AMY↑)
Intra-abdominal diseases other than pancreatitis	Biliary tract disease (P-AMY↑)
	Intestinal obstruction (P-AMY↑)
	Mesenteric infarction (P-AMY↑)
	Perforated peptic ulcer (P-AMY↑)
	Gastritis, duodenitis (P-AMY↑)
	Ruptured aortic aneurysm
	Acute appendicitis (perforated)
	Peritonitis
	Trauma
Genitourinary disease	Ectopic, ruptured tubal pregnancy
	Salpingitis (S-AMY↑)
	Ovarian malignancy (S-AMY↑)
	Renal insufficiency (Mixed)
Miscellaneous	Salivary gland lesions (S-AMY↑)
	Acute alcoholic abuse (S-AMY↑)
	Diabetic ketoacidosis (S-AMY↑)
	Macroamylasemia (S-AMY↑ or P-AMY↑)
	Septic shock (S-AMY↑)
	Cardiac surgery (S-AMY↑)
	Tumors (usually S-AMY↑)
	Drugs (usually S-AMY↑)

*Predominant isoenzyme type is shown in parentheses: *P-AMY,* pancreatic; *S-AMY,* salivary; *Mixed,* either or both isoenzymes may be present.

Hyperamylasemia also occurs in neoplastic disease. Tumors of the lung and serous and mixed (serous and mucinous) carcinomas of the ovary can produce hyperamylasemia (with an S-type isoenzyme mobility) with elevations as high as 50 times the upper reference limit. The AMY isoenzyme in cases of ruptured ectopic pregnancy is not well characterized. In severe cases presenting late, the increased isonzyme may be P-AMY (from pancreatic involvement related to peritonitis) despite the fact that S-AMY is present in fallopian tube. Cases of AMY-producing multiple myeloma have been described.

In 1% of the population, macroamylases are present in sera and may cause hyperamylasemia; these are complexes of ordinary AMY (usually S-type) and IgG or IgA. These macroamylases cannot be filtered through the glomeruli of the kidneys because of their large size (greater than MW 200,000) and are thus retained in the plasma, where their presence may increase AMY activity some twofold to eightfold above the upper reference limit. No clinical symptoms are associated with this disorder, but some cases have been detected during investigation of abdominal pain.

A decrease in serum P-AMY activity (less than the lower reference limit) is highly specific for an exocrine pancreatic insufficiency and can make intubation tests for pancreatic function unnecessary. If, however, P-AMY is normal, reduced pancreatic function cannot be excluded.[42]

Methods for Determination of α-Amylase Activity

Historically, saccharogenic, amyloclastic, and chromolytic starch methods were the assays of choice for determining AMY activity. These assays have been completely displaced in favor of ones with well-defined substrates with shorter glucosyl chains. The use of defined AMY substrates and auxiliary and indicator enzymes in the AMY assay has improved the reaction stoichiometry and has led to more controlled and consistent hydrolysis conditions. Substrates used include small oligosaccharides and 4-nitrophenyl (4-NP)-glycoside substrates.

When hydrolyzed by AMY, small oligosaccharide substrates have been found to give better defined products than do starches. For example, both maltopentaose and maltotetraose showed good stability, consistent hydrolysis products, and unambiguous reaction stoichiometry. Several variations of the reaction rate formulation have been devised.[18]

4-NP-glycoside substrates are prepared by bonding 4-NP to the reducing end of a defined oligosaccharide. If the oligosaccharide is maltoheptaose (G7), the substrate is then 4-NP-G7. AMY splits this substrate to produce free oligosaccharides (G5, G4, and G3) and 4-NP-G2 (9%), 4-NP-G3 (31%), and 4-NP-G4 (60%). P-AMY hydrolyzes the substrate at a greater rate than does S-AMY in the ratio 1.8 : 1. G6, G1, 4-NP-G6, and 4-NP-G5 are not produced in appreciable quantities. In the original assay, the result of combined hydrolysis by AMY in the specimen and by the reagent α-glucosidase (EC 3.2.1.20; maltase) is that more than 30% of the product is free NP. Free NP is detected by its absorbance at 405 nm. α-Glucosidase does not react with any oligosaccharide containing more than four glucose molecules in the chain; G4 is hydrolyzed only very slowly.[70] Problems arose with the use of the 4-NP-glycoside assay with regard to the poor stability of the reconstituted assay mixture, because of slow hydrolysis of the 4-NP-glycoside by α-glucosidase. This effect has been reduced by covalently linking a "blocking" group (i.e., a 4,6-ethylidene group) [ethylidene-protected substrate (EPS)] to the nonreducing end of the molecule. The blocked substrate also shows a different and more advantageous hydrolysis pattern. Thus the ethylidene-4-NP-G7 substrate fragments approximately as 4-NP-G2 (40%), 4-NP-G3 (40%), and 4-NP-G4 (20%). Therefore liberation of 4-NP is increased; however, the reaction rate is reduced in proportion, so these two effects compensate for each other.[37] A novel-type α-glucosidase is also available (recombinant enzyme AGH-211) that completely hydrolyzes nitrophenylated substrates. As a result, cleavage of one α-glucosidic linkage by AMY results in the release of one molecule of 4-NP:

$$\text{5 ethylidene-4-NP-G}_7 + 5\,H_2O \xrightarrow{\alpha\text{-amylase}} \text{2 ethylidene-G}_5 + \text{2 4-NP-G}_2 + \text{2 ethylidene-G}_4 + \text{2 4-NP-G}_3 + \text{ethylidene-G}_3 + \text{4-NP-G}_4$$

$$\text{2 4-NP-G}_2 + \text{2 4-NP-G}_3 + 10\,H_20 \xrightarrow{\alpha\text{-glucosidase}} \text{4 4-NP} + 10\text{ G}$$

The IFCC has optimized this method at 37 °C, recommending it as a reference measurement procedure for AMY.[75]

An alternative method based on the 2-chloro-*p*-nitrophenol (CNP) indicator uses 2-chloro-*p*-nitrophenyl-α-D-maltotrioside (CNP-G3) as a substrate. This assay does not require glucosidases and is considered a "direct" assay. Its disadvantages have been stated to include its low substrate conversion rate compared with G4, G5, and G7 assays; the variation in molar absorptivity of CNP associated with changes in pH, temperature, and protein content; and the presence of the activator, potassium thiocyanate, causing allosteric changes to AMY and precluding the use of antibodies for P-AMY determination.[87]

With the exception of heparin, all common anticoagulants inhibit AMY activity because they chelate Ca^{2+}; citrate, EDTA, and oxalate inhibit it by as much as 15%. Therefore, AMY assays should be performed only on serum or heparinized plasma. AMY is quite stable; activity is fully retained during storage for 4 days at room temperature, for 2 weeks at −4 °C, for 1 year at −25 °C, and for 5 years at −75 °C.

Reference Interval

Using the IFCC recommended method at 37 °C, the serum reference interval was 31 to 107 U/L.[75]

Analytical Methods and Reference Intervals for Amylase Isoenzymes

Methods for AMY isoenzymes based on electrophoresis, ion-exchange chromatography, isoelectric focusing, selective inhibition of the S-AMY by a wheat germ inhibitor, immunoprecipitation by a monoclonal antibody, and immunoinhibition have been introduced. However, only methods based on selective isoenzyme inhibition by monoclonal antibodies have shown sufficient precision, reliability, practicability, and analytical speed to allow the introduction of P-AMY determination into clinical practice.

A double monoclonal antibody assay is commercially available that uses the synergistic action of two immunoinhibitory monoclonal antibodies to S-AMY.[69] After the S-AMY activity is inhibited by the addition of antibodies, uninhibited P-AMY activity is measured using EPS-4-NP-G7 as a substrate. It is an attractive convenience to have this more specific assay available in full automation today on clinical chemistry platforms with reagent costs similar to total AMY, which permits laboratories to abandon the latter.[65]

False-positive P-AMY results have been reported in subjects with macroamylasemia, in whom immunoglobulin complexed to AMY forms diminishes or voids the ability of monoclonal antibodies included in the test to efficiently inhibit S-AMY. Upon electrophoresis, macro-AMY usually forms a broad migrating band, clearly different from the homogeneous bands that are produced by AMY isoenzymes present in serum (Figure 22-6). If electrophoretic separation is not available, precipitation of the macrocomplex by a PEG 6000 solution (240 g/L) represents a good alternative. Residual AMY activity of less than 30% in the supernatant is indicative of macroamylasemia.[12]

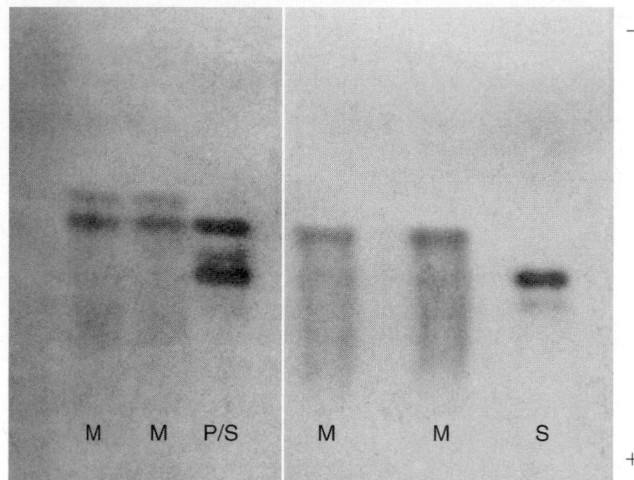

Figure 22-6 Electrophoretic separation of amylase isoenzymes. *M,* Macroamylasemia; *P/S,* mixture of two samples containing, respectively, pancreatic juice and saliva; *S,* saliva. The anodal direction is downward.

In healthy adults, P-AMY represents approximately 40 to 50% of total AMY activity in serum. Using the immunoinhibition method at 37 °C, the reference interval for P-AMY activity in sera from adults was 13 to 53 U/L.[33] Serum P-AMY activity is not demonstrable in most children younger than 6 months, but activity rises slowly thereafter to reach adult concentrations at 5 years of age, reflecting the postnatal development of exocrine pancreatic function. As a consequence, use of this enzyme for the diagnosis of acute pancreatitis in young children should be avoided and the test should be replaced with the measurement of lipase.

Lipase

Human pancreatic lipase (EC 3.1.1.3; triacylglycerol acylhydrolase; LPS) is a single-chain glycoprotein with a molecular weight of 48,000 Da and an isoelectric point of about 5.8. The LPS gene resides on chromosome 10. LPS concentration in the pancreas is about 5000-fold greater than in other tissues, and the concentration gradient between pancreas and serum is ≈20,000-fold.[59] For full catalytic activity and greatest specificity, the presence of bile salts and a cofactor called *colipase,* which is a small molecular weight protein of 10,000 secreted by the pancreas, are required. Human LPS can be fully activated in vitro by colipases from other species (e.g., porcine colipase); this property is used in analytical formulations of the LPS assay.[89]

Lipases are defined as enzymes that hydrolyze glycerol esters of long-chain fatty acids. Only ester bonds at carbons 1 and 3 (α-positions) are attacked, and products of the reaction include 2 moles of fatty acids and 1 mole of 2-acylglycerol (β-monoglyceride) per mole of substrate. The latter is resistant to hydrolysis, probably because of steric hindrance, but it can spontaneously isomerize to the α-form (3-acylglycerol). This isomerization permits the third fatty acid to be split off but at a much slower rate. A scheme for the steps in complete hydrolysis of a molecule of triglyceride to glycerol and three fatty acids is shown here:

$H_2C{-}OFA(1)$
$HC{-}OFA(2)$
$H_2C{-}OFA(3)$
Triglyceride

Lipase, H_2O, $OH^{\ominus}$ →

$H_2C{-}OH$
$HC{-}OFA(2)$
$H_2C{-}OFA(3)$
α,β-Diglyceride + FA(1)OH (Fatty acid I)

Lipase, H_2O, $OH^{\ominus}$ →

$H_2C{-}OH$
$HC{-}OFA(2)$
$H_2C{-}OH$
β-Monoglyceride + FA(3)OH (Fatty acid III)

Isomerization →

$H_2C{-}OH$
$HC{-}OH$
$H_2C{-}OFA(2)$
α-Monoglyceride

Lipase, H_2O, $OH^{\ominus}$ →

$H_2C{-}OH$
$HC{-}OH$
$H_2C{-}OH$
Glycerol + FA(2)OH (Fatty acid II)

LPS acts only when the substrate is present in an emulsified form at the interface between water and the substrate. The rate of LPS action depends on the surface area of the dispersed substrate. Bile acids ensure that the surface of the dispersed substrate remains free of other proteins, including lipolytic enzymes, by lining the surface of the insoluble substrate and the aqueous medium. LPS seems to gain access to the substrate surface in the following manner: Colipase attaches to a micelle of bile salts, thus forming a colipase–bile salt complex that reconfigures the structure of colipase with exposure of a site with high affinity and high specificity for LPS, which therefore attracts LPS and anchors it to the substrate surface, allowing enzyme action to proceed.

Most LPS activity found in serum derives from the pancreas, but some is secreted by gastric, pulmonary, and intestinal mucosa. LPS is a small enough molecule to be filtered through the glomerulus. It is totally reabsorbed by the renal tubules, and it is not physiologically detected in urine. Evidence suggests that pancreatic LPS may exist in at least two isoforms, although the exact nature of these is unknown.[59] Complete absence of LPS has been reported. Such congenital absence results in fat malabsorption and severe steatorrhea.

Clinical Significance

LPS measurement of serum is used to diagnose acute pancreatitis. The clinical sensitivity is 80 to 100% depending on the selected diagnostic cutoff, and the clinical specificity is 80 to 100% depending on the mix of the patient population studied. After an attack of acute pancreatitis, serum LPS activity increases within 4 to 8 hours, peaks at about 24 hours, and decreases within 7 to 14 days. Elevations between 2 and 50 times the upper reference limit have been reported. The increase in serum LPS activity is not necessarily proportional to the severity of the attack.[89]

Acute pancreatitis is sometimes difficult to diagnose because it must be differentiated from other acute intra-abdominal disorders with similar clinical findings, such as perforated gastric or duodenal ulcer, intestinal obstruction, or mesenteric vascular obstruction. In differential diagnosis, elevation of serum LPS activity to greater than 3 times the upper reference limit, in the absence of renal failure, is a more specific diagnostic finding than increases in serum AMY activity.[19] Furthermore, LPS concentrations remain elevated longer than those of AMY do, which is another advantage over AMY measurement in patients with delayed presentation (Figure 22-7). Therefore, it is recommended that LPS should replace AMY as the initial diagnostic test for acute pancreatitis in the emergency department; obtaining both serum AMY and LPS is not warranted.

Obstruction of the pancreatic duct by a calculus or by carcinoma of the pancreas may increase serum LPS activity, depending on the location of the obstruction and the amount of remaining functioning tissue. In patients with a reduced glomerular filtration rate, serum LPS activity is increased. Thus care should be exercised in the interpretation of elevated serum LPS values in the presence of renal disease. Finally, investigation of the biliary tract by endoscopic retrograde pancreatography or treatment with opiates (which causes the sphincter of Oddi to contract) may increase serum LPS activity.

Methods for Measuring Lipase Activity

Many LPS methods have been described; they have used both triglyceride and nontriglyceride substrates and titrimetric, turbidimetric, spectrophotometric, fluorometric, and immunologic techniques. In general, long-chain triglyceride (and some diglyceride) substrates have demonstrated correlation of results with the clinical state that is superior to that seen with methods using other substrates.[38]

In titrimetric methods, LPS catalyzes the hydrolysis of fatty acids from an emulsion of olive oil or oleic acid. The fatty acids liberated are titrated with dilute alkali. Kinetic versions use an automated potentiometric titrator (an instrument commonly referred to as a "pH-stat"). The amount of alkali used is recorded as a function of time and serves as a measure of fatty acid produced during the reaction.

In the turbidimetric method, LPS catalyzes the hydrolysis of fatty acids from an emulsion of oleic acid with a simultaneous decrease in the turbidity of the reaction mixture. Absorbance at 340 nm is read and the ΔA/min is taken as a measure of LPS activity. Turbidities have occasionally been observed to increase rather than decrease during the reaction period. Such increases have frequently been observed in specimens containing rheumatoid factor. The method linearity (≈3 times the upper reference limit) is limited, with many clinical samples needing to be diluted.

Numerous substrates and complex auxiliary and indicator systems are used in spectrophotometric methods. In the Ortho Clinical Diagnostics spectrophotometric reaction rate LPS slide method, the (synthetic) substrate is 1-oleoyl-2,3-diacetylglycerol, and the emulsifier dodecylbenzene sulfonate. LPS activity is measured by a complex auxiliary and indicator enzyme system to produce a colored dye detectable at 540 nm. However, the substrate is likely to be more specific for intestinal than pancreatic LPS and may be subject to interference by postheparin lipase and pancreatic carboxylesterase.

In the enzymatic reaction rate diglyceride assay for LPS, the following sequence of indicator and auxiliary enzymes is used:

$$\text{1,2-Diacylglycerol} + H_2O \xrightarrow[\text{pH 8.7}]{\text{Pancreatic lipase, Colipase}} \text{2-monoacylglycerol} + \text{fatty acid}$$

$$\text{2-monoacylglycerol} + H_2O \xrightarrow{\text{Monoglyceride lipase}} \text{Glycerol} + \text{fatty acid}$$

$$\text{Glycerol} + \text{ATP} \xrightarrow{\text{Glycerol kinase}} \text{L-}\alpha\text{-glycerophospate} + \text{ADP}$$

$$\text{L-}\alpha\text{-glycerophospate} + O_2 \xrightarrow{\text{L-}\alpha\text{-glycerophospate kinase}} \text{Dihydroxyacetone phosphate} + H_2O_2$$

$$2\,H_2O_2 + \text{4-aminoantipyrine} + \text{TOOS} \xrightarrow{\text{Peroxidase}} \text{Quinonediimine dye (colored)} + 2\,H_2O$$

TOOS is sodium *N*-ethyl-*N*-(2-hydroxyl-3-sulfopropyl)-m-toluidine, and its oxidation produces an intensely colored dye detectable at 550 nm. The suggested upper reference limit is 45 U/L at 37 °C.

More recently, a synthetic substrate [1,2-O-dilauryl-rac-glycero-3-glutaric acid-(4-methyl-resorufin)-ester] consisting of two glycerol ether bonds and one ester bond has been proposed, and assays based on its use are currently gaining widespread use. LPS hydrolyzes the ester bond in an alkaline medium to an unstable dicarbonic acid ester that spontaneously hydrolyzes to yield glutaric acid and methylresorufin; this is a bluish-purple chromophore with peak absorption at 580 nm.

1,2-O-Dilauryl-rac-glycero-3-glutaric acid-(4 methyl-resorufin)-ester

Lipase + $OH^{\ominus}$

Spontaneous $OH^{\ominus}$

Glutarate

Red, λ = 580 nm

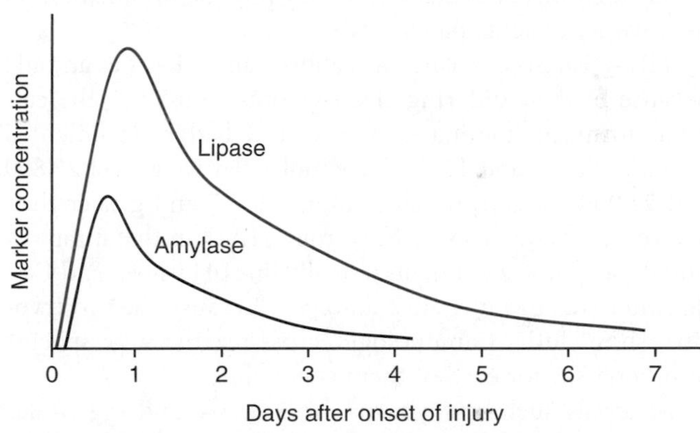

Figure 22-7 Time-dependent changes in serum amylase and lipase after acute pancreatitis.

The rate of methylresorufin formation is directly proportional to the LPS activity of the sample. The upper reference limit is 38 U/L at 37 °C, with no gender- or age-related differences. Compared with previous LPS spectrophotometric methods, this assay principle is based on a direct reaction and appears to have increased specificity for pancreatic LPS.[64]

A newly synthesized thioester (2,3-dibutyrylthio-1-propyl oleate) substrate that is believed to be highly selective for pancreatic LPS has also been proposed, but commercial methods are yet not available to permit its clinical validation.

LPS activity in serum is stable at room temperature for 1 week; sera may be stored for 3 weeks in the refrigerator and for several years if frozen.

Trypsin

Trypsin (EC 3.4.21.4; no systematic name; TRY) is a pancreas-specific serine protease characterized by the presence at the active site of serine and histidine, both of which participate in the catalytic process. TRY hydrolyzes peptide bonds formed by the carboxyl groups of lysine or arginine with other amino acids, although esters and amides involving these amino acids are actually split more rapidly than peptide bonds.[55]

The acinar cells of the human pancreas synthesize two major trypsins (1 and 2) in the form of the inactive proenzymes (or zymogens), trypsinogens-1 and -2. These zymogens are stored in zymogen granules and are secreted into the duodenum under the stimulus of the vagus nerve or the intestinal hormone cholecystokinin-pancreozymin. The two trypsinogens represent approximately 19% of the total protein in pancreatic juice; normally, the pancreas secretes trypsinogen-1 at about twofold to fourfold the concentration of trypsinogen-2, but in pancreatic disease, the ratio of trypsinogen-1 and -2 is reversed. In the intestinal tract, the trypsinogens are converted to the active enzyme TRY by the duodenal enzyme enterokinase or by pre-formed TRY (autocatalysis) (Figure 22-8). When trypsinogens are converted to active TRY, a small peptide is cleaved from the *N*-terminal region of trypsinogen [trypsinogen activation peptide (TAP)]. Determinations of urinary TAP may provide information on the severity of acute pancreatitis.[20]

TRY-1 is also described as cationic and TRY-2 as anionic because of their differing electrophoretic mobility; the cationic form predominates and is the better documented enzyme. TRY-1 and TRY-2 have molecular weights of 25,800 and 22,900 Da and pI values of 4.6 to 6.5 and greater than 6.5, respectively. TRY-2 differs from TRY-1 in that it rapidly undergoes autolysis at neutral or alkaline pH values, and Ca^{2+} does not stabilize it against autolysis. Because the two trypsins show little immunologic cross-reactivity, a specific immunoassay for each of them is possible.

Materials such as soybeans, lima beans, and egg whites contain natural TRY inhibitors—small polypeptides such as α_1-antitrypsin (α_1-protease inhibitor) and α_2-macroglobulin—that combine irreversibly with TRY and inactivate it by blocking the active center. Similar nondialyzable TRY inhibitors [e.g., pancreatic secretory trypsin inhibitor (PSTI)] are present in pancreas, pancreatic juice, serum, and urine. These inhibitors protect plasma and other proteins against hydrolysis by TRY and other proteases if for some reason any appreciable quantity of the enzyme enters the vascular system.[55] The absence of α_1-antitrypsin is associated with an increased tendency toward panlobular emphysema in early life; this example illustrates the effects of uninhibited proteases on organ function.

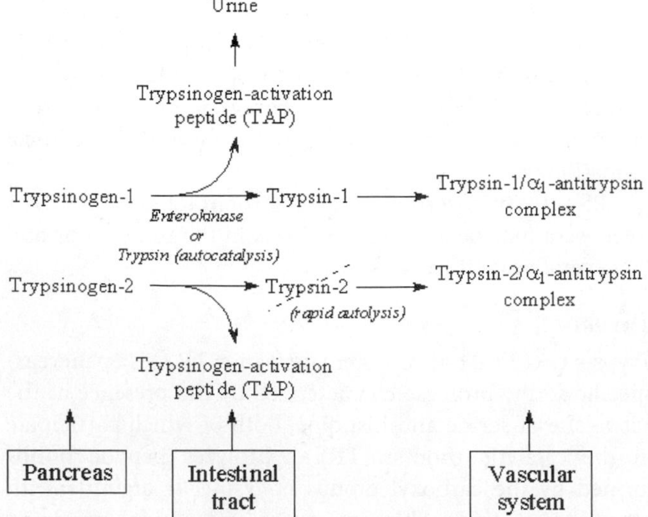

Figure 22-8 A comprehensive representation of the human trypsin system.

Clinical Significance

Trypsin-1 (Cationic Trypsin)[41]

In healthy individuals, free trypsinogen-1 is the major form found in serum. After an attack of acute pancreatitis, serum TRY-1 rises in parallel with serum AMY activity to peak values ranging from 2 to 400 times the upper reference limit. The distribution of the different forms of TRY-1 appears to be related to the type and severity of acute pancreatitis. Thus in the mildest form of acute pancreatitis, 80 to 99% of TRY-1 exists as free trypsinogen-1, with smaller proportions existing as bound TRY-1. In the more severe forms, in which mortality ranges from 20% to more than 50%, the proportion of free trypsinogen-1 may be as low as 30% of the total, with appreciable proportions existing as the α_1-antitrypsin– and α_2-macroglobulin–bound TRY-1.[8]

TRY-1 in serum is elevated in chronic renal failure, as are serum AMY and LPS. Thus renal failure must be ruled out when elevated concentrations are interpreted. In chronic pancreatitis without steatorrhea, plasma concentrations of TRY-1 do not differ from those found in health; when steatorrhea is present, however, fasting concentrations are extremely low. In the relapsing phase of chronic pancreatitis, plasma TRY may be considerably elevated. In carcinoma of the pancreas, TRY concentrations may be high, normal, or even low.

In comparison with P-AMY and LPS measurements, TRY-1 is a more difficult test to perform, requiring several hours to complete. Because TRY estimation has no distinct role in the routine management of patients with acute pancreatitis, this test is considered of limited clinical value.

Cystic fibrosis is a genetic disorder that primarily affects the lungs and digestive system, resulting in the production of thick mucus that blocks ducts in the pancreas, preventing normal transport of trypsinogen. In this condition, plasma TRY concentrations have been reported to be high in neonates; as the disease progresses, activity falls. Newborn screening is done by the measurement of immunoreactive trypsinogen-1 in dried blood specimens. Infants who have a high TRY concentration on initial testing undergo further assessment via a repeat test 1 to 3 weeks later, or by analysis of the initial blood spot for specific DNA mutations.

Trypsin-2 (Anionic Trypsin)

Serum trypsinogen-2 increases more than trypsinogen-1 in acute pancreatitis, the concentrations of the former being on average about 10-fold those of the latter.[31] Consequently, larger amounts of trypsinogen-2 are excreted into urine. Urinary trypsinogen-2 measurement has shown high sensitivity and negative predictive value for the diagnosis of acute pancreatitis on admission to the hospital. However, the positive predictive value of this test is low.

As noted earlier, newly formed TRY is inactivated by complexing with α_1-antitrypsin. Assays of this serum complex with TRY-2 have shown that this determination could be superior to that of trypsinogen-2 or AMY in acute pancreatitis.[24]

Methods for Determination of Trypsin

Early studies used catalytic assays, but it was soon recognized that other proteolytic enzymes present in serum could also hydrolyze the same substrates. A major advance has been the development of commercial immunoassays to specifically quantify TRY in blood. In the case of TRY-1, immunoassays detect trypsinogen-1, TRY-1, and the TRY-1–α_1-antitrypsin complex. They do not detect the TRY-1–α_2-macroglobulin complex, for which different assays are necessary. Free TRY-1 is not usually found in serum; it is always complexed. Because no assay standardization is available, reference limits are method dependent.

A rapid (5 minute) urinary trypsinogen-2 test strip is available, which is based on the use of immunochromatography with monoclonal antibodies. The test is considered positive at urinary trypsinogen-2 concentrations greater than 50 µg/L.

BONE ENZYMES

Bone enzymes are direct products of active osteoblasts (bone ALP) and osteoclasts (tartrate-resistant acid phosphatase).

Alkaline Phosphatase (Bone Isoform)

Bone, liver, and kidney isoforms of ALP are post-translational modifications of the same gene product and are identified by their unique carbohydrate content (see Figure 22-4). They were described previously in the section on liver enzymes. Bone ALP is produced by the osteoblast and has been demonstrated in matrix vesicles deposited as "buds" derived from the cell's membrane. The enzyme therefore is an excellent indicator of global bone formation activity. Genetic inability to produce tissue-nonspecific ALP, including bone isoform, a rare inherited disorder known as hypophosphatasia, results in severe bone disease and impaired bone growth.

Clinical Significance in Bone Disease

Advantages of using bone ALP concentrations in serum as bone formation markers in clinical practice include low diurnal variability and lack of renal function concerns. Among the bone diseases, the highest concentrations of bone ALP are encountered in Paget's disease (osteitis deformans) as a result of the action of osteoblastic cells as they try to rebuild bone that is being resorbed by uncontrolled activity of osteoclasts. Values from 10 to 25 times the upper reference limit are not unusual, and in broad terms the increase reflects the extent of disease. In vitamin D deficiency (osteomalacia and rickets), concentrations two to four times normal may be observed, and these fall slowly to normal on treatment. Primary hyperparathyroidism and secondary hyperparathyroidism are associated with slight to moderate elevations of bone ALP in serum, with the existence and degree of elevation reflecting the presence and extent of skeletal involvement. Very high enzyme concentrations are present in patients with osteogenic bone cancer. Bone ALP can be slightly increased in osteoporosis, but osteoporotic individuals are not clearly distinguished from age-matched controls even if, over the entire population, concentrations are inversely correlated with bone mineral density. Transient elevations may be found during healing of bone fractures. Physiologic bone growth increases bone ALP in serum, and this accounts for the fact that in the sera of growing children, the enzyme concentration is 1.5 to 7 times that in healthy adult serum, the maximum being reached earlier in girls than in boys.

Methods for Determination of Bone Alkaline Phosphatase

In general, separation of tissue-nonspecific ALP forms (i.e., bone and liver) is difficult because of structural similarity. At present, bone ALP in serum can be measured by electrophoretic and immunochemical methods (see the section on liver enzymes). Immunoassays for bone ALP, which measure enzyme activity or mass, are commercially available; cross-reactivity with the liver isoform, however, has been established:

Assay	Type	Cross-Reactivity, %
Beckman Coulter Tandem-R-Ostase	Mass based IRMA	12.7-16.5
Beckman Coulter Tandem-MP-Ostase	Mass based ELISA	8.1-16.2
Metra Alkphase-B	Activity based EIA	5.9-20.0

This general limitation should be borne in mind when test results are interpreted.

With the use of immunoassays measuring bone ALP concentrations, the enzyme is said to be stable at −20 °C for 2 years.

Reference Intervals

When the electrophoretic procedure is used, the reference interval for bone ALP activity in healthy adults is 10 to 50 U/L.[66] Mean (SD) bone ALP concentrations, determined by immunoassays in healthy adults, were 13 µg/L (5).[9]

Acid Phosphatase (Tartrate-Resistant 5b Isoform)

Under the name of acid phosphatase [EC 3.1.3.2; orthophosphoric-monoester phosphohydrolase (acid optimum); ACP] are included all phosphatases with optimal activity below a pH of 7.0.

ACP is present in lysosomes, which are organelles present in all cells with the possible exception of erythrocytes.

Extralysosomal ACPs are also present in many cells. The greatest concentrations of ACP activity occur in prostate, bone (osteoclasts), spleen, platelets, and erythrocytes. The lysosomal and prostatic enzymes are strongly inhibited by dextrorotatory tartrate ions, whereas the erythrocyte and bone isoenzymes are not. Most of the normally low ACP activity of (unhemolyzed) serum is of a tartrate-resistant type (TR-ACP) and probably originates mainly in osteoclasts. Activities of this fraction are increased physiologically in growing children and pathologically in conditions of increased osteolysis and bone remodeling.[46]

At least four ACP-determining genes have been identified and mapped. The erythrocyte ACP gene is located on chromosome 2 and is polymorphic, and a further gene on chromosome 19 encodes the TR-ACP expressed in osteoclasts and other tissue macrophages, such as alveolar macrophages and Kupffer cells (type 5 ACP). Isoenzyme 5 consists of two structurally related isoforms that differ by their carbohydrate content: TR-ACP 5a, which derives mainly from macrophages and dendritic cells, and type 5b, a more specific marker of osteoclastic activity. Genes encoding the tartrate-inhibited lysosomal and prostatic ACPs, mapped to chromosomes 11 and 13 respectively, exhibit considerable homology.[50]

ACPs are unstable, especially at temperatures above 37 °C and at pH above 7.0. Some of the enzyme forms in serum are particularly labile, and more than 30% of ACP activity may be lost in 3 hours at room temperature. Acidification of the serum specimen to a pH below 6.5 aids in stabilizing the enzyme activity.

Clinical Significance

TR-ACP is a potentially useful marker of conditions with a marked osteolytic component. Slight or moderate elevations in serum TR-ACP activity often occur in Paget's disease, in hyperparathyroidism with skeletal involvement, and in the presence of malignant invasion of the bones by cancers such as breast cancer in women. Increased concentrations of the osteoclast-derived ACP are also present in serum in osteoclastoma (giant cell tumor), an osteoclastic neoplasm, and in osteopetrosis (marble bone disease) in which the osteoclasts fail to resorb bone. High concentrations of TR-ACP in the serum of these patients are proportional to the osteoclast number, suggesting that changes in osteoclast function and number do not always go hand in hand.[26] TR-ACP appears to show relatively small dynamic changes in comparison with other markers of bone resorption (e.g., those related to type I collagen metabolism). This may be attributable to the fact that the enzyme is released into the sealed osteoclast microenvironment, rather than directly into the circulation.

Unlike blood concentrations of other markers of bone resorption (e.g., C-telopeptide of type I collagen), TR-ACP is not affected by renal dysfunction. The only nonbone condition in which elevated activities of TR-ACP are found in serum is Gaucher's disease of the spleen, a lysosomal storage disorder. Its source in this disease is the abnormal macrophages in spleen and other tissues, which overexpress this normal macrophage constituent. The hairy cells of hairy cell leukemia (leukemic reticuloendotheliosis) also express the osteoclast-type ACP, providing a useful histologic marker. However, in this condition, the isoenzyme does not enter the plasma in increased amounts.

Although once widely used to detect or monitor carcinoma of the prostate, determination of ACP (tartrate-inhibited) activity in serum has now been replaced by prostate-specific antigen (PSA).

Methods for Determination of Tartrate-Resistant Acid Phosphatase

Continuous-monitoring methods for assay of TR-ACP activity are based on the principle introduced by Hillmann in which α-naphthol released from its phosphate ester forms a colored product with the stabilized diazonium salt of 2-amino-5-chlorotoluene-1,5-naphthalene disulfonate (Fast Red TR). Alcohols, such as 1,5-pentanediol, accelerate the reaction and increase sensitivity by acting as phosphate acceptors in transfer reactions. The addition of sodium tartrate inhibits the sensitive isoenzymes (i.e., prostatic and lysosomal ACPs) if they are present in the sample.

Immunoassays for serum TR-ACP have been developed that preferentially detect isoform 5b. A first method uses a monoclonal antibody to bind serum TR-ACP in a solid-phase format. After the capture, osteoclastic enzyme (type 5b) is specifically determined by measuring its activity at optimal pH 6.1. Another assay uses two monoclonal antibodies generated against purified bone TR-ACP 5b. One of the antibodies captures active intact isoform while the second eliminates interference of inactive 5b fragments in serum. After the immunoreaction, binding TR-ACP 5b activity is measured (fragments absorbed immunocapture enzymatic assay [FAICEA]).

Serum should be immediately separated from erythrocytes and stabilized by the addition of 50 μL of acetic acid (5 mol/L) per milliliter of serum to lower the pH to 5.4, at which the enzyme is stable. Under these conditions, TR-ACP activity is maintained at room temperature for several hours, for up to a week if the serum is refrigerated, and for 4 months if stored at −20 °C. Hemolyzed serum specimens are contaminated with considerable amounts of the erythrocyte tartrate-resistant isoenzyme and should be rejected.

Reference Intervals

In the sera of healthy adults, the reference interval for TR-ACP activity, measured at 37 °C, is 1.5 to 4.5 U/L. Children show higher TR-ACP activities (3.4 to 9.0 U/L).

MISCELLANEOUS ENZYMES

Lactate Dehydrogenase

Lactate dehydrogenase (EC 1.1.1.27; L-lactate: NAD^+ oxidoreductase; LD) is a hydrogen transfer enzyme that catalyzes the oxidation of L-lactate to pyruvate with the mediation of NAD^+ as a hydrogen acceptor.

$$\text{L-Lactate (CH}_3\text{–CH(OH)–COO}^-) + NAD^+ \underset{\text{pH 7.4 to 7.8}}{\overset{\text{Lactate Dehydrogenase, pH 8.8 to 9.8}}{\rightleftharpoons}} \text{Pyruvate (CH}_3\text{–CO–COO}^-) + NADH + H^+$$

As indicated, the reaction is reversible, and the reaction equilibrium strongly favors the reduction of pyruvate to lactate (P → L)—the "reverse reaction."

The pH optimum for the lactate-to-pyruvate (L → P) reaction is 8.8 to 9.8, and an assay reaction mixture, optimized for LD-1 at 37 °C, contains NAD^+, 9 mmol/L, and L-lactate, 80 mmol/L. For the P → L assay, at 37 °C, the pH optimum is 7.4 to 7.8, NADH 300 μmol/L, and pyruvate 0.85 mmol/L. The optimal pH varies with the predominant isoenzymes in the sample and depends on the temperature and on substrate and buffer concentrations. The specificity of the enzyme extends from L-lactate to various related 2-hydroxyacids and 2-oxo-acids. The catalytic oxidation of 2-hydroxybutyrate, the next higher homolog of lactate, to 2-oxobutyrate is referred to as 2-hydroxybutyrate dehydrogenase (HBD) activity. LD does not act on D-lactate, and only NAD^+ serves as a coenzyme.

The enzyme has a molecular weight of 134,000 Da and is composed of four peptide chains of two types: M (or A) and H (or B), each under separate genetic control. The structures of LD-M and LD-H are determined by loci on human chromosomes 11 and 12, respectively. The subunit compositions of the five isoenzymes, in order of decreasing anodal mobility in an alkaline medium, are LD-1 (HHHH; H_4); LD-2 (HHHM; H_3M); LD-3 (HHMM; H_2M_2); LD-4 (HMMM; HM_3); and LD-5 (MMMM; M_4). A different, sixth LDH isoenzyme, LD-X (also called LDH_C), composed of four X (or C) subunits, is present in postpubertal human testes. A seventh LD, called LD-6, has been identified in the sera of severely ill patients.

LD is inhibited by reagents with reactivity against thiol groups, such as mercuric ions and *p*-chloromercuribenzoate, the inhibition being reversed by the addition of cysteine or glutathione. Borate and oxalate inhibit by competing with lactate for its binding site on the enzyme; similarly, oxamate competes with pyruvate for its binding site. Both pyruvate and lactate in excess inhibit enzyme activity, although the effect of pyruvate is greater. Inhibition by either substrate is greater for the H form than for the M form, and substrate inhibition decreases with increases in pH. EDTA inhibits the enzyme perhaps by binding Zn^{2+}; however, the postulated activator role for zinc ions is not fully established.

LD activity is present in many cells of the body and is invariably found only in the cytoplasm of the cell. Enzyme concentrations in various tissues are about 1500 to 5000 times greater than those physiologically found in serum. Therefore, leakage of the enzyme from even a small mass of damaged tissue increases the observed serum activity of LD to a significant extent. Different tissues show different isoenzyme composition. In the heart, kidneys, and erythrocytes, the electrophoretically faster moving isoenzymes LD-1 and LD-2 predominate, whereas in liver and skeletal muscle, the more cathodal LD-4 and LD-5 isoenzymes predominate—although skeletal muscle damage may also result in anodic LD patterns. Isoenzymes of intermediate mobility account for the LD activity from many sources (e.g., spleen, lungs, lymph nodes, leukocytes, platelets).

Clinical Significance

Because of its wide tissue distribution, serum LD elevations occur in a variety of clinical conditions, including myocardial infarction, hepatitis, hemolysis, and disorders of the kidneys, lung, and muscle. Serum LD measurement is, however, relevant only in hematology and oncology.[28]

Hemolytic anemias significantly increase LD concentrations in serum. Marked elevations of LD activity—up to 50 times the upper reference limit—have been observed in the megaloblastic anemias. These anemias, usually resulting from the deficiency of folate or vitamin B_{12}, cause the erythrocyte precursor cell to break down in the bone marrow (ineffective erythropoiesis), resulting in the release of large quantities of LD-1 and LD-2 isoenzymes. These elevations rapidly return to normal after appropriate treatment. For monitoring purposes, LD is relevant in predicting disease activity in leukemia, and the survival rate (probability of survival) and duration in Hodgkin's disease and non-Hodgkin's lymphoma.

Patients with malignant disease often show increased LD activity in serum; up to 70% of patients with liver metastases and 20 to 60% of patients with other nonhepatic metastases (e.g., lymph nodes) have elevated LD activity. Notably elevated LD-1 is observed in germ cell tumors (≈60% of cases) such as teratoma, seminoma of the testis, and dysgerminoma of the ovary.[92] The percentage of patients with increased LD depended on the stage of the disease. LD appears to be a useful predictor of outcome in patients with testicular nonseminomatous germ cell tumors, melanoma, and small cell lung cancer.

Elevations of LD activity (predominant LD-4 and LD-5 isoenzymes) are observed in liver disease, but their routine use in a liver profile appears limited and would not appear to add significantly to the aminotransferase activity investigation.

Macro-LD, usually due to the formation of an autoantibody-enzyme complex that leads to a persistent increase in the amount of circulating enzyme, has been estimated to occur in <1 in 10,000 people. Documentation of a macro-LD (e.g., by the presence of an abnormally migrating band at electrophoresis) should be established in suspected individuals to avoid additional follow-up investigation or unnecessary treatment.

Methods for Determination of Lactate Dehydrogenase Activity

Routine methods for quantitation of total LD activity use kinetic spectrophotometry to measure the interconversion of the coenzyme NAD^+ and NADH at 340 nm. The most widely used procedures employ the L → P reaction, because it is claimed that there is less dependence on the NAD^+ and lactate concentrations and less contamination of NAD^+ with inhibiting products.[4] An L → P reference method, optimized for LD-1, has been developed by the IFCC as a reference procedure for LD at 37 °C.[77]

Serum is the preferred specimen for measuring LD activity. Plasma samples may be contaminated with platelets, which contain high concentrations of LD. Serum should be separated from the clot as soon as possible after the specimen has been obtained. Hemolyzed serum must not be used because erythrocytes contain 4000 times more LD activity than does serum. The different isoenzymes vary in their sensitivity to cold, LD-4 and LD-5 being especially labile. Activity of LD-4 and LD-5 is lost if the samples are stored at −20 °C. Thus serum specimens should be stored at room temperature, at which no loss of activity occurs for at least 3 days.

Reference Intervals

The reference interval for LD activity in adult white subjects, determined at 37 °C with a procedure traceable to the IFCC reference method, was found to be 125 to 220 U/L.[53] LD reference limits are higher in children, with a gradual decrease noted over the whole childhood period.[25]

Methods for Separation and Quantification of Lactate Dehydrogenase Isoenzymes

Electrophoretic separation on agarose gels or cellulose acetate membranes is the procedure most commonly used to demonstrate LD isoenzymes. After the isoenzymes have been separated by electrophoresis, a reaction mixture is layered over the separation medium (typically D,L-lactate, 500 mmol/L, and NAD^+, 13 mmol/L, often dissolved in a suitable pH 8.0 buffer). The NADH generated over the LD zones is detected by its fluorescence, when excited by long-wave ultraviolet light (365 nm), or by its reduction of a tetrazolium salt to form a colored formazan.

Using an agarose gel technique with fluorometric quantitation of generated NADH, the following reference intervals for isoenzymes were obtained (expressed as percent of total LD): LD-1, 14 to 26%; LD-2, 29 to 39%; LD-3, 20 to 26%; LD-4, 8 to 16%; and LD-5, 6 to 16%.

Cholinesterase

Two related enzymes have the ability to hydrolyze acetylcholine. One is acetylcholinesterase (EC 3.1.1.7; acetylcholine acetylhydrolase), which is called *true cholinesterase* or *choline esterase I.* True cholinesterase is found in erythrocytes, the lungs and spleen, nerve endings, and the gray matter of the brain. It is responsible for the prompt hydrolysis of a cetylcholine released at the nerve endings to mediate transmission of the neural impulse across the synapse. Degradation of acetylcholine is required for depolarization of the nerve, so that it is repolarized in the next conduction event.

The other cholinesterase is acylcholine acylhydrolase (EC 3.1.1.8; acylcholine acylhydrolase; CHE), also called pseudocholinesterase, serum cholinesterase, butyrylcholinesterase, or choline esterase II, which is found in the liver, pancreas, heart, white matter of the brain, and serum. Although CHE activity in the human body is about threefold higher than acetylcholinesterase activity, its exact biological role is unknown. A physiologic role for CHE in deactivation of octanoyl ghrelin, a hormone that stimulates feeding and promotes weight gain through its metabolic actions, has been proposed.

The type of reaction catalyzed by both cholinesterases is shown:

$$Br^{\ominus}\ (CH_3)_3N^{\oplus}-CH_2-CH_2-O-C(=O)-CH_3 \xrightarrow[\text{Cholinesterase}]{H_2O \quad H^{\oplus}} CH_3-C(=O)-O^{\ominus} + Br^{\ominus}\ (CH_3)_3N^{\oplus}-CH_2-CH_2OH$$

Acetylcholine bromide → Acetate + Choline bromide

The two enzymes differ in specificity toward some substrates while behaving similarly toward others. The serum enzyme acts on benzoylcholine but cannot hydrolyze acetyl-β-methylcholine; the red cell enzyme acts on the latter but not on the former. The red cell enzyme splits only choline esters; aryl and alkyl esters are not attacked. The red cell enzyme is inhibited by its substrate, acetylcholine, if present at about 10^{-2} mol/L; the serum enzyme is not inhibited by this substrate.

The two enzymes are inhibited by the alkaloids prostigmine and physostigmine, both of which contain quaternary nitrogen (present in choline) in their structures. These two compounds are typical competitive inhibitors, competing with the choline residue of acetylcholine for its binding site on the enzyme surface. Some organic phosphorous compounds, such as diisopropyl fluorophosphate, irreversibly inhibit both enzymes. The phosphoryl group binds very tightly to the enzyme site at which binding of the acyl group normally occurs, thus preventing attachment of the acetylcholine. Both enzymes are also inhibited by a large variety of other compounds, including morphine, quinine, tertiary amines, phenothiazines, pyrophosphate, bile salts, citrate, fluoride, and borate.

CHE in normal sera is separated by electrophoresis into 7 to 12 bands, the number depending on the experimental technique used. The forms of CHE differ in molecular size and appear to be aggregates of different numbers of the same basic unit. Of greater interest are the atypical (genetic) variants of the enzyme, characterized by diminished activity against acetylcholine and other substrates, which are found in the sera of a small fraction of apparently healthy people.

The gene controlling the synthesis of CHE can exist in many allelic forms. Four of the most common forms are designated as E^u, E^a, E^f, and E^s. These four allelic genes can be combined to form one normal and nine abnormal genotypes. At least 40 other forms exist and another gene locus is recognized (E_2). The normal, most common phenotype is designated as E^uE^u, or UU (u for *usual*). The gene E^a is referred to as the *atypical* gene; the sera of people homozygous for this gene (E^aE^a = AA) are only weakly active toward most substrates for CHE and demonstrate increased resistance to inhibition of enzyme activity by dibucaine. The E^f gene (f for *fluoride resistant*) gives rise to a weakly active enzyme but with increased resistance to fluoride inhibition. The E^s gene (s for *silent*) is associated with the absence of enzyme or the presence of a protein with minimal or no catalytic activity. Mutations that give rise to the atypical and fluoride-resistant CHE variants involve a change in the structure of the active center. The variant enzymes (allelozymes) are less effective catalysts than the usual form; the affinity of the enzymes for the substrates is reduced (i.e., K_m is increased), and affinity for competitive inhibitors, such as dibucaine or fluoride, is similarly decreased. This gives rise to the characteristic dibucaine- or fluoride-resistant properties of the genetic variants that are exploited in their characterization.

Homozygous forms, AA and FF, are found in 0.3 to 0.5% of the white population; their incidence among blacks is even lower. Inheritance of increased CHE activity has been reported in a few families. This is apparently due to increased production of the usual allelozyme.

Clinical Significance[40]

Measurements of CHE activity in serum are used (1) as a test of liver function, (2) as an indicator of possible insecticide poisoning, and (3) for the detection of patients with atypical forms of the enzyme who are at risk for prolonged responses to certain muscle relaxants used in surgical procedures.

Measurement of serum CHE activity can serve as a sensitive indicator of the synthetic capacity of the liver. In the absence of genetic causes or known inhibitors, any decrease in CHE activity reflects impaired synthesis of the enzyme by the liver. Serial measurement of CHE has been promoted as an indication of prognosis in patients with liver disease and for monitoring liver function after liver transplantation.

Among the organic phosphorous compounds that inhibit cholinesterase activity are many insecticides, such as parathion, sarin, and tetraethyl pyrophosphate. Workers in agriculture and in organic chemical industries may be subject to poisoning by inhalation of these materials or by direct contact with them. Obviously, if enough material is absorbed to inactivate all the acetylcholinesterase of nervous tissue, death will result. Both cholinesterases are inhibited, but the activity of the serum enzyme falls more rapidly than does that of the erythrocyte enzyme. A 40% drop in CHE activity occurs before the first symptoms are felt, and a drop of 80% is required before neuromuscular effects become apparent. Near-zero concentrations of enzyme activity require emergency treatment with enzyme reactivators such as pyridine-2-aldoxime. Upon retesting, in 3 to 5 days, CHE activity should increase by 15 to 20% if a significant organophosphate-induced inhibition has occurred previously.

Succinyldicholine (suxamethonium) and mivacurium, drugs used in surgery as muscle relaxants, are hydrolyzed by CHE, and their pharmacologic effect normally persists only long enough to meet the needs of the surgical procedure. In patients with low enzyme activities or in those with a weakly active variant, destruction of the drug will not occur rapidly enough, and the patient may enter a period of prolonged paralysis of the respiratory muscles (apnea) requiring mechanical ventilation until the drug effects gradually wear off. Preoperative screening of CHE activity has been advocated to identify patients in whom suxamethonium administration may lead to complications. The degree of drug sensitivity varies with the phenotype of the patient. Total CHE activity is highest in individuals who are homozygous for the usual allele and progressively lower in those who are heterozygous for the usual and a variant allele, those who are homozygous or heterozygous for variant alleles, and those in whom two "silent" alleles are paired and no activity is detected. Subjects who possess one normal allele (i.e., who are heterozygous for the normal and a variant allele) usually produce enough enzyme to protect themselves against suxamethonium sensitivity, whereas patients with paired variant alleles (as homozygotes or heterozygotes) show various degrees of sensitivity. The phenotypes most susceptible to apnea after succinylcholine administration include AA, AS, FF, FS, SS, AF, and to some extent UA. Measurements of total CHE activity and determination of the "dibucaine number" and "fluoride number" are needed to fully characterize CHE variants. The latter values indicate the percentage inhibition of enzyme activity toward specified substrates in the presence of standard concentrations of dibucaine or fluoride. Mutation genotyping may confirm CHE gene abnormalities.

Methods for Determination of Serum Cholinesterase Activity

Many of the contemporary methods use acylthiocholine esters as substrates. The iodide salts of acetylthiocholine, propionylthiocholine, butyrylthiocholine, benzoylthiocholine, and succinylthiocholine all have been used. These substrates are hydrolyzed at approximately the same rate as choline esters, and the thiocholine formed can be measured by reaction with chromogenic disulfide agents, such as 5,5′-dithio-bis(2-nitrobenzoate) (DTNB) (Ellman's reagent). The reaction of the thiocholine product with colorless DTNB forms colored 5-mercapto-2-nitro-benzoic acid, which is measured spectrophotometrically at 410 nm. The clinical question being asked may influence the choice of substrate suitable for measuring the enzyme. Measuring CHE activity using succinyldithiocholine is the method of choice to diagnose succinylcholine sensitivity, purely based on the enzyme activity recorded in serum. This method is, however, well suited for other clinical applications of the test.[44]

Kalow and Genest, using benzoylcholine as a classic substrate, demonstrated the qualitative difference in CHEs. Based on differences such as sensitivity to inhibition by the local anesthetic dibucaine, they developed a simple test to classify the type of CHE as usual, intermediate, or atypical. With 10^{-5} mol/L dibucaine ("dibucaine number"), the usual CHE is inhibited by 80%, but atypical CHE is inhibited by only 20%. Subjects heterozygous for the normal and atypical gene show about 60% inhibition of CHE. To differentiate other genotypes, sodium fluoride can be used as a CHE inhibitor. Molecular biological methods that can be used to identify various CHE genetic defects have been developed and are being used increasingly in clinical laboratories.

Serum is the sample of choice. Enzyme activity in serum is stable for several weeks if the specimen is stored under refrigeration, and for several years if stored at −20 °C. Moderate hemolysis does not interfere if separated serum has been centrifuged to remove red blood cell ghosts.

Reference Intervals

Using the succinyldithiocholine/DTNB method at 37 °C, the reference interval for healthy adults with the usual CHE genotype was estimated to be 33 to 76 U/L for women and 40 to 78 U/L for men, respectively. The median activity in individuals with heterozygous genotype was 22 U/L (range, 5 to 35 U/L), and for atypical homozygotes 1.5 U/L (range, 1 to 4 U/L).[62] A value <23 U/L was approximately five times as likely to occur in a succinyldicholine-sensitive individual as in a normal one.[44] At birth, CHE activity is lower than adult values by about 50%. It increases during the next 3 to 6 years to exceed adult values by about 30%. From the fifth year of life, the activity starts to decrease before it stabilizes at the adult value, which is reached at puberty. The significant CHE decrease (30%) during pregnancy and early puerperium is explained by hemodilution.

CHE phenotyping, based on determination of dibucaine (DN) and fluoride (FN) numbers, has been established:

Phenotype	DN Range	FN Range
UU	≥77	≥55
UF	72-76	≥53
UA	48-72	≥44
AF	45-59	<44
FF	64-69	<44
AA	<35	*

*Redundant for AA phenotype attribution.

ENZYMES AS CARDIOVASCULAR RISK MARKERS

Several cells typical for atherosclerotic plaque secrete enzyme molecules that mirror plaque destabilization and rupture. Their concentrations in the circulation have been shown to be associated with future cardiovascular (CV) events.

Lipoprotein-Associated Phospholipase A_2

Lipoprotein-associated phospholipase A_2 [EC 3.1.1.47; platelet-activating factor (PAF) acetylhydrolase; Lp-PLA_2], a 45,400 Da monomeric protein, is a Ca^{2+}-independent member of the phospholipase A_2 superfamily. It is produced mainly by monocytes, macrophages, T lymphocytes, and mast cells and has been found to be upregulated in atherosclerotic lesions, especially in complex plaque prone to rupture. Lp-PLA_2 has proatherogenic properties by promoting modification of oxidized LDLs. In particular, the enzyme cleaves oxidized phosphatidylcholine components of the lipoprotein particle, generating two potent proinflammatory and proatherogenic mediators, namely, lysophosphatidylcholine (lysoPC) and oxidized free fatty acids. LysoPC serves as a potent chemoattractant for T cells and monocytes, promotes endothelial dysfunction, and stimulates macrophage proliferation, thus enhancing lesion progression.[96]

Clinical Significance

Several prospective epidemiologic studies have reported an association between increased plasma concentrations of Lp-PLA_2 and future coronary and cerebrovascular events.[1] The strength of association varies and is generally modest (hazard ratios <2). However, because some controversy persists as to its independence from LDL cholesterol, no clear recommendation on Lp-PLA_2 clinical usefulness can be given until definitive data document its incremental value above and beyond traditional CV risk factors. Furthermore, no data show that Lp-PLA_2 reduction improves clinical outcomes. Unlike other emerging CV risk markers, Lp-PLA_2 is not an acute-phase reactant and, thus, is unaffected by systemic inflammatory processes.

Methods for Determination of Lipoprotein-Associated Phospholipase A_2

Risk estimates were similar, whether the mass concentration or the activity of the enzyme was measured. A manual ELISA method for Lp-PLA_2 mass concentration has received U.S. Food and Drug Administration (FDA) clearance for use as an aid in CV risk prediction. An immunoturbidimetric method that uses the same monoclonal antibodies has become commercially available, allowing the assay to be run on automated chemistry analyzers. A panel of national experts has recommended that an Lp-PLA_2 concentration >200 μg/L be used as the threshold for higher risk of CV events.

EDTA plasma is the recommended sample for measuring Lp-PLA_2. Average stabilities are up to 4 hours at ambient temperature, 12 hours at 4 °C, and 6 months at −20 °C.

Myeloperoxidase

Myeloperoxidase (EC 1.11.1.7; donor, hydrogen peroxide oxidoreductase; MPO), a member of the heme peroxidase superfamily, is a tetrameric hemoprotein (MW 144,000 Da) consisting of a pair of heavy (57 kDa) and light (15 kDa) chains. It is stored in azurophilic granules of polymorphonuclear neutrophils and monocytes-macrophages and, when released (typically with inflammation), catalyzes the conversion of chloride anion and hydrogen peroxide to hypochlorite (HOCl), a metal ion–independent chlorinating oxidant that possesses potent microbicidal activity, thus having a role in host defense against pathogens.

Paradoxically, MPO may have a causative role in plaque destabilization through its ability to activate latent metalloproteinases (MMPs). Infiltrating macrophages and neutrophils participate in the transformation of stable coronary artery plaques to unstable lesions with a thin fibrous cap through secretion of MMPs and MPO, which degrade the collagen layer that protects atheromas from erosion or abrupt rupture. As a result, plaques that have been highly infiltrated with macrophages have a thin fibrous cap and are vulnerable to erosion or rupture, converting late-stage atherosclerosis into acute CV events. MPO could also be involved in the development of endothelial dysfunction because MPO uses the atheroprotective endothelial nitric oxide as a substrate, thus reducing its bioavailability. Finally, MPO-dependent halides, tyrosyl radicals, and reactive nitrogen species may generate proatherogenic oxidized LDLs, thereby promoting subsequent foam cell formation. This combination of detrimental effects has culminated in the concept that MPO may be an active mediator in atherosclerotic CV disease.[51]

MPO is released into the extracellular fluid and general circulation during inflammatory conditions.

Clinical Significance

Several epidemiologic studies indicate that MPO concentrations in plasma may be an important CV risk marker, especially in patients with unstable coronary artery disease. However, uncertainty remains about the additional benefits conferred by MPO beyond those of standard cardiac biomarkers such as troponin.[73]

Increased MPO is not likely to be specific to cardiac disease, as activation of neutrophils and macrophages can occur in any infectious, inflammatory, or infiltrative disease process.

Methods for Determination of Myeloperoxidase

MPO activity has been measured in blood and tissues by assays using hydrogen peroxide and *o*-dianisidine dihydrochloride as substrates. Mass assays based on sandwich ELISA methods have been developed and made commercially available. One of these assays has been approved by the FDA for use in conjunction with clinical history, electrocardiography, and other cardiac biomarkers to evaluate patients presenting with chest pain at risk of major adverse cardiac events. This assay has been licensed to three other companies and has been made suitable for automated platforms or point-of-care instruments.

MPO is reasonably stable, and EDTA is the preferred anticoagulant.[82] MPO is continuously released from white blood cells in heparinized blood with a spurious increase in MPO concentrations when blood collection tubes are left standing at room temperature. Higher MPO concentrations can also be found in serum owing to leakage of enzyme from leukocytes during coagulation. Samples from individuals positive for anti-MPO antineutrophil cytoplasmic autoantibodies (ANCAs) can show spuriously decreased MPO concentrations.

Reference Intervals

An MPO concentration of 640 pmol/L was reported as the upper reference limit, which is not influenced by gender or age. It should be noted that different assays using different MPO antigens for calibration may generate different results.

Pregnancy-Associated Plasma Protein A

Pregnancy-associated plasma protein A (EC 3.4.24.79; pappalysin-1; PAPP-A) is a high molecular mass (≈200,000 Da) zinc-binding glycoprotein mainly synthesized by the placental syncytiotrophoblast and typically measured during pregnancy for screening of Down syndrome. It was reported to be an insulin-like growth factor (IGF)-dependent IGF-binding protein (IGFBP)-4– and IGFBP-5–specific metalloproteinase produced by different activated cells in unstable plaques and released into the extracellular matrix, thus potentially a proatherosclerotic molecule, through its role in disrupting the integrity of the protective fibrous cap of the atheroma.

In pregnancy, PAPP-A circulates in a heterotetrameric complex consisting of two PAPP-A subunits covalently bound with two subunits of the proform of eosinophil major basic protein (proMBP), its endogenous inhibitor. However, PAPP-A present in human fibroblasts and released during atherosclerotic plaque disruption seems to be in a homodimeric active form, uncomplexed with the inhibitor proMBP (free PAPP-A). This makes it difficult to measure PAPP-A as a CV risk marker with immunoassays that have been designed to detect molecules in pregnancy serum using a sandwich formed by two antibodies: one specific for PAPP-A and one specific for proMBP.[2]

Clinical Significance

Increased PAPP-A concentrations in serum may represent a marker for adverse CV events in both acute coronary syndrome (ACS) and chronic stable angina patients. Unfortunately, the use of assays using different combinations of antibodies by different researchers has led to some controversy regarding the importance of this potential marker of plaque instability. Furthermore, no studies have demonstrated a clear improvement in discrimination or reclassification ability with the use of PAPP-A measurements.[11] In a study evaluating total PAPP-A (free and complex bound) in noncardiac conditions, the marker was increased in one fifth of patients admitted to the hospital with diagnoses other than ACS.[32]

Methods for Determination of Pregnancy-Associated Plasma Protein A

Although it has been suggested that the most appropriate method for analysis would be based on specific detection of the free PAPP-A molecule, most clinical studies evaluating

PAPP-A as a CV risk marker were performed using assays mostly measuring PAPP-A/proMBP complexes. Direct methods are not currently available, as they require antibodies that react exclusively with free PAPP-A. An alternative approach has been to perform two assays in conjunction: one that specifically detects total PAPP-A (free and complexed), and another that specifically detects the PAPP-A-proMBP complex, with the difference representing free PAPP-A. Another approach may be to analyze the enzymatic activity of PAPP-A, which is thought to represent activity of the free molecule only.

Only serum should be used as a sample for measuring PAPP-A, because heparin and other anticoagulants (e.g., EDTA) affect the apparent concentration of PAPP-A in body fluids.[2]

Reference Intervals

Using the previously described two-assay approach, median activities (interquartile range) of free PAPP-A were 0.18 mIU/L (0.63) in serum samples from apparently healthy individuals. Enzyme activities did not correlate with age but were significantly higher in men than in women.[95] However, use of this indirect approach cannot accurately measure the very low activities of the marker found in cardio-healthy people.

REFERENCES

1. Anderson JL. Lipoprotein-associated phospholipase A_2: an independent predictor of coronary artery disease events in primary and secondary prevention. Am J Cardiol 2008;101(Suppl):23F-33F.
2. Apple FS, Wu AHB, Mair J, Ravkilde J, Panteghini M, Tate J, et al. Future biomarkers for detection of ischemia and risk stratification in acute coronary syndrome. Clin Chem 2005;51:810-24.
3. Bais R, Edwards JB. Creatine kinase. CRC Crit Rev Clin Lab Sci 1982;16:291-355.
4. Bais R, Philcox M. Approved recommendation on IFCC methods for the measurement of catalytic concentration of enzymes. Part 8. IFCC method for lactate dehydrogenase (L-lactate: NAD+oxidoreductase, EC 1.1.1.27). International Federation of Clinical Chemistry (IFCC). Eur J Clin Chem Clin Biochem 1994;32:639-55.
5. Beetham R. Biochemical investigation of suspected rhabdomyolysis. Ann Clin Biochem 2000;37:581-7.
6. Bertrand A, Buret J. A one-step determination of serum 5′-nucleotidase using a centrifugal analyzer. Clin Chim Acta 1982;119:275-84.
7. Brancaccio P, Maffulli N, Limongelli FM. Creatine kinase monitoring in sport medicine. Br Med Bull 2007;81-82:209-30.
8. Brodrick JW, Geokas MC, Largman C, Fassett M, Johnson JH. Molecular forms of immunoreactive pancreatic cationic trypsin in pancreatitis patient sera. Am J Physiol 1979;237:E474-80.
9. Broyles DL, Nielsen RG, Bussett EM, Lu WD, Mizrahi IA, Nunnelly PA, et al. Analytical and clinical performance characteristics of Tandem-MP Ostase, a new immunoassay for serum bone alkaline phosphatase. Clin Chem 1998;44:2139-47.
10. Cabrera-Abreu JC, Green A. γ-Glutamyltransferase: value of its measurement in pediatrics. Ann Clin Biochem 2002;39:22-5.
11. Consuegra-Sanchez L, Fredericks S, Kaski JC. Pregnancy-associated plasma protein-A (PAPP-A) and cardiovascular risk. Atherosclerosis 2009;203:346-52.
12. Davidson DF, Watson DJM. Macroenzyme detection by polyethylene glycol precipitation. Ann Clin Biochem 2003;40:514-20.
13. Deutsche Gesellschaft für Klinische Chemie. Proposal of standard methods for the determination of enzyme catalytic concentrations in serum and plasma at 37 °C. III. Glutamate dehydrogenase [L-glutamate: NAD(P)+ oxidoreductase (deaminating), EC 1.4.1.3]. Eur J Clin Chem Clin Biochem 1992;30:493-502.
14. Dolci A, Panteghini M. The exciting story of cardiac biomarkers: from retrospective detection to gold diagnostic standard for acute myocardial infarction and more. Clin Chim Acta 2006;369:179-87.
15. Dufour DR, Lott JA, Nolte FS, Gretch DR, Koff RS, Seeff LB. Diagnosis and monitoring of hepatic injury. II. Recommendations for use of laboratory tests in screening, diagnosis, and monitoring. Clin Chem 2000;46:2050-68.
16. Emdin M, Pompella A, Paolicchi A. Gamma-glutamyltransferase, atherosclerosis, and cardiovascular disease: triggering oxidative stress within the plaque. Circulation 2005;112:2078-80.
17. Fahie-Wilson MN, Burrows S, Lawson GJ, Gordon T, Wong W, Dasgupta B. Prevalence of increased serum creatine kinase activity due to macro-creatine kinase and experience of screening programmes in district general hospitals. Ann Clin Biochem 2007;44:377-83.
18. Foo AY. Amylase measurement—which method? Ann Clin Biochem 1995;32:239-43.
19. Forsmark CE, Baillie J. AGA Institute technical review on acute pancreatitis. Gastroenterology 2007;132:2022-44.
20. Frossard JL. Trypsin activation peptide (TAP) in acute pancreatitis: from pathophysiology to clinical usefulness. JOP J Pancreas (Online) 2001;2:69-77.
21. Goldberg DM. Structural, functional, and clinical aspects of gamma-glutamyltransferase. CRC Crit Rev Clin Lab Sci 1980;12:1-58.
22. Hawkins RC. Assessment of the utility of aldolase determination in serum by monitoring patient outcomes. Biochim Clin 2001;25:331-5.
23. Hayes PC, Bouchier IAD, Beckett GJ. Glutathione S-transferase in humans in health and disease. Gut 1991;32:813-8.
24. Hedström J, Sainio V, Kemppainen E, Haapiainen R, Kivilaakso E, Schröder T, et al. Serum complex of trypsin 2 and α_1 antitrypsin as diagnostic and prognostic marker of acute pancreatitis: clinical study in consecutive patients. Br Med J 1996;313:333-7.
25. Heiduk M, Päge I, Kliem C, Abicht K, Klein G. Pediatric reference intervals determined in ambulatory and hospitalized children and juveniles. Clin Chim Acta 2009;406:156-61.
26. Henriksen K, Tanko LB, Qvist P, Delmas PD, Christiansen C, Karsdal MA. Assessment of osteoclast number and function: application in the development of new and improved treatment modalities for bone diseases. Osteoporosis Int 2007;18:681-5.
27. Hood D, Van Lente F, Estes M. Serum enzyme alterations in chronic muscle disease: a biopsy-based diagnostic assessment. Am J Clin Pathol 1991;95:402-7.
28. Huijgen HJ, Sanders GT, Koster RW, Vreeken J, Bossuyt PM. The clinical value of lactate dehydrogenase in serum: a quantitative review. Eur J Clin Chem Clin Biochem 1997;35:569-75.
29. Ceriotti F, Henny J, Queraltó J, Ziyu S, Özarda Y, Chen B, et al. Common reference intervals for aspartate aminotransferase (AST), alanine aminotransferase (ALT) and γ-glutamyl transferase (GGT) in serum: results from an IFCC multicenter study. Clin Chem Lab Med 2010;48:1593-601.
30. Infusino I, Bonora R, Panteghini M. Traceability in clinical enzymology. Clin Biochem Rev 2007;28:155-61.
31. Itkonen O, Koivunen E, Hurme M, Alfthan H, Schröder T, Stenman U-H. Time-resolved immunofluorometric assays for trypsinogen-1 and -2 in serum reveal preferential elevation of trypsinogen-2 in pancreatitis. J Lab Clin Med 1990;115:712-8.
32. Iversen KK, Teisner AS, Teisner B, Kliem A, Bay M, Kirk V, et al. Pregnancy-associated plasma protein A in non-cardiac conditions. Clin Biochem 2008;41:548-53.
33. Junge W, Wortmann W, Wilke B, Waldenström J, Kurrle-Weittenhiller A, Finke J, et al. Development and evaluation of assays for the determination of total and pancreatic amylase at 37 °C according to the principle recommended by the IFCC. Clin Biochem 2001;34:607-15.
34. Kim WR, Flamm SL, Di Bisceglie AM, Bodenheimer HC. Serum activity of alanine aminotransferase (ALT) as an indicator of health and disease. Hepatology 2008;47:1363-70.

35. Kristensen SR. Mechanisms of cell damage and enzyme release. Dan Med Bull 1994;41:423-33.
36. Kristensen SR, Horder M. Principles of diagnostic enzymology. In: Moss DW, Rosalki SB, eds. Enzyme tests in diagnosis. London: Edward Arnold, 1996:7-24.
37. Kruse-Jarres JD, Kaiser C, Hafkenscheid JCM, Hohenwallner W, Stein W, Bohner J, et al. Evaluation of a new alpha-amylase assay using 4,6-ethylidene-(G_7)-1-4-nitrophenyl-(G_1)-alpha-D-maltoheptaoside as substrate. J Clin Chem Clin Biochem 1989;27:103-13.
38. Lessinger JM, Ferard G. Plasma pancreatic lipase activity: from analytical specificity to clinical efficiency for the diagnosis of acute pancreatitis. Eur J Clin Chem Clin Biochem 1994;32:377-81.
39. Mair J. Tissue release of cardiac markers: from physiology to clinical applications. Clin Chem Lab Med 1999;37:1077-84.
40. McQueen MJ. Clinical and analytical considerations in the utilization of cholinesterase measurements. Clin Chim Acta 1995;237:91-105.
41. Moller-Petersen J. Clinical evaluation of cathodic trypsin-like immunoreactivity in pancreatic diseases in adults. Scand J Clin Lab Invest 1990;50:463-77.
42. Moller-Petersen J, Pedersen JO, Thorsgaard-Pedersen N, Nyboe Andersen B. Serum cathodic trypsin-like immunoreactivity, pancreatic lipase, and pancreatic isoamylase as diagnostic tests of chronic pancreatitis or pancreatic steatorrhea. Scand J Gastroenterol 1988;23:287-96.
43. Morandi L, Angelini C, Prelle A, Pini A, Grassi B, Bernardi G, et al. High plasma creatine kinase: review of the literature and proposal for a diagnostic algorithm. Neurol Sci 2006;27:303-11.
44. Mosca A, Bonora R, Ceriotti F, Franzini C, Lando G, Patrosso MC, et al. Assay using succinyldithiocholine as substrate: the method of choice for the measurement of cholinesterase catalytic activity in serum to diagnose succinylcholine sensitivity. Clin Chem Lab Med 2003;41:317-22.
45. Moss DW. Alkaline phosphatase isoenzymes. Clin Chem 1982;28:2007-16.
46. Moss DW. Changes in enzyme expression related to differentiation and regulatory factors: the acid phosphatase of osteoclasts and other macrophages. Clin Chim Acta 1992;209:131-8.
47. Moss DW. Perspectives in alkaline phosphatase research. Clin Chem 1992;38:2486-92.
48. Moss DW. Physicochemical and pathophysiological factors in the release of membrane-bound alkaline phosphatase from cells. Clin Chim Acta 1997;257:133-40.
49. Moss DW, Edwards RK. Improved electrophoretic resolution of bone and liver alkaline phosphatases resulting from partial digestion with neuraminidase. Clin Chim Acta 1984;143:177-82.
50. Moss DW, Raymond FD, Wile DB. Clinical and biological aspects of acid phosphatase. CRC Crit Rev Clin Lab Sci 1995;32:431-67.
51. Nicholls SJ, Hazen SL. Myeloperoxidase and cardiovascular disease. Arterioscler Thromb Vasc Biol 2005;25:1102-11.
52. Noe DA. Tissue injury. In: Noe DA, ed. The logic of laboratory medicine, 2nd edition. Baltimore: Urban & Schwarzenberg, 2001.
53. Pagani F, Bonora R, Panteghini M. Reference interval for lactate dehydrogenase catalytic activity in serum measured according to the new IFCC recommendation. Clin Chem Lab Med 2003;41: 970-1.
54. Pagani F, Panteghini M. 5′-Nucleotidase in the detection of increased activity of the liver form of alkaline phosphatase in serum. Clin Chem 2001;47:2046-8.
55. Paju A, Stenman UH. Biochemistry and clinical role of trypsinogens and pancreatic secretory trypsin inhibitor. Crit Rev Clin Lab Sci 2006;43:103-42.
56. Panteghini M. Aspartate aminotransferase isoenzymes. Clin Biochem 1990;23:311-9.
57. Panteghini M. Benign inherited hyperphosphatasemia of intestinal origin: report of two cases and a brief review of the literature. Clin Chem 1991;37:1449-52.
58. Panteghini M. Diagnostic application of CK-MB mass determination. Clin Chim Acta 1998;272:23-31.
59. Panteghini M. Electrophoretic fractionation of pancreatic lipase. Clin Chem 1992;38:1712-6.
60. Panteghini M. Hepatic alkaline phosphatase isoenzyme. I. Biochemical and pathophysiological aspects. Giorn It Chim Clin 1990;15:163-71.
61. Panteghini M. Serum isoforms of creatine kinase isoenzymes. Clin Biochem 1988;21:211-8.
62. Panteghini M, Bonora R, Pagani F. An alternative approach to the prevention of succinyldicholine-induced apnoea. J Clin Chem Clin Biochem 1988;26:85-90.
63. Panteghini M, Bonora R, Pagani F. Automated measurement of mitochondrial aspartate aminotransferase by selective proteolysis with proteinase K. Clin Chem 1993;39:2199-200.
64. Panteghini M, Bonora R, Pagani F. Measurement of pancreatic lipase activity in serum by a kinetic colorimetric assay using a new chromogenic substrate. Ann Clin Biochem 2001;38:365-70.
65. Panteghini M, Ceriotti F, Pagani F, Secchiero S, Zaninotto M, Franzini C; for the Italian Society of Clinical Biochemistry and Clinical Molecular Biology (SIBioC) Working Group on Enzymes. Recommendations for the routine use of pancreatic amylase measurement instead of total amylase for the diagnosis and monitoring of pancreatic pathology. Clin Chem Lab Med 2002;40:97-100.
66. Panteghini M, Pagani F. Reference intervals for two bone-derived enzyme activities in serum: bone isoenzyme of alkaline phosphatase (ALP) and tartrate-resistant acid phosphatase (TR-ACP). Clin Chem 1989;35:181-1.
67. Pratt DS, Kaplan MM. Evaluation of abnormal liver-enzyme results in asymptomatic patients. N Engl J Med 2000;342:1266-71.
68. Price CP. Multiple forms of human serum alkaline phosphatase: detection and quantitation. Ann Clin Biochem 1993;30:355-72.
69. Rauscher E, Gerber M. Pancreatic alpha-amylase assay employing the synergism of two monoclonal antibodies. Clin Chim Acta 1989;183:41-4.
70. Rauscher E, Neumann U, Schaich E, von Bulow S, Wahlefeld AW. Optimized conditions for determining activity concentration of alpha-amylase in serum, with 1,4-alpha-D-4-nitrophenylmaltoheptaoside as substrate. Clin Chem 1985;31:14-9.
71. Rees GW, Trull AK, Doyle S. Evaluation of an enzyme-immunometric assay for serum alpha-glutathione S-transferase. Ann Clin Biochem 1995;32:575-83.
72. Rosalki SB, Foo AY. Two new methods for separating and quantifying bone and liver alkaline phosphatase isoenzymes in plasma. Clin Chem 1984;30:1182-6.
73. Schindhelm RK, van der Zwan LP, Teerlink T, Scheffer PG. Myeloperoxidase: a useful biomarker for cardiovascular disease risk stratification? Clin Chem 2009;55:1462-70.
74. Schmidt ES, Schmidt FW. Glutamate dehydrogenase: biochemical and clinical aspects of an interesting enzyme. Clin Chim Acta 1988;43:43-56.
75. Schumann G, Aoki R, Ferrero CA, Ehlers G, Férard G, Gella FJ, et al. IFCC primary reference procedures for the measurement of catalytic activity concentrations of enzymes at 37 °C. Part 8. Reference procedure for the measurement of catalytic concentration of α-amylase. Clin Chem Lab Med 2006;44:1146-55.
76. Schumann G, Bonora R, Ceriotti F, Clerc-Renaud P, Ferrero CA, Férard G, et al. IFCC primary reference procedures for the measurement of catalytic activity concentrations of enzymes at 37 °C. Part 2. Reference procedure for the measurement of catalytic concentration of creatine kinase. Clin Chem Lab Med 2002;40:635-42.
77. Schumann G, Bonora R, Ceriotti F, Clerc-Renaud P, Ferrero CA, Férard G, et al. IFCC primary reference procedures for the measurement of catalytic activity concentrations of enzymes at 37 °C. Part 3. Reference procedure for the measurement of catalytic concentration of lactate dehydrogenase. Clin Chem Lab Med 2002;40:643-8.
78. Schumann G, Bonora R, Ceriotti F, Clerc-Renaud P, Férard G, Ferrero CA, et al. IFCC primary reference procedures for the measurement of catalytic activity concentrations of enzymes at 37 °C. Part 6. Reference procedure for the measurement of catalytic concentration of γ-glutamyltransferase. Clin Chem Lab Med 2002;40:734-8.

79. Schumann G, Bonora R, Ceriotti F, Férard G, Ferrero CA, Franck PFH, et al. IFCC primary reference procedures for the measurement of catalytic activity concentrations of enzymes at 37 °C. Part 4. Reference procedure for the measurement of catalytic concentration of alanine aminotransferase. Clin Chem Lab Med 2002;40:718-24.
80. Schumann G, Bonora R, Ceriotti F, Férard G, Ferrero CA, Franck PFH, et al. IFCC primary reference procedures for the measurement of catalytic activity concentrations of enzymes at 37 °C. Part 5. Reference procedure for the measurement of catalytic concentration of aspartate aminotransferase. Clin Chem Lab Med 2002;40:725-33.
81. Schumann G, Klauke R. New IFCC reference procedures for the determination of catalytic activity concentrations of five enzymes in serum: preliminary upper reference limits obtained in hospitalized subjects. Clin Chim Acta 2003;327:69-79.
82. Shih J, Datwyler SA, Hsu SC, Matias MS, Pacenti DP, Lueders C, et al. Effect of collection tube type and preanalytical handling on myeloperoxidase concentrations. Clin Chem 2008;54:1076-9.
83. Stein P, Rosalki SB, Foo AY, Hjelm M. Transient hyperphosphatasemia of infancy and early childhood: clinical and biochemical features of 21 cases and literature review. Clin Chem 1987;33:313-8.
84. Sunderman FW. The clinical biochemistry of 5′-nucleotidase. Ann Clin Lab Sci 1990;20:123-39.
85. Szasz G, Gerhardt W, Gruber W. Creatine kinase in serum. 3. Further study of adenylate kinase inhibitors. Clin Chem 1977;23:1888-92.
86. Thompson PD, Clarkson P, Karas RH. Statin-associated myopathy. JAMA 2003;289:1681-90.
87. Tietz NW. Support of the diagnosis of pancreatitis by enzyme tests—old problems, new techniques. Clin Chim Acta 1997;257:85-98.
88. Tietz NW, Rinker AD, Shaw LM. IFCC methods for the measurement of catalytic concentration of enzymes. Part 5. IFCC method for alkaline phosphatase (orthophosphoric-monoester phosphohydrolase, alkaline optimum, EC 3.1.3.1). J Clin Chem Clin Biochem 1983;21:731-48.
89. Tietz NW, Shuey DF. Lipase in serum—the elusive enzyme: an overview. Clin Chem 1993;38:1000-10.
90. Tietz NW, Shuey DF. Reference intervals for alkaline phosphatase activity determined by the IFCC and AACC reference methods. Clin Chem 1986;32:1593-4.
91. Visnapuu LA, Karlson LK, Dubinsky EH, Szer IS, Hirsch CA. Pediatric reference ranges for serum aldolase. Am J Clin Pathol 1989;91:476-7.
92. Von Eyben FE. A systematic review of lactate dehydrogenase isoenzyme 1 and germ cell tumors. Clin Biochem 2001;34:441-54.
93. Whitfield JB. Gamma glutamyl transferase. CRC Crit Rev Clin Lab Sci 2001;38:263-355.
94. Whitten RO, Chandler WL, Thomas MGE, Clayson KJ, Fine JS. Survey of alpha-amylase activity and isoamylases in autopsy tissue. Clin Chem 1988;34:1552-5.
95. Wittfooth S, Qin QP, Lund J, Tierala I, Pulkki K, Takalo H, Pettersson K. Immunofluorimetric point-of-care assays for the detection of acute coronary syndrome-related noncomplexed pregnancy-associated plasma protein A. Clin Chem 2006;52:1794-1801.
96. Zalewski A, Macphee C. Role of lipoprotein-associated phospholipase A_2 in atherosclerosis: biology, epidemiology, and possible therapeutic target. Arterioscler Thromb Vasc Biol 2005;25:923-31.

CHAPTER 23

Enzymes of the Red Blood Cell

Wouter W. van Solinge, Ph.D., and Richard van Wijk, Ph.D.

Erythrocytes perform a variety of functions, the most important being the binding, transport, and delivery of oxygen to all tissues. To do so, they must be capable of passage through microcapillaries—a feat that is achieved by modifications of the erythrocyte's biconcave shape. This shape change is possible because, unlike most other cells in the body, the human erythrocyte loses its nucleus and organelles before entering the circulation from the marrow. In addition, remaining RNA in the reticulocyte is lost within the first 2 days in circulation, thereby making further protein synthesis no longer possible.

Normal human red cells survive in the circulation for approximately 120 days, using energy to maintain the electrolyte gradient between plasma and red cell cytoplasm and to keep hemoglobin and the sulfhydryl groups of red cell enzymes and membrane proteins in the reduced state. Because of the absence of a nucleus and mitochondria, the red cell is incapable of generating energy via the (oxidative) Krebs cycle and depends mainly on the anaerobic conversion of glucose by the Embden-Meyerhof pathway (EMP, or direct glycolytic pathway) and the oxidative hexose monophosphate pathway (HMP, or pentose phosphate shunt) (Figure 23-1). Numerous red cell enzymes are involved in these pathways, thereby providing the cell with the necessary high-energy phosphates (primarily ATP) and reducing power (NADH, NADPH).

Deficiencies of any of these red cell enzymes may result in impaired ATP generation or the inability to withstand oxidative stress and, consequently, loss of function of the erythrocyte. By far, a majority of these disorders are hereditary in nature, although acquired deficiencies have been described, mainly in malignant disorders involving the bone marrow.[37] Hereditary enzymatic defects in these pathways are able to (1) disturb the erythrocyte's integrity, (2) shorten its survival, and (3) produce hereditary nonspherocytic hemolytic anemia (HNSHA). In general, deficiencies of enzymes involved in ATP generation lead to chronic hemolytic anemia. Other enzyme deficiencies cause acute episodes of severe hemolysis [e.g., when oxidative stress on the red cell is increased (as in some types of glucose-6-phosphate dehydrogenase deficiency)]. Red cell morphology is, in general, unremarkable, except for the case of pyrimidine-5′-nucleotidase deficiency, which is characterized by prominent stippling (see later).

Many of these enzymes are expressed in other tissues as well but cause notable symptoms predominantly in red blood cells because of the long life span of the erythrocyte after loss of protein synthesis. Once an enzyme is degraded or otherwise becomes nonfunctional, it cannot be replaced by new or other "compensating" proteins because of the lack of a nucleus, mitochondria, ribosomes, and other cell organelles in mature red cells.

Disorders have been described in EMP, HMP, the Rapoport-Luebering cycle, the glutathione pathway (Figure 23-2), purine-pyrimidine metabolism, and methemoglobin reduction. This section describes the clinically important red cell enzymes involved in these metabolic pathways and the disorders associated with defects in these pathways. In addition, diagnostic strategies and pitfalls of laboratory diagnostics for these enzyme deficiencies are explained. The laboratory methods described have been used for decades and are well documented. During the past few years, however, molecular diagnostics have proven to be an indispensable tool in the diagnosis of hereditary red cell enzyme deficiencies.

THE EMBDEN-MEYERHOF PATHWAY

Glucose is the energy source of the red cell. In the normal situation (without increased "oxidative stress"), 90% of glucose is catabolized anaerobically to pyruvate or lactate by the direct glycolytic pathway, or EMP. Although one mole of ATP is used by hexokinase and an additional mole of ATP by phosphofructokinase, the net gain is 2 moles of ATP per mole of glucose, because a total of 4 moles of ATP is formed per mole of glucose by phosphoglycerate kinase and pyruvate kinase. In addition, reducing energy is generated in the form of reduced nicotinamide-adenine dinucleotide in the step catalyzed by glyceraldehyde phosphate dehydrogenase. This reducing energy can be used to reduce methemoglobin

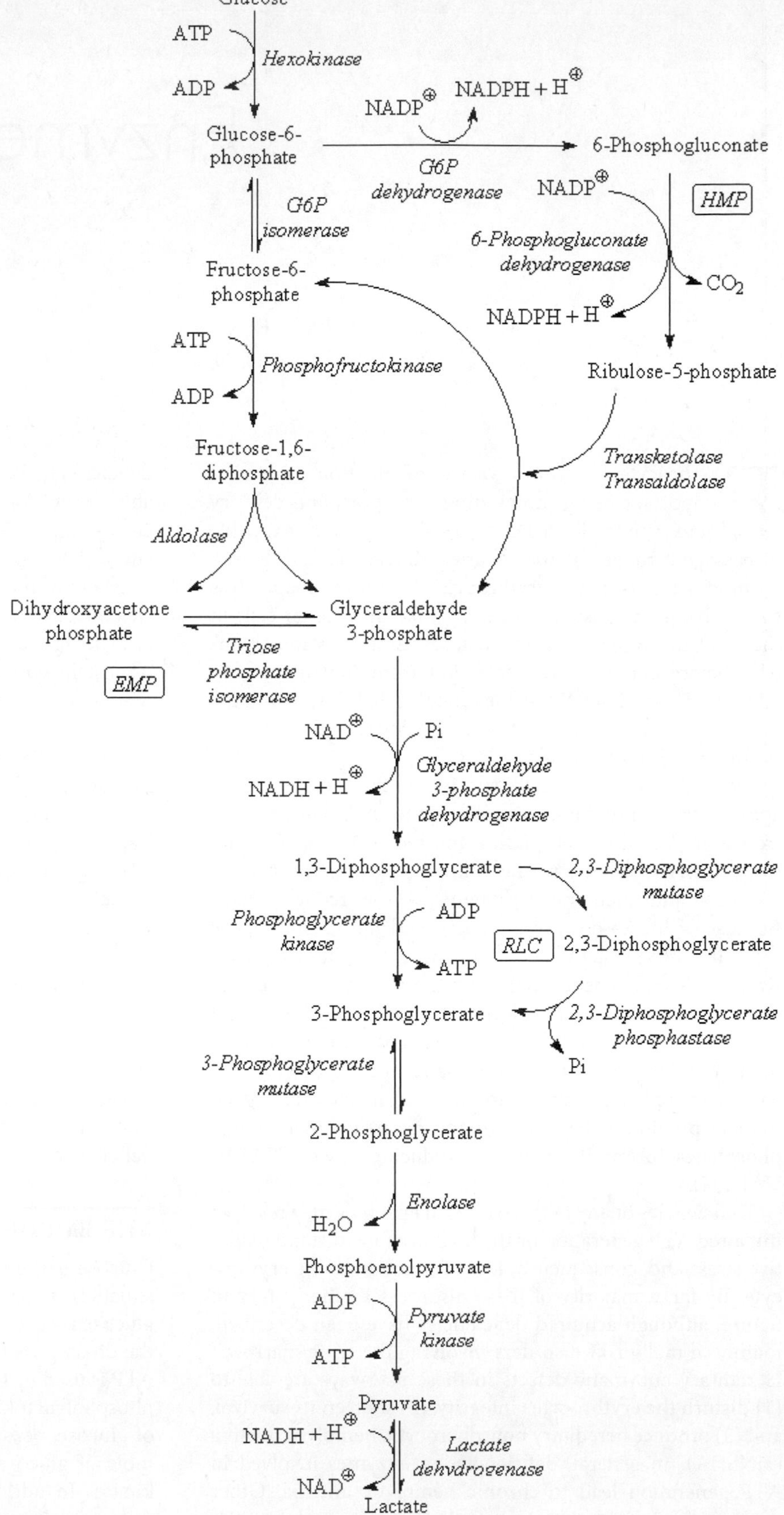

Figure 23-1 Major glycolytic pathways of the erythrocyte. Substrates are in uppercase type, and enzymes are in parentheses. *EMP*, The Embden-Meyerhof pathway; *HMP*, hexose monophosphate pathway or pentose shunt; *RLC*, the Rapoport-Luebering cycle; *ADP*, adenosine diphosphate; *ATP*, adenosine triphosphate; *NAD*$^+$, nicotinamide-adenine dinucleotide; *NADH*, reduced nicotinamide-adenine dinucleotide; *NADP*$^+$, nicotinamide-adenine dinucleotide phosphate; *NADPH*, reduced nicotinamide-adenine dinucleotide phosphate. The step from ribulose 5-phosphate, which is shown as being catalyzed by transketolase and transaldolase, is an abbreviation of this portion of the HMP. Note that diphosphoglycerate and diphosphoglyceric acid are also called bisphophoglycerate and bisphosphoglyceric acid, respectively.

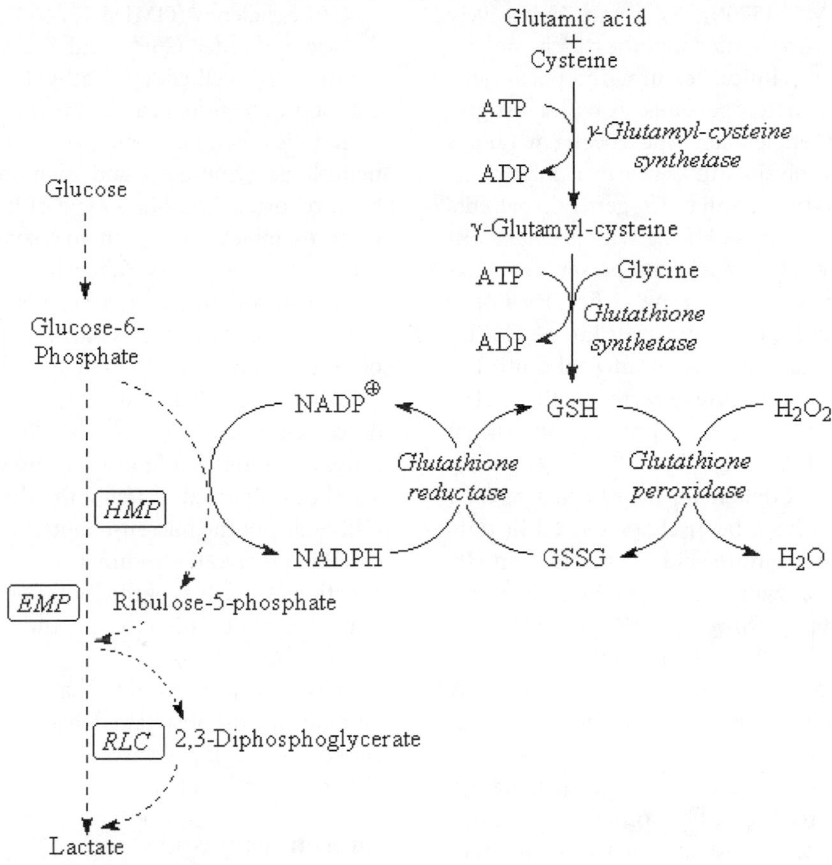

Figure 23-2 Interrelationship of hexose monophosphate and glutathione pathways. *GSH*, Reduced glutathione; *GSSG*, oxidized glutathione.

to hemoglobin by NADH-cytochrome b5 reductase. If this reaction takes place, the end product of the glycolysis is pyruvate. However, if NADH is not reoxidized here, it is used in reducing pyruvate to lactate by lactate dehydrogenase in the last step of the glycolysis.

Although the pathway is reasonably straightforward, it is subjected to a complex mechanism of inhibiting and stimulating factors. Some of the enzymes involved are allosterically stimulated by intermediates of the pathway (e.g., stimulation of pyruvate kinase by fructose diphosphate); others serve as strong inhibitors (e.g., glucose 6-phosphate for hexokinase).

Hexokinase

Hexokinase (HK; EC 2.7.1.1) catalyzes the phosphorylation of glucose to glucose 6-phosphate using ATP as a phosphoryl donor. The activity of HK is significantly higher in reticulocytes than in mature red cells, where it is very low. The HK reaction is one of two rate-limiting steps in this pathway, the other being the phosphofructokinase reaction.

In mammalian tissues, four isozymes of HK with different enzymatic properties exist: HK-I to III with an M_r of 100 kDa, and HK-IV (or glucokinase) with an M_r of 50 kDa. HK-I is the predominant HK isozyme in tissues that depend strongly on glucose for their physiologic functioning, such as brain, muscle, and erythrocytes. HK-I displays unique regulatory properties in its sensitivity to inhibition by physiologic concentrations of the product G6P and, moreover, relief of this inhibition by inorganic phosphate and by high concentrations of glucose.[194] In addition, the enzyme depends on magnesium. HK-I is a homodimer,[7,124] and elucidation of the structures of human and rat HK-I has provided substantial insight into ligand-binding sites and subsequent modes of interaction.[5-7,124,164]

Apart from HK-I, erythrocytes contain a specific subtype of HK: HK-R.[125] Both HKs are encoded by the gene *HK1*, localized on chromosome 10q22 and spanning more than 130 kb.[9] The structure of *HK1* is complex: it encompasses 25 exons that, by tissue-specific transcription, generate multiple transcripts through alternative splicing of different 5′ exons.[9] Erythroid-specific transcriptional control results in the unique red blood cell–specific mRNA that differs from HK-I mRNA at the 5′-untranslated region (5′-UTR) and at the first 63 nucleotides of the coding region.[126,127,158] Consequently, HK-R lacks the porin-binding domain that mediates HK-I binding to mitochondria.[127]

HK deficiency (OMIM 235700)* is a rare, recessively inherited disease with chronic nonspherocytic hemolytic anemia as the predominant clinical feature. The phenotypic expression of the disease is heterogeneous, as with most glycolytic red cell enzyme deficiencies. The spectrum ranges from severe neonatal hemolysis and death to a fully compensated chronic hemolytic anemia. In general, patients benefit from splenectomy. Because HK activity is dependent on red cell age, reticulocytosis, usually present in HK-deficient patients, may obscure the enzyme deficiency. Other age-dependent red cell enzymes (e.g., pyruvate kinase, G6PD) should be measured simultaneously as an internal control to assess the influence of reticulocyte enzyme activity. The *Downeast anemia* mutation in mice represents an animal model of generalized HK deficiency.[142]

Eighteen families with HK deficiency have been described to date, and gene changes have been characterized in only four patients.[32,33,56,90,186] Three amino acid substitutions in HK are known to date to affect enzyme stability (p.Leu529Ser)[32,33] or the enzyme's active site (p.Thr680Ser).[186] The third missense mutation encodes an p.Arg93Gln change and causes aberrant pre-mRNA processing of the *HK1* transcript.[56] A lethal case of HK deficiency was found to be due to an intragenic deletion of 9.5 kb, causing the deletion of exons 5 to 8 of *HK1,* resulting in a null allele.[90] An intriguing mutation was identified in the erythroid-specific promoter. This single NT change downregulates erythroid-specific transcription of *HK1* and, hence, specifically affects HK-R production.[56]

Glucose-6-Phosphate Isomerase

G6P isomerase (GPI; EC 5.3.1.9) [also known as phosphoglucose isomerase (PGI)], catalyzes the interconversion of G6P and fructose 6-phosphate (F6P)—the second step of the EMP. As a result of this reversible reaction, products of the hexose monophosphate pathway can be recycled to G6P. Besides being a housekeeping enzyme of glycolysis, monomeric GPI is identical to neuroleukin and as such exerts lymphokine properties.[101,168] In addition, autoantibodies against GPI seem to be involved in rheumatoid arthritis.[159]

The crystal structure of human GPI has been resolved. The enzyme is a homodimer consisting of two subunits of 63 kDa each. The dimeric form of GPI is a prerequisite for catalytic activity because the active site of the enzyme is composed of polypeptide chains from both subunits.[50,145]

The gene encoding GPI *(GPI)* is located on chromosome 19q13.1 and consists of 18 exons, spanning at least 50 kb, with a cDNA 1.9 kb in length.[197]

*OMIM stands for Online Mendelian Inheritance in Man. It is a World Wide Web database (http://www.ncbi.nlm.nih.gov/omim) developed under the auspices of the National Center for Biotechnology Information (NCBI). It consists of a catalog of human genes and genetic disorders and contains textual information, pictures, and reference information. It also contains links to NCBI's Entre/database of MEDLINE articles and sequence information. Individual disorders may be found by entering OMIM numbers into the search engine of the database.

GPI deficiency (OMIM 172400) is an autosomal recessive disease and, after G6PD and PK deficiency, the third most common red cell enzymopathy. Patients are homozygous or compound heterozygous, showing mild to severe chronic hemolytic anemia. Neonatal death,[80] hydrops fetalis,[115,144] neurologic symptoms, and granulocyte dysfunction[162] have been reported. The phenotype of homozygous GPI-deficient mice resembles that of human enzymopathy.[120] GPI knockout mice die in the embryologic state.[192]

Usually a marked reticulocytosis is seen. Unlike HK, GPI activity in reticulocytes is only marginally higher than that in older cells. Patients generally benefit from splenectomy.

More than 50 families with GPI deficiency have been described worldwide.[47,102,145,148,149] Most mutations are missense mutations, but nonsense and splice-site mutations have also been reported.[102] Using the three-dimensional model of GPI, many of the missense mutations illustrate just how critical the precise three-dimensional structure is for correct function.[145,149] Most of the mutations disrupt key interactions that contribute directly or indirectly to the active site architecture.[48,145]

It is intriguing to note that combined deficiency of GPI and glucose-6-phosphate dehydrogenase appears to be associated with a more favorable clinical outcome than does either deficiency alone.[47]

Phosphofructokinase

6-Phosphofructokinase (PFK; EC 2.7.1.11) catalyzes the phosphorylation of F6P by ATP to fructose 1,6-bisphosphate (FBP; also called fructose 1,6-diphosphate, FDP). This conversion is rate limiting. The enzyme is a homotetramer or heterotetramer with a molecular mass of around 380 kDa. Three distinct subunits have been identified in humans: PFK-M (muscle), PFK-L (liver), and PFK-P (platelet). In erythrocytes, the L and M subunits are expressed; consequently, five forms of phosphofructokinase can be identified that differ in subunit composition: M_4, M_3L_1, M_2L_2, ML_3, and L_4.

The genes encoding PFK-L *(PFKL)* and PFK-M *(PFKM)* are located on chromosomes 21q22.3 and 12q13.3, respectively. The *PFKM* gene spans more than 30 kb, containing 27 exons and at least 3 promoter regions.[128,198]

PFK deficiency is a rare autosomal, recessively inherited disorder. Because red cells contain both M and L subunits, mutations affecting either of the genes coding for these subunits will affect PFK activity. Thus, when the L subunit is affected, RBCs contain only M_4 PFK homotetramers and are partially PFK deficient. In such cases, patients display a mild hemolytic disorder without myopathy. However, when the M subunit is deficient, partial PFK deficiency in red blood cells is accompanied by virtually absent PFK activity in muscle. Consequently, a deficiency in the M subunit due to mutations in the *PFKM* gene causes myopathy and a mild hemolytic disorder (Tarui disease or glycogen storage disease VII, OMIM 610681). PFK-deficient red blood cells display a metabolic block at the PFK step in glycolysis and have decreased concentrations of 2,3-bisphosphoglyceric acid (2,3-BPG, also called 2,3-diphosphoglyceric acid, 2,3-DPG; see later). In PFK-deficient mice, marked alterations in muscle bioenergetics and erythrocyte metabolism interact to produce a complex systemic disorder, indicating that Tarui disease is not simply a muscle glycogenosis.[67]

To date, 15 different mutations associated with PFK deficiency have been identified. Most are missense mutations or mutations affecting pre-mRNA processing.[64,128] Approximately one third of PFK-deficient patients are of Ashkenazi Jewish origin. In this population, the most frequently encountered mutations are an intronic splice-site mutation in intron 5 and a single base pair deletion in exon 22.[143,165] Most other mutations are confined to unique families.

PFK is relatively unstable, and assays should be carried out on fresh blood samples.

Aldolase

Aldolase (fructose-bisphosphate aldolase; EC 4.1.2.13) catalyzes the reversible conversion of fructose 1,6-bisphosphate to glyceraldehyde 3-phosphate and dihydroxyacetone phosphate. The enzyme is a tetramer of identical subunits of 40 kDa. Three isoenzymes have been identified to date: aldolases A, B, and C. Aldolase A is the isoenzyme that is expressed in the RBC, but also in muscle and brain. The flexible C-terminal region of aldolase A has been implicated in the catalytic function of the enzyme.[53,59] Aldolase activity is markedly influenced by red cell age.

The gene for aldolase A *(ALDOA)* is located on chromosome 16p11.2. It spans 7.5 kb and contains 12 exons. Several transcription initiation sites were identified that direct tissue-specific splicing.[82]

Aldolase deficiency (OMIM 611881) is a very rare disease; only six cases have been described.[29,59,99,100,199] The hallmark of aldolase deficiency is chronic hemolytic anemia. In some patients, hemolysis is the sole clinical feature,[99] whereas in other patients, hemolytic anemia is accompanied by myopathy,[29,59,100] rhabdomyolysis,[199] psychomotor retardation,[100] or mental retardation.[29,100]

Triose-Phosphate Isomerase

Triose-phosphate isomerase (TPI; EC 5.3.1.1) is the enzyme of the anaerobic glycolytic pathway with the highest activity. This ubiquitously expressed enzyme catalyzes the interconversion of glyceraldehyde 3-phosphate and dihydroxyacetone phosphate. TPI is active as a dimer, consisting of two identical 27 kDa subunits of 248 amino acids. The three-dimensional structure of the human enzyme has been obtained by crystallography.[109] No isoenzymes are known; only three distinct electrophoretic forms attributable to minor post-translational modifications have been identified.[141,200] In red blood cells, TPI activity is not related to red cell age.

TPI is transcribed from a single gene *(TPI1),* located on chromosome 12p13. The gene spans more than 5 kb and contains 7 exons that encode the 248 amino acids–long TPI subunit.[39]

TPI deficiency (OMIM 190450) is a relatively rare autosomal recessive multisystem disorder, characterized by hemolytic anemia, severe neuromuscular defects, increased susceptibility to infection, and cardiomyopathy.[48,134,161] Patients usually die in childhood, although intriguing exceptions have been reported.[76] Because of metabolic block at the TPI step, a 20- to 60-fold increase in red blood cell concentration of dihydroxyacetone phosphate occurs.[155] Lipid abnormalities have been implicated in the complex pathogenesis of TPI deficiency.[77] To date, 14 mutations have been identified in the gene encoding TPI.[48,133] Mutations result in decreased enzymatic activity and/or dissociation of the TPI dimer into inactive monomers.[133,134] The most common mutation produces a glutamic acid-to-aspartic acid substitution of residue 104—a mutation detected in several unrelated families. Haplotype analyses suggest a single origin for this mutation with the common ancestor in Northern Europe.[160] The other mutations are detected only in individual families. Mutations have been reported in *TPI* promoter sequences of putative regulatory importance, but they exert little if any effect on TPI enzyme activity.[181]

Phosphoglycerate Kinase

Phosphoglycerate kinase (PGK; EC 2.7.2.3) catalyzes the reversible conversion of 1,3-bisphosphoglycerate (also called 1,3-diphosphoglycerate) to 3-phosphoglycerate, thereby generating one molecule of ATP. The reaction can be bypassed by the Rapoport-Luebering shunt at the expense of one molecule of ATP (see later and Figure 23-1). This alternative routing of glycolytic intermediates has been called the *energy clutch* of glycolysis.[96]

In humans, two isoenzymes (PGK-1 and PGK-2) exist. PGK-1 is ubiquitously expressed in all somatic cells; PGK-2 is expressed only in spermatozoa.[118] PGK-1 is a monomeric enzyme consisting of 417 amino acids.[78] The gene encoding PGK-1 *(PGK1)* is located on the long arm of the X chromosome (Xq13). The gene spans 23 kb and is composed of 11 exons.[122]

PGK deficiency (OMIM 311800) is one of the uncommon causes of HNSHA. Sometimes the deficiency manifests only chronic hemolytic anemia, but in many cases, other clinical findings are present, particularly mental retardation and muscle disease; these may occur with or without the anemia.[19] Twenty-eight families with clinical symptoms of severe PGK deficiency have been described, and in 20 of these families the causative mutation is known.[19,167,170] Most of the mutations are missense ones. They are all unique except for the c.491A>T (p.Asp164Val) change, which has been encountered three times, each in the context of a different haplotype,[62] suggesting independent origins of this mutation.[19] One additional PGK variant (PGK München, p.Asp268Asn) does not seem to result in any clinical or biochemical abnormalities.[63] Review of amino acid substitutions in PGK and the crystal structure of pig muscle PGK[61] revealed that most missense mutations occur in three specific regions of the molecule. No correlation could be found, however, between these different locations and clinical expression of the enzyme deficiency.[130,167] Hence, the reason for the range of manifestations in PGK deficiency remains unclear.

Pyruvate Kinase

Pyruvate kinase (PK; EC 2.7.1.40) catalyzes the conversion of phosphoenolpyruvate to pyruvate with concomitant generation of the second molecule of ATP in glycolysis (see Figure 23-1). Pyruvate is crucial for several metabolic pathways, and PK represents one of the major regulatory enzymes of glycolysis. PK is allosterically activated by its substrate and by FBP (fructose 1,6-bisphosphate), and its enzymatic activity strongly depends on red blood cell age. Therefore, because the youngest red blood cells have the highest activity, a deficiency of PK may be masked by reticulocytosis.

PK is a homotetrameric enzyme. In mammals, four isozymes are expressed: PK-M1 is expressed in skeletal muscle, heart, and brain. It is the only PK isozyme that is not allosterically regulated. PK-M2 is expressed in early fetal tissues and in adult tissues including leukocytes and platelets. Both M1 and M2 subunits are produced from a single gene *(PKM2)* by means of alternative splicing.[131,173] PK-L is predominantly expressed in the liver, whereas expression of PK-R is confined to the red blood cell.[89] The PK-L and PK-R subunits are transcribed from a single gene (*PKLR*, for pyruvate kinase, liver, and RBC) located on chromosome 1q21, by the use of tissue-specific promoters.[89,132] The *PKLR* gene consists of 12 exons and is approximately 9.5 kb in size.[104] Exon 1 is exclusively expressed in erythroid cells, whereas expression of exon 2 is confined to the liver. Hence, the PK-R monomer is composed of 574 amino acids.[88] The PK-L subunit comprises 531 amino acids.[174]

In basophilic erythroblasts, both PK-M2 and PK-R isozymes are expressed. During further erythroid differentiation and maturation, the PK-R isozyme progressively replaces PK-M2.[116,117,172] In addition, in the red blood cell, limited proteolytic degradation of the 63 kDa PK-R subunit produces a subset of PK-R monomers of 57 to 58 kDa.[86] Consequently, in young and mature human red blood cells, two distinct species can be distinguished—PK-R1 and PK-R2—that differ in PK-R and "processed" PK-R subunit composition.[187]

The crystal structure of human red cell PK has been elucidated.[184] Each PK-R subunit is composed of four domains: N, A, B, and C. The active site lies in a cleft between the A domain and the flexible B domain. The B domain is capable of rotating with respect to the A domain, generating the "open" or "closed" conformation. The C domain contains the binding site for FBP. In the PK tetramer, subunit interactions at the interfaces between A and C domains, as well as A/B and A/C domain interactions within one subunit, are considered to be key determinants of the allosteric response, involving switching from the low-affinity T-state to the high affinity R-state.[85,114,183,184,196]

Pyruvate kinase deficiency (OMIM 266200) is the most common cause of nonspherocytic hemolytic anemia caused by defective glycolysis. It is an autosomal recessive disease. In the general white population, the allelic frequency is estimated to be around 2%.[25] The prevalence appears to be higher among blacks.[123]

Two major metabolic abnormalities resulting from PK deficiency are ATP depletion and increased levels of 2,3-BPG. The precise mechanisms by which enzyme deficiency leads to a shortened RBC life span are unknown. An important feature, however, involves the selective sequestration of PK-deficient reticulocytes by the spleen.[119] In addition, metabolic disturbances may affect not only red blood cell survival but also the maturation of PK-deficient erythroid progenitors, resulting in ineffective erythropoiesis.[3,4]

PK-deficient patients display a highly variable degree of chronic hemolysis with variable clinical severity. Clinical symptoms range from severe anemia and death at birth, severe transfusion-dependent chronic hemolysis, or moderate hemolysis with exacerbation during infection, to a well-compensated hemolysis without anemia.[204] Splenectomy is, in general, beneficial.[204] PK deficiency has been treated successfully by stem cell transplantation.[175] Gene therapy strategies have been shown to be able to correct the PK-deficient phenotype in mice.[92,121]

To date, more than 190 mutations in *PKLR* have been reported to be associated with pyruvate kinase deficiency (www.pklrmutationdatabase.com). Most (70%) of these mutations are missense mutations affecting conserved residues in structurally and functionally important domains of PK. The most frequently detected mutations are missense mutants c.1456C>T (p.Arg486Trp), c.1529G>A (p.Arg510Gln), and c.994G>A (p.Gly332Ser), and nonsense mutant c.721G>T (p.Glu241X). Evaluating the protein structural context of affected residues using the three-dimensional structure of recombinant human tetrameric PK has provided a rationale for the observed enzyme deficiency and contributes to a better understanding of the genotype-to-phenotype correlation in PK deficiency.[184,185,203] It is important to note that because most PK-deficient patients are compound heterozygous for two different (missense) mutations, up to seven different tetrameric forms of PK may be present in such patients, each with distinct structural and kinetic properties. This complicates genotype-to-phenotype correlations, as it is difficult to infer which mutation is primarily responsible for deficient enzyme function and the clinical phenotype.[185]

Pyruvate kinase deficiency has a protective effect against replication of the malarial parasite in human erythrocytes.[13,58] This protective effect may be related to reduced ATP levels in PK-deficient red blood cells.[12]

Lactate Dehydrogenase

L-Lactate dehydrogenase (LD; EC 1.1.1.27) catalyzes the conversion of pyruvate to lactate—the last step in the EMP. Deficiency of this enzyme is not associated with hematologic disease. LD is described in Chapter 22.

HEXOSE MONOPHOSPHATE PATHWAY

Normally, approximately 10% of glucose is catabolized through the hexose monophosphate pathway (see Figure 23-1). The primary function of this pathway is to reduce 2 moles of $NADP^+$ to NADPH, by means of oxidizing G6P. The amount of glucose passing through this pathway is regulated by the amount of $NADP^+$ that has been made available by the oxidation of NADPH. In the red blood cell, NADPH is required mainly for the regeneration and preservation of the reduced form of glutathione (GSH), which is crucial to the cell in detoxifying hydrogen peroxide and, thereby, protecting against oxidative stress. NADPH also binds to catalase, thereby affecting its activity.[163] Because the red blood cell has no other way of generating NADPH, it depends strongly on the activity of the prime enzyme of NADPH production: glucose-6-phosphate dehydrogenase (G6PD).

Glucose-6-Phosphate Dehydrogenase

Glucose-6-phosphate dehydrogenase (G6PD; EC 1.1.1.49) is expressed in all cells and catalyzes the first step in the hexose monophosphate pathway—the conversion of glucose-6-phosphate to 6-phosphogluconolactone, which is readily converted to 6-phosphogluconate. In the process, 1 mole of NADPH is generated. G6PD activity is much higher in reticulocytes than in mature red blood cells.

The active enzyme is predominantly a homodimer that comprises 59 kDa subunits of 515 amino acids each. Lowering the pH causes a shift from the dimeric to the tetrameric form.[49] In the absence of $NADP^+$, G6PD dissociates into inactive subunits. Each G6PD subunit is built up by two domains. The extensive interface between the two monomers is of crucial importance for enzymatic stability and activity.[11] The importance of $NADP^+$ for stability is explained by the structural $NADP^+$ site, distant from the active site but close to the dimer interface.[11]

The gene coding for G6PD is located on the long arm of the X chromosome (Xq28). It spans 18 kb and consists of 13 exons. Exon 1 is noncoding. The promoter shares many features common to other housekeeping genes.[112]

G6PD deficiency (OMIM 305900) is the most common enzymopathy, affecting an estimated 400 million people worldwide. The parallel between the high frequency of G6PD deficiency and the worldwide distribution of malaria implies that G6PD deficiency confers a selective advantage.[177] This hypothesis is supported by several lines of evidence,[40,108] indicating that the uniform state of G6PD deficiency in hemizygous males, and possibly homozygous females, confers significant protection against severe, life-threatening malaria.[73,157]

G6PD variants have been grouped into five categories according to the level of enzyme activity and clinical manifestations (Table 23-1).[1] More than 400 variants and 140 different mutations have been reported, most of which encode the substitution of a single amino acid. The most common deficient variant is G6PD A–. This variant is characterized by an Asn-to-Asp substitution at codon 126 (c.376A>G), in most cases accompanied by a second mutation encoding a Val-to-Met change at codon 68 (c.202G>A). The second most common variant is G6PD Mediterranean, characterized by a Ser-to-Phe substitution at codon 188 (c.563C>T). Two other polymorphic variants are G6PD Seattle (c.844G>C; p.Asp282His) and G6PD Union (c.1360C>T; p.Arg454Cys).

TABLE 23-1 Classes of Severity of Glucose-6-Phosphate Dehydrogenase (G6PD) Deficiency[1]

Class	Description
Class I	Severe deficiency associated with chronic hemolytic anemia
Class II	Severe deficiency (<10% residual activity), usually without hemolytic anemia
Class III	Moderate to mild deficiency (10 to 60% residual activity) (e.g., G6PD A)
Class IV	Very mild or no deficiency (e.g., G6PD A)
Class V	Increased activity (only one such variant has been described—G6PD Hektoen)

The clinical expression of G6PD deficiency is heterogeneous; five different clinical syndromes can be recognized:
- Drug-induced hemolysis
- Infection-induced hemolysis
- Favism
- Neonatal jaundice (NNJ)
- Chronic nonspherocytic hemolytic anemia (CNSHA)

Most G6PD-deficient individuals are asymptomatic throughout life. They develop acute hemolysis only during periods of increased oxidative stress, elicited by certain drugs,[18] infection, or the ingestion of fava beans. Clinically, such hemolytic episodes are characterized by anemia and jaundice accompanied by increased concentrations of bilirubin and LDH in plasma and reticuloytosis. The exact mechanism by which increased oxidative stress leads to acute hemolysis is unknown, but it results from the inability of G6PD-deficient red blood cells to withstand oxidative damage induced by the triggers mentioned previously. In general, older red blood cells are more susceptible to destruction than young ones. Consequently, they are selectively removed from the circulation, characterizing a self-limited course of hemolysis.[57] The reticulocytosis that is elicited as a result of hemolysis may obscure the enzyme deficiency, as these very young red blood cells have the highest enzyme activity.

Notably, as a result of (skewed) X chromosome inactivation, heterozygous females may be susceptible to the same pathophysiologic phenotype as their hemizygous male counterparts.[30,93,156]

G6PD-deficient neonates who have coinherited a mutation in the uridine-diphosphate-glucuronosyl-transferase-1 (*UGT1A1*) promoter are particularly at risk for developing neonatal jaundice and even kernicterus.[94,205]

A small proportion of G6PD-deficient individuals display the phenotype of chronic nonspherocytic hemolytic anemia. The hemolytic anemia in these class I G6PD-deficient patients may be severe. Mutations associated with class I G6PD deficiency are clustered in exons 10 and 11, designating the subunit interface.[11]

For further reading on the extensive subject of G6PD deficiency, we refer the reader to excellent reviews.[17,41,107,189]

6-Phosphogluconate Dehydrogenase (Decarboxylating) (EC 1.1.1.44)

Even though the oxidation of phosphogluconate to ribulose 5-phosphate by 6-phosphogluconate dehydrogenase generates one mole of NADPH, the few cases of 6-phosphogluconate dehydrogenase deficiency usually are not associated with hemolysis.[42]

Transketolase

Transketolase (EC 2.2.1.1) is decreased in thiamine deficiency. Low values of it have also been found in chronic alcoholism.

RAPOPORT-LUEBERING SHUNT

Red blood cell 2,3-BPG (also called 2,3-DPG) is important in the regulation of the oxygen affinity of hemoglobin.[15,16,180] 2,3-BPG is synthesized and dephosphorylated in the Rapoport-Luebering shunt. Thus, this unique glycolytic bypass represents an important physiologic means for the regulation of oxygen affinity. At the same time, the Rapoport-Luebering shunt provides the red cell with flexibility with regard to the generation of ATP. From an oxygen transport point of view, the Embden-Meyerhof pathway serves principally the generation of 2,3-BPG, because in terms of quantity, it is the principal glycolytic intermediate: the concentration of 2,3-BPG is about equal to the sum of all other glycolytic intermediates. In PK deficiency, 2,3-BPG is increased as a result of the metabolic block at the PK step and of retrograde accumulation of products of glycolysis. Increased 2,3-BPG levels result in decreased oxygen affinity for hemoglobin, so that oxygen is more readily transferred to tissue. This beneficial circumstance is absent in those glycolytic enzyme defects that cause a decrease in 2,3-BPG levels (e.g., HK and GPI deficiency).

Both reactions in the Rapoport-Luebering shunt are catalyzed by one multifunctional protein: 2,3-BPG mutase (BPGM) (EC 5.4.2.4).[81,153] The mutase activity of this enzyme converts the glycolytic intermediate 1,3-BPG to 2,3-BPG. BPGM also has phosphatase activity (2,3-BPG phosphatase [BPGP]; EC 3.1.3.13), converting 2,3-BPG to 3-phosphoglycerate, which then re-enters the glycolytic pathway (see Figure 23-1). In addition, 2,3-BPG may be converted to 2-phosphoglycerate by multiple inositol polyphosphate phosphatase (MIPP1; EC 3.1.3.62), an enzyme that has recently been shown to expand the regulatory capacity of the Rapoport-Luebering shunt.[45]

BPGM is a homodimer with 30 kDa subunits consisting of 258 amino acids. Elucidation of the crystal structure of human BPGM has provided a structural basis for the different enzymatic activities of this enzyme.[190]

The gene for BPGM *(BPGM)* is located on chromosome 7q31-34. It consists of three exons, spanning more than 22 kb.[84] It is expressed only in erythroid tissue during the late stages of differentiation.[84]

BPGM deficiency (OMIM 222800) is a very rare autosomal recessive disorder, resulting in markedly decreased concentrations of 2,3-BPG in erythrocytes. As a result, the oxygen affinity of hemoglobin is increased, causing a decrease in tissue oxygenation and, consequently, erythrocytosis. Only a few cases of BPGM deficiency have been described, all belonging to one, clinically normal French family.[154] Two mutations have been identified in *BPGM*. One single nucleotide substitution predicts the substitution of the highly conserved Arg89 by Cys (BPGM Creteil I).[154] BPGM Creteil II is characterized by a deletion of nucleotide 205, resulting in a shift in the reading frame and, consequently, leading to a premature stop codon.[103]

GLUTATHIONE PATHWAY

Sulfhydryl-containing tripeptide-reduced glutathione (GSH) is present in high concentrations in most mammalian cells.[106] In red blood cells, GSH protects hemoglobin and other critical red blood cell proteins from peroxidative injury. In this process, which involves the reduction of peroxides or oxidized protein sulfhydryl groups, GSH is converted to GSSH (oxidized glutathione) (see Figure 23-2). Enzyme deficiencies in this pathway, except for glutathione peroxidase deficiency, lead to mild chronic nonspherocytic hemolytic anemia, accompanied by drug- and infection-induced hemolytic episodes. The pathogenesis of such enzyme deficiencies is probably similar to the hemolysis that occurs in G6PD deficiency.

γ-Glutamylcysteine Synthetase

γ-Glutamylcysteine synthetase (GCS; EC 6.3.2.2), or glutamate—cysteine ligase, catalyzes the first step in glutathione biosynthesis. The enzyme mediates the formation of γ-glutamylcysteine, ADP, and P_i from glutamate, cysteine, and ATP. This amide linking is the rate-limiting step in glutathione synthesis. There is a feedback inhibition by glutathione. γ-Glutamylcysteine synthetase is a heterodimer composed of a catalytic heavy chain (GCS_h) of 637 amino acids and 73 kDa, and a regulatory light chain (GCS_l) of 274 amino acids and 30 kDa.[69,70]

The genes for GCS_h *(GCLC)* and GCS_l *(GCLM)* are localized on chromosomes 6p12 and 1p21.1, respectively.

Hereditary γ-glutamylcysteine synthetase deficiency is an autosomal recessive disorder that is very rare. Only nine unrelated families have been described. In about half of patients given a diagnosis of γ-glutamylcysteine synthetase deficiency, hemolytic anemia appears to be accompanied by progressive neurologic manifestations.[110] Four families have been characterized at the molecular level.[26,74,110,150] The causative mutation in all these cases affected the heavy subunit of γ-glutamylcysteine synthetase. The homology model of the catalytic subunit, based on the crystal structure of *Saccharomyces cerevisiae,* has been generated to explain the molecular basis of γ-glutamylcysteine synthetase deficiency.[35]

Glutathione Synthase

Glutathione synthase (EC 6.3.2.3; GSH-S) mediates the second irreversible ATP-dependent step in the synthesis of

GSH. The enzyme catalyzes the addition of glycine to the dipeptide γ-glutamylcysteine. Glutathione synthetase is a homodimer of 52 kDa.[65]

The gene for glutathione synthase (*GSS*) is located on chromosome 20q11.2 and contains 12 exons, spanning 23 kb.[191]

Deficiency of glutathione synthetase is rare, but it is the most common abnormality of glutathione metabolism. The disorder is inherited in an autosomal recessive mode. Three distinct clinical forms of GSH-S deficiency can be distinguished on the basis of their severity.[152] The mildest form displays hemolytic anemia as the only clinical manifestation, whereas in the moderate and severe forms, hemolytic anemia is accompanied by metabolic acidosis and 5-oxoprolinuria.[166] Patients with the severe type of GSH-S deficiency develop, in addition, progressive central nervous system damage. Approximately one third of all patients died in childhood, often in the neonatal period.[151]

More than 30 mutations have been described as associated with glutathione synthetase deficiency.[51,52,129,151,166] Most of these mutations are missense ones. To some extent, the type of mutation can predict a mild versus a more severe phenotype.[129]

Glutathione Reductase

Glutathione reductase (glutathione-disulfide reductase; EC 1.8.1.7; GSR) links the glutathione pathway to the hexose monophosphate pathway through reversible oxidation and reduction of NADP.[195] The enzyme maintains high levels of reduced glutathione in the cell and requires flavin adenine dinucleotide (FAD) as a cofactor. Two GSR isoforms exist: a mitochondrial form and a cytoplasmic form, which may be produced by alternative initiation of translation.[135] The active enzyme is a homodimer, linked by a disulfide bridge. Each subunit (522 amino acids; 56 kDa) is divided into four domains, of which domains 1 and 2 bind FAD and NADPH, respectively. Domain 4 is involved in the dimer interface.[95,176]

The gene encoding GSR *(GSR)* is located on chromosome 8p21.1, spans 50 kb, and contains 13 exons.[97]

Because GSR activity is strongly influenced by diet,[20] acquired GSR deficiency is common in malnourished populations. Except when very severe, the deficiency is not associated with hemolysis. Hereditary glutathione reductase deficiency (OMIM 138300) is a very rare autosomal recessive disease. Only two families have been reported. Red blood cells of patients contained no detectable GSR enzymatic activity. Patients from one family[105] presented with favism and were found to be homozygous for a large genomic deletion of 2242 bp.[87] The patient from the other family displayed severe neonatal jaundice without hemolysis and was found to be compound heterozygous for a mutation encoding a premature stop at residue 287 and a Gly-to-Ala substitution at residue 330.[87]

Similar to other rare red blood cell disorders such as PK deficiency, GSR deficiency may provide protection against malaria.[66]

Glutathione Peroxidase

Glutathione peroxidase (GSH Px; EC 1.11.1.9) catalyzes the conversion of hydrogen peroxide to water, thus reducing peroxidative stress to proteins in the cell. It is active as a homotetrameric enzyme consisting of 21 kDa subunits and encoded by the *GPX1* gene on chromosome 3p21.3.[193] Levels of glutathione peroxidase are regulated by selenium.[75,169] Because red blood cells also have high catalase (EC 1.11.1.6) activity to convert H_2O_2 to water and O_2, the activity of GSH-Px is redundant. In fact, deficiencies of catalase or GSH-Px are without clinical consequences.[21]

Low GSH Px activities occur commonly in healthy persons in some population groups,[28] and although association with hemolysis has been reported,[28,72] a clear cause-effect relationship has not been established.

PURINE-PYRIMIDINE METABOLISM

Pyrimidines and purines are needed in the red blood cell for the formation of coenzymes and as active intermediates in carbohydrate and phospholipid metabolism. Because red blood cells cannot synthesize nucleotides de novo, they have evolved nucleotide salvage pathways to effectively preserve them from the reticulocyte stage. Except for pyrimidine 5′-nucleotidase, deficiencies of enzymes affecting these pathways appear to be without functional consequences for the red cell.[136]

5′-Nucleotidase

Pyrimidine-5′-nucleotidases make up a group of enzymes dephosphorylating pyrimidine nucleotides to the corresponding nucleosides and inorganic phosphates. These nucleosides are able to freely diffuse out of the cell; therefore, their accumulation is prevented. Two cytoplasmic forms of the enzyme were identified in the red blood cell: P5′N-1 and P5′N-2. These enzymes are encoded by different genes and have different molecular properties and substrate specificities.[8,137] Because no known disorders are associated with deficiency of P5′N-2, this enzyme will not be further discussed here.

5′-Nucleotidase-1 (P5′N-1; EC 3.1.3.5) is a monomeric 34 kDa protein consisting of 286 amino acids.[171] Enzyme activity is dependent on magnesium ions, and it has optimal substrate specificity for UMP and CMP.[202] P5′N-1 activity is highly dependent on red blood cell age. Its activity is highest in reticulocytes, and a rapid decline occurs during the first few days of maturation, followed by further decline throughout the life span of the red blood cell.[27]

The gene encoding P5′N-1 *(NT5C3)* maps to chromosome 7p14.3, spans about 50 kb, and consists of 11 exons.[111] Three transcripts are created by means of alternative splicing of pre-mRNAs. Only the 286 amino acids–long protein product can be isolated from red blood cells.[91,111]

P5′N-1 deficiency (OMIM 266120) is a relatively common cause of nonspherocytic hemolytic anemia. Its hallmark is the accumulation and precipitation of pyrimidine nucleotides, leading to a shortened red blood cell life span by as yet unknown mechanisms.[188,202] Because of the relatively mild phenotypic expression, many cases may remain undetected.[147] The deficiency is inherited in an autosomal recessive manner. It is the only red cell enzyme deficiency in which red cell morphology is helpful: prominent and characteristic basophilic stippling is visible in blood smears from P5′N-1-deficient patients, representing the accumulation of pyrimidine nucleotides.[182]

Several reports have described mutations associated with P5′N-1 deficiency. To date, 24 patients have been characterized at the molecular level.[44] Although some mutations target different regions of the P5′N structure,[36] they produce similar effects on the molecular properties of the enzyme.[44]

Adenosine Deaminase

Adenosine deaminase (ADA; EC 3.5.4.4) is the enzyme of purine metabolism that deaminates adenosine and 2′-deoxyadenosine to inosine and 2′-deoxyinosine, respectively. Deficiency of ADA leads to severe combined immunodeficiency disease (SCID) without hemolysis.

A hereditary increase in red blood cell ADA activity (OMIM 102730) results in depletion of red cell ATP and, consequently, nonspherocytic hemolytic anemia. It is the only red blood cell enzymopathy that is inherited as an autosomal dominant disorder. Only a few cases have been described, displaying a 30-fold to 70-fold increase in ADA activity. The molecular basis of this disorder has not been elucidated. In patients, high levels of normal ADA mRNA were present, suggesting the mutation of an *in cis* transcriptional regulatory element in close proximity to the gene.[43,46]

For unknown reasons, ADA activity is also increased in patients with Diamond-Blackfan anemia.[71]

Adenylate Kinase

Adenylate kinase (AK; EC 2.7.4.3) catalyzes the reversible interconversion of the adenine nucleotides ATP and AMP to ADP. The gene for AK *(AK1)* has been localized to chromosome 9q34.1, is 12 kb in size, and consists of 7 exons. The mRNA codes for a monomeric enzyme of 194 amino acids.[113]

Adenylate kinase deficiency (OMIM 612631) is a rare autosomal recessive disorder. A small number of cases have been described, displaying moderate to severe hemolytic anemia in some patients, accompanied by mental retardation and psychomotor impairment.[34,179] Because of the absence of hemolytic anemia in a case of complete AK deficiency,[24] the causal relationship of this disorder to hemolytic anemia has been the subject of debate.[23] The study of altered properties of mutant adenylate kinases has provided support for the cause-effect relationship between AK1 mutations and hemolytic anemia.[2]

METHEMOGLOBIN REDUCTION

Hemoglobin can bind oxygen only in the reduced ferrous (Fe^{2+}) state. Thus, when hemoglobin is oxidized to the ferric (Fe^{3+}) state, the capacity to bind oxygen is lost. The oxidized state of hemoglobin, called *methemoglobin,* represents less than 1% of total hemoglobin in healthy red blood cells. To preserve oxygen-binding capacity, the red blood cell keeps hemoglobin in the reduced state. This process strongly depends on the NADH-dependent cytochrome b5/cytochrome b5 reductase system.

Cytochrome b_5 Reductase

Nicotinamide adenine dinucleotide (NADH)-cytochrome b_5 reductase (cb5r; EC 1.6.2.2;) uses the NADH generated by glyceraldehyde-3-phosphate dehydrogenase in the Embden-Meyerhof pathway to reduce the 12 kDa electron transport protein cytochrome b5. In turn, cytochrome b5 reduces methemoglobin to hemoglobin.

The enzyme is present in two different forms. The membrane-bound form is a 35 kDa protein of 301 amino acids that is anchored to the endoplasmic reticulum and the outer mitochondrial membrane.[38] The membrane form has a role in desaturation and elongation of fatty acids, cholesterol biosynthesis, and drug metabolism.[98,138,146]

The second, soluble form of cb5r is a red blood cell–specific protein of 275 amino acids.[79] The two isoforms share an identical hydrophilic C-terminal domain, but the N-terminus of the cytoplasmic form lacks the 25 hydrophobic amino acids that constitute the membrane-binding domain.[201]

Both forms of cb5r are transcribed from the *CYB5R3* gene (previously known as *DIA1*) on chromosome 22q 13-qtr. The gene is 32 kb in length and contains 9 exons.[178] Exon 1 is lacking from the red blood cell–specific mRNA.

NADH-cytochrome b5 reductase deficiency (OMIM 250800) is an autosomal recessive disorder, causing hereditary methemoglobinemia. It was the first identified hereditary enzymopathy.[68] Two distinct clinical forms (types I and II) have been detected.[140] The typically blue color of the skin—cyanosis—due to lack of oxygen in the blood is a prominent feature of both types. In patients with type I methemoglobinemia, the enzyme deficiency is confined to the red blood cells. Patients with type II deficiency are more severely affected. They seldom reach adulthood because of progressive microcephaly.[83]

More than 40 different mutations in *CYBR5R3* have been identified in association with hereditary methemoglobinemia.[10,60,139,140] Some of these mutations are common to both types of methemoglobinemia.[140] The development of a heterologous expression system[54,55] and the three-dimensional models of cb5r[14,31] has allowed the study of cb5r variants and has provided insight into the enzyme's function.

DETECTION OF HEREDITARY RED CELL ENZYME DEFICIENCIES

Other than deficiencies of G6PD and PK, red blood cell enzymopathies are rare or very rare. Therefore, no rationale has been put forth for laboratories that perform such tests only rarely to attempt to identify them. Specimens should be shipped by mail to reference laboratories that specialize in performance of these assays. As a rule, whole blood specimens anticoagulated with EDTA are suitable, and the specimens can be shipped chilled to 4 °C.[22] Exceptions are assays for phosphorylated sugar intermediates, 2,3-BPG, and nucleotide intermediates, which are unstable in freshly drawn blood and require immediate deproteinization in perchloric acid.[22]

Care should be taken to ensure proper removal of leukocytes and platelets because these cells also frequently do contain enzymatic activity, thereby potentially obscuring a deficiency of the red cell enzyme.

Other pitfalls in correct diagnosis of glycolytic enzyme deficiencies include the red blood cell age-dependent behavior of a number of enzymes (in particular, PK, HK, P5′N, and G6PD). For proper evaluation of a single enzyme measurement, its activity should be compared with simultaneous measurement of the activity of a reference enzyme (e.g., HK).

Many patients suffering from severe hemolysis may have already received blood transfusions. In this case, results from red cell enzyme assays must be interpreted with great care, because the presence of donor erythrocytes may obscure an enzyme deficiency. In addition, some mutant enzymes display normal activity in vitro, whereas severe impairment of enzymatic activity may occur in vivo. More sophisticated assays, for example, heat instability tests and enzyme kinetics, are required to identify an enzyme deficiency in those cases.

Over the past few years, most of the genes coding for red cell enzymes have been localized and characterized. This has made molecular diagnostics possible, and many causative mutations have been identified. Molecular diagnostics at the DNA and RNA levels is very attractive in situations in which the diagnosis of enzyme deficiency has been made difficult or impossible by activity measurements, as may occur in transfused patients, as explained previously. In addition, it offers the possibility of prenatal diagnosis. The ability to study the effects of mutations in three-dimensional models of the enzymes and the possibility of expressing recombinant mutant enzymes will lead to a better understanding of the genotype-to-phenotype correlation noted in red blood cell enzymopathies.

METHODS

In this section, methodologic principles and reference values are given for several of the methods used to measure red cell enzymes. Methodologic details of these methods are given in the Evolve site that accompanies this book (http://evolve.elsevier.com/Tietz/textbook).

Method for Determination of Glucose-6-Phosphate Dehydrogenase

Principle

Glucose-6-phosphate dehydrogenase (G6PD) catalyzes the oxidation of glucose-6-phosphate to 6-phosphogluconate with concurrent conversion of $NADP^+$ to NADPH. The activity of G6PD is determined by measurement of the rate of increase in NADPH concentration. Unlike $NADP^+$, NADPH strongly absorbs ultraviolet (UV) light. Therefore, the rate of increase in absorbance at 340 nm is the measure of enzyme activity.

Reference Intervals

The reference interval for G6PD in erythrocytes is 8 to 14 U/g Hb. Values greater than 18 U/g Hb are often encountered in any condition associated with younger than normal RBCs (as in hemolytic anemia not due to G6PD deficiency), but are of no clinical significance.

Method for Screening Erythrocytes for Glucose-6-Phosphate Dehydrogenase Deficiency

In this screening test, $NADP^+$ is reduced to NADPH in the G6PD and 6PGD reactions of the hexose monophosphate pathway. If G6PD activity is low, only a small quantity of NADPH is formed. This is reoxidized to $NADP^+$ by glutathione reductase present in RBCs, and no fluorescence is observed. In the presence of adequate amounts of G6PD, the rate of reduction of $NADP^+$ substantially exceeds the rate of oxidation of NADPH by glutathione reductase, and enough NADPH accumulates in RBCs to be demonstrable by its fluorescence.

Method for Determination of Pyruvate Kinase Activity

Principle

In this assay, the PK reaction is linked with the LD reaction in which NADH is oxidized to NAD^+ in which NADH is oxidized to NAD^+:

$$Phosphoenopyruvate + ADP \xrightarrow{PK} pyruvate + ATP$$
$$Pyruvate + NADH \xrightarrow{LD} lactate + NAD^+ + H^+$$

Because LD is present in excess, the rate of NADH oxidation is limited by the activity of PK. The reaction rate is measured by the rate of decrease in absorbance at 340 nm. Assays are performed at low substrate concentrations with and without the addition of fructose 1,6-bisphosphate, because some PK variants associated with hemolysis have atypical reaction kinetics (and thus may exhibit "normal" activity at high substrate concentrations but lower than normal activity at lower substrate concentrations) or may show absence of enhancement by fructose 1,6-diphosphate, the allosteric activator of PK.

Reference Intervals

Reference intervals for pyruvate kinase are as follows:
- High substrate, 9 to 16 U/g of Hb
- Low substrate, 1.7 to 6.8 U/g of Hb

Method for Determination of Glucose-Phosphate Isomerase Activity

Principle

GPI catalyzes the interconversion of G6P and F6P:

$$F\text{–}6\text{–}P \xleftrightarrow{GPI} G\text{–}6\text{–}P$$
$$NAPH^+ + G\text{–}6\text{–}P \xleftrightarrow{G\text{-}6\text{-}PD} 6\text{–}phosphogluconate + NADPH + H^+$$

In this assay, F6P is used as the substrate for GPI. The GPI reaction is linked to the G6PD reaction. The rate of reduction of $NADP^+$, as indicated by the increase in absorbance at 340 nm, is the measure of GPI activity.

Reference Intervals

The reference interval for GPI is 50 to 70 U/g Hb.

Method for Determination of Erythrocyte Glutathione Concentration

Erythrocyte GSH concentration is diminished in many people who have defects in the hexose monophosphate or GSH synthesis pathway. The GSH stability test, originally devised to permit identification of people susceptible to hemolysis from primaquine (later shown to be the result of G6PD deficiency), remains a useful "stress test" of the intactness of these closely linked pathways. Because deficiencies of GSH synthetase and γ-glutamyl cysteine synthetase are rare disorders, it is not practical for clinical laboratories to contemplate assays for these enzymes unless results of the easily performed GSH stability test are abnormal.

Principle

Virtually all of the nonprotein sulfhydryl groups of RBCs are in the form of reduced GSH. 5,5′-Dithiobis(2-nitrobenzoic acid) (DTNB) is a disulfide chromogen that is readily reduced by sulfhydryl compounds to an intensely yellow compound. The absorbance of the reduced chromogen is measured at 412 nm and is directly proportional to the GSH concentration.

Reference Interval

The reference interval for GSH is 5.5 to 7.5 μmol/g Hb.

Method of Screening for Deficiency of 5′-Nucleotidase Activity

Principle

Pyrimidine-5′-nucleotidase catalyzes the release of phosphate from cytidine-5′-monophosphate and uridine-5′-monophosphate and thus is an enzyme involved in the catabolism of RNA. RNA is a normal constituent of reticulocytes but not of mature RBCs. In the absence (or notable deficiency) of P-5′-N, RNA persists in the RBCs and is manifested by striking basophilic stippling and mild to moderate hemolytic anemia.

Pyrimidine nucleotides, extracted with acid from the RNA remaining in P-5′-N–deficient RBCs, have an absorption peak at 270 nm. This peak is distinct from the peak at 257 nm from purine nucleotides (such as ATP) that are normally present. When P-5′-N is deficient and RNA persists, the P-5′-N deficiency can be inferred by observing a pyrimidine nucleotide peak at 270 nm in an acid extract of RBCs.

Reference Intervals

In normal specimens or in those of any disorder except P-5′-N deficiency, an absorbance curve of low amplitude is present with a peak at about 257 nm (from purines, such as ATP and ADP). No peak is seen at 270 nm. In P-5′-N deficiency, a notably higher amplitude curve is observed, with a peak at 270 nm.

Method for Determination of 2,3-Bisphosphoglycerate in Erythrocytes

Principle

The assay of 2,3-BPG (2,3-DPG) is based on an equilibrium system between 3-phosphoglycerate, 2-phosphoglycerate, and PEP when monophosphoglycerate mutase (MPGM) and enolase are present:

$$\textit{3–Phosphoglycerate} \underset{2,3\text{-}DPG}{\overset{MPGM}{\rightleftharpoons}} \textit{2–phosphoglycerate} \overset{enolase}{\rightleftharpoons} \textit{PEP}$$

The addition of 2,3-DPG (in the sample) shifts the equilibrium so that more 2-phosphoglycerate is converted to 3-phosphoglycerate. This in turn results in the conversion of PEP to 2-phosphoglycerate. The rate of decrease in PEP concentration is measured by the decrease in absorbance at 240 nm, which is proportional to the amount of 2,3-BPG in the specimen.

Reference Intervals

The mean (SD) 2,3-DPG is 12.3 (1.87) μmol/g Hb [0.79 (0.12) mol/mol Hb] or 356 (54) μmol/1012 RBCs [356 (54) amol/RBC].

REFERENCES

1. Anonymous. Glucose-6-phosphate dehydrogenase deficiency. WHO Working Group. Bull World Health Organ 1989;67:601-11.
2. Abrusci P, Chiarelli LR, Galizzi A, Fermo E, Bianchi P, Zanella A, et al. Erythrocyte adenylate kinase deficiency: characterization of recombinant mutant forms and relationship with nonspherocytic hemolytic anemia. Exp Hematol 2007;35:1182-9.
3. Aisaki K, Aizawa S, Fujii H, Kanno J, Kanno H. Glycolytic inhibition by mutation of pyruvate kinase gene increases oxidative stress and causes apoptosis of a pyruvate kinase deficient cell line. Exp Hematol 2007;35:1190-200.
4. Aizawa S, Harada T, Kanbe E, Tsuboi I, Aisaki K, Fujii H, et al. Ineffective erythropoiesis in mutant mice with deficient pyruvate kinase activity. Exp Hematol 2005;33:1292-8.
5. Aleshin AE, Kirby C, Liu X, Bourenkov GP, Bartunik HD, Fromm HJ, et al. Crystal structures of mutant monomeric hexokinase I reveal multiple ADP binding sites and conformational changes relevant to allosteric regulation. J Mol Biol 2000;296:1001-15.
6. Aleshin AE, Zeng C, Bartunik HD, Fromm HJ, Honzatko RB. Regulation of hexokinase I: crystal structure of recombinant human brain hexokinase complexed with glucose and phosphate. J Mol Biol 1998;282:345-57.
7. Aleshin AE, Zeng C, Bourenkov GP, Bartunik HD, Fromm HJ, Honzatko RB. The mechanism of regulation of hexokinase: new insights from the crystal structure of recombinant human brain hexokinase complexed with glucose and glucose-6-phosphate. Structure 1998;6:39-50.
8. Amici A, Emanuelli M, Magni G, Raffaelli N, Ruggieri S. Pyrimidine nucleotidases from human erythrocyte possess phosphotransferase activities specific for pyrimidine nucleotides. FEBS Lett 1997;419:263-7.
9. Andreoni F, Ruzzo A, Magnani M. Structure of the 5′ region of the human hexokinase type I (HKI) gene and identification of an additional testis-specific HKI mRNA. Biochim Biophys Acta 2000;1493:19-26.

10. Arikoglu T, Yarali N, Kara A, Bay A, Bozkaya IO, Tunc B, et al. A novel L218P mutation in NADH-cytochrome b5 reductase associated with type I recessive congenital methemoglobinemia. Pediatr Hematol Oncol 2009;26:381-5.
11. Au SWN, Gover S, Lam VMS, Adams MJ. Human glucose-6-phosphate dehydrogenase: the crystal structure reveals a structural $NADP^+$ molecule and provides insights into enzyme deficiency. Structure Fold Des 2000;8:293-303.
12. Ayi K, Liles WC, Gros P, Kain KC. Adenosine triphosphate depletion of erythrocytes simulates the phenotype associated with pyruvate kinase deficiency and confers protection against *Plasmodium falciparum* in vitro. J Infect Dis 2009;200:1289-99.
13. Ayi K, Min-Oo G, Serghides L, Crockett M, Kirby-Allen M, Quirt I, et al. Pyruvate kinase deficiency and malaria. N Engl J Med 2008;358:1805-10.
14. Bando S, Takano T, Yubisui T, Shirabe K, Takeshita M, Nakagawa A. Structure of human erythrocyte NADH-cytochrome b5 reductase. Acta Crystallogr D Biol Crystallogr 2004;60:1929-34.
15. Bellingham AJ, Huehns ER. Compensatory mechanisms in haemolytic anaemias. Proc R Soc Med 1968;61:1315-6.
16. Benesch RE, Benesch R, Yu CI. The oxygenation of hemoglobin in the presence of 2,3-diphosphoglycerate: effect of temperature, pH, ionic strength, and hemoglobin concentration. Biochemistry 1969;8: 2567-71.
17. Beutler E. G6PD deficiency. Blood 1994;84:3613-36.
18. Beutler E. Disorders of red cells resulting from enzyme abnormalities. In: Lichtman MA, Kipps TJ, Kaushansky K, Beutler E, Seligsohn U, Prchal JT, eds. Williams hematology, 7th edition. New York: McGraw-Hill, 2006:603-31.
19. Beutler E. PGK deficiency. Br J Haematol 2007;136:3-11.
20. Beutler E. Effect of flavin compounds on glutathione reductase activity: in vivo and in vitro studies. J Clin Invest 1969;48:1957-66.
21. Beutler E. Red cell metabolism: a manual of biochemical methods. New York: Grune & Stratton, 1975.
22. Beutler E. Red cell metabolism: a manual of biochemical methods, 3rd edition. Orlando, Fla: Grune & Stratton, 1984.
23. Beutler E. Red cell enzyme deficiencies as non-disease. Biomed Biochim Acta 1983;42:S234-41.
24. Beutler E, Carson D, Dannawi H, Forman L, Kuhl W, West C, et al. Metabolic compensation for profound erythrocyte adenylate kinase deficiency: a hereditary enzyme defect without hemolytic anemia. J Clin Invest 1983;72:648-55.
25. Beutler E, Gelbart T. Estimating the prevalence of pyruvate kinase deficiency from the gene frequency in the general white population. Blood 2000;95:3585-8.
26. Beutler E, Gelbart T, Kondo T, Matsunaga AT. The molecular basis of a case of γ-glutamylcysteine synthetase deficiency. Blood 1999;94:2890-4.
27. Beutler E, Hartman G. Age-related red cell enzymes in children with transient erythroblastopenia of childhood and with hemolytic anemia. Pediatr Res 1985;19:44-7.
28. Beutler E, Matsumoto F. Ethnic variation in red cell glutathione peroxidase activity. Blood 1975;46:103-10.
29. Beutler E, Scott S, Bishop A, Margolis N, Matsumoto F, Kuhl W. Red cell aldolase deficiency and hemolytic anemia: a new syndrome. Trans Assoc Am Physicians 1973;86:154-66.
30. Beutler E, Yeh M, Fairbanks VF. The normal human female as a mosaic of X-chromosome activity: studies using the gene for G-6-PD-deficiency as a marker. Proc Natl Acad Sci USA 1962; 48:9-16.
31. Bewley MC, Marohnic CC, Barber MJ. The structure and biochemistry of NADH-dependent cytochrome b5 reductase are now consistent. Biochemistry 2001;40:13574-82.
32. Bianchi M, Crinelli R, Serafini G, Giammarini C, Magnani M. Molecular bases of hexokinase deficiency. Biochim Biophys Acta 1997;1360:211-21.
33. Bianchi M, Magnani M. Hexokinase mutations that produce nonspherocytic hemolytic anemia. Blood Cells Mol Dis 1995;21:2-8.
34. Bianchi P, Zappa M, Bredi E, Vercellati C, Pelissero G, Barraco F, et al. A case of complete adenylate kinase deficiency due to a nonsense mutation in AK-1 gene (Arg 107 → Stop, CGA → TGA) associated with chronic haemolytic anaemia. Br J Haematol 1999;105:75-9.
35. Biterova EI, Barycki JJ. Mechanistic details of glutathione biosynthesis revealed by crystal structures of *S. cerevisiae* glutamate cysteine ligase. J Biol Chem 2009;284:32700-08.
36. Bitto E, Bingman CA, Wesenberg GE, McCoy JG, Phillips GN Jr. Structure of pyrimidine 5′-nucleotidase type 1: insight into mechanism of action and inhibition during lead poisoning. J Biol Chem 2006;281:20521-9.
37. Boivin P, Galand C, Hakim J, Kahn A. Acquired erythroenzymopathies in blood disorders: study of 200 cases. Br J Haematol 1975;31:531-43.
38. Borgese N, Pietrini G. Distribution of the integral membrane protein NADH-cytochrome b5 reductase in rat liver cells, studied with a quantitative radioimmunoblotting assay. Biochem J 1986;239:393-403.
39. Brown JR, Daar IO, Krug JR, Maquat LE. Characterization of the functional gene and several processed pseudogenes in the human triosephosphate isomerase gene family. Mol Cell Biol 1985;5:1694-706.
40. Cappadoro M, Giribaldi G, O'Brien E, Turrini F, Mannu F, Ulliers D, et al. Early phagocytosis of glucose-6-phosphate dehydrogenase (G6PD)-deficient erythrocytes parasitized by *Plasmodium falciparum* may explain malaria protection in G6PD deficiency. Blood 1998;92:2527-34.
41. Cappellini MD, Fiorelli G. Glucose-6-phosphate dehydrogenase deficiency. Lancet 2008;371:64-74.
42. Caprari P, Caforio MP, Cianciulli P, Maffi D, Pasquino MT, Tarzia A, et al. 6-Phosphogluconate dehydrogenase deficiency in an Italian family. Ann Hematol 2001;80:41-4.
43. Chen EH, Tartaglia AP, Mitchell BS. Hereditary overexpression of adenosine deaminase in erythrocytes: evidence for a *cis*-acting mutation. Am J Hum Genet 1993;53:889-93.
44. Chiarelli LR, Morera SM, Galizzi A, Fermo E, Zanella A, Valentini G. Molecular basis of pyrimidine 5′-nucleotidase deficiency caused by 3 newly identified missense mutations (c.187T>C, c.469G>C and c.740T>C) and a tabulation of known mutations. Blood Cells Mol Dis 2008;40:295-301.
45. Cho J, King JS, Qian X, Harwood AJ, Shears SB. Dephosphorylation of 2,3-bisphosphoglycerate by MIPP expands the regulatory capacity of the Rapoport-Luebering glycolytic shunt. Proc Natl Acad Sci USA 2008;105:5998-6003.
46. Chottiner EG, Cloft HJ, Tartaglia AP, Mitchell BS. Elevated adenosine deaminase activity and hereditary hemolytic anemia: evidence for abnormal translational control of protein synthesis. J Clin Invest 1987;79:1001-5.
47. Clarke JL, Vulliamy TJ, Roper D, Mesbah-Namin SA, Wild BJ, Walker JI, et al. Combined glucose-6-phosphate dehydrogenase and glucosephosphate isomerase deficiency can alter clinical outcome. Blood Cells Mol Dis 2003;30:258-63.
48. Climent F, Roset F, Repiso A, Perez de la Ossa P. Red cell glycolytic enzyme disorders caused by mutations: an update. Cardiovasc Hematol Disord Drug Targets 2009;9:95-106.
49. Cohen P, Rosemeyer MA. Subunit interactions of glucose-6-phosphate dehydrogenase from human erythrocytes. Eur J Biochem 1969;8:8-15.
50. Cordeiro AT, Godoi PH, Delboni LF, Oliva G, Thiemann OH. Human phosphoglucose isomerase: expression, purification, crystallization and preliminary crystallographic analysis. Acta Crystallogr D Biol Crystallogr 2001;57:592-5.
51. Corrons J-L, Alvarez R, Pujades A, Zarza R, Oliva E, Lasheras G, et al. Hereditary non-spherocytic haemolytic anaemia due to red blood cell glutathione synthetase deficiency in four unrelated patients from Spain: clinical and molecular studies. Br J Haematol 2001;112: 475-82.
52. Dahl N, Pigg M, Ristoff E, Gali R, Carlsson B, Mannervik B, et al. Missense mutations in the human glutathione synthetase gene result in severe metabolic acidosis, 5-oxoprolinuria, hemolytic anemia and neurological dysfunction. Hum Mol Genet 1997;6:1147-52.

53. Dalby A, Dauter Z, Littlechild JA. Crystal structure of human muscle aldolase complexed with fructose 1,6-bisphosphate: mechanistic implications. Protein Sci 1999;8:291-7.
54. Davis CA, Barber MJ. Cytochrome b5 oxidoreductase: expression and characterization of the original familial ideopathic methemoglobinemia mutations E255- and G291D. Arch Biochem Biophys 2004;425:123-32.
55. Davis CA, Crowley LJ, Barber MJ. Cytochrome b5 reductase: the roles of the recessive congenital methemoglobinemia mutants P144L, L148P, and R159*. Arch Biochem Biophys 2004;431:233-44.
56. de Vooght KMK, van Solinge WW, van Wesel AC, Kersting S, van Wijk R. First mutation in the red blood cell-specific promoter of hexokinase combined with a novel missense mutation causes hexokinase deficiency and mild chronic hemolysis. Haematologica 2009;94:1203-10.
57. Dern RJ, Beutler E, Alving AS. The hemolytic effect of primaquine. II. The natural course of the hemolytic anemia and the mechanism of its self-limited character. J Lab Clin Med 1954;44:171-5.
58. Durand PM, Coetzer TL. Pyruvate kinase deficiency protects against malaria in humans. Haematologica 2008;93:939-40.
59. Esposito G, Vitagliano L, Costanzo P, Borrelli L, Barone R, Pavone L, et al. Human aldolase A natural mutants: relationship between flexibility of the C-terminal region and enzyme function. Biochem J 2004;380:51-6.
60. Fermo E, Bianchi P, Vercellati C, Marcello AP, Garatti M, Marangoni O, et al. Recessive hereditary methemoglobinemia: two novel mutations in the NADH-cytochrome b5 reductase gene. Blood Cells Mol Dis 2008;41:50-5.
61. Flachner B, Kovari Z, Varga A, Gugolya Z, Vonderviszt F, Naray-Szabo G, et al. Role of phosphate chain mobility of MgATP in completing the 3-phosphoglycerate kinase catalytic site: binding, kinetic, and crystallographic studies with ATP and MgATP. Biochemistry 2004;43:3436-49.
62. Flanagan JM, Rhodes M, Wilson M, Beutler E. The identification of a recurrent phosphoglycerate kinase mutation associated with chronic haemolytic anaemia and neurological dysfunction in a family from USA. Br J Haematol 2006;134:233-7.
63. Fujii H, Chen SH, Akatsuka J, Miwa S, Yoshida A. Use of cultured lymphoblastoid cells for the study of abnormal enzymes: molecular abnormality of a phosphoglycerate kinase variant associated with hemolytic anemia. Proc Natl Acad Sci USA 1981;78:2587-90.
64. Fujii H, Miwa S. Other erythrocyte enzyme deficiencies associated with non-haematological symptoms: phosphoglycerate kinase and phosphofructokinase deficiency. Baillieres Best Pract Res Clin Haematol 2000;13:141-8.
65. Gali RR, Board PG. Sequencing and expression of a cDNA for human glutathione synthetase. Biochem J 1995;310(Pt 1):353-8.
66. Gallo V, Schwarzer E, Rahlfs S, Schirmer RH, van Zwieten R, Roos D, et al. Inherited glutathione reductase deficiency and *Plasmodium falciparum* malaria—a case study. PLoS One 2009;4:e7303.
67. Garcia M, Pujol A, Ruzo A, Riu E, Ruberte J, Arbós A, et al. Phosphofructo-1-kinase deficiency leads to a severe cardiac and hematological disorder in addition to skeletal muscle glycogenolysis. PLoS Genet 2009;5:e1000615.
68. Gibson QH. The reduction of methaemoglobin in red blood cells and studies on the cause of idiopathic methaemoglobinaemia. Biochem J 1948;42:13-23.
69. Gipp JJ, Bailey HH, Mulcahy RT. Cloning and sequencing of the cDNA for the light subunit of human liver gamma-glutamylcysteine synthetase and relative mRNA levels for heavy and light subunits in human normal tissues. Biochem Biophys Res Commun 1995;206: 584-9.
70. Gipp JJ, Chang C, Mulcahy RT. Cloning and nucleotide sequence of a full-length cDNA for human liver gamma-glutamylcysteine synthetase. Biochem Biophys Res Commun 1992;185:29-35.
71. Glader BE, Backer K. Elevated red cell adenosine deaminase activity: a marker of disordered erythropoiesis in Diamond-Blackfan anaemia and other haematologic diseases. Br J Haematol 1988;68:165-8.
72. Gondo H, Ideguchi H, Hayashi S, Shibuya T. Acute hemolysis in glutathione peroxidase deficiency. Int J Hematol 1992;55:215-8.
73. Guindo A, Fairhurst RM, Doumbo OK, Wellems TE, Diallo DA. X-linked G6PD deficiency protects hemizygous males but not heterozygous females against severe malaria. PLoS Med 2007;4:e66.
74. Hamilton D, Wu JH, Alaoui-Jamali M, Batist G. A novel missense mutation in the γ-glutamylcysteine synthetase catalytic subunit gene causes both decreased enzymatic activity and glutathione production. Blood 2003;102:725-30.
75. Harrison PR, Plumb M, Frampton J, Thiele B, Macleod K, Chester J, et al. Regulation of erythroid-specific gene expression. Biomed Biochim Acta 1990;49:S5-10.
76. Hollán S, Fujii H, Hirono A, Hirono K, Karro H, Miwa S, et al. Hereditary triosephosphate isomerase (TPI) deficiency: two severely affected brothers one with and one without neurological symptoms. Hum Genet 1993;92:486-90.
77. Hollán S, Magócsi M, Fodor E, Horányi M, Harsányi V, Farkas T. Search for the pathogenesis of the differing phenotype in two compound heterozygote Hungarian brothers with the same genotypic triosephosphate isomerase deficiency. Proc Natl Acad Sci USA 1997;94:10362-6.
78. Huang IY, Fujii H, Yoshida A. Structure and function of normal and variant human phosphoglycerate kinase. Hemoglobin 1980;4:601-9.
79. Hultquist DE, Passon PG. Catalysis of methaemoglobin reduction by erythrocyte cytochrome B5 and cytochrome B5 reductase. Nat New Biol 1971;229:252-4.
80. Hutton JJ, Chilcote RR. Glucose phosphate isomerase deficiency with hereditary nonspherocytic hemolytic anemia. J Pediatr 1974;85: 494-7.
81. Ikura K, Sasaki R, Narita H, Sugimoto E, Chiba H. Multifunctional enzyme, bisphosphoglyceromutase/2,3-bisphosphoglycerate phosphatase/phosphoglyceromutase from human erythrocytes. Eur J Biochem 1976;66:515-22.
82. Izzo P, Costanzo P, Lupo A, Rippa E, Paolella G, Salvatore F. Human aldolase A gene: structural organization and tissue-specific expression by multiple promoters and alternate mRNA processing. Eur J Biochem 1988;174:569-78.
83. Jaffe ER. Methemoglobin pathophysiology. Prog Clin Biol Res 1981; 51:133-51.
84. Joulin V, Peduzzi J, Romeo PH, Rosa R, Valentin C, Dubart A, et al. Molecular cloning and sequencing of the human erythrocyte 2,3-bisphosphoglycerate mutase cDNA: revised amino acid sequence. EMBO J 1986;5:2275-83.
85. Jurica MS, Mesecar A, Heath PJ, Shi W, Nowak T, Stoddard BL. The allosteric regulation of pyruvate kinase by fructose-1,6-bisphosphate. Structure 1998;6:195-210.
86. Kahn A, Marie J. Pyruvate kinases from human erythrocytes and liver. Methods Enzymol 1982;90:131-40.
87. Kamerbeek NM, van Zwieten R, de Boer M, Morren G, Vuil H, Bannink N, et al. Molecular basis of glutathione reductase deficiency in human blood cells. Blood 2007;109:3560-6.
88. Kanno H, Fujii H, Hirono A, Miwa S. cDNA cloning of human R-type pyruvate kinase and identification of a single amino acid substitution (Thr^{384}→Met) affecting enzymatic stability in a pyruvate kinase variant (PK Tokyo) associated with hereditary hemolytic anemia. Proc Natl Acad Sci USA 1991;88:8218-21.
89. Kanno H, Fujii H, Miwa S. Structural analysis of human pyruvate kinase L-gene and identification of the promoter activity in erythroid cells. Biochem Biophys Res Commun 1992;188:516-23.
90. Kanno H, Murakami K, Hariyama Y, Ishikawa K, Miwa S, Fujii H. Homozygous intragenic deletion of type I hexokinase gene causes lethal hemolytic anemia of the affected fetus. Blood 2002;100:1930.
91. Kanno H, Takizawa T, Miwa S, Fujii H. Molecular basis of Japanese variants of pyrimidine 5′-nucleotidase deficiency. Br J Haematol 2004;126:265-71.
92. Kanno H, Utsugisawa T, Aizawa S, Koizumi T, Aisaki K, Hamada T, et al. Transgenic rescue of hemolytic anemia due to red blood cell pyruvate kinase deficiency. Haematologica 2007;92:731-37.

93. Kaplan M, Hammerman C, Vreman HJ, Stevenson DK, Beutler E. Acute hemolysis and severe neonatal hyperbilirubinemia in glucose-6-phosphate dehydrogenase-deficient heterozygotes. J Pediatr 2001;139:137-40.
94. Kaplan M, Renbaum P, Levy-Lahad E, Hammerman C, Lahad A, Beutler E. Gilbert syndrome and glucose-6-phosphate dehydrogenase deficiency: a dose-dependent genetic interaction crucial to neonatal hyperbilirubinemia. Proc Natl Acad Sci USA 1997;94:12128-32.
95. Karplus PA, Schulz GE. Refined structure of glutathione reductase at 1.54 A resolution. J Mol Biol 1987;195:701-29.
96. Keitt AS. Pyruvate kinase deficiency and related disorders of red cell glycolysis. Am J Med 1966;41:762-85.
97. Kelner MJ, Montoya MA. Structural organization of the human glutathione reductase gene: determination of correct cDNA sequence and identification of a mitochondrial leader sequence. Biochem Biophys Res Commun 2000;269:366-8.
98. Keyes SR, Cinti DL. Biochemical properties of cytochrome b5-dependent microsomal fatty acid elongation and identification of products. J Biol Chem 1980;255:11357-64.
99. Kishi H, Mukai T, Hirono A, Fujii H, Miwa S, Hori K. Human aldolase A deficiency associated with a hemolytic anemia: thermolabile aldolase due to a single base mutation. Proc Natl Acad Sci U S A 1987;84:8623-27.
100. Kreuder J, Borkhardt A, Repp R, Pekrun A, Goettsche B, Gottschalk U, et al. Brief report: inherited metabolic myopathy and hemolysis due to a mutation in aldolase A. N Engl J Med 1996;334:1100-4.
101. Kugler W, Breme K, Laspe P, Muirhead H, Davies C, Winkler H, et al. Molecular basis of neurological dysfunction coupled with haemolytic anaemia in human glucose-6-phosphate isomerase (GPI) deficiency. Hum Genet 1998;103:450-4.
102. Kugler W, Lakomek M. Glucose-6-phosphate isomerase deficiency. Baillieres Best Pract Res Clin Haematol 2000;13:89-101.
103. Lemarchandel V, Joulin V, Valentin C, Rosa R, Galactéros F, Rosa J, et al. Compound heterozygosity in a complete erythrocyte bisphosphoglycerate mutase deficiency. Blood 1992;80:2643-9.
104. Lenzner C, Nürnberg P, Jacobasch G, Thiele B-J. Complete genomic sequence of the human PK-L/R-gene includes four intragenic polymorphisms defining different haplotype backgrounds of normal and mutant PK-genes. DNA Seq 1997;8:45-53.
105. Loos H, Roos D, Weening R, Houwerzijl J. Familial deficiency of glutathione reductase in human blood cells. Blood 1976;48:53-62.
106. Lu SC. Regulation of glutathione synthesis. Mol Aspects Med 2009;30:42-59.
107. Luzzatto L, Mehta A. Glucose 6-phosphate dehydrogenase deficiency. In: Scriver C, Beaudet AL, Sly WS, Valle D, eds. The metabolic and molecular basis of inherited disease, 7th edition. New York: McGraw Hill, 1995:3367-98.
108. Luzzatto L, Usanga EA, Reddy S. Glucose 6-phosphate dehydrogenase deficient red cells: resistance to infection by malarial parasites. Science 1969;164:839-42.
109. Mande SC, Mainfroid V, Kalk KH, Goraj K, Martial JA, Hol WGJ. Crystal structure of recombinant human triosephosphate isomerase at 2.8 A resolution: triosephosphate isomerase-related human genetic disorders and comparison with the trypanosomal enzyme. Protein Sci 1994;3:810-21.
110. Manu Pereira M, Gelbart T, Ristoff E, Crain KC, Bergua JM, Lopez Lafuente A, et al. Chronic non-spherocytic hemolytic anemia associated with severe neurological disease due to γ-glutamylcysteine synthetase deficiency in a patient of Moroccan origin. Haematologica 2007;92:e102-5.
111. Marinaki AM, Escuredo E, Duley JA, Simmonds HA, Amici A, Naponelli V, et al. Genetic basis of hemolytic anemia caused by pyrimidine 5′ nucleotidase deficiency. Blood 2001;97:3327-32.
112. Martini G, Toniolo D, Vulliamy T, Luzzatto L, Dono R, Viglietto G, et al. Structural analysis of the X-linked gene encoding human glucose 6-phosphate dehydrogenase. EMBO J 1986;5:1849-55.
113. Matsuura S, Igarashi M, Tanizawa Y, Yamada M, Kishi F, Kajii T, et al. Human adenylate kinase deficiency associated with hemolytic anemia: a single base substitution affecting solubility and catalytic activity of the cytosolic adenylate kinase. J Biol Chem 1989;264: 10148-155.
114. Mattevi A, Valentini G, Rizzi M, Speranza ML, Bolognesi M, Coda A. Crystal structure of *Escherichia coli* pyruvate kinase type I: molecular basis of the allosteric transition. Structure 1995;3:729-41.
115. Matthay KK, Mentzer WC. Erythrocyte enzymopathies in the newborn. Clin Haematol 1981;10:31-55.
116. Max-Audit I, Kechemir D, Mitjavila MT, Vainchenker W, Rotten D, Rosa R. Pyruvate kinase synthesis and degradation by normal and pathologic cells during erythroid maturation. Blood 1988;72:1039-44.
117. Max-Audit I, Testa U, Kechemir D, Titeux M, Vainchenker W, Rosa R. Pattern of pyruvate kinase isozymes in erythroleukemia cell lines and in normal human erythroblasts. Blood 1984;64:930-6.
118. McCarrey JR, Thomas K. Human testis-specific PGK gene lacks introns and possesses characteristics of a processed gene. Nature 1987;326:501-5.
119. Mentzer WC Jr, Baehner RL, Schmidt-Schönbein H, Robinson SH, Nathan DG. Selective reticulocyte destruction in erythrocyte pyruvate kinase deficiency. J Clin Invest 1971;50:688-99.
120. Merkle S, Pretsch W. Glucose-6-phosphate isomerase deficiency associated with nonspherocytic hemolytic anemia in the mouse: an animal model for the human disease. Blood 1993;81:206-13.
121. Meza NW, Alonso-Ferrero ME, Navarro S, Quintana-Bustamante O, Valeri A, Garcia-Gomez M, et al. Rescue of pyruvate kinase deficiency in mice by gene therapy using the human isoenzyme. Mol Ther 2009;17:2000-9.
122. Michelson AM, Bruns GA, Morton CC, Orkin SH. The human phosphoglycerate kinase multigene family: HLA-associated sequences and an X-linked locus containing a processed pseudogene and its functional counterpart. J Biol Chem 1985;260:6982-92.
123. Mohrenweiser HW. Functional hemizygosity in the human genome: direct estimate from twelve erythrocyte enzyme loci. Hum Genet 1987;77:241-5.
124. Mulichak AM, Wilson JE, Padmanabhan K, Garavito RM. The structure of mammalian hexokinase-1. Nat Struct Biol 1998;5: 555-60.
125. Murakami K, Blei F, Tilton W, Seaman C, Piomelli S. An isozyme of hexokinase specific for the human red blood cell (HK_R). Blood 1990;75:770-5.
126. Murakami K, Kanno H, Miwa S, Piomelli S. Human HK_R isozyme: organization of the hexokinase I gene, the erythroid-specific promoter, and transcription initiation site. Mol Genet Metab 1999;67:118-30.
127. Murakami K, Piomelli S. Identification of the cDNA for human red blood cell-specific hexokinase isozyme. Blood 1997;89:762-6.
128. Nakajima H, Raben N, Hamaguchi T, Yamasaki T. Phosphofructokinase deficiency: past, present and future. Curr Mol Med 2002;2:197-212.
129. Njålsson R, Ristoff E, Carlsson K, Winkler A, Larsson A, Norgren S. Genotype, enzyme activity, glutathione level, and clinical phenotype in patients with glutathione synthetase deficiency. Hum Genet 2005;116:384-9.
130. Noel N, Flanagan JM, Ramirez Bajo MJ, Kalko SG, Manu Mdel M, Garcia Fuster JL, et al. Two new phosphoglycerate kinase mutations associated with chronic haemolytic anaemia and neurological dysfunction in two patients from Spain. Br J Haematol 2006;132:523-29.
131. Noguchi T, Inoue H, Tanaka T. The M_1- and M_2-type isozymes of rat pyruvate kinase are produced from the same gene by alternative RNA splicing. J Biol Chem 1986;261:13807-12.
132. Noguchi T, Yamada K, Inoue H, Matsuda T, Tanaka T. The L- and R-type isozymes of rat pyruvate kinase are produced from a single gene by use of different promoters. J Biol Chem 1987;262:14366-71.
133. Orosz F, Olah J, Ovadi J. Triosephosphate isomerase deficiency: facts and doubts. IUBMB Life 2006;58:703-15.
134. Orosz F, Olah J, Ovadi J. Triosephosphate isomerase deficiency: new insights into an enigmatic disease. Biochim Biophys Acta 2009;1792: 1168-74.

135. Outten CE, Culotta VC. Alternative start sites in the *Saccharomyces cerevisiae* GLR1 gene are responsible for mitochondrial and cytosolic isoforms of glutathione reductase. J Biol Chem 2004;279:7785-91.
136. Paglia DE, Valentine WN. Haemolytic anaemia associated with disorders of the purine and pyrimidine salvage pathways. Clin Haematol 1981;10:81-98.
137. Paglia DE, Valentine WN, Brockway RA. Identification of thymidine nucleotidase and deoxyribonucleotidase activities among normal isozymes of 5′-nucleotidase in human erythrocytes. Proc Natl Acad Sci USA 1984;81:588-92.
138. Passon PG, Hultquist DE. Soluble cytochrome b 5 reductase from human erythrocytes. Biochim Biophys Acta 1972;275:62-73.
139. Percy MJ, Aslan D. NADH-cytochrome b5 reductase in a Turkish family with recessive congenital methaemoglobinaemia type I. J Clin Pathol 2008;61:1122-3.
140. Percy MJ, Lappin TR. Recessive congenital methaemoglobinaemia: cytochrome b(5) reductase deficiency. Br J Haematol 2008;141:298-308.
141. Peters J, Hopkinson DA, Harris H. Genetic and non-genetic variation of triose phosphate isomerase isozymes in human tissues. Ann Hum Genet 1973;36:297-312.
142. Peters LL, Lane PW, Andersen SG, Gwynn B, Barker JE, Beutler E. Downeast anemia *(dea)*, a new mouse model of severe nonspherocytic hemolytic anemia caused by hexokinase (HK_1) deficiency. Blood Cells Mol Dis 2001;27:850-60.
143. Raben N, Sherman J, Miller F, Mena H, Plotz P. A 5′ splice junction mutation leading to exon deletion in an Ashkenazic Jewish family with phosphofructokinase deficiency (Tarui disease). J Biol Chem 1993;268:4963-7.
144. Ravindranath Y, Paglia DE, Warrier I, Valentine W, Nakatani M, Brockway RA. Glucose phosphate isomerase deficiency as a cause of hydrops fetalis. N Engl J Med 1987;316:258-61.
145. Read J, Pearce J, Li X, Muirhead H, Chirgwin J, Davies C. The crystal structure of human phosphoglucose isomerase at 1.6 A resolution: implications for catalytic mechanism, cytokine activity and haemolytic anaemia. J Mol Biol 2001;309:447-63.
146. Reddy VV, Kupfer D, Caspi E. Mechanism of C-5 double bond introduction in the biosynthesis of cholesterol by rat liver microsomes. J Biol Chem 1977;252:2797-801.
147. Rees DC, Duley JA, Marinaki AM. Pyrimidine 5′ nucleotidase deficiency. Br J Haematol 2003;120:375-83.
148. Repiso A, Oliva B, Vives Corrons JL, Carreras J, Climent F. Glucose phosphate isomerase deficiency: enzymatic and familial characterization of Arg346His mutation. Biochim Biophys Acta 2005;1740:467-71.
149. Repiso A, Oliva B, Vives-Corrons JL, Beutler E, Carreras J, Climent F. Red cell glucose phosphate isomerase (GPI): a molecular study of three novel mutations associated with hereditary nonspherocytic hemolytic anemia. Hum Mutat 2006;27:1159.
150. Ristoff E, Augustson C, Geissler J, de Rijk T, Carlsson K, Luo J-L, et al. A missense mutation in the heavy subunit of γ-glutamylcysteine synthetase gene causes hemolytic anemia. Blood 2000;95:1896-7.
151. Ristoff E, Hebert C, Njalsson R, Norgren S, Rooyackers O, Larsson A. Glutathione synthetase deficiency: is gamma-glutamylcysteine accumulation a way to cope with oxidative stress in cells with insufficient levels of glutathione? J Inherit Metab Dis 2002;25:577-84.
152. Ristoff E, Larsson A. Inborn errors in the metabolism of glutathione. Orphanet J Rare Dis 2007;2:16.
153. Rosa R, Gaillardon J, Rosa J. Diphosphoglycerate mutase and 2,3-diphosphoglycerate phosphatase activities of red cells: comparative electrophoretic study. Biochem Biophys Res Commun 1973;51:536-42.
154. Rosa R, Prehu M-O, Beuzard Y, Rosa J. The first case of a complete deficiency of diphosphoglycerate mutase in human erythrocytes. J Clin Invest 1978;62:907-15.
155. Rosa R, Prehu MO, Calvin MC, Badoual J, Alix D, Girod R. Hereditary triose phosphate isomerase deficiency: seven new homozygous cases. Hum Genet 1985;71:235-40.
156. Russo G, Mollica F, Pavone L, Schiliro G. Hemolytic crises of favism in Sicilian females heterozygous for G-6-PD deficiency. Pediatrics 1972;49:854-9.
157. Ruwende C, Khoo SC, Snow RW, Yates SN, Kwiatkowski D, Gupta S, et al. Natural selection of hemi- and heterozygotes for G6PD deficiency in Africa by resistance to severe malaria. Nature 1995;376:246-9.
158. Ruzzo A, Andreoni F, Magnani M. Structure of the human hexokinase type I gene and nucleotide sequence of the 5′ flanking region. Biochem J 1998;331:607-13.
159. Schaller M, Burton DR, Ditzel HJ. Autoantibodies to GPI in rheumatoid arthritis: linkage between an animal model and human disease. Nat Immunol 2001;2:746-53.
160. Schneider A, Westwood B, Yim C, Cohen-Solal M, Rosa R, Labotka R, et al. The 1591C mutation in triosephosphate isomerase (TPI) deficiency: tightly linked polymorphisms and a common haplotype in all known families. Blood Cells Mol Dis 1996;22:115-25.
161. Schneider AS. Triosephosphate isomerase deficiency: historical perspectives and molecular aspects. Baillieres Best Pract Res Clin Haematol 2000;13:119-40.
162. Schroter W, Eber SW, Bardosi A, Gahr M, Gabriel M, Sitzmann FC. Generalised glucosephosphate isomerase (GPI) deficiency causing haemolytic anaemia, neuromuscular symptoms and impairment of granulocytic function: a new syndrome due to a new stable GPI variant with diminished specific activity (GPI Homburg). Eur J Pediatr 1985;144:301-5.
163. Scott MD, Wagner TC, Chiu DT. Decreased catalase activity is the underlying mechanism of oxidant susceptibility in glucose-6-phosphate dehydrogenase-deficient erythrocytes. Biochim Biophys Acta 1993;1181:163-8.
164. Sebastian S, Wilson JE, Mulichak A, Garavito RM. Allosteric regulation of type I hexokinase: a site-directed mutational study indicating location of the functional glucose 6-phosphate binding site in the N-terminal half of the enzyme. Arch Biochem Biophys 1999;362:203-210.
165. Sherman JB, Raben N, Nicastri C, Argov Z, Nakajima H, Adams EM, et al. Common mutations in the phosphofructokinase-M gene in Ashkenazi Jewish patients with glycogenesis VII—and their population frequency. Am J Hum Genet 1994;55:305-13.
166. Shi Z-Z, Habib GM, Rhead WJ, Gahl WA, He X, Sazer S, et al. Mutations in the glutathione synthetase gene cause 5-oxoprolinuria. Nat Genet 1996;14:361-5.
167. Spiegel R, Gomez EA, Akman HO, Krishna S, Horovitz Y, DiMauro S. Myopathic form of phosphoglycerate kinase (PGK) deficiency: a new case and pathogenic considerations. Neuromuscul Disord 2009;19:207-11.
168. Sriram G, Martinez JA, McCabe ERB, Liao JC, Dipple KM. Single-gene disorders: what role could moonlighting enzymes play? Am J Hum Genet 2005;76:911-24.
169. Stadtman TC. Selenocysteine. Annu Rev Biochem 1996;65:83-100.
170. Svaasand EK, Aasly J, Landsem VM, Klungland H. Altered expression of PGK1 in a family with phosphoglycerate kinase deficiency. Muscle Nerve 2007;36:679-84.
171. Swallow DM, Aziz I, Hopkinson DA, Miwa S. Analysis of human erythrocyte 5′-nucleotidases in healthy individuals and a patient deficient in pyrimidine 5′-nucleotidase. Ann Hum Genet 1983;47:19-23.
172. Takegawa S, Fujii H, Miwa S. Change of pyruvate kinase isozymes from M_2- to L-type during development of the red cell. Br J Haematol 1983;54:467-74.
173. Takenaka M, Yamada K, Lu T, Kang R, Tanaka T, Noguchi T. Alternative splicing of the pyruvate kinase M gene in a minigene system. Eur J Biochem 1996;235:366-71.
174. Tani K, Fujii H, Tsutsumi H, Sukegawa J, Toyoshima K, Yoshida MC, et al. Human liver type pyruvate kinase: cDNA cloning and chromosomal assignment. Biochem Biophys Res Commun 1987;143:431-8.

175. Tanphaichitr VS, Suvatte V, Issaragrisil S, Mahasandana C, Veerakul G, Chongkolwatana V, et al. Successful bone marrow transplantation in a child with red blood cell pyruvate kinase deficiency. Bone Marrow Transplant 2000;26:689-90.
176. Thieme R, Pai EF, Schirmer RH, Schulz GE. Three-dimensional structure of glutathione reductase at 2 A resolution. J Mol Biol 1981;152:763-82.
177. Tishkoff SA, Varkonyi R, Cahinhinan N, Abbes S, Argyropoulos G, Destro-Bisol G, et al. Haplotype diversity and linkage disequilibrium at human G6PD: recent origin of alleles that confer malarial resistance. Science 2001;293:455-62.
178. Tomatsu S, Kobayashi Y, Fukumaki Y, Yubisui T, Orii T, Sakaki Y. The organization and the complete nucleotide sequence of the human NADH-cytochrome b5 reductase gene. Gene 1989;80:353-61.
179. Toren A, Brok-Simoni F, Ben-Bassat I, Holtzman F, Mandel M, Neumann Y, et al. Congenital haemolytic anaemia associated with adenylate kinase deficiency. Br J Haematol 1994;87:376-80.
180. Torrance J, Jacobs P, Restrepo A, Eschbach J, Lenfant C, Finch CA. Intraerythrocytic adaptation to anemia. N Engl J Med 1970;283:165-9.
181. Valentin C, Pissard S, Martin J, Héron D, Labrune P, Livet M-O, et al. Triose phosphate isomerase deficiency in 3 French families: two novel null alleles, a frameshift mutation (TPI Alfortville) and an alteration in the initiation codon (TPI Paris). Blood 2000;96:1130-5.
182. Valentine WN, Fink K, Paglia DE, Harris SR, Adams WS. Hereditary hemolytic anemia with human erythrocyte pyrimidine 5′-nucleotidase deficiency. J Clin Invest 1974;54:866-79.
183. Valentini G, Chiarelli L, Fortin R, Speranza ML, Galizzi A, Mattevi A. The allosteric regulation of pyruvate kinase. J Biol Chem 2000;275:18145-52.
184. Valentini G, Chiarelli LR, Fortin R, Dolzan M, Galizzi A, Abraham DJ, et al. Structure and function of human erythrocyte pyruvate kinase: molecular basis of nonspherocytic hemolytic anemia. J Biol Chem 2002;277:23807-14.
185. Van Wijk R, Huizinga EG, Van Wesel ACW, Van Oirschot BA, Hadders MA, van Solinge WW. Fifteen novel mutations in *PKLR* associated with pyruvate kinase (PK) deficiency: structural implications of amino acid substitutions in PK. Hum Mutat 2009;30:446-53.
186. van Wijk R, Rijksen G, Huizinga EG, Nieuwenhuis HK, van Solinge WW. HK Utrecht: missense mutation in the active site of human hexokinase associated with hexokinase deficiency and severe nonspherocytic hemolytic anemia. Blood 2003;101:345-7.
187. van Wijk R, van Solinge WW. The energy-less red blood cell is lost: erythrocyte enzyme abnormalities of glycolysis. Blood 2005;106: 4034-42.
188. Vives I, Corrons JL. Chronic non-spherocytic haemolytic anaemia due to congenital pyrimidine 5′ nucleotidase deficiency: 25 years later. Baillieres Best Pract Res Clin Haematol 2000;13:103-18.
189. Vulliamy TJ, Luzzatto L. Glucose-6-phosphate dehydrogenase deficiency and related disorders. In: Handin RI, Lux SE IV, eds. Blood principles and practice of hematology, 2nd edition. Philadelphia: Lippincott Williams & Wilkins, 2003:1921-50.
190. Wang Y, Wei Z, Bian Q, Cheng Z, Wan M, Liu L, et al. Crystal structure of human bisphosphoglycerate mutase. J Biol Chem 2004;279:39132-8.
191. Webb GC, Vaska VL, Gali RR, Ford JH, Board PG. The gene encoding human glutathione synthetase (GSS) maps to the long arm of chromosome 20 at band 11.2. Genomics 1995;30:617-9.
192. West JD, Flockhart JH, Peters J, Ball ST. Death of mouse embryos that lack a functional gene for glucose phosphate isomerase. Genet Res 1990;56:223-36.
193. Wijnen LM, Monteba-van Heuvel M, Pearson PL, Meera Khan P. Assignment of a gene for glutathione peroxidase (GPX1) to human chromosome 3. Cytogenet Cell Genet 1978;22:232-5.
194. Wilson JE. Hexokinases. Rev Physiol Biochem Pharmacol 1995;126: 65-198.
195. Wong KK, Blanchard JS. Human erythrocyte glutathione reductase: pH dependence of kinetic parameters. Biochemistry 1989;28: 3586-90.
196. Wooll JO, Friesen RHE, White MA, Watowich SJ, Fox RO, Lee JC, et al. Structural and functional linkages between subunit interfaces in mammalian pyruvate kinase. J Mol Biol 2001;312:525-40.
197. Xu W, Lee P, Beutler E. Human glucose phosphate isomerase: exon mapping and gene structure. Genomics 1995;29:732-9.
198. Yamada S, Nakajima H, Kuehn MR. Novel testis- and embryo-specific isoforms of the phosphofructokinase-1 muscle type gene. Biochem Biophys Res Commun 2004;316:580-7.
199. Yao DC, Tolan DR, Murray MF, Harris DJ, Darras BT, Geva A, et al. Hemolytic anemia and severe rhabdomyolysis caused by compound heterozygous mutations of the gene for erythrocyte/muscle isozyme of aldolase, ALDOA$^{(Arg303X/Cys338Tyr)}$. Blood 2004;103:2401-3.
200. Yuan PM, Talent JM, Gracy RW. Molecular basis for the accumulation of acidic isozymes of triosephosphate isomerase on aging. Mech Ageing Dev 1981;17:151-62.
201. Yubisui T, Miyata T, Iwanaga S, Tamura M, Takeshita M. Complete amino acid sequence of NADH-cytochrome b5 reductase purified from human erythrocytes. J Biochem 1986;99:407-22.
202. Zanella A, Bianchi P, Fermo E, Valentini G. Hereditary pyrimidine 5′-nucleotidase deficiency: from genetics to clinical manifestations. Br J Haematol 2006;133:113-23.
203. Zanella A, Fermo E, Bianchi P, Chiarelli LR, Valentini G. Pyruvate kinase deficiency: the genotype-phenotype association. Blood Rev 2007;21:217-31.
204. Zanella A, Fermo E, Bianchi P, Valentini G. Red cell pyruvate kinase deficiency: molecular and clinical aspects. Br J Haematol 2005;130: 11-25.
205. Zangen S, Kidron D, Gelbart T, Roy-Chowdhury N, Wang X, Kaplan M. Fatal kernicterus in a girl deficient in glucose-6-phosphate dehydrogenase: a paradigm of synergistic heterozygosity. J Pediatr 2009;154:616-9.

CHAPTER 24

Tumor Markers

Lori J. Sokoll, Ph.D., F.A.C.B., Alex J. Rai, Ph.D., D.A.B.C.C., F.A.C.B., and Daniel W. Chan, Ph.D., D.A.B.C.C., F.A.C.B

A tumor marker is a substance produced by a tumor or by the host in response to a tumor, which is used to differentiate a tumor from normal tissue, or to detect the presence of a tumor based on measurements in the blood or secretions. Such substances are found in cells, tissues, or body fluids and are measured qualitatively or quantitatively by chemical, immunologic, or molecular biological methods.[246]

Morphologically, cancer tissue has been recognized by pathologists as resembling fetal tissue more than normal adult differentiated tissue. Tumors are graded according to their degree of differentiation as (1) well differentiated, (2) poorly differentiated, or (3) anaplastic (without form). Tumor markers are the biochemical or immunologic counterparts of the differentiation state of the tumor. In general, some tumor markers represent re-expression of substances produced normally by embryogenically closely related tissue (Table 24-1).

Some tumor markers are associated with one type of cancer; others are seen in several cancer types. Many of the better-known markers are also seen in noncancerous conditions. Consequently, these tumor markers are not diagnostic for cancer. However, it is thought that the concentration of tumor markers in blood reflects tumor activity and volume.

Clinically, an ideal tumor marker should be both specific for a given type of cancer and sensitive enough to detect small tumors for early diagnosis or during screening. Unfortunately, few markers are specific for a single individual tumor (tumor-specific markers); most are found with different tumors of the same tissue type (tumor-associated markers). Tumor markers are present in higher quantities in cancer tissue or in blood from cancer patients than in benign tumors or in the blood of healthy subjects. In practice, current tumor markers are most useful for evaluating the progression of disease status after initial therapy and for monitoring subsequent treatment modalities.[21,22]

This chapter begins with general discussions on (1) cancer, (2) the historical background of tumor markers, (3) their clinical applications, (4) how their utility is evaluated, (5) clinical guidelines for their use, and (6) how they are measured. Several clinically relevant tumor markers from each of these categories are then discussed in detail. These are grouped under the general categories of (1) enzymes, (2) hormones, (3) oncofetal antigens, (4) carbohydrate markers, (5) blood group antigens, (6) proteins, (7) receptors, and (8) genes. More detailed information on tumor markers is found in a 2002 textbook on the subject.[71]

CANCER

In 2010, the estimated number of new cancer cases (excluding skin cancer) was 1.53 million. Prostate cancer was the leader among men, and breast cancer was the leader in women, followed by cancer of the lung, colon-rectum, and bladder (men) or uterine corpus (women).[44] Together, diseases of the heart and malignant neoplasms account for 49% of all deaths in the United States. Heart disease remains the leading cause of death in the United States in men and women over the age of 85; however, for those younger than 85 years, cancer has surpassed heart disease as the leading cause of death.[127] Following peak death rates from all cancers in 1990 for men and 1991 for women, death rates decreased by 21.0% in men and 12.3% in women from 1990/1991 to 2006. Death rate reductions in men from lung, prostate, and colorectal cancers accounted for 80% of the decrease, while in women breast and colorectal cancers accounted for 60% of the decrease.[127] These trends support the conclusion that early detection and more effective treatment combined with prevention (e.g., decreasing smoking, improving diet) could reduce the mortality rate of cancer in the future. The American Cancer Society estimates that in 2010, 171,000 deaths are expected to be caused by tobacco use, and one third will likely be related to excess weight, physical inactivity, and poor nutrition.[44]

A simple definition of *cancer* is "a relatively autonomous growth of tissue."[216] Understanding the cause of autonomous growth would clearly facilitate the search for a cure. A *carcinogen* is an agent that causes cancer. A carcinogen may be physical (e.g., radiation), chemical (e.g., a polycyclic hydrocarbon), or biological (e.g., a virus). Exposure to such an agent may cause cancer by producing direct genotoxic effects on deoxyribonucleic acid (DNA) (e.g., as with radiation) or by increasing cell proliferation (e.g., by a hormone), or both (e.g., through the use of tobacco).

TABLE 24-1 Expression of Oncodevelopmental Tumor Markers

		Production of Tumor Markers by Various Tissues		
Marker	**Normal Producing**	**Embryogenically Closely Related**	**Distantly Related**	**Unrelated**
CEA	Colon	Stomach, liver, pancreas	Lung, breast	Lymphoma
AFP	Liver, yolk sac	Colon, stomach, pancreas	Lung	
hCG	Placenta	Germinal tumors	Liver	Epidermal lung
Serotonin	Enteroendocrine carcinoid	Adrenal	Oat cell, lung	Epidermal lung

Modified from Sell S. Cancer markers. In: Moossa AR Schempff SC, Robson MC, eds. Comprehensive textbook of oncology, 2nd edition, volume 1. Baltimore: Williams & Wilkins, 1991:225-38.
AFP, α-Fetoprotein; *CEA*, carcinoembryonic antigen; *hCG*, human chorionic gonadotropin.

Advances in molecular genetics have resulted in a better understanding of the genesis of human cancer. The proliferation of normal cells is thought to be regulated by growth-promoting *oncogenes* and counterbalanced by growth-constraining *tumor suppressor genes*. The development of cancer appears to involve the activation or the altered expression of oncogenes,[1] or the loss or inactivation of a tumor suppressor gene.[297] A pathway to cancer development has been published.[81]

Early detection of cancer offers the best chance for cure. The goal is to diagnose cancer when a tumor is still small enough to be completely removed surgically. Unfortunately, most cancers do not produce symptoms until the tumors are too large to be removed surgically, or until cancerous cells have already spread to other tissue (metastasized).

Although other modes of therapy, such as administration of chemical toxins or irradiation, are effective in destroying most tumor cells, they usually are not curative. The few residual viable tumor cells are able to proliferate, develop resistance to further therapy, and eventually kill the patient.

HISTORICAL BACKGROUND

The first tumor marker reported was the Bence Jones protein. Since its discovery in 1847 by precipitation of a protein in acidified boiled urine,[24] the measurement of Bence Jones protein has been a diagnostic test for multiple myeloma (a tumor of plasma cells). More than 100 years after its discovery, the Nobel Prize–winning studies of Porter and of Edelman and Poulik identified the Bence Jones protein as the monoclonal light chain of immunoglobulin secreted by tumor plasma cells. Monoclonal paraproteins appear as sharp bands in the globulin area in electrophoretic patterns of serum. Multiple myeloma is often diagnosed on the basis of this finding or the finding of an elevated concentration of "monoclonal" immunoglobulin in the serum.[261]

A brief history of tumor markers is shown in Table 24-2.[244] The first period of tumor marker history was the era of the Bence Jones protein. The second era, from 1928 to 1963, included the discovery of hormones, enzymes, isoenzymes, and proteins and their application to the diagnosis of cancer and the beginnings of chromosomal analysis of tumors. Occasionally, such markers were useful in the diagnosis of individual tumors, but the general application of tumor markers for monitoring cancer patients did not start until the third era, with the discovery of α-fetoprotein (AFP) in 1963[2] and carcinoembryonic antigen (CEA) in 1965.[97] The production of such markers during fetal development and in tumors led to use of the term *oncodevelopmental markers*.[85]

The fourth era started in 1975 with the development of monoclonal antibodies and their subsequent use to detect oncofetal antigens and antigens derived from tumor cell lines. Examples include carbohydrate antigens such as CA 125, CA

TABLE 24-2 A Brief History of Tumor Markers

Year	Author	Marker
1846	H. Bence Jones	Bence Jones protein
1928	W. H. Brown	Ectopic hormone syndrome
1930	B. Zondek	hCG
1932	H. Cushing	ACTH
1949	K. Oh-Uti	Deletions of blood group antigens
1959	C. Markert	Isoenzymes
1963	G. I. Abelev	AFP
1965	P. Gold and S. Freeman	CEA
1969	R. Heubner and G. Todaro	Oncogenes
1975	H. Kohler and G. Milstein	Monoclonal antibodies
1980	G. Cooper, R. Weinberg, and M. Bishop	Oncogene probes and transfection
1985	H. Harris, R. Sager, and A. Knudson	Suppressor gene
2001	Multiple investigations	Genomics and proteomics using microarrays, mass spectrometry, neural networks, multiparametric analysis

Modified from Sell S. Cancer markers. In: Moossa AR, Schempff SC, Robson MC, eds. Comprehensive textbook of oncology, 2nd edition, volume 1. Baltimore: Williams & Wilkins, 1991:225-38.
ACTH, Adrenocorticotropic hormone; *AFP*, α-fetoprotein; *CEA*, carcinoembryonic antigen; *hCG*, human chorionic gonadotropin.

15-3, and CA 27.29. Advances in molecular genetics using molecular probes and monoclonal antibodies to detect chromosome or protein alterations, including the study of oncogenes, suppressor genes, and genes involved in DNA repair,[138] have led to the rapid understanding and use of tumor markers at the molecular level. These markers are becoming increasingly useful at the cellular level. For example, mutated *ras* oncogene can be detected in sloughed cellular DNA in fecal material and thus can be used to detect colon cancer.[250] Discovery of the breast cancer susceptibility genes, *BRCA 1* and *BRCA 2,*[177,304] has led to the possibility of screening for familial breast cancer susceptibility in high-risk individuals.[215]

As we begin the 21st century, new technologies are being applied to the discovery of tumor markers and their clinical applications. Notable among these discoveries is the introduction of genomics and proteomics technologies[202] such as the application of complementary DNA (cDNA), protein and tissue microarrays, and the use of mass spectrometry as a diagnostic and discovery tool. Furthermore, the advent of bioinformatic techniques, including neural networks, logistic regression, support vector machines, and other algorithms, is facilitating the use of multiparametric analysis for cancer diagnosis and prognosis, and for prediction of therapy outcomes.[311]

CLINICAL APPLICATIONS

The potential uses of tumor markers are summarized in Table 24-3. In general, tumor markers may be used for (1) diagnosis, prognosis, and prediction; (2) for monitoring the effects of therapy; and (3) as targets for localization and therapy.[246] Ideally, a tumor marker should be produced by tumor cells

TABLE 24-3 Current Applications of Tumor Markers and Their Limitations

Application	Current Usefulness	Comments
Screening for cancer	Limited	1. For screening, you must have a marker that is elevated at early disease stages, when the disease is localized and potentially curable. Most circulating cancer markers (with the exception of PSA) only are elevated notably in the late stages of disease. Thus diagnostic sensitivity is usually low for early-stage disease. 2. With the exception of PSA, most cancer markers are not specific for a particular tissue, and elevations may be due to diseases of other tissue, including benign and inflammatory diseases. Thus diagnostic specificity may be low, leading to many false positives. In screening, there is a necessity for a definitive diagnostic method that will separate true positives from false positives. If this procedure is invasive (e.g., surgery) and/or expensive, patients will not accept it. 3. Screening, even if effective for early cancer diagnosis, must demonstrate benefit to the screened population in terms of survival or other clinical end points.
Diagnosing cancer	Limited	Same as above. Low diagnostic sensitivity and specificity. However, for selected subgroups of high-risk patients in whom the chance of cancer is high (high prevalence), tumor marker analysis may not aid the clinician in ordering more elaborate testing (e.g., imaging techniques, laparoscopic investigations).
Evaluating cancer prognosis	Limited	Most cancer markers have prognostic value, but their accuracy is not good enough to warrant specific therapeutic interventions. For example, higher preoperative concentrations of PSA are associated with capsular penetration, high Gleason score, positive surgical margins, and positive lymph node status, but the decision to treat with two different modalities (e.g., radical prostatectomy vs. nonsurgical approaches) cannot be made based on tumor marker data alone. Same applies to many other cancers.
Prediction of therapeutic response	Important	Despite the importance of using biomarkers in predicting response to specific therapies, very few known markers have such predictive power. These include the steroid hormone receptors for predicting response to antiestrogens and HERr-2/*neu* amplification for predicting response to Herceptin in breast cancer patients. We must have more predictive markers to individualize therapy and maximize clinical response.

Continued

TABLE 24-3 Current Applications of Tumor Markers and Their Limitations—cont'd

Application	Current Usefulness	Comments
Tumor staging	Limited	Same as for prognosis. The data are not good enough for accurate staging unless the value reflects tumor volume.
Detecting tumor recurrence or remission	Controversial	Despite the importance of using biomarkers to detect cancer relapse, current markers are limited by the following: 1. Lead time is short (weeks to a few months) and does not significantly affect outcome, even if therapy is instituted earlier. 2. Therapies for treating recurrent disease are not effective at present. 3. In certain groups of patients, biomarkers are not produced and do not detect relapses. 4. Sometimes biomarkers provide misleading information (e.g., clinical relapses occur without biomarker elevation, or biomarker is elevated nonspecifically, without progressive disease, leading to overtreatment or discontinuation of a current and successful treatment protocol).
Localizing tumor and directing radiotherapeutic agents	Limited	Only a few biomarkers are available for this application, and success is limited at present.
Monitoring the effectiveness of cancer therapy	Important	For patients with advanced disease, who are treated with various modalities, it is important to know if therapy works. In this regard, biomarkers usually provide information that is readily interpretable and more economical, more sensitive, and safer than radiologic or invasive procedures. For certain cancers, this may facilitate increased enrollment of patients into therapeutic clinical trials.

Modified from Diamandis EP. Tumor markers: past, present, and future. In: Diamandis EP, Fritsche HA, Lilja H, Chan DW, Schwartz MK, eds. Tumor markers: physiology, pathobiology, technology, and clinical application. Washington, DC: AACC Press, 2002:5.

and should be detectable in body fluids. It should not be present in healthy people or in benign conditions. Therefore, it could be used for screening for the presence of cancer in asymptomatic individuals in the general population. However, most tumor markers are present in normal, benign, and cancerous tissues and lack specificity. However, if the incidence of cancer is high among certain populations, screening could be feasible. An example is the use of AFP in screening for hepatocellular carcinoma in China and Alaska.[174] Prostate-specific antigen (PSA) has been used in conjunction with digital rectal examination (DRE) for early detection of prostate cancer. Because of elevation of serum PSA in benign prostatic hyperplasia (BPH), PSA velocity and free PSA have been used to improve the detection of prostate cancer.[99]

The clinical staging of cancer is aided by quantification of the marker (i.e., the serum concentration of the marker reflects tumor burden). Marker concentration at the time of diagnosis may be used as a prognostic indicator for disease progression and patient survival. This is possible for an individual patient, but different concentrations of markers produced by different tumors do not usually allow one to determine the prognosis of a tumor from the initial concentration. However, after successful initial treatment, such as surgery, the marker concentration should decrease. The rate of this decrease can be predicted by using the half-life of the marker. For example, the half-life of total PSA is 2 to 3 days, that of human chorionic gonadotropin (hCG) is 12 to 20 hours, and that of AFP is 5 days. If the half-life after treatment is longer than the expected half-life, then treatment has not been successful in removing the tumor. The magnitude of reduction may, however, reflect the degree of success of treatment or the extent of disease involvement.

Targeted therapy in oncology is becoming more effective and will be the therapeutic choice of the future. Tumor markers capable of guiding targeted therapy will improve therapeutic efficacy and will generate less toxicity. Examples in breast cancer are the estrogen and progesterone receptors for the selection of hormonal therapy, HER-2 for the selection of breast cancer patients for trastuzumab (Herceptin) therapy, and Onco*type* DX (Genomic Health, Inc., Redwood City, Calif) for the identification of those patients who most likely will benefit from adjuvant tamoxifen or chemotherapy.

Detecting cancer recurrence may be helpful in initiating early treatment or in changing therapy. The breast cancer marker CA 27.29 has been shown to detect recurrent disease before any clinical evidence is noted in breast cancer patients receiving adjuvant chemotherapy.[54]

Most tumor marker concentrations correlate with effectiveness of treatment and responses to therapy. In breast cancer, the concentration of markers, such as CA 15-3 or CA 27.29, changes with treatment and the clinical outcome of the patient. Concentrations usually increase with progressive disease, decrease with remission, and do not change significantly with stable disease. In reality, tumor marker kinetics in the monitoring of cancer may be more complicated. Marker concentrations in response to treatment may show an initial delay before demonstrating the expected pattern of change.[134]

In addition, antibodies to tumor markers labeled with a radioactive tag are used to localize the tumor masses (radioimmunoscintigraphy)[66] or to provide direction for labeled antibodies to attack the tumor site. Examples include the use of radiolabeled antibodies to CEA to localize colon tumors and the application of labeled antibodies against ferritin to target hepatocellular carcinoma. This approach is also used for treatment by allowing the antibody to bind to the tumor marker epitopes and kill the tumor cell with the dose of radioactivity.[296]

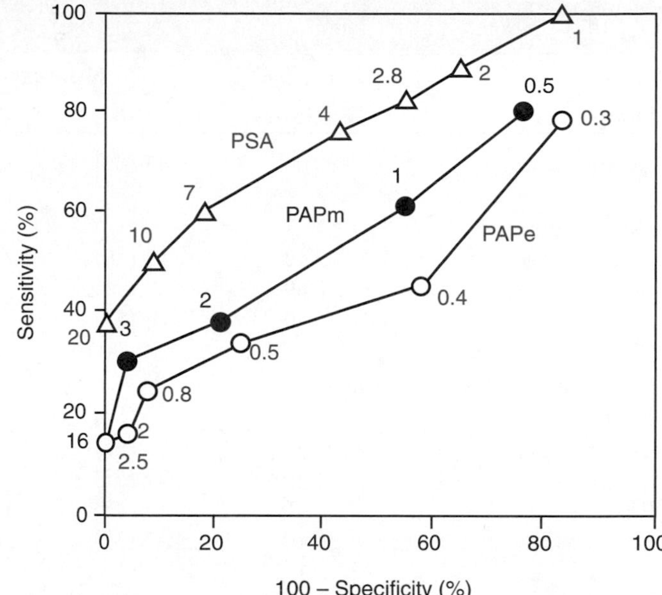

Figure 24-1 Receiver operating characteristic (ROC) curves for prostate-specific antigen (PSA), prostatic acid phosphatase by monoclonal immunoassay (M-PAP), and enzymatic prostatic acid phosphatase (E-PAP). Data for all 128 patients with prostatic disease are plotted, with several quantitative decision cut points (as indicated in the figure) for each assay. Units are µg/L for M-PAP and PSA, and U/L for E-PAP. *(From Rock RC, Chan DW, Bruzek DJ, et al. Evaluation of a monoclonal immunoradiometric assay for prostate-specific antigen. Clin Chem 1987;33:2257-61.)*

EVALUATING CLINICAL UTILITY

To evaluate the clinical usefulness of a tumor marker, it is necessary to establish reference intervals, calculate predictive values, evaluate the distribution of marker concentrations, and determine its role in disease management.

Reference Intervals

Reference intervals of a tumor marker are obtained from a healthy population, preferably using individuals of the same age and sex as those with the cancer of interest.[35] Determination of reference intervals is time-consuming and requires a large healthy population (n = 120 subjects). Statistical analysis based on the mean ± 2 standard deviations (SD) for a population with a Gaussian (normal) distribution is a frequently used method. For a non-Gaussian distribution, the percentile method is a simple approach that is often used (for further discussion of reference intervals, see Chapter 5).

Reference intervals determined using healthy subjects in this fashion are applicable to analytes with physiologically well-defined concentrations. For testing with relatively specific applications, such as the use of tumor markers in the diagnosis and management of cancer, a decision cut point may be more appropriate than the upper limit of the reference population. In most cases, using benign patients as the nondisease group is more appropriate than using a healthy population. The decision cut point can be determined using a predictive value model.

Predictive Value Models

The predictive value model includes the clinical sensitivity and specificity and the predictive value of a test. By varying the decision cut point, clinical sensitivity and specificity will change in opposite directions. An optimal decision cut point can be selected on the basis of strategies outlined in Chapter 3.

A useful approach to evaluating multiple tests for the same analyte or multiple markers for the same type of cancer is the *receiver operating characteristic* (ROC) curve.[253] The ROC curve can be constructed by plotting sensitivity versus 1 minus specificity, or the true-positive rate versus the false-positive rate. The advantage of the ROC curve is the display of performance over the entire range of decision points. One can pinpoint the decision cut point at which optimal sensitivity and specificity can be achieved. By superimposing the ROC curves of several markers, the best predictive marker can be selected. An example is shown in Figure 24-1. Preparation of an ROC curve has been discussed in detail by Zweig and Robertson[314] and is covered in Chapter 3 of this text.

Distribution of Markers

Application of the predictive value model is difficult for analytes that are not diagnostic for a single disease. Concentrations of most, if not all, tumor markers are elevated in more than one disease condition. When the predictive value model is used, it is necessary to select a population that includes groups with and without disease. What patients should be included in these two groups? The decision should be based on the specific clinical questions asked. If the question concerns the diagnostic sensitivity of CEA for active colorectal carcinoma, the disease group should include only those patients with active colorectal carcinoma. Selection of the nondisease group is more challenging. Should healthy individuals and those with benign conditions be included? If so, how many benign condition groups should be included?

TABLE 24-4 CA 549 Distribution

Diagnosis	No. of Patients	Number (and %) of Patients With CA 549 Values, kU/L					
		0-8	>8	>11	>15	>20	>25
Normal women	100	85 (85)	15 (15)	5 (5)	0 (0)	0 (0)	0 (0)
Nonmalignant							
Benign liver	42	19 (45)	23 (55)	11 (26)	3 (7)	0 (0)	0 (0)
Benign breast	69	63 (91)	6 (9)	1 (1)	1 (1)	0 (0)	0 (0)
Pregnancy	30	26 (87)	4 (13)	0 (0)	0 (0)	0 (0)	0 (0)
Nonbreast Metastatic Cancer							
Endometrial	8	7 (88)	1 (12)	1 (12)	1 (12)	1 (12)	0 (0)
Colon	41	25 (61)	16 (39)	7 (17)	3 (7)	1 (2)	1 (2)
Lung	40	22 (55)	18 (45)	13 (33)	11 (28)	6 (15)	6 (15)
Prostate	30	13 (43)	17 (57)	12 (40)	5 (17)	5 (17)	3 (10)
Ovarian	60	22 (37)	38 (63)	30 (50)	21 (35)	15 (25)	10 (17)
Breast Cancer							
Adjuvant	88	61 (69)	27 (31)	10 (11)	6 (9)	4 (5)	0 (0)
Metastatic							
Complete remission	16	11 (69)	5 (31)	3 (19)	1 (6)	1 (6)	1 (6)
Partial remission	52	12 (23)	40 (77)	33 (63)	27 (52)	22 (42)	16 (31)
No Response (Progressive)							
Local	12	5 (42)	7 (58)	5 (42)	3 (25)	2 (17)	2 (17)
Metastasis	94	7 (7)	87 (93)	83 (88)	79 (84)	73 (78)	69 (73)

From Chan DW, Beveridge RA, Bruzek DJ, et al. Monitoring breast cancer with CA 549. Clin Chem 1988;34:2000-4.

Should patients with no evidence of disease be included as well, because they do not have active disease? Values calculated for sensitivity and specificity greatly depend on the types of groups included and on the number of patients in each group (see Chapter 3 for a discussion on the effect of spectrum on sensitivity and specificity).

The distribution of tumor marker concentrations is usually shown as the percentage of patients with elevated concentrations as determined using various cutoffs in healthy, benign, and cancerous groups. When available, international staging criteria should be used to classify cancer patients. Diagnosis should be based on pathologic findings. In breast cancer, for example (Table 24-4), normal women are used as the healthy population for comparison. Nonmalignant or benign groups are selected to include people with the most likely causes of marker elevation: benign liver and breast diseases, and pregnancy. Nonbreast metastatic cancer groups are selected to show the specificity of the marker using endometrial, colon, lung, prostate, ovarian carcinoma, and others.

Grouping all breast cancer patients into a single category is not satisfactory because most markers are elevated in active breast cancer. The adjuvant group consists of patients who had no metastasis, underwent mastectomy and treatment with adjuvant chemotherapy, and have no evidence of disease. The marker concentration is not expected to be elevated. The metastasis group includes patients' complete remission, partial remission, or with progressive breast cancer accompanied by local or distant metastases. The progressive breast cancer group should have the highest percentage of elevated marker concentrations. The partial remission group should have an intermediate percentage of elevated marker concentrations. The complete remission group should have the lowest percentage of elevated marker concentrations.

Disease Management

Most tumor markers are used to monitor treatment and progression of cancer. Selection of patient groups is important to illustrate the usefulness of the marker in various clinical settings. Markers may be used to determine the success of initial treatment (e.g., surgery, radiation), to detect the recurrence of cancer, and to monitor the effectiveness of the treatment modality.

An elevated marker concentration before surgery should fall after a successful operation. The extent of the decrease in marker concentration depends on pretreatment tumor involvement.

With recurrence of cancer after successful initial treatment, the marker concentration may not fall within the expected time according to its half-life. It may fall to a steady concentration that is higher than normal, or it may fall within the reference interval of healthy individuals. A subsequent rise in the marker concentration suggests cancer recurrence.

In monitoring the effectiveness of cancer therapy, marker concentration should increase with the progression of cancer, decrease with the regression of cancer, and not change in the presence of stable disease. When candidate markers are evaluated, all events related to the progression, stability, and regression of disease can be grouped; whether the marker concentration changes in the predicted direction in all these situations can be evaluated next.

The Working Group on Tumor Marker Criteria of the International Society for Oncodevelopmental Biology and Medicine has published the following criteria for the interpretation of changes in tumor markers.[35]

> "If no therapy is given, at least a linear increase in three consecutive samples (i.e., two time intervals) on a log scale should be registered to establish a recurrence. Usual intervals could be three months but are clinically determined. After a first increase, next samples should be taken after 2 to 4 weeks, irrespective of the absolute concentration."

If therapy is given, changes in marker concentrations should reflect the clinical progression of the disease. "Progressive disease is defined by an increase in the marker concentration of at least 25%. Sampling should be repeated within 2 to 4 weeks for additional evidence … The sampling interval during therapy may depend on the type of tumor and should be related to clinical follow-up." A decrease in marker concentration of at least 50% is indicative of partial remission "with the concept that tumor load is related to the changes in serum tumor marker concentrations." The Working Group also provided the general opinion that "a complete remission cannot be determined by marker concentrations, but if tumor marker concentrations are elevated, the clinical decision of complete remission based on conventional methods should be considered incorrect unless an explanation for the presence of the elevated concentration is given."

CLINICAL GUIDELINES

The diagnosis and staging of cancer involve a number of tools, including (1) physical examination, (2) imaging, and (3) laboratory studies. Application of these tools has resulted in several tumor markers that are used for screening, diagnosis, staging, and prognosis, and for directing treatment modalities. However, not all tumor markers are appropriate for all uses, and not all cancers have established tumor markers. Therefore, each type of cancer and each tumor marker must be properly evaluated for use, and clinicians must be educated regarding proper use of tumor markers to conserve resources.

Several national and international groups have released guidelines on the selection and clinical use of tumor markers. These groups include the National Academy of Clinical Biochemistry (NACB), the European Group on Tumor Markers (EGTM), the American Cancer Society (ACS), the American Society for Clinical Oncology (ASCO), and others. All of these groups are composed of experts in the areas being assessed, and a number of criteria are used to form the recommendations, including the level of evidence for the tumor marker and the tumor marker utility grading system (TMUGS).[71] Table 24-5 summarizes the recommendations of several groups.

ANALYTICAL METHODS

Tumor markers are measured by a variety of analytical techniques, including enzyme assay (see Chapters 15 and 22); immunoassay (see Chapter 16); receptor assay and instrumental techniques such as chromatography (see Chapter 13); electrophoresis (see Chapter 12); and mass spectrometry interfaced with liquid or gas chromatographs (see Chapter 13) and microarrays (see Chapter 18). Details of these techniques are found in the indicated chapters. Here we expand on the use of mass spectrometry and microarrays for the assay of protein and genetic tumor markers.

Mass Spectrometry

Mass spectrometry for small molecules has been used in the clinical laboratory for many years. However, developments have allowed for the mass spectrometric identification of high molecular weight compounds, including proteins and nucleic acids. The new ionization technologies were recognized by the Nobel Prize in Chemistry in 2002. These advances triggered investigations toward using the technology for cancer diagnostics or for discovery of new cancer biomarkers. In one approach, sera or other fluids from cancer patients or controls are treated with various adsorbing surfaces, such as ion-exchange, hydrophobic, or metal-binding chips. After excess proteins are washed out, the chips are subjected to mass spectrometric analysis by using MALDI (matrix-assisted laser desorption ionization) or SELDI (surface-enhanced laser desorption ionization)-TOF (time-of-flight) mass spectrometry. This analysis generates many peaks of various M-Z (mass-to-charge) ratios. By comparing these proteomic patterns with patterns obtained from samples from individuals without cancer, and by using sophisticated bioinformatic and computational tools, it is possible to identify patterns that are associated only with cancer. This technology has been investigated for the detection of ovarian,[212,222,312] prostate,[3,214] bladder, and many other cancers,[230] and its use has been reviewed.[202,213,214,267] However, the method has not as yet been prospectively evaluated, and clinical trials are in progress.

A more promising approach is to use this technology to identify novel cancer biomarkers.[155,222,230,312] To date, several molecules have been identified, including (1) apolipoprotein A1, (2) transthyretin fragment, (3) inter-α-trypsin inhibitor, (4) haptoglobin-α subunit, (5) vitamin D–binding protein, and others. Most of these molecules are present in serum at concentrations higher than concentrations of traditional cancer biomarkers. In most cases, these candidate biomarkers are in the process of being validated. OVA1 (Vermillion, Inc., Austin, Tex), a panel of biomarkers for ovarian cancer,[222,312] is the first proteomic IVDMIA (in vitro diagnostic multivariate

TABLE 24-5 Summary of Key Guideline Recommendations*

Cancer Type	NACB	ASCO	ACS	EGTM
Breast	• ER and PR and HER-2 in all cancers for predicting response to therapy • CA 15-3/CA 27.29 and CEA for monitoring advanced disease • Tissue UPA/PAI-1 by ELISA for prognosis in node-negative breast cancer • Onco*type* DX for predicting recurrence in node-negative, ER-positive breast cancer patients receiving adjuvant tamoxifen	• Routine use of CA 15-3, CA 27.29, or CEA alone *not* recommended • Increasing CA 15-3, CA 27.29, and CEA may be used to suggest treatment failure • ER and PR determined for primary lesions. Steroid hormone receptors to be used to select patients for endocrine therapy • HER-2 overexpression or amplification in tissue may be used to select patients for Herceptin (trastuzumab) therapy • Tissue UPA/PAI-1 by ELISA for prognosis in node-negative breast cancer • Onco*type* DX for predicting recurrence/treatment response to tamoxifen in node-negative, ER-positive breast cancer	None	• Steroid receptors in tissue predicting response to hormone therapy • CEA and one *MUC1* gene–related protein in serum for prognosis, follow-up, and monitoring of therapy • HER-2/*neu* in tissue for predicting response to Herceptin (trastuzumab) in patients with advanced disease
Ovarian	CA 125 as an aid in diagnosis and for monitoring therapy, detection of recurrence, and prognosis	None	None	CA 125 as an aid in diagnosis, for monitoring treatment, and for early prediction of recurrence
Prostate	• PSA for early detection (with DRE), prognosis, and monitoring • % fPSA for PSA between 4 and 10 μg/L and negative DRE	None	PSA (DRE optional) screening and detection	• PSA with DRE for screening (studies), case finding, or prognosis • PSA in follow-up and monitoring of therapy • % fPSA for differential diagnosis when PSA is between 4 and 10 μg/L and DRE is negative
Germ cell	• AFP, hCG, LD for diagnosis/case finding, staging/prognosis, recurrence, and monitoring of therapy in testicular tumors • AFP for differential diagnosis of NSGCT	None	None	AFP, hCG, LD, and PLAP[†] for case finding, staging, prognosis, follow-up, and monitoring of therapy. AFP is diagnostic for NSGCT
Colon	CEA for prognosis, postoperative surveillance, and monitoring advanced disease	CEA for prognosis, detecting recurrence, and monitoring therapy	None	CEA for case finding, prognosis, follow-up, and monitoring of therapy

TABLE 24-5 Summary of Key Guideline Recommendations—cont'd

Cancer Type	NACB	ASCO	ACS	EGTM
Lung	CEA and CYFRA 21-1 in NSCLC and NSE and ProGRP in SCLC for differential diagnosis, postoperative surveillance, monitoring of therapy in advanced disease, and detection of recurrence, and CYFRA 21-1 in NSCLC for prognosis	None	None	• NSE in differential diagnosis • CEA, CYFRA 21-1, and/or NSE for follow-up and monitoring of therapy

*"None" indicates that the relevant group has not yet considered this type of cancer.
†Placental alkaline phosphatase (PLAP) is for monitoring of seminomas in nonsmokers only.
ACS, American Cancer Society; *ASCO*, American Society of Clinical Oncology; *EGTM*, European Group on Tumor Markers; *fPSA*, free PSA; *NACB*, National Academy of Clinical Biochemistry; *NSGCT*, nonseminomatous germ cell tumors; *tPSA*, total PSA.
From Sturgeon CM, Duffy MJ, Stenmab UH, et al; National Academy of Clinical Biochemistry. National Academy of Clinical Biochemistry laboratory medicine practice guidelines for use of tumor markers in testicular, prostate, colorectal, breast, and ovarian cancers. Clin Chem 2008;54:e11-79; Harris L, Fritsche H, Mennel R, et al; American Society of Clinical Oncology. American Society of Clinical Oncology 2007 update of recommendations for the use of tumor markers in breast cancer. J Clin Oncol 2007;25:5287-312; Wolf AM, Wender RC, Etzioni RB, et al. American Cancer Society guideline for the early detection of prostate cancer: update 2010. CA Cancer J Clin 2010;60:70-98, available at: http://www.egtm.eu/.

index assay) cleared by the U.S. Food and Drug Administration (FDA).

Microarrays

A microarray uses a solid material such as a microchip of silicon that contains a large number of elements ("spots") in a two-dimensional array. To each of these spots are attached different molecules of immobilized short oligonucleotides (e.g., Affymetrix chips; Affymetrix, Santa Clara, Calif) and cDNAs of various genes, proteins, antibodies, etc.[159,188,237] It is possible to immobilize up to 20,000 to 40,000 elements on such chips; consequently, genome-wide analysis at both messenger ribonucleic acid (mRNA) and protein concentrations is now possible. Commercially available protein microarrays such as the ProtoArrays from Life Technologies Inc. (Carlsbad, Calif) contain as many as 10,000 immobilized proteins. Applications of microarrays include quantitative assessment of gene expression, detection of mutations and polymorphisms (such as single-nucleotide polymorphisms), DNA sequencing, the study of protein expression and protein-protein interactions, and the detection of autoantibodies.

These devices have been used to discover new candidate biomarkers. For example, Welsh and colleagues used microarray analysis of gene expression profiles of normal and cancerous tissues and identified highly overexpressed genes in ovarian and other cancers.[298,299] These overexpressed genes were then to be evaluated further with more quantitative techniques, such as reverse-transcriptase polymerase chain reaction, to confirm the overexpression. Identification of an overexpressed gene can be followed by development of assays to measure the protein and then evaluate it as a serologic or tissue biomarker.[298] Some successes of this process have been reported (e.g., the identification of osteopontin and HE4 as ovarian cancer biomarkers).[116,153]

Another application of microarrays is their use in the classification of cancers based on their gene expression profiles. Numerous examples of subclassifying breast, ovarian, prostate, brain, hematologic, and other cancers using this technology have been described.[133,211] Especially for breast cancer, it has been realized that tissue microarray analysis may stratify patients according to prognosis.[290,291] Van de Vijver and associates showed that a relatively small number of genes (about 70) can be used to classify patients into high- and low-risk groups. This method has been applied clinically to select breast cancer patients for adjuvant chemotherapy.

The application of microarrays for cancer classification and prognosis and for discovery of new cancer biomarkers is relatively new. This method has the potential to revolutionize cancer prognosis and prediction of therapy by using dedicated chips. However, further standardization is necessary.

ENZYMES

Enzymes were one of the first groups of tumor markers identified. Their elevated activities were used to indicate the presence of cancer.[101] Measurement of enzymes was relatively easy using spectrophotometric determination of enzymatic activities. With the introduction of radioimmunoassay (RIA) in the late 1950s, the mass of an enzyme could be measured as a protein antigen instead of its catalytic activity.

With few exceptions, an increase in the activity or mass of an enzyme or isoenzyme is not specific or sensitive enough to be used to identify the type of cancer or the specific organ involvement. An exception is PSA. PSA has mild protease activity and amino acid sequence homology with serine proteases of the kallikrein family.[60,70] It is expressed by normal, benign, hyperplastic, and cancerous prostate glands and minimally by other tissue.[32] Until the application of PSA as a marker for prostate cancer, tumor enzymes had lost most of their popularity for use as cancer markers.[101,243] Enzymes were used historically as tumor markers before the discovery of oncofetal antigens and the advent of monoclonal antibodies.[242] Abnormalities of enzymes as a marker for cancer include expression of the fetal form of the enzyme (isozyme) and ectopic production of enzymes.

Enzymes are present in much higher concentrations inside the cell. Enzymes are released into the systemic circulation as the result of tumor necrosis or following a change in membrane permeability of cancer cells. Increased enzymes are also observed in the blockage of pancreatic or biliary ducts and in renal insufficiency. The intracellular location of the enzyme may determine the rate of release. By the time enzymes are released into the systemic circulation, tumor metastasis may have occurred. Most enzymes are not unique for a specific organ. Therefore, enzymes are most suitable as nonspecific tumor markers. Elevated enzymes may signal the presence of malignancy.

Isoenzymes and multiple forms of enzymes may provide additional organ specificity. Table 24-6 summarizes various enzymes, their associated types of malignancy, and the assays used to measure their activity (Act) or their mass concentration (immunoassay). Enzymes are traditionally measured by their activities. With the introduction of antibody techniques, some enzymes, such as PSA, are measured as protein antigens rather than by their enzyme activity.

Alkaline Phosphatase

Alkaline phosphatase may arise from liver, bone, or placenta. The alkaline phosphatase in the sera of normal adults comes primarily from the liver or biliary tract. Elevated alkaline phosphatase is seen in primary or secondary liver cancer. Quantification may be helpful in evaluating metastatic cancer with bone or liver involvement. Greatest elevations are seen in patients with osteoblastic lesions, such as in those with prostatic cancer with bone metastases. Minimal elevations are seen in patients with osteolytic lesions, such as those with breast cancer with bone metastases.[84,278]

In liver metastases, serum alkaline phosphatase shows a better correlation with the extent of liver involvement than the results of other liver tests. To determine the origin of elevated alkaline phosphatase, tests of other liver enzymes may be performed. Elevations in 5′-nucleotidase or γ-glutamyltransferase suggest that the elevated alkaline phosphatase is of liver, not bone, origin. Determination of alkaline phosphatase isoenzymes may provide additional specificity. The liver isoenzyme is thermally more stable than the bone isoenzyme (see Chapter 22 for a more detailed discussion). Other malignancies, such as leukemia, sarcoma,

TABLE 24-6 Enzymes as Tumor Markers

Enzyme	Assay	Type of Cancer
Alcohol dehydrogenase	Act	Liver
Aldolase	Act	Liver
Alkaline phosphatase	Act	Bone, liver, leukemia, sarcoma
Alkaline phosphatase—placental	Act	Ovarian, lung, trophoblastic, gastrointestinal, seminoma, Hodgkin's
Amylase	Act	Pancreatic, various
Aryl sulfatase B	Act	Colon, breast
Creatine kinase-BB	IMA	Prostate, lung (small cell), breast, colon, ovarian
Esterase	Act	Breast
Galactosyltransferase	Act	Colon, bladder, gastrointestinal, various
γ-Glutamyltransferase	Act	Liver
Hexokinase	Act	Liver
Lactate dehydrogenase	Act	Liver, lymphoma, leukemia, various
Leucine aminopeptidase	Act	Pancreatic, liver
Neuron-specific enolase	IMA	Lung (small cell), neuroblastoma, carcinoid, melanoma, pheochromocytoma, pancreatic
5′-Nucleotidase	Act/IMA	Liver
Prostatic acid phosphatase	Act/IMA	Prostate
PSA	IMA	Prostate
Pyruvate kinase	Act	Liver, various
Ribonuclease	Act	Various (ovarian, lung, large bowel)
Sialyltransferase	Act	Breast, colon, lung
Terminal deoxytransferase	Act	Leukemia
Thymidine kinase	Act/IMA	Various, leukemia, lymphoma, lung (small cell)

Act, Activity; *IMA*, immunoassay.

and lymphoma complicated with hepatic infiltration, may also elevate alkaline phosphatase.

Placental alkaline phosphatase (PALP) is synthesized by the trophoblast and is elevated in the sera of pregnant women. PALP was first identified as the Regan isoenzyme in 1968 by Fishman and colleagues[85] and was recognized as one of the first oncodevelopmental markers, along with AFP and CEA. It is elevated in a variety of malignancies, including ovarian, lung, trophoblastic, and gastrointestinal cancers; seminoma; and Hodgkin's disease.

Creatine Kinase

Creatine kinase catalyzes the phosphorylation of creatine by adenosine triphosphate. CK is a dimer consisting of two subunits—M (muscle) and B (brain)—and three isoenzymes—CK1 (BB), CK2 (MB), and CK3 (MM). CK1 is present in the (1) brain, (2) prostate gland, (3) gastrointestinal tract, (4) lung, (5) bladder, (6) uterus, and (7) placenta. Cardiac muscle has the highest concentration of CK2 (>20%). CK3 is present in skeletal and cardiac muscles.

Elevations in CK1 have been demonstrated in prostate cancer and small cell carcinoma of the lung. Although it is also elevated in other malignancies, such as those of the breast, colon, ovary, and stomach, the clinical usefulness of CK1 as a tumor marker requires further investigation.[243] CK isoenzymes have been included in a prostate cancer panel, "ProstAsure."[14,269] The ProstAsure Index is a neural network–derived algorithm for the early detection of prostate cancer that also includes PSA PAP, and age.

Lactate Dehydrogenase

Lactate dehydrogenase (LD) is an enzyme in the glycolytic pathway that is released as the result of cell damage. Elevation of LD in malignancy is rather nonspecific. It has been demonstrated in a variety of cancers, including liver cancer, non-Hodgkin's lymphoma, acute leukemia, nonseminomatous germ cell testicular cancer, seminoma, neuroblastoma, and other carcinomas, such as breast, colon, stomach, and lung cancer. Serum LD has been shown to correlate with tumor mass in solid tumors and provides a prognostic indicator for disease progression. Its value in the monitoring of therapy is rather limited. The LD isoenzymes provide only marginal specificity for organ involvement. For example, elevation of the LD5 isoenzyme is associated with liver metastases. Elevation of LD5 in the spinal fluid may be an early indication of central nervous system metastases.[243]

Neuron-Specific Enolase

Neuron-specific enolase (NSE) is the γ subunit of the glycolytic enzyme phosphopyruvate hydrolase, which exists as a homodimer ($\gamma\gamma$) and a heterodimer ($\alpha\gamma$). The enzyme is found in neuronal tissue and cells of the diffuse neuroendocrine system. NSE therefore is associated with tumors of neuroendocrine origin. NSE is released into the blood as a result of cell lysis as opposed to secretion. NSE is also released into CSF with neuronal injury. NSE is found in tumors associated with neuroendocrine origin, including small cell lung cancer (SCLC), neuroblastoma, pheochromocytoma, carcinoid, medullary carcinoma of the thyroid, melanoma, and pancreatic endocrine tumor.

Serum NSE concentrations have been measured by immunoassay. Using a cutoff of 12.5 μg/mL, NSE has a clinical sensitivity of 80% in patients with SCLC with a clinical specificity of 80 to 90%. The NSE concentration appears to correlate with stage and provides a useful prognosis for disease progression. The value of NSE in detecting disease relapse has not been proved. Although the findings are mixed, NSE appears to be useful in monitoring chemotherapy and correlates with disease state. Immunostaining of NSE may provide the differential diagnosis between SCLC and other histologic carcinoma types.

Among children with advanced neuroblastoma, more than 90% have been reported to have elevated serum concentrations of NSE. High concentrations of NSE are associated with poor prognosis, and concentrations seem to correlate with the stage of the disease. Monitoring therapy using serum NSE is controversial, particularly with respect to the issue of specificity. However, elevated concentrations of NSE in children with stage IV neuroblastoma were associated with a poorer outcome.[309]

Prostatic Acid Phosphatase

The acid phosphatases include all phosphatases that hydrolyze phosphate esters with an optimum pH of less than 7.0. They are present in the lysozymes of secretory epithelial cells. Although acid phosphatase is produced primarily by the (1) prostate gland, it is also found in (2) erythrocytes, (3) platelets, (4) leukocytes, (5) bone marrow, (6) bone, (7) liver, (8) spleen, (9) kidney, and (10) intestine.

Prostatic acid phosphatase (PAP), with an optimum pH of 5 to 6, is very labile at a pH of greater than 7.0 and a temperature greater than 37 °C. It can be distinguished from other acid phosphatases by using tartrate, which strongly inhibits the prostatic form. Another approach is to select substrates that are more specific for PAP, including thymolphthalein monophosphate (Roy method—most specific) and β-naphthol phosphate. Acid phosphatase was first used as a tumor marker in 1938 by Gutman and colleagues.[101] PAP was measured first by its enzymatic activity, then with the use of counterimmunoelectrophoresis, and subsequently, in the late 1970s, by RIA. Elevated serum PAP may be seen in malignant conditions such as osteogenic sarcoma, multiple myeloma, and bone metastases of other cancers. It also may be elevated in some benign conditions, such as BPH, osteoporosis, and hyperparathyroidism. For clinical use, PAP has been replaced by PSA.[40] PAP is not as sensitive as PSA for detection of early cancer. It is less likely to be elevated in BPH than is PSA. However, as an individual marker, PAP may be useful for disease management in the rare patient whose tumor does not secrete PSA, and it may have utility when combined with other markers for improving prostate cancer detection[15] or predicting recurrence after radical prostatectomy.[108] Currently, the method of choice for PAP is measurement of its enzymatic activity.

KALLIKREINS

Kallikreins constitute a subgroup of the serine protease enzyme family, three members of which have been assigned a specific biological role.

Biochemistry

The human kallikrein (hK) gene locus spans a region of approximately 300 kb of chromosome 19q13.4, which contains 15 tandemly localized kallikrein genes (*KLK1* to *KLK15*) with no intervention from other genes. This is the largest cluster of serine proteases within the human genome. Members of the kallikrein family are identified by various similar features.[73] All have a nearly identical genetic structure (5′ untranslated region, intron-exon size and organization), and the catalytic triad of serine proteases is conserved by all members, with the histidine always occurring near the end of the second exon, the aspartate in the middle of the third exon, and the serine residue at the beginning of the fifth exon. All kallikreins are produced as prepropeptides with a 17 to 20 amino acid signal sequence and a 4 to 9 amino acid activation peptide. They contain 10 to 12 conserved cysteines that form 5 to 6 disulfide bonds. Finally, most if not all genes are under steroid hormone control.

Kallikreins are expressed in a wide variety of tissues, including (1) prostate, (2) breast, (3) ovary, and (4) testis.[306] For example, KLK3 (PSA) is highly expressed in prostate and is discussed in detail later in the chapter. KLK3 also has minor expression in breast, thyroid, salivary glands, lung, and trachea, and KLK11 and KLK12 are highly expressed in more than 10 tissues, with minor expression in at least four others.

Only 3 of the 15 kallikreins have been assigned a specific biological role. The major biological role of hK1 is the release of lysyl-bradykinin (kallidin) from low molecular weight kininogen; however, it has been implicated in the processing of peptide hormones, including proinsulin, low-density lipoprotein (LDL), prorenin, the precursor of atrial natriuretic peptide, and vasoactive intestinal peptide. The role of hK2 has only recently been investigated with seminal plasma hK2 found to cleave seminogelin I and II, but at different sites than hK3 (PSA). Furthermore, a role for hK2 in the regulation of growth factors through the proteolysis of insulin-like growth factor binding protein 3 (IGFBP-3) has been suggested. hK3, also known as PSA, is found not only in prostate tissue (discussed later), but in relatively high concentrations in nipple aspirate fluid, breast cyst fluid, breast milk, amniotic fluid, and tumor extracts.[32] Its presence in these fluids and tissues suggests a biological function in the breast and a possible role in fetal development; however, no specific function in these tissues has been identified to date.

Clinical Applications

The role of kallikreins as tumor markers is rather varied.[79] Several kallikreins have been associated with hormonal malignancies such as (1) prostate, (2) breast, (3) testicular, and (4) ovarian cancers. The roles of hK3 (PSA) and hK2 are discussed in detail later in the chapter. hK6 has been investigated as a serum marker for the diagnosis, prognosis, and monitoring of ovarian cancer,[72] and as a cytosolic marker for prognosis in breast cancer. Serum hK5, hK6, hK10, and hK11 have also been investigated for the diagnosis and monitoring of ovarian cancer,[168,307,308] and a high concentration of cytosolic hK10 in ovarian tumor and breast cells is a poor prognostic marker.[166,167] Kallikrein gene expression is associated with both positive and negative prognoses in various cancers, including prostate, ovarian, and breast cancers.[73]

Analytical Methods

Reverse-transcriptase polymerase chain reaction (RT-PCR), Northern and Western blotting, and immunoassays have been used for detection of kallikrein mRNA and protein in tissue extracts of (1) ovarian, (2) breast, (3) testicular, and (4) prostate tumors. Immunohistochemical techniques have been used for the detection of KLK7 in ovarian tumors and KLK10 in ovarian and testicular tumors. Serum concentrations of KLK3 (PSA) and KLK11 are evaluated by immunoassy.

PROSTATE-SPECIFIC ANTIGEN

Prostate cancer is the leading cancer in older men. When detected early (organ confined), it is potentially curable by radical prostatectomy. Therefore, early detection is important and PSA is widely used for this purpose. It is considered one of the most promising tumor markers available.

In the 1970s, several groups independently discovered prostate antigens for use in forensics and as tumor markers.[257] In 1971, Hara and colleagues identified a protein in seminal plasma that they named *γ-seminoprotein.* Li and Beling isolated the same protein from seminal plasma and called it *protein E1* because it had slow β-mobility in electrophoresis and a molecular weight (MW) of 31,000 Da. In 1978, Sensabaugh characterized this glycoprotein with isoelectric points between 6.5 and 8.0 and MW of approximately 30,000 Da and called it *p30.* In 1979, Wang and coworkers purified a protein from prostatic tissue and called it *prostate-specific antigen.* γ-Seminoprotein, p30, and PSA are biochemically very similar. PSA is found in normal, benign, hypertrophic, and malignant prostatic tissues. Originally, it was thought that PSA was solely expressed in prostate tissue. However, it was later found that PSA also is expressed in numerous other tissues, most notably hormonally regulated tissue such as breast tissue. Low concentrations of PSA are detectable in sera from women as well as in nipple aspirate fluid.

Biochemistry

PSA is a single-chain glycoprotein that is 7% carbohydrate. It has 237 amino acid residues and four carbohydrate side-chains with linkages at amino acid 45 (asparagine), 69 (serine), 70 (threonine), and 71 (serine). The N-terminal amino acid is isoleucine, and the C-terminal residue is proline. Its MW is 28,430 Da,[23] and it has isoelectric points from 6.8 to 7.2 because of its various isoforms. The three-dimensional structure and the antigenic domain of PSA have been characterized.[60]

The complete gene encoding PSA has been sequenced and located on chromosome 19.[165] It is similar to the kallikrein-1 gene with 82% homology. Functionally, PSA is a serine protease of the kallikrein family. It is produced exclusively by epithelial cells of the acini and ducts of the prostate gland. PSA is secreted into the lumina of the prostatic duct. In seminal fluid, PSA cleaves seminal vesicle–specific proteins into several low molecular weight proteins as part of the process of liquefaction of the seminal coagulum. Therefore, PSA possesses chymotrypsin-like and trypsin-like activity. Autodigestion of PSA has been reported at three possible locations: *LYS* 148, *LYS* 185, and *ARG* 85. The addition of protease inhibitors may be important to prevent autohydrolysis of PSA in solution.[60] The PSA promoter contains three androgen response elements and can be activated by androgens, progestins, and glucocorticoids.

Molecular Forms of Prostate-Specific Antigen

PSA exists in two major forms in blood circulation. Most PSA is complexed with the protease inhibitors α_1-antichymotrypsin (ACT) (MW, 100,000 Da) and α_2-macroglobulin (AMG), and a minor component is free PSA (MW, 28,430 Da).[156,275] Most immunoassays measure both free and ACT-complexed PSA but not PSA-AMG, which is sterically inhibited. In human seminal fluid, approximately 60 to 70% of PSA is enzymatically active, and the remainder inactive. Inactive forms of free PSA are composed of three distinct molecular forms: BPSA, pPSA, and iPSA.[178] BPSA is a degraded form of free PSA containing two internal peptide bond cleavages at Lys 145 and Lys 183; BPSA in tissue is relatively localized in the transition zone of the prostate and contributes to free PSA in BPH serum. pPSA is the proenzyme or precursor form of PSA that has a 7 amino acid proleader peptide. Additional truncated forms of pPSA with varying amino acids exist. Activation of pPSA, resulting from cleavage of the leader sequence by hK2 and trypsin, becomes more resistant as the number of amino acids in the pro-leader peptide decreases. pPSA is localized in the peripheral zone of the prostate and contributes to free PSA in cancer serum. iPSA consists of minor variants of intact PSA that is enzymatically inactive as the result of conformational changes.

Physiologic Properties

The metabolic clearance rate of PSA follows a two-compartment model, with initial half-lives of 1.2 and 0.75 hours for free PSA and total PSA and subsequent half-lives of 22 and 33 hours.[206] Because of this relatively long half-life, at least 2 to 3 weeks may be necessary for the serum PSA to return to baseline concentrations after certain procedures, including transrectal biopsy, transurethral resection of the prostate, and radical prostatectomy. Benign prostatic conditions, such as BPH and prostatitis, can also elevate PSA concentrations. Although the DRE typically causes no clinically important effects on serum PSA concentrations in most patients, in some it may lead to a twofold elevation. 5α-Reductase inhibitors, such as finasteride, for treatment of BPH cause a decrease in PSA concentrations of approximately 50%; thus results should be adjusted. Significant physiologic variation in serum PSA concentrations (up to 30%) has also been noted.

Clinical Applications

PSA is an extremely useful tumor marker and is used to detect and monitor treatment of prostate cancer.

Screening and Early Detection of Prostate Cancer

PSA testing by itself is limited in the screening or detection of early prostate cancer because PSA is specific for prostatic tissue but not for prostatic cancer. BPH is a common disease in men 50 years of age and older. Studies have shown that PSA concentrations in patients with BPH are similar yet statistically different from those associated with early prostatic cancer (i.e., those of patients with organ-confined cancer).[193] Unfortunately, the overlap of PSA concentrations between these two groups is so extensive, particularly between 4 and 10 μg/L, that selecting an optimum cutoff of PSA for the recommendation of a prostate biopsy is almost impossible. Results from the Prostate Cancer Prevention Trial showed the presence of prostate cancer over all ranges of PSA.[286] The clinical sensitivity of PSA is 78% at the typically used cutoff of 4.0 μg/L. By lowering the cutoff to 2.8 μg/L, sensitivity increases to 92%, whereas specificity decreases from 33 to 23%. Raising the cutoff to 8 μg/L improves the specificity to 90%.[55] Cutoffs lower than 4 μg/L have been suggested, such as by the National Comprehensive Cancer Network (NCCN).[185]

The use of serum PSA together with DRE is more accurate and sensitive than digital examination alone.[49] DRE testing has been determined to be optional aacording to recent ACS guidelines.[256,303A] PSA for screening is still controversial with recommendations for annual screening put forth by the American Cancer Society (revised in 2010)[256,303A] and by others,[280] and lack of a recommendation by the U.S. Preventive Services Task Force among others. The American Cancer Society[256,303A] emphasizes informed choice utilizing decision-making tools with screening discussions between patients and their physicians at age 50 for men at average risk with a 10-year life expectancy, and at earlier ages for men at high risk. Men at high risk include black men and men with a strong family history of prostate cancer. Definitive recommendations have awaited results from ongoing prospective randomized trials designed to determine whether PSA screening could reduce mortality from prostate cancer. However, initial results from the European Randomized Study of Screening for Prostate Cancer (ERSPC)[241] and the Prostate, Lung, Colorectal, and Ovarian Cancer Screening Trial (PLCO),[10] published in 2009, were conflicting. The European trial showed that PSA screening reduced deaths from prostate cancer by 20%, while in the U.S. study, in which men were followed for a shorter period of time and many of the men in the control arm underwent PSA testing, the rate of death from prostate cancer was low overall and did not differ between men screened and those not screened.

To improve the ability of PSA testing to detect early prostate cancer (clinical sensitivity) and/or spare unnecessary biopsies (clinical specificity), several approaches have been suggested. One approach is to use age-adjusted reference intervals as follows: 0 to 2.5 μg/L for men aged 40 to 49 years, 0 to 3.5 μg/L for those 50 to 59 years, 0 to 4.5 μg/L for men 60 to 69 years, and 0 to 6.5 μg/L for those 70 to 79 years.[194] By lowering the upper limit of the reference interval, more cancer will be detected in younger men, for whom potential cure by radical prostatectomy is most beneficial, although this may increase the overdetection of insignificant tumors. Increasing the upper limit for older men takes into account increases in PSA with aging due to BPH. However, 25% of men with a PSA between 2 and 4 μg/L[16,287] may have cancer, similar to the 4 to 10 μg/L range; thus use of age-specific ranges may result in missed clinically significant tumors in older men.

Another approach is to use PSA density (i.e., divide PSA concentration by prostatic volume as determined by transrectal ultrasonography) to account for more PSA from larger prostates, as in men with BPH.[25] Patients with PSA between 4 and 10 μg/L, a negative DRE result, and elevated PSA density (typical cutoff, 0.15) have increased risk for prostate cancer. The third approach is to use PSA velocity, that is, the rate of PSA increase as a function of time. It is recommended that velocity be calculated using at least three PSA results determined over at least 18 months. Increases in PSA in health, BPH, and prostatic cancer appear to be different, with the highest rate (>0.75 μg/L/y) observed in patients with prostate cancer.[47] Specificity improved to 90% for BPH, and sensitivity is 72% for prostate cancer. The PSA velocity cutoff of 0.75 μg/L/y is recommended for men with a total PSA concentration of 4 to 10 μg/L; lower cutoffs of 0.35 to 0.4 μg/L/y are suggested when PSA concentrations are <4 μg/L.

The most successful approach has been the use of molecular forms of PSA and free PSA. Percent free PSA (free PSA/total PSA*100) has been used to improve the clinical sensitivity and specificity of detecting prostate cancer, particularly for patients in the diagnostic "gray" zone of PSA between 4 and 10 μg/L or between 2 and 20 μg/L.[48,204] Men with cancer have less circulating free PSA (≈10 to 30%) and more PSA bound to protease inhibitors (≈70 to 90%) compared with men without cancer. Percent free PSA results can be interpreted using a single cutoff or a continuum of values to determine the relative risk of prostate cancer in individual men. In biopsied men with a total PSA between 4 and 10 μg/L and a DRE nonsuspicious for cancer, sensitivity for cancer detection is 95% using a %free PSA cutoff of ≤25%. Using this same cutoff (>25%), 20% of biopsied men with benign disease could be spared from biopsy. Percent free PSA may have particular utility in evaluating men who had a previous negative biopsy. A 1996 study of free PSA velocity found that percent free PSA is the earliest serum marker for predicting subsequent diagnosis of prostate cancer.[210] Studies have shown that %pPSA (pPSA/free PSA*100) can represent an improvement over %free PSA for the detection of prostate cancer, with particular utility when total PSA is in the 2.5 to 4.0 μg/L range.[259,260] Complexed PSA (cPSA) showed improved specificity over total PSA for prostate cancer detection in specific PSA subranges in a multicenter clinical trial.[203]

In addition to the approaches described previously, several algorithms using PSA and other analytes, and often clinical and demographic characteristics, have been developed to (1) aid in prostate cancer detection, (2) determine risk for prostate cancer (biopsy outcome), and (3) predict prognosis in men with prostate cancer undergoing therapy. They include nomograms and artificial neural networks. The ProstAsure Index, developed by Zhang, Stamey, and Chan,[14,269] was derived from several parameters, including age, total PSA, creatine kinase isoenzymes, and prostatic acid phosphatase, which were used as inputs for a neural network–derived, nonlinear algorithmic procedure. The resulting zone reflected the probability of prostate cancer and subsequent consideration for prostate biopsy.

Staging of Prostate Cancer

PSA has been found to correlate with clinical stages of prostate cancer.[270] For example, higher PSA concentrations and higher percentages of patients with elevated PSA concentrations are associated with advanced stages. PSA has also been found to correlate with pathologic stages of tumor extension and metastases, cancer volume, and cancer grade (Gleason score). Approximately 80% of men with PSA concentrations <4 μg/L at diagnosis have organ-confined disease; this decreases to 70% and 50% for PSA concentrations of 4 to 10 μg/L and >10 μg/L, respectively. Because significant overlap occurs in PSA concentrations among stages, PSA cannot be used to determine the pathologic stage in a given individual. Therefore, PSA by itself should not be used to decide whether a patient has prostate cancer confined to the organ and therefore is a likely candidate for radical prostatectomy or other treatment, or active surveillance. The concentration of PSA can serve as a guide and is more useful in evaluating the presence of metastases. Patients with PSA concentrations less than 20 μg/L rarely have bone metastases. Studies have shown that PSA can replace the staging radionuclide bone scan in newly diagnosed untreated prostate cancer patients who have a serum PSA concentration <20 μg/L and are asymptomatic. PSA contributes to the prediction of prostate cancer pathologic stage as part of a nomogram (the Partin tables) that also includes clinical stage and biopsy Gleason score. Multivariate logistic regression is used to estimate the probability of organ-confined disease, extraprostatic extension, seminal vesicle involvement, or lymph node involvement.[169]

Monitoring Treatment

The greatest clinical use for PSA is in the monitoring of definitive treatment of prostate cancer. This treatment includes radical prostatectomy, radiation therapy, and antiandrogen therapy.

PSA is produced almost exclusively by prostatic tissue; thus after radical prostatectomy, the PSA concentration should fall below the detection limit of the assay. This may require 2 to 3 weeks owing to the half-life of PSA. If the half-life is longer than usual, it must be assumed that residual tumor is present,[193,270] although detectable PSA may also reflect benign prostatic tissue. Biochemical recurrence has been defined as two postprostatectomy PSA concentrations ≥0.2 µg/L.[99] A cut point of 0.4 µg/L is also used. Increasing PSA after radical prostatectomy is a strong indication of disease recurrence. The time between PSA concentration elevation and clinical evidence of recurrence (metastases) averages 8 years. PSA doubling time is also useful in assessing risk of progression to metastasis with a low likelihood if the doubling time is greater than 10 to 15 months.

Unlike surgery, treatment with external beam radiation does not affect all tissues; therefore, PSA concentrations fall but do not become undetectable. The American Society for Therapeutic Radiology and Oncology (ASTRO) has defined failure as three successive rises above the nadir.[8] The more recent Phoenix guidelines[227] for defining biochemical failure after radiotherapy, which also includes interstitial prostate brachytherapy, advocate a PSA rise of 2.0 µg/L or greater over the nadir.

Hormone therapy includes (1) bilateral orchiectomy, (2) treatment with luteinizing hormone–releasing hormone agonists, and (3) antiandrogen therapy. PSA testing is useful for predicting prognosis and monitoring treatment response to this type of therapy in patients with metastatic prostate cancer. The concentration of PSA is inversely proportional to the survival time and increases with cancer progression, decreases in remission, and remains unchanged in stable disease. Androgen deprivation therapy may have a direct effect on PSA concentration that is independent of the antitumor effect. Production of PSA may be under the influence of androgenic hormones such as dihydrotestosterone. Thus PSA concentrations in patients who receive antiandrogen therapy may have a different meaning than they do in patients receiving other types of therapies.[192]

Analytical Methods

Sandwich immunoassays are used to measure PSA and are commercially available. Most of them use nonisotopic labels, such as enzyme, fluorescence, or chemiluminescence. Most of these assays are automated on an immunoassay system. Different assays and even the same assay with different lots of reagent may produce different results. Such differences are due to changes in (1) assay calibration, (2) production lot variation, (3) assay reaction time, (4) reagent matrices, (5) assay limit of detection, and (6) imprecision. Antibodies react with different PSA epitopes; therefore, some antibodies react dissimilarly with various molecular forms of PSA. Currently, most PSA assays are standardized to the Hybritech (now Beckman Coulter, Inc., Brea, Calif) PSA method or to standards introduced by the World Health Organization in 1999. The two international preparations consist of 100% free PSA (code 96/668) and 90% PSA-ACT complex and 10% free PSA (code 96/670).[58] Because of differences in the molar absorptivities used, PSA results from Hybritech standardized assays are approximately 20% higher than results from WHO standardized assays.

One of the most valuable applications of PSA is the detection of residual or recurrent disease following radical prostatectomy. Traditionally, 0.1 µg/L has been used as the lower limit of detection, which was based on assay analytical characteristics as well as clinical need. Ultrasensitive PSA assays can be defined as those with a functional sensitivity (20% CV) of 0.01 µg/L or lower. One PSA assay has been labeled as a third-generation assay, and many automated assays now achieve limits of detection close to 0.001 µg/L. Although cancer recurrence may be detected earlier, the effect on clinical management is unclear, and no assay has a specific FDA claim for earlier detection of recurrence.

Free PSA is not typically used as a single measurement but is expressed as a ratio or percentage of total PSA. Because of assay differences among manufacturers, total and free PSA should be measured in the same specimen using assays from the same diagnostics company. %fPSA is approved by the FDA as an aid in distinguishing prostate cancer from benign prostatic conditions in men aged 50 and older with a total PSA between 4 and 10 µg/L with a nonsuspicious DRE. The complexed PSA (cPSA) assay (Siemens Healthcare Diagnostics, Deerfield, Ill) measures PSA-ACT and other minor PSA complexes by rendering free PSA nonreactive with a free PSA-specific antibody. The two FDA intended uses are the same as for total PSA: (1) as an aid in the detection of prostate cancer in men aged 50 years or older in conjunction with DRE, and (2) for serial measurements to aid in the management of prostate cancer patients. A cPSA concentration of 3.2 µg/L is equivalent to a PSA cutoff of 4.0 µg/L, and a PSA threshold of 2.5 µg/L corresponds to a cPSA concentration of 2.2 µg/L.

Human Glandular Kallikrein 2

Human kallikrein 2 (hK2) and PSA (human kallikrein 3) are serine proteases that share 80% identity in protein sequence[236] and are almost exclusively found in prostatic epithelium.

Biochemistry

Similar to PSA, hK2 concentrations are 100,000-fold higher in seminal fluid than in serum.[162] hK2 has the ability to form complexes with endogenous antiproteases. One important inhibitor is the protein C inhibitor (PCI), which is the major ligand complexed to hK2 in seminal fluid, but in vitro, hK2 also forms complexes with α_2-antiplasmin, α_2-macroglobulin, ACT, antithrombin III, C1-inactivator, and plasminogen activator inhibitor-1.[179] Gel filtration studies have suggested that hK2 occurs mainly in a free, noncomplexed form in serum, whereas only a minor proportion (5 to 20%) may be complexed with protease inhibitors. In vitro, recombinant hK2 activates proPSA into mature, catalytic active form.

Clinical Applications

Immunohistochemical studies have demonstrated that tissue expression of hK2 shows intense staining in high-grade cancers and lymph node metastases, whereas it shows weaker staining for low-grade cancers and BPH.[65] Serum hK2 alone or hK2*total PSA/free PSA has been shown to be a significantly better predictor of organ-confined disease than tPSA.[103] In addition to the improvement in staging accuracy, hK2 discriminated aggressive, poorly differentiated prostate cancer from less aggressive, well-differentiated prostate cancer.[223] Although serum hK2 is independently indicative of prostate cancer of unfavorable prognosis, a model combining total and free PSA and total hK2 had superior discrimination.[277]

Analytical Methods

Currently, two major hK2 immunoassays are available. Haese and colleagues found notable differences in results when measuring by the two immunoassays for hK2 in identical patient samples.[104] Calibration of the two assays with the use of a common, ek-rhK2–based calibrator resulted in a substantial gain in agreement between the assays.

The Urokinase-Plasminogen Activator System

The urokinase-plasminogen activator system consists of three main components: urokinase-plasminogen activator (uPA, a 53 kDa serine protease), the uPA membrane-bound receptor (uPAR), and the uPA inhibitors, PAI-1 and PAI-2.[9,229]

Biochemistry

The urokinase-plasminogen activator is produced as a single inactive polypeptide, which is activated by cleavage between lysine 158 and isoleucine 159. The cleavage is catalyzed by a number of proteases, including cathepsins B and L and hK2. The active form of uPA consists of an A chain, which interacts with its cell surface receptor, uPAR, and a catalytically active B chain. The most thoroughly characterized activity of uPA is the conversion of plasminogen to active plasmin, which degrades extracellular matrix (ECM) components and activates matrix metalloproteinases (MMPs), which further degrade the ECM and activate and release specific growth factors [fibroblast growth factor (FGF)2 and transforming growth factor (TGF)-β]. The activity of uPA is controlled in vivo by two inhibitor molecules: PAI-1 and PAI-2. PAI-1 and PAI-2 not only act to inhibit uPA but also have a number of other functions, including angiogenesis, cell adhesion and migration, and inhibition of apoptosis.

Clinical Applications

uPA has been used as a prognostic marker in breast cancer and a number of other cancers.

Breast Cancer

uPA was the first protease implicated in metastasis evaluated for prognostic value in humans. At least 20 independent groups have demonstrated that breast cancer patients with high activity of uPA in their primary tumors have a worse disease-free pattern than those patients with low uPA activity.[75] The prognostic impact of uPA appears to be independent of other traditionally used markers, such as (1) axillary node status, (2) tumor size, (3) tumor grade, and (4) estrogen receptor (ER) status. In most studies,[110,310] uPA is a more potent predictor of overall survival than tumor size, tumor grade, or ER status, and is equally powerful as nodal status. Patients who benefit most from uPA measurement are those who are newly diagnosed with histologically negative local nodes. The long-term survival of this group is 70 to 80% with local therapy alone, and no further benefit is gained from adjuvant chemotherapy. uPA may be able to detect the small number of patients most at risk for recurrent disease and spare other cured patients from unnecessary chemotherapy. A prospective, randomized, controlled trial[126] of 674 node-negative breast cancer patients demonstrated that women with high concentrations of uPA and/or PAI-1 had a notably shorter disease-free period than those with low concentrations of both proteins. A pooled analysis of 8377 breast cancer patients showed an independent association between tissue uPA and PAI-1 concentrations in poor relapse-free and overall survival in both lymph node–negative and lymph node–positive patients.[161] ASCO[113] has recommended uPA/PAI, measured by ELISA on 300 mg of breast cancer tissue, to determine prognosis in newly diagnosed node-negative patients; concentrations of both markers may aid in determining the benefit of chemotherapeutic treatment.

Other Cancers

uPA has also demonstrated its usefulness as a prognostic marker in colorectal cancer. For example, in one study,[75] uPA was found to be a marker of disease outcome in patients with tumor invasion but negative node status (Dukes' B stage). High concentrations of uPA were also found to correlate with aggressive disease in both gastric and esophageal cancers. Preliminary studies have implicated uPA as a prognostic marker in (1) ovarian, (2) renal, (3) hepatocellular, (4) pancreatic, (5) urinary, (6) bladder, (7) lung (adenocarcinoma), and (7) cervical cancers and (8) gliomas. Thus uPA may function as a general prognostic marker in cancer.

Analytical Methods

The original assay developed for uPA measured its catalytic activity. This assay has been replaced by enzyme-linked immunosorbent assay (ELISA), and several research and commercially available kits have been developed for detection of uPA and PAI-1 in tumor tissue. Generally, increased concentrations of uPA, PAI-1, or both indicate poor prognosis. A uPA concentration below 3 ng/mg total tissue and a PAI-1 below 14 ng/mg total tissue have a notably better prognosis.[126] Most studies showing a prognostic value for uPA have used ELISA for detection; however, some were performed using immunohistochemistry. Immunohistochemical detection is easier and requires less tissue; however, interpretation is subjective and only semiquantitative.

Cathepsins

The cathepsins are lysosomal proteases; cathepsins B, D, and L have been investigated for their role in tumor development and progression.

Biochemistry

Similar to other proteases, cathepsins are synthesized as high molecular weight precursors that require processing for activation. Cathepsin B (CB) is a thiol-dependent protease normally found in lysosomes; it is activated by cathepsin D (CD) and matrix metalloproteinases. Activated CB in turn can activate uPA and specific metalloproteinases. Cathepsin L (CL) is similar in specificity to CB; however, it shows little activity toward small molecular substrates. Cathepsin D, similar to CB, is a lysosomal protease; however, CD belongs to the aspartyl group of proteases.

Expression and localization of CB appear to be altered in tumors relative to normal tissue. In tumor tissue, CB can be associated with the plasma membrane or secreted. Increased expression has been demonstrated in (1) breast, (2) colorectal, (3) gastric, (4) lung, and (5) prostate carcinomas, (6) gliomas, (7) melanomas, and (8) osteoclastomas, suggesting a link with tumor development and/or progression.[139] Altered localization of CB has been seen in various tumor tissues, such as (1) colon (2) carcinomas, (3) thyroid cancers, (4) gliomas, and (5) breast epithelial tumors. Altered expression and localization are thought to be involved in tissue invasion through ECM degradation and growth promotion. ECM degradation occurs through activation of CB and other proteases, such as MMPs and uPA. In addition to ECM degradation, CB releases growth factors: basic fibroblast growth factor (bFGF), insulin-like growth factor-1 (IGF-1), epidermal growth factor (EGF), and TGF-β associated with the ECM.

Stromal cells were originally thought to be passive bystanders in tumor development; however, evidence suggests an active role. Increased expression of ECM proteases, including CB, has been demonstrated in stromal cells at the border between tumor cells and normal tissue. Expression of both CB and CD is upregulated by various growth factors (bFGF, EGF, IGF-1) and by direct contact with tumor cells. This suggests that as tumor cells invade the stroma, stromal cells are induced to participate directly in matrix degradation.[139] Therefore, detection of CB in stromal cells and tumor cells may have prognostic value.

Clinical Applications

A limited number of studies have associated high values of CB in multiple tumor types with aggressive disease. All, with one exception, are retrospective studies with low numbers of patients. However, in one large study (n = 1500 patients), CB was shown to be an independent prognostic marker for both relapse-free and overall survival in breast cancer patients; however, it is not as good a marker as uPA.

Most data related to the prognostic value of CD are expressed in relation to breast cancer[228]; however, its usefulness in squamous cell carcinoma (SCC) of the head and neck, hepatocellular carcinoma, and gastric adenocarcinoma has been investigated in limited studies. For breast cancer, a 1999 report of 2810 patients confirmed the prognostic value of CD.[86] The authors, using an RIA to detect cytoplasmic CD in tumor tissue, showed that tumors with high CD had notably poorer relapse-free survival than those with low CD concentrations.

In contrast to RIA detection of CD in tissue extracts, immunohistochemical detection has led to conflicting results. Some investigators have reported a significant association between immunohistochemically determined CD and poor outcomes; others have found no relationship. Possible reasons include (1) differences in antibody specificity, (2) different scoring systems used to quantify CD staining, (3) different discrimination cutoff points, and (4) different types of tissue: fresh versus formalin-fixed and paraffin-embedded.[71] Therefore, the prognostic usefulness of CD in SCC and other malignancies needs further study to determine the utility of CD as an independent marker.

The use of CL as a prognostic indicator has been best studied in breast cancer. Most studies measured CL from tumor extracts and correlated high concentrations of CL with a decrease in relapse-free survival. CL appears to be an independent prognostic marker in both node-negative and node-positive breast cancer, especially when combined with other prognostic markers such as CB, CD, node status, and steroid hormone receptor status.

Analytical Methods

Initial assays for detection of CB used chromogenic substrates containing an Arg-Arg sequence and 2-naphthylamide and 7-amino-4-methylcoumarin as chromophores. These early assays lacked specificity and were likely to have suffered from interference by endogenous inhibitors (e.g., cystatins, stefins). CB and CL are now measured by ELISA; however, to date no comparison has been made with older CB methods. Immunohistochemistry has also been used to detect CB in tissue; however, no detailed evaluations have been conducted.

Most studies correlating CD with tumor progression and prognosis have used an immunoassay that detects both the proforms and the mature forms of CD. This assay can be used to measure CD in tissue extract generated for detection of steroid hormone receptors. CD has also been measured by Western blot, by immunohistochemistry, and by activity.

Matrix Metalloproteinases

Matrix metalloproteinases (MMPs) are a family of 23 structurally related zinc-dependent endopeptidases capable of degrading components of the ECM.[195,264]

Biochemistry

Most MMPs are secreted as a zymogen; once activated, their proteolytic activity is inhibited by tissue inhibitors known as tissue inhibitors of metalloproteinases (TIMPs). MMPs have been functionally grouped into four subgroups, based on their ECM specificity: (1) collagenases, (2) gelatinases, (3) stromelysins, and (4) membrane MMPs.

Clinical Applications

MMPs are involved in many functions, including tissue remodeling and wound repair; however, they have also been associated with tumor growth, invasion, and metastasis.[294]

Direct evidence for the role of MMPs in the development and progression of tumors has been provided by mouse knockout studies in which mice lacking various MMPs showed reduced tumorigenesis and progression. Conversely, increased expression is associated with tumor aggressiveness and poor prognosis. Increased expression of MMP-2 and MMP-9 is associated with accelerated tumor progression in (1) oral carcinoma; (2) lung adenocarcinoma; and (3) bladder, (4) ovarian, and (5) papillary thyroid carcinoma. Similarly, increased staining of MMP-3 and MMP-9 is seen in high-grade versus low-grade endometrial sarcoma. In esophageal carcinoma, MMP-7 expression correlates with tumor aggressiveness. In addition, plasma TIMP-1 concentrations have been found to be higher in patients with colon cancer compared with controls and to be improved over CEA for cancer detection.[120,121]

MMPs also act as predictors of recurrence or metastatic risk. Elevated preoperative serum MMP-2 or MMP-3 is predictive of recurrence in patients with advanced urothelial carcinoma. Furthermore, high MMP-2 expression in ovarian tumor cells can predict tumor recurrence. Expression of certain MMPs is predictive of metastatic risk. For example, expression of MMP-1 is associated with lymph node metastasis in cervical cancer and peritoneal metastasis in gastric cancer. MMP inhibition may be a therapeutic strategy for cancer.[195]

Analytical Methods

Gelatin zymography is a technique commonly used to detect MMPs, such as MMP-2 and MMP-9. Zymography is an electrophoretic technique used to identify proteolytic activity in enzymes separated by sodium dodecyl sulfate polyacrylamide gel electrophoresis under nonreducing conditions. The SDS is removed, allowing the MMPs to refold and subsequently digest gelatin at the position of the separated protein. This technique, although tedious, has the advantage of specifically detecting the active form of the protease. MMPs are also detected in tissue sections by immunohistochemistry using specific antibodies, and in tissue extracts and serum by immunoassay.

Tumor-Associated Trypsin Inhibitor

Tumor-associated trypsin inhibitor (TATI) is a 6 kDa trypsin inhibitor that was first identified from the urine of an ovarian cancer patient.

Biochemistry

TATI is identical to the previously identified pancreatic secretory trypsin inhibitor (PSTI), which is also known as the Kazal inhibitor. TATI is strongly expressed by pancreatic acinar cells, together with trypsinogen. It is secreted into the pancreatic juice, where it constitutes 0.1 to 0.8% of the total protein. It is expressed at lower concentrations in other healthy tissue, such as (1) the gastrointestinal and urogenital tracts, (2) the gallbladder, (3) the biliary tract, (4) kidney, (5) lung, (6) liver, and (7) breast. TATI also acts as an acute-phase reactant and is induced under strong inflammatory conditions, as would be expected, as its promoter contains an interleukin (IL)-6 response element. TATI function in vivo is thought to protect against autodigestion of body tissue by trypsinogen secreted by the pancreas and other tissue. TATI is rapidly cleared from the circulation by the kidneys with a half-life of approximately 6 minutes. Therefore, patients with renal disease can have extremely high serum concentrations of TATI (greater than 1000 μg/L).

Clinical Applications

Although pancreatitis, severe injury, and inflammation all can increase its concentration, TATI can still function as a relatively good tumor marker for various cancers. In most cancers, the increase in TATI is due to tumor production; however, inflammation associated with tissue destruction contributes to the overall TATI increase. Serum and urine concentrations correlate well, but because of greater variation in urine, serum is preferred.

Increases in both serum and urine TATI are common in ovarian cancer. In mucinous ovarian cancers, approximately 45% of patients have increased TATI in stage I, and 90 to 100% have increases by stage IV.[273] Fifty-five to 60% of patients with late-stage endometrial cancer have increased serum TATI; however, only 20% show an increase in early stages. TATI is increased in cervical cancer, but squamous cell carcinoma antigen (SCCA) and CEA are better markers.

TATI is useful in gastrointestinal and urologic cancers. As may be expected because of its pancreatic production, TATI is a useful marker for pancreatic cancer and is increased in 75 to 90% of patients. In gastric cancer, TATI is increased in 40 to 65% of patients, and high preoperative concentrations correlate with a poor prognosis. Patients with hepatocellular (60 to 80%) or biliary tract cancer (75 to 100%) show an increase in TATI. The clinical sensitivity of TATI in hepatocellular cancer is similar to that of AFP and is useful in AFP-negative cancers. Colorectal cancers also increase TATI, with approximately 34 to 74% of patients showing an increase. However, CEA is a better marker of disease. In bladder cancer, TATI has been shown to be more useful than other serum markers and is a strong prognostic indicator. In renal cell carcinoma, TATI is a more sensitive marker than CEA, CA 15-3, CA 125, and CA 19-9, and is useful in monitoring disease progression and after surgery.

Analytical Methods

TATI in serum or urine is typically measured by radioimmunoassay. The reference interval for TATI is 3 to 21 μg/L in serum and is method dependent, as a method employing monoclonal antibodies gives a slightly lower reference interval (3.1 to 16 μg/L). The urine concentration is more variable, with a reference interval of 7 to 51 μg/L.

Telomerase

Telomeres are specialized structures at the termini of eukaryotic chromosomes.

Biochemistry

Telomeres are composed of hexanucleotide repeats (TTAGGG) that signal the end of a chromosome and inhibit the DNA repair mechanism from joining the ends of chromosomes together. They also appear to function as a mitotic clock that records the replicative history and sets a finite life span for normal somatic cells. During each replication, cycle telomeric DNA is lost because of inability of the replication machinery to overcome the loss of terminal RNA primers. However, expression of functional telomerase is a mechanism to overcome telomeric DNA loss in germline cells and stem cells. Telomerase is a ribonucleoprotein reverse transcriptase that elongates telomere ends using a segment of its own RNA as a template. Two main components are required for telomerase activity: human telomerase RNA (hTR), which contains the template for reverse transcription, and human telomerase reverse transcriptase (hTERT), which consists of the enzyme's catalytic subunit.

Telomerase is normally active during embryogenesis but is repressed in most somatic cells before or shortly after birth. Germline cells, activated lymphocytes, and other immortal cells show no shortening of telomere length and possess telomerase activity. Thus tumor cells should also show telomerase activity that can act as a specific marker of transformation. In 2009, the Nobel Prize in Physiology or Medicine was awarded for the discovery of telomerase.

Clinical Applications

Telomerase activity has been detected in more than 80% of cancers, including (1) lung, (2) breast, (3) pancreatic, (4) bladder, and (5) many other cancers; however, it does not seem to be necessary for cancer development.[118] Its activity does, however, correlate with tumor progression and prognosis.

Detection of telomerase activity or hTERT mRNA in excretion, secretion, brushings, and washings has been evaluated. In pancreatic secretion samples, which contain freshly exfoliated cells, detection of telomerase activity was associated with cancer detection. Telomerase activity was also found to be useful in distinguishing between adenoma and carcinoma in intraductal papillary-mucinous tumors, which sometimes can be difficult to diagnose. In bronchial brushing samples, the clinical sensitivity of cancer detection is below 70%, and false-positive results are commonly encountered because of contamination with lymphocytes, which contain measurable telomerase activity. Measurement of telomerase may be a useful marker in cervical cancer, because most cervical cancers express telomerase. In cancers such as non–small cell lung cancer, gastric cancer, and neuroblastoma, and adenocarcinomas of the stomach and colon, telomerase activity is upregulated during tumor progression and is useful in the evaluation of malignant grading and patient prognosis.

Analytical Methods

The TRAP (telomeric repeat amplification protocol) assay is a widely used method for detection of telomerase activity. This technique measures the telomerase activity present in cell extracts. Briefly, cellular extract containing telomerase activity is incubated with a telomeric substrate (a short strand of DNA onto which the telomerase will attach the telomeric repeats), followed by polymerase chain reaction (PCR) amplification of the elongated telomere. The PCR product is detected by various methods, including gel electrophoresis, radiometric detection, ELISA, and real-time PCR detection.[117,233]

HORMONES

Hormones have been recognized as tumor markers for more than 50 years. The introduction of specific RIA methods for a particular hormone that has very little cross-reactivity with similar hormones made it possible to monitor the treatment of cancer patients.

With the introduction and use of monoclonal antibodies, measurement of hormones is now accurate and precise. The production of hormones in cancer involves two separate routes. First, the endocrine tissue that normally produces it can produce excess amounts of a hormone. Second, a hormone may be produced at a distant site by a nonendocrine tissue that normally does not produce the hormone. The latter condition is called *ectopic syndrome*. For example, the production of adrenocorticotropic hormone (ACTH) is normotropic by the pituitary and is ectopic by the small cell of the lung. Consequently, elevation of a given hormone is not diagnostic of a specific tumor, because a hormone may be produced by a variety of cancers.

Multiple endocrine neoplasia (MEN) syndromes (MEN-1, MEN-2A, and MEN-2B) are familial disorders inherited in an autosomal dominant fashion that are manifested by both benign and malignant tumors. Various polypeptide hormones, such as (1) ACTH, (2) calcitonin, (3) gastrin, (4) glucagon, (5) insulin, (6) secretin, and (7) vasoactive intestinal polypeptide, may be produced by the pancreatic islet cell and pituitary tumors found in MEN-1 and by medullary thyroid cancer found in MEN-2A and -2B and in familial medullary thyroid cancer (FMTC), a variant of MEN-2A.[145,258] Examples of hormones that are used as tumor markers are listed in Table 24-7. ACTH, calcitonin, and hCG are discussed in greater detail later.

Adrenocorticotropic Hormone

ACTH is a polypeptide hormone with 39 amino acids and an MW of 4500 Da that is produced by corticotropic cells of the anterior pituitary gland (see Chapter 53). In 1928, a patient who had the signs and symptoms of what is now known to be cortisol excess was described as having a small cell carcinoma of the lung.[38] A small number of these carcinomas can produce pro-ACTH, the precursor to ACTH. This precursor has an MW of 22,000 Da, 5% bioactivity, and most of the immunoactivity of ACTH. Traditional RIA measures precursors pro-ACTH and pro-opiomelanocortin (POMC), as well as the intact molecule and ACTH fragments that may be

TABLE 24-7 Hormones as Tumor Markers

Hormone	Type of Cancer
ACTH	Cushing's syndrome, lung (small cell)
Antidiuretic hormone	Lung (small cell), adrenal cortex, pancreatic, duodenal
Bombesin	Lung (small cell)
Calcitonin	Medullary thyroid
Gastrin	Glucagonoma
Growth hormone	Pituitary adenoma, renal, lung
hCG	Embryonal, choriocarcinoma, testicular (nonseminoma)
Human placental lactogen	Trophoblastic, gonads, lung, breast
Neurophysins	Lung (small cell)
Parathyroid hormone	Liver, renal, breast, lung, various
Prolactin	Pituitary adenoma, renal, lung
Vasoactive intestinal peptide	Pancreas, bronchogenic, pheochromocytoma, neuroblastoma

beneficial for ectopic ACTH-producing tumors, whereas reactivity of the immunometric assay depends on the antibodies used and may measure ACTH as well as its precursors.

Elevated plasma concentrations of ACTH could be the result of pituitary or ectopic production. A high concentration of ACTH (>200 ng/L) is suggestive of ectopic origin. Failure of dexamethasone to suppress cortisol is also indicative of ectopic production. About half of the ectopic production of ACTH is a result of small cell carcinoma of the lung. Other conditions that elevate ACTH concentrations have been reported, including pancreatic, breast, gastric, and colon cancer, and benign conditions, such as chronic obstructive pulmonary disease, mental depression, obesity, hypertension, diabetes mellitus, and stress. The value of ACTH in the monitoring of therapy is still unknown.[21]

Calcitonin

Calcitonin is a polypeptide with 32 amino acids; it has an MW of about 3400 Da and is produced by C cells of the thyroid.[13] Normally, calcitonin is secreted in response to increased serum calcium. It inhibits the release of calcium from bone and thus lowers the serum calcium concentration. The serum half-life is about 12 minutes. The concentration in healthy individuals is less than 0.1 μg/L. An elevated concentration is usually associated with medullary carcinoma of the thyroid.

Approximately 75% of MTC cases are sporadic, and 25% are familial. Most familial MEN-2A, MEN-2B, and FMTC cases are the result of mutations of the *RET* proto-oncogene, a receptor tyrosine kinase, and almost all develop MTC. Calcitonin is most useful for diagnosing sporadic MTC or for identifying the index case in familial MTC; genetic testing has supplanted calcitonin for screening family members of the index case. Calcitonin is used for monitoring MTC. Provocative testing with intravenous administration of calcium and/or pentagastrin produces increased calcitonin concentrations and is used to increase the sensitivity and specificity of MTC detection. Microscopic or occult malignancy has been detected in patients having a negative radioisotopic scan and normal thyroid glands on physical examination.

Calcitonin concentrations appear to correlate with indicators of the extent of disease, such as tumor volume and tumor involvement in local and distant metastases. Calcitonin is useful for monitoring treatment and detecting the recurrence of disease.

Calcitonin concentrations are also elevated in some patients with carcinoid tumors and cancers of the lung, breast, kidney, and liver. The usefulness of calcitonin as a tumor marker in these malignancies has not been proven. Calcitonin elevation has been reported in other nonmalignant conditions, such as (1) pulmonary disease, (2) pancreatitis, (3) hyperparathyroidism, (4) pernicious anemia, (5) Paget's disease of bone, and (6) pregnancy.

Human Chorionic Gonadotropin

Elevated hCG concentrations are seen in pregnancy, trophoblastic disease, and germ cell tumor. It is a useful tumor marker for tumors of the placenta (trophoblastic tumors) and for some tumors of the testes. It is also useful for diagnosing and monitoring pregnancy (see Chapter 57 for a discussion of hCG and pregnancy).

Biochemistry

Human chorionic gonadotropin is a glycoprotein secreted by the syncytiotrophoblastic cells of the normal placenta. hCG consists of two dissimilar α and β subunits. The α subunit is common to several other hormones: luteinizing hormone (LH), follicle-stimulating hormone (FSH), and thyroid-stimulating hormone (TSH). The β subunit is unique to hCG, and the 28 to 30 amino acids making up the carboxyl terminal are antigenically distinct. hCG has an MW of 45,000 Da.[289] Additional serum forms, including hyperglycosylated (hCGh) and nicked hCG (hCGn) and the urine form hCGβ core fragment (hCGβcf), have relevant clinical usefulness.[68] The upper reference limit in men and nonpregnant women is 5.0 IU/L. hCG assays with a detection limit <2 IU/L, cross-reactivity with LH <2%, and equimolar recognition of hCG and hCGβ (or a separate assay for hCGβ) are desired for tumor marker use.[280]

Production of the two hCG subunits is under separate genetic control. In early pregnancy, the free β subunit is produced together with intact (a whole molecule of) hCG. In late pregnancy, the free α subunit predominates. Trophoblastic tumors of placental and germ cell origin primarily produce intact hCG, while differential production of the subunits, primarily the free β subunit, has been observed in nontrophoblastic cancer patients.[274]

Clinical Applications

Patients with trophoblastic tumors typically have elevated concentrations of hCG (>1 million IU/L). It is also elevated in 70% of those with nonseminomatous testicular germ cell tumors, and less frequently in those with seminoma. Elevated serum concentrations of hCG[274] are also found in 45 to 60% of (1) biliary and (2) pancreatic cancers and in 10 to 30% of many other cancers, including (3) bladder, (4) renal, (5) prostate, (6) liver, (7) colorectal, (8) non–small cell lung, (9) breast, and (10) head and (11) neck cancers, and (12) hematologic malignancies. Most neuroendocrine tumors produce hCGβ, while carcinoid tumors produce hCGα. Elevations have also been reported in benign conditions, such as cirrhosis, duodenal ulcer, and inflammatory bowel disease.

hCG is useful in identifying patients with trophoblastic tumors and, together with AFP, in detecting nonseminomatous testicular tumors. Concentrations of hCG correlate with tumor volume and disease prognosis. The hyperglycosylated form of hCG may aid in the early detection of new or recurrent active trophoblastic malignancy and may discriminate quiescent gestational trophoblastic disease from active gestational trophoblastic neoplasia/choriocarcinoma.[62] Because hCG does not cross the blood-brain barrier, the normal cerebrospinal fluid-to-serum ratio is 1:60. Higher concentrations in cerebrospinal fluid may indicate metastases to the brain. Furthermore, the response to therapy for patients with central nervous system metastasis may be observed by monitoring the CSF hCG concentration.

hCG is most useful for monitoring treatment and progression of trophoblastic disease.[27] Concentrations of hCG correlate with tumor volume. A patient with an initial hCG concentration greater than 400,000 IU/L is considered at high risk for treatment failure. After surgical removal of the tumor, hCG concentration is expected to decline. The normal half-life of serum hCG is about 12 to 20 hours. Slowly decreasing or persistent concentrations of hCG may indicate the presence of residual disease. During chemotherapy, weekly hCG measurement is recommended. After remission is achieved, yearly hCG measurement is recommended to detect relapse. The detection limit of the assay is important, because any residual hCG activity may indicate the presence of a tumor.

Analytical Methods

Measurement of serum hCG improved greatly in the 1970s. Assay specificity was improved by use of an antibody to the β subunit of hCG that had little cross-reactivity with other glycoprotein hormones, LH, FSH, and TSH. Currently, most hCG assays use an immunometric ("sandwich") format. The hCG assay measures the intact (whole) molecule when an antibody for the α subunit and an antibody for the β subunit are used in the immunometric format. This type of assay does not measure free α or β subunits, because free subunits cannot form a sandwich with both antibodies. The total β-hCG assay measures both intact hCG and free β subunits. As a tumor marker, a total β-hCG assay is preferred, because many cancer patients produce notable amounts of free β subunit. World Health Organization (WHO) international reference reagents (IRRs) for hCG isoforms, including (1) intact hCG, (2) nicked hCG, (3) hCGβ, (4) nicked hCGβ, (5) hCGβcf, and (6) hCGα, have been developed,[30] and studies with these preparations have indicated that varying specificity of these variants in commercial hCG assays contributes to methodologic differences.[279,301] None of the commercially available hCG assays have been approved by the FDA for use as a tumor marker assay. Heterophile antibodies and antianimal antibodies such as human antimouse antibodies (HAMAs) can cause false-positive or -negative results in immunoassays, including those for hCG. Urine hCG testing, among other approaches, can help distinguish true positives from assay interference.

ONCOFETAL ANTIGENS

Oncofetal antigens are proteins produced during fetal life. These proteins are present in high concentration in the sera of fetuses and decrease to low concentration or disappear after birth. In cancer patients, these proteins often reappear, revealing that certain genes are reactivated as the result of the malignant transformation of cells.

Discovery of the oncofetal antigens AFP and CEA in the 1960s revolutionized the modern era of tumor markers. Oncofetal antigens that have been used as tumor markers are listed in Table 24-8.

α-Fetoprotein

AFP is a marker for hepatocellular and germ cell (nonseminoma) carcinoma.[283]

TABLE 24-8 Oncofetal Antigens as Tumor Markers

Name	Nature	Type of Cancer
AFP	Glycoprotein, 70 kDa, 4% CHO	Hepatocellular, germ cell (nonseminoma)
Oncofetal antigen	80 kDa	Colon
Carcinofetal ferritin	Glycoprotein, 600 kDa	Liver
CEA	Glycoprotein, 22 kDa, 50% CHO	Colorectal, gastrointestinal, pancreatic, lung, breast
Pancreatic oncofetal	Glycoprotein, 40 kDa	Pancreatic
Squamous cell antigen	Glycoprotein, 44 to 48 kDa	Cervical, lung, skin, head and neck (squamous)
Tennessee antigen	Glycoprotein, 100 kDa	Colon, gastrointestinal, bladder
Tissue polypeptide antigen	Cytokeratins 8, 18, 19	Various (breast, colorectal, ovarian, bladder)

CHO, Carbohydrate.

Biochemistry

AFP was found first in the sera of mice with liver cancer[2] and later[285] in the sera of humans with hepatocellular carcinoma. AFP is a glycoprotein with a molecular mass of 70 kDa. It consists of a single polypeptide chain and is 4% carbohydrate. AFP is synthesized in large quantities during embryonic development by the fetal yolk sac and liver. It is one of the major proteins in the fetal circulation, but its maximum concentration is about 10% that of albumin. AFP is closely related both genetically and structurally to albumin, having extensive homologies in amino acid sequence. The genes coding for both proteins have been localized to chromosome 4q. As albumin synthesis increases during later fetal development, AFP concentrations in fetal serum begin to decline. They finally reach the trace concentrations found in normal adults 18 months after birth.

For tumor-derived AFP, the composition of carbohydrate on AFP depends on the activity of saccharide transferase within tumor cells. Differences in carbohydrate sidechains on AFP may be determined by the binding of AFP to lectins, such as concanavalin A (Con A) and lens culinaris agglutinin (LCA). Molecular variants of AFP can be separated into the liver type and the yolk sac type; they differ from each other in terms of their carbohydrate moiety. The yolk sac type of AFP contains an additional sugar, *N*-acetylglycosamine; this blocks the Con A binding site on the AFP. Therefore, the yolk sac type of AFP shows a high percentage (50 to 70%) of Con A nonreactive (CNR) fraction, whereas the liver type, which lacks this additional sugar, shows a low CNR fraction (10 to 20%).[57] LCA binds to the fucosylated form of the first core *N*-acetylglucose, which is present in both liver and yolk sac types of tumor-derived AFP, but not in AFP generated by benign liver disease.

Clinical Applications

The serum AFP concentration is less than 10 µg/L in healthy adults.[56] During pregnancy, maternal AFP concentrations increase from 12 weeks' gestation to a peak of about 500 µg/L during the third trimester. Fetal serum AFP reaches a peak of 2 g/L at 14 weeks and then declines to about 70 mg/L at term. The use of AFP for detecting fetuses with neural tube defects is discussed in Chapter 57. In addition to pregnancy, elevated concentrations of serum AFP are associated with benign liver conditions, such as hepatitis and cirrhosis. Most patients with these benign diseases (95%) have AFP concentrations less than 200 µg/L.

Except in the pregnant patient, AFP concentrations greater than 1000 µg/L are indicative of cancer. At these concentrations of AFP, about half of hepatocellular carcinomas may be detected. However, because the serum concentration of AFP correlates with the size of the tumor,[132] detection of hepatocellular carcinoma is more useful at the earlier stages, when the tumor is small enough to be resectable (<5 cm) than when the tumor is large. To detect small tumors, the cutoff for AFP is typically set at a low concentration; a cutoff point of 10 to 20 µg/L has been recommended. However, at this concentration, hepatitis and cirrhosis must be considered as possible causes of elevation.

Screening for hepatocellular carcinoma has been attempted in high-incidence areas, such as Africa, China, Taiwan, Japan, and Alaska.[174] Initial large-scale screening in China using less sensitive techniques (e.g., agglutination and immunodiffusion, which have cutoffs of 400 to 1000 µg/L) was able to detect new cases of this type of cancer. More sensitive immunoassay methods having cutoffs of 10 to 20 µg/L and ultrasonography have been used in Taiwan and Japan with improved sensitivity in detecting hepatocellular carcinoma at earlier stages.

AFP is also useful for determining prognosis and for monitoring therapy for hepatocellular carcinoma.[132] The concentration of AFP is a prognostic indicator of survival. Elevated AFP concentrations (>10 µg/L) and serum bilirubin concentrations greater than 2 mg/dL are associated with shorter survival time.

Differential binding of AFP to the lectin LCA forms the basis of the AFP-L3% test for hepatocellular carcinoma that was cleared by the FDA for clinical use in 2005. Total AFP can be separated into three glycoforms: AFP-L1, AFP-L2, and AFP-L3, based on reactivity to LCA.[152] The L1 fraction of total AFP is present in patients with chronic hepatitis and liver cirrhosis, and it constitutes the majority of total AFP in nonmalignant liver disease. AFP-L1 has low reactivity with LCA. AFP-L2 is mostly derived from yolk sac tumors and has an intermediate affinity to LCA. AFP-L3 is produced by cancer cells and has an additional α-1-6-fucose residue attached at the reducing terminus of *N*-acetylglucosamine. AFP-L3% is calculated as the proportion of measured AFP-L3 to total AFP.

The AFP-L3% test is indicated for use in risk assessment for the development of hepatocellular carcinoma in patients who have chronic liver disease. A cutoff of 10% is used, and those patients with chronic liver disease and an elevated AFP-L3% have a sevenfold increased risk of developing hepatocellular carcinoma within 21 months. The test is useful for early detection, particularly in the AFP range of 20 to 200 µg/L, as has been shown in patients with hepatitis C–related cirrhosis, where hepatocellular incidence was higher in patients with elevated AFP-L3% compared with those with elevated AFP concentrations.[276] AFP-L3% correlates with tumor staging and aggressiveness. Although AFP-L3% is useful in detection and prognosis, it can be used only when AFP concentrations are elevated.

The AFP concentration is a good indicator for monitoring therapy and the change in clinical status. Elevated AFP concentrations after surgery may indicate incomplete removal of the tumor or the presence of metastasis. Falling or rising AFP concentrations after therapy may determine the success or failure of the treatment regimen. A notable increase in AFP concentrations in patients considered free of metastatic tumor may indicate the development of metastasis.

The combination of AFP and hCG is useful in classifying and staging germ cell tumors. Germ cell tumors may be predominantly one type of cell or may be a mixture of seminoma, yolk sac, choriocarcinomatous elements (embryonal carcinoma), and teratoma.[19] Serum concentrations of AFP are elevated in yolk sac tumors, whereas hCG is elevated in choriocarcinoma. Both are elevated in embryonal carcinoma. In seminomas, AFP is not elevated, whereas hCG is elevated in 10 to 30% of patients who have syncytiotrophoblastic cells in the tumor. Neither marker is elevated in teratoma. One or both of the markers are elevated in about 90% of patients with nonseminomatous testicular tumor. Elevations were noted in less than 20% of patients with stage I disease, 50 to 80% with stage II disease, and 90 to 100% with stage III disease. These markers correlate with tumor volume and the prognosis of disease.

The combined use of these markers is useful in monitoring patients with germ cell tumors: elevation of either marker indicates recurrence of disease or development of metastasis. The success of chemotherapy can be assessed by calculating the decrease in concentration of both markers using the half-lives of AFP (5 days) and hCG (12 to 20 hours).

Analytical Methods

Serum AFP is determined by immunometric assay on many automated immunoassay systems. A reference material for AFP [First WHO International Standard (IS)] is available from the National Institute for Biological Standards and Control (NIBSC) in the United Kingdom. AFP is reported using units of ng/mL (μg/L) primarily and kIU/L. One international unit (IU) of AFP is equivalent to 1.21 ng. A detection limit of 1 ng/mL is recommended for clinical use.[280] AFP-L3% is measured using a liquid-phase binding method (LiBASys, Wako Diagnostics, Richmond, Va) that incorporates LCA binding and anion-conjugated antibodies separated by anion-exchange chromatography and detected fluorometrically. AFP-L3% is calculated from the concentration of AFP-L3 fraction and the sum of the two fractions that constitute total AFP.

Carcinoembryonic Antigen

CEA is a marker for colorectal, gastrointestinal, lung, and breast carcinoma. CEA was discovered by Gold and Freeman in 1965 and was known initially as the Gold "antigen."[96] Rabbits were immunized with extracts of human colon cancer tissue, and the resultant antisera were absorbed with extracts of normal human colon. Some antisera reacted with the tumor extracts but not with the extracts of normal tissue. The antigen, which was also found in embryonic tissue, was named *carcinoembryonic antigen*.

Biochemistry

CEA is a glycoprotein with a molecular mass of 150 to 300 kDa; it contains 45 to 55% carbohydrate. It is a single polypeptide chain consisting of 641 amino acids, with lysine in the *N*-terminal position. The heterogeneity of CEA can be demonstrated by using isoelectric focusing to separate the variants.

CEA consists of a large family of related cell surface glycoproteins. CEA proteins are encoded by about 10 genes located on chromosome 19. Up to 36 different glycoproteins have been identified in the CEA family. The major proteins are CEA and nonspecific cross-reacting antigen (NCA).[122] The domain structures of CEA, NCA 50, and the heavy chain of IgG are very similar. Thus CEA is part of the immunoglobulin gene "superfamily."

Clinical Applications

The CEA concentration is elevated in a variety of cancers, such as colorectal (70%), lung (45%), gastric (50%), breast (40%), pancreatic (55%), ovarian (25%), and uterine (40%) carcinomas. Because of the elevations associated with benign disease (i.e., false-positive results) and the number of tumors that do not produce CEA (i.e., false-negative results), CEA testing should not be used for screening.[252]

CEA testing may be useful as an adjunct to clinical staging. Persistently elevated concentrations that are 5 to 10 times the upper reference limit strongly suggest the presence of colon cancer but may be associated with other cancers. In colon cancer, CEA concentrations correlate with the stage of disease. CEA concentrations are elevated in 28% of patients with Dukes' stage A colorectal cancer and in 45% of those with stage B. The pretreatment CEA concentration is prognostic of the development of metastasis. A high concentration of CEA is associated with a greater likelihood of developing metastasis. Evidence suggests that CEA is a cellular adhesion molecule that may potentiate invasion and metastasis.[122]

After successful initial therapy, CEA concentrations decline. During remission, CEA concentrations are stable. Rising CEA concentrations may indicate recurrence of disease. The lead time from CEA elevation to clinical recurrence is about 5 months. A repeat laparotomy can be performed to confirm the relapse, which is detected in 90% of cases. In the monitoring of metastatic colon cancer, CEA is useful in following patients throughout therapy and the clinical course of the disease.

CEA is also useful in monitoring breast, lung, gastric, and pancreatic carcinomas. In breast cancer, elevated CEA is associated with metastatic disease. Early or localized breast cancer does not show CEA elevation and is less sensitive than CA 15-3 and CA 27.29. CEA is most useful in monitoring metastatic breast cancer during therapy and in detecting the development of bone or lung metastasis. An increasing serum CEA concentration may reflect treatment failure when measurable disease is not present.[160] In lung cancer, CEA determination is helpful in diagnosing non–small cell lung carcinoma (>65% of patients have elevated CEA) and in monitoring lung cancer.

Analytical Methods

As with AFP, most assays use the immunometric format for determination of serum CEA. Polyclonal and monoclonal antibodies and combinations of the two types have been used in CEA immunoassays.

In the healthy population, the upper limit of CEA is about 3 μg/L for nonsmokers and 5 μg/L for smokers. Because the concentration of CEA measured is method dependent, values should always be compared using the same method. When methods are changed, all patients who are being monitored should be tested in parallel using both old and new methods. CEA concentration is elevated in some patients with benign conditions, such as cirrhosis (45%), pulmonary emphysema (30%), rectal polyps (5%), benign breast disease (15%), and ulcerative colitis (15%).

CYTOKERATINS

The cytokeratins are a group of approximately 20 proteins that make up the cytoskeletal intermediate filaments of epithelial cells and cells of epithelial origin. The cytokeratins can be grossly divided into two groups: type 1 is smaller and acidic, and type 2 is larger and neutral to basic. Clinically useful members of this family are tissue polypeptide antigen (TPA), tissue polypeptide-specific antigen (TPS), and cytokeratin 19 fragments (CYFRA 21-1).

Tissue Polypeptide Antigen

The discovery of TPA preceded that of AFP and CEA, but TPA is not a specific tumor marker.[31] It was found later that TPA could be identified by antibodies that react with cytokeratins 8, 18, and 19. TPA is produced by both normal and cancerous cells. Elevated serum concentrations of TPA are related to the proliferative activity and turnover of cells, allowing it to be used as a proliferation marker.[39,191] In pregnancy, TPA increases throughout gestation. After pregnancy, the concentration returns to normal after 5 days. TPA is also elevated in inflammatory diseases and in cancer; thus it is not useful for diagnosis. In monitoring of metastatic disease, TPA is useful when combined with CEA and CA 15-3 in breast cancer, with CEA and CA 19-9 in colon cancer, and with CA 125 in ovarian cancer. TPA may be helpful in the differentiation of cholangiocarcinoma (in which TPA concentration is elevated) from hepatocellular carcinoma (in which TPA is not elevated).

Tissue Polypeptide-Specific Antigen

TPS is actually an antigenic site on cytokeratin 18 that is specifically recognized by the M3 monoclonal antibody. This epitope has been proposed as a specific marker of cell proliferation and is detectable in serum using a specific immunoassay. TPS appears to correlate with proliferation activity of lung tumors, irrespective of histology and tumor volume, with increasing TPS concentrations with advancing stage.[29] Elevated concentrations of TPS correlate with a poorer outcome.

Cyfra 21-1

CYFRA 21-1 immunoassays use two monoclonal antibodies—BM 19.21 and KS 19.1—to detect cytokeratin 19 fragments. CYFRA 21-1 is elevated in all types of lung cancer, although it is most sensitive for non–small cell lung cancer, primarily SCC. Concentrations of CYFRA 21-1 positively correlate with advancing stage and are useful in monitoring the disease course and in providing postsurgical follow-up. In a study of non–small cell lung cancer patients, CYFRA 21-1 was shown to independently correlate with decreased survival, nodal status, and tumor stage, and a meta-analysis has further indicated a role for CYFRA 21-1 as a prognostic marker.[217,218] Blood concentrations are not affected by smoking status and may be increased in renal failure, liver cirrhosis, and benign pulmonary disease.[18,240]

Squamous Cell Carcinoma Antigen

As its name implies, SCCA is useful in monitoring a wide variety of SCCs.

Biochemistry

SCCA is a glycoprotein previously referred to as *tumor-associated antigen 4*. Subfractions of SCCA have been separated by isoelectric focusing into neutral and acidic fractions. Molecular weights range from 42,000 to 48,000 Da. Both malignant and nonmalignant squamous cells have been shown to contain the neutral fraction, whereas the acidic fraction is found mainly in malignant cells. The acidic fraction is the one released into the blood circulation. Expression of SCCA appears to correlate with the grade of differentiation of SCCs.[131]

Clinical Applications

SCCA is elevated in a variety of SCCs, including those of the (1) cervix, (2) lung, (3) skin, (4) head, (5) neck, (6) digestive tract, (7) ovaries, and (8) urogenital tract. In general, the concentration of SCCA is proportional to advancing stages of cancer. Screening is not effective, because only a small percentage of patients with early stages of cancer show elevated serum SCCA concentrations. High pretreatment SCCA concentrations appear to be associated with a poor prognosis. SCCA is useful in detecting the recurrence of cancer and in monitoring treatment and disease progression.[131]

Analytical Methods

SCC antigen is measured using immunoassay, including the microparticle enzyme immunoassay on the IMx analyzer (Abbott Diagnostics, Abbott Park, Ill). Healthy, nonpregnant women have SCC antigen concentrations below 1.5 μg/L. Serum SCC antigen concentrations may be elevated (>1.5 μg/L) in certain benign conditions, including pulmonary infection, skin disease, renal failure, and liver disease. SCC antigen is also present in saliva, sweat, and respiratory secretions.

CARBOHYDRATE MARKERS

Carbohydrate-related tumor markers may be (1) antigens on the tumor cell surface, or (2) secreted by the tumor cells.[106,245] Monoclonal antibodies against these antigens have been developed. These markers have been found to be clinically useful as tumor markers and tend to be more specific than naturally secreted markers, such as enzymes and hormones. Biochemically, they are high molecular weight mucins (Table 24-9) or blood group antigens (Table 24-10).

TABLE 24-9 Mucin Tumor Markers

Name	Antigen and Source	Antibody	Type of Cancer
CA 125	Glycoprotein, >200 kDa, OVCA 433	OC 125	Ovarian, endometrial
Episialin			
• CA 15-3	Glycoprotein, 400 kDa, membrane-enriched BRCA	DF3 and 115D8	Breast, ovarian
• CA 549	High-MW glycoprotein	BC4E549, BC4N154	Breast, ovarian
• CA 27.29	High-MW glycoprotein	B27.29	Breast
MCA	350 kDa glycoprotein	b-12	Breast, ovarian
DU-PAN-2	Mucin, 1000 kDa peptide epitope	DU-PAN-2	Pancreatic, ovarian, gastrointestinal, lung

BRCA, Breast cancer.

TABLE 24-10 Blood Group Antigen–Related Cancer Markers

Name	Antigen and Source	Antibody	Type of Cancer
CA 19-9	Sialylated Le^{xa}, SW-1116 colon CA	19-9	Pancreatic, gastrointestinal, hepatic
CA 19-5	Le^{a} and sialylated Le^{ag}	19-5	Gastrointestinal, pancreatic, ovarian
CA 50	Sialylated Le^{a} and afucosyl form	C50	Pancreatic, gastrointestinal, colon
CA 72-4	Sialylated Tn	B27.3, cc49	Ovarian, breast, gastrointestinal, colon
CA 242	Sialylated CHO	C242	Gastrointestinal, pancreatic

CHO, Carbohydrate.

CA 15-3, CA 549, and CA 27.29 assays detect a high molecular weight glycoprotein mucin expressed by the mammary epithelium known as *episialin,* and thus are used as markers for breast carcinoma. Circulating episialin antigen is a heterogeneous molecule. CA 15-3, CA 549, and CA 27.29 assays detect similar yet different epitopes on the episialin. The main differences are the antibodies used for detection. The specific CA 15-3 and CA 27.29 antibodies are described in the following sections.

CA 15-3

CA 15-3 is a marker for breast carcinoma.

Biochemistry

CA 15-3 is detected by a murine monoclonal antibody (MAb) DF3 produced against a membrane-enriched extract of a human breast cancer metastatic to liver. Another monoclonal antibody, 115D8, was developed against the human milk fat globule membrane. Circulating DF3-reactive antigen is a heterogeneous molecule with a molecular mass of 300 to 450 kDa. The gene for this molecule is located on chromosome 1q. cDNA cloning indicates that the DF3 peptide core consists of a highly conserved 60-bp tandem repeat sequence. The polymorphism of the antigen is the result of different numbers of repeats in the peptide core. The DF3 antibody recognizes the epitope within this 20 amino acid repeating sequence of the peptide core. Recognition of the epitope is also affected by glycation.[114]

Clinical Applications

In healthy subjects, the upper limit of CA 15-3 concentrations is 25 kU/L. When this cutoff is used, 5.5% of normal subjects, 23% of patients with primary breast cancer, and 69% of those with metastatic breast cancer have elevated CA 15-3 concentrations.[114] Elevated CA 15-3 concentrations are also found in other malignancies, including pancreatic (80%), lung (71%), breast (69%), ovarian (64%), colorectal (63%), and liver (28%) cancers. CA 15-3 is reported to be elevated in benign disease, although with less frequency [e.g., in benign liver disease (42%) and benign breast disease (16%)].

CA 15-3 should not be used to diagnose primary breast cancer because the incidence of elevation (23%) is fairly low. CA 15-3 is most useful in monitoring therapy and disease progression in metastatic breast cancer patients. Significant change of at least 25% correlates with disease progression in 90% of patients, with regression in 78%. No change correlates with disease stability in 60%.

Analytical Methods

Two antibodies are used in CA 15-3 immunoassays. The MAb 115D8 is attached to a solid support, whereas MAb DF3 is labeled. Assays using alternative antibodies against the same common antigen are also available for clinical use.

CA 549

CA 549 is a marker for breast carcinoma.

Biochemistry

CA 549 is an acidic glycoprotein with an isoelectric point of pH 5.2. By sodium dodecyl sulfate/polyacrylamide gel electrophoresis under reducing conditions, CA 549 can be separated into two species with molecular masses of 400 and 512 kDa. One monoclonal antibody, a murine IgG_1 termed BC4E 549, was raised by immunizing mice with partially purified membrane preparations from the T417 human breast tumor cell line. The other antibody, BC4N 154 (a murine IgM), was developed against human milk fat globule membranes.[37]

Clinical Application

In a population of healthy women, 95% of the population has CA 549 concentrations below 11 kU/L. Pregnancy and benign breast disease show minimum elevation. Some patients with benign liver disease show a slight elevation (see Table 24-4). CA 549 has been shown to be elevated in a variety of non-breast metastatic carcinomas, including ovarian (50%), prostate (40%), and lung (33%) carcinomas.

Similar to CA 15-3, CA 549 is not useful in detecting early breast carcinoma, because the proportion of patients with elevated CA 549 concentrations is low. Using ROC analysis, CA 549 is better than CEA in identifying active breast cancer.[52] CA 549 is useful in detecting recurrence of breast cancer in patients after initial therapy followed by adjuvant therapy. Increasing CA 549 concentration after an initial decrease or stabilization indicates the development of metastases. In the monitoring of advanced breast cancer patients, CA 549 correlates with disease progression and regression and helps detect metastases.[52,53]

CA 27.29

CA 27.29 is a marker for breast carcinoma.

Biochemistry

CA 27.29 is recognized by a monoclonal antibody, B27.29, which is produced against an antigen in ascites of patients with metastatic breast carcinoma. The minimum epitope to which B27.29 reacts is the 8 amino acid sequence (SAPDTRPA) within the 20 amino acid tandem repeating sequence of the mucin core. The reactive sequence of the B27.29 overlaps with the sequence of DF3 used in the CA 15-3 assay. In inhibition studies using labeled MAb, B27.29 effectively competes with DF3 for binding to both CA 27.29 and CA 15-3 antigens.[224]

Clinical Applications

CA 27.29 has been approved by the FDA for clinical use in the detection of recurrent breast cancer in patients with stage II or stage III disease and for monitoring response to therapy in patients with stage IV (metastatic) disease. In a multicenter study over a 2-year period in which 166 breast cancer patients were monitored, 26 patients developed recurrent disease. When two consecutive CA 27.29 antigen test results above 37.7 kU/L (99th percentile) were considered positive, the CA 27.29 assay had a clinical sensitivity of 57.7%, a clinical specificity of 97.9%, a positive predictive value of 83.3%, and a negative predictive value of 92.6% for the detection of recurrent breast cancer. Its performance appeared to be better than that of CA 15-3 in detecting patients with recurrent breast cancer.[54] In a group of metastatic breast cancer patients, CA 27.29 and CA 15.3 showed similar clinical performances.[63]

Analytical Methods

The CA 27.29 immunoassay has both competitive and sandwich formats that incorporate the B27.29 monoclonal antibody. Assays utilizing alternative antibodies against the same common antigen are also available for clinical use.

Mucin-like Carcinoma-Associated Antigen

Mucin-like carcinoma-associated antigen (MCA) is a marker for breast carcinoma.[34]

Biochemistry

MCA was identified on the surface of a breast carcinoma cell line by the monoclonal antibody b-12. MCA is a glycoprotein with a molecular mass of 350 kDa. Epitopes on this molecule are also recognized by DF3 and 115D8 antibodies of the CA 15-3 assay.

Clinical Applications

In a study of 100 healthy women, the upper reference limit for MCA was found to be 14 kU/L. MCA concentrations increase throughout pregnancy. In contrast, CA 15-3 increases only slightly during pregnancy. MCA concentration is elevated in 60% of metastatic breast cancer patients. However, elevated concentrations are also found in (1) ovarian, (2) cervical, (3) endometrial, and (4) prostate carcinoma. Minimum elevation is observed in benign breast disease. MCA concentrations correlate with CA 15-3 concentrations but not with CEA concentrations. In monitoring metastatic breast cancer patients, changes in MCA concentrations parallel changes in CA 15-3 concentrations.

CA 125

CA 125 is a marker for monitoring ovarian cancer.[119,248]

Biochemistry

CA 125 is a high molecular mass (greater than 200 kDa) glycoprotein recognized by the monoclonal antibody OC 125. It contains 24% carbohydrate and is expressed by epithelial ovarian tumors and other pathologic and normal tissues of müllerian duct origin. The molecule has been cloned and designated CA 125/MUC 16.[305] Its physiologic function is unknown.

Bast and associates developed the MAb OC 125 using a cell line (OVCA 433) from a patient with a serous papillary cystadenocarcinoma of the ovary.[136] The OC 125 clone was selected for its reactivity with the OVCA 433 cell line, and for its lack of reactivity with a B-lymphocyte line from the same patient.

Clinical Applications

The primary FDA-indicated use for CA 125 is to monitor response to therapy in patients with epithelial ovarian cancer. The second FDA-indicated use is to detect residual or recurrent disease in patients who have undergone first-line therapy and would be considered for second-look procedures. However, second-look laparotomy is now considered controversial except for use in clinical trials, or when surgical findings would alter disease management. In a healthy population, the upper limit of CA 125 is 35 kU/L. CA 125 is elevated in nonovarian carcinoma, including endometrial, pancreatic, lung, breast, and colorectal and other gastrointestinal tumors. CA 125 is useful for determining the prognosis of endometrial carcinoma. It is also elevated in women in the follicular phase of the menstrual cycle and with benign conditions such as cirrhosis, hepatitis, endometriosis, pericarditis, and early pregnancy. It cannot be used to differentiate ovarian cancer from other malignancies. CA 125 is not useful in screening for ovarian cancer in asymptomatic populations,[125] but screening is recommended in at-risk women with a family history of hereditary ovarian cancer, in conjunction with pelvic examination and ultrasound testing. Strategies to improve the clinical usefulness of CA 125 for screening/early detection of ovarian cancer to achieve needed high sensitivity and very high specificity include combining with transvaginal sonography, assessing changes in concentrations measured over time, and using multimarker panels.[20]

In ovarian carcinoma, CA 125 is elevated in 50% of patients with stage I disease, 90% with stage II, and more than 90% with stages III and IV. The concentration of CA 125 correlates with tumor size and staging. CA 125 is also useful in differentiating benign from malignant disease in patients with palpable ovarian masses. This differentiation is important because surgical intervention for malignant ovarian masses is far more extensive than that for benign masses. Einhorn and colleagues studied 100 patients undergoing diagnostic laparotomy for palpable adnexal masses; of these, 23 were found to have a malignancy.[77] With 35 kU/L used as the cutoff, predictive values for malignant disease were 78% clinical sensitivity, 95% clinical specificity, 82% positive predictive value, and 91% negative predictive value. Preoperative CA 125 concentration less than 65 kU/L is associated with a significantly greater 5-year survival rate (42%) when compared with a concentration greater than 65 kU/L (5%). Postoperative CA 125 concentrations and rate of decline are also predictors of survival. The half-life of CA 125 is normally 4.8 days. A group of patients with a CA 125 half-life of 22 days responded poorly to chemotherapy as compared with another group with a CA 125 half-life of 9 days.

CA 125 is useful for detecting residual disease in cancer patients following initial therapy. The sensitivity of CA 125 for detecting tumors before repeat laparotomy is 50%, and the specificity is 96%. After chemotherapy, CA 125 concentrations provides an indication of disease prognosis. A decrease in the CA 125 concentration by a factor of 10 after the first cycle of chemotherapy is indicative of response. Persistent elevation of CA 125 concentrations after three cycles of chemotherapy indicates a poor prognosis.

In the detection of recurrent metastasis, use of CA 125 concentration as an indicator is about 75% accurate. The lead time from CA 125 elevation to clinically detectable recurrence is about 3 to 4 months. CA 125 correlates with disease progression or regression in 80 to 90% of cases.[125]

Analytical Methods

An immunoradiometric assay for CA 125 was first developed and manufactured by Centocor, Inc., now Fujirebio Diagnostics (Malvern, Pa), which incorporated the OC 125 antibody for both capture and detection, allowing recognition of multiple CA 125 determinants. A second-generation assay (CA 125II) typically uses the monoclonal antibody, M11, as the capture antibody and OC 125 as the conjugate antibody. Other FDA-cleared assays for CA 125, which employ antibodies other than the OC 125 and M11 antibodies, are available on automated immunoassay platforms. Results from different assays are not interchangeable, and individual patients should be monitored with a single assay.

Other Ovarian Cancer Biomarkers

HE4

HE4 is a marker for ovarian cancer.

Biochemistry

The gene for HE4, *Homo sapiens* epididymis specific, *WFDC2*, was initially discovered using microarrays to be overexpressed in epididymal tissue and later in ovarian cancer tissue.[116,153] Tumor expression is histologic dependent with most serous and endometrioid tumors expressing HE4 and only 50% of clear cell and 0% of mucinous tumors.[74] The protein is characterized as part of the four-disulfide core protein family and contains whey acid protein domains (WAPs). These proteins typically are secreted and are protease inhibitors, although this function has not been ascribed to HE4, and its physiologic role is unknown. Subsequent studies have shown that HE4 is not specific for ovarian tumors. Generation of the monoclonal antibodies 2H5 and 3D8 to epitopes on HE4 has allowed development of a sandwich ELISA and measurement in serum.[116]

Clinical Applications

At an HE4 concentration of 150 pM, 95% of healthy women were below this cutoff, while 79% of women with ovarian cancer were above this cutoff. Elevations in other subjects include breast (13%), endometrial (26%), gastrointestinal (16%), and lung cancers (42%), as well as benign gynecologic disease (7%) and other benign disease (24%). The assay is FDA cleared for monitoring recurrence or progressive disease in patients with epithelial ovarian cancer. In serial samples from 80 ovarian cancer patients in which a 25% increase in HE4 concentration was used to define a positive change, 60% of patients with disease progression had an increase greater than 25%, and 75% had a change of 25% or less or did not have disease progression. Results comparing HE4 and CA 125 to distinguish women with ovarian cancer from normal women or those with benign processes appear to depend on the population studied, although combining the two markers may allow more accurate prediction of cancer than use of the individual markers. An algorithm incorporating HE4 and CA 125 has been reported to successfully classify women with a pelvic mass as at high or low risk for epithelial ovarian cancer.

The algorithm was accurate in classifying a high percentage (93.8%) of women with cancer as high risk.[182] The algorithm, termed Risk of Malignancy Index (ROMA), has been marked for use in Europe. HE4 may also have usefulness as a marker in endometrial cancer.[181]

Analytical Methods

HE4 is measured by an enzyme immunoassay, with 2H5 as the capture antibody and 3D8 as the detector antibody (Fujirebio Diagnostics). This assay is not recommended for patients with mucinous or germ cell ovarian cancer.

OVA1: An IVDMIA for Ovarian Cancer

Based on the proteomics biomarker discovery approach using mass spectrometry, Zhang and colleagues identified several proteins that, when combined with CA 125, provide diagnostic value for ovarian cancer. Vermillion Inc. licensed the combination of markers and conducted a clinical trial with 516 patient specimens collected from 27 clinical sites. Data were submitted to the FDA and were cleared for clinical use as the OVA1 test—the first IVDMIA proteomic diagnostic for cancer. The OVA1 test is a qualitative serum test that combines the results of five immunoassays into a single numeric score. The five markers are (1) CA 125, (2) prealbumin (transthyretin), (3) apolipoprotein A1 (Apo A1), (4) transferrin (Tfr), and (5) β2M (beta 2-microglobulin). It is indicated for women who meet the following criteria: over age 18, ovarian adnexal mass present for which surgery is planned, and not yet referred to an oncologist. The OVA1 test is an aid in further assessment of the likelihood that malignancy is present when the physician's independent clinical and radiological evaluation does not indicate malignancy. This test is not intended as a screening or stand-alone diagnostic assay. The OVA1 score is calculated using OvaCalc software (Vermillion Inc.) with values between 0 and 10. Expected values for the probability of malignancy in premenopausal women are (1) high OVA1 ≥5.0, and (2) low OVA1 <5.0, and for postmenopausal women, (1) high OVA1 ≥4.4, and (2) low OVA1 <4.4. The addition of OVA1 to the presurgical clinical assessment improved the sensitivity of predicting malignancy from 72 to 92% for non–gynecologic oncologist (GO) patients and from 78 to 99% for GO patients.

DU-PAN-2

DU-PAN-2 is a marker for pancreatic cancer.[173,176]

Biochemistry

The epitope recognized by the antibody DU-PAN-2 is a mucin. Its molecular mass is between 100 and 500 kDa, and it is 80% carbohydrate. The core protein (cDNA) has been cloned and sequenced, and the predicted amino acid sequence reveals a protein of 126 kDa containing 1295 amino acid residues with 42 tandem repeats. DU-PAN-2 antigen is found mainly in the (1) glandular epithelia of the pancreatic and biliary systems and in the (2) breast and (3) bronchial ducts. Less expression is found in cells of the (4) salivary glands, (5) stomach, (6) colon, and (7) intestine.[173]

Clinical Applications

Serum DU-PAN-2 concentrations are elevated in patients with pancreatic (54 to 61%), biliary tract (44 to 47%), and hepatocellular (44%) carcinomas. Comparative studies between DU-PAN-2 and CA 19-9 concentrations in pancreatic cancer show similar elevations in 70 to 80% of patients. DU-PAN-2 and CA 19-9 concentrations correlate well, except in patients who are Le^{a-b-} and therefore do not express CA 19-9.

Analytical Methods

An RIA assay was developed by Metzgar and coworkers,[173] and an immunoenzymetric assay was developed by Kyowa Medex (Tokyo, Japan). The serum concentration of DU-PAN-2 in a healthy population is less than 100 kU/L. The cutoff used to differentiate the presence of cancer from health is 300 or 400 kU/L.

BLOOD GROUP ANTIGENS

Blood group carbohydrates identified by monoclonal antibodies that have been used as markers of cancers are listed in Table 24-10. These include (1) CA 19-9 (sialylated Le^{xa}), (2) CA 50 (sialylated Le^{x-1}, afucosyl forms), (3) CA 72-4 (sialyl Tn), and (4) CA 242 (sialylated carbohydrate coexpressed with CA 50).

CA 19-9

CA 19-9 is a marker for gastrointestinal cancers and is used primarily to test for pancreatic carcinoma.[146] CA 19-9 has been approved by the FDA for quantitative measurement in serum and as an aid in monitoring pancreatic cancer patients.

Biochemistry

This carbohydrate antigen is a glycolipid, specifically, sialylated lacto-*N*-fucopenteose II ganglioside, that is a sialylated derivative of the Le^a blood group antigen and is denoted as Le^{xa}. Expression of the antigen requires the Lewis gene product, 1,4-fucosyl transferase. CA 19-9 is synthesized by normal human pancreatic and biliary ductular cells and by gastric, colon, endometrial, and salivary epithelia. In serum, it exists as a mucin—a high molecular mass (200 to 1000 kDa) glycoprotein complex. Patients who are genotypically Le^{a-b-} (about 5%) do not express CA 19-9. The monoclonal antibody against CA 19-9 was developed from a human colon carcinoma cell line, SW-1116.[140]

Clinical Applications

The CA 19-9 upper reference limit is 37 kU/L, as determined from the 99th percentile of normal subjects. This cutoff discriminates between pancreatic cancer and benign pancreatic disease with clinical sensitivities of 69 to 93% and clinical specificities of 76 to 99%. Elevated CA 19-9 concentrations (>37 kU/L) are found in patients with pancreatic (80%), hepatobiliary (67%), gastric (40 to 50%), hepatocellular (30 to 50%), colorectal (30%), and breast (15%) cancers. Some patients (10 to 20%) with pancreatitis and other benign gastrointestinal diseases have elevated concentrations up to 120 kU/L. CA 19-9 is useful in monitoring pancreatic and colorectal and gastric cancers. CA 19-9 concentrations correlate with pancreatic cancer staging. With a cutoff of 37 kU/L, 67% of patients with resectable and 87% of those with unresectable pancreatic cancers have elevated concentrations. When the cutoff is raised to 1000 kU/L, 35% of patients with unresectable tumors and only 5% of those with resectable tumors have elevated CA 19-9 concentrations. CA 19-9 is also useful for establishing prognosis for pancreatic cancer at initial diagnosis, as concentrations have independent predictive value for determination of respectability and of overall survival. Elevated or increasing concentrations can indicate recurrence 1 to 7 months before it is detected by radiographs or clinical findings.[272] Unfortunately, early detection of relapse may not be useful because effective therapy for pancreatic cancer is not available.

Analytical Methods

Several companies have produced CA 19-9 immunoassays. Considerable differences among assays are noted,[123] and assay results are not interchangeable for individual patients. Typically, the CA 19-9 antibody is used as both the capture and the signal antibody.

CA 50

CA 50 is a marker for pancreatic and colorectal carcinoma.[105]

Biochemistry

CA 50 is a monoclonal antibody developed against the human colon adenocarcinoma cell line COLO 205. The CA 50 antibody recognizes an epitope on two carbohydrate moieties: sialosylfucosyllactotetraose (sialylated Le^a) and sialosyllactotetraose (sialylated Le^a lacking fucose). This antigen exists as a glycoprotein in serum and also as gangliosides in tissue. Sialylated Le^a is the predominant form of CA 50 in epithelial carcinoma and is recognized by CA 19-9.

Clinical Applications

Elevated CA 50 concentrations have been reported in benign diseases of the pancreas (12 to 46%), biliary tract (35 to 38%), and liver (22 to 59%). In pancreatic cancer, 80 to 97% of patients have elevated concentrations. In colon cancer, elevated concentrations were reported in Dukes' A (19 to 43%), B (30 to 59%), C (53 to 73%), and D (53 to 73%) stages. In digestive tract carcinoma, elevated concentrations were seen in esophageal (41 to 71%), gastric (41 to 78%), biliary (58 to 70%), and hepatocellular (14 to 78%) cancers. Other malignancies were reported to have lower percentages of elevation, including breast, lung, renal, prostate, bladder, and ovarian cancers. Similar performances and good correlations were reported between CA 50 and CA 19-9 concentrations.

Analytical Methods

The original inhibition test has been replaced by an immunoradiometric assay and a time-resolved fluorescent immunoassay. The upper reference interval for healthy subjects varies from 14 to 20 kU/L, depending on the method.

CA 72-4

CA 72-4 is a marker for carcinomas of the gastrointestinal tract and of the ovary.[238]

Biochemistry

The 72-4 assay utilizes the monoclonal antibody B72.3 developed from the membrane-enriched fraction of breast carcinoma in a patient with liver metastasis. The B72.3 reactive antigen was purified and called TAG-72 (tumor-associated glycoprotein). Further purification of TAG-72 from LS-174T human colon carcinoma xenograft produced a new generation of monoclonal antibodies with higher affinity. These antibodies, denoted "cc" for "colon carcinoma," were used in subsequent studies.

Clinical Applications

A cutoff of 6 kU/L is used in the CA 72-4 assay. The following percentages of elevation were observed: in health (3.5%); in benign gastrointestinal disease (6.7%); in gastrointestinal carcinoma (40%); in lung cancer (36%); and in ovarian cancer (24%). A poor clinical correlation between CEA and CA 72-4 concentrations was found in gastric cancer. CEA and CA 72-4 concentrations may be complementary. The plasma clearance of TAG-72 was studied by measuring serial TAG-72 concentrations in patients with primary carcinoma of the breast and with gastric, colorectal, and ovarian cancers. After removal of the tumor, the average time required for the concentration to decrease to 4 kU/L was 23.3 days. This suggests that TAG-72 may be useful in detecting residual tumor in these cancer patients.

Analytical Methods

CA 72-4 is measured using an immunoradiometric assay (IRMA) manufactured by Fujirebio Diagnostics. It uses two monoclonal antibodies that were developed at the National Cancer Institute. B72.3 is the conjugate, whereas cc49 is the capture antibody. An automated eletrochemiluminescence method is also available from Roche Diagnostics (Indianapolis, Ind).

CA 242

CA 242 is a marker for pancreatic and colorectal cancer.[143]

Biochemistry

CA 242 is a monoclonal antibody developed from a human colorectal carcinoma cell line, COLO 205. The antigenic determinant is a sialylated carbohydrate. CA 242 recognizes the epitopes of CA 50 and CA 19-9. CA 242 is found in the apical border of ductal cells of the human pancreas and in epithelial and goblet cells of the colonic mucosa.

Clinical Applications

At a concentration of 20 U/L, elevated CA 242 concentrations were found in 5 to 33% of patients with benign colon, gastric, hepatic, pancreatic, and biliary tract disease; in 68 to 79% of patients with malignant pancreatic cancer; in 55 to 85% of patients with colorectal cancer; and in 44% of patients with gastric cancer. The correlation coefficients *(R^2)* of CA 242, CA 50, and CA 19-9 concentrations in patients with colorectal, liver, pancreatic, and biliary tract disease ranged from 0.81 to 0.95. CA 242 and CEA appeared to have higher percentages of elevation in colorectal cancer than did CA 50 and CA 19-9. CA 242 seems to be less efficient than CA 19-9 or CA 50 in the detection of pancreatic cancer; however, this may depend on the cutoff.

Analytical Methods

An immunometric assay (Fujirebio Diagnostics) uses the C 241 antibody against sialylated Lewis[a] as the capture antibody and the CA 242 antibody as the conjugate. The upper reference limit is 29 U/mL.

PROTEINS

Several proteins having tumor marker potential are listed in Table 24-11. Included in this group of tumor markers are proteins that are not enzymes or hormones, and are not high in carbohydrate content. Additional research is required to assess the clinical usefulness of most of these markers.

Immunoglobulin

Monoclonal immunoglobulin has been used as a marker for multiple myeloma for longer than 100 years.[24] Monoclonal paraproteins appear as sharp bands in the globulin region of serum electrophoretic patterns. More than 95% of patients with multiple myeloma have such an electrophoretic pattern. Appearance of nonmalignant monoclonal immunoglobulins increases with age, reaching 5% in patients older than 75 years. These nonmalignant monoclonal bands are usually lower in concentration than malignant bands and are not associated with Bence Jones protein. Bence Jones protein is a free monoclonal immunoglobulin light chain in the urine. The concentration of monoclonal immunoglobulin at initial diagnosis is a prognostic indicator of disease progression.[261] During treatment, the serum concentration of urinary Bence Jones protein may reflect the success of therapy. Lower concentrations are associated with more favorable outcomes. Serum paraproteins are discussed in Chapter 21.

Bladder Cancer Markers

It is estimated that 600,000 Americans are currently affected by bladder cancer, and 70,000 new cases will be diagnosed each year. Symptoms range from intermittent hematuria to voiding problems or dysuria. The most common type of cell seen is transitional cell carcinoma (TCC), and the most frequent symptom is hematuria. Bladder cancer is staged pathologically and is treated on the basis of the extent of tumor invasion. Carcinoma in situ (stage Tis) and superficial bladder cancers (stages Ta and T1) occur on the epithelial lining and do not invade the muscle layer. Stage Ta tumors are confined to the mucosa, and stage T1 tumors superficially invade the lamina propria. Stage T2 tumors extend into the muscle layer, and T3 tumors invade beyond the muscle layer. Stage T4 tumors have metastasized to local nodes or distant organs.

Urinary Bladder Tumor Markers

Bladder cancer is detected through cystoscopy or cytology of shed cells, or by noncellular markers, such as NMP22, complement factor-H (CFH), and fibronectin.[89,251] Tumor antigens present in urine are the easiest to analyze; however, they cannot be used as the sole mechanism for tumor detection. They should be used in a complementary manner with cystoscopy and cytology. NMP22, in a series of 300 patients with hematuria, with a cutoff of 10 U/mL, detected 100% of

TABLE 24-11 Proteins as Tumor Markers

Name	Nature	Type of Cancer
β_2-Microglobulin	11 kDa	Multiple myeloma, B-cell lymphoma, chronic lymphocytic leukemia, Waldenström's macroglobulinemia
C-peptide	3.6 kDa	Insulinoma
Ferritin	450 kDa iron-binding protein	Liver, lung, breast, leukemia
HER-2/*neu*	97 to 115 kDa, 20% CHO	Breast
Immunoglobulin	160 to 900 kDa, 3 to 12% CHO	Multiple myeloma, lymphomas
Melanoma-associated antigen	90 to 240 kDa	Melanoma
Pancreas-associated antigen	100 kDa, 20% CHO	Pancreatic, stomach
Pregnancy-specific protein 1	10 kDa, 30% CHO	Trophoblastic, germ cell
Pro-gastrin releasing peptide	Amino acid residues 31 to 98	Small cell lung
Prothrombin precursor	Des-γ-carboxy prothrombin	Hepatocellular
Soluble mesothelin-related peptides	Mesothelin/megakaryocyte potentiating factor peptides	Mesothelioma, ovarian
Tumor-associated trypsin inhibitor	6 kDa polypeptide	Lung, gastrointestinal, ovarian

CHO, Carbohydrate.

TABLE 24-12 Comparison of Sensitivity Using Cytology vs. UroVysion for the Detection of Bladder Cancer by Stage

	UroVysion, %	Cytology, %
Stage		
Ta, Grade 1-2	62	23
Ta, Grade 3	83	33
T1, Grade 2	100	100
T1, Grade 3	75	50
T2	100	33
Tis	100	33
Grade		
1	55	18
2	78	44
3	94	41

From Sarosdy MF, Schellhammer P, Bokinsky G, et al. Clinical evaluation of a multi-target fluorescent in situ hybridization assay for detection of bladder cancer. J Urol 2002;168:1950-4.

bladder cancer cases, with a specificity of 85%.[313] In another study, NMP22 and fibronectin were found to have superior clinical sensitivity to that of cytology; however, NMP22 and cytology have the highest clinical specificity.[78] Telomerase, cytokeratins, and survivin have also been evaluated as markers for bladder cancer.

Two bladder cancer–related tests that are fluorescence based have been cleared by the FDA. ImmunoCyt (Scimedx Corporation, Denville, NJ) uses three fluorescently labeled monoclonal antibodies and microscopy to identify bladder cancer markers on cells found in urine. This test appears most useful with cytology in identifying low-grade tumors. UroVysion (Abbott Molecular, Abbott Park, Ill), a fluorescence in situ hybridization (FISH) technique, uses fluorescently labeled probes to detect aneuploidy of chromosomes 3, 7, and 17, and deletion of the 9p21 locus that contains the tumor suppressor p16, which is the most common alteration seen in urothelial carcinoma. Table 24-12 compares cytology with that of UroVysion for the detection of bladder cancer.[235]

Nuclear Matrix Protein (NMP22)

Nuclear matrix proteins (NMPs) make up the internal structure of the nucleus. Their function has been associated with regulating key reactions in the nucleus, such as DNA replication and RNA synthesis. NMPs released by the cancer cell may be different from those in the normal cell. Furthermore, different types of cells may have different NMPs. In one study, soluble NMPs were detected in the sera of cancer patients in higher concentrations than in the sera from normal subjects.[205] In a multicenter follow up study (125 cystoscopies) of 90 patients with 33 pathologically confirmed TCCs of the urinary tract, 70% of 33 recurrences had urinary NMP greater than 10 U/mL. Among patients with NMP less than 10 U/mL, 86% had no malignancy at subsequent cystoscopy.[263]

An ELISA for the measurement of an NMP, called *nuclear mitotic apparatus protein (NuMa)* in urine, has been approved by the FDA for the management of patients with TCC of the urinary tract, to aid in diagnosis of symptomatic patients or those with risk factors and to identify patients with recurrent TCC. This test is called NMP22 and is manufactured by Alere North America, Inc., (Princeton, NJ). A qualitative, immunochromatographic point-of-care version of the test is available as an aid in monitoring patients with a history of bladder cancer.

Bladder Tumor–Associated (BTA) Analytes

A qualitative, lateral flow immunoassay for BTA analytes in urine, termed the BTA *stat* test, has been developed. The antigen detected in the BTA stat assay is human complement factor H–related protein (hCFHrp), which is a variant of human complement factor H (hCFH). hCFH functions in the alternative complement pathway by interacting with complement factor C3b to prevent cell lysis. Bladder tumor–associated antigen may allow tumor cells to evade the host immune system. A multicenter trial compared the BTA *stat* test with voided urine cytology studies in 499 patients undergoing surveillance cystoscopy for recurrent bladder cancer. The BTA *stat* test identified 40% of patients with positive cystoscopy results, and cytology detected 17%. A positive test may provide a higher degree of suspicion for recurrence.[234] A quantitative test in ELISA format, BTA TRAK, is also available. Both tests have FDA-approved indications for use as an aid in conjunction with cystoscopy in the management of bladder cancer patients.

Soluble Mesothelin-Related Peptides (SMRPs)

Mesothelioma is a rare cancer of the mesothelial surfaces of the pleural and peritoneal cavities or the pericardium that is linked to asbestos exposure. Mesothelin is a cell surface glycoprotein expressed on mesothelial cells, and mesothelin fragments, which are soluble mesothelin-related peptides, can be found in the circulation of patients with mesothelial tumor. An ELISA assay has been developed (Mesomark, Fujirebio Diagnostics) that measures serum soluble molecules related to the mesothelin/megakaryocyte potentiating factor (MPF) family of proteins recognized by the monoclonal antibody OV569. The assay also incorporates the 4H3 monoclonal antibody. This test is approved by the FDA under the Humanitarian Device Exemption, which is used for medical devices for diseases affecting fewer than 4000 individuals a year; demonstration of effectiveness is not required. It is intended as an aid in monitoring patients who have been diagnosed with epithelioid mesothelioma. A cutoff of 1.5 nmol/L was derived from the 99th percentile of healthy subjects. In addition to patients with mesothelioma (52%), approximately 10 to 15% of patients with other cancers, including ovarian, lung, colon, and pancreas cancers, may have elevations in SMRP[29] compared with 5% of individuals exposed to asbestos. SMRP increases with increasing stage of malignant pleural mesothelioma.[207] Using ROC analysis, an AUC of 0.81 was obtained to distinguish malignant pleural mesothelioma patients (n = 90) from asbestos-exposed individuals (n = 66) with clinical sensitivity, specificity, and accuracy of 60%, 89%, and 73%, respectively, at a cutoff of 1.9 nmol/L. The AUC for distinguishing malignant pleural mesothelioma from lung cancer (n = 170) was 0.82. SMRPs have also been reported to be higher in malignant pleural mesothelioma pleural effusions compared with benign or other nonmalignant pleural mesothelioma pleural effusions.

Des-γ-Carboxy Prothrombin (PIVKA-II)

Des-γ-carboxy prothrombin (DCP), also called PIVKA-II (proteins induced by vitamin K absence or antagonism II), is an abnormal form of prothrombin and a tumor marker for hepatocellular carcinoma. Prothrombin is a vitamin K–dependent coagulation factor produced in the liver that undergoes a post-translational modification in which the 10 glutamic acid (glu) residues in the N-terminus are carboxylated to form γ-carboxy glutamic acid (gla) to be functional. The γ-glutamyl carboxylase requires vitamin K as a cofactor, and in cases of dietary deficiency or antagonism, such as by warfarin, DCP is produced. Obstructive jaundice with an effect on vitamin K may result in increased DCP. In hepatocellular carcinoma, gene expression of the enzyme is defective, resulting in DCP.

DCP is most commonly used clinically for early detection, monitoring, and recurrence in countries with a high prevalence of hepatocellular carcinoma, such as Japan. When ELISA was used to compare patients with hepatocellular carcinoma versus those with cirrhosis or chronic hepatitis, sensitivity for detection was 48% and specificity 96%.[90] DCP and AFP are independent markers, and in a case control study of patients with hepatocellular carcinoma or cirrhosis,[171] clinical sensitivity for cancer detection in early-stage disease increased to 78% compared with 53% for AFP alone and 61% for DCP alone. DCP correlates with tumor size, although it is less sensitive for detecting small tumors, tumor stage, and prognosis. In the United States, the Wako DCP assay has been FDA cleared as an aid in the risk assessment of patients with chronic liver disease for progression of hepatocellular carcinoma. The liquid phase binding assay (Wako Diagnostics, Richmond, VA) on the Wako LiBASys platform uses separation of monoclonal antibody–bound DCP from serum using anion-exchange chromatography and fluorometric detection. When this assay was used in a prospective study of 334 patients with hepatitis C virus (HCV) cirrhosis, the relative risk of developing hepatocellular carcinoma was 5.7 with a cutoff of 7.5 μg/L. Results from the LiBASys and an electrochemiluminometric assay commonly used in Japan correlate well.[196]

Heat Shock Proteins

Heat shock proteins (HSPs) constitute a conserved group of proteins that were first identified by their ability to be induced by heat and other stressors. Numerous functions have been associated with HSPs, most notably as chaperones to stabilize cellular proteins during periods of unfavorable conditions. HSPs associate with many cellular components, including signal transduction proteins (kinases and phosphatases), steroid receptors, and components of the apoptotic machinery. The ability of HSPs to interact with various cellular components and to protect them from stressors, coupled with the fact that increased expression is seen in a number of tumors, suggests that they may play a role in tumorigenicity. Increased expression of HSP27 is seen in breast cancer, endometrial cancer, and leukemia. HSP70 is increased in breast cancer, endometrial cancer, osteosarcoma, and renal cell tumor. High expression of HSP27 and HSP70 in breast, endometrial, or gastric cancer is correlated with metastasis, poor prognosis, and resistance to chemotherapy.[93] HSP60 and HSP90 are also overexpressed in breast and lung cancers, leukemias, and Hodgkin's disease.

S-100 Proteins

The S-100 proteins constitute a group of at least 19 related calcium-binding proteins. All contain two high-affinity and selective EF-hand calcium-binding domains. Their physiologic role is uncertain; however, some members have been associated with cancer progression, namely, S-100A4, S-100A2, S-100A6, and S-100β.[172] S-100A4 is normally expressed in selected immune cells, with faint expression in keratinocytes, melanocytes, and Langerhans' cells. It is not expressed in breast, colon, thyroid, lung, kidney, or pancreas. Expression of S-100A4 in breast cancer, esophageal-squamous carcinoma, and gastric cancer correlates with a worse outcome and more aggressive disease, and was shown to be an independent marker of prognosis in multivariate analysis. Lack of expression in normal tissue and expression in cancer tissue make it an excellent candidate for routine histologic use as a cancer marker.

S-100β is routinely used as a diagnostic histologic marker of melanoma and melanoma metastases. The measurement of serum concentrations of S-100β has been investigated for monitoring disease recurrence. In the absence of melanoma, serum S-100β concentrations are normally undetectable; however, with recurrent disease, S-100β concentrations rise. With the use of an immunoassay, clinical sensitivity and specificity of 0.29 and 0.93, respectively, with diagnostic accuracy of 0.84, were obtained using a cutoff of 0.12 μg/L.[91] S-100β is a more sensitive and specific marker for recurrent melanoma that is able to detect recurrence earlier than LD or alkaline phosphatase (traditional markers of melanoma recurrence). An automated assay is available on the LIAISON analyzer (DiaSorin, Inc., Stillwater, MN).

Autoantibodies

Autoantibodies are antibodies that specifically recognize self-antigens, or proteins. They are normally thought of in the context of autoimmune disease; however, autoantibodies have been used for the detection and monitoring of cancer.[71] The event that triggers the development of autoantibodies can be an infection that through molecular mimicry breaks self-tolerance in a susceptible individual, or inappropriate expression of a self-antigen, such as a cancer antigen. Various cancers produce proteins or antigens that are recognized by the immune system and are targets for the development of autoantibodies. Detection and monitoring of cancer with the use of circulating tumor markers mainly consists of the detection of proteins or antigens that are not normally present in the circulation, or that notably change in concentration. Various cancers express new antigens (abnormally glycosylated MUC1, detected by CA 15-3) or overexpress existing antigens, such as HER-2/*neu;* autoantibodies that recognize these tumor antigens can also be detected.

Healthy individuals typically do not have autoantibodies or have them at a very low titer, and a change or rise can signify the development of cancer or another disease state. Several cancer antigens have been investigated for their ability to induce detectable autoantibodies, including p53, MUC1, c-myc, and c-erbB-2. For example, accumulation of mutant p53 proteins within tumor cells may lead to the development of autoantibodies. Nine to 48% of primary breast cancer patients have detectable anti-p53 antibodies, as do 11 to 64% of lung cancer patients[71] and almost 100% of ovarian cancer patients. Anti-p53 antibodies have been detected in hepatocellular, bladder, colorectal, gastric, and other cancers.[11]

Many cancers are heterogeneous and do not consistently express tumor markers. It is clear that no single tumor marker will detect all cancers. Therefore, the detection of multiple antigens should increase the clinical sensitivity of cancer detection. This is also the case with autoantibody detection. Using a single autoantibody, detection of primary breast cancer was between 35 and 47%; however, when four autoantibodies were used (p53, MUC1, c-myc, and c-erbB-2), sensitivity was increased to 82%.[71]

Autoantibodies are also useful in prognosis and monitoring of disease. Elevated autoantibodies to p53 are associated with a poor prognosis, independent of tumor-related antigens.[71] This may be due to the fact that expression of the tumor antigen at a distant and/or abnormal site triggers an immune response. The titer of the autoantibodies also tends to follow the amount of tumor antigen, which can provide information about tumor volume. In addition, the concentration of autoantibodies decreases in relation to the antigen load, but will quickly rise again in recurrent disease because of a secondary immune response when the antigen is reintroduced (recurrent disease). Autoantibodies with the greatest potential are used for the early detection of cancer, because a small amount of the antigen has the ability to generate a vigorous humoral immune response; however, more research is needed before autoantibodies will be part of the standard tests ordered.

Markers of Angiogenesis

Angiogenesis, the formation of blood vessels, is a highly regulated and ordered process; however in tumor tissue, this process is disordered. The development of tumors is thought to involve inactivation of tumor suppressor genes and/or uncontrolled activation of oncogenes. Subsequently, another step in the progression toward malignancy has been identified and has been referred to as the *angiogenic switch.*[26,46] The first phase of tumor development is an avascular phase, with a lesion size of 1 to 2 mm. At this point, the tumor is in a vascular steady state. The vascular state occurs next with rapid and unregulated angiogenesis. The architecture of the newly developing vasculature is very different from that of normal vasculature. It is irregularly shaped and dilated and can have dead ends, with irregular blood flow patterns, that make tumors relatively easy to identify histologically.[45] In normal tissue, a balance is noted between proangiogenic signals (VEGF, FGF, PDGFB, EGF, Ets-1, and LPA) and antiangiogenic signals (thrombospondin-1, angiostatin, endostatin, canstatin, and tumstatin).[208] It is believed that in tumors, proangiogenic signals are increased. Therefore, measurement of proangiogenic markers may provide prognostic information related to tumor status.

Increases in blood vascular endothelial growth factor (VEGF) and soluble Tie-2 receptor (sTie2) correlate with the development of metastases, with VEGF being the most powerful predictor of outcome.[59] Ets-1, a transcription factor that activates numerous angiogenic genes, also may serve as a prognostic indicator of uterine cervical cancers. Thrombospondin-1 (TSP-1), an antiangiogenic marker, has been found to be a positive prognostic marker in ductal carcinoma of the breast. Other markers of angiogenesis considered as prognostic markers in cancer have been reviewed.[26]

Thyroglobulin and Antibodies

Biochemistry

Thyroglobulin (Tg) is produced by the thyroid gland as the precursor to thyroid hormone (see Chapter 55).

Clinical Applications

The main use of Tg measurement is as a tumor marker for patients with a diagnosis of differentiated thyroid cancer. Approximately two thirds of these patients have an elevated preoperative Tg concentration. An elevated preoperative concentration of Tg confirms the tumor's ability to secrete Tg and validates the use of postoperative measurement of Tg to monitor for tumor recurrence. Postoperatively, the most sensitive time to detect residual tumor or metastasis is after TSH stimulation. In well-differentiated tumors, a tenfold increase in Tg concentrations is seen after TSH stimulation.[265] Poorly differentiated tumors that do not concentrate iodide may display a blunted response to TSH stimulation. Tg monitoring generally is not useful in patients who do not have elevated preoperative Tg.

Antithyroglobulin antibodies have been proposed to monitor residual disease and/or recurrence. Serial anti-Tg measurements may be an independent prognostic indicator of therapy, because an increase in anti-Tg antibodies may suggest recurrence of the tumor.[266]

Analytical Methods

Immunometric assays (IMAs) and RIAs are the two main methods used for the measurement of Tg. IMA assays have the advantage of having a shorter incubation time and are automatable; however, they suffer from greater interferences. The main interferants in both assays are antithyroglobulin antibodies, which typically cause an underestimation of Tg concentrations in the IMA. Antithyroglobulin antibodies can be measured directly in all patients; if both IMA and RIA are used to measure Tg, a discordant result suggests the presence of antithyroglobulin antibodies.

Chromogranins

Chromogranins are a family of proteins that are major components of the secretory granules of most neuroendocrine cells.

Biochemistry

The granin family consists of three members: (1) chromogranin A (CgA); (2) chromogranin B (CgB); and (3) secretogranin II, III, IV, and V.[83] Chromogranins are found in neuroendocrine cells throughout the body, including the neuronal cells of the central and peripheral nervous systems. Intracellularly located chromogranins have been suggested to play a role in the regulation of secretory granules. In addition, secreted chromogranins can be proteolytically processed to form bioactive peptides. Chromogranin A has been the best studied of the chromogranins, has been shown to be widely expressed by neuroendocrine tissue, and is cosecreted by neuroendocrine cells, along with peptide hormones and neuropeptides. This wide distribution and cosecretion make it an excellent histochemical and plasma marker of neuroendocrine tumors.

Clinical Applications

Both CgA and CgB are useful in detecting various neuroendocrine tumors, including carcinoid tumor, pheochromocytoma, and neuroblastoma. In most cases, CgA is produced at higher concentrations than CgB; however in some cases, CgB is positive when CgA is negative; therefore, both should be measured when possible. In the case of carcinoid tumor, foregut and midgut tumors are normally functional tumors producing serotonin. CgA is as specific for the detection of both foregut and midgut carcinoid tumors as the serotonin metabolite 5-hydroxyindoleacetic acid (5-HIAA), and it is the preferred marker in hindgut tumors, which commonly are nonfunctional.[71] Although nonfunctional tumors have lost the ability to secrete serotonin, they retain the ability to secrete chromogranins. For detection of pheochromocytomas, CgA is at least as sensitive and specific as plasma catecholamines or urinary metanephrines.[28]

Analytical Methods

CgA is measured by immunoassay. Depending on the assay, polyclonal or monoclonal antibodies are used. Care must be taken in choosing an assay because CgA and the other chromogranins are heavily processed after release, which may render them nondetectable by the assay and may produce false-negative results. Therefore, an assay that recognizes both intact and processed molecules may be desirable. Commercial assays for CgB are not yet available.

RECEPTORS AND OTHER MARKERS

Other tumor markers, including catecholamines, polyamines, lipid-associated sialic acid, and receptors, have been used clinically with various degrees of success (Table 24-13). Receptors are probably the most successful of this group of markers. Catecholamines and their metabolites are discussed in Chapter 30.

Estrogen and Progesterone Receptors

Estrogen and progesterone receptors are used in breast cancer as indicators for hormonal therapy.[302] Patients with positive estrogen and progesterone receptors tend to respond to hormonal treatment. Those with negative receptors will be treated using other therapies, such as chemotherapy. Hormone receptors also serve as prognostic factors in breast cancer. Patients positive for hormone receptors tend to survive longer.

Biochemistry

Estrogen receptors (ERs) and progesterone receptors (PRs) are members of the nuclear steroid hormone receptor family, and are involved in hormone-directed transcriptional activation. The general structure of nuclear steroid hormone receptors, including ERs and PRs, consists of a large N-terminal domain containing transcriptional activation domains, a DNA-binding domain, a hinge region, and the hormone-binding domain at the C-terminus. Both ERs and PRs are present in a large protein complex, and upon hormone binding, some members of the complex dissociate, and the receptors bind to their respective response elements and activate transcription.

TABLE 24-13 Other Tumor Markers

Name	Nature	Type of Cancer
Estrogen and progesterone receptors	(Tissue)	Breast
Catecholamine metabolites	(Urine) VMA, HVA, metanephrines	Neuroblastoma, pheochromocytoma
Hydroxyproline	(Urine)	Bone metastasis (breast), multiple myeloma
Lipid-associated sialic acid	Sialic acid bound to lipid	Gastrointestinal, lung, rheumatoid
Polyamine	(CSF)	Brain
	(Urine)	Various
PCA3	(Urine)	Prostate

CSF, Cerebrospinal fluid; *HVA*, homovanillic acid; *VMA*, vanillylmandelic acid.

Estrogen and progesterone each have at least two separate receptors. Estrogen has ERα and ERβ, which are transcribed from separate genes. ERα and ERβ show 96% and 58% homology in their DNA- and hormone-binding domains, respectively, with a more divergent sequence in the N-terminal region.[141] Two forms of PR—PR-A and PR-B—also exist, and both are transcribed from the same gene. PR-A lacks the first 165 amino acids of PR-B.

ERs and PRs are found in target tissue cells, such as the uterus, pituitary gland, hypothalamus, and breast, and appear to be involved in tumor development and progression. Furthermore, ER status and PR status correlate with both prognosis and treatment response; therefore, ER and PR measurement is clinically useful.

Clinical Applications

Measurement of ER content in breast tumor tissue is useful primarily in determining the probability of hormonal therapy and also as a prognostic indicator. ERs and PRs are routinely measured in all newly diagnosed breast cancers. Of patients with carcinoma of the breast, 60% have tumors that are ER positive. ER-positive tumors are seven to eight times more likely to respond to endocrine therapy, such as tamoxifen, toremifene, and droloxifene. Furthermore, the U.S. National Cancer Institute Consensus Statement suggests that all breast cancer patients who have positive ER findings should undergo hormonal treatment regardless of their age, menopausal status, nodal status, or tumor size. Ninety-five percent of patients with ER-negative tumors fail to respond. The greater the ER content of the tumor, the higher the response rate to endocrine therapy. Approximately one third of women with metastatic breast carcinoma obtain an objective remission following various types of endocrine therapy directed at lowering their estrogen concentrations. Such therapy includes oophorectomy, hypophysectomy, and adrenalectomy (ablative therapy), as well as administration of antiestrogens and androgens (additive therapy). As a prognostic indicator, ER positivity suggests a better 5-year outcome; however, after 5 years, ER-negative tumors have a better prognosis.[71]

Occasionally, a tumor is defined as ER negative, but the patient responds to endocrine therapy (false-negative results yielded in an ER assay). False-positive results of ER assays (ER-positive tumor but no response to endocrine therapy) are more common than false-negative results. The most frequent explanation is heterogeneity of tumor with biopsy of a site that is not representative of the other tumor deposits. In addition to this problem, evidence suggests that some tumor cells have receptor defects distal to the initial binding step (e.g., variant cells are able to bind steroid in the cytoplasm but cannot transport the receptor to the nucleus).

In 1996, ERβ was identified as a second ER; it is thought to modulate the activity of ER (now renamed ERα). When bound to hormone, ERα and ERβ signal differently at the activator protein-1 (AP-1) site: ERα activates transcription, and ERβ represses transcription.[198] This ability may have implications as to which isoform of ER is measured and may affect its prognostic use. It was reported that ERβ expression is greatly decreased in breast carcinoma tissue as compared with breast fibroadenoma tissue, but expression of ERα is not. The routinely used ELISA method for quantitation of ER predominantly detects ERα.[71] The fact that ERβ seems to attenuate ERα signaling, coupled with the fact that there is an inverse relationship between ERβ and PR and ERα proteins, suggests a possible mechanism for ER-positive tumors that do not respond to hormonal treatment.[71]

The PR assay is a useful adjunct to the assay of ERs. Because PR synthesis appears to be dependent on estrogen action, measurement of PR activity provides confirmation that all steps of estrogen action are intact. Indeed, metastatic breast cancer patients with both ER- and PR-positive tumors have a response rate of 75% to endocrine therapy, whereas those with ER-positive and PR-negative tumors have a 40% response rate. In addition, only 25% of ER-negative/PR-positive patients respond to endocrine therapy, whereas less than 5% of ER-negative/PR-negative patients respond. The percentage of positive specimens is greater in postmenopausal women than in those who are premenopausal.

Analytical Methods

Immunohistochemistry assay[50,186,232] is used to measure steroid hormone receptors in breast tumor tissue specimens. The classical quantitative biochemical method, the multiple-point dextran-coated (DCC) titration assay, and enzyme immunoassays are obsolete.[280] Immunohistochemical assays are simple and less expensive and can use small amounts of tissue from frozen tissue sections, paraffin-embedded tissue, fine-needle aspirates, and malignant effusions. However, assay interpretations can be subjective, and use of different antibodies can yield different results.

The primary monoclonal antibody is incubated with a thin section of tissue mounted on a microscope slide. Localization and visualization of receptor material are subsequently accomplished by an indirect immunoperoxidase technique. Semiquantitative scoring is based on the percentage of cells with nuclear staining and may include the intensity of staining. Specimens with staining in at least 20% of malignant cells are usually considered to have a favorable response, with 10 to 19% borderline, and <10% unfavorable. Immunohistochemistry is not influenced by the presence of estrogens, antiestrogens, or steroid-binding proteins and can evaluate receptor content specific to malignant cells and not in other nonmalignant breast tissue.

Androgen Receptors

Androgens, namely, testosterone and dihydrotestosterone (DHT), are involved in growth and maintenance of the prostate gland. Testosterone and DHT exert their effects through the androgen receptor, a classical nuclear steroid hormone receptor. The AR activates the transcription of genes containing androgen response elements, and thereby modulates prostate growth and development. The role of the AR in development and progression of prostate cancer is suggested by the fact that antiandrogen therapy is highly but transiently effective, and antiandrogen therapy can stimulate prostate cancer cells, as seen in antiandrogen withdrawal syndrome.

Two polymorphic repeats have been identified: a CAG repeat and a GGN repeat that correlate with prostate cancer development. Shorter CAG repeats are associated with greater cancer risk and increased prostate cancer aggressiveness. Also, mutations have been found that cause inappropriate activation of the AR by estrogens, progestins, glucocorticoids, and antiandrogens that promote prostate cancer cell growth, suggesting that these mutations play a role in cancer progression and development of resistant tumors.

Hepatocyte Growth Factor Receptor (c-Met)

The hepatocyte growth factor (HGF) receptor, also known as c-Met, is a proto-oncogene tyrosine kinase receptor predominantly expressed on healthy epithelial cells. The natural ligand for c-Met is hepatocyte growth factor/scatter factor, and upon activation by its ligand, it induces a wide array of cellular responses, including proliferation, survival, angiogenesis, wound healing, scattering, motility, invasion, and branching morphogenesis. c-Met was originally identified as a fusion gene between the TRP locus and the c-Met locus in a human osteogenic sarcoma cell line treated with a chemical carcinogen. This fusion produced a constitutively active receptor that activates downstream proliferation, survival, and migration pathways.

Involvement of c-Met in the progression of cancer has been investigated in numerous types of tumors. Overexpression of c-Met in (1) prostate, (2) colorectal, (3) breast, and (4) hepatocellular cancers, (5) malignant melanoma, and (6) uterine cervix cancer is associated with increased stage, metastatic potential, and a poor prognosis. Increased mRNA copy number of c-Met in colorectal cancer has been correlated with the depth of invasion.[284] In addition, its increased expression in breast cancer tumors correlates with a shortened survival time and is an independent prognostic marker for HER-2, EGFR, and hormone receptor status.[288] Overall, inappropriate expression and overexpression of c-Met appear to be involved in metastases and invasion and correlate with a worse clinical outcome. Given the potential role that c-Met plays in cancer progression and metastases, it is being studied by various investigators as a potential target for drug therapy.

Epidermal Growth Factor Receptor

The EGFR is a prototype of a family of tyrosine kinase receptors. Natural ligands for the EGFR include epidermal growth factor and transforming growth factor-α. In cancerous tissue, these growth factors promote growth in both a paracrine and autocrine fashion. In an analysis of more than 200 studies completed between 1985 and 2000, it was determined that overexpression of EGFR had prognostic value in several cancers.[187] The EGFR was found to be a strong prognostic indicator in (1) head and neck, (2) ovarian, (3) cervical, (4) bladder, and (5) esophageal cancers. Patients with elevated EGFR showed reduced overall survival in 70% of studies. In breast, colorectal, gastric, and endometrial cancers, elevated EGFR was found to be a moderate prognostic indicator, with 52% of studies showing reduced survival. Because EGFR is implicated in the progression of various tumor types, it represents a potential point of intervention and treatment for these cancers. Several compounds have been developed that inhibit EGFR signaling by blocking ligand binding or inhibiting tyrosine kinase activity. EGFR is identified in tissue by immunohistochemistry and FISH. Detection of the EGFR protein (HER1) in EGFR-expressing cells by immunohistochemistry has been approved by the FDA for use as a companion diagnostic to aid in identifying colorectal cancer patients for treatment with the EGFR inhibitors cetuximab and panitumumab.

GENETIC AND MOLECULAR MARKERS

Cancerous growth is an inheritable characteristic of cells that is thought to be the outcome of genetic changes.[109,262] Multiple genetic alterations may be necessary for the transformation of a cell from a normal state to a cancerous one and, finally, for metastatic spread. Therefore, evaluation of chromosomal changes may fill the gap left by traditional serum biochemical markers in establishing cancer risk and screening for cancer (see Chapters 17 and 37).

Classes of genes implicated in the development of cancer are (1) oncogenes (cell activation genes—Table 24-14) and (2) tumor suppressor genes (genes involved in the recognition and repair of damaged DNA—Table 24-15).[109,297] *Oncogenes* are derived from proto-oncogenes that may be activated by dominant mutations, such as point mutations, insertions, deletions, translocations, or inversions. Most oncogenes code for proteins that function at some stage of activation of cells for proliferation, and their activation leads to cell division. Most oncogenes are associated with hematologic malignancies such as leukemia and, to a lesser extent, solid tumors. Tumor genes of the other class, *tumor suppressor genes,* have been isolated from mostly solid tumors. The oncogenicity of tumor suppressor genes is derived from loss of the gene rather than from their activation, as with oncogenes. Deletion or monosomy may lead to loss of tumor suppressor genes. The major tumor suppressor gene, *p53,* functions to repair damaged DNA through apoptosis (programmed cell death). Repair is mediated by activation of the production of p21, which blocks the cell cycle in late G_1 to allow repair to take place.[129] Loss of function of this gene caused by loss or mutation may result in an impaired DNA repair process, leading to the development of tumorigenesis.

It is expected that knowledge of the sequence of the human genome[147,292] and identification of all genes will allow determination of which genes are differentially or aberrantly expressed in cancer and identification of the role of mutations or rearrangements of these genes in the development and progression of cancer (see Chapter 44). For example, identification of single-nucleotide polymorphisms and other genetic differences between individuals may allow the development of models for predicting individual predisposition to cancer and the deployment of effective prevention strategies,

TABLE 24-14 Some Oncogenes Found in Human Tumors

Oncogene	Function	Product	Type of Cancer
N-*ras* mutation	Signal transduction	Guanine diphosphate (GDP)/ guanine triphosphate (GTP) binding protein	Acute myeloid leukemia, neuroblastoma
K-*ras* mutation	Signal transduction	GDP/GTP binding protein	Leukemia, lymphoma
c-*myc* translocation	Transcription regulation	Binds to DNA	B- and T-cell lymphoma, small cell lung carcinoma
c-*erb* B-2 amplification	Growth factor receptor	Tyrosine kinase	Breast, ovarian, gastrointestinal
c-*abl*/*bcr* translocation	Signal transduction	Tyrosine kinase	Chronic myelocytic leukemia
N-*myc* amplification	Transcription regulation	Binds to DNA	Neuroendocrine
BCL-2	Blocks apoptosis	Mitochondrial membrane protein	Leukemia, lymphoma

TABLE 24-15 Tumor Suppressor Genes: Chromosomal Location and Tumor Types

Chromosome Region	Tumor Type	Gene*
3p	Kidney	*VHL* mutation
5q21	Colorectal	*APC* mutation
9p21	Bladder, glioblastoma, melanoma	*p16 (cdkn2)* mutation
11p13	Wilms' tumor	*WT1* mutation
11p15	Wilms', breast, hepatoblastoma, rhabdomyosarcoma, bladder	Loss of heterozygosity
13q	Breast	*BRCA2*, *RB1*
13q14	Retinoblastoma, osteosarcoma, small cell lung	*RB1* mutation
16q	Breast	*P16* E-cadherin mutation
17q	Neurofibromatosis 1, melanoma, breast	*BRCA1* mutation
17p13	Breast, colorectal, lung, liver, renal cell, bladder, sarcoma	*p53* mutation
18q21	Colorectal	*DCC* mutation
22q	Neurofibromatosis 2, meningioma	*NF2* mutation

*Other genes indicated by loss of heterozygosity include 1p, 8p, 9q, 10q, and others.

such as frequent surveillance, chemoprevention, nutritional and lifestyle modifications, etc.[124]

Advances in technologies (both hardware and software), coupled with robust expansion of nucleotide and protein databases, have led to the development of new tools that allow the simultaneous interrogation of hundreds to thousands of variables simultaneously. In particular, microarray-based analyses are at the forefront of translation to clinical practice. In addition to providing discussion of single gene–based markers that are oncogenes and tumor suppressors, this section on genetic markers ends with discussion of a group of microarray tests that are being used in current clinical practice. Highlighted are four such tests: Amplichip P450 from Roche Diagnostics, Onco*type* Dx from Genomic Health Inc., MammaPrint from Agendia Inc. (Amsterdam Science Park, The Netherlands), and the Tissue of Origin test from Pathwork Diagnostics (Redwood City, Calif). Although relative newcomers to the field of clinical diagnostics, it is anticipated that these organizations will revolutionize the future of cancer therapy by providing biomarkers for better stratification of a patient's disease, and by triaging individuals to the most appropriate therapy based on their genetic makeup. These genetic profiles, which allow for the design of custom-tailored therapies, will help to usher in the new era of personalized medicine.

Oncogenes

Proto-oncogenes are normal cellular genes that are similar to tumor virus genes. Activation of proto-oncogenes is found to be associated with cancer. These genes code for products that are involved in normal cellular processes, such as growth factor signaling pathways. Overexpression of the oncogene will lead to abnormal cell growth, resulting in malignancy. Of the more than 40 proto-oncogenes recognized, only a few have been shown to be useful tumor markers (see Table 24-14).[246]

RAS Genes

The *RAS* genes were first identified as being responsible for the tumorigenic properties of the Harvey (H-*ras*) and Kirsten (K-*ras*) sarcoma viruses, which produce tumors in animals, and provided the first evidence that cellular counterparts in human cells might be involved in the development of human tumors.[17] Proteins coded for by the *ras* genes are located at the inner face of the plasma membrane, as well as in other internal cellular membranes.[82] They bind to guanine nucleotides and function as molecular switches that regulate mitogenic signals from growth factors to the nucleus via signal transduction pathways.[61] *Ras* proteins are activated in association with protein-tyrosine kinase receptors and are required for growth factor proliferation or differentiation of a number of cell types.[163] *NRAS* is found on the short arm of human chromosome 1. Changes in *NRAS* appear to be the critical step in carcinogenesis. The mutated N-*ras* gene is found in neuroblastomas and acute myeloid leukemia. For more information on *RAS* genes in hematopoietic malignancies and myelodysplastic syndromes, see Chapter 44. Mutated *KRAS* is present in 95% of pancreatic cancers, 40% of colon cancers, and 30% of lung and bladder cancers, and in lower percentages in other tumors.[61] A single point mutation at the twelfth K-*ras* codon changes the coded amino acid from glycine to valine in the p21 protein. This mutation is by far the most frequently found in cancer, but other mutations have also been demonstrated, including those at codons 13 and 61.[180] *KRAS* mutations appear to correlate with poor prognosis and shorter disease-free survival in patients with adenocarcinoma of the lung and endometrial carcinoma. Activated *ras* is detected by expression of the *ras* gene product, p21, in cancer tissue. By immunohistochemistry, the *ras* product is found not only in about 40% of colon cancers, but also in colon polyps believed to be premalignant. Higher relative intensity of staining for p21-*ras* may differentiate malignant from normal tissues or benign lesions in (1) breast, (2) pancreas, (3) stomach, (4) lung, (5) uterus, or (6) thyroid tissues.[100] Expression in tissue appears to correlate with stage or grade of the tumor, but p21-*ras* may also be seen in some normal tissue, and other studies show no significant difference between benign and malignant tumors. Use of p21 as a tumor marker in tissue or serum is not well established. Mutations of *ras* oncogenes have been detected in DNA in the stool of symptomatic and asymptomatic patients with colorectal tumors, suggesting a novel, noninvasive paradigm for population screening.[150,250]

Several studies have underscored the importance of *KRAS* mutations in therapeutic regimen selection. As discussed at ASCO 2007-2009 and formalized in a provisional clinical opinion article,[7] individuals with a diagnosis of metastatic colorectal cancer with wild-type *KRAS* tumors are much more likely to benefit from monoclonal antibody treatments targeting the EGFR pathway, such as cetuximab and panitumumab, than individuals whose tumor carries mutated *KRAS* (at codons 12 and 13). Thus, *KRAS* mutation testing is advocated in patients suffering from metastatic colorectal carcinoma who are candidates for anti-EGFR treatments. Further, if the tumor tests positive for mutation at codon 12 or 13, the patient should not receive anti-EGFR treatments.

c-*myc*

The *MYC* gene is the proto-oncogene of avian myelocytoma virus. It binds to DNA and is involved in transcription regulation. The gene product, p62, is located in the nucleus of transformed cells, and expression of c-*myc* correlates with the rate of cell division. The c-*myc* protein is essential for DNA replication and enhances mRNA transcription. Activation of the c *myc* gene is associated with B- and T-cell lymphoma, sarcoma, and endothelioma.[249] In leukemias and lymphomas, increased c-*myc* expression may be due to amplification or chromosomal translocation of the gene. In acute T-cell leukemias, an (8:14) (q24:q11) translocation results in activation of the gene, and is associated with a poor prognosis. A decrease in expression of c-*myc* after initiation of chemotherapy suggests a favorable response. Overexpression of p62 may be seen in 70 to 100% of primary breast cancers with the use of immunohistochemistry, and the intensity of staining is greater with increasing stages of the tumor. Amplification in lung carcinomas and gliomas correlates with clinical aggressiveness. A fivefold to 40-fold higher expression of c-*myc* may be seen in colon cancer when compared with normal mucosa, but the amount of expression does not correlate with progression. A similar relationship has been found for cervical, gastric, liver, and other cancers. Serum concentrations of c-*myc* have been used to detect recurrence, but not to differentiate cancer from benign conditions. Several reviews have highlighted recent developments in application of the c-*myc* tumor marker to breast, cervical, and colorectal cancers.[36,226,231]

Her-2/*neu* (*ERBB2*)

The HER-2/*neu* gene (also known as c-erbB-2, symbol *ERBB2*) is named for its association with neural tumors (*neu*).

Biochemistry

The *ERBB2* gene codes for a 185 kDa transmembrane protein expressed on epithelial cells and belongs to the EGF family of tyrosine kinase receptors. The EGF family includes four members: the EGFR (also known as *ErbB1/HER-1*), *ERBB2* (HER-2/*neu*), *ERBB3*, and *ERBB4*. Members of the EGF family of receptors have the same overall structure consisting of an extracellular ligand-binding domain (ECD), a single transmembrane domain, and an intracellular tyrosine kinase domain. The extracellular domain can undergo proteolytic cleavage by metalloproteases, releasing the ECD (known as p105) into the blood, which can be detected. All are involved in cell proliferation, differentiation, and survival. HER-2/*neu* is normally expressed on the epithelia of numerous organs, including (1) lung, (2) bladder, (3) pancreas, (4) breast, and (5) prostate, and has been found to be elevated in cancer cells.

Clinical Applications

Amplification of *ERBB2* is found in (1) breast, (2) ovarian, and (3) gastrointestinal tumors. In breast cancer, it appears to be as useful a prognostic indicator of overall survival and tumor size as ER and PR expression, but not as good as the number of lymph nodes involved in metastases.[255] Of the three oncogenes—*ERBB2, RAS,* and *MYC*—*ERBB2* has the strongest prognostic value in breast cancer. Herceptin treatment is administered only to those breast cancer patients who have HER2/*neu* amplification.

Serum concentrations of HER2/*neu* are most useful in breast cancer, with some use in ovarian cancer patients.[164] The assay is cleared by the FDA for use in follow-up and monitoring of patients with metastatic breast cancer with a HER-2/*neu* concentration >15 µg/L. Approximately 30% of patients have elevated concentrations. HER2/*neu* concentrations in breast cancer correlate with a worse prognosis and a shorter disease-free state. Elevated HER2/*neu* concentrations also correlate with large tumor size, lymph node positivity, and high grading score. One study of 719 breast cancer patients showed that patients with ER-positive cancers and elevated concentrations of HER2/*neu* derived less clinical benefit from hormonal therapies.[158] Furthermore, the study showed a trend toward improved outcomes with aromatase inhibitors for patients with elevated serum HER2/*neu*. Serum concentrations of HER2/*neu* may also be useful in monitoring the response of breast cancer patients to treatment.

Analytical Methods

Immunohistochemistry is used to detect increased expression of the HER2/*neu* protein. FISH is used for detection of HER2/*neu* gene amplification. ASCO and the College of American Pathologists (CAP) collaborated to develop comprehensive guidelines for HER2/*neu* testing.[303] The ECD of HER2/*neu* in serum is detected by ELISA and automated immunoassay. Both assays use the same monoclonal antibodies, recognizing different epitopes of the ECD, which does not cross-react with any other member of the EGF family. It is important to note that there is no interference from the therapeutic monoclonal antibody, Herceptin, with either assay.[164] The ELISA has a lower detection limit of 1.5 µg/L and an upper limit of 35 µg/L, and the automated immunoassay has a linear range from 0.5 to 350 µg/L. The cutoff for both assays has been set at 15 µg/L.

BCL-2

The product of the *BCL2* oncogene is a 239 amino acid, 25 kDa integral membrane protein that localizes primarily to the mitochondrial membranes and to other cellular membranes. This protein is known to inhibit apoptosis (programmed cell death) and to contribute to survival of cancer cells, especially lymphoma and leukemic cells.[173] The *BCL2* proto-oncogene was identified in follicular lymphomas wherein a 14:18 translocation results in formation of a *BCL-2*–immunoglobulin heavy chain fusion gene. Activation of the *BCL-2* gene through the immunoglobulin promoter results in production of high concentrations of *BCL-2* protein. The protein is normally expressed on cells that have a long life span (e.g., neurons) and on proliferative cells in rapidly renewing cell lineages, such as basal epithelial cells. The *BCL2* oncogene is highly expressed in a variety of hematologic malignancies, including lymphomas, myelomas, and chronic leukemias (malignancies characterized by prolonged cell survival). In the normal colon, *BCL-22*–positive cells are restricted to basal epithelial cells, whereas in dysplastic polyps and carcinomas, many positive cells may be found in parabasal and superficial regions.[254,262] Abnormal expression of the *BCL*-2 gene appears to be an early event in colorectal carcinogenesis. In addition, overexpression of the *BCL2* gene is associated with development of resistance to cytotoxic cancer chemotherapy in a variety of tumors, including epithelial tumors and lymphomas. Thus detection of the *BCL2*-gene product in tumors is an indication of progression. Future studies may determine its usefulness for predicting resistance to chemotherapy. A meta-analysis strongly suggested a prognostic role for BCL-2 (as detected by immmunohistochemistry) in breast cancer, independent of several clinical variables. Additional studies using a large prospective cohort are needed to fully establish its clinical usefulness for this application.[43]

BCR-ABL

Chronic myelogenous leukemia (CML) is a myeloproliferative disorder resulting from the clonal expansion of a transformed multipotent hematopoietic stem cell. In approximately 90% of CML patients, the transforming event is the formation of the Philadelphia chromosome—a balanced translocation between chromosomes 9 and 22 [t(9;22)(q34;q11)] creating the *BCR-ABL* fusion gene. The protein derived from this fusion is a constitutively active cytoplasmic tyrosine kinase that activates several signaling pathways, leading to uncontrolled growth, inhibition of apoptosis, and other aspects of neoplastic transformation.[219]

Detection of the *BCR-ABL* gene is useful in diagnosing CML and in directing treatment, because several strategies target the *BCR-ABL* gene by oligonucleotides (antisense or ribozyme based)[95] or the *BCR-ABL* kinase domain by the tyrosine kinase inhibitor STI571 (also known as Gleevec or Imatinib mesylate). *BCR-ABL* detection by RT-PCR is useful in monitoring minimal residual disease in patients who have undergone bone marrow transplantation. In the subset of acute lymphoblastic leukemia patients who harbor the Philadelphia chromosome, a positive RT-PCR for the *BCR-ABL* gene carries a much higher risk of relapse compared with a negative result. In CML patients after bone marrow transplantation, positive RT-PCR results at 6 to 12 months were associated with a 26-fold elevated risk of relapse, and a positive result at 3 months was not predictive of risk.[221] Also, the amount of BCR-ABL transcript per µg of RNA correlated with risk of relapse; less than 1% of patients with fewer than 50 transcripts per µg of RNA relapsed, and 72% of patients with more than 50 transcripts per µg of RNA relapsed.[157] For more information on BCR-ABL, see Chapter 44.

RET

The *RET* proto-oncogene encodes a tyrosine kinase receptor involved in kidney morphogenesis, maturation of the peripheral nervous system, and differentiation of spermatogonia.[144] RET stands for "rearranged during transfection." The RET receptor exists in a multimeric complex that includes one of four glycosyl-phosphatidylinositol (GPI)-linked coreceptors (GFRα 1, 2, 3, and 4). The complex responds to four ligands: glial-derived neurotrophic factor (GDNF), neurturin (NTN), persephin (PSP), and artemin. Activation of RET appears to occur through dimerization and transphosphorylation of the receptor that recruits numerous signaling molecules. RET, similar to other tyrosine kinase receptors, activates downstream growth pathways, and with uncontrolled signaling, cancer can result.

Inappropriate activation of RET has been extensively studied in (1) papillary thyroid cancer, (2) multiple endocrine neoplasia type 2 (MEN-2), and (3) familial medullary thyroid carcinoma (FMTC).[144] In each, the mechanism of activation of RET is through unregulated dimerization and transphosphorylation of the RET receptor.[6] In the case of papillary thyroid cancer, a genetic event creates a fusion between the *RET* tyrosine kinase domain and a dimerization domain that can be donated by a number of genes. In MEN-2A and FMTC, point mutations of the extracellular domain induce disulfide linkages between receptors, thus inducing dimerization. In MEN-2B, a point mutation in the kinase domain appears to alter the substrate specificity of the tyrosine kinase and presumably leads to inappropriate activation of downstream growth pathways. Specific mutations are highly correlated with disease phenotype and are also important for diagnostic and prognostic purposes. The molecular basis underlying the mutations has provided great insight into separable functional features of this tyrosine kinase protein.[144]

Tumor Suppressor Genes

Several tumor suppressor genes associated with human cancer are listed in Table 24-15. Historically, evidence of tumor suppressor genes was derived from the study of hybrid cells of normal and malignant cells that behaved normally.[271] It was concluded that normal cells contained a gene that suppressed the expression of malignancy.[112] Reversion to malignancy occurred when the cultured cells lost normal chromosomes. The study of tumor suppressor genes may provide a clue as to the development of cancer from normal cell status to benign and cancerous status and to metastasis. The development of colon cancer requires multiple steps that involve several mutations. Loss of a chromosome 5 gene leads to an increase in cell growth. Early adenoma is associated with loss of methyl groups on the DNA strand. With the *RAS* gene mutation and loss of the *DCC* gene on chromosome 18, adenoma advances to the late stage. Carcinoma is found with loss of the *p53* gene on chromosome 17. Finally, metastasis occurs with other chromosome losses.[81] The clinical usefulness of detection of mutations in tumor suppressor genes lies not only in the diagnosis and prognosis of cancer, but also in the prediction of susceptibility when the mutation is carried in the germline, such as with the breast cancer genes *BRCA1* and *BRCA2*.

Retinoblastoma Gene

Retinoblastoma (RB) is a rare tumor of children that occurs both in families and sporadically. The work of Alfred G. Knudson on the familial-specific incidence of RB led to the two-hit hypothesis.[137,138] He reasoned that in the inherited form of the tumor, one mutation was present in the germline and in all cells of the body, the other mutational event occurring somatically in one of the cells of the developing retina. In the sporadic form, both mutations occur somatically in the same developing retinoblast—a relatively rare event. The two-hit hypothesis has served as a model for other tumor suppressor genes. The *RB* gene *(RB1)* has been localized to chromosome 13q by loss of a chromosomal banding region in the peripheral blood lymphocytes of patients with the familial form and by loss of heterozygosity studies in both RBs and some osteosarcomas. However, most tumors do not have gross deletions but point mutations or small insertions and deletions that result in premature truncation of the protein product.[96] The protein product of the *RB1* gene is a nuclear phosphoprotein with a molecular mass of about 105 kDa (p105-RB).[148] This protein binds to a product of a DNA tumor virus, such as the E1A protein of murine tumor virus or the E7 protein of human papillomavirus. When p105-RB is hypophosphorylated, it complexes with transcription factors such as E2F and blocks transcription of genes in S-phase cells. E2F dimerizes with a DP protein and regulates the transcription of several genes involved in DNA synthesis. Inactivation or loss of p105-RB deregulates DNA synthesis and increases cellular proliferation. Thus RB is a tumor suppressor gene, as it suppresses DNA synthesis. Detection of mutations in RB is useful in determining the susceptibility of an individual to development of RB in the familial form, but it is not used as a tumor marker.

p53 Gene

Of particular interest is the *p53* gene,[130,170] *TP53* (tumor protein 53), which lies on chromosome 17q. Native or wild-type p53 is believed to control cell division by regulating entry into the S phase.[129] This controlling effect of p53 protein may be lost by deletion of the gene or production of a competing mutant protein. Seventy-five to 80% of colon carcinomas show deletion in one *TP53* allele and a point mutation in the other allele; thus, no wild-type p53 protein is expressed in these tumors. Allelic deletion of *TP53* occurs only rarely in adenomas (10%), suggesting that p53 inactivation may be a relatively late event in colon carcinogenesis. In addition, up to 70% of breast cancers also have deleted *TP53*. Mutations in *TP53* produce proteins that inactivate the wild-type p53 protein and allow cells to move through the cell cycle and contribute to the autonomous growth of cancer. Several different mutations of *p53* have been found in human cancers.[151] Most point mutations affect one of four regions of the protein (amino acid residues 117 to 142, 171 to 181, 134 to 158, and 270 to 286); three "hot spots" affect residues 175, 248, and 273.[151] In addition, selective guanine-to-thymine mutations are found at codon 249 in human hepatocellular carcinomas taken from patients in high-incidence areas of Africa, and those at codon 197 are associated with aflatoxin exposure. Mutations at codons 245 and 258 are found in Li-Fraumeni syndrome, a rare autosomal dominant syndrome characterized by diverse neoplasms at many different sites in the body.[197,268]

Monoclonal antibodies to mutated p53 proteins have been developed. Wild-type p53 is normally present in very small amounts that are not detected by immunohistochemistry, whereas the mutant protein accumulates and is easily detected. Overexpression of the mutant proteins has been detected in up to 70% of primary colorectal cancers. Overexpression of p53 in breast cancers is associated with poor prognosis, but this association is not as strong as the association with c-*erb*B-2.[187,189] Up to 75% of small cell lung carcinomas appear to overexpress a mutant (missense mutation) protein. Finally, circulating antibodies to mutant p53 proteins have been found in sera from patients with breast and lung cancer and B-cell lymphomas. This antibody response may be useful in this subset of patients for monitoring relapse.[170] Hall and McCluggage review methodologic issues of the different assays for interrogating p53 and its downstream effectors in several clinical contexts.[107]

p21 *(WAF1)*

The wild-type p53 protein activates transcription of various genes, including the *WAF1/CIP1* gene (symbol *CDKN1A* for cyclin-dependent kinase inhibitor 1A). The p21 protein product of the gene binds to and inhibits the cyclin-dependent protein kinases (CDKs) that are active in the G_1 phase of the cell cycle. The cell-cycle arrest function of p53 in response to DNA damage is mediated by p21. Monoclonal antibodies to the p21 protein are now available and are being used to determine whether expression of p21 in tumors may be clinically useful. Recent work assessing the role of p21 suggests that additional data are required before the efficacy of p21 for predicting outcomes in rectal cancer can be validated.[142]

APC

One of the first events in the putative steps of progression of precursor lesions to colon cancer is loss of the adenomatous polyposis coli *(APC)* gene in premalignant polyps.[81] The *APC* gene encodes a 300 kDa protein that may be truncated in cancer cells. The normal function of the *APC* gene product is not known, but it interacts with proteins, such as α- and β-catenin, involved in cell-cell interactions in epithelial cells. This gene is mutated in hereditary colorectal cancer syndromes—polyposis and nonpolyposis types. In the polyposis types, hundreds and even thousands or more benign tumors (polyps) arise before the development of cancer. Among nonpolyposis types, very few polyps are seen, but the elevated risk of cancer is essentially similar. The *APC* gene was detected by an interstitial deletion on chromosome 5q in a patient with hundreds of polyps.[149] More than 80% of individuals with hereditary colorectal cancer have germline mutations in one of the *APC* alleles, including gross deletions or localized mutations. Hereditary forms of colorectal cancer are relatively uncommon, but somatic mutations appear to be of great importance in the development of nonhereditary colorectal cancers. More than 70% of colorectal tumors, regardless of size or histology, have a specific mutation in one of the two *APC* alleles, and mutation may be found in other types of tumors, including breast, esophageal, and brain tumors. The usefulness of loss of the APC protein for diagnosis and prognosis is the subject of ongoing investigation. However, recent evidence suggests the importance of APC functional activity for prognostic purposes, as well as for directing therapy in colorectal cancer.[220]

Neurofibromatosis Type 1

Neurofibromatosis type 1 (NF1), or von Recklinghausen's disease, is a dominantly inherited syndrome manifested mainly by proliferation of cells from the neural crest, resulting in multiple neurofibromas, café au lait spots, and Lisch nodules of the iris.[247] Mutations in the *NF1* gene have been found in about 20% of NF1 patients.[295] The *NF1* gene has been localized to the pericentromeric region of chromosome 17q, band 11. It is a large gene coding for a p300 protein, called *neurofibromin.* This protein has a high degree of similarity to GTPase-activating proteins, and is thought to act as a negative regulator of *Ras.*[300] Although the exact mechanism of action of the protein is not known, it appears likely that loss or inactivation of neurofibromin function leads to alterations in signal transduction pathways regulated by small *ras*-like G proteins, resulting in constitutive signaling from this pathway. Inactivating mutations of *NF1* have also been found in colorectal cancer, melanoma, and neuroblastoma.

WT1

The Wilms' tumor suppressor gene, *WT1,* is located on chromosome 11p13. Its loss plays a causal role in the development of a childhood kidney malignancy, and it is involved in normal and abnormal hematopoiesis.[12] The *WT1* gene encodes a 45 kDa protein that appears to function in transcriptional regulation by suppressing the expression of growth-inducing genes, such as early growth response, insulin-like growth factor-2, and platelet-derived growth factor A chain genes.[102] Other chromosomal changes in Wilms' tumors indicate that mutations of *WT1* may be only one step in the process of carcinogenesis. Thus identification and understanding of one tumor suppressor gene in a given cancer may provide only part of the information eventually required to understand the carcinogenic process.

nm23

The nm23 gene *NME1* was found overexpressed in a nonmetastatic murine melanoma cell line but present in low amounts in a highly metastatic cell line. The *NME1* gene product appears to be elevated in metastatic breast, colon, and prostatic cancer and now is being evaluated as a new marker for metastases.[88]

BRCA1 and *BRCA2*

A subset of breast cancer patients have been shown to have an inherited predisposition to developing breast and ovarian cancer that is inherited as an autosomal dominant trait.[135] Two genetic loci have been identified: *BRCA1* on chromosome 17q, and *BRCA2,* which localizes to 13q12-13.[177,304] *BRCA1* encodes an 1863 amino acid protein that may act as a transcription factor. The ability to detect mutations in *BRCA1* and *BRCA2* in the germline permits the identification of individuals in breast cancer families who carry the mutated gene. It is estimated that as many as 1 in 200 women in the

United States may have a germline mutation in the *BRCA1* gene. This has created an ethical dilemma for physicians, patients, and their families, and for insurance companies and health maintenance organizations, as it is now possible to predict with reasonable certainty that an individual who carries a mutation in one of these genes will develop breast and/or ovarian cancer. What should be done if an otherwise healthy individual is shown to carry a *BRCA* gene mutation? Carriers of a *BRCA1* gene mutation have an 85% risk of developing breast cancer and a 45% risk of developing ovarian cancer by the age of 85.[87] Should such patients have preventive mastectomy or ovariectomy? Should insurance companies and healthcare maintenance organizations have higher rates for carriers? It has always been a goal of cancer research to be able to identify individuals at risk. Now that this is possible, a policy must be developed on how to deal with the information (see Harper[111] or Petty and Killeen[215]). The recently passed GINA legislation (Genetic Information Nondiscriminatory Act) prohibits discrimination based on genetic information and is an important step in the right direction. Although detection of the mutation is not useful as a tumor marker per se, with further understanding of how the mutated gene products act, it may be possible to understand the molecular events for development of some breast and ovarian cancers.

Deleted in Colorectal Carcinoma

The "deleted in colorectal carcinoma" *(DCC)* gene, located on chromosome 18q, encodes a membrane protein of the immunoglobulin superfamily. The exact function of DCC has yet to be elucidated. However, studies have suggested a role in axonal development as a component of the Netrin-1 receptor, and others have suggested a role in promoting apoptosis.[98] Many cellular processes co-opted in oncogenesis are also critical in nervous system development, thus suggesting the possibility of the DCC protein to function in both pathways.[76] In colon cancer, DCC is thought to act as a tumor suppressor; thus deletion or reduced expression correlates with increasing stage and a poorer prognosis.[190] Conversely, loss of *DCC* expression in gastric cancer was associated with a better prognosis and improved tumor cell differentiation.[190] However, the function of DCC and how it fulfills its role as a tumor suppressor are controversial.[175] More work is necessary to determine the exact role of DCC in colon cancer and other cancers.

PTEN

The *PTEN* tumor suppressor gene, located at human chromosome 10q23, is mutated in numerous cancers, and is probably underestimated in terms of its importance in tumor formation and progression.[281] Primary sequence analysis suggested that it encodes a protein tyrosine phosphatase with extensive homology to the cytoskeletal protein tensin.[154] PTEN functions as a phosphatase that negatively regulates phosphoinositide 3-kinase (PI 3-K) signaling by dephosphorylating the D3 position of phosphatidylinositol (3,4,5)-triphosphate [PtdIns(3,4,5)P_3]. PI 3-kinase and its product PtdIns(3,4,5)P_3 are involved in activation of signaling pathways leading to inhibition of apoptosis, cell migration, cell size, and chemotaxis. Mutation or inactivation of *PTEN* allows uncontrolled activation of the downstream pathways, which contribute to tumorigenesis.[183]

Germline mutations in *PTEN* cause the (1) Cowden, (2) Lhermitte-Duclos, (3) Bannayan-Zonana, and (4) Proteus autosomal dominant syndromes, all of which are characterized by the development of hamartomas and an increased likelihood of tumor development, along with other growth-related symptoms. In general, *PTEN* mutation or loss of expression is associated with a more advanced stage and is a poor prognostic indicator in various cancers, including breast, hepatocellular, endometrial, and cervical.

Other Molecular Tests

Single-Nucleotide Polymorphisms

The Human Genome Project identified all of the approximate 25,000 transcriptional units in the human genome and determined the sequences of the 3 billion chemical base pairs that constitute human DNA. A byproduct of the sequencing effort was the identification of a very large number of single-nucleotide polymorphisms (SNPs; single nucleotides that differ between individuals and are inherited), formalized and detailed through the efforts of a related genomic project, the HapMap Project.[124] It has been estimated that one SNP can be found in every approximately 300 bases of human DNA. Most of these SNPs are present in introns, and only a relatively small number (approximately 60,000 of the 2,000,000 SNPs) are within exons. Groups of SNPs (called *haplotypes*) are inherited together in blocks. It has been hypothesized that it may be possible to correlate SNP composition (e.g., various haplotypes) with disease predisposition. Until now, very few SNPs or haplotypes have been associated consistently with human cancers. Many scientists are currently investigating SNPs and are attempting to correlate them with various diseases. Large numbers of SNPs can be surveyed by using hybridization-based technologies such as microarrays, or can be interrogated using targeted approaches utilizing separation techniques such as capillary electrophoresis and mass spectrometry. The hope is to identify characteristic SNPs or haplotypes that can be used for diagnostic purposes or for determining future risk (predisposition) for developing certain diseases.

Cell-Free Nucleic Acids

Circulating DNA and RNA have been recognized since the 1970s, but it was not until the late 1980s that the neoplastic characteristics of DNA were recognized.[128] Circulating DNA and RNA have been proposed as a marker for certain types of cancer.[51,282] To use circulating DNA as a cancer marker, a mechanism must differentiate normal DNA from neoplastic DNA. This is achieved by detecting mutations in circulating DNA that are present in cancer cells (e.g., *ras* mutations that occur in various cancers), by performing microsatellite analysis of circulating DNA, or by detecting common cancer-causing chromosomal translocations. Epigenetic alterations of circulating DNA, such as altered methylation patterns, can also be detected. In recent years, cell free nucleic acids have been detected in bronchial lavage fluid from lung cancer patients and in plasma from colorectal cancer patients.[92,239] Over the next decade, detection of circulating DNA will likely join a growing number of clinically useful markers. In the future, this technology may have the ability to provide a more global picture of the abnormalities present in the patient.

Circulating Tumor Cells

A majority of all cancers are derived from epithelial cells. Under appropriate conditions, these cells break from the primary tumor and shed into the circulation. These circulating tumor cells (CTCs) are very rare (approximately 1 CTC per 5 to 10 million red blood cells and lymphocytes), but they can be captured, enriched, and enumerated. Quantification of CTCs has been demonstrated to be an independent predictor of overall survival and progression-free survival in patients suffering from metastatic breast, colon, and prostate cancers. This technology, as applied using the Veridex CellSearch platform (Veridex LLC, Raritan, NJ),[293] is FDA approved for these applications. It is hoped that this procedure will assist with early detection of disease and enable personalized therapy for targeted management and improved outcomes.

The assay uses a combination of positive and negative selection methods to isolate circulating epithelial cells from whole blood. Specifically, anti-EpCAM antibodies are used to selectively capture epithelial cells from whole blood. This step is followed by a negative selection step using anti-CD45 antibodies to remove white blood cells from the preparation. The remaining cells then are stained for cytokeratin positivity and are analyzed by immunofluorescence microscopy. Cells are enumerated by assessing positivity for cytokeratin, negativity for CD45, and positive DAPI staining. This procedure allows the identification of nucleated epithelial cells from whole blood. Two advantages of this technology are that it is noninvasive, requiring only a blood sample, and it can be performed essentially in real time. Thus, it allows rapid assessment of therapeutic response and hence, adjustment of therapy as needed. For patients not responding to a particular line of therapy, alternative regimens can be prescribed, or dosages can be adjusted as needed. In addition, unnecessary treatment can be avoided. The greatest demonstration of the use of this technology is seen in breast cancer patients.[64] In metastatic breast or prostate cancer, a CTC count of five or more cells per 7.5 mL of blood is associated with a poor prognosis and is predictive of shorter progression-free survival and overall survival. The same is true in metastatic colorectal cancer with a CTC count of three or more cells per 7.5 mL of blood. The CellSearch system has been validated for analytical performance and robustness.[225]

PCA3

PCA3 (prostate cancer gene or antigen 3) is a molecular urine test for prostate cancer. The *PCA3* gene, also known as $PCA3^{DD3}$ or $DD3^{PCA3}$, was first described in 1999.[41] *PCA3* mRNA is noncoding, and its function is unknown. *PCA3* is highly overexpressed in prostate cancer tissue compared with healthy or benign prostate tissue, which has low expression. It is not detectable in healthy tissue or in tumors from bladder, testis, and other organs.[67] PCA3 score correlates with biopsy outcome in men undergoing a first or a repeat biopsy. In a prospective study of 570 men undergoing prostate biopsy, a PCA3 score of 35 yielded 54% clinical sensitivity and 74% specificity for prostate cancer detection.[69] Unlike PSA, PCA3 is independent of prostate volume, and PCA3 scores have been associated with both grade and extent of prostate cancer. In 2006, the PCA3 assay (Gen-Probe PROGENSA; Gen-Probe Inc., San Diego, Calif) received marketing clearance in Europe. Urine specimens for PCA3 are collected following digital rectal exam (DRE) with three strokes per prostate lobe (to release prostate cells) and are mixed with a stabilization buffer to lyse cells and stabilize the RNA. PCA3 and PSA mRNA are quantitated using transcription-mediated nucleic acid amplification. The PCA3 mRNA copy number is normalized with the PSA mRNA housekeeping gene to generate the PCA3 score (PCA3 mRNA/PSA mRNA × 1000).

Microarray-Based Markers

Roche Amplichip P450

The Roche Amplichip P450[80,115] is the first FDA-cleared microarray-based pharmacogenetic assay with application to the clinical management of patients. It detects variations in the cytochrome *P450 2D6* and *2C19* genes, which are involved in the metabolism of many clinically prescribed drugs, including beta blockers, antidepressants, antipsychotics, and, most important for this chapter, chemotherapeutic agents such as tamoxifen and cyclophosphamide. Variation includes the presence of single-nucleotide polymorphisms in the *CYP2D6* and *CYP2C19* genes, as well as deletions and duplications in *CYP2D6*. With this chip, up to 33 2D6 alleles and 3 2C19 alleles can be interrogated simultaneously.

From a technical perspective, the assay is conducted in five steps: (1) PCR amplification of appropriate segments of patient genomic DNA, (2) fragmentation and labeling of the amplified products, (3) hybridization to the microarray and staining of the bound products, (4) scanning of the microarray, and (5) interpretation to give a predicted phenotype based on genotypic results. By determining the patient's genotype, a phenotype is predicted, thus allowing for tailored treatments. The test is used to classify individuals as poor, intermediate, extensive, or ultrarapid metabolizers, and this knowledge can be used to select appropriate therapy. Appropriate triage of patients is useful for optimizing efficacy and minimizing adverse drug reactions.

Drugs that are metabolized through the cytochrome P4502D6 pathway can be inactivated or activated through enzymatic action of 2D6. In the case of inactivation, as exemplified by the antidepressant paroxetine, the following effects may be noted on the basis of patient genotype. Individuals who are poor or intermediate metabolizers of 2D6 may experience toxic side effects as the result of overmedication when given a standard dose. Such individuals may benefit from smaller doses than standard. Extensive metabolizers will be able to properly metabolize their medication with standard doses and should have the expected response to their medication. In contrast, ultrarapid metabolizers metabolize medication quickly and may not respond to standard doses of medication. Such patients may benefit from higher doses of medication. Not all drugs will fit this scenario. In other cases, a drug may be activated through the cytochrome P4502D6 pathway. One example is that of tamoxifen, which is used currently as the standard of care treatment for estrogen receptor–positive (ER+) breast cancer. Tamoxifen is a prodrug that undergoes a series of modifications leading to its activation. Clinically, endoxifen is the most important active metabolite; it has been shown to have 50 to 100 times greater antitumor activity compared with tamoxifen in in vitro assays and higher affinity for the estrogen receptor. Endoxifen is produced by the action of the cytochrome P4502D6 enzyme in the liver.

Poor and intermediate metabolizers of 2d6 will experience suboptimal effects because of reduced endoxifen concentrations. In contrast, ultrarapid metabolizers may experience toxic effects caused by high concentrations of the active metabolite. Because tamoxifen is a prodrug, the effects are the opposite of those given in the previous example, where the drug (paroxetine) is inactivated by CYP2D6.

Similarly, for cytochrome P4502C19, two thoroughly-characterized alleles result in reduced enzymatic activity. These are the *2 and *3 SNPs. 2C19 corresponds to S-mephenytoin hydroxylase and metabolizes many psychiatric medications in use today (e.g., proton pump inhibitors, antiepileptic agents). It is also responsible for metabolism of the chemotherapeutic agent, cyclophosphamide. Genotyping and classification of patients based on 2C19 works similarly to that of 2d6. However, amplifications and deletions of this gene have not been characterized in the scientific literature. Thus, classification of patients is limited to that of poor (at least one reduced functional allele) and extensive metabolizers (at least one wild-type allele).

Onco*type* Dx

The Onco*type* Dx assay, marketed by Genomic Health Inc. Redwood City, CA,[94] determines the expression of 21 genes in breast tissue.[201] It is intended for use in women with early-stage, node-negative, ER-positive breast cancer who will be treated with hormonal therapy.[199,200] The assay provides an assessment of the likelihood of response to chemotherapy and of recurrence within 10 years. The result of this assay is a recurrence score that ranges from 0 to 100. A score above 31 indicates high risk of recurrence, whereas a score of 18 or less indicates low risk of recurrence. Scores greater than 18 but lower than 31 indicate an indeterminate recurrence risk. This test can thus be used for clinical decision making following triaging of patients to the most appropriate therapy—those at high risk can be treated more aggressively, whereas for those at lower risk, standard therapy is recommended. This assay was included in the 2007 American Society of Clinical Oncology (ASCO) clinical guidelines on the use of tumor markers in breast cancer and in the 2008 National Comprehensive Cancer Network (NCCN) breast cancer treatment guidelines.[113,184] Evidence suggests that the test may also be useful in the treatment of postmenopausal women with node-positive, ER-positive, invasive breast cancer.[5]

Agendia MammaPrint

The Agendia MammaPrint assay is the first genomic FDA-cleared IVDMIA (in vitro diagnostic multivariate index assay) used to assess the risk of breast cancer recurrence.[4] It is intended for use in women younger than 60 years of age who are diagnosed with early-stage breast cancer (stage 1 or 2) that is node negative with <5 cm tumors. Assessment is performed on fresh frozen tumor tissue obtained during surgery with samples being sent directly to Agendia Laboratories in The Netherlands. The assay can be used to identify which tumors are most likely to recur after surgery, independent of estrogen receptor status and any prior therapies.

From a technical perspective, the assay measures the expression of 70 genes involved in important signal transduction pathways responsible for breast cancer metastasis. The genes function in various aspects of the metastatic process, including (1) cell cycle progression, (2) angiogenesis, (3) invasion, and (4) cell migration. The assay is based on initial microarray studies performed on samples (both ER positive and negative) with 10-year follow-up data. The analysis identified a 231-gene biomarker signature and after validation was later enriched to capture the 70 most prognostic genes capable of stratifying patients for likelihood of recurrence.[291] This 70-gene biomarker signature has been independently validated in other cohorts.[42] It provides a picture of alterations in gene activity and likelihood of disease spread. Patients are stratified into one of two groups—low risk or high risk—for distant metastasis (there is no intermediate risk group). Because disease can be characterized based on aggressiveness, this knowledge allows a clinician to tailor therapy specifically to the patient. Specifically, for women at low risk based on their MammaPrint score and traditional risk factors, hormonal therapy (such as tamoxifen) may be sufficient. In contrast, for women at high risk based on MammaPrint score and additional risk factors, more aggressive treatment may be recommended, possibly including chemotherapy.

Pathwork Diagnostics Tissue of Origin Test

The tissue of origin test uses gene expression information from tumor samples to reliably determine a cancer's tissue of origin.[209] It is performed on individuals with poorly differentiated or undifferentiated tumors. Such a diagnosis poses a problem because cancer treatment guidelines are dependent on knowing the origin of the primary tumor.[33] In approximately 5% of cancers, the primary tumor site cannot be determined, and therefore the appropriate therapy cannot be selected.

Historically, such assessments have been performed based on immunohistochemical analyses that are subjective, as they are based on pathologist review and interpretation. In contrast, the tissue of origin test measures gene expression using microarrays to interrogate a panel of 1550 genes in addition to 110 control genes. These data are then compared with gene expression patterns from a panel of 15 known tumor tissue types representing 90% of all solid tumors. This comparison results in a similarity score that can aid in determining the most likely tissue of origin. The tissue of origin test uses formalin-fixed paraffin-embedded (FFPE) or frozen specimens. A Clinical Laboratory Improvement Amendments (CLIA)-certified laboratory service is available for this analysis, requiring specimens to be sent directly to Pathwork Diagnostics Laboratory, Redwood City, CA. The in vitro diagnostic kit is FDA cleared for use on frozen samples.

REFERENCES

1. Aaronson SA. Growth factors and cancer. Science 1991;254:1146-53.
2. Abelev GI, Perova SD, Khramkova NI, et al. Production of embryonal alpha-globulins by transplantable mouse hepatomas. Transplantation 1963;1:174-8.
3. Adam B-L, Qu Y, Davies JW, et al. Serum protein fingerprinting coupled with a pattern-matching algorithm distinguishes prostate cancer from benign prostate hyperplasia and healthy men. Cancer Res 2002;62:3609-14.
4. Agendia Inc. MammaPrint. Available at: http://usa.agendia.com/ (accessed May 2, 2011).
5. Albain A, Barlo W, Shak S, et al. Prognostic and predictive value of the 21-gene recurrence score assay in postmenopausal, node-positive, estrogen receptor-positive breast cancer. Lancet Oncol 2010;11:55-65.
6. Alberti L, Carniti C, Miranda C, et al. RET and NTRK1 proto-oncogenes in human diseases. J Cell Physiol 2003;195:168-86.
7. Allegra CJ, Jessup JM, Somerfield MR, et al. American Society of Clinical Oncology provisional clinical opinion: testing for KRAS gene mutations in patients with metastatic colorectal carcinoma to predict response to anti-epidermal growth factor receptor monoclonal antibody therapy. J Clin Oncol 2009;27:2091-6.
8. American Society for Therapeutic Radiology and Oncology Consensus Panel. Consensus statement: guidelines for PSA following radiation therapy. Int J Radiat Oncol Biol Phys 1997;37:1035-41.
9. Andreasen PA, Kjoller L, Christensen L, et al. The urokinase-type plasminogen activator system in cancer metastasis: a review. Int J Cancer 1997;72:1-22.
10. Andriole GL, Grubb RL III, Buys SS, et al. Mortality results from a randomized prostate-cancer screening trial. N Engl J Med 2009;360:1310-9.
11. Angelopoulou K, Diamandis EP, Sutherland DJ, et al. Prevalence of serum antibodies against the p53 tumor suppressor gene protein in various cancers. Int J Cancer 1994;58:480-7.
12. Ariyaratana S, Loeb DM. The role of the Wilms tumour gene (WT1) in normal and malignant haematopoiesis. Expert Rev Mol Med 2007;9:1-17.
13. Austin LA, Heath H. Calcitonin: physiology and pathophysiology. N Engl J Med 1981;304:269-78.
14. Babaian RJ, Fritsche HA, Zhang Z, et al. Evaluation of ProstAsure index in the detection of prostate cancer: a preliminary report. Urology 1998;51:132-6.
15. Babaian RJ, Fritsche H, Ayala A, et al. Performance of a neural network in detecting prostate cancer in the prostate-specific antigen reflex range of 2.5 to 4.0 ng/mL. Urology 2000;56:1000-6.
16. Babaian RJ, Johnston DA, Naccarato W, et al. The incidence of prostate cancer in a screening population with a serum prostate specific antigen between 2.5 and 4.0 ng/ml: relation to biopsy strategy. J Urol 2001;165:757-60.
17. Barak V, Goike H, Panaretakis KW, Einarsson R. Clinical utility of cytokeratins as tumor markers. Clin Biochem 2004;37:529-40.
18. Bar-Sagi D. A Ras by any other name. Mol Cell Biol 2001;21:1441-3.
19. Bartlett NL, Freiha FS, Torti FM. Serum markers in germ cell neoplasms. Hematol Oncol Clin North Am 1991;5:1245-60.
20. Bast RC Jr, Brewer M, Zou C, et al. Prevention and early detection of ovarian cancer: mission impossible? Recent Results Cancer Res 2007;174:91-100.
21. Bates SE. Clinical applications of serum tumor markers. Ann Intern Med 1991;115:623-38.
22. Bates SE, Longo DL. Use of serum tumor markers in cancer diagnosis and management. Semin Oncol 1987;14:102-38.
23. Belanger A, van Halbeek H, Graves HDB, et al. Molecular mass and carbohydrate structure of prostate specific antigen: studies for establishment of an international PSA standard. Prostate 1995;27:187-97.
24. Bence-Jones H. Papers on chemical pathology. Lecture III. Lancet 1847;ii:269-72.
25. Benson MC, Whang IS, Pantuck A, et al. Prostate specific antigen density: a means of distinguishing benign prostatic hypertrophy and prostate cancer. J Urol 1992;147:815-16.
26. Bergers G, Benjamin LE. Tumorigenesis and the angiogenic switch. Nat Rev Cancer 2002;3:401-10.
27. Berkowitz RS, Goldstein DP. Gestational trophoblastic disease. In: Mossa AR, Schimpff SC, Robson MC, eds. Comprehensive textbook of oncology. Baltimore: Williams & Wilkins, 1991:1046-51.
28. Bernini GP, Moretti A, Ferdeghini M, et al. A new human chromogranin "A" immunoradiometric assay for the diagnosis of neuroendocrine tumours. Br J Cancer 2001;84:636-42.
29. Beyer HL, Geschwindt RD, Glover CL, et al. MESOMARK: a potential test for malignant pleural mesothelioma. Clin Chem 2007;53:666-72.
30. Birken S, Berger P, Bidart JM, et al. Preparation and characterization of new WHO reference reagents for human chorionic gonadotropin and metabolites. Clin Chem 2003;49:144-54.
31. Bjorklund B, Bjorklund V. Antigenicity of pooled human malignant and normal tissues by cyto-immunologic techniques: presence of an insoluble heat labile tumor antigen. Arch Allergy 1957;10:153-84.
32. Black MH, Diamandis EP. The diagnostic and prognostic utility of prostate-specific antigen for diseases of the breast. Breast Cancer Res Treat 2000;59:1-14.
33. Bloom G, Yang IV, Boulware D, et al. Multi-platform, multi-site, microarray-based human tumor classification. Am J Pathol 2004;164:9-16.
34. Bombardieri E, Gion M. Mucin-like cancer associated antigen (MCA) as available circulating tumor marker for breast cancer. In: Sell S, ed. Serological cancer markers. Totowa NJ: Humana Press, 1992:341-54.
35. Bonfrer JMG. Working group on tumor marker criteria (WGTMC). Tumour Biol 1990;11:287-88.
36. Bouchalova K, Cizkova M, Cwiertka K, Trojanec R, Hajduch M. Triple negative breast cancer—current status and prospective targeted treatment based on HER1 (EGFR), TOP2A and C-MYC gene assessment. Biomed Pap Med Fac Univ Palacky Olomouc Czech Repub 2009;153:13-7.
37. Bray KR, Koda JE, Gaur PK. Serum concentrations and biochemical characteristics of cancer associated antigen (CA) 549, a circulating breast cancer marker. Cancer Res 1987;47:5853-60.
38. Brown WH. A case of pluriglandular syndrome. Lancet 1928;ii:1022-4.
39. Buccheri G, Ferrigno D. Lung tumor markers of cytokeratin origin: an overview. Lung Cancer 2001;34:S65-9.
40. Bunting PS. Is there still a role for prostatic acid phosphatase? CSCC Position Statement, Canadian Society of Clinical Chemists. Clin Biochem 1999;32:591-4.
41. Bussemakers MJ, van Bokhoven A, Verhaegh GW, et al. DD3: a new prostate-specific gene, highly overexpressed in prostate cancer. Cancer Res 1999;59:5975-9.
42. Buyse M, Loi S, Van't Veer L, et al. Validation and clinical utility of a 70-gene prognostic signature for women with node-negative breast cancer. J Natl Cancer Inst 2006;98:1183-92.
43. Callagy GM, Webber MJ, Pharoah PD, Caldas C. Meta-analysis confirms BCL2 is an independent prognostic marker in breast cancer. BMC Cancer 2008;8:153.

44. Cancer Facts and Figures 2010. Atlanta, Ga: American Cancer Society, 2010:1-62.
45. Cao Y. Tumor angiogenesis and molecular targets for therapy. Front Biosci 2009;14:3962-73.
46. Carmeliet P. Angiogenesis in health and disease. Nat Med 2003;9: 653-60.
47. Carter HB, Pearson JD, Metter EJ, et al. Longitudinal evaluation of prostate specific antigen levels in men with and without prostate disease. JAMA 1992;267:2215-20.
48. Catalona WJ, Partin AW, Slawin KM, et al. Use of the percentage of free prostate-specific antigen to enhance differentiation of prostate cancer from benign prostatic disease: a prospective multicenter clinical trial. JAMA 1998;297:1542-7.
49. Catalona WJ, Smith DS, Ratliff TL, et al. Measurement of prostate specific antigen in serum as a screening test for prostate cancer. N Engl J Med 1991;324:1156-61.
50. Cavaliere A, Bucciarelli E, Sidoni A, et al. Estrogen and progesterone receptors in breast cancer: comparison between enzyme immunoassay and computer-assisted image analysis of immunocytochemical assay. Cytometry 1996;26:204-8.
51. Chan AK, Chiu RW, Lo YM; Clinical Sciences Reviews Committee of the Association of Clinical Biochemists. Cell-free nucleic acids in plasma, serum and urine: a new tool in molecular diagnosis. Ann Clin Biochem 2003;40:122-30.
52. Chan DW, Beveridge RA, Bhargava A, et al. Breast cancer marker CA549: a multicenter study. Am J Clin Pathol 1994;101:465-70.
53. Chan DW, Beveridge RA, Bruzek DJ, et al. Monitoring breast cancer with CA 549. Clin Chem 1988;34:2000-4.
54. Chan DW, Beveridge RA, Muss H, et al. Use of TRUQUANT BR RIA for early detection of breast cancer recurrence in patients with stage II and stage III disease. J Clin Oncol 1997;15:2322-8.
55. Chan DW, Bruzek DJ, Oesterling JE, et al. Prostatic-specific antigen as a marker for prostatic cancer: a monoclonal and a polyclonal immunoassay compared. Clin Chem 1987;33:1916-20.
56. Chan DW, Kelsten M, Rock R, Bruzek D. Evaluation of a monoclonal immunoenzymometric assay for alpha-fetoprotein. Clin Chem 1986;32:1318-22.
57. Chan DW, Maio YC. Affinity chromatographic separation of alpha-fetoprotein variants: development of a minicolumn procedure and application to cancer patients. Clin Chem 1986;32:2143-6.
58. Chan DW, Sokoll LJ. WHO first international standards for prostate-specific antigen: the beginning of the end for assay discrepancies? [Editorial] Clin Chem 2000;46:1291-2.
59. Chin KF, Greenman J, Reusch P, et al. Vascular endothelial growth factor and soluble Tie-2 receptor in colorectal cancer: associations with disease recurrence. Eur J Surg Oncol 2003; 29:497-505.
60. Chu TM. Prostate specific antigen. In: Sell S, ed. Serological cancer markers. Totowa NJ: Humana Press, 1992:99-115.
61. Clark GJ, Der CJ. Ras proto-oncogene activation in human malignancy. In: Garret G, Sell S, eds. Cellular cancer markers. Totowa NJ: Humana Press, 1995:17-52.
62. Cole LA, Butler SA, Khanlian SA, et al. Gestational trophoblastic diseases. 2. Hyperglycosylated hCG as a reliable marker of active neoplasia. Gynecol Oncol 2003;102:151-9.
63. Correale M, Abbate I, Gargano G, et al. Analytical and clinical evaluation of a new tumor marker in breast cancer: CA 27.29. Int J Biol Markers 1992;7:43-6.
64. Cristofanilli M, Budd GT, Ellis MJ, et al. Circulating tumor cells, disease progression, and survival in metastatic breast cancer. N Engl J Med 2004;351:781-91.
65. Darson MF, Pacelli A, Roche P, et al. Human glandular kallikrein 2 expression in prostate adenocarcinoma and lymph node metastases. Urology 1999;53:939-44.
66. De Bie SH, Ferreira TC, Pauwels EKJ, Cleton FJ. Immunoscintigraphy for cancer detection: "a thousand ills require a thousand cures." J Cancer Res Clin Oncol 1992;118:1-15.
67. de Kok JB, Verhaegh GW, Roelofs RW, et al. DD3(PCA3), a very sensitive and specific marker to detect prostate tumors. Cancer Res 2002;62:2695-8.
68. de Medeiros SF, Norman RJ. Human choriogonadotrophin protein core and sugar branches heterogeneity: basic and clinical insights. Hum Reprod Update 2009;15:69-95.
69. Deras IL, Aubin SMJ, Blase A, et al. PCA3—a molecular urine assay for predicting biopsy outcome. J Urol 2008;179:1587-92.
70. Diamandis EP. Prostate-specific antigen: its usefulness in clinical medicine. Trends Endocrinol Metab 1998;8:310-6.
71. Diamandis EP, Fritsche HA, Lilja H, Chan DW, Schwartz MK, eds. Tumor markers: physiology, pathobiology, technology and clinical applications. Washington, DC: AACC Press, 2002.
72. Diamandis EP, Scorilas A, Fracchioli S, et al. Human kallikrein 6 (hK6): a new potential serum biomarker for diagnosis and prognosis of ovarian carcinoma. J Clin Oncol 2003;21:1035-43.
73. Diamandis EP, Yousef GM. Human tissue kallikreins: a family of new cancer biomarkers. Clin Chem 2002;48:1198-205.
74. Drapkin R, von Horsten HH, Lin Y, et al. Human epididymis protein 4 (HE4) is a secreted glycoprotein that is overexpressed by serous and endometrioid ovarian carcinomas. Cancer Res 2005; 65:2162-9.
75. Duffy MJ, Maguire TM, McDermott EW, et al. Urokinase plasminogen activator: a prognostic marker in multiple types of cancer. J Surg Oncol 1999;1:130-5.
76. Duman-Scheel M. Netrin and DCC: axon guidance regulators at the intersection of nervous system development and cancer. Curr Drug Targets 2009;10:602-10.
77. Einhorn N, Bast RC Jr, Knapp RC, et al. Preoperative evaluation of serum CA 125 levels in patients with primary epithelial ovarian cancer. Obstet Gynecol 1986;67:414-6.
78. Eissa S, Swellam M, Sadek M, et al. Comparative evaluation of the nuclear matrix protein, fibronectin, urinary bladder cancer antigen and voided urine cytology in the detection of bladder tumors. J Urol 2002;168:465-9.
79. Emami N, Diamandis EP. Utility of kallikrein-related peptidases (KLKs) as cancer biomarkers. Clin Chem 2008;54:1600-7.
80. F. Hoffmann-La Roche Ltd. AmpliChip CYP450 Test. Available at: http://www.roche.com/products/product-details.htm?type=product&id=17 (accessed May 2, 2011).
81. Fearon ER, Vogelstein B. A genetic model for colorectal tumorigenesis. Cell 1990;61:759-67.
82. Fehrenbacher N, Bar-Sagi D, Philips M. Ras/MAPK signaling from endomembranes. Mol Oncol 2009;3:297-307.
83. Feldman SA, Eiden LE. The chromogranins: their roles in secretion from neuroendocrine cells and as markers for neuroendocrine neoplasia. Endocr Pathol 2003;14:3-23.
84. Fishman WH, Inglis NR, Stolbach LL, Krant MJ. A serum alkaline phosphatase isoenzyme of human neoplastic cell origin. Cancer Res 1968;28:150-4.
85. Fishman WH, Sell S. Onco-developmental gene expression: a preview. In: Fishman WH, Sell S, eds. Onco-developmental gene expression. New York: Academic Press Inc., 1976.
86. Foekens JA, Look MP, Bolt-de Vries J. Cathepsin-D in primary breast cancer: prognostic evaluation involving 2810 patients. Br J Cancer 1999;79:300-7.
87. Ford D, Easton DF, Bishop DT, et al. Risks of cancer in BRCA1-mutation carriers. Breast Cancer Linkage Consortium. Lancet 1994;343:692-5.
88. Freije JM, MacDonald NJ, Steeg PS. Differential gene expression in tumor metastasis: Nm23. Curr Top Microbiol Immunol 1996;213: 215-32.
89. Friedrich MG, Hellstern A, Hautmann SH, et al. Non-invasive urine tests in diagnosis and as prognostic markers for urinary bladder carcinoma: comparison of the BTAstat and NMP 22 tests with immunocytology using monoclonal antibodies against Lewis X and 486p3/12. Urologe A 2003;42:523-30.

90. Fujiyama S, Tanaka M, Maeda S, Ashihara H, Hirata R, Tomita K. Tumor markers in early diagnosis, follow-up and management of patients with hepatocellular carcinoma. Oncology 2002;62(Suppl 1): 57-63.
91. Garbe C, Leiter U, Ellwanger U. Diagnostic value and prognostic significance of protein S-100beta, melanoma-inhibitory activity, and tyrosinase/MART-1 reverse transcription-polymerase chain reaction in the follow-up of high-risk melanoma patients. Cancer 2003;97:1737-45.
92. García-Olmo DC, Domínguez C, García-Arranz M, et al. Cell-free nucleic acids circulating in the plasma of colorectal cancer patients induce the oncogenic transformation of susceptible cultured cells. Cancer Res 2010;70:560-7.
93. Garrido C, Gurbuxani S, Ravagnan L. Heat shock proteins: endogenous modulators of apoptotic cell death. Biochem Biophys Res Commun 2001;286:433-42.
94. Genomic Health Inc. Onco*type* Dx test. Available at: http://www.genomichealth.com/Onco*type*DX/Index.aspx (accessed May 2, 2011).
95. Gewirtz AM. Oligonucleotide therapeutics: clothing the emperor. Curr Opin Mol Ther 1999;1:297-306.
96. Goddard AD, Balakier H, Clanton M, et al. Infrequent genomic rearrangement and normal expression of the putative RB1 gene in retinoblastoma tumors. Mol Cell Biol 1988:8:2082-91.
97. Gold P, Freeman SO. Demonstration of tumor specific antigens in human colonic carcinomata by immunological tolerance and absorption techniques. J Exp Med 1965;121:439-62.
98. Graziano F, Cascinu S, Staccioli MP, et al. Potential role and chronology of abnormal expression of the deleted in colon cancer (DCC) and the p53 proteins in the development of gastric cancer. BMC Cancer 2001;1:9-12.
99. Greene KL, Albertsen PC, Babaian RJ, et al. Prostate specific antigen best practice statement: 2009 update. J Urol 2009;182:2232-41.
100. Gulbis B, Galand P. Immunodetection of the p21-ras products in human normal and preneoplastic tissues and solid tumors: a review. Hum Pathol 1993;24:1271-85.
101. Gutman EB, Sproul EE, Gutman AB. Significance of increased phosphatase activity of bone at the site of osteoplastic metastases secondary to carcinoma of the prostate gland. Am J Cancer 1938;28:485-95.
102. Haber DA, Sohn RL, Buckler AJ, et al. Alternative splicing and genomic structure of the Wilms' tumor gene WT1. PNAS USA 1991;88:9618-22.
103. Haese A, Graefen M, Steuber T, et al. Human glandular kallikrein 2 levels in serum for discrimination of pathologically organ-confined from locally-advanced prostate cancer in total PSA-levels below 10 ng/ml. Prostate 2001;49:101-9.
104. Haese A, Vaisanen V, Finlay JA, et al. Standardization of two immunoassays for human glandular kallikrein 2. Clin Chem 2003;9:601-10.
105. Haglund C, Kuusela P, Roberts P, Jalanko H. CA 50. In: Sell S, ed. Serological cancer markers. Totowa, NJ: Humana Press, 1992:375-86.
106. Hakomori S-I. Tumor associated carbohydrate markers. In: Sell S, ed. Serological cancer markers. Totowa NJ: Humana Press, 1992:207-32.
107. Hall PA, McCluggage WG. Assessing p53 in clinical contexts: unlearned lessons and new perspectives. J Pathol 2006;208:1-6.
108. Han M, Piantadosi S, Zahurak ML, et al. Serum acid phosphatase level and biochemical recurrence following radical prostatectomy for men with clinically localized prostate cancer. Urology 2001;57:707-11.
109. Hanahan D, Weinberg RA. The hallmarks of cancer. Cell 2000;100: 57-70.
110. Harbeck N, Schmitt M, Kates RE, et al. Clinical utility of urokinase-type plasminogen activator and plasminogen activator inhibitor-1 determination in primary breast cancer tissue for individualized therapy concepts. Clin Breast Cancer 2002;3:196-200.
111. Harper PS. Research samples from families with genetic diseases: a proposed code of conduct. Br Med J 1993;306:1391-3.
112. Harris H. The analysis of malignancy by cell fusion: the position in 1988. Cancer Res 1988;48:3302-18.
113. Harris L, Fritsche H, Mennel R, et al; American Society of Clinical Oncology. American Society of Clinical Oncology 2007 update of recommendations for the use of tumor markers in breast cancer. J Clin Oncol 2007;25:5287-312.
114. Hayes DF, Tondini C, Kufe DW. Clinical applications of CA 15-3. In: Sell S, ed. Serological cancer markers. Totowa, NJ: Humana Press, 1992:281-307.
115. Heller T, Kirchheiner J, Armstrong VW, et al. AmpliChip CYP450 GeneChip: a new gene chip that allows rapid and accurate CYP2D6 genotyping. Ther Drug Monit 2006;28:673-7.
116. Hellstrom I, Raycraft J, Hayden-Ledbetter M, et al. The HE4 (WFDC2) protein is a biomarker for ovarian carcinoma. Cancer Res 2003;63:3695-700.
117. Hess JL, Highsmith WE Jr. Telomerase detection in body fluids. Clin Chem 2002;48:18-24.
118. Hiyama E, Hiyama K. Telomerase as tumor marker. Cancer Lett 2003;94:221-33.
119. Hodgall EV, Hodgall CK, Tingulstad S, et al. Predictive values of serum tumour markers tetranectin, OVX1, CASA and CA125 in patients with a pelvic mass. Int J Cancer 2000;89:519-23.
120. Holten-Andersen MN, Christensen IJ, Nielsen HJ, et al. Total levels of tissue inhibitor of metalloproteinases 1 in plasma yield high diagnostic sensitivity and specificity in patients with colon cancer. Clin Cancer Res 2002;8:156-64.
121. Holten-Andersen MN, Fenger C, Nielsen HJ, et al. Plasma TIMP-1 in patients with colorectal adenomas: a prospective study. Eur J Cancer 2004;40:2159-64.
122. Hostetter RB, Augustus LB, Mankarious R, et al. Carcinoembryonic antigen as a selective enhancer of colorectal cancer metastasis. J Natl Cancer Inst 1990;82:380-5.
123. Hotakainen K, Tanner P, Alfthan H, Haglund C, Stenman UH. Comparison of three immunoassays for CA 19-9. Clin Chim Acta 2009;400:123-7.
124. International HapMap Consortium. The International HapMap Project. Nature 2003;426:789-96.
125. Jacobs I, Bast RC. The CA 125 tumor-associated antigen: a review of the literature. Hum Reprod 1989;4:1-12.
126. Janicke F, Prechtl A, Thomssen C. Randomized adjuvant chemotherapy trial in high-risk, lymph node-negative breast cancer patients identified by urokinase-type plasminogen activator and plasminogen activator inhibitor type 1. J Natl Cancer Inst 2001;93:913-20.
127. Jemal A, Siegel R, Xu J, Ward E. Cancer statistics, 2010. CA Cancer J Clin 2010;60:277-300.
128. Johnson PJ, Lo YM. Plasma nucleic acids in the diagnosis and management of malignant disease. Clin Chem 2002;48:1186-93.
129. Kastan MB, Canman CE, Leonard CJ. P53, cell cycle control and apoptosis: implications for cancer. Cancer Metastasis Rev 1995;14:3-15.
130. Kastan MB, Onyekwere O, Sidransky D, Vogelstein B, Craig RW. Participation of p53 protein in the cellular response to DNA damage. Cancer Res 1991;51:6304-11.
131. Kato H. Squamous cell carcinoma antigen. In: Sell S, ed. Serological cancer markers. Totowa NJ: Humana Press, 1992:437-51.
132. Kelsten ML, Chan DW, Bruzek DJ, Rock RC. Monitoring hepatocellular carcinoma by using a monoclonal immunoenzymometric assay for alpha-fetoprotein. Clin Chem 1988;34:76-81.
133. Khan J, Simon R, Bittner M, et al. Gene expression profiling of alveolar rhabdomyosarcoma with cDNA microarrays. Cancer Res 1998;58:5009-13.
134. Kiang DT, Greenberg LJ, Kennedy BJ. Tumor marker kinetics in the monitoring of breast cancer. Cancer 1990;65:193-9.
135. King MC, Rowell S, Love SM. Inherited breast and ovarian cancer. JAMA 1993;269:1975-80.

136. Klug TL, Bast RC, Niloff JM, et al. Monoclonal antibody immunoradiometric assay for an antigenic determinant (CA 125) associated with human epithelial ovarian carcinomas. Cancer Res 1984;44:1048-53.
137. Knudson AG Jr. Mutation and cancer: statistical study of retinoblastoma. PNAS USA 1971;68:820-6.
138. Knudson AG Jr. Hereditary cancer, oncogenes, and anti-oncogenes. Cancer Res 1985;45:1437-81.
139. Koblinski JE, Ahram M, Sloane BF. Unraveling the role of proteases in cancer. Clin Chim Acta 2000;291:113-35.
140. Koprowski HZ, Steplewski K, Mitchell M, et al. Colorectal carcinoma antigens detected by somatic hybridoma antibodies. Cell Genet 1979;5:957-72.
141. Kuiper GG, Enmark E, Pelto-Huikko M, Gustafsson JA. Cloning of a novel receptor expressed in rat prostate and ovary. PNAS USA 1996;93:5925-30.
142. Kuremsky JG, Tepper JE, McLeod HL. Biomarkers for response to neoadjuvant chemoradiation for rectal cancer. Int J Radiat Oncol Biol Phys 2009;74:673-88.
143. Kuusela P, Haglund C, Jalanko H, Roberts PJ. CA 242. In: Sell S, ed. Serological cancer markers. Totowa, NJ: Humana Press, 1992:429-35.
144. Lai AZ, Gujral TS, Mulligan LM. RET signaling in endocrine tumors: delving deeper into molecular mechanisms. Endocr Pathol 2007;18:57-67.
145. Lakhani VT, You YN, Wells SA. The multiple endocrine neoplasia syndromes. Annu Rev Med 2007;58:253-65.
146. Lamerz R. CA19-9: GICA (gastrointestinal cancer antigen). In: Sell S, ed. Serological cancer markers. Totowa, NJ: Humana Press, 1992:309-39.
147. Lander ES, Linton LM, Birren B, et al. Initial sequencing and analysis of the human genome. Nature 2001;409:860-921.
148. Lee W-H, Shew JY, Hong RD, et al. The retinoblastoma susceptibility gene encodes a nuclear phosphoprotein associated with DNA binding activity. Nature 1987;329:642-4.
149. Leppert M, Dobbs M, Scrambler P, et al. The gene for familial polyposis coli maps to the long arm of chromosome 5. Science 1987;238:1411-3.
150. Lev Z, Kislitsin D, Rennert G, Lerner A. Utilization of K-ras mutations identified in stool DNA for the early detection of colorectal cancer. J Cell Biochem Suppl 2000;34:35-9.
151. Levine AJ, Momand J, Finlay CA. The p53 tumour suppressor gene. Nature 1999;351:453-6.
152. Li D, Mallory T, Satomura S. AFP-L3: a new generation of tumor marker for hepatocellular carcinoma. Clin Chim Acta 2001;313:15-9.
153. Li J, Dowdy S, Tipton T, et al. HE4 as a biomarker for ovarian and endometrial cancer management. Expert Rev Mol Diagn 2009;9:555-66.
154. Li J, Yen C, Liaw D, et al. PTEN, a putative protein tyrosine phosphatase gene mutated in human brain, breast, and prostate cancer. Science 1997;275:1943-7.
155. Li JL, Zhang Z, Rosenzweig J, et al. Proteomics and bioinformatics approaches for identification of serum biomarkers to detect breast cancer. Clin Chem 2002;48:1296-304.
156. Lilja H, Christensson A, Dahlen U, et al. Prostate specific antigen in human serum occurs predominantly in complex with alpha-1-antichymotrypsin. Clin Chem 1991;37:1618-25.
157. Lin F, van Rhee F, Goldman JM, et al. Kinetics of increasing BCR-ABL transcript numbers in chronic myeloid leukemia patients who relapse after bone marrow transplantation. Blood 1996;7:4473-8.
158. Lipton A, Ali SM, Leitzel K, et al. Elevated serum Her-2/neu level predicts decreased response to hormone therapy in metastatic breast cancer. J Clin Oncol 2002;20:1467-72.
159. Liotta LA, Espina V, Mehta AI, et al. Protein microarrays: meeting analytical challenges for clinical applications. Cancer Cell 2003;3:317-25.
160. Locker GY, Hamilton S, Harris J, et al. ASCO 2006 update of recommendations for the use of tumor markers in gastrointestinal cancer. J Clin Oncol 2006;24:5313-27.
161. Look MP, van Putten WL, Duffy MJ, et al. Pooled analysis of prognostic impact of urokinase-type plasminogen activator and its inhibitor PAI-1 in 8377 breast cancer patients. J Natl Cancer Inst 2002;94:116-28.
162. Lovgren J, Valtonen-Andre C, Marsal K, et al. Measurement of prostate-specific antigen and human glandular kallikrein 2 in different body fluids. J Androl 1999;20:348-55.
163. Lowe PN, Skinner RH. Regulation of RAS signal transduction in normal and transformed cells. Cell Signal 1994;6:109-23.
164. Luftner D, Luke C, Possinger K. Serum HER-2/neu in the management of breast cancer patients. Clin Biochem 2003;36:233-40.
165. Lundwall A, Lilja H. Molecular cloning of human prostate specific antigen cDNA. FEBS Lett 1987;214:317-22.
166. Luo LY, Diamandis EP, Look MP, et al. Higher expression of human kallikrein 10 in breast cancer tissue predicts tamoxifen resistance. Br J Cancer 2002;86:1790-6.
167. Luo LY, Katsaros D, Scorilas A, et al. Prognostic value of human kallikrein 10 expression in epithelial ovarian carcinoma. Clin Cancer Res 2001;7:2372-9.
168. Luo LY, Katsaros D, Scorilas A, et al. The serum concentration of human kallikrein 10 represents a novel biomarker for ovarian cancer diagnosis and prognosis. Cancer Res 2003;63:807-11.
169. Makarov DV, Trock BJ, Humphreys EB, et al. Updated nomogram to predict pathologic stage of prostate cancer given prostate-specific antigen level, clinical stage, and biopsy Gleason score (Partin tables) based on cases from 2000 to 2005. Urology 2007;69:1095-101.
170. Marks JR, Davidoff AM, Iglehart JD. p53 in human cancer. In: Sell S, ed. Serological cancer markers. Totowa NJ: Humana Press, 1992: 77-110.
171. Marrero JA, Feng Z, Wang Y, et al. Alpha-fetoprotein, des-gamma carboxyprothrombin, and lectin-bound alpha-fetoprotein in early hepatocellular carcinoma. Gastroenterology 2009;137:110-8.
172. Mazzucchelli L. Protein S100A4: too long overlooked by pathologists? Am J Pathol 2002;60:7-13.
173. McDonnell TJ, Marin MC, Hsu B, et al. The BCL-2 oncogene: apoptosis and neoplasia. Radiation Res 1993;136:307-12.
174. McMahon BJ, London T. Workshop on screening for hepatocellular carcinoma. J Natl Cancer Inst 1991;83:916-9.
175. Mehlen P, Furne C. Netrin-1: when a neuronal guidance cue turns out to be a regulator of tumorigenesis. Cell Mol Life Sci 2005;62: 2599-616.
176. Metzgar RS, Sawabu N, Hollingsworth MA. DU-PAN-2: a clinically useful mucin marker of differentiation of pancreatic and other ductal cells and their tumors. In: Sell S, ed. Serological cancer markers. Totowa, NJ: Humana Press, 1992:355-74.
177. Miki Y, Swensen J, Shattuck-Eidens D, et al. A strong candidate for the breast and ovarian cancer susceptibility gene BRCA 1. Science 1994;266:66-71.
178. Mikolajczyk SD, Marks LS, Partin AW, Rittenhouse HG. Free prostate-specific antigen in serum is becoming more complex. Urology 2002;59:797-802.
179. Mikolajczyk SD, Millar LS, Kumar A, et al. Prostatic human kallikrein 2 inactivates and complexes with plasminogen activator inhibitor-1. Int J Cancer 1999;81:438-42.
180. Minamoto T, Mai M, Ronai Z. K-ras mutation: early detection in molecular diagnosis and risk assessment of colorectal, pancreas, and lung cancers—a review. Cancer Detect Prev 2000;24:1-12.
181. Moore RG, Brown AK, Miller MC, et al. Utility of a novel serum tumor biomarker HE4 in patients with endometrioid adenocarcinoma of the uterus. Gynecol Oncol 2008;110:196-201.
182. Moore R, McMeekin DS, Brown AK, et al. A novel multiple marker bioassay utilizing HE4 and CA125 for the prediction of ovarian cancer in patients with a pelvic mass. Gynecol Oncol 2009;112:40-6.
183. Myers MP, Pass I, Batty IH, et al. The lipid phosphatase activity of PTEN is critical for its tumor suppressor function. Proc Natl Acad Sci U S A 1998;95:13513-8.
184. National Comprehensive Cancer Network. Available at: http://www.nccn.org/ (accessed May 2, 2011).

185. National Comprehensive Cancer Network. Practice guidelines in oncology: Prostate cancer early detection, v1. 2010. Available at: http://www.nccn.org/network/business_insights/flash_updates/flash_update_information.asp?FlashID=12 (accessed May 2, 2011).
186. Nichols GE, Frierson HF, Boyd JC, Hanigan MH. Automated immunohistochemical assay for estrogen receptor status in breast cancer using monoclonal antibody CC4-5 on the Ventana ES. Am J Clin Pathol 1996;106:332-8.
187. Nicholson RI, Gee JM, Harper ME. EGFR and cancer prognosis. Eur J Cancer 2001;37:S9-15.
188. Nishizuka S, Chen ST, Gwadry FG, et al. Diagnostic markers that distinguish colon and ovarian adenocarcinomas: identification by genomic, proteomic and tissue array profiling. Cancer Res 2003;63:5243-50.
189. Noguchi M, Mizukami Y, Kinoshita K, et al. c-erbB-2, ras p21, and c-myc expression in breast carcinoma: prognostic value and correlation with clinicopathologic and biologic variables. Int J Oncol 1994;4:255-60.
190. O'Boyle K. The role of the deleted colon cancer (DCC) gene in colorectal and gastric cancer. Cancer Invest 2003;12:484-5.
191. Oehr P, Luthgens ML, Liu Q. Tissue polypeptide antigen and specific TPA. In: Sell S, ed. Serological cancer markers. Totowa NJ: Humana Press, 1992:193-206.
192. Oesterling JE. Prostate specific antigen: a critical assessment of the most useful tumor marker for adenocarcinoma of the prostate. J Urol 1991;145:907-23.
193. Oesterling JE, Chan DW, Epstein JI, et al. Prostate specific antigen in the preoperative and postoperative evaluation of localized prostatic cancer treated with radical prostatectomy. J Urol 1988;139:766-72.
194. Oesterling JE, Jacobsen SJ, Chute GG, et al. Serum prostate specific antigen in a community based population of healthy men: establishment of age-specific reference ranges. JAMA 1993;270:860-4.
195. Overall CM, Lopez-Otin C. Strategies for MMP inhibition in cancer: innovations for the post-trial era. Nat Rev Cancer 2002;2:657-72.
196. Owen WE, Roberts RF, Roberts WL. Performance characteristics of the LiBASys des-gamma-carboxy prothrombin assay. Clin Chim Acta 2008;339:183-5.
197. Ozturk M. p53 mutation in hepatocellular carcinoma after aflatoxin exposure. Lancet 1991;338:1356-9.
198. Paech K, Webb P, Kuiper GG, et al. Differential ligand activation of estrogen receptors ERalpha and ERbeta at AP1 sites. Science 1997;277:1508-10.
199. Paik S, Shak S, Tang G, et al. A multigene assay to predict recurrence of tamoxifen-treated, node-negative breast cancer. N Engl J Med 2004;351:2817-26.
200. Paik S, Tang G, Shak S, et al. Gene expression and benefit of chemotherapy in women with node-negative, estrogen receptor-positive breast cancer. J Clin Oncol 2006;24:3726-34.
201. Paik S. Development and clinical utility of a 21-gene recurrence score prognostic assay in patients with early breast cancer treated with tamoxifen. Oncologist 2007;12:631-5.
202. Palmer-Toy D, Kuzdzal S, Chan DW. Proteomic approaches to tumor marker discovery. In: Diamandis EP, Fritsche HA, Lilja H, Chan DW, Schwartz MK, eds. Tumor markers: physiology, pathobiology, technology and clinical applications. Washington, DC: AACC Press, 2002:391-400.
203. Partin AW, Brawer MK, Bartsch G, et al. Complexed prostate specific antigen improves specificity for prostate cancer detection: results of a prospective multicenter clinical trial. J Urology 2003;170:1787-91.
204. Partin AW, Catalona WJ, Southwick PC, et al. Analysis of percent free prostate specific antigen (PSA) for prostate cancer detection: influence of total PSA, prostate volume and age. Urology 1996;48:55-61.
205. Partin AW, Getzenberg RH, Carmichael MJ, et al. Nuclear matrix protein patterns in human benign prostatic hyperplasia and prostate cancer. Cancer Res 1993;53:744-9.
206. Partin AW, Piantadosi S, Subong ENP, et al. Clearance rate of serum free and total PSA following radical retropubic prostatectomy. Prostate Suppl 1996;7:35-9.
207. Pass HI, Wali A, Tang N, et al. Soluble mesothelin-related peptide level elevation in mesothelioma serum and pleural effusions. Ann Thorac Surg 2008;85:265-72.
208. Pathak AP, Hochfeld WE, Goodman SL, Pepper MS. Circulating and imaging markers for angiogenesis. Angiogenesis 2008;11:321-35.
209. Pathwork Diagnostics. The Pathwork Tissue of Origin laboratory developed test. Available at: http://www.pathworkdx.com/TissueofOriginTest/ (accessed May 2, 2011).
210. Pearson JD, Uderer AA, Metter EJ, et al. Longitudinal analysis of serial measurements of free and total PSA among men with and without prostatic cancer. Urology 1996;48:4-9.
211. Perou CM, Sorlie T, Eisen MB, et al. Molecular portraits of human breast tumours. Nature 2000;406:747-52.
212. Petricoin EF III, Ardekani AM, Hitt BA, et al. Use of proteomic patterns in serum to identify ovarian cancer. Lancet 2002;359:572-7.
213. Petricoin EF III, Ornstein DK, Paweletz CP, et al. Serum proteomic patterns for detection of prostate cancer. J Natl Cancer Inst 2002;94:1576-8.
214. Petricoin EF, Zoon KC, Kohn EC, et al. Clinical proteomics: translating benchside promise into bedside reality. Nature Rev Drug Discov 2002;1:683-95.
215. Petty EM, Killeen AA. BRCA 1 mutation testing: controversies and challenges. Clin Chem 1997;43:6-8.
216. Pitot HC. The language of oncology. In: Pilot HC, ed. Fundamentals of oncology. New York: Marcel Dekker Inc, 1978:16.
217. Pujol JL, Boher JM, Grenier J. Cyfra 21-1, neuron specific enolase and prognosis of non-small cell lung cancer: prospective study in 621 patients. Lung Cancer 2001;31:221-31.
218. Pujol JL, Molinier O, Ebert W, et al. CYFRA 21-1 is a prognostic determinant in non-small-cell lung cancer: results of a meta-analysis in 2063 patients. Br J Cancer 2004;90:2097-105.
219. Quintás-Cardama A, Cortes J. Molecular biology of bcr-abl1-positive chronic myeloid leukemia. Blood 2009;113:1619-30.
220. Quyn AJ, Steele RJ, Carey FA, Näthke IS. Prognostic and therapeutic implications of Apc mutations in colorectal cancer. Surgeon 2008;6:350-6.
221. Radich JP, Gehly G, Gooley T, et al. Polymerase chain reaction detection of the BCR-ABL fusion transcript after allogeneic marrow transplantation for chronic myeloid leukemia: results and implications in 346 patients. Blood 1995;5:2632-8.
222. Rai AJ, Zhang Z, Rosenzweig J, et al. Proteomic approaches to tumor marker discovery: identification of biomarkers for ovarian cancer. Arch Pathol Lab Med 2002;26:1518-26.
223. Recker F, Kwiatkowski MK, Piironen T, et al. Human glandular kallikrein as a tool to improve discrimination of poorly differentiated and non-organ-confined prostate cancer compared with prostate-specific antigen. Urology 2000;55:481-5.
224. Reddish MA, Helbrecht N, Almeida AF, et al. Epitope mapping of Mab within the peptide core of the malignant breast carcinoma associated mucin antigen coded for by the human MUC 1 gene. J Tumor Marker Oncol 1992;7:19-27.
225. Riethdorf S, Fritsche H, Muller V, et al. Detection of circulating tumor cells in peripheral blood of patients with metastatic breast cancer: a validation study of the cell search system. Clin Cancer Res 2007;13:920-8.
226. Riou GF, Bourhis J, Le MG. The c-myc proto-oncogene in invasive carcinomas of the uterine cervix: clinical relevance of overexpression in early stages of the cancer. Anticancer Res 1990;10:1225-31.
227. Roach M 3rd, Hanks G, Thames H Jr, et al. Defining biochemical failure following radiotherapy with or without hormonal therapy in men with clinically localized prostate cancer: recommendations of the RTOG-ASTRO Phoenix Consensus Conference. Int J Radiat Oncol Biol Phys 2006;65:965-74.
228. Rochefort H, Garcia M, Glondu M, et al. Cathepsin D in breast cancer: mechanisms and clinical applications, a 1999 overview. Clin Chim Acta 2000;291:157-70.

229. Rosenberg S. The urokinase-type plasminogen activator system in cancer and other pathological conditions: introduction and perspective. Curr Pharm Des 2003;9:4.
230. Rosty C, Christa L, Kuzdzal S, et al. Identification of hepatocarcinoma-intestine-pancreas/pancreatitis-associated protein I as a biomarker for pancreatic ductal adenocarcinoma by protein biochip technology. Cancer Res 2002;62:1868-75.
231. Rothberg PG. The role of the oncogene c-myc in sporadic large bowel cancer and familial polyposis coli. Semin Surg Oncol 1987;3:152-8.
232. Saccani Jotti G, Johnston SR, Salter J, Detre S, Dowsett M. Comparison of new immunohistochemical assay for estrogen receptor in paraffin wax embedded breast carcinoma tissue with quantitative enzyme immunoassay. J Clin Pathol 1994;47:900-5.
233. Saldanha SN, Andrews LG, Tollefsbol TO. Analysis of telomerase activity and detection of its catalytic subunit, hTERT. Anal Biochem 2003;315:1-21.
234. Sarosdy MF, DeVere White RW, Soloway MS, et al. Results of a multicenter trial using the BTA test to monitor for and diagnose recurrent bladder cancer. J Urol 1995;154:379-84.
235. Sarosdy MF, Schellhammer P, Bokinsky G, et al. Clinical evaluation of a multi-target fluorescent in situ hybridization assay for detection of bladder cancer. J Urol 2002;168:1950-4.
236. Schedlich LJ, Bennetts BH, Morris BJ. Primary structure of a human glandular kallikrein gene. DNA 1987;6:429-37.
237. Schena M, Shalon D, Davis RW, et al. Quantitative monitoring of gene expression patterns with a complementary DNA microarray. Science 1995;270:467-70.
238. Schlom J, Colcher D, Milenic DE, et al. TAG-72 as a tumor marker. In: Sell S, ed. Serological cancer markers. Totowa NJ: Humana Press, 1992:387-416.
239. Schmidt B, Carstensen T, Engel E, Jandrig B, Witt C, Fleischhacker M. Detection of cell-free nucleic acids in bronchial lavage fluid supernatants from patients with lung cancer. Eur J Cancer 2004;40:452-60.
240. Schneider PM, Metzger R, Brabender J, et al. Lung cancer. In: Diamandis, EP, Fritsche, HA, Lilja H, Chan, DW, Schwartz, MK, eds. Tumor markers: physiology, pathobiology, technology, and clinical applications. Washington, DC: AACC Press, 2002:287-305.
241. Schroder FH, Hugosson J, Roobol MJ, et al. Screening and prostate-cancer mortality in a randomized European study. N Engl J Med 2009;360:1320-8.
242. Schwartz MK. Laboratory aids to diagnosis: enzymes. Cancer 1976;37:542-8.
243. Schwartz MK. Enzyme tests in cancer. Clin Lab Med 1982;2:479-91.
244. Sell S. Cancer markers of the 1990s. Clin Lab Med 1990;10:27-31.
245. Sell S. Cancer-associated carbohydrates identified by monoclonal antibodies. Hum Pathol 1991;21:1003-19.
246. Sell S. Cancer markers. In: Moossa AR, Schempff SC, Robson MC, eds. Comprehensive textbook of oncology, 2nd edition, volume 1. Baltimore: Williams & Wilkins, 1991:225-38.
247. Shen MH, Harper PS, Upadhyaya M. Molecular genetics of neurofibromatosis type 1 (NF1). J Med Genet 1996;33:2-17.
248. Shih IM, Sokoll LJ, Chan DW. Ovarian cancer. In: Diamandis EP, Fritsche HA, Lilja H, Chan DW, Schwartz MK, eds. Tumor markers: physiology, pathobiology, technology and clinical applications. Washington, DC: AACC Press, 2002:239-52.
249. Shuin T. C-myc as a tumor marker for primary human cancers. In: Sell S, ed. Serological cancer markers. Totowa, NJ: Humana Press, 1992:53-76.
250. Sidransky D, Tokino T, Hamilton SR, et al. Identification of ras oncogene mutations in the stool of patients with curable colorectal tumors. Science 1992;256:102-5.
251. Siemens DR, Morales A, Johnston B, et al. A comparative analysis of rapid urine tests for the diagnosis of upper urinary tract malignancy. Can J Urol 2003;10:1754-8.
252. Sikorska HM, Fuks A, Gold P. Carcinoembryonic antigen. In: Sell S, ed. Serological cancer markers. Totowa, NJ: Humana Press, 1992: 47-97.
253. Silver HKB, Archibald B-L, Raga J, Coldman AJ. Relative operating characteristic analysis and group modeling for tumor markers: comparison of CA 15.3, carcinoembryonic antigen, and mucin-like carcinoma-associated antigen in breast carcinoma. Cancer Res 1991;51:1904-9.
254. Sinicrope FA, Ruan SB, Cleary KR, et al. bcl-2 and p53 oncoprotein expression during colorectal tumorigenesis. Cancer Res 1995;55:237-41.
255. Slamon DJ, Godolphin W, Jones LA, et al. Studies of the HER-2/neu proto-oncogene in human breast and ovarian cancer. Science 1989;244:707-9.
256. Smith RA, Cokkinides V, Brawley OW. Cancer screening in the United States, 2009: A review of current American Cancer Society guidelines and issues in cancer screening. CA Cancer J Clin 2009;59:27-41
257. Sokoll LJ, Chan DW. PSA: its discovery and biochemical characteristics. Urol Clin North Am 1997;24:253-9.
258. Sokoll LJ, Chan DW. Malignancy-associated endocrine disorders. In: Winter WE, Sokoll LJ, Jialal I , eds. Handbook of diagnostic endocrinology. Washington, DC: AACC Press, 2008:401-31.
259. Sokoll LJ, Chan DW, Mikolajczyk SD, et al. Proenzyme PSA for the early detection of prostate dancer in the 2.5-4.0 ng/mL total PSA range: preliminary analysis. Urology 2003;1:274-6.
260. Sokoll LJ, Wang Y, Feng Z, Kagan J, et al. [-2]proPSA for prostate cancer detection: an NCI Early Detection Research Network validation study. J Urol 2008;180:539-43.
261. Soloman A. Homogeneous (monoclonal) immunoglobulins in cancer. Am J Med 1977;63:169-81.
262. Solomon E, Borrow J, Goddard AD. Chromosome aberrations and cancer. Science 1991;254:1153-60.
263. Soloway MS, Briggman JV, Carpinito GA, et al. Use of a new tumor marker, urinary NMP22, in the detection of occult or rapidly recurring transitional cell carcinoma of the urinary tract following surgical treatment. J Urol 1996;156:363-7.
264. Somerville RPT, Oblander SA, Apte SS. Matrix metalloproteinases: old dogs with new tricks. Genome Biol 2003;4:216.
265. Spencer CA, LoPresti JS, Fatemi S, et al. Detection of residual and recurrent differentiated thyroid carcinoma by serum thyroglobulin measurement. Thyroid 1999;9:435-41.
266. Spencer CA, Wang C, Fatemi S, et al. Serum thyroglobulin autoantibodies: prevalence, influence on serum thyroglobulin measurement and prognostic significance in patients with differentiated thyroid carcinoma. J Clin Endocrinol Metab 1998;83:1121-7.
267. Srinivas PR, Srivastava S, Hannah S, Wright GL Jr. Proteomics in early detection of cancer. Clin Chem 2001;47:1901-11.
268. Srivastava S, Zou Z, Pirollo K, et al. Germ line transmission of a mutated p53 gene in a cancer-prone family with Li-Fraumeni syndrome. Nature 1990;348:747-9.
269. Stamey TA, Barnhill SD, Zhang Z, et al. Effectiveness of ProstAsure in detecting prostate cancer and benign prostatic hyperplasia in men age 50 or older. J Urol 1996;155:436A.
270. Stamey TA, Yang N, Hay AR, et al. Prostatic-specific antigen as a serum marker for adenocarcinoma of the prostate. N Engl J Med 1987;317:909-16.
271. Stanbridge EJ, Cavenee WK. Heritable cancer and tumor suppressor genes: a tentative connection. In: Weinberg RS, ed. Oncogenes and the molecular origins of cancer. Cold Spring Harbor, Mass: Cold Spring Harbor Lab Press, 1989.
272. Steinberg W. The clinical utility of the CA 19-9 tumor-associated antigen. Am J Gastroenterol 1990;85:350-5.
273. Stenman UH. Tumor-associated trypsin inhibitor. Clin Chem 2002;8:1206-9.
274. Stenman UH, Alfthan H, Hotakainen K. Human chorionic gonadotropin in cancer. Clin Biochem 2004;37:549-61.
275. Stenman UH, Leinonen J, Alfthan H. A complex between prostate specific antigen and alpha-1-antichymotrypsin is the major form of prostate specific antigen in serum of patients with prostatic cancer:

assay of the complex improves clinical sensitivity for cancer. Cancer Res 1991;51:222-6.
276. Sterling RK, Jeffers L, Gordon F, et al. Clinical utility of AFP-L3% measurement in North American patients with HCV-related cirrhosis. Am J Gastroenterol 2007;102:2196-205.
277. Steuber T, Vickers AJ, Serio AM, et al. Comparison of free and total forms of serum human kallikrein 2 and prostate-specific antigen for prediction of locally advanced and recurrent prostate cancer. Clin Chem 2007;53:233-40.
278. Stigbrand T, Wahren B. Alkaline phosphatase as tumor markers. In: Sell S, ed. Serological cancer markers. Totowa NJ: Humana Press, 1992:135-49.
279. Sturgeon CM, Berger P, Bidart JM, et al. Differences in recognition of the 1st WHO international reference reagents for hCG-related isoforms by diagnostic immunoassays for human chorionic gonadotropin. Clin Chem 2009;55:1484-91.
280. Sturgeon CM, Duffy MJ, Stenmab UH, et al; National Academy of Clinical Biochemistry. National Academy of Clinical Biochemistry laboratory medicine practice guidelines for use of tumor markers in testicular, prostate, colorectal, breast, and ovarian cancers. Clin Chem 2008;54:e11-79.
281. Sulis ML, Parsons R. PTEN: from pathology to biology. Trends Cell Biol 2003;13:478-83.
282. Swarup V, Rajeswari MR. Circulating (cell-free) nucleic acids—a promising, non-invasive tool for early detection of several human diseases. FEBS Lett 2007;581:795-9.
283. Taketa K. Alpha-fetoprotein in the 1990s. In: Sell S, ed. Serological cancer markers. Totowa, NJ: Humana Press, 1992:31-46.
284. Takeuchi H, Bilchik A, Saha S, et al. c-MET expression level in primary colon cancer: a predictor of tumor invasion and lymph node metastases. Clin Cancer Res 2003;9:1480-8.
285. Tatarinov Y. New data on the embryo-specific antigenic components of human blood serum. Vopr Med Khim 1964;10:584-8.
286. Thompson IM, Goodman PJ, Tangen CM, et al. The influence of finasteride on the development of prostate cancer. N Engl J Med 2003;349:215-24.
287. Thompson IM, Pauler DK, Goodman PJ, et al. Prevalence of prostate cancer among men with a prostate-specific antigen level ≤4.0 ng per milliliter. N Engl J Med 2004;350:2239-46.
288. Tolgay Ocal I, Dolled-Filhart M, D'Aquila TG, et al. Tissue microarray-based studies of patients with lymph node negative breast carcinoma show that met expression is associated with worse outcome but is not correlated with epidermal growth factor family receptors. Cancer 2003;97:1841-8.
289. Vaitukaitis JL. Human chorionic gonadotropin: a hormone secreted for many reasons. N Engl J Med 1979;301:324-6.
290. van de Vijver MJ, He YD, van't Veer LJ, et al. A gene-expression signature as a predictor of survival in breast cancer. N Engl J Med 2002;347:1999-2009.
291. van't Veer LJ, Dai H, van de Vijver MJ, et al. Gene expression profiling predicts clinical outcome of breast cancer. Nature 2002;415:530-6.
292. Venter JC, Adams MD, Myers EW, et al. The sequence of the human genome. Science 2001;291:1304-51.
293. Veridex LLC. Veridex CellSearch circulating tumor cell test. Available at: http://veridex.com/CellSearch/CellSearchHCP.aspx (accessed May 2, 2011).
294. Vihinen P, Kahari VM. Matrix metalloproteinases in cancer: prognostic markers and therapeutic targets. Int J Cancer 2002;99:157-66.
295. Viskochil D, White R, Cawthon RL. The neurofibromatosis type 1 gene. Annu Rev Neurosci 1993;16:183-202.
296. Wawrzynczak EJ. Systemic immunotoxin therapy of cancer: advances and prospects. Br J Cancer 1991;64:624-30.
297. Weinberg RA. Tumor suppressor genes. Science 1991;254:1138-46.
298. Welsh JB, Sapinoso LM, Kern SG, et al. Large-scale delineation of secreted protein biomarkers overexpressed in cancer tissue and serum. PNAS USA 2003;100:3410-5.
299. Welsh JB, Zarrinkar PP, Sapinoso LM, et al. Analysis of gene expression profiles in normal and neoplastic ovarian tissue samples identifies candidate molecular markers of epithelial ovarian cancer. PNAS USA 2001;98:1176-81.
300. Wigler MH. GAPs in understanding Ras. Nature 1990;346:696-9.
301. Whittington J, Fantz CR, Gronowski AM, et al. The analytical specificity of human chorionic gonadotropin assays determined using WHO International Reference Reagents. Clin Chim Acta 2009;411:81-5.
302. Wittliff KL, Pasic R, Bland KI. Steroid and peptide hormone receptors identified in breast tissue. In: Kirby KI, Copeland EM, eds. The breast. Philadelphia: WB Saunders Co, 1990:900-36.
303. Wolff AC, Hammond ME, Schwartz JN, et al. American Society of Clinical Oncology/College of American Pathologists guideline recommendations for human epidermal growth factor receptor 2 testing in breast cancer. J Clin Oncol 2007;25:118-45.
303A. Wolf AM, Wender RC, Etzioni RB, et al. American Cancer Society guideline for the early detection of prostate cancer: update 2010. CA Cancer J Clin 2010;60:70-98.
304. Wooster R, Neuhausen SL, Mangion J, et al. Localization of a breast cancer susceptibility gene, BRCA 2, to chromosome 13q12-13. Science 1994;265:2088-90.
305. Yin BW, Lloyd KO. Molecular cloning of the CA125 ovarian cancer antigen: identification as a new mucin, MUC16. J Biol Chem 2001;276:27371-5.
306. Yousef GM, Diamandis EP. The new human tissue kallikrein gene family: structure, function, and association to disease. Endocr Rev 2001;2:184-204.
307. Yousef GM, Polymeris ME, Grass L, et al. Human kallikrein 5: a potential novel serum biomarker for breast and ovarian cancer. Cancer Res 2003;63:3958-65.
308. Yousef GM, Polymeris ME, Yacoub GM, et al. Parallel overexpression of seven kallikrein genes in ovarian cancer. Cancer Res 2003;63:2223-7.
309. Zeltzer PM, Marangos PJ, Evans AE, Schneider SL. Serum neuron-specific enolase in children with neuroblastoma. Cancer 1986;57:1230-4.
310. Zemzoum I, Kates RE, Ross JS, et al. Invasion factors uPA/PAI-1 and HER2 status provide independent and complementary information on patient outcome in node-negative breast cancer. J Clin Oncol 2003;21:1022-8.
311. Zhang Z. Combining multiple biomarkers in clinical diagnostics: a review of methods and issues. In: Diamandis EP, Fritsche HA, Lilja H, Chan DW, Schwartz MK, eds. Tumor markers: physiology, pathobiology, technology and clinical applications. Washington, DC: AACC Press, 2002:133-9.
312. Zhang Z, Bast RC, Yu Y, et al. Three biomarkers identified from serum proteomic analysis for the detection of early state ovarian cancer. Cancer Res 2004;64:5882-90.
313. Zippe C, Pandrangi L, Agarwal A. NMP22 is a sensitive, cost-effective test in patients at risk for bladder cancer. J Urol 1999;161:62-5.
314. Zweig MH, Robertson EA. Clinical validation of immunoassay: a well-designed approach to a clinical study. In: Chan DW, ed. Immunoassay: a practical guide. San Diego: Academic Press Inc, 1987:97-128.

CHAPTER 25

Kidney Function Tests

Edmund J. Lamb, Ph.D., F.R.C.Path., and Christopher P. Price, Ph.D., F.R.S.C., F.R.C.Path.

The functional unit of the kidney is the nephron, with each kidney containing between 0.4 and 1.2 million nephrons. In nearly all types of renal disease, impaired function of the kidneys is attributed to a diminished number of functioning nephrons rather than to compromised function of individual nephrons. Because glomerular filtration is the initiating phase of all nephron functions, quantitative or qualitative assessment of the glomerular filtration rate (GFR)—or some variable that bears a constant relationship to it—and assessment of the integrity of the filtration barrier generally provide the most useful indices for physicians to assess the severity and progress of kidney damage.

Specific defects in particular functions of the nephrons can also be identified and evaluated. For example, assessment of the maximum concentrating capacity of the kidneys gives an estimate of antidiuretic hormone (ADH)-controlled reabsorption of solute-free water in the distal portion of the tubule. Pinpoint defects, caused by genetically determined deficiencies of specific tubular transport systems or ion channels and giving rise to characteristic biochemical disorders, are considered in Chapter 48.

This chapter describes tests that have proved practical and useful for screening for and diagnosing impaired kidney function in clinical laboratories, and for monitoring the course and management of progressive chronic kidney disease (CKD). In general, where blood markers are discussed, either plasma or serum can be used for most of these tests (the term *serum* is mainly used throughout this chapter). This chapter provides an overview of contemporary methodology with reference intervals and discussion of the clinical utility of the tests.

URINE ANALYSIS

Examination of the urine is often the first step in the assessment of a patient suspected of having, or confirmed as having, deterioration in kidney function. The appearance (color and odor) of urine itself can be helpful; darkening from the pale normal straw color indicates more concentrated urine or the presence of another pigment. Hemoglobin and myoglobin give a pink-red-brown coloration, depending on the concentration. Turbidity in a fresh sample may indicate infection but also may be due to fat particles in a patient with nephrotic syndrome. Excessive foaming of urine when shaken suggests proteinuria. Urine is often chemically evaluated at the point of care with the help of reagent strip tests, which are available for a variety of analytes, or it is microscopically examined.

Reagent Strip (Dipstick) Testing

Over the years, many tests of renal significance have been adapted for use on strips of cellulose or pads of cellulose or strips of plastic that have been coated or impregnated with reagents for the analyte in question. This type of analytical test is commonly known as a *dipstick test.* A reagent strip may contain reagents for just one test per stick or reagents for multiple tests on a single stick. With this type of test, different methods detect substances that overflow into the urine, such as glucose, ketones, bilirubin diglucuronate, and urobilinogen, changes in the concentration of which reflect a change in another organ system in the body. These tests also detect changes in constituents that are more directly linked to alterations brought about by some pathologic condition affecting the kidney or urinary tract. Urine samples for reagent strip testing should be collected in sterile containers, and testing should be performed on fresh urine. Reagent strips should be used only if they have been stored properly desiccated because they can deteriorate in a matter of hours. Strict attention must be paid after sample addition to the timing of reading the absorbance change, which differs between analytes (e.g., from 30 seconds to 2 minutes). Examples of method principles and comments on the performance of tests pertinent to the assessment of kidney function are given in the following sections.

Total Protein

The reagent strip test for total protein includes a cellulose test pad impregnated with tetrabromphenol blue and a citrate pH 3 buffer. The reaction is based on the *protein error of indicators phenomenon,* by which certain chemical indicators demonstrate one color in the presence of protein and another in its absence. Thus tetrabromphenol blue is green in the presence of protein at pH 3 but yellow in its absence. The test has a lower detection limit of 150 to 300 mg/L, depending on the type and proportions of protein present. The reagent is most sensitive to albumin and less sensitive to globulins, Bence Jones protein, mucoproteins, and hemoglobin.[29,109,138] Indeed, it is confusing to note that one commercial application of this principle has been manufactured as Albustix, although the chemical principle underlying this test is identical to those of devices that claim to measure protein.[109]

Although not all patients with CKD will have proteinuria, proteinuria is a common finding in patients with kidney disease, and its presence suggests a poorer prognosis.[129-131,273] Use of a reagent strip assay has been considered an important screening test in any patient suspected of having renal disease. Among patients with suspected or proven CKD, including reflux nephropathy, and early glomerulonephritis, and those with hypertension or previously detected asymptomatic hematuria, annual urinalysis for proteinuria has been accepted as a useful way of identifying patients at risk of progressive kidney disease. Currently, no proven role has been identified for reagent strip protein analysis in the screening of unselected populations.[218,345] For many years, reagent strip testing for proteinuria was deemed inadequate for the detection of CKD among patients with diabetes, in whom urinary albumin loss should be measured specifically (see later); growing consensus suggests that reagent strip testing is also inadequate in other clinical scenarios.

Protein excretion displays considerable biological variability, which may be increased by (1) upright posture, (2) exercise, (3) fever, (4) symptomatic urinary tract infection (UTI),[41] (5) heart failure, and (6) kidney disease. Because standard urine reagent strips rely on estimation of protein concentration, this in turn depends on hydration or how concentrated the urine sample is; these tests therefore give only a rough indication of the presence or absence of pathologic proteinuria. Ralston and associates observed poor specificity for reagent strip analysis in detecting protein loss of 300 mg/d in a rheumatology outpatient population.[258] A pooled analysis of six studies undertaken in obstetric patients reported positive and negative likelihood ratios for "+" protein or greater on reagent strip analysis, for predicting 300 mg/d proteinuria as 0.6 (95%-CI: 0.45 to 0.8) and 3.48 (1.66 to 7.27), respectively,[336] suggesting that reagent strips are not good at ruling in or ruling out significant proteinuria. The Scottish Intercollegiate Guidelines Network (SIGN)[285] and the National Institute for Health and Clinical Excellence (NICE)[216] guard against the use of reagent strips to detect proteinuria. An evidence-based systematic review undertaken by the U.S. National Academy of Clinical Biochemistry (NACB) recommended against routine screening for proteinuria with reagent strip analysis.[214] Academy reviewers found no evidence that the use of urine reagent strip testing for proteinuria at the point of care improved patient outcomes; they described significant evidence of a high false-negative rate and poor negative predictive value compared with laboratory testing. The National Kidney Foundation Kidney Disease Outcomes Quality Initiative (NKF-KDOQI), NACB, SIGN, and NICE concur that these devices may give false-negative results when the urine is dilute.[214,216,218,285] Most authors agree that positive tests require confirmation by laboratory measurement of the protein-to-creatinine ratio (PCR) or the albumin-to-creatinine ratio (ACR) on an early morning or random urine sample.[218] A suitable protocol for the further investigation of patients found to have proteinuria at screening is given in Figure 25-1.

Automated devices capable of reading color changes in reagent strips using reflectance spectrometry have become available. These reduce interoperator variability and improve diagnostic accuracy.[2,275,279,335] A creatinine test pad (using the peroxidase-like activity of transition metal creatinine complexes) has been added to some reagent strip systems to enable a PCR to be reported, thereby reducing the intraindividual variation seen with random urine collections. An evaluation of one such device (Multistix PRO 10LS, Siemens plc, Camberley, Surrey, United Kingdom) read semiquantitatively on the Clinitek Status automated strip reader (Siemens plc) in a renal outpatient setting concluded that the test was suitable for ruling out significant proteinuria (>0.3 g/d).[108]

Albumin

Reagent strip methods are available for the more specific detection of albumin at low concentrations (i.e., in the microalbuminuric range—approximately 20 to 200 mg/L). Both photometric and immunologic methods for detecting albumin have been described for use with urine samples, the former based on binding of bis(3′,3″-diiodo-4′,4″-hydroxy-5′,5″-dinitrophenyl)-3,4,5,6-tetrabromosulfonephthalein (DIDNTB) at pH 1.5.[257] For example, the Clinitek microalbumin reagent strip read on a Clinitek Status analyzer (both products of Siemens) produces semiquantitative ACR results, whereas the DCA 2000+ device (Siemens) is capable of reporting a fully quantitative ACR result. Medicines and Healthcare Products Regulatory Agency reports[200,201] and other published evaluations[238,239] have demonstrated reasonable analytical performance. Good diagnostic performance has been reported in the detection of significant proteinuria in hypertensive pregnancy,[335] in ruling out significant albuminuria (>30 mg/d) in a CKD outpatient population,[107] and in ruling out albuminuria (>3.4 mg/mmol) in a general population.[102]

Hemoglobin

The presence of hemoglobin in the urine may be due to glomerular, tubulointerstitial, or postrenal disease, although the latter two causes are the more common. The presence of blood in the urine is detected by using a phase contrast microscope to determine the presence of red cells in the urine sediment, or by using a reagent strip test. Chemical detection of hemoglobin in urine depends on the peroxidase activity of the protein employing a peroxide substrate and an oxygen acceptor.

For this test, the reagent pad is impregnated with buffered tetramethyl benzidine (TMB) and an organic peroxide. The method depends on detection of the peroxidase activity of hemoglobin, which catalyzes the reaction of cumene hydroperoxide and TMB. The color change ranges from orange through pale to dark green, and red cells, free hemoglobin, and myoglobin are all detected. Two reagent pads are used for the low hemoglobin concentration; if intact red cells are

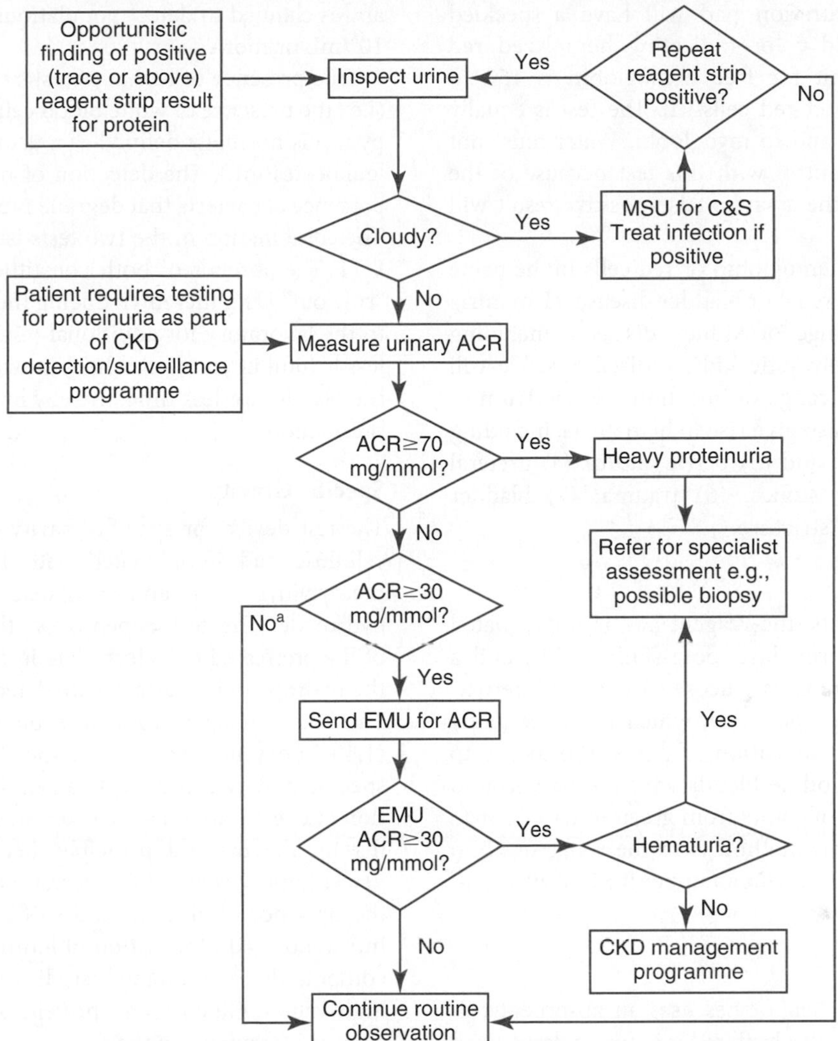

Figure 25-1 Suggested protocol for the further investigation of a nondiabetic individual demonstrating a positive (trace or above) reagent strip test for proteinuria or a quantitative proteinuria test. Reagent strip device results should be confirmed using laboratory testing of the albumin-to-creatinine ratio (ACR) on at least two additional occasions. Patients with two or more positive (≥30 mg albumin/mmol creatinine) tests on early morning samples 1 to 2 weeks apart should be diagnosed as having persistent proteinuria. (The possibility of postural proteinuria should be excluded by examination of an early morning urine.) Protein-to-creatinine ratio (PCR) measurement can be substituted for the ACR: approximate PCR equivalents to ACRs of 30 and 70 mg/mmol are 50 and 100 mg/mmol, respectively. This protocol is adapted from U.K. National Institute for Health and Clinical Excellence (NICE) guidance: other countries and professional organizations have alternate versions (see www.nice.org.uk/CG73 for further information). *C&S,* Culture and sensitivity; *CKD,* chronic kidney disease; *EMU,* early morning urine; *MSU,* midstream urine. [a]In the absence of a systemic disease such as diabetes or hypertension with a borderline increase in albumin (3 to 30 mg/mmol), total protein (15 to 50 mg/mmol) loss without hematuria, or a rise in serum creatinine, a serious primary renal pathology is unlikely. In a diabetic patient, lesser degrees of proteinuria may be significant and should elicit appropriate investigation and management (see "Proteinuria and Albuminuria: Clinical Significance"). *Note:* U.S. guidelines express albuminuria or proteinuria as mg/g creatinine, whereas other guidelines use mg/mmol creatinine. An approximate conversion factor of 0.1136 can be used to convert results in mg/g to mg/mmol (e.g., 30 mg/mmol = 264 mg/g, 70 mg/mmol = 616 mg/g).

present, the low-concentration pad will have a speckled appearance, with a solid color indicating hemolyzed red cells. The detection limit for free hemoglobin is 150 to 600 μg/L, or 5 to 20 intact red cells/μL. The test is equally sensitive to hemoglobin and to myoglobin. Water must not be used as a negative control with this test because of the matrix requirements of the assay; a false-positive result will be obtained.

The presence of free hemoglobin or red cells in the urine indicates the presence of renal or bladder disease. Hematuria can be present in a range of kidney diseases, including glomerular nephritis, polycystic kidney disease, sickle cell disease, vasculitis, and a range of infections. A spectrum of urological diseases may also give rise to hematuria, including (1) bladder, (2) prostate, and (3) pelvic and/or (4) ureteral malignancy, (5) kidney stones, (6) trauma, (7) bladder damage, and (8) ureteral stricture.

Glucose

For glucose measurements, the reagent pad is impregnated with glucose oxidase, peroxidase, potassium iodide, and a blue dye. The reaction employs glucose oxidase and peroxidase to produce hydrogen peroxide, which is subsequently reduced with concurrent oxidation of potassium iodide to release iodine. The free iodine blends with the background color to produce a range of colors from green to dark brown. The detection limit of this method is in the range of 72 to 127 mg/dL (4 to 7 mmol/L), with an upper limit of 2018 mg/dL (111 mmol/L).

Leukocytes

The reagent strip test for leukocytes uses an absorbent cellulose pad impregnated with a buffered mixture of derivatized pyrrole amino acid ester and diazonium salt. Granulocytic leukocytes contain esterases, which catalyze the hydrolysis of the derivatized pyrrole amino acid ester to liberate 3-hydroxy-5-phenylpyrrole. This pyrrole then reacts with a diazonium salt to produce a purple product. The test is claimed to have a detection limit of 5 to 15 cells/μL in urine, and the darkest color block is equivalent to 500 cells/μL or greater. A decrease in the true test result may occur in samples with elevated glucose concentration, high specific gravity, or the presence of cephaloxin, cephalothin, tetracycline, or high concentrations of oxalic acid.

Nitrite

To measure nitrite, the reagent pad is impregnated with *p*-arsanilic acid and tetrahydro-benzo(h)quinolin-3-ol. The reaction is based on arsanilic acid in the presence of nitrite converting to a diazonium salt, which couples with the quinolol to produce a pink color. The detection limit of the test is 61 to 103 μg/dL (13 to 22 μmol/L) nitrite in urine with a normal specific gravity. The test is less sensitive with urine that has a high specific gravity. At urine ascorbic acid concentrations above approximately 25 mg/dL (1.4 mmol/L), a false-negative result may occur at low nitrite concentrations [81 μg/dL (13 μmol/L) or less]. The test measures only nitrite and is claimed to detect populations of bacteria at a value of 10^5/mL or more.

The presence of leukocyte esterase is indicative of pyuria (i.e., the presence of white blood cells in the urine; significant pyuria is normally defined as a urinary white cell count ≥10 leukocytes/mL). The detection of nitrite is indicative of the presence of bacteria that degrade nitrate excreted in the urine. The combination of the two tests is valuable in patients with UTI. The absence of both constituents is a valuable test to "rule out" UTI, thereby reducing the number of samples sent to the laboratory for additional tests. The nitrite test may be less helpful in young children, in whom the urine remains in the bladder for less time, thereby limiting the time for nitrite production.

Specific Gravity

The test device for specific gravity consists of an absorbent cellulose pad impregnated with bromthymol blue, polymethylvinyl ether, and/or maleic anhydride and sodium hydroxide. The test depends on the apparent pK_a change of the pretreated polyelectrolyte in relation to ionic strength; the hydrogen ions released are detected by the pH indicator. The color changes from dark blue at low specific gravity (1.000) to yellow-green at a specific gravity of 1.030. The specific gravity can provide an indication of the concentration of urine; care must be taken with interpretation depending on the method principle, because those devices that detect ionic species will underestimate the specific gravity in the presence of glucose, and so forth. Urine collected after intravenous administration of iodine-containing radiopaque compounds for radiologic studies may give extraordinarily high values. Glucose and protein may also contribute substantial increments to the density of urine, and semiquantitative determination of these substances is necessary for valid interpretation or correction of urine specific gravity measurements. Diabetic patients with uncontrolled hyperglycemia and glucosuria may have high urine specific gravity, even when the normal renal concentrating function is seriously impaired.

pH

To measure the pH of a sample, the test pad is impregnated with indicators, one example being a mixture of methyl red and bromthymol blue. Methyl red in diluted form is red at pH values below 4.2 and yellow at values above 6.2. Bromthymol blue is yellow at pH values below 6.0 and blue at values above 7.6. At a pH within these values, the indicators give shades of orange and green, respectively. Thus the reagent blocks are compared with a color chart, where the lowest pH block at 5.0 is orange and the highest at 8.5 is blue. It is important to recognize that the pH of urine is altered by standing, as is the color of the reagent blocks; therefore careful adherence to the recommended procedure is important. Measurement of urine pH is helpful in the assessment of patients with renal tubular acidosis and in stone formers, although evaluation using a pH electrode may be more informative.

Microscopic Examination of Urine

Microscopic examination of the sediment obtained from centrifugation of a fresh urine sample shows the presence of (1) a few cells (erythrocytes, leukocytes, and cells derived from the kidney and urinary tract), (2) casts [composed predominantly of Tamm-Horsfall glycoprotein (THG)], and (3) possibly fat or pigmented particles. An increase in red cells or casts implies hematuria possibly caused by glomerular disease; white cells or casts imply the presence of white cells in the tubules. Inflammation of the upper urinary tract may result in polymorphonuclear leukocytes and various types of casts; in lower urinary tract inflammation, the casts are not present. In acute glomerulonephritis, hematuria may lead to coloration of the urine and the presence of large numbers of red cells and white cells; as the duration of the disease increases, the amount of sediment diminishes. Nephrologists will often describe urine as having an *active urinary sediment,* or as *bland.* Having an active urinary sediment means that signs (red blood cells, white blood cells, casts) of active kidney inflammation can be detected when urine is examined under the microscope.

New Instrumental Techniques

Flow cytometry and flow imaging systems have been developed for the characterization of erythrocytes in the differential diagnosis of hematuria and as means of improving the recognition of other particulate material in urine. This form of analysis has been used to discriminate between and quantify the particulate matter in a defined volume of urine, bringing the added benefit of better standardization of the technique.[234] Thus the flow imaging method can identify (1) red blood cells, (2) white blood cells, (3) white blood cell clumps, (4) hyaline casts, (5) pathologic casts, (6) squamous epithelial cells, (7) nonsquamous epithelial cells, (8) yeast, (9) crystals, and (10) sperm. These fully automated systems have the potential to replace urinary microscopy because they offer better discriminatory power and quantitation while providing closer agreement between laboratories.[348] The principles of flow cytometry are described in Chapter 10. A flow imaging analyzer, such as the Iris iQ200 (Iris Diagnostics, Chatsworth, Calif), analyzes unspun urine by aspirating sample through a flowcell positioned in a microscope. A digital camera captures the images, and neural network–based particle image recognition software is used to identify and count the particles present from five hundred 884 × 680 μm fields with 0.68 μm resolution. The number of particles for the volume scanned is then calculated. Flow image analysis has been shown to be more accurate than the flow cytometric approach while helping to improve workflow and save valuable technologist time by reducing the number of manual microscopic examinations required.[182,325] However, it has been suggested that manual microscopy may still be required for the assessment of crystals.[197]

Proton nuclear magnetic resonance (NMR) has been investigated as a means of characterizing low molecular weight molecules.[219] Metabolic profiles have been generated, and with the use of sophisticated computer analysis, distinctive patterns of molecules have been associated with damage to specific parts of the nephron. It is expected that this technique will be used to identify individual molecules for which selective assays can then be developed.[219]

QUANTITATIVE ASSESSMENT OF PROTEINURIA: TOTAL PROTEIN AND ALBUMIN

Higher molecular weight proteins are retained within the circulation by the glomerular filter, and lower molecular weight proteins are freely filtered and reabsorbed and catabolized within the tubular cells. Consequently, the appearance of notable amounts of protein in the urine suggests renal disease. Commonly, proteinuria is classified as tubular or glomerular, depending on the pattern of proteinuria observed. A third category, overflow proteinuria, is also recognized in which filtration of excessive amounts of low molecular weight protein exceeds the tubular capacity for reabsorption (Table 25-1). Examples of the latter include Bence Jones proteinuria and myoglobinuria. Proteinuria is a potent risk marker for progressive kidney disease, and reduction of protein excretion is a therapeutic target. This section considers the analytical approach and the rationale used in the quantitation of urinary proteins, with emphasis on total protein and albumin measurement.

Clinical Significance

The clinical significance of proteinuria was discussed earlier (see section on urine analysis) and will be discussed in Chapter 48, along with the physiology and pathophysiology of renal protein handling. Most commonly, proteinuria reflects albuminuria. Several groups have suggested that urinary total protein measurement can be replaced by urine albumin measurement.[12,161,224] This may provide a more specific and sensitive measure of changes in glomerular permeability and is consistent with most,[178,216,218] but not all,[38,285] current national and international guidelines. Strong evidence has linked urinary albumin loss to cardiovascular mortality and kidney disease progression in diabetes.[103] Other evidence suggests that urinary albumin is a more sensitive test to enable detection of glomerular pathology associated with some other systemic diseases, including hypertension and systemic sclerosis.[60,292] In health, relatively small amounts of albumin (less than 30 mg/d) are lost in the urine. Because of this, and because total protein assays are imprecise at low concentrations, relatively large increases in urine albumin loss can occur without a significant measurable increase in urinary total protein. In a methodologic study of urine from patients attending renal transplant, general nephrology, and medicine and obstetric clinics, Newman and colleagues observed increased albumin losses (defined here as >25 mg/d) in 63% of samples that were classified as not having increased total protein loss (defined here as >250 mg/d).[224] Changes in albumin excretion may also reflect overall changes in vascular permeability and therefore may not indicate explicit deterioration in renal function.[99]

TABLE 25-1 Characterization of Proteinuria

Type of Proteinuria	Causes	Examples of Proteins Seen
Glomerular	Increased glomerular permeability	Progressively increasing excretion of higher molecular weight proteins as permeability increases (e.g., albumin, IgG)
Overflow	Increased plasma concentration of relatively freely filtered protein	Bence Jones protein Lysozyme Myoglobin
Tubular	Proximal tubular damage: decreased tubular reabsorptive capacity and/or release of intracellular components (e.g., due to nephrotoxic drugs)	α_1-Microglobulin β_2-Microglobulin Retinol binding protein Enzymuria (e.g., *N*-acetyl-β-D-glucosaminidase, alkaline phosphatase, α-glutathione-S-transferase)
	Decreased nephron number: increased filtered load per nephron	As above
	Distal tubular damage	Tamm-Horsfall glycoprotein π-Glutathione-S-transferase

Concern has been expressed that replacing urinary total protein measurement with albumin measurement may cause tubular proteinuria to be missed.[218]

Microalbuminuria is the term used to describe an increase in urinary excretion of albumin above the reference interval for healthy nondiabetic subjects, but at an excretion that is not generally detectable by less sensitive clinical tests such as reagent strips designed to measure total protein. Approximately, this equates to urinary albumin concentrations between 20 and 200 mg/L. The term *microalbuminuria* is somewhat misleading, in that the albumin being measured is identical in form to that circulating in plasma, and the so-called microalbuminuric range actually refers to increased albumin losses.[206] Nevertheless, the phrase is widely used in clinical practice. Increased urinary albumin loss (microalbuminuria) is considered a clinically important indicator of deteriorating renal function in diabetic subjects. For example, it is now accepted by both European and U.S. diabetes societies that regular screening of urinary albumin loss is valuable in monitoring type 1 and type 2 diabetes.* This recommendation came as a consequence of the widespread availability of sensitive assays for urinary albumin measurement and effective treatments, validated in large multinational trials, along with detailed cost-benefit analyses in the vanguard of evidence-based medicine.

Because large numbers of clinical studies have been performed, guidelines for microalbuminuria screening are now established (Figure 25-2).[19,26,215,217,300] The diagnosis of microalbuminuria requires demonstration of increased albumin loss (increased ACR or increased albumin loss in a timed collection) in at least two of three urine samples collected in the absence of infection or an acute metabolic crisis. Establishing the diagnosis has both prognostic and management implications in the care of patients with diabetes mellitus. The best possible metabolic control of diabetes should be achieved before patients are examined for microalbuminuria, and patients should not be screened during other transitory illnesses. Screening should commence 5 years after diagnosis in patients with type 1 diabetes mellitus and at diagnosis in patients with type 2 diabetes without proteinuria, and should continue on an annual basis up to the age of 75 years. An early morning (preferred) midstream urine sample should be sent to the laboratory for albumin measurement. Exact definitions of microalbuminria differ among national societies.[206] In the United Kingdom, an ACR less than or equal to 23 mg/g (≤2.5 mg/mmol) in a male, or 32 mg/g (≤3.5 mg/mmol) in a female, requires no further investigation until the time of the patient's next annual review.[215] Patients demonstrating ACRs above this cutoff should have urine samples sent to the laboratory on two other occasions (ideally within 1 month) for albumin estimation. Patients demonstrating increased ACRs in one or both of these additional samples have microalbuminuria. It is important to consider other causes of increased albumin excretion, especially in the case of type 1 diabetes present for less than 5 years. These may include nondiabetic renal disease, menstrual contamination, vaginal discharge, uncontrolled hypertension, UTI, heart failure, and strenuous exercise.

Once microalbuminuria has been established, an angiotensin-converting enzyme (ACE) inhibitor or an angiotensin receptor blocker (ARB) is typically prescribed, because these classes of antihypertensive agent have distinct antiproteinuric effects above and beyond their effects on blood pressure. Several major trials have shown such drugs to be effective in reducing not just proteinuria but also the rate of fall in GFR when used in both microalbuminuric and proteinuric diabetes. It has also been suggested that ACE inhibitors should be prescribed for normotensive microalbuminuric patients with diabetes, because the definition of *normotension* as currently used may not reflect the actual intraglomerular pressure, and a lower blood pressure cutoff should be used in such a high-risk group.

Some workers consider that once microalbuminuria is established in a patient with diabetes, it may already be too

*References 19, 141, 209, 215, 217, and 300.

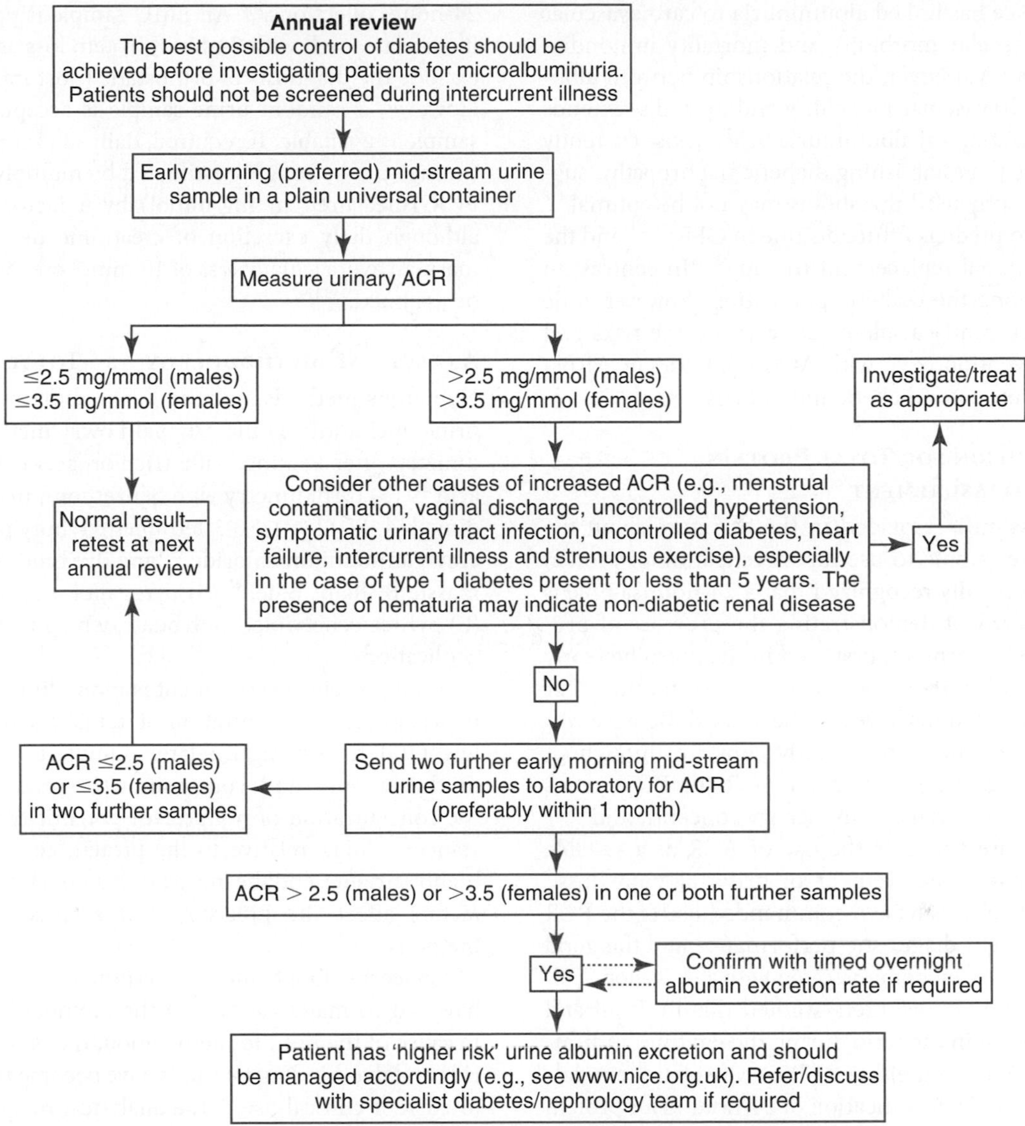

Figure 25-2 Screening for microalbuminuria in diabetes mellitus. Patients demonstrating "higher risk" urine albumin excretion should be managed accordingly. This protocol is adapted from the U.K. National Institute for Health and Clinical Excellence (NICE) guidance: other countries and professional organizations have alternate versions (see www.nice.org.uk and Reference 206 for further information). ***ACR,*** **Albumin-to-creatinine ratio.** ***Note:*** **U.S. guidelines express albuminuria as mg/g creatinine, whereas other guidelines use mg/mmol creatinine. An approximate conversion factor of 0.1136 can be used to convert results in mg/g to mg/mmol (e.g., 2.5 mg/mmol = 22 mg/g, 3.5 mg/mmol = 31 mg/g).**

late to prevent the development of nephropathy,[221] and the use of other, earlier markers may be beneficial. As will be discussed later in the chapter, markers of tubular damage have not, to date, been convincingly shown to demonstrate advantages over urinary albumin in the detection of diabetic nephropathy. Considerable work has been undertaken to look for genetic linkages to the development of nephropathy in persons with diabetes. This work has included studies of polymorphisms of ACE and insulin genes, but as yet no clear relationship has been demonstrated.[280]

Increased urinary albumin loss is common among the general population and probably is not solely attributable to the presence of diabetes. Epidemiologic data from the Third National Health and Nutrition Examination Survey (NHANES III) in the United States suggest that the population prevalence of microalbuminuria is 7.8%.[142] Similar estimates have been reported from population surveys in Australia (6.8%)[9] and The Netherlands (7.2%).[119] In The Netherlands study, even after individuals with diabetes and hypertension were excluded, the population prevalence was still 6.6%. Among patients with risk factors for CKD, prevalences were notably higher. For example, in the NHANES III study, 28.8% of people with diabetes and 16.0% of those with hypertension had microalbuminuria.[142]

Strong evidence has linked albuminuria to cardiovascular and noncardiovascular morbidity and mortality in nondiabetic individuals.* Moreover, the relationship between albuminuria and cardiovascular morbidity and mortality extends down to concentrations of albuminuria below those currently used as thresholds in establishing diabetic nephropathy, suggesting that currently used thresholds may not be optimal.[118] Albuminuria also predicts future decline in GFR[155,230] and the requirement for renal replacement therapy.[326] In contrast to the situation among the diabetic population, however, little information is currently available concerning the risks and benefits of intervention (e.g., with ACE inhibitors or ARBs) in microalbuminuric nondiabetic individuals.

Sample Collection for Total Protein and Albumin Measurement

Extensive discussion is provided in the literature about the appropriate urine sample to use for investigation of protein excretion. It is generally recognized that a 24-hour sample is the definitive means of demonstrating the presence of proteinuria. However, overnight, first void in the morning [early morning urine (EMU)], second void in the morning, or random sample collections have also been used. Because creatinine excretion in the urine is fairly constant throughout the 24-hour period, measurement of ACR (or PCR) ratios allows correction for variations in urinary concentration.[16,148] A body of literature supports the use of ACR as a suitable alternative to timed measurement of urine albumin loss.† Similarly, several authors have recommended use of the PCR based on its excellent diagnostic performance and the good correlation that has been demonstrated with the 24-hour collection.‡ Ginsberg and coworkers studied this in detail and found little variation in the ratio during the daytime, indicating that the first void and either of the two subsequent collections can give a reliable indication of 24-hour urine protein loss.[96] Newman and associates demonstrated a significant reduction in intraindividual variation in the PCR compared with protein excretion in random urines collected throughout the day (a mean reduction to 38.6% from 96.5%).[222] They described a similar experience with albumin loss (a decrease to 52.1% from 80.0%).[222] The ratio to osmolality or to specific gravity to correct for dilution effects associated with changes in water excreted during the day has also been reported.[222] In a systematic review, random urine PCR was shown to perform better as a test for ruling out significant proteinuria than as a rule-in test; the authors suggested that positive PCR results may still require confirmation with a 24-hour collection.[253]

Although the reference point remains the accurately timed 24-hour specimen, it is widely accepted that this is a difficult procedure to control effectively, and that inaccuracies in urinary collection may contribute to errors in estimation of protein losses. In practice, for screening purposes, spot urine ACRs (or PCRs) can be used to rule out the necessity for 24-hour collections.[218] An EMU sample is preferred because it correlates well with 24-hour protein loss and is required to exclude the diagnosis of orthostatic (postural) proteinuria.[218] However, a random urine sample is acceptable if no EMU sample is available. If required, daily albumin or protein loss (in mg) can be roughly estimated by multiplying the ACR or PCR (measured in mg/mmol) by a factor of 10 because, although daily excretion of creatinine depends on muscle mass, an average daily loss of 10 mmol creatinine per day can be assumed.[148,194]

Analytical Methodology – s—Total Protein

Numerous methods are used for measurement of protein in urine, including (1) the original Lowry method,[185] (2) turbidimetry after mixing with trichloroacetic or sulfosalicylic acid,[227] (3) turbidimetry with benzethonium chloride [benzyl dimethyl (2-{2-*p*-1,1,3,3-tetramethyl butylphenoxy}ethoxy) ethyl] ammonium chloride,[198] and dye binding with (4) Coomassie Brilliant Blue,[343] (5) pyrogallol red molybdate,[334] and (6) pyrocatecholviolet-molybdate, which is used in dry-slide applications.

Total protein measurement is more difficult in urine than in serum. The concentration of urinary protein is normally low (100 to 200 mg/L); large sample-to-sample variation in the amount and composition of proteins is common; the concentration of nonprotein potentially interfering substances is high relative to the protein concentration and is highly variable; and the inorganic ion content is high. All these factors affect the precision and accuracy of the various methods.

Concerns about different responses to different proteins have led to many variants of the methods being published. Because of the need for automation, the benzethonium chloride and dye-binding methods have become the most popular in current clinical use.[45] The analytical range of the turbidimetric assays has been of concern, with the equivalent to an "antigen excess" equivalence point being apparent when high protein concentrations give a lower signal because an inadequate amount of denaturant is present relative to protein. This limitation can be overcome by monitoring the rate of turbidity formation.

As with urine reagent strip analysis, turbidimetric and dye binding methods do not provide equal analytical specificity and sensitivity for all proteins. Most approaches tend to react more strongly with albumin than with globulin and other nonalbumin proteins,[199,227,286] although incorporating sodium dodecyl sulfate (SDS) in pyrogallol red reagent is claimed to reduce this issue.[231] Significant interferences include aminoglycosides,[191] nonvisible hematuria,[349] and infused modified gelatin solutions used as plasma expanders,[61] all of which may falsely increase measured urinary total protein concentration.

No reference measurement procedure is listed by the Joint Committee for Traceability in Laboratory Medicine (JCTLM), and no standardized reference material for urinary total protein is available. Because a variable mixture of proteins is measured, it is difficult to define the latter. The variety of

*References 5, 30, 31, 76, 86, 110, 119, and 330.

†References 48, 95, 127, 188, 189, and 206.

‡References 47, 57, 71, 96, 171, 173, 258, 272, and 279.

TABLE 25-2 Characteristics of the Major Urinary Proteins

Protein	Mr, kDa	Free Plasma Concentration, g/L	Diameter, nm	pI	Glomerular Sieving Coefficient	Filtered Load, mg/L*	Urinary Concentration, mg/L†	% Reabsorbed
IgG	150	10	5.5	7.3	0.0001	1	0.1	99
Albumin	66	40	3.5	4.7	0.0002	8	5	99
α_1-Microglobulin	31	0.025	2.9	4.5	≈0.3	7.5	5	99
Retinol binding protein	22	0.025	2.1	4.5	≈0.7	17.5	0.1	99
Cystatin C	12.8	0.01	3.0	9.2	≈0.7	0.7	0.1	99
β_2-Microglobulin	11.8	0.015	1.6	5.6	0.7	1.1	0.1	99

*Concentration in the glomerular filtrate.
†Typical concentrations observed in health.

methods in use means that significant between-laboratory variation is inevitable.[44] This variation tends to diminish at higher concentrations of urinary total protein, presumably in part as albumin becomes the predominant protein. In addition to methodologic differences between various protein assays, calibration differences have been found to be one of the major determinants of intermethod variability.[45,114,190]

Analytical Methodology—Albumin

Urinary albumin is measured by most diagnostic laboratories predominantly by using quantitative immunoturbidimetric or nephelometric approaches capable of detecting albumin at low concentrations. Commercial assays typically have lower limits of quantitation of between 2 and 5 mg/L. As for total protein, no JCTLM reference measurement procedure or standardized reference material is currently available for urinary albumin, although the National Kidney Disease Education Program and the International Federation of Clinical Chemistry and Laboratory Medicine have established a joint committee to address these issues.[203,206] Most commonly, urinary albumin assays are standardized against a serum-based calibrant (CRM 470) distributed by the Institute for Reference Materials and Measurements of the European Commission, as has been recommended by Kidney Disease Improving Global Outcomes (KDIGO).[178] Although intuitively, standardization issues should be more easily addressed than those for total protein measurement, albumin is known to undergo polymerization and fragmentation on storage, when freeze-thawed and when lyophilized.[20,203] Some data have suggested that a significant proportion of albumin present in urine may be nonimmunoreactive,[52,53,187,232] although studies would appear to have refuted this hypothesis as being caused by coeluting proteins in size exclusion high-performance liquid chromatography (HPLC).[288,310,311]

Dry chemistry systems have been developed for the quantitation of albumin in urine.[153,157] For example, in one such device, the urine albumin laterally flows along a porous matrix through an area containing gold particle–labeled antibodies to albumin. In the presence of albumin, these antibody molecules are neutralized and pass through a portion of the matrix containing immobilized albumin to a detection zone, where they appear pink.[157] Point-of-care testing devices for urinary albumin have been discussed previously.

Reference Intervals and Definitions of Proteinuria and Albuminuria

The typical urinary total protein loss is less than 150 mg/d. The proteins lost are made up of albumin (typically <30 mg/d) and some smaller proteins, together with proteins secreted by the tubules, of which THG predominates.[123] Typical concentrations of proteins found in urine are listed in Table 25-2.

No consistent definition of *proteinuria* is available. Proteinuria is commonly detected at the point of care using urine reagent strip devices, and "clinical" proteinuria has sometimes been defined as equivalent to a color change of "+" or greater on the relevant pad on the strip. This equates to approximately 300 mg/L of total protein, or a PCR of 50 mg/mmol, or protein loss of approximately 500 mg/d (assuming an average urine volume of 1.5 L/d). North American guidelines define *proteinuria* as a PCR greater than 23 mg/mmol.[148,218] Australasian guidelines state that the cutoff for abnormal varies between 150 and 300 mg/d, depending on the laboratory.[38] An upper limit of normal loss of 150 mg/d is equivalent to a urinary PCR of 15 mg/mmol (given average daily creatinine excretion of 10 mmol), whereas Scottish guidelines have defined *proteinuria* as a PCR ≥ 100 mg/mmol, approximately equivalent to a loss of 1000 mg/d.[285] In England and Wales, the NICE CKD guideline defines *proteinuria* as a PCR ≥ 50 mg/mmol, or an ACR ≥ 30 mg/mmol (approximately equivalent to a total protein loss of 500 mg/d, or an albumin loss of 300 mg/d).[216] Both Scottish and NICE Guidelines recommend that the classification of CKD should be extended to include a suffix "p" to identify patients with proteinuria at any stage of kidney disease, acknowledging the importance of proteinuria as a risk factor. In the setting of preeclampsia, significant proteinuria is defined as 300 mg or more per day.[59]

Among patients with diabetes, the classification of diabetic nephropathy has been based on urinary albumin loss (commonly expressed as an ACR). In contrast to urinary total protein loss, definitions of *normoalbuminuria, microalbuminuria,* and *macroalbuminuria* are reasonably consistent across international guidelines, allowing for slight differences in units of expression.* In the United Kingdom, patients are categorized as normoalbuminuric (≤2.5 mg/mmol in males, ≤3.5 mg/mmol in females), microalbuminuric (>2.5/3.5 to 29 mg/mmol), and macroalbuminuric or proteinuric (≥30 mg/mmol).[216,217]

The KDIGO classification of CKD is clear in that it requires urinary albumin measurement as a marker of kidney damage to facilitate diagnosis of stage 1 and 2 CKD,[178] with a diagnostic threshold value of 3.4 mg/mmol. In other words, the presence of low-concentration albuminuria (microalbuminuria) in an individual with a GFR of 60 mL/min/1.73 m^2 or less is indicative of CKD irrespective of whether or not diabetes mellitus is present.

QUANTITATIVE ASSESSMENT OF PROTEINURIA: OTHER URINARY PROTEINS

Bence Jones Proteinuria

The presence of immunoglobulin light chains (Bence Jones proteins, 22 kDa) in the urine is an important indication of the presence of myeloma and, in approximately 20% of cases, may occur in the absence of a paraprotein band in the serum.[15] The pathologic significance of these proteins is considered in greater detail in Chapter 44. A variety of tests have been used for the detection of Bence Jones protein, including the classic heat test and the Bradshaw test. To date, electrophoresis supplemented by immunofixation has been the most reliable approach.[15,340] Quantitation of Bence Jones protein excretion may be required when patients with light chain only myeloma are monitored. This has generally been achieved by using a combination of electrophoresis and densitometry,[15] but recently described immunoassays for free light chains in serum and urine may play a role in this setting (see Chapter 44).

Myoglobinuria

Myoglobin is a small (17.8 kDa), heme-containing protein catabolized by endocytosis and proteolysis in the proximal tubule following glomerular filtration. Typically, only 0.01 to 5.0% of filtered protein appears in the urine. However, following rhabdomyolysis, large amounts of myoglobin are released into the plasma, saturating the tubular reabsorptive mechanism. This results in the appearance of notable quantities of myoglobin in the urine (which may color the urine red-brown). Further, myoglobin is directly toxic to the renal tubules and can cause acute tubular necrosis with acute renal failure.[352] Myoglobin will give a positive reaction with hemoglobin reagent strip tests, and basic methods of detection have relied on this principle following removal of hemoglobin (e.g., by ammonium sulfate precipitation), although false-negative and false-positive results were common.[14] Urinary myoglobin is better measured by immunochemical means, although preconcentration of urine may be required.[184] However, for most purposes, evidence that rhabdomyolysis has occurred is better provided by an increase in serum creatine kinase activity not attributable to a cardiac source. Urinary myoglobin measurement provides no additional prognostic or diagnostic information in this setting.[14]

Tubular Proteinuria

In practice, the integrity of the renal tubule is assessed indirectly through measurement of functional change and detection of tissue damage. The most common approach, however, has been the measurement of urinary concentrations of low molecular weight proteins using immunoassay technology. These are freely filtered at the glomerulus and then are reabsorbed and catabolized within the proximal tubule. Consequently, the appearance of notable quantities of these proteins in the urine reflects failure of the tubular reabsorptive mechanisms (see Table 25-1). The most commonly measured proteins are α_1-microglobulin and retinol binding protein (RBP). In the past, there has been considerable study of the excretion of β_2-microglobulin; however, it is an impractical marker because of its instability in urine at a pH less than 6. α_1-Microglobulin (Mr 31 kDa) is also referred to as protein HC because of its human complex–forming capacity with IgA. It is synthesized by the liver, and the free form is readily filtered at the glomerulus.[338] RBP (Mr 22 kDa) is also synthesized by the liver and is found in the plasma as a complex with prealbumin; the protein is the carrier protein for vitamin A.[17,318] For identification of tubular damage, urinary RBP may be more sensitive than α_1-microglobulin, but the higher concentration and excellent stability of the latter in human urine ex vivo facilitate its use as a marker of tubular damage in clinical studies.[143,241] Cystatin C, generally measured in serum as a marker of GFR (discussed later), is also measured in urine as a marker of proximal tubular damage.[116] THG, located in the thick ascending limb of the loop of Henle,[124] has been used as a marker of more distal tubular damage.[243]

Lysozyme is an enzyme that occurs in neutrophilic granulocytes, monocytes, and macrophages, and in several organs of the body, including the spleen, kidney, and gastrointestinal tract. It is freely filtered by the kidney and absorbed by the proximal tubules. Thus lysozymuria is seen in conditions associated with both tubular damage and increased endogenous synthesis. Urinary lysozyme can be measured by a range of methods, including catalytic activity and immunoassay; its primary clinical application has been in the monitoring of patients with monocytic leukemia.[233] The reference interval for the excretion of lysozyme in healthy adults is reported to be 1.3 to 3.6 mg/d.[321]

Tubular damage results in the release of intracellular components into the urinary tract, and measurement of these components reflects the functional integrity of the tubule. A large number of enzymes have been measured in urine. The enzyme *N*-acetyl-β-D-glucosaminidase (NAG) is stable in urine and has been widely used as a marker of tubular

*U.S. guidelines express albuminuria or proteinuria as mg/g creatinine, whereas other guidelines use mg/mmol creatinine. An approximate conversion factor of 0.1136 can be used to convert results in mg/g to mg/mmol (e.g., 200 mg/g = 23 mg/mmol, 30 mg/g = 3.4 mg/mmol).

integrity. Measurement of NAG has been undertaken in a variety of diseases associated with renal injury, including hypertension, drug nephrotoxicity, transplantation, and diabetic nephropathy.[254] It has been used to predict progression to renal failure in patients with idiopathic membranous nephropathy.[13] However, although it is a sensitive marker of kidney damage, it has not generally been shown to provide any unique benefit over other markers of tubular proteinuria. Measurement of α- and *π-glutathione-S-transferase* (EC 2.5.1.18) isoenzymes has been proposed to discriminate between proximal and distal tubular damage, respectively,[151] but the role of these markers in clinical practice has yet to be established. An evaluation of several of these biomarkers in patients presenting to hospital with nonoliguric acute tubular necrosis suggested that urinary cystatin C and α_1-microglobulin were the best predictors of an unfavorable outcome as reflected by the requirement for renal replacement therapy.[116]

Several new markers, including kidney injury molecule-1 (KIM-1)[111] and neutrophil gelatinase-associated lipocalin (NGAL),[64] have emerged as indicators of tubular injury that may be useful early predictors of acute kidney injury (AKI). Whereas increases in serum creatinine concentration may not be seen for several days following AKI, changes in concentrations of these newer biomarkers appear to occur more rapidly (within hours). KIM-1 is a type 1 transmembrane protein that usually is not present in urine but is expressed on the proximal tubule apical membrane in response to injury.[111] Renal expression of NGAL is increased following kidney injury, and in an emergency care setting, has been found to be a better predictor of the presence of AKI than urinary NAG, α_1-microglobulin, α_1-acid glycoprotein, or serum creatinine concentration.[225] Measurement of plasma NGAL concentrations has been found to be useful in predicting AKI.[63] A urinary NGAL assay suitable for use on an automated analyzer has been described.[18]

Several additional markers are available for monitoring the breakdown of basement membrane components, including *collagen* breakdown products[133,347] and *laminin* fragments.[255] However, at present, few of these markers have found a place in the clinical laboratory.

Characterization of Proteinuria

As glomerular damage increases, the permeability of the membrane decreases, with an increasing proportion of higher molecular weight proteins appearing in the urine. The relative clearance of a variety of proteins can be measured to assess the selectivity of the membrane and to provide an assessment of glomerular damage. The *protein selectivity index* is discussed in the third edition of this textbook, but it is generally considered to be of limited value. A commercial semiautomated sodium dodecyl sulfate–agarose gel electrophoresis system (Hydragel, Sebia Electrophoresis, Norcross, Ga) has been introduced for qualitative analysis of urinary proteins. This separates proteins on the basis of their molecular size, enabling visualization of glomerular, tubular, and mixed patterns of proteinuria. This approach has also been used for the detection and quantitation of Bence Jones proteinuria.[169] Panels of protein measurements, including albumin, α_1-microglobulin, IgG, and α_2-macroglobulin, have been employed in the differential diagnosis of prerenal and postrenal disease.[121] This general strategy was extended with the inclusion of reagent strip tests for hematuria, leukocyturia, and proteinuria in the development of an expert system achieving concordance of 98% with clinical diagnosis.[132]

Analytical Methodology—Individual Urinary Proteins

Immunoassay is the preferred method for the accurate and sensitive quantitation of individual proteins (see Chapter 16). A variety of approaches have been used, including (1) immunodiffusion immunoassay, (2) electroimmunoassay, (3) light-scattering assay with particle enhancement, and (4) labeled immunometric assay (e.g., KIM-1, NGAL), but (5) light-scattering immunoassay, with turbidimetric or nephelometric detection of immunoaggregate formation, is the most popular approach. Enzymuria can be measured using a variety of enzyme assay approaches. For example, one method used for the assay of NAG employs the substrate 4-methylumbelliferyl-*N*-acetyl-β-D-glucosaminide with fluorometric measurement of the methylumbelliferone released by the enzyme.[245] Alternative substrates generating products capable of being detected in the visible spectrum have also been described.[351]

CREATININE

Creatinine is a metabolite of creatine.

Biochemistry and Physiology

Creatine is synthesized in the kidneys, liver, and pancreas by two enzymatically mediated reactions. In the first, transamidation of arginine and glycine forms guanidinoacetic acid; in the second, methylation of guanidinoacetic acid occurs with *S*-adenosylmethionine as the methyl donor. Creatine is then transported in blood to other organs such as muscle and brain, where it is phosphorylated to phosphocreatine, a high-energy compound.

Creatine —(Creatine kinase; ATP → ADP)→ Phosphocreatine

Creatine —(Spontaneous; H_2O)→ Creatinine

Phosphocreatine —(Spontaneous; P_i)→ Creatinine

Interconversion of phosphocreatine and creatine is a particular feature of the metabolic processes of muscle contraction. A proportion of free creatine in muscle (thought to be between 1% and 2%/d) spontaneously and irreversibly converts to its anhydride waste product, creatinine. Thus the amount of creatinine produced each day is fairly constant and is related to the muscle mass. In health, the blood concentration of creatinine is also fairly constant, although it may be influenced by diet (see later). Creatinine (Mr 113 Da) is present in all body fluids and secretions and is freely filtered by the glomerulus. Although it is not reabsorbed to any great extent by the renal tubules, a small but notable tubular secretion is present. Creatinine production decreases as the circulating concentration of creatinine increases; several mechanisms for this have been proposed, including feedback inhibition of the production of creatine, reconversion of creatinine to creatine, and conversion to other metabolites.[98,117]

Clinical Significance

The clinical utility of creatinine measurement is considered later in this chapter, together with other GFR markers.

Analytical Methodology

Serum creatinine is measured in virtually all clinical laboratories as a test of kidney function. Most laboratories use adaptations of the same assay for measurements in both serum and urine. Both chemical and enzymatic methods are used to measure creatinine in body fluids.

Chemical Methods: The Jaffe Reaction

Most chemical methods for measuring creatinine are based primarily on the reaction with alkaline picrate. In this reaction, first described by Jaffe in 1886, creatinine reacts with picrate ion in an alkaline medium to yield an orange-red complex. Despite considerable literature on the subject, the reaction mechanism and the structure of the product remain unclear.[329]

The Jaffe reaction is not specific for creatinine. Many compounds have been reported to produce a Jaffe-like chromogen, including (1) protein,[39,49] (2) glucose, (3) ascorbic acid, (4) ketone bodies,[337](5) pyruvate, (6) guanidine, (7) hemoglobin F,[49] (8) blood-substitute products,[3] and (9) cephalosporins[312]; the reader is referred to comprehensive reviews.[28,298] The degree of interference from these compounds is dependent on the exact reaction conditions chosen. The effects of ketones and ketoacids are probably of greatest significance clinically, although the effect is very method dependent. Thus reports on acetoacetate interference vary from a negligible increase to an increase of 3.5 mg/dL (310 μmol/L) in the apparent creatinine concentration at an acetoacetate concentration of 8 mmol/L. Bilirubin is a negative interferent with the Jaffe reaction. The addition of buffering ions, such as borate and phosphate, together with surfactant, has been used to minimize the effects of this interference. A popular maneuver in this context has been the addition of ferricyanide (O'Leary method), which oxidizes bilirubin to biliverdin, hence reducing its interference.[152,228] Noncreatinine chromogens do not generally contribute to measured urinary creatinine concentration.

Several approaches have been used in an attempt to improve the general specificity of the Jaffe reaction. These have included (1) absorption of creatinine into hydrated aluminum silicate (Fuller's earth, Lloyd's reagent) with subsequent elution, (2) acid blanking, (3) use of ion-exchange resins[337] or solvent extraction, and (4) oxidation of interferants with compounds such as cerium sulfate; generally these modifications have not proved practical or sucessful.

The greatest success in terms of common usage and specificity has come from the use of a kinetic measurement approach in combination with careful choice of reactant concentrations. Although manual methods have traditionally been equilibrium methods, with 10 to 15 minutes allowed for color development at room temperature, kinetic assays were developed in a quest both for specificity and for faster and automated analyses. Early studies of interferences in kinetic methods identified two types of noncreatinine chromogens: those whose rates of adduct formation were very rapid in the first 20 seconds after mixing of reagent and sample (e.g., acetoacetate), and those whose rates did not become rapid until 80 to 100 seconds after mixing (e.g., protein). The "window" between 20 and 80 seconds, therefore, was a period in which the rate signal being observed could be attributed predominantly to the creatinine-picrate reaction; (some investigators found 60 seconds as the upper limit of this window). Thus, improved specificity in kinetic assays was achieved by selecting times for rate measurements 20 to 80 seconds after initiation of the reaction (mixing). This approach has been implemented on various automated instruments, and kinetic assays are now the most widely used approach to creatinine measurement. An extensive literature exists on the choice of reactant concentrations and reading interval, and on the choice of wavelength and reaction temperature. Brief comments follow.

Picrate Concentration

The Jaffe reaction is pseudo-first order with respect to picrate up to 30 mmol/L picrate, with most methods employing a concentration between 3 and 16 mmol/L. At concentrations greater than 6 mmol/L, the rate of color development becomes nonlinear, so a two-point fixed interval rather than a multiple data point approach is required.

Hydroxide Concentration

The initial rate of reaction is pseudo-first order with respect to hydroxide concentrations above 0.5 mmol/L; however, at 500 mmol/L, degradation of the Jaffe complex is increased. Furthermore, at hydroxide concentrations greater than 200 mmol/L, the blank absorbance increases notably.

Wavelength

Although the absorbance maximum of the Jaffe reaction is between 490 and 500 nm, improved method linearity and reduced blank values have been reported at other wavelengths, the choice varying with hydroxide concentration.

Temperature

The rate of Jaffe complex formation and the absorptivity of the complex are temperature dependent, with measurable differences observed even between 25 °C and 37 °C. Consequently, temperature control is an important component of assay reproducibility.

"Compensation"

In an attempt to adjust for reaction with noncreatinine chromogens, some manufacturers have introduced so-called "compensated" Jaffe assays, in which a fixed concentration is automatically subtracted from each result. For example, Roche Diagnostics Ltd. (Lewes, Sussex, United Kingdom) has realigned its assays on the Cobas Integra and Hitachi systems by −0.20 mg/dL and −0.32 mg/dL (−18 and −28 μmol/L), respectively. Such assays produce lower results more closely aligned with isotope dilution mass spectrometry (IDMS) reference measurement procedures at concentrations within the reference interval.[159,331] However, they make an assumption that the noncreatinine chromogen interference is a constant between samples; this is clearly an oversimplification, especially when adult and pediatric samples are compared.[49]

Other chemical approaches to the measurement of creatinine have been tried. These include (1) reaction with 1,4-naphthoquinone-2-sulphonate, (2) use of *o*-nitrobenzaldehyde to convert creatinine to methylguanidine and its reaction with α-naphthol and sodium hypochlorite under alkaline conditions,[327] and (3) reaction with 3,5-dinitrobenzoic acid.[236] None of these reactions are widely used in clinical laboratories.

Enzymatic Methods

Enzymes from several metabolic pathways have been investigated for the enzymatic measurement of creatinine. All methods involve a multistep approach leading to a photometric equlibrium. Primarily three approaches are used; they are described in the following paragraphs (Figure 25-3).

Creatininase

The enzyme creatininase (EC 3.5.2.10; creatinine amidohydrolase) catalyzes the conversion of creatinine to creatine. The creatine is then detected with a series of enzyme-mediated reactions involving creatine kinase, pyruvate kinase, and lactate dehydrogenase, with monitoring of the decrease in absorbance at 340 nm (Figure 25-3, *A*). Initiating the reaction with creatininase allows for the removal of endogenous creatine and pyruvate in a preincubation reaction. The kinetics of the reaction is poor, and 30-minute incubation is required to allow the reaction to reach equilibrium. This shortcoming can be overcome by a kinetic approach but with a further reduction in sensitivity. The approach has not been popular, in part because of poor sensitivity, poor precision, and the relatively high cost of reagents.

Creatininase and Creatinase

An alternative, more popular approach has used the enzyme creatinase (EC 3.5.3.3; creatine amidinohydrolase), which yields sarcosine and urea, the former being measured with additional enzyme-mediated steps using sarcosine oxidase (EC 1.5.3.1; yielding glycine, formaldehyde, and hydrogen peroxide) and peroxidase (Figure 25-3, *B*).[89,106] Hydrogen peroxide can be detected through a variety of methods. Care must be taken to watch for interference (e.g., by bilirubin) in the final reaction sequence. This problem has been approached with the addition of potassium ferricyanide (with limited success) or bilirubin oxidase. The potential interference caused by ascorbic acid can be overcome by inclusion of ascorbate oxidase. The influence of endogenous intermediate creatine and urea can be overcome by a preincubation step, initiating the reaction with creatininase. This system has been incorporated in a point-of-care testing device using polarographic detection.[270] An alternative detection system involves measurement of the reduction of nicotanimide adenine dinucleotide (NAD) by formaldehyde in the presence of formaldehyde dehydrogenase (Figure 25-3, *C*).[307]

Creatinine Deaminase

Creatinine deaminase (EC 3.5.4.21; creatinine iminohydrolase) catalyzes the conversion of creatinine to *N*-methylhydantoin and ammonia (Figure 25-3, *D*).[315] Early methods concentrated on the detection of ammonia using glutamate dehydrogenase or the Berthelot reaction.[193] An alternative approach involves the enzyme *N*-methylhydantoin amidohydrolase.[87]

Dry Chemistry Systems

Several multilayer dry reagent methods have been described for the measurement of creatinine using enzyme-mediated reactions. An early "two-slide" approach employed creatinine deaminase, with ammonia diffusing through a semipermeable and optically opaque layer to react with bromphenol blue to obtain an increase in absorbance at 600 nm. A second multilayer film lacking the enzyme was used to quantitate endogenous ammonia, enabling blank correction.[309] A later, more precise, single-slide method used the creatininase-creatinase reaction sequence.[195] Lidocaine metabolites have been reported to interfere with this method.[287] The creatinine deaminase system described previously has been used and adapted for use as a point-of-care testing device (Figure 25-3, *D*).[101] In all cases, the color produced in the film is quantitated by reflectance.

A dry chemistry system has been described in which a nonenzymatic approach was used, based on the reaction with 3,5-dinitrobenzoic acid.[301]

Other Methods

A definitive method employing IDMS was described by Welch et al in 1986.[339] Gas chromatography–IDMS (GC-IDMS) is now accepted as the method of choice for establishing the true concentration of creatinine in serum because of its excellent specificity and low imprecision.[293,303] Three GC-IDMS methods have been approved by the JCTLM as reference measurement procedures for serum creatinine.[212] In these procedures, creatinine must be derivatized before GC

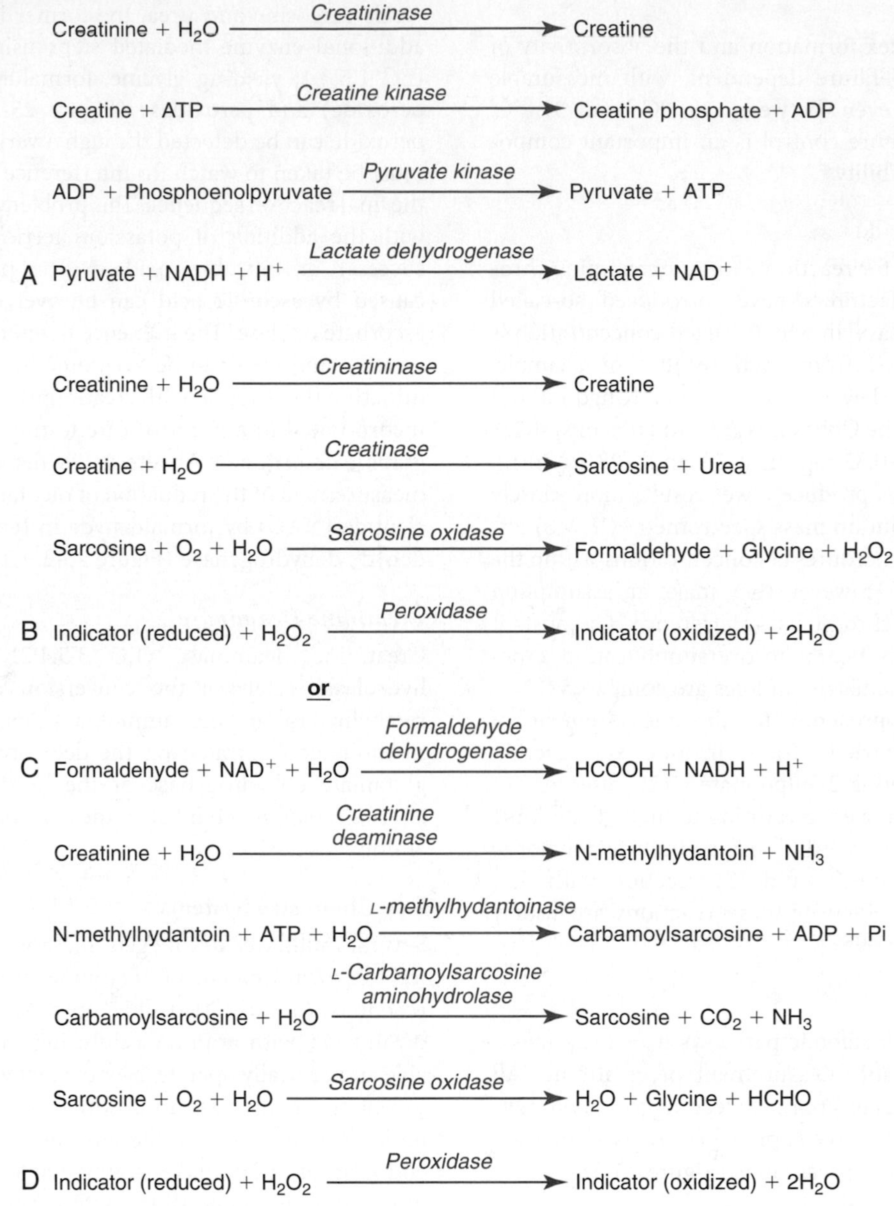

Figure 25-3 Determination of creatinine using a variety of enzymatic methods. For additional details, see text.

analysis because of its polarity. In addition, a cation-exchange cleanup step before GC analysis is necessary because creatine is derivatized into the same chemical species as creatinine. In 2003, a method coupling HPLC with IDMS for the direct quantification of creatinine was reported.[304] This method offered simplicity and improved speed of analysis because only a simple protein precipitation without derivatization is required.

Sensitive and specific approaches to creatinine measurement using HPLC have been described using both cation-exchange[35,112,267] and reversed-phase techniques.[296,299] Separation is followed by quantitation using an on-stream Jaffe reaction,[35] native absorbance of creatinine at ≈230 nm,* or enzymatic detection.[183] All HPLC approaches are reported to be rapid, specific, and precise, and several have been proposed as candidate reference methods.[183,267,320] Thienpont and colleagues reported between-day and within-run imprecision of less than 1% with deviation from GC-IDMS target values of +0.1%.[320] HPLC appears to provide an excellent designated comparison method for in-house use by manufacturers.[212]

A capillary electrophoresis approach to serum creatinine measurement using diode array detection has been described.[354] In addition, a high-performance capillary electrophoresis method[56] and a reagent-free midinfrared method[289] for urinary creatinine measurement have been described.

Quality Issues and Preanalytical Considerations With Creatinine Methods

The method used for measurement of creatinine is complex by virtue of the number of variants of the Jaffe reaction and

*References 4, 112, 237, 267, 296, and 299.

the innovations attempted using enzymatic procedures to overcome the limitations of the former. Although enzymatic methods are more expensive, they are used in dry chemistry systems (with their lower reagent requirement), including some point-of-care testing devices. Kinetic Jaffe approaches predominate in wet chemistry analytical systems. Any laboratorian assessing a new creatinine method (e.g., as part of an analyzer purchase) should review the data for that method on interference due to bilirubin, protein, glucose, and ketones/ketoacids; bilirubin will also be particularly important in enzymatic procedures that generate hydrogen peroxide. Despite criticism of the Jaffe methods, good correlation has been noted invariably between them and enzymatic procedures, with differences likely to be due as much to calibration as to interference.

Creatinine in serum, plasma, or diluted urine is stable for at least 7 days at 4 °C, and serum creatinine is stable during long-term frozen storage (at −20 °C and below) and after repeated thawing and refreezing.[67] However, it should be noted that delayed separation (beyond 14 hours) of serum from erthyrocytes leads to a significant increase in apparent serum creatinine concentration using some kinetic Jaffe (but not enzymatic) assays, possibly as the result of release of noncreatinine chromogens from the red cells.[85,291] Bacterial contamination, which can occur in samples stored for long periods of time, has been reported to falsely lower creatinine values measured using the Jaffe reaction, purportedly as the result of bacterial production of a substance that retards the reaction.[66] Creatinine concentration increases in blood after meals containing cooked meat because of the conversion of creatine to creatinine; ideally, blood for serum creatinine measurement should be obtained in the fasting state.[134,135,196,240,248] Clearly, this latter problem will affect both enzymatic and Jaffe creatinine methods.

Different methods for assaying serum creatinine have varying degrees of accuracy and imprecision. As a result of reaction with noncreatinine chromogens, Jaffe methods often have overestimated true serum creatinine concentrations by up to 20% compared with HPLC or IDMS methods, at physiologic concentrations.[23,39,168] Data from College of American Pathologists (CAP) surveys using a fresh-frozen serum sample have shown that historically most creatinine methods had a positive bias [range, −0.06 to 0.31 mg/dL (−5.3 to 27 μmol/L) at a concentration of 0.90 mg/dL (80 μmol/L)] compared with GC-IDMS reference measurements.[207] The bias varied between different modifications of the Jaffe assay, contributing to interlaboratory variation. Variation in bias was related more to instrument manufacturer than to method principle, suggesting a strong influence of calibration differences on bias. This echoes earlier CAP data demonstrating that systematic differences in the calibration of serum creatinine assays accounted for 85% of observed differences between laboratories.[268] Proficiency studies have demonstrated that although between-laboratory coefficients of variation (CVs) less than 3% are achievable within method groups, overall between-laboratory agreement across methods is much poorer.[39,168] Systematic variation between laboratories of 0.2 to 0.4 mg/dL (18 to 36 μmol/L) has been common,[125,168] with one study reporting a median method group standard deviation of 0.058 mg/dL (5.1 μmol/L) and median CVs of 6.4% at a creatinine concentration of 0.90 mg/dL (80 μmol/L).[207] This is still outside desirable performance standards defined in terms of biological variation.[212,298] Further, interlaboratory and within-laboratory agreement deteriorates as serum creatinine concentration nears the reference interval; the exponential relationship between serum creatinine and GFR means that imprecision at lower creatinine concentrations contributes to greater error in GFR estimation than at higher creatinine concentrations. Additionally, certified reference material is lacking, further contributing to variation between laboratories.

Over the past decade, appreciation of CKD as a major public health issue[38,178,216,218,285] and of its identification using GFR-estimating equations has led to increased focus on the measurement of creatinine. Creatinine-based estimates of GFR (see later) will clearly vary, depending on how accurate the creatinine measurement is that is used in the calculation. The more a method overestimates "true" creatinine, the greater will be the underestimation of GFR, and vice versa. It is no surprise that there have been calls for an international standard to be used when serum creatinine assays are calibrated.[218] Standardized serum matrix reference materials (SRM 967) with known creatinine concentrations [0.80 mg/dL (71 μmol/L) and 4.00 mg/dL (354 μmol/L)] have been prepared by the National Institute of Standards of Technology (NIST) and submitted to the JCTLM for inclusion in a list of standardized reference materials.[212] It is anticipated that use of this material, in combination with IDMS reference methods, will assist reagent manufacturers in achieving better consensus between methods.[235] In practice, most clinical laboratory methods have adjusted their calibration to be traceable to an IDMS reference measurement procedure.[204,205]

Although undoubtedly desirable, it must be recognized that standardization is only one arm of the problem. Standardization will not solve the problem of different reactivity with noncreatinine chromogens across different patient samples, which can be resolved only by the use of highly specific creatinine methods. Wider adoption of enzymatic methods could further improve between-laboratory agreement in creatinine measurement, but these methods are used by a small minority of laboratories at present. For example, of 687 participants in the United Kingdom National External Quality Assessment Scheme for serum creatinine in April 2009, 39% used traditional kinetic Jaffe reactions, 35% used a "compensated" kinetic Jaffe assay, 2% used an equilibrium Jaffe method, 5% used an O'Leary modification of a kinetic Jaffe assay, 6% used an enzymatic assay, and 13% used a dry-slide enzymatic method. In the United States, 2405 laboratories in the CAP Survey in May 2009 used creatinine assays with "traditional" calibration, and 3355 used assays with IDMS-traceable calibration. Overall, 64% used kinetic Jaffe reactions, 8% used "rate-blanked" kinetic Jaffe assays, 4% used an equilibrium Jaffe method, and 23% used an enzymatic assay (including Vitros dry-slide users).

Reference Intervals

Given the previous discussion, reference intervals for serum creatinine have been method dependent; a selection of reported reference values for different methods may be found in the fourth edition of this textbook. A 2008 systematic review of creatinine reference intervals in which studies were included only when, in particular, their calibration was traceable to the reference IDMS procedure; proposed adult reference intervals of 0.72 to 1.18 mg/dL (64 to 104 μmol/L) in men and 0.55 to 1.02 mg/dL (49 to 90 μmol/L) in women.[43] These data were derived using an enzymatic (Roche Diagnostics Ltd.) assay. Reference interval data for children may be found in the same publication.

Urinary creatinine excretion is higher in men (14 to 26 mg/kg/d, 124 to 230 μmol/kg/d) than in women (11 to 20 mg/kg/d, 97 to 177 μmol/kg/d). Creatinine excretion decreases with age: typically, for a 70-kg man, creatinine excretion will decline from approximately 14.5 to 9.1 mmol/d with advancing age from 30 to 80 years.[244] Measurement of urinary creatinine excretion can be a useful indication of the completeness of a timed urine collection. Creatinine excretion is often used as a method of normalizing the urinary excretion of analytes, that is, the excretion of the test analyte (in mmol or grams) is divided by the total amount of creatinine (in mmol or grams) excreted in the same urine specimen. This method is a rough correction for volume differences between patient specimens. Similarly, expressing the concentration of a substance as a ratio to the creatinine concentration is a useful method of adjusting for urinary concentration differences in random ("spot") urine samples. The benefits of this approach in reporting urinary total protein and albumin measurements have been discussed.

UREA

Biochemistry and Physiology

Catabolism of proteins and nucleic acids results in the formation of urea and ammonia, the so-called nonprotein nitrogenous compounds. As ammonia has no role in assessing kidney function, it is discussed in Chapter 32.

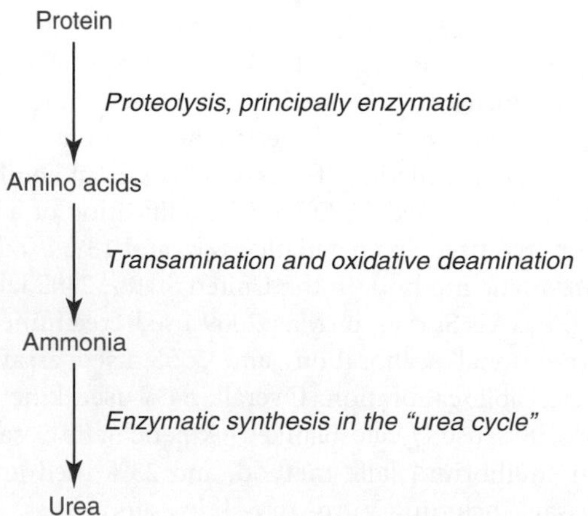

Urea [$CO(NH_2)_2$, Mr 60 Da] is the major nitrogen-containing metabolic product of protein catabolism in humans, accounting for more than 75% of the nonprotein nitrogen eventually excreted. The biosynthesis of urea from amino nitrogen–derived ammonia is carried out exclusively by hepatic enzymes of the urea cycle. During the process of protein catabolism, amino acid nitrogen is converted to urea in the liver by the action of so-called urea cycle enzymes (Figure 25-4).

More than 90% of urea is excreted through the kidneys, with losses through the gastrointestinal tract and skin accounting for most of the remaining minor fraction. Consequently, kidney disease is associated with accumulation of urea in blood. An increase in serum urea concentration characterizes the uremic (azotemic) state. Urea is neither actively reabsorbed nor secreted by the tubules but is filtered freely by the glomeruli. In a normal kidney, 40 to 70% of the highly diffusible urea moves passively out of the renal tubule and into the interstitium, ultimately to re-enter plasma. The back-diffusion of urea is also dependent on urine flow rate, with less entering the interstitium in high-flow states (e.g., pregnancy) and vice versa. Consequently, urea clearance generally

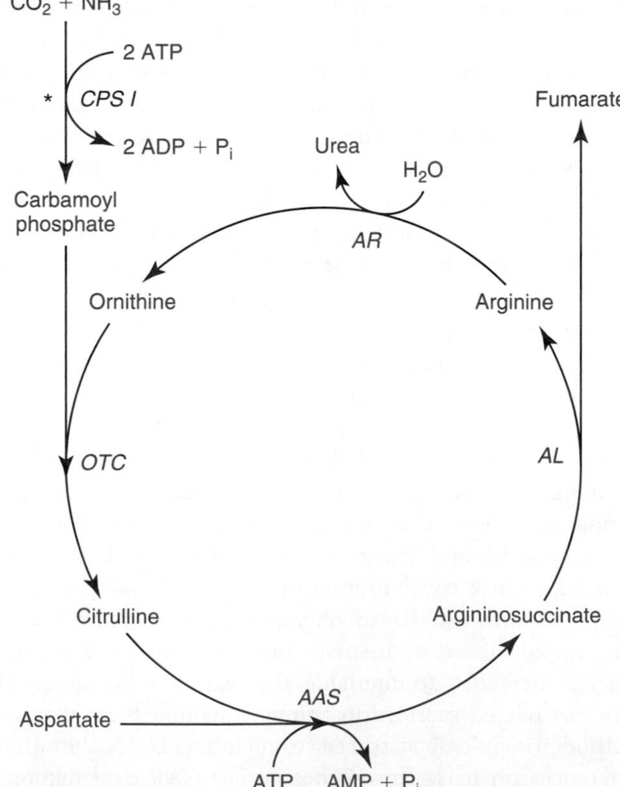

Figure 25-4 The urea cycle pathway. *AAS*, Argininosuccinate synthetase; *ADP*, adenosine diphosphate; *AL*, argininosuccinate lyase; *AR*, arginase; *ATP*, adenosine triphosphate; *CPS I*, carbamyl phosphate synthetase I (N*-acetylglutamate as positive allosteric effector); *OTC*, ornithine transcarbamylase; P_i, inorganic phosphate.**

underestimates GFR. In end-stage renal disease, osmotic diuresis in the remaining functional nephrons limits the back-diffusion of urea, so that urea clearance approaches inulin clearance. Measurement of blood and serum urea has been used for many years as an indicator of kidney function. However, it is generally accepted that creatinine measurement provides better information in this respect. Serum and urinary urea measurement may still provide useful clinical information in particular circumstances, and the measurement of urea in dialysis fluids is widely used in assessing the adequacy of renal replacement therapy (see Chapter 48).

Clinical Significance

Numerous extrarenal factors influence the circulating urea concentration, limiting its value as a test of kidney function. For example, plasma urea concentration is increased by a high-protein diet, increased protein catabolism, reabsorption of blood proteins after gastrointestinal hemorrhage, treatment with cortisol or its synthetic analogs, dehydration, and decreased perfusion of the kidneys (e.g., heart failure). In the prerenal situations already discussed, the plasma creatinine concentration may be normal. In obstructive postrenal conditions (e.g., malignancy, nephrolithiasis, prostatism), both serum creatinine and urea concentrations will be increased, although in these situations, the increase in serum urea is greater than in creatinine because of increased back-diffusion. These considerations give rise to the principal clinical utility of serum urea, which lies in its measurement in conjunction with that of serum creatinine and subsequent calculation of the urea nitrogen-to-creatinine ratio. This can be used as a crude discriminator between prerenal and postrenal azotemia. For a normal individual on a normal diet, the reference interval for the ratio is between 12 and 20 mg urea/mg creatinine (49 and 81 mol urea/mol creatinine). Significantly lower ratios usually denote acute tubular necrosis, low protein intake, starvation, or severe liver disease (decreased urea synthesis). Increased serum urea with *normal* creatinine concentrations giving rise to high ratios may be seen with any of the prerenal states described previously. High ratios associated with *elevated* creatinine concentrations may denote postrenal obstruction or prerenal azotemia superimposed on kidney disease.

Urea clearance is a poor indicator of GFR, as its production rate is dependent on several nonrenal factors, including diet and the activity of the urea cycle enzymes. A high-protein diet causes notable increases in urinary urea excretion. In addition, the variable amount of back-diffusion will influence both serum and urinary urea concentrations.[147] Measurement of urinary urea has little place in clinical diagnosis and management; however, it does provide a crude index of overall nitrogen balance and may be used as a guide to replacement in patients receiving parenteral nutrition. On an average protein diet, urinary excretion expressed as urea nitrogen is 12 to 20 g/d.

Although *blood urea nitrogen* (BUN) continues to be used for ordering the serum urea nitrogen test, this terminology is incorrect and obsolete, because blood is rarely analyzed for urea. The long-established habit of reporting and expressing results of a urea assay in units of urea nitrogen appears to be strongly entrenched in the United States, although the SI system recommends the use of urea, expressed in mmol/L. Thus, it behooves students of clinical chemistry to have in mind the conversion factors for urea to urea nitrogen. Because 60 g (1 g MW) of urea contains 28 g (2 g atomic weight) of nitrogen, the factor is 0.467 for converting urea mass units to those of urea nitrogen, and 2.14 for converting urea nitrogen mass units to those of urea. The factor for converting urea nitrogen in mg/dL to urea in mmol/L is 0.357.

Analytical Methodology

Direct chemical and indirect enzymatic methods are the two principal approaches that have been used to quantify urea in body fluids. Although once widely used, the chemical method has largely been superseded by enzymatic approaches. For a more detailed description of direct urea measurement, the reader is referred to Taylor and Vadgama.[316]

Enzymatic Methods

A vast majority of urea measurements in clinical laboratories are undertaken using enzymatic methods based on preliminary hydrolysis of urea with urease (urea amidohydrolase; EC 3.5.1.5; main source jack bean meal) to generate ammonium ion, which then is quantitated. This approach has been used in equilibrium, rate, conductimetric, and dry chemistry systems.[316]

$$\underset{\text{Urea}}{(H_2N)_2C{=}O} + 2\,H_2O \xrightarrow{\textit{Urease}} 2\,NH_4^{\oplus} + CO_3^{\ominus\ominus}$$

Spectrophotometric approaches to ammonium quantitation include the Berthelot reaction and the enzymatic assay with glutamate dehydrogenase [L-glutamate:NAD(P) oxidoreductase (deaminating); EC 1.4.1.3].[276] This latter approach has been accepted as a reference method[277] and adapted to a variety of analytical platforms.

$$NH_4^{\oplus} + \text{2-Oxoglutarate} \xrightarrow[\text{NADH} + H^{\oplus} \;\rightarrow\; \text{NAD}^{\oplus}]{\textit{Glutamate dehydrogenase}} \text{Glutamate} + H_2O$$

For serum assays, the reaction system is usually formulated with urease, so that the addition of sample containing urea starts the reaction. A decrease in absorbance resulting from the glutamate dehydrogenase reaction is monitored at 340 nm. In another example of a coupled-enzyme assay system for urea, ammonia produced from urea by urease then reacts with glutamate and adenosine triphosphate in the presence of glutamine synthetase (EC 6.3.1.2). Adenosine diphosphate produced in this second enzymatic reaction is then quantitated in third and fourth steps using pyruvate kinase (EC 2.7.1.40) and pyruvate oxidase (EC 1.2.3.3), respectively, thus generating peroxide. In the final step, peroxide reacts with phenol and 4-aminophenazone, catalyzed by peroxidase (EC 1.11.1.7), to yield a quinone-monoamine dye that can be quantitated spectrophotometrically.[174]

Methods for the measurement of urea using dry chemistry systems using the urease approach and a variety of detection methods have been described.[252,297] It is also possible to measure urea using a conductimetric method in which sample and a urease-containing reagent are incubated in a conductivity cell with the rate of change of the conductivity being monitored as the urea is converted to an ionic species. In a potentiometric approach, an ammonium ion-selective electrode is employed and the urease is immobilized on a membrane.[265] This principle has been applied in the NOVA 12 (NOVA Biomedical, Waltham, Mass.),[100] i-STAT (Abbott Point of Core, Princeton, NJ),[208] and AVL OMNI (Roche Diagnostics Ltd., Lewes, East Sussex, United Kingdom) analytical systems. A similar approach has been used to enable real-time monitoring of dialysis efficiency.[92] Alternative enzymatic approaches to the measurement of urea have been described. For example, Morishita and colleagues[210] have described a system incorporating leucine dehydrogenase (EC 1.4.1.9), in addition to urease, which eliminates interference from endogenous ammonium.

The specificity of all of the methods is good, particularly for the urease-glutamate dehydrogenase procedure; however, endogenous ammonia interference must be expected when the protocol employs the sample to initiate the reaction. This may be relevant in aged samples, in some urines, and in particular metabolic disorders. Typically, within-run CVs of less than 3.0% with between-day values of less than 4.0% are achievable in the concentration interval of 14 to 20 mg/dL (5 to 7 mmol/L). Given the high intrinsic biological variation of serum urea, this is well within desired standards of analytical performance.[316]

Other Methods

An improved IDMS method for serum urea measurement has been listed by JCTLM as a reference method.[150] As discussed previously, laboratory urea measurements using standard enzymatic techniques are generally of an acceptable quality for most clinical purposes. New approaches to urea measurement generally are targeted at novel clinical applications, including point-of-care testing. For example, Eddy and Arnold[72] have developed a near-infrared spectroscopy technique for measuring urea in hemodialysis fluids. This would facilitate noninvasive monitoring of dialysis efficacy in real time. A novel enzymatic assay, using luminometric detection, demonstrates sensitivity that would make the method suitable for in vivo monitoring studies using microdialysis techniques.[213]

Reference Intervals

The reference interval for serum urea nitrogen in healthy adults is 6 to 20 mg/dL (2.1 to 7.1 mmol/L expressed as urea). In adults older than 60 years of age, the reference interval is 8 to 23 mg/dL (2.9 to 8.2 mmol/L). Serum concentrations tend to be slightly lower in children and in pregnancy and slightly higher in males than in females.

URIC ACID

In humans, uric acid (2,6,8-trihydroxypurine) is the major product of catabolism of the purine nucleosides, adenosine and guanosine (Figure 25-5).

Biochemistry and Physiology

Purines from the catabolism of dietary nucleic acid are converted to uric acid directly. The bulk of purines excreted as uric acid arise from degradation of endogenous nucleic acids. The daily synthesis rate of uric acid is approximately 400 mg; dietary sources contribute another 300 mg. In men consuming a purine-free diet, the total body pool of exchangeable urate is estimated at 1200 mg; in women it is estimated to be 600 mg. By contrast, patients with gouty arthritis and tissue deposition of urate may have urate pools as large as 18,000 to 30,000 mg.

Overproduction of uric acid may result from increased synthesis of purine precursors. Synthesis and metabolism of the major precursors are illustrated in the outline in Figure 25-5. The second enzymatic step in the synthetic pathway (Figure 25-5, *A*), formation of 5′-phosphoribosylamine, is the first irreversibly committed step in purine biosynthesis. The intracellular concentration of the substrate phosphoribosylpyrophosphate (PRPP) regulates de novo purine synthesis. The enzyme PRPP-amidotransferase is controlled through feedback inhibition by the purine nucleotides that are the final products of the biosynthetic pathway. The first purine nucleotide formed by ring closure is inosine monophosphate (IMP); adenosine and guanosine monophosphates are derived from IMP through enzymatically mediated interconversions. Adenine and guanine nucleotides may then be used as precursors for the corresponding nucleosides that are the building blocks of deoxyribonucleic acid and ribonucleic acid, or, when further phosphorylated, these nucleotides become carriers of high-energy bonds in the form of ATP and guanosine triphosphate.

Catabolism of the nucleotides (Figure 25-5, *B*) begins with removal of their ribose-linked phosphate, a process catalyzed by purine 5′-nucleotidase. Removal of the ribose moiety of inosine and guanosine by the action of purine-nucleoside phosphorylase forms hypoxanthine and guanine, both of which are converted to xanthine. Xanthine is converted to uric acid through the action of xanthine oxidase.

Reutilization of the major purine bases, adenine, hypoxanthine, and guanine, is achieved through "salvage" pathways (Figure 25-5, *C*), in which phosphoribosylation of the free bases leads to resynthesis of the respective nucleotide

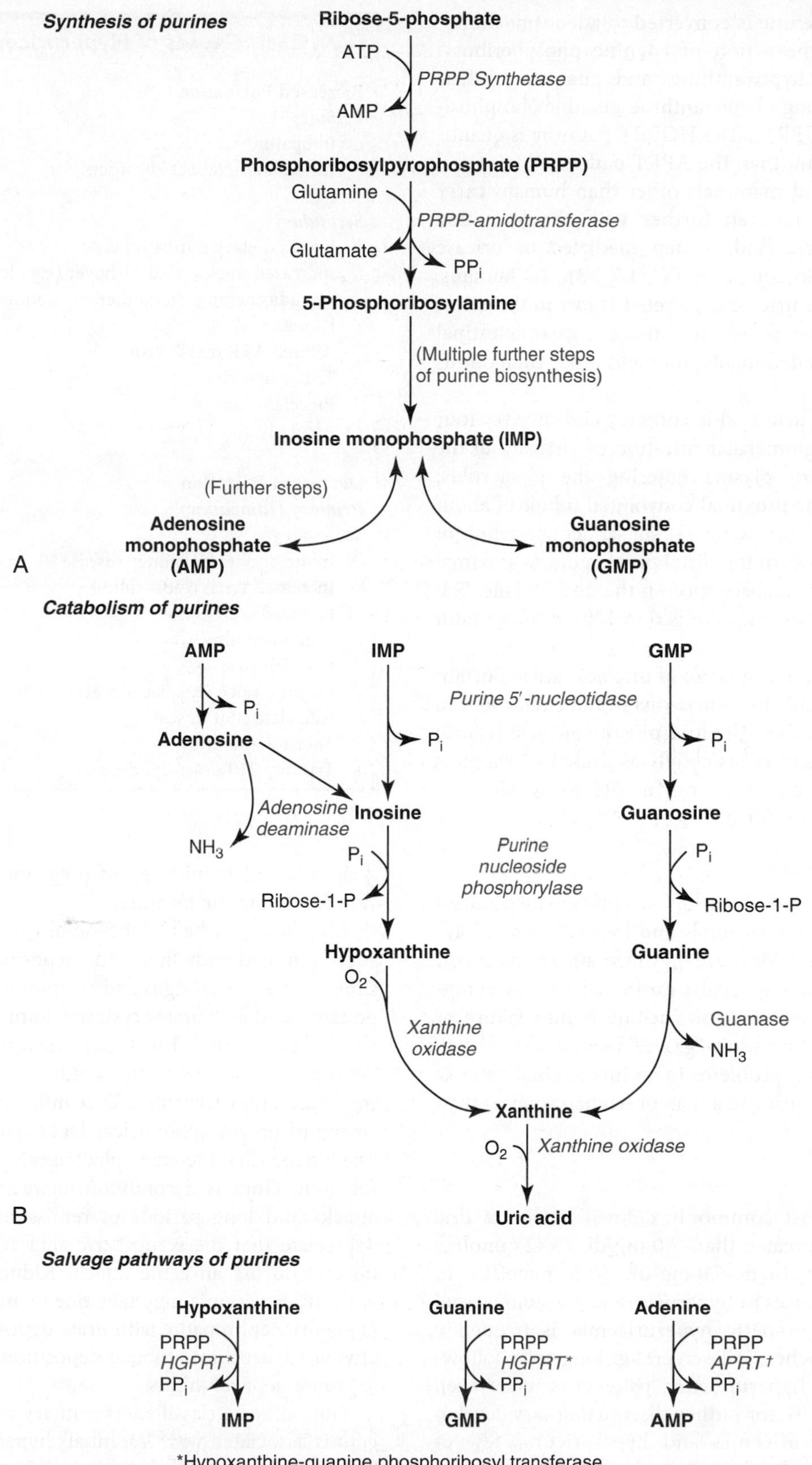

Figure 25-5 Metabolism of purines. A, Synthesis. B, Catabolism. C, Salvage pathways.

monophosphates. Adenine is converted to adenosine monophosphate through the action of adenine phosphoribosyl transferase (APRT), hypoxanthine, and guanine to their monophosphates through hypoxanthine-guanine phosphoribosyl transferase (HGPRT). The HGPRT pathway is quantitatively more important than the APRT pathway.

Lower primates and mammals other than humans carry purine metabolism one step further with the formation of allantoin from uric acid, a step mediated by uricase ([urate: oxygen] oxidoreductase; EC 1.7.3.3). In humans, approximately 75% of uric acid excreted is lost in the urine; most of the remainder is secreted into the gastrointestinal tract, where it is degraded to allantoin and other compounds by bacterial enzymes.

Renal handling of uric acid is complex and involves four sequential steps: (1) glomerular filtration of virtually all the uric acid in capillary plasma entering the glomerulus; (2) reabsorption in the proximal convoluted tubule of about 98 to 100% of filtered uric acid; (3) subsequent secretion of uric acid into the lumen in the distal portion of the proximal tubule; and (4) further reabsorption in the distal tubule. The net urinary excretion of uric acid is 6 to 12% of the amount filtered.

The physicochemical properties of uric acid are important in considering uric acid concentrations in the circulation, in tissue, and in the kidneys. The first pK_a of uric acid is 5.57; above this pH, uric acid exists chiefly as urate ion, which is more soluble than uric acid. At a urine pH below 5.75, uric acid is the preponderant form.

BOX 25-1 Causes of Hyperuricemia

Increased Formation
Primary
- Idiopathic
- Inherited metabolic disorders

Secondary
- Excess dietary purine intake
- Increased nucleic acid turnover (e.g., leukemia, myeloma, radiotherapy, chemotherapy, trauma)
- Psoriasis
- Altered ATP metabolism
- Tissue hypoxia
- Preeclampsia
- Alcohol

Decreased Excretion
Primary (Idiopathic)
Secondary
- Acute or chronic kidney disease
- Increased renal reabsorption
- Reduced secretion
- Lead poisoning
- Preeclampsia
- Organic acids (e.g., lactate, acetoacetate)
- Salicylate (low doses)
- Thiazide diuretics
- Trisomy 21 (Down syndrome)

Clinical Significance

More than 20 inherited disorders of purine metabolism giving rise to both hypouricemias and hyperuricemias have been recognized to date. Most are very rare, and the diagnosis requires support from a specialist purine laboratory. Symptoms that should raise suspicion include kidney failure or stones in a child or young adult, "gravel" in an infant's diaper, unexplained neurologic problems in an infant, child, or adolescent, and gout presenting in a man or woman younger than 30 years old.

Hyperuricemia

Hyperuricemia is most commonly defined by serum uric acid concentrations greater than 7.0 mg/dL (0.42 mmol/L) in men, or greater than 6.0 mg/dL (0.36 mmol/L) in women. The major causes of hyperuricemia are summarized in Box 25-1. Asymptomatic hyperuricemia is frequently detected through biochemical screening; long-term follow-up of asymptomatic hyperuricemic patients is undertaken because many are at risk for kidney disease that may develop as a result of hyperuricemia and hyperuricuria; few of these patients ever develop the clinical syndrome of gout.[284]

Measurement of serum uric acid is predominantly used in the investigation of gout, either as a result of a primary hyperuricemia or caused by other conditions or treatments that give rise to secondary hyperuricemias. It is also used in the diagnosis and monitoring of pregnancy-induced hypertension (preeclamptic toxemia).

Gout occurs when monosodium urate precipitates from supersaturated body fluids; the deposits of urate are responsible for the clinical signs and symptoms. Gouty arthritis may be associated with urate crystals in joint fluid and with deposits of crystals (tophi) in tissues surrounding the joint. The deposits may occur in other soft tissue as well, and wherever they occur, they elicit an intense inflammatory response consisting of polymorphonuclear leukocytes and macrophages. The big toe (first metatarsophalangeal) joint is the classic site for gout. Gout is a condition characterized by occasional attacks and long periods of remission: it is important to appreciate that the serum uric acid concentration is often normal during an acute attack. Kidney disease associated with hyperuricemia may take one or more of several forms: (1) gouty nephropathy with urate deposition in renal parenchyma, (2) acute intratubular deposition of urate crystals, and (3) urate nephrolithiasis.[37]

Gout may be classified as primary or secondary. *Primary gout* is associated with "essential" hyperuricemia, which has a polygenic basis. In more than 99% of cases, the cause is uncertain, but the condition is probably due to a combination of metabolic overproduction of purines (25% of patients have increased PRPP amidotransferase activity), decreased renal excretion (80% of patients show decreased renal tubular secretion of uric acid), and increased dietary intake. Very rarely, primary gout is attributable to inherited defects of enzymes in the pathways of purine metabolism. The *Lesch-Nyhan syndrome* is characterized by a complete deficiency of HGPRT (EC 2.4.2.8), the major enzyme of the purine salvage pathways. This X-linked genetic disorder is manifested clinically by mental retardation, abnormal muscle movements, and behavioral problems (self-mutilation and pathologic aggressiveness). Patients may, in the first weeks of life, have symptoms of crystalluria, acute kidney failure, and gout. Hyperuricemia, hyperuricuria, and markedly decreased activities of HGPRT are present in erythrocytes, fibroblasts, and other cells. Intracellular activities of PRPP and rates of purine synthesis are increased. Neurologic symptoms of this syndrome may be related to decreased availability of purines to the developing brain, which has limited capacity for de novo purine synthesis and therefore relies on the purine salvage pathways to supply it with most of the purine nucleotides it requires. DNA technology has been applied to prenatal diagnosis in the first trimester using chorionic biopsy material. HGPRT assays on cultured fibroblasts obtained by amniocentesis may be used in the second trimester. Partial deficiency of HGPRT (severe X-linked gout) presents in adolescence or early adulthood as early gout, kidney failure, or nephrolithiasis. Increased activities of intracellular PRPP production with consequent increased uric acid concentrations can also occur owing to mutations in PRPP synthetase (EC 2.7.6.1) (phosphoribosyl pyrophosphate synthetase superactivity), which is also inherited as an X-linked recessive trait. An autosomal dominant familial juvenile hyperuricemic nephropathy has been recognized. Glucose-6-phosphatase deficiency leads to hyperuricemia as a result of both overproduction and underexcretion of uric acid.

Secondary gout is a result of hyperuricemia attributable to several identifiable causes. Renal retention of uric acid may occur in acute or chronic kidney disease of any type or as a consequence of administration of drugs; diuretics, in particular, are implicated in the latter instance. Organic acidemia caused by increased acetoacetic acid in diabetic ketoacidosis or to lactic acidosis may interfere with tubular secretion of urate. Increased nucleic acid turnover and a consequent increase in catabolism of purines may be encountered in rapid proliferation of tumor cells and in massive destruction of tumor cells on therapy with certain chemotherapeutic agents.

Management of an acute attack of gout generally involves the use of nonsteroidal anti-inflammatory drugs (NSAIDs). Patients should be advised to avoid foods that have high purine content (e.g., liver, kidney, red meat, sardines) and drugs that affect urate excretion (thiazide diuretics and salicylates). Specific pharmacologic interventions include the use of uricosuric drugs (e.g., probenecid, sulfinpyrazone), which enhance renal excretion of uric acid by blocking carriers in the tubular cells that mediate reabsorption, or the xanthine oxidase inhibitor allopurinol. Measurement of urinary uric acid excretion is an aid in selecting appropriate treatment in this context. Patients excreting less than 600 mg/d (3.6 mmol/d) uric acid are candidates for treatment with uricosuric drugs, which are contraindicated in patients with urate stones or kidney failure. Conversely, patients excreting more than 600 mg/d (3.6 mmol/d) are candidates for treatment with allopurinol. The NSAIDs azapropazone and tiaprofenic acid have a uricosuric effect and so have a place in both long-term and short-term management of gout.

Uric acid kidney stones occur in approximately one in five patients with clinical gout. Although serum and urinary uric acid should be measured in stone formers, many uric acid stone formers do not demonstrate hyperuricuria or hyperuricemia. However, this may reflect the use of reference intervals derived in a purine-rich, westernized society.[278] The cause of uric acid stone formation also involves the passage of a persistently acid urine with loss of the postprandial alkaline tide.[37] Undissociated uric acid (pK_a 5.57) is relatively insoluble, whereas urate at pH 7.0 is greater than 10 times more soluble. Thus, in patients with urinary pH persistently less than 6.0, normal urinary concentrations of uric acid will produce supersaturation. Measurement of urinary pH throughout the day can be useful.[278] Pure uric acid stones account for approximately 8% of all urinary tract stones and, unlike many of the calcium-containing stones, are radiolucent. Allopurinol is the mainstay of treatment of uric acid stones. Hyperuricuria is also a risk factor for calcium stone formation (see Chapter 48). Consequently, attempts to increase urinary pH with potassium alkali salts may be counterproductive as a result of increased calcium stone formation.

Preeclamptic toxemia is associated with increasing serum uric acid concentration, probably caused by uteroplacental tissue breakdown and decreased kidney perfusion.[77] Serum urate measurement can be used as an indicator of the severity of preeclampsia: Redman and coworkers[259] noted that concentrations in excess of 6.0 mg/dL (0.36 mmol/L) at 32 weeks' gestation are associated with a high perinatal mortality rate. More recently, uric acid has been proposed as one of a panel of eight small molecular weight metabolites that could be used for the detection of preeclampsia.[149]

Hypouricemia

Hypouricemia, often defined as serum urate concentrations less than 2.0 mg/dL (0.12 mmol/L), is much less common than hyperuricemia. It may be secondary to any one of a number of underlying conditions. Severe hepatocellular disease with reduced purine synthesis or xanthine oxidase activity is one possibility. Another is defective renal tubular reabsorption of uric acid. Defective reabsorption may be congenital, as in generalized Fanconi's syndrome, or acquired. The reabsorption defect may be acquired acutely because of injection of radiopaque contrast media or chronically because of exposure to toxic agents. Overtreatment of hyperuricemia with allopurinol or uricosuric drugs and cancer chemotherapy with 6-mercaptopurine or azathioprine (inhibitors of de novo purine synthesis) may also cause hypouricemia. Very rarely, hypouricemia may occur as the result of an inherited metabolic defect. Hypouricemia in combination with xanthinuria is rarely encountered and suggests a deficiency of xanthine oxidase, either in isolation or as part of combined molybdenum cofactor deficiency (sulfite oxidase/xanthine oxidase deficiency). Purine nucleoside phosphorylase (EC 2.4.2.1) deficiency and other inherited defects have been described.

Analytical Methodology

Phosphotungstic acid (PTA), uricase, and HPLC-based methods have been described for measuring uric acid.[251] PTA methods are now rarely used; the reader is referred to a review for additional details.[251]

Uricase Methods

Uricase methods are more specific than and have replaced older PTA methods. Uricase [(urate : oxygen) oxidoreductase; EC 1.7.3.3; main sources *Aspergillus flavus, Candida utilis, Bacillus fastidiosus,* and hog liver] is used as a single step or as the initial step to oxidize uric acid. Uricase methods became feasible and popular as a result of the availability of high-quality, low-cost preparations of the bacterial enzyme. Preliminary precipitation of protein is not required. Generally, only guanine, xanthine, and a few other structural analogs of uric acid act as alternative substrates, and then only at concentrations improbable in biological fluids.

Uricase acts on uric acid to produce allantoin, hydrogen peroxide, and carbon dioxide.

Urate + O_2 —Uricase→ Allantoin + H_2O_2 + CO_2

The reaction can be observed in the rate or the equilibrium mode. The *Bacillus fastidiosus* enzyme has the highest Michaelis constant (10×10^{-5} mol/L), and the hog liver has the lowest (1.7×10^{-5} mol/L); the choice of enzyme influences the incubation period required to reach equilibrium and the conditions for a pseudo first-order kinetic approach. The decrease in absorbance as urate is converted may be monitored by a spectrophotometer at 293 nm.[70] However, at this wavelength, most of the absorbance is due to serum proteins. Therefore, there is a high signal-to-noise ratio, which can compromise the precision of the method. A high-quality spectrophotometer with narrow bandpass is necessary, and this is rarely satisfied with automated analyzers.

Most current enzymatic assays for uric acid in serum involve a peroxidase system coupled with one of a number of oxygen acceptors to produce a chromogen.[145,342] For example, one popular method measures hydrogen peroxide with the aid of horseradish peroxidase (donor : hydrogen-peroxide oxidoreductase; EC 1.11.1.7) and an oxygen acceptor to yield a chromogen in the visible spectrum.[88] Its popularity is probably due to the use of less expensive enzymes and greater analytical sensitivity. The most common oxygen acceptor used is 4-aminophenazone, together with phenol or a substituted phenol. The benefit of using substituted phenols is the enhanced molar absorptivity, as follows: phenol $\cong 5.5 \times 10^3$ L • mol/cm, tribromo-phenol $\cong 23.6 \times 10^3$ L • mol/cm, and tribromo-3-hydroxybenzoic acid $\cong 30.0 \times 10^3$ L • mol/cm. Alternative oxygen acceptors include 3-methyl-1-benzothiazoline hydrazone (MBTH), 2,2′-azino-di-(3-ethylbenzothiazoline)-6-sulfonate (ABTS), and *o*-dianisidine.

Although many combinations of oxygen acceptor and phenol have been described, the choice should be guided by minimization of interference and sufficient absorbance to ensure good precision. The use of a substituted phenol yielding a highly absorbing product helps to reduce potential interference by reducing the sample volume requirement. The major interferants to minimize are ascorbic acid and bilirubin. In general, it is necessary to employ ascorbate oxidase (L-ascorbate : oxygen oxidoreductase; EC 1.10.3.3) in uric acid methods.[172] Aminophenazone with a substituted phenol or the addition of ferrocyanide[88,126] has been used to minimize bilirubin interference. Alternatively, use of the oxygen acceptor azure-D2 [3,7-diamino-5-phenothiazine (thionine) derivative], which can be monitored at 600 nm, reduces the spectral but not the chemical[344] interference caused by hyperbilirubinemia.[162] It has also been shown that unknown metabolites in the serum of patients with kidney failure, thought to be phenolic compounds, will interfere by competing with the reagent phenol, giving low recovery of urate.[137] This interference can be overcome by using a phenolic derivative, thereby generating a higher-absorbing product and reducing the sample volume.

Although many methods for the quantitation of uric acid are described in the literature, the most popular methods today employ the uricase-mediated reaction; however, the specificity of this reaction may be compromised by the choice of detector reaction, owing to an interfering enzyme or a molecule that competes in the final absorbance generation step. In practice, reactions that generate a visible end product are preferred because of the higher absorbance obtained; however, care should be taken that interference caused by ascorbate, bilirubin, and unspecified interferants in serum from patients with kidney failure is minimized.

Dry Chemistry Systems

Devices that use uricase in a dry reagent format to measure uric acid have been described. For example, a multilayer film system employs uricase and peroxidase separated by a semipermeable membrane from a leuco dye that is oxidized to form a colored product.[144] A cellulose matrix pad system employs uricase, peroxidase, and MBTH as oxygen acceptors; the system uses a diluted serum sample, which helps to reduce interferences, although ascorbic acid was shown to be a significant interferant.[146] A third system incorporates separation of serum from red cells and uricase, peroxidase, and a substituted phenol to measure uric acid.[42] All three systems use a reflectance meter system to facilitate accurate and precise quantitation of the color change.

Several electrochemical and biosensor systems have been described for the measurement of uric acid. In most cases, uricase is employed, being linked in examples to an oxygen electrode[353] or to a metal-organic probe whose fluorescence is quenched by oxygen.[281] Detection of uric acid has been demonstrated as part of a multianalyte array.[323] A nonenzymatic approach has also been described on a microchip, based on chemiluminescence microflow injection analysis.[113]

HPLC Methods

HPLC methods using ion-exchange or reversed-phase columns have been used to separate and quantify uric acid. The column effluent is monitored at 293 nm to detect the eluting uric acid. HPLC methods are specific and fast, mobile phases are simple, and the retention time for uric acid is less than 6 minutes—reasonable conditions that recommend these methods for reference use.[128] JCTLM-listed reference methods for the assay of uric acid in serum and urine use IDMS.[74,294,303,319]

Reference Intervals

Using an enzymatic method, the reference interval for uric acid has been reported to be 3.5 to 7.2 mg/dL (0.21 to 0.43 mmol/L) for males and 2.6 to 6.0 mg/dL (0.16 to 0.36 mmol/L) for females.[321] The concentration of serum uric acid increases gradually with age, rising about 10% between the ages of 20 and 60 years. A significant rise is seen in women after the menopause; concentrations similar to those in men are reached. During pregnancy, serum uric acid concentrations fall during the first trimester and until about 24 weeks' gestation, when concentrations begin to rise and eventually exceed nonpregnant concentrations.[40,181] Using an enzymatic assay, reference intervals at 32, 36, and 38 weeks' gestation have been reported as 1.9 to 5.5 mg/dL (0.11 to 0.32 mmol/L), 2.0 to 5.8 mg/dL (0.12 to 0.34 mmol/L), and 2.7 to 6.5 mg/dL (0.16 to 0.38 mmol/L), respectively.[181]

Urinary uric acid excretion in individuals on a diet containing purines is 250 to 750 mg/d (1.5 to 4.5 mmol/d). Excretion may decrease by 20 to 25% on a purine-free diet to less than 400 mg/d.

ASSESSMENT OF KIDNEY FUNCTION: ESTIMATION OF GLOMERULAR FILTRATION RATE

The GFR is widely accepted as the best overall measure of kidney function, enabling a statement of the complex functions of the kidney in a single numeric expression.[218] A decrease in GFR precedes kidney failure in all forms of progressive disease. Different kidney pathological conditions can progress to renal failure and dialysis dependency at rates varying from weeks to several decades.[36,262] Symptoms accompanying progressive kidney disease (see Chapter 48) and their correlation with falling GFR will be influenced by this rate of progression. Measuring GFR in established disease is useful in targeting treatment, monitoring progression, and predicting the point at which renal replacement therapy will be required. It is also used as a guide to dosage of renally excreted drugs to prevent potential drug toxicity. Several methods are used to measure the GFR; most involve the ability of the kidneys to clear an exogenous or endogenous marker. Improving methods and the discovery of new markers of GFR and glomerular or tubular damage will continue to provide important contributions to the early diagnosis of renal disease.

The Concept of Clearance

Most of the clinical laboratory information used to assess kidney function is derived from or related to measurement of the clearance of some substance by the kidneys. *Renal clearance of a substance* is defined as the volume of plasma from which the substance is completely cleared (removed) by the kidneys per unit of time.

Provided a substance *S* is in stable concentration in the plasma and is physiologically inert, freely filtered at the glomerulus, and neither secreted, reabsorbed, synthesized, nor metabolized by the kidney, the amount of that substance filtered at the glomerulus is equal to the amount excreted in the urine (i.e., the amount of *S* entering the kidney must exactly equal the amount leaving it). The amount of *S* filtered at the glomerulus equals GFR multiplied by plasma *S* concentration: GFR × PS. The amount of *S* excreted equals the urine *S* concentration (US) multiplied by the urinary flow rate (V, volume excreted per unit time).

Because filtered *S* = excreted *S*,

$$\text{GFR} \times \text{PS} = \text{US} \times \text{V} \quad (1)$$

$$\text{GFR} = (US \times V)/PS \quad (2)$$

where

GFR = the flow rate in milliliters per minute of plasma through the glomerular membranes, estimated as *clearance* in units of milliliters of plasma cleared of a substance per minute

US = urinary concentration of the substance

V = volumetric flow rate of urine in milliliters per minute

PS = plasma concentration of the substance

The term (US × V)/*PS* is defined as the clearance of substance *S* and is an accurate estimate of GFR, provided the aforementioned criteria are satisfied. Inulin satisfies these criteria and has long been regarded as the most accurate (gold standard) estimate of GFR (see later).

Kidney size and GFR are roughly proportional to body size. It is conventional therefore to adjust clearance estimates to a standard body surface area (BSA) of 1.73 m^2, according to the formula devised by Du Bois and Du Bois in 1916[68]:

$$\text{BSA} = \text{Weight (kg)}^{0.425} \times \text{Height (cm)}^{0.725} \times 7.1 \times 10^{-3} \quad (3)$$

A variety of exogenous (radioisotopic and nonradioisotopic) and endogenous markers have been used to estimate clearance (Table 25-3). Measurement of clearance may require accurate measurements of serum and urinary concentrations of the marker used plus a reliable urine collection. For a

TABLE 25-3 Markers of Glomerular Filtration Rate: Hierarchical Arrangement

Hierarchy	Marker	Advantages	Disadvantages
Gold standard	Inulin (sinsitrin) continuous-infusion urinary clearance method	Gold standard	Exogenous Time-consuming[75] Requires timed urine collection Poor specificity of analysis Extrarenal clearance = 0.083 mL/min/kg
Silver standard	Inulin (sinistrin) single-bolus plasma clearance method		Exogenous Time-consuming[75] Poor specificity of analysis Extrarenal clearance = 0.083 mL/min/kg
	^{51}Cr-EDTA	Radioisotopic (simple measurement) Close correlation with inulin clearance[33]	Exogenous Radioisotopic (risks of ionizing radiation) Time-consuming[261] Extrarenal clearance = 0.079 mL/min/kg ^{51}Cr less readily available than ^{99m}Technetium (Tc)
	^{99m}Tc-DTPA	Radioisotopic (simple measurement) Can be used for gamma camera imaging	Exogenous Radioisotopic (risks of ionizing radiation) Time-consuming[73,261] Protein binding
	^{125}I-iothalamate	Radioisotopic (simple measurement)	Exogenous Radioisotopic (risks of ionizing radiation) Not available in all countries Reports of allergic reactions
	Iohexol	Nonradioisotopic	Exogenous Extrarenal clearance = 0.087 mL/min/kg[94,156] Reports of allergic reactions
Bronze standard	Creatinine	Endogenous Inexpensive Can be used to estimate GFR from equations (e.g., MDRD)	Poor sensitivity and specificity
	Cystatin C	Not secreted/reabsorbed Constitutively expressed More sensitive and specific than creatinine	Influence of thyroid function[62,90,139]
Of uncertain clinical use	Creatinine clearance	Endogenous Inexpensive	Requires timed urine collection Inaccurate
	Urea	Endogenous Inexpensive	Poor sensitivity and specificity
	Retinol binding protein (RBP)	Endogenous Not secreted/reabsorbed	Nonrenal influences on production rate
	α_1-Microglobulin	Endogenous Not secreted/reabsorbed	Nonrenal influences on production rate Less freely filtered than RBP

GFR, Glomerular filtration rate; *MDRD,* Modification of Diet in Renal Disease study.

reliable serum measurement, the substance must have reached a steady-state concentration and must not be rapidly changing. For a reliable urine collection, the urine flow must be adequate (several mL/min), the collection period long enough, and complete bladder emptying achieved; this is problematic. Table 25-4 provides some reference data for GFR using a variety of methods.

Exogenous Markers of Glomerular Filtration Rate

Ideally, GFR is measured using exogenous markers, although practical limitations restrict their widespread use. Exogenous markers are also used to determine a GFR that is used to set a benchmark against which deterioration in GFR can be monitored using an endogenous marker such as creatinine.

TABLE 25-4 Glomerular Filtration Rate: Reference Values

Study	Method	Age, y	GFR*, Mean ± SD (Range) mL/min/1.73 m²)	n
Slack and Wilson[295]	Inulin (constant infusion)	20-29		47
		20	118 (90-146)	
		25	115 (88-142)	
		30-39		28
		30	112 (86-138)	
		35	109 (84-134)	
		40-49		30
		40	106 (82-130)	
		45	104 (80-128)	
		50-59		26
		50	101 (78-124)	
		55	99 (75-123)	
		60	96 (73-119)	4
Prescott et al[249]	Inulin (constant infusion)	30 ± 5	100 ± 19	9
		26 ± 8	88 ± 12	10
Prescott et al[249]	Inulin (single injection)	27 ± 6	104 ± 14	27
		27 ± 3	102 ± 20	8
		26 ± 8	95 ± 12	10
Askergren et al[7]	^{51}Cr-EDTA (single injection)	20-63	103 ± 15	26
		20-63	112 ± 13	15
Back et al[11]	Iohexol (single injection)	20-50	100 (78-122)	23
		51-65	83 (58-108)	20
		66-80	72 (52-92)	8
Arvidsson and Hedman[6]	Iohexol (constant infusion) triplicate determinations	19-30	116 ± 10	12
		19-30	117 ± 9	12
		19-30	110 ± 12	12

*All values have been rounded up or down to the nearest whole number.
GFR, Glomerular filtration rate.

Measurement of GFR using an exogenous molecule does enable smaller deteriorations in renal function to be observed, even when the imprecision in measurement is taken into account.

Radioisotopic Markers

Radiopharmaceuticals that have been used include ^{51}Cr-ethylenediaminetetraacetic acid (EDTA),[7,8,21,33,46] ^{99m}Tc-diethylenetriaminepentaacetic acid (DTPA), and ^{125}I-iothalamate. ^{51}Cr-EDTA is preferred to ^{99m}Tc-DTPA and ^{125}I-iothalamate because its clearance is considered to be closest to that of inulin.[22,33] ^{99m}Tc-DTPA offers the advantage that it can also be used for gamma camera imaging. ^{125}I-iothalamate is no longer approved for intravascular use in some countries.[22] GFR measurements may be based on urinary or plasma clearance of the marker. To ensure accuracy when GFR is measured using urinary or plasma clearance methods, it is essential that (1) renal tubular secretion or reabsorption does not contribute to elimination of the compound, (2) plasma protein binding of the radiopharmaceutical is negligible, and (3) no extrarenal elimination of the marker occurs. Incomplete bladder emptying may also contribute to inaccuracy in urinary clearance approaches. ^{99m}Tc-DTPA has been associated with problems of plasma protein binding of the tracer, but more recent formulations have minimized this problem.[22] For research purposes, in patients with low (<30 mL/min) GFR and in patients with ascites or edema, measurement is best performed using a urinary clearance method.[22] From a clinical management perspective, in most patients, urinary or plasma clearance approaches are acceptable.

Constant-infusion or single-bolus injection methods may be used to administer an exogenous marker. In the constant-infusion technique, the fasting subject is required to drink 500 mL of water 1 hour before the study begins, after which he or she is required to take 200 mL every half hour until the end of the study. The subject remains supine throughout the study. An intravenous loading dose of the marker selected is then followed by a constant infusion of a given quantity of marker per minute for 3 hours. After equilibration for 1 hour, blood is taken and urine samples are collected at hourly intervals for 3 hours. This technique can be used with any of the exogenous markers, the dosage being all that will vary between molecules. For example, for inulin, an intravenous loading dose of 2.3 g would be followed by a constant infusion of 18.1 mg/min for 3 hours.

Single-bolus plasma clearance methods have obvious practical advantages compared with the complex continuous-infusion methods. A single dose of the marker [e.g., inulin, 70 mg/kg; iohexol, 5 mL; Ominipaque, 300 mg iodine/mL (Nycomed AS, Oslo, Norway); or ^{51}Cr-EDTA, 50 to 100 μCi) is injected, and venous blood samples are collected at timed intervals (e.g., typically 120, 180, and 240 minutes after the start of the injection for ^{51}Cr-EDTA). The GFR is calculated using knowledge of the amount of marker injected and the decrease in marker concentration (activity) as a function of time. Elimination of the marker is described by a two-compartment model, which comprises an initial equilibration or distribution phase while the marker mixes between vascular and extravascular spaces and is being cleared from the plasma by the kidney. This gives rise to a biexponential clearance curve (Figure 25-6). The first sample should be taken no earlier than 2 hours after injection to avoid inclusion of the fast exponential in the GFR calculation.[81]

GFR is normally calculated using single-exponential analysis by plotting log marker concentration against time and using slope-intercept analysis. The half-life is calculated from the slope *(k)* and the volume of distribution *(C_0)* of the marker just after injection.

$$\text{GFR} = k \times C_0 \tag{4}$$

Because this model ignores the distribution phase, GFR is overestimated. Various corrections are used to adjust for this (e.g., those proposed by Chantler and Barratt[46] and Brochner-Mortensen[32]). For additional details, see Blake and colleagues.[21]

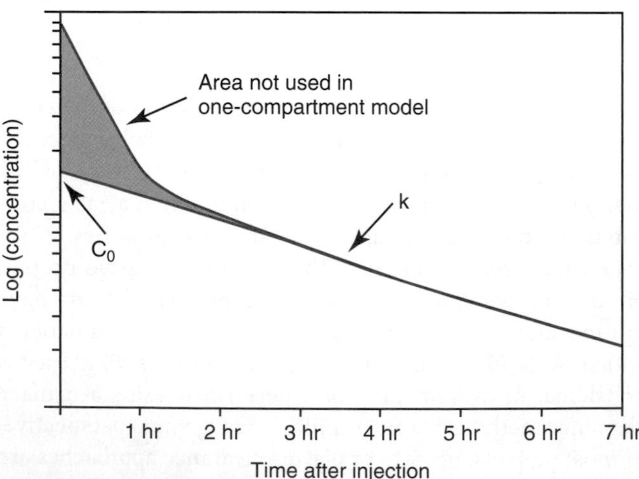

Figure 25-6 Semilog plot used in a single compartmental analysis of the plasma disappearance curve of a glomerular filtration rate (GFR) marker. In this simplified representation of contrast agent elimination, the distribution phase *(colored area)* is neglected, which leads to underestimation of the true area under the curve.

Nonradiosotopic Markers

Nonradioactive compounds used to measure GFR include inulin and iohexol.[73]

Inulin Clearance

The fructose polymer inulin (Mr ≈5000 Da) satisfies the criteria as an ideal marker of GFR. Inulin clearance using a constant-infusion urinary clearance approach has long been regarded as the gold standard measure of GFR. Acceptable single-bolus plasma clearance approaches have also been evaluated.[328] However, lack of availability of simple laboratory methods of measurement remains an impediment to universal usage. Early methods for the measurement of inulin were based on the hydrolysis of inulin with concentrated sulfuric acid and condensation with anthrone to give a green product that could be read at 620 nm. Newer methods have been based on the enzyme inulinase (EC 3.2.17), which converts inulin to fructose; the fructose is then determined with the aid of sorbitol dehydrogenase (EC 1.1.1.14) according to the following reaction sequence[308]:

$$\text{Inulin} \xrightarrow{\text{Inulinase}} \text{Fructose} + \text{NADH} \xrightarrow{\text{Sorbitol dehydrogenase}} \text{Sorbitol} + \text{NAD}$$

The amount of inulin present can be determined from the reduction of nicotinamide-adenine dinucleotide, reduced form (NADH), measured as a decrease in absorbance at 340 nm. The method can be calibrated with inulin or fructose; endogenous fructose in each sample is measured by incubation with an inactivated inulinase reagent. Urine samples require predilution (typically 1 in 40) before analysis. Typical between-run imprecision of less than ±2% for serum and less than ±4% for urine can be obtained with an automated assay.

An alternative method for detecting the fructose produced involves the use of fructokinase (EC 2.7.1.4), phosphoglucose isomerase, and glucose-6-phosphate dehydrogenase (EC 1.1.1.49), measuring in this case the nicotinamide-adenine dinucleotide phosphate, reduced form (NADPH), produced.[249,306]

Iohexol Clearance

Clearance of the nonradioactive x-ray contrast agent iohexol has been proposed as a simpler alternative to inulin clearance in the assessment of GFR.[6,93,94,122,156] Serum iohexol can be measured by HPLC with reversed-phase separation and UV detection, following prior deproteinization with perchloric acid.[156] Analytical imprecision is less than ±3% intraassay and ±5% interassay. Rapid, inexpensive capillary electrophoresis iohexol measurement techniques have been described.[140,266] Single-bolus plasma clearance of iohexol demonstrates excellent agreement with constant-infusion urinary inulin clearance.[94] Biological variability in patients with kidney disease using this technique is approximately 6%.[93] The nonradioisotopic and stable nature of iohexol enables analysis of samples to be delayed and common reference centers to be used for multinational studies. An outpatient procedure based on filter paper blood spots has been described.[226]

Endogenous Markers of Glomerular Filtration Rate

Although the clearance of infused markers is generally considered a more accurate assessment of GFR, to date these procedures have generally been considered too costly and cumbersome for routine use, particularly when GFR must be assessed on a regular basis (e.g., when patients are receiving nephrotoxic drugs). Recognition of CKD as a major public health issue has focused attention on the need for simple and readily available markers of GFR.[216,218] Creatinine and certain low molecular weight proteins (e.g., cystatin C) have been used as endogenous markers of GFR. The use of urea in this context is of limited value[313] and will not be discussed further. Endogenous markers obviate the necessity for injection and require only a single blood sample, simplifying the procedure for the patient, the clinician, and the laboratory. The most widely used endogenous marker of GFR is creatinine, expressed as its serum concentration or as renal clearance. Creatinine as a marker of GFR was first used in 1926 by Rehberg,[260] who exogenously administered creatinine. This led to the work of Popper and Mandel,[247] who in 1937 developed the use of endogenous creatinine clearance.

Creatinine

Most commonly, GFR is assessed by measuring serum creatinine. Creatinine is freely filtered at the glomerulus, and its concentration is inversely related to GFR. As a GFR marker, it is convenient and inexpensive to measure but is affected by (1) age, (2) gender, (3) exercise, (4) certain drugs (e.g., cimetidine,[324] trimethoprim), (5) muscle mass, and (6) nutritional status.[244,298] As previously discussed, significant preanalytical influences and analytical interferences are a problem.[154,298] Further, a small (but significant) and variable proportion of the creatinine appearing in the urine is derived from tubular secretion: typically, 7 to 10% is due to tubular secretion,[202] but this amount is increased in the presence of renal insufficiency. Perhaps most important, serum creatinine remains within the reference interval until notable renal function has been lost (Figure 25-7).[244,290]

Because plasma creatinine is derived from creatine and phosphocreatine breakdown in muscle, the reference interval encompasses the range of muscle mass observed in the

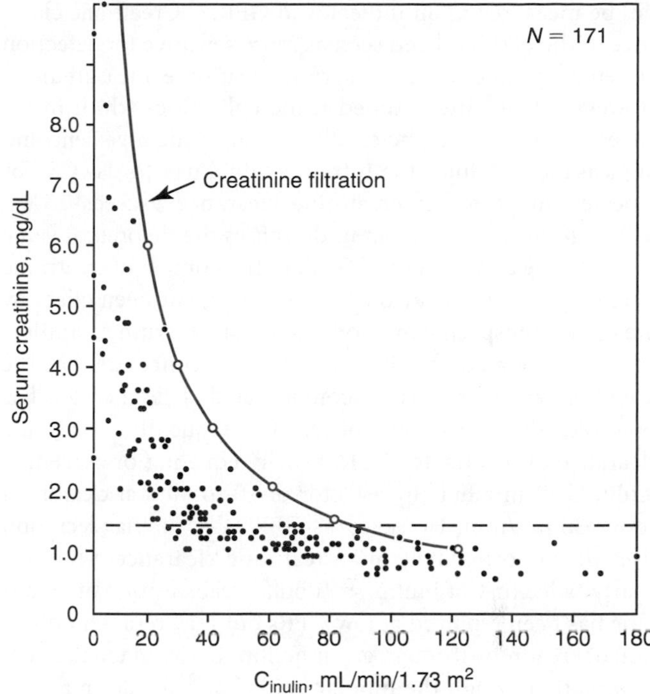

Figure 25-7 The relationship between serum creatinine concentration and glomerular filtration rate (GFR), measured as the clearance of inulin, in 171 patients with glomerular disease. The hypothetical relationship between GFR and serum creatinine is shown as a *continuous line*, assuming that only filtration of creatinine takes place. The *dashed horizontal line* represents the upper limit of a normal serum creatinine (1.4 mg/dL). Because of creatinine secretion and/or a creatinine deficit through gut excretion, the serum creatinine consistently overestimates the GFR. *(From Shemesh O, Golbetz H, Kriss JP, Myers BD. Limitations of creatinine as a filtration marker in glomerulopathic patients. Kidney Int 1985;28:830.)*[290]

reference population used. This limitation contributes to the insensitivity of creatinine as a marker of diminished GFR. Additionally, in patients with CKD, extrarenal clearance of creatinine becomes important when caused by degradation as a result of bacterial overgrowth in the small intestine, further blunting the anticipated increase in plasma creatinine in response to falling GFR.[218] Consequently, serum creatinine measurement will not detect patients with stage 2 CKD (GFR, 60 to 89 mL/min/1.73 m^2) and will fail to identify many patients with stage 3 CKD (GFR, 30 to 59 mL/min/1.73 m^2). Thus, although an elevated serum creatinine concentration generally equates with impaired kidney function, a normal serum creatinine does not necessarily equate with normal kidney function. Because of all these limitations, it is recommended that serum creatinine measurement alone is not used to assess kidney function.[218]

Creatinine Clearance

Because creatinine is endogenously produced and released into body fluids at a reasonably constant rate, its clearance can be measured as an indicator of GFR.[244] Creatinine clearance in the past has been seen as more sensitive for detection of renal dysfunction than serum creatinine measurement. However, it requires a timed urine collection, which introduces its own inaccuracies,[97,242,263] and is inconvenient and unpleasant. In adults, the intraindividual day-to-day CV for repeated measures of creatinine clearance exceeds 25%.[34] Although tubular secretion undermines the theoretical value of creatinine as a marker of GFR, in the context of creatinine clearance, this has previously to some extent been offset by the use of nonspecific methods to measure serum creatinine, which lead to an overestimation of serum concentration. The use of enzymatic assays or "compensated" Jaffe methods has removed this fortuitous offset. Consequently, creatinine clearance overestimates GFR, usually equaling or exceeding inulin GFR in adults by a factor of 10 to 40% at clearances above 80 mL/min. However, as GFR falls, tubular secretion rises disproportionately and creatinine clearance can reach nearly twice that of inulin.[332] Tubular reabsorption of creatinine has been reported at low GFRs but may represent diffusion of creatinine through gap junctions between tubular cells or directly through the tubular epithelial cells, down a concentration gradient.[244] Whatever the mechanism, this further devalues the use of creatinine clearance. Hence at best, creatinine clearance can provide only a crude index of GFR.

Estimating Glomerular Filtration Rate

The mathematical relationship between plasma creatinine and GFR can be improved by correcting for the confounding variables that make this relationship nonlinear. More than 25 different equations have been derived that estimate GFR using serum creatinine corrected for some or all of gender, body size, race, and age.[163,218] These generally produce a better estimate of GFR than serum creatinine alone or measured creatinine clearance,[55,163,165,218,332] and professional societies throughout the world have recommended that such estimates should be used in preference to, or in association with, serum creatinine.[38,178,216,218,285] In adults, two main equations have been used: the Cockcroft and Gault equation and the Modification of Diet in Renal Disease (MDRD) Study equation.

The Cockcroft and Gault equation is one of the earliest of these equations.[50] A full discussion of this equation may be found in the fourth edition of this textbook. It remains widely used, particularly in the context of assessing drug dosages for patients with kidney impairment. However, in addition to several theoretical objections to use of the equation (e.g., females were not included in the original derivation of the equation, and a reference GFR method was not used), the requirement for measurement of body weight has been a major practical impediment to the use of the equation in wider clinical practice.

The era of GFR estimation as a widely used simple clinical tool across both primary and secondary care really began with publication of the MDRD study equation in 1999.[175] The original MDRD equation was developed in a chronic renal insufficiency study in which 1628 predominantly middle-aged patients were enrolled. The equation was later validated against an iothalamate clearance estimate of GFR, and reported GFR is corrected for BSA. It is suitable for use in black African-Americans, and there is no requirement for patient weight. It originally used age, gender, race (black or white), serum creatinine, urea, and albumin as covariables.

$$\begin{aligned}\text{GFR}\,(\text{mL/min}/1.73\,\text{m}^2) = {} & 170 \times [\text{serum creatinine (mg/dL)}]^{-0.999} \\ & \times (\text{age})^{-0.176} \times (0.762 \text{ if patient is female}) \\ & \times (1.180 \text{ if patient is black}) \\ & \times [\text{serum urea nitrogen (mg/dL)}]^{-0.170} \\ & \times [\text{serum albumin (g/dL)}]^{0.318}\end{aligned}$$

or

$$\begin{aligned}\text{GFR}\,(\text{mL/min}/1.73\,\text{m}^2) = {} & 170 \times [\text{serum creatinine } (\mu\text{mol/L}) \\ & \times 0.011312]^{-0.999} \times (\text{age})^{-0.176} \\ & \times (0.762 \text{ if patient is female}) \\ & \times (1.180 \text{ if patient is black}) \\ & \times [\text{serum urea (mmol/L)} \times 2.801]^{-0.170} \\ & \times [\text{serum albumin (g/L)} \times 0.1]^{+0.318}\end{aligned}$$

These workers subsequently also published, in abstract form, an abbreviated version of this equation, which did not require albumin or urea.[179]

$$\begin{aligned}\text{GFR}\,(\text{mL/min}/1.73\,\text{m}^2) = {} & 186 \times [\text{serum creatinine (mg/dL)}]^{-1.154} \\ & \times (\text{age})^{-0.203} \times (1.210 \text{ if patient is black}) \\ & \times (0.742 \text{ if patient is female})\end{aligned}$$

or

$$\begin{aligned}\text{GFR}\,(\text{mL/min}/1.73\,\text{m}^2) = {} & 186 \times [\text{serum creatinine } (\mu\text{mol/L}) \\ & \times 0.011312]^{-1.154} \times (\text{age})^{-0.203} \\ & \times (1.210 \text{ if patient is black}) \\ & \times (0.742 \text{ if patient is female})\end{aligned}$$

Many publications subsequently highlighted the critical susceptibility of the MDRD equation to the bias of the creatinine assay used.[54,211,331,346] The creatinine assay used to derive the MDRD equation was a rate Jaffe method with a positive bias compared with reference creatinine assays. Increasing use of compensated and enzymatic creatinine assays and moves toward standardization of creatinine assays would have limited the accuracy and wider use of the MDRD equation. Subsequently, therefore, the equation has been indirectly restandardized against an IDMS assay, using a Roche enzymatic assay as the reference method.[176,177] In practice, this just required the substitution of a different constant factor.

$$\begin{aligned}\text{GFR}\,(\text{mL/min}/1.73\,\text{m}^2) = {} & 175 \times [\text{serum creatinine (mg/dL)}]^{-1.154} \\ & \times (\text{age})^{-0.203} \times (1.210 \text{ if patient is black}) \\ & \times (0.742 \text{ if patient is female})\end{aligned}$$

or

$$\text{GFR (mL/min/1.73 m}^2) = 175 \times [\text{serum creatinine } (\mu\text{mol/L}) \times 0.011312]^{-1.154} \times (\text{age})^{-0.203} \times (1.210 \text{ if patient is black}) \times (0.742 \text{ if patient is female})$$

In the United States, the National Kidney Disease Education Program (NKDEP) has recommended that laboratories should use the form of the equation with the constant factor 175 or 186 depending on whether their creatinine assay is, or is not, calibrated to an IDMS reference method, respectively (see www.nkdep.nih.gov). In the United Kingdom, it has been recommended that all laboratories should use the IDMS-traceable version of the MDRD equation to estimate GFR, wherever possible using creatinine assays that are specific and zero biased compared with IDMS (e.g., enzymatic assays) and calibrated to a standardized reference material.[216] When such assays are not used, appropriate assay-specific adjustment factors should be employed to minimize between-laboratory variation (e.g., those provided by the U.K. National External Quality Assessment Scheme; www.birminghamquality.org.uk).[160] As discussed previously, during 2009 most clinical laboratory methods moved to calibration that was traceable to an IDMS reference measurement procedure.[204,205] Consequently, most laboratories should now be able to use the IDMS-traceable version of the MDRD equation.[176,177]

Generally, studies have confirmed that the MDRD equation provides a more accurate assessment of GFR than the Cockcroft and Gault equation,[91,246] including among diabetic patients with moderate to severe CKD,[264] although the differences are somewhat marginal and are not universally observed.[163] The most important advantage of the MDRD equation, however, remains its practical advantage of reliance only on readily available data.

However, the MDRD equation is not without its limitations. At higher values of GFR, it shows significant negative bias[246,274] and poor precision[91] compared with reference GFR techniques—a particular limitation in monitoring early diabetic nephropathy.[84,269] Evaluation in older people and South Asians has been limited,[164] and refinements of the equation may be required among Chinese populations.[186,355] Because of its poorer performance at higher values of GFR, several national societies and expert groups have recommended that numeric values of GFR should be reported only up to 60 mL/min/1.73 m^2 using the MDRD equation.[192,212,285] The Chronic Kidney Disease Epidemiology Collaboration (CKD-EPI) has described an equation including log serum creatinine (modeled as a two-slope linear spline with gender-specific knots at creatinine concentrations of 0.9 and 0.7 mg/dL [80 and 62 μmol/L] in males and females, respectively), gender, race, and age on the natural scale.[180] This equation shows reduced bias compared with reference GFR measurements at higher values of GFR, and it has been suggested that the equation should replace the MDRD equation for clinical use.

Serum creatinine is an imperfect marker of GFR; therefore it is not altogether surprising that equations based predominantly upon it are imperfect. Their use cannot circumvent the very significant spectral interferences affecting serum creatinine measurement (i.e., hemolysis, icterus, and lipemia), and the equations are unsuitable for use in patients with AKI, in whom serum creatinine concentrations may change rapidly. In situations where the normal relationship between muscle mass and body size is disturbed, the equations will be inaccurate (e.g., among body builders, amputees, and people with muscle wasting disorders). Notwithstanding this, in general, equations improve the estimation of GFR compared with serum creatinine alone. Future developments could include the use of cystatin C (see later) and creatinine in combination in GFR estimating equations, possibly with the addition of other markers.

Cystatin C (and Other Low Molecular Weight Proteins)

Several proteins with molecular weights of less than 30 kDa are primarily cleared from the circulation by renal filtration and can be considered to be relatively freely filtered at the glomerulus. These include (1) α_2-microglobulin, (2) RBP, (3) α_1-microglobulin, (4) β-trace protein,[256] and (5) cystatin C. These proteins are filtered at the glomerulus, then are reabsorbed (and metabolized) in the proximal tubule or excreted into the urine; thus they are entirely eliminated from the circulation. Therefore they have the potential to meet the criteria for use as a marker of GFR. However, most of these have been shown to have serum concentrations that are influenced by other, nonrenal factors such as inflammation (α_2-microglobulin) and liver disease (RBP, α_1-microglobulin).[10] The relationship between circulating concentrations of these proteins shows the same curvilinear form as serum creatinine, but several groups have demonstrated that cystatin C measurement may offer a more sensitive and specific means of monitoring changes in GFR than serum creatinine.[79,104,158,223]

Cystatin C is a low molecular weight (12.8 kD) protein synthesized by all nucleated cells whose physiologic role is that of a cysteine protease inhibitor.[220] With regard to renal function, its most important attributes are its small size and high isoelectric point (pI 9.2), which enable it to be more freely filtered than previously mentioned proteins at the glomerulus.[104] The gene has been sequenced, and the promoter region has been identified as that of the housekeeping type, with no known regulatory elements. Consequently, the production rate of cystatin C has always been considered to be constant,[1] although several publications suggest an influence of thyroid hormone.[62,90,139] Serum concentrations of cystatin C appear to be relatively unaffected by muscle mass, diet, or gender.[158] No extrarenal routes of elimination are known; clearance from the circulation occurs only by glomerular filtration.[104,136,317]

Cystatin C can be measured by immunodiffusion or rocket electroimmunoassay, but the methods are too insensitive, and any form of labeled immunometric assay is too cumbersome and time-consuming for the response time required. The most practical approaches described are use of a latex particle–enhanced turbidimetric or nephelometric immunoassay; several commercial cystatin C methods are available, including automated applications.[83] An intra-assay precision of less than ±3% can be expected at the upper limit of the reference interval (≈1.00 mg/L), with less than ±4% for the between-day value.[79,158,223,305] Further, cystatin C measurement appears resistant to spectral interferences affecting creatinine assays.[305]

Several reports have documented the correlation between serum cystatin C and creatinine (as a reciprocal), and GFR as assessed by ^{51}Cr-EDTA clearance or using a number of alternative exogenous markers. In almost all studies, the correlation of GFR with cystatin C is superior to that with creatinine.[250] Kyhse-Andersen and associates[158] first demonstrated, using receiver operator analysis, the superiority of cystatin C measurement compared with creatinine for the detection of kidney disease (Figure 25-8); this has been confirmed by meta-analysis.[65]

A further summary receiver operator curve meta-analysis showed an area under the curve of 0.95 for cystatin C and 0.91 for creatinine (P = 0.003).[167] Perhaps more critically, Newman and colleagues found that, in a group of patients with a range of GFRs, the cystatin C concentration increased sooner than creatinine as GFR declined; cystatin C concentration started to increase as GFR fell below about 80 mL/min/1.73 m^2 compared with about 40 mL/min/1.73 m^2 for serum creatinine.[223] Cystatin C therefore is especially useful when the clinician is trying to detect mild to moderate impairment of kidney function.[27,51]

With the emergence of GFR as the primary criterion in the classification of CKD, several authors have developed GFR estimating equations that use cystatin C.[120,166,170,302,341] The equation of Grubb and coworkers was developed in a large patient cohort using an iohexol reference procedure; overall, its performance was only marginally better than that of the MDRD equation[105]:

$$\text{GFR} = 84.69 \times \text{Cystatin C} - 1.680\ (\times 0.948 \text{ if female})$$

Before now, there has been no international standardization of cystatin C measurement, although efforts are under way to address this.[24] This has limited the generalizability of cystatin C–based GFR estimating equations.

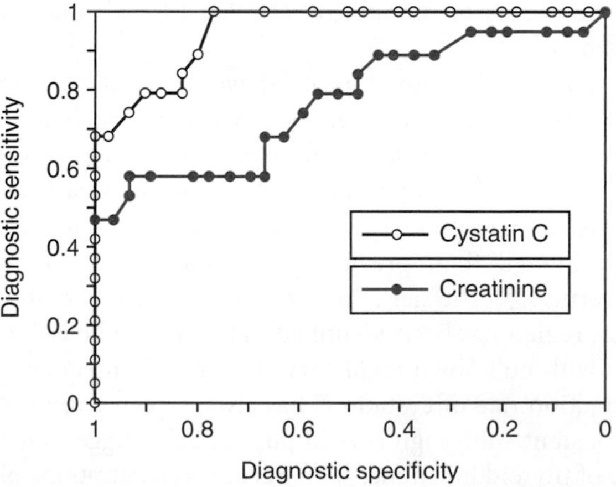

Figure 25-8 Receiver operating characteristic (ROC) curves comparing creatinine and cystatin C in the assessment of glomerular filtration rate (GFR). Nonparametric ROC plots were constructed to assess the diagnostic accuracy of serum concentrations of cystatin C and creatinine in distinguishing between normal and reduced GFR (<80 mL/min per 1.73 m^2) in 51 patients with various renal conditions. *(From Kyhse-Andersen J, Schmidt C, Nordin G, et al. Serum cystatin C, determined by a rapid, automated particle-enhanced turbidimetric method, is a better marker than serum creatinine for glomerular filtration rate. Clin Chem 1994;40:1921.)*

Assessment of Kidney Function at the Extremes of Age

As discussed previously in this chapter, current widely used markers of GFR are imperfect, and the limitations of these tests are accentuated in both pediatric and older populations. At birth, serum creatinine concentrations approximate those of the maternal circulation. Serum creatinine concentrations fall rapidly during the neonatal period, with slower falls observed in premature infants.[271] Serum creatinine concentrations are lower in infants than in adults, despite their lower GFR, reflecting the lower muscle mass (decreased creatinine production rate). The percentage of measured creatinine due to noncreatinine chromogen interference in Jaffe methods is proportionally increased in children, although compensatory adjustments applied to adult samples are probably inappropriate in children, for example, because of their lower total protein concentrations.[49] In the setting of pediatric intensive care medicine, the usefulness of serum creatinine may be further limited by analytical interferences caused by high concentrations of bilirubin and competition with creatinine for tubular secretion by commonly used antibiotics (e.g., trimethoprim, cimetidine). By contrast, serum cystatin C concentrations in infants appear to more closely reflect GFR, being increased in the first 3 months of life and then falling to approximate adult concentrations by age 1 year (Figure 25-9).[25,80]

Further, the diagnostic accuracy of cystatin C for reduced GFR is superior to that of creatinine in children.[115,350] As in adults, equations have been developed to enable GFR estimation in children based predominantly on height and serum creatinine measurement.[58,282] The Schwartz equation has been updated for use with an IDMS-traceable enzymatic creatinine assay. Further, a newly developed "CKiD" study equation has been developed that includes both serum cystatin C and creatinine, in addition to urea, height, and gender.[283] This new equation appears to be more accurate than either version of the original Schwartz equation.

Serum creatinine concentrations in healthy older people are not dissimilar to those in younger people, except among nonagenarians and centenarians, despite the decrease in GFR that occurs, on average, with aging.[322] Possible reasons for this include reduced muscle mass and poorer nutrition. Whatever the reason, the same concentration of serum creatinine may indicate very different degrees of kidney function in younger and older people, and a normal serum creatinine

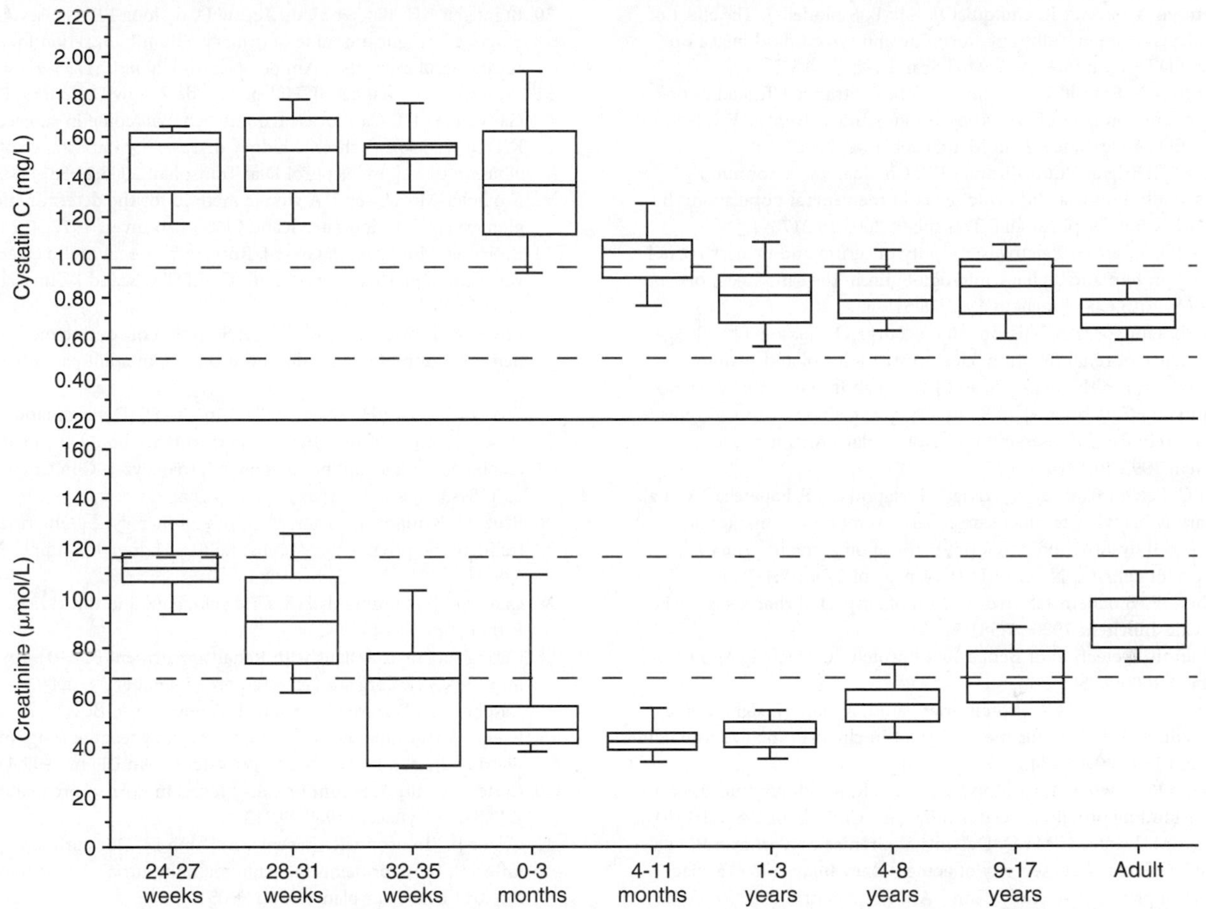

Figure 25-9 Age-related changes in cystatin C and creatinine superimposed upon the reference interval *(horizontal dashed lines)*. Box and Whiskers plot: the box represents the 25th to 75th percentiles with a horizontal line at the median; the whiskers extend to the highest and lowest values. *(From Newman DJ. Cystatin C. Ann Clin Biochem 2002;39:89-104.)*

concentration cannot exclude significant renal impairment. In two large primary care studies,[69,314] GFRs less than 50 mL/min estimated using the Cockcroft and Gault equation were common in patients with normal serum creatinine. This was most pronounced in older age groups (e.g., discordance between normal serum creatinine and reduced GFR was observed in 47% of patients aged 70 years or older, compared with 1.2% of patients aged 40 to 59 years[69]), and the sensitivity of serum creatinine for detecting severely reduced GFR (<30 mL/min/1.73 m^2) was only 46%.[314] As observed in children, serum cystatin C, however, does appear to reflect the age-related decline in kidney function[78,333] and appears to be more sensitive than serum creatinine for detection of reduced GFR.[82,229]

ACKNOWLEDGMENTS

Data on current creatinine method usage in the United Kingdom were provided by Finlay Mackenzie from the United Kingdom National External Quality Assessment Scheme, Birmingham, United Kingdom. Further information about the UKNEQAS estimated GFR scheme may be found at www.bimинghamquality.org.uk/accessed May 5, 2011. We are grateful to the College of American Pathologists for data on current creatinine method usage in the United States (www.cap.org/accessed May 5, 2011).

REFERENCES

1. Abrahamson M, Grubb A, Olafsson I, Lundwall A. Molecular cloning and sequence analysis of cDNA coding for the precursor of the human cysteine proteinase inhibitor cystatin C. FEBS Lett 1987;216: 229-33.
2. Agarwal R, Panesar A, Lewis RR. Dipstick proteinuria: can it guide hypertension management? Am J Kidney Dis 2002;39:1190-5.
3. Ali AC, Mihas CC, Campbell JA. Interferences of o-raffinose cross-linked hemoglobin in three methods for serum creatinine. Clin Chem 1997;43:1738-43.
4. Ambrose RT, Ketchum DF, Smith JW. Creatinine determined by "high-performance" liquid chromatography. Clin Chem 1983;29: 256-9.
5. Arnlov J, Evans JC, Meigs JB, Wang TJ, Fox CS, Levy D, et al. Low-grade albuminuria and incidence of cardiovascular disease events in nonhypertensive and nondiabetic individuals: the Framingham Heart Study. Circulation 2005;112:969-75.
6. Arvidsson A, Hedman A. Plasma and renal clearance of iohexol—a study on the reproducibility of a method for the glomerular filtration rate. Scand J Clin Lab Invest 1990;50:757-61.

7. Askergren A, Brandt R, Gullquist R, Silk B, Strandell T. The effect of fluid deprivation, antidiuretic hormone and forced fluid intake on 51-Cr-EDTA clearance. Acta Med Scand 1981;210:377-80.
8. Askergren A, Brandt R, Gullquist R, Silk B, Strandell T. Studies on kidney function in subjects exposed to organic solvents. IV. Effect on 51-Cr-EDTA clearance. Acta Med Scand 1981;210:373-6.
9. Atkins RC, Briganti EM, Zimmet PZ, Chadban SJ. Association between albuminuria and proteinuria in the general population: the AusDiab Study. Nephrol Dial Transplant 2003;18:2170-4.
10. Ayatse JO, Kwan JT. Relative sensitivity of serum and urinary retinol binding protein and alpha-1 microglobulin in the assessment of renal function. Ann Clin Biochem 1991;28:514-6.
11. Back SE, Ljungberg B, Nilsson-Ehle I, Borga O, Nilsson-Ehle P. Age dependence of renal function: clearance of iohexol and p-amino hippurate in healthy males. Scand J Clin Lab Invest 1989;49:641-6.
12. Ballantyne FC, Gibbons J, O'Reilly DS. Urine albumin should replace total protein for the assessment of glomerular proteinuria. Ann Clin Biochem 1993;30:101-3.
13. Bazzi C, Petrini C, Rizza V, Arrigo G, Napodano P, Paparella M, et al. Urinary *N*-acetyl-beta-glucosaminidase excretion is a marker of tubular cell dysfunction and a predictor of outcome in primary glomerulonephritis. Nephrol Dial Transplant 2002;17:1890-6.
14. Beetham R. Biochemical investigation of suspected rhabdomyolysis. Ann Clin Biochem 2000;37:581-7.
15. Beetham R. Detection of Bence-Jones protein in practice. Ann Clin Biochem 2000;37:563-70.
16. Beetham R, Cattell WR. Proteinuria: pathophysiology, significance and recommendations for measurement in clinical practice. Ann Clin Biochem 1993;30:425-34.
17. Beetham R, Dawnay A, Landon J, Cattell WR. A radioimmunoassay for retinol-binding protein in serum and urine. Clin Chem 1985;31:1364-7.
18. Bennett M, Dent CL, Ma Q, Dastrala S, Grenier F, Workman R, et al. Urine NGAL predicts severity of acute kidney injury after cardiac surgery: a prospective study. Clin J Am Soc Nephrol 2008;3:665-73.
19. Bennett PH, Haffner S, Kasiske BL, Keane WF, Mogensen CE, Parving HH, et al. Screening and management of microalbuminuria in patients with diabetes mellitus: recommendations to the Scientific Advisory Board of the National Kidney Foundation from an ad hoc committee of the Council on Diabetes Mellitus of the National Kidney Foundation. Am J Kidney Dis 1995;25:107-12.
20. Blaabjerg O, Hyltoft Petersen P. Effect of aggregates on albumin standardization. Scand J Clin Lab Invest 1979;39:751-7.
21. Blake GM, Roe D, Lazarus CR. Long-term precision of glomerular filtration rate measurements using ^{51}Cr-EDTA plasma clearance. Nucl Med Commun 1997;18:776-84.
22. Blaufox MD, Aurell M, Bubeck B, Fommei E, Piepsz A, Russell C, et al. Report of the Radionuclides in Nephrourology Committee on renal clearance. J Nucl Med 1996;37:1883-90.
23. Blijenberg BG, Brouwer HJ. The accuracy of creatinine methods based on the Jaffe reaction: a questionable matter. Eur J Clin Chem Clin Biochem 1994;32:909-13.
24. Blirup-Jensen S, Grubb A, Lindstrom V, Schmidt C, Althaus H. Standardization of cystatin C: development of primary and secondary reference preparations. Scand J Clin Lab Invest Suppl 2008;241:67-70.
25. Bokenkamp A, Domanetzki M, Zinck R, Schumann G, Byrd D, Brodehl J. Cystatin C—a new marker of glomerular filtration rate in children independent of age and height. Pediatrics 1998;101:875-81.
26. Borch-Johnsen K, Wenzel H, Viberti GC, Mogensen CE. Is screening and intervention for microalbuminuria worthwhile in patients with insulin dependent diabetes? BMJ 1993;306:1722-5.
27. Bostom AG, Dworkin LD. Cystatin C measurement: improved detection of mild decrements in glomerular filtration rate versus creatinine-based estimates? Am J Kidney Dis 2000;36:205-7.
28. Bowers LD. Kinetic serum creatinine assays I. The role of various factors in determining specificity. Clin Chem 1980;26:551-4.
29. Bowie L, Smith S, Gochman N. Characteristics of binding between reagent-strip indicators and urinary proteins. Clin Chem 1977;23: 128-30.
30. Brantsma AH, Bakker SJ, de Zeeuw D, de Jong PE, Gansevoort RT. Extended prognostic value of urinary albumin excretion for cardiovascular events. J Am Soc Nephrol 2008;19:1785-91.
31. Brantsma AH, Bakker SJ, Hillege HL, de Zeeuw D, de Jong PE, Gansevoort RT. Cardiovascular and renal outcome in subjects with K/DOQI stage 1-3 chronic kidney disease: the importance of urinary albumin excretion. Nephrol Dial Transplant 2008;23:3851-8.
32. Brochner-Mortensen J. A simple method for the determination of glomerular filtration rate. Scand J Clin Lab Invest 1972;30:271-4.
33. Brochner-Mortensen J, Giese J, Rossing N. Renal inulin clearance versus total plasma clearance of ^{51}Cr-EDTA. Scand J Clin Lab Invest 1969;23:301-5.
34. Brochner-Mortensen J, Rodbro P. Selection of routine method for determination of glomerular filtration rate in adult patients. Scand J Clin Lab Invest 1976;36:35-43.
35. Brown ND, Sing HC, Neeley WE, Koetitz SE. Determination of "true" serum creatinine by high-performance liquid chromatography combined with a continuous-flow microanalyzer. Clin Chem 1977; 23:1281-3.
36. Bruzzi I, Benigni A, Remuzzi G. Role of increased glomerular protein traffic in the progression of renal failure. Kidney Int Suppl 1997;62: S29-31.
37. Cameron JS, Simmonds HA. Uric acid, gout and the kidney. J Clin Pathol 1981;34:1245-54.
38. Caring for Australasians with Renal Impairment (CARI). Available at: http://www.cari.org.au/ (accessed on September 22, 2009).
39. Carobene A, Ferrero C, Ceriotti F, Modenese A, Besozzi M, de Giorgi E, et al. Creatinine measurement proficiency testing: assignment of matrix-adjusted ID GC-MS target values. Clin Chem 1997;43:1342-7.
40. Carter J, Child A. Serum uric acid levels in normal pregnancy. Aust N Z J Obstet Gynaecol 1989;29:313-4.
41. Carter JL, Tomson CR, Stevens PE, Lamb EJ. Does urinary tract infection cause proteinuria or microalbuminuria? A systematic review. Nephrol Dial Transplant 2006;21:3031-7.
42. Cattozzo G, Franzini C, Hubbuch A, Tritschler W. Evaluation of determination of uric acid in serum and whole blood with the Reflotron. Clin Chem 1988;34:414-6.
43. Ceriotti F, Boyd JC, Klein G, Henny J, Queralto J, Kairisto V, et al. Reference intervals for serum creatinine concentrations: assessment of available data for global application. Clin Chem 2008;54:559-66.
44. Chambers RE, Bullock DG, Whicher JT. Urinary total protein estimation—fact or fiction? Nephron 1989;53:33-6.
45. Chambers RE, Bullock DG, Whicher JT. External quality assessment of total urinary protein estimation in the United Kingdom. Ann Clin Biochem 1991;28:467-73.
46. Chantler C, Barratt TM. Estimation of glomerular filtration rate from plasma clearance of 51-chromium edetic acid. Arch Dis Child 1972; 47:613-7.
47. Chitalia VC, Kothari J, Wells EJ, Livesey JH, Robson RA, Searle M, et al. Cost-benefit analysis and prediction of 24-hour proteinuria from the spot urine protein-creatinine ratio. Clin Nephrol 2001;55: 436-47.
48. Claudi T, Cooper JG. Comparison of urinary albumin excretion rate in overnight urine and albumin creatinine ratio in spot urine in diabetic patients in general practice. Scand J Prim Health Care 2001;19:247-8.
49. Cobbaert CM, Baadenhuijsen H, Weykamp CW. Prime time for enzymatic creatinine methods in pediatrics. Clin Chem 2009;55: 549-58.
50. Cockcroft DW, Gault MH. Prediction of creatinine clearance from serum creatinine. Nephron 1976;16:31-41.
51. Coll E, Botey A, Alvarez L, Poch E, Quinto L, Saurina A, et al. Serum cystatin C as a new marker for noninvasive estimation of glomerular filtration rate and as a marker for early renal impairment. Am J Kidney Dis 2000;36:29-34.
52. Comper WD, Osicka TM, Clark M, MacIsaac RJ, Jerums G. Earlier detection of microalbuminuria in diabetic patients using a new urinary albumin assay. Kidney Int 2004;65:1850-5.

53. Comper WD, Osicka TM, Jerums G. High prevalence of immuno-unreactive intact albumin in urine of diabetic patients. Am J Kidney Dis 2003;41:336-42.
54. Coresh J, Astor BC, McQuillan G, Kusek J, Greene T, Van Lente F, et al. Calibration and random variation of the serum creatinine assay as critical elements of using equations to estimate glomerular filtration rate. Am J Kidney Dis 2002;39:920-9.
55. Coresh J, Toto RD, Kirk KA, Whelton PK, Massry S, Jones C, et al. Creatinine clearance as a measure of GFR in screenees for the African-American Study of Kidney Disease and Hypertension pilot study. Am J Kidney Dis 1998;32:32-42.
56. Costa AC, da Costa JL, Tonin FG, Tavares MF, Micke GA. Development of a fast capillary electrophoresis method for determination of creatinine in urine samples. J Chromatogr A 2007;1171:140-3.
57. Cote AM, Brown MA, Lam E, von Dadelszen P, Firoz T, Liston RM, et al. Diagnostic accuracy of urinary spot protein:creatinine ratio for proteinuria in hypertensive pregnant women: systematic review. BMJ 2008;336:1003-6.
58. Counahan R, Chantler C, Ghazali S, Kirkwood B, Rose F, Barratt TM. Estimation of glomerular filtration rate from plasma creatinine concentration in children. Arch Dis Child 1976;51:875-8.
59. Davey DA, MacGillivray I. The classification and definition of the hypertensive disorders of pregnancy. Am J Obstet Gynecol 1988;158: 892-8.
60. Dawnay A, Wilson AG, Lamb E, Kirby JD, Cattell WR. Microalbuminuria in systemic sclerosis. Ann Rheum Dis 1992;51: 384-8.
61. de Keijzer MH, Klasen IS, Branten AJ, Hordijk W, Wetzels JF. Infusion of plasma expanders may lead to unexpected results in urinary protein assays. Scand J Clin Lab Invest 1999;59:133-7.
62. den Hollander JG, Wulkan RW, Mantel MJ, Berghout A. Is cystatin C a marker of glomerular filtration rate in thyroid dysfunction? Clin Chem 2003;49:1558-9.
63. Dent CL, Ma Q, Dastrala S, Bennett M, Mitsnefes MM, Barasch J, et al. Plasma neutrophil gelatinase-associated lipocalin predicts acute kidney injury, morbidity and mortality after pediatric cardiac surgery: a prospective uncontrolled cohort study. Crit Care 2007;11:R127.
64. Devarajan P. NGAL in acute kidney injury: from serendipity to utility. Am J Kidney Dis 2008;52:395-9.
65. Dharnidharka VR, Kwon C, Stevens G. Serum cystatin C is superior to serum creatinine as a marker of kidney function: a meta-analysis. Am J Kidney Dis 2002;40:221-6.
66. Dilena BA. Bacterial interference with measurement of creatinine in stored plasma. Clin Chem 1988;34:1007-8.
67. DiMagno EP, Corle D, O'Brien JF, Masnyk IJ, Go VL, Aamodt R. Effect of long-term freezer storage, thawing, and refreezing on selected constituents of serum. Mayo Clin Proc 1989;64:1226-34.
68. Du Bois E, Du Bois D. A formula to estimate the approximate surface area if height and weight be known. Arch Intern Med 1916;17:863-71.
69. Duncan L, Heathcote J, Djurdjev O, Levin A. Screening for renal disease using serum creatinine: who are we missing? Nephrol Dial Transplant 2001;16:1042-6.
70. Duncan PH, Gochman N, Cooper T, Smith E, Bayse D. A candidate reference method for uric acid in serum. I. Optimization and evaluation. Clin Chem 1982;28:284-90.
71. Dyson EH, Will EJ, Davison AM, O'Malley AH, Shepherd HT, Jones RG. Use of the urinary protein creatinine index to assess proteinuria in renal transplant patients. Nephrol Dial Transplant 1992;7:450-2.
72. Eddy CV, Arnold MA. Near-infrared spectroscopy for measuring urea in hemodialysis fluids. Clin Chem 2001;47:1279-86.
73. Effersoe H, Rosenkilde P, Groth S, Jensen LI, Golman K. Measurement of renal function with iohexol: a comparison of iohexol, 99mTc-DTPA, and 51Cr-EDTA clearance. Invest Radiol 1990;25: 778-82.
74. Ellerbe P, Cohen A, Welch MJ, White ET. Determination of serum uric acid by isotope dilution mass spectrometry as a new candidate definitive method. Anal Chem 1990;62:2173-7.
75. Estelberger W, Petek W, Zitta S, Mauric A, Horn S, Holzer H, et al. Determination of the glomerular filtration rate by identification of sinistrin kinetics. Eur J Clin Chem Clin Biochem 1995;33:201-9.
76. Farbom P, Wahlstrand B, Almgren P, Skrtic S, Lanke J, Weiss L, et al. Interaction between renal function and microalbuminuria for cardiovascular risk in hypertension: the Nordic diltiazem study. Hypertension 2008;52:115-22.
77. Fay RA. Uric acid in pregnancy and preeclampsia: an alternative hypothesis. Aust N Z J Obstet Gynaecol 1990;30:141-2.
78. Finney H, Bates CJ, Price CP. Plasma cystatin C determinations in a healthy elderly population. Arch Gerontol Geriatr 1999;29:75-94.
79. Finney H, Newman DJ, Gruber W, Merle P, Price CP. Initial evaluation of cystatin C measurement by particle-enhanced immunonephelometry on the Behring nephelometer systems (BNA, BN II). Clin Chem 1997;43:1016-22.
80. Finney H, Newman DJ, Thakkar H, Fell JM, Price CP. Reference ranges for plasma cystatin C and creatinine measurements in premature infants, neonates, and older children. Arch Dis Child 2000;82:71-5.
81. Fleming JS, Nunan TO. The new BNMS guidelines for measurement of glomerular filtration rate. Nucl Med Commun 2004;25:755-7.
82. Fliser D, Ritz E. Serum cystatin C concentration as a marker of renal dysfunction in the elderly. Am J Kidney Dis 2001;37:79-83.
83. Flodin M, Larsson A. Performance evaluation of a particle-enhanced turbidimetric cystatin C assay on the Abbott CI8200 analyzer. Clin Biochem 2009;42:873-6.
84. Fontsere N, Salinas I, Bonal J, Bayes B, Riba J, Torres F, et al. Are prediction equations for glomerular filtration rate useful for the long-term monitoring of type 2 diabetic patients? Nephrol Dial Transplant 2006;21:2152-8.
85. Ford L, Berg J. Delay in separating blood samples affects creatinine measurement using the Roche kinetic Jaffe method. Ann Clin Biochem 2008;45:83-7.
86. Forman JP, Fisher ND, Schopick EL, Curhan GC. Higher levels of albuminuria within the normal range predict incident hypertension. J Am Soc Nephrol 2008;19:1983-8.
87. Fossati P, Ponti M, Passoni G, Tarenghi G, Melzi d'Eril GV, Prencipe L. A step forward in enzymatic measurement of creatinine. Clin Chem 1994;40:130-7.
88. Fossati P, Prencipe L, Berti G. Use of 3,5-dichloro-2-hydroxybenzenesulfonic acid/4-aminophenazone chromogenic system in direct enzymic assay of uric acid in serum and urine. Clin Chem 1980;26:227-31.
89. Fossati P, Prencipe L, Berti G. Enzymic creatinine assay: a new colorimetric method based on hydrogen peroxide measurement. Clin Chem 1983;29:1494-6.
90. Fricker M, Wiesli P, Brandle M, Schwegler B, Schmid C. Impact of thyroid dysfunction on serum cystatin C. Kidney Int 2003;63:1944-7.
91. Froissart M, Rossert J, Jacquot C, Paillard M, Houillier P. Predictive performance of the modification of diet in renal disease and Cockcroft-Gault equations for estimating renal function. J Am Soc Nephrol 2005;16:763-73.
92. Garred LJ, Canaud B, Bosc JY, Tetta C. Urea rebound and delivered Kt/V determination with a continuous urea sensor. Nephrol Dial Transplant 1997;12:535-42.
93. Gaspari F, Perico N, Matalone M, Signorini O, Azzollini N, Mister M, et al. Precision of plasma clearance of iohexol for estimation of GFR in patients with renal disease. J Am Soc Nephrol 1998;9:310-3.
94. Gaspari F, Perico N, Ruggenenti P, Mosconi L, Amuchastegui CS, Guerini E, et al. Plasma clearance of nonradioactive iohexol as a measure of glomerular filtration rate. J Am Soc Nephrol 1995;6: 257-63.
95. Gatling W, Knight C, Mullee MA, Hill RD. Microalbuminuria in diabetes: a population study of the prevalence and an assessment of three screening tests. Diabet Med 1988;5:343-7.
96. Ginsberg JM, Chang BS, Matarese RA, Garella S. Use of single voided urine samples to estimate quantitative proteinuria. N Engl J Med 1983;309:1543-6.

97. Goldberg TH, Finkelstein MS. Difficulties in estimating glomerular filtration rate in the elderly. Arch Intern Med 1987;147:1430-3.
98. Goldman R. Creatinine excretion in renal failure. Proc Soc Exp Biol Med 1954;85:446-8.
99. Gosling P. Microalbuminuria: a sensitive indicator of non-renal disease? Ann Clin Biochem 1995;32:439-41.
100. Gourmelin Y, Gouget B, Truchaud A. Electrode measurement of glucose and urea in undiluted samples. Clin Chem 1990;36:1646-9.
101. Gray MR, Phillips E, Young DM, Price CP. Evaluation of a rapid specific ward based assay for creatinine in blood. Clin Nephrol 1995;43:169-73.
102. Graziani MS, Gambaro G, Mantovani L, Sorio A, Yabarek T, Abaterusso C, et al. Diagnostic accuracy of a reagent strip for assessing urinary albumin excretion in the general population. Nephrol Dial Transplant 2009;24:1490-4.
103. Gross JL, de Azevedo MJ, Silveiro SP, Canani LH, Caramori ML, Zelmanovitz T. Diabetic nephropathy: diagnosis, prevention, and treatment. Diabetes Care 2005;28:164-76.
104. Grubb A. Diagnostic value of analysis of cystatin C and protein HC in biological fluids. Clin Nephrol 1992;38(Suppl 1):S20-7.
105. Grubb A, Nyman U, Bjork J, Lindstrom V, Rippe B, Sterner G, et al. Simple cystatin C-based prediction equations for glomerular filtration rate compared with the modification of diet in renal disease prediction equation for adults and the Schwartz and the Counahan-Barratt prediction equations for children. Clin Chem 2005;51:1420-31.
106. Guder WG, Hoffmann GE, Hubbuch A, Poppe WA, Siedel J, Price CP. Multicentre evaluation of an enzymatic method for creatinine determination using a sensitive colour reagent. J Clin Chem Clin Biochem 1986;24:889-902.
107. Guy M, Newall R, Borzomato J, Kalra PA, Price C. Diagnostic accuracy of the urinary albumin:creatinine ratio determined by the CLINITEK Microalbumin and DCA 2000+ for the rule-out of albuminuria in chronic kidney disease. Clin Chim Acta 2009;399:54-8.
108. Guy M, Newall R, Borzomato J, Kalra PA, Price C. Use of a first-line urine protein-to-creatinine ratio strip test on random urines to rule out proteinuria in patients with chronic kidney disease. Nephrol Dial Transplant 2009;24:1189-93.
109. Gyure WL. Comparison of several methods for semiquantitative determination of urinary protein. Clin Chem 1977;23:876-9.
110. Hallan S, Astor B, Romundstad S, Aasarod K, Kvenild K, Coresh J. Association of kidney function and albuminuria with cardiovascular mortality in older vs younger individuals: the HUNT II study. Arch Intern Med 2007;167:2490-6.
111. Han WK, Waikar SS, Johnson A, Betensky RA, Dent CL, Devarajan P, et al. Urinary biomarkers in the early diagnosis of acute kidney injury. Kidney Int 2008;73:863-9.
112. Harmoinen A, Sillanaukee P, Jokela H. Determination of creatinine in serum and urine by cation-exchange high-pressure liquid chromatography. Clin Chem 1991;37:563-5.
113. He D, Zhang Z, Huang Y, Hu Y, Zhou H, Chen D. Chemiluminescence microflow injection analysis system on a chip for the determination of uric acid without enzyme. Luminescence 2005;20:271-5.
114. Heick HM, Begin-Heick N, Acharya C, Mohammed A. Automated determination of urine and cerebrospinal fluid proteins with Coomassie Brilliant Blue and the Abbott ABA-100. Clin Biochem 1980;13:81-3.
115. Helin I, Axenram M, Grubb A. Serum cystatin C as a determinant of glomerular filtration rate in children. Clin Nephrol 1998;49:221-5.
116. Herget-Rosenthal S, Poppen D, Husing J, Marggraf G, Pietruck F, Jakob HG, et al. Prognostic value of tubular proteinuria and enzymuria in nonoliguric acute tubular necrosis. Clin Chem 2004;50:552-8.
117. Heymsfield SB, Arteaga C, McManus C, Smith J, Moffitt S. Measurement of muscle mass in humans: validity of the 24-hour urinary creatinine method. Am J Clin Nutr 1983;37:478-94.
118. Hillege HL, Fidler V, Diercks GF, van Gilst WH, de Zeeuw D, van Veldhuisen DJ, et al. Urinary albumin excretion predicts cardiovascular and noncardiovascular mortality in general population. Circulation 2002;106:1777-82.
119. Hillege HL, Janssen WM, Bak AA, Diercks GF, Grobbee DE, Crijns HJ, et al. Microalbuminuria is common, also in a nondiabetic, nonhypertensive population, and an independent indicator of cardiovascular risk factors and cardiovascular morbidity. J Intern Med 2001;249:519-26.
120. Hoek FJ, Kemperman FA, Krediet RT. A comparison between cystatin C, plasma creatinine and the Cockcroft and Gault formula for the estimation of glomerular filtration rate. Nephrol Dial Transplant 2003;18:2024-31.
121. Hofmann W, Regenbogen C, Edel H, Guder WG. Diagnostic strategies in urinalysis. Kidney Int Suppl 1994;47:S111-4.
122. Houlihan C, Jenkins M, Osicka T, Scott A, Parkin D, Jerums G. A comparison of the plasma disappearance of iohexol and 99mTc-DTPA for the measurement of glomerular filtration rate (GFR) in diabetes. Aust N Z J Med 1999;29:693-700.
123. Hoyer JR, Seiler MW. Pathophysiology of Tamm-Horsfall protein. Kidney Int 1979;16:279-89.
124. Hoyer JR, Sisson SP, Vernier RL. Tamm-Horsfall glycoprotein: ultrastructural immunoperoxidase localization in rat kidney. Lab Invest 1979;41:168-73.
125. Hsu CY, Chertow GM, Curhan GC. Methodological issues in studying the epidemiology of mild to moderate chronic renal insufficiency. Kidney Int 2002;61:1567-76.
126. Hullin DA, McGrane MT. Effect of bilirubin on uricase-peroxidase coupled reactions: implications for urate measurement in clinical samples and external quality assessment schemes. Ann Clin Biochem 1991;28:98-100.
127. Hutchison AS, O'Reilly DS, MacCuish AC. Albumin excretion rate, albumin concentration, and albumin/creatinine ratio compared for screening diabetics for slight albuminuria. Clin Chem 1988;34:2019-21.
128. Ingebretsen OC, Borgen J, Farstad M. Uric acid determinations: reversed-phase liquid chromatography with ultraviolet detection compared with kinetic and equilibrium adaptations of the uricase method. Clin Chem 1982;28:496-8.
129. Iseki K, Ikemiya Y, Iseki C, Takishita S. Proteinuria and the risk of developing end-stage renal disease. Kidney Int 2003;63:1468-74.
130. Iseki K, Kinjo K, Iseki C, Takishita S. Relationship between predicted creatinine clearance and proteinuria and the risk of developing ESRD in Okinawa, Japan. Am J Kidney Dis 2004;44:806-14.
131. Ishani A, Grandits GA, Grimm RH, Svendsen KH, Collins AJ, Prineas RJ, et al. Association of single measurements of dipstick proteinuria, estimated glomerular filtration rate, and hematocrit with 25-year incidence of end-stage renal disease in the multiple risk factor intervention trial. J Am Soc Nephrol 2006;17:1444-52.
132. Ivandic M, Hofmann W, Guder WG. Development and evaluation of a urine protein expert system. Clin Chem 1996;42:1214-22.
133. Jackle-Meyer I, Szukics B, Neubauer K, Metze V, Petzoldt R, Stolte H. Extracellular matrix proteins as early markers in diabetic nephropathy. Eur J Clin Chem Clin Biochem 1995;33:211-9.
134. Jacobsen FK, Christensen CK, Mogensen CE, Andreasen F, Heilskov NS. Pronounced increase in serum creatinine concentration after eating cooked meat. Br Med J 1979;1:1049-50.
135. Jacobsen FK, Christensen CK, Mogensen CE, Heilskov NS. Evaluation of kidney function after meals. Lancet 1980;1:319.
136. Jacobsson B, Lignelid H, Bergerheim US. Transthyretin and cystatin C are catabolized in proximal tubular epithelial cells and the proteins are not useful as markers for renal cell carcinomas. Histopathology 1995;26:559-64.
137. James DR, Price CP. Interference in colorimetric reactions for measuring hydrogen peroxide. Ann Clin Biochem 1984;21(Pt 5):398-404.
138. James GP, Bee DE, Fuller JB. Proteinuria: accuracy and precision of laboratory diagnosis by dip-stick analysis. Clin Chem 1978;24:1934-9.

139. Jayagopal V, Keevil BG, Atkin SL, Jennings PE, Kilpatrick ES. Paradoxical changes in cystatin C and serum creatinine in patients with hypo- and hyperthyroidism. Clin Chem 2003;49:680-1.
140. Jenkins MA, Houlihan C, Ratnaike S, Jerums G, Des Parkin J. Measurement of iohexol by capillary electrophoresis: minimizing practical problems encountered. Ann Clin Biochem 2000;37:529-36.
141. Jensen JS, Borch-Johnsen K, Jensen G, Feldt-Rasmussen B. Microalbuminuria reflects a generalized transvascular albumin leakiness in clinically healthy subjects. Clin Sci (Lond) 1995;88:629-33.
142. Jones CA, Francis ME, Eberhardt MS, Chavers B, Coresh J, Engelgau M, et al. Microalbuminuria in the US population: third National Health and Nutrition Examination Survey. Am J Kidney Dis 2002;39: 445-59.
143. Jung K, Pergande M, Priem F, Becker S, Klotzek S. Rapid screening of low molecular mass proteinuria: evaluation of the first immunochemical test strip for the detection of alpha 1-microglobulin in urine. Eur J Clin Chem Clin Biochem 1993;31:683-7.
144. Kadinger CL, O'Kell RT. Clinical evaluation of Eastman Kodak's Ektachem 400 Analyzer. Clin Chem 1983;29:498-501.
145. Kageyama N. A direct colorimetric determination of uric acid in serum and urine with uricase-catalase system. Clin Chim Acta 1971;31:421-6.
146. Karmen A, Lent R. Clinical chemistry testing with the Ames SERALYZER dry reagent system. J Clin Lab Autom 1982;2:284-90.
147. Kassirer JP. Clinical evaluation of kidney function—glomerular function. N Engl J Med 1971;285:385-9.
148. Keane WF, Eknoyan G. Proteinuria, albuminuria, risk, assessment, detection, elimination (PARADE): a position paper of the National Kidney Foundation. Am J Kidney Dis 1999;33:1004-10.
149. Kenny LC, Broadhurst D, Brown M, Dunn WB, Redman CW, Kell DB, et al. Detection and identification of novel metabolomic biomarkers in preeclampsia. Reprod Sci 2008;15:591-7.
150. Kessler A, Siekmann L. Measurement of urea in human serum by isotope dilution mass spectrometry: a reference procedure. Clin Chem 1999;45:1523-9.
151. Kharbanda R, Lauder J, Thomson D, Gouldesbrough DR, Harrison DJ. Heterogeneity of glutathione S-transferase isoenzyme expression in renal disease. Nephrol Dial Transplant 1991;6:695-700.
152. Knapp ML, Mayne PD. Development of an automated kinetic Jaffe method designed to minimise bilirubin interference in plasma creatinine assays. Clin Chim Acta 1987;168:239-46.
153. Kouri T, Solakivi T, Harmoinen A. Performance of NycoCard U-Albumin and Micral-Test rapid methods for detecting microalbuminuria. Eur J Clin Chem Clin Biochem 1994;32:419-23.
154. Kroll MH, Elin RJ. Interference with clinical laboratory analyses. Clin Chem 1994;40:1996-2005.
155. Kronborg J, Solbu M, Njolstad I, Toft I, Eriksen BO, Jenssen T. Predictors of change in estimated GFR: a population-based 7-year follow-up from the Tromso study. Nephrol Dial Transplant 2008;23: 2818-26.
156. Krutzen E, Back SE, Nilsson-Ehle I, Nilsson-Ehle P. Plasma clearance of a new contrast agent, iohexol: a method for the assessment of glomerular filtration rate. J Lab Clin Med 1984;104:955-61.
157. Kutter D, Thoma J, Kremer A, Hansen S, Carl R. Screening for oligoalbuminuria by means of Micral-Test II: a new immunological test strip. Eur J Clin Chem Clin Biochem 1995;33:243-5.
158. Kyhse-Andersen J, Schmidt C, Nordin G, Andersson B, Nilsson-Ehle P, Lindstrom V, et al. Serum cystatin C, determined by a rapid, automated particle-enhanced turbidimetric method, is a better marker than serum creatinine for glomerular filtration rate. Clin Chem 1994;40:1921-6.
159. Lamb EJ. Effect of a compensated Jaffe creatinine method on the estimation of glomerular filtration rate. Ann Clin Biochem 2005;42: 160-1; author reply 161-2.
160. Lamb EJ. United Kingdom guidelines for chronic kidney disease. Scand J Clin Lab Invest Suppl 2008;241:16-22.
161. Lamb EJ, Mackenzie F, Stevens PE. How should proteinuria be detected and measured? Ann Clin Biochem 2009;46:205-17.
162. Lamb EJ, Price CP. Use of azure-D2 for the measurement of uric acid in serum. Eur J Clin Chem Clin Biochem 1995;33:595-601.
163. Lamb EJ, Tomson CR, Roderick PJ. Estimating kidney function in adults using formulae. Ann Clin Biochem 2005;42:321-45.
164. Lamb EJ, Webb MC, O'Riordan SE. Using the modification of diet in renal disease (MDRD) and Cockcroft and Gault equations to estimate glomerular filtration rate (GFR) in older people. Age Ageing 2007;36: 689-92.
165. Lamb EJ, Webb MC, Simpson DE, Coakley AJ, Newman DJ, O'Riordan SE. Estimation of glomerular filtration rate in older patients with chronic renal insufficiency: is the modification of diet in renal disease formula an improvement? J Am Geriatr Soc 2003;51: 1012-7.
166. Larsson A, Malm J, Grubb A, Hansson LO. Calculation of glomerular filtration rate expressed in mL/min from plasma cystatin C values in mg/L. Scand J Clin Lab Invest 2004;64:25-30.
167. Laterza OF, Price CP, Scott MG. Cystatin C: an improved estimator of glomerular filtration rate? Clin Chem 2002;48:699-707.
168. Lawson N, Lang T, Broughton A, Prinsloo P, Turner C, Marenah C. Creatinine assays: time for action? Ann Clin Biochem 2002;39: 599-602.
169. Le Bricon T, Erlich D, Bengoufa D, Dussaucy M, Garnier JP, Bousquet B. Sodium dodecyl sulfate-agarose gel electrophoresis of urinary proteins: application to multiple myeloma. Clin Chem 1998;44:1191-7.
170. Le Bricon T, Thervet E, Froissart M, Benlakehal M, Bousquet B, Legendre C, et al. Plasma cystatin C is superior to 24-h creatinine clearance and plasma creatinine for estimation of glomerular filtration rate 3 months after kidney transplantation. Clin Chem 2000;46:1206-7.
171. Leanos-Miranda A, Marquez-Acosta J, Romero-Arauz F, Cardenas-Mondragon GM, Rivera-Leanos R, Isordia-Salas I, et al. Protein:creatinine ratio in random urine samples is a reliable marker of increased 24-hour protein excretion in hospitalized women with hypertensive disorders of pregnancy. Clin Chem 2007;53:1623-8.
172. Leary NO, Pembroke A, Duggan PF. Adapting the uricase/peroxidase procedure for plasma urate to reduce interference due to haemolysis, icterus or lipaemia. Ann Clin Biochem 1992;29:85-9.
173. Lemann J Jr, Doumas BT. Proteinuria in health and disease assessed by measuring the urinary protein/creatinine ratio. Clin Chem 1987;33:297-9.
174. Lespinas F, Dupuy G, Revol F, Aubry C. Enzymic urea assay: a new colorimetric method based on hydrogen peroxide measurement. Clin Chem 1989;35:654-8.
175. Levey AS, Bosch JP, Lewis JB, Greene T, Rogers N, Roth D. A more accurate method to estimate glomerular filtration rate from serum creatinine: a new prediction equation. Modification of Diet in Renal Disease Study Group. Ann Intern Med 1999;130:461-70.
176. Levey AS, Coresh J, Greene T, Marsh J, Stevens LA, Kusek JW, et al. Expressing the Modification of Diet in Renal Disease Study equation for estimating glomerular filtration rate with standardized serum creatinine values. Clin Chem 2007;53:766-72.
177. Levey AS, Coresh J, Greene T, Stevens LA, Zhang YL, Hendriksen S, et al. Using standardized serum creatinine values in the modification of diet in renal disease study equation for estimating glomerular filtration rate. Ann Intern Med 2006;145:247-54.
178. Levey AS, Eckardt KU, Tsukamoto Y, Levin A, Coresh J, Rossert J, et al. Definition and classification of chronic kidney disease: a position statement from Kidney Disease: Improving Global Outcomes (KDIGO). Kidney Int 2005;67:2089-100.
179. Levey AS, Greene T, Kusek JW, Beck GJ. A simplified equation to predict glomerular filtration rate from serum creatinine. J Am Soc Nephrol 2000;11(Suppl):155A.
180. Levey AS, Stevens LA, Schmid CH, Zhang YL, Castro AF 3rd, Feldman HI, et al. A new equation to estimate glomerular filtration rate. Ann Intern Med 2009;150:604-12.
181. Lind T, Godfrey KA, Otun H, Philips PR. Changes in serum uric acid concentrations during normal pregnancy. Br J Obstet Gynaecol 1984;91:128-32.

182. Linko S, Kouri TT, Toivonen E, Ranta PH, Chapoulaud E, Lalla M. Analytical performance of the Iris iQ200 automated urine microscopy analyzer. Clin Chim Acta 2006;372:54-64.
183. Linnet K, Bruunshuus I. HPLC with enzymatic detection as a candidate reference method for serum creatinine. Clin Chem 1991;37: 1669-75.
184. Loun B, Copeland KR, Sedor FA. Ultrafiltration discrepancies in recovery of myoglobin from urine. Clin Chem 1996;42:965-9.
185. Lowry OH, Rosebrough NJ, Farr AL, Randall RJ. Protein measurement with the Folin phenol reagent. J Biol Chem 1951;193: 265-75.
186. Ma YC, Zuo L, Chen JH, Luo Q, Yu XQ, Li Y, et al. Modified glomerular filtration rate estimating equation for Chinese patients with chronic kidney disease. J Am Soc Nephrol 2006;17:2937-44.
187. Magliano DJ, Polkinghorne KR, Barr EL, Su Q, Chadban SJ, Zimmet PZ, et al. HPLC-detected albuminuria predicts mortality. J Am Soc Nephrol 2007;18:3171-6.
188. Marshall SM. Screening for microalbuminuria: which measurement? Diabet Med 1991;8:706-11.
189. Marshall SM, Alberti KG. Screening for early diabetic nephropathy. Ann Clin Biochem 1986;23:195-7.
190. Marshall T, Williams KM. Total protein determination in urine: elimination of a differential response between the coomassie blue and pyrogallol red protein dye-binding assays. Clin Chem 2000;46: 392-8.
191. Marshall T, Williams KM. Extent of aminoglycoside interference in the pyrogallol red-molybdate protein assay depends on the concentration of sodium oxalate in the dye reagent. Clin Chem 2004;50:934-5.
192. Mathew TH, Johnson DW, Jones GR. Chronic kidney disease and automatic reporting of estimated glomerular filtration rate: revised recommendations. Med J Aust 2007;187:459-63.
193. Mathies JC. Adaptation of the Berthelot color reaction for the determination of urea nitrogen in serum and urine to an ultramicro system. Clin Chem 1964;10:366-9.
194. Mattix HJ, Hsu CY, Shaykevich S, Curhan G. Use of the albumin/creatinine ratio to detect microalbuminuria: implications of sex and race. J Am Soc Nephrol 2002;13:1034-9.
195. Mauck JC, Mauck L, Novros J, Norton GE. Development of a single-slide KODAK EKTACHEM thin film assay for serum and urine creatinine [abstract]. Clin Chem 1986;32:1197-8.
196. Mayersohn M, Conrad KA, Achari R. The influence of a cooked meat meal on creatinine plasma concentration and creatinine clearance. Br J Clin Pharmacol 1983;15:227-30.
197. Mayo S, Acevedo D, Quinones-Torrelo C, Canos I, Sancho M. Clinical laboratory automated urinalysis: comparison among automated microscopy, flow cytometry, two test strips analyzers, and manual microscopic examination of the urine sediments. J Clin Lab Anal 2008;22:262-70.
198. McDowell TL. Benzethonium chloride method for proteins adapted to centrifugal analysis. Clin Chem 1985;31:864-6.
199. McElderry LA, Tarbit IF, Cassells-Smith AJ. Six methods for urinary protein compared. Clin Chem 1982;28:356-60.
200. Medicines and Healthcare Products Regulatory Agency. Point of care devices for the detection and semi-quantitation of microalbuminuria. Victoria, London, United Kingdom: MHRA, 2004.
201. Medicines and Healthcare Products Regulatory Agency. Point of care devices for the quantitation of microalbuminuria. Victoria, London, United Kingdom: MHRA, 2004.
202. Miller BF, Winkler AW. The renal excretion of endogenous creatinine in man: comparison with exogenous creatinine and inulin. J Clin Invest 1938;17:31-40.
203. Miller WG. Urine albumin: recommendations for standardization. Scand J Clin Lab Invest Suppl 2008;241:71-2.
204. Miller WG. Estimating equations for glomerular filtration rate in children: laboratory considerations. Clin Chem 2009;55:402-3.
205. Miller WG. Estimating glomerular filtration rate. Clin Chem Lab Med 2009;47:1017-9.
206. Miller WG, Bruns DE, Hortin GL, Sandberg S, Aakre KM, McQueen MJ, et al. Current issues in measurement and reporting of urinary albumin excretion. Clin Chem 2009;55:24-38.
207. Miller WG, Myers GL, Ashwood ER, Killeen AA, Wang E, Thienpont LM, et al. Creatinine measurement: state of the art in accuracy and interlaboratory harmonization. Arch Pathol Lab Med 2005;129: 297-304.
208. Mock T, Morrison D, Yatscoff R. Evaluation of the i-STAT system: a portable chemistry analyzer for the measurement of sodium, potassium, chloride, urea, glucose, and hematocrit. Clin Biochem 1995;28:187-92.
209. Mogensen CE, Vestbo E, Poulsen PL, Christiansen C, Damsgaard EM, Eiskjaer H, et al. Microalbuminuria and potential confounders: a review and some observations on variability of urinary albumin excretion. Diabetes Care 1995;18:572-81.
210. Morishita Y, Nakane K, Fukatsu T, Nakashima N, Tsuji K, Soya Y, et al. Kinetic assay of serum and urine for urea with use of urease and leucine dehydrogenase. Clin Chem 1997;43:1932-6.
211. Murthy K, Stevens LA, Stark PC, Levey AS. Variation in the serum creatinine assay calibration: a practical application to glomerular filtration rate estimation. Kidney Int 2005;68:1884-7.
212. Myers GL, Miller WG, Coresh J, Fleming J, Greenberg N, Greene T, et al. Recommendations for improving serum creatinine measurement: a report from the Laboratory Working Group of the National Kidney Disease Education Program. Clin Chem 2006;52: 5-18.
213. Naslund B, Stahle L, Lundin A, Anderstam B, Arner P, Bergstrom J. Luminometric single step urea assay using ATP-hydrolyzing urease. Clin Chem 1998;44:1964-73.
214. National Academy of Clinical Biochemistry. Renal Function Testing. Clarke W, Frost SJ, Kraus E, Ferris M, Jaar B, Wu J, Humbertson S, Dyer K, Schmith E, Gallagher K. In: Nichols JH (editor). Evidence-Based Practice for Point-of-Care Testing. Chapter 12. 2007;126-34.
215. National Institute for Health and Clinical Excellence. Type 1 Diabetes: Diagnosis and Management of Type 1 Diabetes in Children, Young People and Adults. Clinical Guideline 15, 2004.
216. National Institute for Health and Clinical Excellence. Chronic Kidney Disease: National Clinical Guideline for Early Identification and Management in Adults in Primary and Secondary Care. Clinical Guideline 73, 2008.
217. National Institute for Health and Clinical Excellence. Type 2 diabetes: the management of type 2 diabetes. Clinical Guideline 66, 2008.
218. National Kidney Foundation. Clinical practice guidelines for chronic kidney disease: evaluation classification and stratification. Am J Kidney Dis 2002;39:S1-266.
219. Neild GH, Foxall PJ, Lindon JC, Holmes EC, Nicholson JK. Uroscopy in the 21st century: high-field NMR spectroscopy. Nephrol Dial Transplant 1997;12:404-17.
220. Newman DJ. Cystatin C. Ann Clin Biochem 2002;39:89-104.
221. Newman DJ, Mattock MB, Dawnay AB, Kerry S, McGuire A, Yaqoob M, et al. Systematic review on urine albumin testing for early detection of diabetic complications. Health Technol Assess 2005;9: iii-vi, xiii-163.
222. Newman DJ, Pugia MJ, Lott JA, Wallace JF, Hiar AM. Urinary protein and albumin excretion corrected by creatinine and specific gravity. Clin Chim Acta 2000;294:139-55.
223. Newman DJ, Thakkar H, Edwards RG, Wilkie M, White T, Grubb AO, et al. Serum cystatin C measured by automated immunoassay: a more sensitive marker of changes in GFR than serum creatinine. Kidney Int 1995;47:312-8.
224. Newman DJ, Thakkar H, Medcalf EA, Gray MR, Price CP. Use of urine albumin measurement as a replacement for total protein. Clin Nephrol 1995;43:104-9.
225. Nickolas TL, O'Rourke MJ, Yang J, Sise ME, Canetta PA, Barasch N, et al. Sensitivity and specificity of a single emergency department measurement of urinary neutrophil gelatinase-associated lipocalin for diagnosing acute kidney injury. Ann Intern Med 2008;148:810-9.

226. Niculescu-Duvaz I, D'Mello L, Maan Z, Barron JL, Newman DJ, Dockrell ME, et al. Development of an outpatient finger-prick glomerular filtration rate procedure suitable for epidemiological studies. Kidney Int 2006;69:1272-5.
227. Nishi HH, Elin RJ. Three turbidimetric methods for determining total protein compared. Clin Chem 1985;31:1377-80.
228. O'Leary N, Pembroke A, Duggan PF. A simplified procedure for eliminating the negative interference of bilirubin in the Jaffe reaction for creatinine. Clin Chem 1992;38:1749-51.
229. O'Riordan SE, Webb MC, Stowe HJ, Simpson DE, Kandarpa M, Coakley AJ, et al. Cystatin C improves the detection of mild renal dysfunction in older patients. Ann Clin Biochem 2003;40:648-55.
230. Obermayr RP, Temml C, Knechtelsdorfer M, Gutjahr G, Kletzmayr J, Heiss S, et al. Predictors of new-onset decline in kidney function in a general middle-european population. Nephrol Dial Transplant 2008;23:1265-73.
231. Orsonneau JL, Douet P, Massoubre C, Lustenberger P, Bernard S. An improved pyrogallol red-molybdate method for determining total urinary protein. Clin Chem 1989;35:2233-6.
232. Osicka TM, Comper WD. Characterization of immunochemically nonreactive urinary albumin. Clin Chem 2004;50:2286-91.
233. Ota H, Yasuma A. Lysozyme activity in hematologic and non-hematologic disorders with special reference to reactive monocytosis associated with chronic infections and inflammatory reactions. Tohoku J Exp Med 1974;114:15-26.
234. Ottiger C, Huber AR. Quantitative urine particle analysis: integrative approach for the optimal combination of automation with UF-100 and microscopic review with KOVA cell chamber. Clin Chem 2003;49:617-23.
235. Panteghini M, Myers GL, Miller WG, Greenberg N. The importance of metrological traceability on the validity of creatinine measurement as an index of renal function. Clin Chem Lab Med 2006;44:1287-92.
236. Parekh AC, Sims C. Serum creatinine assay by use of 3,5-dinitrobenzoates: a critique. Clin Chem 1977;23:2066-71.
237. Paroni R, Arcelloni C, Fermo I, Bonini PA. Determination of creatinine in serum and urine by a rapid liquid-chromatographic method. Clin Chem 1990;36:830-6.
238. Parsons M, Newman DJ, Pugia M, Newall RG, Price CP. Performance of a reagent strip device for quantitation of the urine albumin: creatinine ratio in a point of care setting. Clin Nephrol 1999;51: 220-7.
239. Parsons MP, Newman DJ, Newall RG, Price CP. Validation of a point-of-care assay for the urinary albumin:creatinine ratio. Clin Chem 1999;45:414-7.
240. Pasternack A, Kuhlback B. Diurnal variations of serum and urine creatine and creatinine. Scand J Clin Lab Invest 1971;27:1-7.
241. Payn MM, Webb MC, Lawrence D, Lamb EJ. Alpha1-microglobulin is stable in human urine ex vivo. Clin Chem 2002;48:1136-8.
242. Payne RB. Creatinine clearance: a redundant clinical investigation. Ann Clin Biochem 1986;23:243-50.
243. Pergande M, Jung K, Precht S, Fels LM, Herbort C, Stolte H. Changed excretion of urinary proteins and enzymes by chronic exposure to lead. Nephrol Dial Transplant 1994;9:613-8.
244. Perrone RD, Madias NE, Levey AS. Serum creatinine as an index of renal function: new insights into old concepts. Clin Chem 1992;38: 1933-53.
245. Pocsi I, Taylor SA, Richardson AC, Aamlid KH, Smith BV, Price RG. "VRA-GlcNAc": novel substrate for N-acetyl-beta-D-glucosaminidase applied to assay of this enzyme in urine. Clin Chem 1990;36:1884-8.
246. Poggio ED, Wang X, Greene T, Van Lente F, Hall PM. Performance of the modification of diet in renal disease and Cockcroft-Gault equations in the estimation of GFR in health and in chronic kidney disease. J Am Soc Nephrol 2005;16:459-66.
247. Popper H, Mandel E. Filtrations and reabsorptions leitung in der nierenpathologie. Erg Inn Med Kinder 1937;53:685-95.
248. Preiss DJ, Godber IM, Lamb EJ, Dalton RN, Gunn IR. The influence of a cooked-meat meal on estimated glomerular filtration rate. Ann Clin Biochem 2007;44:35-42.
249. Prescott LF, Freestone S, McAuslane JA. Reassessment of the single intravenous injection method with inulin for measurement of the glomerular filtration rate in man. Clin Sci (Lond) 1991;80:167-76.
250. Price CP, Finney H. Developments in the assessment of glomerular filtration rate. Clin Chim Acta 2000;297:55-66.
251. Price CP, James DR. Analytical reviews in clinical biochemistry: the measurement of urate. Ann Clin Biochem 1988;25:484-98.
252. Price CP, Koller PU. A multicentre study of the new Reflotron system for the measurement of urea, glucose, triacylglycerols, cholesterol, gamma-glutamyltransferase and haemoglobin. J Clin Chem Clin Biochem 1988;26:233-50.
253. Price CP, Newall RG, Boyd JC. Use of protein:creatinine ratio measurements on random urine samples for prediction of significant proteinuria: a systematic review. Clin Chem 2005;51:1577-86.
254. Price RG. The role of NAG (N-acetyl-beta-D-glucosaminidase) in the diagnosis of kidney disease including the monitoring of nephrotoxicity. Clin Nephrol 1992;38(Suppl 1):S14-9.
255. Price RG, Taylor SA, Crutcher E. Assay of laminin fragments in the assessment of renal disease. Kidney Int Suppl 1994;47:S25-8.
256. Priem F, Althaus H, Birnbaum M, Sinha P, Conradt HS, Jung K. Beta-trace protein in serum: a new marker of glomerular filtration rate in the creatinine-blind range. Clin Chem 1999;45:567-8.
257. Pugia MJ, Lott JA, Clark LW, Parker DR, Wallace JF, Willis TW. Comparison of urine dipsticks with quantitative methods for microalbuminuria. Eur J Clin Chem Clin Biochem 1997;35:693-700.
258. Ralston SH, Caine N, Richards I, O'Reilly D, Sturrock RD, Capell HA. Screening for proteinuria in a rheumatology clinic: comparison of dipstick testing, 24 hour urine quantitative protein, and protein/ creatinine ratio in random urine samples. Ann Rheum Dis 1988;47: 759-63.
259. Redman CW, Beilin LJ, Bonnar J, Wilkinson RH. Plasma-urate measurements in predicting fetal death in hypertensive pregnancy. Lancet 1976;1:1370-3.
260. Rehberg P. Studies on kidney function: II. The excretion of urea and chloride analyzed according to a modified filtration reabsorption theory. Biochem J 1926;20:461-82.
261. Rehling M, Moller ML, Thamdrup B, Lund JO, Trap-Jensen J. Simultaneous measurement of renal clearance and plasma clearance of 99mTc-labelled diethylenetriaminepenta-acetate, 51Cr-labelled ethylenediaminetetra-acetate and inulin in man. Clin Sci (Lond) 1984;66:613-9.
262. Remuzzi G, Ruggenenti P, Benigni A. Understanding the nature of renal disease progression. Kidney Int 1997;51:2-15.
263. Ricos C, Jimenez CV, Hernandez A, Simon M, Perich C, Alvarez V, et al. Biological variation in urine samples used for analyte measurements. Clin Chem 1994;40:472-7.
264. Rigalleau V, Lasseur C, Perlemoine C, Barthe N, Raffaitin C, Liu C, et al. Estimation of glomerular filtration rate in diabetic subjects: Cockcroft formula or modification of Diet in Renal Disease study equation? Diabetes Care 2005;28:838-43.
265. Ripamonti M, Mosca A, Rovida E, Luzzana M, Luzi L, Ceriotti F, et al. Urea, creatinine, and glucose determined in plasma and whole blood by a differential pH technique. Clin Chem 1984;30:556-9.
266. Rocco MV, Buckalew VM Jr, Moore LC, Shihabi ZK. Capillary electrophoresis for the determination of glomerular filtration rate using nonradioactive iohexol. Am J Kidney Dis 1996;28:173-7.
267. Rosano TG, Ambrose RT, Wu AH, Swift TA, Yadegari P. Candidate reference method for determining creatinine in serum: method development and interlaboratory validation. Clin Chem 1990;36: 1951-5.
268. Ross JW, Miller WG, Myers GL, Praestgaard J. The accuracy of laboratory measurements in clinical chemistry: a study of 11 routine chemistry analytes in the College of American Pathologists Chemistry Survey with fresh frozen serum, definitive methods, and reference methods. Arch Pathol Lab Med 1998;122:587-608.
269. Rossing P, Rossing K, Gaede P, Pedersen O, Parving HH. Monitoring kidney function in type 2 diabetic patients with incipient and overt diabetic nephropathy. Diabetes Care 2006;29:1024-30.

270. Rowe DJ, Omar H, Barratt SL, Biggs P. An evaluation of blood creatinine measurement by creatinase on the NOVA M7 blood gas analyzer. Clin Chim Acta 2001;307:23-5.
271. Rudd PT, Hughes EA, Placzek MM, Hodes DT. Reference ranges for plasma creatinine during the first month of life. Arch Dis Child 1983;58:212-5.
272. Ruggenenti P, Gaspari F, Perna A, Remuzzi G. Cross sectional longitudinal study of spot morning urine protein:creatinine ratio, 24 hour urine protein excretion rate, glomerular filtration rate, and end stage renal failure in chronic renal disease in patients without diabetes. BMJ 1998;316:504-9.
273. Ruggenenti P, Perna A, Mosconi L, Pisoni R, Remuzzi G. Urinary protein excretion rate is the best independent predictor of ESRF in non-diabetic proteinuric chronic nephropathies. "Gruppo Italiano di Studi Epidemiologici in Nefrologia" (GISEN). Kidney Int 1998;53: 1209-16.
274. Rule AD, Larson TS, Bergstralh EJ, Slezak JM, Jacobsen SJ, Cosio FG. Using serum creatinine to estimate glomerular filtration rate: accuracy in good health and in chronic kidney disease. Ann Intern Med 2004;141:929-37.
275. Rumley A. Urine dipstick testing: comparison of results obtained by visual reading and with the Bayer CLINITEK 50. Ann Clin Biochem 2000;37(Pt 2):220-1.
276. Sampson EJ, Baird MA. Chemical inhibition used in a kinetic urease/glutamate dehydrogenase method for urea in serum. Clin Chem 1979;25:1721-9.
277. Sampson EJ, Baird MA, Burtis CA, Smith EM, Witte DL, Bayse DD. A coupled-enzyme equilibrium method for measuring urea in serum: optimization and evaluation of the AACC study group on urea candidate reference method. Clin Chem 1980;26:816-26.
278. Samuell CT, Kasidas GP. Biochemical investigations in renal stone formers. Ann Clin Biochem 1995;32(Pt 2):112-22.
279. Saudan PJ, Brown MA, Farrell T, Shaw L. Improved methods of assessing proteinuria in hypertensive pregnancy. Br J Obstet Gynaecol 1997;104:1159-64.
280. Schmidt S, Ritz E. The role of angiotensin I-converting enzyme gene polymorphism in renal disease. Curr Opin Nephrol Hypertens 1996;5: 552-5.
281. Schrenkhammer P, Wolfbeis OS. Fully reversible optical biosensors for uric acid using oxygen transduction. Biosens Bioelectron 2008;24: 1000-5.
282. Schwartz GJ, Gauthier B. A simple estimate of glomerular filtration rate in adolescent boys. J Pediatr 1985;106:522-6.
283. Schwartz GJ, Munoz A, Schneider MF, Mak RH, Kaskel F, Warady BA, et al. New equations to estimate GFR in children with CKD. J Am Soc Nephrol 2009;20:629-37.
284. Scott JT. Asymptomatic hyperuricaemia. Br Med J (Clin Res Ed) 1987;294:987-8.
285. Scottish Intercollegiate Guideline Network (SIGN). Diagnosis and management of chronic kidney disease: guideline. Edinburgh, Scotland: SIGN, 2008.
286. Sedmak JJ, Grossberg SE. A rapid, sensitive, and versatile assay for protein using Coomassie brilliant blue G250. Anal Biochem 1977;79: 544-52.
287. Sena SF, Syed D, Romeo R, Krzymowski GA, McComb RB. Lidocaine metabolite and creatinine measurements in the Ektachem 700: steps to minimize its impact on patient care. Clin Chem 1988;34:2144-8.
288. Shaikh A, Seegmiller JC, Borland TM, Burns BE, Ladwig PM, Singh RJ, et al. Comparison between immunoturbidimetry, size-exclusion chromatography, and LC-MS to quantify urinary albumin. Clin Chem 2008;54:1504-10.
289. Shaw RA, Low-Ying S, Leroux M, Mantsch HH. Toward reagent-free clinical analysis: quantitation of urine urea, creatinine, and total protein from the mid-infrared spectra of dried urine films. Clin Chem 2000;46:1493-5.
290. Shemesh O, Golbetz H, Kriss JP, Myers BD. Limitations of creatinine as a filtration marker in glomerulopathic patients. Kidney Int 1985;28: 830-8.
291. Shepherd J, Warner MH, Kilpatrick ES. Stability of creatinine with delayed separation of whole blood and implications for eGFR. Ann Clin Biochem 2007;44:384-7.
292. Shihabi ZK, Konen JC, O'Connor ML. Albuminuria vs urinary total protein for detecting chronic renal disorders. Clin Chem 1991;37: 621-4.
293. Siekmann L. Determination of creatinine in human serum by isotope dilution-mass spectrometry: definitive methods in clinical chemistry, IV. J Clin Chem Clin Biochem 1985;23:137-44.
294. Siekmann L. Determination of uric acid in human serum by isotope dilution-mass spectrometry: definitive methods in clinical chemistry, III. J Clin Chem Clin Biochem 1985;23:129-35.
295. Slack TK, Wilson DM. Normal renal function: CIN and CPAH in healthy donors before and after nephrectomy. Mayo Clin Proc 1976; 51:296-300.
296. Soldin SJ, Hill JG. Micromethod for determination of creatinine in biological fluids by high-performance liquid chromatography. Clin Chem 1978;24:747-50.
297. Spayd RW, Bruschi B, Burdick BA, Dappen GM, Eikenberry JN, Esders TW, et al. Multilayer film elements for clinical analysis: applications to representative chemical determinations. Clin Chem 1978;24:1343-50.
298. Spencer K. Analytical reviews in clinical biochemistry: the estimation of creatinine. Ann Clin Biochem 1986;23:1-25.
299. Spierto FW, MacNeil ML, Culbreth P, Duncan I, Burtis CA. Development and validation of a liquid-chromatographic procedure for serum creatinine. Clin Chem 1980;26:286-90.
300. Stephenson JM, Kenny S, Stevens LK, Fuller JH, Lee E. Proteinuria and mortality in diabetes: the WHO Multinational Study of Vascular Disease in Diabetes. Diabet Med 1995;12:149-55.
301. Stevens JF, Tsang W, Newall RG. Measurement of bilirubin, cholesterol and creatinine in serum and plasma, by solid-phase reflectance spectroscopy. J Clin Pathol 1983;36:598-601.
302. Stevens LA, Coresh J, Levey AS. CKD in the elderly—old questions and new challenges: World Kidney Day 2008. Am J Kidney Dis 2008;51:353-7.
303. Stockl D, Reinauer H. Candidate reference methods for determining target values for cholesterol, creatinine, uric acid, and glucose in external quality assessment and internal accuracy control. I. Method setup. Clin Chem 1993;39:993-1000.
304. Stokes P, O'Connor G. Development of a liquid chromatography-mass spectrometry method for the high-accuracy determination of creatinine in serum. J Chromatogr B Analyt Technol Biomed Life Sci 2003;794:125-36.
305. Stowe H, Lawrence D, Newman DJ, Lamb EJ. Analytical performance of a particle-enhanced nephelometric immunoassay for serum cystatin C using rate analysis. Clin Chem 2001;47:1482-5.
306. Sugita O, Tomiyama Y, Matsuto T, Okada M, Gejyo F, Arakawa M, et al. A new enzymatic method for the determination of inulin. Ann Clin Biochem 1995;32:561-5.
307. Sugita O, Uchiyama K, Yamada T, Sato T, Okada M, Takeuchi K. Reference values of serum and urine creatinine, and of creatinine clearance by a new enzymatic method. Ann Clin Biochem 1992;29: 523-8.
308. Summerfield AL, Hortin GL, Smith CH, Wilhite TR, Landt M. Automated enzymatic analysis of inulin. Clin Chem 1993;39:2333-7.
309. Sundberg MW, Becker RW, Esders TW, Figueras J, Goodhue CT. An enzymic creatinine assay and a direct ammonia assay in coated thin films. Clin Chem 1983;29:645-9.
310. Sviridov D, Drake SK, Hortin GL. Reactivity of urinary albumin (microalbumin) assays with fragmented or modified albumin. Clin Chem 2008;54:61-8.
311. Sviridov D, Meilinger B, Drake SK, Hoehn GT, Hortin GL. Coelution of other proteins with albumin during size-exclusion HPLC: implications for analysis of urinary albumin. Clin Chem 2006;52:389-97.
312. Swain RR, Briggs SL. Positive interference with the Jaffe reaction by cephalosporin antibiotics. Clin Chem 1977;23:1340-2.

313. Swan SK. The search continues—an ideal marker of GFR. Clin Chem 1997;43:913-4.
314. Swedko PJ, Clark HD, Paramsothy K, Akbari A. Serum creatinine is an inadequate screening test for renal failure in elderly patients. Arch Intern Med 2003;163:356-60.
315. Tabata M, Kido T, Totani M, Murachi T. Automated assay of creatinine in serum as simplified by the use of immobilized enzymes, creatinine deiminase, and glutamate dehydrogenase. Anal Biochem 1983;134:44-9.
316. Taylor AJ, Vadgama P. Analytical reviews in clinical biochemistry: the estimation of urea. Ann Clin Biochem 1992;29:245-64.
317. Tenstad O, Roald AB, Grubb A, Aukland K. Renal handling of radiolabelled human cystatin C in the rat. Scand J Clin Lab Invest 1996;56:409-14.
318. Thakkar H, Cornelius J, Dronfield DM, Medcalf EA, Newman DJ, Price CP. Development of a rapid latex enhanced turbidimetric assay for retinol binding protein in urine. Ann Clin Biochem 1991;28(Pt 4):407-11.
319. Thienpont LM, Leenheer AP, Stockl D, Reinauer H. Candidate reference methods for determining target values for cholesterol, creatinine, uric acid, and glucose in external quality assessment and internal accuracy control. II. Method transfer. Clin Chem 1993;39:1001-6.
320. Thienpont LM, Van Landuyt KG, Stockl D, De Leenheer AP. Candidate reference method for determining serum creatinine by isocratic HPLC: validation with isotope dilution gas chromatography-mass spectrometry and application for accuracy assessment of routine test kits. Clin Chem 1995;41:995-1003.
321. Tietz NW. Clinical guide to laboratory tests, 3rd edition. Philadelphia: WB Saunders, 1995.
322. Tietz NW, Shuey DF, Wekstein DR. Laboratory values in fit aging individuals—sexagenarians through centenarians. Clin Chem 1992;38:1167-85.
323. Tsai HC, Doong RA. Simultaneous determination of renal clinical analytes in serum using hydrolase- and oxidase-encapsulated optical array biosensors. Anal Biochem 2004;334:183-92.
324. van Acker BA, Koomen GC, Koopman MG, de Waart DR, Arisz L. Creatinine clearance during cimetidine administration for measurement of glomerular filtration rate. Lancet 1992;340:1326-9.
325. van den Broek D, Keularts IM, Wielders JP, Kraaijenhagen RJ. Benefits of the iQ200 automated urine microscopy analyser in routine urinalysis. Clin Chem Lab Med 2008;46:1635-40.
326. van der Velde M, Halbesma N, de Charro FT, Bakker SJ, de Zeeuw D, de Jong PE, et al. Screening for albuminuria identifies individuals at increased renal risk. J Am Soc Nephrol 2009;20:852-62.
327. Van Pilsum JF, Martin RP, Kito E, Hess J. Determination of creatine, creatinine, arginine, guanidinoacetic acid, guanidine, and methylguanidine in biological fluids. J Biol Chem 1956;222:225-36.
328. van Rossum LK, Mathot RA, Cransberg K, Vulto AG. Optimal sampling strategies to assess inulin clearance in children by the inulin single-injection method. Clin Chem 2003;49:1170-9.
329. Vasiliades J. Reaction of alkaline sodium picrate with creatinine. I. Kinetics and mechanism of formation of the mono-creatinine picric acid complex. Clin Chem 1976;22:1664-71.
330. Verhave JC, Hillege HL, Burgerhof JG, Gansevoort RT, de Zeeuw D, de Jong PE. The association between atherosclerotic risk factors and renal function in the general population. Kidney Int 2005;67:1967-73.
331. Vickery S, Stevens PE, Dalton RN, van Lente F, Lamb EJ. Does the ID-MS traceable MDRD equation work and is it suitable for use with compensated Jaffe and enzymatic creatinine assays? Nephrol Dial Transplant 2006;21:2439-45.
332. Walser M. Assessing renal function from creatinine measurements in adults with chronic renal failure. Am J Kidney Dis 1998;32:23-31.
333. Wasen E, Suominen P, Isoaho R, Mattila K, Virtanen A, Kivela SL, et al. Serum cystatin C as a marker of kidney dysfunction in an elderly population. Clin Chem 2002;48:1138-40.
334. Watanabe N, Kamei S, Ohkubo A, Yamanaka M, Ohsawa S, Makino K, et al. Urinary protein as measured with a pyrogallol red-molybdate complex, manually and in a Hitachi 726 automated analyzer. Clin Chem 1986;32:1551-4.
335. Waugh JJ, Bell SC, Kilby MD, Blackwell CN, Seed P, Shennan AH, et al. Optimal bedside urinalysis for the detection of proteinuria in hypertensive pregnancy: a study of diagnostic accuracy. Br J Obstet Gynaecol 2005;112:412-7.
336. Waugh JJ, Clark TJ, Divakaran TG, Khan KS, Kilby MD. Accuracy of urinalysis dipstick techniques in predicting significant proteinuria in pregnancy. Obstet Gynecol 2004;103:769-77.
337. Weatherburn MW, Trotman RB, Jackson SH. Specific method for serum creatinine determination based on ion exchange chromatography and an automated alkaline picrate reaction—a proposed reference method. Clin Biochem 1978;11:159-66.
338. Weber MH, Verwiebe R. Alpha 1-microglobulin (protein HC): features of a promising indicator of proximal tubular dysfunction. Eur J Clin Chem Clin Biochem 1992;30:683-91.
339. Welch MJ, Cohen A, Hertz HS, Ng KJ, Schaffer R, Van der Lijn P, et al. Determination of serum creatinine by isotope dilution mass spectrometry as a candidate definitive method. Anal Chem 1986;58:1681-5.
340. Whicher JT, Calvin J, Riches P, Warren C. The laboratory investigation of paraproteinaemia. Ann Clin Biochem 1987;24:119-32.
341. White C, Akbari A, Hussain N, Dinh L, Filler G, Lepage N, et al. Estimating glomerular filtration rate in kidney transplantation: a comparison between serum creatinine and cystatin C-based methods. J Am Soc Nephrol 2005;16:3763-70.
342. White RM, Cross RE, Savory J. Enzyme-coupled measurement of uric acid in serum with a centrifugal analyzer. Clin Chem 1977;23:1538-40.
343. Wimsatt DK, Lott JA. Improved measurement of urinary total protein (including light-chain proteins) with a Coomassie brilliant blue G-250-sodium dodecyl sulfate reagent. Clin Chem 1987;33:2100-6.
344. Witte DL, Brown LF, Feld RD. Effects of bilirubin on detection of hydrogen peroxide by use of peroxidase. Clin Chem 1978;24:1778-82.
345. Woolhandler S, Pels RJ, Bor DH, Himmelstein DU, Lawrence RS. Dipstick urinalysis screening of asymptomatic adults for urinary tract disorders. I. Hematuria and proteinuria. JAMA 1989;262:1214-9.
346. Wuyts B, Bernard D, Van den Noortgate N, Van de Walle J, Van Vlem B, De Smet R, et al. Reevaluation of formulas for predicting creatinine clearance in adults and children, using compensated creatinine methods. Clin Chem 2003;49:1011-4.
347. Yagame M, Suzuki D, Jinde K, Saotome N, Sato H, Noguchi M, et al. Significance of urinary type IV collagen in patients with diabetic nephropathy using a highly sensitive one-step sandwich enzyme immunoassay. J Clin Lab Anal 1997;11:110-6.
348. Yasui Y, Tatsumi N, Park K, Koezuka T. Urinary sediment analyzed by flow cytometry. Cytometry 1995;22:75-9.
349. Yilmaz FM, Yucel D. Effect of addition of hemolysate on urine and cerebrospinal fluid assays for protein. Clin Chem 2006;52:152-3.
350. Ylinen EA, Ala-Houhala M, Harmoinen AP, Knip M. Cystatin C as a marker for glomerular filtration rate in pediatric patients. Pediatr Nephrol 1999;13:506-9.
351. Yuen CT, Price RG, Chattagoon L, Richardson AC, Praill PF. Colorimetric assays for *N*-acetyl-beta-D-glucosaminidase and beta-D-galactosidase in human urine using newly-developed omega-nitrostyryl substrates. Clin Chim Acta 1982;124:195-204.
352. Zager RA. Rhabdomyolysis and myohemoglobinuric acute renal failure. Kidney Int 1996;49:314-26.
353. Zhang Y, Wen G, Zhou Y, Shuang S, Dong C, Choi MM. Development and analytical application of an uric acid biosensor using an uricase-immobilized eggshell membrane. Biosens Bioelectron 2007;22:1791-7.
354. Zinellu A, Caria MA, Tavera C, Sotgia S, Chessa R, Deiana L, et al. Plasma creatinine and creatine quantification by capillary electrophoresis diode array detector. Anal Biochem 2005;342:186-93.
355. Zuo L, Ma YC, Zhou YH, Wang M, Xu GB, Wang HY. Application of GFR-estimating equations in Chinese patients with chronic kidney disease. Am J Kidney Dis 2005;45:463-72.

CHAPTER 26

Carbohydrates

*David B. Sacks, M.B., Ch.B., F.R.C.Path.**

Carbohydrates, including sugars and starches, are widely distributed in plants and animals. They perform multiple functions, ranging from being structural components of deoxyribonucleic acid (DNA) and ribonucleic acid (RNA) (*ribose* and *deoxyribose* sugars) to serving as sources of energy *(glucose)*. Glucose is derived from the breakdown of carbohydrates in the diet (grains, starchy vegetables, and legumes) and in body stores (glycogen), and by endogenous synthesis from protein or from the glycerol moiety of triglycerides. When energy intake exceeds expenditure, the excess is converted to fat and glycogen for storage in adipose tissue and liver or muscle, respectively. When energy expenditure exceeds calorie intake, endogenous glucose formation occurs from the breakdown of carbohydrate stores and from noncarbohydrate sources (e.g., amino acids, lactate, glycerol).

The glucose concentration in the blood is maintained within a fairly narrow interval under diverse conditions (feeding, fasting, or severe exercise) by hormones, such as insulin, glucagon, or epinephrine.

Measurement of glucose is one of the most commonly performed analytical procedures. The most frequently encountered disorder of carbohydrate metabolism is high blood glucose concentrations caused by diabetes mellitus, which affects approximately 9% of the U.S. adult population. The incidence of hypoglycemia (low blood glucose) is unknown, but, excluding patients who use exogenous insulin to control blood glucose, it is low.

CHEMISTRY OF CARBOHYDRATES

Carbohydrates are aldehyde or ketone derivatives of polyhydroxy (more than one —OH group), alcohols, or compounds that yield these derivatives on hydrolysis. The term *carbohydrate* refers to hydrates of carbon and is derived from the observation that empirical formulas for these compounds contain approximately one molecule of water per carbon atom. Thus glucose, $C_6H_{12}O_6$, and lactose, $C_{12}H_{22}O_{11}$, are written as $C_6(H_2O)_6$ and $C_{12}(H_2O)_{11}$, respectively. These compounds are not hydrates in the usual chemical sense, however, and noncarbohydrate compounds, such as lactic acid, $CH_3CH(OH)COOH$ or $C_3(H_2O)_3$, can have similar empirical formulas.

Monosaccharides

Monosaccharides, or simple sugars, consist of a single polyhydroxy aldehyde or ketone unit and cannot be hydrolyzed to a simpler form. The backbone is made up of a number of carbon atoms. Sugars containing three, four, five, six, and seven carbon atoms are known as *trioses, tetroses, pentoses, hexoses,* and *heptoses,* respectively. One of the carbon atoms is double bonded to an oxygen atom to form a carbonyl group. An *aldehyde* has the carbonyl group at the end of the carbon chain, whereas if the carbonyl group is at any other position, a *ketone* is formed (Figure 26-1). The simplest carbohydrate is glycol aldehyde, the aldehyde derivative of ethylene glycol. The aldehyde and ketone derivatives of glycerol are, respectively, glyceraldehyde and dihydroxyacetone (see Figure 26-1). Monosaccharides are termed *aldose* or *ketose,* according to the position of the carbonyl group (Figure 26-2).

Compounds that are identical in composition and differ only in spatial configuration are called *stereoisomers.* The carbon atoms in the unbranched chain are numbered, as shown by the numbers at the left of the formula for D-glucose (see Figure 26-2). The designation D or L refers to the position of the hydroxyl group on the carbon atom adjacent to the last (bottom) CH_2OH group. In general, the designation of D or L for a sugar molecule refers to the stereoisomeric forms of the highest-numbered asymmetric carbon atom.* By convention, the D-sugars are written with the hydroxyl group on the right, and the L-sugars are written with the hydroxyl group on the left (see Figure 26-2). Most sugars in the human body are of the D-configuration. Several different structures exist, depending on the relative positions of the hydroxyl groups on the carbon atoms.

**The author gratefully acknowledges the original contributions by Drs. Wendell T. Caraway and Nelson B. Watts on which portions of this chapter are based.*

*Although the D and L designations are retained in this chapter, readers should be aware that in the Cahn-Ingold-Prelog system, a series of sequence rules determine configurations. In this system, the symbols R and S are used to designate configurations instead of D and L.

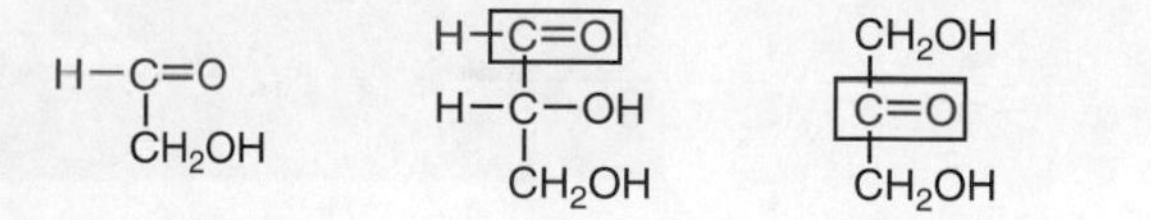

Figure 26-1 Two- and three-carbon carbohydrates.

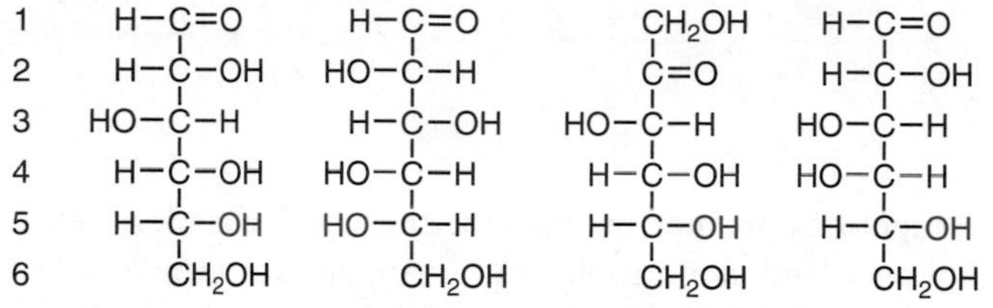

Figure 26-2 Typical six-carbon sugars.

The formula for glucose can be written in the form of aldehyde or enol, a short-lived reactive species. Shift to the enol anion is favored in alkaline solution.

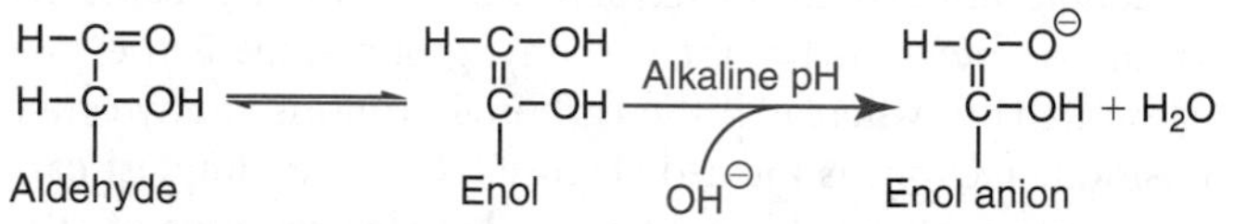

The presence of a double bond and a negative charge in the enol anion makes glucose an active reducing substance that is oxidized by relatively mild oxidizing agents, such as cupric (Cu^{2+}) and ferric (Fe^{3+}) ions. Glucose in hot alkaline solution readily reduces cupric ions to cuprous ions, and the carbonyl carbon is oxidized to carboxylic acid. The color change has been used as a presumptive indication for the presence of glucose, and for many years blood and urine glucose were measured this way. Other sugars reduce cupric ions in alkaline solution.

Aldehyde and alcohol groups react to form hemiacetals. In the case of glucose, the aldehyde group reacts with the hydroxyl group on carbon 5 (Figure 26-3). Note that this ring structure contains an additional asymmetric carbon atom and exists in two stereoisomeric forms. By convention, the form with the hydroxyl group on the right of the first carbon atom is called α-D-glucose, and the form with the hydroxyl group on the left is called β-D-glucose. The common anhydrous crystalline glucose is in the α-D-form. The β-D-form is obtained by crystallization from acetic acid. The two forms differ with respect to optical rotation of polarized light. The specific rotation—$[\alpha]_D^{25°C}$—for the α-D-form is +113°, and for the β-D-form is +19.7°. As a result of mutarotation, either form in aqueous solution gives rise to an equilibrium mixture that has a specific rotation of +52.5°. The equilibrium established at room temperature is such that about 36% of glucose exists in the α-form and 64% in the β-form; only a trace remains in the free aldehyde form. The enzyme glucose oxidase reacts only with β-D-glucose. For this reason, calibrating solutions to be used in glucose oxidase methods for glucose determinations should be permitted to stand at least 2 hours to obtain equilibrium comparable with that in the test samples to be analyzed.

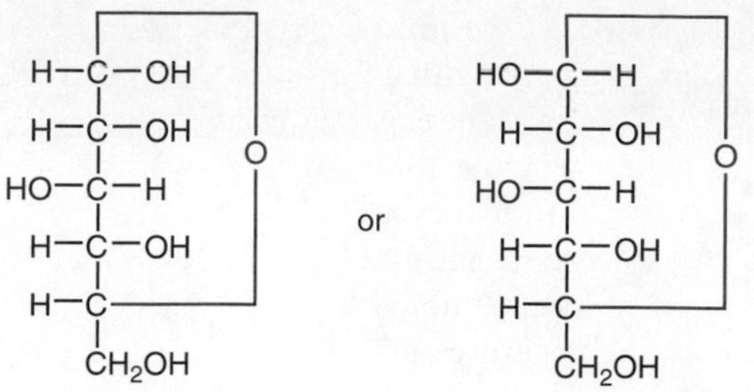

Figure 26-3 Structure of D-glucose (hemiacetal form).

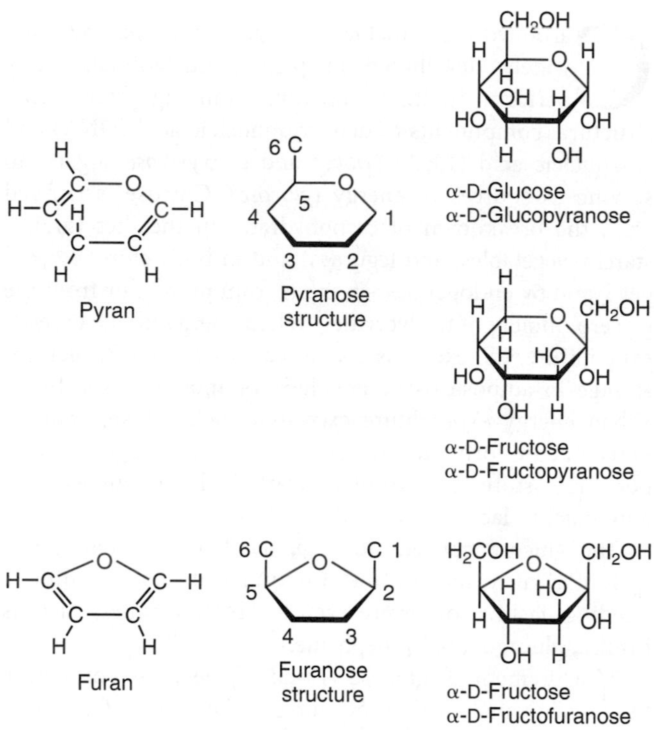

Figure 26-4 The Haworth formula for sugars.

From the ring structures shown in Figure 26-3, it is not apparent why the aldehyde group should react with the distant hydroxyl group on carbon 5. The spatial arrangement of the atoms is better represented by a symmetric ring structure, depicted by the Haworth formula, in which glucose is considered as having the same basic structure as pyran (Figure 26-4). In this formula, the plane of the ring is considered to be perpendicular to the plane of the paper, with heavy lines pointing toward the reader. Hydroxyl groups in position 1 are then below the plane (α-configuration) or above the plane (β-configuration). A six-member ring sugar, containing five carbons and one oxygen, is a derivative of pyran and is called a *pyranose.* When linkage occurs with formation of a five-member ring, containing four carbons and one oxygen, the sugar has the same basic structure as furan and is called a *furanose.* Representative formulas are shown in Figure 26-4. Fructose is shown in two cyclic forms. Fructopyranose is the configuration of free sugar, and fructofuranose occurs whenever fructose exists in combination in disaccharides and polysaccharides, as in sucrose and inulin.

DISACCHARIDES

Two monosaccharides join covalently by an *O-glycosidic bond,* with the loss of a molecule of water, to form a disaccharide. The chemical bond between the sugars always involves the aldehyde or ketone group of one monosaccharide joined to an alcohol group (e.g., maltose) or to an aldehyde or ketone group (e.g., sucrose) of the other monosaccharide. The most common disaccharides are the following:

Maltose = Glucose + Glucose
Lactose = Glucose + Galactose
Sucrose = Glucose + Fructose

Several conventions are followed in the nomenclature of disaccharides (Figure 26-5). The compound is written with the nonreducing end to the left. An *O* precedes the name of the first (left) monosaccharide, emphasizing that the linkage occurs by an oxygen atom. The configuration of the anomeric (carbonyl) carbon is designated α or β. Five- (furanosyl) and six- (pyranosyl) membered rings are distinguished, and carbon atoms joined by the glycosidic bond are identified. Because sucrose has no reducing end, it is written as *O*-α-D-glucopyranosyl-(1 → 2)-β-D-fructofuranose or *O*-β-D-fructofuranosyl-(2 → 1)-α-D-glucopyranose. If the linkage between two monosaccharides is between the aldehyde or ketone group of one molecule and a hydroxyl group of another molecule (as in maltose and lactose), one potentially free ketone or aldehyde group remains on the second monosaccharide. Consequently, the second glucose residue can be oxidized (thus the disaccharide is a reducing sugar) and is capable of existing in α- or β-pyranose form. The reducing power, however, is only approximately 40% of the reducing power of the two single monosaccharides added together, primarily because one of the reducing groups is not available. On the other hand, if the linkage between two monosaccharides involves the aldehyde or ketone groups of both molecules (as in sucrose), a nonreducing sugar results because no free aldehyde or ketone group remains.

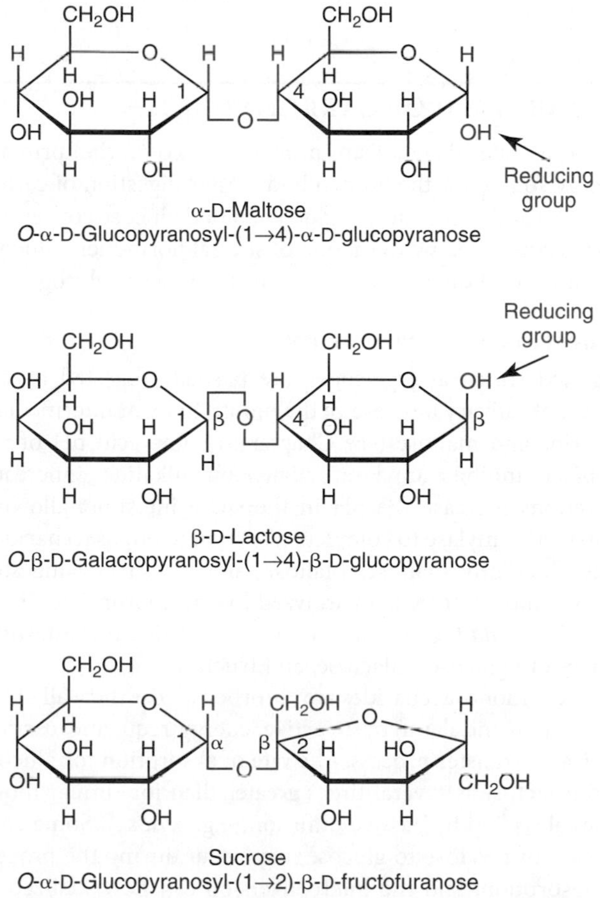

Reducing group
α-D-Maltose
O-α-D-Glucopyranosyl-(1→4)-α-D-glucopyranose

Reducing group
β-D-Lactose
O-β-D-Galactopyranosyl-(1→4)-β-D-glucopyranose

Sucrose
O-α-D-Glucopyranosyl-(1→2)-β-D-fructofuranose

Figure 26-5 Structural formulas of disaccharides.

POLYSACCHARIDES

The linkage of multiple monosaccharide units results in the formation of polysaccharides. The major storage carbohydrates are *starch* in plants and *glycogen* in animals, both of which form granules inside cells. The suffix *-an* attached to the name of a monosaccharide indicates the main type of sugar present in the polysaccharide. Starch and glycogen, for example, are *glucosans,* because they are composed of a series of glucose molecules. Inulin, a polysaccharide found in the tubers of certain plants, consists largely of fructose units and is known as a *fructosan.*

Nearly all starches consist of a mixture of two types of glucosans called *amyloses* and *amylopectins.* The relative proportions of these two glucosans in a starch vary from approximately 20% amylose and 80% amylopectin in wheat, potato, and ordinary corn starch to nearly 100% amylopectin in the starch of waxy corn. On the other hand, a few corn starches are known to contain as much as 75% amylose. Both amylose and amylopectin consist of glucose residues, but their structures exhibit one significant difference. Amylose consists of one long unbranched chain of glucose units linked together by α-1,4-linkages with only the terminal aldehyde group free (Figure 26-6). In amylopectin, most of the units are similarly connected with α-1,4-links, but α-1,6-glycosidic bonds are present every 24 to 30 residues, producing sidechains (see Figure 26-6). Amylopectin contains up to 1 million glucose residues. The structure of glycogen is similar to that of amylopectin, but branching is more extensive in glycogen and occurs every 8 to 12 glucose residues. These branches enhance the solubility of glycogen and allow the glucose residues to be mobilized more readily. Glycogen is most abundant in liver and is found in skeletal muscle as well. The most favorable conformation for α-1,4-linked polymers of D-glucose, such as starch or glycogen, is a tightly coiled helical structure.

The difference in structure between amylose and amylopectin is important when the appropriate starch substrate is selected for amylase determinations (see Chapter 22). The

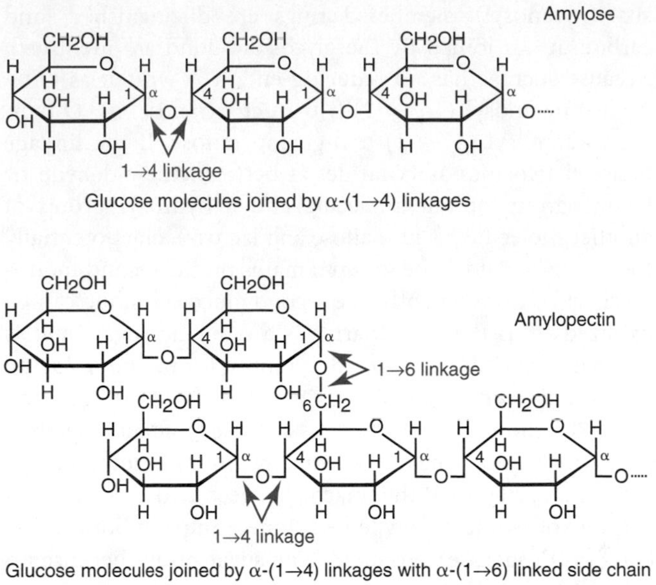

Amylose

1→4 linkage

Glucose molecules joined by α-(1→4) linkages

Amylopectin

1→6 linkage

1→4 linkage

Glucose molecules joined by α-(1→4) linkages with α-(1→6) linked side chain

Figure 26-6 Structures of the polysaccharides amylose and amylopectin.

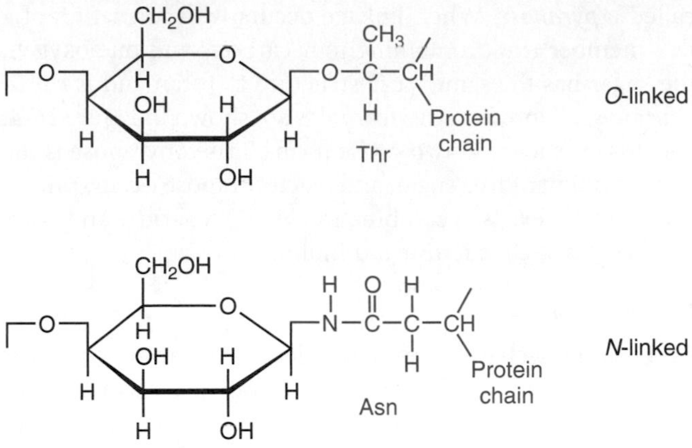

O-linked

N-linked

Figure 26-7 Glycosidic linkages between oligosaccharides and protein.

rate of hydrolysis is affected by structural differences in the starch. α-Amylase from the pancreas hydrolyzes internal α-1,4-glycosidic linkages. This hydrolysis results initially in the production of some maltose and a mixture of dextrins, which subsequently are hydrolyzed to maltose. The β-1,6-linkages are not attacked by α-amylase, and relatively large molecules of so-called residual (limit) dextrins are left after the action of the enzyme on amylopectin. *Dextrins* are the products of partial hydrolysis of starch. They are a complex mixture of molecules of different sizes. Those formed from amylose are unbranched chains, whereas amylopectins produce branched chains of glucose molecules. *Cellulose,* an important structural polysaccharide in plants, is an unbranched polymer of glucose residues joined by β-1,4-linkages. The β-configuration facilitates the formation of long straight chains, producing fibers of high tensile strength. The β-1,4-linkages are not hydrolyzed by α-amylases. Because humans do not have *cellulases,* they are unable to digest vegetable fiber.

Chitin, the principal component of the exoskeleton of arthropods (insects and crustacea), consists of *N*-acetyl-D-glucosamine residues in a β-1,4-linkage. The only chemical difference from cellulose is that the substituent at C-2 is an acetylated amino group instead of a hydroxyl group.

Glycoproteins

Glycosylation is one of the most frequent enzymatic modifications of proteins. Many integral membrane proteins have oligosaccharides covalently attached to the extracellular region, forming *glycoproteins.* In addition, most proteins that are secreted, such as antibodies, hormones, and coagulation factors, are glycoproteins. The number of attached carbohydrates varies among proteins and constitutes 1 to 70% of the weight of the glycoprotein. The oligosaccharides are attached by *O*-glycosidic linkages to the sidechain oxygen of serine and/or threonine residues or by *N*-glycosidic linkages to the sidechain nitrogen of asparagine residues (Figure 26-7).

One of the biological functions of the carbohydrate chains is to regulate the life span of proteins. For example, removal of sialic acid residues from the end of oligosaccharide chains on erythrocytes results in the disappearance of red blood cells from the circulation. Carbohydrates have also been implicated in cell-cell recognition, and in secretion and targeting of proteins to specific subcellular domains. Defects in protein glycosylation have been linked to several forms of congenital muscular dystrophy that are associated with brain abnormalities.[53]

METABOLISM OF CARBOHYDRATES

Carbohydrate metabolism provides glucose, the primary energy source for the human body. After digestion of carbohydrates and absorption of glucose, blood glucose concentration is controlled by the action of several hormones. Glucose is synthesized de novo or stored in the tissue as glycogen.

Digestion and Absorption

Ingested starch and glycogen are partially digested by the action of salivary amylase in the mouth to form intermediate dextrins and maltose (see Chapter 51). The acid pH of the stomach inhibits amylase activity, but alkaline pancreatic secretions increase the pH in the small intestine, allowing pancreatic amylase to complete digestion to oligosaccharides, preponderantly maltose. Maltose, along with any ingested lactose and sucrose, is hydrolyzed by the appropriate disaccharidase (*maltase, lactase,* or *sucrase*) from the intestinal mucosa to glucose, galactose, and fructose.

These monosaccharides are absorbed across the wall of the duodenum and ileum by an active, energy-requiring, carrier-mediated transfer process. The rate of absorption for glucose and galactose is several times greater than for similar molecules absorbed by passive diffusion (e.g., xylose). Some conversion of fructose to glucose may occur during the process of absorption, and the interconversion can be visualized in terms of the enediol form common to both (Figure 26-8).

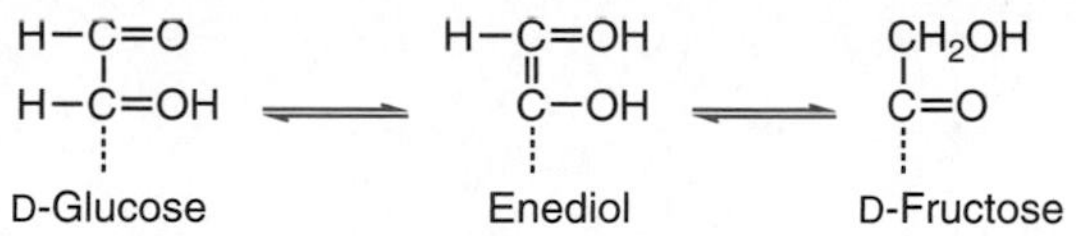

H–C=O H–C=OH	⇌	H–C=OH C–OH	⇌	CH_2OH C=O
D-Glucose		Enediol		D-Fructose

Figure 26-8 Interconversion of glucose and fructose.

Fructose is absorbed more slowly than glucose and galactose by a carrier-mediated process different from glucose and galactose transport mechanisms. The monosaccharides are then transported by the portal vein to the liver.

Intermediary Metabolism

The metabolism of hexoses proceeds according to the body's requirements. This results in (1) energy production by conversion to carbon dioxide and water, (2) storage as glycogen in the liver or as triglyceride in adipose tissue, or (3) conversion to keto acids, amino acids, or protein.

Some steps in the intermediary metabolism of glycogen and hexoses are shown in Figure 26-9. Each step is catalyzed by enzymes. In some cases, different enzymes are responsible for the forward and reverse reactions. For example, the initial phosphorylation of glucose is mediated by glucokinase, but the reverse reaction depends on glucose-6-phosphatase.

Various inborn errors of metabolism (Table 26-1) result from deficiencies or absence of some of the enzymes listed in Figure 26-9. Some of these are discussed later in the chapter. The relationship of carbohydrate metabolism to the production of lactate, ketone bodies, and triglycerides is also depicted in Figure 26-9. The pentose phosphate pathway, also known as the *hexose monophosphate shunt,* is an alternative pathway for glucose metabolism that generates the reduced form of nicotinamide-adenine dinucleotide phosphate (NADPH), which is used in maintaining the integrity of red blood cell membranes, in lipid and steroid biosynthesis, in hydroxylation reactions, and in other anabolic reactions. The complete picture of intermediary metabolism of carbohydrates is complex and is interwoven with the metabolism of lipids and amino acids. For details, readers should consult a biochemistry textbook.

Regulation of Blood Glucose Concentration

The concentration of glucose in the blood is regulated by the complex interplay of multiple pathways, modulated by a number of hormones. *Glycogenesis* is the conversion of glucose to glycogen. The reverse process, namely, the breakdown of glycogen to glucose and other intermediate products, is termed *glycogenolysis.* The formation of glucose from noncarbohydrate sources, such as amino acids, glycerol, or lactate, is termed *gluconeogenesis.* The conversion of glucose or other hexoses into lactate or pyruvate is called *glycolysis.* Further oxidation to carbon dioxide and water occurs through the Krebs (citric acid) cycle and the mitochondrial electron transport chain coupled to oxidative phosphorylation, generating energy in the form of adenosine triphosphate (ATP). Oxidation of glucose to carbon dioxide and water also occurs through the hexose monophosphate shunt pathway, which produces NADPH. Discussion of the hormones that regulate blood glucose is provided in Chapter 46.

TABLE 26-1 Inborn Errors of Carbohydrate Metabolism

Enzyme Deficiency	Disease State
Glucose-6-phosphatase (9)*	Type I GSD (von Gierke disease)
Muscle phosphorylase	Type V GSD (McArdle's disease)
Liver phosphorylase	Type VI GSD (Hers' disease)
Galactose-1-phosphate-uridyl transferase (2)	Galactosemia
Galactokinase (1)	Galactosemia
Uridine diphosphate-galactose-4-epimerase (3)	Galactosemia
Fructokinase (19)	Essential fructosuria
Fructose-1-phosphate aldolase (20)	Hereditary fructose intolerance
Pyruvate kinase (23)	Hemolytic anemia
Glucose-6-phosphate dehydrogenase (10)	Hemolytic disease

*Numbers in parentheses refer to enzymes in Figure 26-9.
GSD, Glycogen storage disease.

HYPOGLYCEMIA

Hypoglycemia is a blood glucose concentration below the fasting value, but it is difficult to define a specific limit.[73] The most widely suggested cutoff is 50 mg/dL, but some authors suggest 60 mg/dL.[8] A transient decline may occur 1.5 to 2 hours after a meal, and it is not uncommon for a plasma glucose concentration as low as 40 mg/dL to be observed 2 hours after ingestion of an oral glucose load. Similarly, extremely low fasting blood glucose values may occasionally be noted without symptoms or evidence of underlying disease. Hypoglycemia is rare in patients who do not have drug-treated diabetes mellitus.[19]

Symptoms of hypoglycemia vary among individuals, and none is specific. Epinephrine produces the classic signs and symptoms of hypoglycemia, namely, (1) trembling, (2) sweating, (3) nausea, (4) rapid pulse, (5) lightheadedness, (6) hunger, and (7) epigastric discomfort. These autonomic (neurogenic) symptoms are nonspecific and may be noted in other conditions, such as hyperthyroidism, pheochromocytoma, or even anxiety. Although controversial, it has been proposed that a rapid decrease in blood glucose may trigger the symptoms even though the blood glucose itself may not reach hypoglycemic values, whereas gradual onset of hypoglycemia may not produce symptoms.[25]

The brain cannot store or produce glucose, and in resting adults the central nervous system (CNS) consumes approximately 50% of the glucose used by the body.[31] Very low concentrations of plasma glucose (<20 or 30 mg/dL) cause severe

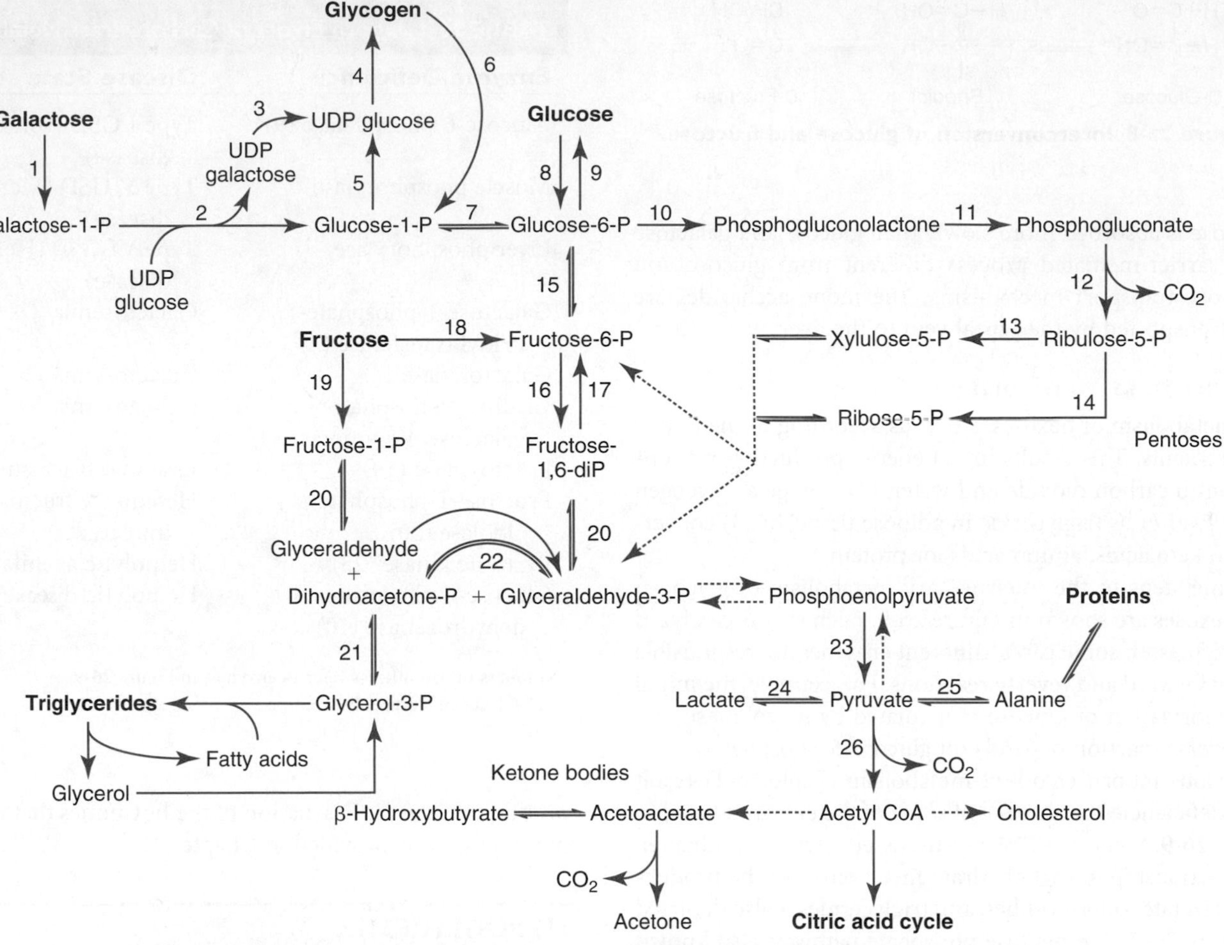

Figure 26-9 Major steps in the intermediary metabolism of carbohydrates. Numbers shown refer to specific enzymes. (- - - - - - - - -), Multistep pathway; (————), single-step pathway.

1. **Galactokinase**
2. **Galactose-1-P-uridyl transferase**
3. **UDP-galactose-4-epimerase**
4. **Glycogen synthetase (plus branching enzyme)**
5. **UDP-glucose pyrophosphorylase**
6. **Glycogen phosphorylase**
7. **Phosphoglucomutase**
8. **Glucokinase (and hexokinase)**
9. **Glucose-6-phosphatase**
10. **Glucose-6-phosphate dehydrogenase**
11. **6-Phosphogluconolactonase**
12. **6-Phosphogluconate dehydrogenase**
13. **Ribulose-5-P-epimerase**
14. **Ribose-5-P-isomerase**
15. **Phosphohexose isomerase**
16. **Phosphofructokinase**
17. **Fructose-1,6-diphosphatase**
18. **Hexokinase (extrahepatic)**
19. **Fructokinase**
20. **Aldolase**
21. **Glycerol phosphate dehydrogenase**
22. **Triose-P-isomerase**
23. **Pyruvate kinase**
24. **Lactate dehydrogenase**
25. **Alanine aminotransferase**
26. **Pyruvate dehydrogenase**

CNS dysfunction. During prolonged fasting or hypoglycemia, ketones may be used as an energy source. The broad spectrum of symptoms and signs of CNS dysfunction range from headache, confusion, blurred vision, and dizziness to seizures, loss of consciousness, and even death; these symptoms are known as *neuroglycopenia.* Restoration of plasma glucose usually produces a prompt recovery, but *irreversible damage may occur.*

The age of onset of hypoglycemia is a convenient way to classify the disorder (Box 26-1), but it should be borne in mind that some overlap occurs among the various groups. For example, some glycogen storage disorders may present in the third decade of life, and hormone deficiencies occur in childhood.

Hypoglycemia in Neonates and Infants

Neonatal blood glucose concentrations are much lower than adult concentrations (mean <35 mg/dL) and decline shortly after birth when liver glycogen stores are depleted. Glucose concentrations as low as 30 mg/dL in a term infant and 20 mg/dL in a premature infant may occur without clinical evidence of hypoglycemia. The more common causes of hypoglycemia in the neonatal period include prematurity, maternal diabetes, gestational diabetes mellitus (GDM), and maternal eclampsia (see Box 26-1; for review, see Haymond).[33] These are usually transient. Hypoglycemia with onset in early infancy is usually less transitory and may be due to inborn errors of metabolism or ketotic hypoglycemia; it usually occurs after fasting or a febrile illness.

Fasting Hypoglycemia in Adults

Hypoglycemia may result from a *decreased* rate of hepatic glucose production or an increased rate of glucose use. Symptoms suggestive of hypoglycemia are fairly common, but hypoglycemic disorders are rare. However, true hypoglycemia usually indicates serious underlying disease and may be life threatening. A precise threshold for establishing hypoglycemia is not always possible, and values as low as 30 mg/dL may be encountered in healthy premenopausal women after a 72-hour fast.[54] Symptoms usually begin at plasma glucose concentrations below 55 mg/dL, and impairment of cerebral function begins when glucose is less than 50 mg/dL.

More than 100 causes of hypoglycemia have been reported. Some of the more common conditions are listed in Box 26-1. Drugs are the most prevalent cause,[72] and a wide variety, including pentamidine, gatifloxacin, and quinine, can produce hypoglycemia. Oral hypoglycemic agents, which have a long half-life (35 hours for chlorpropamide), are the most frequent cause of drug-induced hypoglycemia. Sulfonylureas stimulate secretion of insulin, proinsulin, and C-peptide, and may mimic an insulinoma. Differentiation is made by demonstration of the drug in blood or urine. Surreptitious administration of insulin can be detected by finding low C-peptide concentrations with increased insulin concentrations.

Ethanol produces hypoglycemia by inhibiting gluconeogenesis, and this is aggravated by malnutrition (low glycogen stores) in patients with chronic alcoholism. Decreased glucose production in *hepatic failure* (e.g., viral hepatitis, toxins) caused by impaired gluconeogenesis or glycogen storage may result in hypoglycemia. Because dysfunction of more than 80% of the liver is necessary for hypoglycemia to develop, evidence of liver disease is invariably present. Deficiency of *growth hormone* (especially with coexistent ACTH deficiency), glucocorticoids, thyroid hormone, or glucagon may also produce hypoglycemia. Although a deficiency of glucocorticoids (e.g., Addison's disease) is most consistently associated with hypoglycemia, most glucocorticoid-deficient adults

BOX 26-1 Causes of Hypoglycemia

Neonates
- Small for gestational age/prematurity
- Respiratory distress syndrome
- Maternal diabetes mellitus
- Toxemia of pregnancy
- Other (e.g., cold stress, polycythemia)

Infants
- Ketotic hypoglycemia
- Congenital enzyme defects
- Glycogen storage disease
- Deficiency of gluconeogenic enzymes
- Galactosemia
- Hereditary fructose intolerance
- Leucine hypersensitivity
- Endogenous hyperinsulinism
- Reye's syndrome
- Idiopathic

Adults

Ill or Medicated Individual
- Drugs
  - Insulin or insulin secretagogue
  - Alcohol
  - Others (quinine, indomethacin)
- Critical illness
  - Hepatic, renal or cardiac failure
  - Sepsis (including malaria)
  - Inanation
- Hormone deficiency
  - Cortisol
  - Glucagon and epinephrine

Seemingly Healthy Individual
- Endogenous hyperinsulinism
- Insulinoma
- Functional β-cell disorders
  - Noninsulinoma pancreatogenous hypoglycemia
  - Post gastric bypass hypoglycemia
  - Insulin autoimmune hypoglycemia
  - Antibody to insulin
  - Antibody to insulin receptor
  - Insulin secretagogue
  - Other
- Accidental, surreptitious or malicious hypoglycemia

are not hypoglycemic. Hormonal deficiency causes hypoglycemia in children more frequently than in adults.

Demonstration of a low plasma glucose concentration in the presence of an abnormally high plasma insulin value is highly suggestive of an insulin-producing *pancreatic islet cell tumor.*[27] Because insulin concentrations exhibit a wide range in normal people, absolute hyperinsulinemia occurs in fewer than 50% of patients with insulinomas. Serum insulin concentrations inappropriately high for concurrent plasma glucose have been proposed to increase diagnostic accuracy. Critical diagnostic findings include a plasma insulin concentration of at least 18 pmol/L, plasma C-peptide concentrations greater than or equal to 0.2 nmol/L, and plasma proinsulin concentrations of at least 5.0 pmol/L when fasting plasma glucose is below 55 mg/dL. Ratios employing insulin and glucose have no diagnostic value. Provocative tests [glucagons,[42] tolbutamide,[74] calcium,[40] or suppression tests (infusion of insulin and measurement of C-peptide)], although strongly recommended in the past, generally are not necessary. Intra-arterial calcium stimulation with right hepatic vein sampling for insulin gradients appears to be a sensitive preoperative test for localizing insulinoma, although advances in imaging are making this approach far less common.[26]

Spontaneous production of *antibodies to insulin* may produce hypoglycemia (these antibodies are distinct from those elicited by insulin therapy and from the antibodies detected in certain patients with type 1 diabetes). Anti-insulin antibodies causing hypoglycemia have been reported in Graves' disease, multiple myeloma, systemic lupus erythematosus, and rheumatoid arthritis. This disorder is reported primarily among persons of Japanese or Korean ancestry and is less frequent among whites.[19] Patients exhibit postprandial hyperglycemia and fasting hypoglycemia.[61] Laboratory analysis demonstrates low plasma C-peptide and very high plasma insulin concentrations during hypoglycemia. The high insulin concentrations are believed to be an assay artifact caused by the antibody, and diagnosis is usually made by demonstrating high-titer serum insulin antibodies.

Nonpancreatic neoplasms that cause hypoglycemia are often extremely large mesenchymal neoplasms that appear to overuse glucose but may also have an inhibitory effect on glucose mobilization. Tumors of epithelial origin may cause hypoglycemia, frequently by producing insulin-like growth factor (IGF) II.[22,75]

Hypoglycemia caused by *septicemia* should be relatively easy to diagnose.[56] The mechanism is not well defined, but depleted glycogen stores, impaired gluconeogenesis, and increased peripheral use of glucose may be contributing factors. Glucose tolerance is commonly depressed in renal disease, and hypoglycemia may occur in end-stage *renal failure.*

Some of the conditions producing fasting hypoglycemia are readily apparent, but others require a lengthy diagnostic work-up. Once hypoglycemia is demonstrated, specific tests should be performed to establish the underlying cause. The *oral glucose tolerance test (OGTT) is not an appropriate study for evaluating a patient suspected of having hypoglycemia.*[19]

Postprandial Hypoglycemia

A group of disorders may produce hypoglycemia in the postprandial (fed) state.[34] These include drugs, antibodies to insulin or the insulin receptor, and inborn errors (e.g., fructose-1,6-diphosphatase deficiency). Also included is *reactive hypoglycemia* (referred to as *functional hypoglycemia*), which has been the subject of much debate.[8] Many commentaries and editorials have been published regarding the existence of reactive hypoglycemia (Hofeldt[34] and references listed therein). The general consensus is that no scientific evidence supports the existence of "functional hypoglycemia." It has been proposed that for individuals with vague symptoms after food ingestion, the preferred terminology should be *idiopathic reactive hypoglycemia*[34] or *idiopathic postprandial syndrome.*[73]

At the Third International Symposium on Hypoglycemia,[46] reactive hypoglycemia was defined as a clinical disorder in which the patient has postprandial symptoms suggesting hypoglycemia that occur in everyday life and are accompanied by a blood glucose concentration less than 45 to 50 mg/dL as determined by a specific glucose measurement on arterialized venous or capillary blood, respectively. Patients complain of autonomic symptoms occurring approximately 1 to 3 hours after eating and seem to obtain relief, lasting 30 to 45 minutes, by food intake. These symptoms are rarely due to low blood glucose concentrations (e.g., diabetes mellitus, gastrointestinal dysfunction, hormonal deficiency states). Most of these individuals have postprandial autonomic symptoms without neuroglycopenia in the postprandial state. Some experts in the field state that no true hypoglycemic disorder is characterized solely by autonomic symptoms.[73] A 5- or 6-hour glucose tolerance test was the standard procedure to establish the presence of postprandial hypoglycemia, but its use has been discredited.[8] The test is not reproducible in any particular individual, and low values for plasma glucose may be noted in the absence of symptoms, whereas symptoms may occur with normal glucose concentrations.[15] In addition, patients who have low blood glucose concentrations with autonomic symptoms 3 or 4 hours after an oral glucose load may have identical symptoms with normal blood glucose values after a mixed meal.[15] This may be due in part to anxiety provoked by the stressful environment during the glucose tolerance test. Demonstration of increased plasma epinephrine concentrations at the glucose nadir during an OGTT was reported to differentiate patients with reactive hypoglycemia,[12] but patients studied were identified on the basis of autonomic symptoms and signs, and only 25% demonstrated hypoglycemia. The OGTT should not be used in the diagnosis of reactive hypoglycemia.[76]

Postprandial hypoglycemia is infrequent, and demonstration of hypoglycemia during spontaneously occurring symptomatic episodes is necessary to establish the diagnosis.[61] If this is not possible, a 5-hour meal tolerance test[15] (which simulates the composition of a normal diet) or a *hyperglucidic* (high glucose) breakfast test[8] has been proposed. A protocol for a mixed-meal test can be found in Cryer and associates.[19]

A diagnosis of hypoglycemia has been used to explain a wide variety of disorders that appear unrelated to blood glucose abnormalities.[11] These nonspecific symptoms include fatigue, muscle spasms, palpitations, numbness, tingling, pain, sweating, mental dullness, sleepiness, weakness, and fainting. Behavior abnormalities, poor school performance, and delinquency have been incorrectly attributed to low blood glucose concentrations. Widespread use of the insensitive and nonspecific 5-hour glucose tolerance test caused overdiagnosis of hypoglycemia and led the American Diabetes Association (ADA) to publish a statement to discourage the inappropriate use of the OGTT for the diagnosis of hypoglycemia.[76] Lay publications[78] have supported this recommendation, but it is still important for the medical community to reassure such patients that low blood glucose is not the cause of their symptoms and to deal with specific abnormalities that might underlie patients' complaints or problems. A diagnosis of hypoglycemia should not be made unless a patient meets the criteria of *Whipple's triad of low blood glucose concentration with typical symptoms alleviated by glucose administration.* Demonstration of a plasma glucose concentration >70 mg/dL during a symptomatic episode indicates that the symptoms unequivocally are not the result of hypoglycemia.

Hypoglycemia in Diabetes Mellitus

Hypoglycemia occurs frequently in both type 1 diabetes and type 2 diabetes[20,30] and is the limiting factor in glycemic management of diabetes. Patients using insulin experience approximately one to two episodes of symptomatic hypoglycemia per week, and severe hypoglycemia (i.e., requiring assistance from others or associated with loss of consciousness) affects about 10% of this population per year. In patients practicing intensive insulin therapy (e.g., multiple injections, continuous subcutaneous insulin infusion), these figures are increased twofold to sixfold. The chief adverse event associated with intensive therapy in the Diabetes Control and Complications Trial (DCCT) was a threefold increase in the incidence of severe hypoglycemia.[23] An estimated 2 to 4% of people with type 1 diabetes die from hypoglycemia.[19] Similarly, hypoglycemia occurs in patients with type 2 diabetes (caused by oral hypoglycemic agents or insulin) but is less frequent than in type 1 diabetes. Recent evidence suggests that severe hypoglycemia may have long-term sequelae, including dementia and death from cardiovascular disease. Two pathophysiologic mechanisms contribute to hypoglycemia in patients with diabetes.

Defective Glucose Counter-Regulation

Counter-regulatory responses become impaired in patients with type 1 diabetes,[20] increasing the risk of hypoglycemia. The response of glucagon to hypoglycemia is impaired by an unknown mechanism early in the course of type 1 diabetes. Epinephrine secretory response to hypoglycemia becomes deficient later in the course of the disease. These defects are selective because other stimuli continue to elicit glucagon and epinephrine secretion. Glucose counter-regulation does not appear to be defective in patients with type 2 diabetes.

Hypoglycemia Unawareness

Up to 50% of patients with long-standing (more than 30 years) type 1 diabetes do not experience neurogenic warning symptoms and are prone to more severe hypoglycemia. The mechanism is thought to be associated with a decreased epinephrine response to hypoglycemia. Intensively treated patients with type 1 diabetes require lower plasma glucose concentrations to elicit symptoms of hypoglycemia. Some authors have claimed that human insulin results in an increased incidence of hypoglycemia unawareness, but analysis of 45 studies revealed no significant differences in hypoglycemic episodes between insulin from different species.[67]

Evaluation of Hypoglycemia

The Endocrine Society recently issued guidelines for the evaluation of adult hypoglycemic disorders.[19] These guidelines were cosponsored by the American Diabetes Association, the European Association for the Study of Diabetes, and the European Society of Endocrinology. Patients should be evaluated for hypoglycemia only if Whipple's triad—symptoms and/or signs of hypoglycemia, low plasma glucose concentration, and resolution of symptoms or signs after plasma glucose is raised—is documented.

The *classic diagnostic test is the prolonged fast,* which should be conducted in a hospital.[19] During the fast, the patient should be allowed to drink calorie-free fluids. All nonessential medications should be discontinued, and patients should be active when awake. Samples should be drawn every 6 hours for analysis of plasma glucose, insulin, C-peptide, proinsulin, and β-hydroxybutyrate. When plasma glucose concentration is less than 60 mg/dL, sampling should be performed every 1 to 2 hours. Samples for plasma insulin, C-peptide, and proinsulin should be analyzed only in those samples in which the glucose concentration is <60 mg/dL. The fast should be concluded when plasma glucose concentration falls to less than 45 mg/dL and the patient has symptoms and/or signs of hypoglycemia. If this does not occur, the fast should be terminated after 72 hours. At the conclusion of the fast, blood should be collected for analysis of glucose, insulin, C-peptide, proinsulin, β-hydroxybutyrate, and oral hypoglycemic agents. Then 1 mg of glucagon should be injected intravenously and plasma glucose concentration measured 10, 20, and 30 minutes later. This concludes the protocol, and the patient can be fed. Insulin antibodies should be measured, but not necessarily during hypoglycemia. When a deficiency is suspected, plasma cortisol, growth hormone, or glucagon should be measured at the beginning and end of the fast. A gender difference is observed in plasma glucose concentrations during prolonged fasting, with women exhibiting significantly lower concentrations than men. Low plasma glucose is necessary, but not sufficient, to establish the diagnosis. Absence of symptoms or signs of hypoglycemia during the fast excludes the diagnosis of a hypoglycemic disorder. Symptoms, signs, or both combined

TABLE 26-2 Methods of Glucose Analysis in 5819 Laboratories*

Method	Number†	Percent of Total	Mean, mg/dL	SD	CV, %
Hexokinase					
Photometric (visible)	269	4	135.5	3.2	2.3
Photometric (ultraviolet)	3119	54	135.9	3.5	2.6
Glucose Oxidase					
Photometric	976	17	127.0	2.7	2.1
Oxygen electrode	1431	25	134.9	2.7	2.0
Glucose Dehydrogenase	18	<1	135.8	3.0	2.2

*Results are based on 2009 CAP Survey, Set C-A, Specimen CHM-05 (Copyright 2009 College of American Pathologists; data used with permission). See text for discussion of methods.

†"Number" indicates how many laboratories use the indicated method/type.

CV, Coefficient of variation for all results by all methods of the indicated method/type from all manufacturers. It may include a component of variation attributable to differences in calibrators and to matrix effects.

with concentrations of glucose less than 55 mg/dL, insulin of at least 18 pmol/L, C-peptide of at least 0.2 nmol/L, and proinsulin of at least 5.0 pmol/L document endogenous hyperinsulinism. If β-hydroxybutyrate is 2.7 mmol/L or less and glucose is increased by at least 25 mg/dL after intravenous glucagon (the latter indicating preserved hepatic glycogen stores), hypoglycemia is mediated by insulin or IGF.

Tolbutamide Tolerance Test

Tolbutamide [1-butyl-3-(*p*-tolylsulfonyl)urea] (Orinase) stimulates the normal pancreas to produce insulin. The response of the pancreas to intravenous tolbutamide has been used in the investigation of fasting hypoglycemia. Blood specimens are obtained for glucose and insulin before intravenous injection of 1 g of a water-soluble form of tolbutamide and at 2, 15, 30, 60, 90, and 120 minutes afterwards. Healthy people have a decrease in plasma glucose concentration to about 50% of the fasting value by 30 minutes, with a return to baseline at 120 minutes. Patients with fasting hypoglycemia exhibit a lower glucose nadir, with hypoglycemia persisting up to 2 hours. The insulin response provides further diagnostic information. The peak insulin concentration at 2 minutes is normally less than 150 μIU/mL. This value is increased in patients with islet cell tumors, and an increased insulin concentration at 60 minutes is reported to be the most reliable discriminator.[6] In various conditions such as liver disease, malnutrition, or renal insufficiency, plasma glucose responses to tolbutamide are indistinguishable from those seen with islet cell tumors, *but only patients with insulinoma exhibit exaggerated plasma insulin concentrations.*

DETERMINATION OF GLUCOSE IN BODY FLUIDS

Many analytical procedures are used to measure blood glucose concentrations. In the past, analyses were often performed with relatively nonspecific methods that could produce falsely increased values. Today, almost all common methods are enzymatic (e.g., hexokinase,[9,63] glucose oxidase), and older methods, such as photometric or oxidation reduction techniques, are rarely used. The glucose assays most widely used in the United States may be determined by inspecting proficiency testing surveys conducted by the College of American Pathologists (CAP). Results from 5819 laboratories reported in a survey conducted in 2009 are displayed in Table 26-2. These data show that automated hexokinase methods are used in 58% of participating laboratories. Glucose oxidase is the only other method that is widely used. The most significant change in the past 25 years is the disappearance of the *o*-toluidine method, which was used in the SMA 12/60 Autoanalyzer. It must be emphasized that these data apply only to this CAP survey and are weighted to laboratories participating on a voluntary basis or in compliance with state regulatory agencies. Furthermore, testing performed in physicians' offices is not included. Many kits are commercially available for measuring glucose and are widely used, especially in smaller laboratories. Reference to CAP surveys reveals that all methods exhibit coefficients of variation (CVs) less than or equal to 2.6% for glucose values on lyophilized serum. The method of glucose measurement does not influence the result. Comparison of pooled serum samples measured by ≈6000 clinical laboratories shows that mean glucose concentrations measured by the hexokinase and glucose oxidase methods are essentially the same.[57] However, when evaluated against a reference measurement procedure, significant biases of up to 13% are observed among different methods.

Specimen Collection and Storage

In individuals with a normal hematocrit, fasting whole blood glucose concentration is approximately 10 to 12% lower than plasma glucose. Although glucose concentrations in the water phase of red blood cells and plasma are similar (the erythrocyte plasma membrane is freely permeable to glucose), the water content of plasma (93%) is approximately 11% higher than that of whole blood. In most clinical laboratories, plasma or serum is used for most glucose determinations; methods for self-monitoring of glucose use whole blood samples but may measure the glucose concentration in the plasma phase. Venous plasma is recommended for diagnosis of diabetes.[1,83] Although older methods of analysis reported that glucose concentrations in plasma were 5% lower than in serum,[44] a 2004 study indicated that glucose values measured in serum and plasma are essentially the same.[55] During fasting, capillary blood glucose concentration is only 2 to 5 mg/dL higher than that of venous blood. After a glucose load, however, capillary blood glucose concentrations are 20 to 70 mg/dL (mean ≈30 mg/dL; equivalent to 20 to 25%) higher than concurrently drawn venous blood samples.[43,45]

Glycolysis decreases serum glucose by approximately 5 to 7% in 1 hour (5 to 10 mg/dL) in normal uncentrifuged coagulated blood at room temperature.[13,81] The rate of in vitro glycolysis is higher in the presence of leukocytosis or bacterial contamination, but others have observed a slight decrease.[71] In separated, nonhemolyzed sterile serum, the glucose concentration is generally stable as long as 8 hours at 25 °C and up to 72 hours at 4 °C; variable stability is observed with longer storage periods.[7] Plasma, removed from the cells after moderate centrifugation, contains leukocytes that also metabolize glucose, although cell-free sterile plasma has no glycolytic activity.

Glycolysis has been found to be inhibited and glucose stabilized for as long as 3 days at room temperature by adding sodium fluoride (NaF) or, less commonly, sodium iodoacetate to the specimen.[25] Fluoride ions prevent glycolysis by inhibiting enolase, an enzyme that requires Mg^{2+}. This inhibition is due to the formation of an ionic complex consisting of Mg^{2+}, inorganic phosphate, and fluoride ions; this complex interferes with the interaction of enzyme and substrate. Fluoride is also a weak anticoagulant because it binds calcium; however, clotting may occur after several hours. It is therefore advisable to use a *combined fluoride-oxalate mixture,* such as 2 mg of potassium oxalate ($K_2C_2O_4$) and 2 mg NaF/mL of blood, to prevent late clotting. Other anticoagulants (e.g., EDTA, citrate, heparin) can also be used. Fluoride ions in high concentration inhibit the activity of urease and certain other enzymes; consequently, the specimens are unsuitable for determination of urea in procedures that require urease and for direct assay of some serum enzymes. $K_2C_2O_4$ causes loss of cell water, thereby diluting the plasma. Therefore, samples collected in these tubes should not be used for measurement of analytes other than glucose. Although fluoride maintains long-term blood glucose stability, the rate of decline in the first hour after sample collection is not altered, and glycolysis may continue for up to 4 hours.[13] A 2009 study showed that acidification of blood using citrate buffer inhibits in vitro glycolysis more effectively than fluoride.[29] To minimize glycolysis, the cells should be removed within minutes. Alternatively, the tube should be placed in ice-water slurry and the cells separated within 30 minutes.[83] Neither of these approaches is practical in routine analysis. It may not be necessary to use a fluoride-containing tube if plasma is separated from cells within 30 minutes of blood collection. However, inhibitors of glycolysis are required in patients with greatly increased leukocyte counts (e.g., blast crisis), because differences of up to 65 mg/dL have been observed between glucose values with and without glycolytic inhibitors after 1 to 2 hours of contact with the blood cells.

Cerebrospinal fluid (CSF) may be contaminated with bacteria or other cells and should be analyzed immediately for glucose. If a delay in measurement is unavoidable, the sample should be centrifuged and stored at 4 °C or at −20 °C.

In 24-hour collections of urine, glucose may be preserved by adding 5 mL of glacial acetic acid to the container before starting the collection. The final pH of the urine is usually between 4 and 5, which inhibits bacterial activity. Other preservatives that have been proposed include 5 g of sodium benzoate per 24-hour specimen, or chlorhexidine and 0.1% sodium nitrate ($NaNO_2$) with 0.01% benzethonium chloride. These may be inadequate, and urine should be stored at 4 °C during collection. Urine samples may lose as much as 40% of their glucose after 24 hours at room temperature.[48]

METHODS

Hexokinase and glucose oxidase are the two main types of methods used to measure glucose in body fluids.

Hexokinase Methods

Glucose is phosphorylated by ATP in the presence of hexokinase and Mg^{2+}. The glucose-6-phosphate formed is oxidized by glucose-6-phosphate dehydrogenase (G6PD) to 6-phosphogluconate in the presence of nicotinamide-adenine dinucleotide phosphate (NADPH). The amount of NADPH produced is directly proportional to the amount of glucose in the sample and is measured by absorbance at 340 nm. G6PD derived from yeast is used in the assay with $NADP^+$ as the cofactor. The oxidized form of nicotinamide-adenine dinucleotide (NAD^+) is the cofactor if bacterial *(Leuconostoc mesenteroides)* G6PD is used, and the NADH produced is measured at 340 nm.

$$\text{Glucose} + \text{ATP} \xrightleftharpoons{\textit{Hexokinase}} \text{Glucose-6-phosphate} + \text{ADP}$$

$$\text{Glucose-6-phosphate} \xrightleftharpoons[\text{NADP}^{\oplus}\ (\text{or NAD}^{\oplus}) \;\to\; \text{NADPH} + \text{H}^{\oplus}\ (\text{or NADH})]{\textit{G-6-PD}} \text{6-Phosphogluconate}$$

A reference method based on this principle has been developed and validated.[59] Serum or plasma is deproteinated by adding solutions of barium hydroxide [$Ba(OH)_2$] and zinc sulfate ($ZnSO_4$). The clear supernatant is mixed with a reagent containing ATP, NAD^+, hexokinase, and G6PD, incubated at 25 °C until the reaction is complete, and NADH measured. Calibrators and blanks are carried through the entire procedure, including the deproteination step. Detailed specifications are given for the equipment, materials, and reagents, including tests of enzyme reagent adequacy.

Although highly accurate and precise, the reference method is too exacting and time-consuming for routine use in a clinical laboratory. An alternative approach is to apply the reaction directly to serum or plasma and use a specimen blank to correct for interfering substances that absorb at 340 nm.[58] Because almost all methods are automated and rely on commercially prepared reagents supplied in lyophilized form, only a general discussion of the procedure is presented here.

Serum or plasma may be used. NaF, with an anticoagulant such as EDTA, heparin, oxalate, or citrate, may be used. Hemolyzed specimens containing more than 0.5 g hemoglobin/dL are unsatisfactory because phosphate esters and enzymes released from red blood cells interfere with the assay. Other sources of interference include drugs, bilirubin, and lipemia (triglycerides ≥500 mg/dL cause positive interference). A sample blank is therefore recommended for lipemic and icteric samples. This blank is prepared by adding 10 μL of sample to isotonic saline or buffer instead of reagent. The absorbance of this mixture, read against water at 340 nm, is subtracted. Although fructose interferes in the assay, normal fasting serum has low fructose concentrations. After ingestion of sucrose 2 g/kg of body weight, serum fructose concentration increases up to 8 to 10 mg/dL within 1 hour, and this increase persists for 2 hours. Solutions administered during glucose tolerance testing therefore should not contain any fructose.

Absorbances of sample or calibrator reaction mixtures are measured after the reactions have continued to completion (equilibrium reaction). Although glucose concentrations may be calculated directly, based on the molar absorptivity of NADPH or NADH, inclusion of a set of calibrators is recommended to detect possible deterioration of enzymes, ATP, $NADP^+$, or NAD^+, all of which are unstable. Reagents may also contain substances that react with the coenzymes. The presence of these substances can be evaluated by measuring the increase in absorbance observed in a reagent blank. Reagents are unsuitable for use if the absorbance at 340 nm exceeds 0.35, using water as the blank. The highest calibrator provides a check on the linearity of response and the adequacy of the enzyme reagent. The procedure is linear from 0 to 500 mg/dL. Glucose concentrations that exceed 500 mg/dL should be diluted with isotonic saline and reassayed.

Hexokinase procedures in which indicator reactions produce colored products are available, enabling absorbance to be measured in the visible range.[84] An oxidation reduction system containing phenazine methosulfate (PMS) and a substituted tetrazolium compound, 2-(*p*-iodophenyl)-3-*p*-nitrophenyl-5-phenyltetrazolium chloride (INT), is reacted with NADPH formed in the reaction. The reduced INT is colored with maximum absorbance at 520 nm. The PMS-INT color developer must be refrigerated when not in use and must be protected from exposure to light to retard autoreduction.

Glucose Oxidase Methods

The enzyme glucose oxidase catalyzes the oxidation of glucose to gluconic acid and hydrogen peroxide (H_2O_2):

$$\text{Glucose} + 2H_2O + O_2 \xrightarrow{\text{Glucose Oxidase}} \text{Gluconic Acid} + 2\,H_2O_2$$

Addition of the enzyme peroxidase and a chromogenic oxygen acceptor, such as *o*-dianisidine, results in the formation of a colored compound that is measured:

$$\underset{\text{(Colorless)}}{\text{o} - \text{Dianisidine}} + H_2O_2 \xrightarrow{\text{Peroxidase}} \underset{\text{(Colored)}}{\text{Oxidized o} - \text{Dianisidine}} + 2H_2O$$

Glucose oxidase is highly specific for β-D-glucose. As noted earlier, 36% and 64% of glucose in solution are in α- and β-forms, respectively. Complete reaction of glucose therefore requires mutarotation of the α- to the β form. Some commercial preparations of glucose oxidase contain an enzyme—mutarotase—that accelerates this reaction. Otherwise, extended incubation time allows spontaneous conversion.

The second step, involving peroxidase, *is much less specific than the glucose oxidase reaction.* Various substances, such as uric acid, ascorbic acid, bilirubin, hemoglobin, tetracycline, and glutathione, inhibit the reaction (presumably by competing with the chromogen for H_2O_2), producing lower values. Incorporation of potassium ferrocyanide significantly decreases interference by bilirubin. Most interfering substances can be eliminated by use of a Somogyi filtrate. Acid filtrates cannot be used because peroxides, which cause falsely increased results, may be released. Most modern methods omit the preparation of protein-free filtrates to make the procedure faster and simpler. Some glucose oxidase preparations contain catalase as a contaminant; catalase activity decomposes peroxide and decreases the final color obtained. Calibrators and unknowns should be analyzed simultaneously under conditions in which the rate of oxidation is proportional to the glucose concentration.

In some methods, the final mixture is acidified slightly to stop the reaction, and the intensity of the yellow chromophore is measured at 400 nm. In stronger acid solution, the color becomes pink, with maximum absorbance at 540 nm, and both sensitivity and stability are improved. Other approaches to measure the H_2O_2 produced include the peroxide-mediated oxidative coupling of 3-methyl-2-benzothiazolinone hydrazone (MBTH) with *N,N*-dimethylaniline (DMA) catalyzed by peroxidase,[32] or the oxidative coupling of *p*-aminophenazone (PAP) to phenol.[79] Both procedures have been automated. The MBTH-DMA and PAP procedures are not affected by high concentrations of creatinine, uric acid, or hemoglobin and are performed directly on serum. The chromogen 2-amino-4-hydroxybenzenesulfonic acid produces a yellow color in the presence of peroxidase and H_2O_2.[66] Additional components are not required to produce the color, and the assay can be performed on as little as 2 μL of serum.

Glucose oxidase methods are *suitable for measuring glucose in CSF but not in urine* as urine contains high concentrations of substances that interfere with the peroxidase reaction (such as uric acid), producing falsely low results. The glucose oxidase method therefore should *not be used for urine.* A method in which the urine is first pretreated with an ion-exchange resin to remove interfering substances has been described.

Modified Glucose Oxidase Methods

Some instruments use a polarographic oxygen electrode that measures the rate of oxygen consumption after the sample is added to a solution containing glucose oxidase.[39] Because this measurement involves only the first reaction shown earlier, *interferences encountered in the peroxidase step are eliminated.* To prevent formation of oxygen from H_2O_2 by catalase present in some preparations of glucose oxidase, H_2O_2 is removed by two additional reactions:

$$H_2O_2 + C_2H_5OH \xrightarrow{Catalase} CH_3CHO + 2H_2O$$
$$H_2O_2 + 2\,H^+ + 2\,I^- \xrightarrow{Molybdate} I_2 + 2\,H_2O$$

The latter reaction is effective even when catalase activity has diminished on storage of reagents. The procedure can be applied directly to *urine, serum, plasma,* or *CSF.* However, this approach cannot be used for the *determination of glucose in whole blood* because blood cells consume oxygen.

In the YSI Model 23A (Yellow Springs Instrument Co., Yellow Springs, Ohio), glucose oxidase is immobilized in a thin layer of resinous material sandwiched between two membranes. When a buffered sample is introduced, glucose diffuses through the first polycarbonate membrane and reacts with the enzyme to produce H_2O_2. This diffuses through the second, smaller-pore cellulose acetate membrane and is oxidized at a platinum anode. The current generated is directly proportional to the glucose concentration in the diluted sample.

$$H_2O_2 \rightarrow 2H^+ + O_2 + 2e^-$$

The circuit is completed at a silver cathode, where oxygen is reduced to water.

$$4H^+ + O_2 + 4e^- \rightarrow 2H_2O$$

Any H_2O_2 diffusing back into the sample chamber is destroyed by catalase to prevent interference with the analysis. Determinations may be performed on 25 μL of *plasma, serum,* or *whole blood.* Good precision and correlation with an oxygen consumption rate analyzer have been reported.[17]

The Vitros System (Ortho-Clinical Diagnostics, Raritan, NJ) makes use of dry multilayer films for chemical analyses.[21] Glucose is measured by a glucose oxidase procedure. A 10-μL sample of *serum, plasma, urine, or CSF* is placed on a porous film on top of the layer containing the reagents. Glucose diffuses through the film and reacts with the reagents to produce a colored end product or dye. The intensity of this dye is measured through a lower transparent film by reflectance spectrophotometry. Advantages of this system include small sample size, absence of liquid reagents, and improved stability on storage.

Glucose Dehydrogenase Methods

The enzyme glucose dehydrogenase (β-D-glucose:NAD oxidoreductase; EC 1.1.1.47) catalyzes the oxidation of glucose to gluconolactone. Mutarotase is added to shorten the time necessary to reach equilibrium. The amount of NADH generated is proportional to the glucose concentration.

Glucose dehydrogenase for this assay is isolated from *Bacillus cereus.* The reaction appears to (1) be highly specific for glucose, (2) shows no interference from common anticoagulants and substances normally found in serum, and (3) provides results in close agreement with hexokinase procedures. However, products containing maltose, icodextrin (which is converted to maltose), or galactose spuriously increase results obtained with point-of-care glucose meters that use glucose dehydrogenase pyrrolo-quinoline quinine (GDH-PQQ). Maltose is found in some intravenous immune globulins, and icodextrin is a glucose polymer present in some peritoneal dialysis solutions. These substances do not interfere with glucose measuring systems that use glucose dehydrogenase with NAD as cofactor. Glucose dehydrogenase methods have been adapted to continuous-flow analyzers,[10] including the use of immobilized enzyme,[77] and to a centrifugal analyzer.[51]

Reference Intervals

Although glucose is assayed by several different analytical procedures, reference intervals do not vary significantly among methods. The following values should apply to virtually all currently used glucose assays.

	Sample Fasting Glucose, mg/dL
Plasma/Serum	
Adults	74-99 (4.1-5.5 mmol/L)
Children	60-100 (3.3-5.6 mmol/L)
Premature neonates	20-60 (1.1-3.3 mmol/L)
Term neonates	30-60 (1.7-3.3 mmol/L)
Whole blood	65-95 (3.6-5.3 mmol/L)
CSF	40-70 (2.2-3.9 mmol/L) (60% of plasma value)
Urine	
24 hour	1-15 mg/dL (0.1-0.8 mmol/L)

Note that the ADA criterion[1] of fasting glucose of 126 mg/dL or greater—not the reference interval—is used for the diagnosis of diabetes. Moreover, the threshold for diagnosis of hypoglycemia is variable and is considerably less than the lower limit of the reference interval. There is no sex difference. *Plasma glucose values increase with age from the third to the sixth decade:* fasting, approximately 2 mg/dL per decade; postprandial, 4 mg/dL per decade; and after a glucose challenge, 8 to 13 mg/dL per decade.[60] Fasting plasma glucose does not increase significantly after age 60, but glucose concentrations after a glucose challenge are substantially higher in older individuals.[24] Evidence of an association of increasing insulin resistance with age is inconsistent, and visceral obesity appears to be responsible for the reported decrease in glucose tolerance in middle age.[38,69]

BOX 26-2 Reducing Substances in Urine

Fructose	Ketone bodies
Lactose	Sulfanilamide
Galactose	Oxalic acid
Maltose	Hippuric acid
Arabinose	Homogentisic acid
Xylose	Glucuronic acid
Ribose	Formaldehyde
Uric acid	Isoniazid
Ascorbic acid	Salicylates
Creatinine	Cinchophen
Cysteine	Salicyluric acid
Glucose	

CSF glucose concentrations should be approximately 60% of plasma concentrations and *must always be compared with concurrently measured plasma glucose* for adequate clinical interpretation.

Measurement of Glucose in Urine

Examination of urine for glucose is rapid, inexpensive, and noninvasive and has been used to screen large numbers of samples. The older screening tests detect sugars that reduce copper, producing a color.[35] Unfortunately, these tests react with reducing substances other than glucose (Box 26-2). Qualitative, semiquantitative, and quantitative methods are available for measuring glucose in urine and have essentially replaced the nonspecific tests in adults. *Note:* A reducing sugar method, rather than an enzymatic method specific for glucose, must be used when screening neonates and infants for inborn errors of metabolism that result in the appearance of reducing sugars other than glucose (e.g., galactose, fructose) in the urine.

Qualitative Method

In one such method, using Benedict's reagent (cupric ion complexed to citrate in alkaline solution), reducing substances convert cupric to cuprous ions, forming yellow cuprous hydroxide or red cuprous oxide.

Semiquantitative Methods

Convenient paper test strips are commercially available from a number of manufacturers (Clinistix and Diastix, Siemens Healthcare Diagnostics, Deerfield, Ill; and Chemstrip 2GP, Roche Diagnostics, Branchburg, NJ). All strips use the *glucose-specific enzyme glucose oxidase in a chromogenic assay.* For example, Clinistix has filter paper impregnated with glucose oxidase, peroxidase, and the dye *o*-tolidine. Other dyes, such as tetramethylbenzidine (TMB) have been used. The test end of the strip is moistened with freshly voided urine and examined after 10 seconds. A blue color develops if glucose is present at a concentration of 100 mg/dL or greater. Results are read by comparing the test color with a standard color chart. Automated urinalysis systems capable of analyzing 300 strips per hour are commercially available. The test is more sensitive for glucose than the copper reduction test (Clinitest), which has a detection limit of 250 mg/dL. Despite these claims, evaluation of dipsticks reveals high imprecision at low urine glucose concentrations.[28] Clinitest was reported to detect glucose only when it was above 1 g/L, and only Chemstrip µG could differentiate urine glucose at 300 mg/L (upper limit of reference interval) from 600 mg/L.[4] The sensitivity of the strip has been adjusted to take into account the presence of enzyme inhibitors normally present in urine. Thus a positive test result is obtained with lower concentrations of glucose in water than in urine. For the same reason, misleading high results may be obtained with very dilute specimens.

False-positive results may be produced by contamination of urine with H_2O_2 or a strong oxidizing agent, such as hypochlorite (bleach). Exposure of dipsticks to air gives false-positive readings after 7 days.[18] False-negative results may occur with large quantities of reducing substances, such as ketones, ascorbic acid, and salicylates. In one study of 2000 urine specimens, 11 false-negative enzyme paper tests were encountered. Among the inhibitors identified were ascorbic acid, dipyrone, and meralluride sodium (Mercuhydrin). Several antibiotics contain ascorbic acid as a preservative, which is excreted essentially unchanged. For routine examinations, a negative result by the strip test is usually interpreted to mean that the urine specimen is negative for glucose.

Other strip tests (Keto-Diastix, Siemens Healthcare Diagnostics; and DiaScreen 2GK, Arkray USA, Medina, Minn) are designed for the semiquantitative estimation of both glucose and ketone bodies. The glucose portion of the strip uses the glucose oxidase-peroxidase method. The hydrogen peroxide produced oxidizes iodide to iodine, yielding various intensities of brown that correspond to the concentration of glucose in urine. The detection limit is 100 mg/dL. Diastix and Chemstrip glucose tests are reported to be less inhibited by ascorbic acid than Clinistix.

Quantitative Methods

Applications of various procedures for quantitative determination of glucose in urine were discussed earlier in this chapter under "Determination of Glucose in Body Fluids." Hexokinase or glucose dehydrogenase procedures are recommended for greatest accuracy and specificity. Glucose oxidase procedures that depend only on the consumption of oxygen or the production of H_2O_2 are also reliable. Glucose oxidase procedures that include the H_2O_2-peroxidase reaction are not acceptable.

LACTATE AND PYRUVATE

Lactic acid, an intermediate in carbohydrate metabolism (see Figure 26-9), is derived predominantly from white skeletal muscle, brain, skin, renal medulla, and erythrocytes.

The blood lactate concentration depends on the rate of production in these tissues and the rate of metabolism in the liver and kidneys. Approximately 65% of total basal lactate production is used by the liver, particularly in gluconeogenesis. The *Cori cycle* consists of the conversion of glucose to lactate in the periphery and the reconversion of lactate to glucose in the liver. Extrahepatic removal of lactate occurs by oxidation in red skeletal muscle and the renal cortex. A moderate increase in lactate production results in increased hepatic lactate clearance, but uptake by the liver is saturable when concentrations exceed 2 mmol/L. For example, during strenuous exercise, lactate concentrations may increase significantly, from an average concentration of about 0.9 mmol/L to more than 20 mmol/L within 10 seconds. There is no uniformly accepted concentration for the diagnosis of lactic acidosis, but lactate concentrations exceeding 5 mmol/L and pH less than 7.25 indicate significant lactic acidosis.

Under certain conditions, the ratio of lactate to pyruvate is an indicator of redox status. For example, by rearranging the equation for the equilibrium constant for the reaction catalyzed by lactate dehydrogenase (EC 1.1.1.27), the ratio of lactate to pyruvate is shown to be proportional to the ratio of NADH to NAD^+.

Clinical Significance

Pyruvate is one of the critical metabolites in the cells, most of which originate from glycolysis.[64] It is further metabolized by four enzyme systems, namely, (1) alanine aminotransferase (alanine production), (2) pyruvate carboxylase (the major regulatory enzyme in gluconeogenesis), (3) lactate dehydrogenase (lactate formation), and (4) pyruvate dehydrogenase (see Figure 26-9). The last is a complex of enzymes that decarboxylate pyruvate in the presence of oxygen to acetyl coenzyme A (CoA), allowing entry into the citric acid cycle. Measurement of pyruvate is useful in the evaluation of patients with inborn errors of metabolism who have increased serum lactate concentrations. A lactate-to-pyruvate ratio less than 25 suggests a defect in gluconeogenesis, whereas an increased ratio (≥35) indicates reduced intracellular conditions found in hypoxia. Inborn errors associated with an increased lactate-to-pyruvate ratio include pyruvate carboxylase deficiency and defects in oxidative phosphorylation.[68] A high lactate-to-pyruvate ratio appears to be a sensitive test for detecting mitochondrial muscle toxicity of zidovudine therapy.[14] Pyruvate is also measured in clinical studies evaluating reperfusion after myocardial ischemia. Patients with Alzheimer's disease were reported to have higher CSF pyruvate concentrations than control subjects, and concentrations correlate with the severity of dementia.[62]

Lactic acidosis occurs in two clinical settings: (1) type A (hypoxic), associated with *decreased tissue oxygenation,* such as shock, hypovolemia, and left ventricular failure; and (2) type B (metabolic), associated with *disease* (e.g., diabetes mellitus, neoplasia, liver disease), *drugs and/or toxins* (e.g., ethanol, methanol, salicylates), or *inborn errors of metabolism* (e.g., methylmalonic aciduria, propionic acidemia, fatty acid oxidation defects). Lactic acidosis is not uncommon and occurs in approximately 1% of hospital admissions. It has a mortality rate greater than 60%, and approaches 100% if hypotension is also present. Type A is much more common.

The mechanism of type B lactic acidosis is not known but is speculated to be a primary defect in mitochondrial function with impaired oxygen use. This leads to reduced stores of ATP and NAD^+, with accumulation of NADH and H^+. In the presence of decreased liver perfusion or liver disease, lactate removal from the blood is reduced, thereby aggravating the lactic acidosis.

Measurement of serum lactate in trauma patients on admission to the emergency department does not identify patients at risk of death, but may be useful to identify those patients at low risk of death.[36] Evidence obtained in 2008 from a multicenter trial supports measurement of lactate in fetal scalp blood during labor in the management of intrapartum fetal distress to prevent severe academia at birth.[82]

An uncommon and often undiagnosed cause of lactic acidosis is D-lactic acidosis.[80] It was thought that D-lactate was not produced in human metabolism, but normal individuals have a large capacity to metabolize D-lactate.[80] Moreover, absorption and accumulation of D-lactate from abnormal intestinal bacteria may cause systemic acidosis. This occurs after jejunoileal bypass surgery and manifests as altered mental status (from mild drowsiness to coma) with increased blood concentrations of D-lactate. Virtually all commonly used laboratory assays for lactate use L-lactate dehydrogenase, which does not detect D-lactate. D-Lactate can be measured by gas-liquid chromatography or, more easily, by using a specific D-lactate dehydrogenase (Sigma) from *Lactobacillus leishmanni.*[50] The enzyme assay can be readily automated. Lactate in CSF normally parallels concentrations in the blood, but not in children.[37] With biochemical alterations in the CNS, however, CSF lactate values change independently of blood values. Increased CSF concentrations are noted in cerebrovascular accidents, intracranial hemorrhage, bacterial meningitis, epilepsy, inborn errors of the electron transport chain, and other CNS disorders. In aseptic (viral) meningitis, lactate concentrations in CSF are not usually increased; hence, CSF lactate has been used to help discriminate between viral and bacterial meningitis,[3] but the clinical utility has been questioned. In a few children with inherited metabolic disease, CSF lactate concentrations may be increased despite plasma lactate in the reference interval.[37]

Methods for Measuring Lactate and Pyruvate in Body Fluids

Determination of Lactate in Whole Blood[2,47,49,52]

Principle

Lactate is oxidized to pyruvate by lactate dehydrogenase in the presence of NAD^+. The NADH formed in this reaction is measured by a spectrophotometer at 340 nm and serves as a measure of the lactate concentration.

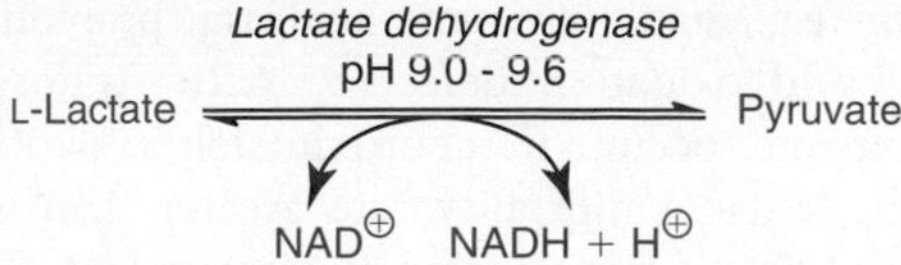

The equilibrium of the reaction normally lies far to the left. However, by using a pH of 9.0 to 9.6 and an excess of NAD^+, and by trapping the reaction product pyruvate with hydrazine, the equilibrium can be shifted to the right. Pyruvate can also be removed by reacting it with L-glutamate in the presence of alanine aminotransferase. Use of tris(hydroxymethyl)-aminomethane (TRIS) buffer results in more rapid completion of a side reaction between NAD^+ and hydrazine and prevents the "creeping" of blank values observed when glycine buffer is used.[47]

Because of its high specificity and simplicity, the enzymatic method is the method of choice for measuring lactate, although other methods may also be used (e.g., gas chromatography,[70] photometry).

The Vitros Analyzer (Ortho-Clinical Diagnostics) uses an assay in which lactic acid is oxidized to pyruvate by lactate oxidase. The H_2O_2 generated oxidizes a chromogen system, and absorbance of the resulting dye complex, measured by a spectrophotometer at 540 nm, is directly proportional to the lactate concentration in the specimen. Each mole of lactate oxidized produces 0.5 mole of dye complex.

$$L-\text{Lactate}+O_2 \xrightarrow{\text{Lactate Oxidase}} \text{Pyruvate}+H_2O_2$$

$$2\,H_2O_2 + \text{4-aminoantipyrine} + \text{1,7-dihydronapthalene} \xrightarrow{\text{Peroxidase}} \text{red dye}$$

Reference Intervals

The reference intervals for lactate are as follows:

LACTATE		
Specimen	**mmol/L**	**mg/dL**
Venous Blood		
At rest	0.5-1.3	5-12
In hospital	0.9-1.7	8-15
Arterial Blood		
At rest	0.36-0.75	3-7
In hospital	0.36-1.25	3-11

Patients in the hospital exhibit a wider range of lactate concentrations with lactic acidosis occurings when blood lactate concentrations exceed 5 mmol/L (45 mg/dL). Severe exercise dramatically increases lactate concentrations, and even movement of leg muscles by patients at bed rest may result in significant increases. Plasma values are about 7% higher than those in whole blood, although differences depend on the procedure used. CSF values are usually similar to blood concentrations, but may change independently in CNS disorders. Age-related reference intervals for CSF lactate (and lactate-to-pyruvate ratios) have been established in children.[5] The upper limit of the reference interval (90th percentile) for CSF lactate in children in hospital from birth to 15.5 years varies continuously from 1.78 to 1.88 mmol/L (16 to 17 mg/dL).[5] Normal 24-hour urine output of lactate is 5.5 to 22 mmol/d.

Determination of Pyruvate in Whole Blood

Principle

The reaction involved in the determination of pyruvate is essentially the reverse of the reaction used in the lactate procedure.

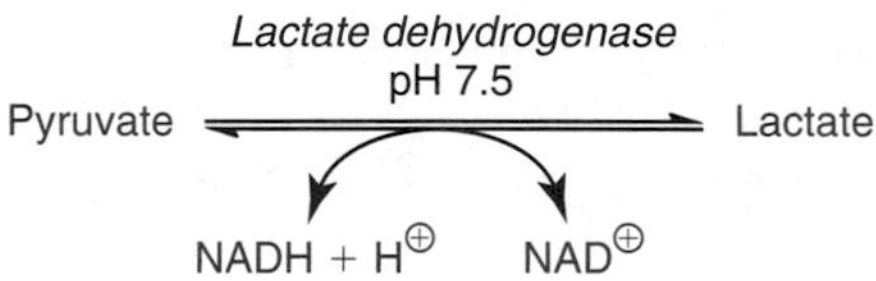

At about pH 7.5, the equilibrium constant strongly favors the reaction to the right. The method is very specific, and 2-oxoglutarate, oxaloacetate, acetoacetate, and β-hydroxybutyrate do not interfere, as with photometric methods.

Reference Intervals

Fasting venous blood, drawn with a patient at rest, has a pyruvate concentration of 0.03 to 0.10 mmol/L (0.3 to 0.9 mg/dL). Arterial blood contains 0.02 to 0.08 mmol/L (0.2 to 0.7 mg/dL). Values for CSF are 0.06 to 0.19 mmol/L (0.5 to 1.7 mg/dL).[65] Age-related reference intervals in CSF have been established in children.[5] Urine output of pyruvate is normally 1 mmol/d or less.

INBORN ERRORS OF CARBOHYDRATE METABOLISM

Deficiency or absence of an enzyme that participates in carbohydrate metabolism may result in accumulation of monosaccharides, which is measured in the urine (see Table 26-1 and Figure 26-9). Most of these conditions are inherited as autosomal recessive traits. Sugars frequently appear in the urine as a result of excessive consumption without underlying disease.

DISORDERS OF GALACTOSE METABOLISM

Galactose is derived from milk in the diet. It resembles glucose in structure, but the hydroxyl group on the fourth carbon has a different spatial arrangement (see Figure 26-2). A deficiency of any of the enzymes that participate in the conversion of galactose to glucose results in *galactosemia.*

Galactose-1-Phosphate Uridyl Transferase Deficiency

Infants with this deficiency fail to thrive on milk because half of the milk sugar, lactose, is galactose. Within a few days of milk ingestion, neonates manifest vomiting and diarrhea. Failure to thrive, liver disease, cataracts, and mental retardation develop later. Hypoglycemia may occasionally develop. The diagnosis should be considered when *the urine demonstrates the presence of a reducing substance that does not react in a glucose oxidase test.* Early detection and treatment (withholding galactose from the diet) are necessary to prevent irreversible changes. Because other reducing sugars may give similar results, galactose should be identified by paper chromatography (discussed later). Diagnosis is suggested by detecting galactose and galactose-1-phosphate in blood and is confirmed by direct assaying of red blood cell transferase activity. A spot test is also available.

Uridine Diphosphate Galactose-4-Epimerase Deficiency

This extremely rare disorder exhibits clinical findings similar to those of transferase deficiency.

Galactokinase Deficiency

This is a milder condition manifested predominantly by cataracts caused by galactitol deposits in the lens. The diagnosis is confirmed by demonstrating normal transferase activity and no galactokinase in red blood cells.

Disorders of Fructose Metabolism

Fructose may appear in the urine after fruit, honey, or syrup is eaten, but it has no significance in these circumstances. Three disorders of fructose metabolism, inherited as autosomal recessive traits, produce fructosuria.

Essential Fructosuria

This rare and harmless defect is due to lack of *fructokinase.*

Hereditary Fructose Intolerance

A *deficiency of fructose-1-phosphate aldolase* produces this rare disorder with hypoglycemia and liver failure. Fructose ingestion inhibits glycogenolysis and gluconeogenesis, producing hypoglycemia. Early detection is important because this condition responds to a diet devoid of sucrose and fructose.

Hereditary Fructose-1,6-Diphosphatase Deficiency

Patients with this deficiency have episodes of apnea and hyperventilation and hypoglycemia, ketosis, and lactic acidosis caused by severe impairment of gluconeogenesis. The condition is diagnosed by demonstrating the enzyme defect in liver biopsy specimens.

Disorders of Pentose Metabolism

Alimentary Pentosuria

Pentoses may be present in the urine after large quantities of fruits such as cherries, plums, or prunes are eaten.

Essential Pentosuria

This is a harmless inborn error caused by a *deficiency of* L*-xylulose reductase,* an enzyme involved in the glucuronic acid pathway.

Other Urinary Sugars

Lactose is sometimes detected in the urine of women during lactation and occasionally towards the end of pregnancy. Patients with *lactase deficiency,* a common disorder caused by a congenital or acquired deficiency of intestinal lactase, exhibit abdominal pain, diarrhea, and lactose in the urine.

Maltose has on rare occasions been detected in the urine of some patients.

Many *reducing substances* other than sugars may be found in urine (see Box 26-2). Ascorbic acid (vitamin C) may be ingested in large quantities or may be present in antibiotic preparations administered intravenously. In either case, excess concentrations usually appear in the urine and contribute significantly to the total reducing substances present.

Methods for Measuring Individual Sugars

Qualitative Tests for Glucose

Techniques for separating and identifying sugars have included (1) fermentation, (2) optical rotation, (3) osazone formation with phenylhydrazine, (4) specific chemical tests, and (5) paper or thin-layer chromatography. The availability of glucose oxidase test strips, specific for glucose, has greatly simplified the differentiation of glucose from other reducing substances. For practical purposes, the *urinary sugars of clinical interest are glucose and galactose.* Urine from infants and children should be tested routinely by both glucose oxidase and copper reduction tests to identify individuals with inborn errors of metabolism. Reducing substances other than glucose should be further identified by chromatographic procedures.

Qualitative Tests for Urinary Sugars Other Than Glucose

Fructose (Selivanoff's Test)

Hot HCl converts fructose to hydroxymethyl furfural (HMF), which links with *resorcinol* to produce a red compound. To make the reagent, dissolve 50 mg of resorcinol in 33 mL of concentrated HCl, and dilute to 100 mL with water. Add 0.5 mL of urine to 5 mL of reagent in a test tube, and bring to a boil. Fructose produces a red reaction within 30 seconds. The test is sensitive to 100 mg fructose/dL, provided there is no excess glucose. A 2-g/dL solution of glucose produces about the same color as 100 mg/dL of fructose after 30 seconds of boiling. A solution of fructose (0.5 g/dL) should be used as a control. With high concentrations of fructose, a red precipitate forms.

Pentoses (Bial's Test)

By heating with HCl, pentoses are converted to furfural, which reacts with orcinol to form green compounds. Dissolve 300 mg of orcinol in 100 mL of concentrated HCl, and add 0.25 mL of ferric chloride solution (10 g/dL). Glucose, if present in the urine, should be removed by fermentation with yeast. Add 0.5 mL of urine to 5 mL of reagent in a test tube, and bring to a boil. Pentoses produce a green reaction. The detection limit of the test is 100 mg pentose/dL. A solution of xylose (0.5 g/dL) should be used as a control.

Glucuronates produce a similar color if the boiling is prolonged. As with Selivanoff's reagent, fructose produces a red reaction.

Identification of Urinary Sugars by Paper Chromatography

Sugars can be separated by ascending or descending chromatography on paper and located after color development with dinitrosalicylic acid. Variable rates of migration depend on the solubility of the sugars in the particular solvent system. Presumptive identification is made by comparing the migration (R_f) value of the unknown to those of reference compounds. One procedure may be performed conveniently in a 6 × 18-inch Pyrex jar with a tightly fitting cover.

Identification of Urinary Sugars by Thin-Layer Chromatography

Urine sugars can be identified by thin-layer chromatographic techniques as described by Young and Jackson.[85] When frequent chromatographic separations are necessary, this method is preferred over paper chromatography because of the shorter time required. If such studies are performed infrequently, paper chromatography is simple, is adequate for most separations, and requires little actual working time.

GLYCOGEN STORAGE DISEASE

Glycogen, although present in most tissue, is stored principally in the liver and skeletal muscle. During fasting, liver glycogen is converted to glucose to provide energy for the whole body. In contrast, skeletal muscle lacks glucose-6-phosphatase, and muscle glycogen can be used only locally for energy. *Glycogen storage disease* is a generic name encompassing at least 10 rare inherited disorders of glycogen storage in tissue (see Table 26-1). The different forms of glycogen storage disease are categorized by numeric type in the chronological sequence in which these defects were identified. Each form is due to a deficiency of a specific enzyme in glycogen metabolism, producing a quantitative or qualitative defect of glycogen storage. Numerous mutations have been identified in patients with these conditions (http://www.ncbi.nim.nih.gov/omim/accessed April 26, 2011). The most common mutations are listed in Table 26-3. Because liver and skeletal muscle have the highest rates of glycogen metabolism, these are the structures most affected. The liver forms (types I, III, IV, and VI) are marked by *hepatomegaly* (caused by increased liver glycogen stores) and *hypoglycemia* (caused by inability to convert glycogen to glucose). Hypoglycemia is manifested by autonomic clinical symptoms (sweating, shakiness, and lightheaded feeling), growth retardation, and laboratory findings of decreased insulin and increased glucagon concentrations in the blood. The muscle forms (types II, IIIA, V, and VII), in contrast, have mild symptoms that *usually appear in young adulthood during strenuous exercise* owing to the inability to provide energy for muscle contraction. Other muscle disorders may exhibit similar symptoms but are readily differentiated by evaluation of glycogen stores. The specific diagnosis of each type is made directly by *demonstrating the enzyme defect in tissue.* A very brief overview is provided here; for a more detailed description, readers should consult Chen and Burchell.[16]

Type I (Glucose-6-Phosphatase Deficiency)

Type I is the most common and severe form, and patients have accumulation of glycogen of normal chemical structure in the liver. The disease is characterized by (1) massive hepatomegaly, (2) growth retardation, (3) fasting hypoglycemia, (4) increased lactic acid concentrations in the blood (caused by excessive glycolysis), (5) hyperuricemia (caused by competitive inhibition by lactate of renal tubular urate secretion and increased uric acid production), and (6) hypertriglyceridemia (increased lipolysis caused by decreased glucose). Glucagon and epinephrine do not produce hyperglycemia but result in increased lactate concentrations. The failure of blood glucose to increase in response to galactose administration (oral or intravenous) is diagnostic. Galactose is normally converted to glucose (see Figure 26-9), but in these patients glucose-6-phosphate cannot be hydrolyzed to glucose. Treatment includes partaking of frequent meals and nasogastric feeding at night to maintain blood glucose concentrations. Glucose-6-phosphatase activity can be assayed in a liver biopsy. Two main subtypes have been identified: type Ia and type Ib.[41] Type 1a (also called *von Gierke disease*) is caused by a deficiency of the glucose-6-phosphatase catalytic subunit, whereas type Ib is due to a defect in the glucose-6-phosphatase transport system. Another form, termed type 1c, was originally attributed to a defect in microsomal phosphate transport, but it is likely that types Ib and Ic represent a single disease.[41] Many mutations have been described in types Ia and Ib.[41]

Individuals with type I glycogen storage disease exhibit decreased availability of liver glycogen demonstrated by decreased or absent blood glucose response to epinephrine administration. An assay based on this phenomenon is known as the *epinephrine tolerance test.* With it, an intramuscular injection of 1 mL of a 1/1000 (1 g/L) solution of epinephrine hydrochloride is given, and blood samples are taken at 30, 45, 60, 90, and 120 minutes. Healthy people increase blood glucose by 35 to 45 mg/dL in 40 to 60 minutes, with a return to the fasting concentration within 2 hours. This test is rarely used because the diagnosis of von Gierke disease is based on failure to increase blood glucose in response to galactose administration, with confirmation by direct assay of glucose-6-phosphatase activity.

Type II (Acid α-Glucosidase Deficiency)

Type II is an autosomal recessive disorder that affects predominantly the heart and skeletal muscle, producing muscle weakness and cardiomegaly. Liver function is normal, and patients do not have hypoglycemia. Two forms are identified: (1) infantile *(Pompe disease),* which usually presents in the first few months of life (presenting symptoms include

TABLE 26-3 Common Mutations in Glycogen Storage Disease*

Nucleotide Change	Amino Acid Change	Frequency	Ethnic Background
GSD Ia			
c.247C→T	p.Arg83Cys	32%	Caucasian
c.247C→T	p.Arg83Cys	93-100%	Jewish
c.248G→A	p.Arg83His	38%	Chinese
c.378_379dupTA	p.130X	50%	Hispanic
c.648G→T	Splicing	88%	Japanese
c.648G→T	Splicing	36%	Chinese
c.562G→C	p.Gly188Arg	21%	Caucasian
GSD Ib			
c.352T→C	p.Trp118Arg	50%	Japanese
c.1042_1043delCT	p.400X	50%	Caucasian
c.1015G→T	p.Gly339Cys	50%	Caucasian
GSD II			
c.32.13T→G	Aberrant splicing	75%	Italian
c.1935C→A	p.Asp645Glu	–	Taiwanese
c.2560C→T	p.Arg854X	–	African American
GSD III			
c.16C→T	p.Gln66X	25%	Caucasian
c.17delAG	p.25X	75%	Caucasian
c.2590C→T	p.Arg864X	10%	Caucasian
c.3682C→T	p.Arg1228X	5%	Caucasian
c.3965delT (3964delT)	p.1348X	7%	African American and Caucasian
c.4455delT	p.1503X	100%	North African Jewish
GSD V			
C→A	p.Arg50X	50-80%	
G→A	p.Gly204Ser	10%	
GSD VII			
G→A	Deletion	65%	Ashkenazi

*Adapted in part from Reference 41.

weakness and respiratory difficulties, and patients usually die from cardiac failure within 1 year), and (2) a juvenile form that is milder and may present in the second or third decade of life with difficulty in walking. More than 200 mutations in the acid α-glucosidase gene are known (http://www.pompecenter.nl/en/). The diagnosis is made by measuring α-glucosidase (acid maltase) activity in skeletal muscle biopsy, peripheral blood cells or cultured skin fibroblasts. Enzyme replacement therapy with recombinant human acid α-glucosidase was approved in 2006.

Type III (Amylo-1,6-Glucosidase Deficiency)

Deficiency of glycogen debranching enzyme results in storage of an abnormal form of glycogen (limit dextrinosis). Both liver and muscle are usually affected (type IIIA), producing hepatomegaly and muscle weakness. Approximately 15% of patients have only liver involvement, without apparent muscle disease (type IIIB). Clinical and biochemical features resemble those of type I disease. Differentiation from type I is seen by a hyperglycemic response to galactose, lower concentrations of urate and lactate in the blood, and increased serum transaminase and creatine kinase activities. Enzyme deficiency can be demonstrated in muscle or liver and occasionally in erythrocytes.

Type IV (Branching Enzyme Deficiency)

Type IV is an extremely rare disorder manifested by production of an abnormal form of unbranched glycogen in all tissues. Patients exhibit hepatosplenomegaly with ascites and liver failure. Abnormal glycogen can be identified in the tissues and muscles; leukocytes or cultured fibroblasts can be used to demonstrate the enzyme deficiency.

Type V (Muscle Phosphorylase Deficiency)

Type V, also called *McArdle disease,* usually presents in the second or third decade with muscle cramps after exercise. Moderate exercise can be sustained, and patients get a "second wind" when symptoms disappear if exercise is continued. Increased plasma creatine kinase activities at rest, failure of ischemic exercise to increase serum lactate concentrations while producing an exaggerated increase in ammonia, myoglobinuria, and diminished activity of muscle phosphorylase establish the diagnosis. Patients respond to oral glucose administration or injections of glucagon.

Type VI (Liver Phosphorylase or Phosphorylase Kinase Deficiency)

Type VI, or *Hers' disease,* is a heterogeneous group of diseases arising from a deficiency of liver phosphorylase or one of the subunits of phosphorylase kinase. It is a rare and relatively benign disorder manifested as hepatomegaly caused by increased deposits of normal glycogen in the liver. Diagnosis is made by measuring enzyme activity in the liver or in red or white blood cells.

Type VII (Muscle Phosphofructokinase Deficiency)

Patients with this rare autosomal recessive disorder have deposits of abnormal glycogen in muscle. Exercise intolerance, unresponsiveness to glucose administration, and hemolysis (caused by decreased glycolysis in erythrocytes) are noted clinically, producing hyperbilirubinemia, pigmenturia, and reticulocytosis. The specific enzyme defect can be demonstrated.

REFERENCES

1. American Diabetes Association. Standards of medical care in diabetes—2009. Diabetes Care 2009;32(Suppl 1):S13-61.
2. Astles R, Williams CP, Sedor F. Stability of plasma lactate in vitro in the presence of antiglycolytic agents. Clin Chem 1994;40:1327-30.
3. Bailey EM, Domenico P, Cunha BA. Bacterial or viral meningitis? Measuring lactate in CSF can help you know quickly. Postgrad Med 1990;88:217-9, 223.
4. Bandi ZL, Myers JL, Bee DE, James GP. Evaluation of determination of glucose in urine with some commercially available dipsticks and tablets. Clin Chem 1982;28:2110-5.
5. Benoist JF, Alberti C, Leclercq S, Rigal O, Jean-Louis R, Ogier de Baulny H, et al. Cerebrospinal fluid lactate and pyruvate concentrations and their ratio in children: age-related reference intervals. Clin Chem 2003;49:487-94.
6. Boehm TM, Lebovitz HE. Statistical analysis of glucose and insulin responses to intravenous tolbutamide: evaluation of hypoglycemic and hyperinsulinemic states. Diabetes Care 1979;2:479-90.
7. Boyanton BL Jr, Blick KE. Stability studies of twenty-four analytes in human plasma and serum. Clin Chem 2002;48:2242-7.
8. Brun JF, Fedou C, Mercier J. Postprandial reactive hypoglycemia. Diabetes Metab 2000;26:337-51.
9. Burrin JM, Price CP. Measurement of blood glucose. Ann Clin Biochem 1985;22(Pt 4):327-42.
10. Bush JL, Campbell J, Sanderson JA. Performance of a glucose procedure based on the glucose dehydrogenase reaction on Technicon continuous flow equipment. Clin Chem 1981;27:1050.
11. Cahill GF Jr, Soeldner JS. "A non-editorial on non-hypoglycemia." N Engl J Med 1974;291:905-6.
12. Chalew SA, McLaughlin JV, Mersey JH, Adams AJ, Cornblath M, Kowarski AA. The use of the plasma epinephrine response in the diagnosis of idiopathic postprandial syndrome. JAMA 1984;251:612-5.
13. Chan AY, Swaminathan R, Cockram CS. Effectiveness of sodium fluoride as a preservative of glucose in blood. Clin Chem 1989;35: 315-7.
14. Chariot P, Monnet I, Mouchet M, Rohr M, Lefaucheur JP, Dubreuil-Lemaire ML, et al. Determination of the blood lactate:pyruvate ratio as a noninvasive test for the diagnosis of zidovudine myopathy. Arthritis Rheum 1994;37:583-6.
15. Charles MA, Hofeldt F, Shackelford A, Waldeck N, Dodson LE Jr, Bunker D, et al. Comparison of oral glucose tolerance tests and mixed meals in patients with apparent idiopathic postabsorptive hypoglycemia: absence of hypoglycemia after meals. Diabetes 1981; 30:465-70.
16. Chen Y-T, Burchell A. Glycogen storage diseases. In: Scriver AL, eds. The metabolic and molecular bases of inherited disease. New York: McGraw-Hill, 1995:935-65.
17. Chua KS, Tan IK. Plasma glucose measurement with the Yellow Springs Glucose Analyzer. Clin Chem 1978;24:150-2.
18. Cohen HT, Spiegel DM. Air-exposed urine dipsticks give false-positive results for glucose and false-negative results for blood. Am J Clin Pathol 1991;96:398-400.
19. Cryer PE, Axelrod L, Grossman AB, Heller SR, Montori VM, Seaquist ER, et al. Evaluation and management of adult hypoglycemic disorders: an Endocrine Society Clinical Practice Guideline. J Clin Endocrinol Metab 2009;94:709-28.
20. Cryer PE, Fisher JN, Shamoon H. Hypoglycemia. Diabetes Care 1994; 17:734-55.
21. Curme HG, Columbus RL, Dappen GM, Eder TW, Fellows WD, Figueras J, et al. Multilayer film elements for clinical analysis: general concepts. Clin Chem 1978;24:1335-42.
22. Daughaday WH. The possible autocrine/paracrine and endocrine roles of insulin-like growth factors of human tumors. Endocrinology 1990;127:1-4.
23. DCCT Research Group. The effect of intensive treatment of diabetes on the development and progression of long-term complications in insulin-dependent diabetes mellitus. N Engl J Med 1993;329: 977-86.
24. DECODE Study Group. Consequences of the new diagnostic criteria for diabetes in older men and women. DECODE Study (Diabetes Epidemiology: Collaborative Analysis of Diagnostic Criteria in Europe). Diabetes Care 1999;22:1667-71.
25. DeFronzo RA, Hendler R, Christensen N. Stimulation of counterregulatory hormonal responses in diabetic man by a fall in glucose concentration. Diabetes 1980;29:125-31.
26. Doppman JL, Chang R, Fraker DL, Norton JA, Alexander HR, Miller DL, et al. Localization of insulinomas to regions of the pancreas by intra-arterial stimulation with calcium. Ann Intern Med 1995;123: 269-73.
27. Fajans SS, Vinik AI. Insulin-producing islet cell tumors. Endocrinol Metab Clin North Am 1989;18:45-74.
28. Froom P, Bieganiec B, Ehrenrich Z, Barak M. Stability of common analytes in urine refrigerated for 24 h before automated analysis by test strips. Clin Chem 2000;46:1384-6.
29. Gambino R, Piscitelli J, Ackattupathil TA, Theriault JL, Andrin RD, Sanfilippo ML, et al. Acidification of blood is superior to sodium fluoride alone as an inhibitor of glycolysis. Clin Chem 2009;55: 1019-21.
30. Gerich JE. Lilly Lecture 1988. Glucose counterregulation and its impact on diabetes mellitus. Diabetes 1988;37:1608-17.
31. Gerich JE. Physiology of glucose homeostasis. Diabetes Obes Metab 2000;2:345-50.
32. Gochman N, Schmitz JM. Application of a new peroxide indicator reaction to the specific, automated determination of glucose with glucose oxidase. Clin Chem 1972;18:943-50.
33. Haymond MW. Hypoglycemia in infants and children. Endocrinol Metab Clin North Am 1989;18:211-52.

34. Hofeldt FD. Reactive hypoglycemia. Endocrinol Metab Clin North Am 1989;18:185-201.
35. Horrocks RH, Manning GB. Partition chromatography on paper: identification of reducing substances in urine. Lancet 1949;1: 1042-5.
36. Hung KK. Best Evidence Topic Report. BET 2: serum lactate as a marker for mortality in patients presenting to the emergency department with trauma. Emerg Med J 2009;26:118-9.
37. Hutchesson A, Preece MA, Gray G, Green A. Measurement of lactate in cerebrospinal fluid in investigation of inherited metabolic disease. Clin Chem 1997;43:158-61.
38. Imbeault P, Prins JB, Stolic M, Russell AW, O'Moore-Sullivan T, Despres JP, et al. Aging per se does not influence glucose homeostasis: in vivo and in vitro evidence. Diabetes Care 2003;26:480-4.
39. Kadish AH. A new and rapid method for the determination of glucose by measurement of rate of oxygen consumption. Clin Chem 1968;14: 116-31.
40. Kaplan EL, Rubenstein AH, Evans R, Lee CH, Klementschitsch P. Calcium infusion: a new provocative test for insulinomas. Ann Surg 1979;190:501-7.
41. Koeberl DD, Kishnani PS, Bali D, Chen YT. Emerging therapies for glycogen storage disease type I. Trends Endocrinol Metab 2009;20: 252-8.
42. Kumar D, Mehtalia SD, Miller LV. Diagnostic use of glucagon-induced insulin response: studies in patients with insulinoma or other hypoglycemic conditions. Ann Intern Med 1974;80:697-701.
43. Kuwa K, Nakayama T, Hoshino T, Tominaga M. Relationships of glucose concentrations in capillary whole blood, venous whole blood and venous plasma. Clin Chim Acta 2001;307:187-92.
44. Ladenson JH, Tsai LM, Michael JM, Kessler G, Joist JH. Serum versus heparinized plasma for eighteen common chemistry tests: is serum the appropriate specimen? Am J Clin Pathol 1974;62:545-52.
45. Larsson-Cohn U. Differences between capillary and venous blood glucose during oral glucose tolerance tests. Scand J Clin Lab Invest 1976;36:805-8.
46. Lefebvre PJ, Andreani D, Marks V. Statement on "post-prandial" or reactive hypoglycemia. In: Andreani D, Marks V, Lefebvre PJ, eds. Hypoglycemia, Serono Symposium. New York: Raven Press, 1987.
47. Livesley B, Atkinson L. Accurate quantitative estimation of lactate in whole blood [Letter]. Clin Chem 1974;20:1478.
48. Lott JA, Turner K. Evaluation of Trinder's glucose oxidase method for measuring glucose in serum and urine. Clin Chem 1975;21: 1754-60.
49. Lubran M. Measurement of lactic and pyruvic acid in biological fluids. In: Sunderman FW, Sunderman FW Jr, eds. Laboratory diagnosis of endocrine diseases. St Louis: Warren H. Green, 1971:401-8.
50. Ludvigsen CW, Thurn JR, Pierpont GL, Eckfeldt JH. Kinetic enzymic assay for D(-)-lactate, with use of a centrifugal analyzer. Clin Chem 1983;29:1823-5.
51. Lutz RA, Fluckiger J. Kinetic determination of glucose with the GEMSAEC (ENI) centrifugal analyzer by the glucose dehydrogenase reaction, and comparison with two commonly used procedures. Clin Chem 1975;21:1372-7.
52. Marbach EP, Weil MH. Rapid enzymatic measurement of blood lactate and pyruvate: use and significance of metaphosphoric acid as a common precipitant. Clin Chem 1967;13:314-25.
53. Martin-Rendon E, Blake DJ. Protein glycosylation in disease: new insights into the congenital muscular dystrophies. Trends Pharmacol Sci 2003;24:178-83.
54. Merimee TJ, Tyson JE. Stabilization of plasma glucose during fasting: normal variations in two separate studies. N Engl J Med 1974;291: 1275-8.
55. Miles RR, Roberts RF, Putnam AR, Roberts WL. Comparison of serum and heparinized plasma samples for measurement of chemistry analytes. Clin Chem 2004;50:1704-5.
56. Miller SI, Wallace RJ Jr, Musher DM, Septimus EJ, Kohl S, Baughn RE. Hypoglycemia as a manifestation of sepsis. Am J Med 1980;68: 649-54.
57. Miller WG, Myers GL, Ashwood ER, Killeen AA, Wang E, Ehlers GW, et al. State of the art in trueness and interlaboratory harmonization for 10 analytes in general clinical chemistry. Arch Pathol Lab Med 2008;132:838-46.
58. Neese JW. Glucose, direct hexokinase method: selected methods. Clin Chem 1982;9:241-8.
59. Neese JW, Duncan P, Bayse D. Development and evaluation of a hexokinase/glucose-6-phosphate dehydrogenase procedure for use as a national glucose reference method. HEW Publication No. (CDC)77-8330. Atlanta, Ga: Centers for Disease Control, 1976.
60. O'Sullivan JB. Age gradient in blood glucose levels: magnitude and clinical implications. Diabetes 1974;23:713-5.
61. Palardy J, Havrankova J, Lepage R, Matte R, Belanger R, D'Amour P, et al. Blood glucose measurements during symptomatic episodes in patients with suspected postprandial hypoglycemia. N Engl J Med 1989;321:1421-5.
62. Parnetti L, Gaiti A, Polidori MC, Brunetti M, Palumbo B, Chionne F, et al. Increased cerebrospinal fluid pyruvate levels in Alzheimer's disease. Neurosci Lett 1995;199:231-3.
63. Passey RB, Gillum RL, Fuller JB, Urry FM, Giles ML. Evaluation and comparison of 10 glucose methods and the reference method recommended in the proposed product class standard (1974). Clin Chem 1977;23:131-9.
64. Pithukpakorn M. Disorders of pyruvate metabolism and the tricarboxylic acid cycle. Mol Genet Metab 2005;85:243-6.
65. Pryce JD, Gant PW, Sau KJ. Normal concentrations of lactate, glucose, and protein in cerebrospinal fluid, and the diagnostic implications of abnormal concentrations. Clin Chem 1970;16:562-5.
66. Reljic R, Ries M, Anic N, Ries B. New chromogen for assay of glucose in serum. Clin Chem 1992;38:522-5.
67. Richter B, Neises G. "Human" insulin versus animal insulin in people with diabetes mellitus. Cochrane Database Syst Rev 2002(3): CD003816.
68. Robinson BH. Lactic acidemia (disorders of pyruvate carboxylase, pyruvate dehydrogenase). In: Shriver CR, Beaudet AL, Sly WS, Agricola BA, Metzger ME, Donahue RE, eds. The metabolic and molecular bases of inherited disease. New York: McGraw-Hill, 1995: 1479-99.
69. Sacks DB, Bruns DE, Goldstein DE, Maclaren NK, McDonald JM, Parrott M. Guidelines and recommendations for laboratory analysis in the diagnosis and management of diabetes mellitus. Clin Chem 2002; 48:436-72.
70. Savory J, Kaplan A. A gas chromatographic method for the determination of lactic acid in blood. Clin Chem 1966;12:559-69.
71. Sazama K, Robertson EA, Chesler RA. Is antiglycolysis required for routine glucose analysis? Clin Chem 1979;25:2038-9.
72. Seltzer HS. Drug-induced hypoglycemia: a review of 1418 cases. Endocrinol Metab Clin North Am 1989;18:163-83.
73. Service FJ. Hypoglycemic disorders. N Engl J Med 1995;332:1144-52.
74. Service FJ, Dale AJ, Elveback LR, Jiang NS. Insulinoma: clinical and diagnostic features of 60 consecutive cases. Mayo Clin Proc 1976;51: 417-29.
75. Shapiro ET, Bell GI, Polonsky KS, Rubenstein AH, Kew MC, Tager HS. Tumor hypoglycemia: relationship to high molecular weight insulin-like growth factor-II. J Clin Invest 1990;85:1672-9.
76. Special report: statement on hypoglycemia. Diabetes 1973;22:137.
77. Sundaram PV, Blumenberg B, Hinsch W. Routine glucose determination in serum by use of an immobilized glucose dehydrogenase nylon-tube reactor. Clin Chem 1979;25:1436-9.
78. The fad disease: hypoglycemia is being diagnosed too often. *Time*, April 7, 1980:71.
79. Trinder P. Determination of glucose in blood using glucose oxidase with an alternative oxygen acceptor. Ann Clin Biochem 1969;6:24-7.
80. Uribarri J, Oh MS, Carroll HJ. D-Lactic acidosis: a review of clinical presentation, biochemical features, and pathophysiologic mechanisms. Medicine (Baltimore) 1998;77:73-82.
81. Weissman M, Klein B. Evaluation of glucose determinations in untreated serum samples. Clin Chem 1958;4:420-2.

82. Wiberg-Itzel E, Lipponer C, Norman M, Herbst A, Prebensen D, Hansson A, et al. Determination of pH or lactate in fetal scalp blood in management of intrapartum fetal distress: randomised controlled multicentre trial. BMJ 2008;336:1284-7.
83. World Health Organization. Definition and diagnosis of diabetes mellitus and intermediate hyperglycemia: report of a WHO/IDF consultation. Geneva: World Health Organization, 2006.
84. Wright WR, Rainwater JC, Tolle LD. Glucose assay systems: evaluation of a colorimetric hexokinase procedure. Clin Chem 1971; 17:1010-5.
85. Young DS, Jackson AJ. Thin-layer chromatography of urinary carbohydrates: a comparative evaluation of procedures. Clin Chem 1970;16:954-9.

CHAPTER 27

Lipids, Lipoproteins, Apolipoproteins, and Other Cardiovascular Risk Factors

*Alan T. Remaley, M.D., Ph.D., Nader Rifai, Ph.D., and G. Russell Warnick, M.S., M.B.A.**

Lipids are ubiquitous in the body tissue and play a vital role in virtually all aspects of life—(1) servinas hormones or hormone precursors, (2) aiding in digestion, (3) providing a source of metabolic fuel and energy storage, (4) acting as functional and structural components in cell membranes, and (5) forming insulation to allow nerve conduction or to prevent heat loss. In this chapter, we have categorized lipids into basic lipids, lipoproteins, and apolipoproteins. We discuss the basic biochemistry, clinical significance, and analytical considerations of each.

BASIC BIOCHEMISTRY

Much attention has been focused on certain lipids and the lipoproteins that transport them in the circulation, mainly because of their strong association with coronary heart disease (CHD). As a consequence, use of the term *lipids* in clinical chemistry and laboratory medicine has virtually become synonymous with lipoprotein metabolism and atherosclerosis—a key step in the pathogenesis of CHD. Much of this association has been recognized through the conduct of large-scale epidemiologic, and clinical studies. In the early 1980s, findings from the Coronary Primary Prevention Trial first demonstrated that a decrease in plasma cholesterol concentration results in a reduction in the incidence of CHD. Subsequently, several secondary prevention trials, using diet or drugs to lower blood cholesterol, have also shown a reduction in cardiovascular death and atherosclerotic clinical events. Based on these trials and other evidence, the National Heart, Lung, and Blood Institute established the National Cholesterol Education Program (NCEP) to increase public awareness about cholesterol; devise strategies for the diagnosis and treatment of hypercholesterolemia in adults, children, and adolescents; and improve the laboratory measurement of lipids. Other international and national organizations have established similar programs to address these issues.

Basic Lipid Biochemistry

The general term *lipid* applies to a class of hydrophobic compounds that are soluble in organic solvents and nearly insoluble in water. Chemically, lipids are usually enriched in carbon and hydrogen and after hydrolysis typically yield fatty acids or complex alcohols, which are usually esterified with fatty acids. Some lipids are more complex, containing other chemical groups, such as sialic, phosphoryl, amino, or sulfate groups. The presence of these charged or polar groups makes these lipids amphipathic, which gives them the property of having an affinity for both water and organic solvents; this is an important feature in their ability to form cell membranes. Lipids can been broadly subdivided into five groups based on their chemical structure (Box 27-1).

Cholesterol

Although every living organism has been found to contain sterols, cholesterol is found almost exclusively in animals, in which it is also the main sterol. Virtually all cells and body fluids contain some cholesterol. Similar to other sterols,

**The authors gratefully acknowledge the contributions by Drs. John Albers and Paul Bachorik on which portions of this chapter are based. Additional portions have been adapted from Rifai N, Kwiterovich PO Jr.: Disorders of lipid and lipoprotein metabolism in children and adolescents. In Soldin SJ, Rifai N, Hick JMB, eds: Biochemical basis of pediatric diseases, 3rd edition. Washington, DC: AACC Press, 1998.*

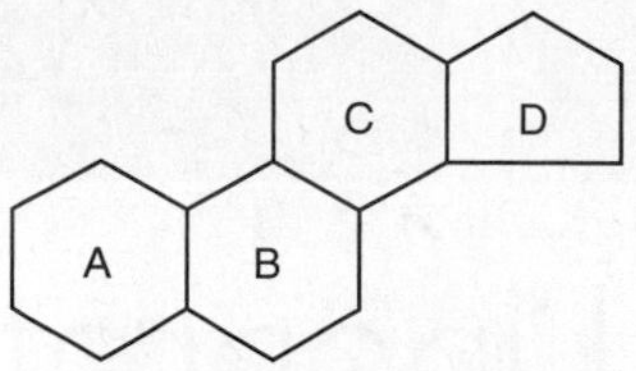

Perhydrocyclopentanophenanthrene (sterane) skeleton

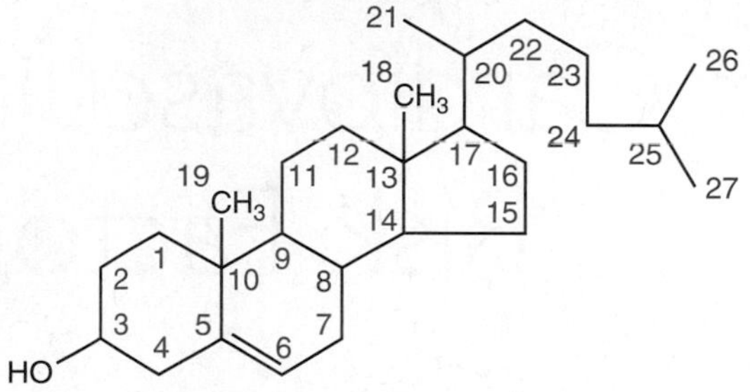

Cholesterol

Figure 27-1 Structure of cholesterol.

BOX 27-1 Classification of Clinically Important Lipids

Sterol Derivatives
- Cholesterol and cholesteryl esters
- Steroid hormones
- Bile acids
- Vitamin D

Fatty Acids
- Short chain (2 to 4 carbon atoms)
- Medium chain (6 to 10 carbon atoms)
- Long chain (12 to 26 carbon atoms)
- Prostaglandins

Glycerol Esters
- Triglycerides, diglycerides, and monoglycerides (acylglycerols)
- Phosphoglycerides

Sphingosine Derivatives
- Sphingomyelin
- Glycosphingolipids

Terpenes (Isoprene Polymers)
- Vitamin A
- Vitamin E
- Vitamin K

cholesterol is a solid alcohol of high molecular weight that possesses a tetracyclic perhydrocyclopentanophenanthrene skeleton. It contains 27 carbon atoms, numbered as shown in Figure 27-1. Knowledge of the sterane skeleton structure and numbering system is important not only to clinical laboratorians but also to practicing clinicians, because cholesterol is the starting point in many different metabolic pathways. These include vitamin D synthesis (see Chapter 52), steroid hormone synthesis (see Chapter 53), and bile acid metabolism (see Chapter 50). Because the enzymes modifying the sterane cholesterol ring or its derivatives are known by their site and type of reaction (e.g., 21-hydroxylase in cortisol synthesis), the diagnosis of many disease states consequently depends on isolating the site of enzyme dysfunction (e.g., 21-hydroxylase deficiency in adrenogenital syndrome).

Cholesterol Absorption

Cholesterol enters the intestinal lumen from three sources: the diet, bile, and the intestine. Animal products—especially meat, egg yolk, seafood, and whole fat dairy products—provide the bulk of dietary cholesterol. Although cholesterol intake varies considerably based on the dietary intake of animal products, the average American diet is estimated to contain approximately 300 to 450 mg of cholesterol per day. A similar amount of cholesterol enters the gut from biliary secretion and from the turnover of intestinal mucosal cells, and possibly from direct intestinal secretions. Practically all cholesterol in the intestinal lumen is present in the unesterified or free form. Esterified cholesterol in the diet is rapidly hydrolyzed in the intestine to free cholesterol and free fatty acids by cholesterol esterases secreted from the pancreas and small intestine.

To be absorbed, unesterified cholesterol first must be solubilized. This occurs through the formation of mixed micelles that contain unesterified cholesterol, fatty acids, monoglycerides (derived from triglycerides), phospholipids, and conjugated bile acids. Formation of mixed micelles promotes cholesterol absorption by both solubilizing the cholesterol and facilitating its transport to the surface of the luminal cell, where it is absorbed by an active process involving the enterocyte protein NPC1L1, which is the drug target for the cholesterol absorption inhibitor ezetimibe. Because of their amphipathic properties, the bile acids act as detergents and are the most important factor affecting micelle formation. In the absence of bile acids, digestion and absorption of both cholesterol and triglyceride are severely impaired, leading to fat malabsorption. The quantity of dietary cholesterol that can be absorbed appears to depend on the amount that can be solubilized by micelles. On average, 30 to 60% of dietary and intestinal cholesterol is absorbed daily. With increments in dietary cholesterol, additional cholesterol is absorbed to a maximum of approximately 1 g/d when oral intake reaches 3 g/d. Absorption of cholesterol and other sterols, such as plant sterols, is limited by the presence of the ABCG5/G8 transporter on enterocytes, which pumps excess sterols back into the lumen for excretion. When this protein is defective, it results in a disease called *sitosterolemia,* which is characterized by a marked increase in plasma and tissue concentrations of plant sterols, such as sitosterol, and an increased risk for CHD. The ability of cholesterol to form micelles is also influenced by the quantity of dietary fat but not its degree of saturation. Increased amounts of fat in the diet results in expansion of mixed micelles, which in turn allows more cholesterol to be solubilized and absorbed. Most cholesterol absorption occurs from the jejunum to the terminal ileum of the small intestine. As absorption of fat and cholesterol occurs in the small intestine, the micelles break up, thus reducing further cholesterol absorption.

After its absorption into the intestinal mucosal cell, cholesterol, together with triglycerides, phospholipids, and a number of specific apoproteins, is assembled into a large lipoprotein called a *chylomicron* (see later section on lipoprotein metabolism, exogenous pathway). One apoprotein component known as apolipoprotein (apo) B-48 is vital in the formation and secretion of chylomicrons. Patients with a rare deficiency in this process develop a disease called *chylomicron retention disorder,* which is characterized by excess lipid in enterocytes and fat malabsorption. Once secreted by enterocytes, chylomicrons enter the lymphatics, which eventually empty into the thoracic duct and enter the systemic venous circulation at the junction of the left subclavian vein and the left internal jugular vein.

Cholesterol Synthesis

Although cholesterol enters the body from the diet, it is also synthesized endogenously by all tissues from acetate. Knowledge of the endogenous cholesterol synthetic pathway has assumed great significance, because drug agents for the treatment of CHD have been sought to suppress or decrease endogenous cholesterol synthesis. The necessity for understanding the fundamental biochemistry of this pathway was originally underscored by the triparanol disaster of 1960. Triparanol is a drug that inhibits the final step in the endogenous cholesterol synthetic pathway—the conversion of desmosterol to cholesterol—but does not inhibit the rate-limiting enzyme of cholesterol synthesis, 3-hydroxy-3-methylglutaryl-CoA (HMG-CoA) reductase (Figure 27-2). When triparanol was used to treat hypercholesterolemia, the drug caused tissue accumulation of desmosterol, resulting in the development of cataracts, alopecia, and accelerated atherosclerosis. Many drugs now used to treat CHD selectively suppress the rate-limiting enzyme HMG-CoA reductase, thereby lowering serum cholesterol concentrations significantly without accumulation of water-insoluble intermediates of cholesterol synthesis, such as desmosterol.

Although essentially all cells have the capacity to synthesize cholesterol from acetyl-CoA, almost 90% of synthesis occurs in the liver and gut; other organs and tissues depend, in part, on cholesterol delivery from the circulation. Cholesterol biosynthesis is best conceptualized as occurring in three stages (Figures 27-2 through 27-4). In the first stage, acetyl-CoA, a key metabolic intermediate that can be derived from carbohydrates, amino acids, and fatty acids, forms the six-carbon thioester HMG-CoA. In the second stage, HMG-CoA is reduced to mevalonate, then is decarboxylated to form five-carbon isoprene units. These isoprene units are condensed to form first a 10-carbon (geranyl pyrophosphate) and then a 15-carbon intermediate (farnesyl pyrophosphate). Two of these C_{15} molecules combine to produce the final product of the second stage—squalene, a 30-carbon acyclic hydrocarbon. The second stage is important, because it contains the step involving the microsomal enzyme HMG-CoA reductase, which is the rate-limiting enzyme in cholesterol biosynthesis. The enzyme that forms farnesyl pyrophosphate, geranyl transferase, is an important second site of regulation in cholesterol synthesis. This degree of inhibition still permits the formation of physiologically important intermediate isoprenoids in the absence of cholesterol synthesis. The third and final stage of synthesis occurs in the endoplasmic reticulum, with many of the intermediate products being bound to a specific carrier protein. Squalene, after initial oxidation, undergoes cyclization to form the four-ring, 30-carbon intermediate, lanosterol. In a series of oxidation-decarboxylation reactions, several sidechains are removed from the pentanophenanthrene structure to form the final 27-carbon molecule of cholesterol.

Cholesterol Esterification

Once synthesized, cholesterol is released into the circulation bound to lipoproteins, such as very low-density lipoprotein (VLDL; see later section on lipoprotein metabolism, endogenous pathway), which is one of the primary lipoproteins secreted by the liver. The major apoprotein found in VLDL is apo B-100. It is produced by the same gene as apo B-48, but represents the full-length product of the apo B gene. Apo B-48 is produced in the intestine by a post-transcriptional editing step, which introduces a stop codon in about the middle of the apo B-100 mRNA transcript, thus resulting in a protein about 48% the length of the full-length apo B-100 protein. The esterification of cholesterol is important, because it serves to enhance the lipid-carrying capacity of the lipoprotein in plasma and prevents intracellular toxicity by free

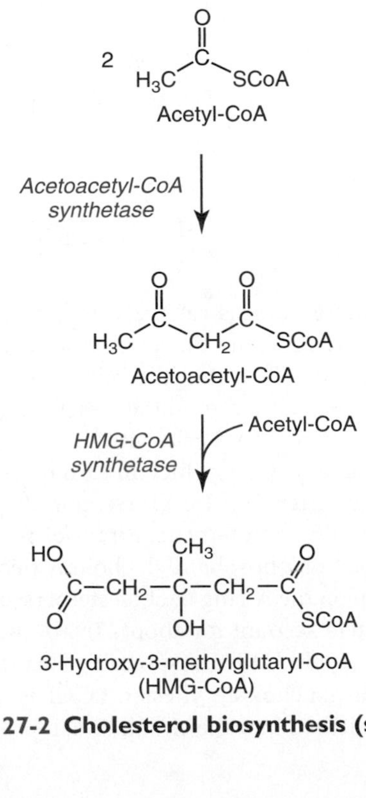

Figure 27-2 Cholesterol biosynthesis (stage I).

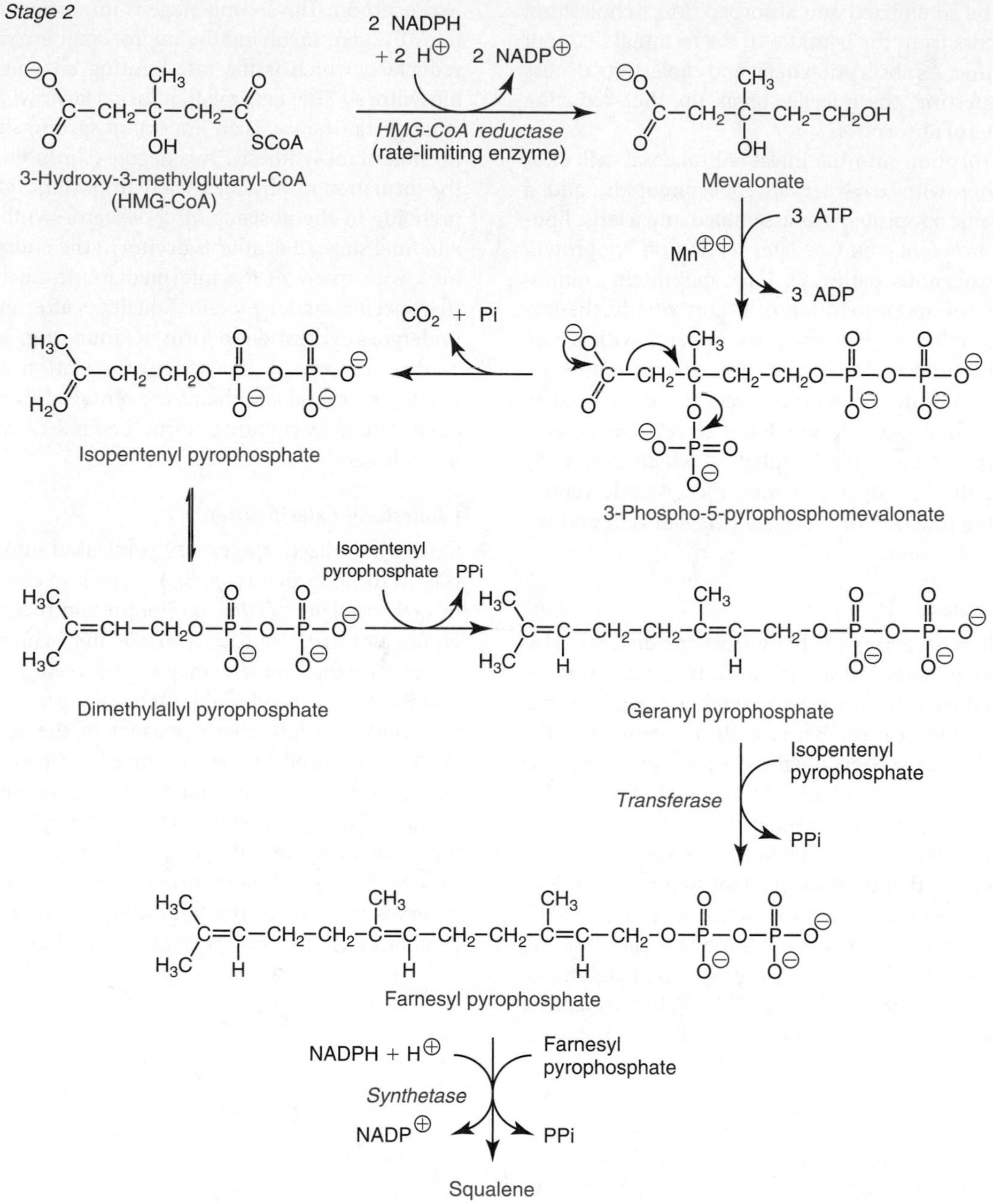

Figure 27-3 Cholesterol biosynthesis (stage 2).

cholesterol. The reaction is catalyzed by lecithin-cholesterol acyltransferase (LCAT) in the plasma and acylcholesterol acyltransferase (ACAT) within the cell. ACAT is an energy-requiring enzyme, and the initial reaction (Figure 27-5) involves activation of a fatty acid with thio coenzyme A (CoASH) to form an acyl-CoA, which in turn reacts with cholesterol to form an ester. The LCAT reaction does not require CoASH and results from fatty acid transfer from the second carbon position of phosphatidyl choline (lecithin) to the hydroxyl group on the A-ring of cholesterol (see Figure 27-5). Cholesteryl esters account for about 70% of the total cholesterol in plasma, and LCAT is responsible for the formation of virtually all plasma cholesteryl ester. LCAT is synthesized in the liver and released into the circulation; it primarily resides on lipoproteins and is activated by apo A-I and other apolipoproteins (see later section on apolipoproteins). The esterification of cholesterol by LCAT on the only polar group of cholesterol makes cholesteryl ester more hydrophobic than cholesterol. This causes the cholesterol on the surface of lipoproteins, once esterified, to partition into the more hydrophobic core of lipoproteins, where triglycerides are also located.

Cholesterol Catabolism

Once a lipoprotein enters the cell, its cholesteryl esters and triglycerides are hydrolyzed by lysosomal acid lipase. Lack or malfunction of this enzyme results in intracellular accumulation of cholesteryl esters and triglycerides, particularly in the

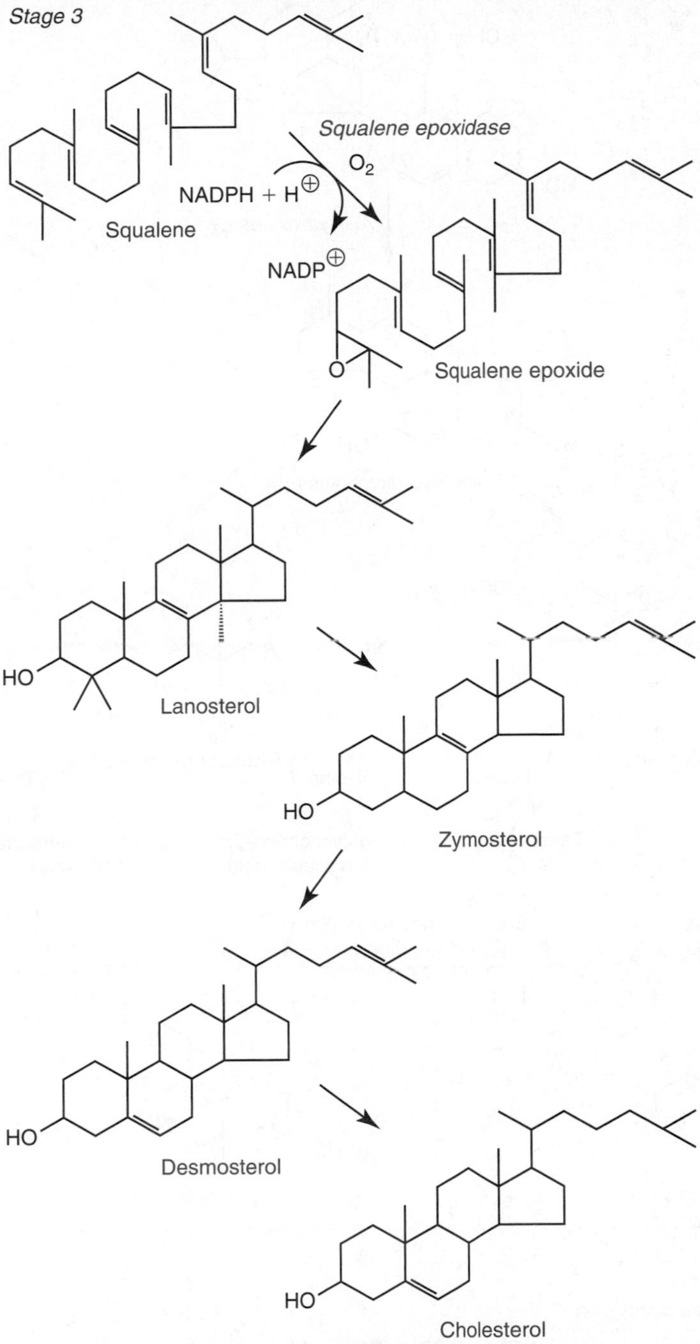

Stage 3

Squalene epoxidase

O_2

NADPH + $H^{\oplus}$

$NADP^{\oplus}$

Squalene

Squalene epoxide

Lanosterol

Zymosterol

Desmosterol

Cholesterol

Figure 27-4 Cholesterol biosynthesis (stage 3).

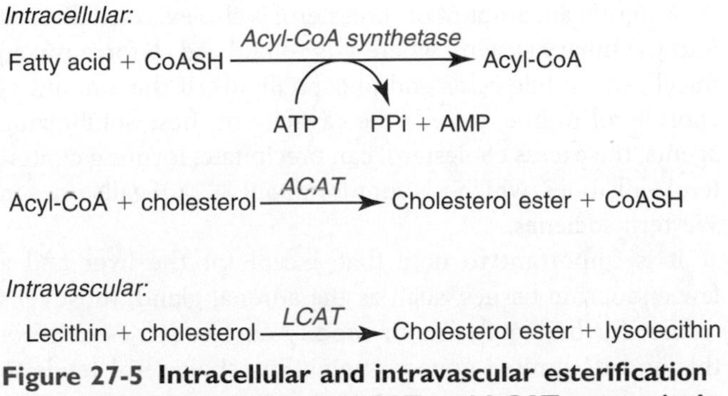

Intracellular:

Fatty acid + CoASH —*Acyl-CoA synthetase*→ Acyl-CoA (ATP → PPi + AMP)

Acyl-CoA + cholesterol —*ACAT*→ Cholesterol ester + CoASH

Intravascular:

Lecithin + cholesterol —*LCAT*→ Cholesterol ester + lysolecithin

Figure 27-5 Intracellular and intravascular esterification of cholesterol mediated by ACAT and LCAT, respectively.

liver, and produces a clinical disorder known as *cholesteryl ester storage disease*, or *Wolman's disease.*

Cholesterol reaching the liver may be secreted unchanged into bile or metabolized to bile acids or resecreted on lipoproteins. Approximately one third of the daily production of cholesterol, or about 400 mg/d, is converted into bile acids (Figure 27-6). Conversion of cholesterol to cholic and chenodeoxycholic acids, the major bile acids in humans, involves shortening of the cholesterol sidechain and hydroxylation of the sterol nucleus. The first step, which is also the rate-limiting step, is hydroxylation of the 7-position of the sterol nucleus, catalyzed by the enzyme 7α-hydroxylase (see Figure 27-6).

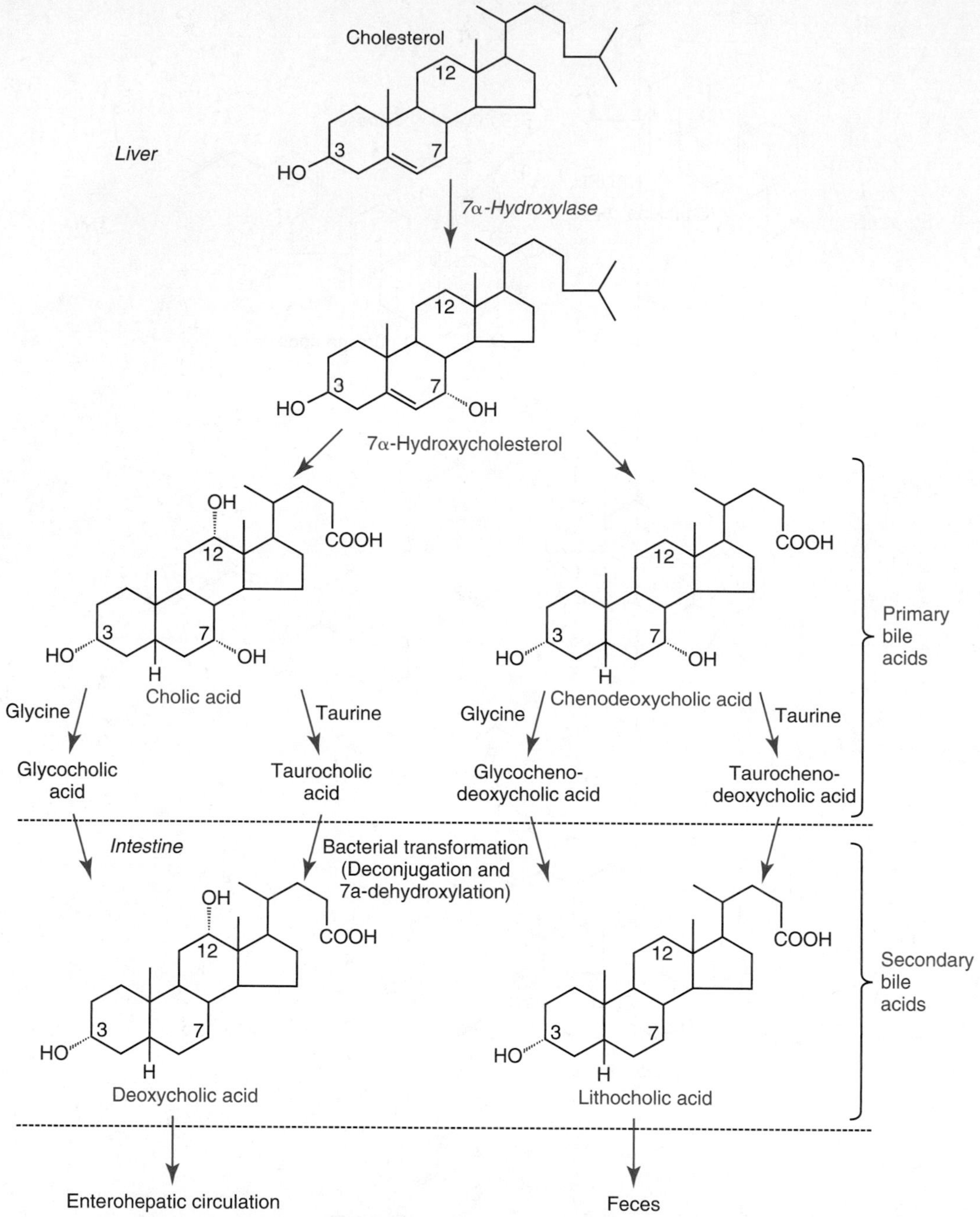

Figure 27-6 Bile acid synthesis.

The bile acids are made more polar after conjugation with glycine or taurine and then are excreted into the bile canaliculi. After reaching the small intestine, the conjugated bile acids play an active part in cholesterol and fat absorption, as discussed previously. Some of the bile acids are deconjugated and converted by bacteria in the intestine to secondary bile acids. Cholic acid is converted to deoxycholic acid, and chenodeoxycholic acid is metabolized to lithocholic acid. About 90% of the bile acids, except lithocholic, are reabsorbed in the lower third of the ileum and returned to the liver by the portal vein, which is called the enterohepatic circulation (see also Chapter 50).

A significant amount of cholesterol is also excreted directly into the biliary system, where it is solubilized to form mixed micelles with bile acids and phospholipids. If the amount of cholesterol in bile exceeds the capacity of these solubilizing agents, the excess cholesterol can precipitate, forming cholesterol gallstones, which account for about 80% of gallstones in Western societies.

It is important to note that except for the liver and a few endocrine tissues, such as the adrenal gland, most cells cannot further catabolize or modify cholesterol. Because of this and its limited aqueous solubility, cholesterol tends to accumulate in cells or extracellular spaces; this is another feature of cholesterol that contributes to its ability to cause atherosclerosis.

Fatty Acids

The fatty acids are one of the simpler molecular forms of lipids. They are generically indicated by the chemical formula RCOOH, where "R" stands for an alkyl chain. Fatty acid chain lengths vary and are commonly classified according to the number of carbon atoms present. Three somewhat arbitrarily defined groups of fatty acids are those containing 2 to 4 carbon atoms (short chain), 6 to 10 carbon atoms (medium chain), and 12 to 26 carbon atoms (long chain). Those of importance in human nutrition and metabolism are of the long-chain class containing an even number of carbon atoms.

Fatty acids are further classified according to their degree of saturation. Saturated fatty acids have no double bonds between carbon atoms, monounsaturated fatty acids contain one double bond, and polyunsaturated fatty acids contain more than one double bond (Figure 27-7). The double bonds in polyunsaturated fatty acids of both animal and plant origin are usually 3 carbon atoms apart. Some fatty acids from marine fish living in deep, cold waters (e.g., salmon), which form oils at room temperature, possess numerous (up to 6) unsaturated bonds and usually are more than 20 carbon atoms long. These fatty acids are prone to oxidation, which occurs at the sites of unsaturation.

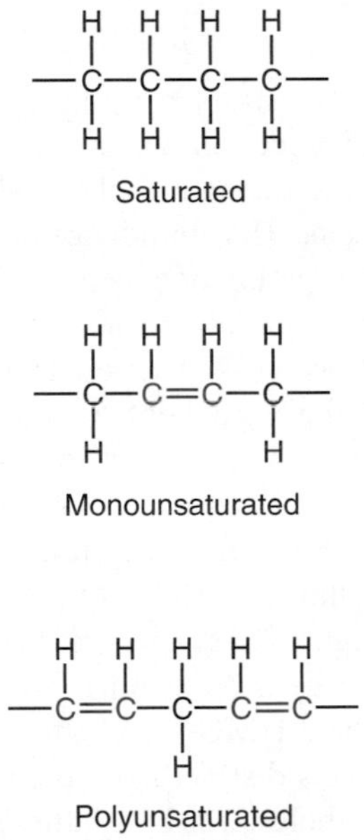

Saturated

Monounsaturated

Polyunsaturated

Figure 27-7 Saturated and unsaturated fatty acids.

Labeling of carbon atoms in fatty acids can take place from the carboxyl terminal (Δ-numbering system) or from the methyl terminal (η- or ω-numbering system; Table 27-1). In addition, carbon atoms may be labeled with Greek symbols, with α being adjacent to the carboxyl group and ω being farthest away. In the Δ-system, fatty acids are abbreviated according to the number of carbon atoms, the number of double bonds, and the position(s) of double bond(s). For example, linoleic acid, which contains 18 carbons and 2 unsaturated bonds between carbons 9 and 10 and between carbons 12 and 13, could be written as C_{18}:2.^{9,12} Using the η- or ω-system, linoleic acid would be abbreviated to C_{18}:2n-6, where only the first carbon forming the unsaturated pair is written. The *Geneva* or *systematic* classification is a third system of nomenclature (see Table 27-1).

In saturated fatty acids, the acyl chain is extended and flexible (i.e., the carbon atoms rotate freely around the longitudinal axis), and each internal carbon atom is fully saturated or, in other words, is covalently linked to two hydrogen molecules. *Cis*-unsaturated fatty acids have a fixed 30° bend in their acyl chains at each double bond, because two hydrogen molecules are missing from the same side of the carbon double bond, thus causing the bend. Lipids containing *cis*-unsaturated fatty acids, such as triglycerides or phospholipids, have lower melting points, because these lipids cannot interact and pack as tightly together by van der Waals interactions. As a consequence, lipids containing *cis*-unsaturated fatty acids, such as olive oil and other plant oils, are usually liquids at room temperature. In mammals, all naturally occurring unsaturated fatty acids are of the *cis* variety. *Trans* unsaturated fatty acids result from a chemical process called *catalytic hydrogenation*, a process used to "harden" unsaturated fats from plant sources in the manufacture of certain

TABLE 27-1 Fatty Acids Commonly Found in Human Tissue

Common Name	Systematic Name	Δ-Numbering	η-(ω) Numbering
Lauric	Dodecanoic	12:0	12:0
Myristic	Tetradecanoic	14:0	14:0
Palmitic	Hexadecanoic	16:0	16:0
Palmitoleic	9-Hexadecenoic	$16:1^{9}$	16:1n-7
Stearic	Octadecanoic	18:0	18:0
Oleic	9-Octadecenoic	$18:1^{9}$	18:1n-9
Linoleic*	9,12-Octadecadienoic	$18:2^{9,12}$	18:2n-6
Linolenic*	9,12,15-Octadecatrienoic	$18:3^{9,12,15}$	18:3n-3
Arachidic	Eicosanoic	20:0	20:0
Arachidonic	5,8,11,14-Eicosatetraenoic	$20:4^{5,8,11,14}$	20:4n-6

*Essential fatty acids.

foods, such as margarine. Although *trans* fatty acids are still unsaturated, one hydrogen is missing from each side of the carbon double bond, making these fatty acids resemble the more linear configuration of the acyl chain of saturated fatty acids, which also makes them solids at room temperature. Epidemiologic and experimental studies have shown that *trans* fatty acids may promote CHD; an effort is under way to reduce the use of catalytic hydrogenation in food processing and to reduce the consumption of *trans* fatty acids in the diet.[203]

Most fats in the human body are derived from the diet, which on the average in Western societies contains up to 40% fat, 90% of which is triglyceride. In addition, humans can synthesize most fatty acids, including saturated, monounsaturated, and some polyunsaturated fats; however, some fatty acids cannot be synthesized. One such fatty acid is linoleic acid ($C_{18}:2^{9,12}$), which is found only in plants. Because it is vital for health and growth and development, it is termed an *essential fatty acid.* Linoleic acid is converted to arachidonic acid, which has an important role in prostaglandin synthesis and in myelinization of the central nervous system.

The fatty acid carboxyl group has a pK_a of approximately 4.8; thus free fatty acid molecules in both plasma and intracellular fluid (pH of 7.4 and 7.0, respectively) exist primarily in an ionized form. Much of the fatty acid in plasma exists as esters with cholesterol or glycerol, or is transported as a free fatty acid–albumin complex or a free fatty acid–prealbumin complex. One molecule of albumin can carry as many as 20 molecules of fatty acid. The normal concentration of free fatty acids in human blood is 0.30 to 1.10 mmol/L, or about 8 to 31 mg/dL of plasma. The flux of free fatty acids through the plasma is very large and is sensitive to physiologic energy demands (exercise and physical work), the concentration of blood glucose, and psychologic stresses that cause liberation of epinephrine.

Fatty Acid Catabolism

Long-chain fatty acids are oxidized in the mitochondria and produce energy by a series of reactions that operate in a repetitive manner to shorten the fatty acid chain by two carbon atoms at a time from the carboxy (—COOH) terminal of the molecule through a process known as β-oxidation. For example, 1 mole of C_{16} fatty acid is converted to 8 moles of acetyl-CoA. Acetyl-CoA does not normally accumulate in the cell but is enzymatically condensed with oxaloacetate, derived largely from carbohydrate metabolism (Figure 27-8), to yield citrate, which is a major component of the tricarboxylic acid cycle, also called *Krebs cycle.* The Krebs cycle serves as a common pathway for the final oxidation of nearly all food material, whether derived from carbohydrate, fat, or protein. It is important to note that the efficiency of the Krebs cycle depends on the availability of sufficient oxaloacetate to serve as an acceptor for acetyl-CoA.

Complete oxidation of a single fatty acid molecule produces a relatively large quantity of energy. For example, the complete oxidation of 1 mole of palmitic acid to carbon dioxide and water produces 16 moles of CO_2, 16 moles of H_2O, and 129 moles of adenosine triphosphate, or 2340 Cal.* Thus the standard free energy for oxidation of palmitic acid is 2340 Cal, whereas the free energy liberated by hydrolysis of 129 moles of ATP is 940 Cal, indicating that the efficiency of energy conservation in fatty acid oxidation is approximately 40% under standard conditions.

By means of suitable enzyme reactions, the chemical energy stored in fatty acids can be released for metabolic processes or stored in the form of high-energy compounds, such as ATP. Triglycerides that contain three fatty acid molecules, therefore, are an efficient storage form for metabolic energy. The amount of energy produced by metabolizing 1 mole of palmitic acid (16 carbon atoms) is approximately twice that produced by metabolizing an equivalent amount (2.5 mole) of glucose (6 carbon atoms per molecule). Carbohydrate storage also requires water for hydration; triglyceride storage does not. In addition to their high intrinsic energy content, triglycerides have a low density (<1 g/mL) and, because of their hydrophobic nature and peripheral distribution in the body, provide excellent insulation.

Ketone Formation

During prolonged starvation, or when carbohydrate metabolism is severely impaired, as in uncontrolled diabetes mellitus (see Chapter 26), the formation of acetyl-CoA exceeds the supply of oxaloacetate. The abundance of acetyl-CoA results from excessive mobilization of fatty acids from adipose tissue and excessive degradation of fatty acids by β-oxidation in the liver. The resulting acetyl-CoA excess is diverted to an alternative pathway in the mitochondria and forms acetoacetic acid, β-hydroxybutyric acid, and acetone—three compounds known collectively as *ketone bodies* (Figure 27-9). The presence of ketone bodies is a frequent finding in severe, uncontrolled diabetes mellitus.

As shown in Figure 27-9, the first product, acetoacetyl-CoA, condenses in the mitochondria with a third molecule of acetyl-CoA to yield HMG-CoA. This pool of HMG-CoA in the mitochondria is distinct from the pool in the cytosol, which is used for cholesterol biosynthesis. The HMG-CoA produced in the mitochondria is cleaved enzymatically to yield acetoacetate and acetyl-CoA. Some of the acetoacetate formed in liver cells is usually reduced to β-hydroxybutyrate. Because acetoacetate is unstable, a further portion decomposes to form carbon dioxide and acetone, the third ketone body found in severe, untreated diabetes mellitus. Ketosis, therefore, develops from excessive production of acetyl-CoA because the body attempts to derive necessary energy from stored fat in the absence of an adequate supply of carbohydrate metabolites (see Chapter 26).

Inadequate incorporation of acetyl-CoA into the Krebs cycle may be further aggravated by inhibition of the oxaloacetate-generating enzyme system through excess

*The unit used in discussing the energy value of food is the calorie (Cal), equal to 1000 calories or 1 kilocalorie (kcal). In the SI system, the unit of energy is the joule (J), and 1 calorie = 4.1868J.

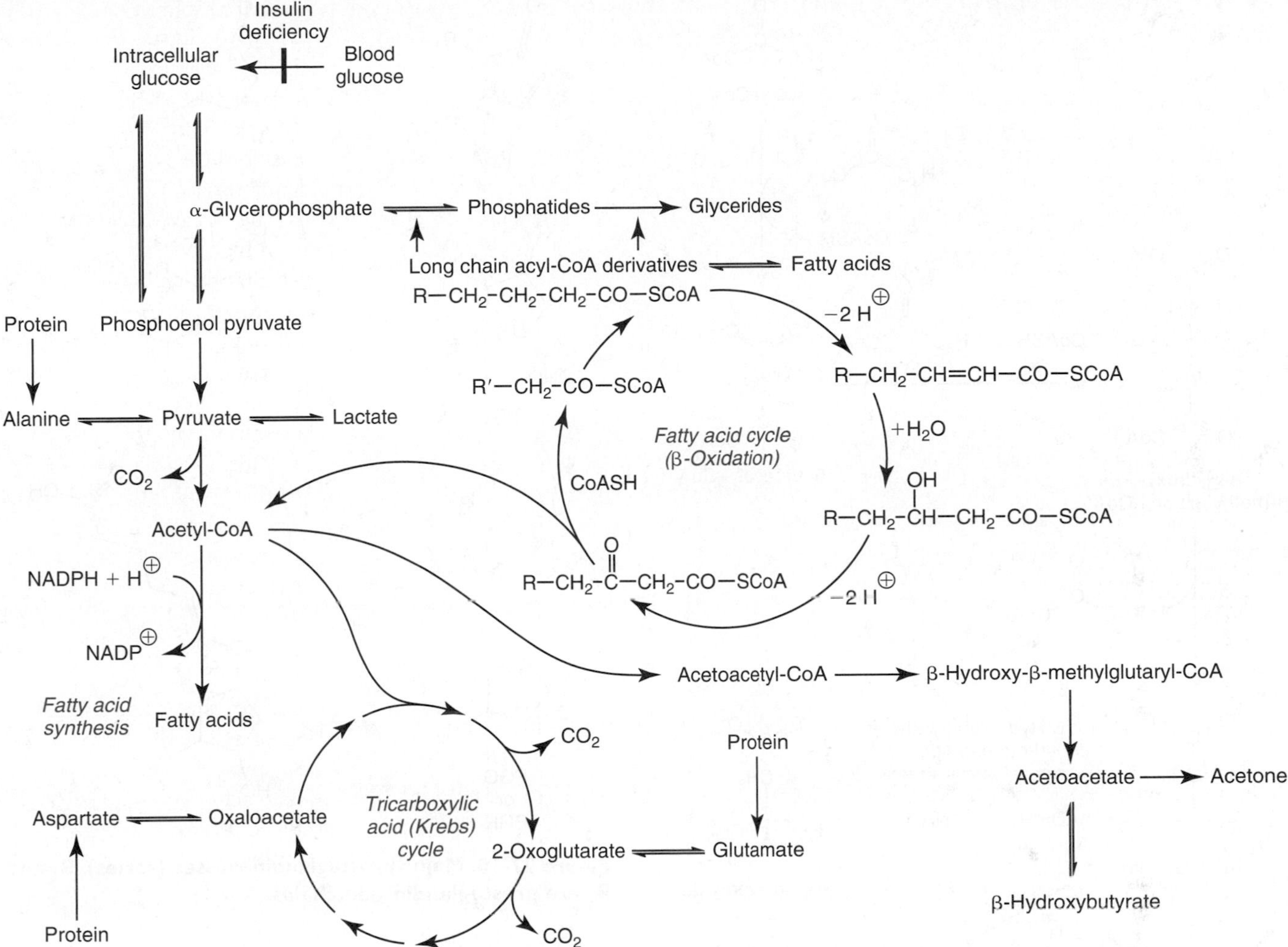

Figure 27-8 Metabolic relations among intermediates of carbohydrate, fat, and protein metabolism. Note that acetyl-CoA is produced from both carbohydrate and fat. The glucogenic amino acids, derived from protein metabolism, enter glycolytic paths as α-keto acids. Ketogenic amino acids enter as acetyl-CoA.

accumulation of palmitic-CoA and other long-chain fatty acid–CoA derivatives in the liver. Skeletal muscle and heart (and brain in prolonged fasting) use ketone bodies by resynthesizing their CoA derivatives and subsequently oxidizing them for the production of energy. Although liver cells are largely responsible for converting fatty acids, they cannot metabolize acetoacetate, because the liver lacks 3-ketoacid CoA transferase, the enzyme required for transferring CoA from succinyl-CoA.

The entire process of ketosis is reversed by restoring adequate metabolism of carbohydrate. In starvation, restoration consists of adequate carbohydrate ingestion; in diabetes mellitus, ketosis can be reversed by insulin administration, which permits circulating blood glucose to be taken up by the cells. With restored concentrations of oxaloacetate, acetyl-CoA can instead enter the Krebs cycle, thus restoring the normal pathway for energy metabolism. Eventually, the release of fatty acids from adipose tissue slows down and is finally reversed. A graphic view of these metabolic reactions is outlined in Figure 27-8, which shows the interrelationship between carbohydrate, fatty acid, and protein metabolism.

Prostaglandins

Prostaglandins and related compounds are derivatives of fatty acids, primarily arachidonate. This group consists of prostaglandins, thromboxanes, some hydroperoxy- and hydroxy-fatty acid derivatives, and leukotrienes. Although their full physiologic role is not completely known, these lipids are known to affect a wide variety of biological functions. In general, they are extremely potent, producing physiologic actions at concentrations as low as 1 μg/L.

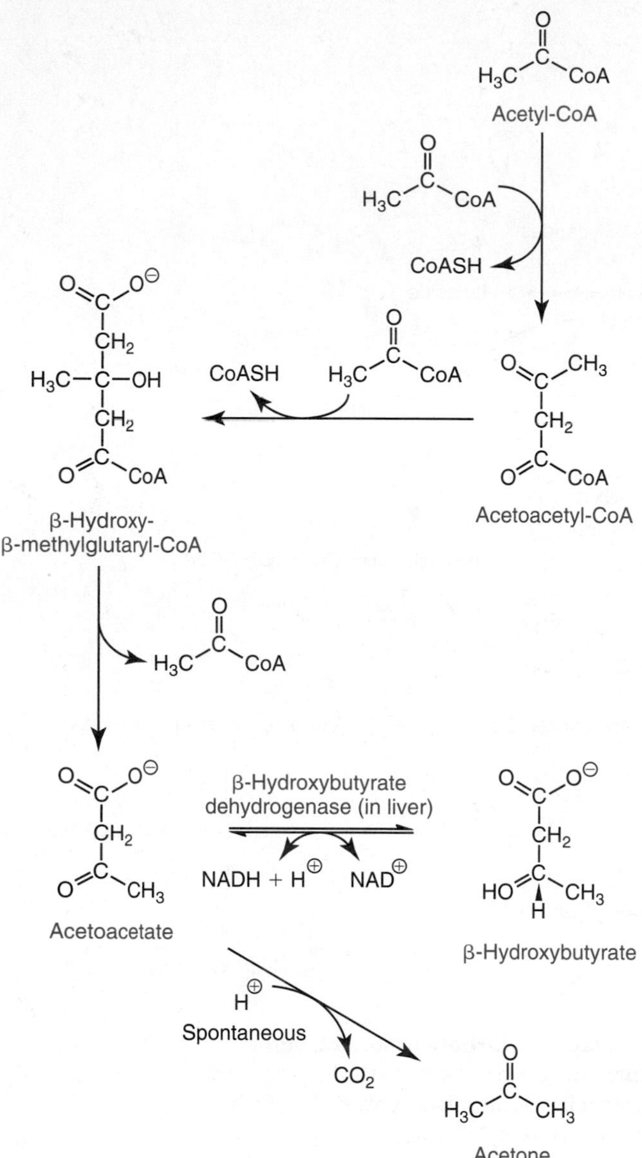

Figure 27-9 Formation of ketone bodies.

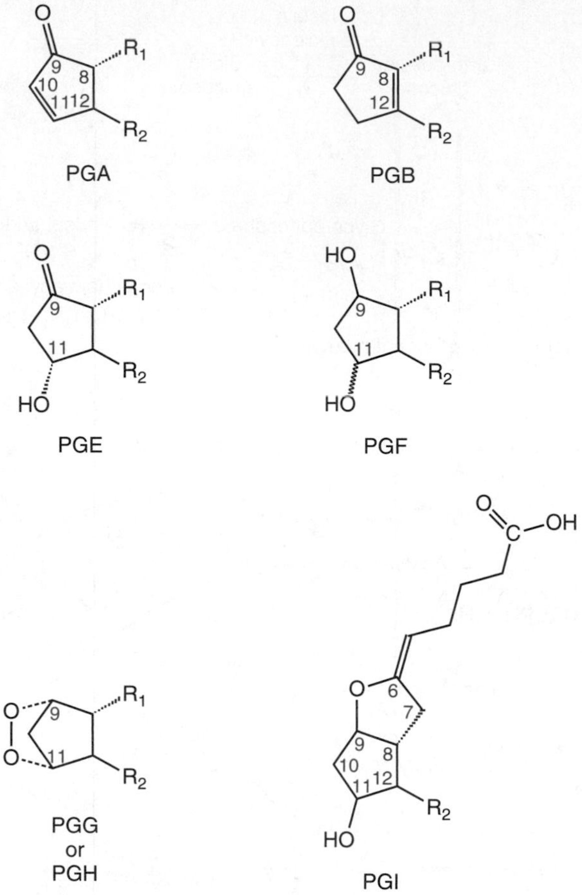

Figure 27-10 Major prostaglandin classes (series). R_1 and R_2 are prostaglandin side chains.

The prostaglandins are a series of C_{20} unsaturated fatty acids containing a cyclopentane ring; the parent fatty acid has been given the trivial name *prostanoic acid.* The seven-carbon chain linked to C-8 of prostanoic acid (R_1) projects below the plane of the ring, whereas the eight-carbon chain attached to C-12 (R_2) projects above the ring.

By convention, prostaglandins are abbreviated *PG,* with the class designated by a capital letter (A, B, E, F, G, H, and I), followed by a number and then in some cases a Greek letter (Figure 27-10). With the exception of PGG and PGH, which have the same ring structure (cyclopentane endoperoxide), the letters refer to different ring structures. PGA and PGB have keto groups at C-9, with the A series having a double bond between C-10 and C-11, and the B series having a double bond between C-8 and C-12. PGE also has a C-9 keto bond but a hydroxyl group at C-11. The F series has hydroxyl groups at both C-9 and C-11. The difference between PGG and PGH, which have identical ring structures, occurs in the sidechain at C-15 in R_2. The G series has a peroxide group, whereas the H series has a hydroxyl group. The I series has a double-ring formation, with the C-9 of the cyclopentane ring linked to C-6 of the sidechain by an oxygen molecule to form a second five-sided ring (see Figure 27-10). The endoperoxide PGs (G and H series) are intermediates in the formation of other PGs.

The number after the capital letter is usually written as a subscript and is used to designate the number of unsaturated bonds in the PG sidechains and not within the ring structure itself. In PGE_1, for example, a double bond exists between C-13 and C-14; in the 2 series (PGE_2), a double bond exists between C-13 and C-14 and between C-5 and C-6; and in the 3 series (PGE_3), an additional double bond occurs between C-17 and C-18. The 2 series is most common. The bond between C-13 and C-14 is always *trans,* whereas bonds between C-5 and C-6 and between C-17 and C-18 are always *cis.* At C-15, all naturally occurring prostaglandins have a hydroxyl group that projects below the plane of the ring. Use of the Greek letter (α or β) applies only to the F series and refers to the hydroxyl group found at C-9. In the α-series, the hydroxyl group projects below the ring plane in the same direction as the C-11 hydroxyl group, whereas the β-series

TABLE 27-2 Naturally Occurring Prostaglandins (PGs)

Primary PG	Other PG
PGE_1	PGA_1
$PGF_{1\alpha}$	PGA_2
PGE_2	19α-$OHPGA_1$
$PGF_{2\alpha}$	19α-$OHPGA_2$
PGG_2	PGB_1
PGH_2	PGB_2
PGI_2	19α-$OHPGB_2$
Thromboxane A_2	PGE_3
Thromboxane B_2	$PGF_{3\alpha}$

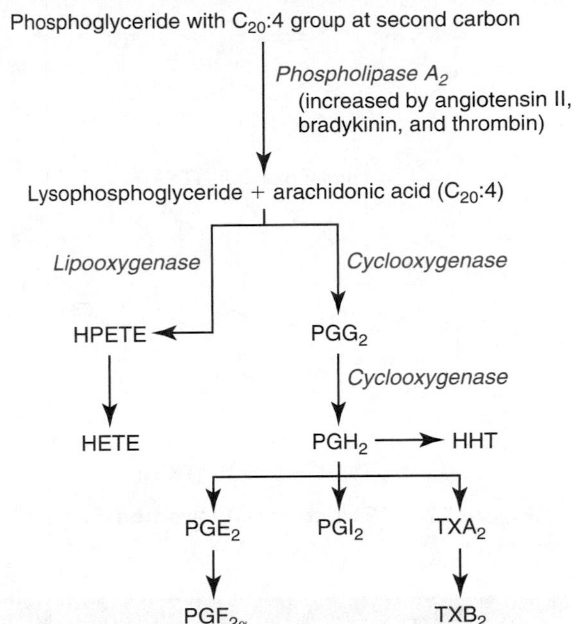

Figure 27-11 Synthesis of prostaglandins from arachidonic precursor. HPETE, HETE, HHT, 12-l-Hydroxy-5,8,10-heptadecatrienoic acid; *PG*, prostaglandin; *TX*, thromboxane.

denotes that the hydroxyl at C-9 is above the plane of the ring. Sixteen naturally occurring prostaglandins have been described (Table 27-2), but only seven, along with two thromboxanes, are commonly found throughout the body, and they are termed the *primary prostaglandins.*

Although prostaglandins have hormone-like actions, they are different from most other hormones in that (1) they are synthesized at the site of action, and (2) they are made in almost all tissues. Linoleic acid ($C_{18}:2^{9,12}$) is the precursor of two of the three 20-carbon fatty acids that form prostaglandins; linolenic acid ($C_{18}:2^{9,12,15}$) is the other precursor. Both of these fatty acids are considered essential because they cannot be synthesized in the body and, therefore, must be present in the diet. The three C_{20} fatty acids subsequently formed are $C_{20}:3^{5,8,11}$ (eicosatrienoic acid), $C_{20}:4^{5,8,11,14}$ (eicosatetraenoic or arachidonic acid), and $C_{20}:5^{8,11,14,17}$(eicosatrienoic acid). These three fatty acids form the PG_1, PG_2, and PG_3 series, respectively.

Once formed, prostaglandins exert very short-lived effects and are rapidly catabolized to inactive forms within a few seconds. Inactivation of prostaglandin appears to be mediated by two enzymes: 15 α-hydroxy-prostaglandin dehydrogenase and Δ^{13}-prostaglandin reductase. Prostaglandins are not stored; instead, precursor C_{20} fatty acids are present in tissue attached to the C-2 (see later section in this chapter on glycerol esters) of phosphoglycerides. When necessary, the C_{20} precursor is hydrolyzed by phospholipase A_2, which is specific for the C-2 position of phosphoglyceride. Release of the C_{20} fatty acid appears to be the rate-limiting step in prostaglandin synthesis and is stimulated by many different agents, such as bradykinin, thrombin, or angiotensin II.

Although it is probable that all prostaglandins follow a similar synthetic pathway, C_{20}:4 (arachidonic acid) has been the most intensively studied and is used to illustrate the pathway (Figure 27-11). Once released, arachidonic acid follows one of two pathways. The lipoxygenase route produces 12-L-hydroperoxy-5,8,10,14 eicosatetraenoic acid (HPETE); HPETE then spontaneously decomposes to 12-L-hydroxy-5,8,10,14 eicosatetraenoic acid (HETE). The alternative pathway is mediated by cyclooxygenase (COX) to produce the endoperoxides PGG_2 and PGH_2. The latter can be degraded to 12-L-hydroxy-5,8,10-heptadecatrienoic acid. What controls the entry into a specific pathway remains speculative; however, it is known that nonsteroidal anti-inflammatory drugs (NSAIDs; aspirin, ibuprofen, and indomethacin) inhibit the COXs, thereby decreasing prostaglandin synthesis. Two isoforms of COX are known: COX-1 and COX-2. COX-1 concentrations in general are constitutively expressed, whereas COX-2 is synthesized in response to inflammation. Certain drugs that inhibit both COXs have nephrotoxic and ulcerogenic side effects. Therefore, newer NSAIDs have been developed that preferentially inhibit COX-2 to reduce side effects, but they have been found to also be associated with an increased incidence of myocardial infarction.[94]

Prostaglandin I_2, or prostacyclin, is derived from arachidonic acid (see Figure 27-11) in the vascular endothelium. It has a powerful vasodilatory action, especially on the coronary arteries, and is responsible for inhibiting platelet aggregation. Thromboxane A_2 is synthesized from arachidonic acid but is also produced by platelets. It has the opposite effect of prostacyclin (i.e., it stimulates the contraction of arterial smooth muscle and enhances platelet aggregation). It has a very short half-life—about 30 seconds—and is rapidly converted to its inactive metabolite, thromboxane B_2. The thromboxanes are slightly different from other prostaglandins in that they contain six-sided rings of five carbon atoms and one oxygen atom (Figure 27-12). Table 27-3 lists some reported functions of the various prostaglandins.

Glycerol Esters (Acylglycerols)

Virtually all complex lipids contain fatty acids, and in most cases they are covalently linked to an alcohol. One of the most

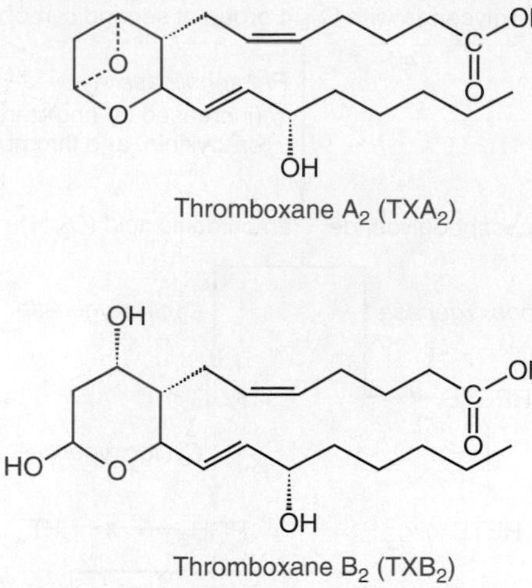

Thromboxane A_2 (TXA_2)

Thromboxane B_2 (TXB_2)

Figure 27-12 Structures of thromboxanes.

TABLE 27-3 Prostaglandin-Mediated Effects

Site of Action	Physiologic Response
Arterial smooth muscle	Alters blood pressure
Uterine muscle	Induces labor, therapeutic abortion
Lower gastrointestinal tract	Increases motility
Bronchial smooth muscle	Bronchospasm
Platelets	Increases coagulability
Capillaries	Increases permeability
Stomach	Enhances gastric acid secretion
Adipose tissue	Inhibits triglyceride lipolysis

common alcohols found in lipids is glycerol, a three-carbon molecule containing three hydroxyl groups.

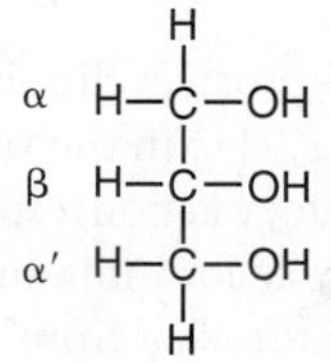

$$\begin{array}{ll} & \text{H} \\ \alpha & \text{H—C—OH} \\ \beta & \text{H—C—OH} \\ \alpha' & \text{H—C—OH} \\ & \text{H} \end{array}$$

The two terminal carbon atoms in the molecule are chemically equivalent and are designated α and α′. The center carbon is labeled β. A common alternative labeling system uses the numeral 1 for the α-carbon, 2 for the β-carbon, and 3 for the α′-carbon.

The class of acylglycerol (glyceride) is determined by the number of fatty acyl groups present; one fatty acid, monoacylglycerols (monoglycerides); two fatty acids, diacylglycerols (diglycerides); three fatty acids, triacylglycerols (triglycerides). In a monoacylglycerol, the fatty acid may be linked to any of the three carbon atoms. By convention, the number system is used to indicate the carbon position (e.g.,

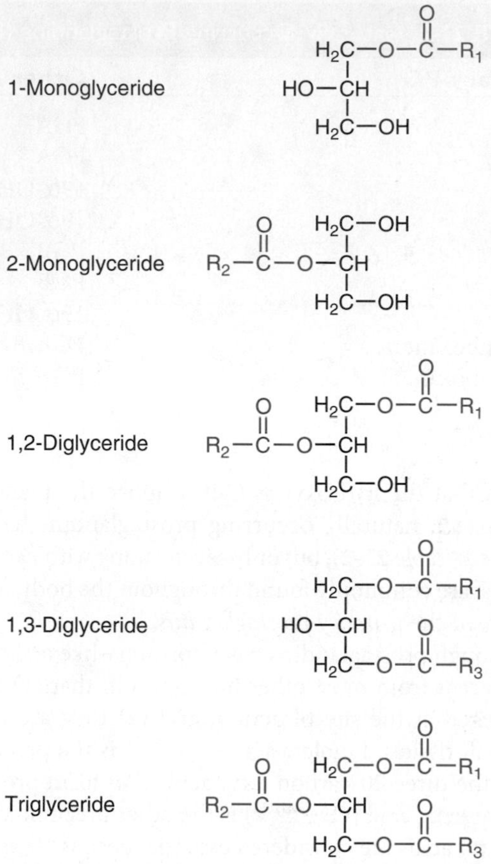

1-Monoglyceride

2-Monoglyceride

1,2-Diglyceride

1,3-Diglyceride

Triglyceride

Figure 27-13 Structure and classification of glycerol esters (acylglycerols). R_1, R_2, and R_3 are fatty acids of varying chain length.

1-monoglyceride indicates a fatty acid attachment to the α-carbon). This numbering system applies to all acylglycerols, including the phosphoglycerides, as shown later. Diglycerides may be 1,2- or 1,3-diglycerides (Figure 27-13).

Triglycerides are the most prevalent glycerol esters encountered in the body and constitute 95% of tissue storage fat; they are the predominant form of glyceryl ester found in plasma. Fatty acid residues found in monoglycerides, diglycerides, or triglycerides vary considerably and usually include combinations of the long-chain fatty acids shown in Table 27-1. Triglycerides from plants (e.g., corn, sunflower seed, safflower oils) tend to have large quantities of *cis*-unsaturated fatty acids, such as C_{18}:2 or linoleic acid, and are liquid at room temperature. Triglycerides from animals, especially ruminants, tend to have C_{12}:0 through C_{18}:0 fatty acid residues (saturated fats) and are solids at room temperature. Rarely, some plant triglycerides, such as coconut oil, are highly saturated and may be solid at room temperature.

Triglycerides are digested in the duodenum and the proximal ileum. Through the action of pancreatic and intestinal lipases and in the presence of bile acids, which activate lipases, they are hydrolyzed to glycerol, monoglycerides, and fatty acids. After absorption, triglycerides are resynthesized in the intestinal epithelial cells and are combined with cholesterol and apo B-48 to form chylomicrons. Another major class of

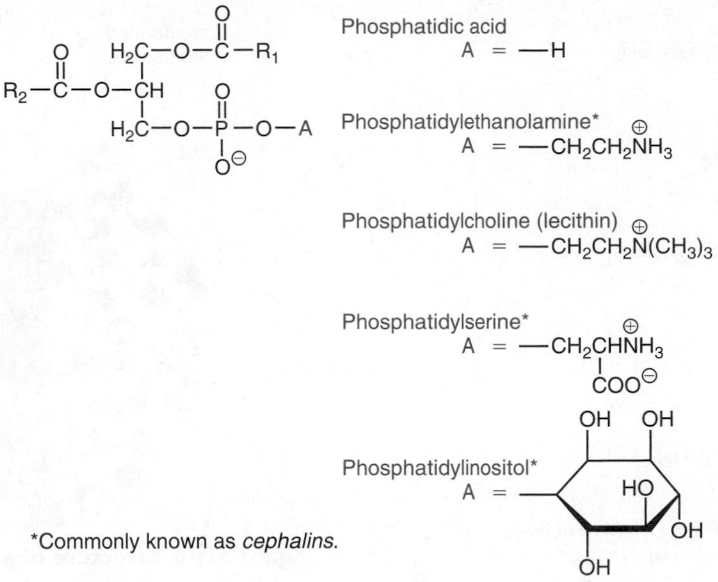

Phosphatidic acid
A = —H

Phosphatidylethanolamine*
A = $—CH_2CH_2NH_3^{\oplus}$

Phosphatidylcholine (lecithin)
A = $—CH_2CH_2N^{\oplus}(CH_3)_3$

Phosphatidylserine*
A = $—CH_2CH(NH_3^{\oplus})COO^{\ominus}$

Phosphatidylinositol*
A =

*Commonly known as *cephalins.*

Figure 27-14 Structures of phosphoglycerides and common alcohol groups associated with them. R_1 and R_2 are fatty acid(s) of varying carbon atom lengths.

glycerol esters consists of those containing phosphoric acid at the third (α′) carbon atom; these esters are called *phosphoglycerides* (Figure 27-14). In their simplest form, the A group is an H atom; the molecule is therefore called a *diacylphosphoglyceride.* Usually, however, the A is an alcohol-derived group, such as choline, serine, inositol, or ethanolamine (see Figure 27-14). If A is choline, the molecule is referred to as *phosphatidylcholine;* if it is ethanolamine, it will be referred to as *phosphatidylethanolamine,* etc. The term *lecithin,* which is an older designation, is a commonly used term for phosphatidylcholines. Because of the wide variety of fatty acid residues at positions R_1 and R_2 (see Figure 27-14), many different types of phospholipids can be formed. These phospholipids are named according to the fatty acid acyl ester attached at C-1 and C-2 of the glycerol. Saturated fatty acids are typically attached to the C-1 position, whereas (poly)unsaturated fatty acids are often present at the C-2 position. In inner mitochondrial membranes, more complex phosphoglycerides known as *cardiolipins* can be found. They are derived from two phosphoglyceride molecules joined by a glycerol bridge.

Sphingolipids

Sphingolipids, a fourth class of lipids found in humans, are derived from the amino alcohol sphingosine (Figure 27-15). This dihydric 18-carbon alcohol contains an amino group at C-17. A fatty acid containing 18 or more carbon atoms can be bound to the amino group through an amide linkage to form *ceramide.* This is the intermediary step in the formation of three important sphingolipids: sphingomyelin, galactosylceramide, and glucosylceramide (see Figure 27-15). The sugar-containing ceramides can have a sulfate group attached (usually on the 2-position of the galactose residue) to form the sulfatides. The glycosyl ceramides can have additional monosaccharide moieties, such as galactose, *N*-acetylgalactosamine, and *N*-acetylneuraminic acid to form complex globosides and gangliosides. These complex sphingolipids form the major lipids of cell membranes, particularly in the central nervous system. Gangliosides, for example, are particularly prevalent in the gray matter of the brain, whereas membrane glycosphingolipids have major roles in cellular interactions, growth, and development. Some glycolipids on red cells form blood group antigens, whereas other glycolipids can be tumor antigens.

Terpenes

Terpenes are polymers of the five-carbon isoprene unit; they form the backbone of vitamins A, E, and K (see Chapter 31) and the dolichols, which play an important role in protein glycosylation.

Lipoproteins

Lipids synthesized in the liver and the intestine must be transported to various tissues to accomplish their metabolic functions. Because of their relative insolubility in aqueous solutions, they are transported in the plasma in macromolecular complexes called *lipoproteins.* Lipoproteins are typically spherical particles with more hydrophobic nonpolar lipids (triglycerides and cholesterol esters) in their core, and more polar or amphipathic lipids (phospholipids and free cholesterol) oriented near the surface as a single monolayer. They also contain one or more specific proteins, called *apolipoproteins,* which usually are located on their surface (Figure 27-16).[266] The association of core lipids with the overlying phospholipid, cholesterol, and protein coat is noncovalent, occurring primarily through hydrogen bonding and van der Waals forces. This binding is loose enough to allow spontaneous exchange of cholesterol, which is more water soluble than the other lipids, among plasma lipoproteins and between cell membranes. The other more hydrophobic lipids require specific transfer proteins to exchange between lipoproteins, such

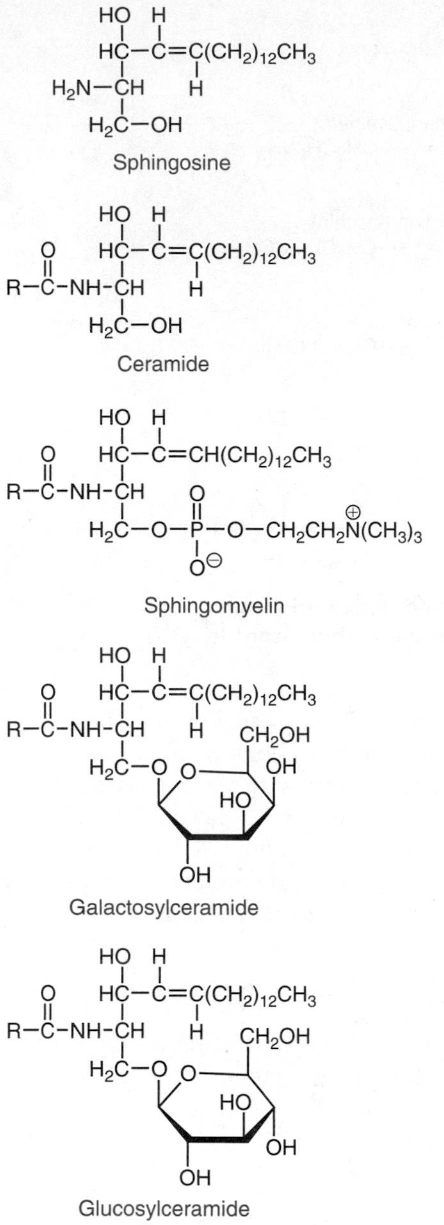

Sphingosine

Ceramide

Sphingomyelin

Galactosylceramide

Glucosylceramide

Figure 27-15 Structures of sphingolipids.

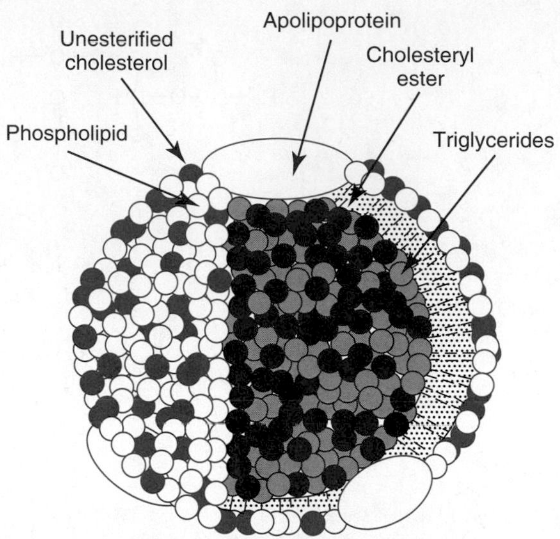

Figure 27-16 Structure of a typical lipoprotein particle.

as cholesteryl ester transfer protein (CETP), which exchanges triglycerides and cholesteryl esters between lipoproteins. Phospholipid transfer protein (PLTP) promotes the transfer of phospholipids between lipoproteins.

Lipoproteins have different physical and chemical properties (Table 27-4) because they contain different proportions of lipids and proteins (Table 27-5). Historically, lipoproteins have been categorized on the basis of differences in their hydrated densities, as determined by ultracentrifugation. Categories include (1) chylomicron, (2) VLDL, (3) intermediate-density lipoprotein (IDL), (4) low-density lipoprotein (LDL), (5) high-density lipoprotein (HDL), and (6) lipoprotein(a) [Lp(a)]. HDL can be further divided by density into two subpopulations: HDL_2 and HDL_3. Lp(a) consists of a distinct class of lipoproteins (see Table 27-4) that are structurally related to LDL, because similar to LDL, it contains one apo B-100 per particle and has a similar lipid composition.[79,177] In contrast to LDL, Lp(a) contains a carbohydrate-rich protein called apo(a), which is covalently bound to apo B-100 through a disulfide linkage. Apo(a) exhibits a significant sequence homology with plasminogen, but unlike plasminogen, Lp(a) is not an active protease. Lp(a) contains a high degree of variation in polypeptide chain length because of a variable number of kringle domains (Figure 27-17). Apo(a) contains 10 distinct classes of kringle 4–like domains that differ from each other in amino acid sequence. Kringle 4 type 1 and kringle 4 types 3 to 10 are present as a single copy, but kringle 4 type 2 is present in variable numbers of repeats (3 to >40) (see Figure 27-17).[157,323]

In the fasting state, most plasma triglycerides are present in VLDL. In the postprandial state, chylomicrons appear transiently and contribute significantly to the total plasma triglyceride concentration. LDL normally carries about 70% of total plasma cholesterol but very little triglyceride (see Table 27-5). HDL contains about 20 to 30% of plasma cholesterol.

Lipoproteins can be separated electrophoretically on agarose or on other solid support material, such as cellulose acetate, paper, or polyacrylamide gels.[224] At a pH of 8.6, HDL migrates with the α-globulins, LDL with the β-globulins, and VLDL and Lp(a) between the α- and β-globulins, in the pre–β-globulin region. IDL forms a broad band between β- and pre–β-globulins. Chylomicrons remain at the point of application. This forms the basis for the following common classification of lipoproteins: pre–β-lipoprotein, VLDL; β-lipoprotein, LDL; and α-lipoprotein, HDL.

Apolipoproteins

Apolipoproteins are the protein components of a lipoprotein. Characteristics and main known functions of the major apolipoproteins are summarized in Table 27-6. Each class of lipoprotein has a variety of apolipoproteins in differing proportions, with the exception of LDL, which contains only apo

TABLE 27-4 Characteristics of Human Plasma Lipoproteins

Variable	Chylomicron	VLDL	IDL	LDL	HDL	Lp(a)
Density, g/mL	<0.95	0.95-1.006	1.006-1.019	1.019-1.063	1.063-1.210	1.040-1.130
Electrophoretic mobility	Origin	Pre-β	Between β and pre-β	β	α	Pre-β
Molecular weight, Da	0.4-30 × 10^9	5-10 × 10^6	3.9-4.8 × 10^6	2.75 × 10^6	1.8-3.6 × 10^5	2.9-3.7 × 10^6
Diameter, nm	>70	27-70	22-24	19-23	4-10	27-30
Lipid-lipoprotein ratio	99:1	90:10	85:15	80:20	50:50	75:27-64:36
Major lipids	Exogenous triglycerides	Endogenous triglycerides	Endogenous triglycerides, cholesteryl esters	Cholesteryl esters	Phospholipids	Cholesteryl esters, phospholipids
Major proteins	A-I	B-100	B-100	B-100	A-I	(a)
	B-48	C-I	E	—	A-II	B-100
	C-I	C-II	—	—	—	—
	C-II	C-III	—	—	—	—
	C-III	E	—	—	—	—

HDL, High-density lipoprotein; *IDL,* intermediate-density lipoprotein; *LDL,* low-density lipoprotein; *Lp(a),* lipoprotein(a); *VLDL,* very low-density lipoprotein.

TABLE 27-5 Chemical Composition (%) of Normal Human Plasma Lipoproteins*

		Surface Components		Core Lipids	
	Cholesterol	Phospholipids	Apolipoproteins	Triglycerides	Cholesteryl Esters
Chylomicrons	2	7	2	86	3
VLDL	7	18	8	55	12
IDL	9	19	19	23	29
LDL	8	22	22	6	42
HDL_2	5	33	40	5	17
HDL_3	4	25	55	3	13

*Surface components and core lipids given as percentage of dry mass.
HDL, High-density lipoprotein; *IDL,* intermediate-density lipoprotein; *LDL,* low-density lipoprotein; *VLDL,* very low-density lipoprotein.
From Havel RJ, Kane JP. Introduction: structure and metabolism of plasma lipoproteins. In: Scriver CR, Beaudet AL, Sly WS, Valle D (eds). The metabolic and molecular bases of inherited diseases, 7th edition, volume II. New York: McGraw-Hill, 1995:1841-50. Reproduced with permission of The McGraw-Hill Companies.

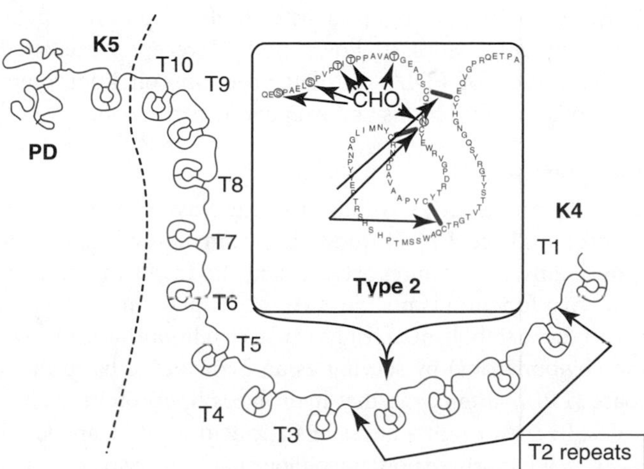

Figure 27-17 Structure of lipoprotein(a).

B-100. Apo A-I is the major protein in HDL. Apo C-I, C-II, C-III, and E are present in various proportions in all lipoproteins except LDL. Apolipoproteins collectively have three major physiologic functions. They are involved in (1) activating important enzymes in the lipoprotein metabolic pathways, (2) maintaining the structural integrity of the lipoprotein complex, and (3) facilitating uptake of lipoprotein into cells through their recognition by specific cell surface receptors.[173] Besides these main apolipoproteins, lipoproteins have been found to weakly bind a large number of plasma proteins, but their relevance is not fully understood.[119]

Apolipoprotein A

Together, apolipoprotein A-I and apo A-II constitute about 90% of total HDL protein. The ratio of apo A-I to A-II in HDL is about 3:1.[41] In addition to being an important structural

TABLE 27-6 Classification and Properties of Major Human Plasma Apolipoproteins

Apolipoprotein	Molecular Weight, Da	Chromosomal Location	Function	Lipoprotein Carrier(s)
Apo A-I	29,016	11	Cofactor LCAT	Chylomicron, HDL
Apo A-II	17,414	1	Not known	HDL
Apo A-IV	44,465	11	Activates LCAT	Chylomicron, HDL
Apo B-100	512,723	2	Secretion of triglyceride from liver binding protein to LDL receptor	VLDL, IDL, LDL
Apo B-48	240,800	2	Secretion of triglyceride from intestine	Chylomicron
Apo C-I	6630	19	Activates LCAT	Chylomicron, VLDL, HDL
Apo C-II	8900	19	Cofactor LPL	Chylomicron, VLDL, HDL
Apo C-III	8800	11	Inhibits apo C-II, activation of LPL	Chylomicron, VLDL, HDL
Apo E	34,145	19	Facilitates uptake of chylomicron remnant and IDL	Chylomicron, VLDL, HDL
Apo(a)	187,000-662,000	6	Unknown	Lp(a)

HDL, High-density lipoprotein; *IDL,* intermediate-density lipoprotein; *LCAT,* lecithin cholesterol acyltransferase; *LDL,* low-density lipoprotein; *Lp(a),* lipoprotein(a); *LPL,* lipoprotein lipase; *VLDL,* very low-density lipoprotein.

component of HDL, apo A-I is a cofactor for LCAT, the enzyme responsible for forming cholesteryl esters in plasma. Some evidence suggests that apo A-II may inhibit LCAT and activate hepatic triglyceride lipase. Apo A-IV is a component of newly secreted chylomicrons, but it is not a major constituent of chylomicron remnants, VLDL, LDL, and HDL. The primary function of apo A-IV is currently unknown, but it has been shown to activate LCAT in vitro,[54] and available data suggest that it plays a role in the intestinal absorption of lipid. Apo A-V is a recently described apolipoprotein.[88] It is relatively low in abundance compared with other apolipoproteins and appears to modulate triglyceride concentrations by a mechanism that currently is not well understood. All these proteins, including most of the other apolipoproteins, contain a structural motif called an *amphipathic helix.* It is an α-helix with approximately half the amino acid residues comprising hydrophobic amino acids, which face toward the neutral lipid core when bound to a lipoprotein particle. The other side of the helix faces outward from the surface of a lipoprotein particle and contains polar or charged amino acids. In general, the binding of amphipathic helices to lipoproteins is relatively weak, thus allowing apolipoproteins to exchange between different lipoproteins during lipoprotein metabolism.

Apolipoprotein B

As already discussed, apolipoprotein B exists in two forms: apo B-100 and apo B-48.[173] Apo B-100, a single polypeptide of more than 4500 amino acids, is the full-length translation product of the apo B gene. In humans, apo B-100 is made in the liver and is secreted into plasma as part of VLDL. Apo B-100 is also the major apolipoprotein of LDL, the end product of VLDL catabolism. Each VLDL particle contains one molecule of apo B-100. In the fasting state, most of the apo B in plasma is apo B-100. Unlike other apolipoproteins, however, apo B-100 cannot move from one lipoprotein particle to another, because in addition to amphipathic helices, it has β-sheets[287]—a structural motif with much higher affinity for lipids. It is for this reason that apo B-100 remains with VLDL as it is transformed by lipolysis of its triglycerides and is eventually converted into LDL. Apo B-48 contains 2152 amino acids and is identical to the amino-terminal portion of apo B-100. Apo B-48 results from post-transcriptional modification of internal apo B-100 messenger ribonucleic acid, in which a single base substitution produces a stop codon corresponding to residue 2153 of apo B-100. Apo B-48 is made in the intestine and is the major apo B component of chylomicrons. Both apo B-100 and apo B-48 play important roles in the secretion of VLDL and chylomicrons, respectively. Apo B-100 is recognized by the LDL receptor in hepatic and peripheral tissues; it allows the LDL receptor-mediated internalization of LDL[44] (see later sections on lipoprotein metabolism, endogenous and exogenous pathways).

Apolipoprotein C

Apolipoproteins C-I, C-II, and C-III are associated with all lipoproteins except LDL. Apo C-I, the smallest of the C apolipoproteins, has been reported to activate LCAT in vitro, but its in vivo function is not clear. Apo C-II plays an important role in the metabolism of triglyceride-rich lipoprotein (VLDL and chylomicrons) by serving as an activator of lipoprotein lipase (LPL), an enzyme that hydrolyzes lipoprotein triglycerides. Because of differences in sialic acid content, apo C-III exists in at least three polymorphic forms.[46] In contrast to apo C-II, apo C-III decreases lipolysis by the inhibition of LPL.

Apolipoprotein E

Apolipoprotein E is a 34-kDa plasma glycoprotein that is found primarily in chylomicrons, VLDL, HDL, and chylomicron and in VLDL remnants. Removal of apo E–bearing lipoproteins is mediated by several different cellular receptors that recognize a cluster of positively charged amino acids in a specific region of apo E. Apo E plays a central role in the metabolism of chylomicrons and VLDL remnants. It regulates and facilitates lipoprotein uptake in the liver through the interaction of chylomicron remnants with chylomicron remnant receptors, and the binding of VLDL remnants to the LDL receptor, as well as probably proteoglycans.[173]

Three common apo E isoforms, designated E_2, E_3, and E_4, were initially distinguished by isoelectric-focusing electrophoresis.[340] These isoforms have amino acid substitutions at residues 112 and 158.[243,340] Apo E_2 has cysteine residues in both positions, and apo E_4 has arginine residues in both positions, whereas apo E_3 has cysteine and arginine at positions 112 and 158, respectively. Apo E_2 exhibits reduced binding affinity for the B and/or E remnant receptor compared with apo E_3, which tends to lead to an accumulation of apo E–containing lipoprotein in the circulation, whereas apo E_4–containing lipoproteins are cleared more rapidly than those containing apo E_3. These isoforms are coded for by three alleles of the apo E gene: ε2, ε3, and ε4. The ε3 allele is most frequent, although relative proportions of the three alleles vary among populations.[67,70,72] These apo E alleles have been shown to contribute significantly to the variability of LDL cholesterol and apo B-100 concentrations within populations.[281] Individuals with at least one ε2 allele tend to have lower concentrations of apo B-100 and LDL cholesterol than do those who are homozygous for the ε3 allele, whereas individuals with at least one ε4 allele tend to have higher concentrations of these analytes. This most likely occurs because increased hepatic uptake of lipoproteins in the presence of the ε4 allele leads to an increase in hepatic cholesterol and downregulation of the LDL receptor. Apo E_4 is also associated with increased cholesterol absorption; in the distant past, this may have offered a selective advantage, but it is a disadvantage with regard to CHD in populations that consume a high-fat diet. Variations at the apo E locus may explain some of the differences observed in plasma lipid and lipoprotein between individual responses to dietary and drug therapy.[230] Finally, the apo E_4 allele has been strongly associated with Alzheimer's disease and other neurologic diseases.[291] This association is likely related to the role of apo E in modulating lipid metabolism in the brain, but the exact connection between apo E_4 and neurologic disease is not known.

Lipoprotein Metabolism

The pathways of lipoprotein metabolism are complex and intersect at several points.[44,110,266] They include exogenous and endogenous pathways based on whether they carry lipids from dietary or hepatic origin (Figures 27-18 and 27-19).

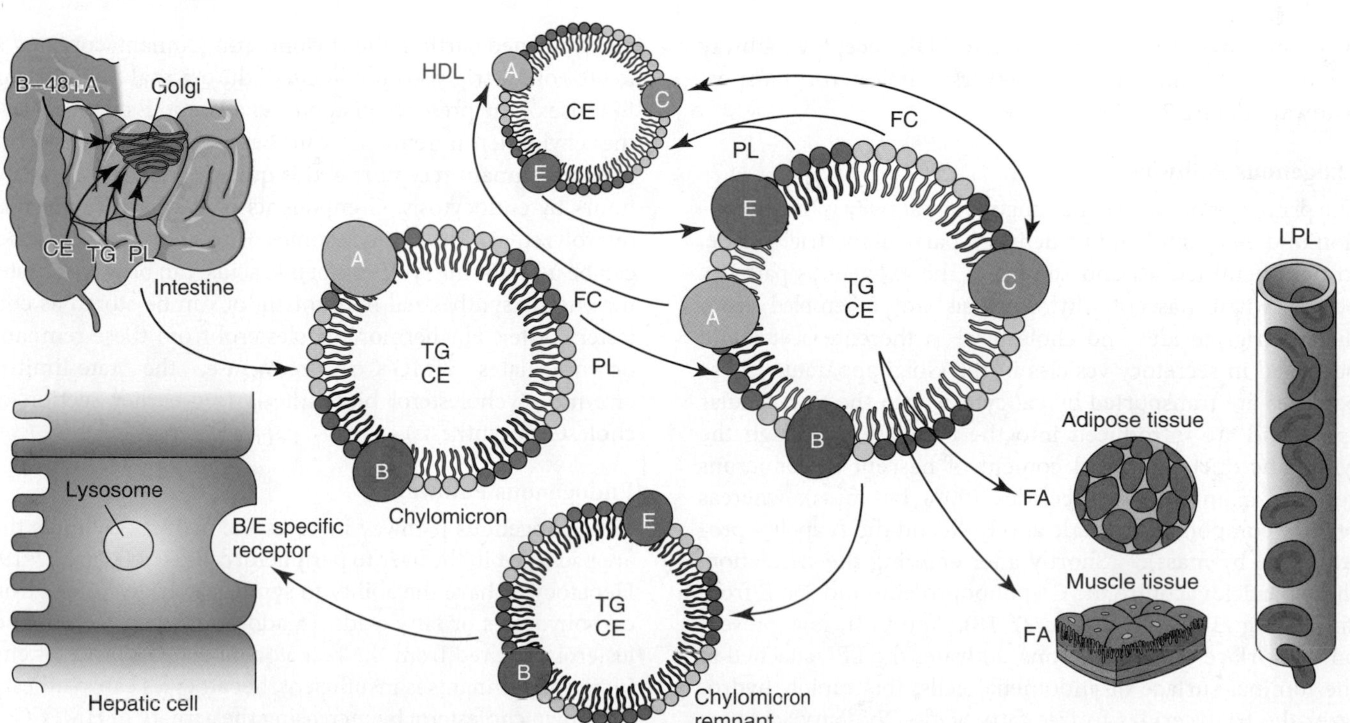

Figure 27-18 Exogenous lipoprotein metabolism pathway. ***A,*** **Apolipoprotein A-I;** ***B,*** **apolipoprotein B-48;** ***C,*** **apolipoprotein C-II;** ***CE,*** **cholesterol ester;** ***E,*** **apolipoprotein E;** ***FA,*** **fatty acid;** ***FC,*** **free cholesterol;** ***HDL,*** **high-density lipoprotein;** ***LPL,*** **lipoprotein lipase;** ***PL,*** **phospholipid;** ***TG,*** **triglyceride.**

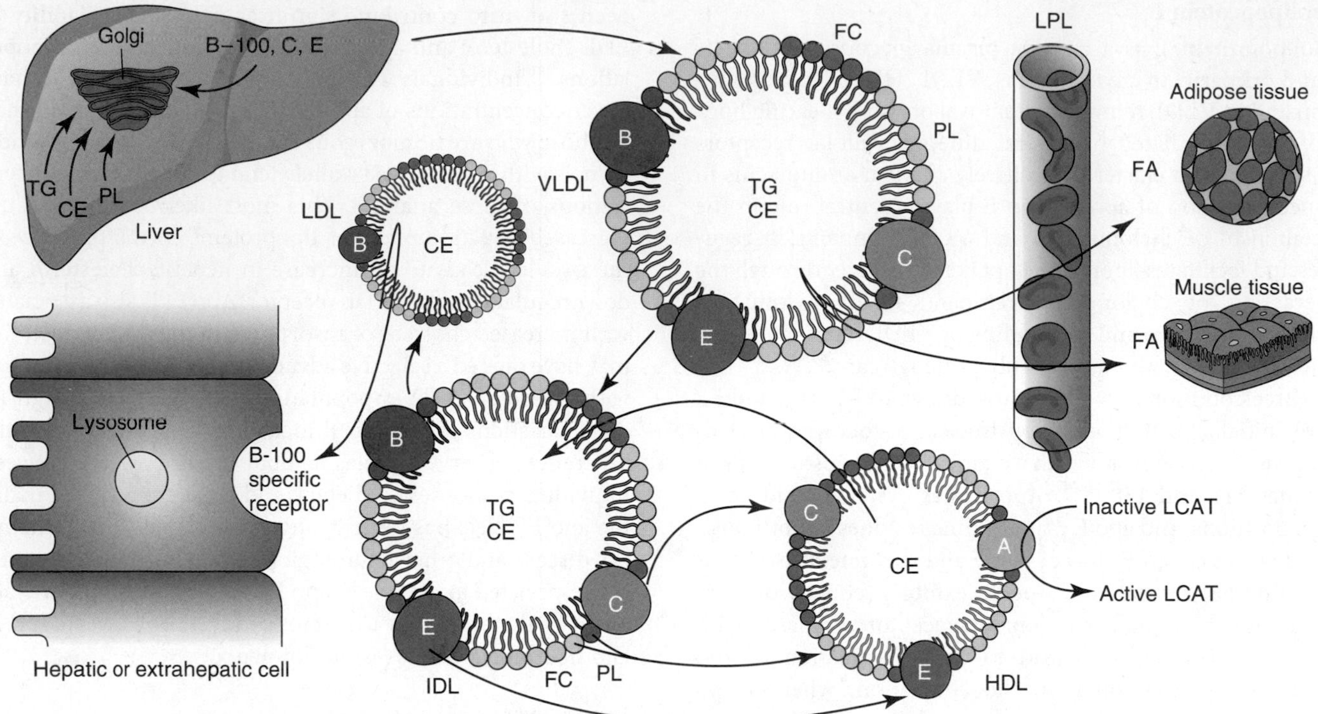

Figure 27-19 Endogenous lipoprotein metabolism pathway. *A,* Apolipoprotein A-I; *B,* apolipoprotein B-100; *C,* apolipoprotein C-II; *CE,* cholesterol ester; *E,* apolipoprotein E; *FA,* fatty acid; *FC,* free cholesterol; *HDL,* high-density lipoprotein; *IDL,* intermediate-density lipoprotein; *LCAT,* lecithin cholesterol acyltransferase; *LDL,* low-density lipoprotein; *LPL,* lipoprotein lipase; *PL,* phospholipid; *TG,* triglyceride; *VLDL,* very low-density lipoproteins.

Also included are the intracellular LDL receptor pathway (Figure 27-20) and the HDL reverse cholesterol transport pathway (Figure 27-21).

Exogenous Pathway

The primary function of the exogenous pathway is the absorption of dietary lipid and its delivery, particularly triglyceride, to peripheral tissues and the liver. The exogenous pathway begins when nascent chylomicrons are assembled from dietary triglycerides and cholesterol in the enterocytes and packaged in secretory vesicles in the Golgi apparatus. These particles are transported by exocytosis into the extracellular space and are introduced into the circulation through the lymphatic duct. The lipid content of nascent chylomicrons consists mainly of triglycerides (90% by mass), whereas protein components include apo B-48 and the A apolipoproteins (2% by mass).[105] Shortly after entering the circulation, these particles acquire the C apolipoproteins and apo E from circulating HDL (see Figure 27-18). Apo C-II, now present on the surface of chylomicrons, activates the LPL attached to the luminal surface of endothelial cells; this rapidly hydrolyzes the triglycerides to free fatty acids. The fatty acids are associated with albumin and can be taken up by muscle cells as an energy source or into adipose cells for storage. Simultaneously, some of the phospholipids and the apo A apolipoproteins are transferred back to HDL during lipolysis. The newly formed particle, the chylomicron remnant, contains 80 to 90% of the triglyceride content of the original chylomicron. Because of the presence of apo B-48 and apo E on its surface, the chylomicron remnant can be recognized by specific hepatic remnant receptors and is quickly internalized within hours by endocytosis. Components of the particle are then hydrolyzed within the lysosomes. The cholesterol released can be used for the synthesis of bile acids, can be incorporated into newly synthesized lipoprotein, or can be stored as cholesteryl ester. Furthermore, cholesterol from these remnants downregulates HMG-CoA reductase, the rate-limiting enzyme of cholesterol biosynthesis (see earlier section on cholesterol synthesis).

Endogenous Pathway

The endogenous pathway involves the delivery of lipids that are packaged in the liver to peripheral cells (see Figure 27-19). Hepatocytes have the ability to synthesize triglycerides from carbohydrates or fatty acids. In addition, when dietary cholesterol acquired from the receptor-mediated uptake of chylomicron remnants is insufficient, hepatocytes can synthesize their own cholesterol by increasing the activity of HMG-CoA reductase. Endogenously made triglycerides and cholesterol are packaged along with apo B-100 into VLDL particles in the endoplasmic reticulum; this involves the microsomal transfer protein. A defective microsomal transfer protein

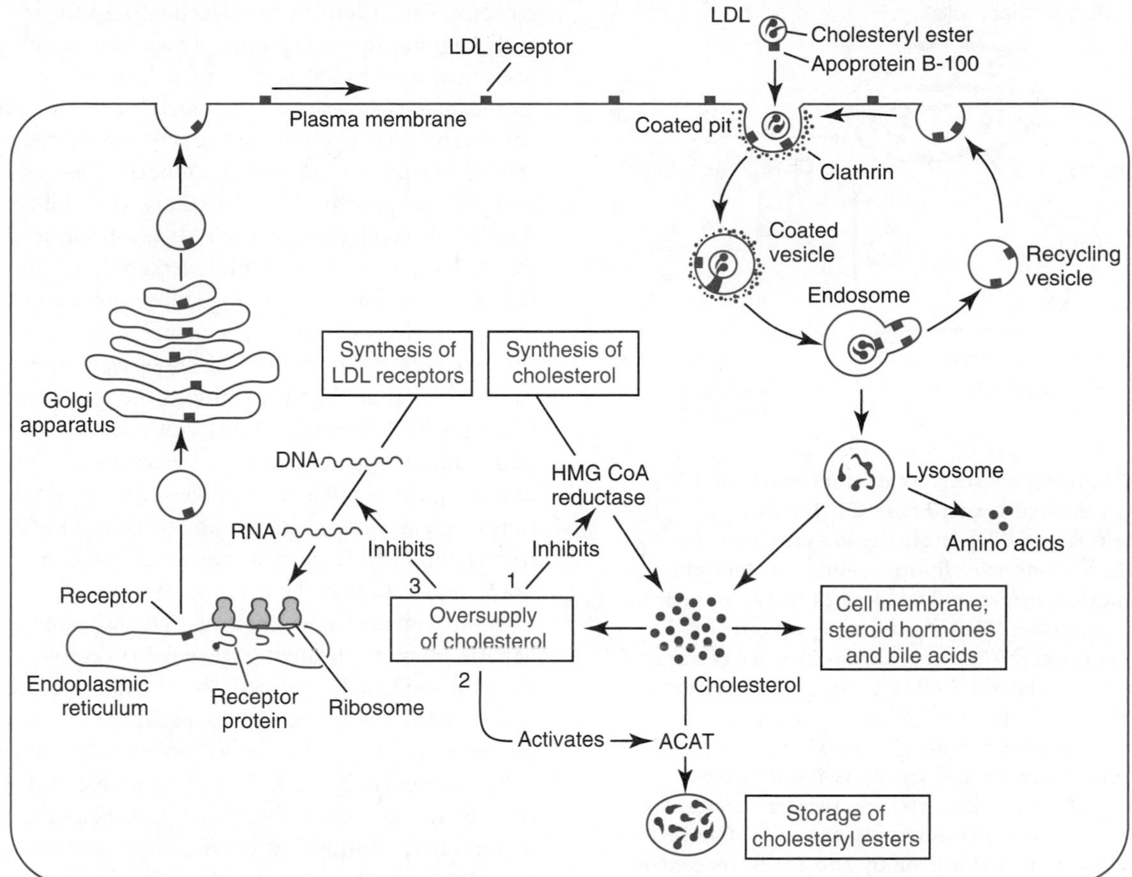

Figure 27-20 Low-density lipoprotein receptor pathway. ***ACAT,*** **Acyl-CoA cholesterol acyltransferase;** ***HMG-CoA reductase,*** **3-hydroxy-3-methylglutaryl coenzyme A reductase;** ***LDL,*** **low-density lipoprotein. Because of the presence of apolipoprotein B-100 on its surface, the LDL particle is recognized by a specific receptor in a coated pit and is taken into the cell in a coated vesicle** ***(top right).*** **Coated vesicles fuse together to form an endosome. The acidic environment of the endosome causes the LDL particle to dissociate from the receptors, which return to the cell surface. LDL particles are taken to a lysosome, where apolipoprotein B-100 is broken down into amino acids and cholesterol ester is converted to free cholesterol for cellular requirements. The cellular cholesterol level is self-regulated. Oversupply of cholesterol will lead to (1) decreased rates of cholesterol synthesis by inhibiting HMG-CoA reductase, (2) increased storage of cholesteryl esters by activating ACAT, and (3) inhibition of manufacture of new LDL receptors by suppressing transcription of the receptor gene into mRNA.** *(From Brown MS, Goldstein JL. How LDL receptors influence cholesterol and atherosclerosis. Sci Am 1984;251:58-66. Copyright 1984 by Scientific American, Inc. All rights reserved.)*

results in the inability to secrete apo B-containing lipoproteins and is referred to as *abetalipoproteimemia.* VLDL is a triglyceride-rich particle (55% by mass) that contains apo B-100, apo E, and small quantities of C apolipoproteins on its surface. Additional C apolipoproteins are transferred from HDL to VLDL after it enters the circulation. As in the case of chylomicron metabolism, apo C-II present on the surface of VLDL activates LPL on endothelial cells, which leads to the hydrolysis of VLDL triglycerides and the release of free fatty acids. It is important to note, however, that the rate of hydrolysis of VLDL triglyceride is significantly lower than that of chylomicron triglyceride. The average residence time of VLDL triglyceride is 15 to 60 minutes, compared with 5 to 10 minutes for chylomicron triglyceride.[118] This difference may be attributed to the fact that VLDL particles are smaller and bind to fewer LPL molecules than do chylomicrons.

During hydrolysis of VLDL triglycerides, C apolipoproteins are transferred back to HDL. VLDL particles are thus converted to VLDL remnants, some of which are taken up by the liver. The rest are converted to smaller, denser particles called *IDL.* Large IDL particles, which also have several molecules of apo E, bind the hepatic remnant receptors and are removed from the circulation. In humans, about 50% of IDL is removed by hepatocytes.

Surface materials from IDL, including some phospholipids, free cholesterol, and apolipoproteins, are transferred to

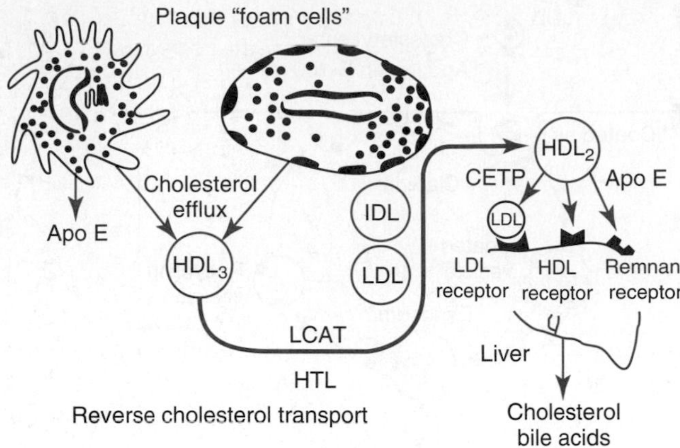

Figure 27-21 Reverse-cholesterol transport pathway. *ABCA1*, ATP binding cassette transporter A1; *ABCG1*, ATP binding cassette transporter G1; *apo A-I*, apolipoprotein A-1; *CETP*, cholesteryl ester transfer protein; *HDL*, high-density lipoprotein; *LCA*, lecithin cholesterol acyltransferase; *LDL*, low-density lipoprotein; *LDL-R*, LDL receptor; *SR-B1*, scavenger receptor B-I; *LDL-R*, LDL receptor. After formation in the liver and intestine, nascent discoidal HDL removes cholesterol from peripheral cells by the ABCA1 transporter. Additional cholesterol can also be removed from HDL by the ABCG1 transporter and by a passive diffusion mechanism. LCAT esterifies the cholesterol content of HDL to prevent it from re-entering the cells. Cholesterol esters are delivered to the liver by the SR-B1 receptor or by the LDL-R after transfer to LDL by CETP. *(Reprinted from Gwynne JT: High density lipoprotein cholesterol levels as a marker of reverse cholesterol transport. Am J Cardiol 64:10G–17G, 1989. Copyright 1989, with permission from Excerpta Medica Inc.)*

HDL, or form HDL de novo in the circulation. Cholesteryl esters are transferred from HDL to LDL by CETP in exchange for triglyceride. The net result of the coupled lipolysis and cholesteryl ester exchange reaction is the replacement of much of the triglyceride core of the original VLDL with cholesteryl esters. IDL undergoes further hydrolysis, in which most of the remaining triglycerides are removed and all apolipoproteins except B-100 are transferred to other lipoproteins; this ultimately leads to the formation of LDL. Most LDL is eventually returned to the liver by the LDL receptor, but when present in excess, it infiltrates into the vessel wall, where it accumulates. This is a key initiation step in the process of atherosclerosis.

Low-Density Lipoprotein Receptor Pathway

The mechanism by which LDL is removed from the circulation is reasonably well understood and primarily occurs via the LDL receptor pathway. Compared with VLDL and chylomicrons, LDL has a relatively long residence time in the circulation of about 3 days.[118] Specific receptors present on plasma membranes recognize and bind apo B-100 associated with LDL (see Figures 27-19 and 27-20). LDL particles then are internalized and fuse with endosomes. Because of the acidic milieu of the endosome, LDL dissociates from the receptor, which returns to the cell surface for reuse, whereas LDL migrates to the lysosome. Once LDL is delivered to the lysosome, apo B-100 is degraded into small peptides and amino acids. Cholesteryl esters are also hydrolyzed, with the cholesterol then available for the synthesis of cell membranes, steroid hormone synthesis in endocrine tissues, or bile acid synthesis in hepatocytes. Cells have the ability to regulate their cholesterol content, most likely because of the cytotoxicity of excess cholesterol. Oversupply of free cholesterol (1) decreases the rate of endogenous cholesterol synthesis by inhibiting the rate-limiting enzyme HMG-CoA reductase; (2) increases the formation of cholesteryl esters, which are catalyzed by ACAT; and (3) inhibits the synthesis of new LDL receptors by suppressing transcription of the receptor gene. Many different intracellular pathways are available for coordinated gene regulation of cholesterol metabolism, but the sterol regulatory element-binding protein (SREBP) transcription factors, which sense intracellular cholesterol concentrations, appear to play the most central role.[289]

Approximately one third of LDL is taken up by extrahepatic tissue through scavenger receptors or non–receptor-mediated pinocytosis. Non–receptor-mediated uptake becomes important as plasma LDL concentrations increase, as in familial hypercholesterolemia (FH). Non–receptor-mediated uptake is not saturable and is not regulated. Scavenger receptors are unregulated and recognize LDL that has been modified in various ways, such as by oxidation. Scavenger receptors are largely found in macrophages; this probably accounts for the accumulation of lipid that occurs in these cells in atherosclerotic plaque. Macrophages that become engorged with cholesteryl esters are called *foam cells,* and are considered the earliest components of the atherosclerotic lesion.

Reverse Cholesterol Transfer Pathway

The reverse cholesterol transport pathway helps the body maintain cholesterol homeostasis by removing excess cholesterol from peripheral cells and delivering it to the liver for excretion. It is mediated mostly by HDL; this in part accounts for the antiatherogenic property of HDL. The pathway begins when HDL is secreted from the liver and intestine as disk-shaped nascent particles that contain phospholipids and apo A-I. Through the extracellular addition of surface components of triglyceride-rich particles, such as phospholipids, cholesterol, and certain apolipoproteins, nascent HDL is converted to spherical particles. Free cholesterol from cell membranes is also transferred to the nascent HDL (see Figure 27-21). This can occur by a passive process called *aqueous diffusion,* but it can also occur by specific energy, requiring transporters.[346] The ABCA1 transporter, which is the defective gene in Tangier disease, promotes the efflux of excess cellular cholesterol and phospholipids to nascent HDL. In contrast, the ABCG1 transporter and the SR-BI receptor promote the efflux of cholesterol to more lipid-rich forms of HDL. Once cholesterol is delivered to HDL by whatever mechanism, it is quickly esterified by the action of LCAT in the presence of its cofactor apo A-I. The size of the HDL particle depends strongly on the quantity of accumulated cholesteryl esters and the activity of LCAT. Lysolecithin, a byproduct of this reaction (see previous discussion), is removed from circulation after binding with albumin. HDL cholesteryl esters are delivered to the liver by one of the following mechanisms: (1) cholesteryl esters are selectively taken up from HDL by the SR-BI receptor, and lipid-depleted forms of HDL are returned to the circulation for further transport; (2) cholesteryl esters are transferred from HDL to apo B-100–containing lipoprotein by a process mediated by cholesterol ester transfer protein; they then are taken up by the liver through receptors for these lipoproteins; or (3) HDL can be taken up in toto by holoparticle receptors, which possibly recognize apo E.[110] These processes constitute the reverse cholesterol transport mechanism by which cellular and lipoprotein cholesterol is delivered back to the liver for reuse or disposal.

Although LDL is the major product resulting from the catabolism of VLDL, some conversion of HDL subfractions also occurs during this process. Surface materials from triglyceride-rich particles that have been transferred to the small circulating HDL_3 are subsequently esterified by LCAT, as described earlier, to create the larger cholesteryl ester–rich HDL_2. It has been shown that in vitro HDL_2 is converted back to HDL_3 in the presence of hepatic LPL.[235] HDL_2 contains twice as many cholesterol molecules per unit of apolipoproteins as does HDL_3.

Reference Lipid, Lipoprotein Cholesterol, and Apolipoprotein Concentrations

At birth, the typical plasma cholesterol concentration is about 66 mg/dL; it is equally distributed among LDL and HDL, with a very small amount in VLDL. Triglyceride concentration is only about 36 mg/dL.[269] Cord blood apo A-I, apo B-100, and Lp(a) have mean concentrations of about 80, 33, and 4 mg/dL, respectively.[267,268] Lipid, lipoprotein cholesterol, and apolipoprotein concentrations rise sharply during the first few months of life, with LDL becoming the predominant carrier of plasma cholesterol, and then remain relatively unchanged until puberty. A profile consisting of total cholesterol of about 155 mg/dL, LDL cholesterol of 90 mg/dL, HDL cholesterol of 53 mg/dL, triglycerides of 55 mg/dL, apo B-100 of 86 mg/dL, and apo A-I of about 130 mg/dL is typical for a normal prepubertal subject. After puberty, triglycerides, LDL cholesterol, and apo B-100 are increased in both sexes, and HDL cholesterol and apo A-I are decreased in men. Lipid concentrations continue to increase throughout adult life, with total and LDL cholesterol and apo B-100 being higher in men than in women up to age 55.[45] Thereafter, women who are not receiving estrogen supplementation have higher total and LDL cholesterol and apo B-100 than their age-matched male counterparts.[111] In contrast to the other lipids, lipoproteins, and apolipoproteins, Lp(a) concentration increases slowly and gradually to reach Lp(a) adult values after the third year of life.[268]

Plasma lipid and lipoprotein concentrations in male and female subjects are presented in Tables 27-7 through 27-10. These reference intervals have been developed using the Lipid Research Clinics (LRC) population. Although reference intervals for apo A-I and B-100 from the Framingham Heart Study, using approved World Health Organization (WHO)/International Federation of Clinical Chemistry and Laboratory Medicine (IFCC) calibrators, were published,[61,63]

TABLE 27-7 Population Distributions for Total Cholesterol, mg/dL*

	Male								Female						
	Percentiles								Percentiles						
Age, y	5	10	25	50	75	90	95	Age, y	5	10	25	50	75	90	95
0-4	114			155			203	0-4	112			156			200
5-9	125	131	141	153	168	183	189	5-9	131	135	150	164	177	189	197
10-14	124	132	144	161	173	191	204	10-14	125	131	142	159	171	191	205
15-19	118	123	135	152	168	183	191	15-19	119	126	140	157	176	198	208
20-24	118	126	142	159	179	197	212	20-24	121	132	147	165	186	220	237
25-29	130	137	154	176	199	223	234	25-29	130	142	158	178	198	217	231
30-34	142	152	161	190	213	237	258	30-34	133	141	158	178	197	215	227
35-39	147	157	176	195	222	248	267	35-39	139	149	165	186	209	233	249
40-44	150	161	179	204	229	251	260	40-44	146	156	172	193	220	241	259
45-49	163	171	188	210	234	255	275	45-49	148	162	182	204	213	256	268
50-54	156	158	189	211	234	262	274	50-54	163	171	188	214	240	267	281
55-59	161	172	188	214	236	260	280	55-59	167	182	201	229	251	270	294
60-64	163	170	191	215	237	262	287	60-64	172	186	207	226	251	282	300
65-69	166	174	192	213	250	275	288	65-69	167	179	212	233	259	282	291
70+	144	160	185	214	236	253	265	70+	173	181	196	226	249	268	280

*To convert to mmol/L, multiply by 0.0259.

From Lipid Research Clinics Program Epidemiology Committee. Plasma lipid distributions in selected North American population: the Lipid Research Clinics Program prevalence study. Circulation 1979;60:427-39; and Lipid Metabolism Branch, Division of Heart, Lung, and Blood Institute. The Lipid Research Clinics population studies data book, volume I. The prevalence study. NIH Publication No. 80-1527. Bethesda, Md: National Institutes of Health, 1980.

TABLE 27-8 Population Distributions for Triglycerides, mg/dL*

	Male								Female						
	Percentiles								Percentiles						
Age, y	5	10	25	50	75	90	95	Age, y	5	10	25	50	75	90	95
0-4	29			56			99	0-4	34			64			112
5-9	28	34	39	48	58	70	85	5-9	32	37	45	57	74	103	126
10-14	33	37	46	58	74	94	111	10-14	39	44	53	68	85	104	120
15-19	38	43	53	68	88	125	143	15-19	36	40	52	64	85	112	126
20-24	44	50	61	78	107	146	165	20-24	37	42	60	80	104	135	168
25-29	45	51	67	88	120	141	204	25-29	42	45	57	76	104	137	159
30-34	46	57	76	102	142	214	253	30-34	40	45	55	73	104	140	163
35-39	52	58	80	109	167	250	316	35-39	40	47	61	83	115	170	205
40-44	56	69	89	123	174	252	318	40-44	45	51	66	88	116	161	191
45-49	56	65	88	119	165	218	279	45-49	44	55	71	94	139	180	223
50-54	63	75	94	128	178	244	313	50-54	53	58	75	103	144	190	223
55-59	60	70	85	117	167	210	261	55-59	59	65	80	111	163	229	279
60-64	56	65	84	111	150	193	240	60-64	57	66	78	105	143	210	256
65-69	54	61	78	108	164	227	256	65-69	56	64	86	118	158	221	260
70+	63	71	87	115	152	202	239	70+	60	68	83	110	141	189	289

*To convert to mmol/L, multiply by 0.0113.
From Lipid Research Clinics Program Epidemiology Committee. Plasma lipid distributions in selected North American population: the Lipid Research Clinics Program prevalence study. Circulation 1979;60:427-39; and Lipid Metabolism Branch, Division of Heart, Lung, and Blood Institute. The Lipid Research Clinics population studies data book, volume I. The prevalence study. NIH Publication No. 80-1527. Bethesda, Md: National Institutes of Health, 1980.

TABLE 27-9 Population Distributions for Low-Density Lipoprotein Cholesterol, mg/dL*

	Male								Female						
	Percentiles								Percentiles						
Age, y	5	10	25	50	75	90	95	Age, y	5	10	25	50	75	90	95
5-9	63	69	80	90	103	117	129	5-9	68	73	88	98	115	125	140
10-14	64	83	82	94	109	123	133	10-14	68	73	81	94	110	126	136
15-19	62	68	80	93	109	123	130	15-19	59	73	78	93	110	129	137
20-24	66	73	85	101	118	138	147	20-24	57	65	82	102	118	141	159
25-29	70	75	96	116	138	157	165	25-29	71	75	90	108	126	148	164
30-34	78	88	107	124	144	166	185	30-34	70	77	91	109	129	146	156
35-39	81	92	110	131	154	176	189	35-39	75	81	96	116	139	161	172
40-44	87	98	115	135	157	173	186	40-44	74	84	104	122	146	165	174
45-49	97	106	120	140	163	185	202	45-49	79	89	105	127	150	173	186
50-54	89	102	118	143	162	185	197	50-54	88	94	111	134	160	186	201
55-59	88	103	123	145	168	191	203	55-59	89	97	120	145	168	199	210
60-64	83	107	121	143	165	188	210	60-64	100	105	126	149	168	191	224
65-69	98	104	125	146	170	199	210	65-69	92	99	125	151	184	205	221
70+	88	100	119	142	164	182	186	70+	96	108	126	147	170	189	206

*To convert to mmol/L, multiply by 0.0259.
From Lipid Research Clinics Program Epidemiology Committee. Plasma lipid distributions in selected North American population: the Lipid Research Clinics Program prevalence study. Circulation 1979;60:427-39.

distributions of these two proteins that better reflect the North American population have become available from the National Health and Nutrition Examination Survey III (NHANES III) (Tables 27-11 and 27-12).[29] Because NHANES was designed to reflect the U.S. population, data for the distribution of these proteins in the main American ethnic groups are available (Table 27-13). Using this information, apo B-100 cut points similar to those recommended for LDL-C can be developed; apo B-100 values that correspond to desirable, borderline high risk, high risk, and very high risk are 88, 115, 132, and 152 mg/dL; apo A-I values that correspond to low and high are 114 and 154 mg/dL.[29] Until Lp(a) measurement is better standardized, the development of appropriate reference intervals is not possible.[17]

TABLE 27-10 Population Distributions for High-Density Lipoprotein Cholesterol, mg/dL*

	Male								Female						
	Percentiles								Percentiles						
Age, y	5	10	25	50	75	90	95	Age, y	5	10	25	50	75	90	95
5-9	38	43	49	55	64	70	75	5-9	36	38	48	52	60	67	73
10-14	37	40	46	55	61	71	74	10-14	37	40	45	52	58	64	70
15-19	30	34	39	46	52	59	63	15-19	35	38	43	51	61	68	74
20-24	30	32	38	45	51	57	63	20-24	33	37	44	51	62	72	79
25-29	31	32	37	44	50	58	63	25-29	37	39	47	55	63	74	83
30-34	28	32	38	45	52	59	63	30-34	36	40	46	55	64	73	77
35-39	29	31	36	43	49	58	62	35-39	34	38	44	53	64	75	82
40-44	27	31	36	43	51	60	67	40-44	34	39	48	56	65	79	88
45-49	30	33	38	45	52	60	64	45-49	34	41	47	58	68	82	87
50-54	28	31	36	44	51	58	63	50-54	37	41	50	62	71	84	92
55-59	28	31	38	46	55	64	71	55-59	37	41	50	60	73	85	91
60-64	30	34	41	49	61	69	74	60-64	38	44	51	61	75	87	92
65-69	30	33	39	49	52	74	75	65-69	35	38	49	62	73	85	96
70+	31	33	40	48	56	70	75	70+	33	38	45	60	71	82	92

*To convert to mmol/L, multiply by 0.0259.
From Lipid Research Clinics Program Epidemiology Committee. Plasma lipid distributions in selected North American population: the Lipid Research Clinics Program prevalence study. Circulation 1979;60:427-39.

TABLE 27-11 Serum Apo A-I Concentrations in Persons Aged ≥4 Years by Sex and Age: Means and Selected Percentiles, United States, 1988-91

	Apo A-I*, mg/dL								
			Percentiles						
Age, y	Mean, (SEM)†	SD	5th	10th	25th	50th	75th	90th	95th
Males‡									
4-5	135 (2)	19	109	112	122	132	149	159	172
6-11	142	20	111	117	126	141	150	168	177
12-19	129	19	99	106	116	128	141	153	165
≥20	136	22	106	111	121	133	147	164	176
20-29	135	21	105	112	121	132	145	164	173
30-39	135	20	105	111	122	132	145	161	173
40-49	136 (2)	25	103	108	119	133	149	164	178
50-59	136 (2)	21	107	111	121	134	147	167	173
60-69	140 (2)	23	111	116	123	136	153	172	184
≥70	138	23	109	114	122	134	150	167	180
Females‡									
4-5	131	18	104	111	118	130	140	155	163
6-11	136	17	110	117	125	135	145	157	166
12-19	136	23	105	111	120	132	146	165	180
≥20	151	27	113	120	132	147	166	186	202
20-29	148 (2)	30	111	117	128	143	164	185	209
30-39	145	24	110	115	126	143	160	173	189
40-49	149 (2)	24	115	122	134	145	165	181	195
50-59	156 (2)	29	117	123	134	152	173	199	211
60-69	157 (2)	28	120	125	138	154	171	191	205
≥70	155 (2)	26	118	124	137	153	171	189	199

*Combined data for total population, including all three ethnic groups.
†All SEMs were 1 mg/dL unless otherwise indicated.
‡Estimates based on 400 to 800 subjects in each age and sex subgroup.
Modified from Bachorik PS, Lovejoy KL, Carroll MD, Johnson CL. Apolipoprotein B and AI distributions in the United States, 1988-1991: results of the National Health and Nutrition Examination Survey III (NHANES III). Clin Chem 1997;43:2364-78.

TABLE 27-12 Serum Apo B-100 Concentrations in Persons Aged ≥4 Years by Sex and Age: Means and Selected Percentiles, United States, 1988-91

			APO B-100*, MG/DL						
			PERCENTILES						
Age, y	Mean, (SEM)†	SD	5th	10th	25th	50th	75th	90th	95th
Males‡									
4-5	79	14	58	0.62	69	79	89	98	103
6-11	79	16	56	0.61	69	76	89	99	105
12-19	78	17	55	0.58	67	75	85	98	110
≥20	107	25	66	0.74	89	106	122	138	150
20-29	91	22	59	0.66	76	88	103	117	130
30-39	106	24	63	0.73	89	107	122	136	143
40-49	112 (2)	24	71	0.82	97	111	126	140	152
50-59	116 (2)	26	75	0.84	98	116	133	149	160
60-69	117 (2)	23	81	0.89	101	116	133	148	156
≥70	110	24	73	0.81	95	109	123	142	152
Females‡									
4-5	82	14	58	0.64	72	82	91	99	104
6-11	82	17	57	0.61	70	81	90	101	113
12-19	81	20	53	0.58	67	79	92	104	119
≥20	103	28	66	0.71	83	99	119	140	153
20-29	91	23	63	0.67	74	86	102	119	132
30-39	93	23	59	0.68	76	89	107	123	132
40-49	99	21	70	0.75	84	96	114	129	136
50-59	116 (2)	29	75	0.84	96	114	133	156	168
60-69	119 (2)	31	75	0.82	98	118	135	156	173
≥70	118	28	79	0.84	98	116	135	152	168

*Combined data for total population, including all three ethnic groups.
†All SEMs were 1 mg/dL unless otherwise indicated.
‡Estimates based on 400 to 800 subjects in each age and sex subgroup.
Modified from Bachorik PS, Lovejoy KL, Carroll MD, Johnson CL. Apolipoprotein B and AI distributions in the United States, 1988-1991: results of the National Health and Nutrition Examination Survey III (NHANES III). Clin Chem 1997;43:2364-78.

TABLE 27-13 Age-Adjusted* Mean Apo A-I and Apo B Concentrations in Persons Aged ≥4 Years by Sex and Age Group, United States, 1988-1991

	MEAN (SEM)† CONC, MG/DL					
	APO A-I			APO B		
Age, y	White	Black	Mexican-American	White	Black	Mexican-American
Males						
All	134	145	135 (2)	99	96	101
4-11	140 (2)	145	139 (2)	79	79	79
12-19	127	139 (2)	131 (3)	78	78	79
≥20	135	146	135 (2)	106	102	109
Females						
All	146	151	144 (2)	97	96	98
4-11	133	142 (2)	132	82	82	81
12-19	122 (2)	144 (2)	140 (4)	80	82	83
≥20	151	154	147 (2)	103	101	105

*Age-adjusted by the direct method to the 1980 U.S. census population.
†All SEMs were 1 mg/dL unless otherwise indicated.
Modified from Bachorik PS, Lovejoy KL, Carroll MD, Johnson CL. Apolipoprotein B and AI distributions in the United States, 1988-1991: results of the National Health and Nutrition Examination Survey III (NHANES III). Clin Chem 1997;43:2364-78.

CLINICAL SIGNIFICANCE

The clinical significance of lipids is primarily associated with CHD but is also associated with other vascular disorders, such as thrombotic stroke and peripheral vascular disease.

Association With Coronary Heart Disease

Increased cholesterol is a critical factor in the pathogenesis of atherosclerotic disease (see also Chapter 47). As early as 1910, Windaus described cholesterol in the lesions of diseased arteries. Subsequently, many studies confirmed that free and esterified cholesterol accumulates in the aorta, coronary arteries, and cerebral vessels, and that the rate of accumulation varies among individuals. The association between serum cholesterol and atherosclerosis in humans was first suggested in 1938, when Muller and Thanhauser each demonstrated familial aggregation of hypercholesterolemia and CHD.[205,313] Additional studies showed that when the total cholesterol concentration is high, the incidence and prevalence of CHD are also high.[101]

However, the relationship between cholesterol and atherosclerotic coronary disease is curvilinear.[109] According to the Multiple Risk Factor Intervention Trial (MRFIT), if a risk ratio of 1.0 is arbitrarily assigned at a cholesterol value of 200 mg/dL, the risk ratio increases to 2.0 at 250 mg/dL and to 4.0 at 300 mg/dL (Figure 27-22). Pathologic studies have helped to explain this curvilinear relationship. When 60% of the surface of coronary arteries is covered with plaque, one enters a critical phase in which any increase in serum cholesterol will markedly increase coronary disease risk. Results of the LRC-Coronary Primary Prevention Trial (CPPT) show that use of the concentration at the 95th percentile of a population distribution is inappropriate to define hypercholesterolemia. Data from this and other studies suggest that risk disproportionately increases as cholesterol concentrations increase; at concentrations of 200 to 240 mg/dL, the risk begins to accelerate at a greater rate. On average, each 1% reduction in cholesterol (2 to 3 mg/dL) results in an ≈2% reduction in CHD incidence—a relationship of considerable clinical and public health significance.[80] In addition, the Cholesterol-Lowering Atherosclerosis Study (CLAS) demonstrated the benefit of cholesterol lowering in people with established disease and even in those with normal or moderately increased cholesterol concentrations (185 to 240 mg/dL).[38] More recent studies have shown that individuals with preexisting disease may actually show reversal of atherosclerosis if they are aggressively treated so that they achieve LDL-C concentrations below 70 mg/dL.[42,222]

Many epidemiologic and clinical studies have shown that other lipids and lipoproteins besides LDL, such as HDL and lipoprotein subfractions, may be useful for predicting CHD risk.[50] For example, several studies have shown that small, dense LDL subfractions may be better correlated with CHD risk than large, less dense LDL subfractions.[26,49] Triglyceride itself may be a risk factor. Initially, a National Institutes of Health consensus conference on triglyceride and CHD failed to establish increased fasting triglyceride concentration as an independent risk factor.[7] However, NCEP and the Adult Treatment Panel III (ATP III) reports[8,11] have given triglycerides greater prominence in CHD risk prediction (see section on diagnosis of lipoprotein disorders, later in this chapter). Furthermore, fat tolerance and the ability to rapidly catabolize ingested triglycerides are reported to correlate well with atherogenic risk.[234] The degree of hypertriglyceridemia appearing after a meal controls the extent to which basal HDL_2 is converted by hepatic lipase to HDL_3. It has also been postulated that chylomicron remnants and IDL, the products of the breakdown of triglyceride-rich lipoprotein,

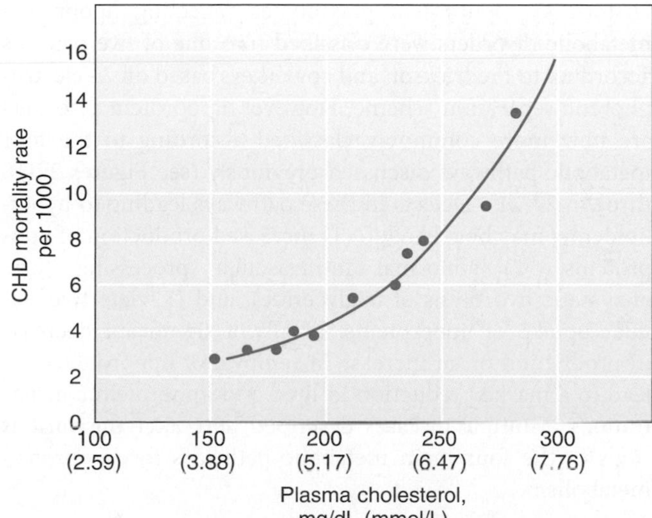

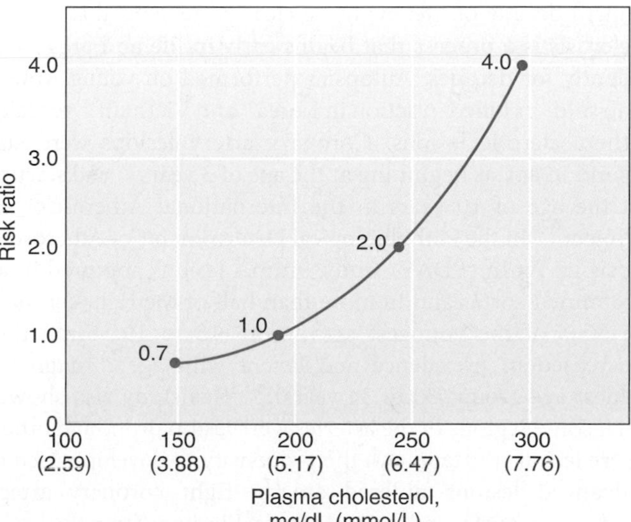

Figure 27-22 Relationship between cholesterol concentration and coronary heart disease mortality, expressed by yearly rate per 1000 and risk ratios [Multiple Risk Factor Intervention Trial (MRFIT) participants].

are important in atherogenesis.[350] They may promote atherosclerosis when their concentrations in plasma are high or their presence in circulation is prolonged by adversely affecting endothelial cell function.

In the early 1970s, Alaupovic suggested that apolipoproteins should be considered when the contribution of lipids and lipoproteins to the development of atherosclerotic disease is evaluated.[15] Several studies showed that in people with CHD, changes in serum concentrations of apo A-I and apo B-100 are similar to those for HDL and LDL, respectively. Apo B-100 values were increased and apo A-I values were decreased in people with CHD compared with those without disease. In many studies, apo A-I and apo B-100 were somewhat better discriminators of people with CHD than the cholesterol concentration of the corresponding lipoprotein,[62,152,172] at least in univariate analyses. Furthermore, these two apolipoproteins were shown to correlate better with the degree of coronary stenosis than LDL and HDL cholesterol.[210] It has been shown that only 14.5% of patients with myocardial infarction younger than the age of 60 years have LDL cholesterol above the 95th percentile. In contrast, 35% of these patients have apo B-100 above the 95th percentile.[295] The measurement of apo B-100 provides information regarding the number of apo B-100–containing particles, because only one apo B molecule is present per lipoprotein particle. If the concentration of LDL cholesterol is normal or slightly increased but apo B-100 is greatly increased, it is likely that the number of small, more atherogenic and dense LDL particles will also be high. Increased serum apo B-100 and decreased apo A-I concentrations were also found in children of parents with premature atherosclerotic disease.[91] Overall, these and other findings[42,106,158] suggest that apolipoproteins may be superior predictors of future CHD, and that tests for apo B and apo A-I are underutilized, most likely because they are still viewed as ancillary tests under most current guidelines for CHD risk prediction.

Although CHD often is not manifested clinically until the fourth decade of life, evidence clearly indicates that atherosclerosis is a process that begins early in life and progresses silently for decades. Autopsies performed on young American soldiers killed in action in Korea[83] and Vietnam[189] revealed atherosclerotic lesions. Coronary artery lesions were also found in aortas beginning at the age of 3 years[300] and starting at the age of 10 years in the International Atherosclerosis Project.[305] In the Pathobiological Determinants of Atherosclerosis in Youth (PDAY) study, intimal lesions appeared in all examined aortas and in more than half of the right coronary arteries of the youngest age group (15 to 19 years); they increased in prevalence and extent with age through the oldest age group (30 to 34 years).[304] This study also showed that some regions of the arteries were lesion prone and others were lesion resistant, and the propensity to develop raised or advanced lesions differed among right coronary artery, abdominal aorta, and thoracic aorta. Findings from the Bogalusa Heart Study[339] showed a correlation between systolic blood pressure, higher total and LDL cholesterol, and lower HDL cholesterol concentrations and the degree of coronary and aortic atherosclerosis in children and adolescents.[36] In the PDAY study, postmortem cholesterol and thiocyanate, a marker for cigarette smoking, predicted the extent of coronary and aortic atherosclerosis, respectively, in autopsies of those aged 14 to 34.[343] Therefore, a direct relation between determinant risk factors and the extent of atherosclerotic lesions in youth seems to exist and suggests that the identification and treatment of children and young adults who may be at high risk for developing CHD offer the possibility of preventing or delaying development of this disease.

Disorders of Lipoprotein Metabolism

Dyslipoproteinemia is diagnosed in most patients using plasma lipid and lipoprotein cholesterol concentrations. Dyslipoproteinemias were previously defined in terms of arbitrary cut points for lipids and lipoprotein; their definition is now based on the relationship between lipoprotein concentrations and risk for CHD (see discussion later in this chapter).

Primary versus Secondary Hyperlipoproteinemia

When hyperlipidemia is evaluated, it first should be determined whether it is from a primary lipoprotein disorder or is secondary to a wide variety of metabolic diseases. The diagnosis of primary hyperlipidemia is made after secondary causes have been ruled out. Causes of secondary hyperlipoproteinemia are listed in Table 27-14. The most commonly seen secondary causes in the first year of life are glycogen storage disease and congenital biliary atresia. Hypothyroidism, nephrotic syndrome, and diabetes mellitus are more prevalent later in childhood. Exogenous factors, such as dietary and alcohol intake, oral contraceptives, diabetes mellitus, and pharmacologic agents [e.g., steroids, isotretinoin (Accutane), and β-blockers], are the main secondary causes of hyperlipidemia in adults.[4,155]

Familial Dyslipoproteinemias

Historically, lipoprotein phenotypes reflecting lipoprotein metabolic disorders were classified into one of five patterns according to Fredrickson and coworkers based on an electrophoretic separation scheme. However, lipoprotein disorders are now more commonly classified according to the four metabolic pathways discussed previously (see Figures 27-18 through 27-21). Defects in these pathways leading to hyperlipidemia may be related to (1) increased production of lipoproteins, (2) abnormal intravascular processing (e.g., enzymatic hydrolysis of triglyceride), and (3) defective cellular uptake of lipoproteins. Finally, a significant decrease in production or an increase in removal of lipoproteins can lead to a marked reduction in lipid and lipoprotein concentrations. Multiple diseases described here alter the various steps of the four main metabolic pathways for lipoprotein metabolism.

Deficiency in Lipoprotein Lipase Activity

This disorder is characterized by marked hyperchylomicronemia and a corresponding hypertriglyceridemia, which can

TABLE 27-14 Causes of Secondary Hyperlipidemia and Dyslipoproteinemia

Disorder	Cause
Exogenous	Drugs: corticosteroids, isotretinoin (Accutane), thiazides, anticonvulsants, beta-blockers, anabolic steroids, certain oral contraceptives
	Alcohol
	Obesity
Endocrine and metabolic	Acute intermittent porphyria
	Diabetes mellitus
	Hypopituitarism
	Hypothyroidism
	Lipodystrophy
	Pregnancy
Storage disease	Cystine storage disease
	Gaucher's disease
	Glycogen storage disease
	Juvenile Tay-Sachs disease
	Niemann-Pick disease
	Tay-Sachs disease
Renal	Chronic renal failure
	Hemolytic-uremic syndrome
	Nephrotic syndrome
Hepatic	Benign recurrent intrahepatic cholestasis
	Congenital biliary atresia
Acute and transient	Burns
	Hepatitis
	Acute trauma (surgery)
	Myocardial infarction
	Bacterial and viral infections
Others	Anorexia nervosa
	Starvation
	Idiopathic hypercalcemia
	Klinefelter's syndrome
	Progeria (Hutchinson-Gilford syndrome)
	Systemic lupus erythematosus
	Werner's syndrome

reach as high as 10,000 mg/dL.[46] As discussed previously, LPL is essential for the hydrolysis of triglyceride and the conversion of chylomicrons to chylomicron remnants. The massive accumulation of chylomicrons in patients is usually related to a defect in lipolysis and an inability to catabolize dietary fat. The concentration of VLDL cholesterol is usually normal, and the concentrations of HDL cholesterol and LDL cholesterol are low (type I pattern). Furthermore, the concentration of apo C-II, the activator of LPL, is normal.

This disorder is usually expressed in childhood. In a review of 43 cases, 35 were manifested before the age of 10.[166,167] It appears that those patients with low to absent LPL activity in all tissues present with symptoms of the disease at an early age, whereas those with a partial deficiency in LPL activity become symptomatic later in life. This disease is usually detected after recurrent episodes of severe abdominal pain and repeated attacks of pancreatitis, which is the greatest source of morbidity in these patients. Eruptive xanthomas and lipemia retinalis are usually present when plasma triglyceride concentrations exceed 2000 and 4000 mg/dL, respectively.[46] The acuteness of the symptoms is directly proportional to the degree of hyperchylomicronemia. It is important to note that patients with this disorder *do not* appear to be predisposed to atherosclerotic disease.

The diagnosis is made by determination of LPL activity in postheparin plasma, because most LPL is firmly bound to proteoglycans on endothelial cells. Intravenously administered heparin binds LPL, causing its dissociation from heparan sulfate, present on the surface of endothelial cells, and its subsequent release to plasma.[125] This autosomal recessive disorder is extremely rare (one per million individuals), but more than 40 insertions and deletions in the LPL gene that lead to absent or truncated LPL protein with defective catalytic activity have been described.[46]

Deficiency in Apolipoprotein C-II

Deficient or defective apo C-II, the required activator for LPL, reduces the activity of this enzyme, impairs chylomicron catabolism, and increases plasma triglycerides (from 500 to 10,000 mg/dL). Those affected by this disorder have less than 10% of the normal concentration of apo C-II, which is the minimum amount necessary for normal LPL activity.[131] Total cholesterol tends to vary considerably (150 to 890 mg/dL) in these patients, but HDL and LDL cholesterol concentrations are often below the 5th percentile. Furthermore, plasma apo A-I, A-II, and B-100 concentrations are also decreased, whereas apo C-III and E concentrations are increased.

Although the clinical symptoms are similar to those seen in patients with LPL deficiency, they are usually milder and are expressed at a later age. The predominant symptom is usually recurrent abdominal pain caused by attacks of pancreatitis. Eruptive xanthomas and lipemia retinalis are not usually seen in these patients. As with LPL deficiency, patients with apo C-II deficiency are not predisposed to atherosclerosis.

The diagnosis is made upon documentation of low LPL activity in postheparin plasma in the absence of added apo C-II. Normal enzymatic activity is restored by the addition of normal apo C-II to the assay mixture. In another approach, the absence of apo C-II can be recognized by using an immunoassay for apo C-II. However, the latter approach may not distinguish between normal subjects and those with normal concentrations of a nonfunctional form of apo C-II. The defective apo C-II disorder is inherited in an autosomal recessive mode, but at an even lower frequency than LPL deficiency. More than 10 structural defects in the apo C-II gene that lead to the absence of apo C-II or the production of a defective apo C-II molecule have been described.[46] Subjects heterozygous for a defective apo C-II gene have normal lipid and lipoprotein profiles, because a sufficient amount of normal apo C-II is usually present to activate LPL.

Familial Combined Hyperlipidemia

About 10 to 15% of patients with premature CHD have familial combined hyperlipidemia (FCHL), thus making it one of the more common forms of dyslipidemia.[99] This disorder is recognized as a distinct phenotype by studying family members of survivors of myocardial infarction. Patients with FCHL can have increased plasma concentrations of total and LDL cholesterol (type IIa) or triglyceride (type IV), or both (type IIb). In all cases, apo B-100 concentrations are increased. The presentation of lipoprotein patterns can vary in an individual over time.[109]

FCHL appears to be caused by overproduction of VLDL and apo B-100, but the underlying molecular defect is not known. Kinetic studies have shown that the rate of flux of apo B-100 from VLDL in FCHL is approximately twice that of normal subjects.[53,66] This causes apo B-100 to be increased (by more than 125 mg/dL) even in subjects with normal LDL cholesterol. Because of the decreased lipid-to-protein ratio in these patients, both VLDL and LDL particles tend to be small and dense. When increased, LDL cholesterol is about 190 mg/dL, but it is lower than that typically seen in heterozygous familial hypercholesterolemia. Triglyceride concentrations are usually between 200 and 400 mg/dL but can be significantly higher. The concentration of HDL cholesterol is usually mildly depressed, particularly in the presence of hypertriglyceridemia. Xanthomas and other clinical symptoms of hyperlipidemia, other than atherosclerosis, are not very common in these patients. The association of FCHL with CHD incidence is high. In addition to increased IDL, the presence of high concentrations of small, dense LDL and low concentrations of HDL cholesterol might explain the increased risk for CHD in this disorder.

Although the mutation(s) responsible for FCHL remain unknown, this disorder is associated with a major gene, apparently interacting with other genes, and it has a prevalence of 1 in 100 persons. Although expression of FCHL is delayed until adolescence, young children from families with premature CHD can present with increased cholesterol or triglyceride, or both.[155]

Hyperapobetalipoproteinemia

This disorder is characterized by increased LDL–apo B-100 concentrations with normal or moderately increased concentrations of LDL cholesterol.[154,293] The ratio of LDL cholesterol to apo B-100 is therefore reduced in these patients (≤1.2).[154] Total cholesterol and triglyceride may be normal but are usually increased, and HDL cholesterol and apo A-I are usually decreased. This disorder appears to be caused by overproduction of VLDL and apo B-100 in the liver, which leads to the formation of atherogenic small and dense LDL.[154] The exact mode of inheritance and the prevalence of this disorder remain unclear; however, about one third of children of a parent with premature CHD or hyperapobetalipoproteinemia will have this disorder.[294] Features common to hyperapobetalipoproteinemia have been reported to occur in patients with FCHL, suggesting metabolic and genetic associations between these two disorders.

Familial Hypertriglyceridemia

The production of large VLDL with abnormally high triglyceride content appears to be responsible for familial hypertriglyceridemia (FHTG).[137] The actual number of VLDL particles produced by the liver, however, is not increased. The cholesterol content of VLDL is also increased, but plasma LDL cholesterol and apo B-100 concentrations are normal. This finding suggests that the conversion of VLDL to LDL is not increased in these patients. Furthermore, plasma HDL cholesterol in FHTG is often dramatically decreased, probably secondary to the hypertriglyceridemia.

The cause of the overproduction of VLDL triglyceride is unknown. Administration of estrogen and corticosteroids aggravates hypertriglyceridemia in these patients and sometimes can lead to acute pancreatitis. The diagnosis of FHTG requires study of other family members to differentiate this disorder from FCHL. This disorder appears to be inherited in an autosomal dominant pattern with delayed expression and an estimated frequency in the population of about 1 : 500 persons, making this a relatively common disorder. About one in five children born to affected parents manifest the phenotype early in life.[96]

Type V Hyperlipoproteinemia

This disorder is characterized by an increase in both chylomicrons and VLDL and has an incidence of about 1 in 500. Although the exact molecular cause of this disorder is not known, the metabolic defect appears to be increased production or decreased removal of VLDL, or a combination of both. The activity of LPL in these patients may be normal or low, and the plasma concentration of apo C-II is normal.[155]

Although this disorder is not usually expressed in childhood, several affected preadolescents have been described.[155] Clinical presentations in adult patients include eruptive xanthomas, lipemia retinalis, pancreatitis, and abnormal glucose tolerance with hyperinsulinism.[46] Premature atherosclerotic complications are not as commonly seen as with FH. This heterogeneous syndrome appears to be inherited in an autosomal dominant mode, but its genetic basis has not yet been fully elucidated.

Dysbetalipoproteinemia (Type III)

This disorder is caused by a primary genetic defect in the removal of remnants of both intestinal chylomicrons and hepatic VLDL.[173] As indicated earlier, apo E present on the surface of lipoprotein remnants interacts with specific hepatic receptors and facilitates the removal of these lipoprotein particles from the circulation. Patients with dysbetalipoproteinemia may be homozygous for a rare mutation in apo E or may be homozygous for the apo E_2 allele.[340] These altered forms of apo E cannot as efficiently bind specific hepatic receptors, leading to the accumulation of lipoprotein remnants. These particles are cholesterol enriched with a density <1.006 g/mL, and are commonly referred to as β-VLDL or floating β-lipoprotein, in plasma.

The disease is characterized by increased plasma cholesterol and triglycerides, and the concentrations of the two lipids are about the same when expressed in milligrams per deciliter. β-VLDL present in type III has been shown to contain both apo B-100 and B-48, and therefore is related to triglyceride-rich lipoprotein remnants of both hepatic and intestinal origin. Both LDL and HDL cholesterol are lower than normal in these patients.[173]

This disorder has a late onset, rarely manifesting itself in childhood.[269] The most distinctive clinical presentation of dyslipoproteinemia is the presence of palmar xanthomas, yellow deposits that occur in the creases of the palms.[140] Tuberous and tuberoeruptive xanthomas also occur but are not unique to this syndrome. Premature atherosclerosis develops in 30% to more than 50% of these patients, particularly in the lower extremities.[306,326]

The apo E_2 alelle occurs in the homozygous state in about 1% of the population in North America; such subjects can exhibit an abnormal form of VLDL called *β-VLDL* or *broad beta,* based on its electrophoretic migration pattern. Overt type III hyperlipoproteinemia, however, occurs in only a small minority—less than 5% of patients homozygous for apo E_2—indicating that occurrence of the defective alleles is necessary but not sufficient to produce type III hyperlipoproteinemia.[321] The penetrance of hyperlipoproteinemia in these patients is modulated by genetic, hormonal, or environmental factors—such as hypothyroidism, glucose intolerance, decreased estrogen concentration after menopause, obesity, and diet—that may lead to decreased LDL receptor activity, increased VLDL production, or increased plasma cholesterol ester transfer protein. Because of the familial nature of this disorder and the predisposition of these patients to hyperlipoproteinemia and premature atherosclerotic disease, family members should be evaluated.

Familial Hypercholesterolemia

Familial hypercholesterolemia (FH) is most often caused by a defect in the LDL receptor gene. As discussed earlier, this cell surface receptor is responsible for the recognition and removal of LDL from the circulation. The defects seen in patients with FH include reduced LDL binding because of defective or absent LDL receptors. In another variant of this disorder, the person may make defective LDL receptors that bind LDL normally but cannot efficiently internalize the LDL particles.[44] FH is characterized clinically by increased plasma LDL cholesterol concentration and cholesterol deposition in skin, tendons, and arteries; it usually is transmitted in an autosomal dominant manner, so that the disease is expressed in the heterozygous and homozygous states. Heterozygous FH is one of the most commonly seen genetic metabolic disorders, with an incidence of 1 in 500 persons in the United States. The prevalence of homozygous FH is about one in a million persons. Mean plasma LDL cholesterol in children and adult heterozygotes is usually two to three times that of normal people of similar age, whereas mean plasma LDL cholesterol of homozygotes is four to six times that of normal subjects.[98] Although the number of LDL particles is increased in these patients, their lipid composition and lipid-to-protein ratio are usually normal.[104] Apo B-100 is increased in proportion to LDL cholesterol. Triglyceride concentration may be normal or slightly increased, and HDL cholesterol concentration is slightly decreased in both heterozygotes and homozygotes.

Hypercholesterolemia is present at birth in most FH patients and persists throughout life. In heterozygotes, xanthomas appear toward the end of the second decade of life, and clinical manifestations of atherosclerotic disease appear during the fourth decade.[285] In homozygotes, the unique yellow-orange cutaneous xanthomas develop by the age of 4, if they are not already present at birth.[140] Tendon xanthomas and atherosclerotic complications begin during childhood. Death from myocardial infarction can occur in homozygotes before the end of the third decade and even earlier, but the prospect for these patients is much better with aggressive lipid-lowering therapy.[4,155]

Although increased plasma LDL cholesterol is indicative of the heterozygous form of FH, it is not sufficient to make the diagnosis; it is now common practice to confirm the diagnosis by sequencing the gene for the LDL receptor. More than 150 different mutations in the LDL receptor gene have been shown to significantly disrupt the normal process of LDL removal from the circulation.[98,123] Heterozygotes possess one normal and one mutant allele at the LDL receptor locus and therefore can remove LDL at about half the normal rate.

Recently, two other rare genetic mutations have been shown to lead to FH. Mutations in PCSK9, which is a hepatic secretory protein, can lead to an autosomal dominant form of FH.[159] PCSK9 normally downregulates expression of the LDL receptor; mutations that cause a gain of function, therefore, can lead to increased concentrations of circulating LDL by decreasing expression of the LDL receptor. Mutations in ARH lead to an autosomal recessive form of FH.[13] ARH is an adapter-like protein that appears to be necessary for proper recycling of the LDL receptor on the plasma membrane.

Familial Defective Apolipoprotein B-100

This disorder results from a mutation in the apo B-100 gene rather than the LDL receptor, resulting in a single substitution of glutamine for arginine at residue 3500 of apo B-100. This substitution reduces the positive charge of apo B-100 and decreases its affinity for the LDL receptor.[297] Other more rare mutations in apo B affecting its binding to the LDL receptor have also been described. Plasma LDL cholesterol in heterozygotes of this disorder can be normal to greatly increased because of inadequate removal of LDL particles by LDL receptors.[324] Those with increased LDL cholesterol have an increased incidence of CHD, but often the disease appears to be less aggressive than FH. Triglyceride and HDL cholesterol concentrations are not usually affected. It is often difficult to differentiate these patients from heterozygous FH patients; however, because the management these two disorders is similar, the distinction is not that clinically important.[137] The frequency of this mutation is 1 : 500 to 1 : 600 hypercholesterolemic persons in populations of European descent,[316] but the mutation is much rarer in non-European populations.

Hypoalphalipoproteinemia

This disorder is characterized by normal plasma lipids and LDL cholesterol, and HDL cholesterol reduced to below the 5th percentile.[269,279] It is associated with an increased incidence of CHD.[314] Several known molecular defects can lead to hypoalphalipoproteinemia. Rarely, patients can have mutations in apo A-I, the main protein component of HDL, which can lead to profoundly low concentrations of HDL.[41,155] These patients typically have corneal clouding and xanthomas, and are at increased risk for development of premature CHD. Heterozygotes exhibit no clinical signs but have about half the normal concentrations of HDL cholesterol and apo A-I. Mutations, such as a rearrangement at the apolipoprotein gene locus that inactivates both apo A-I and C-III, deletion of the entire locus, and an insertion in the apo A-I gene have all been described.[138,155,226]

Tangier disease, so named because it was first observed in patients from Tangier Island in Chesapeake Bay (Eastern United States), is characterized by (1) severely reduced plasma HDL concentration, (2) abnormal HDL composition, and (3) accumulation of cholesteryl esters in many tissues throughout the body.[23,280,284] Kinetic studies have demonstrated that increased catabolism of HDL, rather than a defect in biosynthesis, is the cause of Tangier disease.[280] Tangier disease is caused by mutations in the *ABCA1* (ATP-binding cassette A1) gene on chromosome 9q31 and appears to be inherited in an autosomal dominant fashion. As already mentioned, the ABCA1 transporter is a key protein for the efflux of cholesterol from peripheral cells, particularly from macrophages. ABCA1 is also present in the liver and intestine and is important in the biogenesis of HDL. After lipid-free or lipid-poor apo A-I enters the plasma compartment via secretion from hepatocytes or enterocytes, or by dissociation from a lipoprotein particle, it must acquire additional lipid by the ABCA1 transporter, or it will be quickly catabolized by filtration in the kidney. Plasma cholesterol is usually decreased to about 70 mg/dL in homozygotes and to about 160 mg/dL in heterozygotes. Triglyceride concentrations vary depending on the diet.[23] In homozygotes, plasma HDL cholesterol and apo A-I concentrations are often undetectable; apo A-II is present at less than 10% of its normal concentration and is often found in apo B-100–containing lipoprotein.[24] Heterozygotes are characterized by half-normal concentrations of HDL cholesterol, apo A-I, and apo A-II.

Clinical symptoms of Tangier disease result from the deposition of cholesteryl esters in various tissues in the body. The three major clinical signs are hyperplastic orange tonsils, splenomegaly, and peripheral neuropathy. Other clinical signs that may be seen include hepatomegaly and corneal opacities. Severely reduced HDL cholesterol and enlarged orange tonsils are pathognomonic.[23,155] Current evidence suggests that these patients have an increased incidence of CHD, but they are seemingly less affected than would be expected from their low HDL; this has been attributed to the fact that patients also often have reduced concentrations of LDL.

Mutations in the gene for LCAT, which esterifies cholesterol, can also result in hypoalphalipoproteinemia.[275]

As already discussed, LCAT is important in the proper maturation of HDL. In the absence of LCAT, the primary form of HDL that is found is pre–β-HDL, which is the nascent discoidal form of HDL that is phospholipid rich but cholesterol poor. Because of its small size, this form of HDL is rapidly catabolized, leading to the low concentration of HDL found in these patients. This is an autosomal recessive disorder, but patients with mutations with partial activity develop only cloudy corneas and have a disorder called fish eye disease. Familial LCAT deficiency subjects have near complete absence of LCAT activity and develop not only cloudy corneas but also a mild hemolytic anemia, splenomegaly, and glomerulosclerosis, which is the main cause of morbidity in these patients. It is believed that patients develop renal disease because of the presence of Lp-X. This is an abnormal lipoprotein particle that also sometimes accumulates in liver disease and appears to be trapped by mesangial cells in the glomerulus, leading to fat deposition and eventually to glomerulosclerosis. Unlike other lipoprotein particles, which have a single layer of phospholipids on their surface, Lp-X has a phospholipid bilayer–like structure and can even form multilamellar vesicles with an aqueous core. It is believed that such structures are formed when neutral lipid, such as cholesteryl esters, is insufficient to form the neutral lipid core in lipoproteins. Patients with LCAT deficiency appear to have a modestly increased risk for CHD. Similar to Tangier disease subjects, they may be protected because they often have low LDL cholesterol concentrations, because much of the cholesterol on LDL is ultimately derived from HDL as a consequence of the reverse cholesterol transport pathway.

Diagnosis of Lipoprotein Disorders

On the basis of findings from many different studies, such as the MRFIT and the LRC-CPPT,[1,2,109] hypercholesterolemia in adults is now defined in terms of CHD risk. The National Institutes of Health ATP III of the NCEP[8] has issued its third report for the detection, evaluation, and treatment of hypercholesterolemia.[11] The ATP III built on earlier reports and expanded the indications for intensive cholesterol lowering. In ATP-I, strategies for primary prevention of CHD in subjects with LDL-C ≥160 mg/dL or 130 to 159 mg/dL and multiple risk factors (2+) were addressed. ATP II added new features; for subjects with existing CHD, a lower LDL-C goal of ≤100 mg/dL was established, and the HDL cholesterol value was given greater prominence. ATP III called for intensive LDL-C lowering in several other groups of patients. In this section, only a brief description of ATP III will be presented. Those interested in more detailed information should refer to the executive summary[67] or the complete report (http://www.nhlbi.nih.gov/guidelines/cholesterol/index.htm). An ATP IV report with additional updates is expected in 2012.

For the primary prevention of CHD, adults 20 years of age or older should have their fasting lipoprotein profile (total cholesterol, triglycerides, HDL-C, and LDL-C) measured once every 5 years. If a fasting sample is not available, then only total cholesterol and HDL-C should be considered. In

TABLE 27-15 ATP III Classification of LDL, Total, and HDL Cholesterol, mg/dL

LDL cholesterol	<100	Optimum
	100-129	Near or above optimum
	130-159	Borderline high
	160-189	High
	≥190	Very high
Total cholesterol	<200	Desirable
	200-239	Borderline high
	≥240	High
HDL cholesterol	<40	Low
	≥60	High

ATP, Adult Treatment Panel; *HDL,* high-density lipoprotein; *LDL,* low-density lipoprotein.
Modified from executive summary of the third report of the National Cholesterol Education Program (NCEP) Expert Panel on Detection, Evaluation, and Treatment of High Blood Cholesterol in Adults (Adult Treatment Panel III). JAMA 2001;285:2486-97.

BOX 27-2 Major Risk Factors (Exclusive of LDL Cholesterol)

Cigarette smoking
Hypertension (blood pressure ≥140/90 mm Hg or on antihypertensive medication)
Low HDL cholesterol (<40 mg/dL)*
Family history of premature CHD (CHD in male first-degree relative <55 years; CHD in female first-degree relative <65 years)
Age (men ≥45 years; women ≥55 years)

*HDL cholesterol ≥60 mg/dL counts as a "negative" risk factor; its presence removes one risk factor from the total count.
HDL, High-density lipoprotein; *LDL,* low-density lipoprotein.
Modified from executive summary of the third report of the National Cholesterol Education Program (NCEP) Expert Panel on Detection, Evaluation, and Treatment of High Blood Cholesterol in Adults (Adult Treatment Panel III). JAMA 2001;285:2486-97.

this instance, if total cholesterol is ≥200 mg/dL or HDL-C is ≤40 mg/dL, then a fasting lipoprotein profile is required. The cut points recommended for classification by ATP III are presented in Table 27-15. In addition to LDL-C, other risk determinants, presented in Box 27-2, are used to assess risk and determine goals and modalities of LDL-C–lowering therapy. The highest category of risk consists of those with CHD or CHD risk equivalents (other forms of atherosclerotic disease, such as peripheral arterial disease, abdominal aortic aneurysm, and symptomatic carotid artery disease, diabetes, or multiple risk factors that confer a 10-year risk for CHD >20%, as estimated by the Framingham risk score) (Table 27-16). The Framingham risk score is calculated for intermediate-risk individuals with two or more risk factors but with no history of CHD or risk equivalent. This is done to better estimate the CHD risk of these patients; an algorithm that includes age, gender, total cholesterol, HDL-C, history of hypertension and treatment of hypertension, and cigarette smoking is used. The lowest risk category consists of those subjects having zero to one risk factor, in whom 10-year risk is ≤10%.

TABLE 27-16 Categories of Risk for LDL Cholesterol Goals

Risk Category	LDL Goal, mg/dL
CHD and CHD risk equivalents	<100
Multiple (2+) risk factors*	<130
0-1 risk factor	<160

*Refer to Box 27-2 for list of risk factors.
CHD, Coronary heart disease.
Modified from executive summary of the third report of the National Cholesterol Education Program (NCEP) Expert Panel on Detection, Evaluation, and Treatment of High Blood Cholesterol in Adults (Adult Treatment Panel III). JAMA 2001;285:2486-97.

TABLE 27-17 Clinical Identification of the Metabolic Syndrome

Risk Factor	Defining Level
Abdominal obesity (waist circumference)	
Men	>102 cm (>40 in)
Women	>88 cm (>35 in)
Triglycerides	≥150 mg/dL
High-density lipoprotein cholesterol	
Men	<40 mg/dL
Women	<50 mg/dL
Blood pressure	≥130/≥85 mm Hg
Fasting glucose	≥110 mg/dL

Modified from executive summary of the third report of the National Cholesterol Education Program (NCEP) Expert Panel on Detection, Evaluation, and Treatment of High Blood Cholesterol in Adults (Adult Treatment Panel III). JAMA 2001;285:2486-97.

Although the primary target of risk reduction therapy is LDL-C, the ATP III recognized the metabolic syndrome, a constellation of several risk factors (increased triglycerides, decreased HDL-C, obesity, hypertension, and insulin resistance) as a secondary target of therapy. By definition, those with three or more of these risk factors are considered to have the metabolic syndrome.[11] Specific criteria for clinical identification of the metabolic syndrome are listed in Table 27-17.

The NCEP/Expert Panel on Blood Cholesterol Concentrations in Children and Adolescents[6] and the American Academy of Pediatrics[3,71] defined "high cholesterol" in children and adolescents from families with hypercholesterolemia or premature vascular disease as concentrations greater than the 95th percentile for total and LDL cholesterol in unaffected children (Table 27-18). "Borderline" total and LDL cholesterol concentrations are defined as values between the 75th and 95th percentiles. The NCEP panel referred to total and LDL cholesterol values below the 75th percentile as "desirable." Low HDL cholesterol was also defined as a concentration below 35 mg/dL. Children tend to have higher HDL cholesterol concentrations than adults; therefore, it is important to determine both LDL and HDL cholesterol concentrations before classifying the child as hypercholesterolemic. Unlike the criteria for the risk-based cholesterol classification system used in adults, guidelines for children and adolescents were based on consensus rather than directly on the association with coronary disease, because children as a group have very little disease. When lifetime risk data become available, different cutoffs may be suggested for the pediatric population.

As discussed earlier, universal cholesterol screening is currently recommended for all adults in the United States; however, for children, such a screening program remains highly controversial. According to the NCEP[6] and the American Academy of Pediatrics,[3,71] only children over the age of 2 should be screened for hypercholesterolemia when they have a parent with hypercholesterolemia (>240 mg/dL) or a positive family history (mother, father, uncle, aunt, or grandparent) with early documented CHD (at 55 years or less) such as myocardial infarction, angina pectoris, peripheral vascular disease, cerebrovascular disease, or sudden cardiac death. Children for whom the family history is not known and children with other CHD risk factors, such as obesity, diabetes, and hypertension, should also be screened for cholesterol.[71] Several studies have demonstrated the weakness of this selective approach to screening and have advocated general screening for children. The Bogalusa Heart Study found that by using the selective screening approach, only 50% of white children and 20% of black children with high LDL cholesterol concentrations (>95th percentile) were detected. Furthermore, it has been shown that self-reported cholesterol values among parents are an ineffective means of identifying children with high cholesterol.[249] More than 90% of children with total cholesterol greater than the 75th or 95th percentile were missed when physicians relied on cholesterol values reported by the parents. General screening, however, is expensive and time-consuming, and its effectiveness is limited by the fact that a significant number of children with high cholesterol concentrations will *not* remain hypercholesterolemic as adults.[162,246]

TABLE 27-18 NCEP Classification of Total and LDL Cholesterol in Children and Adolescents*

Category	Total Cholesterol	LDL Cholesterol
Desirable	<170	<110
Borderline	170-199	110-120
High	≥200	≥130

*All values are in mg/dL; to convert to mmol/L, multiply by 0.0259.

Universal screening for those older than 16 has been suggested on the basis of a finding that up to 66% of adolescents with increased LDL cholesterol are missed in a selective screening protocol.[270] When past adolescence, men usually do not start receiving routine healthcare examinations until about the age of 40. Although women typically visit their physicians earlier, this is the result of gynecological needs, and women may not be evaluated for a lipid disorder. Adolescents with increased LDL cholesterol who are missed in the selective screening process may not be identified until two decades later. At that time, the atherosclerotic process may be advanced, and a dietary management approach may not be sufficiently effective. Another possible yet unpopular approach is to do no screening at all. A prudent low-fat diet, such as the one outlined by the American Heart Association (AHA), can be recommended for all children (Table 27-19).[3,71] Such an approach will help prevent unnecessary anxiety, labeling, and overzealous treatment; however, it will miss completely those children with significant hypercholesterolemia, who are most at risk for adult CHD.

Management of Lipoprotein Disorders

Management of Hypercholesterolemia in Adults

According to ATP III, a central element in the clinical prevention of CHD is founded on a public health approach that entails a reduction in saturated fat and cholesterol intake (Table 27-20), increased physical activity, and weight control. Although this therapeutic life-style approach offers the

TABLE 27-19 Current Fat Intake in American Adults, Children, and Adolescents and the American Heart Association Step-One and Step-Two Diets

	Current Intake			
Nutrients	Adults	Children and Adolescents	Step-One	Step-Two
Total fat				
• Percent of total calories	35-36%	36%	<30%	<30%
• Saturated fat	14%	15%	<10%	7%
• Polyunsaturated fat	6%	16%	10%	10%
• Monounsaturated fat	13-14%	15%	10-15%	10-15%
• Cholesterol, mg/d	300-400	400-500	<300	<200

Modified from National Cholesterol Education Program, Lipid Metabolism Branch, Division of Heart, Lung, and Blood Institute. The report of the Expert Panel on Blood Cholesterol Levels in Children and Adolescents. Bethesda, Md: National Institutes of Health, 1991.

opportunity for reducing the morbidity and mortality of CHD in the entire population, more intensified preventive measures for higher-risk individuals are indicated.[11] The primary goal is to reduce one's long-term (>10 years) and short-term risk (<10 years); the target LDL-C value depends on the person's absolute risk (Table 27-21). A more aggressive approach is recommended for those individuals who have already suffered a coronary event and for those with established CHD or those at very high risk of CHD, such as persons with diabetes. Specific models for therapeutic life-style changes and drug therapy in the primary prevention of CHD have been recommended (Figures 27-23 and 27-24). A combination approach of weight reduction, increased physical activity, and appropriate control of lipid concentrations is recommended for the management of patients with metabolic syndrome.

A wide variety of pharmacologic agents are available for cholesterol lowering in adults,[282] including (1) bile acid–binding resins (cholestyramine and colestipol), (2) niacin, (3) gemfibrozil, (4) ezetimibe, and (5) HMG-CoA reductase inhibitors (e.g., atorvastatin, fluvastatin, lovastatin, pravastatin, simvastatin); the latter group has been found to reduce LDL cholesterol by as much as 40%. Some of these drugs are better tolerated by individual patients than others, and all have demonstrated long-term safety. Niacin is the only FDA-approved drug that can significantly raise HDL cholesterol. Its use has been limited by side effects from flushing, although newer formulations have reduced this problem. These drugs can be used individually or in combination.[102,103]

TABLE 27-20 Nutrient Composition of the Therapeutic Life-Style Changes (TLC) Diet

Nutrient	Recommended Intake
Saturated fat	<7% of total calories
Polyunsaturated fat	Up to 10% of total calories
Monounsaturated fat	Up to 20% of total calories
Total fat	25-35% of total calories
Carbohydrate	50-60% of total calories
Fiber	20-30 g/d
Protein	Approximately 15% of total calories
Cholesterol	<200 mg/d
Total calories	Balance energy intake and expenditure to maintain desirable body weight/ prevent weight gain

Modified from executive summary of the third report of the National Cholesterol Education Program (NCEP) Expert Panel on Detection, Evaluation, and Treatment of High Blood Cholesterol in Adults (Adult Treatment Panel III). JAMA 2001;285:2486-97.

Management of Hypercholesterolemia in Children and Adolescents

To lower serum cholesterol concentration in children and adolescents, the NCEP adopted a strategy that combines two complementary approaches: a population approach and an individualized approach.[6,71]

Population Approach

Children and adolescents have relatively high cholesterol concentrations and a high intake of saturated fatty acids and cholesterol (see Table 27-19).[53,71] The population approach attempts to lower the mean cholesterol concentration by instituting population-wide modifications in nutrient intake and eating habits. The AHA Step-One diet is recommended (see Table 27-19). Even a modest decrease in mean cholesterol concentration in children and adolescents, if carried into adulthood, is likely to have a significant impact on lowering the incidence of CHD. The panel did not recommend any dietary changes for infants from birth to 2 years of age, because of concern about the effects of a low-fat diet during early development. Toddlers aged 2 and 3 should start making the transition to the recommended eating pattern. The NCEP

TABLE 27-21 LDL Cholesterol Goals and Cut Points for Therapeutic Life-Style Changes (TLC) and Drug Therapy in Different Risk Categories

Risk Category	LDL Goal, mg/dL	LDL Level at Which to Initiate Therapeutic Life-Style Changes, mg/dL	LDL Level at Which to Consider Drug Therapy, mg/dL
CHD or CHD risk equivalents (10-year risk >20%)	<100	≥100	≥130 (100-129: Drug optional)
2+ Risk factors (10-year risk ≤20%)	<130	≥130	10-Year risk 10-20%: ≥130 10-Year risk <10%: ≥160
0-1 Risk factor (10-year risk <10%)	<160	≥160	≥190 (160-189: LDL-lowering drug optional)

CHD, Coronary heart disease; *LDL,* low-density lipoprotein.
Modified from executive summary of the third report of the National Cholesterol Education Program (NCEP) Expert Panel on Detection, Evaluation, and Treatment of High Blood Cholesterol in Adults (Adult Treatment Panel III). JAMA 2001;285:2486-97.

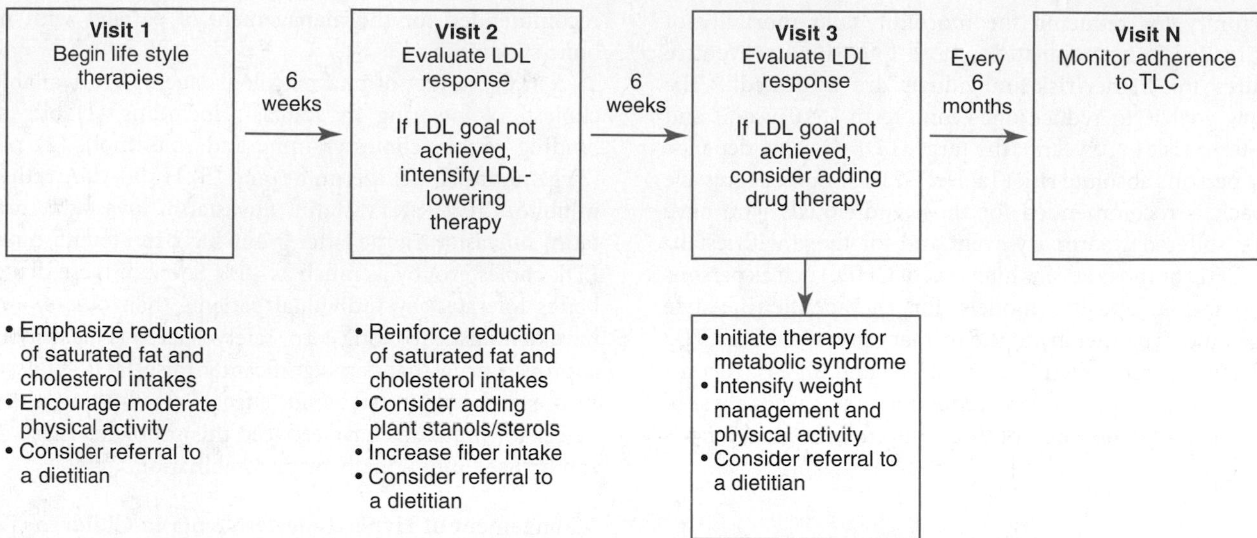

Figure 27-23 Model of steps in therapeutic life-style change. *LDL,* Low-density lipoprotein. *(Modified from Executive summary of the third report of the Expert Panel on Blood Cholesterol Levels in Children and Adolescents, National Cholesterol Education Program. Lipid Metabolism Branch, Division of Heart, Lung, and Blood Institute. NIH Publication No. 01-3670. U.S. Department of Health and Human Services, Public Health Service, National Institutes of Health. Bethesda, Md: National Institutes of Health, 2003.)*

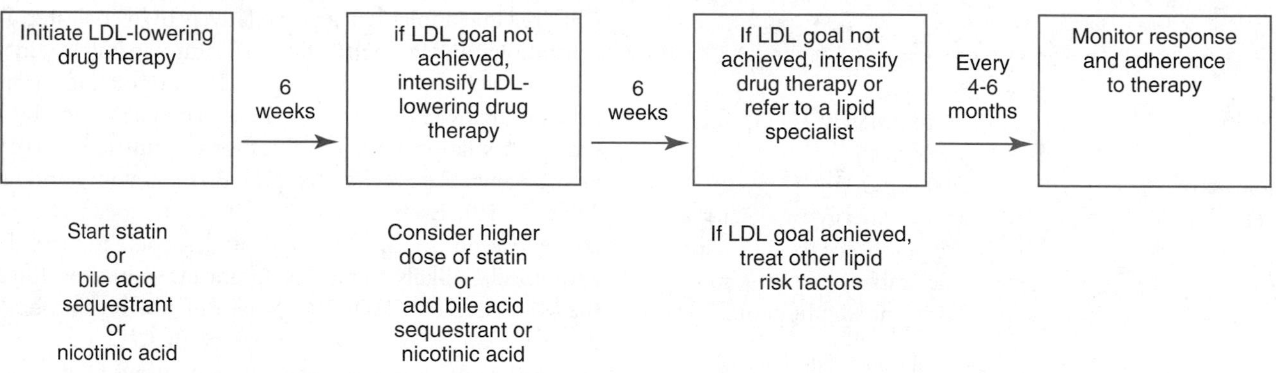

Figure 27-24 Progression of drug therapy in primary prevention. *LDL,* Low-density lipoprotein.

also directed recommendations to schools, health professionals, government agencies, the food industry, and mass media to help influence and modify the eating habits of children and adolescents. The most recent guidelines have stressed the importance of limiting *trans*-fatty acids to less than 1% of total calories consumed.[71] Because of mandatory food labeling requirements and because of local ordinances limiting the use of *trans*-fatty acids, it may now be easier to achieve this goal.

Individualized Approach

Instead of the universal approach used for LDL-C screening in adults, an individualized approach or selective screening is recommended for children older than 2 years of age who may be at risk for cardiovascular disease. Children at risk for cardiovascular disease are recognized because of a family history of hypercholesterolemia or premature cardiovascular disease. It is recommended that such patients be tested for fasting total cholesterol, HDL-C, triglycerides, and LDL-C (Figure 27-25).[6,71] If the family history is not known, or if the child has other risk factors, such as obesity, hypertension or diabetes, it is recommended that they be screened. In general, treatment guidelines for children are less aggressive than those for adults because of concern regarding potential negative consequences of treatment, particularly drug treatment. Under the NCEP guidelines,[12] children with an average LDL cholesterol concentration between 110 and 129 mg/dL are recommended to be placed on the AHA Step-One diet, counseled about other heart disease risk factors, and re-evaluated after 1 year. Those with an average LDL cholesterol concentration greater than 130 mg/dL should also be placed on the AHA Step-One diet and evaluated for secondary causes; their family members should be screened. If after 3 months of initiation of dietary therapy, the LDL cholesterol concentration remains greater than 130 mg/dL, the patient should be placed on the AHA Step-Two diet, which entails further reduction of saturated fatty acid and cholesterol intake (see

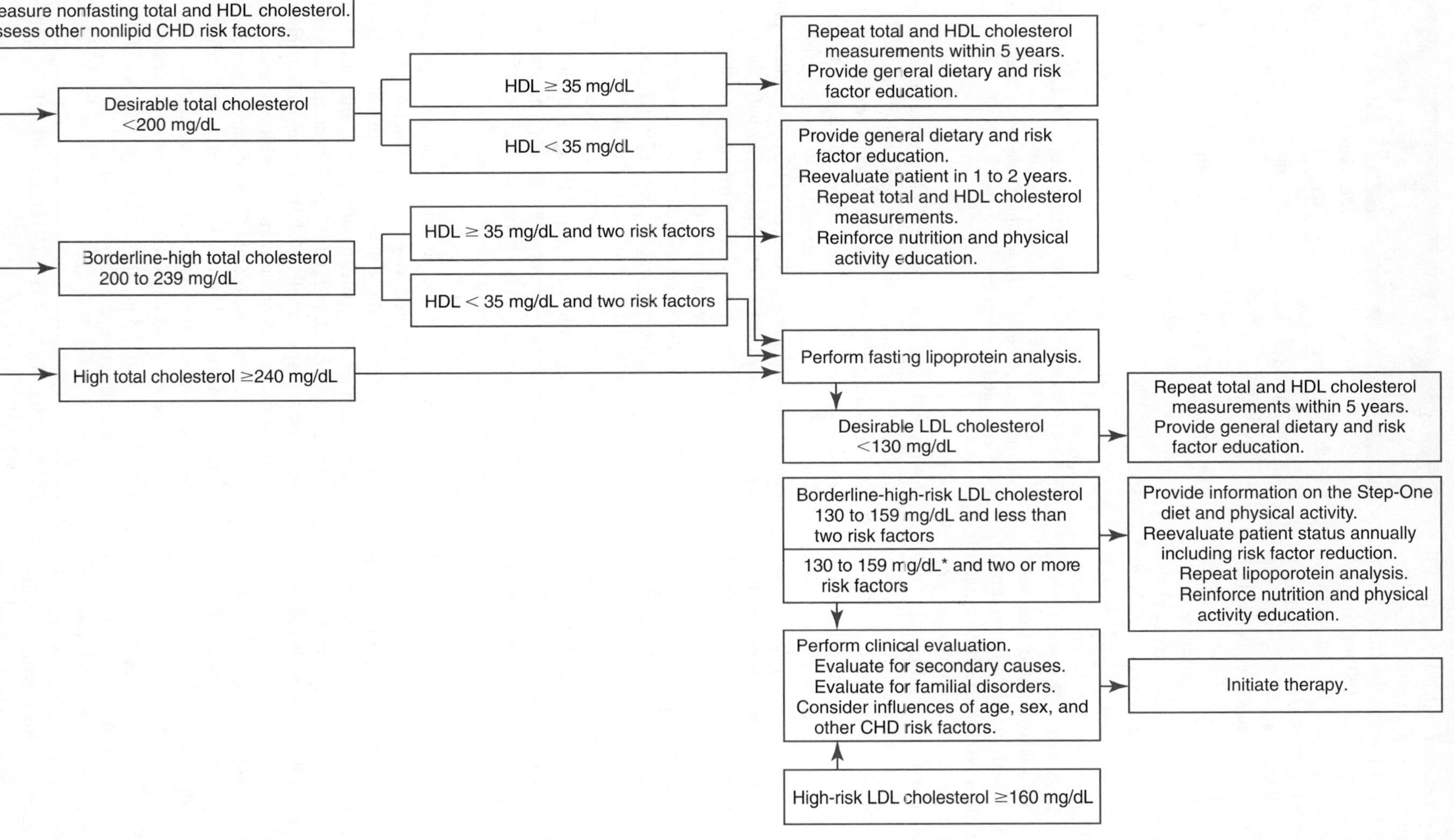

*On the basis of the average of two determinations. If the first two LDL-cholesterol test results differ by more than 30 mg/dL, a third test result should be obtained within 1 to 8 weeks and the average value of the three tests used.

Figure 27-25 Risk assessment flowchart as recommended by the National Cholesterol Education Program Expert Panel on Blood Cholesterol Levels in Children and Adolescents. *(From The report of the Expert Panel on Blood Cholesterol Levels in Children and Adolescents, National Cholesterol Education Program. Lipid Metabolism Branch, Division of Heart, Lung, and Blood Institute. NIH Publication No. 91-2732. U.S. Department of Health and Human Services, Public Health Service, National Institutes of Health. Bethesda, Md: National Institutes of Health, 1991.)*

Table 27-19). Drug therapy was recommended by the NCEP for children 10 years of age and older, if after careful adherence to dietary therapy (6 months to 1 year), the LDL cholesterol concentration remains greater than 190 mg/dL. The action concentration is lower (160 mg/dL) for patients who have a positive family history of premature CHD and for those with two or more other risk factors.

The American Academy of Pediatrics has developed alternative guidelines for lipid screening in children.[71] These guidelines are similar to the older NCEP guidelines, but emphasis is placed on identifying children who may be at risk because they are overweight [overweight is defined as body mass index (BMI) ≥85th percentile for age]. Children with hypertension or diabetes and those who smoke are recommended to be screened with a lipid panel. These additional groups were selected because it was estimated that only between 30% and 60% of children with hypercholesterolemia were being detected when the older NCEP screening criteria of a positive family history of hypercholesterolemia and premature cardiovascular disease were used. Another difference is the greater emphasis of the new guidelines on lowering the fat content of the diet for highest risk subjects. It is recommended to restrict saturated fat to 7% of total calories and to limit cholesterol to 200 mg/d. Finally, more information shows the safety and efficacy of lipid-lowering drug treatment in children, particularly statins, so the American Academy of Pediatrics recommends that subjects 8 years of age and older be considered candidates for drug treatment if their LDL-C is >190 mg/dL after other interventions have been tried. A lower threshold of LDL ≥160 mg/dL should be used in higher-risk subjects with a family history of premature cardiovascular disease, or with *two or more* risk factors, or with diabetes. Subjects younger than 8 years of age but with a marked increase in total cholesterol to greater than 500 mg/dL should be considered as candidates for drug therapy. Children, as well as adults, who have homozygous FH are relatively resistant to drug therapy, particularly statins, because they work in part by upregulating hepatic LDL receptors. Several alternative treatments that have been used include (1) long-term plasmapheresis every 2 weeks or a plasmapheresis-like procedure that selectively removes LDL, (2) partial ileal bypass or portacaval shunt to lower total and LDL cholesterol, and (3) liver transplantation, using livers from donors with functional LDL receptors. An early-stage clinical trial of an antisense oligonucleotide against apo B, which is delivered subcutaneously, has been shown to efficiently lower LDL concentrations in FH patients for several weeks.[129]

Management of Hypertriglyceridemia

Because evidence-based findings have shown triglycerides to be an independent risk factor for CHD in both men and women, greater emphasis is now placed on measurement of this marker and the management of those with increased triglycerides.[11] Furthermore, an *average to low-risk* triglyceride concentration has been redefined from <200 to <150 mg/dL; values of 150 to 199 mg/dL are considered borderline high, 200 to 499 mg/dL high, and ≥500 mg/dL very high. In the general population, several factors are associated with increased triglyceride concentrations, including obesity, cigarette smoking, physical inactivity, and excess alcohol intake, as well as several diseases (e.g., type 2 diabetes, chronic renal failure), drugs (e.g., corticosteroids, estrogens, retinoids), and genetic disorders (e.g., FCHL, FHTG). In clinical practice, hypertriglyceridemia is often associated with the metabolic syndrome. Triglyceride-rich lipoproteins or remnant lipoproteins are currently recognized to be atherogenic. In practice, VLDL cholesterol is often used as a measure of these atherogenic lipoproteins. Therefore, the ATP III suggested the addition of non-HDL cholesterol (total cholesterol–HDL cholesterol) as an indicator for all atherogenic lipoproteins (mainly LDL and VLDL).[11] Non–HDL-C is used as a secondary target of therapy in persons with triglycerides ≥200 mg/dL. The goal for non-HDL cholesterol in those with increased triglycerides is 30 mg/dL above that set for LDL cholesterol. The treatment of hypertriglyceridemia depends on the cause of the increase and the severity. Those with triglycerides <200 mg/dL are treated with weight reduction and increased physical activity; for those at 200 to 499 mg/dL, drug therapy is also considered (fibrate, nicotinic acid, and niacin). In the latter group, the non–HDL-C goal becomes a secondary target of therapy (Table 27-22). Those with triglycerides >500 mg/dL usually are at increased risk of pancreatitis and are treated with a low-fat diet (≤15% of calorie intake), weight reduction, increased physical activity, and triglyceride-lowering drugs. Although nicotinic acid and niacin are usually the drugs of choice, a combination therapy, such as gemfibrozil and resins, or gemfibrozil and an HMG-CoA reductase inhibitor, can also be used.[282]

TABLE 27-22 Comparison of LDL Cholesterol and Non-HDL Cholesterol Goals for Three Risk Categories

Risk Category	LDL Goal, mg/dL	Non-HDL Goal, mg/dL
CHD and CHD risk equivalent (10-year risk for CHD >20%)	<100	<130
Multiple (2+) risk factors and 10-year risk ≤20%	<130	<160
0-1 risk factor	<160	<190

CHD, Coronary heart disease; *HDL,* high-density lipoprotein; *LDL,* low-density lipoprotein.
Modified from executive summary of the third report of the National Cholesterol Education Program (NCEP) Expert Panel on Detection, Evaluation, and Treatment of High Blood Cholesterol in Adults (Adult Treatment Panel III). JAMA 2001;285:2486-97.

MEASUREMENT OF LIPIDS, LIPOPROTEINS, AND APOLIPOPROTEINS

Lipoproteins and their lipid and apolipoprotein constituents have become increasingly important in characterizing the risk of cardiovascular disease, and in the diagnosis and management of disorders of lipoprotein metabolism. In recent decades, our knowledge of such disorders has evolved from an essentially descriptive association between elevated plasma lipids and increased risk for premature cardiovascular disease morbidity and mortality to a much broader understanding of the underlying biochemistry, physiology, and genetic interactions. Remarkable advances have been made in our understanding of the contribution of lipoproteins to the development and progression of arterial lesions. Advances have also been made in the analytical techniques and methods used for measuring lipids, lipoproteins, and apolipoproteins. In this section, we begin with a brief historical perspective on the development of measurement technology; this is followed by a more detailed discussion of pertinent methods.

Historical Perspective and Background

The causal relationship between increased plasma concentrations of LDL and risk of CHD and the efficacy of LDL lowering to reduce risk was widely acknowledged by the mid-1980s. Awareness of the importance of intervention emphasized the necessity for uniform means of defining hyperlipidemia and CHD risk. Previous practice had been to use arbitrarily defined cutoffs based on prevailing lipid and lipoprotein concentrations in the general population or in local populations of "normal patients." Because of the relative nonspecificity of early chemical methods for cholesterol measurement and the different types of methods then in use, significant biases existed between values obtained in different laboratories, and it was not uncommon for "normal" reference intervals to be laboratory specific. Quantitation of the relationship between total or LDL cholesterol concentration and risk for CHD, demonstration of the efficacy of treatment, and development of reference methods and Centers for Disease Control and Prevention (CDC) standardization programs for lipids and lipoproteins[208] made possible the use of risk-related cutoff points (see Tables 27-15 and 27-18). This led to the necessity for uniform definitions of hyperlipidemia based on commonly accepted risk-based lipid and lipoprotein cutoffs and the availability of accurate lipid and lipoprotein measurements.

Consensus Guidelines from Expert Panels

Beginning in the mid-1980s, the NCEP convened expert panels to develop guidelines for diagnosis and treatment of hypercholesterolemia[6,8,11] and for reliable lipid and lipoprotein measurements.[5,9] Two laboratory panels issued recommendations for blood lipids and lipoproteins. The first, the NCEP Laboratory Standardization Panel, focused on measurement of total cholesterol[5]; the second, the NCEP Working Group on Lipoprotein Measurement, addressed measurements of triglycerides, HDL cholesterol, and LDL cholesterol.[9] For more detail, refer to the original reports, both of which include extensive reviews of lipid and lipoprotein methods.[5,9] In 2009 expert recommendations for apo B were published.[62]

Here we summarize the principal considerations and recommendations for clinical lipid and lipoprotein measurements.

Basic Issues

In developing recommendations for lipid and lipoprotein measurement, the NCEP panel considered several basic issues. First, in most of the large-scale clinical and epidemiologic studies that established (1) relationships between lipids and lipoproteins, (2) risk for CHD, and (3) efficacy of cholesterol lowering, measurements were made in standardized laboratories in which the accuracy of measurements was traceable to CDC reference methods. This included studies such as the National Diet Heart Study in the 1960s, various LRC program studies (early 1970s to 1990), Specialized Centers of Research in Atherosclerosis studies (early 1970s to the present), and several NHANES studies conducted between 1960 and 1994.[208]

Second, various methods used in laboratory or nonlaboratory settings should be capable of similar accuracy (i.e., the reliability of the measurements should be independent of how, where, or by whom they were made). Ideally, it should be possible to consider all lipid measurements made in the United States (and eventually globally) as if they had been made in a single laboratory. This premise does *not* require that all laboratories use the same methods; it requires only that all methods be capable of providing values equivalent to those on which the relationships between lipids, lipoproteins, and the risk for CHD were established.

Third, as new methods are developed, particularly those that may be more accurate and precise for various lipoproteins or lipoprotein subfractions, the particular lipoprotein included in the measurement should be specified. This is done to ensure that new methods can be linked to those that were used to establish the known lipoprotein–CHD risk relationships.

To achieve these aims, development of reference methods that could be used as accuracy targets for lipid and lipoprotein measurements was required; also, guidelines for analytical performance were established.

Analytical Challenges

Plasma lipoproteins are heterogeneous and polydisperse macromolecular complexes that vary considerably in size, composition, and function, and consequently present exceptional analytical challenges (see Table 27-4). Traditionally, lipoprotein concentrations have been expressed in terms of their cholesterol content, because methods developed early on for measuring cholesterol and lipoproteins carry virtually all of the cholesterol that circulates in the plasma. This approach simplified the methods used to determine lipoproteins, because the lipoprotein fractions of interest have only to be separated from each other; the other plasma proteins do not have to be removed.

Analytically, cholesterol has a known molecular structure and can be accurately and precisely measured with appropriate chemical or biochemical methods. Triglycerides and the lipoproteins themselves, however, are not unique chemical entities (e.g., triglycerides consist of many possible fatty acyl groups covalently attached to three positions on a glycerol backbone through ester linkages) (see Figure 27-13).

Fatty acyl groups vary in chain length and degree of saturation, leading to a mixture of triglycerides of somewhat different molecular weights. Consequently, triglyceride methods usually measure the glycerol backbone, and triglyceride concentration is then stated only in terms of molar concentration. In the United States, however, lipids have been traditionally expressed in terms of mass concentration (milligrams per deciliter), which is an approximation requiring an assumption about the average molecular weight of the triglyceride mixture. Because palmitate, stearate, and oleate are the major fatty acids in plasma triglycerides and have similar molecular weights, the conversion between molar and mass concentration usually assumes an average triglyceride molecular weight of 885 Da, the molecular weight of tri-oleyl glycerol (olein).

The situation is even more complicated for LDL and HDL. For example, LDL consists of a population of at least seven subparticles varying in size and lipid composition, each containing apo B-100 as the major apolipoprotein component. Thus, LDL has neither a unique molecular weight nor consistent composition of cholesterol or other lipids or proteins. HDL is even more heterogeneous, consisting of at least 12 subclasses, differing in composition, function, and even CHD risk relationships.[25] HDL has been commonly categorized into two major subclasses—HDL_2 and HDL_3—with the larger HDL_2 fraction showing a stronger inverse association with CHD.[266] Because of these characteristics, the exact concentration and composition of a fraction identified as LDL or HDL may vary, depending on how the fraction is isolated. Once isolated, however, the cholesterol content can be measured accurately. A major consideration, therefore, was to define the lipoproteins in a uniform way to afford a common basis for standardization and the assessment of accuracy without inhibiting the development of new methods or necessitating use of the same methods in all laboratories.

Analytical Approach

For more than 50 years, the CDC has maintained reference methods for cholesterol, triglycerides, and HDL cholesterol and has provided standardization programs[208] targeted for the research laboratories. In addition, these reference methods were used to establish the accuracy of lipid and lipoprotein measurements in several population studies, including the LRC prevalence and CPPT studies,[1,2] several NHANES studies conducted by the National Center for Health Statistics since the 1960s,[133] and others. From these studies, cut points for risk characterization in patients were derived. Consequently, and because the standardization programs were already accepted as authoritative by the general laboratory and research communities, the NCEP laboratory panels recommended the CDC reference methods as the basis for defining "accuracy" in the context of recommendations for reliable lipid and lipoprotein measurements.

Use of this approach had several advantages. First, it established the same basis for accuracy that had been used in developing the relationships between lipid and lipoprotein concentration and CHD; second, it provided a reference point by which the accuracy of existing or newly developed methods could be assessed.

Lipids and Lipoproteins

Various technologies have been used to separate and measure plasma lipids and lipoproteins and lipoprotein subfractions, including enzymatic, immunochemical, and chemical precipitation reagents, and physical methods, such as ultracentrifugation, electrophoresis, column chromatography, and others.[10,30] As mentioned earlier, the cholesterol content of any particular lipoprotein class can vary somewhat from individual to individual. Moreover, although different methods of lipoprotein separation may produce similar lipoprotein fractions, they usually do not produce identical fractions, giving rise to systematic biases between methods that purport to measure the same component. The present discussion focuses primarily on accepted reference methods and procedures commonly used in clinical practice for lipid and lipoprotein measurements.

Reference Methods

Reference methods are the "gold standards" or accuracy targets that have been developed for the more common analytes, such as cholesterol, triglycerides, and LDL and HDL cholesterol.[207] The reference method for cholesterol is fully validated and credentialed through the Joint Committee for Traceability in Laboratory Medicine. The other methods, although not formally credentialed, have been accepted by consensus.

Cholesterol

The CDC reference method for cholesterol[64,74,80] is based on a chemical method devised by Abell and associates. In the CDC version of this method,[80] a 0.5-mL aliquot of serum is treated with 5.0 mL of alcoholic KOH (0.36 mol/L) to hydrolyze the cholesteryl esters. Total cholesterol is then extracted from the mixture with 10 mL of hexane for 15 minutes. An aliquot of the extract is dried in vacuo, and the dry residue is treated with 3.2 mL of a mixture of acetic acid, acetic anhydride, and sulfuric acid (Liebermann-Burchard reagent) for color development. After 30 minutes, absorbance is read at 620 nm using pure cholesterol as the calibrator. This method is operated according to a strict protocol requiring replicate measurements in multiple analytical runs. The method exhibits an approximate 1.6% positive bias compared with isotope dilution mass spectrometry, which is considered to be the highest order method for cholesterol and was developed and applied by the National Institute of Standards and Technology.[80] Cholesterol may be expressed in terms of molar (millimoles per liter) or mass (milligrams per deciliter) concentration. Molar concentration is converted to mass concentration using the following equation:

$$\text{mg/dL} = \text{mmol/L} \times 38.7 \quad (1)$$

The CDC reference method, demonstrated to be readily transferable to other laboratories,[64] has been widely adopted by reference laboratories and diagnostic manufacturers as the accuracy target and the basis for calibration in cholesterol measurements.

Triglycerides

In the CDC reference method for triglycerides,[9,207,208] the triglycerides first are extracted quantitatively with chloroform to remove water-soluble interfering substances, such as glucose and glycerol, from the serum. The extract is treated with silicic acid to remove phospholipids, and triglycerides in the extract are subjected to alkaline hydrolysis to produce unesterified fatty acids and glycerol. The glycerol produced is oxidized to produce formaldehyde, which is then reacted with chromotropic acid for color development. Absorbance of chromogen in the reaction mixture is measured at 570 nm:

$$\text{Triglycerides} + \text{KOH} \rightarrow \text{Fatty acids} + \text{Glycerol} \quad (2)$$

$$\text{Glycerol} + \text{Periodate} \rightarrow \text{Formic acid} + \text{Formaldehyde} \quad (3)$$

$$\text{Formaldehyde} + \text{Chromotropic acid} \rightarrow \text{Chromogen} \quad (4)$$

Results may be expressed in terms of molar concentration (millimoles per liter) or mass concentration (milligrams per deciliter). The following equation is used to convert mmol/dL to mg/dL:

$$\text{mg/dL} = \text{mmol/L} \times 88.5 \quad (5)$$

The equation assumes an average molecular weight of 885 g/mol (triolein) for plasma triglycerides. In addition, because of the preliminary extraction and adsorption steps, the CDC reference method measures only the glycerides and does *not* include free glycerol, the so-called triglyceride blank.

To facilitate standardization of triglyceride measurements, a designated comparison method (DCM) has been developed by the Cholesterol Reference Method Laboratory Network (CRMLN), involving similar extraction steps followed by more robust enzymatic quantitation of the triglyceride-derived glycerol.[90] This DCM, established in other reference laboratories, is expected to become the secondary accuracy target for triglycerides.

Because the original reference method of the CDC was complex and not robust, a new reference method for triglyceride based on gas chromatographic isotope dilution mass spectrometry (GC-IDMS) is being developed. In this method, all glycerides (triglycerides, diglycerides, and monoglycerides), as before, are chemically reduced to glycerol, which then is measured by GC-IDMS.

High-Density Lipoprotein Cholesterol

Both a reference method and a designated comparison method have been developed to measure HDL cholesterol.

Reference Method. Because HDL consists of several populations of particles that vary somewhat in their cholesterol content, HDL is commonly defined in terms of the method used to prepare the HDL-containing fraction. The CDC reference method[111,207] uses a combination of ultracentrifugation and polyanion precipitation to prepare the HDL-containing fraction. The cholesterol in this fraction is then quantitated using the CDC reference method for cholesterol. The method is as follows: VLDL and chylomicrons, if present, are first removed by ultracentrifugation of an accurately measured volume of serum for 16.2 hours at 33,700 rpm in a Beckman-type 50.4 rotor. Under these conditions, VLDL and any chylomicrons accumulate as a floating layer at the top of the ultracentrifuge tube (d = 1.006 g/mL). A tube-slicing technique is used to remove the VLDL fraction.[111,207] The infranatant, which contains IDL, LDL, Lp(a), HDL, and the other serum proteins, is recovered quantitatively. The apo B-100–containing lipoproteins in 2 mL of this fraction are precipitated by adding 80 μL of injectable heparin (5000 USP units/mL of 0.15 mol/L NaCl in water) and 100 μL of 1.0 mol/L manganese chloride to water. The precipitate is removed by centrifugation,[111,207] and cholesterol in the clear supernatant is measured. HDL cholesterol may be expressed in molar or mass concentration; molar concentration is converted to mass concentration using equation (1).

Heparin-$MnCl_2$ was selected as the precipitation reagent primarily for historical reasons, because it was the method most commonly used in early studies to establish the relationship between HDL cholesterol concentration and risk for CHD. The ultracentrifugation step was included to prevent interference with sedimentation of the apo B-100–containing lipoproteins by the lighter triglyceride-rich lipoproteins, VLDL, and chylomicrons.

Designated Comparison Method. Only a few laboratories have an ultracentrifuge and the experience required to reliably perform the CDC reference method for HDL cholesterol. Furthermore, ultracentrifugation is expensive and necessitates obtaining an impractically large specimen volume, typically 5.0 mL. As a practical alternative, the CRMLN laboratories developed and validated a modified dextran sulfate (50,000 Da) procedure as a DCM to provide results approximately equivalent to those of the CDC reference method (RM) while avoiding ultracentrifugation.[143] The $MgCl_2$ concentration in the precipitant reagent was decreased slightly from that used in the previously published primary method to increase HDL cholesterol values slightly, achieving closer agreement with the CDC reference method.

Low-Density Lipoprotein Cholesterol

The CDC has also defined a reference method for LDL cholesterol based on the same techniques already described for HDL cholesterol.[207] After ultracentrifugation to remove the VLDL and any chylomicrons present, the bottom fraction (d = 1.006) is subjected to precipitation by heparin and manganese, as described previously. After measurement of cholesterol in the d = 1.006 fraction and in the heparin-Mn^{2+} supernatant solution, LDL cholesterol is calculated by difference. It should be noted that the LDL fraction as measured by this reference method, which is commonly called β-quantification, is a so-called broad-cut fraction, which includes not only LDL but also IDL and Lp(a).

Application of Reference Methods to Standardization

Background

Early efforts in the mid 1980s to achieve general standardization of methods used by clinical laboratories began with a fairly traditional approach with secondary reference materials provided to the laboratory community. The reference materials consisted of lyophilized serum pools with target values assigned on the basis of replicate measurements using the reference methods. However, problems were recognized with this approach, primarily from the confounding effects of matrix changes in the reference materials, making them noncommutable with native clinical samples.[195] Secondary reference materials prepared from pooled serum spiked with artificial analytes, and subjected to freezing and freeze drying, are not always commutable and did not behave like fresh patient specimens with some routine methods. In several notable cases, diagnostic manufacturers used the secondary reference materials to assign presumably reliable targets to their calibrators, but subsequently found that results on patient specimens became inaccurate. The problem was compounded by national proficiency testing programs, which, in an attempt to improve accuracy, began to report reference method target values with similarly prepared survey materials. Laboratories were adjusting calibration to achieve apparent accuracy on the survey materials; however, in some instances, results on actual patient specimens were made inaccurate.

Recognition of these problems focused attention on the issues of "analyte" and "matrix" effects in reference materials.[195] Procedures commonly used in preparing secondary reference materials were inducing changes in the analytes themselves and in the other constituents and fluids surrounding the analytes that made their analyses no longer comparable with measurements in authentic fresh patient specimens. After considerable study and deliberation, the conclusion was reached that the only universally reliable means of transferring accuracy from the reference methods to diagnostic manufacturers and individual laboratories was through direct comparison studies on fresh, representative patient specimens.[338] As a consequence, the CDC and other groups cooperated to organize a network of reference laboratories to provide the reference methods and fresh sample comparison studies.

BOX 27-3 U.S. National Reference Method Laboratory Network Participating Laboratories

Wadsworth Center for Laboratories and Research
New York State Department of Health
Empire State Plaza
Albany, NY 12201
Robert Rej, Ph.D.
clinchem@wadsworth.org
Phone: (518) 474-5101
Fax: (518) 474-9145

Northwest Lipid Research Laboratories
Core Laboratory
2121 N. 35th Street
Seattle, WA 98103
Santica Marcovina, Ph.D.
smm@u.washington.edu
Phone: (206) 685-3331
Fax: (206) 685-3279

The Cholesterol Reference Method Laboratory Network

Because the CDC standardization laboratory maintaining the reference methods did not have the capacity to perform all necessary comparison studies directly, it was obvious that the reference laboratory capability would have to be expanded to accommodate the needs of the industry and the laboratory community. To this end, the CDC and several other interested laboratories cooperated to establish the Cholesterol Reference Method Laboratory Network (CRMLN). Each participating network laboratory underwent stringent protocols to transfer the CDC reference methods and to maintain comparability with the CDC. In turn, the network laboratories performed comparison studies using fresh patient sera with the diagnostic manufacturers and with individual laboratories. Throughout the 1990s, the network was large and active to accommodate the demands of comparison studies. As standardization has steadily improved in subsequent years, the concentration of activity has declined, and the number of domestic U.S. network laboratories has decreased. However, at the same time, the network laboratory program has expanded to include additional international laboratories.

In 2009, the CRMLN included two experienced U.S. laboratories and five international partner laboratories in Canada, Europe, Asia, and South America (Boxes 27-3 and 27-4). The network offers protocols, based on Clinical and Laboratory Standards Institute guidelines, whereby diagnostic manufacturers ensure accuracy by completing comparison studies using the reference methods.[209] A measurement system qualifies for certification by demonstrating agreement within specified limits for total, HDL, and LDL cholesterol and for triglycerides. Based on comparison results, calibrator set points are adjusted if necessary to bring performance into agreement with the reference methods. Diagnostic manufacturers and distributors and instrument partners are encouraged to certify their systems at least every 2 years, and to ensure that every production lot is calibrated to maintain traceability to the accuracy targets; this can be accomplished through ongoing participation in the CDC and/or CRMLN program. The CDC Website (http://www.cdc.gov/labstandards/crmln.html/accessed May 9, 2011) provides details of the program, protocols for comparison studies, contact information for the CDC and/or CRMLN, and a listing of commercial methods that have qualified for certification.

Clinical laboratories can promote standardization by encouraging their reagent suppliers to participate in the CRMLN comparison process. In addition, individual laboratories can make arrangements with a CRMLN laboratory to participate in an abbreviated certification protocol for total cholesterol and to complete comparison studies for the other analytes, especially useful in the case of new or modified systems. The CRMLN program is supported by modest user fees.

BOX 27-4 Cholesterol Reference Method Laboratory Network Participating Laboratories (International)

Erasmus MC
University Medical Center Rotterdam
Lipid Reference Laboratory
3015 GD Rotterdam
The Netherlands
Yolanda B. de Rijke, PhD.
y.derijke@erasmusmc.nl
Phone: 31-10-4636625
Fax: 31-10-4636806

OSAKA Medical Center for Health Science and Promotion
Lipid Reference Laboratory
1-3-2 Nakamichi
Higashinari-ku
Osaka 537-0025 Japan
Masakazu Nakamura, Ph.D.
xnakamura@kenkoukagaku.jp
Phone: 81-6-6973-5582
Fax: 81-6-6973-3574

Canadian External Quality Assessment Laboratory
307-2083 Alma Street
Vancouver
British Columbia V6R 4N6
Canada
David W. Seccombe, M.D., Ph.D.
dseccombe@ceqal.com
Phone: (604) 222-3916
Fax: (604) 222-1373

H.S. Raffaele
Laboratorio Analisi Cliniche
Via Olgettina 60
20132 Milano
Italy
Ferruccio Ceriotti, M.D.
ceriotti.ferruccio@hsr.it
Phone: 39-02-2643-2315 (or 2313)
Fax: 39-02-2643-2640

Fundacíon Bioquímica Argentina
Laboratorio de Referencia y Estandarización en Bioquímica Clínica (LARESBIC)
Calle 6 N 1344
La Plata 1900
Argentina
Daniel Mazziotta, M.D.
dmpeec@netverk.com.ar
Phone: 54-221-4231150
Fax: 54-221-4232021

Beijing Institute of Geriatrics
Beijing Hospital
1 Dahua Road, Post Code 100730
Beijing
P.R. China
Wenxiang Chen, M.D., M.Sc.
chenwenxiang@263.net
Phone: 86-10-6513-0302
Fax: 86-10-6513-2969

Routine Methods

Reference methods are complex, typically time-consuming, and at least partially manual, and require a high degree of expertise for reliable operation. Consequently, simpler and more practical methods have evolved for routine clinical use.

Cholesterol

Enzymatic methods for cholesterol measurement are precise, accurate when calibrated appropriately, and easily adapted for use with modern analyzers. Commercially available cholesterol reagents commonly combine all of the enzymes and other required components into a single photometric reagent. The reagent usually is mixed with a few μL of serum or plasma and incubated under controlled conditions for color development, and absorbance is measured in the visible portion of the spectrum, generally at about 500 nm. The reagents typically use a bacterial cholesteryl ester hydrolase to cleave cholesteryl esters.

$$\text{Cholesteryl ester} + H_2O \xrightarrow{\textit{Cholesteryl ester hydrolase}} \text{Cholesterol} + \text{Fatty acid} \quad \textbf{(6)}$$

The 3-OH group of cholesterol is then oxidized to a ketone in an oxygen-requiring reaction catalyzed by cholesterol oxidase.

$$\text{Cholesterol} + O_2 \xrightarrow{\text{Cholesterol oxidase}} \text{Cholest-4-en-3-one} + H_2O_2 \quad \textbf{(7)}$$

H_2O_2, one of the reaction products, is measured in a peroxidase catalyzed reaction that forms a colored dye:

$$H_2O_2 + \text{Phenol} + \text{4-Aminoantipyrine} \xrightarrow{\text{Peroxidase}} \text{Quinoneimine dye} + 2\,H_2O \quad \textbf{(8)}$$

These methods may be subject to interference from other colored compounds or those that compete with the oxidation reaction or react with peroxide, such as bilirubin, ascorbic acid, and hemoglobin. Assays are usually linear up to about 600 or 700 mg/dL. Reagents have been refined by adding substances such as bilirubin oxidase and dual-wavelength readings to minimize the effects of hemolysis; interference from bilirubin generally is not an issue now in concentrations below 5 mg/dL.[30,74,211] Enzymatic reagents are not entirely specific for cholesterol, because β-hydroxy sterols and plant sterols (e.g., β-sitosterol) can also react. In human serum or plasma, however, this is not a major problem because these interfering sterols are generally present in very low concentrations.

In practice, reagent formulations vary from manufacturer to manufacturer. In most cases, the reagent from a particular manufacturer will have been optimized for use with one or several specific instruments and calibration materials—usually those sold by that manufacturer. Over the past few years, most manufacturers have been supplying calibration materials with assigned values that are traceable to the CDC reference method; this has helped reduce interlaboratory variation. Thus, cholesterol methods are best thought of as "measurement systems" composed of reagent, calibrator (cholesterol standard), and instrument. When a reagent-calibrator-instrument system from a single manufacturer is used, cholesterol measurements within the laboratory usually are accurate within 1 to 3% of reference values, and such systems are routinely operated with coefficients of variation <2.5%. In some cases, however, a reagent from one manufacturer might be used with an instrument from another. In this instance, the responsibility is on the user rather than the manufacturer to ensure that reagent and sample volumes, time and temperature of incubation, and the calibration produce precise and accurate measurements. Although the cholesterol oxidase reagent described previously in this chapter is by far the most common, reagents have been developed using a cholesterol dehydrogenase sequence that may have advantages in some instances.[139] In addition, highly sensitive enzymatic methods have been described for specialized applications.[145] Free or unesterified cholesterol can be readily quantified by deleting the cholesterol esterase from the reagent.

Triglycerides

Triglycerides are commonly measured with enzyme reagents directly in plasma or serum. Reagents combining all required enzymes, cofactors, and buffers are available from various manufacturers; as for cholesterol, such reagents are optimized for use with particular instrument-calibrator systems. Several different enzyme sequences have been used. In all methods, the first step is the lipase-catalyzed hydrolysis of triglycerides to glycerol and fatty acids:

$$\text{Triglyceride} + 3\,H_2O \xrightarrow{\text{Lipase}} \text{Glycerol} + 3\ \text{fatty acids} \quad \textbf{(9)}$$

Glycerol then is phosphorylated in an ATP-requiring reaction catalyzed by glycerokinase:

$$\text{Glycerol} + \text{ATP} \xrightarrow{\text{Glycerokinase}} \text{Glycerophosphate} + \text{Adenosine diphosphate (ADP)} \quad \textbf{(10)}$$

In the most commonly used methods, glycerophosphate is oxidized to dihydroxyacetone and H_2O_2 in a glycerophosphate oxidase–catalyzed reaction,

$$\text{Glycerophosphate} + O_2 \xrightarrow{\text{Glycerophosphate oxidase}} \text{Dihydroxyacetone} + H_2O_2 \quad \textbf{(11)}$$

and the H_2O_2 formed in the reaction is measured as described in reaction (8).

Alternatively, glycerophosphate is measured in a reduced form of nicotinamide-adenine dinucleotide (NADH)-producing reaction, and NADH is measured by a spectrophotometer set at 340 nm or in a diaphorase-catalyzed reaction to form a reaction product whose absorbance is measured at 500 nm:

$$\text{Glycerophosphate} + \text{Nicotinamide-adenine dinucleotide (NAD)} \xrightarrow{\text{Glycerophosphate dehydrogenase}} \text{Dihydroxyacetone phosphate} + \text{NADH} + H^+ \quad \textbf{(12)}$$

$$\text{NADH} + \text{Tetrazolium dye} \xrightarrow{\text{Diaphorase}} \text{Formazan} + \text{NAD}^+ \quad \textbf{(13)}$$

Other methods measure the ADP produced in reaction (10), as shown in equations (14) and (15):

$$\text{ADP} + \text{Phosphoenol pyruvate} \xrightarrow{\text{Pyruvate kinase}} \text{ATP} + \text{Pyruvate} \quad \textbf{(14)}$$

$$\text{Pyruvate} + \text{NADH} + H^+ \xrightarrow{\text{Lactate dehydrogenase}} \text{Lactate} + \text{NAD}^+ \quad \textbf{(15)}$$

Loss of NADH is photometrically measured at 340 nm.

Enzymatic triglyceride methods are fairly specific in that they do not detect glucose or phospholipids. They are linear in the concentration range up to about 700 mg/dL, and when automated they are operated with coefficients of variation up to approximately 3%. The methods are usually calibrated with reference solutions of pure glycerol or with serum-based secondary calibrators. However, because all methods measure the glycerol component, any free glycerol in the sample contributes to the apparent amount of triglyceride. With routine methods, the decision must be made whether to correct for free glycerol by using a method that corrects for the free glycerol blank.

Triglyceride Blanks (Correction for Endogenous Glycerol). Glycerol concentrations in freshly collected serum or plasma in healthy subjects are usually less than 5 to 10 mg/dL. Because this small amount is medically insignificant, the triglyceride blank is usually ignored. Glycerol, however, can be higher in samples with increased triglyceride concentrations and from patients with conditions such as diabetes or those receiving total parenteral nutrition, but even in these conditions, the free glycerol concentration does not generally substantially affect the interpretation of a lipid result. Rarely, glycerol can be markedly increased by 50- to 100-fold in a rare disorder called *hyperglycerolemia,* which is the result of a deficiency in glycerokinase.[186]

Although triglyceride blanks in most cases can be ignored in clinical measurements, they can dramatically affect conclusions about method accuracy.[60] Triglyceride blanking usually requires a separate analysis of glycerol, expressed in terms of equivalent triglyceride concentration, and the measured blank value is subtracted from the total triglyceride measurement.[331] Free glycerol can be measured enzymatically using reactions such as those shown in equations (10) and (11), using a reagent that is identical to the triglyceride reagent but lacking lipase—an approach designated *two-cuvette blanking.* An alternative two-step approach carried out in a single cuvette consumes any free glycerol to produce a colorless product in a preliminary reaction before a lipase enzyme is added to cleave and measure the triglyceride-derived glycerol.

Triglyceride blanking by either of these approaches increases the time and cost of triglyceride analysis.[60] A more common practice, designated *calibration blanking* and used by some manufacturers, involves adjusting calibrator set points to compensate for the average amount of free glycerol in specimens. This is accomplished through a comparison study on actual patient specimens versus the reference method or an accurate equivalent. The calibration blanking approach will underestimate the blank in a few specimens but will give a better and reasonably reliable estimation for most specimens.

Traditionally, triglycerides have been determined on fasting samples obtained from patients after a 10- to 12-hour fast—a practice based on the historical practice in epidemiology studies to achieve a uniform metabolic state. However, patients do not routinely present to physicians' offices in the fasting state, and studies have suggested that triglyceride values measured on nonfasting samples may be more predictive of CHD risk.[225] Postprandial collections are more likely to include remnant lipoproteins that are more atherogenic and reflective of the patient's usual metabolic state. Some national guidelines have been modified to recommend nonfasting collections, and in the future, nonfasting may replace fasting collections. A disadvantage of this approach is that it will preclude the use of calculating LDL-C with the Friedewald equation, because of the presence of chylomicrons and elevated triglycerides.

Phospholipids

Quantitative measurement of phospholipids is rare in routine clinical practice but more common in research (e.g., in studies of dietary influences). The choline-containing phospholipids lecithin, lysolecithin, and sphingomyelin, which account for at least 95% of total phospholipids in serum, are readily measured by an enzymatic reaction sequence using phospholipase D, choline-oxidase, and horseradish peroxidase.[187,310] Kit methods with this enzymatic sequence are available commercially. Before enzymatic reagents became available, the common quantitative method involved extraction and acid digestion with analysis of the total lipid-bound phosphorus.[34]

High-Density Lipoprotein Cholesterol

Under current recommendations for characterizing the cardiovascular disease risk in patients, measurement of the two major cholesterol-carrying lipoproteins, HDL and LDL, is most important. Characterization of the β-VLDL characteristic of the uncommon type III or dysbetalipoproteinemia may be appropriate in a few patients. Measurement of lipoprotein subclasses including IDL or remnant lipoproteins is useful in research and can be helpful in some cases in managing patients.

HDL is classically defined in terms of its density range (1.063 to 1.21g/mL) obtained by ultracentrifugation, which has been used as the standard by which the accuracy of other HDL methods is judged. However, the density range of Lp(a) (1.04 to 1.08 g/mL) overlaps that of HDL (see Table 27-4), so in patients with high Lp(a) concentrations, ultracentrifugation at 1.063 g/mL would overestimate the true HDL concentration. As a consequence, the CDC reference method, described previously, uses precipitation to separate HDL, similar to the approach used for many research determinations.[337] Most routine laboratories now use the newer direct or homogeneous assays, which became available beginning in the early 1990s. The homogeneous assays have advantages in terms of efficiency and convenience, because they are capable of full automation. However, homogeneous assays have been shown to lack specificity, especially on specimens from patients with unusual lipoprotein distributions, and hence cannot be recommended for such patients or for research investigations. Because pretreatment precipitation methods were the standard for decades and preceded the currently more common homogeneous assays, these methods will be reviewed first.

Precipitation Methods. In earlier years, HDL cholesterol was most commonly measured (Box 27-5) in supernatant solutions after precipitation of the apo B-100–containing lipoproteins [VLDL, IDL, Lp(a), LDL, and, when present, chylomicrons] directly from plasma or serum using agents such as polyanions in the presence of divalent cations.[111] As indicated earlier, LDL and HDL are the largest contributors to total cholesterol in healthy people, with LDL accounting for about two thirds and HDL for about one third of the total cholesterol. On average, IDL and Lp(a) each account for only about 2 to 3 mg/dL of the total cholesterol, although their concentrations can be considerably higher in some individuals.

Polyanions bridge positively charged groups on lipoproteins; their action is facilitated in the presence of divalent cations, which interact with negatively charged groups, causing aggregation and a cloudy precipitate. Precipitation is usually complete within 10 to 15 minutes at room temperature; at 2 to 4 °C, a 30-minute incubation period is preferred.

BOX 27-5 Methods for HDL Separation/Quantification

Precipitation (First Generation)
- Heparin-Mn^{2+}
  - 0.46 mmol/L (LRC method)
  - 0.92 mmol/L (recommended for EDTA plasma)
- Dextran sulfate (50 kDa) Mg^{2+} (AACC Selected Method and DCM)
- Phosphotungstate-Mg^{2+}

Facilitated Separation (Second Generation)
- Magnetic with/dextran sulfate-Mg^{2+}

Homogeneous (Third Generation)
- Antibody four-reagent method (International Reagents Corp.)
- Polyethylene glycol modified enzymes w/cyclodextrin (Kyowa Medex)
- Synthetic polymer/detergent (Daiichi)
- Antibodies (Wako)
- Catalase (Denka Seiken)

The precipitate is then sedimented by centrifugation, typically for 45,000 g-min (i.e., the equivalent of 1500 × g for 30 minutes). Centrifugation at higher g-forces (e.g., 10,000 × g) accelerates sedimentation and can actually improve complete precipitation of apo B–containing particles. HDL cholesterol is then measured in the clear supernatant.

Of several polyanion-divalent cation combinations, heparan sulfate with $MnCl_2$ was adopted early on and became common in research laboratories and eventually used in the CDC reference method. With the transition to enzymatic cholesterol assays, residual Mn^{2+} was found to interfere, giving artifactually high results. Techniques were devised to reduce this interference, but additional manipulations were required, making them inconvenient for routine use [e.g., the chelator ethylenediaminetetraacetic acid (EDTA) added to the cholesterol reagent to complex residual manganite],[301] or carbonate was added in a second precipitation step to precipitate excess Mn^{2+}.[32] Most laboratories avoided these tedious approaches, rather adopting alternative precipitants such as dextran sulfate or phosphotungstate with Mg^{2+}.[333] A method that used dextran sulfate with molecular weight of 50 kDa was validated as a selected method; during the 1980s, dextran sulfate became the most common precipitation reagent.

The precipitability of lipoproteins with polyanions and divalent cations depends on the lipid and protein compositions of the particles.[47] Thus, various precipitants differ in precipitating apo B-100–containing lipoprotein completely while leaving most species of HDL in solution,[9,30] resulting in potential biases between reagents. With modern reagent-instrument-calibrator systems, conditions generally are optimized to produce values that closely approximate and are traceable to reference method values. Also, the precipitation methods can be inaccurate under certain conditions (e.g., precipitation of apo B-100–containing lipoprotein can be incomplete in samples with high concentrations of triglyceride-rich lipoproteins). Any residual turbidity in the supernate indicates inadequate sedimentation of the apo B-100–containing lipoprotein, resulting in overestimation of HDL cholesterol. Samples with high triglyceride concentrations (generally those above 400 mg/dL) frequently produce turbid supernatants because the triglycerides can reduce the density of the lipoprotein-precipitating reagent complex to the point that some of the complex remains unsedimented. In cases of extremely high triglyceride concentrations, some of the precipitate may even form a floating layer over a clear or turbid supernatant, in addition to the usual precipitate at the bottom of the centrifuge tube.

Such supernates require additional treatment by one of several techniques. Before precipitation, the sample can be ultracentrifuged and the triglyceride-rich lipoproteins removed as described previously for the reference method. Alternatively, a turbid supernatant sometimes can be cleared by centrifuging for a longer time or at higher g-forces.[332] Or more commonly, the sample can be diluted twofold with saline to reduce the concentration of triglyceride-rich lipoproteins before the precipitant is added. A fourth approach is to pass the turbid supernatant through a 0.45-μm filter to remove the unsedimented precipitate before cholesterol in the filtrate is measured.[332]

HDL cholesterol determination can also be affected by sample matrix effects, which arise from (1) the unusual nature of the sample itself, (2) processing effects, or (3) the addition of anticoagulants or preservatives.[195] For example, HDL cholesterol measurements can be inaccurate and usually are more variable when obtained from lyophilized samples than from fresh or frozen sera.

Additives including anticoagulants, such as citrate and fluoride, can have large osmotic effects that cause water to shift from the cells to the plasma. This dilutes the lipoprotein by 10% or more and produces erroneously low values. EDTA, earlier the preferred anticoagulant for lipoprotein measurements, causes a slight dilution, but has been used because it also inhibits certain oxidative and other changes that can affect some lipoprotein or apolipoprotein measurements. Lipid and lipoprotein concentrations in EDTA plasma tend to be about 3% lower than in serum—an effect that may not be readily noticeable in HDL cholesterol measurements. EDTA, however, complexes some of the Mn^{2+} in the heparin-Mn^{2+} method, and it has been found necessary to use a higher concentration of $MnCl_2$ (0.092 mol/L, final concentration in the reaction system) when the procedure is used with EDTA plasma than with serum (0.046 mol/L).[28,332] Heparin, by virtue of its high molecular weight, and when present in concentrations used for anticoagulation, has no measurable effect on lipid or lipoprotein concentration, and it does not affect HDL cholesterol measurements. A variation of the precipitation method, involving the use of magnetic beads complexed with dextran sulfate, helped reduced interference from high triglyceride samples,[114,216] but it is no longer commercially available.

Homogeneous Assays. A major breakthrough in HDL determination was reported in 1994,[136] with publication of the first of a series of so-called homogeneous methods for lipoproteins (see Box 27-5). Compared with earlier precipitation methods requiring manual pretreatment steps, homogeneous methods were much better suited for the automated systems used in the modern clinical laboratory. Elimination of manual pretreatment was timely, as laboratories were under pressure to reduce operating costs. The fully automated homogeneous methods also improved precision through more consistent pipetting of smaller specimen volumes and precise temperature control and reaction timing, which facilitated achieving the NCEP analytical performance goals.

The first homogeneous assay for HDL cholesterol required four successive reagent additions (International Reagents Corp., Kobe, Japan). The first reagent contained polyethylene glycol, resulting in aggregation of the apo B-100–containing chylomicrons, VLDL, and LDL. The second reagent protected or blocked the aggregated lipoproteins with antibodies to apo B-100 and apo C. The cholesterol reaction enzymes (cholesterol esterase, cholesterol oxidase, and peroxidase) were added in the third reagent, which acted only on the unprotected HDL cholesterol. The fourth reagent stopped the color reaction and solubilized the aggregates with guanidine salts, clearing the reaction mixture for measurement of color. This breakthrough method, even though not suited for all analyzers because of the multiple reagent additions, was capable of full automation, paving the way for subsequent, two-reagent homogeneous methods.

In 1995, a second homogeneous method became available (Kyowa Medex Co., Tokyo, Japan[308]; Roche Diagnostics, Indianapolis, Ind) that used sulfated α-cyclodextrins together with Mg^{2+} to selectively block but not precipitate chylomicrons and VLDL, providing selectivity without the necessity for precipitation. Second, covalently linked polyethylene glycol molecules enhanced the specificities of the enzymes cholesterol esterase and cholesterol oxidase toward the cholesterol in HDL. Polyethylene glycol having an MW of 6000 Da was thought to optimize the specificities at concentrations lower than those used previously to precipitate lipoproteins, implying that modified enzymes were able to distinguish lipoprotein classes on the basis of their size and/or charge. The result was a fully automated homogeneous assay with only two reagent additions applicable for general use. The original kit included the second enzyme-containing reagent in lyophilized form, necessitating reconstitution, but a modification introduced in mid 1998 included both reagents in liquid form.[111] A third modification decreased the Mg^{2+} concentration, apparently to reduce carryover in pipetting.

A synthetic polymer together with a polyanion to block the non-HDL lipoproteins was used in a third homogeneous assay (Daiichi Pure Chemicals Co., Tokyo/Genzyme Corp., Cambridge, Mass).[115,169,216] A detergent was added that exposes only cholesterol in HDL to the enzymes, giving specificity for HDL-C. This method required two reagent additions: the first with the polyanion and polymer-blocking agents, and the second with detergent, enzymes, and substrates. A subsequent modification provided both reagents in liquid form with other changes to improve specificity and decrease potential interference.[112,151,345] A third modification without Mg^{2+} has been reported.[73,130]

A fourth early homogeneous assay was based on immunoinhibition and included two reagents (Wako Pure Chemicals Industry, Osaka, Japan).[163,188,229] The first reagent contained an antibody to human apo B-100 that reacted with apo B-100–containing lipoproteins, chylomicrons, VLDL, and LDL, blocking their reaction to enzymes added in the second reagent. The current formulation included both reagents in liquid form.

A fifth homogeneous method (Denka Seiken Co., Niigata, Japan/Polymedco Inc., Cortlandt Manor, NY/Randox Laboratories Limited, Crumlin, UK) allowed cholesterol esterase and oxidase to react with lipoproteins other than HDL, generating peroxidase, which in turn was scavenged by the enzyme catalase.[215,229] An inhibitor of catalase and a surfactant in a second reagent specifically reacted with HDL cholesterol, producing color through the usual peroxidase sequence.

In subsequent years, the various homogeneous reagents have undergone many additional modifications in attempts to improve their convenience and specificity. Currently, at least seven separate reagent formulations are available.

At least one instrument application for each of the homogeneous assays discussed previously in this chapter has qualified for certification by the CRMLN, implying at least the capability to achieve agreement with the reference method. However, conditions and especially calibration may be different on various instrument applications, and many have not been evaluated. Thus certification for the reagents cannot be considered universally applicable to all distributor versions, instrument applications, and lots. Similarly, published evaluation studies have confirmed that methods can be accurate but may not be so in every commercial application.[208] Laboratories choosing to adopt homogeneous assay applications that have not been certified by the CRMLN are encouraged to confirm that their particular systems are accurate. In addition, an evaluation of all current homogeneous HDL-C and LDL-C assays revealed that many of these assays lack ruggedness because of lack of lipoprotein specificity, especially on specimens with unusual lipoprotein composition.[196]

Specificity and Interference. The accuracy of measuring HDL cholesterol in each individual specimen is a function not only of mean bias or overall inaccuracy of a method related to calibration, but also its specificity for HDL cholesterol and absence of interference by other lipoproteins and constituents of the specimen matrix. CRMLN certification studies and many published evaluation studies undertaken to assess accuracy included only samples from relatively normal subjects. Most studies did not determine performance in samples from patients with extreme hyperlipidemias, such as type III or other conditions such as liver and kidney disease, which often result in unusual lipoproteins with atypical separation characteristics. Only a few studies have included such extreme specimens and have raised questions about the specificity of the homogeneous reagents.* Most studies of interference have used fairly traditional spiking designs; they have been relatively modest in scope and have not properly addressed abnormal lipoprotein composition.[22,114,127,151,215] Hemoglobin below 2 g/L and bilirubin less than 10 mg/dL do not interfere appreciably with any of the homogeneous methods.

Considerations in Choosing a High-Density Lipoprotein Method. Laboratories have had to consider the alternatives in deciding whether to replace a conventional pretreatment method with a homogeneous reagent: improved efficiency on the one hand versus occasional discrepant results on the other. Routine clinical laboratories tend to choose the fully automated methods, often because of unavoidable pressures to improve efficiency. Laboratories performing research and supporting lipid clinics, on the other hand, often choose to retain a conventional precipitation method. An important factor in the latter choice is that a laboratory supporting long-term studies cannot tolerate potential changes and shifts in results that may have occurred because of frequent modifications to the homogeneous reagents.

*References 100, 124, 152, 196, 295, 334, and 342.

BOX 27-6 Methods for LDL Separation/Quantification

β-Quantification
- Ultracentrifugation at density 1.006 kg/L to float and remove VLDL and any chylos
- Measurement of total cholesterol in bottom fraction (LDL-C + HDL-C)
- Precipitation of bottom fraction with heparin/Mn^{2+} to remove LDL
- Measurement of total cholesterol in supernatant, which equals HLD-C
- LDL is calculated by subtracting HDL-C from total cholesterol in bottom fraction; most commonly used by specialty lipid laboratories

Calculation Using Friedewald Formula
- (LDL chol) = (Total chol) − (HDL chol) − (Triglyceride)/5
- Originally proposed for epidemiology studies
- Became the most common method in routine clinical laboratories

Homogeneous Reagents
- LDL solubilization (Kyowa Medex)
- LDL protected/deprotected by surfactants (Daiichi)
- LDL protected/catalase (Wako)
- Non-HDL catalase/LDL azide (Denka Seiken)
- LDL protected by calixarene/cholesterol dehydrogenase (International Reagents Corp.)

Low-Density Lipoprotein Cholesterol

Methods for LDL cholesterol generally quantitate a so-called broad-cut fraction, including not only the primary LDL species in the 1.019 to 1.063 kg/L density range, but also IDL, density 1.006 to 1.019 kg/L, and Lp(a).[218] Therefore, the usual convention for total cholesterol on a fasting sample without cholesterol is based on the following formula:

$$\text{Total cholesterol (chol)} = \text{VLDL chol} + \text{LDL chol} + \text{HDL chol} \quad \textbf{(16)}$$

LDL cholesterol can be measured using both indirect and direct methods, and either approach has been used in major studies that established the relationship between LDL cholesterol concentration and risk for CHD.

Indirect Methods. Indirect methods for measuring LDL cholesterol are based on measuring a number of lipid-related analytes followed by their use in calculating the LDL cholesterol content of a specimen. This includes use of the Friedewald equation and the β-quantification method.

The Friedewald Equation. In the most widely used indirect method (Box 27-6), cholesterol, triglyceride, and HDL cholesterol are measured and LDL cholesterol is calculated from primary measurements using the empirical equation of Friedewald and colleagues[93]:

$$\text{(LDL chol)} = \text{(Total chol)} - \text{(HDL chol)} - \text{(Triglyceride)}/5 \quad \textbf{(17)}$$

where all concentrations are given in mg/dL (triglyceride/2.22 is used when units are expressed in mmol/L). The factor (triglyceride)/5 is an estimate of VLDL cholesterol concentration that is based on the average ratio of triglyceride to cholesterol in VLDL.

Several investigators have evaluated the accuracy of LDL cholesterol estimated by equation (17). For example, DeLong and colleagues recommended use of the expression 0.16 × (triglyceride) as a better estimate of VLDL cholesterol; consequently, the factor (triglyceride)/6 is used in few laboratories.[75] Other factors have been suggested for particular populations,[9] but no single factor has been accurate under all circumstances. However, when the original factor (triglyceride)/5 was compared with a combined ultracentrifugation polyanion precipitation method in about 5000 samples, errors in LDL cholesterol estimated by equation (17) were found to be symmetrically distributed about zero.[334] On balance, the NCEP recommended use of the original factor (triglyceride/5) for estimating LDL cholesterol with equation (17).[9]

In practice, the Friedewald calculation is reasonably accurate, but under several well-known circumstances, the Friedewald equation cannot be used. First, calculation is precluded in samples that have triglyceride concentrations above 400 mg/dL or in those that contain increased quantities of chylomicrons (nonfasting specimens). At high triglyceride concentrations, the factor (triglyceride)/5 as an estimate of VLDL cholesterol concentration is not appropriate, because such samples can also contain chylomicrons, chylomicron remnants, or VLDL remnants, all of which have higher triglyceride/cholesterol ratios and can contribute to errors in estimation. Under these circumstances, use of the factor (triglyceride)/5 would overestimate VLDL cholesterol and therefore underestimate LDL cholesterol. The Friedewald equation has been found to be most accurate in samples with triglyceride concentrations below 200 mg/dL,[334] but the error becomes unacceptably large (i.e., >10%) at triglyceride concentrations greater than 400 mg/dL.

The opposite error can occur if the Friedewald equation is used in patients with type III hyperlipoproteinemia. Type III hyperlipoproteinemia is characterized in part by the presence of β-VLDL not normally present in the blood. Biochemically, as its name implies, β-VLDL occurs in the VLDL density range but has β mobility on electrophoresis and is much richer in cholesterol than the usual VLDL, with a ratio of triglyceride to cholesterol on the order of 3 : 1. Application of the factor (triglyceride)/5 in patients with type III hyperlipidemia would underestimate VLDL cholesterol and in turn would overestimate LDL cholesterol. Thus a patient with type III hyperlipoproteinemia may appear to have an artifactually high LDL cholesterol concentration.

Fortunately, both of these conditions are uncommon. The 95th percentile for fasting plasma triglycerides in the United States is below 300 mg/dL, indicating that only a small percentage of specimens will exceed the 400-mg/dL cutoff. Plasma from fasting subjects does not normally contain chylomicrons; even if present, chylomicrons can be observed visually as a floating "cream" layer in samples that have been

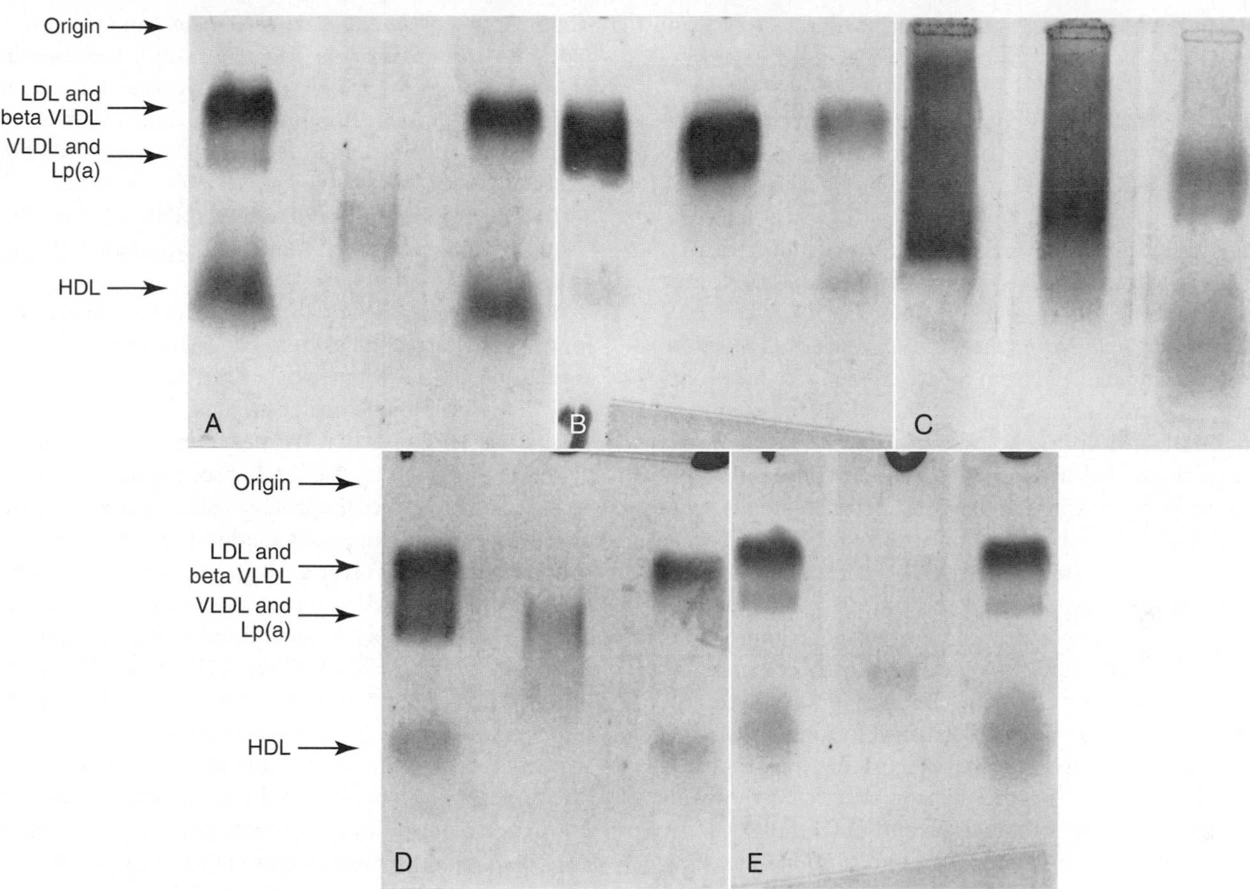

Figure 27-26 Agarose gel electrophoresis of plasma lipoprotein. In each photograph, the samples were applied in the following order, reading from left to right: unfractionated plasma, ultracentrifugal density 1.006 g/mL supernatant solution, ultracentrifugal infranatant solution. A, Pattern seen in normal samples and samples with high LDL cholesterol concentrations. B, Type III hyperlipoproteinemia pattern. C, Severe hypertriglyceridemia, triglyceride = 3840 mg/dL. Note chylomicrons at origin. D, Pattern observed in samples with moderately elevated triglyceride, triglyceride = 281 mg/dL, LDL cholesterol = 145 mg/dL. Note absence of chylomicrons. E, Pattern observed in patients with high concentrations of Lp(a). Note presence of Lp(a) in infranatant solution. This sample had an Lp(a) concentration of 77 mg/dL. *LDL,* Low-density lipoprotein; *Lp(a),* lipoprotein(a); *HDL,* high-density lipoprotein; *VLDL,* very low-density lipoprotein.

allowed to stand undisturbed at 4 °C overnight. Finally, the prevalence of type III hyperlipoproteinemia in the general population is only about 1 to 2 per 1000 persons.[161] On the other hand, as treatments for hyperlipidemia become more effective and more common, patients with very low triglyceride concentrations are encountered. In this instance, the calculation may be distorted and LDL cholesterol overestimated.[283] Nevertheless, because of the ease of the calculation and its reasonable accuracy, calculation of LDL-C has persisted as the most common approach to determining LDL cholesterol in patient management.

β-Quantification (Ultracentrifugation-Polyanion Precipitation). This method is the precursor to the reference methods developed for HDL and LDL and may be used in samples for which the Friedewald equation is unreliable. β-quantification follows the procedure adopted from the NIH Laboratory that was used in the LRC Program, combining preparative ultracentrifugation and polyanion precipitation.[111] An accurately measured aliquot of plasma at native density of 1.006 g/mL is first ultracentrifuged at 105,000 × g for 18 hours at 10 °C. VLDL and, if present, chylomicrons and/or β-VLDL float over the infranatant containing primarily LDL and HDL (Figure 27-26) plus any IDL and Lp(a) that may be present. The floating layer, removed with the aid of a tube slicer, is sometimes analyzed as a check on recovery and may be saved for electrophoretic analysis to determine the presence of β-VLDL. The infranatant solution is remixed and reconstituted to known volume, and its cholesterol content measured. HDL cholesterol is usually measured in a separate aliquot of plasma, but when necessary, an aliquot of the d 1.006 g/mL infranatant can be treated to remove the apo B-100–containing lipoproteins [IDL, LDL, and Lp(a)]; HDL cholesterol is then measured in the clear supernatant. VLDL and LDL cholesterol are calculated as follows:

$$(\text{VLDL chol}) = (\text{Total chol}) - (d > 1.006 \text{ g/mL chol}) \quad (18)$$

$$(\text{LDL chol}) = (d > 1.006 \text{ g/mL chol}) - (\text{HDL chol}) \quad (19)$$

LDL cholesterol measured in this way is unaffected by the presence of chylomicrons or other triglyceride-rich lipoproteins, or by β-VLDL. VLDL cholesterol is usually calculated from equation (18) rather than measured directly in the ultracentrifugal supernatant, because it can be difficult to recover this fraction quantitatively, particularly when triglyceride concentrations are high.

Lipoproteins Included in the "LDL Cholesterol" Measurement. In this context, the term *LDL cholesterol* includes cholesterol in IDL and Lp(a) fractions, as well as the core LDL. Although IDL and Lp(a) cholesterol usually contribute only a few mg/dL to the "total LDL cholesterol" measurement, their contributions can be significant in patients with increased high IDL or Lp(a) concentrations. For example, assuming that cholesterol (i.e., sterol nucleus) constitutes about 30% of the mass of Lp(a), it can be calculated that the Lp(a) cholesterol concentration would contribute about 12 mg/dL, or about 12%, to the LDL cholesterol measurement in a patient with an Lp(a) concentration of 40 mg/dL and an apparent LDL cholesterol concentration of 100 mg/dL. It has been suggested that a more specific measure of LDL cholesterol could be obtained by correcting the measured LDL cholesterol value for the contribution of Lp(a) cholesterol,[134,276] and a similar argument might be made for IDL. However, both IDL and Lp(a) contribute to increased risk for CHD [see later section on Lp(a)]; therefore, although such correction will increase the specificity of methods for LDL cholesterol, per se, it might also give LDL cholesterol values that underestimate cardiovascular risk. Moreover, this might occur more frequently with patients with CHD or those who are at risk for CHD based on their "LDL cholesterol" concentrations. Consequently, the NCEP Working Group on LDL Cholesterol Measurement suggested that LDL cholesterol values should *not* be corrected for the contribution of other atherogenic lipoproteins; this group also recommended that further research should be conducted to establish the individual contributions of IDL, Lp(a), and LDL cholesterol to CHD risk, as reflected in current LDL cholesterol measurements that include all three lipoprotein classes. NCEP guidelines published in 2001 expand on this concept by introducing the term *non-HDL cholesterol,* which includes all of the apo B–containing atherogenic lipoproteins, including not only Lp(a) and IDL, but also VLDL cholesterol, remnant lipoproteins, and chylomicrons for nonfasting samples.[11]

Diagnosis of the Type III Lipoprotein Pattern. The ratio of VLDL cholesterol to plasma triglyceride, expressed in terms of mass, is 0.2 or lower in normal samples and in those from patients with lipoprotein disorders other than type III hyperlipidemia or dysbetalipoproteinemia. In type III hyperlipoproteinemia, the ratio is 0.3 or higher because of the presence of β-VLDL; the elevated ratio can persist even after treatment. In addition, β-VLDL can be observed directly by subjecting the VLDL fraction to agarose gel electrophoresis, where it migrates electrophoretically with LDL rather than VLDL (see Figure 27-26). The combination of a VLDL cholesterol/plasma triglyceride ratio of 0.3 or higher and the observation of β-VLDL in the ultracentrifugal supernatant is considered diagnostic of the type III lipoprotein pattern.

Direct Methods. Selective precipitation and homogeneous immunoassay methods have been used to measure LDL cholesterol directly.

Selective Precipitation. Several direct methods reported for LDL cholesterol measurement are based on selective precipitation with polyvinyl sulfate or heparin at low pH.[132,171,204] LDL cholesterol is then calculated as the difference between total cholesterol and that in the supernatant, or in another variation, directly in the LDL precipitate. It is not clear whether atherogenic lipoproteins other than LDL itself are also detected; these methods might be expected to be subject to similar sources of error as those encountered with precipitation methods for HDL separation. A more specific method used a mixture of polyclonal antibodies to apo A-I and apo E linked to a resin to bind VLDL, IDL, and HDL, with LDL cholesterol measured in a filtrate by the usual methods. This method was reasonably precise and was in good agreement with ultracentrifugation-polyanion precipitation.[116,132,190,239] The reagent was in commercial distribution for several years, but because it required a separate pretreatment step, it was eventually superseded by a new class of direct homogeneous reagents patterned after the homogeneous reagents for HDL cholesterol.

Homogeneous Assays. Following approaches similar to those used with homogeneous methods for HDL cholesterol,[337] homogeneous assays have been developed to measure LDL cholesterol. For example, at least seven homogeneous LDL methods are commercially available (see Box 27-6), which differ by containing different detergents and other chemicals, allowing specific blocking or solubilization of lipoprotein classes to achieve specificity for LDL cholesterol. Most suppliers offer kits with two reagents; these are readily adaptable to most clinical chemistry analyzers.

Sugiuchi and colleagues developed the first homogeneous method for measuring LDL cholesterol[307]—a reagent distributed by Kyowa Medex, Tokyo and Roche Diagnostics, Indianapolis. With this method, LDL was directly measured by suppressing the other lipoproteins (other methods suppressed LDL first and reacted with other lipoproteins before determining LDL cholesterol). The method was formulated in two reagents. The first had $MgCl_2$, dye, buffer (pH 6.75), and α-cyclodextrin sulfate,[308] which has a highly concentrated negative charge to mask cholesterol in chylomicrons and VLDL in the presence of magnesium ions.[307] The second reagent included the enzymes cholesterol oxidase and cholesterol esterase, peroxidase, dye, buffer (pH 6.75), and a polyoxyethylene-polyoxypropylene polyether (POE-POP) to block cholesterol, especially in HDL.[307,308] The molecular mass of POP in the POE-POP molecule and the hydrophobicity index determine selectivity to LDL; 3850 Da was demonstrated to be optimum.[308]

TABLE 27-23 Analytical Performance of Homogeneous LDL-C Assays

			Recovery, %			Accuracy	
	Imprecision, CVs	Dynamic Range, mg/L	LDL	VLDL	IDL	Bias, %	Bias, mg/L
Kyowa	0.7-3.1	2-4100	97-105	16	52-64	0.8-11.2	−60 to −80
Daiichi	<3.1	4-10,000	87	19	31-47	3.9-5.1	−48 to −80
Wako	≤1.2	10-3000	—	—	—	0.4	−15
Denka	<1.8	70-5500	95	10	31	—	—
IRC	≤0.6	?-4000	—	—	—	—	—

A second method by Sekisuie Medical Co. (Tokyo, Japan; formerly Daiichi Pure Chemicals) was also a two-reagent system. The first reagent contained ascorbic acid oxidase, 4-aminoantipyrine, peroxidase, cholesterol oxidase, cholesterol esterase, buffer (pH 6.3), and a detergent, which solubilized all non-LDL lipoproteins, allowing reaction of their cholesterol with the esterase and oxidase enzymes, forming a colorless product. The second reagent contained N,N′-bis-(4-sulfobutyl)-m-toluidine Na_2 (DSBmT), buffer (pH 6.3), and a detergent to specifically release LDL cholesterol. The resulting hydrogen peroxide reacted with N,N′-bis-(4-sulfobutyl)-M-toluidine disodium salt to generate a colored product.

A third method (Wako Pure Chemicals) included a reagent with (1) Good's buffer (pH 6.8), [N-(2-hydroxy-3-sulfopropyl)-3,5-dimethoxyaniline, sodium salt], (2) cholesterol esterase, (3) cholesterol oxidase, (4) catalase, (5) polyanions, and (6) amphoteric surfactants, the latter selectively protecting LDL from enzymatic reaction. The non-LDL cholesterol reacted with esterase and oxidase, producing hydrogen peroxide, which was consumed by catalase. The second reagent included Good's buffer (pH 7.0), 4-aminoantipyrene, peroxidase, sodium azide, and a deprotecting reagent, which removed the protecting agent from LDL, enabling the specific reaction of cholesterol esterase and cholesterol oxidase with its cholesterol, producing hydrogen peroxide and a blue color complex.[85,193]

Non-LDL cholesterol was removed by a fourth method (Denka Seiken, Niigata, Japan/Polymedco Inc., Cortlandt Manor, NY) via a selective reaction with cholesterol oxidase and cholesterol esterase, with the resulting peroxide byproduct eliminated by reaction with catalase (CAT). In this two-reagent method, the first reagent contained $MgCl_2$, cholesterol esterase, cholesterol oxidase, catalase, N-(2-hydroxy-3-sulfopropyl)-3,5-dimethoxyaniline sodium salt, and Emulgen 66 (polyoxyethylene compound; Kao) and Emulgen 90 (both nonionic surfactants) in Good's buffer (PIPES; 100 mmol/L; pH 7.0). Its second reagent contained peroxidase, 4-aminoantipyrine, sodium azide (to inhibit the catalase), and Triton X-100 in Good's buffer. The hydrophilic/lipophilic balance of the detergents was chosen to obtain appropriate selectivity to the lipoproteins.[228]

In a fifth method (International Reagents Corp., Kokusai-Kobe, Japan), its first reagent contained the detergent calixarene, which converts LDL to a soluble complex. Cholesterol esters of HDL-C and VLDL-C were preferentially hydrolyzed by a cholesterol esterase (chromobacterium), cholesterol oxidase, and hydrazine, which divert the accessible cholesterol to cholestenone hydrazone. A second reagent with deoxycholate broke up the LDL-calixarene complex, allowing LDL-C to react with the esterase, a dehydrogenase, and β-NAD to yield cholestenone and β-NADH.

Analytical Performance of LDL Methods. Evaluations of LDL homogeneous assays indicate that CVs are generally <3% and consistently within the NCEP performance target of <4% CV (Table 27-23).[200] By contrast, CVs for the Friedewald calculation have been estimated to approximate 4% in expert laboratories but may be higher in routine clinical laboratories.[218]

With regard to accuracy, all of the homogeneous assays have qualified for certification through the CRMLN program, suggesting agreement with reference methods, at least in relatively normal specimens. Nevertheless, as indicated previously for HDL cholesterol methods, many instrument applications are available, and not all have been evaluated for bias. Factors such as lot-to-lot differences, unique calibrations by distributors, different calibrations from country to country, and reformulations of reagents might affect actual biases.[337] In a 2002 study, four homogeneous assays were compared with the LDL RM; unacceptable total error was found, and the authors recommended caution in adopting the methods.[197] A 2010 study of all current homogenous assays for LDL-C found that these assays work relatively on normolipidemic samples but found frequent discordant results compared with the reference β-quantification procedure for patients with dyslipidemias.[196] Overall, these studies suggest that homogeneous assays interact unequally with different components of the "broad-cut LDL": LDL subclasses, IDL, Lp(a), and Lp-X.* A 2002 study of two homogenous reagents using isolated lipoprotein fractions confirmed the lack of specificity for VLDL and LDL subclasses.[320] The two homogeneous methods included about 20% of isolated VLDL. Also the reagents missed about 30% of IDL and up to 50% of isolated LDL fractions, especially the important smaller and more atherogenic subclasses. Through compensating errors, the inclusion of some VLDL could offset the loss of LDL fractions, so the overall lack of specificity may not be obvious in relatively normal specimens. However, lack of specificity for lipoprotein subclasses and differences among reagents can cause substantial errors in some specimens, depending on the particular lipoprotein profile and the particular reagent characteristics.[196]

*To convert mg/dL of cholesterol to mmol/L, multiply by 0.0259.

Spiking studies, in which potential interfering substances are added to a sample, have demonstrated that these methods are not subject to significant interference from bilirubin and hemoglobin. However, higher concentrations of triglycerides have been shown to interfere, thus increasing apparent LDL cholesterol values; this is not surprising given the reported lack of specificity for LDL and the inclusion of some VLDL in the measurement.[126,214,228] On the other hand, the sulfated α-cyclodextrin used in the Sugiuchi assay to block VLDL cholesterol appeared to cause underestimation of LDL cholesterol.[85,217,307]

A major potential advantage of homogeneous methods over the Friedewald calculation is the ability to use nonfasting specimens, which are convenient in managing patients. Results, judged by mean differences between paired fasting and nonfasting specimens, were promising, but patient classifications were poorer with nonfasting specimens.[217,228,347] Lipoprotein composition is affected by recent diet; changes have been observed even with the more robust ultracentrifugation method. However, the changes in vivo are small, and the convenience of being able to use nonfasting specimens may offset minor effects on accuracy. A recent prospective analysis suggested that LDL cholesterol may not be predictive of CHD risk in nonfasting specimens[201]; more comprehensive studies will be needed to address this question.

Other Considerations in Adopting a Homogeneous LDL Method. Clinical laboratories are faced with the decision whether to implement fully automated homogeneous methods for LDL cholesterol, either replacing or supplementing the traditional Friedewald calculation. The considerations are certainly not as compelling for homogeneous LDL methods as for HDL. Even given the technical disadvantages of the Friedewald method, that is, (1) the necessity for fasting, (2) poor precision from cumulative variations in the three underlying measurements, and (3) well-known limitations in certain patients, it is firmly entrenched in routine practice and likely will be displaced only if homogeneous methods can demonstrate clear advantages. Substantially better analytical performance or overall improved cost-effectiveness in characterizing or monitoring patients has yet to be shown for homogeneous LDL methods. A 2002 review suggests that homogeneous assays can be recommended only to supplement calculation for those patients with elevated triglycerides or other conditions precluding calculation.[218]

Oxidized LDL

In 1983, Brown and Goldstein reported that circulating LDL must undergo some structural modification before it becomes fully proatherogenic.[43] Patients who completely lack LDL receptors accumulate large amounts of cholesterol in their macrophages and form foam cells. The receptors, which recognize the modified LDL, were termed *the scavenger receptors.*[97] Currently, several modifications that enhance the uptake of LDL by macrophages in vitro have been described, such as glycation, self-aggregation, immune complex formation, hydrolysis, and oxidation; the latter has received the greatest attention.[302]

LDL is oxidized in microdomains in the arterial wall, where it is sequestered by proteoglycans and other extracellular matrix constituents and is protected from plasma antioxidants. This process is a free radical–driven lipid peroxidation chain reaction that is initiated by the free radical attacking the double bond associated with polyunsaturated fatty acids (PUFAs), leading to the generation of malonedialdehyde and 4-hydroxynonenal.[14] These intermediate compounds then bind to apo B-100, giving it an increased net negative charge and rendering it unrecognizable by native LDL receptors.

Oxidized LDL (oxLDL) has several proatherogenic properties, including rapid uptake by macrophages to form foam cells, chemoattraction for circulating monocytes, promotion of the differentiation of monocytes into tissue macrophages, and inhibition of the motility of resident macrophages.[302] It is cytotoxic to several types of cells and is immunogenic. Laboratory, clinical, and epidemiologic studies have shown that this oxidation also occurs in vivo. LDL extracted from human atherosclerotic lesions was shown to be oxidatively modified; circulating anti-oxLDL antibodies were detected in serum, with titers correlating with progression of atherosclerotic lesions; the use of various antioxidants (vitamin E and probucol among others) delayed the progression of atherosclerotic lesions.

Several commercial assays specific for various epitopes of oxLDL are currently available (e.g., Mercodia, Uppsala, Sweden).[124] However, at the present time, the clinical relevance of oxLDL has not been established; therefore its routine measurement is not recommended.

Total Lipoproteins and Lipoprotein Subclasses

Several approaches have been used to quantitate all of the lipoproteins and, in some cases, lipoprotein subclasses in a single procedure. Among the earliest methods for characterization of lipoprotein subclasses was analytical ultracentrifugation; the method is tedious, however, and is not widely used today.[170]

Subsequently, other more practical methods were developed. In these procedures, samples are loaded onto a gel and are subjected to an electrical field, causing the negatively charged lipoproteins to move into the gradient, and achieving separation based on particle mobility and/or size. The electropherogram is stained and scanned densitometrically, and areas under the various lipoprotein peaks are reported, usually in relative percents. Relative values can be converted to equivalent lipoprotein cholesterol or apo B concentrations, using assumed average compositions for the particles. Electrophoresis, usually in agarose, for determination of major lipoprotein classes in unfractionated samples is relatively easy to perform but has limited clinical application, such as for detecting β-VLDL in type III hyperlipidemia.[27] Resolution adequate for determination of lipoprotein subclasses can be achieved in gradient gels of polyacrylamide,[336] but this approach is technically more demanding and is performed by only specialized reference laboratories.

Density gradient ultracentrifugation is used to characterize lipoprotein subclasses; it is performed in a vertical rotor with measurement of cholesterol continuously in fractions eluted from the gradient.[56,57,286] Mathematical curve deconvolution derives the component lipoprotein profiles and allows calculation of their concentrations in terms of cholesterol or other constituents. The method can determine concentrations of VLDL, IDL, LDL, Lp(a), and HDL cholesterol. LDL cholesterol subclasses can be expressed separately or can be combined to obtain a measurement similar to that provided by the Friedewald equation or by β-quantification. A disadvantage is that the procedure is technically demanding and requires instrumentation not usually available in routine clinical laboratories.

Nuclear magnetic resonance (NMR) spectroscopy[231,232] detects protons in lipoprotein-associated fatty acyl methyl or methylene groups. Signals from subfractions of VLDL, LDL, and HDL vary by particle size and can be resolved mathematically through deconvolution based on calibration samples with values reported in terms of numbers of lipoprotein particles. A sample can be analyzed quickly using a small volume of serum, and the method can be readily automated. A disadvantage of NMR is its inability to distinguish Lp(a) from LDL particles of the same size. Furthermore, the requirement for expensive specialized equipment and expertise limits application in routine laboratories.

These lipoprotein subclass methods have been compared with relatively poor agreement observed.[84] A method for determining the small, dense fraction of LDL particles that can be adapted to automated chemistry analyzers has been developed more recently.[120] Additional studies will be necessary to better define the relationships between these advanced lipoprotein characterization methods and current reference and routine methods.

Intermediate-Density (Remnant) Lipoproteins

Remnant lipoproteins include the lipolytic products of catabolism of the triglyceride-rich lipoproteins, VLDL and chylomicrons, occurring in the VLDL and LDL ranges. A traditionally defined fraction at the lighter end of the LDL density range, the IDL portion comprises the 1.006 to 1.019 g/mL fraction, which is obtained by sequential ultracentrifugation for quantitation, generally in terms of cholesterol content.

Clinically, remnant lipoproteins have been shown to be predictive of CHD risk.[117] A method used to measure cholesterol in remnant-like particles (RLPs) has become commercially available, using specific antibodies to separate a fraction of lipoprotein remnants. This fraction seems to be particularly indicative of conditions conferring increased CHD risk.[164,191] A fully automated method was recently reported for determination of lipoprotein remnants. However, measurement of triglycerides in nonfasting samples includes the remnant fraction and seems to supersede the need for independent measurement of remnants.[213]

Sources of Variation in Lipid and Lipoprotein Measurements

Lipid and lipoprotein concentrations vary within individuals when measured on several occasions over time. Sources of variation can be broadly categorized as analytical and physiologic or preanalytical. Analytical variations are inherent in the measurements themselves and arise from sample collection procedures, volume measurements, instrument function, reagent formulations, uncertainty in the assignment of values to calibration materials, and other such factors. Normal physiologic variation occurs independently of analytical error and reflects actual changes in concentration that occur through the course of normal, day-to-day living. Such variations result from factors such as change in posture, which causes the redistribution of water between vascular and nonvascular spaces, thereby changing the concentrations of nondiffusible plasma components.[31,194] Recent food intake produces transient increases in plasma triglycerides of 50% or greater and decreases of up to 10 to 15% in LDL and HDL cholesterol, depending on the fat content of the meal.[58,59,342] The shifts result from changes in the lipid composition of lipoproteins that occur as chylomicrons are metabolized. Seasonal changes have also been observed, probably resulting from changes in dietary and exercise patterns throughout the year.[48,100] Normal physiologic variations tend to occur in both directions, causing lipid or lipoprotein concentrations to vary somewhat about a mean value for a particular patient. Other kinds of physiologic conditions cause changes from the patient's usual steady-state concentrations, for example, acute illness or stress, pregnancy, dietary changes that result in weight loss or gain, changes in saturated fat intake, or the effects of treatment with lipid-lowering medications. In these cases, changes tend to occur in one direction, and they are not considered normal physiologic fluctuations. Lipoprotein concentrations eventually return to original steady-state concentrations when the patient recovers, or a new steady state is achieved.

Because normal physiologic variations occur, it is difficult to evaluate a patient based on a single measurement that applies only to the current sample. It is more appropriate to consider the patient's usual range of concentrations and his or her average steady-state concentration. From the laboratory's standpoint, the aim is to provide accurate measurements in the particular sample being measured. For this reason, the laboratory is primarily concerned with minimizing analytical error. From the physician's standpoint, however, the goal is to establish the patient's usual range of concentration for purposes of diagnosis and judge the effects of treatment. This aim is affected primarily by physiologic variation, because physiologic variation contributes the larger proportion of the sample-to-sample variation observed in serial samples from the same patient. Some sources of physiologic variation, such as posture during blood sampling, can be controlled; other factors that cannot be controlled, such as pregnancy, should be considered in interpreting laboratory results.

Analytical Variation

Table 27-24 illustrates the current overall variation of lipid and lipoprotein measurements in more than 100 laboratories participating in an accuracy-based survey conducted by the

TABLE 27-24 Analytical Variation of Lipid and Lipoprotein Measurements*

Analyte	ABL-01/2009	ABL-02/2009	ABL-03/2009
Cholesterol			
Number of laboratories	135	135	134
Mean, mg/dL	150.8	179.2	244.9
CV, %	2.1	2.2	1.8
CDC value	152.6	180.0	244.2
% Bias	−1.18	−0.44	0.29
HDL-C			
Number of laboratories	134	133	135
Mean, mg/dL	31.7	56.6	49.2
CV, %	4.6	3.8	4.7
CDC value	33.9	56.8	49.3
% Bias	−6.49	−0.35	−0.20
	ABL-04/2008	**ABL-05/2008**	**ABL-06/2008**
Triglyceride			
Number of laboratories	142	141	142
Mean, mg/dL	88.8	204.8	225.7
CV, %	3.2	2.4	2.3
CDC value	91	202.5	223.6
% Bias	−2.42	1.14	0.94

*Bias calculated as: (Test mean − CDC value/CDC value) × 100.

CDC, Centers for Disease Control and Prevention measurement done with reference method; *CV,* coefficient of variation; *HDL-C,* high-density lipoprotein cholesterol.

Data from College of American Pathologists Chemistry Survey, Northfield, Ill, 2009.

College of American Pathologists. In this survey, fresh frozen serum is sent to participating laboratories, and the results are compared with the reference method when available. Results from total cholesterol meet the NCEP error goal for bias and imprecision.[5] The average bias was in the range of −01.18 to 0.29%, and CVs were less than 3%. These numbers represent the totals of within- and among-laboratory components of variation, and suggest that reliable cholesterol measurements can be provided by most clinical laboratories. Similarly, the overall bias and precision of various triglyceride assays were relatively good. For HDL cholesterol, most participants used one of the current direct assays, and the avarege bias slightly exceeded the NCEP-recommended bias of ≤5%; the mean CV of the assays also slightly exceeded the ≤4% goal for imprecision. Results for LDL-C are not shown, because freezing of the serum was found to affect the commutability of the material, but the performance of the direct LDL-C assay is comparable with that of the direct HDL-C assay, suggesting the need for improvement.[200] It is important to note that the performance of direct HDL-C and LDL-C assays may not be as good in patients with dyslipidemias or other conditions that may affect the specificity of assays for the lipoprotein being measured.[196]

Physiologic Variation

The normal physiologic component of variation is calculated from the total variation of measurements in serial specimens from the same patients, after adjustment for analytical variation.[39,113,135,181,199] Such estimates differ somewhat from study to study, but after an extensive review of the literature,[5,9] the NCEP panels concerned with lipid and lipoprotein measurement assumed average physiologic CVs (Table 27-25). A wide variety of factors contribute to physiologic variations (Table 27-26). Physiologic variations observed for cholesterol, HDL cholesterol, and LDL cholesterol are similar. Physiologic variation for triglyceride is considerably higher, because fasting triglyceride concentrations can vary widely within an

TABLE 27-25 Physiologic Variation in Lipid and Lipoprotein Concentrations in Serial Specimens from the Same Individual

Component	Physiologic Variation, % CV	Percentage of Variance Contributed by Physiologic Variation*
Total cholesterol	6.5	91
Triglyceride	23.7	98
HDL cholesterol	7.5	69
LDL cholesterol	8.2	81

*Assuming the following analytical CVs: total cholesterol, 2%; triglyceride, 3%; HDL cholesterol, 5%; LDL cholesterol, 4%.

TABLE 27-26 Representative Preanalytical Sources of Variation (Including Biological)

	TC	HDL-C	TG	LDL-C
Intraindividual biological variation of healthy individuals (coefficient of variation)	6.5%	7.5%	23.7%	8.2%
Sampling				
Nonfasting	NC	–	++	–
Prolonged total fasting	++	–	+	+
Posture from standing to:				
Supine	–	—	—	—
Sitting	–	–	–	–
Anticoagulants from serum:				
Plasma	–	–	–	–
Behavioral				
Diet				
Saturated fatty acids (palmitic acid)	+	NC	+	+
Monounsaturated fatty acids	–	NC	–	–
Polyunsaturated fatty acids	—	–	NC	—
Cholesterol intake	+	NC	NC	+
Fish oil	NC	NC	–	NC
Obesity	+	–	++	+
Smoking	+	–	++	+
Exercise (strenuous)	–	+	–	–
Alcohol intake	+	+	++	–
Clinical Sources				
Myocardial infarction				
24 hours	NC	NC	NC	NC
6 weeks	–	–	NC	–
Stroke	–	NC	NC	–
Hypertension diuretics	+	–	++	+
Nephrosis	++	NC	++	++
Diabetes (insulin resistance)	+	–	++	++
Infections	–	–	++	–
Pregnancy, second trimester	+	NC	++	+
Transplantation				
Cyclosporine	++	–	+	++
Prednisone	+	–	++	+

HDL-C, High-density lipoprotein cholesterol; *LDL-C,* low-density lipoprotein cholesterol; *NC,* essentially no change or trend; *TC,* Total cholesterol; *TG,* triglycerides; +, minimal to moderate increase; ++, moderate to high increase; –, minimal to moderate decrease; —, moderate to high decrease.
From Cooper GR, Myers GL, Smith SJ, Schlant RC. Blood lipid measurements: variation and practical utility. JAMA 1992;267:1652-60. Copyright 1992, American Medical Association.

individual. Because the analytical CVs for these assays are relatively small, it can be calculated that, on average, physiologic variations contribute about 70 to 98% of the overall variance of lipid and lipoprotein concentrations (see Table 27-25). For this reason, a patient's usual lipid or lipoprotein concentration cannot be reliably established from a single measurement. NCEP guidelines recommend that for cholesterol, the average of measurements in two serial samples obtained at least 1 week apart should be used; two to three serial specimens are recommended, if feasible, for triglyceride and for HDL and LDL cholesterol.[9]

NCEP Recommendations for Lipid and Lipoprotein Measurements

The following information has been summarized from the NCEP recommendations for lipid and lipoprotein measurement[5,9]:

1. *Database linkage.* Laboratories that provide lipid and lipoprotein measurements should maintain linkage with existing epidemiologic databases relating lipid and lipoprotein concentration to risk for CHD. Because these databases have been established largely on the basis of CDC standardized methods, the methods used for cholesterol,

triglycerides, HDL cholesterol, and LDL cholesterol should give results with accuracy traceable to those used to establish those databases. Accordingly, CDC reference methods for cholesterol, triglycerides, and HDL cholesterol serve as the basis for judging the accuracy of other methods.

2. *Reference methods.* Reference methods should provide serum equivalent values.
3. *Routine methods.* In most cases, lipid and lipoprotein measurements can be made using specimens of serum or plasma. Measurements in EDTA plasma can be converted to serum-equivalent values using the following equation:

$$\text{Equivalent serum value} = \text{Plasma value} \times 1.03 \quad \mathbf{(20)}$$

4. *Cholesterol measurements.* In practice, a fasting or a nonfasting sample is used for cholesterol measurements. Triglycerides, HDL cholesterol, and LDL cholesterol measurements should preferably be made in samples collected after a 12-hour fast. As a convenience to the patient, such measurements are made after a 9-hour fast without introducing unduly large errors into the measurements.
5. *Blood samples.* Blood samples should be collected in the seated position whenever possible. If this is not feasible, the patient should be sampled in the same position on each occasion.
6. *Specimen storage.* Serum or plasma should be removed from cells within 3 hours of venipuncture. Specimens can be stored for up to 3 days at 4 °C; up to several weeks at −20 °C in a non–self-defrosting freezer; and at −70 °C or lower for longer periods.
7. *Serial samples.* Using the mean of several serial measurements for clinical decisions is recommended to average out the effects of physiologic and analytical variation. Measurements therefore should be made in at least two serial samples collected at least 1 week apart, with the values averaged. Three serial samples are preferred for measurement of triglycerides, HDL cholesterol, and LDL cholesterol, but two serial specimens can be used if necessary.
8. *Glycerol blanking.* The NCEP Working Group on Lipoprotein Measurement originally recommended the use of glycerol blanking for triglyceride measurement, but at this time it is not a common practice, because only a limited number of commercial assays of these types are available.
9. *Goals for analytical performance.* The NCEP goals for analytical performance differ slightly from CDC standardization criteria because NCEP goals are stated in terms of total error, which reflects both bias and imprecision,[9] whereas CDC standardization criteria consider each separately. NCEP recommendations for total error are shown in Table 27-27.

These guidelines were established after consideration of degrees of accuracy and imprecision that are achievable in well-controlled research and clinical laboratories.[9] A laboratory can approximate its conformance to the total error recommendations using the following equation:

$$\text{Total error} = \%\ \text{Bias} + 1.96\ \text{X}\ (\text{CVa}) \quad \mathbf{(21)}$$

TABLE 27-27 National Cholesterol Education Program Recommendations for Analytical Performance of Lipid and Lipoprotein Measurements

	Total	Consistent With	
	Error, %	**Bias, %**	**CV, %**
Cholesterol	8.9	≤±3	≤3
Triglycerides	≤15	≤±5	≤5
HDL cholesterol*	≤13	≤±5	≤4
LDL cholesterol	≤12	≤±4	≤4

*When HDL-C <42 mg/dL, the CV criterion is SD ≤1.7.
CV, Coefficient of variation; *HDL,* high-density lipoprotein; *LDL,* low-density lipoprotein.

where % bias is the mean laboratory difference between the measured value for a commutable serum control pool and the reference value for the pool, and CVa is the overall analytical CV for the pool, including within- and among-run variations, and calculated as follows:

$$\frac{\text{Standard deviation}}{\text{Laboratory mean}} \times 100 \quad \mathbf{(22)}$$

Bias should be calculated as the difference from reference values rather than from manufacturers' stated values when these differ.

The individual biases and CVs shown in Table 27-27 should be viewed as examples of conditions under which the total error criteria can be met. A laboratory with less bias can tolerate slightly greater imprecision without exceeding the total error criteria. Conversely, imprecision must be lower if bias increases. For example, a laboratory operating with a bias of 3% and a CV of 3% for cholesterol would have a total error of 3% + (1.96 ∞ 3%), or 8.9%. If, however, bias is only 1%, the CV could be as high as 4% without exceeding the criteria for total error [1% + (1.96 ∞ 4%) = 8.8%]. (In practice, many laboratories can achieve total errors under 6%, assuming a bias of 2% and a CV of 2%.)

It is important to note that the NCEP panel considered that the physician usually does not distinguish between lipid and lipoprotein measurements on the basis of the method used to make the measurements. For this reason, NCEP guidelines do not distinguish between measurements made in the laboratory and those made in alternative settings with desktop analyzers or other methods.

As mentioned previously, CDC standardization criteria consider bias and imprecision separately. For this reason, each of the two criteria must be met to achieve standardization. Current CDC standardization criteria are shown in Table 27-28.

NCEP guidelines as summarized previously are directed primarily to laboratories and users of laboratory measurements. The reader is referred to the original reports for more extensive discussion of these issues.[5,9] The NCEP panels have made many other recommendations to improve lipid and

TABLE 27-28 CDC Standardization Criteria for Lipid and Lipoprotein Measurement

	Bias*†, %	CV‡, %
Cholesterol	≤±3	≤3
Triglycerides	≤±5	≤5
HDL cholesterol*	≤±5	≤4

*With respect to reference values.
†Maximum allowable.
‡CVs shown apply at HDL cholesterol concentrations >42 mg/dL. At lower concentrations, precision criteria are based on standard deviation (SD ≤ 1.7).
CDC, Centers for Disease Control and Prevention; *CV,* coefficient of variation; *HDL,* high-density lipoprotein.

lipoprotein measurements, only several of which are mentioned here. First, it was recommended that manufacturers of calibration materials, control pools, and analytical systems calibrate their materials and methods to provide values with accuracy traceable to reference method values. Many manufacturers are now doing this, which probably accounts for the relatively small interlaboratory biases for total and HDL cholesterol, as reflected in Table 27-24.

APOLIPOPROTEINS

Apolipoproteins are measured by a wide variety of immunoassays, including (1) radioimmunoassay (RIA), (2) ELISA, (3) radial immunodiffusion (RID), (4) immunoturbidimetric assay, and (5) immunonephelometric assay. The concentration of a particular apolipoprotein usually determines the immunotechnique used for its measurement.

Apolipoproteins A-I and B-100

Immunoturbidimetry and immunonephelometry are widely used to measure apo A-I and apo B-100, which are present at relatively high concentrations. According to the CAP Proficiency Testing Survey, all clinical laboratories in the United States that measure apo A-I and apo B-100 use one of these two approaches. Alternatively, more sensitive techniques, such as ELISA and RIA, are perhaps more suitable for those apolipoproteins present at much lower concentrations, such as apo C-I and apo C-II. Additional information about the various analytical techniques used in determination of apolipoprotein concentrations is provided later.

The following paragraphs discuss some unique analytical issues that pertain to apolipoprotein testing.[156]

Presence of a Given Apolipoprotein on Different Lipoproteins

Apolipoprotein B-100, for example, is present on LDL, IDL, VLDL, and Lp(a) particles, which vary significantly in size and composition. To correctly determine the concentration of total apo B-100, the anti–apo B-100 antibody used must be able to recognize apo B-100 present on various lipoprotein classes equally and must display similar kinetic patterns with all of them.[272]

"Masking" Phenomenon

Unlike other plasma proteins, apolipoproteins circulate in the bloodstream as part of a lipoprotein complex. As discussed earlier, lipoprotein particles are heterogeneous spheres consisting of lipids and apolipoproteins. The antigenic sites of these proteins are often covered by lipids.[274,303] To have a maximal antigen-antibody interaction, these epitopes must be unmasked. Nonionic detergents such as Tween 20 or Tween 80 are usually added to the assay buffer to disrupt the lipoprotein particles and make all antigenic sites on the apolipoproteins accessible to the antibodies.

Suitable Antibodies (Polyclonal vs. Monoclonal)

Polyclonal antibodies are widely used in clinical laboratories for the measurement of plasma protein concentrations. However, immunoassays are often sensitive to the nature of the antibody used.[303] The development of polyclonal antibodies is affected by several factors, such as the purity and dose of the antigen used, the species of host animal, and the immunization procedure. Monoclonal antibodies are viewed as a viable alternative to alleviate these problems. However, expression of particular epitopes varies with the lipoprotein particles and among individuals; in addition, the apolipoproteins themselves are polymorphic in nature. Therefore, a single monoclonal antibody might not detect a particular variant. If a monoclonal antibody is used to determine an apolipoprotein, it should be directed to an epitope that is expressed on all polymorphic forms of that particular apolipoprotein. Furthermore, the epitope should be equally reactive to the antibodies, regardless of which lipoprotein class contains it. Alternatively, a mixture of monoclonal antibodies directed at different epitopes of the apolipoprotein may be used. Such mixtures are referred to as *panmonoclonal* antibodies.

Availability of Primary Calibrators

In general, to standardize a particular protein, a purified form of that protein is used as a primary calibrator (see Chapter 21). However, the purified preparation must express the same immunoreactivity as the native protein. Unfortunately, once removed from its natural milieu, apo B-100 is insoluble in aqueous buffers. This phenomenon is attributed to the very hydrophobic nature of apo B-100. An LDL preparation with density of 1.030 to 1.050 g/mL, often referred to as *narrow-cut* LDL, is generally used as the primary standard for apo B-100. The protein concentration of the purified preparation is determined by amino acid analysis. In contrast, freshly purified apo A-I is soluble in aqueous buffers and is suitable as a primary standard.

As indicated earlier, several immunotechniques are used for the quantification of apo A-I and apo B-100. These techniques are affected differently by the analytical issues discussed previously. RIA and ELISA, for example, are normally used for the determination of analytes present at these very low concentrations (nanograms per milliliter). Therefore, large dilutions (up to 40,000-fold) are required when these techniques are applied to apo A-I or apo B-100 measurement, which can result in a substantial analytical error. In addition, these assays are relatively time-consuming and are not easily automated, and RIA requires the use of isotopes. However, the techniques permit the use of monoclonal or polyclonal antibodies and primary or secondary calibrators, and are less affected by the matrix of the specimen, thus permitting the determination of protein concentration in the presence of lipemia. RID is a slow technique. For example, it takes up to 3 days for VLDL to complete migration through the gel. It is also less precise than automated assays and yields lower apo B-100 values than those obtained by other techniques,[65,272] possibly in part because of the relative selectivity of RID for smaller apo B–containing particles. Polyclonal or monoclonal antisera may be used with RID.[156] Immunoturbidimetric and immunonephelometric assays are fully automated and highly precise, and can use polyclonal or multiple monoclonal antibodies. However, they can be affected by the background turbidity of the specimen (e.g., in samples with high triglyceride concentrations). The addition of detergents to the assay buffers reduces nonspecific light scattering; this has helped to diminish this problem.

Considerable effort has been expended over the past decade by national and international organizations in overcoming the problems of apo A-I and B-100 standardization.[65] The Committee on Apolipoproteins of the IFCC embarked on an ambitious international collaborative study aimed at developing secondary serum reference materials that can be used, without influence of matrix bias effects, as master calibrators for all current commercial assays.[176] This program has been successfully completed.[178,179] A lyophilized serum preparation for apo A-I, designated SP1-01, and a liquid-stabilized serum preparation for apo B-100, designated SP3-07, have been approved as international reference materials by the World Health Organization (WHO). An apoA-I value of 150 mg/dL was assigned to SP1-01 by a highly standardized RIA calibrated with purified apo A-I for which the mass value had been determined by amino acid analysis.[178]An accuracy-based apo B-100 value of 122 mg/dL was assigned to SP3-07 using a nephelometric method that was calibrated with freshly isolated LDL, for which the apo B-100 mass value was determined by a standardized sodium dodecyl sulfate–Lowry protein procedure.[179]

The WHO and the IFCC have appointed the CDC to be the repository for the WHO-IFCC First International Reference Reagents for Apolipoproteins A-I and B-100. Dr. Santica Marcovina of Northwest Lipid Research Laboratories (NWLRL) in Seattle, who is the former Chair of the IFCC Apolipoprotein Working Group, uses an IFCC calibration protocol to conduct the standardization and distribution program for manufacturers of instruments and reagents. This protocol involves establishing the linearity of dose response, the parallelism of kinetic responses of standards and calibration sera, and the equality of intercepts for the reference materials and an analysis of fresh frozen sera. NWLRL can be contacted for standardization services and the distribution of apolipoprotein reference materials. These reference materials are also available for reference laboratories in countries where standardized commercial methods are not readily available. It has been shown that through the use of these international reference materials, the analytical performance of apo A-I and apo B-100 measurement, in terms of accuracy and precision, is superior to that of HDL and LDL cholesterol.[178,179] This effort has demonstrated that the use of certified reference materials can significantly reduce the bias of apo A-I and apo B-100 measurements by different immunotechniques. However, an external quality assurance program using fresh or fresh frozen samples and WHO-IFCC–based value assignments is indispensable in monitoring the performance of clinical chemistry laboratories and manufacturers, to ensure that accurate apolipoprotein measurements are made. The NWLRL conducts a quarterly standardization program or Reference Lipoprotein Analysis Basic Survey, which provides the accuracy base for cholesterol, triglyceride, HDL, and LDL cholesterol, and apo A-I and apo B-100. To minimize matrix effects, the survey uses fresh human serum and leads to certification of traceability to the national reference system for cholesterol and to the WHO-IFCC International Reference Reagents for apo A-I and apo B-100.

Apolipoprotein measurements have been shown to further aid in the detection of CHD risk and the diagnosis of hyperlipoproteinemia. For example, measurement of apo B-100 provides a reliable clinical tool by which to identify subjects with increased risk for CHD who may not be readily identified by conventional cholesterol or lipoprotein cholesterol measurements (e.g., subjects with a borderline elevation of LDL cholesterol, subjects with hypertriglyceridemia without an LDL cholesterol elevation). In addition, apo B-100 measurements can assess whether lipid-lowering drugs are effective in lowering the number of atherogenic apo B–containing lipoproteins. However, for apolipoprotein measurements to be used in routine clinical practice, clinically meaningful cutoff values for clinical decision making need to be established, and more information regarding their clinical utility is needed. The use of cutoff values for apo A-I and apo B-100, similar to those recommended by the NCEP for HDL and LDL cholesterol, respectively, has been suggested.[61,63] An apo A-I concentration less than 120 mg/dL may be associated with increased risk of CHD, whereas apo A-I of 160 mg/dL or greater may be protective. Apo B-100 cut points of 100 and 120 mg/dL approximately correspond to the LDL cholesterol cut points of 130 and 160 mg/dL, which fall at approximately the 50th and 75th percentiles, respectively. Alternatively, Sniderman and Cianflone have suggested that apo B-100 values greater than the 75th percentile should be regarded as high risk, and a value greater than the 50th percentile as moderate risk.[295]

Lipoprotein(a)

The structural heterogeneity of Lp(a) as a consequence of apo(a) size heterogeneity has important implications for the accurate measurement of Lp(a) in human plasma.[17,21,177,183,184] Repeated antigenic determinants are present in variable numbers in different Lp(a) particles, and the immunoreactivity of the antibodies directed to these repeated epitopes can vary as a function of apo(a) size. As a consequence, immunoassays using polyclonal antibodies or monoclonal antibodies specifically directed to kringle 4 type 2 epitopes will tend to underestimate apo(a) concentration in samples with apo(a) of smaller size than the apo(a) present in the assay calibrator, and will tend to overestimate the apo(a) concentration in samples with larger apo(a). A detailed evaluation of the effect of apo(a) size heterogeneity on measurement of Lp(a) has been reported.[177] Monoclonal antibody–based assays have the theoretical advantage that the antibodies can be immunochemically characterized and preselected on the basis of their specificity to single epitopes (e.g., those not located in kringle 4 type 2 domain). However, characterization of monoclonal antibodies is a rather complex procedure, and none of the monoclonal antibodies currently used in commercially available assays has been characterized in terms of epitope specificity. An additional disadvantage of monoclonal antibodies is that they cannot be easily used in immunoassays that require precipitation of the antigen-antibody complex.

Assays used to measure Lp (a) in (1) turbidimetric, (2) nephelometric, (3) radiometric, and (4) enzymatic methods. Most of these assays, except for the enzyme immunoassay (ELISA), are based on the use of polyclonal antibodies from various animal species. Commercially available, direct-binding, sandwich-type ELISAs are usually based on the use of a combination of monoclonal and polyclonal antibodies. One approach takes advantage of the presence of both apo(a) and apo B in Lp(a) particles. In this approach, Lp(a) particles are "captured" using a polyclonal or monoclonal antibody to apo(a), and an enzyme-conjugated antibody to apo B-100 is used as the detection antibody. An ELISA method based on this approach has been described and is commercially available.[309] In another approach, both capture and detection antibodies are specific for apo(a). At present, it is not clear which approach would be better with respect to estimating the risk for CHD or stroke, because the pathogenic mechanisms involved have not yet been elucidated. Thus, it is not known whether the risk is associated simply with an increased number of Lp(a) particles in the circulation (as measured using an anti–apo B antibody) or is also related to the presence of polyforms of a particular size [as might be detected more readily with anti-apo(a) detection antibodies]. It is likely that both factors influence the risk.

Historically, Lp(a) concentrations have been reported in terms of total Lp(a) particle mass[16] or, alternatively, in terms of Lp(a) protein.[17] If the aim is to provide Lp(a) values that are independent of apo(a) size, it is recommended that the Lp(a) assay use antibodies directed to an apo(a) domain other than kringle 4 type 2, or to the apo B-100 component of Lp(a). This would allow the values to be expressed in nanomoles per liter.[17] Panmonoclonal mixtures of antibodies to kringle 4 type 2 may be preferred if particular sizes of polyforms contribute to the risk.

At present, Lp(a) measurements are not standardized, and most Lp(a) assays have not been evaluated for their apo(a) size sensitivity. As a result, Lp(a) values reported in clinical studies are difficult to compare. Despite this, a value of about 30 mg/dL of total Lp(a) particle mass has traditionally been used as a cutoff, above which elevated concentrations of Lp(a) are associated with increased risk of CHD. Lp(a) concentrations can also be expressed in terms of particle number and mass of apo(a), apo B-100, or Lp(a) cholesterol. Which approach will best predict the risk for CHD has yet to be determined. At present, Lp(a) values are most commonly expressed in terms of total Lp(a) mass, but this should be confirmed by having the laboratory make the measurements. In view of the current lack of reference methods or standardization procedures for Lp(a), it is difficult to define precise cutoffs that can be used to make clinical decisions. Although less than ideal, one approach would be to establish a reference interval for each assay and report individual results in terms of percentile values within these intervals. In whites, patients with Lp(a) values above the 80th percentile can be considered at increased risk for coronary atherosclerosis. However, because Lp(a) values can vary among ethnic groups, reference values need to be population based. Furthermore, such cutoffs may have to be racially specific. For example, African Americans in general have significantly higher Lp(a) concentrations than whites,[185] but they do not manifest a higher incidence of CHD. An IFCC committee, using an approach similar to that of the apo A-I and B-100 committee, has developed reference materials to be used with all commercially available Lp(a) methods.[311,312] As expected, the use of a common calibrator led to improved harmonization of Lp(a) results but not complete standardization.[180] Only when appropriate antibodies are used can standardization be achieved.

Virtually all retrospective case-control studies in whites have reported a strong association between increased Lp(a) and risk of CHD. In contrast, prospective studies have provided contradictory results, with four of them finding an association between high Lp(a) concentrations and CHD, and three finding no association. Several studies have suggested that apo(a) size isoforms may be related to a high prevalence of CHD (see earlier discussion). The procedure with the greatest resolution and sensitivity for determination of apo(a) phenotypes involves separation of apo(a) on agarose gel electrophoresis, immunoblotting with a specific antibody, and detection with ^{125}I-labeled protein A.[185] This approach identifies at least 34 apo(a) polymorphs. It can be used to express apo(a) size in terms of kringle number, and is consistent with observations on the size variation of the apo(a) gene obtained by pulsed-field gel electrophoresis and genomic blotting.[182]

Apolipoprotein E

As discussed earlier, homozygosity for apo E_2 is characteristic of type III familial hyperlipoproteinemia. Homozygosity for apo E_2 is a necessary but not sufficient condition for expression of the type III hyperlipoproteinemia; a second gene defect or condition appears to be required to cause the characteristic hyperlipidemia. Heterozygosity for some rare apo E mutants may also be associated with type III hyperlipoproteinemia.[322] The study of apo E variants has assumed greater importance in the last few years because of the association between the apo E_4 allele and Alzheimer's disease and dementia.[291]

Traditionally, the determination of apo E isoforms was assessed by isoelectric focusing (IEF) techniques that permit identification of charge variations of the different isoforms. In early studies, IEF was performed on VLDL that had been extracted to remove the lipids. The separated proteins were then stained for protein.[335] This approach is not used as frequently today because it requires a relatively large volume of plasma and because of the expensive and time-consuming step of ultracentrifugation to isolate VLDL. Apo E phenotypes are now assessed by IEF of a small volume of plasma followed by immunoblotting with specific antibodies to apo E. This approach can be applied in the clinical laboratory and is well adapted to large-scale population studies. However, it is important that the samples are analyzed fresh, or if stored, that they are kept at −70 °C before analysis to minimize the introduction of artifacts. Misclassification can occur because of post-translational modifications or nonenzymatic glycation of apo E, the presence of rare variants that have the same charge as the common isoforms, overlooked faint apo E_4 bands, and false-positive apo E_2 bands. Interpretation of the patterns requires significant experience in use of the technique.

The availability of techniques based on the polymerase chain reaction (PCR) permits an analysis of the variation in the nucleotide sequence of the apo E gene (Figure 27-27). One approach for apo E genotyping uses oligonucleotides to amplify apo E gene sequences containing amino acid positions 112 and 158; the amplified products are digested with *Hha*I and are subjected to electrophoresis on polyacrylamide gels.[121] Alternatively, allele-specific oligonucleotide (ASO) primers can be used to specifically amplify E_2, E_3, and E_4 polymorphic sequences of the apo E gene.[107,341] Another approach, the amplification refractory mutation system (ARMS), is based on the strictness of the PCR primer for the 3′ end mismatch and is simple, rapid, and nonisotopic. Reagent costs for the ARMS assay are, however, higher than for the restriction isotyping assay. The single-strand conformation polymorphism (SSCP) method has also been used for apo E genotyping.[82] It can detect unknown apo E mutations but is not very convenient because it requires radiolabeled primers. Because restriction isotyping is rapid, requiring only 1 hour to digest the PCR product and several hours for electrophoresis, and does not require radioactive reagents, it may be the most practical method for apo E genotyping in the diagnostic clinical laboratory. Because of potential errors in interpretation or unpreventable artifacts in the apo E phenotype method, apo E genotyping is more reliable for determining the common apo E alleles and would be the method of choice if DNA or whole blood is available. However, most apo E genotyping methods do not detect rare mutations. Discrepancies of 5 to 20% between results of phenotyping and genotyping have been reported.

OTHER CARDIAC RISK FACTORS

Despite the strong association of lipid concentrations with CHD risk, it has long been recognized that half of all myocardial infarctions occur among individuals without overt hyperlipidemia. In the Women's Health Study (WHS), for example, 77% of future cardiovascular events occurred among those with LDL cholesterol concentrations <160 mg/dL, and 46% occurred among those with LDL cholesterol <130 mg/dL.[264] Furthermore, in a 2003 analysis of more than 120,000 patients, approximately 20% of all coronary events occurred in the absence of any of the major classical risk factors: hyperlipidemia, hypertension, diabetes, and smoking.[141] Another

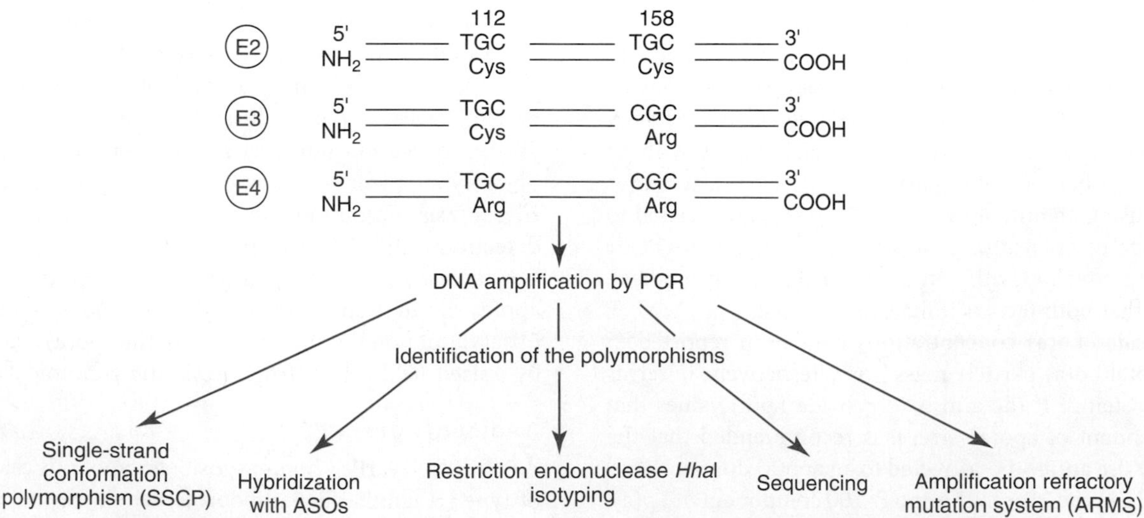

Figure 27-27 Different methods for investigating apolipoprotein E polymorphism at the genomic level. *ASO*, Allele-specific oligonucleotide; *PCR*, polymerase chain reaction. *(From Siest G, Pillot T, Regis-Bailly A, et al. Apolipoprotein E: an important gene and protein to follow in laboratory medicine. Clin Chem 1995;41:1068-86.)*

large study showed that 85 to 95% of participants with CHD had at least one conventional risk factor, but so too did those participants without CHD, despite follow-up for as long as 30 years.[108] These observations raise the question whether only traditional risk factors are adequate to identify all individuals at increased risk of CHD.

A wide variety of nonlipid biochemical markers have been suggested in an effort to better identify those individuals at increased CHD risk, including markers of fibrinolytic and hemostatic function (tissue-type plasminogen activator antigen, plasminogen activator inhibitor-1, fibrinogen, von Willebrand, D-dimer, thrombin-antithrombin III complex, and factors V, VII, and VIII), homocysteine, and markers of inflammation [high-sensitivity C-reactive protein (hsCRP), lipoprotein-associated phospholipase A2 (Lp-PLA$_2$), serum amyloid A, interleukins, adhesion molecules, heat shock proteins, and matrix metalloproteases]. Clinically, use of most of these markers in screening is of limited value for one or more of the following reasons:

1. Lack of standardization among available methods.
2. Inconsistent findings from prospective epidemiologic studies regarding their ability to independently predict future CHD risk (see discussion on homocysteine later in this chapter).
3. Inability to significantly improve prognostic value when added to traditional lipid screening or existing global risk prediction algorithms, such as the Framingham risk score.
4. Unavailability of an appropriate interventional modality that not only modulates the concentration of the biomarker but also reduces the risk associated with increased concentration of that biomarker.

An expert panel of the National Academy of Clinical Biochemistry (NACB) stated in its report on Laboratory Medicine Practice Guidelines for Emerging Biomarkers for Primary Prevention of Cardiovascular Disease that of all examined novel markers, only hsCRP met the previously mentioned criteria for acceptance as a biomarker of risk in the primary prevention setting.[206]

These recommendations were consistent with those stated in the earlier report of the American Heart Association (AHA) and the CDC (AHA/CDC).[236] For this reason, hsCRP is discussed in greater detail in this section. A brief discussion of homocysteine, for historical reasons, is also presented.

High-Sensitivity C-Reactive Protein

Tillet and Francis in 1930 described a substance that was present in the sera of acutely ill patients and was able to bind the cell wall C-polysaccharide of *Streptococcus pneumoniae* and to agglutinate the organisms. In 1941, the substance was shown to be a protein and was given the name *C-reactive protein (CRP)*. CRP was subsequently shown to be an acute-phase reactant that was important in the nonspecific host defense against inflammation, especially infection (see Chapter 21); it is routinely monitored as an indication of infection and autoimmune disease using methods that have detection limits of 3 to 8 mg/L.

Chronic inflammation is an important component in the development and progression of atherosclerosis, and numerous epidemiologic studies have demonstrated that increased serum CRP concentrations are positively associated with the risk of future coronary events, such as coronary artery disease, cerebrovascular disease, or peripheral arterial disease.[148,255,256,259] It has also been shown to be predictive of future events in patients with acute coronary syndromes and in those with stable angina and coronary artery stents.[273]

The use of CRP for these purposes requires the use of hsCRP assays that have detection limits less than 0.3 mg/L.[273] Several automated immunoturbidimetric and immunonephelometric assays are commercially available and are capable of sensitive and precise measurements at low concentrations of CRP. The analytical performance of nine of these assays has been evaluated.[273]

In this section, we summarize the basic biochemistry, clinical significance, and analytical considerations of the measurement of hsCRP. Additional information is presented in Chapter 21.

Biochemistry

CRP consists of five identical, nonglycosylated polypeptide subunits noncovalently linked to form a disk-shaped cyclic polymer with a molecular weight of ≈115 kDa. It contains little or no carbohydrate and is synthesized primarily in the liver. Its production is controlled by interleukin-6, and it binds to polysaccharides present in many bacteria, fungi, and protozoal parasites and polycations, such as histones.

Clinical Significance

Of the markers mentioned previously in this chapter, only hsCRP has fulfilled the required criteria for a novel marker of CHD risk according to the expert panels of the AHA/CDC[236] and the NACB.[206] Here we discuss the roles of hsCRP in CHD, the metabolic syndrome, diabetes, and hypertension, and its possible role in atherogenesis. We conclude with a discussion of possible preventive measures in those individuals with increased concentrations of hsCRP. Comprehensive reviews on this subject have been published.[35,200,251]

Cardiovascular Disease

Prospective epidemiologic studies have consistently shown that a single assay result for hsCRP is a strong predictor of myocardial infarction,[148,153,259,264] stroke,[153,259,264] peripheral vascular disease,[256,265] and sudden cardiac death[18] in individuals without a history of heart disease. The association between hsCRP and future CHD reflects the current understanding of vascular biology, because it is known that chronic inflammation plays a pivotal role in atherogenesis. This association has been observed in studies from around the world involving middle-aged and elderly persons and high- and usual-risk populations.[18,148,153] The association is apparent even in studies with follow-up periods up to 20 years, as seen in the Honolulu Heart Study.[68] In a direct comparison of traditional and novel biochemical markers of CHD risk, hsCRP was the strongest predictor of future coronary events.[259]

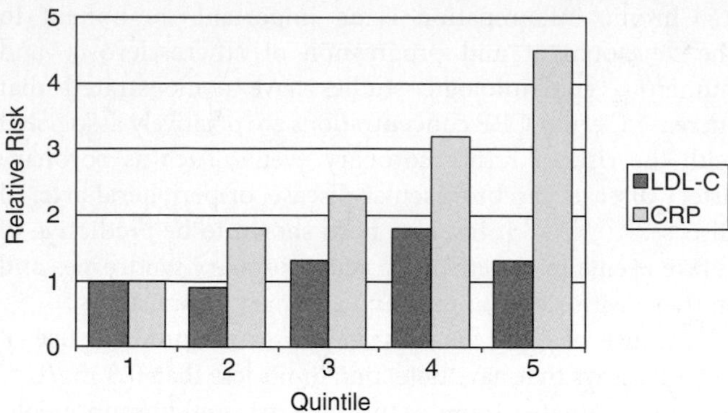

Figure 27-28 Head-to-head comparison of LDL cholesterol and hsCRP in their ability to predict future vascular events. *hsCRP,* High-sensitivity C-reactive protein; *LDL,* low-density lipoprotein cholesterol. *(From Ridker PM, Rifai N, Rose L, Buring JE, Cook NR. Comparison of C-reactive protein and low-density lipoprotein cholesterol levels in the prediction of first cardiovascular events. N Engl J Med 2002;347:1557-65.)*

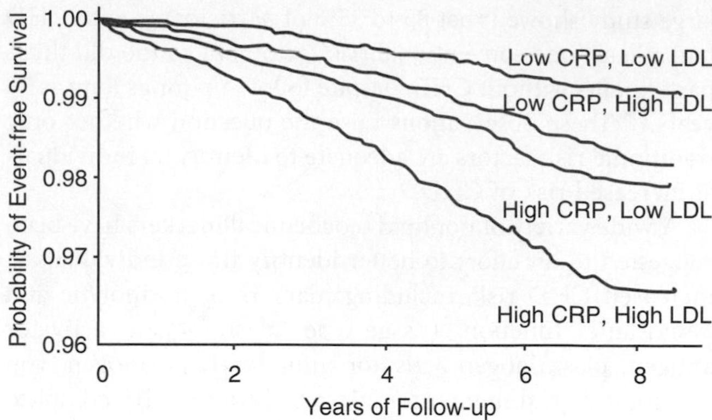

Figure 27-29 Cardiovascular event-free survival according to baseline levels of hsCRP and LDL cholesterol. *(From Ridker PM, Rifai N, Rose L, Buring JE, Cook NR. Comparison of C-reactive protein and low-density lipoprotein cholesterol levels in the prediction of first cardiovascular events. N Engl J Med 2002;347:1557-65.)*

In general, those individuals with hsCRP values in the top quartile of the sample distribution are two to three times more likely to experience a future vascular event than those in the bottom quartile. The association between hsCRP and future vascular events is linear and is independent of age, smoking, hypertension, dyslipidemia, and diabetes. For example, 8-year follow-up data from the Physicians' Health Study and the WHS showed that after adjustment for traditional risk factors, an increase in future cardiovascular risk of 26% was noted for men and 33% for women for each quintile increase in baseline hsCRP.[259]

Although most of the available data on hsCRP and incident CHD have been derived from nested case-control studies, event-free survival data from large cohorts have been published,[261,264] thus enabling estimation of absolute risks rather than relative risks of disease. Data from the WHS, for example, showed hsCRP to be a stronger predictor of risk than LDL cholesterol (Figure 27-28) and demonstrated that event-free survival was poorest for persons with increases in both LDL cholesterol and hsCRP; the best survival was observed for those with low values of both measures.[264] Event-free survival was significantly worse for those with high hsCRP and low LDL cholesterol as compared with those with high LDL cholesterol and low hsCRP (Figure 27-29).

Because hsCRP values minimally correlate with lipid concentrations, and because lipid parameters account for <3 to 5% of the variance in hsCRP measurement, measurement of hsCRP does not replace but instead complements the evaluation of lipids and other classical CHD risk factors in primary prevention settings.[19,261,264] Data from the WHS show that hsCRP adds prognostic information not only at all concentrations of the risk defined by current LDL cut points of the NCEP, but also at all concentrations of the risk specified by the Framingham risk score algorithm—an observation of significant public health implications.[264] Contemporary algorithms were developed for the assessment of global cardiovascular risk in approximately 11,000 men and 25,000 women followed for a median period longer than 10 years (Reynolds risk score).[253,260] Initially, the model was developed in women using 35 different variables, of which only the addition of hsCRP and family history of cardiovascular disease to the traditional Framingham risk components led to improved accuracy in classification; 40 to 50% of women at intermediate risk (5 to 20%, estimated 10-year risk) were reclassified into higher- or lower-risk categories.[253] Similar findings were seen in men, with about 20% of those in intermediate risk being reclassified into higher- or lower-risk categories.[260] However, a 2009 report has cautioned about extending to other ethnic groups the use of algorithms developed in primarily a white population.[69]

Metabolic Syndrome, Diabetes, and Hypertension

Studies have demonstrated a significant association between hsCRP and future risk of metabolic syndrome,[296] diabetes, and hypertension—conditions that confer increased cardiovascular risk. hsCRP values are positively correlated not only with components of the metabolic syndrome that are commonly assessed in clinical practice, such as (1) increased triglycerides, (2) reduced HDL (3) cholesterol, (4) obesity, (5) high blood pressure, and (6) high fasting glucose, but also with other components that are not easily captured in such settings, such as (7) fasting insulin, (8) microalbuminuria, and (9) impaired fibrinolysis.[241] Data from the WHS show that hsCRP measurement improves the cardiovascular risk prediction beyond that of metabolic syndrome status as assessed in clinical practice[252]; those women with metabolic syndrome and hsCRP >3 mg/L were at twice the risk of future coronary events compared with those with metabolic syndrome and hsCRP <3 mg/L. Similar results were observed in the West of Scotland Coronary Prevention Study (WOSCOPS).[277]

Increased hsCRP concentrations have been implicated in the development of type 2 diabetes mellitus. Prospective studies have found strong, graded relationships between hsCRP and incident diabetes, which in many instances persisted after adjustment for body mass index and other covariates.[242] In WOSCOPS, the top quintile of hsCRP was associated with a threefold risk of incident diabetes over a 5-year period compared with the lowest quintile,[92] and in the WHS, the top quartile of hsCRP was associated with a fourfold risk during 4 years of follow-up compared with the lowest quartile.[242] These data support the hypothesis that inflammation, atherothrombosis, and diabetes are tightly interrelated disorders of the immune system.

Accumulating data suggest a link between blood pressure and vascular inflammation, perhaps mediated by angiotensin II.[168] For example, angiotensin II infusion activates nuclear factor κB and leads to increased interleukin-6 expression in human vascular smooth muscle cells.[150] Moreover, cross-sectional studies show graded linear relationships between interleukin-6 and intercellular adhesion molecule-1 and both systolic and diastolic blood pressure.[52] The relationship between blood pressure, hsCRP, and incident cardiovascular events was assessed in the WHS.[37] Despite their strong correlation, hsCRP and blood pressure were independent determinants of future cardiovascular events during an 8-year follow-up period, and hsCRP retained incremental prognostic value at all concentrations of blood pressure. Compared with women with blood pressures lower than 120/75 mm Hg and hsCRP values less than 3 mg/L, those with blood pressures of 160/95 mm Hg or greater and hsCRP values of 3 mg/L or greater were more than eight times as likely to experience a future cardiovascular event. hsCRP also predicts incident hypertension itself. In the same cohort, after adjustment for multiple potential confounders, those women in the highest quintile of hsCRP were at a 50% higher risk of developing hypertension compared with those in the lowest quintile.[288] Moreover, high hsCRP concentration was associated with an increased risk of incident hypertension at all baseline blood pressures and among individuals without traditional CHD risk factors. On the basis of these data, it has been hypothesized that hsCRP may play a critical role in the development of hypertension. Whether or not blood pressure reduction leads to reduced hsCRP values is uncertain and is being tested in an ongoing clinical trial.

Possible Role of CRP in Atherogenesis

It is not clear at present whether CRP is a marker that reflects systemic or vascular inflammation or is an actual participant in atherogenesis. However, findings from pathologic and in vitro studies are increasingly supporting the latter. Recent reports have shown CRP to enhance expression of local endothelial cell surface adhesion molecules,[233] monocyte chemoattractant protein-1,[233] endothelin-1,[325] and endothelial plasminogen activator inhibitor-1[77]; reduce endothelial nitric oxide bioactivity[325]; increase the induction of tissue factor in monocytes[212] and LDL uptake by macrophages[351]; and colocalize with the complement membrane attack complex within atherosclerotic lesions.[315] In addition, it has been demonstrated that expression of human CRP in CRP-transgenic mice directly enhances intravascular thrombosis in both arterial injury and photochemical injury models of endothelial disruption.[315] For a more complete discussion of the possible role of CRP in atherogenesis, as determined by vascular biology experimental studies, refer to the review by Devaraj and colleagues.[76] Investigators in two studies, in which the mendelian randomization approach was used, concluded that hsCRP is not a causal factor in cardiovascular disease.[81,348] Critics of such an approach, however, indicate that when findings from mendelian randomization analysis are positive, they strongly suggest causality, but the opposite is not always true. It is important to remember that whether or not CRP is a causative factor will not preclude or affect its utility as a marker of cardiovascular disease.

Role in Disease Intervention

Although many behavioral interventions known to reduce the risk of clinical cardiovascular events have been linked to lower hsCRP values, it is not definitely known at present whether lowering of hsCRP will necessarily lead to a reduction in vascular events. For example, a reduction not only in hsCRP but also in several proinflammatory cytokines and adhesion molecules was seen in obese premenopausal women assigned to a weight-loss program as compared with women in the control group.[349] Whether these effects translate into reduced risk of subsequent cardiovascular events has not yet been elucidated.

Although no specific drugs are known to lower hsCRP concentrations, several pharmacologic agents have demonstrated cardioprotective ability, such as aspirin and statins, with the latter having the ability to reduce hsCRP values. In the Physicians' Health Study, a large primary prevention trial, reduction in the risk of future myocardial infarction associated with assignment to aspirin was 56% among those with baseline hsCRP concentrations in the highest quartile, and this value declined proportionately with hsCRP values until a reduction of only 14% was noted among those in the lowest quartile, suggesting that aspirin may prevent ischemic events through anti-inflammatory and antiplatelet effects.[255] The effect of aspirin on lowering hsCRP concentrations is uncertain at present.

The ability of statins to lower hsCRP was first described for pravastatin using data accumulated in the Cholesterol and Recurrent Events (CARE) trial.[262,263] These data were initially highly controversial because they suggested that statins have both lipid-lowering and anti-inflammatory effects. However, confirmatory work rapidly showed the effect of statins on hsCRP to be a consistent and important class effect. Studies of atorvastatin, cerivastatin, lovastatin, pravastatin, and simvastatin have shown that median hsCRP concentrations typically decline by 15 to 25% as early as 6 weeks after initiation of therapy.[33] It is important to note that the magnitude of LDL cholesterol reduction caused by statin therapy is minimally correlated with the magnitude of hsCRP reduction.[33]

Data from two large 5-year randomized trials suggest that cardiovascular risk reduction attributable to statin therapy may be most marked for those with increased hsCRP concentrations at baseline. In the CARE trial, the proportion of recurrent events prevented by pravastatin was 54% among persons with increased hsCRP values, but only 25% among persons with lower hsCRP values, even though baseline lipid concentrations were nearly identical in those with and without evidence of inflammation.[263] Similarly, in the Texas Air Force Coronary Atherosclerosis Prevention Study, lovastatin therapy was associated with a 42% reduction in first cardiovascular events among participants with low LDL cholesterol concentrations (<149 mg/dL) but high hsCRP values (>1.6 mg/L).[261]

As a result of these provocative findings, JUPITER, a clinical trial specifically designed to test the efficacy of statins in reducing clinical cardiovascular events among persons with hsCRP of 2 mg/L or greater and LDL cholesterol less than 130 mg/dL, who make up an estimated 25% of the U.S. population, was launched.[250] Approximately 18,000 subjects with such a phenotype were to be randomized to 20 mg of rosuvastatin per day or placebo and followed for a period of 4 years for the occurrence of myocardial infarction, stroke, arterial revascularization, hospitalization for unstable angina, or death from cardiovascular disease (primary end point).[250] However, the safety and efficacy board of the trial terminated it ahead of schedule because its continuation was deemed unethical based on the overwhelmingly positive results. Findings revealed a reduction in the primary trial end point of 44% in those who received rosuvastatin compared with those on placebo[257] (Figure 27-30). The number of subjects with this phenotype who have to be treated with statin to prevent a single coronary event was 25, a number that is similar to those seen in hyperlipidemia trials. Furthermore, using hsCRP less than 2 mg/L and LDL cholesterol less than 70 mg/dL as dual target goals for statin therapy, a reduction of 65% in cardiovascular events was seen; a reduction of 80% in cardiovascular events was noted in those who achieved that concentration of LDL cholesterol but hsCRP less than 1 mg/L[258] (see Figure 27-30). The implications of this trial for the practice of preventive cardiology are currently unfolding.[122,147,200] The concept of dual target goals, using both LDL cholesterol and hsCRP, to optimize statin therapy in patients with acute coronary syndrome has been explored and has been shown to be beneficial[202,223,254] (see Figure 27-30).

ANALYTICAL CONSIDERATIONS

To measure the concentrations required for use in vascular disease assessment, high-sensitivity methods were developed for CRP. Of various techniques used by investigators and manufacturers to improve the sensitivity of CRP assays, the most successful approach has been to amplify the light-scattering properties of the antigen-antibody complex by covalently coupling latex particles to a specific antibody—a procedure that is easily automated using standard laboratory instrumentation. More than 30 hsCRP assays, most of which use this approach, are now commercially available.[165] In a study of nine such assays, all achieved a lowest detection limit of 0.3 mg/L or less, and five had within-laboratory analytical imprecision less than 10% (i.e., reproducibilities greater than 90%).[273] However, hsCRP assays from different laboratories show significant discrepancies in reported results, underscoring the need for additional standardization.[273]

Standardization

Agreement among hsCRP methods is essential because an individual patient's result will be interpreted within the context of nationally established cut points, or patients will be treated to a target value. A standardization program led by the CDC was initiated in 2002 to address this issue.[144] In Phase I, a suitable common calibrator was identified, and in more recently published findings from Phase II, this common calibrator was shown to harmonize patients' results in most commercially available assays.[142]

Biological Variability of CRP

Despite being an acute-phase reactant, hsCRP exhibits a relatively low degree of intraindividual variability in clinically stable patients. In a study of such patients, the use of two independent measurements of hsCRP taken 90 days apart enabled the classification of 90% of participants into the exact or immediately adjacent biomarker tertile, a percentage comparable with that observed for cholesterol (Figure 27-31).[165,227] Furthermore, the age-adjusted correlation between two hsCRP measurements from blood samples drawn 5 years apart was 0.6, a value comparable with that of cholesterol and other lipid parameters.[262] Other groups of investigators reported a 3-year, age-adjusted reliability coefficient of 0.52.[149] Although findings from this epidemiologic study of initially healthy middle-aged men suggest that three independent measurements should be taken to maximize the biomarker's predictive ability,[149] whether serial assessment of hsCRP provides incremental clinical benefit is uncertain. Provided that a value less than 10 mg/L is obtained, the AHA/CDC panel recommends the use of two hsCRP measures taken 2 or more weeks apart, with the average value used to estimate vascular risk.[236] Because hsCRP may reflect subclinical infection, values greater than 10 mg/L should be disregarded initially and the test repeated when the patient has stabilized. Similar recommendations were issued by the NACB expert panel.[206] Furthermore, because hsCRP values are unaffected by food intake and exhibit almost no circadian variation,[192,227] measurements can be made without regard for fasting status or time of day.

Reference Values

Data from several large U.S. and European cohorts indicate that the distribution of circulating hsCRP concentrations appears comparable among men and women not using postmenopausal hormone replacement therapy (HRT),[128,271] with the 50th percentile for both genders being about 1.5 mg/L (Table 27-29). hsCRP concentrations are higher in women who use oral HRT than in women who do not,[264] and increased hsCRP from oral HRT has been associated with increased risk of thrombotic events.[175]

Information on the distribution of hsCRP concentrations in nonwhite populations is sparse. In the nationally

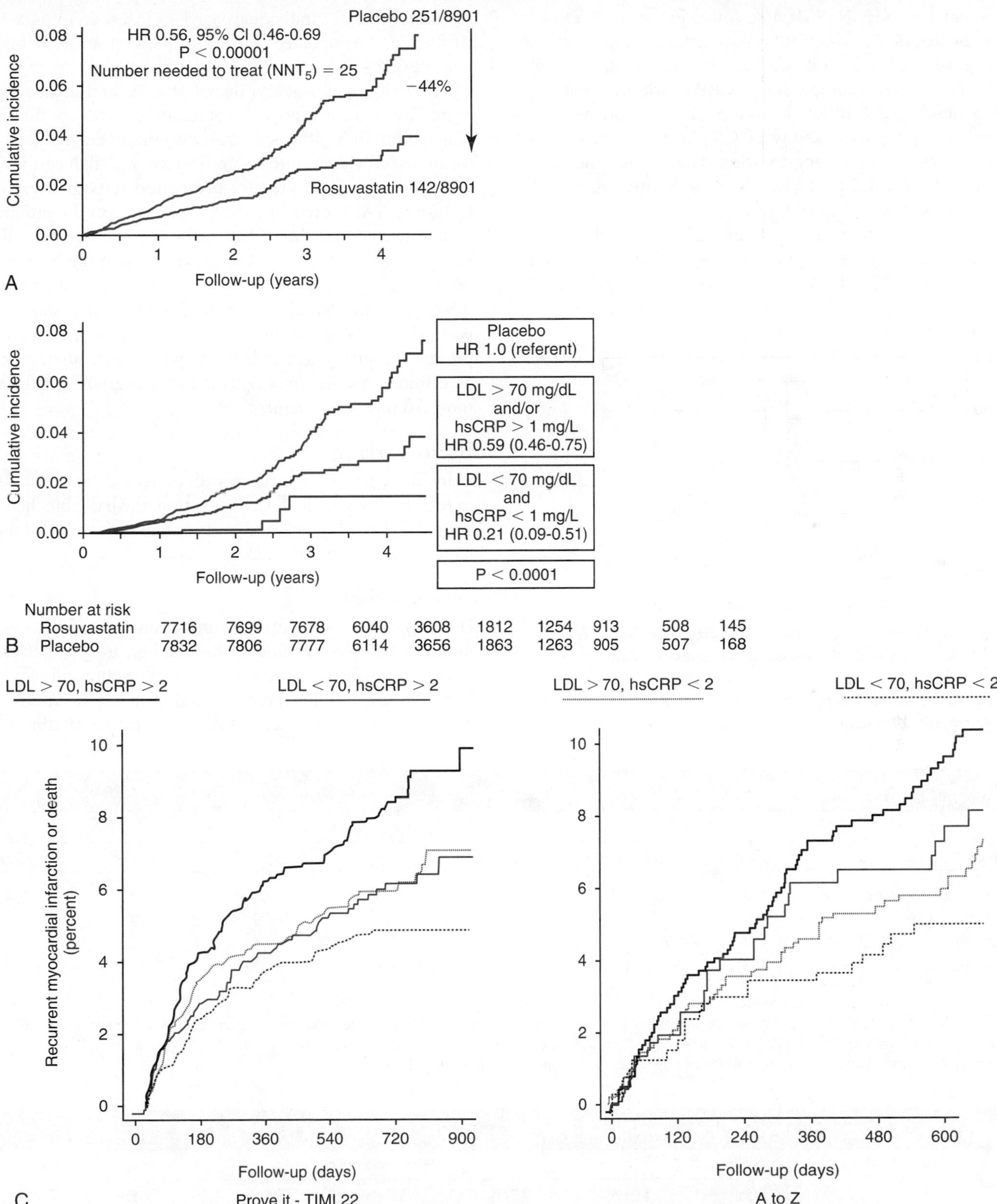

Figure 27-30 A, Cumulative incidence of cardiovascular events in the JUPITER trial. B, Cumulative incidence of cardiovascular events in JUPITER in placebo and statin groups according to achieved LDL cholesterol and hsCRP. C, Cumulative incidence of cardiovascular events in PROVE IT and A to Z in placebo and statin groups, according to achieved LDL cholesterol and hsCRP. (**A** *from N Engl J Med 2008;359:2195-207;* **B** *from Lancet 2009;373:1175-82;* **C** *from Circulation 2006;114:281-8; N Engl J Med 2005;352:20-8.)*

representative NHANES data set, no significant differences were noted in the distribution of hsCRP concentrations among white, black, and Mexican-American men[87] (Table 27-30). Moreover, a comparable hsCRP distribution was seen in Japanese men.[344] Although additional studies on the distribution and prognostic ability of CRP in nonwhite populations are clearly necessary, existing data are insufficient to support the exclusion of any racial or ethnic group from current guidelines for CRP testing.

Most studies have reported only a modest relationship between age (range, 18 to 88 years) and serum hsCRP concentrations.[128,271] In the WHS, for example, median hsCRP concentrations for individuals aged 45 to 54, 55 to 64, 65 to 74, and 75 years or older were 1.31, 1.89, 1.99, and 1.52 mg/L, respectively.[271]

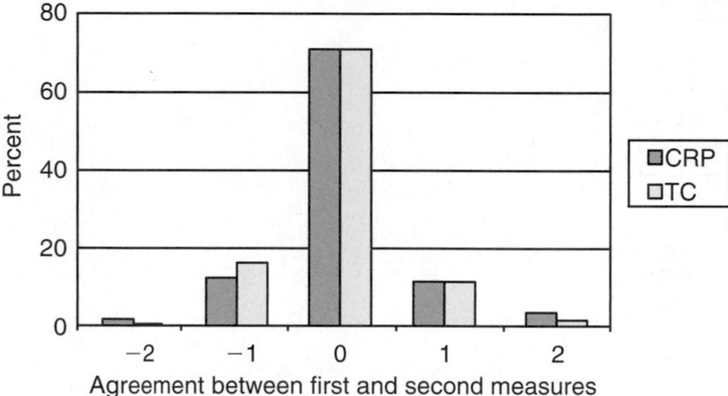

Figure 27-31 Within-person variability: comparison of hsCRP with total cholesterol. *(From Ledue TB, Rifai N. Preanalytic and analytic sources of variations in C-reactive protein measurement: implications for cardiovascular disease risk assessment. Clin Chem 2003;49:1258-71.)*

Reference values of less than 1, 1 to 3, and greater than 3 mg/L, which correspond to approximate tertiles of the CRP distribution in healthy adults, are recommended for classification of individuals into low, moderate, and high cardiovascular risk groups in primary prevention settings by AHA/CDC and NACB expert panels.[206,236] Because of the prognostic additive effect of hsCRP to the lipid screen, an algorithm combining hsCRP and LDL cholesterol using the NCEP cut points has been proposed (Figure 27-32).[271] According to the AHA/CDC and NACB recommendation, hsCRP should be part of the global risk assessment of CHD in the primary prevention setting, and individuals with intermediate risk as determined by the Framingham risk score will benefit the most from its measurement.[206,236]

HOMOCYSTEINE

Many disorders are associated with increased concentrations of total homocysteine.[248] In this section, the basic biochemistry, clinical significance, and measurement of total homocysteine (tHcy) are summarized.

Basic Biochemistry

Homocysteine is a sulfur-containing amino acid with each molecule of homocysteine containing one atom of sulfur. It is formed during the metabolism of methionine and requires folic acid as a cofactor (Figure 27-33). At low concentrations, homocysteine may be anabolized back to methionine in a

TABLE 27-29 Population Distributions of CRP, mg/L

	PERCENTILE						
Population	**5th**	**10th**	**25th**	**50th**	**75th**	**90th**	**95th**
American women*	0.2	0.3	0.6	1.5	3.5	6.6	9.1
American men	0.3	0.4	0.8	1.5	3.2	6.1	8.6
European women*	0.3	0.4	0.9	1.7	3.4	6.2	8.8
European men	0.3	0.6	0.8	1.6	3.3	6.5	8.6

*Only women not taking hormone replacement therapy.
Data from Rifai N, Ridker PM. Population distributions of C-reactive protein in apparently healthy men and women in the United States: implication for clinical interpretation. Clin Chem 2003;49:666-9; Imhof A, Frohlich M, et al. Distributions of C-reactive protein measured by high-sensitivity assays in apparently healthy men and women from different populations in Europe. Clin Chem 2003;49:669-72.

TABLE 27-30 Distributions of CRP Among Men, mg/L

	PERCENTILE						
	5th	**10th**	**25th**	**50th**	**75th**	**90th**	**95th**
White American	0.2	0.4	0.7	1.6	3.4	6.7	12.3
African American	0.1	0.2	0.7	1.7	3.9	8.2	13.2
Mexican American	0.2	0.4	0.6	1.6	3.2	6.3	9.8
Japanese	—	<0.3	0.4	1.6	3.5	7.8	—

Data from Ford ES, Giles WH, Myers GL, et al. Population distribution of high-sensitivity C-reactive protein among US men: findings from National Health and Nutrition Examination Survey 1999-2000. Clin Chem 2003;49:686-90; Yamada S, Gotoh T, Nakashima Y, et al. Distribution of serum C-reactive protein and its association with atherosclerotic risk factors in a Japanese population: Jichi Medical School Cohort Study. Am J Epidemiol 2001;153:1183-90.

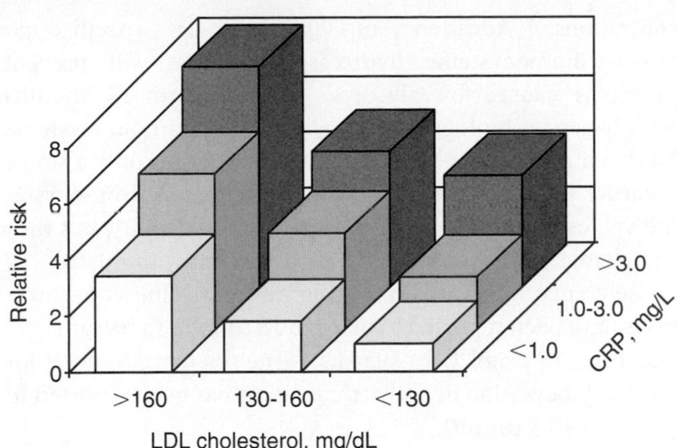

Figure 27-32 Algorithm for risk assessment of CHD risk employing CRP and LDL cholesterol. *(From Rifai N, Ridker PM. Population distributions of C-reactive protein in apparently healthy men and women in the United States: implication for clinical interpretation. Clin Chem 2003;49:666-9.)*

cycle that involves tetrahydrofolate or catabolized to cysteine by enzymes that require vitamin B as a cofactor. Consequently, a deficiency of folic acid or vitamins B_6 and B_{12} can result in increased concentrations of homocysteine (see Chapter 31).[146,278] Homocysteine does not normally accumulate in plasma because it is very unstable in aqueous solution and, when present in excess, undergoes oxidation to homocysteine.

Clinical Significance

Numerous studies have suggested an association between elevated concentrations of circulating homocysteine and various vascular and cardiovascular disorders.[12,55,248,330]

In addition, tHcy concentrations are related to (1) birth defects,[245] (2) pregnancy complications,[329] (3) psychiatric disorders,[220] and (4) mental impairment in the elderly.[292] Clinically, the measurement of tHcy is considered important (1) to diagnose homocystinuria, (2) to identify individuals with or at a risk of developing cobalamin or folate deficiency, and (3) to assess tHcy as a risk factor for cardiovascular disease (CVD) and other disorders.[12,55,248,330]

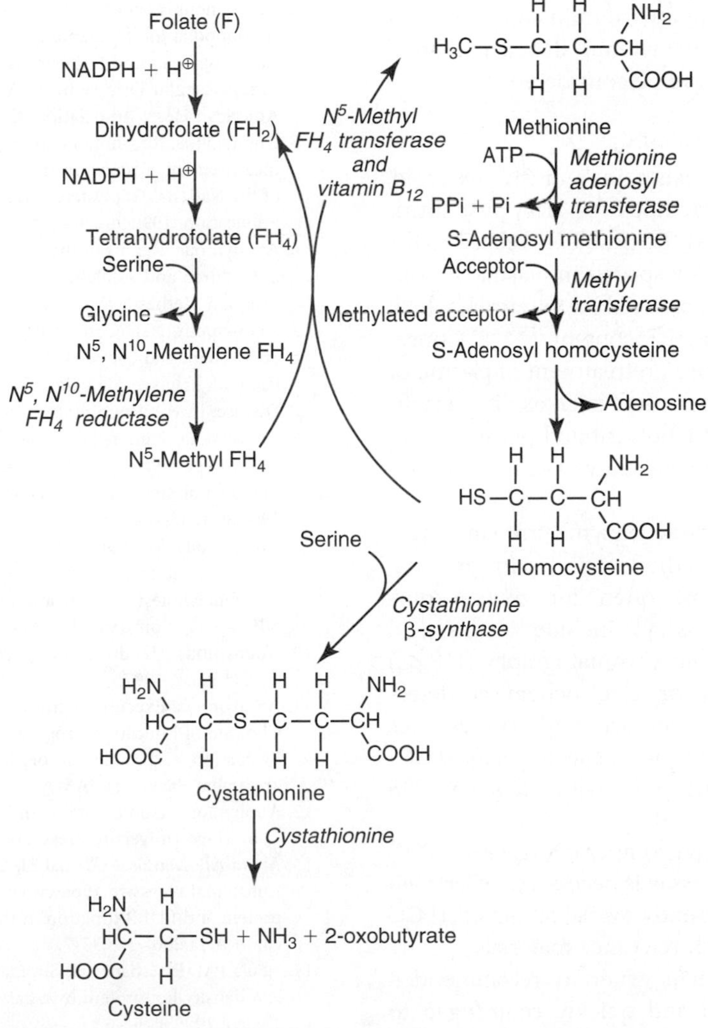

Figure 27-33 Biochemical pathways of the conversion of methionine to homocysteine and cysteine.

Although numerous studies have demonstrated a causal relationship between tHcy and CVD, controversy continues about the clinical significance of this relationship as (1) the methylenetetrahydrofolate reductase 677C>T polymorphism is a strong risk factor for increased tHcy but not for CVD; (2) an apparent discrepancy has been noted between prospective and retrospective case-control studies; and (3) data from controlled clinical trials are lacking.[248]

Because of this concern over the clinical significance of the causal relationship between tHcy and CVD,[40,160,174,246,299] Refsum and colleagues developed the following recommendations[248]:

- Measurement of tHcy in the general population to screen for CVD risk is not recommended.
- In young CVD patients (<40 years), tHcy should be measured to exclude homocystinuria.
- In patients with CVD or persons at high risk for CVD events, a high tHcy concentration should be used as a prognostic factor for CVD events and mortality.
- CVD patients with tHcy greater than 15 µmol/L belong to a high-risk group; it is especially important for them to follow a healthy life-style and to receive optimal treatment for known causal risk factors.
- Increased tHcy combined with low vitamin concentrations should be handled as a potential vitamin deficiency. Other causes of increased tHcy should be considered.

Measurement of Total Homocysteine

Physiologically, homocysteine exists in reduced, oxidized, and protein-bound forms.[198] Methods for tHcy first introduced in the mid 1980s resolved the problems related to the presence of multiple unstable Hcy species in plasma by converting all Hcy species into the reduced form, HcyH, which is measured as an indication of tHcy content.[244,247,298] Consequently, modern methods require pretreatment of plasma or serum specimens with a reducing agent such as dithioerythritol, dithiothreitol, mercaptoethanol, tributyl phosphine, or tris(2-carboxyl-ethyl) phosphine that converts all Hcy species into the reduced form.

Modern tHcy methods include enzyme immunoassays and chromatography-based methods.[240,317,319] In practice, immunoassays[89] are used most often for routine purposes.[237,290] Chromatographic assays include amino acid analysis; high-performance liquid chromatography (HPLC) with ultraviolet, fluorescence, or electrochemical detection[20,86,318,319,327]; capillary electrophoresis with fluorescence detection; gas chromatography-mass spectrometry (GC-MS); and liquid chromatography with tandem MS (MS-MS).[51,78,240,319]

The different tHcy methods give comparable results,[219,238,317] but standardization of the tHcy assay is necessary.[317] Certified reference materials are not currently available, but an IFCC working group is preparing such reference materials.

To obtain accurate results, it is generally recommended that specimens be refrigerated and quickly centrifuged to remove cells.[198] If unspun specimens are allowed to stand at room temperature, glycolysis can double homocysteine concentrations. Addition of fluoride or specific S-adenosylhomocysteine hydrolase inhibitors will prevent problems caused by glycolysis.[198] Short-term (1 month) within-person biological variability of plasma homocysteine has been reported to be approximately 7%; thus only a single measure of homocysteine is commonly done.[95] Homocysteine values do not show much long-term variability, but they can change in response to diet or treatment with folate.[95]

Reference intervals for fasting homocysteine concentrations have been reported to be 13 to 18 µmol/L for serum[221,319] and 10 to 15 µmol/L for plasma.[72] The reference interval for total homocysteine in pediatric patients has been reported to be 3.7 to 10.3 µmol/L.[328]

REFERENCES

1. Anonymous. The Lipid Research Clinics Coronary Primary Prevention Trial results. I. Reduction in incidence of coronary heart disease. JAMA 1984;251:351-64.
2. Anonymous. The Lipid Research Clinics Coronary Primary Prevention Trial results. II. The relationship of reduction in incidence of coronary heart disease to cholesterol lowering. JAMA 1984;251:365-74.
3. Anonymous. American Academy of Pediatrics Committee on Nutrition. Prudent life-style for children: dietary fat and cholesterol. Pediatrics 1986;78:521-5.
4. Anonymous. Diagnosis and treatment of primary hyperlipidemia in childhood: a Joint Statement for Physicians by the Committee on Atherosclerosis and Hypertension in Childhood of the Council of Cardiovascular Disease in the Young and the Nutrition Committee, American Heart Association. Circulation 1986;74:1181A-8A.
5. Anonymous. Recommendations for improving cholesterol measurement: a report from the Laboratory Standardization Panel of the National Cholesterol Education Program. Bethesda, Md: NIH Publication, 1990:90-2964.
6. Anonymous. Report of the Expert Panel on Blood Cholesterol Levels in Children and Adolescents. In: National Cholesterol Education Program. Bethesda, Md: NIH Publication, 1991:91-2732.
7. Anonymous. NIH Consensus Conference. Triglyceride, high-density lipoprotein, and coronary heart disease. NIH Consensus Development Panel on Triglyceride, High-Density Lipoprotein, and Coronary Heart Disease. JAMA 1993;269:505-10.
8. Anonymous. National Cholesterol Education Program. Second report of the Expert Panel on Detection, Evaluation, and Treatment of High Blood Cholesterol in Adults (Adult Treatment Panel II). Circulation 1994;89:1333-445.
9. Anonymous. Recommendations for improving cholesterol measurement: from the Working Group on Lipoprotein Measurement. National Cholesterol Education Program. Bethesda, Md: NIH/NHLBI NIH Publication, 1995:95-3044.
10. Anonymous. Handbook of lipoprotein testing. Washington, DC: AACC Press, 1997.
11. Anonymous. Executive summary of the third report of the National Cholesterol Education Program (NCEP) Expert Panel on Detection, Evaluation, and Treatment of High Blood Cholesterol in Adults (Adult Treatment Panel III). JAMA 2001;285:2486-97.
12. Anonymous. Homocysteine in health and disease. Cambridge, UK: Cambridge University Press, 2001.
13. Abera AB, Marais AD, Raal FJ, Leisegang F, Jones S, George P, et al. Autosomal recessive hypercholesterolaemia: discrimination of ARH protein and LDLR function in the homozygous FH phenotype. Clin Chim Acta 2007;378:33-7.
14. Abuja PM, Esterbauer H. Simulation of lipid peroxidation in low-density lipoprotein by a basic "skeleton" of reactions. Chem Res Toxicol 1995;8:753-63.
15. Alaupovic P. Apoliproproteins and lipoproteins. Atherosclerosis 1971;13:141-6.

16. Albers JJ, Hazzard WR. Immunochemical quantification of human plasma Lp(a) lipoprotein. Lipids 1974;9:15-26.
17. Albers JJ, Marcovina SM. Lipoprotein(a) quantification: comparison of methods and strategies for standardization. Curr Opin Lipidol 1994;5:417-21.
18. Albert CM, Ma J, Rifai N, Stampfer MJ, Ridker PM. Prospective study of C-reactive protein, homocysteine, and plasma lipid levels as predictors of sudden cardiac death. Circulation 2002;105:2595-9.
19. Albert MA, Danielson E, Rifai N, Ridker PM. Effect of statin therapy on C-reactive protein levels: the pravastatin inflammation/CRP evaluation (PRINCE): a randomized trial and cohort study. JAMA 2001;286:64-70.
20. Andersson A, Isaksson A, Brattstrom L, Hultberg B. Homocysteine and other thiols determined in plasma by HPLC and thiol-specific postcolumn derivatization. Clin Chem 1993;39:1590-7.
21. Ariyo AA, Thach C, Tracy R. Lp(a) lipoprotein, vascular disease, and mortality in the elderly. N Engl J Med 2003;349:2108-15.
22. Arranz-Pena ML, Tasende-Mata J, Martin-Gil FJ. Comparison of two homogeneous assays with a precipitation method and an ultracentrifugation method for the measurement of HDL-cholesterol. Clin Chem 1998;44:2499-505.
23. Assmann G, Eckardstein A, Brewer HB Jr. Familial analphaliproteinemia: Tangier disease. In: Scriver C, Beaudet A, Valle D, Sly W, Childs B, Kinzler K, et al, eds. The metabolic and molecular bases of inherited diseases. New York: McGraw-Hill, 2001:2937-81.
24. Assmann G, Herbert PN, Fredrickson DS, Forte T. Isolation and characterization of an abnormal high density lipoprotein in Tangier disease. J Clin Invest 1977;60:242-52.
25. Asztalos BF, Roheim PS, Milani RL, Lefevre M, McNamara JR, Horvath KV, et al. Distribution of ApoA-I-containing HDL subpopulations in patients with coronary heart disease. Arterioscler Thromb Vasc Biol 2000;20:2670-6.
26. Austin MA, Breslow JL, Hennekens CH, Buring JE, Willett WC, Krauss RM. Low-density lipoprotein subclass patterns and risk of myocardial infarction. JAMA 1988;260:1917-21.
27. Bachorik PS. Electrophoresis in the determination of plasma lipoprotein patterns. In: Lewis L, Opplt J, eds. CRC handbook of electrophoresis. Boca Raton, Fla: CRC Press, 1980;7.
28. Bachorik PS, Albers JJ. Precipitation methods for quantification of lipoproteins. Methods Enzymol 1986;129:78-100.
29. Bachorik PS, Lovejoy KL, Carroll MD, Johnson CL. Apolipoprotein B and AI distributions in the United States, 1988-1991: results of the National Health and Nutrition Examination Survey III (NHANES III). Clin Chem 1997;43:2364-78.
30. Bachorik PS, Rifkind BM, Kwiterovich PO. Lipids and dyslipoproteinemia. In: Henry J, ed. Clinical diagnosis and management by laboratory methods. Philadelphia: WB Saunders, 1996:208-36.
31. Bachorik PS, Walker R, Brownell KD, Stunkard AJ, Kwiterovich PO. Determination of high density lipoprotein-cholesterol in stored human plasma. J Lipid Res 1980;21:608-16.
32. Bachorik PS, Walker RE, Virgil DG. High-density-lipoprotein cholesterol in heparin-MnCl2 supernates determined with the Dow enzymic method after precipitation of Mn2+ with HCO3–. Clin Chem 1984;30:839-42.
33. Balk EM, Lau J, Goudas LC, Jordan HS, Kupelnick B, Kim LU, et al. Effects of statins on nonlipid serum markers associated with cardiovascular disease: a systematic review. Ann Intern Med 2003;139:670-82.
34. Bartlett GR. Phosphorus assay in column chromatography. J Biol Chem 1959;234:466-8.
35. Benzaquen LR, Yu H, Rifai N. High sensitivity C-reactive protein: an emerging role in cardiovascular risk assessment. Crit Rev Clin Lab Sci 2002;39:459-97.
36. Berenson GS, Wattigney WA, Tracy RE, Newman WP III, Srinivasan SR, Webber LS, et al. Atherosclerosis of the aorta and coronary arteries and cardiovascular risk factors in persons aged 6 to 30 years and studied at necropsy (The Bogalusa Heart Study). Am J Cardiol 1992;70:851-8.
37. Blake GJ, Rifai N, Buring JE, Ridker PM. Blood pressure, C-reactive protein, and risk of future cardiovascular events. Circulation 2003;108:2993-9.
38. Blankenhorn DH, Nessim SA, Johnson RL, Sanmarco ME, Azen SP, Cashin-Hemphill L. Beneficial effects of combined colestipol-niacin therapy on coronary atherosclerosis and coronary venous bypass grafts. JAMA 1987;257:3233-40.
39. Bookstein L, Gidding SS, Donovan M, Smith FA. Day-to-day variability of serum cholesterol, triglyceride, and high-density lipoprotein cholesterol levels: impact on the assessment of risk according to the National Cholesterol Education Program guidelines. Arch Intern Med 1990;150:1653-7.
40. Booth GL, Wang EE. Preventive health care, 2000 update: screening and management of hyperhomocysteinemia for the prevention of coronary artery disease events. The Canadian Task Force on Preventive Health Care. CMAJ 2000;163:21-9.
41. Breslow JL. Familial disorders of high-density lipoprotein metabolism. In: Scriver C, Beaudet A, Sly W, Valle D, eds. The metabolic and molecular bases of inherited diseases. New York: McGraw-Hill, 1995: 2031-52.
42. Brown G, Albers JJ, Fisher LD, Schaefer SM, Lin JT, Kaplan C, et al. Regression of coronary artery disease as a result of intensive lipid-lowering therapy in men with high levels of apolipoprotein B. N Engl J Med 1990;323:1289-98.
43. Brown MS, Goldstein JL. Lipoprotein metabolism in the macrophage: implications for cholesterol deposition in atherosclerosis. Annu Rev Biochem 1983;52:223-61.
44. Brown MS, Goldstein JL. A receptor-mediated pathway for cholesterol homeostasis. Science 1986;232:34-47.
45. Brown SA, Hutchinson R, Morrisett J, Boerwinkle E, Davis CE, Gotto AM Jr, et al. Plasma lipid, lipoprotein cholesterol, and apoprotein distributions in selected US communities: the Atherosclerosis Risk in Communities (ARIC) study. Arterioscler Thromb 1993;13:1139-58.
46. Brunzell JD, Deeb S. Familial lipoprotein lipase deficiency, apo C-II deficiency, and hepatic lipase deficiency. In: Scriver C, Beaudet A, Sly W, Valle D, eds. The metabolic basis of inherited diseases. New York: McGraw-Hill, 2001:2789-819.
47. Burstein M, Legmann P. Lipoprotein precipitation. Monogr Atheroscler 1982;11:1-131.
48. Buxtorf JC, Baudet MF, Martin C, Richard JL, Jacotot B. Seasonal variations of serum lipids and apoproteins. Ann Nutr Metab 1988;32:68-74.
49. Campos H, Blijlevens E, McNamara JR, Ordovas JM, Posner BM, Wilson PW, et al. LDL particle size distribution: results from the Framingham Offspring Study. Arterioscler Thromb 1992;12:1410-9.
50. Castelli WP, Doyle JT, Gordon T, Hames CG, Hjortland MC, Hulley SB, et al. HDL cholesterol and other lipids in coronary heart disease: the Cooperative Lipoprotein Phenotyping Study. Circulation 1977; 55:767-72.
51. Chace DH, Hillman SL, Millington DS, Kahler SG, Adam BW, Levy HL. Rapid diagnosis of homocystinuria and other hypermethioninemias from newborns' blood spots by tandem mass spectrometry. Clin Chem 1996;42:349-55.
52. Chae CU, Lee RT, Rifai N, Ridker PM. Blood pressure and inflammation in apparently healthy men. Hypertension 2001;38: 399-403.
53. Chait A, Albers JJ, Brunzell JD. Very low density lipoprotein overproduction in genetic forms of hypertriglyceridaemia. Eur J Clin Invest 1980;10:17-22.
54. Chen CH, Albers JJ. Activation of lecithin: cholesterol acyltransferase by apolipoproteins E-2, E-3, and A-IV isolated from human plasma. Biochim Biophys Acta 1985;836:279-85.
55. Christen WG, Ajani UA, Glynn RJ, Hennekens CH. Blood levels of homocysteine and increased risks of cardiovascular disease: causal or casual? Arch Intern Med 2000;160:422-34.

56. Chung BH, Segrest JP, Ray MJ, Brunzell JD, Hokanson JE, Krauss RM, et al. Single vertical spin density gradient ultracentrifugation. Methods Enzymol 1986;128:181-209.
57. Chung BH, Wilkinson T, Geer JC, Segrest JP. Preparative and quantitative isolation of plasma lipoproteins: rapid, single discontinuous density gradient ultracentrifugation in a vertical rotor. J Lipid Res 1980;21:284-91.
58. Cohn JS, McNamara JR, Cohn SD, Ordovas JM, Schaefer EJ. Postprandial plasma lipoprotein changes in human subjects of different ages. J Lipid Res 1988;29:469-79.
59. Cohn JS, McNamara JR, Schaefer EJ. Lipoprotein cholesterol concentrations in the plasma of human subjects as measured in the fed and fasted states. Clin Chem 1988;34:2456-9.
60. Cole TG. Glycerol blanking in triglyceride assays: is it necessary? Clin Chem 1990;36:1267-8.
61. Contois J, McNamara JR, Lammi-Keefe C, Wilson PW, Massov T, Schaefer EJ. Reference intervals for plasma apolipoprotein A-1 determined with a standardized commercial immunoturbidimetric assay: results from the Framingham Offspring Study. Clin Chem 1996;42:507-14.
62. Contois JH, McConnell JP, Sethi AA, Csako G, Devaraj S, Hoefner DM, et al. Apolipoprotein B and cardiovascular disease risk: position statement from the AACC Lipoproteins and Vascular Diseases Division Working Group on Best Practices. Clin Chem 2009;55:407-19.
63. Contois JH, McNamara JR, Lammi-Keefe CJ, Wilson PW, Massov T, Schaefer EJ. Reference intervals for plasma apolipoprotein B determined with a standardized commercial immunoturbidimetric assay: results from the Framingham Offspring Study. Clin Chem 1996;42:515-23.
64. Cooper GR, Smith SJ, Duncan IW, Mather A, Fellows WD, Foley T, et al. Interlaboratory testing of the transferability of a candidate reference method for total cholesterol in serum. Clin Chem 1986;32:921-9.
65. Cooper GR, Smith SJ, Wiebe DA, Kuchmak M, Hannon WH. International survey of apolipoproteins A1 and B measurements (1983-1984). Clin Chem 1985;31:223-8.
66. Cortner JA, Coates PM, Bennett MJ, Cryer DR, Le NA. Familial combined hyperlipidaemia: use of stable isotopes to demonstrate overproduction of very low-density lipoprotein apolipoprotein B by the liver. J Inherit Metab Dis 1991;14:915-22.
67. Couderc R, Mahieux F, Bailleul S, Fenelon G, Mary R, Fermanian J. Prevalence of apolipoprotein E phenotypes in ischemic cerebrovascular disease. A case-control study. Stroke 1993;24:661-4.
68. Curb JD, Abbott RD, Rodriguez BL, Sakkinen P, Popper JS, Yano K, et al. C-reactive protein and the future risk of thromboembolic stroke in healthy men. Circulation 2003;107:2016-20.
69. Cushman M, McClure LA, Howard VJ, Jenny NS, Lakoski SG, Howard G. Implications of increased C-reactive protein for cardiovascular risk stratification in black and white men and women in the US. Clin Chem 2009;55:1627-36.
70. Dallongeville J, Lussier-Cacan S, Davignon J. Modulation of plasma triglyceride levels by apoE phenotype: a meta-analysis. J Lipid Res 1992;33:447-54.
71. Daniels SR, Greer FR. Lipid screening and cardiovascular health in childhood. Pediatrics 2008;122:198-208.
72. Davignon J, Gregg RE, Sing CF. Apolipoprotein E polymorphism and atherosclerosis. Arteriosclerosis 1988;8:1-21.
73. de Keijzer MH, Elbers D, Baadenhuijsen H, Demacker PN. Evaluation of five different high-density lipoprotein cholesterol assays: the most precise are not the most accurate. Ann Clin Biochem 1999;36(Pt 2):168-75.
74. Deacon AC, Dawson PJ. Enzymic assay of total cholesterol involving chemical or enzymic hydrolysis—a comparison of methods. Clin Chem 1979;25:976-84.
75. DeLong DM, Delong ER, Wood PD, Lippel K, Rifkind BM. A comparison of methods for the estimation of plasma low- and very low-density lipoprotein cholesterol. The Lipid Research Clinics Prevalence Study. JAMA 1986;256:2372-7.
76. Devaraj S, Singh U, Jialal I. The evolving role of C-reactive protein in atherothrombosis. Clin Chem 2009;55:229-38.
77. Devaraj S, Xu DY, Jialal I. C-reactive protein increases plasminogen activator inhibitor-1 expression and activity in human aortic endothelial cells: implications for the metabolic syndrome and atherothrombosis. Circulation 2003;107:398-404.
78. Ducros V, Demuth K, Sauvant MP, Quillard M, Causse E, Candito M, et al. Methods for homocysteine analysis and biological relevance of the results. J Chromatogr B Analyt Technol Biomed Life Sci 2002;781:207-26.
79. Durrington PN. Lipoprotein (a). Baillieres Clin Endocrinol Metab 1995;9:773-95.
80. Ellerbe P, Myers GL, Cooper GR, Hertz HS, Sniegoski LT, Welch MJ, et al. A comparison of results for cholesterol in human serum obtained by the reference method and by the definitive, ethod of the national reference system for cholesterol. Clin Chem 1990;36:370-5.
81. Elliot P, Chambers JC, Zhang W, Clarke R, Hopewell JC, Peden JF, et al. Genetic loci associated with C-reactive protein levels and risk of coronary heart disease. JAMA 2009;302:37-48.
82. Emi M, Wu LL, Robertson MA, Myers RL, Hegele RA, Williams RR, et al. Genotyping and sequence analysis of apolipoprotein E isoforms. Genomics 1988;3:373-9.
83. Enos WF, Holmes RH, Beyer J. Landmark article, July 18, 1953. Coronary disease among United States soldiers killed in action in Korea: preliminary report. JAMA 1986;256:2859-62.
84. Ensign W, Hill N, Heward CB. Disparate LDL phenotypic classification among 4 different methods assessing LDL particle characteristics. Clin Chem 2006;52:1722-7.
85. Esteban-Salán M, Guimón-Bardesi A, de La Viuda-Unzueta JM, Azcarate-Ania MN, Pascual-Usandizaga P, Amoroto-Del-Rio E. Analytical and clinical evaluation of two homogeneous assays for LDL-cholesterol in hyperlipidemic patients. Clin Chem 2000;46:1121-31.
86. Evrovski J, Callaghan M, Cole DE. Determination of homocysteine by HPLC with pulsed integrated amperometry. Clin Chem 1995;41: 757-8.
87. Ford ES, Giles WH, Myers GL, Mannino DM. Population distribution of high-sensitivity C-reactive protein among US men: findings from National Health and Nutrition Examination Survey 1999-2000. Clin Chem 2003;49:686-90.
88. Forte TM, Shu X, Ryan RO. The ins (cell) and outs (plasma) of apolipoprotein A-V. J Lipid Res 2009;50(Suppl):S150-5.
89. Frantzen F, Faaren AL, Alfheim I, Nordhei AK. Enzyme conversion immunoassay for determining total homocysteine in plasma or serum. Clin Chem 1998;44:311-6.
90. Franzin M, Ferro C, Ceriotti F, Carobene A, Martini R, Guerra E. Optimization of a designed comparison method (DCM) for triglycerides measurement. Clin Chem Lab Med 1999;37:S260.
91. Freedman DS, Srinivasan SR, Shear CL, Franklin FA, Webber LS, Berenson GS. The relation of apolipoproteins A-I and B in children to parental myocardial infarction. N Engl J Med 1986;315:721-6.
92. Freeman DJ, Norrie J, Caslake MJ, Gaw A, Ford I, Lowe GD, et al. C-reactive protein is an independent predictor of risk for the development of diabetes in the West of Scotland Coronary Prevention Study. Diabetes 2002;51:1596-600.
93. Friedewald WT, Levy RI, Fredrickson DS. Estimation of the concentration of low-density lipoprotein cholesterol in plasma, without use of the preparative ultracentrifuge. Clin Chem 1972;18:499-502.
94. Funk CD, FitzGerald GA. COX-2 inhibitors and cardiovascular risk. J Cardiovasc Pharmacol 2007;50:470-9.
95. Garg UC, Zheng ZJ, Folsom AR, Moyer YS, Tsai MY, McGovern P, et al. Short-term and long-term variability of plasma homocysteine measurement. Clin Chem 1997;43:141-5.
96. Glueck CJ, Mellies MJ, Srivastava L, Knowles HC Jr, Fallat RW, Tsang RC, et al. Insulin, obesity, and triglyceride interrelationships in sixteen children with familial hypertriglyceridemia. Pediatr Res 1977; 11:13-9.

97. Goldstein JL, Ho YK, Basu SK, Brown MS. Binding site on macrophages that mediates uptake and degradation of acetylated low density lipoprotein, producing massive cholesterol deposition. Proc Natl Acad Sci U S A 1979;76:333-7.
98. Goldstein JL, Hobbs HH, Brown MS. Familial hypercholesterolemia. In: Scriver C, Beaudet A, Sly W, Valle D, eds. The metabolic and molecular bases of inherited diseases. New York: McGraw-Hill, 2001:2863-914.
99. Goldstein JL, Schrott HG, Hazzard WR, Bierman EL, Motulsky AG. Hyperlipidemia in coronary heart disease. II. Genetic analysis of lipid levels in 176 families and delineation of a new inherited disorder, combined hyperlipidemia. J Clin Invest 1973;52:1544-68.
100. Gordon DJ, Trost DC, Hyde J, Whaley FS, Hannan PJ, Jacobs DR Jr, et al. Seasonal cholesterol cycles: the Lipid Research Clinics Coronary Primary Prevention Trial placebo group. Circulation 1987;76:1224-31.
101. Gordon T, Kannel WB, Castelli WP, Dawber TR. Lipoproteins, cardiovascular disease, and death. The Framingham Study. Arch Intern Med 1981;141:1128-31.
102. Gotto AM Jr. Management of dyslipidemia. Am J Med 2002;112(Suppl 8A):10S-8S.
103. Gotto AM Jr. Treating hypercholesterolemia: looking forward. Clin Cardiol 2003;26:I21-I28.
104. Gotto AM, Brown WV, Levy RI, Birnbaumer ME, Fredrickson DS. Evidence for the identity of the major apoprotein in low density and very low density lipoproteins in normal subjects and patients with familial hyperlipoproteinemia. J Clin Invest 1972;51:1486-94.
105. Gotto AM Jr, Pownall HJ, Havel RJ. Introduction to the plasma lipoproteins. Methods Enzymol 1986;128:3-41.
106. Gotto AM Jr, Whitney E, Stein EA, Shapiro DR, Clearfield M, Weis S, et al. Relation between baseline and on-treatment lipid parameters and first acute major coronary events in the Air Force/Texas Coronary Atherosclerosis Prevention Study (AFCAPS/TexCAPS). Circulation 2000;101:477-84.
107. Green EK, Bain SC, Day PJ, Barnett AH, Charleson F, Jones AF, et al. Detection of human apolipoprotein E3, E2, and E4 genotypes by an allele-specific oligonucleotide-primed polymerase chain reaction assay: development and validation. Clin Chem 1991;37:1263-8.
108. Greenland P, Knoll MD, Stamler J, Neaton JD, Dyer AR, Garside DB, et al. Major risk factors as antecedents of fatal and nonfatal coronary heart disease events. JAMA 2003;290:891-7.
109. Grundy SM. Cholesterol and coronary heart disease: a new era. JAMA 1986;256:2849-58.
110. Gwynne JT. High-density lipoprotein cholesterol levels as a marker of reverse cholesterol transport. Am J Cardiol 1989;64:10G-7G.
111. Hainline AJ, Karon J, Lippel K. Manual of laboratory operations. Bethesda, Md: U.S. Department of Health and Human Services, 1982.
112. Halloran P, Roetering H, Pisani T, van den BB, Cobbaert C. Reference standardization and analytical performance of a liquid homogeneous high-density lipoprotein cholesterol method compared with chemical precipitation method. Arch Pathol Lab Med 1999;123: 317-26.
113. Harris EK, Kanofsky P, Shakarji G, Cotlove E. Biological and analytic components of variation in long-term studies of serum constituents in normal subjects. II. Estimating biological components of variation. Clin Chem 1970;16:1022-7.
114. Harris N, Galpchian V, Rifai N. Three routine methods for measuring high-density lipoprotein cholesterol compared with the reference method. Clin Chem 1996;42:738-43.
115. Harris N, Galpchian V, Thomas J, Iannotti E, Law T, Rifai N. Three generations of high-density lipoprotein cholesterol assays compared with ultracentrifugation/dextran sulfate Mg^{2+} method. Clin Chem 1997;43:816-23.
116. Harris N, Neufeld EJ, Newburger JW, Ticho B, Baker A, Ginsburg GS, et al. Analytical performance and clinical utility of a direct LDL-cholesterol assay in a hyperlipidemic pediatric population. Clin Chem 1996;42:1182-8.
117. Havel RJ. Determination and clinical significance of triglyceride-rich lipoprotein remnants. In: Rifai N, Warnick GR, Donovan M, eds. Handbook of lipoprotein testing. Washington, DC: AACC Press, 2000:565-80.
118. Havel RJ, Kane JP. Introduction: structure and metabolism of plasma lipoproteins. In: Scriver C, Beaudet A, Sly W, Valle D, eds. The metabolic and molecular bases of inherited diseases. New York: McGraw-Hill, 2001:2705-16.
119. Heinecke JW. The HDL proteome: a marker—and perhaps mediator—of coronary artery disease. J Lipid Res 2009;50(Suppl):S167-71.
120. Hirano T, Ito Y, Saegusa H, Yoshino G. A novel and simple method for quantification of small, dense LDL. J Lipid Res 2003;44:2193-201.
121. Hixson JE, Vernier DT. Restriction isotyping of human apolipoprotein E by gene amplification and cleavage with HhaI. J Lipid Res 1990;31:545-8.
122. Hlatky MA. Expanding the orbit of primary prevention—moving beyond JUPITER. N Engl J Med 2008;359:2280-2.
123. Hobbs HH, Leitersdorf E, Goldstein JL, Brown MS, Russell DW. Multiple crm- mutations in familial hypercholesterolemia: evidence for 13 alleles, including four deletions. J Clin Invest 1988;81:909-17.
124. Holvoet P, Vanhaecke J, Janssens S, Van de WF, Collen D. Oxidized LDL and malondialdehyde-modified LDL in patients with acute coronary syndromes and stable coronary artery disease. Circulation 1998;98:1487-94.
125. Hoogewerf AJ, Cisar LA, Evans DC, Bensadoun A. Effect of chlorate on the sulfation of lipoprotein lipase and heparan sulfate proteoglycans: sulfation of heparan sulfate proteoglycans affects lipoprotein lipase degradation. J Biol Chem 1991;266:16564-71.
126. Horiuchi Y, Takanohashi K, Oikawa S, Numabe A, Hishinuma A, Ieiri T. Measurement of serum low density lipoprotein-cholesterol in patients with hypertriglycemia. Electrophoresis 2000;21:293-6.
127. Hubbard RS, Hirany SV, Devaraj S, Martin L, Parupia J, Jialal I. Evaluation of a rapid homogeneous method for direct measurement of high-density lipoprotein cholesterol. Am J Clin Pathol 1998;110:495-502.
128. Imhof A, Frohlich M, Loewel H, Helbecque N, Woodward M, Amouyel P, et al. Distributions of C-reactive protein measured by high-sensitivity assays in apparently healthy men and women from different populations in Europe. Clin Chem 2003;49:669-72.
129. Ito MK. ISIS 301012 gene therapy for hypercholesterolemia: sense, antisense, or nonsense? Ann Pharmacother 2007;41:1669-78.
130. Izawa S, Okada M, Matsui H, Horita Y. A new direct method for measuring HDL-cholesterol which does not produce any biased values. J Med Pharm Sci 1997;37:1385-8.
131. Jackson RL, Tajima S, Yamamura T, Yokoyama S, Yamamoto A. Comparison of apolipoprotein C-II-deficient triacylglycerol-rich lipoproteins and trioleoylglycerol/phosphatidylcholine-stabilized particles as substrates for lipoprotein lipase. Biochim Biophys Acta 1986;875:211-9.
132. Jialal I, Hirany SV, Devaraj S, Sherwood TA. Comparison of an immunoprecipitation method for direct measurement of LDL-cholesterol with beta-quantification (ultracentrifugation). Am J Clin Pathol 1995;104:76-81.
133. Johnson CL, Rifkind BM, Sempos CT, Carroll MD, Bachorik PS, Briefel RR, et al. Declining serum total cholesterol levels among US adults. The National Health and Nutrition Examination Surveys. JAMA 1993;269:3002-8.
134. Jurgens G, Koltringer P. Lipoprotein(a) in ischemic cerebrovascular disease: a new approach to the assessment of risk for stroke. Neurology 1987;37:513-5.
135. Kafonek SD, Derby CA, Bachorik PS. Biological variability of lipoproteins and apolipoproteins in patients referred to a lipid clinic. Clin Chem 1992;38:864-72.
136. Kakuyama T, Kimura S, Hasiguchi Y. Fully automated determination of HDL-cholesterol from human serum with Hitachi 911. Clin Chem 1994;40:A1104.
137. Kane JP, Havel RJ. Disorders of the biogenesis and secretion of lipoproteins containing the B apolipoprotein. In: Scriver C, Beaudet A, Sly W, Valle D, eds. The metabolic and molecular bases of inherited diseases. New York: McGraw-Hill, 2001:2717-52.

138. Karathanasis SK, Ferris E, Haddad IA. DNA inversion within the apolipoproteins AI/CIII/AIV encoding gene cluster of certain patients with premature atherosclerosis. Proc Natl Acad Sci U S A 1987;84:7198-202.
139. Kayamori Y, Hatsuyama H, Tsujioka T, Nasu M, Katayama Y. Endpoint colorimetric method for assaying total cholesterol in serum with cholesterol dehydrogenase. Clin Chem 1999;45:2158-63.
140. Khachadurian AK, Uthman SM. Experiences with the homozygous cases of familial hypercholesterolemia: a report of 52 patients. Nutr Metab 1973;15:132-40.
141. Khot UN, Khot MB, Bajzer CT, Sapp SK, Ohman EM, Brener SJ, et al. Prevalence of conventional risk factors in patients with coronary heart disease. JAMA 2003;290:898-904.
142. Kimberly MM, Caudill SP, Vesper HW, Monsell EA, Miller WG, Rej R, et al. Standardization of high-sensitivity immunoassays for measurement of C-reactive protein. II. Two approaches for assessing commutability of a reference material. Clin Chem 2009;55:342-50.
143. Kimberly MM, Leary ET, Cole TG, Waymack PP. Selection, validation, standardization, and performance of a designated comparison method for HDL-cholesterol for use in the cholesterol reference method laboratory network. Clin Chem 1999;45:1803-12.
144. Kimberly MM, Vesper HW, Caudill SP, Cooper GR, Rifai N, Dati F, Myers GL. Standardization of immunoassays for measurement of high-sensitivity C-reactive protein. Phase I: evaluation of secondary reference materials. Clin Chem 2003;49:611-6.
145. Kishi K, Ochiai K, Ohta Y, Uemura Y, Kanatani K, Nakajima K, et al. Highly sensitive cholesterol assay with enzymatic cycling applied to measurement of remnant lipoprotein-cholesterol in serum. Clin Chem 2002;48:737-41.
146. Klee GG. Cobalamin and folate evaluation: measurement of methylmalonic acid and homocysteine vs vitamin B(12) and folate. Clin Chem 2000;46:1277-83.
147. Koenig W. Is hsCRP Back on Board? Implications from the JUPITER Trial. Clin Chem 2009;55:216-8.
148. Koenig W, Sund M, Frohlich M, Fischer HG, Lowel H, Doring A, et al. C-reactive protein, a sensitive marker of inflammation, predicts future risk of coronary heart disease in initially healthy middle-aged men: results from the MONICA (Monitoring Trends and Determinants in Cardiovascular Disease) Augsburg Cohort Study, 1984 to 1992. Circulation 1999;99:237-42.
149. Koenig W, Sund M, Frohlich M, Lowel H, Hutchinson WL, Pepys MB. Refinement of the association of serum C-reactive protein concentration and coronary heart disease risk by correction for within-subject variation over time: the MONICA Augsburg Studies, 1984 and 1987. Am J Epidemiol 2003;158:357-64.
150. Kranzhofer R, Schmidt J, Pfeiffer CA, Hagl S, Libby P, Kubler W. Angiotensin induces inflammatory activation of human vascular smooth muscle cells. Arterioscler Thromb Vasc Biol 1999;19:1623-9.
151. Kubono K, Sakurabayashi I, Tsukada Y. Immunoglobulin interference in the homogeneous HDL cholesterol methods. Clin Chem 2000;46:A98.
152. Kukita H, Hiwada K, Kokubu T. Serum apolipoprotein A-I, A-II and B levels and their discriminative values in relatives of patients with coronary artery disease. Atherosclerosis 1984;51:261-7.
153. Kuller LH, Tracy RP, Shaten J, Meilahn EN. Relation of C-reactive protein and coronary heart disease in the MRFIT nested case-control study. Multiple Risk Factor Intervention Trial. Am J Epidemiol 1996;144:537-47.
154. Kwiterovich PO Jr. HyperapoB: a pleiotropic phenotype characterized by dense low-density lipoproteins and associated with coronary artery disease. Clin Chem 1988;34:B71-7.
155. Kwiterovich PO Jr. Diagnosis and management of familial dyslipoproteinemia in children and adolescents. Pediatr Clin North Am 1990;37:1489-523.
156. Labeur C, Shepherd J, Rosseneu M. Immunological assays of apolipoproteins in plasma: methods and instrumentation. Clin Chem 1990;36:591-7.
157. Lackner C, Cohen JC, Hobbs HH. Molecular definition of the extreme size polymorphism in apolipoprotein(a). Hum Mol Genet 1993;2:933-40.
158. Lamarche B, Tchernof A, Mauriege P, Cantin B, Dagenais GR, Lupien PJ, et al. Fasting insulin and apolipoprotein B levels and low-density lipoprotein particle size as risk factors for ischemic heart disease. JAMA 1998;279:1955-61.
159. Lambert G. Unravelling the functional significance of PCSK9. Curr Opin Lipidol 2007;18:304-9.
160. Langman LJ, Cole DE. Homocysteine: cholesterol of the 90s? Clin Chim Acta 1999;286:63-80.
161. LaRosa JC, Chambless LE, Criqui MH, Frantz ID, Glueck CJ, Heiss G, et al. Patterns of dyslipoproteinemia in selected North American populations. The Lipid Research Clinics Program Prevalence Study. Circulation 1986;73:I12-29.
162. Lauer RM, Clarke WR. Use of cholesterol measurements in childhood for the prediction of adult hypercholesterolemia. The Muscatine Study. JAMA 1990;264:3034-8.
163. Lawlor J, Pelczar D, Sane R, Siek G. Performance characteristic of the RDI homogeneous HDL cholesterol assay. Clin Chem 1998;44:A79.
164. Leary ET, Wang T, Baker DJ, Cilla DD, Zhong J, Warnick GR, et al. Evaluation of an immunoseparation method for quantitative measurement of remnant-like particle-cholesterol in serum and plasma. Clin Chem 1998;44:2490-8.
165. Ledue TB, Rifai N. Preanalytic and analytic sources of variations in C-reactive protein measurement: implications for cardiovascular disease risk assessment. Clin Chem 2003;49:1258-71.
166. Lee J, Lauer RM, Clarke WR. Lipoproteins in the progeny of young men with coronary artery disease: children with increased risk. Pediatrics 1986;78:330-7.
167. Lees RS, Wilson DE, Schonfeld G, Fleet S. The familial dyslipoproteinemias. Prog Med Genet 1973;9:237-90.
168. Libby P. Current concepts of the pathogenesis of the acute coronary syndromes. Circulation 2001;104:365-72.
169. Lin MJ, Hoke C, Ettinger B. Evaluation of homogeneous high-density lipoprotein cholesterol assay on a BM/Hitachi 747-200 analyzer. Clin Chem 1998;44:1050-2.
170. Lindgren FT, Elliott HA, Gofman JW. The ultracentrifugal characterization and isolation of human blood lipids and lipoproteins, with applications to the study of atherosclerosis. J Phys Colloid Chem 1951;55:80-93.
171. Lippi U, Graziani MS, Manzato F, Schinella M. Procedure for effective separation of high-density lipoproteins in normal serum and hypertriglyceridemic samples. Clin Biochem 1987;20:313-5.
172. Maciejko JJ, Holmes DR, Kottke BA, Zinsmeister AR, Dinh DM, Mao SJ. Apolipoprotein A-I as a marker of angiographically assessed coronary-artery disease. N Engl J Med 1983;309:385-9.
173. Mahley RW, Innerarity TL, Rall SC Jr, Weisgraber KH. Plasma lipoproteins: apolipoprotein structure and function. J Lipid Res 1984;25:1277-94.
174. Malinow MR, Bostom AG, Krauss RM. Homocyst(e)ine, diet, and cardiovascular diseases: a statement for healthcare professionals from the Nutrition Committee, American Heart Association. Circulation 1999;99:178-82.
175. Manson JE, Hsia J, Johnson KC, Rossouw JE, Assaf AR, Lasser NL, et al. Estrogen plus progestin and the risk of coronary heart disease. N Engl J Med 2003;349:523-34.
176. Marcovina SM, Albers JJ. Apolipoprotein assays: standardization and quality control. Scand J Clin Lab Invest Suppl 1990;198:58-65.
177. Marcovina SM, Albers JJ, Gabel B, Koschinsky ML, Gaur VP. Effect of the number of apolipoprotein(a) kringle 4 domains on immunochemical measurements of lipoprotein(a). Clin Chem 1995;41:246-55.
178. Marcovina SM, Albers JJ, Henderson LO, Hannon WH. International Federation of Clinical Chemistry standardization project for measurements of apolipoproteins A-I and B. III. Comparability of apolipoprotein A-I values by use of international reference material. Clin Chem 1993;39:773-81.

179. Marcovina SM, Albers JJ, Kennedy H, Mei JV, Henderson LO, Hannon WH. International Federation of Clinical Chemistry standardization project for measurements of apolipoproteins A-I and B. IV. Comparability of apolipoprotein B values by use of International Reference Material. Clin Chem 1994;40:586-92.
180. Marcovina SM, Albers JJ, Scanu AM, Kennedy H, Giaculli F, Berg K, et al. Use of a reference material proposed by the International Federation of Clinical Chemistry and Laboratory Medicine to evaluate analytical methods for the determination of plasma lipoprotein(a). Clin Chem 2000;46:1956-67.
181. Marcovina SM, Gaur VP, Albers JJ. Biological variability of cholesterol, triglyceride, low- and high-density lipoprotein cholesterol, lipoprotein(a), and apolipoproteins A-I and B. Clin Chem 1994;40:574-8.
182. Marcovina SM, Hobbs HH, Albers JJ. Relation between number of apolipoprotein(a) kringle 4 repeats and mobility of isoforms in agarose gel: basis for a standardized isoform nomenclature. Clin Chem 1996;42:436-9.
183. Marcovina SM, Koschinsky ML, Albers JJ, Skarlatos S. Report of the National Heart, Lung, and Blood Institute Workshop on Lipoprotein(a) and Cardiovascular Disease: recent advances and future directions. Clin Chem 2003;49:1785-96.
184. Marcovina SM, Morrisett JD. Structure and metabolism of lipoprotein (a). Curr Opin Lipidol 1995;6:136-45.
185. Marcovina SM, Zhang ZH, Gaur VP, Albers JJ. Identification of 34 apolipoprotein(a) isoforms: differential expression of apolipoprotein(a) alleles between American blacks and whites. Biochem Biophys Res Commun 1993;191:1192-6.
186. McCabe E. Disorders of glycerol metabolism. In: Scriver C, Beaudet A, Sly W, Valle D, eds. The Metabolic and molecular bases of inherited diseases. New York: McGraw-Hill, 1995:1631-52.
187. McGowan MW, Artiss JD, Zak B. A procedure for the determination of high-density lipoprotein choline-containing phospholipids. J Clin Chem Clin Biochem 1982;20:807-12.
188. McMillan TA, Warnick GR. Interlaboratory proficiency survey of cholesterol and high-density lipoprotein cholesterol measurement. Clin Chem 1988;34:1629-32.
189. McNamara JJ, Molot MA, Stremple JF, Cutting RT. Coronary artery disease in combat casualties in Vietnam. JAMA 1971;216:1185-7.
190. McNamara JR, Cole TG, Contois JH, Ferguson CA, Ordovas JM, Schaefer EJ. Immunoseparation method for measuring low-density lipoprotein cholesterol directly from serum evaluated. Clin Chem 1995;41:232-40.
191. McNamara JR, Shah PK, Nakajima K, Cupples LA, Wilson PW, Ordovas JM, et al. Remnant lipoprotein cholesterol and triglyceride reference ranges from the Framingham Heart Study. Clin Chem 1998;44:1224-32.
192. Meier-Ewert HK, Ridker PM, Rifai N, Price N, Dinges DF, Mullington JM. Absence of diurnal variation of C-reactive protein concentrations in healthy human subjects. Clin Chem 2001;47:426-30.
193. Miki Y. A homogeneous assay for the selective measurement of LDL-cholesterol in serum: enzymatic selective protection method. Clin Lab 1999;45:398-401.
194. Miller M, Bachorik PS, Cloey TA. Normal variation of plasma lipoproteins: postural effects on plasma concentrations of lipids, lipoproteins, and apolipoproteins. Clin Chem 1992;38:569-74.
195. Miller WG. Matrix effects in the measurement and standardization of lipids and lipoproteins. In: Rifai N, Warnick GR, Dominiczak M, eds. Handbook of lipoprotein testing. Washington, DC: AACC Press, 2000:695-716.
196. Miller WG, Myers GL, Sakurabayashi I, Bachman LM, Caudill SP, Dziekonski A, et al. Seven direct methods for measuring HDL and LDL cholesterol compared with ultracentrifugation reference measurement procedures. Clin Chem 2010;56:977-86.
197. Miller WG, Waymack PP, Anderson FP, Ethridge SF, Jayne EC. Performance of four homogeneous direct methods for LDL-cholesterol. Clin Chem 2002;48:489-98.
198. Miner SE, Evrovski J, Cole DE. Clinical chemistry and molecular biology of homocysteine metabolism: an update. Clin Biochem 1997;30:189-201.
199. Mogadam M, Ahmed SW, Mensch AH, Godwin ID. Within-person fluctuations of serum cholesterol and lipoproteins. Arch Intern Med 1990;150:1645-8.
200. Mora S, Musunuru K, Blumenthal RS. The clinical utility of high-sensitivity C-reactive protein in cardiovascular disease and the potential implication of JUPITER on current practice guidelines. Clin Chem 2009;55:219-28.
201. Mora S, Rifai N, Buring JE, Ridker PM. Fasting compared with nonfasting lipids and apolipoproteins for predicting incident cardiovascular events. Circulation 2008;118:993-1001.
202. Morrow DA, de Lemos JA, Sabatine MS, Wiviott SD, Blazing MA, Shui A, et al. Clinical relevance of C-reactive protein during follow-up of patients with acute coronary syndromes in the Aggrastat-to-Zocor Trial. Circulation 2006;114:281-8.
203. Mozaffarian D, Aro A, Willett WC. Health effects of trans-fatty acids: experimental and observational evidence. Eur J Clin Nutr 2009;63(Suppl 2):S5-21.
204. Mulder K, van LC, Schouten JA, Van Gent CM, Snel MT, Lahey J, et al. An evaluation of three commercial methods for the determination of LDL-cholesterol. Clin Chim Acta 1984;143:29-35.
205. Muller C. Xanthomata, hypercholesterolemia, angina pectoris. Acta Med Scand 1938;75.
206. Myers GL, Christenson RH, Cushman M, Ballantyne CM, Cooper GR, Pfeiffer CM, et al. National Academy of Clinical Biochemistry Laboratory Medicine Practice guidelines: emerging biomarkers for primary prevention of cardiovascular disease. Clin Chem 2009;55:378-84.
207. Myers GL, Cooper GR, Hassemer DJ, Kimberly MM. Standardization of lipid and lipoprotein measurement. In: Rifai N, Warnick GR, Dominiczak M, eds. Handbook of lipoprotein testing. Washington, DC: AACC Press, 2000:717-48.
208. Myers GL, Cooper GR, Winn CL, Smith SJ. The Centers for Disease Control-National Heart, Lung and Blood Institute Lipid Standardization Program. An approach to accurate and precise lipid measurements. Clin Lab Med 1989;9:105-35.
209. Myers GL, Kimberly MM, Waymack PP, Smith SJ, Cooper GR, Sampson EJ. A reference method laboratory network for cholesterol: a model for standardization and improvement of clinical laboratory measurements. Clin Chem 2000;46:1762-72.
210. Naito HK. The association of serum lipids, lipoproteins, and apolipoproteins with coronary artery disease assessed by coronary arteriography. Ann N Y Acad Sci 1985;454:230-8.
211. Naito HK, David JA. Laboratory considerations: determination of cholesterol, triglyceride, phospholipid, and other lipids in blood and tissues. Lab Res Methods Biol Med 1984;10:1-76.
212. Nakagomi A, Freedman SB, Geczy CL. Interferon-gamma and lipopolysaccharide potentiate monocyte tissue factor induction by C-reactive protein: relationship with age, sex, and hormone replacement treatment. Circulation 2000;101:1785-91.
213. Nakajima K, Nakano T, Moon HD, Nagamine T, Stanhope KL, Havel PJ, Warnick GR. The correlation between TG vs remnant lipoproteins in the fasting and postprandial plasma of 23 volunteers. Clin Chim Acta 2009;404:124-7.
214. Nauck M, Graziani MS, Bruton D, Cobbaert C, Cole TG, Lefevre F, et al. Analytical and clinical performance of a detergent-based homogeneous LDL-cholesterol assay: a multicenter evaluation. Clin Chem 2000;46:506-14.
215. Nauck M, Marz W, Jarausch J, Cobbaert C, Sagers A, Bernard D, et al. Multicenter evaluation of a homogeneous assay for HDL-cholesterol without sample pretreatment. Clin Chem 1997;43:1622-9.
216. Nauck M, Marz W, Wieland H. New immunoseparation-based homogeneous assay for HDL-cholesterol compared with three homogeneous and two heterogeneous methods for HDL-cholesterol. Clin Chem 1998;44:1443-51.

217. Nauck M, Rifai N. Analytical performance and clinical efficacy of three routine procedures for LDL cholesterol measurement compared with the ultracentrifugation-dextran sulfate-Mg(2+) method. Clin Chim Acta 2000;294:77-92.
218. Nauck M, Warnick GR, Rifai N. Methods for measurement of LDL-cholesterol: a critical assessment of direct measurement by homogeneous assays versus calculation. Clin Chem 2002;48:236-54.
219. Nexo E, Engbaek F, Ueland PM, Westby C, O'Gorman P, Johnston C, et al. Evaluation of novel assays in clinical chemistry: quantification of plasma total homocysteine. Clin Chem 2000;46:1150-6.
220. Nilsson K, Gustafson L, Faldt R, Andersson A, Brattstrom L, Lindgren A, et al. Hyperhomocysteinaemia—a common finding in a psychogeriatric population. Eur J Clin Invest 1996;26:853-9.
221. Nilsson K, Gustafson L, Faldt R, Andersson A, Hultberg B. Plasma homocysteine in relation to serum cobalamin and blood folate in a psychogeriatric population. Eur J Clin Invest 1994;24:600-6.
222. Nissen SE, Nicholls SJ, Sipahi I, Libby P, Raichlen JS, Ballantyne CM, et al. Effect of very high-intensity statin therapy on regression of coronary atherosclerosis: the ASTEROID trial. JAMA 2006;295:1556-65.
223. Nissen SE, Tuzcu EM, Schoenhagen P, Crowe T, Sasiela WJ, Tsai J, et al. Statin therapy, LDL cholesterol, C-reactive protein, and coronary artery disease. N Engl J Med 2005;352:29-38.
224. Noble RP. Electrophoretic separation of plasma lipoproteins in agarose gel. J Lipid Res 1968;9:693-700.
225. Nordestgaard BG, Benn M, Schnohr P, Tybjaerg-Hansen A. Nonfasting triglycerides and risk of myocardial infarction, ischemic heart disease, and death in men and women. JAMA 2007;298:299-308.
226. Norum RA, Lakier JB, Goldstein S, Angel A, Goldberg RB, Block WD, et al. Familial deficiency of apolipoproteins A-I and C-III and precocious coronary-artery disease. N Engl J Med 1982;306:1513-9.
227. Ockene IS, Matthews CE, Rifai N, Ridker PM, Reed G, Stanek E. Variability and classification accuracy of serial high-sensitivity C-reactive protein measurements in healthy adults. Clin Chem 2001;47:444-50.
228. Okada M, Matsui H, Ito Y, Fujiwara A, Inano K. Low-density lipoprotein cholesterol can be chemically measured: a new superior method. J Lab Clin Med 1998;132:195-201.
229. Okamoto Y, Tanaka S, Nakano H. Direct measurement of HDL cholesterol preferable to precipitation method. Clin Chem 1995;41:1784.
230. Ordovas JM, Lopez-Miranda J, Perez-Jimenez F, Rodriguez C, Park JS, Cole T, et al. Effect of apolipoprotein E and A-IV phenotypes on the low density lipoprotein response to HMG CoA reductase inhibitor therapy. Atherosclerosis 1995;113:157-66.
231. Otvos JD, Jeyarajah EJ, Bennett DW. Quantification of plasma lipoproteins by proton nuclear magnetic resonance spectroscopy. Clin Chem 1991;37:377-86.
232. Otvos JD, Jeyarajah EJ, Bennett DW, Krauss RM. Development of a proton nuclear magnetic resonance spectroscopic method for determining plasma lipoprotein concentrations and subspecies distributions from a single, rapid measurement. Clin Chem 1992;38:1632-8.
233. Pasceri V, Cheng JS, Willerson JT, Yeh ET. Modulation of C-reactive protein-mediated monocyte chemoattractant protein-1 induction in human endothelial cells by anti-atherosclerosis drugs. Circulation 2001;103:2531-4.
234. Patsch JR, Patsch W. Exercise, high density lipoproteins, and fat tolerance. Compr Ther 1984;10:29-33.
235. Patsch JR, Prasad S, Gotto AM Jr, Gatsson-Olivecrona G. Postprandial lipemia: a key for the conversion of high density lipoprotein2 into high density lipoprotein3 by hepatic lipase. J Clin Invest 1984;74: 2017-23.
236. Pearson TA, Mensah GA, Alexander RW, Anderson JL, Cannon RO III, Criqui M, et al. Markers of inflammation and cardiovascular disease: application to clinical and public health practice. A statement for healthcare professionals from the Centers for Disease Control and Prevention and the American Heart Association. Circulation 2003;107:499-511.
237. Pernet P, Lasnier E, Vaubourdolle M. Evaluation of the AxSYM homocysteine assay and comparison with the IMx homocysteine assay. Clin Chem 2000;46:1440-1.
238. Pfeiffer CM, Huff DL, Smith SJ, Miller DT, Gunter EW. Comparison of plasma total homocysteine measurements in 14 laboratories: an international study. Clin Chem 1999;45:1261-8.
239. Pisani T, Gebski CP, Leary ET, Warnick GR, Ollington JF. Accurate direct determination of low-density lipoprotein cholesterol using an immunoseparation reagent and enzymatic cholesterol assay. Arch Pathol Lab Med 1995;119:1127-35.
240. Powers HJ, Moat SJ. Developments in the measurement of plasma total homocysteine. Curr Opin Clin Nutr Metab Care 2000;3:391-7.
241. Pradhan AD, Cook NR, Buring JE, Manson JE, Ridker PM. C-reactive protein is independently associated with fasting insulin in nondiabetic women. Arterioscler Thromb Vasc Biol 2003;23:650-5.
242. Pradhan AD, Manson JE, Rifai N, Buring JE, Ridker PM. C-reactive protein, interleukin 6, and risk of developing type 2 diabetes mellitus. JAMA 2001;286:327-34.
243. Rall SC Jr, Weisgraber KH, Mahley RW. Human apolipoprotein E: the complete amino acid sequence. J Biol Chem 1982;257:4171-8.
244. Rasmussen K, Moller J. Total homocysteine measurement in clinical practice. Ann Clin Biochem 2000;37(Pt 5):627-48.
245. Ray JG, Laskin CA. Folic acid and homocyst(e)ine metabolic defects and the risk of placental abruption, pre-eclampsia and spontaneous pregnancy loss: a systematic review. Placenta 1999;20:519-29.
246. Refsum H, Fiskerstrand T, Guttormsen AB, Ueland PM. Assessment of homocysteine status. J Inherit Metab Dis 1997;20:286-94.
247. Refsum H, Helland S, Ueland PM. Radioenzymic determination of homocysteine in plasma and urine. Clin Chem 1985;31:624-8.
248. Refsum H, Smith AD, Ueland PM, Nexo E, Clarke R, McPartlin J, et al. Facts and recommendations about total homocysteine determinations: an expert opinion. Clin Chem 2004;50:3-32.
249. Resnicow K, Cross D. Are parents' self-reported total cholesterol levels useful in identifying children with hyperlipidemia? An examination of current guidelines. Pediatrics 1993;92:347-53.
250. Ridker PM. Rosuvastatin in the primary prevention of cardiovascular disease among patients with low levels of low-density lipoprotein cholesterol and elevated high-sensitivity C-reactive protein: rationale and design of the JUPITER trial. Circulation 2003;108:2292-7.
251. Ridker PM. C-reactive protein: eighty years from discovery to emergence as a major risk marker for cardiovascular disease. Clin Chem 2009;55:209-15.
252. Ridker PM, Buring JE, Cook NR, Rifai N. C-reactive protein, the metabolic syndrome, and risk of incident cardiovascular events: an 8-year follow-up of 14,719 initially healthy American women. Circulation 2003;107:391-7.
253. Ridker PM, Buring JE, Rifai N, Cook NR. Development and validation of improved algorithms for the assessment of global cardiovascular risk in women: the Reynolds Risk Score. JAMA 2007;297:611-9.
254. Ridker PM, Cannon CP, Morrow D, Rifai N, Rose LM, McCabe CH, et al. C-reactive protein levels and outcomes after statin therapy. N Engl J Med 2005;352:20-8.
255. Ridker PM, Cushman M, Stampfer MJ, Tracy RP, Hennekens CH. Inflammation, aspirin, and the risk of cardiovascular disease in apparently healthy men. N Engl J Med 1997;336:973-9.
256. Ridker PM, Cushman M, Stampfer MJ, Tracy RP, Hennekens CH. Plasma concentration of C-reactive protein and risk of developing peripheral vascular disease. Circulation 1998;97:425-8.
257. Ridker PM, Danielson E, Fonseca FA, Genest J, Gotto AM Jr, Kastelein JJ, et al. Rosuvastatin to prevent vascular events in men and women with elevated C-reactive protein. N Engl J Med 2008;359: 2195-207.
258. Ridker PM, Danielson E, Fonseca FA, Genest J, Gotto AM Jr, Kastelein JJ, et al. Reduction in C-reactive protein and LDL cholesterol and

cardiovascular event rates after initiation of rosuvastatin: a prospective study of the JUPITER trial. Lancet 2009;373:1175-82.
259. Ridker PM, Hennekens CH, Buring JE, Rifai N. C-reactive protein and other markers of inflammation in the prediction of cardiovascular disease in women. N Engl J Med 2000;342:836-43.
260. Ridker PM, Paynter NP, Rifai N, Gaziano JM, Cook NR. C-reactive protein and parental history improve global cardiovascular risk prediction: the Reynolds Risk Score for men. Circulation 2008;118:2243-51.
261. Ridker PM, Rifai N, Clearfield M, Downs JR, Weis SE, Miles JS, et al. Measurement of C-reactive protein for the targeting of statin therapy in the primary prevention of acute coronary events. N Engl J Med 2001;344:1959-65.
262. Ridker PM, Rifai N, Pfeffer MA, Sacks F, Braunwald E. Long-term effects of pravastatin on plasma concentration of C-reactive protein. The Cholesterol and Recurrent Events (CARE) Investigators. Circulation 1999;100:230-5.
263. Ridker PM, Rifai N, Pfeffer MA, Sacks FM, Moye LA, Goldman S, et al. Inflammation, pravastatin, and the risk of coronary events after myocardial infarction in patients with average cholesterol levels. Cholesterol and Recurrent Events (CARE) Investigators. Circulation 1998;98:839-44.
264. Ridker PM, Rifai N, Rose L, Buring JE, Cook NR. Comparison of C-reactive protein and low-density lipoprotein cholesterol levels in the prediction of first cardiovascular events. N Engl J Med 2002;347:1557-65.
265. Ridker PM, Stampfer MJ, Rifai N. Novel risk factors for systemic atherosclerosis: a comparison of C-reactive protein, fibrinogen, homocysteine, lipoprotein(a), and standard cholesterol screening as predictors of peripheral arterial disease. JAMA 2001;285:2481-5.
266. Rifai N. Lipoproteins and apolipoproteins: composition, metabolism, and association with coronary heart disease. Arch Pathol Lab Med 1986;110:694-701.
267. Rifai N, Heiss G. Gender and race differences in cord blood lipoprotein. Circulation 1988;II:481.
268. Rifai N, Heiss G, Doetsch K. Lipoprotein(a) at birth, in blacks and whites. Atherosclerosis 1992;92:123-9.
269. Rifai N, Kwiterovich P Jr. Disorders of lipid and lipoprotein metabolism in children and adolescents. In: Soldin SJ, Rifai N, Hicks JMB, eds. Biochemical bases of inherited disease. Washington, DC: AACC Press, 1995.
270. Rifai N, Neufeld E, Ahlstrom P, Rimm E, D'Angelo L, Hicks JM. Failure of current guidelines for cholesterol screening in urban African-American adolescents. Pediatrics 1996;98:383-8.
271. Rifai N, Ridker PM. Population distributions of C-reactive protein in apparently healthy men and women in the United States: implication for clinical interpretation. Clin Chem 2003;49:666-9.
272. Rifai N, Silverman LM. Immunoturbidimetric techniques for quantifying apolipoproteins CII and CIII. Clin Chem 1986;32:1969-72.
273. Roberts WL, Moulton L, Law TC, Farrow G, Cooper-Anderson M, Savory J, et al. Evaluation of nine automated high-sensitivity C-reactive protein methods: implications for clinical and epidemiological applications. Part 2. Clin Chem 2001;47:418-25.
274. Rosseneu M, Vercaemst R, Steinberg KK, Cooper GR. Some considerations of methodology and standardization of apolipoprotein B immunoassays. Clin Chem 1983;29:427-33.
275. Rousset X, Vaisman B, Amar M, Sethi AA, Remaley AT. Lecithin: cholesterol acyltransferase—from biochemistry to role in cardiovascular disease. Curr Opin Endocrinol Diabetes Obes 2009;16:163-71.
276. Sandkamp M, Funke H, Schulte H, Kohler E, Assmann G. Lipoprotein(a) is an independent risk factor for myocardial infarction at a young age. Clin Chem 1990;36:20-3.
277. Sattar N, Gaw A, Scherbakova O, Ford I, O'Reilly DS, Haffner SM, et al. Metabolic syndrome with and without C-reactive protein as a predictor of coronary heart disease and diabetes in the West of Scotland Coronary Prevention Study. Circulation 2003;108:414-9.
278. Savage DG, Lindenbaum J, Stabler SP, Allen RH. Sensitivity of serum methylmalonic acid and total homocysteine determinations for diagnosing cobalamin and folate deficiencies. Am J Med 1994;96:239-46.
279. Schaefer EJ. Clinical, biochemical, and genetic features in familial disorders of high density lipoprotein deficiency. Arteriosclerosis 1984;4:303-22.
280. Schaefer EJ, Blum CB, Levy RI, Jenkins LL, Alaupovic P, Foster DM, et al. Metabolism of high-density lipoprotein apolipoproteins in Tangier disease. N Engl J Med 1978;299:905-10.
281. Schaefer EJ, Lamon-Fava S, Johnson S, Ordovas JM, Schaefer MM, Castelli WP, et al. Effects of gender and menopausal status on the association of apolipoprotein E phenotype with plasma lipoprotein levels: results from the Framingham Offspring Study. Arterioscler Thromb 1994;14:1105-13.
282. Schaefer EJ, McNamara JR. Overview of the diagnosis and treatment of lipid disorders. In: Rifai N, Dominiczak M, Warnick GR, eds. Handbook of lipoprotein testing. Washington, DC: AACC Press, 1997.
283. Scharnagl H, Nauck M, Wieland H, Marz W. The Friedewald formula underestimates LDL cholesterol at low concentrations. Clin Chem Lab Med 2001;39:426-31.
284. Schmitz G, Assmann G, Robenek H, Brennhausen B. Tangier disease: a disorder of intracellular membrane traffic. Proc Natl Acad Sci U S A 1985;82:6305-9.
285. Schrott HG, Goldstein JL, Hazzard WR, McGoodwin MM, Motulsky AG. Familial hypercholesterolemia in a large kindred: evidence for a monogenic mechanism. Ann Intern Med 1972;76:711-20.
286. Segrest JP, Chung BH, Cone JT, Hughes TA. Coronary heart disease risk: assessment by plasma lipoprotein profiles. Ala J Med Sci 1983;20:76-83.
287. Segrest JP, Jones MK, De LH, Dashti N. Structure of apolipoprotein B-100 in low density lipoproteins. J Lipid Res 2001;42:1346-67.
288. Sesso HD, Buring JE, Rifai N, Blake GJ, Gaziano JM, Ridker PM. C-reactive protein and the risk of developing hypertension. JAMA 2003;290:2945-51.
289. Shimano H. SREBPs: physiology and pathophysiology of the SREBP family. FEBS J 2009;276:616-21.
290. Shipchandler MT, Moore EG. Rapid, fully automated measurement of plasma homocyst(e)ine with the Abbott IMx analyzer. Clin Chem 1995;41:991-4.
291. Siest G, Pillot T, Regis-Bailly A, Leininger-Muller B, Steinmetz J, Galteau MM, et al. Apolipoprotein E: an important gene and protein to follow in laboratory medicine. Clin Chem 1995;41:1068-86.
292. Smith AD. Homocysteine, B vitamins, and cognitive deficit in the elderly. Am J Clin Nutr 2002;75:785-6.
293. Sniderman A, Shapiro S, Marpole D, Skinner B, Teng B, Kwiterovich PO Jr. Association of coronary atherosclerosis with hyperapobetalipoproteinemia [increased protein but normal cholesterol levels in human plasma low density (beta) lipoproteins]. Proc Natl Acad Sci U S A 1980;77:604-8.
294. Sniderman A, Teng B, Genest J, Cianflone K, Wacholder S, Kwiterovich P Jr. Familial aggregation and early expression of hyperapobetalipoproteinemia. Am J Cardiol 1985;55:291-5.
295. Sniderman AD, Silberberg J. Is it time to measure apolipoprotein B? Arteriosclerosis 1990;10:665-7.
296. SoRelle R. Metabolic syndrome: a major predictor of heart disease. Circulation 2004;109:e9010-1.
297. Soria LF, Ludwig EH, Clarke HR, Vega GL, Grundy SM, McCarthy BJ. Association between a specific apolipoprotein B mutation and familial defective apolipoprotein B-100. Proc Natl Acad Sci U S A 1989;86:587-91.
298. Stabler SP, Marcell PD, Podell ER, Allen RH. Quantitation of total homocysteine, total cysteine, and methionine in normal serum and urine using capillary gas chromatography-mass spectrometry. Anal Biochem 1987;162:185-96.
299. Stanger O, Herrmann W, Pietrzik K, Fowler B, Geisel J, Dierkes J, et al. DACH-LIGA homocysteine (German, Austrian and Swiss

Homocysteine Society): consensus paper on the rational clinical use of homocysteine, folic acid and B-vitamins in cardiovascular and thrombotic diseases: guidelines and recommendations. Clin Chem Lab Med 2003;41:1392-403.
300. Stary HC. The sequence of cell and matrix changes in atherosclerotic lesions of coronary arteries in the first forty years of life. Eur Heart J 1990;11(Suppl E):3-19.
301. Steele BW, Koehler DF, Azar MM, Blaszkowski TP, Kuba K, Dempsey ME. Enzymatic determinations of cholesterol in high-density-lipoprotein fractions prepared by a precipitation technique. Clin Chem 1976;22:98-101.
302. Steinberg D, Witztum JL. Is the oxidative modification hypothesis relevant to human atherosclerosis? Do the antioxidant trials conducted to date refute the hypothesis? Circulation 2002;105: 2107-11.
303. Steinberg KK, Cooper GR, Graiser SR, Rosseneu M. Some considerations of methodology and standardization of apolipoprotein A-I immunoassays. Clin Chem 1983;29:415-26.
304. Strong JP, Malcom GT, McMahan CA, Tracy RE, Newman WP III, Herderick EE, et al. Prevalence and extent of atherosclerosis in adolescents and young adults: implications for prevention from the Pathobiological Determinants of Atherosclerosis in Youth Study. JAMA 1999;281:727-35.
305. Strong JP, McGill HC Jr. The pediatric aspects of atherosclerosis. J Atheroscler Res 1969;9:251-65.
306. Stuyt PM, Van't LA. Clinical features of type III hyperlipoproteinaemia. Neth J Med 1983;26:104-11.
307. Sugiuchi H, Irie T, Uji Y, Ueno T, Chaen T, Uekama K, et al. Homogeneous assay for measuring low-density lipoprotein cholesterol in serum with triblock copolymer and alpha-cyclodextrin sulfate. Clin Chem 1998;44:522-31.
308. Sugiuchi H, Uji Y, Okabe H, Irie T, Uekama K, Kayahara N, et al. Direct measurement of high-density lipoprotein cholesterol in serum with polyethylene glycol-modified enzymes and sulfated alpha-cyclodextrin. Clin Chem 1995;41:717-23.
309. Taddei-Peters WC, Butman BT, Jones GR, Venetta TM, Macomber PF, Ransom JH. Quantification of lipoprotein(a) particles containing various apolipoprotein(a) isoforms by a monoclonal anti-apo(a) capture antibody and a polyclonal anti-apolipoprotein B detection antibody sandwich enzyme immunoassay. Clin Chem 1993;39: 1382-9.
310. Takayama M, Itoh S, Nagasaki T, Tanimizu I. A new enzymatic method for determination of serum choline-containing phospholipids. Clin Chim Acta 1977;79:93-8.
311. Tate JR, Berg K, Couderc R, Dati F, Kostner GM, Marcovina SM, et al. International Federation of Clinical Chemistry and Laboratory Medicine (IFCC) Standardization Project for the Measurement of Lipoprotein(a). Phase 2. Selection and properties of a proposed secondary reference material for lipoprotein(a). Clin Chem Lab Med 1999;37:949-58.
312. Tate JR, Rifai N, Berg K, Couderc R, Dati F, Kostner GM, et al. International Federation of Clinical Chemistry standardization project for the measurement of lipoprotein(a). Phase I. Evaluation of the analytical performance of lipoprotein(a) assay systems and commercial calibrators. Clin Chem 1998;44:1629-40.
313. Thanhauser S, Magendantz H. The different clinical groups of xanthomatous diseases: a clinical physiological study of 22 cases. Ann Intern Med 1938;11:1662-746.
314. Third JL, Montag J, Flynn M, Freidel J, Laskarzewski P, Glueck CJ. Primary and familial hypoalphalipoproteinemia. Metabolism 1984;33:136-46.
315. Torzewski J, Torzewski M, Bowyer DE, Frohlich M, Koenig W, Waltenberger J, et al. C-reactive protein frequently colocalizes with the terminal complement complex in the intima of early atherosclerotic lesions of human coronary arteries. Arterioscler Thromb Vasc Biol 1998;18:1386-92.
316. Tybjaerg-Hansen A, Gallagher J, Vincent J, Houlston R, Talmud P, Dunning AM, et al. Familial defective apolipoprotein B-100: detection in the United Kingdom and Scandinavia, and clinical characteristics of ten cases. Atherosclerosis 1990;80:235-42.
317. Ubbink JB. Assay methods for the measurement of total homocyst(e) ine in plasma. Semin Thromb Hemost 2000;26:233-41.
318. Ubbink JB, Hayward Vermaak WJ, Bissbort S. Rapid high-performance liquid chromatographic assay for total homocysteine levels in human serum. J Chromatogr 1991;565:441-6.
319. Ueland PM, Refsum H, Stabler SP, Malinow MR, Andersson A, Allen RH. Total homocysteine in plasma or serum: methods and clinical applications. Clin Chem 1993;39:1764-79.
320. Usui S, Kakuuchi H, Okamoto M, Mizukami Y, Okazaki M. Differential reactivity of two homogeneous LDL-cholesterol methods to LDL and VLDL subfractions, as demonstrated by ultracentrifugation and HPLC. Clin Chem 2002;48:1946-54.
321. Utermann G. Genetic polymorphism of apolipoprotein E: impact on plasma lipoprotein metabolism. In: Crepaldi G, Tiengo A, Baggio G, eds. Obesity and hyperlipidemias. Amsterdam: Elsevier, 1985:1-30.
322. Utermann G, Hees M, Steinmetz A. Polymorphism of apolipoprotein E and occurrence of dysbetalipoproteinaemia in man. Nature 1977; 269:604-7.
323. van der Hoek YY, Wittekoek ME, Beisiegel U, Kastelein JJ, Koschinsky ML. The apolipoprotein(a) kringle IV repeats which differ from the major repeat kringle are present in variably-sized isoforms. Hum Mol Genet 1993;2:361-6.
324. Vega GL, Grundy SM. In vivo evidence for reduced binding of low density lipoproteins to receptors as a cause of primary moderate hypercholesterolemia. J Clin Invest 1986;78:1410-4.
325. Verma S, Li SH, Badiwala MV, Weisel RD, Fedak PW, Li RK, et al. Endothelin antagonism and interleukin-6 inhibition attenuate the proatherogenic effects of C-reactive protein. Circulation 2002;105: 1890-6.
326. Vermeer BJ, Van Gent CM, Goslings B, Polano MK. Xanthomatosis and other clinical findings in patients with elevated levels of very low density lipoproteins. Br J Dermatol 1979;100:657-66.
327. Vester B, Rasmussen K. High performance liquid chromatography method for rapid and accurate determination of homocysteine in plasma and serum. Eur J Clin Chem Clin Biochem 1991;29: 549-54.
328. Vilaseca MA, Moyano D, Ferrer I, Artuch R. Total homocysteine in pediatric patients. Clin Chem 1997;43:690-2.
329. Vollset SE, Refsum H, Irgens LM, Emblem BM, Tverdal A, Gjessing HK, et al. Plasma total homocysteine, pregnancy complications, and adverse pregnancy outcomes: the Hordaland Homocysteine Study. Am J Clin Nutr 2000;71:962-8.
330. Wald DS, Law M, Morris JK. Homocysteine and cardiovascular disease: evidence on causality from a meta-analysis. BMJ 2002;325: 1202.
331. Warnick GR. Enzymatic methods for quantification of lipoprotein lipids. Methods Enzymol 1986;129:101-23.
332. Warnick GR, Albers JJ. A comprehensive evaluation of the heparin-manganese precipitation procedure for estimating high density lipoprotein cholesterol. J Lipid Res 1978;19:65-76.
333. Warnick GR, Benderson J, Albers JJ. Dextran sulfate-Mg2+ precipitation procedure for quantitation of high-density-lipoprotein cholesterol. Clin Chem 1982;28:1379-88.
334. Warnick GR, Knopp RH, Fitzpatrick V, Branson L. Estimating low-density lipoprotein cholesterol by the Friedewald equation is adequate for classifying patients on the basis of nationally recommended cutpoints. Clin Chem 1990;36:15-9.
335. Warnick GR, Mayfield C, Albers JJ, Hazzard WR. Gel isoelectric focusing method for specific diagnosis of familial hyperlipoproteinemia type 3. Clin Chem 1979;25:279-84.
336. Warnick GR, McNamara JR, Boggess CN, Clendenen F, Williams PT, Landolt CC. Polyacrylamide gradient gel electrophoresis of lipoprotein subclasses. Clin Lab Med 2006;26:803-46.
337. Warnick GR, Nauck M, Rifai N. Evolution of methods for measurement of HDL-cholesterol: from ultracentrifugation to homogeneous assays. Clin Chem 2001;47:1579-96.

338. Warnick GR, Spain M, Kloepfer H, Volke TM. Standardization of a commercial (Boehringer Mannheim diagnostics) enzymic method for cholesterol. Clin Chem 1989;35:409-13.
339. Webber LS, Srinivasan SR, Wattigney WA, Berenson GS. Tracking of serum lipids and lipoproteins from childhood to adulthood. The Bogalusa Heart Study. Am J Epidemiol 1991;133:884-99.
340. Weisgraber KH, Innerarity TL, Mahley RW. Abnormal lipoprotein receptor-binding activity of the human E apoprotein due to cysteine-arginine interchange at a single site. J Biol Chem 1982;257:2518-21.
341. Weisgraber KH, Newhouse YM, Mahley RW. Apolipoprotein E genotyping using the polymerase chain reaction and allele-specific oligonucleotide probes. Biochem Biophys Res Commun 1988;157: 1212-7.
342. Wilder LB, Bachorik PS, Finney CA, Moy TF, Becker DM. The effect of fasting status on the determination of low-density and high-density lipoprotein cholesterol. Am J Med 1995;99:374-7.
343. Wissler RW. New insights into the pathogenesis of atherosclerosis as revealed by PDAY. Pathobiological Determinants of Atherosclerosis in Youth. Atherosclerosis 1994;108(Suppl):S3-20.
344. Yamada S, Gotoh T, Nakashima Y, Kayaba K, Ishikawa S, Nago N, et al. Distribution of serum C-reactive protein and its association with atherosclerotic risk factors in a Japanese population. Jichi Medical School Cohort Study. Am J Epidemiol 2001;153:1183-90.
345. Yamamoto A, Nakamura M, Hino K, Saito K, Manabe M. Development of a new homogeneous method for serum HDL-C. Clin Chem 2000;46:A98.
346. Yancey PG, Bortnick AE, Kellner-Weibel G, de la Llera-Moya M, Phillips MC, Rothblat GH. Importance of different pathways of cellular cholesterol efflux. Arterioscler Thromb Vasc Biol 2003;23: 712-9.
347. Yu HH, Markowitz R, De Ferranti SD, Neufeld EJ, Farrow G, Bernstein HH, et al. Direct measurement of LDL-C in children: performance of two surfactant-based methods in a general pediatric population. Clin Biochem 2000;33:89-95.
348. Zacho J, Tybjaerg-Hansen A, Jensen JS, Grande P, Sillesen H, Nordestgaard BG. Genetically elevated C-reactive protein and ischemic vascular disease. N Engl J Med 2008;359:1897-908.
349. Ziccardi P, Nappo F, Giugliano G, Esposito K, Marfella R, Cioffi M, et al. Reduction of inflammatory cytokine concentrations and improvement of endothelial functions in obese women after weight loss over one year. Circulation 2002;105:804-9.
350. Zilversmit DB. Atherogenesis: a postprandial phenomenon. Circulation 1979;60:473-85.
351. Zwaka TP, Hombach V, Torzewski J. C-reactive protein-mediated low density lipoprotein uptake by macrophages: implications for atherosclerosis. Circulation 2001;103:1194-7.

CHAPTER 28

Electrolytes and Blood Gases

Mitchell G. Scott, Ph.D., Vicky A. LeGrys, Ph.D., Dr.A., M.T.(A.S.C.P.), C.L.S.(N.C.A.), and Joshua L. Hood, M.D., Ph.D.

Maintenance of water homeostasis is paramount to life for all organisms. In humans, the maintenance of water homeostasis in various body fluid compartments is primarily a function of the four major electrolytes, Na^+, K^+, Cl^-, and HCO_3^-. These electrolytes also have a role in acid-base balance and heart and muscle function, and serve as cofactors for enzymes. Virtually no metabolic process is independent or unaffected by electrolytes. Abnormal electrolyte concentrations may be the cause or the consequence of a variety of medical disorders. Because of their physiologic and clinical interrelationships, this chapter discusses determination of (1) electrolytes, (2) osmolality, (3) sweat testing, (4) blood gases and pH, and (5) blood oxygenation.

ELECTROLYTES

Electrolytes may be classified as *anions,* negatively charged ions that move toward an anode, or *cations,* positively charged ions that move toward a cathode. Important physiologic electrolytes include Na^+, K^+, Ca^{2+}, Mg^{2+}, Cl^-, HCO_3^-, $H_2PO_4^-$, HPO_4^{2-}, and SO_4^{2-}, and some organic anions, such as lactate. Although amino acids and proteins in solution also carry an electrical charge, they are usually considered separately from electrolytes. Hydrogen ion (H^+) concentration is routinely measured as pH, but its concentration is so low relative to other ions (10^{-9} vs. 10^{-3} mol/L) that for clinical purposes it is not categorized as an electrolyte. The major electrolytes (Na^+, K^+, Cl^-, HCO_3^-) occur primarily as free ions, whereas significant amounts (>40%) of Ca^{2+}, Mg^{2+}, and trace elements are bound by proteins, mainly albumin. Determination of body fluid concentrations of the four major electrolytes (Na^+, K^+, Cl^-, and HCO_3^-) is commonly referred to as an *electrolyte profile.*

Specimens for Electrolyte Determination

Serum and *plasma,* obtained from blood collected by venipuncture into an evacuated tube, are the usual specimens analyzed for electrolytes. Capillary blood, collected in microsample tubes or capillary tubes, or applied directly from a fingerstick to some point-of-care devices, is another sample commonly analyzed. Heparinized whole blood arterial or venous specimens obtained for blood gas and pH determinations may also be used with direct ion-selective electrodes (ISEs). Differences in values between serum and plasma and between arterial and venous samples have been documented, but only the difference between serum and plasma K^+ can be considered clinically significant. Heparin, either lithium or ammonium salt, is required if plasma or whole blood is assayed. Use of plasma or whole blood has the advantage of shortening turnaround time, because it is not necessary to wait for the blood to clot. Furthermore, plasma or whole blood provides a distinct advantage in determining K^+ concentrations, which are invariably higher in serum depending on platelet count.[42,72] Grossly lipemic blood can be a source of analytical error (see "Electrolyte Exclusion Effect"), with some methods making ultracentrifugation of lipemic serum or plasma necessary prior to analysis. Hemolysis of red blood cells will cause erroneously high K^+ results; this problem is usually undetected when whole blood is analyzed. In addition, unhemolyzed specimens that are not promptly processed may have increased K^+ concentrations because of K^+ leakage from red blood cells when whole blood is stored at 4 °C.

Urine collection for Na^+, K^+, or Cl^- assays should be done without the addition of preservatives. Body fluid aspirates, feces, or GI fluid samples may also be submitted for electrolyte analysis.

Sodium

Sodium is the major cation of extracellular fluid. Because it represents approximately 90% of the ≈154 mmol of inorganic cations per liter of plasma, Na^+ is responsible for almost one half the osmotic strength of plasma. It therefore plays a central role in maintaining the normal distribution of water and the osmotic pressure in the extracellular fluid compartment (ECF). The daily diet of the adult male in the United States contains 3 to 6 g (90 to 250 mmol) of Na^+ (7 to 14 g of NaCl), which is nearly completely absorbed from the

GI tract.[84] The body requires only 1 to 2 mmol/d, and the excess is excreted by the kidneys, which are the ultimate regulators of the amount of Na^+ (and thus water) in the body.

Sodium is freely filtered by the kidney glomeruli. Seventy to 80% of the filtered Na^+ load is then actively reabsorbed in the proximal tubules, with Cl^- and water passively following in an iso-osmotic and electrically neutral manner. Another 20 to 25% is reabsorbed in the loop of Henle, along with Cl^- and more water. In the distal tubules, interaction of the adrenal hormone aldosterone with the coupled Na^+-K^+ and Na^+-H^+ exchange systems results directly in the reabsorption of Na^+, and indirectly of Cl^-, from the remaining 5 to 10% of the filtered load. It is the regulation of this latter fraction of filtered Na^+ that primarily determines the amount of Na^+ excreted in the urine. These processes are discussed in detail in Chapter 48.

Specimens

Serum, plasma, and urine may be stored at 4 °C or may be frozen. Erythrocytes contain only one tenth of the Na^+ present in plasma, so hemolysis does not cause significant errors in serum or plasma Na^+ values. Lipemic samples should be ultracentrifuged and the infranatant analyzed unless a direct ISE is used (see "Electrolyte Exclusion Effect").

Fecal and gastrointestinal fluid specimens require preparation before assay. Only liquid stools justify the trouble of analysis, because it is only when liquid feces occur that losses of electrolytes are significant. Immediately after collection, liquid stool specimens should be clarified of particulate matter by filtration through gauze or filter paper and by centrifugation. Because the risk of bacterial contamination of instrument sampling systems is high with fecal samples, special cleaning procedures should follow analysis. If not analyzed immediately, fecal and gastrointestinal fluids should be stored frozen to prevent microbial growth.

Determination of Sodium in Body Fluids

Sodium may be determined by (1) atomic absorption spectrophotometry (AAS), (2) flame emission spectrophotometry (FES), (3) electrochemically with an Na^+-ISE, or (4) spectrophotometrically. Of these methods, ISE methods are by far the most common. Excellent accuracy and coefficients of variation of less than 1.5% are readily achieved with modern equipment, reliable calibrators, and a good quality assurance program. Because sodium and potassium are routinely assayed together, methods for their analysis are described together later in this chapter.

Reference Intervals[87,91]

A typical reference interval for *serum* Na^+ is 136 to 145 mmol/L.[51] The central 95% of Na values from more than 16,000 subjects in the National Health and Nutrition Examination Survey III (NHANES III) was 136 to 146 mmol/L.[54] The interval for premature newborns at 48 hours is 128 to 148 mmol/L, and the value for umbilical cord blood from full-term newborns is ≈127 mmol/L.

Urinary sodium excretion varies with dietary intake, but for an adult male on an average diet containing 7 to 14 g of NaCl per day, an interval of 120 to 240 mmol/d is typical.[84] A large diurnal variation in Na^+ excretion has been noted, with the rate of Na^+ excretion during the night being only 20% of the peak rate during the day. The Na^+ concentration of cerebrospinal fluid is 136 to 150 mmol/L.[94] Mean fecal Na^+ excretion is less than 10 mmol/d.[16]

Potassium

Potassium is the major intracellular cation. In tissue cells, its average concentration is 150 mmol/L, and in erythrocytes, the concentration is 105 mmol/L. High intracellular concentrations are maintained by the Na^+, K^+ adenosine triphosphate (ATP)ase pump, which is fueled by oxidative energy and continually transports K^+ into the cell against a concentration gradient. This pump is a critical factor in maintaining and adjusting the ionic gradients on which nerve impulse transmission and contractility of muscle depend. Diffusion of K^+ out of the cell into the ECF and plasma occurs whenever pump activity is decreased because of (1) depletion of metabolic substrates such as glucose for ATP production; (2) competition for ATP between the pump and other energy-consuming activities of the cell; or (3) slowing of cellular metabolism (as occurs with refrigeration). The importance of these considerations on sample integrity for analysis of K^+ is discussed later.

The body requirement for K^+ is satisfied by an average dietary intake of 2.4 to 4.4 g/d (60 to 120 mmol/d). Potassium absorbed from the gastrointestinal tract is rapidly distributed, with a small amount taken up by cells, and most excreted by the kidneys. Potassium filtered through the glomeruli is almost completely reabsorbed in the proximal tubules and is then secreted in the distal tubules in exchange for Na^+ under the influence of aldosterone. Aldosterone enhances K^+ secretion and Na^+ reabsorption in the distal tubules by an Na^+-K^+ exchange mechanism. The kidneys respond almost immediately to K^+ loading with an increase in K^+ output, so that urine collected during or after a period of high K^+ intake may have K^+ concentrations as high as 100 mmol/L. In contrast, the tubular response to conserve K^+ is very slow in the initial stages of depletion. Unlike the prompt response to conserve Na^+ in deficit states, it can take up to 1 week for the tubules to reduce K^+ excretion to 5 to 10 mmol/d from the typical 50 to 100 mmol/d.

Factors that regulate distal tubular secretion of K^+ include intake of Na^+ and K^+, mineralocorticoid concentration, and acid-base balance. Because renal conservation mechanisms are slow to respond, K^+ depletion can be an early consequence of restricted K^+ intake or loss of K^+ by extrarenal routes such as diarrhea. A diminished glomerular filtration rate is typical of renal failure, and the consequent decrease in distal tubular flow rate is an important factor in the retention of K^+ seen in chronic renal failure. Renal tubular acidosis (RTA) and metabolic and respiratory acidoses and alkaloses also affect renal regulation of K^+ excretion. These topics are discussed in Chapters 48 and 49.

Specimens

Comments made earlier on specimens for Na^+ analysis are generally applicable to those for K^+ analysis. However, some additional points must be made. Potassium concentrations in plasma and whole blood are 0.1 to 0.7 mmol/L lower than those in serum, and most reference intervals for serum K^+ are 0.2 to 0.5 mmol/L higher than those for plasma K^+. The extent of this difference depends on the platelet count, because the additional K^+ in serum is primarily a result of platelet rupture during coagulation.[42,72] This variability in the amount of additional K^+ in serum makes plasma the specimen of choice and emphasizes the necessity of noting on reports whether serum or plasma was assayed and using the appropriate reference interval.

Specimens for determining K^+ concentrations in serum or plasma must be collected by methods that minimize hemolysis, because release of K^+ from as few as 0.5% of erythrocytes can increase K^+ values by 0.5 mmol/L. An increase in K^+ of 0.6% has been estimated for every 10 mg/dL of plasma hemoglobin caused by hemolysis.[13] Thus slight hemolysis (Hb ≈50 mg/dL) can be expected to raise K^+ values by ≈3%, marked hemolysis (Hb ≈200 mg/dL) by 12%, and gross hemolysis (Hb > 500 mg/dL) by as much as 30%. Several correction factors for estimating K^+ in hemolyzed samples have been examined, but routine use of these is not recommended.[65] Therefore it is imperative that any visible hemolysis be noted with reported K^+ values with a comment that results are falsely elevated. If K^+ concentrations are determined by ISE on whole blood specimens using a blood gas instrument or a point-of-care device, increases in K^+ concentrations caused by hemolysis will often be overlooked. Whenever hemolysis is suspected, a portion of the specimen should be centrifuged and visually inspected.

Clinically significant preanalytical errors can occur for K^+ determinations if blood samples are not processed expediently.[41] As mentioned earlier, maintenance of the intracellular-extracellular K^+ gradient depends on the activity of the energy-dependent Na^+-K^+-ATPase. If a whole blood specimen is maintained at 4 °C versus 25 °C before separation, glycolysis is inhibited and the energy-dependent Na^+-K^+-ATPase cannot maintain the Na^+/K^+ gradient. An increase in plasma K^+ will occur as a result of K^+ leakage from erythrocytes and other cells. The increase of K^+ in serum is on the order of 0.2 mmol/L by 1.5 hours at 25 °C, whereas at 4 °C, the increase is considerably greater and has been reported to be as much as 2 mmol/L after 4 hours at 4 °C.[74]

The opposite effect, namely, a falsely decreased K^+ value, can be observed if an unseparated sample is stored at 37 °C, because glycolysis occurs and K^+ shifts intracellularly. Even at room temperature, severe leukocytosis can initially cause falsely decreased K^+ concentrations. The extent of this decrease depends on leukocyte count, temperature, and glucose concentrations but has been reported to be as much as 0.7 mmol/L at 37 °C.[55] This effect is, however, biphasic. Initially, plasma K^+ decreases as a result of glycolysis, but after the glucose substrate is exhausted, K^+ will leak from cells. When the leukocyte count is greater than 100,000/μL and hypokalemia is present (as in acute myeloid leukemia), glycolysis at room temperature may cause the K^+ deficit to seem greater than actuality.[2] In addition to causing pseudohypokalemia,[2] samples from leukemic patients with very high white blood cell counts (>300 × 10^9 cells/L) can result in a pseudohyperkalemia due to WBC rupture.[1] Together, with the effect of glycolysis leading to increased cellular uptake of K^+ followed by K^+ leakage as a result of exhaustion of glucose, or inhibition of glycolysis by refrigeration, the recommendation for reliable K^+ determinations is to collect blood with heparin and to maintain it near 25 °C, then to separate the plasma within minutes by high-speed centrifugation without cooling. In practical terms, separation within 1 hour when samples are maintained at room temperature is unlikely to introduce great error.

Finally, skeletal muscle activity causes K^+ efflux from muscle cells into plasma and can cause a marked elevation in plasma K^+ values. A common example occurs when an upper arm tourniquet is not released before beginning to draw blood after a patient clenches his fist repeatedly. The plasma K^+ values can artificially increase as much as 2 mmol/L because of the muscle activity.[30]

Reference Intervals[87]

Reported reference intervals for the serum of adults vary from 3.5 to 5.1 mmol/L and from 3.7 to 5.9 for newborns. For plasma, a frequently cited interval is 3.4 to 4.8 mmol/L for adults. The central 95% of K^+ values from more than 16,000 subjects in the NHANES III were from 3.4 to 4.7 mmol/L.[54] Cerebrospinal fluid concentrations are ≈70% those of plasma.[94] Urinary excretion of K^+ varies with dietary intake, but a typical range observed in an average diet is 42 to 86 mmol/d for males and 33 to 70 mmol/d for females.[84] Gastric juice contains K^+ at ≈10 mmol/L. Fecal excretion has been reported as 18.2 ± 2.5 mmol/d, but in severe diarrhea, gastrointestinal loss may be as much as 60 mmol/d.[16]

Methods for the Determination of Sodium and Potassium

Although AAS, FES, or spectrophotometric methods have been used for Na^+ and K^+ analyses in the past, most laboratories now use ISE methods. For example, in 2011, of the laboratories reporting proficiency data for Na^+ and K^+ to the College of American Pathologists (CAP), approximately 90 % were using ISE methods.[15]

Flame Emission Spectrophotometry

Although at one time the most common method for Na^+ and K^+ analyses, FES is no longer a common laboratory method. Advances in electrochemistry combined with the large number of maintenance and safety procedures required for FES have essentially led to the demise of this method for electrolyte analysis.

Principle. Samples are diluted in a diluent containing known amounts of lithium (or cesium, if lithium itself is being measured) and are aspirated into a propane-air flame. Sodium, potassium, lithium, and cesium ions, when excited, emit spectra with sharp, bright lines at 589, 768, 671, and 852 nm, respectively. Light emitted from the thermally excited ions is directed through separate interference filters to corresponding photodetectors. The Li^+ or Cs^+ emission signal is used as an internal standard against which the Na^+ and K^+ signals are compared. Details about reagents, procedures, and laboratory safety issues for flame photometry can be found in the third edition of this text.[89]

Ion-Selective Electrodes[63]

Analyzers fitted with ISEs usually contain Na^+ electrodes with glass membranes and K^+ electrodes with liquid ion-exchange membranes that incorporate valinomycin. Simply stated, potentiometry is the determination of change in electromotive force (*E*, potential) in a circuit between a measurement electrode (the ISE) and a reference electrode, as the selected ion interacts with the membrane of the ISE. In instrument applications, the measuring system is calibrated by the introduction of calibrator solutions containing defined amounts of Na^+ and K^+. The potentials of the calibrators are determined, and the $\Delta E/\Delta$ log concentration responses are stored in microprocessor memory as a comparison for calculating unknown concentration when *E* of the unknown is measured. It is important to note that the response of potentiometric electrodes to analytes is a complex process that depends on the composition and thermodynamic and kinetic properties of the sensor membrane, bathing solution, and interface zone between membrane and analyte and between membrane and bathing solution.[11] For simplicity, we classically describe *E* as the sum of the boundary potential *(EPB1)* at the (sample/ion-sensitive film boundary) and *EPB2* at the (membrane/internal contact) boundary, and by the diffusion potential *(ED)* inside the membrane itself. A constant, *C*, is added to account for potential at the internal sensor/contact interface.[11] Thus, we have the equation, $E = EPB1 + ED + EPB2 + C$. For simplicity, we typically assume that *C* and *ED* are zero. Thus, $E = EPB1 + EPB2$. This approximation is appropriate for most modern day electrodes, but the successful development of future solid state ion-selective electrodes (SS-ISEs) containing conducting polymers will require a newer approach to the complexity of *E* determinations. SS-ISEs are based on the covalent binding of ion recognition sites (metal complexing ligands) to a partially oxidized conductive polymer membrane, such as polypyrrole, where pyrrole nitrogens act as electron donors.[67] Thus, ion-selective integration sites are directly coupled with the ion electron transducer (conductive polymer) on the electrode, eliminating internal filling solutions or gels.[10] Development of SS-ISEs will allow for less electrode maintenance and electrode durability and miniaturization.[11] This affords the possibly of constructing microscale or nanoscale sensors.

Frequent calibration, initiated by the user or by microprocessor-controlled uptake of sample from a reservoir of the calibrator, is typical of most current ISE systems. Some instruments are designed to measure Na^+ and K^+ in whole blood, particularly point-of-care testing (POCT) devices and many blood gas analyzers.

Two types of ISE methods are in use and must be distinguished. With *indirect ISE methods,* the sample is introduced into the measurement chamber after mixing with a rather large volume of diluent. Indirect ISE methods are the methods used most commonly on today's automated, high-throughput clinical chemistry systems. Indirect methods were developed early in the history of ISE technology, when dilution was necessary to present a small sample in a volume large enough to adequately cover a large electrode and to minimize the concentration of protein at the electrode surface. With *direct ISE methods,* the sample is presented to the electrodes without dilution. This approach became possible with the miniaturization of electrodes. Direct ISEs are most common in blood gas analyzers and point-of-care devices where whole blood is directly presented to the electrodes. Single-use, thin-film ISEs for Na^+, K^+, and Cl^- are unique applications of a direct ISE method used by Ortho Vitros analyzers (Ortho Diagnostics, Raritan NJ).[25]

Errors observed in the use of ISEs fall into three categories. First are errors caused by lack of selectivity. For instance, many Cl^- electrodes lack selectivity against other halide ions. Most chloride selective membranes use a quaternary ammonium chloride ion exchanger.[73] Any ion that has a hydration energy equivalent to or higher than chloride can interfere with chloride selectivity. Examples include (1) iodide, (2) bromide, (3) thiocyanate, (4) bicarbonate, (5) salicylate, and (6) heparin. By far, bicarbonate is the most common interference, and its ionic activity is taken into account when the Nikolsky-Eisenman equation is used,[73] when the electrical potential difference of the chloride electrode is calculated. Second are errors introduced by repeated protein coating of the ion-sensitive membranes, or by contamination of the membrane or salt bridge by ions that compete or react with the selected ion and thus alter the electrode response. Such errors in ISE measurements necessitate periodic changes of the membrane as part of routine maintenance. Finally, the *electrolyte exclusion effect,* which applies only to indirect methods and is caused by the solvent-displacing effect of lipid and protein in the sample, results in falsely decreased values.[4]

Spectrophotometric Methods

Spectrophotometric methods fall into three categories: those based on enzyme activation and those that detect the spectral shift produced when Na^+ or K^+ binds to a macrocyclic chromophore. These approaches have been applied to smaller instruments. However, the high cost of reagents for these methods and the fact that few problems exist with ISE methods have resulted in small "niche" use of these methods, primarily with smaller instruments used in physicians' offices or clinics.[83]

Kinetic spectrophotometric assays for Na^+ are based on activation of the enzyme β-galactosidase by Na^+ to hydrolyze *o*-nitrophenyl-β-D-galactopyranoside.[75] The rate of production of *o*-nitrophenol (the chromophore) is measured at 420 nm.

o-Nitrophenyl-β-D-galactopyranoside $\xrightarrow[\beta\text{-Galactosidase}]{Na^{\oplus}}$ Galactose + *o*-Nitrophenol (λ_{max} = 420 nm)

K^+-specific enzyme activation assays are illustrated by methods using tryptophanase,[50] one of several K^+-enhanced enzymes.

Macrocyclic ionophores are molecules whose atoms are organized to form a cavity into which metal ions fit and bind with high affinity. Different macrocyclics can be made with cavities tailored to fit the ionic radii of different elements. When chromogenic properties are imparted to these ionophores, spectral shifts occur when the cation is bound. The specificity of many of these ionophores appears sufficient for clinical purposes.[52]

Electrolyte Exclusion Effect[4]

The electrolyte exclusion effect describes the exclusion of electrolytes from the fraction of the total plasma volume that is occupied by solids. The volume of total solids (primarily protein and lipid) in an aliquot of plasma is approximately 7%, so that ≈93% of plasma volume is actually water. The main electrolytes (Na^+, K^+, Cl^-, HCO_3^-) are confined to the water phase. When a fixed volume of total plasma (e.g., 10 μL) is pipetted for dilution before flame photometry or indirect ISE analysis, only 9.3 μL of plasma water that contains the electrolytes is added to the diluent. Thus a concentration of Na^+ determined by flame photometry or indirect ISE to be 140 mmol/L is the concentration in the total plasma volume, *not* in the plasma water volume. In fact, if the plasma contains 93% water, the concentration of Na^+ in plasma water is [140 × (100/93)], or 150 mmol/L. This negative "error" in plasma electrolyte analysis has been recognized for many years.[3] Even though it is the electrolyte concentration in plasma water that is physiologic (the Na^+ concentration of normal saline is indeed 150 mmol/L), it was assumed that the volume fraction of water in plasma is sufficiently constant that this difference could be ignored. In fact, all electrolyte reference intervals are based on this assumption and actually reflect concentrations in total plasma volume and not in water volume. Indeed, virtually all concentrations measured in the clinical chemistry laboratory are related to the total sample volume rather than to the water volume. This electrolyte exclusion effect becomes problematic when pathophysiologic conditions are present that alter the plasma water volume, such as hyperlipidemia or hyperproteinemia. In these settings, falsely low electrolyte values are obtained whenever samples are diluted before analysis, as in flame photometry or with indirect ISE methods[4] (Figure 28-1).

Indirect ISE methods dilute the sample in a diluent of fixed high ionic strength so that for Na^+, the activity coefficient approaches a value of 1. Under these circumstances, the measurement of activity, *(a)*, where $a = \gamma$ (concentration), and γ is the activity coefficient, is tantamount to measurement of concentration. It is the dilution of total plasma volume and the assumption that plasma water volume is constant that render both indirect ISE and flame photometry methods equally subject to the electrolyte exclusion effect. In certain settings, such as ketoacidosis with severe hyperlipidemia[37] or multiple myeloma with severe hyperproteinemia,[56] the negative exclusion effect may be so large that laboratory results lead clinicians to believe that electrolyte concentrations are normal or low when, in fact, the concentration in the water phase may be high or normal, respectively. In severe hypoproteinemia, the effect works in reverse, resulting in falsely high (2 to 4%) Na^+ or K^+ values. Plasma sodium, potassium, and chloride measurements by an indirect ISE were found to be affected by changes in plasma protein concentration when low plasma protein concentrations lead to an observed "pseudohyper" effect, and high plasma concentrations result in a "pseudohypo" effect.[29] The relationship was found to be nonlinear with no ability to calculate an accurate predictive value between changes in plasma protein and electrolyte concentration.

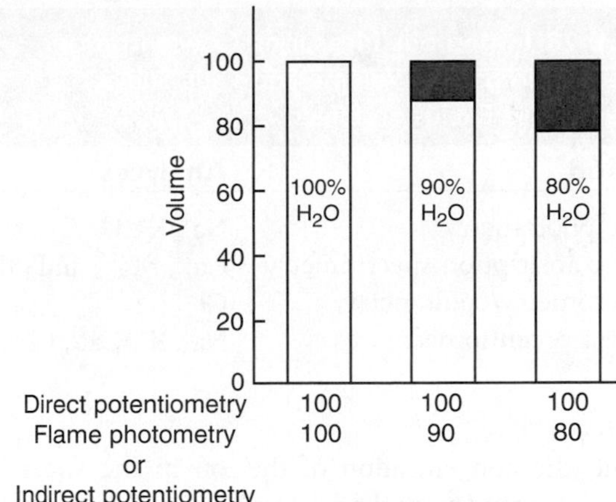

Figure 28-1 Predicted influence of water content on sodium measurements for a 100 mmol/L NaCl solution by direct ion-selective electrode (ISE) versus flame emission photometry or indirect ISE. *Red areas* represent nonaqueous volumes, which could consist of lipids, proteins, or even a slurry of latex or sand particles. *(Adapted from Apple FS, Koch DD, Graves S, Ladenson JH. Relationship between direct-potentiometric and flame-photometric measurement of sodium in blood. Clin Chem 1982;28:1931-5.)*

Direct ISE methods still determine the concentration relative to activity but do not require sample dilution. Because there is no dilution, activity is directly proportional to the concentration in the water phase, not the concentration in the total volume. To make results from direct ISEs equivalent to those from flame photometry and indirect ISEs, most direct ISE methods actually operate in what is commonly referred to as the "flame mode." In this mode, the directly measured concentration in plasma water is multiplied by the average water volume fraction of plasma (0.93). Although the latter may vary widely, as long as the activity of the specific ion is

TABLE 28-1 Methods Measuring Concentration in the Whole Sample Volume and Thus Subject to Electrolyte Exclusion Effect

Method	Analytes
Flame photometry	Na^+, K^+, Li^+
Atomic absorption spectrometry	Ca^{2+}, Mg^{2+}, and others
Amperometry/coulometry	Cl^-
Indirect potentiometry	Na^+, K^+, Ca^{2+}, Cl^-

TABLE 28-2 Methods Measuring Activity, Molality, or Concentration in the Water Phase and Thus Not Subject to Electrolyte Exclusion Effect

Method	Analytes
ISEs with *undiluted* sample	H^+ (pH), Na^+, K^+, Ca^{2+}, Cl^-, Li^+
Gas electrodes	CO_2 (PCO_2), O_2 (PO_2)
	HCO_3^- (calculated from pH and PCO_2)
Freezing point depression	H_2O (osmolality)

ISE, Ion-selective electrode.

constant, the concentration of the ion in the water phase becomes *independent* of the relative proportions of water and total solids if the ion is not bound by proteins. Therefore direct ISE methods are free of electrolyte exclusion effects, and the values determined by direct ISE methods—even in the flame mode—are directly proportional to activity in the water phase and define electrolyte concentrations in a more physiologic and physicochemical sense.

Most clinical chemists and physicians have reached the conclusion that direct ISE methods for electrolyte analysis are the methods of choice. They base their conclusion on the fact that great changes in plasma lipid or protein concentration can be expected in relatively common clinical conditions and in therapies such as parenteral alimentation with lipid emulsions. However, it is clear that results from direct methods will continue to be converted to total plasma volume concentrations by use of the "flame mode," and indeed this is the recommendation of the Clinical Laboratory and Standard Institute (CLSI). This is also a good recommendation in that two thirds of laboratories still use indirect ISE methods.[15] Tables 28-1 and 28-2 summarize methods that are and are not subject to electrolyte exclusion effects, respectively. One approach to improve the physiologic accuracy of electrolyte values from methods subject to the electrolyte exclusion effect consists of centrifugation (100,000 × g) and analysis of the chylomicron-poor infranatant.[3] In situations in which both lipid and protein contents are altered, presenting plasma electrolyte values along with concurrent estimates of plasma water have been suggested. One approach to estimate plasma water (f) is Waugh's empirical equation[95]:

$$f = (991 - 1.03\ L_s - 0.73\ P_s)/1000$$

where P_s is serum total protein and L_s is serum total lipid, both in grams per liter. Alternatively, the best solution is to use a direct ISE method.

Chloride

Chloride is the major extracellular anion. Therefore chloride, similar to Na^+, is significantly involved in the maintenance of water distribution, osmotic pressure, and anion-cation balance in the ECF. In contrast to its high ECF concentrations (≈103 mmol/L), the concentration of Cl^- in the intracellular fluid of erythrocytes is 45 to 54 mmol/L; in the intracellular fluid of most other tissue cells it is only ≈1 mmol/L. In gastric and intestinal secretions, Cl^- is the most abundant anion.

Chloride ions are almost completely absorbed from the intestinal tract. They are filtered from plasma at the glomeruli and are passively reabsorbed, along with Na^+, in the proximal tubules. In the thick ascending limb of the loop of Henle, Cl^- is actively reabsorbed by the chloride pump, which promotes passive reabsorption of Na^+. Loop diuretics such as furosemide and ethacrynic acid inhibit the chloride pump.

Methods for Determination of Chloride in Body Fluids

Chloride is determined by (1) mercurimetric titration, (2) spectrophotometry, (3) coulometric-amperometric titration, or, most commonly today, (4) ISE.

Specimens

Chloride most often is measured in serum or plasma, urine, and sweat. Cl^- is stable in serum and plasma. Even gross hemolysis does not significantly alter serum or plasma Cl^- concentration because the erythrocyte concentration of Cl^- is approximately half of that in plasma. Because very little Cl^- is protein bound, change in posture or stasis, or the use of tourniquets, has little effect on its plasma concentration. Measurement of Cl^- loss in gastric aspirates or intestinal drainages is an adjunct to parenteral replacement therapy. Fecal Cl^- determination may be useful for the diagnosis of congenital hypochloremic alkalosis with hyperchloridorrhea (increased excretion of Cl^- in stool). In this condition, the concentration of Cl^- in feces may reach 180 mmol/L, with undetectable Cl^- in urine.

Mercurimetric Titration

One of the earliest methods for determining Cl^- in biological fluids is mentioned for historical purposes. A protein-free filtrate of specimen is titrated with mercuric nitrate solution in the presence of diphenylcarbazone as an indicator. Free Hg^{2+} combines with Cl^- to form soluble but essentially nonionized mercuric chloride ($HgCl_2$). Excess Hg^{2+} reacts with diphenylcarbazone to form a blue-violet color complex[90]

Spectrophotometric Methods

Spectrophotometric methods based on the reaction of Cl^- with mercuric thiocyanate were common on many automated analyzers in the 1970s and 1980s. Chloride ions react with undissociated mercuric thiocyanate to form undissociated mercuric chloride and free thiocyanate ions. In the presence of perchloric acid, the thiocyanate ions react with ferric ion (Fe^{3+}) to form the highly colored, reddish complex of ferric thiocyanate [$Fe(SCN)_3$] with an absorption peak at 480 nm. High concentrations of globulins in the serum interfere in these methods through turbidity.

Mercurimetric automated methods applied to high-volume testing presented the problem of disposal of reagent waste containing a significant amount of toxic mercury. Consequently, the method is no longer in use.

Coulometric-Amperometric Titration

Reactions in coulometric-amperometric determinations of Cl^- depend on the generation of Ag^+ from a silver electrode at a constant rate and on the reaction of Ag^+ with Cl^- in the sample to form insoluble silver chloride (AgCl)[26]:

$$Ag^+ + Cl^- \rightarrow AgCl$$

After the stoichiometric point is reached, excess Ag^+ in the mixture triggers shutdown of the Ag^+ generation system. A timing device records elapsed time between the start and stop of Ag^+ generation. Because the time interval is proportional to the amount of Cl^- in the sample, the concentration of Cl^- can be calculated.

Applications of the coulometric-amperometric principle (often called the *Cotlove chloridometer technique*)[26] are the most precise methods for measuring Cl^- over the entire range of concentrations found in body fluids. This method is subject to interferences by other halide ions, by CN^- and SCN^- ions, by sulfhydryl groups, and by heavy metal contamination. Maintenance of the systems is crucial for proper operation. Today, less than 1% of ≈5149 laboratories report Cl^- results by using coulometry.[15] However, some laboratories maintain these instruments as backups and for sweat analysis.

Ion-Selective Electrode Methods

Solvent polymeric membranes that incorporate quaternary ammonium salt anion exchangers, such as tri-*n*-octylpropylammonium chloride decanol, are used to construct Cl^--selective electrodes in clinical analyzers.[73] Although they are by far the most common methods for measuring Cl^- in clinical laboratories, these electrodes have been described to suffer from membrane instability and lot-to-lot inconsistency in terms of selectivity to other anions.[73,93] Anions that tend to be problematic include other halides and organic anions, such as SCN^-, which can be particularly problematic because of their ability to solubilize in the polymeric organic membrane of these electrodes.

Approximately 82% of ≈5149 laboratories reporting in a 2008 CAP proficiency test survey for Cl^- used indirect ISE methods.[15]

Reference Intervals[51,91]

Reported reference intervals for Cl^- in the serum or plasma vary from 98 to 107 mmol/L to 100 to 108 mmol/L. The central 95% of Cl^- values from more than 16,000 subjects in NHANES III was 98 to 111 mmol/L.[54] For neonates, the upper limit of the interval extends to 113 mmol/L. Serum values vary little during the day. Spinal fluid Cl^- concentrations are ≈15% higher than those in serum.[94] Urinary excretion of Cl^- varies with dietary intake, but an interval of 110 to 250 mmol/d is typical. Fecal excretion of Cl^- (for eight healthy subjects) has been reported as 3.2 ± 0.7 mmol/d (SEM).[16]

Bicarbonate (Total Carbon Dioxide)

Total carbon dioxide is used here to describe the quantity that is measured most often in automated clinical chemistry analyzers by acidification of a serum or plasma sample and measurement of carbon dioxide released by the process, or by alkalinization and measurement of total bicarbonate. Under certain conditions of collection and specimen handling, total carbon dioxide values determined in this manner will be almost identical to values for the calculated concentration of total carbon dioxide obtained in blood gas analysis (see later section in this chapter on blood gas methods).

Specimens

The same sample types used for Na^+ or K^+ may be assayed. Given a specimen in a vacuum-draw tube, the concentration of total CO_2 is most accurately determined when the assay is done as promptly as possible after collection and centrifugation of the blood in the unopened tube. Ambient air contains far less CO_2 than does plasma, and gaseous dissolved CO_2 will escape from the specimen into the air, with a consequent decrease in the CO_2 value of up to 4 to 5 mmol/L in the course of 1 hour.[88] In practical terms, the logistics of high-volume processing and automated analysis of specimens almost ensures that most CO_2 measurements are done on specimens that have lost some dissolved gaseous CO_2, simply because preservation of anaerobic conditions is not practical between the time plasma is placed on an instrument and the time it is sampled. Thus the term *bicarbonate* may be preferable to *total CO_2*. On the other hand, a sample that is rapidly processed and promptly analyzed has a much smaller error.

Methods for Determination of Serum or Plasma Total Carbon Dioxide

One of the earliest methods for determining total CO_2 was the *manometric method* for total CO_2 content, using the Natelson microgasometer. This has been supplanted in clinical laboratories by automated methods. This method is described in some detail in an earlier edition of this text.[90]

The first step in automated methods is acidification or alkalinization of the sample. Acidifying the sample converts the various forms of CO_2 in plasma to gaseous CO_2 by dilution with an acid buffer. Alkalinizing the sample converts all CO_2 and carbonic acid to HCO_3^-. Methods for total CO_2 measurement with today's automated instruments may be electrode based or enzymatic. In indirect electrode-based methods, the amount of released gaseous CO_2 after acidification is determined by a PCO_2 electrode in the reaction chamber of the CO_2 module. About 32% of laboratories reporting CAP data used an indirect ISE method in 2008.[15] *Direct ISE methods* for total CO_2 are no longer common on automated analyzers. Direct methods for total CO_2 had problems with specificity and are no longer in use. For instance, one direct total CO_2 electrode reacted almost equivalently with nitrate.[27]

In *enzymatic methods* for CO_2, the specimen is first alkalinized to convert all CO_2 and carbonic acid to HCO_3^-. The enzymatic reactions are as follows:

$$\text{Phosphoenolpyruvate} + HCO_3^- \xrightarrow{\text{Phosphoenolpyruvate carboxylase}} \text{Oxaloacetate} + P_i$$

$$\text{Oxaloacetate} + \text{NADH} + H^+ \xrightarrow{\text{Malate dehydrogenase}} \text{Malate} + \text{NAD}^+$$

Decreased absorbance of NADH at 340 nm is proportional to the total CO_2 content.

Reference Intervals[51]

The reference interval for total carbon dioxide in adults is 22 to 28 mmol/L but can be instrument dependent. The central 95% of CO_2 values from more than 16,000 subjects in NHANES III was 21 to 35 mmol/L.[54]

Principles of Osmotic Pressure and Osmosis

Osmometry is a technique for measuring the concentration of solute particles that contribute to the osmotic pressure of a solution. Osmotic pressure governs the movement of solvent (water in biological systems) across membranes that separate two solutions. Different membranes vary in pore size and thus in their ability to select molecules of different size and shape. Examples of biologically important selective membranes are those enclosing the glomeruli and capillary vessels that are permeable to water and to essentially all *small* molecules and ions, but not to large protein molecules. Differences in the concentrations of osmotically active molecules that cannot cross a membrane cause those molecules that can cross the membrane to move to establish an osmotic equilibrium. This movement of solute and permeable ions exerts what is known as *osmotic pressure.*

As an example, consider an aqueous solution of sucrose placed within a sac made up of a membrane permeable only to water, with an open vertical glass tube (a crude manometer) attached to the sac. If the sac is placed into a beaker of distilled water, water will move from the beaker across the membrane into the sucrose solution. The pressure of this solvent movement will cause the sucrose solution to rise up the tube. At equilibrium, the gravitational pressure of the column of solution in the tube equals the osmotic pressure and prevents further net movement of water from the beaker. The height of the rise of the sucrose solution in the manometer tube is a measure of the *osmotic pressure* of the sucrose solution. This is the pressure that would have to be exerted on the sucrose side of the membrane to prevent the flow of water across the membrane.

Osmosis is the process that constitutes the movement of solvent across a membrane in response to differences in osmotic pressure across the two sides of the membrane. Water migrates across the membrane toward the side containing more concentrated solute.

If the sucrose solution in the aforementioned membrane sac were replaced with a sodium chloride solution of the same molarity, the solution in the manometer would reach equilibrium at a point almost twice as high as that observed with sucrose, because sodium chloride dissociates into two ions per molecule. If ion activity is unrestricted, the sodium chloride solution would have twice as many osmotically active particles (osmoles) for the same molecular concentration as the sucrose solution. In reality, the number of active particles is less than this (0.93 for NaCl), as explained later in this chapter. The total number of individual (solute) particles present in a solution per given mass of solvent, regardless of their molecular nature (i.e., nonelectrolyte, ion, or colloid), determines the total osmotic pressure of the solution. In blood plasma, for example, nonelectrolytes such as glucose and urea and, to a much lesser extent, proteins contribute to the osmotic pressure.

Colligative Properties

In addition to increasing osmotic pressure when the solute is added to the solvent, the *vapor pressure* of the solution is *lowered* below that of the pure solvent. As a result of the change in vapor pressure, the *boiling point* of the solution is *raised* above and the *freezing point* of the solution is *lowered* below that of the pure solvent.

These four properties of solutions—(1) increased osmotic pressure, (2) lowered vapor pressure, (3) increased boiling point, and (4) decreased freezing point—are called *colligative properties.* All are directly related to the total number of solute particles per mass of solvent. For instance, a 1-molal solution in water boils at a temperature 0.52 °C higher and freezes at a temperature 1.858 °C lower than pure water. The vapor pressure of this solution is 0.3 mm Hg lower than the vapor pressure of pure water, which is 23.8 mm Hg at 25 °C. The osmotic pressure of the same solution is increased from zero to 17,000 mm Hg (22.4 atmospheres). The term *osmolality* expresses concentrations relative to *mass* of the solvent (1 osmolal solution is defined to contain 1 Osmol/kg H_2O), whereas the term *osmolarity* expresses concentrations per volume of solution (1 osmolar solution is defined to contain 1 Osmol/L solution). Osmolality (Osmol/kg H_2O) is a thermodynamically more exact expression because solution concentrations expressed on a weight basis are temperature independent, whereas those based on volume vary with temperature. Although the term *osmolarity* is often used in the medical literature, *osmolality* is what the clinical laboratory measures.

An electrolyte in solution dissociates into two (in the case of NaCl) or three (in the case of $CaCl_2$) particles; therefore the colligative effects of such solutions are multiplied by the number of dissociated ions formed per molecule. However, because of incomplete electrolyte dissociation and associations between solute and solvent molecules, many solutions do not behave in the ideal case, and a 1-molal solution may give an osmotic pressure lower than theoretically expected. The osmotic activity coefficient is a factor used to correct for deviation from the "ideal" behavior of the system:

$$\text{Osmolality} = \text{osmol}/\text{kg } H_2O = \Phi nC$$

where Φ = osmotic coefficient, n = number of particles into which each molecule in the solution potentially dissociates, and C = molality in mol/kg H_2O. A table of osmotic coefficients of most solutes of biological interest has been compiled.[99]

Glucose has an osmotic coefficient of 1.00, whereas the Φ for sodium chloride is 0.93 at the concentrations found in serum—thus the derivation of 1.86 × Na^+ (mmol) in the formula to calculate plasma osmolality (NaCl potentially contributes two osmotically active particles times 0.93 = 1.86). Ethanol has an osmotic coefficient of 0.83.[38] The total osmolality or osmotic pressure of a solution is equal to the sum of the osmotic pressures or osmolalities of all solute species present. The electrolytes Na^+, Cl^-, and HCO_3^-, which are present in relatively high concentrations, make the greatest contributions to serum osmolality. Nonelectrolytes such as glucose and urea, which are present normally at lower molal concentrations, contribute less, and serum proteins contribute less than 0.5% of the total serum osmolality because even the most abundant protein is present at millimolar concentrations.

Determination of Plasma and Urine Osmolality

Determination of plasma and urine osmolality can be useful in the assessment of electrolyte and acid-base disorders. Comparison of plasma and urine osmolalities can determine the appropriateness and status of water regulation by the kidneys in settings of severe electrolyte disturbances, as might occur in diabetes insipidus or the syndrome of inappropriate antidiuretic hormone (SIADH) (see Chapters 48 and 53). The major osmotic substances in normal plasma are Na^+, Cl^-, glucose, and urea; thus expected plasma osmolality can be calculated from the following empirical equation:

$$\text{mOsmol}/\text{kg} = 1.86[Na^+(\text{mmol}/\text{L})] + \text{Glucose}(\text{mmol}/\text{L}) + \text{Urea}(\text{mmol}/\text{L}) + 9$$

or

$$\text{mOsmol}/\text{kg} = 1.86[Na^+(\text{mmol}/\text{L})] + \text{Glucose}(\text{mg}/\text{dL})/18 + \text{Urea}(\text{mg}/\text{dL})/2.8 + 9$$

The 9 mOsmol/kg added to the previous equation represents the contributions of other osmotically active substances in plasma, such as K^+, Ca^{2+}, and proteins, and 1.86 is two times the osmotic coefficient of Na^+, reflecting the contributions of both Na^+ and Cl^-. Some versions of this equation does not include the plus 9 mOsmol/kg factor. The reference interval for plasma osmolality is 275 to 300 mOsmol/kg.[87] Comparison of measured osmolality versus calculated osmolality can reveal the presence of an *osmolal gap,* which can be important in determining the presence of exogenous osmotic substances. Comparison of calculated and measured osmolalities can also confirm or rule out suspected pseudohyponatremia caused by the electrolyte exclusion effect.

Theoretically, any of the four colligative properties discussed above: (1) vapor pressure, (2) boiling point, (3) freezing point, and (4) osmotic pressure could be used as a basis for the measurement of osmolality. However, freezing point depression is most commonly used in clinical laboratories because of its simplicity. Furthermore, freezing point depression, unlike vapor pressure, is independent of changes in ambient temperature. (The vapor pressure of water is 17.5 mm Hg at 20 °C, 23.8 mm Hg at 25 °C, and 47.1 mm Hg at 37 °C.)

Freezing Point Depression Osmometer

The instrument used is a freezing point depression osmometer, but it is often referred to simply as an osmometer. The components of a freezing point depression osmometer (Figure 28-2) are as follows:

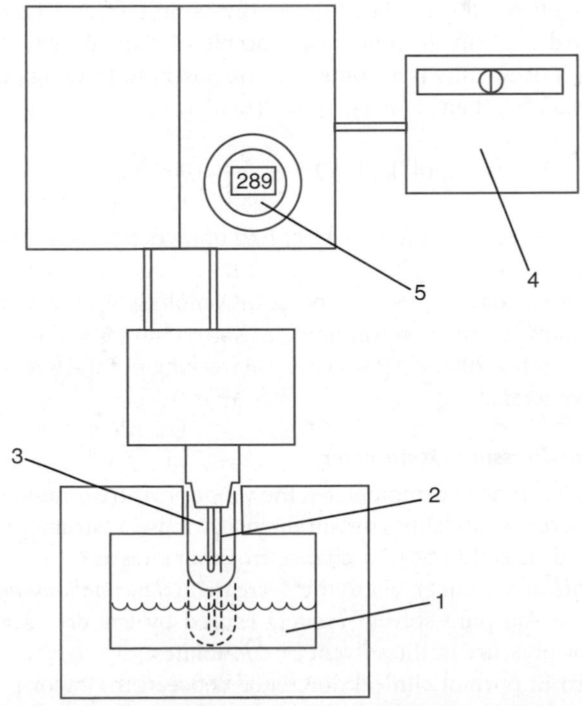

Figure 28-2 Block diagram of a freezing point depression osmometer. *1,* Cooling fluid; *2,* stirring rod; *3,* thermistor; *4,* galvanometer; *5,* potentiometer with direct readout. The test tube is shown above the liquid in the cooling bath *(solid line)* and inside the cooling liquid *(dashed line).*

1. A thermostatically controlled cooling bath or block maintained at −7 °C.
2. A rapid stir mechanism to initiate ("seed") freezing of the sample.
3. A thermistor probe connected to a circuit to measure the temperature of the sample. (The thermistor is a glass bead attached to a metal stem whose resistance varies rapidly and predictably with temperature.)
4. A galvanometer that displays the freezing curve and that is used as a guide when the measuring potentiometer is used.
5. A measuring potentiometer.

In most instruments today, components 4 and 5 are replaced by a light-emitting diode (LED) display that indicates the time course of the freezing curve and the final result.

During analysis, the following steps occur. The sample, in which the thermistor probe and the stirring wire are centered, is lowered into the bath and, with gentle stirring, is supercooled to a temperature several degrees below its freezing point (−7 °C). When the galvanometer (or LED display) indicates that sufficient super cooling has occurred, the sample is raised to a point above the liquid in the cooling bath, and the wire stirrer is changed from a gentle rate of stir to a momentary vigorous amplitude, which initiates freezing of the super-cooled solution. This freezing occurs only to the slush stage, with about 2 to 3% of the solvent solidifying. The released heat of fusion initially warms the solution, and then the temperature plateaus and remains stationary, indicating the equilibrium temperature at which both freezing and thawing of the solution are occurring. At the end of the equilibrium temperature plateau, the galvanometer again indicates decreasing temperature as the sample freezes further toward a complete solid. An example of the calculation to obtain osmolality is as follows: if the observed freezing point is −0.53 °C, then

$$\text{mosmol/kg } H_2O = \frac{-0.53}{-1.86} \times 1000 = 285$$

where −1.86 °C is the molal freezing point depression of pure water.

Day-to-day imprecision of ±2 mOsmol/kg H_2O should be attainable by today's osmometers. More than 98% of laboratories in the 2008 CAP surveys use freezing point depression osmometers.[15]

Vapor Pressure Osmometer

Another type of osmometer is the vapor pressure osmometer. However, osmolality measurement in these instruments is related directly not to a change in vapor pressure (in millimeters of mercury), but to the decrease in *dew point temperature* of the pure solvent (water) caused by the decrease in vapor pressure of the solvent by the solutes.

An important clinical difference between the vapor pressure technique and the freezing point depression osmometer is the failure of the former to include in its measurement of total osmolality any volatile solutes present in the serum. Substances such as ethanol, methanol, and isopropanol are volatile and thus escape from the solution and increase the vapor pressure instead of lowering the vapor pressure of the solvent (water). This makes the use of vapor pressure osmometers impractical for identifying osmolal gaps in acid-base disturbances (see Chapter 49), and use of this type of osmometer cannot be recommended for most clinical laboratories.

SWEAT TESTING

Analysis of sweat for increased chloride concentration is used to confirm the diagnosis of cystic fibrosis (CF). CF is recognized as a syndrome with a wide spectrum of clinical presentations associated with a defect in the cystic fibrosis transmembrane conductance regulator protein (CFTR), a protein that normally regulates electrolyte transport across epithelial membranes. The genetics of CF is discussed in Chapter 40. More than 1600 mutations of CFTR have been identified.[18] Although mutational analysis is available, it is not informative in all cases, and the sweat chloride test remains the standard for diagnostic testing.[35]

The U.S. Cystic Fibrosis Foundation (CFF) bases the diagnosis of CF on the following criteria[35]:

1. The presence of one or more characteristic phenotypic features.
2. *Or* a history of CF in a sibling.
3. *Or* a positive newborn screening test result.
4. *And* laboratory evidence of a CFTR abnormality as documented by elevated *sweat chloride* concentrations on two or more occasions; or identification of two CF-causing mutations; or demonstration of abnormal nasal epithelial ion transport.

To provide appropriate care for CF patients and genetic counseling to their families, it is important that the diagnosis of CF be made accurately and promptly. Newborn screening (NBS) for CF, based on an elevated immunoreactive trypsinogen (IRT) and subsequent DNA mutational analysis or repeat IRT, is mandated throughout the United States. An infant identified by NBS as being at risk for CF must be followed with a sweat chloride test to confirm the diagnosis (Figure 28-3). This practice has led to testing of more infants younger than 1 month of age.

In addition to variable clinical presentation, the diagnosis of CF can be complicated by erroneous sweat testing results. Unreliable methods, technical errors, and errors in interpretation all can lead to false results. In an effort to standardize testing, the Clinical and Laboratory Standards Institute (CLSI) developed the guideline document C34-A3, "Sweat Testing: Sample Collection and Quantitative Chloride Analysis."[22] This CLSI document has been adopted by the CFF for use in its accredited care centers.[35] To encourage acceptable performance of the sweat test, the CAP Laboratory Accreditation Program has incorporated sweat collection and analysis into the Chemistry checklist.

The sweat test occurs in three phases: (1) sweat stimulation by pilocarpine iontophoresis; (2) collection of the sweat onto gauze, filter paper, coil, patch, or capillary tube; and (3) qualitative or quantitative analysis of sweat chloride, sodium, conductivity, or osmolality.

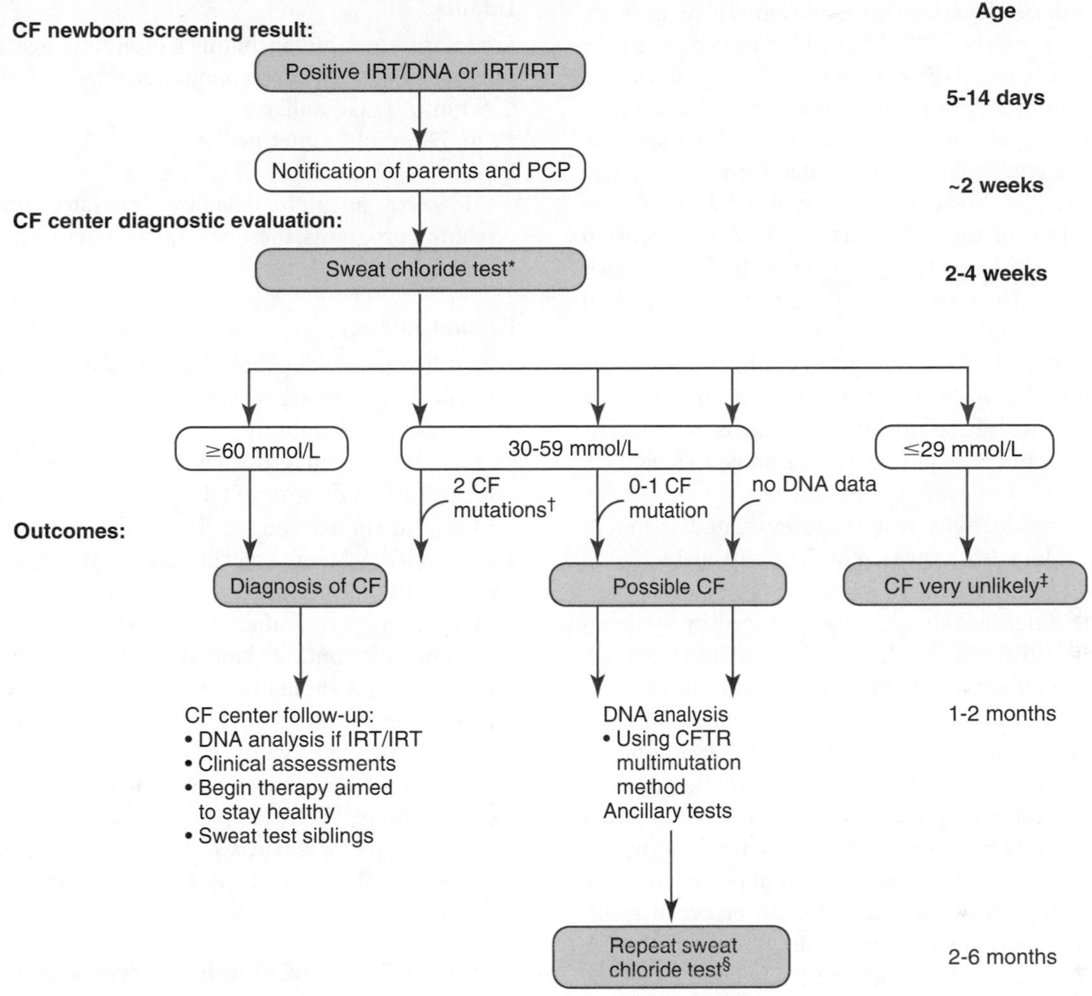

Figure 28-3 Diagnostic algorithm for cystic fibrosis (CF) following newborn screening. *[From Farrell PM, Rosenstein BJ, White TB, Accurso FJ, Castellani C, Cutting GR, et al; Cystic Fibrosis Foundation. Guidelines for diagnosis of cystic fibrosis in newborns through older adults: Cystic Fibrosis Foundation consensus report. J Pediatr 2008;153(2):S4-14.]*

Qualitative Screening Tests

Screening tests may or may not measure the amount of sweat collected and may report a result as positive, negative, or intermediate, or may give an actual concentration of sweat analytes. Patients having a positive or intermediate screening result should be followed with a sweat chloride test. The CFF forbids accredited CF care centers from using screening sweat tests but rather requires those centers to perform quantitative analysis of sweat chloride.[61] Examples of qualitative screening sweat tests currently in use are the (1) Wescor Sweat-Chek and Nanoduct conductivity analyzers (Wescor, Logan, Utah), (2) Advanced Instruments conductivity analyzer (Advanced Instruments, Inc., Norwood, Mass), (3) Orion skin electrode for chloride (Orion Research, Cambridge, Mass), (4) CF Indicator System chloride patch (Polychrome Medical, Brooklyn, Minn), and (5) sweat osmolality measurements. The Nanoduct instrument from Wescor combines pilocarpine iontophoresis with a disposable conductivity cell. Although a variety of systems are in use for sweat testing, several of these methods have documented problems, making them inappropriate for clinical use.[22] For example, the Orion Skin Measuring System and older conductivity analyzers using unheated collection cups are not recommended as diagnostic procedures because problems have been reported with sample evaporation and condensation and the ability to quantify sweat samples adequately.[19,28,60,77,96] The CFF has approved the Macroduct Sweat-Chek (Wescor) for screening at clinical sites, such as community hospitals, using the criteria that a patient having a sweat conductivity ≥50 mmol/L should be referred to an accredited CF care center for a quantitative sweat chloride test.[17,61] Wescor's recommended decision level is higher than that of the CFF; this can lead to confusion between the laboratory and the physician as to the appropriate decision level.[57] The CFF medical advisory committee, in setting the decision limit at 50 mmol/L, did so cautiously, realizing that the goal of screening tests is to tolerate some false-positive results and minimize or prevent false-negative results. Situations with false-positive test results are resolved on further testing, but it would be unacceptable to miss a CF patient.

When sweat conductivity results are evaluated, it should be noted that values from sweat conductivity methods are approximately 15 mmol/L higher than sweat chloride concentration. The difference most likely is caused by the presence of unmeasured anions, such as lactate and bicarbonate.[44] Because of this difference, laboratories must be clear in reporting that the screening test result represents conductivity, not chloride, and must include appropriate sweat conductivity reference intervals. Confusion, anxiety, and the potential for misdiagnosis arise in patients and their families when sweat conductivity is mistakenly evaluated with the use of sweat chloride reference intervals. Sixty-eight percent of laboratories performing sweat conductivity had errors in result reporting that included using inappropriate decision levels, reporting conductivity as chloride, and using conductivity as a diagnostic test, not as a screening test.[57]

Quantitative Confirmatory Tests

According to the CLSI C34-A3 document,[22] a quantitative diagnostic sweat test consists of (1) collecting sweat into gauze, filter paper, or Macroduct coils; (2) evaluating the amount collected in weight (milligrams) or volume (microliters); and (3) measuring the sweat chloride concentration. For diagnostic purposes, the CFF requires laboratories to perform a quantitative analysis of sweat chloride in accordance with the techniques described in the CLSI document C34-A3.[22] Chloride concentration can be determined by coulometric titration using a chloridometer. If a laboratory chooses to quantify sweat chloride using an automated analyzer that employs an ISE, these methods must be systematically validated for accuracy, precision, and, particularly, the lower limit of the analytical measurement range. Instrumentation used for measuring sweat chloride concentration should be able to detect chloride concentration as low as 10 mmol/L on unadulterated sweat. Analysts should not attempt to boost the analytical sensitivity by adding extraneous chloride standard to patients' specimens.

Reference Intervals for Sweat Chloride

Reference intervals for sweat chloride must be stratified by patient age.

Infants

For infants up to and including 6 months of age, the following reference intervals are recommended[22]:

≤29 mmol/L: CF unlikely
30 to 59 mmol/L: intermediate
≥60 mmol/L: indicative of CF

However, as more data are generated from newborn screening programs, these reference intervals may have to be adjusted.

Beyond Infancy

For individuals older than 6 months of age, the following reference intervals are recommended[22]:

≤39 mmol/L: CF unlikely
40 to 59 mmol/L: intermediate
≥60 mmol/L: indicative of CF

The functional upper limit for sweat chloride is 160 mmol/L.[81] Sweat chloride concentrations greater than 160 mmol/L are not physiologically possible and can represent specimen contamination or analytical error. A normal sweat chloride concentration alone is insufficient to rule out the diagnosis; it should be interpreted in light of the clinical picture and with the knowledge that "normal" concentrations have been associated with CF. Some mutations of the CF gene are associated with intermediate or normal sweat chloride concentrations.[35] For example, according to the CFF registry, 3.5% of CF patients had sweat chloride concentrations less than 60 mmol/L, and 1.2% had concentrations less than 40 mmol/L.[61]

Intermediate Sweat Chloride Concentrations

Individuals with intermediate concentrations of sweat chloride should be further evaluated to include more extensive genotyping, clinical assessment, and repeat sweat chloride testing, with recognition of the increasing phenotypic variability of CF.

Decision Limits for Sweat Conductivity

Consensus is lacking regarding the appropriate decision limit for sweat conductivity. The CFF states that a patient with sweat conductivity ≥50 mmol/L should be referred for a confirmatory sweat chloride test. Manufacturers' recommendations may differ.

Sweat Stimulation and Collection

Localized sweating is produced by iontophoresis of the cholinergic drug pilocarpine nitrate into an area of the skin. Iontophoresis uses a small electric current to deliver pilocarpine into the sweat glands from the positive electrode, and an electrolyte solution at the negative electrode completes the circuit. The current source should be battery powered and regularly inspected according to hospital guidelines by qualified personnel for voltage leak and current control.[22] After iontophoresis, sweat is collected onto preweighed gauze pads or filter paper or into Macroduct coils, using techniques to minimize evaporation and contamination. The Centers for Disease Control and Prevention[48] does not list sweat as a potentially infectious material unless it is visibly contaminated with blood.[48] However, laboratory personnel should practice the same standard precautions they would use with any other body fluid. All equipment used in iontophoresis should be disinfected between patients in accordance with procedures consistent with the institution's infection control policies. Disinfectants must not contain bleach, which could contaminate the sweat sample.

Because of transient increases in sweat electrolytes shortly after birth, patients should be at least 48 hours old and preferably at least 2 weeks of age before a sweat test is performed.[22] Symptomatic newborns such as those with meconium ileus can be tested after 48 hours of age; however, the quantity of inconclusive results may be greater at this early age.[33,35] Asymptomatic infants, such as those identified through newborn screening, should be tested when the infant is at least 2 weeks of age, was at least 36 weeks' gestation at birth, and weighs more than 2 kg to maximize the opportunity to collect a sufficient sweat sample.[22,33,35] The patient should be physiologically and nutritionally stable, well hydrated, free of acute illness, and not receiving mineralocorticoids. The inner flexor surface of the forearm is the preferred site for sweat testing. The right or left arm is acceptable. If the arms are unavailable, sweat testing can be performed on the patient's inner thigh; however this area has a lower sweat gland density compared with the forearm.[98] Never allow the current to cross the patient's chest. The skin should be free of cuts, rashes, and inflammation so as to prevent contamination of the sweat sample with serous fluid. For example, sweat testing should never be performed over an area of eczema.[49] The sweat test can be performed on a patient receiving intravenous fluid, as long as good contact between the skin and the electrode is possible, collection techniques do not interfere with venous flow, and intravenous fluids do not contaminate the collection area. Iontophoresis should not be performed on a patient receiving oxygen by an open delivery system. Often such patients can temporarily receive oxygen by way of a face mask or nasal cannula, permitting sweat testing.

If sweat is collected onto gauze or filter paper, the electrodes usually are made of copper and are slightly smaller than the stimulation and collection area. Reagents include U.S. Pharmacopeia (USP) grade 0.2 to 0.5% pilocarpine nitrate solution, a dilute electrolyte solution, and distilled or deionized water. The composition of the electrolyte solution should be selected to prevent contamination with the sweat sample and saline should not be used. A supply of gauze pads, low in electrolyte content, is necessary for cleansing and drying the skin. Before collection, the gauze or filter paper used for sweat collection should be placed into a weighing vial with a secure sealing lid, and the vial should be labeled and weighed using an analytical balance. To minimize contamination, the collection gauze or filter paper and the preweighed vial containing them should never be handled directly. The analyst should always use forceps or powder-free gloves. For a detailed procedure for stimulation and collection, refer to CLSI document C34-A3.[22]

Alternatively, for sweat stimulation, the electrodes and current source can be integrated as in the Wescor Macroduct system, which uses gel reagents containing pilocarpine. The battery-powered iontophoresis system delivers a current of 1.5 mA for 5 minutes. Distilled or deionized water and gauze pads or tissues are necessary for cleaning the skin. With the use of this stimulation system, sweat is collected into a disposable microbore tubing coil collector. After sufficient sweat has been collected, it is transferred from the coil into a sealable microsample cup. When the Macroduct collection system is used, the analyst should not touch or otherwise contaminate the concave collecting surface. For specific procedures using the Macroduct collection system, refer to the manufacturer's instructions.

To standardize and simplify the collection process, it is recommended that the size of the electrodes, reagent pads, and collection material be approximately the same. For example, when a 2 × 2-inch gauze or filter paper collection pad is used, the electrodes should be slightly smaller, about 1.5 × 1.5 inches, and the area of stimulation, represented by the size of the reagent pads, should be the same size as the collection pads, that is, 2 × 2 inches.[61] When the Wescor Macroduct stimulation system and Pilogel are used, sweat should be collected into the coils designed with the system.

Critical Issues Associated With Sweat Collection

The analyst must address several important issues when collecting sweat. These include (1) providing adequate patient education, (2) using appropriate stimulation and collection systems, (3) preventing evaporation and contamination, (4) collecting a sufficient sample, (5) minimizing skin reactions, and (6) obtaining appropriate storage for the sweat sample.

Patient Education

Sweat testing is one of the few clinical chemistry tests involving direct patient contact. Patients and their parents often have questions about the sweat test that their physicians may not have answered. Educational materials on sweat testing have been produced by the CFF in English and Spanish and include both written and video materials.

Appropriate Stimulation and Collection Systems

Sweat should be collected in association with compatible stimulation equipment and should not be hybridized. For example, laboratories using Wescor Pilogel iontophoresis should collect sweat only into the Macroduct coils and not onto gauze or filter paper. Hybridizing the Wescor Pilogel iontophoresis system with gauze or filter paper collection can dramatically alter the minimum collection volume or weight required to ensure adequate sweat gland stimulation and affect the validity of the sweat electrolyte determination.

Evaporation and Contamination

Testing procedures should minimize the opportunity for evaporation and contamination of the sweat sample. For example, only distilled or deionized water should be used in the collection and analysis; "pure" or sterile water should not be used, as it may not be sufficiently free of chloride ions. Detailed instructions on minimizing evaporation and contamination are found in the CLSI sweat testing document.[22]

Specimen Weight and Collection Time

To obtain a valid sweat testing result, determination of and adherence to a minimum sweat weight or volume are critical. The requirement for a minimum amount is physiologic, to ensure an appropriate sweat rate and sweat electrolyte concentration. It is independent of the instrumentation used to measure sweat electrolytes. Unfortunately, this is poorly understood, leading to false-positive and false-negative sweat test results, which have significant implications for patient care. Sweat electrolyte concentration is related to sweat rate. At low sweat rates, sweat electrolyte concentration decreases and the opportunity for sample evaporation is increased.[39] To ensure a valid result, the average sweat rate should exceed 1 g/m^2/min. The minimum acceptable volume or weight depends on the size of the electrode and stimulation area, the type and size of collecting devices, and the length of time the sweat is collected.[61] If a laboratory deviates from standard parameters, the minimum acceptable sweat volume or weight will change. The stimulation and/or collection requirement applies to each site independently, so insufficient samples must not be pooled for analysis.

When the acceptable rate is applied to the parameters described in the CLSI document, the minimum acceptable sample for analysis from a single site using 2 × 2-inch gauze or filter paper for stimulation and collection is 75 mg of sweat collected within 30 minutes. When the Macroduct system is used, the electrodes and stimulation area are smaller, and the minimum acceptable sample is 15 μL collected within 30 minutes. Sweat should be collected for only 30 minutes. If the collection time exceeds 30 minutes, the requirement for the amount of sweat necessary to ensure adequate stimulation would have to be increased. Extending the collection time can allow additional opportunity for sweat evaporation and practically does not significantly increase the sweat yield.

Sufficient Sample Collection

Acquiring the minimum sample should not be a problem for most patients if the laboratorian follows both the procedure in the CLSI document and the manufacturer's recommendations. On average, the percentage of insufficient samples should not exceed 5% for patients older than 3 months of age.[61] If the laboratory collects sweat from two sites (aka bilateral testing), the test is considered QNS (quantity not sufficient) only when both sites are inadequate. The average amount of sweat collected on 2 × 2-inch gauze pads at one CF center is 282 mg, and in Macroduct coils it is 65 μL.[44,58] Insufficient sweat samples can be the result of several factors such as age, race, skin condition, and collection system.[33] Collecting an adequate amount of sweat can be more challenging in patients younger than 1 month of age.[33] For this reason, it is recommended that sweat testing in asymptomatic individuals be performed when the infant is at least 2 weeks of age, is more than 36 weeks' gestation at birth, and weighs more than 2 kg.[35] If an adequate sweat sample is not obtained, the test can be repeated as soon as is practical. To ensure adequate sweat production, the analyst should check that the reagents are within the expiration date, and that the size of the stimulation area corresponds to the size of the collection surface.

Skin Reactions

Burns to the patient's skin after iontophoresis are extremely rare but can occur at either electrode. If the burn occurs at the site of pilocarpine stimulation, sweat should not be collected. Pilocarpine urticaria associated with sweat testing is rare but has been reported.[59]

To minimize the potential for burns, the analyst should:

1. Keep the electrode surfaces clean. Clean copper electrodes after every use with emery cloth to remove surface oxidation.
2. Attach the electrodes firmly. Maintain a wet interface with the skin during iontophoresis. When using liquid reagents on gauze or filter paper, ensure that they are thoroughly saturated. When using gel reagents, apply a drop of distilled or deionized water to the gel surface.
3. Prevent bare metal of the electrode from touching the skin. The gauze or filter paper pads should be slightly larger than the electrodes. When using gel reagents, do not use gel disks that have a crack or a structural defect in them.
4. Limit iontophoretic current. At the beginning of iontophoresis, slowly raise the current, and do not exceed 4.0 mA current.

Storage of Sweat Samples

Sweat samples should be analyzed soon after collection on the same day. However, in unusual circumstances, if there is a significant delay between collection and analysis, the laboratory can store the sweat samples. If sweat is collected into gauze, it should be reweighed promptly and can be stored with a tightly fitting lid up to 72 hours at 4 °C.[22] If sweat is collected in Wescor Macroduct coils, it should be transferred to a 0.2 mL microcentrifuge tube with a tight-fitting cap and stored for up to 72 hours. The sweat should *not* be stored or transported in the microbore tubing.[22]

Sources of Error in Sweat Testing

Unreliable methodology, technical errors, and errors in interpretation all can lead to erroneous sweat test results. Methods that do not quantify sweat collected or that do not have an established minimum sample volume or weight are subject to false-negative results because an adequate sweat rate cannot be ensured.

Other problems with sweat testing include errors of evaporation and contamination, as well as errors in dilution, instrument calibration, sample identification, and result reporting. These errors occur more frequently in institutions performing relatively few tests.[78,92] Laboratories with a low testing volume for sweat analysis should consider discontinuing the test and referring patients to accredited CF care centers for testing and evaluation. Interpretation errors with the sweat test include lack of knowledge about the laboratory method, failure to repeat intermediate results, failure to repeat negative test results when inconsistent with the clinical picture, making a diagnosis on a single positive test result, and failure to repeat testing in patients diagnosed as having CF who do not follow the expected clinical course. Edema, hypoproteinemia, and administration of mineralocorticoids can decrease sweat electrolytes.[40,64]

Sweat Testing Quality Assurance

High-quality sweat testing includes selecting appropriate methods, having a sufficient testing volume to ensure familiarity with the test, and limiting testing personnel to a small number of well-trained individuals. An effective quality assurance program for sweat analysis encompasses (1) preanalytical, (2) analytical, and (3) postanalytical factors.

Preanalytical Quality Assurance

Physicians should be aware of the clinical spectrum of CF and should appropriately order a sweat test on patients suspected of the disorder. Because of the significant preanalytical variation associated with sweat testing, duplicate testing from two body sites is recommended.[35] Most sweat chloride concentrations agree within 5 mmol/L on bilateral testing. Each laboratory should establish a required level of agreement for bilateral results. It has been suggested that when the sweat chloride concentration is less than 60 mmol/L, duplicate tests should agree within 10 mmol/L, and when the chloride concentration exceeds 60 mmol/L, tests should agree within 15 mmol/L.[61] Stimulation and collection procedures should minimize the opportunity for evaporation and contamination of the sweat sample. The patient's skin at the collection site should be free of inflammation or rash.

Analytical Quality Control and Quality Assurance

Analytical methods for sweat testing should be validated and routinely monitored according to local and national regulatory agencies, using sample concentrations and volumes equivalent to patient samples. For quality control, two levels of controls should be performed every day when patient samples are analyzed. One control should reflect the concentration of sweat chloride in a non-CF patient, and the other control should reflect the concentration of sweat chloride found in a CF patient. Controls should be performed in parallel with patient samples, and results should fall within a predetermined interval before patient results can be reported. Short- and long-term quality control should be monitored.

Personnel performing sweat collection and analysis must be carefully trained and periodically evaluated for competency. Sweat testing should include external validation of sweat analysis accuracy through participation in proficiency testing. The CAP offers a proficiency testing program consisting of six specimens per year. Participants receive feedback concerning their performance on these specimens relative to others in their peer group.

BOX 28-1 Reported Diseases or Conditions Other Than Cystic Fibrosis Associated With an Elevated Sweat Electrolyte Concentration

Anorexia nervosa
Atopic dermatitis
Autonomic dysfunction
Celiac disease
Environmental deprivation
Familial cholestasis
Fucosidosis type 1
Glycogen storage disease type 1
Hypogammaglobulinemia
Keratitis, ichthyosis, deafness (KID) syndrome
Mauriac's syndrome (malnutrition of)
Protein-calorie malnutrition
Pseudohypoaldosteronism
Psychosocial failure to thrive
Systemic lupus erythematosus
Trioesphosphate isomerase (TPI) deficiency
Untreated adrenal insufficiency
Untreated hypothyroidism

From Clinical and Laboratory Standards Institute (CLSI). Sweat testing: sample collection and quantitative chloride analysis: approved guideline, 3rd edition. CLSI document C34-A3. Wayne, Pa: Clinical and Laboratory Standards Institute, 2009.

Postanalytical Quality Assurance

Results of the sweat test must be interpreted in light of the patient's clinical presentation by a physician knowledgeable about CF. Several conditions other than CF are associated with elevations in sweat electrolytes, based on the small numbers of patients reported (Box 28-1). These conditions usually are distinguishable from CF based on the patient's clinical presentation, and often, after treatment of the disorder, the sweat test returns to normal.

BLOOD GASES AND pH

Clinical management of respiratory and metabolic disorders often depends on rapid, accurate measurements of oxygen and carbon dioxide in blood. Vigorous measures to support life in patients with cardiopulmonary impairment depend largely on assisted ventilation using mixtures of gases that are tailored in response to laboratory blood gas results. Determination of blood gases also plays an important part in the detection of acid-base imbalances. Modern instruments for blood gas determination are simple to operate and, with meticulous maintenance and quality control, are capable of rapid, very reliable laboratory data. Details of the pathophysiology of blood gases in relation to respiration and acid-base disorders are discussed in detail in Chapter 49.

Nomenclature for this area of analysis has been recommended by the CLSI,[23] but alternative nomenclatures exist and are in common use; these are summarized in Box 28-2.

BOX 28-2 Conversion Factors, Prefixes, Symbols, and Descriptors Used in Discussions of Gases Measured in Blood and Expired Air*

Conversion Factors
1 mm Hg = 0.133 kPa
1 kPa = 7.5 mm Hg
kPa: 1 kilopascal = 1000 pascal. The pascal is the SI derived unit of pressure; it equals 1 Newton/m^2.

General Prefixes
P: partial pressure or tension
Usage: PO_2, PCO_2, PH_2O
Alternative: pO_2
S: saturation fraction
Usage: SO_2
Alternative: sO_2
c: substance concentration
Usage: ctO_2 for concentration of total O_2
Usage: $ctCO_2$ for concentration of total CO_2
Usage: $cHCO_3^-$ for concentration of bicarbonate
d: dissolved gas, used with substance concentration *(c)*
t: total, used with substance concentration *(c)*, thus
$ctCO_2 = cHCO_3^- + cdCO_2$
Specimen origin is indicated by lower case letters. Whole blood and plasma are distinguished by capitals.
a: arterial B: blood
v: venous P: plasma
c: capillary
Usage: PO_2(aB), for partial pressure of O_2 in arterial blood

Prefixes Associated With External Respiration
V: volume of air or blood (unit, L)
$\dot{V}$: volume rate (unit, L/min)
F: substance fraction, also called mole fraction
E: expired air
I: inspired air
A: alveolar air
Usage: $\dot{v}$(A) means alveolar ventilation; $\dot{v}$(B) cardiac output; FO_2(I) fraction of O_2 in inspired air; PO_2(A) partial pressure of O_2 in alveolar air; and PCO_2(E) partial pressure of CO_2 in expired air.

Other Descriptors
BTPS: *B*ody *T*emperature (37 °C or 310.16 K) and ambient *P*ressure, fully *S*aturated (PH_2O = 47 mm Hg or 6.25 kPa)
STPD: *S*tandard *T*emperature (0 °C or 273.16 K) and standard *P*ressure (760 mm Hg or 101.08 kPa) of *D*ry gas
Amb: ambient atmosphere (unit is atm, atmosphere)
B: barometric (atmospheric)
BTPS: Usage: *P*(amb), *P(Amb)*
SVP: *S*aturated *V*apor *P*ressure, the vapor pressure of water. SVP_T means SVP at a specified temperature [e.g., $SVP_{37\,°C}$ = 47 mm Hg; PH_2O(saturated)]
ATPS: *A*mbient *T*emperature and *P*ressure, *S*aturated with water vapor

*This list is not complete but is presented to facilitate interpretation of terms used in the text and to illustrate various forms that may be encountered in the literature.

From Maas AH. IFCC reference methods for measurement of pH, gases and electrolytes in blood: reference materials. Eur J Clin Chem Clin Biochem 1991;29:253-61.

Behavior of Gases

Determination of gas pressures in expired air or blood depends on the application of certain physical principles (Table 28-3). The partial pressure (tension) of a gas dissolved in blood is by definition equal to the partial pressure of the gas in an imaginary ideal gas phase in equilibrium with the blood. At equilibrium, the partial pressure of a gas is the same in erythrocytes and plasma, so that the partial pressure of a gas is the same in whole blood and plasma. The partial pressure of a gas in a gas mixture is defined as the substance fraction of gas (mole fraction) times the total pressure.

Various spaces where gases are present include the ambient environment (room air), the bronchial tree and alveoli of the patient, and the measuring chamber of a laboratory instrument. In all these spaces, atmospheric (barometric) pressure, *P*(Amb), is the prevailing pressure, and partial pressures of each of the gases present in these spaces must add up to the value of *P*(Amb), which will vary with altitude and barometric pressure. Scientific convention reduces measurements of gas volumes made at *P*(Amb) to *S*tandard *T*emperature (0 °C or 273.16 K) and *P*ressure (760 mm Hg or 101.325 kPa) for *D*ry gas (STPD) to make experimental data transferable. However, in blood gas work, the standard is that

TABLE 28-3 Physical Principles Applied in Blood Gas Measurements

Boyle's law: The volume of an ideal gas at a constant temperature varies inversely with the pressure exerted to contain it.	$V \propto 1/P$
Charles' (Gay-Lussac's) law: The volume of an ideal gas at a constant pressure varies directly with its absolute temperature.	$V \propto T$
Avogadro's hypothesis: Equal volumes of different ideal gases at the same temperature and pressure contain the same number of molecules.	$n_i/V_i = n_j/V_j$
Dalton's law: The total pressure exerted by a mixture of ideal gases is the sum of the partial pressures of each of the gases in the mixture.	$P = \Sigma P_i$
Henry's law: The amount of a sparingly soluble gas dissolved in a liquid is proportional to the partial pressure of the gas over the liquid.	$c = \alpha \times P$

measurements of partial pressure are always made at *B*ody *T*emperature (usually 37 °C), at ***P***(Amb), and in the presence of *S*aturated water vapor (PH_2O = 47 mm Hg). Use of this BTPS convention (see Box 28-2) has the following practical effects:

1. It relates laboratory data for blood gases strictly to the geographic location of the patient, so that reference intervals become altitude dependent.
2. It assumes a standard body temperature of 37 °C and that the measuring device also holds the sample of blood at exactly 37 °C. This assumption requires special concern for thermal stability of the instrument. Just as important, it implies that in circumstances such as *imposed* hypothermia, when a patient's temperature is not 37 °C, blood gas values determined at 37 °C might need to be corrected to the actual body temperature to obtain an estimate of blood gas partial pressures in the patient.
3. It recognizes that partial pressures of measured gases in the blood coexist with a constant and standard saturated vapor pressure (SVP), which is identical for both the calibration conditions of the instrument and the measurement conditions of the blood sample.

Boyle's and Charles' laws and Avogadro's hypothesis are combined in what is called the *general gas equation:*

$$P = (nRT)/V$$

where

P = pressure in units of millimeters of mercury (mm Hg) or kilopascals (kPa)
V = volume in liters in which an ideal gas is contained
T = temperature in degrees kelvin (0 °C = 273.16 K)
n = number of moles of gas, and
R = gas constant

The SI unit of P is the pascal (Pa). However, millimeters of mercury (also called *torr*) have continued to remain popular in some countries (see Box 28-2 for conversion factors). Use of SI units does have a practical advantage in that 1 atm almost equals 100 kPa (1atm = 101.325 kPa). Partial pressures expressed in kilopascals therefore are very close estimates of percentages of the gases in the mixture at 1 atm. Pressure, P (or p), may mean total pressure, as in the expression P(Amb) for the mixture of gases in ambient air, or partial pressure in arterial blood, as in PO_2(aB). Numeric value and units of R differ depending on the units used for P, so that:

$$R = 62.36 \text{ mm Hg} \times L° \times K^{-1} \times mol^{-1}$$

or

$$R = 8.31 \text{ kPa} \times L° \times K^{-1} \times mol^{-1}$$

After terms are rearranged and n is evaluated as 1 mol and P as 760 mm Hg, the volume of 1 mol of a pure ideal gas at 0 °C (no water vapor) is 22.4 L. The general gas equation is the justification for accepting partial pressures of gases in blood as estimators of their concentrations. However, PO_2 is related only to the concentration of dissolved O_2 (cdO_2) in the blood and PCO_2 to the concentration of dissolved CO_2 ($cdCO_2$) in the blood (see Henry's law, Table 28-3). In fact, the total concentration of O_2 in blood (ctO_2) is the sum of concentrations of dissolved O_2 and of O_2 bound to hemoglobin, with dO_2 being a small component of tO_2 (see later section on hemoglobin saturation). The total concentration of CO_2 ($ctCO_2$) is defined operationally as the sum of concentrations of dissolved CO_2, carbonic acid, HCO_3^-, undissociated bicarbonate, and carbonate ion.

Dalton's law (see Table 28-3) may be written for room air as follows:

$$P(\text{amb}) = PO_2 + PCO_2 + PN_2 + PH_2O + PX$$

where PX is that of any other gas in the air sample. However, for gases in solution, Dalton's law does not apply as the sum of partial pressures of all dissolved gases may be lower than, equal to, or higher than the measured pressure of the solution. For instance, if the sum of gas tensions is significantly higher than the pressure of the solution, bubbles may form, as they do in the blood of divers surfacing from the deep (giving rise to a condition known as "the bends") or in a cold blood sample being warmed for analysis.

Dalton's law of partial pressures remains important, however, for calibration and control of the measuring devices. Consider a calibrator gas certified to contain 15% O_2 (L/L or mol/mol) and 5% CO_2, the remainder being N_2. The mole fractions (or F) of the gases in the dry mixture are 0.15, 0.05, and 0.80, respectively. This mixture, after saturation with water vapor at 37 °C (to mimic a patient's blood or alveolar air), is introduced into a blood gas instrument's measuring chamber (held at 37 °C to mimic a patient's body temperature) for the purpose of calibrating the instrument for subsequent measurements of gases in patients' samples. If the local barometric pressure, P(Amb), on this occasion is 747 mm Hg, then humidified calibrator gas is present in the chamber at ambient, barometric pressure, such that

$$P(\text{amb}) = 747 \text{ mm Hg} = PO_2 + PCO_2 + PN_2 + PH_2O$$

To set the instrument to the PO_2 and PCO_2 of the calibrator gas, we first must account for PH_2O at 37 °C, which is equal to the SVP of water, 47 mm Hg. Therefore,

$$\begin{aligned} 747 \text{ mm Hg} - PH_2O &= PO_2 + PCO_2 + PN_2 \\ &= 747 - 47 \\ &= 700 \text{ mm Hg} \end{aligned}$$

If P(Amb) corrected for PH_2O represents the sum of partial pressures for the dry gases whose mole fractions we know, we can calculate the exact PO_2 and PCO_2 values for the calibrator gas, under circumstances of measurement, and then enter these calibrator values into the instrument.

The law of partial pressure is also applied in defining gas mixtures used to determine $PO_2(0.5)$ or P_{50} and other derived quantities, and to control instrumentation with tonometered samples. *Henry's law* predicts the amount of dissolved gas in a liquid in contact with a gaseous phase (see Table 28-3).

The coefficient for O_2 in blood, αO_2, is 0.00140 (mol/L)/mm Hg (the corresponding coefficient for the volume-volume relationship is 31 μL/L/mm Hg). Therefore when arterial PO_2 is normal (≈100 mm Hg), the concentration of dissolved O_2 in arterial blood, cdO_2, is 0.140 mmol/L, which is a very small proportion of the ctO_2 content in blood (≈9 mmol/L), the bulk of which is O_2 bound by hemoglobin. Increasing the O_2 fraction of inspired air to 100% or increasing the pressure of inspired air, as in a hyperbaric chamber, forces more O_2 into a solution. In therapy with pure O_2, when PO_2 may rise to 640 mm Hg, the cdO_2 could be as high as 0.9 mmol/L. In hyperbaric treatment, an arterial PO_2 of 2500 mm Hg (≈3.2 atm) is equivalent to a cdO_2 of 3.5 mmol/L. Prediction of concentrations of cdO_2 in these therapies is useful because tissue oxygenation by dissolved O_2 becomes increasingly important when hemoglobin-mediated O_2 delivery is impaired.

The $cdCO_2$ can be calculated in the same way: αCO_2 at 37 °C in plasma = 0.0306 mmol/L/mm Hg. Thus at a PCO_2 of 40 mm Hg, the $cdCO_2 = 40 \times 0.0306 = 1.224$ mmol/L. In the determination of blood gases, PCO_2 is determined along with blood pH. As will be subsequently explained, these two parameters in conjunction with the Henderson-Hasselbalch equation permit the calculation of HCO_3^-, as follows:

$$\log cHCO_3^- = pH - pK' + \log[PCO_2 \times \alpha CO_2(P)]$$

The antilog is then taken to derive $cHCO_3^-$.

Application of the Henderson-Hasselbalch Equation in Blood Gas Measurements

Carbon dioxide and water react to form carbonic acid, which in turn dissociates to hydrogen ions and HCO_3^-.

$$CO_2 + H_2O \xrightleftharpoons{K_{hydration}} H_2CO_3 \xrightleftharpoons{K_{dissociation}} H^{\oplus} + HCO_3^{\ominus}$$

Thus the total concentration of CO_2 ($ctCO_2$), the concentration of bicarbonate ($cHCO_3^-$), the concentration of dissolved CO_2 ($cdCO_2$), and the H^+ ion concentration (cH^+) are interrelated. The constant K for the hydration reaction is 2.29×10^{-3} (pK = 2.64 at 37 °C), whereas the constant K for the dissociation of carbonic acid is 2.04×10^{-4} (pK = 3.69).

In the classical formulation, Henderson (1908), using concentrations for bicarbonate, CO_2, and H^+, and assuming the concentration of water to be constant, combined these two reactions and incorporated the constant K' with a value of 4.68×10^{-7}, and thus a pK' of 6.33 at 37 °C:

$$K' = \frac{cH^+ \times cHCO_3^-}{cdCO_2}$$

The concentration of dissolved CO_2 *includes* the small amount of undissociated (dissolved) carbonic acid. It can be expressed as $cdCO_2 = \alpha \times PCO_2$, where α is the solubility coefficient for CO_2. $cHCO_3^-$ then represents $ctCO_2$ minus $cdCO_2$, which includes carbonic acid. The "bicarbonate" concentration by this definition includes undissociated sodium bicarbonate, carbonate ($NaCO_3$), and carbamate (carbamino-CO_2; $RCNHCOO^-$), which are present in exceedingly small amounts in plasma. If the Henderson equation is rearranged and $cdCO_2$ is replaced by $\alpha \times PCO_2$, the following equation results:

$$cH^+ = K' \times \frac{\alpha \times PCO_2}{cHCO_3^-}$$

In 1916, Hasselbalch showed that a logarithmic transformation of the equation was a more useful form and used the symbols pH (= –log cH^+) and pK' (= –log K'). pH is defined as the negative log of the *activity* of H^+ (aH^+), which is the entity actually measured with pH meters. The resulting Henderson-Hasselbalch equation becomes

$$pH = pK' + \log\frac{cHCO_3^-}{\alpha \times PCO_2}$$

or

$$pH = pK' + \log\frac{ctCO_2 - (\alpha \times PCO_2)}{\alpha \times PCO_2}$$

K' is the apparent overall (combined) dissociation constant for carbonic acid. It is *apparent* because concentrations are used rather than activities and *overall* because both the $cdCO_2$ and the concentration of carbonic acid are used. K' depends not only on the temperature but also on the ionic strength of the solution.

For blood at 37 °C, the normal mean value is pK'(P) = 6.103, with a normal biological standard deviation of about ±0.0015, mainly caused by variations in ionic strength. The solubility coefficient for CO_2 gas, α, also varies with the composition of the solution. For pure water at 37 °C, the solubility coefficient α = (0.0329 mmol) × (L^{-1}) × (mm Hg^{-1}), and for normal plasma at 37 °C, it is (0.0306 mmol) × (L^{-1}) × (mm Hg^{-1}). When pK' and α for normal plasma at 37 °C are inserted, the Henderson-Hasselbalch equation takes the following form:

$$pH = 6.103 + \log\frac{cHCO_3^-}{0.0306 \times PCO_2}$$

or

$$pH = 6.103 + \log\frac{ctCO_2 - 0.0306 \times PCO_2}{0.0306 \times PCO_2}$$

where PCO_2 is measured in millimeters of mercury and $cHCO_3^-$ and $ctCO_2$ are measured in millimoles per liter. By taking the antilogarithm, combining the constants, and expressing [H^+] in nmol/L, the equation becomes

$$cH^+ = 24.1 \times \frac{PCO_2}{cHCO_3^-}$$

If normal values are substituted in the equation,

$$cH^+ = 24.1 \times \frac{40}{24.1}\ \text{nmol/L} = 38.0\ \text{nmol/L}$$

Clearly, by measuring any two of the four parameters—PCO_2 or $cdCO_2$, pH, $ctCO_2$, and $cHCO_3^-$—and by using the Henderson-Hasselbalch equation with the above values for pK' and α, the other two parameters may be calculated. Although used as constants, these values must be recognized as means and are susceptible to biological variation. Changes in ionic strength of ±20% cause changes in pK' between 6.08

and 6.12. Variations in pK' of plasma also occur with temperature (pK will decrease by 0.0026 per 1 °C increase and will decrease slightly with increasing pH). For most clinical purposes, these variations of pK' can be ignored. However, in pathologic cases with markedly deviant ionic strength, the change in pK' may be significant. The value of α is affected by the presence of increased salts or proteins in solution (value decreases) or lipids (value increases). For instance, in lipemic plasma, the value of α may be 0.033 or even higher. Thus, parameters calculated on the assumption that pK' and α are invariant may have significant error under certain pathologic circumstances, and several authors suggest caution in using values calculated from blood gas analyzers in extremely ill patients and in children.[71,76]

For instance, one study showed that in 17 of 51 adult intensive care unit patients, calculated and measured tCO_2 values differed by >10%,[71] whereas another study showed differences >20% in 27 of 107 pediatric intensive care unit patients.[76] The same holds true for comparison of 74 patient blood samples between calculated tCO_2 (using pH and PCO_2) of whole blood by a modern POCT device and measured tCO_2 using an automated analyzer on arterial plasma.[21] Agreement between the devices was significantly correlated ($r = 0.97$, $P < 0.05$) but calculated tCO_2 was highly influenced by PCO_2 values and should be used with caution in managing critically ill patients.[21] Nevertheless, with both pH and PCO_2 measured electrochemically, $cHCO_3^-$, $cdCO_2$, and $ctCO_2$ are routinely calculated by algorithms in most blood gas instruments. One advantage of such a calculated value is that it essentially reflects the *activity* of HCO_3^- in the *water* phase of plasma, and thus it is not affected by the electrolyte exclusion effects, as other indirect measurements of HCO_3^- may be. Additionally, microprocessor algorithms use HCO_3^- values to calculate base excess (BE).[70] BE is defined as the amount of acid required to return the blood pH of a patient to 7.4.

Oxygen in Blood

The total O_2 content (ctO_2) of a blood sample is the sum of the concentrations of hemoglobin-bound O_2 and of dissolved O_2. At a blood ctO_2 of 9 mmol/L, the O_2 associated with hemoglobin as oxyhemoglobin (O_2Hb) is 8.86 mmol/L. The O_2Hb is defined as erythrocyte hemoglobin with O_2 reversibly bound to Fe^{2+} of its heme group. Each mole of hemoglobin-Fe^{2+} binds 1 mol of O_2. In erythrocytes, hemoglobin exists as a tetramer (64,456 g/mol), but when Hb concentration is expressed in moles per liter, it is reported as the concentration of monomer (16,114 g/mol). Thus 1 L of blood with a normal hemoglobin concentration (cHb) of 9.3 mmol/L (≈15 g/dL or 150 g/L) carries 9.3 mmol of O_2 at STPD if all hemoglobin is in the form of O_2Hb.

Thus 1 g of hemoglobin is capable of binding 1.39 mL (0.062 mmol) of O_2 at STPD. This value is referred to as the specific O_2-binding capacity of hemoglobin A (Hb A, the normal adult gene product). Hb A reversibly binds O_2 at its heme moiety and binds biological effectors at other allosteric sites on the molecule. Methemoglobin (MetHb), carboxyhemoglobin (COHb), sulfhemoglobin (SulfHb), and cyanmethemoglobin are forms of hemoglobin that are not capable of reversible binding of O_2 because of chemical alterations of the heme moiety (see Chapter 32). These chemically altered hemoglobins are collectively termed *dyshemoglobins.* Another group of abnormal hemoglobins have genetically determined changes in their amino acid sequence that can alter the allosteric binding properties of the molecule and thus affect O_2 affinity. These hemoglobins are collectively referred to as *hemoglobin variants* or *hemoglobinopathies.* More than 900 hemoglobin variants have been described; only a small fraction are clinically significant, such as sickle cell hemoglobin (Hb S) (see Chapter 32).

Uptake of O_2 by the blood in the lungs is governed primarily by the PO_2 of alveolar air and by the ability of O_2 to diffuse freely across the alveolar membrane into the blood. At the PO_2 normally present in alveolar air (≈102 mm Hg) and with a normal membrane and normal hemoglobin A, more than 95% of hemoglobin will bind O_2. At a PO_2 > 110 mm Hg, more than 98% of normal hemoglobin A binds O_2. When all hemoglobin is saturated with O_2, further increase in the PO_2 of alveolar air simply increases the concentration of dO_2 in the arterial blood. Delivery of O_2 by the blood to the tissue is governed by the large gradient between PO_2 of the arterial blood and that of the tissue cells, and by the dissociation of O_2Hb in the erythrocytes at the lower PO_2 of the blood-tissue cell interface.

Three properties of arterial blood are essential to ensure adequate O_2 delivery to the tissue:

1. Arterial PO_2 must be sufficiently high (≈90 mm Hg) to create a diffusion gradient from the arterial blood to the tissue cells. Low arterial PO_2 *(hypoxemia)* results in tissue O_2 starvation *(hypoxia).*
2. The O_2-binding capacity of the blood must be normal (i.e., the concentration of hemoglobin capable of binding and releasing O_2 must be normal). Decreased Hb concentration will cause so-called anemic hypoxia.
3. The hemoglobin must be able to bind O_2 in the lungs yet release it at the tissue. In other words, the affinity of hemoglobin for O_2 must be normal. Too great an affinity of hemoglobin for O_2 may cause "affinity-based" tissue hypoxia, in which O_2 is not released at the capillary-tissue interface.

The PO_2 at the venous end of the capillaries should stay around 38 mm Hg; thus the normal arteriovenous difference in PO_2 is 50 to 60 mm Hg. This corresponds to a normal delivery of ≈2.3 mmol of O_2 to the tissue per liter of blood.

Hemoglobin Oxygen Saturation

Before the factors that affect Hb affinity for O_2 are discussed, it is important to define the concept of hemoglobin oxygen saturation (SO_2):

$$SO_2 = \frac{\text{Oxygen Content}}{\text{Oxygen Capacity}}$$

This is the fraction (percentage) of functional hemoglobin that is saturated with oxygen and is essentially an indirect means of estimating the PO_2. However, at least three different approaches exist for determining oxygen "saturation," and although each is distinct, they are often used interchangeably to determine "oxygen saturation." These three terms—hemoglobin oxygen saturation (SO_2), fractional oxyhemoglobin (FO_2Hb), and estimated oxygen saturation (O_2Sat)—have distinct definitions previously set by the CLSI.[23] Ambiguous use of these three terms occurs because in healthy subjects with normal amounts of normal hemoglobin, the values for all three entities are very similar. However, the assumptions made for normal, healthy subjects can lead to erroneous conclusions in seriously ill patients and those with dyshemoglobins or hemoglobin variants when these values are used interchangeably.

Spectrophotometric methods are used to determine O_2Hb and HHb,[68] and SO_2 is calculated according to

$$SO_2 = \frac{cO_2Hb}{cO_2Hb + cHHb}$$

where cO_2Hb is the concentration of oxyhemoglobin, $cHHb$ is the concentration of deoxyhemoglobin, and the sum of oxyhemoglobin and deoxyhemoglobin represents all hemoglobin capable of reversibly binding O_2. SO_2 is usually expressed as a percent in the United States, but it may also be expressed as a decimal fraction of 1.00.

SO_2 most often is determined by simple pulse oximetry, a spectrophotometric approach that can determine oxyhemoglobin and reduced hemoglobin (HHb) but not COHb, MetHb, or SulfHb. These devices measure absorbance at 660 and 940 nm for which O_2Hb and HHb have unique absorbance patterns.[46] These are usually bedside monitors used for monitoring HbO_2 saturation, and they serve this purpose extremely well. However, use of SO_2 in the initial evaluation of a patient with dyshemoglobins or other abnormal hemoglobins can be very misleading. For instance, in a comatose patient with 15% COHb, the SO_2 by simple pulse oximetry might read 0.95, whereas the fraction of oxyhemoglobin in reality would be only 0.80. Thus it seems reasonable to assess for the presence of dyshemoglobins before SO_2 is used for clinical purposes. The reference interval for SO_2 from healthy adults is 0.94 to 0.98 (94 to 98%). Recent experimental pulse oximeters can measure some of the dyshemoglobins such as COHb and metHb.[6]

Another expression of oxygen "saturation" is fractional oxyhemoglobin (FO_2Hb), which is calculated as

$$FO_2Hb = (cO_2Hb / cHHb + cCOHb + cMethHb + cSulfHb)$$

This value requires determination of all hemoglobin species and can be performed on a co-oximeter present in many modern blood gas analyzers. These instruments prepare a hemolysate from whole blood by sonication, and by spectrophotometry they determine the total amount of hemoglobin and the percent of each of the aforementioned species. This is accomplished by using monochromatic light at 6 to 128 fixed wavelengths between 535 and 670 nm and measuring absorbance at each of the wavelengths. Newer co-oximeters use a diode array and 128 wavelengths. Because each species of hemoglobin has its own absorbance pattern, a microcomputer can calculate the percent of each one. The reference interval for FO_2Hb is 0.90 to 0.95 (90 to 95%).

Finally, the microprocessors of many blood gas instruments can estimate the oxygen saturation from measured pH, PO_2, and hemoglobin with the use of empirical equations.[86] If used at all, this value should be clearly referred to as an *estimated oxygen saturation,* but it frequently is reported as and referred to as "O_2Sat." Calculated values such as "O_2Sat" should be interpreted with reservation because the algorithm assumes normal O_2 affinity of the hemoglobin, normal 2,3-diphosphoglycerol (2,3-DPG) concentrations, and the absence of dyshemoglobins. Such calculated estimates have been found to vary by as much as 6% saturation from measured values.[79]

Decreases in arterial FO_2Hb may indicate a low arterial PO_2 or an impaired ability of hemoglobin to bind O_2. The amount of O_2 that the blood can carry is determined by three major factors: (1) the PO_2, which reflects how much O_2 is dissolved in the blood; (2) the amount of normal hemoglobin available in erythrocytes; and (3) the affinity of available hemoglobin for O_2. Decreases in PO_2 indicate a reduced ability of O_2 to diffuse from alveolar air into the blood. This may be due to hypoventilation or to increased venoarterial shunting that is secondary to cardiac or pulmonary insufficiency. In either case, the result is a right-to-left shunting of blood that has not reached equilibrium with alveolar air. This results in a decreased PO_2 and an increased PCO_2. Decreases in the concentration of total hemoglobin can result from a decreased number of erythrocytes that contain a normal concentration of hemoglobin (normochromic anemia) or a decreased mean cell concentration of hemoglobin in the erythrocytes (hypochromic anemia). Decreased FO_2Hb hemoglobin can also occur as a result of poisonings that convert part of the hemoglobin into the species COHb, MetHb, SulfHb, or cyanmethemoglobin, which cannot properly bind or exchange O_2. Clinically, it is important to distinguish between arterial hypoxemia (decreased arterial PO_2 and decreased FO_2Hb caused by decreased availability of O_2) and cyanosis (decreased FO_2Hb caused by abnormally high concentrations of reduced hemoglobin or chemically altered hemoglobin incapable of carrying O_2). Note that in the cyanosis setting, measurement of SO_2 or an estimated SO_2 ("O_2Sat") could be normal if cyanosis is due to the presence of metHb or COHb.[46] The oxygen concentration of blood (ctO_2) is the sum of O_2 bound to hemoglobin and cdO_2. Blood gas analyzers determine ctO_2 by the following calculation[23]:

$$ctO_2(\text{mL/dL}) = FO_2Hb \times bO_2 \times ctHb(\text{g/dL}) + (\alpha O_2) \times (PO_2)$$

where bO_2 equals 1.39 mL/g Hb and α, the solubility coefficient of O_2 at 37 °C, and STPD = 0.00314 (mL/dL)/mm Hg = 0.00140 (mmol/L)/mm Hg. Note that this calculation is based on FO_2Hb and $ctHb$. If SO_2 is used, it is necessary to use the effective hemoglobin concentration (i.e., to subtract the concentration of any dyshemoglobins present from the concentration of $ctHb$). Thus on initial patient presentation, determination of any dyshemoglobins may be necessary to obtain an accurate value for ctO_2 for its use in subsequent calculations.

Hemoglobin-Oxygen Dissociation

The degree of association or dissociation of O_2 with hemoglobin is determined by PO_2 and the affinity of hemoglobin for O_2. When the SO_2 of blood is determined over a range of PO_2 and is plotted against PO_2, a sigmoidal curve called the *O_2 dissociation curve* is obtained. The *shape* of the curve is affected by the increasing efficiency with which HHb molecules bind more O_2 once some O_2 has been bound (*cooperativity;* see also Chapter 32). The *location* of the curve relative to the PO_2 required to achieve a particular concentration of SO_2 in the blood is a function of the affinity of hemoglobin for O_2.

The affinity of hemoglobin for O_2 depends on five factors: temperature, pH, PCO_2, concentration of 2,3-DPG, and the presence of minor hemoglobins such as COHb and metHb. Dissociation of O_2 in relation to 2,3-DPG concentration and abnormal hemoglobin proteins, such as fetal hemoglobin (Hb F), thalassemias, and other hemoglobinopathies, is discussed in Chapter 32. Note that increases of 2,3-DPG shift the SO_2-PO_2 relationship to the right. This chapter describes the effects of temperature, pH, and PCO_2 on dissociation behavior.

The graph in Figure 28-4 shows the effect of plasma pH on the O_2 dissociation curve (the Bohr effect). Similar graphs can be made for variations of PCO_2 and temperature. The shifting locations of the curves are described in the third column of the chart in Figure 28-4, with increasing affinity for O_2 shifting the curve to the left. These sigmoidal curves, however, are difficult to use when quantitative estimates of the amount of shift are desired, when the PO_2 at which 50% of Hb is binding O_2 (P_{50}) is calculated. The Hill logit-log transform (illustrated as the Hill plot, Figure 28-4, *B*) converts the curvilinear dissociation function into a linear function. The slope of the linear function is essentially constant at 2.7 for an SO_2 between 40% and 80%.

The linear transforms of the dissociation curves have allowed linear coefficients of change (fourth column of the chart in the legend to Figure 28-4) to be determined for each of the factors that shift dissociation curves, and hence the lines on the Hill plot. These coefficients find application for correcting measured PO_2 or calculated P_{50} for the effects of different body temperatures, PCO_2, pH, and 2,3-DPG concentrations.

Determination of P_{50}

P_{50} is defined as the PO_2 at which the hemoglobin of the blood is half saturated with O_2. The measured value of P_{50} differs from the standard value of P_{50} by some amount determined by the extent that pH differs from 7.40, PCO_2 differs from 40 mm Hg, temperature differs from 37 °C, and 2,3-DPG differs from 5.0 mmol/L. The value of P_{50} therefore becomes a measure of change of hemoglobin affinity because of the factors that affect it. A procedure for determining P_{50} uses the principle that

$$\log P_{50} = \log PO_2 - \operatorname{logit} SO_2 / 2.7$$

where logit SO_2 = log[SO_2/(1 − SO_2)] and 2.7 is the Hill slope.[53,80,82]

The P_{50} reference interval for adults, measured at 37 °C and corrected to pH(P) of 7.4, is 25 to 29 mm Hg. For newborn infants, the interval is 18 to 24 mm Hg because of the presence of Hb F.

Clinical Significance

Increased values for P_{50} indicate displacement of the O_2 dissociation curve to the right (i.e., decreased affinity of the hemoglobin for O_2). The chief causes are hyperthermia, acidemia, hypercapnia, high concentrations of 2,3-DPG, and the presence of a hemoglobin variant with decreased O_2 affinity. The physiologic effects of decreased affinity of hemoglobin are small. The affinity is still sufficient to bind adequate amounts of O_2 in the lungs, and the low affinity facilitates dissociation of O_2Hb at the peripheral tissues. Indeed, in anemia, low affinity (as a result of increases in 2,3-DPG) is a desirable compensatory mechanism. The compensatory responses in healthy individuals to alter the P_{50} can be remarkable. For instance, in fully acclimatized (70 days) high-altitude climbers (Mt. Everest) full cognition was maintained without supplemental oxygen at an altitude of 8400 m and an average $P(a)O_2$ of only 25 mm Hg.[43]

Low values for P_{50} signify displacement of the O_2 dissociation curve to the left (i.e., increased affinity of hemoglobin). The main causes are hypothermia, acute alkalemia, hypocapnia, low 2,3-DPG, and a hemoglobin variant. The physiologic consequence of increased affinity of hemoglobin for O_2 is less efficient dissociation of O_2Hb at the peripheral tissue and lower tissue PO_2.

Tonometry

Tonometry is the process of exposing a sample to a gas phase in such a way that each gas in the gaseous phase partitions to an equilibrium between liquid and gas. Equilibration by tonometry uses gases of known fractional composition, humidified at 37 °C to give a saturated water vapor pressure of 47 mm Hg. The PCO_2 or PO_2 of such gases is calculated according to Dalton's law (see section on behavior of gases). Tonometry is used to treat blood samples for various special studies that are rarely requested in most hospital settings and to prepare quality control material in whole blood. Direct determination of P_{50} and of standard bicarbonate are two applications of tonometry.

Additional detail on tonometry and its applications can be found in a previous edition of this textbook.[90] Reference conditions for tonometry have been recommended by a committee of the International Federation of Clinical Chemistry and Laboratory Medicine (IFCC).[14]

Determination of PCO_2, PO_2, and pH

The instruments used for determination of PCO_2, PO_2, and pH are highly automated. Proper specimen collection and handling are critical for accurate determinations.

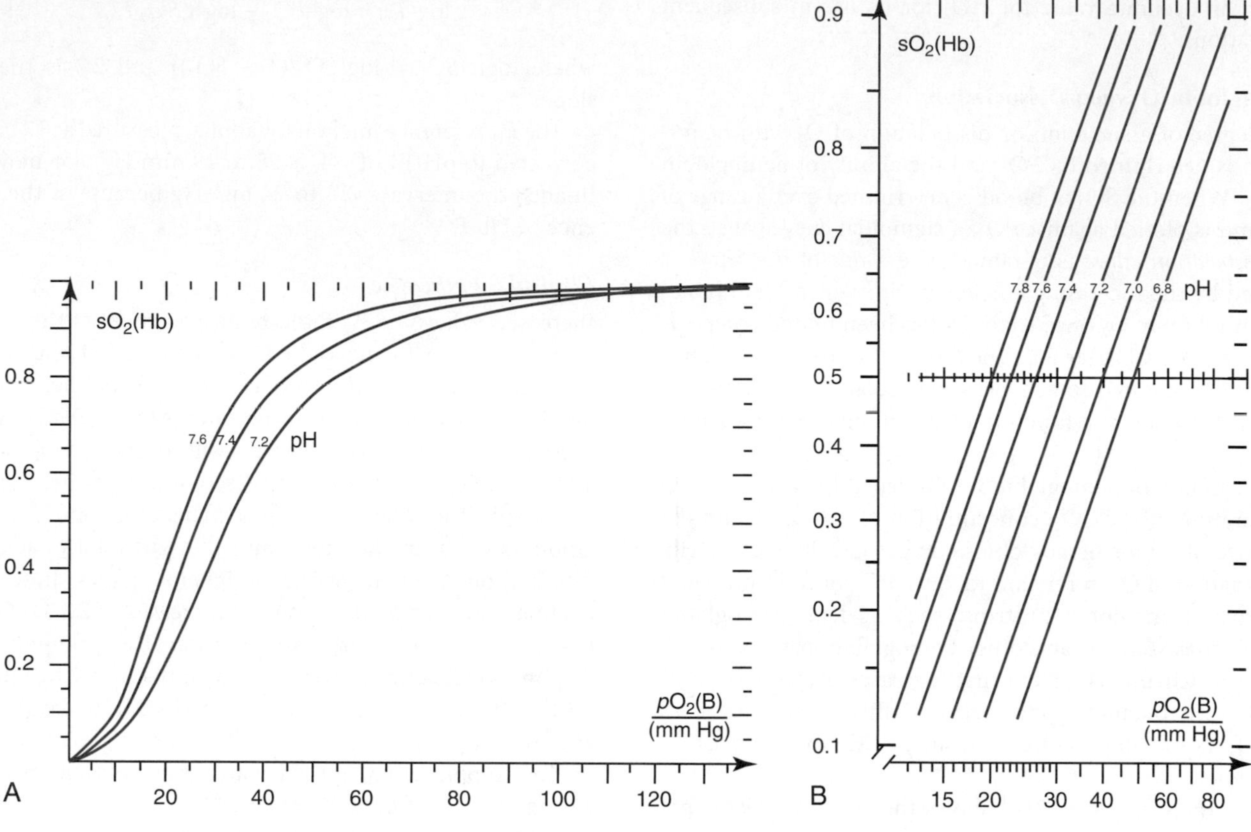

C

Deviation from standard conditions	Shift in dissociation curve	Affinity of hemoglobin for O_2	Coefficient of change*
pH(P) > 7.4 pH(P) < 7.4	← →	↑ ↓	$\frac{\Delta \log PO_2}{\Delta pH(P)} = -0.46$
Temperature >37 °C <37 °C	 → ←	 ↓ ↑	$\frac{\Delta \log PO_2}{\Delta T} = +0.024\ K^{-1}$
PCO_2 > 40 mm Hg PCO_2 < 40 mm Hg	→ ←	↓ ↑	$\frac{\Delta \log PO_2}{\Delta \log PCO_2} = +0.02$
*c*DPG(E) >normal <normal	 → ←	 ↓ ↑	$\frac{\Delta \log PO_2}{\Delta (cDPG(E)/c^*)} = +0.04$

Figure 28-4 A, Oxygen dissociation curves for human blood with different plasma pH but constant PCO_2 of 40 mm Hg, a 2,3-diphosphoglycerol (2,3-DPG) concentration in erythrocytes of 5.0 mmol/L, and temperature at 37 °C. B, A Hill plot. Conditions are the same as in A. The coefficients given in this chart form the basis for the correction of measured PO_2. The effect of pH(P) to shift the dissociation curve is called the *Bohr effect;* the coefficient above for $\Delta \log PO_2/\Delta pH(P)$ applies to conditions when the PCO_2 is 40 mm Hg, and changes in pH(P) are due to changes in concentrations of noncarbonic acids and bases. If, however, the changes in pH(P) are being caused by changes in PCO_2, then the absolute value of the coefficient is greater (i.e., $\Delta \log PO_2/\Delta pH[P] = -0.49$). The coefficients for the Bohr effect are specified for PO_2 of whole blood but use the pH of plasma, pH(P). The coefficient for DPG effect is based on the DPG concentration in the erythrocytes, cDPG(E). c* = 1 mmol/L.

Specimens

Whole blood is the most likely specimen for a clinical laboratory to receive for gas analysis. Differences in measured blood gas values between arterial and venous blood are most pronounced for PO_2. In fact, PO_2 is the only clinical reason for arterial collections. PO_2 is generally ≈60 mm Hg lower in venous blood after O_2 is released in the capillaries, whereas PCO_2 is 2 to 8 mm Hg higher in venous blood. pH generally is only 0.02 to 0.05 pH units lower in a venous sample.

Quality assurance of blood analysis for gases and pH is dependent on control of preanalytical error (i.e., on proper collection and handling of the specimen) and on control of the analytical instrument and testing process. Placement of indwelling catheters with heparin locks for short- and long-term intravenous therapies is common. Failure to flush the lock properly with blood (≈5 mL) has unpredictable effects on measured quantities and often is indicated by bizarre, nonphysiologic results.

Arterial or venous specimens are best collected anaerobically with lyophilized heparin anticoagulant in 1 to 3 mL sterile syringes. Although in theory, glass syringes are preferred to prevent gas exchange through the syringe wall, most blood gas syringes today are plastic, and the gas exchange that occurs within 1 hour is trivial. Lyophilized heparin is preferable to liquid heparin because liquid heparin, which has atmospheric PO_2 and PCO_2 values, dilutes the sample, with the effect being greatest when the syringe is not completely filled. An increasing ratio of liquid heparin to blood can have an increasingly marked effect on measured PCO_2 and the parameters calculated from it. In one study, dilution with 10% volume of liquid heparin having an atmospheric PCO_2 of 0.25 mm Hg led to a 10 to 20 mm Hg decrease in blood PCO_2.[45]

Anaerobic technique for collection means no exposure of blood to atmospheric air. The PCO_2 of air is about 0.25 mm Hg; this is much less than that of blood (≈40 mm Hg). Thus the CO_2 content and PCO_2 of blood exposed to air will decrease, and blood pH, which is a function of PCO_2, will rise. The PO_2 of atmospheric air (≈155 mm Hg) is ≈60 mm Hg higher than that of arterial blood and ≈100 mm Hg higher than that of venous blood. Therefore blood from patients breathing room air that is exposed to atmospheric air gains O_2, and blood with PO_2 >150 mm Hg, as occurs in patients undergoing O_2 therapy, loses O_2. Blood can also be exposed to air simply from the air in the needle and the syringe hub dead space. Error will be minimal if the resulting bubble is ejected immediately after drawing by holding it tip up and ejecting a small drop of blood. The potential effect of small bubbles on blood gas results was clearly demonstrated in one study in which a 100 μL bubble of room air was added to ten 2 mL blood samples with PO_2 values between 25 and 40 mm Hg. In these samples, PO_2 increased an average of 4 mm Hg in only 2 minutes, whereas PCO_2 decreased 4 mm Hg.[69] Before analysis, mixing of the sample by simple but vigorous rolling of the syringe between the palms should be done to establish a homogeneous sample.

Arterialized capillary blood is sometimes an acceptable alternative to arterial blood when an arterial cannula is not available, or when repeated arterial puncture must be prevented. Freely flowing cutaneous blood originates in the arterioles and corresponds closely to arterial blood in composition. However, arterialized capillary blood is not acceptable when systolic blood pressure is less than 95 mm Hg, in cases of vasoconstriction, in patients on O_2 therapy, in newborns during the first few hours after birth, or in newborns with respiratory distress syndrome. Capillary puncture should be preceded by warming of the selected skin puncture site for 10 minutes to achieve vasodilation and adequate blood flow. For collection from the finger of a child or an adult or from an infant's heel, warming may be accomplished by immersing the arm or leg in water warmed to 42 °C. The first blood drop to appear should be wiped away, and subsequent free-forming drops should be taken up in a capillary collection tube containing lyophilized heparin. Only free-flowing blood provides a satisfactory sample, and taking up the drops as soon as they form minimizes aerobic exposure. Appropriate capillary tubes hold 70 to 300 μL of blood, and larger-diameter tubes require mixing. A flea (a slender wire approximately 5 mm in length) is immediately inserted after filling, and a magnet is used to move the flea back and forth.

Transport and analysis of specimens should be prompt. However, delayed analysis of up to 1 hour will have a minimal effect on reported values from most samples. The pH of freshly drawn blood decreases on standing at a rate of 0.04 to 0.08 pH unit/h at 37 °C, 0.02 to 0.03/h at 22 °C, and <0.01/h at 4 °C. The decrease in pH is accompanied by a corresponding decrease in glucose and an equivalent increase in lactate. PCO_2 increases by ≈5 mm Hg/h at 37 °C, by 1 mm Hg/h at 22 °C, and by only ≈0.5 mm Hg/h at 2 to 4 °C. The primary cause of these changes is glycolysis by leukocytes, platelets, and reticulocytes. In freshly drawn blood with a normal PO_2 that is maintained anaerobically, cell respiration causes PO_2 to decrease at a rate of ≈2 mm Hg/h at room temperature and 5 to 10 mm Hg/h at 37 °C. Adverse effects of glycolysis and respiration on pH, $ctCO_2$, PO_2, and PCO_2 of blood can best be prevented by analysis within 30 minutes after collection. If analysis must be delayed longer than 30 minutes, the syringe should be immersed in a mixture of ice and water until analysis is possible. Under these conditions, changes are negligible because glycolysis is inhibited. With today's blood gas instrumentation, introduction of a chilled sample carries little risk of low-temperature effect on measurements, because thermal equilibration to 37 °C is rapid and complete.

The aforementioned small changes in values that can be expected with delays in analysis are true *only* when the white blood cell count (WBC) is normal or is only slightly elevated. Glycolysis and the resulting effects on pH, PO_2, and PCO_2 increase dramatically with markedly elevated WBC, such as occurs in leukemia. Experiments have shown that PO_2 decreases by 20 mm Hg in just 2 minutes and by 40 mm Hg in only 5 minutes with WBC values >100,000/μL.[20,47] Indeed, for samples with these types of WBC values, it is very difficult to overcome this effect. Even after the sample is immersed in ice, thermal equilibrium takes several minutes, allowing significant PO_2 loss before the contents reach 4 °C. The only alternative to obtaining accurate blood gas values on such patients is immediate analysis performed by using a point-of-care device or by taking the blood gas analyzer to the patient.

Instrumentation

Reference methods for blood gas and electrolyte determinations have been described in detail by the IFCC.[62] A schematic diagram characteristic of a typical instrument is shown in Figure 28-5. Electrochemical principles and structural features of electrodes are discussed in Chapter 11.

Operation of a traditional blood gas instrument begins with the operator presenting a blood specimen at the sample probe. The sample is taken through the probe by a peristaltic pump that loads the chamber with 60 to 150 μL of the sample. The sample then resides in the chamber long enough to allow thermal equilibration and completion of measurements. On completion of measurement, the pump pushes the sample to waste, while output is made available on a display, a printed tape, and often a laboratory information system.

Because electrodes are not stable over long periods of time, frequent calibration of pH, PCO_2, and PO_2 is required. The instrument (see Figure 28-5) is designed so that a manually actuated or a microprocessor actuated valve admits calibrator gases, standard buffers, or a sample to a small chamber (C) maintained at 37 ± 0.1 °C. Most instruments contain a barometer so that barometric pressure *P*(Amb) is always known to the microprocessor during calibration. In the calibration phase of the instrument, a high pH standard buffer and a low pH standard buffer are alternately admitted into the chamber or gas mixtures with high and low fractional concentrations of O_2 and CO_2, and electronic responses of the upper and lower limits of the linear curves are set. Most modern instruments are designed to be self-calibrating with microprocessor-controlled timed intervals of calibration.

Other instruments perform point-of-care or bedside testing.[34] Almost all manufacturers now produce small, portable, stand-alone, easy-to-operate instruments designed for "satellite lab" operations; several hand-held devices that use disposable electrodes are also available.[34] Such instruments often combine measurement systems for blood gases and pH with ISEs for electrolytes, glucose, urea nitrogen, and hematocrit or hemoglobin. Although design and construction may

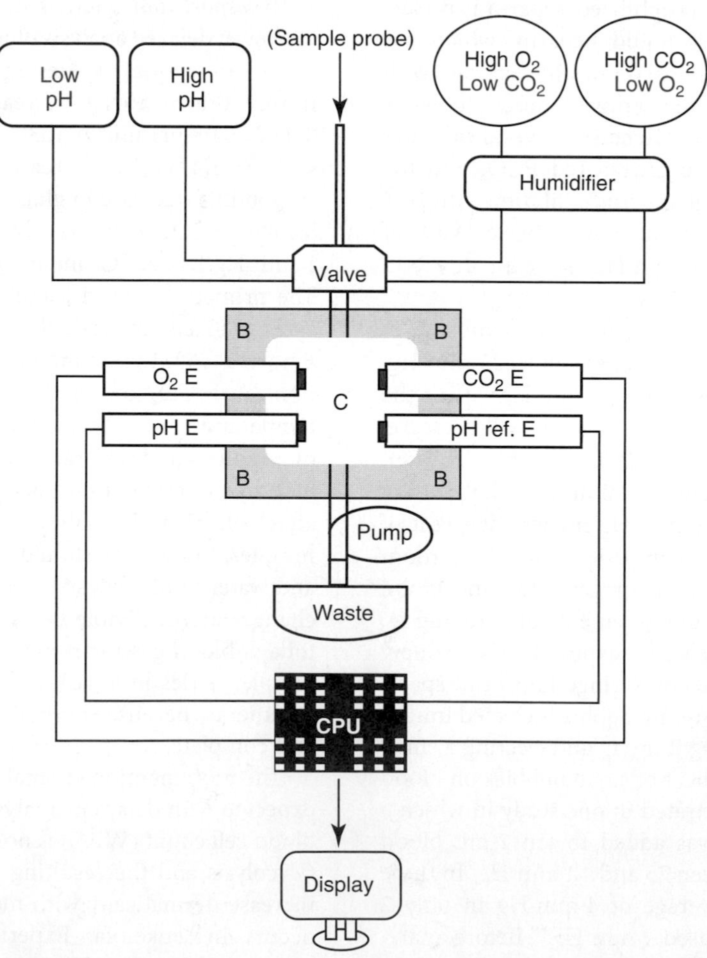

Figure 28-5 Diagram of blood gas instrumentation. *B*, Constant temperature bath at 37 °C; *C*, chamber; *CPU*, computer; *E (electrodes)*, pH and gas standards are shown at top of diagram.

differ significantly from those used in laboratory instrumentation, the principles of analysis are not novel. Readers are referred to the manufacturers' literature and to Chapter 20 for a discussion of POCT.

Electrodes

The tip of the pH measuring electrode is made of H^+-sensitive glass (see Chapter 11), and aside from miniaturization, most pH measuring and reference electrodes differ little from those of free-standing pH meters. The membrane of the PCO_2 electrode usually consists of Teflon or silicone rubber approximately 25 μm thick. The electrolyte solution is a thin film containing sodium bicarbonate at 0.005 mol/L and sodium chloride (NaCl) at 0.1 mol/L saturated with AgCl. A spacer of nylon net or cellophane lies between the solution and the H^+-sensitive glass of the measuring element proper. As CO_2 diffuses from the sample into the electrolyte solution, the slight rise in (H^+) from its hydration reaction is measured as ΔpH by an especially sensitive potentiometer and is transformed electronically to Δlog PCO_2. The membrane of a PO_2 electrode in a standard blood gas analyzer is usually ≈20 μm thick polypropylene. The electrolyte solution is a thin film of phosphate buffer saturated with AgCl but also containing KCl; it is in contact with the polarized platinum cathode and the Ag/AgCl anode. As O_2 diffuses into the electrolyte, it reacts with the cathode to cause current to flow; the generated current is measured.

Maintenance of Instrumentation

Sophistication of contemporary equipment and availability of high-quality calibrator materials have made reliable and accurate determination of blood pH and gases primarily a matter of meticulous maintenance, adherence to the manufacturer's recommended procedures, and control of the equipment and proper collection and handling of specimens. Software programs of the instrument's microprocessor often provide display warnings and diagnostic routines that alert the operator and assist in troubleshooting. The frequency with which maintenance should be scheduled is in direct proportion to the volume of analyses performed in the laboratory. The manufacturer's suggested schedule should be considered a minimum guideline, with reliance on experience to indicate maintenance frequency.

Cleanliness of the sample chamber and path is especially important. Automatic flushing to cleanse the sample chamber and path after each blood sample measurement is a feature of most instruments without disposable electrodes. When it is not, manual modes of flushing recommended by the manufacturer should be faithfully practiced. Despite proper flushing, however, complete or partial clogging of the chamber or path or both may occur. Frequency of clogging is often related to the number of heparinized capillary blood samples that are analyzed. Fibrin threads and small clots may be present in the specimen or may form while the sample resides in the warm chamber. If allowed to remain, they can affect subsequent measurements or calibrations by interfering with contact of blood, buffers, or gases with electrode membranes. Visibility of the path through the heat sink is helpful for detecting clogs, dirt, and bubbles. Bubbles that fail to rinse out can be a particular problem if they settle on an electrode.

Quality Assurance and Quality Control

Elements of good quality assurance of blood gas and pH measurements include (1) proper maintenance of the instrument, (2) use of control materials, (3) verification of electrode linearity, (4) checking of barometer accuracy, and (5) accurate measurement of temperature.

External quality assurance (proficiency testing) mandated by federal law in the United States [Clinical Laboratory Improvement Amendments (CLIA) '88] has assumed new importance for quality control of blood gas analysis. These rules became effective in January 1991, and set criteria for satisfactory interlaboratory performance are as follows: pH, target value ±0.04; PO_2, target value ±3 SD; and PCO_2, target value ±8% or ±5 mm Hg, whichever is greater. The risks of failure in a testing event are greatest for PCO_2, according to a computer model.[32] The significance of proficiency testing and the penalties for failure place strong incentives on faithful performance of internal control measures and effective response to failures of quality control. At the same time, pressures to control costs have raised the question of how many concentrations of control materials are necessary to monitor intralaboratory performance effectively and how often this should be done. The facile answer is as many concentrations and as often as it takes to maintain confidence in the measurement systems. The regulatory answer in the United States per CLIA '88 is one concentration of control every 8 hours, with the entire range of control concentrations covered in every 24 hour period. The CAP requires at least two concentrations of controls every 8 hours. In many laboratories, however, the practical answer is to run on every instrument in use, at least once per shift, three concentrations of control for pH, PO_2, and PCO_2, always on completion of maintenance and troubleshooting procedures. Newer analyzers, particularly the smaller satellite laboratory and point-of-care instruments, frequently have an "auto quality control (QC)" feature or use "electronic QCs."[97] Auto QC consists of onboard QC material that is automatically analyzed by the instrument at designated intervals that fulfill regulatory requirements. Electronic QC, which is most common in devices with disposable electrode cartridges, consists of cartridges that verify the electronic specification of the instruments. In 1999, the CLSI published a guideline for electronic QC and other alternative QC approaches for devices that use disposable electrodes.[24] For further discussion of these issues, see Chapter 20 on POCT.

Blood-Based and Fluorocarbon-Based Control Materials

Commercial blood-based control material usually consists of tanned human erythrocytes suspended in buffered medium and sealed in vials with a gas mixture of known O_2 and CO_2 content. Nonblood fluorocarbon materials with O_2-carrying properties similar to those of blood are also available. These products usually are made at three concentrations of pH,

PCO_2, and PO_2. Unopened, these types of control materials have the advantages of a long shelf life in the refrigerator: 20 to 28 days for tanned erythrocytes and even longer for the others. The buffered medium allows for control of pH along with control of PO_2 and PCO_2. Within-day and day-to-day consistency in the lifetime of a given lot have been reported to be excellent; within-day coefficients of variation over the range of concentrations were 1 to 2% for pH, PCO_2, and PO_2.

Aqueous Fluid Control Materials

These materials consist of a buffered medium sealed in vials with gas mixtures; the fluid is equilibrated with the gas by vigorous shaking by hand immediately before the vial is opened, and a sample is admitted to the instrument. Coefficients of variation of 0.1% for pH, 2.5% for PCO_2, and 3.2% for PO_2 are common for these types of materials. The disadvantages of aqueous controls stem from their dissimilarity to blood. Lower viscosity and surface tension confer different washout characteristics and impair their ability to reflect clogging. Greater electrical conductivity reduces their effectiveness in detecting inadequate grounding, and lower thermal coefficients make them slower to detect failures of temperature control. These disadvantages are most apparent with respect to PO_2, where a fluorocarbon-based matrix is superior. Nevertheless, aqueous commercial controls are far and away the most common. Tonometered controls have been used as adjuncts to commercial controls, but this is done rarely because of the reliability and ease of use of modern blood gas analyzers. For details of using tonometered whole blood, see a previous edition of this textbook.[90]

Sources of Analytical Error

General causes of analytical error include calibration of the instrument with incorrect set points for pH buffers or calibrator gases, degraded calibration materials, failure of temperature control of the measurement chamber, and a dirty sample chamber or path. Incorrect calibration may arise from wrong entries made for buffer or gas values into the microprocessor, from incorrect manual calculations of PCO_2 and PO_2 values by Dalton's law for calibrator gases, or from using gases that are dry because the humidification device is not working properly. Measurements of PO_2 are particularly sensitive to temperature error. To keep systematic error to 1 to 2%, the temperature control at 37 °C must be within ±0.1 °C. Built-in barometers can be checked by contacting nearby meteorologic stations. Gases other than O_2 present in a blood sample may affect performance of the PO_2 electrode. The anesthetic gases halothane and nitrous oxide have a direct effect because both can be reduced at the polarized cathode in competition with O_2. Under most circumstances, however, these effects are small and can be ignored.

Reference Intervals

Reference intervals for arterial blood PO_2, SO_2, PCO_2, and pH are extensively described in Chapter 60. Values for PO_2 and PCO_2 will decrease with increasing altitude, but compensatory mechanisms keep pH values the same. The P_{50} corrected to pH 7.40 is 18 to 24 mm Hg for newborns and 24 to 29 mm Hg for adults.

PCO_2 values decrease with altitude above sea level at a rate of 3 mm Hg/km (5 mm Hg/mile). A physiologic change occurs with change in posture; PCO_2 is 2 to 4 mm Hg higher for a sitting or standing person than for one in the supine position. During pregnancy, PCO_2 falls gradually to a mean of about 28 mm Hg just before term.

Temperature Correction of Measured pH, PCO_2, and PO_2

In the Henderson-Hasselbalch equation, pK' and α are used as constants for a temperature of 37 °C. The temperature-controlled sample chamber of an instrument is specified to be 37 ± 0.1 °C, and it is at that temperature that all measurements of pH and partial pressure of gases are made. The body temperature of a febrile patient may be elevated to 40 to 41 °C, or a patient may be made hypothermic for some surgeries and have a temperature as low as 23 °C. Most blood gas instruments on keyboard entry of a patient's actual temperature can calculate and present temperature-corrected pH and PCO_2. Algorithms used by some manufacturers in their instruments have been listed[5]; these are very similar or identical to the algorithms shown in Table 28-4 and specified by the CLSI.[23] Correction of pH and PCO_2 to the actual temperature of the patient is usually omitted in states of hyperthermia. However, significant disagreement exists with respect to hypothermic states.[9] Two basic strategies are used by anesthetists in managing hypothermic patients. In the pH-stat method, the measured pH is corrected to the actual body temperature of the patient and then is maintained as close to 7.4 as possible by introducing 3 to 5% CO_2 into the inhaled ventilator gas. Alternatively, in the α-stat strategy, uncorrected values are used to keep pH and PCO_2 close to the 37 °C reference value. In most situations, the α-stat method is used, primarily because it is technically easier to perform. However, in children undergoing deep hypothermia and circulatory arrest, the pH-stat strategy has been shown to be more effective in protecting the brain, and it is the recommended strategy.

The equation shown in Table 28-4 illustrates the complexity of the calculation used to correct PO_2 to the patient's body temperature.[23] Complexity is unavoidable because at PO_2 < 100 mm Hg ($SO_2 \leq 0.95$), the hemoglobin-oxygen dissociation curve is shifted to the left by the decrease in temperature

TABLE 28-4 Temperature Correction Formulas Recommended by the CLSI[23]

pH	$pH(T) = pH(37\ °C) - [0.147 + 0.0065 \times (pH\{37\ °C\} - 7.40) \times (T - 37\ °C)]$
PCO_2	$PCO_2\ (T) = PCO_2\ (37\ °C) \times 10^{[0.019 \times (T - 37\ °C)]}$
PO_2	$pO_2(T) = pO_2(37\ °C) \times 10^{\left(\frac{5.49\times10^{-11}\times pO_2^{3.88}+0.071}{9.72\times10^{-9}\times pO_2^{3.88}+2.30}\right)\times(T\text{-}37\ °C)}$

and by the concomitant rise in pH (see Figure 28-5). For temperature corrections of PO_2 between 100 and 400 mm Hg, accurate formulas become even more complicated. The most accurate calculation of the temperature variation of PO_2 is made by iterative calculations when the only necessary parameters are the temperature coefficients of the P_{50} and the solubility coefficient of O_2 (αO_2). Several analyzers perform such calculations. Temperature-corrected values should always be reported with the original 37 °C values.

Continuous and Noninvasive Monitoring of Blood Gases

Obtaining arterial, venous, or capillary blood is an invasive procedure, and test results reflect conditions pertaining only to a single point in time. Repetitive sampling in intensive or acute care management carries risks, including infection and vascular complications. In premature infants particularly, repeated sampling imposes an undesirable blood loss. Decisive action during intensive cardiopulmonary care or cardiac surgery often demands continuous monitoring or discrete real-time data for blood gases.

Extensive discussion of noninvasive and continuous modes of monitoring is beyond the purview of this text. However, laboratorians must be aware of them, because blood samples and standard analytical equipment remain the reference for monitoring the effectiveness of such devices, and because responsibility for quality assessment and review for them is often assigned to the clinical laboratory. Indeed, some agencies, such as the CAP, have developed guidelines for laboratory oversight of "alternative test systems" that include transcutaneous and in vivo monitoring devices. Such guidelines state that "in some cases traditional approaches to management, quality control, etc. may not be directly applicable but that systems must be in place to ensure that accurate results are generated."

Pulse oximeters that continuously monitor SO_2Hb are common and are generally reliable.[46] Older pulse oximeters were susceptible to error depending on placement and motion, but technology has made these devices very reliable.[12,31] Transcutaneous monitoring of PCO_2 and PO_2 is a noninvasive continuous monitoring approach that has been around for longer than 30 years and has had particular value and general success in neonatal and pediatric care.[8] These devices consist of gel-encased self-adhesive electrodes that heat the skin to 43 to 44 °C to arterialize the capillaries and facilitate diffusion of O_2 through the skin.[85] Although the electrodes differ considerably in appearance from those used on blood gas instrumentation, they operate on exactly the same electrochemical principle.

Transcutaneous monitoring of PO_2 can vary widely depending on whether the site of application reflects arterial, capillary, or venous blood flow. However, because there is little difference between arterial and venous PCO_2, transcutaneous monitoring of PCO_2 is less problematic, and pulse oximeters can often serve as a surrogate for PO_2. Transcutaneous monitoring works best in areas of thin skin, thus its popularity in neonates and in settings of normovolemia. Additionally, hypovolemia can make pulse oximeter devices less reliable.[36] Nevertheless, their correlations with arterial co-oximetry are reasonable (r values ranging from 0.7 to 0.8), and they have been recommended for trending and monitoring. Transcutaneous monitoring can also be used to monitor local tissue perfusion after certain surgical procedures and trauma.[85]

In addition to monitoring PO_2 and PCO_2, new inline devices that also monitor pH, electrolytes, glucose, and hematocrit have been introduced to the market.[7] These consist of a single-use inline cartridge consisting of six conventional electrodes. The cartridge is attached to an arterial line and upon operator command withdraws ≈1.5 mL of blood into the cartridge, where analysis takes place. The analytical time is about 60 seconds, after which the blood is returned via the arterial line. Cartridges undergo two-point calibration before they are placed in service, and a single-point calibration is used to flush the sensors after each analysis. Analysis can be repeated every 5 minutes, and it is claimed that cartridges can be used for up to 72 hours. In a multicenter study, results from 1414 paired sample measurements showed good agreement and correlation for results from an inline monitor compared with traditional laboratory methods.[7] The future of such devices will likely depend on costs versus benefits for patient care and outcomes.

Although POCT testing and transcutaneous devices have been invaluable for quickly monitoring PO_2 levels in critically ill patients, development of implantable xerogel (nanoporous solid gel formed by drying without shrinkage)-coated oxygen sensors may be critical for future care management.[66] The idea of using implantable oxygen sensors in critically ill patients has been around for a while, but development has been hindered by biocompatibility issues such as platelet adhesion and activation on the sensor surface or vasoconstriction at the sensor implant site.[66] To overcome biocompatibility issues, nitric oxide–releasing xerogel films have been developed that contain hydrophilic polyurethane (HPU) that increases oxygen permeability while preventing vasoconstriction and platelet adhesion through nitric oxide release. Although still in early developmental stages, such sensors are promising. They demonstrate a rapid and repeatable linear response to oxygen and high sensitivity of ≈6 nAmp/mm Hg.[66] Moreover, HPU xerogel oxygen sensors stably release nitric oxide for longer than 48 hours in in vitro test situations. It is hoped that continued development of HPU xerogel coatings will lead to increased nitric oxide release capability for intravascular applications where numerous nitric oxide scavengers exist.

REFERENCES

1. Abraham B, Fakhar I, Tikaria A, Hocutt L, Marshall J, Swaminathan S, et al. Reverse pseudohyperkalemia in a leukemic patient. Clin Chem 2008;54:449-51.
2. Adams PC, Woodhouse KW, Adela M, Parnham A. Exaggerated hypokalemia in acute myeloid leukemia. Br Med J 1962;282:1034-5.
3. Albrink MJ, Hald PM, Man EB, Peters JP. The displacement of serum water by the lipids of hyperlipemic serum: a new method for the rapid determination of serum water. J Clin Invest 1955;34:1483-8.

4. Apple FS, Koch DD, Graves S, Ladenson JH. Relationship between direct potentiometric and flame photometric measurement of sodium in blood. Clin Chem 1982;28:1931-5.
5. Ashwood ER, Kost G, Kenny M. Temperature correction of blood-gas and pH measurements. Clin Chem 1983;29:1877-85.
6. Barker SJ, Curry J, Redford D, Morgan S. Measurement of carboxyhemoglobin and methemoglobin by pulse oximetry: a human volunteer study. Anesthesiology 2006;105:892-7.
7. Billman GF, Hughes AB, Dudell GG, Waldman E, Adcock LM, Hall DM, et al. Clinical performance of an in-line, ex vivo point-of-care monitor: a multicenter study. Clin Chem 2002;48:2030-43.
8. Binder N, Atherton H, Thorkelsson T, Hoath SB. Measurement of transcutaneous carbon dioxide in low birthweight infants during the first two weeks of life. Am J Perinatol 1994;11:237-41.
9. Bisson J, Younker J. Correcting arterial blood gases for temperature: (when) is it clinically significant? Nurs Crit Care 2006;11:232-8.
10. Bobacka J. Conducting polymer-based solid state ion-selective electrodes. Electroanalysis 2006;18:7-18.
11. Bobacka J, Ivaska A, Lewenstam A. Potentiometric ion sensors. Chem Rev 2008;108:329-51.
12. Bohnhorst B, Peter CS, Poets CF. Pulse oximeters' reliability in detecting hypoxemia and bradycardia: comparison between a conventional and two new generation oximeters. Crit Care Med 2000;28:1565-8.
13. Brydon WG, Roberts LB. The effect of haemolysis on the determination of plasma constituents. Clin Chim Acta 1972;41:435-8.
14. Burnett RW, Covington AK, Maas AH, Muller-Plathe O, Weisberg HF, Wimberley PD, et al. IFCC document stage 3, draft 1, dated 1989 02 01. An approved IFCC recommendation. IFCC method (1988) for tonometry of blood: reference materials for pCO2 and pO2. International Federation of Clinical Chemistry Scientific Division. Committee on pH, Blood Gases and Electrolytes. Clin Chim Acta 1989;185:S17-24.
15. CAP. Comprehensive chemistry survey set C-A: CAP surveys. Chicago, Ill: College of American Pathologists, 2008.
16. Caprilli R, Sopranzi N, Colaneri O, Levi Della Vida M, de Magistris L. Salt-losing diarrhoea in idiopathic proctocolitis. Scand J Gastroenterol 1978;13:331-5.
17. CFF (Cystic Fibrosis Foundation) center director committee. Update I. Bethesda, Md: CFF, 1990.
18. CFF (Cystic Fibrosis Foundation). Cystic fibrosis mutation database. Available at: http://www.genet.sickkids.on.ca/accessed May /10/2011.
19. CFF (Cystic Fibrosis Foundation). Problems in sweat testing: report on GAP conference. Bethesda, Md: CFF, 1975.
20. Chillar RK, Belman MJ, Farbstein M. Pseudohypoxemia due to leukemia and thrombocytosis. N Engl J Med 1980;302:584.
21. Chittamma A, Vanavanan S. Comparative study of calculated and measured total carbon dioxide. Clin Chem Lab Med 2008;46:15-7.
22. CLSI (Clinical and Laboratory Standards Institute). C34-A3. Sweat testing: sample collection and quantitative chloride analysis: approved guideline, 3rd edition. Wayne, Pa: CLSI, 2009.
23. CLSI (Clinical and Laboratory Standards Institute). C46-A2. Blood gas and pH analysis and related measurements. Wayne, Pa: CLSI, 2009.
24. CLSI (Clinical and Laboratory Standards Institute). EP-18. Quality management for unit-use testing. Wayne, Pa: CLSI, 1999.
25. Costello P, Kubasik NP, Brody BB, Sine HE, Bertsch JA, D'Souza JP. Multilayer film analysis: evaluation of ion-selective electrolyte slides. Clin Chem 1983;29:129-32.
26. Cotlove E. Determination of chloride in biological materials. In: Glick D, ed. Methods of biochemical analysis, volume 12. New York: Interscience Publishers, 1964:277-391.
27. Daoud EW, McClellan AC, Scott MG. Positive interferences with the Ektachem total CO_2 assay from therapy with topical cerous nitrate. Clin Chem 1990;36:1521-2.
28. Denning CR, Huang NN, Cuasay LR, Shwachman H, Tocci P, Warwick WJ, et al. Cooperative study comparing three methods of performing sweat tests to diagnose cystic fibrosis. Pediatrics 1980;66:752-7.
29. Dimeski G, Barnett RJ. Effects of total plasma protein concentration on plasma sodium, potassium and chloride measurements by an indirect ion selective electrode measuring system. Crit Care Resusc 2005;7: 12-5.
30. Don BR, Sebastian A, Cheitlin M, Christiansen M, Schambelan M. Pseudohyperkalemia caused by fist clenching during phlebotomy. N Engl J Med 1990;322:1290-2.
31. Durbin CG Jr, Rostow SK. More reliable oximetry reduces the frequency of arterial blood gas analyses and hastens oxygen weaning after cardiac surgery: a prospective, randomized trial of the clinical impact of a new technology. Crit Care Med 2002;30:1735-40.
32. Ehrmeyer SS, Laessig RH. A computer model to translate federal proficiency testing peformance standards for pH/blood gases into intralaboratory precision and accuracy requirements. In: Moran RF, VanKessel AL, eds. Methodology and clinical applications of blood gases, pH, electrolytes and sensor technology IFCC, volume 12. Utrecht, The Netherlands: MVI Publishing, 1990:3-18.
33. Eng W, LeGrys VA, Schechter MS, Laughon MM, Barker PM. Sweat-testing in preterm and full-term infants less than 6 weeks of age. Pediatr Pulmonol 2005;40:64-7.
34. Erickson KA, Wilding P. Evaluation of a novel point-of-care system, the i-STAT portable clinical analyzer. Clin Chem 1993;39:283-7.
35. Farrell PM, Rosenstein BJ, White TB, Accurso FJ, Castellani C, Cutting GR, et al. Guidelines for diagnosis of cystic fibrosis in newborns through older adults: Cystic Fibrosis Foundation consensus report. J Pediatr 2008;153:S4-14.
36. Fernandez M, Burns K, Calhoun B, George S, Martin B, Weaver C. Evaluation of a new pulse oximeter sensor. Am J Crit Care 2007;16: 146-52.
37. Frier BM, Steer CR, Baird JD, Bloomfield S. Misleading plasma electrolytes in diabetic children with severe hyperlipidaemia. Arch Dis Child 1980;55:771-5.
38. Geller RJ, Spyker DA, Herold DA, Bruns DE. Serum osmolal gap and ethanol concentration: a simple and accurate formula. J Toxicol Clin Toxicol 1986;24:77-84.
39. Gibson LE, Disant Agnese PA. Studies of salt excretion in sweat: relationships between rate, conductivity, and electrolyte composition of sweat from patients with cystic fibrosis and from control subjects. J Pediatr 1963;62:855-67.
40. Goldman AS, Travis LB, Dodge WF, Daeschner CW. Falsely negative sweat tests in children with cystic fibrosis complicated by hypoproteinemic edema. J Pediatr 1961;59:301.
41. Goodman JR, Vincent J, Rosen I. Serum potassium changes in blood clots. Am J Clin Pathol 1954;24:111-3.
42. Graber M, Subramani K, Corish D, Schwab A. Thrombocytosis elevates serum potassium. Am J Kidney Dis 1988;12:116-20.
43. Grocott MP, Martin DS, Levett DZ, McMorrow R, Windsor J, Montgomery HE. Arterial blood gases and oxygen content in climbers on Mount Everest. N Engl J Med 2009;360:140-9.
44. Hammond KB, Turcios NL, Gibson LE. Clinical evaluation of the macroduct sweat collection system and conductivity analyzer in the diagnosis of cystic fibrosis. J Pediatr 1994;124:255-60.
45. Hansen JE, Simmons DH. A systematic error in the determination of blood PCO2. Am Rev Respir Dis 1977;115:1061-3.
46. Haymond S, Cariappa R, Eby CS, Scott MG. Laboratory assessment of oxygenation in methemoglobinemia. Clin Chem 2005;51:434-44.
47. Hess CE, Nichols AB, Hunt WB, Suratt PM. Pseudohypoxemia secondary to leukemia and thrombocytosis. N Engl J Med 1979;301: 361-3.
48. Centers for Disease Control and Prevention (CDC). Guideline for isolation precautions: preventing transmission of infectious agents in healthcare settings, 2007. Available at: www.cdc.gov/hicpac/2007IP/2007isolationPrecautions.html/accessed May 11, 2011.
49. Kibel MA. Sweat tests in cystic fibrosis. Lancet 1978;2:1050.
50. Kimura S, Asari S, Hayashi S, Yamaguchi Y, Fushimi R, Amino N, et al. New enzymatic method with tryptophanase for determining potassium in serum. Clin Chem 1992;38:44-7.

51. Kratz A, Ferraro M, Sluss PM, Lewandrowski KB. Case records of the Massachusetts General Hospital: laboratory reference values. N Engl J Med 2004;351:1548-63.
52. Kumar A, Chapoteau E, Czech BP, Gebauer CR, Chimenti MZ, Raimondo O. Chromogenic ionophore-based methods for spectrophotometric assay of sodium and potassium in serum and plasma. Clin Chem 1988;34:1709-12.
53. Kwant G, Oeseburg B, Zijistra WG. Reliability of the determination of whole-blood oxygen affinity by means of blood-gas analyzers and multi-wavelength oximeters. Clin Chem 1989;35:773-7.
54. Lacher DA, Hughes JP, Carroll MD. Estimate of biological variation of laboratory analytes based on the Third National Health and Nutrition Examination Survey. Clin Chem 2005;51:450-2.
55. Ladenson JH. Non-analytical sources of variation in clinical chemistry results. In: Sonnenwirth AC, Jarett L, eds. Gradwohl's clinical laboratory methods and diagnosis. St Louis: CV Mosby, 1980:149-92.
56. Ladenson JH, Apple FS, Aguanno JJ, Koch DD. Sodium measurements in multiple myeloma: two techniques compared. Clin Chem 1982;28: 2383-6.
57. LeGrys VA. Common errors in sweat testing reporting for cystic fibrosis. Lab Med 2002;33:21-3.
58. LeGrys VA. Trends and methodology in sweat testing. Lab Med. 1990;21:155-8.
59. LeGrys VA, Retsch-Bogart GZ. Urticaria associated with the pilocarpine iontophoresis sweat test. Pediatr Pulmonol 1997;24:296-7.
60. LeGrys VA, Wood RE. Incidence and implications of false-negative sweat test reports in patients with cystic fibrosis. Pediatr Pulmonol 1988;4:169-72.
61. LeGrys VA, Yankaskas JR, Quittell LM, Marshall BC, Mogayzel PJ Jr. Diagnostic sweat testing: the Cystic Fibrosis Foundation guidelines. J Pediatr 2007;151:85-9.
62. Maas AH. IFCC reference methods for measurement of pH, gases and electrolytes in blood: reference materials. Eur J Clin Chem Clin Biochem 1991;29:253-61.
63. Maas AH, Siggaard-Andersen O, Weisberg HF, Zijlstra WG. Ion-selective electrodes for sodium and potassium: a new problem of what is measured and what should be reported. Clin Chem 1985;31:482-5.
64. MacLean WC Jr, Tripp RW. Cystic fibrosis with edema and falsely negative sweat test. J Pediatr 1973;83:86-8.
65. Mansour MM, Azzazy HM, Kazmierczak SC. Correction factors for estimating potassium concentrations in samples with in vitro hemolysis: a detriment to patient safety. Arch Pathol Lab Med 2009;133:960-6.
66. Marxer SM, Robbins ME, Schoenfisch MH. Sol-gel derived nitric oxide-releasing oxygen sensors. Analyst 2005;130:206-12.
67. McNeill R, Siudak R, Wardlaw JH, Weiss DE. Electronic conduction in polymers. Aust J Chem 1963;16:1056-75.
68. Moran RF. The laboratory assessment of oxygenation. J Intern Fed Clin Chem 1993;5:147.
69. Mueller RG, Lang GE. Blood gas analysis: effect of air bubbles in syringe and delay in estimation. Br Med J (Clin Res Ed) 1982;285:1659-60.
70. Nakamaru K, Hatakeyama N, Yamada M, Yamazaki M. Comparison of bicarbonate and base excess values analyzed by four different blood gas analyzers. J Anesth 2007;21:429-32.
71. Natelson S, Nobel D. Effect of the variation of pK′ of the Henderson-Hasselbalch equation on values obtained for total CO2 calculated from pCO2 and pH values. Clin Chem 1977;23:767-9.
72. Nijsten MW, de Smet BJ, Dofferhoff AS. Pseudohyperkalemia and platelet counts. N Engl J Med 1991;325:1107.
73. Oesch U, Ammann D, Simon W. Ion-selective membrane electrodes for clinical use. Clin Chem 1986;32:1448-59.
74. Oliver TK Jr, Young GA, Bates GD, Adamo JS. Factitial hyperkalemia due to icing before analysis. Pediatrics 1966;38:900-2.
75. Quiles R, Fernandez-Romero JM, Fernandez E, Luque de Castro MD, Valcarcel M. Automated enzymatic determination of sodium in serum. Clin Chem 1993;39:500-3.
76. Rosan RC, Enlander D, Ellis J. Unpredictable error in calculated bicarbonate homeostasis during pediatric intensive care: the delusion of fixed pK′. Clin Chem 1983;29:69-73.
77. Rosenstein B. Sweat testing in CF: not to be taken lightly. J Respir Dis 1982;3:71-6.
78. Rosenstein BJ, Langbaum TS. Misdiagnosis of cystic fibrosis: need for continuing follow-up and reevaluation. Clin Pediatr 1987;26:78-82.
79. Salyer JW, Chatburn RL, Dolcini DM. Measured vs calculated oxygen saturation in a population of pediatric intensive care patients. Resp Care 1989;34:342-8.
80. Samaja M, Mosca A, Luzzana M, Rossi-Bernardi L, Winslow RM. Equations and nomogram for the relationship of human blood p50 to 2,3-diphosphoglycerate, CO2, and H+. Clin Chem 1981;27:1856-61.
81. Schulz IJ. Micropuncture studies of the sweat formation in cystic fibrosis patients. J Clin Invest 1969;48:1470-7.
82. Siggaard-Anderson M, Siggaard-Anderson O. Oxygen status algorithm, version 3, with some applications. Acta Anaesthesiol Scand Suppl 1995;107:13-20.
83. Southgate HJ, Colliss JS, Short SM. Comparison of a colorimetric potassium method with flame photometry and ion-selective electrodes. Ann Clin Biochem 1991;28(Pt 4):412-3.
84. Stamler J, Elliott P, Chan Q, for the INTERMAP Research Group. INTERMAP appendix tables. J Hum Hypertens 2003;17:665-758.
85. Tatevossian RG, Wo CC, Velmahos GC, Demetriades D, Shoemaker WC. Transcutaneous oxygen and CO_2 as early warning of tissue hypoxia and hemodynamic shock in critically ill emergency patients. Crit Care Med 2000;28:2248-53.
86. Thomas LJ Jr. Algorithms for selected blood acid-base and blood gas calculations. J Appl Physiol 1972;33:154-8.
87. Tietz NW. Clinical guide to laboratory tests, 5th edition. Philadelphia, Pa: WB Saunders, 2005.
88. Tietz NW, ed. Fundamental of clinical chemistry, 2nd edition. Philadelphia, Pa: WB Saunders, 1976.
89. Tietz NW, ed. Textbook of clinical chemistry, 3rd ed. Philadelphia, Pa: WB Saunders, 1999, (pp 1059 to 1060).
90. Tietz NW, ed. Textbook of clinical chemistry, 1st ed. Philadelphia, Pa: WB Saunders, 1986.
91. Tietz NW, ed. Textbook of clinical chemistry and molecular diagnostics, 4th ed. Philadelphia, Pa: WB Saunders, 2006.
92. Tocci PM, McKey RM Jr. Laboratory confirmation of the diagnosis of cystic fibrosis. Clin Chem 1976;22:1841-4.
93. Wang T, Diamandis EP, Lane A, Baines AD. Variable selectivity of the Hitachi chemistry analyzer chloride ion-selective electrode toward interfering ions. Clin Biochem 1994;27:37-44.
94. Watson MA, Scott MG. Clinical utility of biochemical analysis of cerebrospinal fluid. Clin Chem 1995;41:343-60.
95. Waugh WH. Utility of expressing serum sodium per unit of water in assessing hyponatremia. Metabolism 1969;18:706-12.
96. Webster HL. Laboratory diagnosis of cystic fibrosis. Crit Rev Clin Lab Sci 1983;18:313-38.
97. Westgard JO. Electronic quality control, the total testing process, and the total quality control system. Clin Chim Acta 2001;307:45-8.
98. Wilke K, Martin A, Terstegen L, Biel SS. A short history of sweat gland biology. Int J Cosmet Sci 2007;29:169-79.
99. Wolf AV. Aqueous solutions and body fluids. New York: Hoeber Medical Division, Harper and Row, 1966.

CHAPTER 29

Hormones

Michael Kleerekoper, M.D., F.A.C.B., F.A.C.P., M.A.C.E.*

A hormone is a chemical substance produced in the body by an organ, cells of an organ, or scattered cells, having a specific regulatory effect on the activity of an organ or organs.[15] Hormones are produced at one site in the body and exert their action(s) at distant sites through what is called the *endocrine* system. It is increasingly recognized that many hormones exert actions locally through what is termed the *paracrine* system. Finally, some hormones exert their action on the cells of origin, regulating their own synthesis and secretion via an *autocrine* system. The classic endocrine hormones include insulin, thyroxine, and cortisol. Neurotransmitters and neurohormones are examples of the paracrine system, and certain growth factors that stimulate synthesis and secretion of true hormones from the same cell are examples of an autocrine system.

Table 29-1 lists hormones that are commonly measured in clinical practice plus a few others to illustrate concepts. Biochemical, clinical, and analytical information for specific hormones may be found in Chapters 26 and 46 through 57.

CLASSIFICATION

Hormones are classified as (1) polypeptides or proteins, (2) steroids, or (3) derivatives of amino acids.

Polypeptide or Protein Hormones

Adrenocorticotropic hormone (ACTH), insulin, and parathyroid hormone (PTH) are examples of polypeptide or protein hormones. They are generally water soluble and circulate freely in plasma as the whole molecule or as active or inactive fragments. The half-life of these hormones in plasma is short (≤10 to 30 minutes), and wide fluctuations in their concentration may be seen in several physiologic and pathologic circumstances. These hormones initiate their response by binding to cell membrane receptors (on or in the membrane) and exciting a "second messenger" system, which continues the specific actions of these hormones.

Steroid Hormones

Steroid hormones (e.g., cortisol, estrogen) are hydrophobic and insoluble in water. These hormones circulate in plasma, reversibly bound to transport proteins (e.g., cortisol-binding globulin, sex hormone-binding globulin) with only a small fraction free, or unbound available to exert physiologic action.[5,8,17] The half-life of steroid hormones is 30 to 90 minutes. Free steroid hormones, being hydrophobic, enter the cell by passive diffusion and bind with intracellular receptors in the cytoplasm or the nucleus.[3]

Amino Acid–Related Hormones

Thyroxine and catecholamine are examples of hormones that are derived from amino acids; they are water soluble and circulate in plasma bound to proteins (thyroxine) or free (catecholamines). Thyroxine binds avidly to three binding proteins and has a half-life of about 7 to 10 days; free and unbound catecholamines such as epinephrine have a very short half-life of a minute or less. As do the water-soluble peptide and protein hormones, these hormones interact with membrane-associated receptors and use a second messenger system.

RELEASE AND ACTION OF HORMONES

The physiologic functions of hormones have been broadly categorized into those that (1) affect growth and development, (2) exert homeostatic control of metabolic pathways, and (3) regulate the production, use, and storage of energy. The descriptions that follow illustrate examples of these functions and mechanisms of control of hormone secretion.

Growth and Development

Normal growth and development of the whole human organism is dependent on the complex integrative function of many hormones, including gonadal steroids (estrogen and androgen), growth hormone, cortisol, and thyroxine. Several pituitary hormones are responsible specifically for the growth and development of endocrine glands themselves, and thus are responsible for control of synthesis and secretion of other hormones. Those other hormones can provide negative feedback on secretion of the pituitary hormones. Other regulators of secretion of the pituitary hormones include circadian rhythms and a hypothalamic pulse generator that controls the

Text continued on page 842

The author gratefully acknowledges the original contribution by Dr. Ronald J. Whitley on which portions of this chapter are based.

TABLE 29-1 Major Hormones and Frequently Measured Hormone Precursors and Cytokines

Endocrine Organ and Hormone	Chemical Nature of Hormone	Major Sites of Action	Principal Actions
Hypothalamus			
Thyrotropin-releasing hormone (TRH)	Peptide (3aa, Glu-His-Pro)[a]	Anterior pituitary	Release of TSH and prolactin (PRL)
Gonadotropin-releasing hormone (Gn-RH) or luteinizing hormone-releasing hormone (LH-RH)	Peptide (10aa)	Anterior pituitary	Release of LH and FSH
Corticotropin-releasing hormone (CRH)	Peptide (41aa)	Anterior pituitary	Release of ACTH and β-lipotropic hormone (LPH)
Growth hormone-releasing hormone (GH-RH)	Peptides (40, 44aa)	Anterior pituitary	Release of growth hormone (GH)
Somatostatin[b] (SS) or growth hormone-inhibiting hormone (GH-IH)	Peptides (14, 28aa)	Anterior pituitary	Suppression of secretion of many hormones [e.g., GH, TSH, gastrin, vasoactive intestinal polypeptide (VIP), gastric inhibitory polypeptide (GIP), secretin, motilin, glucagon, and insulin]
Prolactin-releasing peptide	Peptide (20aa)	Anterior pituitary	Release of PRL
Prolactin-releasing/inhibiting factor	Dopamine	Anterior pituitary	Suppression of synthesis and secretion of PRL
Anterior Pituitary Lobe			
Thyrotropin or thyroid-stimulating hormone (TSH)	Glycoprotein, heterodimer[c] (α, 92aa; β, 112aa)	Thyroid gland	Stimulation of thyroid hormone formation and secretion
Follicle-stimulating hormone (FSH)	Glycoprotein, heterodimer[c] (α, 92aa; β, 117aa)	Ovary	Growth of follicles with LH, secretion of estrogens, and ovulation
		Testis	Development of seminiferous tubules; spermatogenesis
Luteinizing hormone (LH)	Glycoprotein, heterodimer[c] (α, 92aa; β, 121aa)	Ovary	Ovulation; formation of corpora lutea; secretion of progesterone
		Testis	Stimulation of interstitial tissue; secretion of androgens
PRL	Peptide (199aa)	Mammary gland	Proliferation of mammary gland; initiation of milk secretion; antagonist of insulin action
Growth hormone (GH) or somatotropin	Peptide (191aa)	Liver	Production of IGF-1 (promoting growth)
		Liver and peripheral tissues	Anti-insulin and anabolic effects
Corticotropin or adrenocorticotropin (ACTH)	Peptide (39aa)	Adrenal cortex	Stimulation of adrenocortical steroid formation and secretion
β-Endorphin (β-END)[b,h]	Peptide (31aa)	Brain	Endogenous opiate; raising of pain threshold and influence on extrapyramidal motor activity
Chorionic gonadotropin (CG) or choriogonadotropin	Glycoprotein, heterodimer[c] (α, 92aa; β, 145aa)		
α-Melanocyte-stimulating hormone (α-MSH)	Peptide (13aa)	Skin	Dispersion of pigment granules, darkening of skin
Leu-enkephalin (LEK)[b,h] and met-enkephalin (MEK)[b,h]	Peptide (5aa)	Brain	Same as β-endorphin

TABLE 29-1 Major Hormones and Frequently Measured Hormone Precursors and Cytokines—cont'd

Endocrine Organ and Hormone	Chemical Nature of Hormone	Major Sites of Action	Principal Actions
Posterior Pituitary Lobe			
Vasopressin or ADH	Peptide (9aa)	Arterioles Renal tubules	Elevation of blood pressure; water reabsorption
Oxytocin	Peptide (9aa)	Smooth muscles (uterus, mammary gland)	Contraction; action in parturition and in sperm transport; ejection of milk
Pineal Gland			
Serotonin or 5-hydroxytryptamine (5-HT)	Indoleamine	Cardiovascular, respiratory, and gastrointestinal systems; brain	Neurotransmitter; stimulation or inhibition of various smooth muscles and nerves
Melatonin	Indoleamine	Hypothalamus	Suppression of gonadotropin and GH secretion; induction of sleep
Thyroid Gland			
Thyroxine (T_4) and triiodothyronine (T_3)	Iodoamino acids	General body tissue	Stimulation of oxygen consumption and metabolic rate of tissue
Calcitonin or thyrocalcitonin	Peptide (32aa)	Skeleton	Uncertain in humans
Parathyroid Gland			
Parathyroid hormone (PTH) or parathyrin	Peptide (84aa)	Kidney	Increased calcium reabsorption, inhibited phosphate reabsorption; increased production of 1,25-dihydroxycholecalciferol
		Skeleton	Increased bone resorption
Adrenal Cortex			
Aldosterone	Steroid	Kidney	Salt and water balance
Androstenedione[d]	Steroid	Hormone precursor	Converted to estrogens and testosterone
Cortisol	Steroid	Many	Metabolism of carbohydrates, proteins, and fats; anti-inflammatory effects; others
Dehydroepiandrosterone (DHEA) and dehydroepiandrostenedione sulfate (DHEAS)	Steroids	Hormone precursors	Converted to estrogens and testosterone
17-Hydroxyprogesterone	Steroid	Hormone precursor	Converted to cortisol
Adrenal Medulla			
Norepinephrine and epinephrine	Aromatic amines	Sympathetic receptors	Stimulation of sympathetic nervous system
Epinephrine		Liver and muscle, adipose tissue	Glycogenolysis Lipolysis
Ovary			
Activin A	Peptides[e] 2 β_A subunits	Pituitary, ovarian follicle	Stimulates release of FSH; enhances FSH action; inhibits androgen production by theca cells
Activin B	Peptides[e] 2 β_B subunits beta	See activin A above	See activin A above
DHEA and DHEAS	Steroids	Hormone precursors	Converted to androstenedione

Continued

TABLE 29-1 Major Hormones and Frequently Measured Hormone Precursors and Cytokines—cont'd

Endocrine Organ and Hormone	Chemical Nature of Hormone	Major Sites of Action	Principal Actions
Ovary—cont'd			
Estrogens	Phenolic steroids	Female accessory sex organs	Development of secondary sex characteristics
		Bone	Control of skeletal maturation et al
Follistatin	Peptides (288aa, 315aa)	Pituitary, ovarian follicles	Inhibits FSH synthesis and secretion by binding activin
Inhibin A	Peptide (α subunit and β_A subunit)	Hypothalamus, ovarian follicle	Inhibits FSH secretion; stimulates theca cell androgen production
Inhibin B	Peptide (α subunit and β_B subunit)	See inhibin A above	See inhibin A above
Progesterone	Steroid	Female accessory reproductive structure	Preparation of the uterus for ovum implantation, maintenance of pregnancy
Relaxin	Peptide[f]	Uterus	Inhibition of myometrial contraction
Testis			
Inhibin B	See above	Anterior pituitary, hypothalamus	Control of LH and FSH secretion
Testosterone	Steroid	Male accessory sex organs	Development of secondary sex characteristics, maturation, and normal function
Placenta			
Estrogens	See above	See above	See above
Progesterone	See above	See above	See above
Relaxin	See above	See above	See above
Chorionic gonadotropin (CG) or choriogonadotropin	Glycoprotein, heterodimer[c](α, 92aa; β, 145aa)	Same as LH	Same as LH; prolongation of corpus luteal function
Placental growth hormone (GH-V)	Peptides (22 and 26 kDa)	Same as GH	Same as GH
Chorionic somatomammotropin (CS) or placental lactogen (PL)	Peptide (191aa)	Same as PRL	Same as PRL
Pancreas			
Amylin	Peptide (37aa)	Pancreas	Inhibits glucagon and insulin secretion
Glucagon	Peptide (29aa)	Liver	Glycogenolysis
Insulin	Peptide[g]	Liver, fat, muscle	Regulation of carbohydrate metabolism; lipogenesis
Pancreatic polypeptide (PP)	Peptide (36aa)	Gastrointestinal tract	Increased gut motility and gastric emptying; inhibition of gallbladder contraction
Somatostatin (SS)[h]	Peptide (14aa)	Pancreas	Inhibition of secretion of insulin, glucagon
Gastrointestinal Tract			
Gastrin[h]	Peptide (17aa)	Stomach	Secretion of gastric acid, gastric mucosal growth
Ghrelin[h] (GHRP)	Peptide (28aa)	Anterior pituitary	Secretion of GH
Secretin	Peptide (27aa)	Pancreas	Secretion of pancreatic bicarbonate and digestive enzymes

TABLE 29-1 Major Hormones and Frequently Measured Hormone Precursors and Cytokines—cont'd

Endocrine Organ and Hormone	Chemical Nature of Hormone	Major Sites of Action	Principal Actions
Cholecystokinin-pancreozymin (CCK-PZ)[h]	Peptide (33aa)	Gallbladder and pancreas	Stimulation of gallbladder contraction and secretion of pancreatic enzymes
Motilin	Peptide (22aa)	Gastrointestinal tract	Stimulation of gastrointestinal motility
VIP[h]	Peptide (28aa)	Gastrointestinal tract	Neurotransmitter; relaxation of smooth muscles of gut and of circulation; increased release of hormones and secretion of water and electrolytes from pancreas and gut
Gastric inhibitory peptide (GIP)	Peptide (42aa)	Gastrointestinal tract	Inhibition of gastric secretion and motility; increase in insulin secretion
Glucagon-like peptide-1	Peptide (30-31aa)	Gastrointestinal tract	Increase insulin and decrease glucagon secretion; inhibit gastric emptying
Bombesin[h]	Peptide (14aa)	Gastrointestinal tract	Stimulation of release of various hormones and pancreatic enzymes, smooth muscle contractions and hypothermia, changes in cardiovascular and renal function
Neurotensin[h]	Peptide (13aa)	Gastrointestinal tract and hypothalamus	Uncertain
Substance P (SP)[h]	Peptide (11aa)	Gastrointestinal tract and brain	Sensory neurotransmitter, analgesic; increase in contraction of gastrointestinal smooth muscle; potent vasoactive hormone; promotion of salivation, increased release of histamine
Kidney			
1,25-$(OH)_2$ cholecalciferol	Sterol	Intestine Bone	Facilitation of absorption of calcium and phosphorus; increase in bone resorption in conjunction with PTH
		Kidney	Increase in reabsorption of filtered calcium
Erythropoietin	Peptide (165aa)	Bone marrow	Stimulation of red cell formation
Renin-angiotensin-aldosterone system	Peptides (renin, 297aa; Ang I, 10aa; Ang II, 8aa, produced from Ang I by angiotensin converting enzyme)	Renin (from kidney) catalyzes hydrolysis of angiotensinogen (from liver, 485aa) to ang I in the intravascular space	Ang II increases blood pressure and stimulates secretion of aldosterone (see adrenal)
Liver			
IGF-1, formerly called somatomedin	Peptide (70aa)	Most cells	Stimulation of cellular and linear growth
IGF-2	Peptide (67aa)	Most cells	Insulin-like activity

Continued

TABLE 29-1 Major Hormones and Frequently Measured Hormone Precursors and Cytokines—cont'd

Endocrine Organ and Hormone	Chemical Nature of Hormone	Major Sites of Action	Principal Actions
Thymus			
Thymosin and thymopoietin	Peptides (28, 49aa)	Lymphocytes	Maturation of T lymphocytes
Heart			
Atrial natriuretic peptide (ANP, Atriopeptin)	Peptide with an intrachain disulfide bond (28aa)	Vascular, renal, and adrenal tissues	Regulation of blood volume and blood pressure
B-type natriuretic peptide (BNP)	Peptide with an intrachain disulfide bond (32aa)	Vascular, renal, and adrenal tissues	Regulation of blood volume and blood pressure
Adipose Tissue			
Adiponectin	Peptide oligomers of 30 kDa subunits	Muscle Liver	Increases fatty acid oxidation Suppresses glucose formation
Leptin	Peptide (167aa)	Hypothalamus	Inhibition of appetite, stimulation of metabolism
Resistin	Peptide (94aa)	Liver	Insulin resistance
Multiple Cell Types			
Estrogens	See above	See above	See above
Galanin	Peptide (30aa)	Brain, pancreas, gastrointestinal (GI) tract	Regulates food intake, memory, and cognition; inhibits endocrine and exocrine secretions of pancreas; delays gastric emptying; prolongs colonic transport times
Parathyroid hormone-related peptide (PTH-RP)	Peptides (139, 141, 173aa)	Kidney, bone	Physiologic function conjectural; PTH-like actions; tumor marker
Growth factors (e.g., epidermal growth factor, fibroblast growth factor, transforming growth factor family, platelet-derived growth factor, nerve growth factors)	Peptides	Many	Stimulation of cellular growth
Monocytes/Lymphocytes/Macrophages			
Cytokines (e.g., interleukins 1 to 18, tumor necrosis factor, interferons)	Peptides	Many	Stimulation or inhibition of cellular growth; other

[a]*aa*, Amino acid residues.
[b]Also produced by gastrointestinal tract and pancreas.
[c]Glycoprotein hormones composed of two dissimilar peptides. The α-chains are similar in structure or identical; the β-chains differ among hormones and confer specificity.
[d]Androstenedione is also produced in the ovary and testis.
[e]Each activin and inhibin is found in multiple forms.
[f]Two chains linked by two disulfide bonds: α, 24aa; β, 29aa.
[g]Two chains linked by two disulfide bonds: α, 21aa; β, 30aa.
[h]Also produced in the brain.

pulsatile secretion of gonadotropins. Examples of hormones of the anterior pituitary gland include the following:

- Gonadotropins [luteinizing hormone (LH) and follicle-stimulating hormone (FSH)] that regulate the development, growth, and function of the ovary and testis (see Chapter 56). Ovarian and testicular hormones in turn regulate pubertal growth; development and maintenance of secondary sex characteristics; growth, development, and maintenance of the skeleton and muscles; and distribution of body fat.

- ACTH that regulates growth of the adrenal glands and synthesis and secretion of adrenal gland hormones (see Chapters 53 and 54).
- Thyroid-stimulating hormone (TSH) that regulates growth of the thyroid gland and iodination of amino acids to produce the thyroid hormones triiodothyronine and thyroxine (see Chapter 55).[1]

Homeostatic Control of Metabolic Pathways

The metabolic pathways under hormonal control are diverse and complex. The following important examples illustrate the feedback control of hormone secretion, which is critical for homeostasis:

- Regulation of blood glucose: In response to a glucose load, insulin is promptly released from the pancreas, which regulates the dispersal of glucose into cells (fat, muscle, liver, and brain) for the metabolism necessary to produce energy from glucose (see Chapter 26). As circulating glucose concentrations thus return to preload concentrations, insulin secretion slows. Several counter-regulatory hormones come into play to further regulate this process to ensure that blood glucose concentrations do not become too low. These include glucagon, cortisol, epinephrine, and growth hormone. Recent attention has focused on a group of gastrointestinal hormones termed *incretins* (see Chapter 46) that are released during eating and stimulate insulin secretion from the pancreas in advance of any measurable increase in blood glucose. Incretins also affect the rate of absorption of nutrients from the gut by slowing down the rate of gastric emptying. Another mechanism by which incretins have a role in the regulation of blood glucose is by delaying release of the counter-regulatory hormone glucagon from the alpha cells of the pancreatic islets. The most studied incretins are glucagon-like peptide-1 (GLP-1) and gastric inhibitory peptide (GIP).
- Regulation of serum calcium (see Chapter 52): The calcium-sensing receptor (CaSR) on the parathyroid gland recognizes the ambient concentration of ionized calcium, which in turn regulates the synthesis and secretion of PTH. When ionized calcium concentrations fall (so imperceptibly that most analytical methods could not detect the change), PTH synthesis and secretion are stimulated. This additional PTH will attempt to restore serum ionized calcium by enhancing renal tubular reabsorption of calcium and calcium efflux from the skeleton. PTH also catalyzes the synthesis of the renal hormone calcitriol (1,25-dihyroxycholecalciferol), which acts on the gut to increase intestinal absorption of calcium. These very rapid responses of PTH and calcitriol quickly restore ionized calcium to concentrations where the CaSR is no longer activated, and PTH and calcitriol synthesis and secretion return to basal rates.
- Water and electrolyte metabolism is regulated by aldosterone from the adrenal gland, renin from the kidney, and vasopressin [antidiuretic hormone (ADH)] from the posterior pituitary gland (see Chapters 48, 53, and 54).

Regulation of the Production, Use, and Storage of Energy

Under normal conditions, regulation of energy production, use, and storage is under tight hormonal control. Under conditions of changing demands that require more energy (e.g., exercise, starvation, infection or trauma, emotional stress), many hormones are upregulated to control not only circulating levels of nutrients but also the metabolism of these nutrients into necessary energy. This very complex activity, which may involve hormones from different organs, as already alluded to in the preceding section, is under neurologic control, with numerous neuroendocrine hormones participating actively in this integrative metabolic process, which affects most organs in the body and modulates, for example, heart rate, sweating, fertility, and reproduction.

ROLE OF HORMONE RECEPTORS

The "unique" or specific action of a hormone on its target tissue is a function of the interaction between the hormone and its receptor. As discussed previously, several types of hormone-receptor interactions may occur.[3,5,8,17] The hormone-receptor complex provides the very high specificity of the action of the hormone, allowing the target tissue to accumulate the hormone from among all the molecules to which it is exposed. This is essential because hormones generally circulate in picomolar or nanomolar concentrations (10^{-9} to 10^{-12} mol/L).

Hormone receptors may be on the cell surface or may be intracellular within the cytoplasm or nucleus.

Cell-Surface Receptors

Peptide hormones bind to cell surface receptors, and the conformational change resulting from this binding activates an effector system, which in turn is responsible for the downstream actions of the hormone (Figure 29-1).[11,12] For most peptide hormones, the intracellular effector that is activated by the hormone-receptor interaction is a specific G-protein (guanyl-nucleotide–binding protein),[4,10,13,18] and the receptors are called G-protein–coupled receptors (GPCRs; Figure 29-2). GPCRs are hepta-helical molecules with seven membrane-spanning domains. The amino terminus is extracellular, and the carboxy terminus is intracellular. The major structural classes of GPCRs have been identified, each containing receptors for specific subsets of hormones (Figure 29-3). Group I is the largest group, containing receptors for many peptide hormones and catecholamines. Group II contains receptors for the family of gastrointestinal hormones (secretin, glucagons, and vasoactive intestinal polypeptide). Group III contains the CaSR and the glutamate receptor. Stimulation of a G-protein initiates the intracellular processes of signal transduction that characterize the specific action of the hormone. G-proteins are composed of α, β, and γ subunits and are classified according to the α subunit, of which 20 have been identified to date (see Figure 29-3). G-proteins may stimulate adenylate cyclase (G_S type of G-proteins) or may inhibit adenylate cyclase (G_i type). The many classes of

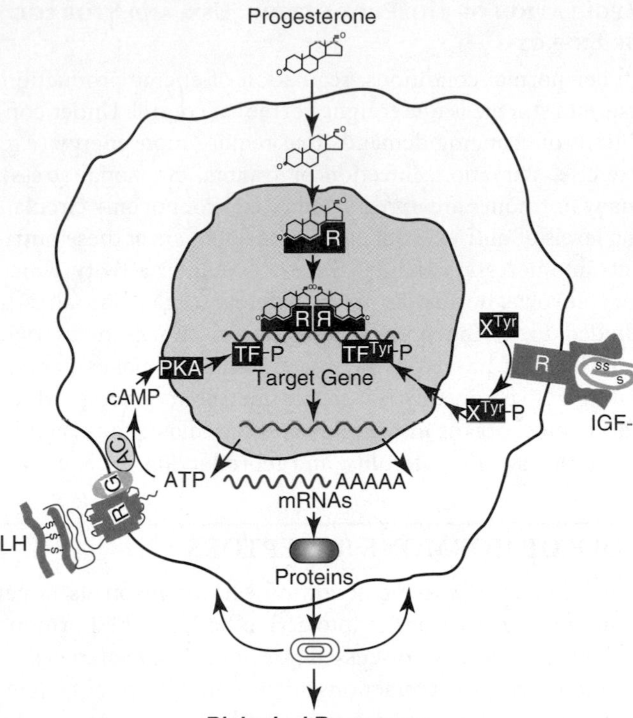

Figure 29-1 Hormonal signaling by cell surface and intracellular receptors. Receptors for the water-soluble polypeptide hormones, luteinizing hormone (LH) and insulin-like growth factor (IGF)-1, are integral membrane proteins located at the cell surface. They bind the hormone using extracellular sequences and transduce a signal through the generation of second messengers—cyclic adenosine monophosphate (cAMP) for the LH receptor and tyrosine-phosphorylated substrates for the IGF-1 receptor. Although effects on gene expression are indicated, direct effects on cellular proteins (e.g., ion channels) are also observed. In contrast, the receptor for the lipophilic steroid hormone progesterone resides in the cell nucleus. It binds the hormone and becomes activated and capable of directly modulating target gene transcription. ***Tf,*** **Transcription factor;** ***R,*** **receptor molecule.** *(From Conn PM, Melmed S. Textbook of endocrinology. Towanta NJ: Humana Press, 1997.)*

GPCRs and G-proteins briefly described in this section provide some insight into the mechanisms responsible for the specificity of hormone action. Some nonpeptide hormones also use cell surface receptors.

Intracellular Receptors

Lipid-soluble hormones such as progesterone (see Figure 29-1) are transported in plasma bound to carrier proteins, with only a small fraction of the hormone being in the free or unbound state. The free hormone enters the cell via passive diffusion and binds to intracellular receptors in the cytoplasm or, more often, the nucleus (see Figure 29-1). These receptors are characterized by a hormone-binding domain, a deoxyribonucleic acid (DNA)-binding domain, and an amino-terminal variable domain. Just as the interaction of protein or polypeptide hormones with cell surface receptors changes the conformation of the receptor protein, the binding of a lipid-soluble hormone with its specific hormone-binding domain on the intracellular receptor changes the molecular conformation of the intracellular receptor. This conformational change, or activation of the receptor, enables the hormone-receptor complex to bind to specific regulatory DNA sequences of a target gene, permitting control of specific gene expression (see Figure 29-1).[7]

POSTRECEPTOR ACTIONS OF HORMONES

Cell surface and intracellular receptors have different postreceptor actions.

Cell Surface Receptors

Once GPCRs are occupied by a hormone, G-protein subunits begin a cascade of activation of specific enzymes that generate molecules that serve as second messengers to effect the hormone response. The best known of these are adenylyl cyclase, which generates cyclic adenosine monophosphate (cAMP), and phospholipase C, which generates both inositol 1,4,5-trisphosphate (IP_3) and diacylglycerol (see Figure 29-2). The production of second messengers and the subsequent magnitude of the effect of the hormone are functions of the amount of hormone bound to the GPCR. The binding of a small number of hormone molecules on the cell surface leads to the production of many molecules of the second messenger, thus amplifying the signal sent by the hormone (which can be thought of as the first messenger).

cAMP-dependent protein kinases (PKAs) are a family of enzymes that, in the presence of cAMP, phosphorylate a number of intracellular enzymes and other proteins to activate or inactivate the function of these enzymes and proteins, thereby regulating their function. As a further means of regulating hormone action, these cAMP-dependent kinases consist of two catalytic and two regulatory subunits (C and R, respectively, in Figure 29-4). The regulatory subunits exist as a dimer that can bind two molecules of cAMP, and the binding of cAMP releases the catalytic subunits, which then are activated as phosphorylating enzymes. When cAMP is removed from the regulatory subunit, this dimer is not able to associate two catalytic subunits and amplify the signal of the hormone.

Phospholipase C (Figure 29-2) acts on inositol phospholipids within the cell membrane to produce IP_3, which opens up ion channels to facilitate entry of calcium into the cytoplasm, where it acts as a messenger, and diacylglycerol, which modulates protein kinase C activity.

The insulin receptor represents a somewhat different class of cell surface receptors that contain intrinsic hormone-activated tyrosine kinase activity and do not otherwise involve a second messenger.[16] The insulin receptor, the prototype of this type of receptor, consists of two α and two β subunits joined by disulfide bridges. The extracellular hormone-binding domains are the α subunits, and the β subunits are intracellular. They contain an ATP-binding site and a catalytic

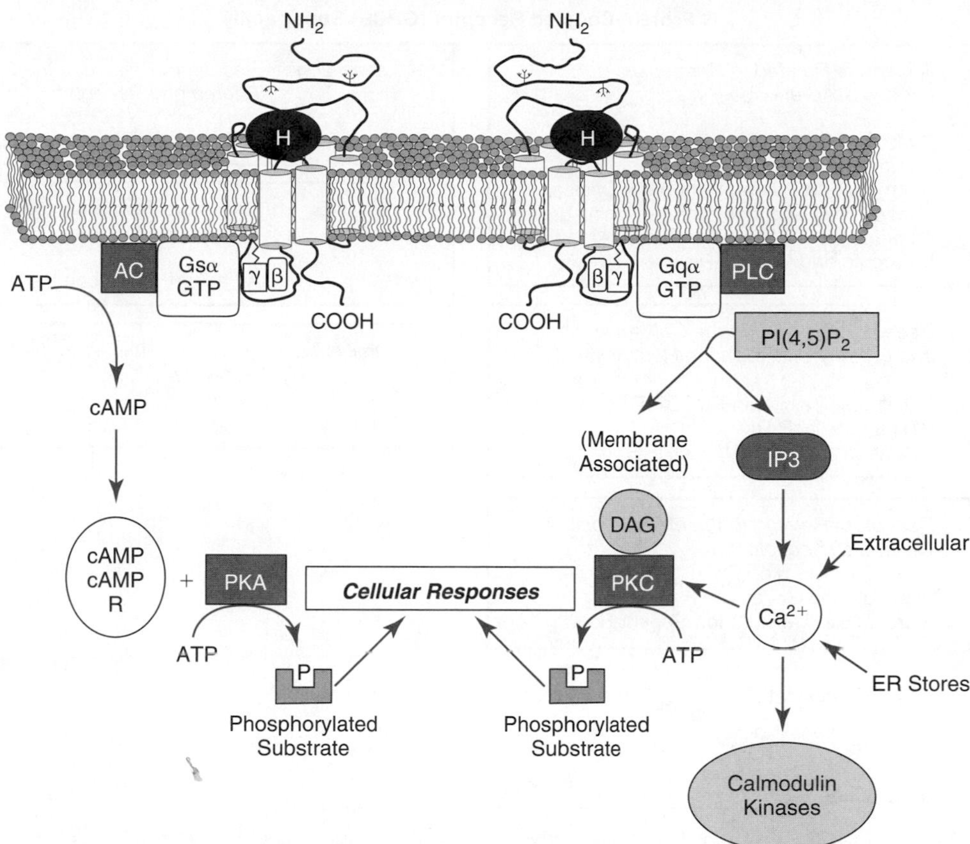

Figure 29-2 Signal transduction by cell surface receptors that are coupled to G-proteins. Two seven-transmembrane domains, coupled to different G-proteins (G_S and G_q), are shown. Activation of GS leads to stimulation of the effector enzyme adenylate cyclase and production of a cyclic adenosine monophosphate (cAMP) second messenger, causing the activation of protein kinase A (PKA) and the initiation of potential phosphorylation cascades. Activation of G_q leads to stimulation of the effector enzyme phospholipase C-β and the production of inositol 1,4,5-trisphosphate (IP_3) and diacylglycerol (DAG) second messengers, one effect of which is to activate protein kinase C (PKC) and initiate a potential phosphorylation cascade. *(From Conn PM, Melmed S, eds. Textbook of endocrinology. Towanta NJ: Humana Press, 1997.)*

kinase domain through which tyrosine kinase is activated immediately upon insulin binding to the receptor.

Because hormones largely serve a regulatory function, there are of necessity many self-limiting steps in the previous processes. Without these self-limiting processes, hormone action would continue unabated. For cAMP, cessation of hormone action involves the inactivation of G-protein stimulation of adenylate cyclase by guanosine triphosphatase (GTPase) (Figure 29-5). In the absence of hormone interaction with the GPCR (basal or unstimulated state), G_S is bound to guanosine diphosphate (GDP). Once the hormone is bound to the receptor, GDP is released from G_s and is replaced by GTP, and the G_s-GTP complex activates adenylate cyclase. The G_s-GTP complex is inactivated by GTPase, restoring the G_S-GDP state, which cannot stimulate formation of cAMP until further hormone binding to the GPCR takes place. Within a few minutes (or less) of hormone-GPCR interaction and the initiation of hormone action, the receptor is phosphorylated by protein kinase A and protein kinase C. This phosphorylation of the hormone receptor permits internalization of the complex from the cell surface into the cytoplasm where dephosphorylation occurs, permitting degradation of the hormone and recycling of the GPCR to its original transmembrane location, awaiting coupling with more hormone.

Intracellular Receptors

As noted, lipid-soluble hormones bind to the hormone-binding domain of cytosolic or nuclear receptors.[11,12] This results in a conformational change that enables the hormone-receptor complex to bind to specific regulatory DNA sequences in the 5′ end of the target gene.[7] The binding specificity of the (hormone-bound) receptor for specific regions of the DNA of the target gene is determined by zinc finger structures in the receptor's DNA-binding domain. It is the binding of the hormone-receptor complex to DNA regulatory elements that enhances or represses gene transcription. The messenger ribonucleic acid (RNA) that is enhanced or

G Protein-Coupled Receptor (GPCR) Superfamily

Family A:	*Receptors Related to Rhodopsin and the β-Adrenergic Receptor*
Group I:	Olfactory, Adenosine, Melanocortin Rs
Group II:	Adrenergic, Muscarinic, Serotonin, DA Rs
Group III:	Neuropeptide Rs and Vertebrate Opsins
Group IV:	Bradykinin R and Invertebrate Opsins
Group V:	Peptide and GP Hormone, Chemokine Rs
Group VI:	Melatonin and Orphan Rs

Family B:	*Receptors Related to the Calcitonin and Parathyroid Hormone Receptors*
Group I:	Calcitonin, Calcitonin-like, CRF Rs
Group II:	PTH and PTHrP Rs
Group III:	Glucagon, Secretin, VIP, GHRH Rs

Family C:	*Receptors Related to the Metabotropic Glutamate Receptors*
Group I:	Metabotropic Glutamate Rs
Group II:	Extracellular Calcium Ion Sensor Rs

Family D:	*Receptors Related to the STE2 Pheromone Receptor*
Group I:	Alpha Factor Pheromone Rs

Family E:	*Receptors Related to the STE3 Pheromone Receptor*
Group I:	A Factor Pheromone Rs

Family F:	*Receptors Related to the cAMP Receptor*
Group I:	Dictyostelium cAR1-4 Rs

A

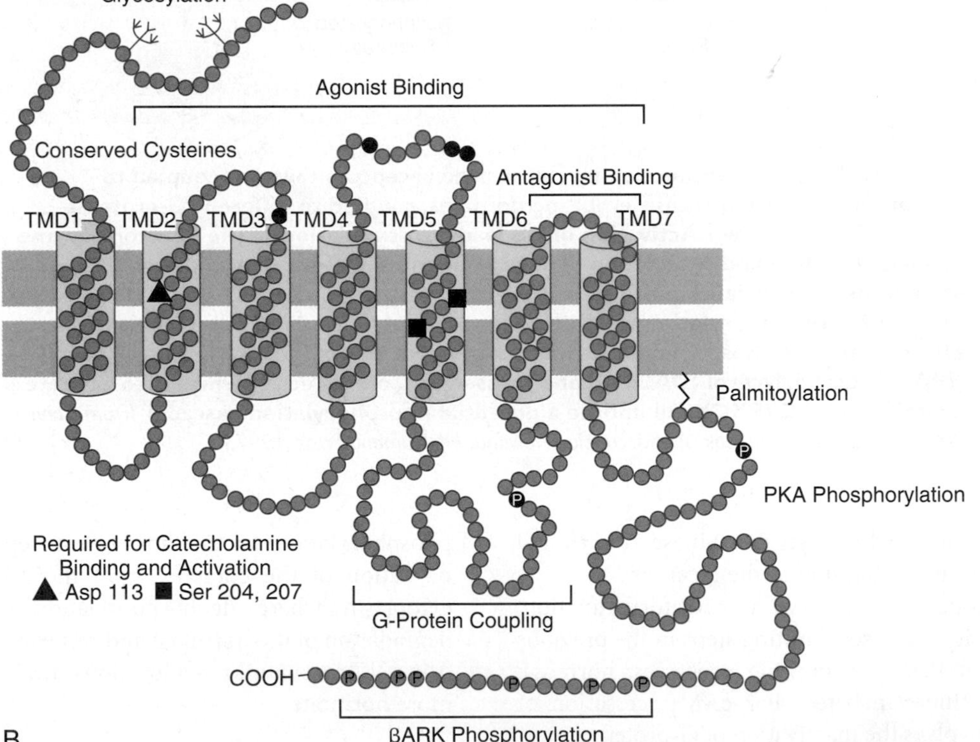

B

Figure 29-3 Classification and basic architecture of cell surface receptors that couple to G-proteins. A, Lists the major families and groups of G-protein–coupled receptors (GPCRs). The mammalian receptors are confined to families A, B, and C. Family A is the largest and includes the diverse odorant receptors and prototypic GPCRs such as rhodopsin and the β-adrenergic receptor. B, Shows a schematic structure of one of the most extensively characterized GPCRs, the β-adrenergic receptor. Major structural features are indicated and are expanded on in the text. *(From Conn PM, Melmed S, eds. Textbook of endocrinology. Towanta NJ: Humana Press, 1997.)*

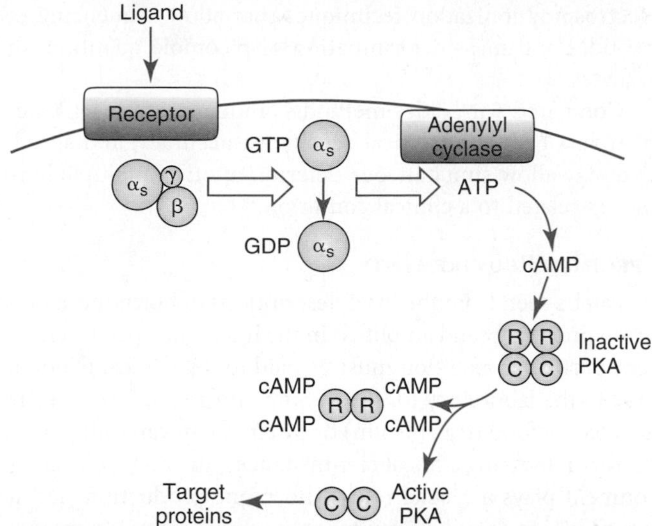

Figure 29-4 Signaling by G_S. The alpha, beta, and gamma subunits of G_s are shown. The alpha subunit, when bound to GTP, activates adenylyl cyclase which catalyzes the formation of cyclic AMP (cAMP) from ATP. Then cAMP binds to the regulatory subunit (R) of protein kinase A (PKA, cyclic AMP-dependent protein kinase), releasing PKA's catalytic subunit (C) and thus leading to phosphorylation of target proteins. *(Image from Conn PM, Melmed S, eds. Textbook of endocrinology. Towanta NJ: Humana Press, 1997.)*

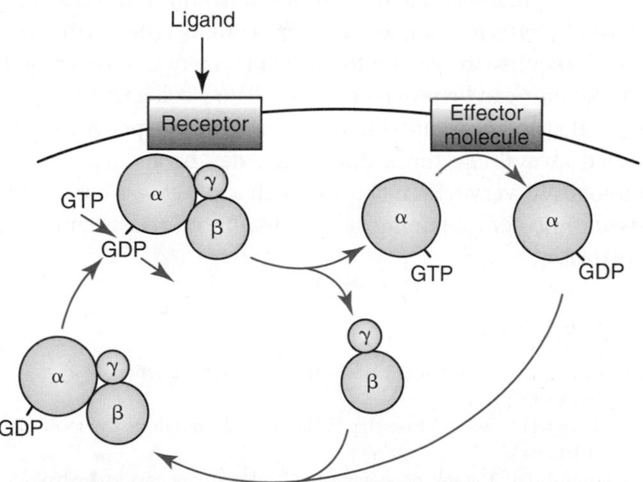

Figure 29-5 The G-protein cycle. The alpha, beta, and gamma subunits of G_s are shown. The alpha subunit, when bound to GTP, activates the effector molecule (such as adenylyl cyclase, see Figure 29-4). GTP then is hydrolyzed to GDP, stopping the activation of the effector molecule and leading to reformation of the GDP-bound state of the G protein. *(Image from Conn PM, Melmed S, eds. Textbook of endocrinology. Towanta NJ: Humana Press, 1997.)*

diminished by hormone receptor binding to the target gene regulates the synthesis of specific proteins that mediate the hormone's physiologic actions. The system is further regulated by the presence or absence of coactivators or corepressors of gene expression. In addition, many actions of hormones that bind to intracellular receptors are rapid and do not depend on synthesis of protein, suggesting that these hormone-receptor complexes exert actions by mechanisms different from binding to DNA.

From these descriptions, one can begin to deduce both the complexity and the specificity of hormone action, in terms of an "on and/or off" concept and in terms of an "effect size" concept.

CLINICAL DISORDERS OF HORMONES

Although several chapters of this textbook detail a variety of endocrine disorders, a brief introduction is appropriate here. In general, endocrine diseases may result from a deficiency or an excess of a single hormone or several hormones, or from resistance to the action of hormones. Hormone deficiency can be congenital or acquired, and hormone excess can result from endogenous overproduction (from within the body) or exogenous overmedication. Hormone resistance can occur at several levels but can most simply be characterized as receptor mediated, postreceptor mediated, or at the level of the target tissue. The clinical manifestations will depend on the hormone system affected and the type of abnormality.

Diabetes mellitus (DM) is an example of an endocrine disorder; it is the most common endocrine disorder in the United States (see Chapter 46). It is classified as type 1 or type 2. DM type 1 results from failure of the pancreas to secrete insulin even though the pancreas is otherwise normal. Type 2, the most common form of DM, results from end-organ resistance to the action of insulin, which, in this case, is secreted from the pancreas in abundant amounts and circulates at high concentrations. Secondary DM occurs when a nonendocrine disease such as pancreatitis destroys the pancreas, including the insulin-secreting cells. The biochemical hallmark of DM is hyperglycemia.

In contrast to diabetes, there are uncommon, insulin-producing tumors of the pancreas (insulinomas) in which the production of insulin is not regulated by the blood glucose concentration and the biochemical hallmark of the tumors is hypoglycemia. Thus hyperglycemia can be present when there is insulin deficiency or insulin excess, and insulin excess can accompany both hyperglycemia and hypoglycemia. This simple illustration underscores the homeostatic and/or regulating nature of the endocrine system.

MEASUREMENTS OF HORMONES AND RELATED ANALYTES

Hormones are measured by a variety of analytical techniques, including bioassay, receptor assay, immunoassay, and instrumental techniques such as mass spectrometry interfaced with liquid or gas chromatography. A general overview of these techniques is given here. Analytical details for individual hormones using such techniques are found in the discussion of the individual hormones in their respective chapters.

Bioassay Techniques

Bioassays are based on observations of physiologic responses specific for the hormone being measured. In vivo bioassays usually involve the injection of test materials (such as blood or urine from a patient) into suitably prepared animals; target gland responses such as growth or steroidogenesis are then measured. In vitro bioassays involve the incubation of tissue, membranes, dispersed cells, or permanent cell lines in a defined culture medium, with subsequent measurement of an appropriate hormone response. Most in vitro bioassays measure responses proximal or distal to a second messenger such as stimulation of cAMP formation. Bioassays tend to be imprecise and are rarely necessary in clinical medicine.

Receptor-Based Assays

Receptor assays depend on the in vitro interaction of a hormone with its biological receptor. In this type of assay, unlabeled hormone displaces trace amounts of radioactively labeled hormone from receptor sites. A second approach is to measure a response, such as production of cAMP, when a test sample is added to a preparation that includes the receptor and necessary cofactors. In general, receptor assays are simpler to perform and have greater sensitivity than bioassays. Receptor assays also have an advantage over immunoassays in that they reflect the biological function of a hormone, namely, the capacity to combine with specific receptor sites. By contrast, immunoassays may measure active hormone and inactive prohormone, hormone polymer, and metabolites when all share a common antigenic determinant or set of determinants. In general, receptor assays are not as sensitive as immunoassays, and enzymes in the biological specimen may degrade the receptor or destroy the labeled tracer. The added complexity and lability of receptor preparations also contribute to the limited application of these assays in the routine clinical laboratory.

Immunoassay Techniques

Immunoassays employing antibodies are widely used to quantify hormones (see Chapter 16). Currently labeled antibody (immunometric) assays with nonisotopic labels are the method of choice for measuring most hormones, especially peptides and proteins. Immunometric assays use saturating concentrations of two or more antibodies (often monoclonal) that are prepared against different epitopes of the protein molecule. One of the two antibodies is usually attached to a solid phase separation system and extracts the hormone from the serum specimen. The second antibody is linked to a signal molecule, which is then measured. The resultant signal is used to quantify the bound hormone.

Instrumental Techniques

Mass spectrometers (see Chapter 14) coupled with gas and liquid chromatographs (see Chapter 13) are powerful qualitative and quantitative analytical tools that are widely used to measure hormones.[2,6,9,14] Technical advancements in mass spectrometry have resulted in the development of matrix-assisted laser desorption/ionization (MALDI) and electrospray ionization techniques that allow sequencing of peptides and mass determination of picomole quantities of analytes.

Compared with older methods, tandem mass spectrometry offers greater analytical sensitivity, accuracy, and speed, and may allow simultaneous determination of multiple hormones related to a clinical condition.[14]

Specimen Requirements

As can be seen from the brief descriptions of hormone action given previously and amplified in the hormone-specific chapters, particular attention must be paid to the clinical material sent to the laboratory for assay. Some hormones are directly affected by food (e.g., insulin) or by circadian variability (e.g., cortisol). In many clinical circumstances, the metabolic environment plays a crucial role in hormone production, and it is essential to obtain a simultaneous sample for measurement of both the hormone and the molecule(s) regulated by that hormone. An isolated measurement of plasma insulin without concurrent knowledge of the plasma glucose, or measurement of parathyroid hormone independent of serum calcium, is of little if any value. When a patient is evaluated for possible hormone deficiency or hormone excess, it is often necessary to perform a stimulation or suppression test. Most hormone assays can be performed on plasma or serum, and many can be performed on urine samples, usually a 24 hour collection. Increasingly, saliva has become a convenient body fluid for hormone analysis, particularly for hormones secreted in a diurnal rhythm such as cortisol. Unlike blood sampling, which requires the patient to present to a blood drawing facility, patients can be provided with salivary collection material such that they can provide to the laboratory specimens collected at multiple times during the day or at unusual (but biologically very relevant) times such as 11 PM—a commonly used time for obtaining a specimen for measurement of cortisol.

REFERENCES

1. Brent GA. The molecular basis of thyroid hormone action. N Engl J Med 1994;331:847-53.
2. Chace DH. Mass spectrometry in the clinical laboratory. Chem Rev 2001;101:445-77.
3. Edwards DP. The role of co-activators and co-repressors in the biology and mechanism of action of steroid hormone receptors. J Mammary Gland Biol Neoplasia 2000;5:307-24.
4. Farfel Z, Bourne HR, Iiri T. The expanding spectrum of G protein disease. N Engl J Med 1999;340:1012-20.
5. Funder JW. Mineralocorticoids, glucocorticoids, receptors and response elements. Science 1993;259:1132-3.
6. Giese RW. Measurement of endogenous estrogens: analytical challenges and recent advances. J Chromatogr A 2003;1000:401-12.
7. Glass CK. Differential recognition of target genes by nuclear receptor monomers, dimers, and heterodimers. Endocr Rev 1994;15:391-407.
8. Klinge CM. Estrogen receptor interaction with estrogen response elements. Nucleic Acids Res 2001;29:2905-19.
9. Lagerstedt SA, O'Kane DJ. Measurement of plasma free metanephrine and normetanephrine by liquid chromatography-tandem mass spectrometry for diagnosis of pheochromocytoma. Clin Chem 2004;50:603-11.
10. Lefkowitz RJ. G proteins in medicine. N Engl J Med 1995;332:186-7.

11. Mangelsdorf DJ, Thummel C, Beato M, Herrlich P, Schutz G, Umesono K, et al. The nuclear receptor superfamily: the second decade. Cell 1995;83:835-9.
12. McKenna NJ, Lanz RB, O'Malley BW. Nuclear receptor coregulators: cellular and molecular biology. Endocr Rev 1999;20:321-44.
13. Neer EJ. Heterotrimeric G proteins: organizers of transmembrane signals. Cell 1995;80:249-57.
14. Nelson RE, Grebe SK, O'Kane DJ, Singh RJ. Liquid chromatography-tandem mass spectrometry assay for simultaneous measurement of estradiol and estrone in human plasma. Clin Chem 2004;50:373-84.
15. Newman WA. Dorland's illustrated medical dictionary, 30th edition. Philadelphia, Pa: WB Saunders, 2003.
16. Olefsky JM. The insulin receptor: a multifunctional protein. Diabetes 1990;39:1009-16.
17. Pike AC, Brzozowski AM, Hubbard RE. A structural biologist's view of the oestrogen receptor. J Steroid Biochem Mol Biol 2000; 74:261-8.
18. Vaughan M. Signaling by heterotrimeric G proteins minireview series. J Biol Chem 1998;273:667-13.

CHAPTER 30

Catecholamines and Serotonin

Graeme Eisenhofer, Ph.D.,
Ronald J. Whitley, Ph.D., D.A.B.C.C.,
and Thomas G. Rosano, Ph.D., D.A.B.C.C, D.A.B.F.T.

Catecholamines and serotonin are biogenic amines that serve as transmitters of neuronal or hormonal signals in a wide range of physiologic processes. Dopamine, norepinephrine, and epinephrine are naturally occurring catecholamines with important roles as neurotransmitters in the brain or sympathetic nervous system, or as hormones produced by the adrenal medulla and other peripheral cellular systems. They are critical in maintaining the body's homeostasis and in responding to acute and chronic stress through an orchestration of cardiovascular, metabolic, glandular, and visceral organ activities. Serotonin serves as a neurotransmitter in the central nervous system and as a modulator of vascular and gastrointestinal functions. Abnormal production of catecholamines or serotonin is a hallmark of several neuroendocrine tumors for which clinical signs and symptoms reflect the pharmacologic properties of the secreted amines. Clinical measurement of biogenic amines and their metabolites aids in detection and monitoring of these tumors, and analytical advances in recent years have produced sensitive and specific laboratory methods available for clinical practice. This chapter provides an overview of important aspects of biochemistry, pathophysiology, and analytical methods for clinical assessment of catecholamines, serotonin, and their metabolites.

CHEMICAL STRUCTURE

The catecholamines produced naturally in humans—including *dopamine, norepinephrine* (noradrenaline), and *epinephrine* (adrenaline)—are phenylethylamines with hydroxyl groups on positions three and four of the benzene ring and an ethylamine sidechain on position one (Figure 30-1). Hydroxyl and methyl substitutions on the ethylamine sidechain distinguish the individual catecholamines in both structure and function. The catecholamines demonstrate varying degrees of alkaline instability in biological fluids, and their dihydroxybenzene or catechol structure is sensitive to oxidative formation of quinones in the presence of air and light. Several pharmaceutical and designer drugs with the basic phenylethylamine structure also have effects on related neuroeffector systems; such drugs are commonly referred to as *sympathomimetic agents.*

Serotonin with its indoleamine structure is distinct from the catecholamines (see Figure 30-1), and is an important naturally occurring biogenic amine produced widely in animal and plant kingdoms. Serotonin is structurally related to melatonin, the principle indoleamine produced by the pineal gland. A number of natural or synthetic congeners of serotonin have biological effects ranging from cerebral vasoconstriction (e.g., sumatripan) to psychoactive hallucinogenic actions (e.g., *N,N*-dimethyltryptamine).

Although structurally distinct, the catecholamines and serotonin have related biometabolism, and each serves as an important monoamine neurotransmitter or neurohormone in health and disease.

BIOSYNTHESIS, RELEASE, AND METABOLISM

The catecholamines and serotonin share similar pathways of biosynthesis and metabolism, including in some steps the same enzymes. Catecholamines and serotonin are sequestered and stored in vesicular granules from which they are released into the extracellular environment by calcium-dependent exocytosis. Termination of the physiologic effects of both the catecholamines and serotonin is dependent on active uptake processes, facilitated by specific plasma membrane transport proteins. Irreversible inactivation occurs after cellular uptake by metabolism, primarily by deamination and *O*-methylation for catecholamines, and by deamination for serotonin.

Biosynthesis

Catecholamines are synthesized from the amino acid, tyrosine, and serotonin from tryptophan (Figure 30-2). The rate-limiting step in catecholamine biosynthesis involves conversion of tyrosine to 3,4-dihydroxyphenylalanine (L-dopa) by the enzyme, tyrosine hydroxylase.[191] A related enzyme, tryptophan hydroxylase, catalyzes conversion of tryptophan to 5-hydroxytryptophan in the first step of serotonin synthesis. In contrast to tyrosine hydroxylase, which is encoded by

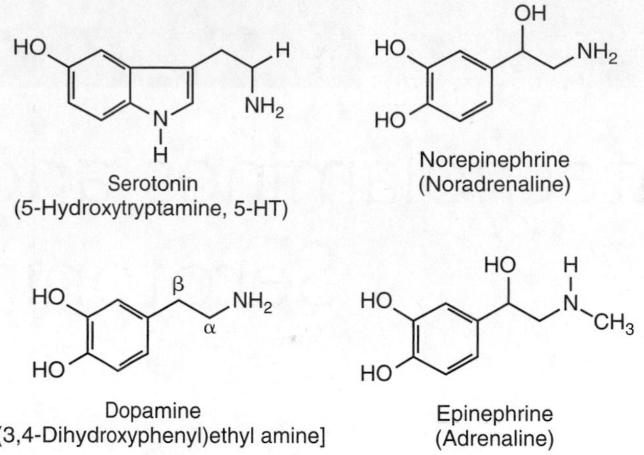

Figure 30-1 Chemical structure of the catecholamines and serotonin.

one gene, tryptophan hydroxylase is encoded by two genes and exists as two distinct isoforms; one of these isoforms is expressed in the central nervous system and the other at peripheral sites of serotonin synthesis, including the gut, pineal gland, spleen, and thymus.[258]

Tissue sources of catecholamines are principally dependent on the presence of tyrosine hydroxylase, which is largely confined to dopaminergic and noradrenergic neurons of the central nervous system, and to sympathetic nerves and chromaffin cells of the adrenal medulla and paraganglia in the periphery. Similarly, sources of serotonin are largely dependent on the presence of tryptophan hydroxylase in central nervous system serotonergic neurons, the pineal gland, and some peripheral endocrine tissues, particularly enterochromaffin cells of the digestive tract. Platelets also contain large amounts of serotonin; however, this is derived from serotonin synthesized in enterochromaffin cells of the gastrointestinal tract.[242]

Both tyrosine and tryptophan hydroxylases belong to a small family of mono-oxygenases that also includes phenylalanine hydroxylase; all three enzymes require tetrahydrobiopterin as a substrate to drive the hydroxylation reaction.[79] Deficiencies in the enzymes responsible for formation and recycling of tetrahydrobiopterin result in variant forms of phenylketonuria and hyperphenylalaninemia characterized by low concentrations of monoamine neurotransmitters and severe neurologic abnormalities.[130]

Conversion of L-dopa to dopamine and of 5-hydroxytryptophan to serotonin is catalyzed by aromatic-L-amino acid decarboxylase (see Figure 30-2), an enzyme with a wide tissue distribution and broad substrate specificity for aromatic amino acids and requiring pyridoxal-5-phosphate as a cofactor. The dopamine and serotonin formed in the cytoplasm are then transported into vesicular storage granules, where the amines are available for exocytotic release as the principal neurotransmitters of central nervous system dopaminergic and serotonergic neurons. The dopamine formed in noradrenergic neurons and chromaffin cells is further converted to norepinephrine by dopamine β-hydroxylase, a copper-containing enzyme requiring molecular oxygen and ascorbic acid for activity. The enzyme has a unique presence in vesicular storage granules, bound to the vesicular membrane or present in the soluble matrix core. The noradrenergic neurochemical phenotype of central noradrenergic neurons and peripheral sympathetic nerves depends on both translocation of dopamine into storage granules and the presence of dopamine β-hydroxylase.

The additional presence of phenylethanolamine *N*-methyltransferase (PNMT) in adrenal medullary chromaffin cells leads to further conversion of norepinephrine to epinephrine (see Figure 30-2). Because PNMT is a cytosolic enzyme, this step depends on leakage of norepinephrine from vesicular storage granules into the cell cytoplasm, where the amine is available for *N*-methylation. Epinephrine is then translocated into chromaffin granules, where it is stored awaiting release.

Melatonin is synthesized from serotonin in the pineal gland by two highly specific enzymes, the first step catalyzed by serotonin-*N*-acetyltransferase and the second by hydroxyindole-*O*-methyltransferase (see Figure 30-2). Synthesis of melatonin in the pineal gland is regulated by the 24-hour light/dark cycle, resulting in pronounced diurnal fluctuations in production, with higher melatonin concentrations at night associated with induction of sleep.

Conversion of tyrosine to L-dopa by tyrosine hydroxylase and conversion of tryptophan to 5-hydroxytrytophan by tryptophan hydroxylase represent pivotal points for regulating synthesis and maintaining stores of catecholamines and serotonin in response to changes in monoamine turnover associated with variations in exocytotic release. Rapid activation of tyrosine hydroxylase is achieved by phosphorylation of serine residues at the regulatory domain, under the control of multiple Ca^{2+} and cyclic adenosine monophosphate (cAMP)-dependent pathways influenced by changes in nerve activity and actions of peptides and other coactivators.[192,275] Feedback inhibition by catecholamines provides a further mechanism for short-term regulation of enzyme activity. Long-term regulation involves induction of synthesis of the enzyme at the transcriptional level. Similar mechanisms are involved in the regulation of tryptophan hydroxylase, although these differ for the two isoforms expressed at central nervous system and peripheral sites of serotonin synthesis.[190] Synthesis of serotonin is also controlled by the availability of tryptophan precursor derived exclusively from the diet.[271] Tyrosine, in contrast, is additionally derived by hydroxylation of phenylalanine.

Administration of catecholamine metabolic precursors and drugs that block catecholamine biosynthetic pathways has several therapeutic uses. Alpha-methyl-L-tyrosine or metyrosine (Demser®) is an analog of tyrosine that inhibits tyrosine hydroxylase, thereby decreasing catecholamine stores. The drug is occasionally used to control high blood pressure in patients with pheochromocytoma. Alpha-methyl-L-dopa (Aldomet®) is an analog of L-dopa and a prodrug that is converted to alpha-methyl-dopamine and alpha-methyl-norepinephrine. The antihypertensive actions of the agent

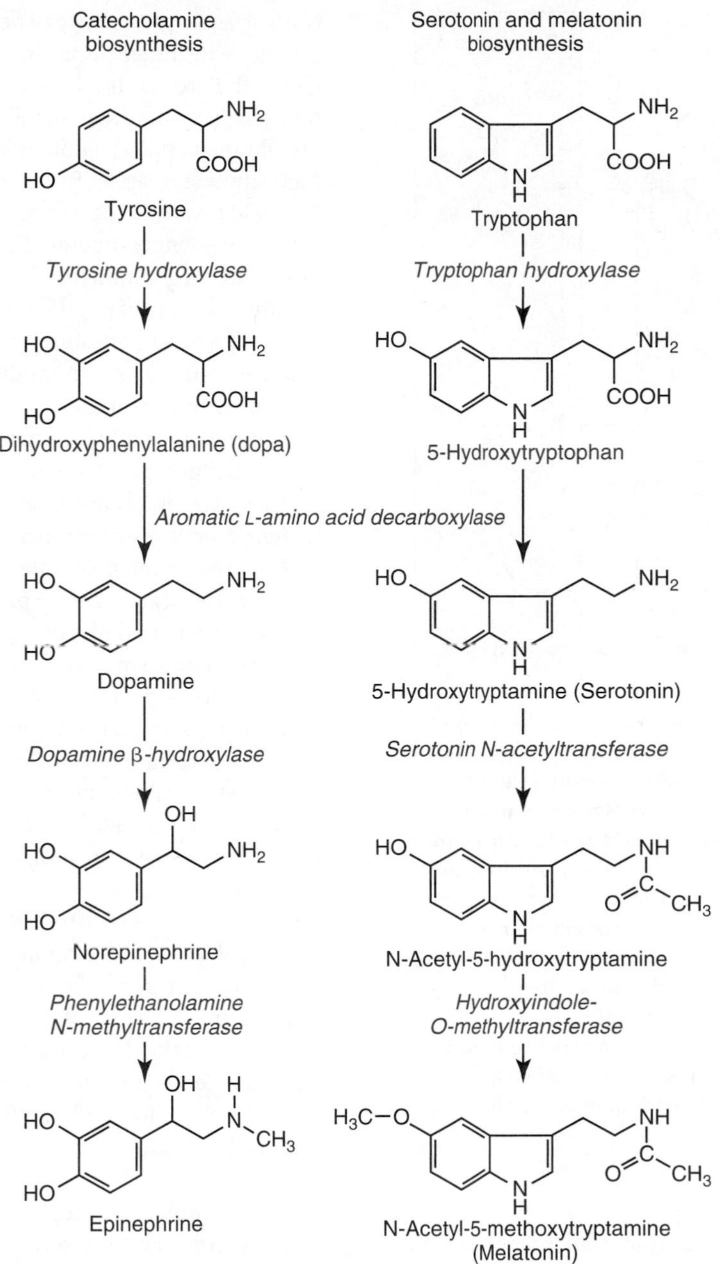

Figure 30-2 Biosynthesis of catecholamines and serotonin, and metabolism of serotonin to melatonin.

appear to result from central nervous system–mediated inhibition of sympathetic outflow. L-Dopa is used to treat Parkinson's disease and usually is coadministered with an inhibitor of peripheral L-aromatic amino acid decarboxylase, such as carbidopa or beserazide.

Storage and Release

Storage of catecholamines and serotonin in vesicular granules is facilitated by two vesicular monoamine transporters.[108] Both transporters have a wide specificity for different monoamine substrates.

The driving force for vesicular monoamine transport is provided by an adenosine triphosphate–dependent vesicular membrane proton pump, which maintains an H^+ electrochemical gradient between the cytoplasm and granule matrix.[230] Disruption of this gradient in situations of energy depletion and lowered intracellular pH—such as occur with ischemia, anoxia, or cyanide poisoning—results in a rapid and massive loss of monoamines from storage vesicles into the neuronal cytoplasm.

Contrary to usual depictions, vesicular stores of catecholamines and serotonin do not exist in a static state until exocytotic release. Rather, vesicular stores of monoamines exist in a highly dynamic equilibrium with the surrounding cytoplasm, with passive outward leakage of monoamines into the cytoplasm counterbalanced by inward active transport under

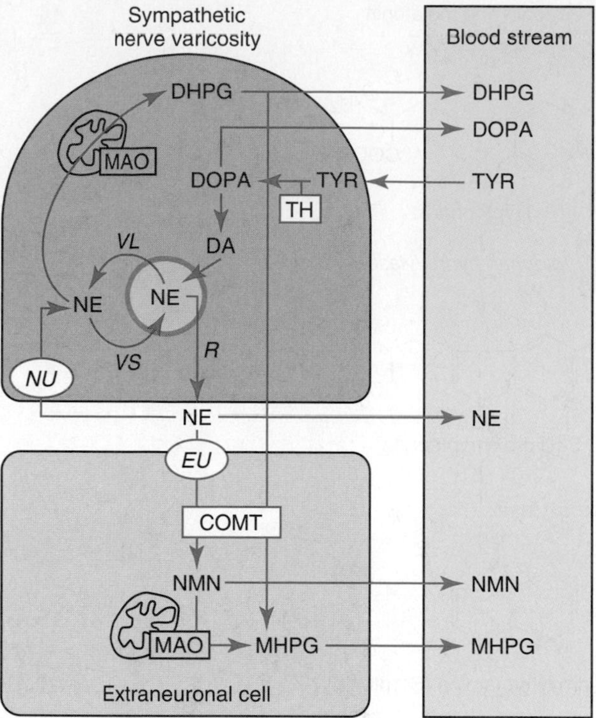

Figure 30-3 Schematic diagram illustrating the dynamics of synthesis, exocytotic release (R), neuronal reuptake (NU), extraneuronal uptake (EU), vesicular leakage (VL), vesicular sequestration (VS), and metabolism of norepinephrine (NE) in sympathetic nerve endings in relation to extraneuronal tissue and the bloodstream. Relative magnitudes of the various processes are reflected by the relative sizes of arrows. *COMT,* Catechol-*O*-methyltransferase; *DA,* dopamine; *DHPG,* 3,4-dihydroxyphenylglycol; L-*dopa,* 3,4-dihydroxyphenylalanine; *MAO,* monoamine oxidase; *MHPG,* 3-methoxy-4-hydroxyphenylglycol; *NMN,* normetanephrine; *TH,* Tyrosine hydroxylase; *TYR,* tyrosine.

the control of vesicular monoamine transporters (Figure 30-3). The magnitude and highly dynamic nature of this process can be appreciated by consideration of the effects of reserpine, a drug that blocks the ability of vesicular monoamine transporters to move monoamines from the cytoplasm into vesicles. Leakage of monoamines from vesicles is then no longer counterbalanced by vesicular translocation, and stores of monoamines are rapidly depleted.

Monoamines share the acid environment of the storage granule matrix with adenosine triphosphate (ATP), peptides, and proteins, the best known of which are the chromogranins.[247] The chromogranins are ubiquitous components of secretory vesicles; their widespread presence among endocrine tissues has led to their measurement in plasma as useful, albeit relatively nonspecific, markers of neuroendocrine tumors, including pheochromocytomas and carcinoid tumors.[199]

The process of exocytosis occurs at specialized locations on nerve endings or sympathetic varicosities dictated by the cell surface expression of specialized docking proteins that interact with other proteins on the surface of secretory vesicles.[20] The process is stimulated by an influx of Ca^{2+}, which in neurons is primarily controlled by nerve impulse–mediated membrane depolarization, and in adrenal medullary cells by acetylcholine release from innervating splanchnic nerves. The wide variety of voltage-, receptor-, G-protein–, and second messenger–operated Ca^{2+} channels provide numerous points for regulation of Ca^{2+}-triggered exocytosis. Consequently, a variety of peptides, neurotransmitters, and humoral factors provide additional mechanisms for stimulation of exocytosis or may act to modulate nerve impulse–stimulated release of monoamines. Dopamine, norepinephrine, and serotonin also modulate their own release through occupation of autoreceptors. Regulation of monoamine release and synthesis is closely coordinated, thereby ensuring appropriate replenishment of the amines lost through exocytosis.[193]

Neuronal release of catecholamines and serotonin may also occur by calcium-independent nonexocytotic processes involving increased loss of monoamines from storage vesicles into the cytoplasm and reversal of normal inward carrier-mediated transport to outward transport of monoamines into the extracellular environment. Examples of this process include the release of catecholamines induced by the sympathomimetic amines, tyramine and amphetamine. Excessive release of catecholamines, which accompanies hypoxic ischemia, occurs in part through a similar mechanism.

Uptake and Metabolism

Because the enzymes responsible for metabolism of catecholamines have intracellular locations, the primary mechanism limiting the life span of catecholamines in the extracellular space is uptake by active transport, not metabolism by enzymes (see Figure 30-3). Uptake is facilitated by transporters that belong to two large families of proteins with mainly neuronal or extraneuronal locations.[62] Neuronal uptake of monoamines involves the dopamine transporter at dopaminergic neurons, the norepinephrine transporter at noradrenergic neurons, and the serotonin transporter at serotonergic neurons. These same transporters are also present at some non-neuronal locations, including adrenal chromaffin cells, endothelial cells of the lungs, specialized cells of the gastrointestinal tract, and some blood cells such as platelets. However, most extraneuronal uptake of monoamines is facilitated by a second set of proteins belonging to the organic cation transporter family. These latter transporters are expressed exclusively at extraneuronal locations and act on a broader range of substrates than the plasma membrane monoamine transporters expressed at neuronal locations.

The neuronal monoamine transporters provide the principal mechanism for rapid termination of the signal in neuronal transmission, whereas transporters at extraneuronal locations are more important for limiting the spread of the signal and for clearance of catecholamines from the bloodstream. For norepinephrine released by sympathetic nerves, about 90% is removed back into nerves by neuronal uptake, 5% is removed by extraneuronal uptake, and 5% escapes these

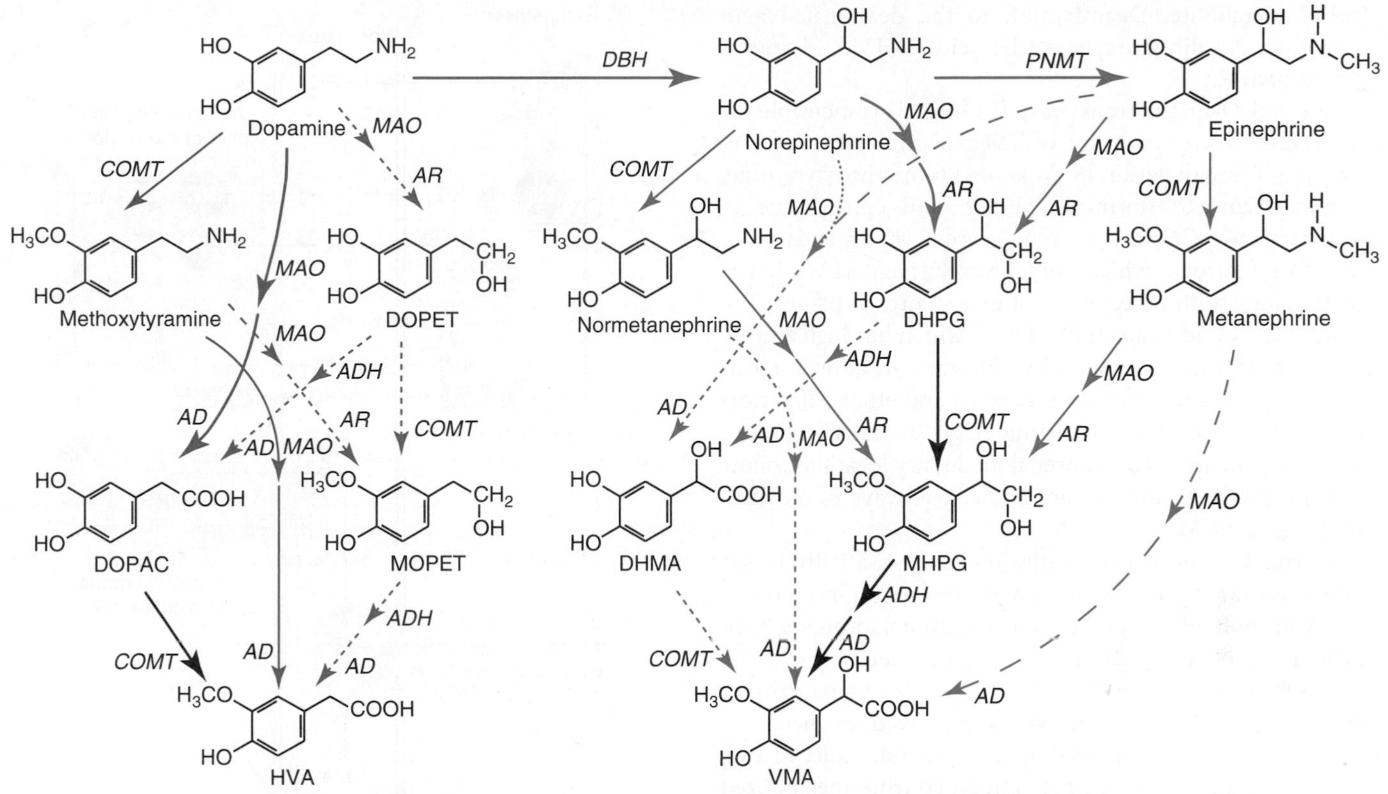

Figure 30-4 Pathways of metabolism of catecholamines. Enzymes responsible for each pathway are shown at the heads of arrows. *Solid arrows* indicate the major pathways, whereas *dotted arrows* indicate pathways of negligible importance. Pathways of sulfate conjugation—which are particularly important for metabolism of dopamine, normetanephrine, metanephrine, 3-methoxytyramine, and 3-methoxy-4-hydroxyphenylglycol—are not shown. *AR*, Aldose or aldehyde reductase; *AD*, aldehyde dehydrogenase; *ADH*, alcohol dehydrogenase; *COMT*, catechol-O-methyltransferase; *DBH*, dopamine β-hydroxylase; *DHMA*, 3,4-dihydroxymandelic acid; *DHPG*, 3,4-dihydroxyphenylglycol; *DOPAC*, 3,4-dihydroxyphenylacetic acid; *DOPET*, 3,4-dihydroxyphenylethanol; *HVA*, homovanillic acid; *MAO*, monoamine oxidase; *MHPG*, 3-methoxy-4-hydroxyphenylglycol; *MOPET*, 3-methoxy-4-hydroxyphenylethanol; *PNMT*, phenylethanolamine-N-methyltransferase; *VMA*, vanillylmandelic acid.

processes to enter the bloodstream. In contrast, for epinephrine released by adrenal chromaffin cells directly into the bloodstream, about 90% is removed by extraneuronal monoamine transport processes. The presence of these highly active transport processes means that monoamines are rapidly cleared from the bloodstream with a circulatory half-life of less than 2 minutes.

In addition to terminating the actions of released monoamines, the plasma membrane monoamine transporters at neuronal locations function in sequence with vesicular monoamine transporters to recycle catecholamines for re-release (see Figure 30-3). Thus most of the norepinephrine released and recaptured by sympathetic nerves is sequestered back into storage vesicles, thereby substantially reducing the requirements for synthesis of new transmitter.

Plasma membrane monoamine transporters also function as part of metabolizing systems, requiring the additional actions of enzymes for irreversible inactivation of the released amines. For both neuronal and extraneuronal metabolizing systems, inactivation of catecholamines and serotonin occurs in a series arrangement with uptake followed by metabolism.

Metabolism of catecholamines occurs by a multiplicity of pathways catalyzed by an array of enzymes, resulting in a wide variety of metabolites (Figure 30-4).[67] Deamination of catecholamines by monoamine oxidase (MAO) yields reactive aldehyde intermediates that are further metabolized to deaminated acids by aldehyde dehydrogenase, or to deaminated glycols by aldehyde or aldose reductase. The aldehyde intermediate formed from dopamine is a good substrate for aldehyde dehydrogenase, but not aldehyde or aldose reductase. In contrast, the aldehyde intermediate formed from the β-hydroxylated catecholamines—norepinephrine and epinephrine—is a good substrate for aldehyde or aldose reductase, but is a poor substrate for aldehyde dehydrogenase. Therefore, norepinephrine and epinephrine are preferentially deaminated to 3,4-dihydroxyphenylglycol (DHPG), the alcohol metabolite. Deamination to the deaminated acid metabolite, 3,4-dihydroxymandelic acid (DHMA), is not a favored pathway.

Catechol-*O*-methyltransferase (COMT) is responsible for the second major pathway of catecholamine metabolism, catalyzing *O*-methylation of dopamine to methoxytyramine, norepinephrine to normetanephrine, and epinephrine to metanephrine. COMT is not present in monoamine-producing neurons, which contain exclusively MAO, but is present along with MAO in most extraneuronal tissues. The membrane-bound isoform of COMT, which has high affinity for catecholamines, is especially abundant in adrenal chromaffin cells. As a result of the preceding and other differences in the expression of metabolizing enzymes, catecholamines produced at neuronal and adrenal medullary locations follow different neuronal and extraneuronal pathways of metabolism (Figure 30-5).

Neuronal deamination pathways are quantitatively far more important than extraneuronal pathways for metabolism of the catecholamines synthesized at neuronal locations, such as the norepinephrine produced in sympathetic nerves. The reasons for this are twofold: first, much more norepinephrine released by sympathetic nerves is removed by neuronal uptake than by extraneuronal uptake; second, under resting conditions, much more of the norepinephrine metabolized intraneuronally is derived from transmitter leaking from storage vesicles than from transmitter recaptured after exocytotic release. Thus, most of the norepinephrine produced in the body is metabolized initially to DHPG, mainly from transmitter deaminated intraneuronally after leakage from storage vesicles or after release and reuptake. Most circulating DHPG is derived from sympathetic nerves, with relatively small contributions from the brain (<5%) and the adrenals (<7%).

DHPG is further *O*-methylated by COMT in non-neuronal tissues to 3-methoxy-4-hydroxyphenylglycol (MHPG), a metabolite also produced to a limited extent by deamination of normetanephrine and metanephrine (see Figure 30-5). The latter *O*-methylated metabolites are produced in much smaller amounts compared with DHPG, and only at extraneuronal locations; their single largest source is adrenal chromaffin cells, which account for more than 90% of circulating metanephrine and 24 to 40% of circulating normetanephrine.[56] Within the adrenals, normetanephrine and metanephrine are produced in a similar manner to the production of DHPG within sympathetic nerves, from norepinephrine and epinephrine leaking from storage granules into the chromaffin cell cytoplasm.

The MHPG produced from DHPG and metanephrines may be sulfate-conjugated or metabolized to vanillylmandelic acid (VMA), the latter pathway catalyzed by the sequential actions of hepatic alcohol dehydrogenase and aldehyde dehydrogenase. At least 90% of the VMA formed in the body is produced in the liver, mainly from hepatic uptake and metabolism of circulating DHPG and MHPG.[57]

In contrast to production of VMA, production of homovanillic acid (HVA) from dopamine depends mainly on

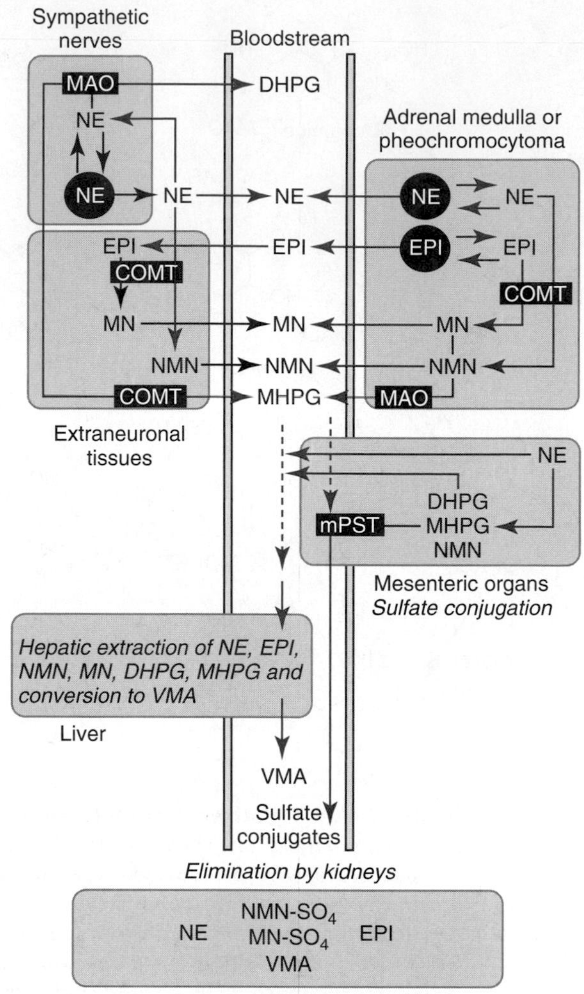

Figure 30-5 Schematic diagram illustrating regional pathways of norepinephrine and epinephrine metabolism. Most norepinephrine is released and metabolized within sympathetic nerves, including up to one half produced in sympathetic nerves of mesenteric organs. Sulfate conjugation of catecholamines and catecholamine metabolites, particularly 3-methoxy-4-hydroxyphenylglycol (MHPG), occurs mainly in mesenteric organs, whereas production of vanillylmandelic acid (VMA) occurs mainly in the liver. COMT, Catechol-O-methyltransferase; *DHPG*, 3,4-dihydroxyphenylglycol; *EPI*, epinephrine; *MAO*, monoamine oxidase; *MHPG*, 3-methoxy-4-hydroxyphenylglycol; *MHPG-SO₄*, 3-methoxy-4-hydroxyphenylglycol sulfate; *MN*, metanephrine; *MN-SO₄*, metanephrine sulfate; *NE*, norepinephrine; *NMN*, normetanephrine; *NMN-SO₄*, normetanephrine sulfate; *SULT1A3*, sulfotransferase type 1A3; *VMA*, vanillylmandelic acid.

O-methylation of the deaminated metabolite of dopamine, 3,4-dihydroxyphenylacetic acid (DOPAC), and to a lesser extent on deamination of methoxytyramine, the *O*-methylated metabolite of dopamine (see Figure 30-4). As a result, HVA is formed in multiple tissues, with about 30% of circulating

TABLE 30-1 Average Urinary Excretion of Catecholamines and Metabolites*

	Amount Excreted, mmol/d (mg/d)	Percent of Total from Parent Catecholamines
Epinephrine (free)	0.03 (5)	0.1†
Norepinephrine (free)	0.18 (30)	0.5†
Epinephrine and norepinephrine (conjugated)	0.59 (100)	1.7†
Metanephrine (free and conjugated)	0.33 (65)	1.0†
Normetanephrine (free and conjugated)	0.55 (100)	1.6†
Dihydroxyphenylglycol (free and conjugated)	1.26 (215)	3.7†
3-Methoxy-4-hydroxyphenylglycol (free and conjugated)	10.9 (2000)	32.0†
Vanillylmandelic acid (free)	20.2 (4000)	59.3†
Dopamine (free)	1.50 (225)	From DOPA‡
Dopamine (conjugated)	2.80 (700)	5.7§
Methoxytyramine (free and conjugated)	0.80 (130)	1.6§
Dihydroxyphenylacetic acid (free and conjugated)	7.5 (1300)	15.3§
Homovanillic acid	37.9 (6900)	77.3§

*Average values in human subjects derived from published data.[138]
†Percent derived from norepinephrine and epinephrine.
‡Urinary free dopamine is derived mainly from renal decarboxylation of circulating L-dopa.
§Percent derived from dopamine.

and urinary HVA arising from mesenteric organs and up to 20% from the brain.

With the exception of VMA, all catecholamines and their metabolites are metabolized to sulfate conjugates by a specific sulfotransferase isoenzyme (SULT1A3). In humans, a single amino acid substitution confers the enzyme with particularly high affinity for dopamine and the *O*-methylated metabolites of catecholamines, including normetanephrine, metanephrine, and methoxytyramine.[39] The SULT1A3 isoenzyme is found in high concentrations in gastrointestinal tissues, which therefore represent a major source of sulfate conjugates.

In humans, VMA and the sulfates and glucuronide conjugates of MHPG represent the main end products of norepinephrine and epinephrine metabolism (Table 30-1). HVA and conjugates of HVA are the main metabolic end products of dopamine metabolism. These end products and the other conjugates are eliminated mainly by urinary excretion. As a result, their circulatory clearance is slow and plasma concentrations are high relative to those of the precursor amines.

Serotonin is not a substrate for COMT and follows simpler pathways of metabolism than those for catecholamines (Figure 30-6). Deamination of serotonin to the aldehyde intermediate is preferentially followed by oxidation to 5-hydroxyindoleacetic acid (5-HIAA) catalyzed by aldehyde dehydrogenase. Reduction to 5-hydroxytryptophol (5-HTOL) normally represents a relatively minor pathway, so that the major urinary excretion product of serotonin metabolism is 5-HIAA. Metabolism through these pathways is altered by consumption of ethyl alcohol, which through changes in redox state leads to increased formation of 5-HTOL. Increases in ratios of 5-HTOL to 5-HIAA in urine thereby provide a marker of alcohol abuse.[41]

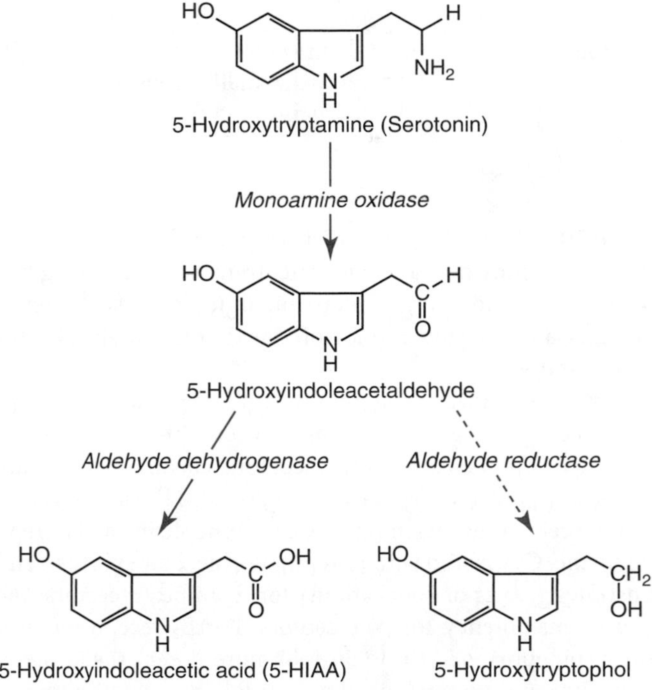

Figure 30-6 Metabolism of serotonin to 5-hydroxyindoleacetic acid (5-HIAA) and 5-hydroxytryptophol.

PHYSIOLOGY OF CATECHOLAMINE AND SEROTONIN SYSTEMS

The physiologic and behavioral actions of catecholamines and serotonin provide a foundation for understanding disorders of monoamine excess or deficiency. Major sites of catecholamine and serotonin synthesis and action are listed in

TABLE 30-2 Locations of Monoamine Production and Action in the Body

Monoamine Type	Site of Monoamine Production	Mode of Transmission	Site of Monoamine Action
Epinephrine	Adrenal medulla (chromaffin cells)	Hormonal	Cardiac muscle, smooth muscle, and widespread effects on cellular metabolism
Norepinephrine	Sympathetic ganglia and varicosities of autonomic nervous system	Neuroeffector cell junction	Effector tissue including cardiac muscle, smooth muscle, vascular endothelium, and exocrine glands
	Adrenal medulla (chromaffin cells)	Hormonal	Primarily cardiac and smooth muscle
	Brain stem (locus coeruleus and reticular formation)	Neuronal synapse	Widespread CNS neuronal connections
Dopamine	Midbrain (substantia nigra)	Neuronal synapse	Neuronal connections in cerebral striatum
	Midbrain (ventral tegmentum)	Neuronal synapse	Cerebral mesolimbic and mesocortical neuronal connections
	Diencephalon (hypothalamus)	Neuronal synapse	Pituitary gland
	Retina	Neuronal synapse	Neuronal connections within the retina
	Olfactory bulb	Neuronal synapse	Neuronal connections within the olfactory bulb
	Gastrointestinal tract	Autocrine/paracrine	Regulation of bicarbonate secretion, gut motility, sodium in exocrine secretions
	Kidney (derived from circulating L-dopa)	Autocrine/paracrine	Regulation of natriuresis
Serotonin	Brain stem (raphe nucleus)	Neuronal synapse	Widespread CNS neuronal connections
	GI (enterochromaffin cells)	Hormonal (paracrine)	Gastrointestinal smooth muscle
	GI (enterochromaffin cells)	Platelet uptake/release	Platelets, vascular smooth muscle

Table 30-2 for both central and peripheral nervous systems. The table provides an anatomic framework showing the locations of adrenergic, dopaminergic, and serotonergic systems and varying modes of signal transmission by the monoamines.

Catecholamines and serotonin regulate physiologic events at the cellular level through interaction with families of cell surface receptors. Adrenergic receptors, classified as α_1 (subtypes $\alpha_{1a,b,d}$), α_2 (subtypes $\alpha_{2a,b,c}$), β_1, β_2, and β_3 subcategories, initiate cellular events in response to epinephrine and norepinephrine. Compared with norepinephrine, epinephrine demonstrates greater or equal affinity for α_1 and α_2 receptors, and equivalent potency for β_1 receptors. For β_2 receptor activation, epinephrine is 10- to 50-fold more potent than norepinephrine, and norepinephrine is 10-fold more active toward β_3 receptors.[113]

Dopamine has known pharmacologic reactivity with α_1- and α_2-adrenergic receptors but transmits central and peripheral nerve signals primarily by selective interaction with a family of dopaminergic receptors designated as D_1, D_2, D_3, D_4, and D_5 subtypes.[178] An even larger family of serotonergic receptor subtypes (5-$HT_{1A,B,D,E,F}$, 5-$HT_{2A\text{-}C}$, 5-HT_3, 5-HT_4, 5-$HT_{5A\text{-}B}$, 5-HT_6, 5-HT_7) have been identified by histologic and molecular techniques.[118] Receptors, including α_2-adrenergic 5-HT_{1A}, 5-HT_{1B}, and 5-HT_{1D}, may serve as autoreceptors by turning off the release of their respective neurotransmitters via a negative feedback mechanism. The major physiologic effects of catecholamines and serotonin are explained in part by these diverse receptor interactions, which occur in function-specific locations throughout the vasculature and organ systems of the body.

Central Nervous System

Norepinephrine, dopamine, and serotonin represent only about 1 to 2% of all neurotransmitters in the brain but have important functions in autonomic (involuntary), somatic (voluntary), and information processing systems. As neurotransmitters, they are produced primarily in regions of the brain stem (medulla oblongata, pons, midbrain) by neurons with axons that project to defined, sometimes widespread, areas of the brain or spinal cord. Although our understanding of central adrenergic, dopaminergic, and serotonergic systems is incomplete, their role in central nervous system function and dysfunction is increasingly evident and has important diagnostic and therapeutic implications.

Most norepinephrine synthesis in the brain takes place in the locus coeruleus of the pons and in the reticular formation of the medulla oblongata. About half of the norepinephrine is produced in the locus coeruleus by only a small nucleus of neurons capable of responding in unison to sensory input signals.[194] Norepinephrine-producing neurons in the lower brain stem send highly diffuse axonal projections throughout the brain as high as the cerebral cortex. They also send descending fibers to the spinal cord, where they synapse with preganglionic sympathetic neurons that communicate with the peripheral sympathetic nervous system. The norepinephrine-producing neurons of the brain stem process incoming sensory signals. They also participate in regulating the activity of the sympathetic nervous system.[208]

The locus coeruleus serves as part of the brain's redundant arousal system. Neuronal discharge of norepinephrine from this brain stem region stimulates cortical activation, in addition to behavioral arousal, that occurs via increased muscle tone.[124,125] The stimulant effect of amphetamine can be explained by the pharmacologic enhancement of norepinephrine release with associated cortical and muscle stimulation. A predominant physiologic function of norepinephrine systems in the brain is response to stress. Stress-induced stimuli activate brain stem production of norepinephrine with synaptic release and neuroactivation throughout many areas of the brain and spinal cord.

Dopamine accounts for more than half the catecholamine production of the brain, but its distribution and functions are markedly different from those of norepinephrine. Dopaminergic neurotransmission is involved in processing sensory signals and in regulating hormonal release. Dopaminergic neurons in the retina and olfactory bulb have ultrashort projections that transmit signals within these neuronal centers for vision and smell. Neurons in the arcuate nucleus of the hypothalamus have projecting fibers that release dopamine in the portal vessels, exerting key neuroendocrine inhibition on prolactin and thyroid stimulating hormone release, as well as effects on other hormones of the pituitary gland.[251]

Dopamine is also produced by neurons in the substantia nigra and the ventral tegmentum. The ventral tegmental area modulates diverse forebrain functions such as cognitive activity through axonal projections to the prefrontal cortex and reward seeking behavior via axonal fibers sent to limbic structures of the brain.[231] Consequently, disturbances in dopamine production and release from these areas of the brain are involved in several important neurologic and psychiatric disorders, with dopamine receptors serving as key pharmacologic targets for antipsychotic drugs.[201] In addition, dopaminergic neurons in the substantia nigra project into the striatum to form the nigrostriatal system, which regulates the initiation and maintenance of motor function. Control by this system over extrapyrimidal (involuntary) movement is evidenced by loss of motor control when nigrostriatal neurons degenerate in Parkinson's disease.[200]

Serotonin, similar to norepinephrine, is produced by small clusters of neurons in the brain stem regions, but serves a diverse range of behavioral and physiologic functions.[245] Neurons in the raphe nuclei of the pons and upper brain stem are a primary source of brain serotonin and project axonal fibers throughout the brain and spinal cord. Physiologic and behavioral processes that may be influenced by this extensive serotoninergic system include memory, learning, feeding behavior, sleep patterns, thermoregulation, pain modulation, cardiovascular function, and hypothalamic regulation of pituitary hormones. Each of the 14 known subtypes of serotonin receptors have distinct patterns of distribution in the brain and account for diverse cognitive, behavioral, and physiologic responses.[4,124] Raphe projections to the subcortical regions of the cerebral hemisphere (amygdala and hippocampus) activate receptors that influence mood and anxiety.

Development of numerous pharmacologic agents for manipulation of serotonin concentrations and selective receptor responses in the brain clearly indicates the importance of the central serotoninergic system as a drug target.[126] Increased synaptic concentrations of serotonin in the brain produce a quiet satiated waking state, providing a therapeutic target for anxiolytic and antidepressant drugs. Buspirone, for example, reduces anxiety through activation of serotonin autoreceptors in the subcortical areas of the brain, thus reducing serotonin release. Hypoactivity of the serotoninergic system, on the other hand, plays an important role in depression. Selective serotonin reuptake inhibitors such as fluoxetine, paroxetine, and sertraline are effective agents in the treatment of this form of central serotoninergic deficiency.

Serotonin is also involved in hormonal regulation. Serotonin-releasing nerve fibers that originate in the raphe nuclei and terminate in the hypothalamus exert a circadian influence on pituitary-adrenal function by stimulating hypothalamic corticotropin-releasing hormone, as well as by signaling other hormonal events mediated by enhanced prolactin and growth hormone release.[251] Serotonin also influences overall blood flow to the brain as evidenced by the vasoconstrictor effects of the amine on carotid vasculature and the beneficial pharmacologic effects of a serotoninergic agonist, sumatriptan, in the treatment of migraine.

The functions of serotonin and catecholamines in the central nervous system are diverse and complex, with important implications for numerous clinical disorders; however, direct assessment of central neurotransmitters by clinical laboratory methods remains limited. Nevertheless, many clinical laboratory tests of metabolic and hormonal function are directly influenced by functions of central noradrenergic, dopaminergic, and serotoninergic systems. Also, many therapeutic and illicit drugs that modulate central monoamine neurotransmission are monitored by laboratory techniques in a wide range of clinical settings.

Sympathetic Nervous System

Norepinephrine is the principal neurotransmitter of the sympathetic branch of the autonomic nervous system. Sympathetic nerve transmission operates below the level of consciousness in controlling the physiologic functions of many organs and tissues of the body (Figure 30-7). The sympathetic nervous system plays a particularly important role in regulating cardiovascular function in response to postural, exertional, thermal, and mental stress. With sympathetic activation, heart rate is increased, peripheral arterioles are constricted, skeletal arterioles are dilated, and blood pressure is elevated. In addition, sympathetic nerve stimulation dilates pupils, inhibits smooth muscles of the intestines, bronchi, and

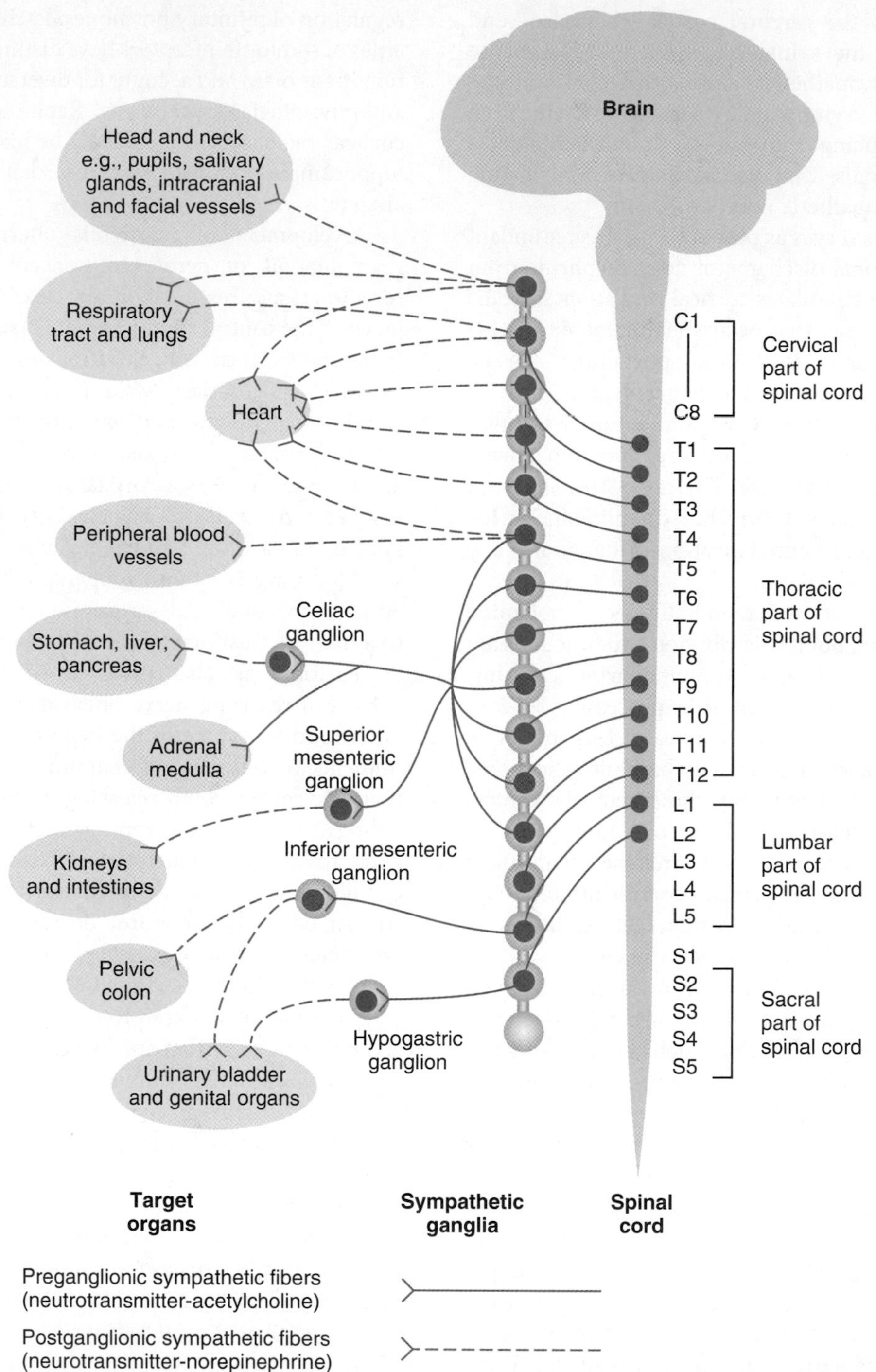

Figure 30-7 Schematic diagram of sympathetic division of the autonomic nervous system. Preganglionic cholinergic fibers *(solid lines)* from the spinal cord project to the paravertebral sympathetic chain, the visceral peripheral ganglia, and the adrenal medulla, whereas postganglionic noradrenergic fibers *(dashed lines)* project from sympathetic ganglia to sympathetically-innervated target organs.

bladder, and closes the sphincters. Sympathetic signals work in balance with the parasympathetic branch of the autonomic nervous system to maintain a stable internal environment.

The hypothalamus, which integrates the autonomic and neuroendocrine systems, has a controlling influence over sympathetic outflow from brain stem centers and the spinal cord. Afferent or incoming sensory signals originate from pressure, stretch, chemical, pain, and temperature receptors located in visceral organs and vessels. Afferent nerve impulses enter the central nervous system to form the efferent component of local reflex arcs within the spinal cord or to ascend to higher centers such as the hypothalamus, where afferent signals are integrated with other neural pathways. Efferent or outgoing responses are transmitted by preganglionic sympathetic neurons that exit the spinal cord and converge on sympathetic ganglia chains along the spinal column or in visceral ganglia (see Figure 30-7). These preganglionic neurons release the neurotransmitter acetylcholine to regulate multiple postganglionic projections. Terminal branches of postganglionic fibers that project from these ganglia into target organs have varicosities that form a rich ground plexus for synaptic contact with a large number of effector cells in glands and muscle fibers.

Most sympathetic postganglionic nerves liberate norepinephrine as their neurotransmitter. In limited locations, sympathetic nerve endings release acetylcholine, such as sweat glands that undergo a noradrenergic-to-cholinergic switch during development.[229] Preganglionic sympathetic fibers also innervate the adrenal medulla, stimulating release of epinephrine from chromaffin cells.

The relative contributions of individual organs to overall sympathetic activity have been inferred from data on the release of norepinephrine into plasma.[3,56,73] Plasma norepinephrine is derived primarily from postganglionic sympathetic neurons with little contribution from the central nervous system. In the resting state, the overall rate of norepinephrine spillover into the systemic circulation is on the order of 200 to 600 ng/min. Because of intervening neuronal and extraneuronal removal processes, this spillover represents less than 10% of the total norepinephrine released by sympathetic nerves. Turnover of norepinephrine, representing loss due mainly to metabolism, is driven primarily in the resting state by leakage of norepinephrine from vesicles into the neuronal axoplasm.[68]

Major contributors to basal sympathetic outflow, based on spillover measurements, include the GI tract (≈37%), kidneys (≈25%), and skeletal muscle (≈11%). The adrenals, heart, liver, lungs, and skin each contribute less than 10%. Alterations in norepinephrine spillover occur in response to physiologic and pathologic states. Exercise, overeating, low salt intake, upright position, mental stress, and aging increase sympathetic outflow. Increased spillover is also found in disorders such as cardiac failure, hypertension, and depression. Reduction in baseline norepinephrine overflow from the heart has also been shown in autonomic insufficiency and syncope, consistent with sympathetic denervation or depressed sympathetic activity in these disorders.

The physiologic response to sympathetic activity in individual organs is dependent not only on the rate of neurotransmitter release from postganglionic nerve varicosities but also on the types of adrenergic receptors and their locations in tissues. Vascular and organ-specific responses are classified in Table 30-3 according to interactions with adrenergic receptors. In peripheral target organs, α_1- and β_1-adrenergic receptors appear strategically located in the immediate vicinity of nerve terminals for rapid postsynaptic smooth muscle contraction, secretion, and endocrine activation via signals from the brain. Postsynaptic β_2-adrenergic receptors in the heart also allow rapid sympathetic neuroactivation.

TABLE 30-3 Direct Effects of Adrenergic Activation on Some Organ Systems Based on Receptor Subtype

Receptor Subtype (Relative Potency)	Tissue Location	Response
α_1 (NE ≤ E)	Heart	Increased force
	Arterioles	Constriction
	Veins	Constriction
	Pupils	Dilation
	Adrenergic sweat glands	Secretion
	GI sphincters	Contraction
	Urinary bladder sphincter	Contraction
	Uterus in pregnancy	Contraction
	Spleen capsule	Contraction
	Penis	Ejaculation
α_2 (NE ≤ E)	Arterioles	Constriction
	Adipocytes	Inhibit lipolysis
	GI motility and tone	Decreased
	Intestinal secretions	Inhibit
	Pancreatic islet cell secretion	Inhibit
	Platelet aggregation	Stimulate
β_1 (NE = E)	Heart	Increased rate and force
	Kidney	Renin release
	Adipocytes	Stimulate lipolysis
β_2 (NE << E)	Heart	Increased rate and force
	Arterioles	Dilation
	Gallbladder and ducts	Relaxation
	GI motility and tone	Decreased
	Adipocytes	Stimulate lipolysis
	Bronchial muscle	Dilation
β_3 (NE > E)	Adipocytes	Stimulate lipolysis

E, Epinephrine; *NE*, norepinephrine.
Modified from published data.[143] The distribution of the six α_1 ($\alpha_{1a,b,d}$) and α_2 ($\alpha_{2a,b,c}$) subtypes is not completely understood and therefore is not included in the table. For receptor locations in the central nervous system, refer to von Bohlen und Halbach O, Dermietzel R. Neurotransmitters and neuromodulators: handbook of receptors and biological effects. Darmstadt: Wiley-VCH Verlag GmbH, 2002.[256]

Extrajunctional α_2 and β_2 receptors that are remote from sympathetic nerve terminals in vascular smooth muscle or platelets may be preferentially influenced by circulating catecholamines such as epinephrine produced by the adrenal gland.[113]

An earlier concept of the sympathetic nervous system functioning primarily as an all-or-none responder to fight or flight has been challenged by studies indicating organ-specific responses to sympathetic activation.[146,186] Thermal and pain sensors, for example, result in a sympathetic response that differs markedly from the physiologic response to baroreceptor signals produced by changes in blood pressure. An increase in environmental temperature reduces sympathetic tone in peripheral vascular beds, thereby resulting in vasodilatation and increased heat loses by radiation from the surface of the body. Pain receptor stimulation from surgical incision in anesthetized humans causes a proportionate increase in cutaneous vasoconstriction.[234] During changes from supine to upright posture, however, baroreceptors signal both cardiac and vascular responses via the sympathetic nerves. In the heart, sympathetic release of norepinephrine increases the rate and force of cardiac muscle contractions, ultimately increasing cardiac output. In skin and mucosa, sympathetic activation causes vasoconstriction with a resultant increase in blood pressure and redistribution of blood to visceral organs. Therefore, although global sympathetic activation clearly operates in extreme conditions of stress, the differential control of sympathetic output enables an appropriate patterning of physiologic responses according to different behavioral and environmental stressors.

Adrenal Medullary System

Although often considered a part of the sympathetic nervous system, the adrenal medulla produces and secretes a different catecholamine, epinephrine, with different functions from the norepinephrine secreted by sympathetic nerves.[64] The adrenal medulla and sympathetic nerves are also regulated separately, often in divergent directions in response to different forms of stress. This makes it appropriate to consider the two systems separately.

The human adrenals overlie the superior poles of the kidneys. Each gland consists of an outer part, the lipid-rich cortex, and a thin inner central medulla containing chromaffin cells. The adrenal medulla is up to 2 mm thick and accounts for about one tenth of the entire weight of the gland. Blood is supplied to the adrenal medulla by direct arterial supply and through vessels draining from the cortex to the medulla. The latter supply provides an important source of adrenocortical steroids for regulation of adrenal medullary function. Neural input to the adrenal medulla includes direct innervation by cholinergic fibers that pass through the sympathetic paravertebral chain from preganglionic sympathetic cell bodies of the spinal cord.

A characteristic feature of adrenal medullary chromaffin cells is the presence of numerous catecholamine storage granules ranging in size from 100 to 300 nm in diameter. These granules turn brown when exposed to potassium bichromate solutions, ammoniacal silver nitrate, or osmium tetroxide as a result of the oxidation and polymerization of epinephrine and norepinephrine. This process is known as the *chromaffin reaction,* hence the terms *chromaffin cells* and *chromaffin granules.* At least two types of adrenal medullary chromaffin cells have been identified in most animal species: (1) norepinephrine-producing chromaffin cells possess dense-core granules eccentrically located in the vesicle, while (2) cells storing epinephrine have less electron-dense homogenous granules.

The human adrenal medulla produces mainly epinephrine, which, as a hormone, is secreted directly into the bloodstream to act on cells distant from sites of release. Both the proximity of sites of norepinephrine and epinephrine release to adrenoceptors and differences in potencies of action on α- and β-adrenergic receptors contribute to differences in adrenoceptor-mediated responses to the two catecholamines. Consequently, epinephrine exerts its effects on different populations of adrenoceptors than norepinephrine. As a circulating hormone, epinephrine acts potently on β_2-adrenergic receptors of the skeletal muscle vasculature, causing vasodilatation. In contrast, norepinephrine released locally within the vasculature causes α_1-adrenoceptor–mediated vasoconstriction. Increases in circulating epinephrine during stress may contribute to skeletal muscle vasodilatory responses, but do not significantly contribute to other cardiovascular changes, including increases in heart rate. Thus, despite the potent hemodynamic actions of epinephrine, the adrenal medulla appears to play a minimal role in cardiovascular regulation compared with sympathetic nerves.

Epinephrine released from the adrenals is more important as a metabolic than as a hemodynamic regulatory hormone.[38] In particular, epinephrine stimulates lipolysis, ketogenesis, thermogenesis, and glycolysis and raises plasma glucose concentrations by stimulating glycogenolysis and gluconeogenesis. Epinephrine also has potent effects on pulmonary function, causing β_2-adrenoceptor–mediated dilatation of airways. Circulating norepinephrine, in minor part derived from the adrenal medulla and functioning as a hormone, may have additional metabolic actions, but appears to have little importance for cardiovascular regulation compared to the higher concentrations of the amine at sympathoneuroeffector sites.

Despite the apparent importance of the adrenal medulla in homeostasis, particularly in the regulation of metabolism, the medulla in contrast to the adrenal cortex is not vital for survival. Studies in adrenalectomized subjects clearly show that both hemodynamic and glucose counter-regulatory responses to insulin hypoglycemia, exercise, and other manipulations remain intact, despite the absence of epinephrine responses.[112] This contrasts with the severe disturbances of blood pressure regulation that accompany loss of sympathetic nerves.

In contrast to the sympathetic nervous system, the adrenal medulla makes a relatively minor contribution to the overall production and turnover of catecholamines (Table 30-4). However, because PNMT is expressed mainly in adrenal chromaffin cells, more than 90% of circulating epinephrine is derived from the adrenal medulla. This contrasts with circulating norepinephrine, more than 90% of which is derived from sympathetic nerves.

Apart from catecholamines, adrenal medullary chromaffin cells produce, store and secrete a wide array of neuropeptides and proteins. Peptides include (1) enkephalins, (2) β-endorphin, (3) neuropeptide Y, (4) substance P, (5) vasoactive intestinal peptide, (6) neurotensin, (7) galanin, (8) atrial natriuretic peptide, (9) pituitary adenylate cyclase–activating

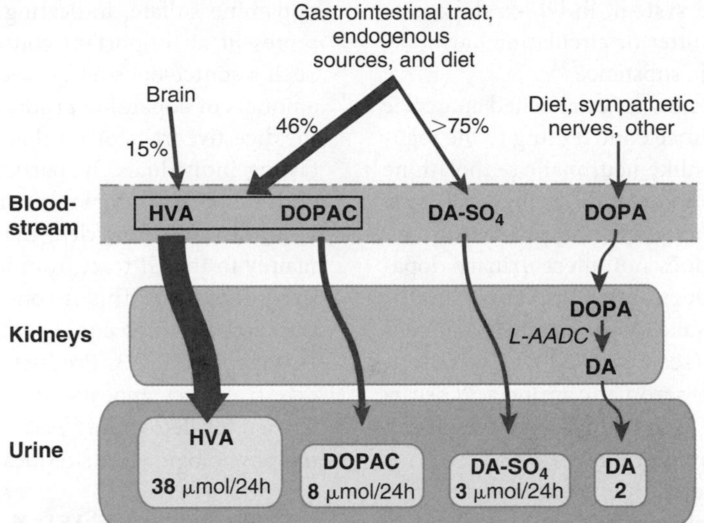

Figure 30-8 Schematic diagram illustrating the main sources of dopamine (DA) and the principal metabolites of dopamine—homovanillic acid (HVA), dihydroxyphenylacetic acid (DOPAC), and dopamine-sulfate (DA-SO4)—in plasma and urine. The brain makes a relatively minor contribution, whereas dopamine synthesized in the gastrointestinal tract or derived from the diet contributes substantially to dopamine metabolites in the bloodstream and urine. This contrasts with the free dopamine excreted in urine, which is derived almost entirely from renal extraction of circulating L-dihydroxyphenylalanine (L-dopa) and local decarboxylation to dopamine by L-aromatic amino acid decarboxylase (L-AADC).

TABLE 30-4 Contribution of the Adrenals to Circulating Catecholamines and Metabolites

	Adrenals (pmol/min)*	Total Body (pmol/min)†	Adrenal Contribution, %
Catecholamines			
Epinephrine	979	1075	91
Norepinephrine	274	3953	7
Dopamine	6	>290	<2
Metabolites			
Metanephrine	449	494	91
Normetanephrine	91	392	23
DHPG	665	13,964	5
DOPAC	300	>4120	<7

*Values represent rates of entry (spillovers) of catecholamines and metabolites into the venous drainage of the adrenal glands derived from clinical studies involving sampling of adrenal venous blood.[56]

†Values represent spillovers of catecholamines and metabolites into the circulation from all organs and tissues of the bodies derived from clinical studies involving regional blood sampling and kinetics analyses.[56,57,96]

peptide, (10) adrenomedullin, and (11) corticotrophin. These peptides are secreted together with the catecholamines and may be involved in local autocrine or paracrine regulation of adrenal medullary and cortical function. The major soluble proteins within chromaffin vesicles belong to the family of granins, which consist of several secretory acidic glycoproteins, the major representative being chromogranin A.

Peripheral Dopaminergic System

Dopamine usually is thought of as a neurotransmitter in the brain or as an intermediate in the production of norepinephrine and epinephrine in the periphery. It has been presumed that these sources account for the large quantities of dopamine and dopamine metabolites excreted in urine. However, the contribution of the brain to circulating concentrations and urinary excretion of dopamine metabolites is now known to be relatively minor.[67] Also, the dopamine formed in sympathetic nerves and in the adrenal medulla is mainly converted to norepinephrine. Most of the dopamine and dopamine metabolites in the circulation and excreted into urine are therefore derived from other sources (Figure 30-8). Accumulating evidence indicates the presence of a third peripheral catecholamine system, in which dopamine functions not as a neurotransmitter or circulating hormone, but as an autocrine or paracrine substance.[92]

In the kidneys, dopamine is now an established autocrine and/or paracrine effector substance contributing to the regulation of sodium excretion.[24] Unlike neuronal catecholamine systems, the production of dopamine in the kidneys is largely independent of local synthesis of L-dopa by tyrosine hydroxylase. Thus, renal denervation does not affect urinary dopamine excretion. Instead, production of dopamine in the kidneys depends mainly on uptake by proximal tubular cells of L-dopa from the circulation (see Figure 30-8). The L-dopa is then converted to dopamine by aromatic amino acid decarboxylase, the activity of which is upregulated by a high-salt diet and downregulated by a low-salt diet.

The presence of a renal dopamine paracrine/autocrine system explains the considerable amount of free dopamine excreted in the urine.[19] Most derives from renal uptake and decarboxylation of circulating L-dopa and reflects the plasma concentrations of this amino acid and the function of the renal dopamine paracrine/autocrine system.

Although the kidneys represent the major source of urinary free dopamine, this source does not account for the larger quantities of excreted dopamine metabolites such as HVA and dopamine sulfate. Findings of large arterial-to-portal venous increases in plasma concentrations of dopamine and its metabolites have indicated that substantial amounts of dopamine are produced and metabolized in the GI tract and other mesenteric organs.[59]

The substantial production and metabolism of dopamine in the human GI tract appear to reflect functions of dopamine as an enteric neuromodulator or paracrine/autocrine substance. Dopamine and dopamine receptor agonists stimulate bicarbonate secretion and protect against ulcer formation, whereas dopamine antagonists augment secretion of gastric acid and promote ulcer development.[81] Dopamine also appears to influence (1) GI motility, (2) sodium transport, and (3) gastric and intestinal submucosal blood flow. In the pancreas, dopamine may modulate the secretion of digestive enzymes and bicarbonate.

Morphologic studies have demonstrated the presence of cells in the GI tract that contain dopamine and express components of dopamine signaling pathways, including catecholamine biosynthetic enzymes and specific dopamine receptors and transporters.[175] In the stomach, tyrosine hydroxylase is expressed in epithelial cells, including acid-secreting parietal cells. In the small intestine, cells of the lamina propria, including immune cells, also express tyrosine hydroxylase. The enzyme is additionally found in pancreatic exocrine cells.

The high rates of dopamine production by mesenteric organs cannot be accounted for by local extraction and decarboxylation of circulating L-dopa. Thus, unlike the kidneys, where dopamine is produced mainly from circulating L-dopa, in the GI tract, production of dopamine requires the presence of tyrosine hydroxylase or other sources of L-dopa.

Consumption of food increases plasma concentrations of L-dopa, dopamine, and dopamine metabolites, particularly dopamine sulfate, indicating that dietary constituents may represent an important source of peripheral dopamine.[50,94] Such a source does not, however, account for the substantial amounts of dopamine produced in peripheral tissues outside the digestive tract, or for that produced in digestive tissues of fasting individuals. In particular, plasma concentrations of both L-dopa and dopamine sulfate remain high, even after a 3-day fast. It is now clear that dopamine sulfate is produced mainly in the GI tract from both dietary and locally synthesized dopamine. This is consistent with findings that the GI tract contains high concentrations of the sulfotransferase isoenzyme, SULT1A3. Production of sulfate conjugates in the digestive tract appears to provide an enzymatic *gut-blood barrier,* for detoxifying dietary biogenic amines and delimiting physiologic effects of locally produced dopamine.

Enteric Nervous System

The enteric nervous system (ENS) is defined as an independent and integrated system of neurons and supporting cells located in the gastrointestinal tract, gallbladder, and pancreas. It is the largest division of the autonomic nervous system and contains about the same number of neurons as the spinal cord. The ENS is composed of two networks or plexuses of intrinsic neurons: the myenteric plexus and the submucous plexus. Both are embedded in the wall of the gut and extend from the esophagus to the anus. These networks contain more than 100 million sensory neurons, interneurons, and motor neurons. The myenteric plexus lies between the longitudinal and circular layers of intestinal smooth muscle and controls propulsive movements (peristalsis). The submucous plexus innervates glandular epithelium, intestinal endocrine cells, and submucosal blood vessels. This network senses the environment within the lumen, regulates local blood flow, and controls epithelial cell secretion.

The ENS is connected to the central nervous system by extrinsic parasympathetic and sympathetic motor neurons, and by extrinsic spinal and vagal sensory neurons. Through these bidirectional connections, the ENS can be monitored and modified.[98,102] Despite the presence of these extrinsic nerve connections, the ENS can function autonomously in some intestinal regions.

Neural transmission within the ENS is controlled by a large variety of neurotransmitters and neuromodulatory peptides, such as (1) serotonin, (2) norepinephrine, (3) acetylcholine, (4) ATP, and (5) nitric oxide. Most of these substances are also found in the brain. In addition to its function as a neurotransmitter within the ENS, serotonin acts as a local paracrine molecule, participating in mucosal sensory transduction.

More than 95% of the body's serotonin is located within the GI tract, and most is synthesized and stored in enterochromaffin cells in the gut mucosa. Serotonin is released from these cells in response to mechanical or chemical stimuli, such as the passage of food; this in turn stimulates both intrinsic (via $5\text{-}HT_{1P}$ and $5\text{-}HT_4$ receptors) and extrinsic (via $5\text{-}HT_3$) vagal sensory nerve fibers.[86] Intrinsic sensory neurons activated by serotonin stimulate the peristaltic reflex and secretion, whereas extrinsic sensory neurons initiate bowel sensations such as nausea, vomiting, abdominal pain, and bloating. The paracrine actions of serotonin are terminated by uptake into epithelial cells by the same serotonin transporter present in serotonergic neurons.

Serotonin modulates numerous physiologic and behavioral systems in the human body and is involved in a wide variety of clinical disorders. In the ENS, for example, serotonin plays pivotal roles in the pathogenesis of the carcinoid syndrome and the irritable bowel syndrome.[37,117] Differences in serotonin receptor subtypes provide a strong rationale for using pharmaceutical agents that selectively act on serotonin receptors in the treatment of these clinical disorders.

CLINICAL APPLICATIONS

Catecholamines and serotonin have important roles in health and disease. For example, increased plasma concentrations of catecholamines are associated with (1) psychic stress, (2) a fall in blood pressure or blood volume, (3) thyroid hormone deficiency, (4) congestive heart failure, and (5) arrhythmias. Low concentrations of catecholamines are seen in patients with pure autonomic failure or catecholamine biosynthetic deficiency states. Increased concentrations of circulating serotonin have been implicated in several pathologic conditions, including (1) chronic tension headache, (2) hypertension, (3) schizophrenia, (4) Duchenne's muscular dystrophy, and (5) preeclampsia.

Although investigational measurements of catecholamines, serotonin, and their metabolites are commonly used to assess numerous pathophysiologic processes, clinical laboratory measurements of the amines and their metabolites in plasma or urine are directed primarily at diagnosis of neuroendocrine tumors. Catecholamine-producing chromaffin cell tumors include pheochromocytomas, paragangliomas, and neuroblastomas; carcinoids are serotonin-secreting tumors. Measurements of catecholamines and their metabolites in plasma or urine are also useful in the diagnosis or evaluation of numerous disorders featuring autonomic dysfunction.

Pheochromocytoma

Pheochromocytomas are catecholamine-producing neuroendocrine tumors arising from chromaffin cells of the adrenal medulla or extra-adrenal paraganglia.[157] Those arising from extra-adrenal chromaffin tissue are referred to as *extra-adrenal pheochromocytomas* or *paragangliomas.* The same term, *paragangliomas,* is also used to refer to tumors arising from parasympathetic tissue in the head and neck, most of which do not produce significant quantities of catecholamines. About 85% of pheochromocytomas arise from the adrenal medulla, and about 15% arise from extra-adrenal chromaffin tissue (paragangliomas).

Pheochromocytomas and catecholamine-producing paragangliomas are treacherous tumors that almost invariably cause devastating cardiovascular complications and death if not recognized and properly treated. Autopsy studies continue to indicate that most pheochromocytomas remain undetected throughout life, contributing to premature death.[172] In many cases, presenting signs and symptoms may be misdiagnosed as another condition (e.g., preeclampsia in the pregnant patient with hypertension) with tragic consequences.[167] To think of the tumor therefore remains the critical first step in diagnosis.

The presence of a pheochromocytoma is usually suspected because of signs and symptoms that reflect the biological effects of catecholamines released by the tumor. Hypertension is the most common sign and can be sustained or paroxysmal. Symptoms include (1) headache, (2) palpitations, (3) diaphoresis, (4) pallor, (5) dyspnea, (6) nausea, (7) attacks of anxiety, and (8) generalized weakness. Although headache, palpitations, and sweating are nonspecific symptoms, their presence with hypertension should arouse immediate suspicion of the tumor. Signs and symptoms that occur in paroxysms reflect episodic catecholamine secretion. Paroxysmal attacks usually last less than an hour with intervals between attacks varying widely; these attacks may be as infrequent as once every few months. Pronounced but transient symptoms usually accompany such attacks; symptoms usually are less pronounced when hypertension is sustained. For additional details on the clinical presentation and other aspects of pheochromocytoma, the reader is referred to the texts of Manger and Gifford[165] and Pacak and colleagues.[204]

Pheochromocytomas are rare, occurring in less than 0.2% of patients with hypertension. However, because of the high prevalence of hypertension and the wide spectrum of symptoms produced by pheochromocytoma, many of which occur in other clinical conditions, pheochromocytoma must be considered in many patients with and without hypertension. Patients with a high risk for pheochromocytoma, in whom testing may be carried out independently of the presence of signs and symptoms, include those with a predisposing germline mutation, a previous history of the tumor, or the finding of an adrenal incidentaloma.

Most pheochromocytomas are sporadic, but a significant number occur in several familial tumor syndromes. Mutations in nine genes to date have been identified as responsible for familial pheochromocytoma: (1) the von Hippel-Lindau *(VHL)* gene, leading to VHL syndrome; (2) the *RET* gene, leading to multiple endocrine neoplasia type 2 (MEN-2); (3) the neurofibromatosis type 1 *(NF-1)* gene, associated with von Recklinghausen's disease; (4) genes encoding succinate dehydrogenase complex assembly factor 2 (SDHAF2) and the four subunits of succinate-dehydrogenase (SDHA, *SDHB, SDHC,* and *SDHD*) associated with familial paragangliomas and pheochromocytomas; and finally (5) the gene for transmembrane protein 27 (TMEM27).

Mutation testing, now routinely available for many of the above genes, has indicated that germline mutations are responsible for 30% or more of all pheochromocytomas—well in excess of the 10% of tumors previously thought to be hereditary. Between 12% and 24% of tumors with no obvious syndrome or family history appear to be due to otherwise unsuspected germline mutations.[1,195] Mutation testing therefore should be considered in all patients with pheochromocytoma, independently of the presence of any obvious syndrome or family history. Conversely, patients with identified germline mutations should undergo routine periodic screening for pheochromocytoma, independently of the presence of signs and symptoms of catecholamine excess.

Although most pheochromocytomas are benign, about 15% are malignant. A higher risk of malignant pheochromocytoma has been noted in patients with large or extra-adrenal primary tumors.[66] The risk for malignancy is particularly significant in patients with mutations of the *SDHB* gene.[1] Diagnosis of malignant pheochromocytoma is not possible based on histopathologic features, but instead requires evidence of metastatic lesions (e.g., in liver, lungs, lymphatic nodes, and bones). Metastases can occur more than 20 years after removal of an apparently benign solitary tumor. Therefore, all patients with a previous history of the tumor are at risk for recurrent or malignant disease and should undergo periodic screening for the tumor.

Adrenal masses are present in 6% or more of the older population. Most are benign adenomas, but up to 10% represent pheochromocytomas. With escalation in the use of computed tomography and magnetic resonance imaging, an increasing frequency of incidental findings of adrenal masses has been reported during imaging procedures for unrelated conditions. These adrenal incidentalomas represent another situation in which biochemical testing for pheochromocytoma is recommended, irrespective of the presence of the usual signs and symptoms of the tumor.[101]

It is imperative that appropriate biochemical tests are employed for accurate diagnosis both once a tumor is suspected and in situations involving routine screening. Biochemical testing has traditionally relied on measurements of urinary catecholamines, metanephrines, and VMA.[222] Most patients with hypertension and symptoms due to active pheochromocytomas have large increases in these analytes, making the tumor relatively easy to diagnose. Problems occur in those patients in whom hypertension is paroxysmal and in whom catecholamine secretion between episodes may be negligible. False-negative test results are also commonly encountered in patients with *silent pheochromocytomas,* in whom testing is carried out not because of signs or symptoms, but because of an adrenal incidentaloma or as part of a routine surveillance plan for recurrent or hereditary pheochromocytoma. In one study involving 35 patients with hereditary pheochromocytoma, rates of false-negative results for plasma and urinary catecholamines, urinary total metanephrines, and urinary VMA ranged from 29 to 53%; among the 35 patients, 6 (17%) had normal results on all four tests.[61]

Recognition that free metanephrines are produced by metabolism of catecholamines within chromaffin cells, including pheochromocytoma tumor cells, provided the rationale for development of these measurements as a new test to diagnose chromaffin cell tumors.[63] Improved diagnostic performance of free metanephrines over other analytes is explained by several factors: (1) production of free metanephrines occurs secondary to leakage of catecholamines from storage vesicles into the chromaffin cell cytoplasm by a process that occurs continuously and independently of variations in catecholamine release by tumors; (2) normally only small quantities of metanephrines are produced in the body, and these compared to the parent amines are relatively unresponsive to sympathoadrenal activation; and (3) VMA and the metanephrines commonly measured in urine are different metabolites from the free metanephrines measured in plasma, and they are produced in different parts of the body by metabolic processes not directly related to the tumor itself.

As reviewed elsewhere,[99,203] the high diagnostic sensitivity of plasma free metanephrines has been confirmed by five independent groups. A sixth Australian group, reporting a diagnostic sensitivity for the test of 100%, has provided further independent support for superiority of the test over other available diagnostic tests.[110] In the largest of all six independent studies—involving biochemical testing in more than 1000 patients, including 214 with pheochromocytoma—measurements of plasma free metanephrines and urinary fractionated metanephrines provided the highest diagnostic sensitivities[156]; however, measurements of plasma free metanephrines provided higher diagnostic specificity than measurements of urinary fractionated metanephrines. It is important to note that receiver operating characteristic curves show that a single test of plasma free metanephrines provided greater diagnostic efficacy than all other tests, even when carried out in combination (Figure 30-9).

With issues of sensitivity and specificity in mind, and with consideration of the potential dangers and rarity of pheochromocytoma, the most important consideration in selecting a biochemical test is the reliability of the test for detecting and thus excluding the tumor. With pheochromocytoma, a missed diagnosis due to false-negative results can have catastrophic consequences for the patient. In contrast, false-positive results can be refuted by additional tests. Therefore, suitably sensitive biochemical tests remain the first choice in the initial work-up of a patient suspected of harboring a pheochromocytoma.

Based on these considerations, a now widely endorsed recommendation is that initial testing for pheochromocytoma should always include measurement of plasma free metanephrines or urinary fractionated metanephrines, or both.[99,203] A lag has been reported in the shift from measurements of catecholamines to metanephrines,[207,264] but this is expected, and measurements of metanephrines nevertheless are starting to supplant urinary and plasma catecholamines as first-line tests for the diagnosis of pheochromocytoma.

Measurements of the parent catecholamines in urine or plasma remain important for providing supportive information, but a negative result for these tests cannot be used to exclude pheochromocytoma. In contrast, negative results for measurements of plasma free metanephrines reliably exclude almost all catecholamine-producing pheochromocytomas. Exceptions include small or microscopic (<1 cm) tumors in asymptomatic patients encountered during routine screening and tumors that synthesize predominantly dopamine. However, the latter tumors are extremely rare, have an unusual clinical presentation, and may be diagnosed by additional

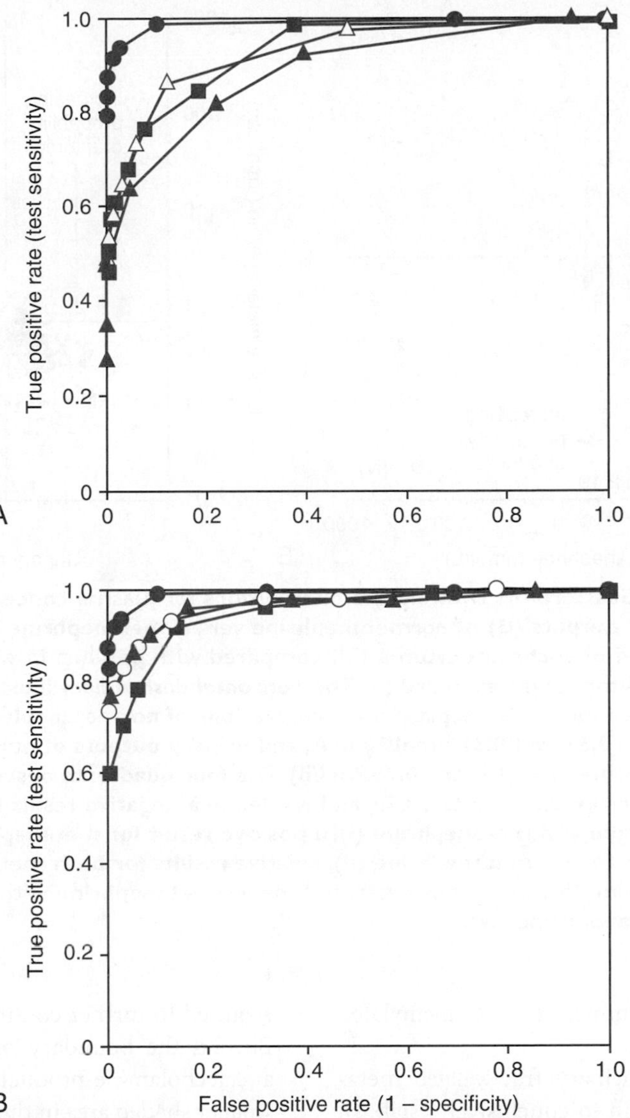

Figure 30-9 Receiver operating characteristic (ROC) curves determined from biochemical tests of catecholamine excess in 214 patients with confirmed pheochromocytomas and 644 patients in whom pheochromocytomas were excluded. The data in A show relationships between rates of true-positive test results (i.e., diagnostic sensitivity) and rates of false-positive test results (i.e., 1 − specificity) for measurements of plasma free metanephrines (●—●) compared with plasma catecholamines (■—■), urinary catecholamines (△—△), and urinary VMA (▲—▲). B shows the ROC curve for measurements of plasma free metanephrines (●—●) compared with ROC curves for combinations of tests for urinary fractionated metanephrines and catecholamines (○—○), urinary fractionated metanephrines and plasma catecholamines (▲—▲), and the combination of urinary total metanephrines (sum of normetanephrine and metanephrine) and urinary catecholamines (■—■). The larger area under the curve for measurements of plasma free metanephrines than for all other tests or combinations of tests indicate that measurements of plasma free normetanephrine and metanephrine provide a superior method for diagnosis of pheochromocytoma compared with all other examined tests or combinations of tests. *(Data adapted from Lenders JW, Pacak K, Walther MM, Linehan WM, Mannelli M, Friberg P, et al. Biochemical diagnosis of pheochromocytoma: which test is best? JAMA 2002;287:1427-34.)*

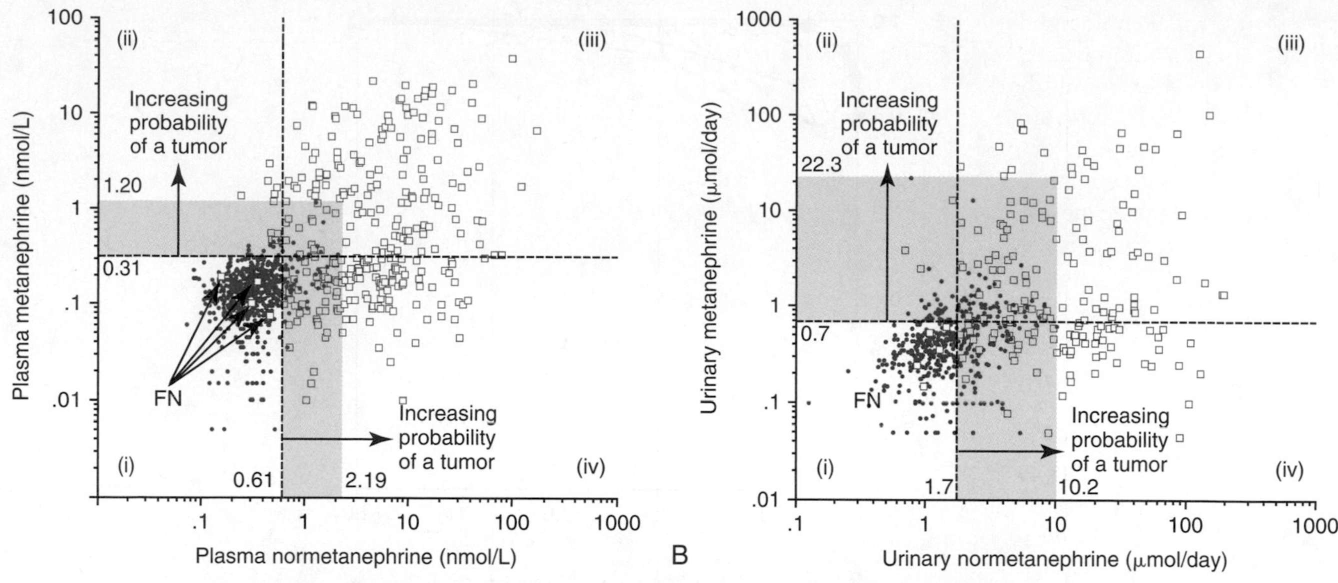

Figure 30-10 Scatterplots showing the distributions for plasma concentrations (A) or urinary outputs (B) of normetanephrine versus metanephrine in patients with confirmed pheochromocytoma (□) compared with patients in whom pheochromocytoma was excluded (•). The *horizontal dashed lines* illustrate the upper reference intervals for plasma concentrations of normetanephrine and metanephrine (0.61 and 0.31 nmol/L) in A, and urinary outputs of normetanephrine and metanephrine in B (1.8 and 0.7 μmol/d). The four quadrants described by these reference intervals (quadrants i, ii, iii, and iv) define a negative result for both normetanephrine and metanephrine (i), a positive result for metanephrine with a negative result for normetanephrine (ii), positive results for both metanephrine and normetanephrine (iii), and a positive result for normetanephrine with a negative result for metanephrine (iv).

measurements of methoxytyramine, the *O*-methylated metabolite of dopamine.[69]

Increases in plasma free or urinary fractionated metanephrines are usually large enough to conclusively establish the presence of most cases of pheochromocytoma, but a major remaining problem involves test results in the "gray area," which are not sufficiently elevated to reliably confirm pheochromocytoma (Figure 30-10). The problems involved in distinguishing false-positive from true-positive results are common to all biochemical tests of catecholamine excess; false-positive results must always be expected when the test reference interval is set at anything less than the 100% confidence intervals of a reference population. For pheochromocytoma, the large number of patients tested, very few of whom have the tumor, compounds this problem. The low pretest prevalence of pheochromocytoma means that false-positive biochemical results outnumber true-positive results, making it difficult to unequivocally confirm the tumor in the vast majority of patients with positive results. In such patients, additional biochemical testing is usually necessary.

The shaded areas beyond the upper reference intervals shown in Figure 30-10 indicate the plasma concentrations or urinary outputs of metanephrines where positive results are of insufficient magnitude to allow false-positive and true-positive results to be reliably distinguished. Among patients with test results in the shaded area, follow-up testing is usually required to further confirm or exclude pheochromocytoma. Beyond the boundary of shaded areas, the probability of a catecholamine-producing tumor approaches 100%. The smaller shaded area in the figure for measurements of plasma free metanephrines compared with urinary fractionated metanephrines indicates that pheochromocytoma can be unequivocally confirmed in a larger proportion of patients using measurements of plasma metanephrines than using urinary metanephrines. This conversely implies that more follow-up testing is required after measurements of urinary fractionated metanephrines than after measurements of plasma free metanephrines.

Before additional biochemical testing is initiated, consideration should be given to eliminating possible causes of false-positive results.[65] Such results may occur because of inappropriate sampling conditions, such as blood sampled without an overnight fast or a preceding 20-minute period of supine rest.[158] Medications leading to direct analytical interference or that influence the physiologic disposition of catecholamines and their metabolites represent other leading causes of false-positive results. Tricyclic antidepressants and phenoxybenzamine (dibenzyline) are particularly problematic, in one study accounting for 41% of all false-positive elevations in plasma normetanephrine, and for 44 to 45% of all false-positive elevations in urinary and plasma norepinephrine.[65]

After potential confounding influences of medications or other causes of false-positive results have been eliminated, some consideration should be given to the choice of additional biochemical tests and patterns of results needed to more firmly establish or refute the diagnosis of pheochromocytoma. When initial testing reveals elevations in plasma normetanephrine, metanephrine, or both amines, this finding may be corroborated by a similar pattern of results after additional measurements of urinary normetanephrine and metanephrine. Conversely, when initial testing yields positive results for urinary fractionated metanephrines, additional measurements of plasma free metanephrines are useful.

Patterns of increases in plasma free metanephrines and catecholamines also are useful for confirming pheochromocytoma in patients for whom initial tests of free metanephrines are positive but insufficiently elevated for a firm diagnosis.[65] More specifically, patients with pheochromocytoma usually have larger relative increases in metanephrines than in the parent catecholamines, whereas patients with false-positive results due to sympathoadrenal activation usually have larger increases in catecholamines than in metanephrines.

When biochemical testing continues to yield equivocal results, the clonidine suppression test may be useful for further confirming or excluding pheochromocytoma. As originally introduced by Bravo and associates,[17] this test was designed to distinguish patients with increases in plasma catecholamines due to pheochromocytoma from those with increases due to sympathetic activation. By activating α_2-adrenoceptors in the brain and on sympathetic nerve endings, clonidine suppresses norepinephrine release by sympathetic nerves. Decreases in elevated plasma norepinephrine after clonidine therefore suggest sympathetic activation, whereas lack of a decrease suggests pheochromocytoma.

A problem with the clonidine suppression test is that patients with normal or mildly increased plasma concentrations of norepinephrine may have clonidine-induced decreases in plasma norepinephrine, despite the presence of a pheochromocytoma.[65,239] Such patients represent those in whom it is most difficult to conclusively diagnose pheochromocytoma. Additional measurements of plasma normetanephrine before and after clonidine overcome this limitation.[65]

In a study involving 48 patients with and 49 patients without pheochromocytoma, lack of decrease in and elevated plasma concentrations of norepinephrine or normetanephrine after clonidine confirmed pheochromocytoma with high specificity (98 to 100%). However, of 48 patients with pheochromocytoma, 16 had normal concentrations or decreases in norepinephrine after clonidine. In contrast, plasma normetanephrine remained elevated after clonidine in all but two patients, indicating higher sensitivity (96% vs. 67%) and more reliable diagnosis using normetanephrine than norepinephrine responses to clonidine. Box 30-1 outlines the clonidine suppression test protocol, along with these added testing recommendations.

BOX 30-1 Protocol for Clonidine Suppression Test

Principle: Clonidine activates α_2-adrenergic receptors in the brain and sympathetic nerve endings to suppress norepinephrine release by sympathetic nerves without effect on catecholamine release from pheochromocytomas.

Indication: The test is used to discriminate patients with pheochromocytomas from patients with false-positive test results for plasma norepinephrine or normetanephrine.

Procedure: The test is best performed in the morning after an overnight fast. The patient remains recumbent throughout the entire procedure. A forearm venous cannula is placed for baseline and 3-hour blood sampling during the procedure. After at least 20 minutes of supine rest, a baseline blood sample is drawn in a heparinized tube. Clonidine, 4.3 μg/kg of body weight, is then given orally, and a repeat blood sample is drawn 3 hours later. The samples are analyzed for plasma catecholamines, with plasma normetanephrine measurement also recommended.

Interpretation: For optimum clinical specificity, a positive result highly suggestive of a pheochromocytoma includes elevation of norepinephrine and normetanephrine at 3 hours and failure to suppress norepinephrine by more than 50% and normetanephrine by more than 40% below the baseline plasma concentration.

Modified from Bravo et al.[17] with additional recommendations for normetanephrine testing and interpretation from Eisenhofer et al.[65]

Neuroblastoma

Neuroblastomas are malignant neoplasms characterized in most cases by overproduction of catecholamines and their metabolites.[150,184] Similar to pheochromocytomas, neuroblastomas are derived from neural crest blastic precursors. However, neuroblastomas are more primitive tumors than pheochromocytomas and do not express a chromaffin phenotype. Unlike pheochromocytomas, neuroblastomas occur almost exclusively in children, accounting for approximately 7 to 10% of childhood cancer and the most common malignancy diagnosed in the first year of life.[103-105]

The incidence of neuroblastoma is approximately 10 cases per million children, resulting worldwide in about 10,000 new cases per year.[170] Although familial cases have been reported,[144] the vast majority of neuroblastomas develop sporadically.[150,184]

The anatomic location of the primary tumor in neuroblastoma is predicted by the neuroblast origins. Most tumors are intra-abdominal, arising in the adrenal gland or the upper abdomen; less frequent locations include the chest, neck, and pelvis. Approximately 60% of neuroblastomas are extra-adrenal, compared with only about 15% of pheochromocytomas. Metastases in disseminated neuroblastoma may involve bone marrow, bone, lymph nodes, liver, and, less frequently, the skin, testis, and intracranial structures.

The biological behavior of neuroblastoma varies from regression and maturation to an aggressive course with unfavorable outcome. Neuroblastoma is most notable for a subset of cases with complete regression or maturation to ganglioneuroma, a benign neoplasm. The high rate of neuroblastoma detection in infant screening programs compared with clinically diagnosed cases has been explained by spontaneous tumor maturation.[116] Mass screening programs and use of prenatal and postnatal ultrasound of the abdomen have led to an increase in early identification of neuroblastoma[5,137] and to reports of "wait and see" treatment options.[82,272] Although cautious delay in treatment has provided further evidence of regressive tumor behavior, investigation of potential early biomarkers that may identify aggressive tumor and assist in treatment decisions is ongoing.[120,243]

The clinical stage of the disease (localized vs. disseminated) is an important prognostic factor. Patients with early, more localized stages of disease and infants younger than 1 year of age with a localized primary tumor or dissemination limited to skin, liver, and/or bone marrow are considered to have a better prognosis than those at other stages.[18] Age at diagnosis is also important in predicting the course of the disease, with infants diagnosed in the first year of life having better survival rates than those diagnosed later.[33] Other factors, including expression of the N-myc (also known as MYCN) proto-oncogene and unfavorable histologic classification, have been associated with an aggressive course of the disease. Unfortunately, the overall incidence of metastatic neuroblastoma at the time of diagnosis is approximately 60%, and the need for earlier detection of children with progressive disseminating tumors remains a diagnostic challenge.

Hypertension and other signs of catecholamine excess are uncommon in neuroblastoma. Patients commonly present with a tumor mass and clinical signs caused by compression effects on neighboring structures or by hematologic abnormalities from bone marrow involvement. The low incidence of hypertension and other signs of catecholamine excess may be attributed to the characteristic pattern of tumor storage and release of catecholamines and their metabolites. Catecholamine storage capacity in neuroblastoma cells is limited, as is evidenced by electron microscopic findings of few secretory granules.[122] Inefficient storage, coupled with excessive production of catecholamines, may lead to an increase in the intracellular metabolism of the catecholamines and the release of mainly inactive metabolites. Hypertension, although rare, does occur in some patients with neuroblastoma, and an abundance of secretory granules has been noted in neuroblastoma tissue from some tumors.[179,260]

Laboratory evidence of a functional catecholamine-producing tumor is important in clinical evaluation when neuroblastoma is suspected. Catecholamine and metabolite production patterns, however, may differ markedly among patients with the tumor. Neuroblastoma cells have the capacity to synthesize dopamine and norepinephrine, depending on their degree of metabolic maturity, but usually lack PNMT and do not produce epinephrine. Because of variability in catecholamine production and metabolism in neuroblastomas, no single reliable marker of catecholamine overproduction is currently known; consequently, a combination of analytes is required for diagnostic evaluation.

VMA and HVA are the most widely used analytes both in the clinical setting and in screening programs for diagnosis of neuroblastoma. Elevated urinary excretion of HVA and VMA is the result of excessive tumor production of dopamine and norepinephrine. A small diurnal variation in HVA and VMA excretion and a positive correlation between random and 24-hour urine test results allow the convenient use of random urine specimens, with results expressed as the ratio of catecholamine metabolite to creatinine concentrations. Clinical sensitivity in the range of 90% has been reported for urinary HVA and VMA testing by some centers.[149,250] Others, however, report a lower rate of neuroblastoma detection. In a large prospective neuroblastoma screening program, in which the population with negative screening results was tracked for occurrence of neuroblastoma, an elevation in VMA, HVA, or both acid metabolites detected only 73% of tumors.[228] Patients with early-stage disease have the highest rate of false-negative test results,[213] and screening programs generally have been unsuccessful in reducing the rate of metastatic neuroblastoma in the population.[116]

Additional markers of catecholamine overproduction have been used to improve the biochemical detection of neuroblastoma. Free dopamine may be abnormal in urine from patients with neuroblastoma.[44,197,221] Combined testing for VMA, HVA, and dopamine may therefore improve tumor detection, and in 1993, an international consensus report on neuroblastoma diagnosis added dopamine to the list of acceptable measurements by which to document the adrenergic nature of the tumor.[18] In a study of 114 children with a clinical diagnosis of neuroblastoma, the combined use of urinary VMA, HVA, and dopamine detected 91.2% of cases, while clinical sensitivity for individual measurements of VMA (80.7%), HVA (71.9%), and dopamine (61.3%) was lower.[243]

As outlined earlier, most free dopamine in urine is derived from the renal decarboxylation of circulating L-dopa[19]; thus increases in urinary dopamine most probably reflect increases in circulating L-dopa, concentrations of which can also be elevated in patients with neuroblastoma.[72,90] Measurement of the *O*-methylated metabolites, especially normetanephrine, has also been explored.[21] In one study comparing measurements of catecholamines—the *O*-methylated metabolites, VMA and HVA—clinical sensitivity for detection of neuroblastoma was 97 to 100% when results of normetanephrine testing were coupled with VMA among infants, or with HVA in children older than 1 year.[183] Nevertheless, even with an extended panel of catecholamine and metabolite measurements, a low incidence of tumors with completely normal biochemical test results must be considered.

The pattern of catecholamine metabolism is associated with important biological and genetic prognostic factors in neuroblastoma.[274] Lower excretion rates of VMA, HVA, dopamine, and norepinephrine are found more often in infants with early stages of the disease; this may explain the lower diagnostic sensitivity of VMA and HVA testing reported in infants with early-stage neuroblastoma.[33]

The relative excretion of catecholamines and their metabolites may point to an unfavorable outcome in neuroblastoma.

Immature metabolic patterns have been observed in neuroblastoma tumor tissue, based on excretion of dopamine or HVA relative to norepinephrine or VMA. A high ratio of HVA to VMA, of dopamine to VMA, or of dopamine to norepinephrine indicates a relative deficiency in beta hydroxylation, with a reduction in tumor cell conversion of dopamine to norepinephrine. This immature metabolic pattern has been associated with aggressive tumor behavior and other unfavorable prognostic factors.[123,274]

An investigation into the diagnostic and prognostic usefulness of the relative excretion of VMA, HVA, and dopamine has been reported by Strenger and coworkers.[243] In their study of 114 children with neuroblastoma, they reaffirmed that elevations in VMA are associated with more favorable prognostic factors (e.g., age <12 months, no MYCN amplification, no 1p deletion, stages 2 and 4s), and that elevations in dopamine predict unfavorable tumor features. When expressed as a dopamine-to-VMA ratio, stage 4 versus stage 4s was differentiated with 80% sensitivity and 91% specificity. Future studies are needed to determine whether catecholamines and their metabolites, in addition to their use in diagnosis, may serve as additional biomarkers of tumor behavior and prognosis.

Finally, clinical specificity in detecting neuroblastoma with catecholamine and metabolite measurements may be influenced by the choice of laboratory methods, dietary interference, and other catecholamine overproduction conditions. Significant advances in the analytical specificity and availability of newer mass spectrometric methods have reduced many of the exogenous interferences that hampered interpretation with earlier methods.

Carcinoids

Carcinoids are the most common tumors arising from the diffuse neuroendocrine system of the GI tract and pancreas. Derived primarily from enterochromaffin cells, these tumors belong to the larger family of neuroendocrine cancers known as gastroenteropancreatic neuroendocrine tumors (GET-NET). Carcinoids are widely distributed in the body, but are found with greatest frequency in the GI (64%) and respiratory (28%) tracts.[142] Carcinoids were previously classified as APUDomas (endocrine tumors of *a*mine *p*recursor *u*ptake and *d*ecarboxylation) because of the ability of enterochromaffin cells to take up and decarboxylate amino acid precursors of biogenic amines. In this regard, carcinoid tumors share certain pathologic and biological similarities with pheochromocytomas. However, the APUD classification is no longer adequate to describe the morphologic spectrum of carcinoids.

Carcinoid tumors are traditionally classified according to their presumed origin from the embryonic foregut (bronchus, lung, stomach, duodenum, and pancreas), midgut (ileum, jejunum, appendix, and proximal colon), or hindgut (rectum and distal colon).[141] The most common sites for these tumors are the bronchus and/or lung (25%), ileum and/or jejunum (20%), rectum (14%), and appendix (5%).[180] A revised classification system takes into account variations in histopathologic characteristics.[28,241] In this scheme, the term *carcinoid* is used synonymously with the term *well-differentiated neuroendocrine tumor.*

The overall incidence of clinically significant carcinoids in the United States was previously estimated to vary from 1 to 2 cases per 100,000 persons; more recent estimates indicate that the incidence may be as high as 5 per 100,000—an increase presumed to reflect improved recognition and diagnosis.[181,209] Carcinoid tumors may develop in all age groups, but they appear most frequently in adults, with a mean age of 63 years for tumors of the small intestine and respiratory tract. Clinically, most patients are asymptomatic until metastases are present. Bowel obstruction and abdominal pain are the most frequent presenting symptoms. However, the clinical manifestations of these tumors are extremely varied and are often obscure (e.g., flushing, diarrhea, steatorrhea, wheezing, dyspepsia, ulcers, hypoglycemia, heart disease, deep vein thrombosis, anorexia, nausea, vomiting, constipation, hypotension, fainting, skin disorders, dumping syndrome, pernicious anemia, autoimmune disorders, diabetes, gallbladder disease). These variable presentations reflect the diverse secretory products produced by the tumors, which frequently lead to confusion and delay in achieving the correct diagnosis.[181] Consequently, the average time from symptom onset to diagnosis is usually longer than 9 years.

The usual carcinoid tumor is solid and yellow-tan in appearance. Tumor cells exhibit a monotonous morphology, with pink granular cytoplasm and round nuclei with infrequent mitoses. Most carcinoids can be recognized by their reactions to silver stains and to neuroendocrine cell markers such as chromogranin and neuron-specific enolase. Ultrastructurally, carcinoids possess numerous membrane-bound, electron-dense neurosecretory granules. These granules contain peptide hormones and bioactive amines, which occasionally can be identified by immunocytochemical techniques.

Carcinoid tumors show aggressive malignant behavior depending on the origin, depth of penetration, and size of the primary tumor. Most rectal carcinomas are found incidentally at endoscopy. They often measure less than 1 cm and have a low rate of metastasis, even though they may show extensive local spread. Carcinoids of the appendix are seen in about 1 in every 300 appendectomies. Almost all measure less than 1 cm, and distant metastasis is rare. By contrast, 90% of intestinal carcinoids that penetrate halfway through the muscle wall will have spread to lymph nodes and distant sites at the time of diagnosis. More than 70% of intestinal carcinoids 1 to 2 cm in diameter metastasize to the liver. Fortunately, most carcinoid tumors grow slowly and do not cause clinically significant disease. Patients may live for many years. The 5-year survival rate of patients with carcinoids in the appendix is about 98%. Patients with carcinoids in the small intestine have a 5-year survival rate of about 60%.[181]

As with normal gut endocrine cells, carcinoids synthesize, store, and release a variety of peptide hormones, proteins, and biogenic amines. One of the most thoroughly characterized of the latter substances is serotonin [5-hydroxytryptamine

(5-HT)]. Carcinoid tumors also produce and secrete numerous other biologically active substances, including (1) histamine, (2) kallikrein, (3) bradykinins, (4) tachykinins, (5) prostaglandins, (6) chromogranin A, (7) dopamine, and (8) norepinephrine. Production of these substances often varies in relation to the tissue origin of the tumor.[198] For example, midgut carcinoids release large quantities of serotonin into the circulation, whereas tumors derived from the foregut secrete primarily 5-hydroxytryptophan (5-HTP) (a serotonin precursor) and histamine rather than serotonin.[134] Primary hindgut carcinoids usually show no 5-HT or 5-HTP secretory activity. In some instances, carcinoid tumors may coexist with other neuroendocrine tumors that produce gastrin, insulin, adrenocorticotropic hormone (ACTH), and catecholamines. Several different genetic syndromes may be associated with carcinoids, including MEN-1 and neurofibromatosis.[162]

Secretion of vasoactive substances into the systemic circulation plays an important role in development of the carcinoid syndrome. The full-blown syndrome associated with the humoral manifestations of these tumors is striking but uncommon, occurring in less than 10% of patients with carcinoids, and usually occurring only after metastasis to the liver and release of these substances directly into the systemic circulation.[218]

The classic clinical presentation of the carcinoid syndrome includes pronounced flushing (especially on the face and neck), diarrhea, bronchoconstriction, and eventual right-sided valvular heart failure. Overproduction of serotonin is found in 90 to 100% of patients with the carcinoid syndrome and is thought to be responsible for the diarrhea through its known stimulatory effects on gut motility and fluid secretion. Serotonin receptor antagonists relieve the diarrhea in most cases. The pathophysiology of carcinoid flushing is not yet known, but tachykinins, bradykinins, and histamine may be mediators. Somatostatin analogs reduce circulating concentrations of these vasodilators. The causative agents of bronchoconstriction are unknown, but tachykinins and bradykinins are likely mediators.

The clinical chemical evaluation of the carcinoid syndrome continues to rely on measurements of serotonin and its metabolites in body fluids and chromogranin A (CgA) in serum.[135] The latter is ubiquitously distributed in neuroendocrine cells and is a useful general marker for many neuroendocrine tumors, not just carcinoids. In patients with the typical carcinoid syndrome, 5-HTP is converted to serotonin and is stored in tumor secretory granules and in platelets. A small amount of serotonin remains free in plasma, but most is converted by monoamine oxidase to 5-HIAA, which is excreted in urine in free and conjugated forms.

Patients with midgut tumors often have increased blood and platelet serotonin concentrations and increased urinary 5-HIAA. However, some patients with foregut carcinoid tumors can hydroxylate tryptophan but lack the aromatic L-amino acid decarboxylase and secrete 5-HTP rather than serotonin into the bloodstream. Patients with these tumors have normal or low serotonin concentrations in blood and in platelets, but urinary serotonin concentrations are increased because 5-HTP is converted to serotonin in the kidney; urinary 5-HIAA concentrations may be slightly elevated. Patients with hindgut carcinoids often have low (or absent) hydroxylase and decarboxylase activities and may produce only small amounts of 5-HT, 5-HTP, or 5-HIAA. In contrast, serum CgA measurements are elevated in most patients with hindgut tumors, as well as in 80 to 90% of patients with metastatic cancers of the midgut and foregut.[162]

Patients with serotonin-producing midgut carcinoid tumors usually have striking increases in urinary 5-HIAA excretion (at least tenfold), but occasionally elevations are smaller. False-positive elevations can occur if the patient ingests serotonin-rich foods or medications such as bananas, pineapples, chocolate, walnuts, pecans, kiwi fruit, plums, avocados, and cough medicines containing guaifenesin.[76,133] Conversely, alcohol, aspirin, and other drugs can suppress 5-HIAA concentrations. Patients should avoid these agents during 24-hour urine collections. Incomplete or excess 24-hour urine collections may be assessed more accurately in terms of a creatinine ratio. Fasting plasma 5-HIAA has been proposed as a convenient replacement for urine collections.[52]

The upper limit of the reference interval for urinary 5-HIAA excretion may be as low as 6 mg/d (30 μmol/d) if dietary and medicinal intakes are controlled. A cutoff value of 15 mg/d (80 μmol/d) may be used to reduce false-positive results.[196] At an intermediate value of 10.7 mg/d (56 μmol/d), urinary 5-HIAA has a reported 77% sensitivity and 97% specificity for carcinoid disease.[25] To exclude the presence of a carcinoid tumor, lower cutoff values may be preferred (higher sensitivity); to confirm the presence of a carcinoid tumor, higher cutoff values (higher specificity) would be indicated. Two or more 24-hour urine collections may be needed to confirm a diagnosis if 5-HIAA secretion is intermittent.[269]

Most physicians rely on serial measurements of 5-HIAA and CgA for diagnosis and follow-up of carcinoid syndrome.[269] But when a patient strongly suspected for carcinoid syndrome shows normal or borderline increases in these tests, documentation of elevated serotonin concentrations in platelets, plasma, whole blood, or urine may help establish the diagnosis.[132] In a symptomatic patient, a blood or serum serotonin concentration greater than 400 ng/mL (>2280 nmol/L) is consistent with a carcinoid.[269] Platelet serotonin has been reported to be more sensitive than urinary 5-HIAA for detecting carcinoids that produce small or moderate amounts of serotonin, such as foregut and hindgut carcinoids and midgut carcinoids with a low tumor volume.[173] Also, platelet serotonin concentrations are not affected by the patient's diet. The storage capacity of platelets can be saturated at high serotonin secretion rates, however, and blood serotonin concentrations fluctuate widely over time. Concentrations of serum CgA and urinary 5-HIAA better correlate with tumor burden and often are preferred for monitoring patients with extensive disease and high serotonin production. The presence of a functioning carcinoid can be excluded if CgA, 5-HT, and 5-HIAA are all normal.

Serum CgA may be a more sensitive diagnostic marker of carcinoid tumor than urinary 5-HIAA or blood serotonin.[199,276] However, increased concentrations of circulating CgA are not specific to carcinoids, and elevations are seen in other neuroendocrine tumors. False-positive elevations can be found in various conditions, including impaired renal function, liver failure, and congestive heart disease. Proton pump inhibitors represent another important cause of false-positive elevations of serum CgA. Serum CgA correlates with treatment response and is a sensitive means for detecting residual or recurrent disease. CgA also generally correlates with tumor burden and therefore can be used to predict prognosis, particularly in patients with midgut tumors.

Plasma concentrations of neuron-specific enolase, neuropeptide K, and substance P have been suggested as other diagnostic and prognostic markers in carcinoid tumors. These general neuroendocrine markers are investigational at this time and are not recommended for routine use.[74] Nevertheless, for many of the related gastroenteropancreatic (GEP) neuroendocrine tumors—in particular, the less common insulinomas, pancreatic polypeptide tumors (PPomas), gastrinomas, etc—it is usually necessary to reach the final diagnosis using measurements of specific peptide hormones carried out with appropriate preparation of patients and under carefully controlled conditions of blood sampling.[47]

Dysautonomias and Related Genetic Disorders

Dysautonomias are conditions in which altered function of the autonomic nervous system adversely affects health.[95] Such conditions vary from more common transient episodes in otherwise healthy people (e.g., neurocardiogenic syncope) to progressive neurodegenerative diseases (e.g., multiple system atrophy) and to even more rare genetic disorders such as dopamine β-hydroxylase deficiency (Table 30-5).

TABLE 30-5 Disorders Featuring Altered Sympathetic Nervous System Function (Dysautonomias) or Altered Adrenal Medullary Function

Inhibition/Interruption		Activation
Dysautonomias		
Neurocardiogenic syncope	*Common*	Obesity
Diabetic autonomic neuropathy	↓	Essential hypertension
Parkinson's disease		Congestive heart failure
Hyperthyroidism		Intracranial bleeding
Multiple system atrophy		Renovascular hypertension
Postural tachycardia syndrome		Sleep apnea
Quadriplegia		Hypothyroidism
Amyloidosis		Baroreflex failure
Pure autonomic failure		Guillain-Barré syndrome
Familial dysautonomia*		NE transporter deficiency*
Dopamine β-hydroxylase deficiency*	*Rare*	
Adrenal Medullary Dysfunction		
Obesity	*Common*	Neurocardiogenic syncope
Diabetes type 1	↓	Panic disorder
Addison's disease		Pheochromocytoma
Congenital adrenal hyperplasia*	*Rare*	Adrenal medullary hyperplasia

*Denotes genetic disorders.
Genetic disorders (not included above): tyrosine hydroxylase deficiency; dopa-responsive dystonia; dihydropteridine reductase deficiency; aromatic L-amino acid decarboxylase deficiency; Menkes' disease; monoamine oxidase deficiency.

Dysautonomias also vary from mechanistically straightforward disorders in which altered autonomic function plays a primary pathophysiologic role (e.g., pure autonomic failure) to conditions in which altered autonomic function worsens an independent pathophysiologic state (e.g., cardiac failure) and to more mysterious disorders in which involvement of the autonomic nervous system is less clear (e.g., chronic fatigue syndrome). Abnormalities of blood pressure control represent a common presenting clinical feature of most dysautonomias. In those involving inhibition or interruption of sympathetic outflow, the presenting clinical feature is usually hypotension, particularly orthostatic hypotension. In those involving sympathetic activation, there is often hypertension—and in some, excessive increases in heart rate upon standing.

In most dysautonomias, altered or deranged sympathetic nervous function is evident from measurements of plasma or urinary concentrations of norepinephrine or norepinephrine metabolites. The most well-known dysautonomias, in which measurements of norepinephrine provide useful and even crucial information for diagnosis, involve the autonomic failure syndromes, particularly pure autonomic failure and multiple system atrophy.[131] The most important debilitating clinical manifestation in both conditions is orthostatic hypotension. In their most severe forms, patients are unable to remain in the upright posture for even a few minutes.

The basis of both pure autonomic failure and multiple system atrophyisorder involves failure of neurogenic vasoconstrictor responses secondary to defective sympathoneural release of norepinephrine. In pure autonomic failure, the lesion is postganglionic, involving degeneration of sympathetic nerves and lack of norepinephrine release, whereas in multiple system atrophy, the lesion is preganglionic and sympathetic nerves are present but do not release norepinephrine appropriately. The two syndromes therefore can be diagnosed based on measurements of catecholamines. In both, increases in plasma concentrations of norepinephrine are usually absent or significantly attenuated in response to assumption of upright posture. In pure autonomic failure, concentrations of norepinephrine and its metabolites are usually decreased, reflecting loss of sympathetic nerves. In contrast, in multiple system atrophy, resting concentrations of catecholamines and catecholamine metabolites may be normal or even increased.

Abnormalities in plasma or urinary concentrations of catecholamines in most of the more common disorders featuring abnormalities of autonomic function (e.g., obesity, diabetes, panic disorder) are usually subtle and are not easily interpreted. Plasma or urinary concentrations of catecholamines and catecholamine metabolites in such conditions have been measured mainly for investigational purposes to better characterize and understand the disorders. Resulting improved understanding of such disorders, combined with advances in measurement techniques and improved ability to interpret different patterns of neurochemical results, will likely lead to increasing use of measurements of catecholamines and catecholamine metabolites for routine diagnostic and prognostic purposes. This is becoming particularly apparent for conditions that have a hereditary basis or are due to de novo mutations of specific genes, in which advances in molecular genetics are enabling precise identification of the genetic abnormality.[93]

Familial dysautonomia, dopamine β-hydroxylase deficiency, norepinephrine transporter deficiency, and congenital adrenal hyperplasia include dysautonomias or conditions associated with adrenal medullary dysfunction in which specific genetic abnormalities have been identified. In other disorders involving mutations of genes coding for proteins involved in catecholamine synthesis and metabolism, clinical manifestations do not always clearly involve sympathoadrenal systems or may be so globally severe that abnormalities of autonomic or adrenal medullary function are obscured (see Table 30-5).

Deficiencies of tyrosine hydroxylase or of enzymes involved in production of tetrahydrobiopterin cofactor (e.g., dopa-responsive dystonia) usually result in presentation of severe neurologic abnormalities in early childhood. Depending on the exact mutation, deficiencies of tyrosine hydroxylase can involve moderate to severe loss of enzyme activity, most accurately diagnosed by low cerebrospinal fluid (CSF) concentrations of catecholamine metabolites such as MHPG and HVA, but normal concentrations of 5-HIAA.[15,16]

In the autosomal dominant form of dopa-responsive dystonia (Segawa disease), failure to synthesize tetrahydrobiopterin cofactor leads to a similar clinical and neurochemical phenotype as in the rarer tyrosine hydroxylase deficiency syndrome.[232] In contrast to classical forms of tetrahydrobiopterin deficiency, characterized by phenylketonuria (e.g., dihydropteridine reductase deficiencies), deficiencies of guanosine triphosphate (GTP) cyclohydrolase responsible for dopa-responsive dystonia are not accompanied by hyperphenylalaninemia and require diagnosis by measurements of pterins and pterin metabolism, in addition to measurements of catecholamine metabolites.[10]

Patients with aromatic L–amino acid decarboxylase deficiency present with clinical and biochemical manifestations that overlap those of the tyrosine hydroxylase deficiency states described previously. However, this deficiency state is characterized by additional decreases in CSF and urinary concentrations of 5-HIAA.[119] Also, concentrations of L-dopa in urine, plasma, and cerebrospinal fluid are increased and not decreased, as in the other deficiency states. Concentrations of 5-hydroxytryptophan are similarly increased.

The major clinical feature of patients with deficiency of dopamine β-hydroxylase is orthostatic hypotension caused by reduced synthesis and release of norepinephrine by sympathetic nerves.[7] The deficiency is characterized neurochemically by decreased concentrations of norepinephrine and norepinephrine metabolites and increased concentrations of dopamine and dopamine metabolites. Diagnosis is best achieved from an increased ratio of plasma dopamine to norepinephrine. Copper deficiency in Menkes' disease is due to defects in the gene coding for a copper-transporting adenosine triphosphatase.[129] Because dopamine β-hydroxylase is a copper-dependent enzyme, the deficiency is associated with decreased activity of the enzyme and reduced production of norepinephrine from dopamine. Prompt diagnosis at childbirth is essential for copper replacement therapy and is best achieved through measurement of the ratio of plasma concentrations of DOPAC to DHPG.

Congenital adrenal hyperplasia is a relatively common genetic disorder that occurs secondary to deficiencies of certain enzymes, usually 21-hydroxylase, responsible for synthesis of cortisol.[174] The disorder is characterized clinically by adrenal insufficiency with or without salt wasting, virilization, and, in girls, genital ambiguity resulting from increased androgen concentrations. As a result of the importance of adrenocortical steroids for adrenal medullary function, including maintenance of PNMT expression, the disorder is also characterized by adrenal medullary hypofunction and decreased epinephrine release and intra-adrenal metabolism to metanephrine. Decreased plasma concentrations of metanephrine provide a biomarker of disease severity that may be useful for prognosis and in treatment decisions.[29]

Isolated deficiencies of MAO A and B are extremely rare and are associated with distinct clinical and neurochemical phenotypes.[155] Deficiency of MAO A is associated with a behavioral disorder characterized by increased aggressiveness. Plasma and urinary concentrations of deaminated metabolites of catecholamines are severely decreased, whereas concentrations of normetanephrine and metanephrine are increased. An increased ratio of plasma normetanephrine to DHPG has therefore been proposed to provide a sensitive marker for the deficiency state. In contrast, deficiency of MAO B is associated with a mild phenotype; the only biochemical alteration is increased urinary excretion of phenylethylamine.

ANALYTICAL METHODOLOGY

In clinical practice, laboratory determinations of catecholamines, serotonin, and their metabolites in biological fluids are performed primarily for diagnosis and follow-up of patients with pheochromocytomas, neuroblastomas, and

GEP tumors, including carcinoids. For evaluation of pheochromocytomas, most laboratories now offer measurements of urinary fractionated or plasma free metanephrines or both, with measurements of catecholamines in urine or plasma available as supporting measurements. For detection of neuroblastoma, urinary HVA and VMA remain the most commonly ordered tests in clinical practice, but other catecholamine metabolites and dopamine are also measured. Diagnostic evaluation of patients with carcinoid tumors routinely involves measurement of 5-HIAA, with measurement of serotonin in platelets and urine also advocated.

Numerous methods have been developed for the determination of catecholamines, serotonin, and their metabolites in biological samples. Early fluorometric, spectrophotometric, and radioenzymatic assays have largely been superseded by modern techniques employing liquid chromatography (LC) that enable fractionation of different analytes and higher analytical specificity. These methods are emphasized here. For information on earlier fluorometric, spectrophotometric, and radioenzymatic assays, the reader is referred to an earlier article by Rosano and coworkers.[222]

Beginning in the early 1980s, analytical methods involving high-performance liquid chromatography (HPLC), coupled with electrochemical or fluorometric detection, increasingly provided the mainstay method for laboratories specializing in measurements of biogenic amines. Once equipment has been purchased and trained personnel are in place, HPLC methods offer reliable, reproducible, and relatively rapid measurements of reasonably large numbers of samples at minimum cost per sample. Problems with interference from drugs or dietary constituents usually can be identified by careful inspection of chromatograms. Consistent sources of interference can be remedied by simple changes to chromatographic conditions. A large number of different HPLC methods have been described for measurements of monoamines and their metabolites, all requiring a preanalytical extraction step to concentrate (plasma) and clean up (plasma and urine) the sample.

In addition, advances in coupling mass spectrometry with liquid phase separation methods—in particular, liquid chromatography with tandem mass spectrometry (LC-MS/MS)—have ushered in a new era for analytical laboratories, including those specializing in measurements of biogenic amines and metabolites. The extended capabilities of mass spectrometry have been made possible largely through development in the mid-1980s of electrospray ionization and other techniques, enabling analytes to be delivered to the mass spectrometer in an aqueous rather than a gaseous phase.[88]

Development of tandem mass spectrometry (MS/MS) represents a further breakthrough, enabling analyses of relationships between "parent precursor ions" in the first stage and "daughter fragment ions" in the second stage of the instrument.[88] For targeted quantitative analyses, the filtering capabilities and multiple reaction monitoring (MRM) made possible with MS/MS triple quadrupole instruments provide not only high selectivity, but also improved signal-to-noise ratios. *High analytical specificity* means that sample purification and chromatographic resolution need not be as rigorous as for other procedures. This enables considerably shortened chromatographic run times (i.e., higher sample throughput) and simplified sample purification and analyte extraction procedures. Improvements in analytical sensitivity coupled with the high specificity offered by LC-MS/MS are now well recognized to offer critical advances over standard HPLC and immunoassay procedures, which are subject to analytical interference or do not allow precise and accurate identification of structurally related compounds.

Fusion of LC-MS/MS with other technologies—such as multiplexing parallel LC systems, turboflow technology, and automated online sample processing—provides additional advantages in laboratory medicine for efficient and accurate high-throughput quantitative analyses. The addition of an automated online sample extraction system minimizes time spent on sample preparation and allows multiple applications to be efficiently handled by one instrument[48]; this additional versatility provides further justification for a single LC-MS/MS system that can take over the jobs of multiple standard HPLC systems.

With recognition of all the advantages of LC-MS/MS over other methods, many laboratories are rapidly moving to this new technology. This is particularly appropriate for the high-throughput laboratory, where the large capital expenditure on instruments can be easily justified. For smaller hospital-based laboratories, the high instrument costs present a major obstacle. Versatility in multiple applications that may be handled by a single instrument and continuing reductions in instrument costs may provide partial solutions.

Catecholamines and Metabolites

Collection and Storage of Samples

The conditions under which plasma or urine samples are collected and stored can be crucial to the reliability and interpretation of test results. Release of catecholamines from sympathetic nerves and the adrenal medulla can be markedly increased in response to changes from supine to upright posture and during states of mental or physiologic stress.

Because plasma free metanephrines are less responsive to changes in sympathoadrenal outflow than parent catecholamines,[55] it has been suggested that there is less need for the stringent sampling conditions required for measurements of catecholamines. However, it has been clearly demonstrated that plasma concentrations of normetanephrine are 30% higher and metanephrine about 12% higher in seated compared with supine positions.[50,158] These metabolites are rapidly cleared from the circulation, have short half-lives, and show prompt decreases in plasma concentrations after assumption of the supine position (Figure 30-11). Therefore, to minimize the possibility of false-positive results, it is recommended that subjects should be resting in the supine position for at least 30 minutes before blood is collected for measurements of plasma free metanephrines. Alternatively, if blood collected with the patient in the seated position returns a positive test result, then consideration should be given to repeat sampling in the supine position.[158]

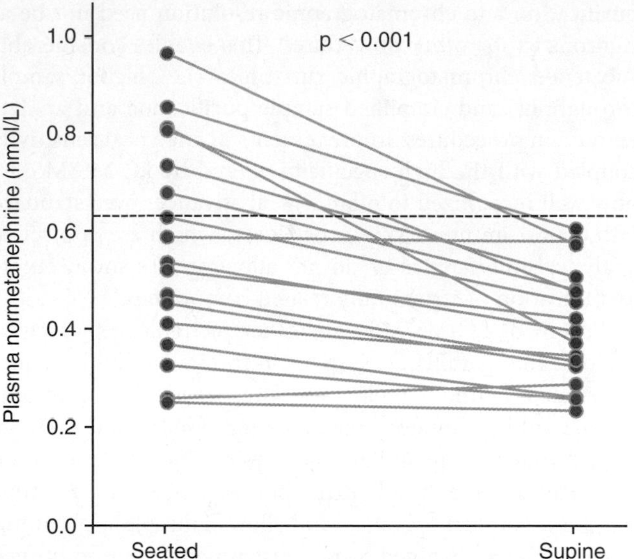

Figure 30-11 Plasma concentrations of free normetanephrine measured in blood samples taken from 17 healthy volunteers, first in the seated position, and then after 30 minutes' rest in the supine position. The *dotted horizontal line* indicates the upper reference intervals (0.61 nmol/L and 112 pg/mL) determined from the 95% confidence intervals of plasma normetanephrine concentrations in a separate population of 178 hypertensive and normotensive volunteers, with samples taken in the supine position as described elsewhere.[61]

Because of the rigid sampling conditions required for blood collections, many clinicians prefer 24-hour collections of urine to blood sampling. Urine collections in particular are more convenient for clinical staff to implement. However, 24-hour collections of urine are not always easily, conveniently, or reliably collected by patients, particularly pediatric patients. Also, influences of diet and sympathoadrenal activation associated with physical activity or changes in posture are not as easily controlled for as they are for blood collections.

To avoid possible errors resulting from incomplete 24-hour urine collections or uncontrolled influences of physical activity, some investigators advocate spot or overnight urine collections.[109,206] Correction for differences in duration of collection is achieved by normalizing catecholamine or catecholamine metabolite excretion against urinary creatinine excretion. Additional considerations for urine collected under these conditions include dietary protein, muscle mass, level of physical activity, and time of day, all of which influence creatinine excretion and may further confound interpretation of results.

Studies on the stability of catecholamines in urine and plasma have yielded mixed results and variable recommendations on appropriate preservatives and methods of collection.[12,224,261] In general, however, catecholamines are unstable in biological fluids, and appropriate precautions must be taken to minimize degradation. Nevertheless, the elaborate techniques for sample preservation recommended previously now appear to be largely unnecessary.

Variable findings on stability of urinary catecholamines may be explained by interindividual differences in the chemistry of patient samples, with auto-oxidation particularly prevalent at alkaline pH, and deconjugation prevalent at low pH—two processes with opposing effects on concentrations of free amines.[26,267] The general recommendation is that catecholamines in urine samples are best preserved with hydrochloric acid (HCl) to maintain urine acid. Aliquots are best stored frozen over protracted periods of time at −80 °C to further minimize auto-oxidation and deconjugation. Blood samples are best collected into tubes containing heparin or ethylenediaminetetraacetic acid (EDTA) as an anticoagulant and stored on ice before centrifugation at 4 °C, with separation of plasma for further storage at −80 °C.

In general, the metabolites of catecholamines are more stable than their parent amines.[26,267] Nevertheless, some consideration should be given to differences in the susceptibility of different metabolites to auto-oxidation and deconjugation. Urinary fractionated metanephrines usually are measured after a deconjugation step and therefore largely reflect sulfate conjugates, which are present in urine and plasma at much higher concentrations than free metabolites. These sulfate-conjugated metabolites appear to be relatively stable in urine. so there is little need for acidification during 24-hour collections.[267] For measurements of free metanephrines, this may be a problem, and consideration should be given to the likely confounding influence of deconjugation under acid conditions.

As outlined by Willemsen and colleagues,[267] use of EDTA and sodium metabisulphite ($Na_2S_2O_5$) instead of HCl as stabilizers should minimize deconjugation during initial collection, while still protecting catecholamines from auto-oxidation. Once the 24-hour collection is received, the urine can be acidified to pH 4.0 and stored frozen until assayed. Significant degradation of metabolites in urine has been noted after long-term storage up to 9 months at −18 °C.[46] Therefore, long-term storage at −80 °C remains recommended for both urine and plasma samples.

Studies on the stability of free metanephrines in urine are lacking. In samples of blood or plasma, however, it is clear that the metabolites are unstable if samples are left at room temperature for any length of time beyond 15 minutes for whole blood and a few hours for plasma.[266] At 4 °C, the free metanephrines are stable in whole blood for a few hours and in plasma for a longer period. Thus, for measurements of plasma free metanephrines, blood samples should be stored at 4 °C (e.g., on ice) before refrigerated centrifugation. The plasma may be stored refrigerated for up to 3 days before assay, but should be frozen for longer periods of storage.

Interferences from and Influences of Diet and Drugs

Dietary constituents or drugs can cause direct analytical interference in assays or can influence the physiologic processes that determine plasma and urinary concentrations of catecholamines and catecholamine metabolites. In the former circumstances, interference can be highly variable, depending on the particular measurement method used. The high analytical specificity offered by mass spectrometry–based methods provides a major advantage for these methods over other methods. In the latter circumstances, interference usually is of a more general nature and independent of the measurement method (Table 30-6).

Because of chromatographic interferences from dietary constituents, such as dihyrocaffeic acid,[89] blood sampling for measurements of catecholamines by HPLC is most appropriately carried out after an overnight fast. Such dietary constituents are unlikely to pose a problem for measurements by LC-MS/MS. Nevertheless, emerging evidence indicates other confounding influences of diet that are independent of the method of measurement.

High concentrations of catecholamines in numerous food products (e.g., fruits, vegetables, nuts), although well established to cause large increases in plasma and urinary concentrations of sulfate-conjugated catecholamines,[71,94,133] until

TABLE 30-6 Drug-Induced Increases in Catecholamines and Metanephrines

	CATECHOLAMINES		METANEPHRINES	
	NE	EPI	NMN	MN
Tricyclic Antidepressants				
Amitriptyline (Elavil), imipramine (Tofranil), nortriptyline (Aventyl)	+++	–	+++	–
α-Blockers (Nonselective)				
Phenoxybenzamine (Dibenzyline)	+++	–	+++	–
α-Blockers (α_1-Selective)				
Doxazosin (Cardura), terazosin (Hytrin), prazosin (Minipress)	+	–	–	–
β-Blockers				
Atenolol (Tenormin), metoprolol (Lopressor), propranolol (Inderal), labetalol* (Normodyne)	+	+	+	+
Calcium Channel Antagonists				
Nifedipine (Procardia), amlodipine (Norvasc), diltiazem (Cardizem), verapamil (Calan)	+	+	–	–
Vasodilators				
Hydralazine (Apresoline), isosorbide (Isordil, Dilatrate), minoxidil (Loniten)	+	–	Unknown	
Monoamine Oxidase Inhibitors				
Phenelzine (Nardil), tranylcypromine (Parnate), selegiline (Eldepryl)	–	–	+++	+++
Sympathomimetics				
Ephedrine, pseudoephedrine (Sudafed), amphetamines, albuterol (Proventil)	++	++	++	++
Stimulants				
Caffeine (coffee*, tea), nicotine (Tobacco), theophylline	++	++	Unknown	
Miscellaneous				
Levodopa, carbidopa (Sinemet)*	++	–	Unknown	
Cocaine	++	++	Unknown	

+++, Substantial increase; ++, moderate increase; +, mild increase if any; –, little or no increase.
*Indicates a drug that can also cause direct analytical interference with some methods.
Adapted from Young WF Jr. Pheochromocytoma: issues in diagnosis and treatment. Compr Ther 1997;23:319-26[273]; Eisenhofer G, Goldstein DS, Walther MM, Friberg P, Lenders JW, Keiser HR, et al. Biochemical diagnosis of pheochromocytoma: how to distinguish true- from false-positive test results. J Clin Endocrinol Metab 2003;88:2656-66.

recently have not been recognized as a confounding variable for measurements of other catecholamine metabolites. As shown by de Jong and associates,[50] dietary catecholamines can cause large increases in plasma concentrations and urinary outputs of the sulfate conjugates of normetanephrine and methoxytyramine. Concentrations of free methoxytyramine are also affected. Therefore, collection of blood samples after an overnight fast continues to be recommended as the simplest solution to avoid dietary influences on plasma measurements. This, however, is not practical for measurements of the urinary metabolites, for which other dietary restrictions may need to be considered.

Development of new drugs, variations in assay techniques, and continuing improvements in analytical procedures often make it difficult to identify which directly interfering medications should be avoided for a given analytical test. More readily identifiable and generalized sources of interference that are independent of the particular assay method tend to be associated with drugs that have primary actions on catecholamine systems. Because of the importance of these systems as therapeutic targets, such drugs represent a relatively common source of false-positive results.

Tricyclic antidepressants in particular are a major source of false-positive results for measurements of norepinephrine and normetanephrine in plasma or urine.[65] Presumably this is due to the primary inhibitory actions of these agents on monoamine reuptake. The result is increased escape of norepinephrine from sympathetic nerve terminals into the bloodstream.

Other medications that can cause significant interference, but that are less commonly encountered during testing for pheochromocytoma, include L-dopa, Sinemet, α-methyldopa (Aldomet®), and MAO inhibitors. L-Dopa used alone or in combination with carbidopa (Sinemet®) for the treatment of Parkinson's disease is an alumina-extractable catechol and the direct precursor of dopamine. The drug therefore can interfere directly with catecholamine assays and is converted by catecholamine synthesizing and metabolizing enzymes to catecholamine products and metabolites with additional interfering actions.[31,216] Similarly, the antihypertensive agent α-methyldopa is metabolized by catecholamine biosynthetic and metabolizing enzymes to α-methyldopamine, α-methylnorepinephrine, and other products, which in some but not all assays can result in significant interference.[42,189]

Because cellular uptake and not metabolism is the main determinant of catecholamine clearance, inhibitors of MAO have little effect on plasma or urinary catecholamines.[62] However, by blocking the main pathway for catabolism of the O-methylated catecholamine metabolites, MAO inhibitors can cause substantial increases in plasma concentrations and urinary excretion of normetanephrine and metanephrine.[58,257]

Reference Intervals

As indicated from the results of interlaboratory proficiency testing, measured values for monoamines and metabolites in identical samples can vary considerably among different laboratories, depending on differences in analytical methods and calibrators.[100,211,237] Establishment of and participation in interlaboratory quality assurance programs can be useful in improving consistency of calibrators and assay results among laboratories.[100,211] However, until such consistency is achieved, it remains important that laboratories appropriately establish their own method-specific reference intervals in suitably selected and sized populations according to the guidelines given in Chapter 5. The reference intervals outlined in this chapter or in kit method package inserts may serve as a general guide.

It is important to note that reference intervals should be established using the same precautions outlined earlier for collections of diagnostic samples from patients. In particular, for plasma free metanephrines, reference intervals should be established in blood samples taken after at least 30 minutes of supine rest.[158]

Plasma concentrations of plasma free normetanephrine in samples taken from subjects in the seated position on average are 30% higher than concentrations determined in the supine position (see Figure 30-11). Thus, reference intervals can also be expected to be 30% higher. It might be argued that this should not pose a problem so long as samples are consistently taken in one position or another. This argument, however, ignores the fact that production of metanephrines by a tumor is autonomous of changes in sympathoadrenal activity.

The high diagnostic sensitivity of plasma free metanephrines reflects the strong signal produced by catecholamine-producing tumors relative to the background noise associated with production of metabolites from sympathoadrenal sources. Increasing the background noise by sampling in the seated position instead of in the recommended supine position will decrease the relative strength of the diagnostic signal from a catecholamine-producing tumor. Reduced diagnostic sensitivity and increased numbers of false-negative results can therefore be expected when blood samples for both reference intervals and diagnostic tests are collected in the seated instead of the supine position.[158] An example is illustrated in Figure 30-12. To optimize the diagnostic signal produced by a catecholamine-producing tumor, blood samples collected for reference intervals and diagnostic testing should be collected under conditions of low baseline sympathoadrenal activity, with subjects in the supine position.

Influences of dietary biogenic amines are a particularly important consideration when reference intervals are established for measurements of serotonin and 5-HIAA. Although a biogenic amine free diet does not appear to be important for measurements of free normetanephrine and metanephrine, emerging evidence indicates that such a diet may be an important consideration for measurements of the deconjugated metabolites in both urine and plasma.[50] Because both free and deconjugated methoxytyramine are affected by dietary catecholamines, the simplest precaution for plasma tests of the free metabolites is an overnight fast. For urine measurements of free and deconjugated metabolites, a longer period of an amine free diet may be required.

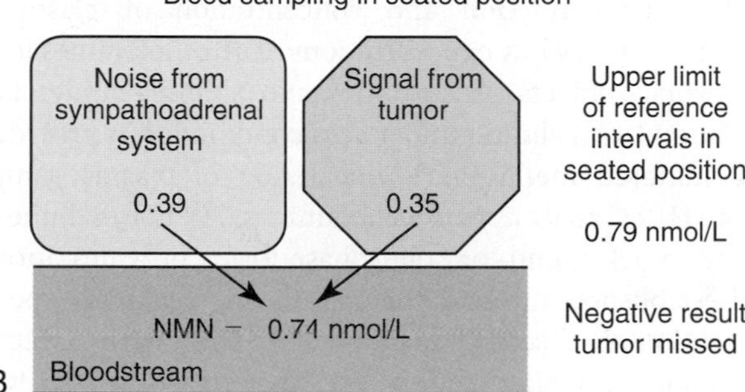

Figure 30-12 Mathematical explanation illustrating the importance of blood sampling in the supine position for establishing reference intervals for plasma concentrations of free metanephrines.

Reference intervals should also be established with due consideration of frequency distributions (see Chapter 5). Concentrations of catecholamines and metanephrines in 24-hour urine specimens and plasma are not normally distributed.[106,154,223] Normalization of distributions, usually achievable by logarithmic transformation, can be used to establish valid reference intervals. Alternatively, nonparametric methods may be used.[106]

A certain proportion of false-positive results must always be expected depending on how confidence intervals are set and how many analytes are used in the test. For pairs of test results commonly used for diagnosis of pheochromocytoma (e.g., normetanephrine and metanephrine), it can be expected that the proportion of false-positive results will exceed that determined by the reference percentiles set for each test. However, proportions of false-positive results usually tend to be even higher than expected; this is likely due to reduced control over sampling conditions and sources of interference or differences in clinical characteristics of reference and patient populations.

Because of the normally very low pretest prevalence of catecholamine-producing tumors and the resulting high proportion of false-positive compared with true-positive results, some investigators have advocated using decision limits above the upper reference limits of diagnostic tests to maximize diagnostic specificity and to minimize false-positive results.[140,226] However, this is always done at the expense of decreased diagnostic sensitivity. Because of the dangers of a missed diagnosis, it is therefore recommended that reference intervals for plasma or urinary fractionated metanephrines should be established primarily to ensure optimum diagnostic sensitivity, with specificity a secondary consideration.[99,203]

Use of appropriately matched reference populations can be important for effective diagnosis of monoamine-producing tumors among different populations of patients tested for such tumors. Urinary and plasma concentrations of catecholamines and metanephrines show different reference intervals in hypertensive or hospitalized patients compared with normotensive healthy volunteers,[187,223] in children compared with adults,[187,215,221,262] and in males compared with females.[55,85]

Patients with hypertension tend to have higher plasma and 24-hour urinary concentrations of catecholamines and metanephrines than normotensive patients.[55,152] Use of reference intervals established in hypertensive rather than normotensive populations therefore minimizes the likelihood of false-positive results in patients most commonly tested for pheochromocytoma because of high blood pressure and symptoms of catecholamine excess. However, these same reference intervals may not be necessarily appropriate for patients with pheochromocytoma who are normotensive and asymptomatic and are tested for the tumor because of a hereditary predisposition or the finding of an adrenal incidentaloma. In some of these patients, the tumor may be too small to produce large enough quantities of catecholamines and their *O*-methylated metabolites for a positive test result using reference intervals established in hypertensive, hospital patient populations. For such patient populations, use of reference intervals established in normotensive healthy volunteers may be more appropriate.

Reference intervals for plasma and urinary catecholamines and catecholamine metabolites also differ according to gender and age. Females have lower plasma concentrations of epinephrine and metanephrine than males.[55] Similarly, 24-hour urinary outputs of catecholamines and metanephrines are lower in women than in men[85,128]; for epinephrine, this difference remains significant when values are normalized for creatinine excretion.[85] Plasma concentrations of norepinephrine and normetanephrine increase with advancing age in adults, whereas plasma concentrations of epinephrine and metanephrine are little affected.[55,227] Age-related increases in 24-hour urinary outputs of norepinephrine and normetanephrine have also been reported.[128,152] In general, the influences of age and gender on adult reference intervals are relevant to consider only for patients with borderline normal or abnormal biochemical test results.

Age is particularly important to consider in children. Because of the dynamic changes that occur throughout childhood, and because of the difficulty of obtaining complete urine collections, a standard practice for biochemical testing in children is to normalize excretion of catecholamines and metanephrines to that of creatinine. When this is done, ratios of urinary catecholamines or metanephrines to creatinine show a decrease with age throughout childhood.[22,168,215] Therefore, it is imperative that age-appropriate reference intervals are used for urinary outputs of catecholamines and catecholamine metabolites in children. For measurements of metanephrines and catecholamines in plasma, the differences are less dramatic than in urine, but nevertheless should be considered. For children, upper reference intervals for plasma normetanephrine and noradrenaline are lower than for adults, whereas for metanephrine and epinephrine, upper limits are higher in children than in adults.[262]

Another patient population in which the usual reference intervals are often invalid, and in which diagnosis of a catecholamine-producing tumor can prove particularly difficult involves patients with renal failure.[13,70,246] In end-stage renal failure, urine collections may be impossible; even in less severely affected patients, results of 24-hour urine testing are difficult to interpret. Impaired renal function results in dramatic increases in plasma concentrations of VMA and sulfate-conjugated metanephrines, rendering these tests invalid.[70,111,185] In contrast, because the circulatory clearance of plasma catecholamines and free metanephrines is largely independent of renal function, measurements of these analytes in plasma represent the most appropriate tests for diagnosis of pheochromocytoma in renal failure.[70] Nevertheless, plasma concentrations of catecholamines and free metanephrines tend to be elevated more in patients with renal failure than in normal and hypertensive populations. Also, diet- and medication-associated interferences with chromatographic analysis tend to be much more pronounced in patients with renal failure, making it difficult to obtain reliable results using HPLC methods. LC-MS/MS methods should provide advantages in this context.

Plasma Catecholamines and Metanephrines

Highly sensitive, specific, and reliable assay methods are required for measuring the normally very low concentrations of free catecholamines and their *O*-methylated metabolites in plasma. Plasma concentrations of dopamine and its *O*-methylated metabolite, methoxytyramine, are particularly low, making accurate measurements of these analytes especially difficult.

The sulfate-conjugated metabolites of the catecholamines and metanephines are present in plasma at higher concentrations than the free forms. Plasma concentrations of dopamine sulfate in particular are more than 100-fold higher than those of free dopamine, and plasma concentrations of the sulfate conjugates of normetanephrine, metanephrine, and methoxytyramine are 20- to 30-fold higher than concentrations of the free metabolites.[60,96] Rather than reflecting differences in rates of formation, the higher plasma concentrations of the sulfate conjugates reflect their relatively slow circulatory clearance by renal extraction and elimination in the urine. This contrasts with the free catecholamines and their *O*-methylated metabolites, all of which are cleared rapidly from the bloodstream by active extraneuronal uptake mechanisms.[62]

Although the catecholamines and their *O*-methylated metabolites are more easily measured in their deconjugated than in their free form, measurements in the free form are preferred because this avoids the potential confounding influences of diet or impaired renal function. The more rapid circulatory clearances and correspondingly much shorter plasma half-lives of the free than the conjugated forms mean that only relatively short periods of supine rest are required to reach the low baseline concentrations useful for exclusion of catecholamine-producing tumors. This also makes such measurements useful for investigations of rapid changes in the disposition of catecholamines produced, released and metabolized by the sympathetic nervous and adrenal medullary systems.

HPLC assays currently remain the most accepted and commonly employed method for accurate determination of catecholamines in plasma. However, these methods require preliminary extraction and concentration of plasma to measure the very low concentrations of catecholamines found in normal subjects. Adsorption onto alumina under basic conditions with elution under acid conditions has provided a time-honored method for preparation of plasma samples before HPLC analysis of catecholamines.[54,171] Use of diphenylborate in gel, liquid, or solid-phase forms provides another well-established method that allows for relatively specific adsorption of catecholamines.[114,217,254] Solid-phase extraction techniques utilizing cation exchange or other matrices provide other methods that have become increasingly popular for purification of plasma samples.[53,163,225] Ultrafiltration also has been used for sample preparation.[252]

Many HPLC procedures analyze the derived plasma extracts using reversed-phase chromatography with ion-pairing reagents; others use cation-exchange HPLC columns to separate the extracted amines. Electrochemical detection (EC) using amperometric or coulometric measurement is commonly used to quantify the catecholamines.[54,225] HPLC separation can also be coupled with fluorescence detection,[254] but precolumn or postcolumn derivatization techniques are required to enhance sensitivity and specificity.

Reflecting increased recognition of the importance of metanephrines for diagnosis of catecholamine-producing tumors, numerous new methods are available for measurement of these metabolites in plasma. In addition to the earlier described HPLC-EC procedures,[153] immunoassay methods[84,159] and LC-MS/MS procedures are now available.[48,148] All are undergoing continuing modification to improve their reliability for measurement of low concentrations of free metanephrines in plasma.

Modifications to the original HPLC-EC method for measurement of plasma free metanephrines, as initially described in 1993,[153] include improvements to the procedures for cation-exchange sample purification or coulometric detection that minimize analytical interferences.[110,219] Other improvements to instrumentation have enabled measurement of extremely low plasma concentrations of methoxytyramine, in addition to routinely measured normetanephrine and metanephrine.[69]

As outlined elsewhere,[236] the need for labor-intensive and time-consuming sample preparation procedures represents a major limiting factor for HPLC-EC measurements of plasma free metanephrines. This, together with relatively long chromatographic run times of up to 40 minutes, severely limits throughput of samples. Introduction of LC-MS/MS methods for measurements of plasma free metanephrines, initially described in 2004 by Lagerstedt and colleagues[148] and then by several other groups,[48,169] represents a major advance in addressing many of the shortcomings of HPLC-EC procedures.

The higher analytical specificity offered by LC-MS/MS methods avoids the analytical interferences that can plague HPLC-EC methods; it also means that the preanalytical sample cleanup need not be as rigorous as for HPLC-EC methods. To minimize ion suppression, some preanalytical cleanup remains necessary, but in one outlined procedure, all that was required was an isopropanol protein precipitation step followed by evaporation of the supernatant.[169] In another procedure, sample preparation was performed using an automated online system.[48] Continuing technical advances in instrumentation providing increased analytical sensitivity also make it possible to use smaller volumes of plasma and yet still measure methoxytyramine. This advance now makes it possible to assess these analytical methods in infants with neuroblastoma, a patient population for which sample volumes are important limiting factors for diagnostic tests involving blood sampling.[238]

A further advance of importance for many routine laboratories is the high sample throughput possible with LC-MS/MS procedures. Sample run times of less than 8 minutes compared with longer than 30 minutes for HPLC-EC procedures enable a more than four-fold increase in the numbers of samples that can be run by a single LC-MS/MS instrument. Because of these advances, it has been relatively easy for high-throughput commercial laboratories to justify the costs of LC-MS/MS instruments. Consequently, most such laboratories now utilize LC-MS/MS for measurements of plasma free metanephrines.

As indicated by interlaboratory proficiency programs, the analytical performance of immunoassays appears to be less than optimal compared with HPLC-EC and LC-MS/MS methods.[211] Difficulties in obtaining L-isomers of the metanephrines for calibration of stereo-specific immunoassays have presented a problem likely contributing to large differences in measured concentrations of free metanephrines by immunoassays compared with HPLC-EC and LC-MS/MS procedures.

Representative reference intervals for plasma concentrations of catecholamines are shown in Table 30-7; those for free and deconjugated (free plus conjugated) metanephrines in normotensive and hypertensive adults and in normotensive children are shown in Table 30-8.

Plasma L-Dopa, DOPAC, and DHPG

HPLC measurements of plasma catechols usually are limited to dopamine, norepinephrine, and epinephrine. However, with an alumina adsorption extraction procedure, it is possible to simultaneously measure several other catechols by HPLC.[54] These catechols include (1) DHPG, the deaminated metabolite of norepinephrine and epinephrine; (2) DOPAC, the deaminated metabolite of dopamine; and (3) 3,4-dihydroxyphenylalanine (L-dopa), the immediate precursor of dopamine. All are present in plasma at concentrations many-fold higher than the catecholamines, making their detection relatively simple once appropriate chromatographic separation is achieved.

Each of the above catechols provide unique and useful clinical information about the function of peripheral catecholamine systems.[97] DHPG in plasma is almost exclusively derived from deamination of norepinephrine in sympathetic nerves. These measurements therefore provide information about the activity of MAO. Decreases in plasma DHPG combined with reciprocal increases in normetanephrine, as assessed by plasma DHPG/normetanephrine ratios, provide a particularly useful method for identifying patients with deficiencies of MAO.[155] DHPG is derived in part from deamination of the norepinephrine recaptured by sympathetic

TABLE 30-7 Reference Intervals for Plasma Catecholamines in Normotensive and Hypertensive Adults and in Normotensive Children

	Norepinephrine	Epinephrine	Dopamine
Hypertensive Adults			
pg/mL	101-711	3-111	1-42
nmol/L	0.60-4.21	0.02-0.61	0.01-0.28
Normotensive Adults			
pg/mL	78-466	2-87	1-33
nmol/L	0.46-2.76	0.01-0.48	0.01-0.22
Normotensive Children			
pg/mL	96-294	3-90	1-30
nmol/L	0.57-1.74	0.02-0.49	0.01-0.20

Note: The above reference intervals were determined after an overnight fast with subjects resting for 30 minutes in the supine position before blood sampling. Reference intervals may vary according to mode of sample collection, method of measurement, and source of calibrators. The laboratory performing the measurements should establish its own independent reference intervals. The above reference intervals therefore serve as a general guide but should not be used for diagnostic decision making.

TABLE 30-8 Reference Intervals for Plasma Free and Deconjugated Normetanephrine (NMN) and Metanephrine (MN) in Normotensive and Hypertensive Adults and in Normotensive Children

	Free Metanephrines		Deconjugated Metanephrines	
	NMN	MN	NMN	MN
Hypertensive Adults				
pg/mL	24-141	12-72	755-5623	327-2042
nmol/L	0.13-0.77	0.06-0.37	4.1-30.7	1.7-10.4
Normotensive Adults				
pg/mL	18-101	12-67	624-3041	328-1837
nmol/L	0.10-0.55	0.06-0.34	3.4-16.6	1.7-9.3
Normotensive Children				
pg/mL	22-83	10-95	851-2398	380-1995
nmol/L	0.12-0.45	0.05-0.48	4.7-13.1	1.9-10.1

Note: The above reference intervals were determined after an overnight fast with subjects resting for 30 minutes in the supine position before blood sampling. Reference intervals may vary according to mode of sample collection, method of measurement, and source of calibrators. The laboratory performing the measurements should establish its own independent reference intervals. The above reference intervals therefore serve as a general guide but should not be used for diagnostic decision making.

nerves and in part from leakage of the transmitter from storage vesicles into the sympathetic axoplasm. Provided appropriate procedures are employed to distinguish the two sources, measurements of DHPG can be used to evaluate norepinephrine transporter function and to assess the state of sympathoneural transmitter stores.

Approximately 8% of the L-dopa synthesized in sympathetic nerves is not converted to dopamine, but instead escapes into the bloodstream. Plasma concentrations of L-dopa therefore provide information about the activity of tyrosine hydroxylase, the rate-limiting enzyme in catecholamine synthesis.[91] Changes in plasma L-dopa also occur in a variety of disorders that feature derangements in catecholamine synthesis. Patients with neuroblastomas can have extremely high plasma L-dopa concentrations.[72,90] Small amounts of circulating L-dopa appear to be derived from melanocytes, where amino acid is produced during phase I melanogenesis. Thus highly elevated plasma L-dopa concentrations occur in patients with melanoma, particularly when this is associated with development of metastases.[160] Increases in plasma L-dopa occur in patients with deficiencies of aromatic L-amino acid decarboxylase, and decreases occur in inherited disorders featuring impaired tyrosine hydroxylase activity.[93]

Although simultaneous measurements of plasma L-dopa, DHPG, and the catecholamines offer considerable clinical utility, adoption of the method in the routine clinical chemistry laboratory is limited by several technical problems. First, separation of all the catechols and of DHPG from the solvent front requires relatively low mobile phase concentrations of organic modifiers. This consequently leads to long chromatographic run times that limit high throughput of more of the commonly requested catecholamines. Second, interference from uric acid presents a problem for measurement of DHPG by most amperometric detectors. This problem can be overcome by using a coulometric electrode system for irreversible oxidation of uric acid with detection of catechols at a reducing instead of the more commonly used oxidizing potential. Third, recoveries of DHPG, L-dopa, and DOPAC from alumina tend to be lower than that of the catecholamines, presenting some problem regarding their accurate measurement. This latter problem is resolved by the use of minimum quantities of alumina, close attention to types and strengths of acids used in the elution of catechols from alumina, and additional correction for differences in recoveries from the internal standard.[115]

Alternatives to simultaneous measurements of the various plasma catechols include methods of individual measurements more suitable for specific applications. Examples include HPLC measurements of L-dopa and 3-*O*-methyldopa in Parkinson's disease or malignant melanoma.[6,160]

Representative reference intervals for plasma concentrations of L-dopa, DOPAC, and DHPG in normotensive adults are shown in Table 30-9.

Urinary Catecholamines and Metanephrines

The catecholamines and their O-methylated metabolites are excreted in urine as free amines and as sulfate conjugates in proportions that largely reflect their circulating concentrations in plasma. The notable exception is urinary free dopamine, which is largely derived from renal extraction of circulating L-dopa and conversion in the kidney to free dopamine.[19] Thus, whereas concentrations of free dopamine in plasma are lower than those of norepinephrine and epinephrine, concentrations of free dopamine in urine considerably exceed those of norepinephrine and epinephrine.

Urinary catecholamines are commonly measured in the free form. In contrast, urinary metanephrines are usually measured after an acid hydrolysis step, so that these

TABLE 30-9 Reference Intervals for Plasma Concentrations of L-Dopa, DOPAC, and DHPG in Normotensive and Hypertensive Adults and in Normotensive Children

	L-Dopa	DOPAC	DHPG
Hypertensive Adults			
pg/mL	1048-2485	595-2742	446-1591
nmol/L	6.24-14.79	3.27-15.07	2.62-9.36
Normotensive Adults			
pg/mL	1099-1552	762-2916	567-1284
nmol/L	6.54-9.24	4.19-16.02	3.34-7.55
Normotensive Children			
pg/mL	1107-2545	695-4399	529-1215
nmol/L	6.59-15.15	3.82-24.17	3.11-7.15

Note: The above reference intervals were determined after an overnight fast with subjects resting for 30 minutes in the supine position before blood sampling. Reference intervals may vary according to mode of sample collection, method of measurement, and source of calibrators. The laboratory performing the measurements should establish its own independent reference intervals. The above reference intervals therefore serve as a general guide but should not be used for diagnostic decision making.

measurements reflect both free and conjugated metabolites, but mainly the latter, the predominant form in both plasma and urine. These procedural differences in part reflect the results of early studies, indicating consistently clear influences of dietary catecholamines on plasma and urinary concentrations of conjugated catecholamines, but inconsistent influences on urinary metanephrines.[23,36,182] In 2009, de Jong and coworkers[50] established that dietary catecholamines are capable of causing substantial increases in urinary excretion of deconjugated normetanephine, without appreciably affecting excretion of free normetanephrine. Such effects of diet may explain findings of higher rates of false-positive results for measurements of urinary fractionated metanephrines than plasma free metanephrines,[156] providing additional incentive for investigations of urinary free metanephrines as an alternative to standard measurements of urinary deconjugated metanephrines.[14]

HPLC-EC methods that allow selective quantification of urinary epinephrine, norepinephrine, and dopamine continue to serve as the principal approach used by routine clinical laboratories for measurements of urinary catecholamines. Numerous preanalytical cleanup techniques have been described for preparing samples of urine into a form suitable for analysis.[270] An alumina extraction procedure typically is coupled with ion-exchange or adsorption chromatography. Alumina pretreatment usually involves a batch extraction technique in which catechols first are adsorbed at pH 8.6 and then are eluted with boric acid, which forms a complex with *cis*-diol groups. Purification on boric acid affinity gels provides an alternative procedure for selective adsorption of catecholamines.

Analysis of urinary catecholamines and metanephrines by electrochemical detection with ion-pairing adaptations of reversed-phase chromatography is the most common method, and ion pairing with alkyl sulfonates or sulfates is generally used to enhance retention of cationic amine moieties on lipophilic stationary phases.[187,222] Potential analytical interference, depending on chromatographic conditions, has been reported with α-methyldopa,[187] acetaminophen,[268] labetalol,[77] and captopril.[34] Most of the analytical interferences discussed here can be avoided by tandem mass spectrometry methods, which offer the added advantage of high-throughput capability.[145]

Selective quantification of metanephrine and normetanephrine by HPLC-EC techniques provides a valuable method for measurements of urinary fractionated metanephrines.[235,265] However, it can be expected that HPLC-EC techniques will increasingly be superseded by high-throughput mass spectrometric methods that additionally offer considerably improved analytical specificity.[35,248,263]

Isolation of metanephrines from the urine for HPLC-EC techniques usually is accomplished through ion-exchange chromatography. Weak cation-exchange resins are used primarily, although some procedures use a combination of strong and weak cation exchange to enhance recovery. Differential solvent extraction methods (e.g., using ethyl acetate and cyclohexane) can also be applied to remove potential interference. Column conditions and stationary phases vary; typical applications include reversed-phase chromatography with ion-pairing reagents and silica-based cation-exchange chromatography. Analytical interferences that may falsely increase the HPLC-based estimation of normetanephrine or metanephrine have been reported for viloxazine,[8] acetaminophen,[45] labetalol,[77] and buspirone.[32] Methenamine has been reported to cause an unusual form of interference related to a decrease in the signal strength of the internal standard, 4-*O*-methytyramine, leading to falsely elevated increases in both normetanephrine and metanephrine.[255]

Use of LC-MS/MS avoids the analytical interference problems already discussed and enables faster analytical run times and less arduous preanalytical cleanup steps. Whiting examined five different types of solid-phase extraction cartridges and identified one cartridge that, in combination with diphenyl-boronate as a complexing agent, allowed elution of both catecholamines and metanephrines in a form suitable for direct injection into the LC-MS/MS system.[263] This method thereby allows simultaneous determination of urinary metanephrines and catecholamines, all quantified within 6 minutes of sample injection.

Representative reference intervals for free catecholamines, based on 24-hour outputs[187] and creatinine excretion[221] in normotensive children and adults, are shown in Table 30-10; those for deconjugated metanephrine and normetanephrine in children and adults are shown in Table 30-11. Diagnostic testing based on overnight rather than on 24-hour urine collections for measurements of catecholamines and metanephines provides an alternative strategy that minimizes the potentially confounding influences of posture, ambulation,

TABLE 30-10 Reference Intervals for Urinary Free Catecholamines

	Age, y	Epinephrine	Norepinephrine	Dopamine
Daily excretion, µg/24 h (nmol/24 h)	0-1	≤2.5 (≤14)	≤10 (≤59)	≤85 (≤555)
	1-2	≤3.5 (≤19)	1-17 (6-100)	10-140 (65-914)
	2-4	≤6.0 (≤33)	4-29 (24-171)	40-260 (261-1697)
	4-7	0.2-10 (1-55)	8-45 (47-266)	65-400 (424-2612)
	7-10	0.2-10 (1-55)	13-65 (77-384)	65-400 (424-2612)
	10-15	0.5-20 (3-109)	15-80 (89-473)	65-400 (424-2612)
	>15	0.5-20 (3-109)	15-80 (89-473)	65-400 (424-2612)
Excretion relative to creatinine, µg/g creatinine	0-1	≤0.38	≤0.31	≤1.29
	1-4	≤0.08	≤0.29	≤1.22
	4-10	≤0.09	≤0.11	≤0.72
	10-18	≤0.06	≤0.11	≤0.45
	>18	≤0.04	≤0.11	≤0.35

Note: Reference intervals may vary according to mode of sample collection, method of measurement, and source of calibrators. The laboratory performing the measurements should establish its own independent reference intervals. The above reference intervals therefore serve as a general guide but should not be used for diagnostic decision making.

TABLE 30-11 Reference Intervals for Urinary Deconjugated Metanephrine and Normetanephrine

	Metanephrine		Normetanephrine	
Age	µg/d	µg/g Creatinine	µg/d	µg/g Creatinine
0-3 mo	5.9-37	202-708	47-156	1535-3355
4-6 mo	6.1-42	156-572	31-111	737-2194
7-9 mo	12.0-41	150-526	42-109	592-1046
10-12 mo	8.5-101	148-651	23-103	271-1117
1-2 y	6.7-52	40-526	32-118	350-1275
2-6 y	11-99	74-504	50-111	104-609
6-10 y	54-138	121-319	47-176	103-452
10-16 y	39-242	46-307	53-290	96-411
Adult	74-297		105-354	

Note: Reference intervals may vary according to mode of sample collection, method of measurement, and source of calibrators. The laboratory performing the measurements should establish its own independent reference intervals. The above reference intervals therefore serve as a general guide but should not be used for diagnostic decision making.

exercise, and mental stress–associated increases in sympathoadrenal activity during waking hours.[206] For such investigations, reference intervals must be established that take into account diurnal variations in the excretion of catecholamines and metanephrines.

Urinary Vanillylmandelic Acid and Homovanillic Acid

In humans, vanillylmandelic acid (VMA) is the major end product of norepinephrine and epinephrine metabolism excreted in urine.[67] VMA is not significantly conjugated; therefore, it is measured without a hydrolysis step. More than 94% of the VMA excreted in urine is formed in the liver, where the presence of alcohol dehydrogenase leads to oxidation of MHPG derived from portal venous inflow (60%) or produced locally by *O*-methlylation of DHPG after removal from the bloodstream by the liver (28%).[57] Because most MHPG is derived from DHPG, and since DHPG is derived almost exclusively from deamination of norepinephrine within sympathetic nerves, very little VMA is derived from circulating catecholamines or metanephrines. Consequently, VMA provides a relatively poor diagnostic marker for pheochromocytoma.[156] In practice, VMA is now used most frequently in combination with urinary homovanillic acid (HVA) in the detection and monitoring of neuroblastoma.

HVA, in contrast to VMA, is not produced to any appreciable extent in the liver[59]—a difference attributable to dependence of its formation on the combined actions of catechol-O-methyltransferase and monoamine oxidase, without the requirement of any additional action of hepatic alcohol dehydrogenase.[67] HVA is produced and excreted in

TABLE 30-12 Reference Intervals for Urinary VMA and HVA

Age, y	VMA, mg/g Creatinine	HVA, mg/g Creatinine
0-3 mo	3.0-18.9	6.4-35.0
3-6 mo	2.9-21.8	12.5-32.1
6-12 mo	4.9-16.9	9.0-31.4
1-2 y	2.5-15.5	5.7-27.3
2-5 y	2.1-10.3	2.7-23.5
5-10 y	1.1-7.6	1.1-16.5
10-15 y	1.1-5.6	1.1-9.7
15-20 y	0.7-4.3	1.4-5.8
20-25 y	0.4-4.6	0.6-5.2

Note: Reference intervals may vary according to mode of sample collection, method of measurement, and source of calibrators. The laboratory performing the measurements should establish its own independent reference intervals. The above reference intervals therefore serve as a general guide but should not be used for diagnostic decision making.

urine in both free and conjugated forms at up to twice the rate for VMA. About 30% of HVA appears to be derived from dopamine metabolized in the gastrointestinal tract and 12% in the brain[59,67]; the source of the remaining HVA is unclear.

Earlier spectrophotometric methods for determination of VMA and HVA have largely been replaced by gas chromatography or, more commonly, by HPLC methods of analysis. In addition, gas chromatographic methods with flame ionization or mass spectrometric detection have been described for determinations of urinary VMA and HVA.[75,233,249] HPLC is, however, the most frequently used chromatographic method, featuring isocratic reversed-phase separation with electrochemical, spectrophotometric, fluorometric, or postcolumn detection.[9,83,220] Anion-exchange chromatography has been used effectively to isolate VMA and HVA from urine prior to HPLC analysis.[9] Mass screening for neuroblastoma using filter paper sample collection and transport has also been reported with simultaneous liquid chromatography measurement of VMA and HVA. HPLC applications are relatively free of interference and may provide simultaneous measurement of additional metabolites.[11,27,43,87,205]

LC-MS/MS methods have been developed for determination of urinary VMA,[164] as well as for combined determinations of urinary VMA, HVA, and 5-HIAA.[161] For the latter method, the sample preparation before injection on the LC-MS/MS instrument simply involves dilution and centrifugation. The minimal sample preparation step represents a significant advance, reflecting the high analytical specificity allowed by tandem mass spectrometric methods, the relatively high urinary concentrations of the acid metabolites, and consequent minimal problems associated with ion suppression,

Urinary VMA and HVA may be measured in 24-hour urine samples or in random urine specimens corrected for urinary output for creatinine. Because of the challenge in collecting 24-hour specimens in neonates and pediatric patients, testing of random urine for VMA, HVA, and creatinine is the predominant practice. Reference intervals for both timed and random specimens have been reported in a number of studies, usually with limited subjects and age intervals. A few larger reference interval studies have been reported.[78,212,215] Data from a 2009 study of 865 outpatients categorized into nine age groups from birth to early adult years, with age-specific 95% reference intervals for VMA and HVA measurement in acidified random urine collections, are listed in Table 30-12.[215]

Serotonin and Metabolites

Serotonin

A variety of specific and precise analytical methods are available for the determination of serotonin in body fluids and platelets.[135] HPLC with fluorometric[2,25,147] or electrochemical[151,214] detection is the most frequently used chromatographic method. HPLC techniques have been developed for measuring serotonin separately or have been adapted for simultaneous measurement of metabolically related indoles such as 5-HTP and 5-HIAA. Preliminary extraction and deproteinization are required before analysis, with several choices available. Solvent partition has been largely replaced by methods that employ cation-exchange resins. Other solid-phase extraction procedures have also been employed to isolate serotonin, such as reversed-phase chromatography using disposable cartridges of octadecylsilyl (ODS)-silica. Several methods simply deproteinize with perchloric acid or trichloroacetic acid before injecting the sample directly onto the HPLC column.

Most HPLC assays employ ODS (C18) reversed-phase columns, although strong cation-exchange columns have also been used. Chromatography is usually performed with an isocratic mobile phase at an acid pH that contains an organic modifier and perhaps an ion-pair reagent. Serotonin is protonated in the pH range of 3 to 6, and addition of an anionic ion-pair reagent creates an uncharged conjugate, which enhances the affinity of serotonin for the hydrophobic stationary phase. For measurements of very small amounts of serotonin or for specialized projects, HPLC with amperometric or coulometric detection is often favored over fluorometric detection. Serotonin is readily oxidized electrochemically, and the current that flows is proportional to concentration. For serotonin, the oxidation potential is below 0.6 V; this reduces the risk of electrochemical interference by other compounds. If other tryptophan metabolites are analyzed simultaneously, however, higher oxidation potentials are required.

To enhance analytical sensitivity, some HPLC procedures incorporate precolumn derivatization with fluorescent[127] and chemiluminescent[121] reagents, thereby achieving detection limits in the femtomole range. Completely automated analyses of serotonin have been described, and some systems incorporate direct injection and online solid-phase extraction.[136] Mass spectrometric methods offer considerably improved specificity and expanded linear range while permitting simultaneous determination of related indoles.[40] For laboratories that may not have the equipment, staff, or experience to measure serotonin by HPLC or LC-MS/MS methods, alternative technologies based on radioimmunoassay (RIA) and enzyme immunoassay (EIA) are available as commercial test kits.

Serotonin has been measured in (1) whole blood, (2) serum, (3) platelet-rich plasma, (4) platelet-poor plasma (i.e., platelet-free plasma), (5) isolated platelet pellets, (6) urine, and (7) CSF. Most blood serotonin is stored in the platelets and is easily released during sample preparation. For whole blood serotonin, venous blood (10 mL) is drawn into a tube containing potassium EDTA as an anticoagulant, gently mixed, placed on ice, and transferred to a storage tube containing an antioxidant such as ascorbic acid. The latter stabilizes serotonin, which is sensitive to light, oxygen, and high (or low) pH. An aliquot of blood is then removed for a platelet count; alternatively, a simultaneous EDTA blood sample can be collected. Blood serotonin samples are stored frozen at −20 °C, preferably within 2 hours after collection.

Platelet-rich plasma samples are prepared from whole blood by centrifuging at 120×g for 30 minutes at 4 °C[173] or at 200×g for 15 minutes at room temperature.[214] To prevent lowering of the serotonin concentration, platelet-rich plasma is prepared within 1 hour after the blood is collected and placed on ice. An aliquot of platelet-rich plasma is removed for a platelet count. Platelet-poor plasma and platelet pellets are prepared from measured aliquots of the platelet-rich sample plasma by centrifuging at 4500×g for 10 minutes at 4 °C[202] or at 1000×g for 30 minutes at room temperature.[214] To reduce the probability of platelet rupture, samples should never be frozen before the cell-free plasma is obtained. Plasma and pellets are stored frozen at −20 °C and are analyzed within 1 to 2 weeks after collection.

Serum samples are conveniently collected in serum separation tubes (SSTs). Blood clotting releases serotonin from platelets; samples should be centrifuged within 1 hour after collection and stored frozen at −20 °C. Twenty-four- hour urine samples are collected in 2-L brown polypropylene bottles containing 250 mg each of sodium metabisulfite and EDTA as preservatives. Samples are acidified to pH 4 with acetic acid before freezing.

Whole blood measurement of serotonin is popular because time-consuming isolation of platelets is not required. In general, serotonin concentrations in whole blood, collected with EDTA anticoagulant, better represent peripheral blood concentrations than serum serotonin, although the latter are often recommended for pediatric patients. Whole blood serotonin concentrations, expressed in nmol/L, are higher while standing than supine because of an increase in platelets.[214] For meaningful comparisons, whole blood serotonin determinations should be corrected for platelet count. Several types of anticoagulants have been studied for their ability to prevent release of serotonin from platelets; potassium EDTA gave better results than citrate in platelet-free plasma.[176] Serotonin measurements in whole blood, serum, or platelet-rich plasma are not significantly influenced by short-term ingestion of serotonin- or tryptophan-rich foods.[133] Similar to 5-HIAA, urinary serotonin concentrations are markedly affected by diet. Medications that may affect serotonin concentrations include lithium, MAO inhibitors, methyldopa, morphine, and reserpine. Serotonin reuptake inhibitors, such as fluoxetine, may deplete platelet serotonin concentrations. Platelet serotonin is age dependent; elderly subjects have higher values than newborns but lower values than children and adults.[80] Representative reference intervals are shown in Table 30-13.

5-Hydroxyindoleacetic Acid (5-HIAA)

Earlier spectrophotometric and fluorometric procedures for quantifying 5-HIAA in urine and plasma have been replaced by more selective and specific methods, including (1) gas chromatography, (2) immunoassays, (3) HPLC, and (4) LC-MS/MS. In practice, HPLC continues to be the most widespread method for measuring 5-HIAA in the clinical

TABLE 30-13 Reference Intervals for Serotonin in Whole Blood, Serum, Urine, CSF, Platelets, and Platelet-Rich or -Poor Plasma

Sample Type	Metric Units	Conversion Factor	Molar Units
Whole blood	50-200 ng/mL	×5.68	280-1140 nmol/L
	88-1230 ng/10^9 platelets	×0.00568	0.5-7.0 nmol/10^9 platelets
Serum	30-200 ng/mL	×5.68	170-1140 nmol/L
Urine	≤200 μg/24 h	×5.68	≤1140 nmol/24 h
	38-101 μg/g creatinine	×0.653	25-66 μmol/mol creatinine
CSF	1.0-2.1 ng/mL	×5.68	5.7-12.0 nmol/L
Platelet-rich plasma	670 ± 150 ng/10^9 platelets	×0.00568	3.81 ± 0.87 nmol/10^9 platelets
Isolated platelets	620 ± 233 ng/10^9 platelets	×0.00568	3.52 ± 1.32 nmol/10^9 platelets
Platelet-poor plasma	0.93 ± 0.67 ng/mL	×5.68	5.3 ± 3.8 nmol/L

Note: Reference intervals may vary according to mode of sample collection, method of measurement, and source of calibrators. The laboratory performing the measurements should establish its own independent reference intervals. The above reference intervals therefore serve as a general guide but should not be used for diagnostic decision making.

laboratory. Numerous HPLC methods have been described for measuring 5-HIAA, separately or in combination with other clinically interesting substances.[51] Most procedures employ reversed-phase, paired-ion separations under optimized isocratic conditions. Alkyl-bonded silica, such as ODS (C18), is often used as the hydrophobic stationary phase, and an organic-aqueous buffer mixture at an acid pH is frequently used as the polar mobile phase.

Electrochemical detection using amperometric or coulometric measurement is preferred for specific measurement of small quantities of 5-HIAA. Similar to serotonin, the oxidation potential for 5-HIAA is below 0.6 V and must be optimized for each application. Very few interfering compounds are electrochemically active at such low voltage potentials.[30] But if detection of 5-HIAA with other indoles and catecholamines is desired, then hydrodynamic voltammograms for each analyte should be studied to select the minimum potential that achieves maximum specificity.[253] Combining fluorometric and electrochemical detection also improves specificity.[244] Some HPLC systems use fluorometric detection, with or without derivatization, for a less demanding measurement of 5-HIAA.[240]

Preliminary extraction of 5-HIAA may be required as an initial purification step before HPLC analysis. Organic solvents, anion-exchange resins, and other solid-phase extraction procedures have all been used.[259] Automated methods have been described that incorporate online solid-phase extraction to reduce analysis time and increase sample throughput.[188] For many systems, direct injection of urine onto the analytical column is a common practice[11,107]; for this, samples are often merely diluted with a buffer and centrifuged to minimize contamination of the HPLC system. Methods that analyze 5-HIAA without prior sample cleanup rely on the selectivity of the HPLC separation combined with fluorescence or electrochemical detection to provide the requisite specificity.

Alternative technologies based on immunoassay and tandem mass spectrometry are available for quantifying 5-HIAA in urine. For the immunoassay procedure, dichloromethane is used to convert 5-HIAA to its methyl ester during sample preparation. This methylated derivative competes with biotin-labeled 5-HIAA for a limited number of binding sites of an antibody immobilized on microtiter plates. After incubation, the wells are washed to remove unbound biotin-labeled HIAA and then are incubated with antibiotin alkaline phosphatase before a *p*-nitrophenyl phosphate substrate is added. The amount of biotinylated HIAA bound to the antibody is inversely proportional to the 5-HIAA concentration.

LC-MS/MS methods for determination of 5-HIAA in urine have been developed using solid-phase extraction and quantification against stable isotope-labeled internal standards.[49,139,210] Methods for the combined determination of 5-HIAA, VMA, and HVA have also been described.[161,166] With these procedures, sample preparation is automated, chromatographic interferences are eliminated, and analytical time is reduced (2 to 6 minutes per sample).

Sample collection and storage protocols are an important consideration in testing plasma or urine by the instrumental techniques discussed previously. For determination of 5-HIAA in plasma, a blood specimen is collected with heparin as an anticoagulant after an overnight fast. The separated plasma is stored frozen at −20 °C until analysis, because plasma stored at 4 °C for 7 days shows an 8% average increase in 5-HIAA concentration.[25] For urinary measurement of 5-HIAA, two 24-hour specimen collections are recommended.[74] Concentrations in random urine are extremely variable, but shorter (or longer) collection times may be acceptable provided results are expressed per milligram of creatinine.[276] Because 5-HIAA is light sensitive, urine should ideally be collected in a 2-L brown polypropylene container. Because 5-HIAA is unstable at alkaline pHs, a stabilizing preservative is recommended to prevent urine from becoming alkaline (e.g., 0.5 g boric acid; 10 mL HCl, 6 mol/L; 25 mL glacial acetic acid). Most important, the specimen should be refrigerated during collection and kept in the dark. On receipt in the laboratory, the urine specimen is thoroughly mixed and the total volume measured and recorded. If the specimen is not collected with an acid preservative, then the pH of the urine may now be adjusted to between 2 and 3 by the addition of HCl. Acidified urine can be stored at 4 °C for 2 to 4 weeks and for longer periods of time at −20 °C.

Dietary instruction for the patient may reduce potential exogenous interferences. For example, dietary sources of 5-hydroxyindoles (e.g., walnuts, bananas, avocados, eggplants, pineapples, plums, tomatoes) should be restricted 3 to 4 days before and during urine collection. If possible, patients should abstain from all known medications that may cause an apparent increase (glycerol guaiacolate, mephenesin, phenacetin, and acetaminophen) or decrease (methenamine, phenothiazine tranquilizers, homogentisic acid, acetic acid, and levodopa) in 5-HIAA concentrations.[177] Whereas serotonin-containing foods clearly alter urinary 5-HIAA results, fasting plasma 5-HIAA results are not affected by foods high in hydroxyindole content. Representative reference intervals used in interpretation of plasma and urinary 5-HIAA are shown in Table 30-14.

TABLE 30-14 Reference Intervals for Plasma and Urinary 5-HIAA in Adults

Sample Type	Metric Units	Conversion Factor	Molar Units
Urine	≤7 mg/d	×5.23	6-37 μmol/d
	≤6.6 mg/g creatinine	×0.592	≤3.9 μmol/mmol creatinine
Plasma	5.2-13.4 ng/L	×5.23	27-70 nmol/L

Note: Reference intervals may vary according to mode of sample collection, method of measurement, and source of calibrators. The laboratory performing the measurements should establish its own independent reference intervals. The above reference intervals therefore serve as a general guide but should not be used for diagnostic decision making.

REFERENCES

1. Amar L, Bertherat J, Baudin E, Ajzenberg C, Bressac-de Paillerets B, Chabre O, et al. Genetic testing in pheochromocytoma or functional paraganglioma. J Clin Oncol 2005;23:8812-8.
2. Anderson GM, Feibel FC, Cohen DJ. Determination of serotonin in whole blood, platelet-rich plasma, platelet-poor plasma and plasma ultrafiltrate. Life Sci 1987;40:1063-70.
3. Aneman A, Eisenhofer G, Olbe L, Dalenback J, Nitescu P, Fandriks L, et al. Sympathetic discharge to mesenteric organs and the liver: evidence for substantial mesenteric organ norepinephrine spillover. J Clin Invest 1996;97:1640-6.
4. Barnes NM, Sharp T. A review of central 5-HT receptors and their function. Neuropharmacology 1999;38:1083-152.
5. Bessho F, Hashizume K, Nakajo T, Kamoshita S. Mass screening in Japan increased the detection of infants with neuroblastoma without a decrease in cases in older children. J Pediatr 1991;119:237-41.
6. Betto P, Ricciarello G, Giambenedetti M, Lucarelli C, Ruggeri S, Stocchi F. Improved high-performance liquid chromatographic analysis with double detection system for L-dopa, its metabolites and carbidopa in plasma of parkinsonian patients under L-dopa therapy. J Chromatogr 1988;459:341-9.
7. Biaggioni I, Goldstein DS, Atkinson T, Robertson D. Dopamine-beta-hydroxylase deficiency in humans. Neurology 1990;40:370-3.
8. Bieva CJ, Ladmirant IH, Scheirs I, Dardenne JP. Administered viloxazine interferes in liquid-chromatographic assay of normetanephrines. Clin Chem 1987;33:1677-8.
9. Binder SR, Sivorinovsky G. Measurement of urinary vanilmandelic acid and homovanillic acid by high-performance liquid chromatography with electrochemical detection following extraction by ion-exchange and ion-moderated partition. J Chromatogr 1984;336:173-88.
10. Bonafe L, Thony B, Leimbacher W, Kierat L, Blau N. Diagnosis of dopa-responsive dystonia and other tetrahydrobiopterin disorders by the study of biopterin metabolism in fibroblasts. Clin Chem 2001;47:477-85.
11. Bonfigli AR, Coppa G, Testa R, Testa I, De Sio G. Determination of vanillylmandelic, 5-hydroxyindoleacetic and homovanillic acid in urine by isocratic liquid chromatography. Eur J Clin Chem Clin Biochem 1997;35:57-61.
12. Boomsma F, Alberts G, van Eijk L, Man in't Veld AJ, Schalekamp MA. Optimal collection and storage conditions for catecholamine measurements in human plasma and urine. Clin Chem 1993;39: 2503-8.
13. Box JC, Braithwaite MD, Duncan T, Lucas G. Pheochromocytoma, chronic renal insufficiency, and hemodialysis: a combination leading to a diagnostic and therapeutic dilemma. Am Surg 1997;63:314-16.
14. Boyle JG, Davidson DF, Perry CG, Connell JM. Comparison of diagnostic accuracy of urinary free metanephrines VMA, and catecholamines and plasma catecholamines for diagnosis of pheochromocytoma. J Clin Endocrinol Metab 2007;92:4602-8.
15. Brautigam C, Wevers RA, Jansen RJ, Smeitink JA, de Rijk-van Andel JF, Gabreels FJ, et al. Biochemical hallmarks of tyrosine hydroxylase deficiency. Clin Chem 1998;44:1897-1904.
16. Brautigam C, Steenbergen-Spanjers GC, Hoffmann GF, Dionisi-Vici C, van den Heuvel LP, Smeitink JA, et al. Biochemical and molecular genetic characteristics of the severe form of tyrosine hydroxylase deficiency. Clin Chem 1999;45:2073-8.
17. Bravo EL, Tarazi RC, Fouad FM, Vidt DG, Gifford RW Jr. Clonidine-suppression test: a useful aid in the diagnosis of pheochromocytoma. N Engl J Med 1981;305:623-6.
18. Brodeur GM, Pritchard J, Berthold F, Carlsen NL, Castel V, Castelberry RP, et al. Revisions of the international criteria for neuroblastoma diagnosis, staging, and response to treatment. J Clin Oncol 1993;11:1466-77.
19. Brown MJ, Allison DJ. Renal conversion of plasma DOPA to urine dopamine. Br J Clin Pharmacol 1981;12:251-3.
20. Burgoyne RD, Morgan A. Secretory granule exocytosis. Physiol Rev 2003;83:581 632.
21. Candito M, Thyss A, Albertini M, Deville A, Politano S, Mariani R, et al. Methylated catecholamine metabolites for diagnosis of neuroblastoma. Med Pediatr Oncol 1992;20:215-20.
22. Canfell PC, Binder SR, Khayam-Bashi H. Pediatric reference intervals for normetanephrine/metanephrine. Clin Chem 1986;32: 222-3.
23. Cardon PV, Guggenheim FG. Effects of large variations in diet on free catecholamines and their metabolites in urine. J Psychiatr Res 1970;7: 263-73.
24. Carey RM. Theodore Cooper Lecture. Renal dopamine system: paracrine regulator of sodium homeostasis and blood pressure. Hypertension 2001;38:297-302.
25. Carling RS, Degg TJ, Allen KR, Bax ND, Barth JH. Evaluation of whole blood serotonin and plasma and urine 5-hydroxyindole acetic acid in diagnosis of carcinoid disease. Ann Clin Biochem 2002;39: 577-82.
26. Chan EC, Wee PY, Ho PC. Evaluation of degradation of urinary catecholamines and metanephrines and deconjugation of their sulfoconjugates using stability-indicating reversed-phase ion-pair HPLC with electrochemical detection. J Pharm Biomed Anal 2000;22:515-26.
27. Chan YP, Siu TS. Simultaneous quantitation of catecholamines and O-methylated metabolites in urine by isocratic ion-pairing high-performance liquid chromatography with amperometric detection. J Chromatogr 1988;459:251-60.
28. Chang S, Choi D, Lee SJ, Lee WJ, Park MH, Kim SW, et al. Neuroendocrine neoplasms of the gastrointestinal tract: classification, pathologic basis, and imaging features. Radiographics 2007;27: 1667-79.
29. Charmandari E, Eisenhofer G, Mehlinger SL, Carlson A, Wesley R, Keil MF, et al. Adrenomedullary function may predict phenotype and genotype in classic 21-hydroxylase deficiency. J Clin Endocrinol Metab 2002;87:3031-7.
30. Chou PP, Jaynes PK. Determination of urinary 5-hydroxyindole-3-acetic acid using solid-phase extraction and reversed-phase high-performance liquid chromatography with electrochemical detection. J Chromatogr 1985;341:167-71.
31. Collinson PO, Kind PR, Slavin B, Weg MW, Sandler M. False diagnosis of phaeochromocytoma in patients on Sinemet. Lancet 1984;1:1478-9.
32. Cook FJ, Chandler DW, Snyder DK. Effect of buspirone on urinary catecholamine assays. N Engl J Med 1995;332:401.
33. Cotterill SJ, Pearson AD, Pritchard J, Foot AB, Roald B, Kohler JA, et al. Clinical prognostic factors in 1277 patients with neuroblastoma: results of The European Neuroblastoma Study Group "Survey" 1982-1992. Eur J Cancer 2000;36:901-8.
34. Crawford GA, Gyory AZ, Gallery ED, Kelly D. HPLC of urinary catecholamines in the presence of labetalol, captopril, and alpha-methyldopa. Clin Chem 1990;36:1849.
35. Crockett DK, Frank EL, Roberts WL. Rapid analysis of metanephrine and normetanephrine in urine by gas chromatography-mass spectrometry. Clin Chem 2002;48:332-7.
36. Crout JR, Sjoerdsma A. The clinical and laboratory significance of serotonin and catechol amines in bananas. N Engl J Med 1959;261: 23-6.
37. Crowell MD. Role of serotonin in the pathophysiology of the irritable bowel syndrome. Br J Pharmacol 2004;141:1285-93.
38. Cryer PE. Adrenaline: a physiological metabolic regulatory hormone in humans? Int J Obes Relat Metab Disord 1993;17(Suppl 3):S43-6; discussion S68.
39. Dajani R, Hood AM, Coughtrie MW. A single amino acid, glu146, governs the substrate specificity of a human dopamine sulfotransferase, SULT1A3. Mol Pharmacol 1998;54:942-8.
40. Danaceau JP, Anderson GM, McMahon WM, Crouch DJ. A liquid chromatographic-tandem mass spectrometric method for the analysis

of serotonin and related indoles in human whole blood. J Anal Toxicol 2003;27:440-4.

41. Das SK, Dhanya L, Vasudevan DM. Biomarkers of alcoholism: an updated review. Scand J Clin Lab Invest 2008;68:81-92.
42. Davidson DF. Urinary catecholamine assay by HPLC: in vitro interference by some drugs. Ann Clin Biochem 1988;25(Pt 5):583-4.
43. Davidson DF. Simultaneous assay for urinary 4-hydroxy-3-methoxy-mandelic acid, 5-hydroxyindoleacetic acid and homovanillic acid by isocratic HPLC with electrochemical detection. Ann Clin Biochem 1989;26(Pt 2):137-43.
44. Davidson DF. Elevated urinary dopamine in adults and children. Ann Clin Biochem 2005;42:200-7.
45. Davidson FD. Paracetamol-associated interference in an HPLC-ECD assay for urinary free metadrenalines and catecholamines. Ann Clin Biochem 2004;41:316-20.
46. Davis BA. Effects of long-term storage on the concentrations of the unconjugated acidic metabolites of the trace amines, indoleamines and catecholamines. J Chromatogr 1988;433:23-30.
47. de Herder WW. Biochemistry of neuroendocrine tumours. Best Pract Res Clin Endocrinol Metab 2007;21:33-41.
48. de Jong WH, Graham KS, van der Molen JC, Links TP, Morris MR, Ross HA, et al. Plasma free metanephrine measurement using automated online solid-phase extraction HPLC tandem mass spectrometry. Clin Chem 2007;53:1684-93.
49. de Jong WH, Graham KS, de Vries EG, Kema IP. Urinary 5-HIAA measurement using automated on-line solid-phase extraction-high-performance liquid chromatography-tandem mass spectrometry. J Chromatogr B Analyt Technol Biomed Life Sci 2008;868:28-33.
50. de Jong WH, Eisenhofer G, Post WJ, Muskiet FA, de Vries EG, Kema IP. Dietary influences on plasma and urinary metanephrines: implications for diagnosis of catecholamine-producing tumors. J Clin Endocrinol Metab 2009;94:2841-9.
51. Deacon AC. The measurement of 5-hydroxyindoleacetic acid in urine. Ann Clin Biochem 1994;31(Pt 3):215-32.
52. Degg TJ, Allen KR, Barth JH. Measurement of plasma 5-hydroxyindoleacetic acid in carcinoid disease: an alternative to 24-h urine collections? Ann Clin Biochem 2000;37(Pt 5):724-6.
53. Dutton J, Hodgkinson AJ, Hutchinson G, Roberts NB. Evaluation of a new method for the analysis of free catecholamines in plasma using automated sample trace enrichment with dialysis and HPLC. Clin Chem 1999;45:394-9.
54. Eisenhofer G, Goldstein DS, Stull R, Keiser HR, Sunderland T, Murphy DL, et al. Simultaneous liquid-chromatographic determination of 3,4-dihydroxyphenylglycol, catecholamines, and 3,4-dihydroxyphenylalanine in plasma, and their responses to inhibition of monoamine oxidase. Clin Chem 1986;32:2030-3.
55. Eisenhofer G, Friberg P, Pacak K, Goldstein DS, Murphy DL, Tsigos C, et al. Plasma metadrenalines: do they provide useful information about sympatho-adrenal function and catecholamine metabolism? Clin Sci (Lond) 1995;88:533-42.
56. Eisenhofer G, Rundquist B, Aneman A, Friberg P, Dakak N, Kopin IJ, et al. Regional release and removal of catecholamines and extraneuronal metabolism to metanephrines. J Clin Endocrinol Metab 1995;80:3009-17.
57. Eisenhofer G, Aneman A, Hooper D, Rundqvist B, Friberg P. Mesenteric organ production, hepatic metabolism, and renal elimination of norepinephrine and its metabolites in humans. J Neurochem 1996;66:1565-73.
58. Eisenhofer G, Lenders JW, Harvey-White J, Ernst M, Zametkin A, Murphy DL, et al. Differential inhibition of neuronal and extraneuronal monoamine oxidase. Neuropsychopharmacology 1996;15:296-301.
59. Eisenhofer G, Aneman A, Friberg P, Hooper D, Fandriks L, Lonroth H, et al. Substantial production of dopamine in the human gastrointestinal tract. J Clin Endocrinol Metab 1997;82:3864-71.
60. Eisenhofer G, Coughtrie MW, Goldstein DS. Dopamine sulphate: an enigma resolved. Clin Exp Pharmacol Physiol Suppl 1999;26:S41-53.
61. Eisenhofer G, Lenders JW, Linehan WM, Walther MM, Goldstein DS, Keiser HR. Plasma normetanephrine and metanephrine for detecting pheochromocytoma in von Hippel-Lindau disease and multiple endocrine neoplasia type 2. N Engl J Med 1999;340:1872-9.
62. Eisenhofer G. The role of neuronal and extraneuronal plasma membrane transporters in the inactivation of peripheral catecholamines. Pharmacol Ther 2001;91:35-62.
63. Eisenhofer G, Huynh TT, Hiroi M, Pacak K. Understanding catecholamine metabolism as a guide to the biochemical diagnosis of pheochromocytoma. Rev Endocr Metab Disord 2001;2:297-311.
64. Eisenhofer G, Ehrhart-Bornstein M, Bornstein SR. The adrenal medulla: physiology and pathophysiology. In: Bolis CL, Licinio J, Govoni S, eds. Handbook of the autonomic nervous system in health and disease. New York: Marcel Dekker Inc, 2003:185-224.
65. Eisenhofer G, Goldstein DS, Walther MM, Friberg P, Lenders JW, Keiser HR, et al. Biochemical diagnosis of pheochromocytoma: how to distinguish true- from false-positive test results. J Clin Endocrinol Metab 2003;88:2656-66.
66. Eisenhofer G, Bornstein SR, Brouwers FM, Cheung NK, Dahia PL, De Krijger RR, et al. Malignant pheochromocytoma: current status and initiatives for future progress. Endocr Relat Cancer 2004;11: 423-36.
67. Eisenhofer G, Kopin IJ, Goldstein DS. Catecholamine metabolism: a contemporary view with implications for physiology and medicine. Pharmacol Rev 2004;56:331-49.
68. Eisenhofer G, Kopin IJ, Goldstein DS. Leaky catecholamine stores: undue waste or a stress response coping mechanism? Ann N Y Acad Sci 2004;1018:224-30.
69. Eisenhofer G, Goldstein DS, Sullivan P, Csako G, Brouwers FM, Lai EW, et al. Biochemical and clinical manifestations of dopamine-producing paragangliomas: utility of plasma methoxytyramine. J Clin Endocrinol Metab 2005;26:1925-39.
70. Eisenhofer G, Huysmans F, Pacak K, Walther MM, Sweep FC, Lenders JW. Plasma metanephrines in renal failure. Kidney Int 2005; 67:668-77.
71. Eldrup E, Moller SE, Andreasen J, Christensen NJ. Effects of ordinary meals on plasma concentrations of 3,4-dihydroxyphenylalanine, dopamine sulphate and 3,4-dihydroxyphenylacetic acid. Clin Sci (Lond) 1997;92:423-30.
72. Eldrup E, Clausen N, Scherling B, Schmiegelow K. Evaluation of plasma 3,4-dihydroxyphenylacetic acid (DOPAC) and plasma 3,4-dihydroxyphenylalanine (DOPA) as tumor markers in children with neuroblastoma. Scand J Clin Lab Invest 2001;61:479-90.
73. Esler M, Jennings G, Lambert G, Meredith I, Horne M, Eisenhofer G. Overflow of catecholamine neurotransmitters to the circulation: source, fate, and functions. Physiol Rev 1990;70:963-85.
74. Ezzat S, Asa SL, Taupenot L, O'Connor DT, Lambert EA, Oberg K. National Academy of Clinical Biochemistry guidelines for the use of tumor markers in neoplasms of the dispersed neuroendocrine system. In: Fleisher M, Dnistrian A, Sturgeon C, Lamerz R, Witliff J, eds. Guidelines and recommendations for use of tumor markers in the clinic. Washington, DC: AACC Press, 2003.
75. Fauler G, Leis HJ, Huber E, Schellauf C, Kerbl R, Urban C, et al. Determination of homovanillic acid and vanillylmandelic acid in neuroblastoma screening by stable isotope dilution GC-MS. J Mass Spectrom 1997;32:507-14.
76. Feldman JM, Lee EM. Serotonin content of foods: effect on urinary excretion of 5-hydroxyindoleacetic acid. Am J Clin Nutr 1985;42: 639-43.
77. Feldman JM. Falsely elevated urinary excretion of catecholamines and metanephrines in patients receiving labetalol therapy. J Clin Pharmacol 1987;27:288-92.
78. Fitzgibbon M, FitzGerald RJ, Tormey WP, O'Meara A, Kenny D. Reference values for urinary HMMA, HVA, noradrenaline, adrenaline, and dopamine excretion in children using random urine samples and HPLC with electrochemical detection. Ann Clin Biochem 1992;29(Pt 4):400-4.

79. Fitzpatrick PF. Tetrahydropterin-dependent amino acid hydroxylases. Annu Rev Biochem 1999;68:355-81.
80. Flachaire E, Beney C, Berthier A, Salandre J, Quincy C, Renaud B. Determination of reference values for serotonin concentration in platelets of healthy newborns, children, adults, and elderly subjects by HPLC with electrochemical detection. Clin Chem 1990;36:2117-20.
81. Flemstrom G, Safsten B. Role of dopamine and other stimuli of mucosal bicarbonate secretion in duodenal protection. Dig Dis Sci 1994;39:1839-42.
82. Fritsch P, Kerbl R, Lackner H, Urban C. "Wait and see" strategy in localized neuroblastoma in infants: an option not only for cases detected by mass screening. Pediatr Blood Cancer 2004;43:679-82.
83. Fujita K, Maruta K, Ito S, Nagatsu T. Urinary 4-hydroxy-3-methoxymandelic (vanillylmandelic) acid, 4-hydroxy-3-methoxyphenylacetic (homovanillic) acid, and 5-hydroxy-3-indoleacetic acid determined by liquid chromatography with electrochemical detection. Clin Chem 1983;29:876-8.
84. Gao YC, Lu HK, Luo QY, Chen LB, Ding Y, Zhu RS. Comparison of free plasma metanephrines enzyme immunoassay with (131)I-MIBG scan in diagnosis of pheochromocytoma. Clin Exp Med 2008;8:87-91.
85. Gerlo EA, Schoors DF, Dupont AG. Age- and sex-related differences for the urinary excretion of norepinephrine, epinephrine, and dopamine in adults. Clin Chem 1991;37:875-8.
86. Gershon MD. Review article: roles played by 5-hydroxytryptamine in the physiology of the bowel. Aliment Pharmacol Ther 1999;13(Suppl 2):15-30.
87. Gironi A, Seghieri G, Niccolai M, Mammini P. Simultaneous liquid-chromatographic determination of urinary vanillylmandelic acid, homovanillic acid, and 5-hydroxyindoleacetic acid. Clin Chem 1988;34:2504-6.
88. Glish GL, Vachet RW. The basics of mass spectrometry in the twenty-first century. Nat Rev Drug Discov 2003;2:140-50.
89. Goldstein DS, Stull R, Markey SP, Marks ES, Keiser HR. Dihydrocaffeic acid: a common contaminant in the liquid chromatographic-electrochemical measurement of plasma catecholamines in man. J Chromatogr 1984;311:148-53.
90. Goldstein DS, Stull R, Eisenhofer G, Sisson JC, Weder A, Averbuch SD, et al. Plasma 3,4-dihydroxyphenylalanine (dopa) and catecholamines in neuroblastoma or pheochromocytoma. Ann Intern Med 1986;105:887-8.
91. Goldstein DS, Udelsman R, Eisenhofer G, Stull R, Keiser HR, Kopin IJ. Neuronal source of plasma dihydroxyphenylalanine. J Clin Endocrinol Metab 1987;64:856-61.
92. Goldstein DS, Mezey E, Yamamoto T, Aneman A, Friberg P, Eisenhofer G. Is there a third peripheral catecholaminergic system? Endogenous dopamine as an autocrine/paracrine substance derived from plasma DOPA and inactivated by conjugation. Hypertens Res 1995;18(Suppl 1):S93-9.
93. Goldstein DS, Lenders JW, Kaler SG, Eisenhofer G. Catecholamine phenotyping: clues to the diagnosis, treatment, and pathophysiology of neurogenetic disorders. J Neurochem 1996;67:1781-90.
94. Goldstein DS, Swoboda KJ, Miles JM, Coppack SW, Aneman A, Holmes C, et al. Sources and physiological significance of plasma dopamine sulfate. J Clin Endocrinol Metab 1999;84:2523-31.
95. Goldstein DS, Robertson D, Esler M, Straus SE, Eisenhofer G. Dysautonomias: clinical disorders of the autonomic nervous system. Ann Intern Med 2002;137:753-63.
96. Goldstein DS, Eisenhofer G, Kopin IJ. Sources and significance of plasma levels of catechols and their metabolites in humans. J Pharmacol Exp Ther 2003;305:800-11.
97. Goldstein DS, Eisenhofer GF, Kopin IJ. Sources and significance of plasma levels of catechols and their metabolites in humans. J Pharmacol Exp Ther 2003;305:800-11.
98. Goyal RK, Hirano I. The enteric nervous system. N Engl J Med 1996;334:1106-15.
99. Grossman A, Pacak K, Sawka A, Lenders JW, Harlander D, Peaston RT, et al. Biochemical diagnosis and localization of pheochromocytoma: can we reach a consensus? Ann N Y Acad Sci 2006;1073:332-47.
100. Grouzmann E, Mathian B, Buclin T. Calibration of fractionated metanephrines in urine: still an issue? Clin Chem 2008;54:1738-9.
101. Grumbach MM, Biller BM, Braunstein GD, Campbell KK, Carney JA, Godley PA, et al. Management of the clinically inapparent adrenal mass ("incidentaloma"). Ann Intern Med 2003;138:424-9.
102. Grundy D, Schemann M. Enteric nervous system. Curr Opin Gastroenterol 2007;23:121-6.
103. Gurney JG, Davis S, Severson RK, Fang JY, Ross JA, Robison LL. Trends in cancer incidence among children in the United States. Cancer 1996;78:532-41.
104. Gurney JG, Ross JA, Wall DA, Bleyer WA, Severson RK, Robison LL. Infant cancer in the U.S.: histology-specific incidence and trends, 1973 to 1992. J Pediatr Hematol Oncol 1997;19:428-32.
105. Hasegawa T, Hirose T, Ayala AG, Ito S, Tomaru U, Matsuno Y, et al. Adult neuroblastoma of the retroperitoneum and abdomen: clinicopathologic distinction from primitive neuroectodermal tumor. Am J Surg Pathol 2001;25:918-24.
106. Heider EC, Davis BG, Frank EL. Nonparametric determination of reference intervals for plasma metanephrine and normetanephrine. Clin Chem 2004;50:2381-4.
107. Helander A, Beck O, Wennberg M, Wikstrom T, Jacobsson G. Determination of urinary 5-hydroxyindole-3-acetic acid by high-performance liquid chromatography with electrochemical detection and direct sample injection. Anal Biochem 1991;196:170-3.
108. Henry JP, Sagne C, Bedet C, Gasnier B. The vesicular monoamine transporter: from chromaffin granule to brain. Neurochem Int 1998;32:227-46.
109. Heron E, Chatellier G, Billaud E, Foos E, Plouin PF. The urinary metanephrine-to-creatinine ratio for the diagnosis of pheochromocytoma. Ann Intern Med 1996;125:300-3.
110. Hickman PE, Leong M, Chang J, Wilson SR, McWhinney B. Plasma free metanephrines are superior to urine and plasma catecholamines and urine catecholamine metabolites for the investigation of phaeochromocytoma. Pathology 2009;41:173-7.
111. Hoeldtke RD, Israel BC, Cavanaugh ST, Krishna GG. Effect of renal failure on plasma dihydroxyphenylglycol, 3-methoxy-4-hydroxyphenylglycol, and vanillymandelic acid. Clin Chim Acta 1989;184:195-6.
112. Hoelzer DR, Dalsky GP, Schwartz NS, Clutter WE, Shah SD, Holloszy JO, et al. Epinephrine is not critical to prevention of hypoglycemia during exercise in humans. Am J Physiol 1986;251:E104-10.
113. Hoffman B, Taylor P. Neurotransmission: the autonomic and somatic motor nervous system. In: Hardman JG, Limbird LE, Gilman AG, editors. Goodman and Gilman's, The Pharmacological Basis of Therapeutics. Tenth Edition ed. New York: McGraw-Hill, 2001: 115-54.
114. Hollenbach E, Schulz C, Lehnert H. Rapid and sensitive determination of catecholamines and the metabolite 3-methoxy-4-hydroxyphen-ethyleneglycol using HPLC following novel extraction procedures. Life Sci 1998;63:737-50.
115. Holmes C, Eisenhofer G, Goldstein DS. Improved assay for plasma dihydroxyphenylacetic acid and other catechols using high-performance liquid chromatography with electrochemical detection. J Chromatogr B Biomed Appl 1994;653:131-8.
116. Honjo S, Doran HE, Stiller CA, Ajiki W, Tsukuma H, Oshima A, et al. Neuroblastoma trends in Osaka, Japan, and Great Britain 1970-1994, in relation to screening. Int J Cancer 2003;103:538-43.
117. Horwitz BJ, Fisher RS. The irritable bowel syndrome. N Engl J Med 2001;344:1846-50.
118. Hoyer D, Martin G. 5-HT receptor classification and nomenclature: towards a harmonization with the human genome. Neuropharmacology 1997;36:419-28.
119. Hyland K, Clayton PT. Aromatic L-amino acid decarboxylase deficiency: diagnostic methodology. Clin Chem 1992;38:2405-10.
120. Iehara T, Hosoi H, Akazawa K, Matsumoto Y, Yamamoto K, Suita S, et al. MYCN gene amplification is a powerful prognostic factor even in infantile neuroblastoma detected by mass screening. Br J Cancer 2006;94:1510-5.

121. Ishida J, Takada M, Hitoshi N, Iizuka R, Yamaguchi M. 4-Dimethylaminobenzylamine as a sensitive chemiluminescence derivatization reagent for 5-hydroxyindoles and its application to their quantification in human platelet-poor plasma. J Chromatogr B Biomed Sci Appl 2000;738:199-206.
122. Itoh T, Omori K. Biosynthesis and storage of catecholamines in pheochromocytoma and neuroblastoma cells. J Lab Clin Med 1973;81:889-96.
123. Izbicki T, Bozek J, Perek D, Wozniak W. Urinary dopamine/noradrenaline and dopamine/vanillylmandelic acid ratios as a reflection of different biology of adrenergic clones in children's neuroblastic tumors. J Pediatr Surg 1991;26:1230-4.
124. Jones BE. Arousal systems. Front Biosci 2003;8:s438-51.
125. Jones BE. Modulation of cortical activation and behavioral arousal by cholinergic and orexinergic systems. Ann N Y Acad Sci 2008;1129: 26-34.
126. Jones BJ, Blackburn TP. The medical benefit of 5-HT research. Pharmacol Biochem Behav 2002;71:555-68.
127. Kai M, Iida H, Nohta H, Lee MK, Ohta K. Fluorescence derivatizing procedure for 5-hydroxytryptamine and 5-hydroxyindoleacetic acid using 1,2-diphenylethylenediamine reagent and their sensitive liquid chromatographic determination. J Chromatogr B Biomed Sci Appl 1998;720:25-31.
128. Kairisto V, Koskinen P, Mattila K, Puikkonen J, Virtanen A, Kantola I, et al. Reference intervals for 24-h urinary normetanephrine, metanephrine, and 3-methoxy-4-hydroxymandelic acid in hypertensive patients. Clin Chem 1992;38:416-20.
129. Kaler SG, Holmes CS, Goldstein DS, Tang J, Godwin SC, Donsante A, et al. Neonatal diagnosis and treatment of Menkes disease. N Engl J Med 2008;358:605-14.
130. Kaufman S. Genetic disorders involving recycling and formation of tetrahydrobiopterin. Adv Pharmacol 1998;42:41-3.
131. Kaufmann H, Biaggioni I. Autonomic failure in neurodegenerative disorders. Semin Neurol 2003;23:351-63.
132. Kema IP, de Vries EG, Schellings AM, Postmus PE, Muskiet FA. Improved diagnosis of carcinoid tumors by measurement of platelet serotonin. Clin Chem 1992;38:534-40.
133. Kema IP, Schellings AM, Meiborg G, Hoppenbrouwers CJ, Muskiet FA. Influence of a serotonin- and dopamine-rich diet on platelet serotonin content and urinary excretion of biogenic amines and their metabolites. Clin Chem 1992;38:1730-6.
134. Kema IP, de Vries EG, Slooff MJ, Biesma B, Muskiet FA. Serotonin, catecholamines, histamine, and their metabolites in urine, platelets, and tumor tissue of patients with carcinoid tumors. Clin Chem 1994;40:86-95.
135. Kema IP, de Vries EG, Muskiet FA. Clinical chemistry of serotonin and metabolites. J Chromatogr B Biomed Sci Appl 2000;747:33-48.
136. Kema IP, Meijer WG, Meiborg G, Ooms B, Willemse PH, de Vries EG. Profiling of tryptophan-related plasma indoles in patients with carcinoid tumors by automated, on-line, solid-phase extraction and HPLC with fluorescence detection. Clin Chem 2001;47:1811-20.
137. Kerbl R, Urban CE, Ambros IM, Dornbusch HJ, Schwinger W, Lackner H, et al. Neuroblastoma mass screening in late infancy: insights into the biology of neuroblastic tumors. J Clin Oncol 2003;21: 4228-34.
138. Kopin IJ. Catecholamine metabolism: basic aspects and clinical significance. Pharmacol Rev 1985;37:333-64.
139. Kroll CA, Magera MJ, Helgeson JK, Matern D, Rinaldo P. Liquid chromatographic-tandem mass spectrometric method for the determination of 5-hydroxyindole-3-acetic acid in urine. Clin Chem 2002;48:2049-51.
140. Kudva YC, Sawka AM, Young WF Jr. Clinical review 164. The laboratory diagnosis of adrenal pheochromocytoma: the Mayo Clinic experience. J Clin Endocrinol Metab 2003;88:4533-9.
141. Kulke MH, Mayer RJ. Carcinoid tumors. N Engl J Med 1999;340: 858-68.
142. Kulke MH. Clinical presentation and management of carcinoid tumors. Hematol Oncol Clin North Am 2007;21:433-55; vii-viii.
143. Kurz T, Yamada KA, DaTorre SD, Corr PB. Alpha 1-adrenergic system and arrhythmias in ischaemic heart disease. Eur Heart J 1991; 12(Suppl F):88-98.
144. Kushner BH, Gilbert F, Helson L. Familial neuroblastoma: case reports, literature review, and etiologic considerations. Cancer 1986;57:1887-93.
145. Kushnir MM, Urry FM, Frank EL, Roberts WL, Shushan B. Analysis of catecholamines in urine by positive-ion electrospray tandem mass spectrometry. Clin Chem 2002;48:323-31.
146. Kvetnansky R, Sabban EL, Palkovits M. Catecholaminergic systems in stress: structural and molecular genetic approaches. Physiol Rev 2009;89:535-606.
147. Kwarts E, Kwarts J, Rutgers H. A simple paired-ion liquid chromatography assay for serotonin in cerebrospinal fluid, platelet-rich plasma, serum and urine. Ann Clin Biochem 1984;21(Pt 5): 425-9.
148. Lagerstedt SA, O'Kane DJ, Singh RJ. Measurement of plasma free metanephrine and normetanephrine by liquid chromatography-tandem mass spectrometry for diagnosis of pheochromocytoma. Clin Chem 2004;50:603-11.
149. Laug WE, Siegel SE, Shaw KN, Landing B, Baptista J, Gutenstein M. Initial urinary catecholamine metabolite concentrations and prognosis in neuroblastoma. Pediatrics 1978;62:77-83.
150. Lee KL, Ma JF, Shortliffe LD. Neuroblastoma: management, recurrence, and follow-up. Urol Clin North Am 2003;30:881-90.
151. Lee MS, Cheng FC, Yeh HZ, Liou TY, Liu JH. Determination of plasma serotonin and 5-hydroxyindoleacetic acid in healthy subjects and cancer patients. Clin Chem 2000;46:422-3.
152. Lehmann M, Keul J. Urinary excretion of free noradrenaline and adrenaline related to age, sex and hypertension in 265 individuals. Eur J Appl Physiol Occup Physiol 1986;55:14-8.
153. Lenders JW, Eisenhofer G, Armando I, Keiser HR, Goldstein DS, Kopin IJ. Determination of metanephrines in plasma by liquid chromatography with electrochemical detection. Clin Chem 1993;39:97-103.
154. Lenders JW, Keiser HR, Goldstein DS, Willemsen JJ, Friberg P, Jacobs MC, et al. Plasma metanephrines in the diagnosis of pheochromocytoma. Ann Intern Med 1995;123:101-9.
155. Lenders JW, Eisenhofer G, Abeling NG, Berger W, Murphy DL, Konings CH, et al. Specific genetic deficiencies of the A and B isoenzymes of monoamine oxidase are characterized by distinct neurochemical and clinical phenotypes. J Clin Invest 1996;97:1010-9.
156. Lenders JW, Pacak K, Walther MM, Linehan WM, Mannelli M, Friberg P, et al. Biochemical diagnosis of pheochromocytoma: which test is best? JAMA 2002;287:1427-34.
157. Lenders JW, Eisenhofer G, Mannelli M, Pacak K. Phaeochromocytoma. Lancet 2005;366:665-75.
158. Lenders JW, Willemsen JJ, Eisenhofer G, Ross HA, Pacak K, Timmers HJ, et al. Is supine rest necessary before blood sampling for plasma metanephrines? Clin Chem 2007;53:352-4.
159. Lenz T, Zorner J, Kirchmaier C, Pillitteri D, Badenhoop K, Bartel C, et al. Multicenter study on the diagnostic value of a new RIA for the detection of free plasma metanephrines in the work-up for pheochromocytoma. Ann N Y Acad Sci 2006;1073:358-73.
160. Letellier S, Garnier JP, Spy J, Bousquet B. Determination of the L-DOPA/L-tyrosine ratio in human plasma by high-performance liquid chromatography: usefulness as a marker in metastatic malignant melanoma. J Chromatogr B Biomed Sci Appl 1997; 696:9-17.
161. Lionetto L, Lostia AM, Stigliano A, Cardelli P, Simmaco M. HPLC-mass spectrometry method for quantitative detection of neuroendocrine tumor markers: vanillylmandelic acid, homovanillic acid and 5-hydroxyindoleacetic acid. Clin Chim Acta 2008;398:53-6.
162. Lips CJ, Lentjes EG, Hoppener JW. The spectrum of carcinoid tumours and carcinoid syndromes. Ann Clin Biochem 2003;40:612-27.
163. Machida M, Sakaguchi A, Kamada S, Fujimoto T, Takechi S, Kakinoki S, et al. Simultaneous analysis of human plasma catecholamines by high-performance liquid chromatography with a reversed-phase

triacontylsilyl silica column. J Chromatogr B Analyt Technol Biomed Life Sci 2006;830:249-54.
164. Magera MJ, Thompson AL, Matern D, Rinaldo P. Liquid chromatography-tandem mass spectrometry method for the determination of vanillylmandelic acid in urine. Clin Chem 2003;49:825-6.
165. Manger WM, Gifford RW. Clinical and experimental pheochromocytoma, 2nd edition. Cambridge, Mass: Blackwell Science, 1996.
166. Manini P, Andreoli R, Cavazzini S, Bergamaschi E, Mutti A, Niessen WM. Liquid chromatography-electrospray tandem mass spectrometry of acidic monoamine metabolites. J Chromatogr B Biomed Sci Appl 2000;744:423-31.
167. Mannelli M, Bemporad D. Diagnosis and management of pheochromocytoma during pregnancy. J Endocrinol Invest 2002;25:567-71.
168. Marchese N, Canini S, Fabi L, Famularo L. Paediatric reference values for urinary catecholamine metabolites evaluated by high performance liquid chromatography and electrochemical detection. Eur J Clin Chem Clin Biochem 1997;35:533-37.
169. Marney LC, Laha TJ, Baird GS, Rainey PM, Hoofnagle AN. Isopropanol protein precipitation for the analysis of plasma free metanephrines by liquid chromatography-tandem mass spectrometry. Clin Chem 2008;54:1729-32.
170. Massimo L. Neuroblastoma: a challenge for pediatric oncology of the third millennium. Ann N Y Acad Sci 2002;963:59-62.
171. Maycock PF, Frayn KN. Use of alumina columns to prepare plasma samples for liquid-chromatographic determination of catecholamines. Clin Chem 1987;33:286-7.
172. McNeil AR, Blok BH, Koelmeyer TD, Burke MP, Hilton JM. Phaeochromocytomas discovered during coronial autopsies in Sydney, Melbourne and Auckland. Aust N Z J Med 2000;30:648-52.
173. Meijer WG, Kema IP, Volmer M, Willemse PH, de Vries EG. Discriminating capacity of indole markers in the diagnosis of carcinoid tumors. Clin Chem 2000;46:1588-96.
174. Merke DP, Chrousos GP, Eisenhofer G, Weise M, Keil MF, Rogol AD, et al. Adrenomedullary dysplasia and hypofunction in patients with classic 21-hydroxylase deficiency. N Engl J Med 2000;343:1362-8.
175. Mezey E, Eisenhofer G, Hansson S, Harta G, Hoffman BJ, Gallatz K, et al. Non-neuronal dopamine in the gastrointestinal system. Clin Exp Pharmacol Physiol Suppl 1999;26:S14-22.
176. Middelkoop CM, Dekker GA, Kraayenbrink AA, Popp-Snijders C. Platelet-poor plasma serotonin in normal and preeclamptic pregnancy. Clin Chem 1993;39:1675-8.
177. Mills KC. Serotonin syndrome: a clinical update. Crit Care Clin 1997;13:763-83.
178. Missale C, Nash SR, Robinson SW, Jaber M, Caron MG. Dopamine receptors: from structure to function. Physiol Rev 1998;78:189-225.
179. Misugi K, Misugi N, Newton WA Jr. Fine structural study of neuroblastoma, ganglioneuroblastoma, and pheochromocytoma. Arch Pathol 1968;86:160-70.
180. Modlin IM, Lye KD, Kidd M. A 5-decade analysis of 13,715 carcinoid tumors. Cancer 2003;97:934-59.
181. Modlin IM, Oberg K, Chung DC, Jensen RT, de Herder WW, Thakker RV, et al. Gastroenteropancreatic neuroendocrine tumours. Lancet Oncol 2008;9:61-72.
182. Moleman P. Effect of diet on urinary excretion of unconjugated catecholamines and some of their metabolites in healthy control subjects and depressed patients. Clin Chim Acta 1990;189:19-24.
183. Monsaingeon M, Perel Y, Simonnet G, Corcuff JB. Comparative values of catecholamines and metabolites for the diagnosis of neuroblastoma. Eur J Pediatr 2003;162:397-402.
184. Morgenstern BZ, Krivoshik AP, Rodriguez V, Anderson PM. Wilms' tumor and neuroblastoma. Acta Paediatr Suppl 2004;93:78-84; discussion 84-75.
185. Mornex R, Peyrin L, Pagliari R, Cottet-Emard JM. Measurement of plasma methoxyamines for the diagnosis of pheochromocytoma. Horm Res 1991;36:220-6.
186. Morrison SF. Differential control of sympathetic outflow. Am J Physiol Regul Integr Comp Physiol 2001;281:R683-98.
187. Moyer TP, Jiang NS, Tyce GM, Sheps SG. Analysis for urinary catecholamines by liquid chromatography with amperometric detection: methodology and clinical interpretation of results. Clin Chem 1979;25:256-63.
188. Mulder EJ, Oosterloo-Duinkerken A, Anderson GM, De Vries EG, Minderaa RB, Kema IP. Automated on-line solid-phase extraction coupled with HPLC for measurement of 5-hydroxyindole-3-acetic acid in urine. Clin Chem 2005;51:1698-1703.
189. Munion GL, Seaton JF, Harrison TS. HPLC for urinary catecholamines and metanephrines with alpha-methyldopa. J Surg Res 1983;35:507-14.
190. Murphy KL, Zhang X, Gainetdinov RR, Beaulieu JM, Caron MG. A regulatory domain in the N terminus of tryptophan hydroxylase 2 controls enzyme expression. J Biol Chem 2008;283:13216-24.
191. Nagatsu T, Levitt M, Udenfriend S. Tyrosine hydroxylase: the initial step in norepinephrine biosynthesis. J Biol Chem 1964;239:2910-7.
192. Nagatsu T. Tyrosine hydroxylase: human isoforms, structure and regulation in physiology and pathology. Essays Biochem 1995;30: 15-35.
193. Nagatsu T, Stjarne L. Catecholamine synthesis and release: overview. Adv Pharmacol 1998;42:1-14.
194. Nestler EJ, Alreja M, Aghajanian GK. Molecular control of locus coeruleus neurotransmission. Biol Psychiatry 1999;46:1131-9.
195. Neumann HP, Bausch B, McWhinney SR, Bender BU, Gimm O, Franke G, et al. Germ-line mutations in nonsyndromic pheochromocytoma. N Engl J Med 2002;346:1459-66.
196. Nuttall KL, Pingree SS. The incidence of elevations in urine 5-hydroxyindoleacetic acid. Ann Clin Lab Sci 1998;28:167-74.
197. O'Meara A, Tormey W, FitzGerald RJ, Fitzgibbon M, Kenny D. Interpretation of random urinary catecholamines and their metabolites in neuroblastoma. Acta Paediatr 1994;83:88-92.
198. Oberg K. Neuroendocrine gastrointestinal tumours. Ann Oncol 1996;7:453-63.
199. Oberg K, Stridsberg M. Chromogranins as diagnostic and prognostic markers in neuroendocrine tumours. Adv Exp Med Biol 2000;482: 329-37.
200. Obeso JA, Rodriguez-Oroz M, Marin C, Alonso F, Zamarbide I, Lanciego JL, et al. The origin of motor fluctuations in Parkinson's disease: importance of dopaminergic innervation and basal ganglia circuits. Neurology 2004;62:S17-30.
201. Olijslagers J, Werkman T, McCreary A, Kruse C, Wadman W. Modulation of midbrain dopamine neurotransmission by serotonin, a versatile interaction between neurotransmitters and significance for antipsychotic drug action. Curr Neuropharmacol 2006;4:59-68.
202. Ortiz J, Artigas F, Gelpi E. Serotonergic status in human blood. Life Sci 1988;43:983-90.
203. Pacak K, Eisenhofer G, Ahlman H, Bornstein SR, Gimenez-Roqueplo AP, Grossman AB, et al. Pheochromocytoma: recommendations for clinical practice from the First International Symposium. Nat Clin Pract Endocrinol Metab 2007;3:92-102.
204. Pacak K, Eisenhofer G, Lenders JW. Pheochromocytoma: diagnosis, localization and treatment, 1st edition. Oxford: Wiley-Blackwell, 2007.
205. Parker NC, Levtzow CB, Wright PW, Woodard LL, Chapman JF. Uniform chromatographic conditions for quantifying urinary catecholamines, metanephrines, vanillylmandelic acid, 5-hydroxyindoleacetic acid, by liquid chromatography, with electrochemical detection. Clin Chem 1986;32:1473-6.
206. Peaston RT, Lennard TW, Lai LC. Overnight excretion of urinary catecholamines and metabolites in the detection of pheochromocytoma. J Clin Endocrinol Metab 1996;81:1378-84.
207. Peaston RT, Ball S. Biochemical detection of phaeochromocytoma: why are we continuing to ignore the evidence? Ann Clin Biochem 2008;45:6-10.
208. Pedrino GR, Rosa DA, Korim WS, Cravo SL. Renal sympathoinhibition induced by hypernatremia: involvement of A1 noradrenergic neurons. Auton Neurosci 2008;142:55-63.

209. Perez EA, Koniaris LG, Snell SE, Gutierrez JC, Sumner WE 3rd, Lee DJ, et al. 7201 carcinoids: increasing incidence overall and disproportionate mortality in the elderly. World J Surg 2007;31:1022-30.
210. Perry H, Keevil B. Online extraction of 5-hydroxyindole acetic acid from urine for analysis by liquid chromatography-tandem mass spectrometry. Ann Clin Biochem 2008;45:149-52.
211. Pillai D, Ross HA, Kratzsch J, Pedrosa W, Kema I, Hoad K, et al. Proficiency test of plasma free and total metanephrines: report from a study group. Clin Chem Lab Med 2009;47:786-90.
212. Premel-Cabic A, Turcant A, Allain P. Normal reference intervals for free catecholamines and their acid metabolites in 24-h urines from children, as determined by liquid chromatography with amperometric detection. Clin Chem 1986;32:1585-7.
213. Pritchard J, Barnes J, Germond S, Hartman O, de Kraker J, Lewis I, et al. Stage and urinary catecholamine metabolite excretion in neuroblastoma. European Neuroblastoma Study Group. Lancet 1989;2:514-5.
214. Pussard E, Guigueno N, Adam O, Giudicelli JF. Validation of HPLC-amperometric detection to measure serotonin in plasma, platelets, whole blood, and urine. Clin Chem 1996;42:1086-91.
215. Pussard E, Neveux M, Guigueno N. Reference intervals for urinary catecholamines and metabolites from birth to adulthood. Clin Biochem 2009;42:536-9.
216. Quinn N, Carruthers M. False positive diagnosis of phaeochromocytoma in a patient with Parkinson's disease receiving levodopa. J Neurol Neurosurg Psychiatry 1988;51:728-9.
217. Raggi MA, Sabbioni C, Casamenti G, Gerra G, Calonghi N, Masotti L. Determination of catecholamines in human plasma by high-performance liquid chromatography with electrochemical detection. J Chromatogr B Biomed Sci Appl 1999;730:201-11.
218. Robertson RG, Geiger WJ, Davis NB. Carcinoid tumors. Am Fam Physician 2006;74:429-34.
219. Roden M, Raffesberg W, Raber W, Bernroider E, Niederle B, Waldhausl W, et al. Quantification of unconjugated metanephrines in human plasma without interference by acetaminophen. Clin Chem 2001;47:1061-7.
220. Rosano TG, Brown HH. Liquid-chromatographic assay for urinary 3-methoxy-4-hydroxymandelic acid, with use of a periodate oxidative monitor. Clin Chem 1979;25:550-4.
221. Rosano TG. Liquid-chromatographic evaluation of age-related changes in the urinary excretion of free catecholamines in pediatric patients. Clin Chem 1984;30:301-3.
222. Rosano TG, Swift TA, Hayes LW. Advances in catecholamine and metabolite measurements for diagnosis of pheochromocytoma. Clin Chem 1991;37:1854-67.
223. Ross GA, Newbould EC, Thomas J, Bouloux PM, Besser GM, Perrett D, et al. Plasma and 24 h-urinary catecholamine concentrations in normal and patient populations. Ann Clin Biochem 1993;30(Pt 1):38-44.
224. Rumley AG. The in vitro stability of catecholamines in whole blood. Ann Clin Biochem 1988;25(Pt 5):585-6.
225. Sabbioni C, Saracino MA, Mandrioli R, Pinzauti S, Furlanetto S, Gerra G, et al. Simultaneous liquid chromatographic analysis of catecholamines and 4-hydroxy-3-methoxyphenylethylene glycol in human plasma: comparison of amperometric and coulometric detection. J Chromatogr A 2004;1032:65-71.
226. Sawka AM, Jaeschke R, Singh RJ, Young WF Jr. A comparison of biochemical tests for pheochromocytoma: measurement of fractionated plasma metanephrines compared with the combination of 24-hour urinary metanephrines and catecholamines. J Clin Endocrinol Metab 2003;88:553-8.
227. Sawka AM, Thabane L, Gafni A, Levine M, Young WF Jr. Measurement of fractionated plasma metanephrines for exclusion of pheochromocytoma: can specificity be improved by adjustment for age? BMC Endocr Disord 2005;5:1.
228. Schilling FH, Spix C, Berthold F, Erttmann R, Fehse N, Hero B, et al. Neuroblastoma screening at one year of age. N Engl J Med 2002;346: 1047-53.
229. Schotzinger RJ, Landis SC. Cholinergic phenotype developed by noradrenergic sympathetic neurons after innervation of a novel cholinergic target in vivo. Nature 1988;335:637-9.
230. Schuldiner S, Shirvan A, Linial M. Vesicular neurotransmitter transporters: from bacteria to humans. Physiol Rev 1995;75:369-92.
231. Schultz W, Tremblay L, Hollerman JR. Reward prediction in primate basal ganglia and frontal cortex. Neuropharmacology 1998;37:421-9.
232. Segawa M. Hereditary progressive dystonia with marked diurnal fluctuation. Brain Dev 2000;22(Suppl 1):S65-80.
233. Seviour JA, McGill AC, Dale G, Craft AW. Method of measurement of urinary homovanillic acid and vanillylmandelic acid by gas chromatography-mass spectrometry suitable for neuroblastoma screening. J Chromatogr 1988;432:273-7.
234. Shimoda O, Ikuta Y, Nishi M, Uneda C. Magnitude of skin vasomotor reflex represents the intensity of nociception under general anesthesia. J Auton Nerv Syst 1998;71:183-9.
235. Shoup RE, Kissinger PT. Determination of urinary normetanephrine, metanephrine, and 3-methoxytyramine by liquid chromatography, with amperometric detection. Clin Chem 1977;23:1268-74.
236. Singh RJ. Advances in metanephrine testing for the diagnosis of pheochromocytoma. Clin Lab Med 2004;24:85-103.
237. Singh RJ, Grebe SK, Yue B, Rockwood AL, Cramer JC, Gombos Z, et al. Precisely wrong? Urinary fractionated metanephrines and peer-based laboratory proficiency testing. Clin Chem 2005;51:472-3; discussion 473-4.
238. Singh RJ, Eisenhofer G. High-throughput, automated, and accurate biochemical screening for pheochromocytoma: are we there yet? Clin Chem 2007;53:1565-7.
239. Sjoberg RJ, Simcic KJ, Kidd GS. The clonidine suppression test for pheochromocytoma: a review of its utility and pitfalls. Arch Intern Med 1992;152:1193-7.
240. Skrinska V, Hahn S. High-performance liquid chromatography of 5-hydroxyindole-3-acetic acid in urine with direct sample injection. J Chromatogr 1984;311:380-4.
241. Solcia E, Klöppel G, Sobin LH. Histological typing of endocrine tumours. In: World Health Organization, ed. International histological classification of tumours, 2nd edition. Berlin, Germany: Springer, 2000.
242. Stoltz JF. Uptake and storage of serotonin by platelets. In: VanHoutte PM, ed. Serotonin and the cardiovascular system. New York: Raven Press, 1985:37-42.
243. Strenger V, Kerbl R, Dornbusch HJ, Ladenstein R, Ambros PF, Ambros IM, et al. Diagnostic and prognostic impact of urinary catecholamines in neuroblastoma patients. Pediatr Blood Cancer 2007;48:504-9.
244. Stroomer AE, Overmars H, Abeling NG, van Gennip AH. Simultaneous determination of acidic 3,4-dihydroxyphenylalanine metabolites and 5-hydroxyindole-3-acetic acid in urine by high-performance liquid chromatography. Clin Chem 1990;36:1834-7.
245. Struder HK, Weicker H. Physiology and pathophysiology of the serotonergic system and its implications on mental and physical performance. Part I. Int J Sports Med 2001;22:467-81.
246. Stumvoll M, Radjaipour M, Seif F. Diagnostic considerations in pheochromocytoma and chronic hemodialysis: case report and review of the literature. Am J Nephrol 1995;15:147-51.
247. Taupenot L, Harper KL, O'Connor DT. The chromogranin-secretogranin family. N Engl J Med 2003;348:1134-49.
248. Taylor RL, Singh RJ. Validation of liquid chromatography-tandem mass spectrometry method for analysis of urinary conjugated metanephrine and normetanephrine for screening of pheochromocytoma. Clin Chem 2002;48:533-9.
249. Tuchman M, Crippin PJ, Krivit W. Capillary gas-chromatographic determination of urinary homovanillic acid and vanillylmandelic acid. Clin Chem 1983;29:828-31.
250. Tuchman M, Ramnaraine ML, Woods WG, Krivit W. Three years of experience with random urinary homovanillic and vanillylmandelic acid levels in the diagnosis of neuroblastoma. Pediatrics 1987;79: 203-5.

251. Tuomisto J, Mannisto P. Neurotransmitter regulation of anterior pituitary hormones. Pharmacol Rev 1985;37:249 332.
252. Ueyama J, Kitaichi K, Iwase M, Takagi K, Hasegawa T. Application of ultrafiltration method to measurement of catecholamines in plasma of human and rodents by high-performance liquid chromatography. J Chromatogr B Analyt Technol Biomed Life Sci 2003;798:35-41.
253. Vaarmann A, Kask A, Maeorg U. Novel and sensitive high-performance liquid chromatographic method based on electrochemical coulometric array detection for simultaneous determination of catecholamines, kynurenine and indole derivatives of tryptophan. J Chromatogr B Analyt Technol Biomed Life Sci 2002;769:145-53.
254. van der Hoorn FA, Boomsma F, Man in 't Veld AJ, Schalekamp MA. Determination of catecholamines in human plasma by high-performance liquid chromatography: comparison between a new method with fluorescence detection and an established method with electrochemical detection. J Chromatogr 1989;487:17-28.
255. van Laarhoven HW, Willemsen JJ, Ross HA, Beex LV, Lenders JW, Sweep FC. Pitfall in HPLC assay for urinary metanephrines: an unusual type of interference caused by methenamine intake. Clin Chem 2004;50:1097-9.
256. von Bohlen und Halbach O, Dermietzel R. Neurotransmitters and neuromodulators: handbook of receptors and biological effects. Darmstadt: Wiley-VCH Verlag GmbH, 2002.
257. Waldmeier PC, Antonin KH, Feldtrauer JJ, Grunenwald C, Paul E, Lauber J, et al. Urinary excretion of O-methylated catecholamines, tyramine and phenyl-ethylamine by volunteers treated with tranylcypromine and CGP 11305 A. Eur J Clin Pharmacol 1983;25:361-8.
258. Walther DJ, Peter JU, Bashammakh S, Hortnagl H, Voits M, Fink H, et al. Synthesis of serotonin by a second tryptophan hydroxylase isoform. Science 2003;299:76.
259. Warburton R, Keevil B. Urinary 5-hydroxyindole-acetic acid by high-performance liquid chromatography with electrochemical detection. Ann Clin Biochem 1997;34(Pt 4):424-6.
260. Weinblatt ME, Heisel MA, Siegel SE. Hypertension in children with neurogenic tumors. Pediatrics 1983;71:947-51.
261. Weir TB, Smith CC, Round JM, Betteridge DJ. Stability of catecholamines in whole blood, plasma, and platelets. Clin Chem 1986;32:882-3.
262. Weise M, Merke DP, Pacak K, Walther MM, Eisenhofer G. Utility of plasma free metanephrines for detecting childhood pheochromocytoma. J Clin Endocrinol Metab 2002;87:1955-60.
263. Whiting MJ. Simultaneous measurement of urinary metanephrines and catecholamines by liquid chromatography with tandem mass spectrometric detection. Ann Clin Biochem 2009;46:129-36.
264. Whiting MJ, Doogue MP. Advances in biochemical screening for phaeochromocytoma using biogenic amines. Clin Biochem Rev 2009;30:3-17.
265. Willemsen JJ, Ross HA, Wolthers BG, Sweep CG, Kema IP. Evaluation of specific high-performance liquid-chromatographic determinations of urinary metanephrine and normetanephrine by comparison with isotope dilution mass spectrometry. Ann Clin Biochem 2001;38:722-30.
266. Willemsen JJ, Sweep CG, Lenders JW, Ross HA. Stability of plasma free metanephrines during collection and storage as assessed by an optimized HPLC method with electrochemical detection. Clin Chem 2003;49:1951-3.
267. Willemsen JJ, Ross HA, Lenders JW, Sweep FC. Stability of urinary fractionated metanephrines and catecholamines during collection, shipment, and storage of samples. Clin Chem 2007;53:268-72.
268. Wilson SP, Kamin DL, Feldman JM. Acetaminophen administration interferes with urinary metanephrine (and catecholamine) determinations. Clin Chem 1985;31:1093-4.
269. Wu A. Tietz clinical guide to laboratory tests, 4th edition. Philadelphia, Pa: Saunders Elsevier, 2006.
270. Wu AH, Gornet TG. Preparation of urine samples for liquid-chromatographic determination of catecholamines: bonded-phase phenylboronic acid, cation-exchange resin, and alumina adsorbents compared. Clin Chem 1985;31:298-302.
271. Wurtman RJ, Hefti F, Melamed E. Precursor control of neurotransmitter synthesis. Pharmacol Rev 1980;32:315-35.
272. Yoneda A, Oue T, Imura K, Inoue M, Yagi K, Kawa K, et al. Observation of untreated patients with neuroblastoma detected by mass screening: a "wait and see" pilot study. Med Pediatr Oncol 2001; 36:160-2.
273. Young WF Jr. Pheochromocytoma: issues in diagnosis and treatment. Compr Ther 1997;23:319-26.
274. Zambrano E, Reyes-Mugica M. Hormonal activity may predict aggressive behavior in neuroblastoma. Pediatr Dev Pathol 2002;5: 190-9.
275. Zigmond RE, Schwarzschild MA, Rittenhouse AR. Acute regulation of tyrosine hydroxylase by nerve activity and by neurotransmitters via phosphorylation. Annu Rev Neurosci 1989;12:415-61.
276. Zuetenhorst JM, Korse CM, Bonfrer JM, Peter E, Lamers CB, Taal BG. Daily cyclic changes in the urinary excretion of 5-hydroxyindoleacetic acid in patients with carcinoid tumors. Clin Chem 2004;50:1634-9.

CHAPTER 31

Vitamins and Trace Elements

*Alan Shenkin, Ph.D., and Norman B. Roberts, M.Sc., Ph.D., C.Chem.**

Adequate supplies of vitamins and trace elements are critical in maintaining the health and development of humans. These nutrients occupy the attention of those concerned with the physical well-being of a public made increasingly aware of the need for maintaining the quality and the quantity of their dietary intake. The general principle regarding assessment of nutritional status is to determine the extent to which the metabolic demand for nutrients has been or is currently being met by the supply. In clinical practice, this requires balancing supply and demand.

Accurate assessment of supply and intake is a complex procedure. In practice, a crude estimate of intake is obtained from a careful clinical history taken by an experienced practitioner or from a food frequency questionnaire that summarizes the content of the individual's diet over several days, depending on how frequently particular typical foods are consumed.[60] A more accurate quantitative assessment usually requires a minimum of 3 days' recording of a complete dietary diary, which is subsequently analyzed using a computer program with reference tables of the nutritional contents of most foods.[450] Unfortunately, estimates of portion size, amounts consumed, and actual nutritional composition of the food consumed may be inaccurate. In addition, the disease process affects the amount actually consumed and absorbed, further reducing the accuracy of the estimate of nutritional intake.

The requirements for most nutrients to maintain health have been characterized and made available in reports from the Institute of Medicine (IOM) of the National Academies (http://www.iom.e).[186-190] However, the effects of disease may increase demands. For example, hypermetabolism, as a result of trauma or infection, increases the need for protein and energy and for the vitamin and trace element cofactors necessary for their metabolism.[585] Increased losses from the gut, kidney, and skin, or through dialysis, may also increase the overall demand for these nutrients.

An estimate of supply also is obtained from a careful dietary history, especially if performed by a dietitian, together with knowledge of any artificial nutritional supplements or therapy that may have been provided enterally or intravenously. Table 31-1 summarizes the Recommended Dietary Allowance (RDA) used in the United States and the Population Reference Intakes (from the European community) for vitamins and trace elements. These amounts are expected to be present in the normal diet of healthy adults. Table 31-1 also summarizes the amounts present in 2000 kcal of most tube feeds used in nutritional support. It is clear that the amounts used enterally are greater than the oral amounts recommended in health so as to meet increased needs resulting from preexisting deficiencies and increased ongoing requirements resulting from disease. The amounts recommended for supply during intravenous nutrition are also summarized in Table 31-1. For the trace elements, these amounts are generally less than the oral and/or enteral requirements to allow for reduced absorption enterally. For the vitamins, these amounts are usually greater than the oral and/or enteral requirements to allow for the effects of disease.

In an attempt to improve accuracy of assessment of nutritional status, clinicians often turn to the laboratory to obtain a result that may reflect the net balance of supply and demand.[583,585] Clinical laboratorians need to be aware of when such tests are useful and how to place the results of laboratory tests into the context of the clinical situation of the patient. It is important to be aware of the limitations of laboratory tests, especially in acutely ill patients.

NUTRITIONAL ASSESSMENT AND MONITORING

In this brief overview, the nutrients used in nutritional assessment and in monitoring will be briefly discussed.*

**The authors gratefully acknowledge the original contributions of Donald B. McCormick, Harry L. Green, George G. Klee, and David B. Milne, on which portions of this chapter are based.*

TABLE 31-1 Oral and Intravenous Micronutrient Intakes for Adults

	RDA (USA)	PRI (Europe)	Amount in 2000 kcal Tube Feed[580]	IV Intake[9,10,260,578]
Vitamins				
A, µg	900	700	1000-2160	1000
D, µg	5-15	0-10	8.5-14.6	5
E, mg	15	0.4/g PUFA	20-64	10
K, µg	120	100-200	150	
Thiamine, mg	1.2	1.1	1.4-3.4	6
Riboflavin, mg	1.3	1.6	2-6	3.6
Pyridoxine, mg	1.3	1.5	2-13.8	6
Niacin, mg	16	18	18-45	40
Folate, µg	400	200	340-880	600
B_{12}, µg	2	1.4	3-15	5
Pantothenic acid, µg	5*	3-12†	7-20	15
Biotin, µg	30*	15-100	100-660	60
Ascorbic acid, mg	90	45	100-300	200
Trace Elements				
Zinc, mg	11	9.5	13-36	3.2-6.5
Copper, mg	0.9	1.1	2-3.4	0.3-1.3
Selenium, µg	55	55	30-130	40-100
Chromium, µg	25	30-200	10-20	
Molybdenum, µg	45*	74-240	19	
Manganese, mg	2-3*	1-10†	2.4-8	0.05-0.2

*Adequate intake.
†Acceptable range.
PRI, Population reference intake (Europe)[517]; *RDA,* recommended dietary allowance (U.S.).[186,188,190]
Reference intakes for infants and children are age and weight dependent and are summarized in various sources.[186,188,190,225,589]

Protein-Energy Status

In clinical practice, only a few laboratory tests are of value in the assessment of protein-energy status[583,587] and it is particularly important to recognize that serum protein concentrations are not helpful in sick patients with any form of inflammatory process (see Chapter 21). Although serum albumin is often measured and reported as an indicator of protein-energy status, factors such as increased transcapillary escape[182] and reduced hepatic synthesis make it of little value as a nutritional marker. Serum albumin is, however, a valuable prognostic marker and is frequently used as part of prognostic indices.[97] Short half-life proteins such as transthyretin (TTR) (prealbumin) also may be of value in patients with no inflammatory response.[182,286] Although some workers have suggested that TTR may reflect protein-energy status in patients with an inflammatory response,[149] it seems more likely that it helps to identify the patient who is at risk of becoming malnourished as a result of their illness.[586]

Assessment of nitrogen balance may be used to obtain information on recent protein-energy status. This requires careful 24-hour urine collection and estimation of total nitrogen content,[335] or urea nitrogen (from which total nitrogen usually can be approximately estimated).[208] With a reasonable calculation of protein (nitrogen) intake, intake minus urine output (together with some unmeasured losses) gives an estimate of nitrogen balance. In practice, however, such measurements are now rarely required except when (1) patients appear to have excessive losses, (2) they are failing to respond to what appears to be adequate nutritional support therapy, or (3) a novel therapy is being evaluated for its effectiveness in limiting catabolism or stimulating anabolism.

Vitamin and Trace Element Status

Measurements of vitamin and trace element concentrations are frequently helpful in nutritional assessment. The relative value of such tests is increased by the fact that clinical assessment of their status is often poor.

Although requirements for vitamins and trace elements in health are known (see Table 31-1), the effects of illness on

*Various anthropometric and biochemical techniques and methods are used to assess nutritional status. They are discussed in an earlier edition of this textbook. (Veldee MS. Nutritional assessment, therapy, and monitoring. In: Burtis CA, Ashwood ER, eds. Tietz textbook of clinical chemistry, 3rd edition. Philadelphia: WB Saunders, 1999:1380-8.)

these requirements are poorly understood and quantified. However, it is now apparent that as an individual develops progressively more severe depletion in vitamin or trace element status, they pass through a series of stages with biochemical or physiologic consequences. The metabolic or physiologic penalty of such suboptimal nutritional status usually is not clear, but the assumption remains that suboptimal metabolism is likely to have detrimental effects [e.g., subclinical deficiency of folic acid is associated with an increase in serum homocysteine concentration, which has been proposed to be an independent risk factor for coronary artery disease (see Chapter 27)], although folate supplements do not reduce this risk.[389] Similarly, subclinical deficiency of chromium may be associated with impaired glucose tolerance in certain types of diabetes.[13]

The time course for development of a subclinical deficiency state varies for each individual vitamin and trace element and depends on the nature and quantity of body stores. Moreover, the extent of depletion necessary before significant biochemical, physiologic, or histologic changes occur is poorly characterized. The consequences of an inadequate intake are clearly delineated in Figure 31-1, which shows progression from optimal tissue status through a period of initial depletion until a period of subclinical deficiency is reached with a variety of biochemical and nonspecific physiologic effects. In some cases, certain nonspecific histologic changes may put the individual at risk of tissue damage or neoplastic change. It is only with persistent mismatch of intake and demand that eventually a full blown clinical deficiency state develops.

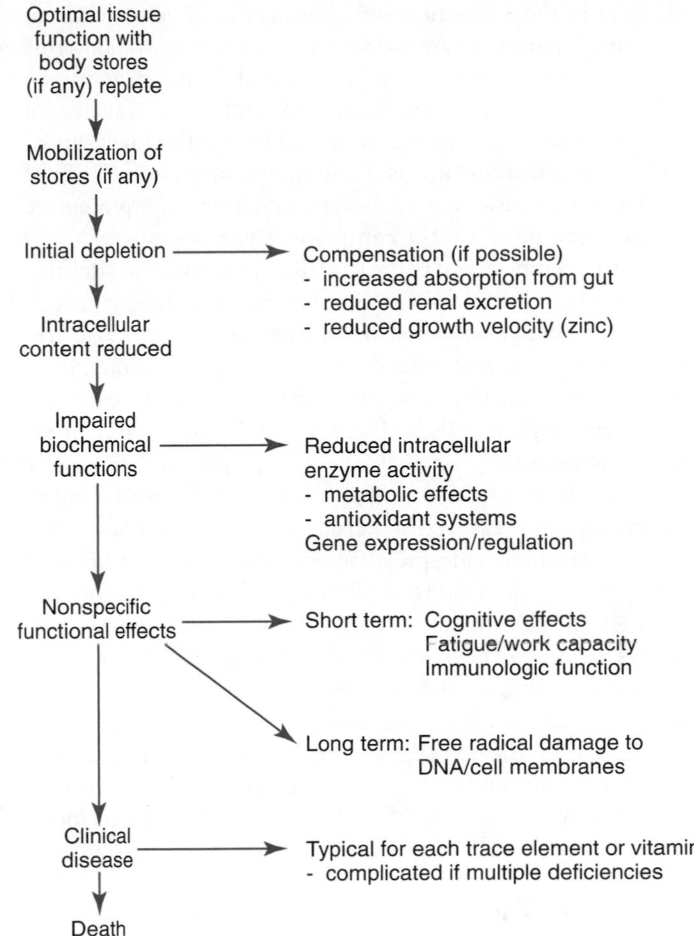

Figure 31-1 Consequences of inadequate mineral or trace element intake. *(From Shenkin A, Allwood MC. Trace elements and vitamins in adult intravenous nutrition. In: Rombeau JL, Rolandelli RH, eds. Clinical nutrition: parenteral nutrition. Philadelphia: WB Saunders, 2001:60-79.)*

Enzymes or Metabolites

Determination of the effective functioning of particular enzymes or metabolic pathways may be useful in demonstrating adequacy of nutritional status. Enzymes in plasma may be helpful in this regard [e.g., glutathione peroxidase as an index of selenium status and red cell enzymes such as transketolase (thiamine), glutathione reductase (riboflavin) or transaminase (pyridoxine), or glutathione peroxidase (selenium) are all used]. Methyltetrahydrofolate reductase is involved in the metabolism of homocysteine; hence assessment of plasma homocysteine is a useful measure of folate status obtained through indirect assessment of the action of this enzyme system.

Markers of Antioxidant Status

In practice, it is practically impossible to measure all biologically active antioxidants in human samples; therefore the concept of a "global" assessment of antioxidant capacity has proved attractive. Several methods have been developed for use in assessing this capacity and in conducting clinical research.[600] Most of these methods use one of two main approaches to measurement: (1) quenched or delayed production of a stable, measurable radical species; or (2) the reductant properties of antioxidants against a radical cation or a metal ion.[554] These are usually standardized with the water-soluble vitamin E analog Trolox. An example of the former is the total radical-trapping antioxidant parameter (TRAP) assay, which uses the stable radical species 2,2′-azinobis(3-ethylbenzthiazoline sulfonate) ($ABTS^+$), and an example of the latter is the ferric reducing ability of plasma (FRAP) assay.[47] Because these methods use different reaction principles, the same antioxidant can make different contributions to each assay, and it is for this reason that the use of more than one method is recommended for any study.[503] Vitamins that have contributed to plasma antioxidant capacity include ascorbate (up to 24% of measured capacity), α-tocopherol (up to 10% of measured capacity), and β-carotene, although at typical plasma concentrations of around 0.5 μmol/L, the contribution of β-carotene—as with most fat-soluble vitamins—to a total antioxidant capacity of around 1000 μmol/L is minimal.

A disadvantage of many methods of total antioxidant capacity measurement is the variable contribution of common plasma constituents, particularly albumin and urate, to the measured concentration.[215] Changes in circulating concentrations of these molecules caused by acute-phase changes or changes in renal function can alter measured values without reflecting changes in antioxidant vitamin concentration. This problem is typically resolved by the use of the *antioxidant gap,* a derived value that subtracts the Trolox equivalence of albumin and urate from the measured total antioxidant capacity.[422] Another drawback is the nonphysiologic conditions of study; hence new approaches to genomic and proteomic studies may allow a more comprehensive assessment.[331]

In an attempt to assess the functional adequacy of vitamins and trace elements involved in antioxidant pathways, products of oxidative metabolism can be measured. Those frequently used are malondialdehyde and F_2 isoprostanes, both of which give an indication of oxidation of polyunsaturated fatty acids within cells.[352] Increasing the provision of individual antioxidants or cocktails of vitamins and trace elements can lead to reduction in production of these metabolites, which can be measured in serum or urine. Such tests have not yet reached widespread application primarily because interpretation of results is difficult. Also, the appropriate amount of oxidative activity that is linked to particular outcomes has not yet been identified. This is especially important in that few clinical studies have demonstrated benefit from provision of increased quantities of antioxidants.[46] Most studies have indicated that antioxidant supplements (usually vitamin C and/or vitamin E) have no beneficial effect or indeed may be harmful,[63,90] although antioxidant-rich foods may be beneficial.[691]

Analytical Factors

Numerous analytical factors must be considered when the status of each nutrient is assessed. These include reference intervals, concentrations of markers in plasma and tissue, and their measurement in urine.

Reference Intervals

As for all laboratory tests, interpretation of tests of nutritional status requires access to relevant reference intervals and an understanding of factors that may alter them. Ethnic origin and geographic variation might affect the typical diet and its chemical composition; also, the fiber or phytate content may alter the bioavailability of minerals. In early infancy, the liver matures, leading to an increase in serum copper, whereas dietary changes in milk and weaning are associated with changes in plasma selenium. Seasonal variations may alter the reference intervals of vitamins, especially vitamin D. The time of sampling is also important, because zinc and iron concentrations tend to be higher in fasting than fed individuals and therefore are usually lower in the afternoon.

Plasma Concentrations

Concentrations of vitamins and trace elements are measured most often in plasma or serum; this provides a reliable index of status for only a few of them (e.g., vitamin B_{12}, vitamin D). For others (e.g., folate, selenium), their concentrations may reflect only the adequacy of recent intake. Excessive provision of elements, such as manganese and chromium, may be detected by high serum concentrations.[579]

For some vitamins or trace elements, serum measurement is limited in value, especially in seriously ill patients. In part, this is a result of the lack of correlation between the amount of nutrient in the plasma compartment and the amount within the intracellular compartment in most body tissue. For example, substantial stores of particular vitamins or trace elements may be present in individual tissue (e.g., vitamin A in the liver), but mobilization into the plasma is affected by the availability of appropriate binding proteins or by metabolism. Also, differences in the content of individual vitamins or trace elements have been noted between tissues, and the serum concentration will not reflect these differences. Furthermore and particularly important is the fact that the concentration in plasma can alter rapidly when a systemic inflammatory response syndrome (SIRS) [previously known as the acute-phase response (APR)] results from trauma or infection, leading to redistribution of metals between body compartments[582]; increased synthesis of metallothionein leads to uptake of zinc into the liver and increased synthesis of ferritin, causing uptake of iron.[135,529] The result is a fall in plasma concentrations of both zinc and iron. These changes in plasma concentration clearly do not reflect changes in whole body status.

Changes in the binding proteins in plasma also occur as a result of the disease process. Because serum albumin falls in association with any acute illness, this inevitably leads to a fall in plasma zinc concentration. Similarly, a reduction in retinol-binding protein concentration as part of SIRS or protein malnutrition, leads to a fall in serum retinol concentrations, whatever the quantity of retinol stores within the liver.

Some patients may be relatively stable, with little SIRS after injury, infection, or other inflammatory disease. If this is the case, it may be possible to interpret the plasma concentrations of elements such as zinc, copper, and iron, or of vitamins such as vitamin C or B_6, that would be affected by SIRS.[372] Of particular relevance is the trend in concentration of a trace element or vitamin in relation to the magnitude of SIRS changes.[211] Therefore, repeated measurement of a rapid response acute-phase protein, such as C-reactive protein (CRP), together with trace elements, may be helpful to include as part of the nutritional assessment.

Tissue Concentrations

Tissue concentrations of vitamins or trace elements are rarely measured in nutritional assessment because of lack of availability of suitable tissue; however, when such tissue is available, measurement may be helpful (e.g., copper analysis on liver biopsy of patients with suspected Wilson's disease).

More commonly, certain types of cells may be obtained from blood samples and can provide useful information. For example, red cell folate is commonly used as a marker of folate status, and leukocyte vitamin C is a better marker of vitamin C status than plasma concentration.[550] Because of the difficulty of preparation of pure populations of cells, cellular measurements usually are used only within a research environment.

Urine Measurements

For most vitamins and trace elements, their measurement in urine is rarely helpful because most are not under homeostatic control, and excretion may be a direct reflection of intake rather than active retention in the face of whole body deficiency. High concentrations of excretion of certain water-soluble vitamins or trace elements may indicate ingestion of large quantities of supplements.

VITAMINS

Vitamins are organic compounds required in trace amounts (microgram to milligram quantities per day) in the diet for health, growth, and reproduction. It is commonly understood that vitamins are natural materials that are isolated from organisms (such as plants that synthesize most of these compounds) or are chemically synthesized. Additionally, synthetic analogs and derivatives of vitamins are designed to serve as inhibitors (e.g., amethopterin as an antifolate), and others substitute in part for the natural vitamin (e.g., 8-ethylriboflavin for riboflavin). Only small amounts of vitamins are required for the functional, often catalytic (coenzymatic), roles they serve, in contrast to the relatively large amounts of such macronutrients as protein, lipid, and carbohydrate, which constitute the bulk of the ingesta that serve primarily as sources of energy and reconstitution of body mass.

Historically, vitamin groups such as A, B, and D bear an Arabic subscript number following the letter to designate structural and functional similarity [e.g., A_1 (retinol) and A_2 (3-dehydroretinol)] or to indicate the approximate order in which they were identified as members of the so-called B-complex [e.g., B_1 (thiamine) and B_2 (riboflavin)]. Common chemical names, which are being used more often, give a better indication of the types of compounds involved. These often reflect the presence of some specific atom (*thia*mine), the prime functional group (pyridox*amine*), or even a larger portion of the molecular structure (phyllo*quinone*). Parts of some names reflect functional properties (chole*calciferol*).

Another classification pertains to the relative solubility of vitamins. Those of the *fat-soluble* group (A, D, E, and K) are more soluble in organic solvents, whereas B-complex group vitamins and vitamin C are *water soluble.* This general separation based on solubility is useful not just for purposes of noting gross physical properties but also as a reminder that fat-soluble vitamins are absorbed, transported, and stored for longer periods of time and in a manner generally similar to that used for fats. Most water-soluble vitamins share the fate of other solutes more compatible with an aqueous, physiologic medium; this includes a lesser tendency to be retained for long periods of time in the body and greater loss by way of urinary excretion. Additionally, a general functional difference exists, in that water-soluble vitamins function as coenzymes for several important enzymatic reactions in both mammals and microorganisms. By contrast, fat-soluble vitamins generally do not function as coenzymes and are rarely used by microorganisms.

Table 31-2 provides a list of 13 known vitamins and vitameric groups essential to humans.

Vitamin A

Vitamin A serves many important functions in the body, with its role in vision being of particular significance.

Chemistry

Vitamin A is the nutritional term for the group of compounds with a 20-carbon structure containing a methyl-substituted cyclohexenyl ring (β-ionone ring) and an isoprenoid side-chain (Figure 31-2), with a hydroxyl group (retinol), an aldehyde group (retinal), a carboxylic acid group (retinoic acid), or an ester group (retinyl ester) at the terminal C15.

Retinol, the principal vitamin A vitamer, can be oxidized reversibly to retinal—which shares all the biological activity of retinol—or further oxidized to retinoic acid, which shows some of its biological activity. The principal storage forms of vitamin A are retinyl esters, particularly palmitate. The term *retinoids* refers to retinol, its metabolites, and synthetic analogs with similar structure. Included in the vitamin A family are some dietary carotenoids (C40 polyisoprenoid compounds) that are classified as provitamin A because they are cleaved biologically to yield retinol. Although around 1000 compounds with carotenoid structure have been identified,[395] only about 50 possess provitamin A activity, with the principal dietary compounds being β-carotene, α-carotene, and β-cryptoxanthin. Vitamin A compounds are yellowish oils or low-melting-point solids (depending on isomeric purity) that are practically insoluble in water but are soluble in organic solvents and mineral oil. Vitamin A is sensitive to oxygen and to ultraviolet light, which induces a greenish fluorescence with an absorbance peak at 325 nm. The structure for the most common and effective provitamin A, *β-carotene,* is given in Figure 31-2. This compound is an orange-to-purple, water-insoluble solid that is oxidized in air to inactive products. The other carotenes, cryptoxanthin and β-apocarotenals, are asymmetric with only one β-ionone ring and yield less vitamin A activity.

Dietary Sources

Pre-formed vitamin A is obtained from animal-derived foods, such as liver, other organ meats, and fish oils. Other sources are full cream milk, butter, and fortified margarines. The provitamin A carotenoids are obtained from yellow to orange fruits and vegetables and from green leafy vegetables. Good sources are pumpkin, carrots, tomatoes, apricots, grapefruit, lettuce, and most green vegetables.[385] The U.S. National Health and Nutrition Examination Survey (NHANES II) indicated that approximately 25% of the vitamin A requirement was provided by carotenoids and about 75% by pre-formed retinol.[67]

Absorption, Transport, Metabolism, and Excretion

Pre-formed vitamin A, most often in the form of retinyl ester, or carotenoids are subject to emulsification and mixed micelle formation by the action of bile salts before they are

TABLE 31-2 Vitamins Required by the Human

Common Name	Trivial Chemical Name	General Roles	Symptoms of Deficiency or Disease	Direct and Indirect Assays
Fat Soluble				
Vitamin A	Retinol, retinal, retinoic acid	Vision, growth, reproduction	Nyctalopia, xerophthalmia, keratomalacia	Photometric, HPLC, fluorimetric, RIA
Vitamin D_2, D_3	Ergocalciferol, cholecalciferol	Modulation of Ca^{2+} metabolism, calcification of bone and teeth	Rickets (young), osteomalacia (adult)	CPB, HPLC, RIA
Vitamin E	Tocopherols, tocotrienols	Antioxidant for unsaturated lipids, neurologic and reproductive functions	Lipid peroxidation, including red blood cell fragility, hemolytic anemia (premature, newborn)	Photometric, HPLC, erythrocyte hemolysis
Vitamin K_1, K_2	Phylloquinones, menaquinones	Blood clotting, osteocalcins	Increased clotting time, hemorrhagic disease (infant)	HPLC, prothrombin time, RIA (abnormal prothrombin, PIVKA)
Water Soluble				
Vitamin B_1	Thiamine	Carbohydrate metabolism, nervous function	Beriberi, Wernicke-Korsakoff syndrome	Fluorimetric, transketolase, HPLC
Vitamin B_2	Riboflavin	Oxidation-reduced reactions	Angular stomatitis, dermatitis, photophobia	Fluorimetric, HPLC, glutathione reductase
Vitamin B_6	Pyridoxine, pyridoxal, pyridoxamine	Amino acid, phospholipid, and glycogen metabolism	Epileptiform convulsions, dermatitis, hypochromic anemia	HPLC, aspartate transaminase, urine pyridoxic acid
Niacin, niacinamide	Nicotinic acid, nicotinamide	Oxidation-reduction reactions	Pellagra	Fluorometric, HPLC, nicotinamide coenzymes
Folic acid	Pteroylglutamic acid	Nucleic acid and amino acid biosynthesis	Megaloblastic anemia, neural tube defects	CPB, microbiological, homocysteine
Vitamin B_{12}	Cyanocobalamin	Amino acid and branched-chain keto acid metabolism	Pernicious and megaloblastic anemia, neuropathy	CPB, microbiological, RIA, methylmalonate
Biotin	—	Carboxylation reactions	Dermatitis	Microbiological, CPB, carboxylases, avidin binding
Pantothenic acid	—	General metabolism, acetyl and acyl transfer	Burning feet syndrome	Microbiological, RIA, CPB/HPLC
Vitamin C	Ascorbic acid	Connective tissue formation, antioxidant	Scurvy	Photometric, HPLC, enzymatic

CPB, Competitive protein binding; *HPLC*, high-performance liquid chromatography; *PIVKA*, protein induced by vitamin K absence or antagonism; *RIA*, radioimmunoassay.

transported into the intestinal cell. Here the retinyl esters are moved across the mucosal membrane and hydrolyzed to retinol within the cell to be then re-esterified by cellular retinol-binding protein II and packaged into chylomicra, which then enter the mesenteric lymphatic system and pass into the systemic circulation.[445] A small amount of the ingested retinoid is converted into retinoic acid in the intestinal cell. The efficiency of absorption of pre-formed vitamin A is high at between 70% and 90%.[593]

Carotenoids, also in micellar form, are absorbed into the duodenal mucosal cells by passive diffusion. The efficiency of absorption of carotenoids is much lower than for vitamin

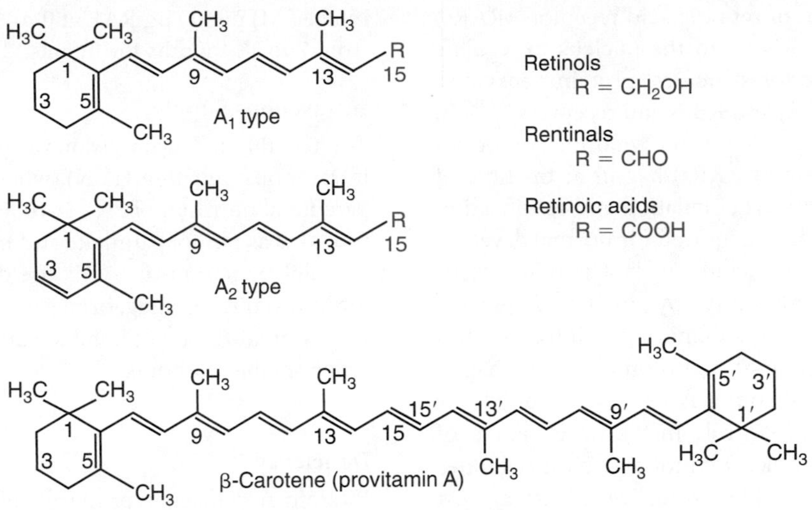

A$_1$ type

A$_2$ type

β-Carotene (provitamin A)

Retinols
R = CH_2OH

Rentinals
R = CHO

Retinoic acids
R = COOH

Figure 31-2 Vitaminic forms of A$_1$, A$_2$, and β-carotene.

A—between 9% and 22%[461]—and is subject to a large number of variables, including carotenoid type, the amount in the meal, matrix properties, nutrient status, and genetic factors.[621] Once inside the mucosal cell, β-carotene is principally converted to retinal by the enzyme β-carotene-15,15′-dioxygenase. The retinal is converted by retinal reductase to retinol and esterified. β-Carotene can also be cleaved eccentrically to β-apocarotenals, which can be further degraded to retinal or retinoic acid. The newly synthesized retinyl esters, from both pre-formed vitamin A and carotenoids, along with exogenous lipids and nonhydrolyzed carotenoids, then pass with chylomicrons via the lymphatic system to the liver, where uptake by parenchymal cells again involves hydrolysis. In the liver, retinol is bound with retinol-binding protein (RBP) (MW ≅ 21,000 Da) and transthyretin (thyroxine-binding prealbumin) (MW ≅ 55,000 Da) in a 1:1:1 complex of sufficient size to prevent loss by glomerular filtration and is returned to the circulation, or it may be stored as esters within the stellate cells. Delivery of retinol to the tissue is controlled by the availability of the vitamin A–protein complex in the circulation, although this control mechanism can be bypassed by large doses of retinol.

Retinoic acid from the intestinal mucosa is transported bound to serum albumin via the portal vein. Retinoic acid cannot be significantly reduced to retinal but is rapidly metabolized in tissue, such as liver, to yield more polar catabolites (e.g., 5,6-epoxyretinoic acid) and conjugates, such as retinoyl β-glucuronide, that are excreted. A small amount of retinoic acid undergoes enterohepatic circulation after intestinal hydrolysis of the glucuronide is excreted in the bile.

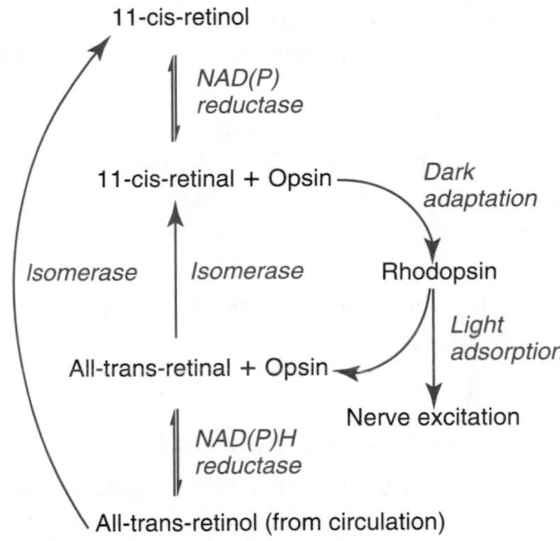

Figure 31-3 Participation of A vitamers in the visual cycle.

Functions

The participation of retinal in vision is considered the most important physiologic function of vitamin A. All-*trans*-retinol is the predominant circulating form of vitamin A. Cells of the retina isomerize this to the 11-*cis* alcohol that is reversibly dehydrogenated to 11-*cis* retinal. This sterically hindered geometrical isomer of the aldehyde combines as a lysyl-linked Schiff base with suitable proteins (e.g., opsin) to generate photosensitive pigments, such as rhodopsin. Illumination of such pigments causes photoisomerization and the release of all-*trans*-retinal and the protein, a process that couples the large conformational change with ion flux and optic nerve transmission. The all-*trans*-retinal is isomerized to the 11-*cis* isomer, which combines with the liberated protein to reconstitute the photo pigment in a visual cycle, as shown in Figure 31-3. The pyridine nucleotide–dependent dehydrogenase (reductase) can also reduce the all-*trans*-retinal to all-*trans*-retinol.

Other functions of vitamin A include its role in reproduction, growth, and embryonic development, as well as in immune function; many of these functions are mediated through the binding of retinoic acid to specific nuclear receptors that regulate genomic expression. In normal growth, and in maintenance of the integrity of epithelial cells, retinoic acid acts through the activation of retinoic acid receptors (RARs) and retinoid X receptors (RXRs) in the nucleus to regulate various genes that encode for structural proteins, enzymes, extracellular matrix proteins, and RBPs and receptors.[142,387] In vertebrate embryonic development, the vitamin A requirement (mediated via RARs and RXRs) begins at the time of formation of the primitive heart circulation and specification of the hindbrain,[709] and is later required for normal development of the limbs, heart, eyes, and ears.[151] Vitamin A deficiency impairs innate immunity by impeding normal regeneration of mucosal barriers damaged by infection, and by diminishing the function of neutrophils, macrophages, and natural killer cells. Vitamin A is also required for adaptive immunity and plays a role in the development of both T-helper cells and B cells. Retinol and its metabolites and synthetic retinoids provide protective effects against the development of certain types of cancer by blocking tumor promotion, by inhibiting proliferation, by inducing apoptosis, by inducing differentiation, or by performing a combination of these actions.[433,458] Finally, synthetic retinoids have been used successfully, both topically and systemically, to treat severe acne and other skin disorders of abnormal keratinization.

Some caution is required regarding the use of vitamin A or β-carotene supplements in the general population. Although synthetic retinoids are of value in treating certain forms of leukemia,[433] they appear to provide no benefit in reducing the incidence of gastrointestinal cancer and indeed may increase the incidence of lung cancer and mortality in certain other cancers.[63,474]

Requirements and Reference Nutrient Intakes

Historical studies in adult humans have suggested that intakes of retinol of 500 to 600 μg/d are required to maintain adequate blood concentrations and to prevent all deficiency symptoms. The relative contributions of β-carotene and other provitamin A carotenoids toward achieving this goal have undergone much revision as our knowledge has developed. In the older system of international units (IU), now largely redundant, a ratio for equivalence of activity of 1 : 2 : 4 for retinol:β-carotene : other provitamin A carotenoids was used, but this was superseded in 1967 by the retinol equivalent (RE), devised by a Food and Agriculture/World Health Organization Expert Committee and proposing an equivalence ratio of 1 : 6 : 12. However, studies using stable isotopes of β-carotene[653] led the Food and Nutrition Board of the U.S. Institute of Medicine to recommend the retinol activity equivalent (RAE) as the basis of calculation of retinol intake. In this system, a ratio equivalence of 1 : 12 : 24 is recommended (i.e., 12 μg β-carotene or 24 μg mixed carotenoids has the same biological activity as 1 μg retinol). With this system, current RDAs for vitamin A are 900 μg RAE for men 19 years and older; 700 μg RAE for women 19 years and older, with up to 770 μg RAE/d in pregnancy and up to 1300 μg RAE/d in lactation; 300 to 900 μg RAE for children 1 to 18 years, dependent on age and sex; and an adequate intake (AI) of 400 μg RAE at 0 to 6 months and 500 μg RAE from 7 to 12 months for infants.[190]

Intravenous Supply

The recommended provision of vitamin A to adults during intravenous nutrition (IVN), whether this is partial or total parenteral nutrition (TPN), is 1000 μg retinol. This is usually provided as retinol palmitate and may be supplied with other fat-soluble vitamins in a mixture dissolved in a fat emulsion for intravenous feeding, or may be designed to be compatible with a mixture of all vitamins suitable for addition to other water-soluble nutrients.[578]

Deficiency

Vitamin A deficiency primarily affects infants and children, and its prevalence is subject to World Health Organization (WHO) surveillance.[692] Risk factors include poverty, low birth weight, poor sanitation, malnutrition, infection, and parasitism. Because hepatic accumulation of vitamin A occurs during the last trimester of pregnancy, preterm infants are relatively vitamin A deficient at birth. Providing a daily oral intake of vitamin A that meets the RDA of 400 μg RAE is therefore important. Infants with birth weights of less than 1500 g (those under 30 weeks' gestation) have virtually no hepatic vitamin A stores and are at risk of vitamin A deficiency. Various workers have observed that (1) bronchopulmonary dysplasia (BPD), a debilitating, chronic lung disease that mimics some histologic features of vitamin A deficiency, is common in premature infants; (2) intramuscular injections of 630 μg RAE every 2 days can reduce the incidence of BPD; (3) blood concentrations of vitamin A decline during TPN, often reaching concentrations of 10 to 15 μg/dL (normal, 20 to 65 μg/dL) unless adequate supplements are given; and (4) vitamin A (retinol) delivered in TPN solutions may be adsorbed into the inner walls of plastic administration sets; however, this loss can be minimized by the use of ethylene vinyl acetate rather than polyvinyl chloride.[225,577]

Fat malabsorption, particularly caused by celiac disease or chronic pancreatitis, and protein-energy malnutrition predispose to vitamin A deficiency. Liver disease diminishes RBP synthesis, and ethanol abuse leads to both hepatic injury and competition with retinol for alcohol dehydrogenase, which is necessary for the oxidation of retinol to retinal and retinoic acid.[353] Vitamin A deficiency may lead to anemia, although the precise mechanism is not known.[568]

Clinical features of vitamin A deficiency include degenerative changes in eyes and skin and poor dark adaptation or *night blindness* (nyctalopia) followed by degenerative changes in the retina. X*erophthalmia* is seen to occur when the conjunctiva becomes dry with small gray plaques with foamy surfaces (Bitot's spots). These lesions are reversible with vitamin A administration. More serious effects of deficiency are known as *keratomalacia* and cause ulceration and necrosis of the cornea that lead to perforation, prolapse, endophthalmitis, and blindness. Usually, associated skin changes include dryness, roughness, papular eruptions, and follicular hyperkeratosis. The general change consists of atrophy of certain specialized epithelia, followed by metaplastic hyperkeratinization.

Toxicity

Although vitamin A metabolism is tightly regulated, toxic effects of hypervitaminosis A have occurred as a result of ingestion of excess vitamin, or as a side effect of inappropriate therapy.[485,682] Hypervitaminosis A occurs after liver storage of retinol and its esters exceeds 3000 μg/g tissue, with ingestion of more than 30,000 μg/d for months or years, or if plasma vitamin A concentrations exceed 140 μg/dL (4.9 μmol/L). The elderly are more susceptible to vitamin A toxicity at lower doses, as exposure to retinyl esters is longer because of delayed postprandial clearance of lipoproteins.[537] Symptoms of acute toxicity from a single massive dose present as abdominal pain, nausea, vomiting, severe headaches, dizziness, sluggishness, and irritability, followed within a few days by desquamation of the skin and recovery. Chronic toxicity from moderately high doses taken for protracted periods is characterized by bone and joint pain, hair loss, dryness and fissures of the lips, anorexia, benign intracranial hypertension, weight loss, and hepatomegaly. Administration of doses up to threefold the RDA for several years resulted in classic histologic changes of hepatotoxicity in 41 patients.[214] Osteoporosis and hip fracture are associated with vitamin A intakes only twice the RDA.[485] Infants given excess vitamin A over months to years can develop intracranial features, typically bulging fontanelle, and skeletal abnormalities at doses of 5500 to 6750 μg/d.[487]

Epidemiologic and experimental evidence has supported the view that high vitamin A intake in humans, acting via 13-*cis*-retinoic acid, is teratogenic.[343] The critical period of susceptibility is the first trimester of pregnancy, and primary abnormalities derive from the cranial neural crest (CNC) cells. A 1995 study of almost 23,000 pregnant women found that those who ingested more than 4500 μg/d of pre-formed vitamin A were at greater risk of delivering infants with malformations of CNC cell origin than were women consuming less than 1500 μg/d.[532] A further intriguing association, supported in part by epidemiologic studies, is that observed between excessive vitamin A intake and reduction in bone mineral density (BMD). Studies of Scandinavian women show that consistent loss of BMD at four sites was associated with increased intake of pre-formed vitamin A.[408] Intake amounts of vitamin A exceeding 1500 μg/d were associated with these changes, although studies in the United States have showed no increase in bone mineral loss at pre-formed vitamin A intakes up to 2000 μg/d.[274]

The findings of these and other studies led the Food and Nutrition Board of the U.S. Institute of Medicine to recommend a tolerable upper intake amount of 3000 μg/d of pre-formed vitamin A for men 19 years and older, with lower concentrations for women of childbearing age, infants, children, and adolescents. Carotenemia results from chronic excessive intake of carotene-rich foods, principally carrots. This condition, in which yellowing of the skin is observed, is benign, because the excess carotene is deposited rather than converted to vitamin A.

Laboratory Assessment of Status

Although measurement of the plasma concentration of vitamin A is the most convenient and widely used assessment of vitamin A status, it is not an ideal indicator because it does not decline until liver stores become critically depleted, which is thought to occur at a concentration of approximately 20 μg/g liver. Early chemical methods, which may remain in use if high-performance liquid chromatography (HPLC) is not available, include the Carr-Price photometric method, which uses antimony trichloride in chloroform as the reagent, and the later Neeld-Pearson method, which uses trifluoroacetic acid to produce a blue pigment with the conjugated double bonds of vitamin A (and the carotenoids). To improve specificity and sensitivity, later methods used solvent extraction and other separation techniques with fluorometric or spectrophotometric measurement. HPLC has brought enhanced (1) specificity, (2) lowered limits of detection (<0.07 μmol/L), (3) accuracy (using primary standards, reference materials, and quality assurance schemes), and (4) reproducibility (between batch coefficients of variation of 10% or better).[632] Both normal-phase and reversed-phase techniques have been used.[123,403]

In the normal-phase HPLC, compounds to be separated are adsorbed to microparticulate silica gel and are eluted in the order of least polar to most polar. Acceptable separation and quantitative yields of neutral and charged retinoids are obtained. Reversed-phase HPLC is preferable for acid-sensitive compounds such as 5,6-epoxyretinoic acid. Photometric, electrochemical, and mass spectrophotometric detectors have been used.

Because retinol circulates in plasma as a 1 : 1 : 1 complex with RBP and TTR, both of these hepatically produced proteins have been measured as indicators of vitamin A status. RBP has been measured by radial immunodiffusion or nephelometry (see Chapter 21), but its circulating concentration may be limited by inadequate dietary protein, energy, or zinc, all of which are necessary for RBP synthesis. Another confounding factor in the assessment of vitamin A status is the effect of the SIRS. Both RBP and TTR are negative acute-phase proteins; thus inflammatory changes will result in transient falls in both proteins and plasma retinol. To distinguish inflammatory from nutritional causes of reduced plasma retinol concentrations, it may be necessary to measure CRP.[564]

Because circulating retinol concentrations do not always correlate with total body stores of vitamin A, indirect tests have been used to assess these stores. The relative-dose-response test, described first by Loerch and associates,[366] requires two blood samples to be collected—one before and one 5 hours after a physiologic dose of vitamin A. In vitamin A–depleted subjects, a rapid, large, and sustained rise in serum retinol concentration contrasts with a lower, more shallow rise in vitamin A–sufficient subjects. A modified relative-dose-response test [using 3,4-didehydroretinyl (DR)

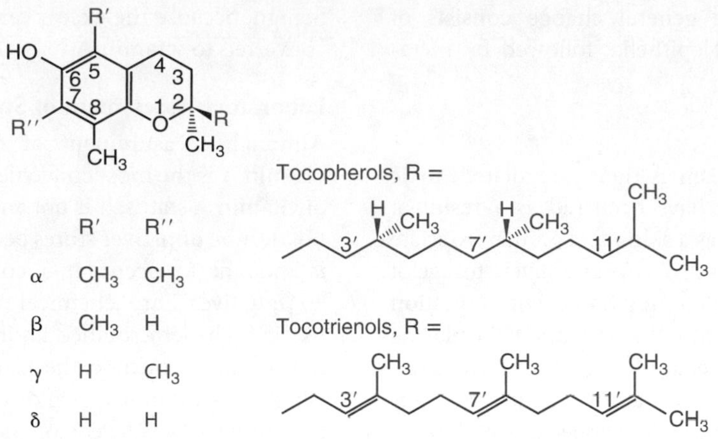

Figure 31-4 Vitaminic forms of vitamin E.

acetate rather than retinyl acetate and measuring the DR : retinol ratio after 5 hours] has been used by other workers to assess the vitamin A status of preschool Indonesian children[622] and also in a population of well-nourished American children.[623] Quantitative assessment of total body stores may be made by using deuterated retinol dilution techniques, but these require long periods (about 3 weeks) for equilibration. Ribaya-Mercado and colleagues developed a predictive mathematical formula that does not require serum isotope equilibration, allowing blood sampling 3 days after isotope dosing.[520]

Reference Intervals

Guidance reference intervals for serum vitamin A are 20 to 40 μg/dL (0.70 to 1.40 μmol/L) for 1- to 6-year-old children; 26 to 49 μg/dL (0.91 to 1.71 μmol/L) for 7- to 12-year-old children; 26 to 72 μg/dL (0.91 to 2.51 μmol/L) for 13- to 19-year-old adolescents; and 30 to 80 μg/dL (1.05 to 2.80 μmol/L) for adults.[365] Values above 30 μg/dL (1.05 μmol/L) are associated with appreciable reserves in the liver and correlate well with vitamin A intake. Within the reference interval, values for men are generally about 20% higher than those for women.

By HPLC, the reference interval for serum β-carotene is 10 to 85 μg/dL (0.19 to 1.58 μmol/L).[633] Elevated concentrations are found in hypothyroid patients, in whom conversion to vitamin A is decreased, and in patients with hyperlipemia associated with diabetes mellitus.

Vitamin D

Vitamin D plays an essential role as a hormone in the control of calcium and phosphorous metabolism. It is discussed in detail in Chapter 52.

Vitamin E

Vitamin E is an antioxidant that acts as a scavenger for molecular oxygen and free radicals. It also has a role in cellular respiration.

Chemistry

Vitamin E is the nutritional term for the group of naturally occurring tocopherols and tocotrienols that have biological activity similar to RRR-α-tocopherol (formerly D-α-tocopherol).[416] Both groups have a common 6-chromanol nucleus substituted with methyl groups at positions 2 and 8 and with a phytyl tail of isoprenoid units at position 2. The isoprenoid chain is saturated in the tocopherols but is unsaturated at positions 3′, 7′, and 11′ for tocotrienols (Figure 31-4). The Greek letter prefixes α, β, γ, and δ indicate the presence or absence of methyl groups at positions 5 and 7. The tocopherols have three asymmetric carbon atoms in the isoprenoid chain, giving eight optical isomers. The naturally occurring tocopherols occur as the RRR forms, whereas the synthetic compounds are of the racemic SR forms. Synthetic vitamin E contains about 12.5% of RRR-α-tocopherol, together with seven other tocopherol isomers that are less biologically active. Tocopherol and tocotrienols are viscous oils at room temperature, soluble in fat solvents and insoluble in aqueous solutions, although there exists a water-soluble analog (Trolox-6-hydroxy-2,5,7,8-tetramethylchroman-2-carboxylic acid). Also, tocopherol and tocotrienols are stable to acid and heat in the absence of oxygen, but are labile to oxygen in alkaline solutions and to ultraviolet light.

Dietary Sources

The principal sources of dietary vitamin E are oils and fats, particularly wheat germ oil and sunflower oil, grains, and nuts.[35] Meats, fruits, and vegetables contribute little vitamin E. Gamma-tocopherol is the major form of vitamin E in many plant seeds in the U.S. diet, but it is present at only one quarter to one tenth of the concentration of α-tocopherol in human plasma.[303]

Absorption, Transport, Metabolism, and Excretion

In the presence of bile, vitamin E is absorbed from the small intestine. Most forms of vitamin E are absorbed nonselectively and are secreted in chylomicron particles along with

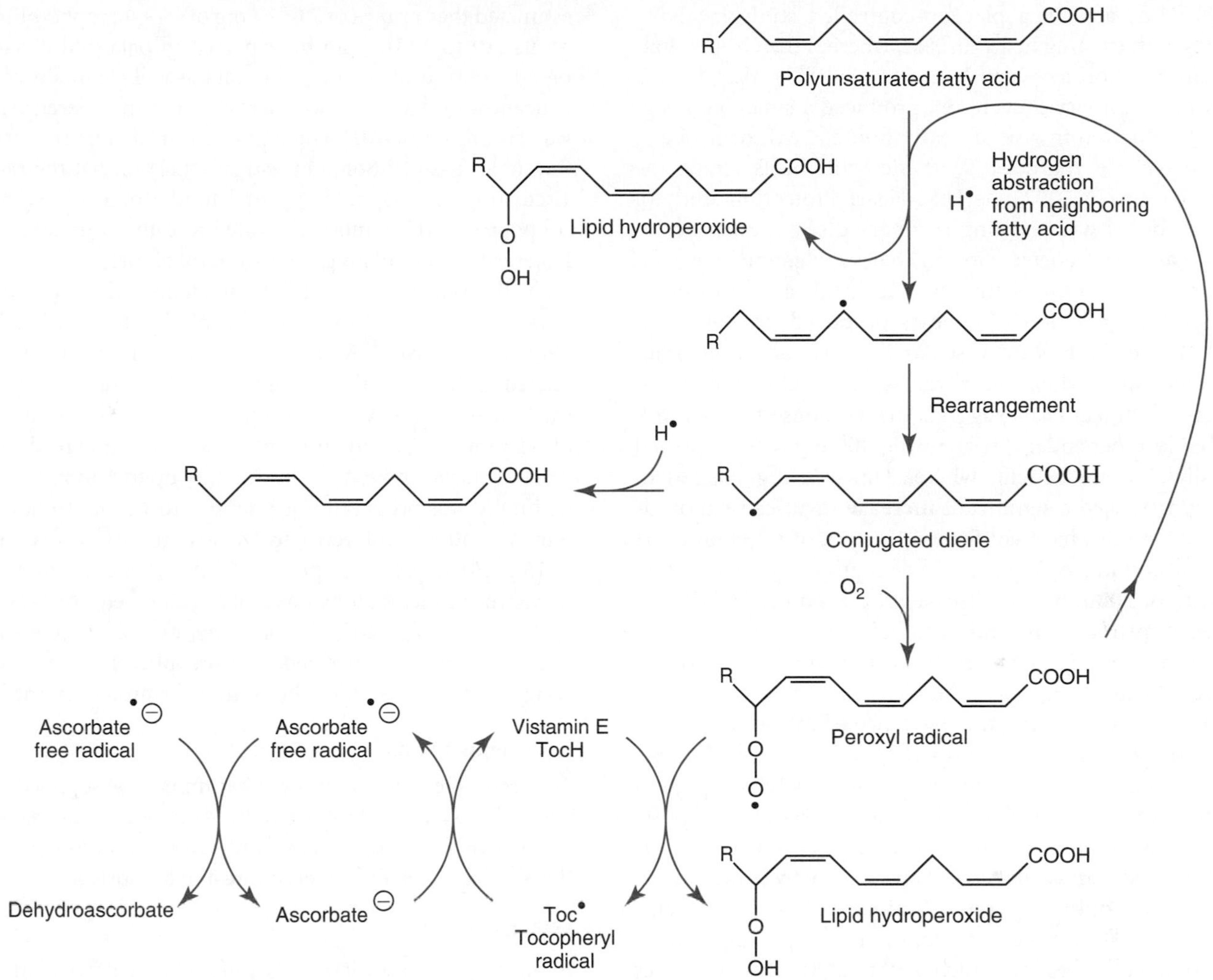

Figure 31-5 Lipoperoxidation and synergistic action of vitamin E and ascorbate.

triacylglycerol and cholesterol. Some of this chylomicron-bound vitamin E is transported and delivered to the peripheral tissue (mainly adipose tissue) with the aid of lipoprotein lipase. The liver takes up the chylomicron remnants where α-tocopherol is incorporated into very low-density lipoproteins (VLDLs) by α-tocopherol transfer protein (α-TTP), enabling further distribution of α-tocopherol throughout the body. Plasma vitamin E is further delivered to the tissue by low-density lipoprotein (LDL) and high-density lipoprotein (HDL).[303] The specificity of α-TTP for α-tocopherol is probably responsible for its preferential storage in most tissue. Vitamin E is excreted via the bile, in the urine as tocopheronic acid and its β-glucuronide conjugate, as carboxyethyl hydroxychromans (CEHC), and by unknown routes.[561] The future direction of vitamin E research has been reviewed.[85]

Functions

Historically, vitamin E has been recognized as necessary for neurologic and reproductive functions, for protection of the red cell from hemolysis, and for prevention of retinopathy in premature infants.[85] Inhibition of free radical chain reactions of lipid peroxidation is the most thoroughly defined role of vitamin E.[302] This occurs mainly within the polyunsaturated fatty acids of membrane phospholipids. Tocopherols and tocotrienols inhibit lipid peroxidation largely because they scavenge lipid peroxyl radicals faster than the radical can react to adjacent fatty acid sidechains or membrane proteins. The resultant tocopheryl or tocotrienyl radicals may then react with additional peroxyl radicals to produce tocopherones (nonradicals), or they may be regenerated by transfer of an electron to ascorbate to form the ascorbyl radical. Thus vitamins E and C act synergistically to reduce lipid peroxidation (Figure 31-5).[115] Moreover, intracellular and extracellular concentrations of vitamin C may critically control the amount of biologically active vitamin E within the cell membrane.[59] Some epidemiologic surveys have shown an association between reduced vitamin E intake (and other dietary factors) and increased incidence of chronic disease, particularly cardiovascular disease and cancer, although intervention studies have produced mixed results. The Cambridge Heart Antioxidant Study[606] showed a significant 47% reduction in nonfatal myocardial infarction (MI) in the vitamin E treatment (400 or 800 IU/d) arm of a placebo-controlled study involving subjects with existing heart disease, whereas the Gruppo Italiano Studio Sopravvivenza Infarcto (GISSI) trial,[231] also involving secondary prevention, produced a small but insignificant reduction in risk of death, nonfatal MI, or stroke in those given 300 mg/d of synthetic vitamin E versus the control group. In 2002, the U.K. Heart Protection Study of 20,536 subjects with existing coronary disease, other occlusive disease, or diabetes showed that supplementation with vitamin E (600 mg), vitamin C (250 mg), and β-carotene (20 mg) over a period of 5 years produced no significant reduction in any type of vascular disease, cancer, or other major outcome, when compared with placebo.[256] A meta-analysis of clinical trials suggests that response to vitamin E may be dose dependent; trials using 400 mg or less showed very slight or no benefit, whereas those using more than 400 mg/d showed a significant **increase** in all-cause mortality. Other studies have confirmed the lack of effect on heart disease[133] and in slowing the rate of cognitive decline.[313] Any influence of vitamin E on disease progression may therefore be seen in primary prevention rather than secondary intervention, but growing concern has arisen about the possible harmful effects of high-dose supplements. Vitamin E has no proven effect in reducing the incidence of various cancers[63]

Beyond its antioxidant properties, α-tocopherol inhibits protein kinase C and 5-lipoxygenase and activates protein phosphatase 2A and diacylglycerol kinase at the post-translational amount. Some genes (coding for CD36, α-TTP, α-tropomyosin, and collagenase) are affected by α-tocopherol at the transcriptional concentration. α-Tocopherol also induces inhibition of cell proliferation, platelet aggregation, and monocyte adhesion, which are thought to be the result of direct interaction of α-tocopherol with cell components.[85,521] α-Tocopherol reduces inflammatory mediator production.[98] Properties independent of α-tocopherol have been ascribed to γ-tocopherol. These include inhibition of cyclo-oxygenase activity, thus conferring anti-inflammatory properties, and the natriuretic property of its main metabolite, γ-CEHC [2,7,8-trimethyl-2-(β-carboxyethyl)-6-hydroxychroman], not shared by α-CEHC.[303]

Requirements and Reference Nutrient Intakes

The requirement for vitamin E is related to the polyunsaturated fatty acid content of cellular structures and therefore depends on the nature and quantity of dietary fat that affect such composition. Hence the minimum adult requirement for vitamin E is not certain but is probably not more than 3 to 4 mg (4.5 to 6 IU) of RRR-α-tocopherol/d for those who ingest a diet containing the minimum of essential fatty acids (3% of calories).[188] Because vitamin E activity is derived from a series of tocopherols and tocotrienols in usual mixed diets, calculations are used that are based on their abundance and activity relative to the biologically most active RRR-α-tocopherol. The milligrams of β-tocopherol are multiplied by 0.5, those of γ-tocopherol by 0.1, and those of α-tocotrienol by 0.3. Their sum plus milligrams of α-tocopherol accounts for the milligrams of α-tocopherol equivalents. It has been estimated that a range of 7 to 13 mg of α++-tocopherol equivalents (10 to 20 IU) can be expected in balanced diets supplying 1800 to 3000 kcal. This intake will maintain plasma concentrations of total tocopherols within the reference interval of 0.5 to 1.2 mg/dL, which ensures an adequate concentration in all tissue.[58] Some investigators claim that the ratio of circulating α-tocopherol to total lipids (or triglycerides or β-lipoproteins) is a more accurate indicator of tissue vitamin E status than circulating α-tocopherol alone.

In the year 2000, the RDA for vitamin E for adults was increased by 50% from 10 to 15 mg/d by the U.S. Food and Nutrition Board.[188] Most European reference intakes are related to the polyunsaturated fatty acid intake.[517] Changes in the United States were accompanied by some debate, with critics arguing that this amount could not be met by the usual North American diet.[273,636] For infants up to 6 months, an AI of 4 mg/d was proposed, for infants 7 to 12 months an AI of 5 mg/d, and for children 1 to 18 years the RDA was set at 6 to 15 mg/d, dependent upon age.[188] Another departure in the newer recommendations was that the daily requirement must be met by RRR-α-tocopherol alone, as the other forms of vitamin E are not converted to α-tocopherol and are poorly recognized by the α-tocopherol transfer protein in the liver.

Intravenous Supply

The recommended amount of vitamin E to be supplied intravenously to adults as α-tocopherol is 10 mg.[260] This is rather lower than the oral provision, but takes into account the fact that it is completely delivered into the bloodstream.

Deficiency

Premature and low birth weight infants are particularly susceptible to development of vitamin E deficiency, because placental transfer is poor and infants have such limited adipose tissue where much of the vitamin is normally stored.[58] Signs of deficiency include (1) irritability, (2) edema, and (3) hemolytic anemia. Anemia reflects the shortened life span of erythrocytes with fragile membranes; it does not respond to iron therapy, which may aggravate the condition. Although symptoms of vitamin E deficiency are rare in children and adults, deficiency can occur in some conditions. Fat malabsorption states, such as cystic fibrosis and chronic cholestasis in children, can cause neuropathy[597] and hemolytic anemia,[683] as can the genetic disorder abetalipoproteinemia (within which vitamin E is transported).[438] Mutations of the gene coding for α-TTP lead to very low plasma α-tocopherol concentrations and cause neurologic symptoms, including cerebellar ataxia.[560] Plasma concentrations may be normalized only by administering large amounts (up to 2 g/d) of vitamin E. Low concentrations of vitamin E may exist without clinical signs, and may occur acutely as a result of oxidative stress, as in major trauma or SIRS.[59]

Toxicity

Excess vitamin E intake usually is achieved only by dietary supplementation. Such supplementation is contraindicated in subjects with coagulation defects caused by vitamin K deficiency and in those receiving anticoagulant drugs. The U.S. Food and Nutrition Board has recommended a tolerable upper limit of 1000 mg/d of vitamin E for adults 19 years and older, based on the absence of hemorrhagic toxicity in animal models,[188] although this has been challenged on the grounds that in those regularly taking aspirin, this intake may be associated with increased risk of bleeding.[273] A comprehensive review of tolerance and safety of vitamin E suggested that intakes up to 3000 mg/d were safe, and reversible side effects of gastrointestinal symptoms, increased creatinuria, and impairment of blood coagulation are seen at intakes of 1000 to 3000 mg/d.[318] However, as noted earlier, long-term use of intakes greater than 400 mg/d may cause increased mortality.

Laboratory Assessment of Status

Assessment of vitamin E status has been achieved by functional methods such as (1) protection of erythrocyte hemolysis on addition of peroxide,[167] (2) inhibition of lipid peroxidation products [malondialdehyde, thiobarbituric acid–reactive substances (ethane or pentane)],[651] or (3) direct measurement of vitamin E concentration in tissues (erythrocytes, lymphocytes, or platelets) or serum. Early direct methods used photometric or fluorometric measurement often based on the Emmerie-Engel procedure, in which tocopherol is oxidized to tocopheryl quinone by $FeCl_3$, and the resultant Fe^{2+} is coupled with α,α'-dipyridyl to form a red color. Later, chromatographic methods were used, including thin layer and gas liquid, which had the ability to separate the tocopherols and the tocotrienols, but these methods were labor intensive and time consuming. HPLC is currently the method of choice for quantitation of tocopherols in serum, as it offers the advantages of accuracy (through the use of primary standards) and reproducibility (between-batch coefficients of variation of 7% or better) and the ability to quantitate multiple analytes, including vitamin A and some carotenoids, in a single analytical run.[703] Both α- and γ-tocopherols are the principal vitamers seen, although others may be detected with minor modifications to the analytical conditions.

Reference Intervals

Guidance reference intervals for serum or plasma (heparin) vitamin E are 0.1 to 0.5 mg/dL (2.3 to 11.6 μmol/L) for premature neonates; 0.3 to 0.9 mg/dL (7 to 21 μmol/L) for children (1 to 12 years)[365]; 0.6 to 1.0 mg/dL (14 to 23 μmol/L) for adolescents (13 to19 years); and 0.5 to 1.8 mg/dL (12 to 42 μmol/L) for adults.[656]

VITAMIN K

Vitamin K promotes clotting of the blood, is required for the conversion of several clotting factors and prothrombin, and is of growing interest in bone metabolism.

Chemistry

Compounds in the vitamin K series are 2-methyl-1,4-napthoquinones, which are substituted with sidechains at carbon 3. *Phylloquinon* (K_1 type) synthesized in plants and *menaquinones* (K_2 type) of bacterial origin are the two principal natural classes of vitamin K (Figure 31-6). The principal vitamin K_1 (phylloquinone) bears a saturated, phytol, 20-carbon sidechain derived from four isoprenoid units; this is the main K vitamin produced by plants and is the major dietary form for humans.[575] K_2 shows greater variation, but an all-*trans*-farnesylgeranylgeranyl, 35-carbon chain of 7 isoprenoid units is typical; these are produced in humans by the large bowel bacterial mass, although their contribution to vitamin K status remains a matter of dispute. Several synthetic analogs and derivatives have been used in human nutrition; most relate to or derive from *menadione* (K_3), which lacks a sidechain substituent at position 3, but can be converted to menaquinone (MK) (e.g., MK-4, where 4 is the number of isoprenoid sidechains) through addition of the sidechain in the liver. The K vitamins are insoluble in water but dissolve in organic fat solvents. They are destroyed by alkaline solutions and reducing agents and are sensitive to ultraviolet light.

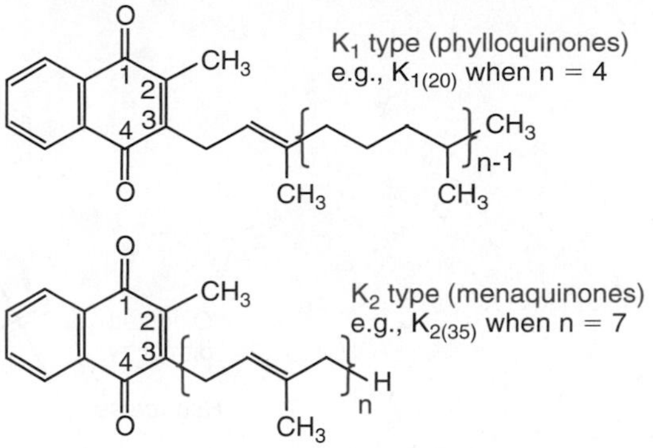

K_1 type (phylloquinones) e.g., $K_{1(20)}$ when n = 4

K_2 type (menaquinones) e.g., $K_{2(35)}$ when n = 7

Figure 31-6 Vitaminic forms of vitamin K.

Dietary Sources

The main dietary sources of the phylloquinones are green vegetables, margarines, and plant oils, whereas some menaquinones can be obtained from cheese, other milk products, and eggs.[563]

Absorption, Transport, Metabolism, and Excretion

Absorption of natural vitamin K from the small intestine into the lymphatic system is facilitated by bile, as is true for other fat-soluble materials. The efficiency of absorption varies from 15 to 65%, as reflected by recovery in lymph within 24 hours. Vitamins K_1 and K_2 are bound to chylomicrons for transport from mucosal cells to the liver. Menadione (K_3) is more rapidly and completely absorbed from the gut before entering the portal blood. In liver, intracellular distribution is seen mostly in the microsomal fraction, where phenylation of menadione to form K_2 occurs. Release of vitamin K to the bloodstream allows association with circulating β-lipoproteins for transport to other tissue. Significant concentrations of vitamin K have been noted in the spleen and skeletal muscle.

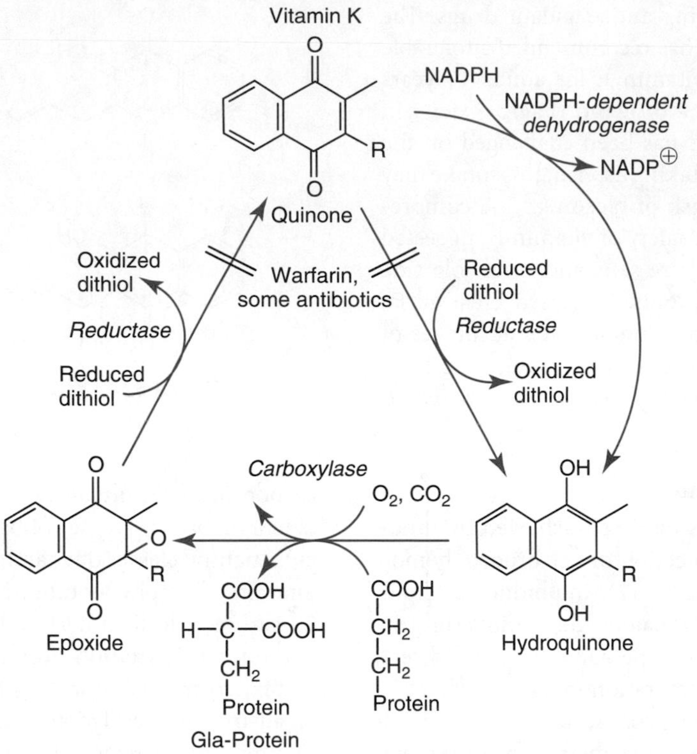

Figure 31-7 Metabolic cycling of vitamin K, the effect of warfarin, and the formation of γ-carboxyglutamyl (GLA) proteins.

Within metabolically active and vitamin K–using tissue, especially liver, a microsomal vitamin K cycle exists (Figure 31-7). The vitamin (quinone) is normally reduced by a thiol-sensitive flavoprotein system to the hydroquinone, which then can couple to the oxygen and carbon dioxide with the use of γ-carboxylation of glutamyl residues in specific proteins (e.g., prothrombin).[176] The 2,3-epoxide of vitamin K that is subsequently formed is reduced to the starting vitamin K quinones—a process that can be antagonized by such vitamin K antagonists as warfarin.

Only traces of urinary metabolites of vitamins K_1 and K_2 appear in urine; a considerable portion of vitamin K_3 (menadione) is conjugated at the hydroquinone concentration to form β-glucuronide and sulfate esters, which are excreted.

Functions

The essential and most thoroughly defined role of vitamin K is as a cofactor to vitamin K–dependent carboxylase, an enzyme necessary for the post-translational conversion of specific glutamyl residues in target proteins to γ-carboxyglutamyl (Gla) residues. This γ-carboxylation increases the affinity of these proteins for calcium.[51] The antihemorrhagic function of vitamin K depends on the formation of the Gla proteins prothrombin (factor II), proconvertin (factor VII), plasma thromboplastin component (factor IX), and Stuart factor (factor X), which, together with two other hemostatic vitamin K–dependent proteins, proteins C and S, and Ca^{2+}, initiate a process to form thrombin that then catalyzes the conversion of fibrinogen to a fibrin clot.[449]

Proteins that contain γ-carboxyglutamyl are also abundant in bone tissue, with osteocalcin accounting for up to 80% of the total γ-carboxyglutamyl content of mature bone. Epidemiologic studies[71,178] have shown an association between low vitamin K intakes and hip fracture risk, but not BMD measurements. Intervention studies have shown that vitamin K can increase BMD in osteoporotic subjects and can reduce fracture rates,[590] although these studies have used menaquinone-4 in pharmacologic rather than physiologic doses. The improvement in bone markers was accompanied by a significant fall in the concentration of undercarboxylated osteocalcin in treated groups. Evidence indicates that vitamins K and D may act synergistically in maintaining bone density.[293,575]

A further major Gla protein, matrix Gla protein (MGP)—containing five residues of γ-carboxyglutamic acid—is found in vascular smooth muscle, bone, and many soft tissues (heart, kidney, and lungs). It is thought that MGP accumulates at sites of calcification, including calcified aortic valves and bone, and is a potent inhibitor of calcification. In experimental studies with mice lacking the gene coding for MGP, calcification of the arteries was observed that led to hemorrhagic death of the animals as a result of blood vessel rupture.[377] Several other Gla proteins have been identified, and putative roles have been assigned[576]

Requirements and Reference Nutrient Intakes

Although the human gut bacteria synthesize large quantities of menaquinones, and such compounds are found in the liver in concentrations up to 10 times those of phylloquinones, absorption of these compounds has been difficult to demonstrate, and dietary restriction of vitamin K leads to evidence of inadequacy, as demonstrated by undercarboxylation of vitamin K–dependent proteins.[176] Thus dietary reference intakes for vitamin K have been revised by the Food and Nutrition Board of the U.S. Institute of Medicine. Current recommendations are 120 µg/d for men older than 18 years; 90 µg/d for women older than 18 years, including those pregnant or lactating; 30 to 75 µg/d for children 1 to 18 years, dependent on age; 2.0 µg/d for infants up to 6 months; and 2.5 µg/d for infants between 7 and 12 months, with the latter requirements met by mature breast milk.[190] Dietary intake of phylloquinone in North American and most European populations studied has been estimated at around 150 µg/d for subjects older than 55 years and around 80 µg/d for younger subjects, although intakes in the Netherlands have been reported to be two to three times higher than these estimates.[563]

Intravenous Supply

In the United States, whether vitamin K should be included in preparations of vitamins for use in TPN is controversial. Although this has been standard in Europe for many years,[581] the long-standing recommendation from the American Medical Association was not to include vitamin K, because this would complicate the provision of adequate warfarin therapy in those patients who require anticoagulation.[9] However, the 2003 requirements of the U.S. Food and Drug Administration (FDA) specified that vitamin K should be included in vitamin supplements for both infants and adults, making the judgment that the physiologic and practical benefits of regular provision outweigh any problems in readjusting warfarin dosage.[260] The recommended intravenous (IV) adult dose is 150 µg/d, which is provided as phytonadione.

Deficiency

Although vitamin K deficiency in the adult is uncommon, the risk is increased for fat malabsorption states such as (1) bile duct obstruction, (2) cystic fibrosis, and (3) chronic pancreatitis and liver disease.[337] Risk is also increased by the use of drugs that interfere with vitamin K metabolism, such as the coumarin anticoagulants (e.g., warfarin) and antibiotics containing the *N*-methylthiotetrazole sidechain (e.g., cephalosporin).[574] Other at-risk groups are hospitalized patients with poor nutrient intakes or those receiving TPN, when fat-soluble vitamin supplements may not fully meet requirements. Conversely, ingestion of supraphysiologic doses of vitamins A and E has been reported to induce vitamin K deficiency, probably through competitive mechanisms.[473] Defective blood coagulation and demonstration of abnormal noncarboxylated prothrombin are at present the only well-established signs of vitamin K deficiency.

Hemorrhagic disease of the newborn can develop readily because of (1) poor placental transfer of vitamin K, (2) hepatic immaturity leading to inadequate synthesis of coagulation proteins, and (3) the low vitamin K content of early breast milk. Prothrombin concentrations during this period are only about 25% of adult concentrations. Severe diarrhea and antibiotics used to suppress diarrhea readily exacerbate the situation, so prothrombin concentrations can drop below 5% of the adult concentration and bleeding can occur. This condition is routinely prevented by the prophylactic administration of 0.5 to 1.0 mg of phylloquinone intramuscularly, or 2.0 mg given orally, immediately after birth.

Toxicity

The use of high doses of naturally occurring vitamin K (K_1 and K_2) appears to have no untoward effect; however, menadione (K_3) treatment can lead to the formation of erythrocyte cytoplasmic inclusions known as Heinz bodies and hemolytic anemia.[441] With severe hemolysis, increased bilirubin formation and undeveloped capacity for its conjugation may produce kernicterus in the newborn.

Because no adverse effects associated with vitamin K consumption from food or supplements have been reported in humans or animals, the U.S. Institute of Medicine has reported that a quantitative risk assessment cannot be performed, and thus an upper limit (UL) cannot be derived for vitamin K.[190]

Laboratory Assessment of Status

A wide range of biochemical and functional tests are available for vitamin K status.[576] Because of its relatively low plasma concentration (approximately 50 times lower than vitamin D and at least 10^3 times lower than vitamin A or E), vitamin K has long presented an analytical challenge. For this reason, vitamin K status has traditionally been assessed by functional methods, primarily by its effect on clotting time. The *prothrombin time (PT)* is assessed by adding a portion of tissue thromboplastin to recalcified plasma and measuring the clotting time against a normal control sample. In vitamin K deficiency, the PT may rise above 30 seconds (normal, 10 to 14 seconds), and at least 2 seconds beyond the control time. Attempts at cross-laboratory standardization led to the introduction of the International Normalized Ratio (INR), by which PT can be expressed as a fraction of the control time. A more sensitive (1000-fold) assessment of vitamin K status with respect to prothrombin can be made by the immunoassay of des-γ-carboxy prothrombin, or undercarboxylated prothrombin, PIVKA-II (protein induced by vitamin K absence or antagonism).[66] PIVKA-II has proved to be a useful marker of subclinical vitamin K deficiency. Another measurement of deficient γ-carboxylation, plasma undercarboxylated osteocalcin, has been shown to correlate individually with PIVKA-II and plasma phylloquinone concentrations and has a better correlation with plasma phylloquinone than PIVKA-II.[599] In this study of biochemical indices of vitamin K nutritional status in a healthy adult population, and in a later one looking at changes in response to dietary phylloquinone,[598] the urinary γ-carboxyglutamic acid : creatinine ratio was measured by derivatization, HPLC separation, and fluorometric detection and was shown to be sensitive to changes in dietary phylloquinone intake. This marker may have advantages in epidemiologic surveys as a less invasive sample.

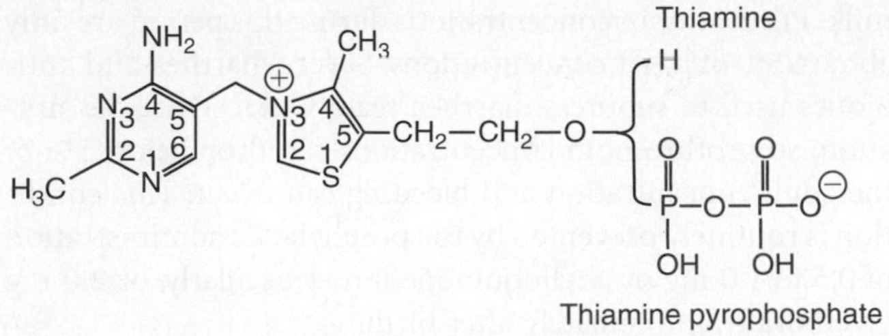

Figure 31-8 Thiamine and the pyrophosphate coenzyme.

Direct measurement of plasma phylloquinone is probably the best indicator of vitamin K status and has been shown to correlate with intake.[598] HPLC methods have been reviewed[573] and typically require 0.5 to 2.0 mL of serum or plasma. Protein precipitation and lipid extraction (often into hexane) followed by solvent evaporation, preparative HPLC (to isolate vitamin K from other lipids), re-evaporation of the vitamin K–rich fraction, dilution in the mobile phase, and further HPLC, with electrochemical or fluorometric detection[299] often after postcolumn reduction, are required. Typical between-batch imprecision values are coefficients of variation (CVs) of 11 to 18% with limits of detection lower than 50 pmol/L. An External Quality Assessment Scheme (EQAS) is available in the United Kingdom.

Reference Interval

A guidance reference interval for plasma vitamin K is 0.13 to 1.19 ng/mL (0.29 to 2.64 nmol/L).[633]

Vitamin B_1—Thiamine

Thiamine, also known as vitamin B_1, forms the coenzyme thiamine pyrophosphate (TPP). It is required for the essential decarboxylation reactions catalyzed by the pyruvate and 2-oxoglutarate complexes.

Chemistry

The structure of *thiamine* (vitamin B_1) [3-(4-amino-2-methylpyrimidyl-5-methyl)-4-methyl-5-(β-hydroxyethyl)thiazole] is that of a pyrimidine ring, bearing an amino group, linked by a methylene bridge to a thiazole ring (Figure 31-8). The thiazole has a primary alcohol sidechain at C5, which can be phosphorylated in vivo to produce thiamine phosphate esters, the most common of which is thiamine pyrophosphate (TPP) [also known as thiamine diphosphate (cocarboxylase)]. Monophosphate and triphosphate esters also occur. The basic vitamin is isolated or synthesized and handled as a solid thiazolium salt (e.g., thiamine chloride hydrochloride). Thiamine is somewhat heat labile, particularly in alkaline solutions, where base attacks occur at C2 of the thiazolium ring.

Dietary Sources

Small amounts of thiamine and its phosphates are present in most plant and animal tissues, but more abundant sources include unrefined cereal grains, liver, heart, kidney, and lean cuts of pork. The enrichment of flour and derived food products, particularly breakfast cereals, has considerably increased the availability of this vitamin.

Absorption, Transport, Metabolism, and Excretion

Thiamine absorption occurs primarily in the proximal small intestine[342] by a saturable (thiamine transporter) process at low concentration (1 μmol/L or lower) and by simple passive diffusion beyond that, although percentage absorption diminishes with increased dose. Absorbed thiamine undergoes intracellular phosphorylation, mainly to the pyrophosphate, but at the serosal side, 90% of transferred thiamine is present in the free form.[522] Thiamine uptake is enhanced by thiamine deficiency and is reduced by thyroid hormone, diabetes, and ethanol ingestion. The gene for the specific thiamine transporter has been identified, and the transporter cloned.[183] Thiamine is carried by portal blood to the liver. The free vitamin occurs in the plasma, but the coenzyme, TPP, is the primary cellular component. Approximately 30 mg is stored in the body, with 80% as pyrophosphate, 10% as triphosphate, and the rest as thiamine and its monophosphate. About half of body stores are found in skeletal muscle, with much of the remainder in heart, liver, kidneys, and nervous tissues (including the brain, which contains most of the triphosphate).

The three tissue enzymes known to participate in the formation of phosphate esters are (1) thiaminokinase (a pyrophosphokinase), which catalyzes formation of TPP and adenosine monophosphate (AMP) from thiamine and adenosine triphosphate (ATP); (2) TPP-ATP phosphoryltransferase (cytosolic 5′-adenylic kinase),[317] which forms the triphosphate and adenosine diphosphate from TPP and ATP; and (3) thiamine triphosphatase, which hydrolyzes TPP to the monophosphate. Although thiaminokinase is widely distributed in the body, phosphoryl transferase and the membrane-associated triphosphatase are found mainly in nervous tissue.

With the use of labeled thiamine probes, a study of thiamine metabolism at normal loads produced an estimated half-life of thiamine of 9.5 to 18.5 days, and showed a large number of breakdown products in the urine.[19] Several of these urinary catabolites are shown in Figure 31-9.

Functions

Thiamine is required by the body as the pyrophosphate (TPP) in two general types of reactions: (1) the oxidative decarboxylation of 2-oxo acids catalyzed by dehydrogenase complexes, and (2) the formation of α-ketols (ketoses) as catalyzed by transketolase and as the triphosphate (TTP) within the nervous system. TPP functions as the Mg^{2+}-coordinated coenzyme for so-called active aldehyde transfers in multienzyme dehydrogenase complexes that affect decarboxylative conversion of α-keto (2-oxo) acids to acyl-coenzyme A (acyl-CoA) derivatives, such as pyruvate dehydrogenase and α-ketoglutarate dehydrogenase. These are often localized in the mitochondria, where efficient use in the Krebs tricarboxylic acid (citric acid) cycle follows.

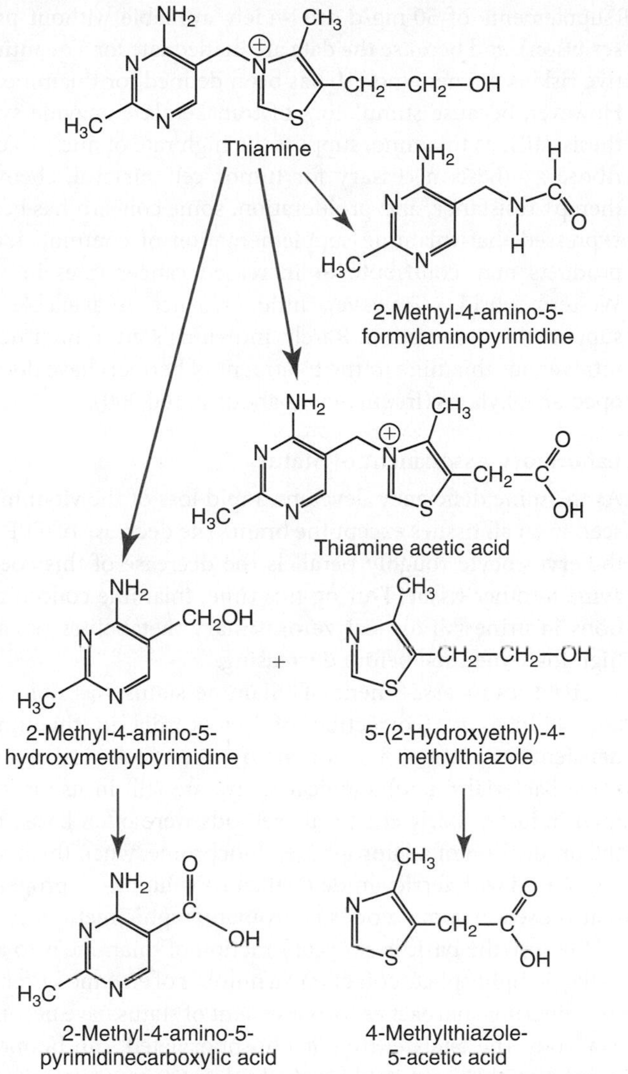

Figure 31-9 Principal urinary catabolites of thiamine.

Three types of subunit proteins constitute such dehydrogenase complexes: (1) a TPP-dependent decarboxylase, which converts the 2-oxo acid to an α-hydroxyalkyl–TPP complex; (2) a transacylase core, which contains lipoyl residues that are acylated by the α-hydroxyalkyl–TPP; and (3) a flavin adenine dinucleotide (FAD)-dependent dihydrolipoyl dehydrogenase, which reoxidizes the reduced lipoyl residues produced after transfer of their acyl functions to reduced CoA. In addition to energy and an ultimate ATP supply derived from reactions in the Krebs cycle, the initial pyruvate dehydrogenase–catalyzed step provides acetyl-CoA as a biosynthetic precursor to other essential compounds, such as lipids and acetylcholine of the parasympathetic nervous system.

Transketolase is a TPP-dependent enzyme found in the cytosol of many tissues, especially liver and blood cells, in which principal carbohydrate pathways exist. In the pentose phosphate pathway, which additionally supplies reduced nicotinamide-adenine dinucleotide phosphate (NADPH) necessary for biosynthetic reactions, this enzyme catalyzes the reversible transfer of a glycoaldehyde moiety from the first two carbons of a donor ketose phosphate to the aldehyde carbon of an aldose phosphate.

Although thiamine as its pyrophosphate contributes to nervous system composition and function in such essential reactions as energy production and biosynthesis of lipids and acetylcholine, a further specific, noncofactor role for thiamine has been proposed in excitable cells. Here, TTP is thought to be involved in the regulation of ion channels, specifically, chloride channels of large unitary conductance, the so-called maxi-Cl channels.[55] TTP may also have more basic metabolic functions, including acting as a phosphate donor for the phosphorylation of proteins, suggesting a potential role in cell signaling. A subacute necrotizing encephalomyelopathy is seen in patients with Leigh syndrome, resulting from the presence of an inhibitor of TPP-ATP phosphoryl transferase[620] and consequent reduction in TTP concentration.

Requirements and Reference Nutrient Intakes

Because thiamine is necessary mainly for the metabolism of carbohydrates, fats, and alcohol, a direct correlation of need with the amount of metabolizable food intake has been noted. A greater requirement is present under situations in which metabolism is increased (e.g., in normal conditions of increased muscular activity, pregnancy, and lactation; in abnormal cases of protracted fever, post trauma, and hyperthyroidism). Clinical signs of deficiency in adults can be prevented with intakes of thiamine above 0.15 to 0.2 mg/1000 kcal, but 0.35 to 0.4 mg/1000 kcal may be closer to a concentration necessary to maintain urinary excretion and TPP-dependent erythrocyte transketolase activity within normal reference intervals.[186] With further consideration of average caloric intakes and activities in different age groups, the most recent recommendations of RDA are 1.2 mg/d for males 19 years and older and 1.1 mg/d for females 19 years and older.[186] The requirement for pregnant women increases early in pregnancy and then remains constant; an additional allowance of 0.3 mg/d is recommended. The lactating woman secretes 0.1 to 0.2 mg of thiamine/d in milk, so an additional 0.3-mg/d allowance is suggested. Based on the thiamine content of human milk and with an increment considered to provide a margin of safety, 0.2 mg/d is the allowance for infants up to 6 months, and 0.3 mg/d for infants 7 to 12 months. Increases above this are suggested for growing children.

Intravenous Supply

Traditionally, the intravenous recommendation was 3 mg/d for adults, usually provided as thiamine hydrochloride, but also as thiamine mononitrate or tetrahydrate. In the 2000 FDA recommendations, this was increased to 6 mg/d,[260] with recognition of the likelihood of increased demands for thiamine caused by hypercatabolism in such patients and the very serious potential complications of deficiency.[660]

Deficiency

Causes of thiamine deficiency include inadequate intake caused by diets largely dependent on milled, nonenriched grains such as rice and wheat, or the ingestion of raw fish containing microbial thiaminases,[164] which hydrolytically destroy the vitamin in the gastrointestinal tract. Tea may contain antithiamine factors that have been detected in certain other plant extracts. Chronic alcoholism often leads to thiamine deficiency caused by reduced intake, impaired absorption, impaired use, and reduced storage,[629] and may lead clinically to the Wernicke-Korsakoff syndrome. Other at-risk groups include those receiving parenteral nutrition without adequate thiamine supplementation,[444] elderly patients taking diuretics,[611] and patients undergoing long-term renal dialysis.[279]

Beriberi is the disease resulting from thiamine deficiency. Clinical signs of thiamine deficiency primarily involve the nervous and cardiovascular systems.[620] In the adult, symptoms most frequently observed include mental confusion, anorexia, muscular weakness, ataxia, peripheral paralysis, ophthalmoplegia, edema (wet beriberi), muscle wasting (dry beriberi), tachycardia, and an enlarged heart. In infants, symptoms appear suddenly and severely, often involving cardiac failure and cyanosis. Commonly, the distinction between wet (cardiovascular) and dry (neuritic) manifestations of beriberi relate to duration and severity of the deficiency, the degree of physical exertion, and caloric intake.[684] The wet or edematous condition results from severe physical exertion and high carbohydrate intake, whereas the dry or polyneuritic form stems from relative inactivity with caloric restriction during the chronic deficiency. The three major physiologic derangements that typically involve the cardiovascular system are peripheral vasodilatation leading to a high-output state, biventricular myocardial failure, and retention of sodium and water, leading to edema. Nervous system involvement includes peripheral neuropathy, Wernicke's encephalopathy, and the amnesic psychosis of Korsakoff's syndrome. More rarely, but especially in seriously ill patients in hospitals, an acute form of cardiac failure has been described (Shoshin beri-beri), which may be fatal, but can be successfully and rapidly reversed with high-dose intravenous thiamine.[660]

Several thiamine-responsive disorders are caused by genetic mutation. In thiamine-responsive megaloblastic anemia (TRMA), the gene has been mapped and cloned and designated "*SLC19A2*" as a member of the solute carrier gene superfamily. Mutations of this gene, the product of which is a membrane protein that transports thiamine with submicromolar affinity, have been found in all TRMA kindreds studied.[452] Thiamine-responsive pyruvate dehydrogenase complex deficiency, presenting with lactic acidosis, can be caused by a point mutation within the thiamine pyrophosphate–binding region,[443] and a thiamine-responsive branched-chain keto acid dehydrogenase complex deficiency, presenting as a form of maple syrup urine disease, is caused by mutations in the E1 α-subunit of the enzyme complex.[693] Therapeutic doses of 5 to 20 mg of thiamine daily have proved beneficial in these cases.

Toxicity

Because no reports have described adverse effects from consumption of excess thiamine from food and supplements (supplements of 50 mg/d are widely available without prescription), and because the data are inadequate for a quantitative risk assessment, no UL has been defined for thiamine.[186] However, because stimulators of transketolase enzyme synthesis, such as thiamine, support the high rate of nucleic acid ribose synthesis necessary for tumor cell survival, chemotherapy resistance, and proliferation, some concern has been expressed that thiamine supplementation of common food products may contribute to increased cancer rates in the Western world.[74] However, little evidence is available to support this assumption. Rarely, individuals given high-dose intravenous thiamine in the treatment of beriberi have developed anaphylaxis (frequency of about 1 : 100,000).

Laboratory Assessment of Status

As thiamine deficiency develops, rapid loss of the vitamin is seen from all tissues except the brain. The decrease of TPP in the erythrocyte roughly parallels the decrease of this coenzyme in other tissue. During this time, thiamine concentrations in urine fall to near zero; urinary metabolites remain high for some time before decreasing.

Historically, assessment of thiamine status was done by animal bioassay (correction of bradycardia in thiamine-deficient rats). Later, it was done by microbiological assays; some bacterial microbiological assays are still in use in the food industry. Early chemical methods were often based on the production of a fluorophore, thiochrome, when thiamine is oxidized with ferricyanide in alkaline solution—a property that is used in some modern chromatographic methods.

Because the basic biological function of thiamine is to act as the pyrophosphate cofactor in a number of enzyme systems, two differing approaches to assessment of status have become available. The analyte, free or phosphorylated, can be measured directly in a suitable body fluid or tissue, or its properties as an enzymatic cofactor can be exploited in a functional assay. Both approaches have their advantages and disadvantages, and consensus as to which is the more useful has not been achieved; the two are probably complementary, each supplying some, but not all, of the information necessary to assess thiamine adequacy (Table 31-3).

The most commonly used enzyme for the functional assay is transketolase. Transketolase catalyzes two reactions in the pentose phosphate pathway (Figure 31-10). As an enzyme within the erythrocyte, transketolase is independent of nonspecific changes in the extracellular plasma. As vitamin B_1 deficiency becomes more severe, (1) thiamine becomes limiting in the body cells, (2) the amount of the coenzyme is depleted, and (3) transketolase activity subsequently diminishes. The *TPP effect* measures the extent of depletion of the transketolase enzyme for coenzyme by assaying enzyme activity before and after TPP supplementation. The percent increase in activity is defined as the TPP effect, or the activation coefficient. Several methods are available to measure transketolase activity. In the Brin procedure,[86] activities of holo forms and apo forms of transketolase in erythrocyte hemolysates are measured before and after addition of TPP, by spectrophotometric determinations of the amount of

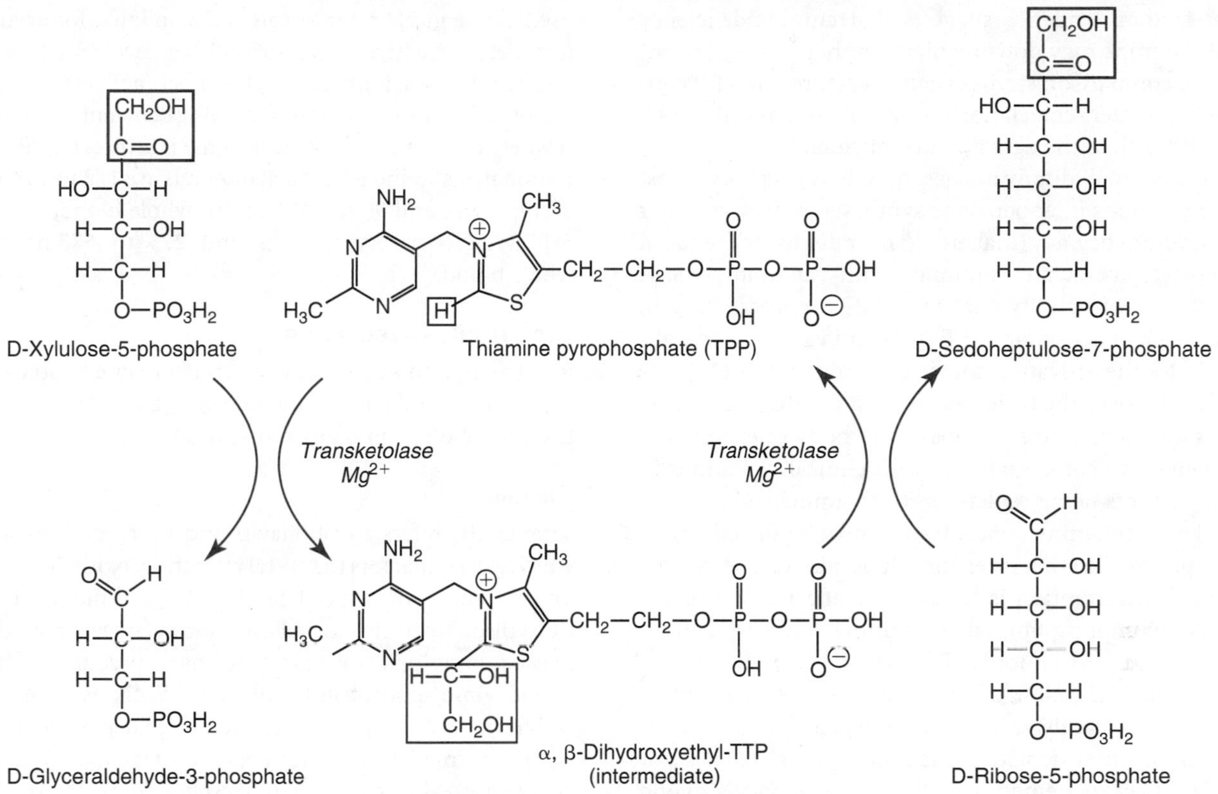

Figure 31-10 The transketolase reaction.

TABLE 31-3 Relative Merits of Direct (Erythrocyte Thiamine Pyrophosphate) or Functional (Erythrocyte Transketolase) Measurements in Assessing Thiamine Status

	Erythrocyte Thiamine Pyrophosphate	Erythrocyte Transketolase Activation
Advantages	Pure standard available Precise and robust method More stable when frozen Depletes at rates similar to other organs Method (HPLC) allows measurement of other forms of thiamine Can detect tissue accumulation	May correlate better with clinical conditions in repleted patients Large database established
Disadvantages	May normalize very early with parenteral treatment	Depletion of apoenzyme may be non-nutritional (e.g., liver disease, diabetes) Variants may have abnormal binding May be influenced by cofactor deficiencies (e.g., magnesium) Difficult to standardize, less robust Derived activation coefficient reduces precision

HPLC, High-performance liquid chromatography.

ribose-5′-phosphate used or hexose-6-phosphate formed. This method is reliable but time-consuming. In an alternative method, the rate of formation of glyceraldehyde-3-P is measured indirectly by a coupled reaction in a system containing excess triosephosphate isomerase (TIM), glycerolphosphate dehydrogenase (GD), and NADH.[550] Glyceraldehyde-3-P is converted by TIM to dihydroxyacetone-P, which, in the presence of GD and NADH, is reduced to glycerol-1-P. The rate of NADH oxidation, measured at 340 nm, is proportional to the transketolase activity. Kinetic methods such as these have been automated with consequent improvements in throughput and precision.

The transketolase activation test basically consists of two tests: (1) measurement of basal activity, and (2) assessment of the degree to which basal activity can be increased by exogenous thiamine pyrophosphate; each may be influenced by different factors. Evidence suggests that chronic deficiency states of thiamine may downregulate synthesis of the apoenzyme.[527] In comparison studies against erythrocyte TPP concentrations, better correlations were obtained with basal activity rather than the activation coefficient.[26]

Other potential disadvantages of the transketolase test include reductions in apoenzyme synthesis in diseases other than thiamine deficiency (diabetes,[199] liver disease[172]), reduced apoenzyme-to-coenzyme binding with apotransketolase variants,[309] lack of stability relative to TPP on processing and storage,[505] lack of a standard or EQAS, and variations in published ULs for the activation coefficient from 15.5 to 40%. The main advantages of the transketolase test are that it is widely used, has a relatively large database and body of experience, and is claimed to correlate better with clinical conditions in alcoholic patients being repleted with thiamine.[275]

Circulating thiamine concentration may be directly measured in plasma, erythrocytes, or whole blood. The plasma (or serum) concentration is thought to reflect recent intake and is mainly unphosphorylated thiamine at low concentration (around 10 to 20 nmol/L). Because the erythrocyte contains approximately 80% of the total thiamine content of whole blood[558] (mainly as the pyrophosphate) and erythrocyte thiamine stores deplete at a similar rate to other major organs, HPLC measurement of TPP in erythrocytes is a good indicator of body stores. Typical HPLC methods include a protein precipitation step; precolumn or postcolumn formation of the fluorophore; thiochrome, usually with alkaline ferricyanide; and isocratic separation.[615] The method is easily standardized with pure thiamine pyrophosphate; it has good precision (interbatch CVs of 5 to 8%) and acceptable limits of detection (around 10 nmol/L), and the analyte is stable at −70 °C for at least 7 months and at room temperature for 48 hours.[26] Whole blood samples may be analyzed in a similar manner to washed erythrocytes and may provide the advantage of simpler sample handling, but they are subject to variable plasma dilution. However, a good correlation has been obtained between erythrocyte and whole blood TPP concentrations, particularly when whole blood TPP included a correction for hemoglobin (Hb). Rapid HPLC methods for measuring both thiamine and its phosphate esters have been described.[375]

Determination of the urinary excretion of thiamine in a 4-hour specimen, especially with comparison of excretion before and after a test load, is helpful in differentiating among extremes of thiamine status. However, as with most assessments based on the quantity of water-soluble vitamins in urine, excretion can be influenced considerably by dietary intake, absorption, and other factors. Measurements of certain urinary metabolites, notably thiamine acetic acid, have been suggested as reflecting thiamine status.[447]

Reference Intervals

Reference intervals for thiamine and its esters depend on whether (1) erythrocytes, whole blood, or plasma is used as a sample; (2) cellular concentrations are expressed per liter of packed red cells or grams of Hb; and (3) mass or SI units are used. Some guidance intervals are as follows: for erythrocyte transketolase activity, 0.75 to 1.30 U/g Hb (48.4 to 83.9 kU/mol Hb) is used; for percent TPP effect (activation), 0 to 15% is normal, 16 to 25% is marginally deficient, and >25% is severely deficient with clinical signs. For direct TPP concentration measurements, typical intervals are 173 to 293 nmol/L erythrocytes and 90 to 140 nmol/L whole blood,[184] or 280 to 590 ng/g Hb in erythrocytes and 275 to 675 ng/g Hb in whole blood.[615]

Vitamin B_2—Riboflavin

Riboflavin, also known as vitamin B_2, is an essential component of FAD and flavin mononucleotide (FMN)—coenzymes that are involved in many redox reactions.

Chemistry

Vitamin B_2 refers to riboflavin and its related metabolites, which act as cofactors to several reduction-oxidation enzymes. The parent compound [riboflavin, 7,8-dimethyl-10-(1′-D-ribityl)isoalloxazine] is a yellow fluorescent compound whose major physiologic role is to act as a precursor for FMN (riboflavin-5′-phosphate) and FAD. FMN is formed from riboflavin by flavokinase-catalyzed phosphorylation, and FAD is formed from FMN and ATP by the action of FAD synthetase, also called *pyrophosphorylase* (Figure 31-11). FAD is further converted by covalent bonding to form various tissue flavoproteins.[415] Flavins are stable during exposure to heat but are decomposed by light, which causes photodegradation of the D-ribitol sidechain at position 10 of the isoalloxazine ring system to yield ultimately lumiflavin (7,8,10-trimethylisoalloxazine) under alkaline conditions and lumichrome (7,8-dimethylalloxazine) at all pH values, especially in neutral-to-acidic solutions. Flavins are chemically and biologically reduced to nearly colorless compounds that rapidly reoxidize on exposure to air (oxygen).

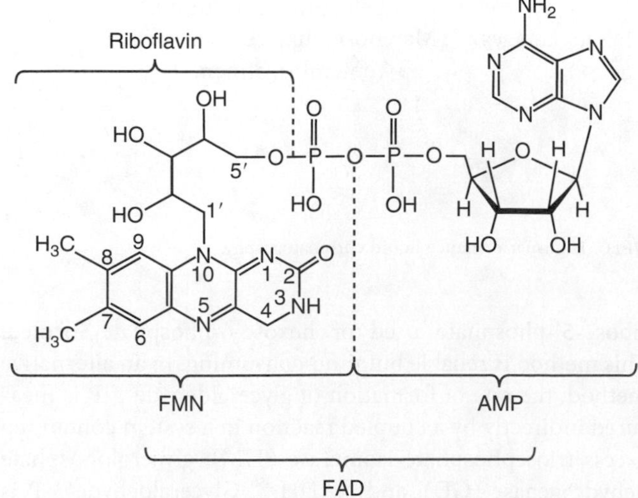

Figure 31-11 Riboflavin and flavin mononucleotide (FMN) as components of flavin adenine dinucleotide (FAD).

Dietary Sources

Rich sources of the coenzyme forms of the vitamin include liver, kidney, and heart. Many vegetables are also good sources, but cereals are rather low in flavin content. Current practices of fortification and enrichment of cereal products have made these significant contributors to the daily requirement. Milk from cows[534] and from humans[533] is a good source of the vitamin, but considerable loss can occur from exposure to light during pasteurization and bottling, or as a result of irradiation to increase vitamin D content.

Absorption, Transport, Metabolism, and Excretion

Most dietary riboflavin is taken in as a complex of food protein with the coenzymes FMN and FAD. These coenzymes are released from noncovalent attachment to proteins as a consequence of gastric acidification. Nonspecific action of pyrophosphatase and phosphatase on the coenzyme occurs in the upper gut.[400] The vitamin is primarily absorbed in the proximal small intestine by a saturable transport system that is rapid and proportional to intake before leveling off at doses near 27 mg riboflavin/d.[706] Bile salts appear to facilitate uptake, and a modest amount of the vitamin circulates via the enterohepatic system.[524] Active transport at lower concentrations of intake was thought to be sodium ion–dependent and to involve phosphorylation, although later work has suggested that uptake is independent of sodium ions.[543] The transport of flavins in human blood involves loose binding to albumin and tight binding to numerous globulins, with major binding noted to several classes of immunoglobulins (IgA, IgG, and IgM).[287] Pregnancy increases the concentration of carrier protein for riboflavin, which results in a higher rate of riboflavin uptake at the maternal surface of the placenta.[140] Uptake of riboflavin into the cells of organs such as liver is facilitated, possibly requiring a specific carrier at physiologic concentrations, but it can occur by diffusion at higher concentrations.[76] Metabolic interconversions of flavins at the cellular concentration are outlined in Figure 31-12.

Conversion of riboflavin to coenzymes occurs within the cellular cytoplasm of most tissue but particularly in the small intestine, liver, heart, and kidney. The obligatory first step is the ATP-dependent phosphorylation of the vitamin catalyzed by flavokinase. The FMN product can be complexed with specific apoenzymes to form several functional flavoproteins, but the larger quantity is further converted to FAD in a second ATP-dependent reaction catalyzed by FAD synthetase (pyrophosphorylase). Biosynthesis of flavocoenzymes, particularly at the flavokinase step, probably is tightly regulated. Thyroxine and triiodothyronine stimulate FMN and FAD synthesis in mammalian systems.[349] FAD is the predominant flavocoenzyme present in tissue, where it is complexed mainly with numerous flavoprotein dehydrogenases and oxidases. Some FAD (<10%) can become covalently linked to any of five specific amino acid residues of a few important apoenzymes.[158] Examples include 8α-*N*(3)-histidyl FAD within succinate dehydrogenase and 8α-*S*-cysteinyl FAD within monoamine oxidase, both of mitochondrial localization. Turnover of covalently attached flavocoenzymes requires intracellular proteolysis, and further degradation of the coenzymes involves nonspecific pyrophosphatase cleavage of FAD to FMN and AMP, and further action by nonspecific phosphates on FMN and AMP. Because there is little storage of riboflavin as such, urinary excretion reflects dietary intake. Milk contains reasonable quantities of the vitamin and lesser amounts of coenzyme, principally FMN. Smaller quantities of sidechain degradation products such as lumichrome, 10-formylmethylflavin and 10-(2′-hydroxyethyl)flavin, and ring-altered compounds are excreted; this may largely result from the action of intestinal microorganisms.[116] Traces of 8α-flavin peptides and catabolites are found in urine and feces.

Functions

Riboflavin and its coenzyme derivatives are involved in a large variety of chemical reactions. These derivatives are capable of one- and two-electron transfer processes and play a pivotal role in coupling the two-electron oxidation of most organic substrates to the one-electron transfer of the respiratory chain,[392] thus being involved in energy production. They also function as electrophiles and nucleophiles, with covalent intermediates of flavin and substrate frequently involved in catalysis. Flavoproteins catalyze dehydrogenation reactions, hydroxylations, oxidative decarboxylations, deoxygenations, and reductions of oxygen to hydrogen peroxide.[524] The chemical versatility of the flavoproteins is clearly controlled by specific interactions with the proteins with which they are bound.[392] Other major functions of riboflavin include drug metabolism in conjunction with the cytochrome P450 enzymes and lipid metabolism.

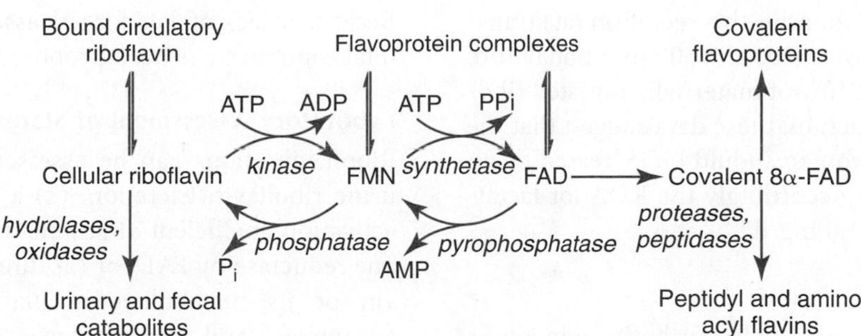

Figure 31-12 Cellular interconversions of flavins.

Flavins also have pro-oxidative and antioxidative functions. They are thought to contribute to oxidative stress through their ability to produce superoxide[392] and to catalyze the production of hydrogen peroxide. As an antioxidant, FAD is a coenzyme to glutathione reductase in the regeneration of reduced glutathione from oxidized glutathione, which is necessary for the removal of lipid peroxides. Riboflavin deficiency is associated with increased lipid peroxidation.[157] Flavins have also been linked with apoptosis[392] and have homocysteine-lowering properties; FAD is a cofactor to methylenetetrahydrofolate reductase (MTHFR) in the remethylation of homocysteine.[428] An interaction between folate, riboflavin, and the genotype of MTHFR is apparent, especially in colorectal cancer.[495] Other possible therapeutic uses of riboflavin include prophylaxis of migraine attacks[555] and treatment of lactic acidosis caused by the use of nucleoside reverse transcriptase inhibitors in patients with the acquired immunodeficiency syndrome[195] or by genetic defects in the mitochondrial respiratory chain, as seen in Leigh disease.[472] Riboflavin is also effective in treating the lipid storage myopathy associated with mutations of *ETFDH* (electron-transferring flavoprotein dehydrogenase).[677]

Requirements and Reference Nutrient Intakes

Riboflavin status has been assessed on the basis of the relationship of dietary intake to overt signs of hyporiboflavinosis, urinary excretion of the vitamin, erythrocyte riboflavin content, and erythrocyte glutathione reductase activity.[186] Calculations have been based on protein allowances, energy intakes, and metabolic body size, but these do not differ significantly because they are interdependent. At least 0.5 mg of riboflavin/1000 kcal is required by the adult, and 0.6 mg/1000 kcal constitutes the allowance suggested for all ages. Based on considerations such as these, the current RDA has been set at 1.3 mg/d for men 19 to 70 years of age and older, and 1.1 mg/d for women in the same age group. Children 1 to 3 years old have an RDA of 0.5 mg/d, increasing to 0.6 mg/d up to age 8. From 8 to 18 years, RDAs progressively approach adult concentrations. Because pregnant women tend to excrete less riboflavin as pregnancy progresses and additionally exhibit FAD stimulation of erythrocyte glutathione reductase activity, recommended allowances call for an additional 0.3 mg/d during pregnancy. During lactation, between 18 and 80 μg of riboflavin is secreted daily into every 100 mL of human milk. If it is assumed that an infant will ingest an average of 750 mL of milk/d during its first 6 months and 600 mL/d for the next 6 months, this secretion rate translates into an ingestion of between 100 and 600 μg riboflavin/d. Further, if it is assumed that 70% of maternally ingested riboflavin is used for milk production, these data suggest that the present RDA for lactating women should be increased by an additional 400 to 500 μg/d. Accordingly the RDA for lactating women has been set at 1.6 mg/d.[186]

Intravenous Supply

The recommended intravenous supply of riboflavin in adults is 3.6 mg/d.[9] Riboflavin in TPN mixtures may be subject to degradation under exposure to ultraviolet light, so bags containing riboflavin should contain fat emulsion or should be covered to provide protection from light.[578]

Deficiency

Although riboflavin has a wide distribution in foodstuffs, many people live for long periods on low intakes; consequently, minor signs of deficiency are common in many parts of the world. In addition to poor intake, functional deficiency can be induced by diseases such as hypothyroidism and adrenal insufficiency, which inhibit the conversion of riboflavin to its coenzyme derivatives, and by drugs such as chlorpromazine, imipramine, and amitriptyline, which have a similar tricyclic structure to riboflavin—the anticancer drug doxorubicin and the antimalarial quinacrine.[156,484] Excess ethanol ingestion interferes with both digestion and absorption of riboflavin.[490]

Because flavin coenzymes are widely distributed in intermediary metabolism, the consequences of deficiency may be widespread. Because riboflavin coenzymes are involved in the metabolism of folic acid, pyridoxine, vitamin K, and niacin,[524] deficiency will affect enzyme systems other than those requiring flavin coenzymes. With increasing riboflavin deficiency, tissue concentrations of FMN and FAD will fall, as does flavokinase activity, thus further decreasing FMN concentrations. FMN concentrations are decreased proportionately more than FAD concentrations. Decreases in the activities of enzymes requiring FMN generally follow the fall in tissue concentrations, whereas FAD-dependent enzymes are more variably affected.

The deficiency syndrome is characterized by (1) sore throat; (2) hyperemia; (3) edema of the pharyngeal and oral mucous membranes; (4) cheilosis; (5) angular stomatitis; (6) glossitis (magenta tongue); (7) seborrheic dermatitis; and (8) normochromic, normocytic anemia associated with pure red blood cell aplasia of the bone marrow. However, some of these symptoms, such as glossitis and dermatitis, when encountered in the field may be seen to have resulted from other complicating deficiencies.

Toxicity

Probably as a result of its limited solubility and limited gastric absorption, no adverse effects have been associated with ingestion of riboflavin appreciably above RDA amounts. One study reported no short-term side effects in 49 patients treated with 400 mg/d of riboflavin with meals for at least 3 months.[555] Because of lack of data for risk assessment, no tolerable upper intake amount has been proposed for riboflavin.[186]

Laboratory Assessment of Status

Riboflavin status can be assessed by (1) determination of urine riboflavin excretion, (2) a functional assay using the activation coefficient of stimulation of the enzyme glutathione reductase by FAD, or (3) direct measurement of riboflavin or its metabolites in plasma or erythrocytes. The advantages and disadvantages of functional and direct methods were discussed in the section on thiamine.

Urinary riboflavin has been measured using fluorometric and microbiological procedures, but for specificity, HPLC combined with fluorometric detection is the method of choice.[116] Under conditions of adequate intake, the amount excreted per day is more than 120 µg or 80 µg/g creatinine. The rate of excretion expressed as µg/g creatinine is greater for children than for adults. Conditions causing negative nitrogen balance and the administration of antibiotics and certain psychotropic drugs (phenothiazine derivatives) increase urinary riboflavin as a consequence of tissue depletion and displacement. A load return test may augment reliability but is more cumbersome.

A method commonly used to assess riboflavin status uses the determination of FAD-dependent glutathione reductase activity in freshly lysed erythrocytes.[550] This enzyme-based assay has been chosen for most surveys of riboflavin status. Most methods measure the rate of change of absorbance at 340 nm caused by the oxidation of NADPH and have been automated to give rapid throughputs and CVs of less than 2% within the run, although some have used fluorescence detection with increased sensitivity.[100] Potential problems include that (1) in long-standing riboflavin deficiency, apoenzyme activity may be reduced, possibly leading to a misleading activation coefficient calculation; and (2) in patients with glucose-6-phosphate deficiency, a misleadingly low activation coefficient may be measured, possibly caused by enhanced binding of FAD to the apoenzyme.[501] Methodologic variation can lead to substantial differences in results.[268]

Direct measurement of riboflavin, FMN, and FAD in plasma or erythrocytes may be made by HPLC, usually with fluorescence detection after protein precipitation,[100] or by capillary zone electrophoresis with laser-induced fluorescence detection (CZE-LIF).[486] In a study of riboflavin status, with FMN and FAD concentrations in plasma and erythrocytes from elderly subjects at baseline and after low-dose riboflavin supplementation obtained using activation coefficient measurements and CE-LIF, it was concluded that concentrations of all B_2 vitamers except plasma FAD are potential indicators of vitamin B_2 status, and that plasma riboflavin and erythrocyte FMN may be useful in assessment of vitamin B_2 status in population studies.[282] In critically ill patients, red cell FAD may be a more sensitive marker of status than plasma FAD.[506]

Reference Intervals

The reference interval for erythrocyte riboflavin using a fluorometric method[332] is 10 to 50 µg/dL (266 to 1330 nmol/L).[633] The reference interval for serum or plasma concentrations of riboflavin has been quoted as 4 to 24 µg/dL (106 to 638 nmol/L)[203,633]; however, a lower interval of 5 to 28 nmol/L was reported using HPLC.[282] Similar intervals were found by liquid chromatography with tandem mass spectrometry.[419] Guidance reference intervals for the activation coefficient of erythrocyte glutathione reductase by FAD are 1.20 (adequacy), 1.21 to 1.40 (marginal deficiency), and 1.41 and above (deficiency).[33]

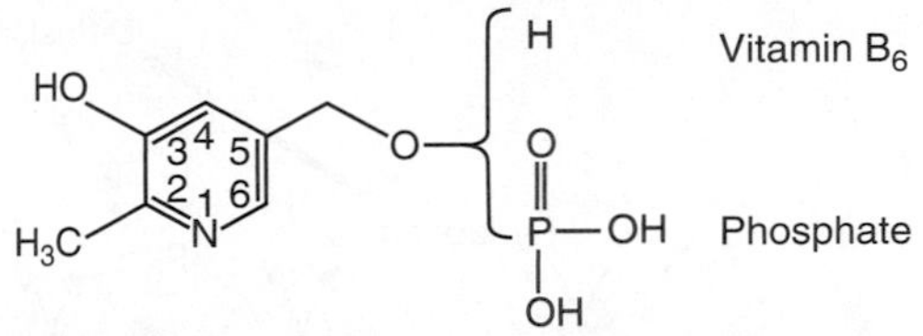

Figure 31-13 Free and phosphorylated forms of vitamin B_6. R = CH_2OH for pyridoxine, CH_2NH_2 for pyridoxamine, and CHO for pyridoxal.

Vitamin B_6—Pyridoxine, Pyridoxamine, and Pyridoxal

Pyridoxine (pyridoxol), pyridoxamine, and *pyridoxal* are the three natural forms of vitamin B_6. They are converted to pyridoxal phosphate, which is required for synthesis, catabolism, and interconversion of amino acids.

Chemistry

The vitamin B_6 group comprises three natural forms: *pyridoxine* (pyridoxol) *(PN), pyridoxamine (PM),* and *pyridoxal (PL),* which are 4-substituted 2-methyl-3-hydroxyl-5-hydroxymethyl pyridines (Figure 31-13). During metabolic conversion, each vitamer becomes phosphorylated at the 5-hydroxymethyl substituent. Although both pyridoxamine-5′-phosphate (PMP) and pyridoxal-5′-phosphate (PLP; P-5′-P) interconvert as coenzyme forms during aminotransferase (transaminase)-catalyzed reactions, PLP is the coenzyme form that participates in a large number of B_6-dependent enzyme reactions.

Dietary Sources

Vitamin B_6 is widely distributed in animal and plant tissues, where the phosphorylated forms, particularly PLP, predominate. Meats, poultry, and fish are good sources, as are yeast, certain seeds, bran, and bananas; somewhat more limited sources are milk, eggs, and green leafy vegetables.[314] In the United States and in some other countries, fortified ready-to-eat cereals are the main dietary source of vitamin B_6. The common commercial form of the vitamin is pyridoxine hydrochloride, which is a water-soluble, white, crystalline solid. Solutions of B_6 vitamers are decomposed by light, especially in the ultraviolet region, at neutral to alkaline pH. The reactive aldehyde function of PLP leads to significant loss during thermal processing of foods.[228]

Absorption, Transport, Metabolism, and Excretion

Food sources of animal origin contain mainly PLP with some PMP, whereas plant sources also contain pyridoxine-5′-glucoside, which is absorbed in a different manner. The phosphorylated sources are hydrolyzed by the intraluminal action of intestinal alkaline phosphatase, but pyridoxine-5′-glucoside is less effectively hydrolyzed by nonspecific glycosidase within cells, and some pyridoxine-5′-glucoside can be absorbed intact and hydrolyzed in various tissues.[399] The nonphosphorylated vitamers are readily absorbed by the mucosal cells through a process of passive diffusion, which does not

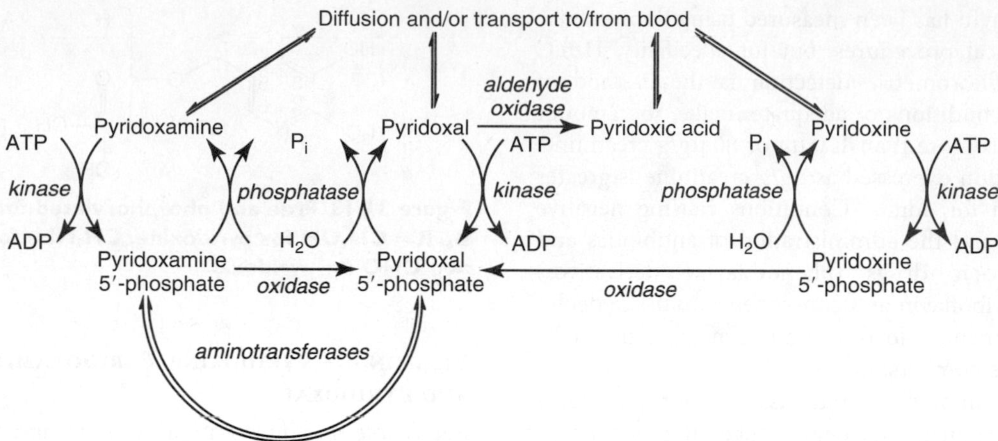

Figure 31-14 Metabolism of vitamin B_6.

appear to be limited by load, although a carrier mechanism may also exist.[542] Here, as in other cells requiring vitamin B_6, the unphosphorylated vitamers may be "metabolically trapped" as phosphorylated forms by cytoplasmic pyridoxal kinase, which is responsible for catalyzing the ATP-dependent phosphorylation of all three vitamin forms. Transport to the liver via the portal vein is done by the unphosphorylated form.

Figure 31-14 shows the intracellular metabolism of vitamin B_6. Most cells contain a cytosolic FMN-dependent, pyridoxine (pyridoxamine)-5′-phosphate oxidase responsible for catalyzing the oxygen-dependent conversion of pyridoxine phosphate and pyridoxamine phosphate to PLP (and hydrogen peroxide). PLP can enter directly into subcellular organelles such as hepatocyte mitochondria and can bind for catalytic function with numerous specific apoenzymes throughout the cell. In addition, the erythrocyte traps PLP as a conjugate Schiff base with hemoglobin.[406] Vitamin B_6 in muscle accounts for 80% of body stores, mostly as PLP bound to glycogen phosphorylase.[64] Total body stores of vitamin B_6 are thought to be about 1 mmole.

Release of free vitamin, mainly pyridoxal, occurs when physiologic nonsaturating concentrations of vitamin are absorbed. Here the phosphates are hydrolyzed by nonspecific alkaline phosphatase located on the plasma membrane of cells. Some PLP is released into the circulation by the liver.[638] Because the reactive aldehyde is capable of forming Schiff bases with amino groups, PLP in plasma is more tightly complexed to proteins—mostly albumin—than is pyridoxal, which forms an intramolecular hemiacetal between the 4-formyl and 5-hydroxymethyl functions. Although PLP is the principal tissue form of vitamin B_6 and pyridoxal constitutes much of the circulating vitamin, the main catabolite excreted in urine is 4-pyridoxic acid (4-PA), which is formed by the action of the FAD-dependent general liver aldehyde oxidase, and especially by NAD-specific aldehyde dehydrogenase, which is found in most tissues.

Functions

As coenzyme PLP, vitamin B_6 functions in more than 100 reactions that embrace the metabolism of macronutrients, such as proteins, carbohydrates, and lipids.[399] Especially diverse are PLP-dependent enzymes that are involved in amino acid metabolism. By virtue of the ability of PLP to condense its 4-formyl substituent with the α-amino group of an amino acid to form an azomethine (Schiff base) linkage, a conjugated double-bond system, extending from the α-carbon of the amino acid to the pyridinium nitrogen in PLP, results in reduced electron density about the α-carbon. This configuration potentially weakens each of the bonds from the amino acid α-carbon to the adjoined hydrogen, carboxyl, and sidechain functions. A given apoenzyme then locks in a particular configuration of the coenzyme-substrate compound, such that maximal overlap of the bond to be broken will occur with the resonant, coplanar, electron-withdrawing system of the coenzyme complex. Aminotransferases affect rupture of the α-hydrogen bond with the ultimate formation of a 2-oxo acid and pyridoxamine-5′-phosphate; this reversible reaction provides an interface between amino acid metabolism and that of ketogenic and glucogenic reactions (see Chapter 22).

Other examples of PLP-requiring enzymes are the amino acid decarboxylases that lead to formation of amines, including several that are functional in nervous tissue (e.g., epinephrine, norepinephrine, serotonin, γ-aminobutyrate); cysteine desulfhydrase and serine hydroxymethyltransferase, which use PLP to effect the loss or transfer of amino acid sidechains; phosphorylase, which catalyzes phosphorolysis of the α-1,4-linkages of glycogen; and cystathione β-synthase in the transsulfuration pathway of homocysteine. Additionally, the biosynthesis of heme depends on the early formation of 5-aminolevulinate from PLP-dependent condensation of glycine and succinyl-CoA, followed by decarboxylation; an important role in lipid metabolism is the PLP-dependent condensation of L-serine with palmitoyl-CoA to form 3-dehydrosphinganine, a precursor of sphingomyelins. Therapeutically, vitamin B_6 has been used for the treatment of some intractable seizures in neonates and infants and for the treatment of other vitamin B_6–responsive inborn errors of metabolism[45] and the carpal tunnel syndrome.[271]

Requirements and Reference Nutrient Intakes

Requirements for vitamin B_6 are complicated by (1) differences in protein intake, (2) the probable provision of a fraction of the necessary quantity through bacterial synthesis in the intestinal tract, (3) the use of alcohol and oral contraceptives, and (4) the infrequent cases in which extra requirements are apparent.[185,351] Estimates of requirements with some margin of safety have been based on the production and cure of clinical signs of deficiency but more often on biochemical parameters. The latter include determination of the urinary excretion of vitamin B_6 and 4-PA or xanthurenic acid after a tryptophan load test, plasma concentrations of PLP, and red blood cell transaminase activity.[186] A ratio of 0.016 mg of vitamin B_6/g of protein intake has been suggested for normal adults and may be extrapolated to children and adolescents. Recent recommendations have proposed RDAs of 0.5 mg/d for children 1 to 3 years, 0.6 mg/d for children 4 to 8 years, 1.0 mg/d for children 9 to 13 years, 1.3 mg/d for boys 14 to 18 years, 1.3 mg/d for men to age 50 years, and 1.7 mg/d for men older than 50 years. Girls 14 to 18 years of age have an RDA of 1.2 mg/d; women 19 to 50 years, 1.3 mg/d; and women older than 50 years, 1.5 mg/d.[186] An addition of 0.6 mg B_6/d is suggested for pregnant women to match the increased protein allowance that occurs during gestation. During lactation, an additional 0.5 mg/d is recommended to accommodate for extra protein intake and to provide a concentration of 0.10 to 0.25 mg/L of the vitamin in milk, which is adequate for the breast-fed infant.

Intravenous Supply

The recommended intravenous supply of vitamin B_6 for adults has been increased from 4 mg/d to 6 mg/d to ensure adequate amounts in patients who are sometimes receiving large amino acid intakes.[260] This is usually provided as pyridoxine hydrochloride.

Deficiency

A deficiency of vitamin B_6 alone is uncommon; it is more usual to expect the problem to occur in association with deficits in other vitamins of the B-complex. As with other water-soluble vitamins that function as coenzymes, the relative affinity of the coenzyme for a given apoenzyme and the extent to which a particular holoenzyme-catalyzed reaction is essential are reflected in progressive symptoms of deficiency of the vitamin. Investigations into the consequences of vitamin B_6 deficiency in the human patient use diets deficient in the vitamin and/or diets containing an antagonist, usually 4′-deoxypyridoxine.[127] However, in some instances, drug interactions have led to hypovitaminosis of B_6.[401] The antituberculosis drug isoniazid (isonicotinic acid hydrazide) forms hydrazones with pyridoxal and PLP. As with other *carbonyl reagents,* not only do such compounds cause loss by displacement and urinary excretion, but the Schiff bases formed with pyridoxal inhibit pyridoxal kinase,[402] and the PLP Schiff bases may additionally inhibit some PLP-dependent enzymes.[638] Penicillamine (β-dimethyl cysteine), used in the treatment of patients with Wilson's disease in an attempt to decrease the damaging concentrations of copper found in liver, inactivates PLP by forming a thiazolidine derivative.[298] Other drugs that can cause vitamin B_6 deficiency include the antiparkinsonian drugs benserazide and carbidopa, which react by forming hydrazones,[44] and theophylline.[217]

Several vitamin B_6–responsive inborn errors of metabolism[45] are known, including (1) cases of infantile convulsions where the apoenzyme for glutamate decarboxylase has poor affinity for the coenzyme; (2) a type of chronic anemia wherein the number but not the morphologic abnormality of erythrocytes is improved by pyridoxine supplementation; (3) xanthurenic aciduria in which affinity of the mutant kynureninase for PLP is decreased; (4) primary cystathioninuria caused by similarly defective cystathionase; and (5) homocystinuria, in which less of the normal cystathionine synthetase is present. In these cases, increased concentrations (200 to 1000 mg/d) of administered vitamin B_6 are required for life.[530] Low vitamin B_6 status (together with low vitamin B_{12} and folate status) in humans has been linked to hyperhomocysteinemia and is an independent risk factor for cardiovascular disease.[139,339]

Biochemical markers of vitamin B_6 deficiency occur early and become more marked as the deficiency progresses.[550] Plasma concentrations of PLP and urinary output of B_6 and 4-PA are decreased within 1 week of removal of the vitamin from the diet. Because liver kynureninase activity is decreased, xanthurenic acid is increased in urine. Aminotransferase activity in serum and red blood cells also decreases. Clinically, electroencephalographic abnormalities appear within 3 weeks, and epileptiform convulsions are a common finding in young vitamin B_6–deficient subjects. In addition, skin changes occur, including dermatitis with cheilosis and glossitis. Hematologic manifestations may include a decrease in the number of circulating lymphocytes and possibly a normocytic, microcytic, or sideroblastic anemia.

Toxicity

Although no adverse effects have been observed with high intakes of vitamin B_6 from food sources, high oral supplemental doses have been found to have neurotoxic and photosensitive effects. The first reported cases in humans were a series of seven patients who had taken between 2 and 6 g pyridoxine/d for up to 40 months. Four of these patients were unable to walk, and all showed severe sensory neuropathy of the extremities, although most of the symptoms were reversed on stopping the pyridoxine.[552] None of the subsequent studies showed any evidence of sensory nerve damage at intakes below 200 mg/d. Based on the end point of development of sensory neuropathy, 1998 recommendations have set a tolerable upper intake amount of 100 mg/d for adults.[186]

Laboratory Assessment of Status

As with the other B vitamins that act as coenzymes, biochemical assessment of vitamin B_6 can be made by direct chemical analysis of the vitamer or its metabolites, or by functional means. Measurements that have been used are PLP in plasma or red cells, its metabolite 4-PA in urine or plasma, the activity and activation coefficient of the red cell aminotransferases (aspartate and alanine), and the tryptophan load metabolite excretion test.[33] Because no single marker adequately reflects status, a combination of these markers offers the best approach.

Direct assessment was originally performed by microbiological techniques using specific strains of *Saccharomyces carlsbergensis* for all three natural vitamers, *Enterococcus faucium* for pyridoxal and pyridoxamine, and *Lactobacillus casei* for pyridoxal. Concentrations of 20 µg vitamin B_6/g creatinine in urine are considered indicative of marginal or inadequate dietary intake of the vitamin. Plasma PLP and plasma or urine 4-PA are most commonly measured by HPLC, PLP with fluorescence detection following precolumn fluorophore formation as a semicarbazone[643] or a pyridoxic acid phosphate,[420] and 4-PA with its natural fluorescence. During deficiency, the concentration of 4-PA will drop well below the normal concentration of at least 0.8 mg/d in urine. Using ion-pair reversed-phase chromatography,[72] plasma vitamin B_6 vitamers (PLP, PL, PN, PMP, PM, and 4-PA) were measured in 90 patients undergoing coronary angiography before and after treatment with pyridoxine 40 mg daily for up to 84 days. PLP, 4-PA, and to a lesser degree PL were found to be the predominant B_6 metabolites in pretreatment plasma. After treatment, PN was also detectable, and PN and PL showed the largest increases in concentration. Increases in plasma concentrations of PLP, PL, and 4-PA occurred within 3 days of supplementation and were steady for the remainder of the study period. In critical illness, plasma PL and PLP are low, and the relationship between them is disturbed, whereas this is less pronounced in red and white blood cells, suggesting that intracellular PLP concentrations are more reliable than plasma measurements in such patients.[655] Other direct measurements have used recombinant enzyme technology. A homogeneous, nonradioactive recombinant enzymatic method for PLP has been described that uses 5 µL of plasma, has a detection limit of 5 nmol/L, and may be applicable to adaptation to an automated analyzer.[243]

Functional assessment of vitamin B_6 status may be made by measuring the activity of red cell aspartate (or alanine) aminotransferase and its activation coefficient on incubation with PLP, although because the apoenzyme is highly unsaturated with PLP, the results obtained have greater variability than those derived by corresponding methods for vitamins B_1 and B_2 and thus are considered less useful. Activation coefficients of less than about 1.5 for aspartate aminotransferase and 1.2 for alanine aminotransferase are considered normal, but this may depend somewhat on the assay method used. Measurement of urinary tryptophan metabolites, particularly xanthurenic acid, following an oral load (2 to 5 g) of L-tryptophan, is one of the most common indices used in studies of vitamin B_6 nutriture, because changes can be recognized early and measurements are relatively easy. Amounts of xanthurenate well above normal (about 25 mg/d) are seen in vitamin B_6 deficiency. Concentrations of other metabolites, such as kynurenic acid and 3-hydroxykynurenine, are increased.

Reference Intervals

A guidance reference interval for plasma PLP is 5 to 30 ng/mL (20 to 121 nmol/L).[518] Plasma concentrations less than 5 ng/mL (20 nmol/L) are judged deficient. Guidance values for other vitamin B_6 metabolites have been published elsewhere.[550]

Vitamin B_{12}—Cyanocobalamin

Vitamin B_{12}, also known as cyanocobalamin, is a water-soluble hematopoietic vitamin that is required for the maturation of erythrocytes.

Chemistry

Vitamin B_{12} is one of the most structurally complex small molecules produced by nature, whose biosynthetic pathway has been extensively studied and elucidated.[674] The generic term *vitamin B_{12}* refers to a group of physiologically active substances chemically classified as cobalamins or corrinoids. They are composed of tetrapyrrole rings surrounding central cobalt atoms and nucleotide sidechains attached to the cobalt. The cobalamin tetrapyrrole ring, exclusive of cobalt and other sidechains, is called a *corrin.* All compounds containing this corrin nucleus are corrinoids. The cobalt-corrin complex is termed *cobamide.* In cobalamins, 5,6-dimethylbenzimidazole riboside is bound to the cobalt atom by one of its imidazole nitrogens, and its 2′-ribose carbon is linked with an ester of aminoisopropanol and propionic acid to the corrin ring (Figure 31-15).

Cobalamins differ in the nature of additional side groups bound to cobalt. Examples include methyl (methylcobalamin), 5′-deoxyadenosine [deoxyadenosyl (short form, adenosyl), cobalamin, or coenzyme B_{12}], hydroxyl

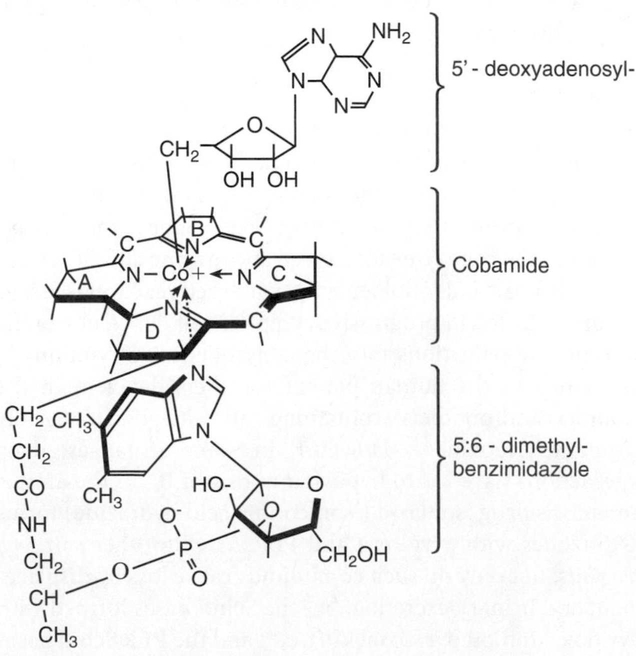

Figure 31-15 The structure of 5′-deoxyadenosyl cobalamin. *(Modified from Chanarin I. The megaloblastic anemias, 2nd edition. Oxford: Blackwell Scientific, 1979.)*

(hydroxocobalamin), H_2O (aquocobalamin, or vitamin B_{12b}), and cyanide (cyanocobalamin). Cyanocobalamin is a stable compound that forms dark red, needle-like crystals; it is the reference compound for measuring serum cobalamin concentration. Less stable serum cobalamins may be converted to this compound for quantitation. The predominant physiologic form of cobalamin in serum is methylcobalamin, whereas that in cytosols is adenosylcobalamin. It is recommended that the term *vitamin B_{12}* be used as the generic descriptor for all corrinoids exhibiting qualitatively the biological activity of cyanocobalamin.[144] Cyanocobalamin has a molecular weight of 1355 Da and a solubility of 12 g/L in water at 20 °C. It is soluble in lower alcohols and aliphatic acids, but is insoluble in acetone, ether, and chloroform. It is gradually destroyed on exposure to light.[144] Aqueous solutions of cyanocobalamin exhibit a distinctive absorption spectrum with maxima at 278, 361, and 550 nm, and with absorptivity coefficients of 115, 207, and 63, respectively, at these maxima. The spectrum is independent of pH but changes when cyanocobalamin binds to intrinsic factor (IF). Because of its stability in aqueous solutions and its distinct absorption spectrum, accurate concentrations of cyanocobalamin is prepared and used as calibrators for the measurement of serum cobalamin concentrations.

Dietary Sources

All vitamin B_{12} is ultimately the product of microbial synthesis. Because plants do not use the vitamin, the main dietary sources are meat and meat products, dairy products, fish and shellfish, and fortified ready-to-eat cereals.[186]

Absorption, Transport, Metabolism, and Excretion

The uptake of vitamin B_{12} from the intestine into the circulation is a complex mechanism, involving five separate vitamin B_{12}–binding molecules, receptors, and transporters.[538] Vitamin B_{12} released from food in the stomach is bound to haptocorrin (R protein, a salivary protein) and travels with it into the intestine, where the haptocorrin is digested by pancreatic enzymes. Liberated vitamin B_{12} then binds to IF, a glycoprotein with a molecular weight of approximately 50 kDa that is produced by the gastric mucosa. When the vitamin B_{12}–IF complex reaches the distal ileum, it is bound by receptors on the surface of mucosal epithelial cells and then enters the cells. The vitamin B_{12}–IF complex is dissociated within the mucosal epithelial cells, with vitamin B_{12} then binding with transcobalamin II (TcII). The B_{12}-TcII complex is then transported across the cell membrane while bound to a TcII receptor and is released into the plasma of the mucosal capillaries and subsequently to the blood in the portal vein.[240]Almost all vitamin B_{12} is taken up by hepatocytes as the blood in the portal vein passes through the liver. It is stored in the liver and is released to plasma to meet physiologic demands. If the quantity of vitamin B_{12} exceeds the capacity of hepatocyte receptors, most of the excess is excreted by the kidneys. Normally, approximately 1 mg of vitamin B_{12} is stored in the liver—a quantity equivalent to the daily metabolic requirement for 2000 days. Thus when the dietary supply of vitamin B_{12} is interrupted or mechanisms of absorption are impaired, vitamin B_{12} deficiency does not become evident for 5 years or longer.

IF, a glycoprotein with a molecular weight of approximately 50 kDa, is secreted by the parietal cells of the stomach. Many other substances bind vitamin B_{12}, but no other known substance has the property of transporting it across the intestinal wall. One molecule of IF binds one molecule of vitamin B_{12}. Gastric secretion of IF is stimulated by food, histamine, and gastrin; it is inhibited by vagal blockade. The ileal receptor for the IF–vitamin B_{12} complex has an association constant of approximately 5×10^9 mol/L between pH 6.4 and 8.4. Binding does not appear to be specific for the configuration of the vitamin B_{12} molecule, because complexes of IF with various analogs of vitamin B_{12} bind equally well to the ileal receptors.

The most important vitamin B_{12} transport protein in plasma is TcII, a β-globulin. It is synthesized mainly in the liver but also in other tissue. TcII is a polypeptide with a molecular weight of approximately 43 kDa; it has a single vitamin B_{12}–binding site per molecule.[566] TcII is less specific for vitamin B_{12} than is IF; it also binds cobalamins that are physiologically inactive. TcII transports vitamin B_{12} to receptors on cell membranes throughout the body. Binding is very rapid: if TcII–vitamin B_{12} is injected intravenously, it is almost completely cleared in one passage through tissue, mostly by the liver.[240] The TcII–vitamin B_{12} complex enters the cell by pinocytosis. Lysosomal proteolysis degrades TcII and releases the vitamin B_{12}. Unbound vitamin B_{12} can enter the tissue cells, but the process is much less efficient.[240]

Two types of vitamin B_{12} binders are found in human gastric juice—one with slow (S) and one with rapid (R) mobility in zone electrophoresis. The slow component is IF, and the rapid component is R protein. Immunologically identical R proteins are found in plasma, amniotic fluid, milk, saliva, ascitic fluid, and granulocytes. However, this granulocyte-derived protein is differentiated from the other R proteins electrophoretically. It is called *transcobalamin III,* whereas the R protein from other sources is designated *transcobalamin I.* Collectively, these two binders are called *cobalophilins.* They are glycoproteins with molecular weights between 60 and 150 kDa. Heterogeneity of R proteins may be due to variations in the carbohydrate moieties (sialic acid residues) rather than in the apoproteins. They have one binding site per molecule and bind vitamin B_{12} analogs to some extent. In gastric juice at pH 2, the cobalophilins have much greater affinity than IF and bind almost all vitamin B_{12}. It has been postulated that cobalophilins aid in host defense against bacteria by depriving them of access to vitamin B_{12}. However, the physiologic function of these proteins is unknown.

Vitamin B_{12} is continually secreted in the bile, but most is reabsorbed and is available for metabolic functions. If circulating vitamin B_{12} concentrations exceed the binding capacity of the blood, the excess will be excreted in the urine, but in most circumstances, the highest losses of vitamin B_{12} occur through the feces.

1. Adenosylcobalamin-dependent, L-methylmalonyl–CoA mutase reaction

L-methylmalonyl-CoA ⇌ Succinyl-CoA

2. Methylcobalamin-dependent, methionine synthase reaction

CH_3-Cob(III)alamin + homocysteine → Cob(I)alamin + methionine

Cob(I)alamin + 5-methyltetrahydrofolate → CH_3-Cob(III)alamin + tetrahydrofolate

Figure 31-16 Participation of cobalamin coenzymes in human metabolism.

Functions

Vitamin B_{12} is required in coenzyme form for more than 12 different enzyme systems.[40] In humans it is required in (1) adenosylcobalamin, coenzyme to L-methylmalonyl-CoA mutase in the conversion of L-methylmalonyl CoA to succinyl-CoA; and (2) methylcobalamin, coenzyme to methionine synthase in the conversion of homocysteine to methionine. In the former reaction (Figure 31-16), the mutase is a mitochondrial matrix enzyme that binds 2 moles of adenosyl-cobalamin (Cbl)/dimer[376] and participates in a complex reaction using radical chemistry.[29] The conversion of L-methylmalonyl-CoA to succinyl-CoA links propionyl-CoA, which is formed from amino acids such as valine, isoleucine, and methionine with odd-chain fatty acids with the tricarboxylic acid (TCA) cycle. Congenital defects of mutase synthesis or inability to synthesize adenosyl-Cbl results in life-threatening methylmalonic aciduria and metabolic ketoacidosis. In the latter reaction (see Figure 31-16), methylcobalamin serves as an intermediate in the transfer of a methyl group from 5-methyltetrahydrofolate to homocysteine for the formation of methionine. Methionine is required for protein synthesis and as the methyl donor, *S*-adenosylmethionine. Congenital defects in methionine synthase or the synthesis of methyl-Cbl results in severe hyperhomocysteinemia.[174]

Requirements and Reference Nutrient Intakes

Total body stores of vitamin B_{12} are estimated to be between 2 and 5 mg in the adult man,[4] of which about 1 mg is in the liver and a smaller amount in the kidney. A daily obligatory loss of vitamin B_{12} of about 0.1% of body pool is believed to occur, irrespective of size,[264] suggesting that a daily requirement to maintain stores would be 2 to 5 μg. The daily diet of Western countries contains between 5 and 30 μg of vitamin B_{12}, with average ingestion of 7 to 8 μg/d by adult men and 4 to 5 μg/d by adult women. Additional small amounts may be available from vitamin B_{12} synthesis by intestinal microorganisms. Of the amount ingested, between 1 and 5 μg is absorbed.

The RDA for vitamin B_{12} is based on the amount necessary for maintenance of hematologic status and normal serum vitamin B_{12} concentrations; it assumes 50% absorbance of ingested vitamin B_{12}. The RDA for adults (19 to 50 years) has been set at 2.4 μg/d, with an increase to 2.6 μg/d in pregnancy and to 2.8 μg/d in lactation. RDAs for children are 0.9 μg/d at 1 to 3 years, 1.2 μg/d at 4 to 8 years, 1.8 μg/d at 9 to 13 years, and 2.4 μg/d at 14 to 18 years. Because 10% to 30% of older persons may be unable to absorb naturally occurring vitamin B_{12}, it is recommended that those older than 50 years meet their RDA mainly by consuming foods fortified with vitamin B_{12} or with a vitamin B_{12}–containing supplement.[186]

Intravenous Supply

The recommended intravenous intake for adults is 5 μg/d as cyanocobalamin—an amount in excess of the oral recommendation that will more than meet requirements.[9]

Deficiency

Deficiency of vitamin B_{12} in humans is associated with megaloblastic anemia and neuropathy. The most common cause of vitamin B_{12} deficiency is *pernicious anemia,* an autoimmune disease in which chronic atrophic gastritis results from antibodies to gastric parietal cells and IF, directed against gastric parietal cell H^+/K^+-ATPase.[634] One population study showed that 1.9% of persons older than 60 years have undiagnosed pernicious anemia, although the diagnosis is made most commonly in young to middle-aged black women (mean age, 53 years) and in middle-aged to elderly whites.[103] Pernicious anemia may also occur in children because of failure of IF secretion or secretion of biologically inactive IF. Other groups at risk for vitamin B_{12} deficiency include those (1) older than 65 years of age; (2) with malabsorption; (3) who are vegetarians; (4) with autoimmune disorders; and (5) taking prescribed medication known to interfere with vitamin absorption or metabolism, including nitrous oxide, phenytoin, dihydrofolate reductase inhibitors, metformin, and proton pump inhibitors; as well as (6) infants with suspected metabolic disorders.

Intestinal malabsorption of vitamin B_{12} may be caused by gastrectomy or ileal resection, with an inverse relationship noted between the length of ileum resected and absorption of vitamin B_{12}. Other causes of malabsorption include tropical sprue, inflammatory disease of the small intestine, intestinal stasis with overgrowth of colonic bacteria, which consume vitamin B_{12} ingested by the host, and human immunodeficiency virus (HIV) infection. Another cause of vitamin B_{12} malabsorption is failure to extract cobalamin from food. Some patients fail to absorb cobalamin bound to food, whereas absorption of non–food-bound cobalamin in the Schilling test is unimpaired. This is particularly a problem in patients with compromised gastric status[103] or early in the course of development of pernicious anemia.

Vegetarians have a lower intake of vitamin B_{12} than omnivores, and although clinical signs of deficiency are uncommon, biochemical markers of status indicate functional vitamin B_{12} deficiency. In a study of 66 lactovegetarians or lacto-ovovegetarians, 29 vegans, and 79 omnivores, the incidence of low holotranscobalamin II was 77%, 92%, and 11%, respectively, in the three groups; of elevated methylmalonic acid (MMA), 68%, 83%, and 5%; and of elevated total homocysteine, 38%, 67%, and 16%.[263] A large number of disorders are associated with cobalamin deficiency in infancy or childhood. Of these, the most commonly encountered is the Imerslund-Graesbeck syndrome, a condition that is characterized by inability to absorb vitamin B_{12}, with or without IF, and proteinuria. It appears to be due to an inability of intestinal mucosa to absorb the vitamin B_{12}–IF complex. The second most common of these is congenital deficiency of gastric secretion of IF. Very rarely, congenital deficiency of vitamin B_{12} in a breast-fed infant is due to deficiency of vitamin B_{12} in maternal breast milk resulting from unrecognized pernicious anemia in the mother. This is rare because most women with undiagnosed and untreated pernicious anemia are infertile. Additionally, some rare methylmalonic acidemias (acidurias) caused by inborn errors in homocysteine and methionine metabolism are responsible for disorders of vitamin B_{12} status.[173]

The hematologic effects of vitamin B_{12} deficiency are indistinguishable from those of folate deficiency. Classical morphologic changes in the blood, in approximate order of appearance, are as follows: hypersegmentation of neutrophils, macrocytosis, anemia, leukopenia, and thrombocytopenia, with megaloblastic changes in bone marrow accompanying peripheral blood changes. The cause of the hematologic abnormalities is thought to be an imbalance of decreased deoxyribonucleic acid (DNA) synthesis and adequate ribonucleic acid (RNA) synthesis caused by the secondary block in folate metabolism caused by vitamin B_{12} deficiency.[7] Many immature cells die in the bone marrow, possibly by apoptosis, leading to the release of bilirubin and lactate dehydrogenase (LD) into the blood. This is termed *ineffective erythropoiesis.* All bone marrow lesions can be reversed by vitamin B_{12} treatment.

In addition to hematologic changes, vitamin B_{12} deficiency can lead to a demyelinating disorder of the central nervous system in man. Serious and often irreversible neurologic disorders can occur, such as burning pain or loss of sensation in the extremities, weakness, spasticity and paralysis, confusion, disorientation, and dementia. This condition has been given the name *subacute combined degeneration of the spinal cord.* Neurologic symptoms may occur without any discernible hematologic changes in the blood; indeed an intriguing inverse relationship between the hematologic and the neurologic has been observed.[255] The incidence of neurologic complications is between 75% and 90% of all individuals with clinically observable vitamin B_{12} deficiency; in about 25% of cases, these may be the only clinical manifestation of deficiency. The mechanism of the disorder is uncertain, although indirect evidence suggests that disorders of both enzyme systems requiring vitamin B_{12} coenzymes are necessary before neurologic symptoms occur.[174] The response of neurologic symptoms to vitamin B_{12} replacement is often dependent on the duration of the symptoms. Vitamin B_{12} deficiency may be associated with other mainly gastrointestinal complications, such as glossitis of the tongue, appetite and weight loss, flatulence and constipation, mental changes, and infertility.[7] Interest in a possible link between vitamin B_{12} status and cognitive decline is increasing, but data remain inconclusive even though supplements of vitamin B_{12} and folate may normalize homocysteine concentrations.[667]

Toxicity

No adverse effects have been associated with excess vitamin B_{12} intake from food or supplements in healthy people. Daily oral doses of up to 2 mg of cyanocobalamin have been used for treatment of deficiency in those who tolerate oral supplementation.[344] Data in the literature are insufficient to propose a tolerable upper intake amount for vitamin B_{12}.[186]

Laboratory Assessment of Status

Both direct and indirect (functional) methods are available for assessment of vitamin B_{12} status. Indirect tests include assays for urinary and serum concentrations of MMA, plasma homocysteine, the deoxyuridine suppression test, and the vitamin B_{12} absorption test. Cytochemical staining of red blood cell (RBC) precursors and the test for IF blocking antibodies are other ancillary methods of assessing vitamin B_{12} status.

A comprehensive review of methods for measuring vitamin B_{12} in various biological samples has been published.[340] Microbiological, competitive protein binding (CPB), and immunometric assays have been used for quantitation of serum vitamin B_{12}. Microbiological assays have largely been replaced by the other, more convenient and precise methods, although they remain reference methods for the determination of biologically active vitamin B_{12}. The most widely used procedures use *Euglena gracilis, Lactobacillus leishmannii,* or a mutant of *Escherichia coli,* although each of these organisms is susceptible to growth inhibition by antibiotics or other drugs, such as methotrexate, that may be present in a patient's serum. Furthermore, these assays require at least 24 hours to establish adequate growth of the microorganism. However, use of microtiter enzyme-linked immunosorbent assay (ELISA) plate technology has enhanced the utility of some microbiological assays.[321]

Commercial kits are available for CPB assays of vitamin B_{12}. The vitamin B_{12} binder used is often nonhuman IF, usually obtained from hog stomach. If the IF is not highly purified, it may contain R proteins, which bind not only vitamin B_{12} but also related metabolically inactive compounds, yielding higher values. IF therefore must be highly purified or must have cobinamide (a vitamin B_{12} analog) added to the IF to saturate all binding sites on the R proteins. Cobinamide is not bound by IF.

In a widely used CPB assay, vitamin B_{12} (cobalamin) competes with ^{57}Co-labeled cobalamin for a limited number of binding sites on IF. Some assays require a preliminary step in which the specimen is boiled in a buffered solution containing dithiothreitol, KCN, and ^{57}Co-labeled tracers to release vitamin B_{12} from endogenous binding proteins. Alternatively, other procedures irreversibly denature endogenous binding proteins by increasing the pH from 12 to 13 and then readjusting the pH to 9.3 before the binding reagent is added. Subsequent separation of bound and free folate and vitamin B_{12} is achieved by contact with dextran-coated charcoal, which absorbs the free (unbound) molecules, leaving protein-bound vitamin B_{12} in the solution.

Most immunometric methods use solid-phase separation by immobilizing the IF binder on beads or magnetic particles. The free vitamin B_{12} then remains in the supernatant, and the bound analytes become part of the solid-phase suspension. For simultaneous folate/vitamin B_{12} measurement, a gamma-scintillation counter that discriminates between the energy levels of ^{57}Co (for vitamin B_{12}) and ^{125}I (for folate) must be used.

Multiple automated and semiautomated systems are available for measuring vitamin B_{12} and folate, using, for example, chemiluminescence as a signal. The assays are standardized with 7.5-minute incubation, magnetic particle separation, and an acridium ester signal. The precision of automated systems allows specimens to be analyzed in singlet while CVs less than those found for the mean of duplicates of radioimmunoassays are maintained.

Indirect tests assess the functional adequacy of vitamin B_{12}. Serum methylmalonic acid concentration is increased when lack of adenyl-Cbl causes a block in the conversion of methylmalonyl-CoA to succinyl-CoA. It is a sensitive test of status, being often the first analyte to be raised in subclinical vitamin B_{12} deficiency.[551] It has a further advantage in that it is unaffected by folate deficiency. Early methods for methylmalonic acid lacked sensitivity and specificity; this situation has been resolved by the adoption of gas chromatographic–mass spectrometric methods,[604] although these methods require specialized handling. Plasma total homocysteine concentration is a sensitive indicator of vitamin B_{12} status because methyl-Cbl is required for the remethylation of homocysteine to methionine, but it is not specific, being elevated in deficiencies of folate and vitamin B_6 and vitamin B_{12}. Plasma concentrations of total homocysteine can be reliably measured by HPLC with fluorescent or electrochemical detection, and with enzymatic and capillary gas chromatography–mass spectroscopy methods.[550] Plasma samples for homocysteine analysis must be obtained soon after venipuncture to reduce preanalytical increases that may occur on standing, although these can be minimized by the use of a fluoride–ethylenediaminetetraacetic acid (EDTA) tube. Increased screening of plasma total homocysteine concentrations as an independent risk factor for cardiovascular disease (see Chapter 27) may lead to identification of additional cases of subclinical vitamin B_{12} deficiency.

The measurement of holotranscobalamin II is potentially useful as a specific marker of biologically available vitamin B_{12}, because only cobalamin bound to TcII is specifically available for uptake by all cells. Other methods have been described for the measurement of holotranscobalamin in serum, using an immobilized monoclonal antibody to human transcobalamin, followed by measurement of released cobalamin by CPB[645] or an automated assay by enzyme immunoassay.[77] Another method uses magnetic beads coated with cobalamin to precipitate apotranscobalamin, followed by measurement of holotranscobalamin in the supernatant by ELISA.[453] Although these methods are claimed to be precise and simple to perform, there remains doubt over interpretation of the measured concentrations[104] and their sensitivity and specificity in the diagnosis of vitamin B_{12} deficiency.[367]

The deoxyuridine suppression test measures the effects of prior addition of deoxyuridine on uptake of radiolabeled thymidine into the DNA of cultured bone marrow cells, peripheral blood lymphocytes, or whole blood. Normal samples that contain vitamin B_{12} can convert deoxyuridine to thymidine and therefore do not take up as much thymidine. Samples from patients who are deficient in vitamin B_{12} show less suppression than those from normal patients. Because it is relatively time-consuming, the deoxyuridine suppression test is not widely available for use as a diagnostic test.[618]

The Schilling test is primarily a test of vitamin B_{12} absorption and not of status, but it permits differentiation of causes of vitamin B_{12} deficiency (pernicious anemia or intestinal malabsorption). The proportion absorbed from orally administered ^{57}Co- or ^{58}Co-labeled vitamin B_{12} is measured by determining radioactivity in feces, urine, or serum or by externally scanning the liver. The usual procedure is to measure radioactivity in a 24-hour urine sample, which is collected after oral administration of 0.5 μg of radioactive Co-labeled vitamin B_{12} after an overnight fast. In normal individuals, 8% or more of the dose administered is excreted in the urine, whereas in people with pernicious anemia, less than 7% (often 0 to 3%) is excreted. A confirmatory test for lack of IF requires ingestion of vitamin B_{12} and IF.[84]

Reference Intervals

Depending on the laboratory and the procedure used, reference intervals vary widely. The WHO, in its report in 1968, defined a serum vitamin B_{12} concentration less than 150 ng/L (110 pmol/L) as deficient, and a concentration of 201 ng/L (147 pmol/L) or higher[681] as acceptable. A dietary and nutritional survey of British adults in 1990 published a reference interval of 206 to 678 ng/L (151 to 497 pmol/L).[227] Changes in serum vitamin B_{12} concentration as a function of age in healthy adults have been the subject of contradictory reports. Data from a study population in the United States (Framingham Study) showed an increased prevalence (40.5% of 222 subjects) of low serum vitamin B_{12} concentration (<258 pmol/L) in elderly subjects in comparison with a control group of younger subjects (17.9% incidence).[360] Vitamin B_{12} concentrations within the reference interval may not necessarily reflect adequate vitamin B_{12} status, because serum concentrations may be maintained at the expense of tissue stores. Conversely, low serum vitamin B_{12} concentrations may not be indicative of vitamin B_{12} deficiency. Most of the vitamin B_{12} in serum is bound to TcI, which is released by granulocytes and has no functional role in the transport of vitamin B_{12} to cells. Low serum vitamin B_{12} concentration may be due to a reduction in TcI as a consequence of low total granulocyte mass. This has been observed in benign neutropenia, multiple myeloma, and leukemic reticuloendotheliosis and may be expected in other conditions in which the bone marrow is hypoplastic, aplastic, or replaced by malignant cells.

Elevated MMA and low holotranscobalamin may be found in patients with normal vitamin B_{12}; hence holotranscobalamin is a better predictor of B_{12} than total B_{12}.[262] Serum methylmalonic acid concentrations below 376 nmol/L have been considered acceptable in an elderly U.S. population,[360] as have concentrations below 320 nmol/L in a group of older Dutch subjects.[649] Reference values for holotranscobalamin have been variable but are in the range of 19 to 134 pmol/L[77] and are age and gender dependent.[514]

VITAMIN C—ASCORBIC ACID

Vitamin C (L-ascorbic acid) serves as a reducing agent in several important hydroxylation reactions in the body.

Chemistry

As shown in Figure 31-17, the term *vitamin C* refers to all molecules that exhibit antiscorbutic properties in humans and includes both ascorbic acid and its oxidized form, dehydroascorbic acid (DHA). The vitamin C redox system comprises these molecules and the free radical intermediate, monodehydroascorbic acid,[305] the product of one-electron oxidation of ascorbic acid. L-ascorbic acid is the enol form of 2-oxo-L-gulofuranolactone, the enolic hydroxyl on ring carbon 3 having a pK_a of 4.2 and conferring its acidic nature. The vitamin is a white, crystalline solid that is readily soluble in water. Acidic solutions (below pH 3) show absorption maximum at 245 nm, whereas solutions of the ionized material (above pH 5) have an absorption peak at 265 nm. Ascorbic acid is a relatively strong reductant with an E'_0 (pH 7) of +0.58 volt. The dehydro form is more labile than the reduced form to hydrolytic ring opening to yield 2,3-diketo-L-gulonic acid, which is not antiscorbutic.

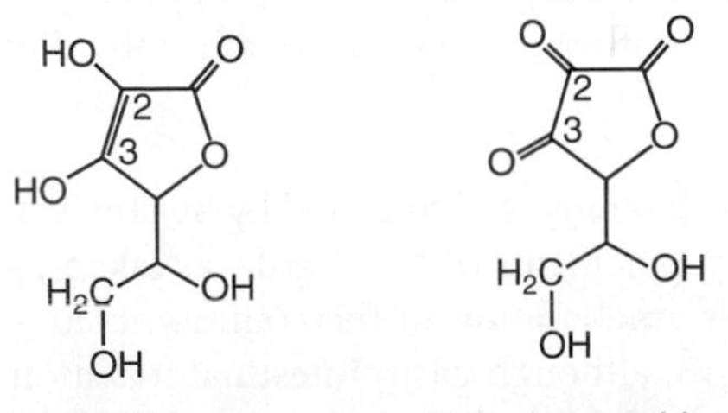

Figure 31-17 L-Ascorbic and dehydroascorbic acids. *(Modified from Row PB. Inherited disorders of folate metabolism. In: Stanbury JB, Wyngaarden DS, eds. The metabolic bases of inherited disease, 5th edition. New York: McGraw-Hill, 1983.)*

Dietary Sources

Plants and most animals possess the ability to synthesize the vitamin from D-glucose via the lactones of D-glucuronic and L-gulonic acids; however, some mammals, including the human, lack L-gulonolactone oxidase, the enzyme that catalyzes the formation of 2-keto-L-gulonolactone, which spontaneously tautomerizes to L-ascorbic acid. Excellent sources of the vitamin include citrus fruits, berries, melons, tomatoes, green peppers, broccoli, brussel sprouts, and leafy green vegetables.[609] Losses during processing, especially with heat and aerobic conditions, can be considerable.

Absorption, Transport, Metabolism, and Excretion

Gastrointestinal absorption of ascorbic acid occurs through a combination of sodium-dependent active transport at low concentrations[542] and simple diffusion at high concentrations.[536] Between 70% and 90% of a usual dietary intake of ascorbic acid (up to 180 mg/d) is absorbed, falling to 50% or less at loads greater than 1 g/d.[312] The absorbed ascorbic acid moves rapidly from the intestinal cell into the blood through a process of facilitated diffusion.[383] Ascorbate uptake by cells is mediated by specific transporters—ascorbate by the sodium-dependent transporters SVCT 1 and SVCT 2, and DHA via the facilitated-diffusion glucose transporters GLUT 1, 3, and 4.[357] Vitamin C is found in most tissues, but glandular tissues, such as pituitary, adrenal cortex, corpus luteum, and thymus, have the highest amounts, and the retina has 20 to 30 times the plasma concentration. DHA, once transported intracellularly, is reduced to ascorbate; in plasma, vitamin C exists predominantly as the ascorbate ion. Many cells, particularly hepatic cells, neutrophils, mononuclear phagocytes, osteoblasts, and erythrocytes, are capable of DHA uptake and recycling to ascorbate, which maintains a human body pool of up to 2 g.[312] The biological half-life of vitamin C in an individual ranges from 8 to 40 days, with an average of about 16 days. Vitamin C is conserved during periods of low intake, with absorption becoming maximum with minimum urinary excretion. Excretion of unchanged ascorbate occurs increasingly with increased dosage, with almost all of an injected dose of more than 500 mg excreted over 24 hours.[356] DHA that is not recycled may be irreversibly delactonized to 2,3-diketogulonic acid and further degraded to oxalic acid for urine excretion. Other catabolic products of 2,3-diketogulonic acid are L-lyxonic acid, L-xylose, and L-threonic acid.

Functions

Ascorbic acid acts as a cofactor for a number of mixed function oxidases in processes in which it promotes enzyme activity by maintaining metal ions in their reduced form (particularly iron and copper). Its most clearly established and critical functional role is as a cofactor for protocollagen hydroxylase, the enzyme responsible for hydroxylation of prolyl and lysyl residues within nascent peptides in connective tissue proteins.[305] Among these are collagen and related proteins, which make up the intercellular material of cartilage, dentin, and bone. Ascorbate is also involved in

(1) carnitine biosynthesis, serving as a cofactor to 6-*N*-trimethyl-L-lysine hydrolase; (2) γ-butyrobetaine hydrolase, which converts γ-butyrobetaine to carnitine; (3) degradation of tyrosine via 4-OH phenylpyruvate dioxygenase; (4) synthesis of adrenal hormones via dopamine β-hydroxylase; (5) biosynthesis of corticosteroids and aldosterone; (6) hydroxylation of cholesterol in the formation of bile acids; and (7) folate metabolism and leukocyte functions. Nonheme iron absorption, as Fe^{2+}, is also enhanced by simultaneous ingestion of the vitamin.[281] More recently identified functions include nucleic acid and histone dealkylation and proteoglycan deglycanation.[384]

Ascorbic acid is one of the most effective water-soluble antioxidants in biological fluids[200] and is capable of scavenging physiologically important reactive oxygen species and reactive nitrogen species. Both ascorbate and the ascorbyl radical have low reduction potentials[91] and react with most other biologically relevant radicals. The ascorbyl radical is relatively stable because of resonance stabilization of the unpaired electron. Ascorbate can regenerate other small molecule antioxidants, including α-tocopherol, reduced glutathione, urate, and β-carotene, from their respective radical species, and therefore may prevent oxidative damage to biological macromolecules, including DNA, lipids, and proteins. Concern has been raised that in certain situations of vitamin supplementation, ascorbic acid may act as a pro-oxidant.[493] Indeed, although pro-oxidants usually are harmful, pharmacologic doses of ascorbate may have beneficial pro-oxidant activity in the treatment of certain diseases.[118] However, this has been disputed by other workers.[105] It has also been recognized that dehydroascorbate has important intracellular properties that are different from, but sometimes complementary to, those of ascorbate.[685]

Requirements and Reference Nutrient Intakes

The amount of vitamin C sufficient to alleviate and cure the clinical signs of scurvy is only 10 mg/d, which is probably near the minimum requirement in man. This amount, however, is not adequate to maintain near saturation of tissue in the adult human male, who has a body pool of 1.5 to 2 g and shows clinical symptoms of deficiency when this total pool falls below about 300 mg.[27] Acknowledgment of functions of vitamin C beyond the antiscorbutic, particularly the antioxidant, function has led to the development of the concept of the optimal nutrition state, along with the intake required to achieve this. Current recommendations of the U.S. Institute of Medicine regarding estimated average requirements and RDAs have reflected this approach.[188] The RDA for adult males older than 19 years and beyond 70 years has been set at 90 mg/d, and the corresponding RDA for women at 75 mg/d. To provide for fetal needs, an additional 10 mg/d is recommended for the pregnant woman to offset the decrease in plasma vitamin C concentration during pregnancy. A lactating woman should receive an additional 45 to 50 mg/d because an average of 18 to 22 mg may be secreted in 600 to 700 mL of milk. Children 1 to 3 years of age have an RDA of 15 mg/d; those 4 to 8 years, an RDA of 25 mg/d; boys aged 9 to 13, an RDA of 45 mg/d; and those 14 to 18 years, an RDA of 75 mg/d. Corresponding values for girls are 45 and 65 mg/d, respectively. No RDA is given for infants up to 1 year old; instead, adequate intake amounts of 40 mg/d up to 6 months and 50 mg/d from 7 to 12 months are recommended. Some special groups, such as smokers, should take an additional 35 mg/d.[378]

Intravenous Supply

The recommended IV intake for adult patients receiving TPN was 100 mg for many years,[9] but this has been increased to 200 mg/d.[260] This change reflects the expected increased requirements for wound healing and for antioxidant activity.

Deficiency

Protracted deficiency of vitamin C leads to the classic disease of scurvy, which still occurs in developed countries. Those most at risk of the disease include (1) elderly men, particularly those who live alone; (2) those with alcohol dependence and smokers; (3) those taking unbalanced diets; (4) some mentally ill patients; (5) renal failure patients undergoing peritoneal dialysis or hemodialysis; and (6) some patients with cancer. Lack of vitamin C causes an inability to form adequate intercellular substance in connective tissue and is reflected in swollen, tender, and often bleeding or bruised loci at joints and in other areas where structurally weakened tissue cannot withstand stress. Infantile scurvy, also known as *Barlow's disease,* exhibits a bayonet-rib syndrome. The gums are livid and swollen, cutaneous bleeding often begins on the lower thighs as perifollicular hemorrhages, and large spontaneous bruises (ecchymoses) may arise almost anywhere on the body. Ocular hemorrhages, drying of salivary and lacrimal glands, parotid swelling, femoral neuropathy, edema of the lower extremities, and psychologic disturbances have also been described. Some scorbutic patients may develop anemia, display radiologic changes characteristic of osteoporosis, or die suddenly from heart failure. Diseases of vitamin C deficiency that might reflect its role as an antioxidant include increased risk of coronary heart disease, as demonstrated in a cohort of Finnish men,[464] and increased risk of death by stroke in a cohort of elderly British individuals.[210] An important meta-analysis showed that dietary vitamin C intake, but not vitamin C from supplements, correlated inversely with coronary heart disease, suggesting that benefit is derived from other components of a healthy diet.[697]

Toxicity

Vitamin C is generally well tolerated by healthy subjects, and ingestion of supplements of 2 to 4 g/d—as taken by some for prevention or amelioration of the common cold—is usually without hazard, although gastrointestinal irritation has been experienced.[270] Other potential but rare adverse effects include increased oxalate excretion and kidney stone formation, increased uric acid excretion, excess iron absorption, lowered vitamin B_{12} concentrations, systemic conditioning and "rebound" scurvy, and pro-oxidant effects in the presence of free Fe^{3+} or Cu^{2+} ions.[172] Ingestion of amounts of vitamin C above 200 mg/d shows little increase in plasma steady-state concentrations, which suggests that overload of vitamin C is unlikely. Consideration of such data has led the Food and Nutrition Board of the U.S. Institute of Medicine to propose a tolerable upper intake amount for vitamin C of 2 g/d for adults older than 19 years.[152]

Laboratory Assessment of Status

At present, no useful functional tests of vitamin C adequacy are available; thus laboratory assessment of status is made by direct measurement of plasma, urine, or tissue concentrations of ascorbic acid, total vitamin C, or (rarely) metabolite. Because ascorbic acid is readily oxidized by dissolved oxygen at a neutral pH, plasma samples should be treated with a metal-chelating and protein-precipitating acid, such as metaphosphoric acid, soon after a phlebotomy. Samples so treated may be stored at −80 °C for several years.[33] Plasma ascorbate concentration is considered a reliable indicator of ascorbate intake[296] and has been measured photometrically by oxidation with 2,4-dinitrophenylhydrazine to form the red *bis*-hydrazone, or with 2,4-dichlorophenol-indophenol, which is reduced to a colorless form.[609] A more specific approach is to use the enzyme ascorbate oxidase to convert ascorbate to dehydroascorbate, which then is coupled with *o*-phenylene diamine to form a product that is measured fluorometrically[668] or at 340 nm on an automated analyzer.[350] HPLC methods offer the potential advantage of specificity but generally are time-consuming. Detection may be done by precolumn derivatization to the fluorescent quinoxaline, or by electrochemical or coulometric means. Care must be taken during the analysis to prevent oxidation of the ascorbate before detection, because a sulfhydryl donor, such as dithiothreitol or homocysteine, should be added to the sample and mobile phase.[33] With suitable sample preparation, ascorbic acid, total vitamin C, and, by difference, DHA may be measured together with HPLC[386] or gas chromatography–mass spectrometry.[147] Leukocyte ascorbic acid is considered to be a better indicator of body stores than plasma ascorbate, but its use has not been widely adopted because of the large sample volume requirement, the difficulty involved in automating the analysis, the influence of fluctuating leukocyte numbers, and the relative difficulty of the analysis. Urinary excretion and RBC concentrations have not been found to be specific and useful indices of vitamin C status; however, urinary concentrations of ascorbic acid, especially following a load test, can be helpful in the clinical diagnosis of scurvy. Interpretation of results in seriously ill patients with SIRS is limited by the acute fall in plasma and leukocyte ascorbic acid seen in injury or infection. This represents transient redistribution because even without supplements, the concentration returns to normal in a few days.[372]

Reference Intervals

With adequate intake of vitamin C, plasma concentrations of total vitamin (ascorbic acid plus dehydroascorbic acid) are between 0.4 and 1.5 mg/dL (23 to 85 μmol/L). The lower limit value may be seen in some cases with subclinical vitamin C deficiency and in older individuals. A value lower than 0.2 mg/dL (11 μmol/L) is considered deficient. The guidance reference interval for vitamin C concentration is 20 to 53 μg/10^8 leukocytes (1.14 to 3.01 fmol/leukocyte). A value of less than 10 μg/10^8 leukocytes (0.57 fmol/leukocyte) is considered deficient.[609]

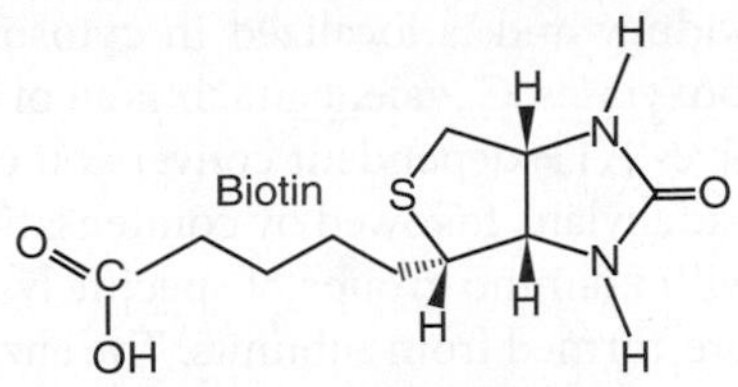

Figure 31-18 Biotin.

BIOTIN

Biotin (also known as vitamin H) is the prosthetic group for a number of carboxylation reactions (e.g., pyruvate, acetyl-CoA, propionyl Co-A, decarboxylases).

Chemistry

Biotin is *cis*-tetrahydro-2-oxothieno[3,4-*d*]-imidazoline-4-valeric acid (Figure 31-18). The vitamin in most organisms occurs mainly bound to protein. The ε-amino group of the lysyl side chain of protein is linked via an amide function involving the carboxyl group of the valeryl sidechain of biotin. In addition, some biotin is linked noncovalently as a complex with avidin, a protein in egg white.

Dietary Sources

Good sources of biotin include liver, kidney, pancreas, eggs, yeast, and milk. Cereal grains, fruits, most vegetables, and meat are poor sources.[130] The ureido ring and the ionizable carboxyl group of biotin allow modest solubility of the white crystalline solid in aqueous solution, especially at an alkaline pH. Oxidizing agents convert the thioether to sulfoxides and sulfones, which do not have biotin activity.

Absorption, Transport, Metabolism, and Excretion

Biotin in the diet is largely protein bound, and digestion of these proteins by gastrointestinal enzymes produces biotinyl peptides, which may be further hydrolyzed by intestinal biotinidase to release biotin. Avidin, a protein found in raw egg whites, binds biotin tightly and prevents its absorption. The peptide biocytin (ε-*N*-biotinyl lysine) is resistant to hydrolysis by proteolytic enzymes in the intestinal tract but together with biotin is readily absorbed.[707] A biotin carrier, the sodium-dependent multivitamin transporter (SMVT) for which pantothenic acid and lipoate compete,[542] is located in the intestinal brush border membrane and transports biotin against a sodium ion concentration gradient. The enzyme biocytinase (biotin amidohydrolase) in plasma and erythrocytes catalyzes the hydrolysis of biocytin to yield free biotin. Biotin is cleared from the circulating blood more rapidly in deficient than in normal mammals; it is taken up by such tissues as liver, muscle, and kidney and is localized in cytosolic and mitochondrial carboxylases. Covalent attachment of biotin to apoenzymes involves ATP-dependent conversion of the vitamin to biotinyl-5′-adenylate, followed by condensation of the biotinyl moiety with ε-amino groups of specific lysyl residues in apoenzymes pre-formed from subunits. The enzymes responsible for catalyzing the formation of the ε-*N*-biotinyl-L-lysyl (biocytinyl) moiety of proteins are holoenzyme synthetases.

About half of absorbed biotin is excreted as the metabolites bisnorbiotin, occurring from β-oxidation of the valeric acid sidechain, and biotin sulfoxide, occurring from oxidation of sulfur in the heterocyclic ring.[705] Circulating plasma and urinary excretion patterns show a ratio of 3:2:1 for biotin, bisnorbiotin, and biotin sulfoxide. Minor metabolites are bisnorbiotin methyl ketone and biotin sulfone. Careful balance studies in humans, where perhaps only 1 mg is the total body content, show that urinary excretion of biotin often exceeded dietary intake, and that in all cases, fecal excretion was as much as three to six times greater than dietary intake because of microfloral biosynthesis.

Functions

The principal biochemical function of biotin in humans is as a cofactor for carboxylation reactions. Five carboxylases are currently found in human tissue[541]; one of these, an acetyl-CoA carboxylase, is inactive and may act as a storage vehicle for biotin.[591] The others are carboxylases for acetyl-CoA, propionyl-CoA, β-methylcrotonyl-CoA, and pyruvate. These enzymes operate via a common mechanism, which involves phosphorylation of bicarbonate by ATP to form carbonyl phosphate, followed by transfer of the carboxyl group to the sterically less hindered nitrogen of the biotin moiety. The resulting *N*(1)-carboxybiotinyl enzyme can then exchange the carboxylate function with a reactive center in a substrate. With cytosolic acetyl-CoA carboxylase, the product is malonyl-CoA, used for fatty acid biosynthesis. In mitochondria, pyruvate carboxylase catalyzes the formation of oxaloacetate, which, together with acetyl-CoA, forms citrate. The other carboxylases are involved in the metabolism of odd-numbered fatty acids and branched-chain fatty acids.[705] Research showing altered gene expression during biotin deficiency and new enzymatic activities of the enzyme biotinidase is confirming earlier suggestions of a role for biotin in the regulation of gene expression.[404]

Requirements and Reference Nutrient Intakes

At present, scientific data are insufficient to allow recommendations of RDAs for biotin. Intestinal microflora makes a significant contribution to the body pool of available biotin, making determination of the dietary requirement difficult. Mean urinary excretion, reflective of dietary intake, varies from 6 to 50 μg/d for adults who ingest 28 to 100 μg/d. Consideration of urinary excretion of both biotin and the metabolite 3-hydroxyisovalerate[432] has led to recommendations on AI, rather than requirements.[186] The suggested AI for adults 19 years and older is 30 μg/d; for adolescents 14 to 18 years, 25 μg/d; for children 9 to 13 years, 20 μg/d; for children 4 to 8 years, 12 μg/d; for children 1 to 3 years, 8 μg/d; and for infants younger than 1 year, 0.7 μg/kg of body weight. An additional 5 μg/d is recommended for the lactating mother. Those receiving hemodialysis or peritoneal dialysis, or with a biotinidase deficiency, would require more.

Intravenous Supply

The recommended supply of biotin for adults during TPN is 60 μg/d.[9]

Deficiency

Biotin deficiency is uncommon but may be seen (1) with prolonged consumption of raw egg whites, (2) in TPN without biotin supplementation, and (3) in patients with a genetic deficiency of biotinidase. The first two situations may be complicated by effects on gut flora that produce biotin.[541] Symptoms include anorexia, nausea, vomiting, glossitis, pallor, depression, and a dry scaly dermatitis.[102] Based on urinary excretion patterns of 3-hydroxyisovaleric acid (Figure 31-19), concern has been expressed about marginal biotin deficiency in pregnancy, because this has been shown to be teratogenic in several mammalian species.[431] Significantly lowered urinary excretion or circulating blood concentrations have been found in alcoholic individuals, in patients with achlorhydria, and among the elderly and some athletes.[70] Finally, rather rare genetic enzyme defects, such as those associated with holoenzyme synthetase (reflected in

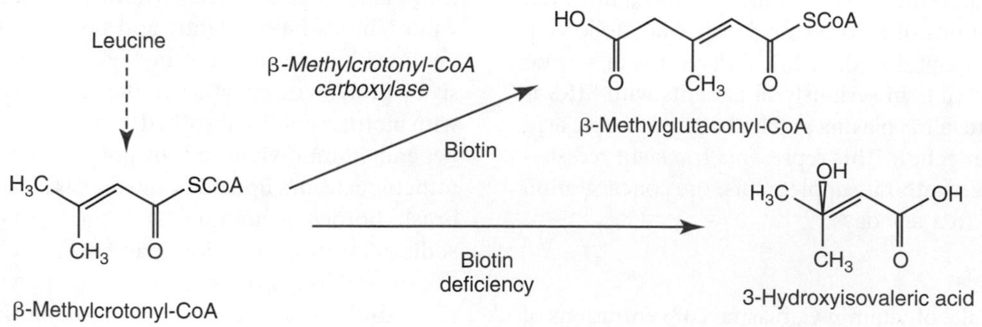

Figure 31-19 Formation of 3-hydroxyisovaleric acid under conditions of biotin deficiency.

inadequate conversion of apocarboxylases to holocarboxylases) and propionyl-CoA carboxylase (reflected in a distinguishing acidemia), have been reported.[705]

Toxicity

No adverse effects of biotin in doses up to 300 times normal dietary intake have been reported, as in patients with biotinidase deficiency.[686] Tolerable upper intake amounts for biotin have not been set because the data are insufficient.[186]

Laboratory Assessment of Status

Traditionally, biotin has been measured in biological samples by microbiological assay, where whole blood is first digested with papain or acid hydrolysis to release free biotin, samples of which are added to a biotin-deficient medium inoculated with a test organism such as *Lactobacillus plantarum*.[557] Other methods for unbound biotin include avidin-binding assays, where a competitive protein-binding radioassay is set up with ^{3}H-labeled biotin, and nonradioactive enzyme-linked sorbent assays, using streptavidin as the binding agent.[557,675] Generally, the biotin content of red cells is similar to that of plasma for a given method, but agreement between methods is often poor, which may relate to the specificity of the methods employed.[550] Urinary excretion of biotin and 3-hydroxyisovaleric acid appears to be a better indicator of biotin status than blood concentrations. This was shown in a study of experimental biotin deficiency, when both urinary biotin and metabolites, measured by HPLC separation followed by an avidin-binding assay, and urinary 3-hydroxyisovaleric acid, measured by gas chromatography–mass spectrometry, showed significant changes, whereas serum biotin concentration did not.[432] Functional markers of biotin status are being increasingly investigated. Lymphocyte propionyl-CoA carboxylase, measured by an optimized assay that is based on the incorporation of labeled $H^{14}CO_3^-$, has been shown to be an early and sensitive indicator of biotin deficiency in a rat model,[430] in patients on prolonged TPN without biotin,[659] and in children with protein-energy malnutrition.[658]

Reference Intervals

Typical reference interval values for whole blood biotin by a microbiological method are 0.5 to 2.20 nmol/L, with a mean of 1.31 nmol/L. Deficiency is considered likely below 0.5 nmol/L.[557] Reference values for other metabolites and fluids have been published elsewhere.[550]

Folic Acid

Folic acid serves as a carrier of one-carbon groups in many metabolic reactions. It is required for the biosynthesis of compounds such as choline, serine, glycine, purines, and deoxythymidine monophosphate (dTMP).

Chemistry

Folate and *folic acid* are generic terms for a family of compounds that function as coenzymes in the processing of one-carbon units and that are derived from pteroic acid *(Pte)*, to which one or more molecules of glutamic acid are attached. Pteroic acid is composed of a pteridine ring joined to a *p*-aminobenzoic acid residue (Figure 31-20). In basic solution, this substance has absorption maxima at 256, 282, and 365 nm and is fluorescent. When pteroic acid is conjugated

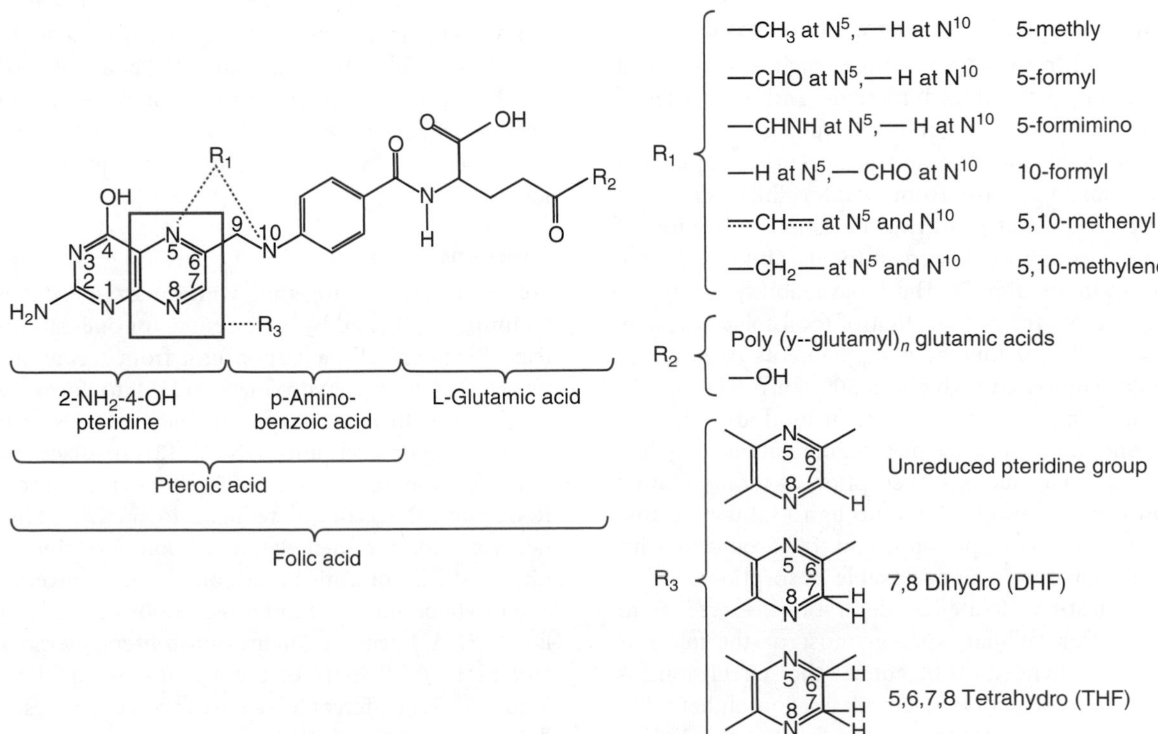

Figure 31-20 Structure and relationships of folic acid and its derivatives.

with one molecule of L-glutamic acid, pteroylglutamic acid (PteGlu) is formed; this can be reduced to dihydrofolic acid (H_2PteGlu or DHF/FH_2) with hydrogens in positions 7 and 8, or to tetrahydrofolate (H_4PteGlu or THF/FH_4) with hydrogens in positions 5, 6, 7, and 8. Only the reduced forms are biologically active. Other folate derivatives have multiple glutamic acid residues ($H_4PteGlu_n$), when *n*, the number of glutamate residues, may be 1 to 7. Biochemically, these polyglutamates are similar to monoglutamates, but the former function as the natural coenzymes. Multiple forms of folic acid occur with substitutions of functional groups such as methyl, formyl, methylene, hydroxymethyl, and others at nitrogen atoms in the pteroic acid residue, usually N^5 or bridging N^5 and N^{10}. Although various forms of folic acid are normally present in human serum and other body fluids, the principal form is 5-methyltetrahydrofolate. This is slowly oxidized in alkaline solution, but the process is reversed by adding ascorbic acid. It is relatively stable in acid solutions but is unstable when exposed to light.

Dietary Sources

The principal food sources of folate are liver, spinach, and other dark green leafy vegetables, legumes such as kidney and lima beans, and orange juice, although in countries where cereal fortification with folate is established, cereal is often the major source of dietary folate.[24] Since the U.S. FDA program of fortification of all enriched grain products with folic acid (140 μg/100 g) began, in 1996, study populations have shown a doubling of mean plasma folate concentrations and significant falls in total homocysteine concentrations, with a substantial reduction in the incidence of neural tube defects.[525]

Absorption, Transport, Metabolism, and Excretion

Folate is absorbed from dietary sources such as those listed previously, mainly as reduced methyl- and formyl-tetrahydropteroylpolyglutamates. The bioavailability of folate from food sources is variable and is dependent on factors such as incomplete release from plant cellular structure, entrapment in food matrix during digestion, inhibition of deglutamation by other dietary constituents, and possibly the degree of polyglutamation.[547] The bioavailability of supplemental folic acid is greater than that of food folate and may be as high as 100% for folic acid supplements taken on an empty stomach compared with about 50% for food folates.[186] Polyglutamate forms of folate present in food are first converted to monoglutamates, by pteroylpolyglutamate hydrolase, in the intestinal mucosa. Absorption of monoglutamyl folates at low concentration occurs through a saturable transport process with an acidic pH optimum (pH around 5), with an additional, apparently nonsaturable absorption mechanism when intestinal folate concentrations exceed 5 to 10 μmol/L.[391] After cellular uptake, most of the folate is reduced and methylated and enters the circulation as 5-methyltetrahydrofolate (THF), circulating loosely bound to albumin or to a lesser degree to a high-affinity folate-binding protein. Uptake by certain cells (kidney, placenta, and choroid plexus) occurs by membrane-associated folate-binding proteins that act as folate receptors, and the reduced folate carrier, a member of the SLC19 family, facilitates uptake by most tissue.[393] Once within the cell, 5-methyl THF is demethylated and converted to the polyglutamyl form by folylpolyglutamate synthase, which helps to retain folate within the cell, because it is unable to cross cell membranes. For release into the circulation, the polyglutamates are reconverted to monoglutamates by polyglutamate hydrolase.

Folic acid and vitamin B_{12} metabolism is linked by the reaction that transfers a methyl group from 5-methyltetrahydrofolate to cobalamin. In cases of cobalamin deficiency, folate is "trapped" as 5-methyltetrahydrofolate and is "metabolically dead." It cannot be recycled as tetrahydrofolate back into the folate pool to serve as the main one-carbon unit acceptor for many biochemical reactions. Eventually, cellular depletion of methylenetetrahydrofolate ensues, causing a reduction in thymidylic acid synthesis, which, in turn, results in megaloblastic anemia and neuropathies. This concept is supported by the fact that tetrahydrofolate corrects megaloblastic anemia in patients with congenital methylmalonic aciduria and homocystinuria, whereas it is not corrected with methyltetrahydrofolate. However, some investigators have suggested that vitamin B_{12} is required for the conversion of folic acid to the formyl form, and that formyltetrahydrofolates are natural substrates for forming folate polyglutamates.

Protein-free plasma folate is filtered at the glomerulus, and most is reabsorbed by the proximal renal tubules. Consequently, intact urinary folate represents only a small percentage of intake. Folate is predominately excreted by catabolism following cleavage of the C9-N10 bond to produce *p*-aminobenzoylpolyglutamates, which then are hydrolyzed to monoglutamates and *N*-acetylated before excretion. Biliary excretion of folate has been estimated at about 100 μg/d, but much of this is reabsorbed in an enterohepatic circulation. Fecal losses have been studied by radiolabeling and have been found to be similar in type and quantity to urinary losses.[338]

Functions

Folate coenzymes, together with coenzymes derived from vitamins B_{12}, B_6, and B_2, are essential for one-carbon metabolism. Biochemically, a carbon unit from serine or glycine is transferred to tetrahydrofolate (THF) to form methylene-THF, which then is (1) used in the synthesis of thymidine (and incorporation into DNA), (2) oxidized to formyl-THF for use in the synthesis of purines (precursors of RNA and DNA), or (3) reduced to methyl-THF, which is necessary for the methylation of homocysteine to methionine. Much of this methionine is converted to *S*-adenosylmethionine, a universal donor of methyl groups to DNA, RNA, hormones, neurotransmitters, membrane lipids, and proteins.[567] Some of these reactions are illustrated in Figure 31-21. Different folates are involved in these reactions, depending on the chemical state of the single carbon fragments transferred:

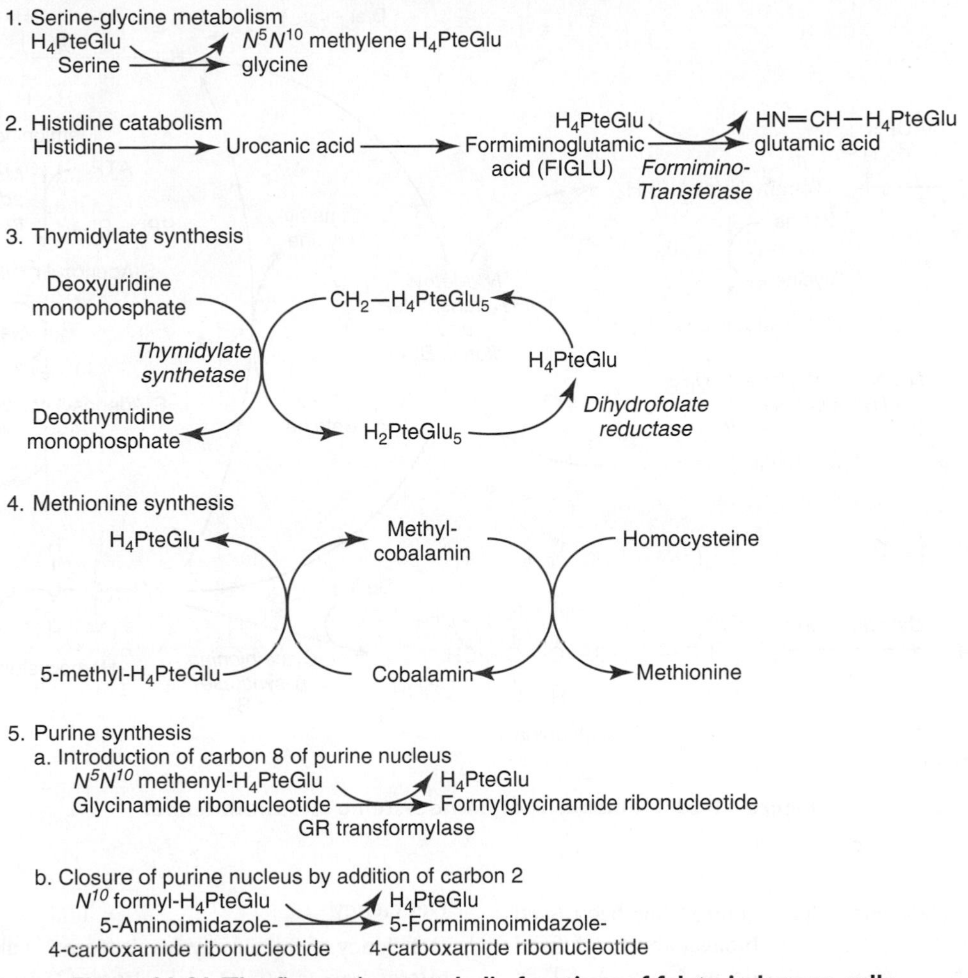

Figure 31-21 The five major metabolic functions of folate in human cells.

Reaction	Group Transferred	Folic Acid Derivative
Serum/glycine metabolism	Methylene ($-CH_2-$)	N^5,N^{10}-methylene THF/FH_4
Histidine catabolism	Formimino ($-CHNH$)	N^5-formimino THF/FH_4
Thymidylate synthesis	Methylene ($-CH_2-$)	N^5,N^{10}-methylene THF/FH_4
Methionine synthesis	Methyl ($-CH_3$)	N^5-methyl THF/FH_4
Purine synthesis	Methenyl ($-CH-$)	N^5,N^{10}-methyenyl THF/FH_4
	Formyl ($-CHO$)	N^{10}-formyl THF/FH_4

Interconversion of these forms of folic acid takes place through various electron transfer reactions facilitated by specific enzyme systems and coenzymes, such as reduced forms of flavin-adenine dinucleotide ($FADH_2$) and NADPH. Conversion between the N^5-,N^{10}-methylene form and N^{10}-formyl forms is readily reversible, but the reduction of methylene to methyl and the reduction of free tetrahydrofolate to formyltetrahydrofolate are essentially irreversible. Conversion of N^5-methyltetrahydrofolate back to free tetrahydrofolate may require cobalamin.

The role of folic acid in the metabolism of homocysteine has received much interest.[699] Elevation of plasma homocysteine concentration has been postulated to be an independent risk factor for coronary artery disease[644] and cerebrovascular disease (see Chapter 27).[435] The involvement of folate in its coenzyme forms with homocysteine and methionine metabolism is summarized in Figure 31-22. Folate is the principal micronutrient determinant of homocysteine status,[348] and supplementation with folate has been used as a treatment modality to reduce circulating homocysteine concentrations. Primary (fasting) homocysteinemia can be treated with 0.5 to 5.0 mg/d of folic acid,[652] with an expectation of an approximate 25% fall in baseline concentration.[224] Trials of homocysteine-lowering therapy with folic acid have not, however, led to a reduction in cardiovascular disease.[389]

Requirements and Reference Nutrient Intakes

Based on folate concentrations in liver biopsy samples, and given that the liver contains about half of all body stores, total body stores of folate are estimated to be between 12 and 28 mg.[680] Kinetic studies that show both fast-turnover and very-slow-turnover folate pools indicate that about 0.5 to 1% of body stores are catabolized or excreted daily,[229] suggesting a minimum daily requirement of between 60 and 280 μg to replace losses. In calculating nutritional requirements, the

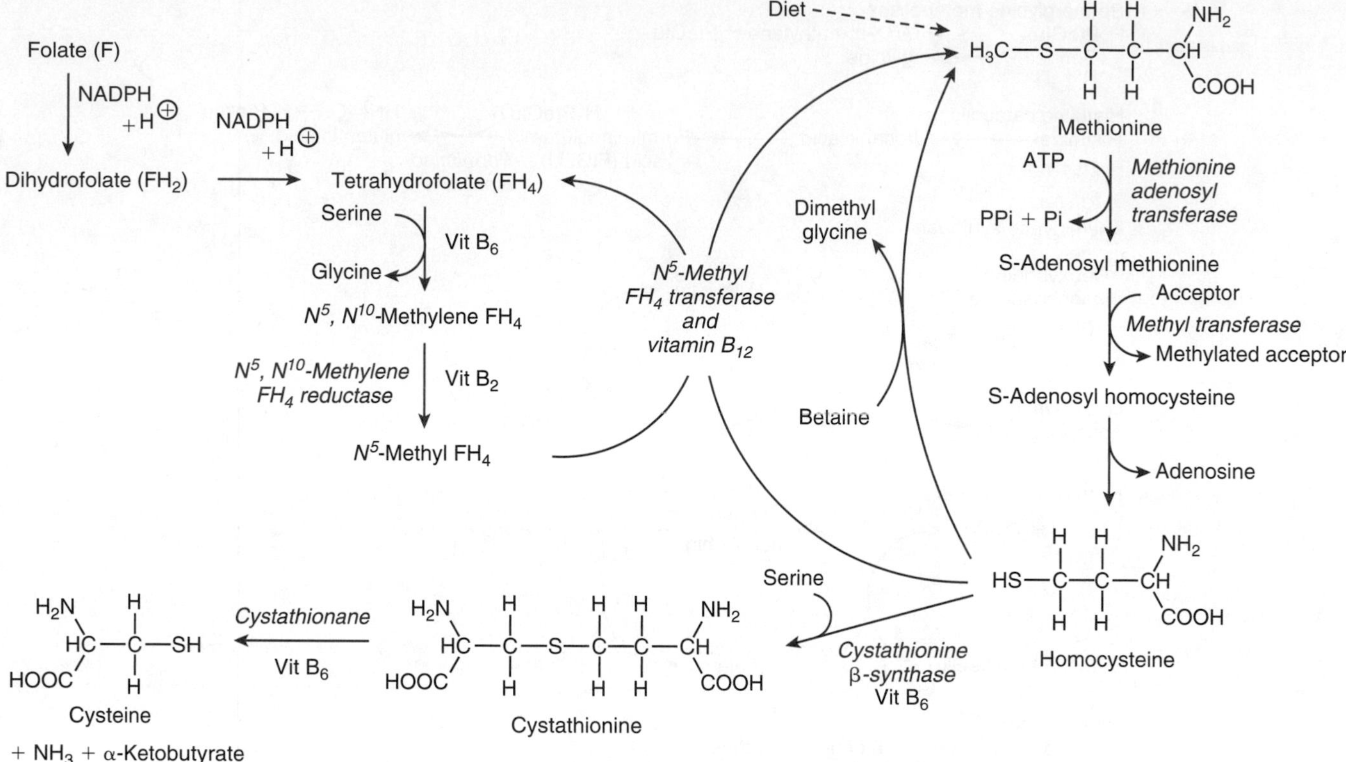

Figure 31-22 Metabolism of homocysteine and methionine.

concept of dietary folate equivalents (DFEs) has been used to adjust for the nearly 50% lower bioavailability of food folate compared with supplemental folic acid, such that 1 μg DFE = 0.6 μg of folic acid from fortified food = 1 μg of food folate = 0.5 μg folic acid supplement taken on an empty stomach.[186] Before the fortification program of cereal grains with folic acid conducted between 1988 and 1994, the median intake of folate from food in the United States was approximately 250 μg/d; this figure is expected to increase by about 100 μg/d after fortification. Recommendations on dietary reference intakes by the U.S. Institute of Medicine made in 1998 have shifted the emphasis away from prevention of deficiency and toward the concept of optimal health.[186] Awareness of the contribution of micronutrient intake to genomic stability has also increased.[171] Current RDAs of the U.S. Institute of Medicine are 400 μg/d DFE for adults 19 years and older and for adolescents between 14 and 18 years; 300 μg/d DFE for children 9 to 13 years; 200 μg/d DFE for children 4 to 8 years; and 150 μg/d DFE for children 1 to 3 years. Adequate intake for infants 0 to 6 months is set at 65 μg/d DFE, and for infants 7 to 11 months, 80 μg/d DFE. Based on maintenance of erythrocyte folate concentrations during pregnancy, the RDA for pregnant women of all ages is set at 600 μg/d DFE, and for lactating women of all ages 500 μg/d DFE.[25,186]

Intravenous Supply

The previous adult recommendation for an intravenous supply of folic acid of 400 μg/d has been increased to 600 μg/d as part of the requirements set by the FDA.[260]

Deficiency

Deficiency of folate may result from (1) absence of intestinal microorganisms (gut sterilization), (2) poor intestinal absorption (e.g., after surgical resection, in celiac disease or sprue), (3) insufficient dietary intake (including chronic alcoholism), (4) excessive demands (as in pregnancy, liver disease, and malignancies), (5) administration of antifolate drugs (e.g., methotrexate), and (6) anticonvulsant therapy (that increases folate requirements, especially during pregnancy).[359] Inadequate folate intake leads first to decreased serum folate concentration, then to a decrease in erythrocyte folate concentration and an increase in plasma homocysteine, and then to megaloblastic changes in the bone marrow and other tissues.[186] Megaloblastic anemia (characterized by large, abnormally nucleated erythrocytes in the bone marrow) is the major clinical manifestation of folate deficiency, although sensory loss and neuropsychiatric changes may also occur. Deficiencies of folate and iron may coexist in malnourished people, in which case macrocytosis of RBCs, otherwise typical of folic acid deficiency, is not observed.

Pregnancy brings increased demand to folate stores because of increased DNA synthesis, and one-carbon transfer reactions and low serum folate concentrations in pregnancy are associated with adverse outcomes, including preterm delivery, infant low birth weight, and fetal growth retardation.[556] Additionally, many observational studies have confirmed a reduction in risk of neural tube defects (NTDs) with periconceptual folic acid supplementation.[75] In a large controlled intervention trial conducted in two regions of China and involving approximately 250,000 women, a daily supplement of 400 μg of folic acid taken at least 80% of the time was associated with an 85% risk reduction of NTD in an area of high baseline frequency, and a 40% reduction in an area of low baseline frequency.[52] Current suggestions are that women planning pregnancy should take at least 400 μg/d, although a daily intake of 5 mg of folic acid is recommended, especially for those with a previous history of NTD.[669]

Although the cause of NTD is probably multifactorial, involving more than one aspect of folate use,[31] one factor that contributes to this and other folate-requiring conditions is genetic polymorphism. The most extensively studied polymorphic alleles are those of 5,10-methyleneterahydofolate reductase (MTHFR), the enzyme responsible for the irreversible reduction of 5,10-MTHF to 5-methyltetrahydrofolate (5-MTHF), the methyl donor of homocysteine to methionine. A single-point C-to-T mutation at base pair 677 (C677T), causing substitution of valine for alanine, leads to a thermolabile protein with reduced enzymatic activity. The homozygous T/T enzyme has an incidence of around 12% in Asian and white populations and loss of enzyme activity of about 50%; the heterozygous C/T variant can have an incidence of up to 50% in some populations, with a lesser degree of enzyme inactivity.[78] Folate appears to have a protective effect on colorectal cancer development[177] but is associated with increased risk of gastric cancer, and may be associated with lung cancer.[69] This is clearly an important area, both for pathogenesis and for potential therapy, on which much future research will focus.

The C/T variant and a second with an A-to-C substitution at base pair 1298 (A1298C), with its effects on folate metabolism and intracellular folate availability, may increase the risk of chromosomal aberrations; its link with leukemia has been reviewed.[526] An additional enzyme involved in folate metabolism, methionine synthase, has been shown to have at least two relatively prevalent polymorphisms, although these are thought to be benign.[117] Absorption of folate from polyglutamyl folate food sources is thought to be reduced by a variant of glutamate carboxypeptidase II because of a H475Y substitution.[148]

Lower than normal serum folate concentrations have been reported in patients with psychiatric disorders. In two studies, about one third of psychiatric patients had low RBC folate concentrations, with most of the low values being reported in depressed patients. Another study reported an inverse correlation between serum folate concentrations and the duration of depressive illness. Limited evidence suggests that folate may have a role as a supplement to other treatments for depression.[625]

Toxicity

No adverse effects have been reported from the consumption of folate-fortified foods, thus any signs of toxicity are associated with supplemental folate. Most of the limited evidence suggests that excessive folate supplementation, typically in doses up to 10 mg/d (although some have given 500 mg/d), can precipitate or exacerbate neuropathy in vitamin B_{12}–deficient subjects, and it is this end point that has been used to set a tolerable upper intake concentration of 1 mg/d from fortified foods or supplements for adults.[186] One recognized complication of folate supplementation is that it "masks" vitamin B_{12} deficiency, because the associated anemia responds to folate alone. This may delay treatment of the deficiency, allowing neurologic abnormalities to progress.

Laboratory Assessment of Status

Folate status may be reliably assessed by direct measurement of serum and erythrocyte or whole blood concentrations, and its metabolic function as a coenzyme may be assessed by metabolite concentrations such as plasma homocysteine (see Chapters 21 and 27). Serum folate concentrations are considered indicative of recent intake and not of tissue stores, but serial measurements have been used to confirm adequate intake. Whole blood and erythrocyte folate concentrations are more indicative of tissue stores and have been shown to have a moderate correlation with liver folate concentrations taken through a biopsy.[186] Because folate is taken up only by the developing erythrocyte in the bone marrow and not by the mature cell, erythrocyte concentrations reflect folate status over the 120-day life span of the cell. Urine folate excretion is not considered to be a sensitive indicator of folate status.[550]

CPB assays have now largely replaced microbiological procedures for the measurement of serum, whole blood, or erythrocyte folate, although the use of microtiter 96-well plates has enabled a microbiological assay using *Lactobacillus casei* to be partially automated.[466] The binder used in the CPB folate assay is a protein that occurs naturally in milk, called β-lactoglobulin or milk folate binder; it is commonly used together with a radioactive ^{125}I-folate label, although nonisotopic fluorescence and bioluminescence labels are becoming more popular. One commercial assay uses selective protein binding coupled with ion capture, followed by fluorescence assay. A comparison of frequently used laboratory analyzers shows marked variation.[479] However, because problems of standardization and intermethod agreement persist with CPB assays, more specific analytical techniques have been developed, including HPLC with electrochemical or mass-spectrometric detection.[33]

Several analytes are known to be indicative of folate metabolism. Plasma total homocysteine increases when a deficiency of 5-MTHF is present, such that the methylation of homocysteine to methionine is compromised. However, although plasma homocysteine is considered a sensitive functional indicator, it is not specific, because its concentration can be influenced by deficiency of other vitamins (B_6 and B_{12}) involved in the metabolism of homocysteine. Similarly, the methylation of DNA is dependent on adequate 5-MTHF. A sensitive new method for the rapid detection of abnormal methylation patterns among global DNA patterns has been reported and may have promise as a functional marker,[494] as may measurement of the degree of uracil incorporation into DNA, with 5,10-methylene THF required for the conversion of deoxyuridine monophosphate (dUMP) to dTMP by thymidylate synthetase.[68]

Reference Intervals

Because of methodologic differences, reference values for folate are method dependent. Data collected from the National Health and Nutritional Examination Survey of 1988 to 1994 in the United States, in which almost 3000 blood samples were analyzed, revealed reference intervals of 2.6 to 12.2 μg/L (6.0 to 28.0 nmol/L) for serum folate and 103 to 411 μg/L (237 to 945 nmol/L) for erythrocyte folate. However, a more recent analysis conducted since mandatory supplementation of cereal grain products has yielded values of 13.1 to 74.3 nmol/L for serum folate, and 347 to 1167 nmol/L for erythrocyte folate.[488] This demonstrates the importance of establishing local, or at least national, reference values. Biochemical deficiency has been defined as a concentration of <3 μg/L (<6.7 nmol/L) for serum folate and <140 μg/L (<322 nmol/L) for erythrocyte folate.[510,596]

Niacin and Niacinamide

Niacin and niacinamide (nicotinamide and nicotinic acid amide) are converted to the ubiquitous redox coenzymes nicotinamide-adenine dinucleotide $(NAD)^+$ and nicotinamide-adenine dinucleotide phosphate $(NADP)^+$.

Chemistry

The term *niacin* refers to nicotinic acid (pyridine-3-carboxylic acid), its amide nicotinamide, and derivatives that show the same biological activity as nicotinamide. A distinction between the two primary vitamin forms has to be considered, however, when some aspects of their metabolism and especially their different pharmacologic actions at high doses are considered. Structures of both vitamers and the two coenzyme forms containing the nicotinamide moiety are given in Figure 31-23.

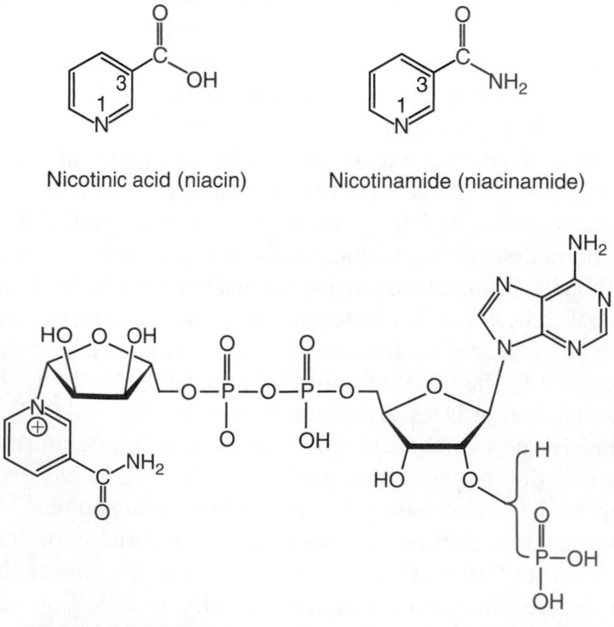

Nicotinic acid (niacin)

Nicotinamide (niacinamide)

Figure 31-23 Niacin, niacinamide, and coenzyme.

Dietary Sources

Nicotinamide-adenine dinucleotide (NAD; diphosphopyridine nucleotide) and nicotinamide-adenine dinucleotide phosphate (NADP; also termed *triphosphopyridine nucleotide*) represent most of the niacin activity found in good sources that include yeast, lean meats, liver, and poultry.[114] Milk, canned salmon, and several leafy green vegetables contribute lesser amounts but are still sufficient to prevent deficiency. Additionally, some plant foodstuffs, especially cereals, such as corn and wheat, contain niacin bound to various peptides and sugars in forms that nutritionally are not readily available (niacinogens or niacytin).[294] Because tryptophan is a precursor of niacin, protein provides a considerable portion of the niacin equivalent. As much as two thirds of niacin required by adults can be derived from tryptophan metabolism via nicotinic acid ribonucleotide to NAD and NADP. It has been found that 60 mg of tryptophan can provide the equivalent of 1 mg of niacin in the adult. In countries where fortification of processed cereals is practiced, this may provide up to 20% of niacin intake.[294]

Free forms of the vitamin are white, stable solids that are soluble in water. Oxidized coenzymes are labile to alkali, whereas reduced (dihydro) coenzymes are labile to acid. Reduction of oxidized coenzymes commonly occurs through the addition of a hydride ion to the *para* (4) position of the nicotinamide ring, with simultaneous formation of a solvated proton. NADH and NADPH (but not NAD and NADP) absorb light in the near ultraviolet region (339 nm). This forms the basis for many biochemical assays.

Absorption, Transport, Metabolism, and Excretion

Dietary NAD and NADP are hydrolyzed by enzymes, such as NAD glycohydrolase, in the intestinal mucosa to release nicotinamide, which, together with any nicotinic acid, is rapidly absorbed in the stomach and the intestine by Na^+-dependent facilitated diffusion at low concentrations and passive diffusion at higher concentrations.[39] Nicotinamide is the main circulating form in the plasma post absorption or following release from hydrolyzed liver NAD; it can be taken up by most tissues requiring NAD by simple diffusion.

Once inside blood, kidney, brain, and liver cells, both nicotinic acid and nicotinamide are converted to coenzyme forms. The first step involves the cytosolic phosphoribosyltransferase-catalyzed reaction of nicotinate or nicotinamide with 5-phosphoribosyl-1-pyrophosphate to form pyrophosphate and nicotinic acid ribonucleotide or nicotinamide ribonucleotide, respectively.[397] An additional source of nicotinic acid ribonucleotide is the action of quinolate phosphoribosyltransferase on quinolinate formed from tryptophan. The efficiency of this pathway is under nutritional and hormonal regulation, with deficiency of vitamin B_6 (riboflavin) and iron slowing the conversion—and protein, tryptophan, energy, and niacin restriction increasing the efficiency.[294] Nicotinic acid ribonucleotide from whatever source is converted to deamido-NAD by an adenylyltransferase-catalyzed attachment of the AMP moiety from ATP; the deamido compound subsequently reacts with glutamine and a cytosolic ATP-dependent synthetase step to yield NAD, glutamate, and phosphate. Nicotinamide mononucleotide is directly converted by adenylyltransferase to NAD. NADP is formed by kinase-catalyzed phosphorylation of NAD. In the tissue, most of the vitamin is present as nicotinamide in NAD and NADP, although the liver may contain a significant fraction of free vitamin. Little storage of niacin as such occurs.

Excess niacin is excreted mainly as the *N*-methylnicotinamide (NMN) after methylation in the liver and as the two oxidation products of NMN, *N*-methyl-2-pyridone-5-carboxamide, and *N*-methyl-4-pyridone-carboxamide.[437]

Functions

Niacin is essential as the coenzymes NAD and NADP in which nicotinamide acts as an electron acceptor or a hydrogen donor in a large number of redox reactions. Many enzymes function as dehydrogenases and catalyze such diverse reactions as the conversion of alcohols (often sugars and polyols) to aldehydes or ketones, hemiacetals to lactones, aldehydes to acids, and certain amino acids to keto acids.[397] The common mechanism of operation involves the stereospecific abstraction of a hydride ion from substrate, with *para* addition to one or the other side of carbon 4 in the pyridine ring of the nucleotide coenzyme. The second hydrogen of the substrate group oxidized is concomitantly removed as a proton and ultimately is exchanged as a hydronium ion. Most dehydrogenases using NAD or NADP function reversibly. Glutamate dehydrogenase, for example, favors the oxidative direction, whereas others, such as glutathione reductase, preferentially catalyze reduction. In addition to redox reactions, NAD is a substrate for three classes of enzymes that cleave the β-*N*-glycosylic bond of NAD to free nicotinamide and catalyze the transfer of adenosine diphosphate (ADP)-ribose.[346] One such enzyme, poly (ADP-ribose) polymerase-1 (PARP-1), is involved in base excision repair and is thought to be important for genomic stability.[235] Nicotinic acid, when used as a pharmaceutical agent, has important antiatherogenic properties. It effectively lowers triglycerides, raises HDL cholesterol, and shifts LDL particles to a less atherogenic phenotype.[290]

Requirements and Reference Nutrient Intakes

Requirements for niacin are expressed as niacin equivalents (NEs), which take account of the contributions of tryptophan derived from protein. Earlier estimates of niacin requirements were based on energy expenditure, reflecting the biological function of niacin coenzymes in the oxidation of fuel molecules. However, current recommendations merely reflect the fact that different age groups and sexes have, on average, different energy expenditures, and that no directly relevant studies have linked energy intake or expenditure with niacin requirement.[186] The median intake of pre-formed niacin from food in the United States is 28 mg for men and 18 mg for women. A study of two Canadian populations showed corresponding values of 41 mg and 28 mg/d. Additionally, the average U.S. diet supplies between 0.7 and 1.1 g of tryptophan/d.[446] Based on niacin metabolite excretion data, current RDA for males 19 years to older than 70 years is 16 mg/d of NE, and for women of the same age, 14 mg/d. An increase of 4 NE/d during pregnancy is recommended, and an increase of 3 NE daily for lactation will offset the preformed niacin lost in milk. Human milk contains approximately 0.17 mg of niacin and 22 mg of tryptophan/dL, or 70 kcal; these amounts are adequate to meet the niacin needs of the infant. Adequate intakes of 2 mg/d of pre-formed niacin and 4 mg/d NE have been extrapolated from adult requirements for infants 0 to 6 months and 7 to 12 months, respectively. RDAs are set at 6 mg/d for children 1 to 3 years, 8 mg/d for children 4 to 8 years, 12 mg/d for boys and girls 9 to 13 years, 14 mg/d for girls 14 to 18 years, and 16 mg/d for boys 14 to 18 years.[186]

Intravenous Supply

The recommended supply for adult patients receiving TPN is 40 mg/d in the form of nicotinamide.[9] This increase above the oral recommendations will ensure adequate intake to match increased energy expenditure.

Deficiency

Pellagra is the classic deficiency disease of the human that has been most often found among those who subsist chiefly on corn (maize), which is low in both niacin and tryptophan concentrations.[528] Although its pathogenesis has been attributed to a deficiency of these two factors, other associated complicating factors include lack of pyridoxal-5-phosphate, FAD, and iron, which are functional in the conversion of tryptophan to niacin, and the presence of mycotoxins elaborated by mold infestations, mainly by *Fusarium*.[622] Pellagra is an occasional secondary manifestation of *carcinoid syndrome*, in which up to 60% of tryptophan is catabolized to 5-OH tryptophan and serotonin; of *Hartnup disease*, an autosomal recessive disorder in which several amino acids, including tryptophan, are poorly absorbed; and of treatment with the antituberculous drug isoniazid, which competes with pyridoxal-5-phosphate.

The typical presentation of pellagra is that of a chronic wasting disease associated with dermatitis, dementia, and diarrhea. The characteristic erythematous dermatitis is bilateral and symmetric and occurs on skin areas exposed to sunlight. Mental changes include fatigue, insomnia, and apathy, all of which precede an encephalopathy characterized by confusion, disorientation, hallucination, loss of memory, and eventually frank organic psychoses. Diarrhea, when it occurs, reflects widespread inflammation of the intestinal mucous surfaces, including a bright red tongue; other gastrointestinal manifestations include achlorhydria, glossitis, stomatitis, and vaginitis.

Toxicity

Although no toxic effects have been associated with niacin intake from naturally occurring foods, the use of supplements and of pharmacologic doses of niacin has produced adverse effects in some subjects. In disorders of reduced tryptophan availability, such as Hartnup syndrome and carcinoid syndrome, daily niacin doses of 40 to 200 mg may be required, and in the treatment of dyslipidemias, nicotinic acid in doses up to 6 g daily may be used. Such doses are commonly associated with vascular dilation or "flushing," a burning, tingling sensation of the face (that may be reddened), arms, and chest that is thought to be mediated by prostaglandins. This may be modulated by gradual increments of the drug and by taking it with meals. Other side effects of high-dose niacin treatment are pruritus, nausea, vomiting, and diarrhea, although these symptoms often abate with continued therapy. Additional effects include abnormal glucose tolerance, hyperuricemia, peptic ulcer, hepatomegaly, jaundice, and increased serum aminotransferases. In a study of 814 patients taking a combination extended-release niacin preparation (maximum dose, 2 g), flushing caused intolerance in 10% of those studied, hepatotoxicity was seen in 0.5%, and myopathy was not reported.[434] The symptoms of flushing have been taken as an end point sign in the formulation of a tolerable upper intake amount for niacin. This has been set at 35 mg/d for adults 19 years and older, with lower amounts for children and adolescents.[186]

Laboratory Assessment of Status

At present, no blood markers are commonly used as indicators of niacin status. Most assessments of niacin nutriture have been based on measurement of the two urinary metabolites, *N*′-methylnicotinamide and *N*′-methyl-2-pyridone-5-carboxamide. Normally, adults excrete 20 to 30% of their niacin in the form of methylnicotinamide and 40 to 60% as the pyridone. An excretion ratio of pyridone to methylnicotinamide of 1.3 to 4.0 is thus normal, but latent niacin deficiency is indicated by a value below 1.0. As depletion occurs, pyridone is absent for weeks before clinical signs are noted, and methylnicotinamide excretion falls to a minimum at about the time that clinical signs become evident.[550] HPLC methods are currently the methods of choice,[588] although some capillary electrophoresis methods have been developed.[292] However, measurement of 2-pyridone and *N*′-methylnicotinamide concentrations in plasma may provide a more reliable metabolite ratio than urine measurements. An approach that may prove valuable is the ratio of NAD to NADP in erythrocytes.[570] NAD concentrations respond to the niacin status, whereas NADP concentrations remain relatively constant under different conditions of niacin status. The niacin number is NAD/NADP × 100. Enzyme assays are used with alcohol dehydrogenase for NAD and with isocitrate dehydrogenase for NADP.[205] A niacin number less than 130 would be indicative of risk of developing niacin deficiency.

Reference Intervals

A guidance reference interval for the excretion rate of N^1-methylnicotinamide is 2.4 to 6.4 mg/d (17.5 to 46.7 μmol/d) or 1.6 to 4.3 mg/g creatinine (11.7 to 31.4 μmol/g creatinine).[550]

Pantothenic Acid

Pantothenic acid is a component of coenzyme A (CoA) that is required for the metabolism of fat, protein, and carbohydrate via the citric acid cycle.

Chemistry

Pantothenic acid is of ubiquitous occurrence in nature, where it is synthesized by most microorganisms and plants from pantoic acid (D-2,4-dihydroxy-3,3-dimethylbutyric acid) derived from L-valine, and from β-alanine derived from L-aspartate. Addition of cysteamine at the C-terminal end and phosphorylation at C4 of pantoic acid form 4′-phosphopantetheine, which serves as a covalently attached prosthetic group of acyl carrier proteins; when attached to ribose 3′-phosphate and adenine, CoA is formed, as shown in Figure 31-24. Pantothenic acid is hygroscopic, viscous oil that is easily destroyed by heat, especially at extremes of pH. The most common commercial synthetic form is the calcium salt.

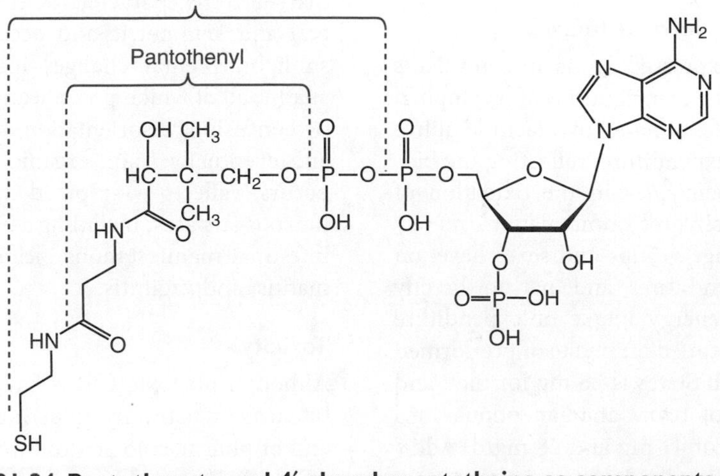

Figure 31-24 Pantothenate and 4′-phosphopantetheine as components of CoA.

Dietary Sources

Pantothenic acid is widely distributed in foods, mostly within CoA-containing compounds, and is particularly abundant in animal sources, legumes, and whole grain cereals. Excellent food sources (100 to 200 μg/g dry weight) include egg yolk, kidney, liver, and yeast. Fair sources (35 to 100 μg/g) include broccoli, lean beef, skimmed milk, sweet potatoes, and molasses. More than one half of the pantothenate in wheat may be lost during manufacture of flour, and up to one third is lost during cooking of meat.[186,492]

Absorption, Transport, Metabolism, and Excretion

Pantothenic acid is taken in as dietary CoA compounds and 4′-phosphopantetheine and is hydrolyzed by pyrophosphatase and phosphatase in the intestinal lumen to dephospho-CoA, phosphopantetheine, and pantetheine, which are further hydrolyzed to pantothenic acid. The vitamin is primarily absorbed as pantothenic acid through a saturable process at low concentrations and through simple diffusion at higher ones. The saturable process is facilitated by a sodium-dependent multivitamin transporter, for which biotin and lipoate compete.[500] After absorption, pantothenic acid enters the circulation and is taken up by cells in a manner similar to its intestinal adsorption. The synthesis of CoA from pantothenate is regulated by pantothenate kinase, which itself is subject to negative feedback from the products CoA and acyl-CoA.[613] The steps involved were outlined previously. Pantothenic acid is excreted in the urine after hydrolysis of CoA compounds by enzymes that cleave phosphate and the cysteamine moieties. Only a small fraction of pantothenate is secreted into milk, and even less into colostrum.

Functions

Pantothenic acid has two major metabolic roles—the first as part of CoA, and the other as the prosthetic group of the acyl-carrier protein (ACP). In the former role, CoA is primarily involved in acetyl and acyl transfer reactions in catabolic processes of carbohydrate, lipid, and protein chemistry. Examples of these are the acetylation of sugars, phospholipid, isoprenoid, and steroid biosynthesis and protein acetylation.[421] Acetyl-CoA that derives from the metabolism of carbohydrates, fats, and amino acids can acetylate compounds, such as choline and hexosamines, to produce essential biochemicals; it can also condense with other metabolites, such as oxaloacetate, to supply citrate and cholesterol. As the 4′-phosphopantetheine moiety of ACP, the phosphodiester-linked prosthetic group uses the sulfhydryl terminus to exchange with malonyl-CoA to form an ACP-S malonyl thioester, which can chain elongate during fatty acid biosynthesis.[398] Pantothenic acid protects rats against some of the deleterious effects of gamma radiation[594] and may also protect lymphocytes from ultraviolet light–induced apoptosis.[595] Pantothenic acid used pharmaceutically may provide the benefits of lowering cholesterol, enhancing athletic performance, and relieving symptoms of rheumatoid arthritis.[421]

Requirements and Reference Nutrient Intakes

A dietary intake of pantothenic acid in humans of 4 to 7 mg/d seems sufficient for normal health.[319] Urinary excretion of pantothenic acid in a typical American diet averages 2.6 mg/d,[624] but may vary from 2 to 7 mg/d in adults consuming 5 to 7 mg/d and is strongly dependent on intake; another 1 to 2 mg/d is lost in feces. The primary criterion used to estimate adequate intake for pantothenic acid is whether its intake is adequate to replace urinary excretion. It has been set at 5 mg/d for adolescents 14 to 18 years and for adults.[186] Children 1 to 13 years have AIs extrapolated from adult values, and infants have AIs reflecting intake from human milk, which contains approximately 2 mg/L. An additional 1 mg/d is suggested in pregnancy, and an additional 2 mg/d is suggested for lactating mothers.

Intravenous Supply

The recommended intravenous supply for adults is 15 mg/d of dexpanthenol.[9]

Deficiency

The widespread availability of pantothenic acid in food is commensurate with its many roles and makes uncomplicated dietary deficiency of pantothenate unlikely in humans. Symptoms have been produced in a few volunteers who received ω-methylpantothenic acid as an antagonist[269] and in people fed semisynthetic diets virtually free of pantothenate.[204] Subjects became irascible and developed postural hypotension and rapid heart rate on exertion, epigastric distress with anorexia and constipation, numbness and tingling of the hands and feet, hyperactive deep tendon reflexes, and weakness of finger extensor muscles. The eosinopenic response to adrenocorticotropic hormone was impaired. More severe deficiency in animals leads to adrenal cortical failure. Historically, pantothenic acid deficiency has been associated with the syndrome of "burning feet," experienced by prisoners in the second World War in Asia and relieved only by pantothenic acid supplementation—not by other B-group vitamins.[218]

Toxicity

No reports have described adverse effects, with the exception of occasional mild diarrhea, with oral pantothenic acid given in doses as high as 20 g/d.[613] In the absence of evidence of toxicity, a tolerable upper intake amount has not been derived for pantothenic acid.

Laboratory Assessment of Status

No convenient or reliable functional tests of pantothenic acid status are available; thus assessment is made by direct measurement of whole blood or urine pantothenic acid concentrations. Urine measurements are perhaps the easiest to conduct and interpret, and concentrations are closely related to dietary intake.[550] Whole blood measurements are preferred to plasma, which contains only free pantothenic acid and is insensitive to changes in pantothenic acid intake. Concentrations of pantothenic acid in all of the fluids already described can be measured by microbiological assay, most commonly using *Lactobacillus plantarum*. Whole blood must first be treated with an enzyme preparation to release pantothenic acid from CoA.[28] Some techniques that have been used to measure pantothenic acid in human samples include radioimmunoassay[694] and gas chromatography.[562] Other techniques that have been developed include gas chromatography–mass spectrometry[30] and a stable isotope dilution assay.[540] CoA and ACP have been measured by enzymatic methods.[123]

Reference Intervals

Urinary excretion of less than 1 mg/d of pantothenic acid is considered abnormally low. Suspicion of inadequate intake is further supported if whole blood concentrations are less than 100 μg/L. A guidance reference interval for pantothenic acid in whole blood or serum is 344 to 583 μg/L (1.57 to 2.66 μmol/L),[159] and for urinary excretion 1 to 15 mg/d (5 to 68 μmol/d).[694]

TRACE ELEMENTS

The term *trace element* was originally used to describe the residual amount of inorganic analyte quantitatively determined in a sample. More sensitive methods allow accurate determination of most inorganic micronutrients present at very low concentrations in body fluids and tissue. Those present in body fluids (μg/dL) and in tissue (mg/kg) are, however, still widely referred to as "trace elements," and those found at ng/dL or μg/kg as "ultratrace elements." The corresponding dietary requirements are quoted in mg/d or μg/d, respectively.

The biological effects of deficiency disease define the essential trace elements. For example, an element is considered essential when signs and symptoms induced by a deficient diet are uniquely reversed by an adequate supply of the particular trace element under investigation.

For iron, iodine, cobalt (as cobalamins), selenium, copper, and zinc, there are clinical examples of reversible deficiency disease. Enough is known about the biochemical functions of these elements to explain their importance in human nutrition. For others, such as manganese, chromium, molybdenum, and vanadium, their importance remains to be fully accepted in clinical practice. Still other elements, such as bromine, fluorine, cadmium, lead, strontium, lithium, and tin, have been claimed by at least one investigator to be essential for one or more animal species, as demonstrated by dietary deprivation studies. It should be noted that several of these metals are toxic at higher concentrations (see Chapter 36).

Classification

This wide range of biologically active elements has led to a suggestion for classification beyond "essentiality" into the additional categories of "pharmacologically beneficial," "nutritionally beneficial," and "possibly essential."[455]

Pharmacologically Beneficial

Trace elements in this category would include fluoride used for protection against dental caries, lithium salts used in the treatment of manic depression, and strontium ranelate for the treatment of osteoporosis. Dosages required for a beneficial pharmacologic effect greatly exceed the amounts of these elements normally found in food.

Nutritionally Beneficial or Possibly Essential

For some trace elements, continued suboptimal dietary intake—in the presence of physiologic, nutritional, or other metabolic stress—may eventually have a detrimental effect. Additional dietary supplementation may then have a "health restorative" effect. Such effects are most clearly demonstrated in experimental animals. Examples include the effects of boron in the presence of vitamin D depletion[280] and the need for increased vanadium with an experimentally induced deficient or excessive supply of dietary iodine.[648]

Various reviews have investigated epidemiologic evidence of the involvement of trace elements, especially copper, zinc, and selenium, in influencing cancer risk; it is clear that evidence is relatively weak, and the need for more detailed study remains.[691]

A systematic review of most of the trace and toxic elements measured in plasma or whole blood in hemodialysis patients suggested that zinc and selenium were consistently below normal values, whereas copper and chromium were within reference limits. The authors recommended more careful monitoring of this group of patients, for whom intake is easily compromised.[635]

Dose-Effect Relationships

At low intakes of recognized essential trace elements, deficiency disease may be seen; with increasing dietary supply, a plateau region of optimal supply is reached. Still higher intakes will result in adverse toxic effects. The concentration window separating beneficial dietary intake from toxic intake varies depending on the element in question and on the nature of the chemical species present in the diet. This is similar to the dose-effect relationship described for organic micronutrients (Figure 31-25). Therefore the RDA is set at amounts that are sufficient to prevent deficiency. A tolerable upper intake value that will prevent toxicity has been proposed for the inorganic micronutrients of known importance to human health.[190]

Reversal of clinical signs and symptoms by supplementation with a single trace element or with micronutrient mixtures has been used as indirect evidence of a preexisting deficiency. Growth velocities in children, regain of lean body mass, rate of wound healing, resistance to infection, and alterations in cognitive function can be assessed. However, many confounding factors, in particular the presence of disease or of other nutritional deficits, can affect the interpretation of changes in these indices.

Reductions in metalloenzyme activity induced by the deficiency may be partially or wholly restored by effective treatment. Reversal of hematologic and immune function

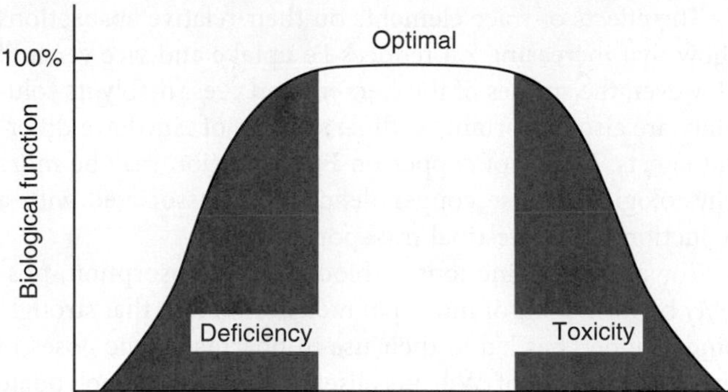

Figure 31-25 Model of the relationship between tissue concentration and intake of an essential nutrient and dependent biological function.

laboratory abnormalities can also be addressed, as can hormonal changes induced by the deficiency.

Overview of Chemistry

Knowledge of the chemistry of trace elements is important, as this not only will affect awareness of role and function but will be essential in understanding possible mechanisms of action. All elements (with the possible exception of selenium) behave in the charged ionized form, and the relative ease with which they are able to pass from one state to another is key in the role they exert in their respective metalloproteins. Thus, iron exists as Fe^{2+} and Fe^{3+} but functions only as the 2^+ ion in carrying oxygen in Hb. Transport of Fe occurs as the Fe^{3+} state in transferrin, so any elements that are in this oxidation state will compete for transport (e.g., Mn^{3+}, Al^{3+}, Cr^{3+}).[436] Also, if transferrin is saturated with Fe, these other ions will seek alternative complexing moieties (e.g., albumin or organo acids, as with citric acid).[334]

The elements zinc and copper exert their effects through dynamic switching between the 2^+ and 1^+ states, whereas Cr exists commonly as the 3^+ ion, and the valency (VI) state as CrO_4 2^-, which is readily reduced to the 3^+ state. The Cr^{3+} form is given as a supplement, often as picolinate. The distribution of these two ions is different, with the chromate ion tending to be taken in by cells, whereas Cr^{3+} ions are held in the plasma probably while attached to transferrin.[212] Selenium is rarely present as the selenite ion (SeO^{2-}), in fact probably only in supplements or intravenous (IV) solutions, and is more likely to exist in selenoproteins as the amino acid selenocysteine or selenomethionine. Nevertheless, one functional aspect of selenium is that it allows oxidation to occur during transfer from reduced Se to the peroxide form.

Similarly, the bioavailability of these elements from foods and drinks will depend on their chemical state; solubilities could be critical, particularly at the alkaline pH of the intestine. The Fe^{2+} ion is much more soluble than Fe^{3+}, but the latter is more likely to be present in oxidizing conditions of the gastrointestinal tract; hence to maintain solubility and intestinal absorption, iron is usually taken as the Fe^{2+} salt with a reducing agent, vitamin C. Formation of the more soluble complexes has been shown to be important in elemental absorption with citric and other organic acids.[307] It is likely that formation of these organo complexes will affect the bioavailability of trace elements, as absorption will be facilitated through organic acid transporters.[616] Hence trace elements are given as supplements, often as salts of citrate.

It is important to understand how metals are transported, and when an excess will result in toxicity. Thus in iron overload, transferrin becomes saturated, and the excess iron is probably complexed with other proteins, especially the bioavailable citrate complex, which leads to increased cellular uptake and storage-associated damage.[442]

Metals are transported into and carried from cells and then are excreted. Initially, they are taken with food when complexation with protein or organic acids is likely. One can envisage that free metal ions are unlikely to exist in solution, except in model experimental solutions. Metal absorption therefore takes place through the naturally occurring complexes found in food (e.g., Fe Haem, Fe citrate).[345] These compounds behave differently from free uncomplexed ions in test solution or in vivo. Thus ferric (Fe^{3+}) ions are much less soluble and are poorly absorbed compared with soluble ferric citrate complexes.

To improve understanding of trace elements and how they function, we need always to consider the ionic forms, relative solubilities, possible organo complex formation, and resultant speciation. This approach will provide a proper basis from which to understand physiologic function, as well as relevant approaches to measurement.

Trace elements interact with available ligands, mainly the electron donors nitrogen, sulfur, and oxygen, to form a wide variety of chemical complexes or species. Some metals such as Fe, Cu, Mo, and Cr are stable in more than one valence state and participate in biologically important oxidation-reduction reactions.[197] The transition metals with an incompletely filled 3d orbital (Fe, Cu, and Co) coordinate with a large number of groups to form stable complexes. Zinc lies at the end of the first transition series in the periodic table. Zn^{2+}, with a complete 3d electron shell, is a particularly stable ion with unique biological functions. Reviews of the biological chemistry of the essential elements are available.[180,428]

Biochemistry/Homeostasis

Most aspects of intermediary metabolism require essential trace elements in the form of metalloenzymes that have a number of catalytic properties. Specific metalloproteins are required for the transport and safe storage of very reactive metal ions such as Fe^{3+} or Cu^{2+}. Examples include metallothionein (Cu, Zn), transferrin, ferritin and hemosiderin (Fe), and ceruloplasmin (Cu).

Homeostatic controls are required to regulate the supply of essential trace elements to tissue cells in the face of varying dietary intakes. These involve regulation of intestinal absorption, specific transport systems in peripheral blood, uptake and storage mechanisms in tissue, and control of excretion. The principal excretory route for some important trace metals (Zn, Cu) is in feces, both by regulation of initial absorption and by resecretion into the intestinal tract in bile and other intestinal fluids. In essence, if zinc homeostasis is used as an example, it can be seen that the more the intake, the greater the overall excretion associated with increasing overall element retention.[327]

For the halides (iodide and fluoride), excess intake is excreted primarily in urine. For others (Se, B, Mo, and Cr), urinary output is also important. Loss of trace elements by other routes, such as through hair and/or nails, by skin cell desquamation, and in sweat, is generally minor; published studies have reported such measured losses.[295] Similarly, menstrual iron loss or seminal fluid zinc loss could be important in specialized studies.

Combinations of poor dietary supply, intestinal malabsorption caused by the antagonistic effects of other trace elements, and blockage of uptake by substances such as phytate—together with increased excretory losses as a result of disease, injury, and infection—can result in overt, symptomatic trace element deficiency disease. Liver disease, inflammatory bowel disease, and renal disease will affect trace element absorption and excretion to a variable extent and may cause an acquired deficiency disease.

Catabolic responses to injury, infection, and malignant disease can result in increased essential trace element losses in feces and in urine; burn injury causes extensive loss in exudates through the damaged skin.[48]

If postsurgical patients, especially those with short bowel syndrome, require prolonged periods of nasogastric tube feeding or intravenous feeding and are treated with nutrient regimens lacking sufficient inorganic micronutrients, they will develop symptomatic deficiency disease. Clinical cases of trace element deficiency have been described for copper, zinc, selenium, and chromium.[584]

Inborn Errors

Although genetic defects in the metabolism of trace elements are rare, they are nonetheless important because of the information they provide as to homeostatic control mechanisms. This information has led to the development of effective therapeutic strategies. The most commonly investigated disorders are those affecting iron (hemochromatosis), copper (Wilson's disease and Menkes' syndrome), zinc (acrodermatitis enteropathica), and molybdenum (molybdenum cofactor disease).

Interactions

The physiologic interaction between different essential trace elements and with the other essential major minerals can have significant effects on health. Such interactions are mostly considered as affecting the intestinal bioavailability of nutrients from various diets. Both synergistic and antagonistic effects on bioavailability have been given a theoretical basis by the observation that ions with similar electronic configurations in their outer orbit are likely to interact competitively. For example, strong interaction between zinc and copper has been noted, as well as between molybdenum and tungsten.[266]

The effects of trace elements on their relative absorptions show that increasing Zn reduces Fe uptake and vice versa.[531] However, the species of the element and presumably its solubility are also important, as different salts of zinc have different effects. Effects of copper on Fe absorption may be more physiologic, because copper deficiency is associated with a reduction in Fe intestinal transporters.[572]

The ability of zinc ions to block copper absorption, possibly by formation of intestinal metallothionein that strongly binds copper, has led to their use in pharmacologic doses in the management of Wilson's disease.[83] Similarly, molybdate ion can form insoluble copper-molybdate complexes in the intestine that limit copper absorption. The detrimental effects of organic phosphate (phytic acid) in limiting zinc absorption are aggravated by excessive dietary calcium, probably through formation of a highly insoluble Ca-Zn-phytate complex. The subject of these and other interactions has been reviewed.[467]

Synergistic interactions occur in other tissues and can have important biological and clinical consequences. For example, the interaction between selenium and iodine has been investigated. It is known that deiodinases are selenoproteins, and that they remove iodine from T_4 to produce the biologically active T_3. Also, the selenoprotein glutathione peroxidase is active in the thyroid in the destruction of excess hydrogen peroxide; it is therefore important in thyroid hormone production. In certain areas of the world, combined selenium and iodine deficiency can occur and can affect treatment; provision of selenium may be necessary to correct hypothyroidism, but this also may precipitate its onset.[21]

Selenium deficiency in experimental animal studies is exacerbated by vitamin E depletion. The antioxidant properties of tocopherol and glutathione peroxidase are similar and can, to some extent, overlap, although this is highly species dependent.[610]

Zinc and vitamin A are interrelated, and it appears that zinc depletion limits the bioavailability of vitamin A. Low zinc reduces vitamin A binding protein and hence reduces vitamin A transport and intake.[509] Controlled studies found that combined zinc and vitamin A supplementation is more clinically effective than vitamin A alone or zinc alone in controlling diarrhea and minimizing respiratory infection.[508]

Experimentally, it is usual to conduct animal and human studies using depletion of one essential element at a time. It is likely that in vivo, circumstances causing depletion of one essential element will be accompanied by varying degrees of depletion of other micronutrients, and that the possibility of interactions and synergistic effects should be considered when therapies are designed.

Laboratory Assessment of Trace Element Status

As understanding of underlying biochemical intracellular mechanisms increases for a particular trace element, the determination of active species becomes of increased importance.[626] For iodine, assay of the thyroid hormones and of their control and feedback systems has largely replaced direct determination of the element. Cobalamin (vitamin B_{12}) is measured in body fluids by immunoassay rather than by a nonspecific cobalt determination. This process is gradually being extended to other trace elements, because metalloenzymes and protein species are proposed as indices of Fe, Zn, Cu, and Se status.

Biological parameters have been thoroughly described for assessing iron status, whereas zinc and copper biomarkers are not routinely used.[242] Nonetheless, some new markers are being identified (e.g., zinc-induced metallothionein monocyte mRNA relates to low zinc intake).[373]

For several of the "ultratrace" elements (Cr, Mo, and V), insufficient information is currently available as to the critical molecular species underlying their biological actions. Direct methods of determining total trace element concentrations in biological samples are therefore required. This can pose severe analytical difficulties and may require specialist laboratory facilities, with use of appropriate techniques to reduce sample contamination.[423]

Dietary intakes of trace elements have been assessed for individual patients or population groups by direct dietary analysis and by documentation of dietary histories. Estimated intakes are then compared with current dietary reference values.

Direct measurement of total dietary intake over several days, together with measurement of all outputs in urine, in feces, or by other routes, has been used to estimate positive or negative balance. Because of the intrinsic difficulty of ensuring complete collection of all materials with minimal contamination, metabolic balance studies can have systematic errors.[411]

Net intake is estimated by using exogenous and endogenous labeling of representative diets with radioisotopes or stable isotopes of the trace element under investigation. These research methods can provide valuable insights as to the bioavailability of nutrients and the efficiency of uptake by the intestinal tract from particular diets.[483]

Analytical Considerations

Analytical factors that have to be considered in the measurement of trace elements include (1) specimen requirements, (2) preanalytical factors, (3) collection equipment, and (4) analytical methods.

Specimen Requirements

Direct determination of trace elements is done in many types of specimens, including whole blood, blood plasma or serum, leukocytes, urine, saliva, CSF, breast milk, and sweat. Tissue samples may be obtained by needle biopsy (liver, bone) or following an autopsy. Hair and nail samples offer a noninvasive means of sampling tissue and are used to assess toxic metal exposure. Measurements of hair and nails for essential elements may be of value on a group basis during studies of severely depleted populations but are of limited value in the investigation of individual hospital patients. Problems of external contamination from environmental pollution, cosmetics, shampoos, and other sources are difficult to control.[237]

The samples most commonly submitted for direct trace element analysis consist of whole blood, blood plasma, or serum. Plasma protein concentrations of the relevant carrier proteins transferrin (Fe), albumin (Zn), ceruloplasmin (Cu), and selenoprotein P (Se) provide useful additional information.

The concentration of essential trace elements in nucleated cells can be determined in various types of leukocytes and in platelets; this is a direct measure of intracellular trace element concentrations. However, separation of different types of white cells and platelets in whole blood is subject to serious problems of contamination before trace element analysis.[425]

Studies have suggested variability in blood cell compartment concentrations in different patient groups.[161] Moreover, of relevance especially in research studies, different tissues may have markedly different concentrations of individual elements.[390] An improved understanding of how the metals are distributed and function in vivo, and how best these properties can be investigated, is now part of the approach of metallomics.[417]

Problems caused by prolonged storage of samples can arise, and short-term storage at 4 to 10 °C with rapid turnaround analytical time is good practice. Repeated freezing and thawing of blood plasma and other types of material can lead to precipitation of proteins and nonhomogeneous samples.

Preanalytical Factors

Numerous variables can affect trace element determinations before analysis of the sample is undertaken, and these require careful control.[181] Guidelines giving details of sample collection procedures and procedures for limitation of contamination in a variety of sample types are available for essential and toxic trace elements.[364,423] Age, sex, ethnic origin, time of sampling in relation to food intake, time of day and year, history of medication, tobacco usage, and other factors should be recorded when reference intervals are established from healthy control populations.

For hospital patients with infection, and after accidental injury or post surgery, the systemic inflammatory response will affect the concentration of essential elements in circulating blood, independently of nutritional status. For example, the acute-phase reaction causes increased permeability of capillaries and transfer of certain plasma carrier proteins and their trace metals into interstitial space. Hepatic synthesis of some plasma proteins, so-called acute-phase proteins, is also induced, so that these proteins increase in concentration in plasma, together with any metals that they carry (e.g., ceruloplasmin, copper). Moreover, marked changes are noted in the kinetics of elements, with altered rates of transfer to and from the tissue. Knowledge of the effect of disease on metal kinetics and distribution is therefore essential.[582]

Collection Equipment

The choice of container for samples is important, in that contamination from rubber, cork, and colored plastics can be a problem. For blood plasma, collection plastic tubes with lithium heparin as an anticoagulant are suitable for most analyses. For blood serum, plain glass containers are used. For the ultratrace metals (Mn, Cr), special arrangements have to be made to collect blood via plastic cannulae or silanized steel needles; then the sample is placed into acid washed containers. "Trace metal" vacutainers are available commercially (see Chapter 7).

It is not recommended to use acid washed plastic bottles, as these may release elements combined within the plastic. It is better simply to wash any container thoroughly with ultrapure water. A wash with dilute acid through glass containers and collection systems may be acceptable. Blanks should always be checked before any collection system is used.

To avoid contamination from the needle during venous sampling, it is recommended that samples for the ultratrace elements (e.g., Mn, Ni, Co, Cr) are taken last (assuming a minimal sample collection of three), as this will ensure washout of the needle, thereby reducing any contamination.

For random urine samples and for tissue biopsy samples, a plain plastic container with no added preservative is preferable. For 24-hour urine collections, polyethylene bottles with no chemical additives are used. On receipt in the laboratory, the sample volume should be measured and aliquots stored at 4 °C or −15 °C before analysis.[73] It is important that urine should not be collected into disposable fiber or stainless steel containers.

For additional details and advice, specialist laboratories should be consulted [e.g., in the United States, the U.S. Department of Agriculture (USDA), Beltsville Agricultural Research Center (BARC), Washington, DC[462]; U.S. Department of Agriculture, Agriculture Research Service, Human Nutrition Research Center, Grand Forks, ND].[426] U.K. and European readers may wish to consult the Supra Area Assay Service[549] or the Scottish Trace Element and Vitamin Laboratory.[637] These sites have links to other specialist laboratories.

Analytical Methods

An analytical method used for determination of trace and ultratrace elements in biological specimens must be (1) sensitive, (2) specific, (3) precise, (4) accurate, and (5) relatively fast. The detection limits of such methods are very important because concentrations of trace or ultratrace elements in some samples are in the nanogram per gram to microgram per gram range. In practice, the concentration of a trace or ultratrace element should be at least 10 times the detection limit of the method, thus ensuring sufficient accuracy and precision.

Analytical techniques used for clinical trace metal analysis include spectrophotometry, atomic absorption spectrophotometry (AAS), inductively coupled plasma optical emission (ICP-OES), and inductively coupled plasma mass spectrometry (ICP-MS). Other techniques, such as neutron activation analysis (NAA) and x-ray fluorescence (XRF), and electrochemical methods, such as anodic stripping voltammetry (ASV), are used less commonly. For example, NAA requires a nuclear irradiation facility and is not readily available, and ASV requires completely mineralized solutions for analysis (this is a time-consuming process).

Spectrophotometry

The principles of spectrophotometric measurement are discussed in Chapter 10. When applied to analysis of trace elements, spectrophotometric methods are based on the use of a color-forming reagent; however, they are not specific for a particular metal. Interferences also occur in hemolyzed, lipemic, and icteric samples. In practice, the technique is not sensitive enough for all but the more abundant trace elements, such as iron, zinc, and copper. Many spectrophotometric methods for zinc and copper have been described,[81,272] and kits for them are available commercially.

Atomic Absorption Spectrophotometry

Atomic absorption spectrophotometry (AAS), a widely used method for determination of Zn and Cu in serum, has largely replaced less specific spectrophotometric methods. (The principles of AAS are detailed in Chapter 10 and elsewhere,[61] and Delves has written a useful review on the application of AAS to clinical pathology.[145])

The technique is not sensitive enough to measure Cu in urine; the more sensitive but technically more demanding technique of electrothermal atomization atomic absorption spectrometry (ETA-AAS) is required. Sample volumes as small as 10 μL are sequentially volatilized and are atomized in a graphite tube. This technique is useful in situations where the sample volume is limiting (e.g., premature babies), or with elements for which a more sensitive method is required, such as selenium or manganese. Significant analytical error can result from nonspecific optical absorption in the graphite tube caused by volatilization of matrix components along with analyte atoms. Optical background correction systems using a deuterium lamp or employing the Zeeman effect are standard components of ETA-AAS instrumentation (see Chapter 10). Flame and electrothermal types of AS are widely used, but these are single-element techniques; therefore, methods used for different elements have to be run sequentially, which can be wasteful in terms of time and sample.

Inductively Coupled Plasma-Optical Emission Spectrometry

ICP-OES is replacing AAS in some laboratories. Major changes to ICP-OES instrumentation that have led to this trend in replacement include (1) use of conventionally or radially viewed plasmas, which now can be viewed axially, thereby greatly improving sensitivity; (2) replacement of monochromators with echelle spectrometers; (3) replacement of photomultiplier detectors with charge-coupled detectors (CCDs), which have the ability to capture the whole echellogram, thereby delivering truly simultaneous analysis over the entire spectrum; and (4) use of vacuum or argon purged optics, allowing measurement down to and including the primary aluminum line at 167 nm.

With up-to-date ICP-OES, the elements Ca, Mg, Zn, Cu, Fe, and Al are all determined in a single analysis.[507] Apart from its multielement capabilities and increased sensitivity, ICP-OES offers a wide dynamic range (e.g., three orders of magnitude for most elements) that allows simultaneous analyses to be obtained on a single diluted aliquot of sample. The high temperature of the plasma (7500 °C) renders the technique largely free of chemical interferences, but matrix effects, background, and spectral interferences are greater than those in AAS. This is especially true of axially viewed plasma, in which emission from metal oxides may be observed. However, it is expected that sophisticated algorithms built into the software of modern instruments will overcome most problems. Axially and radially viewed ICP has been compared with respect to signal : background ratio, matrix effects, and sodium and calcium interferences.[80]

Inductively Coupled Plasma-Mass Spectrometry

ICP-MS is more widely used in trace element analysis because of its (1) relative ease of use, (2) wide analytical application,[257] and (3) competitive price of instrument purchase. This technique is more sensitive than ETA-AAS or ICP-OES and is now the method of choice for ultratrace elements. The spectra are simpler than those of ICP-OES, but problems still exist, in particular, interferences in the assay from the production of polyatomics formed within high-temperature plasma, so-called isobaric interference (i.e., ions of the same mass as the analyte ion).[394] Polyatomic interferences are more likely at masses less than 80. Improvements in analysis through sample modification, with the use of alternative mass ions, or with dynamic reaction cell technology to remove these interferences have been reported.[34] Modification of the geometry of inlet cones into the mass spectrometer side of the instrument can result in reduction of polyatomics with improved signal-to-noise response, particularly for analyte ions of low concentration (e.g., manganese).

Another improvement in mass ion discrimination is the use of a sector field inductively coupled plasma mass spectrometer (SFICPMS). This technique uses an electric and/or magnetic field to affect the path and/or velocity of charged particles in some way. These sector instruments bend the trajectories of the ions as they pass through the mass analyzer, according to their mass : charge ratios, deflecting further the more charged and faster-moving, lighter ions. The analyzer can be used to select a narrow range of m/z (with high resolution >3000) or to scan through a range of m/z to catalog the ions present, thus providing optimum signal to noise for the elemental mass of interest.[106] Commercial control solutions for trace elements will be increasingly referenced to stated values obtained by this technique (ICPMS-SF) as a definitive analytical procedure.

Because ICP-MS can be used to measure stable isotopes, it is used for conducting stable isotope tracer experiments and isotope dilution analysis. The principles of mass spectrometry are discussed in Chapter 14, and several textbooks on ICP-MS are available. Clinical applications of ICP-MS have been described and reviewed.[504]

Accelerator Mass Spectrometry

Accelerator mass spectrometry (AMS) differs from other forms of mass spectrometry in that it accelerates ions to extraordinarily high kinetic energies before mass analysis.[258] This makes possible the detection of naturally occurring, long-lived radioisotopes such as ^{10}Be, ^{36}Cl, ^{26}Al, and ^{14}C. Their typical isotopic abundance varies from 10^{-12} to 10^{-18}. The special property of AMS compared with other mass spectrometric methods is its power to separate a rare isotope from an abundant neighboring mass (e.g., ^{14}C from ^{12}C). For this reason, the technique is particularly useful in drug kinetic studies where only very small amounts of actual labeled drug are required (i.e., at low μg concentration).[236]

Other Techniques

Other techniques have been applied to elemental analysis, including x-ray–based techniques that have lower limits of detection at the μg/g concentration achievable for most sample materials. For thin sections of tissue, femto gram concentrations have been detected and reported for μ-SRXRF stations installed at second-generation synchrotrons; by using this technique, it is possible to map the three-dimensional (3D) orientation of metal in tissues (e.g., bone).[300]

Speciation Methods of Assessment

Speciation methods involve techniques to separate the chemical complexes of individual elements present in any particular medium; these are now regarded as crucial for an understanding of the absorption, utilization, and function of elements and how we deal with problems of excess and potential toxicity.[513] Because the most common fluid for consideration in clinical chemistry is blood/plasma, to speciate the element, an important starting point is to separate the plasma proteins and establish the elements within each protein fraction. Separative procedures involve high-performance ion-exchange chromatography and fast protein liquid chromatography; they allow separation of protein constituents [e.g., albumin (α), transferrin (β), and globulin (γ) zones of plasma proteins]. Aliquots of these fractions are analyzed by sensitive techniques such as graphite furnace (GF)-AAS, ICP-OES, or ICP-MS.

Recent developments have coupled separative with analytical procedures, in particular with ICP-OES or ICP-MS, and are known collectively as *hyphenated techniques.* This application has enabled the analysis of several elements and study of their distribution in plasma in various abnormal clinical states (e.g., uremia).[37] The low limit of detection of ICP-MS has enabled the low sample requirement of capillary electrophoresis to be coupled in this way.[418]

Coupling of analytical procedures such as ICP-MS with ion-exchange chromatography specifically configured to measure the elements attached to small molecules (e.g., organic acids) will allow chemical speciation not only of the organo complexes but also of chemically ionized states of the elements in solution. Such techniques are important in speciation analysis and have been applied to our understanding of metal complexes (e.g., aluminium) likely to be relevant in absorption.[53] Relatively little work has been carried out on the organo speciation of metals such as Fe, Zn, and Cu in physiologic solutions.

A study using double-focusing ICP-MS with low limits of detection on the speciation/distribution of metals Co, Cr, and Ni, released as a result of metal damage after total hip arthroplasty, indicated different protein interactions.[476] Cobalt ions showed affinity to both albumin and transferrin, whereas Cr (presumably as 3^+ ions) was preferentially bound to transferrin. Most of the total element content (>90%) was attached in some way to protein.

Speciation of the small molecular weight species of manganese in CSF showed that the citrate complex was predominant; other ion complexes were also detected, but in relatively low amounts (e.g., malate, lactate, various amino acids such as histidine).[418]

It is possible to model such speciation in physiologic fluids using established affinity constants and commercial computer programs.[334] Such a model predicts that the major small species of elements will be complexed with citric acid (e.g., iron); obviously this will affect cellular uptake of the elements.

The European Virtual Institute for Speciation Analysis (EVISA) is a service provider in the field of speciation analysis. The EVISA Web portal (www.speciation.net) is a primary source for all those seeking information about chemical species with respect to analysis, biological activity (toxicity, nutritional value, metabolism), legislation (laws, rules, standards), and research in related fields.

Quality Assurance Considerations

Because methods of trace element analysis are not standardized and are disposed to matrix effects and contamination problems, quality assurance measures must be incorporated into trace element analysis schemes. An effective quality assurance scheme for trace or ultratrace element analyses requires incorporation of the following into each batch of analysis: (1) reagent blanks, (2) replicate analyses to assess precision, (3) calibrators of trace elements of interest in the expected concentration range of specimens analyzed, and (4) a control or reference solution with known or certified concentrations of trace elements to be determined to assess accuracy and batch-to-batch precision. The reference material should be of the same matrix type and should contain approximately the same amount of analyte as the specimen. Many different control or reference materials that contain certified amounts of trace elements are available. For quality control of trace element determination in tissue specimens, reference materials of different biological matrices that have certified values for most macro and trace elements are available from the National Institute of Standards and Technology, Office of Standard Reference Materials, in Washington, DC (see Chapter 9).

It is recommended that laboratories that measure trace elements should participate in one or more EQAS. Organizations that provide such schemes are listed in Box 31-1, and compilations of reference intervals have been published.[194,662]

Individual Trace Elements

Trace elements discussed in this chapter include chromium, cobalt, copper, fluoride, iron, manganese, molybdenum, selenium, and zinc.

Chromium

Chromium occurs naturally in various crustal materials. It is a transitional element with many industrial uses and is discharged into the environment as industrial waste. The function and biochemistry of chromium have been reviewed.[665]

Chemistry

Chromium (atomic number 24, atomic weight 51.99) is a transition metal that occurs in biology with valence 3^+ or 6^+, each having markedly different properties. Trivalent Cr^{3+} is a d^3 cation that usually forms octahedral complexes with slow ligand exchange. The element has no redox or acid-base properties.[197] It is considered an essential trace element that enhances the action of insulin.[413] Hexavalent Cr^{6+} is a strong oxidant that can cause tissue damage,[647] although toxic Cr(VI) is normally rapidly reduced to Cr^{3+} during contact with foodstuffs and gastric contents.

A biologically active form of Cr^{3+} found in brewer's yeast, known as glucose tolerance factor (GTF). The structure of the Cr^{3+} bioactive molecule is thought to be an octahedral chromium complex, with two molecules of nicotinic acid having four coordination sites linked to glutamic acid, glycine, and cysteine, but attempts to isolate and purify the substance have not been successful. It is not clear whether GTF in brewer's yeast is better used than inorganic chromium in relation to insulin activation.[471]

Dietary Sources

Estimates of the amount of chromium in foodstuffs vary, in part because of analytical difficulties, but also because of contamination caused by contact with stainless steel during food processing, storage, and cooking. Processed meats, whole grain products, green beans, broccoli, and some spices are relatively good sources, but fruit and dairy products are not. Foodstuffs with high amounts of sucrose or fructose are intrinsically low in chromium; furthermore, these sugars may promote urine loss. The estimated dietary intake for adults in the United States varies from 20 to 30 μg/d. Supplements containing chromium are taken by about 8% of adults in the United States; the NHANES III survey estimated that this added 23 μg Cr/d.[190]

Absorption, Transport, Metabolism, and Excretion

Intestinal absorption of Cr^{3+} is low, ranging from 0.4 to 2.5%, so fecal output mainly consists of unabsorbed dietary chromium. In a 2001 study, 1.7% of a Cr^{3+} dose was absorbed as the chloride, whereas Cr^{6+} (chromate) fractional absorption was from 3.9 to 12.0%. This variation was probably related to lack of conversion of Cr^{6+} to the Cr^{3+} form, and the rapid appearance of both Cr^{3+} and Cr^{6+} in the blood suggests that both must be absorbed from the stomach, as well as from the intestine.[469]

BOX 31-1 Organizations Providing Proficiency Testing and Quality Assurance Programs for Trace Element Testing Laboratories

The College of American Pathologists
325 Waukegan Road
Northfield, IL 60093-2750
USA
Contact: Survey Coordinator
www.cap.org
Phone: (800) 323-4040

Laboratoire de Toxicologie Humaine
Institute National de Sante Publique du Quebec
945, Ave Wolfe, Sainte-Foy Quebec G1V 5B3
Canada
ctq@inspq.qc.ca
www.inspq.qc.ca
Phone: (418) 650-5115
Fax: (418) 654-2148

Societe Francaise de Biologie Clinique (SFBC)
Laboratoire de Biochemie C
CHRU Grenoble- B.P. 217
38043 Grenoble Cedex 9
France
INRS-Service TMPC-B.P.27
54501 Vandoevre-les-Nancy
francois.baruthio@inrs.fr
Phone: (33) 83 50 20 00
Fax: (33) 83 50 20 19

SKZL (Foundation for Quality Assessment in Clinical Laboratories), Section Multi Component Analysis
Beatrix Park 1,
NL-7101 BN Winterswijk,
The Netherlands
Phone + 31 543 544774
Fax: +31 543 524265

Trace Elements Proficiency Testing Program
New York State Department of Health
Wadsworth Centre, PO Box 509,
Albany, NY 12201-0509
USA
lead@wadsworth.org
www.wadsworth.org/testing/Lead/index.htm
Phone: (518) 474-5475
Fax: (518) 473-7586

Guildford Trace Elements External Quality Assessment Scheme (TEQUAS)
Robens Institute, University of Surrey
Guildford GU2 5XH
UK
A.Taylor@surrey.ac.uk
Phone: +44 1483 502742
Fax: +44 1483 503517

METOS Scheme, Department of Clinical Biochemistry, National Institutes of Health
Viale Regina Elena, 299-00161 Roma
Italy
m.patria@iss.it
Phone: +39 6 49902559/31
Fax: + 39 6 4461961/8380

Institut und Poliklinik fur Arbeits-, Sozial-und Umweltmedizin
Schillerstr. 25, D-91054
Erlingen
Germany
Tobias.weiss@rzmail.uni-erlangen.de
www.g-equas.de
Phone: 09131-85 22 37 4
Fax: 09131-85 61 26

Absorption is increased marginally by ascorbic acid, amino acids, oxalate, and other dietary factors. After absorption, chromium binds to plasma transferrin with an affinity similar to that of iron.[245] It then concentrates in human liver, spleen, other soft tissue, and bone.[358] Urine chromium output is around 0.2 to 0.3 μg/d; the amount excreted to some extent is dependent on intake. Paradoxically, urine output appears to be relatively increased at low dietary amounts. Thus 2% is lost in urine at an intake of 10 μg/d, but only 0.5% at an intake of 40 μg/d.[14] Running and resistive exercises increase urine chromium excretion.[15,535]

Functions

Severely chromium-deficient rats have (1) impaired growth; (2) reduced life span; (3) corneal lesions; and (4) alterations in carbohydrate, lipid, and protein metabolism. Supplementation with inorganic chromium restored glucose tolerance in these animals. Repetition of laboratory studies on experimental animals by other groups yielded inconsistent results. Claims of benefit from chromium supplementation in diabetic patients, in the elderly, and in malnourished children were published but were not confirmed by others. It was later realized that chromium concentrations measured by earlier methods were orders of magnitude too high because of contamination of samples before analysis. Also ineffective background optical correction was used in the graphite furnace AAS systems then available.[657] However, many of the important biological observations made in those early investigations have since been confirmed using more accurate analytical techniques.[412]

The biochemical mechanism that allows chromium to potentiate the actions of insulin receptors on cell membranes has been intensively investigated.[663] It is now suggested that a low molecular weight intracellular octapeptide (LMWCr), also known as chromodulin, binds Cr^{3+} and enhances the response of insulin receptors. Chromodulin binds four Cr^{3+} ions and then locates on cell membranes near to the site of insulin receptors. The structure of chromodulin has been examined by a variety of advanced spectroscopic techniques, and the complex has been shown to possess a unique type of multinuclear assembly, with chromium centers having an octahedral coordination with oxygen-based ligands.[297]

Chromodulin, first described in the1980s, has been isolated from liver, kidney, and other tissues in several species of experimental animals. Its proposed mode of action consists of the following: (1) inactive insulin receptors on cell membranes are converted to an active form by binding circulating insulin; (2) this binding stimulates movement into cells of chromium bound to plasma transferrin; (3) chromium then binds to apoLMWCr, converting it to an active form that then binds to the insulin receptors and potentiates kinase activity; and (4) as plasma glucose and insulin fall to normoglycemic concentrations, the LMWCr factor is released from the cell to terminate its effects.[663] It is thought that released chromodulin is the naturally occurring form of chromium in urine.[126]

Requirements and Reference Nutrient Intakes

Because evidence has been insufficient to set an estimated average requirement (EAR), an adequate intake based on estimated intakes has been set at 35 μg Cr/d for men and 25 μg Cr/d for women. No tolerable upper limit was set for dietary Cr^{3+} intake.[190]

Intravenous Supply

It is now advised that patients on short-term TPN (<1 to 3 months) should receive 10 to 20 μg Cr/d. Those on long-term TPN who are clinically and biochemically stable may be receiving enough chromium via contamination of their nutrients.[11]

Commercial multielement intravenous additives usually contain about 10 to 30 μg Cr. When high concentrations of glucose (20 to 50%) are given intravenously as the main energy source, increased loss of chromium in urine may occur. Urinary losses could be monitored (although this is rarely done) and input increased, especially if signs of unexplained glucose intolerance are seen. However, reports have indicated that excessive amounts of chromium may have been given to children and adults during TPN, with possible detrimental effects on renal function.[238,354]

Deficiency

Clinical signs of human chromium deficiency were clearly described first in patients receiving parenteral nutrition for a prolonged period using a nutritional regimen that did not supply sufficient chromium.[11] Only a few case histories[301] have been published. All patients had similar presentations, with previously stable patients developing insulin-resistant glucose intolerance, weight loss, and in some cases neurologic deficits. Addition of substantial amounts of Cr^{3+} to the intravenous regimen (150 to 200 μg/d) reversed glucose intolerance and reduced insulin requirements with eventual improvement in neurologic disorders.

These cases, although rare, influenced the U.S. Food and Nutrition Board to designate chromium as an essential trace element.[190] It is not clear why so few cases of clinical chromium deficiency have been reported in comparison with zinc, copper, and selenium, but this fact might be related to chromium contamination of infusion fluids, especially in the amino acid mixture.[579]

Clinical Significance

Chromium is thought to play a role in impaired glucose tolerance, diabetes, and cardiovascular disease.

Impaired Glucose Tolerance and Diabetes. More than 15% of adults aged 40 to 74 are thought to have impaired glucose tolerance; it has been suggested that poor chromium nutritional status may be a factor.[190] Tissue chromium concentrations of patients with diabetes tend to be lower than in controls.[278] However, the variability of dietary chromium intake and the lack of an easily usable laboratory or clinical marker to identify those patients with poor chromium status create difficulties. A controlled trial of higher doses (250 μg and 1000 μg of chromium) given as chromium picolinate was conducted in China on 180 type 2 diabetic subjects. This trial reported improvements in glucose handling and reduction in glycosylated hemoglobin.[13] Benefit was also found in previous studies on populations of malnourished children in Jordan, Nigeria, and Turkey. It is possible that other interacting dietary depletions may aggravate chromium deficiency in these populations.[413]

It has been suggested that a short-term dosage of <1000 μg Cr/d may be a useful additional treatment for type 2 diabetes. Not all patients respond to chromium supplements—clinical response correlates with baseline insulin sensitivity, fasting glucose, and glycated hemoglobin[108]—but in such patients, insulin resistance is improved.[278] Monitoring of kidney function and clinical assessment of dermatologic changes are advised.[539] Anderson maintains that chromium supplementation has been shown to improve glucose handling in all the main types of diabetes,[12] but this is not a widely held view. Chromium therapy in the control and prevention of diabetes is of considerable interest and is the subject of much controversy. However, recommendations of the American Diabetes Association state that "at the present, benefit from chromium supplementation in persons with diabetes has not been conclusively demonstrated."[107]

Glucose Intolerance in the Elderly. Glucose intolerance is age related, and chromium supplementation trials in the elderly have been conducted with variable results.[471] An inability to determine which of the elderly trial subjects were initially chromium depleted makes it difficult to interpret the findings. If the observations can be confirmed, and if an age-related decrease is seen in chromium concentrations in hair, sweat, and blood serum, additional studies on the elderly are needed.[143]

Cardiovascular Disease. Chromium depletion has long been thought to be associated with increased cardiovascular risk.[410] A double-blind 12-week study of 23 healthy adult men showed that 200 μg chromium (as chromium chloride) increased HDL cholesterol and decreased insulin concentrations.[519] Other reports of favorable lipid responses to chromium supplementation have also been published.[2,261] Abnormal lipid profiles have been found in patients with type 2 diabetes and may be associated with increased risk of cardiovascular disease. However, additional larger-scale studies are necessary to confirm the effects of chromium on risk factors for cardiovascular disease.[471]

Studies in animal models have shown that intramuscular injection of chromium reduces the size of lipid deposits in the coronary vasculature of hypercholesterolemic rabbits.[1] Lipid deposits in the ascending aorta were similarly reduced, as were serum cholesterol concentrations. Chromium concentrations were extremely high (3258 to 4513 μg/L) compared with untreated animals (3.2 to 6.3 μg/L), and kidney function tests and histopathology were normal.[502] These findings suggest an interesting possibility—that high chromium may be beneficial as a treatment option for removal of atherosclerotic lesions in human patients.

Toxicity

Hexavalent chromium (Cr^{6+}) is a recognized carcinogen, and industrial exposure to fumes and dusts containing this metal is associated with increased incidence of lung cancer, dermatitis, and skin ulcers. Environmental health risks arise from soil contamination by Cr^{6+} waste disposal sites left by the leather tanning and dyestuff industries.[647] Cr^{6+} is more efficiently absorbed than Cr^{3+}, and its toxicity and carcinogenic effects involve reduction to Cr^{6+} and Cr^{3+} by cysteine, with formation of intracellular DNA adducts.[708] Cr^{3+}species are relatively nontoxic in part because of their poor intestinal absorption and rapid excretion in urine.

However, chromium picolinate is a widely used dietary supplement, and this compound has been reported to cause renal and hepatic damage when used at high doses.[113] Patients with preexisting renal or liver disease may be at particular risk for adverse effects. Vincent[664] has found that chromium picolinate has a different intracellular pathway compared with other forms of Cr^{3+}. Benefits from chromium picolinate may be related to diabetes control,[13] but claims that this supplement can promote body fat loss and muscle mass gain have not been substantiated.[664]

In addition, markedly increased concentrations (up to 1000-fold) have been observed in both plasma (12 μg/L; 620 nmol/L) and urine (50 μg/L; 2600 nmol/L) in patients with problem hip prostheses.[137] These may be raised in any patient receiving chrome-cobalt prostheses.[382] No harmful effects of these high concentrations have been observed.

Laboratory Assessment of Status

A beneficial response of glucose-intolerant patients to chromium supplementation is presently the only means of confirming chromium deficiency. No practicable method of assessing intracellular chromium depletion is yet available, and no consistently reliable animal model has been identified for chromium deficiency. Furthermore, it has been known from early animal experiments that circulating chromium is not in equilibrium with physiologically important reserves.[412] It has been shown in late pregnancy that serum chromium concentration does not correlate with glucose intolerance, insulin resistance, or serum lipids.[233]

A possibly useful test has been proposed that uses radioactive $^{51}Cr^{6+}$ to label red cells. The ion is then reduced to Cr^{3+}, and the amount bound to cell membranes is dependent on the amount of Cr^{3+} initially present, which, in turn, is a reflection of the adequacy of chromium nutritional status. The test was applied to 25 patients with type 2 diabetes and 35 controls. No difference was found, and it was concluded that chromium nutrition has only a minor role in this condition.[676]

Direct determination of chromium in the diet, in oral and intravenous nutritional support regimens, and in blood plasma or serum can be carried out only if great care is taken to prevent contamination before and during analysis.[471] Sample collection procedures have to avoid any contact with stainless steel, so all-plastic phlebotomy systems or siliconized steel needles should be used, and samples should be stored in acid washed containers. Acid digestion of diet samples in sealed pressure vessels using microwave heating may be necessary to reduce background effects and to prevent loss of volatile chromium compounds. Specialist trace element laboratories employing ICP-MS and stable chromium isotopes now offer improved analytical sensitivity and allow tracer methods for metabolic studies.[483]

Detection of increased amounts of chromium in urine provides confirmation of recent occupational or environmental exposure to excess chromium. It also may be useful for monitoring urine chromium in trials that use pharmacologic dosages of chromium, both to confirm compliance and to detect potential toxicity. This is possible using available graphite furnace AAS instrumentation.[241]

Reference Values

Very low values are now considered as normal for serum (0.1 to 0.2 μg/L, 2 to 3 nmol/L) and for urine (<0.2 μg/L, <3 nmol/L). Thus detection of deficiency by direct analysis is difficult.[471,657]

Cobalt

Cobalt is essential for humans only as an integral part of vitamin B_{12} (cobalamin). No other function for cobalt in the human body is known. Details of vitamin B_{12} biochemistry and function were discussed earlier in the chapter. The microflora of the human intestine cannot use cobalt to synthesize physiologically active cobalamin. The human vitamin B_{12} requirement must be supplied by the diet. Free (nonvitamin B_{12}) cobalt does not interact with the body vitamin B_{12} pool.

Cobalt status is usually assessed through measurement of vitamin B_{12} or cobalamin; with evidence of effects of exposure by the metal ion Co^{2+} itself, awareness of the importance of changes in physiologic concentration is necessary. Normal values in plasma are less than 1 μg/L and in urine usually less than 2 μg/g creatinine.[704] Increased exposure from industrial uses, particularly with hard metal saw blades, leads to high mean urinary Co concentrations. Increases are also associated with hip prostheses for which concentrations can be markedly raised with no evidence of overt toxicity.[137]

Copper

Copper (Cu) is an important trace element that is associated with a number of metalloproteins. It is present in biological systems in both 1^+ and 2^+ valence states.

Chemistry

Copper (atomic number 29, atomic weight 63.54) has Cu^{1+} and Cu^{2+} oxidation states in biological systems; facile exchange between these ions gives the element important redox properties. Because of their high electron affinities, these ions are most strongly bound to organic molecules of all essential trace metals. Copper in biological material is complexed with proteins, peptides, and other organic ligands. An elaborate series of binding and transport proteins inside cells protects the genome from copper-generated free radical attack.[361] This keeps the concentration of free copper in the cytoplasm very low ($\cong 10^{-15}$ mol/L). Copper bioinorganic chemistry evolved concurrently with that of molecular oxygen. Numerous blue-colored copper-containing proteins, most of which are oxidases, are located outside the cytoplasm on the surface of cell membranes or in vesicles. However, the copper metalloenzyme superoxide dismutase (SOD) protects against random free radical damage both in the cytoplasm and in blood plasma. Paradoxically, it was the ability of copper ions to generate free radicals that led to the evolutionary development of the extracellular matrix by polymerization and cross-linking of low molecular weight substrates. This allowed the formation of collagen, chitin, and other structural proteins essential for the development of multicellular life forms.[197]

Dietary Sources

The copper content of food is variable and can be affected by application to crops of copper-containing fertilizers and fungicidal sprays. Also, the use of copper-containing cooking vessels contributes to total intake. The metal is most plentiful in organ meats, such as liver and kidney, with relatively high amounts also found in shellfish, nuts, whole grain cereals, bran, and all cocoa-containing products. Lesser amounts of copper are found in white meats and in dairy products, especially cow's milk. The median intake of copper in the United States is around 1.0 to 1.6 mg/d.[190] Intake mainly from meat and vegetables in the older adult (>60 years) is prone to be low, particularly among low-income groups and those with less education; continual assessment of the nutriture is needed in this group.[380]

Absorption, Transport, Metabolism, and Excretion

Copper absorption occurs mainly in the small intestine, although gastric uptake has been shown to occur to a lesser extent. Some copper may be incorporated by inhalation and skin absorption. The extent of intestinal copper absorption varies with dietary copper content and is around 50% at low copper intakes (<1 mg Cu/d) but only 20% at higher intakes (>5 mg Cu/d).[640] Copper intestinal uptake is pH dependent and relatively efficient. Absorption is reduced by other dietary components such as zinc (via metallothionein), molybdate, and iron, and is increased by amino acids and by dietary sodium.[244]

Absorbed copper is transported to the liver in portal blood bound to albumin, where it is incorporated by hepatocytes into cuproenzymes and other proteins and then is exported in peripheral blood to tissue and organs. Although two thirds of the 80 to100 mg total body copper content is located in the skeleton and muscle, the liver is the key organ in copper homeostasis.[640] More than 90% of copper exported from the liver into peripheral blood is in the form of the glycoprotein ceruloplasmin, which has a blue color when separated from other plasma proteins. Its structure can be studied by electron paramagnetic resonance spectroscopy and other spectroscopic techniques.[381] It is a positive acute-phase reactant that is increased during infection and after tissue injury. Ceruloplasmin also is increased in pregnancy and during use of oral contraceptives, leading to a rise in serum copper concentration. A smaller amount of copper in plasma (<10%) is bound to albumin by specific peptide sequences, and this copper is in equilibrium with plasma amino acids. This fraction may be important for cellular uptake.

An overview of copper metabolism is illustrated in Figure 31-26.[230] Between 0.5 and 2.0 mg of copper/d is excreted via bile into feces. Patients with cholestatic jaundice or other forms of liver dysfunction therefore are at risk for copper accumulation caused by failure of excretion. Copper losses in urine and sweat account for less than 3% of dietary intake. Urine copper output is normally less than 60 μg/d.

Functions

Copper, a catalytic component of numerous enzymes, is also a structural component of other important proteins in humans, animals, plants, and microorganisms.[244] Some of those considered of potential importance in human biochemistry are briefly described in the following sections. Only small amounts of copper are present in biological fluids, and essentially none of it exists in a free ion form. These properties and the low redox potential of copper dictate special structural and mechanistic features in copper transporters.[316]

Energy Production. Cytochrome c oxidase is a multisubunit complex containing copper and iron. Located on the external face of mitochondrial membranes, the enzyme catalyzes four-electron reduction of molecular oxygen, establishing a high-energy proton gradient across the inner mitochondrial membrane that is necessary for ATP production. Cytochrome c and cytochrome c oxidase are essential for oxidative phosphorylation that serves as the basis of intracellular energy production.

Connective Tissue Formation. Protein-lysine 6-oxidase (lysyl oxidase) is a cuproenzyme that is essential for stabilization of extracellular matrixes, specifically, for enzymatic cross-linking of collagen and elastin. Complex mechanisms involve the deamination of lysine and hydrolysine residues at specific extracellular sites. The enzyme is highly associated

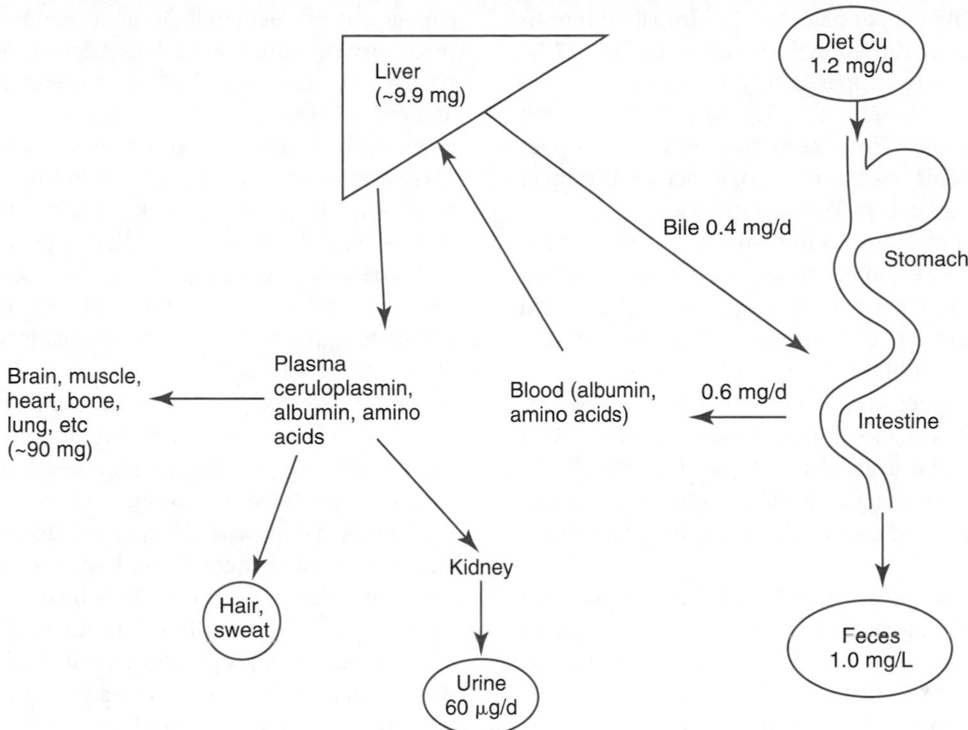

Figure 31-26 Metabolism of copper. *(Modified from Harris ED. Copper. In: O'Dell BL, Sunde RA, eds. Handbook of nutritionally essential mineral elements. New York: Marcel Dekker, 1997:231-73.)*

with connective tissue and is located in the aorta, dermal connective tissue, fibroblasts, and cytoskeleton of many other cells.

Iron Metabolism. Copper-containing enzymes, namely, ferroxidase I (ceruloplasmin) and ferroxidase II, and hephaestin in the enterocyte oxidize ferrous iron to ferric iron. This allows incorporation of Fe^{3+} into transferrin and eventually into hemoglobin. Ferroxidase II is a yellow protein, the importance of which in iron metabolism is not as well characterized as that of ceruloplasmin.

Central Nervous System. Dopamine mono-oxygenase (DMO) is an enzyme that requires copper as a cofactor and uses ascorbate as an electron donor. This enzyme catalyzes the conversion of dopamine to norepinephrine, the important neurotransmitter. Soluble and membrane bound forms of the enzyme are present, with the latter found in chromaffin granules of the adrenal cortex. Monoamine oxidase, one of the numerous amine oxidases, is a copper-containing enzyme that catalyzes the degradation of serotonin in the brain and is also involved in the metabolism of catecholamines.

Formation of the phospholipids necessary for myelin sheath formation is affected by cytochrome c oxidase depletion. It is now known that the prion protein (PrP) binds Cu^{2+} and may be involved in copper regulation within the brain.[95] Also, a dysfunction in copper homeostasis has been shown in Alzheimer's disease, with an excess of fragmentation of ceruloplasmin in cerebrospinal fluid. This was related to increased proteolysis of ceruloplasmin, indicating an inflammatory process rather than a causative effect of copper on tau protein precipitation.[602]

Melanin Synthesis. Tyrosinase is a copper-containing enzyme that is present in melanocytes and catalyzes the synthesis of melanin. Starting with L-dopa as a substrate, tyrosinase catalyzes multiple oxidative steps to produce the melanin biopigments, pheomelanin and eumelanin.

Antioxidant Functions. Both intracellular and extracellular SODs are Cu- and Zn-containing enzymes, able to convert superoxide radicals to hydrogen peroxide, which can be removed subsequently by catalase and other antioxidant defenses. The plasma protein ceruloplasmin also binds copper ions and thus prevents oxidative damage from free copper ions, which can generate hydroxyl radicals.

Regulation of Gene Expression and Intracellular Copper Handling. Copper-dependent proteins act as transcription factors for specific genes, such as those regulating SOD, and catalase. Metallothionein synthesis is controlled by copper-responsive transcription factors; this protein is important in regulating the intracellular distribution of copper.[642] Additional specialized proteins act as "copper chaperones" to deliver copper to intracellular sites and to prevent oxidative damage by free copper ions.[179]

Inborn Errors of Copper Metabolism. Menkes' syndrome is caused by a defective gene that regulates the metabolism of copper in the body. Wilson's disease is inherited as an autosomal recessive trait having a defect in the metabolism of copper, with accumulation of copper in the liver, brain, kidney, cornea, and other tissues. Investigation of these rare genetic defects has been of great value in uncovering details on the control of copper transport. Copper-transporting P-type ATPases, known as ATP7A and ATP7B, are essential factors in maintaining copper balance.[136,679] Impaired intestinal transport of copper caused by a mutation in the *ATP7A* gene leads to the severe copper deficiency disease seen in Menkes' syndrome. Defects in the *ATP7B* gene affect both incorporation of copper into ceruloplasmin and copper excretion via bile. This results in a toxic accumulation of copper and forms the basis of Wilson's disease.

Another genetic defect results in failure of hepatic synthesis of ceruloplasmin (aceruloplasminemia), which is a neurodegenerative disease. Retinal damage, secondary iron overload, and insulin-dependent diabetes present in the fourth to fifth decade of life.[247,259]

Angiogenesis. Copper plays an essential role in promoting angiogenesis, as was shown in the stimulation of blood vessel formation in the avascular cornea of rabbits.[246] On x-ray fluorescence microscopy (XFM), highly vascularized ductal carcinomas showed copper clustering in putative neoangiogenic areas.[180]

Various clinical trials have established that Cu privation by diet or by Cu chelators diminishes a tumor's ability to mount an angiogenic response. These data have shed new light on the functional role of Cu in microvessel development and, of equal importance, have stimulated new nutritional models of cancer therapeutic intervention. The use of Tetrathio molydate can directly and reversibly downregulate copper delivery to secreted metalloenzymes, which suggests that proteins involved in metal regulation might be fruitful drug targets.[8] Initial observations in animal models of breast cancer were encouraging,[481] but later studies showed no benefit at least in neuroglioblastoma.[79]

Requirements and Reference Nutrient Intakes

The recommended dietary intake of Cu for adults is 0.9 mg/d. This is close to the lower limit of 1.0 mg/d found in dietary surveys and has led to suggestions that marginal copper depletion could be found in the U.S. population.[330] The tolerable upper limit is 10 mg/d.[190]

Intravenous Supply

The usual adult supply of copper given intravenously varies from 0.3 to 1.3 mg/d (5 to 20 μmol/d), with higher amounts required in those patients with preexisting depletion or biliary losses and lower amounts in those with cholestasis.

Deficiency

Malnourished Infants. When malnourished infants with a history of chronic diarrhea were rehabilitated using a formula based on cow's milk, they developed iron-resistant anemia, neutropenia, and other hematologic disorders and bone lesions. Copper supplementation of milk feeds reversed these abnormalities, and the addition of 2.5 mg Cu/d is now advised.[134]

Premature Infants. Most of the accumulation of copper in the fetal liver occurs in the last 3 months of pregnancy, and premature infants fed formula lacking sufficient copper are at risk of deficiency disease because they lack adequate liver copper stores. Hematologic abnormalities and easily fractured brittle bones have been described.[370] Radiographic changes in infants with copper deficiency include osteopenia and metaphyseal spurs.[230] As noted earlier, formulas based on cow's milk require copper supplementation. Monitoring of plasma copper is advisable, and results should be related to postnatal age: at 4 weeks, mean values are 42 μg/dL (6.6 μmol/L), rising to 55 μg/dL (8.7 μmol/L) by 14 weeks.[96]

Nutritional Support. Adults and children fed intravenously without the addition of sufficient copper to the nutrient regimen develop symptomatic copper deficiency. Hematologic changes of hypochromic anemia and neutropenia are reversed by copper supplementation.[206,207] Similar effects have been reported during prolonged enteral feeding via jejunostomy.[99] Children may develop the typical bone changes mentioned previously.

Menkes' Syndrome. History and aspects of the diagnosis and therapy of this condition have been reviewed.[311] It is a rare condition (1/100,000 live births), the mutation is X-linked, and it typically occurs in male infants at 2 to 3 months. Such infants present with loss of previously normal development, hypotonia, seizures, and failure to thrive. Physical changes in the hair (pili torti) and in facial appearance, as well as neurologic abnormalities, suggest the diagnosis. Low concentrations of copper in plasma, liver, and brain occur because of impaired intestinal copper absorption. Local first-line tests would provide findings of plasma copper <10 μmol/L and ceruloplasmin <220 mg/L, along with demonstration of pili torti by microscopic examination of the hair. Additional tests can demonstrate failure of isotopic copper egress from cultured fibroblasts and show plasma catecholamine abnormalities. Placental copper measurement and direct mutation analysis are additional investigative procedures. Deficiency of the copper enzyme DMO in CSF is thought to be an important finding that allows early diagnosis. The effectiveness of therapy with parenteral copper histidine is debatable, although success has been claimed in less severely affected cases, especially if treatment is started early.[122]

Malabsorption Syndromes. Patients at risk include those with celiac disease, tropical sprue, cystic fibrosis, and short bowel syndrome. Excessive intake of oral zinc supplements can cause anemia and hematologic abnormalities in the absence of occult blood loss.[234,284] Copper deficiency is caused by zinc induction of metallothionein in the intestinal mucosa, which then sequesters dietary copper, blocking its absorption.

Cardiovascular Disease. Animal studies show that severe copper deficiency causes cardiac damage, but the abnormality differs from that seen in human cardiovascular disease. The myocardium is hypertrophied and may rupture in animal models. Coronary artery pressure is decreased, but in human ischemic disease, it is increased.[141] The role of copper in human cardiovascular disease is controversial, although much supporting evidence for a positive link with low dietary copper intake has been published.[330]

Epidemiologic surveys have shown that increased plasma copper values are a positive cardiovascular risk factor. A U.S. study of 4400 adult men and women found that those with plasma copper values in the two highest quartiles had the greatest risk of dying from cardiovascular disease.[192] An increase in plasma ceruloplasmin and hence plasma copper may be a nonspecific response to the inflammation of arteries found in arteriosclerosis. It is known that the ceruloplasmin hepatic messenger RNA (mRNA) increases during inflammation, and that this is induced by interleukin-6. Insulin is also known to be involved in the transcriptional regulation of ceruloplasmin synthesis.[216,569]

Anemia. Copper deficiency is an established cause of hematologic abnormalities but is frequently misdiagnosed. Patients with copper deficiency can present with a combination of hematologic and neurologic abnormalities that may masquerade as a myelodysplastic syndrome. Records between 1970 and 2005 of patients excluding Wilson's disease with hypocupremia (mean, 0.23; range, 0 to 0.69 μg/mL; normal plasma zinc) identified various hematologic abnormalities on bone marrow examination, including (1) vacuoles in myeloid precursors, (2) iron-containing plasma cells, and (3) a decrease in granulocyte precursors and ring sideroblasts.[239] Thus copper deficiency is an uncommon but very treatable cause of hematologic abnormalities.

Neuropathy. Copper deficiency is an increasingly recognized cause of gait unsteadiness. A case report of copper deficiency due to celiac disease suggested that ataxia associated with celiac disease was likely due to a copper deficiency myeloneuropathy.[222]

A case of copper deficiency–associated myeloneuropathy has been described whereby the patient was malabsorbing copper with low plasma copper (0.37 μmol/L; reference interval, 12 to 20 μmol/L), probably as a result of excess zinc intake (plasma zinc 34.4 μmol/L; reference interval, 10 to 18 μmol/L).[565]

Toxicity

As mentioned previously, Wilson's disease is a genetic disorder of copper metabolism that causes an increase in copper to toxic concentrations.[168,221] Problems of diagnosis and appropriate laboratory investigations have been reviewed.[175,209] It is suggested that ceruloplasmin oxidase activity and serum free copper concentration should be monitored in patients on long-term decoppering therapy to prevent iatrogenic copper deficiency.[121]

The incidence of Wilson's disease is estimated to be 1/30,000 live births with a carrier frequency of 1/90 in the general population. The presentation is highly variable, so adolescents or young adults with otherwise unexplained liver disease or neurologic symptoms should be screened, especially when a family history of suspected Wilson's disease is reported. Initial local investigations would include plasma copper and ceruloplasmin, which usually will be low (<50 μg/dL, 8 μmol Cu/L, and less than 200 mg/L ceruloplasmin). Although the total plasma copper is decreased, the non–ceruloplasmin-bound fraction is increased, allowing deposition of copper in the brain, eyes, and kidneys.

Slit-lamp eye examination may detect copper deposits in the eye (Kayser-Fleischer rings), and abnormalities in liver function tests may be noted with an increased urine copper output (>500 μg Cu/L). Liver biopsy for copper analysis is useful in suspected cases, and results above 250 μg/g Cu dry weight are usually found (normal, 8 to 40 μg Cu/g dry weight). Failure of copper incorporation into plasma ceruloplasmin can be demonstrated using an oral dose of stable ^{65}Cu isotope.[379] This may be helpful in excluding Wilson's disease when other tests are equivocal. Gene tracking and mutation detection are now possible, but because several hundred mutations exist, this may not be informative.

Diagnosis can be difficult in patients with Wilson's disease who present with acute liver failure.[545,605] Prompt diagnosis is important in that urgent liver transplantation may be required.[553] In these cases, greatly increased plasma copper will be found but without an appropriately increased ceruloplasmin. The unbound plasma copper fraction can increase to more than 80% of total plasma copper (normal, 5 to 10%). Excess copper is released from the necrotic liver and causes intravascular hemolysis and renal failure.[468]

The chronic form of Wilson's disease is treated by oral chelating agents, such as penicillamine and trientine, that remove excess copper from tissue and increase urine copper excretion.[670] Oral administration of zinc salts or ammonium molybdate, which blocks copper intestinal absorption, has been successful.[83] Treatment with ammonium tetra thio molybdate, however, has been shown to cause pituitary atrophy in animals treated for copper overload. This was thought to be a result of significant accumulation of total molybdenum in the pituitary, so care must be used in administration of this therapy.[253]

Toxicity can also arise directly from copper contamination of diet and water supplies. Acute poisoning has been recorded following accidental or intentional ingestion of copper sulfate. Guidelines for the maximum copper content of drinking water have been suggested and vary from about 1 to 3 mg Cu/L. Children may be genetically sensitive to copper in drinking water and may develop chronic liver disease,[440] as is found in Indian children exposed to a copper-contaminated diet.[619] Environmental aspects of copper toxicity and its impact upon human health have been reviewed.[163,185]

Laboratory Assessment of Status

Several well-controlled dietary deprivation studies have demonstrated the utility of the clinical laboratory in providing measures of copper status. For example, plasma copper and ceruloplasmin assays are convenient and widely used to confirm severe copper deficiency. However, they are not sensitive indicators in marginal copper depletion.[251]

Because about 90% of plasma copper is bound to ceruloplasmin, factors that increase the hepatic synthesis of ceruloplasmin, such as an acute-phase response or the oral contraceptive pill, will increase plasma copper independently of dietary copper intake.[216,569] In premature infants with liver immaturity and low ceruloplasmin synthesis, plasma copper values below 30 μg/L (<5 μmol Cu/L) suggest the necessity for increased copper input.

Dietary depletion studies using low-copper diets have demonstrated a decrease in plasma copper and then a return upon dietary supplementation; however, plasma copper values remained largely within the reference interval.[640] It is suggested that the ratio of immunologically to enzymatically measured ceruloplasmin may be a useful index of marginal copper depletion. This ratio, which is the specific activity of ceruloplasmin, will be low in marginal copper depletion. Apoceruloplasmin increases in blood serum during copper depletion; this will contribute to the total ceruloplasmin assay. The enzymatic activity decreases even in marginal copper depletion. The specific activity of ceruloplasmin is therefore sensitive to copper status and is not affected by age, sex, or hormonal influences.[423] In a study of copper depletion, a low-copper diet (0.57 mg/d) was fed to 12 postmenopausal women for 35 days, followed by supplementation for 35 days (2 mg/d).[424] Responsive markers were red cell SOD, platelet cytochrome oxidase, red cell glutathione peroxidase, and clotting factor VIII. Although of potential value for detecting marginal copper depletion, these measurements are not in widespread use because of sample instability and lack of standardized methods.[423] It has been suggested that interpretation of a copper value can be properly assessed only by an adjusted copper : ceruloplasmin ratio.[641]

Urine copper is decreased during dietary deprivation, but the change from an already low basal value is small, and difficulties in reliable collection and with sample contamination make this of limited use.

Clinically, copper status should be investigated initially by measurement of serum copper and assessment of the acute-phase reaction and should be interpreted in light of clinical and drug information.

Reference Intervals

For adults, plasma copper is usually in the interval 70 to 140 μg/dL (10 to 22 μmol/L). Values in women of childbearing age and especially in pregnancy are higher. For adults, a plasma copper below 50 μg/dL (8 μmo/L) and for infants below 30 μg/dL (5 μmol/L) indicates probable copper depletion. Adjusting the copper concentration to account for variations in ceruloplasmin is unfortunately problematic, as it depends on the accuracy of an immunoassay. It is not surprising therefore that problems have been encountered, with negative values for free copper being produced.[641]

The most reliable procedure consists of using plasma ultrafiltration when a reference interval of 0 to 10 μg/dL (0 to 1.6 μmol/L) has been reported in 137 healthy adult (20 to 59 years) blood donors.[405] Free copper concentrations for patients diagnosed with Wilson's disease were at least sixfold greater than the upper limit.

Urine copper output is normally less than 60 μg/24 h (<1.0 μmol/24 h), and values above 200 μg/24 h (3 μmol/L) are found in Wilson's disease. A copper concentration in a liver biopsy sample >250 μg Cu/g dry weight (normally 8 to 40 μg/g dry weight) is indicative of Wilson's disease, in the absence of other causes of cholestatic disease.

Urine copper output in response to an oral penicillamine test greater than 25 μmol/24 h is thought to be diagnostic of Wilson's disease (WD). However, a postpenicillamine Cu >25 μmol/24 h was observed in 29 of 38 patients with WD and in 4 of 60 controls, indicating that the test is valuable in the diagnosis of WD with active liver disease, but is unreliable in excluding the diagnosis in asymptomatic siblings.[439]

Manganese

Manganese is present in biological systems bound to protein in the 2^+ or 3^+ valence state. It is associated mainly with the formation of connective and bony tissue, with growth and reproductive functions, and with carbohydrate and lipid metabolism.

Chemistry

Mn (atomic number 25, atomic weight 54.94) is a first transition series metal ($3d^5s^2$) and is next to iron in the periodic table. Of 11 oxidation states available chemically to Mn, only Mn^{2+} and Mn^{3+} are found in biological systems, most often bound to protein. The Mn^{2+} ion with an unpaired electron is paramagnetic and can be detected in tissue by magnetic resonance imaging. The bioinorganic chemistry of manganese is complex, and detailed accounts have been published.[197,347]

Dietary Sources

Manganese-rich sources include whole grain foods, nuts, leafy vegetables, soy products, and teas. Average intake in the United States is about 2 mg/d, with median values for adult men of 2.2 mg/d (range, 0.3 to 8.3 mg/d), and for women of 1.8 mg/d (range, 0.3 to 5.9 mg/d) (NHANES III). Vegetarian diets containing large quantities of whole grains and nuts can supply more than 10 mg/d.[190]

Absorption, Transport, Metabolism, and Excretion

Dietary manganese is absorbed from the small intestine by mechanisms that may have a common pathway to that of iron. Manganese absorption is increased at low dietary intakes and is decreased at higher intakes, with tracer studies suggesting absorption efficiencies of 2 to 15%. Diets high in iron, calcium, magnesium, phosphates, fiber, phytic acid, oxalate, and tannins from tea can reduce the absorption of manganese.

Once absorbed manganese is transported in portal blood to the liver bound to albumin, it is exported to other tissues bound to transferrin and possibly to α_2-macroglobulin. Excretion of manganese occurs primarily via bile into feces, with urine output being very low and not sensitive to dietary intake.[347]

Functions

Manganese, which is a constituent of many important metalloenzymes, acts as a nonspecific enzyme activator. Mn^{2+} ions can be replaced by Mg^{2+}, Co^{2+}, and other cations during the activation of some enzymes.[347] Some important manganese-dependent enzymes are discussed in the following sections.

Superoxide Dismutase. Manganese-dependent SOD is a mitochondrial enzyme that is an important factor in limiting oxygen toxicity; it is one of the best studied enzymes in human biochemistry. The enzyme catalyzes the breakdown of the superoxide radical O_2^- to H_2O_2, which is then removed by catalase and glutathione peroxidase. The half-life of this enzyme in blood serum is longer than that of cytoplasmic Cu, Zn SOD.

Pyruvate Carboxylase. This enzyme has manganese firmly in its structure and acts in combination with phosphoenol pyruvate (PEP) carboxykinase, an enzyme that is activated by manganese ions. These enzymes are required to catalyze the formation of PEP, from pyruvate, a key reaction in the hepatic synthesis of glucose.

Arginase. Arginase is the terminal enzyme in the urea cycle, hydrolyzing L-arginine to urea and ornithine and completing the deamination of amino acids. Arginase is most concentrated in the liver, but is also found in other tissues. The structure of the enzyme isolated from rat liver shows that it has a unique binuclear manganese cluster.[315] The activity of arginase affects the production of nitric oxide by limiting the availability of L-arginine required for synthesis of nitric oxide synthetase. This relationship has been investigated in a number of diverse diseases, including asthma and schizophrenia.[414,696]

Glycosyl Transferases. These enzymes are responsible for the sequential addition of carbohydrate molecules to proteins to form proteoglycans, and ultimately connective tissue and cartilage. Therefore, they are important for the structural integrity of bone and skin, and for normal wound healing.

Requirements and Reference Nutrient Intakes

Because of lack of information on manganese dietary requirements, the U.S. Food and Nutrition Board has set an adequate intake amount for adults at 2.3 mg/d for males and 1.8 mg/d for females. A tolerable upper intake limit of 11 mg/d was set for adults based on no observed effect for Western diets. For infants, the UL could not be set because of lack of data. Concern has arisen about the potential toxicity of manganese for infants whose immature hepatic development reduces the biliary excretion of excess manganese. Therefore, the only dietary source of manganese in the age group (0 to 12 months) should be a normal diet or a formula.[190]

Deficiency

Overt manganese deficiency has not been documented in humans eating natural diets. However, in numerous animal studies, signs of experimentally induced manganese deficiency include impaired growth and reproductive function, skeletal abnormalities, impaired glucose tolerance, and impaired cholesterol synthesis.[347] A child on long-term TPN lacking manganese developed signs of bone demineralization and impaired growth that were reversed by supplementation.[460] A volunteer male was deprived of vitamin K and inadvertently of manganese when fed a diet with only 0.34 mg Mn/d for 6.5 months. Effects included a low plasma cholesterol, dermatitis, color changes in the hair, and reduced blood-clotting function not responsive to vitamin K. Supplementation with manganese gradually reversed these symptoms.[154] Seven young men fed experimental diets low in manganese developed skin lesions and low plasma cholesterol.[202]

Prolidase deficiency in infants is a rare genetic disorder that causes (1) skin ulceration, (2) mental retardation, (3) increased urinary excretion of iminodipeptides, (4) recurrent infections, and (5) splenomegaly; it is known to be associated with abnormalities of manganese biochemistry. Red cells have an increased amount of manganese, although serum manganese is normal. Red cell arginase activity is less than half of normal, suggesting a defect in the supply of manganese for enzyme activation.[368,371]

Various unrelated medical conditions have been observed to be associated with lowered serum or whole blood manganese. These include osteoporosis, diabetes mellitus, and epilepsy.[265] The clinical relevance of such observations is uncertain.

Toxicity

The occupational health hazard from prolonged exposure to manganese-containing dust or fumes is well recognized (see Chapter 36). Neurologic symptoms resembling Parkinson's disease develop slowly over a period of months or years. Health risks resulting from long-term, low-concentration manganese exposure have been reviewed.[226]

Of concern is the possibility that patients with severe liver disease may have neurologic and behavioral signs of manganese neurotoxicity resulting from failure to excrete manganese in bile. Manganese deposition in the globus pallidus during liver failure results in T_1-weighted magnetic resonance signal hypersensitivity. By causing deficits in neurotransmitter production, manganese ions may be partially responsible for symptoms of postsystemic hepatic encephalopathy.[254] Deposition of manganese in the brain has been demonstrated in children with biliary atresia[285] and in adult cirrhotic patients.[601]

Patients receiving manganese intravenously during TPN, especially those with cholestasis, have shown evidence of manganese retention and deposition in the midbrain and brain stem. Typical symptoms include a Parkinsonian-like tremor and abnormalities of gait.[160] Children have been observed to accumulate manganese in the globus pallidus and brain stem, but with nonspecific symptoms.[475] A study on adults compared the effects of increasing doses of manganese of 0, 1, 2, and 20 μmol/d in patients receiving home parenteral nutrition.[614] A high correlation was found between blood manganese, magnetic resonance imaging (MRI) intensity, and T_1 values in the globus pallidus. A dose of 1 μmol/d (55 μg/d) caused no abnormalities in MRI measurements, and blood manganese remained within the reference interval.

In a study of 30 patients receiving long-term home IV nutrition, whole blood manganese was increased (>11.6 μg/L, 210 nmol/L) in 26 patients, and plasma manganese (>4 μg/L,

23 nmol/L) in 23 patients. No patients had signs of neurologic disease. In a control group of patients with cholestatic disease but not receiving IVN, whole blood manganese was within the reference interval.[672] This suggests that cholestasis alone will not lead to increased blood manganese, and the main reason for high blood concentrations in patients on IV nutrition is excess provision; this is made worse if cholestasis also exists. Infants (0 to 12 months) requiring IVN are at particular risk because of immature hepatic function. In a group of 57 children receiving IVN,[170] 11 had both cholestasis and increased blood manganese, and 1 had a movement disorder. Four of these 11 patients died, and whole blood manganese was very high (34 to 101 μg/L, 615 to 1840 nmol/L) among the 7 survivors. Manganese supplements were reduced or withdrawn, and after 4 months, blood manganese had declined to 35 μg/L (643 nmol/L). During the same period, serum bilirubin declined significantly. The long-term outcome of manganese deposition has been investigated in two children on long-term TPN who initially had MRI scan abnormalities and raised whole blood manganese.[310] After reduction of manganese input, they were followed for a 3-year period with improvement in MRI scan abnormalities and a fall in whole blood manganese. No neurologic signs were found, and children developed normally. It is now recommended that only 1 μg Mn/kg (18 nmol/kg) should be administered during TPN in infants, and no more than 1 to 2 μmol/d (55 to 110 μg/d) in adults.

All patients requiring prolonged IVN, especially those who have cholestasis, should be monitored for evidence of manganese retention.

Laboratory Assessment of Status

It is necessary to balance the need for adequate manganese nutrition against potential risk from toxicity.[226] This necessitates monitoring of manganese status in at-risk patients. Whole blood manganese concentrations are not responsive to dietary depletion, but measurements of serum manganese, lymphocyte Mn SOD activity, and blood arginase are potentially useful when possible nutritional depletion is assessed, although these are rarely performed in clinical practice. Whole blood manganese and serum manganese in combination with brain MRI scans and neurologic assessment are used to detect excessive exposure. Manganese in whole blood and plasma or serum can be determined by standard graphite furnace AAS methods.[423,478]

Plastic cannulae should be used for phlebotomy, and hemolysis should be prevented during sample separation. Whole blood has about 10 times as much manganese as plasma or serum and is not as affected by contamination from steel needles during sample collection. This makes measurement of whole blood manganese the most widely used method in clinical laboratory practice for monitoring manganese status.

Whole blood values are used to indicate chronic exposure related to the red blood cell cycle, whereas plasma concentrations although lower will increase in response to acute exposure typical of changes post absorption/infusion.

Reference Intervals

The reference interval for serum manganese is 0.5 to 1.3 μg/L (9 to 24 nmol/L). The reference interval for whole blood manganese is 5 to 15 μg/L (90 to 270 nmol/L). Increases in serum manganese to >1.6 μg/L (>30 nmol/L) or in blood manganese to >20 μg/L (>360 nmol/L) are indices of manganese retention.

Molybdenum

The essential need for molybdenum by animals and humans is based on its incorporation into metalloenzymes.

In plants, Mo is part of the nitrogen fixation and nitrate assimilation process and therefore is fundamental to life. The functional chemical species is the molybdate ion, and its production in the environment is the rate-limiting factor.[276]

Chemistry

Molybdenum (atomic number 42, atomic weight 96.4) is a metal in the second transition series. The element can have a number of oxidation states, but the most stable in biological systems is Mo^{6+} as found in molybdate (MoO_4^{2-}). Molybdenum has the highest atomic number of the essential trace metals. A close parallel can be seen between molybdenum, tungsten, and vanadium chemistry. Molybdenum enzymes are ecologically vital, facilitating important carbon, nitrogen, and sulfur cycles.[197]

Dietary Sources

Legumes, such as peas, lentils, and beans, are good sources, along with grains and nuts, whereas meats, fruits, and many vegetables are relatively poor sources.[190] Average dietary intake for U.S. adults is 76 to 109 μg Mo/d.

Absorption, Transport, Metabolism, and Excretion

Molybdenum is efficiently absorbed over a wide range of dietary intakes, mainly as molybdate, although competitive inhibition of absorption by sulfate reduces intestinal uptake. Concentrations in whole blood are about 1.0 μg/L (10 nmol/L), and some 80 to 90% or more of molybdenum in whole blood is bound to red cell proteins. Transport of the smaller amount in blood plasma may involve α_2-macroglobulin.[190] Urine output directly reflects the dietary intake of molybdenum, with stable isotope studies at high and low concentrations of intake indicating renal homeostatic regulation.[639,678]

Functions

Several important mammalian enzymes, such as sulfite oxidase, xanthine dehydrogenase, and aldehyde oxidase, require molybdenum as a cofactor.[409] This organic component is a molybdopterin complex.[328] Sulfite oxidase is probably the most important enzyme in relation to human health. This enzyme catalyzes the last step in the degradation of sulfur amino acids, oxidizing sulfite to sulfate and transferring electrons to cytochrome c. Xanthine dehydrogenase and aldehyde oxidase hydroxylate numerous heterocyclic substances, such as purines, pteridines, and others.[304]

Requirements and Reference Nutrient Intakes

The RDA for Mo has been set at 45 μg Mo/d for adults, which is below the estimated average dietary intake.[190]

Deficiency

Molybdenum deficiency has not been observed in healthy people consuming a normal diet. A single case report[3] described a patient receiving prolonged parenteral nutrition during treatment for severe Crohn's disease who developed an intolerance to intravenous amino acids, especially L-methionine. Clinical signs included tachycardia, visual defects, neurologic irritability, and eventually coma. Symptoms improved on discontinuation of amino acid infusion. Biochemical abnormalities included high plasma methionine and low plasma uric acid concentrations. Increased urinary sulfite and thiosulfate and other abnormalities of urinary sulfur output were reported, with low excretion of uric acid and xanthine metabolites, suggesting defects in sulfite oxidase and xanthine oxidase. Treatment with ammonium molybdate (300 μg/d) improved the clinical and biochemical abnormalities.

Lack of additional reports of this nature suggests that for most patients, sufficient molybdenum is present as a contaminant in TPN fluids. Nonetheless, it is now common to include a small amount of molybdenum (19 μg/d, 0.2 μmol/d) in trace element additive mixtures.

Very rare recessive inherited diseases result from defects in the biosynthesis of molybdenum cofactor; in most cases, they lead to early childhood death. First symptoms include failure to thrive and seizures; in later stages, lens dislocations are noted, together with cerebral atrophy. Disease-causing mutations have been located, and the possibility of gene therapy is being investigated.[515,516]

Biochemical diagnosis has been made by detection of excess sulfite in urine using the Merckoquant Sulfite Dipstick test (Merck KGaA, Darmstadt, Germany). Samples should not be evaluated until at least 10 days after birth and should be tested within 10 minutes of collection. Another type of molybdenum cofactor deficiency can be confirmed by finding a low plasma uric acid. Specialized centers offer biochemical prenatal diagnosis on chorionic villous samples.[328]

Toxicity

Molybdenum compounds have low toxicity in humans. Reports have described increased blood uric acid in those with occupational exposure and in Armenian populations that have an abnormally high dietary intake (10 to 15 mg Mo/d). A single report of acute toxicity from self-administration of 300 to 800 μg Mo/d was not confirmed by later studies on healthy men given as much as 1500 μg Mo/d for 24 days.[265]

Excess molybdenum intake induces copper deficiency in ruminants by blockading copper absorption through formation of an insoluble thiomolybdate-copper complex. This has suggested the use of ammonium molybdate in the management of Wilson's disease.[83] Speculation suggests that blockade of copper absorption using molybdate may influence new blood vessel formation (angiogenesis) during tumor growth.[82]

Laboratory Assessment of Status

Whole blood and serum or plasma molybdenum concentrations are too low to be used for the detection of deficiency. However, urinary output is responsive to increases or decreases in input. Measuring urate or sulfite in the urine is the most available means of confirming molybdenum cofactor disorder or possible molybdenum deficiency by detecting changes in sulfur and purine metabolism. Until recently, only neutron activation analysis (NAA) had sufficient sensitivity to measure molybdenum in biological samples.[661] With the availability of ICP-MS, studies using stable molybdenum isotopes are now possible; this technique has been used to investigate absorption and excretion of molybdenum during depletion and repletion studies.[639]

Reference Intervals

About 0.5 μg Mo/L (5 nmol/L) is present in plasma or serum, along with about 1 μg Mo/L (10 nmol/L) in whole blood.[661] Urine molybdenum values determined by ICP-MS vary from 40 to 60 μg/L, with the amount determined influenced by recent dietary intake.[291]

Selenium

Selenium (Se) is a constituent of the enzyme glutathione peroxidase that is considered an essential element for humans; it is believed to be closely associated with vitamin E in its functions.

Chemistry

Selenium (atomic number 34, atomic weight 78.96) is a nonmetal that has several chemical forms and valences. Selenium is in group VI of the periodic table; therefore it has a bioinorganic chemistry that is related to sulfur.[197,610] The most important biologically active compounds contain selenocysteine, where selenium is substituted for sulfur in cysteine. Now considered to be the twenty-first amino acid, selenocysteine is incorporated into proteins by the specific codon UGA, which was previously thought to be solely a stop codon.[252] Selenomethionine is synthesized by plants but not in animals or humans. Because it is biologically identical to methionine, sharing the same metabolic pathways, selenomethionine is nonspecifically incorporated into the general protein pool and is present in major proteins such as albumin and hemoglobin. Selenium in selenomethionine makes up about half of the total dietary intake and is made available for selenocysteine synthesis when the methionine pathways catabolize selenomethionine. Ingested selenium compounds, selenate, selenite, selenocysteine, and selenomethionine, are metabolized largely via selenide that may be associated with a chaperone protein before being converted to selenophosphate, which is an important precursor in the synthesis of selenocysteine proteins (Figure 31-27).[610]

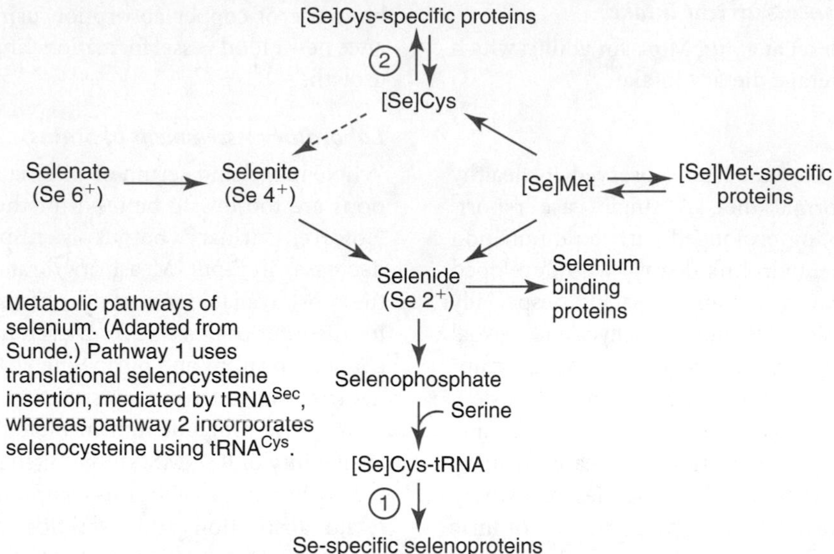

Figure 31-27 Metabolic pathways of selenium.

Dietary Sources

Selenium enters the food chain mainly as selenomethionine from plants that take the element up from the soil but do not appear to use it. The soil content of selenium is highly variable and can be low in volcanic soils when soluble salts are leached out by ground water. Soils in parts of China and New Zealand are particularly low in selenium. Acid soils, where insoluble selenium complexes can be formed with iron and aluminium, occur in some parts of Europe, resulting in low available soil selenium. The geographic source of plant and animal food-stuffs determines the amount of dietary intake. In the United States and Canada, wheat and other cereal products are a good source of selenium; average intakes in North America range from 80 to 220 μg Se/d, whereas in the United Kingdom, dietary intake is about 30 to 60 μg/d.[32] Intakes in China are as low as 11 μg/d and in New Zealand 28 μg/d.[92]

Absorption, Transport, Metabolism, and Excretion

Intestinal absorption of various dietary forms of selenium is efficient but is not regulated. The inorganic salts selenite and selenate used as dietary supplements and in food fortification are almost completely absorbed, but much of the selenate ion is rapidly excreted in urine.[196] Selenium from inorganic salts is more rapidly incorporated into glutathione peroxidase and other selenoproteins than selenium from organic sources containing selenomethionine. However, selenium-enriched yeast containing the organic forms is considered less toxic and is widely used as a dietary supplement.[188]

Contradictory data[94] have indicated that increased selenium concentration correlated with the amount of selenomethionine administered but not the selenite, and neither glutathione peroxidase activity nor selenoprotein P concentration responded to selenium supplementation. Also, plasma selenium seems to reflect the selenomethionine, and selenium in the form of selenomethionine was much better absorbed than selenite. This would suggest that a yeast complex is the better supplement.

This study also suggested a revision of safe upper amounts of selenium intake as greater than 800 μg selenium/d for at least 16 weeks with no toxic signs.

Whole body selenium is about 15 mg, as estimated by direct tissue analysis and radioisotope techniques, with the tissue concentration of selenium being highest in the kidney and the liver, followed by the other organs. Radioisotope-labeled selenium accumulates initially in the liver, kidneys, and lungs. Selenium present in some selenocysteine proteins appears to be a functional reserve. When dietary selenium is limited, synthesis of glutathione peroxidase (GSHP)x-1 is downregulated, making selenium available for synthesis of other proteins.[188]

The concentrations of selenium in whole blood and in plasma and/or serum are related to dietary intake. About 50 to 60% of total plasma selenium is present as the protein selenoprotein P, a highly basic protein having multiple histidine residues and about 10 atoms of selenium per molecule.[610] Around 30% of plasma selenium is present as glutathione peroxidase (GSHPx-3); the remainder is incorporated into albumin as selenomethionine.[249]

Urinary output of selenium is the major route of excretion and reflects recent dietary intake. The amounts excreted vary widely, ranging from less than 20 μg Se/L to more than 1000 μg Se/L, depending on the geographic origins of the food.[6]

Functions

More than 30 biologically active selenocysteine-containing proteins have been identified; more than 15 have been purified and their biological function investigated.[88,610] Some of the most important ones are listed in the next sections.

Glutathione Peroxidase (GSHPx). This enzyme has four isoforms: GSHPx-1 in red cells, GSHPx-2 in gastrointestinal mucosa, blood plasma GSHPx-3, and GSHPx-4 located in the cell membrane. These enzymes use the reducing power of glutathione to remove an oxygen atom from hydrogen peroxide and lipid hydroperoxides. They may also be involved in regulation and formation of arachidonic metabolites derived from hydroperoxides.[20]

Iodothyronine Deiodinase. Type I, II, and III isoforms of this enzyme are responsible for conversion of the precursor hormone T_4 to the active hormone T_3.[88,333] Type I, thyroxine-5-deiodinase, is located in the liver, kidney, and muscle and is responsible for more than 90% of plasma T_3 production. Pituitary, brain, and brown adipose tissue contain the Type II and III deiodinases.[610]

Thioredoxin Reductases. Three isoforms catalyze the NADPH-dependent reduction of thioredoxin and are important in maintaining the intracellular redox state.

Selenophosphate Synthetase. This enzyme is required for the intracellular synthesis of selenoproteins via a monoselenium phosphate intermediate.

Selenoprotein P. This protein is the major selenium-containing protein in blood plasma; it may be a transport protein for the element, and it has an antioxidant function.[93]

Selenoprotein W. This selenoprotein is found in skeletal muscle that is reduced in concentration in white muscle disease in animals.[610] Deficiencies in the production of these selenoproteins, especially the glutathione peroxidases, are likely to be related to signs and symptoms of selenium deficiency disease.

Requirements and Reference Nutrient Intakes

It is now proposed that the RDA for selenium should be set at 55 μg/d for adults.[188] On this basis, dietary surveys in North America do not indicate that selenium deficiency is likely in the general population. However, in many countries in Europe, intakes are now close to or below 55 μg/d, and selenium dietary provision may now be suboptimal.[511]

Intravenous Supply

Uncertainty continues about the most appropriate intake, but given the previous figures for dietary requirement, intravenous requirement is unlikely to be less than 40 μg/d (0.5 μmol/d), and in many adult patients, especially the more seriously ill, it may be 100 μg/d (1.3 μmol/d) or more.

Deficiency

The role of selenium in human medicine has been reviewed.[92,333,511] Animal studies in the 1950s demonstrated the nutritionally beneficial effects of selenium by showing that there was a selenium-responsive liver necrosis in vitamin E–deficient rats. Important selenium-dependent diseases are seen in farm animals, such as white muscle disease in sheep and cattle, and myopathy of cardiac and skeletal muscle in lambs and calves. In these animals, some cause of oxidative stress, such as increased physical activity or vitamin E deficiency—together with dietary selenium deficiency—is required to elicit the disease.

Severe Deficiency. Symptomatic selenium deficiency has been well characterized in Keshan disease, and nutritional depletion in hospital patients.

Keshan Disease. Conclusive evidence of a role for selenium in human nutrition came with publication of the results of large-scale trials in China that show the protective effects of selenium supplementation on children and young adults suffering from an endemic cardiomyopathy. This was observed in areas of the country (Keshan region) with low soil selenium concentrations.[610]

Kashin-Beck Disease. A type of severe arthritis is described in parts of China and neighboring areas of Russia where soil selenium is particularly low. However, trials of selenium supplementation were not conclusive, and other unidentified factors may be present.

Nutritional Depletion in Hospital Patients. Selenium was one of the last essential trace elements to be accepted as nutritionally important, with more attention given to its potential toxicity. Initially, inadequate selenium provision in specialized diets was used to treat inborn errors[650] and during long-term parenteral nutrition,[654] leading to cases of deficiency. Symptomatic cases continue to be reported, although the need for selenium supplementation during nutritional support is well established. Symptoms of severe deficiency include muscle weakness.[322] Cases involving cardiomyopathy, which is usually fatal and resembles Keshan disease,[701] and macrocytosis and pseudoalbinism in children[666] have been described.

Marginal Deficiencies. Marginal selenium deficiencies are thought to be involved in thyroid function, immune function, reproductive disorders, mood, inflammatory conditions, cardiovascular disease, viral virulence, and cancer chemoprevention.

Thyroid Function. Selenium and other trace elements are necessary for normal thyroid function because the important deiodinase enzymes are selenoproteins.[21,333] Three children with biochemical and clinical signs of hypothyroidism were successfully treated with oral selenium therapy.[491] Although the deiodinases are not thought to be significantly affected in marginal selenium depletion, it has been observed that endemic goiter in Sri Lanka, which is resistant to iodine supplementation, occurs in areas with low soil selenium.[193] Similarly, endemic thyroid disease in Zaire may be related to the combination of iodine and selenium depletion. Care must be taken because the stimulation of thyroid hormone metabolism may induce hypothyroidism.

The low T_3 syndrome observed after major trauma may also be related to changes in selenium status affecting the activity of iodothyronine deiodinase, with selenium supplements reversing most of the biochemical abnormalities found in thyroid function tests.[49]

The exact role of selenium in thyroid function, however, continues to be controversial. A study of a New Zealand population with both marginal selenium status and mild iodine deficiency showed that additional selenium improved GPx activity but not the thyroid hormone status of older New Zealanders.[631] Also, no significant treatment effects were found for TSH, free T_3, free T_4, or the ratio of T_3 to T_4. It was concluded that no synergistic action of selenium and iodine occurs. A study in the United Kingdom had reached a similar conclusion—that selenium supplementation had no effect on thyroid status.[512]

Immune Function. Deficiency of selenium is accompanied by loss of immunocompetence, and this is related to the reduction of selenoproteins in the liver, spleen, and lymph nodes. Both cell-mediated immunity and B-cell function are impaired.

Considerable selenium losses in wound exudates following severe burns have been recorded, and supplementation with a mixture of selenium, zinc, and copper leads to a reduction in respiratory infection.[50] Supplementation, even in apparently selenium-adequate individuals, has some immune function stimulatory effects, including improvement in natural killer cell activity and increases in interleukin (IL)-2 receptor expression.[511] It has been speculated that the increased infection rates in patients with acquired immunodeficiency syndrome (AIDS) may be related to selenium depletion, and this may even influence the progression from HIV positivity to the AIDS syndrome.[36]

It has been suggested that antioxidant nutrient deficiencies may hasten the progression of HIV disease by impairing antioxidant defenses; it was shown that well-nourished subjects are able to mount a compensatory antioxidant response to HIV infection.[607] However, the role of selenium in particular was equivocal in that among HIV-infected women from Dar es Salaam, Tanzania, selenium supplements given during and after pregnancy did not improve HIV disease progression or pregnancy outcomes.[341]

Reproductive Disorders. Adequate selenium supply is necessary for successful reproduction in a variety of farm animals. Various studies have looked at the situation in humans. Male fertility could be affected by selenium depletion in so far as it is necessary for testosterone synthesis and for maintenance of sperm viability.[511]

Mood. The brain is reported to receive a priority supply of selenium during dietary depletion and/or repletion studies in animals, and the turnover of neurotransmitters is altered. This has led to extensive studies on the role of selenium and other antioxidants in senility of the elderly, in epilepsy in children, and in Alzheimer's disease. Marginal selenium depletion has been associated with anxiety, confusion, and hostility, and improvements have been claimed following supplementation.[511]

Inflammatory Conditions. Many conditions associated with inflammation and increased oxidative stress could be influenced by selenium status. Positive effects from supplementation studies in arthritis and in pancreatitis have been reported. Low serum selenium values are found in asthma, and some limited clinical trial studies show benefits from supplementation.[511] In a trial in patients in intensive care with SIRS, high-dose selenium supplements over 9 days were associated with reduced mortality in the most severely ill.[18] However, these results have not been confirmed in all studies[427]; hence definitive recommendations regarding high-dose supplements in intensive care cannot yet be made.[17]

Cardiovascular Disease. The protective role of selenium against cardiovascular disease has been extensively investigated, but with no conclusive findings.[165,511] The low soil selenium concentration in Finland resulted in low selenium content in locally grown food. This, together with concerns about the high incidence of coronary disease in parts of the country, led to selenium fortification of agricultural fertilizers. Although an impressive decline in coronary disease mortality was found between 1972 and 1992, the benefits were linked primarily to other major diet and life-style changes.[489]

Viral Virulence. It is now considered possible that an unusually virulent strain of the Coxsackie virus is part of the cause of cardiomyopathy in selenium-depleted regions of China. This is consistent with marked seasonal variations in the incidence of the disease.

It is known that nutritional depletion will impair immune responses and will increase the lethalness of viruses and other infectious agents. A series of experimental studies on mice have shown that a nonlethal form of Coxsackie B (CVB 3/O) converted to a virulent strain when inoculated into selenium-deficient mice.[43] Inoculation of selenium-adequate mice with the mutated virus then caused myocarditis. Sequencing of DNA from the altered virus showed that six nucleotide changes corresponded to nucleotide sequences in the genome of a virulent strain of the virus. Further evidence came from experiments with GSPHx knockout mice. More than half of these mice infected with the nonlethal CVB/3O virus developed myocarditis, but none of the wild-type controls were affected. The virus recovered from these affected mice showed genome changes similar to those seen in virulent strains of the virus. It is thought that the selenium-deficient host altered the viral pathogen, probably involving oxidative stress in the tissue of depleted animals. Additional animal studies[42] have demonstrated that a mild strain of influenza virus exhibits increased virulence when given to selenium-deficient mice. New viruses continue to appear through the evolution of existing viruses, and these may be lethal strains. RNA viruses are known to mutate easily and lack proofreading systems and repair mechanisms.[41,355,451]

It is speculated that a similar process occurs in regions of the world, such as parts of Africa, where the human population has depletions of selenium and other micronutrients and is intermittently exposed to viral disease. As yet, no direct evidence indicates that similar processes occur in human populations. However, an epidemic of optic and peripheral neuropathy in Cuba that affected more than 50,000 individuals was shown to be associated with deficiencies of several micronutrients, including selenium. Supplementation of the population with a multicomponent micronutrient mixture coincided with subsidence of the disease.[41]

Cancer Chemoprevention. Although it is not primarily a nutritional issue, interest in the role of selenium supplementation in the prevention of certain types of cancer continues. Experimental work on animals shows that chemical carcinogenesis is modified by selenium. Also, epidemiologic surveys have found a link between cancer incidence and soil selenium content, suggesting a higher incidence of certain cancers in individuals with a low selenium intake.[132] Large-scale trials in

China, conducted on more than 130,000 individuals, compared one township (20,847 people) at high risk for viral hepatitis B and liver cancer with four control townships in the same area. The high-risk population received selenium-enriched table salt, and in an 8-year follow-up, the average incidence of liver cancer was reduced by 35%. No reduction in incidence was seen in control populations. Studies on 226 people with chronic hepatitis B found that a controlled trial of selenium-enriched yeast reduced the development of liver cancer during a 2-year follow-up period.[700]

For some years, it was hoped that selenium supplementation above the minimum dietary requirement may have a role in cancer prevention, particularly in relation to prostatic cancer.[125] This was based essentially on secondary analyses of two randomized controlled trials,[131,132] and supportive epidemiologic and preclinical data indicated the potential of selenium and vitamin E for preventing prostate cancer and other cancers (e.g., lung, colorectal). The mechanism was not established, but in selenium-adequate subjects, it was suggested that excess selenium may produce a low molecular weight methylated selenium compound that has chemopreventive properties.[131,132] However, the large selenium and vitamin E cancer prevention study known as the Selenium and Vitamin E Cancer Prevention Trial (SELECT)[329] has reported and concluded that selenium or vitamin E, alone or in combination at the doses and formulations used, did not prevent prostate cancer in this population of relatively healthy men.[362]

Toxicity

Areas of China and the United States have large amounts of selenium in the soil, and locally produced food contains excess selenium. Clinical signs of selenosis include garlic odor in the breath, hair loss, and nail damage.[188] The tolerable upper limit has been set at 400 μg/d for adults and less for children. Cases of toxicity from self-administered dosages have been reported. Because of a manufacturing error, 13 individuals taking supplements containing 27.3 mg (27,300 μg)/tablet showed clinically significant selenium toxicity.[265]

Symptoms of selenium toxicity vary among individuals and are dependent on a number of factors such as dose, type, and form of selenium ingested and length of time the product was used. Symptoms of selenium poisoning can include significant hair loss, muscle cramps, nausea, vomiting, diarrhea, joint pain, fatigue, fingernail changes, and blistering skin. Patients have reported that symptoms typically occur within 5 to 10 days after daily ingestion of these supplements begins. After use of the product is discontinued, symptoms of selenium toxicity may last for several weeks, but they should improve eventually without treatment for the poisoning. Nail changes are the most common sign of chronic selenium poisoning.[463] The nails become brittle, and white spots and longitudinal streaks appear on the surface. Fragile nails and similar changes obviously are not specific for selenosis; other causes include fungal infection, psoriasis, and arsenic exposure. As yet, no proven antidote for selenium poisoning is known.

Laboratory Assessment of Status

Early animal studies and human population surveys used whole blood as the main indicator of selenium status. Whole blood selenium can be determined after acid digestion using a fluorometric method.[250] The more convenient carbon furnace atomic absorption spectroscopy (CFAAS) assay for plasma and/or serum selenium is now the most widely used procedure,[213] although ICP-MS, without the need for dynamic cell reaction to remove polyatomic interference from argon mass 80, is probably the preferred procedure in routine laboratories.[592]

The main components of plasma selenium are extracellular glutathione peroxidase (GSHPx-3) and selenoprotein P. Red cell GSPHx-1 and plasma GSPHx-3 are assayed by enzymatic methods using a variety of peroxide substrates,[610] with tertiary-butyl peroxide being a commonly used substrate, because it is not as affected by catalase as is hydrogen peroxide.[56] The values obtained are dependent on the substrate used and the reaction conditions. During selenium supplementation studies, the plateau reached in plasma GSPHx-3 activity has been used to assess minimum dietary requirements.[188]

The effects of different forms of inorganic and organic selenium supplementation on GSPHx activity in blood lymphocytes, granulocytes, platelets, and erythrocytes have been described in a trial on 45 human volunteers.[89] Some changes were acute and transient, whereas cytosolic GSHPx activity (GSHPx-1) increased gradually in both treatment groups over 28 days.

In patients receiving TPN at home, the time course for development of deficiency and repletion of enzyme activity has been studied.[128] After 1 year on TPN without selenium supplements, all patients had low plasma selenium and red cell GSHPx, and cellular metabolism of exogenous hydrogen peroxide was impaired. With replacement of selenium as selenious acid, a rapid increase in GSHPx-3 was seen within the first 24 hours, and normal concentrations were reached within 1 to 2 weeks. Platelet GSHPx also returned to normal in 1 to 2 weeks, whereas polymorph GSHPx was more variable but normalized in about 3 weeks. Red cell GSHPx took 3 to 4 months to recover, consistent with the need for formation of these cells in the presence of selenium.

The major selenium-containing plasma protein selenoprotein P can be determined by immunologic methods.[5] The production of monoclonal antibodies to selenoprotein P has been described[544] and used to study the structure and function of the protein and to quantify it. It is also possible to separate selenoprotein P from other plasma proteins by heparin affinity chromatography followed by CFAAS selenium analysis.[249] Selenoprotein P concentration in plasma responds rapidly to supplementation and has been used in nutritional studies of Chinese populations to confirm the adequacy of intake.[267]

Plasma selenoprotein P, plasma GSPHx-3, and total plasma selenium concentration are all lowered by the acute-phase response to injury or infection.[454] This effect should be considered when plasma selenium values are interpreted in postoperative patients or those with infection or inflammatory disease. Hair and nail selenium analysis can be useful as a measure of long-term dietary selenium intake. Because selenium is a sulfur analog, it is incorporated into the sulfur-rich keratin of hair and nails. One study showed a correlation between toenail selenium, blood selenium, and dietary intake.[369] In a study of a 10-year-old child receiving TPN who developed selenium-responsive muscle weakness, hair analysis was used to help assess selenium dosage.[627] An analytical method using microwave-assisted acid digestion of hair and nails, followed by CFAAS selenium analysis, has been described.[248] In a small study using this procedure, values for hair and nail selenium in healthy U.K. people were found to be 0.32 to 0.76 μg/g (n = 25) and 0.17 to 0.66 μg/g (n = 27), respectively. However, for population studies, use of selenium-containing hair preparations will affect hair selenium results; this would have to be carefully assessed and controlled.

Urine selenium output is mainly a reflection of recent dietary input and has not been extensively employed in population surveys.

In summary, many possible markers for selenium status have been identified. In practice, measurement of plasma selenium or GSHPx provides a good estimate of status and in particular, the adequacy of recent intake, provided values are interpreted with knowledge of changes in the acute-phase response. For a better index of long-term intake, platelet, red cell, or neutrophil GSHPx or hair or nail selenium can also be measured. The value of various biological parameters in assessing selenium status has been systematically reviewed; these parameters were shown to change in response to selenium treatment, although no single parameter was regarded as optimal.[22]

Reference Intervals

The reference interval for selenium in whole blood, plasma or serum, hair, and nails should be established locally, because these indices are affected by dietary selenium intake. Plasma selenium adult values lie in the interval 63 to 160 μg/L (0.8 to 2.0 μmol/L). Values less than 40 μg Se/L (0.5 μmol/L) indicate probable selenium depletion.

Values in children are lower and in the United Kingdom are as follows: 16 μg/L to 71 μg/L (0.2 to 0.9 μmol/L) for those younger than 2 years old; 40 μg/L to 103 μg/L (0.5 to 1.3 μmol/L) for 2- to 4-year-olds; and 55 μg/L to 134 μg/L (0.7 to 1.7 μmol/L) for 4- to 16-year-olds.[628] Cutoff values of less than 8 μg/L (0.1 μmol/L) in neonates are strongly suggestive of selenium depletion. Increased plasma values are found in suspected selenium toxicity, and results above 5 μmol/L (400 μg/L) are an indication of excess intake.

In cases of toxicity (selenosis), serum concentrations were as high as 1400 μg/L with no obvious effects, and acute fatal poisonings were seen with selenium at up to 30,000 μg/L.[463] However, the nature of the selenium compound is important, as most reports that describe acute selenium poisoning involve ingestion of inorganic compounds such as selenious acid, which is found in gun-bluing agents, and fatalities that occur within the first day are associated with postmortem blood selenium concentrations greater than 1400 μg/L.

In an earlier study of patients with selenosis from eating vegetables containing grossly elevated selenium contents, blood concentrations were 1300 to 7500 μg/L; normal concentrations were 95 μg/L and suggested selenium deficiency concentrations at 27 μg/L.[695]

Red cell glutathione peroxidase activity (GSHPx-1) in adults varies from 13 to 25 U/g Hb, whereas values in children are slightly lower.[628] Local age-related reference intervals are again required.

Zinc

The discovery of a variety of zinc (Zn)-related clinical disorders has directly demonstrated the importance of zinc in human nutrition. It is second to iron as the most abundant trace element in the body.

Chemistry

Zn (atomic number 30, atomic weight 65.37) lies at the end of the first transition series. Zn^{2+} with a filled 3d electron shell is a particularly stable ion. The bioinorganic chemical features of zinc, which underlie the very diverse biological functions of this trace metal, include its relatively high abundance compared with other trace elements. Zinc has fast ligand exchange kinetics and flexible coordination geometry, and it is a good electron acceptor (strong Lewis acid) with no redox reactions. It has been hypothesized that zinc ions, present in the cytoplasm at 10^{-11} moles and in equilibrium with numerous zinc metalloenzymes and transcription factors, can act as a "master hormone," particularly in relation to cell division and growth.[197] No naturally colored zinc complexes have been identified; this may have delayed recognition of the biological importance of zinc until suitable atomic spectroscopic methods were developed that could be applied to biological samples and used as probes to identify and study metalloproteins.[109]

Dietary Sources

Zinc is widely distributed in food mainly bound to proteins. The bioavailability of dietary zinc is dependent on the digestion of these proteins to release zinc and allow it to bind to peptides, amino acids, phosphate, and other ligands within the intestinal tract. The most available dietary sources of zinc are red meat and fish, whereas white meat and flesh from young animals provide less zinc. Wheat germ and whole bran are good sources, but their zinc content is reduced by milling and food processing. The median intake for men in the United States is about 14 mg/d and for women 9 mg/d.[190]

The intake distribution from various foods showed that intake was potentially poor in the older than 60 years age group because of a diet deficient in legumes and meat.

Absorption, Transport, Metabolism, and Excretion

The net intestinal uptake of zinc is regulated by control of absorption efficiency in the face of variable dietary zinc input and varies from 20 to 50% of the dietary content. At an intake of 12.2 mg Zn/d, fractional absorption was 26%, but at the very low intake of 0.23 mg Zn/d, this increased to 100%. These and other measurements were made on 12 male volunteers using stable ^{67}Zn tracer to assess zinc homeostasis and plasma zinc kinetics.[326] Estimates of zinc absorption have also been compared using four different stable isotope techniques.[374] It was concluded that a double isotopic tracer ratio method is accurate and is recommended as a practicable procedure. When this method was used, the fraction of dietary zinc absorbed was equivalent to 30% ± 10%. Fine control of net absorption is attained by secretion of endogenous zinc into the intestinal lumen from pancreatic fluid and other intestinal fluids.[325] Such losses range from less than 1 mg/d on a low-zinc diet to more than 5 mg/d on a zinc-rich diet. The ability to conserve dietary zinc by limiting intestinal loss can allow a positive metabolic balance, even at low dietary zinc intakes. Interaction with other dietary constituents, such as phytate, calcium, and iron, reduces the net absorption of zinc significantly, so that diets high in phytate and calcium reduce the growth rate of young rats. In essence, the greater the intake, the greater the overall excretions, but with increasing overall retention.[327]

New insights into mammalian zinc metabolism have been acquired through the identification and characterization of zinc transporters. These proteins all have transmembrane domains and are encoded by two solute-linked carrier (SLC) gene families: *ZnT (SLC30)* and *Zip (SLC39)*. At least 9 ZnT and 15 Zip transporters are present in human cells. They appear to have opposite roles in cellular zinc homeostasis. ZnT transporters reduce intracellular zinc availability by promoting zinc efflux from cells or into intracellular vesicles; Zip transporters increase intracellular zinc availability by promoting extracellular zinc uptake and, perhaps, vesicular zinc release into the cytoplasm.

Both ZnT and Zip transporter families exhibit unique tissue-specific expression, differential responsiveness to dietary zinc deficiency and excess, and differential responsiveness to physiologic stimuli via hormones and cytokines.[363]

A study of patients who had previously undergone ileostomy confirmed regulated expression of plasma membrane zinc transporters in the human intestine and suggested that regulated control of zinc uptake is dependent on body status.[138] In human diets, leavening of bread and exposure of cereals to wet heat lower the phytate content, thus increasing zinc availability. Other factors, such as dietary fiber and a constituent of beans, also lower zinc intestinal absorption but to a lesser extent.[119] Iron at supplemental dosages (up to 65 mg/d) may decrease zinc absorption, so that pregnant and lactating women taking iron may require zinc supplementation.[465] The effects of zinc and iron on their relative intestinal absorption have been reviewed.[336]

Absorbed zinc is transported to the liver by the portal circulation, where active incorporation into metalloenzymes and plasma proteins, such as albumin and α_2-macroglobulin, occurs. Blood plasma contains less than 1% of the total body content of zinc and lies within a narrow concentration interval (80 to 120 μg/dL, 12 to 18 μmol/L). About 80% of plasma zinc is associated with albumin, and most of the rest is tightly bound in the high molecular protein α_2-macroglobulin.[191] The zinc on albumin is in equilibrium with plasma amino acids (mostly histidine and cysteine), and this small (<1%) ultrafilterable fraction may be important in cellular uptake mechanisms (Figure 31-28).[119]

The total adult body content of zinc is about 2 to 2.5 g, and the metal is present in the cells of all metabolically active tissues and organs. About 55% of the total is found in muscle, and approximately 30% in bone.[119] The prostate, semen, and the retina have particularly high local concentrations of zinc. Almost all zinc in a red cell is present in the form of carbonic anhydrase, so that red cell zinc concentration is about 10 times higher than in plasma. Hemolysates normally have about 50 μg Zn/g Hb, and total leukocyte zinc is normally about 100 ± 25 μg/10^{10} cells.

Fecal excretion includes both unabsorbed dietary zinc and zinc resecreted into the gut. The total amount normally equals the total dietary intake and is on the order of 10 to 15 mg/d in healthy populations. In contrast, urine output of zinc is normally only about 0.5 mg/d, but this can increase markedly during catabolic illness. The release of intracellular contents from skeletal muscle has been established as the source of excess urinary zinc in the postoperative period, using a labeled zinc radiotracer. Two patients took an oral dose of 5 μ Ci radioactive ^{65}Zn about a month before elective surgery for total hip replacement, allowing incorporation of the tracer into skeletal muscle. Urine output of radioactive zinc, total zinc, and total nitrogen was measured before operation and daily for 3 weeks after surgery. A large increase in the excretion of all of these was observed, with peaks occurring at 10 days. Good correlation was noted between radioactive zinc and total zinc in the urine of both patients, suggesting skeletal muscle as the source.[169] Urine zinc also increases more than threefold during short-term total starvation, as a result of release from skeletal muscle and excretion of ketone bodies.[162]

Dietary intakes of zinc are lower in the elderly because of reduced energy requirements; it is not clear whether aging influences adaptive homeostatic mechanisms, or how aging affects the function, expression, or gene regulatory responses to zinc of zinc transporters.[165] However, in a study of aged mice, zinc supplementation reversed some age-related thymic defects, indicating that this may be of considerable benefit in improving immune function and overall health in elderly populations.[688] Further, advancing age, particularly very old age, is associated with an increase in the percentage of cells with short telomeres, resulting in cells that have a tendency toward premature apoptosis. These observations have been related to impaired production of zinc metallothionein and possibly zinc deficiency, and therefore are of significance as prognostic factors in age-related disease.[124]

Functions

General. More than 300 zinc metalloenzymes occur in all six categories of enzyme systems. Important examples in

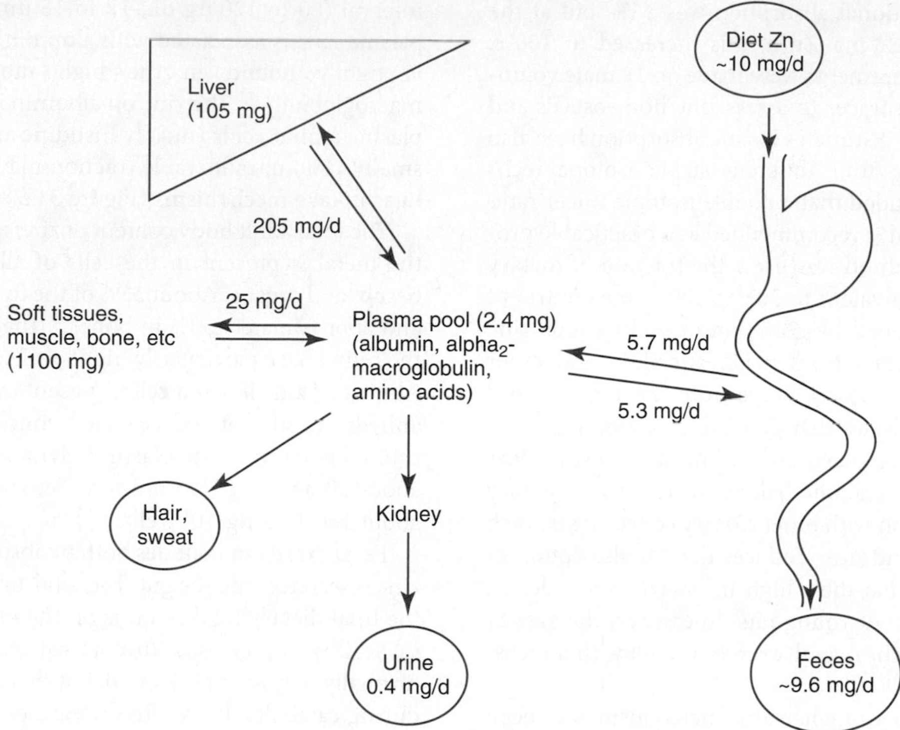

Figure 31-28 Summary of zinc metabolism.

human tissue include (1) carbonic anhydrase, (2) alkaline phosphatase, (3) RNA and DNA polymerases, (4) thymidine kinase carboxypeptidases, and (5) alcohol dehydrogenase.[396] The key roles of zinc in protein and nucleic acid synthesis explain the failure of growth and impaired wound healing observed in individuals with zinc deficiency. In some enzymes, such as Cu and Zn superoxide dismutase, structural stability is ensured by zinc protein binding and the catalytic activity of the enzyme by the active copper site. Classifications of zinc enzymes and their structure and mode of action have been detailed in various texts.[119,197] Proteins can form domains able to bind tetrahedral zinc atoms by coordination with histidine and cysteine to form folded structures that have become known as "zinc fingers." These biologically active molecules have important roles in gene expression by acting as DNA-binding transcription factors; they play a key role in developmental biology and in the regulation of steroid, thyroid, and other hormone synthesis.[166,646] Zinc binding to the metal response factor MTF1 activates metallothionein (MT) expression. This multifunctional, low molecular weight protein (9000 to 10,000 Da) has a high content of cysteine and reversibly binds zinc. MT is important in intracellular zinc trafficking and helps to maintain intracellular zinc concentrations. Hepatic synthesis of MT is induced by interleukin-1, interleukin-6, and glucocorticoids in response to infection, trauma, and other stressors.[119,559]

Prostate Function. Secretion by the prostate of large amounts of zinc (resultant concentration, 1 to 2 mmol/L) is key to the function of sperm, maintaining both vitality and an antibacterial environment.[689] The mechanism of this aspect of zinc function is regulation of motility through interaction of Zn^{2+} ions with semenogelin (Sg1) during semen coagulum formation at ejaculation, as well as during liquefaction of the coagulum in the female reproductive tract.[698] However, the determination of zinc in seminal plasma did not discriminate on the basis of actual sperm fertility. Nevertheless, other studies[129] have implicated seminal Zn with parameters of semen quality, in that decreased seminal Zn can be a risk factor for sperm abnormality and idiopathic male infertility, and smokers in particular are susceptible to Zn deficiency in their seminal fluid. These data suggest that poor Zn nutrition may be an important risk factor for low quality of sperm and idiopathic male infertility. Routine determination of Zn concentrations during infertility investigation therefore is recommended.

Seminal plasma zinc concentrations are virtually normal in chronic prostatitis and adenoma, whereas with prostatic neoplasm, a highly significant decrease (100-fold) in zinc secretion has been noted.[702] Prostate cancer cells do not secrete zinc because of a reduced capacity for accumulation of intracellular zinc caused by the decrease in ZIP1 protein expression and the intracellular redistribution of intracellular transporter ZIP3.[277] These neoplastic cells are extremely sensitive to the Zn^{2+} ion; direct tumor injection causes marked cell death and therefore may represent a possible chemo prevention therapy.[571]

Requirements and Reference Nutrient Intakes

In the United States, the dietary reference intake (DRI) for zinc is 11 mg/d for men and 8 mg/d for women. Infants and young children need smaller amounts. Increased amounts are required during pregnancy and lactation. Strict vegetarians may need as much as 50% more zinc per day because of increased phytic acid and fiber in their diet.[190]

Intravenous Supply

Stable adult patients require 2.5 to 4.0 mg/d (40 to 60 μmol/d), but in those who are depleted or who have increased gastrointestinal losses, the requirement is about 6 mg/d (100 μmol/d).

Clinical Deficiency

As might be expected from the multiple biochemical functions of zinc, the clinical presentation of deficiency disease is varied, nonspecific, and related to the degree and duration of depletion.[496] Signs and symptoms include depressed growth with stunting; increased incidence of infection, possibly related to alterations in immune function; diarrhea; altered cognition; defects in carbohydrate use; reproductive teratogenesis; skin lesions; alopecia; eyesight defects; and other adverse clinical outcomes.

Effects on Growth. It has been claimed that dietary zinc deficiency is prevalent in countries worldwide where a cereal-based diet high in phytate and fiber but low in animal protein is common.[498] This condition could affect as many as 2 billion people and may be a major public health issue, comparable with recognized deficiencies of iron and iodine. In children, reduced growth and other developmental abnormalities are reversible by zinc supplementation. A meta-analysis of some 37 intervention trials shows that zinc supplementation has a significant effect on linear growth and weight regain.[87] Studies have also shown that lean tissue retention and protein synthesis are increased if zinc is added to therapeutic regimens used in famine relief, especially when soya-based formulations with a high phytate content were used as a protein source.[219]

It is known that the zinc in human breast milk is efficiently absorbed because of the presence of factors such as picolinate and citrate. However, the total quantity of zinc in breast milk is related to maternal nutritional status, and a physiologic decline in the zinc content of "mature milk" is noted after about 6 months' lactation. Although cases of symptomatic zinc deficiency have been reported in breast-fed infants,[288] the need for zinc supplementation for women in low-income countries during pregnancy is controversial. Reduction of neonatal morbidity and incidence of infection has been reported in some studies, but the large-scale introduction of zinc supplementation for pregnant women requires more controlled trials.[477]

Acrodermatitis Enteropathica. Acrodermatitis enteropathica (AE) is characterized by periorificial and acral dermatitis, alopecia, and diarrhea. Patients with this disorder have abnormally low blood zinc concentrations (<30 μg/dL); symptoms are reversed by oral zinc supplementation, with this being diagnostic. This formerly fatal condition is an autosomal recessive inborn error affecting zinc absorption from the intestinal mucosa. The gene defect involves ZIP4, a zinc transporter that plays an important role in zinc homeostasis.[16]

Parenteral Nutrition. When clinical techniques were developed for TPN in the 1960s and 1970s, early sources of amino acids were based on whole protein hydrolysates that had zinc and other trace elements present as contaminants. When these were replaced by mixtures of synthetic amino acids in the 1980s, this necessitated the addition of trace element additives. Some patients requiring intravenous feeding after surgery are likely to be significantly zinc depleted because of poor oral intake before and after surgery. They also may have increased zinc losses from the intestinal tract via diarrhea and in urine from catabolism of muscle during periods of negative nitrogen balance. Diarrhea, mental depression, dermatitis, delayed wound healing, and alopecia are seen during the anabolic period of weight regain when zinc is insufficient in the nutritional regimen to support tissue repair.[320] Provision of adequate zinc intravenously to achieve a positive zinc balance is associated with improvement in nitrogen balance.[687] Routine provision of 100 μmol/d (6.5 mg) in the PN regimen is normally adequate in stable patients,[587] but increased amounts of zinc and other micronutrients are required in the most severely injured patients.[585]

Infectious Disease. Zinc depletion impairs immunity[496] and has a direct effect on the gastrointestinal tract[608]; this increases the severity of enteric infections. A placebo-controlled trial of zinc supplementation (10 to 20 mg/d) of 1240 children aged 6 to 30 months was conducted in North India. A substantial reduction in the incidence of severe and prolonged diarrhea was reported in the treated group.[57] A review of controlled trials of zinc supplementation of children in low-income countries found significant clinical benefits.[65] Six of nine trials claimed improvement in cases of persistent diarrhea; in five trials in respiratory disease, a lower rate of infection was described. Some caution is required with the doses of zinc employed. In a study of severely malnourished children, those treated with doses of 3 to 6 mg Zn/kg had significantly increased mortality compared with those given 1.0 to1.5 mg Zn/kg.[153] Interaction with vitamin A is important; in populations at risk of zinc and vitamin A deficiency, provision of zinc alone increased the incidence of respiratory infection, but when vitamin A was added, respiratory infections were decreased.[509]

Other Conditions. Other groups of individuals are considered to be at risk from a marginal dietary deficiency or from an acquired deficiency secondary to disease. These groups would include female adolescents during pregnancy and lactation. Also affected may be patients with malabsorption syndrome, inflammatory bowel disease, alcoholic liver disease, and anorexia nervosa.[325] A significant proportion of cases of sickle cell anemia have clinical signs and symptoms, along with some laboratory abnormalities of zinc deficiency. These patients respond well to zinc supplementation.[497]

Subclinical Effects of Deficiency

When zinc deficiency is not severe enough to cause clinical signs and symptoms, it still may have a subclinical affect on immune function, the synthesis and action of hormones, and neurologic function.

Immune Function. Patients with zinc deficiency in the Middle East were known to die before the age of 25 because of various infections and parasitic disease. In zinc deficiency, a reduction in the activity of serum thymulin, the thymus-specific hormone involved in T-cell function, and an imbalance between Th1 and Th2 helper cells are noted. The lytic activity of natural killer cells also decreases. Moreover, zinc is necessary for intracellular binding of tyrosine kinase to the T-cell receptors CD4 and CD8, which are required for T-lymphocyte activation. These complex changes result in impairment of cell-mediated immunity and may serve as the basis for increased infection rates seen in marginal zinc depletion.[496]

Lowering of plasma zinc in the acute-phase response associated with inflammatory conditions is thought related to increased intake into tissue. For example, in the liver, this occurs by upregulation of the zinc transporter Zip-4. Thus zinc deficiency is frequently observed during autoimmune disease, indicating that modulating zinc homeostasis could be a promising approach by which to counteract inflammation and autoimmunity.[523]

It has been suggested that zinc supplements may be beneficial in reducing the severity or duration of the common cold. Studies have been inconsistent, putative benefits small, and, given the doses of zinc used, a high incidence of side effects was encountered.[388]

Hormones. Zinc is thought to have a role in the synthesis and actions of many hormones via zinc transcription factors. Zinc depletion is associated with low circulating concentrations of testosterone, free T_4, insulin-like growth factor (IGF)-1, and thymulin.[496] Both plasma IGF-1 and growth velocity are increased in zinc-supplemented children.[459] Production of testosterone has been shown to be improved in patients given zinc supplements when initial plasma concentrations indicated zinc deficiency.[499] Hence zinc may play an important role in modulating serum testosterone concentrations in normal men.

Neurologic Effects. Severe zinc deficiency is known to affect mental well-being, with varying degrees of confusion and depression consistent with zinc enzymes having important activity in brain development and function. The history of zinc in relation to the brain and possible relevance to human disease have been reviewed.[548]

Zinc has been shown to be a neurosecretory product or cofactor and is highly concentrated in the synaptic vesicles of a specific contingent of neurons, called "zinc-containing" neurons.[198] Zinc in the vesicles probably exceeds 1 mmol/L in concentration and is only weakly coordinated with any endogenous ligand. Zinc-containing neurons are found almost exclusively in the forebrain, where in mammals they have evolved into a complex and elaborate associational network that interconnects most of the cerebral cortices and limbic structures. Alterations in zinc homeostasis may be associated with brain dysfunction, including brain inflammatory status.[429] Zinc ion dyshomeostasis may also play a role in the aging neuron through deterioration of synapses.[54]

Toxicity

Clinical effects of ingestion of a zinc-contaminated diet include abdominal pain, diarrhea, nausea, and vomiting (see Chapter 36). Single doses of 225 to 450 mg of Zn can induce vomiting, with milder forms of gastrointestinal upset reported at 50 to 150 mg Zn/d (dosages that were initially used in therapy). More than 60 mg Zn/d can result in copper depletion by causing intestinal blockade of intestinal absorption. The U.S. Nutrition Board has set the tolerable upper amount of intake for adults at 40 mg/d.[190]

It is also important to know that Zn^{2+} ions themselves may be toxic, as shown from cell culture experiments with neurones[324] indicating the importance of the compartmentation of zinc within cells. Apparent lack of toxicity in vivo may be related to cellular protection afforded by extra production of the zinc-complexing protein metallothionein.[480]

Laboratory Assessment of Status

Although plasma zinc determination is insensitive to dietary zinc intake and is subject to a variety of influences, it remains the most widely used laboratory test to confirm severe deficiency and to monitor adequacy of zinc provision, especially when interpreted together with changes in serum albumin and the acute-phase response. No practicable laboratory procedures have been established for clearly identifying populations with marginal zinc depletion. Clinical and biochemical responses to zinc supplementation therefore are used to postulate a marginally zinc-depleted state. Thus, in contrast to iron, for which a number of indicators of metabolism/function are available, an effective measure to assess the functional zinc status of humans has remained elusive. Nevertheless various factors have been used, such as metallothionein (MT), zinc transporter proteins, and cytokine gene expression (as transcript abundance), in which zinc supplementation of human subjects indicated enhanced production.[23]

A systematic review confirmed that among healthy individuals, plasma and urinary and hair zinc are reliable biomarkers of zinc status in suitable samples.[373]

Plasma Zinc. Plasma samples are preferred to serum for zinc analysis because of possible zinc contamination from erythrocytes, platelets, and leukocytes during clotting and centrifugation. Plasma zinc concentrations are most commonly measured by FAAS, although spectrophotometric methods are available.

A study using stable zinc isotope tracers during experimental induction of acute zinc depletion (0.23 mg Zn/d) found that the plasma zinc concentration took 5 weeks to decline to 65% of baseline values, and that the observed fall was caused by a reduction in zinc release from the slowest zinc pool.[326] Care has to be taken in controlling numerous preanalytical factors that will lower plasma zinc independently of dietary intake. These include collection of sample in relation to meals, time of day, and use of steroid-based medications, such as the contraceptive pill. Any cause of hypoalbuminemia will also lower plasma zinc. Plasma albumin is a negative acute-phase reactant that is redistributed into interstitial space from the plasma pool during infection, after trauma, and in chronic disease. The induction of hepatic MT synthesis during the acute-phase response and subsequent sequestering of zinc further lower the plasma concentration.[582] It is therefore essential to consider plasma zinc results along with plasma albumin and plasma CRP or another marker of the acute-phase response.

Knowledge of bioavailable zinc is of fundamental importance. Five cases of hyperzincemia (between 5 and 10 times the upper limit of normal) were recorded in patients with apparent zinc deficiency, indicating extremely low bioavailable free zinc.[546] Presentation signs included recurrent infections, hepatosplenomegaly, arthritis, anemia, and persistently raised CRP. A binding protein that effectively sequestered functional zinc was identified as calprotectin, and the observations were subsequently explained as a new disease entity of dysregulation of calprotectin.

Blood Cell Zinc. Some investigators have suggested that the zinc content of white cells and platelets better reflects tissue zinc.[630,671] The zinc content of neutrophils, lymphocytes, and platelets has been shown to decline more rapidly than plasma zinc in experimental studies of zinc depletion in humans.[496] However, the relatively large volume of blood required and problems with contamination make large-scale application to patients in hospital or to population surveys difficult, especially in studies involving children. Erythrocyte zinc has been suggested as an alternative; however, in a study of low-income black women (n = 580) stratified by total daily zinc intake during pregnancy, no changes in erythrocyte zinc were found, although plasma zinc increased with intake.[448]

Zinc in Hair. Low hair zinc has been associated with poor growth in children, and has been used as a criterion for initiating supplementation studies.[190] However, variables such as hair growth rate and external contamination from hair dyes and cosmetics can cause inconsistent results. Results from individual patients are difficult to interpret.

Zinc-Dependent Enzymes. Despite the large number of zinc metalloenzymes that have been identified, no single enzyme assay has yet found acceptance as an indicator of zinc status. This may be a result of avid retention of zinc by these enzymes, even in the face of dietary zinc depletion, and of difficulties with reproducible measurements of activity. However, bone-specific alkaline phosphatase, extracellular SOD, and lymphocyte and plasma 5-nucleotidase appear to be responsive to zinc intake.[690]

Metallothionein. Determination of metallothionein in red cells and MT mRNA in circulating monocytes is considered of probable value because metallothionein falls in zinc deficiency. However, clinical use of these measurements has not yet been confirmed by large-scale investigations of depleted populations.[690]

Urine Zinc. A slight fall in the urine excretion of zinc has been noted during dietary deficiency. Difficulties of sample contamination during collection make this of limited practical value. However, increased urine zinc is an important source of loss in the severely injured catabolic patient, although measurement is rarely required except in research studies. Urine output increases with amino acid infusion given during TPN.

Zinc Speciation

Relatively few studies have explored the actual chemical species present in physiologic fluids. However, studies on wound fluids regarded as an important site of zinc wound healing have revealed complex interactions.[306] Most Zn ions were present as charged species, and the major species was a citrate complex.

Reference Intervals

Serum zinc concentrations are generally 5 to 15% higher than those of plasma because of osmotic fluid shifts from the blood cells when various anticoagulants are used. Plasma zinc concentrations exhibit both circadian and postprandial fluctuations. Concentrations are decreased after food and are higher in the morning than in the evening.

A reference interval for clinical guidance is 80 to 120 μg/dL (12 to 18 μmol/L).

Fasting morning values of plasma zinc below 70 μg/dL (10.7 μmol/L) on more than one occasion require further investigation. Results below 30 μg/dL (5 μmol/L) suggest likely deficiency. Urine zinc excretion lies in the range from 0.2 to 1.3 mg/24 h (3 to 21 μmol/24 h).

Other Possibly Essential Elements

More than 15 additional trace elements are considered by some investigators to have a potentially important role in human medicine. A review by Nielsen considers these in detail and discusses emerging concepts of "essentiality."[419] The clinical laboratory will consider some, such as lead, cadmium, arsenic, aluminium, and nickel, primarily as toxic elements (see Chapter 36). Others, such as lithium and fluoride, are classified as pharmacologically beneficial, and monitoring of dosage may be required. Some elements can be considered "nutritionally beneficial" and are reported to produce "restorative health effects" at lower dosages. Evidence is derived mainly from animal studies, when dietary depletion of the element is combined with other metabolic, hormonal, or physiologic "stressors."

For a few elements (boron, silicon, and vanadium), circumstantial evidence is considered strong, although no agreed biochemical mechanism has been established. The 2006 DRI report[190] discusses the nutritional aspects of arsenic, boron, nickel, silicon, and vanadium. For boron, silicon, and vanadium, it was noted that measurable responses in humans have been observed during variations in the dietary intake of these elements. These and other elements have been promoted by the supplement industry, and the clinical chemist may be asked for advice and possibly for monitoring of dosage in cases of suspected toxicity. AAS, ICP-OES, and ICP-MS methods can be applied to the determination of most of these elements in biological samples.[423]

Contamination of TPN solutions by small amounts of metals, such as Al, Pb, Cd and Ni, could also be a problem, as could the lack of others, such as Si, B, and V, when very long-term nutritional support is required.

Fluoride

Fluoride (Fl) is the most widely used of the "pharmacologically beneficial trace elements" in the area of public health. Dental caries has been described as the last major epidemic of preventable bacterial disease, and dental decay leads to tooth loss, nutritional problems, and systemic infection.[110]

Dietary Sources

Many studies over the past 50 years have established that addition of fluoride to drinking water reduces the incidence of tooth decay; more than 60% of the U.S. population now uses fluoridated water. Clinical studies from 1950 to 1980 in 20 different countries found that adding fluoride to community water supplies, within the interval 0.7 mg/L to 1.2 mg/L, reduced the incidence of caries by 40 to 50% in primary (infant) teeth and by 50 to 60% in permanent teeth.[146] The subject is controversial, and "mass medication" with fluoride has been opposed. Reviews of the benefits and risks associated with the use of fluoride are available.[111,265]

Fluoride supplementation of salt, sugar, and milk has been used in areas where fluoride is not added to water supplies.

Function

The fluoride ion can be exchanged for hydroxyl in the crystal structure of apatite, a main component of skeletal bone and teeth. This stabilizes the regenerating tooth surface. Fluoride is available from saliva and may be released from dental plaque at low pH.[111] Initially, benefit was considered to involve solely the erupting teeth of children, but topical effects on adult teeth are now thought to reduce decay. Initial evidence from small studies suggests that pharmacologic doses of fluoride may reduce the incidence of bone fracture in patients with osteoporosis. However, a meta-analysis of fluoride therapy from 11 controlled studies on 1429 subjects found that although this increased lumbar bone density, the incidence of vertebral fracture was not significantly decreased.[265] Another study showed that sodium fluoride was more effective than etidronate at increasing lumbar bone mass, but no differences were observed in the incidence of fracture. The problem with fluoride is the potential for excess, and monitoring was thought essential; a higher incidence of side effects, mainly gastrointestinal symptoms and lower extremity pain syndrome, was observed in the fluoride group.[232]

Absorption, Transport, Metabolism, and Excretion[112]

Fluoride ions are absorbed from both the stomach and the small intestine. Soluble salts are efficiently absorbed, and a peak increase of fluoride occurs in blood plasma within 1 hour of ingestion. Ions are rapidly cleared from plasma into tissue in exchange with anions, such as hydroxyl, citrate, and carbonate. At least 95% of the 2.6 g of total body fluoride is located in bones and teeth. Almost 90% of excess fluoride is excreted in urine.

Toxicity

Dental fluorosis, the mottling of enamel in the erupting teeth of children, is now estimated to affect around 20% of the population. This can be a disfiguring condition, and it occurs in a greater proportion of children than initially expected.[673] This is possibly due to ingestion of fluoride-containing toothpaste by children. It is suggested that "pediatric" toothpastes with lower fluoride content should be made available in areas where fluoridation of the water supply exists.[111]

Occupational exposure to inhaled fluoride dusts among cryolite workers during aluminium refining has resulted in severe bone abnormalities, but safety equipment now limits such exposure. No cases of skeletal fluorosis are attributed to the use of controlled fluoridation of water supplies.[112] However, skeletal fluorosis may occur in areas of the world where naturally occurring drinking water has high concentrations of fluoride, such as China and the Indian subcontinent. It is thought that exposure to fluoride intakes of 10 to 25 mg/d for 10 years or longer may result in skeletal fluorosis, but other nutritional factors may make these populations more susceptible.[265]

Numerous diverse adverse effects have been attributed to water fluoridation. Investigators have found no convincing evidence of increased rates of cancer, heart disease, kidney disease, liver disease, presenile dementia, birth defects, or Down syndrome.[265]

Laboratory Assessment of Status

Laboratory analysis of drinking water may be required to assess possible fluoride excess in natural well waters, and may also be necessary during incidents of failure of the equipment used to treat drinking water. Determination of fluoride in urine can be used to assess exposure to different sources of fluoride.[323] For drinking water and urine, direct determination using a fluoride-specific electrode is employed. For food, feces, and tissue, prior separation of fluoride from the sample matrix is required, using a Conway diffusion procedure.[112] The combination of the fluoride electrode with flow injection has allowed the use of a rapid and sensitive method for serum and urine fluoride analysis.[289]

Reference Intervals

Concentrations of fluoride in body fluids and tissue vary widely, depending on the fluoride content of drinking water and input from diet, toothpaste, and mouth rinses. For urine, a guideline interval is 0.2 mg/L to 3.2 mg/L (10.5 to 168 μmol/L).

Boron

Boron (B) has not been officially designated as essential to human health, although it is considered an essential macronutrient for plants.

Function

Boron normally present in living organisms as the borate ion (BO_3^{3-}) does have essential properties in plants that affect cell wall integrity.[470] However, it still is not known to have any specific physiologic function in humans, although various studies have suggested that it may be a bioactive beneficial element.[456] Responses to dietary deprivation of boron have been described with alterations in calcium metabolism, brain function, and energy production.[455] Responses from low dietary boron intake (0.25 mg/2000 kcal) for 63 days and the effects of supplementation with 3.0 mg/d have included increases in 25-hydroxycholecalciferol, decreases in calcitonin, decreased serum glucose, and increased serum triglycerides, among other biochemical changes.[455] Some of these effects were more evident when dietary copper was marginal and magnesium inadequate. Further research is needed to clarify the role of boron in human and animal physiology and to establish a dietary requirement.[150]

Dietary Sources

It is thought that the acceptable safe range of boron intake is from 1 to 13 mg/d, and evidence suggests that some people are consuming less than 1 mg/d. Plant foods, especially fruits, leafy vegetables, nuts, and legumes are good sources; whereas meat, fish, and dairy products are not.[455] Average daily intakes of dietary boron in the United Kingdom are variable (2.8 ∀ 1.5 mg), and intakes are higher than in the United States (1.5 ∀ 0.4 mg).

Absorption, Transport, Metabolism, and Excretion

Dietary boron is efficiently absorbed as boric acid, $B(OH)_3$, and is efficiently excreted into urine, with about 85 to 100% of an oral dose of borate appearing in urine over a 5- to 7-day period. The oral toxicity of boron is relatively low; it has been estimated that safe population mean intakes are <13 mg/d, and that individuals are at risk of toxicity when intakes continually exceed 100 mg/d for up to 6 days. The richest food sources of boron are nuts and dried fruits (15 to 30 mg/kg) and wine (8.5 mg/L). The use of boric acid food additives is now prohibited, except for caviar at 4000 mg/kg. Thus a toxic intake of boron could be provided by 200 g nuts plus 20 g caviar, or by 25 g low-fat crisps plus 12 L of wine.

Laboratory Assessment of Status

Problems with contamination and loss of volatile boron compounds during sample preparation have limited the reliable documentation of boron concentrations in human tissue and body fluids.[155] A complex technique involving a porous graphite column—inductively coupled plasma–atomic emission spectrophotometry (ICP-AES)—and an ICP time-of-flight mass spectrometer (TOF-MS) has been developed for investigation of boron neutron capture in cancer therapy.[612] Adaptation of this method to nutritional studies of boron should be possible.

Normal concentrations in plasma of less than 30 μg/L were established by ICP-AES,[617] the recommended procedure for assay because of the low atomic mass (10) of boron. Excretion in urine is normally less than 1 mg/d and up to 5 mg/L with boron intake of 0.33 to 3.33 mg/d.[38]

Silicon

Silicon (Si) is a nonmetallic element that has an atomic weight of 28; it is a member of group IV C, Si, Ge, etc. Similar to elements in this group, it forms tetrahedral types of complexes and a multitude of polymer types. Silica is used to refer to the naturally occurring materials composed principally of silicon dioxide. The term *silicone* refers to any of a large group of siloxane polymers that do not occur naturally and are based on the structure of alternating oxygen and silicon (…-Si-O-Si-O-Si-O-…), with organic side groups attached to the four-coordinate silicon atoms. In some cases, organic side groups can be used to link two or more of these -Si-O- backbones together. By varying -Si-O- chain lengths, side groups, and cross-linking, silicones can be synthesized with a wide variety of properties and compositions. These compounds have a variety of uses from parchment coatings to sealant and breast implants. Silicon is widely distributed in nature and is the second most abundant element, accounting for approximately 28% of the earth's crust. Silicon is always found in nature as the oxide silica or as a silicate and plays an important role in cell structural organization.

Dietary Sources

Soluble silica (orthosilicic acid) is ubiquitous in the diet (20 to 50 mg Si/d) and in natural waters (0.8 to 44 mg Si/L),[603] and, unlike crystalline silica (quartz), it has no associated toxicity. Silicon is widely distributed in plants and is an essential element for structural integrity. Amorphous silica is incorporated as an anticaking agent at concentrations up to 2% in a variety of foods. Beer can also be rich in silicon with up to 20 mg/L content. No values have been suggested for the recommended intake of silicon.

Absorption, Transport, Metabolism, and Excretion

The absorption of silicon seems to be dependent on its polymeric nature; the smaller the molecule (i.e., monomeric orthosilicic acid), the more effective is absorption, whereas the larger polymer forms are poorly absorbed.[603] Passive nonfacilitated transport appears to occur and is probably based on size-related simple diffusion. The efficiency of absorption is up to 60% of an ingested load, with most excreted renally within 24 hours of exposure. As yet, little evidence suggests retention in any tissue-specific site.

Functions and Clinical Significance

In veterinary and laboratory animals, silicon has been shown to be important in the synthesis of collagen and bone. The few supplementation studies in humans have indicated associated increases in trabecular bone volume and bone mineral density.[308] Silica deprivation experiments in the 1970s in growing chicks and rats suggested that silica is essential for normal growth and development, although this remains to be confirmed. Birchall suggested that soluble silica is essential for living organisms, because it binds endogenous aluminum and thereby prevents its toxicity,[62] although this remains unproven. Nielsen has reviewed the case for silicon in intravenous nutrition.[457]

Laboratory Assessment of Status

Normal fasting plasma concentrations of silicon are less than 12 μmol/L.[101] These are raised in renal failure, particularly in patients on hemodialysis, up to above 150 μmol/L and can be higher, depending on the content of dialysis water.[482] Urine silicon excretion depends on intake and varies from 100 to 1000 μmol/24 h. Toxicity from silicon has never been reported, although increased concentrations (>3 mmol/L) have resulted in the formation of silica stones.[283]

Vanadium

Vanadium, a group V trace element that belongs to the first transition series of elements, is ubiquitously distributed. It can exist in four valency states—2, 3, 4, and 5; thus, its chemistry is complex. Vanadium occurs in neutral solutions as metavanadate (VO_3^-), the predominant species in body fluids, and enters cells by an anion transport system. Exogeneously administered vanadyl sulfate and ammonium vanadate have been found to bind serum transferrin tightly, indicating that this protein may serve as a vanadium transporter. Although the vanadium requirement of fewer organisms has been established, its essential value in humans remains to be proven.[201]

Although most foods contain low concentrations of vanadium (<1 ng/g), food is the major source of exposure to vanadium for the general population; however, absorption of vanadium salts from the gastrointestinal tract is poor. Excretion of vanadium by the kidneys is rapid, with a biological half-life of 20 to 40 hours. Estimated daily intake of the U.S. population ranges from 10 to 60 μg. Vanadyl sulfate is a supplement that is commonly used to enhance weight training in athletes at doses up to 60 mg/d. In general, the toxicity of vanadium compounds is low. Most of the toxic effects of vanadium compounds result from local irritation of the eyes and upper respiratory tract, rather than from systemic toxicity.

Functional Aspects

Vanadium plays a limited role in biology. Nevertheless a vanadium-containing nitrogenase is used by some nitrogen-fixing microorganisms. Clinical interest in the vanadate compounds involves their potential role in the treatment of diabetes. Various studies have suggested that these compounds reduce the requirement for insulin by activating the cellular response without the presence of insulin, in effect mimicking its action.[407] Different oxidation states for vanadate (V^{5+}) and vanadyl (V^{4+}; i.e., vanadyl sulfate) mimic the rapid responses of insulin through alternative signaling pathways not involving insulin receptor activation. The insulin-like effects of vanadium may be initiated by inhibiting phosphotyrosine phosphatases (PTPases) and stimulating protein tyrosine kinase activity, implying that cells (adipose cells in particular) contain distinct vanadyl V^{4+}(V^{4+})-sensitive and vanadate V^{5+}(V^{5+})-sensitive PTPases. However, in a study population (n = 16) with type 2 diabetes, no dose relationship was noted between the drug administered and glucose regulation after administration of vanadyl sulfate.[220]

Amounts given in such trials are much greater than the suggested normal intake, suggesting that vanadium compounds are more likely to work as alternative therapies, rather than indicating the essential function of the element. The possibility of using vanadium compounds is focused on cytotoxicity and cancer treatment.

Assessment of Laboratory Status

Plasma and urine concentrations are usually measured by GF-AAS or ICP-AES. Use of ICP-MS revealed a number of urinary vanadium compounds in healthy volunteers (n = 95) of 1 to 10 μg/L.[223] Detection of the vanadate ion using size exclusion chromatography coupled with ICP-MS with a dynamic reaction cell yielded normal serum concentrations of less than 0.05 μg/L.[120] Studies with high-resolution ICP-MS also showed whole blood concentrations less than 0.05 μg/L (i.e., near detection limits), indicating that careful sampling techniques are required for confident use of analysed concentrations.

REFERENCES

1. Abraham AS, Brooks BA, Eylath U. Chromium and cholesterol-induced atherosclerosis in rabbits. Ann Nutr Metab 1991;35:203-7.
2. Abraham AS, Brooks BA, Eylath U. The effects of chromium supplementation on serum glucose and lipids in patients with and without non-insulin-dependent diabetes. Metabolism 1992;41:768-71.
3. Abumrad NN, Schneider AJ, Steel D, Rogers LS. Amino acid intolerance during prolonged total parenteral nutrition reversed by molybdate therapy. Am J Clin Nutr 1981;34:2551-9.
4. Adams JF, Tankel HI, MacEwan F. Estimation of the total body vitamin B12 in the live subject. Clin Sci 1970;39:107-13.
5. Akesson B, Bellew T, Burk RF. Purification of selenoprotein P from human plasma. Biochim Biophys Acta 1994;1204:243-9.
6. Alaejos MS, Romero CD. Urinary selenium concentrations. Clin Chem 1993;39:2040-52.
7. Allen RH. Megaloblastic anemias. In: Goldman L, Bennett JC, eds. Cecil textbook of medicine. Philadelphia: WB Saunders, 2000:859-67.
8. Alvarez HM, Xue Y, Robinson CD, Canalizo-Hernandez MA, Marvin RG, Kelly RA, et al. Tetrathiomolybdate inhibits copper trafficking proteins through metal cluster formation. Science 2010;327:331-4.
9. American Medical Association Department of Foods and Nutrition. Multivitamin preparations for parenteral use: a statement by the Nutrition Advisory Group. J Parenter Enteral Nutr 1979;3:258-62.
10. American Medical Association Department of Foods and Nutrition. Working conference on parenteral trace elements. Bull N Y Acad Med 1984;60:1115-212.
11. Anderson RA. Chromium and parenteral nutrition. Nutrition 1995; 11:83-6.
12. Anderson RA. Chromium in the prevention and control of diabetes. Diabetes Metab 2000;26:22-7.
13. Anderson RA, Cheng N, Bryden NA, Polansky MM, Cheng N, Chi J, et al. Elevated intakes of supplemental chromium improve glucose and insulin variables in individuals with type 2 diabetes. Diabetes 1997;46:1786-91.
14. Anderson RA, Kozlovsky AS. Chromium intake, absorption and excretion of subjects consuming self-selected diets. Am J Clin Nutr 1985;41:1177-83.

15. Anderson RA, Polansky MM, Bryden NA, Roginski EE, Patterson KY, Reamer DC. Effect of exercise (running) on serum glucose, insulin, glucagon, and chromium excretion. Diabetes 1982;31:212-6.
16. Andrews GK. Regulation and function of Zip4, the acrodermatitis enteropathica gene. Biochem Soc Trans 2008;36:1242-6.
17. Andrews PJ. Selenium and glutamine supplements: where are we heading? A critical care perspective. Curr Opin Clin Nutr Metab Care 2010;13:192-7.
18. Angstwurm MW, Engelmann L, Zimmermann T, Lehmann C, Spes CH, Abel P, et al. Selenium in intensive care (SIC): results of a prospective randomized, placebo-controlled, multiple-center study in patients with severe systemic inflammatory response syndrome, sepsis, and septic shock. Crit Care Med 2007;35:118-26.
19. Ariaey-Nejad MR, Balaghi M, Baker EM, Sauberlich HE. Thiamin metabolism in man. Am J Clin Nutr 1970;23:764-78.
20. Arthur JR. The glutathione peroxidases. Cell Mol Life Sci 2000;57: 1825-35.
21. Arthur JR, Beckett GJ. Thyroid function. Br Med Bull 1999;55:658-68.
22. Ashton K, Hooper L, Harvey LJ, Hurst R, Casgrain A, Fairweather-Tait SJ. Methods of assessment of selenium status in humans: a systematic review. Am J Clin Nutr 2009;89:2025S-39S.
23. Aydemir TB, Blanchard RK, Cousins RJ. Zinc supplementation of young men alters metallothionein, zinc transporter, and cytokine gene expression in leukocyte populations. Proc Natl Acad Sci U S A 2006;103:1699-704.
24. Bailey LB, Moyers S, Gregory JF III. Folate. In: Bowman BA, Russell RA, eds. Present knowledge in nutrition. Washington, DC: ILSI Press, 2001:214-29.
25. Bailey LB. New standard for dietary folate intake in pregnant women. Am J Clin Nutr 2000;71:1304S-7S.
26. Baines M, Davies G. The evaluation of erythrocyte thiamin diphosphate as an indicator of thiamin status in man, and its comparison with erythrocyte transketolase activity measurements. Ann Clin Biochem 1988;25(Pt 6):698-705.
27. Baker EM, Hodges RE, Hood J, Sauberlich HE, March SC, Canham JE. Metabolism of 14C- and 3H-labeled L-ascorbic acid in human scurvy. Am J Clin Nutr 1971;24:444-54.
28. Ball GFM. Pantothenic acid: water-soluble vitamin assays in human nutrition. New York: Chapman and Hall, 1994.
29. Banerjee R, Vlasie M. Controlling the reactivity of radical intermediates by coenzyme B(12)-dependent methylmalonyl-CoA mutase. Biochem Soc Trans 2002;30:621-4.
30. Banno K. Measurement of pantothenic acid and hopantenic acid by gas chromatography-mass spectroscopy. Methods Enzymol 1997; 279:213-9.
31. Barber RC, Lammer EJ, Shaw GM, Greer KA, Finnell RH. The role of folate transport and metabolism in neural tube defect risk. Mol Genet Metab 1999;66:1-9.
32. Barclay MN, MacPherson A, Dixon J. Selenium content of a range of UK foods. J Food Compos Anal 1995;8:307-8.
33. Bates CJ. Vitamin analysis. Ann Clin Biochem 1997;34(Pt 6):599-626.
34. Batista BL, Rodrigues JL, Nunes JA, Souza VC, Barbosa F Jr. Exploiting dynamic reaction cell inductively coupled plasma mass spectrometry (DRC-ICP-MS) for sequential determination of trace elements in blood using a dilute-and-shoot procedure. Anal Chim Acta 2009;639:13-8.
35. Bauernfeind JC. The tocopherol content of food and influencing factors. CRC Crit Rev Food Sci Nutr 1977;8:337-82.
36. Baum MK, Miguez-Burbano MJ, Campa A, Shor-Posner G. Selenium and interleukins in persons infected with human immunodeficiency virus type 1. J Infect Dis 2000;182(Suppl 1):S69-73.
37. Bayon MM, Cabezuelo A, Gonzalez EB, Alonso IG, Sans-Medel A. Capabilities of fast protein liquid chromatography coupled to a double focussing inductively couple plasma mass spectrometer for trace metal speciation in human serum. J Anal Atom Spectros 1999;14:947-51.
38. Beattie JH, Peace HS. The influence of a low-boron diet and boron supplementation on bone, major mineral and sex steroid metabolism in postmenopausal women. Br J Nutr 1993;69:871-84.
39. Bechgaard H, Jespersen S. GI absorption of niacin in humans. J Pharm Sci 1977;66:871-2.
40. Beck WS. Cobalamin (Vitamin B12). In: Rucker RB, Suttie JW, McCormick DB, Machlin LJ, eds. Handbook of vitamins. New York: Marcel Dekker Inc, 2001:463-512.
41. Beck MA. Nutritionally induced oxidative stress: effect on viral disease. Am J Clin Nutr 2000;71:1676S-81S.
42. Beck MA, Levander OA, Handy J. Selenium deficiency and viral infection. J Nutr 2003;133:1463S-7S.
43. Beck MA, Shi Q, Morris VC, Levander OA. Rapid genomic evolution of a non-virulent coxsackievirus B3 in selenium-deficient mice results in selection of identical virulent isolates. Nat Med 1995;1:433-6.
44. Bender DA. Effects of benserazide, carbidopa and isoniazid administration on tryptophan-nicotinamide nucleotide metabolism in the rat. Biochem Pharmacol 1980;29:2099-104.
45. Bender DA. Non-nutritional uses of vitamin B6. Br J Nutr 1999;81: 7-20.
46. Bender DA. Daily doses of multivitamin tablets. BMJ 2002;325:173-4.
47. Benzie IF, Strain JJ. The ferric reducing ability of plasma (FRAP) as a measure of "antioxidant power": the FRAP assay. Anal Biochem 1996;239:70-6.
48. Berger MM, Cavadini C, Chiolero R, Dirren H. Copper, selenium, and zinc status and balances after major trauma. J Trauma 1996; 40:103-9.
49. Berger MM, Reymond MJ, Shenkin A, Rey F, Wardle C, Cayeux C, et al. Influence of selenium supplements on the post-traumatic alterations of the thyroid axis: a placebo-controlled trial. Intensive Care Med 2001;27:91-100.
50. Berger MM, Spertini F, Shenkin A, Wardle C, Wiesner L, Schindler C, et al. Trace element supplementation modulates pulmonary infection rates after major burns: a double-blind, placebo-controlled trial. Am J Clin Nutr 1998;68:365-71.
51. Berkner KL. The vitamin K-dependent carboxylase. J Nutr 2000;130: 1877-80.
52. Berry RJ, Li Z, Erickson JD, Li S, Moore CA, Wang H, et al. Prevention of neural-tube defects with folic acid in China. China-U.S. Collaborative Project for Neural Tube Defect Prevention. N Engl J Med 1999;341:1485-90. Erratum in N Engl J Med 1999;341:1864.
53. Berthon B. Aluminium speciation in relation to aluminium bioavailability, metabolism and toxicity. Coordinated Chemical Reviews 2002;228:319-41.
54. Bertoni-Freddari C, Fattoretti P, Casoli T, DiStefano G, Giorgetti B, Balietta M. Brain aging: the zinc connection. Exp Gerontol 2008;43: 389-93.
55. Bettendorff L. A non-cofactor role of thiamine derivatives in excitable cells? Arch Physiol Biochem 1996;104:745-51.
56. Beutler E, Blume KG, Kaplan JC, Lohr GW, Ramot B, Valentine WN. International Committee for Standardization in Haematology: recommended methods for red-cell enzyme analysis. Br J Haematol 1977;35:331-40.
57. Bhandari N, Bahl R, Taneja S, Strand T, Molbak K, Ulvik RJ, et al. Substantial reduction in severe diarrheal morbidity by daily zinc supplementation in young north Indian children. Pediatrics 2002;109:e86.
58. Bieri JG, Evarts RP. Tocopherols and polyunsaturated fatty acids in human tissues. Am J Clin Nutr 1975;28:717-20.
59. Biesalski HK. Vitamin E requirements in parenteral nutrition. Gastroenterology 2009;137:S92-104.
60. Bingham SA, Welch AA, McTaggart A, Mulligan AA, Runswick SA, Luben R, et al. Nutritional methods in the European Prospective Investigation of Cancer in Norfolk. Public Health Nutr 2001;4:847-58.
61. Bings NH, Bogaerts A, Broekaert JA. Atomic spectroscopy. Anal Chem 2002;74:2691-711.
62. Birchall JD. The essentiality of silicon in biology. Chem Soc Rev 1995; 24:351-7.
63. Bjelakovic G, Nikolova D, Simonetti RG, Gluud C. Systematic review: primary and secondary prevention of gastrointestinal cancers with antioxidant supplements. Aliment Pharmacol Ther 2008;28:689-703.

64. Black AL, Guirard BM, Snell EE. The behavior of muscle phosphorylase as a reservoir for vitamin B6 in the rat. J Nutr 1978;108:670-7.
65. Black RE. Zinc deficiency, infectious disease and mortality in the developing world. J Nutr 2003;133:1485S-9S.
66. Blanchard RA, Furie BC, Kruger SF, Waneck G, Jorgensen MJ, Furie B. Immunoassays of human prothrombin species which correlate with functional coagulant activities. J Lab Clin Med 1983;101:242-55.
67. Block G, Dresser CM, Hartman AM, Carroll DM. Nutrient sources in the American Diet: quantitative data from the NHANES-II Survey. I. Vitamins and minerals. Am J Epidemiol 1985;122:13-26.
68. Blount BC, Mack MM, Wehr CM, MacGregor JT, Hiatt RA, Wang G, et al. Folate deficiency causes uracil misincorporation into human DNA and chromosome breakage: implications for cancer and neuronal damage. Proc Natl Acad Sci U S A 1997;94:3290-5.
69. Boccia S, Boffetta P, Brennan P, Ricciardi G, Gianfagna F, Matsuo K, et al. Meta-analyses of the methylenetetrahydrofolate reductase C677T and A1298C polymorphisms and risk of head and neck and lung cancer. Cancer Lett 2009;273:55-61.
70. Bonjour JP. Biotin in man's nutrition and therapy—a review. Int J Vitam Nutr Res 1977;47:107-18.
71. Booth SL, Tucker KL, Chen H, Hannan MT, Gagnon DR, Cupples LA, et al. Dietary vitamin K intakes are associated with hip fracture but not with bone mineral density in elderly men and women. Am J Clin Nutr 2000;71:1201-8.
72. Bor MV, Refsum H, Bisp MR, Bleie O, Schneede J, Nordrehaug JE, et al. Plasma vitamin B6 vitamers before and after oral vitamin B6 treatment: a randomized placebo-controlled study. Clin Chem 2003; 49:155-61.
73. Bornhorst JA, Hunt JW, Urry FM, McMillin GA. Comparison of sample preservation methods for clinical trace element analysis by inductively coupled plasma mass spectrometry. Am J Clin Pathol 2005;123:578-83.
74. Boros LG. Population thiamine status and varying cancer rates between western, Asian and African countries. Anticancer Res 2000;20:2245-8.
75. Botto LD, Moore CA, Khoury MJ, Erickson JD. Neural-tube defects. N Engl J Med 1999;341:1509-19.
76. Bowman BB, McCormick DB, Rosenberg IH. Epithelial transport of water-soluble vitamins. Annu Rev Nutr 1989;9:187-99.
77. Brady J, Wilson L, McGregor L, Valente E, Orning L. Active B12: a rapid, automated assay for holotranscobalamin on the Abbott AxSYM analyzer. Clin Chem 2008;54:567-73.
78. Brattstrom L, Wilcken DE, Ohrvik J, Brudin L. Common methylenetetrahydrofolate reductase gene mutation leads to hyperhomocysteinemia but not to vascular disease: the result of a meta-analysis. Circulation 1998;98:2520-6.
79. Brem S, Grossman SA, Carson KA, New P, Phuphanich S, Alavi JB, et al. Phase 2 trial of copper depletion and penicillamine as antiangiogenesis therapy of glioblastoma. Neuro Oncol 2005;7: 246-53.
80. Brenner IB, Zander A, Cole M, Wiseman A. Comparison of axially and radially viewed inductively coupled plasmas for multi-element analysis: effect of sodium and calcium. J Anal Atom Spectrom 1997;12:897-906.
81. Brenner AJ, Harris ED. A quantitative test for copper using bicinchonic acid. Anal Biochem 1995;226:80-4.
82. Brewer GJ. Copper control as an antiangiogenic anticancer therapy: lessons from treating Wilson's disease. Exp Biol Med (Maywood) 2001;226:665-73.
83. Brewer GJ, Hedera P, Kluin KJ, Carlson M, Askari F, Dick RB, et al. Treatment of Wilson disease with ammonium tetrathiomolybdate: III. Initial therapy in a total of 55 neurologically affected patients and follow-up with zinc therapy. Arch Neurol 2003;60:379-85.
84. Brigden ML. Schilling test still useful in pernicious anemia? Postgrad Med 1999;106:37-8.
85. Brigelius-Flohe R. Widened horizon of vitamin E research. Mol Nutr Food Res 2010;54:581.
86. Brin M, Tai M, Ostashever AS, Kalinsky H. The effect of thiamine deficiency on the activity of erythrocyte hemolysate transketolase. J Nutr 1960;71:273-81.
87. Brown KH, Peerson JM, Rivera J, Allen LH. Effect of supplemental zinc on the growth and serum zinc concentrations of prepubertal children: a meta-analysis of randomized controlled trials. Am J Clin Nutr 2002;75:1062-71.
88. Brown KM, Arthur JR. Selenium, selenoproteins and human health: a review. Public Health Nutr 2001;4:593-9.
89. Brown KM, Pickard K, Nicol F, Beckett GJ, Duthie GG, Arthur JR. Effects of organic and inorganic selenium supplementation on selenoenzyme activity in blood lymphocytes, granulocytes, platelets and erythrocytes. Clin Sci (Lond) 2000;98:593-9.
90. Bruckdorfer KR. Antioxidants and CVD. Proc Nutr Soc 2008;67: 214-22.
91. Buettner GR. The pecking order of free radicals and antioxidants: lipid peroxidation, alpha-tocopherol, and ascorbate. Arch Biochem Biophys 1993;300:535-43.
92. Burk RF. Selenium: recent clinical advances. Curr Opin Gastroenterol 2001;17:162-6.
93. Burk RF, Hill KE, Motley AK. Selenoprotein metabolism and function: evidence for more than one function for selenoprotein P. J Nutr 2003;133:1517S-20S.
94. Burk RF, Norsworthy BK, Hill KE, Motley AK, Byrne DW. Effects of chemical form of selenium on plasma biomarkers in a high-dose human supplementation trial. Cancer Epidemiol Biomarkers Prev 2006;15:804-10.
95. Burns CS, Aronoff-Spencer E, Legname G, Prusiner SB, Antholine WE, Gerfen GJ, et al. Copper coordination in the full-length, recombinant prion protein. Biochemistry 2003;42:6794-803.
96. Burns J, Forsyth JS, Paterson CR. Factors associated with variation in plasma copper levels in preterm infants of very low birth weight. Eur J Pediatr 1993;152:240-3.
97. Buzby GP, Mullen JL, Matthews DC, Hobbs CL, Rosato EF. Prognostic nutritional index in gastrointestinal surgery. Am J Surg 1980;139:160-7.
98. Calder PC, Albers R, Antoine JM, Blum S, Bourdet-Sicard R, Ferns GA, et al. Inflammatory disease processes and interactions with nutrition. Br J Nutr 2009;101(Suppl 1):S1-45.
99. Camblor M, De La Cuerda C, Bretón I, Pérez-Rus G, Alvarez S, García P. Copper deficiency with pancytopenia due to enteral nutrition through jejunostomy. Clin Nutr 1997;16:129-31.
100. Capo-Chichi CD, Gueant JL, Feillet F, Namour F, Vidailhet M. Analysis of riboflavin and riboflavin cofactor levels in plasma by high-performance liquid chromatography. J Chromatogr B Biomed Sci Appl 2000;739:219-24.
101. Carlisle EM. Silicon as an essential trace element in animal nutrition. In: Evered D, O'Connor M, eds. Silicon biochemistry. Chichester: John Wiley, 1986:123-39.
102. Carlson GL, Williams N, Barber D, Shaffer JL, Wales S, Isherwood D, et al. Biotin deficiency complicating long-term total parenteral nutrition in an adult patient. Clin Nutr 1995;14:186-90.
103. Carmel R. Subtle and atypical cobalamin deficiency states. Am J Hematol 1990;34:108-14.
104. Carmel R. Measuring and interpreting holo-transcobalamin (holo-transcobalamin II). Clin Chem 2002;48:407-9.
105. Carr A, Frei B. Does vitamin C act as a pro-oxidant under physiological conditions? FASEB J 1999;13:1007-24.
106. Case CP, Ellis L, Turner JC, Fairman B. Development of a routine method for the determination of trace metals in whole blood by magnetic sector inductively coupled plasma mass spectrometry with particular relevance to patients with total hip and knee arthroplasty. Clin Chem 2001;47:275-80.
107. Cefalu WT, Hu FB. Role of chromium in human health and in diabetes. Diabetes Care 2004;27:2741-51.
108. Cefalu WT, Rood J, Pinsonat P, Qin J, Sereda O, Levitan L, et al. Characterization of the metabolic and physiologic response to chromium supplementation in subjects with type 2 diabetes mellitus. Metabolism 2010;59:755-62.

109. Centre for Biochemical and Biophysical Science and Medicine, 2003. Available at: www.hms.harvard.edu/bbsm/vallee.htm.
110. Centers for Disease Control. Achievements in public health 1900-1999: fluoridation of drinking water to prevent dental caries. MMWR 1999;48:933-40.
111. Centers for Disease Control. Recommendations for using fluoride to prevent and control dental caries in the United States. MMWR 2001; 50:1-42.
112. Cerklewski FL. Fluoride. In: O'Dell BL, Sunde RA, eds. Handbook of nutritionally essential mineral elements. New York/Basel/Hong Kong: Marcel Dekker, 1997:583-602.
113. Cerulli J, Grabe DW, Gauthier I, Malone M, McGoldrick MD. Chromium picolinate toxicity. Ann Pharmacother 1998;32: 428-31.
114. Cervantes-Laureen D, McElvaney NG, Moss J. Niacin. In: Shils ME, Olson JA, Shike M, Ross AC, eds. Modern nutrition in health and disease. Baltimore, Md: Williams and Wilkins, 1999:401-11.
115. Chan AC. Partners in defense, vitamin E and vitamin C. Can J Physiol Pharmacol 1993;71:725-31.
116. Chastain JL, McCormick DB. Flavin catabolites: identification and quantitation in human urine. Am J Clin Nutr 1987;46:830-4.
117. Chen LH, Liu ML, Hwang HY, Chen LS, Korenberg J, Shane B. Human methionine synthase: cDNA cloning, gene localization, and expression. J Biol Chem 1997;272:3628-34.
118. Chen Q, Espey MG, Sun AY, Lee JH, Krishna MC, Shacter E, et al. Ascorbate in pharmacologic concentrations selectively generates ascorbate radical and hydrogen peroxide in extracellular fluid in vivo. Proc Natl Acad Sci U S A 2007;104:8749-54.
119. Chesters JK. Zinc. In: O'Dell BL, Sunde RA, eds. Handbook of nutritionally essential mineral elements. New York/Basel/Hong Kong: Marcel Dekker, 1997:185-230.
120. Chéry CC, De Cremer K, Cornelis R, Vanhaecke F, Moens L. Optimisation of ICP-dynamic reaction cell-MS as specific detector for the speciation analysis of vanadium at therapeutic levels in serum. J Anal Atom Spectros 2003;18:1113-8.
121. Chloe M, Mak CM, Lam C-W. Diagnosis of Wilson's disease: a comprehensive review. Crit Rev Clin Lab Sci 208;45:263-90.
122. Christodoulou J, Danks DM, Sarkar B, Baerlocher KE, Casey R, Horn N, et al. Early treatment of Menkes disease with parenteral copper-histidine: long-term follow-up of four treated patients. Am J Med Genet 1998;76:154-64.
123. Chytil F, McCormick DB. Vitamins and coenzyme: methods in enzymology. Orlando, Fla: Academic Press Inc, 1986:Part H.
124. Cipriano C, Tesei S, Malavolta M, Giacconi R, Muti E, Costarelli L, et al. Accumulation of cells with short telomeres is associated with impaired zinc homeostasis and inflammation in old hypertensive participants. J Gerontol A Biol Sci Med Sci 2009;64:745-51.
125. Clark LC, Combs GF Jr, Turnbull BW, Slate EH, Chalker DK, Chow J, et al. Effects of selenium supplementation for cancer prevention in patients with carcinoma of the skin: a randomized controlled trial. Nutritional Prevention of Cancer Study Group. JAMA 1996;276: 1957-63.
126. Clodfelder BJ, Emamaullee J, Hepburn DD, Chakov NE, Nettles HS, Vincent JB. The trail of chromium(III) in vivo from the blood to the urine: the roles of transferrin and chromodulin. J Biol Inorg Chem 2001;6:608-17.
127. Coburn SP. The chemistry and metabolism of the vitamin B6 antagonist, 4-deoxypyridine. Boca Raton, Fla: CRC Press, 1981.
128. Cohen HJ, Brown MR, Hamilton D, Lyons-Patterson J, Avissar N, Liegey P. Glutathione peroxidase and selenium deficiency in patients receiving home parenteral nutrition: time course for development of deficiency and repletion of enzyme activity in plasma and blood cells. Am J Clin Nutr 1989;49:132-9.
129. Colagar AH, Marzony ET, Chaichi MJ. Zinc levels in seminal plasma are associated with sperm quality in fertile and infertile men. Nutr Res 2009;29:82-8.
130. Combs GF. Biotin: the vitamins: fundamental aspects in nutrition and health. San Diego, Calif: Academic Press, 1992:350-65.
131. Combs GF Jr, Clark LC, Turnbull BW. An analysis of cancer prevention by selenium. Biofactors 2001;14:153-9.
132. Combs GF Jr, Gray WP. Chemopreventive agents: selenium. Pharmacol Ther 1998;79:179-92.
133. Cook NR, Albert CM, Gaziano JM, Zaharris E, MacFadyen J, Danielson E, et al. A randomized factorial trial of vitamins C and E and beta carotene in the secondary prevention of cardiovascular events in women: results from the Women's Antioxidant Cardiovascular Study. Arch Intern Med 2007;167:1610-8.
134. Cordano A. Clinical manifestations of nutritional copper deficiency in infants and children. Am J Clin Nutr 1998;67:1012S-6S.
135. Cousins RJ, Leinart AS. Tissue-specific regulation of zinc metabolism and metallothionein genes by interleukin 1. FASEB J 1988;2:2884-90.
136. Cox DW, Moore SD. Copper transporting P-type ATPases and human disease. J Bioenerg Biomembr 2002;34:333-8.
137. Cozma I, Elmigy M, Miller D, Sheehan TM, Roberts NB. Release of cobalt and chromium in complicated metal on metal hip arthroplasties. Ann Clin Biochem 2009;46:17.
138. Cragg RA, Phillips SR, Piper JM, Varma JS, Campbell FC, Mathers JC, et al. Homeostatic regulation of zinc transporters in the human small intestine by dietary zinc supplementation. Gut 2005;54:469-78.
139. Cravo ML, Gloria LM, Selhub J, Nadeau MR, Camilo ME, Resende MP, et al. Hyperhomocysteinemia in chronic alcoholism: correlation with folate, vitamin B-12, and vitamin B-6 status. Am J Clin Nutr 1996;63:220-4.
140. Dancis J, Lehanka J, Levitz M. Placental transport of riboflavin: differential rates of uptake at the maternal and fetal surfaces of the perfused human placenta. Am J Obstet Gynecol 1988;158:204-10.
141. Danks DM. Copper deficiency in humans. Annu Rev Nutr 1988;8:235-57.
142. Davidovici BB, Tuzun Y, Wolf R. Retinoid receptors. Dermatol Clin 2007;25:525-30, viii.
143. Davies S, McLaren HJ, Hunnisett A, Howard M. Age-related decreases in chromium levels in 51,665 hair, sweat, and serum samples from 40,872 patients—implications for the prevention of cardiovascular disease and type II diabetes mellitus. Metabolism 1997;46:469-73.
144. Davis RE. Clinical chemistry of vitamin B12. Adv Clin Chem 1985;24:163-216.
145. Delves HT. Atomic absorption spectroscopy in clinical analysis. Ann Clin Biochem 1987;24(Pt 6):529-51.
146. DePaola DP. Nutrition in relation to dental medicine. In: Shils ME, Olson JA, Shihe M, Ross AC, eds. Modern nutrition in health and disease. Baltimore, Md: Williams and Wilkins, 1999:1099-124.
147. Deutsch JC, Kolhouse JF. Ascorbate and dehydroascorbate measurements in aqueous solutions and plasma determined by gas chromatography-mass spectrometry. Anal Chem 1993;65:321-6.
148. Devlin AM, Ling EH, Peerson JM, Fernando S, Clarke R, Smith AD, et al. Glutamate carboxypeptidase II: a polymorphism associated with lower levels of serum folate and hyperhomocysteinemia. Hum Mol Genet 2000;9:2837-44.
149. Devoto G, Gallo F, Marchello C, Racchi O, Garbarini R, Bonassi S, et al. Prealbumin serum concentrations as a useful tool in the assessment of malnutrition in hospitalized patients. Clin Chem 2006;52:2281-5.
150. Devrian TA. The physiological effects of dietary boron. Crit Rev Food Sci Nutr 2003;43:219-31.
151. Dickman ED, Smith SM. Selective regulation of cardiomyocyte gene expression and cardiac morphogenesis by retinoic acid. Dev Dyn 1996;206:39-48.
152. Dietary Antioxidants and Related Compounds Panel. Dietary reference intakes for vitamin C, vitamin E, selenium and carotenoids. Washington, DC: National Academy Press, 2000.
153. Doherty CP, Sarkar MA, Shakur MS, Ling SC, Elton RA, Cutting WA. Zinc and rehabilitation from severe protein-energy malnutrition: higher-dose regimens are associated with increased mortality. Am J Clin Nutr 1998;68:742-8.
154. Doisy EA Jr. Micronutrient controls on biosynthesis of clotting proteins and cholesterol. In: Hemphill DD, ed. Trace substances in

environmental health. Columbia, Mo: University of Missouri, 1973: 193-9.
155. Downing RG, Strong PL, Hovanec BM, Northington J. Considerations in the determination of boron at low concentrations. Biol Trace Elem Res 1998;66:3-21.
156. Dutta P. Disturbances in glutathione metabolism and resistance to malaria: current understanding and new concepts. J Soc Pharm Chem 1993;2:11-48.
157. Dutta P, Seirafi J, Halpin D, Pinto J, Rivlin R. Acute ethanol exposure alters hepatic glutathione metabolism in riboflavin deficiency. Alcohol 1995;12:43-7.
158. Edmondson DE, Newton-Vinson P. The covalent FAD of monoamine oxidase: structural and functional role and mechanism of the flavinylation reaction. Antioxid Redox Signal 2001;3:789-806.
159. Eissenstat BR, Wyse BW, Hansen RG. Pantothenic acid status of adolescents. Am J Clin Nutr 1986;44:931-7.
160. Ejima A, Imamura T, Nakamura S, Saito H, Matsumoto K, Momono S. Manganese intoxication during total parenteral nutrition. Lancet 1992;339:426.
161. Ekmekcioglu C, Prohaska C, Pomazal K, Steffan I, Schernthaner G, Marktl W. Concentrations of seven trace elements in different hematological matrices in patients with type 2 diabetes as compared to healthy controls. Biol Trace Elem Res 2001;79:205-19.
162. Elia M, Crozier C, Neale G. Mineral metabolism during short-term starvation in man. Clin Chim Acta 1984;139:37-45.
163. Environmental health criteria: copper. Geneva, Switzerland: World Health Organization (WHO), 1998.
164. Evans WC. Thiaminases and their effect on animals. In: Munson PL, Glover J, Diczfalusy E, Olson RE, eds. Vitamins and hormones. New York: Academic Press Inc, 1975:467-504.
165. Fairweather-Tait SJ, Harvey LJ, Ford D. Does ageing affect zinc homeostasis and dietary requirements? Exp Gerontol 2008;43: 382-8.
166. Falchuk KH. The molecular basis for the role of zinc in developmental biology. Mol Cell Biochem 1998;188:41-8.
167. Farrell PM, Bieri JG, Fratantoni JF, Wood RE, di Sant'Agnese PA. The occurrence and effects of human vitamin E deficiency: a study in patients with cystic fibrosis. J Clin Invest 1977;60:233-41.
168. Fatemi N, Sarkar B. Molecular mechanism of copper transport in Wilson disease. Environ Health Perspect 2002;110(Suppl 5):695-8.
169. Fell GS, Fleck A, Cuthbertson DP, Queen K, Morrison C, Bessent RG, et al. Urinary zinc levels as an indication of muscle catabolism. Lancet 1973;1:280-2.
170. Fell JM, Reynolds AP, Meadows N, Khan K, Long SG, Quaghebeur G, et al. Manganese toxicity in children receiving long-term parenteral nutrition. Lancet 1996;347:1218-21.
171. Fenech M. Micronutrients and genomic stability: a new paradigm for recommended dietary allowances (RDAs). Food Chem Toxicol 2002; 40:1113-7.
172. Fennelly J, Frank O, Baker H, Leevy CM. Red blood cell-transketolase activity in malnourished alcoholics with cirrhosis. Am J Clin Nutr 1967;20:946-9.
173. Fenton WA, Rosenberg LE. Disorders of proprionate and methylmalonate metabolism. In: Scriver CS, Beaudet AL, Sly WS, Valle D, eds. The metabolic and molecular basis of inherited disease. New York: McGraw-Hill, 1995:1423-49.
174. Fenton WA, Rosenberg LE. Inherited disorders of cobalamin transport and metabolism. In: Scriver CR, Beaudet AL, Sly WS, Valle DR, eds. The metabolic and molecular bases of inherited disease. New York: McGraw-Hill, 1995:3129-49.
175. Ferenci P, Caca K, Loudianos G, Mieli-Vergani G, Tanner S, Sternlieb I, et al. Diagnosis and phenotypic classification of Wilson disease. Liver 2003;23:139-42.
176. Ferland G. Vitamin K. In: Bowman BA, Russell RA, eds. Present knowledge in nutrition. Washington, DC: ILSI Press, 2001: 164-72.
177. Fernandez-Peralta AM, Daimiel L, Nejda N, Iglesias D, Medina Arana V, González-Aguilera JJ. Association of polymorphisms MTHFR C677T and A1298C with risk of colorectal cancer, genetic and epigenetic characteristic of tumors, and response to chemotherapy. Int J Colorectal Dis 2010;25:141-51.
178. Feskanich D, Weber P, Willett WC, Rockett H, Booth SL, Colditz GA. Vitamin K intake and hip fractures in women: a prospective study. Am J Clin Nutr 1999;69:74-9.
179. Field LS, Luk E, Culotta VC. Copper chaperones: personal escorts for metal ions. J Bioenerg Biomembr 2002;34:373-9.
180. Finney L, Mandava S, Ursos L, Zhang W, Rodi D, Vogt S, et al. X-ray fluorescence microscopy reveals large-scale relocalization and extracellular translocation of cellular copper during angiogenesis. Proc Natl Acad Sci U S A 2007;104:2247-52.
181. Fisher GL, Davies LG, Rosenblatt LS. The effects of container composition, storage duration, and temperature on serum mineral levels, Symposium on Accuracy in Trace Analysis, 6th IMR Symposium, June 14-17, 1994, Bergen.
182. Fleck A, Raines G, Hawker F, Trotter J, Wallace PI, Ledingham IM, et al. Increased vascular permeability: a major cause of hypoalbuminaemia in disease and injury. Lancet 1985;1:781-4.
183. Fleming JC, Tartaglini E, Steinkamp MP, Schorderet DF, Cohen N, Neufeld EJ. The gene mutated in thiamine-responsive anaemia with diabetes and deafness (TRMA) encodes a functional thiamine transporter. Nat Genet 1999;22:305-8.
184. Floridi A, Pupita M, Palmerini CA, Fini C, Alberti FA. Thiamine pyrophosphate determination in whole blood and erythrocytes by high performance liquid chromatography. Int J Vitam Nutr Res 1984;54:165-71.
185. Food and Agriculture Organisation, World Health Organisation. Joint FAO/WHO expert consultation on human vitamin and mineral requirements. Bangkok, Thailand: FAO/WHO, 1998.
186. Food and Nutrition Board. Dietary reference intakes for thiamin, riboflavin, niacin, vitamin B6, folate, vitamin B12, pantothenic acid, biotin, and choline. Washington, DC: National Academy Press, 1998.
187. Food and Nutrition Board. Dietary reference intakes for calcium, phosphorus, magnesium, vitamin D, and fluoride. Washington, DC: National Academy Press, 1999.
188. Food and Nutrition Board. Dietary reference intakes for vitamin C, vitamin E, selenium, and carotenoids. Washington, DC: National Academy Press, 2000.
189. Food and Nutrition Board. Dietary reference intakes for energy, carbohydrate, fiber, fat, fatty acids, cholesterol, protein, and amino acids. Washington, DC: National Academy Press, 2006.
190. Food and Nutrition Board. The essential guide to nutrient requirements. Washington, DC: National Academy Press, 2002.
191. Foote JW, Delves HT. Albumin bound and alpha 2-macroglobulin bound zinc concentrations in the sera of healthy adults. J Clin Pathol 1984;37:1050-4.
192. Ford ES. Serum copper concentration and coronary heart disease among US adults. Am J Epidemiol 2000;151:1182-8.
193. Fordyce FM, Johnson CC, Navaratna UR, Appleton JD, Dissanayake CB. Selenium and iodine in soil, rice and drinking water in relation to endemic goitre in Sri Lanka. Sci Total Environ 2000;263:127-41.
194. Forrer R, Gautschi K, Lutz H. Simultaneous measurement of the trace elements Al, As, B, Be, Cd, Co, Cu, Fe, Li, Mn, Mo, Ni, Rb, Se, Sr, and Zn in human serum and their reference ranges by ICP-MS. Biol Trace Elem Res 2001;80:77-93.
195. Fouty B, Frerman F, Reves R. Riboflavin to treat nucleoside analogue-induced lactic acidosis. Lancet 1998;352:291-2.
196. Francesconi KA, Pannier F. Selenium metabolites in urine: a critical overview of past work and current status. Clin Chem 2004;50: 2240-53.
197. Frausto Da Silva JJR, Williams RJP. The biological chemistry of the elements. In: The inorganic chemistry of life, 2nd edition. New York: Oxford University Press, 2001.
198. Frederickson CJ, Suh SW, Silva D, Frederickson CJ, Thompson RB. Importance of zinc in the central nervous system: the zinc-containing neuron. J Nutr 2000;130:1471S-83S.

199. Fredrich W. Thiamine. Vitamins. Berlin: de Gruyter, 1988:341-94.
200. Frei B, Stocker R, England L, Ames BN. Ascorbate: the most effective antioxidant in human blood plasma. Adv Exp Med Biol 1990;264: 155-63.
201. French RJ, Jones PJ. Role of vanadium in nutrition: metabolism, essentiality and dietary considerations. Life Sci 1993;52:339-46.
202. Friedman BJ, Freeland-Graves JH, Bales CW, Behmardi F, Shorey-Kutschke RL, Willis RA, et al. Manganese balance and clinical observations in young men fed a manganese-deficient diet. J Nutr 1987;117:133-43.
203. Fritz I, Said H, Harris C, et al. A new sensitive assay for plasma riboflavin using high performance liquid chromatography. J Am Coll Nutr 1987;6:454.
204. Fry PC, Fox HM, Tao HG. Metabolic response to a pantothenic acid deficient diet in humans. J Nutr Sci Vitaminol (Tokyo) 1976;22: 339-46.
205. Fu CS, Swendseid ME, Jacob RA, McKee RW. Biochemical markers for assessment of niacin status in young men: levels of erythrocyte niacin coenzymes and plasma tryptophan. J Nutr 1989;119:1949-55.
206. Fuhrman MP, Herrmann V, Masidonski P, Eby C. Pancytopenia after removal of copper from total parenteral nutrition. JPEN J Parenter Enteral Nutr 2000;24:361-6.
207. Fujita M, Itakura T, Takagi Y, Okada A. Copper deficiency during total parenteral nutrition: clinical analysis of three cases. JPEN J Parenter Enteral Nutr 1989;13:421-5.
208. Fuller NJ, Elia M. Inadequacy of urinary urea for estimating nitrogen balance. Ann Clin Biochem 1990;27(Pt 5):510-1.
209. Gaffney D, Fell GS, O'Reilly DS. ACP Best Practice No. 163. Wilson's disease: acute and presymptomatic laboratory diagnosis and monitoring. J Clin Pathol 2000;53:807-12.
210. Gale CR, Martyn CN, Winter PD, Cooper C. Vitamin C and risk of death from stroke and coronary heart disease in cohort of elderly people. BMJ 1995;310:1563-6.
211. Galloway P, McMillan DC, Sattar N. Effect of the inflammatory response on trace element and vitamin status. Ann Clin Biochem 2000;37(Pt 3):289-97.
212. Gao M, Levy LS, Braithwaite RA, Brown SS. Monitoring of total chromium in rat fluids and lymphocytes following intratracheal administration of soluble trivalent or hexavalent chromium compounds. Hum Exp Toxicol 1993;12:377-82.
213. Gardiner PH, Littlejohn D, Halls DJ, Fell GS. Direct determination of selenium in human blood serum and plasma by electrothermal atomic absorption spectrometry. J Trace Elem Med Biol 1995;9:74-81.
214. Geubel AP, De Galocsy C, Alves N, Rahier J, Dive C. Liver damage caused by therapeutic vitamin A administration: estimate of dose-related toxicity in 41 cases. Gastroenterology 1991;100:1701-9.
215. Ghiselli A, Serafini M, Natella F, Scaccini C. Total antioxidant capacity as a tool to assess redox status: critical view and experimental data. Free Radic Biol Med 2000;29:1106-14.
216. Gitlin JD. Transcriptional regulation of ceruloplasmin gene expression during inflammation. J Biol Chem 1988;263:6281-7.
217. Glenn GM, Krober MS, Kelly P, McCarty J, Weir M. Pyridoxine as therapy in theophylline-induced seizures. Vet Hum Toxicol 1995;37: 342-5.
218. Glusman M. The syndrome of "burning feet" (nutritional myalgia) as a manifestation of nutritional deficiency. Am J Med 1947;3: 211-23.
219. Golden BE, Golden MH. Effect of zinc on lean tissue synthesis during recovery from malnutrition. Eur J Clin Nutr 1992;46:697-706.
220. Goldfine AB, Patti ME, Zuberi L, Goldstein BJ, LeBlanc R, Landaker EJ, et al. Metabolic effects of vanadyl sulfate in humans with non-insulin-dependent diabetes mellitus: in vivo and in vitro studies. Metabolism 2000;49:400-10.
221. Gollan JL, Gollan TJ. Wilson disease in 1998: genetic, diagnostic and therapeutic aspects. J Hepatol 1998;28(Suppl 1):28-36.
222. Goodman BP, Mistry DH, Pasha SF, Bosch PE. Copper deficiency myeloneuropathy due to occult celiac disease. Neurologist 2009;15: 355-6.
223. Goullé J-P, Mahieu L, Castermant J, Neveu N, Bonneau L, Lainé G, et al. Metal and metalloid multi-elementary ICP-MS validation in whole blood, plasma, urine and hair: reference values. Forensic Sci Int 2005;153:39-44.
224. Graham IM, O'Callaghan P. Vitamins, homocysteine and cardiovascular risk. Cardiovasc Drugs Ther 2002;16:383-9.
225. Greene HL, Hambidge KM, Schanler R, Tsang RC. Guidelines for the use of vitamins, trace elements, calcium, magnesium, and phosphorus in infants and children receiving total parenteral nutrition: report of the Subcommittee on Pediatric Parenteral Nutrient Requirements from the Committee on Clinical Practice Issues of the American Society for Clinical Nutrition. Am J Clin Nutr 1988;48:1324-42.
226. Greger JL. Nutrition versus toxicology of manganese in humans: evaluation of potential biomarkers. Neurotoxicology 1999;20:205-12.
227. Gregory J, Foster K, Tyler H, Wiseman M. The dietary and nutritional survey of British adults. Office of Population Censuses and Surveys, Social Survey Division. London: HMSO, 1990.
228. Gregory JF, Kirk JR. Vitamin B6 in foods: assessment of stability and bioavailability. Human vitamin B6 requirements. Washington, DC: National Academy of Sciences, 1978.
229. Gregory JF III, Williamson J, Liao JF, Bailey LB, Toth JP. Kinetic model of folate metabolism in nonpregnant women consuming [2H2] folic acid: isotopic labeling of urinary folate and the catabolite para-acetamidobenzoylglutamate indicates slow, intake-dependent, turnover of folate pools. J Nutr 1998;128:1896-906.
230. Grunebaum M, Horodniceanu C, Steinherz R. The radiographic manifestations of bone changes in copper deficiency. Pediatr Radiol 1980;9:101-4.
231. Gruppo Italiano per lo Studio della Sopravvivenza nell'Infarto Miocardico. Dietary supplementation with n-3 polyunsaturated fatty acids and vitamin E after myocardial infarction: results of the GISSI-Prevenzione trial. Lancet 1999;354:447-55.
232. Guanabens N, Farrerons J, Perez-Edo L, Monegal A, Renau A, Carbonell J, et al. Cyclical etidronate versus sodium fluoride in established postmenopausal osteoporosis: a randomized 3 year trial. Bone 2000;27:123-8.
233. Gunton JE, Hams G, Hitchman R, McElduff A. Serum chromium does not predict glucose tolerance in late pregnancy. Am J Clin Nutr 2001;73:99-104.
234. Gyorffy EJ, Chan H. Copper deficiency and microcytic anemia resulting from prolonged ingestion of over-the-counter zinc. Am J Gastroenterol 1992;87:1054-5.
235. Hageman GJ, Stierum RH. Niacin, poly(ADP-ribose) polymerase-1 and genomic stability. Mutat Res 2001;475:45-56.
236. Hah SS. Recent advances in biomedical applications of accelerator mass spectrometry. J Biomed Sci 2009;16:54.
237. Hair Analysis Panel Discussion. Exploring the state of the science, 2003. Available at: www.astdr.cdc.gov/HAC/hair_analysis.
238. Hak EB, Storm MC, Helms RA. Chromium and zinc contamination of parenteral nutrient solution components commonly used in infants and children. Am J Health Syst Pharm 1998;55:150-4.
239. Halfdanarson TR, Kumar N, Li CY, Phyliky RL, Hogan WJ. Hematological manifestations of copper deficiency: a retrospective review. Eur J Haematol 2008;80:523-31.
240. Hall CA. The transport of vitamin B12 from food to use within the cells. J Lab Clin Med 1979;94:811-6.
241. Halls DJ, Fell GS. Faster determination of chromium in urine by atomic absorption spectrometry. J Anal Atom Spectrom 1988;3:105-9.
242. Hambidge M. Biomarkers of trace mineral intake and status. J Nutr 2003;133(Suppl 3):948S-55S.
243. Han Q, Xu M, Tang L, Tan X, Tan X, Tan Y, et al. Homogeneous, nonradioactive, enzymatic assay for plasma pyridoxal 5-phosphate. Clin Chem 2002;48:1560-4.
244. Harris ED. Copper. In: O'Dell BL, Sunde RA, eds. Handbook of nutritionally essential mineral elements. New York/Basel/Hong Kong: Marcel Dekker, 1997:231-73.
245. Harris DC. Different metal-binding properties of the two sites of human transferrin. Biochemistry 1977;16:560-4.

246. Harris ED. A requirement for copper in angiogenesis. Nutr Rev 2004; 62:60-4.
247. Harris ZL. Aceruloplasminemia. J Neurol Sci 2003;207:108-9.
248. Harrison I, Littlejohn D, Fell GS. Determination of selenium in human hair and nail by electrothermal atomic absorption spectrometry. J Anal Atom Spectros 1995;10:215-9.
249. Harrison I, Littlejohn D, Fell GS. Distribution of selenium in human blood plasma and serum. Analyst 1996;121:189-94.
250. Harrison I, Littlejohn D, Fell GS. Improved molecular fluorescence method for the determination of selenium in biological samples. Analyst 1996;121:1641-6.
251. Harvey LJ, Ashton K, Hooper L, Casgrain A, Fairweather-Tait SJ. Methods of assessment of copper status in humans: a systematic review. Am J Clin Nutr 2009;89:2009S-24S.
252. Hatfield DL, Gladyshev VN. How selenium has altered our understanding of the genetic code. Mol Cell Biol 2002;22:3565-76.
253. Haywood S, Dincer Z, Jasani B, Loughran MJ. Molybdenum-associated pituitary endocrinopathy in sheep treated with ammonium tetrathiomolybdate. J Comp Pathol 2004;130:21-31.
254. Hazell AS, Butterworth RF. Hepatic encephalopathy: an update of pathophysiologic mechanisms. Proc Soc Exp Biol Med 1999;222: 99-112.
255. Healton EB, Savage DG, Brust JC, Garrett TJ, Lindenbaum J. Neurologic aspects of cobalamin deficiency. Medicine (Baltimore) 1991;70:229-45.
256. Heart Protection Study Collaborative Group. MRC/BHF heart protection study of antioxidant vitamin supplementation in 20,536 high-risk individuals: a randomised placebo-controlled trial. Lancet 2002;360:23-33.
257. Heitland P, Koster HD. Biomonitoring of 37 trace elements in blood samples from inhabitants of northern Germany by ICP-MS. J Trace Elem Med Biol 2006;20:253-62.
258. Hellborg R, Skog G. Accelerator mass spectrometry. Mass Spectrom Rev 2008;27:398-427.
259. Hellman NE, Gitlin JD. Ceruloplasmin metabolism and function. Annu Rev Nutr 2002;22:439-58.
260. Helphingstine CJ, Bistrian BR. New Food and Drug Administration requirements for inclusion of vitamin K in adult parenteral multivitamins. JPEN J Parenter Enteral Nutr 2003;27:220-4.
261. Hermann J, Arquitt A, Stoecker BJ. Effect of chromium supplementation on plasma lipids, apolipoproteins and glucose in elderly subjects. Nutr Res 1994;14:671-4.
262. Herrmann W, Obeid R, Schorr H, Geisel J. The usefulness of holotranscobalamin in predicting vitamin B12 status in different clinical settings. Curr Drug Metab 2005;6:47-53.
263. Herrmann W, Schorr H, Obeid R, Geisel J. Vitamin B-12 status, particularly holotranscobalamin II and methylmalonic acid concentrations, and hyperhomocysteinemia in vegetarians. Am J Clin Nutr 2003;78:131-6.
264. Heyssel RM, Bozian RC, Darby WJ, Bell MC. Vitamin B12 turnover in man: the assimilation of vitamin B12 from natural foodstuff by man and estimates of minimal daily dietary requirements. Am J Clin Nutr 1966;18:176-84.
265. Higden J. An evidence-based approach to vitamins and minerals. New York/Stuttgart: Thieme, 2003.
266. Hill CH, Matrone G. Chemical parameters in the study of in vivo and in vitro interactions of transition elements. Fed Proc 1970;29:1474-81.
267. Hill KE, Xia Y, Akesson B, Boeglin ME, Burk RF. Selenoprotein P concentration in plasma is an index of selenium status in selenium-deficient and selenium-supplemented Chinese subjects. J Nutr 1996;126:138-45.
268. Hill MH, Bradley A, Mushtaq S, Williams EA, Powers HJ. Effects of methodological variation on assessment of riboflavin status using the erythrocyte glutathione reductase activation coefficient assay. Br J Nutr 2009;102:273-8.
269. Hodges RE, Bean WB, Ohlson MA, Bleiler R. Human pantothenic acid deficiency produced by omega-methyl pantothenic acid. J Clin Invest 1959;38:1421-5.
270. Hoffer A. Ascorbic acid and toxicity. N Engl J Med 1971;285:635-6.
271. Holm G, Moody LE. Carpal tunnel syndrome: current theory, treatment, and the use of B6. J Am Acad Nurse Pract 2003;15:18-22.
272. Homsher R, Zak B. Spectrophotometric investigation of sensitive complexing agents for the determination of zinc in serum. Clin Chem 1985;31:1310-3.
273. Horwitt MK. Critique of the requirement for vitamin E. Am J Clin Nutr 2001;73:1003-5.
274. Houtkooper LB, Ritenbaugh C, Aickin M, Lohman TG, Going SB, Weber JL, et al. Nutrients, body composition and exercise are related to change in bone mineral density in premenopausal women. J Nutr 1995;125:1229-37.
275. Howard JM. Assessment of vitamin B(1) status. Clin Chem 2000;46: 1867-8.
276. Howarth RW, Cole JJ. Molybdenum availability, nitrogen limitation, and Phytoplankton growth in natural waters. Science 1985;229:653-5.
277. Huang L, Kirschke CP, Zhang Y. Decreased intracellular zinc in human tumorigenic prostate epithelial cells: a possible role in prostate cancer progression. Cancer Cell Int 2006;6:10.
278. Hummel M, Standl E, Schnell O. Chromium in metabolic and cardiovascular disease. Horm Metab Res 2007;39:743-51.
279. Hung SC, Hung SH, Tarng DC, Yang WC, Chen TW, Huang TP. Thiamine deficiency and unexplained encephalopathy in hemodialysis and peritoneal dialysis patients. Am J Kidney Dis 2001;38:941-7.
280. Hunt CD. The biochemical effects of physiologic amounts of dietary boron in animal nutrition models. Environ Health Perspect 1994;102(Suppl 7):35-43.
281. Hunt JR, Mullen LM, Lykken GI, Gallagher SK, Nielsen FH. Ascorbic acid: effect on ongoing iron absorption and status in iron-depleted young women. Am J Clin Nutr 1990;51:649-55.
282. Hustad S, McKinley MC, McNulty H, Schneede J, Strain JJ, Scott JM, et al. Riboflavin, flavin mononucleotide, and flavin adenine dinucleotide in human plasma and erythrocytes at baseline and after low-dose riboflavin supplementation. Clin Chem 2002;48: 1571-7.
283. Ichiyanagi O, Sasagawa I, Adachi Y, Suzuki H, Kubota Y, Nakada T. Silica urolithiasis without magnesium trisilicate intake. Urol Int 1998;61:39-42.
284. Igic PG, Lee E, Harper W, Roach KW. Toxic effects associated with consumption of zinc. Mayo Clin Proc 2002;77:713-6.
285. Ikeda S, Sera Y, Yoshida M, Ohshiro H, Uchino S, Oka Y, et al. Manganese deposits in patients with biliary atresia after hepatic porto-enterostomy. J Pediatr Surg 2000;35:450-3.
286. Ingenbleek Y, Young VR. Significance of transthyretin in protein metabolism. Clin Chem Lab Med 2002;40:1281-91.
287. Innis WS, McCormick DB, Merrill AH Jr. Variations in riboflavin binding by human plasma: identification of immunoglobulins as the major proteins responsible. Biochem Med 1985;34:151-65.
288. Inoue K, Kito M, Kato S, Osawa M, Okuda H, Yabuta K, et al. A case of acquired zinc deficiency in a mature breast-fed infant. J Perinat Med 1998;26:495-7.
289. Itai K, Tsunoda H. Highly sensitive and rapid method for determination of fluoride ion concentrations in serum and urine using flow injection analysis with a fluoride ion-selective electrode. Clin Chim Acta 2001;308:163-71.
290. Ito MK. Niacin-based therapy for dyslipidemia: past evidence and future advances. Am J Manag Care 2002;8:S315-22.
291. Iversen BS, Menne C, White MA, Kristiansen J, Christensen JM, Sabbioni E. Inductively coupled plasma mass spectrometric determination of molybdenum in urine from a Danish population. Analyst 1998;123:81-5.
292. Iwaki M, Murakami E, Kakehi K. Chromatographic and capillary electrophoretic methods for the analysis of nicotinic acid and its metabolites. J Chromatogr B Biomed Sci Appl 2000;747:229-40.
293. Iwamoto J, Takeda T, Ichimura S. Effect of combined administration of vitamin D3 and vitamin K2 on bone mineral density of the lumbar spine in postmenopausal women with osteoporosis. J Orthop Sci 2000;5:546-51.

294. Jacob RA. Niacin. In: Bowman BA, Russell RM, eds. Present knowledge in nutrition. Washington, DC: ILSI Press, 2001:199-206.
295. Jacob RA, Sandstead HH, Munoz JM, Klevay LM, Milne DB. Whole body surface loss of trace metals in normal males. Am J Clin Nutr 1981;34:1379-83.
296. Jacob RA, Skala JH, Omaye ST. Biochemical indices of human vitamin C status. Am J Clin Nutr 1987;46:818-26.
297. Jacquamet L, Sun Y, Hatfield J, Gu W, Cramer SP, Crowder MW, et al. Characterization of chromodulin by X-ray absorption and electron paramagnetic resonance spectroscopies and magnetic susceptibility measurements. J Am Chem Soc 2003;125:774-80.
298. Jaffe IA. The antivitamin B6 effect of penicillamine: clinical and immunological implications. Adv Biochem Psychopharmacol 1972;4:217-26.
299. Jakob E, Elmadfa I. Rapid HPLC assay for the assessment of vitamin K1, A, E and beta-carotene status in children (7-19 years). Int J Vitam Nutr Res 1995;65:31-5.
300. Janssens K, Vincze L, Vekemans B, Williams CT, Radtke M, Haller M, et al. The non-destructive determination of REE in fossilized bone using synchrotron radiation induced K-line X-ray microfluorescence analysis. Fresenius J Anal Chem 1999;363:413-20.
301. Jeejeebhoy KN, Chu RC, Marliss EB, Greenberg GR, Bruce-Robertson A. Chromium deficiency, glucose intolerance, and neuropathy reversed by chromium supplementation, in a patient receiving long-term total parenteral nutrition. Am J Clin Nutr 1977;30:531-8.
302. Jialal I, Grundy SM. Effect of combined supplementation with alpha-tocopherol, ascorbate, and beta carotene on low-density lipoprotein oxidation. Circulation 1993;88:2780-6.
303. Jiang Q, Christen S, Shigenaga MK, Ames BN. Gamma-tocopherol, the major form of vitamin E in the US diet, deserves more attention. Am J Clin Nutr 2001;74:714-22.
304. Johnson JL. Molybdenum. In: O'Dell BL, Sunde RA, eds. Handbook of nutritionally essential mineral elements. New York/Basel/Hong Kong: Marcel Dekker, 1997:413-38.
305. Johnston CS. Vitamin C. In: Bowman BA, Russell RM, eds. Present knowledge in nutrition. Washington, DC: ILSI Press, 2001.
306. Jones PW, Taylor DM, Williams DR. Analysis and chemical speciation of copper and zinc in wound fluid. J Inorg Biochem 2000;81:1-10.
307. Jovani M, Alegria A, Barbera R, Farre R, Lagarda MJ, Clemente G. Effect of proteins, phytates, ascorbic acid and citric acid on dialysability of calcium, iron, zinc and copper in soy-based infant formulas. Nahrung 2000;44:114-7.
308. Jugdaohsingh R, Tucker KL, Qiao N, Cupples LA, Kiel DP, Powell JJ. Dietary silicon intake is positively associated with bone mineral density in men and premenopausal women of the Framingham Offspring cohort. J Bone Miner Res 2004;19:297-307.
309. Kaczmarek MJ, Nixon PF. Variants of transketolase from human erythrocytes. Clin Chim Acta 1983;130:349-56.
310. Kafritsa Y, Fell J, Long S, Bynevelt M, Taylor W, Milla P. Long-term outcome of brain manganese deposition in patients on home parenteral nutrition. Arch Dis Child 1998;79:263-5.
311. Kaler SG. Metabolic and molecular bases of Menkes disease and occipital horn syndrome. Pediatr Dev Pathol 1998;1:85-98.
312. Kallner A, Hartmann D, Hornig D. Steady-state turnover and body pool of ascorbic acid in man. Am J Clin Nutr 1979;32:530-9.
313. Kang JH, Cook NR, Manson JE, Buring JE, Albert CM, Grodstein F. Vitamin E, vitamin C, beta carotene, and cognitive function among women with or at risk of cardiovascular disease: the Women's Antioxidant and Cardiovascular Study. Circulation 2009;119:2772-80.
314. Kant AK, Block G. Dietary vitamin B-6 intake and food sources in the US population: NHANES II, 1976-1980. Am J Clin Nutr 1990;52:707-16.
315. Kanyo ZF, Scolnick LR, Ash DE, Christianson DW. Structure of a unique binuclear manganese cluster in arginase. Nature 1996;383:554-7.
316. Kaplan JH, Lutsenko S. Copper transport in mammalian cells: special care for a metal with special needs. J Biol Chem 2009;284:25461-5.
317. Kaplowitz T. Thiamin triphosphate synthesis in animals. In: Kobayashi T, ed. Proceedings of the 1st International Congress on Vitamins and Biofactors in Life Sciences. Tokyo: Centre for Academic Publications Japan, 1992:383-6.
318. Kappus H, Diplock AT. Tolerance and safety of vitamin E: a toxicological position report. Free Radic Biol Med 1992;13:55-74.
319. Kathman JV, Kies C. Pantothentic acid status of free living adolescents and young adults. Nutr Res 1984;4:245-50.
320. Kay RG, Tasman-Jones C, Pybus J, Whiting R, Black H. A syndrome of acute zinc deficiency during total parenteral alimentation in man. Ann Surg 1976;183:331-40.
321. Kelleher BP, Broin SD. Microbiological assay for vitamin B12 performed in 96-well microtitre plates. J Clin Pathol 1991;44:592-5.
322. Kelly DA, Coe AW, Shenkin A, Lake BD, Walker-Smith JA. Symptomatic selenium deficiency in a child on home parenteral nutrition. J Pediatr Gastroenterol Nutr 1988;7:783-6.
323. Ketley CE, Cochran JA, Lennon MA, O'Mullane DM, Worthington HV. Urinary fluoride excretion of young children exposed to different fluoride regimes. Community Dent Health 2002;19:12-7.
324. Kim YH, Kim EY, Gwag BJ, Sohn S, Koh JY. Zinc-induced cortical neuronal death with features of apoptosis and necrosis: mediation by free radicals. Neuroscience 1999;89:175-82.
325. King JC, Keen CL. Zinc. In: Shils ME, Olson JA, Shihe M, Ross AC, eds. Modern nutrition in health and disease. Baltimore, Md: Williams and Wilkins, 1999:223-39.
326. King JC, Shames DM, Lowe NM, Woodhouse LR, Sutherland B, Abrams SA, et al. Effect of acute zinc depletion on zinc homeostasis and plasma zinc kinetics in men. Am J Clin Nutr 2001;74:116-24.
327. King JC, Shames DM, Woodhouse LR. Zinc homeostasis in humans. J Nutr 2000;130:1360S-6S.
328. Kisker C, Schindelin H, Rees DC. Molybdenum-cofactor-containing enzymes: structure and mechanism. Annu Rev Biochem 1997;66:233-67.
329. Klein EA, Lippman SM, Thompson IM, Goodman PJ, Albanes D, Taylor PR, et al. The selenium and vitamin E cancer prevention trial. World J Urol 2003;21:21-7.
330. Klevay LM. Trace element and mineral nutrition in ischemic heart disease. In: Bogden JD, Klevay LM, eds. Clinical nutrition of the essential trace elements and minerals. Totowa, NJ: Humana Press, 2000:251-71.
331. Knasmuller S, Nersesyan A, Misik M, Gerner C, Mikulits W, Ehrlich V, et al. Use of conventional and -omics based methods for health claims of dietary antioxidants: a critical overview. Br J Nutr 2008;99 (E Suppl 1):ES3-52.
332. Knoblock E, Hodr R, Janda J, Herzmann J, Houdkova V. Spectrofluorimetric micromethod for determining riboflavin in the blood of newborn babies and their mothers. Int J Vitam Nutr Res 1979;49:144-51.
333. Köhrle J, Gärtner R. Selenium and thyroid. Best Pract Res Clin Endocrinol Metab 2009;23:815-27.
334. Konigsberger LC, Konigsberger E, May PM, Hefter GT. Complexation of iron(III) and iron(II) by citrate: implications for iron speciation in blood plasma. J Inorg Biochem 2000;78:175-84.
335. Konstantinides FN. Nitrogen balance studies in clinical nutrition. Nutr Clin Pract 1992;7:231-8.
336. Kordas K, Stoltzfus RJ. New evidence of iron and zinc interplay at the enterocyte and neural tissues. J Nutr 2004;134:1295-8.
337. Krasinski SD, Russell RM, Furie BC, Kruger SF, Jacques PF, Furie B. The prevalence of vitamin K deficiency in chronic gastrointestinal disorders. Am J Clin Nutr 1985;41:639-43.
338. Krumdieck CL, Fukushima K, Fukushima T, Shiota T, Butterworth CE Jr. A long-term study of the excretion of folate and pterins in a human subject after ingestion of 14C folic acid, with observations on the effect of diphenylhydantoin administration. Am J Clin Nutr 1978;31:88-93.
339. Kuller LH, Evans RW. Homocysteine, vitamins, and cardiovascular disease. Circulation 1998;98:196-9.
340. Kumar SS, Chouhan RS, Thakur MS. Trends in analysis of vitamin B12. Anal Biochem 2010;398:139-49.

341. Kupka R, Mugusi F, Aboud S, Msamanga GI, Finkelstein JL, Spiegelman D, et al. Randomized, double-blind, placebo-controlled trial of selenium supplements among HIV-infected pregnant women in Tanzania: effects on maternal and child outcomes. Am J Clin Nutr 2008;87:1802-8.
342. Laforenza U, Patrini C, Alvisi C, Faelli A, Licandro A, Rindi G. Thiamine uptake in human intestinal biopsy specimens, including observations from a patient with acute thiamine deficiency. Am J Clin Nutr 1997;66:320-6.
343. Lammer EJ, Chen DT, Hoar RM, Agnish ND, Benke PJ, Braun JT, et al. Retinoic acid embryopathy. N Engl J Med 1985;313:837-41.
344. Lane LA, Rojas-Fernandez C. Treatment of vitamin B(12)-deficiency anemia: oral versus parenteral therapy. Ann Pharmacother 2002;36: 1268-72.
345. Latunde-Dada GO, Simpson RJ, McKie AT. Recent advances in mammalian haem transport. Trends Biochem Sci 2006;31:182-8.
346. Lautier D, Lagueux J, Thibodeau J, Menard L, Poirier GG. Molecular and biochemical features of poly (ADP-ribose) metabolism. Mol Cell Biochem 1993;122:171-93.
347. Leach RM, Harris ED. Manganese. In: O'Dell BL, Sunde RA, eds. Handbook of nutritionally essential mineral elements. New York/ Basel/Hong Kong: Marcel Dekker, 1997.
348. Lee BJ, Lin PT, Liaw YP, Chang SJ, Cheng CH, Huang YC. Homocysteine and risk of coronary artery disease: folate is the important determinant of plasma homocysteine concentration. Nutrition 2003;19:577-83.
349. Lee SS, McCormick DB. Thyroid hormone regulation of flavocoenzyme biosynthesis. Arch Biochem Biophys 1985;237: 197-201.
350. Lee W, Roberts SM, Labbe RF. Ascorbic acid determination with an automated enzymatic procedure. Clin Chem 1997;43:154-7.
351. Leklem JE. Vitamin B6. In: Ziegler EE, Filer LJ, eds. Present knowledge in nutrition. Washington, DC: ILSI Press, 1996:174-83.
352. Lemineur T, Deby-Dupont G, Preiser JC. Biomarkers of oxidative stress in critically ill patients: what should be measured, when and how? Curr Opin Clin Nutr Metab Care 2006;9:704-10.
353. Leo MA, Lieber CS. Alcohol, vitamin A, and beta-carotene: adverse interactions, including hepatotoxicity and carcinogenicity. Am J Clin Nutr 1999;69:1071-85.
354. Leung FY, Galbraith LV. Elevated serum chromium in patients on total parenteral nutrition and the ionic species of contaminant chromium. Biol Trace Elem Res 1995;50:221-8.
355. Levander OA. Involvement of selenium in the regulation of viral virulence. ML Moxon Honorary Lectures, Special Circular, 2003: 167-99. Available at: ohioline.ag.ohio-state.edu/sc167/sc_08.
356. Levine M, Conry-Cantilena C, Wang Y, Welch RW, Washko PW, Dhariwal KR, et al. Vitamin C pharmacokinetics in healthy volunteers: evidence for a recommended dietary allowance. Proc Natl Acad Sci U S A 1996;93:3704-9.
357. Liang WJ, Johnson D, Jarvis SM. Vitamin C transport systems of mammalian cells. Mol Membr Biol 2001;18:87-95.
358. Lim TH, Sargent T III, Kusubov N. Kinetics of trace element chromium(III) in the human body. Am J Physiol 1983;244: R445-54.
359. Lindenbaum J, Allen RH. Clinical spectrum and diagnosis of folate deficiency. In: Bailey LB, ed. Folate in health and disease. New York: Marcel Dekker, 1995:43-74.
360. Lindenbaum J, Rosenberg IH, Wilson PW, Stabler SP, Allen RH. Prevalence of cobalamin deficiency in the Framingham elderly population. Am J Clin Nutr 1994;60:2-11.
361. Linder MC. Copper and genomic stability in mammals. Mutat Res 2001;475:141-52.
362. Lippman SM, Klein EA, Goodman PJ, Lucia MS, Thompson IM, Ford LG, et al. Effect of selenium and vitamin E on risk of prostate cancer and other cancers: the Selenium and Vitamin E Cancer Prevention Trial (SELECT). JAMA 2009;301:39-51.
363. Liuzzi JP, Cousins RJ. Mammalian zinc transporters. Annu Rev Nutr 2004;24:151-72.
364. Lockitch G, Fasset JD, Gerson B, et al. Control of preanalytical variation in trace element determinations. Approved Guideline NCCLS 1997;17:1-30.
365. Lockitch G, Halstead AC, Wadsworth L, Quigley G, Reston L, Jacobson B. Age- and sex-specific pediatric reference intervals and correlations for zinc, copper, selenium, iron, vitamins A and E, and related proteins. Clin Chem 1988;34:1625-8.
366. Loerch JD, Underwood BA, Lewis KC. Response of plasma levels of vitamin A to a dose of vitamin A as an indicator of hepatic vitamin A reserves in rats. J Nutr 1979;109:778-86.
367. Loikas S, Lopponen M, Suominen P, Moller J, Irjala K, Isoaho R, et al. RIA for serum holo-transcobalamin: method evaluation in the clinical laboratory and reference interval. Clin Chem 2003;49:455-62.
368. Lombeck I, Wendel U, Versieck J, van Ballenberghe L, Bremer HJ, Duran R, et al. Increased manganese content and reduced arginase activity in erythrocytes of a patient with prolidase deficiency (iminodipeptiduria). Eur J Pediatr 1986;144:571-3.
369. Longnecker MP, Stampfer MJ, Morris JS, Spate V, Baskett C, Mason M, et al. A 1-y trial of the effect of high-selenium bread on selenium concentrations in blood and toenails. Am J Clin Nutr 1993;57: 408-13.
370. Lonnerdal B. Copper nutrition during infancy and childhood. Am J Clin Nutr 1998;67:1046S-53S.
371. Lopes I, Marques L, Neves E, Silva A, Taveira M, Pena R, et al. Prolidase deficiency with hyperimmunoglobulin E: a case report. Pediatr Allergy Immunol 2002;13:140-2.
372. Louw JA, Werbeck A, Louw ME, Kotze TJ, Cooper R, Labadarios D. Blood vitamin concentrations during the acute-phase response. Crit Care Med 1992;20:934-41.
373. Lowe NM, Fekete K, Decsi T. Methods of assessment of zinc status in humans: a systematic review. Am J Clin Nutr 2009;89:2040S-51S.
374. Lowe NM, Woodhouse LR, Matel JS, King JC. Comparison of estimates of zinc absorption in humans by using 4 stable isotopic tracer methods and compartmental analysis. Am J Clin Nutr 2000;71:523-9.
375. Lu J, Frank EL. Rapid HPLC measurement of thiamine and its phosphate esters in whole blood. Clin Chem 2008;54:901-6.
376. Ludwig ML, Matthews RG. Structure-based perspectives on B12-dependent enzymes. Annu Rev Biochem 1997;66:269-313.
377. Luo G, Ducy P, McKee MD, Pinero GJ, Loyer E, Behringer RR, Karsenty G. Spontaneous calcification of arteries and cartilage in mice lacking matrix GLA protein. Nature 1997;386:78-81.
378. Lykkesfeldt J, Christen S, Wallock LM, Chang HH, Jacob RA, Ames BN. Ascorbate is depleted by smoking and repleted by moderate supplementation: a study in male smokers and nonsmokers with matched dietary antioxidant intakes. Am J Clin Nutr 2000;71:530-6.
379. Lyon TD, Fell GS, Gaffney D, McGaw BA, Russell RI, Park RH, et al. Use of a stable copper isotope (65Cu) in the differential diagnosis of Wilson's disease. Clin Sci (Lond) 1995;88:727-32.
380. Ma J, Betts NM. Zinc and copper intakes and their major food sources for older adults in the 1994-96 continuing survey of food intakes by individuals (CSFII). J Nutr 2000;130:2838-43.
381. Machonkin TE, Zhang HH, Hedman B, Hodgson KO, Solomon EI. Spectroscopic and magnetic studies of human ceruloplasmin: identification of a redox-inactive reduced Type 1 copper site. Biochemistry 1998;37:9570-8.
382. Maezawa K, Nozawa M, Yuasa T, Aritomi K, Matsuda K, Shitoto K. Seven years of chronological changes of serum chromium levels after Metasul metal-on-metal total hip arthroplasty. J Arthroplasty 2010;25: 1196-200.
383. Malo C, Wilson JX. Glucose modulates vitamin C transport in adult human small intestinal brush border membrane vesicles. J Nutr 2000;130:63-9.
384. Mandl J, Szarka A, Banhegyi G. Vitamin C: update on physiology and pharmacology. Br J Pharmacol 2009;157:1097-110.
385. Mangels AR, Holden JM, Beecher GR, Forman MR, Lanza E. Carotenoid content of fruits and vegetables: an evaluation of analytical data. J Am Diet Assoc 1993;93:284-9.

386. Margolis SA, Paule RC, Ziegler RG. Ascorbic and dehydroascorbic acids measured in plasma preserved with dithiothreitol or metaphosphoric acid. Clin Chem 1990;36:1750-5.
387. Marrill J, Idres N, Capron CC, Nguyen E, Chabot GG. Retinoic acid metabolism and mechanism of action: a review. Curr Drug Metab 2003;93:284-9.
388. Marshall I. Zinc for the common cold (Cochrane Review). In: The Cochrane Library. Oxford: Update Software, 2003:4.
389. Marti-Carvajal AJ, Sola I, Lathyris D, Salanti G. Homocysteine lowering interventions for preventing cardiovascular events. Cochrane Database Syst Rev 2009;CD006612.
390. Martin BJ, Lyon TD, Fell GS. Comparison of inorganic elements from autopsy tissue of young and elderly subjects. J Trace Elem Electrolytes Health Dis 1991;5:203-11.
391. Mason JB. Intestinal transport of monoglutamyl folates in mammalian systems. In: Picciano MF, Stokstad ELR, Gregory JF, eds. Folic acid metabolism in health and disease. New York: Wiley-Liss, 1990:47-64.
392. Massey V. The chemical and biological versatility of riboflavin. Biochem Soc Trans 2000;28:283-96.
393. Matherly LH, Goldman DI. Membrane transport of folates. Vitam Horm 2003;66:403-56.
394. May TW, Wiedmeyer RH. A table of polyatomic interferences in ICP-MS. Atomic Spectroscopy 1998;19:150-5.
395. Mayne ST. Beta-carotene, carotenoids, and disease prevention in humans. FASEB J 1996;10:690-701.
396. McCall KA, Huang C, Fierke CA. Function and mechanism of zinc metalloenzymes. J Nutr 2000;130:1437S-46S.
397. McCormick DB. Biochemistry of coenzymes. In: Meyers RA, ed. Encyclopedia of molecular biology and molecular medicine. New York: Wiley-VCH, 1996:396-406.
398. McCormick DB. Biochemistry of coenzymes: pantothenic acid. In: Meyers RA, ed. Encyclopedia of molecular biology and molecular medicine. New York: Wiley-VC, 1996:390-395.
399. McCormick DB. Biochemistry of coenzymes: pyridoxine B6. In: Meyers RA, ed. Encyclopedia of molecular biology and molecular medicine. New York: Wiley-VCH, 1996:396-406.
400. McCormick DB. Riboflavin. In: Shils ME, Olson JA, Shihe M, Ross AC, eds. Modern nutrition in health and disease. Baltimore, Md: Williams and Wilkins, 1999:391-9.
401. McCormick DB. Vitamin B6. In: Bowman BA, Russell RA, eds. Present knowledge in nutrition. Washington, DC: ILSI Press, 2001:207-13.
402. McCormick DB, Snell BA. Pyridoxal phosphokinases: II. Effect of inhibitors. J Biol Chem 1961;236:2085-8.
403. McCormick DB, Wright LD. Vitamins and coenzyme: methods in enzymology. New York: Academic Press Inc, 1980:part F.
404. McMahon RJ. Biotin in metabolism and molecular biology. Annu Rev Nutr 2002;22:221-39.
405. McMillin GA, Travis JJ, Hunt JW. Direct measurement of free copper in serum or plasma ultrafiltrate. Am J Clin Pathol 2009;131:160-5.
406. Mehansho H, Henderson LM. Transport and accumulation of pyridoxine and pyridoxal by erythrocytes. J Biol Chem 1980;255: 11901-7.
407. Mehdi MZ, Pandey SK, Theberge JF, Srivastava AK. Insulin signal mimicry as a mechanism for the insulin-like effects of vanadium. Cell Biochem Biophys 2006;44:73-81.
408. Melhus H, Michaelsson K, Kindmark A, Bergstrom R, Holmberg L, Mallmin H, et al. Excessive dietary intake of vitamin A is associated with reduced bone mineral density and increased risk for hip fracture. Ann Intern Med 1998;129:770-8.
409. Mendel RR. Cell biology of molybdenum. Biofactors 2009;35:429-34.
410. Mertz W. Trace minerals and atherosclerosis. Fed Proc 1982;41:2807-12.
411. Mertz W. Use and misuse of balance studies. J Nutr 1987;117:1811-3.
412. Mertz W. Chromium research from a distance: from 1959 to 1980. J Am Coll Nutr 1998;17:544-7.
413. Mertz W. Interaction of chromium with insulin: a progress report. Nutr Rev 1998;56:174-7.
414. Meurs H, Maarsingh H, Zaagsma J. Arginase and asthma: novel insights into nitric oxide homeostasis and airway hyperresponsiveness. Trends Pharmacol Sci 2003;24:450-5.
415. Mewies M, McIntire WS, Scrutton NS. Covalent attachment of flavin adenine dinucleotide (FAD) and flavin mononucleotide (FMN) to enzymes: the current state of affairs. Protein Sci 1998;7:7-20.
416. Meydani M. Vitamin E. Lancet 1995;345:170-5.
417. Meyer JA, Spence DM. A perspective on the role of metals in diabetes: past findings and possible future directions. Metallomics 2010;1: 32-42.
418. Michalke B, Berthele A, Mistriotis P, Ochsenkuhn-Petropoulou M, Halbach S. Manganese speciation in human cerebrospinal fluid using CZE coupled to inductively coupled plasma MS. Electrophoresis 2007;28:1380-6.
419. Midttun O, Hustad S, Schneede J, Vollset SE, Ueland PM. Plasma vitamin B-6 forms and their relation to transsulfuration metabolites in a large, population-based study. Am J Clin Nutr 2007;86:131-8.
420. Millart H, Lamiable D. Determination of pyridoxal 5′-phosphate in human serum by reversed phase high performance liquid chromatography combined with spectrofluorimetric detection of 4-pyridoxic acid 5′-phosphate as a derivative. Analyst 1989;114:1225-8.
421. Miller JW, Rogers LM, Rucker RB. Pantothentic acid. In: Bowman BA, Russell RA, eds. Present knowledge in nutrition. Washington, DC: ILSI Press, 2001:253-60.
422. Miller NJ, Johnston JD, Collis CS, Rice-Evans C. Serum total antioxidant activity after myocardial infarction. Ann Clin Biochem 1997;34(Pt 1):85-90.
423. Milne DB. Laboratory assessment of trace elements and mineral status. In: Bogden JD, Klevay LM, eds. Laboratory assessment of trace elements and minerals. Totawa, NJ: Humana Press, 2000:69-90.
424. Milne DB, Nielsen FH. Effects of a diet low in copper on copper-status indicators in postmenopausal women. Am J Clin Nutr 1996; 63:358-64.
425. Milne DB, Ralston NV, Wallwork JC. Zinc content of cellular components of blood: methods for cell separation and analysis evaluated. Clin Chem 1985;31:65-9.
426. Mineral Analysis Laboratory Grand Forks Human Nutrition Center, 2003. Available at: www.gfhnrc.ars.usda.gov.
427. Mishra V, Baines M, Perry SE, McLaughlin PJ, Carson J, Wenstone R, et al. Effect of selenium supplementation on biochemical markers and outcome in critically ill patients. Clin Nutr 2007;26:41-50.
428. Moat SJ, Ashfield-Watt PA, Powers HJ, Newcombe RG, McDowell IF. Effect of riboflavin status on the homocysteine-lowering effect of folate in relation to the MTHFR (C677T) genotype. Clin Chem 2003;49:295-302.
429. Mocchegiani E, Malavolta M. Zinc dyshomeostasis, ageing and neurodegeneration: implications of A2M and inflammatory gene polymorphisms. J Alzheimers Dis 2007;12:101-9.
430. Mock DM, Mock NI. Lymphocyte propionyl-CoA carboxylase is an early and sensitive indicator of biotin deficiency in rats, but urinary excretion of 3-hydroxypropionic acid is not. J Nutr 2002;132:1945-50.
431. Mock DM, Quirk JG, Mock NI. Marginal biotin deficiency during normal pregnancy. Am J Clin Nutr 2002;75:295-9.
432. Mock NI, Malik MI, Stumbo PJ, Bishop WP, Mock DM. Increased urinary excretion of 3-hydroxyisovaleric acid and decreased urinary excretion of biotin are sensitive early indicators of decreased biotin status in experimental biotin deficiency. Am J Clin Nutr 1997;65:951-8.
433. Montrone M, Martorelli D, Rosato A, Dolcetti R. Retinoids as critical modulators of immune functions: new therapeutic perspectives for old compounds. Endocr Metab Immune Disord Drug Targets 2009;9:113-31.
434. Moon YS, Kashyap ML. Niacin extended-release/lovastatin: combination therapy for lipid disorders. Expert Opin Pharmacother 2002;3:1763-71.
435. Morris MS. Folate, homocysteine, and neurological function. Nutr Clin Care 2002;5:124-32.

436. Moshtaghie AA, Badii A, Hassanzadeh MFT, Kharazi H. Manganese and iron binding to human transferrin. Iranian J Pharmaceut Res 2010;6:101-6.
437. Mrochek JE, Jolley RL, Young DS, Turner WJ. Metabolic response of humans to ingestion of nicotinic acid and nicotinamide. Clin Chem 1976;22:1821-7.
438. Muller DP, Lloyd JK. Effect of large oral doses of vitamin E on the neurological sequelae of patients with abetalipoproteinemia. Ann N Y Acad Sci 1982;393:133-44.
439. Muller T, Koppikar S, Taylor RM, Carragher F, Schlenck B, Heinz-Erian P, et al. Re-evaluation of the penicillamine challenge test in the diagnosis of Wilson's disease in children. J Hepatol 2007;47:270-6.
440. Muller T, Muller W, Feichtinger H. Idiopathic copper toxicosis. Am J Clin Nutr 1998;67:1082S-6S.
441. Munday R, Smith BL, Munday CM. Effects of butylated hydroxyanisole and dicumarol on the toxicity of menadione to rats. Chem Biol Interact 1998;108:155-70.
442. Musilkova J, Kriegerbeckova K, Krusek J, Kovar J. Specific binding to plasma membrane is the first step in the uptake of non-transferrin iron by cultured cells. Biochim Biophys Acta 1998;1369:103-8.
443. Naito E, Ito M, Yokota I, Saijo T, Matsuda J, Ogawa Y, et al. Thiamine-responsive pyruvate dehydrogenase deficiency in two patients caused by a point mutation (F205L and L216F) within the thiamine pyrophosphate binding region. Biochim Biophys Acta 2002;1588:79-84.
444. Nakasaki H, Ohta M, Soeda J, Makuuchi H, Tsuda M, Tajima T, et al. Clinical and biochemical aspects of thiamine treatment for metabolic acidosis during total parenteral nutrition. Nutrition 1997;13:110-7.
445. Napoli JL. A gene knockout corroborates the integral function of cellular retinol-binding protein in retinoid metabolism. Nutr Rev 2000;58:230-6.
446. National Research Council. Recommended dietary allowances, 10th edition. Washington, DC: National Academy of Sciences, 1989.
447. Neal RA. Vitamin deficiencies: thiamin. In: Hansen RG, Munro HN, eds. National Institute of Health Proceedings of Workshop on Problems of Assessment and Alleviation of Malnutrition in the United States, 1970, Nashville, Tenn.
448. Neggers YH, Goldenberg RL, Tamura T, Johnston KE, Copper RL, DuBard M. Plasma and erythrocyte zinc concentrations and their relationship to dietary zinc intake and zinc supplementation during pregnancy in low-income African-American women. J Am Diet Assoc 1997;97:1269-74.
449. Nelsestuen GL, Shah AM, Harvey SB. Vitamin K-dependent proteins. Vitam Horm 2000;58:355-89.
450. Nelson M. Methods and validity of dietary assessment. In: Garrow JS, James WPT, Ralph A, eds. Human nutrition and dietetics. Edinburgh: Churchill Livingstone, 2000:311-31.
451. Nelson HK, Shi Q, Van Dael P, Schiffrin EJ, Blum S, Barclay D, et al. Host nutritional selenium status as a driving force for influenza virus mutations. FASEB J 2001;15:1846-8.
452. Neufeld EJ, Fleming JC, Tartaglini E, Steinkamp MP. Thiamine-responsive megaloblastic anemia syndrome: a disorder of high-affinity thiamine transport. Blood Cells Mol Dis 2001;27:135-8.
453. Nexo E, Christensen AL, Hvas AM, Petersen TE, Fedosov SN. Quantification of holo-transcobalamin, a marker of vitamin B12 deficiency. Clin Chem 2002;48:561-2.
454. Nichol C, Herdman J, Sattar N, O'Dwyer PJ, St J, O'Reilly D, Littlejohn D, et al. Changes in the concentrations of plasma selenium and selenoproteins after minor elective surgery: further evidence for a negative acute phase response? Clin Chem 1998;44:1764-6.
455. Nielsen FH. Possibly essential trace elements. In: Bogden JD, Klevay LM, eds. Clinical nutrition of the essential trace elements and minerals. Totawa, NJ: Humana Press, 2000:11-36.
456. Nielsen FH. Is boron nutritionally relevant? Nutr Rev 2008;66:183-91.
457. Nielsen FH. Micronutrients in parenteral nutrition: boron, silicon, and fluoride. Gastroenterology 2009;137:S55-60.
458. Niles RM. Recent advances in the use of vitamin A (retinoids) in the prevention and treatment of cancer. Nutrition 2000;16:1084-9.
459. Ninh NX, Thissen JP, Collette L, Gerard G, Khoi HH, Ketelslegers JM. Zinc supplementation increases growth and circulating insulin-like growth factor I (IGF-I) in growth-retarded Vietnamese children. Am J Clin Nutr 1996;63:514-9.
460. Norose N, Terai M, Norose K. Manganese deficiency in a child with very short bowel syndrome receiving long-term parenteral nutrition. J Trace Elem Exp Med 1992;5:100-1.
461. Novotny JA, Dueker SR, Zech LA. Compartmental analysis of the dynamics of B-carotene metabolism in an adult volunteer. J Lipid Res 1995;36:1825-38.
462. Nutrient Requirements and Functions Laboratory Beltsville Agriculture Research Centre, 2003. Available at: www.barc.usda.gov/bhnrc/nrfl/nrflres.html.
463. Nuttall KL. Evaluating selenium poisoning. Ann Clin Lab Sci 2006;36:409-20.
464. Nyyssonen K, Parviainen MT, Salonen R, Tuomilehto J, Salonen JT. Vitamin C deficiency and risk of myocardial infarction: prospective population study of men from eastern Finland. BMJ 1997;314:634-8.
465. O'Brien KO, Zavaleta N, Caulfield LE, Wen J, Abrams SA. Prenatal iron supplements impair zinc absorption in pregnant Peruvian women. J Nutr 2000;130:2251-5.
466. O'Broin S, Kelleher B. Microbiological assay on microtitre plates of folate in serum and red cells. J Clin Pathol 1992;45:344-7.
467. O'Dell BL, Sunde RA. Handbook of nutritionally essential minerals. New York/Basel/Hong Kong: Marcel Dekker, 1997.
468. O'Donnell JG, Watson ID, Fell GS, Allison ME, Russell RI, Mills PR. Wilson's disease presenting as acute fulminant hepatic failure. Scott Med J 1990;35:118-9.
469. O'Flaherty EJ, Kerger BD, Hays SM, Paustenbach DJ. A physiologically based model for the ingestion of chromium(III) and chromium(VI) by humans. Toxicol Sci 2001;60:196-213.
470. O'Neill MA, Warrenfeltz D, Kates K, Pellerin P, Doco T, Darvill AG, et al. Rhamnogalacturonan-II, a pectic polysaccharide in the walls of growing plant cell, forms a dimer that is covalently cross-linked by a borate ester: in vitro conditions for the formation and hydrolysis of the dimer. J Biol Chem 1996;271:22923-30.
471. Offenbacker GE, Xavier P-S, Stoecker BJ. Chromium. In: O'Dell BL, Sunde RA, eds. Handbook of nutritionally essential mineral elements. New York/Basel/Hong Kong: Marcel Dekker, 1997:389-412.
472. Ogle RF, Christodoulou J, Fagan E, Blok RB, Kirby DM, Seller KL, et al. Mitochondrial myopathy with tRNA(Leu(UUR)) mutation and complex I deficiency responsive to riboflavin. J Pediatr 1997;130:138-45.
473. Olson RE. The function and metabolism of vitamin K. Annu Rev Nutr 1984;4:281-337.
474. Omenn GS, Goodman GE, Thornquist MD, Balmes J, Cullen MR, Glass A, et al. Effects of a combination of beta carotene and vitamin A on lung cancer and cardiovascular disease. N Engl J Med 1996;334:1150-5.
475. Ono J, Harada K, Kodaka R, Sakurai K, Tajiri H, Takagi Y, et al. Manganese deposition in the brain during long-term total parenteral nutrition. JPEN J Parenter Enteral Nutr 1995;19:310-2.
476. Ordonez YN, Bontes-Byron M, Blanco-Gonsolaz E, Paz-Jimenrez J, Tejerina-Lobo JM, Pena-Lopez JM, et al. Metal release in patients with total hip arthroplasty by DF-ICP-MS and their association with serum proteins. J Anal Atom Spectros 2009;24:1037-43.
477. Osendarp SJ, West CE, Black RE. The need for maternal zinc supplementation in developing countries: an unresolved issue. J Nutr 2003;133:817S-27S.
478. Ottaway JM, Halls DJ. Determination of manganese in biological materials. Pure Appl Chem 1986;1307-16.
479. Owen WE, Roberts WL. Comparison of five automated serum and whole blood folate assays. Am J Clin Pathol 2003;120:121-6.
480. Palmiter RD. Protection against zinc toxicity by metallothionein and zinc transporter 1. Proc Natl Acad Sci U S A 2004;101:4918-23.
481. Pan Q, Kleer CG, van Golen KL, Irani J, Bottema KM, Bias C, et al. Copper deficiency induced by tetrathiomolybdate suppresses tumor growth and angiogenesis. Cancer Res 2002;62:4854-9.

482. Parry R, Plowman D, Delves HT, Roberts NB, Birchall JD, Bellia JP, et al. Silicon and aluminium interactions in haemodialysis patients. Nephrol Dial Transplant 1998;13:1759-62.
483. Patterson KY, Veillon C. Stable isotopes of minerals as metabolic tracers in human nutrition research. Exp Biol Med (Maywood) 2001;226:271-82.
484. Pelliccione N, Pinto J, Huang YP, Rivlin RS. Accelerated development of riboflavin deficiency by treatment with chlorpromazine. Biochem Pharmacol 1983;32:2949-53.
485. Penniston KL, Tanumihardjo SA. The acute and chronic toxic effects of vitamin A. Am J Clin Nutr 2006;83:191-201.
486. Perez-Ruiz T, Martinez-Lozano C, Sanz A, Bravo E. Determination of riboflavin, flavin mononucleotide and flavin adenine dinucleotide in biological tissues by capillary zone electrophoresis and laser-induced fluorescence detection. Electrophoresis 2001;22:1170-4.
487. Persson B, Tunell R, Ekengren K. Chronic vitamin A intoxication during the first half year of life. Acta Paediatr Scand 1965;54:49-60.
488. Pfeiffer CM, Caudill SP, Gunter EW, Osterloh J, Sampson EJ. Biochemical indicators of B vitamin status in the US population after folic acid fortification: results from the National Health and Nutrition Examination Survey 1999-2000. Am J Clin Nutr 2005; 82:442-50.
489. Pietinen P, Vartiainen E, Seppanen R, Aro A, Puska P. Changes in diet in Finland from 1972 to 1992: impact on coronary heart disease risk. Prev Med 1996;25:243-50.
490. Pinto J, Huang YP, Rivlin RS. Mechanisms underlying the differential effects of ethanol on the bioavailability of riboflavin and flavin adenine dinucleotide. J Clin Invest 1987;79:1343-8.
491. Pizzulli A, Ranjbar A. Selenium deficiency and hypothyroidism: a new etiology in the differential diagnosis of hypothyroidism in children. Biol Trace Elem Res 2000;77:199-208.
492. Plesofsky-Vig N. Pantothentic acid. In: Shils ME, Olson JA, Shihe M, Ross AC, eds. Modern nutrition in health and disease. Baltimore, Md: Williams and Wilkins, 1999:423-32.
493. Podmore ID, Griffiths HR, Herbert KE, Mistry N, Mistry P, Lunec J. Vitamin C exhibits pro-oxidant properties. Nature 1998;392:559.
494. Pogribny I, Yi P, James SJ. A sensitive new method for rapid detection of abnormal methylation patterns in global DNA and within CpG islands. Biochem Biophys Res Commun 1999;262:624-8.
495. Powers HJ, Hill MH, Welfare M, Spiers A, Bal W, Russell J, et al. Responses of biomarkers of folate and riboflavin status to folate and riboflavin supplementation in healthy and colorectal polyp patients (the FAB2 Study). Cancer Epidemiol Biomarkers Prev 2007;16: 2128-35.
496. Prasad AS. Effects of zinc deficiency on immune functions. J Trace Elements Exp Med 2000;13:1-20.
497. Prasad AS. Zinc deficiency in patients with sickle cell disease. Am J Clin Nutr 2002;75:181-2.
498. Prasad AS. Zinc deficiency. BMJ 2003;326:409-10.
499. Prasad AS, Mantzoros CS, Beck FW, Hess JW, Brewer GJ. Zinc status and serum testosterone levels of healthy adults. Nutrition 1996;12:344-8.
500. Prasad PD, Ganapathy V. Structure and function of mammalian sodium-dependent multivitamin transporter. Curr Opin Clin Nutr Metab Care 2000;3:263-6.
501. Prentice AM, Bates CJ, Prentice A, Welch SG, Williams K, McGregor IA. The influence of G-6-PD activity on the response of erythrocyte glutathione reductase to riboflavin deficiency. Int J Vitam Nutr Res 1981;51:211-5.
502. Price Evans DA, Tariq M, Dafterdar R, Al Hussaini H, Sobki SH. Chromium chloride administration causes a substantial reduction of coronary lipid deposits, aortic lipid deposits, and serum cholesterol concentration in rabbits. Biol Trace Elem Res 2009;130:262-72.
503. Prior RL, Cao G. In vivo total antioxidant capacity: comparison of different analytical methods. Free Radic Biol Med 1999;27:1173-81.
504. Pruszkowski E, Neubauer K, Thomas R. An overview of clinical applications by inductively coupled plasma mass spectrometry. Atom Spectros 1998;19:115.
505. Puxty JA, Haskew AE, Ratcliffe JG, McMurray J. Changes in erythrocyte transketolase activity and the thiamine pyrophosphate effect during storage of blood. Ann Clin Biochem 1985;22(Pt 4): 423-7.
506. Quasim T, McMillan DC, Talwar D, Vasilaki A, St JO, Kinsella J. The relationship between plasma and red cell B-vitamin concentrations in critically-ill patients. Clin Nutr 2005;24:956-60.
507. Rahil-Khazen R, Henriksen H, Bolann BJ, Ulvik RJ. Validation of inductively coupled plasma atomic emission spectrometry technique (ICP-AES) for multi-element analysis of trace elements in human serum. Scand J Clin Lab Invest 2000;60:677-86.
508. Rahman MM, Vermund SH, Wahed MA, Fuchs GJ, Baqui AH, Alvarez JO. Simultaneous zinc and vitamin A supplementation in Bangladeshi children: randomised double blind controlled trial. BMJ 2001;323:314-8.
509. Rahman MM, Wahed MA, Fuchs GJ, Baqui AH, Alvarez JO. Synergistic effect of zinc and vitamin A on the biochemical indexes of vitamin A nutrition in children. Am J Clin Nutr 2002;75:92-8.
510. Raiten DJ, Fisher KD. Assessment of folate methodology used in the Third National Health and Nutrition Examination Survey (NHANES III, 1988-1994). J Nutr 1995;125:1371S-98S.
511. Rayman MP. The importance of selenium to human health. Lancet 2000;356:233-41.
512. Rayman MP, Thompson AJ, Bekaert B, Catterick J, Galassini R, Hall E, et al. Randomized controlled trial of the effect of selenium supplementation on thyroid function in the elderly in the United Kingdom. Am J Clin Nutr 2008;87:370-8.
513. Reeder RJ, Schoonen MAA, Lanzirotti A. Metal speciation in bioaccessibility and bioavailability. Rev Miner Geochem 2006;64: 59-113.
514. Refsum H, Smith AD. Homocysteine, B vitamins, and cardiovascular disease. N Engl J Med 2006;355:207-11.
515. Reiss J. Genetics of molybdenum cofactor deficiency. Hum Genet 2000;106:157-63.
516. Reiss J, Johnson JL. Mutations in the molybdenum cofactor biosynthetic genes MOCS1, MOCS2, and GEPH. Hum Mutat 2003;21:569-76.
517. Reports of the Scientific Committee for Food, Commission of the European Communities. 31st Series, 1992. Office for Official Publications of the European Communities, Luxembourg.
518. Reynolds RD. Nationwide assay of vitamin B6 in human plasma by different methods. Fed Proc 1983;42:665.
519. Riales R, Albrink MJ. Effect of chromium chloride supplementation on glucose tolerance and serum lipids including high-density lipoprotein of adult men. Am J Clin Nutr 1981;34:2670-8.
520. Ribaya-Mercado JD, Solon FS, Dallal GE, Solomons NW, Fermin LS, Mazariegos M, et al. Quantitative assessment of total body stores of vitamin A in adults with the use of a 3-d deuterated-retinol-dilution procedure. Am J Clin Nutr 2003;77:694-9.
521. Ricciarelli R, Zingg JM, Azzi A. The 80th anniversary of vitamin E: beyond its antioxidant properties. Biol Chem 2002;383:457-65.
522. Rindi G, Laforenza U. Thiamine intestinal transport and related issues: recent aspects. Proc Soc Exp Biol Med 2000;224:246-55.
523. Rink L, Haase H. Zinc homeostasis and immunity. Trends Immunol 2007;28:1-4.
524. Rivlin RS. Riboflavin. In: Bowman BA, Russell RM, eds. Present knowledge in nutrition. Washington, DC: ILSI Press, 2001:191-8.
525. Robbins JM, Tilford JM, Bird TM, Cleves MA, Reading JA, Hobbs CA. Hospitalizations of newborns with folate-sensitive birth defects before and after fortification of foods with folic acid. Pediatrics 2006;118:906-15.
526. Robien K, Ulrich CM. 5,10-Methylenetetrahydrofolate reductase polymorphisms and leukemia risk: a HuGE minireview. Am J Epidemiol 2003;157:571-82.
527. Rodriguez MR. [Importance of water-soluble vitamins as regulatory factors of genetic expression]. Rev Invest Clin 2002;54:77-83.
528. Roe DA. A plague of corn. Ithaca, NY: Cornell University Press, 1973.

529. Rogers JT, Bridges KR, Durmowicz GP, Glass J, Auron PE, Munro HN. Translational control during the acute phase response: ferritin synthesis in response to interleukin-1. J Biol Chem 1990;265:14572-8.
530. Rosenberg LE. Vitamin-responsive inherited diseases affecting the nervous system. Res Publ Assoc Res Nerv Ment Dis 1974;53:263-72.
531. Rossander-Hulten L, Brune M, Sandstrom B, Lonnerdal B, Hallberg L. Competitive inhibition of iron absorption by manganese and zinc in humans. Am J Clin Nutr 1991;54:152-6.
532. Rothman KJ, Moore LL, Singer MR, Nguyen US, Mannino S, Milunsky A. Teratogenicity of high vitamin A intake. N Engl J Med 1995;333:1369-73.
533. Roughead ZK, McCormick DB. Flavin composition of human milk. Am J Clin Nutr 1990;52:854-7.
534. Roughead ZK, McCormick DB. Qualitative and quantitative assessment of flavins in cow's milk. J Nutr 1990;120:382-8.
535. Rubin MA, Miller JP, Ryan AS, Treuth MS, Patterson KY, Pratley RE, et al. Acute and chronic resistive exercise increase urinary chromium excretion in men as measured with an enriched chromium stable isotope. J Nutr 1998;128:73-8.
536. Rumsey SC, Levine M. Absorption, transport and disposition of ascorbic acid in humans. J Nutr Biochem 1998;9:116-30.
537. Russell RM. The vitamin A spectrum: from deficiency to toxicity. Am J Clin Nutr 2000;71:878-84.
538. Russell-Jones GJ, Alpers DH. Vitamin B12 transporters. Pharm Biotechnol 1999;12:493-520.
539. Ryan GJ, Wanko NS, Redman AR, Cook CB. Chromium as adjunctive treatment for type 2 diabetes. Ann Pharmacother 2003;37:876-85.
540. Rychlik M. Quantification of free and bound pantothentic acid in foods and blood plasma by a stable isotope dilution assay. J Agric Food Chem 2000;48:1175-81.
541. Said HM. Biotin: the forgotten vitamin. Am J Clin Nutr 2002;75: 179-80.
542. Said HM. Recent advances in carrier-mediated intestinal absorption of water-soluble vitamins. Annu Rev Physiol 2004;66:419-46.
543. Said HM, Ma TY. Mechanism of riboflavin uptake by CaCo-2 human intestinal epithelial cells. Am J Physiol 1994;266:G15-G21.
544. Saito Y, Watanabe Y, Saito E, Honjoh T, Takahashi K. Production and application of monoclonal antibodies to human selenoprotein P. J Health Sci 2001;47:346-52.
545. Sallie R, Katsiyiannakis L, Baldwin D, Davies S, O'Grady J, Mowat A, et al. Failure of simple biochemical indexes to reliably differentiate fulminant Wilson's disease from other causes of fulminant liver failure. Hepatology 1992;16:1206-11.
546. Sampson B, Fagerhol MK, Sunderkotter C, Golden BE, Richmond P, Klein N, et al. Hyperzincaemia and hypercalprotectinaemia: a new disorder of zinc metabolism. Lancet 2002;360:1742-5.
547. Sanderson P, McNulty H, Mastroiacovo P, McDowell IF, Melse-Boonstra A, Finglas PM, et al. Folate bioavailability: UK Food Standards Agency workshop report. Br J Nutr 2003;90:473-9.
548. Sandstead HH, Frederickson CJ, Penland JG. History of zinc as related to brain function. J Nutr 2000;130:496S-502S.
549. SAS Trace Element Laboratories, 2003. Available at: www.sas-centre.org.
550. Sauberlich HE. Laboratory tests for the assessment of nutritional status, 2nd edition. Boca Raton, Fla: CRC Press, 1999.
551. Savage DG, Lindenbaum J, Stabler SP, Allen RH. Sensitivity of serum methylmalonic acid and total homocysteine determinations for diagnosing cobalamin and folate deficiencies. Am J Med 1994;96:239-46.
552. Schaumburg H, Kaplan J, Windebank A, Vick N, Rasmus S, Pleasure D, et al. Sensory neuropathy from pyridoxine abuse: a new megavitamin syndrome. N Engl J Med 1983;309:445-8.
553. Schilsky ML, Scheinberg IH, Sternlieb I. Liver transplantation for Wilson's disease: indications and outcome. Hepatology 1994;19: 583-7.
554. Schlesier K, Harwat M, Bohm V, Bitsch R. Assessment of antioxidant activity by using different in vitro methods. Free Radic Res 2002;36: 177-87.
555. Schoenen J, Lenaerts M, Bastings E. High-dose riboflavin as a prophylactic treatment of migraine: results of an open pilot study. Cephalalgia 1994;14:328-9.
556. Scholl TO, Johnson WG. Folic acid: influence on the outcome of pregnancy. Am J Clin Nutr 2000;71:1295S-303S.
557. Schrijver J, van Breederode N, van ben Berg H, Bitsch R. Biotin in whole blood by microbiological assay: biotin in plasma or urine by RIA. In: Fidanza F, ed. Nutritional status assessment: a manual for population studies. London: Chapman & Hall, 1991:296-303.
558. Schrijver J, Speek AJ, Klosse JA, van Rijn HJ, Schreurs WH. A reliable semiautomated method for the determination of total thiamine in whole blood by the thiochrome method with high-performance liquid chromatography. Ann Clin Biochem 1982;19:52-6.
559. Schroeder JJ, Cousins RJ. Interleukin 6 regulates metallothionein gene expression and zinc metabolism in hepatocyte monolayer cultures. Proc Natl Acad Sci U S A 1990;87:3137-41.
560. Schuelke M, Mayatepek E, Inter M, Becker M, Pfeiffer E, Speer A, et al. Treatment of ataxia in isolated vitamin E deficiency caused by alpha-tocopherol transfer protein deficiency. J Pediatr 1999;134:240-4.
561. Schultz M, Leist M, Petrzika M, Gassmann B, Brigelius-Flohe R. Novel urinary metabolite of alpha-tocopherol, 2,5,7,8-tetramethyl-2(2′-carboxyethyl)-6-hydroxychroman, as an indicator of an adequate vitamin E supply? Am J Clin Nutr 1995;62:1527S-34S.
562. Schulze zur WE, Hesse C, Hotzel K. [The gas chromatographic determination pantothenic acid in urine (author's transl)]. Z Klin Chem Klin Biochem 1974;12:498-503.
563. Schurgersl LJ, Geleijnse JM, Grobee DE, et al. Nutritional intake of vitamin K1 (phylloquinone) and K2 (memoquinone) in the Netherlands. J Nutr Environ Med 1999;9:115-22.
564. Schweigert FJ. Inflammation-induced changes in the nutritional biomarkers serum retinol and carotenoids. Curr Opin Clin Nutr Metab Care 2001;4:477-81.
565. Scurr C, Sampson B, Ball J, Gabriel C. Copper deficiency myeloneuropathy in a patient with haemachromatosis: a case report. Cases J 2009;2:6168.
566. Seetharam B, Li N. Transcobalamin II and its cell surface receptor. Vitam Horm 2000;59:337-66.
567. Selhub J. Folate, vitamin B12 and vitamin B6 and one carbon metabolism. J Nutr Health Aging 2002;6:39-42.
568. Semba RD, Bloem MW. The anemia of vitamin A deficiency: epidemiology and pathogenesis. Eur J Clin Nutr 2002;56:271-81.
569. Seshadri V, Fox PL, Mukhopadhyay CK. Dual role of insulin in transcriptional regulation of the acute phase reactant ceruloplasmin. J Biol Chem 2002;277:27903-11.
570. Shah GM, Shah RG, Veillette H, Kirkland JB, Pasieka JL, Warner RR. Biochemical assessment of niacin deficiency among carcinoid cancer patients. Am J Gastroenterol 2005;100:2307-14.
571. Shah MR, Kriedt CL, Lents NH, Hoyer MK, Jamaluddin N, Klein C, et al. Direct intra-tumoral injection of zinc-acetate halts tumor growth in a xenograft model of prostate cancer. J Exp Clin Cancer Res 2009;28:84.
572. Sharp P. The molecular basis of copper and iron interaction. Proc Nutr Soc 2004;63:563-9.
573. Shearer MJ. Measurement of phylloquinone (vitamin K1) in serum and plasma by HPLC. In: Fidanza F, ed. Nutritional status assessment: a manual for population studies. London: Chapman and Hall, 1991:214-20.
574. Shearer MJ. Vitamin K metabolism and nutriture. Blood Rev 1992;6:92-104.
575. Shearer MJ. The roles of vitamins D and K in bone health and osteoporosis prevention. Proc Nutr Soc 1997;56:915-37.
576. Shearer MJ. Vitamin K in parenteral nutrition. Gastroenterology 2009;137:S105-18.
577. Shenai JP, Kennedy KA, Chytil F, Stahlman MT. Clinical trial of vitamin A supplementation in infants susceptible to bronchopulmonary dysplasia. J Pediatr 1987;111:269-77.
578. Shenkin A, Allwood MC. Trace elements and vitamins in adult intravenous nutrition. In: Rombeau JL, Rolandelli RH, eds. Clinical

nutrition: parenteral nutrition. Philadelphia: WB Saunders, 2001: 60-79.
579. Shenkin A, Fell GS, Halls DJ, et al. Essential trace element provision to patients receiving home intravenous nutrition in the United Kingdom. Clin Nutr 1986;5:91-7.
580. Shenkin A. Adult micronutrient requirements. In: Payne-James J, Grimble G, Silk D, eds. Artificial nutrition support in clinical practice. London: GMM, 2001:193-212.
581. Shenkin A. Vitamin and essential trace element recommendations during intravenous nutrition: theory and practice. Proc Nutr Soc 1986;45:383-90.
582. Shenkin A. Trace elements and inflammatory response: implications for nutritional support. Nutrition 1995;11:100-5.
583. Shenkin A. Impact of disease on markers of macronutrient status. Proc Nutr Soc 1997;56:433-41.
584. Shenkin A. Micronutrients in adult nutritional support: requirements and benefits. Curr Opin Clin Nutr Metab Care 1998;1:15-9.
585. Shenkin A. Micronutrients in the severely-injured patient. Proc Nutr Soc 2000;59:451-6.
586. Shenkin A. Serum prealbumin: is it a marker of nutritional status or of risk of malnutrition? Clin Chem 2006;52:2177-9.
587. Shenkin A, Cederblad G, Elia M, Isaksson B; International Federation of Clinical Chemistry. Laboratory assessment of protein-energy status. Clin Chim Acta 1996;253:S5-59.
588. Shibata K, Onodera M, Kawada T, Iwai K. Simultaneous micro-determination of serotonin and 5-hydroxyindole-3-acetic acid with 5-hydroxy-*N*-omega-methyltryptamine, as an internal standard, in biological materials by high-performance liquid chromatography with electrochemical detection. J Chromatogr 1988;430:381-7.
589. Shils ME, Brown RO. Parenteral nutrition. In: Shils ME, Olson JA, Shike M, Ross AC, eds. Modern nutrition in health and disease. Baltimore, Md: Williams & Wilkins, 1999:1657-88.
590. Shiraki M, Shiraki Y, Aoki C, Miura M. Vitamin K2 (menatetrenone) effectively prevents fractures and sustains lumbar bone mineral density in osteoporosis. J Bone Miner Res 2000;15:515-21.
591. Shriver BJ, Roman-Shriver C, Allred JB. Depletion and repletion of biotinyl enzymes in liver of biotin-deficient rats: evidence of a biotin storage system. J Nutr 1993;123:1140-9.
592. Sieniawski CE, Mensikov R, Delves HT. Determination of total selenium in serum, whole blood and erythrocytes by ICP-MS. J Anal Atom Spectros 1999;14:109-12.
593. Sivakumar B, Reddy V. Absorption of labelled vitamin A in children during infection. Br J Nutr 1972;27:299-304.
594. Slyshenkov VS, Omelyanchik SN, Moiseenok AG, Trebukhina RV, Wojtczak L. Pantothenol protects rats against some deleterious effects of gamma radiation. Free Radic Biol Med 1998;24:894-9.
595. Slyshenkov VS, Piwocka K, Sikora E, Wojtczak L. Pantothenic acid protects jurkat cells against ultraviolet light-induced apoptosis. Free Radic Biol Med 2001;30:1303-10.
596. Snow CF. Laboratory diagnosis of vitamin B12 and folate deficiency: a guide for the primary care physician. Arch Intern Med 1999;159:1289-98.
597. Sokol RJ, Butler-Simon N, Heubi JE, Iannaccone ST, McClung HJ, Accurso F, et al. Vitamin E deficiency neuropathy in children with fat malabsorption: studies in cystic fibrosis and chronic cholestasis. Ann N Y Acad Sci 1989;570:156-69.
598. Sokoll LJ, Booth SL, O'Brien ME, Davidson KW, Tsaioun KI, Sadowski JA. Changes in serum osteocalcin, plasma phylloquinone, and urinary gamma-carboxyglutamic acid in response to altered intakes of dietary phylloquinone in human subjects. Am J Clin Nutr 1997;65:779-84.
599. Sokoll LJ, Sadowski JA. Comparison of biochemical indexes for assessing vitamin K nutritional status in a healthy adult population. Am J Clin Nutr 1996;63:566-73.
600. Somogyi A, Rosta K, Pusztai P, Tulassay Z, Nagy G. Antioxidant measurements. Physiol Meas 2007;28:R41-55.
601. Spahr L, Butterworth RF, Fontaine S, Bui L, Therrien G, Milette PC, et al. Increased blood manganese in cirrhotic patients: relationship to pallidal magnetic resonance signal hyperintensity and neurological symptoms. Hepatology 1996;24:1116-20.
602. Squitti R, Barbati G, Rossi L, Ventriglia M, Dal Forno G, Cesaretti S, et al. Excess of nonceruloplasmin serum copper in AD correlates with MMSE, CSF [beta]-amyloid, and h-tau. Neurology 2006;67:76-82.
603. Sripanyakorn S, Jugdaohsingh R, Dissayabutr W, Anderson SH, Thompson RP, Powell JJ. The comparative absorption of silicon from different foods and food supplements. Br J Nutr 2009;102:825-34.
604. Stabler SP, Marcell PD, Podell ER, Allen RH, Lindenbaum J. Assay of methylmalonic acid in the serum of patients with cobalamin deficiency using capillary gas chromatography-mass spectrometry. J Clin Invest 1986;77:1606-12.
605. Steindl P, Ferenci P, Dienes HP, Grimm G, Pabinger I, Madl C, et al. Wilson's disease in patients presenting with liver disease: a diagnostic challenge. Gastroenterology 1997;113:212-8.
606. Stephens NG, Parsons A, Schofield PM, Kelly F, Cheeseman K, Mitchinson MJ. Randomised controlled trial of vitamin E in patients with coronary disease: Cambridge Heart Antioxidant Study (CHAOS). Lancet 1996;347:781-6.
607. Stephensen CB, Marquis GS, Douglas SD, Kruzich LA, Wilson CM. Glutathione, glutathione peroxidase, and selenium status in HIV-positive and HIV-negative adolescents and young adults. Am J Clin Nutr 2007;85:173-81.
608. Sturniolo GC, Mestriner C, D'Inca RD. Trace element and mineral nutrition in gastrointestinal disease. In: Bogden JD, Klevay LM, eds. Clinical nutrition of the essential trace elements and minerals. Totowa, NJ: Humana Press, 2000:289-307.
609. Suaberlich HE. Vitamin C. In: Laboratory tests for the assessment of nutritional status. Boca Raton, Fla: CRC Press, 1999.
610. Sunde RA. Selenium. In: O'Dell BL, Sunde RA, eds. Handbook of nutritionally essential mineral elements. New York/Basel/Hong Kong: Marcel Dekker, 1997:493-557.
611. Suter PM, Vetter W. Diuretics and vitamin B1: are diuretics a risk factor for thiamin malnutrition? Nutr Rev 2000;58:319-23.
612. Svantesson E, Capala J, Markides KE, Pettersson J. Determination of boron-containing compounds in urine and blood plasma from boron neutron capture therapy patients: the importance of using coupled techniques. Anal Chem 2002;74:5358-63.
613. Tahiliani AG, Beinlich CJ. Pantothentic acid in health and disease. Vitam Horm 1991;46:165-228.
614. Takagi Y, Okada A, Sando K, Wasa M, Yoshida H, Hirabuki N. Evaluation of indexes of in vivo manganese status and the optimal intravenous dose for adult patients undergoing home parenteral nutrition. Am J Clin Nutr 2002;75:112-8.
615. Talwar D, Davidson H, Cooney J, O'Reilly D. Vitamin B(1) status assessed by direct measurement of thiamin pyrophosphate in erythrocytes or whole blood by HPLC: comparison with erythrocyte transketolase activation assay. Clin Chem 2000;46:704-10.
616. Tamai I, Sai Y, Ono A, Kido Y, Yabuuchi H, Takanaga H, et al. Immunohistochemical and functional characterization of pH-dependent intestinal absorption of weak organic acids by the monocarboxylic acid transporter MCT1. J Pharm Pharmacol 1999;51: 1113-21.
617. Tamat SR, Moore DE, Allen BJ. Determination of boron in biological tissues by inductively coupled plasma atomic emission spectrometry. Anal Chem 1987;59:2161-4.
618. Tamura T, Soong SJ, Sauberlich HE, Hatch KD, Cole P, Butterworth CE Jr. Evaluation of the deoxyuridine suppression test by using whole blood samples from folic acid-supplemented subjects. Am J Clin Nutr 1990;51:80-6.
619. Tanner MS. Role of copper in Indian childhood cirrhosis. Am J Clin Nutr 1998;67:1074S-81S.
620. Tanphaichitr V. Thiamine. In: Shils ME, Olson JA, Shihe M, Ross AC, eds. Modern nutrition in health and disease. Baltimore, Md: Williams and Wilkins, 1999:381-90.
621. Tanumihardjo SA. Factors influencing the conversion of carotenoids to retinol: bioavailability to bioconversion to bioefficacy. Int J Vitam Nutr Res 2002;72:40-5.

622. Tanumihardjo SA, Koellner PG, Olson JA. The modified relative-dose-response assay as an indicator of vitamin A status in a population of well-nourished American children. Am J Clin Nutr 1990;52:1064-7.
623. Tanumihardjo SA, Muhilal Yuniar Y, Permaesih D, Sulaiman Z, Karyadi D, Olson JA. Vitamin A status in preschool-age Indonesian children as assessed by the modified relative-dose-response assay. Am J Clin Nutr 1990;52:1068-72.
624. Tarr JB, Tamura T, Stokstad EL. Availability of vitamin B6 and pantothenate in an average American diet in man. Am J Clin Nutr 1981;34:1328-37.
625. Taylor MJ, Carney S, Geddes J, Goodwin G. Folate for depressive disorders. Cochrane Database Syst Rev 2003;CD003390.
626. Templeton DM. The importance of trace element speciation in biomedical science. Anal Bioanal Chem 2003;375:1062-6.
627. Terada A, Nakada M, Nakada K, Yamate N, Tanaka Y, Yoshida M, et al. Selenium administration to a ten-year-old patient receiving long-term total parenteral nutrition (TPN): changes in selenium concentration in the blood and hair. J Trace Elem Med Biol 1996;10:1-5.
628. Thomas AG, Miller V, Shenkin A, Fell GS, Taylor F. Selenium and glutathione peroxidase status in paediatric health and gastrointestinal disease. J Pediatr Gastroenterol Nutr 1994;19:213-9.
629. Thompson AD. Mechanisms of vitamin deficiency in chronic alcohol misuse and the development of the Wernicke-Korsakoff syndrome. Alcohol Alcohol 2000;35(Suppl 1):2-7.
630. Thompson RP. Assessment of zinc status. Proc Nutr Soc 1991;50: 19-28.
631. Thomson CD, Campbell JM, Miller J, Skeaff SA, Livingstone V. Selenium and iodine supplementation: effect on thyroid function of older New Zealanders. Am J Clin Nutr 2009;90:1038-46.
632. Thurnham DI, Smith E, Flora PS. Concurrent liquid-chromatographic assay of retinol, alpha-tocopherol, beta-carotene, alpha-carotene, lycopene, and beta-cryptoxanthin in plasma, with tocopherol acetate as internal standard. Clin Chem 1988;34:377-81.
633. Tietz NW. Clinical guide to laboratory tests. Philadelphia: WB Saunders, 1995.
634. Toh BH, van Driel IR, Gleeson PA. Pernicious anemia. N Engl J Med 1997;337:1441-8.
635. Tonelli M, Wiebe N, Hemmelgarn B, Klarenbach S, Field C, Manns B, et al. Trace elements in hemodialysis patients: a systematic review and meta-analysis. BMC Med 2009;7:25.
636. Traber MG. Vitamin E: too much or not enough? Am J Clin Nutr 2001;73:997-8.
637. Trace element and micronutrient unit, NHS Scotland, 2003. Available at: www.trace-element.org.uk.
638. Tryfiates GP. Vitamin B6 metabolism and role in growth. Westport, Conn: Food and Nutrition Press Inc, 1980.
639. Turnlund JR, Keyes WR, Peiffer GL. Molybdenum absorption, excretion, and retention studied with stable isotopes in young men at five intakes of dietary molybdenum. Am J Clin Nutr 1995;62:790-6.
640. Turnlund JR, Keyes WR, Peiffer GL, Scott KC. Copper absorption, excretion, and retention by young men consuming low dietary copper determined by using the stable isotope 65Cu. Am J Clin Nutr 1998;67:1219-25.
641. Twomey PJ, Viljoen A, House IM, Reynolds TM, Wierzbicki AS. Relationship between serum copper, ceruloplasmin, and non-ceruloplasmin-bound copper in routine clinical practice. Clin Chem 2005;51:1558-9.
642. Uauy R, Olivares M, Gonzalez M. Essentiality of copper in humans. Am J Clin Nutr 1998;67:952S-9S.
643. Ubbink JB, Serfontein WJ, de Villiers LS. Stability of pyridoxal-5-phosphate semicarbazone: applications in plasma vitamin B6 analysis and population surveys of vitamin B6 nutritional status. J Chromatogr 1985;342:277-84.
644. Ueland PM, Refsum H, Beresford SA, Vollset SE. The controversy over homocysteine and cardiovascular risk. Am J Clin Nutr 2000;72:324-32.
645. Ulleland M, Eilertsen I, Quadros EV, Rothenberg SP, Fedosov SN, Sundrehagen E, et al. Direct assay for cobalamin bound to transcobalamin (holo-transcobalamin) in serum. Clin Chem 2002;48:526-32.
646. Urnov FD. A feel for the template: zinc finger protein transcription factors and chromatin. Biochem Cell Biol 2002;80:321-33.
647. U.S. Department of Health and Human Services. Case studies in environmental medicine: chromium toxicity. Course SS3048, Agency for Toxic Substances and Disease Registry. Publication No. ASTDR-HE-CS-2001-0005. Atlanta, Ga: ATSDR, 2000.
648. Uthus EO, Nielsen FH. Effect of vanadium, iodine and their interaction on growth, blood variables, liver trace elements and thyroid status indices in rats. Magnes Trace Elem 1990;9:219-26.
649. van Asselt DZ, de Groot LC, van Staveren WA, Blom HJ, Wevers RA, Biemond I, et al. Role of cobalamin intake and atrophic gastritis in mild cobalamin deficiency in older Dutch subjects. Am J Clin Nutr 1998;68:328-34.
650. van Bakel MM, Printzen G, Wermuth B, Wiesmann UN. Antioxidant and thyroid hormone status in selenium-deficient phenylketonuric and hyperphenylalaninemic patients. Am J Clin Nutr 2000;72:976-81.
651. Van Gossum A, Shariff R, Lemoyne M, Kurian R, Jeejeebhoy K. Increased lipid peroxidation after lipid infusion as measured by breath pentane output. Am J Clin Nutr 1988;48:1394-9.
652. van Guldener C, Stehouwer CD. Homocysteine-lowering treatment: an overview. Expert Opin Pharmacother 2001;2:1449-60.
653. van Lieshout M, West CE, van Breemen RB. Isotopic tracer techniques for studying the bioavailability and bioefficacy of dietary carotenoids, particularly beta-carotene, in humans: a review. Am J Clin Nutr 2003;77:12-28.
654. van Rij AM, McKenzie JM, Thomson CD, Robinson MF. Selenium supplementation in total parenteral nutrition. JPEN J Parenter Enteral Nutr 1981;5:120-4.
655. Vasilaki AT, McMillan DC, Kinsella J, Duncan A, O'Reilly DS, Talwar D. Relation between pyridoxal and pyridoxal phosphate concentrations in plasma, red cells, and white cells in patients with critical illness. Am J Clin Nutr 2008;88:140-6.
656. Vatassery GT, Krezowski AM, Eckfeldt JH. Vitamin E concentrations in human blood plasma and platelets. Am J Clin Nutr 1983;37:1020-4.
657. Veillon C. Analytical chemistry of chromium. Sci Total Environ 1989;86:65-8.
658. Velazquez A, Teran M, Baez A, Gutierrez J, Rodriguez R. Biotin supplementation affects lymphocyte carboxylases and plasma biotin in severe protein-energy malnutrition. Am J Clin Nutr 1995;61:385-91.
659. Velazquez A, Zamudio S, Baez A, Murguia-Corral R, Rangel-Peniche B, Carrasco A. Indicators of biotin status: a study of patients on prolonged total parenteral nutrition. Eur J Clin Nutr 1990;44:11-6.
660. Velez RJ, Myers B, Guber MS. Severe acute metabolic acidosis (acute beriberi): an avoidable complication of total parenteral nutrition. JPEN J Parenter Enteral Nutr 1985;9:216-9.
661. Verseick J, Cornelis R. Normal levels of trace elements in human blood plasma or serum. Anal Chim Acta 1980;116:217-54.
662. Versieck J, Cornelis R. Trace element in human plasma or serum. Boca Raton, Fla: CRC Press, 1989.
663. Vincent JB. The biochemistry of chromium. J Nutr 2000;130:715-8.
664. Vincent JB. The potential value and toxicity of chromium picolinate as a nutritional supplement, weight loss agent and muscle development agent. Sports Med 2003;33:213-30.
665. Vincent JB. Recent developments in the biochemistry of chromium(III). Biol Trace Elem Res 2004;99:1-16.
666. Vinton NE, Dahlstrom KA, Strobel CT, Ament ME. Macrocytosis and pseudoalbinism: manifestations of selenium deficiency. J Pediatr 1987;111:711-7.
667. Vogel T, Li-Youcef N, Kaltenbach G, Andres E. Homocysteine, vitamin B12, folate and cognitive functions: a systematic and critical review of the literature. Int J Clin Pract 2009;63:1061-7.
668. Vuilleumier JP, Keck E. Fluorimetric assay of vitamin C in biological materials, using a centrifugal analyser with fluorescence attachment. J Micronutr Anal 1989;5:25-34.
669. Wald NJ, Law MR, Morris JK, Wald DS. Quantifying the effect of folic acid. Lancet 2001;358:2069-73.

670. Walshe JM. Treatment of Wilson's disease: the historical background. QJM 1996;89:553-5.
671. Wang H, Prasad AS, Dumouchelle F. Zinc in platelets, lympohocytes and granulocytes by flameless atomic absorption spectrophotometry. J Micronutrient Anal 1989;5:181-90.
672. Wardle CA, Forbes A, Roberts NB, Jawhari AV, Shenkin A. Hypermanganesemia in long-term intravenous nutrition and chronic liver disease. JPEN J Parenter Enteral Nutr 1999;23:350-5.
673. Warren JJ, Levy SM. Current and future role of fluoride in nutrition. Dent Clin North Am 2003;47:225-43.
674. Warren MJ, Raux E, Schubert HL, Escalante-Semerena JC. The biosynthesis of adenosylcobalamin (vitamin B12). Nat Prod Rep 2002;19:390-412.
675. Wellenberg GJ, Banks JN. Enzyme linked sorbent assay to quantify d-biotin in blood. J Sci Fd Agric 1993;63:1-5.
676. Wells IC, Claassen JP, Anderson RJ. A test for adequacy of chromium nutrition in humans: relation to type 2 diabetes mellitus. Biochem Biophys Res Commun 2003;303:825-7.
677. Wen B, Dai T, Li W, Zhao Y, Liu S, Zhang C, et al. Riboflavin responsive lipid storage myopathy caused by ETFDH gene mutations. J Neurol Neurosurg Psychiatry 2010;81:231-6.
678. Werner E, Roth P, Heinrichs U, Giussani A, Cantone MC, Zilker TH, et al. Internal biokinetic behaviour of molybdenum in humans studied with stable isotopes as tracers. Isotopes Environ Health Stud 2000;36: 123-32.
679. Wessling-Resnick M. Understanding copper uptake at the molecular level. Nutr Rev 2002;60:177-9.
680. Whitehead VM. Polygammaglutamyl metabolites of folic acid in human liver. Lancet 1973;1:743-5.
681. WHO Scientific Group. Nutritional anaemias. World Health Organisation Technical Report Series No. 405. Geneva, Switzerland: World Health Organisation, 1968.
682. Wiegand VW, Hartmann S, Hummler H. Safety of vitamin A: recent results. Int J Vitam Nutr Res 1998;68:411-6.
683. Wilfond BS, Farrell PM, Laxova A, Mischler E. Severe hemolytic anemia associated with vitamin E deficiency in infants with cystic fibrosis: implications for neonatal screening. Clin Pediatr 1994;33: 2-7.
684. Wilson JD. Disorders of vitamins: deficiency, excess, and errors of metabolism. In: Petersdorf RG, Adams RD, Braunwald E, et al, eds. Harrison's principles of internal medicine. New York: McGraw-Hill Book Company, 1991.
685. Wilson JX. The physiological role of dehydroascorbic acid. FEBS Lett 2002;527:5-9.
686. Wolf B, Heard GS. Biotinidase deficiency. In: Barness L, Oski F, eds. Advances in pediatrics. Chicago: Medical Book Publishers, 1991: 1-21.
687. Wolman SL, Anderson GH, Marliss EB, Jeejeebhoy KN. Zinc in total parenteral nutrition: requirements and metabolic effects. Gastroenterology 1979;76:458-67.
688. Wong CP, Song Y, Elias VD, Magnusson KR, Ho E. Zinc supplementation increases zinc status and thymopoiesis in aged mice. J Nutr 2009;139:1393-7.
689. Wong WY, Flik G, Groenen PM, Swinkels DW, Thomas CM, Copius-Peereboom JH, et al. The impact of calcium, magnesium, zinc, and copper in blood and seminal plasma on semen parameters in men. Reprod Toxicol 2001;15:131-6.
690. Wood RJ. Assessment of marginal zinc status in humans. J Nutr 2000;130:1350S-4S.
691. World Cancer Research Fund. Food, nutrition and physical activity and the prevention of cancer: a global perspective, 2007. World Cancer Research Fund, London, UK.
692. World Health Organisation. The global prevalence of vitamin A deficiency. 1995. Geneva. Micronutrient Series document WHO/ NUT/95.3.
693. Wynn RM, Davie JR, Chuang JL, Cote CD, Chuang DT. Impaired assembly of E1 decarboxylase of the branched-chain alpha-ketoacid dehydrogenase complex in type IA maple syrup urine disease. J Biol Chem 1998;273:13110-8.
694. Wyse BW, Wittwer C, Hansen RG. Radioimmunoassay for pantothenic acid in blood and other tissues. Clin Chem 1979;25:108-10.
695. Yang GQ, Wang SZ, Zhou RH, Sun SZ. Endemic selenium intoxication of humans in China. Am J Clin Nutr 1983;37:872-81.
696. Yanik M, Vural H, Kocyigit A, Tutkun H, Zoroglu SS, Herken H, et al. Is the arginine-nitric oxide pathway involved in the pathogenesis of schizophrenia? Neuropsychobiology 2003;47:61-5.
697. Ye Z, Song H. Antioxidant vitamin intake and the risk of coronary heart disease: meta-analysis of cohort studies. Eur J Cardiovasc Prev Rehabil 2008;15:26-34.
698. Yoshida K, Kawano N, Yoshiike M, Yoshida M, Iwamoto T, Morisawa M. Physiological roles of semenogelin I and zinc in sperm motility and semen coagulation on ejaculation in humans. Mol Hum Reprod 2008;14:151-6.
699. Young IS, Woodside JV. Folate and homocysteine. Curr Opin Clin Nutr Metab Care 2000;3:427-32.
700. Yu SY, Zhu YJ, Li WG. Protective role of selenium against hepatitis B virus and primary liver cancer in Qidong. Biol Trace Elem Res 1997; 56:117-24.
701. Yusuf SW, Rehman Q, Casscells W. Cardiomyopathy in association with selenium deficiency: a case report. JPEN J Parenter Enteral Nutr 2002;26:63-6.
702. Zaichick VY, Sviridova TV, Zaichick SV. Zinc in the human prostate gland: normal, hyperplastic and cancerous. Int Urol Nephrol 1997; 29:565-74.
703. Zaman Z, Fielden P, Frost PG. Simultaneous determination of vitamins A and E and carotenoids in plasma by reversed-phase HPLC in elderly and younger subjects. Clin Chem 1993;39:2229-34.
704. Zeiner M, Ovari M, Zaray G, Steffan I. Reference concentrations of trace elements in urine of the Budapestian population. Biol Trace Elem Res 2004;101:107-15.
705. Zempleni J. Biotin: present knowledge in nutrition. In: Bowman BA, Russell RA, eds. Present knowledge in nutrition. Washington, DC: ILSI Press, 2001.
706. Zempleni J, Galloway JR, McCormick DB. Pharmacokinetics of orally and intravenously administered riboflavin in healthy humans. Am J Clin Nutr 1996;63:54-66.
707. Zempleni J, Mock DM. Bioavailability of biotin given orally to humans in pharmacologic doses. Am J Clin Nutr 1999;69:504-8.
708. Zhitkovich A, Quievryn G, Messer J, Motylevich Z. Reductive activation with cysteine represents a chromium(III)-dependent pathway in the induction of genotoxicity by carcinogenic chromium(VI). Environ Health Perspect 2002;110(Suppl 5):729-31.
709. Zile MH. Function of vitamin A in vertebrate embryonic development. J Nutr 2001;131:705-8.

CHAPTER 32

Hemoglobin, Iron, and Bilirubin

*Trefor Higgins, M.Sc., John H. Eckfeldt, M.D., Ph.D., James C. Barton, M.D., and Basil T. Doumas, Ph.D.**

Hemoglobin (Hb), iron (Fe), and bilirubin are analytes that may be viewed collectively in terms of a manufacturing process in which the raw material (iron) is incorporated with other raw materials in a multistage complex process leading to a finished product (Hb). This finished product has a limited life span, after which degradation into the waste product (bilirubin) occurs. Within this process many exquisite biochemical control, conservation, and synthesis mechanisms are found. This process may be disrupted by a deficiency in the supply of raw material, lack of control or synthesis mechanisms, excessive loss of finished product, or excessive conversion to or deficiency in the elimination of waste products. These disruptions are manifest in the clinical disorders of iron deficiency anemias, liver disease, and various genetic diseases, including Crigler-Najjar and Gilbert syndromes, hemoglobinopathies, and thalassemias.

Reliable analytical methods for the measurement of these analytes were among the first to be developed for routine use in the clinical laboratory. Laboratory analysis has contributed significantly to our understanding of the physiologic role of these analytes and continues to be crucial in the diagnosis of diseases associated with disruptions in supply, synthesis, and elimination of these parameters.

HEMOGLOBIN

Hb is a hemoprotein whose primary function is to transport oxygen from the lungs to the body tissue. It was first isolated in 1849 and was the first oligomeric protein to be characterized by ultracentrifugation and to have (1) its molecular mass accurately determined; (2) its physiologic function described; and (3) following the 25-year study of Max Perutz and colleagues in Cambridge, its structure defined by x-ray crystallography.[H61] In 1949, Linus Pauling and H. Itano[H60] showed that Hb from patients with sickle cell disease differed from normal Hb by having two to four additional net positive charges. Later, the reasons for the charge difference were elucidated by locating the single amino acid difference between Hb from normal individuals and Hb from those with sickle cell disease.[H40-H43]

Biochemistry

Hemoglobin is a globular protein with a diameter of 6.4 nm and a molecular mass of approximately 64,500 Da. As shown in Figure 32-1, Hb consists of four globin subunits (two alpha and two non-alpha β-, γ-, or δ-chains) with each looped about itself to form a pocket or cleft in which the heme group nestles. Normally, this heme pocket is formed entirely by nonpolar (hydrophobic) amino acids. The heme moiety (see Figure 32-1) is suspended within this pocket by an attachment of its iron atom to the imidazole group of the proximal histidine [position 92 of the β-chain (β92) or position 87 of the α-chain (α87)]. The imidazole group of the distal histidine (β63 or α58) is also in contiguity with the iron of heme, but it appears to swing into and out of this position to permit the passage of O_2 into and out of the Hb molecule. The four iron atoms are in the divalent state, whether Hb is oxygenated or deoxygenated.

Globin Structure of Normal and Fetal Hemoglobin

In normal human adults, Hb A is composed of two normal α- and two normal β-polypeptide chains and is represented symbolically as $\alpha_2\beta_2$; it represents at least 96% of the total Hb contained in a sample of whole blood. Hb A_2 is typically about 2.5 to 3.0% of total Hb; it contains two α- and two δ-chains and is designated as $\alpha_2\delta_2$. HbA2′ is considered a variant of Hb A_2 and is the result of a glycine-to-arginine substitution in the 16th position of the δ-chain; it occurs in 1 to 2% of African Americans. It rarely forms more than 3% of the total hemoglobin. *Fetal Hb (Hb F)* predominates during fetal life but rapidly diminishes during the first year of postnatal life. In normal adults, less than 1% of Hb is Hb F. It consists of two α- and two γ-chains ($\alpha_2\gamma_2$).

**The authors gratefully acknowledge the original contributions of Virgil F. Fairbanks and George G. Klee (hemoglobin and iron) Ph.D., and Keith G. Tolman and Robert Rej (bilirubin), upon which portions of this chapter are based.*

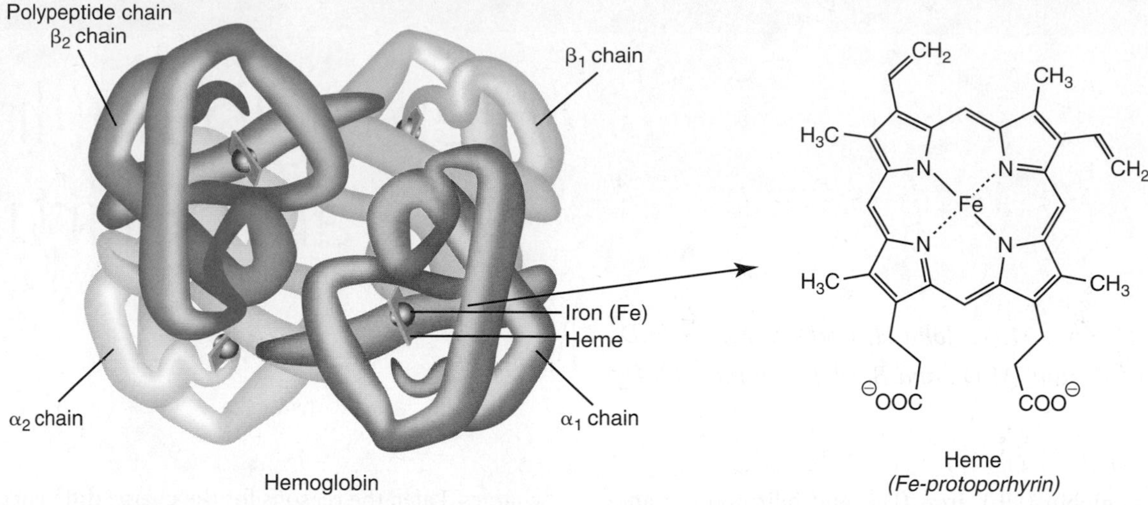

Figure 32-1 Model of the Hb tetramer with the α-chain subunits facing the reader. Each subunit contains a molecule of heme attached to an atom of iron.

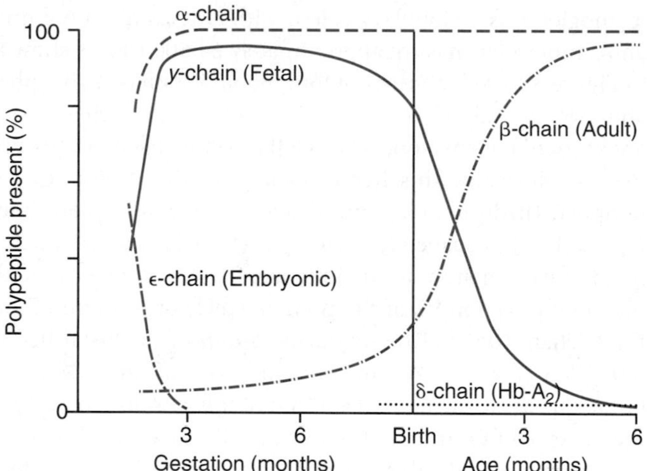

Figure 32-2 Changes in relative proportions of globin chains at various stages of embryonic, fetal, and postnatal life. *(Reprinted from Huehns ER, Dance N, Beaven GH, Hecht F, Motulsky AG. Human embryonic hemoglobins. Cold Spring Harbor Symp Quant Biol 1965;29:327-31.)*

In early embryonic life, the yolk sac produces the globin chains zeta (ζ) and epsilon (ε). These globin chains combine to form the major embryonic hemoglobins Hb Gower 1($\zeta_2\varepsilon_2$) and 2($\alpha_2\varepsilon_2$) and Hb Portland 1($\zeta_2\gamma_2$) and 2($\zeta_2\beta_2$). Production of the ζ-chain ceases at a gestational age of approximately 4 months.

Production of α- and γ-chains starts at about 6 weeks' gestation, with Hb F (fetal hemoglobin, $\alpha_2\gamma_2$) increasing in concentration to become the major Hb found in the fetus (Figure 32-2). Glycine or alanine may be found at position 136 of the γ-chain in the fetus, giving rise to two distinct γ-chains designated Gγ and Aγ, respectively. Formation of Hb A ($\alpha_2\beta_2$) commences at about 28 weeks' gestation, and at birth it can form up to 15% of the total Hb, with the remainder of the Hb consisting mainly of Hb F with a very small amount of Hb A_2. Production of the γ-chain declines after birth, and normal adult Hb F concentrations are usually obtained by 1 year of age but may be elevated until 2 years of age.

Protein Structure

As with all proteins, the function of Hb is dictated by its primary, secondary, tertiary, and quaternary structures.

Primary Structure. The α- and non–α-globin chains of Hb are 141 and 146 amino acid residues in length, respectively. Some sequence homology has been noted, with 64 individual amino acid residues in identical positions in both α- and β-chains. The β-chain differs from the δ- and γ-chains by 39 and 10 residues, respectively. The amino terminal of the β-globin chain is the site of attachment of glucose (Hb A_{1c}), urea, and salicylate.[H13] The carboxy terminal amino acid of the β-chain is tyrosine and can function as a part of salt bridges. Although no disulfide bonds are present, six SH groups are noted (from cysteine at positions α104, β93, and β112). The γ-chain has a glycine amino terminal, and the alkali resistance of Hb F is attributed to the presence of threonine and tryptophan at positions 112 and 130 of the γ-chain, respectively. The γ-chain is unique in that it is the only globin chain to be susceptible to acetylation, and acetylated Hb F is a prominent feature in cord and neonatal blood and may form as much as 25% of the total Hb.

Secondary Structure. Approximately 75 to 80% of polypeptide chains of the α- and non–α-chains are arranged in helices, with the remainder forming nonhelical turns. The β-chain of Hb A is arranged into eight helices identified as A through H. In contrast, the α-chain is missing an equivalent of the D helix and so has only seven helices. Nomenclature within the helices identifies the helix and the position within the helix of the amino acid residue (e.g., F3 is the third amino residue in the F helix). Amino acid residues in the peptide chains that join adjacent helices are described by the identification of two adjacent helices and the position of residues within the joining peptide. For example, EF3 would be the third residue in the peptide joining the E and F helices.

Tertiary Structure. The tertiary structure of Hb refers to the arrangement of helices into a three-dimensional, pretzel-like structure. The heme group, located in a crevice between the E and F helices, is attached to histidine residues in each globin chain. This attachment is essential to maintaining the secondary and tertiary structure of the globin chains.

Quaternary Structure. The quaternary structure of Hb results from the attachment of the four globin chains to each other. Strong $\alpha_1\beta_1$ and $\alpha_2\beta_2$ dimeric bonds hold the molecule in a stable form. The tetrameric $\alpha_1\beta_2$ and $\alpha_2\beta_1$ bonds make significant contributions to the stability of the structure. Shifting, rotation, and sliding in the quaternary structure result in a number of physiologic effects, including the sigmoid-oxygen dissociation curve and the Bohr effect (described in greater detail later in this chapter).

Modified Hemoglobins

In addition to the Hbs discussed previously, carboxyhemoglobin, methemoglobin, and sulfhemoglobin are other Hbs whose structure has been environmentally or chemically modified.

Each of the modified Hbs has a characteristic spectral pattern, as shown in Figure 32-3. These spectral characteristics form the basis of analysis in the many co-oximeters and blood gas analyzers that provide, in a single analysis, the simultaneous quantitative measurement of carboxyhemoglobin, methemoglobin, and sulfhemoglobin. The spectral scans are performed using multidiode arrays covering a number of wavelengths followed by patented calculations that discriminate between normal and modified Hbs.

Carboxyhemoglobin

Carboxyhemoglobin is formed by the preferential attachment of carbon monoxide instead of oxygen to Hb. Carboxyhemoglobin concentrations (usually expressed as a carboxyhemoglobin saturation) have been known to reach 20% in individuals who are exposed to significant workplace concentrations of carbon monoxide. For example, police directing traffic at busy intersections and workers in radiator and welding shops have high carboxyhemoglobin concentrations at the end of the working day. The ability to perform heavy manual work or complex tasks is impaired at carboxyhemoglobin concentrations of 10% or less.[H14] Faulty home furnaces and automobile exhaust systems have been known to produce large amounts of carbon monoxide, sometimes with tragic results. Carboxyhemoglobin saturation varying from 15 to 25% may be associated with dizziness, headaches, and nausea, and greater than 50% saturation is considered life threatening.[H71] Following removal of the exposed individual from the carbon monoxide source, a slow decline in carboxyhemoglobin saturation occurs in keeping with the half-life of 4 to 5 hours at sea level.[H72]

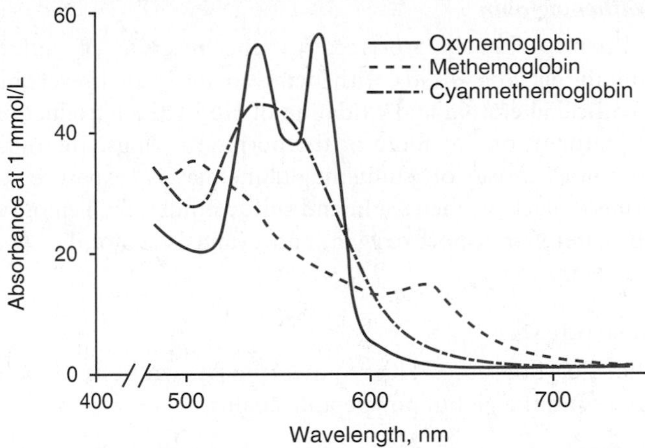

Figure 32-3 Spectrophotometric absorption curves for oxyhemoglobin, methemoglobin, and cyanmethemoglobin (authors' data). Oxyhemoglobin and cyanmethemoglobin are used in measuring the Hb concentration. The peak at 630 nm, which is distinctive for methemoglobin, is abolished by addition of cyanide, and the resultant decrease in absorbance is directly proportional to the methemoglobin concentration. All heme proteins exhibit their maximum absorbance in the Soret band region of 400 to 440 nm. Because the absorbance of Hb in the Soret region is approximately 10 times the absorbance at 540 nm, the Soret peaks have been omitted from this diagram. The absorbance curve for methemoglobin is greatly influenced by small changes in pH. The curve given here was obtained at a pH of 6.6.

Methemoglobin

The iron of heme is normally in the reduced ferrous state (Fe^{2+}). Under alkaline conditions, the iron is oxidized to the ferric state (Fe^{3+}) by toxic agents, such as nitrates (found in some well waters), aniline dyes, chlorates, drugs—such as quinones, phenacetin, and sulfonamides—or local anesthetics, such as procaine, benzocaine, and lidocaine. This oxidation converts the heme to hematin[H79] and the Hb to methemoglobin. Patients with methemoglobin are cyanotic because methemoglobin is unable to reversibly bind oxygen. Methemoglobin is normally reduced to Hb in the cell by the reduced form of the nicotinamide-adenine dinucleotide (NADH)-cytochrome reductase system.

Hereditary methemoglobinemia is a rare condition first described in Europeans but later found in individuals of many racial backgrounds. Familial methemoglobinemia in an autosomal recessive mode of transmission is due to a deficiency in the enzyme NADH-cytochrome b5 reductase. Hb variants, Hb M Saskatoon, Hb Freiburg, and Hb St. Louis stabilize the ferric iron state and are associated with an autosomal dominant familial methemoglobinemia. Methemoglobinemia is treated by the administration of ascorbic acid or methylene blue.

Sulfhemoglobin

Sulfhemoglobin is produced by the reaction of sulfur-containing compounds with heme to form an irreversible chemical alteration and oxidation of Hb by the introduction of sulfur in one or more of the porphyrin rings. The most common cause of sulfhemoglobinemia is exposure to drugs[H10] such as phenacetin and sulfonamides. Sulfhemoglobin cannot transport oxygen, and cyanosis is noted at low concentrations.

Biosynthesis

The biosynthesis of Hb requires the biosynthesis of both heme and the globin polypeptide chains.

Heme Biosynthesis

Heme, ferrous protoporphyrin IX, consists of four pyrrole rings surrounding an iron atom with four of the six electron pairs of iron attached to the nitrogen atoms in the pyrrole rings (see Chapter 33). One of the remaining electron pairs attaches to a histidine residue in a globin chain, and the other pair is available for binding and transporting an oxygen molecule. The latter electron pair is protected from oxidation by the surrounding nonpolar amino acid residues of the globin chain. Hemin results from the relatively easy oxidation of the iron of heme from the ferrous to the ferric state.[H79] To remain electrically neutral, a halide molecule, usually chloride, becomes attached to hemin. In alkaline solution, hematin is formed by the replacement of the halide atom of hemin by a hydroxyl group.

The biosynthesis of heme, shown schematically in Figure 32-4, takes place primarily in the bone marrow and the liver and is an eight-step process with each step involving a different genetically controlled enzyme. Details of this process are given in Chapter 33.

Heme synthesis is controlled by a regulatory negative feedback loop in which heme inhibits the activity of ferrochelatase and the acquisition of iron from the transport protein transferrin. The decrease in iron acquisition leads to a decrease in iron uptake into the cell with a subsequent decrease in δ-aminolevulinic acid and heme production. Iron deficiency and increased erythropoietin synthesis lead to the combination of the iron regulatory proteins with the iron-responsive elements in the transferrin receptor protein messenger ribonucleic acid (mRNA). This combination in turn leads to protection of the mRNA from degradation with subsequent increased uptake of iron into erythroid cells caused by the increased expression of transferrin receptors on the cell membrane.

Globin Synthesis

The genes that control the α-like and ζ-globin chains are located in a cluster on chromosome 16 at position 16p13.3, which is near to the chromosome 16 telomere (Figure 32-5). The α-like gene extends over 28 kb and contains, reading from the upstream (5′) end to the downstream (3′) end of the DNA segment, an embryonic α-like ζ-globin gene, a hypervariable region (HVR), a pseudo(ψ)–ζ-gene, a pair of pseudo (ψ)–α-genes, a pair of functional α-globin genes, an unexpressed α-like θ gene, and finally another hypervariable region. Alpha-thalassemia arises from the deletion of one or more α-globin genes. Deletion of all four genes with subsequent production of Hb Bart's is incompatible with life.

The β-, γ-, and δ-globin genes are clustered closely together on chromosome 11. Reading from the 5′ end, the gene sequence is an ε-gene followed by two γ-genes (designated Gγ and Aγ, respectively), a pseudo–ψβ-gene, a δ-gene, and another β-gene. Therefore two genes determine the γ-chain, with one gene each determining the δ- and β-chains. Substantial variability is seen between individuals and groups in the α- and β-genes, with the most frequent being multiples of the ζ-, ψζ-, and α-genes.

In common with all genes, the globin genes consist of exons (coding sequences) and introns (intervening noncoding sequences), with codons (triplets of nucleotides) coding for specific amino acids. The globin genes have three exons and two introns with a promoter region (specific for the globin chain) at the 5′ end of each gene. The transcription and translation processes are the same as in any other synthesis of amino acid chains.

Physiologic Role

The iron of heme is in the ferrous state and is able to combine reversibly with oxygen to act as the major oxygen-carrying moiety. The term *cooperativity* is used to describe the interaction of globin chains in such a way that oxygenation of one heme group enhances the probability of oxygenation of the other heme group. The *Bohr effect* refers to reduction of oxygen affinity with a decrease in pH from the physiologic range (7.35 to 7.45) to 6.0 and is another result of this cooperativity. As the pH of the tissue decreases as a result of the presence of the end products of anaerobic metabolism, CO_2 and carbonic acid, the delivery of oxygen to the exercising tissue is enhanced. The O_2 dissociation curve of normal blood hemoglobin is sigmoidal (Figure 32-6). Physiologically, the carbon dioxide reversibly combines with the amino terminal groups of Hb to form carbamated Hb, facilitating the removal of about 10% of the CO_2 formed as a result of metabolism in the tissue to the lungs. Removal and transport of CO_2 from the tissue are enhanced by the preference for the attachment of more CO_2 by carbamated Hb.

Clinical Significance

The thalassemias and hemoglobinopathies are clinical disorders related to Hb pathophysiology. Although they may have similar clinical manifestations[H19] such as anemia of varying severity,[H17] they form two distinct disease groups of genetic origin. For example, the thalassemias originate from insufficient globin chain production instigated by a variety of causes, including gene deletion and nonsense mutations, or from mutations that affect the transcription or stability of mRNA products. The name *thalassemia* is derived from the Greek word for "sea," *thalassa,* because all early cases of β-thalassemia were described in children of Mediterranean origin.

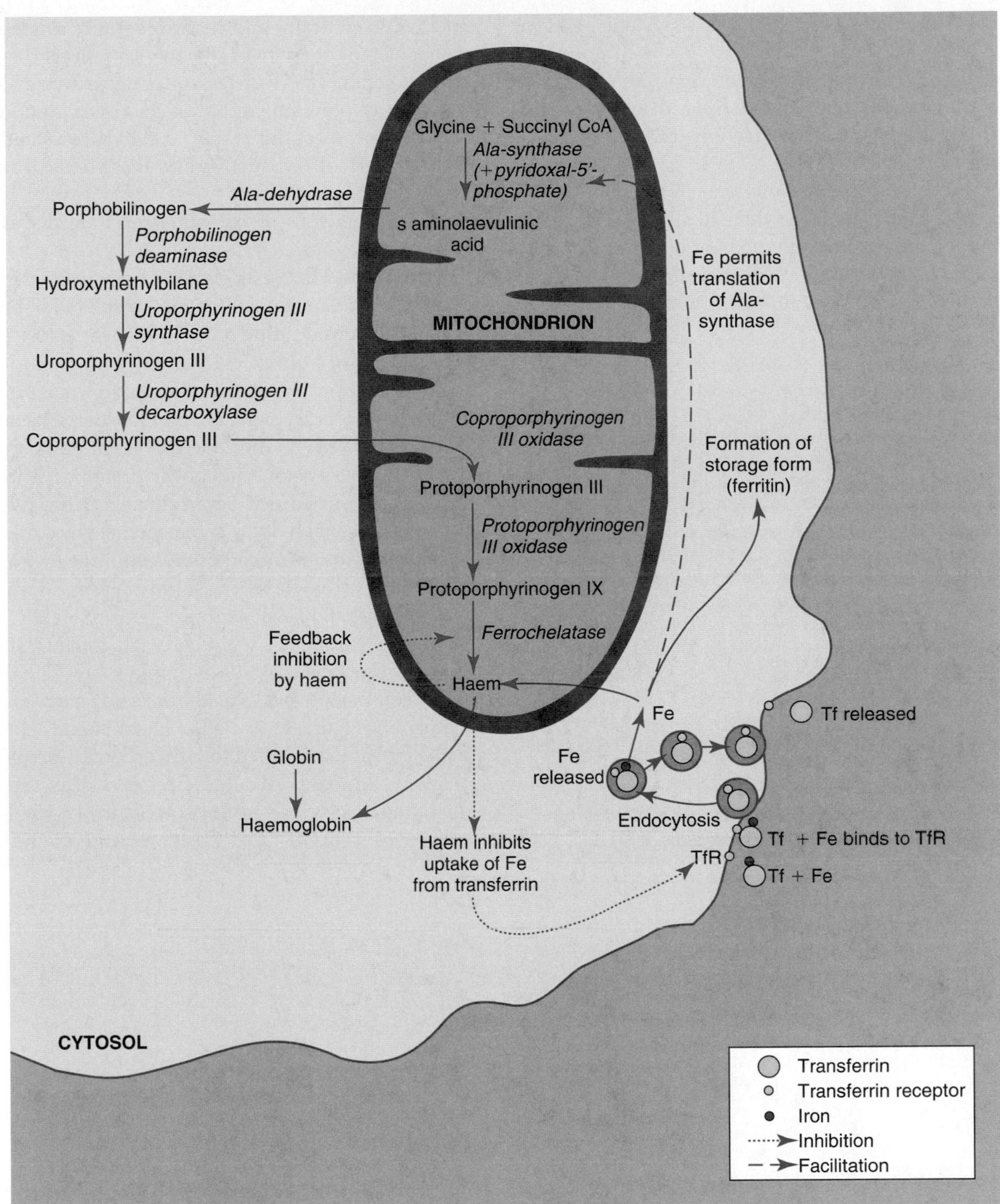

Figure 32-4 Heme synthesis. *(From Bain BJ. Haemoglobinopathy diagnosis. London: Blackwell, 2001.)*

Hemoglobinopathies, the most common single gene disorder in the world, are structural Hb variants arising from mutations in the globin genes, which result in substitutions or disruptions in the normal amino acid residue sequence in one or more of the globin chains of Hb.

Thalassemias

Thalassemias are identified by the globin chain in which a production deficiency occurs. For example, α- and β-thalassemias result from a deficiency in α- and β-globin chain production, respectively. They are further classified depending on the extent of globin chain production and the resultant severity of the anemia.

α-Thalassemias

The α-thalassemias arise from deficiencies in production of the α-globin chains and are caused by deletions or (less frequently) point mutations in one or more of the four α-globin genes. By convention, the term α^0*-thalassemia* is used when the two deleted α-globin chain genes are in the same gene cluster. This is sometimes described as a *cis* deletion and is written as (–/αα). The term *α⁺-thalassemia* is used when the two deleted α-globin chain genes are on opposite gene clusters. It is sometimes described as a *trans* deletion and is written (-α/-α). A single α-gene deletion (αα/-α) is called *α-thalassemia silent.*

Thalassemias causing point mutations are much less frequent, currently numbering fewer than 40. The conventional nomenclature for these point mutations of α-thalassemias is $\alpha^T\alpha$ or $\alpha\alpha^T$. The α-thalassemias vary in clinical presentation from conditions that are incompatible with life to slight anemia or clinically and hematologically single-gene silent deletions. The severity of the anemia reflects the number of deleted genes. The α-thalassemias occur worldwide and are particularly prevalent in South East Asia, Southern China, Mediterranean countries (particularly Greece and the Greek Cypriot part of Cyprus), India, the Middle East, and the islands of the South Pacific.

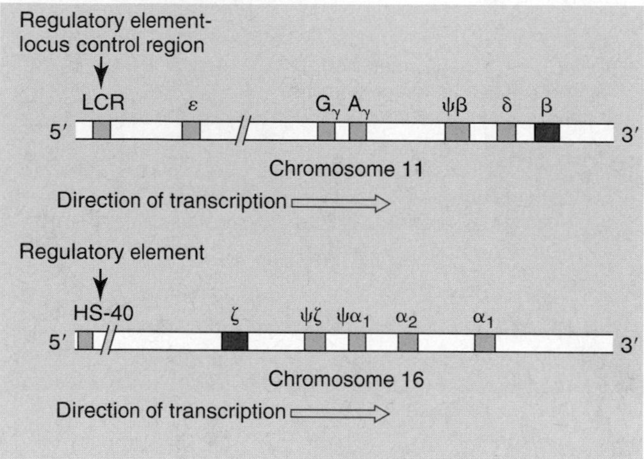

Figure 32-5 Globin α- and β-gene clusters. *(From Bain BJ. Haemoglobinopathy diagnosis. London: Blackwell, 2001.)*

Individual types of α-thalassemias are discussed in the following sections.

Hb Bart's. Hb Bart's results from deletion of all four α-globin genes with subsequent inability to produce any α-globin chains, leading to failure of synthesis of Hb A, F, or A_2. In the fetus, an excess number of γ-globin chains join together to form unstable tetramers known as Hb Bart's (γ^4). Mothers who carry a fetus with Hb Bart's usually present clinically between 20 and 26 weeks' gestation with pregnancy-induced hypertension and polyhydramnios. Ultrasound of the fetus shows hydrops. Severe anemia (Hb usually <80 g/L) is noted on a fetal blood sample obtained by cordocentesis. It is important to rule out other causes for the hydropic fetus by performing serologic testing for *t*oxoplasmosis, *r*ubella, *c*ytomegalovirus, and *h*erpes simplex testing.

High-performance liquid chromatography (HPLC) analysis of a cordocentesis blood sample shows one or two very sharp and narrow peaks at the injection point on the chromatogram (Figure 32-7, *a*). The major band is Hb Bart's with a smaller band attributed to Hb Portland. Complete absence of Hb F is noted. Alkaline electrophoresis shows a band migrating at or close to the solvent front (Hb Bart's) with another band in the Hb A position (Hb Portland).

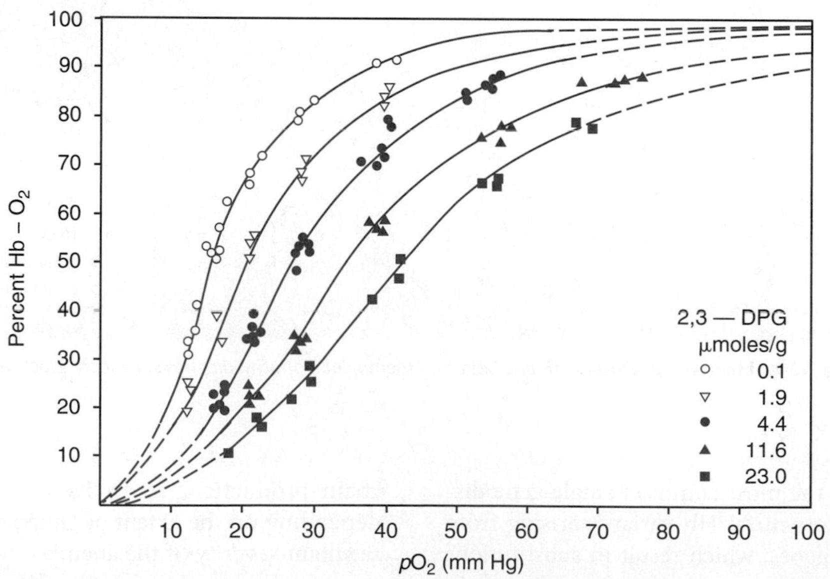

Figure 32-6 Normal oxygen dissociation curve of Hb. Changes in 2,3-diphosphoglycerate (2,3-DPG) concentration in the erythrocyte greatly influence the position of the curve. As the concentration of 2,3-DPG increases, the curve shifts to the right. *[From Duhm J. The effect of 2,3-DPG and other organic phosphates on the Donnan equilibrium and the oxygen affinity of human blood. In: Roth M, Astrup P, eds. Oxygen affinity of hemoglobin and red cell acid base status (Alfred Benzon Symposium, IV). Copenhagen, Denmark: Alfred Benzon Foundation, 1972.]*

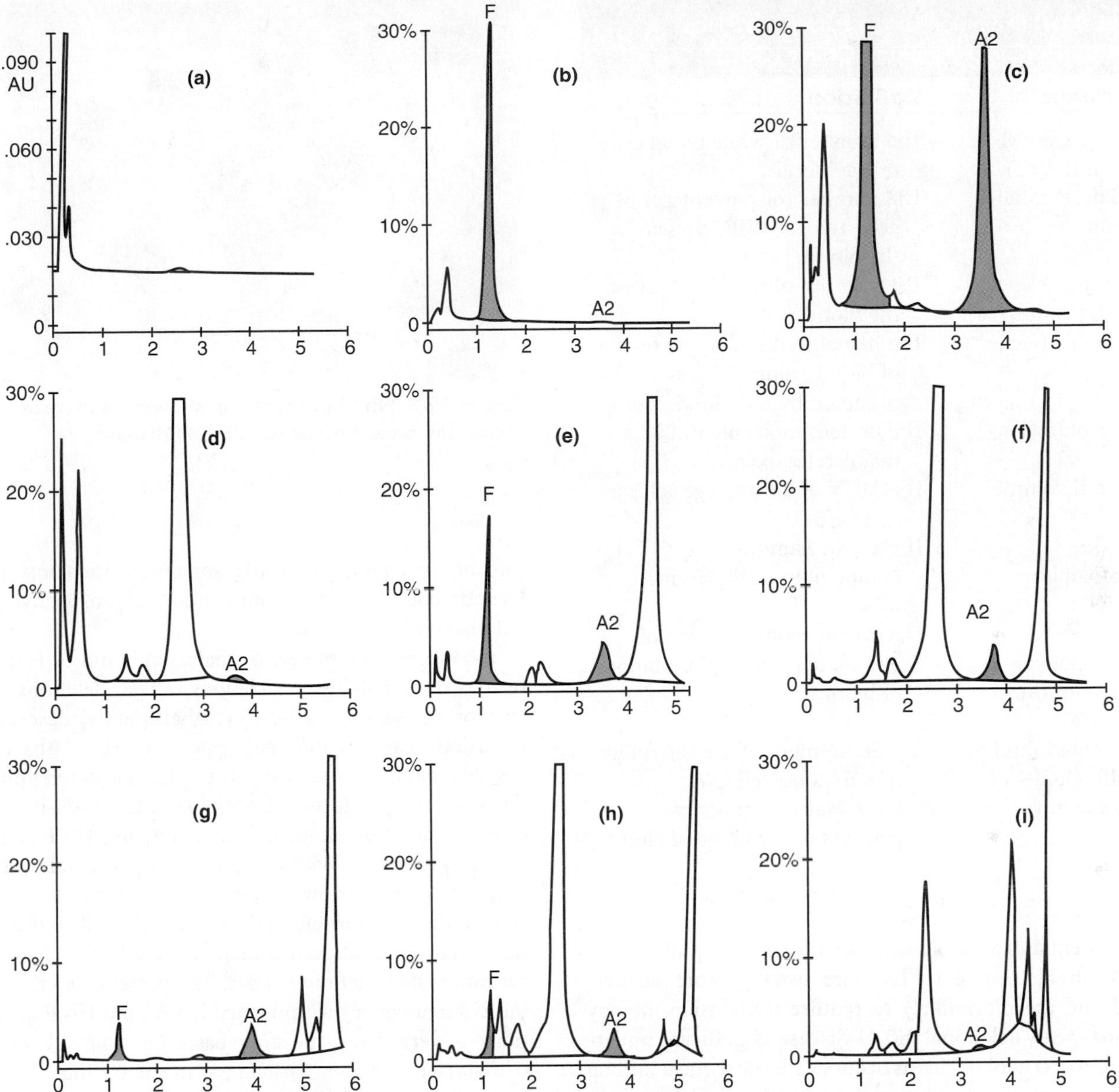

Figure 32-7 High-performance liquid chromatography (HPLC) chromatograms obtained on the Bio-Rad Variant β-Thal short program for (a) Hb Bart's; (b) β^0-thalassemia major; (c) B^+-thalassemia homozygous E; (d) Hb H; (e) homozygous S; (f) S trait; (g) homozygous C; (h) C trait; and (i) Hb S-Hb G Philadelphia. *(From Clarke GM, Trefor N, Higgins TN. Laboratory investigation of hemoglobinopathies and thalassemias: review and update. Clin Chem 2000;46:1284-90.)*

Hb Bart's hydrops fetalis is almost invariably fatal[H18] with some fetuses dying in utero and others surviving a few hours after birth. Treatment using intrauterine transfusion has had very limited success, with potential complications in the children of growth retardation and severe brain damage, which may be related to long-standing intrauterine anemia.

Laboratory investigation of the parents of fetuses with Hb Bart's shows a normal HPLC pattern with normal Hb F and A_2 quantification. Parental analysis typically shows a decreased concentration of Hb and decreased MCH and MCV with the blood smear showing hypochromic, microcytic red cells. The Hb H test may be positive in one or both parents. A two α-gene *cis*-deletion (-/αα) or a three gene deletion (-/-α) is seen in genetic testing of both parents. This requirement restricts the incidence of Hb Bart's to a much smaller population than would be expected based on the worldwide distribution of two α-gene deletions, as the presence of *trans* deletions in both parents would not give rise to a four gene deletion in the offspring. Hb Bart's is relatively common in South East Asia, particularly in Thailand, the Philippines, and Hong Kong, where there is a high prevalence of the –SEA deletion.

Hb H Disease. This disorder is usually caused by a three α-globin gene deletion (-/-α) and is characterized by a

TABLE 32-1 Definition of the Parameters That Constitute a Complete Blood Count (CBC)

Parameter	Definition
White blood cell count (WBC)	The number of white blood cells in the blood
WBC differential count	The number (or percentage) of each type of WBC present in the blood
Red blood cell (RBC) count	The number of red blood cells in the blood
Hematocrit (Hct)	The hematocrit is the proportion of blood volume that is occupied by red blood cells.
Hemoglobin (Hb)	The protein molecule in RBCs that carries oxygen
Mean cell volume (MCV)	The MCV is the average volume of an RBC.
Mean cell hemoglobin (MCH)	The average amount of hemoglobin in the average RBC
Mean cell hemoglobin concentration (MCHC)	The average concentration of hemoglobin in a given volume of blood
Red cell distribution width (RCDW)	A measurement of the variability of red blood cell size
Platelet count	The calculated number of platelets in a volume of blood

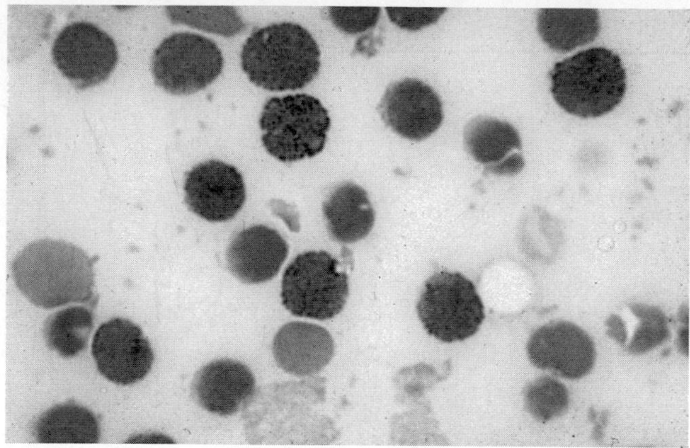

Figure 32-8 Hb H preparation showing punctate inclusions on a patient with Hb H disease.

chronic anemia of variable severity. Individuals with nondeletional Hb H disease ($\alpha^T\alpha$/-) are usually more severely affected and are more likely to require transfusion therapy than those with deletional Hb H disease. Significant underproduction of α-globin chains occurs with subsequent joining of free β-globin chains to form the insoluble β-globin chain tetramer Hb H. HPLC analysis of a hemolysate from an individual with Hb H disease shows two bands with low retention times forming a doublet together with a normal Hb A band. Hb F and Hb A_2 concentrations are within the reference interval (see Figure 32-7, *d*). Electrophoresis at alkaline pH shows a fast moving band together with a band in the Hb A position that possibly has reduced staining when compared with other samples run concurrently. The complete blood count (CBC) (Table 32-1) shows a moderately reduced concentration of Hb and markedly reduced mean corpuscular volume (MCV) and mean corpuscular hemoglobin (MCH), increased red cell distribution width (RDW), and slightly raised red blood cell (RBC) count. Iron studies are normal, although the ferritin concentration may be elevated. The Hb H preparation is positive, with many cells having typical punctate inclusions (Figure 32-8).

Iron therapy is not indicated, and transfusion therapy is usually unnecessary except in acute illness, in pregnancy, and with exposure to oxidant drugs, which destabilizes Hb H, causing precipitation of the somewhat insoluble protein. Genetic counseling is recommended to prospective parents who have Hb H disease.

α-Thalassemia Minor. α-Thalassemia minor is the result of a two α-chain gene deletions. These deletions may be seen on the same gene (-/αα,α^0-thalassemia) described as a *cis* deletion or on different genes (-α/-α, α^+-thalassemia) described as a *trans* deletion. The CBC of affected individuals shows a mildly reduced Hb with low MCV and MCH. HPLC analysis shows no abnormal Hb peaks, and Hb F and Hb A_2 concentrations are within the reference interval. The Hb H preparation may show a rare cell with punctate inclusions. Iron studies are normal. In the routine clinical laboratory, the diagnosis of α-thalassemia major is based on exclusion criteria rather than definitive tests. The presence of thalassemic indices in a patient with normal Hb A_2 and Hb F quantifications is very often the only basis for many diagnoses of α-thalassemia major, particularly in the setting of a positive family history. A photometric enzyme-linked immunosorbent assay (ELISA) for the identification of adult carriers of the (–SEA) α^0-thalassemia deletion has been described.[H51] This method is based on the measurement of minuscule quantities of embryonic ζ-cells present in these adult carriers. Not all α-thalassemia deletions have continued ζ-chain production, and so a negative test is not diagnostic of α-thalassemia major. This test could be useful in screening individuals at risk for giving birth to a fetus with Hb Bart's hydrops fetalis.

α-Thalassemia Silent. α-Thalassemia trait describes a single α-globin chain gene deletion (-α/αα). A single α-globin gene deletion is frequently clinically and hematologically silent. A CBC of an individual with this trait shows a normal or marginally decreased Hb concentration, MCV, and MCH. Iron studies are normal, and no abnormal Hb peaks are seen on HPLC analysis.

In Table 32-2, the effects of various α-thalassemias on the percentage of β-chain hemoglobin variants are shown.[H52] In general, the percentage of hemoglobin variant decreases as a

TABLE 32-2 Effects of α Thalassemia on the Percentage of β-Chain Variant Hemoglobin in Heterozygotes

	AS	AC	AE
αα/αα	41.0 ± 1.8	43.8 ± 1.5	30.0 ± 1.5
αα/α–	35.4 ± 1.6	37.5 ± 1.4	27.0 ± 2.0
α^{-}/α^{-} or $\alpha\alpha/^{-}$	28.1 ± 1.4	32.2 ± 0.8	22.0 ± 2.0

Adapted from Bunn HF, Forget BG, eds. Hemoglobin: molecular genetics and clinical aspects. Philadelphia: Saunders, 1986.

percentage of total hemoglobin as the number of α-chain deletions increases.

β-Thalassemias

The β-thalassemias result from a reduction in the synthesis of the β-globin chain[H58] and are commonly found in (1) the Mediterranean region; (2) Africa; (3) the Middle East; (4) South East Asia—especially the Southern provinces of China including Hong Kong, the Indian subcontinent, the Malay peninsula, Burma, and Indonesia.[H78] Frequency of gene distribution is estimated at 3 to 10% in some populations. The high frequency of β-thalassemia in the tropics is thought to reflect an advantage of heterozygotes against *Plasmodium falciparum* malaria. More than 200 β-thalassemia mutations have been described; however, in each ethnic group a relatively small number of mutations account for the majority of cases (the ratio most often quoted is that 20 or fewer mutations account for 80% or more of cases). Clinical manifestations of β-thalassemia range from mild anemia to severe life-threatening disease requiring lifelong transfusions.

β^0-Thalassemia (β-Thalassemia Major). This is sometimes called Cooley's anemia, after the physician who in 1925 first described the condition in the children of Italian and Greek immigrants in New York by noting that these children (1) failed to grow, (2) had frequent infections, (3) appeared pale and malnourished, (4) had splenomegaly, and (5) had facial bone changes.

β-Thalassemia major results from mutations that interfere with translation or are involved in the initiation, elongation, or termination of globin chain synthesis. Mutations that interfere with translation account for almost 50% of all β-thalassemia mutations. Included in this are frame shift or nonsense mutations that produce premature termination codons, resulting in incomplete translation of the β-globin gene and nonproduction of the β-globin chain, leading to β^0-thalassemia.

Clinical presentation usually occurs at younger than 1 year of age with features such as small size for age, abdominal girth expansion, and failure to thrive. Physical examination of the subject may reveal frontal bossing[H63] (an unusually prominent forehead) caused by thickening of the cranial bones, pallor, and prominence of the cheek bones, which, in older children, obscures the base of the nose and exposes the teeth. These features are a result of marrow expansion (up to a 30-fold increase) caused by ineffective erythropoiesis with

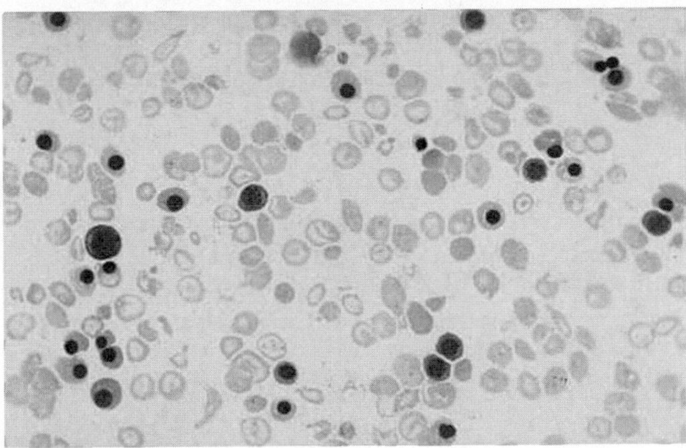

Figure 32-9 Peripheral blood smear of an individual with β^0-thalassemia. *(Courtesy Dr. G. Clarke, Dynacare Kasper Medical Laboratories.)*

production of highly unstable α-globin tetramers leading to increased plasma volume and the formation of extramedullary erythropoietic tissue, especially in the thorax and the paraspinal region. The spleen, liver, and heart may be enlarged also because of extramedullary hematopoiesis.

Typical CBC results include severe anemia with Hb concentration between 30 and 65 g/L, MCV 48 to 72 fL, and MCH 230 to 320 g/L. On the peripheral blood smear, a characteristic markedly abnormal RBC morphology is noted; this includes a large number of microcytes, numerous target cells, which may have a bridge joining the central and peripheral pigment zones, polychromasia, and occasional spherocytes, schistocytes, and nucleated red cells. When a patient's red blood cells are of unequal size (anisocytosis), the diameter of the RBC varies from 3 to 15 μm with little pigment, and shape distortion is noted, along with prominent basophilic stippling. RBC osmotic fragility is frequently observed. Typical peripheral blood on a patient with β^0 thalassemia is shown in Figure 32-9.

White blood cell (WBC) and platelet counts are usually normal. Ferritin is usually within the upper half of the reference interval, and total bilirubin is mildly elevated with a borderline elevation in the conjugated fraction. Urinalysis frequently shows increased urobilinogen or urobilin concentration, and urine is often dark brown to black because of the presence of dipyroles and mesobilifuscin. The latter features reflect ineffective hematopoiesis with intramedullary red cell destruction. HPLC analysis (see Figure 32-7, *b*) shows a major Hb F peak with absence of an Hb A peak and variable Hb A_2 (interval, 1 to 5.9%; mean, 1.7%) peak. Electrophoresis at alkaline and acid pH shows a dominant band in the F position on both gels.[H2]

Family studies on both parents and siblings should be performed, and the classical β-thalassemia minor pattern described later in the chapter should be found in the parents. Siblings may be normal or may have β-thalassemia minor. A family case history is seen in Figure 32-10.

Transfusion together with iron chelation is the only therapy, and splenectomy is frequently performed. Following

TEST/REF	INDEX PAT 7 MO F	MOTHER 33 YRS	FATHER 40 YRS	SIBLING 3 YR F
Hb	¯72 G/L	¯114	¯132	122
REF	105-135	120-160	135-175	115-135
RBC	¯3.23 (10^{12}/L)	5.19	↑6.61	4.42
REF	3.70-5.30	4.10-5.20	4.50-6.00	3.90-5.30
MCV	¯69 fL	¯68	¯63	80
REF	70-86	80-100	80-100	75-87
MCH	¯22 pg	¯22	¯20	28
REF	26-35	26-35	26-35	26-35
HbA	¯0.00	0.94	↑0.93	0.96
REF	0.94-0.98	0.94-0.98	0.94-0.98	0.94-0.98
HbA2	0.030	↑0.054	↑0.058	0.030
REF	<0.03	<0.03	<0.03	<0.03
HbF	0.97	<0.01	<0.01	<0.01
REF	<0.10	<0.01	<0.01	<0.01

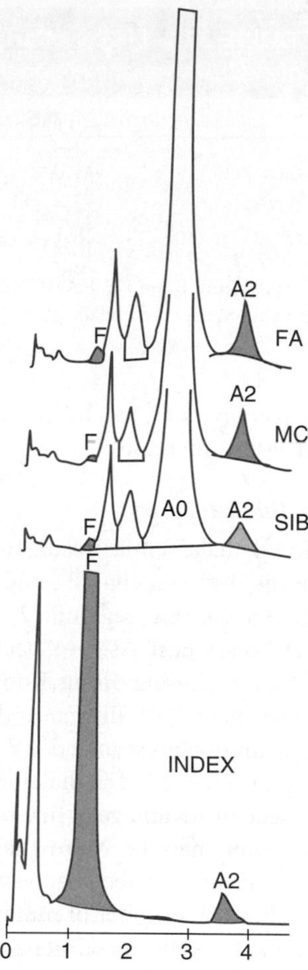

Figure 32-10 High-performance liquid chromatography (HPLC) chromatograms and complete blood count (CBC) results from a family study of a child with β^0-thalassemia. *(From Berendt HL, Blakney GB, Clarke GM, Higgins TN. A case of β-thalassemia major detected using HPLC in a child of Chinese ancestry Clin Biochem 2000;33:311-3.)*

splenectomy inclusion, bodies consisting of denatured α-chains can be observed in the blood smear after staining with methyl violet. Puberty is often delayed, incomplete, or completely absent. In boys, active spermatogenesis may occur and Leydig cell function is normal. In the older, chronically transfused patient, iron overload is a common feature. Diabetes mellitus and hypoparathyroidism are frequent sequelae. Numerous cardiopulmonary conditions, including pericarditis and myocardial hemosiderosis, are the leading causes of death in transfused patients, and are frequently associated with β^0-thalassemia.

β^+-Thalassemia (β-Thalassemia Intermedia). With this disorder, a significant reduction in the production of β-globin chain occurs with subsequent reduction in the quantity of Hb A present; this is attributed to a wide variety of genotypes. Many different causes of β^+-thalassemia have been identified, with variations in one or two β-globin genes. Clinical severity in individuals with variations in two β-globin chains is much less than when variation is seen in only one gene, a condition sometimes called *dominant β-thalassemia*. The severity of clinical features is reduced with coinheritance of α-thalassemia. β^+-Thalassemia is found in Mediterranean countries, especially in the Eastern Mediterranean.

Clinical presentation varies from symptoms similar to β^0-thalassemia to those associated with β-thalassemia trait. Transfusions usually are not necessary, and hydroxyurea therapy is frequently used to increase the production of Hb F and to mitigate disease symptoms.

HPLC analysis shows a large Hb F peak with a reduced Hb A peak. Hb A_2 is above the reference interval at concentrations greater than those associated with β-thalassemia minor. Bands in the A and F positions are seen on electrophoresis at both alkaline and acid pH. Hb is significantly reduced (60 to 100 g/L). The peripheral blood smear shows the same features seen in β^0-thalassemia, including anisocytosis, hypochromia, target cells, basophilic stippling, and nucleated RBCs.

β-Thalassemia Minor (β-Thalassemia Trait). Patients with β-thalassemia minor are very often asymptomatic, except at times of hematopoietic stress, such as infection or pregnancy, when they may require, in extreme situations, blood transfusions because of the development of anemia.

The CBC on patients with β-thalassemia trait shows low normal or decreased Hb concentration and hematocrit, decreased MCV (<72 fL) and MCH (<27 pg), and normal RDW. The discriminant factor is <60 pg (see following "Analytical Methods" section for definition). However, for patients with liver disease and β-thalassemia, MCV and MCH may be at the low end of the reference interval.

The peripheral blood smear shows microcytic RBCs with occasional hypochromia, poikilocytosis, and target cells.

The diagnosis of β-thalassemia minor, with appropriate indices in the CBC, is dependent on the finding of a raised Hb A_2 (>3.5%). Hb A_2 and Hb A_2' should be added together to obtain an accurate Hb A_2 value for the investigation of β-thalassemia minor. Hb A_2 may be elevated in HIV-positive women without hypochromic microcytic indices,[H39] hyperthyroidism, and megoblastic anemia, and with some unstable hemoglobins.[H70] Iron-depleted individuals should become iron replete before a definitive diagnosis of β-thalassemia is made, because Hb A_2 may be falsely low. HPLC is the preferred method for this quantification; densitometric scanning of the Hb A_2 band on an alkaline electrophoresis gel is not recommended because of poor precision and accuracy.[H70] In 30 to 40% of all cases of β-thalassemia minor, Hb F will also be elevated (>1.0%). The life span of the RBC may be reduced, and diabetic individuals may show a lower Hb A_{1c} compared with normal individuals with equivalent glycemic control. The β-thalassemia mutation may be identified by Southern blot using mutation-specific probes or by gap–polymerase chain reaction (PCR).

δβ-Thalassemia. Deletion of both δ- and β-genes results in δβ-thalassemia. Both heterozygous and homozygous conditions have been described. It is found in a variety of ethnic groups but is most prevalent in countries of the Eastern Mediterranean, especially Greece and Italy, and is the result of one of eight mutations that have been described to date. CBC analysis shows a reduced concentration of Hb (80 to 135 g/L) with reduced MCV and MCH and sometimes an increased RDW. HPLC analysis shows an Hb A peak with a normal or reduced Hb A_2 concentration and a raised Hb F concentration (between 5 and 20%), with the highest HbF concentration seen in the Sardinian type of δβ-thalassemia. Hb Lepore sometimes is incorrectly classified as a δβ-thalassemia because of a reduction in the production of both δ- and β-globin chains, or as an Hb variant because of the presence of an abnormal globin chain.

Hereditary Persistence of Fetal Hemoglobin (HPFH). The term *hereditary persistence of Hb F* is used to describe a group of genetic conditions in which the concentration of Hb F is increased above the upper limit of the reference interval because of a reduction in β-globin synthesis and a compensatory increase in δ-globin synthesis. Two major classes of HPFH have been described: heterocellular and deletional. Several deletional variants of HPFH have been described, including Greek, Indian, Italian, Corfu, and black.

In black HPFH, the Hb F is raised to between 10 and 36% of the total Hb with normal Hb A_2 concentrations. Hb, MCV, and MCH are within the reference intervals. This condition is clinically innocuous and asymptomatic. Similarly, no clinical abnormalities are associated with Greek HPFH, although the concentration of Hb F is in the range of 15 to 25%.

Nondeletional HPFH, sometimes named heterocellular HPFH, describes a group of presentations in which the increase in Hb F is distributed heterogeneously among the red cells in otherwise normal individuals. The Hb F concentration varies between 1 and 13% of total Hb heterozygotes and between 19 and 21% of homozygotes. No clinical or hematologic abnormalities are noted.

Hemoglobinopathies

If only single point mutations are considered, 1695 possible hemoglobin variants are known; 733 were identified by mid-2007.[H48] Currently, more than 900 hemoglobinopathies have been described, but only 9 have some clinical significance. Recent migration from regions with a high frequency of hemoglobinopathies (South East Asia or Africa) to regions (Western Europe, Central and South America, and Canada) that had low frequencies has increased the incidence of hemoglobinopathy in these areas to such an extent that some western European countries have introduced neonatal testing for hemoglobin variants. The incidental finding of a hemoglobinopathy during HPLC analysis for Hb A_{1c} has increased both the number and the incidence of Hb variants.[H16,H75] Several Hb variants (e.g., Hb Rambam, Niigata, Camden) interfere with HPLC methods for quantifying Hb A_{1c} (for a more extensive list, see Elder[H23]), and one Hb variant was found as the result of interference in pulse oximetry measurements.[H81]

Nomenclature

Hb variants are named using (1) letters (Hbs S, D, E, etc.), (2) the family name of the index case (Hb Lepore), (3) the place of discovery of the variant or place of origin of the propositus (Hb Edmonton), or (4) the name of the river (Hb Saale) flowing through the city in which the propositus lived. In some cases, both a letter and a name are used, as in Hb J-Baltimore, indicating that the Hb is classified as having electrophoretic mobility similar to that of other J Hbs but differs from them in amino acid sequence and was originally discovered in Baltimore. The term *AS trait* (sometimes abbreviated to *S trait*) is used to describe a heterozygous state in which one of the β-globin chains is S and the other is A. In instances in which no normal β-globin chain is present (e.g., Hb SD), the β-globin chain present in the higher concentration is usually, although not always, placed first. A systematic nomenclature system is now used alongside the variant name to describe the affected chain and location on the chain and the amino acid substitution. For example, Hb Spanish Town [$\alpha 27(\beta 8)^{Glu \rightarrow Val}$], a Hb variant named after a district in Kingston, Jamaica, and found in Jamaicans of African descent, results from a substitution of valine for glutamic acid in position 27 of the α-globin chain, which is located in position 8 of the B helix of the α-chain.

Classification of Hemoglobin Variants

Hb variants are classified according to the type of mutation.[H52] Single point mutations in α-globin chains give rise to substitution of one amino acid residue. As an example, Hb San Diego [β109(G11)$^{Val\rightarrow Met}$] has a methionine residue instead of the normal valine at position 109 of the β-chain. Hemoglobin C Harlem [β6(A3)$^{Glu\rightarrow Val}$; β73(E17)$^{Asp\rightarrow Asn}$] is an example of an Hb variant in which two amino acid residues are substituted, namely, valine replacing glutamic acid at position 6 and asparagine replacing aspartic acid at position 73 of the β-chain. Hemoglobin C Harlem is electrophoretically similar to Hb C but behaves like Hb S in every other aspect, including clinical manifestation. *Deletion* Hb variants arise from the deletion of one to five amino acid residues in the globin chain. Hb Vicksburg [β75(E19)$^{Leu\rightarrow 0}$] is an example in this category of Hb having a deletion of leucine in position 75 of the β-chain. *Insertion* Hbs arise from insertion of one to three amino acid residues into the globin chain. Hemoglobin Grady is an example in this category with an insertion of a three amino acid residue sequence (glutamine-phenylalanine-threonine) between positions 118 and 119 of the α-chain. *Deletion-insertion* Hbs arise from the deletion of a portion of the normal amino acid residue sequence and the insertion of another sequence, with resultant lengthening or shortening of the globin chain. An example of this type of Hb variant is Hb Montreal, in which the three normal amino acid residues between positions 72 and 76 of the β-globin chain are replaced with a four amino acid residue sequence. *Elongation* Hbs result from a single base pair mutation or frameshift at the 3′ end of exon 3 or the 5′ end of exon 1 of the α_2- or the β-globin chain. The elongation hemoglobin, Hb Constant Spring (named after an ethnic Chinese family from the Constant Spring district of Jamaica), has an additional 31 amino acid residues joined at position 142 (the carboxy terminal) of the α-chain. *Fusion* Hbs result from the fusion of an α- or β-globin chain with a portion of another globin chain. Hemoglobin Lepore-Hollandia results from the fusion of the first 22 amino acid residues of the δ-chain with the amino acid sequence from position 50 onward of normal β-globin. For the latter four categories, the systematic name is long and cumbersome, prompting universal use of the variant name rather than the systematic nomenclature.

Types of Hemoglobin Variants

In α-chain variants, the variant usually forms less than 25% of the total Hb (Hb G Philadelphia is an exception) because the mutation typically occurs in only one of the four genes that code for the α-globin chain. For β-chain variants in the heterozygous state, the variant forms more than 25% but less than 50% of the total Hb. Based on the mutation of only one of the β-globin chain genes, the β-chain variant should form 50% of total Hb. However, if the amino acid substitution results in a net negative charge to the β-variant chain, then the variant chain competes more effectively for α-chains and the % hemoglobin variant is greater than Hb A (e.g., HbN-Baltimore). The converse is true; a decrease in negative charge results in a % variant hemoglobin less than Hb A (e.g., Hb S). This information can be used to categorize an unknown Hb variant as an α- or β-globin chain variant and in preliminary hemoglobin variant identification.

Hb VarDatabase is a relational database of Hb variants and thalassemia mutations and may be accessed at the Website http://globin.cse.psu.edu/hbvar/menu.html/accessed June 22, 2011.

Laboratories should maintain a bank of hematologic and chromatographic data for hemoglobin variants found in their facilities.

Hemoglobin S [β6(A3)$^{Glu\rightarrow Val}$]. Hb S in the heterozygous or homozygous state is the most widespread of the Hb variants and arises from a substitution of valine for glutamic acid at position 6 in the A helix of the β-globin chain. Hb S is found in high frequency in West and North Africa, the Middle East (especially Saudi Arabia), and the Indian subcontinent. Approximately 8% of African Americans are heterozygous for Hb S, and homozygous Hb S is found in 1 in 500 newborns in this group. Four haplotypes originating from different geographic locations have been described. The widespread distribution of the single point gene mutation responsible for the synthesis of Hb S in areas where *P. falciparum* malaria is endemic is due to protection of Hb S heterozygotes from the worst manifestations of the malaria.

Homozygous Hemoglobin S (Hb SS). In homozygous Hb S, a valine-for-glutamic acid substitution occurs on both β-globin chains because of the inheritance of mutated β-globin chain genes from both parents. This condition is described as "sickle cell anemia" or "sickle cell disease" because of the sickle-shaped RBCs that occur when a "sickle cell crisis" occurs. It sometimes is written as $\beta^S\beta^S$.[H65]

HPLC analysis (see Figure 32-7, *e*) of a hemolysate of an individual homozygous for Hb S shows no Hb A peak and a small Hb A_2 peak. The apparent Hb A_2 concentration may be falsely increased because of the presence of glycated Hb S. Hemoglobin S forms 85 to 90% of the total Hb. The Hb F concentration is variable, with females having higher concentrations than men, and is somewhat, although not exclusively, haplotype dependent. The highest Hb F concentrations (10 to 25%) are found in individuals from the Middle East and the Indian subcontinent with the Arab-Indian haplotype. Low Hb F concentrations (5 to 6%) are found in the West African Cameroon (sometimes called Senegal) haplotype. The remaining haplotypes, the Benin and Bantu, have Hb F concentrations in the range of 6 to 7%. Increased concentrations of Hb F mitigate to some extent the clinical manifestations of sickle cell anemia. Electrophoresis (Figure 32-11) at both alkaline and acid pH shows a single large band in the Hb S position with small bands at the Hb A_2 and Hb F positions. The sickle cell screen test is positive.

CBC analysis of an individual homozygous for Hb S indicates a moderate to a major decrease in Hb concentration (60 to 100 g/L) with normal to increased MCV and MCH. In individuals with a concurrent thalassemia, the Hb is further decreased and both MCV and MCH are lowered. In the neonate the peripheral blood smear shows occasional sickle and target cells and Howell-Jolly bodies. As a patient's

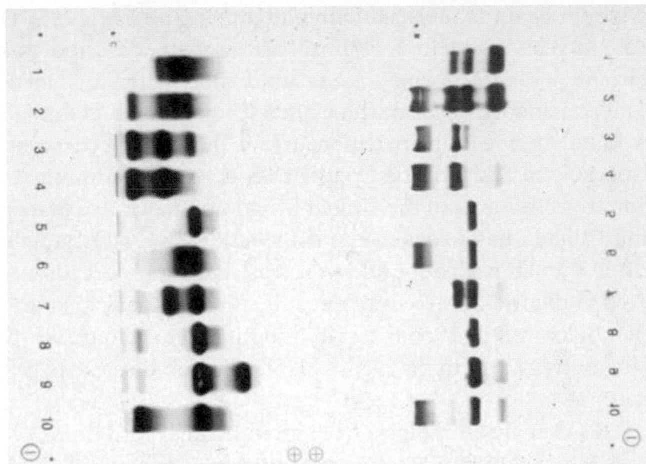

Figure 32-11 Alkaline *(left)* and acid *(right)* electrophoresis of various hemoglobinopathies. *Lane 1,* Hb S, Hb FA control. *Lane 2,* HB S, Hb F, HbCA control. *Lane 3,* Transfused SC disease. *Lane 4,* SC disease. *Lane 5,* Hb A (normal). *Lane 6,* Hb Presbyterian. *Lane 7,* Hb S. *Lane 8,* Raised Hb A_2 (β-thalassemia trait). *Lane 9,* Hb J Baltimore. *Lane 10,* Hb C.

age increases, these features of hyposplenism become increasingly evident. In the adult the percentage of sickle cells observed can be as great as 30 to 40%. In the setting of a sickle cell crisis, fewer sickle cells may be present than when individuals are clinically well. Howell-Jolly bodies, target cells, Pappenheimer bodies, boat-shaped cells, and nucleated RBCs are noted. The platelet count and neutrophil counts are elevated. Sometimes blister cells in which the Hb appears to be present in only one half of the cell are observed.

Treatment of children with homozygous HbS includes the use of hydroxyurea with an increase in the quantity of HbF sometimes to 25%. In adults, transfusion is the usual treatment, and the patient is retransfused when the Hb A concentration falls to 20% of the total hemoglobin.

Heterozygous Hemoglobin S (Hb S Trait). HPLC analysis (see Figure 32-7, *f*) of a hemolysate of a blood sample from an individual who is heterozygous for Hb S shows peaks in the Hb A and S positions, with 40% of the total Hb found in the Hb S peak. Hb S concentrations less than 30% are suggestive of coinheritance of α-thalassemia. Hb F concentration is variable. Electrophoresis (see Figure 32-11) at both alkaline and acid pH shows bands in the A and S positions.

CBC analysis from an individual who is heterozygous for Hb S shows a slightly decreased concentration of Hb, and sickle cells are not typically seen on the peripheral blood film. Patients are often asymptomatic, and the first time an individual is diagnosed as heterozygous for Hb S (sickle cell trait) is often when an Hb A_{1c} analysis is requested on the individual, or when a family study is initiated for genetic counseling. In the United States, neonatal screening programs are designed specifically to detect both heterozygous and homozygous Hb S in newborns. Although individuals with sickle cell trait are clinically asymptomatic, genetic counseling should be considered because coinheritance of two β-globin gene abnormalities may contribute to a sickle cell disorder. α- and β-Thalassemia can be coinherited with heterozygous Hb S.

Hemoglobin SC (Hb SC Disease). SC disease arises when both β-globin chains are substituted at position 6 with valine (Hb S) or lysine (Hb C). On HPLC and capillary electrophoresis, analysis peaks are noted in the S and C positions, with the S peak forming the majority of the Hb present.

Electrophoresis (see Figure 32-11) at both alkaline and acid pH shows bands in the S and C positions, and the sickling test is positive.

Hemoglobin SD. Hb S may be coinherited with Hb D (SD disease). Individuals with this disease have similar but milder clinical presentation when compared with that of sickle cell disease (Hb SS). HPLC analysis shows two peaks—one in the Hb S position forming approximately 38 to 42% of the total Hb, and the other in the Hb D position forming 43 to 45% of the total Hb. The Hb F concentration is usually within the reference interval, although concentrations as high as 14% have been observed in some individuals with SD disease. Alkaline electrophoresis shows a band in the S position. Acid electrophoresis shows bands in the S and A positions. The sickling test is positive. CBC analysis shows a greatly decreased concentration of Hb with normal to slightly elevated MCV. Target, boat-shaped, nucleated, red, and sickle cells—together with anisocytosis and poikilocytosis—are noted on the peripheral blood smear.

Hemoglobin S/O Arab. Coinheritance of Hb S and Hb O Arab presents a similar or somewhat milder clinical presentation to sickle cell disease and is found in the Middle East and North Africa.

Hemoglobin S/G Philadelphia. One or more abnormal α-globin chains can combine with Hb S. In African Americans and West Africans, the combination of Hb G Philadelphia [$\alpha68(E17)^{Asn\rightarrow Lys}$] with Hb S is prevalent. HPLC analysis (see Figure 32-7, *i*) on blood samples from these individuals shows at least two major peaks and two smaller peaks. The two major peaks are due to combinations of the normal α-chain with the normal β-chain and the abnormal α-chain with the normal β-chain. The two smaller peaks are due to combinations of the normal α-chain with the abnormal β-chain and the abnormal α-chain with the abnormal β-chain. Electrophoresis at alkaline pH shows major bands in the A and S positions with a minor band in the C position. At acid pH, bands are seen in the A and S positions. CBC analysis gives a slightly decreased Hb concentration with normal MCV and MCH. α- or β-Thalassemia can be coinherited with Hb G Philadelphia and Hb S. In these cases, CBC analysis results in markedly decreased MCV and MCH with reduced Hb concentration.

Double heterozygosity Hb G Philadelphia/Hb S occurs in 1 in 125,500 African Americans. On HPLC of patients with Hb G Philadelphia/Hb S trait, four bands are noted, representing four different hemoglobin species, namely, normal

α-chain with normal β-chain, abnormal α-chain with normal β-chain, normal α-chain with abnormal β-chain, and abnormal α-chain with abnormal β-chain. Hemoglobin electrophoresis at alkaline pH shows bands in the A, S, and C positions. At acid, pH bands are noted in the A and S positions. In African Americans, the Hb G Philadelphia mutation occurs with an α-chain deletion, which is *cis* to the mutated alle ($\alpha^G/\alpha\alpha$). This results in a change in the amount of mutated α-chain (α^G) from the usual 25 to around 30%. No clinical or hematologic manifestations are noted with Hb G Philadelphia/Hb S.

Hemoglobin C [$\beta 6(A3)^{Glu \rightarrow Lys}$]. Hb C arises from a substitution of lysine for glutamic acid at position 6 of the β-globin chain. Hb C may be found in the homozygous (Hb C disease, $\beta^C\beta^C$) or heterozygous (Hb C trait) state. Hb C is commonly found in West Africa and the Caribbean. It is the second most commonly studied, after Hb S, of all Hb variants. HPLC analysis (see Figure 32-7, *g*) on samples from individuals with homozygous Hb C shows a large peak in the C position, with Hb C forming 90 to 95% of the total Hb. Hb F concentrations are variable. Glycated Hb C is found as a small peak eluting before the Hb C peak. The ratio of the elution times of glycated Hb C to Hb C is the same as that of Hb A_{1c} and Hb A. Electrophoresis at alkaline and acid pH shows a single band in the C position.

Mild to moderate anemia is the most common clinical presentation. CBC analysis shows normal or slightly decreased Hb concentrations with a normochromic and normocytic red cell morphology. An increase in polychromasia may be present, and the reticulocytes may contribute to an increase in the MCV. The peripheral blood smear shows numerous target cells with occasional nucleated RBCs and characteristic irregular contracted red cells (sometimes called *pyknocytes*). Hb C crystals may be seen, and bilirubin concentrations may be slightly elevated. Red cell survival and osmotic fragility are decreased.

Heterozygous Hemoglobin C (Hb C Trait). HPLC analysis (see Figure 32-7, *h*), capillary electrophoresis, and electrophoresis at both alkaline and acid pH (see Figure 32-11) on blood samples from individuals who are heterozygous for Hb C reveal bands in the A and C positions, with Hb C forming 38 to 45% of the total Hb. CBC analysis may show target cells and generally is normochromic with the MCV near the lower limit of the reference interval.

Heterozygous Hb C individuals are usually asymptomatic. Genetic counseling may be useful when prospective parents have abnormalities in the β-globin gene.

Hb C may be coinherited with both α- and β-thalassemia, and the concentration of Hb C is related to the number of functioning α-genes. With only two functioning α-genes, the Hb C concentration can fall to 32% of the total Hb. Coinheritance of Hb C with β^0- or β^+-thalassemia results in moderately severe anemia with splenomegaly. The Hb F concentration is often increased.

Hemoglobin D Punjab [$\beta 121(GH4)^{Glu \rightarrow Gln}$]. Hb D Punjab is an Hb variant in which glutamic acid at position 121 of the β-globin chain is replaced with glutamine. The names Hb D Los Angeles and Hb D Punjab are used to describe this variant, with the former name used more often in North America and the latter in the United Kingdom. Hb D Punjab is found in the Punjab region of the Indian subcontinent, especially in Sikhs of the Lycus Valley. Large-scale immigration from this area to the United Kingdom, the United States, and Canada has widened the distribution of Hb D Punjab. Hb D Punjab is also found in Caucasians whose foreparents lived in the Indian subcontinent at the time of the British Raj. Hemoglobin D Punjab is found in both heterozygous (Hb D Punjab trait) and homozygous (Hb D Punjab disease, $\beta^D\beta^D$) states.

HPLC analysis of blood from an individual with homozygous Hb D Punjab shows normal or marginally raised Hb F and Hb A_2 peaks with a large peak in the Hb D position forming more than 90% of the total Hb. Electrophoresis at alkaline pH shows a band in the S position, which migrates to the A position in acid electrophoresis. CBC analysis shows a mild decrease in Hb concentrations, MCV, and MCH with target cells observed in the blood smear. Patients present clinically with mild anemia.

HPLC analysis on individuals with Hb D Punjab trait shows two peaks—one at the A position and the other at the D position—with Hb D forming 30 to 40% of the total Hb. The Hb F and Hb A_2 concentrations are within or slightly above the reference intervals. Electrophoresis at alkaline pH shows two bands—one in the A position and the other in the S position. On electrophoresis at acid pH, a single band in the A position is noted. HPLC is the preferred method for identification of Hb D because a similar electrophoretic pattern, on both alkaline and acid pH, is seen with Hb G. CBC analysis is unremarkable except for the presence of target cells on the blood smear.

Individuals with Hb D Punjab trait are clinically asymptomatic.

Coinheritance of Hb D Punjab (both heterozygous and homozygous states) with β-thalassemia is common. CBC analysis on these patients shows decreased concentrations of Hb with markedly decreased MCV and MCH. Target and irregular contracted cells together with hypochromia and anisocytosis are seen on the blood smear. Quantification of Hb A_2 in individuals with coinheritance of Hb D Punjab and β-thalassemia presents a challenge to the laboratory in that HPLC analysis underestimates the Hb A_2 concentration because of an unstable rising baseline in these individuals. Although not normally recommended, quantification of Hb A_2 by densitometry on alkaline electrophoresis may be the only method available to many laboratories. CBC analysis shows a greatly decreased concentration of Hb with low MCV and MCH. The blood smear shows target cells (erythrocytes with increased surface area-to-volume ratio that appear as a target with a bull's eye) and contracted cells with hypochromia and anisocytosis.

Individuals with coinheritance of Hb D Punjab and β-thalassemia present with a notable compensated anemia.

Hemoglobin D Iran [b22(B4)$^{Glu \rightarrow Gln}$]. Hb D Iran is a β-globin chain variant in which glutamine replaces glutamic acid at position 22 of the β-globin chain.

On HPLC analysis, peaks are seen in the A and A_2 positions with quantification for Hb A_2 far above that normally expected. Alkaline electrophoresis shows two bands—one in the A position and the other in the S position. On acid electrophoresis, a single band in the A position is noted. Individuals with Hb D Iran are asymptomatic.

Hemoglobin E [b26(B8)$^{Glu \rightarrow Lys}$]. Hb E is a β-chain variant with lysine replacing glutamic acid at position 26 of the β-globin chain. More individuals have the Hb variant Hb E than any other variant. Hb E is found in both homozygous and heterozygous states and may be combined with β-thalassemia. It is widespread in the Far East, including Southern China, Cambodia, Thailand, and Laos. Hb E is increasingly found in the United States and Canada and is caused by emigration from this area. It may be thought of as the "thalassemic variant," as some of the features of the CBC resemble thalassemia especially in the homozygous state.

HPLC analysis of blood from individuals with homozygous Hb E (Hb E disease, $\beta^E\beta^E$) shows a single peak (>90% of the total Hb) coeluting with Hb A_2. Hemoglobin F is within or marginally above the reference interval. On alkaline electrophoresis, a single band is noted in the C position, which migrates to the A position in acid electrophoresis. CBC analysis shows normal to marginally decreased Hb concentrations with low MCV and MCH. Target cells are noted in the peripheral blood smear. Iron studies are normal.

Homozygous Hb E individuals are usually asymptomatic, although slight anemia may be present.

HPLC analysis of blood from individuals with heterozygous Hb E reveals two peaks—one in the A position and the other in the A_2 position. Hb E forms approximately 30% of the total Hb. Capillary electrophoresis resolves Hb E from Hb A_2. Hb A_2 is higher in patients with Hb E than in patients without a hemoglobin variant or thalassemia as the result of decreased synthesis of the abnormal β-globin chain, allowing for increased binding between the excess α-globin and δ-globin chains producing Hb A.[H36-H37] CBC analysis shows normal Hb concentrations and occasionally low MCV. Target cells are noted in the peripheral blood smear. Iron studies are normal.

Heterozygous Hb E individuals are usually asymptomatic, although slight anemia may be present.

Coinheritance of Hb E and thalassemia produces an anemia of variable severity. HPLC on a patient with coinheritance of β-thalassemia and homozygous E is shown in Figure 32-7, *C*. Coinheritance of homozygous Hb E and β-thalassemia leads to a severe anemia with greatly reduced Hb concentrations, MCV, and MCH with increased Hb F concentration. Numerous target cells are noted on the peripheral blood smear, together with microcytosis, anisocytosis, hypochromia, and a few nucleated red cells. Iron studies are normal. In the most severe cases, the clinical presentation is similar to that of β^0-thalassemia, and transfusion may be the only therapy. Coinheritance of heterozygous Hb E with α-thalassemia produces a less severe anemia with low Hb and MCV and MCH. Target cells are noted on the peripheral blood smear, together with microcytosis and hypochromia. Patients who are pregnant may need to be monitored closely, although transfusion is not usually required.

Quantification of Hb A_2, which is important in the diagnosis of possible coinheritance of β-thalassemia with Hb E, provides a challenge to the laboratory in that Hb E and Hb A_2 coelute. Molecular studies are the only satisfactory method by which to establish coinheritance of Hb E and β-thalassemia, although the severity of the disease, family studies, and increased Hb F may lead to suspicion of coinheritance.

Hemoglobin O Arab [b121(GH4)$^{Glu \rightarrow Lys}$]. Hb O Arab is a β-chain variant with lysine replacing glutamic acid at position 121 of the β-globin chain. Hb O Arab is found in a wide variety of ethnic groups in North Africa and Eastern Europe and is not confined, nor is it even common, among Arab populations. Hb O Arab has been found in both heterozygous and homozygous states.

HPLC analysis of blood from an individual with homozygous Hb O Arab shows a single band between the S and C positions, with Hb O Arab forming more than 90% of the total Hb. Electrophoresis at alkaline pH shows a band close to the C position. On electrophoresis at acid pH, a band is seen between the A and S positions (but closer to A). CBC analysis shows a normal or marginally low Hb concentration, MCV, and MCH. The peripheral blood smear shows slight microcytosis.

No unusual hematologic features are noted in individuals with heterozygous Hb O Arab. HPLC analysis on blood from these individuals shows two peaks—one in the A position and the other eluting close to the C position and forming 30 to 40% of the total Hb. Electrophoresis at alkaline electrophoresis shows bands in the A and close to the C position. On acid electrophoresis, two bands are noted—one in the A position and the other in a position between the A and S positions.

Hybrid Hemoglobins. Hybrid Hbs, or crossover Hbs, describe a group of Hb variants in which one of the globin chains is a hybrid of amino acid sequences of two other globin chains. The term *crossover Hb* is sometimes used because there is a point in the amino acid sequence at which there is crossover from the amino acid sequence of one globin chain to another globin chain. Individuals with these hybrid Hb variants present with clinical features and laboratory findings, particularly in their CBC, that are similar to those of thalassemia. Production of the hybrid globin chain is reduced. Hb Lepore is the prototypical hybrid Hb.

Hemoglobin Lepore. Hb Lepore is classified as a δβ-hybrid Hb variant on the basis that the non–α-chain is a hybrid of δ- and β-globin chains. It is unique in that it is the only hemoglobinopathy named after the family name of the index case. δβ-Hybrid Hbs arise because there are deletions of part of the 3′ portion of the δ-globin gene and in the 5′ portion of the β-globin chain with resultant formation of a δβ-fusion gene. Three distinct variations of Hb Lepore have been described. In Hb Lepore-Hollandia [δβ-hybrid (δ through 22; β from 50)], a variant found in Canada and Papua New Guinea, fusion occurs of the first 22 amino acid residues of the δ-globin chain with the amino acids from position 50 onward of the β-globin chain. In Hb Lepore-Baltimore [δβ-hybrid (δ through 50: β from 86)], found mainly in individuals of Spanish ancestry, the first 50 amino acid residues of the δ-globin chain are fused with amino acid residues from position 86 of the β-globin chain. In Hb Lepore-Boston-Washington [δβ-hybrid (δ through 87; β from 116)], the most common Hb Lepore, the first 87 amino acid residues of the δ-globin chain are fused with amino acid residues from position 116 onward of the β-globin chain. Hb Lepore-Boston-Washington, sometimes called Hb Lepore-Boston, is found mainly in individuals of Italian descent, although it has been found in individuals from Eastern Europe.

HPLC analysis of blood from individuals with Hb Lepore shows greatly elevated Hb A_2 concentration with marginally reduced Hb A. The Hb A_2 concentration is usually greater than 10% of the total Hb and is falsely increased because of the coelution of Hb A_2 and Hb Lepore. Electrophoresis at alkaline pH shows a band in the S position for Hb Lepore-Boston-Washington and in a position between the A and S positions for the other Hb Lepore variants. At acid pH, a single band is present in the A position for all Hb Lepore variants. Hb A_2 and Hb Lepore are resolved on capillary electrophoresis.

CBC analysis shows greatly reduced concentrations of Hb, MCV, and MCH in Hb Lepore homozygotes. Hematologic findings are very similar to those of β-thalassemia major or intermedia. CBC analysis on heterozygotes shows slightly reduced MCV and MCH. Hematologic findings are very similar to those of β-thalassemia trait. Iron studies are normal in both heterozygotes and homozygotes. The similarity of the hematology in Hb Lepore and in β-thalassemia makes careful review of the HPLC and electrophoretic analysis essential. A greatly elevated Hb A_2 by HPLC analysis and a small band in the S position on electrophoresis at alkaline pH suggest Hb Lepore.

Elongation Hemoglobins. Elongation Hbs, of which there are 13, including seven α-chain and six β-chain variants, result from lengthening of the C or N terminus of either globin chain. The most important, from a clinical perspective, are the five C terminal α-chain variants in which the terminal codon TAA is changed and an amino acid sequence is added. The prototypical elongation Hb is Hb Constant Spring. In this variant, the C terminal TAA codon is changed to CAA in the α_2-gene, and a 31 amino acid sequence is added at the C terminal end to give an α-globin chain length of 173 amino acid residues, rather than the normal 142 residue length. This increase in length results in instability of the Hb variant, and synthesis of this elongated globin chain is reduced. Hemoglobin Constant Spring is found in South East Asia, especially in Vietnam, Cambodia, and Laos, and is found in both heterozygous and homozygous states.

Patients with Hb Constant Spring present with slightly reduced Hb, MCV, and MCH with hypochromia and microcytosis in the peripheral blood smear. Iron studies are often normal.

The instability of Hb Constant Spring presents a challenge to the laboratory diagnosis of this variant. The blood used for analytical procedures should be as fresh as possible. Samples older than 24 hours should not be used. HPLC analysis of blood from individuals with Hb Constant Spring demonstrates a small peak in the C position, which forms approximately 4 to 6% of the total Hb in the homozygote and 1 to 3% in the heterozygote. On electrophoresis at alkaline pH, a small band migrating cathodally to the application point may be seen. This electrophoretic mobility is unique in that it is the only Hb variant that moves toward the cathode rather than the anode.

Hemoglobin Constant Spring is commonly found in combination with α^0-thalassemia, especially the -^{SEA} mutation. The clinical presentation of this combination results in a severe form of Hb H disease.

Analytical Methods

The laboratory plays a crucial role in detection and characterization of the hemoglobinopathies and thalassemias discussed in the next sections.[H1] Several recommendations have been put forth for the laboratory investigation of abnormal Hbs and thalassemias.[H12,H30,H44] For example, in 1978 the International Committee for Standardization in Hematology expert panel on abnormal Hbs published recommendations for the laboratory investigation of these conditions.[H45] In its initial investigation, (1) a CBC, (2) electrophoresis at pH 9.2, (3) tests for solubility and sickling, and (4) quantification of Hb A_2 and Hb F were recommended. If an abnormal Hb was found as a result of these initial tests, further tests including electrophoresis at pH 6.2, globin chain separation, and isoelectric focusing were recommended by the panel. If the presence of an unstable Hb or Hb with altered oxygen affinity was suspected, then heat and isopropanol stability tests were recommended. Although new techniques have replaced some of these tests, the approach of using multiple assays in the initial investigation of hemoglobinopathies and thalassemias is an accepted practice that is used in many laboratories involved in the investigation of these disorders. In addition to these tests, the iron status of the patient should be ascertained by measurement of ferritin or by the iron/total iron-binding capacity/saturation index. Information on the ethnicity and/or nationality of the patient, when allowed under patient confidentiality rules, may provide useful information because thalassemias (e.g., β-thalassemia in individuals of Mediterranean origin) and certain hemoglobinopathies (e.g., Hb S trait and homozygous S in African Americans) are associated with particular ethnic and/or national groups.

The 2010 guidelines of the British Committee for Standards in Haematology[H31] for the laboratory diagnosis of hemoglobinopathies recommend that qualification for genetic counseling requires identification of hemoglobins S, C, D Punjab, O Arab, E, Lepore, and H and the detection of carriers of α^0-thalasssemia and β-thalasssemia traits. To accomplish this, it is recommended that "all ethnic groups" be screened for β thalassemia trait when the mean cell (or corpuscular) hemoglobin (MCH) is less than 27 pg. All ethnic groups, except for Northern European Caucasians, should be screened for hemoglobin variants. Selected ethnic groups should be screened for α^0-thalassemia trait when the MCH is less than 25. Recommended methods include HPLC and hemoglobin electrophoresis for identification of hemoglobin variants, and HPLC and microcolumn chromatography for quantification of hemoglobin A_2. Electrophoresis is not recommended for the quantification of HbA^2 In addition, it is recommended that two methods, based on different analytical principle, be used to establish a presumptine identification of the hemoglobin variant. A flow chart, as shown in Figure 32-12, is suggested for identification of α^0-, β-, and δβ-thalassemia traits and hemoglobin variants.

Preferred Specimen

The preferred blood sample for use in detection and characterization of the hemoglobinopathies is one collected with K or Na salts of ethylenediaminetetraacetic acid (EDTA) as the anticoagulant. To minimize the formation of degradation products, which are especially noticeable as small bands eluting with similar retention time as Hb A_{1c} and Hb F on HPLC analysis, testing should be performed within 5 days of collection and samples should be stored at 4 °C.

Techniques

Analytical techniques used to measure RBCs and their indices, Hb, and related compounds include (1) determination of CBC; (2) electrophoresis; (3) immunoassay; (4) separation techniques such as HPLC, capillary electrophoresis, and mass spectrometry; (5) molecular techniques such as deoxyribonucleic acid (DNA) analysis; and (6) specific tests for specific variants.

Complete Blood Count

A CBC of a whole blood sample consists of (1) numbers of RBCs (erythrocytes), (2) numbers of white blood cells, (3) numbers of platelets, (4) a measure of Hb, (5) estimates of red cell volume, and (6) estimation of white blood cell subtypes (see Table 32-1). [*Note:* A CBC is also known as a full **blood** count **(FBC),** a full **blood** examination (FBE), or a **blood** panel.] Knowledge of red cell indices[H24,H56] and the information obtained from microscopic examination of a peripheral blood film is vital to the diagnosis of both α- and β-thalassemias. Hemoglobinopathies have a lesser impact on red cell indices but may present abnormal red cell morphology on peripheral blood films. In thalassemias, the Hb concentration and the MCV, an index of cell size, are decreased, sometimes markedly, whereas in hemoglobinopathies, both are often normal. One study recommends that an MCV of less than 72 fL (reference interval ≈80 to 100 fL)[H50] is maximally sensitive and specific for the presumptive diagnosis of thalassemia. However, an MCH less than 27 pg (reference interval ≈26 to 35 pg)[H55] has been recommended as the decision point for further investigation for iron deficiency anemia and thalassemia. The rationale for the selection of MCH over MCV as the decision point for further investigation is the potential increase of up to 5 fL in MCV in samples older than 24 hours.

The RBC count may be in the upper half of or above the reference interval in thalassemias but within the reference interval in most hemoglobinopathies without a coinherited thalassemia. In contrast, the RBC count is low in iron deficiency anemias and anemia of chronic disease and is proportionally related to the decrease in Hb concentration. The RDW, a measure of variation in the size of the RBC (anisocytosis), tends to be above the reference interval in iron deficiency anemias and other microcytic anemias. The RDW in thalassemias is usually within or very close to the reference interval, reflecting the uniformity of red cell size. However, in Hb H disease and δβ-thalassemia, the RDW is moderately increased.

In thalassemias, the RBCs in the peripheral blood smear are hypochromic and microcytic. Characteristic sickle- or crescent-shaped RBCs are seen (Figure 32-13) in the peripheral blood smear of patients who are homozygous for Hb S (sickle cell disease), and targets are seen in blood smears from patients who are homozygous for Hb E (see Figure 32-13) and Hb C. In addition, microspherocytes (erythrocytes whose diameter is less than normal, but whose thickness is increased) and crystalline inclusions (Hb C cells) have been found in peripheral blood smears from individuals who are homozygous for Hb C. These findings are less uniformly present than the typical morphologic features of sickle cell disease.

Several formulas, based on parameters from the CBC, may be used to calculate a thalassemic index and have been used to differentiate iron deficiency from thalassemia.[H50] Although none have proved to be totally satisfactory in all clinical situations or to add significant information over the use of MCV alone in selecting cases for further investigation, many laboratories use these calculations as an adjunct to CBC parameters. The most commonly used formulas are the following:

$$\text{Mentzler Index (MI)} = \frac{\text{MCV}}{\text{RBC}}$$

$$\text{Discriminant Factor (DF)} = (\text{MCV})^2 \times \frac{RDW}{Hb \times 100}$$

$$\text{Shine and Lal Index (S \& L)} = \text{MCV}^2 \times \frac{\text{MCH}}{100}$$

$$\text{Srivastava Index (SI)} = \frac{\text{MCH}}{\text{RBC}}$$

$$\text{RDW Index (RDWI)} = \frac{\text{MCV} \times \text{RDW}}{\text{RBC}}$$

where

MCV = mean cell volume
RBC = red blood cell count
RDW = red blood cell distribution width
Hb = hemoglobin
MCH = mean cell hemoglobin

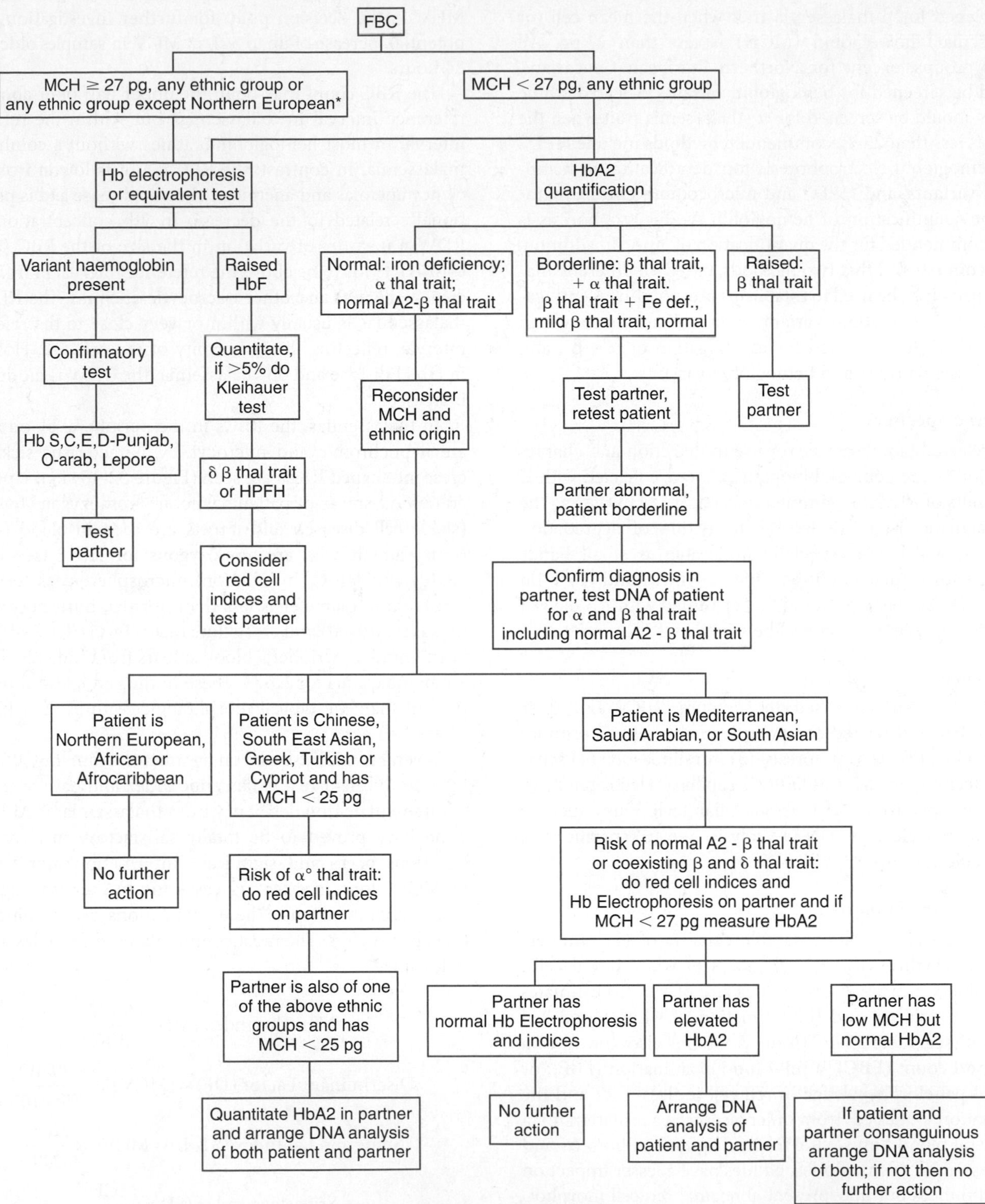

Figure 32-12 Flowchart demonstrating procedure for diagnosis of ∀⁰-, β-, and *β-thalassemia trait and clinically significant hemoglobin variants in pregnant women ("patients") and their partners. Selective screening is acceptable in low-incidence areas but only if accurate information on ethnic origin is available. *FBC,* Full blood count; *Hb,* hemoglobin; *Hb S, C, E, D, F, Punjab, Arab, Lepore,* various types of hemoglobin; *MCH,* mean cell hemoglobin; *thal,* thalassemia. *(Adapted from Guidelines for the laboratory diagnosis of haemoglobinopathies. The Working Party of the General Haematology Task Force of the British Committee for Standards in Haematology. Brit J Haematol 1998;101:783-92.)*

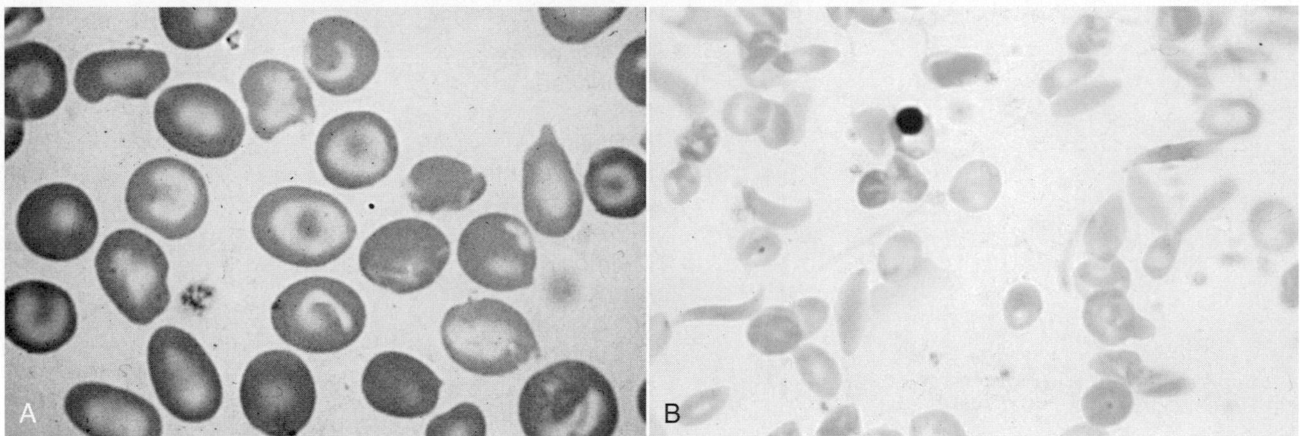

Figure 32-13 Peripheral blood smear from patients with (A) homozygous Hb E and (B) homozygous Hb S.

In using these formulas, it is not possible to use a single cutpoint to distinguish between iron repletion, iron deficiency, and thalassemia. The use of two cutpoints, one to distinguish iron replete status from deficiency and another to distinguish iron deficiency from thalassemia, is recommended.

CBC parameters are very often the first indication that the patient might have a thalassemia or a hemoglobinopathy; however, these data are not sufficient to allow even a presumptive diagnosis. In addition, the iron status of the patient, as measured with ferritin or iron/iron-binding/saturation index tests (see the next section), helps in differentiating iron deficiency anemia from anemia of chronic disease and thalassemia. However, ferritin is elevated in acute-phase reactions, and iron deficiency can mask an underlying thalassemia.

An algorithm based on MCV, MCH, Hb A_2, and Hb F quantifications has been advocated to better discriminate between β-thalassemia minor, iron deficiency, δβ-thalassemia, and HPFH.[H57]

Electrophoresis

Electrophoresis (see Chapter 12) under alkaline conditions (pH 9.2) is the most common initial screening method for the detection and preliminary identification of hemoglobinopathies.[H7] Several media, including paper and cellulose acetate, have been used, although agarose[H5] is now the medium of choice and the one usually supplied commercially. A pH 9.2 barbital buffer is the most common buffer system. Visualization of separated Hb bands is achieved by using a protein-binding stain, such as Amido Black or Ponceau S. Hemoglobin bands stain blue with Amido Black and reddish pink with Ponceau S. Following clearing of excess stain, Hb bands on the agarose media are clearly seen against the clear background. The left panel of Figure 32-11 shows an alkaline electrophoresis gel stained with Amido Black. Quantification by densitometry of Hb A_2 and F bands on alkaline electrophoresis, although commonly performed by laboratories, is not recommended by the College of American Pathologists in the hemoglobinopathy survey critiques[H49] because of high analytical imprecision resulting from limitations of densitometry in quantifying faint bands. Scanning densitometry is not adequate for Hb A_2 quantification because the precision requirement is 10 times greater than is needed for hemoglobin variant quantification and cannot be met by densitometric methods.[H70]

At alkaline pH, Hbs migrate according to electrical charge, with Hb H moving the fastest (closest to the anode). The order of migration (fastest to slowest) is Hb H, Hb N, Hb I, Hb J, Hb A, Hb F, Hb S, and Hb C. Hemoglobins D and G co-migrate with Hb S, and Hbs E, O, and A_2 co-migrate with Hb C. Hemoglobin Constant Spring migrates slightly toward the cathode. An easy way to remember the sequence is Hb A goes to the Anode, wheras Hb C migrates to the Cathode. Hb F and S follow after Hb A in alphabetical order.

Electrophoresis at pH 6.4 using a citrate buffer is performed when an abnormal band is noted on alkaline Hb electrophoresis. Agarose is the preferred medium, with Acid Violet the preferred stain. In the right panel of Figure 32-11, the same Hb variants performed on agarose electrophoresis at pH 6.4 and stained with Acid Violet are shown. The order of migration (cathode to anode, fastest to slowest) is Hb F, Hb A, Hb S, and Hb C. Hemoglobins D, G, I, J, O, A_2, and E co-migrate with Hb A.

Based on positions of the bands in acid and alkaline electrophoresis, a presumptive identification of the Hb variant may be made. For example, bands are found on alkaline electrophoresis in both A and C positions. On acid electrophoresis if bands are found in the A and C positions, then a presumptive identification of Hb C trait may be made, as this pattern is characteristic. However, if a band is found only in the A position on acid electrophoresis, then a presumptive identification of Hb E may be made. If bands are found in the C position on alkaline electrophoresis and between the S and A positions on acid electrophoresis, then a presumptive identification of Hb O may be made. Further testing is required to determine whether the Hb O is Hb O Arab, O Indonesia, or O Padova. Fairbanks[H25] described a numbering system for the most common Hb bands on alkaline electrophoresis

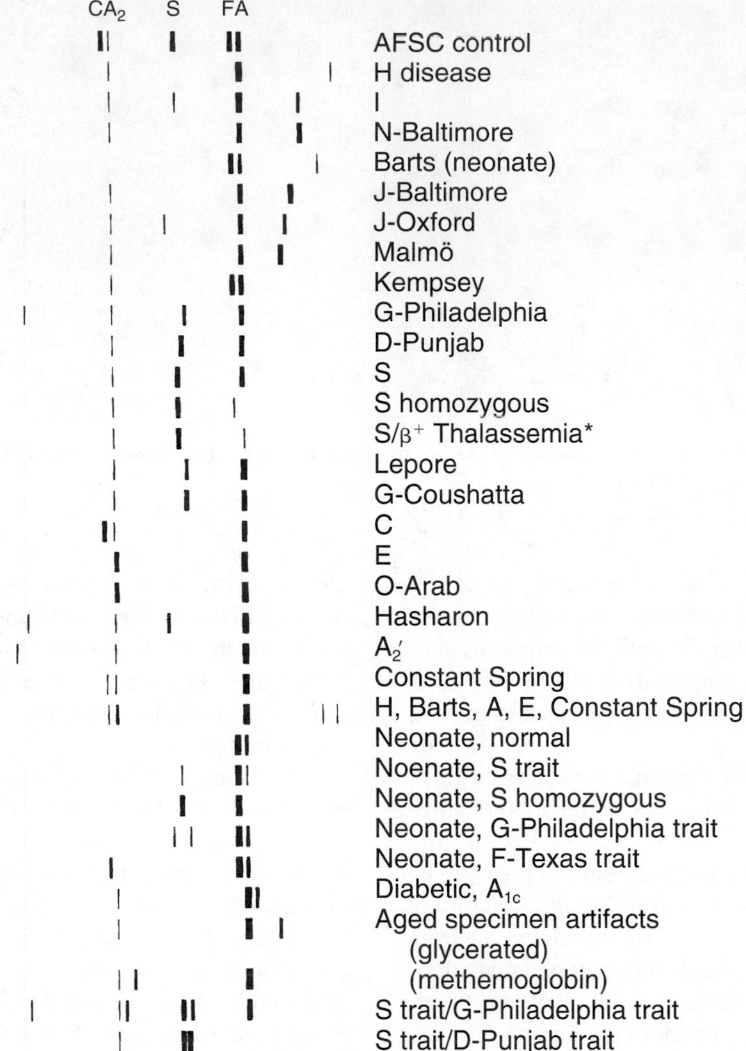

Figure 32-14 A diagram of isoelectric focusing patterns for a variety of Hb variants. The conditions shown represent heterozygotes (traits) unless otherwise indicated. The width of the bars approximates the relative density of the bands observed. The acid anodic (pH 6) side is to the right, and the alkaline cathodic (pH 8) side is to the left. The same pattern is observed in homozygous patients with Hb S disease who have received Hb A by transfusion.

(Hb H is position 1, Hb A is position 5, Hb S is position 9, and Hb Cis position 13) that allowed the position of a band to be described more exactly than the commonly used descriptive term "between S and A positions." Unfortunately, this system has not found universal acceptance. Laboratories should keep a bank of electrophoretic data obtained to help in future identification of unusual Hb variants.

Specific types of electrophoresis that are used for Hb analysis include isoelectric focusing, electrophoresis, and capillary electrophoresis.

Isoelectric Focusing Electrophoresis. Isoelectric focusing electrophoresis (IEF)[H15] has greater resolving power than conventional electrophoresis, but it is more expensive, time-consuming, and technique dependent to perform (see Chapter 12). Commercial IEF gels are made of cellulose acetate or polyacrylamide with the pH gradient produced by the inclusion of amphoteric materials of different pH in bands in the gel. Locations of the Hb bands are identified using stains similar to those used in conventional electrophoresis. The bands or zones produced by IEF (Figure 32-14) are more clearly defined than with those seen with conventional electrophoresis, and reliable quantification of separated Hbs may be made at high concentrations using densitometry. Quantification of Hb A_2 and Hb F at low concentrations, however, is imprecise and is not recommended. The Hb elution pattern in IEF is similar to that of alkaline Hb electrophoresis, except that Hb D and Hb G are resolved from each other and from Hb S. Historically, IEF has been used extensively to identify and characterize Hb variants; however, it is less frequently used now because of the previously mentioned limitations.

Capillary Isoelectric Focusing Electrophoresis. Capillary isoelectric focusing electrophoresis[H20,H29,H33,H68,H74] combines the detection sensitivity of capillary electrophoresis (see Chapter 12) with the resolution qualities and existing extensive data on Hb variant separation by immunoelectrophoresis (IEP) and the automated sampling and digital data acquisition techniques developed for chromatography. With this approach, the hemolysate is introduced into the capillary chamber using low-pressure injection and then is focused at high voltage (typically ≈30 kV and 0.5 to 1.5 μA), during which it is essential to maintain adequate cooling. The separated Hbs are then eluted, using low-pressure and simultaneous voltage, past a single-wavelength spectrophotometric detector set to read at 415 nm or a dual-wavelength detector set at 415 and 450 nm. In routine use, the Hbs are typically separated within 15 minutes, but the elution time may be extended if the presence of abnormal Hb is suspected. Hb variants[H33] are identified by comparison of isoelectric point (pI) values and migration times of the unknown, using Hb A as the reference peak, with known controls and published data. Quantification is based on integration of the measured absorbance of the bands, and accurate results have been obtained for Hb A_2 and Hb F concentrations.

Capillary Electrophoresis. The introduction of commercial capillary electrophoresis instrumentation for the separation of hemoglobins has made this technique available to clinical laboratories.[H29] Separation in an alkaline buffer at specific pH using high voltages is based on charge difference, electrolyte pH, and electro-osmotic flow. Hemoglobin measurement is commonly performed at a wavelength of 415 nm and identification is based on retention time. All common hemoglobin variants are separated, and quantification of HbF and Hb A_2 is performed in a single analytical run.[H20,H53,H54] Cotton and Mario[H20] initially described the application of this technique to the identification of hemoglobin variants and quantification of Hb A_2; others have described the usefulness of the technique in the clinical laboratory.[H36,H46,H80] Advantages of capillary electrophoresis over HPLC include quantification of Hb A_2 in the presence of Hb E (due to incomplete resolution of Hb A_2 from Hb E in HPLC), quantification of Hb H, and identification of Hb Lepore.

High-Performance Liquid Chromatography

HPLC using a column packed with cation-exchange resin[H26,H27,H59] provides, in a single analytical protocol, the quantification of Hbs F and A_2 (see Chapter 13 for a detailed discussion of HPLC). With it, the initial identification of an Hb variant on the basis of elution time may be made. It has also been used to detect α-thalassemia phenotypes.

After injection and subsequent adsorption onto the particles of cation-exchange resin, molecules of Hb are eluted using gradient elution. Detection of eluted Hbs is achieved by monitoring the effluent solvent stream using a dual-wavelength photometer (usually set to measure at wavelengths of 415 and 690 nm). The technique is precise for the quantification of both Hb F and Hb A_2, and presumptive identification of the common Hb variant may be made. These features have made HPLC the method of choice for hemoglobinopathy and thalassemia screening for many laboratories, including those performing neonatal hemoglobinopathy screening. Figure 32-7 shows the separation on a commercial system of nine Hb variants.

Several commercial methods are available but lack the resolution achieved by noncommercial methods. A noncommercial HPLC method has been described with the retention time and relative concentration of 40 common Hb variants listed.[H59] This system (1) requires a longer time of analysis, (2) provides superior resolution, and (3) overcomes the problem of coelution of several Hb variants that occurs with commercial systems. For example, with one commercial system, Hbs E, Osu-Christianborg, G-Coushatta, Lepore, and G-Copenhagen coelute with Hb A_2, making Hb A_2 quantification and definitive identification of the Hb variants impossible.[H19,H35]

Other chromatographic problems, such as rising baseline, have resulted in falsely low Hb A_2 concentration in Hb D patients.[H22,H66] This may be corrected mathematically to produce a more accurate result. Patients with Hb S have falsely increased Hb A_2 concentrations; this was originally thought to be caused by the coelution of glycated Hb S with Hb A_2.[H73] Subsequent studies have shown that the increase in Hb A_2 in patients with HbS is due to coelution of carbamylated Hb S species.[H82] Diagnosis of coinheritance of β-thalassemia with Hb S may be compromised by this false increase in Hb A_2. However, knowledge of the concentration of Hb A_2 is not essential in making the diagnosis of β^0- or β^+-thalassemia in these patients. In the case of β^0-thalassemia (β-thalassemia major), no δ-globin chain is produced, and the electrophoretic pattern and HPLC closely resemble those of a homozygous Hb S patient (large Hb F and Hb S peaks with no Hb A peak). In β^+-thalassemia (β-thalassemia intermedia), the concentration of Hb S is greater than that of Hb A, a situation that otherwise is seen only in recently transfused patients who have sickle cell disease. Coinheritance of β-thalassemia minor and Hb S may be diagnosed in these patients by setting the upper limit of the reference interval at 5.0%.[H38] Capillary zone electrophoresis and microcolumn methods have been described that eliminate the interference of glycated Hb S with Hb A_2 quantification.

The use of relative elution time rather than absolute elution time in initial identification of an unknown Hb variant is useful and recommended. The reference Hb ideally is one that is found in low concentrations in most individuals. In this regard, Hb A_2 is probably most useful as a reference point despite the number of coeluting Hb variants.

The elution time of the Hb may change slightly with increasing Hb variant concentration. For example, Hb F concentrations obtained by HPLC are often lower than those obtained from alkaline denaturation and/or spectrophotometric methods that are often quoted in standard hematology texts and used for the diagnosis of juvenile myelomonocytic leukemia (JMML) and monosomy 7 syndrome. Caution should be used in interchanging Hb F concentrations obtained by HPLC with those obtained by other methods.

It should be noted that hemoglobinopathies may interfere with glycated hemoglobin (GHb) analysis, as results may be falsely increased or decreased, depending on the particular method and the hemoglobinopathy.[H13,H64] Hemoglobin variants that cannot be separated from Hb A or Hb A_{1c} will produce spuriously increased or decreased results by ion-exchange HPLC.

Electrospray Mass Spectroscopy

Electrospray mass spectrometry (see Chapter 14) is becoming the method of choice[H11] for the complete characterization of newly discovered Hb variants.[H4-H6,H16,H35,H48,H62,H75,H82] By using this method, the mass of the variant, whether it is an α- or a β-chain variant, as well as the possible location and identity of the amino acid residue substitution and the quantity of variant present can be derived.

To analyze a sample with this technique, the globin chains first are separated and then are isolated by semipreparative HPLC. The isolated fractions are further concentrated using a variety of techniques, including membrane filtration. The fraction containing the mutant globin chain is digested using specific endopeptidases that selectively cut at certain amino acid residues of the globin chain. The resultant digested peptide fragments are further separated by preparative HPLC and the mutant peptide sequenced using Edman degradation. Another portion of the digested globin chains is entered into the electrospray mass spectrometer, and the resultant mass spectrum provides information on the mass of the mutant globin chain, which can be used to provisionally identify the substituted amino acid. For Hb Rambam,[H5] the mass spectrum of the β-globin chains shows the mass of the normal β-chain to be 15,867 Da and the mass of the mutant β-chain to be 15,925 Da. The increase in mass of 58 in the mutant β-globin chain may be attributed to a change in amino acid residue from glycine (75 Da) to aspartic acid (133 Da).

Tandem mass spectroscopy has been used for newborn screening for sickle cell disease[H8,H47] and for the characterization of Hb A_2.[H21]

DNA Analysis

DNA analysis is used in the investigation of thalassemias and hemoglobinopathies to identify, in populations with a known high incidence of disease, those specific individuals at risk and who may benefit from genetic counseling. For example, DNA analysis has been used to do the following:

1. Diagnose α^0- and α^+-thalassemia.[H3,H9,H77]
2. Investigate potentially life-threatening disorders of Hb synthesis in the fetus; it is performed at less than 10 weeks' gestation on chorionic villus[H57] samples.
3. Characterize the β-thalassemia genotype.[H28,H34,H67,H76]
4. Screen at-risk populations for clinically significant Hb variants.[H28,H69]
5. Distinguish between conditions that have similar laboratory and clinical presentations but are the result of different genetic conditions.

The Southern blot analysis of genomic DNA using α- and ζ-primers is widely used in the investigation of α-thalassemias, especially in the identification of individuals with α^0-thalassemia. Polymerase chain reaction (PCR), using allele-specific primers, is used by reference laboratories in the identification of common β-thalassemia mutations and some hemoglobinopathies. Gene sequencing information may supplement these techniques in some cases.

Specific Tests

Tests that are used to measure Hbs and related analytes include those for Hb H, Hb S, unstable Hbs, and globin chains.

Determining Hemoglobin H

Hb H, an insoluble tetramer consisting of four β-globin chains, arises in α-thalassemia in which decreased production of α-globin chains is caused by nonexpression of three of the four α-globin genes and a subsequent excess of β-globin chains. If these tetramers are oxidized, precipitation occurs, which may be viewed microscopically. In the laboratory, this oxidation is achieved by staining unfixed cells with freshly prepared methylene blue or brilliant cresyl blue at 37 °C. Inclusion of positive and negative controls with each batch of Hb H preparations is essential because substantial batch-to-batch variability is seen in the dye.[H32] Controversy is ongoing regarding the necessity to perform this test on freshly collected blood, and whether the test should be performed in all suspected α-thalassemia cases.

In Hb, H disease, 30 to 100% of the red cells contain inclusions, which have been described as looking like "golf balls." In α-thalassemia silent (one functional α-gene), as few as one cell with inclusions per 1000 to 10,000 red cells may be seen, and the diagnosis of α-thalassemia silent or minor cannot be made definitively in the absence of Hb H inclusions. The presence of Hb H inclusions may serve as confirmation of a presumptive diagnosis of α^0-thalassemia (α-thalassemia major) or Hb H disease.

Precipitate patterns resembling Hb H inclusions may arise from staining of reticulin and Howell-Jolly bodies and other protein and nucleic acid entities. Hb H inclusions may be very rare and difficult to detect when reticulocytosis is increased.

Hb H detection by this method is laborious to perform and is subjective. However, for detection of the two α-gene *cis* deletion (-/αα) of α^0-thalassemia, the test is reported to have a clinical sensitivity of 0.47 and a specificity of 0.99.[H51]

Use of molecular tests in selected groups with suspected α-thalassemia, for example, in females of childbearing age, is becoming the standard, rather than use of the H prep, in all age groups.

Sickling Tests

Sickling tests are useful in confirming the presence of Hb S in a sample following initial electrophoresis at alkaline pH. When Hb S is oxygenated, it is fully soluble. When Hb S is deoxygenated, polymerization occurs, forming deformed red

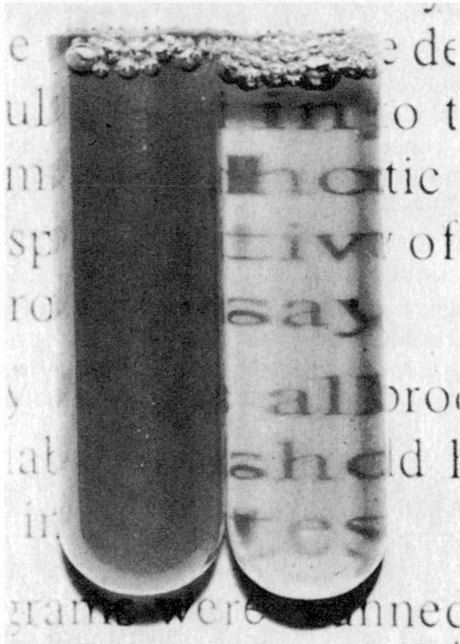

Figure 32-15 Solubility test for Hb S. Deoxyhemoglobin S *(left tube)* is insoluble in 2.3 mol/L phosphate buffer. By contrast, normal hemolysate *(right tube)* is sufficiently transparent that print can easily be read through it.

cells with a characteristic rigid sickle shape. In the laboratory, deoxygenation and lysis of RBCs is achieved by the use of a solution of sodium metabisulfite in a phosphate buffer. Addition of the sodium metabisulfite reagent to an Hb S–containing blood sample causes turbidity. This turbidity is visualized by holding a lined card or a card with writing on it behind the reaction test tube (Figure 32-15). In positive samples, lines or letters cannot be seen, whereas in negative samples, lines or letters are clearly visible. Both a positive and a negative control should be used with each test. The hematocrit of the blood sample to be tested should be measured, and if less than 15% the amount of blood used in the test should be doubled, because low Hb concentration is a cause of falsely negative sickling screens. Lipemic samples and samples with a monoclonal protein (M-protein) may give a false-positive result. Hb C Harlem and Hb Memphis [$\alpha 23(B4)^{Glu\psi Gln}$] also give a positive result in this procedure; therefore it is essential to identify the Hb in all positive tests by other techniques. The test is subjective and the combination of two identification techniques, such as HPLC and alkaline electrophoresis, may eliminate the necessity to perform this test on a routine basis.

Tests for Unstable Hemoglobins

These tests use heat or isopropanol to precipitate the unstable Hb and must be performed on fresh blood. More than 100 unstable Hbs are mainly the result of the interchange of nonpolar amino acid residues for polar amino acid residues in positions in the α- or β-globin chain associated with the heme cleft. Hb Hasharon [$\alpha 47(CD)^{Asp\psi His}$], an Hb variant found in Ashkenazi Jews, results from substitution of the nonpolar amino acid residue histidine for the polar aspartic acid residue at position 47 of the α-chain. In conventional nomenclature, Hb Hasharon should be written as $\alpha 47(CE5)^{Asp\psi His}$; however, to maintain uniformity with β-, γ-, and δ-globin chains, the term *CD* is used to designate the corresponding interhelical segment of the α-chain, which does not have a D segment.

Nonpolar isopropanol weakens the internal bonds within Hb, decreasing the stability of the Hb molecule. Normal hemoglobin (Hb A) precipitates within 40 minutes at 37 °C in the presence of a 17% solution of isopropanol with a pH 7.4 TRIS buffer. Unstable Hbs usually precipitate within 5 minutes under these conditions. Both a positive and a negative control should be included with each analysis, although a positive control may not always be readily available. An umbilical cord blood or neonatal sample, not fresh, may be an acceptable alternative as a positive control. At the time of reading, the negative control should be clear, and the positive control should have some flocculation.

Normal Hb is stable when heated to 50 °C. However, unstable Hbs precipitate to varying extents when similarly treated. A hemolysate of the sample in a pH 7.4 TRIS-phosphate buffer is divided into two aliquots. One is stored at 4 °C, the other is heated at 50 °C for 2 hours. Both samples are centrifuged and Hb quantification is performed on each supernatant. Quantification of the unstable Hb is calculated using the following formula:

$$\%\ \text{Unstable hemoglobin} = \frac{\text{Hb}\,(4\,°\text{C}) - \text{Hb}\,(50\,°\text{C})}{\text{Hb}\,(4\,°\text{C})} \times 100$$

Frequently, both heat and isopropanol stability tests are performed when a suspected unstable Hb variant is investigated. Unstable Hb variants may not appear on HPLC or electrophoresis, especially if the variant is unstable enough to precipitate before analysis by these techniques.

Globin Chain Analysis

Globin chain analysis by electrophoresis and HPLC has been replaced by mass spectroscopy; however, the techniques used to dissociate the globin chains—urea and dithiothretiol treatment—are still used.

IRON

In healthy individuals, very small quantities of iron are present in most cells of the body, in plasma, and in other extracellular fluids. Physiologically, iron stores are rigorously conserved with less than 0.1% of the body iron content lost daily, mostly as the result of desquamation, minor trauma, and menses. Body iron stores are replenished daily by controlled absorption of iron in quantities that equal iron losses.

Biochemistry

Distribution

Body iron is distributed into different compartments that include (1) hemoglobin (Hb), (2) storage iron (ferritin and hemosiderin), (3) myoglobin, (4) a labile iron pool, (5) other

TABLE 32-3 Average Iron Content of Compartments in an Average 70-kg Male (Based on Estimates)

Compartment	Iron Content, mg	Total Body Iron, %
Hb iron	2000	67
Storage iron (ferritin, hemosiderin)	1000	27
Myoglobin iron	130	3.5
Labile pool	80	2.2
Other tissue iron	8	0.2
Transport iron (apotransferrin and transferring)	3	0.08

From Fairbanks VF, Beutler E. Iron metabolism. In: Beutler E, Lichtman MA, Coller BS, Kipps TJ, Seligsohn U, eds. Williams hematology. New York: McGraw-Hill, 2001:295-304.

tissue iron, and (6) transport iron (transferrin and apotransferrin). An estimate of the average amount of iron contained in each of these compartments for a 70-kg male is listed in Table 32-3.

Hemoglobin

The red cell volume in a 70-kg male is about 2 liters, with each milliliter containing approximately 1 mg of iron. Therefore, the body contains approximately 2 g of iron incorporated into Hb.[I13]

Storage Iron

Iron is stored in the body in the form of ferritin and a partially degraded form of *ferritin* known as hemosiderin.

Ferritin. Ferritin consists of a protein shell surrounding an iron core,[I11,I48] and hemosiderin is formed when ferritin is partially degraded in secondary lysosomes.[I11,I100] Ferritin consists of an apoferritin protein shell and an interior ferric oxyhydroxide $(FeOOH)_x$ crystalline core. The apoferritin shell is composed of 24 ferritin chains that may be classified as L (light) or H (heavy), the proportions of which vary in different tissues. The diameter of the shell is 12 to 13 nm, and that of its interior cavity is 7 to 8 nm. Only ferrous iron is taken up by ferritin, and it is oxidized to ferric iron by a catalytic site on the ferritin H-chain. The H-chains contain small intrasubunit channels that may facilitate entry of iron into the storage cavity of the molecule. Across species, the exact composition of the FeOOH core crystal differs somewhat, and it contains different amounts of phosphates. In humans, it is a ferrihydrite $(5Fe_2O_3{\bullet}9H_2O)$. Release of iron from ferritin is probably nonenzymatic and may involve reduction by reduced flavin mononucleotide or other substances. The resultant Fe^{2+} leaves the crystal and diffuses out through a pore of the ferritin shell.

Ferritin is present in nearly all cells of the body and provides a reserve of iron that is readily available for formation of Hb and other heme proteins. This stored iron is shielded from body fluids and thus is unable to cause oxidative damage, as would occur if it were in a free ionic form. In men, the total body content of stored iron, mostly as ferritin, is approximately 800 mg; in healthy women, iron stores are typically lower (≤200 mg). In serum, minute quantities of ferritin are present in concentrations proportional to total body stored iron. Serum ferritin differs from tissue ferritin in that it is glycosylated, contains mostly L-chains, and is iron-poor (mostly apoferritin). Liver injury and many other pathologic processes not associated with iron overload may cause release of relatively large amounts of ferritin into plasma, leading to hyperferritinemia.

Hemosiderin. *Hemosiderin* is aggregated, partially deproteinized ferritin that is formed when ferritin is partially degraded in secondary lysozomes. In contrast to ferritin, hemosiderin is insoluble in aqueous solutions—a difference that has been used traditionally to distinguish these two iron storage compounds. Iron is only slowly released from hemosiderin, possibly because it occurs in relatively large aggregates and therefore has a much smaller surface-to-volume ratio. Like ferritin, hemosiderin is found predominantly in cells of the liver, spleen, and bone marrow.

Tissue Iron

Numerous cellular enzymes and coenzymes require iron as an integral part of the molecule or as a cofactor. These include *peroxidases* and *cytochromes,* all of which are heme proteins, like Hb. Other enzymes, such as *aconitase* and *ferredoxin,* have iron that is coordinated with sulfur in a so-called iron-sulfur cluster. Nearly half of the enzymes of the *Krebs cycle* contain iron. These enzymes and coenzymes, which occur in all nucleated cells of the body, are referred to collectively as the *tissue iron compartment.* In health, the tissue iron compartment comprises approximately 8 mg. Although small, this compartment is metabolically critical, and some iron enzyme activities diminish early in the course of iron deficiency.[I36]

Myoglobin

Myoglobin closely resembles a single Hb subunit. Because myoglobin does not form tetramers, it lacks the allosteric oxygen-binding properties of Hb.

Labile Pool

Approximately 80 mg of iron is found in the labile pool. This compartment has no clear anatomic location; it is a concept derived from kinetic measurements with radiolabeled iron.[I54]

Transport

Iron is transported from one organ to another by the plasma protein, *apotransferrin.* This β_1-globulin has an approximate molecular mass of 75 kDa and two iron-binding sites per molecule. Each site can bind one Fe^{3+} ion together with one ion of HCO_3^-. The apotransferrin- Fe^{3+} complex is called *transferrin.* Normally, approximately 2.5 mg of iron bound to transferrin circulates in the plasma of adults. Under abnormal conditions, as in patients with severe thalassemia, untreated hemochromatosis, or other severe iron overload disorders, a small amount of iron that is not bound to apotransferrin also occurs in the plasma.[120,149] When transferrin binds to the specific *transferrin receptor* of cell surface membranes, the transferrin-receptor complex is internalized into a vacuole that becomes acidified, releasing the iron from transferrin (see Figure 32-5). The apotransferrin then is transported back to the cell surface and released, ready to transport additional iron. This series of reactions has been designated the *transferrin cycle.* The transferrin receptor forms a complex with the human hemochromatosis protein (also known as the HFE protein), producing minor kinetic changes in transferrin binding[158,176] and in hepatic production of hepcidin, a peptide hormone produced by the liver that regulates iron homeostasis in humans and other mammals.

Studies have indicated that hepcidin deficiency underlies most known forms of hereditary hemochromatosis.[143]

Regulation of Iron Homeostasis

Regulation of body iron content is achieved almost entirely by modulating the amount of iron absorbed from the duodenum and the proximal jejunum. Daily iron loss from the body depends minimally upon the magnitude of iron stores. Iron stores are rigorously conserved, so that less than 0.1% of the body iron content is lost daily, mostly as the result of desquamation, minor trauma, and menses. Body iron stores are replenished daily by controlled absorption of iron in quantities that equal iron losses.

The average daily American diet contains 10 to 15 mg of iron, mostly in the form of the heme proteins Hb and myoglobin ingested as meat. In the past, a significant component of iron in the diet consisted of inorganic iron leached from iron utensils, although fractional absorption of such extraneous iron is low. Normally, approximately 1 mg of iron is absorbed each day by men and postmenopausal women, and 3 mg daily in women during the reproductive years. Absorption occurs principally in the duodenum. Heme is absorbed directly via heme receptors on the microvillous surfaces of absorptive enterocytes. Inorganic iron must be in the ferrous state (Fe^{2+}). Ferric iron is converted to the ferrous form by reducing agents in the luminal contents of the gut, by duodenal cytochrome reductase B (DCytB), or by STEAP ferrireductase proteins.

The mechanism by which the body normally regulates its iron content is complex and incompletely understood. Nonetheless, many proteins influence iron homeostasis, and mutations in genes that encode these proteins may result in iron overload or in iron deficiency (Table 32-4). A widely adopted schema of the participation of some of the proteins in iron transport across the intestinal mucosal cell is illustrated in Figure 32-16.

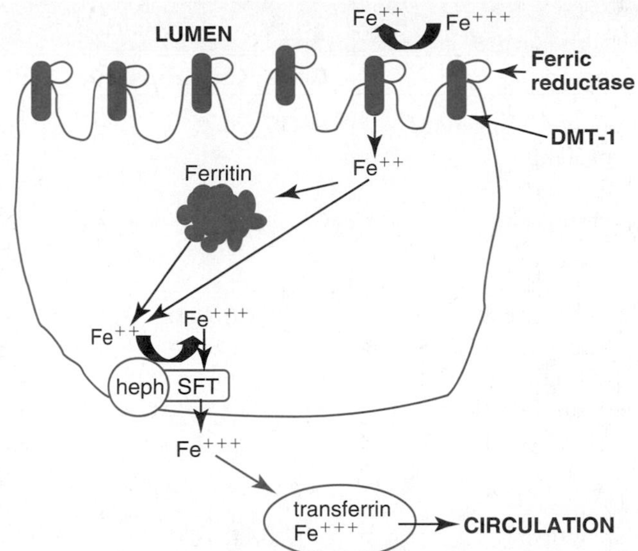

Figure 32-16 Schematic representation of some of the steps that may occur when iron is transported from the intestinal lumen to the blood. *DMT-1,* Divalent metal transporter-1; *Heph,* hephaestin; *SFT,* stimulator of iron transport.

Clinical Significance

Iron deficiency and iron overload are the major disorders of iron metabolism. In addition, many heritable disorders are known in which abnormal distribution of iron or abnormal production of iron-related proteins may play a primary or secondary role. The latter include such disorders as (1) hereditary hyperferritinemia–cataract syndrome,[184] (2) aceruloplasminemia,[147,170,193] (3) GRACILE (growth retardation, aminoaciduria, cholestasis, iron overload, lactacidosis, and early death) syndrome,[138] (4) neuroferritinopathy,[123] (5) pantothenate kinase–associated neurodegeneration (formerly Hallervorden-Spatz disease),[145] (6) atransferrinemia,[117,156] and possibly (7) neurodegenerative disorders such as Parkinsonism and Alzheimer's disease.[177,190]

Iron Deficiency

Iron deficiency is one of the most prevalent disorders of humans.[126] It is particularly a disorder of children, young women, and older persons, but it can occur in people of all ages and social strata. In children, iron deficiency is frequently caused by dietary deficiency, because milk has a low iron content and iron requirements for growth and development are high. In adults, iron deficiency is almost always the result of chronic blood loss or childbearing.[136]

Many different measurements have been advocated for the diagnosis of iron deficiency. Originally, emphasis was placed on the red blood cell indices; hypochromic anemia was generally considered to be a synonym for iron deficiency in the first half of the twentieth century. Subsequently, techniques such as staining of marrow with Perls' Prussian Blue to allow visualization of ferric iron and measurement of (1) serum iron, (2) iron-binding capacity, (3) serum ferritin, and (4) erythrocyte protoporphyrin were used for their utility in diagnosing iron deficiency. Circulating transferrin receptor and reticulocyte Hb concentrations also have diagnostic value. Of all these tests, stainable marrow iron is probably the most reliable but the least practical, except for patients who present complex diagnostic problems. Even this technique can be misleading (1) when the sample size or observer skill

TABLE 32-4 Proteins That Have a Primary Effect on Iron Homeostasis in Man

Protein	Gene; Chromosome	Effect of Deficiency	References
Bone morphogenetic protein-2	*BMP2;* 20q2	Dysregulation of hepcidin production through altered *HAMP* promoter binding; modifier of *HFE* hemochromatosis	I64
Ceruloplasmin	*CP;* 3q23-q24	Decreased oxidation of ferrous iron, decreased iron binding to transferrin; iron overload of basal ganglia, retina, and liver	I47 I70 I93
Divalent metal transporter-1 (DMT1)	*SLC11A1;* 2q35	Iron-deficient erythropoiesis, parenchymal iron overload	I65
Ferritin heavy (H) chain	*FTH;* 11q12-q13	Decreased H-chain synthesis; iron overload	I55
Ferritin light (L) chain	*FTL;* 19q13.3-q13.4	Hyperferritinemia with cataracts (mutations of iron-responsive element); hypoferritinemia and iron overload of basal ganglia (coding region mutations)	I28 I84
Ferroportin	*SLC40A1;* 2q32	Abnormal response to hepcidin action; parenchymal iron overload "gain-of-function" mutations; macrophage iron overload ("loss-of-function" mutations)	I30 I72 I99 I102
Hemojuvelin	*HJV;* 1q21	Dysregulation of hepcidin production through altered bone morphogenetic protein signaling; parenchymal iron overload; modifier of *HFE* hemochromatosis	I3 I25 I64 I75
Hepcidin	*HAMP;* 19q13	Decreased binding to ferroportin; parenchymal iron overload; modifier of *HFE* hemochromatosis	I34 I53 I63 I85
HFE	*HFE;* 6p21.3	Dysregulation of hepcidin; parenchymal iron overload; decreased risk of iron deficiency	I14 I37
Matripase-2	*TMPRSS6;* 2q12-q13	Upregulation of hepcidin, impaired iron absorption, iron-resistant iron deficiency	I81 I89
Transferrin	*TF;* 3q21	Iron-deficient erythropoiesis, parenchymal iron overload	I16 I56
Transferrin receptor-2	*TFR2;* 7q22	Dysregulation of hepcidin; parenchymal iron overload	I24 I32 I59 I67

HFE, Human hemochromatosis protein.

is insufficient,[I4] (2) in patients treated with parenteral iron supplements, (3) where stainable iron may be present in the face of deficiency,[I73] and (4) in patients with myeloproliferative disorders.[I27,I91]

Although most methods readily identify severe, uncomplicated iron deficiency, the large number of tests advocated for the diagnosis of iron deficiency reflects the fact that none by itself is sufficient to detect mild iron deficiency or iron deficiency in a clinically complex setting. Receiver operating characteristic (ROC) curves confirm that no one method is superior, and that studies differ in the conclusions that they draw regarding advantages of one method over another.[I39,I61,I96,I97]

Iron refractory or familial iron deficiency may be due to mutations in the *TMPRSS6* gene, which encodes matripase-2, a protein essential for normal hepcidin regulation.[I81,I89] In neuroferritinopathy, serum ferritin concentrations were below the reference interval for iron deficiency in 82% of males, all postmenopausal females, and 23% of premenopausal females; Hb and serum iron concentrations were typically normal. Thus, subnormal serum ferritin measures are very prevalent in persons with neuroferritinopathy; they mimic iron deficiency and provide a useful screening test in routine practice.[I28] Reports of the association of the transferrin mutation *G277S* with iron deficiency are conflicting.[I1,I60,I81,I86,I89]

Iron Overload

Hemochromatosis and some types of anemia associated with ineffective erythropoiesis are associated with multisystem iron overload due to increased absorption that affects the liver, heart, pancreas, and joints. Subnormal or inappropriately low action of the hepatic polypeptide hepcidin is central to the increased iron absorption and iron overload that occur in these conditions.[I43] Other heritable disorders such as aceruloplasminemia, neuroferritinopathy, or Friedreich's ataxia cause deleterious iron overload in parts of the brain, although nonbrain iron overload also occurs in patients with aceruloplasminemia.[I23,I71,I88] *Hemosiderosis* and *siderosis* are terms best used to describe iron overload at the tissue level. Examples include relatively innocuous deposition of iron at sites of bleeding or inflammation and the life-threatening iron overload of cardiac myocytes that occurs in some persons with hemochromatosis or severe β-thalassemia. Hyperferritinemia without iron overload may be caused by common liver disorders, neoplasms, acute or chronic inflammation, and hereditary hyperferritinemia–cataract syndrome.

Race/ethnicity factors (especially in Native Africans, African Americans, and Asians) are also associated with higher mean concentrations of serum ferritin than are typical of whites, but the basis of this phenomenon is incompletely understood.[I5,I46]

Hemochromatosis

Hemochromatosis is a group of heritable disorders that increase the susceptibility to develop primary iron overload, because iron is absorbed in quantities that exceed unavoidable loss. Some persons with severe iron overload due to hemochromatosis have the "classic triad" of bronzing of the skin due to increased skin iron and melanin content, cirrhosis due to iron-induced hepatocyte injury, and diabetes mellitus due to iron-induced injury of pancreatic β-cells and liver disease. Other manifestations of severe iron overload include cardiomyopathy, hypogonadotrophic hypogonadism, and characteristic arthropathy. Anemia and iron-induced neurologic injury are uncommon in hemochromatosis. The term *juvenile hemochromatosis* is used to describe rare forms of hemochromatosis characterized by severe iron overload, heart failure, and hypogonadotrophic hypogonadism in children, adolescents, and adults younger than 30 years of age. Nonetheless, specific types of hemochromatosis are best designated by the name of the gene in which causative mutations have been detected.

HFE Hemochromatosis. This is the most prevalent type of hemochromatosis, and it occurs predominantly in Caucasians of European descent. This disorder is the "classical" type of hemochromatosis previously called *hereditary* or *idiopathic hemochromatosis;* it accounts for more than 80% of the hemochromatosis cases diagnosed in European whites. *HFE* hemochromatosis, transmitted as an autosomal recessive trait, is caused by common mutations in the *HFE* gene[I37]; *HFE* is tightly linked to human leukocyte antigen (HLA)-A and -B genes on chromosome 6p. The most common deleterious *HFE* mutation is C282Y (nt.845G → A).[I37] This mutation occurs as a polymorphism is European whites, of whom approximately 10% are C282Y heterozygotes. Approximately 1 in 200 European whites are *HFE* C282Y homozygotes. Other common mutations in *HFE* include H63D and S65C, but these mutations are infrequently associated with severe iron overload.

HFE protein associates with the transferrin receptor and modulates hepatic expression of hepcidin.[I43,I58,I76] Thus, abnormal HFE protein caused by common *HFE* mutations can lead to augmentation of iron absorption by the small intestine. Clinically significant iron overload occurs almost exclusively in adults but is rarely severe before the fourth decade. The biochemical penetrance of *HFE* C282Y homozygosity is fairly high; more than 50% of homozygotes have elevated transferrin saturation values and/or serum ferritin concentrations, and about 10% have elevated serum alanine aminotransferase.[I14,I16] A high proportion of homozygotes diagnosed in families of probands are seriously affected,[I22,I74] whereas sufficient penetrance to cause severe iron overload (serum ferritin >1000 μg/L) in C282Y homozygotes discovered in screening programs is very low (1 to 5%).[I2,I16,I52,I78] Without doubt, some C282Y homozygotes, largely those diagnosed in medical care, suffer reduced longevity that is directly attributable to complications of severe iron overload.[I69] Nonetheless, life span is normal in most C282Y homozygotes identified in population screening.[I15]

Hemojuvelin (HJV) Hemochromatosis. This rare disorder is characterized by early age of onset and severe multiorgan iron overload. Although the patterns of parenchymal iron deposition in *HFE* and *HJV* hemochromatosis are similar, cardiac damage and hypogonadotrophic hypogonadism occur much earlier and are more prevalent in *HJV* than in *HFE* hemochromatosis.[I33] Testicular atrophy and amenorrhea are the most common presenting symptoms of *HJV* hemochromatosis. Many patients also have or develop diabetes mellitus, arthropathy, and cutaneous hyperpigmentation. Heart failure and arrhythmia due to cardiomyopathy are the predominant causes of death. Untreated subjects have high transferrin saturation values and severe hyperferritinemia.[I33] Most reported patients have had European ancestry. *HJV* hemochromatosis is transmitted as an autosomal recessive disorder. Affected persons have two deleterious mutations of the hemojuvelin gene *(HJV)* on chromosome 1q; a high proportion are compound heterozygotes.[I75] Penetrance is relatively high. Consanguinity in *HJV* hemochromatosis kinships is common. Worldwide, the most common deleterious *HJV* mutation is *G320V* (nt.959G →T); many other *HJV* mutations are "private" alleles. In health, bone morphogenetic protein (BMP) signaling by hemojuvelin regulates hepcidin expression through BMP-responsive elements located in the proximal and distal hepcidin *(HAMP)* promoter.[I3,I25] Thus, a major pathophysiologic attribute of *HJV* hemochromatosis is dysregulation of hepcidin.

***HAMP* Hemochromatosis.** Hepcidin structure and function are critical to normal iron homeostasis. Accordingly, some persons with hemochromatosis phenotypes have deleterious promoter or coding region mutations of the *HAMP* gene on chromosome 19q13.[I85] Iron phenotypes resemble those of *HFE* or *HJV* hemochromatosis. Digenic inheritance has been described in most *HAMP* hemochromatosis cases;

patients usually have *HFE* C282Y heterozygosity or homozygosity, in addition to heterozygosity for an *HAMP* mutation.[153,163] In a consanguineous Australian kinship, homozygosity for *HAMP* C78T (nt.233G →A) caused severe iron overload.[134] Heterozygosity for a deleterious *HAMP* mutation alone does not always cause an iron overload phenotype.

TFR2 Hemochromatosis. *TFR2* hemochromatosis is a rare autosomal recessive disorder characterized by elevated serum iron measures, parenchymal iron deposition, and complications of iron overload.[124] In some kinships, severe iron overload occurs in children or young adults and thus resembles that of *HJV* hemochromatosis. In others, the *TFR2* hemochromatosis phenotype appears in adulthood and therefore resembles that of *HFE* hemochromatosis. Most patients have European or Asian ancestry. Consanguinity in *TFR2* hemochromatosis kinships is common. Penetrance is moderate or high. Some pathogenic mutations, especially *TFR2* Y250X and R455Q, have appeared in individuals or kindreds who were not closely related.[132,159] Most other known deleterious *TFR2* mutations are "private." Many patients are compound heterozygotes for two different *TFR2* mutations. The *TFR2* gene (chromosome 7q22) encodes transferrin receptor-2, a protein that continues to mediate uptake of transferrin-bound iron by the liver after the classical transferrin receptor is downregulated by iron overload. The mediator of increased iron absorption in *TFR2* hemochromatosis is hepcidin dysregulation.[167]

Ferroportin *(SLC40A1)* Hemochromatosis. Ferroportin, the receptor for hepcidin, occurs as a multimer on the surfaces of cells responsible for gathering and recycling iron: enterocytes (basolateral surfaces), macrophages, hepatocytes, and placental syncytiotrophoblasts.[168] Hepcidin participates in regulation of plasma iron and tissue distribution of iron by post-translational regulation of ferroportin. Mutations in the *SLC40A1* gene that encodes ferroportin cause an uncommon, heterogeneous group of iron overload disorders characterized by an autosomal dominant pattern of inheritance.[130] In many ferroportin hemochromatosis kinships, serum iron measures and complications of iron overload typical of other types of hemochromatosis are relatively uncommon. *SLC40A1* mutations cause two major iron overload phenotype patterns, each depending on the particular mutation and its effect on the function of the transcribed ferroportin protein. "Gain-of-function" ferroportin mutations cause a disorder that resembles *HFE* or *HJV* hemochromatosis phenotypes: elevated transferrin saturation, hyperferritinemia, and a predominance of parenchymal iron overload, especially in hepatocytes. Typical examples include *SLC40A1* N144D and N144H.[172,199] "Loss-of-function" ferroportin mutations cause a disorder characterized by normal or subnormal transferrin saturation, hyperferritinemia, and a predominance of iron deposition in macrophages in the liver, spleen, and other sites. The most common known "loss-of-function" *SLC40A1* allele is V162del.[1102] Ferroportin hemochromatosis has been described worldwide in a variety of race/ethnicity groups. *SLC40A1* Q248H occurs as a common polymorphism in persons of Native African descent, but is not associated with increased risk to develop iron overload.[16]

African Iron Overload and African American Iron Overload. African iron overload occurs in 14 to 18% of Bantu-speaking Natives in many sub-Saharan Africa countries.[118] Previously known as Bantu siderosis, this type of nontransfusion iron overload is due primarily to the ingestion of large quantities of iron contained in traditional beer, although unconfirmed evidence suggests that an African iron overload gene does exist.[144] Some patients develop potentially harmful iron deposits in the liver, spleen, pancreas, and other organs, predominantly in macrophages. Affected persons have normal or elevated transferrin saturation and elevated serum ferritin concentrations. Persons with severe iron overload have reduced longevity and increased risks of malignancy.[118] A similar disorder occurs in African Americans, although it is recognized infrequently, perhaps because the iron overload is typically less severe than iron overload in African Natives.[19] A role for excessive dietary iron in the causation of nontransfusion iron overload in most African American cases has not been suspected or demonstrated. Some cases are due to *HFE* genotypes typical of Caucasian hemochromatosis, to mutations of other hemochromatosis-associated genes, or to types of hemoglobinopathy or thalassemia.[17]

Iron Overload Due to Anemia With Ineffective Erythropoiesis

Some types of heritable and acquired anemia are associated with ineffective erythropoiesis, a factor that stimulates iron absorption, and with iron overload. Recent discoveries demonstrate that GDF15 (growth/differentiation factor-15) concentrations are increased in such patients.[141,180,194,195] GDF15, a member of the transforming growth factor-beta superfamily, is produced by erythroblasts,[198] downregulates hepcidin expression, and thus increases iron absorption. Types of anemia with increased GDF15 expression include β-thalassemia major (with or without coinheritance of Hb E), pyruvate kinase deficiency, congenital dyserythropoietic anemia, and refractory anemia with ringed sideroblasts due to myelodysplasia. It is presumed that GDF15 expression also occurs in patients with X-linked sideroblastic anemia. In patients with these types of anemia, the prevalence of common *HFE* mutations is similar to that in the corresponding general population; therefore hemochromatosis alleles are not major contributors to increased iron absorption or to iron overload phenotypes. Chronic erythrocyte transfusion may exacerbate iron overload through increased absorption in persons with these types of anemia.

Secondary Iron Overload

Acquisition of iron from nondietary sources in amounts that exceed the body's limited excretory capacity can cause iron overload. Chronic erythrocyte transfusion is the most common cause. In some patients with ineffective erythropoiesis and increased *GDF15* expression, transfusion exacerbates iron overload due to increased absorption. This is especially prevalent in patients with β-thalassemia major. Among such

TABLE 32-5 Characteristics of Some Chromogens Used in Iron Assays

CHROMOGEN		Absorbance Maximum of Fe^{2+} Complex, nm	Molar Absorbance of Fe^{2+} Complex
Common Name	Chemical Name		
Bathophenanthroline disulfonate, sodium	4,7-bis(4-phenyl sulfonic acid)-1,10-phenanthroline, sodium salt	534	22.14×10^3
Tripyridyl triazine	2,4,6-tripyridyl-*s*-triazine	593	22.6×10^3
Ferrozine	3-(2-pyridyl)-5,6-bis(4-phenyl sulfonic acid) 1,2,4 triazine	562	28.0×10^3
Terosite	2,6-bis(4-phenyl-2,2-pyridyl)-4-phenyl pyridine	583	30.2×10^3

Modified from Carter P. Spectrophotometric determination of serum iron at the submicrogram level with a new reagent (ferrozine). Anal Biochem 1971;40:450-8.

patients, cardiac siderosis is the most common cause of death.[I19] Transfusion iron overload develops in many persons with sickle cell disease and causes clinical disease in some, especially hepatic iron overload and cirrhosis.[I21,I31] In sickle cell disease, erythropoiesis is mildly ineffective,[I101] but the predominant cause of iron overload is chronic transfusion.[I21] In the past, iron overload was a common complication of chronic hemodialysis due to the administration of excessive iron dextran,[I79] a problem now avoidable with erythropoietin supplementation and prudent ferritin monitoring.[I42] Iron overload also occurs in persons without renal insufficiency as a result of the administration of excessive intravenous or intramuscular iron supplements.[I12,I87] Chronic transfusion is usually the sole cause of iron overload in persons treated for (1) severe aplastic anemia, (2) Blackfan-Diamond syndrome, (3) Fanconi's anemia, (4) acute leukemia, (5) autoimmune hemolytic anemias, and (6) myelodysplasia without ringed sideroblasts.

In Bantu-speaking Native Africans, the daily consumption of traditional beer that contains large amounts of iron is an essential factor in the development of African iron overload.[I18,I44] Rarely does iron overload develop in persons who ingest large quantities of supplemental iron in misguided attempts to correct anemia due to noniron factors. Some of these patients have hemochromatosis-associated mutations.[I10] Hematite miners and other workers chronically exposed to iron ore dust may develop iron overload of the lungs and adjacent lymph nodes, but serum iron measures are usually normal.[I57]

Analytical Methods

Several methods are used to measure iron and related analytes. These include methods for serum iron, iron-binding capacity, transferrin saturation, and serum ferritin.

Methods for Serum Iron, Iron-binding Capacity, and Transferrin Saturation[I40,I50,I51,I83]

Principle

With serum iron assays, iron is (1) released from transferrin by decreasing the pH of the serum, (2) reduced from Fe^{3+} to Fe^{2+}, and (3) complexed with a chromogen such as bathophenanthroline or ferrozine. Such iron-chromogen complexes have an extremely high absorbance in the visible region that is proportional to iron concentration. Optical characteristics of bathophenanthroline, of ferrozine, and of alternative chromogens are shown in Table 32-5. The assay may be performed manually or in automated fashion by any of several commercially available methods.

The serum total iron-binding capacity (TIBC) is determined by the addition of sufficient Fe^{3+} to saturate iron-binding sites of transferrin. Excess Fe^{3+} is removed [e.g., by adsorption with light magnesium carbonate ($MgCO_3$) powder, a silica column, or ion-exchange resin], and the assay for iron content is then repeated. From this second measurement, the TIBC is obtained. Transferrin saturation is calculated as follows:

$$\text{Transferrin saturation}\,(\%) = (100 \times \text{serum iron})/\text{TIBC}$$

Modern automated chemistry analyzers now measure unsaturated iron-binding capacity (UIBC) and calculate TIBC, rather than measure it directly. UIBC is measured by adding a known excess concentration of iron to serum. The iron rapidly binds to all available previously unsaturated binding sites on transferrin. By leaving the pH near neutral, only the iron that did not bind to transferrin is measured upon addition of iron-binding chromogen. A blank with no added serum is also measured, and the UIBC for each serum sample is determined as the difference in the absorbance produced by the serum-free iron blank and the absorbance produced by the residual non–transferrin-bound iron in each serum-containing solution. TIBC is then calculated by adding the UIBC to the serum iron. Transferrin saturation can be computed as described above. The advantage of the UIBC approach is that it can be fully automated, because no separation steps are required to remove the non–transferrin-bound iron, unlike all of the traditional TIBC approaches.

Reference Intervals

Reference intervals for serum iron differ by as much as 35% between commercial methods. Therefore, a generic reference interval is not valid. Many commercially available methods appear to underestimate the true value of serum iron concentration by 25% or more, and some appear to be unreliable at quantifying concentrations of serum iron less than 30 μg/dL (5 μmol/L). Methods that include deproteinization, by precipitation or by dialysis, consistently appear to provide results that are substantially higher than those results obtained by methods that do not include a step of deproteinization. From a practical standpoint, if an automated commercial method is used, a laboratory should independently define its own reference intervals.

Clinical Relevance

The serum iron concentration refers to the Fe^{3+} bound to serum transferrin and does not include the iron contained in serum as free Hb. The serum iron concentration is decreased in many but not all patients with iron deficiency anemia and chronic inflammatory disorders such as acute infection, immunization, and myocardial infarction (Table 32-6). Erythropoietic response to specific hematinic therapy for anemias of other causes (e.g., treatment of pernicious anemia with cyanocobalamin) decreases serum iron concentration through increased efficiency of iron incorporated into developing erythroblasts. Acute or recent hemorrhage, including that caused by blood donation, results in low serum iron concentration. Menstruation is a common circumstance that decreases serum iron concentration. Use of hormonal contraceptives raises serum iron concentration; after cessation of hormonal contraceptive intake, serum iron concentrations decrease by as much as 30% concurrently with uterine bleeding.

Supranormal concentrations of serum iron occur in iron-loading disorders such as hemochromatosis, in patients with aplastic anemia, in acute iron poisoning in children, and after oral ingestion of iron medication or parenteral iron administration or acute hepatitis. For example, one 0.3-g tablet of ferrous sulfate ingested by an adult may raise the serum iron concentration by 300 to 500 μg/dL (50 to 90 μmol/L).

Because only about one third of the iron-binding sites of transferrin are occupied by Fe^{3+} in normal subjects, serum transferrin has considerable reserve iron-binding capacity (UIBC). The TIBC is a measurement of the maximum concentration of iron that transferrin can bind. The serum TIBC varies in disorders of iron metabolism. It is increased in many persons with iron deficiency and is decreased in those with chronic inflammatory disorders or malignancies. In many persons with untreated hemochromatosis, the TIBC is slightly decreased.

Comments and Precautions

1. Except when atomic absorption spectroscopy is used, hemolysis has very little effect on serum iron assay results because Hb iron is not released from heme by acid treatment. However, when serum specimens show marked hemolysis, a small amount of iron may be liberated from Hb. Such specimens should be rejected.
2. Many factors influence serum iron concentration and TIBC. Various physiologic or pathologic conditions that

TABLE 32-6 Conditions Known to Affect Serum Iron Concentration, Total Iron-Binding Capacity, and Transferrin Saturation

Condition	Effect
Diurnal variation	Normal values in morning; low values in midafternoon; very low values near midnight
Menstrual cycle	Premenstrually, elevated values (SI increased by 10 to 30%); at menstruation, low values (SI decreased by 10 to 30%)
Pregnancy	May elevate SI owing to increased progesterone; may lower SI owing to iron deficiency
Ingestion of iron (including iron-fortified vitamins)	High values; may raise SI by +54 μmol/L (+300 μg/dL) and Tsat to 100%
Oral contraceptives (progesterone-like)	High values; may raise SI to >36 μmol/L (>200 μg/dL) and Tsat to 75%; also elevates TIBC
Iron contamination of syringe, vacutainer tube, or other glassware (phenomenon may be rare, sporadic, very difficult to prove)	High values [e.g., SI >30 μmol/L (>170 μg/dL)]; Tsat of 75 to 100%
Iron dextran injection	Very high values; SI may be >180 μmol/L (>1000 μg/dL), Tsat 100%, probably from circulating iron dextran; effect may persist for several weeks
Hepatitis	Very high values; SI may be >180 μmol/L (>1000 μg/dL) owing to hyperferritinemia from hepatocyte injury
Acute inflammation (respiratory infection), abscess, immunization, myocardial infarction	Low or normal SI; normal or low Tsat
Chronic inflammation or malignancy	Low or normal SI; normal or low Tsat
Iron deficiency	Low or normal SI; low or normal Tsat; increased TIBC
Iron overload (hemochromatosis)	High SI; high Tsat; normal or low TIBC

SI, Serum iron concentration; *TIBC,* total iron binding capacity; *Tsat,* transferrin saturation.
From Fairbanks VF. Laboratory testing for iron status. Hosp Pract 1991;26:19.

affect these measures are listed in Table 32-6. Day-to-day variation is great in many healthy people. Diurnal variation in serum iron concentrations has been noted. Values are lower in the afternoon than in the morning and are very low in the evening [as low as 10 to 20 µg/dL (2 to 4 µmol/L) in healthy individuals]. Because many causes of low serum iron concentration are known, results must be interpreted with caution. Furthermore, values of serum iron concentration and TIBC are normal in many people with mild iron deficiency.

3. Because iron is ubiquitous in the environment, scrupulous care is necessary to ensure that glassware, water, and reagents do not become contaminated with extraneous iron.
4. Serum transferrin concentration may be estimated from the TIBC by the following relationship:

$$\text{Serum transferrin (g/L)} = 0.007 \times \text{TIBC } (\mu\text{g/dL})$$

The relationship is not entirely linear, because a small portion of iron in serum is bound to proteins other than transferrin. Therefore, calculated TIBC values are slightly higher than the amount of transferrin-bound iron. However, these small differences are of no practical consequence. Immunoassays are available for assay of serum transferrin concentration. Results of the immunologic measurement of transferrin concentration correlate with those of the TIBC assay, but transferrin measurement has little clinical utility. A slight advantage for the immunoassay of transferrin is that the required volume per specimen is much smaller.

Methods for Serum Ferritin

Principles

Serum ferritin is measured by any of several methods, including (1) immunoradiometric, (2) ELISA, (3) immunochemiluminescent, and (4) immunofluorometric methods. Reagents for this assay are available in kit form and in automated immunoassay instruments from several manufacturers.

Reference Intervals

Reference intervals for serum ferritin concentrations are summarized in Table 32-7. Nonetheless, much variation in reference intervals has been observed with different methods for serum ferritin. Consequently, reference intervals must be determined for each laboratory.

TABLE 32-7 Reference Intervals for Serum Ferritin

	ng/mL	µg/L
Newborn	25-200	25-200
1 mo	200-600	200-600
2 to 5 mo	50-200	50-200
6 mo to 15 y	7-140	7-140
Adult man	20-250	20-250
Adult woman	20-200	20-200
Iron overload[182]		
• Adult male	>400	>400
• Adult female	>200	>200

Clinical Relevance

Ferritin is present in the blood in very low concentration. Although ferritin is an acute-phase reactant, the serum ferritin concentration roughly reflects the body iron content in many subjects. Most serum ferritin consists of iron-poor, glycosylated L-chains and thus is largely apoferritin. The plasma ferritin concentration declines very early in the development of iron deficiency, long before changes are observed in blood Hb concentration, erythrocyte size, or serum iron concentration. Accordingly, the serum ferritin concentration is a sensitive indicator of iron deficiency uncomplicated by other concurrent disease. Alternatively, many disorders result in increased serum ferritin concentration.[182] These disorders include chronic infections; chronic inflammatory disorders, such as rheumatoid arthritis or renal disease; common liver conditions (e.g., alcoholism, viral hepatitis B or C, nonalcoholic fatty liver); heart disease; and numerous malignancies, especially lymphomas, leukemias, breast cancer, and neuroblastoma. In patients with these disorders who also have iron deficiency, serum ferritin concentration is often normal. An increase in plasma ferritin concentration occurs as a result of ferritin release due to hepatocellular injury of diverse causes. Plasma ferritin concentration is also increased in patients with iron overload of any cause and is used to gauge the effectiveness of phlebotomy therapy. As a screening test for detection of early iron overload, measurement of serum ferritin concentration is less sensitive than measurement of transferrin saturation (or UIBC), or *HFE* mutation analysis.

Comments and Precautions

1. Replicate same-day assays on the same specimen should have a coefficient of variation (CV) of ±4% for ferritin concentrations of 100 to 300 µg/L and ±10% for ferritin concentrations of 10 to 20 µg/L.
2. The precision of many analytical methods decreases at very high serum ferritin concentrations. Consequently, manufacturers' directions for diluting specimens with very high ferritin concentrations should be followed scrupulously.
3. A high-dose hook effect that is similar to a prozone phenomenon formerly complicated interpretation of many serum ferritin assays. For example, specimens with a ferritin concentration greater than 1000 µg/L could exhibit a normal serum ferritin concentration. Fortunately, almost all currently available reagents avoid the hook effect when serum ferritin concentration is high.

Method for Red Cell Volume and Hemoglobin Content

MCV and mean corpuscular hemoglobin concentration (MCHC) are the red cell indices used to characterize the blood of patients with anemia. MCV is most commonly measured by electrical impedance changes as red cells flow through a very small orifice, which is used in combination with automated spectrophotometric measurement of hemoglobin concentration to compute MCHC. Alternatively, laser light scattering has been used to measure the Hb content and its concentration of individual red cells.[I66] Low MCV and MCHC are early indicators of iron deficiency. However, their usefulness is limited in patients with MCV values greater than 100 fL, although in others they compare favorably with other measurements of iron status.[I29,I35,I61,I92] Values of MCV are elevated in many persons with untreated *HFE* hemochromatosis. This is due predominantly to increased iron delivery to developing erythroid cells in subjects whose transferrin saturation with iron is significantly elevated.[I8,I62]

Method for Serum Transferrin Receptor

Cell membranes of developing erythroid cells in bone marrow are rich in transferrin receptors to which the iron-transferrin complex binds as a normal attribute of the transferrin cycle. The number of transferrin receptors increases in the presence of iron deficiency and decreases in iron excess. These variations in the quantity of transferrin receptors in erythropoietic tissue are also reflected in changes in soluble serum transferrin receptor, which can be measured by a variety of standard immunoassay techniques. To a large extent, serum transferrin receptor concentrations reflect the rate of erythropoietic activity, regardless of the iron status of the patient.

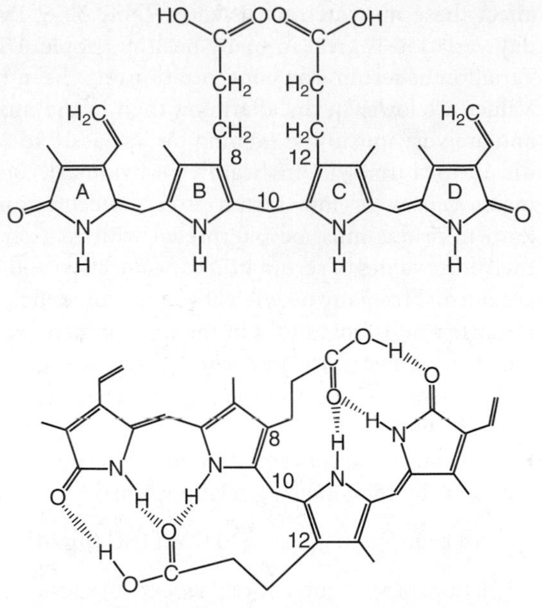

Figure 32-17 ***Top,*** **A linear molecular representation of unconjugated bilirubin.** ***Bottom,*** **The preferred structure of unconjugated bilirubin IXa, Z,Z configuration. The folded ridge-tile structure is stabilized by six hydrogen bonds formed between the two carboxyl groups of the sidechains and the two carbonyl- and four imino-groups. The "ridge" involves carbon atoms 8 through 12.**

BILIRUBIN

Bilirubin is the orange-yellow pigment derived from senescent red blood cells. It is extracted and biotransformed mainly in the liver and is excreted in bile and urine. The chemistry, biochemistry, and analytical methods for bilirubin and related compounds are reviewed in this section.

Chemistry

Bilirubin was discovered by Virchow in 1849 in blood extravasates; he called the yellow pigment "hematoidin." The term *bilirubin* was coined by Stadeler in 1864, and in 1874 Tarchanoff demonstrated the direct association of bile pigments with hemoglobin. In 1942, Fisher and Plieninger synthesized bilirubin IXα and proposed the structure shown in the upper portion of Figure 32-17. This linear tetrapyrrolic structure of the bilirubin molecule was accepted for longer than 30 years. However, important chemical properties of the bilirubin molecule are its insolubility in water and its solubility in a variety of nonpolar solvents. The solubility of bilirubin in nonpolar, lipid solvents is not predicted from this linear tetrapyrrole structure, because the two propionic acid sidechains would be expected to make the bilirubin molecule highly polar and therefore water soluble.

The overall chemical structure of bilirubin was established by x-ray crystallography.[B7] According to this work, bilirubin assumes a ridge-tiled configuration stabilized by six intramolecular hydrogen bonds. Two additional important structural features have also been noted: (1) a so-called Z-Z *(trans)* conformation for the double bonds between carbons 4 and 5 and 15 and 16, and (2) an involuted hydrogen-bonded structure in which the propionic acid–carboxylic acid groups are hydrogen-bonded to the nitrogen atoms of the pyrrole rings (Figure 32-17, *bottom*). These bonds stabilize the Z-Z configuration of bilirubin and prevent its interaction with polar groups in aqueous media. When exposed to light, the Z-Z configuration is converted to the E-E *(cis)* conformation and to other combinations, namely, 4E-15Z and 4Z-15E. The E-E conformation and other E-containing isomers do not permit the degree of internal hydrogen bonding that occurs in the Z-Z conformation and therefore are more water soluble than in the Z-Z conformation. Thus light-exposed forms of bilirubin are more water soluble and are readily excreted in the bile. This is the rationale for irradiating jaundiced newborns with 450 nm light.[B33]

The bilirubin molecule in the crystalline state takes, as mentioned earlier, the form of a ridge tile rather than a linear tetrapyrrole, with the ridge being along the line C8-C10-C12. In this configuration, rings A and B lie in one plane and rings C and D in another, with a 98° angle between the two rings. The preferred conformation of bilirubin in aqueous solution at pH 7.4 is not known, but the occurrence of a hydrogen-bonded structure in aqueous solution would explain some of the unique chemical properties of bilirubin IXα. For example, the addition of hydrogen bond–breaking chemicals such as caffeine, methanol, ethanol, urea, or surface active agents is required for unconjugated bilirubin to react with diazo reagent. These reagents likely act by breaking internal hydrogen bonds of the bilirubin molecule, allowing it to react with diazotized sulfanilic acid or other diazo compounds. In contrast, bilirubin IXα monoglucuronide and diglucuronide are soluble in water and react readily with diazo reagents. The bulky glucuronic acid moiety precludes conjugated bilirubin from undergoing internal hydrogen bond formation. Bilirubin glucuronides, being water soluble, are readily excreted in the bile and urine, whereas unconjugated bilirubin is not.

Bilirubin deriving from natural sources consists almost entirely (99%) of the isomer IXα. Bilirubins IXβ and IXδ, arising from cleavage of the β- and δ-methene bridges, consist of less than 0.5% of bilirubin isolated from bile. However, bilirubin reference materials available from commercial sources and from the National Institute of Standards and Technology (Standard Reference Material 916a) contain variable quantities of IIIα and XIIIα isomers.[B31] The two isomers are formed by cleavage of bilirubin IXα at the central methylene bridge; subsequent recombination of the two different dipyrrole units gives a mixture of the three isomers. This isomerization of bilirubin occurs in aqueous solution at acidic or neutral pH, but not when bilirubin is bound to albumin.[B32]

Biochemistry

Bilirubin IXα is produced from the catabolism of protoporphyrin IX by a microsomal heme oxygenase. The tetrapyrrolic product of the ring opening at the α-methene bridge is the green pigment biliverdin, which is subsequently reduced to bilirubin by the reduced form of nicotinamide adenine dinucleotide phosphate (NADPH)-dependent, cytosolic enzyme biliverdin reductase (Figure 32-18). For each mole of heme catabolized by this pathway, one mole each of carbon monoxide, bilirubin, and ferric iron is produced. Daily bilirubin production from all sources in man averages from 250 to 300 mg. Approximately 85% of the total bilirubin produced is derived from the heme moiety of hemoglobin released from senescent erythrocytes that are destroyed in the reticuloendothelial cells of the liver, spleen, and bone marrow. The remaining 15% is produced from RBC precursors destroyed in the bone marrow (so-called ineffective erythropoiesis) and from the catabolism of other heme-containing proteins, such as myoglobin, cytochromes, and peroxidases.

In blood, bilirubin is bound to albumin ($K_d \approx 10^{-8}$ mol/L) and is transported to the liver. Bilirubin then dissociates from albumin by an unknown process at the sinusoidal membrane of the hepatocyte. It is transported across the membrane (Figure 32-19). Once inside the liver cells, bilirubin is reversibly bound to soluble proteins known as *ligandins* or *protein Y.* Ligandins are cytosolic proteins of the glutathione-S-transferase gene family and constitute ≈5% of the total protein of human liver cytosol. Ligandin also binds a variety of other compounds, such as steroids, bromsulphthalein (BSP), indocyanine green, and some carcinogens. Ligandin likely plays an important role in the processing of these compounds; it may increase the net efficiency of uptake by retarding the reflux of these substances back to plasma.

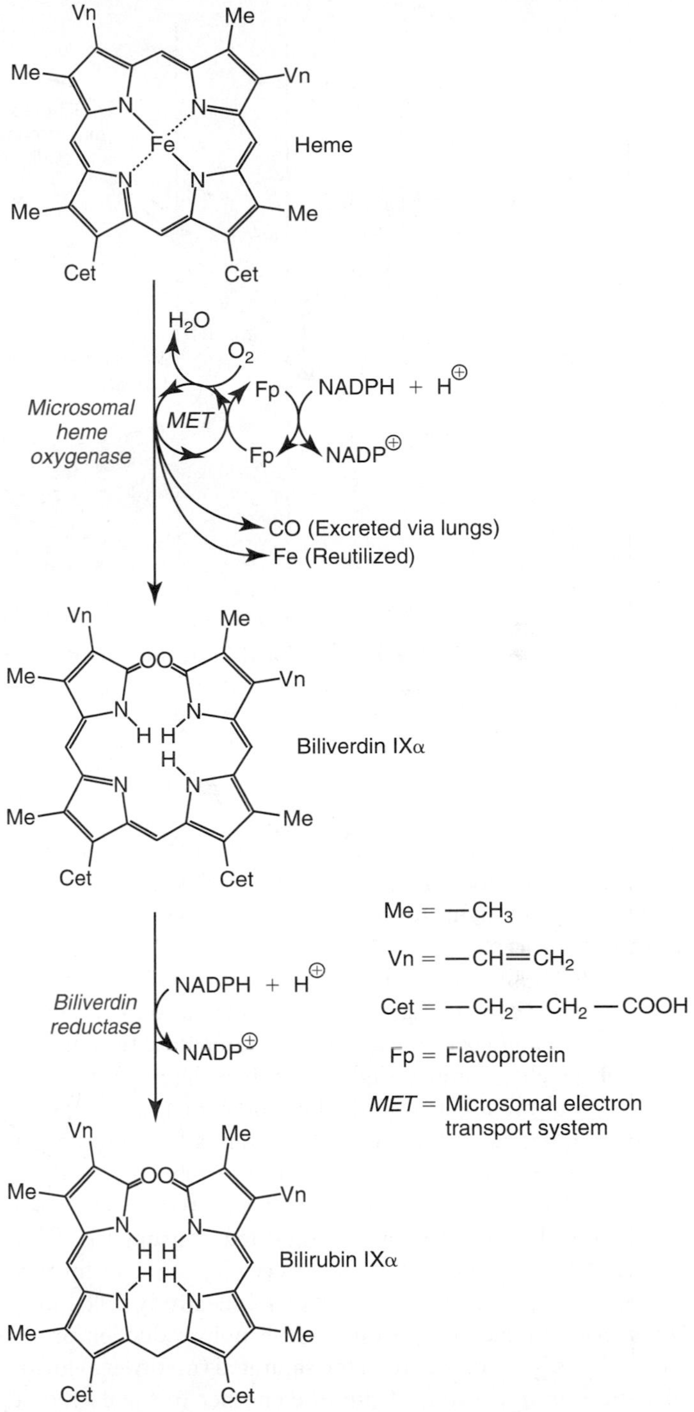

Vn Me Me Vn Fe N N N N Heme Me Me Cet Cet

H_2O O_2 Fp NADPH + $H^{\oplus}$

Microsomal heme oxygenase *MET* Fp $NADP^{\oplus}$

CO (Excreted via lungs)
Fe (Reutilized)

Biliverdin IXα

Biliverdin reductase NADPH + $H^{\oplus}$ $NADP^{\oplus}$

Bilirubin IXα

Me = $-CH_3$
Vn = $-CH{=}CH_2$
Cet = $-CH_2-CH_2-COOH$
Fp = Flavoprotein
MET = Microsomal electron transport system

Figure 32-18 Catabolism of heme to bilirubin IXα. *(From Berlin NI, Berk PD. Quantitative aspects of bilirubin metabolism for hematologists. Blood 1981;57:983-99.)*

Inside the hepatocytes, bilirubin is rapidly conjugated with glucuronic acid to produce bilirubin monoglucuronide and diglucuronide, which then are excreted into bile (see Figure 33-19). The microsomal enzyme bilirubin uridine diphosphate (UDP)–glucuronyltransferase (EC 2.4.1.17) catalyzes the formation of bilirubin monoglucuronide. It is not certain whether conversion of the monoglucuronide to the diglucuronide is catalyzed by the same enzyme or by another

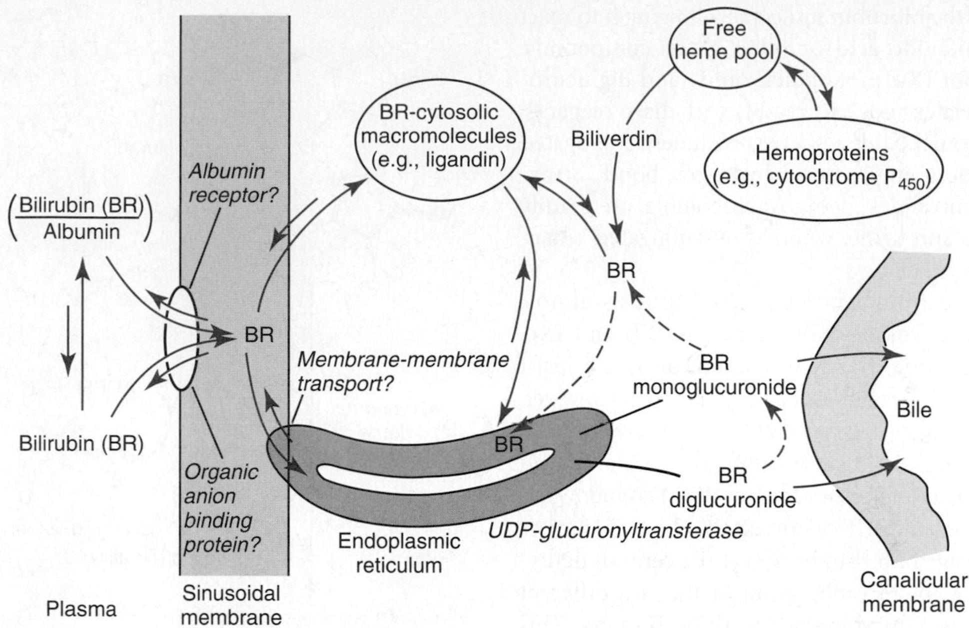

Figure 32-19 Bilirubin uptake, metabolism, and transport in the hepatocyte. *(From Gollan JL, Schmid R. In: Popper H, Schaffner F, eds. Progress in liver diseases, vol 7, Chapter 15. Philadelphia: WB Saunders, 1982.)*

enzyme located in or near the canaliculus. The excretion of conjugated bilirubin into bile against a marked concentration gradient is thought to be an energy-dependent, active-transport process.

In adults, virtually all bilirubin excreted in bile is in the form of glycosidic conjugates; glucuronides account for ≈95% of them, and glucosides and xylosides constitute the remainder. Of the glucuronides, diglucuronide is the major fraction (≈90%) and monoglucuronide the minor fraction (≈10%).

Bilirubin glucuronides are not substantially reabsorbed in the intestine. Rather, they are hydrolyzed by the catalytic action of β-glucuronidase from the liver, intestinal epithelial cells, and bacteria. This unconjugated bilirubin is then reduced by anaerobic intestinal microbial flora to form a group of three colorless tetrapyrroles collectively called *urobilinogens.* In each of these three bilirubin reduction products, all bridge carbons are in the saturated (methylene) form. The urobilinogens differ from one another in the degree of hydrogenation of the vinyl sidechains and in the two end pyrrole rings; urobilinogens contain 6, 8, or 12 more hydrogen atoms than does bilirubin and are named *stercobilinogen, mesobilinogen,* or *urobilinogen,* respectively. Up to 20% of the urobilinogen produced daily is reabsorbed from the intestine and enters the enterohepatic circulation. Most of the reabsorbed urobilinogen is taken up by the liver and is re-excreted in the bile; a small fraction (2 to 5%) enters the general circulation and appears in urine. In the lower intestinal tract, the three urobilinogens are spontaneously oxidized at the middle methylene bridge to produce the corresponding bile pigments stercobilin, mesobilin, and urobilin, which are orange-brown and the major pigments of stool. Approximately 50% of the conjugated bilirubin excreted in bile is metabolized to products other than the urobilinogens. The detailed structure of these metabolites has not been characterized.

Clinical Significance

Jaundice is a condition characterized by hyperbilirubinemia and deposition of bile pigment in the skin, mucous membranes, and sclera with a resulting yellow appearance of the patient; it is also called *icterus.* Defects in bilirubin metabolism resulting in jaundice can occur at each step of the metabolic pathway (see Figure 32-19). The disorders are usually classified as (1) inherited disorders of bilirubin metabolism, and (2) jaundice of the newborn. All of these disorders are characterized by elevations in conjugated or unconjugated bilirubin in the absence of other abnormal liver tests. It is only in these disorders that bilirubin fractionation is clinically useful.

Patients are occasionally seen with isolated elevations in bilirubin concentration. In most cases, this is due to inherited disorders of bilirubin metabolism, familial hyperbilirubinemia, or hemolysis. It is not difficult to establish hemolysis as the cause of hyperbilirubinemia because the patient with severe hemolysis will have many other disease manifestations. An algorithm for differentiating familial causes of hyperbilirubinemia is presented in Figure 32-20.

Inherited Disorders of Bilirubin Metabolism

Inherited disorders of bilirubin metabolism include Gilbert, Crigler-Najjar (types I and II), Lucey-Driscoll, Dubin-Johnson, and Rotor syndromes.

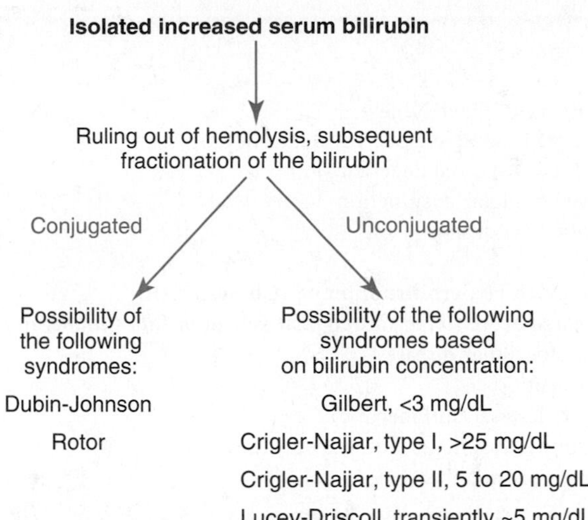

Figure 32-20 Algorithm for differentiating the familial causes of hyperbilirubinemia.

Gilbert Syndrome

Gilbert syndrome is a benign condition manifested by mild unconjugated hyperbilirubinemia. This abnormality, affecting 3 to 5% of the population, is clinically important because it is often misdiagnosed as chronic hepatitis. The serum concentration of bilirubin fluctuates between 1.5 and 3 mg/dL (26 and 51 μmol/L) and tends to increase with fasting. Hepatic glucuronyltransferase activity is low as a consequence of a mutation in the bilirubin-UDP-glucuronosyltransferase *(UGT1A1)* gene. In the vast majority of patients, this mutation is a repeat in the promoter, so that there are seven rather than the "normal" six ATs. Occasionally, subjects are encountered with five or eight repeats; the transcription of the gene is inversely proportional to the number of repeats,[B2] so that bilirubin concentrations tend to be higher in those patients with the largest number of repeats in the promoter. In Asia, Gilbert syndrome is sometimes found to be caused by a single point mutation in exon 1 of the *UGT1A1* gene.[B17] Gilbert syndrome is easily distinguished from chronic hepatitis by the absence of anemia and bilirubin in urine, and by normal liver function tests. The condition is probably inherited as an autosomal recessive trait. Despite the fact that total biliary bilirubin is reduced, the ratio of bilirubin monoglucuronide to diglucuronide is increased, suggesting that a defect is also present in the conversion of bilirubin monoglucuronide to diglucuronide.

Patients with Gilbert syndrome may be predisposed to acetaminophen toxicity because acetaminophen is primarily metabolized by glucuronidation. The diagnosis is usually made by chance on routine medical examination or when jaundice occurs following an intercurrent infection or fasting. Special diagnostic tests are occasionally necessary and include demonstrating a rise in bilirubin on fasting and a fall in bilirubin upon taking phenobarbital. No treatment is needed, but patients must be reassured that they do not have liver disease.

Crigler-Najjar Syndrome (Type I)

Crigler-Najjar syndrome type I, a rare disorder caused by complete absence of UDP-glucuronyltransferase, is manifested by very high concentrations of unconjugated bilirubin often exceeding 20 mg/dL (340 μmol/L). It is inherited as an autosomal recessive trait. Most patients die of severe brain damage caused by kernicterus (encephalopathy related to increased serum bilirubin that leads to permanent brain damage) within the first year of life. Phlebotomy and plasmapheresis can reduce the serum bilirubin, but encephalopathy usually develops. Early liver transplantation is the only effective therapy.

Crigler-Najjar Syndrome (Type II)

This rare autosomal dominant disorder is characterized by a partial deficiency of UDP-glucuronyltransferase. Unconjugated bilirubin is usually 5 to 20 mg/dL (85 to 340 μmol/L). Unlike the Crigler-Najjar syndrome type I, type II responds dramatically to phenobarbital and a normal life is expected.

Lucey-Driscoll Syndrome

Lucey-Driscoll syndrome is a familial form of unconjugated hyperbilirubinemia caused by a circulating inhibitor of bilirubin conjugation. The hyperbilirubinemia is mild and lasts for the first 2 to 3 weeks of life.

Dubin-Johnson Syndrome

Dubin-Johnson syndrome is due to a rare autosomal recessive disorder and is characterized by jaundice with predominantly elevated conjugated bilirubin and a minor elevation of unconjugated bilirubin. Excretion of various conjugated organic anions and bilirubin, but not bile salts, into bile is impaired, reflecting the underlying defect in canalicular excretion. Intravenous cholangiography does not show the gallbladder, but a ^{99m}Tc-hepatobiliary iminodiacetic acid (HIDA) scan does. A derangement in the excretion of urinary coproporphyrin occurs, and the normal ratio of coproporphyrin I to III is reversed. The liver has a characteristic greenish black appearance, and liver biopsy reveals a dark brown pigment in hepatocytes and Kupffer cells that looks like lipofuscin but probably is melanin. Serum alanine aminotransferase and alkaline phosphatase are usually normal, and pruritus is absent. The condition is benign, although patients may develop jaundice during pregnancy or while taking oral contraceptives.

Rotor Syndrome

Rotor syndrome is another form of conjugated hyperbilirubinemia similar to Dubin-Johnson syndrome but without pigment in the liver. The gallbladder is seen on intravenous cholecystography. Total urinary coproporphyrins are elevated, with about two thirds being coproporphyrin I. The prognosis is excellent.

Jaundice in the Neonate

Disorders that cause jaundice in the neonate are classified as unconjugated or conjugated hyperbilirubinemia (Box 32-1).[B37]

BOX 32-1 Physiologic Classification of Jaundice

Unconjugated Hyperbilirubinemia

Increased Production of Unconjugated Bilirubin from Heme

Hemolysis
- Hereditary
- Acquired

Ineffective erythropoiesis

Rapid turnover of increased red blood cell (RBC) mass (in the neonate)

Decreased Delivery of Unconjugated Bilirubin (in Plasma) to Hepatocyte

Right-sided congestive heart failure

Portacaval shunt

Decreased Uptake of Unconjugated Bilirubin Across Hepatocyte Membrane

Competitive inhibition
- Drugs
- Others

Gilbert syndrome

Sepsis, fasting

Decreased Storage of Unconjugated Bilirubin in Cytosol (Decreased Y and Z Proteins)

Competitive inhibition

Fever

Decreased Biotransformation (Conjugation)

Neonatal jaundice (physiologic)

Inhibition (drugs)

Hereditary (Crigler-Najjar)
- Type I (complete enzyme deficiency)
- Type II (partial deficiency)

Hepatocellular dysfunction

Gilbert syndrome

Conjugated Hyperbilirubinemia (Cholestasis)

Decreased Secretion of Conjugated Bilirubin Into Canaliculi

Hepatocellular disease
- Hepatitis
- Cholestasis (intrahepatic)

Dubin-Johnson and Rotor syndromes

Drugs (estradiol)

Decreased Drainage

Extrahepatic obstruction
- Stones
- Carcinoma
- Stricture
- Atresia

Sclerosing cholangitis

Intrahepatic obstruction
- Drugs
- Granulomas
- Primary biliary cirrhosis
- Bile duct paucity
- Tumors

Unconjugated Hyperbilirubinemia

Unconjugated hyperbilirubinemia poses a risk for development of kernicterus (acute bilirubin encephalopathy), especially in low birth weight infants. Kernicterus refers to a neurologic syndrome that results in brain damage owing to deposition of bilirubin in the basal ganglia and brain stem nuclei. In term infants, the early symptoms of kernicterus are poor feeding, lethargy, and vomiting; later, opisthotonos (backward arching of the trunk), seizures, and death may follow. Seventy percent of affected infants die within the first week, and those remaining have severe brain damage. This syndrome can be prevented by phototherapy and exchange transfusion in infants with elevated unconjugated bilirubin concentrations.

Causes of unconjugated hyperbilirubinemia in the neonate are physiologic jaundice of the newborn, hemolytic disease, and breast milk hyperbilirubinemia.

Guidelines for Assessing Risk. In 2004, the Subcommittee on Hyperbilirubinemia of the American Academy of Pediatrics issued new guidelines for the management of jaundice in the neonate.[B41] These guidelines became necessary because newborns are currently discharged between 36 and 72 hours after birth, and severe hyperbilirubinemia may not be present at discharge. The time-honored bilirubin concentration of 20 mg/dL (34 μmol/L), which was considered critical and required action (e.g., phototherapy, exchange transfusion), is now being abandoned and replaced by monitoring the increase in bilirubin concentration from the time of birth until the time of discharge from the hospital. In practice, it is now recommended that a plot of bilirubin concentration (mg/dL) versus time (hours) should be constructed and compared with the similar plot found in Figure 2 of reference B41 (http://pediatrics.aappublications.org/cgi/reprint/114/1/297/accessed June 23, 2011).

Physiologic Jaundice of the Newborn. Babies frequently become jaundiced within a few days of birth; this condition is known as *physiologic jaundice of the newborn.* Bilirubin concentrations reach a peak within 3 to 5 days of birth and remain elevated for less than 2 weeks. Bilirubin is usually less than 5 mg/dL, with 90% unconjugated. Factors contributing to physiologic jaundice include (1) an increased bilirubin load in the newborn because the RBCs have a shortened life span; (2) the appearance of "shunt" bilirubin, which is bilirubin derived from ineffective erythropoiesis or non-RBC sources; (3) decreased conjugation of bilirubin owing to a relative lack of glucuronyl transferase (conjugating enzyme) in the first few days following birth; (4) increased absorption of bilirubin in the intestine caused by β-glucuronidase in meconium, which hydrolyzes bilirubin conjugates to unconjugated bilirubin that can be passively reabsorbed; and (5) exposure of breast-feeding infants to pregnanediol, nonesterified fatty acids, and other inhibitors of bilirubin conjugation present in breast milk.

Bilirubin concentrations of 13 mg/dL (222 μmol/L) or greater occurred in 6% of 2297 infants who weighed more than 2500 g.[B28] Physiologic jaundice generally is not harmful, but bilirubin concentrations above 10 mg/dL (170 μmol/L), coupled with prematurity, low serum albumin, acidosis, and substances that compete for the binding sites of albumin (e.g., ceftriaxone, sulfisoxazole, aspirin), may increase the risk for kernicterus. Physiologic jaundice of the newborn is treated with phototherapy; the infant is exposed to light of approximately 450 nm that disrupts intramolecular hydrogen bonds in the bilirubin molecule and yields several photoisomers that are more water soluble than the Z,Z-isomer and thus are excreted in the bile.[B33] Exchange transfusions are rarely necessary.

Hemolytic Disease. Hemolytic disease of the newborn results from maternal-fetal incompatibility of Rhesus blood factors in which the maternal Rh-negative blood becomes sensitized by a previous pregnancy with an Rh-positive fetus or an Rh-positive blood transfusion. The infant becomes jaundiced with unconjugated bilirubin in the first or second day of life and is susceptible to kernicterus. The diagnosis is confirmed by a Coombs' test with Rh-positive blood in the infant and Rh-negative blood in the mother. Other rare, inherited hemolytic anemias such as glucose-6-phosphate dehydrogenase (G6PD) deficiency may also lead to unconjugated hyperbilirubinemia.

Breast Milk Hyperbilirubinemia. This type of hyperbilirubinemia affects about 30% of breast-fed newborns. It is due to α-glucuronidase in breast milk, which hydrolyzes conjugated bilirubin in the intestine. The unconjugated bilirubin, being more lipophilic, is passively absorbed. The condition lasts for a few weeks and is treated by discontinuation of breast-feeding.

Conjugated Hyperbilirubinemias

These syndromes are characterized by hyperbilirubinemia in which conjugated bilirubin exceeds 1.5 mg/dL (26 μmol/L). The most important are idiopathic neonatal hepatitis and biliary atresia. Diagnosing the cholestatic syndromes may be difficult. The family history may be helpful in diagnosing α_1-antitrypsin deficiency, cystic fibrosis, galactosemia, hereditary fructose intolerance, and tyrosinosis. Serum tyrosine and α_1-antitrypsin concentrations should be obtained. If galactosemia is suspected, the diagnosis is confirmed by absence of the enzyme UDP galactose-1-phosphate uridyl transferase in cells and tissues such as RBCs and liver. Serologic tests may be necessary for hepatitis A, B, and C, and for adenovirus, Coxsackie virus, cytomegalovirus, herpes simplex, rubella, and *Toxoplasma*. Liver biopsy may be performed, but the liver tends to look similar, with giant cells and extramedullary erythropoiesis dominating, in hepatitis and cholestatic syndromes. The typical features of periportal red hyaline globules seen with periodic acid–Schiff (PAS) stain that are characteristic for α_1-antitrypsin deficiency usually are not seen early in the course of the disorder. An HIDA isotope scan is essential for determining the patency of the biliary tree. Percutaneous or endoscopic cholangiography may be done in patients with equivocal HIDA scan results.

Conjugated hyperbilirubinemia is seen fairly often in the newborn as a complication of parenteral nutrition.

Idiopathic Neonatal Hepatitis

About 75% of cases of hepatitis in the neonate are idiopathic giant cell hepatitis, a disorder of unknown origin characterized by cholestatic jaundice. A familial trend may reflect an autosomal recessive inheritance. Jaundice appears within the first 2 weeks. The child initially appears well and gains weight. The liver and spleen then become enlarged, and stools become pale. Serum aminotransferases are usually 400 U/L; the prothrombin time is prolonged. Liver biopsy reveals characteristic giant cells with hepatocyte acinar formation. Cholestasis is prominent. It is important to rule out extrahepatic biliary obstruction, such as occurs in biliary atresia, with an HIDA scan.

Treatment is supportive, with adequate nutrition and correction of hypoprothrombinemia. The prognosis is favorable, with 90% of infants surviving without sequelae.

Biliary Atresia

Biliary atresia is a heterogeneous group of acquired disorders that involve the extrahepatic or intrahepatic bile ducts. Possible causes include cytomegalovirus, reovirus III, Epstein-Barr virus, rubella virus, α_1-antitrypsin deficiency, Down syndrome, and trisomy 17 or 18.

Extrahepatic biliary atresia may involve all or part of the extrahepatic biliary tree. The gallbladder is usually absent. Involvement of the hepatic or common duct leads to the characteristic syndrome of severe cholestatic jaundice. It occurs in 1 in 10,000 births, with females more commonly affected than males. Jaundice and pruritus usually appear in the first week. Stools are pale and the urine is tea colored. Jaundice is deep, but the aminotransferases are only mildly elevated. If jaundice persists beyond 14 days of age, a direct or conjugated bilirubin measurement must be performed to exclude biliary atresia. If it is elevated, the urine should be tested for bile and the stool color inspected; if the stool is not green or yellow, biliary atresia is likely. Early identification of this condition is essential if these infants are to benefit from the operation of portoenterostomy, which should be performed no later than 60 days after birth.[B15] If portoenterostomy is not successful, liver transplantation is the treatment of choice. Children rarely live beyond 3 years unless the lesion is surgically correctable.

Intrahepatic biliary atresia is characterized by a paucity of intrahepatic bile ducts. Jaundice usually appears within the first few days of life. Serum bilirubin is elevated and serum cholesterol may be very high, leading to the formation of xanthomas. The hepatic histology is nonspecific, showing bile duct paucity, giant cells, inflammation, and fibrosis. Survival into adolescence is common, although growth is usually retarded.

A syndromic variant, *Alagille syndrome,* has similar features but is an autosomal dominant condition with a characteristic triangular face, skeletal abnormalities, retinal pigmentation, and pulmonary stenosis.

Treatment of intrahepatic biliary atresia includes intramuscular replacement of vitamins A, D, and E. Medium-chain triglycerides that do not need bile acids for absorption provide calories in patients with partial atresia. Cholestyramine may relieve pruritus. Ursodeoxycholic acid reduces serum enzyme activities and relieves pruritus in some patients.

Analytical Methods

Several analytical techniques are used to measure bilirubin and metabolites in serum, urine, and feces. Measurement of bilirubin in amniotic fluid is discussed in Chapter 57.

Serum Bilirubin

The reaction of bilirubin with diazotized sulfanilic acid, known as the *diazo reaction,* discovered by Ehrlich in 1883 and applied to the measurement of bilirubin in serum and bile by van den Bergh and Muller in 1916, is the basis of the most widely used methods for measuring bilirubin. The observation that in sera from jaundiced infants the reaction was slow and required an accelerator to proceed, and that it was rapid in bile and in adult sera without addition of ethanol, led to the terms *indirect* and *direct* bilirubin, respectively. The chemical nature of direct and indirect bilirubins was elucidated by Billing, Cole, and Lathe in the mid-1950s.[B5] By open-column reversed-phase chromatography on siliconized kieselguhr (cellite or diatomaceous earth), investigators isolated three bilirubin fractions—unconjugated bilirubin (indirect reacting fraction) and bilirubin monoglucuronide and diglucuronide (direct reacting fractions). Kuenzle and colleagues[B19] were the first to successfully use an open-column chromatography technique that did not involve a deproteinization step. They obtained four bilirubin fractions—unconjugated bilirubin (α-bilirubin), monoconjugated bilirubin (β-bilirubin), diconjugated bilirubin (γ-bilirubin), and a fraction bound strongly to protein (δ-bilirubin). The last fraction was clearly distinct from the albumin-bilirubin complex that exists in serum.

Diazo Methods

The most widely used chemical methods for bilirubin measurement are those based on the coupling of bilirubin with a diazo compound.[B25] In this reaction (Figure 32-21), diazotized sulfanilic acid (the diazo reagent) reacts with bilirubin to produce two azodipyrroles (azopigments), which are reddish purple at neutral pH and blue at low or high pH values. Van den Bergh and Muller[B42] applied this reaction to the quantitation of bilirubin in serum. They described the fraction of bilirubin that reacted with the diazo reagent in the

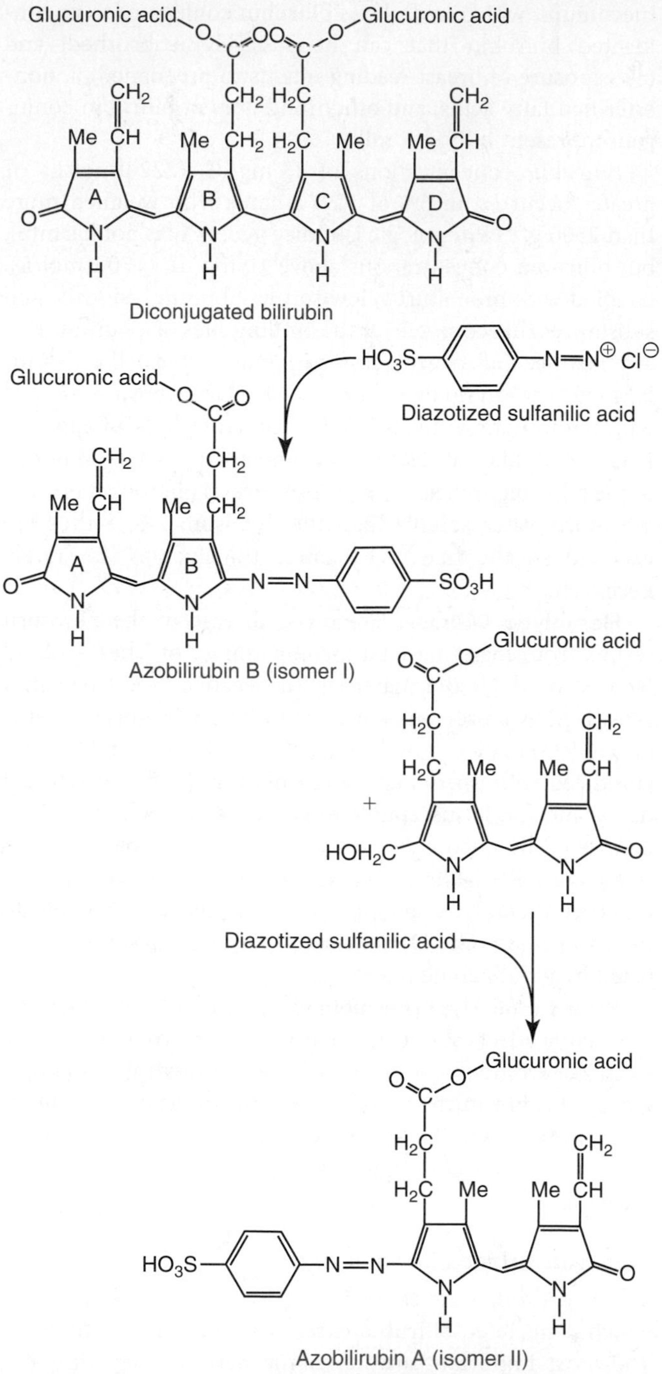

Figure 32-21 The reaction of bilirubin glucuronide with diazotized sulfanilic acid to produce isomers I and II of azobilirubin B. Unconjugated bilirubin reacts in the same way to produce isomers I and II of azobilirubin A.

absence of alcohol as the direct bilirubin fraction and used the term *indirect bilirubin* for the difference between total bilirubin (found after the addition of alcohol to the reaction mixture) and the direct bilirubin fraction. Numerous variations of the van den Bergh method have been developed. All use one of a variety of "accelerators," which, like alcohol, facilitate the reaction of unconjugated (indirect) bilirubin with the diazo reagent; the most commonly used accelerators are caffeine,[B16] dyphylline,[B34] and several surface active agents. The diazo method of Malloy and Evelyn,[B30] which uses methanol as an accelerator, has substantial matrix effects, negative interference by hemoglobin, turbidity due to protein precipitation by methanol, and a long reaction time.[B10] This method, which has been virtually abandoned, is mentioned here for historical reasons only.

The diazo method described by Jendrassik and Grof in 1938[B16] and later modified by Doumas and colleagues[B11] gives results for serum total bilirubin that are reproducible and reliable.[B8,B26,B36] In this procedure, an aqueous solution of caffeine and sodium benzoate serves as the accelerator. Studies on the mechanism by which the caffeine-benzoate solution facilitates the reaction of unconjugated bilirubin with the diazo reagent have provided strong, albeit indirect, evidence that caffeine, and perhaps benzoate, displaces unconjugated bilirubin from its association sites on albumin. This occurs by (1) formation of hydrogen bonds between bilirubin and caffeine,[B14,B20] thus making bilirubin water soluble, or (2) complex formation and disruption of the bilirubin internal hydrogen bonds. With the use of samples prepared by addition of unconjugated bilirubin and authentic human diconjugated (with glucuronic acid) bilirubin to low-bilirubin pooled sera—and a nuclear magnetic resonance technique—Lo and Wu[B24] have shown that the modified Jendrassik-Grof total bilirubin assay detects unconjugated and diconjugated bilirubin quantitatively (as unconjugated bilirubin equivalents). This method has acceptable transferability among laboratories[B8,B36,B39] and is currently the method of choice.

Other methods for determining bilirubin include direct spectrophotometric measurement of total bilirubin in serum using analysis of a two-component system by measuring absorbance at two wavelengths and solving a system of two simultaneous equations. This approach is applicable to sera from healthy neonates because only unconjugated bilirubin is present in such sera. Correction for oxyhemoglobin is necessary because it is invariably present in sera from neonates. (For further details, see "Analytical Methods" in this book's accompanying Evolve site/.)

Calibrators for Bilirubin Measurements

A number of instrument manufacturers are using bovine serum, instead of human serum, as the protein base for preparing fluids for calibrating methods for total and direct bilirubin; the protein base is enriched with unconjugated bilirubin or ditaurobilirubin or both. Unconjugated bilirubin in human serum reacts completely with the reference method and with diazo methods available in commonly used clinical analyzers; however, its reaction in bovine serum from commercial sources is incomplete and unpredictable.[B27] That makes virtually impossible the assignment of accurate bilirubin values to calibrators, the protein base of which is commercial bovine serum. In human serum, ditaurobilirubin was underestimated by two of seven clinical analyzers tested; the calibrators of these two analyzers were made in bovine serum. Ditaurobilirubin in commercial bovine serum was underestimated by all analyzers and by the reference method; in human serum, it was underestimated by two analyzers only. The practice of using bilirubin calibrators in bovine sera must be abandoned because it compromises the accuracy of bilirubin measurements in jaundiced neonates. However, fresh bovine serum (obtained from a slaughterhouse) had only a small effect on the measurement of unconjugated bilirubin or ditaurobilirubin.

High-Performance Liquid Chromatography

HPLC methods have been developed for relatively rapid separation and quantification of the four bilirubin fractions. HPLC has been helpful in separating and detecting the various bilirubin photoisomers produced during phototherapy in newborns and thus in elucidating the mechanism by which phototherapy lowers the concentration of bilirubin in newborn blood.[B33,B44] Several HPLC methods are available for analysis of bilirubin fractions. In the method of Blanckaert,[B6] bilirubin conjugates, but not unconjugated bilirubin, are converted to the corresponding bilirubin methyl esters by base-catalyzed transesterification in methanol followed by extraction with chloroform. With this procedure, the α-, β-, and γ-bilirubin fractions are recoverable, but the δ-fraction (δ-bilirubin) remains in the denatured protein pellet that is produced by the chloroform extraction. In the HPLC method of Lauff and coworkers,[B22] all four bilirubin fractions remain in solution after a step that involves salting out globulins with sodium sulfate. Both methods require the use of dim incandescent or yellow light to minimize photodegradation of the various bilirubin species. A simple and fast HPLC method has been published by Adachi and associates[B1]; this method uses a Micronex RP-30 column (Sekisui Chemical Co., Mount Laurel, NJ), which does not require salting out of globulins or chemical transformation of bilirubin conjugates. This method separates serum bilirubin into five fractions; the fifth fraction eluted between the monoglucuronide and the unconjugated bilirubin is the Z,E or the E,Z photoisomer. The elution sequence is the same as in the procedure of Lauff.[B22]

Additional studies indicated that the δ-bilirubin fraction consists of one or more bilirubin species that are covalently bound to albumin.[B23] Existence of covalent linkage is supported by the fact that the associated bilirubin species are not released from the albumin fraction by treatment with strong acid or base or a variety of strong denaturing agents, by hydrolysis with proteolytic enzymes, or by boiling in methanol. δ-Bilirubin reacts directly (without a promoter) with diazotized sulfanilic acid. The discovery of δ-bilirubin has solved the mystery of the persisting high bilirubin concentrations, mostly direct reacting, in patients with intrahepatic or obstructing jaundice long after hepatitis has subsided or obstruction has been relieved. It is the slowest fraction to clear from serum because it follows the catabolism of albumin, which has a half-life of approximately 17 to 19 days.

HPLC has been very helpful in elucidating the nature of the bilirubin species occurring naturally in blood or formed during phototherapy. Clinically, it offers little, if any, aid to the physician in the differential diagnosis of jaundice, because knowing the percentage of each of the bilirubin fractions in blood is of no diagnostic value. It cannot be considered as a reference method for measuring total bilirubin in blood because its accuracy and precision are inadequate. The method is calibrated with unconjugated bilirubin with the untested assumption that the other three bilirubin fractions have molar absorptivities identical to that of the calibrator,[B21] when in fact this is not known. Furthermore, errors in measurement of the four species may be cumulative and may result in a large total error; also, the method is insensitive at total bilirubin concentrations below 1 mg/dL (17 μmol/L) and is too laborious for routine clinical analysis. Some of the δ-bilirubin may be lost during pretreatment of samples.

A capillary electrophoresis method for measuring the different types of bilirubin has been developed by Wu and his associates.[B43]

Enzymatic Methods

Enzymatic methods for total and direct bilirubin and for bilirubin conjugates with glucuronic acid are based on the oxidation of bilirubin with bilirubin oxidase to biliverdin with molecular oxygen.[B35] At a pH near 8 and in the presence of sodium cholate and sodium dodecylsulfate, all four bilirubin fractions are oxidized to biliverdin, which is further oxidized to purple and finally colorless products. The decrease in absorbance at 425 or 460 nm is proportional to the concentration of total bilirubin. Results obtained by the bilirubin oxidase method were in good agreement with those obtained by the Jendrassik-Grof procedure.[B38] Direct bilirubin is measured at pH 3.7 to 4.5; at this pH range, the enzyme oxidizes bilirubin conjugates and δ-bilirubin, but not unconjugated bilirubin.[B9,B18] At pH 10, the enzyme oxidizes selectively the two glucuronides.[B12,B18] δ-Bilirubin is not oxidized at all, and only 5% of unconjugated bilirubin is measured as conjugates.[B12]

Transcutaneous Measurement of Bilirubin

A noninvasive approach for measuring bilirubin was introduced in 1980 by Yamanouchi and colleagues.[B45] The first bilirubinometer (icterometer) was a reflectance photometer, which used two filters to correct for the color of Hb and required measurements at eight body sites. Efforts to improve the accuracy of such measurements have been successful and led to the development of devices of acceptable performance. Reports indicate that at least one of these devices (Bili*Check* SpectR$_x$ Inc., Norcross, Ga) provides results that are within ±2 mg/dL (34.2 μmol/L) of those obtained using a serum diazo procedure.[B3,B40] Another study found that the Bili*Check* underestimated serum bilirubin when its concentration was greater than 10 mg/dL (170 μmol/L).[B13]

Although transcutaneous bilirubin measurements may not substitute for laboratory quantitative determinations, they provide instantaneous information, reduce the necessity for serum bilirubin determinations, spare infants the trauma of heelsticks, and save money.[B29] Furthermore, they are useful in determining whether in a jaundiced infant it is necessary to draw blood before initiating treatment, such as phototherapy or exchange transfusion (currently this is extremely rare). Another application is predicting those babies who require follow-up according to the "hour-specific" serum bilirubin nomogram developed by Bhutani and coworkers.[B4]

See also "Guidelines for Assessing Risk," earlier in this chapter.

Urine Bilirubin

Because only conjugated bilirubin is excreted in urine, its presence indicates conjugated hyperbilirubinemia. The most commonly used method for detecting bilirubin in urine involves the use of a dipstick impregnated with a diazo reagent. Dipstick methods are capable of detecting bilirubin concentrations as low as 0.5 mg/dL.

A fresh urine specimen is required because bilirubin is unstable when exposed to light and room temperature, and it may be oxidized to biliverdin (which is diazo negative) at the normally acidic pH of the urine. If the test is delayed, the sample must be protected from light and stored at 2 to 8 °C for no longer than 24 hours. The reagent strip (ChemStrip, Roche Diagnostics, Indianapolis, Inc.; Multistix, Siemens Healthcare Diagnostics, Deerfield, Ill) is immersed in the urine specimen for no longer than 1 second and is read 60 seconds later. During this time, bilirubin reacts with a diazo reagent, yielding a pink to red-violet color, the intensity of which is proportional to the bilirubin concentration. The reaction mechanism for urinary conjugated bilirubin is the same as that described in Figure 32-21, except that 2,6-dichlorobenzene-diazonium-tetrafluoroborate is substituted for diazotized sulfanilic acid in the Chemstrip, and 2,4-dichloroaniline diazonium salt in the Multistix. Another commonly used test, more sensitive than the Multistix, is the Ictotest reagent tablet (Siemens Healthcare Diagnostics); in this semiquantitative procedure, the diazo reagent is *p*-nitrobenzenediazonium-*p*-toluenesulfonate.

Chemstrip and Multistix strips for bilirubin in urine are highly specific tests and have a low incidence of false-positive results. However, medications that color the urine red or that give a red color in an acid medium, such as phenazopyridine, can produce a false-positive reading. Large quantities of ascorbic acid or of nitrite also worsen the detection limit of the test. In practice, bilirubin is rarely measured in urine.

Urobilinogen in Urine and Feces

The measurement of urobilinogen in urine is of no diagnostic value in the assessment of liver disease. The same applies to the measurement of urobilinogen in fecal 72-hour or 96-hour specimens. Both tests are obsolete and do not deserve to be presented. A brief description of both tests is found in the third edition of this textbook on page 1137.

REFERENCES

Hemoglobin References

H1. Bains B. Laboratory techniques for the identification of abnormalities of globin chain synthesis. In: Bain BJ, ed. Haemoglobinopathy diagnosis. London: Blackwell Science, 2001:20-48.

H2. Berendt HL, Blakney GB, Clarke G, Higgins TN. A case of beta thalassemia major detected using HPLC in a child of Chinese ancestry. Clin Biochem 2000;33:311-3.

H3. Berfstrome Jones AC, Doon A. Evaluation of a single-tube multiplex polymerase chain reaction screen for detection of common alpha thalassemia genotypes in a clinical laboratory. Am J Clin Path 2002; 118:18-24.

H4. Bissé E, Schauber C, Zorn N, Epting T, Eigel A, Van Dorselaer A, et al. Hemoglobin Görwihl [alpha2beta(2)5(A2)Pro→Ala], an electrophoretically silent variant with impaired glycation. Clin Chem 2003;49:137-43.

H5. Bissé E, Zorn N, Eigel A, Lizama M, Huaman-Guillen P, März W. Hemoglobin Rambam (beta69[E 13]Gly→Asp), a pitfall in the assessment of diabetic control-characterization by electrospray mass spectrometry and HPLC. Clin Chem 1998;44:2172-7.

H6. Bissé E, Zorn N, Heinrichs I, Eigel A, Van Dorsselaert A, Weiland H, et al. Characterization of a new electrophoretically silent hemoglobin variant. J Biol Chem 2000;275:21380-4.

H7. Blouquit Y, Delanoe GJ, Lacombe C, Arous N, Cayre Y, Peduzzi J, et al. Structural study of hemoglobin Hazebrouck, beta 38(C4) Thr—Pro: a new abnormal hemoglobin with instability and low oxygen affinity. FEBS Lett 1984;172:155-8.

H8. Boemer F, Ketelsegers O, Minon J-M, Bours V, Schoos R. Newborn screening for sickle cell disease using tandem mass spectrometry. Clin Chem 2008;54:2036-41.

H9. Bowie LJ, Reddy PL, Nagabhushan M, Sevigny P. Detection of α thalassemia by multiplex polymerase chain reaction. Clin Chem 1994;40:2260-6.

H10. Brandebury RO, Smith HL. Sulfhemoglobinemia: a study of 63 clinical cases. Am Heart J 1951;42:582.

H11. Brennan SO. Fifty-eight years of hemoglobin analysis. Clin Chem 2008;54: 8-10.

H12. British Committee for Standards in Haematology. Guidelines for hemoglobinopathy screening. Clin Lab Haematol 1988;10:87-94.

H13. Bry L, Chen PC, Sacks DB. Effects of hemoglobin variants and chemically modified derivatives on assays for glycohemoglobin. Clin Chem 2001;47:153-63.

H14. Buchwald H. A rapid and sensitive method for estimating carbon monoxide in blood and its application in problem areas. J Am Ind Hygiene Assoc 1969;30:564-9.

H15. Campbell M, Henthorn JS, Davies SC. Evaluations of cation-exchange HPLC compared with isoelectric focusing for neonatal hemoglobinopathy screening. Clin Chem 1999;45:969-75.

H16. Caruso D, Du Riva L, Giavarini F, Galli G, Brambilla S, Luraschi P, et al. A hemoglobin variant found during glycohemoglobin measurement, identified as Hb Toulon [alpha77(EF6)Pro—Hia] by random mass spectroscopy. Hemoglobin 2002;26:197-9.

H17. Cazzola M, May A, Bergamaschi G, Cerani P, Ferrillo S, Bishop DF. Absent phenotypic expression of X-linked sideroblastic anemia in one of two brothers with a novel ALAS2 mutation. Blood 2002;100:4236-8.

H18. Chur DH, Waye JS. Hydrops fetalis caused by alpha thalassemia: an emerging health care problem. Blood 1998;91:2213-22.

H19. Clarke GM, Higgins TN. Laboratory investigation of hemoglobinopathies and thalassemias: review and update. Clin Chem 2000;46:1284-90.

H20. Cotton F, Lin C, Fontaine B, Gulbu B, Jansens J, Ventongen F. Evaluation of a capillary electrophoresis method for routine determination of hemoglobins A2 and F. Clin Chem 1999;46:237-43.

H21. Daniel YA, Turner C, Haynes RM, Hunt BJ, Dalton RN. Quantification of hemoglobin A2 by tandem mass spectrometry. Clin Chem 2007;53:11448-54.

H22. Dash S. HbA2 in subjects with HbD. Clin Chem 1998;44:2381-2.

H23. Elder GE, Lappin TRJ, Horne AB, Fairbanks VF, Jones RT, Winter PC, et al. Hemoglobin Old Dominion/Burton-upon-Trent, β143 (H21) his→tyr, codon 143 CAC→TAC—a variant with altered oxygen affinity—compromises the measurement of glycated hemoglobin in diabetes mellitus: structure, function and DNA sequence. Mayo Clin Proc 1998;73:321-8.

H24. Fairbanks VF. Commentary: should whole-body red cell mass be measured or calculated. Blood Cells Mol Dis 2000;26:32-6.

H25. Fairbanks V. Tables of hemoglobin variants. In: Fairbanks VF, ed. Hemoglobinopathies and thalassemias. New York: BC Decker, 1980: 247-60.

H26. Fucharoen S, Winichagoon P. Thalassemia and abnormal hemoglobin. Int J Hematol 2002;(Suppl 2):83-9.

H27. Fucharoen S, Winichagoon P, Wisedpanichkiy BS-N, Sriphanich R, Oncoung W, Wuangsapaya W, et al. Prenatal and post natal diagnosis of thalassemias and hemoglobinopathies by HPLC. Clin Chem 1998; 44:740-8.

H28. Gemignani F, Perra C, Landi S, Canzian F, Kury A, Tõnisson N, et al. Reliable detection of beta thalassemia and G6PD mutations by a DNA microarray. Clin Chem 2002;48:2051-4.

H29. Gerritsma J, Sinnige D, Drieze C, Sittrop B, Houtsma P, Hulshort-Jansen N, et al. Qualitative and quantitative analysis of hemoglobin variants using capillary zone electrophoresis. Ann Clin Biochem 2000;37:380-9.

H30. Guidelines for the investigation of the alpha and beta thalassemia traits: the thalassemia Working Party of the BCSH General Hematology Task Force. J Clin Pathol 1994;47:289-95.

H31. Significant haemoglobinopathies: guidelines for screening and diagnosis. Working group: On behalf of the British Committee for Standards in hematology. British Journal of Hematology 2010;149:35-49.

H32. Hall RB, Haga JA, Guerra CG, Castleberry SM, Hichman JR. Optimizing the detection of hemoglobin H disease. Lab Med 1995;26: 736-41.

H33. Hempe JM, Craver RD. Separation of hemoglobin variants with similar change by capillary isoelectric focussing: value of isoelectric point for identification of common and uncommon hemoglobin variants. Electrophoresis 2000;21:738-43.

H34. Herrmann MM, Dobrowolski SF, Wittwer CT. Rapid beta globin genotyping by multiplexing probable melting temperature and color. Clin Chem 2000;46:425-8.

H35. Higgins TN, Guo N. MALDI-TOF MS/microwave-assisted acid hydrolysis identification of HbG Coushatta. Clin Biochem 2009;42: 99-107.

H36. Higgins TN, Khajuria A, Mack M. Quantification of HbA2 in patients with and without β thalassemia and in the presence of HbS, HbC, HbE and HbD Punjab. Am J Clin Path 2009;131:357-62.

H37. Higgins TN, Khajuria A, Mack M. Comparison of two methods for the quantification and identification of hemoglobin variants. Clin Biochem 2009;42:701-5.

H38. Howanitz JH, Howanitz PJ, Chauhan YP. Influences of CBC results and HPLC hemoglobin S measurements on criteria for diagnosis of beta thalassemia. Clin Chem 2003;496:A18.

H39. Howard J, Henthorn JS, Murphy S, Davies SC. Implications of increased haemoglobin A2 in HIV positive women in the antenatal setting. J Clin Pathol 2005;58:556-8.

H40. Ingram VM. A specific chemical difference between globins of normal and sickle-cell anemia hemoglobins. Nature 1956;178:792-4.

H41. Ingram VM. Gene mutations in human hemoglobin: the chemical difference between normal and sickle cell hemoglobin. Nature 1957;180:326-8.

H42. Ingram VM. The chemical difference between normal and sickle cell hemoglobin. Biochem Biophys Acta 1959;36:402-11.

H43. Ingram VM. The comparison of normal human and sickle-cell hemoglobin by "Finger Printing." Biochem Biophys Acta 1958;28:539-45.

H44. International Committee for Standardization in Haematology. ISCH Expert Panel for neonatal screening of haemologlobinopathies. Clin Lab Haematol 1988;10:335-45.

H45. International Committee for Standardization in Haematology. Recommendations for a system for identifying abnormal hemoglobins. Blood 1978;50:1065-7.

H46. Karen DF, Hedstrom D, Gulbranson R, Ou C-N, Bak R. Comparison of Sebia capillarys electrophoresis with the Primus high-pressure liquid chromatography in the evaluation of hemoglobinopathies. Am J Clin Path 2008;130;824-31.

H47. Kiernan UA, Black JA, Williams P, Nelson RW. High-throughput analysis of hemoglobin from neonates using matrix-assisted laser desorption/ionization time-of-flight mass spectrometry. Clin Chem 2002;48:9479.

H48. Kleinert P, Schmid M, Zurbriggen K, Speer O, Schmugge M, Roschitzki B, et al. Mass spectrometry: a tool for enhanced detection of hemoglobin variants. Clin Chem 2008;54:69-76.

H49. Lafferty J. College of American Pathologists hemoglobinopathy survey (HG-B). Chicago, Ill: College of American Pathologists, 1999.

H50. Lafferty JD, Crowther MA, Ali MA, Levine ML. The evaluation of various mathematical RBC indices and their efficacy in discriminating between thalassemic and non-thalassemic microcytosis. Am J Clin Path 1996;106:201-5.

H51. Lafferty JD, Crowther MD, Waye JS, Chui DHK. A reliable screening test to identify adult carriers of the (–SEA) alpha-thalassemia deletion A. J Clin Path 2000;114:927-31.

H52. Lehmann H. Hemoglobin variants. In: Bunn HF, Forget BG, eds. Hemoglobin: molecular genetics and clinical aspects. Philadelphia: Saunders, 1986.

H53. Mario N, Baudin B, Aussel C, Giboudeau J. Capillary isoelectric focussing and high-performance cation-exchange chromatography compared for qualitative and quantitative analysis of hemoglobin variants. Clin Chem 1997;43:2137-42.

H54. Mario N, Baudin B, Janssens J, Vanbourdolle M. Capillary zone electrophoresis for the diagnosis of congenital hemoglobinopathies. Clin Chem 1999;45:285-8.

H55. Milner PF, Gooden HM. Rapid citrate-agar electrophoresis in routine screening for hemoglobinopathies using a simple hemolysate. Am J Clin Path 1975;64:58-64.

H56. Mohandas N, Kim YR, Tycko DH, Orlik J, Wyatt J, Groner W. Accurate and independent measurement of volume and hemoglobin concentration of individual red cells by laser light scattering. Blood 1986;68:506-13.

H57. Old JM. Screening and genetic diagnosis of haemoglobin disorders. Blood Rev 2003;17:43-53.

H58. Olivieri NF. The beta-thalassemias. N Engl J Med 1999;341:99-109.

H59. Ou C-N, Rognerud CL. Diagnosis of hemoglobinopathies electrophoresis vs HPLC. Clin Chem Acta 2001;313:187-94.

H60. Pauling L, Itano HA, Singer SJ, Wells IC. Sickle cell anemia, a molecular disease. Science 1949;110:543-8.

H61. Peurtz MF, Muirhead H, Cox J, Goaman LCG. Three dimensional Fourier synthesis of horse oxyhemoglobin at 2.8A resolution: the atomic model. Nature 1968;219:133-9.

H62. Reynolds TM, Harvey TC, Green BN, Smith A, Hartland AJ. Hemoglobin Wayne in a British family: identification by electrospray ionization/mass spectrometry. Clin Chem 2002;48:2261-3.

H63. Rioya L, Grot R, Garabedian M, Cournot-Witmer G. Bone disease in children with homozygous beta thalassemia. Bone Miner 1990;8: 69-86.

H64. Sacks DS. Hemoglobin variants and hemoglobin A1c analysis: problem solved? Clin Chem 2003;49:1245-7.

H65. Sarnaik SA. Sickle cell diseases: current therapeutic options and potential pitfalls in preventive therapy for transcranial Doppler abnormalities. Pediatr Radiol 2005;35:223-8.

H66. Schendl WJ, Lipp RW, Trinker M, Hopmeirer P. Hemoglobin D [β121(GH4)Glu→Gln] causing falsely low and high HbA2 values in HPLC. Clin Chem 1998;44:1999-2000.

H67. Shaji RV, Edison ES, Poonkuzhali B, Srivastava A, Chandy M. Rapid detection of beta-globin gene mutations and polymorphisms by temporal temperature gradient gel electrophoresis. Clin Chem 2003;49:777-81.

H68. Shihabi ZK, Hinsdale ME. Simplified hemoglobin chain detection by capillary electrophoresis. Electrophoresis 2005;26:581-5.

H69. Simsek M, Darr S, Ojeli H, Bayami R. Improved diagnosis of sickle cell mutation by a robust amplification refractory polymerase chain reaction. Clin Biochem 1999;32:677-80.

H70. Sternberg MH, Adams JG. Hemoglobin A2: origin, evolution and aftermath. Blood 1991;78:2165-77.

H71. Stewart RD. The effect of carbon monoxide on humans. Ann Rev Pharm 1975;15:405-22.

H72. Stewart RD, Baretta LR, Platte LR, Stewart EB, Kalbfleisch JH, Van Yserloo B, et al. Carboxyhemoglobin levels in American blood donors. J Am Med Assoc 1974;229:1187-95.

H73. Suh DD, Krauss JS, Bures K. Influence of hemoglobin S adducts on HbA2 quantification by HPLC. Clin Chem 1996;42:1113-4.

H74. Tian H, Emrich CA, Scherer JR, Mathies RA, Andersen PS, Larsen LA, et al. High-throughput single-strand conformation polymorphism analysis on a microfabricated capillary array electrophoresis device. Electrophoresis 2005;26:1834-42.

H75. Wallace C, Arfay AA, Salkie ML, Crockford PM. Spurious levels of glycated hemoglobin due to the presence of unsuspected hemoglobin variants Can J Diab Care 1994;18:16-20.

H76. Wang W, Kham SKY, Yeo G-H, Quah T-C, Chong SS. Multiplex minisequencing screen for common Southeast Asian and Indian beta thalassemia mutations. Clin Chem 2003;49:209-13.

H77. Wang W, Ma ESK, Chan AYY, Chui DHK, Chong SS. Multiple minisequencing screen for seven Southeast Asian non-deletional alpha-thalassemia mutations. Clin Chem 2003;49:800-3.

H78. Weatherall DJ, Clegg JB. Thalassemia: a global public health problem. Nat Med 1996;2:847-9.

H79. Wright RO, Lewander WJ, Woolf AD. Methemoglobinemia: etiology, pharmacology, and clinical management. Ann Emerg Med 1999;34:646-56.

H80. Yang Z, Chaffin CH, Easley PL, Thigpen B, Reddy VVB. Prevalence of elevated hemoglobin A2 measured by the CAPILLARYS system. Am J Clin Path 2009;131:42-8.

H81. Zur B, Hornung A, Breuer J, Doll U, Bernhardt C, Ludwig M, et al. A novel hemoglobin, Bonn, causes falsely decreased oxygen saturation measurements in pulse oximetry. Clin Chem 1998;54: 594-6.

H82. Zurbriggen K, Schmudde M, Schmid M, Durka S, Klienert P, Kuster T, et al. Analysis of minor hemoglobins by matrix-assisted laser desorption/ionization time-of-flight mass spectrometry. Clin Chem 2005;51:989-96.

Iron References

I1. Aisen P. The G277S mutation in transferrin does not disturb function. Br J Haematol 2003;121:674-5.

I2. Asberg A, Hveem K, Kruger O, Bjerve KS. Persons with screening-detected haemochromatosis: as healthy as the general population? Scand J Gastroenterol 2002;37:719-24.

I3. Babitt JL, Huang FW, Wrighting DM, Xia Y, Sidis Y, Samad TA, et al. Bone morphogenetic protein signaling by hemojuvelin regulates hepcidin expression. Nat Genet 2006;38:531-9.

I4. Barron BA, Hoyer JD, Tefferi A. A bone marrow report of absent stainable iron is not diagnostic of iron deficiency. Ann Hematol 2001; 80:166-9.

I5. Barton JC, Acton RT, Dawkins FW, Adams PC, Lovato L, Leiendecker-Foster C, et al. Initial screening transferrin saturation values, serum ferritin concentrations, and HFE genotypes in whites and blacks in the Hemochromatosis and Iron Overload Screening Study. Genet Test 2005;9:231-41.

I6. Barton JC, Acton RT, Lee PL, West C. *SLC40A1 Q248H* allele frequencies and *Q248H*-associated risk of non-HFE iron overload in persons of sub-Saharan African descent. Blood Cells Mol Dis 2007; 39:206-11.

I7. Barton JC, Acton RT, Rivers CA, Bertoli LF, Gelbart T, West C, et al. Genotypic and phenotypic heterogeneity of African Americans with primary iron overload. Blood Cells Mol Dis 2003;31:310-9.

I8. Barton JC, Bertoli LF, Rothenberg BE. Peripheral blood erythrocyte parameters in hemochromatosis: evidence for increased erythrocyte hemoglobin content. J Lab Clin Med 2000;135:96-104.

I9. Barton JC, Edwards CQ, Bertoli LF, Shroyer TW, Hudson SL. Iron overload in African Americans. Am J Med 1995;99:616-23.

I10. Barton JC, Lee PL, West C, Bottomley SS. Iron overload and prolonged ingestion of iron supplements: clinical features and mutation analysis of hemochromatosis-associated genes in four cases. Am J Hematol 2006;81:760-7.

I11. Bell SH, Weir MP, Dickson DP, Gibson JF, Sharp GA, Peters TJ. Mossbauer spectroscopic studies of human haemosiderin and ferritin. Biochim Biophys Acta 1984;787:227-36.

I12. Ben Hariz M, Goulet O, De Potter S, Girot R, Rambaud C, Colomb V, et al. Iron overload in children receiving prolonged parenteral nutrition. J Pediatr 1993;123:238-41.

I13. Beutler E. Production and destruction of erythrocytes. In: Beutler E, Lichtman MA, Coller BS, Kipps TJ, Seligsohn U, eds. Williams hematology. New York: McGraw-Hill, 2001:413-7.

I14. Beutler E, Felitti V, Gelbart T, Ho N. The effect of *HFE* genotypes on measurements of iron overload in patients attending a health appraisal clinic. Ann Intern Med 2000a;133:329-37.

I15. Beutler E, Felitti VJ. The C282Y mutation does not shorten life span. Arch Intern Med 2002a;162:1196-7.

I16. Beutler E, Felitti VJ, Koziol JA, Ho NJ, Gelbart T. Penetrance of *845G→A (C282Y)* HFE hereditary haemochromatosis mutation in the USA. Lancet 2002b;359:211-8.

I17. Beutler E, Gelbart T, Lee P, Trevino R, Fernandez MA, Fairbanks VF. Molecular characterization of a case of atransferrinemia. Blood 2000b;96:4071-4.

I18. Bloom PD, Burstein GR, Gordeuk VR. Iron overload in African Americans. In: Barton JC, Edwards CQ, eds. Hemochromatosis: genetics, pathophysiology, diagnosis and treatment. Cambridge: Cambridge University Press, 2000:475-83.

I19. Borgna-Pignatti C, Cappellini MD, De Stefano P, Del Vecchio GC, Forni GL, Gamberini MR, et al. Survival and complications in thalassemia. Ann N Y Acad Sci 2005;1054:40-7.

I20. Breuer W, Ermers MJ, Pootrakul P, Abramov A, Hershko C, Cabantchik ZI. Desferrioxamine-chelatable iron, a component of serum non-transferrin-bound iron, used for assessing chelation therapy. Blood 2001;97:792-8.

I21. Brown K, Subramony C, May W, Megason G, Liu H, Bishop P, et al. Hepatic iron overload in children with sickle cell anemia on chronic transfusion therapy. J Pediatr Hematol Oncol 2009;31:309-12.

I22. Bulaj ZJ, Ajioka RS, Phillips JD, LaSalle BA, Jorde LB, Griffen LM, et al. Disease-related conditions in relatives of patients with hemochromatosis. N Engl J Med 2000;343:1529-35.

I23. Burn J, Chinnery PF. Neuroferritinopathy. Semin Pediatr Neurol 2006;13:176-81.

I24. Camaschella C, Roetto A, Cali A, De Gobbi M, Garozzo G, Carella M, et al. The gene *TFR2* is mutated in a new type of haemochromatosis mapping to 7q22. Nat Genet 2000;25:14-5.

I25. Casanovas G, Mleczko-Sanecka K, Altamura S, Hentze MW, Muckenthaler MU. Bone morphogenetic protein (BMP)-responsive elements located in the proximal and distal hepcidin promoter are critical for its response to HJV/BMP/SMAD. J Mol Med 2009;87:471-80.

I26. Centers for Disease Control and Prevention. Iron deficiency—United States, 1999-2000. MMWR Morb Mortal Wkly Rep 2002;51:897-9.

I27. Cervantes F, Rozman C, Brugues R, Llanas I. Iron stores in chronic granulocytic leukaemia at presentation. Scand J Haematol 1984;32: 469-74.

I28. Chinnery PF, Crompton DE, Birchall D, Jackson MJ, Coulthard A, Lombes A, et al. Clinical features and natural history of neuroferritinopathy caused by the *FTL1* 460InsA mutation. Brain 2007;130:110-9.

I29. Chuang CL, Liu RS, Wei YH, Huang TP, Tarng DC. Early prediction of response to intravenous iron supplementation by reticulocyte haemoglobin content and high-fluorescence reticulocyte count in haemodialysis patients. Nephrol Dial Transplant 2003;18: 370-7.

I30. Cremonesi L, Forni GL, Soriani N, Lamagna M, Fermo I, Daraio F, et al. Genetic and clinical heterogeneity of ferroportin disease. Br J Haematol 2005;131:663-70.

I31. Darbari DS, Kple-Faget P, Kwagyan J, Rana S, Gordeuk VR, Castro O. Circumstances of death in adult sickle cell disease patients. Am J Hematol 2006;81:858-63.

I32. De Gobbi M, Barilaro MR, Garozzo G, Sbaiz L, Alberti F, Camaschella C. *TFR2* Y250X mutation in Italy. Br J Haematol 2001; 114:243-4.

I33. De Gobbi M, Roetto A, Piperno A, Mariani R, Alberti F, Papanikolaou G, et al. Natural history of juvenile haemochromatosis. Br J Haematol 2002;117:973-9.

I34. Delatycki MB, Allen KJ, Gow P, MacFarlane J, Radomski C, Thompson J, et al. A homozygous *HAMP* mutation in a multiply consanguineous family with pseudo-dominant juvenile hemochromatosis. Clin Genet 2004;65:378-83.

I35. Enders HM. Evaluating iron status in hemodialysis patients. Nephrol Nurs J 2002;29:366-70.

I36. Fairbanks VJ, Brandhagen DJ. Disorders of iron storage and transport. In: Beutler E, Lichtman MA, Coller BS, Kipps TJ, Seligsohn U, eds. Williams hematology. New York: McGraw-Hill, 2001:489-502.

I37. Feder JN, Gnirke A, Thomas W, Tsuchihashi Z, Ruddy DA, Basava A, et al. A novel MHC class I-like gene is mutated in patients with hereditary haemochromatosis. Nat Genet 1996;13:399-408.

I38. Fellman V. The GRACILE syndrome, a neonatal lethal metabolic disorder with iron overload. Blood Cells Mol Dis 2002;29:444-50.

I39. Fernandez-Rodriguez AM, Guindeo-Casasus MC, Molero-Labarta T, Dominguez-Cabrera C, Hortal C, Perez-Borges P, et al. Diagnosis of iron deficiency in chronic renal failure. Am J Kidney Dis 1999;34: 508-13.

I40. Fielding J. Iron. In: Cook JD, eds. Methods in hematology. New York: Churchill Livingstone, 1980:15-43.

I41. Finkenstedt A, Bianchi P, Theurl I, Vogel W, Witcher DR, Wroblewski VJ, et al. Regulation of iron metabolism through GDF15 and hepcidin in pyruvate kinase deficiency. Br J Haematol 2009;144:789-93.

I42. Fishbane S, Kalantar-Zadeh K, Nissenson AR. Serum ferritin in chronic kidney disease: reconsidering the upper limit for iron treatment. Semin Dial 2004;17:336-41.

I43. Ganz T. Hepcidin and its role in regulating systemic iron metabolism. Hematology Am Soc Hematol Educ Program 2006;507: 29-35.

I44. Gordeuk V, Mukiibi J, Hasstedt SJ, Samowitz W, Edwards CQ, West G, et al. Iron overload in Africa: interaction between a gene and dietary iron content. N Engl J Med 1992;326:95-100.

I45. Gregory A, Hayflick SJ. Neurodegeneration with brain iron accumulation. Folia Neuropathol 2005;43:286-96.

I46. Harris EL, McLaren CE, Reboussin DM, Gordeuk VR, Barton JC, Acton RT, et al. Serum ferritin and transferrin saturation in Asians and Pacific Islanders. Arch Intern Med 2007;167:722-6.

I47. Harris ZL, Takahashi Y, Miyajima H, Serizawa M, MacGillivray RT, Gitlin JD. Aceruloplasminemia: molecular characterization of this disorder of iron metabolism. Proc Natl Acad Sci U S A 1995;92: 2539-43.

I48. Harrison PM, Arosio P. The ferritins: molecular properties, iron storage function and cellular regulation. Biochim Biophys Acta 1996; 1275:161-203.

I49. Hershko C, Peto TE. Non-transferrin plasma iron. Br J Haematol 1987;66:149-51.

I50. International Committee for Standardization in Haematology. The measurement of total and unsaturated iron binding capacity in serum. Br J Haematol 1978;38:281-94.

I51. Iron Panel of the International Committee for Standardization in Haematology. Revised recommendations for the measurements of the serum iron in human blood. Br J Haematol 1990;75:615-6.

I52. Jackson HA, Carter K, Darke C, Guttridge MG, Ravine D, Hutton RD, et al. *HFE* mutations, iron deficiency and overload in 10,500 blood donors. Br J Haematol 2001;114:474-84.

I53. Jacolot S, Le Gac G, Scotet V, Quere I, Mura C, Ferec C. HAMP as a modifier gene that increases the phenotypic expression of the *HFE* pC282Y homozygous genotype. Blood 2004;103:2835-40.

154. Kakhlon O, Cabantchik ZI. The labile iron pool: characterization, measurement, and participation in cellular processes(1). Free Radic Biol Med 2002;33:1037-46.
155. Kato J, Fujikawa K, Kanda M, Fukuda N, Sasaki K, Takayama T, et al. A mutation in the iron-responsive element of H ferritin mRNA, causing autosomal dominant iron overload. Am J Hum Genet 2001; 69:191-7.
156. Knisely AS, Gelbart T, Beutler E. Molecular characterization of a third case of human atransferrinemia. Blood 2004;104:2607.
157. Laflamme L, Blank VL. Age-related accident risks: longitudinal study of Swedish iron ore miners. Am J Ind Med 1996;30:479-87.
158. Lebron JA, Bennett MJ, Vaughn DE, Chirino AJ, Snow PM, Mintier GA, et al. Crystal structure of the hemochromatosis protein HFE and characterization of its interaction with transferrin receptor. Cell 1998; 93:111-23.
159. Lee PL, Barton JC. Hemochromatosis and severe iron overload associated with compound heterozygosity for *TFR2* R455Q and two novel mutations TFR2 R396X and G792R. Acta Haematol 2006;115: 102-5.
160. Lee PL, Halloran C, Trevino R, Felitti V, Beutler E. Human transferrin G277S mutation: a risk factor for iron deficiency anaemia. Br J Haematol 2001;115:329-33.
161. Mast AE, Blinder MA, Lu Q, Flax S, Dietzen DJ. Clinical utility of the reticulocyte hemoglobin content in the diagnosis of iron deficiency. Blood 2002;99:1489-91.
162. McLaren CE, Barton JC, Gordeuk VR, Wu L, Adams PC, Reboussin DM, et al. Determinants and characteristics of mean corpuscular volume and hemoglobin concentration in white *HFE* C282Y homozygotes in the hemochromatosis and iron overload screening study. Am J Hematol 2007;82:898-905.
163. Merryweather-Clarke AT, Cadet E, Bomford A, Capron D, Viprakasit V, Miller A, et al. Digenic inheritance of mutations in *HAMP* and *HFE* results in different types of haemochromatosis. Hum Mol Genet 2003;12:2241-7.
164. Milet J, Dehais V, Bourgain C, Jouanolle AM, Mosser A, Perrin M, et al. Common variants in the *BMP2, BMP4,* and *HJV* genes of the hepcidin regulation pathway modulate *HFE* hemochromatosis penetrance. Am J Hum Genet 2007;81:799-807.
165. Mims MP, Guan Y, Pospisilova D, Priwitzerova M, Indrak K, Ponka P, et al. Identification of a human mutation of DMT1 in a patient with microcytic anemia and iron overload. Blood 2005;105:1337-42.
166. Mohandas N, Kim YR, Tycko DH, Orlik J, Wyatt J, Groner W. Accurate and independent measurement of volume and hemoglobin concentration of individual red cells by laser light scattering. Blood 1986;68:506-13.
167. Nemeth E, Roetto A, Garozzo G, Ganz T, Camaschella C. Hepcidin is decreased in *TFR2* hemochromatosis. Blood 2005;105:1803-6.
168. Nemeth E, Tuttle MS, Powelson J, Vaughn MB, Donovan A, Ward DM, et al. Hepcidin regulates cellular iron efflux by binding to ferroportin and inducing its internalization. Science 2004;306:2090-3.
169. Niederau C, Fischer R, Purschel A, Stremmel W, Haussinger D, Strohmeyer G. Long-term survival in patients with hereditary hemochromatosis. Gastroenterology 1996;110:1107-19.
170. Nittis T, Gitlin JD. The copper-iron connection: hereditary aceruloplasminemia. Semin Hematol 2002;39:282-9.
171. Nittis T, Gitlin JD. Role of copper in the proteosome-mediated degradation of the multicopper oxidase hephaestin. J Biol Chem 2004;279:25696-702.
172. Njajou OT, de Jong G, Berghuis B, Vaessen N, Snijders PJ, Goossens JP, et al. Dominant hemochromatosis due to N144H mutation of *SLC11A3*: clinical and biological characteristics. Blood Cells Mol Dis 2002;29:439-43.
173. Olsson S, Lundvall O, Weinfeld A. Availability of iron stores built up by iron dextrin as studied with desferrioxamine and phlebotomy. Acta Med Scand 1972;191:49-56.
174. Olynyk JK, Cullen DJ, Aquilia S, Rossi E, Summerville L, Powell LW. A population-based study of the clinical expression of the hemochromatosis gene. N Engl J Med 1999;341:718-24.
175. Papanikolaou G, Samuels ME, Ludwig EH, MacDonald ML, Franchini PL, Dube MP, et al. Mutations in *HFE2* cause iron overload in chromosome 1q-linked juvenile hemochromatosis. Nat Genet 2004;36:77-82.
176. Parkkila S, Waheed A, Britton RS, Bacon BR, Zhou XY, Tomatsu S, et al. Association of the transferrin receptor in human placenta with HFE, the protein defective in hereditary hemochromatosis. Proc Natl Acad Sci U S A 1997;94:13198-202.
177. Perry RT, Gearhart DA, Wiener HW, Harrell LE, Barton JC, Kutlar A, et al. Hemoglobin binding to A beta and HBG2 SNP association suggest a role in Alzheimer's disease. Neurobiol Aging 2008;29:185-93.
178. Phatak PD, Ryan DH, Cappuccio J, Oakes D, Braggins C, Provenzano K, et al. Prevalence and penetrance of *HFE* mutations in 4865 unselected primary care patients. Blood Cells Mol Dis 2002;29:41-7.
179. Pitts TO, Barbour GL. Hemosiderosis secondary to chronic parenteral iron therapy in maintenance hemodialysis patients. Nephron 1978;22:316-21.
180. Ramirez JM, Schaad O, Durual S, Cossali D, Docquier M, Beris P, et al. Growth differentiation factor 15 production is necessary for normal erythroid differentiation and is increased in refractory anaemia with ring-sideroblasts. Br J Haematol 2009;144:251-62.
181. Ramsay AJ, Hooper JD, Folgueras AR, Velasco G, Lopez-Otin C. Matriptase-2 (TMPRSS6): a proteolytic regulator of iron homeostasis. Haematologica 2009;94:840-9.
182. Reeves WB, Haurani FI. Clinical applicability and usefulness of ferritin measurements. Ann Clin Lab Sci 1980;10:529-35.
183. Rice EW, Fenner HE. Study of the ICSH proposed reference method for serum iron assay: obtaining optically clear filtrates and substitution of ferrozine. Clin Chim Acta 1974;53:391-3.
184. Roetto A, Bosio S, Gramaglia E, Barilaro MR, Zecchina G, Camaschella C. Pathogenesis of hyperferritinemia cataract syndrome. Blood Cells Mol Dis 2002;29:532-5.
185. Roetto A, Papanikolaou G, Politou M, Alberti F, Girelli D, Christakis J, et al. Mutant antimicrobial peptide hepcidin is associated with severe juvenile hemochromatosis. Nat Genet 2003;33:21-2.
186. Sarria B, Navas-Carretero S, Lopez-Parra AM, Perez-Granados AM, Arroyo-Pardo E, Roe MA, et al. The G277S transferrin mutation does not affect iron absorption in iron deficient women. Eur J Nutr 2007; 46:57-60.
187. Saven A, Beutler E. Iron overload after prolonged intramuscular iron therapy. N Engl J Med 1989;321:331-2.
188. Schulz JB, Boesch S, Burk K, Durr A, Giunti P, Mariotti C, et al. Diagnosis and treatment of Friedreich ataxia: a European perspective. Nat Rev Neurol 2009;5:222-34.
189. Silvestri L, Guillem F, Pagani A, Nai A, Oudin C, Silva M, et al. Molecular mechanisms of the defective hepcidin inhibition in *TMPRSS6* mutations associated with iron-refractory iron deficiency anemia. Blood 2009;113:5605-8.
190. Sipe JC, Lee P, Beutler E. Brain iron metabolism and neurodegenerative disorders. Dev Neurosci 2002;24:188-96.
191. Sokal JE, Sheerin KA. Decreased stainable marrow iron in chronic granulocytic leukemia. Am J Med 1986;81:395-9.
192. Stoffman N, Brugnara C, Woods ER. An algorithm using reticulocyte hemoglobin content (CHr) measurement in screening adolescents for iron deficiency. J Adolesc Health 2005;36:529.
193. Takahashi Y, Miyajima H, Shirabe S, Nagataki S, Suenaga A, Gitlin JD. Characterization of a nonsense mutation in the ceruloplasmin gene resulting in diabetes and neurodegenerative disease. Hum Mol Genet 1996;5:81-84.
194. Tamary H, Shalev H, Perez-Avraham G, Zoldan M, Levi I, Swinkels DW, et al. Elevated growth differentiation factor 15 expression in patients with congenital dyserythropoietic anemia type I. Blood 2008;112:5241-4.
195. Tanno T, Bhanu NV, Oneal PA, Goh SH, Staker P, Lee YT, et al. High levels of GDF15 in thalassemia suppress expression of the iron regulatory protein hepcidin. Nat Med 2007;13:1096-101.
196. Tessitore N, Solero GP, Lippi G, Bassi A, Faccini GB, Bedogna V, et al. The role of iron status markers in predicting response to

intravenous iron in haemodialysis patients on maintenance erythropoietin. Nephrol Dial Transplant 2001;16:1416-23.
I97. van Tellingen A, Kuenen JC, de Kieviet W, van Tinteren H, Kooi ML, Vasmel WL. Iron deficiency anaemia in hospitalised patients: value of various laboratory parameters: differentiation between IDA and ACD. Neth J Med 2001;59:270-9.
I98. Vaulont S, Labie D. [Erythroblast-derived GDF15 suppresses hepcidin in thalassemia]. Med Sci (Paris) 2008;24:139-41.
I99. Wallace DF, Clark RM, Harley HA, Subramaniam VN. Autosomal dominant iron overload due to a novel mutation of ferroportin1 associated with parenchymal iron loading and cirrhosis. J Hepatol 2004;40:710-3.
I100. Weir MP, Gibson JF, Peters TJ. Biochemical studies on the isolation and characterization of human spleen haemosiderin. Biochem J 1984;223:31-8.
I101. Wu CJ, Krishnamurti L, Kutok JL, Biernacki M, Rogers S, Zhang W, et al. Evidence for ineffective erythropoiesis in severe sickle cell disease. Blood 2005;106:3639-45.
I102. Zoller H, McFarlane I, Theurl I, Stadlmann S, Nemeth E, Oxley D, et al. Primary iron overload with inappropriate hepcidin expression in V162del ferroportin disease. Hepatology 2005;42:466-72.

Bilirubin References

B1. Adachi Y, Inufusa H, Yamashita M, Kambe A, Yamazaki K, Sawada Y, et al. Clinical application of serum bilirubin fractionation by simplified liquid chromatography. Clin Chem 1988;34:385-8.
B2. Beutler E, Gelbart T, Demina A. Racial variability in the UDP-glucuronosyltransferase 1 (UGT1A1) promoter: a balanced polymorphism for regulation of bilirubin metabolism? Proc Natl Acad Sci U S A 1998;95:8170-4.
B3. Bhutani VK, Gourley GR, Adler S, Kreamer B, Dalin C, Johnson LH. Noninvasive measurement of total serum bilirubin in a multiracial predischarge newborn population to assess the risk of severe hyperbilirubinemia. Pediatrics 2000;106:E17.
B4. Bhutani VK, Johnson L, Sivieri EM. Predictive ability of a predischarge hour-specific serum bilirubin for subsequent significant hyperbilirubinemia in healthy term and near-term newborns. Pediatrics 1999;103:6-14.
B5. Billing BH, Cole PG, Lathe GH. The excretion of bilirubin as a glucuronide giving the direct van den Bergh reaction. Biochemical J 1957;65:774-83.
B6. Blanckaert N. Analysis of bilirubin and bilirubin mono- and di-conjugates: determination of their relative amounts in biological samples. Biochem J 1980;185:115-28.
B7. Bonnett R, Davis E, Hursthouse MB. The structure of bilirubin. Nature 1976;262:327-8.
B8. Doumas BT, Perry BW, McComb RB, Kessner A, Vader HL, Vink KL, et al. Molar absorptivities of bilirubin (NIST SRM 916a) and its neutral and alkaline azopigments. Clin Chem 1990;36:1968-701.
B9. Doumas BT, Perry B, Jendrzejczak B, Davis L. Measurement of direct bilirubin by use of bilirubin oxidase. Clin Chem 1987;33:1349-53.
B10. Doumas BT, Perry BW, Sasse EA, Straumfjord JV. Standardization in bilirubin assays: evaluation of selected methods and stability of bilirubin solutions. Clin Chem 1973;19:984-93.
B11. Doumas BT, Poon PKC, Perry BW, Jendzejczak B, McComb RB, Schaffer R, et al. Candidate reference method for determination of total bilirubin in serum: development and validation. Clin Chem 1985;31:1779-89.
B12. Doumas BT, Yein F, Perry B, Jendrzejczak B, Kessner A. Determination of the sum of bilirubin sugar conjugates in plasma by bilirubin oxidase. Clin Chem 1999;45:1255-60.
B13. Engle WD, Jackson GL, Sendelbach D, Manning D, Frawley WH. Assessment of a transcutaneous device in the evaluation of neonatal hyperbilirubinemia in a primarily Hispanic population. Pediatrics 2002;110:61-7.
B14. Franzini C, Cattozzo G. Low affinity complex between bilirubin and caffeine. Clin Chem 1987;33:597-9.
B15. Hussein M, Howard ER, Mieli-Vergani G, Mowat AP. Jaundice at 14 days of age: exclude biliary atresia. Arch Dis Child 1991;66:1177-9.
B16. Jendrassik L, Grof P. Vereinfachte photometrische Methoden zur Bestimmung des Blutbilirubins. Biochem Z 1938;297:81-9.
B17. Koiwai O, Nishizawa M, Hasada K, Aono S, Adachi Y, Mamiya N, et al. Gilbert's syndrome is caused by a heterozygous missense mutation in the gene for bilirubin UDP-glucuronosyltransferase. Hum Mol Genet 1995;4:1183-6.
B18. Kosaka A, Yamamoto C, Morishita Y, Nakane K. Enzymatic determination of bilirubin fractions in serum. Clin Biochem 1987:20:451-8.
B19. Kuenzle CC, Maier C, Rutner JR. The nature of four bilirubin fractions from serum and of three bilirubin fractions from bile. J Lab Clin Med 1966;67:294-306.
B20. Landis JB, Pardue HL. Kinetics of the reaction of unconjugated and conjugated bilirubins with *p*-diazobenzenesulfonic acid. Clin Chem 1978;24:1690-9.
B21. Lauff JJ, Kasper ME, Ambrose RT. Quantitative liquid chromatographic estimation of bilirubin species in pathological serum. Clin Chem 1983;29:800-5.
B22. Lauff JJ, Kasper ME, Ambrose RT. Separation of bilirubin species in serum and bile by high performance reverse-phase liquid chromatography. J Chromatogr 1981;226:391-402.
B23. Lauff JJ, Kasper ME, Wu TW, Ambrose RT. Isolation and preliminary characterization of a fraction of bilirubin in serum that is firmly bound to protein. Clin Chem 1982;28:629-37.
B24. Lo DH, Wu TW. Assessment of the fundamental accuracy of the Jendrassik and Grof total and direct bilirubin assays. Clin Chem 1983;29:31-6.
B25. Lo SF, Doumas BT, Ashwood ER. Performance of bilirubin determinations in US laboratories—revisited. Clin Chem 2004;50:190-4.
B26. Lo SF, Jendrzejczak B, Doumas BT. Laboratory performance in neonatal bilirubin testing using commutable specimens: a progress report on a College of American Pathology study. Arch Pathol Lab Med 2008;132:1781-5.
B27. Lo SF, Jendrzejczak B, Hubbard L, Doumas BT. Bovine serum-based bilirubin calibrators are inappropriate for some diazo methods. Clin Chem 2010;56:869-72.
B28. Maisels MJ, Gilford K. Normal bilirubin levels in the newborn and the effect of breast feeding. Pediatrics 1986;78:837-45.
B29. Maisels MJ, Kring E. Transcutaneous bilirubinometry decreases the need for serum bilirubin measurements and saves money. Pediatrics 1997;99:599-601.
B30. Malloy HT, Evelyn KA. The determination of bilirubin with the photoelectric colorimeter. J Biol Chem 1937;119:481-90.
B31. McDonagh AF, Assisi F. Commercial bilirubin: a trinity of isomers. FEBS Lett 1971;18:315-7.
B32. McDonagh AF, Assisi F. The ready isomerization of bilirubin IX-α in aqueous solution. Biochem J 1972;129:797-800.
B33. McDonagh AF, Palma LA, Lightner DA. Blue light and bilirubin excretion. Science 1980;208:145-51.
B34. Michaelsson M. Bilirubin determination in serum and urine. Scand J Clin Lab Invest 1961;13(Suppl 56).
B35. Murao S, Tanaka N. Isolation and identification of a microorganism producing bilirubin oxidase. Agric Biol Chem 1982:46:2031-4.
B36. National Institute of Standards and Technology. Certificate of Analysis: Standard Reference Material 916a, Bilirubin. Gaithersburg, Md: National Institute of Standards and Technology, 2001.
B37. Newman TB, Liljestrand P, Escobar GJ. Combining clinical risk factors with serum bilirubin levels to predict hyperbilirubinemia in newborns. Arch Pediatr Adolesc Med 2005;159:113-9.
B38. Perry B, Doumas BT, Buffone G, Glick M, Ou CN, Ryder K. Measurement of total bilirubin by use of bilirubin oxidase. Clin Chem 1986;32:329-32.
B39. Perry BW, Doumas BT, Bayse DD, Butler T, Cohen A, Fellows N, et al. A candidate reference method for determination of bilirubin in serum: test for transferability. Clin Chem 1983;29:297-301.

B40. Robertson A, Kazmierczak S, Vos P. Improved transcutaneous bilirubinometry: comparison of SpectRx Bili Check and Minolta Jaundice Meter JM-102 for estimating total serum bilirubin in a normal newborn population. J Perinatol 2002;22:12-4.

B41. Subcommittee on Hyperbilirubinemia. Management of hyperbilirubinemia in the newborn infant 35 or more weeks of gestation. Pediatrics 2004;114:297-316.

B42. van den Bergh AAH, Muller P. Uber eine direkte und eine indirekte Diazo-reaktion auf Bilirubin. Biochem Z 1916;77:90-103.

B43. Wu N, Sweedler JV, Lin M. Enhanced separation and deletion of serum bilirubin species by capillary electrophoresis using a mixed anionic surfactant-protein buffer system with laser-induced fluorescence detection. J Chromatogr B Biomed Appl 1994;654: 185-91.

B44. Wu TW, Dappen GM, Powers DM, Lo DH, Rand RN, Spayd RW. The Kodak Ektachem clinical chemistry slide for measurement of bilirubin in newborns: principles and performance. Clin Chem 1982; 28:2366-72.

B45. Yamanouchi I, Yamauchi Y, Igarashi I. Transcutaneous bilirubinometry: preliminary studies of noninvasive bilirubin meter in the Okayama National Hospital. Pediatrics 1980;65:195-202.

CHAPTER 33

The Porphyrias and Other Disorders of Porphyrin Metabolism

Michael N. Badminton, M.B., Ch.B, Ph.D., F.R.C.Path., Sharon D. Whatley, Ph.D., Allan C. Deacon, Ph.D., F.R.C.Path., and George H. Elder, M.D., F.R.C.P., F.R.C.Path.

The porphyrias are a group of uncommon, inherited disorders of heme biosynthesis.[3,102] Each porphyria results from a partial deficiency of one of the enzymes of the pathway converting 5-aminolevulinate (ALA) to heme or, in one rare disorder, an increase in activity of the rate-controlling enzyme of erythroid heme synthesis. Each functional abnormality is associated with a specific pattern of overproduction, accumulation, and excretion of the intermediates of the pathway. These intermediates are excreted in excessive amounts in urine, feces, or both. The clinical consequences depend on the nature of the heme precursors that accumulate. In the acute porphyrias, excess porphyrin precursors [ALA and porphobilinogen (PBG)] are associated with potentially fatal acute neurovisceral attacks that often are provoked by (1) various commonly prescribed drugs, (2) hormonal factors, (3) alcohol, (4) starvation, (5) stress, or (6) infection. In the nonacute porphyrias, and in those acute porphyrias in which both acute neurovisceral attacks and skin lesions occur, accumulation of porphyrins results in photosensitization of sun-exposed skin. Diagnosis depends on laboratory investigation to demonstrate the pattern of heme precursor accumulation specific for each type of porphyria and requires examination of appropriate specimens for the key metabolites using adequately sensitive and specific methods. Technical advances in the field of molecular genetics have made it possible to investigate all porphyrias at the molecular level. Although rarely essential for diagnosis of symptomatic cases, DNA analysis is now the method of choice for the investigation of families with porphyria and continues to provide new information about the pathology of these disorders. Abnormalities of porphyrin excretion and accumulation also occur in a wide variety of other disorders that are collectively far more common than the porphyrias. Recognition of these secondary porphyrin disorders is important to avoid diagnostic errors.

PORPHYRIN CHEMISTRY

Before porphyrin synthesis and disorders of porphyrin metabolism are discussed, porphyrin structure, nomenclature, and chemical characteristics are reviewed.

Structure and Nomenclature

The basic porphyrin structure consists of four monopyrrole rings connected by methene bridges to form a tetrapyrrole ring (Figure 33-1).[16] Many porphyrin compounds are known, but only a limited number are of clinical interest. The porphyrin compounds of relevance to the porphyrias (Table 33-1) differ in the substituents occupying peripheral positions 1 through 8. Variation in the distribution of the same substituents around the peripheral positions of the tetrapyrrole ring gives rise to porphyrin isomers, which usually are depicted by Roman numerals (e.g., I, II, III). The reduced form of a porphyrin, known as a *porphyrinogen* (see Figure 33-1), differs by the absence of six hydrogens (four from the methylene bridges and two from ring nitrogens). Porphyrinogens are unstable in vitro and are spontaneously oxidized to the corresponding porphyrins. Under the lower oxygen tension of the cell, porphyrinogens are sufficiently stable to act as intermediates of the heme biosynthetic pathway; aromatization to protoporphyrin at the penultimate step requires an enzyme.

Chelation of Metals

The arrangement of four nitrogen atoms in the center of the porphyrin ring enables porphyrins to chelate various metal ions. Protoporphyrin that contains iron is known as heme; ferroheme refers specifically to the Fe^{2+} complex and ferriheme to Fe^{3+}. Ferriheme associated with a chloride counter ion is known as hemin, or hematin when the counter ion is hydroxide.

Spectral Properties

Porphyrins were named from the Greek root for "purple" ("porphyra") and owe their color to the conjugated double-bond structure of the tetrapyrrole ring. The porphyrinogens have no conjugated double bonds and therefore are colorless. Porphyrins show particularly strong absorbance near 400 nm, often called the Soret band. When exposed to light in the 400-nm region, porphyrins display a characteristic orange-red fluorescence in the range of 550 to 650 nm. Absorbance and fluorescence are altered by substituents around the porphyrin ring and by metal binding. Zinc chelation shifts the fluorescence emission peak of protoporphyrin to shorter wavelengths and reduces the fluorescence intensity. The strong binding of iron alters the character of protoporphyrin to the extent that heme lacks significant fluorescence.

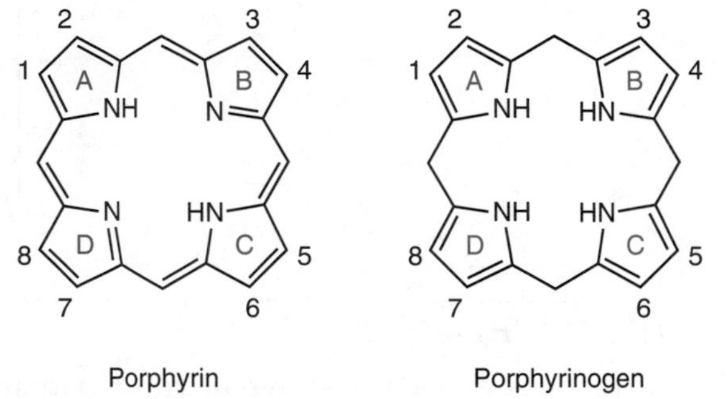

Porphyrin   Porphyrinogen

Figure 33-1 Porphyrin and porphyrinogen structures: numbers 1 to 8 represent various substituents, the nature and order of which determine the type of porphyrin or porphyrinogen (see Table 33-1). Numbering system and ring designations are based on the Fischer system. A revised system formulated by the International Union of Pure and Applied Chemistry–International Union of Biochemistry (IUPAC-IUB) Joint Commission on Biochemical Nomenclature is appropriate for more complex needs. Because of increasing complexity, this Roman numeral designation is no longer recommended above IV.[86]

Solubility

Porphyrins are only marginally soluble in water. The differing solubilities of individual porphyrins are of importance not only in the design of analytical methods for their extraction and fractionation but in determining the route of excretion from the body. At pH 7, the carboxyl groups are ionized, and the molecule has a net negative charge. Below pH 2, the pyrrole nitrogens and the carboxyl groups become protonated so that the molecule has a net positive charge. At physiologic pH, the solubility of a given porphyrin is determined by the number of substituent carboxyl groups. Uroporphyrin has eight carboxylate groups and is the most soluble porphyrin in aqueous media. Protoporphyrin has only two carboxylate groups and is essentially insoluble in water, but it dissolves readily in lipid environments and binds readily to the hydrophobic regions of proteins such as albumin. Coproporphyrin, with four carboxylate groups, has intermediate solubility.

Traditional extraction methods for porphyrins have two steps: first, extraction into an acidified organic solvent, followed by a second or back extraction into aqueous acid. The initial extraction takes advantage of the fact that at pH 3 to 5 (near to their isoelectric point) porphyrins are less soluble in aqueous media and move into the organic phase. Coproporphyrin and protoporphyrin are readily extracted into diethyl ether, but the more highly carboxylated porphyrins (uroporphyrin and heptacarboxylate porphyrin) require the use of a more hydrophilic solvent such as cyclohexanone or butanol. The back extraction induces porphyrin compounds to move back into the aqueous solution by decreasing the pH to less than 2. This pH shift causes protonation of the pyrrolenine nitrogen and carboxylate groups, thereby reversing the solubility characteristics of porphyrins. Compounds such as

TABLE 33-1 Substituents Around the Macrocycle in Porphyrins of Clinical Importance

Position	1	2	3	4	5	6	7	8
Uroporphyrin-I	C_m	C_{et}	C_m	C_{et}	C_m	C_{et}	C_m	C_{et}
Uroporphyrin-III	C_m	C_{et}	C_m	C_{et}	C_m	C_{et}	C_{et}	C_m
Heptacarboxylate porphyrin-III	C_m	C_{et}	C_m	C_{et}	C_m	C_{et}	C_{et}	Me
Hexacarboxylate porphyrin-III	Me	C_{et}	C_m	C_{et}	C_m	C_{et}	C_{et}	Me
Pentacarboxylate porphyrin-III	Me	C_{et}	Me	C_{et}	C_m	C_{et}	C_{et}	Me
Coproporphyrin-III	Me	C_{et}	Me	C_{et}	Me	C_{et}	C_{et}	Me
Coproporphyrin-I	Me	C_{et}	Me	C_{et}	Me	C_{et}	Me	C_{et}
Isocoproporphyrin	Me	Et	Me	C_{et}	C_m	C_{et}	C_{et}	Me
Dehydroisocoproporphyrin	Me	Vn	Me	C_{et}	C_m	C_{et}	C_{et}	Me
Deethylisocoproporphyrin	Me	H	Me	C_{et}	C_m	C_{et}	C_{et}	Me
Protoporphyrin	Me	Vn	Me	Vn	Me	C_{et}	C_{et}	Me
Pemptoporphyrin	Me	H	Me	Vn	Me	C_{et}	C_{et}	Me
Deuteroporphyrin	Me	H	Me	H	Me	C_{et}	C_{et}	Me
Mesoporphyrin	Me	Et	Me	Et	Me	C_{et}	C_{et}	Me

C_m, Carboxymethyl ($-CH_2COOH$); *C_{et}*, carboxyethyl ($-CH_2CH_2COOH$); *Et*, ethyl ($-CH_2CH_3$); *Me*, methyl ($-CH_3$); *Vn*, vinyl ($-CH{=}CH_2$).

heme and chlorophyll, in which the pyrrole nitrogens are tightly bound to iron and magnesium, respectively, remain uncharged at low pH and trapped in the organic layer.

HEME BIOSYNTHESIS

The complex tetrapyrrole ring structure of heme is built up in a stepwise fashion from the very simple precursors succinyl–coenzyme A (CoA) and glycine (Figure 33-2).[21] The pathway is present in all nucleated cells. From measurements of total bilirubin production,[8] it has been estimated that daily synthesis of heme in humans is 5 to 8 mmol/kg body weight. Of this, 70 to 80% occurs in the bone marrow and is used for hemoglobin synthesis. Approximately 15% is synthesized in other tissues, mainly the liver and is used to produce cytochrome P450, mitochondrial cytochromes, and other hemoproteins. The pathway is compartmentalized, with some steps occurring in the mitochondrion and others in the cytoplasm. Several carriers that transfer intermediates across the mitochondrial membrane have now been identified.[50,112a] Although all are potential sites for pathogenic mutations, only one such mutation has been identified: a mutation in the erythroid-specific mitochondrial glycine transporter SLC25A38 that causes nonsyndromic autosomal recessive sideroblastic anemia.[50]

Enzymes of Heme Biosynthesis

The genes for all enzymes of human heme biosynthesis have been characterized (Table 33-2). The structures of human hydroxymethylbilane synthase (HMBS) , uroporphyrinogen-III synthase (UROS), uroporphyrinogen decarboxylase (UROD), coproporphyrinogen oxidase (CPOX), ferrochelatase (FECH), bacterial 5-aminolevulinate synthase (ALAS), 5-aminolevulinic acid dehydratase (ALAD), and protoporphyrinogen oxidase (PPOX) have been determined by x-ray crystallography.[5,19,35,44,73,80,131,135]

5-Aminolevulinate Synthase (EC 2.3.1.37) (ALAS)

ALAS, the initial enzyme of the pathway, catalyzes the formation of ALA from succinyl-CoA and glycine. The enzyme is mitochondrial and requires a cofactor of pyridoxal phosphate, which forms a Schiff base with the amino group of glycine at the enzyme surface. The carbanion of the Schiff base displaces CoA from succinyl-CoA with the formation of α-amino-β-ketoadipic acid, which is then decarboxylated to ALA. The activity of ALAS is rate limiting as long as the catalytic capacities of other enzymes in the pathway are normal.

5-Aminolevulinic Acid Dehydratase (EC 4.2.1.24) (ALAD)

ALAD (also known as porphobilinogen synthase) is a cytoplasmic enzyme that catalyzes the formation of the monopyrrole PBG from two molecules of ALA with elimination of two molecules of water. The enzyme requires zinc ions as a cofactor and reduced sulfhydryl groups at the active site and therefore is susceptible to inhibition by lead.

Hydroxymethylbilane Synthase (EC 2.5.1.61) (HMBS)

HMBS (also known as PBG deaminase) is a cytoplasmic enzyme that catalyzes the formation of one molecule of the linear tetrapyrrole 1-hydroxymethylbilane (HMB; also known as preuroporphyrinogen) from four molecules of PBG with the release of four molecules of ammonia.[124] The enzyme has two molecules of its own substrate: PBG, attached covalently to the apoenzyme as a prosthetic group.[115] The enzyme is susceptible to allosteric inhibition by intermediates farther down the heme biosynthetic pathway, notably coproporphyrinogen-III and protoporphyrinogen-IX.[85]

Uroporphyrinogen-III Synthase (EC 4.2.1.75) (UROS)

UROS is a cytoplasmic enzyme that rearranges and cyclizes HMB to form uroporphyrinogen-III.[124] Each pyrrole ring of HMB contains a methylcarboxylate and an ethylcarboxylate substituent, which are in the same orientation. By the rotation of zero, one, or two alternate or two adjacent pyrrole rings, it is possible to arrive at four different isomers. Apart from closing the ring structure, the enzyme rotates the D-ring via a spirane intermediate,[7] producing the type III isomer—an essential reaction because only this isomer contributes to

TABLE 33-2 Human Enzymes and Genes of Heme Biosynthesis

Enzyme	Monomer Mol Mass, kDa*†	Chromosomal Location of Gene	Gene Size, kb	No. of Exons	Expression
ALAS1	70.6	3p21.1	17	12	Ubiquitous
ALAS2	64.6	Xp11.21	22	11	Erythroid cells
ALAD	36.3	9q34	13	13	Ubiquitous and erythroid-specific mRNAs
HMBS	37.0	11q24.1-24.2	10	15	Ubiquitous and erythroid-specific isoforms
UROS	29.5	10q25.2-26.3	34	10	Ubiquitous and erythroid-specific mRNAs
UROD	40.8	1p34	3	10	Ubiquitous
CPOX	40.3	3q12	14	7	Ubiquitous
PPOX	50.8	1q21-23	5	13	Ubiquitous
FECH	47.8	18q21.3	45	11	Ubiquitous

*ALAD is a homo-octamer, and HMBS and UROS are monomers; all other enzymes are homodimers.

†Molecular masses for ALAS1, ALAS2, CPOX, and FECH include presequences that are cleaved during mitochondrial import.

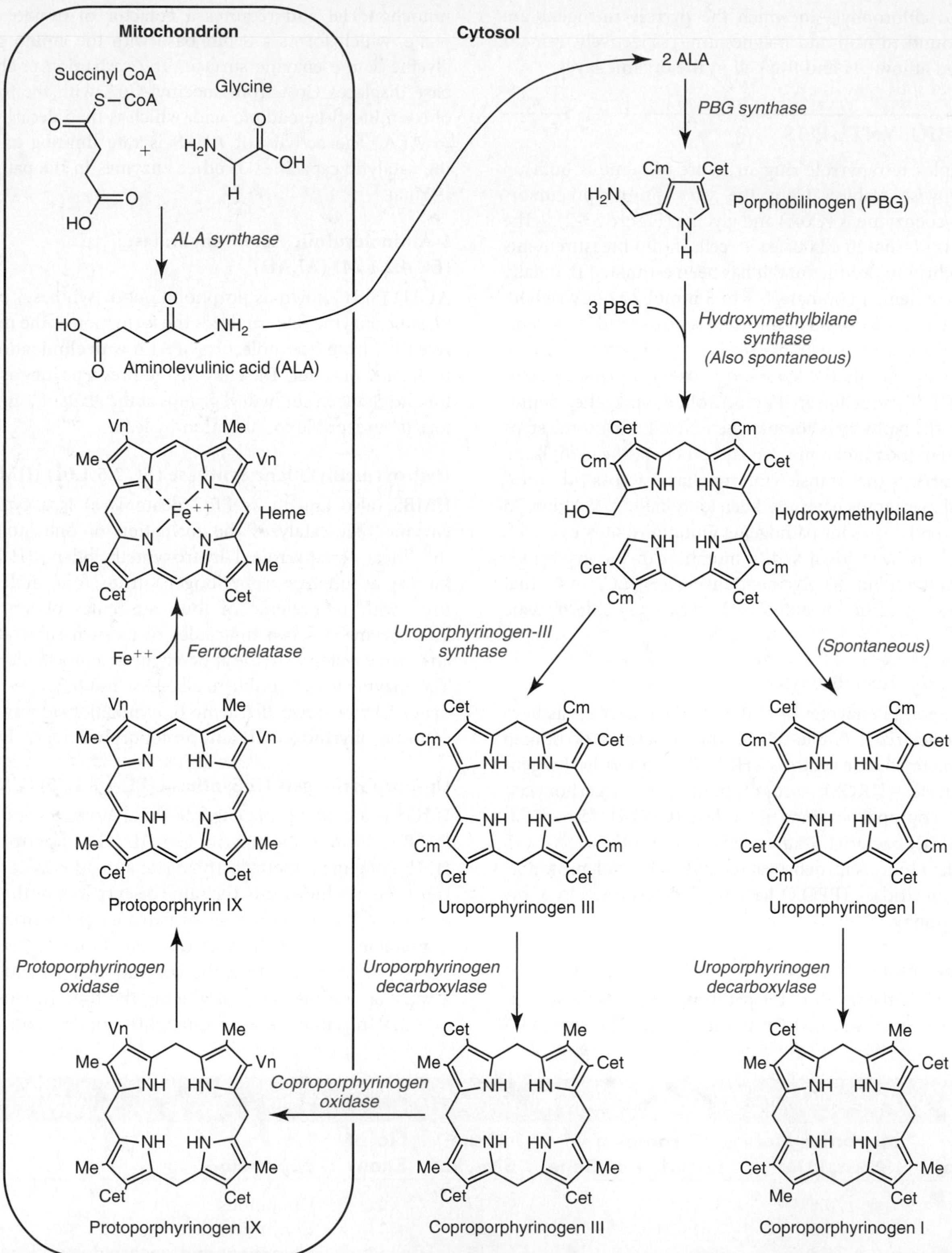

Figure 33-2 Biosynthetic pathway of porphyrins and heme. ***C_{et}***, **$—CH_2CH_2COOH$;** ***C_m***, **$—CH_2COOH$;** ***Me***, **$—CH_3$;** ***Vn***, **$—CH{=}CH_2$.**

heme biosynthesis. HMB is unstable, and in those porphyrias in which excess HMB accumulates, cyclization occurs nonenzymatically with the formation of the type I isomer. Normally, only minimum amounts of uroporphyrinogen-I are formed.

Uroporphyrinogen Decarboxylase (EC 4.1.1.37) (UROD)

This is the last cytoplasmic enzyme in the pathway, and it catalyzes the decarboxylation of all four carboxymethyl groups to form the tetracarboxylic coproporphyrinogen. The enzyme will use I and III isomers of uroporphyrinogen as substrate. Decarboxylation commences on ring D and proceeds stepwise through rings A, B, and C with formation of heptacarboxylate, hexacarboxylate, and pentacarboxylate intermediates at a single active site.[95] Decreased UROD activity causes accumulation of these intermediates in addition to its substrate, uroporphyrinogen. At high substrate concentrations, decarboxylation occurs by a random mechanism.[78]

Coproporphyrinogen Oxidase (EC 1.3.3.3) (CPOX)

CPOX, which is located in the intermembrane space of mitochondria, catalyzes the sequential oxidative decarboxylation of the 2- and 4-carboxyethyl groups to vinyl groups to produce the more lipophilic protoporphyrinogen-IX, with formation of a tricarboxylic intermediate, harderoporphyrinogen.[71] Oxygen is required as the oxidant. The enzyme requires sulfhydryl groups for activity, making it a target for inhibition by metals.[133] The enzyme is specific for the type III isomer, so that metabolism of the I-series of porphyrins does not occur beyond coproporphyrinogen-I. The product of the enzyme differs from the substrate in that replacement of two of the carboxyethyl groups by vinyl groups introduces a third substituent into the molecule. Therefore the number of possible isomeric forms is increased, and conventionally the numbering system changes, so that the III isomer becomes the IX isomer. In UROD-deficient states, one of the ethylcarboxylate groups of the accumulated pentacarboxylate porphyrinogen is decarboxylated by CPOX to form the isocoproporphyrin series of porphyrins.

Protoporphyrinogen Oxidase (EC 1.3.3.4) (PPOX)

PPOX, a flavoprotein located in the inner mitochondrial membrane, catalyzes the removal of six hydrogens (four from methylene bridges and two from ring nitrogens) to form protoporphyrin-IX. This involves a three-step, six-electron flavin adenine dinucleotide (FAD)-dependent oxidation that consumes molecular oxygen.[21] Nonenzymatic oxidation also occurs in vitro. However, under the low oxygen tension in the cell, PPOX is essential for oxidation to occur. The protoporphyrin produced is the only porphyrin that functions in the heme pathway. Other porphyrins are produced by nonenzymatic oxidation and represent porphyrinogens that have irreversibly escaped from the pathway.

Ferrochelatase (EC 4.99.1.1) (FECH)

FECH (also known as heme synthase) is an iron-sulfur protein located in the inner mitochondrial membrane.[135] This enzyme inserts ferrous iron into protoporphyrin to form heme. During this process, two hydrogens are displaced from the ring nitrogens. Other metals in the divalent state also act as substrates, yielding the corresponding chelate (e.g., incorporation of Zn^{2+} into protoporphyrin to yield zinc protoporphyrin). In iron-deficient states, Zn^{2+} successfully competes with Fe^{2+} in developing red cells, so that the concentration of zinc protoporphyrin in erythrocytes increases. Some other dicarboxylic porphyrins also serve as substrates (e.g., mesoporphyrin). Integration of the final stages of erythroid heme biosynthesis may be facilitated by interaction between FECH and proteins involved in iron import.[18a]

EXCRETION OF HEME PRECURSORS

Typically, only minute quantities of heme precursors accumulate in the body. The route of excretion largely depends on solubility. The porphyrin precursors ALA and PBG are water soluble and are excreted almost exclusively in urine. Uroporphyrinogen, with eight carboxylate groups, is readily water soluble and is also excreted via the kidney. The last intermediate of the pathway, protoporphyrin (and also protoporphyrinogen), which has only two carboxylate groups, is insoluble in water and is excreted in the feces via the biliary tract. The other porphyrins are of intermediate solubility and appear in both urine and feces. Coproporphyrinogen-I is taken up and excreted by the liver in preference to the III isomer, so that coproporphyrinogen-I predominates in feces and coproporphyrinogen-III in urine. All porphyrinogens in the urine or feces are slowly oxidized to the corresponding porphyrins. Reference intervals for porphyrins and their precursors in urine, feces, and blood are given in Table 33-3.

Once in the gut, porphyrins are susceptible to modification by gut flora. The two vinyl groups of protoporphyrin are reduced to ethyl groups, hydrated to hydroxyethyl groups, or removed, giving rise to a variety of secondary porphyrins. Gut flora can also metabolize heme (whether dietary heme, as components from cells sloughed off from the lining of the gut, or heme resulting from gastrointestinal bleeding) to produce a variety of dicarboxylic porphyrins.[9] In addition, some bacteria are capable of de novo synthesis of porphyrins.

REGULATION OF HEME BIOSYNTHESIS

Heme supply in all tissues is controlled by the activity of mitochondrial ALAS, the first enzyme of the pathway. Two isoforms of ALAS are known. The ubiquitous isoform, ALAS1, is encoded by a gene on chromosome 3p21 and is expressed in all tissues. Because it has a half-life of only about an hour, changes in its rate of synthesis produce short-term alterations in enzyme concentration and cellular ALAS activity. Synthesis of ALAS1 is under negative feedback control by heme.[82] In the liver, but not most other tissues, ALAS1 is induced by a wide variety of drugs and chemicals that induce microsomal cytochrome P450–dependent oxidases (CYPs). This effect is thought to be mediated mainly by direct transcriptional activation by drug-responsive nuclear receptors,[118]

TABLE 33-3 Adult Reference Intervals

Specimen	Analyte	Reference Interval
Urine	Porphobilinogen	<10 μmol/L[24]
		<1.5 μmol/mmol creatinine[11]
	Total porphyrin	20-320 nmol/L[24]
		<35 nmol/mmol creatinine[11]
	Uroporphyrin	0.8-3.1 nmol/mmol creatinine[9]
	Heptacarboxylate porphyrin	<0.9 nmol/mmol creatinine[9]
	Coproporphyrin-I	1.2-5.7 nmol/mmol creatinine[9]
	Coproporphyrin-III	4.8-23.8 nmol/mmol creatinine[9]
	% Coproporphyrin-III*	68-86[9]
Feces	Total porphyrin	10-200 nmol/g dry wt[77]
	Coproporphyrin-I	1.1-5.5 nmol/g feces[9]
	Coproporphyrin-III	0.2-2.5 nmol/g feces[9]
	Coproporphyrin-III/I ratio	0.3-1.4[130]
	Total dicarboxylate porphyrin	0.5-12.8 nmol/g feces[9]
Erythrocytes	Total porphyrin	0.4-1.7 μmol/L erythrocytes

*Percentage of total coproporphyrin.

TABLE 33-4 The Main Types of Human Porphyria

Disorder	Defective Enzyme	Prevalence*	Neurovisceral Crises	Skin Lesions	Inheritance
Acute Porphyrias					
ALA dehydratase deficiency porphyria (ADP)	ALAD	–	+	–	AR
AIP	HMBS	1-2:100,000	+	–	AD
HCP	CPO	1-2:10^6	+	+†‡	AD
VP	PPOX	1:250,000	+	+†‡	AD
Nonacute Porphyrias					
CEP	UROS	1:10^6	–	+‡	AR
PCT	UROD	1:25,000	–	+‡	Complex (20% AD)
EPP (FECH-deficient)	FECH	1:140,000	–	+§	AR
EPP (XLDPP)	ALAS2	0.15:10^6	–	+§	XLD

*Estimated prevalence of clinically overt disease in the United Kingdom.
†Skin lesions and neurovisceral crises may occur alone or together.
‡Fragile skin, bullae.
§Acute photosensitivity without fragile skin, bullae.
AD, Autosomal dominant; *AR,* autosomal recessive; *XLD,* X-linked dominant.

rather than occurring secondary to depletion of an intracellular regulatory heme pool as a consequence of use of heme for CYP assembly. Induction of ALAS1 is prevented by heme, which acts by destabilizing messenger ribonucleic acid (mRNA) for ALAS1, by blocking mitochondrial import of pre-ALAS1, and possibly by inhibiting transcription.[64] In addition, ALAS1 activity is regulated by PGC-1α; an effect that forms a link between the rate of hepatic heme synthesis and nutritional status.[51]

The erythroid isoform, ALAS2, is encoded by a gene on chromosome Xq21-22 and is expressed only in erythroid cells. Its activity is regulated by two distinct mechanisms.[101] Transcription is enhanced during erythroid differentiation by the action of erythroid-specific transcription factors, and mRNA concentrations are regulated by iron. Iron deficiency in erythroid cells promotes specific binding of iron regulatory proteins to an iron-responsive element in the 5′ untranslated region (UTR) of ALAS2 mRNA with consequent inhibition of translation.

THE PORPHYRIAS

The porphyrias are a group of metabolic disorders that result from decreased or, in one rare form of erythropoietic protoporphyria, increased activities of the enzymes of heme biosynthesis[3,102] (Table 33-4). All are inherited in monogenic

TABLE 33-5 The Porphyrias: Patterns of Overproduction of Heme Precursors During Clinically Overt Phase of Disease

Porphyria	Urine PBG/ALA	Urine Porphyrins	Fecal Porphyrins	Erythrocyte Porphyrins	Plasma Fluorescence Emission Peak
ADP	ALA	Copro-III	Not increased	ZPP	–
AIP	PBG>ALA	Mainly uroporphyrin from PBG	Normal or increased[a] Copro-I/III ratio normal	Not increased	615-622 nm[b]
CEP	Not increased	Uro-I, Copro-I	Copro-I	ZPP, Proto, Copro-I, Uro-I	615-620 nm
PCT	Not increased	Uro, Hepta[c]	Isocopro, Hepta	Not increased	615-622 nm
HCP	PBG>ALA[d]	Copro-III, uroporphyrin from PBG	Copro-III, Copro-III/I ratio increased	Not increased	615-622 nm[b]
VP	PBG>ALA[d]	Copro-III, uroporphyrin from PBG	Proto IX>Copro-III[e] X-porphyrin	Not increased	624-628 nm
EPP (FECH-deficient)	Not increased	Not increased	±Proto[f]	Proto	626-634 nm[g]
EPP (XLDPP)	Not increased	Not increased	Proto	Proto, ZPP[h]	626-634 nm

[a]Slight increase only unless uroporphyrin is present.[107]
[b]Not always increased during acute attack.
[c]Other methylcarboxylate-substituted porphyrins are increased to a smaller extent; uroporphyrin is a mixture of type I and III isomers; heptacarboxylate porphyrin is mainly type III.
[d]PBG and ALA may be normal when only skin lesions are present.
[e]Coproporphyrin-III/I ratio may be increased, but increase is usually less than in overt HCP.[107]
[f]Not increased in about 40% of patients.
[g]Protoporphyrin bound to globin (if hemolysis is seen in the sample) has a peak at 626 to 628 nm.
[h]Zn-protoporphyrin 20 to 60% of total protoporphyrin.

patterns, apart from some forms of porphyria cutanea tarda (PCT) and rare erythropoietic porphyrias associated with malignant myeloid disorders. Each type of porphyria is defined by the association of characteristic clinical features with a specific pattern of accumulation of heme precursors that reflects increased formation of the substrate of the enzyme that is partially deficient or becomes secondarily rate-limiting in that type of porphyria (Table 33-5). Defects that cause porphyria have been identified in all enzymes of the pathway except for ALAS1. Mutations that decrease ALAS2 activity cause nonsyndromic X-linked sideroblastic anemia[13]; those that increase activity cause an X-linked erythropoietic protoporphyria.[129]

The porphyrias are characterized clinically by two main features: skin lesions on sun-exposed areas and acute neurovisceral attacks, typically comprising (1) abdominal pain, (2) peripheral neuropathy, and (3) mental disturbance. The skin lesions are caused by porphyrin-catalyzed photodamage, of which singlet oxygen is the main mediator.[100] Acute attacks are associated with increased formation of ALA from induced activity of hepatic ALAS1 and partial hepatic heme deficiency, often in response to induction of hepatic CYPs by drugs and other factors. The relationship of these biochemical changes to the neuronal dysfunction that underlines all clinical features of the acute attack is uncertain.[76,87] The observation that correction of the metabolic defect in the liver by transplantation is curative[113] and that domino transfer of the affected organ to an unaffected recipient causes acute attacks indistinguishable from those suffered by the donor,[113a] suggests that their primary cause is release of a neurotoxin(s), probably ALA,[36] formed in the liver.

In Table 33-4, the porphyrias are classified as acute, in which acute neurovisceral attacks occur, or nonacute. Porphyrias also are classified as hepatic or erythropoietic, according to the main site of overproduction of heme precursors. The main hepatic porphyrias are (1) acute intermittent porphyria (AIP), (2) hereditary coproporphyria (HCP), (3) variegate porphyria (VP), and (4) PCT. Erythropoietic porphyrias include congenital erythropoietic porphyria (CEP) and erythropoietic protoporphyria (EPP). Porphyrias also may be classified as cutaneous or acute porphyrias; however, it should be noted that even with these classifications, some porphyrias are difficult to place.

Acute Porphyrias

The acute porphyrias include (1) ALA dehydratase deficiency porphyria (ADP), (2) AIP, (3) VP, and (4) HCP. These disorders are autosomal dominant except for the very rare disorder, ADP, which is autosomal recessive.

Biochemistry and Molecular Genetics

The inherited defect in each of the autosomal dominant acute porphyrias (see Table 33-4) is a mutation leading to complete or near complete inactivation of one of the pairs of allelic genes that encode the enzyme whose partial deficiency causes the disorder. Enzyme activities are therefore half of normal in all tissues in which they are expressed, reflecting the activity of the normal gene *trans* to the mutant allele. Heme supply is maintained at normal or near normal concentrations by upregulation of ALAS1, with a consequent increase in the substrate concentration for the defective enzyme. These compensatory changes vary between tissues; they are most prominent in the liver and are undetectable in most other organs and between individuals. Thus in all autosomal dominant acute porphyrias, some individuals show no evidence of overproduction of heme precursors, and others have biochemically manifest disease with or without clinical symptoms.

Low clinical penetrance (the frequency of expression of an allele when it is present in the genotype) is a prominent feature of all the autosomal dominant acute porphyrias.[3,102] Family studies indicate that many affected individuals are asymptomatic throughout life. Surveys of blood donors suggest that the AIP gene may be present in as many as 1 in 1675 of the population.[90] For all three disorders, the gene frequency is sufficiently high for rare "homozygous" variants of AIP, HCP, or VP to occur in individuals who are homozygotes or compound heterozygotes for disease-specific mutations,[32,71] and for the same person to have two separate types of porphyria. About 25% of patients with overt acute porphyria have no family history of the disease. Such sporadic presentation is a reflection of the high prevalence and low penetrance of mutations in the population; acute porphyria caused by de novo mutation is uncommon.

All the autosomal dominant acute porphyrias show extensive allelic heterogeneity. More than 340 disease-specific mutations have been identified in the *HMBS* gene in AIP, about 50 in the *CPOX* gene in HCP, and more than 150 in the *PPOX* gene in VP (Human Gene Mutation Database: www.hgmd.org). About 3% of families with AIP have *HMBS* mutations that only impair expression of the ubiquitous isoform and therefore do not decrease activity in erythroid cells. All other mutations in the autosomal dominant acute porphyrias affect all tissues. Most are restricted to one or a few families, but founder mutations are present in some populations and explain the high frequency of VP in South Africans of Dutch descent and of AIP in Sweden.[56,72]

Unlike the other acute porphyrias, ADP is an autosomal recessive disorder. Patients are compound heterozygotes or homozygotes for a range of mutations in the *ALAD* gene.[29] The prevalence of heterozygous carriers may be as high as 2% in some populations.[79]

Clinical Features

The life-threatening, acute neurovisceral attacks that occur in AIP, VP, and HCP are clinically identical.[3,102] Acute attacks are more common in women, usually occurring first between the ages of 15 and 40, and are very rare before puberty. The main clinical features are summarized in Table 33-6. The clinical features of ADP, which has been reported in only six patients, are similar but may start in childhood.[79,102]

TABLE 33-6 Clinical Features of an Acute Neurovisceral Attack of Porphyria

Symptom/Sign	Percent of Acute Attacks
Abdominal pain	97
Nonabdominal pain	25
Vomiting	85
Constipation	46
Psychologic symptoms	8
Convulsions	5
Muscle weakness	8
Sensory loss	2
Hypertension (diastolic >85 mm Hg)	64
Tachycardia (>80/min)	65
Hyponatremia (<135 nmol/L)	37

Data from Elder GH, Hift RJ. Treatment of acute porphyria. Hosp Med 2001;62:422-8.

Acute attacks almost always start with abdominal pain that rapidly becomes very severe but is not accompanied by other signs of an acute surgical condition.[55,97] Pain may also be present in the back and thighs and may occasionally be most severe in these regions. Signs of autonomic neuropathy, such as vomiting, constipation, tachycardia, and hypertension, are frequent. When convulsions occur, they may be caused by hyponatremia. Pain may dissipate within a few days, but in severe cases a predominant motor neuropathy develops that may progress to flaccid quadriparesis.[97] Persistent pain and vomiting may lead to weight loss and malnutrition. The acute phase may be accompanied by mental confusion with abrupt changes in mood, hallucinations, and other psychotic features. However, these mental disturbances disappear with remission. Persistent psychiatric illness is not a feature of the acute porphyrias, although mild anxiety or depression may be present in some patients.[88] Abdominal pain usually resolves within 2 weeks, but recovery from neuropathy may take many months and is not always complete. Most patients have one or a few attacks followed by complete recovery and prolonged remission. About 5% have repeated acute attacks, which in women may be premenstrual.

Precipitating factors have been identified in about two thirds of patients who present with acute attacks. The most important are (1) drugs; (2) alcohol, especially binge drinking; (3) the menstrual cycle; (4) calorie restriction; (5) infection; and (6) stress. Acute attacks may complicate a small proportion of pregnancies in affected patients. Drugs are frequent precipitants of acute attacks in VP, and hormonal factors appear more important in AIP.[55] Drugs known to provoke acute attacks include barbiturates, sulfonamides, progestogens, and some anticonvulsants, but many others have been implicated in the precipitation of acute attacks (http://www.drugs-porphyria.org).

Skin lesions similar to those of PCT and other bullous porphyrias are present in about 80% of patients with clinically manifest VP (see Table 33-4). About 60% of patients with this condition present with skin lesions alone. The skin is less commonly affected in HCP; skin lesions without an acute attack are uncommon and usually are provoked by intercurrent cholestasis.

Long-term complications of acute porphyria include chronic renal failure, hypertension, and primary hepatocellular carcinoma.[3,102]

Treatment

As soon as an attack of acute porphyria is suspected as the cause of illness, drugs and other potential provoking agents should be withdrawn and supportive treatment started using drugs that are known to be safe.[34,55,102] Opiates are usually required to control pain. Addition of chlorpromazine or promazine may help to reduce the requirement for analgesics. Patients are prone to severe hyponatremia, and careful administration of any intravenous fluids, with avoidance of hypotonic solutions, is essential. If hyponatremia develops, it should be corrected slowly because patients with acute porphyria are particularly susceptible to cerebral edema and osmotic demyelination. Adequate caloric intake must be maintained, preferably by giving carbohydrate-rich supplements orally or if necessary via a nasogastric tube. When vomiting prevents enteral administration, 100 g of dextrose per day given intravenously as a 5% solution in normal saline should suffice.

Unless the attack is mild and is clearly resolving, specific treatment with intravenous heme should be started as soon as the diagnosis has been established.[34,55,102] This treatment increases the concentration of heme in the liver, thus decreasing the activity of ALAS1 and the formation of ALA and PBG. The effect of treatment may be monitored by measuring these metabolites, but this is not essential because clinical improvement is the required end point. Heme administration will not reverse an established neuropathy. If heme preparations are not available, hepatic ALA synthase activity can be decreased by carbohydrate loading,[14] but this treatment is less effective than intravenous heme and is more difficult to administer.

Repeated attacks are difficult to control. Cyclic premenstrual attacks in women may be prevented by suppression of ovulation with gonadorelin analogs, but many patients require repeated courses of intravenous heme.[3,34,102] Orthotopic liver transplantation leads to immediate and prolonged remission with restoration of PBG excretion to normal.[113]

Management of Families

Diagnosis of autosomal dominant acute porphyria should be followed by investigation of the patient's family to identify affected, often asymptomatic, relatives, so that they can be advised to avoid drugs and other factors known to provoke potentially fatal acute attacks (http://www.drugs-porphyria.org). Presymptomatic diagnosis also has the benefit that specific treatment can be started promptly if an attack does develop without delay while a diagnosis is sought. Although attacks are very rare before puberty, children should be tested at as young an age as is practicable to ensure that their status is known by the time they reach puberty and to enable the very low risk for affected children to be further reduced. Counseling to reduce the risk of an acute attack should include comprehensive information about the disease, including specific advice to guide selection of safe drugs, and provision of jewelry or some other means to identify the individual as having an acute porphyria. Where available, patients should be made aware of the relevant national patient support group.

Nonacute Porphyrias

The nonacute porphyrias include PCT, CEP, and EPP.

Porphyria Cutanea Tarda

PCT is by far the most common porphyria.[31] The annual incidence of new cases in the United Kingdom is between 2 and 5 per million of the population. The disease occurs at all ages in both sexes with onset usually during the fifth and sixth decades.

Clinical Features

Lesions on sun-exposed skin, particularly the backs of the hands, the forearm, and the face, are present in all patients. These lesions are identical to those seen in the other bullous porphyrias (see Table 33-4). Increased mechanical fragility of the skin, with trivial trauma leading to erosions, is present in virtually all patients. Subepidermal bullae, milia, hypertrichosis of the face, and patchy pigmentation are also common.

Erosions and bullae heal slowly to leave atrophic scars, milia, and depigmented areas. Patchy or diffuse sclerodermatous changes are less common and, unlike the other skin lesions, may affect areas of the trunk that are not exposed to sun.

Skin lesions are often the first sign of underlying liver cell damage. Clinically, overt liver disease is uncommon, but minor alterations in biochemical tests of liver function are present in more than 50% of patients. Needle biopsy of the liver reveals hepatic siderosis in most patients, usually accompanied by minor histopathologic abnormalities such as mild fatty infiltration, focal necrosis of hepatocytes, and inflammation of portal tracts. Cirrhosis is present in less than 15% of patients, but carries a high risk of hepatocellular carcinoma.

This combination of skin lesions with liver damage is strongly associated with alcohol abuse, estrogens, infection with hepatotropic viruses, particularly hepatitis C (HCV), and mutations in the hemochromatosis *(HFE)* gene.[15,30,31] PCT may complicate HIV infection.[30] Hepatic iron overload and at least one of the other associated factors are present in almost all patients. Between 8% and 79% of patients have antibodies to HCV, with prevalence highest in the United States and southern Europe and lowest in Western Europe. About 20% of patients of Northern European descent are homozygous for the C282Y mutation in the *HFE* gene, but in spite of having the genotype of genetic hemochromatosis, very few patients have clinical signs or symptoms of iron overload. However, increased serum ferritin concentrations and other biochemical indicators of iron overload are common in PCT irrespective of the HFE genotype, suggesting that the origin of hepatic iron overload is multifactorial. PCT may occur in association with other disorders, notably chronic renal failure, systemic lupus erythematosus, and hematologic malignancies. In addition, rare cases of a PCT-like syndrome resulting from production of porphyrins by primary hepatic tumors have been described.[91]

Pathogenesis and Molecular Genetics

PCT results from a decrease in activity of UROD in the liver, which leads to overproduction of uroporphyrin and other carboxymethyl-substituted porphyrinogens. These autooxidize to porphyrins, which accumulate in the liver and skin, where they act as photosensitizers and are excreted in urine and bile. Two main types of PCT can be identified by measurement of UROD activity in liver and extrahepatic tissue, and by analysis of the *UROD* gene. About 80% of patients have the sporadic (type I) form of PCT, in which the enzyme defect is restricted to the liver and the *UROD* gene appears to be normal. Typically, no family history of PCT is reported, but rare cases are clustered in families (type III PCT). The rest have familial (type II) PCT. In this form, mutation of one *UROD* gene leads to half-normal UROD activity in all tissues, which is inherited in an autosomal dominant manner. As with the other autosomal dominant porphyrias, clinical penetration of familial PCT is low with considerable allelic heterogeneity; each of the more than 85 mutations is described as present in only one or a few families, except in Norway, where the high prevalence of PCT has been attributed to a founder effect.[1] A rare variant of familial PCT, hepatoerythropoietic porphyria (HEP), in which *UROD* mutations, some of which have also been found in familial PCT, are present on both alleles, has been described.[31,32] PCT may also be caused by exposure to certain polyhalogenated aromatic hydrocarbons, such as hexachlorobenzene and 2,3,7,8-tetrachlorodibenzo-*p*-dioxin.[31]

In families with familial PCT, a decrease of 50% in enzyme activity is not by itself sufficient to cause clinically overt disease. Further inactivation of UROD in the liver seems to be required, and the process responsible for this inactivation appears also to be responsible for inactivation of hepatic UROD in sporadic PCT and in toxic PCT caused by chemicals. The inactivation process decreases catalytic activity without impairing enzyme concentration, is iron dependent, and is reversible. Current evidence from experimental models of PCT suggests that UROD is inactivated by a porphomethene inhibitor that is produced by iron-dependent oxidation of a substrate of the UROD reaction, possibly mediated by hepatic CYPs, particularly CYP1A2.[93]

Treatment

In addition to protection of the skin from sunlight, two specific treatments may be used for PCT: depletion of hepatic iron stores by repeated phlebotomy or other means, and low-dose oral chloroquine.[110] In patients with chronic renal failure and PCT, hepatic iron stores can be decreased by erythropoietin with or without phlebotomy.

Congenital Erythropoietic Porphyria

CEP is the least common but most severe of the cutaneous porphyrias.[38,121] The prevalence is less than one per million in the United Kingdom. This disorder is also known as Günther disease.

Clinical Features

The clinical features vary in severity from hydrops fetalis with death in utero—through onset in infancy of severe skin lesions with transfusion-dependent hemolytic anemia—to mild skin lesions, resembling PCT, that do not start until adult life. Late-onset cases may also develop in association with hematologic malignancy, particularly myelodysplasia.[65]

Most patients present in early infancy. Blisters on skin exposed to the sun or other sources of ultraviolet A (UVA) and near visible radiation and reddish-brown staining of diapers by urinary porphyrins are common early signs. The skin lesions resemble those of PCT but are more severe and persistent throughout life. With age, progressive scarring, particularly if erosions become infected, and atrophic changes lead to photomutilation with erosions of the terminal phalanges; destruction of ears, nose, and eyelids; and alopecia. Accumulation of porphyrin in bone is visible as erythrodontia—brownish-red teeth that fluoresce in UVA light. The skin changes are usually accompanied by hemolytic anemia and splenomegaly. Hemolysis may be fully compensated or mild, but in some patients, anemia is severe enough to require repeated transfusion.

Molecular Pathology

CEP is an autosomal recessive disease. Patients are homoallelic or heteroallelic for mutations in the *UROS* gene or, rarely, the *GATA1* gene, that decrease UROS activity (see Table 33-2).[27,94] Decreased UROS activity leads to massive overproduction of uroporphyrinogen-I and other isomer-I series of porphyrins, mainly in the bone marrow. Porphyrins accumulate in erythroid cells and are released into the plasma as these cells die. Most patients are heteroallelic unless their parents are consanguineous. More than 30 separate mutations have been identified, with C73R being the most common.[27,121] Some correlation has been noted between genotype and severity of disease.[27,40] Patients who are homozygous for C73R have particularly severe disease; in compound heterozygotes, the effect of C73R is modified by the nature of the mutation on the other allele.

Treatment

Protection against sunlight and prevention of skin infection are essential. Sunscreen ointments may occasionally provide some benefit, but physical avoidance of UVA radiation is usually necessary. Blood hypertransfusion, hydroxyurea and intravenous heme have been used to suppress erythropoiesis and porphyrin formation, oral activated charcoal to decrease the enterohepatic circulation of porphyrin, and antioxidant preparations to ameliorate the effects of porphyrin accumulation, but none has been shown to have a reliable long-term effect.[27,38,121] Hemolytic anemia may require repeated transfusion and infusion of deferoxamine or other procedures to prevent iron overload.

At present the only curative treatment is allogeneic bone marrow transplantation. Family donors are usually screened for *UROS* mutations, although the current evidence indicates that transplantation using a heterozygous carrier is effective. Gene therapy by introduction of a normal *UROS* gene into the patient's hematopoietic stem cells remains under development.[104]

Erythropoietic Protoporphyria

EPP is characterized by life-long acute photosensitivity caused by accumulation of protoporphyrin-IX in the skin.[20,120] The absence of fragile skin, subepidermal bullae, and hypertrichosis distinguish it clinically from all other cutaneous porphyrias.

Clinical Features

Patients present with acute photosensitivity. Symptoms normally start between birth and the age of 6 years, with median age of onset at 1 year, and both sexes are equally affected.[58] When a child within an EPP family reaches the age of 14, the risk of developing acute photosensitivity becomes very low. Onset after the age of 40 years is very rare; most cases are associated with myelodysplasia and are caused by acquired somatic mutation of *FECH*.[46] Diagnosis is often delayed; the median age at diagnosis was 12 years in one series.[58]

Exposure to sun is followed, usually within 5 to 30 minutes, by an intensely painful, burning, prickling, itching sensation in the skin, most frequently on the face and the backs of the hands. Symptoms persist for several hours or occasionally for days and are not relieved by shielding the skin from light. Patients characteristically seek relief by plunging their hands into water or covering their skin with wet towels. Young children may become very distressed by the pain. The skin may appear normal throughout, although there is often erythema, which may be followed by edematous swelling with crusting. These changes usually subside within a few hours, so that by the time the child reaches the physician, nothing remains to be seen, and the episode may be dismissed as severe sunburn. Subsequent exposure to sunlight provokes a similar reaction. Recurrent episodes lead to chronic skin changes that often are minor and difficult to detect. Typical lesions are shallow linear scars over the bridge of the nose and elsewhere on the face; the skin may become thickened and waxy, especially over the knuckles. Seasonal palmar keratoderma is present in about 3% of patients.[58] Symptoms tend to be more severe during spring and summer and may improve during pregnancy.

The most severe complication of EPP is progressive hepatic failure that is caused by accumulation of protoporphyrin in the liver.[4] About 20% of patients have abnormal biochemical tests of liver function, particularly increased aspartate aminotransferase, but only 2 to 5% of patients develop liver failure. EPP may also increase the risk of cholelithiasis, because the formation of gallstones is promoted by high concentrations of protoporphyrin in the bile. Erythropoiesis is impaired in all patients with a downward shift in hemoglobin concentration, so that about 50% of women and 30% of men have a mild microcytic anemia.[60] Biochemical evidence of vitamin D deficiency is present in up to 50% of patients.[117]

Molecular Pathology and Genetics

EPP is a clinical syndrome that results from increased formation of protoporphyrin mainly or exclusively in the bone marrow. The toxic effects of protoporphyrin on the skin and other tissues are directly responsible for its main clinical manifestations.[120] Accumulation of protoporphyrin in the liver is the result of failure of the liver to excrete the increased load it receives through release of protoporphyrin from erythrocytes and their immediate precursors.[4]

In most patients, overproduction of protoporphyrin results from decreased activity of FECH. FECH-deficient EPP is an autosomal recessive disease. In most families, photosensitive individuals are compound heterozygotes for a *FECH* mutation that abolishes or severely decreases FECH activity and a hypomorphic *FECH* IVS3-48C allele.[33,48,128] This allele is a polymorphic *FECH* variant that shows marked variation in frequency between populations, ranging from less than 1% in West Africans through around 10% in Western Europeans to 45% in Japanese. Substitution of a T nucleotide by a C nucleotide at a polymorphic site in intron 3 (IVS3-48C/T) enhances use of an alternative splice site, leading to increased formation of an unstable, untranslated mRNA and reduction of *FECH* expression by about 30%.[48] Together, these two functional defects decrease FECH activity to below the threshold of about 35% of normal at which protoporphyrin accumulation and clinical symptoms occur. In populations where the hypomorphic allele is common, EPP families show pseudodominant inheritance. In about 4% of families with FECH-deficient EPP, clinically affected individuals are heteroallelic or homoallelic for *FECH* mutations and tend to have lower enzyme activities than those in whom an *FECH* mutation is *trans* to the IVS3-48C allele.[33] To date, all patients with seasonal palmar keratoderma have been found to have this form of EPP.[59] FECH-deficient EPP may show less allelic heterogeneity than other porphyrias,[128] but most mutations in *FECH* are restricted to one or a few families; more than 130 have been identified.

In about 2% of families with protoporphyria, overproduction of protoporphyrin is caused by gain-of-function mutations in *ALAS2* [X-linked dominant protoporphyria (XLDPP)], which lead to formation of protoporphyrin in excess of the amount required for hemoglobinization.[129] XLDPP is inherited in an X-linked pattern with expression of disease in males and most females. The risk of liver disease is substantially greater in XLDPP and in patients with dysfunctional *FECH* variants on both alleles, particularly those without palmar keratoderma, than in compound heterozygotes for the hypomorphic allele.[33] Among patients with *FECH* mutations *trans* to a IVS3-48C allele, some evidence suggests an association between null mutations and severe liver disease, but this association is too weak to be of any practical use.[33]

Treatment

Acute photosensitivity has been controlled by avoidance of sunlight, suitable clothing, and reflectant sunscreens, if these are cosmetically acceptable. Some patients are helped by production of a photoprotectant tan by measures such as narrowband ultraviolet B (UVB) phototherapy or dihydroxyacetone ointment.[89,120] Oral β-carotene, which acts as a singlet oxygen quencher, may be effective in some patients, but little support for its use has been gained from clinical trials.[89] Doses should be sufficient to maintain a plasma concentration of 6 to 8 μg/L.[120] Patients should be monitored for vitamin D deficiency.[117]

At present, no reliable method is known for predicting liver failure in EPP. All patients should have at least annual biochemical tests of liver function. Persistent abnormalities should be investigated by liver biopsy and further treatment considered if even mild hepatocellular necrosis and fibrosis are present.[4] Once liver failure becomes irreversible, orthotopic liver transplantation is the only treatment, but protoporphyrin may reaccumulate in the transplanted liver.[4] Reaccumulation can be prevented by bone marrow transplantation.[123]

Abnormalities of Porphyrin Metabolism Not Caused by Porphyria

Abnormalities of porphyrin metabolism may occur in a number of diseases other than the porphyrias. These disorders are more often the cause of abnormal porphyrin metabolism than porphyria and need to be considered when data from patients in whom porphyria is suspected are interpreted.[54,83]

Lead and Other Heavy Metals

Lead exposure increases urinary ALA and coproporphyrin-III excretion and causes accumulation of Zn-protoporphyrin in erythrocytes. The definitive test for lead toxicity is measurement of blood lead, but occasionally lead exposure is responsible for porphyria-like symptoms and may be an unexpected finding when patients are evaluated for suspected porphyria.[63] Increased ALA excretion occurs secondary to inhibition of ALAD caused by lead displacing zinc at its catalytic center. Two isoenzymes (ALAD1 and ALAD2) are produced from the *ALAD* gene by alternative splicing activated by two nontranslated codominant alleles 1 and 2.[62] The ALAD2 isoenzyme is more electronegatively charged than ALAD1, so that its affinity for lead is higher.[126] As a consequence, individuals with the ALAD2 genotype are more susceptible to lead toxicity.[116] In addition, individuals who are heterozygous for ALAD deficiency appear to be at increased risk from lead exposure.

Lead also causes increased excretion of coproporphyrin-III in urine. *CPOX* requires sulfhydryl groups for activity and so is potentially a target for inhibition by lead. Increased concentrations of red cell zinc-protoporphyrin (ZPP) associated with lead exposure are probably not caused by inhibition of *FECH* because inhibition of this enzyme requires higher lead concentrations than those usually encountered following lead exposure. Lead exposure may lead to an intramitochondrial deficiency of ferrous iron, so that zinc replaces iron as a substrate for *FECH*.[108] Once formed, erythrocyte ZPP remains elevated for the life of the red cell. Because the half-life of an erythrocyte is longer than that of blood lead, monitoring of lead workers requires both whole-blood lead and ZPP testing. ZPP measurement also has the advantage that no interference from lead contamination occurs via the skin when the blood sample is collected, especially if a fingerprick sample is used. Coproporphyrinuria has also been reported following exposure to arsenic and other heavy metals.[54]

Secondary Coproporphyrinuria: Hepatobiliary and Other Disorders

Coproporphyrinuria secondary to excess alcohol intake, liver dysfunction, or drugs is by far the commonest abnormality of porphyrin excretion. Alcohol increases the excretion of coproporphyrin-III in normal subjects, and coproporphyrin excretion is frequently increased in chronic alcoholism.[84,111]

In cholestatic jaundice, hepatitis, and cirrhosis, impaired biliary excretion of coproporphyrin-I leads to its appearance in the urine with reversal of the normal coproporphyrin-isomer ratio so that the I isomer predominates.[54,83] Impaired biliary excretion is also probably the cause of the coproporphyrinuria that may accompany severe infections, other acute illnesses, and the administration of some drugs.

Coproporphyrinuria is also a feature of inherited forms of jaundice. In the Dubin-Johnson syndrome, overall urinary excretion of coproporphyrin is normal, but coproporphyrin-I is increased and excretion of coproporphyrin-III is reduced. In Rotor syndrome, urinary excretion of coproporphyrin-I is increased with normal coproporphyrin-III excretion, and in Gilbert disease, urinary excretion of both isomers is increased.[54]

Increased Fecal Porphyrin Concentration

The dicarboxylic porphyrin fraction of feces contains protoporphyrin and other dicarboxylic porphyrins derived from it by bacterial reduction or removal of vinyl side groups. Additional protoporphyrin and other dicarboxylic porphyrins have been formed by the action of gut flora on heme-containing proteins derived from the diet or from gastrointestinal hemorrhage.[9,106] Even minor gastrointestinal hemorrhage, particularly if it occurs high in the gut (which may not give rise to a positive occult blood test) can markedly increase the concentration of dicarboxylic porphyrins in feces. Confusion with EPP may occur when associated iron deficiency increases erythrocyte total porphyrin, and when skin lesions from some other cause are present, or with VP when coexisting liver disease causes coproporphyrinuria. Porphyria is excluded when no porphyrin fluorescence is detectable on fluorescence emission spectroscopy of plasma, and fecal coproporphyrin excretion is normal. Porphyrins may come directly from the diet, and one report described consumption of brewer's yeast, producing a fecal porphyrin profile indistinguishable from VP.[75]

Increased Plasma Porphyrin Concentration: Renal and Other Disorders

Plasma porphyrin concentrations may be increased when hepatobiliary or renal excretion of porphyrins is impaired.[24] In end-stage renal failure, concentrations are often markedly increased; clearance of porphyrins by dialysis is inefficient.[37,114] Dermatologic problems are common in patients undergoing dialysis, and skin lesions may resemble those of PCT.[43] Concentrations of porphyrins in the plasma of dialysis patients, although often much higher than normal, rarely approach those found in patients with active skin lesions caused by PCT. It seems unlikely that the skin lesions are related to the increased porphyrin concentrations. However, PCT is itself an uncommon complication of end-stage renal failure. Because such patients are often anuric, careful evaluation of plasma and fecal porphyrins is required to distinguish PCT and those acute porphyrias in which skin lesions may occur, from the dermatosis of renal failure.[45] Although plasma porphyrin concentrations are usually higher in chronic renal failure with PCT than in renal failure alone, unequivocal diagnosis of PCT in this situation may be achieved by fractionation of plasma porphyrins by high-performance liquid chromatography (HPLC) or, preferably, by fecal porphyrin analysis.[45]

Hematologic Disorders

In iron deficiency anemia, zinc acts as an alternative substrate for FECH, leading to increased erythrocyte ZPP. Increased red cell protoporphyrin (mostly ZPP) may also occur in sideroblastic, megaloblastic, and hemolytic anemias.[69,83]

Hereditary Tyrosinemia Type I

Succinylacetone, which accumulates in this disease, has a structural resemblance to ALA and is therefore a competitive inhibitor of ALAD. Consequently, its substrate ALA accumulates, and excess amounts are excreted in urine. Patients with hereditary tyrosinemia suffer neurologic crises very similar to attacks of acute porphyria, and some have been treated with heme infusions.[103]

LABORATORY DIAGNOSIS OF PORPHYRIA

Laboratory investigation is essential for identification of the porphyrias because none have clinical features that are sufficiently distinctive to allow diagnosis on clinical grounds alone. In patients with current symptoms caused by porphyria, it should always be possible to demonstrate excessive production of heme precursors. Diagnosis depends on demonstrating specific patterns of overproduction of heme precursors (see Table 33-5) and is usually straightforward, provided appropriate specimens are examined for the relevant intermediates using adequately sensitive techniques.[12,22,24,119] Acute attacks of porphyria are always associated with excess excretion of PBG, except in ADP, where only ALA is increased. Patients with cutaneous symptoms caused by porphyria always show evidence of increased accumulation or excretion of porphyrins. DNA and enzyme analyses give no information about disease activity, are rarely necessary to confirm the diagnosis in clinically overt porphyria, and are mainly of use for family studies in the autosomal dominant acute porphyrias and in EPP.

Patients With Symptoms of Porphyria

Strategies for the laboratory investigation of patients suspected on clinical grounds of having porphyria depend on the mode of presentation.

Patients With Current or Past Symptoms Consistent With an Acute Neurovisceral Attack

Strategies used when patients with acute neurovisceral symptoms that depend on the clinical setting are tested include (1) investigating the acute attack, (2) diagnosing the cause, and (3) investigating possible acute porphyria when the patient is in remission.

Investigation During a Suspected Acute Attack

The essential investigation in any patient with a suspected attack of acute porphyria is measurement of urinary PBG by an adequately sensitive and specific method.[11,24]

PBG excretion is always increased during an acute attack of AIP, HCP, or VP to a concentration that usually exceeds 10 times the upper reference limit.[61] Normal PBG excretion, at a time when symptoms are present, provides very strong evidence against any type of acute porphyria as their cause, except for the very rare ADP, in which ALA is increased. In AIP, PBG excretion usually remains elevated for weeks or even months after an attack. However, in VP or HCP, PBG may rapidly return to normal (sometimes within days) once the attack starts to resolve. Therefore, if a suspected attack is entering remission, or if clinical suspicion of acute porphyria persists, analysis of fecal and plasma porphyrins, with measurement of ALA if these are normal, is advisable, even if PBG excretion is normal. Increased urinary PBG requires careful evaluation, because although the patient clearly has an acute porphyria, the disease may not be the cause of current symptoms. Some patients with AIP have very high rates of PBG excretion in the absence of symptoms, and poor correlation has been noted between urinary PBG and symptoms, with no "threshold" above which symptoms appear. PBG excretion increases during an acute attack, but detection of this change requires information about the patient's baseline excretion. Even though a high urinary PBG excretion increases the likelihood that porphyria is responsible for symptoms, the final diagnosis must always be made on clinical grounds.

If increased urinary PBG is found by a qualitative and/or semiquantitative screening test, confirmation by a specific, quantitative method, preferably using the same urine sample, is essential to exclude possible false positives.

Testing for ALA is often performed along with testing for PBG. Both are typically elevated in the autosomal dominant acute porphyrias, although ALA is increased to a lesser extent.[61,102] Measurement of ALA allows lead poisoning and ADP to be detected, but the risk of missing these conditions is very low if total urinary porphyrin is measured in addition to PBG. In addition, measurement of ALA is more susceptible to interference.[66]

Measurement of urinary total porphyrin should not be used to screen for acute porphyria. False positives due to secondary coproporphyrinuria are common,[98] and although in vitro polymerization of PBG to uroporphyrin usually increases the urinary porphyrin concentration when excess PBG is present, false negatives may occur.

Failure to correctly diagnose an attack of acute porphyria not only delays appropriate life-saving treatment but may cause the patient to be subjected to the risk of unnecessary surgery or administration of drugs that may further aggravate the attack with potentially fatal consequences. Alternatively, a false diagnosis of porphyria may be just as serious because of delayed vital surgery or other treatment, and may also lead to analgesic (including opiate) misuse and dependency.

Differentiation Between the Acute Porphyrias

Management of the attack is the same regardless of the type of porphyria, so further investigation is not a matter of urgency. However, differentiation between the acute porphyrias is essential for the selection of appropriate tests for use in family studies; the absence of skin lesions does not exclude VP or HCP (see Table 33-4).

Once the diagnosis of acute porphyria has been established by demonstration of an unequivocal increase in urinary PBG excretion, various strategies have been developed for distinguishing the different types of acute porphyria.[12,22,119,130] One approach involves the combined use of fluorescence emission spectroscopy of plasma and fecal porphyrin analysis. The presence of a plasma fluorescence emission peak around 626 nm confirms VP (see Table 33-5).[53] This investigation is always abnormal in VP when symptoms are present. Although excretion of fecal protoporphyrin (and other dicarboxylate porphyrins) and, to a lesser extent, coproporphyrin-III is increased in VP, fecal porphyrin analysis is not essential for the diagnosis of this condition, unless plasma fluorescence scanning is unavailable (see Table 33-5), but it does provide additional confirmation of the diagnosis if this is required. In AIP and HCP, the plasma fluorescence scan may be normal or may show a peak around 620 nm. These two disorders can readily be distinguished by fecal porphyrin analysis. In AIP, the total fecal porphyrin concentration is often normal, whereas it is increased in HCP. However, total fecal porphyrin is increased in some patients with AIP, particularly if a method that extracts uroporphyrin in addition to ether-soluble porphyrins is used.[107] If total fecal porphyrin is raised, porphyrins should be fractionated by an HPLC technique, preferably one capable of resolving coproporphyrin isomers.[74] In HCP, coproporphyrin-III and the coproporphyrin isomer-III/I ratio are elevated, and protoporphyrin-IX is minimally raised or normal. In AIP, coproporphyrin-III excretion and the isomer ratio are normal (see Table 33-5).[130] Analysis of urinary porphyrins is unhelpful for differentiating between the acute porphyrias.

Enzyme measurements are not required for diagnosis of the acute porphyrias, except in patients with atypical presentations that suggest the possibility of a homozygous variant. Enzyme assay of red cell for *HMBS* activity is not sensitive enough and lacks specificity for the diagnosis of AIP.[61,130] Activities in patients with AIP may overlap those in normal subjects, particularly if the patient is acutely ill, and are normal in the 3% of patients with mutations that affect only the ubiquitous isoform. Assays of leukocyte coproporphyrinogen oxidase or protoporphyrinogen oxidase (the enzymes deficient in HCP and VP, respectively) are technically difficult and are not essential for diagnosis.

Investigation of an Asymptomatic Patient With Past Symptoms Consistent With an Acute Attack

Diagnosis may be less straightforward when a patient presents for investigation after all clinical symptoms have resolved. Again, the essential initial investigation consists of measurement of urinary PBG by a specific quantitative method; screening tests are too insensitive for this purpose. If PBG excretion is increased, the type of porphyria is identified, as described previously. When PBG excretion is normal, further investigation is required, including measurement of urinary ALA. Excretion of urinary PBG and ALA is within the reference interval in about 20% of AIP patients during clinical remission.[61] In VP and HCP, excretion of PBG and ALA is usually normal in the absence of symptoms, but the plasma fluorescence scan in VP and the fecal coproporphyrin-isomer ratio in HCP remain abnormal for years after the onset of full clinical remission.[42,53] If all these tests are normal, ADP is excluded and the likelihood of VP or HCP is very low; mutational analysis of the *CPOX* and *PPOX* genes is indicated only if clinical suspicion remains high. Therefore, the patient is likely to have AIP in remission or to have had a nonporphyric illness with symptoms mimicking those of acute porphyria. Mutational analysis of *HMBS*, supplemented by assay of HMBS activity in mutation-negative patients, helps to distinguish these possibilities.[130]

Patients With Cutaneous Symptoms

Skin lesions of cutaneous porphyrias are always accompanied by overproduction of porphyrins.

Patients With Acute Photosensitivity Without Skin Fragility or Bullae

Often, patients in this group will be children and will have EPP or acute photosensitivity caused by a disorder other than porphyria. For suspected EPP, the essential investigation consists of measurement of erythrocyte porphyrin concentration using a sensitive fluorometric method. Screening tests using solvent extraction of blood or fluorescence microscopy of erythrocytes are unreliable. If the erythrocyte porphyrin concentration is within the reference interval, EPP is excluded. If the concentration is increased, it is important to determine whether the increase is caused by free protoporphyrin, as in EPP, or ZPP, as in iron deficiency and lead toxicity. This requires extraction with a neutral solvent, such as ethanol[39] or acetone,[52] to prevent the demetalation caused by strong acids, followed by fluorescence spectroscopy or HPLC to distinguish free protoporphyrin from ZPP (fluorescence emission maxima 630 nm and 587 nm, respectively).

In FECH-deficient EPP, ZPP is typically less than 15% of the total erythrocyte porphyrin. The combination of a markedly increased total porphyrin with more than 15% of ZPP suggests XLDPP.[129] The plasma porphyrin concentration is increased in all forms of EPP (see Table 33-5), but not in lead poisoning, iron deficiency, or other anemias associated with an increased total erythrocyte porphyrin concentration. Thus, plasma fluorescence scanning is a useful additional investigation, particularly in the uncommon patients with EPP in whom erythrocyte porphyrin concentrations are only marginally increased. Measurement of fecal protoporphyrin is not essential for the diagnosis of EPP (see Table 33-5) and should never be used as the primary diagnostic investigation. DNA analysis is required to confirm the diagnosis of XLDPP in patients with an increased percentage of ZPP. It is also the most reliable way to identify patients who have dysfunctional *FECH* variants, other than IVS3-48C, on both alleles, and who may therefore have an increased risk of developing liver disease. Assay of FECH activity in lymphocytes has also been used for this purpose.[48]

Once the diagnosis of EPP has been established, all patients should be investigated for the presence of protoporphyric liver disease using biochemical tests of liver function. Persistently increased serum aminotransferase activities indicate the need for further investigation. Patients in whom these tests are normal or only minimally altered should be monitored by regular testing at least annually.

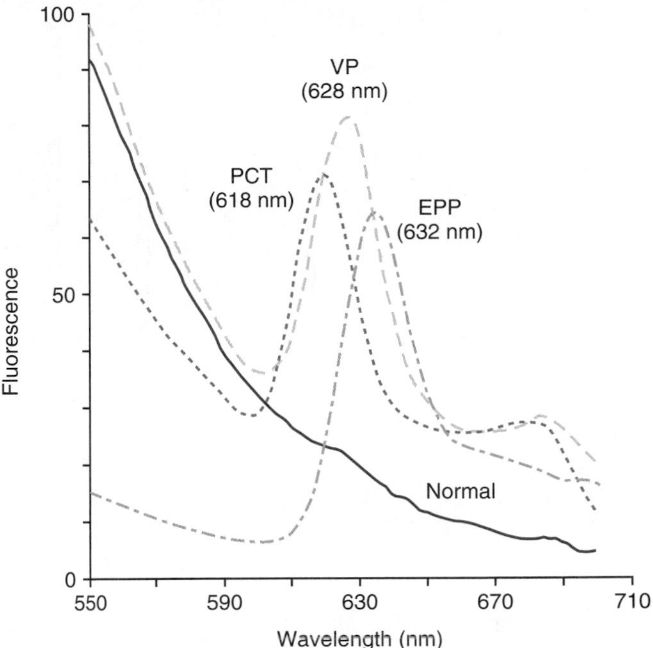

Figure 33-3 Fluorescence emission spectra (excitation, 405 nm) of dilutions in phosphate-buffered saline (PBS) of plasma from a normal individual and from patients with various porphyrias.

Patients With Bullae/Fragility/Scarring

Clinically indistinguishable skin lesions occur in PCT, VP, HCP, CEP (see Table 33-4), HEP, and other rare variants.[32] In addition, identical skin lesions characterize the pseudoporphyria caused by some drugs and the use of sunbeds, in which porphyrin metabolism is normal.[54] Initial investigations should include measurement of total urinary porphyrins and fluorescence emission spectroscopy of plasma.[24,42] If the latter is unavailable, fecal porphyrins should be analyzed. Most patients will have PCT or VP. A plasma emission peak around 626 nm identifies VP (see Table 33-5; Figure 33-3) and no further investigations are necessary. An emission peak at around 618 to 620 nm usually indicates PCT but is not specific for this disorder (see Table 33-5 and Figure 33-3). It is possible to differentiate PCT from other bullous porphyrias, apart from HEP, by fractionation of urinary or fecal porphyrins, using HPLC or other techniques that identify individual porphyrins (Figure 33-4). Confirmation of the diagnosis of CEP requires fractionation of urinary and fecal porphyrins, preferably using a technique that separates porphyrin isomers and measurement of erythrocyte porphyrins. Identification of *UROS* mutations may help in assessment of prognosis. PCT in young children needs to be distinguished from HEP by measurement of erythrocyte porphyrins and UROD activity and by mutational analysis of *UROD*. Suspected homozygous VP and other rare cutaneous porphyrias similarly require intensive investigation.

A normal plasma fluorescence scan excludes porphyria as the cause of any active skin lesions.[42] If clinical suspicion persists, total plasma and fecal porphyrins should be measured and the fecal porphyrin pattern determined. Normal findings exclude all bullous porphyrias. Patients may present for investigation after their skin lesions have healed. In PCT, excretion and plasma porphyrin concentrations return to normal during remission, with the proportions of individual porphyrins in urine and feces remaining abnormal for longer than total porphyrin concentrations. Thus, in a patient whose skin lesions have healed, and whose total urinary and fecal porphyrin concentrations are within the reference interval, determination of individual porphyrins may reveal the diagnosis. The plasma fluorescence scan in VP and fecal coproporphyrin-III excretion in HCP remain abnormal during clinical remission.

All patients with PCT should be screened for associated risk factors through testing for the C282Y mutation in the hemochromatosis *(HFE)* gene in patients of northern European descent. Although inherited deficiency of UROD is an important risk factor, determination of the type of PCT is not essential for the management of individual patients.

Asymptomatic Relatives of Patients With Porphyria

Depending on the type of porphyria, investigation of asymptomatic relatives may be beneficial.

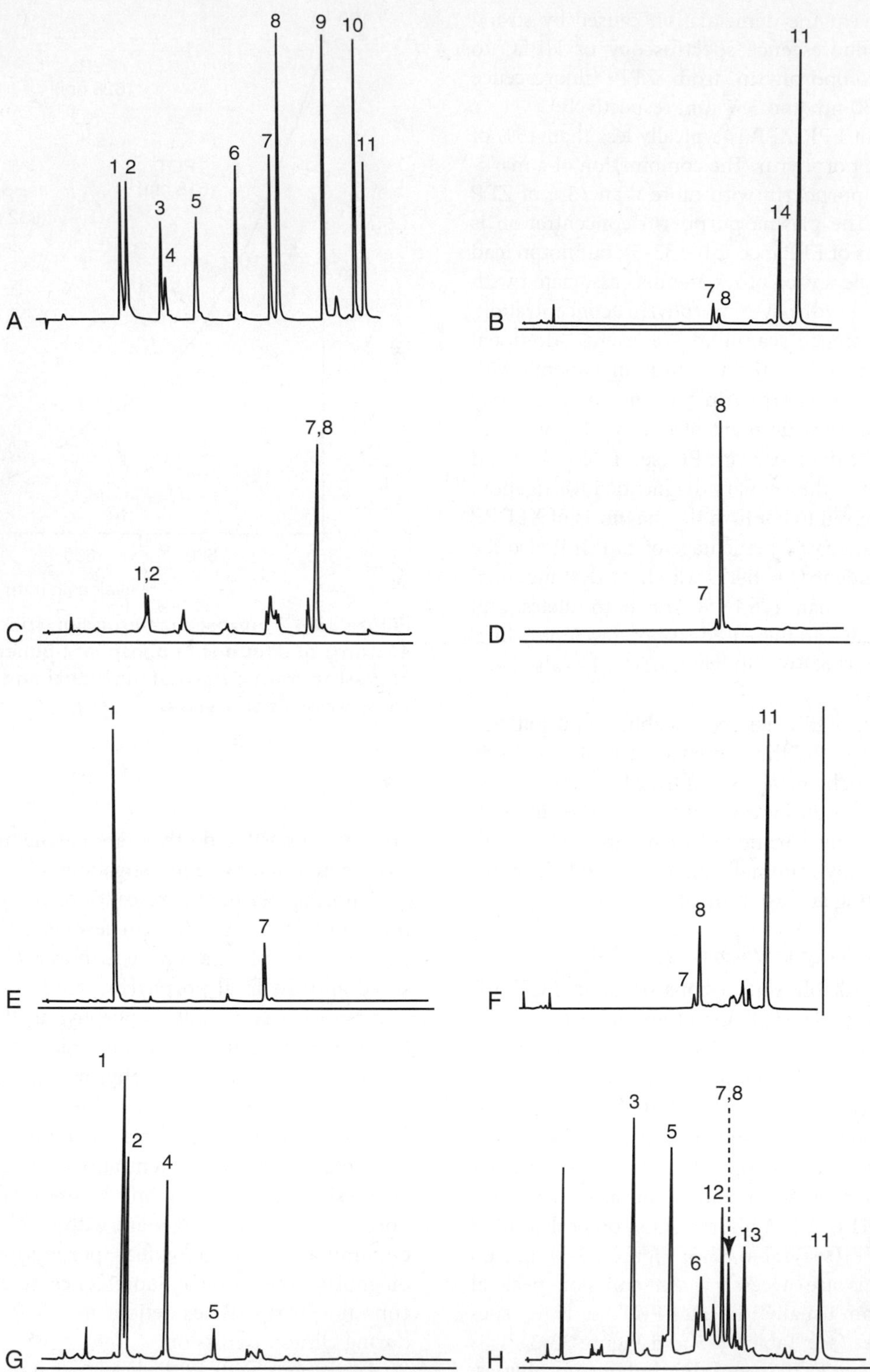

Figure 33-4 Representative high-performance liquid chromatography (HPLC) chromatograms for (A) working standard, (B) normal feces, (C) normal urine, (D) feces—hereditary coproporphyria, (E) urine—congenital erythropoietic porphyria, (F) feces—variegata porphyria, (G) urine—porphyria cutanea tarda, and (H) feces—porphyria cutanea tarda chromatographic conditions. Peaks are *(1)* uroporphyrin-I, *(2)* uroporphyrin-III, *(3)* heptacarboxylate porphyrin-I, *(4)* heptacarboxylate porphyrin-III, *(5)* hexacarboxylate porphyrin, *(6)* pentacarboxylate porphyrin, *(7)* coproporphyrin-I, *(8)* coproporphyrin-III, *(9)* deuteroporphyrin-IX, *(10)* mesoporphyrin-IX, *(11)* protoporphyrin-IX, *(12)* hydroxyisocoproporphyrin, *(13)* isocoproporphyrin, and *(14)* pemptoporphyrin-IX.

TABLE 33-7 Presymptomatic Diagnosis of Autosomal Dominant Acute Porphyrias: Metabolite Measurements in Asymptomatic Individuals With Porphyria Proven by Mutational Analysis

Porphyria	Metabolite	No. of Individuals	Sensitivity	Specificity
AIP	Urine PBG*	98†	59%	100%
HCP	Fecal copro isomer-I/III ratio‡	28§	96%	100%
VP	Plasma porphyrin fluorescence	112†	64%	100%

*Greater than 10.2 μmol/L.
†Aged 15 years or more.
‡Greater than 1.4.
§Aged 7 years or more.

Presymptomatic Diagnosis of Autosomal Dominant Acute Porphyrias

Screening of family members to identify asymptomatic individuals who have inherited AIP, VP, or HCP and therefore are at risk for acute attacks is an essential part of the management of families with these disorders. Screening may be carried out by metabolite measurement, enzyme assay, DNA analysis, or a combination of these approaches. The most sensitive metabolite assays for the presymptomatic diagnosis of each disorder are listed in Table 33-7. These tests are almost always normal before puberty, except in HCP (see Table 33-7),[2,10] and therefore are not suitable for the evaluation of children. In addition, urinary PBG excretion in AIP and the plasma fluorescence scan in VP may often be normal in asymptomatic adults shown by DNA analysis to be affected (see Table 33-7). Measurement of the activity of the defective enzyme is more sensitive, but diagnostic accuracy is limited by the overlap between activities in individuals with disease and in the normal population. Assay of erythrocyte HMBS activity has been widely used for the presymptomatic diagnosis of AIP.[61]

Mutation detection by DNA analysis is now the method of choice for family studies. It is specific and much more sensitive than biochemical methods[130] and offers the additional advantage of enabling asymptomatic disease to be excluded with certainty. In the few families in which a mutation is not identified, erythrocyte HMBS assay in AIP or gene tracking using intragenic single-nucleotide polymorphisms (SNPs) may be helpful. Gene tracking requires at least two unequivocally affected family members and certainty that the correct gene is being tracked.

EPP

In EPP caused by mutations in the *FECH* gene, testing of the unaffected parent for the presence of the hypomorphic *FECH IVS3-48C* allele is helpful in assessing the risk that a future child will have clinically overt disease; the presence of this allele increases the risk from about 1 in 100 to 1 in 4.[49] In addition, asymptomatic individuals from EPP families may wish to know whether they have inherited a severe *FECH* mutation and thus have the potential to transmit the disease. FECH assay and/or mutation identification is required for this purpose; erythrocyte protoporphyrin concentrations are rarely unequivocally abnormal in such individuals. In XLDPP, mutational analysis of the *ALAS2* gene is required to identify female carriers, not all of whom have clinically overt disease.

Other Porphyrias

Family investigation has a more limited role in the clinical management of other porphyrias. In PCT, the autosomal dominant familial form has been identified by erythrocyte UROD assay or mutational analysis, but as yet little evidence suggests that family studies are necessary unless requested by anxious relatives.[1]

In the autosomal recessive porphyrias, CEP and ADP, screening of families for asymptomatic carriers is not normally helpful, because the low carrier frequency in the general population makes the risk of transmission to the next generation very low. For severe homozygous or compound heterozygous porphyrias, such as CEP, ADP, HEP, and homozygous AIP, prenatal diagnosis may be indicated and has been reported for CEP[121] and HEP.[41]

ANALYTICAL METHODS

The analytical methods used in conjunction with porphyrias are described here briefly.

Methods for Metabolites

The metabolite methods include those for ALA; PBG; and urinary, fecal, plasma, and blood porphyrins.

Specimen Collection and Stability

For porphyrin analysis, all samples must be protected from light, as urinary porphyrin concentrations have been observed to decrease by up to 50% if kept in the light for 24 hours. Urinary porphyrins and PBG are best analyzed in fresh, random (10 to 20 mL) samples collected without preservative. Very dilute urine (creatinine <2 mmol/L) is unsuitable for analysis.

Urine often is of normal color in the nonacute porphyrias, except in CEP, when it is usually red, occasionally to such an extent that it is mistaken for hematuria. During an acute attack, urine may be a red-brown color because of the presence of uroporphyrin and other pigments formed by the nonenzymatic polymerization of PBG.

Twenty-four-hour urine collections (1) offer little advantage, (2) delay diagnosis, and (3) increase the risk of losses during the collection period. PBG and porphyrins are stable in urine in the dark at 4 °C for up to 48 hours, and for at least a month at −20 °C. Specimens for ALA estimation should be promptly refrigerated. Urine specimens have been stored at 4 °C in the dark for at least 2 weeks without significant loss of ALA,[105] and frozen specimens are stable for weeks. Whereas PBG is more stable around pH 8 to 9, ALA is more stable around pH 3 to 4, although more acidic environments notably reduce ALA stability.

About 5 to 10 g wet weight of feces is adequate for porphyrin measurements. Diagnostically, important changes in concentration are unlikely to occur within 36 hours at room temperature, and samples are stable for many months at −20 °C.

Blood, anticoagulated with ethylenediaminetetraacetic acid (EDTA), shows no loss of protoporphyrin for up to 8 days at room temperature and for at least 8 weeks at 4 °C in the dark.

External Quality Assessment

Comparison of analyses between specialist laboratories has revealed differences in analytical quality that may influence their ability to diagnose and monitor porphyria. External quality assessment (EQA) and internal quality control are therefore essential to secure acceptable analytical quality for constituents used for these purposes. EQA schemes for the more common analyses are available in some countries and may accept participants from other countries. The European Porphyria Network(EPNET) (www.europe-porphyria.org) is running a clinical EQA scheme that is open to specialist laboratories throughout the world.

Methods for Porphyrin Precursors

The water-soluble metabolites, PBG and ALA, are excreted by the kidney and usually are measured in the urine in the clinical laboratory. Both have been measured in plasma by HPLC–mass spectrometry and fluorometric enzyme assays.[22,109]

Porphobilinogen

Most methods for PBG are based on the reaction of Ehrlich's reagent (dimethylaminobenzaldehyde in acidic solution) with the α-methene carbon of the pyrrole ring to form a colored product variously described as "rose red" or "magenta," which has a characteristic absorption spectrum with a peak at 553 nm and a shoulder at 540 nm. Porphyrins do not contain any α-methene hydrogens and so do not react. Some other substances in urine may react with the reagent to give red products, notably urobilinogen, may inhibit the reaction, or are pigmented themselves and so mask the red chromogen.[22,136] All need to be removed. This is best achieved by ion-exchange chromatography (first described by Mauzerall and Granick[81]), but methods for accurate quantification of PBG based on this procedure are time-consuming.

Qualitative screening tests in which urine is reacted directly with Ehrlich's reagent and is assessed visually for the formation of red chromogen (e.g., the Watson-Schwartz[125] and Hoesch[70] tests) are convenient but have been criticized for poor detection limits and interferences, even when solvent extraction has been used to separate the PBG-Ehrlich compound from the urobilinogen-Ehrlich complex.[23,112]

The Mauzerall-Granick method has been modified in attempts to produce an alternative that is acceptable for screening purposes. Buttery and Stuart[17] avoided the use of columns by employing batch-wise treatment with resin, and visually compared the final color with that of a surrogate calibrator. Blake and colleagues[11] eliminated the centrifugation steps by using resin-filled syringes with detachable filters and compared the final color with a variety of artificial calibrators. These modifications reduced the time taken to perform the test to 10 minutes and produced a semiquantitative result. A commercial kit based on Blake's method is available (Thermo Scientific PBG Kit, Pittsburgh, Pa) and has been found to be more analytically sensitive and specific for initial screening than the qualitative solvent extraction procedures.[26] A 2002 modification used resin-filled nylon sacs instead of columns.[47]

If a qualitative or semiquantitative screening test is used, it is essential to include appropriate controls and to confirm all positive test results using a specific quantitative method. The procedure described uses commercially available ion-exchange columns, but some laboratories may prefer to prepare an ion-exchange resin themselves. PBG in the resin eluate reacts with Ehrlich's reagent to form a colored product that is scanned in a spectrometer. Reference intervals are given in Table 33-3. Scanning the spectrum of the product is essential if interferences are to be identified. Imipenem, for example, often gives a peak at 580 nm with Ehrlich's reagent.[122] The coefficient of variation at the cutoff of 9 μmol/L is approximately ±10%, but the method is less precise at lower concentrations. Urinary PBG that is raised at least two to three times the upper reference limit is diagnostic of an acute porphyria, but it is important that individual laboratories determine a cut point above which further investigation is required.

5-Aminolevulinic Acid

It is possible to measure ALA directly,[22,109] but it is more usually converted into an Ehrlich's-reacting pyrrole through condensation with a reagent such as acetylacetone after separation from PBG by two-stage anion-exchange chromatography.[81] A method for measurement of PBG and ALA, based on that of Mauzerall and Granick,[81] is available commercially (Bio-Rad Laboratories, Hercules, Calif). A photometric method has been proposed for more rapid testing.[18] Compared with PBG procedures, interferences are more common with ALA. For example, the acetylacetone derivatization step forms a compound with penicillin that reacts with Ehrlich's reagent.[66]

Analysis of Porphyrins in Urine and Feces

Methods for porphyrin fractionation are complex and time-consuming and are not available in every laboratory. Consequently, simple qualitative screening tests are often used to differentiate the majority of specimens that do not require further investigation from the few that justify fractionation of the individual porphyrins. Screening tests in which extracts of urine or feces are examined visually for typical red-pink fluorescence of porphyrins are not sensitive analytically and should not be used.[23] Methods based on spectrophotometric scanning of acidified urine or fecal extracts for the presence of the Soret band are recommended and yield semiquantitative information.[24] Quantitative fluorometric methods are also available.[11]

All methods for the fractionation of porphyrins are based on the different solubilities of individual porphyrins caused by their different β-substituents and, to a lesser extent, on the substituent order around the macrocycle. Methods include (1) differential extraction with solvents, (2) paper and thin-layer chromatography, and (3) HPLC. Solvent extraction methods should not be used because they yield only limited and sometimes misleading information.[25] Reversed-phase HPLC, the current method of choice, separates all porphyrins of clinical interest, including isomers and metal chelates, without the need for prior methylation. Spectrophotometric or fluorometric detection has been used; the latter method is more sensitive and specific.

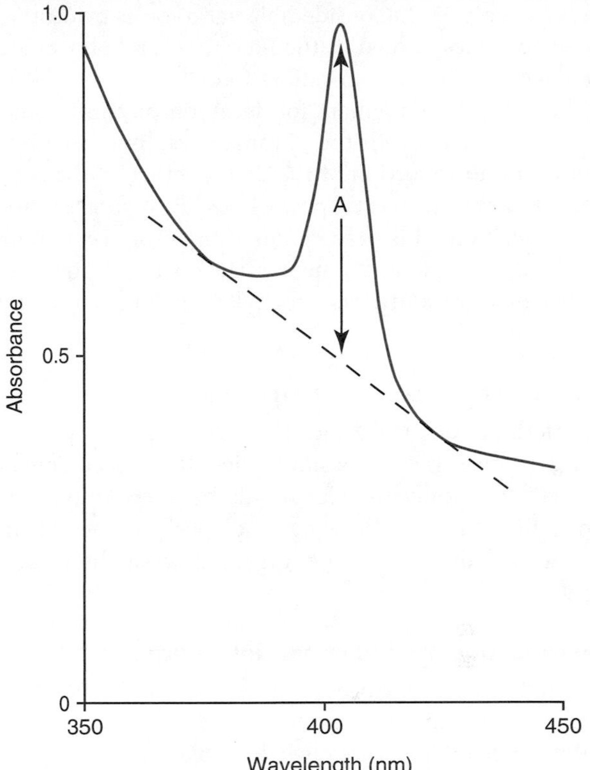

Figure 33-5 Absorption spectrum of acidified urine showing the procedure for measurement of corrected absorbance *(A)* of the porphyrin peak.

Semiquantitative Method for Total Porphyrin in Urine

This simple method for total urine porphyrins[24] uses scanning spectrometry. A typical spectrum is shown in Figure 33-5.

Reference values are given in Table 33-3. This method is reproducible but is only semiquantitative. The detection limit depends on the amount of background absorbance, but concentrations of approximately 50 nmol/L should be detected in urine of normal color. Ideally, concentrations should be expressed as a ratio to creatinine concentration to correct for urine concentration. Very occasionally, urine contains substances that produce very high background absorbance, making identification of any peak in the 400-nm region difficult. Such samples require analysis by alternative methods, such as HPLC. Increased concentrations require further investigation to identify individual porphyrins; porphyria should not be diagnosed on the basis of increased total porphyrin alone.

Semiquantitative Method for Total Porphyrin in Feces

This simple method for total fecal porphyrins uses scanning spectrometry after extraction.[77] Reference values are given in Table 33-3. The expression of concentration on a dry weight basis corrects for the moisture content of feces. Total fecal porphyrin determined by this method, unlike most of those based on solvent extraction, includes uroporphyrin.[107] Very occasionally, feces contain substances that produce very high background absorbance, making identification of any peak in the 400-nm region difficult. Such samples require analysis by alternative methods, such as HPLC.

Increased total fecal porphyrin concentration requires further investigation by fractionation, identification, and quantification of individual porphyrins using a technique, such as reversed-phase HPLC, which resolves coproporphyrin-I and -III isomers. Porphyria should never be diagnosed on the basis of raised total fecal porphyrin alone.

HPLC Fractionation of Porphyrins in Urine and Feces

This method for fractionation of urinary and fecal porphyrins uses sample preparation, HPLC separation, and fluorometric detection.[74] Samples are assayed with and without addition of calibrator to assist with fluorometric peak identification.

Figure 33-4 shows typical profiles from patients with various types of porphyria. For diagnostic purposes, quantification of individual porphyrins is rarely necessary, particularly if the concentrations are clearly elevated. Table 33-5 shows expected findings in the various types of porphyria, and reference values for individual porphyrin fractions are given in Table 33-3. Considerable variation is evident in the reference values quoted in the literature, probably as a consequence of difficulties in calibration.

The extraction method for fecal porphyrins results in some interference with the chromatography caused by dissolution of a proportion of the diethyl ether in the aqueous phase. As a result, an extra peak elutes just before the uroporphyrin position. This peak contains any uroporphyrin in the sample, up to 50% of the heptacarboxylate porphyrins, and smaller quantities of hexacarboxylate and pentacarboxylate porphyrins.

Methods for Blood Porphyrins

The methods described later require a spectrofluorometer with a red-sensitive photomultiplier. If such equipment is not available locally, samples should be referred to a specialized laboratory. Erythrocyte and plasma measurements are rarely required for the urgent assessment of acutely ill patients.

Determination of Erythrocyte Total Porphyrin

This method for erythrocyte total porphyrin uses double extraction and fluorometry.[11,96]

Reference intervals are given in Table 33-3. Total erythrocyte porphyrin concentrations are increased in (1) EPP, (2) CEP, (3) the rare homozygous variants of the autosomal dominant porphyrias, (4) iron deficiency, (5) hemolytic anemia, (6) some other forms of anemia, and (7) lead poisoning. A total porphyrin concentration within the reference interval excludes EPP. Distinction between EPP and other causes of increased erythrocyte total porphyrin concentration requires differentiation between protoporphyrin and its zinc chelate, because the acidic condition of this assay dissociates the zinc chelate and provides only a measure of total porphyrin.

Qualitative Determination of Zinc-Protoporphyrin and Protoporphyrin

This qualitative method for ZPP and protoporphyrin uses extraction and fluorometry.[39]

Emission peaks for ZPP and free protoporphyrin are 587 nm and 630 nm, respectively. In EPP, the concentration of free protoporphyrin greatly exceeds that of ZPP, except in the 2% of patients with XLDPP in whom ZPP concentration may constitute up to 60% of the greatly increased concentration of total porphyrin.[129] In lead poisoning, iron deficiency, and other anemias, ZPP is the main component (Figure 33-6). With experience, this test can be used to screen for EPP without the necessity for quantitative analysis. It is possible to quantify both ZPP and protoporphyrin by measuring the peak heights at 587 nm and 630 nm above a constructed baseline, if calibrator solutions of both protoporphyrins are prepared, provided allowance is made for a contribution of fluorescence from ZPP at the maximum wavelength for free protoporphyrin. A limitation of this method is that the efficiency of the extraction of ZPP is only about 50%. Hematofluorometers specifically designed to measure ZPP concentrations are unsuitable for measurement of the concentration of free protoporphyrin and should not be used to screen for EPP.

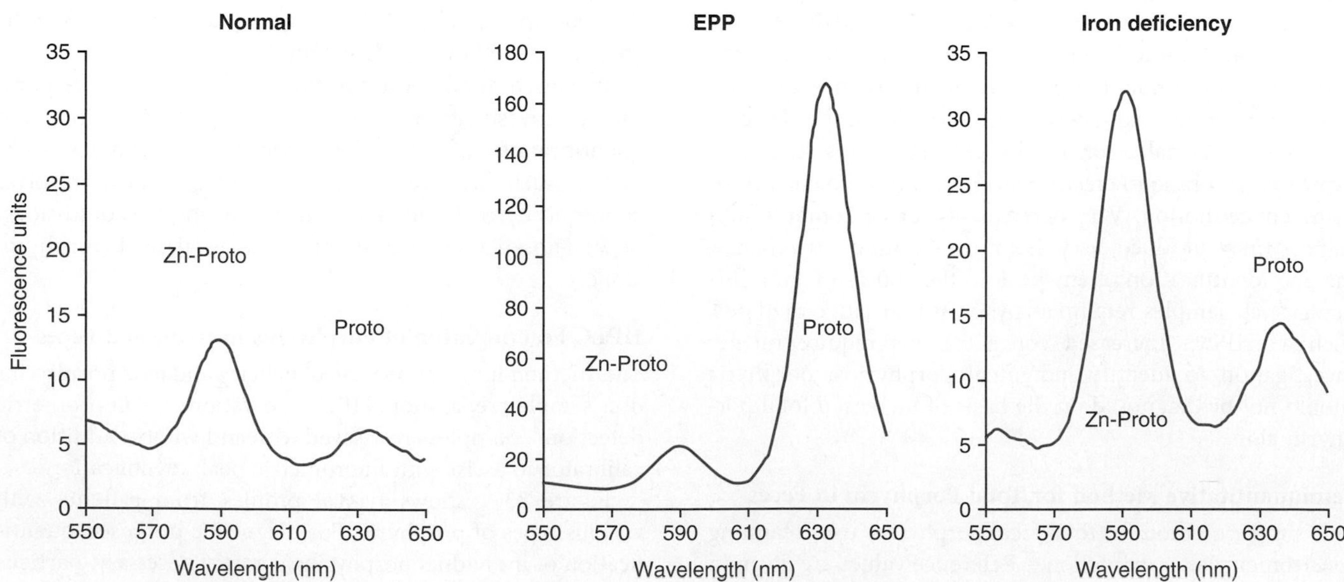

Figure 33-6 Fluorescence emission spectra (excitation at 405 nm) of ethanolic extracts of erythrocytes from a normal individual and from patients with erythropoietic protoporphyria (EPP) or iron deficiency. Note that different scales are used.

Analysis of Plasma Porphyrins

Plasma porphyrins may be determined by fluorescence emission spectroscopy of saline-diluted plasma[99] or deproteinized extracts, or by HPLC.[57] The fluorescence emission method, which offers the advantages of simplicity and inclusion of porphyrins that are bound covalently to plasma proteins, is detailed in the following sections.

Fluorescence Emission Spectroscopy of Plasma Porphyrins

This method determines the fluorescence emission spectrum of saline-diluted plasma excited at 405 nm.[99]

Figure 33-3 shows typical fluorescence emission maximum wavelengths for various porphyrias. In VP, the plasma contains porphyrin covalently bound to protein with a fluorescence emission maximum at 624 to 628 nm.[53,99] In other porphyrias, porphyrin is noncovalently bound to albumin and hemopexin.[67] In freshly separated plasma, protoporphyrin has a fluorescence emission peak around 632 nm. If separation is delayed, binding to globin released from red cells decreases the peak toward 626 nm. Apart from porphyrias (see Table 33-5), the plasma porphyrin concentration may be increased in conditions in which porphyrin excretion is impaired, such as renal failure and cholestasis.

Enzyme Measurements

Assay of individual enzymes of the heme biosynthetic pathway is rarely required for the assessment of patients with symptoms of porphyria. However, measurement of enzyme activities is useful for family studies when it is not possible to identify the individual mutation, or when DNA analysis is not available, and for the identification of uncommon subtypes such as nonerythroid AIP and "homozygous" forms of autosomal dominant porphyrias. Erythrocytes are a convenient source of cytoplasmic enzymes (ALAD, HMBS, UROS, and UROD), but assay of the mitochondrial enzymes (CPO, PPOX, and FECH) requires nucleated cells such as lymphocytes, Epstein-Barr virus (EBV)-transformed lymphoblasts, or cultured fibroblasts.[22] Assays for enzymes that use porphyrinogens as substrates are difficult because the substrate (1) is unstable; (2) has to be prepared fresh, and, particularly with protoporphyrinogen; (3) undergoes nonenzymatic oxidation during the assay. However, erythrocyte HMBS measurement is relatively straightforward and is the most widely used of these enzyme assays.

Assay of Erythrocyte Hydroxymethylbilane Synthase Activity

The enzymatic assay measures the rate of formation of porphyrinogens from PBG by hemolyzed erythrocytes. The reference interval [mean ± 2 standard deviations (SD)] is 20 to 42 nmol uroporphyrin per milliliter of erythrocytes per minute at 37 °C.[134]

Measurement of erythrocyte HMBS activity discriminates between individuals with AIP and their unaffected relatives, with a likelihood ratio of 3.4.[61] Although activities are usually below the reference interval in AIP, some overlap is noted between activities in AIP and healthy individuals, and activities are within the reference interval in the uncommon nonerythroid form.[61,130] In addition, erythrocyte HMBS activity declines sharply with erythrocyte age and is markedly influenced by the proportions of reticulocytes and young cells in peripheral blood. Therefore, HMBS assay should not be used for presymptomatic diagnosis of AIP in patients who (1) are hematologically abnormal, (2) have received a recent blood transfusion, or (3) are younger than 1 year old. Activity may increase in acutely ill patients, for example, during an acute attack of porphyria,[68] and may also be increased or decreased in disorders other than porphyria, including liver disease and chronic alcohol abuse.[61] In France, the prevalence of abnormally low HMBS activities in the general population is about 1 in 800.[90]

DNA Analysis

DNA analysis is required in the porphyrias mainly (1) for family screening, (2) for identifying the pattern of inheritance in families with EPP, and (3) as an aid in assessing prognosis in CEP. Its use as a front-line diagnostic investigation is largely restricted to exclusion of an acute porphyria in patients without current symptoms or biochemical abnormalities, and to the investigation of rare atypical cases. Screening of families for porphyria by DNA analysis is a two-stage process. First, the mutation that causes porphyria in the family under investigation needs to be identified by analysis of DNA from a family member in whom the diagnosis of a specific type of porphyria has been established unequivocally. Second, that patient's relatives are then screened for the mutation. The first part of this process is the more complex. Because most mutations are restricted to one or a few families, identification of a mutation in a new family almost always requires analysis of all exons with their flanking intronic sequences and the promoter region. Only in those countries where founder mutations predominate, as with, for example, VP in South Africa[56] and AIP in Sweden,[72] is initial testing for a single mutation useful.

Analysis of a gene for the presence of a mutation is most commonly carried out using direct sequencing of genomic DNA. DNA extraction, polymerase chain reaction (PCR) amplification, and sequencing are carried out by standard methods using the appropriate amplification and sequencing primers. Primer sequences have been published for the *HMBS*, *PPOX*, *CPOX*,[130] and *UROS*[132] genes or are available from the authors for the *UROD*,[6] *FECH*,[92] and *ALAD*[29] genes. If no mutation is identified by direct sequencing, gene dosage analysis should be carried out to search for large deletions undetectable by standard sequencing protocols. PCR-based methods for gene dosage analysis include quantitative fluorescent PCR, multiplex ligation probe amplification, and real-time quantitative PCR (see Chapter 17). Sufficient patients have now been identified with gross deletions in porphyria genes[28,127,130] to indicate that a method for gene dosage analysis should be included in routine protocols for mutation analysis. Nonclassified variants continue to be identified in the porphyria genes, and these need to be assessed individually (CMGS: http://cmgsweb.shared.hosting.zen.co.uk/BPGs/Best_Practice_Guidelines.htm). However, proof that a missense mutation causes disease may require expression and characterization of the mutant enzyme in a prokaryotic or eukaryotic vector.

Once the mutation that causes porphyria in a family has been identified, relatives are screened for its presence by direct sequencing of the region containing the mutation, or by some other mutation-specific method (see Chapter 17). The *FECH IVS3-48C* allele is readily identified by direct sequencing.

The clinical sensitivity of mutation detection in the acute porphyrias is high, provided gene dosage analysis is included in the analysis, for example, it is 98% for *HMBS*, 100% for *PPOX*, and 97% for *CPOX*.[130] Investigation of a large number of unrelated patients with EPP identified *FECH* or *ALAS2* mutations in 94% of them[128]; indirect evidence suggests that sensitivity for mutation detection in the *UROD* gene is around 95%[1]; at least 10% of mutant *UROS* alleles are undetected by current methods.[121]

REFERENCES

1. Aarsand AK, Boman H, Sandberg S. Familial and sporadic porphyria cutanea tarda: characterization and diagnostic strategies.Clin Chem 2009;55:795-803.
2. Allen KR, Whatley SD, Degg TJ, Barth JH. Hereditary coproporphyria: comparison of molecular and biochemical investigations in a large family. J Inherit Metab Dis 2005;28:779-85.
3. Anderson KE, Sassa S, Bishop DF, Desnick RJ. Disorders of heme biosynthesis: X-linked sideroblastic anemia and the porphyrias. In: Scriver CR, Beaudet AL, Sly WS, Valle D, eds. The metabolic and molecular basis of inherited disease, 8th edition. New York: McGraw-Hill, 2000:2961-3062.
4. Anstey AV, Hift RJ. Liver disease in erythropoietic protoporphyria: insights and implications for management. Postgrad Med J 2007;83:739-48.
5. Astner I, Schulze JO, van den Heuvel J, Jahn D, Schubert WD, Heinz DW. Crystal structure of 5-aminolevulinate synthase, the first enzyme of heme biosynthesis, and its link to XLSA in humans. EMBO J 2005;24:3166-77.
6. Badenas C, To-Figueras J, Phillips JD, Warby CA, Muñoz C, Herrero C. Identification and characterization of novel uroporphyrinogen decarboxylase gene mutations in a large series of porphyria cutanea tarda patients and relatives. Clin Genet 2009;75:346-53.
7. Battersby AR, Fookes CJ, Matcham GW, McDonald E. Biosynthesis of the pigments of life: formation of the macrocycle. Nature 1980;285:17-21.
8. Berk PD, Rodkey FL, Blaschke TF, Collison HA, Waggoner JG. Comparison of plasma bilirubin turnover and carbon monoxide production in man. J Lab Clin Med 1974;83:29-36.
9. Beukeveld GJ, Wolthers BG, van Saene JJ, de Haan TH, de Ruyter-Buitenhuis LW, van Saene RH. Patterns of porphyrin excretion in feces as determined by liquid chromatography: reference values and the effect of flora suppression. Clin Chem 1987;33:2164-70.
10. Blake D, McManus J, Cronin V, Ratnaike S. Fecal coproporphyrin isomers in hereditary coproporphyria. Clin Chem 1992;38:96-100.
11. Blake D, Poulos V, Rossi R. Diagnosis of porphyria—recommended methods for peripheral laboratories. Clin Biochem Rev 1992; 13(Suppl 1):S1-24.
12. Bonkovsky HL, Barnard GF. Diagnosis of porphyric syndromes: a practical approach in the era of molecular biology. Semin Liver Dis 1998;18:57-65.
13. Bottomley SS. Sideroblastic anemias. In: Greer JP, Foerster J, Lukens JN, Rogers GM, Paraskevas F, Glader BE, eds. Wintrobe's clinical hematology. Philadelphia: Lippincott Williams & Wilkins, 2004:1012-33.
14. Brodie MJ, Moore MR, Thompson GG, Goldberg A. The treatment of acute intermittent porphyria with laevulose. Clin Sci Mol Med 1977;53:365-71.
15. Bulaj ZJ, Phillips JD, Ajioka RS, Frankilin MR, Griffen LM, Guinee DJ, et al. Hemochromatosis genes and other factors contributing to the pathogenesis of porphyria cutanea tarda. Blood 2000;95:1565-71.
16. Burnham BF. The chemistry of porphyrins. Semin Haematol 1968;5:296-322.
17. Buttery JE, Stuart S. Measurement of porphobilinogen in urine by a simple resin method with use of a surrogate standard. Clin Chem 1991;37:2133-6.
18. Buttery JE, Stuart S, Panall PR. An improved direct method for the measurement of urinary δ-aminolevulinic acid. Clin Biochem 1995;28:477-80.

18a. Chen W, Dailey HA, Paw BH. Ferrochelatase forms an oligomeric complex with mitoferrin-1 and Abcb 10 for erythroid heme biosynthesis. Blood 2010;116:628-30.

19. Corradi HR, Corrigall AV, Boix E, Mohan CG, Sturrock ED, Meissner PN, et al. Crystal structure of protoporphyrinogen oxidase from *Myxococcus xanthus* and its complex with the inhibitor acifluorfen. J Biol Chem 2006;281:38625-33.
20. Cox TM. Protoporphyria. In: Kadish KM, Smith KM, Guilard R, eds. The porphyrin handbook. Volume 14. Medical aspects of porphyrias. Amsterdam: Academic Press, 2003:121-50.
21. Dailey HA. Enzymes of heme biosynthesis. J Biol Inorg Chem 1997;2:411-7.
22. De Rooij FW, Edixhoven A, Wilson JHP. Porphyria: a diagnostic approach. In: Kadish KM, Smith KM, Guilard R, eds. The porphyrin handbook. Volume 14. Medical aspects of porphyrias. Amsterdam: Academic Press, 2003:211-46.
23. Deacon AC. Performance of screening tests for porphyria. Ann Clin Biochem 1998;25:392-7.
24. Deacon AC, Elder GH. ACP best practice no. 165: front line tests for the investigation of suspected porphyria. J Clin Pathol 2001;54:500-7.
25. Deacon AC, Ledden JA. Limitations of solvent fractionation techniques for urinary and faecal porphyrins. Ann Clin Biochem 1998;35:314-6.
26. Deacon AC, Peters TJ. Identification of acute porphyria: evaluation of a commercial screening test for porphobilinogen. Ann Clin Biochem 1998;35:726-32.
27. Desnick RJ, Aplin KH. Congenital erythropoietic porphyria: advances in pathogenesis and treatment. Br J Haematol 2002;117:779-95.
28. Di Pierro E, Besana V, Moriondo V, Brancaleoni V, Tavazzi D, Casalgrandi G, et al. A large deletion on chromosome 11 in acute intermittent porphyria. Blood Cells Mol Dis 2006;37:50-4.
29. Doss MO, Stauch T, Gross U, Renz M, Akagi R, Doss-Frank M, et al. The third case of Doss porphyria (delta-amino-levulinic acid dehydratase deficiency) in Germany. J Inherit Metab Dis 2004;27:529-36.
30. Egger NG, Goeger DE, Payne DA, Miskovsky EP, Weinman SA, Anderson KE. Porphyria cutanea tarda: multiplicity of risk factors including HFE mutations, hepatitis C, and inherited uroporphyrinogen decarboxylase deficiency. Dig Dis Sci 2002;47:419-26.
31. Elder GH. Porphyria cutanea tarda and related disorders. In: Kadish KM, Smith KM, Guilard R, eds. The porphyrin handbook. Volume 14. Medical aspects of porphyrias. Amsterdam: Academic Press, 2003:67-92.
32. Elder GH. Hepatic porphyrias in children. J Inherit Metab Dis 1997;20:237-46.

33. Elder GH, Gouya L, Whatley SD, Puy H, Badminton MN, Deybach J-C. The molecular genetics of erythropoietic protoporphyria. Cell Mol Biol (Noisy-le-grand) 2009;15:118-26.
34. Elder GH, Hift RJ. Treatment of acute porphyria. Hosp Med 2001;62: 422-8.
35. Erskine PT, Senior A, Awan SJ, Lambert R, Lewis G, Tickle IJ, et al. X-ray structure of 5-aminolaevulinate dehydratase, a hybrid aldolase. Nat Struct Biol 1997;4:1025-31.
36. Felitsyn N, McLeod C, Shroads AL, Stacpoole PW, Notterpek L. The heme precursor delta-aminolevulinate blocks peripheral myelin formation. J Neurochem 2008;106:2068-79.
37. Fontanellas A, Coronel F, Santos JL, Herrero JA, Moran MJ, Guerra P, et al. Heme biosynthesis in uremic patients on CAPD or hemodialysis. Kidney Int 1994;45:220-3.
38. Fritsch C, Bolsen K, Ruzicka T, Goerz G. Congenital erythropoietic porphyria. J Am Acad Dermatol 1997;36:594-610.
39. Garden JS, Mitchell DG, Jackson KW. Improved ethanol extraction procedure for determining zinc protoporphyrin in whole blood. Clin Chem 1977;23:264-9.
40. Ged C, Moreau-Gaudry F, Richard E, Robert-Richard E, de Verneuil H. Congenital erythropoietic porphyria: mutation update and correlations between genotype and phenotype. Cell Mol Biol (Noisy-le-grand) 2009;55:53-60.
41. Ged C, Ozalla D, Herrero C, Lecha M, Mendez M, de Verneuil H, et al. Description of a new mutation in hepatoerythropoietic porphyria and prenatal exclusion of a homozygous fetus. Arch Dermatol 2002;138:957-60.
42. Gibbs NK, Traynor N, Ferguson J. Biochemical diagnosis of the cutaneous porphyrias: five years experience of plasma spectrofluorimetry. Br J Dermatol 1995;135(Suppl 45):18.
43. Gibson GE, McGinnity E, McGrath PM, Carmody M, Walshe J, Donohoe J, et al. Cutaneous abnormalities and metabolic disturbance of porphyrins in patients on maintenance dialysis. Clin Exp Dermatol 1997;22:124-7.
44. Gill R, Kolstoe SE, Mohammed F, Al D-Bass A, Mosely JE, Sarwar M, et al. Structure of human porphobilinogen deaminase at 2.8 Å: the molecular basis of acute intermittent porphyria. Biochem J 2009;420: 17-25.
45. Glynne P, Deacon AC, Goldsmith D, Pusey C, Clutterbuck E. Bullous dermatoses in end-stage renal failure: porphyria or pseudoporphyria? Am J Kidney Dis 1999;34:155-60.
46. Goodwin RG, Kell WJ, Laidler P, Long CC, Whatley SD, McKinley M, et al. Photosensitivity and acute liver injury in myeloproliferative disorder secondary to late-onset protoporphyria caused by deletion of a ferrochelatase gene in hematopoietic cells. Blood 2006;107:60-2.
47. Gorchein A. Testing for porphobilinogen in urine. Clin Chem 2002; 48:564-6.
48. Gouya L, Martin-Schmitt C, Robreau A-M, Austerlitz F, Da Silva V, Brun P, et al. Contribution of a single-nucleotide polymorphism to the genetic predisposition for erythropoietic protoporphyria. Am J Hum Genet 2006;78:2-14.
49. Gouya L, Puy H, Robreau AM, Lamoril J, Da Silva V, Grandchamp B, et al. The penetrance of autosomal dominant erythropoietic protoporphyria is modulated by expression of wild type FECH. Nat Genet 2002;30:23-7.
50. Guernsey DL, Jiang H, Campagna DR, Evans SC, Ferguson M, Kellogg MD, et al. Mutations in mitochondrial carrier family gene SLC25A38 cause nonsyndromic autosomal recessive congenital sideroblastic anemia. Nat Genet 2009;41:651-3.
51. Handschin C, Lin J, Rhee J, Peyer AK, Chin S, Wu PH, et al. Nutritional regulation of hepatic heme biosynthesis and porphyria through PGC-1α. Cell 2005;122:505-15.
52. Hart D, Piomelli S. Simultaneous quantitation of zinc protoporphyrin and free protoporphyrin in erythrocytes by acetone extraction. Clin Chem 1981;27:220-2.
53. Hift RJ, Davidson BP, van der Hooft C, Meissner DM, Meissner PN. Plasma fluorescence scanning and fecal porphyrin analysis for the diagnosis of variegate porphyria: precise determination of sensitivity and specificity with detection of protoporphyrinogen oxidase mutations as a reference standard. Clin Chem 2004;50:915-23.
54. Hift R, Meissner P. Miscellaneous abnormalities in porphyrin production and disposal. In: Kadish KM, Smith KM, Guilard R, eds. The porphyrin handbook. Volume 14. Medical aspects of porphyrias. Amsterdam: Academic Press, 2003:151-68.
55. Hift RJ, Meissner PN. An analysis of 112 acute porphyric attacks in Cape Town, South Africa. Medicine 2005;84:48-60.
56. Hift RJ, Meissner D, Meissner PN. A systematic study of the clinical and biochemical expression of variegate porphyria in a large South African family. Br J Dermatol 2004;151:465-71.
57. Hindmarsh JT, Oliveras L, Greenway DC. Plasma porphyrins in the porphyrias. Clin Chem 1999;45:1070-6.
58. Holme SA, Anstey AV, Finlay AY, Elder GH, Badminton MN. Erythropoietic protoporphyria in the United Kingdom: clinical features and effect on quality of life. Br J Dermatol 2006;155:574-81.
59. Holme SA, Whatley SD, Roberts AG, Anstey AV, Elder GH, Ead RD, et al. Seasonal palmar keratoderma in erythropoietic protoporphyria indicates autosomal recessive inheritance. J Invest Dermatol 2009;129: 599-605.
60. Holme SA, Worwood M, Anstey AV, Elder GH, Badminton MN. Erythropoiesis and iron metabolism in dominant erythropoietic protoporphyria. Blood 2007;110:4108-10.
61. Kauppinen R, Fraunberg M. Molecular and biochemical studies of acute intermittent porphyria in 196 patients and their families. Clin Chem 2002;48:1891-900.
62. Kaya AH, Plewinska M, Wong DM, Desnick RJ, Wetmur JG. Human delta-aminolaevulinate dehydratase (ALAD) gene: structure and alternative splicing of the erythroid and housekeeping mRNAs. Genomics 1994;19:242-8.
63. Kean RW, Deacon AC, Delves HT, Moreton JA, Frost PG. Indian herbal remedies for diabetes as a cause of lead poisoning. Postgrad Med J 1994;70:113-4.
64. Kolluri S, Sadlon TJ, May BK, Bonkovsky HL. Haem repression of the housekeeping 5-aminolevulinic acid synthase gene in the hepatoma cell line LMH. Biochem J 2005;392:173-80.
65. Kontos A, Ozog D, Bichakjian C, Lim HW. Congenital erythropoietic porphyria associated with myelodysplasia presenting in a 72-year old man: report of a case and review of the literature. Br J Dermatol 2003; 148:160-4.
66. Kornfield JM, Ullman WW. Penicillin interference with the determination of δ-aminolevulinic acid. Clin Chim Acta 1973;46: 187-90.
67. Koskelo P, Muller-Eberhard U. Interaction of porphyrins with proteins. Semin Hematol 1977;14:221-6.
68. Kostrewska E, Gregor A. Increased activity of porphobilinogen deaminase in erythrocytes during attacks of acute intermittent porphyria. Ann Clin Res 1986;18:195-8.
69. Labbe RF, Rettmer RL. Zinc protoporphyrin: a product of iron-deficient erythropoiesis. Semin Hematol 1989;26:40-6.
70. Lamon J, With T, Redeker A. The Hoesch test: bedside screening for urinary PBG inpatients with suspected porphyria. Clin Chem 1974;20: 1438-40.
71. Lamoril J, Puy H, Gouya L, Rosipal R, Da Silva V, Grandchamp B, et al. Neonatal hemolytic anemia due to inherited harderoporphyria: clinical characteristics and molecular basis. Blood 1998;91:1453-7.
72. Lee JS, Anvret M. Identification of the most common mutation within the porphobilinogen deaminase gene in Swedish patients with acute intermittent porphyria. Proc Natl Acad Sci U S A 1991;88: 10912-5.
73. Lee DS, Flachsová E, Bodnárová M, Demeler B, Martásek P, Raman CS. Structural basis of hereditary coproporphyria. Proc Natl Acad Sci U S A 2005;102:14232-7.
74. Lim CK, Peters TJ. Urine and faecal porphyrin profiles by reversed-phase high-performance liquid chromatography in the porphyrias. Clin Chim Acta 1984;139:55-63.

75. Lim CK, Rideout JM, Peters TJ. Pseudoporphyria associated with consumption of brewer's yeast. Br Med J 1984;288:1640-2.
76. Lin CS, Krishnan AV, Lee MJ, Zagami AS, You HL, Yang CC, et al. Nerve function and dysfunction in acute intermittent porphyria. Brain 2008;131:2510-9.
77. Lockwood WH, Poulos V, Rossi E, Curnow DH. Rapid procedure for fecal porphyrin assay. Clin Chem 1985;31:163-7.
78. Luo J, Lim CK. Order of uroporphyrinogen-III decarboxylations on incubation of porphobilinogen and uroporphyrinogen-III with erythrocyte uroporphyrinogen decarboxylase. Biochem J 1993;289: 519-23.
79. Maruno M, Furuyama K, Akagi R, Horie Y, Meguro K, Garbaczewski L, et al. Highly heterogeneous nature of delta-aminolevulinate dehydratase (ALAD) deficiencies in ALAD porphyria. Blood 2001;97: 972-8.
80. Matthews MA, Schubert HL, Whitby FG, Alexander KJ, Schadick K, Bergonia HA, et al. Crystal structure of human uroporphyrinogen III synthase. EMBO J 2001;21:5832-9.
81. Mauzerall D, Granick S. The occurrence and determination of delta-aminolevulinic acid and porphobilinogen in urine. J Biol Chem 1956;219:435-46.
82. May BK, Dogra SC, Sadlon TJ, Bhasker CR, Cox TC, Bottomley SS. Molecular regulation of heme biosynthesis in higher vertebrates. Prog Nucleic Acid Res Mol Biol 1995;51:1-51.
83. McColl KE, Goldberg A. Abnormal porphyrin metabolism in diseases other than porphyria. Clin Hematol 1980;9:427-45.
84. McColl KE, Thompson GC, Moore MR, Goldbert A. Acute alcohol ingestion and haem biosynthesis in healthy subjects. Eur J Clin Invest 1980;10:107-12.
85. Meissner P, Adams P, Kirsch R. Allosteric inhibition of human lymphoblast and purified PBG-deaminase by protoporphyrinogen and coproporphyrinogen. J Clin Invest 1991;91:1436-44.
86. Merritt JE, Loening KL. Nomenclature of tetrapyrroles. Eur J Biochem 1982;108:1-30.
87. Meyer UA, Schuurmans MM, Lindberg RL. Acute porphyrias: pathogenesis of neurological manifestations. Semin Liver Dis 1998;18: 43-52.
88. Millward LM, Kelly P, Deacon A, Senior V, Peters TJ. Self-rated psychosocial consequences and quality of life in the acute porphyrias. J Inherit Metab Dis 2001;24:733-47.
89. Minder EI, Schneider-Yin X, Steurer J, Bachmann LM. A systematic review of treatment options for dermal photosensitivity in erythropoietic protoporphyria. Cell Mol Biol (Noisy-le-grand) 2009;55:84-97.
90. Nordmann Y, Puy H, Da Silva V, Simonin S, Robreau AM, Bonaiti C, et al. Acute intermittent porphyria: prevalence of mutations in the porphobilinogen deaminase gene in blood donors in France. J Intern Med 1997;242:213-7.
91. O'Reilly K, Snape J, Moore MR. Porphyria cutanea tarda resulting from primary hepatocellular carcinoma. Clin Exp Dermatol 1988;13: 44-8.
92. Parker M, Corrigall AV, Hift RJ, Meissner PN. Molecular characterisation of erythropoietic protoporphyria in South Africa. Br J Dermatol 2008;159:182-91.
93. Phillips JD, Bergonia HA, Reilly CA, Franklin MR, Kushner JP. A porphomethene inhibitor of uroporphyrinogen decarboxylase causes porphyria cutanea tarda. Proc Natl Acad Sci U S A 2007;104: 5079-84.
94. Phillips JD, Steensma DP, Pulsipher MA, Spangrude GJ, Kushner JP. Congenital erythropoietic porphyria due to a mutation in GATA1: the first trans-acting mutation causative for a human porphyria. Blood 2007;109:2618-21.
95. Phillips JD, Warby CA, Whitby FG, Kushner JP, Hill CP. Substrate shuttling between active sites of uroporphyrinogen decarboxylase is not required to generate coproporphyrinogen. J Mol Biol 2009;389: 306-14.
96. Piomelli S. Free erythrocyte porphyrin in the detection of undue absorption of lead and of iron deficiency. Clin Chem 1977;23:264-9.
97. Pischik E, Kauppinen R. Neurological manifestations of acute intermittent porphyria. Cell Mol Biol (Noisy-le-grand) 2009;55:72-83.
98. Pischik E, Kazakov V, Kauppinen R. Is screening for urinary porphobilinogen useful among patients with acute polyneuropathy or encephalopathy? J Neurol 2008;255:974-9.
99. Poh-Fitzpatrick MB. A plasma fluorescence marker for variegate porphyria. Arch Dermatol 1980;116:543-7.
100. Poh-Fitzpatrick MB. Clinical features of the porphyrias. Clin Dermatol 1998;16:251-64.
101. Ponka P. Tissue-specific regulation of iron metabolism and heme synthesis: distinct control mechanisms in erythroid cells. Blood 1997;89:1-25.
102. Puy H, Gouya L, Deybach J-C. Porphyrias. Lancet 2010;375:924-37.
103. Rank JM, Pascual-Leone A, Payne W, Glock M, Freese D, Sharp H, et al. Hematin therapy for the neurologic crisis of tyrosinemia. J Pediatr 1991;118:136-9.
104. Robert-Richard E, Moreau-Gaudry F, Lalanne M, Lamrissi-Garcia I, Cario-André M, Guyonnet-Dupérat V, et al. Effective gene therapy of mice with congenital erythropoietic porphyria is facilitated by a survival advantage of corrected erythroid cells. Am J Hum Genet 2008;82:113-24.
105. Roels H, Lauwerys R, Buchet JP, Berlin A, Smeets J. Comparison of four methods for determination of δ-aminolevulinic acid in urine, and evaluation of critical factors. Clin Chem 1974;20:753-60.
106. Rose IS, Young GP, St John DJ, Deacon MC, Blake D, Henderson RW. Effect of ingestion of hemoproteins on fecal excretion of hemes and porphyrins. Clin Chem 1989;35:2290-6.
107. Rossi E. Increased fecal porphyrins in acute intermittent porphyria. Clin Chem 1999;45:281-3.
108. Rossi E, Attwood PV, Garcia-Webb P. Inhibition of human lymphocyte coproporphyrinogen oxidase activity by metals, bilirubin and haemin. Biochim Biophys Acta 1992;1135:262-8.
109. Sardh E, Harper P, Andersson DE, Floderus Y. Plasma porphobilinogen as a sensitive biomarker to monitor the clinical and therapeutic course of acute intermittent porphyria attacks. Eur J Intern Med 2009;20:201-7.
110. Sarkany RE. The management of porphyria cutanea tarda. Clin Exp Dermatol 2001;26:225-32.
111. Schoenfeld N, Mamet R, Leibovici L, Lanir A. Alcohol-induced changes in urinary aminolevulinic acid and porphyrins: unrelated to liver disease. Alcohol 1996;13:59-63.
112. Schreiber WE, Jamani A, Pudek MR. Screening tests for porphobilinogen are insensitive. Am J Clin Pathol 1989;92:644-9.
112a. Schultz IJ, Chen C, Paw BH, Hamza I. Iron and porphyrin trafficking in heme biogenesis. J Biol Chem 2010; 285:26753-9.
113. Seth AK, Badminton MN, Mirza D, Russell S, Elias E. Liver transplantation for porphyria: who, when, and how? Liver Transpl 2007;13:1219-27.
113a. Dowman JK, Gunson BK, Newsome PN, Bramhall S, Badminton MN Liver transplantation from donors with acute intermittent porphyria. Ann Intern Med. 2011;154(8):571-2.
114. Seubert S, Seubert A, Rumpf KW, Kiffe H. A porphyria cutanea tarda-like distribution pattern of porphyrins in plasma, hemodialysate, hemofiltrate, and urine of patients on chronic hemodialysis. J Invest Dermatol 1985;85:107-9.
115. Shoolingin-Jordan PM, Warren MJ, Awan SJ. Dipyrromethane cofactor assembly of porphobilinogen deaminase: formation of apoenzyme and preparation of holoenzyme. Methods Enzymol 1997;281:327-36.
116. Sithisarankul P, Schwartz BS, Lee BK, Kelsey KT, Strickland PT. Aminolevulinate dehydratase genotype mediates plasma levels of the neurotoxin, 5-aminolevulinic acid, in lead exposed workers. Am J Ind Med 1997;32:15-20.
117. Spelt JM, de Rooij FW, Wilson JM, Zandbergen AA. Vitamin D deficiency in patients with erythropoietic protoporphyria. J Inherit Metab Dis 2009 Jan 10. Epub ahead of print.
118. Thunell S. (Far) Outside the box: genomic approach to acute porphyria. Physiol Res 2006;55(Suppl 2):S43-66.

119. Thunell S, Harper P, Brock A, Peterson NE. Porphyrins, porphyrin metabolism and porphyrias. II. Diagnosis and monitoring in the acute porphyrias. Scan J Clin Lab Invest 2000;60:541-59.
120. Todd DJ. Erythropoietic protoporphyria. Br J Dermatol 1994;131: 751-66.
121. Verneuil H, de Ged C, Moreau-Gaudry F. Congenital erythropoietic porphyria. In: Kadish KM, Smith KM, Guilard R, eds. The porphyrin handbook. Volume 14. Medical aspects of porphyrias. Amsterdam: Academic Press, 2003:43-66.
122. Verstraeten L, Ledoux MC, Moos B, Callebaut B, Cornu G, Hassoun A. Interference of Tienam in the colorimetric determination of 5-aminolevulinic acid and porphobilinogen in serum and urine. Clin Chem 1992;38:2557-8.
123. Wahlin S, Harper P. Bone marrow transplantation in erythropoietic protoporphyria. J Invest Dermatol. In press.
124. Warren MJ, Scott AI. Tetrapyrrole assembly and modification into the ligands of biologically functional cofactors. Trends Biochem Sci 1990; 15:486-91.
125. Watson CJ, Schwartz S. A simple test for urinary porphobilinogen. Proc Soc Exp Biol 1941;47:393-4.
126. Wetmur JG, Kaya AH, Plewinska M, Desnick RJ. Molecular characterization of the human aminolaevulinate dehydratase 2 (ALAD2) allele: implications for molecular screening of individuals for genetic susceptibility to lead poisoning. Am J Hum Genet 1991;49: 757-63.
127. Whatley SD, Mason NG, Holme SA, Anstey AV, Elder GH, Badminton MN. Gene dosage analysis identifies large deletions of the FECH gene in 10% of families with erythropoietic protoporphyria. J Invest Dermatol 2007;127:2790-4.
128. Whatley SD, Mason NG, Holme SA, Anstey AV, Elder GH, Badminton MN. Molecular epidemiology of erythropoietic protoporphyria in the United Kingdom. Br J Dermatol 2010;162: 642-6.
129. Whatley SD, Ducamp S, Gouya L, Grandchamp B, Beaumont C, Badminton MN, et al. C-terminal deletions in the ALAS2 gene lead to gain of function and cause X-linked dominant protoporphyria without anemia or iron overload. Am J Hum Genet 2008;83:408-14.
130. Whatley SD, Mason NG, Woolf JR, Newcombe RG, Elder GH, Badminton MN. Diagnostic strategies for autosomal dominant acute porphyrias: retrospective analysis of 467 unrelated patients referred for mutational analysis of the HMBS, CPOX, or PPOX gene. Clin Chem 2009;55:1406-14.
131. Whitby FG, Phillips JD, Kushner JP, Hill CP. Crystal structure of human uroporphyrinogen decarboxylase. EMBO J 1998;17:2463-71.
132. Wiederholt T, Poblete-Gutiérrez P, Gardlo K, Goerz G, Bolsen K, Merk HF, et al. Identification of mutations in the uroporphyrinogen III cosynthase gene in German patients with congenital erythropoietic porphyria. Physiol Res 2006;55(Suppl 2):S85-92.
133. Woods JS, Miller HD. Quantitative measurement of porphyrins in biological tissues and evaluation of tissue porphyrins during toxicant exposures. Fundam Appl Toxicol 1993;21:291-7.
134. Wright DJ, Lim CK. Simultaneous determination of hydroxymethylbilane synthase and uroporphyrinogen-III synthase in erythrocytes by HPLC. Biochem J 1983;213:85-8.
135. Wu CK, Dailey HA, Rose JP, Burden A, Sellers VM, Wang BC. The 2.0 Å structure of human ferrochelatase, the terminal enzyme of heme biosynthesis. Nat Struct Biol 2000;8:156-60.
136. Young D. Effect of drugs on clinical laboratory tests, 5th edition. Volume 1. Listing by test. Washington: AACC Press, 2000:642-3.

USEFUL WEBSITES

American Porphyria Foundation: http://www.porphyriafoundation.com
European Porphyria Network: http://www.porphyria-europe.org
Nordic Drug Database: http://www.drugs-porphyria.com
South African Porphyria Centre: http://www.porphyria.uct.ac.za

CHAPTER 34

Therapeutic Drugs and Their Management

Christine L. H. Snozek, Ph.D.,
Gwendolyn A. McMillin, Ph.D., D.A.B.C.C.(C.C.,T.C.),
and Thomas P. Moyer, Ph.D.

Physicians have long recognized the limitations of empirical drug dosing, such as standard or fixed dose regimens, and have responded with their clinical judgment and knowledge of basic pharmacology to individualize each patient's drug dosage. Approximately 40 years ago, quantification of drugs in blood or serum, known as *therapeutic drug monitoring,* became a standard of practice in cardiology, infectious diseases, neurology, and psychiatry, and more recently in transplantation, to facilitate dose adjustments to attain optimal drug response. Therapeutic drug monitoring offered the physician a scientific rather than empirical approach to selecting a drug regimen to optimize therapy. Now known as *therapeutic drug management (TDM),* this multidiscipline clinical activity facilitates selection of the drug to which the patient responds best, as well as the optimal dose, and allows assessment of therapeutic compliance and efficacy. It also facilitates detection of drug-drug interactions and is the basis for defining drug-induced toxicity. Laboratory testing to support TDM may include (1) detection of risk factors (e.g., pharmacogenomics; see Chapter 43) that qualify or disqualify a person for a particular therapy, based on the likelihood of predictable pharmacokinetics, toxicity, and response; and (2) quantification of drug and/or drug metabolite concentrations in a biological fluid to assess pharmacokinetics or biomarkers indicative of response. The medical professionals involved in TDM include the ordering physician, the clinical laboratorian (the chemical pathologist, the clinical chemist), the clinical pharmacologist, the pharmacist, and the nurse who handles medication delivery and monitoring.

Once a therapeutic regimen has been selected and initiated, the practice of TDM facilitates optimum therapy by providing the prescribing physician with objective information about drug disposition; TDM describes a patient's pharmacokinetic status at the moment of specimen collection. Pharmacokinetics is the science that describes the relationship between drug dose and the time course of drug absorption, distribution, and elimination that results in a specific drug concentration in biological systems. Clinical pharmacokinetics involves the application of mathematical relationships to predict whether a drug concentration quantified at a specific time reflects distribution and metabolism of a defined population for a unique patient. Pharmacokinetics that deviates from that typical for a specific population may indicate genetic variants, drug-drug or drug-food interaction, organ failure, or patient noncompliance. Clinical pharmacokinetics can also be applied to predict appropriate change in dose or dosing interval to allow for safe and effective treatment and to attain optimal response to the drug as quickly as possible. It is important therefore for the clinician and the laboratorian to understand how to quantify drugs in biological specimens and how these results are used to achieve effective drug therapy. As mentioned earlier, TDM is a multidisciplinary approach that relies on the cooperative efforts of the physician, nurse, pharmacologist, pharmacist, and clinical laboratorian.

Knowledge of the impact of genetics on drug disposition developed rapidly in the late 1990s and continues to develop in the 2000s. This knowledge field as it relates to drug disposition has become known as pharmacogenomics (PG). TDM and PG are highly interactive disciplines used in conjunction to elucidate the overall pharmacokinetic status of an individual patient. Although the basic concepts of PG are outlined elsewhere in this text (see Chapter 43), the specific aspects of the discipline that relate to the interpretation of TDM results are explained in this chapter. Reviews by O'Kane[142] and Weinshilboum[208] and the Internet Website offered by Flockhart[63] are good sources of additional information.

To be effective, TDM requires the acquisition of a valid specimen followed by timely determination of the drug concentration in the specimen and interpretation of results in the context of dose, time of last dose, and other drugs present. Results should be reported or collated with the dosing schedule so that they may be interpreted in a pharmacokinetic context.

This chapter focuses on the role of the laboratory in the discipline of drug monitoring. Excellent descriptions of the roles of the physician and the consulting pharmacologist are presented in Melmon and Morrelli's *Basic Principles in Therapeutics,*[129] Goodman and Gilman's *The Pharmacological Basis of Therapeutics,*[30] Burton and colleagues' *Applied Pharmacokinetics and Pharmacodynamics: Principles of Therapeutic Drug Monitoring,*[34] and Mandell and colleagues' *Principles and Practice of Infectious Diseases.*[122] The *Physicians' Desk Reference* (PDR), published annually by Medical Economics of Montvale, New Jersey, is also an excellent source of dosing guidance and pharmacokinetic information.

DEFINITIONS

Pharmacology comprises that body of knowledge surrounding chemical agents and their effects on living processes. This is a broad field that has traditionally been confined to drugs useful in the prevention, diagnosis, and treatment of disease. *Pharmacotherapeutics* is that part of pharmacology concerned primarily with the application or administration of drugs to patients for the purpose of prevention and treatment of disease. For this aspect of medical practice to be effective, the pharmacodynamic and pharmacokinetic properties of drugs should be understood.

Pharmacodynamics describes response to drugs (what the drug does to the body) and encompasses the processes of interaction of pharmacologically active substances with target sites, and the biochemical and physiologic consequences that lead to therapeutic or adverse effects.[54] For many drugs, the ultimate effect or mechanism of action at the molecular concentration is understood poorly, if at all. However, effects at the cellular or organ system concentration or in the whole body are relatively well understood and usually can be related to the dose of the drug.

Pharmacokinetics describes how drugs are received and handled by the body (what the body does to the drug) and includes the processes of uptake of drugs by the body, the biotransformations they undergo, the distribution of the drugs and their metabolites in tissue, and the elimination of the drugs and their metabolites from the body. Clinical pharmacokinetics is the discipline that applies the principles of pharmacokinetics to safe and effective therapeutic management of an individual patient. It is this aspect of pharmacology that most strongly influences the interpretation of TDM results and that is dealt with in greater detail in this chapter.

Note that the term *pharmacology* relates to broad knowledge of the systemic effects of a drug; *pharmacodynamics* refers to the interaction of a drug at its site of action, whereas *pharmacokinetics* is a mathematical description of drug disposition. These terms are quite different and should not be used interchangeably.

Figure 34-1 illustrates the conceptual relationship between pharmacodynamics and pharmacokinetics. The former relates drug concentration at the site of action to the observed magnitude of the effect (desirable or undesirable). Pharmacokinetics, on the other hand, relates dose, dosing interval, and route of administration (regimen) to drug concentration

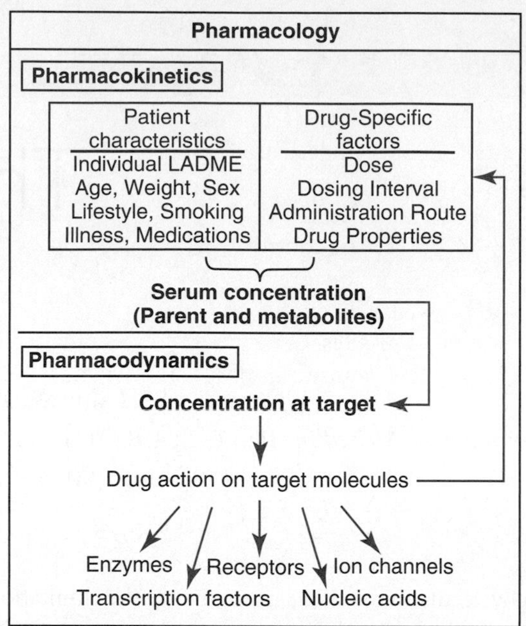

Figure 34-1 Conceptual relationship between pharmacodynamics and pharmacokinetics. Many drug- and patient-specific factors determine both the serum concentration of a therapeutic compound and its metabolites. Serum concentration in turn is related to the amount of drug present at the target site, resulting in effects on a variety of molecules (several examples are shown) to induce a pharmacologic response. The efficacy and degree of response provide feedback to allow optimization of the dosing regimen for an individual patient.

in the blood over time. For more complete discussions of these basic concepts, the reader is encouraged to review standard textbooks of pharmacology.[30,129,167] *Toxicology* is the subdiscipline of pharmacology concerned with adverse effects of chemicals on living systems. Toxic effects and mechanisms of action may be different from therapeutic effects and mechanisms for the same drug. Similarly, at the high dose of drugs at which toxic effects may be produced, rate processes are frequently altered compared with those at therapeutic doses. For these reasons, the terms *toxicodynamics* and *toxicokinetics* are now applied to these special situations.

BASIC CONCEPTS

The pharmacologic effect of a drug is elicited by direct interaction of the drug with a receptor controlling a specific function or by drug-mediated alteration of the physiologic process regulating the function; this is known as the *mechanism of action.* In a given tissue, the site at which a drug acts to initiate events leading to a specific biological effect is called the *site of action* of the drug. For most drugs, the intensity and duration of the observed pharmacologic effect are proportional to the concentration of the drug at the receptor, predicted by pharmacokinetics.

Mechanism of Action

The *mechanism of action* of a drug is the biochemical or physical process that occurs at the site of action to produce the pharmacologic effect. Drug action is usually mediated through a receptor. Cellular enzymes and structural or transport proteins are important examples of drug receptors. Nonprotein macromolecules may also bind drugs, resulting in altered cellular functions controlled by membrane permeability or DNA transcription. Some drugs are chemically similar to important natural endogenous substances and may compete for binding sites. Other drugs may block formation, release, uptake, or transport of essential substances. And some may produce an effect by interacting with relatively small molecules to form complexes that actively bind to receptors. These and other examples of receptor binding are more completely discussed in pharmacology texts.[30,129,167]

Although the exact molecular interactions that describe the mechanism of action remain obscure for many drugs, theoretical models have been developed to explain them. One concept postulates that a drug binds to intracellular macromolecular receptors through ionic and hydrogen bonds and van der Waals forces. This theoretical model further postulates that if the drug-receptor complex is sufficiently stable and is able to modify the target system, an observable pharmacologic response will occur. As Figure 34-2 illustrates, the response is dose dependent until a maximum effect is reached. The plateau may be due to saturation at the receptor or overload of a transport or clearance process.

The utility of monitoring drug concentration is based on the premise that pharmacologic response correlates with the concentration of the drug at the site of action (receptor). Measurement of the concentration at the receptor site in a patient is technically impractical, if not impossible, thus surrogate measures must be used. Because of individual variation in pharmacokinetics, the administered dose is often a poor predictor of the concentration at the receptor and the pharmacodynamic response. However, studies have shown that for many drugs, a strong correlation exists between the serum drug concentration and the observed pharmacologic effect. It is recognized that pharmacodynamic effects may vary between individuals, despite similar serum drug concentrations. For this reason, use of appropriate biomarkers may complement TDM and improve prediction of individual responses to drug therapy; although clinically validated biomarkers have not yet been identified for many therapeutic areas, this is an area of continued research interest.

Years of relating blood concentrations to drug effects have demonstrated the clinical utility of drug concentration information. Nevertheless one must always keep in mind that a serum drug concentration does not necessarily equal the concentration at the receptor; it merely reflects it. However, for pharmacokinetic studies, it is assumed that changes in drug concentration in blood (or serum) versus time are proportional to changes in local concentrations at the receptor site or in body tissue. This assumption is sometimes called the *property of kinetic homogeneity* and is applicable to all pharmacokinetic models in postabsorptive and postdistributive phases of the time course. Figure 34-3 illustrates that property for a hypothetical compound. Parallel concentrations (log C) are expected in blood at the receptor and in tissue as time passes. Concepts depicted in Figure 34-3 are hypothetical; the absolute concentration of a drug in various tissues is highly variable from drug to drug.

The property of kinetic homogeneity is an important assumption in TDM because it is the basis on which all therapeutic and toxic concentration reference values are

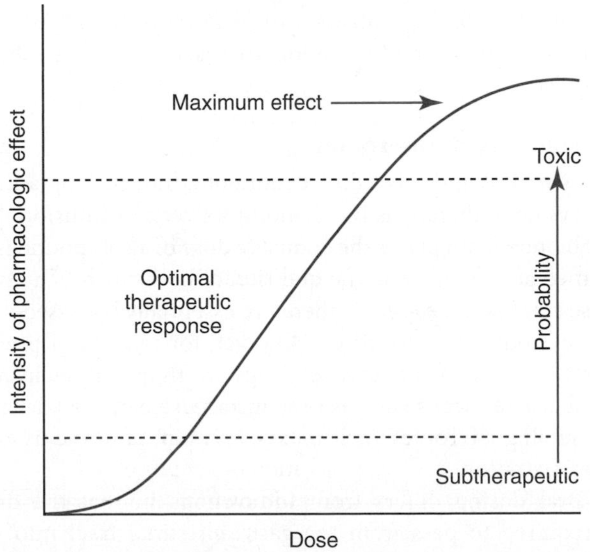

Figure 34-2 The dose-effect relationship. The probability of increasing pharmacologic response and risk of toxicity parallels concentration for most drugs. The plateau (maximum effect) is likely due to saturation at the receptor.

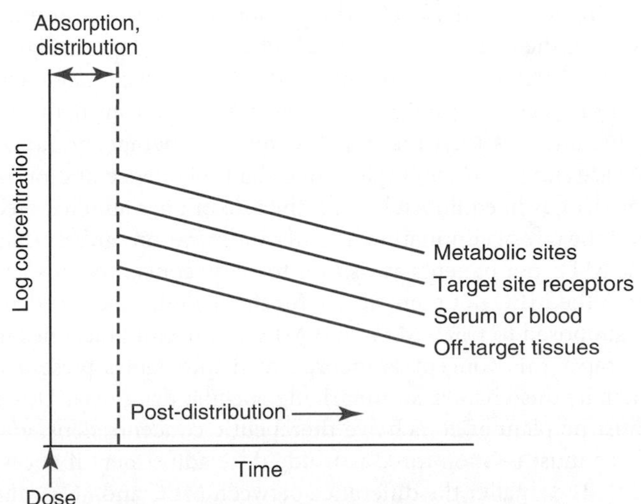

Figure 34-3 Property of kinetic homogeneity. The blood concentration of a drug is assumed to correlate with, although perhaps not equal, the concentration at the receptor site and in various tissues.

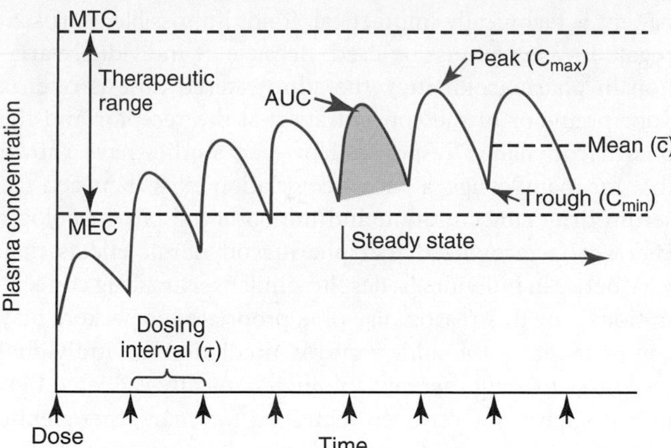

Figure 34-4 Peak, mean, and trough drug concentrations increase with multiple identical doses administered once each half-life until they reach steady state. For most drugs, it takes five to seven half-lives to reach steady state. At steady state, optimal peak and trough concentrations are less than the MTC and greater than the MEC. The range of values between MEC and MTC is referred to as the *therapeutic range*. *AUC*, Area under the concentration-time curve; *MEC*, minimum effective concentration; *MTC*, minimum toxic concentration. *(Modified from Gilman AG, Goodman L, Gilman A, eds. The pharmacological basis of therapeutics, 6th edition. New York: Macmillan, 1980. Reproduced with permission of The McGraw-Hill Companies.)*

established. Measurable concentration ranges collectively define a *therapeutic range* (Figure 34-4) that represents the relationship between *minimum effective concentration* (MEC) and *minimum toxic concentration* (MTC). In the optimal dosing cycle, the *trough blood concentration* (the lowest concentration achieved just before the next dose) should not fall below the MEC, and the *peak blood concentration* (the highest concentration achieved within the dosing cycle) should not rise higher than the MTC. This is usually achieved by administering the drug once every half-life, denoted by τ in Figure 34-4. Multiple dosing regimens should achieve *steady-state* serum drug concentrations consistently greater than the MEC and less than the MTC within the therapeutic range. *Steady state* is the point at which the body concentration of the drug is in equilibrium with the rate of dose administered and the rate of elimination. Blood concentrations greater than the MTC put patients at risk for toxicity; concentrations less than the MEC put them at risk for the disorder that the drug is supposed to treat. MTC and MEC are useful guidelines in therapy; this concept is incorporated into tables presented later in this chapter summarizing specific drug data. Doses must be planned to achieve therapeutic concentrations, and these must be monitored to guide dose adjustment if necessary. The smaller the difference between MEC and MTC, the smaller the therapeutic index and the more likely TDM will be necessary. The key concept to remember is that MEC and MTC define the therapeutic range for most drugs. In contrast to the concept of reference intervals in clinical chemistry, no protocol has been generally accepted for establishing the therapeutic range of a drug. For some therapeutic agents, the onset of toxicity may occur before maximal clinical response; for others, there may exist a threshold above which no further clinical improvement is seen, but which is not associated with adverse effects. The therapeutic range, therefore, represents the range of drug concentrations within which the probability of the desired clinical response is relatively high, and the probability of unacceptable toxicity or failure to achieve further clinical benefit is relatively low.

Antibiotic administration and management deviate from the principles outlined in the previous paragraph. Antibiotics typically are dosed to achieve a *peak blood concentration* that exceeds the minimal inhibitory concentration (MIC) sufficient to kill the infecting organism, but is never greater than the MTC. Antibiotics are administered at intervals much longer than the half-life to allow the antibiotic concentration to decay away to allow the host to recover; the ideal *trough blood concentration* of many antibiotics is nondetectable. Also, antibiotics do not achieve steady state because they do not accumulate.

Pharmacokinetics

Drug Disposition

Pharmacokinetics is the mathematical description of the physiologic disposition of xenobiotics (drugs, poisons, etc.) or endogenous chemicals. The key processes involved in drug disposition include liberation, absorption, distribution, metabolism, and excretion, commonly referred to by the acronym LADME. These processes are affected by several factors specific to the individual receiving the drug, including disease state, comedication, and demographic elements such as age, weight, and gender (Box 34-1). Such factors contribute to interindividual and intraindividual variability in both drug concentration and pharmacologic response, as summarized in Figure 34-5. The processes of drug absorption, distribution, metabolism, and excretion are discussed in the following sections.

Liberation and Absorption

The simplest and most direct route of administering a drug for systemic therapy is intravenous delivery, as infusion into the bloodstream places the complete dose of a compound into immediate circulation. The question of how much of a given dose reaches the patient is therefore essentially bypassed with intravenous administration. However, for reasons of practicality and patient preference, drugs are frequently delivered by alternate means such as oral, intramuscular, transdermal, or sublingual routes; the most common of these is oral administration.

Oral dosing differs from intravenous in that the drug is required to pass from the gastrointestinal tract into the vascular system through a process known as *absorption.* To be absorbed, a compound must dissociate from its dosing formulation into digestive fluids (i.e., the process of liberation), then cross both gastrointestinal and vascular biological membranes by passive diffusion or, less commonly, by active

BOX 34-1 Factors That Influence Drug Disposition in Humans

Demographic Factors
- Age category (premature infant, neonate, infant, child, adolescent adult, elderly adult)
- Weight (obesity, malnourishment)
- Gender
- Race
- Genetic constitution (metabolic enzyme polymorphisms)

Disease-Related Factors
- Liver disease (cirrhosis, hepatitis, cholestasis)
- Kidney disease
- Thyroid disorders (hypothyroidism or hyperthyroidism)
- Cardiovascular disease (arrhythmias, congestive heart failure)
- Gastrointestinal disease or disorder (sprue or other malabsorption syndromes, peptic ulcer, colitis)
- Cancer
- Surgery
- Burns
- Volume status (e.g., dehydration)
- Nutritional status (cachectic or anorexic state)

Extracorporeal Factors
- Hemodialysis
- Peritoneal dialysis
- Cardiopulmonary bypass
- Hypothermia or hyperthermia

Chemical and Environmental Factors Influencing:

Absorption of Drug
- Food or coadministered drug affecting extent and rate of absorption
- Immediate- or extended-release formulation
- Gastric pH and motility
- Activity of transporters (e.g., P-glycoprotein) and GI metabolic enzymes (e.g., CYP3A4)

Distribution of Drug
- Coadministered drug affecting binding to plasma proteins or tissue receptors
- Changes in physiologic composition (e.g., rapid weight loss)
- Pregnancy, aging, or other condition affecting plasma proteins and body composition

Metabolism of Drug
- Food, herbs, or drugs competing for metabolism
- Coadministration of drug that induces metabolic enzymes (e.g., phenobarbital)
- Coadministration of drug that inhibits metabolic enzymes (e.g., cimetidine)

Excretion of Drug
- Coadministration of drug that competes for renal tubular secretory paths (e.g., probenecid, penicillin)
- Changes in urinary flow rate
- Coadministration of compounds that enhance tubular reabsorption (e.g., sodium bicarbonate, phenobarbital)

transport. The ability to negotiate these steps determines the rate and extent of drug absorption and is affected greatly by the nature of the drug itself (e.g., solubility, pK_a), the formulation matrix (e.g., immediate- or sustained-release), and the physiologic environment (e.g., pH, gastrointestinal motility).

Most drugs are weak acids or bases that are able to assume ionized or nonionized forms depending on the surrounding pH. The pK_a or ionization constant of a compound reflects the pH at which the equilibrium between these forms shifts direction. Passive diffusion across lipid membranes requires the drug to be nonionized; thus absorption will occur most readily at a pH where the nonionized form is favored (i.e., below the pK_a of an acidic drug or above the pK_a of a basic drug). For this reason, alterations in gastrointestinal pH (e.g., antacid use) can affect the ability of a compound to enter the circulation. Likewise, use of absorptive resins (e.g., cholestyramine) or medications that influence gastrointestinal motility (e.g., opiates) can change the extent or rate of drug absorption, as can diseases that adversely affect gastrointestinal function.

The rate of absorption is also an important consideration for oral administration. Absorption of a drug generally occurs much more rapidly than its elimination; however, the oral formulation of many agents can be manipulated to produce sustained-release products. These prolong the apparent rate of drug absorption, generally with the intent of allowing less frequent dosing or of lessening the variability in plasma drug concentrations between doses.

The amount of drug absorbed relative to the quantity given is referred to as its *bioavailability* (f). This is calculated as the ratio of drug exposure after equivalent doses of oral and intravenous forms, where exposure is measured as the area under the curve (AUC) of plasma drug concentration over time:

$$f = \frac{AUC_{oral}}{AUC_{iv}} \quad (1)$$

Thus, the better a drug is absorbed, the more its exposure (AUC) after oral dosing resembles exposure after intravenous administration, up to a maximum of 100% bioavailability or identical exposure for the two formulations. To be useful as an oral agent, a compound must be absorbed rapidly and extensively enough to provide therapeutically effective concentrations. This typically corresponds to bioavailability greater than 50%, although exceptions to this general rule are certainly known. In some cases, poor bioavailability is advantageous, as with medications (e.g., antibiotics) whose site of action is the gastrointestinal lumen; in this situation, lack of absorption would prevent systemic exposure while still permitting effective therapy.

In addition to the steps required for absorption, the bioavailability of a compound can be affected by *first-pass metabolism,* which reflects the activity of metabolic enzymes in the intestine and liver. After absorption from the gastrointestinal lumen, drugs can be metabolized in intestinal cells before reaching the bloodstream; furthermore, drugs absorbed from the small intestine are transported via the portal vein directly

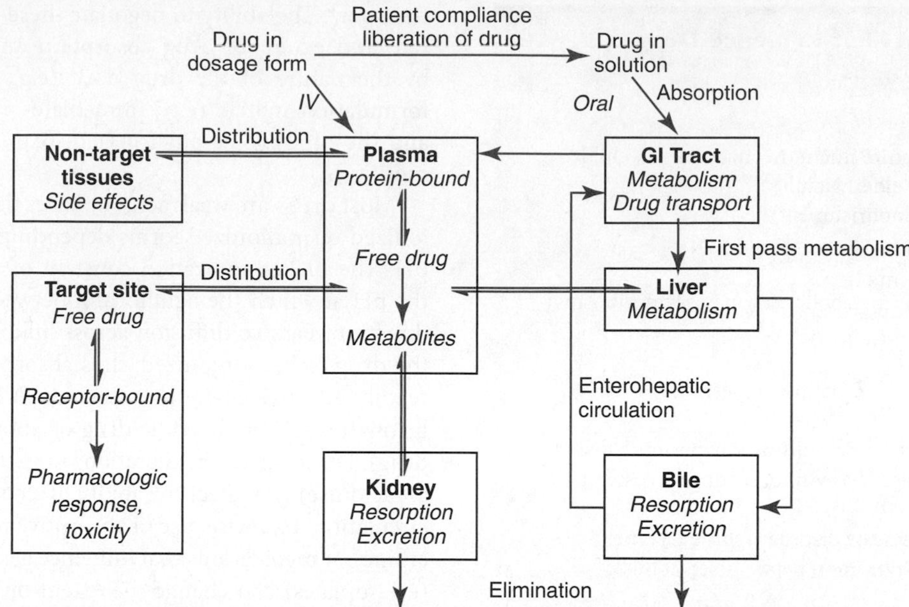

Figure 34-5 Factors affecting plasma drug concentration. *Absorption:* Patients must comply with administration, and the drug must be formulated to ensure bioavailability from the gastrointestinal (GI) tract or other site of absorption. First-pass metabolism occurs for many drugs absorbed via the GI. *Distribution:* The drug may be found in both target and nontarget tissues. Interaction with a receptor or other target molecule is generally required for response, which can include intended (therapeutic), unintended (side), or toxic effects. *Metabolism:* Conversion of the drug to pharmacologically active or inactive compounds may occur in tissue other than the liver. *Elimination:* Excretion in urine or feces is most common, but can also occur via saliva, expired air, breast milk, or other means.

to the liver, where they are exposed to hepatic metabolic enzymes. Thus, first-pass metabolism in the intestine and liver after absorption can preclude entry into the systemic circulation. Similarly, gastrointestinal transporters such as *p*-glycoprotein can expel an absorbed drug before it is able to reach the bloodstream. For these reasons, some drugs that are well absorbed nevertheless have low bioavailability.

Distribution

Once in the bloodstream, drugs undergo a process termed *distribution.* This is the spread of a compound from its point of entry (e.g., digestive tract, infusion catheter) throughout the systemic circulation and into various tissues. Some drugs remain primarily in the blood plasma (e.g., ibuprofen, warfarin); others localize extensively to tissue (e.g., amiodarone, chloroquine). The distribution of a drug to a particular site in the body depends on numerous factors, including drug size, degree of ionization, lipid solubility, extent of protein binding, body composition, and perfusion of the tissue in which the drug accumulates. In general, drugs that distribute extensively tend to be lipophilic, as this facilitates passage through cell membranes; widely distributed compounds often show relatively slow clearance because of the need to remove drug stored in tissue. Alteration of parameters related to distribution can affect the disposition of a drug. For example, rapid weight loss in an acutely ill patient may release drugs previously distributed to adipocytes, leading to elevated serum concentrations and possible toxicity.

Many drugs bind to one or more plasma proteins, most notably albumin, globulins such as α_1-acid glycoprotein (AAG), and lipoproteins. In general, acidic drugs associate primarily with albumin, whereas basic drugs preferentially bind globulins and lipoproteins. An equilibrium exists between the amount of drug that is *protein-bound* and the amount *free,* that is, not bound to protein; disturbances in serum proteins related to pathologic (e.g., stress response, malnutrition) and physiologic (e.g., pregnancy, aging) settings can shift the balance of this equilibrium. Free drug is more readily accessible to cell membranes, drug receptors, and elimination mechanisms; thus the free fraction is considered the active component of the drug responsible for its biological effects. Changes in equilibrium between free and bound drug can greatly affect the physiologic response to that compound. Serum free drug concentrations have been estimated using ultrafiltration or ultracentrifugation techniques; measurement in oral fluid (saliva) has been proposed as an alternative to ultrafiltration but is unacceptable for most compounds.[47]

The fact that many drugs and endogenous molecules (e.g., fatty acids) bind to albumin and other serum proteins creates the potential for one compound to be displaced by another as they compete for limited binding sites. Factors determining whether this displacement occurs include the relative affinity for the binding protein and the concentrations of the compounds involved. For example, elevations in fatty acids can displace weakly bound drugs without affecting strongly bound drugs. Similarly, the antiepileptic agents valproic acid and phenytoin compete for the same binding sites on albumin; the higher concentration of valproic acid allows it to displace phenytoin, increasing the free fraction of the latter. Finally, some agents (e.g., valproic acid) can saturate all available protein-binding sites at therapeutic concentrations, leading to rapid elevations in free drug concentrations if the dose exceeds the point of saturation. It is important to recognize in such situations that the total drug concentration may remain unchanged, even in the setting of clinically significant elevations in the free fraction.

Physiologic states or diseases that alter serum composition (e.g., pH, electrolyte balance) can also affect the equilibrium of free and bound drugs. Thus in many situations, patients may experience adverse effects, even severe toxicity, as a direct consequence of increased free drug concentrations. For highly protein-bound drugs (typically more than 60 to 70% bound), clinically significant changes in the free fraction can go unnoticed if only the total (i.e., protein-bound plus free) concentration is monitored; the total amount of drug in serum may not change, or may even decrease, in situations that significantly elevate free concentrations. For example, in healthy individuals, the total concentration of phenytoin comprises (on average) 90% protein-bound and 10% free drug; a total plasma phenytoin of 15 mg/L in a healthy person would correspond to a free phenytoin concentration of approximately 1.5 mg/L. Uric acid competes with phenytoin for protein binding; thus uremic patients can have free fractions of 20 to 30% of the total phenytoin concentration. In other words, in uremia, the same total phenytoin (15 mg/L) could correspond to a free concentration of 4.5 mg/L, a potentially toxic concentration. Measurement of free drug concentrations is required to manage such situations.

Situations involving alterations in protein concentration can also affect the equilibrium between free and protein-bound drug. Acute stress response is one such setting, especially for basic drugs bound to globulins. AAG is a stress response protein, so its concentrations increase notably after physiologic insult; the rise in circulating AAG may necessitate increases in drug dosage to account for the shift in equilibrium toward the protein-bound state. In contrast, hypoalbuminemia is common in pregnancy and in the elderly. Management of these conditions requires careful attention to clinical presentation and, if available, free drug measurements. Elderly patients in particular may manifest atypical signs of toxicity, notably cognitive changes such as confusion; thus analysis of free drug concentrations may be especially helpful in their care.

Metabolism

Metabolism is the process by which the body alters the chemical structure of a compound, whether endogenous or exogenous. In the context of drug therapy, metabolism is typically thought to enhance excretion of xenobiotics, most commonly by increasing water solubility. It is important to note that this does not necessarily coincide with deactivation or detoxification of the drug. Acetaminophen hepatotoxicity, for example, is the result of a minor metabolite (*N*-acetyl-*p*-benzoquinone imine) rather than the parent compound. Many drug metabolites are themselves active; an excellent example of this is seen with tamoxifen, a selective estrogen receptor modulator used in breast cancer therapy (Figure 34-6). Not only is tamoxifen active, but three of its metabolites display equal (*N*-desmethyltamoxifen) or greater (4-hydroxytamoxifen and endoxifen) anticancer activity compared with the parent drug.[71] Some therapeutics [e.g., acetylsalicylate (aspirin), codeine, tamoxifen] are delivered as inactive or low-activity compounds, called *prodrugs*, which require metabolism by the body to exert the desired physiologic effect. Active metabolites must be considered when the clinical effect of a medication is assessed.

Most drug metabolism in humans is the result of enzymatic activity; metabolic enzymes are expressed ubiquitously in tissues and blood components, but the greatest preponderance by far is found in hepatocytes. Hepatic metabolism varies with age: in neonates and very young infants (<1 year), the liver is immature and metabolic activity is slow. The metabolic rate accelerates as a child ages, reaching a peak around puberty and declining thereafter. Age-specific differences in dosing are often necessary to accommodate this variability in hepatic metabolism. In contrast, the current understanding of extrahepatic metabolism is poor, although undeniably important for certain settings (e.g., intestinal modification of ingested agents, lung detoxification of inhaled compounds).[146] Tissue-specific metabolism may also play a role in interindividual differences in response to drug therapy.[67]

Metabolism can be described using similar mathematical models (e.g., Michaelis-Menten kinetics) to those applied to other enzymatic processes; readers are referred to Chapter 15 for a discussion of enzyme kinetics, although a brief description of *first-order* and *zero-order* processes is appropriate here. Most drugs exhibit first-order metabolism, that is, the rate of their metabolism is proportional to the drug concentration. This occurs when the available metabolic capacity exceeds the amount of drug present; thus the rate of biotransformation primarily depends on how rapidly drug molecules associate with enzyme active sites. Compounds displaying first-order metabolism show a log-linear association of concentration versus time, meaning that a given *fraction* of drug is metabolized per unit time. This forms the basis for a half-life (i.e., the time required to remove 50% of the drug present), as will be discussed in the following sections.

Several agents (e.g., ethanol, salicylate, phenytoin, theophylline) do not follow first-order kinetics. Physiologically relevant concentrations of these drugs approach or exceed normal metabolic capacity; thus the availability of enzyme to bind substrate becomes the rate-limiting factor. This situation, where the rate of metabolism is independent of drug concentration, is termed zero-order or *nonlinear* kinetics (Figure 34-7). The most familiar example of zero-order drug

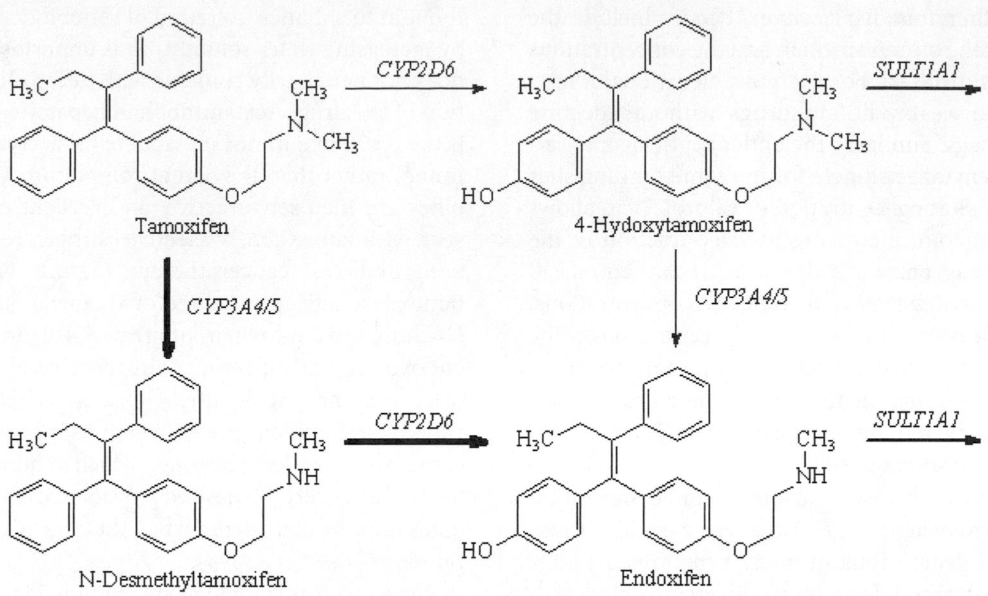

Tamoxifen
CYP2D6
4-Hydoxytamoxifen
SULT1A1
CYP3A4/5
CYP3A4/5
N-Desmethyltamoxifen
CYP2D6
Endoxifen
SULT1A1

Figure 34-6 Tamoxifen and metabolites. Parent tamoxifen is converted to its major metabolite, *N*-desmethyltamoxifen *(thick arrow)*, with a smaller fraction undergoing hydroxylation to 4-hydroxytamoxifen *(thin arrow)*. Both of these metabolites can be converted to endoxifen; all four compounds are active. Both endoxifen and 4-hydroxytamoxifen are eliminated via sulfation. The primary enzymes responsible for metabolism are shown at each step.

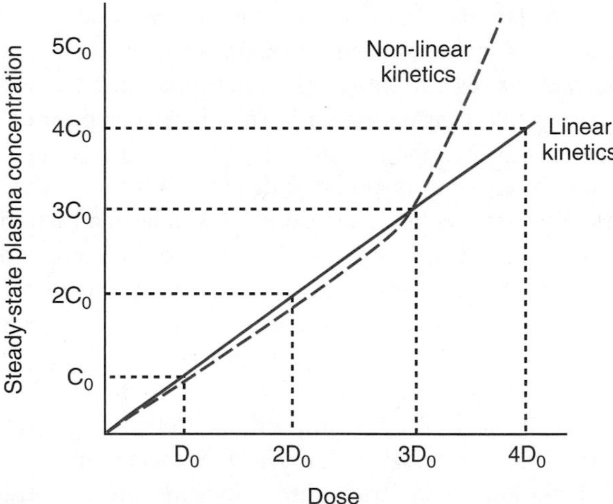

Figure 34-7 Nonlinear response to dose changes. Drugs with linear kinetics *(solid line)* display serum steady-state concentrations *(C)* that vary proportionately with dose *(D)*. In contrast, for drugs with nonlinear kinetics *(dotted line)*, an increase in dose may result in a disproportionate elevation in serum steady-state concentrations.

kinetics is the oft quoted clearance estimate for alcoholic beverages: roughly one drink is eliminated per hour, regardless of the number of drinks consumed. Thus, in contrast to first-order metabolism of a set fraction of drug per unit time, zero-order kinetics affects a given *concentration* of drug per unit time. Although comparatively few drugs display nonlinear behavior at therapeutic concentrations, many will convert to zero-order kinetics in overdoses where available metabolic capacity becomes overwhelmed. An important factor to consider with zero-order behavior is that small dose increases create disproportionately large elevations in serum concentrations because of lack of excess metabolic capacity to accommodate additional drug entering the system.

Metabolic processes can be generalized into two major categories: *phase I* and *phase II* metabolism. Phase I consists of chemical modifications such as oxidation, reduction, hydrolysis, or removal of a nonpolar group (e.g., demethylation); phase II processes involve conjugation of the xenobiotic to a water-soluble moiety such as glucuronic acid, sulfate, or glutathione. The names phase I and phase II indicate a convenient grouping system rather than the order in which steps occur; although some compounds do undergo phase I metabolism followed by phase II, others undergo phase II first, while still others proceed through only one type of metabolic reaction. Most compounds have several possible metabolic pathways that require both phase I and phase II reactions. So-called phase III metabolism refers to the activity of transporters such as P-glycoprotein, which are key regulators of drug activity and metabolism but do not themselves alter chemical structure.

The most important enzymes in phase I metabolism are the cytochrome P450 (CYP) family, with just a few CYP isoenzymes accounting for biotransformation of the vast majority of current pharmaceuticals. Those isoenzymes (CYP2D6, CYP3A4/5, and CYP2C9/10) account for less than half the mass of CYP proteins expressed in the liver[176]; thus there is ample opportunity for substrate competition for enzyme binding sites. Coadministration of drugs or "herbal" products that are metabolized by the same CYPs creates the potential for exceeding available enzymatic capacity, resulting in decreased metabolism of all substrates of that enzyme, whether exogenous or endogenous. Such *drug-drug interactions* can often be managed by adjusting the dose of one or both compounds, so long as the physician is aware of the interaction.

Drug-metabolizing enzymes are subject to a great deal of interindividual variability, both at the concentration of genetic polymorphisms and at transcriptional or post-translational concentrations. Pharmacogenetics studies the effects of genetic variation in *CYP*s and other metabolic enzymes; this topic is covered extensively in Chapter 43 and thus will not be discussed here. At the environmental concentration, metabolic activity can be induced or inhibited by a wide variety of drugs, herbal products, and foods. *Induction* refers to an increase in metabolic activity, typically as a result of enhanced expression of genes encoding drug-metabolizing enzymes. An example of this is the upregulation of *CYP3A4* by the herbal product St. John's Wort; use of this product has been linked to accelerated metabolism of other CYP3A4 substrates including oral contraceptives and immunosuppressive drugs, leading to unintended pregnancies and transplant rejection.[123] Intentional induction of enzymes can be performed therapeutically, as with the use of phenobarbital to induce expression of the glucuronide transferase UGT1A1, an enzyme whose reduced activity results in hyperbilirubinemia (i.e., Gilbert or Crigler-Najjar syndrome).[163]

Inhibition of metabolic activity is more common than enzyme induction. Inhibition can occur by simple substrate competition, where more than one compound must compete for a limited number of enzyme binding sites. This slows the metabolic rate of both substrates, although the difference in metabolism may be more apparent for one of the involved drugs, particularly if one compound has stronger affinity for the enzyme or is present in greater concentration. Other forms of inhibition (e.g., noncompetitive, uncompetitive) directly affect the inherent enzymatic function of a given molecule by binding to the active site or elsewhere on the protein, thus preventing normal metabolic reactions. Mechanisms of enzyme inhibition are discussed in detail in Chapter 15.

Many compounds found in therapeutic drugs (e.g., antiretrovirals, antifungals), herbal products (e.g., saw palmetto, Ginkgo biloba), and common foods (e.g., garlic, green tea) have been reported to inhibit metabolic enzymes. The site of inhibition can be important. For example, grapefruit juice potently inhibits CYP3A4 in intestinal cells.[81] Reduced metabolism in the gut actually increases bioavailability with less influence on elimination; this can greatly affect CYP3A4 substrates with variable absorption, such as the immunosuppressive drug cyclosporine. Several algorithms are available to predict potential drug-drug interactions, using current information on metabolic enzyme (mainly CYP) inhibitors, inducers, and substrates.[55,68,74]

Excretion

Excretion (or elimination) is the final removal of drugs from the body. This can occur by numerous routes, including secretion into sweat, breath, and breast milk, incorporation into hair and nails, or even crossing the placenta into the fetal bloodstream. However, by far the most common means of drug elimination is excretion into urine or stool, depending on the water solubility of the compound. The rate of elimination into urine can be estimated using the glomerular filtration rate (e.g., calculated from serum creatinine).

Clearance can also be measured directly for a particular drug. This requires multiple samples from the same patient and is infrequently done, except for therapeutic agents with a narrow window between efficacy and toxicity. An example of this is the alkylating agent busulfan, used in high doses to ablate bone marrow precursor cells prior to hematopoietic stem cell transplant. Given the delicate balance between effective ablation (leading to successful transplant engraftment) and excessive treatment (leading to serious complications such as veno-occlusive disease of the liver), serial measurements of busulfan are used clinically to assess exposure to the drug and to individualize subsequent doses.[126]

Urine can be a useful matrix for drug testing; it is readily collected in a noninvasive manner, is relatively poor in protein and other analytical interferences, and generally shows higher drug concentrations because of the ability of the kidneys to concentrate compounds filtered from the blood. For these reasons, it is the most common matrix for drugs of abuse testing and other toxicologic applications (see Chapter 35). However, it is important to note that the correlation between urine drug concentrations and serum concentrations is poor at best. This is the result of wide variability in several factors that can affect renal drug elimination, including patient hydration status, urine pH, and circadian fluctuations in renal function. Although it may be possible to normalize urine drug concentrations somewhat with 24-hour urine samples and correction to a marker of renal function such as creatinine, in practice urine is rarely used for TDM purposes. In select exceptions such as assessing patient compliance in pain clinics,[137] samples are obtained frequently, serum concentrations are poorly related to therapeutic efficacy, and risk of drug diversion or misuse is relatively high.

Pharmacokinetic Models

The processes of drug absorption, distribution, metabolism, and elimination are not completely independent steps, but rather occur in an overlapping fashion, often simultaneously, within the body. This is especially true of those agents that are administered serially, as a subsequent dose is typically given before the first dose has been completely eliminated. Thus, it is necessary to have mathematical means of estimating factors such as the amount of drug present at a given time, the rate of clearance of a drug from the system, and the overall exposure to a drug for a given dose. Pharmacokinetic models have been developed to permit such calculations, and the practical aspects of some common models will be discussed here. Readers are referred to previous versions of this chapter for more comprehensive explanation of the derivation of the equations that follow.

Compartmental Models

The concept of physiologic compartments is used to envision the systemic distribution of a drug. A compartment is not a true corollary to a particular organ or fluid; rather, each compartment can be thought of as a representation of those regions of the body (e.g., fluids, various tissues) to which a compound partitions with similar affinity. To clarify this, contrast two dissimilar therapeutic agents: one, a drug such as ibuprofen that remains preferentially in the plasma, and the other, a drug like digoxin that distributes extensively into lipid-rich organs. For the former, an administered dose distributes throughout the systemic circulation with minimal partitioning into tissues; thus, only the pool of drug in the blood needs to be considered when factors such as clearance rate are estimated. Such a compound is well described by a one-compartment model (Figure 34-8), where the compartment in this example is roughly analogous to the systemic circulation.

Alternatively, digoxin exhibits extensive tissue distribution. After absorption of an administered dose, this agent too will rapidly spread throughout the vasculature (the first compartment). However, because of its lipophilic nature, the drug will undergo a second, typically slower process of partitioning into various organs. This step requires passive or active transport into the tissue, thus its kinetics (e.g., rates of entry into, and departure from, tissues) differs from the initial distribution into the bloodstream. This is modeled with a second compartment, approximating the tissue stores of the compound. Because the only fraction of drug available for transport to sites of metabolism and elimination (e.g., liver and kidneys) is in the circulatory system, removal of distributed drug requires re-entry from the secondary "tissue" compartment back into the "blood" compartment (see Figure 34-8). Thus, the presence of a tissue-bound store of drug can greatly increase the amount of time required to fully eliminate a compound. Note that a drug that distributes to tissue can also be modeled reasonably accurately using a single compartment, so long as the drug exhibits similar kinetics in the tissues and fluids involved; the compartments are not true corollaries to regions of the body, merely representations of the number of distinct pools of drug.

The number of compartments included in the model can be extended to three or more; for example, a third compartment could represent sites of extended storage, as seen with strongly lipophilic drugs distributed into adipocytes. For many drugs, increasing the number of compartments will enhance the accuracy of the model. However, each additional compartment increases the complexity of the equations used to describe expected kinetics for the drug of interest. For simplicity, only the one- and two-compartment models will be discussed here.

In a one-compartment model, only a single pool of distributed drug is present within the body, and the rate of elimination is governed by metabolism or clearance from that pool. With a first-order process, a certain percentage of drug is removed per unit time; this is commonly expressed as the *half-life* ($t_{1/2}$), which is a measure of the amount of time required to eliminate 50% of the available drug. Compounds that display zero-order kinetics do not have a true half-life because a constant amount of drug is eliminated per unit time, rather than a constant fraction of the total. However, for a given quantity of a drug with nonlinear kinetics, an *apparent half-life* can be defined that reflects the time required to eliminate 50% of the initial concentration. Note that the apparent half-life changes with alterations in the total amount of drug present (i.e., increasing with higher concentrations and decreasing with lower concentrations).

Drug concentration following first-order elimination decreases in a log-linear fashion, as is shown graphically in Figure 34-9. The slope of the line describing the decline is the *elimination constant, k,* which is a measure of overall elimination that includes loss of drug into urine or feces, loss due to metabolism, and so on. The elimination constant is related to half-life according to the following formula:

$$t_{1/2} = \frac{0.693}{k} \tag{2}$$

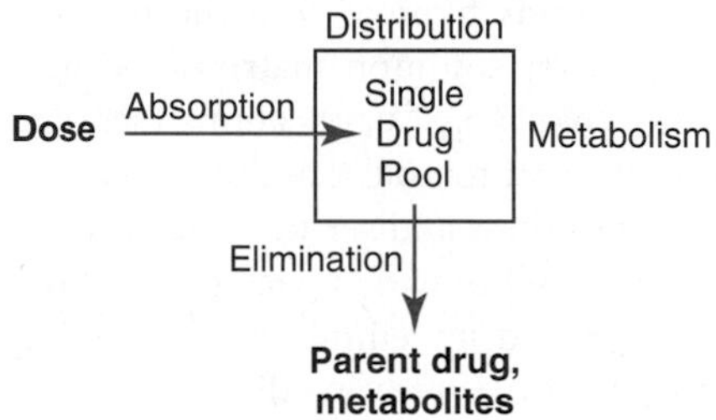

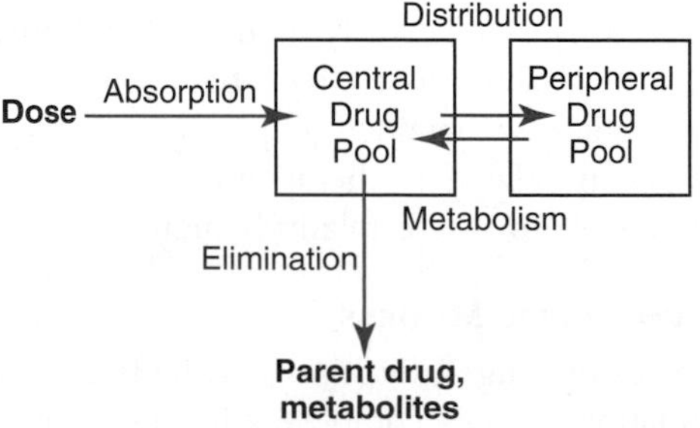

Figure 34-8 One- and two-compartment pharmacokinetic models. For a one-compartment model *(top)*, an administered dose is considered as being contained within a single pool of drug in the body. All pharmacokinetic processes affect that single pool. For a two-compartment model *(bottom)*, pharmacokinetic estimates must consider the equilibration of drug between the central and peripheral compartments. Final elimination from the body generally occurs from the pool of drug contained in the central compartment, thus peripherally distributed drug must re-enter the central compartment to be removed.

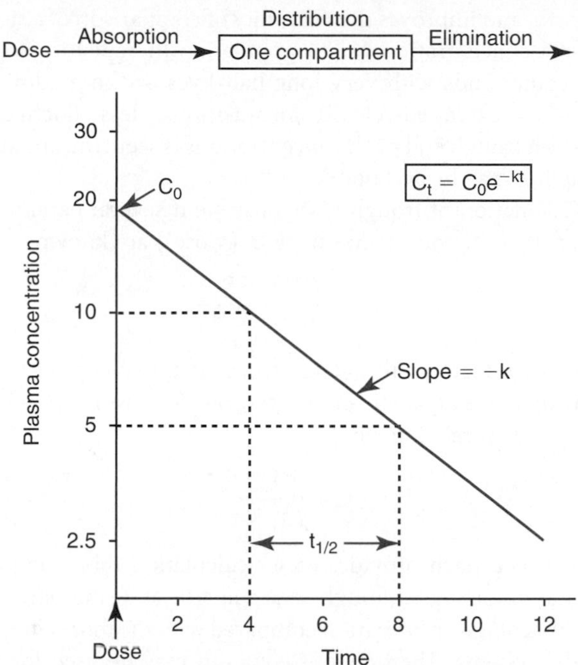

Figure 34-9 Drug concentration in plasma after administration of a dose, for a one-compartment model. Monoexponential decline from the original concentration (C_0) is described by the elimination constant (*k*), which is related to the drug half-life ($t_{1/2}$). Drug concentration at any time (C_t) can be estimated with knowledge of C_0, *k*, and the time (*t*).

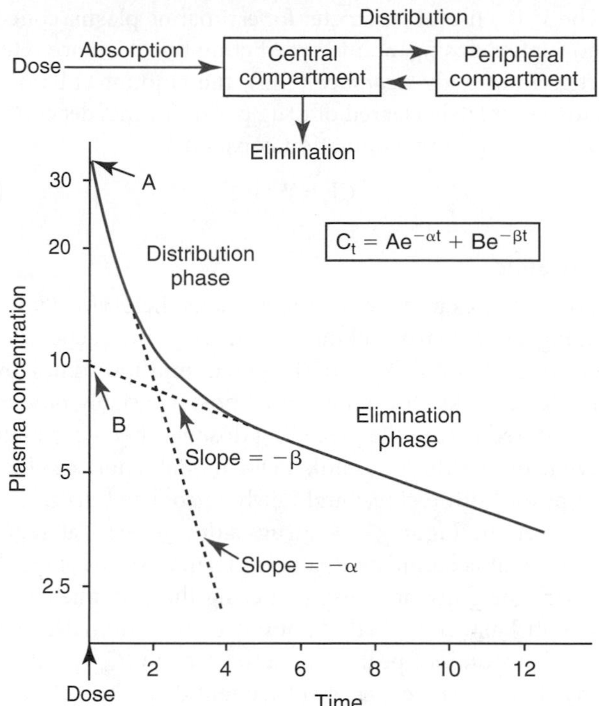

Figure 34-10 Drug concentration in plasma after administration of a dose for a two-compartment model. Decline from the original concentration (C_0) is affected by both the distribution phase (characterized by the constant α) and the elimination phase (characterized by the constant β).

In this model, the concentration of drug at any time (C_t) following a single dose can be calculated from the original concentration (C_0), the elimination constant, and the time (*t*):

$$C_t = C_0e^{-kt} \tag{3}$$

In a two-compartment model, the kinetics of distribution and elimination are distinct from one another, in contrast to the simpler one-compartment model. As shown in Figure 34-10, the initial plasma concentration of drug declines rapidly as the compound equilibrates between the two compartments. This is termed the *distribution phase*. As equilibrium between the two compartments is approached, the dominant kinetic mechanism becomes the elimination of drug from the plasma pool. This is termed the *elimination phase*. In general, the elimination process is slowed by the need for drug to leave the tissue compartment before it can be cleared from the body. The slopes fitted to the two phases reflect the distribution (α) and elimination (β) constants, which in turn determine corresponding half-lives for each phase. The distribution half-life is commonly called the *alpha half-life,* while the elimination half-life is the *beta half-life*. Calculation of concentration following a single dose incorporates both phases, as is evident in the following equation:

$$C_t = Ae^{-\alpha t} + Be^{-\beta t} \tag{4}$$

As discussed earlier, it is possible for a one-compartment model to describe a variety of drugs, ranging from water-soluble compounds found almost exclusively in the blood, to more lipophilic molecules that simply show similar kinetics in tissues and fluids. To account for differences in the extent of distribution, a *volume of distribution* (V_d) can be determined for each drug. The V_d is defined by the relationship between a single dose (D_0) corrected for bioavailability (*f*) and the plasma concentration (C_0) observed after dosing:

$$V_d = \frac{D_0 \, X f}{C_0} \tag{5}$$

The V_d is not an actual physiologic volume; rather, it is a calculated parameter that can be much larger than the volume of a human body. A helpful description is that the V_d is the volume of fluid theoretically required to dilute a given dose to its known concentration if the drug were present only in the blood. If the majority of a compound enters tissue, its plasma concentration will be low, resulting in a higher calculated V_d. Thus a large V_d reflects extensive distribution, and a small V_d suggests that the drug is preferentially retained in the vasculature.

The value of V_d in an individual depends on many of the factors that determine distribution of a compound, including drug lipophilicity, body composition, protein binding, and so forth. Thus, although it is commonly provided as an average value, V_d can show substantial interindividual variability. V_d can be expressed as a volume (e.g., in liters) or as a volume per unit body weight (e.g., L/kg).

The V_d is a useful parameter for estimating plasma concentrations after dosing, and for predicting the clearance rate of a drug. Total body *clearance* (Cl_T), the amount of blood or plasma completely cleared of drug per unit time, depends on both the V_d and the elimination constant *k:*

$$Cl_T = V_d k \tag{6}$$

Steady State

Although the example of a single dose is helpful for understanding basic pharmacokinetic principles, in practice TDM is performed for drugs administered multiple times over many days, weeks, or even years. Almost invariably, doses are administered before the preceding dose has been completely eliminated; thus to be useful, TDM models must be able to account for both residual and newly introduced drug.

As seen in Figure 34-4, drugs administered at regular intervals will accumulate to a point termed *steady state,* that is, where the amount of drug entering the systemic circulation is in balance with the amount being eliminated. Each dose still produces a peak *(C_{max})* and a trough *(C_{min})*, but once steady state is reached, each subsequent dose should provide an identical profile of drug concentration versus time. For the purposes of this discussion, the dosing interval (τ) will be assumed to equal the half-life, although this is not universally true in practice.

Assuming doses are given at each half-life, a drug with first-order kinetics will require more than five doses to approach steady-state concentrations (>95% of C_{ss}). Similarly, at the end of therapy, five to seven half-lives after the last dose must pass for more than 95% of the steady-state concentration to be eliminated. Reaching steady state can be more complicated for drugs with very long half-lives, such as the antiarrhythmic agent amiodarone ($t_{1/2}$ = 25 days). The time to steady state would be prohibitively long if such a compound were administered only once per half-life; thus such agents are usually given in a larger, initial bolus known as a *loading dose* to rapidly elevate plasma concentrations closer to steady-state concentrations.

Particular caution must be used with drugs that display nonlinear kinetics. Recall that elimination of such compounds is not affected by the drug concentration; thus an increase in the administered dose is not countered by a corresponding enhancement in clearance. Therefore, a drug with zero-order properties will respond disproportionately to changes in dosing; for example, doubling the dose will result in greater than twofold elevation in plasma concentrations. In addition, because the apparent half-life changes with alterations in the amount of drug present, the time required to reach a new steady-state concentration varies compared with a drug with linear kinetics (e.g., prolonged after a dose increase because of the longer apparent half-life).

Once steady state is achieved, TDM measurements are generally made at trough, that is, immediately before a scheduled dose. The rationale for this is that trough sampling minimizes interpatient variability in absorption, distribution, and so forth, and improves the reliability of comparison of a single plasma concentration versus population therapeutic ranges. For compounds with very long half-lives or those administered as extended-release formulations, less fluctuation between trough and peak concentrations is seen; thus random sampling may be acceptable.

Calculation of trough C_{ss} is possible if several parameters [D_0, *f*, V_d, *k*, τ, and *t* (time since last dose)] are known:

$$C_{SS} = \frac{(D_0 \times f)e^{-kt}}{V_d(1 - e^{-kt})} \tag{7}$$

If these factors are not known, it is possible to estimate a median steady-state concentration *(C)* using a model-independent relationship:

$$C = \frac{D_{0 \times f}}{Cl_T \times \tau} \tag{8}$$

This approach provides easier calculation than compartmental modeling, although with the risk of losing pertinent pharmacologic information compared with the more complex model systems. The previous equation may be used for any drug but is most relevant when the half-life of the drug is considerably greater than the dosing interval.

CLINICAL AND ANALYTICAL CONSIDERATIONS

A robust TDM program offers clinicians the means to better manage patients and has the potential to improve patient quality of life through optimizing dose, supporting compliance, and minimizing toxicity. The practice of TDM has been expanded and enhanced by advancements in rapid, sensitive, and specific analytical techniques for a wide variety of therapeutic agents.

Clinical Utility

The best candidate drugs for TDM are those meeting one or more of the following criteria: (1) a narrow therapeutic index; (2) used for long-term therapy; (3) correlation between serum concentration and clinical response; (4) wide interindividual or intraindividual variability in pharmacokinetics; (5) absence of a biomarker associated with therapeutic outcome; or (6) administered with other, potentially interacting compounds. Ideally, TDM allows determination of a baseline drug concentration at a time when the patient is responding well clinically and is known to be compliant; this baseline therapeutic concentration can then be used over time to assess compliance, address physiologic or pathologic changes, and maintain optimal dosing for each individual patient. Single measurements of serum drug concentrations should always be interpreted in the context of clinical presentation, length of therapy, comedications, and other factors capable of affecting serum concentrations.

Chronic pharmacologic therapy is a necessary component in managing many conditions. Some therapeutic agents have convenient biomarkers or clinical indicators of their efficacy; for example, statin treatment can be assessed by quantifying cholesterol, and antihypertensive therapy can be evaluated by following blood pressure. However, for many drugs, biomarkers and clinical indicators are absent or are not visible until after the onset of therapeutic failure (e.g., transplant rejection resulting from inadequate immunosuppression). Such drugs are frequently managed using TDM, particularly when the condition for which they are prescribed involves the potential for serious risk to the patient, as with antiseizure therapy or post-transplant immunosuppression. Even for agents with available biomarkers, use of TDM can often assist clinical decision making; if a patient on antiarrhythmic therapy fails to improve cardiac rhythm, TDM may be able to clarify whether the patient requires a different dose, is refractory to that particular drug, or is simply noncompliant.

The ability to detect noncompliance is a major asset of consistent use of TDM. The World Health Organization estimates that only half of patients on long-term drug therapy comply with the prescribed regimen; noncompliance may be a result of taking the medication erratically, too often, too infrequently, or not at all. The cost of medication noncompliance is estimated at more than $100 billion in the United States alone.[59] Patients at particular risk include the elderly, who frequently must manage several drug regimens for comorbidities; those with conditions prone to reducing ability or will to comply (e.g., severe depression); and individuals whose conditions include asymptomatic periods, wherein patients feel better and forget or do not feel the need to continue treatment. Without routine TDM, noncompliance with therapy may remain unnoticed until symptoms resume (e.g., renewed seizure activity in an epileptic individual) or the treatment fails (e.g., rejection of a transplanted organ).

Serum drug concentrations are useful in many stages of treatment. Initial selection and dosing of a drug may be guided by TDM, particularly if wide interpatient variability in absorption, metabolism, or other parameters of drug disposition is noted. Without measuring drug concentrations, it is difficult to discern which patients respond poorly to therapeutic concentrations of a particular drug and which ones simply are not within the therapeutic range. Similarly, the presence of comorbidities (e.g., hepatic failure, renal dysfunction) or comedications can complicate the process of establishing an effective dose; population pharmacokinetics often does not adequately address comorbidities or drug interactions, necessitating TDM for such patients.

Routine TDM is also helpful for detecting and managing alterations in drug disposition within an individual. Such changes can occur with physiologic processes (e.g., puberty, pregnancy, aging); however, they may also reflect development or progression of a pathologic state. Conditions as seemingly simple as weight loss or as complex as severe illness can radically affect the disposition of a drug within a single patient; these changes can occur rapidly and may be very difficult to manage clinically. Both acute and chronic shifts in pharmacokinetic behavior can be addressed more effectively with TDM because dose adjustments can be guided by each individual patient's serum drug concentrations.

Analytical Concerns

A wide variety of analytical techniques are available to facilitate TDM, including numerous permutations of immunoassay methods such as enzyme multiplied immunoassay technique (EMIT), fluorescent polarization immunoassay (FPIA), cloned enzyme donor immunoassay (CEDIA), and chromatographic techniques such as gas chromatography–mass spectrometry (GC-MS), liquid chromatography–mass spectrometry/mass spectrometry (LC-MS/MS), and high performance liquid chromatography–ultraviolet (HPLC-UV). These methods are discussed in Chapters 13 and 16. Immunoassays provide rapid results and ready automation; chromatographic techniques improve specificity and limits of detection, although at a lower throughput. Unfortunately, commercial immunoassays are not available for many of the newer-generation drugs. LC-MS/MS is progressively replacing other HPLC-based methods; it displays greater selectivity and fewer analytical interferences, allowing development of multianalyte assays with higher throughput and less influence from metabolites or other potentially coeluting compounds. The choice of analytical method typically depends on the availability of resources (e.g., technologist expertise, laboratory funding) and the clinical demand for turnaround.

TDM analysis embodies many of the same concerns as other areas of clinical chemistry: the need for accurate, reproducible methods; the requirement for quality assurance and proficiency testing programs; and the necessity of establishing target ranges (i.e., therapeutic indices) and critical values (e.g., toxic concentrations). Certain preanalytical and analytical issues are of particular importance for drug assays. For example, some pharmaceuticals adsorb to the gel matrix in serum or plasma separator tubes, causing falsely low apparent drug concentrations and making these collection devices unacceptable for many tests. Similarly, the time of blood draw relative to administration of the drug is often a key factor in the interpretation of TDM results. Most TDM protocols require sampling at trough (i.e., immediately before the next scheduled dose), particularly for compounds with short half-lives or variable pharmacokinetics.

Other considerations for TDM include the determination of which metabolites and which drug fractions (e.g., free or protein-bound) are clinically relevant. Active metabolites should be quantified, and if the parent compound is also active (i.e., not a prodrug), the concentrations of parent and metabolite should be considered together in interpretation of the results. Inactive metabolites are often of interest as well. They may be associated with toxicity that is independent of the drug's intended activity (e.g., the acetaminophen metabolite *N*-acetyl-*p*-benzoquinone imine) or may serve as a reservoir for conversion to active drug (e.g., the glucuronide conjugate of the immunosuppressant mycophenolic acid). Metabolites often accumulate at a different rate than the parent drug; thus inactive metabolites may provide longer detection windows or in vivo assessment of an individual's metabolic capacity.

TDM of drugs with extensive protein binding may benefit from monitoring of free drug concentrations. In reasonably healthy individuals free of conditions affecting protein concentrations (e.g., pregnancy, malnutrition) or of comedications capable of altering the free versus bound equilibrium, analysis of free drug concentrations typically is not necessary. However, illness, physiologic alterations, or changes in comedications may shift the balance of free drug concentrations; similarly, free drug measurements are helpful in managing digoxin overdose treated with a drug-binding agent that nullifies but does not remove the excess digoxin. Equilibrium dialysis is the reference method for most free drug assays but is extremely time-consuming. In practice, ultrafiltration is used to remove larger molecules, including protein-bound drug; removal is followed by analysis of the remaining unbound fraction.

Finally, one further issue of clinical and analytical relevance to TDM is the format in which concentration units are expressed. Measured therapeutic drug concentrations are often expressed in units of micrograms per milliliter (μg/mL) or milligrams per liter (mg/L). However, it is recognized that use of the abbreviation μ could adversely affect patient safety.[29] For example, in prescribing medication, a handwritten "μg" can be mistaken for mg (milligram), resulting in a thousandfold overdose of drug, which clearly has the potential to harm a patient. As part of the National Patient Safety Goals initiative, the U.S. Joint Commission (formerly the Joint Commission on Accreditation of Healthcare Organizations) has identified common abbreviations that might be misinterpreted and therefore should not be used in healthcare, especially when medication is prescribed.[2] Of relevance to the clinical laboratory is the use of μg as the abbreviation for microgram. Although μg is not currently on the list of abbreviations to be avoided, it is among a group of notations that are reviewed yearly and considered for inclusion on the "Do Not Use" list.[1,2,29]

Institutions accredited by the Joint Commission now use "mcg" rather than μg when prescribing medication. Some clinical laboratories have likewise chosen to use mcg in reporting concentrations, although other laboratories continue to use μg in laboratory reports, as this practice does not pose the same risks as those inherent in prescribing medication. The Joint Commission states that the "Do Not Use" list of abbreviations does not currently apply to preprogrammed health information technology systems such as laboratory information systems, electronic medical records, or computerized provider order entry systems.[1] Complicating the issue, many national and international organizations [e.g., the Unified Code for Units of Measure (http://unitsofmeasure.org/) and the American Medical Association Manual of Style (http://www.amamanualofstyle.com/)] recommend or mandate the use of μ as the symbol for "micro." It should be noted that if concentrations are reported in units of mg/L, this obviates any problem with the use of μg/mL without affecting the numeric value. Drug concentrations in this chapter are provided as mg/L (equivalent to μg/mL) or μg/L (equivalent to ng/mL) unless conventionally reported in molar units.

SPECIFIC DRUG GROUPS

Drugs that are routinely monitored are conveniently classified by the type of therapy they support (e.g., control of epilepsy or infection, management of respiratory or cardiac function, suppression of immune response). The following discussion is organized in accordance with classifications commonly recognized. Note that some drugs, such as salicylate and nitroprusside (assessed by the quantification of thiocyanate), are discussed in Chapter 35.

Antiepileptics

Many drugs are available for treating seizures (Table 34-1). In general, antiepileptic drugs prevent or minimize seizures by augmenting inhibitory processes, for example, by enhancing γ-aminobutyric acid (GABA)-mediated neurotransmission or inhibiting excitatory processes (e.g., voltage- or ligand-gated ion channels, glutamate-mediated neurotransmission) in the brain. Therefore, it is not surprising that some of these drugs are also used as sedatives; to treat neuropathic pain, migraine headaches, and psychiatric conditions; and to manage addictions.[186] The discussion presented here is limited to application of antiepileptic TDM to support management of seizures, based on widely accepted consensus documents[96,98,145,192] and information provided in individual drug labeling.

Antiepileptic drugs were among the first class of drugs monitored to establish appropriate dosing, in part because both underdosing and overdosing can be manifested by seizure activity, making it difficult to titrate and optimize dose clinically. In addition, therapeutic and toxic effects of early drugs such as phenobarbital and phenytoin were shown to relate to serum concentrations. TDM provided a vehicle through which noncompliance and drug-drug interactions could be identified. In 1971 a workshop produced an authoritative reference book regarding TDM of antiepileptic drugs.[213] Several books and consensus documents evolved from this and subsequent workshops held in locations worldwide. As many laboratories began to develop analytical methods to support TDM of antiepileptic drugs, it was recognized that substantial variation existed in results among laboratories.[151] Through international cooperation, antiepileptic drug quality control programs were established that helped promote consistency harmonization and improved quality of results. The introduction of commercially available semiautomated assays for TDM in the 1980s further improved standardization of laboratory testing and enhanced accessibility of testing for patients.[211,212] However, essentially no new drugs were introduced for seizure control between 1980 and 1990. Therefore, antiepileptic drugs are frequently described as first-generation

TABLE 34-1 Pharmacokinetic Parameters of Antiepileptic Drugs

Drug	Recommended[145,207] Therapeutic Range, mg/L	Mean Time to Steady State, d	Observed Range of Half-Life in Adults, h[†]	Mean Volume of Distribution, L/kg	Mean Oral Bioavailability, %	Protein Binding, %	Important Metabolizing Enzymes
Carbamazepine	4-12	2-4	8-12	1.4	70	75	CYP3A4
Clonazepam	0.02-0.07	3-10	17-56	3.2	>90	85	CYP3A4
Ethosuximide	40-100	7-10	30-60	0.7	>90	0	CYP3A4
Felbamate	30-60	3-4	14-21	0.8	>90	25	CYP3A4
Gabapentin	2-20	1-2	5-9	0.9	Variable	0	NA
Lamotrigine	2.5-15	3-6	20-30	1.2	>90	55	NA
Levetiracetam	12-46	1-2	6-8	0.6	>90	0	NA
Monohydroxy oxcarbazepine (MHD)*	3-35	2-3	8-15	0.8	>90	40	NA
Phenobarbital	10-40	12-24	70-140	0.7	>90	50	CYP2C19
Phenytoin	10-20 (free: 1.0-2.0)	5-17	30-100	0.6	80	90	CYP2C9, 2C19
Primidone	5-10	2-4	3-22	0.7	>90	20	CYP2C9, 2C19
Tiagabine	0.02-0.2	1-2	5-9	1.4	>90	96	CYP3A4
Topiramate	5-20	4-5	20-30	0.7	80	15	NA
Valproic acid	50-100	2-4	11-20	0.2	>90	90	CYP2C9, 2C19, 2B6, 2E1, 2A6
Vigabatrin	0.8-36	1-2	5-8	0.8	60	0	NA
Zonisamide	10-40	9-12	50-70	1.4	65	50	CYP2C19, 3A4

*Active metabolite not available as a unique drug.
[†]Based on average half-life and no interfering medications.
NA, Not applicable.

or classical (introduced clinically prior to 1990), versus newer or second-generation (introduced clinically after 1990). Many additional antiepileptic drugs are currently in development and showing promise,[20] but they are not discussed here.

Professional organizations, such as those represented by the International League Against Epilepsy, continue to actively produce and review guidelines for TDM of all currently used antiepileptic drugs, most recently in 2008.[145] Although therapeutic ranges and toxic thresholds are proposed for all antiepileptic drugs, the overwhelming caution is to "treat the patient, not the level." Most antiepileptic therapy is administered long-term, possibly life-long, meaning that dosing requirements will change with age, stage of development, and clinical status. In addition to comparing steady-state concentrations of antiepileptic drugs versus proposed therapeutic ranges and toxic thresholds, TDM for antiepileptics is used early in therapy to ensure that steady-state concentrations have been achieved before efficacy is evaluated, particularly for drugs that exhibit nonlinear and/or variable pharmacokinetics. With maintenance therapy, TDM is useful to identify and manage drug-drug interactions, to manage changes in dose or drug formulation, and to evaluate compliance, particularly when signs of therapeutic failure or toxicity are evident.[97] In general, older antiepileptic drugs are monitored more frequently than the newer drugs, in part because of the wide availability of automated immunoassays. In general, immunoassay procedures target a single analyte (usually the parent drug) and are fast, inexpensive, and available for a wide variety of analyzers. When immunoassays are not available, or in certain clinical situations wherein higher sensitivity and specificity than can be accomplished through existing immunoassays is required, chromatographic methods are applied to support antiepileptic TDM.[112] Chromatographic methods are particularly valuable in situations wherein pharmacologically active metabolites are important to monitor with parent drug, when no commercial methods are available, or when commercial methods are fraught with poor specificity. Another advantage of chromatographic methods is that simultaneous analyses of multiple drugs and active drug metabolites can be accomplished to monitor polypharmacy, but also to improve the efficiency of operations in the laboratory.[102]

Some antiepileptics are extensively bound to circulating plasma proteins. As with most drugs, only the unbound (free) fraction of drug is able to pass through membranes to exert pharmacologic activity, and many drug-drug interactions occur as a result of competition for protein-binding sites. For patients with unpredictable protein concentrations, or for whom drug-drug interactions are a significant concern, it may be appropriate to provide TDM for the free fraction of drug. For example, if the proportion of drug bound to proteins changes from 95 to 80%, the amount of active (free) drug in circulation will increase dramatically, while the total drug concentration for that patient may not change. As such, risk of toxicity could be missed and TDM results could be misinterpreted, particularly for pregnant women and elderly persons with poor nutritional status who are managed with multiple medications.[39] Most analytical techniques are designed to measure total drug concentrations and do not distinguish between free and bound drug concentrations. To accommodate TDM of free drug concentrations, protein-bound drug can be separated and removed from plasma using physical or chemical techniques. Resulting free drug concentrations can be determined by immunoassays or chromatographic techniques, with calibration and sensitivity designed to accommodate lower concentrations than those observed when total drug concentrations are measured.[128] In theory, measurement of drugs in oral fluid (saliva) could approximate free drug concentrations. Antiepileptic TDM using saliva is of interest because of the convenience of specimen collection, particularly at the time of a seizure, and for children. Oral fluid testing is not currently done routinely. However, oral fluid may become an important specimen type of the future. When a standardized method of saliva stimulation is used, a linear relationship between drug concentrations and dose has been observed for some drugs such as valproic acid, but not for others such as carbamazepine.[121]

Key attributes of TDM support for specific antiepileptic drugs that are currently in use are provided here, organized along the following historical lines.

1. *Traditional and still widely used:* Antiepileptic drugs introduced before 1990 and currently in use include carbamazepine, phenytoin, phenobarbital, primidone, clonazepam, diazepam, ethosuximide, fosphenytoin, and valproic acid.
2. *Contemporary:* Antiepileptic drugs introduced after 1990 and currently in use include felbamate, gabapentin, levetiracetam, lamotrigine, oxcarbazepine, pregabalin, tiagabine, topiramate, vigabatrin, and zonisamide.
3. *Historical and not widely used:* Bromides, methsuximide, ethotoin, and mephobarbital.

Traditional Antiepileptics, Still Widely Used

Benzodiazepines

Benzodiazepines are a diverse class of drugs that, similar to barbiturates, reduce neuronal excitation through agonist activity at the $GABA_A$ receptor (increasing the duration of chloride flow into the synapse). Although many benzodiazepines have antiseizure activity, those used most often in management of seizures include diazepam (proprietary name Valium) and clonazepam (proprietary name Klonopin). Both drugs are available in a wide variety of formulations and are sold under other names. Diazepam is frequently administered by the rectal or intravenous route in emergency situations, such as to gain control of status epilepticus. Diazepam is not used for long-term control of seizure disorders because tolerance at the $GABA_A$ receptor develops rapidly, and the drug becomes ineffective within 2 to 3 days. Because tolerance to clonazepam does not develop rapidly, it is used to manage absence seizures, infantile spasms, akinetic seizures, and Lennox-Gastaut syndrome. The remaining discussion will focus on clonazepam.

Clonazepam is rapidly and completely absorbed after oral dosing, and peak plasma concentrations occur after 1 to 4 hours. Clonazepam has a relatively high volume of distribution (3.2 L/kg). Protein binding is approximately 85%.

Clonazepam is extensively metabolized by CYP3A4 as well as by glucuronidation and sulfation reactions. As such, modulators of CYP3A4 will affect plasma concentrations of clonazepam. The 7-amino-clonazepam metabolite has some pharmacologic activity and is present in approximately equal concentrations to parent drug at steady state. The half-life of clonazepam is 17 to 56 hours for adults, and 23 to 33 hours for children. Clearance is increased by coadministration of enzyme-inducing drugs and other antiepileptics such as carbamazepine and phenytoin.

Serum concentrations of clonazepam increase in a linear fashion with doses for both children and adults; however, serum concentrations are not well correlated with efficacy or toxicity because of the development of tolerance that occurs to some extent with long-term administration. For patients that respond to clonazepam, serum concentrations are generally reported to fall within the range of 15 to 60 μg/L.[53,91] The proposed therapeutic range is 20 to 70 μg/L. At concentrations higher than 80 μg/L, no additional seizure protection is observed, and toxicity (drowsiness and ataxia) ensues.

Carbamazepine

Carbamazepine (proprietary name Tegretol) is available under other names and in generic form. Similar to phenytoin, carbamazepine modulates the synaptic sodium channel, which prolongs inactivation, reducing the ability of the neuron to respond at high frequency.[30] The physiologic effect of this action is reduction in central synaptic transmission, aiding in control of abnormal neuronal excitability. Carbamazepine is used in the treatment of generalized tonic-clonic, partial, and partial-complex seizures. Carbamazepine also has an antidiuretic effect, reducing concentrations of antidiuretic hormone, although it is unlikely that this contributes to antiepileptic activity.

After oral administration, carbamazepine is slowly but erratically absorbed with wide individual formulation–based variability. Approximately 75% of the drug is protein bound. For this reason, determination of protein-free carbamazepine concentrations for patients with abnormally low or unpredictable concentrations of albumin is sometimes clinically important. The volume of distribution is modest at 1 to 2 L/kg. The elimination half-life early after the first dose varies from 18 to 55 hours for adults and from 3 to 32 hours for children. During maintenance dosing, the half-life is 8 to 20 hours for adults, 10 to 14 hours for children, and 30 to 50 hours in elderly patients. The reduced half-life with long-term therapy is explained somewhat by the induction of CYP3A4. Because hepatic metabolism is the principal means by which plasma concentration is reduced, any reduction in liver function results in drug accumulation. The active metabolite of carbamazepine is carbamazepine-10,11-epoxide formed by the action of CYP3A4. This metabolite has been found to accumulate in children and exists in concentrations equivalent to carbamazepine. Monitoring of ratios may be useful for evaluating compliance and drug-drug interactions. Cross-reactivity of this metabolite in commercial immunoassays is variable and should be considered when carbamazepine TDM is provided. Because carbamazepine is metabolized by CYP3A4, drugs that induce this enzyme (erythromycin, oxcarbazepine, phenytoin, and St. John's Wort) increase the rate of clearance of carbamazepine. Coadministration of erythromycin, phenytoin, or valproic acid increases the rate of metabolism of carbamazepine, reducing the blood concentration. Itraconazole and grapefruit juice interfere with CYP3A4 activity, increasing carbamazepine concentrations.

The therapeutic concentration range for optimal pharmacologic effect of carbamazepine is 4 to 12 mg/L. Toxicity associated with excessive carbamazepine may occur at plasma concentrations in excess of 15 mg/L (or free carbamazepine >3 mg/L) and is characterized by symptoms of blurred vision, paresthesia, nystagmus, ataxia, drowsiness, and diplopia.[186] Side effects unrelated to plasma concentration include development of an urticarial rash, which usually disappears on discontinuation of the drug, and hematologic depression (leukopenia, thrombocytopenia, and aplastic anemia).

Ethosuximide

Ethosuximide (proprietary name Zarontin) is used for the treatment of absence seizures characterized by brief loss of consciousness. Ethosuximide reduces the flow of calcium through T-type calcium channels in the synapse of thalamic neurons. Because thalamic neurons are the main source of 3-Hz spike-wave rhythms in absence seizures, reduction of calcium flow slows the rate of these seizure-inducing pulses. Ethosuximide is a chiral molecule that is used clinically as a racemic mixture.

Ethosuximide is readily absorbed from the gastrointestinal tract with near complete bioavailability. Several formulations are available, a fact that influences the time to peak concentrations; for example, liquid suspension is absorbed faster than capsules. Peak concentrations also vary with age and occur faster in adults (1 to 4 hours) than in children (3 to 7 hours). Ethosuximide is not protein bound, has a V_d of 0.7 L/kg, and undergoes extensive metabolism. In children, its half-life is approximately 33 hours, although this may be prolonged to as long as 60 hours in adults. The drug is cleared in a linear fashion, primarily by metabolism mediated by CYP3A4 (hydroxyethyl metabolite) and the glucuronide. Drug-drug interactions occur primarily as a result of enzyme induction or through CYP3A4. Valproic acid is reported to exert variable effects on ethosuximide concentrations.

The established therapeutic range of ethosuximide is 40 to 100 mg/L, although it is not uncommon that higher concentrations are required. Toxicity related to an excessive blood concentration of ethosuximide is rare. Symptoms of gastrointestinal distress, lethargy, dizziness, and euphoria may be encountered early in therapy, but patients usually become tolerant to these symptoms.

Phenobarbital

Phenobarbital is a broad-spectrum antiepileptic drug that was introduced clinically in 1912 under the name Luminal. It is now known by a wide variety of proprietary names, is given alone or in combination with many other drugs, and is still used today to manage all but absence seizure types. It is known to reduce synaptic transmission, resulting in decreased excitability of the entire nerve cell, inducing sedation. Phenobarbital potentiates synaptic inhibition through action on the $GABA_A$ receptor by increasing the duration of chloride flow into the synapse. The end result is an increase in seizure threshold with inhibition of the spread of discharges from epileptic foci.

Serum concentrations of phenobarbital are well correlated with dose; however, pharmacokinetics is widely variable. Absorption of oral phenobarbital is near complete, but the rate of absorption is age dependent—rapid in adults, slow in children. Thus, the time at which peak plasma concentrations are reached ranges from 4 to 10 hours after the dose. Phenobarbital is 40 to 60% bound to plasma proteins, wherein protein binding is higher in adults than in children. Children have larger V_d values than adults, although V_d is generally about 0.6 to 1.0 L/kg. CYP2C19 is the primary hepatic enzyme involved in metabolism, producing an elimination half-life of 70 to 140 hours; metabolism is also age dependent (children average 70 hours, geriatric patients 100 hours). Phenobarbital is metabolized by CYP2C19 to *p*-hydroxyphenobarbital, which is largely excreted as the glucuronide. Drug-drug interactions are common. For example, phenobarbital concentrations increase with coadministration of phenytoin, valproic acid, felbamate, and oxcarbazepine. Phenobarbital concentrations decrease with coadministration of other barbiturates, alcohol, rifampin, or carbamazepine. When renal or hepatic function is decreased, patients experience decreased clearance of the drug and a prolonged half-life. Phenobarbital is also recognized to induce hepatic enzymes, which will affect the concentrations of other coadministered medications.

The widely recognized therapeutic range for phenobarbital for adults is between 15 and 40 mg/L. The predominant side effect observed in adults at blood concentrations greater than 40 mg/L is sedation, although tolerance to this effect develops with long-term therapy. Actual optimal concentrations will vary and may not be realized until tolerance to the sedative effects has occurred. Because of the long elimination half-life of phenobarbital, the blood concentration does not change rapidly. Therefore, blood for TDM can be collected at any time of day, once steady state has been achieved.

Primidone

Primidone (proprietary name Mysoline) is metabolized to phenobarbital. Both compounds have antiseizure activity. The mechanism of action of this drug is similar to that described for phenobarbital, and the therapeutic effect is due partially to the accumulation of its major metabolite, phenobarbital, created by the action of CYP2C19. A second metabolite of primidone, phenylethylmalonamide (PEMA), created by the action of CYP2C9, also has some antiepileptic activity.

Primidone is rapidly and nearly completely absorbed after oral administration. Once absorbed, it is not highly protein bound, and it has a half-life of approximately 10 hours; however, because the pharmacokinetics are variable, the half-life may vary from 3 to 22 hours.[42] Disposition of the drug is known to be affected by drugs that alter CYP2C19 and 2C9 metabolism and by diseases that alter phenobarbital disposition. Coadministration of acetazolamide with primidone results in decreased gastrointestinal absorption of primidone and subsequent diminished plasma concentrations. Primidone administered in association with phenytoin produces a modest elevation of the phenobarbital-to-primidone ratio because phenytoin competes with the hepatic hydroxylating enzymes associated with the metabolism of phenobarbital. Coadministration of valproic acid, for the same reasons outlined for phenobarbital, causes a modest increase in both primidone and phenobarbital serum concentrations.

The optimal therapeutic concentration of primidone has been established as 5 to 10 mg/L. Because phenobarbital is an active metabolite of primidone, concurrent analysis of phenobarbital is required for complete interpretation of results. The previously defined therapeutic range for phenobarbital applies to adequate primidone therapy. Phenobarbital concentrations rise gradually over a period of 1 to 2 weeks after therapy is initiated. Toxicity due to accumulation of primidone occurs at serum concentrations greater than 15 mg/L and usually is associated with symptoms of sedation, nausea, vomiting, diplopia, dizziness, and ataxia, and a phenobarbital concentration greater than 40 mg/L. In addition to detection of drug-drug interactions, evaluating the ratio of phenobarbital to primidone may assist with detection of noncompliance.

Phenytoin

Phenytoin (diphenylhydantoin), most commonly available as Dilantin, but also available under other names and in generic form, is used in the treatment of primary or secondary generalized tonic-clonic seizures, partial or complex-partial seizures, and status epilepticus. The drug is not effective for absence seizures. Phenytoin interferes with sodium channel activity by prolonging inactivation, which reduces the ability of the neuron to respond at high frequency.[30] The physiologic effect of this action is reduction in central synaptic transmission, which aids in control of abnormal neuronal excitability.

The pharmacokinetics of phenytoin are complex and unpredictable as the result of variable absorption, high (>90%) protein binding, saturable metabolism, and drug-drug interactions. Absorption of oral phenytoin is slow and sometimes is incomplete. A wide selection of drug preparations contribute to variable and sometimes poor bioavailability, but V_d is 0.6 to 0.7 L/kg. Phenytoin is not readily soluble in aqueous solutions. When administered by intramuscular injection, most of the dose precipitates at the site of injection and then is slowly absorbed. A prodrug called fosphenytoin (Cerebyx) allows intramuscular injection and rapid conversion to and liberation of phenytoin.[157] Monitoring of fosphenytoin is accomplished through the use of routine phenytoin assays. However, specimens collected shortly after administration of fosphenytoin may not accurately reflect active drug concentrations; interpretation of TDM for fosphenytoin should be performed after phenytoin concentrations reach steady state.

Phenytoin is metabolized by hepatic microsomal hydroxylating enzymes CYP2C19 and 2C9. The principal metabolite is 5-(*p*-hydroxyphenyl)-5-phenylhydantoin, which is excreted principally as a glucuronide. Hepatic metabolism of phenytoin may become saturated within the therapeutic range. Once metabolism is saturated, small dose increments result in large changes in blood concentration; this phenomenon partially explains the wide variation in dose among patients that is required to achieve a therapeutic effect. Because of this saturation phenomenon, first-order kinetics does not apply to phenytoin at plasma concentrations in excess of 5 mg/L (or lower in select patients), and half-life can vary tremendously. It is noteworthy that some commercially available immunoassays exhibit cross-reactivity for phenytoin metabolites and may generate falsely elevated results.[185] In addition, various drug interactions result in alteration of the disposition of phenytoin. Alcohol, carbamazepine, barbiturates, and rifampin induce CYP2C19 and 2C9; this induction results in increased metabolism of phenytoin, reduced serum concentration of both total and free phenytoin, and reduced pharmacologic effect. Drugs such as chloramphenicol, cimetidine, disulfiram, isoniazid, omeprazole, and topiramate compete with phenytoin metabolism, resulting in an increase in both total and free phenytoin concentrations and enhancement of the pharmacologic effect. Salicylate, valproic acid, phenylbutazone, sulfisoxazole, and sulfonylureas compete with phenytoin for serum protein-binding sites. The end result is diminished total serum concentration of phenytoin, while the free phenytoin concentration and the pharmacologic effect remain approximately the same.

The optimal therapeutic concentration for seizure control without side effects is 10 to 20 mg/L. In a large population study, Buchthal and colleagues[31] found a 50% response rate in patients with plasma concentrations greater than 10 mg/L and 86% suppression of seizure activity at concentrations exceeding 15 mg/L. Free phenytoin concentrations of 1 to 2 mg/L are optimal.[207] Total phenytoin concentrations greater than 20 mg/L usually do not enhance seizure control and often are associated with nystagmus and ataxia. Total phenytoin plasma concentrations greater than 35 mg/L have been shown to precipitate seizure activity. A side effect of phenytoin not related to plasma concentration is development of gingival hyperplasia.

Valproic Acid

Valproic acid (brand names Depakene and Depakote, but also available under other names and in generic form) is used for the treatment of absence seizures. It has also been shown to be useful against tonic-clonic and partial seizures when used in conjunction with other antiepileptic agents, such as phenobarbital or phenytoin. The drug inhibits the enzyme GABA transaminase, resulting in an increase in the concentration of GABA in the brain. GABA is a potent inhibitor of presynaptic and postsynaptic discharges in the central nervous system. Valproic acid also modulates the synaptic sodium channel by prolonging inactivation, which reduces the ability of the neuron to respond at high frequency. This action gives it some activity against tonic-clonic seizures.[30]

Valproic acid is rapidly and almost completely absorbed after oral administration and has a very low V_d (0.1 to 0.5 L/kg). Peak concentrations occur 1 to 4 hours after an oral dose of conventional tablets and solutions, but they are extended for enteric-coated and sustained-release formulations, as well as when taken with food. Valproic acid is highly protein bound (>90%), but the extent of protein binding decreases with increasing concentration, leading to nonlinear kinetics in some patients. The metabolism of valproic acid is extensive, involving β-oxidation (≈30% of dose) and production of several glucuronide conjugates (≈40% of dose). The clinical significance of these metabolites is not well understood.[95,145] The half-life is shortened from approximately 20 hours with the initial dose to approximately 12 hours as steady state is achieved. The half-life is shorter still in children than in adults, with the exception of neonates with hepatic disease, in whom the half-life becomes prolonged. Relatively poor correlation has been noted between dose and serum concentrations. Valproic acid modulates the pharmacokinetics of many other antiepileptic drugs. For example, it inhibits the clearance of phenobarbital and competes with phenytoin for protein-binding sites. The free phenytoin concentration remains approximately the same, but total phenytoin in the plasma is decreased. Other drugs that induce hepatic oxidative enzymes result in increased valproic acid clearance, requiring a higher dose to maintain effective therapeutic concentrations.

The minimum effective therapeutic concentration of valproic acid is 50 mg/L. Concentrations greater than 100 mg/L have been associated with hepatic toxicity and acute toxic encephalopathy. Free concentrations are sometimes clinically useful. Glycine has been observed to accumulate in patients taking valproic acid therapy.

Contemporary Antiepileptics

Felbamate

Felbamate (Felbatol), which was approved for primary or adjunctive therapy of partial seizures, exerts efficacy through several mechanisms, including potentiation of GABA-ergic neurotransmission and inhibition of glutamate excitation due to interaction with the *N*-methyl-D-aspartate (NMDA) receptor. Felbamate is particularly effective in controlling Lennox-Gastaut syndrome. However, its use is limited to those patients who fail other drug treatments, because felbamate carries with it a substantial risk of aplastic anemia and liver failure that is not related to the blood concentrations. Biweekly monitoring of complete blood count, serum aminotransferases, and bilirubin is recommended to detect early onset of these side effects.

Felbamate is completely absorbed from the gastrointestinal tract with peak concentrations observed 2 to 6 hours after administration. The drug is only 25% bound to plasma proteins and has a volume of distribution less than 1.0 L/kg. It is eliminated by hepatic metabolism (CYP3A4), with its half-life ranging from 14 to 21 hours.[30,52] Felbamate saturates metabolism when the concentration exceeds 120 mg/L and is inducible, shifting elimination kinetics from first order to zero order. Half-life is also affected by other drugs and is substantially shorter in children, who may exhibit felbamate clearance 40 to 65% higher than in adults. The proposed therapeutic range for felbamate is narrow, ranging from 30 to 60 mg/L.[145] An intermediate metabolite, an atropaldehyde, has been implicated in the idiosyncratic adverse events associated with felbamate.

Gabapentin

Gabapentin (Neurontin) is a chemical analog of GABA that promotes the release of GABA. It does not interact directly with the GABA receptor, nor does it inhibit glutamic acid decarboxylase, the enzyme that usually controls cellular concentrations of GABA. The mechanism of action is somewhat unclear but is thought to be most related to interactions with voltage-gated calcium channels. A chemically and mechanistically related drug, pregabalin (Lyrica) is used primarily for managing neuropathic pain. Gabapentin has proved effective in the treatment of drug-resistant partial seizures, so it is primarily considered adjuvant therapy.[156]

Absorption of oral gabapentin is mediated by the L-amino transport system in the small intestines through a saturable process. Thus, bioavailability is dose dependent. Peak concentrations are observed 2 to 3 hours after a dose. Absorption is reduced by concomitant use of antacids. Pregabalin does not require active absorption and exhibits far more predictable and linear pharmacokinetics. Gabapentin is less than 10% bound to plasma proteins, and the volume of distribution is 0.65 to 1.4 L/kg. Gabapentin is not metabolized and does not induce or inhibit metabolic enzymes. The elimination half-life is 5 to 9 hours, and elimination is proportional to renal clearance. Approximately 30% higher doses are required in children.

The minimum effective concentration of gabapentin is 2 mg/L, and the optimally effective therapeutic serum concentration of gabapentin is reported as between 2 and 20 mg/L.[21,52] Side effects observed in adults at serum concentrations greater than 12 mg/L are somnolence, ataxia, dizziness, and fatigue.

Lamotrigine

Lamotrigine (Lamictal) is a broad-spectrum antiepileptic drug that is widely used. Lamotrigine is thought to act through multiple mechanisms, including blocking sodium and calcium channels to reduce repetitive nerve firings induced by depolarization of spinal cord neurons, and reducing glutamate release.

Lamotrigine is completely absorbed from the gastrointestinal tract after oral administration, with peak concentrations occurring at 1 to 3 hours. A linear relationship between dose and serum concentrations is observed, volume of distribution is 0.9 to 1.5 L/kg, and binding to plasma proteins is moderate (≈55%). Lamotrigine is extensively metabolized and is eliminated primarily as the glucuronide ester. Half-life ranges from 20 to 30 hours. Autoinduction reduces serum concentrations by ≈20% with approximately 2 weeks of therapy. Enzyme-inducing drugs such as phenobarbital, phenytoin, or carbamazepine also result in reduced lamotrigine concentrations. Clearance is greater in children and increases up to 300% in pregnancy.

The proposed therapeutic range for lamotrigine is between 2.5 and 15 mg/L. Dizziness, ataxia, diplopia, blurred vision, nausea, and vomiting are signs of toxicity that have been reported, although these effects are rare when plasma concentrations are less than 15 mg/L. Lamotrigine is a potent inhibitor of dihydrofolate reductase. Folate concentrations are decreased when this drug is administered. If folate replacement is not implemented, rash and anemia may be experienced when lamotrigine is within the therapeutic range. Lamotrigine, similar to carbamazepine, has also been associated with the development of severe rash (Stevens-Johnson syndrome) in approximately 1% of patients.

Levetiracetam

Levetiracetam (Keppra) is a broad-spectrum antiepileptic that has been found useful for managing focal and generalized seizures. The primary mechanism of action is unique and appears to be mediated through interactions with synaptic vesicle protein SV2A, which is involved in the release of neurotransmitters from presynaptic terminals. This drug is chiral, and its antiepileptic activity is highly enantioselective.[93]

Levetiracetam is 100% bioavailable following an oral dose and reaches maximum concentration in approximately 1 hour. Although absorption is slowed by food, a good correlation between dose and serum concentrations has been reported. Levetiracetam is less than 10% bound to plasma proteins, has a volume of distribution of 0.5 to 0.7 L/kg, and is not extensively metabolized. Renal function and age are the major determinants of elimination kinetics. The possibility of in vitro metabolism (after specimen is collected) by blood esterases has been proposed, so plasma should be separated from cells promptly. The half-life ranges from 16 to 18 hours for newborns and from 6 to 8 hours in healthy adults. No pharmacokinetic interactions have been noted between levetiracetam and other antiepileptic drugs.

The minimal effective serum concentration of levetiracetam for seizure control is 3 mg/L, but the effective concentration is not well defined. The predose therapeutic concentration range proposed in a 2008 consensus document is 12 to 46 mg/L.[145] Toxicity effects known to be associated with levetiracetam use include decreased RBC count and hematocrit, decreased neutrophil count, somnolence, asthenia, and dizziness. These toxicities may be associated with blood concentrations in the therapeutic range.

Oxcarbazepine

Oxcarbazepine (Trileptal) is a 10-keto analog of carbamazepine that is useful in managing partial and generalized seizures. Oxcarbazepine is a chiral prodrug that is metabolized to 10-hydroxy-10,11-dihydrocarbamazepine, known commonly as monohydroxycarbamazepine (MHD), the metabolite responsible for the therapeutic effect. MHD, similar to carbamazepine, blocks sodium channels; MHD also exhibits inhibitory activity at calcium channels.

Oxcarbazepine is rapidly and completely absorbed, with peak concentrations observed at 1 to 2 hours; food has no effect on rate or extent of absorption. The half-life of oxcarbazepine is approximately 2 hours. Concentrations of MHD peak at 3 to 5 hours, protein binding is approximately 40%, and the V_d is less than 1.0 L/kg. Concentrations of the *S*-enantiomer of MHD are much higher than those of the *R*-enantiomer because conversion is stereoselective. The metabolism of MHD is extensive; about 96% of the dose is excreted in the urine as metabolites. Most of the dose is eliminated and recovered as the glucuronide ester of oxcarbazepine or MHD. Metabolism does not involve inducible enzymes, however, so drug-drug interactions are minimal compared with carbamazepine. Because carbamazepine activates the uridine diphosphate glucuronosyltransferase (UGT) enzyme system, patients taking carbamazepine concomitantly with oxcarbazepine have significantly lower MHD concentrations than those not receiving carbamazepine. The elimination half-life for MHD is 8 to 15 hours. Because MHD is cleared predominantly by the kidney, the dose for patients with creatinine clearance less than 30 mL/min should be half that given to patients with normal renal function.[72] MHD selectively induces CYP3A4 enzymes and may inhibit CYP2C19.

Optimal response is reported when predose MHD concentration is in the range of 3 to 35 mg/L. Toxicities include hyponatremia, dizziness, somnolence, diplopia, fatigue, nausea, vomiting, ataxia, abnormal vision, abdominal pain, tremor, dyspepsia, and abnormal gait. These toxicities may be transient and may be observed when blood concentrations are in the therapeutic range, although the incidence is highest in patients with serum MHD concentration greater than 30 mg/L. Serum sodium concentration less than 125 mmol/L and decreased thyroxine (T_4) have also been seen in patients treated with MHD. To prevent peaks in MHD, it is suggested that dosing be split throughout the day.

Tiagabine

Tiagabine (Gabitril) is indicated as adjunctive therapy in adults and children for the treatment of partial seizures. It is frequently administered to patients receiving at least one concomitant antiepileptic drug. Tiagabine is a nipecotic acid derivative that blocks reuptake of GABA into presynaptic neurons, permitting more GABA to be available for receptor binding on the surface of postsynaptic cells. This drug has been found particularly effective in patients with drug-resistant epilepsy associated with glial tumors.

Tiagabine is rapidly and completely absorbed, reaching peak concentration approximately 45 minutes following an oral dose in the fasting state. Administration with food is recommended to reduce fluctuations in plasma concentrations between doses. Pediatric patients reach peak concentration at approximately 2.4 hours.[79] Tiagabine pharmacokinetics is linear over the typical dose range. This drug is highly (≈96%) bound to human plasma proteins, mainly to serum albumin and AAG. The volume of distribution is 1.0 L/kg, and it is extensively metabolized, with a major route mediated by CYP3A4. Half-life is approximately 5 to 9 hours and is extended to 12 to 16 hours in patients with compromised liver function. Children require higher doses because of accelerated clearance. This drug does not induce or inhibit metabolism of other drugs but is subject to drug-drug interactions through both protein-binding interactions and enzyme-inducing drugs. For example, coadministration with valproic acid reduces protein binding to 94%, increasing the free fraction of tiagabine by 40%.[17] Naproxen and salicylates are also known to displace tiagabine from protein-binding sites.

A proposed therapeutic range for tiagabine is 20 to 200 saliva µg/L.[145] Serum concentrations greater than 800 µg/L may be associated with adverse effects such as asthenia, ataxia, difficulty concentrating, and depression. Timing of specimen collection is critical for TDM of tiagabine because of the rapid absorption and relatively short half-life.

Topiramate

Topiramate (Topamax) is a broad-spectrum antiepileptic drug that exerts activity through several mechanisms. It has sodium and calcium channel blocking activity, potentiates the activity of GABA, and inhibits glutamate release. Because of this range of activities, topiramate blocks seizure spread rather than raising seizure potential.

Topiramate is routinely administered orally, is absorbed rapidly, and peaks at 2 to 4 hours. Although time to peak concentration is delayed by food, the peak concentration is not affected, and the relationship between dose and serum concentration is linear. Topiramate is minimally bound (≈15%) to plasma proteins, and V_d is 0.6 to 0.8 L/kg. Approximately 50% of topiramate is metabolized, with a serum half-life of 20 to 30 hours in adults, less in children. Topiramate inhibits CYP2C19 and induces CYP3A4, although serum concentrations of other anticonvulsant drugs are not significantly affected by concurrent administration of topiramate. Enzyme-inducing medications reduce serum topiramate concentrations; serum concentrations are increased by amitriptyline, lithium, and sumatriptan. As with other renally eliminated anticonvulsant drugs, patients with impaired renal function exhibit decreased renal clearance.

Most studies have reported a therapeutic range for topiramate of 5.0 to 20 mg/L, yet considerable overlap is seen in serum concentrations between responders and nonresponders. Concentrations less than 2.0 mg/L indicate that the dose is suboptimal or was administered too infrequently.[148] Adverse side effects (cognitive, emotional, physical) are related to serum concentrations in some patients.

Vigabatrine

Vigabatrine (Flexyx, Sabril) is a structural analog of GABA that acts as a suicidal inhibitor of GABA-transaminase, the enzyme responsible for GABA metabolism. This drug is effective for managing infantile spasm associated with tuberous sclerosis and refractory partial epilepsies and is used outside the United States. However, because of irreversible visual field impairment that occurs in approximately one third of patients, this drug is not widely used within the United States. Because of the mechanism of action, the value of TDM is limited to compliance testing in most cases.

Zonisamide

Zonisamide (proprietary name Zonegran) is a sodium and calcium channel blocker. It binds to the GABA receptor but does not produce a chloride influx. Therefore, zonisamide is a broad-spectrum antiepileptic. Zonisamide has weak inhibitory activity on carbonic anhydrase, is a free radical scavenger, and promotes dopaminergic and serotonergic neurotransmission, but these actions are not likely to contribute to its antiepileptic activity.

Peak concentrations of zonisamide are observed 2 to 6 hours after dose administration. Pharmacokinetics becomes nonlinear at high concentrations. As with many other antiepileptic drugs, children generally require higher doses than adults. It is 50% bound to plasma proteins but has high affinity for red cell protein components. The V_d is 0.8 to 1.6 L/kg. The relatively long half-life (50 to 70 hours) is shortened considerably (25 to 35 hours) when enzyme-inducing drugs are also administered. Zonisamide is extensively metabolized, with a primary pathway mediated by CYP2C19 and CYP3A4. Thus, coadministration with CYP-inducing drugs such as phenobarbital, phenytoin, or carbamazepine results in reduced zonisamide concentration.[64] Zonisamide does not inhibit CYP isozymes, nor does it undergo autoinduction.

The proposed therapeutic range of zonisamide is 10 to 40 mg/L, but overlap in plasma concentrations between responders and nonresponders occurs. Adverse effects on cognition are reported at concentrations that exceed 30 mg/L. Toxicity is likely at concentrations that exceed 70 mg/L.

Historical and Not Widely Used

Bromides, ethotoin, mephobarbital, and methsuximide have antiepileptic activity. However, they are used very infrequently and TDM is uncommon. Previous editions of this text describe TDM for these drugs.

Antimicrobial Agents

Antimicrobial agents include a wide range of compounds with very different target organisms, mechanisms of activity, and pharmacokinetics. Efficacy of therapy is dependent on both the drug and the infectious agent, thus TDM for these compounds requires knowledge not only of the pharmacologic and toxicologic characteristics of the drug itself, but also of the nature of the infection it is intended to treat.

Antibacterials

Bacterial susceptibility to antibiotics is commonly measured in terms of the minimum inhibitory concentration (MIC), that is, the concentration of drug sufficient to inhibit growth of an organism.[164] The MIC varies widely for different strains of the same species, thus cultures must be obtained from each patient to ascertain not only the organism involved but also its vulnerability to a panel of agents. TDM for antibiotics often involves relating some aspect of the serum concentration of drug [AUC, maximum plasma concentration of the drug (C_{max}), or time above a given concentration] to the MIC measured for the specific infectious agent being treated. Pharmacokinetic details of antibacterials are summarized in Table 34-2.

Aminoglycosides

Aminoglycoside antibiotics inhibit protein synthesis to kill aerobic, gram-negative bacteria. Because oral absorption is poor, aminoglycosides are administered intravenously or by intramuscular injection. Elimination is largely renal, almost entirely as the unchanged parent drug; the presence of kidney dysfunction is therefore a concern with use of these agents and may necessitate adjusting dose or dosing intervals.[80,164] Aminoglycosides are associated with the risk of serious toxicity. The most common concentration-related adverse effects are nephrotoxicity (renal tubular necrosis) and potentially irreversible ototoxicity (auditory nerve degeneration) leading to hearing loss. Aminoglycosides include amikacin, gentamicin, and tobramycin, among many others.

Several studies have shown that efficacy of these drugs correlates well with the ratio of the C_{max} relative to the MIC of the organism; this characteristic is termed *concentration-dependent* killing. Ratios of C_{max}/MIC ≥ 10 are preferred for optimal effect against sensitive bacteria.[160,164] In contrast, toxicity is best averted when trough concentrations are allowed to decline substantially.[80] This does not adversely affect therapeutic efficacy, because aminoglycosides show a considerable *postantibiotic effect,* that is, they continue to enhance bactericidal activity after the drug has been cleared from the body.[164]

A popular dosing strategy for aminoglycosides is extended-interval administration, which provides large, less-frequent doses to drive C_{max} above the organism MIC with adequate time for substantial drug elimination to minimize toxicity.[164] Serum concentrations do not reach steady state in extended-interval dosing. Peak concentrations should rise well above the MIC (and often above previously published "toxic" limits for more-frequent administration protocols), but trough concentrations will decline to near-undetectable concentrations. For these reasons, TDM is less routine for extended-interval dosing, although it is still common for patients with renal disease, sepsis, cystic fibrosis, or other conditions necessitating individualized therapy rather than application of population-derived protocols.[13,45]

If administered more frequently, aminoglycoside TDM samples should be drawn at peak (1 hour post infusion) and at trough (immediately predose, or at minimum 10 to 12 hours post infusion) to monitor both efficacy and risk of toxicity, respectively.[80] In practice, one or both of these samples is often replaced by the use of a nomogram, Bayesian model, or other predictive protocol.[13] However, publications have highlighted the prevalence of suboptimal use of antibiotics, including failure of these predictive models to

TABLE 34-2 Pharmacokinetic Parameters of Antibiotics

Drug	Therapeutic Targets*	Mean Half-life, h	Mean Volume of Distribution, L/kg	Mean Oral Bioavailability, %	Protein Binding, %	Enzymes Inhibited or Induced
Aminoglycosides[80]						
Amikacin	C_{max}: 25-35 C_{min}: 1-8	2.3	0.3	NA	5	
Gentamicin	C_{max}: 5-12 C_{min}: <1	2.5	0.3	NA	5	
Tobramycin	C_{max}: 5-12 C_{min}: <1	2	0.3	NA	<10	
Glycopeptides[13,168]						
Vancomycin (aggressive dosing)	C_{min} > 10 mg/L C_{min} > 15 mg/L	5.5	0.4	NA	30	
Teicoplanin (aggressive dosing)	C_{min} > 10 mg/L C_{min} > 20 mg/L	100	1.2		90	
Antituberculars[147]						
p-Aminosalicylic acid	C_{min}: 1-8 mg/L	1.25	0.25	60	55	
Cycloserine	C_{max}: 20-35 mg/L	10	0.2	80		
Ethambutol	C_{min}: <8 mg/L	3.1	1.6	77	20	
Pyrazinamide	C_{min}: >20 mg/L	6	0.6	70	10	
Rifampicin	C_{min}: 2.5-40 mg/L	3.5	1	90	75	CYP 2B6, 2C9, 2C19, 2D6, 3A4
Fluoroquinolones[147]						
Ciprofloxacin	AUC: MIC > 30 (gram-positive) AUC: MIC > 125 (gram-negative)	3.5	2.2	60	40	CYP 1A2, 3A4
Levofloxacin	AUC: MIC > 25 (most infections) AUC: MIC > 100 (severe infections)	7	1.25	99	30	

*The optimal parameter for determining therapeutic efficacy varies by drug class [e.g., ratio of peak concentration *(C_{max})* to minimum inhibitory concentration *(MIC)* for aminoglycosides, or ratio of area under the curve *(AUC)* to MIC for fluoroquinolones.
C_{min}, Minimum concentration of a drug; *NA,* data not available.

consistently achieve sufficient concentrations above the MIC, or to allow adequate drug clearance in patients with renal dysfunction or other atypical pharmacokinetic parameters (e.g., elderly, septic patients).[85,139,160] Ineffective antibacterial treatment fails to rid patients of infection at the risk of avoidable toxicity; it also enhances the development of antibiotic-resistant bacterial strains; thus, TDM-based management of aminoglycoside therapy is recommended to optimize patient outcomes.

Glycopeptides

Vancomycin and teicoplanin (available in Europe) are glycopeptide antibiotics with activity against antibiotic-resistant bacteria, including methicillin-resistant *Staphylococcus aureus* (MRSA).[164,168] Teicoplanin is generally considered to have minimal toxicity at therapeutic concentrations[46]; it is important to note that early concerns of vancomycin-related nephrotoxicity and ototoxicity were likely due to impurities in early formulations of the drug.[168]

More recent studies evaluating current preparations of vancomycin (>90% pure) show much lower (although not absent) risk for adverse effects, unless administered with other agents capable of damaging hearing or renal function, such as aminoglycosides.

TDM of vancomycin has been associated with improved therapy and reduced risk of toxicity; however, until recently, the optimal TDM protocol has remained contested. Recent guidelines[168] suggest that the preferred monitoring parameter for vancomycin is the trough serum concentration, obtained immediately before the fourth dose. For most infections, trough vancomycin concentrations should be maintained above 10 mg/L, depending on the MIC of the pathogen; the target parameter for optimal therapy is an AUC/MIC ratio greater than 400. For more severe infections, such as MRSA endocarditis, more aggressive dosing is required and trough concentrations should be sustained in the range of 15 to 20 mg/L. Peak vancomycin concentrations do not appear to be helpful in monitoring risk of toxicity.[168] In contrast to vancomycin, teicoplanin efficacy appears to correlate better with the time spent above the MIC [(teicoplanin) > MIC].[46] TDM of teicoplanin is not routinely necessary. However, in patients with renal dysfunction, atypical pharmacokinetics, or comedications associated with nephrotoxicity or ototoxicity, frequent TDM of both glycopeptide antibiotics should be considered.[13]

Tuberculosis Therapy

Management of tuberculosis (TB) typically involves an initial intensive treatment with several agents followed by months of continuation therapy to eliminate residual disease.[147] Most patients respond well to such protocols; cure rates are high with acceptably low concentrations of adverse effects. However, certain populations present therapeutic challenges, including those with drug-resistant disease (e.g., isoniazid-resistant or multidrug-resistant TB), individuals with comorbidities (e.g., diabetes mellitus, renal failure), and patients with HIV, wherein the disease affects immune response while treatment disrupts the disposition of comedications (see later, "Antiretrovirals").[43,116,147]

First-line agents for TB include isoniazid, rifampicin, pyrazinamide, ethambutol, and streptomycin. These compounds are generally effective with minimal toxicity.[116] Second-line therapy involves compounds that are less effectual or are poorly tolerated; second-line agents include cycloserine, *p*-aminosalicylic acid, and levofloxacin or other fluoroquinolones. Trough concentrations often are too low to be readily measured, thus peak sampling is preferred. One protocol suggests obtaining a 2-hour sample (close to the serum peak for several primary agents) followed by a 6-hour sample to ascertain delayed absorption, malabsorption, or atypical elimination.[116] Samples should be processed immediately to eliminate issues of drug instability ex vivo (e.g., rifampicin degradation in serum).

Rifampicin and related rifamycin drugs (e.g., rifabutin, rifapentine) are known inducers of most major hepatic phase I enzymes, including CYP2B6, CYP2C8/9/19, CYP2D6, and CYP3A4/5/7.[147] Rifampicin is one of the most potent enzyme inducers characterized to date; thus its use can be a significant concern in patients with comedications. It also presents a particular concern in patients with HIV, as many antiretroviral agents inhibit or induce those same enzymes.[43] Resources for TDM in large TB practices are increasing alongside the recognition that TDM is key to managing both drug-drug interactions and multidrug-resistant TB; achieving optimal drug concentrations is essential to successful therapy and preventing the development of other resistant strains.[147]

Other Antibiotics

Analytical methods to detect many other types of antibiotics have been described, but little consensus has been reached as to the best practices for using TDM to optimize efficacy and minimize toxicity for most of these agents.[13,164] Fluoroquinolones (e.g., ciprofloxacin) and β-lactams (e.g., penicillins), display little correlation between serum concentration and toxicity. The efficacy of many of these common antibiotics follows a *time-dependent* rather than a concentration-dependent pattern (i.e., serum concentrations must simply remain above the MIC for a certain percentage of time to obtain killing); thus measurement of drug peak or trough concentrations is not routinely necessary.[164] TDM is recommended for management of patients with renal dysfunction, severe hepatic disease, or suspicion of atypical pharmacokinetics (e.g., poor absorption, altered distribution).[13,80] Several specific antibiotic classes were reviewed extensively in the previous version of this chapter, to which readers are referred for further information.

Antifungal Agents

The incidence of fungal infection is increasing as is the prevalence of susceptible immunocompromised individuals (e.g., transplant recipients, HIV-positive patients).[73] The most common pathogens are species of *Candida* yeasts or *Aspergillus* molds. Recent advances have expanded the number of fungicidal drugs available to combat such infections; however, the relative novelty of these agents is accompanied by a scarcity of data regarding optimal use of TDM for patient management. This section will discuss TDM of an older antifungal, 5-flucytosine, and several newer triazole compounds. Pharmacokinetic details of antifungals are summarized in Table 34-3.

5-Flucytosine

One of the first antifungals developed, the pyrimidine analog 5-flucytosine (Ancobon), is a broad-spectrum agent that is coadministered with another fungicidal drug (typically amphotericin B) to prevent emergence of resistant pathogen populations.[7] Toxicity of 5-flucytosine is well correlated with serum concentrations greater than 100 mg/L and presents as myelosuppression (e.g., thrombocytopenia) or hepatic dysfunction evidenced by elevated transaminases.[7,73]

Evidence for the utility of TDM for 5-flucytosine is more convincing than evidence for most other antifungal agents. Its bioavailability is excellent, but its renal elimination

TABLE 34-3 Pharmacokinetic Parameters of Antifungal Drugs

Drug	Therapeutic Targets*[7,73]	Toxic Level, mg/L	Mean Half-life, h	Mean Volume of Distribution, L/kg	Mean Oral Bioavailability, %	Protein Binding, %	CYP Enzymes Inhibited or Induced
Routine TDM Recommended							
5-Flucytosine	C_{max}: >25 mg/L	C_{max}: >100 mg/L	4.5	0.75	85	<4	NA
Itraconazole	C_{min}: >0.5 mg/L		40	14	55	99	3A4, 2C9
+ Hydroxyitraconazole	C_{min}: >1 mg/L	NA	30	NA	NA	99	NA
Posaconazole	C_{min}: >1.25 mg/L		24	>100	High, varies	98	3A4
Voriconazole	C_{min}: 1-6 mg/L	>6	6	4.6	96	60	2C9, 3A4, 2C19
TDM Useful for Select Patients							
Amphotericin B	C_{max}: MIC > 40	>5	15 days	4	10	>90	NA
Fluconazole	AUC: MIC > 25	>20	30	0.75	>90	10	2C9, 3A4, 2C19
Echinocandins	C_{min}: 1-2.5 mg/L	NA	10-24	0.1-0.5	<10	>95	NA

*The optimal parameter for determining therapeutic efficacy varies by drug class [e.g., peak concentration *(C_{max})* for 5-flucytosine, trough concentration *(C_{min})* for itraconazole, or ratio of area under the curve *(AUC)* to minimum inhibitory concentration *(MIC)* for fluconazole].
NA, Data not available; *TDM,* therapeutic drug management.

is variable and may be affected by the nephrotoxicity of amphotericin B. TDM is therefore recommended at the onset of therapy (to ensure that concentrations are within the target range) and in patients with renal dysfunction or evidence of toxicity.[73] Because of its short half-life, the drug is administered in multiple doses daily; it is recommended to draw TDM samples at peak serum concentrations, roughly 2 hours after a dose.[13] Target concentrations for efficacy appear to vary with the pathogen and the extent of infection but are approximately 30 to 80 mg/L for most patients.[73]

Triazoles

The triazole group of antifungal drugs includes fluconazole (Diflucan), itraconazole (Sporanox), voriconazole (Vfend), and posaconazole (Noxafil). These broad-spectrum compounds kill by inhibiting synthesis of the major fungal sterol, ergosterol.[101] All triazoles are available for oral or intravenous administration, except posaconazole, which currently is approved only in the oral formulation. Bioavailability can vary greatly, thus specific recommendations have been put forth for taking these agents while fasting (voriconazole), with acidic food such as a cola (itraconazole), or with a high-fat meal (posaconazole). Efficacy of triazoles correlates best with the ratio of drug AUC to pathogen MIC and appears optimal for eliminating invasive fungal infections when AUC/MIC is greater than 25. Target concentrations for prophylactic therapy are likely lower than for invasive infections but have not been as well characterized.[73]

All triazole agents are known to inhibit one or more of the CYP enzymes (specifically, CYP3A4, CYP2C9, or CYP2C19); thus their administration can greatly affect serum concentrations of other drugs (e.g., immunosuppressants).[7,170] As substrates of these same enzymes, triazole antifungals are subject to induction or inhibition of metabolism; thus comedication with interacting compounds is a common rationale for performing TDM on triazoles.[118] Currently, relatively few institutions are able to perform such TDM analyses; bioassay has historically been the most common method used, but newer assays are HPLC or LC-MS/MS based.[89]

Of the individual compounds, fluconazole is the only triazole for which routine TDM does not appear necessary. Fluconazole concentrations are reasonably predictable based on dose, thus TDM is recommended only for special populations (e.g., children), or when concerns of poor absorption or noncompliance arise.[73,89] In contrast, itraconazole shows widely variable absorption and nonlinear kinetics, making TDM necessary for optimal therapy.[7] The major metabolite, hydroxyitraconazole, shows comparable antifungal effect to the parent compound, and must therefore be included in nonbioassay methods. Recommended steady-state trough concentrations for itraconazole are greater than 0.5 mg/L (HPLC) or greater than 5 mg/L (bioassay); no upper limit has been defined given the poor correlation of serum concentration with toxicity.[89]

The newer triazoles, voriconazole and posaconazole, show broader spectra of activity and are effective against fluconazole- and itraconazole-resistant fungi.[28,101] As with itraconazole, absorption of these two triazoles is extremely variable and can be greatly affected by food intake. Voriconazole shows nonlinear kinetics; posaconazole generally follows linear kinetics but can convert to nonlinear behavior (saturation) at high doses. Both agents show progressively greater risk of toxicity as serum concentrations increase, but there does not appear to be a single cutoff that clearly delineates toxic concentrations from nontoxic.[89] Recommended steady-state trough concentrations for voriconazole are 1 to 6 mg/L; targets for posaconazole are as yet poorly defined, although concentrations greater than 1.5 mg/L appear to be effective against invasive fungal infections.[89,101]

Other Antifungal Agents

Concentrations of amphotericin B or the echinocandin antifungals (e.g., caspofungin, anidulafungin, micafungin) are not commonly measured for TDM.[73] These agents show poor correlation between efficacy or toxicity and serum concentrations; thus their use is best monitored by clinical parameters specific to known adverse effects (e.g., amphotericin B–induced nephrotoxicity).

Antiretrovirals

The prevalence of infection with HIV has led to the development of several classes of drugs targeting this disease, collectively termed *antiretroviral agents.*[182] The major categories include nucleoside/nucleotide reverse transcriptase inhibitors (NRTIs), non-nucleoside reverse transcriptase inhibitors (NNRTIs), protease inhibitors (PIs), and entry/fusion inhibitors. Current guidelines for treatment of antiretroviral-naive patients recommend the use of drug combinations termed *highly active antiretroviral therapy (HAART).*[106] This generally involves the use of two NRTIs, plus one or more agents from the other categories. Management of previously treated individuals can be more complex, as therapeutic options tend to be limited by viral strains with resistance to specific agents, or patients who are intolerant of certain drugs. Clinical response is assessed by monitoring viral load (i.e., the number of copies of HIV RNA) and the count of $CD4^+$ T-lymphocytes.

Several factors indicate that TDM of antiretrovirals can aid long-term patient management.[22] First, these agents exhibit wide interindividual variability in serum drug concentrations for a given dose, suggesting that there is risk of undertreatment or toxicity if serum concentrations are not assessed. Second, both the success of therapy and the prevention of viral drug resistance depend heavily on patient compliance. Third, several antiretroviral agents are capable of inhibiting or inducing various CYP isoforms. Patients generally are on multiple medications for HIV, opportunistic infections, and comorbidities; thus there is ample opportunity for drug interaction.[23] Finally, for special populations, including pediatric patients, pregnant women, and those with liver damage (e.g., due to hepatitis coinfection), optimizing HIV treatment is even more complex.[182,199] U.S. and British guidelines encourage use of TDM for antiretroviral therapy in these special populations; recommendations for routine use remain controversial, given the conflicting results reported for TDM trials.

Successful use of TDM requires analytical methods capable of quantitating drugs of interest without interference from other compounds.[182] This is extremely important for antiretrovirals, given the large number of medications commonly administered to HIV-positive patients. Where available, LC-MS/MS methods are generally preferred for their ability to specifically monitor multiple agents with minimal interference.[94,135] However, the complexity and expense of LC-MS/MS can prevent its use in many laboratories, notably in the developing world, where HIV infection rates are highest. For this and other reasons, assays for antiretroviral TDM are currently performed at only a few sites, although the need for better availability is well recognized. Efforts to expand access to testing are under way, such as measuring drug concentrations from dried blood spots to facilitate sample transport and minimize infection risk.[94] Pharmacokinetic details of antiretrovirals are summarized in Table 34-4.

Protease Inhibitors

PIs inhibit viral propagation by interfering with the processing of HIV polypeptide precursors, thus disrupting a step that is mandatory for formation of mature viral particles and continuation of the infection cycle.[103] Oral bioavailability tends to vary greatly depending on formulation and food intake. Most PIs are highly protein bound, and in vivo efficacy (which involves entry into cells) may require higher serum concentrations than those predicted by in vitro measures of viral susceptibility. PIs in current use include indinavir, saquinavir, atazanavir, lopinavir, nelfinavir, and ritonavir; nelfinavir has an active metabolite, M8, which should be included in TDM considerations.[103,182]

Most of these agents are CYP substrates, and several are capable of modulating the activity of specific CYPs. Enzyme inducers (e.g., lopinavir, nelfinavir) and inhibitors (e.g., atazanavir, ritonavir) may affect their own metabolism, as well as that of comedications. This has been exploited therapeutically in so-called boosted regimens, wherein a PI is administered alongside low-dose ritonavir—a potent CYP3A4 inhibitor—to prolong exposure to the first agent.[103,106] This strategy enhances the efficacy of the boosted PI, allowing use of less drug (likely reducing expense) while potentially minimizing toxicity, because the AUC of the PI is increased without a dramatic rise in peak concentrations.

Particularly for treatment-experienced patients, current antiretroviral TDM assesses both the amount of drug present and the susceptibility of the HIV isolate to that agent. This strategy, termed the *inhibitory quotient (IQ),* has been expressed as the phenotypic IQ [C_{min}/IC_{50} (half maximal inhibitory concentration)], the virtual IQ (vIQ; C_{min}/virtual IC_{50}), the genotypic IQ (gIQ; C_{min}/number of mutations), and a normalized IQ based on population susceptibility.[22,94] Although additional studies are required to delineate the preferred measure of IQ, it appears that the use of IQ to optimize antiretroviral therapy is more successful than examination of pharmacologic or virologic parameters alone.[199] Effective IQ concentrations are drug specific and likely regimen specific (e.g., boosted vs. nonboosted); thus target IQs for individual agents must be carefully assessed.

Non-nucleoside Reverse Transcriptase Inhibitors

NNRTIs specifically target the reverse transcriptase enzyme that transcribes viral RNA into DNA, thus preventing viral incorporation into the host genome.[182] Unlike the NRTIs, these agents are not nucleoside or nucleotide analogs, and they do not bind reverse transcriptase at its active site. Compared with PIs, NNRTIs appear to display less marked interindividual variability in serum concentrations, but evidence suggests that their use can be improved by robust TDM.[9,182] Common NNRTIs include efavirenz and nevirapine.

Efavirenz and nevirapine induce metabolic activity via CYP3A4 and CYP2B6, the same enzymes responsible for NNRTI metabolism.[106] Management of drug interactions therefore is one of the more obvious reasons to request TDM for these agents.[9] Much like the PIs, target concentrations for TDM of NNRTIs are still being defined; use of IQ strategies appears helpful in achieving effective clinical responses, particularly in treatment-experienced patients. Some evidence suggests that high serum NNRTI concentrations correlate with onset of toxicity, specifically, central nervous system effects in the case of efavirenz, or liver enzyme elevations and rash for nevirapine.[106] Although the association of serum concentration with toxicity has been challenged, TDM-guided dose reduction trials have successfully decreased adverse effects, supporting the utility of TDM in optimizing NNRTI therapy.[162]

Other Antiretroviral Drugs

NRTIs include both nucleoside and nucleotide analogs, which inhibit viral replication by competing with natural nucleotides to terminate the growth of viral DNA strands.[106] NRTIs include some of the first anti-HIV therapies devised, such as zidovudine, didanosine, and stavudine, as well as several newer agents (e.g., abacavir, tenofovir). Studies addressing TDM for NRTIs provide mixed results, but in general TDM is less helpful for these drugs than for other antiretrovirals. Relatively poor correlation has been found between serum NRTI concentrations and efficacy, largely because these compounds must undergo intracellular phosphorylation for activity.[199] Their metabolism occurs via routes similar to those of endogenous nucleic acids; thus minimal risk of drug interactions is associated with CYPs and other common metabolic enzymes.

Entry/fusion inhibitors, the newest group of antiretrovirals, target the ability of the virus to infect host cells.[182] Entry inhibitors such as maraviroc specifically bind and block access to host proteins (e.g., CCR5, CD4) that the virus hijacks to gain entry to cells; the fusion inhibitor enfuvirtide mimics portions of the HIV fusion mechanism to

TABLE 34-4 Pharmacokinetic Parameters of Antiretroviral Drugs

Drug	Minimum Effective Concentration (C_{min}, mg/L)[106,199]	Minimum Toxic Concentration (C_{max}, mg/L)[106]	Mean Half-life, h	Mean Volume of Distribution, L/kg	Mean Oral Bioavailability, %	Protein Binding, %	CYP Enzymes Involved in Metabolism	CYP Enzymes Inhibited or Induced
Protease Inhibitors								
Amprenavir	>0.2	>8	8	6	NA	90	3A4	3A4
Atazanavir	NA	NA	7	2	NA	86	3A4	3A4, 1A2, 2C9
Fosamprenavir	NA	NA	8	6	NA	90	3A4	3A4
Indinavir	>0.1	>10	2	2.5	30	60	3A4	3A4
Lopinavir (boosted)	>4	NA	5	0.6	NA	98	3A4	3A4
Nelfinavir	>1	>6	4	5	20-80	98	3A4, 2C19, 2C9, 2D6	3A4
Ritonavir	>2	>22	4	0.4	60	98	3A4, 2D6	3A4, 2D6
Saquinavir	>0.25	>6	7	10	NA	98	3A4	3A4
Non-Nucleoside Reverse Transcriptase Inhibitors								
Efavirenz	1-4	>4	50	3	NA	99	3A4, 2B6	3A4
Nevirapine	>3.5	>12	25	1.2	93	60	3A4, 2B6	3A4, 2B6
Other Antiretrovirals								
Abacavir	NA	NA	1.5	0.85	83	50	NA	NA
Didanosine	NA	NA	1.6	1	40	<5	NA	NA
Emtricitabine	NA	NA	10		93	<4	NA	NA
Lamivudine	>0.4	NA	9	1.3	86	<36	NA	NA
Stavudine	NA	NA	1	0.5	86	0	NA	NA
Zalcitabine	NA	NA	1.2		85		NA	NA
Zidovudine	>0.2	NA	1.1	1.5	60	<25	NA	NA
Tenofovir	NA	NA	17	0.6	25	0	NA	NA

NA, Data not available.

prevent complete fusion with the target cell. Data are currently insufficient to guide recommendations for TDM, and very few assays are available.

Antineoplastics

Treatment of cancer is based on clinical protocols that often utilize a series of drugs or combinations of drugs. Drugs used for conditioning and for primary and adjuvant chemotherapy may be mechanistically distinct and, in fact, may have been developed for other purposes (e.g., immunosuppression, infection). The standard of care in dosing most chemotherapy agents is based on body surface area (mg/m^2), yet tremendous pharmacokinetic and pharmacodynamic variability is observed, and therapeutic monitoring of most of the drugs utilized is not common. However, the potential benefit of monitoring deserves attention because there exist few other medical situations in which the need for optimal dosing is equal. The temporal opportunity for efficacy of cancer chemotherapy is limited, and risk of toxicity is high. Factors contributing to pharmacokinetic and pharmacodynamic variability include genetic variation (germline and somatic), physiologic and clinical status, and drug-drug interactions. In addition, many chemotherapeutic agents are prodrugs that require biotransformation to exert therapeutic effects, and strong evidence suggests that interpatient and intrapatient variability in biotransformation reactions is a major contributor to both toxicity and treatment failure. For some chemotherapeutics, pretherapeutic testing may have utility in identifying individuals at risk of therapeutic failure or significant toxicity. Herein a discussion of therapeutic monitoring for treatment with busulfan, methotrexate, and 6-mercaptopurine is presented. Table 34-5 lists pharmacokinetic parameters for antimetabolites.

Busulfan

Busulfan is a chemotherapeutic drug that inhibits the growth of malignant cells by alkylating DNA. An orally administered formulation was introduced in 1953 as a possible treatment for chronic myelogenous leukemia and was largely replaced by the introduction of an IV formulation (Busulfex). The clinical utility of oral busulfan was compromised by its wide variability in distribution[84] and clearance.[76] Busulfan is currently used in hematopoietic stem cell transplant preparative regimens to maximize an antitumor effect. Studies have shown that high-dose oral busulfan combined with 2 or 4 days of cyclophosphamide, prior to bone marrow transplant, is an effective alternative to cyclophosphamide and total body irradiation.[105,172] In addition to being an effective antitumor agent, the busulfan-cyclophosphamide regimen has been reported to minimize the risk of secondary tumor development and growth retardation in children when compared with irradiation. As such, busulfan is also used to treat malignant and nonmalignant bone marrow disorders, such as acute and chronic leukemias, myelodysplastic syndromes, β-thalassemia major, polycythemia vera, and sickle cell anemia, as well as inborn errors of metabolism and severe immune deficiencies.

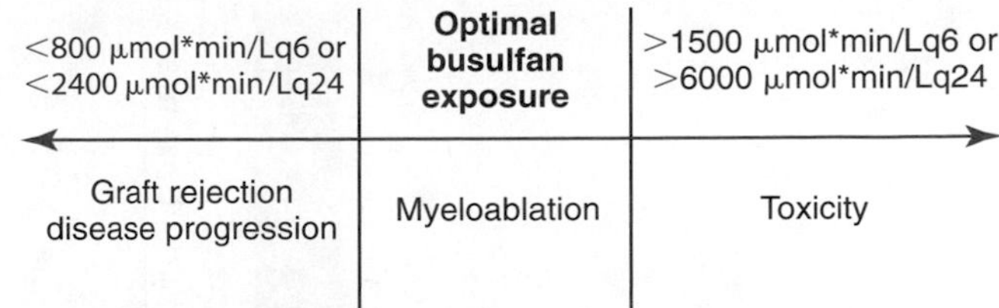

Figure 34-11 Busulfan therapeutic values. Optimal target values for myeloablation with busulfan are based on area under the curve (AUC) measurements and depend on the administration regimen. Four-times-daily dosing (q6) and once-daily dosing (q24) are the most common busulfan protocols. AUC measurements below target ranges are associated with unsuccessful transplant outcomes, and exceeding target ranges incurs risk for toxicity.

A well-accepted dosing paradigm for IV busulfan to replace the historical 1-mg/kg PO dosing consists of 0.8 mg/kg IV (adult) and 1.0 mg/kg IV (children), administered as a 2-hour infusion every 6 hours for 16 doses (4 days), followed by 2 days of 60 mg/kg/d or 4 days of 50 mg/kg/d of cyclophosphamide. The busulfan dose is normalized to body weight to reduce variability in clearance among patients. Despite hope that TDM may not be required by implementation of the IV formulation, TDM is still required to account for pharmacokinetic variables not overcome by IV administration and to address the narrow therapeutic range of this drug (Figure 34-11).[24,127] Busulfan pharmacokinetics is affected by age, weight, disease status, hepatic function, and drug interactions. The optimal range of therapeutic area under the plasma concentration versus time curve (AUC) for standard dosed busulfan is 900 to 1350 µmol•min/L. Patients with busulfan concentrations below the therapeutic range are thought of as having an increased risk of relapse as well as of rejection, even though the immunosuppressive capability of busulfan is controversial.[181] Conversely, patients with plasma concentrations greater than 1500 µmol•min/L have an increased risk of severe treatment-related toxicity, such as sinusoidal obstruction syndrome (SOS; previously called veno-occlusive disease of the liver) and oral mucositis.[76,84]

Once-daily dosing of busulfan for adults at 3.2 mg/kg IV has been proposed to replace the four-times-daily dosing protocols that were originally designed on the basis of convenience of oral dosing (0.8 mg/kg IV). Pharmacokinetic variables and rates of complications are not significantly different between the protocols. The AUC generated by once-daily dosing is approximately four times that observed with four-times-daily dosing, indicating that overall daily exposure using either of the dosing protocols is similar.[169] In one study, a 3.6-fold range of AUC was observed among 51 patients, supporting the continued need for TDM to optimize dose. Further, progression-free survival was associated with an AUC greater than 2400 µmol•min/L but less than 6000 µmol•min/L.[65] Once-daily administration of busulfan to children has also proved successful.[10] Another change in conditioning protocols is to combine busulfan with

TABLE 34-5 Pharmacokinetic Parameters of Antineoplastic Drugs

Drug	Minimum Effective Concentration	Minimum Toxic Concentration	Mean Half-Life, h	Mean Volume of Distribution, L/kg	Mean Protein Binding, %	Important Metabolizing Enzymes
Busulfan, 6 h dose[181]	AUC: >900 µmol•min/L	AUC: >1350 µmol•min/L	2.6	0.99	10	SULT
Busulfan, 24 h dose[65]	AUC: >2400 µmol•min/L	AUC: >6000 µmol•min/L	2.6	0.99	10	SULT
Methotrexate[161]						
At 24 hours	<10 µmol/L	>10 µmol/L	1.8	0.55	46	None
At 48 hours	<1 µmol/L	>1 µmol/L	8.4	0.55	46	None
At 72 hours	<0.1 µmol/L	>0.1 µmol/L	>10	0.55	46	None
Azathioprine	NA	NA	0.2	0.8	0	
6-Mercaptopurine	NA	NA	0.9	0.56	19	TPMT
Tamoxifen[26]	NA		15	55	>98	CYP2D6, CYP3A4/5
Endoxifen	>50 nmol/L	Not defined				

AUC, Area under the curve; *NA,* not applicable.

fludarabine instead of cyclophosphamide. In contrast to cyclophosphamide, fludarabine is not associated with SOS and has a sufficiently long plasma half-life to accommodate once-daily dosing; this simplifies and shortens conditioning protocols.[6,50]

Methotrexate

Methotrexate has proved useful in the (1) management of acute lymphoblastic leukemia in children; (2) management of choriocarcinoma and related trophoblastic tumors in women[61]; (3) management of carcinomas of the breast, tongue, pharynx, and testes; (4) maintenance of remission in leukemia; and (5) treatment of severe, debilitating psoriasis. High-dose methotrexate administration followed by leucovorin rescue is effective in treatment of carcinoma of the lung and osteogenic sarcoma. Intrathecal administration is effective in treating meningeal leukemia or lymphoma.

Methotrexate inhibits DNA synthesis by decreasing the availability of pyrimidine nucleotides. Methotrexate competitively inhibits the enzyme dihydrofolate reductase, thus decreasing the concentrations of the tetrahydrofolate essential to the methylation of the pyrimidine nucleotides and consequently the rate of pyrimidine nucleotide synthesis. Leucovorin, a folate analog, is used to rescue host cells from methotrexate inhibition; as a synthetic substrate for dihydrofolate reductase, leucovorin administration allows resumption of tetrahydrofolate-dependent synthesis of pyrimidines and reinitiation of DNA synthesis. Methotrexate is a nonspecific cytotoxin, and prolongation of blood concentrations appropriate to killing tumor cells may lead to severe, unwanted cytotoxic effects such as myelosuppression, gastrointestinal mucositis, and hepatic cirrhosis.

Serum concentrations of methotrexate are commonly monitored during high-dose therapy (>50 mg/m^2) to identify the time at which active intervention by leucovorin rescue should be initiated. Criteria for serum concentrations indicative of a potential for toxicity after single-bolus, high-dose therapy are as follows[161]:

1. Methotrexate concentration greater than 10 μmol/L 24 hours after dose.
2. Methotrexate concentration greater than 1 μmol/L 48 hours after dose.
3. Methotrexate concentration greater than 0.1 μmol/L 72 hours after dose.

Characteristically, serum concentrations are monitored at 24, 48, and 72 hours after the single dose, and leucovorin is administered when methotrexate concentrations are inappropriately high for a postdose phase. The route of elimination for methotrexate is primarily renal excretion. During the period of high serum concentrations, particular attention must be paid to maintaining output of a large volume of alkaline urine. The pK_a of methotrexate is 5.5; thus small decreases in urine pH result in significant reduction in its solubility. Keeping urinary pH alkaline diminishes the risks of intratubular precipitation of the drug and obstructive nephropathy during the treatment period. Monitoring serum concentrations therefore provides the basis for decisions related to timing of initiation and continuance of leucovorin treatment and for management of urinary pH.

Methotrexate has been measured in biological specimens using a wide variety of techniques. Radioimmunoassay (RIA) and folate reductase inhibition techniques have been used, but nonisotopic immunoassays are now the method of choice.[4] Liquid chromatographic procedures have also been developed to allow for coanalysis of the drug and its metabolites.[16]

Low-dose methotrexate, as is used to manage rheumatoid arthritis, Crohn's disease, psoriasis, or inflammatory bowel disease, is not typically monitored because analytical methods are not sensitive enough to monitor once-weekly dosing, and because methotrexate concentrations have not been shown to correlate well with disease control.[203] However, recent literature suggests that measurement of polyglutamated forms of methotrexate in erythrocytes is useful. Specifically, steady-state concentrations of long-chain polyglutamate forms have been shown to correlate with efficacy of methotrexate; both proposed therapeutic ranges and analytical methods are beginning to emerge.[27,92]

Thiopurines

The thiopurine drug mercaptopurine and its prodrug azathioprine are used as to treat neoplasias such as leukemia, as well as Crohn's disease, irritable bowel syndrome, and psoriasis.[217] Thiopurines are metabolized to the pharmacologically active 6-thioguanine-nucleotides (6-TGNs), which are responsible for the therapeutic and toxic effects of the parent drugs. The enzyme thiopurine *S*-methyltransferase (TPMT) opposes the transformation of 6-mercaptopurine or 6-thioguanine to 6-TGN; therefore patients with TPMT deficiency are at risk for thiopurine drug-induced toxicity, such as myelosuppression. Approximately 0.5% of Caucasians are homozygous for an allele variant of *TPMT* that expresses no activity. Patients expressing minimal TPMT activity shunt thiopurine to an alternate metabolic pathway, resulting in accumulation of thiopurine nucleosides, which cause cytotoxicity. Patients at risk for thiopurine intoxication can be identified by monitoring TPMT phenotypic enzymatic activity,[209] genotype,[208] or thiopurine nucleotide concentration.[150] A good correlation demonstrated between 6-TGN and 6-methylated (6-MMPN) metabolites and genotype (Figure 34-12) could be used to optimize dosing.[51]

Other Antineoplastic Agents

Tamoxifen is a selective estrogen receptor modulator used in breast cancer therapy. Tamoxifen must be metabolized by CYP2D6 and CYP3A4/5 to endoxifen for the estrogen receptor activity of tamoxifen to be expressed (see Figure 34-6).[71] Endoxifen has 100 times greater estrogen receptor modulator activity as compared with tamoxifen.[26,99]

For various reasons, purine and pyrimidine drugs have not been routinely monitored outside of clinical trials. Cytosine arabinoside; 5-fluorouracil; 5-fluorodeoxyuridine and its monophosphate, 5-azacytidine; and 2,2 difluorodeoxycytidine, all of which are antimetabolites like methotrexate, have

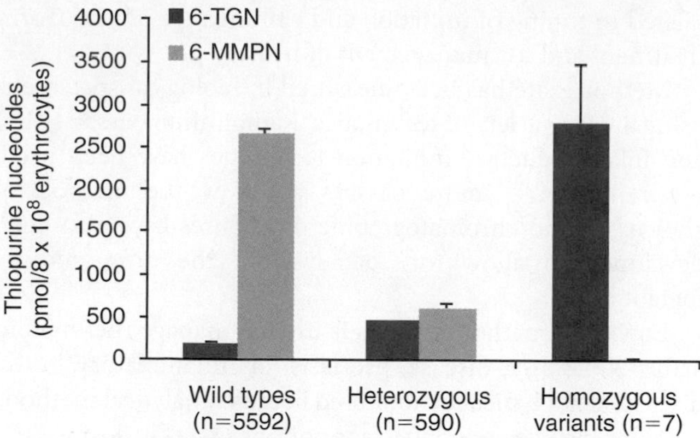

Figure 34-12 Thiopurine therapeutic drug management (TDM) relative to thiopurine *S*-methyltransferase (TPMT) genotype. The profile of thiopurine-containing nucleotides [6-thioguanine-nucleotides (6-TGNs), 6-methylated metabolites (6-MMPNs)] in erythrocytes correlates with TPMT genotype and is a potential biomarker. *(Modified from Figure 4A of Dervieux T, Meyer G, Barham R, Matsutani M, Barry M, Boulieu R, et al. Liquid chromatography-tandem mass spectrometry analysis of erythrocyte thiopurine nucleotides and effect of thiopurine methyltransferase gene variants on these metabolites in patients receiving azathioprine/6-mercaptopurine therapy. Clin Chem 2005;51:2074-84.)*

been extensively studied. Analytical methods have been developed, but little relationship between circulating blood concentration and therapeutic efficacy has been found to justify routine monitoring. Alkylating agents such as cyclophosphamide are metabolically converted to active compounds with life spans of only seconds before they interact with tissue and are destroyed. Measurement of active metabolite would be extremely useful but is impractical. Actinomycin and doxorubicin have toxic effects (bone marrow suppression and dermatitis) that are both immediate and long acting and that appear to relate not to a circulating blood concentration but to dose mass and length of exposure. Definition of specific dosing regimens for these drugs is currently of greater concern than is control of circulating concentration. Cisplatin, easily measurable by platinum analysis, causes renal toxicity that may be related to both blood concentrations and length of exposure, although monitoring is not common.

Cardioactive Drugs

Many agents used to treat various cardiovascular conditions are predominantly assessed for efficacy by biomarkers (e.g., monitoring cholesterol for statin therapy) or by clinical measures (e.g., blood pressure for antihypertensives). For many of these drugs, the therapeutic window is sufficiently wide to obviate the requirement for TDM, or poor correlation is noted between serum concentration and clinical effect or toxicity. Although laboratory measurements for such agents are still useful in ascertaining compliance for such agents, this section will focus on cardioactive medications for which TDM has been shown to be clinically useful in optimizing therapy or preventing toxicity. Pharmacokinetic parameters of select cardioactive drugs are listed in Table 34-6.

The major cardioactive drugs requiring TDM are the antiarrhythmic agents and the glycoside digoxin. These compounds have benefited from well-established monitoring guidelines[197] for over a decade; the guidelines are still valid, and the essential importance of TDM for cardioactive therapeutics has not diminished. However, prescription trends for cardioactive agents have shifted in recent years, resulting in fewer prescriptions for older, relatively difficult-to-manage drugs.[60] Key points pertaining to current TDM recommendations are summarized here; for additional information, readers are referred to the previous edition of this chapter, wherein specific cardioactive agents were described in excellent detail.

Antiarrhythmic Agents

Arrhythmias, disturbances of the normal cardiac sinus rhythm, can be associated with substantial morbidity and mortality; atrial fibrillation is the most common form of serious arrhythmia.[36] A variety of agents are available to treat atrial fibrillation and other medically significant arrhythmias. Many of these drugs act via regulation of cation channels (Na^+, K^+, or Ca^{2+}) and are associated with the potential for serious side effects and drug-drug interactions.[37] Monitoring of clinical parameters (e.g., thyroid function tests for amiodarone therapy) is essential but can be complemented by TDM measurements.[37,179,197] Antiarrhythmic agents for which TDM is commonly performed tend to show onset of toxicity at concentrations only slightly above or even coincident with the upper range of the therapeutic window.

The antiarrhythmic agents are classified according to function.[37,197] Class I compounds primarily affect sodium channel function, although several members of the class have other activities as well. Moderate Na^+ channel blockers (i.e., class IA agents) include quinidine, procainamide, and disopyramide; procainamide should be monitored in conjunction with its active metabolite, *N*-acetylprocainamide. Many of these agents can be measured by immunoassays compatible with high-throughput autoanalyzers, making TDM convenient for most providers.[197] However, the use of class IA agents has fallen off in recent years, most notably in the case of quinidine.[60] This trend may reflect cardiac toxicity associated with these agents, including risk of a potentially lethal arrhythmia, torsades de pointes.[36]

Class IB agents (weak Na^+ channel blockers) include lidocaine, tocainide, and mexiletine; these agents are used in acute management of cardiac conditions (e.g., life-threatening ventricular arrhythmia, digitalis toxicity) but are less likely to be used in settings requiring prolonged TDM. Serum concentrations are typically measured to ensure adequate therapy and to minimize toxicity.[37] Of note, lidocaine binds primarily to AAG, which is often elevated in acute situations such as myocardial infarction, possibly affecting free concentrations of the drug.[197]

Use of strong Na^+ channel blockers (class IC agents) has increased slowly over time, possibly in part because of their

TABLE 34-6 Pharmacokinetic Parameters of Cardioactive Drugs

Drug	Therapeutic Range,[197] mg/L*	Minimum Toxic Concentration, mg/L	Mean Half-life, h	Mean Volume of Distribution, L/kg	Mean Oral Bioavailability, %	Protein Binding, %	Enzymes Involved in Metabolism
Amiodarone	0.5-2	>2.5	45 days	60	45	99	CYP3A4, 2C8
Digitoxin	0.01-0.03	>0.045	150	0.5	80	90	CYP3A4
Digoxin	0.5-2 μg/L	>3 μg/L	40	5	70	25	CYP3A4
(in heart failure)	0.5-0.8 μg/L						
Disopyramide	2-5	>7	8	0.6	83	65	CYP2D6, 3A4
Flecainide	0.2-1	>1	14	5	70	45	CYP2D6
Lidocaine	1.5-5	6	1.8	1.1	35	70	CYP2D6, 3A4, Pg
Mexiletine	0.5-2	>2	10	5	90	60	CYP2D6, 1A2
Procainamide	4-8	>10	6	1.9	83	20	NAT
N-acetylprocainamide	10-20	>40	8	NA	NA	NA	NA
Quinidine	2-5	>6	6	3	80	85	CYP3A4
Sotalol	1-3	NA	12	2	60	NA	NA

NA, Data not available.
*Except where noted.

comparatively lower association with torsades de pointes [a form of polymorphic ventricular tachycardia associated with a long QT interval on electrocardiogram (ECG)] or other serious arrhythmias.[36,60] Class IC agents include flecainide and propafenone. TDM for these agents is primarily recommended to prevent concentration-dependent toxicity (flecainide) and to ensure adequate concentrations after first-pass metabolism (propafenone).[37]

Class III antiarrhythmics, which act primarily via K^+ channel blockade, include amiodarone, dofetilide, and sotalol. Amiodarone (Cordarone, Pacerone) has rapidly gained popularity for the management of atrial fibrillation[60]; it is less prone to inducing arrhythmia than many of the class I agents but is nonetheless associated with adverse events such as pulmonary fibrosis, hepatic failure (both uncommon, but serious), and disruption of thyroid function (relatively common, but generally manageable).[179] Most of these complications are related to the extent of exposure to amiodarone and may reverse after reduction or elimination of the drug. TDM for amiodarone should include measurement of its active metabolite, desethylamiodarone, although recommended therapeutic ranges tend to address only the parent drug.[37]

Acceptance of TDM for cardioactive agents is not universal,[180,193] although the benefits of a robust program have been shown.[37,197] Common situations that call strongly for the use of TDM include management of patients with comorbidities such as renal failure (not uncommon in the elderly populations most prone to arrhythmia) and those experiencing physiologic change, for example, rapid weight fluctuations. In addition, many antiarrhythmic agents affect both metabolic (e.g., CYP enzymes) and transporter (e.g., P-glycoprotein) activities; thus the potential for serious drug-drug interactions is very real.[36]

Digoxin

Obtained from *Digitalis* plants such as foxglove, digoxin (Lanoxin) is a cardiac glycoside used in treatment of arrhythmias and heart failure. Cardiac glycosides (i.e., cardioactive agents containing one or more sugar moieties) are a group of related compounds found in a variety of plants, many of which are poisonous (e.g., oleandrin, the toxic component of oleander).[48,174] Thus it is not surprising that digoxin use is accompanied by the risk of serious toxicity, necessitating the use of TDM to avert such concerns.

Digoxin is thought to act through several mechanisms, including inhibition of the Na^+-K^+-ATPase that regulates cation flux in myocardial cells. Its direct and indirect activities coordinate to slow heart rate, increase the strength and velocity of cardiac contraction, and regulate nervous (sympathetic) and endocrine (renin-angiotensin) systems, affecting cardiovascular function.[66] Digoxin use has declined in recent years, but the drug is still prescribed,[60] particularly in congestive heart failure where it is successful in relieving symptoms although without substantial improvement in mortality,[66] and for treatment of atrial rhythm disturbances.

Clinical response to digoxin is thought to correlate better with tissue concentrations than with serum concentrations. The relationship between tissue and serum stores can be highly variable, thus serum measurements are an unreliable predictor of efficacy. The practice of titrating dose to target serum concentrations is now discouraged, following large studies showing that low digoxin concentrations (<0.9 mg/L) can produce adequate clinical responses.[66]

However, TDM remains essential in assessing risk of digoxin toxicity, particularly in patients with suspicious symptoms.[66,180] Certain populations (e.g., women, the elderly) are at increased risk for elevated digoxin concentrations and thus toxicity, which begins with nonspecific effects (nausea, vomiting, anorexia) but can progress to severe, potentially lethal cardiac manifestations (tachycardia, ventricular fibrillation).[115] A greenish-yellow visual distortion has been described; although relatively uncommon, this is highly suspicious for digoxin toxicity. Patients with serum electrolyte imbalance (high calcium, low magnesium, or low potassium) or renal dysfunction are predisposed to developing toxicity, even at digoxin concentrations within the therapeutic window.[115,183]

If samples are collected at the appropriate time, high serum digoxin correlates with toxicity. Digoxin distributes extensively into tissue, a process that requires several hours after a dose is administered. For this reason, TDM samples must be drawn at least 8 hours after the last dose (i.e., the time of peak *tissue* concentration); serum drawn earlier will provide elevated results that are not representative of the true serum concentration after distribution. Similarly, because of its long half-life, digoxin requires 8 to 10 days after a dose adjustment to reach steady state.[183] Reviews of current TDM practices have shown that digoxin sampling is often performed inappropriately, leading to potential confusion and mismanagement of patients.[180,197]

Digoxin-binding agents (e.g., Digibind, Digifab) are available for treatment of toxicity.[174,197] These are modified antibodies specific to digoxin that sequester the drug to prevent its physiologic effects. It should be noted that these agents only mildly enhance elimination of digoxin; thus the antidote-bound drug remains in serum for some time after treatment. For this reason, assays measuring total digoxin concentrations will still reflect the sum of digoxin bound to antidote plus serum protein-bound digoxin. The active fraction (i.e., that which is not bound to the antidote antibody fragments) can be determined by measuring free digoxin concentrations.[47,197]

As a substrate for CYP3A4 and P-glycoprotein, digoxin is subject to a variety of drug-drug interactions, particularly in the setting of heart disease, where many patients require multiple medications. It is interesting to note that herbal products not only can affect digoxin therapy (e.g., induction of CYP3A4-mediated metabolism by St. John's Wort) but can also interfere with common analytical methods used to detect digoxin.[48] Certain traditional herbal therapies containing a closely related cardiac glycoside can cause false elevation of immunoassay results for digoxin; similarly, patients experiencing oleander poisoning can show positive digoxin results due to antibody cross-reactivity.[47,197] There is a positive clinical utility for antibody cross-reactivity, however, as it has been shown that digoxin-binding antidotes can successfully treat poisoning by oleander or related plants.[155]

Digitoxin, a cardiac glycoside that is closely related to digoxin, is similarly effective in therapy of congestive heart failure. Its use is less prevalent in the United States but remains common in some European countries.[15] The mechanism of action and clinical efficacy of digitoxin are similar to those of digoxin; however, its pharmacokinetic parameters may be preferable for certain patients. Specifically, digitoxin undergoes hepatic metabolism, and its elimination is less heavily dependent on renal function than digoxin, which is excreted largely unchanged in urine. Thus patients with renal disease do not accumulate digitoxin; however, hepatic metabolism presents the potential for additional drug-drug interactions. Digitoxin and other cardiac glycosides are now being studied as potential anticancer agents, although few studies have progressed beyond preclinical trials.[140]

Immunosuppressants

Immunosuppressants, drugs capable of suppressing immune responses, are used to treat autoimmune disease, allergies, multiple myeloma, and chronic nephritis, and in organ transplantation. Therapeutic ranges and toxic thresholds are proposed and are widely utilized to optimize dosing of these drugs. TDM is important for optimizing immunosuppressant therapy because serious consequences of underdosing (e.g., graft rejection) and overdosing (e.g., risk of opportunistic infections) are known. TDM can also prevent drug-related toxicity (e.g., kidney damage) and can be used to evaluate compliance.

Patterns of use of immunosuppressive drugs in transplant patients have changed through the decades.[3] From 1954 to 1962, referred to as the Experimental Era, few transplants were performed. The incidence of acute rejection during the first year following transplant surgery was 80%, and 1-year graft survival was 40%; the search was on to find acceptable immunosuppression techniques. The successful use of azathioprine combined with corticosteroid from 1962 to 1983, the Azathioprine Era, made widespread kidney transplantation possible. However, the rates and severity of acute rejection remained high (65% acute rejection), as was the rate of graft loss (60% with 1-year survival). The Cyclosporine Era (1983 to 1995) provided for significant improvement in outcomes (45% acute rejection, 85% with 1-year survival), and routine transplantation of organs other than kidneys was instituted with a relatively fixed drug regimen. Recognition, in early clinical trials, that cyclosporine has a narrow therapeutic index and highly variable pharmacokinetics in renal transplant patients led to the development of immunoassay and HPLC methods for quantification. It was during this era that TDM of cyclosporine became a standard of practice, which set the stage for the evolution of this practice with the other major maintenance immunosuppressants. The introduction of tacrolimus in 1994 and mycophenolate mofetil in 1995 opened the most recent era. The introduction of sirolimus in 1999 and everolimus in 2004 provided major additions to this era.

Drug regimens used in the current era for maintenance immunosuppression vary widely according to the transplanted organ type and the specific clinical scenario. All immunosuppressant drugs have narrow therapeutic indices, and their pharmacokinetics are highly variable in transplant patients, particularly in the early post-transplant period. Frequent (sometimes daily) monitoring during the early post-transplant stage of therapy requires rapid response from the laboratory until a stable therapeutic dosing strategy is established. TDM support during the maintenance stage of therapy, often a few weeks post transplant and potentially lifelong afterward, remains important but is often performed only periodically to verify compliance, to respond to anticipated changes in pharmacokinetics, or as otherwise indicated clinically. Consensus guidelines and position papers regarding immunosuppression TDM methods and application are common. Interest in application of LC-MS/MS methods to immunosuppressive TDM is prominent in today's literature[109,191,194,214] because of increased sensitivity and specificity compared with common immunoassay methods, and multianalyte capabilities. Note that, because of metabolite cross-reactivity of the detection antibodies on which commercially available immunoassays are based, therapeutic ranges for immunosuppressant drugs may vary with the analytical technique. Values obtained by immunoassay may be 20 to 60% higher than those obtained by chromatographic techniques such as HPLC or LC-MS/MS.[100] The therapeutic ranges and toxic thresholds provided within this chapter are intended to provide general guidelines but should not be applied to clinical practice without consideration of the analytical technique used, and the circumstances surrounding the patient, such as the clinical indication, the clinical status of the patient, time post transplant (for tissue or organ transplant recipients), time of specimen collection relative to drug administration, and comedications. In general, therapeutic ranges are higher in the immediate post-transplant period (0 to 3 months) and are lower during maintenance therapy. They may also be lower for combination therapies and specialized protocols, such as those designed to minimize calcineurin inhibitors.[58,133]

Monitoring drug concentrations and optimizing dose are traditionally based on adjusting dose to achieve steady-state concentrations that fall within target ranges. These target ranges are established through experience for a specific clinical scenario or population and do not necessarily ensure that immunosuppression is adequate, nor that the patient will escape drug-related toxicity. Indeed, controlled pharmacokinetics does not equate to clinical response. Therefore, interest in developing biomarkers to evaluate the pharmacodynamics of immunosuppressive therapy is growing.[200] Peripheral biomarkers that describe immune events and overall immunosuppression, used in combination with TDM, would complement and further personalize immunosuppressant drug therapy.

One approach to pharmacodynamic monitoring has been to measure the activity of target enzymes to evaluate response to cyclosporine, sirolimus, and mycophenolic acid.[32,75,82] Although it detects change in activity due to drug interactions, this approach does not reflect the downstream immunosuppression that is anticipated. Markers of cell activation status, including proliferation and apoptosis markers, have also been proposed. For example, flow cytometric analysis of cell surface antigens that may correlate with cell activation status has been described.[11] Thresholds for adequacy of immunosuppression, possible infection, and acute rejection need to be defined, as do guidelines for interpretation of proportional changes in patient values. A commercial assay, based on incubating patient blood with a mitogen (phytohemagglutinin) and measuring adenosine triphosphate concentrations in CD4+ T cells, is available for evaluating cell proliferation status. The utility of this assay in predicting acute rejection or infection is controversial.[19,83,165] Monitoring non–T-cell mediated events associated with rejection, such as antibody-mediated rejection, has also been proposed, such as through antibody neutralization assays or identification of more specific protein biomarkers.[153] Nonetheless, pharmacodynamic monitoring has great potential to augment the therapeutic management of immunosuppressants and could become a prominent component of therapeutic management in the future.

Discussion here will focus on the common immunosuppressants currently monitored clinically to support initiation and maintenance of immunosuppression in solid organ and bone marrow transplant patients, including two calcineurin inhibitors (cyclosporine, tacrolimus), an inosine-5′-monophosphate dehydrogenase (IMPDH) inhibitor (mycophenolate mofetil), and two mammalian target of rapamycin (mTOR) inhibitors (sirolimus and everolimus). Pharmacokinetic parameters for immunosuppressants are summarized in Table 34-7.

Calcineurin Inhibitors

Cyclosporine

Cyclosporine, also known as Cyclosporin A ,Cicloral, Gengraf, Neoral, Restasis, and Sandimmune, is a fat-soluble cyclic peptide composed of 11 amino acids, some of novel structure, isolated from the fungus *Trichoderma polysporum*. It is available in many formulations and brand names (e.g., Sandimmune Neoral, Gengraf). The compound has been shown effective in suppressing acute rejection in recipients of allograft organ transplants, and is approved for use in renal, cardiac, hepatic, pancreatic, and bone marrow transplants. Although not discussed further here, cyclosporine is also used to treat keratoconjunctivitis sicca, and to manage immune-mediated conditions such as psoriasis and rheumatoid arthritis.

Cyclosporine is considered a calcineurin inhibitor, but in reality, it provides immunosuppression by blocking the activation of T lymphocytes via a multifaceted mechanism.[149] Cyclosporine crosses the lymphocyte membrane freely, where it forms a pharmacologically active complex with the intracellular immunophilin receptor cyclophilin. This complex, but not cyclosporine by itself, inhibits the Ca^{2+}/calmodulin-activated form of serine/threonine phosphatase calcineurin, thereby inhibiting the activation of nuclear factor of activated T (NFAT) in T cells.[158] Inhibition of NFAT activation mediated by cyclosporine leads to the downregulation of transcription of genes for cytokines such as interleukin (IL)-2, IL-3, IL-4, and IL-12; inflammatory mediators such as tissue necrosis factor-alpha (TNF-α); and growth factors such as granulocyte and/or macrophage colony-stimulating factor. Inhibition of calcineurin by the cyclosporine-cyclophilin complex produces other important intracellular effects that contribute to the overall immunosuppressive effect. The intracellular mechanism(s) by which cyclosporine produces side effects—such as acute nephrotoxic effects including reduced renal blood flow, afferent arteriolar vasoconstriction, decreased glomerular filtration rate, and increased renal vascular resistance—remains unknown but appears to be related to altered release of vasoactive factors and effects on transcriptional regulation.[35]

Cyclosporine formulations are not bioequivalent and cannot be used interchangeably. Formulations are described as "modified" (Gengraf, Neoral) or "nonmodified" (Sandimmune), wherein the modified forms (microemulsion formulations) are better absorbed. However, all formulations are considered to have erratic and incomplete absorption after oral administration, ranging from 5 to 60%, and averaging 30%.[90,152] Peak concentrations are reached in 2 to 6 hours after oral administration with the nonmodified formulations, and in 1 to 2 hours with the modified forms. With the nonmodified form, a second peak is sometimes observed at 5 to 6 hours after administration. Cyclosporine is highly protein bound (≈90%), primarily to lipoprotein concentrates in erythrocytes, and has a relatively high volume of distribution (V_d = 3 to 5 L/kg). Cyclosporine undergoes extensive metabolism mediated by CYP3A4. Many of the 31 known metabolites of cyclosporine are inactive.[216] One of the major metabolites, hydroxylated at the number 1 amino acid, retains approximately 10% of the immunosuppressive activity of the parent compound. The combination of variable expression of CYP3A4 and the associated multidrug efflux pump known as P-glycoprotein in the small intestine is thought to form a natural barrier to the absorption of cyclosporine after oral administration, and is thought to explain much of the extensive interpatient range of bioavailability. Because many other drugs are substrates for these two systems, the gastrointestinal tract is an important site for drug-drug interactions. Elimination of cyclosporine is biphasic and is primarily biliary. Terminal half-life is variable with formulation and patient, ranging from 5 to 18 hours for the modified forms and from 10 to 27 hours for the nonmodified forms.

TDM is best performed with whole blood. The degree of concentration in erythrocytes is temperature dependent in vitro; for this reason, measurement of plasma concentration is not recommended.[87,214] Whole blood concentration of the parent drug (cyclosporine) correlates with the degree of immunosuppression and toxicity, but a poor relationship is seen between dose and blood concentration. Immunoassay methods were historically nonspecific because polyclonal

TABLE 34-7 Pharmacokinetic Parameters of Immunosuppressant Drugs

Drug[49,58,133,143,171]	Minimum Effective Concentration, MEC, µg/L	Minimum Toxic Concentration, MTC*, µg/L	Average Half-life, h	Average Volume of Distribution, L/kg	Average Oral Bioavailability, %	Average Protein Binding, %	Important Metabolizing Enzymes
Cyclosporin A†	50	350*	8.4	3-5	30	90	CYP 3A4, Pg
Everolimus	3	15*	24	NA	16	74	CYP 3A4, Pg
Mycophenolic acid	1.3 mg/L	12 mg/L	18	4	94	97	UGT
Sirolimus	4	20*	62	12	10	90	CYP 3A4, Pg
Tacrolimus	3	20*	21	0.85	15	85	CYP 3A4, Pg

*Trough (predose) concentrations. The minimum effective and toxic concentrations are intended to provide general guidelines but should not be applied to clinical practice without consideration of the analytical technique used, the clinical indication, the clinical status of the patient, time post transplant (for tissue or organ transplant recipients), time of specimen collection relative to drug administration, and comedications. In general, therapeutic ranges are higher in the immediate post-transplant period (0 to 3 months) and lower during maintenance therapy. They may also be lower for combination therapies and specialized protocols.

†Refers to data for Neoral.

NA, Data not available; *UGT,* uridine diphosphate glucuronosyltransferase.

antibodies were approximately 30% cross-reactive with several metabolites, leading to falsely elevated concentrations in some patients. This finding was corroborated by a study conducted by the College of American Pathologists.[184] Immunoassays based on monoclonal antibodies provide better specificity but still may not be as specific as methods based on HPLC or LC-MS/MS.

Conventional therapeutic trough blood concentrations of cyclosporine for renal transplants are 150 to 300 μg/L immediately post transplant, and 100 to 200 μg/L thereafter. Efforts to minimize toxicity have led to evaluation of lower cyclosporine target ranges, such as 50 to 100 μg/L. Rates of acute rejection have not been different with low-dose versus conventional dosing; hence, prescribing patterns are being redefined to minimize cyclosporine exposure.[49] Higher target concentrations are commonly used for cardiac, hepatic, and pancreatic transplants.

Although trough concentration monitoring of cyclosporine was shown to be less effective than interval AUC of the drug in providing a precise estimate of drug exposure, the impracticality of measuring a full AUC using a series of samples collected over the 12-hour dose interval prevented this more accurate and precise determination of cyclosporine exposure from ever becoming a widely used monitoring test. Another approach is based on the association of most of the variability in cyclosporine pharmacokinetics during the first few hours following oral administration. This approach measures either the area under the blood cyclosporine concentration-time curve in the first 4 hours post dose,[14] or the blood cyclosporine concentration at 2 hours post dose, known as *C2 monitoring.*[44] It has been reported that patients with C2 concentrations higher than 1300 μg/L during the first week post kidney transplant were free of acute rejection, although specific target ranges for C2 monitoring are not well established.[56] However, C2 monitoring is logistically challenging and has not been proven to improve outcomes over traditional predose monitoring.[108]

Many drugs alter the disposition of cyclosporine. Drugs that inhibit CYP3A enzyme activity and block P-glycoprotein have been found to decrease cyclosporine metabolism and reduce the barrier to absorption from the gastrointestinal tract, thereby causing increased blood concentration.[5,78] Examples include the calcium channel blockers verapamil, diltiazem, and nicardipine; azole antifungal drugs fluconazole, itraconazole, voriconazole, and ketoconazole; and antibiotics, such as erythromycin. All prolong the metabolism of cyclosporine and reduce the barrier to absorption sufficiently to increase the risk of nephrotoxicity. Coadministration of phenytoin, phenobarbital, carbamazepine, and rifampin results in induction of CYP3A enzymes and P-glycoprotein, which, respectively, increases the rate at which cyclosporine is metabolized in the gastrointestinal tract and liver along with the countertransport of the drug, thereby reducing significantly the bioavailability of the parent drug. Intravenous administration of sulfadimidine and trimethoprim decreases cyclosporine concentrations.

Tacrolimus

Tacrolimus (proprietary names Prograf, Advagraf, and Protopic, and formerly known as FK506) is a macrolide lactone isolated from *Streptomyces tsukubaensis* in 1984; it is a potent immunosuppressant that consists of a 23-member carbon ring and a hemiketal-masked α,β-diketoamide function. Structurally, tacrolimus is similar to the other macrolides sirolimus and everolimus. Tacrolimus is approved for prophylaxis of organ rejection in patients receiving allogeneic liver transplants and for use as an immunosuppressant in kidney transplantation. This potent immunosuppressant has been used effectively in other solid organ transplant patients, for prevention of graft-versus-host disease in allogeneic stem cell transplant recipients, and in pancreatic islet transplantation, as well as for atopic dermatitis.

As with cyclosporine, tacrolimus exerts its immunosuppressive effects following the formation of a complex with immunophilins. The complex of tacrolimus and FK-BP12 in lymphocytes suppresses the synthesis of cytokines and inflammatory mediators by the same mechanisms as with cyclosporine (see cyclosporine section for details and references). Tacrolimus is administered in much lower doses than cyclosporine because of its substantially higher potency.

Absorption from the small intestine is generally low, averaging 25%, but is highly variable from patient to patient and with time post transplant.[202] Low tacrolimus bioavailability, as with cyclosporine, is probably due to the presence of CYP3A4 and P-glycoprotein in the small intestinal enterocytes.[41] Peak concentrations are observed 0.5 to 4 hours after administration. The distribution in blood is characterized by extensive uptake by the cells. The whole blood-to-plasma ratio varies from 15 to 35, but the V_d is 1 to 2 L/kg if based on blood. Approximately 99% of tacrolimus in plasma is bound to proteins, primarily α_1-acid glycoprotein, lipoproteins, albumin, and globulins.[218] The major route of elimination is fecal excretion of metabolites. The elimination half-life of tacrolimus is variable, averaging 8 to 12 hours, but it can range from 4 to 41 hours. As with cyclosporine, CYP3A4 is primarily responsible for tacrolimus metabolism; nine metabolites have been identified, including one active metabolite, 31-O-desmethyl tacrolimus. This metabolite is generally present at very low concentrations and therefore is negligible in most patients. An exception, however, is seen in liver transplant patients with hyperbilirubinemia, in whom significant high bias in the immunoassay results may occur because of metabolite accumulation that results from impaired bile clearance.

TDM for tacrolimus is similar to that for cyclosporine. The relationship between tacrolimus dose, trough blood concentration, and clinical outcomes—including acute rejection, nephrotoxicity, and toxicity requiring dose reduction—was investigated in a prospective multicenter study in liver transplant patients.[201] A significant inverse correlation between tacrolimus trough blood concentration and risk of acute rejection during the first week following liver transplantation was shown using logistic regression analysis. Nephrotoxicity and other side effects were significantly correlated with increasing tacrolimus trough blood concentrations during this period. Receiver operator characteristic curve analyses showed that tacrolimus trough blood concentrations could differentiate between toxicity and nonevents. However, these relationships are somewhat controversial. Despite the fact that tacrolimus exposure is best predicted by the AUC, most TDM occurs with single predose blood samples and, as with cyclosporine, whole blood is the preferred specimen.[204] The originally proposed therapeutic range for tacrolimus was 5 to 20 μg/L, although efficacy has been demonstrated at lower concentrations, particularly for protocols designed to minimize renal toxicity by lowering concentrations of calcineurin inhibitors. The European consensus conference of 2007 recommended that laboratories seek methods with lower limits of quantification of 1 μg/L or less, to support sparing protocols that lower and narrow the limits of therapeutic to 3 to 7 μg/L.[49,204] As with cyclosporine, many drugs alter the disposition of tacrolimus through interaction with CYP3A4 or P-glycoprotein. A comprehensive review on this subject has been published.[41]

IMPDH Inhibitor: Mycophenolate Mofetil

Mycophenolate mofetil (MMF) (proprietary names CellCept and Myfortic) is the 2-morpholinoethyl ester prodrug form of the active immunosuppressant mycophenolic acid (MPA). The latter is a fermentation product of several *Penicillium* species that has antifungal, antibacterial, antitumor, and immunosuppressive activity in animal models. Following demonstration of its immunosuppressive efficacy in human renal transplant patients and in combination with cyclosporine and corticosteroids, formal clinical trials were conducted. In 1995, MMF was approved by the U.S. Food and Drug Administration (FDA) for this use. MMF is also used with cardiac and liver transplantation, particularly for patients who do not tolerate cyclosporine or tacrolimus well, to treat Crohn's disease, and to manage psoriasis.

MPA is a reversible and uncompetitive inhibitor of IMPDH. A very important characteristic of proliferating lymphocytes is the greatly increased rate of de novo purine biosynthesis. The sustained and markedly increased rate of guanine nucleotide production catalyzed by IMPDH is the rate limiting step in de novo purine biosynthesis that cannot be provided by the salvage pathway in proliferating lymphocytes. Thus the proliferative response of activated T cells is dependent on a continuous and increased supply of intracellular guanine nucleotide pool. T-cell proliferation is arrested by the suppression of guanine nucleotide production when IMPDH is inhibited by MPA. The mechanism of action whereby MPA produces its immunosuppressive effects in proliferating T lymphocytes is thus clearly distinct from that of the calcineurin and mTOR inhibitors.

MMF has near complete bioavailability after oral administration and is rapidly hydrolyzed by widely distributed esterases in blood and tissues to produce MPA. MPA usually reaches maximal concentrations within an hour of oral administration of MMF. Distribution of the drug is rapid and is essentially complete in most patients within 2 to 3 hours of oral administration.[33] In whole blood, more than 99.9% of the drug is in the plasma compartment and is highly protein bound.[141] The volume of distribution for MPA is 4 L/kg, and the half-life is, on average, 18 hours. Clearance of MPA is affected by (1) glucuronidation, (2) enterohepatic circulation (EHC), and (3) the quantity of its free fraction. EHC is considered to be a significant contributor to the dose interval kinetics of MPA, especially the postdistribution phase of the concentration-time curve. The contribution of EHC to the MPA AUC is about 37%, ranging from 10 to 61%, based on the effects of concomitant administration of cholestyramine.[33] The appearance of a secondary MPA concentration peak anywhere from 4 to 12 hours following the morning dose of MMF is believed to result from EHC. The rate-limiting step in the clearance of MPA is its conversion to the phenolic glucuronide metabolite mycophenolic acid glucuronide (MPAG) via the catalytic action of UGT in the liver, gastrointestinal tract, and possibly other tissues such as kidney. MPAG is the primary metabolite of MPA and is pharmacologically inactive.[111] The acyl glucuronide and 7-O-glucoside are metabolites that are produced in much smaller quantities than MPA or MPAG.[178] The glucoside metabolite has no pharmacologic activity, but the acyl glucuronide is under evaluation for its potential toxic effects.[177] MPAG is cleared by the kidney and accumulates to as much as several hundred-fold higher plasma concentration as the steady-state trough concentration of MPA in uremic patients.

The specimen of choice for TDM of MPA is plasma or serum. A well-accepted therapeutic range for predose MPA is 1.0 to 3.5 mg/L when combined with cyclosporine, and 1.9 to 4.0 mg/L when combined with tacrolimus. The therapeutic range based on AUC measurements is 30 to 60 mg/h•L.[175,198] Timing of specimen collection relative to drug administration is important in ensuring that MMF is fully hydrolyzed in vivo. It has been shown that MMF can become hydrolyzed in vitro, which may lead to determinations that overestimate the proportion of active MPA in vivo.[177] Because MPA is avidly and extensively bound to albumin in plasma, investigators have studied the utility of monitoring the free fraction for patients with poor kidney function, hypoalbuminemia, and hyperbilirubinemia. In stable transplant patients, the MPA free fraction ranges from 1 to 3%.[141] Increased free fraction will cause enhanced clearance of MPA, resulting in lower total MPA concentrations that return to baseline values when the condition that caused the change in free fraction becomes normal. In chronic renal failure, the total MPA concentration is often within the guidelines for effective immunosuppression, but the free concentrations can be substantially elevated, placing the patient at increased risk for over-immunosuppression.[87] It is hypothesized that chronic uremia causes a reduction in intrinsic clearance that results in zero-order kinetics for MPA elimination. Severely decreased creatinine clearance (<25 mL/min) is associated with reduced exposure to MPA, and moderate loss of renal function appears to increase MPA AUC.

The primary sites and effects of drug-drug interactions involving other medications and MPA are likely to include decreased absorption in the gastrointestinal tract, inhibition of EHC, and inhibition of transport of the primary phenolic glucuronide metabolite. Meal consumption just before oral intake of MMF delays absorption, causing a reduction in maximal concentration of about 25%. Administration of antacids containing magnesium and aluminum hydroxides has been reported to reduce peak concentration of MPA by 33% and AUC by 17%. The two interactions with the greatest reported effects are cholestyramine and ferrous sulfate.[33,134] Cholestyramine produces a 40% reduction in the MPA AUC when coadministered with MMF. The common iron supplement ferrous sulfate lowers the MPA AUC by about 90%. Metronidazole, norfloxacin, and rifampin are among the other drugs that reduce exposure to MPA. Long-term effects of these drug interactions are under investigation. It has been suggested that corticosteroids cause enhanced clearance of MPA via induction of UGT activity. This is based on the observed 33% increase in the dose-corrected MPA trough concentration in a cohort of stable renal transplant patients at 12 months, following corticosteroid withdrawal, compared with the value at 6 months during maintenance therapy with corticosteroids.[38] Inhibition of multidrug resistance protein 2 (MRP2) activity through coadministration of cyclosporine reduces the secondary peak and the overall AUC of MPA.[62,114]

Inhibition of transport of MPAG from liver into bile is the presumed mechanism for the significant lowering of MPA concentration and raising of MPAG concentration by concomitant cyclosporine.[198] This drug-drug interaction results in MPA AUC values, adjusted for MMF dose, that are approximately 45% higher in patients on concomitant tacrolimus versus those on concomitant cyclosporine.

Immunoassays are now available to support TDM, although most TDM currently occurs through the use of chromatographic assays. A new functional method that uses IMPDH, the natural target receptor of MPA, is also available. Inhibition of IMPDH activity by MPA in an aliquot of patient serum or plasma is the basis for this method.[25]

mTOR Inhibitors

Sirolimus

Sirolimus (proprietary name Rapamune, formerly known as Rapamycin) is a macrocyclic antibiotic with immunosuppressive activity.[88] It is a fermentation product of the Actinomycete *Streptomyces hygroscopicus,* which was isolated from soil samples collected on Rapa Nui (Easter Island) following a search for novel antifungal agents. Structurally, sirolimus is a lipophilic macrocyclic lactone composed of a 31-member macrolide ring. It was shown to possess antifungal, antitumor, and immunosuppressive activity in animal model studies. Subsequently, following discovery of its efficacy for the prophylaxis of acute rejection in renal transplant patients, formal clinical trials were undertaken; in 1999, sirolimus was approved for this indication by the FDA. In 2007, the FDA approved an intravenous prodrug called temsirolimus (Torisel), which is metabolized to sirolimus by CYP3A4 and is indicated for the treatment of advanced renal cell carcinoma.[110]

Sirolimus inhibits T-lymphocyte activation and proliferation by inhibiting the mTOR through a mechanism of action unique from calcineurin or IMPDH inhibitors. The complex of sirolimus and the intracellular immunophilin FK-BP12 modulates the immune response by combining with the specific cell-cycle regulatory protein mTOR and inhibiting its activation, and inhibiting progression from the G_1 to the S phase of the cell cycle.[120]

Formulations of sirolimus are not bioequivalent, although tablet and solution formulations were shown to be clinically equivalent.[124] Sirolimus is rapidly absorbed from the gastrointestinal tract, with average time to reach maximal concentration in whole blood of about 2 hours. The average bioavailability of sirolimus is 15%.[221] As with calcineurin inhibitors, the low bioavailability is attributable to extensive intestinal and hepatic metabolism by CYP3A4 and to countertransport by the multidrug efflux pump P-glycoprotein in the gastrointestinal tract. This absorption barrier varies considerably from patient to patient and within patients and is the site of clinically important drug-drug and drug-food interactions. Sirolimus distributes primarily into red blood cells (95%), with only 3% and 2% distributing into plasma and other blood cellular components, respectively. Extensive and avid binding of sirolimus to the ubiquitously distributed intracellular FK-binding proteins accounts for the high blood-to-plasma sirolimus concentration ratio. Approximately 92% of the sirolimus within the plasma fraction is bound to circulating protein, primarily albumin. Metabolism of sirolimus by the human body is driven by oxidative metabolism by CYP3A4 in the gastrointestinal tract and liver. At least seven metabolites are characterized as 41-O- and 7-O-demethyl, hydroxy, hydroxy-demethylated, and didemethylated sirolimus, which are thought to be pharmacologically inactive. Elimination occurs primarily through the biliary tract, with average half-life of 62 hours in adults and substantially shorter (≈11 hours) in children.[173,190]

The specimen of choice for sirolimus TDM is whole blood. The relationship between predose sirolimus concentrations has been investigated in renal transplant patients who received concomitant full-dose cyclosporine and corticosteroid therapy. According to this study, the minimum effective sirolimus concentration, below which a significant increase in risk for acute rejection is seen, is 4 to 5 μg/L.[104] The threshold concentration of 13 to 15 μg/L has been identified, above which the risks for concentration-related side effects of thrombocytopenia (<100,000 platelets/mm^3), leukopenia (<4000 leukocytes/mm), and hypertriglyceridemia (>300 mg/dL serum triglycerides) are increased. In general, a well-accepted range is 4 to 12 μg/L when sirolimus is used in conjunction with cyclosporine and corticosteroids. Alternative ranges proposed include 5 to 10 μg/L when sirolimus is combined with MMF and corticosteroids, and 12 to 20 μg/L when used with just corticosteroids.[143,188] Drug-drug interactions revolving around CYP3A4 and P-glycoprotein, as described earlier, apply for sirolimus as well and have been reviewed extensively.[220]

Chromatographic methods with ultraviolet (UV) and mass spectrometric detection have been validated and are used in laboratories worldwide.

Everolimus

Everolimus (proprietary names Afinitor and Certican) also known as SDZ RAD and RAD001, is a structural analog of sirolimus with potent immunosuppressive activity when used in conjunction with cyclosporine. The primary difference between everolimus and sirolimus is the half-life, which is approximately half that of sirolimus, theoretically leading to more rapid attainment of steady-state concentrations. Everolimus is a semisynthetic lipophilic macrocyclic lactone macrolide. Similar to sirolimus, everolimus forms a complex with intracellular immunophilin FK-BP12 that modulates the immune response by combining with the specific cell-cycle regulatory protein mTOR and inhibiting its activation. This inhibition results in suppression of cytokine-driven T-lymphocyte proliferation, inhibiting progression from the G_1 to the S phase of the cell cycle. Everolimus is metabolized through oxidation by CYP3A4 in the gastrointestinal tract and liver. At least 20 metabolites have been identified.[118] Cyclosporine inhibits the metabolism of everolimus, requiring everolimus dose reduction when coadministered. Everolimus does not affect cyclosporine metabolism. A review of drug-drug interactions observed with everolimus has been published.[113] The primary side effect of concern with everolimus therapy is hyperlipidemia and thrombocytopenia of concentrations >8 μg/L.[57]

Everolimus is administered orally as an oral microsuspension. Everolimus is rapidly absorbed from the gastrointestinal tract, with the average time to reach maximal concentration in whole blood of about 3 hours. Low bioavailability is predicted by extensive intestinal and hepatic metabolism by CYP3A4 and countertransport by the multidrug efflux pump P-glycoprotein in the gastrointestinal tract. This absorption barrier varies considerably from patient to patient and within patients and is the site of clinically important drug-drug and drug-food interactions. Peak concentrations are observed in adults approximately 30 minutes after dosing. The apparent elimination half-life of everolimus is 32 hours.[107] Proportionality between dose and blood concentration increases with increasing dose,[57] and higher dosing appears to increase bioavailability. Steady-state trough blood concentration on a 3-mg/d dose in an adult is likely to be in the range of 5 to 20 μg/L.[57,138] The proposed therapeutic dose for kidney transplant patients comedicated with cyclosporine is 1.5 mg/d, and the target therapeutic range is 3 to 8 μg/L.[113,171] In addition, recommendations for the use of everolimus in heart transplantation have been published.[166]

The specimen of choice for supporting TDM of everolimus is currently predose whole blood. Everolimus can be determined by immunoassay or by multiple HPLC methods with UV or mass spectrometric detection.[191,194]

Pain Management

Chronic noncancer pain affects approximately one in three Americans during a lifetime, and is the leading cause of health-related absenteeism. Escalating medical costs and lost productivity, as well as increased risk of depressive and anxiety disorders associated with chronic pain, have created a tremendous social burden. Pharmacologic management of pain involves mechanistically diverse drugs, including antiepileptics, tricyclic antidepressants, muscle relaxants, benzodiazepines, anesthetics, and opioids. Therapeutic ranges for these drugs in the management of pain have not been established, although thresholds for analgesic efficacy have been proposed for some drugs.[8] However, use of TDM to evaluate compliance with prescribed medications and to detect noncompliance, such as use of nonprescribed medications, has become common and is recommended in the guidelines of the American Society of Interventional Pain Physicians.[195] Of particular interest is detection of compliance with opioid therapy, because safety concerns, risk of drug diversion, risk of drug abuse, and tolerance to the analgesic properties of these drugs require sometimes dramatic escalation in dosing for continued efficacy. Nonprescribed medications of particular interest include other opioids or benzodiazepines and classical drugs of abuse (e.g., marijuana, cocaine, amphetamines). However, conventional drugs of abuse tests designed for occupational or forensic purposes may not meet the needs of medical testing because conventional tests have relatively high cutoff concentrations and may not detect drugs of interest such as oxycodone and methadone. Compliance monitoring is most commonly accomplished with random urine specimens, although patients who cannot provide a urine specimen (e.g., dialysis patients) and patients for whom pharmacokinetic evaluations are desired may be monitored with serum or plasma specimens.

Opioids

Drugs that produce analgesia through interaction with opioid receptors found in the central nervous system are referred to as *opioids.* Opioids include opiates, those drugs derived naturally from the opium poppy plant (e.g., codeine, morphine), semisynthetic opiates (e.g., hydromorphone, hydrocodone, oxycodone, oxymorphone, heroin), and fully synthetic opioids (e.g., fentanyl, methadone, tramadol, propoxyphene, buprenorphine, meperidine). These drugs are widely used to manage chronic pain and are monitored to detect compliance, diversion, and use of nonprescribed opioids.[40,195]

Laboratories that provide testing for opioids to verify compliance must implement very specific and sensitive analytical methods. Many common immunoassays for opiates do not detect all opioids and may have inadequate sensitivity for testing with random urine specimens, particularly when serum or plasma specimens are tested. Concentrations of various opioids relative to prescribed doses, individual drug pharmacokinetics, dosing intervals, and consideration of complex metabolism must be considered for accurate assessment of compliance.[137] Figure 34-13 depicts the complexity of opioid metabolism.

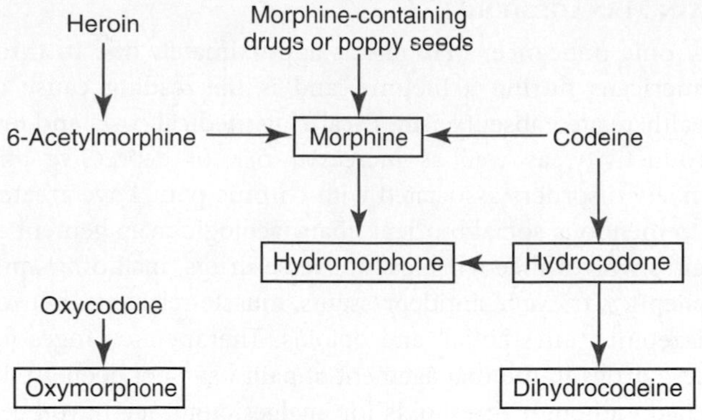

Figure 34-13 Opiate metabolism. Metabolic relationships between several of the major natural and semisynthetic opiates are shown. Drugs appearing in boxes could be present in patient specimens as a result of administration of that compound (i.e., parent drug), or as a metabolic product resulting from administration of a related agent.

Psychiatric Therapies

Psychiatry is one area of clinical practice that has largely embraced the use of TDM. Therapy in psychiatric illness fits many of the criteria for monitoring: treatment is usually long term; efficacy can be difficult to assess from clinical indicators alone; and the toxicity of many psychoactive drugs is concentration dependent and preventable. Compliance rates are often lower in mental disorders than in nonpsychological illnesses,[196] supporting the rationale for measuring psychotropic drug concentrations. In addition, several psychiatric agents exhibit significant drug-drug interactions and effects on metabolic enzyme activity, making serum concentrations difficult to predict in combination therapy.

Antidepressants

Antidepressants are the therapy of choice for endogenous depression, that is, depressive behavior lacking an apparent organic or societal cause. These agents are also used to treat a variety of other psychological and mood-related conditions, including anxiety disorders, obsessive-compulsive behavior, eating disorders, substance abuse, insomnia, and chronic pain.[210] Their primary mechanism for activity is believed to be modulation of monoamine neurotransmitters (catecholamines) such as serotonin, norepinephrine, and dopamine in the central nervous system.[119]

Published guidelines strongly recommend TDM for most tricyclic antidepressants and venlafaxine, on the basis of well-established correlations between serum concentration and clinical effect (response or toxicity).[12] TDM of other antidepressants can still be useful in evaluating individual pharmacokinetics, assessing compliance, managing comedication, and caring for patients with renal or hepatic disease. Pharmacologic parameters of antidepressants are shown in Table 34-8.

Tricyclic Antidepressants

For one of the first drug classes available to treat depression, the tricyclic antidepressants (TCAs), strong evidence supports the utility of monitoring serum concentrations to improve patient management and reduce toxicity.[70,117,132] In general, TCA pharmacokinetic parameters are unfavorable: bioavailability is often low; the drugs are extensively protein bound and distribute widely into tissue; and metabolism depends on enzymes that can be inhibited or induced, with ample opportunity for drug interactions.[210] Despite their troublesome pharmacokinetics, TCAs are effective agents with a manageable safety profile, justifying their continued use. Common TCAs include amitriptyline (Elavil), clomipramine (Anafranil), desipramine (Norpramin), doxepin, imipramine (Tofranil), and nortriptyline (Pamelor), among others.

Several TCAs have active metabolites that must be included in TDM measurements [e.g., amitriptyline (active metabolite, nortriptyline), clomipramine (norclomipramine), imipramine (desipramine), and doxepin (nordoxepin)]. Most of these metabolites have comparable antidepressant activity to the parent drug; clomipramine is an interesting exception in that the parent and the metabolite preferentially affect reuptake of serotonin and norepinephrine, respectively.[210] TCAs generally show an initial positive correlation between increasing serum concentration and clinical improvement; however, they exhibit a threshold concentration past which clinical progress may decline because of return of symptoms (e.g., mood worsening) or development of toxicity. This pattern is termed an *inverted U correlation* between clinical response and increasing drug concentration, and has been best described for nortriptyline.[18]

Adverse responses to TCA excess follow an anticholinergic pattern, that is, dry mouth, fever, urinary retention, agitation, confusion, and seizures.[117] Additional cardiovascular complications include hypotension and electrocardiographic changes (QRS widening) that are characteristic of TCA overdose.[144] Serum concentrations correlate with the risk of toxicity but are poor predictors of cardiovascular changes or seizures.

The combination of TCAs with other regulators of monoamine neurotransmitters can create the potential for serotonin toxicity. Detailed reviews of this potentially life-threatening response are available[69]; briefly, increased synaptic serotonin leads to neuromuscular hyperactivity, fever, tachycardia, tachypnea, and agitation, and severe toxicity produces dangerously high fever (>38.5 °C), confusion, and seizures. A variety of medications regulate serotonin concentrations and have the potential to induce serotonin toxicity, including other antidepressants and antipsychotics (see later), anti-Parkinson agents, migraine therapies, and several drugs of abuse such as MDMA (3,4-methylenedioxymethamphetamine; Ecstasy), amphetamine, and cocaine.[69] Use of more than one of these drugs increases the risk of serotonin toxicity, and coadministration of agents that lower the seizure threshold may worsen its severity.

TABLE 34-8 Pharmacokinetic Parameters of Antidepressant Drugs

Drug	Recommended[12] Therapeutic Range, μg/L	Minimum Toxic Concentration, μg/L	Mean Half-life, h	Volume of Distribution, L/kg	Oral Bioavailability, %	Protein Binding, %	CYP Enzymes Involved in Metabolism
Routine TDM Strongly Recommended							
Amitriptyline + nortriptyline	80-200	>500 (sum)	21	15	50	95	2D6, 2C19, 2C9, 1A2, 3A4
Clomipramine + norclomipramine	175-450	>400 (sum)	21	12	36-62	96	2C19, 3A4, 2D6
Desipramine	100-300	>400	22	24-60	35-51	90	2D6
Imipramine + desipramine	175-300	>400 (sum)	12	18	40	90	2D6, 2C19, 1A2, 3A4
Nortriptyline	70-170	>500	30	18	50	92	2D6, 3A4
Venlafaxine + desmethylvenlafaxine	195-400	>1000 (sum)	5	6.5	92	27	2D6, 3A4
TDM Recommended for Select Patients							
Citalopram	30-130	>500	33	12	80	80	2C19, 2D6, 3A4
Doxepin + nordoxepin	50-150	>500	17	20	27	68-85	2D6, 2C19, 2C9, 1A2
Escitalopram	15-80	>250	22	15	80	56	2C19, 3A4
Fluoxetine + norfluoxetine	120-300	>1000	55	35	60	95	2D6, 2C9
Fluvoxamine	150-300	>650	17	5	53	77	1A2, 2D6
Maprotiline	125-200	>300	40	16	79-87	89	2D6, 1A2
Mianserin	15-70	>500	20	20	70	90	1A2, 2D6, 3A4
Mirtazapine	40-80	>1000	22	4.5	50	85	1A2, 2D6, 3A4
Moclobemide	300-1000	>5000	2.5	1.2	70	50	2C19
Paroxetine	70-120	>350	21	13	90	95	2D6
Reboxetine	10-100	NA	1.5	14	95	97	3A4
Sertraline	10-50	>300	26	25-50	>44	98	2D6, 2C9, 2C19, 3A4
Trazodone	650-1500	>4000	7	1	75	93	
Trimipramine	150-350	>500	25	35	40	94	
Viloxazine	20-500	NA	3.5	1	85	88	

NA, Not applicable; *TDM,* therapeutic drug management.

Selective Serotonin Reuptake Inhibitors

Selective serotonin reuptake inhibitors (SSRIs) are second-generation antidepressants whose primary activity is modulation of synaptic serotonin concentrations. In general, their toxicity profile is better than that of older antidepressants,[132,159] although serotonin toxicity is a greater potential risk for SSRIs than for most other drugs; additionally, coadministration of SSRIs with first-generation antidepressants of the monoamine oxidase (MAO) inhibitor class can produce significant risk for serotonin-induced toxicity.[69] SSRIs include citalopram (Celexa), escitalopram (*S*-citalopram; Lexapro), fluoxetine (Prozac, Sarafem), fluvoxamine (Luvox), paroxetine (Paxil), and sertraline (Zoloft); many other compounds are nonselective regulators of serotonin but are not strictly considered SSRIs.

The structural dissimilarities of this class of compounds lead to notable differences in pharmacokinetics. In general, SSRIs show good absorption and intermediate half-lives (12 to 36 hours), except for fluoxetine, which displays a long and variable half-life of several days.[159] Most SSRIs are substrates for multiple CYP enzymes, resulting in complex metabolic pathways; in addition, significant risk for drug-drug interactions is present, as several SSRIs display inhibition of metabolic enzymes ranging from mild (e.g., the effect of citalopram on CYP2D6) to potent (e.g., fluoxetine on CYP2D6).[187] This self-regulation of SSRI metabolism, in addition to other pharmacokinetic variables, leads to extremely wide interindividual variability in serum concentrations at a given dose of drug.

The usefulness of TDM is less well established for SSRIs than for TCAs, given that comparatively weaker correlation has been noted between serum concentrations and clinical efficacy or risk of toxicity.[131,159] However, assessment of SSRI compliance through TDM has shown cost savings by preventing both hospitalizations and time away from work due to disease relapse.[12] In addition, select groups may receive greater benefit from TDM than the general population: monitoring serum SSRI concentrations in elderly patients allowed a substantial number of doses to be lowered, saving drug costs without reducing clinical efficacy.[119]

Serotonin and Norepinephrine Reuptake Inhibitors

As their name implies, serotonin and norepinephrine reuptake inhibitors (SNRIs) act primarily via modulation of intrasynaptic concentrations of those two neurotransmitters.[132] Similar to the SSRIs, this class of antidepressants has the potential to cause serotonin toxicity when given alone or in combination with other monoamine regulators.[69] SNRIs include venlafaxine (Effexor) and duloxetine (Cymbalta); the opioid analgesic tramadol is also believed to act in part through SNRI-like modulation of neurotransmitter concentrations.[130]

Venlafaxine was recently included in guidelines strongly recommending measurement of serum concentrations for TDM.[12] Its active metabolite, O-desmethylvenlafaxine, is itself an antidepressant of the SSRI class. Clinical improvement correlates with serum concentrations of the parent and the metabolite; in addition, venlafaxine shows concentration-related toxicity, including hypertension and severe arrhythmia (particularly in CYP2D6 poor metabolizers), suggesting that serious adverse responses might be prevented with routine TDM.

Other Antidepressants

Several other classes of antidepressants are known, including reuptake inhibitors selective for norepinephrine (NRI; e.g., reboxetine) or for more than one neurotransmitter (e.g., buproprion, which regulates both norepinephrine and dopamine).[210] Some newer agents with varying degrees of antidepressant activity function as catecholamine receptor antagonists (e.g., trazodone). Older antidepressants include MAO inhibitors, which have fallen in popularity with the availability of better tolerated alternatives, and tetracyclic antidepressants (e.g., maprotiline, mirtazapine). Although analytical methods have been developed for many of these compounds, the primary clinical uses for TDM include assessing nonresponders, confirming compliance, and managing comorbidities (e.g., renal or hepatic dysfunction).[12]

Neuroleptic Agents

Neuroleptics are used to treat patients with mental illness involving a psychotic component, including schizophrenia and bipolar disorder, as well as other neurologic conditions such as Tourette's syndrome.[136] Most antipsychotics in current use act by antagonism or partial agonism of specific dopamine receptors (D_2-like receptors)[77]; this section also discusses TDM for the mood stabilizer lithium. Several of the neuroleptic agents have numerous metabolites, some of which are active, but with one exception (risperidone), current guidelines do not include active metabolites in TDM interpretations.[12] The existence of multiple metabolites can create difficulty with immunoassay reliability; thus chromatographic methods are the preferred analytical platform where available.[154,215] A review of antipsychotic analytical methods has been published.[219] Pharmacologic parameters of antipsychotics are shown in Table 34-9.

Classical Antipsychotics

Older antipsychotic agents successfully treat the "positive" aspects of psychotic disorders (e.g., hallucinations, delusions) but are less effective in managing "negative" aspects such as social withdrawal.[77] Many of these agents are associated with potentially severe cardiac toxicity, prolactin elevation, and development of extrapyramidal symptoms (i.e., involuntary motor activity) such as tardive dyskinesia, that is, uncontrollable repetition of purposeless facial motions that can persist after cessation of therapy. Antipsychotics are associated with a rare but potentially fatal condition, neuroleptic malignant syndrome, which is characterized by muscle rigidity, fever, unstable blood pressure, and poor mental status; risk of this syndrome may be increased with concomitant SSRI use.[189]

According to current recommendations, the classical neuroleptics with evidence to recommend TDM include haloperidol, thioridazine, and several phenothiazines (e.g.,

TABLE 34-9 Pharmacokinetic Parameters of Antipsychotics

Drug	Recommended[12] Therapeutic Range, μg/L*	Mean Half-life, h	Mean Volume of Distribution, L/kg	Mean Oral Bioavailability, %	Protein Binding, %	CYP Enzymes Involved in Metabolism
Routine TDM Strongly Recommended						
Chlorpromazine	30-300	12	21	32	96	NA
Clozapine	350-600	13	5	40	95	1A2, 2C19, 3A4, 2D6
Fluphenazine	0.5-2	13	11	3	99	NA
Haloperidol	5-17	18	18	60	92	NA
Olanzapine	20-80	33	16	80	93	1A2, 2D6
Perphenazine	0.6-2.4	10	20	20	92	2D6
Risperidone +	20-60	20	1	80	89	2D6, 3A4
9-hydroxyrisperidone		NA	NA	NA	77	NA
Thioridazine	200-2000	6.5	18	NA	98	2D6
Lithium	0.5-1.2 mmol/L	24	1	99	0	NA
TDM for Select Patients						
Amisulpride	100-400	12	5.8	50	17	NA
Pimozide	15-20	55	NA	NA	50	3A4, 2D6, 1A2
Quetiapine	70-170	6	10	100	83	3A4, 2D6
Ziprasidone	50-120	9	1.5	60	99	3A4
Zuclopentixol	4-50	20	20	NA	98	NA

*Except where noted.
NA, Data not available; *TDM,* therapeutic drug management.

chlorpromazine, fluphenazine, perphenazine).[12] Consensus guidelines suggest that TDM is best used for optimizing quality of life for patients receiving classical antipsychotics; concentration-dependent toxicity (specifically, extrapyramidal symptoms and seizures) is rarely a threat to patient safety, whereas life-threatening adverse responses (e.g., neuroleptic malignant syndrome) are generally unrelated to serum concentration. The goal of antipsychotic TDM is to maintain patients at the minimum effective concentration for clinical response. Marked interindividual variability is noted in serum drug concentrations at a given dose, suggesting that steady-state serum analysis is the preferred means to protect drug-refractory patients from inadequate therapy.

Atypical Antipsychotics

The desire to minimize extrapyramidal side effects associated with classical neuroleptics led to the development of a newer generation of compounds termed the *atypical antipsychotics.*[77] This nomenclature is somewhat deceiving, as their mechanism of action is similar to that of older agents, namely, modulation of dopamine receptors; studies show that serum antipsychotic concentrations better predict dopamine receptor occupancy than does dose.[125] It is thought that atypical antipsychotics show reduced influence on areas of the brain involved in motor control, hence the reduction in extrapyramidal effects compared with classical neuroleptics.[77] Clozapine is the prototype of the atypical agents, which also include olanzapine, risperidone, quetiapine, and amisulpride.

Clozapine (Clozaril), olanzapine (Zyprexa), and risperidone (Risperdal) are the only atypical antipsychotics strongly recommended for routine TDM, although some studies show promise for monitoring other drugs in the class.[12,86] Clozapine has at least two clinically relevant active metabolites: norclozapine and clozapine-*N*-oxide. Toxicity associated with clozapine therapy includes several potentially fatal conditions, including severe myocarditis (particularly at the start of therapy), dose-dependent risk of seizures, and agranulocytosis; this last necessitates monitoring of white blood cell counts throughout clozapine treatment.[77]

Most newer antipsychotics show improved safety profiles, without the risk of agranulocytosis seen with clozapine, and with reduced incidence of the sedation and hyperprolactinemia that characterize the classical neuroleptics.[77] Several atypical agents are metabolized by CYP isoforms; this creates the potential for drug interactions with commonly coprescribed medications such as antidepressants or antiepileptics.[187]

Risperidone is converted to an active metabolite, 9-hydroxyrisperidone, primarily by CYP2D6; both the parent and the metabolite should be measured for TDM purposes.[12,187] The minimal effective concentration for risperidone therapy is still debated, but a threshold concentration has been well defined above which extrapyramidal effects appear (74 µg/L).[125] Similar to risperidone, olanzapine is comparatively safer and better tolerated than older neuroleptics; its most notable adverse effect is pronounced weight gain. Good correlation has been noted between serum olanzapine concentration and clinical efficacy, supporting the use of TDM.[12,125]

Lithium

The monovalent cation lithium (Eskalith) has been used for decades as a mood-stabilizing agent in the treatment of bipolar disorder and other conditions with a manic component.[205] Its pharmacokinetics is relatively favorable in that it is rapidly and completely absorbed, exhibits moderate distribution (1 L/kg) without protein binding, has a convenient half-life (24 hours) for dosing, and is excreted in urine without undergoing metabolism. Purely renal elimination prevents hepatic drug interactions, but certain drugs (e.g., diuretics, nonsteroidal anti-inflammatory agents) and physiologic conditions (e.g., excessive activity, renal disease, aging) can affect lithium excretion.[205]

Lithium exhibits a narrow therapeutic window, with toxic concentrations (>1.5 mmol/L) very near the upper threshold for effective therapy (up to 1.2 mmol/L).[12] The severity of toxicity is concentration related: early signs include lethargy, muscle weakness and tremors, and speech difficulties; concentrations greater than 2.5 mmol/L can produce signs of severe intoxication, including muscle rigidity and life-threatening seizures.[206] Lithium is most commonly measured by automated spectrophotometry, although ion-selective electrodes, atomic absorption spectrometry, and inductively coupled plasma mass spectrometry methods are also available.

BRONCHODILATORS

Drugs used as bronchodilators include the β-adrenergic agonists, theophylline and caffeine, although the latter two are being used less and less.

β-Adrenergic Agonists

β-Adrenergic agonists, such as albuterol, bitolterol, isoproterenol, metaproterenol, pirbuterol, and terbutaline in inhaled form, have become the treatment of choice for a short-acting approach to relief of asthma. These drugs are very effective at providing rapid bronchodilation without significant cardiac or systemic effects. Because they are administered in the vapor form, have a short time of action, and produce little toxicity, measurement of blood concentrations offers little clinical benefit; patient response provides a convenient way by which to monitor therapy.

Theophylline

Theophylline, available under many proprietary names, relaxes bronchial smooth muscles to relieve or prevent asthma. The therapeutic effect of theophylline is likely due to antagonism of adenosine receptors in smooth muscle, whereas the toxic effects are due to inhibition of cyclic nucleotide phosphodiesterase. With increased use of β-adrenergic agonists, and because of the considerable associated toxicity, theophylline is now considered an alternative therapy used only in the treatment of persistent asthma and neonatal apnea.

Theophylline is readily absorbed after oral, rectal, or parenteral administration. If the drug is taken orally without food, the blood concentration peaks within 2 hours. If it is administered with food or as the slow-release formula, peak concentrations occur 3 to 5 hours after the dose. Once absorbed, it is 50% protein bound. Theophylline is metabolized by CyP1A2, which is highly active in children and in adults who smoke. In these people, the half-life ranges from 3 to 4 hours.

Nonsmoking adults in good health have an elimination half-life averaging 9 hours. The half-life in neonates and in adults with congestive heart failure can be prolonged to 20 to 30 hours, depending on the degree of liver immaturity or loss of liver function. Coadministration of cimetidine, ciprofloxacin, and ticlopidine will reduce the clearance of theophylline.

Theophylline clearance is a function of a metabolic process that is dose dependent. At serum concentrations greater than 20 mg/mL, small dose increases lead to disproportionately large increases in serum concentration and intoxication. Symptoms of theophylline toxicity include nausea, vomiting, headache, diarrhea, irritability, and insomnia. Transient central nervous system stimulation occurring at initial administration is not directly related to blood concentration.

This effect diminishes with long-term use. Serious toxicity characterized by cardiac arrhythmias and seizures is usually associated with serum concentrations in excess of 30 mg/mL. Once seizure activity begins, the final prognosis is very poor. Morbidity is reported in nearly all patients, and mortality can be as high as 50%.

Immunoassay is the standard method for the determination of theophylline. Theophylline, caffeine, and dyphylline have been simultaneously quantified by HPLC.

Caffeine

A minor metabolite of theophylline in adults, caffeine has been shown to accumulate to significant concentrations in neonates. Caffeine itself is an effective inhibitor of apnea, which may explain the lower therapeutic concentration required for control of neonatal apnea. Therapy with caffeine alone has been demonstrated as effective in the treatment of neonatal apnea; it is gaining popularity because of the long half-life of caffeine in neonates (>30 hours). Caffeine is metabolized by CyP1A2; this enzyme is not active in neonates. The optimal therapeutic concentration of caffeine in this situation ranges from 8 to 14 mg/mL.

Caffeine is measured by HPLC or immunoassay.

REFERENCES

1. Anonymous. Facts about the Joint Commission's "Do Not Use" list, updated June 9, 2009. Available at: http://www.jointcommission.org/PatientSafety/DoNotUseList/facts_dnu.htm (accessed on February 2, 2010).

2. Anonymous. The Joint Commission: official "Do Not Use" list, updated March 5, 2009. Available at: http://www.jointcommission.org/NR/rdonlyres/2329F8F5-6EC5-4E21-B932-54B2B7D53F00/0/06_dnu_list.pdf (accessed on February 2, 2010).
3. Anonymous. Immunosuppression practice and trends. UNOS Market Share Report, Chapter 4, 2005. Available at: www.unos.org (accessed February 2, 2010).
4. Albertioni F, Rask C, Eksborg S, Poulsen JH, Pettersson B, Beck O, et al. Evaluation of clinical assays for measuring high-dose methotrexate in plasma. Clin Chem 1996;42:39-44.
5. Ambudkar SV, Dey S, Hrycyna CA, Ramachandra M, Pastan I, Gottesman MM. Biochemical, cellular, and pharmacological aspects of the multidrug transporter. Annu Rev Pharmacol Toxicol 1999;39: 361-98.
6. Andersson BS, de Lima M, Thall PF, Wang X, Couriel D, Korbling M, et al. Once daily i.v. busulfan and fludarabine (i.v. Bu-Flu) compares favorably with i.v. busulfan and cyclophosphamide (i.v. BuCy2) as pretransplant conditioning therapy in AML/MDS. Biol Blood Marrow Transplant 2008;14:672-84.
7. Andes D, Pascual A, Marchetti O. Antifungal therapeutic drug monitoring: established and emerging indications. Antimicrob Agents Chemother 2009;53:24-34.
8. Atkinson JH, Patel SM, Meyer JM, Slater MA, Zisook S, Capparelli E. Is there a therapeutic window with some antidepressants for analgesic response? Curr Pain Headache Rep 2009;13:93-9.
9. Back D, Gibbons S, Khoo S. An update on therapeutic drug monitoring for antiretroviral drugs. Ther Drug Monit 2006;28:468-73.
10. Bartelink IH, Bredius RG, Ververs TT, Raphael MF, van Kesteren C, Bierings M, et al. Once-daily intravenous busulfan with therapeutic drug monitoring compared to conventional oral busulfan improves survival and engraftment in children undergoing allogeneic stem cell transplantation. Biol Blood Marrow Transplant 2008;14:88-98.
11. Barten MJ, Tarnok A, Garbade J, Bittner HB, Dhein S, Mohr FW, et al. Pharmacodynamics of T-cell function for monitoring immunosuppression. Cell Prolif 2007;40:50-63.
12. Baumann P, Hiemke C, Ulrich S, Eckermann G, Gaertner I, Gerlach M, et al. The AGNP-TDM expert group consensus guidelines: therapeutic drug monitoring in psychiatry. Pharmacopsychiatry 2004; 37:243-65.
13. Begg EJ, Barclay ML, Kirkpatrick CM. The therapeutic monitoring of antimicrobial agents. Br J Clin Pharmacol 2001;52(Suppl 1):35S-43S.
14. Belitsky P, Dunn S, Johnston A, Levy G. Impact of absorption profiling on efficacy and safety of cyclosporin therapy in transplant recipients. Clin Pharmacokinet 2000;39:117-25.
15. Belz GG, Breithaupt-Grogler K, Osowski U. Treatment of congestive heart failure—current status of use of digitoxin. Eur J Clin Invest 2001;31(Suppl 2):10-7.
16. Belz S, Frickel C, Wolfrom C, Nau H, Henze G. High-performance liquid chromatographic determination of methotrexate, 7-hydroxymethotrexate, 5-methyltetrahydrofolic acid and folinic acid in serum and cerebrospinal fluid. J Chromatogr B Biomed Appl 1994; 661:109-18.
17. Benedetti MS. Enzyme induction and inhibition by new antiepileptic drugs: a review of human studies. Fundam Clin Pharmacol 2000;14: 301-19.
18. Bengtsson F. Therapeutic drug monitoring of psychotropic drugs: TDM "nouveau." Ther Drug Monit 2004;26:145-51.
19. Bhorade SM, Janata K, Vigneswaran WT, Alex CG, Garrity ER. Cylex ImmuKnow assay levels are lower in lung transplant recipients with infection. J Heart Lung Transplant 2008;27:990-4.
20. Bialer M, Johannessen SI, Kupferberg HJ, Levy RH, Perucca E, Tomson T. Progress report on new antiepileptic drugs: a summary of the Eighth Eilat Conference (EILAT VIII). Epilepsy Res 2007;73:1-52.
21. Blum RA, Comstock TJ, Sica DA, Schultz RW, Keller E, Reetze P, et al. Pharmacokinetics of gabapentin in subjects with various degrees of renal function. Clin Pharmacol Ther 1994;56:154-9.
22. Boffito M, Acosta E, Burger D, Fletcher CV, Flexner C, Garaffo R, et al. Current status and future prospects of therapeutic drug monitoring and applied clinical pharmacology in antiretroviral therapy. Antivir Ther 2005;10:375-92.
23. Boffito M, Acosta E, Burger D, Fletcher CV, Flexner C, Garaffo R, et al. Therapeutic drug monitoring and drug-drug interactions involving antiretroviral drugs. Antivir Ther 2005;10:469-77.
24. Booth BP, Rahman A, Dagher R, Griebel D, Lennon S, Fuller D, et al. Population pharmacokinetic-based dosing of intravenous busulfan in pediatric patients. J Clin Pharmacol 2007;47:101-11.
25. Brandhorst G, Marquet P, Shaw LM, Liebisch G, Schmitz G, Coffing MJ, et al. Multicenter evaluation of a new inosine monophosphate dehydrogenase inhibition assay for quantification of total mycophenolic acid in plasma. Ther Drug Monit 2008;30:428-33.
26. Brauch H, Murdter TE, Eichelbaum M, Schwab M. Pharmacogenomics of tamoxifen therapy. Clin Chem 2009;55:1770-82.
27. Brooks AJ, Begg EJ, Zhang M, Frampton CM, Barclay ML. Red blood cell methotrexate polyglutamate concentrations in inflammatory bowel disease. Ther Drug Monit 2007;29:619-25.
28. Bruggemann RJ, Donnelly JP, Aarnoutse RE, Warris A, Blijlevens NM, Mouton JW, et al. Therapeutic drug monitoring of voriconazole. Ther Drug Monit 2008;30:403-11.
29. Brunetti L, Santell JP, Hicks RW. The impact of abbreviations on patient safety. Jt Comm J Qual Patient Saf 2007;33:576-83.
30. Brunton LL, Lazo JS, Parker KL, eds. Goodman and Gilman's the pharmacological basis of therapeutics, 11th edition. New York: McGraw-Hill Professional, 2005.
31. Buchthal F, Svensmark O, Schiller PJ. Clinical and electroencephalographic correlations with serum levels of diphenylhydantoin. Arch Neurol 1960;2:624-30.
32. Budde K, Glander P, Bauer S, Braun K, Waiser J, Fritsche L, et al. Pharmacodynamic monitoring of mycophenolate mofetil. Clin Chem Lab Med 2000;38:1213-6.
33. Bullingham RE, Nicholls AJ, Kamm BR. Clinical pharmacokinetics of mycophenolate mofetil. Clin Pharmacokinet 1998;34:429-55.
34. Burton ME, Shaw LM, Schentag JJ, Evans WE, eds. Applied pharmacokinetics and pharmacodynamics: principles of therapeutic drug monitoring, 4th edition. Philadelphia, Pa: Lippincott, Williams, & Wilkins, 2006.
35. Busauschina A, Schnuelle P, van der Woude FJ. Cyclosporine nephrotoxicity. Transplant Proc 2004;36:229S-33S.
36. Camm AJ. Safety considerations in the pharmacological management of atrial fibrillation. Int J Cardiol 2008;127:299-306.
37. Campbell TJ, Williams KM. Therapeutic drug monitoring: antiarrhythmic drugs. Br J Clin Pharmacol 2001;52(Suppl 1):21S-34S.
38. Cattaneo D, Perico N, Gaspari F, Gotti E, Remuzzi G. Glucocorticoids interfere with mycophenolate mofetil bioavailability in kidney transplantation. Kidney Int 2002;62:1060-7.
39. Chan K, Beran RG. Value of therapeutic drug level monitoring and unbound (free) levels. Seizure 2008;17:572-5.
40. Chou R, Fanciullo GJ, Fine PG, Adler JA, Ballantyne JC, Davies P, et al. Clinical guidelines for the use of chronic opioid therapy in chronic noncancer pain. J Pain 2009;10:113-30.
41. Christians U, Jacobsen W, Benet LZ, Lampen A. Mechanisms of clinically relevant drug interactions associated with tacrolimus. Clin Pharmacokinet 2002;41:813-51.
42. Cloyd JC, Miller KW, Leppik IE. Primidone kinetics: effects of concurrent drugs and duration of therapy. Clin Pharmacol Ther 1981;29:402-7.
43. Cohen JM, Whittaker E, Walters S, Lyall H, Tudor-Williams G, Kampmann B. Presentation, diagnosis and management of tuberculosis in HIV-infected children in the UK. HIV Med 2008;9: 277-84.
44. Cole E, Midtvedt K, Johnston A, Pattison J, O'Grady C. Recommendations for the implementation of Neoral C(2) monitoring in clinical practice. Transplantation 2002;73:S19-22.
45. Coulthard KP, Peckham DG, Conway SP, Smith CA, Bell J, Turnidge J. Therapeutic drug monitoring of once daily tobramycin in cystic fibrosis—caution with trough concentrations. J Cyst Fibros 2007;6: 125-30.

46. Darley ES, MacGowan AP. The use and therapeutic drug monitoring of teicoplanin in the UK. Clin Microbiol Infect 2004;10:62-9.
47. Dasgupta A. Usefulness of monitoring free (unbound) concentrations of therapeutic drugs in patient management. Clin Chim Acta 2007; 377:1-13.
48. Dasgupta A. Herbal supplements and therapeutic drug monitoring: focus on digoxin immunoassays and interactions with St. John's wort. Ther Drug Monit 2008;30:212-7.
49. de Jonge H, Naesens M, Kuypers DR. New insights into the pharmacokinetics and pharmacodynamics of the calcineurin inhibitors and mycophenolic acid: possible consequences for therapeutic drug monitoring in solid organ transplantation. Ther Drug Monit 2009;31:416-35.
50. de Lima M, Couriel D, Thall PF, Wang X, Madden T, Jones R, et al. Once-daily intravenous busulfan and fludarabine: clinical and pharmacokinetic results of a myeloablative, reduced-toxicity conditioning regimen for allogeneic stem cell transplantation in AML and MDS. Blood 2004;104:857-64.
51. Dervieux T, Meyer G, Barham R, Matsutani M, Barry M, Boulieu R, et al. Liquid chromatography-tandem mass spectrometry analysis of erythrocyte thiopurine nucleotides and effect of thiopurine methyltransferase gene variants on these metabolites in patients receiving azathioprine/6-mercaptopurine therapy. Clin Chem 2005; 51:2074-84.
52. Devinsky O, Vazquez B, Luciano D. New antiepileptic drugs for children: felbamate, gabapentin, lamotrigine, and vigabatrin. J Child Neurol 1994;9(Suppl 1):S33-45.
53. Dreifuss FE, Penry JK, Rose SW, Kupferberg HJ, Dyken P, Sato S. Serum clonazepam concentrations in children with absence seizures. Neurology 1975;25:255-8.
54. Duffus J. Glossary for chemists of terms used in toxicology. Pure Appl Chem 1993;65:2003-122.
55. Ecker GF, Stockner T, Chiba P. Computational models for prediction of interactions with ABC-transporters. Drug Discov Today 2008;13: 311-7.
56. Einollahi B, Taheri S, Lessan-Pezeshki M, Pourfarziani V, Hosseini MS, Nemati E, et al. Approach to a target value for 2-hours post dose cyclosporine (C2) during the first week post renal transplantation. Ann Transplant 2009;14:18-22.
57. Eisen HJ, Tuzcu EM, Dorent R, Kobashigawa J, Mancini D, Valantine-von Kaeppler HA, et al. Everolimus for the prevention of allograft rejection and vasculopathy in cardiac-transplant recipients. N Engl J Med 2003;349:847-58.
58. Ekberg H, Tedesco-Silva H, Demirbas A, Vitko S, Nashan B, Gurkan A, et al. Reduced exposure to calcineurin inhibitors in renal transplantation. N Engl J Med 2007;357:2562-75.
59. Ellwood M, Lichtenfeld L, Parker RM, Tuncer D, Solis P, Fusco-Walker SJ, et al. Enhancing prescription medicine adherence: a national action plan. Bethesda, Md: National Council on Patient Information and Education, 2007.
60. Fang MC, Stafford RS, Ruskin JN, Singer DE. National trends in antiarrhythmic and antithrombotic medication use in atrial fibrillation. Arch Intern Med 2004;164:55-60.
61. Ferrari S, Sassoli V, Orlandi M, Strazzari S, Puggioli C, Battistini A, et al. Serum methotrexate (MTX) concentrations and prognosis in patients with osteosarcoma of the extremities treated with a multidrug neoadjuvant regimen. J Chemother 1993;5:135-41.
62. Filler G, Lepage N, Delisle B, Mai I. Effect of cyclosporine on mycophenolic acid area under the concentration-time curve in pediatric kidney transplant recipients. Ther Drug Monit 2001;23:514-9.
63. Flockhart D. Available at: http://medicine.iupui.edu/flockhart/table.htm.
64. Fukuoka N, Tsukamoto T, Uno J, Kimura M, Morita S. Influence of coadministered antiepileptic drugs on serum zonisamide concentrations in epileptic patients: quantitative analysis based on suitable transforming factor. Biol Pharm Bull 2003;26:1734-8.
65. Geddes M, Kangarloo SB, Naveed F, Quinlan D, Chaudhry MA, Stewart D, et al. High busulfan exposure is associated with worse outcomes in a daily i.v. busulfan and fludarabine allogeneic transplant regimen. Biol Blood Marrow Transplant 2008;14:220-8.
66. Gelow JM, Fang JC. Update in the approach to and management of heart failure. South Med J 2006;99:1346-55; quiz 56-7, 84.
67. Gervasini G, Carrillo JA, Benitez J. Potential role of cerebral cytochrome P450 in clinical pharmacokinetics: modulation by endogenous compounds. Clin Pharmacokinet 2004;43:693-706.
68. Ghanbari F, Rowland-Yeo K, Bloomer JC, Clarke SE, Lennard MS, Tucker GT, et al. A critical evaluation of the experimental design of studies of mechanism based enzyme inhibition, with implications for in vitro-in vivo extrapolation. Curr Drug Metab 2006;7:315-34.
69. Gillman PK. A review of serotonin toxicity data: implications for the mechanisms of antidepressant drug action. Biol Psychiatry 2006;59: 1046-51.
70. Gillman PK. Tricyclic antidepressant pharmacology and therapeutic drug interactions updated. Br J Pharmacol 2007;151:737-48.
71. Goetz MP, Kamal A, Ames MM. Tamoxifen pharmacogenomics: the role of CYP2D6 as a predictor of drug response. Clin Pharmacol Ther 2008;83:160-6.
72. Gonzalez-Esquivel DF, Ortega-Gavilan M, Alcantara-Lopez G, Jung-Cook H. Plasma level monitoring of oxcarbazepine in epileptic patients. Arch Med Res 2000;31:202-5.
73. Goodwin ML, Drew RH. Antifungal serum concentration monitoring: an update. J Antimicrob Chemother 2008;61:17-25.
74. Grime KH, Bird J, Ferguson D, Riley RJ. Mechanism-based inhibition of cytochrome P450 enzymes: an evaluation of early decision making in vitro approaches and drug-drug interaction prediction methods. Eur J Pharm Sci 2009;36:175-91.
75. Grinyo JM, Cruzado JM, Millan O, Caldes A, Sabate I, Gil-Vernet S, et al. Low-dose cyclosporine with mycophenolate mofetil induces similar calcineurin activity and cytokine inhibition as does standard-dose cyclosporine in stable renal allografts. Transplantation 2004;78: 1400-3.
76. Grochow LB, Jones RJ, Brundrett RB, Braine HG, Chen TL, Saral R, et al. Pharmacokinetics of busulfan: correlation with veno-occlusive disease in patients undergoing bone marrow transplantation. Cancer Chemother Pharmacol 1989;25:55-61.
77. Grunder G, Hippius H, Carlsson A. The 'atypicality' of antipsychotics: a concept re-examined and re-defined. Nat Rev Drug Discov 2009;8: 197-202.
78. Guengerich FP. Cytochrome P-450 3A4: regulation and role in drug metabolism. Annu Rev Pharmacol Toxicol 1999;39:1-17.
79. Gustavson LE, Boellner SW, Granneman GR, Qian JX, Guenther HJ, el-Shourbagy T, et al. A single-dose study to define tiagabine pharmacokinetics in pediatric patients with complex partial seizures. Neurology 1997;48:1032-7.
80. Hammett-Stabler CA, Johns T. Laboratory guidelines for monitoring of antimicrobial drugs. National Academy of Clinical Biochemistry. Clin Chem 1998;44:1129-40.
81. Harris RZ, Jang GR, Tsunoda S. Dietary effects on drug metabolism and transport. Clin Pharmacokinet 2003;42:1071-88.
82. Hartmann B, Schmid G, Graeb C, Bruns CJ, Fischereder M, Jauch KW, et al. Biochemical monitoring of mTOR inhibitor-based immunosuppression following kidney transplantation: a novel approach for tailored immunosuppressive therapy. Kidney Int 2005;68: 2593-8.
83. Hashimoto K, Miller C, Hirose K, Diago T, Aucejo F, Quintini C, et al. Measurement of CD4+ T-cell function in predicting allograft rejection and recurrent hepatitis C after liver transplantation. Clin Transplant 2010;24:701-8.
84. Hassan M, Oberg G, Ehrsson H, Ehrnebo M, Wallin I, Smedmyr B, et al. Pharmacokinetic and metabolic studies of high-dose busulphan in adults. Eur J Clin Pharmacol 1989;36:525-30.
85. Herring AR, Williamson JC. Principles of antimicrobial use in older adults. Clin Geriatr Med 2007;23:481-97.
86. Hiemke C, Dragicevic A, Grunder G, Hatter S, Sachse J, Vernaleken I, et al. Therapeutic monitoring of new antipsychotic drugs. Ther Drug Monit 2004;26:156-60.

87. Holt DW, Armstrong VW, Griesmacher A, Morris RG, Napoli KL, Shaw LM. International Federation of Clinical Chemistry/International Association of Therapeutic Drug Monitoring and Clinical Toxicology working group on immunosuppressive drug monitoring. Ther Drug Monit 2002;24:59-67.
88. Holt DW, Denny K, Lee TD, Johnston A. Therapeutic monitoring of sirolimus: its contribution to optimal prescription. Transplant Proc 2003;35:157S-61S.
89. Hope WW, Billaud EM, Lestner J, Denning DW. Therapeutic drug monitoring for triazoles. Curr Opin Infect Dis 2008;21:580-6.
90. Hoppu K, Jalanko H, Laine J, Holmberg C. Comparison of conventional oral cyclosporine and cyclosporine microemulsion formulations in children with a liver transplant. Transplantation 1996; 62:66-71.
91. Hosoda N, Miura H, Takanashi S, Shirai H, Sunaoshi W. The long-term effectiveness of clonazepam therapy in the control of partial seizures in children difficult to control with carbamazepine monotherapy. Jpn J Psychiatry Neurol 1991;45:471-3.
92. Hroch M, Tukova J, Dolezalova P, Chladek J. An improved high-performance liquid chromatography method for quantification of methotrexate polyglutamates in red blood cells of children with juvenile idiopathic arthritis. Biopharm Drug Dispos 2009;30:138-48.
93. Isoherranen N, Yagen B, Soback S, Roeder M, Schurig V, Bialer M. Pharmacokinetics of levetiracetam and its enantiomer (R)-alpha-ethyl-2-oxo-pyrrolidine acetamide in dogs. Epilepsia 2001; 42:825-30.
94. Ivanovic J, Nicastri E, Ascenzi P, Bellagamba R, De Marinis E, Notari S, et al. Therapeutic drug monitoring in the management of HIV-infected patients. Curr Med Chem 2008;15:1925-39.
95. Johannessen CU, Johannessen SI. Valproate: past, present, and future. CNS Drug Rev 2003;9:199-216.
96. Johannessen SI, Battino D, Berry DJ, Bialer M, Kramer G, Tomson T, et al. Therapeutic drug monitoring of the newer antiepileptic drugs. Ther Drug Monit 2003;25:347-63.
97. Johannessen SI, Landmark CJ. Value of therapeutic drug monitoring in epilepsy. Expert Rev Neurother 2008;8:929-39.
98. Johannessen SI, Tomson T. Pharmacokinetic variability of newer antiepileptic drugs: when is monitoring needed? Clin Pharmacokinet 2006;45:1061-75.
99. Johnson MD, Zuo H, Lee KH, Trebley JP, Rae JM, Weatherman RV, et al. Pharmacological characterization of 4-hydroxy-*N*-desmethyl tamoxifen, a novel active metabolite of tamoxifen. Breast Cancer Res Treat 2004;85:151-9.
100. Johnston A, Holt DW. Therapeutic drug monitoring of immunosuppressant drugs. Br J Clin Pharmacol 1999;47:339-50.
101. Juang P. Update on new antifungal therapy. AACN Adv Crit Care 2007;18:253-60; quiz 61-2.
102. Juenke J, McMillin GA. Analytical support of classical anticonvulsant drug monitoring beyond immunoassay: application of chromatographic methods. In: Dasgupta A, ed. Advances in chromatographic techniques for therapeutic drug monitoring. Boca Raton, Fla: CRC Press, 2009;87-103.
103. Justesen US. Protease inhibitor plasma concentrations in HIV antiretroviral therapy. Dan Med Bull 2008;55:165-85.
104. Kahan BD, Napoli KL, Kelly PA, Podbielski J, Hussein I, Urbauer DL, et al. Therapeutic drug monitoring of sirolimus: correlations with efficacy and toxicity. Clin Transplant 2000;14:97-109.
105. Kapoor N, Kirkpatrick D, Blaese RM, Oleske J, Hilgartner MH, Chaganti RS, et al. Reconstitution of normal megakaryocytopoiesis and immunologic functions in Wiskott-Aldrich syndrome by marrow transplantation following myeloablation and immunosuppression with busulfan and cyclophosphamide. Blood 1981;57:692-6.
106. Kappelhoff BS, Crommentuyn KM, de Maat MM, Mulder JW, Huitema AD, Beijnen JH. Practical guidelines to interpret plasma concentrations of antiretroviral drugs. Clin Pharmacokinet 2004;43: 845-53.
107. Kirchner GI, Meier-Wiedenbach I, Manns MP. Clinical pharmacokinetics of everolimus. Clin Pharmacokinet 2004;43:83-95.
108. Knight SR, Morris PJ. The clinical benefits of cyclosporine C2-level monitoring: a systematic review. Transplantation 2007;83:1525-35.
109. Koal T, Deters M, Casetta B, Kaever V. Simultaneous determination of four immunosuppressants by means of high speed and robust on-line solid phase extraction-high performance liquid chromatography-tandem mass spectrometry. J Chromatogr B Analyt Technol Biomed Life Sci 2004;805:215-22.
110. Konings IR, Verweij J, Wiemer EA, Sleijfer S. The applicability of mTOR inhibition in solid tumors. Curr Cancer Drug Targets 2009;9: 439-50.
111. Korecka M, Nikolic D, van Breemen RB, Shaw LM. The apparent inhibition of inosine monophosphate dehydrogenase by mycophenolic acid glucuronide is attributable to the presence of trace quantities of mycophenolic acid. Clin Chem 1999;45:1047-50.
112. Kouno Y, Ishikura C, Homma M, Oka K. Simple and accurate high-performance liquid chromatographic method for the measurement of three antiepileptics in therapeutic drug monitoring. J Chromatogr 1993;622:47-52.
113. Kovarik JM, Beyer D, Schmouder RL. Everolimus drug interactions: application of a classification system for clinical decision making. Biopharm Drug Dispos 2006;27:421-6.
114. Kuypers DR. Influence of interactions between immunosuppressive drugs on therapeutic drug monitoring. Ann Transplant 2008;13:11-8.
115. Leibundgut G, Pfisterer M, Brunner-La Rocca HP. Drug treatment of chronic heart failure in the elderly. Drugs Aging 2007;24:991-1006.
116. Li J, Burzynski JN, Lee YA, Berg D, Driver CR, Ridzon R, et al. Use of therapeutic drug monitoring for multidrug-resistant tuberculosis patients. Chest 2004;126:1770-6.
117. Linder MW, Keck PE Jr. Standards of laboratory practice: antidepressant drug monitoring. National Academy of Clinical Biochemistry. Clin Chem 1998;44:1073-84.
118. Lipp HP. Antifungal agents—clinical pharmacokinetics and drug interactions. Mycoses 2008;51(Suppl 1):7-18.
119. Lundmark J, Bengtsson F, Nordin C, Reis M, Walinder J. Therapeutic drug monitoring of selective serotonin reuptake inhibitors influences clinical dosing strategies and reduces drug costs in depressed elderly patients. Acta Psychiatr Scand 2000;101:354-9.
120. MacDonald A, Scarola J, Burke JT, Zimmerman JJ. Clinical pharmacokinetics and therapeutic drug monitoring of sirolimus. Clin Ther 2000;22(Suppl B):B101-21.
121. Maldonado EF, Fernandez FJ, Trianes MV, Wesnes K, Petrini O, Zangara A, et al. Cognitive performance and morning levels of salivary cortisol and alpha-amylase in children reporting high vs. low daily stress perception. Span J Psychol 2008;11:3-15.
122. Mandell GR, Bennett JE, Dolin R, eds. Principles and practice of infectious diseases, 7th edition. New York: Churchill Livingstone, 2009.
123. Mannel M. Drug interactions with St John's wort: mechanisms and clinical implications. Drug Saf 2004;27:773-97.
124. Mathew TH, Van Buren C, Kahan BD, Butt K, Hariharan S, Zimmerman JJ. A comparative study of sirolimus tablet versus oral solution for prophylaxis of acute renal allograft rejection. J Clin Pharmacol 2006;46:76-87.
125. Mauri MC, Volonteri LS, Colasanti A, Fiorentini A, De Gaspari IF, Bareggi SR. Clinical pharmacokinetics of atypical antipsychotics: a critical review of the relationship between plasma concentrations and clinical response. Clin Pharmacokinet 2007;46:359-88.
126. McCune JS, Gibbs JP, Slattery JT. Plasma concentration monitoring of busulfan: does it improve clinical outcome? Clin Pharmacokinet 2000; 39:155-65.
127. McCune JS, Holmberg LA. Busulfan in hematopoietic stem cell transplant setting. Expert Opin Drug Metab Toxicol 2009;5:957-69.
128. McMillin GA, Juenke J, Dasgupta A. Effect of ultrafiltrate volume on determination of free phenytoin concentration. Ther Drug Monit 2005;27:630-3.
129. Melmon M, Morelli H, Hoffman B, Nierenberg D, eds. Melmon and Morelli's clinical pharmacology: basic principles in therapeutics, 4th edition. New York: McGraw-Hill, 2000.

130. Minami K, Uezono Y, Ueta Y. Pharmacological aspects of the effects of tramadol on G-protein coupled receptors. J Pharmacol Sci 2007; 103:253-60.
131. Mitchell PB. Therapeutic drug monitoring of psychotropic medications. Br J Clin Pharmacol 2001;52(Suppl 1):45S-54S.
132. Mitchell PB. Therapeutic drug monitoring of non-tricyclic antidepressant drugs. Clin Chem Lab Med 2004;42:1212-8.
133. Moore J, Middleton L, Cockwell P, Adu D, Ball S, Little MA, et al. Calcineurin inhibitor sparing with mycophenolate in kidney transplantation: a systematic review and meta-analysis. Transplantation 2009;87:591-605.
134. Morii M, Ueno K, Ogawa A, Kato R, Yoshimura H, Wada K, et al. Impairment of mycophenolate mofetil absorption by iron ion. Clin Pharmacol Ther 2000;68:613-6.
135. Moyer TP, Temesgen Z, Enger R, Estes L, Charlson J, Oliver L, et al. Drug monitoring of antiretroviral therapy for HIV-1 infection: method validation and results of a pilot study. Clin Chem 1999;45:1465-76.
136. Musenga A, Saracino MA, Sani G, Raggi MA. Antipsychotic and antiepileptic drugs in bipolar disorder: the importance of therapeutic drug monitoring. Curr Med Chem 2009;16:1463-81.
137. Nafziger AN, Bertino JS Jr. Utility and application of urine drug testing in chronic pain management with opioids. Clin J Pain 2009;25: 73-9.
138. Nashan B. Review of the proliferation inhibitor everolimus. Expert Opin Investig Drugs 2002;11:1845-57.
139. Neef C, Touw DJ, Harteveld AR, Eerland JJ, Uges DR. Pitfalls in TDM of antibiotic drugs: analytical and modelling issues. Ther Drug Monit 2006;28:686-9.
140. Newman RA, Yang P, Pawlus AD, Block KI. Cardiac glycosides as novel cancer therapeutic agents. Mol Interv 2008;8:36-49.
141. Nowak I, Shaw LM. Mycophenolic acid binding to human serum albumin: characterization and relation to pharmacodynamics. Clin Chem 1995;41:1011-7.
142. O'Kane DJ, Weinshilboum RM, Moyer TP. Pharmacogenomics and reducing the frequency of adverse drug events. Pharmacogenomics 2003;4:1-4.
143. Oellerich M, Armstrong VW. The role of therapeutic drug monitoring in individualizing immunosuppressive drug therapy: recent developments. Ther Drug Monit 2006;28:720-5.
144. Pacher P, Kecskemeti V. Cardiovascular side effects of new antidepressants and antipsychotics: new drugs, old concerns? Curr Pharm Des 2004;10:2463-75.
145. Patsalos PN, Berry DJ, Bourgeois BF, Cloyd JC, Glauser TA, Johannessen SI, et al. Antiepileptic drugs—best practice guidelines for therapeutic drug monitoring: a position paper by the subcommission on therapeutic drug monitoring, ILAE Commission on Therapeutic Strategies. Epilepsia 2008;49:1239-76.
146. Pavek P, Dvorak Z. Xenobiotic-induced transcriptional regulation of xenobiotic metabolizing enzymes of the cytochrome P450 superfamily in human extrahepatic tissues. Curr Drug Metab 2008;9:129-43.
147. Peloquin CA. Therapeutic drug monitoring in the treatment of tuberculosis. Drugs 2002;62:2169-83.
148. Perucca E. Pharmacokinetic profile of topiramate in comparison with other new antiepileptic drugs. Epilepsia 1996;37(Suppl 2):S8-13.
149. Pette M, Pette DF, Muraro PA, Martin R, McFarland HF. In vitro modulation of human, autoreactive MBP-specific CD4 + T-cell clones by cyclosporin A. J Neuroimmunol 1997;76:91-9.
150. Pike MG, Franklin CL, Mays DC, Lipsky JJ, Lowry PW, Sandborn WJ. Improved methods for determining the concentration of 6-thioguanine nucleotides and 6-methylmercaptopurine nucleotides in blood. J Chromatogr B Biomed Sci Appl 2001;757:1-9.
151. Pippenger CE, Penry JK, White BG, Daly DD, Buddington R. Interlaboratory variability in determination of plasma antiepileptic drug concentrations. Arch Neurol 1976;33:351-5.
152. Pollard S, Nashan B, Johnston A, Hoyer P, Belitsky P, Keown P, et al. A pharmacokinetic and clinical review of the potential clinical impact of using different formulations of cyclosporin A, Berlin, Germany, November 19, 2001. Clin Ther 2003;25:1654-69.
153. Pomfret EA, Feng S, Hale DA, Magee JC, Mulligan M, Knechtle SJ. The Art and science of immunosuppression: the fifth annual American Society of Transplant Surgeons' state-of-the-art winter symposium. Am J Transplant 2006;6:275-80.
154. Raggi MA, Mandrioli R, Sabbioni C, Pucci V. Atypical antipsychotics: pharmacokinetics, therapeutic drug monitoring and pharmacological interactions. Curr Med Chem 2004;11:279-96.
155. Rajapakse S. Management of yellow oleander poisoning. Clin Toxicol (Phila) 2009;47:206-12.
156. Ramsay RE. Clinical efficacy and safety of gabapentin. Neurology 1994;44:S23-30; discussion S1-2.
157. Ramsay RE, Wilder BJ, Uthman BM, Garnett WR, Pellock JM, Barkley GL, et al. Intramuscular fosphenytoin (Cerebyx) in patients requiring a loading dose of phenytoin. Epilepsy Res 1997;28:181-7.
158. Rao A, Luo C, Hogan PG. Transcription factors of the NFAT family: regulation and function. Annu Rev Immunol 1997;15:707-47.
159. Rasmussen BB, Brosen K. Is therapeutic drug monitoring a case for optimizing clinical outcome and avoiding interactions of the selective serotonin reuptake inhibitors? Ther Drug Monit 2000;22:143-54.
160. Rea RS, Capitano B, Bies R, Bigos KL, Smith R, Lee H. Suboptimal aminoglycoside dosing in critically ill patients. Ther Drug Monit 2008;30:674-81.
161. Relling MV, Fairclough D, Ayers D, Crom WR, Rodman JH, Pui CH, et al. Patient characteristics associated with high-risk methotrexate concentrations and toxicity. J Clin Oncol 1994;12:1667-72.
162. Rendon A, Nunez M, Jimenez-Nacher I, Gonzalez de Requena D, Gonzalez-Lahoz J, Soriano V. Clinical benefit of interventions driven by therapeutic drug monitoring. HIV Med 2005;6:360-5.
163. Ritter JK, Kessler FK, Thompson MT, Grove AD, Auyeung DJ, Fisher RA. Expression and inducibility of the human bilirubin UDP-glucuronosyltransferase UGT1A1 in liver and cultured primary hepatocytes: evidence for both genetic and environmental influences. Hepatology 1999;30:476-84.
164. Roberts JA, Lipman J. Antibacterial dosing in intensive care: pharmacokinetics, degree of disease and pharmacodynamics of sepsis. Clin Pharmacokinet 2006;45:755-73.
165. Rossano JW, Denfield SW, Kim JJ, Price JF, Jefferies JL, Decker JA, et al. Assessment of the Cylex ImmuKnow cell function assay in pediatric heart transplant patients. J Heart Lung Transplant 2009;28: 26-31.
166. Rothenburger M, Zuckermann A, Bara C, Hummel M, Struber M, Hirt S, et al. Recommendations for the use of everolimus (Certican) in heart transplantation: results from the second German-Austrian Certican Consensus Conference. J Heart Lung Transplant 2007;26: 305-11.
167. Rowland M, Tozer T. Clinical pharmacokinetics: concepts and application. Philadelphia: Lea & Febiger, 1995.
168. Rybak M, Lomaestro B, Rotschafer JC, Moellering R Jr, Craig W, Billeter M, et al. Therapeutic monitoring of vancomycin in adult patients: a consensus review of the American Society of Health-System Pharmacists, the Infectious Diseases Society of America, and the Society of Infectious Diseases Pharmacists. Am J Health Syst Pharm 2009;66:82-98.
169. Ryu SG, Lee JH, Choi SJ, Lee JH, Lee YS, Seol M, et al. Randomized comparison of four-times-daily versus once-daily intravenous busulfan in conditioning therapy for hematopoietic cell transplantation. Biol Blood Marrow Transplant 2007;13:1095-105.
170. Saad AH, DePestel DD, Carver PL. Factors influencing the magnitude and clinical significance of drug interactions between azole antifungals and select immunosuppressants. Pharmacotherapy 2006; 26:1730-44.
171. Sanchez-Fructuoso AI. Everolimus: an update on the mechanism of action, pharmacokinetics and recent clinical trials. Expert Opin Drug Metab Toxicol 2008;4:807-19.
172. Santos GW, Tutschka PJ, Brookmeyer R, Saral R, Beschorner WE, Bias WB, et al. Marrow transplantation for acute nonlymphocytic leukemia after treatment with busulfan and cyclophosphamide. N Engl J Med 1983;309:1347-53.

173. Schachter AD, Meyers KE, Spaneas LD, Palmer JA, Salmanullah M, Baluarte J, et al. Short sirolimus half-life in pediatric renal transplant recipients on a calcineurin inhibitor-free protocol. Pediatr Transplant 2004;8:171-7.
174. Schoner W, Scheiner-Bobis G. Endogenous and exogenous cardiac glycosides and their mechanisms of action. Am J Cardiovasc Drugs 2007;7:173-89.
175. Shaw LM, Figurski M, Milone MC, Trofe J, Bloom RD. Therapeutic drug monitoring of mycophenolic acid. Clin J Am Soc Nephrol 2007; 2:1062-72.
176. Shimada T, Yamazaki H, Mimura M, Inui Y, Guengerich FP. Interindividual variations in human liver cytochrome P-450 enzymes involved in the oxidation of drugs, carcinogens and toxic chemicals: studies with liver microsomes of 30 Japanese and 30 Caucasians. J Pharmacol Exp Ther 1994;270:414-23.
177. Shipkova M, Armstrong VW, Kiehl MG, Niedmann PD, Schutz E, Oellerich M, et al. Quantification of mycophenolic acid in plasma samples collected during and immediately after intravenous administration of mycophenolate mofetil. Clin Chem 2001;47:1485-8.
178. Shipkova M, Armstrong VW, Wieland E, Niedmann PD, Schutz E, Brenner-Weiss G, et al. Identification of glucoside and carboxyl-linked glucuronide conjugates of mycophenolic acid in plasma of transplant recipients treated with mycophenolate mofetil. Br J Pharmacol 1999;126:1075-82.
179. Siddoway LA. Amiodarone: guidelines for use and monitoring. Am Fam Physician 2003;68:2189-96.
180. Sidwell A, Barclay M, Begg E, Moore G. Digoxin therapeutic drug monitoring: an audit and review. N Z Med J 2003;116:U708.
181. Slattery JT, Sanders JE, Buckner CD, Schaffer RL, Lambert KW, Langer FP, et al. Graft-rejection and toxicity following bone marrow transplantation in relation to busulfan pharmacokinetics. Bone Marrow Transplant 1995;16:31-42.
182. Slish JC, Catanzaro LM, Ma Q, Okusanya OO, Demeter L, Albrecht M, et al. Update on the pharmacokinetic aspects of antiretroviral agents: implications in therapeutic drug monitoring. Curr Pharm Des 2006;12:1129-45.
183. Smellie WS, Coleman JJ. Pitfalls of testing and summary of guidance on safety monitoring with amiodarone and digoxin. BMJ 2007;334:312-5.
184. Soldin SJ, Steele BW, Witte DL, Wang E, Elin RJ. Lack of specificity of cyclosporine immunoassays: results of a College of American Pathologists study. Arch Pathol Lab Med 2003;127:19-22.
185. Soldin SJ, Wang E, Verjee Z, Elin RJ. Phenytoin overview—metabolite interference in some immunoassays could be clinically important: results of a College of American Pathologists study. Arch Pathol Lab Med 2003;127:1623-5.
186. Spina E, Perugi G. Antiepileptic drugs: indications other than epilepsy. Epileptic Disord 2004;6:57-75.
187. Spina E, Santoro V, D'Arrigo C. Clinically relevant pharmacokinetic drug interactions with second-generation antidepressants: an update. Clin Ther 2008;30:1206-27.
188. Stenton SB, Partovi N, Ensom MH. Sirolimus: the evidence for clinical pharmacokinetic monitoring. Clin Pharmacokinet 2005;44:769-86.
189. Stevens DL. Association between selective serotonin-reuptake inhibitors, second-generation antipsychotics, and neuroleptic malignant syndrome. Ann Pharmacother 2008;42:1290-7.
190. Straatman LP, Coles JG. Pediatric utilization of rapamycin for severe cardiac allograft rejection. Transplantation 2000;70:541-3.
191. Streit F, Armstrong VW, Oellerich M. Rapid liquid chromatography-tandem mass spectrometry routine method for simultaneous determination of sirolimus, everolimus, tacrolimus, and cyclosporin A in whole blood. Clin Chem 2002;48:955-8.
192. Striano S, Striano P, Capone D, Pisani F. Limited place for plasma monitoring of new antiepileptic drugs in clinical practice. Med Sci Monit 2008;14:RA173-8.
193. Takada M, Goto T, Kotake T, Saito M, Kawato N, Nakai M, et al. Appropriate dosing of antiarrhythmic drugs in Japan requires therapeutic drug monitoring. J Clin Pharm Ther 2005;30:5-12.
194. Taylor PJ. Therapeutic drug monitoring of immunosuppressant drugs by high-performance liquid chromatography-mass spectrometry. Ther Drug Monit 2004;26:215-9.
195. Trescot AM, Helm S, Hansen H, Benyamin R, Glaser SE, Adlaka R, et al. Opioids in the management of chronic non-cancer pain: an update of American Society of the Interventional Pain Physicians' (ASIPP) guidelines. Pain Physician 2008;11:S5-62.
196. Trivedi MH, Lin EH, Katon WJ. Consensus recommendations for improving adherence, self-management, and outcomes in patients with depression. CNS Spectr 2007;12:1-27.
197. Valdes R Jr, Jortani SA, Gheorghiade M. Standards of laboratory practice: cardiac drug monitoring. National Academy of Clinical Biochemistry. Clin Chem 1998;44:1096-109.
198. van Gelder T, Le Meur Y, Shaw LM, Oellerich M, DeNofrio D, Holt C, et al. Therapeutic drug monitoring of mycophenolate mofetil in transplantation. Ther Drug Monit 2006;28:145-54.
199. van Luin M, Kuks PF, Burger DM. Use of therapeutic drug monitoring in HIV disease. Curr Opin HIV AIDS 2008;3:266-71.
200. van Rossum HH, de Fijter JW, van Pelt J. Pharmacodynamic monitoring of calcineurin inhibition therapy: principles, performance, and perspectives. Ther Drug Monit 2010;32:3-10.
201. Venkataramanan R, Shaw LM, Sarkozi L, Mullins R, Pirsch J, MacFarlane G, et al. Clinical utility of monitoring tacrolimus blood concentrations in liver transplant patients. J Clin Pharmacol 2001;41: 542-51.
202. Venkataramanan R, Swaminathan A, Prasad T, Jain A, Zuckerman S, Warty V, et al. Clinical pharmacokinetics of tacrolimus. Clin Pharmacokinet 1995;29:404-30.
203. Visser K, Katchamart W, Loza E, Martinez-Lopez JA, Salliot C, Trudeau J, et al. Multinational evidence-based recommendations for the use of methotrexate in rheumatic disorders with a focus on rheumatoid arthritis: integrating systematic literature research and expert opinion of a broad international panel of rheumatologists in the 3E Initiative. Ann Rheum Dis 2009;68: 1086-93.
204. Wallemacq P, Armstrong VW, Brunet M, Haufroid V, Holt DW, Johnston A, et al. Opportunities to optimize tacrolimus therapy in solid organ transplantation: report of the European Consensus Conference. Ther Drug Monit 2009;31:139-52.
205. Wang PW, Ketter TA. Pharmacokinetics of mood stabilizers and new anticonvulsants. Psychopharmacol Bull 2002;36:44-66.
206. Waring WS. Management of lithium toxicity. Toxicol Rev 2006;25: 221-30.
207. Warner A, Privitera M, Bates D. Standards of laboratory practice: antiepileptic drug monitoring. National Academy of Clinical Biochemistry. Clin Chem 1998;44:1085-95.
208. Weinshilboum R. Inheritance and drug response. N Engl J Med 2003; 348:529-37.
209. Weinshilboum RM, Sladek SL. Mercaptopurine pharmacogenetics: monogenic inheritance of erythrocyte thiopurine methyltransferase activity. Am J Hum Genet 1980;32:651-62.
210. Wille SM, Cooreman SG, Neels HM, Lambert WE. Relevant issues in the monitoring and the toxicology of antidepressants. Crit Rev Clin Lab Sci 2008;45:25-89.
211. Williams J, Bialer M, Johannessen SI, Kramer G, Levy R, Mattson RH, et al. Interlaboratory variability in the quantification of new generation antiepileptic drugs based on external quality assessment data. Epilepsia 2003;44:40-5.
212. Wilson JF, Tsanaclis LM, Williams J, Tedstone JE, Richens A. Evaluation of assay techniques for the measurement of antiepileptic drugs in serum: a study based on external quality assurance measurements. Ther Drug Monit 1989;11:185-95.
213. Woodbury DM, Penfy JK, Schmidt RP, eds. Antiepileptic drugs. Amsterdam: North-Holland Publishing, 1972.
214. Yang Z, Peng Y, Want S. Immunosuppressants: pharmacokinetics, methods of monitoring and role of high performance liquid chromatography/mass spectrometry. Clin Appl Immunol Rev 2005;5: 405-30.

215. Yasui-Furukori N, Furukori H, Saito M, Inoue Y, Kaneko S, Tateishi T. Poor reliability of therapeutic drug monitoring data for haloperidol and bromperidol using enzyme immunoassay. Ther Drug Monit 2003; 25:709-14.
216. Yatscoff RW, Rosano TG, Bowers LD. The clinical significance of cyclosporine metabolites. Clin Biochem 1991;24:23-35.
217. Yip JS, Woodward M, Abreu MT, Sparrow MP. How are azathioprine and 6-mercaptopurine dosed by gastroenterologists? Results of a survey of clinical practice. Inflamm Bowel Dis 2008;14: 514-8.
218. Zahir H, Nand RA, Brown KF, Tattam BN, McLachlan AJ. Validation of methods to study the distribution and protein binding of tacrolimus in human blood. J Pharmacol Toxicol Methods 2001;46:27-35.
219. Zhang G Jr, Bartlett MG. Bioanalytical methods for the determination of antipsychotic drugs. Biomed Chromatogr 2008;22:671-87.
220. Zimmerman JJ. Exposure-response relationships and drug interactions of sirolimus. AAPS J 2004;6:e28.
221. Zimmerman JJ, Kahan BD. Pharmacokinetics of sirolimus in stable renal transplant patients after multiple oral dose administration. J Clin Pharmacol 1997;37:405-15.

CHAPTER 35

Clinical Toxicology

Loralie Langman, Ph.D., F.C.A.C.B., D.A.B.C.C.(C.C., M.B., T.C.), D.A.B.F.T., Laura Bechtel, Ph.D., D.A.B.C.C., and Christopher P. Holstege, M.D.

Toxicology is a broad, multidisciplinary science whose goal is to determine the effects of chemical agents on living systems. Innumerable potential toxins can inflict harm, including pharmaceuticals, herbals, household products, environmental agents, occupational chemicals, drugs of abuse, and chemical terrorism threats. Each year millions of human exposure cases are reported to the American Association of Poison Control Centers.[96] The Centers for Disease Control has reported that poisoning (both intentional and unintentional) is one of the top 10 causes of injury-related death in the United States in all adult age groups. From the beginnings of written history, poisons and their effects have been well described. Paracelsus (1493-1541) correctly noted that "Alle Ding sind Gift, und nichts ohn Gift; allein die Dosis macht, daß ein Ding kein Gift ist," which means, "Everything is a poison; there is nothing which is not. The dose differentiates a poison." As life in the modern era has become more complex, so has the study of poisons and their treatments.

This chapter provides a general overview of Clinical Toxicology and the laboratory services necessary to support the care of poisoned patients. Because a comprehensive discussion of all aspects of toxicology is beyond the scope of this chapter, the clinical significance and toxicity of only a select number of common drugs, drugs of abuse, and other chemicals are discussed.

BASIC INFORMATION

In practice, it is neither possible nor necessary to test for all of the hundreds or thousands of clinical toxins that may be encountered. In reality up to 24 drugs or agents account for 80% or more of cases of intoxication treated in most emergency departments.[588] Moreover, some drugs are encountered very infrequently in some locations but with relatively high frequency in others. For example, phencyclidine (PCP) use is almost nonexistent in some areas but is responsible for a relatively high number of intoxications in a few large metropolitan cities. Thus the scope of clinical toxicology testing provided by the laboratory will depend on the pattern of local drug use and on the available resources of the institution and should be developed in consultation with the appropriate clinical staff.

The value of drug and/or substance testing (screening) is well established (1) in the workplace, (2) for some athletic competitions, (3) to monitor drug use during pregnancy, (4) to evaluate drug exposure and/or withdrawal in newborns, (5) to monitor patients in pain management and drug abuse treatment programs, and (6) to aid in the prompt diagnosis of toxicity for a select number of drugs or agents for which a specific antidote or treatment modality is required (Table 35-1). In many other instances of drug toxicity, the value of drug screening, especially on an emergency basis, is more controversial.[94,411,552,695]

Approaches to drug testing vary from the provision of just a few specific tests (e.g., acetaminophen, salicylate, ethanol, digoxin, iron) to testing for additional targeted groups of drugs (e.g., stimulant panel and coma panel) or to a more comprehensive general drug screen that might include hundreds of drugs and/or substances. For all of these situations, it is imperative that the laboratory communicate with the physician concerning the scope (and limitation) of the service and the proper timing and selection of specimens; when possible, the laboratory should assist with interpretation of results. At a minimum, the laboratory request slip should clearly state the drugs that it has the capability of detecting. Otherwise, the report of a "negative" result for a drug screen could be misleading.

Clinical Considerations

To operate effectively, the laboratory should be closely associated with the healthcare team directly managing the patient. Through close and collaborative work, clinical information provided will help to guide appropriate ordering of tests and to ensure that interpretation of results is complete and accurate. For example, the team caring for the patient should provide the following information with the laboratory request:

1. The time and date of the suspected exposure along with the time and date of sample collection.
2. History from the patient or witnesses that might aid in identification of the toxin.
3. Assessment of the physical state of the patient at the time of presentation.

Such information is useful to guide test selection and interpretation of results.

TABLE 35-1 Antidote or Specific Treatment for Intoxication

Toxin	Antidote/ Treatment[14,68,185,251,722]
Acetaminophen	*N*-Acetylcysteine
Aluminum, iron	Deferoxamine
Anticholinergic agents	Physostigmine
Arsenic	Dimercaprol; 2,3-dimercaptosuccinic acid; D-penicillamine
Barbiturates	Multiple-dose oral activated charcoal; alkaline diuresis (phenobarbital only)
Benzodiazepines	Flumazenil
Beta-blockers	Glucagon
Calcium channel blockers	Calcium; glucagon; high-dose insulin infusion
Carbamazepine	Multiple-dose oral activated charcoal; charcoal hemoperfusion
Carbon monoxide	Oxygen
Cyanide	Amyl nitrite, sodium nitrite, sodium thiosulfate; hydroxocobalamin
Digoxin	Anti-digoxin Fab fragments
Ethylene glycol, methanol	Fomepizole (4-methylpyrazol) or ethanol; hemodialysis
Isoniazid	Pyridoxine
Lead	Calcium disodium edetate; dimercaprol; 2,3-dimercaptosuccinic acid
Lithium	Hemodialysis
Mercury	Dimercaprol; 2,3-dimercaptosuccinic acid; D-penicillamine
Methanol	Fomepizole (4-methylpyrazol) or ethanol; hemodialysis; folate
Nitrites, nitrates	Methylene blue
Opioids	Naloxone
Organophosphate or carbamate	Atropine; pralidoxime (controversial for carbamates)
Salicylates	Bicarbonate; hemodialysis
Theophylline	Multiple-dose oral activated charcoal; hemodialysis
Tricyclic antidepressants	Bicarbonate; benzodiazepines

Analytical Considerations

Because of the wide range of drugs of interest, no single analytical technique is adequate for broad-spectrum drug detection. Therefore several analytical approaches in combination are generally required. These may include simple, inexpensive, and rapid spot tests; immunoassays (see Chapter 16); and chromatographic and/or mass spectrometric techniques (see Chapters 13 and 14), including thin-layer chromatography (TLC), high-performance liquid chromatography (HPLC), gas chromatography (GC), gas chromatography-mass spectrometry (GC-MS or GC-MS/MS), and liquid chromatography-mass spectrometry (LC-MS or LC-MS/MS).[772] Currently, GC-MS is the most widely used definitive confirmatory procedure, although LC-MS/MS is becoming more popular. Confirmatory testing is mandatory for forensic drug testing (e.g., workplace drug testing).

Speed of analysis, or turnaround time (TOT), and availability are critical issues in clinical toxicology. A drug analysis that requires several hours to complete or that is not available at all hours of the day is of little value in a clinical emergency. Alternatively, a rapid test that provides false information could result in erroneous diagnostic and therapeutic decisions. For numerous agents, quantitative determinations guide management during a clinical emergency. These agents include (1) acetaminophen, (2) carbamazepine, (3) digoxin, (4) ethanol, (5) ethylene glycol, (6) iron, (7) isopropanol, (8) lithium, (9) methanol, (10) phenobarbital, (11) phenytoin, (12) salicylate, (13) valproic acid, and (14) theophylline, and in whole blood, (15) carboxyhemoglobin and (16) methemoglobin. Results for these determinations should be available within 1 hour of specimen receipt.[860]

Proper selection of analytical methods and interpretation of results require knowledge of the pharmacology and pharmacokinetics of the toxins of interest. For example, the potential hepatotoxicity of acetaminophen is related to the concentration of unmetabolized drug. Conversely, delta-9-tetrahydrocannabinol (THC)—a metabolite of marijuana—is measured in urine as an indication of marijuana use.

Clinical Evaluation

Primary Survey

When a healthcare team initially evaluates a patient who presents with a potential toxicologically induced health problem, the final diagnosis is often determined by (1) reviewing the history, (2) performing a directed physical examination, (3) using ancillary tests (e.g., electrocardiogram, radiology), and (4) applying a rational approach to laboratory testing. Often no specific antidote or treatment is available for a poisoned patient and careful supportive care is the most important intervention.[234]

All patients who present with potential toxicity should be thoroughly assessed, and it is imperative that the clinician follow a standard "ABC" approach with attention to "airway, breathing, and circulation" respectively. The patient's airway should be open and unblocked and adequate ventilation ensured. If the patient's airway is not secure and endotracheal tube intubation is considered, the first diagnostic test that should be performed is a rapid bedside glucose concentration. Hypoglycemia can result in coma or new-onset seizures, thereby mimicking a toxic etiology. In addition, numerous toxins are clinically associated with hypoglycemia (e.g., sulfonylureas, iron, *Mentha pulegium*). Clinical effects induced by hypoglycemia can be rapidly reversed with intravenous glucose, thus preventing unnecessary and costly procedures and testing.

Too often healthcare providers are lulled into a false sense of security when a patient presents with altered mental status and oxygen saturations on pulse oximetry that are adequate on high-flow oxygen. If the patient has inadequate ventilation or a poor gag reflex, then the patient may be at risk for progressive CO_2 narcosis or aspiration, respectively, and yet may be maintaining adequate oxygen saturation on supplemental oxygen. It is imperative that the healthcare team avoid common complications of poisonings such as aspiration pneumonitis.[138,359] An arterial blood gas (ABG) can rapidly aid the healthcare team in determining the need for intubation and mechanical ventilation. The ABG can also provide valuable information regarding the patient's acid-base status and can help the clinician begin to generate a differential diagnosis. For example, in the scenario of a febrile toxic patient who presents with an altered mental status, a normal ABG (lack of acidosis) immediately rules-out uncoupling of oxidative phosphorylation as a cause of that patient's fever. Finally, an ABG with co-oximetry can rapidly assist in determining other toxic etiologies, such as carbon monoxide poisoning (depending on the timing of the blood draw in relation to the exposure) and methemoglobinemia.

The initial treatment of hypotension in all toxic patients consists of the administration of intravenous fluids.[340] The patient's pulmonary status should be closely monitored to ensure that pulmonary edema does not develop as fluids are infused. Symptomatic toxic patients should be placed on continuous cardiac monitoring with pulse oximetry, and the healthcare team must perform frequent neurologic checks to ensure continued protection of the airway. Acutely poisoned patients should receive a large-bore peripheral intravenous line, and all symptomatic patients should have a second line placed in the peripheral or central venous system, depending on the severity of their clinical status. At this time in patient care, blood can be drawn and sent for appropriate laboratory diagnostic testing. Placement of a urinary catheter should be considered early in the care of hemodynamically unstable poisoned patients to monitor urinary output as an indicator of adequate perfusion. A rapid bedside urine dipstick (photometric chemical assay) provides helpful information rapidly as healthcare team members await further laboratory testing. For example, a urine specific gravity will give insight into the patient's initial hydration status, and the appearance of tea-colored urine positive for blood may indicate the presence of myoglobinuria in a comatose patient with rhabdomyolysis.

Secondary Survey

Upon completion of the primary survey, the healthcare team should be assured that the patient's airway is open and unblocked (also described as a patent airway), the ventilatory effort is adequate, and blood pressure is sustained in an appropriate range. At this point in management, the secondary survey can be performed. The secondary survey involves a thorough examination of the entire patient. For adequate access to a toxic patient, the patient must be completely undressed. Exposure of the patient ensures that a complete physical examination is performed.[234] If the patient is not completely undressed, an important diagnostic clue may be missed. For example, skin lesions consistent with pressure necrosis on the back of a comatose patient may indicate the need to obtain a blood creatine phosphokinase activity or a urine myoglobin concentration. A comatose drug abuser may have attached transdermal drug patches (e.g., fentanyl, clonidine) in atypical locations (e.g., gluteal sulcus) that when found can rapidly lead to a diagnosis, avoiding the need for further laboratory testing. Besides completing a thorough physical review of all organ systems, the secondary survey involves reviewing items brought with the patient (e.g., medication bottles, drug paraphernalia). Searching carefully through the patient's clothing may assist in providing clues that change the plan for specific laboratory tests or explain specific laboratory findings. For example, the discovery of a cough and cold product in the patient's pocket that contains dextromethorphan could explain the clinical presentation of an agitated patient with hyperreflexia whose initial urine toxicology screen was positive for phencyclidine but later was found negative on confirmation.

Toxic Syndromes

Toxic syndromes ("toxidromes") are clinical syndromes that are essential for the successful recognition of poisoning patterns. A *toxidrome* is the constellation of clinical signs and symptoms that suggests a specific class of poisoning. An important component of the secondary survey is to determine whether a specific toxic syndrome is present.[234] The most commonly encountered toxidromes include (1) anticholinergic, (2) cholinergic, (3) opioid, (4) sedative-hypnotic, and (5) sympathomimetic (Table 35-2). Many toxidromes have several overlapping features. For example, anticholinergic findings are highly similar to sympathomimetic findings, with one exception being the effects on sweat glands: anticholinergic agents produce warm, flushed dry skin, but sympathomimetic agents produce diaphoresis. Toxidrome findings may also be affected by individual variability, comorbid conditions, and coingestants. For example, tachycardia associated with sympathomimetic or anticholinergic toxidromes may be absent in a patient who is concurrently taking beta-antagonist medications. Additionally, although toxidromes may be applied to classes of drugs, one or more toxidrome findings may be absent for some individual agents within these classes. For instance, meperidine is an opioid analgesic, but it does not induce miosis, which helps to define the "classic" opioid toxidrome. When accurately identified, the toxidrome may provide invaluable information for diagnosis and subsequent treatment, although the many limitations impeding acute toxidrome diagnosis must be carefully considered.

Anticholinergic

Characteristics of the anticholinergic syndrome have long been taught using the old medical adage, "dry as a bone, blind as a bat, red as a beet, hot as a hare, and mad as a hatter," which corresponds with a symptomatic person's anhidrosis,

TABLE 35-2 Symptoms of the Important Toxidromes

Toxidrome	Symptom
Anticholinergic	Agitation
	Blurred vision
	Decreased bowel sounds
	Dry skin
	Fever
	Flushing
	Hallucinations
	Ileus
	Lethargy/coma
	Mydriasis
	Myoclonus
	Psychosis
	Seizures
	Tachycardia
	Urinary retention
Cholinergic	Diarrhea
	Urination
	Miosis
	Bradycardia
	Bronchorrhea
	Emesis
	Lacrimation
	Salivation
Opioid	Bradycardia
	Decreased bowel sounds
	Hypotension
	Hypothermia
	Lethargy/coma
	Miosis
	Shallow respirations
	Slow respiratory rate
Sedative-hypnotic	Ataxia
	Blurred vision
	Confusion
	Diplopia
	Dysesthesias
	Hypotension
	Lethargy/coma
	Nystagmus
	Respiratory depression
	Sedation
	Slurred speech
Sympathomimetic	Agitation
	Diaphoresis
	Excessive motor activity
	Excessive speech
	Hallucinations
	Hypertension
	Hyperthermia
	Insomnia
	Restlessness
	Tachycardia
	Tremor

mydriasis, flushing, fever, and delirium, respectively. Depending on the dose and time post exposure, various central nervous system effects may manifest from an anticholinergic agent. Restlessness, apprehension, abnormal speech, confusion, agitation, tremor, picking movements, ataxia, stupor, and coma all have been described following exposure to various anticholinergics. When manifesting delirium, the individual will often stare into space and mutter, fluctuating between occasional lucid intervals with appropriate responses and then descriptions of vivid hallucinations. Phantom behaviors, such as plucking or picking in the air or at garments, are characteristic. Hallucinations are prominent, and they may be benign, entertaining, or terrifying to the patient experiencing them. Exposed patients may have conversations with hallucinated figures and/or they may misidentify persons they typically know well. Simple tasks typically performed well by the exposed person may become difficult. Motor coordination, perception, cognition, and new memory formation are altered.

Mydriasis causes photophobia. Impairment of near vision occurs because of loss of accommodation and reduced depth of field secondary to ciliary muscle paralysis and pupillary enlargement. Tachycardia and exacerbated heart rate responses to exertion are expected. Systolic and diastolic blood pressure may show moderate elevation. A decrease in capillary tone may cause skin flushing. Intestinal motility slows, resulting in nausea, vomiting, and decreased bowel sounds. All glandular cells become inhibited, resulting in dry mucous membranes of the mouth and inhibition of sweating with resultant dry skin. Urination may be difficult, and urinary retention may occur. The exposed patient's temperature may become elevated from an inability to sweat and dissipate heat. In warm climates, this may result in marked hyperthermia.

Numerous substances can cause the anticholinergic syndrome. More common agents include antihistamines, atropine, cyclic antidepressant drugs, phenothiazines, anti-Parkinson's drugs, cyclobenzaprine, scopolamine, and several plants such as *Datura stramonium* (Jimson weed).

Cholinergic

Acetylcholine is a neurotransmitter found throughout the central nervous system, including (1) the sympathetic and parasympathetic autonomic ganglia, (2) the postganglionic parasympathetic nervous system, and (3) the skeletal muscle motor end plate. Acetylcholine binds to and activates muscarinic and nicotinic receptors. Activating muscarinic receptors stimulates or inhibits cellular function at visceral smooth muscle, cardiac muscle, and secretory glands. Alternatively, nicotinic receptors are present at postsynaptic membranes in autonomic ganglia and at skeletal muscle motor end plates. The enzyme acetylcholinesterase (AChE) regulates the activity of acetylcholine within the synaptic cleft. Acetylcholine binds to the active site of AChE, where the enzyme rapidly hydrolyzes acetylcholine to choline and acetic acid. These hydrolyzed products rapidly dissociate from AChE, so that the enzyme is free to act on another molecule.

The respiratory effects of cholinergic poisoning tend to be dramatic and are considered to be the major factor leading to the death of its victims. Respiratory failure typically occurs as a triad of increased airway resistance, neuromuscular failure, and depression of central respiratory centers. Profuse watery nasal discharge, marked salivation, bronchorrhea, and bronchoconstriction result in a prolonged expiratory phase, cough, and wheezing. Because of the widespread presence of cholinergic receptors in the brain, cholinergic poisoning can produce great variation in neurologic signs and symptoms, including centrally mediated respiratory failure, coma, and seizures. Cholinergic cardiotoxicity can result in two clinical scenarios: a period of intense sympathetic activity that results in sinus tachydysrhythmias, or a period of increased parasympathetic tone that leads to bradydysrhythmias, prolongation of the PR interval, and atrioventricular block. Muscular symptoms may be vague and may consist of muscular weakness and difficulty with ambulation that can progress to muscular fasciculations and subsequent paralysis. Cholinergic agents cause constriction of both the sphincter muscle of the iris and the ciliary muscle of the lens, as well as stimulation of the lacrimal gland, resulting in lacrimation and miosis. The dermal sweat glands are innervated by sympathetic muscarinic receptors. When these receptors are stimulated, profuse sweating occurs. Cholinergic gastrointestinal and genitourinary symptoms may result in nausea, vomiting, abdominal cramps, tenesmus, and involuntary defecation and urination. Two mnemonics have been developed to help recall cholinergic clinical effects: DUMB BELS (diarrhea, urination, miosis, bradycardia, and bronchorrhea-bronchoconstriction, emesis, lacrimation, sweating-salivation)[415] and SLUDGE (salivation, lacrimation, urination, defecation, GI distress, emesis-eye findings, miosis).[145]

Agents that cause these cholinergic clinical effects include organophosphate and carbamate insecticides (cholinesterase inhibitors), certain species of mushrooms that contain muscarine, and the nictonic receptor agonists nicotine, lobeline, and conine.

Opioid

Opioids can induce coma, respiratory depression, bradycardia, hypotension, hypothermia, miosis, pulmonary edema, decreased bowel sounds, and decreased reflexes. Common causes of this syndrome, in which central nervous system depression and miosis are the cardinal two signs, include morphine, codeine, diacetylmorphine, oxycodone, hydrocodone, hydromorphone, and methadone. Meperidine and propoxyphene toxicity has been associated with mydriasis and not with miosis. Numerous drugs can mimic the opioid syndrome by inducing coma, respiratory depression, and miosis, including clonidine, oxymetazoline, and antipsychotics.

Sympathomimetic

Norepinephrine is the neurotransmitter for postganglionic sympathetic fibers (adrenergic) that enervate skin, eyes, heart, lungs, gastrointestinal tract, exocrine glands, and some neuronal tracts in the central nervous system. Physiologic responses to activation of the adrenergic system are complex and depend on the type of receptor (α_1, α_2, β_1, β_2) activated; some are excitatory and others have opposing inhibitory responses. Stimulation of the sympathetic nervous system produces central nervous system excitation (agitation, anxiety, tremors, delusions, and paranoia), tachycardia, seizures, hypertension, mydriasis, hyperpyrexia, and diaphoresis. In severe cases, cardiac arrhythmias and coma may occur. Examples of drugs that produce a sympathomimetic response include amphetamines, cocaine, phencyclidine, ephedrine, cathine, methcathinone, and pseudoephedrine.

Hyperthermic Syndromes

Toxin-induced hyperthermic syndromes are potentially devastating and require rapid management. Even though the patient's temperature is one of the *vital* signs, the temperature often is not obtained in clinical practice. Fever in a poisoned patient can be associated with several hyperthermic syndromes: sympathomimetic toxicity, uncoupling of oxidative phosphorylation, serotonin syndrome, neuroleptic malignant syndrome, malignant hyperthermia, anticholinergic poisoning, and withdrawal syndromes.[692] Sympathomimetics, such as amphetamines and cocaine, may produce hyperthermia as the result of excess serotonin and dopamine, leading to thermal deregulation.[372] Uncoupling of oxidative phosphorylation, as seen in severe salicylate poisoning, occurs when the process of oxidative phosphorylation is disrupted, leading to heat generation and a reduced ability to aerobically generate adenosine-5′-triphosphate (ATP).[409] Serotonin syndrome occurs when a relative excess of serotonin is present at both peripheral and central serotonergic receptors.[360] Patients may present with hyperthermia, alterations in mental status, and neuromuscular abnormalities (rigidity, hyperreflexia, clonus), although individual variability is noted in these findings. Serotonin syndrome is associated with drug interactions such as those associated with the combination of monoamine oxidase inhibitors and meperidine, but it may also occur with single-agent therapeutic dosing or overdosing of serotonergic agents. Neuroleptic malignant syndrome is a condition caused by relative deficiency of dopamine within the central nervous system.[717] It has been associated with dopamine receptor antagonists and the withdrawal of dopamine agonists such as levodopa/carbidopa products. Clinically, it may be difficult to distinguish from serotonin syndrome and other hyperthermic emergencies. Malignant hyperthermia occurs when genetically susceptible individuals are exposed to depolarizing neuromuscular blocking agents or volatile general anesthetics. Anticholinergic poisoning may result in hyperthermia through impairment of normal cooling mechanisms such as sweating. Withdrawal syndromes can produce excessive adrenergic responses (e.g., sedative-hypnotic withdrawal, ethanol withdrawal) and subsequent heat generation. It should be noted that opioid withdrawal is not associated with fever or altered mental status. Overall, differentiating between the toxic hyperthermic syndromes may be challenging, and additional causes of hyperthermia such as heat stroke and infection should be explored.

SCREENING PROCEDURES FOR DETECTION OF DRUGS

Screening procedures are designed for the relatively rapid and generally qualitative detection of drugs or other toxic substances. In general, screening tests have adequate clinical sensitivity but may not be highly specific. Thus, a negative result yielded by a screening procedure may rule out with reasonable certainty the presence of clinically significant concentrations of a particular analyte. Because of possible interferences, a positive result should be considered "presumptive positive" and should be confirmed by an alternate procedure of greater specificity. Screening procedures may be designed to detect a particular drug or drug class. Tests for such purposes include simple visual color tests (spot tests) and immunoassays.

Spot Tests

Spot tests are rapid, easily performed, noninstrumental qualitative procedures that provide presumptive evidence for the presence of tested drugs. Any positive response must be followed by testing with a more specific method. They are potentially valuable to rule out the presence of drugs or to suggest (but not prove) the presence of a drug of a particular group. Spot tests are less frequently employed now because many have been largely replaced by rapid immunoassays that may be performed at the point of care or in the central laboratory.

Ferric Chloride and Trinder Tests

Two bedside tests have been proposed for rapid identification of the patient with salicylate toxicity. Both involve simply applying a few drops of a prepared reagent to a small sample of a patient's urine and watching for a characteristic color change. The first such reagent is ferric chloride ($FeCl_3$). Applying a few drops of a 10% solution of ferric chloride to 1 mL of urine containing even very small amounts of salicylate will produce a characteristic purple color caused by the formation of an iron-salicylate complex.[337] This color change also will occur if the urine in question contains acetoacetic acid and phenylpyruvic acid.[250] The urine Trinder spot test uses a reagent composed of mercuric chloride, ferric nitrate, concentrated hydrogen chloride, and deionized water.[421] Applying 1 mL of this solution to 1 mL of urine with salicylates present will also lead to a purple color change.[250]

One study exploring the salicylate question[254] examined the use of the ferric chloride test in 187 patients presenting to the emergency department. These ferric chloride tests were subsequently followed with serum salicylate concentrations. The sensitivity of the ferric chloride was 93.2% for salicylate concentrations ≥3.0 mg/dL and 93.8% for concentrations ≥30.0 mg/dL. Specificity was 88.8% and 75.4%, respectively. Three false negatives were reported, one of which had a toxic salicylate concentration of 34 mg/dL. King and associates evaluated the clinical utility of the Trinder reagent.[421] Investigators enlisted 12 volunteers who ingested 975 mg of aspirin. The sensitivity of the test in this study was 100% with two false positives from controls.

Weiner and colleagues examined the application of these two bedside tests in patients presenting to the emergency department with suspected drug overdose with or without unexplained metabolic acidosis.[827] Both reagents were added to urine samples from all 180 patients enrolled, and confirmatory serum salicylate concentrations were drawn. Different from the previous studies, however, any darkening of color was regarded as a positive test. Twenty of these patients (11%) had salicylate concentrations ≥5 mg/dL. Both tests were 100% sensitive for recognizing these patients. The specificities for both tests were relatively low (Trinder with 73% and ferric chloride with 71%).

Overall both of these tests can be used for rapid bedside testing. Each is relatively inexpensive and, when color change is interpreted as suggested by Weiner and coworkers, has a low limit of detection. Positive tests indicate the possible presence of salicylate and not toxicity. Both tests should be followed with determination of serum salicylate concentrations to confirm toxicity and quantitate the salicylate concentration.

Urine Fluorescence

Automotive antifreeze is a major source of ethylene glycol exposure. Sodium fluorescein is added to the antifreeze to aid in identifying cooling system leaks. Some have suggested that fluorescein excreted in the urine of a patient who has ingested antifreeze would fluoresce with the aid of a Wood's lamp.[818] Unfortunately, it seems that little advantage is derived by checking for urinary fluorescence by Wood's lamp in those suspected of ethylene glycol poisoning.[120,818]

Anion Gap

Obtaining a basic metabolic panel in all poisoned patients is recommended and is an important initial screening test. When low serum bicarbonate is discovered on a metabolic panel, the clinician should determine whether an elevated anion gap exists. The formula most commonly used for the anion gap (AG) calculation is as follows[124]:

$$AG = [Na^+] - [Cl^- + HCO_3^-]$$

This equation allows one to determine whether serum electroneutrality is being maintained. The primary cation (sodium) and anions (chloride and bicarbonate) are represented in the equation.[364] Other contributors to this equation are "unmeasured."[267] Other serum cations are not commonly included in this calculation because either their concentrations are relatively low (e.g., potassium) or assigning a number to represent their respective contribution is difficult (e.g., magnesium, calcium).[267] Similarly, a multitude of other serum anions (e.g., sulfate, phosphate, organic anions) are also difficult to measure and quantify in an equation.[267,364] These "unmeasured" ions represent the anion gap calculated using the previous equation. The reference interval for this anion gap is accepted to be 8 to 16 mmol/L,[267] but it has been suggested that because of changes in the technique used to measure chloride, the interval should be lowered to 6 to 14 mmol/L.[364] Practically speaking, an increase in the anion

BOX 35-1 Common Causes of Increased Anion Gap (MUDILE)

Methanol
Uremia
Diabetic ketoacidosis
Iron, inhalants (i.e., carbon monoxide, cyanide, toluene), isoniazid, ibuprofen
Lactic acidosis
Ethylene glycol, ethanol ketoacidosis
Salicylates, starvation ketoacidosis, sympathomimetics

gap beyond an accepted reference interval, accompanied by a metabolic acidosis, represents an increase in unmeasured endogenous (e.g., lactate) or exogenous (e.g., salicylates) anions.[124] A list of the more common causes of this phenomenon is organized in the classic MUDILES pneumonic (Box 35-1). Note: The "P" has been removed from the older acronym of MUDPILES, because paraldehyde is no longer available.

It is imperative that clinicians who admit poisoned patients initially presenting with an increased anion gap metabolic acidosis investigate the cause of that acidosis. Many symptomatic poisoned patients may have an initial mild metabolic acidosis upon presentation caused by processes resulting in elevated serum lactate. However, with adequate supportive care including hydration and oxygenation, the anion gap acidosis should improve. If, despite adequate supportive care, an anion gap metabolic acidosis worsens in a poisoned patient, the clinician should consider continued absorption of exogenous acids (e.g., salicylate), formation of acidic metabolites (e.g., ethylene glycol, methanol, toluene metabolites), and cellular ischemia with worsening lactic acidosis (e.g., cyanide) as potential causes.

Electrocardiogram

Interpretation of the electrocardiogram (ECG) in the poisoned patient can significantly facilitate appropriate laboratory testing, diagnosis, and management of the poisoned patient, because numerous drugs can cause ECG changes.[832] Despite the fact that drugs have widely varying indications for therapeutic use, many unrelated drugs share common cardiac electrocardiographic effects if taken in overdose. Potential toxins can be placed into broad classes on the basis of their cardiac effects. For example, agents that block cardiac potassium efflux channels and agents that block cardiac fast sodium channels can lead to characteristic changes in cardiac indices consisting of QRS prolongation and QT prolongation, respectively. The recognition of specific ECG changes associated with other clinical data (toxidromes) can be potentially lifesaving.[341]

Radiographic Studies

Radiologic testing is sometimes used to diagnose complications associated with poisonings, such as aspiration pneumonitis and anoxic brain injury. The use of radiology has also been advocated to detect the presence of potentially radiopaque poisons. For example, O'Brien and associates studied the detectability of 459 different tablets and capsules using plain radiography.[596] Investigators used a ferrous sulfate tablet as a control in grading the radiopacity of other tablets. Overall, of the wide variety of pills tested, only 6.3% were graded as having radiopacity the same as or greater than ferrous sulfate; 29.6% were regarded as having at least moderate opacity; and the largest remaining portion of pills (64%) was regarded as no more than minimally detectable. Based on this and other studies, the indiscriminate use of plain abdominal x-rays is not justified, and a negative film should not be relied upon to rule out potential toxic pill ingestion, especially if enough time is given to allow the pills to dissolve.

Osmol Gap

The main osmotically active constituents of serum are Na^+, Cl^-, HCO_3^-, glucose, and urea. Several empirical formulas based on measurement of these substances have been used to estimate the serum osmolality.[276,539,606,617,662] In practice, one has not shown itself to be superior to the others, yet each equation demonstrates significant differences in the osmol gap reference interval.[443] Therefore, reference intervals must be validated on appropriate patient populations. Two commonly used formulas (in conventional and SI units) are presented here:

$$\text{OSMc (mOsm/kg)} = 2\ \text{Na (mmol/L)} + \text{glucose (mg/dL)}/18 + \text{urea (mg/dL)}/2.8$$

$$\text{OSMc (mOsm/kg)} = 2\ \text{Na (mmol/L)} + \text{glucose (mmol/L)} + \text{urea (mmol/L)}$$

or

$$\text{OSMc (mOsm/kg)} = 1.86\ \text{Na (mmol/L)} + \text{glucose (mg/dL)}/18 + \text{urea (mg/dL)}/2.8 + 9$$

$$\text{OSMc (mOsm/kg)} = 1.86\ \text{Na (mmol/L)} + \text{glucose (mmol/L)} + \text{urea (mmol/L)} + 9$$

The difference between the actual osmolality (OSMm), measured by freezing-point depression, and the calculated osmolality (OSMc) is referred to as delta-osmolality, or the osmol gap (OSMg).

$$\text{OSMg} = \text{OSMm} - \text{OSMc}$$

Elevated OSMg implies the presence of unmeasured osmotically active substances.[427] Volatile alcohols (ethanol, methanol, isopropanol, acetone, and ethylene glycol) when present at significant concentrations, increase serum osmolality, thus resulting in an increased OSMg. The calculation of OSMg is commonly used as a screen.[276] However, it is important to remember that volatile alcohols are not detected when osmolality is measured with a vapor pressure osmometer. Therefore, for the purpose of determining the OSMg, only osmolality measurements based on freezing-point depression are acceptable.

What constitutes a normal osmol gap is widely debated. Traditionally, a normal gap has been defined as 10 mOsm/kg or less. The original source of this value is an article by Smithline and Gardner,[742] which declared that this number was pure convention. Further clinical study has not shown this assumption to be correct. However, large variability is seen in the normal population.[456,558] Researchers have found the OSMg to vary from −9 to +5 mOsm/kg[288]; from −13.5 to +8.9[536]; and from −10 to +20 mOsm/kg,[1] depending on the population studied. An important point to consider is that the day-to-day coefficient of variance of sodium was 1%. This analytical variance alone may account for the variation found in patients' osmol gaps.[1]

One would expect that each 100 mg/dL (21.7 mmol/L) of ethanol (molecular weight = 46.068 g/mol) in serum results in an approximate increase of 21.7 mOsm/kg.[640] However, this is not found to be the case. Applying a correction factor of 0.83 to the ethanol value will more closely approximate the contribution of ethanol to the OSMg.[276] By considering this effect of ethanol on the serum osmolality, it is possible to determine what portion of an increased osmol gap is due to ethanol. The contribution of ethanol to the measured osmolality can be calculated (ethanol, mg/dL/4.6 × 0.83) and included in the preceding formula for delta osmolality calculation. However, it has been observed that ethanol and methanol do not follow a completely predictable relationship with OSMg. In severe ethanol and methanol intoxication, OSMg increases with increasing concentration, making it appear that something is present besides the alcohol.[276,469,539,606,662]

A significant residual osmol gap (>10 mOsm/kg) after the correction for ethanol would suggest the possible presence of isopropanol, methanol, acetone, or ethylene glycol. This information, in conjunction with the presence or absence of metabolic acidosis or serum acetone, is helpful to the clinician when specific measurements of alcohols other than ethanol and of ethylene glycol are not available on an emergency basis (Table 35-3). It must be realized that ketones (diabetics) and substances administered to patients such as polyethylene glycol (burn cream),[98] mannitol (osmotic diuretic), and propylene glycol (solvent for diazepam and phenytoin) may increase serum osmolality.

For the diagnosis of ethanol intoxication, OSMg poisoning has lost its usefulness because ethanol is measured quickly on most chemistry analyzers. However, because other toxic alcohols can be measured only by chromatographic techniques, it is still useful. Unfortunately, OSMg as a screening method is insensitive to low, yet clinically significant, concentrations of ethylene glycol (<50 mg/dL), and methanol (<30 mg/dL).[616]

Immunoassay

Different types of immunoassays are useful in screening specimens for drugs (see Chapters 16 and 34). In some cases, these assays are relatively specific for a single drug (LSD), but in others, several drugs of a similar class are detected (e.g., opiates). The detection limit for various members of a class of drugs or the degree of cross-reactivity for similar drugs varies, and each manufacturer of immunoassay reagents should be consulted for specific information. These assays are easy to perform; many are available for use on automated instrumentation and may be able to provide "semiquantitative" results. Several portable, noninstrumental, immunoassay-based drug detection devices are available for use in point-of-care testing (POCT). For the vast majority of drugs of abuse, immunoassays are the methods of choice for initial screening. However, for a more comprehensive drug screening, chromatographic procedures complement immunoassays.

Planar Chromatography

Planar chromatography, commonly known as thin-layer chromatography (TLC), is a versatile procedure that requires no instrumentation and thus is operationally relatively simple and inexpensive (see Chapter 13). With this technique, a large number of drugs may be detected; it may be applied to the analysis of serum, gastric contents, or urine. Urine, however, is the specimen of choice because most drugs and drug metabolites are present in urine in relatively high concentrations. However, application of TLC to drug screening requires considerable experience and skill to recognize drug and metabolite patterns and various color hues for detection; it has largely been replaced by other chromatographic techniques. For a more comprehensive description, refer to previous editions of this textbook.[78]

Gas Chromatography

Also known as gas liquid chromatography, GC is relatively rapid, is capable of resolving a broad spectrum of drugs, and is widely used for qualitative and quantitative drug analysis.[392] Capillary columns, because of their high efficiency, are analytical columns that are commonly used for drug detection by GC (see Chapter 13). In many instances, nonderivatized

TABLE 35-3 Laboratory Findings Characteristic of Ingestion of Alcohols

Alcohol	Serum Osmol Gap	Metabolic Acidosis With Anion Gap	Serum Acetone	Urine Oxalate
Ethanol	+	−	−	−
Methanol	+	+	−	−
Isopropanol	+	−	+	−
Ethylene glycol	+	+	−	+

drugs have good GC properties when capillary columns are used; in some instances, derivatization to a less polar or more volatile compound is necessary. Common detectors for drug detection by GC are flame ionization and alkali flame ionization (nitrogen phosphorus) detectors and mass spectrometers, which provide the greatest accuracy of identification. Numerous methods for general drug screening by GC-MS spectrometry have been published, but one comprehensive method can be adapted to multiple body fluids and tissues.[392]

High-Performance Liquid Chromatography

The resolving power of HPLC (see Chapter 13) for separating widely divergent chemical constituents has been applied to the complex challenge of comprehensive drug screening in biological fluids. Advantages of HPLC over GC include the ability to analyze polar and thermally labile drugs without derivatization. The advent of diode array detectors that provide a spectral scan of compounds as they elute from the column greatly increased the discriminatory power of this technique.[82,500,661,785] LC-MS or LC-MS/MS currently plays a limited role in comprehensive screening but is rapidly gaining in popularity.*

Point of Care (POC) Drug Testing

Numerous POC drug test devices for urine (and oral fluid) are designed for easy, rugged, and portable use by nontechnical personnel. Although these devices are relatively simple to use, proper training of nonlaboratory users is important for optimal performance (see Chapter 20).[279,445] These noninstrumental immunoassay test devices are designed for use at the site of collection; results are available within minutes and are variously configured to detect only one drug or many drugs simultaneously. The spectrum of drugs tested includes tricyclic antidepressants, barbiturates, benzodiazepines, methadone, MDMA (methylenedioxymethamphetamine), MDA (methylenedioxyamphetamine), MDEA (methylenedioxyethylamphetamine), oxycodone, and the traditional SAMHSA (Substance Abuse and Mental Health Services Administration) or NIDA (National Institute on Drug Abuse) 5 (amphetamine, cocaine, marijuana, opiates, and phencyclidine). As previously cited, such devices are also available for measurement of acetaminophen and salicylate in serum or whole blood. Evaluations for some of these test devices for urine and oral fluid[558,639] have been published. A comprehensive review of on-site drug testing is also available.[629] The assay principles of these POC test devices include the following:

- Sequential competitive binding microparticle capture immunoassay
- Homogeneous microparticle capture immunochromatography
- Solid-phase competitive sequential enzyme immunoassay
- Latex-agglutination-inhibition immunoassay

*References 281, 282, 446, 511, 523, and 794.

A more detailed description of these methods can be found in Chapter 16 and in the package insert for each specific test kit.

PHARMACOLOGY AND ANALYSIS OF SPECIFIC DRUGS AND TOXIC AGENTS

The toxic, pharmacologic, biochemical, and analytical characteristics of several individual drugs and toxins are discussed in this section.

Agents That Cause Cellular Hypoxia

Carbon monoxide and methemoglobin-forming agents interfere with oxygen transport, resulting in cellular hypoxia. Cyanide interferes with oxygen use and therefore causes an apparent cellular hypoxia.

Carbon Monoxide

Carbon monoxide (CO) is a colorless, odorless, tasteless gas that is a product of incomplete combustion of carbonaceous material. Common exogenous sources of carbon monoxide include cigarette smoke, gasoline engines, and improperly ventilated home heating units. Small amounts of carbon monoxide are produced endogenously in the metabolic conversion of heme to biliverdin.[458] This endogenous production of carbon monoxide is accelerated in hemolytic anemias.[496]

Toxic Effects

When inhaled, carbon monoxide combines tightly with the heme Fe^{2+} of hemoglobin to form carboxyhemoglobin. The binding affinity of hemoglobin for carbon monoxide is about 250 times greater than that for oxygen. Therefore high concentrations of carboxyhemoglobin limit the oxygen content of blood. Moreover, the binding of carbon monoxide to a hemoglobin subunit increases the oxygen affinity for the remaining subunits in the hemoglobin tetramer. Thus at a given tissue PO_2 value, less oxygen dissociates from hemoglobin when carbon monoxide is also bound, shifting the hemoglobin-oxygen dissociation curve to the left. Consequently, carbon monoxide not only decreases the oxygen content of blood, it also decreases oxygen availability to tissue, thereby producing a greater degree of tissue hypoxia than would result from an equivalent reduction in oxyhemoglobin due to hypoxia alone.[368,778] Carbon monoxide may also bind to other heme proteins, such as myoglobin and mitochondrial cytochrome oxidase a_3; this may limit oxygen use when tissue PO_2 is very low.[368,778]

The toxic effects of carbon monoxide are a result of hypoxia. Organs with high oxygen demand, such as heart and brain, are most sensitive to hypoxia and thus account for the major clinical sequelae of carbon monoxide poisoning. It must be emphasized that the carboxyhemoglobin concentration, although helpful in diagnosis, does not always correlate with the clinical findings or prognosis.[569,702] Factors other than carboxyhemoglobin concentration that contribute to toxicity include length of exposure, metabolic activity, and underlying disease, especially cardiac or cerebrovascular disease.

Moreover, low carboxyhemoglobin concentrations relative to the severity of poisoning may be observed if the patient was removed from the carbon monoxide–contaminated environment several hours before blood sampling.[318]

An insidious effect of carbon monoxide poisoning is the delayed development of neuropsychiatric sequelae, which may include personality changes, motor disturbances, and memory impairment. These manifestations do not correlate with the length of exposure or with the maximum blood carboxyhemoglobin concentration.[45]

Treatment for carbon monoxide poisoning involves removal of the individual from the contaminated area and administration of oxygen. The half-life ($t_{1/2}$) of carboxyhemoglobin in the body is variable, and attempts to determine the exact elimination $t_{1/2}$ for CO based on the inhaled oxygen concentration have not been validated. Hyperbaric oxygen therapy for CO is highly debated, and current position papers have found no evidence to support its use.[101]

Analytical Methods

Carbon monoxide may be released from hemoglobin and then measured by GC, or it may be determined indirectly as carboxyhemoglobin by spectrophotometry. Gas chromatographic methods are accurate and precise even for very low concentrations of carbon monoxide. Spectrophotometric methods are rapid, convenient, accurate, and precise, except at very low concentrations of carboxyhemoglobin (<2 to 3%).

Gas chromatographic methods measure the carbon monoxide content of blood. When blood is treated with potassium ferricyanide, carboxyhemoglobin is converted to methemoglobin, and carbon monoxide is released into the gas phase. Measurement of the released carbon monoxide may be performed by GC using a molecular sieve column and a thermal conductivity detector.[213] A lower detection limit is achieved by incorporating a reducing catalyst (e.g., nickel) between the GC column and the detector to convert carbon monoxide to methane. The methane may then be detected with a flame ionization detector.[307] A very low detection limit may be achieved with the use of a heated mercuric oxide reaction chamber between the GC column and an ultraviolet light detector. As carbon monoxide elutes from the column, it reacts with mercuric oxide to form mercury gas, which has a high molar absorptivity at 254 nm.[809] In practice, the carbon monoxide binding capacity is also determined after an aliquot of the blood specimen is treated with carbon monoxide to saturate the hemoglobin. The results are then expressed as percent of carboxyhemoglobin:

$$\%\ \text{HbCO} = \frac{\text{CO}_{\text{content}}}{\text{CO}_{\text{capacity}}} \times 100$$

GC methods are accurate and precise and are considered to be reference procedures. Normal values for carboxyhemoglobin in rural nonsmokers are about 0.5%; for urban nonsmokers, 1 to 2%; and for smokers, 5 to 6%.[49] Values may be increased by about 3% in cases of hemolytic anemia.[496]

Spectrophotometric methods rely on the characteristic spectral absorption properties of carboxyhemoglobin.[197,879] Among several such methods, the most popular are based on automated, multiwavelength measurements of several hemoglobin species. These methods are rapid and convenient for the determination of carboxyhemoglobin and other hemoglobin species. Spectrophotometric methods generally compare favorably with gas chromatographic procedures at carboxyhemoglobin concentrations greater than 2 to 3%, but their precision is poor below these concentrations.[809] Therefore, they are sufficiently accurate and precise for measurement of carbon monoxide after exogenous exposure but are too insensitive to detect the increased endogenous production of carbon monoxide that occurs in hemolytic anemia.

Fetal hemoglobin has slightly different spectral properties than adult hemoglobin. Consequently, falsely high carboxyhemoglobin values of 4 to 7% may occur when blood from neonates is measured by some spectrophotometric methods utilizing fewer wavelengths.[810] Moreover, erroneous results may occur with lipemic specimens, with bilirubin, and in the presence of methylene blue (see section on "Methemoglobin-Forming Agents").

Cyanide

Cyanide is a chemical group that consists of one atom of carbon bound to one atom of nitrogen by three molecular bonds (C≡N). Inorganic cyanides (also known as cyanide salts) contain cyanide in the anion form (CN^-) and are used in numerous industries, such as metallurgy, photographic developing, plastic manufacturing, fumigation, and mining. Organic compounds that have a cyano group bonded to an alkyl residue are called *nitriles*. For example, methyl cyanide is also known as acetonitrile (CH_3CN). Hydrogen cyanide (HCN) is a colorless gas at standard temperature and pressure with a reported bitter odor. Cyanogen gas, a dimer of cyanide, reacts with water and breaks down into the cyanide anion. Many plants, such as *Manihot* spp. (cassava), *Linum* spp., *Lotus* spp., *Prunus* spp., *Sorghum* spp., and *Phaseolus* spp., contain cyanogenic glycosides. Iatrogenic cyanide poisoning may occur during use of nitroprusside as a vasodilator given to reduce blood pressure and afterload. Each nitroprusside molecule contains five cyanide molecules, which are slowly released in vivo. If endogenous sulfate stores are depleted, as in the malnourished or postoperative patient, cyanide may accumulate even with therapeutic nitroprusside infusion rates (2 to 10 mcg/kg/min).

Toxic Effects

Hydrocyanic acid binds to hemoglobin. The hydrocyanic acid bound in the erythrocyte is in equilibrium with free hydrocyanic acid in the serum at a ratio of 10 : 1. Cyanide in serum readily crosses all biological membranes and avidly binds to heme iron (Fe^{3+}) in the cytochrome a-a_3 complex within mitochondria.[715,803] When bound to cytochrome a-a_3, cyanide is a competitive inhibitor that causes decoupling of oxidative phosphorylation. Patients exposed to toxic concentrations of cyanide exhibit rapid onset of symptoms typical of cellular hypoxia—flushing, headache, tachypnea, dizziness,

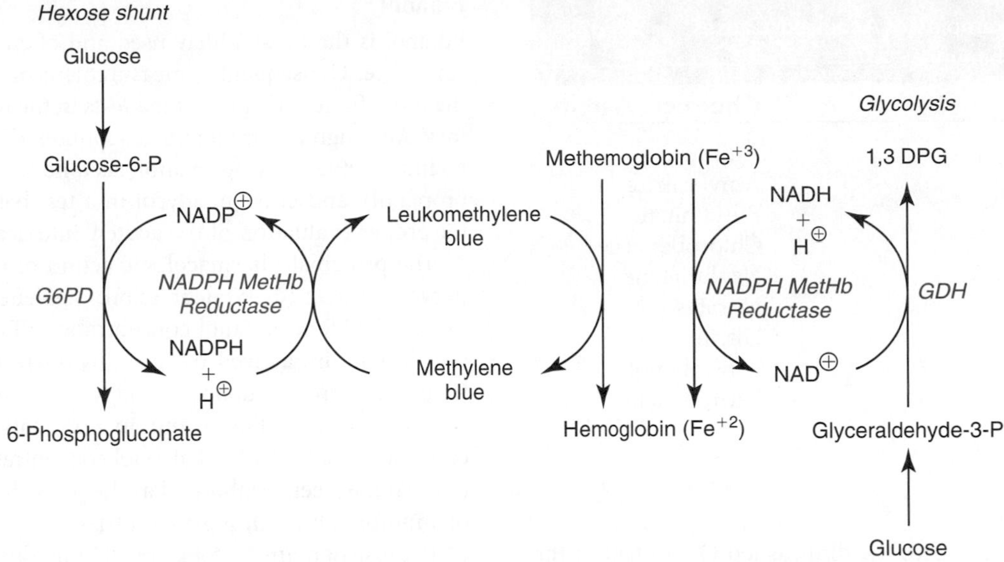

Figure 35-1 Enzymatic pathways for methemoglobin reduction.

and respiratory depression—which progress rapidly to coma, seizures, complete heart block, and death if the dose is sufficiently large.

Hydroxycobalamin or the cyanide antidote kit should be administered as soon as cyanide poisoning is suspected. Hydroxocobalamin, a vitamin B_{12} precursor, is a metalloprotein with a central cobalt atom that complexes cyanide, forming cyanocobalamin (vitamin B_{12}). Cyanocobalamin is eliminated in the urine or releases the cyanide moiety at a rate sufficient to allow detoxification by rhodanese. The cyanide antidote kit contains amyl nitrite, sodium nitrite, and sodium thiosulfate. Thiosulfate donates the sulfur atoms necessary for rhodanese-mediated cyanide biotransformation to thiocyanate. The mechanism of nitrite is less clear. The traditional rationale relies on the ability of nitrite to generate methemoglobin. Because cyanide has a higher affinity for methemoglobin than for cytochrome a_3, cytochrome oxidase function is restored.

Analytical Methods

Following microdiffusion, whole blood CN^- is measured by photometric analysis[179] or by headspace gas chromatography.[111]

With the spectrophotometric method, a sealed, two-well microdiffusion cell is used to separate hydrocyanic acid from blood by mixing a sample of whole blood with strong acid in a sealed chamber and allowing the hydrocyanic acid gas generated to be absorbed into a strong base located in another part of the sealed chamber. One well of the cell contains the blood specimen and strong acid (unmixed until the cell is sealed), and the other well contains a strong base to absorb the hydrocyanic acid gas. After the hydrocyanic acid is collected in the aqueous base medium, pyridine, barbituric acid, and chloramine-T are added to generate a red complex, with the intensity of the color proportional to the concentration of CN^-. A good quality spectrophotometer is required to measure the absorbance. Quick and easy methods for plasma thiocyanate analysis have been described.[802]

Methemoglobin-Forming Agents

The heme iron in hemoglobin is normally present in the ferrous state (Fe^{2+}). When oxidized to the ferric state (Fe^{3+}), methemoglobin is formed, and this form of hemoglobin cannot bind oxygen (Figure 35-1). The principal physiologic system that maintains hemoglobin iron in the reduced state is nicotinamide adenine dinucleotide (NADH)-methemoglobin reductase. The NADH for this enzyme is supplied by normal glycolysis (Embden-Meyerhof pathway). A minor pathway for methemoglobin reduction involves nicotinamide adenine dinucleotide phosphate (NADPH)-methemoglobin reductase, and the NADP for this enzyme reaction is derived from the hexose-monophosphate shunt. Congenital methemoglobinemia may result from a deficiency of NADH-methemoglobin reductase or, more rarely, from hemoglobin variants (hemoglobin M) in which heme iron is both more susceptible to oxidation and more resistant to reduction by the methemoglobin reductase system.

Toxic Effects

An acquired (toxic) methemoglobinemia may be caused by various drugs and chemicals (Table 35-4). The normal percentage of methemoglobin is <1.5% of total hemoglobin. In otherwise healthy individuals, methemoglobin percentages up to 20% may cause slate-gray cutaneous discoloration, cyanosis, and chocolate-brown blood. Percentages between 20% and 50% may cause dyspnea, exercise intolerance, fatigue, weakness, and syncope. More severe symptoms of dysrhythmias, seizures, metabolic acidosis, and coma are associated with methemoglobin percentages of 50 to 70%, and >70% may be lethal.[659,858] All of these symptoms are a consequence

TABLE 35-4 Examples of Acquired Causes of Methemoglobinemia

Drugs	Chemical Agents
Amyl nitrite	Aniline
Benzocaine	Amyl nitrite
Chloroquine	Butyl nitrite
Dapsone	Chlorobenzene
Nitroglycerin	Naphthalene
Phenacetin	Nitrates
Phenazopyridine	Nitrites
Primaquine	Nitrophenol
Sulfonamides	Nitrous oxide

of hypoxia associated with the diminished O_2 content of the blood, and with a decreased O_2 dissociation from hemoglobin species in which some, but not all, subunits contain heme iron in the ferric state (i.e., shift of dissociation curve to the left). The PO_2 is normal in these patients, and therefore so is the calculated hemoglobin oxygen saturation. Thus, a normal PO_2 in a cyanotic patient is a significant indication for the possible presence of methemoglobinemia. Direct measurement of methemoglobin is important in these cases and may be performed by the manual spectrophotometric method of Evelyn and Malloy[235] or by automated multiwavelength measurements with a co-oximeter (see section on "Carbon Monoxide").

Specific therapy for toxic methemoglobinemia involves the administration of methylene blue, which acts as an electron transfer agent in the NADPH-methemoglobin reductase reaction, thereby increasing the activity of this system severalfold.[649,658] Methylene blue and sulfhemoglobin cause spectral interference in the measurement of methemoglobin with some co-oximeters[412,875] but not with the Evelyn-Malloy method.[412]

Analytical Methods

Methemoglobin is measured in blood manually,[235,412] or by automated multiwavelength measurements with a co-oximeter.[325] Methemoglobin interferes with the noninvasive pulse oximetry method, measuring the absorbance of light at 660 nm (oxyhemoglobin) and 940 nm (deoxyhemoglobin). Because methemoglobin is not stable at room temperature, specimens should be kept on ice or refrigerated but not frozen.[412] The stability of methemoglobin at 4 °C has not been well studied. Some sources indicate significant decreases in methemoglobin concentration after 4 to 8 hours,[470] whereas others report little or no change after 24 hours.[412] Freezing results in an increase in methemoglobin concentration.[412]

Alcohols of Toxicologic Interest

Several alcohols are toxic and medically important.[197A] They include ethanol, methanol, isopropanol, acetone, and ethylene glycol.

Ethanol

Ethanol is the most widely used and often abused chemical substance. Consequently, measurement of ethanol is one of the more frequently performed tests in the toxicology laboratory. Although less frequently encountered, it is important to include methanol, isopropanol, acetone (a metabolite of isopropanol), and ethylene glycol in a test battery for alcohols for proper evaluation of the acutely intoxicated patient.

The principal pharmacologic action of ethanol is central nervous system (CNS) depression. CNS effects vary depending on the blood ethanol concentration (Table 35-5) but are also heavily influenced by an individual's tolerance. Symptoms vary from euphoria and decreased inhibitions, to increased disorientation and incoordination, and then to coma and death. A blood alcohol concentration of 80 mg/dL (0.08%) has been established as the *per se* limit for operation of a motor vehicle in most countries.

Because of many factors, not all individuals experience the same degree of CNS dysfunction at similar blood alcohol concentrations. Moreover, the CNS actions of ethanol are more pronounced when the blood ethanol concentration is increasing (absorptive phase) than when it is declining (elimination phase), in part because of the phenomenon of acute tolerance.[291] In addition, heavy alcohol use leads to a more chronic form of tolerance. When consumed with other CNS depressant drugs, ethanol exerts a potentiation or synergistic depressant effect. This can occur at relatively low alcohol concentrations, and numerous deaths have resulted from combined ethanol and drug ingestion.[274]

The pharmacologic mechanisms for the CNS depressant actions of ethanol are complex and incompletely understood, but probably involve both enhancement of major inhibitory neurons and impairment of excitatory neurons. The principal CNS inhibitory neuronal system is mediated by the neurotransmitter γ-aminobutyric acid (GABA). When GABA binds to its postsynaptic receptor subtype $GABA_A$, this oligomeric ion-gated complex "opens" to allow inward flux of Cl, leading to membrane hyperpolarization and subsequent decreased electrical response. This GABA-mediated inhibitory response is enhanced by ethanol and sedative, hypnotic, and anesthetic agents, including barbiturates, benzodiazepines, and volatile anesthetics.[248] Neuronal nicotinic acetylcholine receptors also may be prominent molecular targets of alcohol.[576] Both enhancement and inhibition of nicotinic acetylcholine receptor function have been reported depending on receptor subunit concentration and the concentrations of ethanol tested. Ethanol also inhibits the function of the *N*-methyl-D-aspartate (NMDA)- and kainate-receptor subtypes; AMPA receptors are largely resistant to alcohol.[119]

The aforementioned chronic tolerance to ethanol is considered to be mediated by ethanol-induced increased responsiveness and upregulation in the synthesis of NMDA receptors, attained by concomitant downregulation and desensitization through phorphorylation of $GABA_A$ and glutamate receptors.[248,452,819] Largely because of these adaptive changes, abrupt withdrawal from chronic, heavy ethanol use leads to a physical abstinence syndrome that has prominent

TABLE 35-5 Stages of Acute Alcoholic Influence/Intoxication

Blood Alcohol Concentration, g/100 mL or mg/dL	Influence	Clinical Signs/Symptoms
0.01-0.05	Subclinical	Influence/effects not apparent or obvious Behavior nearly normal by ordinary observation Impairment detectable by special tests
0.03-0.12	Euphoria	Mild euphoria, sociability, talkativeness Increased self-confidence; decreased inhibitions Diminution of attention, judgment, and control Some sensorimotor impairment Slowed information processing Loss of efficiency in finer performance tests Impairment of perception, memory
0.09-0.25	Excitement	Emotional instability; loss of critical judgment comprehension Decreased sensory response; increased reaction time Reduced visual acuity, peripheral vision, and glare recovery Sensorimotor incoordination; impaired balance Drowsiness
0.18-0.30	Confusion	Disorientation, mental confusion; dizziness Exaggerated emotional states (fear, rage, grief, etc.) Disturbances of vision (diplopia, etc.) and of perception of color, form, motion, dimensions Increased pain threshold Increased muscular incoordination; staggering gait; slurred speech Apathy, lethargy
0.25-0.40	Stupor	General inertia; approaching loss of motor functions Markedly decreased response to stimuli Marked muscular incoordination; inability to stand or walk Vomiting; incontinence of urine and feces Impaired consciousness; sleep or stupor
0.35-0.50	Coma	Complete unconsciousness; coma; anesthesia Depressed or abolished reflexes Subnormal temperature Impairment of circulation and respiration Possible death
0.45 +	Death	Death from respiratory arrest

Modified from Dubowski KM, Gadsden RH Sr, Poklis A. The stability of ethanol in human whole blood controls: an interlaboratory evaluation. J Anal Toxicol. 1997 Oct;21(6):486-91.

features of CNS excitation. Included among these withdrawal symptoms are anxiety, irritability, insomnia, muscle tremor and cramps, seizures, hallucinations, and increased temperature, blood pressure, and heart rate.

Ethanol is metabolized principally by liver alcohol dehydrogenase to acetaldehyde, which is subsequently oxidized to acetic acid by aldehyde dehydrogenase (Figure 35-2). The rate of elimination of ethanol from blood approximates a zero-order process. This rate varies among individuals, averaging about 15 mg/dL/h for males and 18 mg/dL/h for females.[210,211] At both low (<20 mg/dL)[813] and high (>300 mg/dL) ethanol concentrations, elimination becomes more nearly first-order; it is accelerated at high concentrations.[81] The elimination rate is also influenced by drinking practices (e.g., alcoholics have increased elimination rates caused by enzyme induction).[847]

Ethanol is a teratogen, and alcohol consumption during pregnancy can result in the birth of a baby with fetal alcohol spectrum disorder (FASD). FASD is an umbrella term that describes the variety of effects that can occur in an individual whose mother drank alcohol during pregnancy (http://www.nofas.org/accessed June 13, 2011). These effects may include physical, mental, behavioral, and/or learning disabilities with possible lifelong implications and are 100% preventable when a woman completely abstains from alcohol during her pregnancy.

Methanol

Methanol is used as a solvent in several commercial products, as a constituent of antifreeze and window cleaning fluids, and as a component of canned fuel. It may be consumed

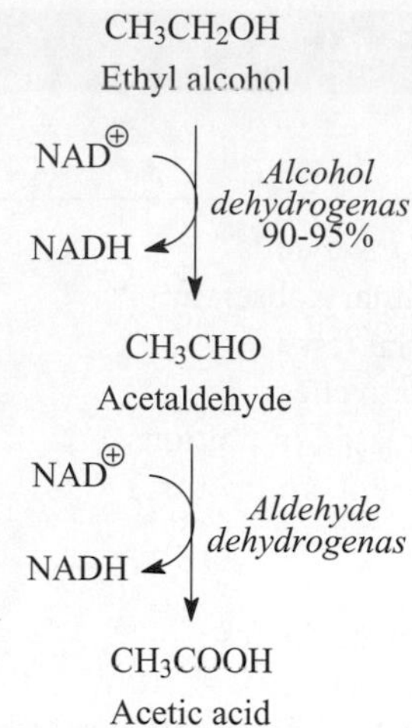

Figure 35-2 Metabolism of ethanol.

intentionally by alcoholics as an ethanol substitute or accidentally when present as a contaminant in illegal whiskey. Accidental ingestions have occurred in children.

The CNS effects of methanol are substantially less severe than those of ethanol. Methanol is oxidized by liver alcohol dehydrogenase (at about one tenth the rate of ethanol) to formaldehyde. Formaldehyde in turn is rapidly oxidized by aldehyde dehydrogenase to formic acid, which may cause serious acidosis and optic neuropathy, resulting in blindness or death.[513,534] Serum formate concentrations correlate better with the degree of acidosis and the severity of CNS and ocular toxicity than do serum methanol concentrations.[718] Therefore, some investigators recommend the measurement of serum formate to assess the severity of toxicity and to guide appropriate therapy in cases of methanol ingestion. The mainstay of therapy for methanol toxicity includes the administration of ethanol or fomepizole as a competitive alcohol dehydrogenase inhibitor, either folate or folinic acid, and dialysis.

Isopropanol and Acetone

Isopropanol is readily available to the general population as a 70% aqueous solution for use as rubbing alcohol. It has about twice the CNS depressant action as ethanol, but it is not as toxic as methanol.[58] Isopropanol has a short $t_{1/2}$ of 2.5 to 3.0 hours,[58] as it is rapidly metabolized by alcohol dehydrogenase to acetone, which is eliminated much more slowly ($t_{1/2}$, 3 to 6 hours).[47] Therefore concentrations of acetone in serum often exceed those of isopropanol during the elimination phase following isopropanol ingestion. Acetone has CNS depressant activity similar to that of ethanol, and because of its longer $t_{1/2}$, it may prolong the apparent CNS effects of isopropanol.[47,58] Supportive care is the mainstay of treatment, with rare reports of dialysis in severe intoxication.

Ethylene Glycol

Ethylene glycol, present in antifreeze products, may be ingested accidentally or for the purpose of inebriation or suicide. Because it tastes sweet, some animals are attracted to it. Veterinarians are often familiar with ethylene glycol toxicity because of cases involving dogs or cats that drank radiator fluid.

Ethylene glycol itself is relatively nontoxic, and its initial CNS effects resemble those of ethanol.[386] However, metabolism of ethylene glycol by alcohol dehydrogenase (ADH) results in the formation of numerous acid metabolites, including lactate, oxalic acid and glycolic acid.[53,386] These acid metabolites are responsible for much of the toxicity of ethylene glycol.[334,371] Serum concentrations associated with death from ethylene glycol ingestion have been observed to vary from 0.06 to 4.3 g/L,[53,651] highlighting the lack of correlation between ethylene glycol concentration and severity of toxicity. It is thus impossible to define a serum ethylene glycol concentration associated with a high probability of death. The serum concentration of glycolic acid correlates more closely with clinical symptoms and mortality than does the concentration of ethylene glycol.[334,651] Because of the rapid elimination of ethylene glycol ($t_{1/2}$, 2 to 5 hours),[53] its serum concentration may be low or undetectable at a time when glycolic acid remains elevated.[257,334,651] Thus the determination of ethylene glycol and glycolic acid provides useful clinical and confirmatory analytical information in cases of ethylene glycol ingestion. The mainstay of therapy for ethylene glycol toxicity includes administration of ethanol or fomepizole as a competitive alcohol dehydrogenase inhibitor and dialysis.

Analysis of Ethanol

Serum, plasma, and whole blood are suitable blood-related specimens for the determination of ethanol. The venipuncture site should be cleansed with an alcohol-free disinfectant, such as aqueous benzalkonium chloride.

Serum/Plasma and Blood Ethanol

Alcohol distributes into the aqueous compartments of blood; because the water content of serum is greater than that of whole blood, higher alcohol concentrations are obtained with serum as compared with whole blood. Experimentally, the serum-to-whole blood ethanol ratio is 1.18 (1.10 to 1.35)[628] and varies slightly with hematocrit.[846] Therefore, laboratories that perform alcohol determinations should make clear the choice of specimen.

Because of the volatile nature of alcohols, specimens should be kept capped to avoid evaporative loss. Blood may be stored, when properly sealed, for 14 days at room temperature or at 4 °C, with or without preservative.[848] For longer storage or for nonsterile postmortem specimens, sodium fluoride should be used as a preservative to prevent a decrease or occasionally an increase (via fermentation) in ethanol concentration.

To measure ethanol in serum/plasma, enzymatic analysis is the method of choice for many laboratories. In this method, ethanol is measured by oxidation to acetaldehyde with NAD, a reaction catalyzed by ADH. With this reaction, the formation of NADH, measured at 340 nm, is proportional to the amount of ethanol in the specimen[268]:

$$\text{Ethanol} + \text{NAD} \xrightarrow{\text{ADH}} \text{Acetaldehyde} + \text{NADH}$$

Under most assay conditions, ADH is reasonably specific for ethanol, with interferences by isopropanol, acetone, methanol, and ethylene glycol of typically <1%. However, spuriously increased results for ethanol have been described in the presence of high concentrations of lactate dehydrogenase (LDH) and lactate.[34,590] This phenomenon is a result of the production of NADH by LDH:

$$\text{Lactate} + \text{NAD} \xrightarrow{\text{LDH}} \text{Pyruvate} + \text{NADH}$$

Serum (or plasma) is the most common specimen for ethanol analysis by ADH methods; this method also performs well with urine or oral fluid, although in some methods, whole blood may be used directly[117] or a precipitation step may be required before analysis to avoid interference from hemoglobin.[269] Results from these methods generally compare closely with those from gas chromatographic methods.[117,291] For more information about these methods, see "Analysis of Volatile Alcohols" section, later.

Estimation of Blood Alcohol

During the early part of the twentieth century, Dr. Erik M.P. Widmark, a Swedish physician, did much of the foundational research regarding alcohol pharmacokinetics in the human body. In addition, he developed an algebraic equation that allows one to estimate the amount of alcohol consumed by an individual or the associated blood alcohol concentration when the values of the other variables are given[489,840]:

$$N = W \bullet \rho \bullet [C_t + \beta \bullet t]/(d \bullet Z)$$

N = number of drinks
W = body weight (kg)
ρ (rho) = volume of distribution (L/kg) (0.68 for males, 0.55 for females)
C_t = blood alcohol concentration (kg/L)
β = rate of ethanol elimination (0.15 g/L/h)
t = time since first drink (h)
d = specific gravity of alcohol (0.8)
Z = amount of ethanol alcohol per drink (L) (15 mL of ethanol in a standard drink)

Typically one wants to calculate the amount of ethanol consumed or the associated ethanol concentration. Note that it may be necessary to convert the units from those more commonly reported. It is important to remember that this formula is applicable only after completion of alcohol absorption, and when equilibrium has been reached between blood and body tissue.

Frequently the time since the first drink is unknown; the formula can be modified to estimate the number of drinks in an individual's system at the time of the test.

$$N = W \bullet \rho \bullet [C_t]/(d \bullet Z)$$

The rate of elimination in the average person is commonly estimated at 0.015 g/100 mL/h (range, 0.010 to 0.030 g/100 mL/h).[553] Retrograde extrapolation is an estimation of a subject's alcohol concentration at a prior time, derived from a blood alcohol concentration measured at a later time. This process may be applied when certain assumptions are made concerning absorption rates, elimination rates, and patterns of alcohol consumption, including drinking duration and volume consumed. Unfortunately, to be forensically useful and scientifically valid, such extrapolations may require facts about the person and that person's alcohol consumption, as well as related information that often is not available. Consequently, significant legal debate surrounds the validity and accuracy of retrograde extrapolation.

Breath Ethanol

Statutory laws for driving under the influence of alcohol were originally based on the concentration of ethanol in venous whole blood. Because the collection of blood is invasive and requires intervention by medical personnel, the determination of alcohol in expired air (breath) has long been the mainstay of evidential alcohol measurements.[321,389,516] Clinical interest in determination of breath alcohol at the point of care is growing. The fundamental principle for use of breath analysis is that alcohol in capillary alveolar blood rapidly equilibrates with alveolar air in a ratio of approximately 2100:1 (blood:breath). This blood-to-breath ratio may actually be closer to 2300:1 but in any case is variable. Nevertheless, in the United States, evidential breath alcohol measurements are based on the ratio of 2100:1. The lower blood-to-breath ratio will predict a slightly lower than actual blood alcohol concentration; its use therefore is not prejudicial. To alleviate confusion and uncertainty surrounding the conversion from breath to blood alcohol concentration, the traffic laws in many countries specify per se limits for blood and/or breath.

Before breath alcohol analysis, a deprivation period of 15 minutes is required to allow for clearance of any residual alcohol that may have been present in the mouth (e.g., very recent drinking, use of alcohol-containing mouthwash, vomiting of alcohol-rich gastric fluid). Duplicate tests, performed 5 to 10 minutes apart and within 20 mg/dL (0.02%) are used as an additional safeguard against mouth alcohol contamination.

During the period of active alcohol absorption, generally 30 to 60 minutes depending on a variety of factors,[592,728] and before peak blood alcohol concentration is obtained, the alcohol concentration in arterial blood will be initially higher than that in peripheral venous blood, and the converse is true in the postabsorptive phase.[391] Because end-expiratory air equilibrates with pulmonary alveolar/capillary blood, the breath alcohol concentration more closely reflects that of arterial alcohol[483]; however, the difference between arterial and venous blood is within the analytical error of most assays.

Determination of ethanol in expired air requires specialized breath alcohol analyzers. Several commercial evidential breath alcohol measurement devices are available. Principles of measurement used in such analyzers include (1) infrared absorption spectrometry (most common), (2) dichromate-sulfuric acid oxidation-reduction (photometric), (3) GC (flame ionization or thermal conductivity detection), (4) electrochemical oxidation (fuel cell), and (5) metal oxide semiconductor sensors.[321,389] Breath alcohol devices also may be used for the medical evaluation of patients at the point of care (e.g., emergency department).

Oral Fluid Ethanol

Because oral fluid (saliva) may be easily and noninvasively collected, interest is growing in its use for ethanol measurements and for the detection of drugs of abuse, but it is not a frequently used sample for ethanol determinations (see section below on "Detection of Drugs of Abuse Using Other Types of Specimens").

Urine Ethanol

Urine has been used as an alternative, less invasive specimen for the determination of alcohol use. During the postabsorptive phase following alcohol ingestion, the concentration of alcohol in urine is roughly 1.3 times that in blood.[52,115] However, the use of urine alcohol measurements to estimate blood concentrations is discouraged because the ratio of 1.3 is highly variable, and, perhaps more important, the urine alcohol concentration may better reflect an average of the blood alcohol concentration during the period in which urine is collected in the bladder. The detection of alcohol in urine represents ingestion of alcohol within the previous 8 to 12 hours.

Ethylglucuronide

Ethylglucuronide (EtG) is a phase II metabolite of ethanol formed through the UDP-glucuronosyl transferase–catalyzed conjugation of ethanol with glucuronic acid.[182] Because of its long urinary elimination time, its specificity for ethanol exposure, and the low detection limits of assays, the use of EtG has been proposed as a marker of recent ethanol intake in a variety of clinical and legal settings, including medical monitoring for relapse, emergency department patient evaluation, postmortem assessment, and transportation accident investigation.[613,864] However, challenges associated with factors such as establishing appropriate cutoff concentrations capable of distinguishing between drinking and nonbeverage sources of ethanol exposure, nonuniform laboratory reporting limits, sample stability, and microbial activity substantially complicate accurate interpretation of results.[613]

Analysis of Volatile Alcohols (Methanol, Isopropanol, and Acetone)

Methanol poisoning can be lethal if not recognized early. Unfortunately, in some instances, a latent period can be as long as 12 to 24 hours[728] before toxicity is recognized, making laboratory identification of this poisoning critical. Development of gas chromatographic methods for volatiles in 1964[217,333] was a significant step in the recognition and treatment of this very toxic alcohol.

Flame ionization GC remains the most common method for the detection and quantitation of volatile alcohols in biological samples.[52] Not only does it distinguish between ethanol, methanol, isopropanol, and acetone, it has the capability to measure concentrations as low as 10 mg/dL (0.01%). Specimens are prepared by a variety of methods; the two most common are direct injection and headspace analysis. Direct injection involves injection of a sample prepared by diluting it with an aqueous solution of internal standard (thus reducing the amount of matrix introduced into the GC). Repeated injection of biological aqueous matrix into the GC will cause buildup on the injector and front of the analytical column, requiring frequent maintenance and column replacement. This can be alleviated by the use of headspace injection. The volatility of the alcohols is used to separate them from the matrix. Specifically, the "Gas Law" states that at a given temperature, the amount of volatile substance in the air space above the liquid—headspace—is proportional to the concentration of the volatile alcohol in the solution. Therefore, the sample in the headspace allows calculation of the concentration in the specimen.

Headspace gas chromatographic analysis is another excellent method for the measurement of methanol, isopropanol, acetone, and ethanol. In addition, an adaptation of this technique may be used to measure formate, the toxic metabolite of methanol, after esterification to methyl formate. Conversely, direct injection GC is the method of choice for ethylene glycol, because it has a higher boiling point and is not as amenable to headspace analysis. A modification of the GC procedure described in 2005 has the potential of combining both toxic alcohols in a single GLC analysis.[405] Methods that simultaneously measure ethylene glycol and glycolic acid have the advantage of being free from interference by propylene glycol (a diluent for parenteral drugs) or 2,3-butanediol (may be present in serum from some alcoholics).[652,867] Similar techniques are used to measure volatile alcohols in blood, serum, oral fluid, urine, other clinical specimens, and postmortem specimens (e.g., vitreous fluid, skeletal muscle).

Analgesics (Nonprescription)

Analgesics are substances that relieve pain without causing loss of consciousness. When used in excess, analgesics such as acetaminophen and salicylate can result in a toxic response.

Acetaminophen

Acetaminophen has analgesic and antipyretic actions. In common with the group of drugs referred to as nonsteroidal anti-inflammatory drugs (NSAIDs; e.g., aspirin, ibuprofen, indomethacin), the pharmacologic actions of acetaminophen are related to its competitive inhibition of cyclooxygenase enzymes. This results in decreased production of prostaglandins, which are important mediators of inflammation, pain (low to moderate), and fever.[106] Contrary to other NSAIDs, acetaminophen has very weak anti-inflammatory activity—a consequence of its weak inhibition of peripheral tissue cyclooxygenase compared with that in the brain. In normal doses, acetaminophen is safe and effective, but it may cause severe hepatic toxicity or death when consumed in overdose quantities. Less frequently, nephrotoxicity may also occur. The initial clinical findings in acetaminophen toxicity are relatively mild and nonspecific (nausea, vomiting, and

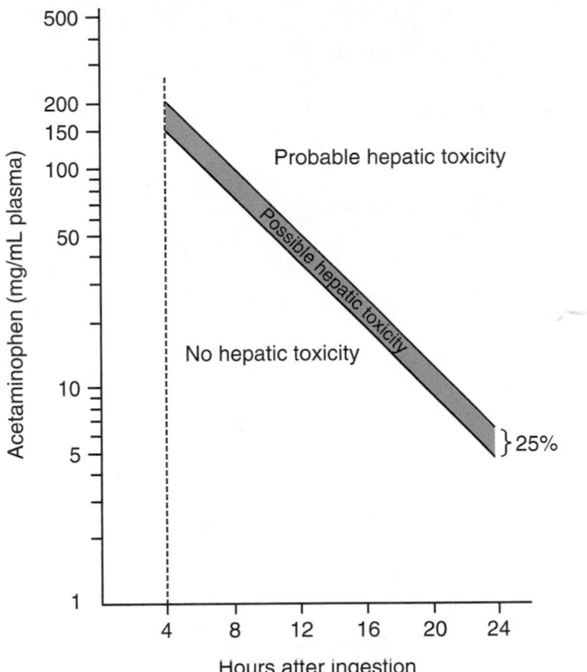

Figure 35-3 Rumack-Matthew nomogram. *(From Rumack BH, Matthew H. Acetaminophen poisoning and toxicity. Pediatrics 1975;55:871-6. Reproduced by permission of Pediatrics.)*

abdominal discomfort) and thus are not predictive of impending hepatic necrosis, which typically begins 24 to 36 hours after toxic ingestion and becomes most severe by 72 to 96 hours.[636] Although uncommon with severe overdose, coma and metabolic acidosis may occur before development of hepatic necrosis.[246] Antidotal therapy with *N*-acetylcysteine (NAC; Mucomyst) (see later) is most effective when administered before hepatic injury occurs, as signified by elevations of AST and ALT. Thus the measurement of serum acetaminophen concentration becomes paramount for proper assessment of the severity of overdose and for appropriate decision making for antidotal therapy. The Rumack-Matthew nomogram relates serum acetaminophen concentration and time following acute ingestion to the probability of hepatic necrosis (Figure 35-3).[691]

Several qualifications pertain to the use of this nomogram. First, blood samples should not be obtained earlier than 4 hours after ingestion to ensure that absorption is complete. Second, the nomogram applies only to acute and not to chronic ingestion. Toxicity from chronic ingestion of acetaminophen or other drugs is cumulative and typically occurs at lower blood concentrations than in acute overdose. Third, the nomogram is not useful if the time of ingestion is unknown or is considered unreliable. In this case, when the exact time of ingestion is unknown, clinicians should err on the side of treating with NAC until the acetaminophen concentration is nondetectable and no transaminase elevation is seen. Fourth, if acetaminophen is ingested with another substance that may delay absorption (i.e., an anticholinergic), the patient should be clinically monitored for clinical effects. If, for example, no anticholinergic signs or symptoms develop after the 4-hour acetaminophen concentration is measured, one may assume that absorption will not be delayed and the concentration can be plotted normally. If however, the patient develops anticholinergic signs and symptoms, and the acetaminophen concentration is detectable, that patient should be treated with NAC as absorption is most likely delayed, and the concentration should not be plotted. Fifth, alcoholic patients, fasting or malnourished patients, and patients on long-term therapy with microsomal enzyme-inducing drugs (anticonvulsants) may have increased susceptibility to acetaminophen hepatotoxicity,[92,133,731,836] presumably as a result of induction of cytochrome P450 (see later) and, in the case of alcoholics or fasting patients, depletion of glutathione (see later). In these cases, it has been proposed that the decision line in the nomogram should be lowered by 50 to 70%.[731,736] Others do not advocate any change in the therapeutic decision line for such patients with acute ingestion. These risk factors may be more important in chronic acetaminophen poisoning. Although therapeutic guidelines for chronic acetaminophen poisoning have not been established, it is recommended to administer NAC if the AST is elevated or acetaminophen is given at >10 µg/mL.[330]

Acetaminophen is normally metabolized in the liver to glucuronide (50 to 60%) and sulfate (≈30%) conjugates.[255] A smaller amount (≈10%) is metabolized by a cytochrome P450 mixed-function oxidase pathway that is thought to involve formation of a highly reactive intermediate (Figure 35-4), *N*-acetylbenzoquinoneimine (NAPQI).[545] This intermediate normally undergoes electrophilic conjugation with glutathione and then subsequent transformation to cysteine and mercapturic acid conjugates of acetaminophen. With acetaminophen overdose, the sulfation pathway becomes saturated; consequently, a greater portion is metabolized by the P450 mixed-function oxidase pathway. When the tissue stores of glutathione become depleted, arylation of cellular molecules by the benzoquinoneimine intermediate leads to hepatic necrosis.[545]

Specific therapy for acetaminophen overdose is the administration of NAC, which probably acts as a glutathione substitute.[103] NAC may also provide substrate to replenish hepatic glutathione[175] or to enhance sulfate conjugation,[480] or both. The time of administration of NAC is critical. Maximum efficacy is observed when NAC is administered within 8 hours, but efficacy then declines sharply between 18 and 24 hours after ingestion.[732] The antidote provides definite beneficial effects even after liver injury has occurred, presumably through its ability to improve tissue oxygen delivery and use.[322] NAC can be given by both oral and intravenous routes. Oral dosing consists of a 140-mg/kg loading dose followed by 70 mg/kg every 4 hours for 17 doses. Intravenous dosing consists of a 150-mg/kg loading dose followed by 50 mg/kg over 4 hours, then 100 mg/kg infused over 16 hours. If serum acetaminophen analytical services are not available locally within 8 hours of suspected ingestion, treatment with NAC should begin.

An area of some controversy is whether acetaminophen screening should be performed on all intentional overdose

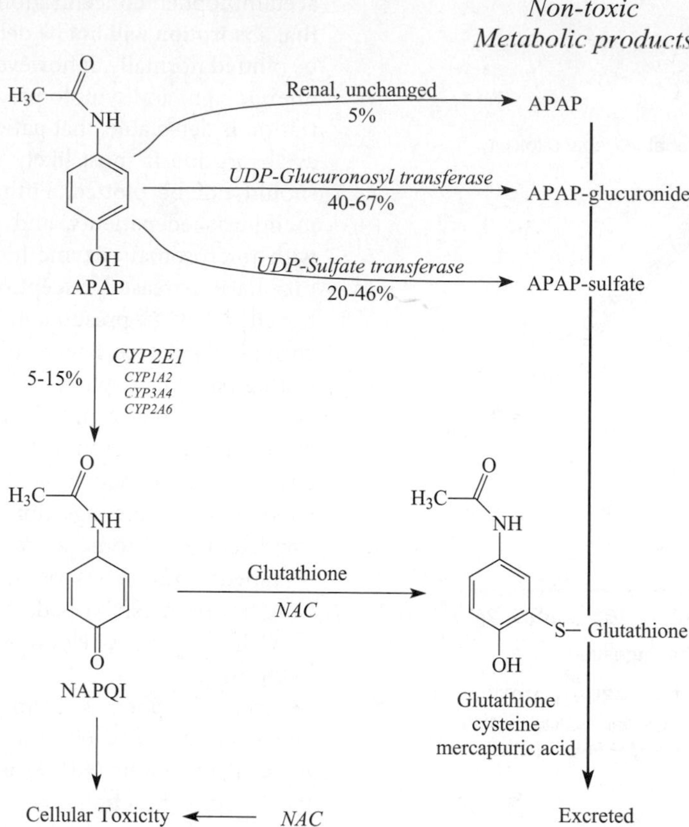

Figure 35-4 Pathways of acetaminophen metabolism. APAP (*N*-acetyl-*p*-aminophenol/acetaminophen), NAPQI (*N*-acetyl-*p*-benzo-quinone imine), and NAC (*N*-acetyl-L-cysteine).

patients.[75] One of the most worrisome aspects of acetaminophen poisoning is that initial clinical symptoms (e.g., nausea, vomiting, abdominal pain) may be vague or even absent in the first 24 hours.[76] This possible delay in diagnosis is particularly problematic because the antidote, NAC, has been shown to be most effective when initiated within the first 8 hours.[732] Studies looking at the issue of universal acetaminophen screening recommend screening all patients with suicidal ingestion and those with altered mental status in whom ingestion is suspected.[31,750]

Many spectrophotometric methods are available for the determination of acetaminophen.[95,842] In general, these methods are relatively easy to perform but are subject to various interferences such as bilirubin or bilirubin byproducts absorbing at similar wavelengths.[95,648] Some methods measure the nontoxic metabolites and the potentially toxic parent acetaminophen, and thus may produce especially misleading results. Therefore, only methods specific for parent acetaminophen should be used.[650] Immunoassays are widely used for this purpose, as they are rapid, easily performed, and accurate. A different spectrophotometric approach uses arylacylamide amidohydrolase to hydrolyze acetaminophen (but not conjugates) to *p*-aminophenol and acetate. Subsequent formation of the absorbing species depends on the reaction of generated *p*-aminophenol with 8-hydroxyquinoline[560] or o-cresol.[657] Arylacylamide amidohydrolase methods are susceptible to interference by NAC,[526] bilirubin, and immunoglobulin (Ig)M monoclonal immunoglobulins.[351] Most chromatographic methods are very accurate and are considered reference procedures.[748] A qualitative, one-step lateral flow immunoassay (cutoff of 25 µg/mL) may be suitable for point-of-care application, yet it has a low positive predictive value.[184]

Salicylate

Acetylsalicylic acid (aspirin) has analgesic, antipyretic, and anti-inflammatory properties. These therapeutic benefits derive from its ability to inhibit biosynthesis of prostaglandins by acetylation of active site serine and subsequent irreversible inhibition of cyclooxygenase enzymes (COX-1; COX-2 isoenzymes).[106] Salicylate, the metabolite of aspirin, also reduces prostaglandin synthesis by uncertain mechanisms. Because of these therapeutic benefits and the general lack of serious side effects at normal doses, aspirin is widely available and frequently consumed. Therapeutic serum salicylate concentrations are generally lower than 60 mg/L for analgesic-antipyretic effects, and 150 to 300 mg/L for anti-inflammatory actions.[106]

Aspirin also interferes with platelet aggregation and thus prolongs bleeding time. The platelet inhibitory effect is a consequence of the ability of aspirin to acetylate and irreversibly inhibit platelet cyclooxygenase, thereby reducing the formation of thromboxane A_2, a potent mediator of platelet aggregation. Platelets have little or no capacity for protein synthesis; therefore, the duration of this enzyme inhibition is the normal life span of the platelets (8 to 11 days).[686] Because of this platelet inhibitory activity, low-dose aspirin has been recommended as prophylactic therapy for some individuals at risk for thromboembolic disease.[621,753] An epidemiologic association has been noted between aspirin ingestion and Reye syndrome in children and adolescents with viral infection (e.g., varicella, influenza).[353] Therefore, aspirin use is contraindicated in these patients.

Absorption of normal doses of regular aspirin from the GI tract is generally rapid, with peak serum concentration achieved within 2 hours.[106] This peak value may be delayed for 12 hours or longer for enteric-coated or slow-release formulations.[447] Moreover, toxic doses of aspirin may form concretions or bezoars and produce pylorospasm, thereby delaying absorption. Serum salicylate in such instances may not reach maximum concentration for 6 hours or longer[200]—an important consideration when assessment of the severity of toxicity is based on such measurements.

Once absorbed, aspirin has a very short half-life ($t_{1/2}$ = 15 minutes) because of its rapid hydrolysis to salicylate. Salicylate is eliminated mainly by conjugation with glycine to form salicyluric acid, and to a lesser extent with glucuronic acid to form phenol and acyl glucuronides.[649] A very small amount is hydroxylated to gentisic acid. These metabolic pathways may become saturated even at high therapeutic doses. Consequently, serum salicylate concentration may increase disproportionately with dosage. At high therapeutic or toxic doses, the salicylate elimination half-life is prolonged (15 to 30 hours vs. 2 to 3 hours at low dose) and a much larger portion of the dose is excreted in urine as salicylate.[106]

Salicylates directly stimulate the central respiratory center and thereby cause hyperventilation and respiratory alkalosis. Moreover, salicylates cause uncoupling of oxidative phosphorylation. As a result, heat production (hyperthermia), oxygen consumption, and metabolic rate may be increased. In addition, salicylates enhance anaerobic glycolysis but inhibit the Krebs cycle and transaminase enzymes, all of which lead to accumulation of organic acids and thus to metabolic acidosis.[798]

The primary acid-base disturbance observed with salicylate overdosage depends on age and severity of intoxication. Respiratory alkalosis predominates in children over age 4 and in adults, except in very severe cases that may progress through a mixed respiratory alkalosis–metabolic acidosis to metabolic acidosis. Among 97 adult patients who had plasma salicylate concentrations greater than 700 mg/L, 19% were found to have respiratory alkalosis, 61% had combined respiratory alkalosis and metabolic acidosis, and 15% had metabolic acidosis. Mortality was associated with acidemia.[129] In children younger than age 4, the initial period of respiratory alkalosis is very brief and therefore may not be observed; in such cases, metabolic acidosis predominates.[798] CNS depression is more pronounced when acidemia is severe, which is a consequence of increased brain uptake of nonionized salicylic acid. Respiratory acidosis, a result of severe CNS depression or pulmonary edema, may sometimes occur and is indicative of a poor prognosis.

Salicylates remain readily available in numerous over-the-counter products. In any patient with a history of salicylate ingestion or possessing characteristic signs or symptoms of salicylate poisoning, a serum salicylate concentration should be obtained. Early identification of salicylate toxicity can be lifesaving.

Following acute salicylate overdose, patients initially may be asymptomatic, especially if that product is enteric coated. Salicylate toxic patients may develop nausea, vomiting, abdominal pain, tinnitus, tachypnea, oliguria, and altered mental status ranging from lethargy to coma.[767] Chronic intoxication can present in a similar fashion as acute exposures, yet such exposures typically are more insidious and therefore are often misdiagnosed.[250]

Interpretation of salicylate concentrations as a guide for clinical management decisions can be difficult. Perhaps the most well-known attempt at utilizing salicylate concentrations to predict the severity of salicylate toxicity was the nomogram developed by Done.[200] After examining both the clinical symptoms and the salicylate concentrations in patients who had a single acute overdose, Done created a nomogram that predicted severity of poisoning based on the salicylate concentration drawn at a given time from ingestion. This tool has significant limitations. Because this nomogram as originally developed was based on only 38 pediatric patients, its utility for acute adult overdose is not known. One of the assumptions allowing the creation of this nomogram was that salicylates are eliminated by first-order kinetics. It has since been well established that some of the pathways for elimination of salicylates become saturated in overdose and follow zero-order kinetics.[579] One study demonstrated significant disagreement between the clinical severity predicted by the nomogram and the severity judged by physicians.[214] Therefore, we no longer recommend its use in the management of the salicylate-poisoned patient.

Use of salicylate concentrations to guide management must be done cautiously and only in conjunction with careful evaluation of a patient's clinical status. One group of investigators examined 97 patients who experienced significant exposure to this agent. Patients who did not survive the ingestion and patients with reasonably high serum concentrations (≥700 mg/L) were included in this study.[129] Although toxic concentrations alone were of poor prognostic value, the investigators did identify certain clinical findings that predicted a poor prognosis, including pulmonary edema, fever, coma, and acidosis. The absorptive phase of salicylates can be unpredictable (delayed or erratic) as a result of bezoar formation, enteric-coated product, gastric outlet obstruction, or pylorospasm.[250] Therefore, a concentration drawn soon after the original ingestion may not be reflective of the potential peak concentration. Initial serial concentrations should be performed every 2 hours while the patient is monitored clinically. When the concentrations begin to decline and the patient's clinical status is improved, concentrations can be measured less frequently.

The units reported with each concentration should be documented before management decisions are made. Laboratories may alternatively report concentrations in terms of mg/dL and mg/L. This important distinction, which involves a tenfold difference in concentration, is infamous for causing confusion. In extreme cases of these miscommunications, hemodialysis has been ordered for patients thought to have astronomically high salicylate concentrations that were later proven to be nontoxic.[312]

The need to screen all intentional overdose patients for salicylates is highly debated.[127,128,750] Diagnosis of salicylate poisoning based solely on clinical examination is not without pitfalls. Although large, acute ingestions are usually detected through history and clinical symptoms, chronic salicylate toxicity often is more difficult to diagnose. Numerous cases have been reported pertaining to a delayed or mistaken diagnosis in the face of significant salicylate toxicity. In these cases, patients presented with nonspecific symptoms such as fever, abdominal pain, and encephalopathy and subsequently were misdiagnosed with surgical abdomen, myocardial infarction, sepsis, encephalitis, and alcoholic ketoacidosis.[142,250,465,626] One study revealed that delayed diagnosis (at times up to 72 hours) of chronic salicylate poisoning is associated with higher morbidity and mortality rates compared with diagnosis on admission.[18] Another study involving salicylate-related fatalities in Ontario revealed that symptoms and signs of salicylate poisoning were apparently missed even in patients who were alert on presentation.[533] The "classic" finding of ototoxicity was described by one group of investigators to be neither sensitive nor specific of serum salicylate concentration.[316] Characteristic laboratory findings as well may not be reliable. Although a wide anion gap metabolic acidosis with respiratory alkalosis is often encountered in association with salicylate poisoning, one study involving 20 elderly patients with chronic salicylate poisoning revealed that 35% cases presented with a normal anion gap and PCO_2.[36]

Because products containing salicylates are readily available, the clinical effects of salicylate toxicity are nonspecific, and lack of metabolic acidosis does not rule out the potential for salicylate toxicity, clinicians should have a low threshold for obtaining serum salicylate concentrations.

Treatment for salicylate intoxication is directed toward (1) decreasing further absorption, (2) increasing elimination, and (3) correcting acid-base and electrolyte disturbances. Activated charcoal binds aspirin and prevents its absorption. Elimination of salicylate may be enhanced by alkaline diuresis and in severe cases by hemodialysis.[798] Sodium bicarbonate may be given to alleviate metabolic acidosis. Indications for hemodialysis include serum salicylate >1000 mg/L, severe CNS depression, intractable metabolic acidosis, hepatic failure with coagulopathy, and renal failure.[252]

A urine drug screen may be helpful in detecting the presence of drugs included as part of combination medications with aspirin (e.g., antihistamines, sympathomimetic amines, propoxyphene) or that otherwise are coingested.

Classic methods for the measurement of salicylate in serum are based on the method of Trinder (see "Spot Tests").[782] These procedures rely on the reaction between salicylate and Fe^{3+} to form a colored complex that is measured at 540 nm. To lessen endogenous background interference, a protein precipitation step or a serum blank is necessary. Nevertheless, blank readings equivalent to about 20 to 25 mg/L are generally observed. Moreover, interference by salicylate metabolites, endogenous compounds, and some drugs, especially structurally related drugs such as diflunisal (difluorophenyl salicylate),[704] may occur. Azide, present as a preservative in some commercial control sera, also causes interference. Despite these limitations, photometric methods continue to be successfully used to assess salicylate overdose. The Trinder method results agreed very closely with those of a reference HPLC procedure.[375] However, significant interference with the Trinder method was observed for one patient, who consumed an overdose of dichloralphenazone. Thus for best interpretation of test results, as much information as possible should be obtained regarding drug ingestion history.

Other methods for salicylate quantitation include fluorescent polarization immunoassay[406] and a salicylate hydroxylase–mediated photometric procedure.[561,649] These procedures are subject to some of the same interferences as the Trinder method, but the salicylate hydroxylase method is considered more specific[561] and has been adapted to automated analyzers. Gas and liquid chromatographic methods are the most specific methods for salicylate,[125,665] but their general availability, especially for emergency use, is limited and probably is not necessary. A qualitative, one-step lateral flow immunoassay (cutoff of 100 μg/mL) is commercially available for point-of-care application but has a low positive predictive value (0.47).[184]

Agents Related to the Anticholinergic Toxidrome[125]

The tricyclic antidepressants, the phenothiazines, and the antihistamines have divergent therapeutic applications; however in overdose, they often share similar anticholinergic and antihistaminic toxidromes as principal components of their overall toxic effects.

Tricyclic Antidepressants

Tricyclic antidepressants (TCAs), so named because of their three-ring structure (Figure 35-5), represent a class of drugs frequently prescribed for the treatment of depression (see Chapter 34). The TCAs have been largely supplanted by the newer, less toxic selective serotonin reuptake inhibitors (SSRIs) and other atypical agents, which now are accepted broadly as drugs of first choice, particularly for medically ill or potentially suicidal patients and for the elderly and the young.[97,249,605,730,838] Fatalities are much less common since modern antidepressants have widely replaced these drugs. However, because of their continued use and narrow therapeutic range, and because of the nature of the illness for which they are typically prescribed, TCAs are frequently associated with severe or fatal toxicity.[187,479,632]

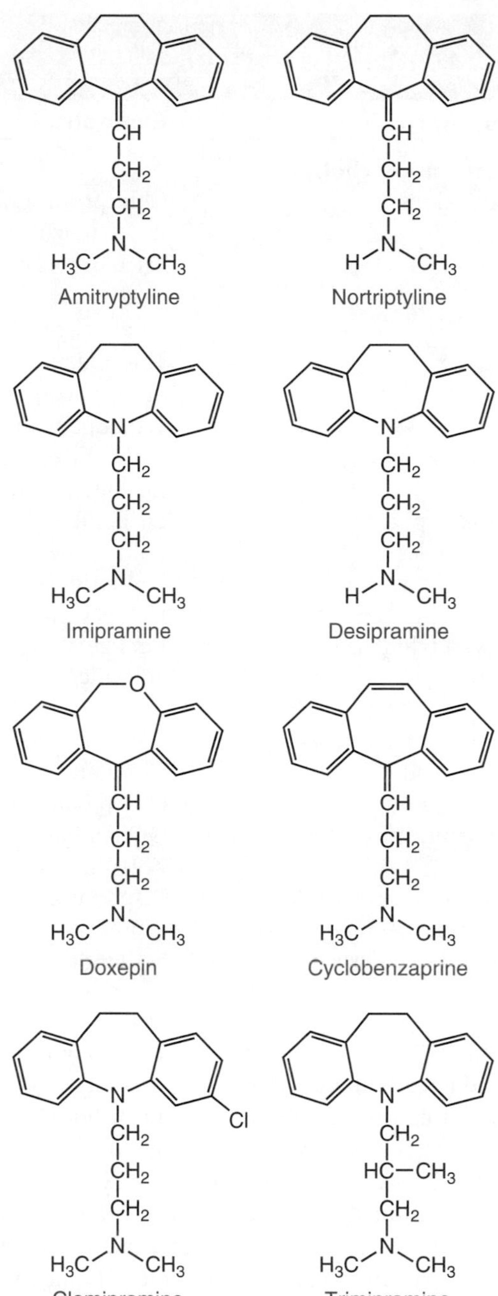

Figure 35-5 Structure of tricyclic antidepressants and related drugs.

Tricyclic antidepressants block neuronal uptake of serotonin and/or norepinephrine.[19] In general, TCAs with secondary-amine side chains or the *N*-demethylated (nor) metabolites of agents with tertiary-amine moieties (e.g., desipramine, norclomipramine, nordoxepin, nortriptyline) are relatively selective inhibitors of norepinephrine transport.[19,38] However, tertiary TCAs (amitriptyline, doxepin, and imipramine) are less selective and inhibit the reuptake of serotonin.[19,38] Clomipramine, a notable exception, is relatively selective against serotonin.[38] Among the TCAs, trimipramine is exceptional in that it lacks prominent inhibitory effects at monoamine transport, and its clinical actions remain unexplained.[38]

The TCAs have many other pharmacologic actions that apparently do not contribute to the therapeutic effects but do contribute to the side effects. For example, most TCAs have at least moderate affinity for α_1-adrenergic receptors, much less for α_2, and virtually none for β-receptors,[38] leading to hypotension, dizziness, and sedation.[19] TCAs also have sedative effects that may be related to antihistamine activity.[19] Tertiary amines produce greater sedation than secondary amines. TCAs also exert central and peripheral anticholinergic effects (dry skin and mouth, flushing, hyperpyrexia, dilated pupils, constipation, urinary retention, and decreased GI motility) through their interaction with M1 muscarinic receptors.[19]

Cardiovascular toxicity, the most serious manifestation of TCA overdose, accounts for the majority of fatalities. Cardiovascular effects include orthostatic hypotension, sinus tachycardia, and variable prolongation of cardiac conduction times with the potential for arrhythmias, particularly with overdose.[38] The anticholinergic effect, mediated through M1 blockade, and sympathomimetic effects contribute to cardiac dysrhythmias.[19] In mild overdose, these effects result in tachycardia and a slight increase in blood pressure. With more severe overdose, serious arrhythmias and conduction delays may develop, of which the most distinct feature is prolongation of the QRS interval in the electrocardiogram. Cardiac output decreases coupled with peripheral vasodilatation (α_1-adrenergic blockade) lead to life-threatening hypotension. Death often results from arrhythmias or hypotension. Cardiotoxic manifestations may occur within a few hours of overdose, or they may be delayed. It is important to recognize that a patient's symptoms (perhaps initially only mild anticholinergic effects) are due to tricyclic antidepressants, so that a proper period of monitoring for delayed and possibly catastrophic cardiotoxicity is followed.

In general antidepressants are associated with several clinically important drug interactions,[471] and they potentiate the effects of alcohol and probably other sedatives.[38] Virtually any agent with serotonin-potentiating activity, including TCAs, can interact dangerously or even fatally with monoamine oxidase (MAO) inhibitors (particularly long-acting MAO inhibitors).[233] The resulting reactions are referred to as *serotonin syndrome*.[754]

Some tolerance to the sedative and autonomic effects of TCAs tends to develop with continued drug use.[38] Occasionally, patients show physical dependence, with malaise, chills, muscle aches, and sleep disturbance following abrupt discontinuation, particularly of high doses.[38] Some withdrawal effects may reflect increased cholinergic activity following its inhibition.[38] Some of these reactions have been confused with clinical worsening of depressive symptoms. Emergence of agitated or manic reactions has been observed after abrupt discontinuation of TCAs.[38]

TCAs are oxidized by hepatic cytochrome P450 (CYP) microsomal enzymes, followed by conjugation with glucuronic acid.[38] The *N*-demethylated metabolites of several tricyclic antidepressants are pharmacologically active and may accumulate in concentrations approaching or exceeding those of the parent drug, to contribute variably to overall pharmacodynamic activity (see Chapter 34).

Analytical Methods

Tricyclic antidepressants are measured by chromatographic or immunoassay methods (see Chapters 13 and 16). Immunoassays are rapid and relatively easy to perform but may be subject to interference by other drugs, such as chlorpromazine,[615] thioridazine,[694] cyclobenzaprine,[615] and diphenhydramine,[746] and are not able to necessarily identify which TCA is being quantitated. In cases of overdose, qualitative identification (serum or urine) is sufficient, because the severity of intoxication is more reliably indicated by an increase in the QRS interval than by the serum concentration.[79]

Cyclobenzaprine, a tricyclic amine structurally very similar to amitriptyline (see Figure 35-5), is used as a centrally acting skeletal muscle relaxant. Similar to amitriptyline, cyclobenzaprine causes sedation, produces central and peripheral muscarinic blockade, and potentiates adrenergic actions. In overdose, cyclobenzaprine may cause a typical anticholinergic toxidrome and cardiac arrhythmias, hypotension, and coma. The analytical distinction between amitriptyline and cyclobenzaprine is often difficult. Cyclobenzaprine cross-reacts with immunoassays for tricyclic antidepressants and can coelute or comigrate with amitriptyline in HPLC and TLC. However, cyclobenzaprine and amitriptyline have different ultraviolet spectra; therefore, they may be distinguished by HPLC using a diode array detector by multiwavelength scanning or dual-wavelength discrimination.[196,644] However, amitriptyline and cyclobenzaprine are well resolved using capillary column GC and may be distinguished by careful examination of their respective mass spectra.[853]

Antipsychotic Drugs

The antipsychotic drugs are generally used for primary psychiatric disorders such as (1) schizophrenia, (2) bipolar disorder, (3) schizoaffective disorder, and (4) psychotic depression. In addition to their psychotherapeutic effects, these drugs have a number of other actions, so that certain members of this group are used as antiemetics (prochlorperazine), as antihistaminics (promethazine),[685] and for sedation or potentiation of analgesia and general anesthesia.[38] Antipsychotic compounds are traditionally divided and subdivided according to their chemical structure (Table 35-6 and Figure 35-6).[456,685]

The exact mechanism of action of antipsychotic drugs is not known; however, the primary pharmacologic effect of all antipsychotic drugs is thought to be blockade of D2 receptors in the central nervous system.[38,456,673] The idea comes from studies showing that the ability of classical antipsychotics to reduce psychotic symptoms correlates with their affinity for the D2 receptor.[456] However, the drugs are pharmacologically "dirty" and bind to many other receptors, including histamine (H_1, H_2), $GABA_A$, muscarinic receptors, α_1- and α_2-adrenoreceptors, and sodium and potassium voltage-gated ion channels.[100,109,751,758] The atypical antipsychotics on the other hand have a different mechanism that my involve other dopamine receptors, serotonin receptors, or both.[456]

TABLE 35-6 Examples of Classical and Atypical Antipsychotics

Antispychotics	Examples[39,100,456,685]
Classical Antipsychotics	
Phenothiazines	Chlorpromazine
	Promethazine
	Trichlorperazine
	Perphenazine
	Fluphenazine
	Thioridazine
	Mesoridazine
	Trifluoperazine
Thioxanthines	Flupenthizol
	Zuclopenthixol
Dibenzoxazepine	Loxapine
Dihydroindoles	Molindone
Butyrophenones	Droperidol
	Haloperidol
Diphenylbutylpiperidines	Pimozide
Benzamides	Sulpride
Atypical Antipsychotics	
Dibenzdiazepine derivatives	Clozapine
	Olanzapine
Benzothiapine derivatives	Quetiapine
	Zotepine
Bezisoxazole derivatives	Risperidone
Benzoisthioazoyl piperazine	Ziprasidone
Imidazolindone derivatives	Setindole

The principal manifestations of phenothiazine toxicity involve the CNS and the cardiovascular system.[38,65,494] The presentation for most of these drugs is qualitatively similar to that following TCA overdose, but in general they are less toxic. The most common effects in significant phenothiazine overdose include (1) sedation, (2) hypotension, (3) small pupils, (4) anticholinergic effects, and (5) ECG changes.[100,102,109] Phenothiazines are relatively safe and rarely cause death when ingested alone. More severe toxicity occurs when phenothiazines are coingested with tricyclic antidepressant drugs or other CNS depressant drugs, such as ethanol, opioids, barbiturates, or benzodiazepines.

All of the neuroleptic drugs are metabolized in the liver. Many have active metabolites and complex metabolic pathways. The main enzymes involved in metabolism are cytochrome P450 (CYP) enzymes, specifically CYP1A2, CYP2D6, and CYP3A4.[109,183,780] Many sources of variation are found in CYP-mediated metabolism; however, where multiple enzymes are involved, such variability has only a relatively small effect on clearance and drug concentrations.

Toxicity is strongly correlated with peak serum concentrations and thus usually occurs within the first 4 to 6 hours after

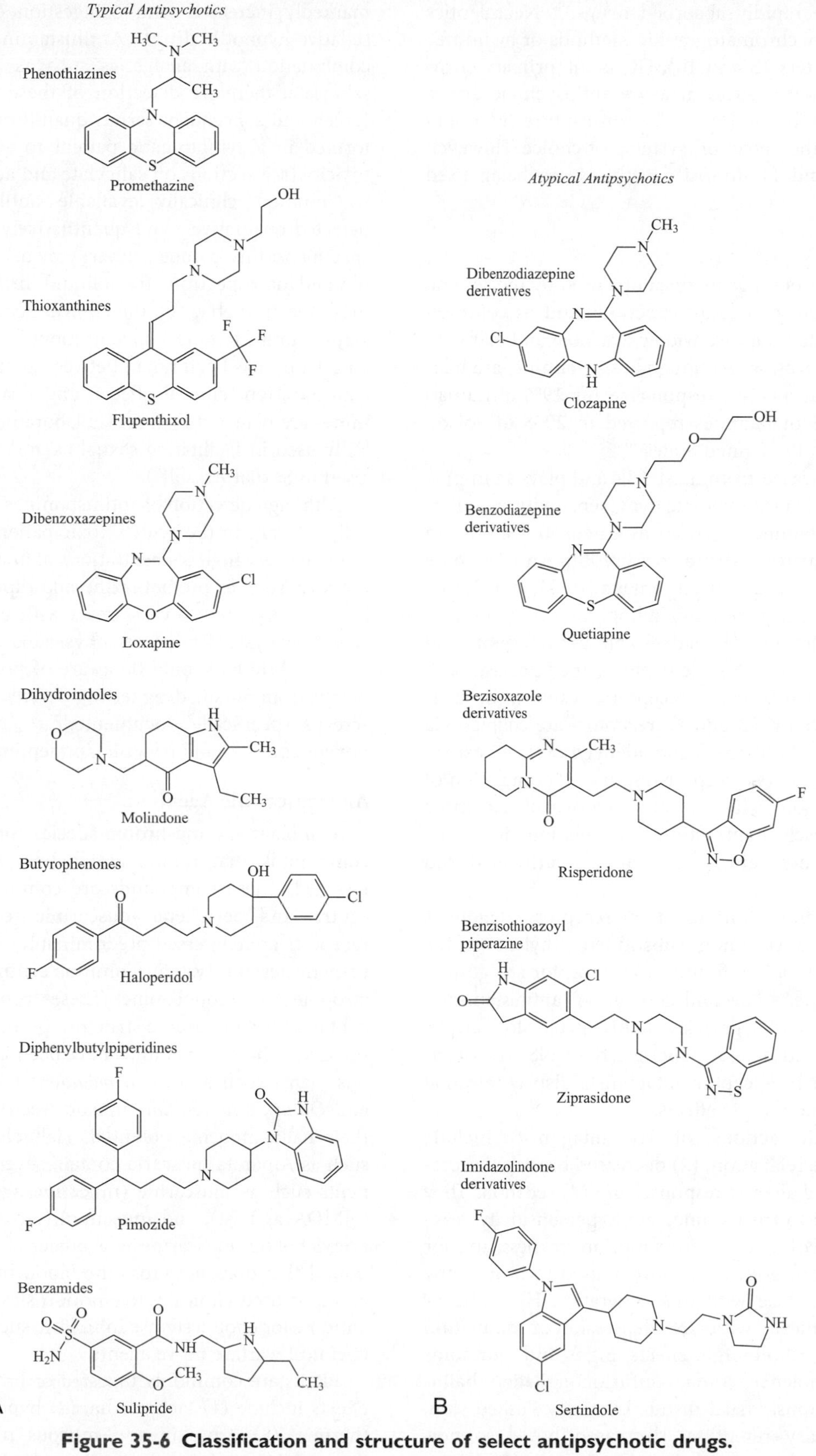

Typical Antipsychotics

Phenothiazines

Promethazine

Thioxanthines

Flupenthixol

Dibenzoxazepines

Loxapine

Dihydroindoles

Molindone

Butyrophenones

Haloperidol

Diphenylbutylpiperidines

Pimozide

Benzamides

Sulipride

A

Atypical Antipsychotics

Dibenzodiazepine derivatives

Clozapine

Benzodiazepine derivatives

Quetiapine

Bezisoxazole derivatives

Risperidone

Benzisothioazoyl piperazine

Ziprasidone

Imidazolindone derivatives

Sertindole

B

Figure 35-6 Classification and structure of select antipsychotic drugs.

ingestion of these rapidly absorbed drugs.[100] Neuroleptics may be detected by chromatographic methods or by immunoassay (see Chapters 13 and 16). GC is the primary chromatographic method used to measure antipsychotic drugs, and nitrogen phosphorus (NP), electron capture (EC), and MS detectors are the detection systems of choice. However, HPLC, LC-MS, and LC-MS/MS methods are being used more commonly.

Antihistamines

Antihistamines are popular medications used by the general public for treatment of allergic reactions and as common sleep aids. Antihistamines are widely available and many do not require a prescription. Although antihistamines are relatively safe, these agents are responsible for 19% of human exposures and 6% of fatalities reported in 2008 to Poison Control Centers in the United States.[96]

Histamine is released from mast cells and plays an important physiologic role in immediate hypersensitivity and allergic responses. Histamine functions as a neurotransmitter in the CNS and stimulates gastric acid secretion. Antihistamine drugs currently available clinically antagonize H_1 and H_2 histamine receptors. First-generation liphophilic antihistamines, such as diphenhydramine (Benadryl), bind H_1 receptors and exhibit peripheral and CNS system effects; they can also bind to muscarinic and adrenergic receptors, resulting in their anticholinergic activity. H_1 and H_2 receptors are coupled via G-proteins to phospholipase C and adenylyl cyclase, respectively.[777] The principal H_2 receptor response is stimulation of gastric acid secretion, whereas other actions of histamine (e.g., smooth muscle contraction, vasodilation, increased capillary permeability, pain, itching) are primarily mediated by H_1 receptors.

The broad binding affinities of H_1 receptor antagonists are attributed to a common substituted ethylene amine ($—CH_2CH_2NR_2—$) moiety found in H_1 receptor antagonists and in acetylcholine.[649] "Second-generation" antihistamines, such as fexofenadine (Allegra), are highly specific for peripheral H_1 receptors and do not penetrate the CNS. Therefore, second-generation H_1 receptor antagonists display minimal sedative and anticholinergic effects.

The therapeutic actions of H_1 antagonists include (1) smooth muscle relaxation, (2) decreased bronchial secretions, (3) decreased allergic response, and (4) sedation. They are therefore used to treat immediate hypersensitivity reactions, as cold remedies, to suppress motion sickness, and for sedation. The H_2 antagonists are widely used to treat peptic ulcer disease. Overdose with first-generation H_1 antihistamines presents clinically with CNS depression or stimulation and peripheral anticholinergic effects. Signs and symptoms may include somnolence, coma, confusion, agitation, hallucinations, convulsions, visual disturbance, dry flushed skin, dry mouth, urinary retention, decreased bowel sounds, hypertension, and supraventricular arrhythmias.[777,866]

Acute toxic effects are rarely observed when extremely high doses of second-generation H_1 and H_2 antihistamine are ingested. However, clinical effects such as sedation can be markedly increased with coingestion of alcohol or other sedative-hypnotic drugs. Antihistamines are available in combination with analgesics such as acetaminophen and salicylate; therefore detection of these analgesics by urine screen and subsequent serum quantification should be performed in a symptomatic patient to assess their potential toxicity (see sections on salicylate and acetaminophen).

Common clinically available antihistamines can be detected qualitatively and quantitatively in blood and urine specimens; this is done primarily by using gas chromatography and mass spectrometry or liquid chromatography tandem mass spectrometry. Yet, the clinical necessity of quantitative serum antihistamine concentrations is questionable. Poor correlation has been noted between patient age, dose, blood concentration, clinical effects, and death.[37,260,654] Antihistamines are detected by forensic laboratories as agents potentially used in facilitating sexual assault (see section, "Drugs Used in Sexual Assault").

Although detection of antihistamines is not typically clinically relevant in the acutely toxic patient, it is important to note that very high concentrations of first-generation antihistamines, such as promethazine and diphenhydramine, have been documented to cross-react with urine drug immunoscreen analyses. Therefore, physicians and medical review officers (MROs) should be aware of potential false-positive results from on-site drug testing devices, as well as immunoscreens specifically documented in amphetamine,[199] propoxyphene,[646,711] and tricyclic antidepressants.[247,795,839]

Antimuscarinic Agents

Several plant and mushroom species contain antimuscarinic compounds that mimic anticholinergic symptoms when ingested. These compounds are competitive antagonists at central and peripheral muscarinic receptors. Muscarinic receptors are expressed predominantly within the parasympathetic nervous system. Common centrally acting agents are atropine and scopolamine. These tropane alkaloid agents contain a tertiary amine structure permitting penetration of the CNS. These compounds have been isolated from numerous plants such as *Atropa belladonna* (Deadly nightshade) and *Datura stramonium* (Jimson weed) and are abused for their hallucinogenic potential. Hallucinogenic mushrooms such as Amanita muscaria contain several bioactive components such as muscarine (mucarine agonist), ibotenic acid (NMDA agonist), and muscimol ($GABA_A$ agonist). Unlike acetylcholine, muscarine is a quaternary ammonium compound that does not cross the blood-brain barrier. Scopolamine is used clinically for motion sickness. Atropine is an antidote for cholinesterase inhibitors such as insecticides and chemical warfare nerve agents.

Plants are commonly ingested or brewed as tea. Clinical effects include (1) tachycardia, (2) hypertension, (3) hyperthermia, (4) dry skin and mucous membranes, (5) skin flushing, (6) diminished bowel sounds, (7) urinary retention, (8) agitation, (9) disorientation, and (10) hallucination.[612,671] The effects of muscarine often last longer than those of acetylcholine, because it lacks an ester bond required for acetylcholinesterase hydrolysis. Patients are clinically managed on the basis of clinical presentation, rather than by identification of ingested plants or drug-specific testing.[482] Testing for atropine and scopolamine can be performed by liquid chromatography–tandem mass spectrometry and is available in some clinical laboratories. Although HPLC techniques may be used to identify muscarine, no clinical techniques are yet available.

Agents Related to Cholinergic Syndrome

Agents inducing cholinergic syndrome are diverse and act by producing uncontrolled acetylcholine transmission through inactivation of cholinesterase enzymes or direct stimulation of acetylcholine receptors. Acetylcholine is an essential neurotransmitter that affects parasympathetic synapses (autonomic and CNS), sympathetic preganglionic synapses, and the neuromuscular junction (see also prior section, "Toxic Syndromes"). Clinical manifestations in cholinergic syndrome include muscarinic, nicotinic, and central effects (see Table 35-2). The duration of acetylcholine action is controlled by acetylcholinesterase and butyrylcholinesterase (pseudocholinesterase). Acetylcholinesterase is found in red blood cells, nervous tissue, and skeletal muscle. Butyrylcholinesterase is found in plasma, liver, heart, pancreas, and brain.

Organophosphate (e.g., Malathion, Parathion, Diazinon, Dursban) and carbamate (e.g., Sevin, Furadan) insecticides (Figure 35-7), as well as military nerve agents [e.g., Sarin (GB), Soman (GD), Tabun (GA) (VX)], exert their toxicity by inhibiting the action of acetylcholinesterase and thereby causing a pronounced cholinergic response.[43,118,145] Acetylcholinesterase inhibition is the consequence of phosphorylation (organophosphates) or carbamylation (carbamates) of

Organophosphate insecticide

$R_1R_2P(=O)X$ or $R_1R_2P(=S)X$

R_1, R_2 = for example, —O—CH_3, —O—CH_2—CH_3

X = for example, —F, —CN, —O—C_6H_4—NO_2

Carbamate insecticide

CH_3—NH—C(=O)—O—X

X = for example, [naphthyl ring]

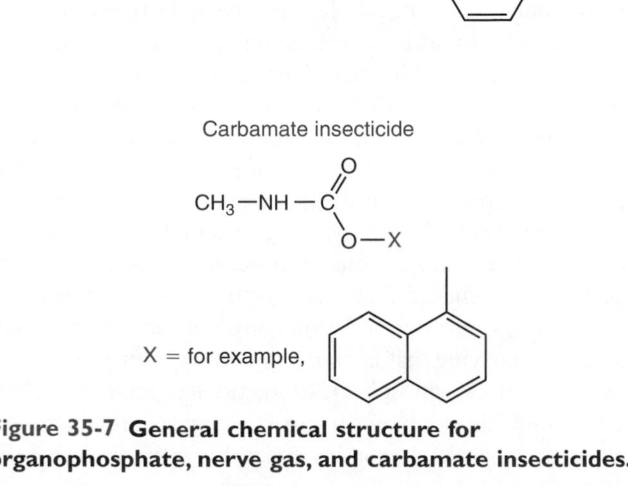

Figure 35-7 General chemical structure for organophosphate, nerve gas, and carbamate insecticides.

the cholinesterase-active site serine hydroxyl group. Acetylcholinesterase enzyme activity can be reactivated by administering an "oxime" drug, or through de novo cellular synthesis of enzyme.

Organophosphate and Carbamate Compounds

Organophosphate insecticides are toxic because they inactivate acetylcholinesterases that are required for hydrolyzing acetylcholine at nerve junctions. Nerve agents are also organophosphorus inhibitors of acetylcholinesterases, yet these agents are more potent than their pesticide counterparts.[566] Nerve agents share a similar structural backbone observed in organophosphate insecticides (see Figure 35-7).

Excess synaptic acetylcholine stimulates muscarinic receptors (peripheral and CNS) and stimulates but then depresses or paralyzes nicotinic receptors. Activation of peripheral muscarinic receptors causes signs and symptoms described by the mnemonics SLUDGE or DUMB BELS, defined earlier. CNS neurotoxic effects include (1) restlessness, (2) agitation, (3) lethargy, (4) confusion, (5) slurred speech, (6) seizures, (7) coma, (8) cardiorespiratory depression, and (9) death. Stimulation or paralysis of nicotinic receptors at the neuromuscular junction causes muscle fasciculations, cramping, weakness, and respiratory muscle paralysis; stimulation of nicotinic receptors at sympathetic ganglia results in hypertension, tachycardia, pallor, and mydriasis.

The actual signs and symptoms observed with these toxins depend on the balance of muscarinic and nicotinic receptor activation. Although miosis (muscarinic action) is most common, it may not always be present, and indeed mydriasis (nicotinic action) may occur. Likewise, tachycardia (nicotinic effect) may be present rather than bradycardia (muscarinic action). Death most commonly results from respiratory failure, a consequence of nicotinic receptor–mediated muscle paralysis, combined with muscarinic-facilitated bronchorrhea, bronchoconstriction, and CNS depression.

Organophosphate inhibition is a consequence of phosphorylation of the serine hydroxyl group at the active site of the cholinesterase enzyme catalytic triad (Ser-Glu-His). The partially electropositive phosphorus is attracted to the partially electronegative serine (see Figure 35-7). The negatively charged glutamate present in the catalytic triad attracts the organophosphate leaving group and forms an alkylphosphoryl serine bond, creating a "transition state." Subsequent hydrolysis results in irreversible dealkylation ("aging") of the AChE.[9] Aging proceeds at variable rates depending on the size and branching of the alkyl groups (24 to 48 hours) to form a phosphoryl oxyanion serine bond that is completely resistant to even pharmacologically mediated hydrolysis.

Although carbamates are structurally different from organophosphates (see Figure 35-7), carbamates exert their toxicity at the active site of AChE but inhibit enzyme activity through carbamylation rather than phosphorylation of the serine hydroxyl group. In contrast to the phosphoryl-serine bond, the carbamyl-serine bond undergoes spontaneous hydrolysis, and regeneration of enzyme activity occurs in hours rather than days.[265] Carbamates exhibit poor CNS

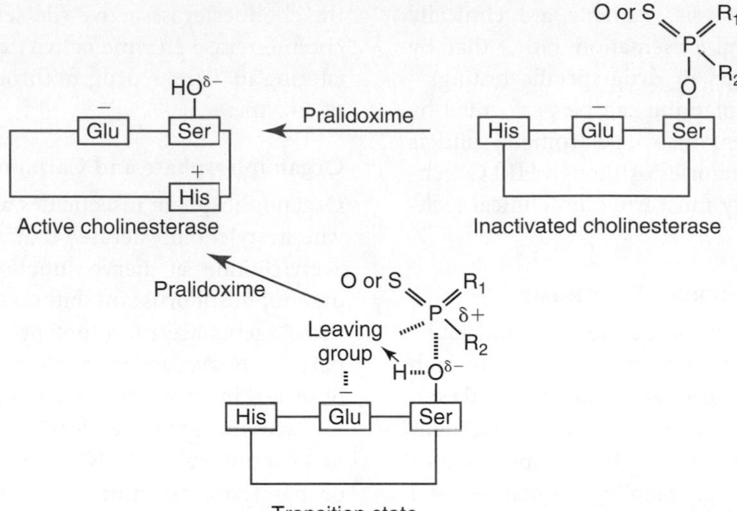

Figure 35-8 Reactivation of inactivated acetylcholinesterase by pralidoxime. The partially electropositive phosphorus of the organophosphate/nerve agent is attracted to the partially electronegative serine present in the catalytic triad of the acetylcholinesterase enzyme. The negatively charged glutamate in the catalytic triad attracts the leaving group of the organophosphate, creating a "transition state" compound. Pralidoxime can mediate regeneration of acetylcholinesterase in the transition state. Formation of the dealkylated "aged" acetylcholinesterase does not reactivate.

penetration and have a shorter duration of action; therefore neurotoxicity is usually less severe. Oximes are not recommended for carbamate toxicity and may exacerbate symptoms by stabilizing the carbamylation of acetylcholinesterase enzymes.[220]

Specific therapy for organophosphate and carbamate insecticide poisoning includes administration of atropine to block the muscarinic (but not nicotinic) actions of acetylcholine. In addition, pralidoxime is given to reactivate cholinesterase. Pralidoxime binds to the cholinesterase catalytic site and, via nucleophilic attack by its oxime group, dephosphorylates or decarbamylates the serine group (see Figures 35-7 and 35-8). Pralidoxime is ineffective in reactivating the "aged" form of the phosphorylated enzyme. Administration of pralidoxime may not be necessary in cases of carbamate insecticide poisoning because carbamylated cholinesterase spontaneously reactivates within a few hours. In fact, pralidoxime is considered contraindicated in these cases by some authors, because cholinesterase inhibition by carbaryl (Sevin), but not by other carbamates, may be enhanced by pralidoxime. Others administer pralidoxime in either case because the particular insecticide ingested may not be known.[118,145] A more potent bisquaternary oxime, obidoxime, is available outside the United States.

Administration of a site-directed nucleophile [pyridine-2-aldoxime chloride (2-PAM)] targets AChE reactivation during the transition state. Oxime antidotes such as 2-PAM contain a quaternary nitrogen that binds to the choline-binding site of AChE, positioning the oxime for nucleophilic attack, and by transferring the phosphoryl group from the serine hydroxyl group to itself, it releases free, active enzyme.[844,845] 2-PAM is not effective on aged AChE, so it must be administered as soon as possible after intoxication. Reactivation of aged AChE requires de novo cellular synthesis of enzyme (days).

Diagnosis of organophosphate and carbamate toxicity depends mainly on exposure history, physical presentation, clinical suspicion, and laboratory support. Treatment requires immediate attention and should not rely on laboratory confirmation. Yet cholinesterase activity is often monitored by clinicians in occupational exposure, acute intentional and accidental exposure, and response to therapy.

Three neurologic sequelae of organophosphate poisoning may occur after the initial cholinergic crisis has responded to atropine and oxime therapy in what is referred to as the *intermediate syndrome.*[719] Paralysis of proximal limb muscles, neck flexors, cranial nerves, and respiratory muscles may occur 24 to 96 hours following cholinergic resolution. Respiratory muscle paralysis may be severe enough to result in death. This phenomenon, caused by excessive nicotinic receptor stimulation, may result from redistribution of lipophilic organophosphates from adipose tissue and/or from inadequate oxime therapy. In another syndrome, organophosphate-induced delayed neuropathy (OPIDN),[3] weakness of extremities, ataxia, and eventually paralysis may occur 1 to 3 weeks following severe intoxication. Respiratory muscles are not affected. It is believed that this peripheral neuropathy is the consequence of phosphorylation and inhibition of an axonal membrane enzyme that is designated *neuropathy target esterase.* Alternatively, phosphorylation and activation of a Ca^{2+}/calmodulin kinase may in turn enhance proteolysis of neuronal cytoskeletal proteins and cause structural changes in neurofilaments, resulting in impaired axonal transport.[3] Finally, extrapyramidal symptoms similar to those of Parkinson's disease have very rarely occurred several days after cholinergic crisis resolution. A favorable response was observed with an antiparkinsonian agent.[27]

Cholinesterase activity is measured to assess exposure and to monitor reactivation during treatment. Acetylcholinesterase and butyrylcholinesterase enzyme activity are typically monitored using spectrophotometric analyses (see Chapter 22). Acetylcholinesterase activity present at nerve junctions is similar to that present in red blood cells and is an appropriate index of neurotoxicity.[773] This assay is more sensitive than serum cholinesterase activity and often is used to confirm exposure and to predict enzyme reactivation during treatment. A different cholinesterase, butyrylcholinesterase (pseudocholinesterase), is present in serum and is also inhibited by these insecticides. The activity of butyrylcholinesterase declines then returns to normal more rapidly than is observed for the red cell enzyme. Serum butyrylcholinesterase can be readily measured on hemolyzed samples and in clinical laboratories without isolation of red blood cells. However, interindividual variability is high; therefore pre-exposure activities are optimal when butyrylcholinesterase activities are interpreted.[515] Because butyrylcholinesterases are synthesized in the liver, this assay is particularly sensitive to conditions such as pregnancy and liver disease (acute and chronic hepatitis, cirrhosis, malignancy).[535] Thus red cell cholinesterase activity theoretically should correlate more closely with the degree of neurotoxicity. In acute poisoning, symptoms generally begin when cholinesterase activity is inhibited by about 50% of the lower limits of normal, and this degree of inhibition is of diagnostic value. However, the degree of cholinesterase inhibition generally does not correlate well with the clinical severity of poisoning. Interpretation of test results is made more difficult by considerable individual variability of normal activities. The presence of urinary organophosphate and carbamate metabolites is generally measured by GC-MS[670] and GC-MS/MS.[91] These methods are labor intensive and are typically reserved for monitoring chronic occupational exposure to specific agents rather than for emergency management of acute toxicity.

Drugs of Abuse

Drug use and abuse are widespread in society, and public awareness has been heightened as to their impact on public safety and on lost productivity in industry.[197A] To resolve these issues, governmental, industrial, educational, and sports agencies are increasingly requiring drug testing of prospective and existing employees, students, and participants in professional and amateur athletics. Moreover, drug abuse during pregnancy is a matter of concern, both medically and socially.[15] Testing for drugs of abuse may be a medical requirement for (1) organ transplantation candidates, (2) pain management clinics, (3) drug abuse treatment programs, and (4) psychiatric programs.[635] Drug testing for these purposes represents a significant activity for toxicology laboratories.

Testing for drugs of abuse usually involves testing a single urine specimen for various drugs. It should be noted, however, that a single urine drug test detects only fairly recent drug use and it does not differentiate casual use from chronic drug abuse. The latter requires sequential drug testing and clinical evaluation. Moreover, urine drug testing alone cannot determine the degree of impairment, the dose of drug taken, or the exact time of use. Many of these issues were described in detail at the 1987 Arnold O. Beckman Conference[212] and in a report by the Committee on Substance Abuse Testing.[453] Because of these and other limitations of testing for drugs in urine, integrating the use of alternate biological specimens for drug testing is a matter of growing interest (see section on alternate specimens).

Drug testing results for nonmedical purposes may provide the sole evidence for punitive action or denial of individual rights. Therefore this testing should be considered a forensic toxicology activity, requiring the highest standards of analytical methods, specimen security, and documentation.[239] Moreover, laboratories engaged in this testing should be appropriately certified by the Substance Abuse and Mental Health Service Administration (SAMHSA) of the U.S. Department of Health and Human Services (DHHS) or the Forensic Urine Drug Testing program sponsored jointly by the American Association for Clinical Chemistry and the College of American Pathologists.

Several techniques are used by persons attempting to mask or adulterate drugs to avoid detection. These tactics may include the exchange of urine from a drug-free individual or dilution of the urine specimen by excessive consumption of water, use of a diuretic, or simple addition of water to the specimen to reduce drug concentrations to below cutoff limits. Also, readily available adulterants, such as detergent, bleach, salt, alkali, ammonia, tetrahydrozoline, or acid, may be added to the specimen after collection in an attempt to interfere with immunoassay screening procedures. Other more sophisticated adulterants specifically marketed to avoid drug detection include glutaraldehyde (Urine Aid; Clear Choice), nitrite (Klear; Whizzies), chromate (Urine Luck; Sweet Pee's Spoiler), and a combination of peroxide and peroxidase (Stealth). These adulterants also interfere with immunoassays to variable degrees, and the oxidizing agents (nitrite, chromate, and peroxide/peroxidase) may result in destruction of morphine, codeine, and the principal metabolite resulting from marijuana use, thus interfering with their GC-MS confirmation and with immunoassays.[154]

Direct observation of urine collection is the most stringent means to guard against specimen exchange or adulteration. However, an individual's right to privacy and dignity must be weighed against the need for the highest degree of certainty of specimen integrity. Alternative measures to prevent specimen adulteration include (1) limitations on clothing or other personal belongings allowed in the specimen collection area, (2) addition of coloring agent to toilet water, and (3) inactivation of the hot water tap. In addition, several validity checks for specimen integrity may be made at the collection site and at the testing site. Validity testing criteria have been

TABLE 35-7 U.S. Government Drug Detection Cutoff Concentrations[105]

Drug or Drug Class	Screening, ng/mL HHS/DOT[239]	Screening, ng/mL DOD[597]	Confirmation, ng/mL HHS/DOT[239]	Confirmation, ng/mL DOD[597]
Amphetamines	1000	500		
Designer amphetamines		500		
Amphetamine			500	100†
Methamphetamine			500*	100*†
MDA				500
MDMA				500
MDEA				500
Cannabinoids	50	50		
THC-COOH			15	15
Cocaine metabolites	300	150		
Benzoylecgonine			150	100
Opiates	2000	2000		
Morphine			2000	4000
Codeine			2000	2000
6-Acetylmorphine		10	10	10
Oxycodone/Oxymorphone		100		
Oxycodone				100
Oxymorphone				100
PCP	25	25	25	25

*Also requires the presence of amphetamine (≥200 ng/mL).
†Requires chiral analysis; *S*(+)-amphetamine/methamphetamine.
DOD, Department of Defense; *DOT,* Department of Transportation; *GC-MS,* gas chromatography–mass spectrometry; *HHS,* U.S. Department of Health and Human Services.

established by the DHHS for the drug testing program mandated for U.S. federal employees.[239] According to these criteria, the specimen must be examined for unusual color, odor, foaming, or precipitate, and its temperature should be 90 to 100 °F (32 to 38 °C) when determined within 4 minutes of collection. A specimen is reported as dilute when the specific gravity is >1.0010 but <1.0030 and the creatinine is >2 mg/dL but ≤20 mg/dL. A substituted specimen is defined by a specific gravity ≤1.0010 or ≥1.0200 and a creatinine <2 mg/dL. Adulterated urine has pH <3 or ≥11 or nitrite >500 µg/mL (much lower concentrations occur with some urinary tract infections), or may be confirmed if a specific adulterant is detected and confirmed. A specimen is invalid if the pH is ≥3 and <4.5 or ≥9 and <11, if the creatinine and specific gravity are inconsistent, if nitrite is >200 and <500 µg/mL, or if the presence of other adulterants is suspected. In such cases, the urine specimen is rejected and generally is not tested for drugs. The finding of a substituted or an adulterated specimen is deemed equivalent to a refusal to test and would result in removal of the individual from safety-sensitive duties. Numerous commercial reagents for validity testing are available in both test strip and liquid forms.

Urine should be collected in tamper-proof specimen cups, and a chain of custody maintained to identify all individuals involved in specimen collection, transfer, and testing. Specimens that test positive should be stored frozen for a minimum of 1 year. Detailed information on the collection and processing of specimens for drug testing has been presented in the federal rules for employee drug testing[239] and in the federal regulations promulgated by the Department of Transportation[10] and the Nuclear Regulatory Commission (http://www.nrc.gov/reading-rm/doc-collections/cfr/part026/full-text.html; accessed on July 20, 2010).

Workplace drug testing generally is restricted to alcohol (see section on alcohols) and a few drugs that have high abuse potential, some of which are illicit (Tables 35-7 and 35-8). Depending on the nature of the testing program, testing may be provided for a select number of the following drug classes: *amphetamines,* barbiturates, benzodiazepines, *cannabinoids, cocaine,* LSD, *opiates,* synthetic opioids, and *PCP* (drugs in italics are required for testing by the National Institute of Drug Abuse). Testing programs for participants[86] engaged in athletic competition typically are much more extensive and include assays for a larger group of drugs, including stimulants, β-blockers, diuretics, and anabolic steroids.[5]

Initial screening tests for the previously listed drugs are typically immunoassays (see Chapter 16). These assays are calibrated at established cutoff concentrations. Specimens yielding responses greater than the cutoff (threshold) value are considered positive, whereas values below the cutoff are considered negative. Cutoff values are not synonymous with assay detection limits. Instead, the cutoff is established higher than the detection limit (to ensure reliable measurement) but

TABLE 35-8 Suggested Cutoff Concentrations for Different Matrices[110]

Initial Test	Urine, ng/mL	Oral Fluid, ng/mL	Sweat, ng/patch	Hair, pg/mg
THC metabolite[a]	50	4[b]	4	1
Cocaine metabolite	150	20	25	500
Opiates[c]	2000	40	25	200
PCP	25	10	20	300
Amphetamines[d]	500	50	25	500
MDMA	500	50	25	500
Confirmatory test				
THC parent		2	1	
THC metabolite	15			0.05
Cocaine				500[e]
Benzoylecgonine (BE)	100[e,f]	8[e,f]	25[e,f]	50[e]
Morphine	2000	40	25	200
Codeine	2000	40	25	200
6-AM	10[g]	4	25	200[g,h]
PCP	25	10	20	300
Amphetamine	250	50	25	300
Methamphetamine	250[i]	50[j]	25[j]	300[k]
MDMA	250	50	25	300
MDA	250	50	25	300
MDEA	250	50	25	300

[a]Δ9-THC-COOH.
[b]Parent and metabolite.
[c]Initial test for 6-AM allowed at cutoffs of 10 ng/mL (urine), 4 ng/mL (oral fluid), 25 ng/patch (sweat), and 200 pg/mg (hair).
[d]S(++)-methamphetamine calibrator.
[e]Cocaine ≥ cutoff and BE/cocaine ≥0.05 or cocaethylene ≥50 pg/mg or norcocaine ≥50 pg/mg.
[f]Cocaine or BE.
[g]May be reported alone if initial and confirmatory tests are above cutoffs.
[h]Must contain morphine ≥200 ng/mg.
[i]Must contain amphetamine ≥100 ng/mL.
[j]Must contain amphetamine ≥limit of detection (LOD).
[k]Must contain amphetamine ≥50 ng/mg.

low enough to detect drug use within a reasonable time frame.

Immunoassays may demonstrate limited specificity within certain drug classes. Similar drugs may result in a positive test, for example, pseudoephedrine, present in cold medications, may produce a positive response in immunoassays designed to detect amphetamine and methamphetamine. Therefore, it is imperative that positive screening tests be confirmed by an alternate, more definitive test. The most widely accepted method for drug confirmation is GC-MS. For further discussion of this technique, the reader is referred to Chapter 13. Liquid chromatography–tandem mass spectrometry is also used for rapid detection and confirmation of drugs of abuse.[223,593]

For confirmation, quantitative drug measurements are performed using selective ion monitoring with GC-MS. Cutoff values for confirmation are established at or generally below cutoff values for the initial screening tests (see Table 35-7). The result may be reported as positive or negative relative to the cutoff value. However, the actual concentration may be helpful when morphine and codeine results are interpreted, and when individuals enrolled in drug treatment programs are monitored. In the latter case, subjects who test positive but who have decreasing values on sequential testing may be judged abstinent, whereas those whose values suddenly increase are likely noncompliant. For this purpose, it is essential to normalize the drug concentration-to-urine creatinine concentration (nanograms of drug per milligram of creatinine). This will help compensate for fluctuations in absolute drug concentration related to physiologic variation in urine dilution or concentration.[71,505] In the following sections, the pharmacologic and analytical aspects of commonly measured drugs will be discussed.

Barbiturates

Since antiquity, alcoholic beverages and potions containing laudanum (an alcoholic herbal preparation containing opium) and various herbals have been used to induce sleep. In the middle of the nineteenth century, bromide was the first agent to be introduced specifically as a sedative-hypnotic. The success of barbital in 1903 and phenobarbital (Figure 35-9) in 1912[130] spawned the synthesis and testing of more than 2500 barbiturate derivatives, of which approximately 50 were distributed commercially. Today, about a dozen are in medical use. The barbiturates were so dominant that fewer than a

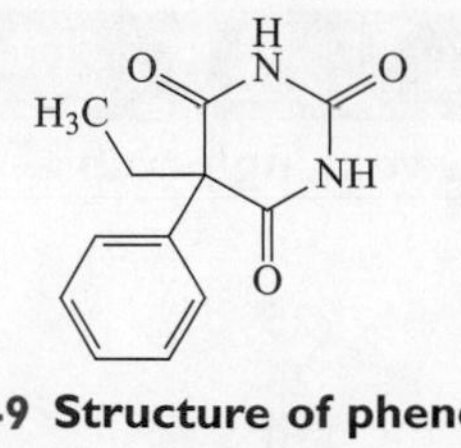

Figure 35-9 **Structure of phenobarbital.**

TABLE 35-9 Half-life and Significant Active Metabolites of Select Barbiturates

Drug[725]	Half-life[46]	Active Metabolite
Ultra-Short-Acting		
thiopental	6-46 h	pentobarbital
methohexital	1.2-2.1 h	
thiamylal	0.6-0.8 h initial	
	12-34 h terminal	
Short-Acting and Intermediate-Acting		
pentobarbital	15-48 h	
secobarbital	22-29 h	
butalbital	35-88 h	
aprobarbital	14-34 h	
amobarbital	15-40 h (dose dependent)	
butabarbital	34-42 h	
Long-Acting		
phenobarbital	2-6 d	
mephobarbital	48-52 h	phenobarbital

dozen other sedative-hypnotics were marketed successfully before 1960.

The antianxiety properties of the barbiturates are less than those exerted by the benzodiazepines.[130] Because of their low therapeutic index and high potential for abuse, they have been largely replaced by the much safer benzodiazepines. Nevertheless, barbiturates continue to be available as sedative-hypnotics or for use in combination with analgesic, antihypertensive, antiasthmatic, antispasmodic, or antidiuretic drugs. The combination of barbiturates, such as butalbital, with analgesic preparations is ironic. Not only do barbiturates lack analgesic properties, but at low doses they antagonize the effects of analgesics.[130] Phenobarbital is effective as an anticonvulsant drug (see Chapter 34), and short- and ultra-short-acting barbiturates are used for IV anesthesia. The classification of barbiturates as "ultra short acting," "short-acting," "intermediate-acting," and "long-acting" refers to the duration of effect and not to the elimination half-life (Table 35-9). The duration of action is determined by the rate of distribution into brain and subsequent redistribution to other tissues.[130] Anesthetic doses of barbiturates, such as pentobarbital, are used to reduce intracranial pressure from cerebral edema associated with head trauma, surgery, or cerebral ischemia.[512] Therefore appropriate analytical methods are necessary to monitor serum pentobarbital concentrations in these circumstances.

Barbiturates continue, although much less frequently than in the past, to be subject to abuse. Because of their rapid onset and short duration of action, the short- to intermediate-acting barbiturates that are used as sedative-hypnotics (amobarbital, butabarbital, butalbital, pentobarbital, and secobarbital) are most commonly abused. The longer-acting barbiturates (mephobarbital and phenobarbital), used primarily for their anticonvulsant properties, are rarely abused. The detection period in urine following ingestion of barbiturates varies with different assays and depends on the pharmacologic properties of the drugs. Short- to intermediate-acting barbiturates generally may be detected for 1 to 4 days following use; long-acting barbiturates, such as phenobarbital, may be detected for several weeks after long-term use.[299]

Barbiturates act throughout the CNS; nonanesthetic doses preferentially suppress polysynaptic responses, suppress CNS neuronal activity, and thus have sedative and hypnotic properties.[310] The site of inhibition occurs primarily at synapses where neurotransmission is mediated by GABA acting at $GABA_A$ receptors. This CNS suppression is a result of barbiturate-enhanced activation of the inhibitory GABA-ergic neuronal system.[130] Postsynatic $GABA_A$ receptors are multisubunit transmembrane Cl conductance channels that when activated by GABA open to allow flow of Cl into the neuron, with subsequent hyperpolarization and inhibition of electrical transmission. High doses of barbiturates increase neural chloride conductance independent of GABA.[130] Mechanisms underlying the actions of barbiturates on $GABA_A$ receptors appear to be distinct from those of GABA or the benzodiazepines, and they promote the binding of benzodiazepines.[16,130] In addition, barbiturates suppress excitatory glutamate-responsive AMPA (alpha-amino-3-OH-4-isoxozole propionic acid) ion-gated receptor subtypes. Taken together, the findings that barbiturates activate inhibitory $GABA_A$ receptors and inhibit excitatory AMPA receptors explain their CNS-depressant effects.[706]

The barbiturates produce all degrees of depression of the CNS, ranging from mild sedation to general anesthesia. Barbiturates reversibly depress the activity of all excitable tissues. The CNS is exquisitely sensitive, and even when barbiturates are given in anesthetic concentrations, direct effects on peripheral excitable tissues are weak. However, serious deficits in cardiovascular and other peripheral functions occur in acute barbiturate intoxication.[130] Severe intoxication results in coma, hypothermia, hypotension, and cardiorespiratory arrest.[130] Pharmacodynamic (functional) and pharmacokinetic tolerance to barbiturates can occur. With long-term administration of gradually increasing doses, pharmacodynamic tolerance continues to develop over a period of weeks to months, depending on the dosage schedule, whereas pharmacokinetic tolerance reaches its peak in a few days to a week. Tolerance to effects on mood, sedation, and hypnosis occurs more readily and is greater than tolerance to anticonvulsant and lethal effects; thus, as tolerance increases, the therapeutic index decreases.[130]

The barbiturates undergo extensive hepatic metabolism. The metabolic elimination of barbiturates is more rapid in young people than in the elderly and in infants, and half-lives are increased during pregnancy in part because of the expanded volume of distribution. Chronic liver disease, especially cirrhosis, often increases the half-life of the biotransformable barbiturates. Repeated administration, especially of phenobarbital, shortens the half-life of barbiturates that are metabolized as a result of induction of microsomal enzymes.[130] Oxidation of radicals at C5 is the most important biotransformation that terminates biological activity.[130] Oxidation results in the formation of alcohols, ketones, phenols, or carboxylic acids, which may appear in the urine as such or as glucuronic acid conjugates.[130] For phenobarbital and amobarbital, *N*-glycosylation is an important metabolic pathway. Other biotransformations include *N*-hydroxylation, desulfuration of thiobarbiturates to oxybarbiturates, opening of the barbituric acid ring, and *N*-dealkylation of *N*-alkylbarbiturates to active metabolites (e.g., mephobarbital to phenobarbital). Except for the less lipid-soluble aprobarbital and phenobarbital, nearly complete metabolism and/or conjugation of barbiturates in the liver precedes their renal excretion.[130] As a result, only a relatively small amount of an administered barbiturate dose is excreted in urine as a parent drug; notable exceptions are phenobarbital and aprobarbital. About 25% of phenobarbital and nearly all of aprobarbital are excreted unchanged in the urine. Their renal excretion can be increased greatly by osmotic diuresis and/or alkalinization of urine.[130] Nevertheless, the parent drugs, rather than hydroxy or carboxylic acid metabolites, are targeted for detection in urine screening and confirmation procedures. This analytical approach is generally successful for barbiturates because these drugs are ingested in sufficiently high doses to allow detection of unmetabolized drug in urine.

Analytical Methods

Screening. Numerous commercial immunoassays for barbiturates are available. Most use antibodies directed toward secobarbital, and although the degree of cross-reactivity of other barbiturates varies with each assay, most have sufficient cross-reactivity to detect the major therapeutically used barbiturates.[475,485]

Confirmation Testing. Numerous confirmation methods for barbiturates have been described. These include GC with flame ionization detection,[358,833,843] nitrogen phosphorous detection[769] and MS,* capillary electrophoresis-ultraviolet (UV),[195,383,825] liquid chromatography using ultraviolet (LC-UV) detection,[413,506] and LC-MS[328,394] and mass spectrometry.[546] GC-MS has merits attributable to high resolution and precise retention times with sharp peaks; however, the detection limit of GC-MS for barbiturates is compromised by adsorption at its NH group.[698] To overcome this problem, derivatization prior to injection is widely used, but this procedure is time-consuming.[42,537,872] On-column methylation is a rapid and sensitive method,[769] but phenobarbital cannot be distinguished from mephobarbital after methylation.

*References 42, 366, 537, 574, 575, 641, and 872.

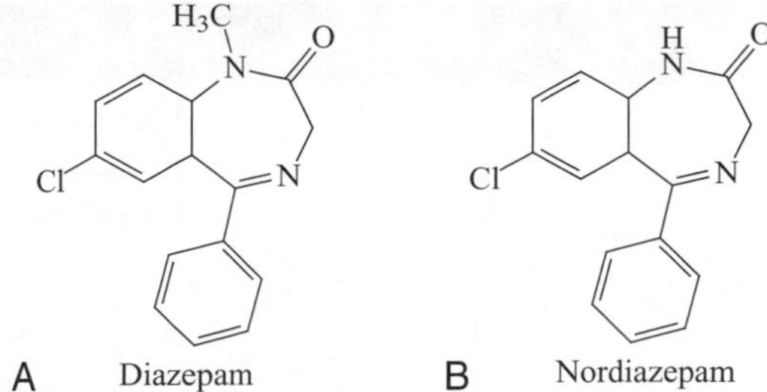

Figure 35-10 Structure of (A) diazepam and (B) nordiazepam.

Benzodiazepines

Benzodiazepines are any of a group of compounds having a common molecular structure and acting similarly as depressants of the CNS. The term *benzodiazepine* refers to the portion of the structure composed of a benzene ring fused to a seven-membered diazepine ring and a phenyl ring attached to the 5-position of the diazepine ring.[130,475] The prototype benzodiazepines are diazepam and nordiazepam (*N*-desmethyl diazepam) (Figure 35-10). Fifteen members of this group are presently marketed in the United States, and about 20 additional benzodiazepines are marketed in other countries[725]; the most common of these are listed in Table 35-10.

Pharmacologic Response

As a class of drugs, benzodiazepines are among the most commonly prescribed drugs in the Western hemisphere because of their (1) efficacy, (2) safety, (3) low addiction potential, (4) minimal side effects, and (5) high public demand for sedative and anxiolytic agents. They have largely replaced barbiturates for sedative-hypnotic use because they have fewer side effects and liver enzyme inductions and are safer in overdose.[130,238,475,499] New-generation sedative-hypnotics such as zolpidem (Ambien), eszopiclone (Lunesta), and zaleplon (Sonata) modulate the $GABA_A$ receptor, as do benzodiazepines, yet they are structurally different, permitting unique physiologic properties that will be discussed in a subsequent section (see "Drugs Used in Sexual Assault").

Long-term benzodiazepine use poses a risk for the development of dependence and abuse,[852,855,856] particularly for those agents with the shortest half-life, the highest potency (alprazolam, triazolam), and the greatest lipophilicity (diazepam).[727,789] Regular use will produce tolerance to most of the adverse effects of benzodiazepines.[207] Consequently, some of the sedative and other adverse effects of benzodiazepines discussed earlier may wane with repeated drug use.[207] Tolerance may take weeks or months to develop, although this will depend on the dose of drugs used, the frequency of administration, and the pharmacokinetic half-life of the drug. Drugs with short half-lives are more likely to produce a quicker onset of tolerance.[207]

The benzodiazepines given by themselves or in combination with other drugs, particularly narcotic analgesics

TABLE 35-10 Half-life of Select Benzodiazepines

Drug[725]	Half-life, h[46]	Significant Phase I Metabolites
Short-Acting		
Midazolam	1-4	α-hydroxy-midazolam
Estazolam	10-24	3-hydroxy-estazolam
Flurazepam	1-3 47-100 (*N*-desalkyl-flurazepam)	hydroxy-ethyl-flurazepam *N*-desalkyl-flurazepam*
Temazepam	3-13	
Triazolam	1.8-3.9	α-hydroxy-triazolam
Intermediate-Acting		
Flunitrazepam†	9-25	7-amino-flunitrazepam
Long-Acting Agents		
Diazepam	21-37	Nordiazepam* Oxazepam* Temazepam*
Quazepam	39-53	3-hydroxy-quazepam *N*-desalkyl-2-oxo-quazepam 2-oxo-3-hydroxy-quazepam
Alprazolam	6-27	α-hydroxy-alprazolam
Chlordiazepoxide	6-27	nordiazepam* oxazepam*
Clonazepam	19-60	7-amino-clonazepam
Clorazepate‡	2 31-97 (nordiazepam)	nordiazepam* oxazepam*
Lorazepam	9-16	
Oxazepam	4-11	

*Active metabolite.
†Not available in the United States.
‡Converted to nordiazepam by gastric HCl.

(opioids), are among the most widely abused drugs. Their ability to suppress or dampen withdrawal symptoms and to boost the effects of heroin has made them a favored drug type among the drug-using population.[207] They are also widely used by the cocaine-using population, especially clonazepam to increase the seizure threshold.[207] They are commonly seen in drug-facilitated sexual assault cases. Drinks spiked with a benzodiazepine are commonly used to administer drugs. The most common benzodiazepines used in drug-facilitated sexual assaults are flunitrazepam, midazolam, temazepam, and clonazepam, although almost all members of the class are suitable.[207]

Although the benzodiazepines exert qualitatively similar clinical effects, important quantitative differences in their pharmacodynamic spectra and pharmacokinetic properties have led to varying patterns of therapeutic application. Several distinct mechanisms of action are thought to contribute to the sedative-hypnotic, muscle relaxant, anxiolytic, and anticonvulsant effects of the benzodiazepines, and specific subunits of the $GABA_A$ receptor are responsible for specific pharmacologic properties of benzodiazepines.[130]

All the benzodiazepines are well absorbed, with the exception of clorazepate; this drug is decarboxylated rapidly in gastric juice to *N*-desmethyldiazepam (nordazepam), which subsequently is absorbed.[130] Benzodiazepines are rapidly distributed to the CNS. Subsequently, benzodiazepines are more slowly redistributed from the CNS to more poorly perfused tissue, such as adipose tissue and muscle. The rate of this redistribution is an important determinant of the duration of action of benzodiazepines and, similar to that for GI absorption, is largely determined by drug lipophilicity, with the more lipophilic drugs, such as midazolam and triazolam, having the shortest duration of action. These drugs cross the placental barrier and are secreted into breast milk.[130]

Benzodiazepines may be divided into four categories based on their elimination half-lives: (1) ultra-short-acting; (2) short-acting agents, with half-lives less than 6 hours; (3) intermediate-acting agents, with half-lives of 6 to 24 hours; and (4) long-acting agents, with half-lives greater than 24 hours.[130] These pharmacokinetic properties in part determine the primary clinical applications for some benzodiazepines. For instance, midazolam ($t_{1/2}$, 1 to 4 hours) is used for preanesthetic sedation or for sedation for endoscopic procedures because of its rapid onset and short duration of action. Benzodiazepines useful in treating anxiety generally have intermediate to long elimination half-lives (alprazolam and diazepam), and those primarily used as anticonvulsants (clonazepam) have the longest. Elimination half-life clearly is not the sole determinant of duration of action of benzodiazepines, and in some cases, the rate of drug redistribution from the CNS may be a more important factor.[26]

Benzodiazepines undergo hepatic oxidation (phase I) and conjugation (phase II), often forming metabolites with pharmacologic activity (see Table 35-10). Cytochrome P450 enzymes, particularly CYP3A4 and CYP2C19, are frequently involved.[130] Following these reactions, conjugation with glucuronic acid occurs; these glucuronidated metabolites constitute the major urinary products of benzodiazepines.[130,475,688,789,855] Drugs and other agents that are inhibitors of CYP3A4 (erythromycin, clarithromycin, ritonavir, itraconazole, ketoconazole, nefazodone, and grapefruit juice) affect the metabolism of benzodiazepines.[203] However, benzodiazepines apparently do not significantly induce the synthesis of hepatic cytochrome P450 enzymes; their long-term administration usually does not result in accelerated metabolism of other drugs.

Nordazepam is a major metabolite common to the biotransformation of diazepam, clorazepate, and prazepam; it is formed from chlordiazepoxide via an intermediate metabolite demoxepam.[130] Some benzodiazepines, such as oxazepam and lorazepam, are conjugated directly and do not undergo phase I metabolism. In some cases, metabolic transformations occur before the drug reaches significant concentrations in the systemic circulation. For example, clorazepate is decarboxylated to nordiazepam by stomach acid, and flurazepam and prazepam are converted to active metabolites by hepatic first-pass metabolism.[130,238]

Because active metabolites of some benzodiazepines are biotransformed more slowly than are the parent compounds, the duration of action of many benzodiazepines bears little relationship to the half-life of elimination of the drug that has been administered (see Table 35-10). For example, the half-life of flurazepam in plasma is 1 to 3 hours, but that of a major active metabolite (*N*-desalkylflurazepam) is 50 hours or longer.[54] Conversely, with benzodiazepines that lack active metabolites (oxazepam, lorazepam, temazepam, triazolam, and midazolam), the half-life is an important determinant of their duration of action. Additional factors that influence the duration of benzodiazepine action are hepatic metabolism and acute tolerance, resulting in decreased response to benzodiazepines with continued drug exposure.

Virtually all results of the pharmacologic effects of benzodiazepines are caused by their actions on the CNS. The most prominent of these effects are (1) sedation, (2) hypnosis, (3) decreased anxiety, (4) muscle relaxation, (5) anterograde amnesia, and (6) anticonvulsant activity. Only two effects of these drugs result from peripheral actions: (1) coronary vasodilation, seen after intravenous administration of therapeutic doses of certain benzodiazepines; and (2) neuromuscular blockade, seen only with very high doses. Ethanol increases both the rate of absorption of benzodiazepines and the associated CNS depression. Except for additive effects with other sedative or hypnotic drugs, reports of clinically important pharmacodynamic interactions between benzodiazepines and other drugs have been infrequent.

Benzodiazepines are believed to exert most of their effects by interacting with inhibitory neurotransmitter receptors directly activated by GABA. GABA receptors are membrane-bound proteins that are divided into two major subtypes: $GABA_A$ and $GABA_B$ receptors. The ionotropic $GABA_A$ receptors are responsible for most inhibitory neurotransmission in the CNS. Binding enhances GABA-mediated chloride transmembrane conductance, which results in hyperpolarization and diminished neural electrical discharge. Ultimately, this reduces the arousal of the cortical and limbic systems in the CNS.[207] Benzodiazepines also depress the electrical after-discharge in the amygdala, hippocampus, and septum components of the limbic system that affect emotions.[207] In contrast are the metabotropic $GABA_B$ receptors. Benzodiazepines act at $GABA_A$ but not $GABA_B$ receptors by binding directly to a specific site that is distinct from that of GABA binding. Multiple $GABA_A$ receptors are known, and benzodiazepines seem to interact with many of these subtypes, which could account for the varied pharmacologic use of these drugs.[475] Unlike barbiturates, benzodiazepines do not activate $GABA_A$ receptors directly but rather require GABA to express their effects as they only modulate the effects of GABA. Benzodiazepines modulate GABA binding, and GABA alters benzodiazepine binding in an allosteric fashion.[130] The remarkable safety of benzodiazepines compared with barbiturates is probably related to this effect.

Benzodiazepines and related compounds also act as agonists, partial agonists, inverse agonists, or antagonists. Agonists and partial agonists increase the amount of chloride current generated by $GABA_A$ receptor activation, and inverse agonists decrease it. The vast majority of effects of agonists and inverse agonists can be reversed or prevented by the benzodiazepine antagonist flumazenil, which competes for binding to the $GABA_A$ receptor.

Benzodiazepines occasionally have paradoxical effects and sometimes cause garrulousness, anxiety, irritability, tachycardia, and sweating. Amnesia, euphoria, restlessness, hallucinations, and hypomanic behavior have been reported to occur during use of various benzodiazepines. The release of bizarre uninhibited behavior has been noted in some users, whereas hostility and rage may occur in others; collectively, these are sometimes referred to as *disinhibition* or *dyscontrol reactions*. Paranoia, depression, and suicidal ideation occasionally may accompany the use of these agents. Such paradoxical or disinhibition reactions are rare and appear to be dose related.[130] Valproate and benzodiazepines given in combination may cause psychotic episodes.[130]

One benzodiazepine, flunitrazepam (Rohypnol), is approved for use in many countries but not the United States. However, it has illegally entered the United States and has been illicitly sold to the drug-abusing community. In addition, because of its potent sedative-hypnotic action, especially in combination with alcohol, and its ability to induce short-term (anterograde) amnesia, it has gained notoriety for drug-facilitated crimes.

Long-acting benzodiazepines (diazepam, chlordiazepoxide, and clorazepate) are given in relatively large doses and may be detected for several days to weeks or even months following long-term use. Short-acting benzodiazepines (alprazolam and triazolam) are used in lower doses and might be detected only for a few days.

The treatment of benzodiazepine toxicity is primarily supportive. Flumazenil may be used in select cases and is a competitive inhibitor of the benzodiazepine site on the GABA complex. It finds its greatest utility in the reversal of benzodiazepine-induced sedation from minor surgical procedures. However, flumazenil should not be administered as a nonspecific coma-reversal drug and should be used with extreme caution after intentional benzodiazepine overdose because it has the potential to precipitate withdrawal in benzodiazepine-dependent individuals and/or to induce seizures in those at risk.

Analytical Methods

Benzodiazepines are measured using a variety of techniques. However, their structural diversity and wide variations in potency provide a challenge for laboratories to detect all relevant members in one analytical scheme. Reviews of analysis of benzodiazepines have been published.[205,206,522] These cover the techniques used to screen for the presence of the class of drugs and to confirm the presence of one or more members.

Screening. Screening techniques using immunoassay kits will rarely be able to detect all members of the class because of differing immunoreactivities among active drug and metabolites. This seems to apply to the more potent members (i.e., lorazepam, triazolam, clonazepam).[205] Several commercial immunoassay systems are available for the detection of a wide variety of benzodiazepines and metabolites, but they differ somewhat in their ability to detect the various benzodiazepines, their metabolites, and glucuronide conjugates. Cross-reactivity in screening immunoassays of the various benzodiazepines and their metabolites varies considerably from manufacturer to manufacturer, and screening assays are not able to distinguish between the individual benzodiazepines. Most assays are calibrated to the common metabolite oxazepam, temazepam, or nordiazepam.[300] However, the large number of different functional groups that may be present on the benzodiazepine nucleus makes it difficult to detect all drugs in this class, and some compounds such as midazolam, chlordiazepoxide, and flunitrazepam may not be detected by many assays.* Other factors, such as low doses and short half-lives, make the detection of some benzodiazepines especially challenging. In the absence of sufficiently sensitive or specific immunoassays, direct analysis by a confirmatory method is warranted in suspected cases.

It should be noted that benzodiazepines may be identified and quantified in serum, but such quantitative information is not warranted in cases of benzodiazepine overdose because serum concentrations are not predictive of severity of intoxication.[238] However, a urine or serum immunoassay screening test for benzodiazepines is valuable in the evaluation of patients with an unknown cause of CNS depression.

Confirmation Testing. Analysts need to be aware that the specimen type will dictate the target substance. Blood analyses invariably will target the parent benzodiazepine and perhaps the major active metabolite (e.g., nordiazepam for diazepam and other analogs metabolized to nordiazepam). This applies similarly to analyses targeted for saliva.[638A] In urine, a metabolite is often the required target species.[207]

Benzodiazepines and their metabolites have been extracted from biological specimens by liquid-liquid extraction (LLE) or solid-phase extraction (SPE). When urine specimens are analyzed, a hydrolysis step is necessary to cleave the glucuronide conjugates.[475] Enzymatic hydrolysis is preferred over acid hydrolysis because some benzodiazepines are unstable and rearrange to form benzophenones.[475]

Many benzodiazepines are analyzed without derivatization by GC; these include diazepam, nordiazepam, flurazepam, and alprazolam. Drugs that are more polar, such as those with hydroxyl groups (oxazepam, temazepam, and lorazepam) or a nitro group (clonazepam, nitrazepam), display poor chromatographic characteristics and require derivatization.[475] Chlordiazepoxide is thermally unstable and may degrade at high temperatures in the GC.[475] Some consider GC-MS as the definitive confirmation method[207]; however, LC with UV detection (240 nm) has been used to detect benzodiazepines and metabolites without derivatization. LC-MS and LC-MS/MS are becoming increasingly useful and popular methods for benzodiazepines.[433,466,530,546,800,801,828,869]

*References 156, 273, 699, 743, 821, and 824.

Cannabinoids

Cannabinoids are a group of C_{21} compounds found in the marijuana plant *Cannabis sativa*. Cannabis is the most extensively abused drug in the world[176] and it has been used as a medicinal and an illicit psychotropic agent for centuries. The main psychotropic effects are (1) euphoria, (2) distorted perceptions, (3) relaxation, and (4) a feeling of well-being.[298,306] Since 1996, 13 states have legalized cannabis for medical conditions such as glaucoma, chemotherapy-related nausea and vomiting, migraine, and anorexia. In 2005, the Gonzales *vs.* Raich ruling permitted the federal government to ban the nonmedical and medical use of cannabis.

Delta-9-tetrahydrocannabinol (THC), the primary psychoactive component of the *C. sativa* plant (Figure 35-11), binds to endogenous cannabinoid receptors, CB1 (neuronal) and CB2 (immune cells).[305,614,637] These transmembrane receptors are G-protein–coupled receptors that mediate signal transduction through inhibition of adenylate cyclase and calcium ions, and activation of potassium ion channels.[259,345] The distribution pattern of CB1 receptors in the CNS accounts for most of the clinical effects of THC such as mood, memory, cognition, pain, and appetite.[365,467,759] CB2 may regulate immune and inflammatory processes.

THC is typically consumed by smoking the plant leaves, flower buds, and sometimes stems. THC also has been extracted from the glandular hairs of cannabis flowers and produced as a resin (hashish). Hashish is often a more potent form and has been mixed into foods, brewed as tea then ingested, or smoked. Hemp oil also has been extracted from cannabis seeds for use in soaps, body care products, and dietary supplements and is used because of its high essential fatty acid content, but negligible THC content.

Pharmacologic Response

When marijuana is smoked, THC rapidly diffuses into the plasma in seconds and is distributed multiphasically. First, it distributes to highly vascularized tissues in minutes because of its lipophilic nature.[12] THC then is redistributed back into the bloodstream, undergoes hepatic metabolism, and slowly accumulates into less vascularized and fatty tissues.[304,448] After cessation of marijuana smoking, THC and its metabolites are slowly released from fat stores.[570]

The main psychotropic effects after inhalation of marijuana occur within minutes and persist for several hours. The peak plasma concentration of THC is dependent on the dose

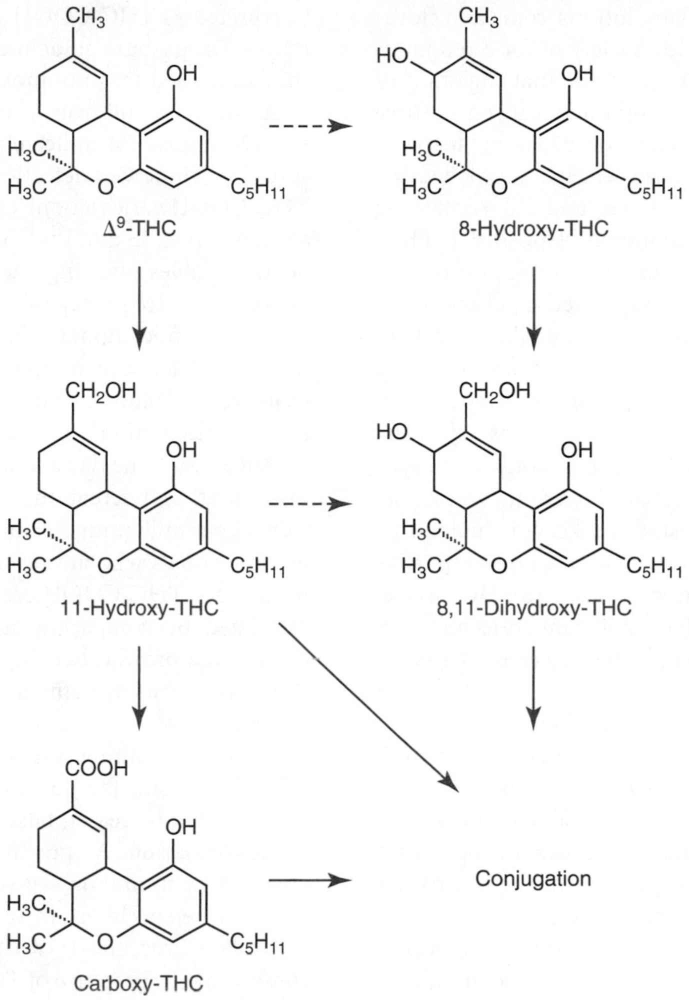

Figure 35-11 Principal metabolic route for delta-9-tetrahydrocannabinol (THC) in humans.

and occurs during the early acute phase (6 to 10 minutes). Numerous factors contribute to the variability in dose, such as (1) method of consumption, (2) depth of inhalation, (3) exposure frequency, and (4) cannabis potency.[231,567,647] Onset of clinical symptoms and peak plasma concentrations after oral ingestion of THC is slower (2 to 6 hours) than after inhalation, primarily as the result of first-pass hepatic clearance.[6,816] The intensity of clinical effects described for smoked cannabis occurs during multiple phases: acute (0 to 60 minutes), postacute (60 to 150 minutes), and residual (>150 minutes). THC blood concentrations accurately reflect clinical psychotropic effects observed during the early postacute phase after smoking cannabis.[304,598,811] Therefore, plasma concentrations of THC can be monitored to discriminate between intoxication and prior use of cannabis. The ratio of THC to 11-nor-delta-9-tetrahydrocannabinol-9-carboxylic acid (THC-COOH) metabolite has been used to estimate the time of exposure to marijuana.[548] This approach may be useful in naive users but is unreliable in chronic abusers of marijuana.

Although marijuana is the most frequently used illicit drug, it does have some limited legitimate medicinal use. Dronabinol (Marinol) contains synthetic THC and is used to treat anorexia and nausea in patients with acquired immunodeficiency syndrome (AIDS) and those with nausea and vomiting associated with chemotherapy, or asthma and glaucoma.[532] Measurement in urine of the principle THC metabolite THC-COOH, present in cannabis but not in dronabinol, has been proposed as a means to distinguish ingestion of marijuana from ingestion of Marinol.[228]

Analytical Methods

An immunoassay method is typically used to screen for potential cannabinoid use in workplace drug testing, athlete drug testing, and clinical specimens. A presumptive positive sample should be confirmed by quantitative GC-MS. Confirmation of quantitative concentrations of the parent compound, THC, is typically reserved for forensic samples.

Screening. Legitimate concern has been raised concerning the potential for false-positive results from dietary sources and "passive inhalation" of sufficient sidestream marijuana smoke from nearby users, resulting in a positive urine cannabinoid test. Hemp seeds and oil are produced from the same *Cannabis sativa* plant that is harvested for drug use.

Hemp has been used to make soaps, lotions, rope, and clothing, and as an ingredient in a wide variety of food products. In the mid-1990s, several studies reported that ingestion of single or multiple doses of hemp products caused positive results in cannabinoid screens and confirmatory analyses. Since 1998, the U.S. Federal Government has prohibited the importation of *Cannabis sativa* seeds and oil containing greater than 0.3% THC to reduce human exposure to THC. The concentration of THC consumed in drug use is 2 to 20%.[231,473] Subsequent studies have suggested that these measures were successful in reducing potential positive cannabinoid drug screen results from dietary sources.[473] Yet, immunoscreens and GC-MS analyses of urine specimens from volunteers exposed to very low doses of THC (0.39 mg/d) have tested positive for cannabinoids.[293,308]

Numerous studies have been conducted to investigate exposure to THC from second-hand smoke, concluding that the SAMHSA cutoff is sufficient to separate moderate passive exposure from first-hand inhalation exposure to THC. Several of these studies demonstrated that significant concentrations of TCH-COOH (<10 ng/mL) could be detected in passive inhalers housed in unventilated confined facilities, but most were below the assay cutoff.[463,565] Individuals that tested positive (>20 ng/mL cutoff, immunoassay) were exposed to multiple marijuana cigarettes in an unventilated car containing ≤3500 L of air.[559,633] Therefore, it is improbable that a passive inhaler would be able to sustain exposure to significant THC concentrations long enough to produce a positive drug screen. Nevertheless, as a precaution against passive inhalations resulting in a positive test, some laboratories screen for urine cannabinoids at a cutoff concentration of 100 ng/mL THC-COOH equivalents. However, at this cutoff value, test sensitivity in one study was only 47% when compared with that for GC-MS (cutoff value, 15 ng/mL THC-COOH). Test sensitivity increased to 93% at a cutoff value of 20 ng/mL THC-COOH equivalents.[735] The U.S. federally mandated screening cutoff was reduced from 100 ng/mL to 50 ng/mL THC-COOH equivalents.[761] One study demonstrated that such a reduction in screening cutoff resulted in a 23 to 54% increase in test sensitivity, depending on the immunoassay, with only a slight decrease (1.0 to 2.6%) in test specificity.[349] A 1997 study suggests that consideration should be given to lowering the values listed for THC-COOH (see Table 35-7).[849]

TCH is metabolized by CYP2D6 liver enzymes to greater than 100 metabolites. The main active metabolite, 11-hydroxy-delta-9-THC, is further oxidized to the most abundant inactive THC-COOH (see Figure 35-11).[348,567] Immunoassay screens have been designed to detect cannabis use in urine samples using antibody reagents developed against the inactive THC-COOH metabolite; these reagents cross-react with numerous other THC metabolites. Therefore the presence of multiple cannabinoid metabolites in a patient specimen will have an additive effect in immunoscreen analyses. Quantitative results based on these metabolites are 1.5 to 8 times greater than the actual concentration of THC-COOH as determined by GC-MS.[387] Therefore immunoassay results are interpreted as THC-COOH equivalents. The National Institute on Drug Abuse guidelines specify that a 50-ng/mL cutoff should be used for immunoscreens.

A positive result from a urine cannabinoid screen or confirmation does not indicate intoxication or degree of exposure. The window of detection for the urine concentration of THC-COOH varies among casual (2 to 7 days)[567] and chronic abusers (up to 73 days)[226,457] of marijuana and is dose dependent. Variables affecting the duration of detection include (1) dose, (2) frequency of exposure, (3) route of exposure, (4) body composition, (5) fluid excretion, and (6) method of detection. Therefore, monitoring of abstinence is particularly challenging. Dilution of urine due to normal biological fluctuations (hydration) or ingested adulterants has caused a negative result one day and a positive on the next. To correct for hydration fluctuations, urine concentrations of THC-COOH per milligram creatinine are normalized for monitoring individuals who are resuming cannabis use. Using these normalized THC-COOH:creatinine concentrations, a ratio is calculated by comparing any normalized urine specimen (U2) with a previously collected normalized urine specimen (U1). "New use" is defined as a U2/U1 ratio of ≥0.5 to 1.5 collected from urine specimens taken more than 24 hours apart and containing THC-COOH concentrations >15 ng/mL.[166,258,738] Using the 1.5 cutoff rate results in decreased false-positives, but increased false-negative decisions.[738]

Confirmation. A positive screening result for THC obtained by immunoassay is confirmed by GC-MS analysis of the urine specimen. In the United States, the Division of Workplace Programs (DWP) in SAMHSA set the cutoff for confirming the presence of TCH-COOH metabolite at 15 ng/mL (GC-MS).[110]

Opiates (Opioids)

The term *opioid* describes a wide range of compounds encompassing the natural and semisynthetic opiates—essentially variations on the structure of morphine—and fully synthetic opioids with minimal structural homology to the natural alkaloids (Figure 35-12).[630] The defining characteristic of this class of drugs is their morphine-like antinociceptive activity stemming from interaction with opioid receptors, which play a major role in pain perception.[309,745] Other compounds that are somewhat loosely referred to as "opioids" include receptor antagonists and mixed agonist/antagonists, as well as other opium-derived alkaloids such as papaverine that are not known to bind opioid receptors.[874]

Pharmacologic Response

For pain management, opioid therapy is a mainstay in treating acute needs such as postsurgical analgesia, and in relieving moderate to severe chronic pain.[320] In the latter case, opioids are well accepted in the setting of cancer-related pain, but the propriety and effectiveness of their use in nonmalignant chronic pain are controversial.[320] Most opioids have both substantial addictive capacity and potentially life-threatening side effects; thus the benefits of their use in non–end-stage patients must be carefully weighed against the chance of

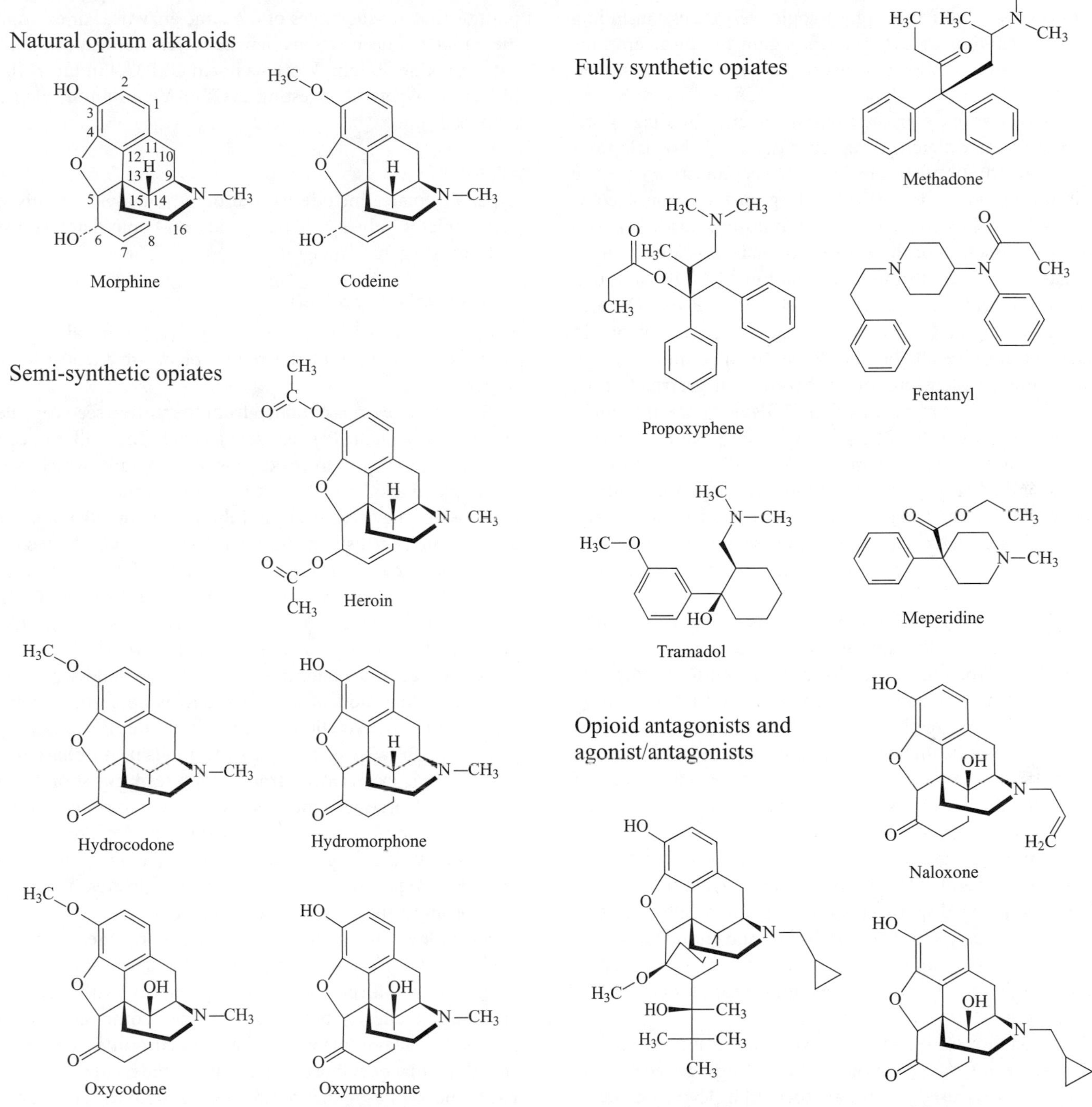

Figure 35-12 Structure of common opioids.

rather serious consequences. In addition, the development of tolerance and the risk of prescription diversion complicate even further the process of monitoring long-term opioid therapy for compliance and efficacy.

The hallmark of opioids is their ability to interact with the family of opioid receptors that are variably distributed throughout the body; opioid receptor agonists typically produce analgesia, and antagonists block this response.[309,620] The biochemistry of opioid receptor binding, regulation, and signaling is complex and has been reviewed in detail elsewhere.[309,620,815] A general overview is presented here.

The classical opioid receptors are divided into the mu, delta, and kappa (μ, δ, and κ, or MOR, DOR, and KOR, respectively) subfamilies,[309] which exhibit considerable overlap in ligand specificity and downstream signaling.[309,620] A related protein, the ORL-1/nociceptin receptor, has also been described as an opioid receptor, although its characterization lags behind that of the other receptors.[550] Finally, the sigma receptor family will interact with some opioids but produces very different physiologic responses, including cardiac excitation and tachypnea; sigma receptors are now considered to be completely distinct from the classical opioid receptors.[620]

Opioids also have preferential or selective binding to one or more of the different receptor classes. It is possible for a compound to stimulate one opioid receptor subtype while inhibiting another, as with mixed agonist/antagonist compounds.[309,620] The effect of ligand binding varies between receptor classes. Morphine-like analgesia is thought to be mediated primarily through stimulation of MOR, although compounds with preferential binding to DOR or KOR also produce analgesia.[309,620] Other classical sequelae of opioid treatment are also attributable to MOR, including sedation and inhibition of respiratory function and gastrointestinal transit.[270,309,591] In contrast, neither DOR nor KOR is thought to affect respiration; DOR agonists do not produce sedation or reduce gastrointestinal motility.[309] KOR and its endogenous ligand dynorphin are implicated in response to addiction to numerous drugs such as opioids; KOR gene polymorphisms have been linked to susceptibility to alcohol dependence, supporting a role for this receptor in addictive behavior.[501,502,790,791]

In addition to undesirable side effects, a major concern in long-term opioid therapy is the development of tolerance.[215,309,620] Tolerant individuals may require many-fold increases in dose to achieve the same concentration of analgesia, which can greatly complicate interpretation of serum results and establishment of a therapeutic window. Tolerance to a particular opioid is thought to be a consequence of altered regulation of the opioid receptor(s) to which that compound binds; for this reason, cross-tolerance can occur when multiple drugs interact with the same receptor.[215,309,620,689] In addition, several of the enzymes involved in opioid metabolism (see later) display substrate-dependent alterations in activity. Although substrate inhibition and induction represent different phenomena than tolerance, the clinical effect can be similar and may necessitate modification of the therapeutic regimen.

The metabolism of opioids is varied, but numerous biotransformations are common to these drugs. Several of the most commonly used opiates are formed in vivo by metabolism of other compounds, as is seen with codeine demethylation resulting in conversion to morphine.[309,492] This interconversion is a frequent source of confusion and must be considered when the results of opiate screens are interpreted; specific details will be outlined later for key opioids with active metabolites.

One of the more important CYP enzymes, CYP2D6, is particularly notable for its role in variable clinical response to opioids; it will be discussed in greater detail in a later section. Many additional CYP enzymes are involved in opioid metabolism, including CYP3A and CYP2C isoforms, among others.[492] It is important to note that several of these enzymes are subject to substrate inhibition and/or induction.[243] Substrate-dependent changes in metabolic activity are affected by other drugs, herbal supplements, or endogenous compounds that are substrates of the same enzyme. For example, methadone concentrations may be lower than expected in a patient taking St. John Wort—a noted CYP3A4 inducer—but higher in a patient ingesting a CYP3A4 inhibitor such as grapefruit juice.[243]

Types

Types of opiates include natural opium alkaloids, semisynthetic opiates, fully synthetic opioids, and opioid antagonists and mixed agonist/antagonists.

Natural Opium Alkaloids

Morphine and codeine are examples of natural opiates. The juice and seeds of the poppy plant are their primary source.

Source. Opium is obtained from the unripe seed capsules of the poppy plant, *Papaver somniferum*. The milky juice is dried and powdered to make powdered opium, which contains several alkaloids. Only a few—morphine, codeine, and papaverine—have clinical usefulness. These alkaloids are divided into two distinct chemical classes: *phenanthrenes* and *benzylisoquinolines*. The principal phenanthrenes are morphine (10% of opium), codeine (0.5%), and thebaine (0.2%). The principal benzylisoquinolines are papaverine (1%), which is a smooth muscle relaxant and *noscapine* (6%).[309]

Poppy seeds contain morphine and to a lesser extent codeine.[631] Ingestion of bakery products containing poppy seeds leads to excretion of morphine (and codeine) in urine.[324,757] Because of first-pass metabolism, no pharmacologic effect is experienced from poppy seed ingestion. Consumption of large amounts has been known to result in urine morphine concentrations up to 2000 ng/mL for a period of 6 to 12 hours after ingestion. In practice, it is obvious that caution is required when the results of a positive urine test for morphine and codeine are interpreted.

Morphine. The archetypical opiate, morphine, is used as the basis of comparison for relative characterizations of the opioid class. Morphine interacts primarily with MOR to mediate its effects, but it also shows some affinity for KOR.[309] Its major metabolites are glucuronide conjugates, including inactive morphine-3-glucuronide (M3G; ≈60%), active morphine-6-glucuronide (M6G; ≈10%), and a small amount of morphine-3,6-diglucuronide.[155,850] Free hydroxyl groups, such as the 3- and 6-hydroxy moieties of morphine, are frequently glucuronidated by enzymes of the uridine diphosphate glucuronyl transferase (UGT) family.[309,492] UGT2B7 is the isoform primarily responsible for morphine glucuronidation in humans[155]; other UGT enzymes such as UGT1A1 and UGT1A8 metabolize morphine in vitro, but their relevance in vivo remains uncertain.[599] Most morphine glucuronides are excreted in the feces, where substantial enterohepatic circulation of conjugated and intestinally deconjugated morphine occurs. The detection time for morphine is usually 48 hours, but this varies with individual differences in metabolism excretion and route and frequency of use.[414]

With long-term administration and when morphine concentrations are high, a minor fraction is converted to hydromorphone (up to 2.5% of the urine morphine concentration).[163] M6G has greater MOR agonist activity than morphine and appears to contribute less to unwanted side effects.[309,492,604] However, the relative importance of morphine and M6G in analgesia and adverse responses remains controversial.[850] The elimination half-life for glucuronides is longer than for morphine.[287] Therefore, glucuronides accumulate in serum to greater concentrations than morphine, and in patients with renal insufficiency, morphine glucuronides are thought to significantly contribute to opioid toxicity, as patients are unable to excrete the water-soluble metabolites.[309,638]

Codeine. Because of its antitussive and analgesic properties, codeine is one of the most frequently prescribed opiates in the world; it is frequently combined with nonopiate analgesic agents such as aspirin and acetaminophen. Therefore, detection of salicylate or acetaminophen along with codeine in the urine of patients who display an opiate toxidrome should lead to the measurement of salicylate or acetaminophen in serum to assess its toxicity. Alternatively, empirical quantitative serum acetaminophen and salicylate determinations are appropriate for patients with the opioid toxidrome. Codeine has only about one tenth the analgesic potency of morphine and shows poor affinity for MOR, with only a fraction of the pain-relieving capacity of morphine; therefore, it is generally considered a prodrug.[50] Analgesia is attributed to the small fraction (<10%) of codeine converted to morphine by CYP2D6 via O-demethylation, although some studies suggest that the predominant (≈80%) metabolite, codeine-6-glucuronide, may be capable of mediating CNS effects independently of morphine.[492] Both codeine and morphine may be detected in urine following codeine ingestion; however, after 30 hours only morphine may be detectable.[170] Codeine is also converted to an inactive metabolite, norcodeine (10%), and long-term high-dose administration leads to metabolism to the active compound hydrocodone (up to 11% of the urine codeine concentration).[492,610] During the early phase of excretion, codeine and conjugates predominate, but after this time, morphine conjugates are the major product. Approximately 3 days after codeine use, morphine and its conjugates are the only metabolites detected.[50,414]

Genetic variation may play a significant role in the metabolism of codeine and several other opioids. More than 60 alleles have been described for CYP2D6, with resultant enzymatic activity varying from essentially zero, in the case of null alleles, to many times higher than normal, in the case of amplified alleles (http://www.cypalleles.ki.se/cyp2d6.htm; accessed on July 23, 2010).[73,355] Thus, at the same codeine dose, patients with minimal CYP2D6 activity (poor metabolizers) would likely receive inadequate analgesia because of lack of conversion to morphine; however, patients with very high CYP2D6 activity (ultra-rapid metabolizers) would be at risk for adverse responses to excessive morphine.[221,309] Without knowledge of the CYP2D6 genotype, these clinical presentations can be confusing; the possibility of pharmacogenetic effects is therefore important to consider when appropriate dosing, patient compliance, and potential diversion or illicit use are assessed.

Semisynthetic Opiates

Heroin, hydrocodone, hydromorphone, oxycodone, and oxymorphone are examples of semisynthetic opiates.

Heroin. Heroin is a synthetic opiate that is made from morphine and is also called *diacetylmorphine* or *diamorphine;* it has an analgesic potency two to three times that of morphine[414] because of its better penetration across the blood-brain barrier. Heroin is no longer legally produced in the United States, but it is still used elsewhere for fast-acting analgesia.[284] The two acetyl groups enhance CNS distribution,[684] providing a rapid effect when first-pass metabolism is bypassed (e.g., intravenous administration). Heroin itself is rarely found in body fluids because of its extremely short half-life (2 to 6 minutes).[55,414] The metabolite, 6-acetylmorphine, is hydrolyzed to morphine,[55,357] and although it has a longer half-life (6 to 25 minutes),[55] it is detectable in urine only for about 8 hours after administration.[414] Both 6-acetylmorphine and morphine are pharmacologically active, with 6-MAM being four to six times more potent than morphine.[414] Other than the presence of its unique metabolite 6-monoacetylmorphine (6-MAM), which is definitive for heroin use, the metabolic profile of heroin resembles that of morphine.[683] Given that acetylcodeine is a common contaminant of heroin, both morphine and low concentrations of codeine are frequently detected in urine following heroin use.

Hydrocodone. Hydromorphone has about six times the potency and greater oral bioavailability than codeine,[57] but it is thought to be more toxic than codeine.[756] Hydrocodone is *O*-demethylated to hydromorphone, *N*-demethylated to form norhydrocodone, and C6-keto-reduced to form approximately equal amounts of 6-alpha- and 6-beta-hydrocol.[37,38] Similar to codeine, hydrocodone is metabolized by CYP2D6 to an active metabolite (hydromorphone) and therefore may be subject to pharmacogenetic variability in patients with abnormal CYP2D6 activity.[744]

It has been suggested that most of the pharmacologic effects of hydrocodone actually result from the hydromorphone formed during metabolism.[756] However, studies are somewhat contradictory. Hydrocodone may provide effective pain relief even in the absence of CYP2D6- mediated conversion to hydromorphone.[29] It remains unclear whether this is due primarily to the activity of hydrocodone itself or to that of other active metabolites.[56]

Hydromorphone. Oral hydromorphone is five to seven times more potent than morphine.[57] Although it is used as an analgesic in its own right with potency somewhat higher than hydrocodone,[29] hydromorphone is also an active metabolite of hydrocodone.[163] Similar to morphine, hydromorphone is metabolized in large part to a 3-glucuronide by UGT2B7, but also to a lesser extent by UGT1A3.[28,401] Hydromorphone lacks a free hydroxyl group at the 6-position, thus there is no metabolite analogous to M6G.[28,401] Two minor metabolites of hydromorphone—dihydromorphine and dihydroisomorphine—have demonstrated pharmacologic activity, but their contribution may be minimal because of the small amount formed.[57,756]

Oxycodone. Oxycodone is a potent analgesic with high oral bioavailability[62,309] that is frequently formulated in combination with aspirin or acetaminophen. Therefore, the detection of salicylate or acetaminophen along with oxycodone in the urine of patients who display an opiate toxidrome should lead to measurement of serum salicylate or acetaminophen concentration to assess toxicity. Noncombination oxycodone is also available in immediate- and extended-release dosage forms. The latter (OxyContin) is a very effective oral analgesic for patients with chronic pain (e.g., cancer patients). The pills may be chewed, crushed, snorted, or solubilized for IV injection to permit immediate availability of the entire dose, which is intended for extended release over a 12-hour period. This misuse has led to widespread misuse, more frequent emergency department visits, and increased mortality in the United States.[756]

Although its own strong analgesic activity precludes oxycodone from being considered a prodrug, it is converted to a highly active metabolite, oxymorphone, through the activity of CYP2D6.[674] This conversion appears to be less of a concern for CYP2D6 poor metabolizers, in whom oxycodone itself still provides analgesia, than for ultra-rapid metabolizers, who could be at increased risk for adverse effects.[191]

Oxymorphone. Oxymorphone provides potent analgesia with minimal interaction with CYP enzymes, although it is also a substrate for CYP2C9 and CYP3A4.[126] The majority of oxymorphone is metabolized by UGT2B7 to the 3-glucuronide; a minor metabolite, 6-hydroxyoxymorphone, is an active analgesic with a steady-state area under the curve (AUC) similar to the parent compound. Oxymorphone is a metabolite of oxycodone that is formed via CYP2D6.[28,401]

Fully Synthetic Opioids

Fentanyl, meperidine, methadone, propoxyphene, and tramadol are examples of fully synthetic opioids.

Fentanyl. Fentanyl is an alipophilic drug with numerous routes of administration that is used in applications ranging from anesthesia to rapid management of breakthrough pain.[619] Fentanyl provides the structural backbone for a number of related, ultra-short-acting opioids, including remifentanil and sufentanil. Norfentanyl, the primary metabolite, is generated by CYP3A and is inactive[765]; the high potency of fentanyl and the clinical insignificance of its metabolites make it a preferred analgesic for patients with major organ failure.[619] Transdermal fentanyl patches are used for longer-term administration and are gaining popularity among drug abusers, although nonstandard application of the patch (e.g., chewing, extraction) carries substantial risk for overdose.[774]

Meperidine. Originally synthesized as an anticholinergic, meperidine has analgesic potency comparable with or somewhat lower than that of morphine.[462] One major metabolite, normeperidine, also has analgesic activity; normeperidine is thought to be responsible for the serotonergic toxicity of meperidine, particularly in patients receiving concomitant monoamine oxidase inhibitors.[309,462] Meperidine use has declined in recent years in favor of alternatives such as fentanyl.

Methadone. A relatively long-acting opiate, methadone is used both for analgesia and in the treatment of opioid addiction.[309] It is thought to provide (1) milder withdrawal, (2) somewhat lower potential for abuse, and (3) reduced exposure to the risks of illicit intravenous drug use.[216] Methadone has affinity for both MOR and DOR,[504] the latter of which may explain its apparent utility in patients whose pain no longer responds to other opioids.[177] Substantial interindividual and intraindividual variability in metabolism and elimination has been noted; both urine pH and seemingly self-inducible metabolism substantially influence the pharmacokinetics of this compound, as do commonly coadministered drugs such as benzodiazepines and antiretrovirals.[309] Although a large fraction of methadone is excreted unchanged, measurement of a metabolite such as EDDP (2-ethylidene-1,5-dimethyl-3,3-diphenylpyrrolidine) in the setting of addiction treatment provides evidence for patient compliance rather than an exogenously spiked sample.[271,278,280] EDDP excretion is less pH dependent than is clearance of the parent drug.[59,309,414] Use of the methadone/EDDP ratio to assess compliance has been suggested but is complicated by the pharmacokinetic variability already described.[271,278,280]

Propoxyphene. A relatively weak analgesic, propoxyphene is less potent than codeine but carries the significant risk of atypical adverse effects such as cardiac arrhythmia and seizure. The incidence of such negative responses is particularly high in the elderly.[44] In July 2009, the U.S. Food and Drug Administration (FDA) required manufacturers to strengthen the black box warning to address the increased risk of overdose (http://www.fda.gov/NewsEvents/Newsroom/PressAnnouncements/ucm170769.htm, accessed on June 14, 2011), and in November of 2010 recommends against the continued use of the drug (http://www.fda.gov/Drugs/DrugSafety/ucm234338.htm; accessed on June 14, 2011) and announced that prescription containing medications were being withdrawn form the US market (http://www.fda.gov/NewsEvents/Newsroom/PressAnnouncements/2010/ucm234350.htm, accessed on June 14, 2011) However, its nonmedical abuse remains common.[264]

Tramadol. Unlike the majority of opioid agonists, tramadol has low abuse potential and therefore is unscheduled.[663] It has low affinity for opioid receptors and mediates analgesia through opioid-independent regulation of neurotransmitter uptake; however, its main active metabolite (O-desmethyltramadol, or M1) is a potent opioid receptor agonist.[492] These mechanisms are thought to work synergistically to provide greater total pain relief than the sum of each individual component. Metabolism to M1 occurs via CYP2D6; thus opioid-like effects are subject to genetic variability, as with codeine.[663] However, because of its effects on neurotransmission, tramadol has the potential to cause serotonergic toxicity even in patients lacking CYP2D6.[492] In fact, several synthetic phenylpiperidine opioids (tramadol, methadone, dextromethorphan, and propoxyphene) have been associated with increased risk of serotonin toxicity caused by weak reuptake inhibition of monoamines when used in combination with serotonin reuptake inhibitors, monoamine oxidase inhibitors, and amphetamine-type stimulants.[40,89,149,283]

Opioid Antagonists and Mixed Agonist/Antagonists

These clinically useful compounds produce very different physiologic responses, depending on the situation. For example, in opioid-naive patients, mixed agonist/antagonists (MAAs) provide MOR-mediated analgesia with less risk of an adverse reaction, but the same dose in an opioid-tolerant patient may precipitate immediate withdrawal. In medical usage, coadministration of low-dose antagonists or MAAs alleviates minor opioid-induced side effects and appears useful in preventing opioid tolerance. In opioid addiction treatment, the addition of a low-dose antagonist to maintenance therapy seems to minimize subjective "feel-good" effects without substantially worsening withdrawal symptoms.

Buprenorphine, naloxone, and naltrexone are examples of opioid antagonists and mixed agonist/antagonists.

Buprenorphine. A semisynthetic derivative of thebaine, buprenorphine is a MOR partial agonist and a KOR antagonist. Low doses provide analgesia through MOR activation, but unlike full agonists, pain relief has a maximal threshold or "ceiling effect."[820] Buprenorphine is available as sublingual tablets (with or without naloxone) for the treatment of opioid dependence.[264] Buprenorphine is metabolized via *N*-dealkylation by CYP3A4 to the active compound, norbuprenorphine, both of which can be further conjugated to inactive glucuronides by UGT1A1.[28,29] CYP3A4 and UGT1A1 are subject to environmental and genetic variability, although the effects of these factors on buprenorphine are not well characterized.[309] The drug is eliminated primarily in feces, with only a small amount in urine, and is usually detectable for 1 to 3 days.[414]

Naloxone. The prototypical opioid antagonist naloxone binds nonspecifically to all three receptor types, with the greatest effect at MOR and the least effect at DOR.[309,781] Its efficacy is much greater by intravenous administration as compared with oral and sublingual routes.[263,264] This characteristic is advantageous in deterring misuse of prescribed opioids: oral or sublingual opioid/naloxone formulations provide the desired benefit when taken properly, but when diverted for intravenous use cause opioid antagonism and may precipitate withdrawal.[263,264]

Naloxone is commonly used in comatose patients as a therapeutic and diagnostic agent. The standard dosage regimen is 0.4 mg/mL administered slowly, preferably intravenously, with the dose increased until the desired end point is achieved, namely, restoration of respiratory function, ability to protect the airway, and improved level of consciousness. Naloxone has been known to precipitate profound withdrawal symptoms in opioid-dependent patients. Its clinical efficacy lasts for as little as 45 minutes. Therefore, patients are at risk for recurrence of narcotic effect. This is particularly true for patients exposed to opioids with long elimination half-lives, such as methadone and sustained-release opioid products. Patients should be observed for resedation for at least 4 hours after reversal with naloxone. Because naloxone is via the kidney eliminated, patients with renal dysfunction may have delayed resedation past the 4 hours and should therefore be observed for a longer period of time.

Naltrexone. Commonly used for the treatment of alcoholism, naltrexone is a potent antagonist of all three opioid receptors.[781] Its combined formulation with opioid agonists is less common than are naloxone/opioid combinations; however, the greater oral bioavailability of naltrexone suggests that it may be useful in applications where poor oral delivery limits the utility of naloxone.[264]

Analytical Methods. Many different immunoassay methods are used to screen for opiates. Gas chromatography (GC) with mass spectroscopic detection (GC-MS) is the technique of choice for confirmation of a positive screening test.

Screening Assays. Given their relatively rapid turnaround time and ability to identify several opiates, immunoassays are the methods of choice to screen urine samples for their opiate content. For clinical application, a cutoff of 300 ng/mL morphine (or morphine equivalents) is commonly used to distinguish negative from positive urine specimens, whereas a cutoff of 2000 ng/mL is mandated by SAMHSA for workplace drug screening. Antibodies in opiate abuse screens commonly target morphine, because commercial immunoassay development has largely been driven by detection of illicit heroin use. Wide variability in cross-reactivity to other congeners has been noted; thus some opiates or opioids (see Figure 35-12) with high abuse potential such as oxycodone are often poorly detected.[485,669,739] To address this problem, several immunoassays are commercially available for individual synthetic opioids, such as fentanyl. Finally, analytical interferences are also a problem with opiate immunoassays.* Other general opiate screening methods are available, including thin-layer chromatography, but these techniques are more labor intensive and may not provide adequate turnaround time for stat or emergency testing. In this setting, point-of-care devices are being used more frequently.[178,547,861]

In pain management programs, urine drug testing is often used to monitor compliance, diversion, or substitution for prescribed drugs. Based on the results of such tests, an individual may be dismissed from the program. It is important for drug-testing laboratories to communicate relevant aspects of the metabolic interconversion of opiates to physicians responsible for these programs. Monitoring compliance for oxycodone in pain management programs is problematic because of the low cross-reactivity of oxycodone in most opiate immunoassays. In this instance, a false-negative opiate immunoassay test may lead to an accusation of oxycodone diversion. Direct determination of oxycodone by a confirmatory method (GC-MS, LC-MS, LC-MS/MS) is more appropriate to monitor compliance for this drug.

*References 35, 181, 538, 669, 740, and 793.

Confirmation Testing. For compound-specific confirmation assays, GC with mass spectroscopic detection (GC-MS) has historically been considered the method of choice. Analysis of specific opioids is typically performed using GC or LC. GC generally results in longer run times and is often incompatible with larger metabolites such as glucuronide conjugates. LC systems require large quantities of organic solvents and are not considered acceptable for federal testing. A wide variety of detectors are available for both GC and LC; MS or tandem MS is often preferred for the structural and mass-specific information provided. Analytical and technical considerations are discussed in detail later.

Sample Preparation and Extraction. The matrix and rationale for opioid testing influence the choice of method. Analysis of urine requires hydrolysis to recover glucuronide- or sulfate-conjugated metabolites of various opioids. Hydrolysis is performed by acidification (e.g., concentrated hydrochloric acid at 115 to 120 °C for 15 minutes)[162,623,757] or by enzymatic treatment with β-glucuronidase alone[90,157,491] or in combination with arylsulfatase.[72] Acid hydrolysis is simpler and more rapid, and typically provides greater recovery than enzymatic methods, although a few studies have shown better recovery of some analytes with glucuronidase.[194] Acidification, however, destroys the metabolite 6-MAM, preventing conclusive determination of heroin use; it also partially degrades morphine.[244] For this reason, drugs-of-abuse testing for opiates typically employs enzymatic hydrolysis, regardless of its generally poorer analytical performance.

Serum analysis is performed with or without a hydrolysis step; if a hydrolysis step is included, results reflect the sum of parent drug and metabolites, that is, "total" drug concentration. For detection of illicit drug use, total concentrations are typically sufficient. However, omitting hydrolysis to preserve conjugated metabolites can be useful, for example, when both the parent and the metabolite are active compounds, as with morphine and M6G.

Methods of analysis from serum or urine were initially developed using liquid-liquid extraction (LLE),* although solid-phase extraction (SPE)[72,286,347,714,826] is now often preferred. Some methods do not derivatize prior to GC analysis,[113,519] but this typically results in poor chromatographic properties. Although the number of derivatizing agents described in the literature is relatively limited, great variability in experimental conditions has been noted.†

Gas Chromatography. Several GC-MS methods have been developed to quantitate various combinations of morphine, other opiates, and their metabolites from extracts of human urine.[162,266,551] GC-MS is considered the reference method for determination of most natural and semisynthetic opiates, particularly in forensic settings, although other detectors are available and have been used for GC applications. Various GC-MS methods have been described for the identification and determination of opiates. Some investigators use chemical ionization,[144,161,204,627] but electron impact mode is more common. The GC is typically equipped with a 12- or 15-m fused-silica capillary column with a polar stationary phase of cross-linked dimethylsilicone, phenyl methyl silicone, or 95% dimethyl-5% polysiloxane.[72,90,131,227,240] Because of structural similarities between many opiates, particularly natural and semisynthetic opiates, assays must be evaluated for interference from metabolites and congeners. The degree of overlap is such that the fragmentation patterns of various opioids can resemble one another greatly, as is seen with the mass spectra of the trimethylsilane (TMS) derivatives of hydromorphone, morphine, and norcodeine.[290] Chromatographic resolution of these compounds must be carefully optimized to provide reliable characterization, particularly because many structurally related opiates are commercially available and are part of the same metabolic pathways.

Although acetyl derivatives have the advantage of being stable for up to 72 hours when stored at room temperature in ethyl acetate, incomplete derivatization may occur when acetyl-donating agents are used.[90,240] Both morphine and 6-MAM are converted to diacetylmorphine (heroin); thus acetyl derivatization does not permit distinction between morphine, 6-MAM, and heroin. In addition to diacetylmorphine, a small amount of 3-monoacetylmorphine (3-MAM) is formed by acetylating agents; although clinically insignificant, 3-MAM shares the m/z 285 ion with deuterated (d3) d3-acetylcodeine and interferes with analysis of these compounds.[303]

In contrast to acetylating agents, TMS creates single derivatives for most opiates, although TMS derivatives are sensitive to moisture.[131] Several analytical interferences are associated with TMS: codeine and norcodeine derivatives coelute on gas chromatography, while 6-MAM produces an additional peak that coelutes with morphine and increases with room temperature storage.[140] Like TMS, pentafluoropropionic anhydride (PFP) derivatives are moisture-sensitive; however, no breakdown products are detected after storage for 24 hours.[303] The addition of pentafluoropropanol (PFPOH) improves the yield of PFP derivatives and allows morphine and 6-MAM to be clearly distinguished.[240,714]

Liquid Chromatography. Despite the long-standing role of GC in opiate analysis, LC methods are common and are often analytically advantageous. One notable example is that LC provides the ability to analyze glucuronide-conjugated metabolites as well as parent compounds. In addition, LC methods are able to measure polar metabolites without prior derivatization,[86] and on-column extraction is possible with some LC systems. As with GC, a variety of detectors are available for LC. For example, HPLC methods for opioid analysis have been described using fluorescence (FD), ultraviolet-visible (UV), electrochemical (EC), and diode array detection (DAD), alone and in various combinations. In addition, several analytical methods for morphine and its glucuronide

*References 90, 157, 218, 390, 468, 623, and 625.

†References 72, 90, 131, 157, 193, 240, 303, 324, 564, 623, 625, and 757.

metabolites exist for LC-MS or LC-MS/MS with different MS interfaces.*

Analytical methods also include common opioids such as methadone[682] or buprenorphine,[8] or other nonopioid drugs of abuse such as cocaine, amphetamines, and lysergic acid diethylamide (LSD).[86,158,830]

For TDM testing, several reports have focused on quantitation of multiple opioids used therapeutically (e.g., in palliative care). For example, in one study, an LC-MS/MS method was developed that was capable of measuring 11 opioids and 5 metabolites, namely, buprenorphine, codeine, fentanyl, hydromorphone, methadone, morphine, oxycodone, oxymorphone, piritramide, tilidine, and tramadol, with the metabolites bisnortilidine, morphine glucuronides, norfentanyl, and nortilidine.[568] In another study, a combination screening and confirmation method was developed that could be used to identify fentanyl, alfentanil, remifentanil, and sufentanil and their respective *N*-dealkylated or de-esterified metabolites by LC-MS/MS.[771] Metabolite profiling is another growing area in TDM testing, especially for compounds with known active metabolites such as tramadol.[313]

Drugs of Abuse Related to the Sympathomimetic Syndrome

Several stimulants and hallucinogens chemically related to phenylethylamine are referred to collectively as amphetamine-type stimulants (ATSs). They are considered to be sympathomimetic drugs, meaning that they mimic endogenous transmitters in the sympathetic nervous system.[487] Other drugs related to the sympathomimetic syndrome include cocaine and LSD.

Amphetamines

Amphetamine and methamphetamine (Figure 35-13) are CNS stimulant drugs that have limited legitimate pharmacologic use,[343] including narcolepsy, obesity, and attention-deficit hyperactivity disorders. They produce an initial euphoria and have a high abuse potential. Other sympathomimetic amines that have high potential for abuse include the "designer" amphetamines—ephedrine, pseudoephedrine, phenylpropanolamine, and methylphenidate (Ritalin).

Amphetamine and Methamphetamine

These drugs are sympathomimetic amines that have a stimulating effect on both the central and peripheral nervous systems. In the brain, a primary action is to elevate the concentrations of extracellular monoamine neurotransmitters (dopamine, serotonin, norepinephrine) by promoting presynaptic release from the nerve endings[497,687,835] rather than blockade of reuptake.[595] Amphetamine and methamphetamine are substrates for the dopamine, serotonin, and norepinephrine transporters. Once in the cell, they interfere with the vesicular monoamine transporter (VMAT) and MAO,[296,835] depleting synaptic vesicles of their neurotransmitter content. As a consequence, concentrations of dopamine (or other transmitter amines) in the cytoplasm increase and quickly become sufficient to cause release into the synapse by reversal of the plasma membrane dopamine transporter (DAT/ SLC6A3). Normal vesicular release of dopamine consequently is decreased (because synaptic vesicles contain less transmitter), while nonvesicular release is increased. Similar mechanisms apply to other biogenic amines (serotonin and norepinephrine).[497,762]

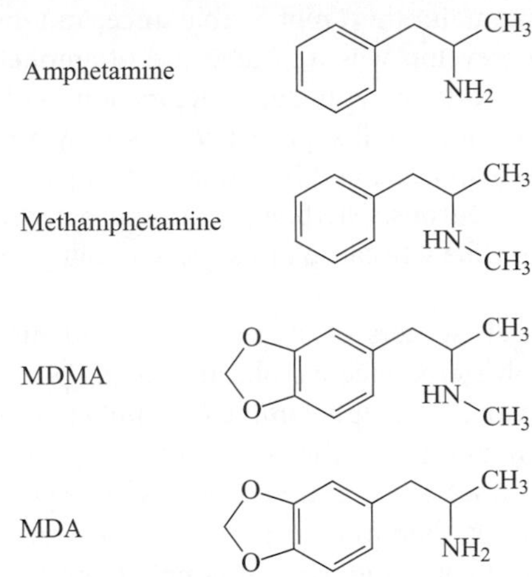

Figure 35-13 Select amphetamine-type stimulants.

Amphetamine cardiovascular activation is thought to be due to the release of norepinephrine from sympathetic nerve endings.[292,835] Stereotyped repetitive behavior and some aspects of locomotor activity induced by amphetamine probably are a consequence of the release of dopamine from dopaminergic nerve terminals, particularly in the neostriatum.[835] The anorectic effect and at least a component of its locomotor-stimulating action are mediated by release of norepinephrine.[835] With higher doses, dopamine release in the mesolimbic system and enhanced release of 5-hydroxytryptamine (5-HT; serotonin) in tryptaminergic neurons may be responsible for disturbances of perception and frank psychotic behavior.[224,835] High doses also lead to decreases in brain concentrations of the neurotransmitters dopamine and 5-HT, as well as a reduction in the activity of enzymes responsible for their synthesis (tyrosine dehydroxylase and tryptophan hydroxylase, respectively).[487]

Amphetamine and methamphetamine (1) increase blood pressure, heart rate, body temperature, and motor activity, (2) relax bronchial muscle, and (3) depress the appetite. Abuse of these drugs may lead to strong psychologic dependence, marked tolerance, and mild physical dependence associated with tachycardia, increased blood pressure, restlessness, irritability, insomnia, personality changes, and a severe form of chronic intoxication psychosis similar to schizophrenia. These unpleasant responses reinforce repetitive use of the

*References 77, 83-85, 407, 562, 571, 611, 707, 724, 786, 873, and 876.

drugs to maintain the "high." Tolerance and psychologic dependence develop with repeated use of amphetamines.[343] Long-term effects may include depression and impaired memory and motor skills, probably caused by a decrease in dopamine transporters and by damage to dopaminergic and serotonergic neurons. Methamphetamine has greater CNS efficacy, most likely because of its greater ability to penetrate the CNS.[556]

The optical isomers of amphetamine and methamphetamine exhibit stereoselective pharmacologic properties. The CNS activity of S(+) amphetamine (D-amphetamine) is three to four times greater than that of R(−) amphetamine (L-amphetamine), but the latter drug has more potent cardiovascular effects than the former.[48,343] The CNS effects of S(+) methamphetamine (D-methamphetamine) are about 10 times greater than those of R(−) methamphetamine (L-methamphetamine), but the latter drug has greater vasoconstrictive properties than the former.[245,343] Because of minimal CNS activity and thus low abuse potential, R(−) methamphetamine is included in some nonprescription nasal inhalants (e.g., Vick's) for its vasoconstrictive properties.

The main metabolic pathways of amphetamine and methamphetamine include (1) aromatic hydroxylation, (2) aliphatic hydroxylation, (3) *N*-demethylation, (4) oxidative deamination, (5) *N*-oxidation, and (6) conjugation of nitrogen.[442] Amphetamine itself is extensively metabolized to a variety of metabolites, including norephedrine and *p*-hydroxyamphetamine, both of which are pharmacologically active, and may be glucuronidated prior to excretion.[487] Amphetamine is metabolized in a stereoselective manner such that the elimination half-life for R(−) amphetamine may be as much as 40% longer than that for S(+) amphetamine.[112,823] Methamphetamine is metabolized in liver primarily by hydroxylation and, to a lesser extent, by *N*-demethylation to amphetamine. Overall metabolism, including formation of amphetamine, is enantioselective.[70,112] Thus when racemic methamphetamine is ingested, urine specimens contain relatively more R(−) methamphetamine than S(+) methamphetamine, but a greater amount of S(+) amphetamine than R(−) amphetamine.[151,350]

In addition to hepatic metabolism, amphetamine is eliminated as unchanged drug in urine. Elimination is dependent on urine pH, and although typically about 30% of a dose is excreted unchanged, this may vary from as much as 74% in acid urine to as little as 1% in alkaline urine.[48] Therefore, elimination half-life (renal excretion and hepatic metabolism) also varies with urine pH from 7 to 14 hours at acid pH to 18 to 34 hours at alkaline pH.[253,556] These effects of urine pH on the elimination of unchanged amphetamines are a consequence of tubular reabsorption of nonionized amphetamine (pK_a, 9.9). Similarly methamphetamine is eliminated in urine in a pH-dependent manner similar to that used for amphetamine.

Pharmacogenetics may play a role in the differences seen in the metabolism/elimination of these drugs. CYP2D6 is responsible for the 4-hydroxylation of amphetamine and methamphetamine and the *N*-demethylation of methamphetamine.[33,442,464,481] However, the effects of methamphetamine are not reliably predicted from serum concentrations.[676]

Designer Amphetamines

The terms "designer drugs" and "club drugs" originated in the 1980s.[488] These drugs include derivatives of amphetamines and the new benzylpiperazine, phenylpiperazine; pyrolidinophenone types have gained popularity and notoriety among people who participate in all-night dance parties (raves) and who visit nightclubs.[22,525,779] Most designer drugs produce feelings of euphoria and energy and a desire to socialize[402]; they also promote social and physical interactions. They are used at these events to enhance energy for prolonged partying and/or dancing, and to distort or enhance visual and auditory sensations. The moniker "club drug" does not imply that recreational use is restricted to this social environment. In this context, designer drugs mistakenly have the reputation of being safe; several experimental studies in rats and humans and epidemiologic studies have revealed risks to humans such as life-threatening serotonin syndrome, hepatotoxicity, neurotoxicity, psychopathology, and the abuse potential of such drugs.[402,525,529]

Some of the more common designer amphetamines are listed in Box 35-2; however, only a few will be discussed here.

MDMA (3,4-Methylenedioxymethamphetamine) and MDA (3,4-Methylenedioxyamphetamine). MDMA (also known as "Ecstasy") is categorized as a stimulant as a result of its sympathomimetic effects, including (1) peripheral vasoconstriction, (2) bronchodilation, (3) cardiorespiratory stimulation, (4) pupillary dilation, and (5) appetite suppression. The drug is a sympathomimetic; however, it has significantly fewer CNS stimulant properties than methamphetamine.[488] It also is categorized as an empathogen-entactogen.[488,563]

Similar to amphetamine and methamphetamine, MDMA causes release of biogenic amines by reversing the action of their respective transporters. It has a preferential affinity for the serotonin transporter and therefore most strongly increases the extracellular concentration of serotonin.[497] This release is so profound that marked presynaptic intracellular depletion occurs for 24 hours after a single dose. With repetitive administration, concentrations of 5-HT, 5-hydroxyindoleacetic acid (5-HIAA), and tryptophan hydroxylase, and serotonin transporter density are reduced.[618] Some suggest that serotonin depletion may become permanent; this has triggered a debate on its neurotoxicity. Although direct proof from animal models for neurotoxicity remains weak, several studies have reported long-term cognitive impairment in heavy users of MDMA.[497]

MDMA is a chiral compound in which the S(+)-enantiomer possesses greater pharmacologic activity. MDMA undergoes demethylation to MDA,[542] with the rate of conversion of S(+)-MDMA to S(+)-MDA exceeding that of R(−)-MDMA to R(−)-MDA. Consequently, the concentrations in urine of R(−)-MDMA and S(+)-MDA are greater than those for S(+)-MDMA and R(−)-MDA subsequent to ingestion of racemic MDMA.[236,331]

BOX 35-2 Designer Drugs Related to Phenylethylamine, Benzylpiperazine, Phenylpiperazine, and Pyrrolidinophenone[87,139,385,509,525,770]

Phenylethylamines
- 3,4-Methylenedioxymethamphetamine (MDMA; Ecstasy)
- 3,4-Methylenedioxyethylamphetamine (MDEA; "Eve")
- 3,4-Methylenedioxyamphetamine (MDA), which is also a metabolite of MDMA
- Paramethoxyamphetamine (PMA)
- Paramethoxymethamphetamine (PMMA)
- 2,5-Dimethoxy-4-methylamphetamine (DOM)
- 2,5-Dimethoxy-4-methylthioamphetamine (DOT)
- 4-Iodo-2,5-dimethoxyamphetamine (DOI)
- 2,5-Dimethoxy-4-bromo-amphetamine (DOB)
- 2,5-Dimethoxy-4-bromo-methamphetamine (MDOB)
- 3,4-(Methylenedioxyphenyl)-2-butanamine (BDB)
- *N*-Methyl-1-(3,4-methylenedioxy-phenyl)-2-butanamine (MBDB)
- 6-Chloro-3,4-methylenedioxymethamphetamine (Cl-MDMA)
- 3,4-Methylenedioxymethcathinone
- 4-Bromo-2,5-diemthoxy-phenylethylamine (2C-B)
- 2,5-Dimethoxy-4ethylthio-phenylethylamine (2C-T-2)
- 2,5-Dimethoxy-4 propylthio-phenylethylamine (2C-T-7)

Benzylpiperazines
- 1-Benzylpiperazine (BZP)
- 1-(3,4-Methylenedioxybenzyl)-piperazine (MDBP)

Phenylpiperazines
- 1-(3-Trifluoromethylphenyl)piperazine (TFMPP)
- 1-(3-Chlorophenyl)piperazine (mCPP)
- 1-(4-Methoxyphenyl)piperazine (MeOPP)

Pyrrolidinophenone
- α-Pyrrolidinopropiophenone (PPP)
- 4-Methoxy-α-pyrrolidinopropiophenone (MOPPP)
- 3,4-Methylenedioxy-α-pyrrolidinopropiophenone (MDPPP)
- 4-Methyl-α-pyrrolidinopropiophenone (MPPP)
- 4-Methyl-α-pyrrolidinohexanophenone (MPHP)

MDMA is *N*-demethylated in humans to MDA, via CYP1A2, and to a significantly lesser extent by CYP2D6.[488] Although extensive and poor MDMA metabolizers have been identified, the contribution of these polymorphisms to MDMA toxicity is unclear, because the metabolism may be saturable even at normal doses, resulting in greater dose-proportional excretion of the parent drug.[189] The saturable kinetics does, however, suggest that beyond a certain threshold, small increases in dose may result in larger increases in plasma concentration, and consequently greater risk of toxicity.[488]

MDEA (3,4-Methylenedioxyethylamphetamine). MDEA is an empathogen-entactogen drug of the phenethylamine family that produces distinctive emotional and social effects similar to those of MDMA. On the street, it is known as "Love." MDEA undergoes oxidative cleavage of the methoxy rings but also *N*-de-ethylation.[60,442] MDEA also undergoes de-ethylation to MDA, with the rate of conversion of S(+)-MDEA to S(+)-MDA exceeding that of R(−)-MDEA to R(—)-MDA.[541]

The MDEA enantiomers have different pharmacokinetic properties. They include *S*-MDEA, which produces elevated mood and impairment in conceptually driven cognition, and *R*-MDEA, which produces increased depression and enhanced visual feature processing[541]; a generally higher affinity toward *S*-MDEA than *R*-MDEA is seen.[541]

PMA (Paramethoxyamphetamine) and PMMA (Paramethoxymethamphetamine). PMA and PMMA are methoxylated phenylethylamine derivatives with effects similar to but more potent than those of MDMA; they are frequently sold on this basis.[385] PMA is a metabolite of PMMA,[680] but it is also an especially toxic designer amphetamine that has resulted in several deaths from its unsuspected ingestion as an ecstasy substitute.[444]

PMA is 10 times more active than MDMA in elevating brain serotonin concentrations and inhibiting serotonin uptake, but it has only a few effects on the dopamine system.[186,327,783,784] Inhibition of MAO A is a further pharmacologic property of PMA.[297] These pharmacologic properties are thought by some to be responsible for the higher rate of death seen with PMA compared with other substituted amphetamines.[404] Multiple deaths have been associated with its use; symptoms usually mimic serotonin syndrome and include hyperthermia, tachycardia, seizures, cardiac dysrhythmias, and coma.[143,241,374]

Ephedrine and Pseudoephedrine

These amines are diastereoisomers that possess two asymmetrical carbon atoms and exist as four isomers designated as 1R,2S- and 1S,2R-ephedrine and 1R,2R- and 1S,2S-pseudoephedrine.[302] The 1R,2S-ephedrine (ephedrine) and 1S,2S-pseudoephedrine (pseudoephedrine) isomers occur naturally in various plants of the *Ephedra* genus.

Ephedrine and pseudoephedrine have been used as nasal decongestants, bronchodilators, and CNS stimulants, and for the treatment of obesity.[25,403,486,835] Ephedrine is both an α- and a β-adrenergic receptor agonist; in addition, it enhances the release of norepinephrine from sympathetic neurons and is considered a mixed-acting sympathomimetic drug.[835] Many dietary supplements contain ephedra, the herbal form of ephedrine. These products are widely marketed for energy enhancement or weight loss[51,395] and are used by some athletes to enhance performance. Adverse effects such as hypertension, tremors, myocardial infarction, seizures, and stroke have resulted in fatalities.[141,317,837] Because of this, the FDA banned the sale of dietary supplements containing ephedra in 2004.[835] However, herbal products containing ephedra remain in use in other countries.

Pseudoephedrine is used primarily as a decongestant because of its vasoconstrictive properties (α-adrenergic action).[64] It also is used as a nasal decongestant and precursor for the illicit synthesis of methamphetamine. Because of this, the quantity per purchase of products containing these drugs is now restricted in many places.

PPA (Phenylpropanolamine)

PPA was widely available in a number of nonprescription cold medications and diet control products. Adverse effects are similar to those described for ephedrine. In response to an FDA warning of increased risk of hemorrhagic stroke, especially in women, PPA has been withdrawn from the market by most manufacturers.[63] PPA is also a metabolite of ephedrine and pseudoephedrine.[51,64]

Methylphenidate (Ritalin)

Methylphenidate (MPH) is a phenethylamine derivative with psychostimulant properties similar to S(+) amphetamine. It is commonly used to treat attention-deficit hyperactivity disorder (ADHD) and narcolepsy.[61,497] Its pharmacologic properties are essentially the same as those of the amphetamines.[835] Like many of its related amphetamine-type stimulants, it exists as an isomer, as (R,R)-methylphenidate (D-MPH), and as (S,S)-methylphenidate (L-MPH).[510] The pharmacologic actions of MPH are almost solely performed by the D-isomer.[510] Methylphenidate is rapidly metabolized favoring L-MPH over D-MPH,[510] such that the more potent D-MPH has a half-life of about 6 hours, and the less potent L-MPH has a half-life of about 4 hours.[835] Diversion and abuse of methylphenidate have been increasing among children and adults because of its stimulant and purported aphrodisiac properties. In overdose, the clinical effects of methylphenidate are similar to those of amphetamine and produce signs of generalized CNS stimulation that may lead to convulsions.[497]

Analytical Methods. The initial screening test for amphetamines and related drugs is typically immunoassay. For confirmation of a presumptive positive test, a quantitative drug measurement is performed using GC-MS.

Immunoassay. Most "amphetamine" immunoassays have been designed to detect amphetamine/methamphetamine; others have been designed to detect MDMA and MDA; and others to more broadly capture the ATS group—all with varying cross-reactivities.[346,799] Many older immunoassays lacked the ability to distinguish between the isoforms.[645] Currently, many use antibodies specific for S(+) amphetamine (D-amphetamine) and/or S(+) methamphetamine (D-methamphetamine). The degree of cross-reactivity of these antibodies varies, with antibodies raised to immunogens protein-linked to the amphetamine molecule through the phenyl ring having better cross-reactivity than those linked through the sidechain.[488]

Not all amphetamine immunoassays were suitable for detection of the amphetamine-derived designer drugs PMA, PMMA, and MDEA,[367,472,766,871] and especially not for the new piperazine-derived substances.[188,752] Alternatively, other chemically related compounds such as pseudoephedrine have been shown to produce positive results.[860] Additionally, many psychotropic medications have been reported to interfere with immunoassays.[556,734] Immunoassays from different manufacturers can have very different "interference" profiles, which the pathologist and the laboratory scientist must understand and relay to clinicians.

Regarding methylphenidate, it should be noted that its detection by urine drug immunoassay is problematic, as it does not cross-react well with amphetamine immunoassays; detection of the parent drug is made difficult by its generally low concentration; and ritalinic acid, present in much higher concentration, is difficult to extract and analyze by GC; it is unstable upon storage even when frozen.[61]

Confirmatory Methods. All positive immunoassay results should be confirmed by a second independent method, but what may be more significant is that if the other designer amphetamines (see Box 35-2) are suspected, a negative immunoassay screen cannot rule out the presence of these drugs. Fortunately, numerous GC- and LC-based methods for identification and quantitation of these drugs in biological samples have been put forth.[418,640,808]

Amphetamine-type stimulants are considered volatile and are lost during a dry-down or evaporation step, if this is part of the procedure. This loss is avoided by the addition of a small amount of hydrochloric acid during the evaporation step, or the addition of a less volatile "keeper" solvent such as dimethylformamide (DMF).[487] Also, because of their extreme volatility at the high temperatures encountered in GC-MS, derivatization prior to analysis lowers the limit of detection. Although many derivatives are available for GC-MS use, the most commonly used include heptafluorobuic anhydride (HFBA), pentafluoropropionic anhydride (PFPA), trifluoroacetic anhydride (TFAA), and 4-carbethoxyhexfluorobutyryl chloride (4-CB). However, the 4-CB derivative in the presence of ephedrine/pseudoephedrine may generate methamphetamine,[775] which leads to the DHHS rule to have amphetamine also detected to report a positive methamphetamine result.[556]

Methamphetamine is a prototypical basic drug (pK_a 9.9) that is readily extracted from biological material into organic solvents at alkaline pH. It is readily soluble in chloroform, *N*-butyl chloride, ethyl acetate, and diethyl ether, and is extracted in most common protocols designed to isolate alkaloidal and basic drugs. It also readily extracts back into acid, and back into organic solvents without significant loss.[487] Most published methods for analysis of members of the amphetamine class in urine, plasma, and blood use LLE or SPE.[488]

Methamphetamine is readily analyzed by GC; this is the most popular method in use today for analysis of methamphetamine in biological material. Its poor UV absorption properties make it an unsuitable candidate for HPLC with UV detection, and it has no native fluorescence and no significant oxidative electrochemical properties at low voltages.[487] Liquid chromatography may be used for MDMA analysis and offers an advantage over GC in that MDMA and its polar metabolites can be quantified simultaneously without derivatization.[488]

The molecular weight of methamphetamine, the low intensity of its mass fragments in electron impact mode, and

TABLE 35-11 Prescription Drugs That Are Metabolized to Amphetamine or Methamphetamine

Drug		Drugs Detected[153,487,681]
Adderall	amphetamine	amphetamine
Dexedrin	D-amphetamine	D-amphetamine
Deprenyl	selegiline	L-methamphetamine L-amphetamine
Didrex	benzphetamine	methamphetamine amphetamine

the structural similarity of many endogenous and exogenous compounds result in its mass spectrum not being highly characteristic.[487] The issue of lack of specificity of the methamphetamine mass spectrum is resolved by derivatization.[792] Many methods have been published for analysis of amphetamine, methamphetamine, and related compounds.* Unfortunately, routine GC-MS also does not distinguish between the two isomers and necessitates the use of chiral chromatography to differentiate between them. Chiral discrimination of methamphetamine isomers may be necessary to distinguish the use of nonprescription nasal inhalants [R(−) methamphetamine] from the illicit use of methamphetamine [S(+) and R(−)] or other prescription medications, as indicated in Table 35-11. Some immunoassays have high specificity for S(+)isoforms. However, definitive enantio-discrimination requires the use of a chiral derivatization reagent conventional GC-MS,[150,245,350,667] or possibly chiral separation by LC-MS or LC-MS/MS. Also, care must be taken in interpreting the results of drug screens. Several other prescription drugs available in the United States and Canada that are metabolized to amphetamine or methamphetamine are listed in Table 35-11.

Regarding methylphenidate, its confirmation by GC-MS is complicated by the fact that it does not form a stable *N,O*-ditrimethylsilyl derivative. However, after sequential reactions with MSTFA [*N*-methyl-*N*-(trimethylsilyl)trifluoroacetamide] and MBTFA [*N*-methyl-bis (trifluoroacetamide)] to form the *N*-trifluoroacetyl, *O*-trimethylsilyl ester,[222] it is possible to measure methylphenidate by GC-MS. Ritalinic acid may be isolated from urine using a dehydration procedure, then methylated with dimethylformamide dimethyl acetal, and the resulting methylphenidate analyzed by GC-MS. Last, ritalinic acid may be analyzed directly by LC-tandem mass spectrometry,[508] or by GC-MS, after sequential reactions with MSTFA and MBTFA to form the *N*-trifluoroacetyl, *O*-trimethylsilyl ester,[222] or after methylation to re-form methylphenidate.

Cocaine

Cocaine is an alkaloid found in *Erythroxylon coca,* which grows principally in the northern South American Andes and to a lesser extent in India, Africa, and Java.[361,362] In clinical medicine, it is used mainly for local anesthesia and vasoconstriction in nasal surgery, and to dilate pupils in ophthalmology. Sigmund Freud famously proposed its use to treat depression and alcohol dependence, but the realities of cocaine addiction quickly brought this idea to an end.[497] Cocaine abuse has a long history and is rooted in the drug culture in the United States.[21] Cocaine is still one of the most common illicit drugs of abuse.[18,361] According to the National Survey on Drug Use and Health, the rate of past year use for cocaine (powder and crack combined) among individuals aged 12 and older has remained stable since 2002; 2.1 million users were reported in 2007.[107]

Cocaine is sold on the street in two forms: a hydrochloride salt (powder) and a free-base product known as "crack." The hydrochloride salt form of cocaine is administered by nasal insufflation ("snorting") or, less frequently, intravenously. "Crack" is a free-base form that has not been neutralized by an acid to make the hydrochloride salt. It comes as a rock crystal that is heated and its vapors smoked. The term refers to the crackling sound heard when it is heated.[361]

It should be noted that the use of "crack" cocaine is not to be confused with "free-basing," which is a process in which the user purifies cocaine HCl by mixing an aqueous solution of cocaine with baking soda or ammonia and adding diethyl ether, thereby extracting the free form of the drug into the organic solvent, which is then evaporated to dryness. The drug can then be smoked. However, because of the extremely flammable nature of diethyl ether, and therefore the risk of igniting any remaining ether, "free-basing" is no longer commonly practiced.[361]

Chemically, cocaine is methylbenzoylecognine (COC), an ester of benzoic acid and the amino alcohol (methylecognine) that contains a tropine moiety.[362] Its metabolism is complex (Figure 35-14) and occurs via both nonenzymatic hydrolysis and enzymatic transformation in the plasma and liver, where it is rapidly metabolized to benzoylecgonine (BE) and ecogonine methyl ester, both of which are inactive.[361] COC contains two ester moieties; the alkyl ester is hydrolyzed to its major metabolite BE via spontaneous hydrolysis at physiologic and alkaline pH.[361] It has been shown that COC is also hydrolyzed to BE by liver carboxylesterases.[192] BE is considered to be a pharmacologically inactive metabolite, but because its half-life is longer than that of COC, it is the most commonly monitored analyte in urine for determination of COC use.

BE is further metabolized to minor metabolites such as m-hydroxybenzoylecgonine (m-HOBE) and p-hydroxybenzoylecgonine (p-HOBE).[362,441] Of these, m-HOBE has been shown to be an important metabolite in the meconium of cocaine-exposed babies.[474,555] Positive BE results in urine are sometimes challenged in legal and administrative proceedings on the grounds that the presence of BE is due to the addition of COC to the urine sample with subsequent in vitro hydrolysis to BE. However, m-HOBE is believed to arise exclusively via in vivo metabolism[435]; therefore, its presence confirms COC use. Additionally, in adults, m-HOBE has a longer half-life and has the potential to be detected for longer

*References 2, 198, 275, 331, 487, 488, 524, and 723.

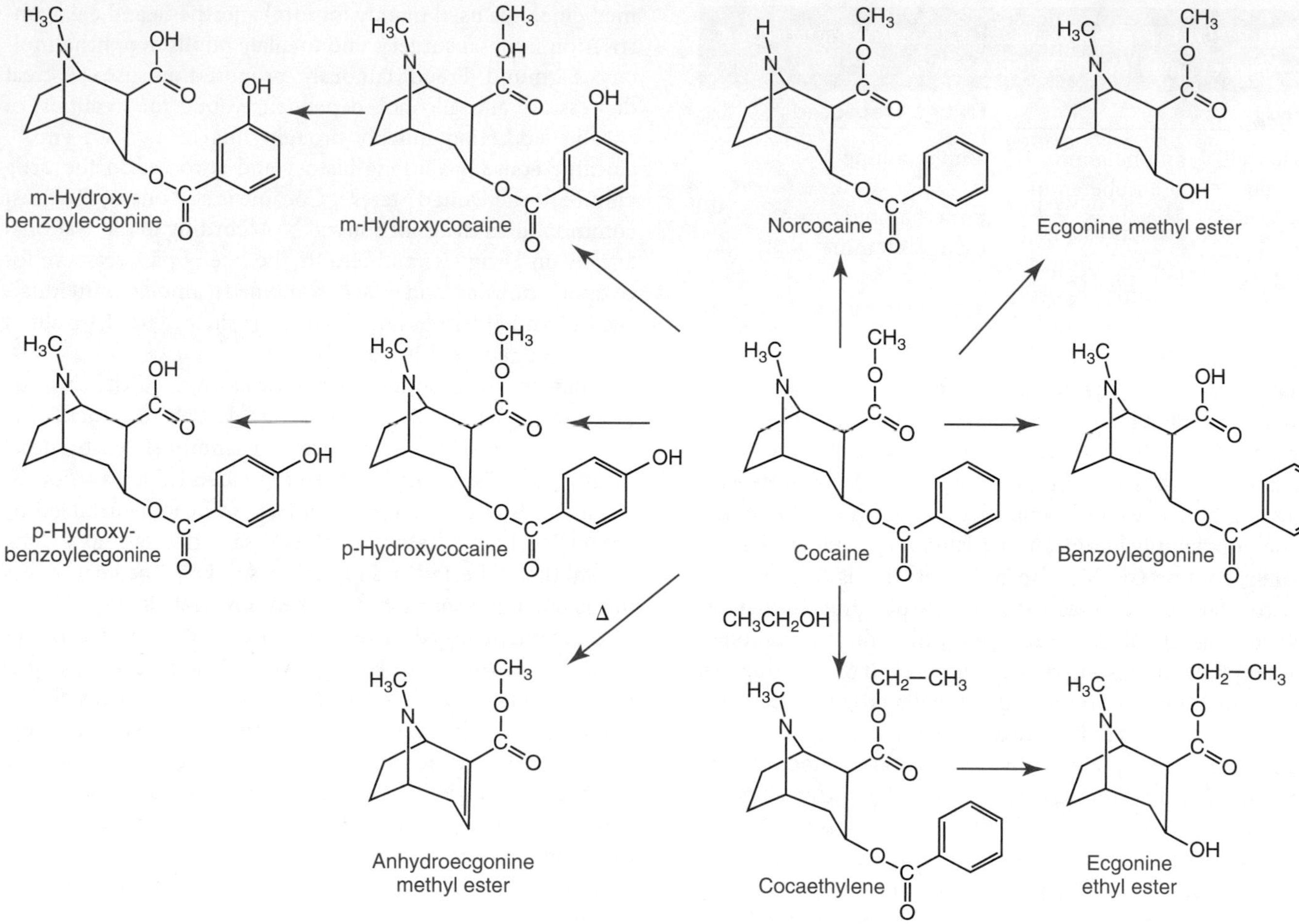

Figure 35-14 Metabolism of cocaine.

periods of time[168,441] than BE; it has been useful in the clinical management of patients because it expands the detection window. It should be noted that cocaethylene possesses the same CNS stimulatory activity as cocaine in experimental animals.

Norcocaine (NC) is an *N*-demethylated metabolite of COC produced by liver cytochrome P450; it is of clinical interest because of its conversion into hepatotoxic metabolites.[361,437,438] NC is subsequently metabolized to hydroxylnorcocaine and then to norcocaine-nitroxide.[438] Although the mechanism for hepatotoxicity is not well understood, it appears to be related to one or more of the *N*-oxidative metabolites. In animals, these metabolites have been reported to inhibit mitochondrial respiration leading to ATP depletion and subsequent cell death.[80] Norcocaine concentrations have been shown to be present in greater concentrations in cholinesterase-deficient subjects[354] and in simultaneous cocaine and ethanol users.[237]

Anhydroecgonine methyl ester (AEME; methyl ecgonidine) has been identified as a unique COC metabolite after smoked COC ("crack") administration. Anhydroecgonine ethyl ester (AEEE; ethyl ecgonidine) has been identified in COC smokers who also use ethyl alcohol.[164,381,741]

Pharmacologic Response

Cocaine has cardiovascular effects and is a potent CNS stimulant that elicits a state of increased alertness and euphoria[361] with actions similar to those of amphetamine but of shorter duration.[123] These CNS effects are thought to be largely associated with the ability of cocaine to block dopamine reuptake at nerve synapses, thereby prolonging the action of dopamine in the CNS. It is this response that leads to recreational abuse of cocaine. Cocaine also blocks the reuptake of norepinephrine at presynaptic nerve terminals; this produces a sympathomimetic response (including an increase in blood pressure, heart rate, and body temperature). Cocaine is effective as a local anesthetic and vasoconstrictor of mucous membranes and therefore is used clinically for nasal surgery, rhinoplasty, and emergency nasotracheal intubation.

The CNS and cardiovascular effects of cocaine exhibit acute tolerance; its effects are more pronounced when the concentration of cocaine in blood is increasing than when it is at a similar but decreasing concentration.[13,378] Thus, a clockwise hysteresis is observed when the blood concentration of cocaine is plotted against its CNS or cardiovascular effects over time. This phenomenon mitigates against attempts to correlate isolated blood concentration values with psychomotor effects. Because rate of change is probably more significant than absolute concentration, the psychomotor stimulant effects of cocaine are dependent both on dose and on route of administration, with IV administration and smoking resulting in the most rapid rates of increase in concentration.

Acute cocaine toxicity produces a sympathomimetic response that may result in (1) mydriasis, (2) diaphoresis, (3) hyperactive bowel sounds, (4) tachycardia, (5) hypertension, (6) hyperthermia, (7) hyperactivity, (8) agitation, (9) seizures, or (10) coma. Sudden death due to cardiotoxicity may occur following cocaine use. Death may also occur following the sequential development of hyperthermia, agitated delirium, and respiratory arrest. Excited delirium and extreme physical activity may lead to rhabdomyolysis, acute renal failure, and disseminated intravascular coagulopathy.

COC is frequently used with other drugs, most commonly ethanol. In simultaneous COC and ethanol use, liver methylesterase catalyzes the conversion of COC to BE and the transesterification of COC to CE in the presence of ethyl alcohol.[326,361,377] This reaction occurs about 3.5 times faster than hydrolysis to BE.[99] COC administered with ethanol produced greater euphoria and enhanced perception of well-being relative to COC.[361,528] CE appears to be equipotent to cocaine with regard to dopamine transporter affinity[326] but is less potent than cocaine pharmacologically.[323,634] As a consequence, large amounts of COC and ethanol may be ingested, placing users at greater risk for toxicity than if either drug were used alone. The elimination half-life for cocaethylene is longer than that for cocaine.[369,378] This longer elimination half-life may contribute to the toxicity of cocaethylene. Additionally, with simultaneous administration of COC and ethanol, the production of NC may be increased, along with the potential for toxicity.[237,362,441] It has been suggested that simultaneous COC and ethanol use carries an 18- to 25-fold increase in risk for immediate death over COC alone.[20,361,528,796]

Analytical Methods

The elimination half-life for cocaine varies from 0.5 to 1.5 hours, for ecgonine methyl ester from 3 to 4 hours, and for benzoylecgonine from 4 to 7 hours.[5-7] The principal urinary metabolites are benzoylecgonine and ecgonine methyl ester. Only small amounts of cocaine are excreted in urine. The elimination half-life for cocaethylene is 2.5 to 6 hours,[19,218,221] which is considerably longer than that for cocaine. This longer elimination half-life may contribute to the toxicity of cocaethylene.

BE excretion is detectable for 1 to 3 days following cocaine use. However, for chronic heavy cocaine users, the detection time may extend to 10 to 22 days following the last dose,[831] apparently because of tissue storage of cocaine. Ordinarily, cocaine may be detected in urine by chromatographic methods for only about 8 to 12 hours after use, but in heavy chronic users, this detection period may last 4 to 5 days.[169] These facts should be considered when the results of urine drug testing for individuals in drug treatment programs are interpreted. A positive urine drug test for benzoylecgonine beyond 3 days after the last dose does not necessarily indicate continued use. For such purposes, it is better to monitor quantitatively the urinary excretion of benzoylecgonine, normalized to creatinine, over time.[768] Drug abstinence would be indicated by decreasing urinary excretion of cocaine metabolites. However, creatinine normalization may not always reliably indicate reuse.[656]

The initial screening test for cocaine (BE) is typically immunoassay. For confirmation of a presumptive positive, BE is quantified by GC-MS.

Screening. The half-life of cocaine is 0.5 to 1.5 hours, of ecgonine methyl ester 3 to 4 hours, and of BE 4 to 7 hours.[376] Thus, BE is the analyte of choice in screening for cocaine use.[362] The initial screening test for BE is typically immunoassay, and screening immunoassays frequently apply a 300-ng/mL cutoff.

Confirmation. Most confirmation assays offer quantification of both parent drug and metabolite. Numerous methods have been described for the measurement of COC and various metabolites. GC techniques for analysis of COC and its metabolites require derivatization, especially of polar metabolites. Early detection techniques have included flame ion detection (FID), EC, and nitrogen-phosphorous detector (NPD).* GC-MS is the method of choice for many laboratories.† Some methods have included not only COC and BE, but also clinically and forensically relevant secondary metabolites such as m-HOBE, CE, NC, AEME, and AEEE.[164,399,435,622] The use of LC-based separation techniques that detect COC, BE, and CE has been described previously, including LC-UV detection,[517,543,760] as well as LC-DAD.[147] LC-MS/MS methods have also been described, including COC, BE, and m-HOBE,‡ along with other relevant secondary metabolites such as CE, NC, AEME, and AEEE.[460] Reports have suggested that AEME is not a truly unique indicator of smoked cocaine use, because it has been reported to be produced in the injector port of a GC[370,495,776] at high temperatures. However, less than 1% generation of AEME occurs if the injector port of the GC is maintained at 250 °C.[164] In an LC method, high temperatures are not present in the injector or in any other part of the LC; therefore, AEME is not generated, and its presence identifies a smoked route of COC use.

Lysergic Acid Diethylamide (LSD)

LSD shares structural features with serotonin (5-hydroxytryptamine; Figure 35-15), a major CNS neurotransmitter and neuromodulator.[32,857] LSD is synthesized from D-lysergic acid, a naturally occurring ergot alkaloid found in the fungus *Claviceps purpurea,* which grows on wheat and other grains. During synthesis, some LSD epimerizes to iso-LSD, which is inactive.[649]

*References 373, 379, 440, 603, 807, and 817.

†References 174, 190, 335, 363, 733, and 747.

‡References 242, 380, 384, 436, 578, 677, and 763.

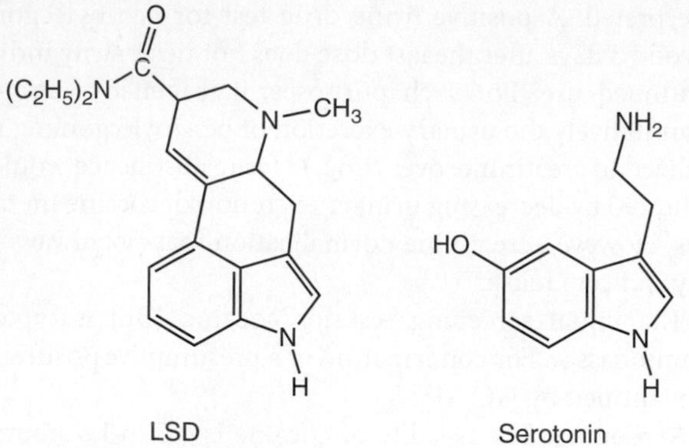

Figure 35-15 Chemical structure of lysergic acid diethylamide (LSD) and serotonin.

Pharmacologic Response

LSD is an extremely potent psychedelic ergot alkaloid derived from the fungus, *Claviceps purpurea*.[32] The drug LSD binds to serotonin receptors in the CNS and acts as a serotonin agonist. The principal psychological effects of LSD are perceptual distortions of color, sound, distance, and shape; depersonalization and loss of body image; and rapidly changing emotions from ecstasy to depression or paranoia. These hallucinogenic actions of LSD are stereoselective, elicited only by the D-isomer. A resurgence has occurred in the use of LSD, previously popular as a drug of abuse during the 1960s. The Department of Defense includes LSD among the drugs for which urine testing is required (see Table 35-7).

The physiologic effects of LSD are related to its sympathomimetic actions and include mydriasis (most frequent and consistent), tachycardia, increased body temperature, diaphoresis, and hypertension; at higher doses, parasympathomimetic actions may be observed [e.g., salivation, lacrimation, nausea, vomiting (muscarinic actions)]. Neuromuscular effects may include paresthesia, muscle twitches, and incoordination (nicotinic actions).[32,857]

The most common adverse effects of LSD are panic attacks. In addition, unpredictable recurrence of hallucinations (flashbacks) may occur weeks or months after last drug use, and LSD may elicit psychotic reactions (thought disorders, hallucinations, depression, and depersonalization). LSD is used illicitly because of its hallucinogenic effects. No evidence suggests that repeated LSD use results in dependence or withdrawal symptoms.[32,857]

Popular dosage forms include powder, gelatin capsule, tablet, and LSD-impregnated sugar cubes, filter paper, or postage stamps. The drug is rapidly absorbed from the GI tract; the effects begin within 40 to 60 minutes, peak at about 2 to 4 hours, and subside by 6 to 8 hours. The elimination $t_{1/2}$ is about 3 hours. The metabolism of LSD in humans is incompletely understood, but 2-oxo-3-hydroxy-LSD is present in urine at concentrations 10- to 43-fold greater than LSD.[642,643,649,672] *N*-demethyl-LSD is also present in urine specimens, but at concentrations approximately equivalent to those of LSD. The other metabolites are among those identified in animals, but as yet not conclusively identified in man.[649] Iso-LSD is not a metabolite but is formed by nonenzymatic epimerization of LSD during synthesis or storage of urine at alkaline pH and elevated temperature.[700]

The clinical effects of LSD ingestion are usually benign and require no medical intervention. However, panic attacks may be severe and require treatment with diazepam; LSD-induced psychosis has been treated with haloperidol. Rare cases of massive overdose have resulted in life-threatening hyperthermia, rhabdomyolysis, acute renal failure, hepatic failure, disseminated intravascular coagulation (DIC), respiratory arrest, and coma. Few if any well-documented deaths directly related to LSD ingestion have been reported.

Analytical Methods

Because of the very high potency of LSD, and therefore a low typical dose (20 to 80 μg) and rapid and extensive metabolism, only about 1 to 2% of the drug is excreted unchanged in urine.[672] Thus, detection of LSD presents an especially difficult analytical challenge. Even with sensitive assays, the detection window for LSD is generally only 12 to 24 hours.[672]

Immunoassays are targeted to detect LSD at the usual cutoff concentration of 500 pg/mL. Confirmation is typically performed by GC-MS[256,624] at the U.S. Department of Defense established cutoff concentration of 200 pg/mL. Although the metabolites 2-oxo-3-hydroxy-LSD and *N*-demethyl LSD generally cross-react only when present at about 100 to 200 times the amount in LSD,[841] other metabolites may potentially account for some instances of nonconfirmed positive immunoassay response.[152,859] However, true false-positive results due to various therapeutic drugs may occur.[152,675,841] The detection window may be extended, perhaps twofold to threefold, by including 2-oxo-3-hydroxy-LSD in the confirmatory test, using sensitive techniques such as GC-MS-MS,[672] LC-MS-MS,[643] or LC-MS.[434,642] Likewise, detection of iso-LSD in addition to LSD may extend the detection interval.[146] Urine specimens should be protected from sunlight, bright fluorescent light, or elevated temperature at alkaline pH to avoid degradation of LSD[478] and 2-oxo-3-hydroxy-LSD or epimerization of LSD to iso-LSD.[478,700]

Drugs Used in Sexual Assault

Drug-facilitated sexual assault (DFSA) is defined as voluntary or surreptitious use of alcohol, drugs, and/or chemical agents to incapacitate an individual and facilitate sexual assault.[315] In addition to alcohol, the drugs most often implicated in drug-facilitated sexual assault include (1) choral hydrate, (2) flunitrazepam, (3) nonbenzodiazepine sedative-hypnotics, (4) gamma-hydroxybutyric acid (GHB), (5) dextramethorphan, (6) ketamine, (7) phencyclidine, and (8) benzodiazepines, and nonprescription medications such as (9) antihistamines and (10) anticholinergics (Box 35-3). These drugs share similar characteristics that are desired by an assailant such as fast onset, colorlessness, tastelessness, and easy access. Similar clinical effects permit the victim to be easily incapacitated. They include impaired judgment, confusion, reduced inhibitions, sedation, hypnosis, loss of muscle coordination, and sometimes anterograde amnesia. These

BOX 35-3 Examples of Agents Used in Drug-Facilitated Sexual Assault

Anticholinergics
Antihistamines
Barbiturates
Benzodiazepines
Chloral hydrate
Dextromethorphan
Ethanol
γ-Hydroxybutyrate (GHB)
Ketamine
Opioids
Sedative-hypnotics

effects are intensified when they are coadministered willingly or involuntarily with other psychotropic medications that produce CNS depression. This is a common occurrence in reported cases of sexual assault or rape.[232,336]

Choral Hydrate

Anecdotal reports concerning assailants dosing beverages with incapacitating compounds to assault their victims date back to the early nineteenth century. An infamous example is the saloon proprietor Mickey Finn. He was alleged to have drugged his customers with the addition of chloral hydrate to their ethanol-based beverages and to have subsequently robbed them.

Chloral hydrate is classified as a nonbarbiturate hypnotic. It is an inexpensive transparent crystalline compound that easily dissolves in beverages. It was first synthesized in 1832 and was one of the original "depressants" developed for the specific purpose of inducing sleep. This drug is still used today in pediatric medicine for sedating children before diagnostic procedures. Abuse and misuse of this drug and subsequent introduction of newer sedatives (barbiturates and benzodiazepines) led to its decline for medicinal purposes.

Pharmacologic Effects

The clinical diagnosis of chloral hydrate intoxication is difficult to differentiate from alcohol, benzodiazepine, and barbiturate intoxication, as all share similar clinical effects. Although the exact mechanism of action of chloral hydrate has not been determined, it is a general CNS depressant that has sedative effects with minimal analgesic effects when administered independently. At low doses (<20 mg/kg), symptoms may include relaxation, dizziness, slurred speech, confusion, disorientation, euphoria, irritability, and hypersensitivity rash. At higher doses (>50 mg/kg), chloral hydrate causes hypotension, hypothermia, hypoventilation, tachydysrhythmias, nausea, vomiting, diarrhea, headache, and amnesia.[690] Onset of action is rapid (10 to 20 minutes). The elimination half-life of choral hydrate is 4 to 12 hours.[93,690] If coingested with alcohol, the metabolism of chloral hydrate may be seriously impaired. Because both ethanol and chloral hydrate are metabolized by CYP2E1 and alcohol dehydrogenase, coingestion may not only exacerbate their clinical effects, but may also prolong their duration of action.[93,587]

Analytical Methods

Chloral hydrate is not detected on routine, commercially available drug screens. Quantification of chloral hydrate and its metabolites trichloroethanol (TCE), TCE-glucuronide, and trichloroacetic acid is detected in plasma using HPLC-MS and capillary gas chromatography with electron-capture detection (GC-ECD),[352,546,710] or GC-flame ion detection (GC-FID).[393] Typical therapeutic concentrations are 2 to 12 µg/mL. Chloral hydrate metabolites have been detected as low as 10 ng/mL using GC-ECD.[352]

Flunitrazepam

It is estimated that 8% of sexual assault cases are positive for benzodiazepines.[232,336,582,581] Flunitrazepam (Rohypnol) is the most frequently reported benzodiazepine used in DFSA, partially because of the development and implementation of specific toxicologic tests in response to increased public awareness, resulting in a testing bias.[219,232,600,705,729] Other benzodiazepines that have been reported in sexual assault victims are diazepam, triazolam, temazepam, tetrazepam, and clonazepam.[4,134,398,507,581]

Flunitrazepam is a fast-acting sedative-hypnotic categorized as a Schedule I drug in the United States. Because it is still licensed for use in Europe, Asia, and Latin America for sedation and treatment of insomnia, sexual predators can acquire this drug through illegal trafficking.[822] Sexual assault predators use flunitrazepam because it can be easily dissolved into a beverage, it is relatively tasteless and odorless, it will quickly incapacitate their victims, and routine drug screens do not detect its presence.

Pharmacologic Effects

Flunitrazepam is more potent than diazepam because of its slower dissociation from the GABA receptor.[137,520,521] It is rapidly absorbed and distributed into tissues upon oral administration. Onset of its sedative, amnesic, hypnotic, and disinhibitory effects can occur within 20 to 30 minutes.[520] Flunitrazepam has a long half-life (≈26 hours), permitting an extended window of detection in blood and urine.

Although the effects of flunitrazepam occur rapidly when used alone, it is often coingested with alcohol, which amplifies its effects.[209,720] Initial symptoms may consist of dizziness, disorientation, lack of coordination, and slurred speech, all of which mimic alcohol intoxication. Another unique effect is anterograde amnesia as early as 15 minutes after oral administration.[294] Rapid alternation of hot and cold flashes may be followed precipitously by loss of consciousness. Large doses (>2 g) have produced aspiration, muscular hypotonia, hypotension, bradycardia, coma, and death.[134,507,716]

Analytical Methods

The detection of flunitrazepam is especially challenging because of the low therapeutic and illicit doses and the low degree of cross-reactivity of most immunoassays with the principal urinary metabolite, 7-aminoflunitrazepam.[518,699,743] As for other benzodiazepines, prior glucuronidase hydrolysis may improve immunoassay detection. Enzyme-linked immunosorbent assay (ELISA) methods with high selectivity for 7-aminoflunitrazepam and low limits of detection have been developed.[821,824] Direct analysis or confirmation of 7-aminoflunitrazepam by GC-MS or LC-MS/MS is indicated in suspected cases of flunitrazepam ingestion.[230,824,863] Flunitrazepam metabolites are detectable as early as 7 days in hair samples (HPLC-MS/MS).[134] Deposition and stability of a drug in hair samples are variable, depending on the route of exposure and the chemical characteristics.

Nonbenzodiazepine Sedative-Hypnotics

Zopiclone, eszopiclone (Lunesta), zolpidem (Ambien), and zaleplon (Sonata) belong to a new generation of sedative-hypnotics that are structurally different from benzodiazepines (Figure 35-16). Similar to benzodiazepines, these drugs modulate the $GABA_A$ receptor chloride channel by binding to the benzodiazepine (BZ) receptors, otherwise known as the $omega_1$ (ω_1) receptors, in the brain[812] without binding to peripheral BZ receptors.[703,721] Therefore, these drugs have fewer muscle relaxant properties.[721]

Most of the nonbenzodiazepine sleep aids are available through a prescription as a Schedule IV drug and are readily prescribed, shared, and sold illegally. The rapid-onset and amnesic properties of this class of drugs can result in disinhibition, passivity, and retrograde amnesia, making it a favored DFSA drug. These drugs require only a low dosage to cause an effect and are rapidly metabolized. Because of the amnesic properties of these drugs, victims are often confused following the event and may be delayed in reporting their sexual assault. Commonly utilized drug screens do not test for these substances.

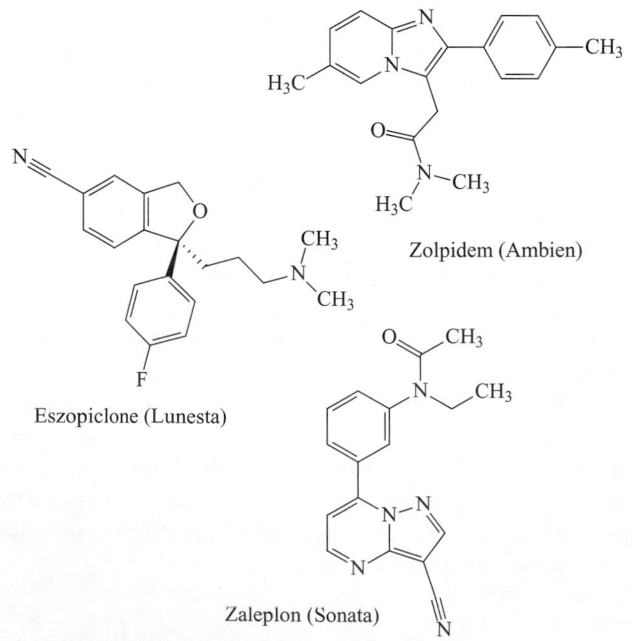

Figure 35-16 Chemical structures of the nonbenzodiazepine sedative-hypnotics (zolpidem, eszopiclone, zaleplon).

Recognition of these new-generation sleep aids as agents potentially used in facilitating sexual assault has been reported in the United States, the United Kingdom, and France for over a decade.[17,232,295,336,716] Yet only two published reports in the United States tested sexual assault victims for the presence of zolpidem.[429,805]

All may produce additive CNS-depressant effects when coadministered with other psychotropic medications such as anticonvulsants, antihistamines, ethanol, and other drugs that produce CNS depression.

Pharmacologic Effects

Examples of nonbenzodiazepine sedative-hypnotics include (1) zolpidem, (2) zaleplon, (3) eszopiclone, and (4) zopiclone.

Zolpidem. The pharmacologic effects of Zolpidem (Ambien) are believed to result from its interaction with a specific subtype of $GABA_A$ receptor complex consisting of α_1-subunits.[319] It is available as an immediate- or extended-release tablet. After an average oral dose of 10 to 15 mg, onset of effects occurs in 10 and 30 minutes. Clinical effects peak at approximately 1.5 hours for immediate release, duration is about 6 to 8 hours for both immediate- and extended-release preparations, and the $t_{1/2}$ is approximately 2.5 hours.[23] Evidence of minimal respiratory depression is noted when used as a single agent, but it may produce additive CNS-depressive effects and death when coadministered with other sedatives.[289]

Zaleplon. Zaleplon (Sonata) is available as an immediate-release tablet or capsule. After an average oral dose of 10 to 15 mg onset of effects occurs in approximately 10 to 30 minutes. Although the $t_{1/2}$ for zaleplon is about 1 hour, the duration of clinical effects may persist for longer than 6 hours. This may be due to the higher affinity of zaleplon for specific α_2- and α_3-subunits of the GABA receptor, in contrast to zolpidem or zopiclone.[277] At higher doses (>40 to 60 mg), its use may cause increased central nervous system effects and impaired motor skills.[690]

Eszopiclone. The exact mechanism of action of eszopiclone (Lunesta) is unknown, but its effect is believed to result from interaction with $GABA_A$ receptor complexes containing α_1- to α_5-subunits.[319] After an average dose of 2 to 3 mg onset of effects occurs in approximately 30 minutes. Both immediate- and extended-release forms are available. The clinical effects of eszopiclone are longer in duration compared with those of zopiclone or zolpidem, with a $t_{1/2}$ of 6 hours.[703]

Zopiclone. Zopiclone is not currently available in the United States. It is the racemic mixture of two stereoisomers; the active stereoisomer is eszopiclone. Therefore, clinical effects are similar to those of eszopiclone.

Analytical Methods

Because of the amnesic properties of these drugs, victims often may not report their sexual assault for several days. Therefore, sensitive analytical techniques are necessary to detect these drugs and their metabolites in urine or hair samples after a single dose. Although these drugs do not cross-react with most benzodiazepine immunoassays, specific reagent systems (ELISA) directed against the non-benzodiazepine hypnotics are available.[668] Screening and confirmation are performed by GC-MS or LC-MS/MS.

γ-Hydroxybutyrate, 1,4-butanediol, and γ-butyrolactone

γ-Hydroxybutyrate (GHB) and its synthetic precursor compounds, 1,4-butanediol (1,4-BD) and γ-butyrolactone (GBL), are Schedule I agents in the United States, and availability is restricted in numerous other countries. GHB is illegally purchased as an odorless and colorless liquid form, or as an off-white powder that easily dissolves in liquids. When ingested, GHB stimulates dopamine release, leading to pleasurable effects such as euphoria, muscle relaxation, and heightened sexual desire.[74,180] It also has CNS depressant effects, resulting in sedation and hypnosis. Because GHB was reported to enhance growth hormone release, it has been used by body builders and athletes as a steroid alternative. Athletes have used GHB as a sleep aid because they believe it promotes rapid recovery from vigorous repetitive competition. These properties and the availability of GHB in dietary supplements have led to growing recreational abuse of the drug. GHB has become popular as a euphorigenic club drug, most often used in combination with alcohol, and also with MDMA or cocaine, to "mellow" their adverse stimulant properties. Its rapid onset and hypnotic and short-term amnestic properties have resulted in the use of GHB for drug-facilitated sexual assault (date rape drug).[201,295,716,737] Publications estimate that 4% of alleged sexual assault cases in the United States are positive for GHB.[225,232,716,729]

GHB is a naturally occurring substance produced in the brain. GHB is reversibly metabolized to GABA through multiple endogenous enzymes (Figure 35-17).[202,503,797] Illicit consumption of GHB, or the synthetic GHB precursor compound 1,4-BD or GBL, will promote GABA activity.[202] In addition to increased metabolism to GABA, GHB has direct effects on the CNS by binding GHB-specific receptors and $GABA_B$ receptors.[74,410,439,862] The latter are G-protein–coupled receptors distinct from the $GABA_A$ receptors for depressant drugs, such as benzodiazepines and barbiturates. Of note, patients with GHB overdose do not respond to the opioid antagonist naloxone or to the benzodiazepine antagonist flumazenil.

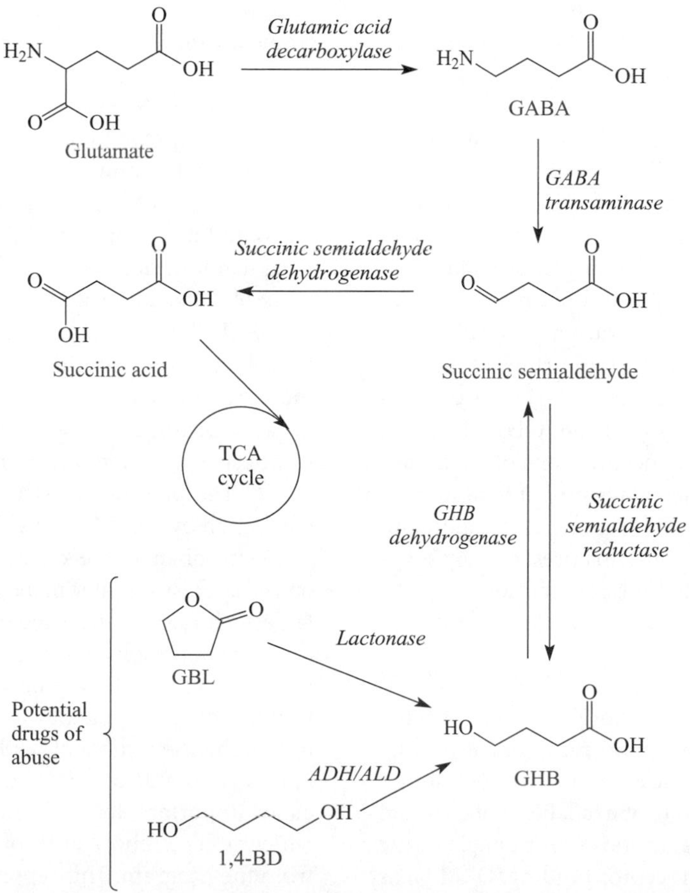

Figure 35-17 Metabolism of γ-hydroxybutyrate. γ-Hydroxybutyrate (GHB) and its synthetic precursor compounds, 1,4-butanediol (1,4-BD) and γ-butyrolactone (GBL), are often used illicitly. These drugs are endogenously metabolized to γ-aminobutyric acid (GABA). GHB and GABA mediate GABA receptors.

Fomepizole, an inhibitor of alcohol dehydrogenase, is likely beneficial for patients who ingest 1,4-butanediol.[878] GHB is suggested to increase dopamine concentrations in the substantia nigra, to potentiate the endogenous opioid system, and to mediate GABA transmission.[202]

Pharmacologic Effects

Onset of GHB effects occurs in approximately 15 to 30 minutes, depending on the dose (average, 1 to 5 g) and the chemical purity. The duration of response is short, typically 1 to 3 hours for normal dose and 2 to 4 hours with excessive doses. The clinical effects are dose dependent and typically last 3 to 6 hours. A low dose (<1 g) produces mild symptoms such as CNS depression, amnesia, hypotonia, and reduced inhibitions (similar to alcohol). Larger doses (1 to 2 g) cause increased somnolence, drowsiness, dizziness, bradycardia, and bradypnea. High doses (>2 g) often interfere with motor coordination and balance and may induce significant respiratory depression and bradypnea, Cheyne-Stokes respiration, nausea, and vomiting, diminished cardiac output, seizures, coma, and death.[289,514,804] Periods of agitation may be interspersed between times of apnea and unresponsiveness. It is uncertain whether this agitation is a direct GHB effect or a consequence of coingested stimulant drugs. Deaths have been reported but are almost always associated with coingestion of alcohol or other drugs.

Analytical Methods

GHB is metabolized rapidly ($t_{1/2}$ ≈30 minutes) and currently is not detected on immunoscreens. GHB is identified on urine and serum specimens using GC-FID or GC-MS.[225,430,531] Because GBH is metabolized rapidly, timely sample collection is an important facet of GBH assay; plasma samples should be collected within 6 to 8 hours after ingestion, and urine samples within 10 to 12 hours. Urine and plasma concentrations may exhibit endogenous concentrations of GHB within 8 to 12 hours after ingestion (<1 mg/dL in urine; <4 mg/L in blood/plasma).[868] Samples approaching endogenous concentrations make it difficult to legally associate GHB doping in sexual assault cases. Exogenous concentrations of GHB have been detected in hair samples at 7 days post intoxication.[295] Timely presentation of the patient for medical attention and physician recognition of GHB symptoms presented by sexually assaulted victims are essential for prosecution of sexual offenders.

Dextromethorphan

Dextromethorphan (DXM) is structurally related to the opioids, but it does not bind to opioid receptors at normal dose and thus is devoid of analgesic activity.[585] The (−) isomer of dextromethorphan, levorphan (not available in the United States), is a potent opioid analgesic and is an example of the stereoselective nature of opioid receptor binding. DXM lacks analgesic activity but does have antitussive activity comparable with that of codeine. At high doses, DXM binds opioid receptors to produce miosis, respiratory depression, and CNS depression. High doses may also cause lethargy, agitation, ataxia, nystagmus, diaphoresis, and hypertension.[594,851,870]

DXM is present in various over-the-counter (OTC) cough medications, often in combination with antihistamines, nasal decongestants, guaifenesin, aspirin, and acetaminophen. Potential toxicity from OTC combination medications must be considered when DXM is consumed in large doses to achieve euphoric effects.[41,432] Abuse of DXM, especially by adolescents and teenagers, who refer to it as "Dex, Robos, Skittles," has become widespread. Abusers describe feelings of euphoria, dissociative effects such as a sense of floating, and hallucinations. Discontinuation of the drug is frequently followed by dysphoria and depression.

Pharmacologic Effects

Dextromethorphan is metabolized to dextrophan[649] by the cytochrome P450 isozyme 2D6 (CYP2D6), which exhibits genetic polymorphisms. Dextrophan may be responsible for the more pleasant psychotropic effects of high-dose dextromethorphan, whereas the parent drug may cause dysphoria, sedation, and ataxia.[870] Thus, poor metabolizers (deficient in CYP2D6 activity) may be less prone and extensive metabolizers more prone to continue the abuse of dextromethorphan. Dextrophan and to a lesser degree DXM bind to the PCP- and ketamine-binding site on the NMDA receptor, causing sedation; this may account for their similar dissociative psychotropic actions[585] (see phencyclidine and ketamine sections).

Analytical Methods

Clinically approved doses of DXM are not detected by most clinical opiate immunoassays,[755] but larger doses may cross-react.[740] However, ELISA assays are now available to detect DXM and its major metabolite, dextrorphan.[678] Some toxicologic laboratories have used the cross-reactivity of DXM with phencyclidine antibodies to screen for the presence of DXM.[709] Because most preparations contain dextromethorphan as the bromide salt, excessive ingestion of dextromethorphan may result in bromide poisoning and in a negative serum anion gap consequent to the disproportionate response to bromide with common methods of chloride analysis.[586] The presence of DXM or dextrophan in a sample is confirmed by GC-MS or LC-MS/MS.

Dextrophan is the enantiomer of levorphanol, a potent opioid agonist available in the United States (Levo-Dromoran). Unless chiral analytical techniques are used, these enantiomers are not resolved. Drug testing laboratories that use conventional chromatographic techniques should not report a finding of levorphanol only, but should instead report dextrophan/levorphanol, with a comment on their isomeric relationship and on the origin of dextrophan. This is especially important for pain management drug screening, in which a false report of levorphanol may result in dismissal from the program. This report duality is advisable even when parent dextromethorphan is also detected. Savvy abusers of levorphanol conceivably may coingest dextromethorphan to conceal use of levorphanol. If such is suspected, chiral resolution of dextrophan and levorphanol would then be necessary.

Ketamine and Phencyclidine

Ketamine and phencyclidine (PCP) are potent analgesics and general anesthetics used in veterinary medicine. PCP is listed as a Schedule II drug in the U.S. Federal Controlled Substance Act and is not approved for human use. Ketamine is a Schedule III drug, commonly used as an anesthetic in pediatric medicine for short surgical procedures. Both drugs have been used illicitly in human cases of drug abuse, as well as in cases of drug-facilitated sexual assault.

On the street, ketamine and PCP are sold under a variety of names. They are available as a colorless, odorless liquid, or as a white powder. Either form can be easily disguised in a victim's beverage. More commonly, these powdered agents are sprinkled onto marijuana or tobacco and smoked.

Pharmacologic Effects

Ketamine and PCP share similar structural features[649] and pharmacologic actions. They are classified as dissociative anesthetics because they produce rapid-acting dissociation of perception, consciousness, movement, and memory.[171,342,601] The effects are dose dependent and vary between individuals. Some individuals experience effects similar to the psychosis observed in schizophrenia.[11,664] An anesthetic dose produces profound analgesia, but the individual is awake yet incapacitated, with limited voluntary limb movement. Ketamine has about one tenth the potency of PCP, a shorter duration of action, and less prominent emergentce reactions, especially in children. Both PCP and ketamine have been associated with psychologic disturbances.

The mechanism of action for these compounds consists of complex integration of neurologic pathways. They bind and antagonize the excitatory glutaminergic system by binding to NMDA receptors. They also decrease GABA transmission, disrupt cortical activity, and increase dopamine and norepinephrine synaptic reuptake. These actions can produce clinical effects such as euphoria, elevated blood pressure, tachycardia, and bronchodilation, all of which are consequences of inhibition of dopamine and norepinephrine synaptic reuptake.[461,601] At a higher dose, GABA-ergic and central nicotinic actions may produce sedation, lethargy, coma, and respiratory depression. Additionally, central and peripheral muscarinic and nicotinic responses may cause miosis or mydriasis, diaphoresis, increased salivation, bronchorrhea, blurred vision, and urinary retention.

Phencyclidine. PCP [1-(1-**p**henyl**c**yclohexyl)-**p**iperidine] was synthesized in 1926 and was clinically utilized as a general anesthetic. Because of adverse side effects experienced by some individuals, such as acute psychosis and dysphoria during emergence from PCP-induced anesthesia, clinical use was discontinued. PCP is used recreationally for its mind-altering "out of body" experience. Recreational use of PCP declined in the 1980s but has re-emerged in recent years. Presentation of adverse effects such as (1) dysphoria, (2) ataxia, (3) nystagmus, (4) agitation, (5) anxiety, (6) paranoia, (7) amnesia, (8) seizures, (9) muscle rigidity, (10) hostility, (11) delirium, (12) delusions, and (13) hallucinations is unpredictable. LSD users can experience "flashbacks of the drug experience." Flashbacks occur suddenly, often without warning, and may occur within a few days or more than a year after LSD use.

The onset of action for PCP is fast for intravenous and inhalation routes (2 to 5 minutes) and slower following oral administration (30 to 60 minutes).[172,173] Clinical effects typically last 4 to 6 hours, yet psychotic episodes have been reported to last a month.[11,664] The relationship between dosage, clinical effects, and serum concentrations is not a reliable predictor of the degree of PCP intoxication.[601] PCP has a pK_a between 8.5 and 9.4, is highly lipophilic, and distributes to the brain and fat tissues. An ion-trapping phenomenon occurs after oral, IV, or inhalation dosing. PCP enters acidic gastric fluid after oral administration, where concentrations may be 20 to 50 times greater than in serum, then undergoes gastroenterohepatic recirculation.[857] Ion trapping also occurs in cerebrospinal fluid (CSF), causing it to cross back into the blood; CSF may accumulate to concentrations six to nine times greater than those observed in serum.[544] These properties may contribute to the waxing and waning of clinical effects and prolonged excretion. PCP has a large V_d of 5 to 7 L/kg, a long elimination $t_{1/2}$ (20 to 50 hours), a long duration of action (24 to 48 hours), and prolonged urinary excretion after the last dose (1 to 2 weeks; longer with long-term use).[857]

With repeated use of PCP, psychologic dependence may develop, but tolerance or withdrawal syndrome is not profound. A sense of superhuman strength coupled with lack of pain perception may lead to excessive physical exertion and accidental or intentionally induced trauma. Thus PCP-related deaths most often are secondary to these adverse behavioral drug effects. Treatment of PCP toxicity is supportive. Severe agitation or seizures may respond to diazepam; severe psychoses may require a neuroleptic drug, such as haloperidol. For the most serious cases, continuous nasogastric suction to help remove PCP may be beneficial; urine acidification to hasten elimination has been advocated by some but is controversial.[601]

Ketamine. Ketamine was discovered during subsequent studies characterizing PCP analogs. Liquid ketamine is rapidly injected intramuscularly. The liquid or powder form can be easily disguised in a victim's beverage; this has resulted in its use in DFSA.[716,737] Ketamine powder can even be sprinkled onto marijuana or tobacco and smoked.

Ketamine produces effects similar to those of phencyclidine. Onset of clinical effects is rapid and is dependent on dose and route of administration. Anesthesia effects via intramuscular injection take as little as 20 to 30 seconds, oral ingestion about 30 minutes,[301] and nasal insufflation approximately 10 minutes.[332,493,690] Its hallucinatory effects may be short-acting (<1 hour) but so intense that the victim may have trouble discerning reality.[737]

Ketamine has a $t_{1/2}$ of 2 to 3 hours.[148] Ketamine is metabolized to norketamine, which has about one third the activity of ketamine, and to dehydronorketamine, which also may be active.[649] Duration of anesthetic effects is dose dependent (usually <1 hour), and effects on the senses, judgment, and coordination can have a longer duration (≈6 to 24 hours). At higher doses, ketamine causes delirium, amnesia, dissociative anesthesia, hallucinations, delirium, hypersalivation, nystagmus, impaired motor function, hypertension, and potentially fatal respiratory problems. Effects on blood pressure and respiratory depression are significantly enhanced when coingested with alcohol.

Analytical Methods

Initial screening for PCP is typically done by immunoassay. Confirmation of a presumptive positive test is performed by GC-MS.[253] No immunoassays are available to detect ketamine at this time. Ketamine and its active metabolites are detected in urine samples using GC-MS or LC-MS analyses.[557]

Immunoassay. Quantification of PCP in serum is not helpful in the diagnosis or management of PCP toxicity because the correlation between drug concentration and drug effects is low.[601] However, qualitative identification of PCP in urine is useful to help diagnose PCP toxicity. For this purpose, PCP-specific immunoassays are rapid and generally are more sensitive than thin-layer chromatography. Whether or not PCP is included in a general urine drug screen depends on applicable regulations and on the prevalence of PCP use in the local community. In some locations, the prevalence of PCP use may be too low to warrant routine screening for PCP. Immunoassays for PCP are generally reliable; false positives have been reported because of high concentrations of dextromethorphan,[104,709] diphenhydramine,[476] and thioridazine.[490,814] Immunoassay-positive specimens should be confirmed using GC-MS.[253]

Gas Chromatography–Mass Spectrometry. PCP is required to be included in U.S. Government–regulated drug abuse screening programs (see Table 35-7); nongovernmental screening programs may elect to include PCP in drug abuse screens, depending on the local probability of PCP use. Initial screening by immunoassay, if positive, is followed by confirmation using GC-MS. Ketamine and its active metabolites norketamine and dehydronorketamine are detected in urine samples using GC-MS[132,420] or LC-MS analyses.[557]

Detection of Drugs of Abuse Using Other Types of Specimens

The collection of biological samples for the purpose of determining exposure to various agents is dominated by blood and urine. Blood is considered invasive, and the collection of urine may require some invasion of privacy and loss of dignity; urine specimens are subject to adulteration or manipulation to evade detection. For these reasons, alternate biological specimens have been investigated.[116,197A] Cutoff values had been proposed by SAMHSA[110] for some of the matrices and are listed in Table 35-8. However, current guidelines for Federal Workplace Drug Testing have determined that urine will continue to be the only biological fluid approved for testing.[239] An additional review conducted by DHHS is expected.

Meconium, oral fluid, hair, and sweat have been investigated as alternative types of samples for drug analysis.

Meconium

Illicit drug use during pregnancy is a major social and medical issue. Drug abuse during pregnancy is associated with significant perinatal complications, including a high incidence of (1) stillbirth, (2) meconium-stained fluid, (3) premature rupture of the membranes, (4) maternal hemorrhage (abruptio placentae or placenta previa), and (5) fetal distress.[607] In the neonate, the mortality rate and morbidity (e.g., asphyxia, prematurity, low birth weight, hyaline membrane disease, infection, aspiration pneumonia, cerebral infarction, abnormal heart rate and breathing patterns, drug withdrawal) are increased.[607]

Unfortunately, identification of the drug-exposed mother or her neonate is not easy. Maternal admission of the use of drugs is often inaccurate principally because of denial about addiction or fear of the consequences stemming from such admission. Likewise, many infants who have been exposed to drugs in utero may appear normal at birth and show no overt manifestations of drug effects. Thus, identification of the drug-exposed mother or her infant requires a high index of suspicion. Drug testing, on the other hand, is an objective means of determining drug exposure in both mother and infant. In infants, drug testing is necessary to document proof of the infant's exposure to illicit drugs. Urine testing of the mother or newborn can detect only recent drug use (within a few days before birth), and urine collection from newborns may be problematic.

The first intestinal discharge from newborns is meconium, which is a viscous, dark green substance composed of intestinal secretions, desquamated squamous cells, lanugo hair, bile pigments, and blood. Meconium also contains pancreatic enzymes, free fatty acids, porphyrins, interleukin-8, and phospholipase A_2 primary bile acids with a small quantity of secondary bile acids. Water is the major liquid constituent, making up 85 to 95% of meconium.[7] Meconium is derived from the Greek word "mekonion," meaning poppy juice or opium. Aristotle is credited with noting the relationship between the presence of meconium in amniotic fluid and a sleepy fetal state in utero.[7] Meconium begins to form during the second trimester and continues to accumulate until birth; drugs taken by the mother can be detected in the meconium of the newborn.[608]

The disposition of drug in meconium is not well understood. The proposed mechanism is that the fetus excretes drug into bile and amniotic fluid. Drug accumulates in meconium by direct deposition from bile or through swallowing of amniotic fluid.[229,608] The first evidence of meconium in the fetal intestine appears at approximately the 10th to 12th week of gestation; meconium slowly moves into the colon by the 16th week of gestation.[7] Therefore, the presence of drugs in meconium has been proposed to be indicative of in utero drug exposure up to 5 months before birth—a longer historical measure than is possible by urinalysis.[608]

Meconium has been used for detection of prenatal drug use, showing an improved drug detection rate compared with urine.[114,477,572,608] The collection of meconium is noninvasive, making sample collection easy,[693] and is more successful than urine collection.[527] The amount collected is usually sufficient for complete analysis, including confirmation. Meconium testing does have some limitations. Meconium is usually passed by full-term newborns within 24 to 48 hours, after which transition from a blackish-green color to a yellow color indicates the beginning of passage of neonatal stool. Infants with low birth weight (<1000 g) have been shown to pass their first meconium at a median age of 3 days. Thus, meconium collection is missed because of delayed passage, and meconium may not be available soon after birth for early detection of intrauterine drug exposure.

In the clinical laboratory, meconium is an unfamiliar matrix; it is a sticky material that is more difficult to work with than urine. Meconium drug screening has been adapted to various analytical techniques, including radioimmunoassay, enzyme immunoassay, and fluorescence polarization immunoassay. Urine drugs-of-abuse screening assays frequently use meconium extracts and therefore must be investigated for possible effects of matrix on accuracy, precision, and assay linearity. However, some other immunoassays screening methods have been used.

Radioimmunoassay (RIA), fluorescence polarization immunoassay (FPIA), enzyme multiplied immunoassay technique (EMIT), and enzyme-linked immunosorbent assay (ELISA) have been used for detection of drugs in meconium, but ELISA is rapidly becoming the method of choice for screening.[272] The sample preparation for the ELISA screen is usually a simple buffer extraction versus a lengthy and more laborious sample preparation procedure for the other immunoassay methods.

As with any immunoassay-based drug screen, confirmation by MS is critical. Confirmation assays for meconium are more difficult than those for urine. Recovery of drugs from meconium is sometimes low (30 to 50%). A variety of GC-MS, LC-MS, and LC-MS/MS methods and their advantages and disadvantages have been described elsewhere[272,477,555] and will not be discussed here.

Many questions remain to be answered about the disposition of drugs in meconium. Some debate continues as to which are the most appropriate drug analytes to measure in meconium; Table 35-12 attempts to summarize the current knowledge. Meconium drug testing is growing but is far less standardized than urine drug testing. Assay cutoff limits and units (ng/g meconium or ng/mL of extract) may vary; suitable reference or control materials are not yet available.

Meconium should be sent to the laboratory for processing as soon as it is collected to prevent possible loss of drugs. Meconium, allowed to stand at room temperature for 24 hours, showed a decrease in cocaine and cannabinoid concentrations.[607] However, suspending meconium in an organic solvent, such as buffered methanol, may prevent decreases for as long as 72 hours.[607] For prolonged storage, meconium should be frozen. Drugs are stable in meconium, frozen at −15 °C, for as long as 9 months.[607]

TABLE 35-12 Drugs and Metabolites of Significance in Meconium

Drug Class	Confirmation Compound[69,229,474,555]
Cocaine	cocaine
	benzoylecgonine
	cocaethylene
	m-hydroxybenzoylecgonine
Opiates	morphine
	codeine
	6-monoacetylmorphine (6-MAM)
	hydromorphone
	hydrocodone
	oxycodone
Cannabinoids	9-carboxy-11-nor-delta-9-THC
	11-hydroxy-delta-9-tetrahydrocannabinol
	8,11-dihydroxy-delta-9-tetrahydrocannabinol
Amphetamines	amphetamine
	methamphetamine
	MDMA
	MDA
	MDEA
Ethanol	fatty acid ethyl esters
PCP	PCP

Overinterpretation of meconium data is a dangerous practice. It is clear that matrix effects are associated with the analysis of meconium, as they are with each biological fluid or tissue.[474] Another important confounding factor is possible contamination of the meconium specimen by urine. Numerous reports have described the specificity and sensitivity of different analytes with the use of different testing methods.[454,455,527,607,609] A tremendous, and potentially inappropriate, value has been placed on a meconium result. On occasion, decisions about treatment or custody of the infant have been based solely on meconium drug screen results. It is critical to remember that a positive test could indicate intrauterine drug exposure. However, a negative result does not rule it out. It is clear that additional work is necessary to address these important issues and to improve our understanding of the disposition of drugs in meconium.[474]

Oral Fluid

Reports concerning the appearance of organic solutes in saliva have been included in the scientific literature for longer than 70 years.[726] Analysis of saliva for drugs was first used almost 30 years ago for the purpose of therapeutic drug monitoring.[344] It has since been evaluated for use in forensic toxicology, with recognition of its advantages over other biological matrices.[638A] Most studies on saliva in humans use whole saliva. The term "oral fluid" is preferred for the specimen collected from the mouth. Oral fluid is a complex fluid consisting not only of secretions from the three major pairs of salivary glands (parotid, submandibular, and sublingual), but also secretions from the minor glands (labial, buccal, and palatal), bacteria, sloughed epithelial cells, gingival fluid, food debris, and other particulate matter.[338] The concentration of drug from each secretion and the relative contributions of the various glands to the final fluid may vary.[726]

Biologically, before any drug circulating in plasma can enter the oral fluid, it must pass through the capillary wall, the basement membrane, and the membrane of the salivary gland epithelial cells. However, this fluid is not a simple ultrafiltrate of plasma, as has sometimes been suggested, but rather a complex fluid formed by different mechanisms, including ultrafiltration through pores in the membrane, active transport against a concentration gradient, and passive diffusion.*

Ethanol was the first drug of abuse to be investigated in oral fluid[261]; since then, many additional studies have expanded on our knowledge of this drug in it. Ethanol appears to reach a higher peak concentration in oral fluid than in peripheral blood. Because distribution of ethanol in the body is considered to occur by passive diffusion, under equilibrium conditions, ethanol content will be dependent upon the water content of the fluid or tissue being measured. The content in saliva therefore will be higher than that found in blood or serum. On a theoretical basis, the saliva-to-blood (S/B) ethanol ratio should be 1.17; however, lower ratios have been found in the postabsorption phase.[159,388]

In recent years, great interest has been expressed in the use of oral fluid testing for roadside drug screening, for monitoring the compliance of individuals on drug maintenance programs, and for workplace drug testing (see Table 35-8). Low concentrations of drugs and metabolites necessitate sensitive screening methods, which typically are immunoassays.[431] Again, the low concentrations of drugs have necessitated that confirmatory methods be equally as sensitive. Many confirmatory methods have been developed for oral fluid testing of abused drugs, including GC-MS, LC-MS and LC-MS/MS.† Specimens can be monitored for cannabinoids, cocaine, opiates, amphetamines, phencyclidine, methadone, barbiturates, and benzodiazepines. Interpretation of the presence and concentrations of these drugs in saliva and information on their use have been extensively reviewed elsewhere.[159,208,400,417,708]

Several advantages are associated with monitoring oral fluid as contrasted with monitoring plasma or serum concentrations.[749] Collection of oral fluid is considered to be a noninvasive procedure, and some of the risks associated with the drawing of blood are avoided. Furthermore, for the patient, fear, anxiety, and discomfort that may accompany the drawing of blood are diminished. Although some training and explanation are necessary to ensure proper gathering of oral fluid samples, the level of training needed for blood sampling is not required. In principle, oral fluid drug concentration is related to plasma free drug concentration, except when buccal contamination may have occurred because of oral ingestion, smoking, or snorting of the drug. Therefore oral fluid has the potential to show a relation between behavior/impairment and drug concentration, making it a possible medium for monitoring drug intoxication or for conducting therapeutic drug management.[431,459] On a related note, one significant disadvantage of oral fluid is that the window of detection is about equivalent to that of blood or serum and is short compared with that in urine.[712,713,749] Another disadvantage is the small volume of sample collected. The problem of small sample size can be overcome by using methods that simultaneously extract multiple drug groups.[431,865]

Hair

For more than 30 years, hair has been analyzed for trace metals, including lead, arsenic, and mercury. This was achieved using atomic absorption spectroscopy (see Chapters 10 and 36). At first, the examination of hair for organic substances, specifically drugs, was not possible because the analytical methods were not sensitive enough.[424] Baumgartner and associates in 1979[66] published the first report on the detection of morphine in the hair of heroin abusers using RIA. Since that time, interest in analysis of hair for the purpose of detecting drug use has increased.[67,356,416,422]

It is generally accepted that drugs enter hair by at least three mechanisms: (1) from blood that supplies the growing hair follicle, (2) through sweat and sebum, and (3) via the external environment.[396,424] The exact mechanism by which chemicals are incorporated into hair is not known. It has been suggested that passive diffusion may be augmented by binding of the drug to intracellular components of hair cells such as the hair pigment melanin. Specific binding of basic drugs to hair components is likely to involve both electrostatic attraction and weaker forces, such as van der Waals attraction. Neutral and acidic drugs presumably bind through weaker forces and possibly by other mechanisms.[160]

Factors that may affect how efficiently drugs are incorporated into hair are not well established but may include rate of hair growth, anatomic location of hair, hair color (melanin content), and hair texture (thick or fine, porous or not); these are determined by genetic factors and by the effects of various hair treatments.[424] For example, in vitro substantially higher binding was found with hair from black men than with hair from blond white men, suggesting that melanin pigment plays an important role in drug binding.[397] Studies have demonstrated that after the same dosage is given, black hair incorporates much more of the drug than is incorporated

*References 24, 105, 311, 338, 419, 498, 666, 806, and 877.

†References 136, 167, 262, 314, 382, 399, 408, 426, 427, 554, 577, 589, 602, 679, 701, 707, 708, 712, 764, and 854.

by blond hair.[329,339,449] This may lead to bias in hair testing for drugs of abuse and discussions about possible genetic variability of drug deposition in hair and is still under evaluation.

Drugs, when deposited in hair, are generally present in relatively low concentrations (pg/ng/µg/mg); thus sensitive analytical techniques are required for detection. Immunoassay procedures have been modified for use with hair.[424] Although GC-MS is generally the method of choice,[696] various GC-MS/MS or LC-MS/MS methods may be used for targeted analysis of low-dose compounds such as fentanyl, buprenorphine, and flunitrazepam.[450,451,697,787,829] These methods are also useful in the detection of some drugs or metabolites typically present in hair at trace concentrations such as THC-COOH[135,788] or in retrospective detection of drugs administered as single doses.[430,580,581,583]

As mentioned, external exposure to drugs causes them to be detected in hair, and because it is unlikely that anyone would intentionally or accidentally apply drugs of abuse to his or her own hair, the most crucial issue facing hair analysts today is technical and evidentiary false positives.[424] False positives may be caused during collection or after collection. Externally deposited substances easily contaminate the hair because of its high surface-to-volume ratio. Substances deposited in hair from the environment are loosely bound to the surface of the hair, and thus are removed by appropriate decontamination procedures. These usually involve a washing step.[67,424] It is fundamental to be able to distinguish between passive exposure (environmental contamination) and active consumption; consequently, decontamination procedures for hair are compulsory.[88] Needless to say, hair analysis is a complex scientific undertaking, and a comprehensive review on this topic has been published.[655]

Hair is advantageous as a biological specimen because it is easily obtained, with less embarrassment; it is not easily altered or manipulated to avoid drug detection. Hair also differs from other human materials used for toxicological analysis such as blood or urine in that it has a substantially longer detection window. Once deposited in hair, drugs are very stable, and analysis can be performed even after centuries.[653]

Hair also differs from other human materials used for toxicological analysis such as blood or urine because of its substantially longer detection window (months to years). Hair grows at a relatively constant rate. The average rate of hair growth is usually stated to be 0.44 mm per day (range, 0.38 to 0.48 mm/d) for men and 0.45 mm per day (range, 0.40 to 0.55/d) for women in the vertex region of the scalp.[573] The rate of hair growth depends on anatomic location, race, gender, and age. Scalp hair grows faster than pubic or axillary hair (≈0.3 mm/d), which in turn grows faster than beard hair (≈0.27 mm/d).[88] It is generally accepted that sectional hair analysis can be used to prove drug history.[88] Numerous forensic applications in which hair analysis was used to document the case have been described in the literature; these include (1) differentiation between a drug dealer and a drug consumer, (2) chronic poisoning, (3) crime under the influence of a drug, (4) child sedation and abuse, (5) suspicious death, (6) child custody, (7) abuse of drugs in jail, (8) body identification, (9) survey of drug addicts, (10) chemical submission, (11) obtaining a driver's license, and (12) doping control.[423,431,549,834]

Sweat

Drugs may be excreted in sweat, with the parent drug generally present in a greater amount than metabolites.[356,417] Moreover, sweat excretion may be an important mechanism by which drugs enter hair.[165]

Sweat patch collection devices that resemble an adhesive bandage may be worn for several days to several weeks; during this time, drug, if present, accumulates in the absorbent pad in the patch, while water vapor escapes through the semipermeable covering.[428] Thus sweat drug testing offers the possibility of monitoring drug use over extended periods of time without the need for frequent collection of urine.[108] Sweat drug testing would be particularly advantageous for monitoring drug use in correctional institutions or in drug rehabilitation programs.[425]

Athletes and Drug Testing

"Doping" in athletic competitions has a history of abuse in a variety of sports for centuries. Regulation of performance-enhancing substances was initiated in 1967 in response to the death of Danish cyclist, Knud Jensen, at the 1960 Olympic Games in Rome. After decades of reform between universal governments and sporting agencies, the World Anti-Doping Agency (WDA) was established in 1999. Currently, 36 facilities around the world are accredited by the International Organization for Standardization (ISO) for detecting drug use among competitive athletes.[122] Prohibited drugs are substances or methods that conform to two of three criteria: (1) performance enhancing, (2) may endanger the athlete's health, (3) go against the spirit of the sport. "In-competition" testing was established to detect drugs (stimulants, narcotics, cannabinoids, glucocorticosteroids) taken at the time of a competition to temporarily enhance performance. "Out-of-competition" testing is performed to detect substances and methods such as anabolic-androgenic steroids (AAS), hormones, hormone modulators, oxygen transfer enhancement, and gene transfer, whose performance-enhancing effects have a gradual onset to allow for more intense and efficient training; they can be abruptly discontinued before competition.[5,122]

Most testing for prohibited substance abuse is performed by GC-MS. Specialized testing such as isoelectric focusing ("double blotting") was implemented at the 2002 Salt Lake City Olympics to discriminate between endogenous and recombinant forms of erythropoietin.[121] Erythrocyte phenotyping by flow cytometry is used to detect homologous blood transfusions.[30,285,484] Limited windows of detection and individual biological variability for specific substances (especially hormones) are challenges faced when novel analytical methods are developed and validated. Tracking of specific clinical biomonitors (such as hormone or hormone-responsive protein concentrations) over an athlete's performance career, termed *biological passport* and *longitudinal profiling*, is currently under investigation.[584,660]

REFERENCES

1. Aabakken L, Johansen KS, Rydningen EB, Bredesen JE, Ovrebo S, Jacobsen D. Osmolal and anion gaps in patients admitted to an emergency medical department. Hum Exp Toxicol 1994;13:131-4.
2. Aalberg L, DeRuiter J, Noggle FT, Sippola E, Clark CR. Chromatographic and mass spectral methods of identification for the side-chain and ring regioisomers of methylenedioxymethamphetamine. J Chromatogr Sci 2000;38:329-37.
3. Abou-Donia MB, Lapadula DM. Mechanisms of organophosphorus ester-induced delayed neurotoxicity: type I and type II. Annu Rev Pharmacol Toxicol 1990;30:405-40.
4. Adamowicz P, Kala M. Date-rape drugs scene in Poland. Przegl Lek 2005;62:572-5.
5. Agency WA-D. The 2009 prohibited list. Geneva, Switzerland: International Organization for Standardization, 2009.
6. Agurell S, Halldin M, Lindgren JE, Ohlsson A, Widman M, Gillespie H, et al. Pharmacokinetics and metabolism of delta 1-tetrahydrocannabinol and other cannabinoids with emphasis on man. Pharmacol Rev 1986;38:21-43.
7. Ahanya SN, Lakshmanan J, Morgan BL, Ross MG. Meconium passage in utero: mechanisms, consequences, and management. Obstet Gynecol Surv 2005;60:45-56; quiz 73-4.
8. Al-Asmari AI, Anderson RA. Method for quantification of opioids and their metabolites in autopsy blood by liquid chromatography-tandem mass spectrometry. J Anal Toxicol 2007;31:394-408.
9. Aldridge WN. Some properties of specific cholinesterase with particular reference to the mechanism of inhibition by diethyl p-nitrophenyl thiophosphate (E 605) and analogues. Biochem J 1950;46:451-60.
10. Allen MJ. Procedures for transportation workplace drug testing programs. Fed Reg 1989;54:49854-84.
11. Allen RM, Young SJ. Phencyclidine-induced psychosis. Am J Psychiatry 1978;135:1081-4.
12. Alozie SO, Martin BR, Harris LS, Dewey WL. 3H-Delta-9-tetrahydrocannabinol, 3H-cannabinol and 3H-cannabidiol: penetration and regional distribution in rat brain. Pharmacol Biochem Behav 1980;12:217-21.
13. Ambre JJ, Belknap SM, Nelson J, Ruo TI, Shin SG, Atkinson AJ Jr. Acute tolerance to cocaine in humans. Clin Pharmacol Ther 1988;44:1-8.
14. American Academy of Clinical Toxicology; European Association of Poisons Centres and Clinical Toxicologists. Position statement and practice guidelines on the use of multi-dose activated charcoal in the treatment of acute poisoning. J Toxicol Clin Toxicol 1999;37:731-51.
15. American College of Obstetricians and Gynecologists. Committee opinion no. 422: at-risk drinking and illicit drug use: ethical issues in obstetric and gynecologic practice. Obstet Gynecol 2008;112:1449-60.
16. Amin J, Weiss DS. GABAA receptor needs two homologous domains of the beta-subunit for activation by GABA but not by pentobarbital. Nature 1993;366:565-9.
17. Anderson IB, Kim SY, Dyer JE, Burkhardt CB, Iknoian JC, Walsh MJ, et al. Trends in gamma-hydroxybutyrate (GHB) and related drug intoxication: 1999 to 2003. Ann Emerg Med 2006;47:177-83.
18. Anderson RJ, Potts DE, Gabow PA, Rumack BH, Schrier RW. Unrecognized adult salicylate intoxication. Ann Intern Med 1976;85:745-8.
19. Anderson WH. Therapeutic drugs II: antidepressants. In: Levine B, ed. Principles of forensic toxicology, 2nd edition. Washington, DC: AACC Press, 2003:297-314.
20. Andrews P. Cocaethylene toxicity. J Addict Dis 1997;16:75-84.
21. Andrinolo D, Michea LF, Lagos N. Toxic effects, pharmacokinetics and clearance of saxitoxin, a component of paralytic shellfish poison (PSP), in cats. Toxicon 1999;37:447-64.
22. Anonymous. An overview of club drugs, Drug Intelligence Brief, DEA, February 2000.
23. Anonymous. Ambien CR (zolpidem tartrate extended-release) prescribing information. Bridgewater, NJ: Sanofi-Aventis US LLC, January 2008a.
24. Araki Y. Nitrogenous substances in saliva. I. Protein and non-protein nitrogens. Jpn J Physiol 1951;2:69-78.
25. Arch JR, Ainsworth AT, Cawthorne MA, Piercy V, Sennitt MV, Thody VE, et al. Atypical beta-adrenoceptor on brown adipocytes as target for anti-obesity drugs. Nature 1984;309:163-5.
26. Ariano RE, Kassum DA, Aronson KJ. Comparison of sedative recovery time after midazolam versus diazepam administration. Crit Care Med 1994;22:1492-6.
27. Arima H, Sobue K, So M, Morishima T, Ando H, Katsuya H. Transient and reversible parkinsonism after acute organophosphate poisoning. J Toxicol Clin Toxicol 2003;41:67-70.
28. Armstrong SC, Cozza KL. Pharmacokinetic drug interactions of morphine, codeine, and their derivatives: theory and clinical reality, part I. Psychosomatics 2003;44:167-71.
29. Armstrong SC, Cozza KL. Pharmacokinetic drug interactions of morphine, codeine, and their derivatives: theory and clinical reality, part II. Psychosomatics 2003;44:515-20.
30. Arndt PA, Kumpel BM. Blood doping in athletes—detection of allogeneic blood transfusions by flow cytofluorometry. Am J Hematol 2008;83:657-67.
31. Ashbourne JF, Olson KR, Khayam-Bashi H. Value of rapid screening for acetaminophen in all patients with intentional drug overdose. Ann Emerg Med 1989;18:1035-8.
32. Babu KM, Ferm RP. Hallucinogens. In: Goldfrank LR, Flomenbaum NE, Hoffman RS, Howland MA, Lewin NA, Nelson L, eds. Goldfrank's toxicologic emergencies, 8th edition. New York, NY: McGraw-Hill, 2006:1202-11.
33. Bach MV, Coutts RT, Baker GB. Involvement of CYP2D6 in the in vitro metabolism of amphetamine, two N-alkylamphetamines and their 4-methoxylated derivatives. Xenobiotica 1999;29:719-32.
34. Badcock NR, O'Reilly DA. False-positive EMIT-ST ethanol screen with post-mortem infant plasma. Clin Chem 1992;38:434.
35. Baden LR, Horowitz G, Jacoby H, Eliopoulos GM. Quinolones and false-positive urine screening for opiates by immunoassay technology. JAMA 2001;286:3115-9.
36. Bailey RB, Jones SR. Chronic salicylate intoxication: a common cause of morbidity in the elderly. J Am Geriatr Soc 1989;37:556-61.
37. Baker AM, Johnson DG, Levisky JA, Hearn WL, Moore KA, Levine B, et al. Fatal diphenhydramine intoxication in infants. J Forensic Sci 2003;48:425-8.
38. Baldessarini R. Drug therapy of depression and anxiety disorders (Chapter 17). In: Brunton LL, Lazo JS, Parker KL, eds. Goodman & Gilman's the pharmacological basis of therapeutics, 11th edition. New York, NY: McGraw-Hill, 2006.
39. Baldessarini RJ, Tarazi FI. Pharmacotherapy of psychosis and mania (Chapter 18). In: Brunton LL, Lazo JS, Parker KL, eds. Goodman & Gilman's the pharmacological basis of therapeutics, 11th edition. New York, NY: McGraw-Hill, 2006.
40. Bamigbade TA, Davidson C, Langford RM, Stamford JA. Actions of tramadol, its enantiomers and principal metabolite, O-desmethyltramadol, on serotonin (5-HT) efflux and uptake in the rat dorsal raphe nucleus. Br J Anaesth 1997;79:352-6.
41. Banerji S, Anderson IB. Abuse of Coricidin HBP cough and cold tablets: episodes recorded by a poison center. Am J Health Syst Pharm 2001;58:1811-4.
42. Barbour AD. GC/MS analysis of propylated barbiturates. J Anal Toxicol 1991;15:214-5.
43. Bardin PG, van Eeden SF, Moolman JA, Foden AP, Joubert JR. Organophosphate and carbamate poisoning. Arch Intern Med 1994;154:1433-41.
44. Barkin RL, Barkin SJ, Barkin DS. Propoxyphene (dextropropoxyphene): a critical review of a weak opioid analgesic that should remain in antiquity. Am J Ther 2006;13:534-42.

45. Bartlett R. Carbon monoxide poisoning. In: Haddad L, Shannon M, Winchester J, eds. Clinical management of poisoning and drug overdose, 3rd edition. Philadelphia, Pa: WB Saunders, 1998:885-98.
46. Baselt RC. In: Baselt RC, ed. Disposition of toxic drugs and chemical in man, 8th edition. Foster City, Calif: Biomedical Publications, 2008.
47. Baselt RC. Acetone. In: Baselt RC, ed. Disposition of toxic drugs and chemical in man, 8th edition. Foster City, Calif: Biomedical Publications, 2008:15-7.
48. Baselt RC. Amphetamine. In: Baselt RC, ed. Disposition of toxic drugs and chemical in man, 8th edition. Foster City, Calif: Biomedical Publications, 2008:83-6.
49. Baselt RC. Carbon monoxide. In: Baselt RC, ed. Disposition of toxic drugs and chemical in man, 8th edition. Foster City, Calif: Biomedical Publications, 2008.
50. Baselt RC. Codeine. In: Baselt RC, ed. Disposition of toxic drugs and chemical in man, 8th edition. Foster City, Calif: Biomedical Publications, 2008:355-60.
51. Baselt RC. Ephedrine. In: Baselt RC, ed. Disposition of toxic drugs and chemical in man, 8th edition. Foster City, Calif: Biomedical Publications, 2008:542-4.
52. Baselt RC. Ethanol. In: Baselt RC, ed. Disposition of toxic drugs and chemical in man, 8th edition. Foster City, Calif: Biomedical Publications, 2008:561-5.
53. Baselt RC. Ethylene glycol. In: Baselt RC, ed. Disposition of toxic drugs and chemical in man, 8th edition. Foster City, Calif: Biomedical Publications, 2008:578-82.
54. Baselt RC. Flunitrazepam. In: Baselt RC, ed. Disposition of toxic drugs and chemical in man, 8th edition. Foster City, Calif: Biomedical Publications, 2008:633-5.
55. Baselt RC. Heroin. In: Baselt RC, ed. Disposition of toxic drugs and chemical in man, 8th edition. Foster City, Calif: Biomedical Publications, 2008:730-5.
56. Baselt RC. Hydrocodone. In: Baselt RC, ed. Disposition of toxic drugs and chemical in man, 8th edition. Foster City, Calif: Biomedical Publications, 2008:745-6.
57. Baselt RC. Hydromorphone. In: Baselt RC, ed. Disposition of toxic drugs and chemical in man, 8th edition. Foster City, Calif: Biomedical Publications, 2008:750-2.
58. Baselt RC. Isopropanol. In: Baselt RC, ed. Disposition of toxic drugs and chemical in man, 8th edition. Foster City, Calif: Biomedical Publications, 2008:789-91.
59. Baselt RC. Methadone. In: Baselt RC, ed. Disposition of toxic drugs and chemical in man, 8th edition. Foster City, Calif: Biomedical Publications, 2008:941-5.
60. Baselt RC. Methylenedioxyethylamphetamine. In: Baselt RC, ed. Disposition of toxic drugs and chemical in man, 8th edition. Foster City, Calif: Biomedical Publications, 2008:995-6.
61. Baselt RC. Methylphenidate. In: Baselt RC, ed. Disposition of toxic drugs and chemical in man, 8th edition. Foster City, Calif: Biomedical Publications, 2008:1008-11.
62. Baselt RC. Oxycodone. In: Baselt RC, ed. Disposition of toxic drugs and chemical in man, 8th edition. Foster City, Calif: Biomedical Publications, 2008:1166-8.
63. Baselt RC. Phenylpropanolamine. In: Baselt RC, ed. Disposition of toxic drugs and chemical in man, 8th edition. Foster City, Calif: Biomedical Publications, 2008:1252-4.
64. Baselt RC. Pseudoephedrine. In: Baselt RC, ed. Disposition of toxic drugs and chemical in man, 8th edition. Foster City, Calif: Biomedical Publications, 2008:1344-6.
65. Bass R. The antipsychotic drugs. In: Haddad L, Shannon M, Winchester J, eds. Clinical management of poisoning and drug overdose, 3rd edition. Philadelphia, Pa: WB Saunders, 1998:780-93.
66. Baumgartner AM, Jones PF, Baumgartner WA, Black CT. Radioimmunoassay of hair for determining opiate-abuse histories. J Nucl Med 1979;20:748-52.
67. Baumgartner WA, Hill V. Hair analysis for drugs of abuse: decontamination issues. In: Sunshine I, ed. Recent developments in therapeutic drug monitoring and clinical toxicology, New York: Marcel Dekker Inc, 1992:577-97.
68. Bayer MJ, McKay C. Advances in poison management. Clin Chem 1996;42:1361-6.
69. Bearer CF, Lee S, Salvator AE, Minnes S, Swick A, Yamashita T, Singer LT. Ethyl linoleate in meconium: a biomarker for prenatal ethanol exposure. Alcohol Clin Exp Res 1999;23:487-93.
70. Beckett AH, Rowland M. Urinary excretion of methylamphetamine in man. Nature 1965;206:1260-1.
71. Bell R, Taylor EH, Ackerman B, Pappas AA. Interpretation of urine quantitative 11-nor-delta-9 tetrahydrocannabinol-9-carboxylic acid to determine abstinence from marijuana smoking. J Toxicol Clin Toxicol 1989;27:109-15.
72. Bermejo AM, Ramos I, Fernandez P, Lopez-Rivadulla M, Cruz A, Chiarotti M, et al. Morphine determination by gas chromatography/mass spectroscopy in human vitreous humor and comparison with radioimmunoassay. J Anal Toxicol 1992;16:372-4.
73. Bernard S, Neville KA, Nguyen AT, Flockhart DA. Interethnic differences in genetic polymorphisms of CYP2D6 in the U.S. population: clinical implications. The Oncologist 2006;11:126-35.
74. Bernasconi R, Mathivet P, Bischoff S, Marescaux C. Gamma-hydroxybutyric acid: an endogenous neuromodulator with abuse potential? Trends Pharmacol Sci 1999;20:135-41.
75. Bertholf RL, Johannsen LM, Bazooband A, Mansouri V. False-positive acetaminophen results in a hyperbilirubinemic patient. Clin Chem 2003;49:695-8.
76. Bizovi K, Smilkstein M. Acetaminophen. In: Goldfrank L, Flomenbaum N, Lewin N, Howland M, Hoffman R, Nelson L, eds. Goldfrank's toxicologic emergencies, 7th edition. New York, NY: McGraw-Hill, 2002:480-501.
77. Blanchet M, Bru G, Guerret M, Bromet-Petit M, Bromet N. Routine determination of morphine, morphine 3-beta-D-glucuronide and morphine 6-beta-D-glucuronide in human serum by liquid chromatography coupled to electrospray mass spectrometry. J Chromatogr A 1999;854:93-108.
78. Blanke R, Decker W. Analysis of toxic substances. In: Tietz N, ed. Textbook of clinical chemistry, 1st edition. Philadelphia, Pa: WB Saunders, 1986:1670-744.
79. Boehnert MT, Lovejoy FH Jr. Value of the QRS duration versus the serum drug level in predicting seizures and ventricular arrhythmias after an acute overdose of tricyclic antidepressants. N Engl J Med 1985;313:474-9.
80. Boess F, Ndikum-Moffor FM, Boelsterli UA, Roberts SM. Effects of cocaine and its oxidative metabolites on mitochondrial respiration and generation of reactive oxygen species. Biochem Pharmacol 2000;60:615-23.
81. Bogusz M, Pach J, Stasko W. Comparative studies on the rate of ethanol elimination in acute poisoning and in controlled conditions. J Forensic Sci 1977;22:446-51.
82. Bogusz M, Wu M. Standardized HPLC/DAD system, based on retention indices and spectral library, applicable for systematic toxicological screening. J Anal Toxicol 1991;15:188-97.
83. Bogusz MJ. Liquid chromatography-mass spectrometry as a routine method in forensic sciences: a proof of maturity. J Chromatogr 2000;748:3-19.
84. Bogusz MJ, Maier RD, Driessen S. Morphine, morphine-3-glucuronide, morphine-6-glucuronide, and 6-monoacetylmorphine determined by means of atmospheric pressure chemical ionization-mass spectrometry-liquid chromatography in body fluids of heroin victims. J Anal Toxicol 1997;21:346-55.
85. Bogusz MJ, Maier RD, Erkens M, Driessen S. Determination of morphine and its 3- and 6-glucuronides, codeine, codeine-glucuronide and 6-monoacetylmorphine in body fluids by liquid chromatography atmospheric pressure chemical ionization mass spectrometry. J Chromatogr 1997;703:115-27.
86. Bogusz MJ, Maier RD, Kruger KD, Kohls U. Determination of common drugs of abuse in body fluids using one isolation procedure

and liquid chromatography—atmospheric-pressure chemical-ionization mass spectrometry. J Anal Toxicol 1998;22:549-58.
87. Bossong MG, Van Dijk JP, Niesink RJ. Methylone and mCPP, two new drugs of abuse? Addict Biol 2005;10:321-3.
88. Boumba VA, Ziavrou KS, Vougiouklakis T. Hair as a biological indicator of drug use, drug abuse or chronic exposure to environmental toxicants. Int J Toxicol 2006;25:143-63.
89. Bowdle TA. Adverse effects of opioid agonists and agonist-antagonists in anaesthesia. Drug Saf 1998;19:173-89.
90. Bowie LJ, Kirkpatrick PB. Simultaneous determination of monoacetylmorphine, morphine, codeine, and other opiates by GC/MS. J Anal Toxicol 1989;13:326-9.
91. Bravo R, Driskell WJ, Whitehead RD Jr, Needham LL, Barr DB. Quantitation of dialkyl phosphate metabolites of organophosphate pesticides in human urine using GC-MS-MS with isotopic internal standards. J Anal Toxicol 2002;26:245-52.
92. Bray GP, Harrison PM, O'Grady JG, Tredger JM, Williams R. Long-term anticonvulsant therapy worsens outcome in paracetamol-induced fulminant hepatic failure. Hum Exp Toxicol 1992;11:265-70.
93. Breimer DD. Clinical pharmacokinetics of hypnotics. Clin Pharmacokinet 1977;2:93-109.
94. Brett AS. Implications of discordance between clinical impression and toxicology analysis in drug overdose. Arch Intern Med 1988;148:437-41.
95. Bridges RR, Kinniburgh DW, Keehn BJ, Jennison TA. An evaluation of common methods for acetaminophen quantitation for small hospitals. J Toxicol Clin Toxicol 1983;20:1-17.
96. Bronstein AC, Spyker DA, Cantilena LR Jr, Green JL, Rumack BH, Heard SE. The American Association of Poison Control Centers' National Poison Data System (NPDS): 25th annual report. Clin Toxicol 2008;46:927-1057.
97. Brown WA, Khan A. Which depressed patients should receive antidepressants? CNS Drugs 1994;1:341-7.
98. Bruns DE, Herold DA, Rodeheaver GT, Edlich RF. Polyethylene glycol intoxication in burn patients. Burns 1982;9:49-52.
99. Brzezinski MR, Abraham TL, Stone CL, Dean RA, Bosron WF. Purification and characterization of a human liver cocaine carboxylesterase that catalyzes the production of benzoylecgonine and the formation of cocaethylene from alcohol and cocaine. Biochem Pharmacol 1994;48:1747-55.
100. Buckley NA. Antipsychotic drugs (neuroleptics). In: Dart RC, ed. Medical toxicology. Philadelphia, Pa: Lippincott Williams & Wilkins, 2004:861-70.
101. Buckley NA, Eddleston M, Szinicz L. Oximes for acute organophosphate pesticide poisoning. Cochrane Database Syst Rev 2005(1):CD005085.
102. Buckley NA, Whyte IM, Dawson AH. Diagnostic data in clinical toxicology—should we use a Bayesian approach? J Toxicol Clin Toxicol 2002;40:213-22.
103. Buckpitt AR, Rollins DE, Mitchell JR. Varying effects of sulfhydryl nucleophiles on acetaminophen oxidation and sulfhydryl adduct formation. Biochem Pharmacol 1979;28:2941-6.
104. Budai B, Iskandar H. Dextromethorphan can produce false positive phencyclidine testing with HPLC. Am J Emerg Med 2002;20:61-2.
105. Burgen AS. The secretion of non-electrolytes in the parotid saliva. J Cell Physiol 1956;48:113-38.
106. Burke A, Smyth E, FitzGerald GA. Analgesic-antipyretic and antiinflammatory agents: pharmacotherapy of gout (Chapter 26). In: Brunton LL, Lazo JS, Parker KL, eds. Goodman & Gilman's the pharmacological basis of therapeutics, 11th edition. New York, NY: McGraw-Hill, 2006.
107. Burkhart KK. Intravenous propranolol reverses hypertension after sympathomimetic overdose: two case reports. J Toxicol Clin Toxicol 1992;30:109-14.
108. Burns M, Baselt RC. Monitoring drug use with a sweat patch: an experiment with cocaine. J Anal Toxicol 1995;19:41-8.
109. Burns MJ. The pharmacology and toxicology of atypical antipsychotic agents. J Toxicol Clin Toxicol 2001;39:1-14.
110. Bush DM. The U.S. mandatory guidelines for federal workplace drug testing programs: current status and future considerations. Forensic Sci Int 2008;174:111-9.
111. Calafat AM, Stanfill SB. Rapid quantitation of cyanide in whole blood by automated headspace gas chromatography. J Chromatogr B Analyt Technol Biomed Life Sci 2002;772:131-7.
112. Caldwell J. The metabolism of amphetamines in mammals. Drug Metab Rev 1976;5:219-80.
113. Caldwell R, Challenger H. A capillary column gas-chromatographic method for the identification of drugs of abuse in urine samples. Ann Clin Biochem 1989;26(Pt 5):430-43.
114. Callahan CM, Grant TM, Phipps P, Clark G, Novack AH, Streissguth AP, et al. Measurement of gestational cocaine exposure: sensitivity of infants' hair, meconium, and urine. J Pediatr 1992;120:763-8.
115. Caplan YH. Blood, urine, and other fluid and tissue specimens for alcohol analyses. In: Garriott JC, ed. Medicolegal aspects of alcohol. Tucson, Ariz: Lawyers & Judges Publishing, 1996:137-50.
116. Caplan YH, Goldberger BA. Alternative specimens for workplace drug testing. J Anal Toxicol 2001;25:396-9.
117. Caplan YH, Levine B. Evaluation of the Abbott TDx-radiative energy attenuation (REA) ethanol assay in a study of 1105 forensic whole blood specimens. J Forensic Sci 1987;32:55-61.
118. Carlton FB, Simpson WMJ, Haddad LM. The organophosphates and other insecticides. In: Haddad LM, Shannon MW, Winchester JF, eds. Clinical management of poisoning and drug overdose, 3rd edition. Philadelphia, Pa: WB Saunders, 1999:836-45.
119. Carta M, Ariwodola OJ, Weiner JL, Valenzuela CF. Alcohol potently inhibits the kainate receptor-dependent excitatory drive of hippocampal interneurons. Proc Natl Acad Sci U S A 2003;100:6813-8.
120. Casavant MJ, Shah MN, Battels R. Does fluorescent urine indicate antifreeze ingestion by children? Pediatrics 2001;107:113-4.
121. Catlin DH, Breidbach A, Elliott S, Glaspy J. Comparison of the isoelectric focusing patterns of darbepoetin alfa, recombinant human erythropoietin, and endogenous erythropoietin from human urine. Clin Chem 2002;48:2057-9.
122. Catlin DH, Fitch KD, Ljungqvist A. Medicine and science in the fight against doping in sport. J Intern Med 2008;264:99-114.
123. Catterall WA, Mackie K. Local anesthetics (Chapter 14). In: Brunton LL, Lazo JS, Parker KL, eds. Goodman & Gilman's the pharmacological basis of therapeutics, 11th edition. New York, NY: McGraw-Hill, 2006.
124. Chabali R. Diagnostic use of anion and osmolal gaps in pediatric emergency medicine. Pediatr Emerg Care 1997;13:204-10.
125. Cham BE, Johns D, Bochner F, Imhoff DM, Rowland M. Simultaneous liquid-chromatographic quantitation of salicylic acid, salicyluric acid, and gentisic acid in plasma. Clin Chem 1979;25:1420-5.
126. Chamberlin KW, Cottle M, Neville R, Tan J. Oral oxymorphone for pain management. Ann Pharmacother 2007;41:1144-52.
127. Chan TY, Chan AY. Use of a plasma salicylate assay service in a medical unit in Hong Kong: a follow-up study. Vet Hum Toxicol 1996;38:278-9.
128. Chan TY, Chan AY, Ho CS, Critchley JA. The clinical value of screening for salicylates in acute poisoning. Vet Hum Toxicol 1995;37:37-8.
129. Chapman BJ, Proudfoot AT. Adult salicylate poisoning: deaths and outcome in patients with high plasma salicylate concentrations. Q J Med 1989;72:699-707.
130. Charney DS, Mihic SJ, Harris RA. Hypnotics and sedatives (Chapter 16). In: Brunton LL, Lazo JS, Parker KL, eds. Goodman & Gilman's the pharmacological basis of therapeutics, 11th edition. New York, NY: McGraw-Hill, 2006.
131. Chen BH, Taylor EH, Pappas AA. Comparison of derivatives for determination of codeine and morphine by gas chromatography/mass spectrometry. J Anal Toxicol 1990;14:12-7.
132. Cheng PS, Fu CY, Lee CH, Liu C, Chien CS. GC-MS quantification of ketamine, norketamine, and dehydronorketamine in urine specimens and comparative study using ELISA as the preliminary

test methodology. J Chromatogr B Analyt Technol Biomed Life Sci 2007;852:443-9.
133. Cheung L, Potts RG, Meyer KC. Acetaminophen treatment nomogram. N Engl J Med 1994;330:1907-8.
134. Cheze M, Duffort G, Deveaux M, Pepin G. Hair analysis by liquid chromatography-tandem mass spectrometry in toxicological investigation of drug-facilitated crimes: report of 128 cases over the period June 2003-May 2004 in metropolitan Paris. Forensic Sci Int 2005;153:3-10.
135. Chiarotti M, Costamagna L. Analysis of 11-nor-9-carboxy-delta(9)-tetrahydrocannabinol in biological samples by gas chromatography tandem mass spectrometry (GC/MS-MS). Forensic Sci Int 2000;114:1-6.
136. Chikhi-Chorfi N, Pham-Huy C, Galons H, Manuel N, Lowenstein W, Warnet JM, et al. Rapid determination of methadone and its major metabolite in biological fluids by gas-liquid chromatography with thermionic detection for maintenance treatment of opiate addicts. J Chromatogr 1998;718:278-84.
137. Chiu TH, Rosenberg HC. Comparison of the kinetics of [3H] diazepam and [3H]flunitrazepam binding to cortical synaptosomal membranes. J Neurochem 1982;39:1716-25.
138. Christ A, Arranto CA, Schindler C, Klima T, Hunziker PR, Siegemund M, et al. Incidence, risk factors, and outcome of aspiration pneumonitis in ICU overdose patients. Intensive Care Med 2006;32:1423-7.
139. Christophersen AS. Amphetamine designer drugs—an overview and epidemiology. Toxicol Lett 2000;112-113:127-31.
140. Christophersen AS, Biseth A, Skuterud B, Gadeholt G. Identification of opiates in urine by capillary column gas chromatography of two different derivatives. J Chromatogr 1987;422:117-24.
141. Chua SS, Benrimoj SI. Non-prescription sympathomimetic agents and hypertension. Med Toxicol Adverse Drug Exp 1988;3:387-417.
142. Chui PT. Anesthesia in a patient with undiagnosed salicylate poisoning presenting as intraabdominal sepsis. J Clin Anesth 1999;11:251-3.
143. Cimbura G. PMA deaths in Ontario. Can Med Assoc J 1974;110:1263-7.
144. Clarke PA, Foltz RL. Quantitative analysis of morphine in urine by gas chromatography-chemical ionization-mass spectrometry, with (N-C2H3)morphine as an internal standard. Clin Chem 1974;20:465-9.
145. Clarke RF. Insecticides: organic phosphorus compounds and carbamates. In: Flomenbaum NE, Goldfrank LR, Hoffman RS, Howland MA, Lewin NA, Nelson LS, eds. Goldfrank's toxicologic emergencies, 8th edition. New York, NY: McGraw-Hill, 2006:1497-512.
146. Clarkson ED, Lesser D, Paul BD. Effective GC-MS procedure for detecting iso-LSD in urine after base-catalyzed conversion to LSD. Clin Chem 1998;44:287-92.
147. Clauwaert KM, Van Bocxlaer JF, Lambert WE, De Leenheer AP. Liquid chromatographic determination of cocaine, benzoylecgonine, and cocaethylene in whole blood and serum samples with diode-array detection. J Chromatogr Sci 1997;35:321-8.
148. Clements JA, Nimmo WS, Grant IS. Bioavailability, pharmacokinetics, and analgesic activity of ketamine in humans. J Pharm Sci 1982;71:539-42.
149. Codd EE, Shank RP, Schupsky JJ, Raffa RB. Serotonin and norepinephrine uptake inhibiting activity of centrally acting analgesics: structural determinants and role in antinociception. J Pharmacol Exp Ther 1995;274:1263-70.
150. Cody JT. Determination of methamphetamine enantiomer ratios in urine by gas chromatography-mass spectrometry. J Chromatogr 1992;580:77-95.
151. Cody JT, Schwarzhoff R. Interpretation of methamphetamine and amphetamine enantiomer data. J Anal Toxicol 1993;17:321-6.
152. Cody JT, Valtier S. Immunoassay analysis of lysergic acid diethylamide. J Anal Toxicol 1997;21:459-64.
153. Cody JT, Valtier S. Detection of amphetamine and methamphetamine following administration of benzphetamine. J Anal Toxicol 1998;22:299-309.
154. Cody JT, Valtier S. Effects of Stealth adulterant on immunoassay testing for drugs of abuse. J Anal Toxicol 2001;25:466-70.
155. Coffman BL, Rios GR, King CD, Tephly TR. Human UGT2B7 catalyzes morphine glucuronidation. Drug Metab Dispos 1997;25:1-4.
156. Colbert DL. Drug abuse screening with immunoassays: unexpected cross-reactivities and other pitfalls. Br J Biomed Sci 1994;51:136-46.
157. Combie J, Blake JW, Nugent TE, Tobin T. Morphine glucuronide hydrolysis: superiority of beta-glucuronidase from *Patella vulgata*. Clin Chem 1982;28:83-6.
158. Concheiro M, de Castro A, Quintela O, Lopez-Rivadulla M, Cruz A. Determination of drugs of abuse and their metabolites in human plasma by liquid chromatography-mass spectrometry: an application to 156 road fatalities. J Chromatogr B Analyt Technol Biomed Life Sci 2006;832:81-9.
159. Cone EJ. Saliva testing for drugs of abuse. Ann N Y Acad Sci 1993;694:91-127.
160. Cone EJ. Mechanisms of drug incorporation into hair. Ther Drug Monit 1996;18:438-43.
161. Cone EJ, Darwin WD. Simultaneous determination of hydromorphone, hydrocodone and their 6alpha- and 6beta-hydroxy metabolites in urine using selected ion recording with methane chemical ionization. Biomed Mass Spectrom 1978;5:291.
162. Cone EJ, Darwin WD, Buchwald WF. Assay for codeine, morphine and ten potential urinary metabolites by gas chromatography–mass fragmentography. J Chromatogr 1983;275:307-18.
163. Cone EJ, Heit HA, Caplan YH, Gourlay D. Evidence of morphine metabolism to hydromorphone in pain patients chronically treated with morphine. J Anal Toxicol 2006;30:1-5.
164. Cone EJ, Hillsgrove M, Darwin WD. Simultaneous measurement of cocaine, cocaethylene, their metabolites, and "crack" pyrolysis products by gas chromatography-mass spectrometry. Clin Chem 1994;40:1299-305.
165. Cone EJ, Hillsgrove MJ, Jenkins AJ, Keenan RM, Darwin WD. Sweat testing for heroin, cocaine, and metabolites. J Anal Toxicol 1994;18:298-305.
166. Cone EJ, Lange R, Darwin WD. In vivo adulteration: excess fluid ingestion causes false-negative marijuana and cocaine urine test results. J Anal Toxicol 1998;22:460-73.
167. Cone EJ, Oyler J, Darwin WD. Cocaine disposition in saliva following intravenous, intranasal, and smoked administration. J Anal Toxicol 1997;21:465-75.
168. Cone EJ, Sampson-Cone AH, Darwin WD, Huestis MA, Oyler JM. Urine testing for cocaine abuse: metabolic and excretion patterns following different routes of administration and methods for detection of false-negative results. J Anal Toxicol 2003;27:386-401.
169. Cone EJ, Weddington WW Jr. Prolonged occurrence of cocaine in human saliva and urine after chronic use. J Anal Toxicol 1989;13:65-8.
170. Cone EJ, Welch P, Paul BD, Mitchell JM. Forensic drug testing for opiates, III. Urinary excretion rates of morphine and codeine following codeine administration. J Anal Toxicol 1991;15:161-6.
171. Contreras PC, DiMaggio DA, O'Donohue TL. Evidence for an endogenous peptide ligand and antagonist for PCP receptors. Prog Clin Biol Res 1985;192:495-8.
172. Cook CE, Brine DR, Jeffcoat AR, Hill JM, Wall ME, Perez-Reyes M, et al. Phencyclidine disposition after intravenous and oral doses. Clin Pharmacol Ther 1982;31:625-34.
173. Cook CE, Brine DR, Quin GD, Wall ME, Perez-Reyes M, Di Guiseppi SR. Smoking of phencyclidine: disposition in man and stability to pyrolytic conditions. Life Sci 1981;29:1967-72.
174. Corburt MR, Koves EM. Gas chromatography/mass spectrometry for the determination of cocaine and benzoylecgonine over a wide concentration range (<0.005-5 mg/dL) in postmortem blood. J Forensic Sci 1994;39:136-49.
175. Corcoran GB, Todd EL, Racz WJ, Hughes H, Smith CV, Mitchell JR. Effects of N-acetylcysteine on the disposition and metabolism of acetaminophen in mice. J Pharmacol Exp Ther 1985;232:857-63.

176. Costa A, Chawla S, Me A, le Pichon T. World drug report: United Nations Office on Drugs and Crime. New York, NY: United Nations Publication, 2008.
177. Crews JC, Sweeney NJ, Denson DD. Clinical efficacy of methadone in patients refractory to other mu-opioid receptor agonist analgesics for management of terminal cancer pain: case presentations and discussion of incomplete cross-tolerance among opioid agonist analgesics. Cancer 1993;72:2266-72.
178. Crouch DJ, Frank JF, Farrell LJ, Karsch HM, Klaunig JE. A multiple-site laboratory evaluation of three on-site urinalysis drug-testing devices. J Anal Toxicol 1998;22:493-502.
179. Cruz-Landeira A, Lopez-Rivadulla M, Concheiro-Carro L, Fernandez-Gomez P, Tabernero-Duque MJ. A new spectrophotometric method for the toxicological diagnosis of cyanide poisoning. J Anal Toxicol 2000;24:266-70.
180. Curry SC, Mills KC, Buha A. Neurotransmitters and neuromodulators. In: Flomenbaum G, Hoffman RS, Howland MA, Lewin NA, Nelson LS, eds. Goldfrank's toxicologic emergencies, 8th edition. New York: McGraw Hill, 2006:214-48.
181. Daher R, Haidar JH, Al-Amin H. Rifampin interference with opiate immunoassays. Clin Chem 2002;48:203-4.
182. Dahl H, Stephanson N, Beck O, Helander A. Comparison of urinary excretion characteristics of ethanol and ethyl glucuronide. J Anal Toxicol 2002;26:201-4.
183. Dahl ML. Cytochrome p450 phenotyping/genotyping in patients receiving antipsychotics: useful aid to prescribing? Clin Pharmacokinet 2002;41:453-70.
184. Dale C, Aulaqi AA, Baker J, Hobbs RC, Tan ME, Tovey C, et al. Assessment of a point-of-care test for paracetamol and salicylate in blood. QJM 2005;98:113-8.
185. Dart RC. Part 1. General approach to the poisoned patient. Section 5. Antidotes and specific therapies. In: Dart RC, ed. Medical toxicology, 3rd edition. Philadelphia: Lippincott Williams & Wilkins, 2004:160-268.
186. Daws LC, Irvine RJ, Callaghan PD, Toop NP, White JM, Bochner F. Differential behavioural and neurochemical effects of para-methoxyamphetamine and 3,4-methylenedioxymethamphetamine in the rat. Prog Neuropsychopharmacol Biol Psychiatry 2000;24:955-77.
187. Dawson AH. Cyclic antidepressants drugs. In: Dart RC, ed. Medical toxicology. Philadelphia, Pa: Lippincott Williams & Wilkins, 2004:834-51.
188. de Boer D, Bosman IJ, Hidvegi E, Manzoni C, Benko AA, dos Reys LJ, et al. Piperazine-like compounds: a new group of designer drugs-of-abuse on the European market. Forensic Sci Int 2001;121: 47-56.
189. de la Torre R, Farre M, Ortuno J, Mas M, Brenneisen R, Roset PN, et al. Non-linear pharmacokinetics of MDMA ('ecstasy') in humans. Br J Clin Pharmacol 2000;49:104-9.
190. de la Torre R, Ortuno J, Gonzalez ML, Farre M, Cami J, Segura J. Determination of cocaine and its metabolites in human urine by gas chromatography/mass spectrometry after simultaneous use of cocaine and ethanol. J Pharmaceut Biomed Anal 1995;13:305-12.
191. de Leon J, Dinsmore L, Wedlund P. Adverse drug reactions to oxycodone and hydrocodone in CYP2D6 ultrarapid metabolizers. J Clin Psychopharmacol 2003;23:420-1.
192. Dean RA, Christian CD, Sample RH, Bosron WF. Human liver cocaine esterases: ethanol-mediated formation of ethylcocaine. FASEB J 1991;5:2735-9.
193. Delbeke FT, Debackere M. Urinary concentrations of codeine and morphine after the administration of different codeine preparations in relation to doping analysis. J Pharmaceut Biomed Anal 1991;9: 959-64.
194. Delbeke FT, Debackere M. Influence of hydrolysis procedures on the urinary concentrations of codeine and morphine in relation to doping analysis. J Pharmaceut Biomed Anal 1993;11:339-43.
195. Delinsky DC, Srinivasan K, Solomon HM, Bartlett MG. Simultaneous capillary electrophoresis determination of barbiturates from meconium. J Liquid Chromatogr Relat Technol 2002;25:113-23.
196. Demorest DM. Distinguishing cyclobenzaprine from amitriptyline and imipramine by liquid chromatography with UV multi-wavelength or full-spectrum detection: blood levels of cyclobenzaprine in emergency screens. J Anal Toxicol 1987;11:133-4.
197. Dennis RC, Valeri CR. Measuring percent oxygen saturation of hemoglobin, percent carboxyhemoglobin and methemoglobin, and concentrations of total hemoglobin and oxygen in blood of man, dog, and baboon. Clin Chem 1980;26:1304-8.
197A. Dasgupa A, ed. Alcohol and Drugs of Abuse Testing. Washington D.C., AACC Press, 2009:1-319.
198. Di Pietra AM, Gotti R, Del Borrello E, Pomponio R, Cavrini V. Analysis of amphetamine and congeners in illicit samples by liquid chromatography and capillary electrophoresis. J Anal Toxicol 2001;25: 99-105.
199. Dietzen DJ, Ecos K, Friedman D, Beason S. Positive predictive values of abused drug immunoassays on the Beckman Synchron in a veteran population. J Anal Toxicol 2001;25:174-8.
200. Done AK. Salicylate intoxication: significance of measurements of salicylate in blood in cases of acute ingestion. Pediatrics 1960;26: 800-7.
201. Dorandeu AH, Pages CA, Sordino MC, Pepin G, Baccino E, Kintz P. A case in south-eastern France: a review of drug facilitated sexual assault in European and English-speaking countries. J Clin Forensic Med 2006;13:253-61.
202. Drasbek KR, Christensen J, Jensen K. Gamma-hydroxybutyrate—a drug of abuse. Acta Neurol Scand 2006;114:145-56.
203. Dresser GK, Spence JD, Bailey DG. Pharmacokinetic-pharmacodynamic consequences and clinical relevance of cytochrome P450 3A4 inhibition. Clin Pharmacokinet 2000;38:41-57.
204. Drost RH, van Ooijen RD, Ionescu T, Maes RA. Determination of morphine in serum and cerebrospinal fluid by gas chromatography and selected ion monitoring after reversed-phase column extraction. J Chromatogr 1984;310:193-8.
205. Drummer OH. Methods for the measurement of benzodiazepines in biological samples. J Chromatogr 1998;713:201-25.
206. Drummer OH. Chromatographic screening techniques in systematic toxicological analysis. J Chromatogr 1999;733:27-45.
207. Drummer OH. Benzodiazepines—effects on human performance and behavior. Forensic Sci Rev 2002;14:1-14.
208. Drummer OH. Review: pharmacokinetics of illicit drugs in oral fluid. Forensic Sci Int 2005;150:133-42.
209. Drummer OH, Syrjanen ML, Cordner SM. Deaths involving the benzodiazepine flunitrazepam. Am J Forensic Med Pathol 1993;14: 238-43.
210. Dubowski KM. Human pharmacokinetics of alcohol. Alcohol Tech Rep 1976:55-63.
211. Dubowski KM. Absorption, distribution and elimination of alcohol: highway safety aspects. J Studies Alcohol 1985;10:98-108.
212. Dubowski KM. Proceedings of the 1987 Arnold O. Beckman Conference. Clin Chem 1987;33:5B-112B.
213. Dubowski KM, Luke JL. Measurement of carboxyhemoglobin and carbon monoxide in blood. Ann Clin Lab Sci 1973;3:53-65.
214. Dugandzic RM, Tierney MG, Dickinson GE, Dolan MC, McKnight DR. Evaluation of the validity of the Done nomogram in the management of acute salicylate intoxication. Ann Emerg Med 1989;18:1186-90.
215. DuPen A, Shen D, Ersek M. Mechanisms of opioid-induced tolerance and hyperalgesia. Pain Manag Nurs 2007;8:113-21.
216. Durakovic Z, Gjurasin M, Plavsic F. [Poisoning by a large dose of digitalis]. Arh Hig Rada Toksikol 1984;35:277-84.
217. Duritz G, Truitt EB Jr. A rapid method for the simultaneous determination of acetaldehyde and ethanol in blood using gas chromatography. Q J Studies Alcohol 1964;25:498-510.
218. Dutt MC, Lo DS, Ng DL, Woo SO. Gas chromatographic study of the urinary codeine to morphine ratios in controlled codeine consumption and in mass screening for opiate drugs. J Chromatogr 1983;267:117-24.
219. Dyer JK. Drug facilitated sexual assault: a review of 24 incidents. J Toxicol Clin Toxicol 2004;42:519.

220. Eddleston M, Dawson A, Karalliedde L, Dissanayake W, Hittarage A, Azher S, et al. Early management after self-poisoning with an organophosphorus or carbamate pesticide—a treatment protocol for junior doctors. Crit Care 2004;8:R391-7.
221. Eichelbaum M, Evert B. Influence of pharmacogenetics on drug disposition and response. Clin Exp Pharmacol Physiol 1996;23:983-5.
222. Eichhorst J, Etter M, Lepage J, Lehotay DC. Urinary screening for methylphenidate (Ritalin) abuse: a comparison of liquid chromatography-tandem mass spectrometry, gas chromatography-mass spectrometry, and immunoassay methods. Clin Biochem 2004;37:175-83.
223. Eichhorst JC, Etter ML, Rousseaux N, Lehotay DC. Drugs of abuse testing by tandem mass spectrometry: a rapid, simple method to replace immunoassays. Clin Biochem 2009;42:1531-42.
224. Ellinwood EH Jr, Kilbey MM. Fundamental mechanisms underlying altered behavior following chronic administration of psychomotor stimulants. Biol Psychiatry 1980;15:749-57.
225. Elliott SP, Burgess V. Clinical urinalysis of drugs and alcohol in instances of suspected surreptitious administration ("spiked drinks"). Sci Justice 2005;45:129-34.
226. Ellis GM Jr, Mann MA, Judson BA, Schramm NT, Tashchian A. Excretion patterns of cannabinoid metabolites after last use in a group of chronic users. Clin Pharmacol Ther 1985;38:572-8.
227. ElSohly HN, Stanford DF, Jones AB, ElSohly MA, Snyder H, Pedersen C. Gas chromatographic/mass spectrometric analysis of morphine and codeine in human urine of poppy seed eaters. J Forensic Sci 1988;33: 347-56.
228. ElSohly MA, deWit H, Wachtel SR, Feng S, Murphy TP. Delta9-tetrahydrocannabivarin as a marker for the ingestion of marijuana versus Marinol: results of a clinical study. J Anal Toxicol 2001;25: 565-71.
229. ElSohly MA, Feng S. Delta 9-THC metabolites in meconium: identification of 11-OH-delta 9-THC, 8 beta,11-diOH-delta 9-THC, and 11-nor-delta 9-THC-9-COOH as major metabolites of delta 9-THC. J Anal Toxicol 1998;22:329-35.
230. ElSohly MA, Feng S, Salamone SJ, Wu R. A sensitive GC-MS procedure for the analysis of flunitrazepam and its metabolites in urine. J Anal Toxicol 1997;21:335-40.
231. ElSohly MA, Ross SA, Mehmedic Z, Arafat R, Yi B, Banahan BF 3rd. Potency trends of delta9-THC and other cannabinoids in confiscated marijuana from 1980-1997. J Forensic Sci 2000;45:24-30.
232. ElSohly MA, Salamone SJ. Prevalence of drugs used in cases of alleged sexual assault. J Anal Toxicol 1999;23:141-6.
233. Ener RA, Meglathery SB, Van Decker WA, Gallagher RM. Serotonin syndrome and other serotonergic disorders. Pain Med 2003;4:63-74.
234. Erickson TB, Thompson TM, Lu JJ. The approach to the patient with an unknown overdose. Emerg Med Clin North Am 2007;25:249-81; abstract vii.
235. Evelyn KA, Malloy HT. Microdetermination of oxyhemoblobin, methemoglobin, and sulfhemoglobin in a single sample of blood. J Biol Chem 1938;126:655-62.
236. Fallon JK, Kicman AT, Henry JA, Milligan PJ, Cowan DA, Hutt AJ. Stereospecific analysis and enantiomeric disposition of 3,4-met hylenedioxymethamphetamine (Ecstasy) in humans. Clin Chem 1999;45:1058-69.
237. Farre M, de la Torre R, Llorente M, Lamas X, Ugena B, Segura J, et al. Alcohol and cocaine interactions in humans. J Pharmacol Exp Ther 1993;266:1364-73.
238. Farrell SE, Roberts JR. Benzodiazepines. In: Haddad LM, Shannon MW, Winchester JF, eds. Clinical management of poisoning and drug overdose, 3rd edition. Philadelphia, Pa: WB Saunders, 1998: 609-27.
239. Federal Register 49 CFR Part 40. Procedures for transportation workplace drug and alcohol testing programs. Updated as of August 31, 2009.
240. Fehn J, Megges G. Detection of O6-monoacetylmorphine in urine samples by GC/MS as evidence for heroin use. J Anal Toxicol 1985;9: 134-8.
241. Felgate HE, Felgate PD, James RA, Sims DN, Vozzo DC. Recent paramethoxyamphetamine deaths. J Anal Toxicol 1998;22:169-72.
242. Feng J, Wang L, Dai I, Harmon T, Bernert JT. Simultaneous determination of multiple drugs of abuse and relevant metabolites in urine by LC-MS-MS. J Anal Toxicol 2007;31:359-68.
243. Ferrari A, Coccia CP, Bertolini A, Sternieri E. Methadone—metabolism, pharmacokinetics and interactions. Pharmacol Res 2004;50:551-9.
244. Fish F, Hayes TS. Hydrolysis of morphine glucuronide. J Forensic Sci 1974;19:676-83.
245. Fitzgerald RL, Ramos JM Jr, Bogema SC, Poklis A. Resolution of methamphetamine stereoisomers in urine drug testing: urinary excretion of R(−)-methamphetamine following use of nasal inhalers. J Anal Toxicol 1988;12:255-9.
246. Flanagan RJ, Mant TG. Coma and metabolic acidosis early in severe acute paracetamol poisoning. Hum Toxicol 1986;5:179-82.
247. Fleischman A, Chiang VW. Carbamazepine overdose recognized by a tricyclic antidepressant assay. Pediatrics 2001;107:176-7.
248. Fleming M, Mihic SJ, Harris RA. Ethanol (Chapter 22). In: Brunton LL, Lazo JS, Parker KL, eds. Goodman & Gilman's the pharmacological basis of therapeutics, 11th edition. New York, NY: McGraw-Hill, 2006.
249. Flint AJ. Choosing appropriate antidepressant therapy in the elderly: a risk-benefit assessment of available agents. Drugs Aging 1998;13:269-80.
250. Flomenbaum NE. Salicylates. In: Goldfrank LR, Flomenbaum NE, Lewin NA, Howland MA, Hoffman RS, Nelson LS, eds. Goldfrank's toxicologic emergencies, 7th edition. New York, NY: McGraw-Hill, 2002:507-27.
251. Flomenbaum NE. Principles of managing the poisoned or overdosed patient. In: Flomenbaum NE, Goldfrank LR, Hoffman RS, Howland MA, Lewin NA, Nelson LS, eds. Goldfrank's toxicologic emergencies, 8th edition. New York, NY: McGraw-Hill, 2006:42-50.
252. Flomenbaum NE. Salicylates. In: Flomenbaum NE, Goldfrank LR, Hoffman RS, Howland MA, Lewin NA, Nelson LS, eds. Goldfrank's toxicologic emergencies, 8th edition. New York, NY: McGraw-Hill, 2006:550-64.
253. Foltz RL, Fentiman AF Jr, Foltz RB. GC/MS assays for abused drugs in body fluids. NIDA Res Monogr 1980;32:1-198.
254. Ford M, Tomaszewski C, Kerns W, Kirk M, Eichhorst A. Bedside ferric chloride urine test to rule out salicylate intoxication. Vet Hum Toxicol 1994;36:364.
255. Forrest JA, Clements JA, Prescott LF. Clinical pharmacokinetics of paracetamol. Clin Pharmacokinet 1982;7:93-107.
256. Francom P, Andrenyak D, Lim HK, Bridges RR, Foltz RL, Jones RT. Determination of LSD in urine by capillary column gas chromatography and electron impact mass spectrometry. J Anal Toxicol 1988;12:1-8.
257. Fraser AD, MacNeil W. Colorimetric and gas chromatographic procedures for glycolic acid in serum: the major toxic metabolite of ethylene glycol. J Toxicol Clin Toxicol 1993;31:397-405.
258. Fraser AD, Worth D. Urinary excretion profiles of 11-nor-9-carboxy-delta9-tetrahydrocannabinol. Study III: a delta9-THC-COOH to creatinine ratio study. Forensic Sci Int 2003;137:196-202.
259. Freund TF, Katona I, Piomelli D. Role of endogenous cannabinoids in synaptic signaling. Physiol Rev 2003;83:1017-66.
260. Frick S, Roos M, Fattinger K. How much is too much? Oligosymptomatic presentation after 11.5 g of diphenhydramine. Hum Exp Toxicol 2007;26:131-3.
261. Friedemann T. The excretion of ingested ethyl alcohol in saliva. J Lab Clin Med 1938;29:1007-14.
262. Fucci N, De Giovanni N, Chiarotti M, Scarlata S. SPME-GC analysis of THC in saliva samples collected with "EPITOPE" device. Forensic Sci Int 2001;119:318-21.
263. Fudala PJ, Bridge TP, Herbert S, Williford WO, Chiang CN, Jones K, et al. Office-based treatment of opiate addiction with a sublingual-tablet formulation of buprenorphine and naloxone. N Engl J Med 2003;349:949-58.

264. Fudala PJ, Johnson RE. Development of opioid formulations with limited diversion and abuse potential. Drug Alcohol Depend 2006; 83(Suppl 1):S40-7.
265. Fukuto TR. Mechanism of action of organophosphorus and carbamate insecticides. Environ Health Perspect 1990;87:245-54.
266. Fuller DC, Anderson WH. A simplified procedure for the determination of free codeine, free morphine, and 6-acetylmorphine in urine. J Anal Toxicol 1992;16:315-8.
267. Gabow PA. Disorders associated with an altered anion gap. Kidney Int 1985;27:472-83.
268. Gadsden RH Jr, Taylor EH, Steindel SJ. Ethanol in biological fluids by enzymic analysis. In: Frings C, Faulkner W, eds. Selected methods of emergency toxicology. Washington, DC: AACC Press, 1986: 63-5.
269. Gadsden RH Sr. Study of forensic and clinical source hemoglobin interference with the duPont ACA ethanol method. Ann Clin Lab Sci 1986;16:399-406.
270. Gallagher RM, Rosenthal LJ. Chronic pain and opiates: balancing pain control and risks in long-term opioid treatment. Arch Phys Med Rehabil 2008;89:S77-82.
271. Galloway FR, Bellet NF. Methadone conversion to EDDP during GC-MS analysis of urine samples. J Anal Toxicol 1999;23:615-9.
272. Gareri J, Klein J, Koren G. Drugs of abuse testing in meconium. Clin Chim Acta 2006;366:101-11.
273. Garretty DJ, Wolff K, Hay AW, Raistrick D. Benzodiazepine misuse by drug addicts. Ann Clin Biochem 1997;34(Pt 1):68-73.
274. Garriott JC. Pharmacology and toxicology of ethyl alcohol. In: Garriott JC, ed. Medicolegal aspects of alcohol. Tucson, Ariz: Lawyers & Judges Publishing, 1996:35-63.
275. Geiser L, Cherkaoui S, Veuthey JL. Simultaneous analysis of some amphetamine derivatives in urine by nonaqueous capillary electrophoresis coupled to electrospray ionization mass spectrometry. J Chromatogr A 2000;895:111-21.
276. Geller RJ, Spyker DA, Herold DA, Bruns DE. Serum osmolal gap and ethanol concentration: a simple and accurate formula. J Toxicol Clin Toxicol 1986;24:77-84.
277. George CF. Pyrazolopyrimidines. Lancet 2001;358:1623-6.
278. George S, Braithwaite RA. A pilot study to determine the usefulness of the urinary excretion of methadone and its primary metabolite (EDDP) as potential markers of compliance in methadone detoxification programs. J Anal Toxicol 1999;23:81-5.
279. George S, Braithwaite RA. Use of on-site testing for drugs of abuse. Clin Chem 2002;48:1639-46.
280. George S, Parmar S, Meadway C, Braithwaite RA. Application and validation of a urinary methadone metabolite (EDDP) immunoassay to monitor methadone compliance. Ann Clin Biochem 2000;37(Pt 3): 350-4.
281. Gergov M, Ojanpera I, Vuori E. Simultaneous screening for 238 drugs in blood by liquid chromatography-ion spray tandem mass spectrometry with multiple-reaction monitoring. J Chromatogr B Analyt Technol Biomed Life Sci 2003;795:41-53.
282. Gergov M, Robson JN, Ojanpera I, Heinonen OP, Vuori E. Simultaneous screening and quantitation of 18 antihistamine drugs in blood by liquid chromatography ionspray tandem mass spectrometry. Forensic Sci Int 2001;121:108-15.
283. Gillman PK. Monoamine oxidase inhibitors, opioid analgesics and serotonin toxicity. Br J Anaesth 2005;95:434-41.
284. Giovannelli M, Bedforth N, Aitkenhead A. Survey of intrathecal opioid usage in the UK. Eur J Anaesthesiol 2008;25:118-22.
285. Giraud S, Robinson N, Mangin P, Saugy M. Scientific and forensic standards for homologous blood transfusion anti-doping analyses. Forensic Sci Int 2008;179:23-33.
286. Gjerde H, Fongen U, Gundersen H, Christophersen AS. Evaluation of a method for simultaneous quantification of codeine, ethylmorphine and morphine in blood. Forensic Sci Int 1991;51:105-10.
287. Glare PA, Walsh TD. Clinical pharmacokinetics of morphine. Ther Drug Monit 1991;13:1-23.
288. Glasser L, Sternglanz PD, Combie J, Robinson A. Serum osmolality and its applicability to drug overdose. Am J Clin Pathol 1973;60:695-9.
289. Gock SB, Wong SH, Nuwayhid N, Venuti SE, Kelley PD, Teggatz JR, et al. Acute zolpidem overdose—report of two cases. J Anal Toxicol 1999;23:559-62.
290. Goldberger BA, Cone EJ. Confirmatory tests for drugs in the workplace by gas chromatography-mass spectrometry. J Chromatogr A 1994;674:73-86.
291. Goldstein DB. Pharmacology of alcohol. New York, NY: Oxford University Press, 1983.
292. Goldstein DS, Nurnberger J Jr, Simmons S, Gershon ES, Polinsky R, Keiser HR. Effects of injected sympathomimetic amines on plasma catecholamines and circulatory variables in man. Life Sci 1983;32: 1057-63.
293. Goodwin RS, Gustafson RA, Barnes A, Nebro W, Moolchan ET, Huestis MA. Delta(9)-tetrahydrocannabinol, 11-hydroxy-delta(9)-tetrahydrocannabinol and 11-nor-9-carboxy-delta(9)-tetrahydrocannabinol in human plasma after controlled oral administration of cannabinoids. Ther Drug Monit 2006;28:545-51.
294. Goulle JP, Anger JP. Drug-facilitated robbery or sexual assault: problems associated with amnesia. Ther Drug Monit 2004;26:206-10.
295. Goulle JP, Cheze M, Pepin G. Determination of endogenous levels of GHB in human hair: are there possibilities for the identification of GHB administration through hair analysis in cases of drug-facilitated sexual assault? J Anal Toxicol 2003;27:574-80.
296. Green AL, el Hait MA. Inhibition of mouse brain monoamine oxidase by (+)-amphetamine in vivo. J Pharm Pharmacol 1978;30:262-3.
297. Green AL, el Hait MA. p-Methoxyamphetamine, a potent reversible inhibitor of type-A monoamine oxidase in vitro and in vivo. J Pharm Pharmacol 1980;32:262-6.
298. Green B, Kavanagh D, Young R. Being stoned: a review of self-reported cannabis effects. Drug Alcohol Rev 2003;22:453-60.
299. Green KB, Isenschmid DS. Medical review officer interpretation of urine drug test results. In: Liu R, Goldberger B, eds. Handbook of workplace drug testing. Washington, DC: AACC Press, 1995:321-53.
300. Green KB, Isenschmid DS. Medical review officer interpretation of urine drug testing results. Forensic Sci Rev 1995;7:41-60.
301. Green SM, Johnson NE. Ketamine sedation for pediatric procedures. Part 2: review and implications. Ann Emerg Med 1990;19:1033-46.
302. Griffith RK, Johnson EA. Adrenergic drugs. In: Foye WO, Lemke TL, Williams DA, eds. Principles of medicinal chemistry. Baltimore, Md: Williams & Wilkins, 1995:345-65.
303. Grinstead GF. A closer look at acetyl and pentafluoropropionyl derivatives for quantitative analysis of morphine and codeine by gas chromatography/mass spectrometry. J Anal Toxicol 1991;15:293-8.
304. Grotenhermen F. Pharmacokinetics and pharmacodynamics of cannabinoids. Clin Pharmacokinet 2003;42:327-60.
305. Grotenhermen F. Pharmacology of cannabinoids. Neuroendocrinol Lett 2004;25:14-23.
306. Grotenhermen F, Leson G, Berghaus G, Drummer OH, Kruger HP, Longo M, et al. Developing limits for driving under cannabis. Addiction 2007;102:1910-7.
307. Guillot JG, Weber JP, Savoie JY. Quantitative determination of carbon monoxide in blood by head-space gas chromatography. J Anal Toxicol 1981;5:264-6.
308. Gustafson RA, Levine B, Stout PR, Klette KL, George MP, Moolchan ET, et al. Urinary cannabinoid detection times after controlled oral administration of delta9-tetrahydrocannabinol to humans. Clin Chem 2003;49:1114-24.
309. Gutstein HB, Akil H. Opioid analgesics (Chapter 21). In: Brunton LL, Lazo JS, Parker KL, eds. Goodman & Gilman's the pharmacological basis of therapeutics, 11th edition. New York, NY: McGraw-Hill, 2006.
310. Haddad LM, Winchester JF. Barbiturates. In: Haddad L, Shannon M, Winchester J, eds. Clinical management of poisoning and drug overdose. Philadelphia, Pa: WB Saunders, 1998:521-7.

311. Haeckel R, Hanecke P. Application of saliva for drug monitoring: an in vivo model for transmembrane transport. Eur J Clin Chem Clin Biochem 1996;34:171-91.
312. Hahn IH, Chu J, Hoffman RS, Nelson LS. Errors in reporting salicylate levels. Acad Emerg Med 2000;7:1336-7.
313. Hakala KS, Kostiainen R, Ketola RA. Feasibility of different mass spectrometric techniques and programs for automated metabolite profiling of tramadol in human urine. Rapid Commun Mass Spectrom 2006;20:2081-90.
314. Hall BJ, Satterfield-Doerr M, Parikh AR, Brodbelt JS. Determination of cannabinoids in water and human saliva by solid-phase microextraction and quadrupole ion trap gas chromatography/mass spectrometry. Anal Chem 1998;70:1788-96.
315. Hall JA, Moore CB. Drug facilitated sexual assault—a review. J Forensic Leg Med 2008;15:291-7.
316. Halla JT, Atchison SL, Hardin JG. Symptomatic salicylate ototoxicity: a useful indicator of serum salicylate concentration? Ann Rheum Dis 1991;50:682-4.
317. Haller CA, Benowitz NL. Adverse cardiovascular and central nervous system events associated with dietary supplements containing ephedra alkaloids. N Engl J Med 2000;343:1833-8.
318. Hampson NB, Hauff NM. Carboxyhemoglobin levels in carbon monoxide poisoning: do they correlate with the clinical picture? Am J Emerg Med 2008;26:665-9.
319. Hanson SM, Morlock EV, Satyshur KA, Czajkowski C. Structural requirements for eszopiclone and zolpidem binding to the gamma-aminobutyric acid type-A (GABAA) receptor are different. J Med Chem 2008;51:7243-52.
320. Harden RN. Chronic pain and opiates: a call for moderation. Arch Phys Med Rehabil 2008;89:S72-6.
321. Harding P. Methods for breath analysis. In: Garriott JC, ed. Medicolegal aspects of alcohol. Tucson, Ariz: Lawyers & Judges Publishing, 1996:181-217.
322. Harrison PM, Wendon JA, Gimson AE, Alexander GJ, Williams R. Improvement by acetylcysteine of hemodynamics and oxygen transport in fulminant hepatic failure. N Engl J Med 1991;324:1852-7.
323. Hart CL, Jatlow P, Sevarino KA, McCance-Katz EF. Comparison of intravenous cocaethylene and cocaine in humans. Psychopharmacology 2000;149:153-62.
324. Hayes LW, Krasselt WG, Mueggler PA. Concentrations of morphine and codeine in serum and urine after ingestion of poppy seeds. Clin Chem 1987;33:806-8.
325. Haymond S, Cariappa R, Eby CS, Scott MG. Laboratory assessment of oxygenation in methemoglobinemia. Clin Chem 2005;51:434-44.
326. Hearn WL, Flynn DD, Hime GW, Rose S, Cofino JC, Mantero-Atienza E, et al. Cocaethylene: a unique cocaine metabolite displays high affinity for the dopamine transporter. J Neurochem 1991;56:698-701.
327. Hegadoren KM, Greenshaw AJ, Baker GB, Martin-Iverson MT, Lodge B, Soin S. 4-Ethoxyamphetamine: effects on intracranial self-stimulation and in vitro uptake and release of 3H-dopamine and 3H-serotonin in the brains of rats. J Psychiatry Neurosci 1994;19: 57-62.
328. Heller DN. Liquid chromatography/mass spectrometry for timely response in regulatory analyses: identification of pentobarbital in dog food. Anal Chem 2000;72:2711-6.
329. Henderson GL, Harkey MR, Zhou C, Jones RT, Jacob P 3rd. Incorporation of isotopically labeled cocaine into human hair: race as a factor. J Anal Toxicol 1998;22:156-65.
330. Hendrickson R, Bizovi KE. Acetaminophen. In: Goldfrank LR, Flomenbaum NE, Lewin NA, Howland MA, Hoffman RS, Nelson LS, eds. Goldfrank's toxicologic emergencies, 8th edition. New York, NY: McGraw-Hill, 2006:523-43.
331. Hensley D, Cody JT. Simultaneous determination of amphetamine, methamphetamine, methylenedioxyamphetamine (MDA), methylenedioxymethamphetamine (MDMA), and methylenedioxyethylamphetamine (MDEA) enantiomers by GC-MS. J Anal Toxicol 1999;23:518-23.
332. Hersack RA. Ketamine's psychological effects do not contraindicate its use based on a patient's occupation. Aviat Space Environ Med 1994; 65:1041-6.
333. Hessel DW, Modglin FR. The quantitative determination of ethanol and other volatile substances in blood by gas-liquid partition chromatography. J Forensic Sci 1964;9:255-64.
334. Hewlett TP, McMartin KE, Lauro AJ, Ragan FA Jr. Ethylene glycol poisoning: the value of glycolic acid determinations for diagnosis and treatment. J Toxicol Clin Toxicol 1986;24:389-402.
335. Hime GW, Hearn WL, Rose S, Cofino J. Analysis of cocaine and cocaethylene in blood and tissues by GC-NPD and GC-ion trap mass spectrometry. J Anal Toxicol 1991;15:241-5.
336. Hindmarch I, ElSohly M, Gambles J, Salamone S. Forensic urinalysis of drug use in cases of alleged sexual assault. J Clin Forensic Med 2001;8:197-205.
337. Hoffman RJ, Nelson LS, Hoffman RS. Use of ferric chloride to identify salicylate-containing poisons. J Toxicol Clin Toxicol 2002;40:547-9.
338. Hold K, de Boer D, Zuidema J, Maes RA. Saliva as an analytical tool in toxicology. Int J Drug Testing 1995;1:1-36.
339. Hold KM, Borges CR, Wilkins DG, Rollins DE, Joseph RE Jr. Detection of nandrolone, testosterone, and their esters in rat and human hair samples. J Anal Toxicol 1999;23:416-23.
340. Holstege C, Baer A, Brady WJ. The electrocardiographic toxidrome: the ECG presentation of hydrofluoric acid ingestion. Am J Emerg Med 2005;23:171-6.
341. Holstege CP, Dobmeier S. Cardiovascular challenges in toxicology. Emerg Med Clin North Am 2005;23:1195-217.
342. Honey CR, Miljkovic Z, MacDonald JF. Ketamine and phencyclidine cause a voltage-dependent block of responses to L-aspartic acid. Neurosci Lett 1985;61:135-9.
343. Hornbeck CL, Czarny RJ. Retrospective analysis of some L-methamphetamine/L-amphetamine urine data. J Anal Toxicol 1993;17:23-5.
344. Horning MG, Brown L, Nowlin J, Lertratanangkoon K, Kellaway P, Zion TE. Use of saliva in therapeutic drug monitoring. Clin Chem 1977;23:157-64.
345. Howlett AC, Barth F, Bonner TI, Cabral G, Casellas P, Devane WA, et al. International Union of Pharmacology. XXVII. Classification of cannabinoid receptors. Pharmacol Rev 2002;54:161-202.
346. Hsu J, Liu C, Liu CP, Tsay WI, Li JH, Lin DL, et al. Performance characteristics of selected immunoassays for preliminary test of 3,4-methylenedioxymethamphetamine, methamphetamine, and related drugs in urine specimens. J Anal Toxicol 2003;27:471-8.
347. Huang W, Andollo W, Hearn WL. A solid phase extraction technique for the isolation and identification of opiates in urine. J Anal Toxicol 1992;16:307-10.
348. Huestis MA, Henningfield JE, Cone EJ. Blood cannabinoids. I. Absorption of THC and formation of 11-OH-THC and THCCOOH during and after smoking marijuana. J Anal Toxicol 1992;16:276-82.
349. Huestis MA, Mitchell JM, Cone EJ. Lowering the federally mandated cannabinoid immunoassay cutoff increases true-positive results. Clin Chem 1994;40:729-33.
350. Hughes RO, Bronner WE, Smith ML. Detection of amphetamine and methamphetamine in urine by gas chromatography/mass spectrometry following derivatization with (−)-menthyl chloroformate. J Anal Toxicol 1991;15:256-9.
351. Hullin DA. An IgM paraprotein causing a falsely low result in an enzymatic assay for acetaminophen. Clin Chem 1999;45:155-7.
352. Humbert L, Jacquemont MC, Leroy E, Leclerc F, Houdret N, Lhermitte M. Determination of chloral hydrate and its metabolites (trichloroethanol and trichloracetic acid) in human plasma and urine using electron capture gas chromatography. Biomed Chromatogr 1994;8:273-7.
353. Hurwitz ES, Barrett MJ, Bregman D, Gunn WJ, Schonberger LB, Fairweather WR, et al. Public Health Service study on Reye's syndrome and medications: report of the pilot phase. N Engl J Med 1985;313:849-57.

354. Inaba T, Stewart DJ, Kalow W. Metabolism of cocaine in man. Clin Pharmacol Ther 1978;23:547-52.
355. Ingelman-Sundberg M. Genetic polymorphisms of cytochrome P450 2D6 (CYP2D6): clinical consequences, evolutionary aspects and functional diversity. Pharmacogenom J 2005;5:6-13.
356. Inoue T, Seta S, Goldberger BA. Analysis of drugs in unconventional samples. In: Liu R, Goldberger B, eds. Handbook of workplace drug testing. Washington, DC: AACC Press, 1995:131-58.
357. Inturrisi CE, Max MB, Foley KM, Schultz M, Shin SU, Houde RW. The pharmacokinetics of heroin in patients with chronic pain. N Engl J Med 1984;310:1213-7.
358. Ioannides C, Chakraborty J, Parke D. Improvement of barbiturate gas chromatography by formic acid: possible mechanism. Chromatographia 1974;7:351-6.
359. Isbister G, Downes F, Sibbritt D, Dawson A, Whyte I. Aspiration pneumonitis in an overdose population: frequency, predictors, and outcomes. Crit Care Med 2004;32:88-93.
360. Isbister GK, Buckley NA, Whyte IM. Serotonin toxicity: a practical approach to diagnosis and treatment. Med J Aust 2007;187:361-5.
361. Isenschmid DS. Cocaine: effects on human performance and behavior. Forensic Sci Rev 2002;14:61-100.
362. Isenschmid DS. Cocaine. In: Levine B, ed. Principles of forensic toxicology, 2nd edition. Washington, DC: AACC Press, 2003:207-28.
363. Isenschmid DS, Levine BS, Caplan YH. A method for the simultaneous determination of cocaine, benzoylecgonine, and ecgonine methyl ester in blood and urine using GC/EIMS with derivatization to produce high mass molecular ions. J Anal Toxicol 1988;12:242-5.
364. Ishihara K, Szerlip HM. Anion gap acidosis. Semin Nephrol 1998;18: 83-97.
365. Iversen L. Cannabis and the brain. Brain 2003;126:1252-70.
366. Iwai M, Hattori H, Arinobu T, Ishii A, Kumazawa T, Noguchi H, et al. Simultaneous determination of barbiturates in human biological fluids by direct immersion solid-phase microextraction and gas chromatography-mass spectrometry. J Chromatogr B Analyt Technol Biomed Life Sci 2004;806:65-73.
367. Iwersen-Bergmann S, Schmoldt A. Direct semiquantitative screening of drugs of abuse in serum and whole blood by means of CEDIA DAU urine immunoassays. J Anal Toxicol 1999;23:247-56.
368. Jackson DL, Menges H. Accidental carbon monoxide poisoning. JAMA 1980;243:772-4.
369. Jacob P 3rd, Jones RT, Benowitz NL. Formation and elimination kinetics of cocaethylene in humans. Clin Pharmacol Ther 1993;53:174.
370. Jacob P 3rd, Lewis ER, Elias-Baker BA, Jones RT. A pyrolysis product, anhydroecgonine methyl ester (methylecgonidine), is in the urine of cocaine smokers. J Anal Toxicol 1990;14:353-7.
371. Jacobsen D, Ovrebo S, Ostborg J, Sejersted OM. Glycolate causes the acidosis in ethylene glycol poisoning and is effectively removed by hemodialysis. Acta Med Scand 1984;216:409-16.
372. Jaehne EJ, Salem A, Irvine RJ. Pharmacological and behavioral determinants of cocaine, methamphetamine, 3,4-met hylenedioxymethamphetamine, and para-methoxyamphetamine-induced hyperthermia. Psychopharmacology 2007;194:41-52.
373. Jain NC, Chinn DM, Budd RD, Sneath TS, Leung WJ. Simultaneous determination of cocaine and benzoyl ecgonine in urine by gas chromatography with on-column alkylation. J Forensic Sci 1977;22:7-16.
374. James RA, Dinan A. Hyperpyrexia associated with fatal paramethoxyamphetamine (PMA) abuse. Med Sci Law 1998;38:83-5.
375. Jarvie DR, Heyworth R, Simpson D. Plasma salicylate analysis: a comparison of colorimetric, HPLC and enzymatic techniques. Ann Clin Biochem 1987;24(Pt 4):364-73.
376. Jatlow P. Cocaethylene: pharmacologic activity and clinical significance. Ther Drug Monit 1993;15:533-6.
377. Jatlow P, Elsworth JD, Bradberry CW, Winger G, Taylor JR, Russell R, et al. Cocaethylene: a neuropharmacologically active metabolite associated with concurrent cocaine-ethanol ingestion. Life Sci 1991; 48:1787-94.
378. Jatlow PI. Drug of abuse profile: cocaine. Clin Chem 1987;33: 66B-71B.
379. Javaid JI, Dekirmenjian H, Brunngraber EG, Davis JM. Quantitative determination of cocaine and its metabolites benzoylecgonine and ecgonine by gas-liquid chromatography. J Chromatogr 1975;110: 140-9.
380. Jeanville PM, Estape ES, Needham SR, Cole MJ. Rapid confirmation/quantitation of cocaine and benzoylecgonine in urine utilizing high performance liquid chromatography and tandem mass spectrometry. J Am Soc Mass Spectrom 2000;11:257-63.
381. Jenkins AJ, Goldberger BA. Identification of unique cocaine metabolites and smoking by-products in postmortem blood and urine specimens. J Forensic Sci 1997;42:824-7.
382. Jenkins AJ, Oyler JM, Cone EJ. Comparison of heroin and cocaine concentrations in saliva with concentrations in blood and plasma. J Anal Toxicol 1995;19:359-74.
383. Jiang T-F, Wang Y-H, Lu Z-H, Yue M-E. Direct determination of barbiturates in urine by capillary electrophoresis using a capillary coated dynamically with polycationic polymers. Chromatographia 2007;65:611-5.
384. Johansen SS, Bhatia HM. Quantitative analysis of cocaine and its metabolites in whole blood and urine by high-performance liquid chromatography coupled with tandem mass spectrometry. J Chromatogr B Analyt Technol Biomed Life Sci 2007;852:338-44.
385. Johansen SS, Hansen AC, Muller IB, Lundemose JB, Franzmann MB. Three fatal cases of PMA and PMMA poisoning in Denmark. J Anal Toxicol 2003;27:253-6.
386. Jolliff HA, Sivilotti ML. Ethylene glycol. In: Dart RC, ed. Medical toxicology. Philadelphia, Pa: Lippincott Williams & Wilkins, 2004:1223-30.
387. Jones AB, ElSohly HN, Arafat ES, ElSohly MA. Analysis of the major metabolite of delta 9-tetrahydrocannabinol in urine. IV: a comparison of five methods. J Anal Toxicol 1984;8:249-51.
388. Jones AW. Distribution of ethanol between saliva and blood in man. Clin Exp Pharmacol Physiol 1979;6:53-9.
389. Jones AW. Measurement of alcohol in blood and breath for legal purposes. In: Crow KE, Batt RD, eds. Human metabolism of alcohol, vol I. Pharmacokinetics, medicolegal aspects, and general interests. Boca Raton, Fla: CRC Press, 1989:71-99.
390. Jones AW, Blom Y, Bondesson U, Anggard E. Determination of morphine in biological samples by gas chromatography-mass spectrometry: evidence for persistent tissue binding in rats twenty-two days post-withdrawal. J Chromatogr 1984;309:73-80.
391. Jones AW, Lindberg L, Olsson SG. Magnitude and time-course of arterio-venous differences in blood-alcohol concentration in healthy men. Clin Pharmacokinet 2004;43:1157-66.
392. Jones G. Post-mortem toxicology. In: Moffat A, ed. Clarke's analysis of drugs and poisons, 3rd edition. London, UK: Pharmaceutical Press, 2004:95-108.
393. Jones GR, Singer PP. An unusual trichloroethanol fatality attributed to sniffing trichloroethylene. J Anal Toxicol 2008;32:183-6.
394. Jones JJ, Kidwell H, Games DE. Application of atmospheric pressure chemical ionisation mass spectrometry in the analysis of barbiturates by high-speed analytical countercurrent chromatography. Rapid Commun Mass Spectrom 2003;17:1565-72.
395. Josefson D. Herbal stimulant causes US deaths. BMJ 1996;312:1441.
396. Joseph RE Jr, Hold KM, Wilkins DG, Rollins DE, Cone EJ. Drug testing with alternative matrices II. Mechanisms of cocaine and codeine deposition in hair. J Anal Toxicol 1999;23:396-408.
397. Joseph RE Jr, Su TP, Cone EJ. In vitro binding studies of drugs to hair: influence of melanin and lipids on cocaine binding to Caucasoid and Africoid hair. J Anal Toxicol 1996;20:338-44.
398. Joynt BP. Triazolam blood concentrations in forensic cases in Canada. J Anal Toxicol 1993;17:171-7.
399. Jufer RA, Walsh SL, Cone EJ. Cocaine and metabolite concentrations in plasma during repeated oral administration: development of a human laboratory model of chronic cocaine use. J Anal Toxicol 1998; 22:435-44.

400. Kadehjian L. Legal issues in oral fluid testing. Forensic Sci Int 2005; 150:151-60.
401. Kadiev E, Patel V, Rad P, Thankachan L, Tram A, Weinlein M, et al. Role of pharmacogenetics in variable response to drugs: focus on opioids. Exp Opin Drug Metab Toxicol 2008;4:77-91.
402. Kalant H. The pharmacology and toxicology of "ecstasy" (MDMA) and related drugs. CMAJ 2001;165:917-28.
403. Kalix P. The pharmacology of psychoactive alkaloids from ephedra and catha. J Ethnopharmacol 1991;32:201-8.
404. Kaminskas LM, Irvine RJ, Callaghan PD, White JM, Kirkbride P. The contribution of the metabolite p-hydroxyamphetamine to the central actions of p-methoxyamphetamine. Psychopharmacology 2002;160: 155-60.
405. Kapur BM, Vandenbroucke A, Cogionis B, Losner K. Rapid analysis of toxic alcohols. Clin Chem 2005;51:A155.
406. Karnes HT, Beightol LA. Evaluation of fluorescence polarization immunoassay for quantitation of serum salicylates. Ther Drug Monit 1985;7:351-4.
407. Katagi M, Nishikawa M, Tatsuno M, Miki A, Tsuchihashi H. Column-switching high-performance liquid chromatography-electrospray ionization mass spectrometry for identification of heroin metabolites in human urine. J Chromatogr 2001;751:177-85.
408. Kato K, Hillsgrove M, Weinhold L, Gorelick DA, Darwin WD, Cone EJ. Cocaine and metabolite excretion in saliva under stimulated and nonstimulated conditions. J Anal Toxicol 1993;17:338-41.
409. Katz KD, Curry SC, Brooks DE, Gerkin RD. The effect of cyclosporine A on survival time in salicylate-poisoned rats. J Emerg Med 2004;26: 151-5.
410. Kaupmann K, Cryan JF, Wellendorph P, Mombereau C, Sansig G, Klebs K, et al. Specific gamma-hydroxybutyrate-binding sites but loss of pharmacological effects of gamma-hydroxybutyrate in GABA(B) (1)-deficient mice. Eur J Neurosci 2003;18:2722-30.
411. Kellermann AL, Fihn SD, LoGerfo JP, Copass MK. Impact of drug screening in suspected overdose. Ann Emerg Med 1987;16:1206-16.
412. Kelner MJ, Bailey DN. Mismeasurement of methemoglobin ("methemoglobin revisited"). Clin Chem 1985;31:168-9.
413. Kepczynska E, Bojarski J, Haber P, Kaliszan R. Retention of barbituric acid derivatives on immobilized artificial membrane stationary phase and its correlation with biological activity. Biomed Chromatogr 2000;14:256-60.
414. Kerrigan S, Goldberger BA. Opioids. In: Levine B, ed. Principles of forensic toxicology, 2nd edition. Washington, DC: AACC Press, 2003:187-205.
415. Keyes DC, Dart RC. Initial diagnosis and treatment of the poisoned patient. In: Dart RC, ed. Medical toxicology. Philadelphia, Pa: Lippincott Williams & Wilkins, 2004:21-31.
416. Kidwell DA, Blank D. Hair analysis: techniques and potential problems. In: Sunshine I, ed. Recent developments in therapeutic drug monitoring and clinical toxicology. New York, NY: Marcel Dekker, 1992:555-63.
417. Kidwell DA, Holland JC, Athanaselis S. Testing for drugs of abuse in saliva and sweat. J Chromatogr 1998;713:111-35.
418. Kikura-Hanajiri R, Hayashi M, Saisho K, Goda Y. Simultaneous determination of nineteen hallucinogenic tryptamines/beta-calbolines and phenethylamines using gas chromatography-mass spectrometry and liquid chromatography-electrospray ionisation-mass spectrometry. J Chromatogr B Analyt Technol Biomed Life Sci 2005;825:29-37.
419. Killmann SA, Thaysen JH. The permeability of the human parotid gland to a series of sulfonamide compounds, para-aminohippurate and inulin. Scand J Clin Lab Invest 1955;7:86-91.
420. Kim EM, Lee JS, Choi SK, Lim MA, Chung HS. Analysis of ketamine and norketamine in urine by automatic solid-phase extraction (SPE) and positive ion chemical ionization-gas chromatography-mass spectrometry (PCI-GC-MS). Forensic Sci Int 2008;174:197-202.
421. King JA, Storrow AB, Finkelstein JA. Urine Trinder spot test: a rapid salicylate screen for the emergency department. Ann Emerg Med 1995;26:330-3.
422. Kintz P. Drug testing in hair. Boca Raton, Fla: CRC Press, 1996.
423. Kintz P. Hair testing and doping control in sport. Toxicol Lett 1998; 102:109-13.
424. Kintz P. Value of hair analysis in postmortem toxicology. Forensic Sci Int 2004;142:127-34.
425. Kintz P, Brenneisen R, Bundeli P, Mangin P. Sweat testing for heroin and metabolites in a heroin maintenance program. Clin Chem 1997; 43:736-9.
426. Kintz P, Samyn N. Determination of "Ecstasy" components in alternative biological specimens. J Chromatogr 1999;733:137-43.
427. Kintz P, Samyn N. Use of alternative specimens: drugs of abuse in saliva and doping agents in hair. Ther Drug Monit 2002;24:239-46.
428. Kintz P, Tracqui A, Jamey C, Mangin P. Detection of codeine and phenobarbital in sweat collected with a sweat patch. J Anal Toxicol 1996;20:197-201.
429. Kintz P, Villain M, Dumestre-Toulet V, Ludes B. Drug-facilitated sexual assault and analytical toxicology: the role of LC-MS/MS. A case involving zolpidem. J Clin Forensic Med 2005;12:36-41.
430. Kintz P, Villain M, Ludes B. Testing for the undetectable in drug-facilitated sexual assault using hair analyzed by tandem mass spectrometry as evidence. Ther Drug Monit 2004;26:211-4.
431. Kintz P, Villain M, Ludes B. Testing for zolpidem in oral fluid by liquid chromatography-tandem mass spectrometry. J Chromatogr B Analyt Technol Biomed Life Sci 2004;811:59-63.
432. Kirages TJ, Sulc HP, Mycyk MB. Severe manifestations of coricidin intoxication. Am J Emerg Med 2003;21:473-5.
433. Kleinschnitz M, Herderich M, Schreier P. Determination of 1,4-benzodiazepines by high-performance liquid chromatography-electrospray tandem mass spectrometry. J Chromatogr B Biomed Appl 1996;676:61-7.
434. Klette KL, Horn CK, Stout PR, Anderson CJ. LC-MS analysis of human urine specimens for 2-oxo-3-hydroxy LSD: method validation for potential interferants and stability study of 2-oxo-3-hydroxy LSD under various storage conditions. J Anal Toxicol 2002;26:193-200.
435. Klette KL, Poch GK, Czarny R, Lau CO. Simultaneous GC-MS analysis of meta- and para-hydroxybenzoylecgonine and norbenzoylecgonine: a secondary method to corroborate cocaine ingestion using nonhydrolytic metabolites. J Anal Toxicol 2000;24:482-8.
436. Klingmann A, Skopp G, Aderjan R. Analysis of cocaine, benzoylecgonine, ecogonine methyl ester, and ecgonine by high-pressure liquid chromatography-API mass spectrometry and application to a short-term degradation study of cocaine in plasma. J Anal Toxicol 2001;25:425-30.
437. Kloss MW, Rosen GM, Rauckman EJ. N-demethylation of cocaine to norcocaine: evidence for participation by cytochrome P-450 and FAD-containing monooxygenase. Mol Pharmacol 1983;23:482-5.
438. Kloss MW, Rosen GM, Rauckman EJ. Cocaine-mediated hepatotoxicity: a critical review. Biochem Pharmacol 1984;33:169-73.
439. Koek W, Carter LP, Lamb RJ, Chen W, Wu H, Coop A, France CP. Discriminative stimulus effects of gamma-hydroxybutyrate (GHB) in rats discriminating GHB from baclofen and diazepam. J Pharmacol Exp Ther 2005;314:170-9.
440. Kogan MJ, Verebey KG, DePace AC, Resnick RB, Mule SJ. Quantitative determination of benzoylecgonine and cocaine in human biofluids by gas-liquid chromatography. Anal Chem 1977;49:1965-9.
441. Kolbrich EA, Barnes AJ, Gorelick DA, Boyd SJ, Cone EJ, Huestis MA. Major and minor metabolites of cocaine in human plasma following controlled subcutaneous cocaine administration. J Anal Toxicol 2006; 30:501-10.
442. Kraemer T, Maurer HH. Toxicokinetics of amphetamines: metabolism and toxicokinetic data of designer drugs, amphetamine, methamphetamine, and their N-alkyl derivatives. Ther Drug Monit 2002;24:277-89.
443. Krahn J, Khajuria A. Osmolality gaps: diagnostic accuracy and long-term variability. Clin Chem 2006;52:737-9.
444. Kraner JC, McCoy DJ, Evans MA, Evans LE, Sweeney BJ. Fatalities caused by the MDMA-related drug paramethoxyamphetamine (PMA). J Anal Toxicol 2001;25:645-8.

445. Kranzler HR, Stone J, McLaughlin L. Evaluation of a point-of-care testing product for drugs of abuse: testing site is a key variable. Drug Alcohol Depend 1995;40:55-62.
446. Kratzsch C, Peters FT, Kraemer T, Weber AA, Maurer HH. Screening, library-assisted identification and validated quantification of fifteen neuroleptics and three of their metabolites in plasma by liquid chromatography/mass spectrometry with atmospheric pressure chemical ionization. J Mass Spectrom 2003;38:283-95.
447. Krenzelok EP, Kerr F, Proudfoot AT. Salicylate toxicity. In: Haddad LM, Shannon MW, Winchester JD, eds. Clinical management of poisoning and drug overdose, 3rd ed. Philadelphia, Pa: WB Saunders, 1998:675-87.
448. Kreuz DS, Axelrod J. Delta-9-tetrahydrocannabinol: localization in body fat. Science 1973;179:391-3.
449. Kronstrand R, Forstberg-Peterson S, Kagedal B, Ahlner J, Larson G. Codeine concentration in hair after oral administration is dependent on melanin content. Clin Chem 1999;45:1485-94.
450. Kronstrand R, Nystrom I, Josefsson M, Hodgins S. Segmental ion spray LC-MS-MS analysis of benzodiazepines in hair of psychiatric patients. J Anal Toxicol 2002;26:479-84.
451. Kronstrand R, Nystrom I, Strandberg J, Druid H. Screening for drugs of abuse in hair with ion spray LC-MS-MS. Forensic Sci Int 2004;145: 183-90.
452. Kumar S, Fleming RL, Morrow AL. Ethanol regulation of gamma-aminobutyric acid A receptors: genomic and nongenomic mechanisms. Pharmacol Ther 2004;101:211-26.
453. Kwong TC, Chamberlain RT, Frederick DL, Kapur BM, Sunshine I. Critical issues in urinalysis of abused substances: report of the Substance-Abuse Testing Committee. Review. Clin Chem 1988;34: 605-32.
454. Kwong TC, Ryan RM. Detection of intrauterine illicit drug exposure by newborn drug testing. National Academy of Clinical Biochemistry. Clin Chem 1997;43:235-42.
455. Kwong TC, Shearer D. Detection of drug use during pregnancy. Obstet Gynecol Clin North Am 1998;25:43-64.
456. Lacy TL, Nichols JH. Therapeutic drugs III: neuroleptic (antipsychotic) drugs. In: Levine B, ed. Principles of forensic toxicology, 2nd edition. Washington, DC: AACC Press, 2003:315-25.
457. Lafolie P, Beck O, Blennow G, Boreus L, Borg S, Elwin CE, et al. Importance of creatinine analyses of urine when screening for abused drugs. Clin Chem 1991;37:1927-31.
458. Landaw SA, Winchell HS. Endogenous production of carbon-14 labeled carbon monoxide: an in vivo technique for the study of heme catabolism. J Nucl Med 1966;7:696-707.
459. Langman LJ. The use of oral fluid for therapeutic drug management: clinical and forensic toxicology. Ann N Y Acad Sci 2007;1098: 145-66.
460. Langman LJ, Bjergum MW, Williamson CL, Crow FW. Sensitive method for detection of cocaine and associated analytes by liquid chromatography: tandem mass spectrometry in urine. J Anal Toxicol 2009;33:447-455.
461. Large CH. Do NMDA receptor antagonist models of schizophrenia predict the clinical efficacy of antipsychotic drugs? J Psychopharmacol 2007;21:283-301.
462. Latta KS, Ginsberg B, Barkin RL. Meperidine: a critical review. Am J Ther 2002;9:53-68.
463. Law B, Mason PA, Moffat AC, King LJ, Marks V. Passive inhalation of cannabis smoke. J Pharm Pharmacol 1984;36:578-81.
464. Law MY, Slawson MH, Moody DE. Selective involvement of cytochrome P450 2D subfamily in in vivo 4-hydroxylation of amphetamine in rat. Drug Metab Dispos 2000;28:348-53.
465. Leatherman JW, Schmitz PG. Fever, hyperdynamic shock, and multiple-system organ failure: a pseudo-sepsis syndrome associated with chronic salicylate intoxication. Chest 1991;100:1391-6.
466. LeBeau MA, Montgomery MA, Miller ML, Burmeister SG. Analysis of biofluids for gamma-hydroxybutyrate (GHB) and gamma-butyrolactone (GBL) by headspace GC-FID and GC-MS. J Anal Toxicol 2000;24:421-8.
467. Ledent C, Valverde O, Cossu G, Petitet F, Aubert JF, Beslot F, et al. Unresponsiveness to cannabinoids and reduced addictive effects of opiates in CB1 receptor knockout mice. Science 1999;283:401-4.
468. Lee HM, Lee CW. Determination of morphine and codeine in blood and bile by gas chromatography with a derivatization procedure. J Anal Toxicol 1991;15:182-7.
469. LeGatt DF, Audette RJ, Blakney G, Vaughan D. Excess serum osmolality after ingestion of methanol: the exception, not the rule. Clin Chem 1991;37:1802-4.
470. Leikin J, Paloucek F. Methemoglobin, blood. In: Leikin J, Paloucek F, eds. Leikin & Paloucek's poisoning & toxicology handbook, 4th edition. Hudson, Ohio: Lexi-Comp, 2008:1047.
471. Leipzig RM, Mendelowitz A. Adverse psychotropic drug interactions. In: Kane JM, Lieberman JA, eds. Adverse effects of psychotropic drugs. New York, NY: Guilford Press, 1992:13-76.
472. Lekskulchai V, Mokkhavesa C. Evaluation of Roche Abuscreen ONLINE amphetamine immunoassay for screening of new amphetamine analogues. J Anal Toxicol 2001;25:471-5.
473. Leson G, Pless P, Grotenhermen F, Kalant H, ElSohly MA. Evaluating the impact of hemp food consumption on workplace drug tests. J Anal Toxicol 2001;25:691-8.
474. Lester BM, ElSohly M, Wright LL, Smeriglio VL, Verter J, Bauer CR, et al. The maternal lifestyle study: drug use by meconium toxicology and maternal self-report. Pediatrics 2001;107:309-17.
475. Levine B. Central nervous system depressants. In: Levine B, ed. Principles of forensic toxicology, 2nd edition. Washington, DC: AACC Press, 2003:157-72.
476. Levine BS, Smith ML. Effects of diphenhydramine on immunoassays of phencyclidine in urine. Clin Chem 1990;36:1258.
477. Lewis DE, Moore CM, Leikin JB, Koller A. Meconium analysis for cocaine: a validation study and comparison with paired urine analysis. J Anal Toxicol 1995;19:148-50.
478. Li Z, McNally AJ, Wang H, Salamone SJ. Stability study of LSD under various storage conditions. J Anal Toxicol 1998;22:520-5.
479. Liebelt EL, Francis PD. Cyclic antidepressants. In: Goldfrank LR, Flomenbaum NE, Lewin NA, Howland MA, Hoffman RS, Nelson LS, eds. Goldfrank's toxicologic emergencies, 7th edition. New York, NY: McGraw-Hill, 2002:847-64.
480. Lin JH, Levy G. Sulfate depletion after acetaminophen administration and replenishment by infusion of sodium sulfate or N-acetylcysteine in rats. Biochem Pharmacol 1981;30:2723-5.
481. Lin LY, Di Stefano EW, Schmitz DA, Hsu L, Ellis SW, Lennard MS, et al. Oxidation of methamphetamine and methylenedioxy-methamphetamine by CYP2D6. Drug Metab Dispos 1997;25: 1059-64.
482. Lin TJ, Nelson LS, Tsai JL, Hung DZ, Hu SC, Chan HM, et al. Common toxidromes of plant poisonings in Taiwan. Clin Toxicol 2009;47:161-8.
483. Lindberg L, Brauer S, Wollmer P, Goldberg L, Jones AW, Olsson SG. Breath alcohol concentration determined with a new analyzer using free exhalation predicts almost precisely the arterial blood alcohol concentration. Forensic Sci Int 2007;168:200-7.
484. Lippi G, Banfi G. Blood transfusions in athletes: old dogmas, new tricks. Clin Chem Lab Med 2006;44:1395-402.
485. Liu RH. Evaluation of common immunoassay kits for effective workplace drug testing. In: Liu R, Goldberger B, eds. Handbook of workplace drug testing. Washington, DC: AACC Press, 1995:67-129.
486. Liu YL, Toubro S, Astrup A, Stock MJ. Contribution of beta 3-adrenoceptor activation to ephedrine-induced thermogenesis in humans. Int J Obes Relat Metab Disord 1995;19:678-85.
487. Logan BK. Methamphetamine: effects on human performance and behavior. Forensic Sci Rev 2002;14:133-51.
488. Logan BK, Cooper FA. 3,4-Methylenedioxymethamphetamine: effects on human performance and behavior. Forensic Sci Rev 2003;15:11-28.
489. Logan BK, Gullberg RG. Alcohol, drugs and driving. In: Moffat AC, Osselton MD, Widdop B, eds. Clarke's analysis of drugs and poisons, 3rd ed. Grayslake, Ill: Pharmaceutical Press, 2004:53-67.

490. Long C, Crifasi J, Maginn D. Interference of thioridazine (Mellaril) in identification of phencyclidine. Clin Chem 1996;42:1885-6.
491. Lora-Tamayo C, Tena T, Tena G. Concentrations of free and conjugated morphine in blood in twenty cases of heroin-related deaths. J Chromatogr 1987;422:267-73.
492. Lotsch J. Opioid metabolites. J Pain Symptom Manage 2005;29:S10-24.
493. Louon A, Lithander J, Reddy VG, Gupta A. Sedation with nasal ketamine and midazolam for cryotherapy in retinopathy of prematurity. Br J Ophthalmol 1993;77:529-30.
494. LoVecchio F, Lewin LA. Antipsychotics. In: Goldfrank LR, Flomenbaum NE, Lewin NA, Howland MA, Hoffman RS, Nelson LS, eds. Goldfrank's toxicologic emergencies, 7th edition. New York, NY: McGraw-Hill, 2002:875-84.
495. Lukaszewski T, Jeffery W. Impurities and artifacts of illicit cocaine. J Forensic Sci 1980;25:499-508.
496. Lundh B, Cavallin-Stahl E, Mercke C. Heme catabolism, carbon monoxide production and red cell survival in anemia. Acta Med Scand 1975;197:161-71.
497. Lüscher C. Drugs of abuse (Chapter 32). In: Katzung BG, ed. Basic & clinical pharmacology, 11th edition. New York, NY: McGraw-Hill, 2009.
498. Macheras P, Rosen A. Is monitoring of drug in saliva reliable for bioavailability testing of a protein-bound drug? A theoretical approach. Pharm Acta Helv 1984;59:34-6.
499. Mackler SA, Schweizer E. Benzodiazepines as anxiolytic agents: the risks of long-term treatment. Hosp Pract 1992;27:109-12, 15-6.
500. Maier RD, Bogusz M. Identification power of a standardized HPLC-DAD system for systematic toxicological analysis. J Anal Toxicol 1995;19:79-83.
501. Maisonneuve IM, Ho A, Kreek MJ. Chronic administration of a cocaine "binge" alters basal extracellular levels in male rats: an in vivo microdialysis study. J Pharmacol Exp Ther 1995;272:652-7.
502. Maisonneuve IM, Kreek MJ. Acute tolerance to the dopamine response induced by a binge pattern of cocaine administration in male rats: an in vivo microdialysis study. J Pharmacol Exp Ther 1994;268:916-21.
503. Maitre M. The gamma-hydroxybutyrate signalling system in brain: organization and functional implications. Prog Neurobiol 1997;51: 337-61.
504. Mancini I, Lossignol DA, Body JJ. Opioid switch to oral methadone in cancer pain. Curr Opin Oncol 2000;12:308-13.
505. Manno J. Interpretation of urinalysis results. In: Hawks R, Chiang C, eds. Urine testing for drugs of abuse. National Institute on Drug Abuse, Research Monograph 73. Publication (ADM) 87-1481. Washington, DC: U.S. Department of Health and Human Services, 1986:65-71.
506. Mao Y, Carr PW. Separation of barbiturates and phenylthiohydantoin amino acids using the thermally tuned tandem column concept. Anal Chem 2001;73:1821-30.
507. Marc B, Baudry F, Vaquero P, Zerrouki L, Hassnaoui S, Douceron H. Sexual assault under benzodiazepine submission in a Paris suburb. Arch Gynecol Obstet 2000;263:193-7.
508. Marchei E, Farre M, Pellegrini M, Rossi S, Garcia-Algar O, Vall O, et al. Liquid chromatography-electrospray ionization mass spectrometry determination of methylphenidate and ritalinic acid in conventional and non-conventional biological matrices. J Pharmaceut Biomed Anal 2009;49:434-9.
509. Maresova V, Hampl J, Chundela Z, Zrcek F, Polasek M, Chadt J. The identification of a chlorinated MDMA. J Anal Toxicol 2005;29:353-8.
510. Markowitz JS, Patrick KS. Differential pharmacokinetics and pharmacodynamics of methylphenidate enantiomers: does chirality matter? J Clin Psychopharmacol 2008;28:S54-61.
511. Marquet P. Is LC-MS suitable for a comprehensive screening of drugs and poisons in clinical toxicology? Ther Drug Monit 2002;24:125-33.
512. Marshall LF, Smith RW, Shapiro HM. The outcome with aggressive treatment in severe head injuries. Part II: acute and chronic barbiturate administration in the management of head injury. J Neurosurg 1979;50:26-30.
513. Martin-Amat G, McMartin KE, Hayreh SS, Hayreh MS, Tephly TR. Methanol poisoning: ocular toxicity produced by formate. Toxicol Appl Pharmacol 1978;45:201-8.
514. Marwick C. Coma-inducing drug GHB may be reclassified. JAMA 1997;277:1505-6.
515. Mason HJ, Lewis PJ. Intra-individual variation in plasma and erythrocyte cholinesterase activities and the monitoring of uptake of organo-phosphate pesticides. J Soc Occup Med 1989;39:121-4.
516. Mason MF, Dubowski KM. Breath as a specimen for analysis for ethanol and other low molecular weight alcohols. In: Garriott JC, ed. Medicolegal aspects of alcohol. Tucson, Ariz: Lawyers & Judges Publishing, 1996:171-80.
517. Masoud AN, Krupski DM. High-performance liquid chromatographic analysis of cocaine in human plasma. J Anal Toxicol 1980;4:305-10.
518. Mastrovitch TA, Bithoney WG, DeBari VA, Nina AG. Point-of-care testing for drugs of abuse in an urban emergency department. Ann Clin Lab Sci 2002;32:383-6.
519. Masumoto K, Tashiro Y, Matsumoto K, Yoshida A, Hirayama M, Hayashi S. Simultaneous determination of codeine and chlorpheniramine in human plasma by capillary column gas chromatography. J Chromatogr 1986;381:323-9.
520. Mattila MA, Larni HM. Flunitrazepam: a review of its pharmacological properties and therapeutic use. Drugs 1980;20:353-74.
521. Mattila MA, Saila K, Kokko T, Karkkainen T. Comparison of diazepam and flunitrazepam as adjuncts to general anaesthesia in preventing arousal following surgical stimuli. Br J Anaesth 1979;51: 329-37.
522. Maurer HH. Systematic toxicological analysis of drugs and their metabolites by gas chromatography-mass spectrometry. J Chromatogr 1992;580:3-41.
523. Maurer HH. Current role of liquid chromatography-mass spectrometry in clinical and forensic toxicology. Anal Bioanal Chem 2007;388:1315-25.
524. Maurer HH, Bickeboeller-Friedrich J, Kraemer T, Peters FT. Toxicokinetics and analytical toxicology of amphetamine-derived designer drugs ('Ecstasy'). Toxicol Lett 2000;112-113:133-42.
525. Maurer HH, Kraemer T, Springer D, Staack RF. Chemistry, pharmacology, toxicology, and hepatic metabolism of designer drugs of the amphetamine (ecstasy), piperazine, and pyrrolidinophenone types: a synopsis. Ther Drug Monit 2004;26:127-31.
526. Mayer M, Salpeter L. More on interference of N-acetylcysteine in measurement of acetaminophen. Clin Chem 1998;44:892-3.
527. Maynard EC, Amoruso LP, Oh W. Meconium for drug testing. Am J Dis Child 1991;145:650-2.
528. McCance-Katz EF, Price LH, McDougle CJ, Kosten TR, Black JE, Jatlow PI. Concurrent cocaine-ethanol ingestion in humans: pharmacology, physiology, behavior, and the role of cocaethylene. Psychopharmacology 1993;111:39-46.
529. McCann UD, Szabo Z, Scheffel U, Dannals RF, Ricaurte GA. Positron emission tomographic evidence of toxic effect of MDMA ("Ecstasy") on brain serotonin neurons in human beings. Lancet 1998;352:1433-7.
530. McClean S, O'Kane E, Hillis J, Smyth WF. Determination of 1,4-benzodiazepines and their metabolites by capillary electrophoresis and high-performance liquid chromatography using ultraviolet and electrospray ionisation mass spectrometry. J Chromatogr A 1999;838: 273-91.
531. McCusker RR, Paget-Wilkes H, Chronister CW, Goldberger BA. Analysis of gamma-hydroxybutyrate (GHB) in urine by gas chromatography-mass spectrometry. J Anal Toxicol 1999;23:301-5.
532. McGuigan M. Cannabinoids. In: Goldfrank LR, Flomenbaum NE, Hoffman RS, Howland MA, Lewin NA, Nelson LS, eds. Goldfrank's toxicologic emergencies, 8th edition. New York, NY: McGraw-Hill, 2006:1212-30.
533. McGuigan MA. A two-year review of salicylate deaths in Ontario. Arch Intern Med 1987;147:510-2.
534. McMartin KE, Ambre JJ, Tephly TR. Methanol poisoning in human subjects: role for formic acid accumulation in the metabolic acidosis. Am J Med 1980;68:414-8.

535. McQueen MJ. Clinical and analytical considerations in the utilization of cholinesterase measurements. Clin Chim Acta 1995;237:91-105.
536. McQuillen KK, Anderson AC. Osmol gaps in the pediatric population. Acad Emerg Med 1999;6:27-30.
537. Meatherall R. GC/MS confirmation of barbiturates in blood and urine. J Forensic Sci 1997;42:1160-70.
538. Meatherall R, Dai J. False-positive EMIT II opiates from ofloxacin. Ther Drug Monit 1997;19:98-9.
539. Meatherall R, Krahn J. Excess serum osmolality gap after ingestion of methanol. Clin Chem 1990;36:2004-7.
540. Meng QH, Adeli K, Zello GA, Porter WH, Krahn J. Elevated lactate in ethylene glycol poisoning: true or false? Clin Chim Acta 2010;411: 601-4.
541. Meyer MR, Maurer HH. Enantioselectivity in the methylation of the catecholic phase I metabolites of methylenedioxy designer drugs and their capability to inhibit catechol-O-methyltransferase-catalyzed dopamine 3-methylation. Chem Res Toxicol 2009;22:1205-11.
542. Meyer MR, Peters FT, Maurer HH. The role of human hepatic cytochrome P450 isozymes in the metabolism of racemic 3,4-methylenedioxy-methamphetamine and its enantiomers. Drug Metab Dispos 2008;36:2345-54.
543. Miller RL, DeVane CL. Determination of cocaine, benzoylecgonine and ecgonine methyl ester in plasma by reversed-phase high-performance liquid chromatography. J Chromatogr 1991;570:412-8.
544. Misra AL, Pontani RB, Bartolomeo J. Persistence of phencyclidine (PCP) and metabolites in brain and adipose tissue and implications for long-lasting behavioural effects. Res Commun Chem Pathol Pharmacol 1979;24:431-45.
545. Mitchell JR, Thorgeirsson SS, Potter WZ, Jollow DJ, Keiser H. Acetaminophen-induced hepatic injury: protective role of glutathione in man and rationale for therapy. Clin Pharmacol Ther 1974;16: 676-84.
546. Miyaguchi H, Kuwayama K, Tsujikawa K, Kanamori T, Iwata YT, Inoue H, Kishi T. A method for screening for various sedative-hypnotics in serum by liquid chromatography/single quadrupole mass spectrometry. Forensic Sci Int 2006;157:57-70.
547. Moeller KE, Lee KC, Kissack JC. Urine drug screening: practical guide for clinicians. Mayo Clin Proc 2008;83:66-76.
548. Moeller MR, Doerr G, Warth S. Simultaneous quantitation of delta-9-tetrahydrocannabinol (THC) and 11-nor-9-carboxy-delta-9-tetrahydrocannabinol (THC-COOH) in serum by GC/MS using deuterated internal standards and its application to a smoking study and forensic cases. J Forensic Sci 1992;37:969-83.
549. Moeller MR, Fey P, Sachs H. Hair analysis as evidence in forensic cases. Forensic Sci Int 1993;63:43-53.
550. Mollereau C, Parmentier M, Mailleux P, Butour JL, Moisand C, Chalon P, et al. ORL1, a novel member of the opioid receptor family: cloning, functional expression and localization. FEBS Lett 1994;341: 33-8.
551. Montagna M, Stramesi C, Vignali C, Groppi A, Polettini A. Simultaneous hair testing for opiates, cocaine, and metabolites by GC-MS: a survey of applicants for driving licenses with a history of drug use. Forensic Sci Int 2000;107:157-67.
552. Montague RE, Grace RF, Lewis JH, Shenfield GM. Urine drug screens in overdose patients do not contribute to immediate clinical management. Ther Drug Monit 2001;23:47-50.
553. Montgomery MR, Reasor MJ. Retrograde extrapolation of blood alcohol data: an applied approach. J Toxicol Environ Health 1992;36: 281-92.
554. Moolchan ET, Cone EJ, Wstadik A, Huestis MA, Preston KL. Cocaine and metabolite elimination patterns in chronic cocaine users during cessation: plasma and saliva analysis. J Anal Toxicol 2000;24: 458-66.
555. Moore C, Negrusz A, Lewis D. Determination of drugs of abuse in meconium. J Chromatogr 1998;713:137-46.
556. Moore KA. Amphetamines/sympathomimetic amines. In: Levine B, ed. Principles of forensic toxicology, 2nd edition. Washington, DC: AACC Press, 2003:245-64.
557. Moore KA, Sklerov J, Levine B, Jacobs AJ. Urine concentrations of ketamine and norketamine following illegal consumption. J Anal Toxicol 2001;25:583-8.
558. Moore L, Wicks J, Spiehler V, Holgate R. Gas chromatography-mass spectrometry confirmation of Cozart RapiScan saliva methadone and opiates tests. J Anal Toxicol 2001;25:520-4.
559. Morland J, Bugge A, Skuterud B, Steen A, Wethe GH, Kjeldsen T. Cannabinoids in blood and urine after passive inhalation of Cannabis smoke. J Forensic Sci 1985;30:997-1002.
560. Morris HC, Overton PD, Ramsay JR, Campbell RS, Hammond PM, Atkinson T, et al. Development and validation of an automated enzyme assay for paracetamol (acetaminophen). Clin Chim Acta 1990;187:95-104.
561. Morris HC, Overton PD, Ramsay JR, Campbell RS, Hammond PM, Atkinson T, et al. Development and validation of an automated, enzyme-mediated colorimetric assay of salicylate in serum. Clin Chem 1990;36:131 5.
562. Mortier KA, Maudens KE, Lambert WE, Clauwaert KM, Van Bocxlaer JF, Deforce DL, et al. Simultaneous, quantitative determination of opiates, amphetamines, cocaine and benzoylecgonine in oral fluid by liquid chromatography quadrupole-time-of-flight mass spectrometry. J Chromatogr B Analyt Technol Biomed Life Sci 2002;779:321-30.
563. Mueller PD, Korey WS. Death by "ecstasy": the serotonin syndrome? Ann Emerg Med 1998;32:377-80.
564. Mule SJ, Casella GA. Rendering the "poppy-seed defense" defenseless: identification of 6-monoacetylmorphine in urine by gas chromatography/mass spectroscopy. Clin Chem 1988;34:1427-30.
565. Mule SJ, Lomax P, Gross SJ. Active and realistic passive marijuana exposure tested by three immunoassays and GC/MS in urine. J Anal Toxicol 1988;12:113-6.
566. Munro N. Toxicity of the organophosphate chemical warfare agents GA, GB, and VX: implications for public protection. Environ Health Perspect 1994;102:18-38.
567. Musshoff F, Madea B. Review of biologic matrices (urine, blood, hair) as indicators of recent or ongoing cannabis use. Ther Drug Monit 2006;28:155-63.
568. Musshoff F, Trafkowski J, Kuepper U, Madea B. An automated and fully validated LC-MS/MS procedure for the simultaneous determination of 11 opioids used in palliative care, with 5 of their metabolites. J Mass Spectrom 2006;41:633-40.
569. Myers RA, Britten JS. Are arterial blood gases of value in treatment decisions for carbon monoxide poisoning? Crit Care Med 1989;17: 139-42.
570. Nahas G, Leger C, Tocque B, Hoellinger H. The kinetics of cannabinoid distribution and storage with special reference to the brain and testis. J Clin Pharmacol 1981;21:208S-14S.
571. Naidong W, Lee JW, Jiang X, Wehling M, Hulse JD, Lin PP. Simultaneous assay of morphine, morphine-3-glucuronide and morphine-6-glucuronide in human plasma using normal-phase liquid chromatography-tandem mass spectrometry with a silica column and an aqueous organic mobile phase. J Chromatogr 1999;735:255-69.
572. Nair P, Rothblum S, Hebel R. Neonatal outcome in infants with evidence of fetal exposure to opiates, cocaine, and cannabinoids. Clin Pediatr 1994;33:280-5.
573. Nakahara Y. Hair analysis for abused and therapeutic drugs. J Chromatogr 1999;733:161-80.
574. Namera A, Yashiki M, Iwasaki Y, Ohtani M, Kojima T. Automated procedure for determination of barbiturates in serum using the combined system of PrepStation and gas chromatography-mass spectrometry. J Chromatogr B Biomed Appl 1998;716:171-6.
575. Namera A, Yashiki M, Okada K, Iwasaki Y, Ohtani M, Kojima T. Automated preparation and analysis of barbiturates in human urine using the combined system of PrepStation and gas chromatography-mass spectrometry. J Chromatogr 1998;706:253-9.
576. Narahashi T, Aistrup GL, Marszalec W, Nagata K. Neuronal nicotinic acetylcholine receptors: a new target site of ethanol. Neurochem Int 1999;35:131-41.

577. Navarro M, Pichini S, Farre M, Ortuno J, Roset PN, Segura J, de la Torre R. Usefulness of saliva for measurement of 3,4-methylenedioxymethamphetamine and its metabolites: correlation with plasma drug concentrations and effect of salivary pH. Clin Chem 2001;47:1788-95.
578. Needham SR, Jeanville PM, Brown PR, Estape ES. Performance of a pentafluorophenylpropyl stationary phase for the electrospray ionization high-performance liquid chromatography-mass spectrometry-mass spectrometry assay of cocaine and its metabolite ecgonine methyl ester in human urine. J Chromatogr 2000;748:77-87.
579. Needs CJ, Brooks PM. Clinical pharmacokinetics of the salicylates. Clin Pharmacokinet 1985;10:164-77.
580. Negrusz A, Bowen AM, Moore CM, Dowd SM, Strong MJ, Janicak PG. Deposition of 7-aminoclonazepam and clonazepam in hair following a single dose of Klonopin. J Anal Toxicol 2002;26:471-8.
581. Negrusz A, Gaensslen RE. Analytical developments in toxicological investigation of drug-facilitated sexual assault. Anal Bioanal Chem 2003;376:1192-7.
582. Negrusz A, Juhascik M, Gaensslen RE. Estimate of the incidence of drug-facilitated sexual assault in the U.S. U.S. Department of Justice, 2005.
583. Negrusz A, Moore CM, Hinkel KB, Stockham TL, Verma M, Strong MJ, et al. Deposition of 7-aminoflunitrazepam and flunitrazepam in hair after a single dose of Rohypnol. J Forensic Sci 2001;46:1143-51.
584. Nelson AE, Ho KK. A robust test for growth hormone doping—present status and future prospects. Asian J Androl 2008;10:416-25.
585. Nelson LS. Opioids. In: Flomenbaum NE, Goldfrank LR, Hoffman RS, Howland MA, Nelson LS, eds. Goldfrank's toxicologic emergencies, 8th edition. New York, NY: McGraw Hill, 2006:590-613.
586. Ng YY, Lin WL, Chen TW, Lin BC, Tsai SH, Chang CC, et al. Spurious hyperchloremia and decreased anion gap in a patient with dextromethorphan bromide. Am J Nephrol 1992;12:268-70.
587. Ni YC, Wong TY, Lloyd RV, Heinze TM, Shelton S, Casciano D, et al. Mouse liver microsomal metabolism of chloral hydrate, trichloroacetic acid, and trichloroethanol leading to induction of lipid peroxidation via a free radical mechanism. Drug Metab Dispos 1996;24:81-90.
588. Nice A, Leikin JB, Maturen A, Madsen-Konczyk LJ, Zell M, Hryhorczuk DO. Toxidrome recognition to improve efficiency of emergency urine drug screens. Ann Emerg Med 1988;17:676-80.
589. Niedbala RS, Kardos KW, Fritch DF, Kardos S, Fries T, Waga J, et al. Detection of marijuana use by oral fluid and urine analysis following single-dose administration of smoked and oral marijuana. J Anal Toxicol 2001;25:289-303.
590. Nine JS, Moraca M, Virji MA, Rao KN. Serum-ethanol determination: comparison of lactate and lactate dehydrogenase interference in three enzymatic assays. J Anal Toxicol 1995;19:192-6.
591. Noble M, Tregear SJ, Treadwell JR, Schoelles K. Long-term opioid therapy for chronic noncancer pain: a systematic review and meta-analysis of efficacy and safety. J Pain Symptom Manage 2008;35:214-28.
592. Norberg A, Jones AW, Hahn RG, Gabrielsson JL. Role of variability in explaining ethanol pharmacokinetics: research and forensic applications. Clin Pharmacokinet 2003;42:1-31.
593. Nordgren HK, Beck O. Direct screening of urine for MDMA and MDA by liquid chromatography-tandem mass spectrometry. J Anal Toxicol 2003;27:15-9.
594. Nordt SP. "DXM": a new drug of abuse? Ann Emerg Med 1998;31:794-5.
595. O'Brien CP. Drug addiction and drug abuse (Chapter 23). In: Brunton LL, Lazo JS, Parker KL, eds. Goodman & Gilman's the pharmacological basis of therapeutics, 11th edition. New York, NY: McGraw-Hill, 2006.
596. O'Brien RP, McGeehan PA, Helmeczi AW, Dula DJ. Detectability of drug tablets and capsules by plain radiography. Am J Emerg Med 1986;4:302-12.
597. Office of the Assistant Secretary of Defense for Health Affairs: Status of drug use in the Department of Defense personnel: fiscal year 2007. Drug testing statistical report, 2008.
598. Ohlsson A, Lindgren JE, Wahlen A, Agurell S, Hollister LE, Gillespie HK. Plasma delta-9 tetrahydrocannabinol concentrations and clinical effects after oral and intravenous administration and smoking. Clin Pharmacol Ther 1980;28:409-16.
599. Ohno S, Kawana K, Nakajin S. Contribution of UDP-glucuronosyltransferase 1A1 and 1A8 to morphine-6-glucuronidation and its kinetic properties. Drug Metab Dispos 2008;36:688-94.
600. Ohshima T. A case of drug-facilitated sexual assault by the use of flunitrazepam. J Clin Forensic Med 2006;13:44-5.
601. Olmedo R. Phencyclidine and ketamine. In: Goldfrank L, Flomenbaum N, Howland M, Lewin N, Hoffman R, Nelson L, eds. Goldfrank's toxicologic emergencies, 8th edition. New York, NY: McGraw Hill, 2006:1231-43.
602. Ortelli D, Rudaz S, Chevalley AF, Mino A, Deglon JJ, Balant L, et al. Enantioselective analysis of methadone in saliva by liquid chromatography-mass spectrometry. J Chromatogr A 2000;871:163-72.
603. Ortuno J, de la Torre R, Segura J, Cami J. Simultaneous detection in urine of cocaine and its main metabolites. J Pharmaceut Biomed Anal 1990;8:911-4.
604. Osborne R, Joel S, Trew D, Slevin M. Morphine and metabolite behavior after different routes of morphine administration: demonstration of the importance of the active metabolite morphine-6-glucuronide. Clin Pharmacol Ther 1990;47:12-9.
605. Oshima A, Higuchi T. Treatment guidelines for geriatric mood disorders. Psychiatry Clin Neurosci 1999;53(Suppl):S55-9.
606. Osterloh JD, Kelly TJ, Khayam-Bashi H, Romeo R. Discrepancies in osmolal gaps and calculated alcohol concentrations. Arch Pathol Lab Med 1996;120:637-41.
607. Ostrea EM Jr. Understanding drug testing in the neonate and the role of meconium analysis. J Perinat Neonat Nurs 2001;14:61-82; quiz 105-6.
608. Ostrea EM Jr, Brady MJ, Parks PM, Asensio DC, Naluz A. Drug screening of meconium in infants of drug-dependent mothers: an alternative to urine testing. J Pediatr 1989;115:474-7.
609. Ostrea EM Jr, Knapp DK, Tannenbaum L, Ostrea AR, Romero A, Salari V, et al. Estimates of illicit drug use during pregnancy by maternal interview, hair analysis, and meconium analysis. J Pediatr 2001;138:344-8.
610. Oyler JM, Cone EJ, Joseph RE Jr, Huestis MA. Identification of hydrocodone in human urine following controlled codeine administration. J Anal Toxicol 2000;24:530-5.
611. Pacifici R, Pichini S, Altieri I, Caronna A, Passa AR, Zuccaro P. High-performance liquid chromatographic-electrospray mass spectrometric determination of morphine and its 3- and 6-glucuronides: application to pharmacokinetic studies. J Chromatogr B Biomed Appl 1995;664:329-34.
612. Palmer M, Betz JM. Plants. In: Goldfrank LR, Flomenbaum NE, Hoffman RS, Howland MA, Lewin NA, Nelson L, eds. Goldfrank's toxicologic emergencies, 8th edition. New York, NY: McGraw Hill, 2006:1577-602.
613. Palmer RB. A review of the use of ethyl glucuronide as a marker for ethanol consumption in forensic and clinical medicine. Semin Diagn Pathol 2009;26:18-27.
614. Pandey R, Mousawy K, Nagarkatti M, Nagarkatti P. Endocannabinoids and immune regulation. Pharmacol Res 2009;60:85-92.
615. Pankey S, Collins C, Jaklitsch A, Izutsu A, Hu M, Pirio M, et al. Quantitative homogeneous enzyme immunoassays for amitriptyline, nortriptyline, imipramine, and desipramine. Clin Chem 1986;32:768-72.
616. Pappas AA, Gadsden RH Jr, Porter WH, Mullins RE. Osmolality of serum for evaluating the acutely intoxicated patient. In: Frings C, Faulkner W, eds. Selected methods of emergency toxicology. Washington, DC: AACC Press, 1986:85-8.
617. Pappas AA, Gadsden RH Sr, Taylor EH. Serum osmolality in acute intoxication: a prospective clinical study. Am J Clin Pathol 1985;84:74-9.
618. Parrott AC. Human psychopharmacology of Ecstasy (MDMA): a review of 15 years of empirical research. Hum Psychopharmacol 2001;16:557-77.

619. Pasero C. Fentanyl for acute pain management. J Perianesth Nurs 2005;20:279-84.
620. Pasternak GW. Multiple opiate receptors: deja vu all over again. Neuropharmacology 2004;47(Suppl 1):312-23.
621. Patrono C. Aspirin as an antiplatelet drug. N Engl J Med 1994;330: 1287-94.
622. Paul BD, Lalani S, Bosy T, Jacobs AJ, Huestis MA. Concentration profiles of cocaine, pyrolytic methyl ecgonidine and thirteen metabolites in human blood and urine: determination by gas chromatography-mass spectrometry. Biomed Chromatogr 2005;19: 677-88.
623. Paul BD, Mell LD Jr, Mitchell JM, Irving J, Novak AJ. Simultaneous identification and quantitation of codeine and morphine in urine by capillary gas chromatography and mass spectroscopy. J Anal Toxicol 1985;9:222-6.
624. Paul BD, Mitchell JM, Burbage R, Moy M, Sroka R. Gas chromatographic-electron-impact mass fragmentometric determination of lysergic acid diethylamide in urine. J Chromatogr 1990;529:103-12.
625. Paul BD, Mitchell JM, Mell LD Jr, Irving J. Gas chromatography/ electron impact mass fragmentometric determination of urinary 6-acetylmorphine, a metabolite of heroin. J Anal Toxicol 1989;13:2-7.
626. Paul BN. Salicylate poisoning in the elderly: diagnostic pitfalls. J Am Geriatr Soc 1972;20:387-90.
627. Pawula M, Barrett DA, Shaw PN. An improved extraction method for the HPLC determination of morphine and its metabolites in plasma. J Pharmaceut Biomed Anal 1993;11:401-6.
628. Payne JP, Hill DW, Wood DG. Distribution of ethanol between plasma and erythrocytes in whole blood. Nature 1968;217:963-4.
629. Peace MR, Poklis JL, Tarnai LD, Poklis A. An evaluation of the OnTrak Testcup-er on-site urine drug-testing device for drugs commonly encountered from emergency departments. J Anal Toxicol 2002;26:500-3.
630. Peat M. Workplace drug testing. In: Anthony M, Osselton MD, Brian W, eds. Clarke's analysis of drugs and poisons, vol 3. London, UK: Pharmaceutical Press, 2004:68-79.
631. Pelders MG, Ros JJ. Poppy seeds: differences in morphine and codeine content and variation in inter- and intra-individual excretion. J Forensic Sci 1996;41:209-12.
632. Pentel PR, Keyler DE, Haddad LM. Tricyclic antidepressants and selective serotonin reuptake inhibitors. In: Haddad LM, Shannon MW, Winchester JF, eds. Clinical management of poisoning and drug overdose. Philadelphia, Pa: WB Saunders, 1998:437-51.
633. Perez-Reyes M, Di Guiseppi S, Mason AP, Davis KH. Passive inhalation of marihuana smoke and urinary excretion of cannabinoids. Clin Pharmacol Ther 1983;34:36-41.
634. Perez-Reyes M, Jeffcoat AR, Myers M, Sihler K, Cook CE. Comparison in humans of the potency and pharmacokinetics of intravenously injected cocaethylene and cocaine. Psychopharmacology 1994;116:428-32.
635. Perrone J, De Roos F, Jayaraman S, Hollander JE. Drug screening versus history in detection of substance use in ED psychiatric patients. Am J Emerg Med 2001;19:49-51.
636. Perry H, Shannon MW. Acetaminophen. In: Haddad LM, Shannon MW, Winchester JF, eds. Clinical management of poisoning and drug overdose, 3rd edition. Philadelphia, Pa: WB Saunders, 1998: 664-74.
637. Pertwee RG. The pharmacology of cannabinoid receptors and their ligands: an overview. Int J Obes 2006;30(Suppl 1):S13-8.
638. Peterson GM, Randall CT, Paterson J. Plasma levels of morphine and morphine glucuronides in the treatment of cancer pain: relationship to renal function and route of administration. Eur J Clin Pharmacol 1990;38:121-4.
638A. Pfaffe T, Cooper-White J, Beyerlein P, Karam Kostner K, Punyadeera C. Diagnostic potential of saliva: current state and future applications. Clin Chem 2011;57:675-87.
639. Pichini S, Navarro M, Farre M, Ortuno J, Roset PN, Pacifici R, et al. On-site testing of 3,4-methylenedioxymethamphetamine (ecstasy) in saliva with Drugwipe and Drugread: a controlled study in recreational users. Clin Chem 2002;48:174-6.
640. Pichini S, Pujadas M, Marchei E, Pellegrini M, Fiz J, Pacifici R, et al. Liquid chromatography-atmospheric pressure ionization electrospray mass spectrometry determination of "hallucinogenic designer drugs" in urine of consumers. J Pharmaceut Biomed Anal 2008;47:335-42.
641. Pocci R, Dixit V, Dixit VM. Solid-phase extraction and GC/MS confirmation of barbiturates from human urine. J Anal Toxicol 1992;16:45-7.
642. Poch GK, Klette KL, Anderson C. The quantitation of 2-oxo-3-hydroxy lysergic acid diethylamide (O-H-LSD) in human urine specimens, a metabolite of LSD: comparative analysis using liquid chromatography-selected ion monitoring mass spectrometry and liquid chromatography-ion trap mass spectrometry. J Anal Toxicol 2000;24:170-9.
643. Poch GK, Klette KL, Hallare DA, Manglicmot MG, Czarny RJ, McWhorter LK, et al. Detection of metabolites of lysergic acid diethylamide (LSD) in human urine specimens: 2-oxo-3-hydroxy-LSD, a prevalent metabolite of LSD. J Chromatogr 1999;724:23-33.
644. Poklis A, Edinboro LE. REMEDi drug profiling system readily distinguishes between cyclobenzaprine and amitriptyline in emergency toxicology urine specimens. Clin Chem 1992;38: 2349-50.
645. Poklis A, Moore KA. Response of EMIT amphetamine immunoassays to urinary desoxyephedrine following Vicks inhaler use. Ther Drug Monit 1995;17:89-94.
646. Poklis A, Poklis JL, Tarnai LD, Backer RC. Evaluation of the Triage PPY on-site testing device for the detection of dextropropoxyphene in urine. J Anal Toxicol 2004;28:485-8.
647. Policy ONDC. Study finds highest levels of THC in U.S. marijuana to date. Washington, DC: Office of National Drug Control Policy, 2007.
648. Polson J, Wians FH Jr, Orsulak P, Fuller D, Murray NG, Koff JM, et al. False positive acetaminophen concentrations in patients with liver injury. Clin Chim Acta 2008;391:24-30.
649. Porter W. Clinical toxicology. In: Burtis CA, Bruns DE, eds. Tietz textbook of clinical chemistry, 4th edition. St Louis, Mo: Elsevier Saunders, 2006:1287-369.
650. Porter WH. In acetaminophen assay, only unconjugated drug should be measured. Clin Chem 1984;30:1884-5.
651. Porter WH, Rutter PW, Bush BA, Pappas AA, Dunnington JE. Ethylene glycol toxicity: the role of serum glycolic acid in hemodialysis. J Toxicol Clin Toxicol 2001;39:607-15.
652. Porter WH, Rutter PW, Yao HH. Simultaneous determination of ethylene glycol and glycolic acid in serum by gas chromatography-mass spectrometry. J Anal Toxicol 1999;23:591-7.
653. Pragst F, Balikova MA. State of the art in hair analysis for detection of drug and alcohol abuse. Clin Chim Acta 2006;370:17-49.
654. Pragst F, Herre S, Bakdash A. Poisonings with diphenhydramine—a survey of 68 clinical and 55 death cases. Forensic Sci Int 2006;161: 189-97.
655. Pragst F, Rothe M, Spiegel K, Sporkert F. Illegal and therapeutic drug concentrations in hair segments: a timetable of drug exposure. Forensic Sci Rev 1998;10:81-111.
656. Preston KL, Epstein DH, Cone EJ, Wtsadik AT, Huestis MA, Moolchan ET. Urinary elimination of cocaine metabolites in chronic cocaine users during cessation. J Anal Toxicol 2002;26:393-400.
657. Price CP, Hammond PM, Scawen MD. Evaluation of an enzymic procedure for the measurement of acetaminophen. Clin Chem 1983;29:358-61.
658. Price D. Methemoglobinemia. In: Goldfrank LR, Flomenbaum NE, Lewin NA, Howland MA, Hoffman RS, Nelson LS, eds. Goldfrank's toxicologic emergencies, 7th edition. New York, NY: McGraw-Hill, 2002:1438-49.
659. Price D. Methemoglobin inducers. In: Goldfrank LR, Flomenbaum NE, Hoffman RS, Howland MA, Lewin NA, Nelson L, eds. Goldfrank's toxicologic emergencies, 8th edition. New York, NY: McGraw Hill, 2006:1734-45.

660. Prommer N, Sottas PE, Schoch C, Schumacher YO, Schmidt W. Total hemoglobin mass—a new parameter to detect blood doping? Med Sci Sports Exerc 2008;40:2112-8.
661. Puopolo PR, Volpicelli SA, Johnson DM, Flood JG. Emergency toxicology testing (detection, confirmation, and quantification) of basic drugs in serum by liquid chromatography with photodiode array detection. Clin Chem 1991;37:2124-30.
662. Purssell RA, Pudek M, Brubacher J, Abu-Laban RB. Derivation and validation of a formula to calculate the contribution of ethanol to the osmolal gap. Ann Emerg Med 2001;38:653-9.
663. Raffa RB. Basic pharmacology relevant to drug abuse assessment: tramadol as example. J Clin Pharm Ther 2008;33:101-8.
664. Rainey JM Jr, Crowder MK. Prolonged psychosis attributed to phencyclidine: report of three cases. Am J Psychiatry 1975;132:1076-8.
665. Rance MJ, Jordan BJ, Nichols JD. A simultaneous determination of acetylsalicylic acid, salicylic acid and salicylamide in plasma by gas liquid chromatography. J Pharm Pharmacol 1975;27:425-9.
666. Rasmussen F. Salivary excretion of sulphonamides and barbiturates by cows and goats. Acta Pharmacol Toxicol (Copenh) 1964;21:11-9.
667. Rasmussen LB, Olsen KH, Johansen SS. Chiral separation and quantification of R/S-amphetamine, R/S-methamphetamine, R/S-MDA, R/S-MDMA, and R/S-MDEA in whole blood by GC-EI-MS. J Chromatogr B Analyt Technol Biomed Life Sci 2006;842:136-41.
668. Reidy L, Gennaro W, Steele BW, Walls HC. The incidence of Zolpidem use in suspected DUI drivers in Miami-Dade Florida: a comparative study using immunalysis Zolpidem ELISA KIT and gas chromatography-mass spectrometry screening. J Anal Toxicol 2008; 32:688-94.
669. Reisfield GM, Salazar E, Bertholf RL. Rational use and interpretation of urine drug testing in chronic opioid therapy. Ann Clin Lab Sci 2007;37:301-14.
670. Remaley AT, Hicks DG, Kane MD, Shaw LM. Laboratory assessment of poisoning with a carbamate insecticide. Clin Chem 1988;34:1933-6.
671. Renner UD, Oertel R, Kirch W. Pharmacokinetics and pharmacodynamics in clinical use of scopolamine. Ther Drug Monit 2005;27:655-65.
672. Reuschel SA, Percey SE, Liu S, Eades DM, Foltz RL. Quantitative determination of LSD and a major metabolite, 2-oxo-3-hydroxy-LSD, in human urine by solid-phase extraction and gas chromatography-tandem mass spectrometry. J Anal Toxicol 1999;23:306-12.
673. Richelson E. Preclinical pharmacology of neuroleptics: focus on new generation compounds. J Clin Psychiatry 1996;57(Suppl 11):4-11.
674. Riley J, Eisenberg E, Muller-Schwefe G, Drewes AM, Arendt-Nielsen L. Oxycodone: a review of its use in the management of pain. Curr Med Res Opin 2008;24:175-92.
675. Ritter D, Cortese CM, Edwards LC, Barr JL, Chung HD, Long C. Interference with testing for lysergic acid diethylamide. Clin Chem 1997;43:635-7.
676. Riviere GJ, Gentry WB, Owens SM. Disposition of methamphetamine and its metabolite amphetamine in brain and other tissues in rats after intravenous administration. J Pharmacol Exp Ther 2000;292:1042-7.
677. Robandt PP, Reda LJ, Klette KL. Complete automation of solid-phase extraction with subsequent liquid chromatography-tandem mass spectrometry for the quantification of benzoylecgonine, m-hydroxybenzoylecgonine, p-hydroxybenzoylecgonine, and norbenzoylecgonine in urine—application to a high-throughput urine analysis laboratory. J Anal Toxicol 2008;32:577-85.
678. Rodrigues WC, Wang G, Moore C, Agrawal A, Vincent MJ, Soares JR. Development and validation of ELISA and GC-MS procedures for the quantification of dextromethorphan and its main metabolite dextrorphan in urine and oral fluid. J Anal Toxicol 2008;32:220-6.
679. Rodriguez-Rosas ME, Medrano JG, Epstein DH, Moolchan ET, Preston KL, Wainer IW. Determination of total and free concentrations of the enantiomers of methadone and its metabolite (2-ethylidene-1,5-dimethyl-3,3-diphenyl-pyrrolidine) in human plasma by enantioselective liquid chromatography with mass spectrometric detection. J Chromatogr A 2005;1073:237-48.
680. Rohanova M, Balikova M. Studies on distribution and metabolism of para-methoxymethamphetamine (PMMA) in rats after subcutaneous administration. Toxicology 2009;259:61-8.
681. Romberg RW, Needleman SB, Snyder JJ, Greedan A. Methamphetamine and amphetamine derived from the metabolism of selegiline. J Forensic Sci 1995;40:1100-2.
682. Rook EJ, Hillebrand MJ, Rosing H, van Ree JM, Beijnen JH. The quantitative analysis of heroin, methadone and their metabolites and the simultaneous detection of cocaine, acetylcodeine and their metabolites in human plasma by high-performance liquid chromatography coupled with tandem mass spectrometry. J Chromatogr B Analyt Technol Biomed Life Sci 2005;824:213-21.
683. Rook EJ, Huitema AD, van den Brink W, van Ree JM, Beijnen JH. Population pharmacokinetics of heroin and its major metabolites. Clin Pharmacokinet 2006;45:401-17.
684. Rook EJ, van Ree JM, van den Brink W, Hillebrand MJ, Huitema AD, Hendriks VM, et al. Pharmacokinetics and pharmacodynamics of high doses of pharmaceutically prepared heroin, by intravenous or by inhalation route in opioid-dependent patients. Basic Clin Pharmacol Toxicol 2006;98:86-96.
685. Ropper A, Samuels M. Disorders of the nervous system caused by drugs, toxins, and other chemical agents (Chapter 43). In: Ropper A, Samuels M, eds. Adams and Victor's principles of neurology, 9th edition. New York, NY: McGraw-Hill, 2009.
686. Roth GJ, Majerus PW. The mechanism of the effect of aspirin on human platelets. I. Acetylation of a particulate fraction protein. J Clin Invest 1975;56:624-32.
687. Rothman RB, Baumann MH. Monoamine transporters and psychostimulant drugs. Eur J Pharmacol 2003;479:23-40.
688. Rothschild AJ, Shindul R, Viguera A, Murray M, Brewster S. Comparison of the frequency of behavioral disinhibition on alprazolam, clonazepam, or no benzodiazepine in hospitalized psychiatric patients. J Clin Psychopharmacol 2000;20:7-11.
689. Rozenfeld R, Abul-Husn NS, Gomez I, Devi LA. An emerging role for the delta opioid receptor in the regulation of mu opioid receptor function. Sci World J 2007;7:64-73.
690. Rumack B, Toll L, Gelman C. Micromedex healthcare series, vol 129. Englewood, Colo: Micromedex, 2006.
691. Rumack BH, Matthew H. Acetaminophen poisoning and toxicity. Pediatrics 1975;55:871-6.
692. Rusyniak DE, Sprague JE. Hyperthermic syndromes induced by toxins. Clin Lab Med 2006;26:165-84, ix.
693. Ryan RM, Wagner CL, Schultz JM, Varley J, DiPreta J, Sherer DM, et al. Meconium analysis for improved identification of infants exposed to cocaine in utero. J Pediatr 1994;125:435-40.
694. Ryder KW, Glick MR. The effect of thioridazine on the Automatic Clinical Analyzer serum tricyclic anti-depressant screen. Am J Clin Pathol 1986;86:248-9.
695. Rygnestad T, Aarstad K, Gustafsson K, Jenssen U. The clinical value of drug analyses in deliberate self-poisoning. Hum Exp Toxicol 1990;9:221-30.
696. Sachs H, Kintz P. Testing for drugs in hair: critical review of chromatographic procedures since 1992. J Chromatogr 1998;713: 147-61.
697. Sachs H, Uhl M, Hege-Scheuing G, Schneider E. Analysis of fentanyl and sufentanil in hair by GC/MS/MS. Int J Legal Med 1996;109: 213-5.
698. Saka K, Uemura K, Shintani-Ishida K, Yoshida K. Determination of amobarbital and phenobarbital in serum by gas chromatography-mass spectrometry with addition of formic acid to the solvent. J Chromatogr B Analyt Technol Biomed Life Sci 2008;869:9-15.
699. Salamone SJ, Honasoge S, Brenner C, McNally AJ, Passarelli J, Goc-Szkutnicka K, et al. Flunitrazepam excretion patterns using the Abuscreen OnTrak and OnLine immunoassays: comparison with GC-MS. J Anal Toxicol 1997;21:341-5.
700. Salamone SJ, Li Z, McNally AJ, Vitone S, Wu RS. Epimerization studies of LSD using 1H nuclear magnetic resonance (NMR) spectroscopy. J Anal Toxicol 1997;21:492-7.

701. Samyn N, van Haeren C. On-site testing of saliva and sweat with Drugwipe and determination of concentrations of drugs of abuse in saliva, plasma and urine of suspected users. Int J Legal Med 2000;113:150-4.
702. Sanchez R, Fosarelli P, Felt B, Greene M, Lacovara J, Hackett F. Carbon monoxide poisoning due to automobile exposure: disparity between carboxyhemoglobin levels and symptoms of victims. Pediatrics 1988;82:663-6.
703. Sanna E, Busonero F, Talani G, Carta M, Massa F, Peis M, et al. Comparison of the effects of zaleplon, zolpidem, and triazolam at various GABA(A) receptor subtypes. Eur J Pharmacol 2002;451:103-10.
704. Sarma L, Wong SH, DellaFera S. Diflunisal significantly interferes with salicylate measurements by FPIA-TDx and UV-VIS aca methods. Clin Chem 1985;31:1922-3.
705. Saum CA, Inciardi JA. Rohypnol misuse in the United States. Subst Use Misuse 1997;32:723-31.
706. Saunders PA, Ho IK. Barbiturates and the GABAA receptor complex: progress in drug research. Fortsch Arzneimittelforsch 1990;34:261-86.
707. Schanzle G, Li S, Mikus G, Hofmann U. Rapid, highly sensitive method for the determination of morphine and its metabolites in body fluids by liquid chromatography-mass spectrometry. J Chromatogr 1999;721:55-65.
708. Schepers RJ, Oyler JM, Joseph RE Jr, Cone EJ, Moolchan ET, Huestis MA. Methamphetamine and amphetamine pharmacokinetics in oral fluid and plasma after controlled oral methamphetamine administration to human volunteers. Clin Chem 2003;49:121-32.
709. Schier J. Avoid unfavorable consequences: dextromethorpan can bring about a false-positive phencyclidine urine drug screen. J Emerg Med 2000;18:379-81.
710. Schmitt TC. Determination of chloral hydrate and its metabolites in blood plasma by capillary gas chromatography with electron capture detection. J Chromatogr B Analyt Technol Biomed Life Sci 2002;780:217-24.
711. Schneider S, Wennig R. Interference of diphenhydramine with the EMIT II immunoassay for propoxyphene. J Anal Toxicol 1999;23:637-8.
712. Schramm W, Craig PA, Smith RH, Berger GE. Cocaine and benzoylecgonine in saliva, serum, and urine. Clin Chem 1993;39:481-7.
713. Schramm W, Smith RH, Craig PA, Kidwell DA. Drugs of abuse in saliva: a review. J Anal Toxicol 1992;16:1-9.
714. Schuberth J, Schuberth J. Gas chromatographic-mass spectrometric determination of morphine, codeine and 6-monoacetylmorphine in blood extracted by solid phase. J Chromatogr 1989;490:444-9.
715. Schulz V. Clinical pharmacokinetics of nitroprusside, cyanide, thiosulphate and thiocyanate. Clin Pharmacokinet 1984;9:239-51.
716. Scott-Ham M, Burton FC. Toxicological findings in cases of alleged drug-facilitated sexual assault in the United Kingdom over a 3-year period. J Clin Forensic Med 2005;12:175-86.
717. Seitz DP, Gill SS. Neuroleptic malignant syndrome complicating antipsychotic treatment of delirium or agitation in medical and surgical patients: case reports and a review of the literature. Psychosomatics 2009;50:8-15.
718. Sejersted OM, Jacobsen D, Ovrebo S, Jansen H. Formate concentrations in plasma from patients poisoned with methanol. Acta Med Scand 1983;213:105-10.
719. Senanayake N, Karalliedde L. Neurotoxic effects of organophosphorus insecticides: an intermediate syndrome. N Engl J Med 1987;316:761-3.
720. Seppala T, Nuotto E, Dreyfus JF. Drug-alcohol interactions on psychomotor skills: zopiclone and flunitrazepam. Pharmacology 1983;27(Suppl 2):127-35.
721. Lunesta (eszopiclone) product information. Marlborough, Mass: Sepracor, 2005.
722. Shannon M, Haddad L. The emergency management of poisoning. In: Haddad L, Shannon M, Winchester J, eds. Clinical management of poisoning and drug overdose, 3rd edition. Philadelphia, Pa: WB Saunders, 1998:2-31.
723. Shima N, Kamata H, Katagi M, Tsuchihashi H, Sakuma T, Nemoto N. Direct determination of glucuronide and sulfate of 4-hydroxy-3-methoxymethamphetamine, the main metabolite of MDMA, in human urine. J Chromatogr B Analyt Technol Biomed Life Sci 2007;857:123-9.
724. Shou WZ, Pelzer M, Addison T, Jiang X, Naidong W. An automatic 96-well solid phase extraction and liquid chromatography-tandem mass spectrometry method for the analysis of morphine, morphine-3-glucuronide and morphine-6-glucuronide in human plasma. J Pharmaceut Biomed Anal 2002;27:143-52.
725. Sides GD. QT interval prolongation as a biomarker for torsades de pointes and sudden death in drug development. Dis Markers 2002;18:57-62.
726. Siegel IA. The role of saliva in drug monitoring. Ann N Y Acad Sci 1993;694:86-90.
727. Simpson RJ, Power KG, Wallace LA, Butcher MH, Swanson V, Simpson EC. Controlled comparison of the characteristics of long-term benzodiazepine users in general practice. Br J Gen Pract 1990;40:22-6.
728. Sivilotti ML. Ethanol, isopropanol, and methanol. In: Dart RC, ed. Medical toxicology. Philadelphia, Pa: Lippincott Williams & Wilkins, 2004:1211-23.
729. Slaughter L. Involvement of drugs in sexual assault. J Reprod Med 2000;45:425-30.
730. Small GW. Treatment of geriatric depression. Depression Anxiety 1998;8(Suppl 1):32-42.
731. Smilkstein MJ, Douglas DR, Daya MR. Acetaminophen poisoning and liver function. N Engl J Med 1994;331:1310-1; author reply 1-2.
732. Smilkstein MJ, Knapp GL, Kulig KW, Rumack BH. Efficacy of oral N-acetylcysteine in the treatment of acetaminophen overdose: analysis of the national multicenter study (1976 to 1985). N Engl J Med 1988;319:1557-62.
733. Smirnow D, Logan BK. Analysis of ecgonine and other cocaine biotransformation products in postmortem whole blood by protein precipitation-extractive alkylation and GC-MS. J Anal Toxicol 1996;20:463-7.
734. Smith-Kielland A, Olsen KM, Christophersen AS. False-positive results with Emit II amphetamine/methamphetamine assay in users of common psychotropic drugs. Clin Chem 1995;41:951-2.
735. Smith DE, Gutgesell ME, Schwartz RH, Thorne MM, Bogema S. Federal guidelines for marijuana screening should have lower cutoff levels: a comparison of results from immunoassays and gas chromatography-mass spectrometry. Arch Pathol Lab Med 1989;113:1299-300.
736. Smith JA, Hine ID, Beck P, Routledge PA. Paracetamol toxicity: is enzyme induction important? Hum Toxicol 1986;5:383-5.
737. Smith KM. Drugs used in acquaintance rape. J Am Pharm Assoc 1999;39:519-25; quiz 81-3.
738. Smith ML, Barnes AJ, Huestis MA. Identifying new cannabis use with urine creatinine-normalized THCCOOH concentrations and time intervals between specimen collections. J Anal Toxicol 2009;33:185-9.
739. Smith ML, Hughes RO, Levine B, Dickerson S, Darwin WD, Cone EJ. Forensic drug testing for opiates. VI. Urine testing for hydromorphone, hydrocodone, oxymorphone, and oxycodone with commercial opiate immunoassays and gas chromatography-mass spectrometry. J Anal Toxicol 1995;19:18-26.
740. Smith ML, Shimomura ET, Summers J, Paul BD, Nichols D, Shippee R, et al. Detection times and analytical performance of commercial urine opiate immunoassays following heroin administration. J Anal Toxicol 2000;24:522-9.
741. Smith RM. Ethyl esters of arylhydroxy- and arylhydroxymethoxycocaines in the urines of simultaneous cocaine and ethanol users. J Anal Toxicol 1984;8:38-42.
742. Smithline N, Gardner KD Jr. Gaps—anionic and osmolal. JAMA 1976;236:1594-7.
743. Snyder H, Schwenzer KS, Pearlman R, McNally AJ, Tsilimidos M, Salamone SJ, et al. Serum and urine concentrations of flunitrazepam

and metabolites, after a single oral dose, by immunoassay and GC-MS. J Anal Toxicol 2001;25:699-704.
744. Somogyi AA, Barratt DT, Coller JK. Pharmacogenetics of opioids. Clin Pharmacol Ther 2007;81:429-44.
745. Sora I, Takahashi N, Funada M, Ujike H, Revay RS, Donovan DM, et al. Opiate receptor knockout mice define mu receptor roles in endogenous nociceptive responses and morphine-induced analgesia. Proc Natl Acad Sci U S A 1997;94:1544-9.
746. Sorisky A, Watson DC. Positive diphenhydramine interference in the EMIT-ST assay for tricyclic antidepressants in serum. Clin Chem 1986;32:715.
747. Spanbauer AC, Moody DE, Foltz RL, Walsh SL. A gas chromatographic-positive ion chemical ionization-mass spectrometric method for determination of cocaine, benzoylecgonine, ecgonine methyl ester, and norcocaine in plasma: detection of norcocaine in plasma after oral administration of cocaine. J Anal Toxicol 2000;24: 453-5.
748. Speed DJ, Dickson SJ, Cairns ER, Kim ND. Analysis of paracetamol using solid-phase extraction, deuterated internal standards, and gas chromatography-mass spectrometry. J Anal Toxicol 2001;25:198-202.
749. Spiehler V. Drugs in saliva. In: Moffat A, Osselton MD, Widdop B, eds. Clarke's analysis of drugs and poisons, vol 3. London, UK: Pharmaceutical Press, 2004:109-23.
750. Sporer KA, Khayam-Bashi H. Acetaminophen and salicylate serum levels in patients with suicidal ingestion or altered mental status. Am J Emerg Med 1996;14:443-6.
751. Squires RF, Saederup E. Mono N-aryl ethylenediamine and piperazine derivatives are GABAA receptor blockers: implications for psychiatry. Neurochem Res 1993;18:787-93.
752. Staack RF, Fritschi G, Maurer HH. Studies on the metabolism and toxicological detection of the new designer drug N-benzylpiperazine in urine using gas chromatography-mass spectrometry. J Chromatogr B Analyt Technol Biomed Life Sci 2002;773:35-46.
753. Steering Committee of the Physicians' Health Study Research Group. Final report on the aspirin component of the ongoing Physicians' Health Study. N Engl J Med 1989;321:129-35.
754. Sternbach H. The serotonin syndrome. Am J Psychiatry 1991;148: 705-13.
755. Storrow AB, Wians FH Jr, Mikkelsen SL, Norton J. Does naloxone cause a positive urine opiate screen? Ann Emerg Med 1994;24:1151-3.
756. Stout PR, Farrell LJ. Opioids: effects on human performance and behavior. Forensic Sci Rev 2003;15:30-59.
757. Struempler RE. Excretion of codeine and morphine following ingestion of poppy seeds. J Anal Toxicol 1987;11:97-9.
758. Studenik C, Lemmens-Gruber R, Heistracher P. Proarrhythmic effects of antidepressants and neuroleptic drugs on isolated, spontaneously beating guinea-pig Purkinje fibers. Eur J Pharm Sci 1999;7:113-8.
759. Sugiura T, Waku K. Cannabinoid receptors and their endogenous ligands. J Biochem 2002;132:7-12.
760. Sukbuntherng J, Walters A, Chow HH, Mayersohn M. Quantitative determination of cocaine, cocaethylene (ethylcocaine), and metabolites in plasma and urine by high-performance liquid chromatography. J Pharm Sci 1995;84:799-804.
761. Sullivan M. Mandatory guidelines for federal workplace drug testing programs, vol 53. Federal Register 1988;119:70-89.
762. Sulzer D, Sonders MS, Poulsen NW, Galli A. Mechanisms of neurotransmitter release by amphetamines: a review. Prog Neurobiol 2005;75:406-33.
763. Sun QR, Xiang P, Yan H, Shen M. [Simultaneous analyses of cocaine and its metabolite benzoylecgonine in urine by LC-MS/MS]. Fa Yi Xue Za Zhi 2008;24:268-72.
764. Suzuki S, Inoue T, Hori H, Inayama S. Analysis of methamphetamine in hair, nail, sweat, and saliva by mass fragmentography. J Anal Toxicol 1989;13:176-8.
765. Tateishi T, Krivoruk Y, Ueng YF, Wood AJ, Guengerich FP, Wood M. Identification of human liver cytochrome P-450 3A4 as the enzyme responsible for fentanyl and sufentanil N-dealkylation. Anesth Analg 1996;82:167-72.
766. Taylor EH, Oertli EH, Wolfgang JW, Mueller E. Accuracy of five on-site immunoassay drugs-of-abuse testing devices. J Anal Toxicol 1999;23:119-24.
767. Temple AR. Acute and chronic effects of aspirin toxicity and their treatment. Arch Intern Med 1981;141:364-9.
768. Tennant F, Shannon J. Quantitative urine testing: a new tool for diagnosing and treating cocaine use. Postgrad Med 1989;86:107-14.
769. Terada M, Shinozuka T, Bai H, Islam MN, Tun Z, Honda K, et al. Simultaneous determination of barbiturate drugs in human serum by wide-bore capillary gas chromatography with nitrogen-phosphorus detection. Jpn J Forensic Toxicol 1995;13:223-31.
770. Theobald DS, Fehn S, Maurer HH. New designer drug, 2,5-dimethoxy-4-propylthio-beta-phenethylamine (2C-T-7): studies on its metabolism and toxicological detection in rat urine using gas chromatography/mass spectrometry. J Mass Spectrom 2005;40: 105-16.
771. Thevis M, Geyer H, Bahr D, Schanzer W. Identification of fentanyl, alfentanil, sufentanil, remifentanil and their major metabolites in human urine by liquid chromatography/tandem mass spectrometry for doping control purposes. Eur J Mass Spectrom 2005;11:419-27.
772. Thevis M, Opfermann G, Schanzer W. Liquid chromatography/ electrospray ionization tandem mass spectrometric screening and confirmation methods for beta2-agonists in human or equine urine. J Mass Spectrom 2003;38:1197-206.
773. Thiermann H, Szinicz L, Eyer P, Zilker T, Worek F. Correlation between red blood cell acetylcholinesterase activity and neuromuscular transmission in organophosphate poisoning. Chem Biol Interact 2005;157-158:345-7.
774. Thomas S, Winecker R, Pestaner JP. Unusual fentanyl patch administration. Am J Forensic Med Pathol 2008;29:162-3.
775. Thurman EM, Pedersen MJ, Stout RL, Martin T. Distinguishing sympathomimetic amines from amphetamine and methamphetamine in urine by gas chromatography/mass spectrometry. J Anal Toxicol 1992;16:19-27.
776. Toennes SW, Fandino AS, Kauert G. Gas chromatographic-mass spectrometric detection of anhydroecgonine methyl ester (methylecgonidine) in human serum as evidence of recent smoking of crack. J Chromatogr 1999;735:127-32.
777. Tomassoni AW. Antihistamines and decongestants. In: Goldfrank LR, Flomenbaum NE, Hoffman RS, Howland MA, Lewin NA, Nelson L, eds. Goldfrank's toxicologic emergencies, 8th edition. New York, NY: McGraw-Hill, 2005.
778. Tomaszewski C. Carbon monoxide. In: Goldfrank LR, Flomenbaum NE, Hoffman RS, Howland MA, Lewin NA, Nelson L, eds. Goldfrank's toxicologic emergencies, 8th edition. New York, NY: McGraw Hill, 2006:1689-704.
779. Tong T, Boyer EW. Club drugs, smart drugs, raves, and circuit parties: an overview of the club scene. Pediatr Emerg Care 2002;18:216-8.
780. Trenton A, Currier G, Zwemer F. Fatalities associated with therapeutic use and overdose of atypical antipsychotics. CNS Drugs 2003;17:307-24.
781. Trescot AM, Datta S, Lee M, Hansen H. Opioid pharmacology. Pain Physician 2008;11:S133-53.
782. Trinder P. Rapid determination of salicylate in biological fluids. Biochem J 1954;57:301-3.
783. Tseng LF. Effects of para-methoxyamphetamine and 2,5-dimethoxyamphetamine on serotonergic mechanisms. Arch Pharmacol 1978;304:101-5.
784. Tseng LF, Menon MK, Loh HH. Comparative actions of monomethoxyamphetamines on the release and uptake of biogenic amines in brain tissue. J Pharmacol Exp Ther 1976;197:263-71.
785. Turcant A, Premel-Cabic A, Cailleux A, Allain P. Toxicological screening of drugs by microbore high-performance liquid chromatography with photodiode-array detection and ultraviolet spectral library searches. Clin Chem 1991;37:1210-15.
786. Tyrefors N, Hyllbrant B, Ekman L, Johansson M, Langstrom B. Determination of morphine, morphine-3-glucuronide and morphine-6-glucuronide in human serum by solid-phase extraction and liquid

chromatography-mass spectrometry with electrospray ionisation. J Chromatogr A 1996;729:279-85.

787. Uhl M. Determination of drugs in hair using GC/MS/MS. Forensic Sci Int 1997;84:281-94.
788. Uhl M, Sachs H. Cannabinoids in hair: strategy to prove marijuana/hashish consumption. Forensic Sci Int 2004;145:143-7.
789. Uhlenhuth EH, Balter MB, Ban TA, Yang K. International study of expert judgment on therapeutic use of benzodiazepines and other psychotherapeutic medications. IV. Therapeutic dose dependence and abuse liability of benzodiazepines in the long-term treatment of anxiety disorders. J Clin Psychopharmacol 1999;19:23S-9S.
790. Unterwald EM, Ho A, Rubenfeld JM, Kreek MJ. Time course of the development of behavioral sensitization and dopamine receptor up-regulation during binge cocaine administration. J Pharmacol Exp Ther 1994;270:1387-96.
791. Unterwald EM, Rubenfeld JM, Kreek MJ. Repeated cocaine administration upregulates kappa and mu, but not delta, opioid receptors. Neuroreport 1994;5:1613-6.
792. Valtier S, Cody JT. Evaluation of internal standards for the analysis of amphetamine and methamphetamine. J Anal Toxicol 1995;19:375-80.
793. van As H, Stolk LM. Rifampicin cross-reacts with opiate immunoassay. J Anal Toxicol 1999;23:71.
794. Van Bocxlaer JF, Clauwaert KM, Lambert WE, Deforce DL, Van den Eeckhout EG, De Leenheer AP. Liquid chromatography-mass spectrometry in forensic toxicology. Mass Spectrom Rev 2000;19:165-214.
795. Van Hoey N. Effect of cyclobenzaprine on tricyclic antidepressant assays. Ann Pharmacother 2005;39:1314-7.
796. Vanek VW, Dickey-White HI, Signs SA, Schechter MD, Buss T, Kulics AT. Concurrent use of cocaine and alcohol by patients treated in the emergency department. Ann Emerg Med 1996;28:508-14.
797. Vayer P, Mandel P, Maitre M. Conversion of gamma-hydroxybutyrate to gamma-aminobutyrate in vitro. J Neurochem 1985;45:810-4.
798. Veltri JC, Thompson MIB. Salicylates. In: Stoutakis V, ed. Clinical toxicology of drugs: principles and practice. Philadelphia, Pa: Lea & Febiger, 1982:227-43.
799. Verstraete AG, Heyden FV. Comparison of the sensitivity and specificity of six immunoassays for the detection of amphetamines in urine. J Anal Toxicol 2005;29:359-64.
800. Verweij AM, Hordijk ML, Lipman PJ. Liquid chromatographic-thermospray tandem mass spectrometric quantitative analysis of some drugs with hypnotic, sedative and tranquillising properties in whole blood. J Chromatogr B Biomed Appl 1996;686:27-34.
801. Verweij AM, Lipman PJ, Zweipfenning PG. Quantitative liquid chromatography, thermospray/tandem mass spectrometry (LC/TSP/MS/MS) analysis of some thermolabile benzodiazepines in whole-blood. Forensic Sci Int 1992;54:67-74.
802. Vesey CJ, Kirk CJ. Two automated methods for measuring plasma thiocyanate compared. Clin Chem 1985;31:270-4.
803. Vesey CJ, Wilson J. Red cell cyanide. J Pharm Pharmacol 1978;30:20-6.
804. Viera AJ, Yates SW. Toxic ingestion of gamma-hydroxybutyric acid. South Med J 1999;92:404-5.
805. Villain M, Cheze M, Tracqui A, Ludes B, Kintz P. Windows of detection of zolpidem in urine and hair: application to two drug facilitated sexual assaults. Forensic Sci Int 2004;143:157-61.
806. Vining RF, McGinley RA. Hormones in saliva. Crit Rev Clin Lab Sci 1986;23:95-146.
807. von Minden DL, D'Amato NA. Simultaneous determination of cocaine and benzoylecgonine in urine by gas-liquid chromatography. Anal Chem 1977;49:1974-7.
808. Vorce SP, Sklerov JH. A general screening and confirmation approach to the analysis of designer tryptamines and phenethylamines in blood and urine using GC-EI-MS and HPLC-electrospray-MS. J Anal Toxicol 2004;28:407-10.
809. Vreman HJ, Mahoney JJ, Van Kessel AL, Stevenson DK. Carboxyhemoglobin as measured by gas chromatography and with the IL 282 and 482 co-oximeters. Clin Chem 1988;34:2562-6.
810. Vreman HJ, Ronquillo RB, Ariagno RL, Schwartz HC, Stevenson DK. Interference of fetal hemoglobin with the spectrophotometric measurement of carboxyhemoglobin. Clin Chem 1988;34:975-7.
811. Wachtel SR, ElSohly MA, Ross SA, Ambre J, de Wit H. Comparison of the subjective effects of delta(9)-tetrahydrocannabinol and marijuana in humans. Psychopharmacology 2002;161:331-9.
812. Wagner J, Wagner ML, Hening WA. Beyond benzodiazepines: alternative pharmacologic agents for the treatment of insomnia. Ann Pharmacother 1998;32:680-91.
813. Wagner JG, Wilkinson PK, Sedman AJ, Kay DR, Weidler DJ. Elimination of alcohol from human blood. J Pharm Sci 1976;65:152-4.
814. Walberg CB, Gupta RC. Quantitation of phencyclidine in urine by enzyme immunoassay. J Anal Toxicol 1982;6:97-9.
815. Waldhoer M, Bartlett SE, Whistler JL. Opioid receptors. Annu Rev Biochem 2004;73:953-90.
816. Wall ME, Sadler BM, Brine D, Taylor H, Perez Reyes M. Metabolism, disposition, and kinetics of delta-9-tetrahydrocannabinol in men and women. Clin Pharmacol Ther 1983;34:352-63.
817. Wallace JE, Hamilton HE, King DE, Bason DJ, Schwertner HA, Harris SC. Gas-liquid chromatographic determination of cocaine and benzoylecgonine in urine. Anal Chem 1976;48:34-8.
818. Wallace KL, Suchard JR, Curry SC, Reagan C. Diagnostic use of physicians' detection of urine fluorescence in a simulated ingestion of sodium fluorescein-containing antifreeze. Ann Emerg Med 2001;38:49-54.
819. Wallner M, Hanchar HJ, Olsen RW. Ethanol enhances alpha 4 beta 3 delta and alpha 6 beta 3 delta gamma-aminobutyric acid type A receptors at low concentrations known to affect humans. Proc Natl Acad Sci U S A 2003;100:15218-23.
820. Walsh SL, Preston KL, Stitzer ML, Cone EJ, Bigelow GE. Clinical pharmacology of buprenorphine: ceiling effects at high doses. Clin Pharmacol Ther 1994;55:569-80.
821. Walshe K, Barrett AM, Kavanagh PV, McNamara SM, Moran C, Shattock AG. A sensitive immunoassay for flunitrazepam and metabolites. J Anal Toxicol 2000;24:296-9.
822. Waltzman ML. Flunitrazepam: a review of "roofies." Pediatr Emerg Care 1999;15:59-60.
823. Wan SH, Matin SB, Azarnoff DL. Kinetics, salivary excretion of amphetamine isomers, and effect of urinary pH. Clin Pharmacol Ther 1978;23:585-90.
824. Wang PH, Liu C, Tsay WI, Li JH, Liu RH, Wu TG, et al. Improved screen and confirmation test of 7-aminoflunitrazepam in urine specimens for monitoring flunitrazepam (Rohypnol) exposure. J Anal Toxicol 2002;26:411-8.
825. Wang QL, Fan LY, Zhang W, Cao CX. Sensitive analysis of two barbiturates in human urine by capillary electrophoresis with sample stacking induced by moving reaction boundary. Anal Chim Acta 2006;580:200-5.
826. Wasels R, Belleville F, Paysant P, Nabet P, Krakowski I. Determination of morphine in plasma by gas chromatography using a macrobore column and thermoionic detection after Extrelut column extraction: application to follow-up morphine treatment in cancer patients. J Chromatogr 1989;489:411-18.
827. Weiner AL, Ko C, McKay CA Jr. A comparison of two bedside tests for the detection of salicylates in urine. Acad Emerg Med 2000;7:834-6.
828. Weinmann W, Lehmann N, Muller C, Wiedemann A, Svoboda M. Identification of lorazepam and sildenafil as examples for the application of LC/ionspray-MS and MS-MS with mass spectra library searching in forensic toxicology. Forensic Sci Int 2000;113:339-44.
829. Weinmann W, Muller C, Vogt S, Frei A. LC-MS-MS analysis of the neuroleptics clozapine, flupentixol, haloperidol, penfluridol, thioridazine, and zuclopenthixol in hair obtained from psychiatric patients. J Anal Toxicol 2002;26:303-7.
830. Weinmann W, Svoboda M. Fast screening for drugs of abuse by solid-phase extraction combined with flow-injection ionspray-tandem mass spectrometry. J Anal Toxicol 1998;22:319-28.

831. Weiss RD, Gawin FH. Protracted elimination of cocaine metabolites in long-term high-dose cocaine abusers. Am J Med 1988;85:879-80.
832. Wells K, Williamson M, Holstege CP, Bear AB, Brady WJ. The association of cardiovascular toxins and electrocardiographic abnormality in poisoned patients. Am J Emerg Med 2008;26:957-9.
833. Welton B. Analysis of nanogram levels of barbiturates. Chromatographia 1970;3:211-5.
834. Wennig R. Potential problems with the interpretation of hair analysis results. Forensic Sci Int 2000;107:5-12.
835. Westfall TC, Westfall DP. Adrenergic agonists and antagonists (Chapter 10). In: Brunton LL, Lazo JS, Parker KL, eds. Goodman & Gilman's the pharmacological basis of therapeutics, 11th edition. New York, NY: McGraw-Hill, 2006.
836. Whitcomb DC, Block GD. Association of acetaminophen hepatotoxicity with fasting and ethanol use. JAMA 1994;272:1845-50.
837. White LM, Gardner SF, Gurley BJ, Marx MA, Wang PL, Estes M. Pharmacokinetics and cardiovascular effects of ma-huang *(Ephedra sinica)* in normotensive adults. J Clin Pharmacol 1997;37:116-22.
838. Whittington CJ, Kendall T, Fonagy P, Cottrell D, Cotgrove A, Boddington E. Selective serotonin reuptake inhibitors in childhood depression: systematic review of published versus unpublished data. Lancet 2004;363:1341-5.
839. Wians FH Jr, Norton JT, Wirebaugh SR. False-positive serum tricyclic antidepressant screen with cyproheptadine. Clin Chem 1993;39:1355-6.
840. Widmark EMP. Principles and applications of medicolegal alcohol determination. Davis, Calif: Biomedical Publications, 1981.
841. Wiegand RF, Klette KL, Stout PR, Gehlhausen JM. Comparison of EMIT II, CEDIA, and DPC RIA assays for the detection of lysergic acid diethylamide in forensic urine samples. J Anal Toxicol 2002;26:519-23.
842. Wiener K. A review of methods for plasma paracetamol estimation. Ann Clin Biochem 1978;15:187-96.
843. Williams AJ, Jones TW, Cooper JD. A rapid method for the determination of therapeutic barbiturate levels in serum using gas-liquid chromatography. Clin Chim Acta 1973;43:327-32.
844. Wilson IB, Ginsburg B. A powerful reactivator of alkylphosphate-inhibited acetylcholinesterase. Biochim Biophys Acta 1955;18:168-70.
845. Wilson IB, Ginsburg S. Reactivation of acetylcholinesterase inhibited by alkylphosphates. Arch Biochem 1955;54:569-71.
846. Winek CL, Carfagna M. Comparison of plasma, serum, and whole blood ethanol concentrations. J Anal Toxicol 1987;11:267-8.
847. Winek CL, Murphy KL. The rate and kinetic order of ethanol elimination. Forensic Sci Int 1984;25:159-66.
848. Winek CL, Paul LJ. Effect of short-term storage conditions on alcohol concentrations in blood from living human subjects. Clin Chem 1983;29:1959-60.
849. Wingert WE. Lowering cutoffs for initial and confirmation testing for cocaine and marijuana: large-scale study of effects on the rates of drug-positive results. Clin Chem 1997;43:100-3.
850. Wittwer E, Kern SE. Role of morphine's metabolites in analgesia: concepts and controversies. AAPS J 2006;8:E348-52.
851. Wolfe TR, Caravati EM. Massive dextromethorphan ingestion and abuse. Am J Emerg Med 1995;13:174-6.
852. Wolff K, Hay A, Raistrick D. Methadone in saliva. Clin Chem 1991;37:1297-8.
853. Wong EC, Koenig J, Turk J. Potential interference of cyclobenzaprine and norcyclobenzaprine with HPLC measurement of amitriptyline and nortriptyline: resolution by GC-MS analysis. J Anal Toxicol 1995;19:218-24.
854. Wood M, De Boeck G, Samyn N, Morris M, Cooper DP, Maes RA, De Bruijn EA. Development of a rapid and sensitive method for the quantitation of amphetamines in human plasma and oral fluid by LC-MS-MS. J Anal Toxicol 2003;27:78-87.
855. Woods JH, Katz JL, Winger G. Benzodiazepines: use, abuse, and consequences. Pharmacol Rev 1992;44:151-347.
856. Woods JH, Winger G. Abuse liability of flunitrazepam. J Clin Psychopharmacol 1997;17:1S-57S.
857. Wright R, Woolf A. Phencyclidine. In: Haddad L, Shannon M, Winchester J, eds. Clinical management of poisoning and drug overdose, 3rd edition. Philadelphia, Pa: WB Saunders, 1998:552-9.
858. Wright RO, Lewander WJ, Woolf AD. Methemoglobinemia: etiology, pharmacology, and clinical management. Ann Emerg Med 1999;34:646-56.
859. Wu AH, Feng YJ, Pajor A, Gornet TG, Wong SS, Forte E, Brown J. Detection and interpretation of lysergic acid diethylamide results by immunoassay screening of urine in various testing groups. J Anal Toxicol 1997;21:181-4.
860. Wu AH, McKay C, Broussard LA, Hoffman RS, Kwong TC, Moyer TP, et al. National Academy of Clinical Biochemistry Laboratory Medicine practice guidelines: recommendations for the use of laboratory tests to support poisoned patients who present to the emergency department. Clin Chem 2003;49:357-79.
861. Wu AH, Wong SS, Johnson KG, Callies J, Shu DX, Dunn WE, et al. Evaluation of the triage system for emergency drugs-of-abuse testing in urine. J Anal Toxicol 1993;17:241-5.
862. Wu Y, Ali S, Ahmadian G, Liu CC, Wang YT, Gibson KM, et al. Gamma-hydroxybutyric acid (GHB) and gamma-aminobutyric acid B receptor (GABABR) binding sites are distinctive from one another: molecular evidence. Neuropharmacology 2004;47:1146-56.
863. Wu YH, Tan JY, Xia Y. [Determination of 7-aminoflunitrazepam, the major metabolite of flunitrazepam in urine by high performance thin-layer chromatography]. Se Pu 2002;20:182-4.
864. Wurst FM, Skipper GE, Weinmann W. Ethyl glucuronide—the direct ethanol metabolite on the threshold from science to routine use. Addiction 2003;98(Suppl 2):51-61.
865. Wylie FM, Torrance H, Anderson RA, Oliver JS. Drugs in oral fluid. Part I. Validation of an analytical procedure for licit and illicit drugs in oral fluid. Forensic Sci Int 2005;150:191-8.
866. Wyngaarden JB, Seevers MH. The toxic effects of antihistaminic drugs. JAMA 1951;145:277-82.
867. Yao HH, Porter WH. Simultaneous determination of ethylene glycol and its major toxic metabolite, glycolic acid, in serum by gas chromatography. Clin Chem 1996;42:292-7.
868. Yeatman DT, Reid K. A study of urinary endogenous gamma-hydroxybutyrate (GHB) levels. J Anal Toxicol 2003;27:40-2.
869. Yuan H, Mester Z, Lord H, Pawliszyn J. Automated in-tube solid-phase microextraction coupled with liquid chromatography-electrospray ionization mass spectrometry for the determination of selected benzodiazepines. J Anal Toxicol 2000;24:718-25.
870. Zawertailo LA, Kaplan HL, Busto UE, Tyndale RF, Sellers EM. Psychotropic effects of dextromethorphan are altered by the CYP2D6 polymorphism: a pilot study. J Clin Psychopharmacol 1998;18:332-7.
871. Zhao H, Brenneisen R, Scholer A, McNally AJ, ElSohly MA, Murphy TP, et al. Profiles of urine samples taken from Ecstasy users at Rave parties: analysis by immunoassays, HPLC, and GC-MS. J Anal Toxicol 2001;25:258-69.
872. Zhao H, Wang L, Qiu Y, Zhou Z, Zhong W, Li X. Multiwalled carbon nanotubes as a solid-phase extraction adsorbent for the determination of three barbiturates in pork by ion trap gas chromatography-tandem mass spectrometry (GC/MS/MS) following microwave assisted derivatization. Anal Chim Acta 2007;586:399-406.
873. Zheng M, McErlane KM, Ong MC. High-performance liquid chromatography-mass spectrometry-mass spectrometry analysis of morphine and morphine metabolites and its application to a pharmacokinetic study in male Sprague-Dawley rats. J Pharmaceut Biomed Anal 1998;16:971-80.
874. Zollner C, Stein C. Opioids: handbook of experimental pharmacology. New York, NY: Springer-Verlag, 2007:31-63.
875. Zoppi F, Brenna S, Fumagalli C, Marocchi A. Discrimination among dyshemoglobins: analytical approach to a toxicological query. Clin Chem 1996;42:1300-2.
876. Zuccaro P, Ricciarello R, Pichini S, Pacifici R, Altieri I, Pellegrini M, et al. Simultaneous determination of heroin 6-monoacetylmorphine,

morphine, and its glucuronides by liquid chromatography—atmospheric pressure ionspray-mass spectrometry. J Anal Toxicol 1997;21:268-77.
877. Zuidema J, van Ginneken CA. Clearance concept in salivary drug excretion. Part I. Theory. Pharm Acta Helv 1983;58: 88-93.
878. Zvosec DL, Smith SW, McCutcheon JR, Spillane J, Hall BJ, Peacock EA. Adverse events, including death, associated with the use of 1,4-butanediol. N Engl J Med 2001;344:87-94.
879. Zwart A, van Kampen EJ, Zijlstra WG. Results of routine determination of clinically significant hemoglobin derivatives by multicomponent analysis. Clin Chem 1986;32:972-8.

CHAPTER 36

Toxic Metals

Thomas P. Moyer, Ph.D.

Metals have been recognized as toxins for centuries. For example, arsenic (As) poisoning was a favored way to dethrone royalty in the Renaissance era, and mercury (Hg) poisoning was common in eighteenth century Europe, where it was associated with the generation of felt from beaver pelts to make the popular top hat. This resulted in behavioral changes and common use of the phrase "mad as a hatter."

This chapter explores these and other toxic metals and the role of the clinical laboratory in diagnosing and monitoring toxicity associated with exposure to them.

ASSESSMENT OF METAL POISONING

Important questions to address when considering metal toxicity today are listed in Box 36-1. These questions are addressed generally in the first section of this chapter. In the second section, the unique characteristics of the more common metals known to be associated with toxicity are discussed. Readers are referred to *The Handbook on the Toxicology of Metals*[101] for details on rare metal toxicities.

Prevalence of Metal-Based Toxicity

As the twenty-first century begins, one would expect that metal toxicities would be thoroughly known and avoidable. However, humans frequently still encounter elemental toxins, and chronic, low-concentration exposure occurs more frequently in individuals than in large population groups. Concern continues regarding low-concentration exposure to lead and the effect such exposure has on mental development in the young. As is common in our environment, individuals are occasionally exposed because of lack of knowledge of the household products they are using. Many insecticides contain As as an active ingredient; careless use of these products has led to significant exposure. As is frequently identified as the cause of peripheral neuropathy among patients who have been unwittingly exposed. Ground water contaminated with As in the Bengal basin of Bangladesh, exceeding World Health Organization (WHO) safety limits because of leaching from bedrock, presents a serious health risk to the large population living in that region. Cadmium (Cd) is used to manufacture brightly colored paint pigments; painters who fail to use adequate respiratory protection while using abrasive materials to remove paint, or while spray painting with cadmium-containing products, can experience significant exposure. Cd is also significantly present in tobacco products.[61] Studies indicate that apoptotic pathways are initiated by metals such as As, Cd, chromium (Cr) , nickel (Ni), and beryllium (Be); and possibly lead (Pb), antimony (Sb), and cobalt (Co).[108]

Although rare, manufacturing errors have caused the production of products that contain toxic metals. For example, in the early 1960s, a Canadian beer brewery accidentally contaminated a large lot of its product with Co. The product was sold to and consumed by the public, resulting in an outbreak of renal disease and cardiomyopathy. In this type of situation, the Public Health Service is often called in to identify the cause of an outbreak of unusual symptoms. The clinical laboratory should be prepared to support these types of investigations.

The incidence of metal poisoning in a large population attributable to As, Cd, Pb, or mercury (Hg) poisoning appears to be of the same scale as the more common inborn errors of metabolism, such as neonatal hypothyroidism and phenylketonuria, and is the same order of magnitude as the incidence of adult-onset hemochromatosis, a disease for which mandatory screening has been suggested. Screening for these diseases is indicated because they are treatable, and treatment significantly reduces long-term morbidity.[92] The same is true for metal toxicities. When identified early, disease caused by metal exposure is readily treatable with good outcomes. Conversely, if exposure is not identified and reduced, serious and sometimes irreparable damage to the nervous, renal, and cardiovascular systems can occur.

Diagnosing Toxicity

Confirming the diagnosis of metal toxicity is difficult because signs and symptoms are similar to those of a number of non–element-dependent diseases. Diagnosis of metal toxicity requires demonstration of *all* of the following factors: (1) a source of metal exposure must be evident, (2) the patient must demonstrate signs and symptoms typical of the metal, and (3) abnormal metal concentration in the appropriate tissue must be evident. If one of these features is absent, one cannot make a conclusive diagnosis of metal toxicity. The laboratory plays a key role in this process, and appropriate specimen collection coupled with accurate analysis can make a major difference in correct diagnosis.

In clinical practice, analysis of toxic elements should always be considered in the clinical work-up of the patient with (1) renal disease of unexplained origin, (2) bilateral peripheral neuropathy, (3) acute changes in mental function, (4) acute inflammation of the nasal or laryngeal epithelium, or (5) a history of exposure. Certain elements should be considered as the active, causative, or deficient agent in specific circumstances (Table 36-1).

Classification of Metals

Some metals are essential for life (see Chapter 31), but if an individual's exposure exceeds a certain threshold, toxicity may develop. Some nonessential metals are toxic even at low concentrations. Review of the periodic table provides some insight into the determination of a metal's potential toxicity (Figure 36-1).

BOX 36-1 Pertinent Questions Relative to Metal Toxicity

1. Is the metal of concern toxic?
2. What is the prevalence associated with the metal of concern?
3. What are the signs and symptoms of exposure to that metal?
4. Is the degree of exposure known?
5. Are adequate analytical techniques available to measure the metal?
6. Are appropriate body fluids and tissues and analytical techniques available to identify and quantify the metal?

TABLE 36-1 Conditions That Involve Metal Toxicity

Metal	Condition
Aluminum	Dialysis, encephalopathy, or dementia
Arsenic	Bilateral pain radiating from feet to legs or peripheral neuropathy, or unexplained impaired renal function
Cadmium	Impaired renal function in aerosol painters
Copper-zinc deficiency	Impaired wound healing
Gadolinium	Nephrogenic systemic fibrosis
Lead	Children younger than 2 years living in older homes, or unexplained gastric upset, anemia, or impaired renal function at any age
Mercury	Acute changes in behavior, impaired speech, visual field constriction, hearing loss, and somatosensory disorders
Manganese	Onset of parkinsonism younger than age 50
Selenium (deficiency)	Patients undergoing total parenteral nutrition
Thallium	Acute hair loss
Zinc (deficiency)	Burn patients exhibiting erythema

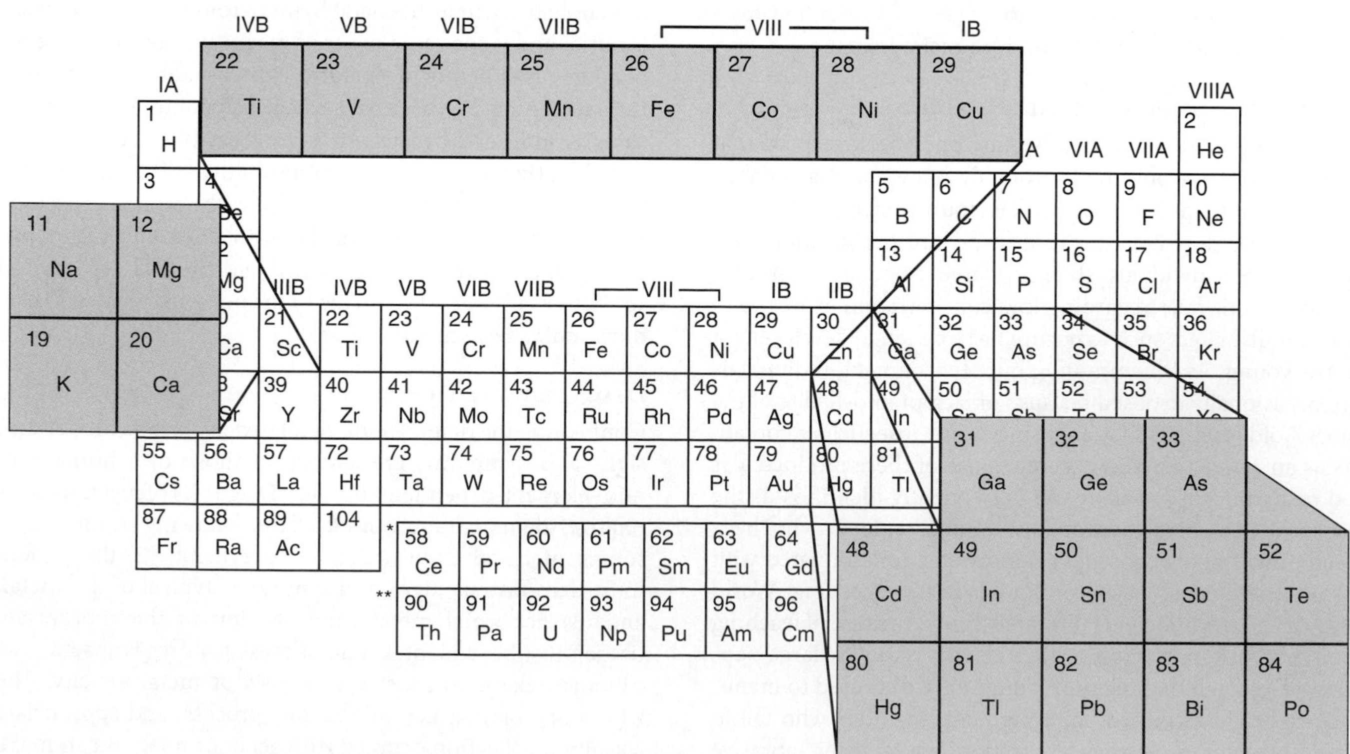

Figure 36-1 Periodic table, with emphasis on toxic elements.

Elements in rows 3 and 4 of groups 1 and 2 of the periodic table are essential elements. The gastrointestinal tract and the dermis are very effective at regulating the body burden of these compounds—patients rarely experience toxicity from one of these elements unless the element is injected directly into the vascular system. Elements in groups 6 through 12 in row 4 of the periodic table are essential for life but are required at low concentrations; many are protein cofactors required for enzymatic activity. The gastrointestinal tract and the dermis regulate intake to some degree, but overload will induce passive diffusion that can lead to excessive concentrations and toxicity. Elements in rows 5 and below are classified as nonessential (or if essential, are required at picomolar concentrations or less). As one moves from right to left across the periodic table, the elements become more prevalent and therefore have greater potential to induce toxicity. Elements in groups 13 through 16 in rows 4 through 6 are of particular interest as toxins, because they have electron configuration that allows them to bond covalently with sulfur. Later in this chapter, this characteristic is identified as a significant factor in the mechanism of action of this group of metals. These include As, Cd, Pb, Hg, and thallium (Tl)—all toxins of considerable concern. Elements in group 17 (halides) are essential for life but are toxic when present in excess. The inert elements that constitute group 18 are toxic in the gas phase because they can cause anoxia; their inert characteristic is the very cause of their toxicity.

Occupational Monitoring

Employees are frequently monitored when working in an environment where exposure to toxic metals is a possibility.[101] The most common form of monitoring involves quantification of airborne concentrations of metals in the production process. Threshold limit values (TLVs) for airborne concentrations and time interval exposure concentrations are defined by the U.S. National Institute for Occupational Safety and Health (NIOSH) to ensure worker safety. Workers may also be monitored by quantification of biological samples. The most common sample used is a random urine sample, and results are expressed in concentration units for the metal of interest per gram of creatinine to normalize for excretion volume variances. Cd, Cr, and Pb have defined urine excretion concentrations set by a U.S. federal agency to ensure worker safety.[15,26,80] Additional technical and regulatory information about toxic metals is available at the Occupational Safety and Health Administration (OSHA) Website at http://www.osha.gov/SLTC/metalsheavy/index.html/ accessed June 2, 2011.

The WHO and OSHA have defined blood concentrations for Pb that are designed to warn employers when workers are overexposed.[113] Safety limits for other metals have been set by professional organizations, such as the American Conference of Governmental Hygienists.[36]

Analytical Methods

Analytical techniques used to measure metals in biological fluid includes (1) atomic absorption spectrometry with flame (AA-F) or electrothermal atomization furnace (AA-ETA), (2) inductively coupled plasma emission spectroscopy (ICP-ES), (3) inductively coupled plasma mass spectrometry (ICP-MS), and (4) high-performance liquid chromatography–inductively coupled plasma mass spectrometry (LC-ICP/MS). These tecniques are specific, sensitive, and provide the clinical laboratory with the capability to measure a broad array of metals at clinically significant concentrations. For example, ICP-MS is used to measure several metals simultaneously.[13,88,100] Photometric assays have been used in the past but require large volumes of sample and have limited specificity. Spot tests are also available but should be considered obsolete because they are error prone, often yielding false-positive results.

SPECIFIC METALS

Certain metals are known to be toxic when humans are exposed to elevated concentrations; five metals are listed in the top 20 of the 2007 CERCLA (Comprehensive Environmental Response, Compensation, and Liability Act) Priority List of Hazardous Substances.[21] They include As (No. 1), Pb (No. 2), Hg (No. 3), Cd (No. 7), and Cr (No. 18). Other metals of concern include aluminum (Al), Be, Co, copper (Cu), gadolinium (Gd), iron (Fe), manganese (Mn), Ni, platinum (Pt), selenium (Se), silicon (Si), silver (Ag), and Ti. The Agency for Toxic Substances and Disease Registry (ATSDR) provides toxicologic profiles for many of these metals on its Website.[2] These hazardous substances are ranked on the basis of their frequency of occurrence, toxicity, and potential for human exposure.

Several of these metals are also considered essential trace elements and are discussed in Chapter 31. Risk assessments for essentiality versus toxicity for Cr, Cu, iodine (I), Fe, Mn, molybdenum (Mo), Se, and zinc (Zn) have been performed by several U.S. governmental and private organizations.[52,98]

Aluminum

In 1972, Alfrey and colleagues first described an encephalopathy that was observed in patients undergoing prolonged hemodialysis for renal failure.[1] The disease was characterized by abnormal speech, myoclonic jerks, and convulsions. Patients with these signs also showed a predominance of osteomalacic fractures. Subsequently, it was found that exposure of patients in renal failure to Al (1) laden dialysis water, (2) containing oral phosphate binders, and (3) laden albumin administered during dialysis is the primary cause of these signs of Al toxicity. Aluminum is also a developmental toxicant if administered parenterally.[37]

Under normal physiologic conditions, the usual daily dietary intake of Al is 5 to 10 mg, which is completely excreted. This excretion is accomplished by avid filtration of Al from the blood by the glomerulus of the kidney. Patients in renal failure lose this ability and are candidates for Al toxicity. The dialysis process is not highly effective at eliminating Al and can be a significant source of exposure. Furthermore, it is a common practice to administer Al-based gels orally to patients in renal failure to reduce the amount of phosphate absorbed from their diet to avoid excessive phosphate accumulation.[104] A small fraction of this Al may be absorbed and patients in renal failure accumulate this Al. Following dialysis, albumin may be administered to replace that which is removed during dialysis. Some albumin products have high Al content resulting from the pharmaceutical purification process of passing the product through Al silicate filters.

Aluminum (1) accumulates in blood if not filtered by the kidney; (2) avidly binds to proteins, such as transferrin; and (3) rapidly distributes throughout the body. Deposition of it in bone interrupts physiologic calcium exchange; the calcium in bone becomes unavailable for resorption into blood, a process under the physiologic control of parathyroid hormone (PTH) and 1,25-dihydroxy vitamin D (see Chapter 52). The normal physiologic action of PTH on bone is blunted in patients with renal failure because their renal cells are not synthesizing the 1,25-dihydroxy vitamin D required for normal PTH action. It is typical for patients in renal failure to have high serum PTH values and low serum calcium; this represents secondary hyperparathyroidism, the normal physiologic response to vitamin D deficit. Deposition of Al at the bone mineralization front and binding to parathyroid calcium receptors interfere with this physiologic process. The usual parathyroid response to these conditions decreases secretion of PTH. The result is lower-than-expected serum PTH concentration for the degree of renal disease present.

In addition, a biochemical profile that characterizes Al overload disease has been defined.[87] In human subjects with normal renal function, serum Al concentration is typically lower than 6 μg/L, but patients in renal failure invariably have serum Al concentrations significantly higher. Clinical guidelines published in 2006[91] suggest that patients with no signs or symptoms of osteomalacia or encephalopathy are likely to have serum Al concentrations <20 μg/L and PTH whole molecule concentrations 150 to 300 ng/L, typical for secondary hyperparathyroidism associated with renal failure.[119] Patients with signs and symptoms of osteomalacia or encephalopathy typically have serum Al concentrations >60 μg/L, and PTH concentrations <65 ng/L indicate Al-related bone disease. Patients with serum Al concentrations >20 and <60 μg/L were identified as candidates for likely onset of Al-related bone disease; these patients required aggressive efforts to reduce their daily Al exposure. Efforts to reduce Al intake include (1) switching from Al-containing phosphate binders to calcium-containing phosphate binders, (2) ensuring that dialysis water contains less than 10 μg/L of Al, and (3) ensuring that albumin used during postdialysis therapy is Al-free.

Interest in the role of Al in Alzheimer's disease (AD) was raised when Perl observed that Al accumulates in the neurofibrillary tangle of patients with AD.[107] He concluded that the focal accumulation of Al had an association with neurofibrillary degeneration in the hippocampal neurons that might play a role in the development of AD. Although a cause-and-effect relationship between accumulation of Al in brain and AD has yet to be conclusively demonstrated,[11A,112] studies have clearly shown an increased concentration of Al in the brain.[90] It is possible that accumulation of Al in the neurofibrillary tangle of AD patients is a secondary finding associated with the disease but not directly related to the cause. Also, the neurofibrillary tangle has a higher than normal affinity for Al that may explain increased accumulation of Al in brain tissue of Alzheimer's patients.

Aluminum-related bone disease has been diagnosed and treated with deferoxamine, an avid chelator of both iron and Al.[31] The deferoxamine infusion test is useful for the ultimate diagnosis of Al overload disease, and the drug has demonstrated utility for treating acute Al overload.[31,40]

Preanalytical considerations related to collection of specimen for Al analysis are significant. Most of the common evacuated blood collection devices used in phlebotomy today have rubber stoppers that are made of Al silicate. Puncture of the rubber stopper for blood collection is sufficient to contaminate the sample with Al and produce an abnormal concentration of Al. Typically, blood collected in standard evacuated blood tubes will be contaminated by 20 to 60 μg/L of Al; this is readily demonstrated by collecting blood from a healthy volunteer into a standard evacuated phlebotomy tube. Special evacuated blood collection tubes are required for Al testing.[94] These tubes are readily available from commercial suppliers and should always be used. Failure to pay attention to this issue can result in the generation of abnormal results because of sample contamination, which leads to misinterpretation and misdiagnosis.

Analysis of Al is routinely performed by inductively coupled plasma (ICP) mass spectrometry (ICP-MS). Alternatively, atomic absorption spectrometry with electrothermal atomization may be employed, but considerable attention must be paid to matrix interferences.

Antimony

Sb compounds have been known since ancient Egyptian times and were used as cosmetics by the women of that era. In the sixteenth century, Sb preparations were thought to be wonder drugs that in the nineteenth century were prescribed for a number of conditions. Today antimony compounds are used to treat parasitic diseases such as leishmaniasis, schistosomiasis, and bilharziasis.[18,126]

Pure metallic Sb is very brittle; however, alloys of Sb are used in various fields of technology. For example, addition of Sb to lead, tin, and copper increases the hardness of these metals when used as electrodes, bullets, type metal for printing, and ball bearings. Other uses include fire-resistant chemicals, pigments, and dyes.

Antimony is not an essential metal. Workplace exposure to Sb dust over a period of years leads to pneumoconiosis. The size of the dust particles of Sb trioxide significantly increases the occurrence of pneumoconiosis, with smaller particles being more dangerous.[126] The workers at greatest danger are those in underground facilities and metal production. Smoking may also contribute to respiratory problems. Symptoms of acute exposure include (1) a metallic taste,

(2) headache, (3) nausea, and (4) dizziness; and after a short interval, (5) vomiting, (6) diarrhea, and (7) intestinal spasms. In chronic intoxication, adverse health effects include (1) cardiac arrhythmias, (2) upper respiratory and ocular irritation, (3) spontaneous abortion, (4) premature birth, and (5) dermatitis.[35] Lymphocytosis, eosinophilia, and a reduction in leukocyte and platelet counts are also seen and indicate damage to the liver and spleen. Evidence supports increased risk for the development of lung cancer in Sb smelter workers, but the effect may be multifactorial and may be due, for example, to the presence of arsenic in the work environment.[30] It is important to remember that when intoxication occurs with metallic Sb, the effect is caused not only by Sb, but also by the lead, arsenic, and other metals that may accompany it.

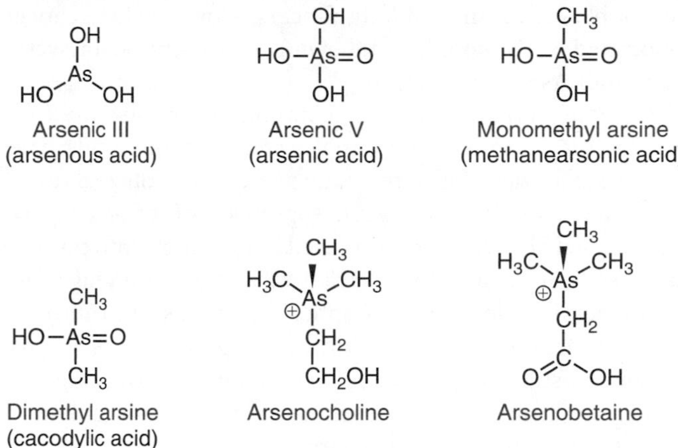

Figure 36-2 Structures of arsenic species.

Arsenic

As is perhaps the best known of the metal toxins, having gained notoriety from its extensive use by Renaissance nobility as an antisyphilitic agent and an antidote against acute arsenic poisoning; long-term administration of low arsenic doses protects against acute poisoning by massive doses—an historic example of hepatic enzyme induction. This agent was memorably used in the well-known tale "Arsenic and Old Lace"[73] as a means of terminating undesirable acquaintances. Currently, As is still a dangerous toxicant as evidenced by the Bangladesh incident wherein several hundred persons were poisoned by drinking ground water contaminated with As leaching from bedrock. As discussed earlier, As is listed as the No. 1 toxicant on the 2007 U.S. CERCLA Priority List of Hazardous Substances,[21] and it is still used extensively in insecticides.

Arsenic exists in numerous toxic and nontoxic forms.[93] The toxic forms include (1) the inorganic species As^{3+}, also denoted as As(III); (2) the more toxic As^{5+}, also known as As(V), and their partially detoxified metabolites; (3) monomethylarsine (MMA); and (4) dimethylarsine (DMA). Detoxification occurs in the liver as As^{5+} is reduced to As^{3+} and then is methylated to MMA and DMA. As a result of these detoxification steps, As^{3+} and As^{5+} are found in the urine shortly after ingestion, whereas MMA and DMA are the species that predominate longer than 24 hours after ingestion. Urinary As^{3+} and As^{5+} concentrations peak in urine at approximately 10 hours and return to normal 20 to 30 hours after ingestion. Urinary MMA and DMA concentrations normally peak at about 40 to 60 hours and return to baseline 6 to 20 days after ingestion.[93] In a large U.S. population study, for all participants aged >6 years, dimethylarsinic acid and arsenobetaine had the greatest contribution to the quantity of total urinary arsenic. Aarsenobetaine was the primary contributor to high total urinary arsenic concentrations.[16,33,45]

The half-life of inorganic As in blood is 4 to 6 hours, and the half-life of the methylated metabolites is 20 to 30 hours. Blood concentrations of As are elevated for only a short time after administration, after which As rapidly disappears into the large body phosphate pool. Abnormal blood As concentrations in the 5 to 50 ng/mL range are detected after exposure.[55] The structures of these and related As species are shown in Figure 36-2.

Nontoxic forms of As are present in many foods. Arsenobetaine and arsenocholine are the two most common forms of organic As that are found in food.[59] The foods that most commonly contain significant concentrations of organic As are shellfish and other predators in the seafood chain (e.g., cod, haddock). In the large U.S. population study, for all participants aged >6 years, dimethylarsinic acid and arsenobetaine had the greatest contribution to the total urinary arsenic. Arsenobetaine was the primary contributor to high total urinary arsenic concentrations.[16] Arsenic excretion in normal people who have ingested arsenobetaine-containing foods is >120 μg per 24-hour specimen. Following ingestion, arsenobetaine and arsenocholine undergo rapid renal clearance to become concentrated in the urine. Arsenobetaine and arsenocholine are completely excreted within 1 to 2 days after ingestion, and no residual toxic metabolites are present. The apparent half-life of organic As is 4 to 6 hours. Consumption of seafood before collection of a urine sample for As testing is likely to result in an elevated concentration of As in the urine; this can be clinically misleading.

The toxicity of As is due to three different mechanisms, two of which are related to energy transfer. Arsenic avidly binds to dihydrolipoic acid, a necessary cofactor for pyruvate dehydrogenase. Absence of the cofactor inhibits the conversion of pyruvate to acetyl coenzyme A—the first step in gluconeogenesis. Arsenic competes with phosphate for reaction with adenosine diphosphate (ADP), resulting in formation of the lower-energy adipic acids (ADPAs) rather than adenosine triphosphate (ATP). Arsenic also binds with any hydrated sulfhydryl group on protein, distorting the three-dimensional configuration of the protein, thus causing it to lose activity. British antilewisite (BAL) is an effective antidote for treating As intoxication; the active agent in BAL is dimercaprol, a sulfhydryl-reducing agent. This suggests that the primary mechanism of action of the toxicity of As is related to sulfhydryl binding. Arsenic also interferes with the activity of several enzymes of the heme biosynthetic pathway.[49] Arsenic is also a known carcinogen[24] as evidence suggests increased risk of bladder, skin, and lung cancers, as well as lung cancer associated with smoking, following consumption of water with high As contamination.[11,115]

Of note, is the fact that As compounds are also used for therapeutic reasons. For example, arsenic compounds have been used for decades in the management of protozoal infections such as trypanosomiasis. A preparation of arsenic trioxide called Fowler's agent was used in the nineteenth century as a health tonic and for a variety of ailments ranging from skin disease to leukemia. Arsphenamine was used intravenously to treat syphilis, yaws, and some protozoal infections. Arsenic is still a key ingredient of certain herbal remedies, and arsenic trioxide is currently used in the management of refractory promyelocytic leukemia.

To distinguish among toxic inorganic species and nontoxic organic species of As of seafood origin, high-performance liquid chromatography (HPLC) techniques that separate the various species of As in biological fluids and tissues have been developed.[16] A typical finding in a urine specimen with total 24-hour excretion of As of 350 μg/24 hours is that more than 95% is present as the organic nontoxic seafood species, and less than 5% is present as the inorganic toxic species. Such a finding indicates that the elevated total As concentration was likely due to ingestion of seafood.

Hair analysis is frequently used to document time of As exposure.[76] Arsenic circulating in the blood will bind to protein by formation of a covalent complex with sulfhydryl groups of the amino acid cysteine. Because As has a high affinity for keratin, which has high cysteine content, the As concentration in hair or nails is greater than in other tissue. Several weeks after exposure, transverse white striae, called *Mees' lines*, may appear in the fingernails; this event is caused by denaturation of keratin by metals such as As, Cd, Pb, and Hg. Because hair grows at a rate of approximately 0.5 cm/mo, hair collected from the nape of the neck can be used to document recent exposure. Axillary or pubic hair is used to document long-term (6 months to 1 year) exposure. Hair As >1 μg/g dry weight indicates excessive exposure. In one study, the highest hair As observed was 210 μg/g dry weight in a case of chronic exposure that was the cause of death.[63]

Blood is the least useful specimen for identifying As exposure. Blood As concentrations are elevated for only a short time after administration[55] and rapidly disappear into the large body phosphate pool, because the body treats As like phosphate, incorporating it wherever phosphate would be incorporated. Absorbed As is rapidly circulated and distributed into tissue storage sites. Abnormal blood As concentrations are detected for only a few hours (<4 hours) after ingestion. This test is useful only to document an acute exposure when the As is likely to be >20 ng/mL for a short period of time. Typically, serum As is <40 ng/mL.

Arsenic has been accurately analyzed by ICP-MS. The specimen is prepared in dilute acid containing gallium as an internal standard and is aspirated directly into the argon plasma. Mass response from the argon plasma is monitored for As (75 m/z), gallium (70 m/z), and $^{16}O^{35}Cl$ (51 m/z) to allow for correction for $^{40}Ar^{35}Cl$ (75 m/z) interference. The operator must be aware of the potential for interference from argon chloride. A correction is made by accounting for chloride by measuring 51 m/z and subtracting that residual from 75 m/z.[100] Urine is the sample of choice for As analysis because As is excreted predominantly by the kidney, where it becomes concentrated.

Beryllium

Be is an alkaline earth metal found in the earth's crust at an approximate concentration of 3 to 5 mg/kg; it is poisonous and is not necessary for human health. Beryllium alloys are lightweight, stiff, and highly electrically conductive. Beryllium metal and alloys and Be ceramics are used in a wide range of applications, including dental appliances, golf clubs, nonsparking tools, wheelchairs, satellite and spacecraft manufacture, circuit board production, and nuclear power, and in weapons as a neutron modulator.

The general population is exposed to low concentrations of Be through food and drinking water; these exposures are of no clinical consequence. The major route by which Be enters the body is via the respiratory tract, and industrial exposure usually occurs from inhalation and ingestion of Be dust. Inhaled Be compounds are cleared very slowly from the lungs. Soluble compounds are absorbed to a much greater degree than other such as Be oxide, which are much less soluble. Beryllium salts are strongly acidic when dissolved in water, and this is thought to have a major toxic effect on human tissue. Absorbed Be accumulates in the skeleton. Renal clearance is very slow. Beryllium inhibits a variety of enzyme systems, including alkaline phosphatase, acid phosphatase, phosphoglycerate mutase, hexokinase, and lactate dehydrogenase.[114]

Acute exposure to Be is rare, is usually caused by an industrial accident or explosion, and typically results in chemical pneumonitis. Chronic Be exposure in the workplace has led to occupational health concerns because of its potential to cause a progressive and potentially fatal respiratory condition called *chronic Be disease (CBD)*. This disease, also known as berylliosis, is characterized by the formation of granulomas resulting from an immune reaction to Be particles in the lung.[34,67] To reduce the number of workers currently exposed to beryllium in the course of their work at the U.S. Department of Energy (DOE) facilities or among its contractors, the DOE has established a chronic beryllium disease prevention program (CBDPP) to minimize the concentrations of, and the potential for exposure to, beryllium, and has put forth medical surveillance requirements to ensure early detection of the disease (http://www.hss.energy.gov/healthsafety/wshp/be/ accessed June 2, 2011).

Studies have suggested that the size of the Be particles affects not only the site of deposition but also the amount deposited. This in turn may influence the clearance rate and thus the time of contact between the immune cells and Be.[74] Several years ago, researchers noted that blood and lung cells from CBD patients proliferated when exposed to Be in culture. This assay has been refined and is offered as the Be lymphocyte proliferation test (BeLPT). Unfortunately, because of the nature of the test and the variability from lab to lab, the BeLPT has been known to produce false-negative and problematic results.[34,86] Efforts are under way by several groups to standardize the assay. Despite these issues, the BeLPT in bronchoalveolar cells is part of the current "gold standard" diagnosis for CBD.[114] Quantification of Be in serum or urine is not useful in making this diagnosis. Air analysis (TLV) is the preferred method of exposure evaluation.[75]

Cadmium

Cd is a byproduct of zinc and lead smelting. It is used (1) in industry in electroplating, (2) in the production of rechargeable batteries, (3) as a common pigment in organic-based paints, and (4) in tobacco products. Breathing the fumes of Cd vapors leads to nasal epithelial deterioration and pulmonary congestion resembling chronic emphysema. Spray painting of organic-based paints without the use of protective breathing apparatus is a common source of chronic exposure. Auto repair mechanics represent a work group that has significant opportunity for exposure to Cd.

The toxicity of Cd resembles that of As, Hg, and Pb in that it attacks the kidney; renal dysfunction with proteinuria of slow onset (over a period of years) is the typical presentation. Chronic exposure to Cd causes accumulated renal damage.[15,33,101] Breathing the fumes of Cd vapors leads to nasal epithelial deterioration and pulmonary congestion resembling chronic emphysema. Cadmium toxicity is expressed via formation of protein-Cd adducts that change the conformational structure of the protein, causing it to denature. This protein denaturation occurs at the site of highest concentration—in the alveoli if exposure is due to dust inhalation, and in the proximal tubule of the kidney because this is a major route of excretion.

NIOSH regulations mandate that employees exposed to Cd in the workplace must be monitored using quantification of urine Cd and creatinine, with the results in μg of Cd expressed per gram of creatinine.[95] This is based on the finding that renal damage caused by Cd exposure is detected by increased Cd excretion relative to creatinine. Cadmium excretion >3 μg Cd/g of creatinine indicates significant exposure to Cd. Results >15 μg Cd/g of creatinine are considered indicative of severe exposure. Urine Cd is a more specific measure of Cd exposure than are other markers of renal function, such as β_2-microglobulin, retinol-binding protein, and *N*-acetyl glucosaminidase.[33,95]

Normal blood Cd concentration is less than 5 ng/mL, with most concentrations in the interval of 0.5 to 2 ng/mL. Moderately increased blood Cd (3 to 7 ng/mL) may be associated with tobacco use.[61] Acute toxicity is observed when the blood concentration exceeds 50 ng/mL. Usual daily excretion of Cd is less than 3 μg/d. Collection of urine samples using a rubber catheter has been known to result in elevated results because rubber contains trace amounts of Cd that are extracted as urine passes through it. Brightly colored plastic urine collection containers should be avoided because the pigment in the plastic may be Cd-based. Cadmium concentrations also increase with age and may be involved with senescence.[9] Cadmium is usually quantified by atomic absorption spectrometry, but it has been accurately quantified by ICP-MS.[100]

Chromium

Occupational exposure to Cr represents a significant health hazard.[77,103] Chromium is used extensively (1) in the manufacture of stainless steel, (2) in chrome plating, (3) in the tanning of leather, (4) as a dye for printing and textile manufacture, (5) as a cleaning solution, and (6) as an anticorrosive in cooling systems. The toxic form of Cr is Cr^{6+} [Cr(VI)], which is rare; a strong oxidizing environment is required to convert the common form Cr^{3+} [Cr(III)] to Cr^{6+}, as might be found when Cr^{3+} is exposed to high temperatures in the presence of oxygen or during high-voltage electroplating. Inhalation of the vapors of Cr^{6+} causes erosion of the epithelium of the nasal passages and produces squamous cell carcinomas of the lung.[120] Cr^{6+} is highly lipid soluble and readily crosses cell membranes, whereas Cr^{3+} is rather insoluble and does not readily cross membranes. Clinically, monitoring biological specimens for Cr^{6+} is neither practical nor clinically useful to detect Cr toxicity, because the instant it enters a cell, it is reduced to nontoxic Cr^{3+}.[77] Instead, monitoring the air at the manufacturing site for Cr^{6+} is the usual way to test for Cr^{6+} exposure.

Quantification of total Cr in urine can be used to assess exposure to total Cr. NIOSH has proposed <30 μg chromium/g creatinine as the concentration of concern, but this concentration does not indicate that the specific exposure was to Cr^{6+}. The presence of chromium in erythrocytes is suggestive of exposure to Cr^{6+} within the past 120 days, because Cr^{6+} crosses biological membranes but Cr^{3+} does not.[25] Increased serum chromium concentrations are observed in association with orthopedic implants made from chromium alloys.[72,82] ICP-MS is the preferred technology for quantification of Cr in body fluids.

Cobalt

Co is widely distributed in the environment and is the essential cofactor in vitamin B_{12}. Quantification of active vitamin B_{12} (see Chapter 31) is the usual way to assess nutritional status; quantification of serum, blood, or urine Co concentration is not typical for assessing vitamin B_{12} status. Cobalt deficiency has not been reported in humans.

Cobalt is found in metal alloys that (1) are very hard, (2) have high melting points, and (3) are resistant to oxidation. Cobalt is not highly toxic, but large exposures will produce (1) pulmonary edema, (2) allergy, (3) nausea, (4) vomiting, (5) hemorrhage, and (6) renal failure. Occupational exposure occurs during production and machining of these metal alloys and has been known to result in interstitial lung disease. Cardiomyopathy and renal failure are symptomatic of acute Co exposure; this was exemplified by an incidence of mass population exposure to Co when beer contaminated with the metal was consumed.[124] Chronic exposure may cause (1) pulmonary syndrome, (2) skin irritation, (3) allergy, (4) gastrointestinal irritation, (5) nausea,

(6) cardiomyopathy, (7) hematologic disorders, and (8) thyroid abnormalities. Cobalt exposure alone may not lead to toxicity and must be considered within the context of exposure to multiple metals.[83] Quantification of urinary Co is an effective means of identifying individuals with excessive exposure; the National Health and Nutrition Examination Survey (NHANES/http://www.cdc.gov/nchs/nhanes.html/ accessed June 2, 2011) reported that the geometric mean of cobalt excretions in a large population was 0.54 μg/g creatinine in children and 0.34 μg/g creatinine in adults. Serum cobalt concentrations are increased above normal (>1 μg/L) in patients with orthopedic implants made from cobalt alloys.[72,82] Cobalt is quantified in biological tissues by atomic absorption spectrometry or by ICP-MS.

Copper

The homeostasis and analysis of Cu are discussed in Chapter 31. Copper ingestion has been known to cause serious toxicity,[46] and exposure may be caused by common pesticides. Copper arsenate is one of the active agents in marine antifouling paints and in the wood preservative used with green "treated" wood; copper arsenate wood products have been taken off the market in the United States because of this concern. Ingestion of copper produces severe gastrointestinal pain with erosion of the epithelial layer of the gastrointestinal tract, hemolytic anemia, centrilobular hepatitis with jaundice, and renal damage. The classical presentation of Cu toxicosis is represented by the genetic disease of Cu accumulation known as Wilson's disease.[85] This disease is typified by hepatocellular damage (increased transferases) and/or changes in mood and behavior caused by accumulation of Cu in central neurons. Evaluation of serum and urine copper concentration is useful in diagnosing Wilson's disease (see Chapter 21). Because most Cu circulating in blood is bound to ceruloplasmin, and ceruloplasmin formation is decreased in Wilson's disease, serum copper concentration is less than normal (reference interval for serum Cu, 0.7 to 1.4 μg/mL), while urinary Cu concentrations are increased to 15 to 60 μg/L in Wilson's disease. Increased hepatic Cu >2.0 (adjusted for age and reported as the hepatic iron index) is diagnostic for Wilson's disease.[85] Increased serum Cu is observed in patients prescribed estrogen. Excess Zn ingestion interferes with absorption of copper and leads to copper deficiency, which is characterized by myeloneuropathy.[123]

Gadolinium

Gd is a chemical element found in image contrast agents that are used during magnetic resonance imaging (MRI) and magnetic resonance angiography (MRA) procedures. These agents have come under scrutiny by the U.S. Food and Drug Administration (FDA) (http://www.fda.gov/ accessed June 2, 2011) because gadolinium-based contrast agent (GBCA) is thought to be involved in nephrogenic systemic fibrosis (NSF), a debilitating disorder characterized by edema, plaques, discoloration, and severe thickening of the skin, resulting in contractures and immobility. In addition to GBCA exposure, other proposed contributing factors and associations with NSF include (1) renal insufficiency, (2) pharmaceutical erythropoietin usage, (3) hypocalcemia acidosis, (4) low serum albumin concentrations, and (5) high serum ferritin concentrations.[125,130] Exposure to GBCA during a condition of low glomerular filtration rate (GFR) appears to be the most consistent risk factor.[8,29] Because GBCA is excreted by the kidney, exposure is prolonged in patients with renal insufficiency[68]; it is thought that extended exposure permits transmetallation to occur; this allows free gadolinium to come in contact with proteins and other cellular components. Although several different attempted therapies have been administered, some leading to moderate disease regression, no known cure is uniformly effective.[71] Gadolinium accumulates in tissues affected by NSF,[62] but it is not detectable in the skin of patients with normal renal function after exposure to GBCA.[12]

Iron

The homeostasis and analysis of iron (Fe) are reviewed in Chapter 32. Iron supplements are used frequently to maintain an adequate body burden of Fe. Occasionally, ingestion exceeds the needed daily requirement, resulting in Fe toxicity. For example, ingestion of more than 0.5 g of Fe has been known to produce severe irritation of the epithelial lining of the gastrointestinal tract, resulting in hemosiderosis, which may develop into hepatic cirrhosis. The presence of Fe >350 μg/dL or transferrin >125 micromole/L in serum corroborates this diagnosis.[132]

Lead

Lead (Pb) is a metal commonly found in the environment. It is an acute and a chronic toxin. Lead is present at high concentration (up to 35% w/w) in many paints manufactured before 1972. The Pb content of paints intended for household use was limited to <0.5% in 1978, but Pb is still found in paint products intended for nondomestic use and in artists' pigments. Ceramic products for use in homes available from noncommercial suppliers (e.g., local artists) have been known to contain significant amounts of Pb; lead is leached from the ceramic by weak acids such as vinegar and fruit juices. Leaded crystal contains up to 10% Pb, which is leached during long-term storage of acidic fluids such as fruit juice. Lead is also found (1) in dirt from areas adjacent to homes painted with Pb-based paints and (2) on highways, where it has accumulated from the use of leaded gasoline in automobiles. Use of leaded gasoline has diminished significantly since the introduction of unleaded gasoline, which has been required in personal automobiles in the United States since 1978. Lead is also found in soil near abandoned industrial sites where Pb may have been used. Water transported through Pb or Pb-soldered pipe contains some Pb, with higher concentrations found in water that is weakly acidic. Some foods (e.g., moonshine distilled in Pb pipes) and some traditional home medicines also contain Pb.[60] Exposure to Pb from any of these sources by ingestion, inhalation, or dermal contact has been known to cause significant toxicity.

A typical diet in the United States contributes approximately 3 μg of Pb per day, of which 1 to 10% is absorbed;

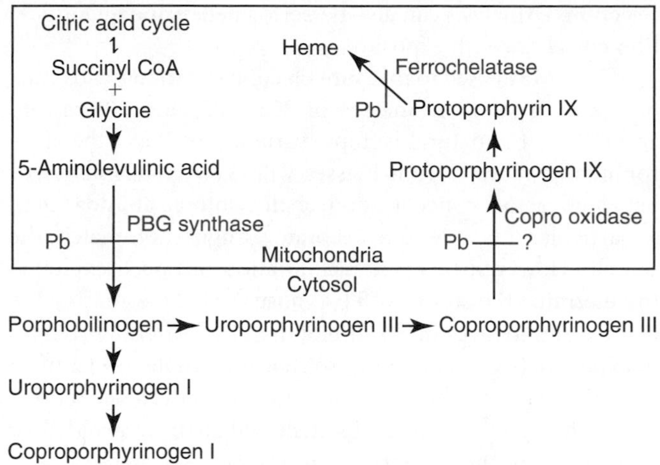

Figure 36-3 Erythropoietic effects of lead.

children may absorb as much as 50% of the dietary intake. The fraction of Pb absorbed is enhanced by nutritional deficiency. Most of the daily intake is excreted in the stool after direct passage through the gastrointestinal tract. Although a significant fraction of the absorbed Pb is rapidly incorporated into bone and erythrocytes, Pb is ultimately distributed among all tissues. Lipid-dense tissues, such as the central nervous system, are particularly sensitive to organic forms of Pb. Erythrocyte turnover of Pb occurs within approximately 120 days. Lead is ultimately excreted in bile or urine.

Lead expresses its toxicity by several mechanisms that are described graphically in Figure 36-3. It avidly inhibits amino levulinic acid dehydratase (ALAD), one of the enzymes that catalyze synthesis of heme from porphyrin. Inhibition of ALAD causes accumulation of protoporphyrin in erythrocytes (see Chapter 33), which is a significant marker for Pb exposure. Anemia caused by lack of heme is frequently observed in Pb toxicity. Lead also is an electrophile that avidly forms covalent bonds with the sulfhydryl group of cysteines in proteins. Thus proteins in all tissues exposed to Pb will have Pb bound to them. Keratin in hair contains a high fraction of cysteine relative to other amino acids and avidly binds Pb; hair analysis for Pb is a good marker for exposure. Some proteins become labile as Pb binds with them because Pb causes the tertiary structure of the protein to change; cells of the nervous system are particularly susceptible to this effect. Some Pb-bound proteins change their tertiary configuration sufficiently that they become antigenic; renal tubular cells are particularly susceptible to this effect because they are exposed to relatively high Pb concentrations during clearance.[33]

The development of Pb toxicity follows a progressive pattern. Figure 36-4 describes this progression through a series of symptoms.[19] The finding that Pb contributes significantly to decreased intellectual capability in the very young is of particular concern.[69,89] Young children are particularly prone to the effects of Pb because they have greater opportunity for exposure.[5] Children tend to spend a lot of time on the floor. In older homes that have been previously treated

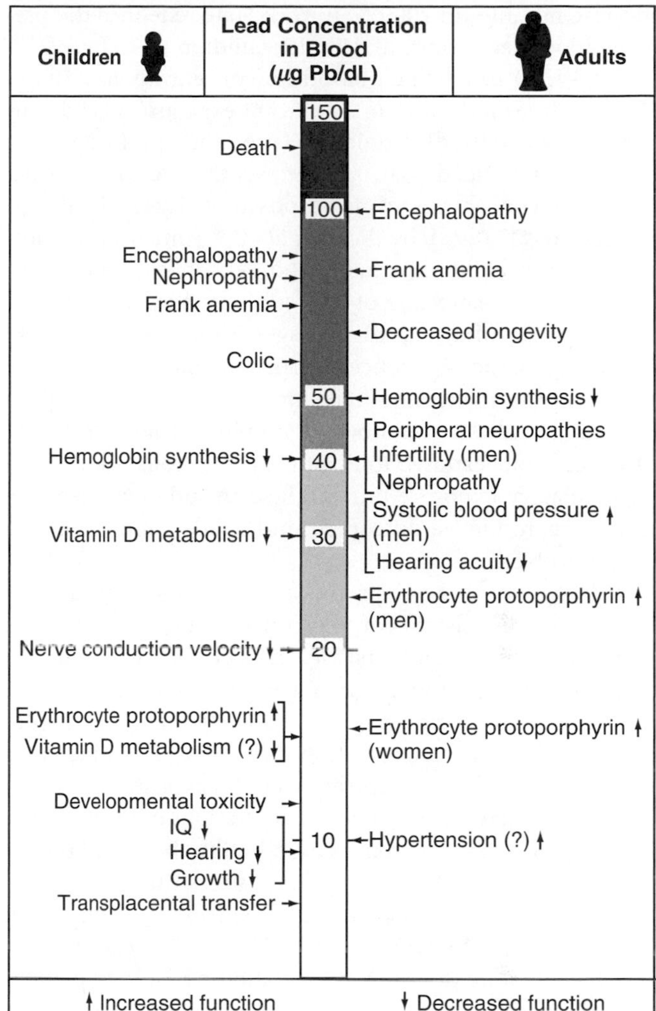

Figure 36-4 Effects of inorganic lead on children and adults (lowest observable adverse effect concentrations). *(From Royce SE, Needleman HL, eds. Case studies in environmental medicine: lead toxicity. Washington, DC: U.S. Public Health Service, ATSDR, 1990.)*

with Pb-based paints, Pb-laden paint chips and dust accumulate on the floor, which children are likely to ingest.

The definitive test for Pb toxicity is measurement of blood Pb.[113] Over the past 3 decades, studies have shown an inverse relationship between blood Pb concentrations and children's IQ at increasingly lower Pb concentrations. In response, the Centers for Disease Control and Prevention (CDC) has continued to lower the upper limit of normal for children, which is now stated at less than 10 μg/dL (http://www.cdc.gov/nceh/lead/ accessed June 2, 2011). It is important to note that the median blood Pb concentration in children fell from 15 μg/dL in 1978 to 2 μg/dL in 1999.[110] Consequently, renewed interest in determining safe blood Pb concentrations resulted in additional studies.[69,89] These studies assessed intellectual impairment in children with Pb concentrations below 10 μg/dL. Preliminary data have revealed an inverse relationship between Pb concentrations and children's IQ even at blood Pb concentrations <10 μg/dL.[17,69,89] Based on these findings, in 2009 New York State redefined the preferred blood lead concentration for children to <5 μg/dL.[102]

The WHO has defined blood Pb concentrations >30 μg/dL in adults as indicative of significant exposure.[44] Lead concentrations >60 μg/dL require chelation therapy. In 2000, the CDC recommended that, as a preventive health measure, blood Pb concentrations in exposed workers should be reduced to <25 μg/dL by the year 2010.[58] Similar to the situation seen in children, adult blood Pb concentrations have dropped to a mean value of 1.4 μg/dL for ages 20 to 49 and a mean value of 1.9 μg/dL for ages 50 to 69.[99] Given the decreasing blood Pb concentrations in adults, it may be important to revisit the recommendations regarding Pb exposure. Studies have shown a number of adverse health effects in adults exposed to Pb at concentrations below existing regulatory exposure limits. These include hypertension, adverse reproductive outcomes, and subtle central nervous system problems.[53]

Although erythrocyte protoporphyrin concentrations are not a sensitive indicator of low-concentration Pb exposure, they are definitive markers for Pb overdose. For example, an erythrocyte protoporphyrin concentration greater than 60 μg/dL is a significant indicator of Pb exposure (see Chapter 33). Serum ALAD concentrations are also a useful indicator for medium to high concentrations of Pb exposure; however, they do not correlate with low concentrations of Pb exposure. Serum Pb analysis is of very limited utility because Pb concentrations are abnormal only for a short time after exposure.[22] The National Health and Nutrition Examination Survey (NHANES) reported a median urine excretion of 3 μg/L lead or 2.4 μg lead per g creatinine in a large population.[97] Quantification of urine excretion rates before or after chelation therapy has been used as an indicator of Pb exposure.[122] Normally, the hair Pb content is lower than 5 μg/g; hair Pb concentration >5 μg/g indicates significant Pb exposure. Blood Pb concentrations have the strongest correlation with toxicity.

Avoidance of continued exposure to Pb is paramount when blood Pb concentrations exceed acceptable limits. Oral dimercaprol has become a standard therapy and is being used in the outpatient setting for all except those with the most severe Pb poisoning.[10] Although chelation therapy is effective in reducing blood Pb concentrations, a 2003 study indicated that chelation therapy given to preschool children with Pb concentrations in the range of 20 to 44 μg/dL showed no beneficial effect on tests of cognition or behavior.[110] Thus, prevention is the best therapeutic option.

Analysis of Pb is routinely performed by ICP-MS,[13] electrothermal atomic absorption spectrometry,[14] or anodic stripping voltammetry.[134] Because Pb is concentrated in the erythrocytes, ethylenediaminetetraacetic acid (EDTA) anticoagulated blood is the specimen of choice for Pb analysis. Sodium heparin may also be used; however, samples that are not analyzed within 48 hours are frequently clotted and must be rejected. Care must be taken when obtaining capillary blood. Surface contamination, insufficient collection volume, or inadequate mixing with EDTA results in frequent sample rejection. Urinalysis can also be performed; urine quantification correlates with exposure.

If ICP-MS is used to measure Pb concentrations, care must be taken to sum the masses of 206, 207, and 208 m/z to account for the natural isotopic variation of Pb in the environment. Failure to sum masses will skew results above or below the actual concentration, as the isotopic abundance of a particular mass in the calibrator might not match the sample. However, this isotopic variation has been exploited to determine the source of Pb exposure. By determining the relative abundances of Pb in blood and of potential sources of exposure (e.g., paint chips, soil), it is possible to identify a matching pattern. The exposure source with the same ratio of major Pb isotopes as the blood should then be avoided or removed from the patient's environment.

Manganese

Mn is ubiquitous in the environment and is used as (1) a binding agent in red brick, (2) an anticorrosive in most steel alloys, (3) a cleaning agent for glassware, and (4) a common pigment in paints and glazes. Humans exhibit toxicity to Mn when exposed to large quantities of dust containing the metal, which occurs in mining, ore crushing, the machining of Mn alloys, and the construction and destruction of brick. Manganese exposure during metal welding has been suggested to cause neurologic disease, but this finding was not substantiated in a large study.[116] After chronic exposure, Mn accumulates in the substantia nigra of the brain, causing a Parkinson-like neurodegenerative disorder known as manganism.[117] Manganese toxicity is also a concern in newborns and children receiving long-term parenteral nutrition.[41]

Blood or urine Mn concentrations are good indicators of exposure.[117] Adult reference values for blood Mn are 0.4 to 1.1 ng/mL (7.0 to 20.0 nmol/L) for serum or plasma and 7.7 to 12.1 ng/mL (140 to 220 nmol/L) for whole blood. Typical daily excretion of Mn in urine varies from 0.2 to 0.5 μg/d. However, approximately 5% of healthy individuals excrete up to 2 μg of the metal per day, probably because of greater than average exposure.

Most of the Mn in daily diets is not absorbed. Because Mn-containing dust is common, contamination of urine with the metal occurs easily. Trace contamination of acid preservatives used for stabilizing the urine has also been observed. Manganese is quantified by electrothermal atomization atomic absorption spectrometry and ICP-MS.

Mercury

Metallic mercury is a liquid at room temperature; its elemental symbol, Hg, is derived from the Greek word *hydrargyrias*, meaning "water silver" (http://emedicine.medscape.com/article/819872-overview/ accessed June 2, 2011). As mentioned earlier, mercury is listed as No. 3 on the 2007 CERCLA Priority List of Hazardous Substances.

Hg is widely found in the environment[81] and occurs both naturally and as the result of industrial processes, with the single largest source of Hg being its natural out-gassing from granite rock.[6] Hg is also found in deposits throughout the world, mostly as cinnabar (mercuric sulfide), which is the source of the red pigment vermilion.

In the past, Hg was extensively used in the manufacture of devices such as thermometers, barometers, manometers, and sphygmomanometers. However, concerns about its toxicity have resulted in the phasing out of Hg-based instruments, which have been replaced with alcohol-filled, digital, or thermistor-based ones. It is still used as a dental amalgam and in lighting as mercury vapor lamps, although these are being replaced by sodium vapor bulbs. Hg is used in the pulp and paper industry as a whitener, as a catalyst in the synthesis of plastics, and as a potent fungicide in antifouling and latex paints.

Mercury is essentially nontoxic in its elemental form (Hg^0). In the absence of any chemical or biological system that chemically alters Hg^0, it is possible to consume it orally with no significant side effects. However, once Hg^0 is chemically modified to the ionized, inorganic species, Hg^{2+}, it becomes toxic. Further bioconversion to an alkyl Hg, such as methyl Hg (CH_3Hg^+), yields a very toxic species of Hg that is highly selective for lipid-rich tissue, such as the neuron.[28] The relative order of toxicity is as follows:

$$Hg^0 <<<< Hg^{2+} << \text{Monomethyl-Hg}\,(CH_3Hg^+)\text{ or Dimethyl-Hg}\,[(CH_3)_2Hg]$$

Chemically, it is possible to convert Hg from its elemental state to its ionized state; in industry, this is frequently accomplished by exposing Hg^0 to a strong oxidant, such as chlorine. Elemental Hg is also bioconverted to both Hg^{2+} and alkyl Hg by microorganisms that exist both in the normal human gut and in the bottom sediment of lakes and rivers. When Hg^0 enters bottom sediment, it is absorbed by bacteria, fungi, and related microorganisms; these organisms metabolically convert it to Hg^{2+}, CH_3Hg^1, $(CH_3)_2Hg$, and similar species. Consequently, the methyl mercurials are accumulated in the aquatic food chain and reach their highest concentrations in predatory fish.[20,27]

As a consequence of accumulation of methylmercury in the aquatic food chain, most human exposure to mercury happens through the eating of contaminated fish, shellfish, and sea mammals. In adults, cases of methylmercury poisoning are characterized by the focal degeneration of neurons in regions of the brain such as the cerebral cortex and the cerebellum. Depending on the degree of in utero exposure, methylmercury may result in effects ranging from fetal death to subtle neurodevelopmental delays. Consequently, because pregnant women, women of childbearing age, and young children are particularly at risk, the FDA recommends that they avoid eating shark, swordfish, mackerel, and tilefish (http://www.fda.gov/food/foodsafety/product-specificinformation/seafood/foodbornepathogens contaminants/methylmercury/ucm115662.html/ accessed June 2, 2011.[43] Mercury toxicity is expressed in three ways. First, Hg^{2+} avidly reacts with sulfhydryl groups of protein, causing a change in the tertiary structure of the protein with subsequent loss of the biological activity associated with that protein; because Hg^{2+} becomes concentrated in the kidney during regular clearance processes, this is the target organ that experiences the greatest toxicity. Second, with the tertiary change noted previously, some proteins become immunogenic, eliciting a proliferation of β-lymphocytes that generate immunoglobulins to bind the new antigen (collagen tissues are particularly sensitive to this). Third, alkyl Hg species, such as methylmercury, are particularly lipophilic and avidly bind to proteins in lipid-rich tissue, such as neurons; myelin is particularly susceptible to disruption by this mechanism.[27] Mercury has also been found to alter porphyrin excretion patterns.[131]

Experience with Hg poisoning has been gained from investigation of the 1951 to 1963 industrial dumping of Hg-laden waste sludge into Minamata Bay, Japan. Fish in Minamata Bay became heavily laden with Hg through the food chain. The local human population, whose diet was dependent on fish from the bay, exhibited symptoms of methylmercury poisoning, which include (1) ataxia, (2) impaired speech, (3) visual field constriction, (4) hearing loss, and (5) somatosensory change, characterized histologically by cerebral cortex necrosis. Collectively, these symptoms have become known as Minamata disease.[42]

In the late 1980s, the public became concerned about exposure to Hg from dental amalgams.[81,109] However, later studies have failed to confirm a causal relationship.[4,56] Basic to the initial concerns was the fact that restorative dentistry used an Hg-silver amalgam for approximately 90 years as a filling material. In 1989, Hahn showed that a small (2 to 20 μg/d) release of Hg^0 from amalgam occurs when it is mechanically manipulated, such as by chewing.[54] The normal bacterial flora present in the mouth converts a fraction of Hg^{2+} to CH_3Hg^+; the latter has been shown to be incorporated into body tissue. In addition, the habit of gum chewing can cause release of Hg from dental amalgams at concentrations greatly above normal. Hanson noted in 1991 the release of up to 100 μg/d of Hg in several human subjects who had the typical placement of dental amalgams (weighing approximately 800 mg each) after chewing gum for 8 hours.[57] In 2010, the FDA issued rules that classify dental amalgam, reclassify dental mercury, and specify special controls for dental amalgam, mercury, and amalgam alloy (21 CFR Part 872/http://www.fda.gov/ accessed June 2, 2011).

Concerns have been raised about the possible relationship between Hg exposure from vaccines and autistic disorders. In the United States, the prevalence of autism has risen from 1 in approximately 2500 in the mid-1980s to 1 in approximately 300 children in the mid-1990s.[50,108A] Some investigators believe that this rise occurs because of the Hg that is present in vaccines as the preservative thimerosal (sodium ethyl mercury thiosulfate).[7,32,50] However, this causality has been questioned by numerous other studies, which have not been able to confirm this relationship.[118] In 2001, the Committee on Immunization Safety Review of the Board on Health Promotion and Disease Prevention of the Institute of Medicine[127] initiated a study to review the connection between Hg-containing vaccines and neurodevelopmental disorders, including autism. The Committee has issued several reports; in its eighth and final report, put forth in 2004, the Committee reported that the hypothesis was biologically plausible, but that evidence was insufficient to accept or reject a causal connection. At that time, the Committee recommended a comprehensive research program.[127] The findings of this report have been challenged,[51] and thimerosal has been removed from most vaccines in the United States.

The reader should note that the issue of linking Hg exposure from vaccines with autistic disorders became highly controversial and resulted in the Journal Lancet retracting the article linking autism to MMR (Measles, Mumps, and Rubella) vaccines.[38A,39A,104A] However, the senior author involved with this publication has challenged this retraction.[38B]

Dietary sources also contribute to Hg body burden, as many foods contain Hg. For example, commercially distributed fish considered safe for consumption contain less than 0.3 μg/g, but some game fish contain more than 2 μg/g and, if consumed on a regular basis, contribute to significant body Hg loads.

Of note is the fact that Hg compounds have been used for therapeutic reasons. For example, Hg has been used (1) in medications that were touted as cures for syphilis and dysentery, (2) to treat constipation, and (3) as diuretics.

Analysis of blood, urine, and hair for Hg concentrations is used to determine exposure. The quantity of Hg found in blood and urine correlates with the degree of toxicity, and hair analysis has been used historically to document the time of peak exposure. However, it should be noted that hair analysis for metals in general is difficult because of contamination. Normal whole blood Hg concentration is usually lower than 10 μg/L. Individuals who have mild occupational exposure (e.g., dentists) may routinely have whole blood Hg concentrations up to 15 μg/L.[39] Significant exposure is indicated when the whole blood Hg concentration is greater than 50 μg/L (if exposure is to methylmercury) or greater than 200 μg/L (if exposure is to Hg^{2+}). The WHO safety standard for daily exposure of Hg is 45 μg/d; daily urine excretion exceeding 50 μg/d indicates significant exposure. Normally, hair contains less than 1 μg/g of Hg; greater amounts indicate increased exposure. Treatment with BAL or penicillamine will mobilize Hg, allowing for its excretion in the urine. Therapy is usually monitored by following urinary excretion of Hg; therapy may be terminated after the daily urine excretion rate falls below 50 μg/L.

Nickel

Ni is frequently used (1) in the production of metal alloys (which are popular for their anticorrosive and hardness properties), (2) in Ni-based rechargeable batteries, and (3) as a catalyst in the hydrogenation of oils. Nickel alloyed with transition metals is considered nontoxic, except that it will induce inflammation at the point of contact. Nickel oxides and sulfides and aqueous solution of Ni in the oxidation state of 1^+, 2^+, or 3^+ are considered group I carcinogens.[47,129] If Ni is essential for life, it is only so at very low concentrations, below the detection limit of most analytical techniques (see Chapter 31). Nickel carbonyl [$Ni(CO)_4$], used in petroleum refining, is one of the most toxic chemicals known to humans[3] as it is absorbed after inhalation, readily crosses all biological membranes, and noncompetitively inhibits ATPase and RNA polymerase. Patients exposed to Ni carbonyl exhibit rapid onset of pulmonary congestion and inability to oxygenate hemoglobin, followed by development of lesions of the lung, liver, kidney, adrenal glands, and spleen.[70]

Patients undergoing dialysis are exposed to Ni and accumulate Ni in blood and other organs. No adverse health effects have been associated with this exposure. Nickel is quantified by AA-ETA or ICP-MS.

Platinum

A variety of Pt-containing antineoplastic agents are used in chemotherapy, typified by cisplatin (*cis*-dichlorodiammineplatinum dihydrate).[38,128] All of these compounds have some nephrotoxicity that is related to the concentration of Pt circulating in the blood.[79] Although it is not common to measure Pt concentrations in all patients receiving cisplatin therapy, quantification of Pt concentrations in patients with reduced renal function helps to identify whether Pt is the cause of the compromised renal function. Peak serum concentrations greater than 1 μg/mL but less than 1.5 μg/mL correlate with little nephrotoxicity and good therapeutic response.[48] Both AA-ETA and ICP-MS are used to measure Pt.

Selenium

Se is an essential element (see Chapter 31) and may play a role in mitigating biological damage caused by oxidative damage.[64,105] It is a cofactor required to maintain glutathione peroxidase activity, an enzyme that catalyzes the degradation of organic hydroperoxides. Absence of Se correlates with loss of glutathione peroxidase activity and is associated with damage to cell membranes caused by the accumulation of free radicals. In a situation of Se deficiency associated with loss of glutathione peroxidase activity, the serum concentration is less than 40 ng/mL.[121]

In humans, cardiac muscle is the tissue most susceptible to Se deficiency; with cell membrane damage, normal cells are replaced with fibroblasts.[23] This condition, known as *cardiomyopathy*, is characterized by an enlarged heart consisting of predominantly nonfunctioning fibrotic tissue.

The geographic source of plant and animal foodstuffs determines the amount of dietary intake. In the United States and Canada, wheat and other cereal products are a good source of selenium; average intakes in North America range from 80 to 220 μg Se/d, whereas in the United Kingdom, dietary intake is about 30 to 60 μg/d. Intakes in China are as low as 11 μg/d, and in New Zealand 28 μg/d (see Chapter 31). Symptoms of selenium toxicity vary among individuals and are dependent on a number of factors such as the dose, type, and form of selenium ingested, and the length of time the product was used. Symptoms of selenium poisoning include significant hair loss, muscle cramps, nausea, vomiting, diarrhea, joint pain, fatigue, fingernail changes, and blistering skin. The tolerable upper limit has been set at 400 μg/d for adults and less for children.[133]

Selenium deficiency among people who consume food only from a particular region has been related to the low soil content of the metal in that region; the soil of the Keshan region of China is noted for this characteristic.[133] Children living in the Keshan region who receive no Se supplement develop cardiomyopathy. Deficiency is also related to use of total parenteral nutrition, which is administered to patients who have no functional bowel (e.g., those who have undergone surgical removal of the small and large intestines because of cancer) or who have acute inflammatory bowel disease, such as Crohn's disease (see Chapter 51). Selenium supplementation to raise serum concentration to above 90 ng/mL is the usual practice in these patients, and serum monitoring is performed on a semiannual basis to ensure the adequacy of supplementation.

Selenium toxicity has been observed in animals when daily intake exceeds 400 μg/d.[133] Teratogenic effects are frequently noted in the offspring of animals living in regions where Se soil content is high, such as in south central South Dakota and the northern coastal regions of California. Selenium toxicity in humans is not known to be a significant problem except in acute overdose cases, and Se is not classified as a human teratogen. Selenium is found in many over-the-counter vitamin preparations because its antioxidant activity is thought to be anticarcinogenic.

Selenium is quantified by ICP-MS or by atomic absorption spectrometry after the specimen has been mixed with matrix modifier.

Silicon

Si is the most abundant element in the earth's environment; it constitutes 26% of the earth's crust. From the toxicologic viewpoint, several forms of Si are of interest, including asbestos (amorphous oxides of Si) and methylated polymers of Si (e.g., silicone).

Inhalation of asbestos-containing dust leads to deposition of asbestos fibers in the pulmonary alveoli.[96,106] These fibers are needle-shaped spicules approximately 150 micrometer in length and up to 15 micrometer in diameter. When these fibers are inhaled, they deposit in the alveoli, where they are surrounded by macrophages and become coated with protein and mucopolysaccharide to form "asbestos bodies." The diagnosis of asbestosis is made by interpretation of a chest x-ray by a qualified radiologist, demonstration of asbestos in sputum, and documentation of asbestos bodies in a lung biopsy by electron microscopy.[111] Direct analysis of lung tissue for Si is not useful because all lung tissue is infiltrated with Si, most of which is not asbestos. Thus, direct analysis for Si cannot distinguish asbestosis from normal background Si.

Methylated polymers of Si (silicone) are used in breast implants. Concern as to the safety of such devices has been a subject of debate. A recent Medscape report states, "A great deal of recent safety research combined with more than 40 years of clinical experience has proven the value and relative safety of breast implants. To date, no convincing evidence exists of any systemic disorder that can be attributed to silicone" (http://emedicine.medscape.com/article/1275451-overview/ accessed June 2, 2011).[96A]

Silver

Clinical interest in Ag analysis is limited to two applications: (1) monitoring burn patients treated with Ag sulfadiazine, and (2) monitoring patients treated with Ag-containing nasal decongestants. In both cases, Ag deposits in many organs, including the subepithelium of the skin and mucous membranes, producing a syndrome called *argyria* (graying of the skin). Argyria is associated with (1) growth retardation, (2) hemopoiesis, (3) cardiac enlargement, (4) degeneration of the liver, and (5) destruction of renal tubules. The customary concentration of serum Ag is less than 2 ng/mL. Typical Ag concentrations observed in serum of unaffected patients during treatment range up to 300 ng/mL, and their urine output has been found to be as high as 550 μg/d.[78]

Thallium

Tl is a byproduct of lead smelting. Interest in Tl derives primarily from its former use as a rodenticide; accidental exposure represents the most likely source of exposure. Additionally, environmental concerns are growing because thallium is a waste product of coal combustion and the manufacturing of cement. Thallium is rapidly absorbed via ingestion, inhalation, and skin contact. It is considered to be as toxic as lead and mercury and has similar sites of action. The mechanism of Tl toxicity consists of (1) competition with potassium at cell receptors to affect ion pumps, (2) inhibition of DNA synthesis, (3) binding to sulfhydryl groups on proteins in neural axons, and (4) concentration in renal tubular cells to cause necrosis. Patients exposed to high doses of Tl (>1 g) demonstrate alopecia (hair loss), peripheral neuropathy and seizures, and renal failure. Typical serum concentrations are less than 10 ng/mL, and daily urine excretion is less than 10 μg/d. Exposed patients have been observed to have serum concentrations as high as 50 μg/mL, with urine output in excess of 500 μg/d.[65]

Titanium

Ti is the ninth most abundant element in the earth's crust. No evidence indicates that titanium is an essential element (see Chapter 31). In part because of the formation propensity of titanium oxide, the element is considered to be nontoxic. Average daily oral intake through food consumption is 0.1 to 1 mg/d, which accounts for more than 99% of exposure. Gastrointestinal absorption of titanium is low (approximately 3%), and most ingested titanium is rapidly excreted in the urine and stool. The total body burden of titanium is usually in the range of 9 to 15 mg, a significant portion of which is contained in the lung. Titanium dust entering the respiratory tract is nonirritating and is almost completely nonfibrogenic in humans.[66]

Titanium-containing alloys are used in artificial joints, prosthetic devices, and implants. Titanium dioxide allows osseointegration between an artificial medical implant and bone. Despite their wide use, exposure to these materials has not been linked to toxicity. However, as implant wear occurs, a significant increase in detectable serum titanium becomes evident. Although titanium concentrations are not a measure of toxicity, they are useful in determining whether implant breakdown is occurring.[84] Serum titanium <1.0 ng/mL suggests that a prosthetic device is in good condition. Serum concentrations >3 ng/mL in a patient with a titanium-based implant suggest prosthesis wear. An increased serum titanium concentration in the absence of corroborating clinical information does not independently predict prosthesis wear or failure.

Vanadium

V is naturally found in minerals and rocks and is considered an essential element for mammals (see Chapter 31), although conclusive evidence for humans is lacking. V is recovered from minerals or is derived as a byproduct of iron, titanium, and uranium refining. Vanadium compounds are used in dyes, photography, and ceramics, and in the production of special glasses. V is also a component of many fiber mesh prosthetic devices.

The main source of V intake for the general population is food, with an estimated daily intake of 20 μg, of which most is not absorbed and excreted in the feces. Absorption through the inhalation route results in more effective uptake. The clearance half-life is not well documented, but it appears to be on the order of several days. V has been recognized as an occupational hazard for many years. Elevated atmospheric V concentration can result from burning fossil fuels with a high V content. Inhalation and ingestion are the primary exposure routes. V exposure can result in a metallic taste and so-called "green tongue." Sensitization has been known to result in asthma or eczema.

Because the kidney is primarily responsible for V elimination, increased serum concentrations are observed in dialysis patients and those with compromised renal function. Serum V values <1.0 ng/mL are typical; values >5.0 ng/mL indicate probable exposure. Elevated serum V concentrations have been observed in patients with joint replacement; concentrations are likely to be increased above the reference interval in patients with metallic joint prosthesis.[84] A modest increase (1 to 2 ng/mL) in serum V concentration is likely to be associated with a prosthetic device in good condition. Serum concentrations >5 ng/mL in a patient with a vanadium-based implant suggests significant prosthesis wear. Increased serum trace element concentrations in the absence of corroborating clinical information do not independently predict prosthesis wear.

REFERENCES

1. Alfrey A, Mitchell J, Burks J. Syndrome of dyspraxia and multifocal seizures associated with chronic hemodialysis. Trans Am Soc Artif Intern Organs 1972;18:257-61.
2. Agency for Toxic Substances and Disease Registry (ATSDR) documents. Available at: http://www.atsdr.cdc.gov/toxpro2.html/ accessed June 2, 2011.
3. Barcelous DB. Nickel. J Toxicol Clin Toxicol 1999;37:239-58.
4. Bates MN, Fawcett J, Garrett N, Cutress T, Kjellstrom T. Health effects of dental amalgam exposure: a retrospective cohort study. Int J Epidemiol 2004;33:894-902.
5. Bellinger DC. Lead. Pediatrics 2004;113:1016-22.
6. Berlin M, Zalups R, Fowler B. Mercury. Amsterdam: Academic Press, 2007:675-729.
7. Bernard S, Enayati A, Roger H, Binstock T, Redwood L. The role of mercury in the pathogenesis of autism. Mol Psychiatry 2002;7(Suppl 2):S42-3.
8. Bhave G, Lewis JB, Chang SS. Association of gadolinium based magnetic resonance imaging contrast agents and nephrogenic systemic fibrosis. J Urol 2008;180:830-5; discussion 835.
9. Bin QH, Garfinkel D. The cadmium toxicity hypothesis of aging: a possible explanation for the zinc deficiency hypothesis of aging. Med Hypotheses 1994;42:380-4.
10. Blanusa M, Varnai VM, Piasek M, Kostial K. Chelators as antidotes of metal toxicity: therapeutic and experimental aspects. Curr Med Chem 2005;12:2771-94.
11. Boffetta P, Nyberg F. Contribution of environmental factors to cancer risk. Br Med Bull 2003;68:71-94.

11A. Bondy SC. The neurotoxicity of environmental aluminum is still an issue. Neurotoxicology. 2010 Sep;31(5):575-81.

12. Boyd AS, Zic JA, Abraham JL. Gadolinium deposition in nephrogenic fibrosing dermopathy. J Am Acad Dermatol 2007;56:27-30.
13. Burritt M, Butz J. Modified from Forrer R, Gutaschi K, Lutz H. Simultaneous measurement of trace element A1, As, B, Be, Cd, Co, Cu, Fe, Li, Mn, Mo, Ni, Rb, Se, Sr. and Zn in human serum and their reference ranges by ICP-MS. Biol Trace Elem Res 2001;80:77-93.
14. Butcher D. Advances in electrothermal atomization atomic absorption spectrometry: instrumentation, methods, and application. Applied Spectroscopy Reviews 2006;41:15-34.
15. Occupational Safety and Health Administration. Cadmium-OSHA. Available at: http://www.osha.gov/SLTC/cadmium/evaluation.html/ accessed June 2, 2011.
16. Caldwell KL, Jones RL, Verdon CP, Jarrett JM, Caudill SP, Osterloh JD. Levels of urinary total and speciated arsenic in the US population: National Health and Nutrition Examination Survey 2003-2004. J Exp Sci Environ Epidemiol 2009;19:59-68.
17. Canfield RL, Henderson CR Jr, Cory-Slechta DA, Cox C, Jusko TA, Lanphear BP. Intellectual impairment in children with blood lead concentrations below 10 microg per deciliter. N Engl J Med 2003; 348:1517-26.
18. Carrio J, de Colmenares M, Riera C, Gallego M, Arboix M, Portus M. *Leishmania infantum:* stage-specific activity of pentavalent antimony related with the assay conditions. Exp Parasitol 2000;95:209-14.
19. Case studies in environmental medicine: lead toxicity. Washington, DC: U.S. Public Health Service, ATSDR, 2010 (http://www.atsdr.cdc.gov/csem/lead/accessed June 29, 2011).
20. Castoldi AF, Coccini T, Manzo L. Neurotoxic and molecular effects of methylmercury in humans. Rev Environ Health 2003;18:19-31.
21. Comprehensive Environmental Response, Compensation, and Liability Act/CERCLA 2007. Available at: http://www.atsdr.cdc.gov/cercla/07list.html/accessed June 2, 2011.
22. Chalevelakis G, Bouronikou H, Yalouris AG, Economopoulos T, Athanaselis S, Raptis S. Delta-aminolaevulinic acid dehydratase as an index of lead toxicity: time for a reappraisal? Eur J Clin Invest 1995; 25:53-8.
23. Chariot P, Bignani O. Skeletal muscle disorders associated with selenium deficiency in humans. Muscle Nerve 2003;27:662-8.
24. Chiou HY, Hsueh YM, Liaw KF, Horng SF, Chiang MH, Pu YS, et al. Incidence of internal cancers and ingested inorganic arsenic: a seven-year follow-up study in Taiwan. Cancer Res 1995;55:1296-300.
25. National Institute for Occupational Safety and Health. Chromium-NIOSH. Available at: http://www.cdc.gov/niosh/review/public/144/default.html/accessed June 2, 2011.
26. Occupational Safety and Health Administration. Chromium-OSHA. Available at: http://www/cdc.gov.nisoh/review/public/144/default.html/accessed June 2, 2011.

27. Clarkson TW, Magos L, Myers GJ. The toxicology of mercury—current exposures and clinical manifestations. N Engl J Med 2003;349:1731-7.
28. Costa LG, Aschner M, Vitalone A, Syversen T, Soldin OP. Developmental neuropathology of environmental agents. Annu Rev Pharmacol Toxicol 2004;44:87-110.
29. Cowper SE, Robin HS, Steinberg SM, Su LD, Gupta S, LeBoit PE. Scleromyxoedema-like cutaneous diseases in renal-dialysis patients. Lancet 2000;356:1000-1.
30. Criteria Group for Occupational Standards. Scientific basis for Swedish occupational standards XXI: consensus for antimony compounds. In: Halsa AO, ed. University of Gothenburg, Gothenburg, Sweden, XXX. 2000:1-14.
31. D'Haese PC, Couttenye MM, Goodman WG, Lemoniatou E, Digenis P, Sotornik I, et al. Use of the low-dose desferrioxamine test to diagnose and differentiate between patients with aluminium-related bone disease, increased risk for aluminium toxicity, or aluminium overload. Nephrol Dial Transplant 1995;10:1874-84.
32. Davidson PW, Myers GJ, Weiss B. Mercury exposure and child development outcomes. Pediatrics 2004;113:1023-9.
33. de Burbure C, Buchet J-P, Leroyer A. Renal and neurological effects of cadmium, lead, mercury, and arsenic in children: evidence of early effects and multiple interactions at environmental exposure levels. Environ Health Perspect 2006;114:584-90.
34. Deubner DC, Goodman M, Iannuzzi J. Variability, predictive value, and uses of the beryllium blood lymphocyte proliferation test (BLPT): preliminary analysis of the ongoing workforce survey. Appl Occup Environ Hyg 2001;16:521-6.
35. Dickerson O. Antimony, arsenic and their compounds, 3rd edition. St Louis, Mo: Mosby-Year Book, 1994:466-73.
36. Documentation of the 2011 threshold limit values and biological exposure indices www.acgih.org/store/accessed June 2, 2011.
37. Domingo JL. Reproductive and developmental toxicity of aluminum: a review. Neurotoxicol Teratol 1995;17:515-21.
38. Dubey S, Schiller JH. Chemotherapy for advanced non-small cell lung cancer. Hematol Oncol Clin North Am 2004;18:101-14.
38A. Dyer C. Wakefield was dishonest and irresponsible over MMR research, says GMC. BMJ 2010 Jan 29;340:c593. doi: 10.1136/bmj.c593.
38B. Dyer O. Wakefield tells GMC he was motivated by concern for autistic children. BMJ 2008 Apr 5;336(7647):738.
39. Echeverria D, Heyer NJ, Martin MD, Naleway CA, Woods JS, Bittner AC Jr. Behavioral effects of low-level exposure to elemental Hg among dentists. Neurotoxicol Teratol 1995;17:161-8.
39A. Eggertson L. Lancet retracts 12-year-old article linking autism to MMR vaccines. CMAJ. 2010 Mar 9;182(4):E199-200. Epub 2010 Feb 8.
40. Eknoyan G, Levin A, Levin N. Clinical practice guidelines for bone metabolism and disease in chronic kidney disease. Am J Kid Dis 2003;42:S7-201.
41. Erikson KM, Thompson K, Aschner J, Aschner M. Manganese neurotoxicity: a focus on the neonate. Pharmacol Ther 2007;113: 369-77.
42. Eto K. Minamata disease. Neuropathology 2000;20(Suppl):S14-9.
43. Evans EC. The FDA recommendations on fish intake during pregnancy. J Obstet Gynecol Neonatal Nurs 2002;31:715-20.
44. Fewtrell LJ, Pruss-Ustun A, Landrigan P, Ayuso-Mateos JL. Estimating the global burden of disease of mild mental retardation and cardiovascular diseases from environmental lead exposure. Environ Res 2004;94:120-33.
45. Fowler B, Chou C-H, Jones R, Chen C-J. Arsenic. Amsterdam: Academic Press, 2007:367-406.
46. Gaetke LM, Chow CK. Copper toxicity, oxidative stress, and antioxidant nutrients. Toxicology 2003;189:147-63.
47. Galanis A, Karapetsas A, Sandaltzopoulos R. Metal-induced carcinogenesis, oxidative stress and hypoxia signalling. Mutat Res 2009;674:31-5.
48. Gamelin E, Allain P, Maillart P, Turcant A, Delva R, Lortholary A. Long-term pharmacokinetic behavior of platinum after cisplatin administration. Cancer Chemother Pharmacol 1995;37:97-102.
49. Garcia-Vargas GG, Hernandez-Zavala A. Urinary porphyrins and heme biosynthetic enzyme activities measured by HPLC in arsenic toxicity. Biomed Chromatogr 1996;10:278-84.
50. Geier DA, Geier MR. An assessment of the impact of thimerosal on childhood neurodevelopmental disorders. Pediatr Rehabil 2003;6: 97-102.
51. Geier DA, Sykes LK, Geier MR. A review of thimerosal (Merthiolate) and its ethylmercury breakdown product: specific historical considerations regarding safety and effectiveness. J Toxicol Environ Health B Crit Rev 2007;10:575-96.
52. Goldhaber S. Trace element risk assessment: essentiality vs. toxicity. Regul Toxicol Pharmacol 2003;38:232-42.
53. Hage FG, Venkataraman R, Zoghbi GJ, Perry GJ, DeMattos AM, Iskandrian AE. The scope of coronary heart disease in patients with chronic kidney disease. J Am Coll Cardiol 2009;53:2129-40.
54. Hahn LJ, Kloiber R, Vimy MJ, Takahashi Y, Lorscheider FL. Dental "silver" tooth fillings: a source of mercury exposure revealed by whole-body image scan and tissue analysis. FASEB J 1989;3:2641-6.
55. Hall M, Chen Y, Ahsan H, Slavkovich V, van Geen A, Parvez F, Graziano J. Blood arsenic as a biomarker of arsenic exposure: results from a prospective study. Toxicology 2006;225:225-33.
56. Hansen G, Victor R, Engeldinger E, Schweitzer C. Evaluation of the mercury exposure of dental amalgam patients by the Mercury Triple Test. Occup Environ Med 2004;61:535-40.
57. Hanson M, Pleva J. The dental amalgam issue: a review. Experientia 1991;47:9-22.
58. Healthy People 2010. Understanding and improving health. XXX, Washington, DC: U.S. Department of Health and Human Services, 2000 (http://web.health.gov/healthypeople/document/accessed June 2, 2011).
59. Heinrich-Ramm R, Mindt-Prufert S, Szadkowski D. Arsenic species excretion after controlled seafood consumption. J Chromatogr B Analyt Technol Biomed Life Sci 2002;778:263-73.
60. Herbal Product Warning. Available at: http://www.nyc.gov/html/doh/downloads/pdf/lead/lead-herbalmed.pdf/ accessed June 2, 2011
61. Hertz-Picciotto I, Hu SW. Contribution of cadmium in cigarettes to lung cancer: an evaluation of risk assessment methodologies. Arch Environ Health 1994;49:297-302.
62. High WA, Ayers RA, Cowper SE. Gadolinium is quantifiable within the tissue of patients with nephrogenic systemic fibrosis. J Am Acad Dermatol 2007;56:710-2.
63. Hindmarsh JT, McCurdy RF. Clinical and environmental aspects of arsenic toxicity. Crit Rev Clin Lab Sci 1986;23:315-47.
64. Hoberg J, Alexander J. Selenium. In: Nordberg G, Bowler B, Nordberg M, Friberg L, eds. Handbook on the toxicology of metals. Amsterdam: Academic Press, 2007:783-807.
65. Ibrahim D, Froberg B, Wolf A, Rusyniak DE. Heavy metal poisoning: clinical presentations and pathophysiology. Clin Lab Med 2006;26:67-97, viii.
66. Jacobs J, Skipor A, Patterson L, Hallab N, Paprosky W, Black J, et al. Metal release in patients who have a primary total hip arthroplasty. J Bone Joint Surg Am 1998;80:1447-58.
67. Jakubowski M, Palczynski C. Beryllium. In: Nordberg G, Bowler B, Nordberg M, Friberg L, eds. Handbook on the toxicology of metals. Amsterdam: Academic Press, 2007:415-31.
68. Joffe P, Thomsen HS, Meusel M. Pharmacokinetics of gadodiamide injection in patients with severe renal insufficiency and patients undergoing hemodialysis or continuous ambulatory peritoneal dialysis. Acad Radiol 1998;5:491-502.
69. Jusko TA, Henderson CR, Lanphear BP, Cory-Slechta DA, Parsons PJ, Canfield RL. Blood lead concentrations <10 microg/dL and child intelligence at 6 years of age. Environ Health Perspect 2008;116:243-8.
70. Kasprzak KS, Sunderman FW Jr, Salnikow K. Nickel carcinogenesis. Mutat Res 2003;533:67-97.
71. Kay J, Bazari H, Avery LL, Koreishi AF. Case records of the Massachusetts General Hospital. Case 6-2008: a 46-year-old woman with renal failure and stiffness of the joints and skin. N Engl J Med 2008;358:827-38.

72. Keegan GM, Learmonth ID, Case CP. A systematic comparison of the actual, potential, and theoretical health effects of cobalt and chromium exposures from industry and surgical implants. Crit Rev Toxicol 2008;38:645-74.
73. Kesserling J. Arsenic and old lace: a comedy. New York: Random House Inc, 1941.
74. Kolanz M, Madl A, Kelsh M, Kent M, Kalmes R, Paustenbach D. A comparison and critique of historical and current exposure assessment method for beryllium: implications for evaluating risk of chronic beryllium disease. Appl Occup Environ Hyg 2001;6: 593-614.
75. Kreiss K, Day GA, Schuler CR. Beryllium: a modern industrial hazard. Annu Rev Public Health 2007;28:259-77.
76. Kumar N, Moyer T. Neurotoxic metals. In: Noseworthy JH, ed. Neurological therapeutics: principles and practice, vol 2. Abingdon: Informa Healthcare, 2006:1716-35.
77. Langard S, Costa M. Chromium. In: Nordberg G, Bowler B, Nordberg M, Friberg L, eds. Handbook on the toxicology of metals. Amsterdam: Academic Press, 2007:487-510.
78. Lansdown AB. Critical observations on the neurotoxicity of silver. Crit Rev Toxicol 2007;37:237-50.
79. Launay-Vacher V, Rey JB, Isnard-Bagnis C, Deray G, Daouphars M. Prevention of cisplatin nephrotoxicity: state of the art and recommendations from the European Society of Clinical Pharmacy Special Interest Group on Cancer Care. Cancer Chemother Pharmacol 2008;61:903-9.
80. Occupational Safety and Health Administration. Lead-OSHA. Available at: http://www.osha.gov/pls/oshaweb/owadisp.show_document?p_table=STANDARDS&p_id=10030/accessed June 2, 2011.
81. Lee R, Middleton D, Caldwell K, Dearwent S, Jones S, Lewis B, et al. A review of events that expose children to elemental mercury in the United States. Environ Health Perspect 2009;117:871-8.
82. Lhotka C, Szekeres T, Steffan I, Zhuber K, Zweymuller K. Four-year study of cobalt and chromium blood levels in patients managed with two different metal-on-metal total hip replacements. J Orthop Res 2003;21:189-95.
83. Lison D. Cobalt. In: Nordberg G, Bowler B, Nordberg M, Friberg L, eds. Handbook on the toxicology of metals. Amsterdam: Academic Press, 2007:511-28.
84. Liu TK, Liu SH, Chang CH, Yang RS. Concentration of metal elements in the blood and urine in the patients with cementless total knee arthroplasty. Tohoku J Exp Med 1998;185:253-62.
85. Ludwig J, Moyer TP, Rakela J. The liver biopsy diagnosis of Wilson's disease: methods in pathology. Am J Clin Pathol 1994;102:443-6.
86. Maier LA. Beryllium health effects in the era of the beryllium lymphocyte proliferation test. Appl Occup Environ Hyg 2001;16: 514-20.
87. McCarthy JT, Milliner DS, Kurtz SB, Johnson WJ, Moyer TP. Interpretation of serum aluminum values in dialysis patients. Am J Clin Pathol 1986;86:629-36.
88. Michalke B. Element speciation definitions, analytical methodology, and some examples. Ecotoxicol Environ Saf 2003;56:122-39.
89. Miranda ML, Kim D, Galeano MA, Paul CJ, Hull AP, Morgan SP. The relationship between early childhood blood lead levels and performance on end-of-grade tests. Environ Health Perspect 2007;115: 1242-7.
90. Miu AC, Benga O. Aluminum and Alzheimer's disease: a new look. J Alzheimers Dis 2006;10:179-201.
91. Moe S, Drueke T, Cunningham J, Goodman W, Martin K, Olgaard K, et al. Definition, evaluation, and classification of renal osteodystrophy: a position statement from Kidney Disease: Improving Global Outcomes (KDIGO). Kidney Int 2006;69:1945-53.
92. Moyer T, Burritt M, Butz J. Toxic metals. In: Burtis C, Ashwood E, Bruns D, eds. Tietz fundamentals of clinical chemistry. St Louis, Mo: Saunders Elsevier, 2008:603-13.
93. Moyer TP. Testing for arsenic. Mayo Clin Proc 1993;68:1210-1.
94. Moyer TP, Mussmann GV, Nixon DE. Blood-collection device for trace and ultra-trace metal specimens evaluated. Clin Chem 1991;37: 709-14.
95. Navas-Acien A, Silbergeld EK, Sharrett R, Calderon-Aranda E, Selvin E, Guallar E. Metals in urine and peripheral arterial disease. Environ Health Perspect 2005;113:164-9.
96. Neuberger JS, Field RW. Occupation and lung cancer in nonsmokers. Rev Environ Health 2003;18:251-67.
96A. Neuhann-Lorenz C, Fedeles J, Eisenman-Klein M, Kinney B, Cunningham BL. Eighth IQUAM consensus conference position statement: transatlantic innovations, April 2009. Plast Reconstr Surg. 2011 Mar;127(3):1368-75.
97. NHANES 2011. http://www.cdc.gov/exposurereport/pdf/Updated_Tables.pdf.
98. NHANES 2011. http://www.cdc.gov/exposurereport/.
99. NHANES (National Health and Nutrition Examination Survey). Hyattsville, Md: U.S. Department of Health and Human Services, Centers for Disease Control and Prevention, National Center for Health Statistics, 1999.
100. Nixon D, Moyer T. Routine clinical determination of lead, arsenic, cadmium, mercury, and thallium in urine and whole blood by inductively coupled plasma mass spectrometry. Spectrochim Acta 1996;51B:13-25.
101. Nordberg G, Nogawa K, Nordberg M, Friberg L. Cadmium. In: Nordberg G, Fowler B, Nordberg M, Friberg L, eds. Handbook on the toxicology of metals, 3rd edition. Amsterdam: Academic Press, 2007:445-86.
102. New York State Department of Health. Lead poisoning prevention. Available at: www.health.state.ny.us/environmental/lead/accessed on June 1, 2011.
103. O'Brien TJ, Ceryak S, Patierno SR. Complexities of chromium carcinogenesis: role of cellular response, repair and recovery mechanisms. Mutat Res 2003;533:3-36.
104. Paige NM, Nagami GT. The top 10 things nephrologists wish every primary care physician knew. Mayo Clin Proc 2009;84:180-6.
104A. Patil RR. MMR vaccination and autism: Learnings and implications. Hum Vaccin 2011 Feb 1;7(2). [Epub ahead of print].
105. Patrick L. Toxic metals and antioxidants: Part II. The role of antioxidants in arsenic and cadmium toxicity. Altern Med Rev 2003;8:106-28.
106. Pelucchi C, Pira E, Piolatto G, Coggiola M, Carta P, La Vecchia C. Occupational silica exposure and lung cancer risk: a review of epidemiological studies 1996-2005. Ann Oncol 2006;17:1039-50.
107. Perl DP, Brody AR. Alzheimer's disease: x-ray spectrometric evidence of aluminum accumulation in neurofibrillary tangle-bearing neurons. Science 1980;208:297-9.
108. Pulido M, Parrish A. Metal-induced apoptosis: mechanisms. Mutat Res 2003;533:227-41.
108A. Ratajczak HV. Theoretical aspects of autism: causes–a review. J Immunotoxicol. 2011;8(1):68-79.
109. Roberts HW, Charlton DG. The release of mercury from amalgam restorations and its health effects: a review. Oper Dent 2009;34:605-14.
110. Rogan WJ, Ware JH. Exposure to lead in children—how low is low enough? N Engl J Med 2003;348:1515-6.
111. Roggli VL, Pratt PC, Brody AR. Asbestos content of lung tissue in asbestos associated diseases: a study of 110 cases. Br J Ind Med 1986;43:18-28.
112. Rondeau V. A review of epidemiologic studies on aluminum and silica in relation to Alzheimer's disease and associated disorders. Rev Environ Health 2002;17:107-21.
113. Roper W, Houk V, Falk H, Binder S. Preventing lead poisoning in young children: a statement by the Centers for Disease Control. Atlanta, Ga: Centers for Disease Control, U.S. Department of Health and Human Services, 1991.
114. Rossman M. Beryllium. In: Seiler H, Sigel A, Sigel H, eds. Handbook on metals in clinical and analytical chemistry. New York: Marcel Dekker, 1994:259-67.

115. Rossman TG. Mechanism of arsenic carcinogenesis: an integrated approach. Mutat Res 2003;533:37-65.
116. Santamaria AB, Cushing CA, Antonini JM, Finley BL, Mowat FS. State-of-the-science review: does manganese exposure during welding pose a neurological risk? J Toxicol Environ Health B Crit Rev 2007;10:417-65.
117. Saric M, Lucchini R. Manganese. In: Nordberg G, Bowler B, Nordberg M, Friberg L, eds. Handbook on the toxicology of metals. Amsterdam: Academic Press, 2007:645-74.
118. Schultz ST. Does thimerosal or other mercury exposure increase the risk for autism? A review of current literature. Acta Neurobiol Exp (Wars) 2010;70:187-95.
119. Schwarz C, Sulzbacher I, Oberbauer R. Diagnosis of renal osteodystrophy. Eur J Clin Invest 2006;36(Suppl 2):13-22.
120. Shelnutt SR, Goad P, Belsito DV. Dermatological toxicity of hexavalent chromium. Crit Rev Toxicol 2007;37:375-87.
121. Skelton JA, Havens PL, Werlin SL. Nutrient deficiencies in tube-fed children. Clin Pediatr 2006;45:37-41.
122. Soden SE, Lowry JA, Garrison CB, Wasserman GS. 24-Hour provoked urine excretion test for heavy metals in children with autism and typically developing controls, a pilot study. Clin Toxicol 2007;45: 476-81.
123. Spain RI, Leist TP, De Sousa EA. When metals compete: a case of copper-deficiency myeloneuropathy and anemia. Nat Clin Pract Neurol 2009;5:106-11.
124. Sullivan J, Parker M, Carson SB. Tissue cobalt content in "beer drinkers' myocardiopathy." J Lab Clin Med 1968;71:893-911.
125. Swaminathan S, Ahmed I, McCarthy JT, Albright RC, Pittelkow MR, Caplice NM, et al. Nephrogenic fibrosing dermopathy and high-dose erythropoietin therapy. Ann Intern Med 2006;145:234-5.
126. Tylenda C, Fowler B. Antimony. In: Nordberg G, Bowler B, Nordberg M, Friberg L, eds. Handbook on toxicology of metals. Amsterdam: Academic Press, 2007:353-65.
127. Vaccines and autism. In: Press TNA, ed. Report of immunization safety review committee. New York, NY: Institute of Medicine of the National Academies, 2004/ http://www.nap.edu/. openbook.php?record_id=10997/accessed June 2, 2011.
128. van Wijk FH, van der Burg ME, Burger CW, Vergote I, van Doorn HC. Management of recurrent endometrioid endometrial carcinoma: an overview. Int J Gynecol Cancer 2009;19:314-20.
129. VirSinghRana S. Metals and apoptosis: recent developments. J Trace Elem Med Biol 2008;22:262-84.
130. Wiginton CD, Kelly B, Oto A, Jesse M, Aristimuno P, Ernst R, et al. Gadolinium-based contrast exposure, nephrogenic systemic fibrosis, and gadolinium detection in tissue. AJR Am J Roentgenol 2008;190: 1060-8.
131. Woods JS. Altered porphyrin metabolism as a biomarker of mercury exposure and toxicity. Can J Physiol Pharmacol 1996;74:210-5.
132. Wu AH, McKay C, Broussard LA, Hoffman RS, Kwong TC, Moyer TP, et al. National Academy of Clinical Biochemistry laboratory medicine practice guidelines: recommendations for the use of laboratory tests to support poisoned patients who present to the emergency department. Clin Chem 2003;49:357-79.
133. Yang G, Zhou R. Further observations on the human maximum safe dietary selenium intake in a seleniferous area of China. J Trace Elem Electrolytes Health Dis 1994;8:159-65.
134. Yantasee W, Lin Y, Hongsirikarn K, Fryxell GE, Addleman R, Timchalk C. Electrochemical sensors for the detection of lead and other toxic heavy metals: the next generation of personal exposure biomonitors. Environ Health Perspect 2007;115:1683-90.

SECTION IV

Molecular Diagnostics and Genetics

CHAPTER 37

Principles of Molecular Biology

Rossa W. K. Chiu, M.B.B.S., Ph.D., F.H.K.A.M.(Pathology), F.R.C.P.A., and Y. M. Dennis Lo, M.A., D.M., D.Phil., F.R.C.P.,(Lond. & Edin.), F.R.C.Path., F.R.S.

Molecular diagnostics represents one of the most rapidly developing areas in clinical chemistry. Advances in the field have been made possible by our improved understanding of molecular biology and genetics and of their relationships with human diseases, and by the development of powerful technologies for analysis of nucleic acids.[21] The chapters in this section attempt to provide an overview of important advances in molecular diagnostics. Fundamental concepts in molecular biology are reviewed in this chapter. Molecular diagnostic techniques are discussed in Chapters 38 and 39. The subsequent chapters focus on key areas of molecular diagnostics, specifically, inherited diseases (see Chapter 40), identity assessment (see Chapter 41), infectious diseases (see Chapter 42), pharmacogenetics (see Chapter 43), and hematologic malignancies (see Chapter 44). Last, molecular diagnostic applications based on analysis of plasma nucleic acids are discussed in Chapter 45.

LANDMARK DEVELOPMENTS IN GENETICS AND MOLECULAR DIAGNOSTICS

Amazing developments in biotechnology have taken place in the late twentieth century. For example, we have witnessed dramatic progress in sequencing of the human genome, cloning of organisms, and progress in stem cell research and gene therapy. Many of these advances would not have been possible without the many earlier landmark discoveries that unveiled the mysteries of genetics and paved the way for modern molecular diagnostics.[32] Genetics began modestly when Mendel experimented with garden peas. His findings, published in 1866 and suggesting the concepts of alleles and genes as units of heredity, essentially captured the most fundamental concepts in inheritance. In 1910, Morgan revealed that the units of heredity are contained within chromosomes, but it was Avery in 1944 who confirmed through studies on bacteria that it was DNA that carried the genetic information. Franklin and Wilkins studied DNA by x-ray crystallography, which subsequently led to unraveling of the double-helical structure of DNA by Watson and Crick in 1953. In the 1960s, Smith demonstrated that DNA can be cleaved by restriction enzymes, which Arber had discovered earlier; this facilitated the subsequent development of recombinant DNA technologies. Nathans furthered the work on restriction enzymes and was the first to construct a genetic map. In 1975, the Southern blot was invented, which allowed the detection of specific DNA sequences. Soon after, in 1977, DNA-sequencing methods were developed, and the first complete DNA sequence of an organism, a bacteriophage, was published. Cloning of the first human gene mutation, a β-thalassemia mutation, was achieved by Orkin and associates in 1980. Prenatal genetic diagnosis of sickle cell disease was shown to be feasible by Chang and Kan in 1981. Mullis and coworkers developed the polymerase chain reaction in 1985. The existence of functional small noncoding RNAs (ncRNAs) in organisms was first realized in 1993. DNA microarrays, which allow the simultaneous interrogation of many DNA/cDNA loci by nucleic acid hybridization, became a reality in 1996. Remarkably, the draft human genome sequence was released in 2001 and completed in 2003.[33,60] Massively parallel genomic sequencing became an accessible laboratory tool from 2005[41] and vastly accelerated the pace of molecular biology research in a way that was not achievable before.

This brief account describes a fraction of the many great discoveries that shaped modern genetics and molecular diagnostics. Although the explosive accumulation of genetic knowledge has translated into escalating clinical demands for molecular diagnostics, improved molecular diagnostic techniques have reciprocally led to the discovery of new genetic knowledge. An understanding of the fundamental aspects of molecular biology as outlined in this chapter is required for the effective implementation and interpretation of molecular diagnostics. This chapter begins with an overview of the essential principles of molecular biology, which is followed by a more in-depth discussion of key aspects, starting with the Watson and Crick model of DNA, through to discussion of the greatest biotechnological achievement of humankind of our time—the Human Genome Project—and beyond.

THE ESSENTIALS

On the simplest level, genes can be defined as segments of deoxyribonucleic acid (DNA) that encode for proteins or ribonucleic acid (RNA) products with biological functions. DNA is a biological substance that carries genetic information and is a polymer of nucleotides or bases. Genetic information is reproduced from parent to daughter cells during cell division through the process of DNA replication. When genes are expressed ("switched on"), the DNA sequence is transcribed into RNA. RNA molecules (RNAs) are polymers of ribonucleotides that exist in a number of functional forms. RNA molecules that act as intermediates for protein production are termed *messenger RNA (mRNA)*. RNA molecules that serve a direct biological function without coding for a protein are collectively termed *ncRNAs*.[58] mRNA is the product of a transcribed nucleotide sequence and is in turn translated into a protein, which is a polymer of amino acids. Each amino acid is encoded by a triplet nucleotide code, termed a *codon*. The human genetic code comprises 64 codons encoding for 21 amino acids and 3 stop codons. mRNA codons are read by the anticodon regions of transfer RNA (tRNA) molecules, which are small RNAs that bring the corresponding amino acid to the growing polypeptide chain. The polypeptide chain is synthesized by ribosomes, which are macromolecular complexes containing ribosomal RNA (rRNA) and a protein component with catalytic function.

Most human cells contain two full copies/versions of the haploid human genome, which is organized and packaged into 23 pairs of chromosomes (diploid genome). A chromosome is a highly ordered structure of a single DNA molecule with specialized structural features, namely, one centromere and two telomeres. Every individual inherits one copy/version of the human genome from his or her father and another from the mother. Thus, the human genome contains two copies, termed *alleles*, of each autosomal gene. Although a gene sequence may encode for a specific protein or RNA with defined functions, alleles of genes may demonstrate sequence variations that in turn contribute to variations in the functional characteristics of the gene product between individuals. The primary nucleotide sequences of the two gene alleles form the *genotype*, whereas the expressed function or biological effect of the gene product is termed the *phenotype*. Thus one could study a human disease or trait at the genetic level through determination of the allelic sequence of a gene (i.e., genotyping) or at the functional level (i.e., phenotyping). Examples of phenotyping include the investigation of enzyme concentrations or activities, ABO blood groups, electrophoretic mobility of hemoglobin variants, RNA expression levels, and others. The choice of genotyping or phenotyping for making a diagnosis depends on the specific diagnostic application and the strength of the association between a genotype and its consequential phenotype.

NUCLEIC ACID STRUCTURE AND ORGANIZATION

An intimate relationship has been observed between nucleic acid structure and function. The physiologic function of nucleic acid is facilitated by its "strategically designed" structure. Although an alteration in the structure of nucleic acids would lead to an altered function, an altered function, on the other hand, may be seen as an altered structure. Thus, a discussion of nucleic acid structure is pertinent to further discussion on nucleic acid function.

Molecular Compositions and Structures of DNA and RNA

DNA

The physicochemical properties and functions of nucleic acids are largely governed by the compositions and structures of DNA and RNA. A single molecule of DNA is a polymer consisting of a backbone of invariant composition and side groups arranged in a variable sequence (Figures 37-1 and 37-2). The polymer is synthesized from monomers (nucleotides) composed of the sugar deoxyribose, a phosphate residue, and a purine or pyrimidine base. The purines are adenine (A) and guanine (G), and the pyrimidines are cytosine (C) and thymine (T) (see Figure 37-1). The four nucleotide building blocks of DNA are abbreviated dATP (deoxyadenosine-triphosphate), dGTP (deoxyguanosine-triphosphate), dCTP (deoxycytidene-triphosphate), and dTTP (deoxythymidene-triphosphate), respectively. Nucleotides are joined by phosphodiester bonds that link the 5′-phosphate group of one to the 3′-hydroxyl group of the next (see Figure 37-2). No 3′-3′ or 5′-5′ linkages are present; thus the sugar and phosphate moieties compose the nonspecific portions of the molecule. The sequence of the bases varies from molecule to molecule and uniquely identifies each DNA polymer, which, as discussed later, determines the identity and function of the protein or RNA products that the DNA encodes.

Although the purines and pyrimidines are of different compositions and sizes, when in the proper orientation, adenine forms two hydrogen bonds with thymine, and guanine forms three hydrogen bonds with cytosine, to form planar structures of similar dimensions (see Figure 37-1). This combined with the fact that the base portion of each nucleotide is hydrophobic contributes to the energetically favorable secondary structure of DNA as it is found in its native form: a right-handed, double-stranded helix. The planar base pairs stack in the inside of the helix, 10 bases per turn, whereas the hydrophilic sugar-phosphate backbone forms noncovalent bonds with surrounding water molecules. For the two DNA polymers to form the proper hydrogen bonds between the bases, two requirements must be fulfilled: the polymers must run in opposite directions (antiparallel) as defined by the free hydroxyl groups at each end (3′-5′ vs. 5′-3′), and the sequences of each molecule must be such that A:T and G:C hydrogen bonds are always formed (base

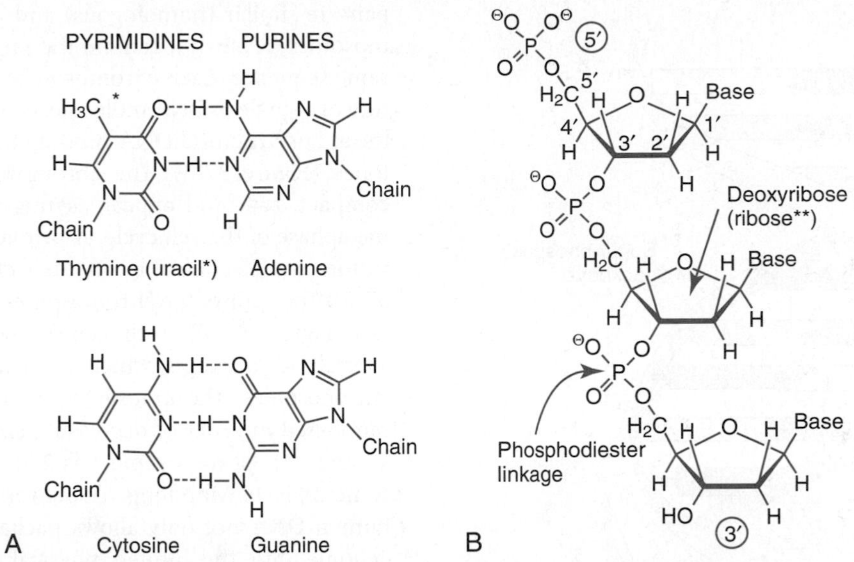

Figure 37-1 A, Purine and pyrimidine bases and the formation of complementary base pairs. *Dashed lines* indicate the formation of hydrogen bonds. (*In RNA, thymine is replaced by uracil, which differs from thymine only in its lack of the methyl group.) B, A single-stranded DNA chain. Repeating nucleotide units are linked by phosphodiester bonds that join the 5′ carbon of one sugar to the 3′ carbon of the next. Each nucleotide monomer consists of a sugar moiety, a phosphate residue, and a base. (In RNA, the sugar is ribose, which adds a 2′-hydroxyl to deoxyribose.)** *(Modified from Piper MA, Unger ER. Nucleic acid probes: a primer for pathologists. Chicago, Ill: ASCP Press, 1989.)*

pairing). Two DNA strands that meet this requirement are called *complementary.*

Owing to base pairing and the double-helical conformation, double-stranded DNA (dsDNA) is an exceptionally stable molecule. Retention of base pairs in the inner portion of the helix prevents disruption by water molecules. The helical conformation places each monomer in an identical orientation within the molecule and forms the same secondary bonds as every other monomer. This secondary bonding contributes to the overall stability. Because the base pairs are of similar size, the helix retains a constant angle of rotation and avoids distortion. All of these features dictate that all dsDNA molecules, regardless of base sequence, retain the same shape and size within a pH range of approximately 4 to 9. Outside these limits, the base pair bonds are disrupted and the helix unwinds.

RNA

RNA is chemically very similar to DNA but differs in important ways. The sugar unit is ribose with an added hydroxyl group at the 2′ position, and the methylated pyrimidine uracil (U) replaces thymine. RNA exists in various functional forms but mostly as a single-stranded polymer that is much shorter than DNA and that has an irregular three-dimensional structure. Despite their irregular shape, RNA conformations are not random structures, and the folding mechanism of RNA molecules is complex.[1,53] The secondary structure adopted by an RNA molecule is to a large extent related to its nucleotide sequence. RNA molecules fold sequentially from 5′ to 3′ to form stable submotifs dictated by their primary sequence. One such example is the hairpin loop structure of precursor miRNAs (see below section on ncRNAs). RNA molecules may adopt further tertiary folding. An RNA molecule has the potential to be folded into a number of different conformations, but usually only one conformation is functional.[53] The folding process is influenced by ions, cofactors, and proteins.[1] Once an RNA molecule adopts a conformation most favored by its immediate cellular environment, it rarely switches to another conformation.[1] RNA molecules can further interact with other RNA or protein molecules to form complex quaternary structures, such as ribonucleoproteins, that are essential to certain cellular processes.

Chromosome Structure

DNA molecules are extremely long and in the eukaryotic cell are maintained in orderly and compact three-dimensional structures. Each diploid human cell contains two full sets of the human genome, with each copy consisting of approximately 3.2 billion nucleotides. This vast amount of genetic material is organized into 23 homologous chromosome pairs, with each pair contributed by a homolog of maternal origin and one of paternal origin. The two chromosomes of each

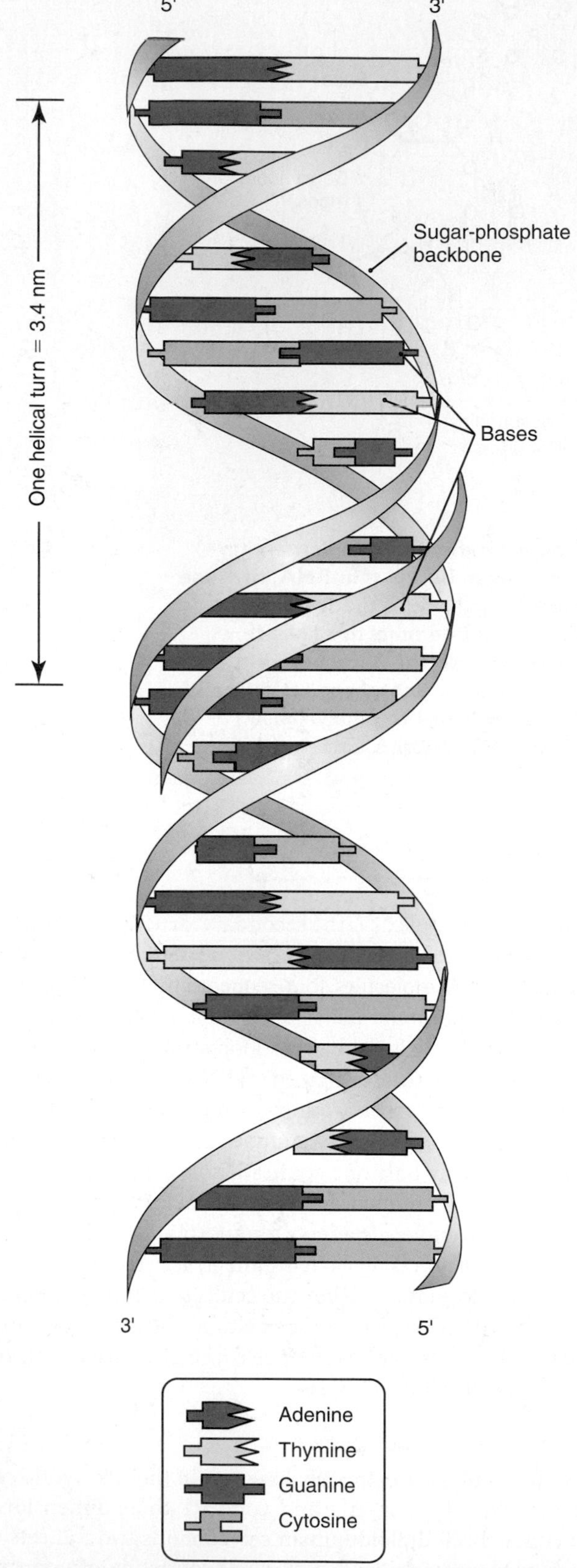

Figure 37-2 The DNA double helix, with sugar-phosphate backbone and pairing of the bases in the core-forming planar structures. *(From Jorde LB, Carey JC, Bamshad MJ, editors: Medical genetics, 4th edition, Philadelphia: Mosby, 2010.)*

pair are similar (homologous) and, except for the sex chromosomes (X and Y), contain the same genes arranged in the same sequence. Each chromosome is a highly ordered structure of a single dsDNA molecule, compacted many times with the aid of structural DNA-binding proteins, for example, histones (Figure 37-3). The chromosomes are in their most compact state and appear as finger-like structures during metaphase of the cell cycle. A primary constriction, the centromere, is also notable on each chromosome (see Figure 37-3). The ends of the chromosomes are termed the *telomeres* (see Figure 37-3). Both centromeres and telomeres have specialized functions, which are discussed later. The nonsex chromosomes, the *autosomes*, in the human genome are numbered in order of decreasing size (except chromosomes 21 and 22). Chromosome 1 is 250 Mbp long, and chromosome 21 is 48 Mbp long. The chromosomal arrangement of human DNA not only allows packaging of the vast human genome into the limited physical dimensions of the cell nucleus, but also governs one of the mendelian laws of inheritance on independent assortment whereby genes located on different chromosomes recombine at random from one generation to the next.

Chromatin Packing

Nuclear DNA in conjunction with its associated structural proteins, including histone and nonhistone proteins, is known as chromatin. Chromatin is arranged and organized in a hierarchical fashion whereby the degree of packing or condensation increases with higher levels of structural organization.[9,23,51] The nucleosome represents the most basic level of chromatin organization and is present as repeated units along the full length of each chromosome. Each nucleosome unit consists of a nucleosome core particle and 20 to 80 base pairs of linker DNA, which spans between adjacent nucleosomes, resembling what has been referred as "beads on a string" (Figure 37-4). A nucleosome core particle involves 147 base pairs of dsDNA tightly wound 1.65 times around an octamer of histone proteins, two each of four histone proteins, namely, H2A, H2B, H3, and H4.[9,23] Amino termini or "tails" of these histone molecules protrude from the nucleosomal core. The histone tails are subjected to covalent modifications, including acetylation, methylation, phosphorylation, and ubiquitination.[34] The linker DNA segments are associated with the linker histone H1. Nucleosomes are further packed in successive levels of complexity by up to a factor of 10,000[23]; in the most compact stage, chromatin appears as discrete mitotic chromosomes seen in the metaphase of a cell cycle, as described earlier. The orderly process of chromatin condensation involves DNA methylation, histone modifications, ncRNAs, and sequence-specific DNA binding proteins.

Chromatin packing serves the function of containing the genome within the nucleus, but this could potentially render the genetic code inaccessible to various cellular machineries.[23] However, this is not the case because chromatin condensation is not a static process but a dynamic one that changes in a coordinated fashion during the cell cycle. In general, chromatin is much less condensed during interphase,

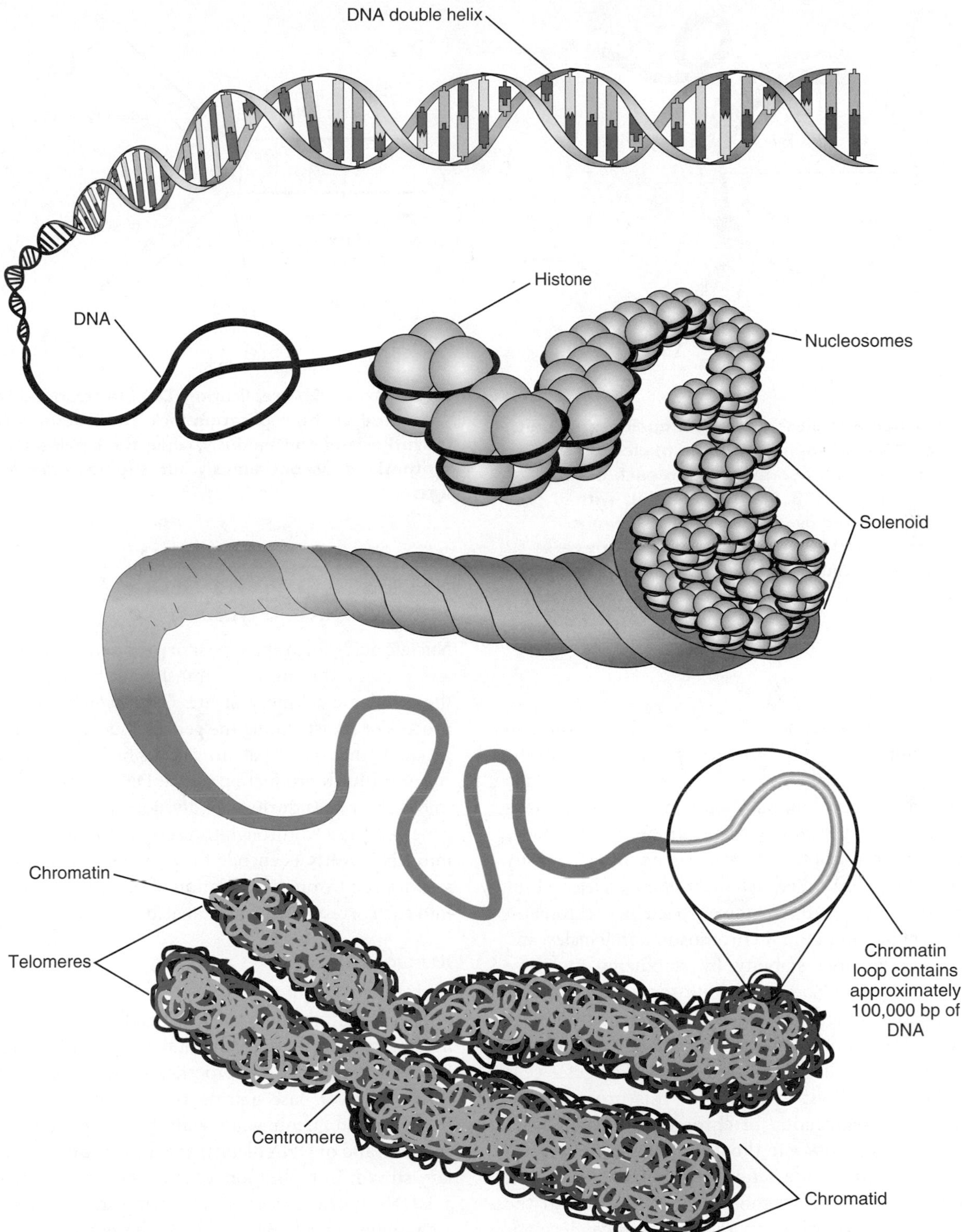

Figure 37-3 Structural organization of human chromosomal DNA. Double-stranded DNA is wound around histones to form nucleosomes. Nuclear DNA in conjunction with its associated structural proteins is known as *chromatin*. Chromatin in its most compact state forms chromosomes. The primary constriction of a chromosome is the centromere, and the chromosome's ends are the telomeres. *(From Jorde LB, Carey JC, Bamshad MJ, editors: Medical genetics, 4th edition, Philadelphia: Mosby, 2010.)*

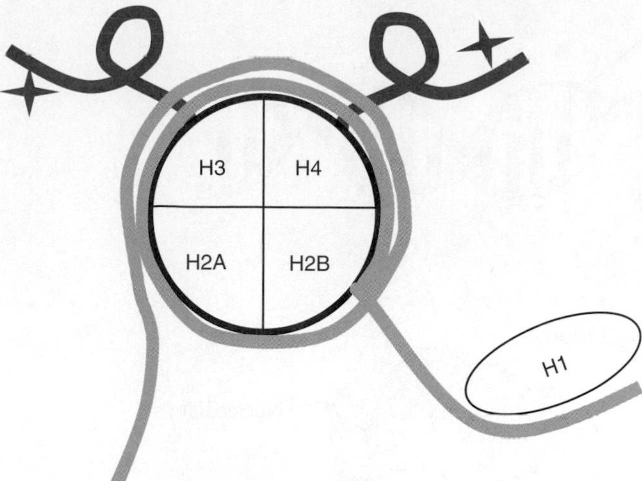

Figure 37-4 Schematic illustration of a nucleosome unit. A segment of DNA is wound around a nucleosome core particle consisting of an octamer of two each of the histone proteins H2A, H2B, H3, and H4. Tails with modifications *(indicated by a red star)* are shown to protrude from H3 and H4. Adjacent nucleosomes are separated by a segment of linker DNA and the linker histone, H1.

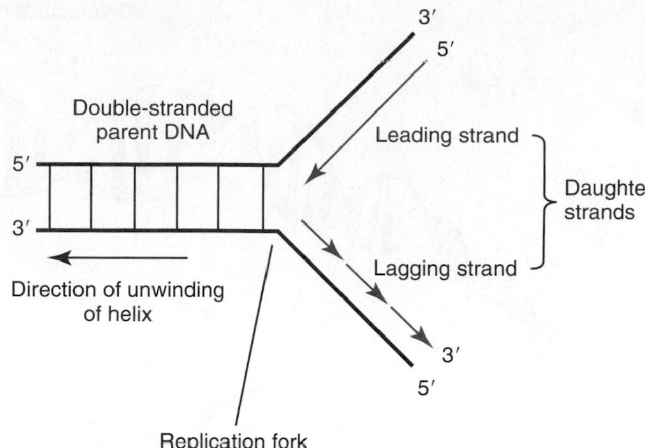

Figure 37-5 DNA replication. Double-stranded DNA is separated at the replication fork. The leading strand is synthesized continuously, while the lagging strand is synthesized discontinuously but is joined later by DNA ligase.

at which time DNA is replicated. The extent of chromatin condensation during interphase varies among regions of the genome. Genomic regions that are rich in genes generally open up to become less compactly organized during interphase and are termed *euchromatin*. Regions that are gene-poor or that span transcriptionally silent genes remain mostly densely packed and are called *heterochromatin*. Heterochromatin is important for maintenance of specialized chromatin structures, inactivation of the X chromosome in females, and maintenance of genome stability by stabilizing repetitive DNA sequences.[19,30] Eukaryote chromosomes contain two specialized regions of heterochromatin, namely, centromeres and telomeres. Centromeres play an important role in directing the movement of chromosomes between daughter cells during cell division.[2] Poor execution of this process could result in incorrect segregation of chromosomes, leading to chromosomal gains or losses in the daughter cells. Telomeres contain repetitive nucleotide sequences that are located on and protect the ends of chromosomes. Alterations in the lengths of telomeres contribute to aging and cancer development.[5] Genomic regions that remain condensed during the cell cycle, such as centromeres, telomeres, and the inactivated X chromosome in female cells, are termed *constitutive heterochromatin*. On the contrary, some other heterochromatin domains are scattered throughout the genome and are able to respond dynamically in various cellular states. Those regions are termed *facultative heterochromatin* and are associated with regulation of gene expression.[19,30] Functional implications of the structural organization of chromatin will be discussed further in the following sections.

NUCLEIC ACID PHYSIOLOGY AND FUNCTIONAL REGULATION

Nucleic acids form the repository for hereditary information and provide the means of translating that information into the cellular machinery of life. *Gene expression* refers to the process of transforming the genetic blueprint into functional products that participate in various biological processes of a cell. Faithful reproduction of the DNA content from parent to daughter cells during cell division is termed *replication*. A gene is expressed through transcription of its DNA sequence into RNA. mRNAs encode for proteins, and a polypeptide is synthesized through translation of the mRNA base sequence into the corresponding amino acid sequence.

Replication

Each time a cell divides, the entire DNA content of that cell must be faithfully duplicated, so that the total complement of hereditary information (the human genome) is retained in each daughter cell. This process is called replication. Owing to the laws of base pairing (i.e., adenine pairs only with thymine, and guanine only with cytosine), the sequence of a single strand of DNA dictates the sequence of its complementary strand. In replication, each of the two parent strands of a dsDNA molecule serves as the template for the synthesis of a daughter strand (Figure 37-5). The process is called *semi-conservative* because each of the duplicated dsDNA molecules produced in this manner is composed of one parent (conserved) strand and one daughter strand. For replication to occur, the original double-stranded helix must be separated. This is an energetically unfavorable event that is accomplished with a combination of DNA-specific proteins and enzymes, and synthesis of both daughter strands proceeds as the parent strands separate. Replication is initiated at multiple sites (origins of replication) during this process, but each origin of replication is used only once during a single cell cycle.

Daughter strands are synthesized by DNA polymerase III, an enzyme that reads the parent template and attaches nucleotides to the growing daughter strand according to the base pairing rules of dsDNA. DNA polymerase III begins synthesis at the replication fork (see Figure 37-5), the point of strand separation, with a short RNA primer that base pairs to the parent template. Later, this primer is excised and replaced with DNA by the DNA repair enzyme, DNA polymerase I. Because DNA polymerase III synthesizes DNA only in the 5′-3′ direction, one daughter strand, the leading strand, is synthesized continuously, whereas the other, the lagging strand, must be synthesized discontinuously in short segments (see Figure 37-5). Fragments on the discontinuous strand are then joined by the DNA ligase enzyme. Many other proteins are involved in unwinding and stabilizing the parent strands for synthesis, in protecting single-stranded regions, in recognizing initiation sites, and in synthesizing the RNA primer. In addition to synthetic capabilities, the DNA polymerases possess an exonuclease or "proofreading" function: when an incorrect nucleotide is added to the growing polymer, a conformational change brings the chain in contact with the exonuclease portion of the enzyme, which cuts out ("excises") the incorrect nucleotide. This helps maintain the integrity of the original DNA sequence. In fact, it has been estimated that one nucleotide error could occur for every 10^5 nucleotides incorporated into the growing strand. However, the proofreading function of DNA polymerase works in concert with a set of DNA repair mechanisms that detect and correct DNA replication errors in such a way that the resultant error rate of DNA replication is reduced to one error per 10^9 to 10^{10} nucleotides replicated.[39] Given that 3 billion base pairs are present in the human genome, about 0.3 to 3 errors occur per cell division.

Transcription

DNA carries information that specifies the production of RNA molecules and proteins that can execute biological functions. The segment of the genome that specifies the production of a functional product, that is, a protein or ncRNA, is termed a *gene*. In short, a gene is a functional unit of the genome. On the most basic level, the span of a gene encompasses the nucleotide sequence that specifies its ncRNA product or the amino acid sequence of its protein product. However, a series of processes determines the timing and rate of expression of each gene. Those processes that control gene expression act via regulatory regions of the genome. Thus, it is customary to define a gene to be inclusive of such associated regulatory elements.[17,49] An important regulatory region is the promoter of a gene, which, as will be discussed later, is the genomic region where regulatory factors act in concert to activate expression of said gene. Previously, it was generally thought that the promoter region laid immediately 5′ to the start of the protein-coding portion of a gene. Yet, recent evidence demonstrates that regions showing properties of a promoter could be found within the protein-coding portion of genes, toward the 3′ end, or lying at a substantial distance between coding sequences.[28] In addition, the same promoter region could trigger the expression of different DNA segments both 5′ or 3′ to it.[28] Hence, it has become increasingly difficult to precisely define the physical boundaries of individual genes.[17,49]

When a gene is expressed, the DNA sequence is first transcribed into RNA. The process of transferring the sequence information from DNA to RNA is called *transcription*. Regulation of transcription is the primary mechanism that cells use to control gene expression.[59] Similar to replication, transcription requires separation of duplex DNA strands and uses a polymerase to copy the template DNA strand. For transcription, the polymerase is RNA polymerase II, which first binds to specific sequences in the promoter, called the *core promoter*, upon initiation of gene expression. Core promoters that have been identified to date generally occur within a hundred bases around the initiation site of transcription, known as the *transcription start site*, where the first ribonucleotide unit is paired with the template DNA (uracil pairs with adenine). Several nucleotide sequence motifs or patterns have now been recognized among core promoters.[26] For example, one of the best studied core promoter motifs, the TATA box, refers to a short stretch of nucleotides rich in thymine and adenine in repeating patterns. It is typically located between 24 to 31 nucleotides "upstream" (i.e., at the 5′ end) of the transcription start site.[59] Some other core promoter elements are located just downstream to the transcription start site. Research has suggested that the various core promoter elements may have different strength and efficiency in activating gene expression.[59]

To initiate transcription, a series of protein cofactors, known as *general transcription factors*, is required to bind to RNA polymerase II to form an assembly known as the *preinitiation complex*, which, in turn, acts on the gene by interacting with the core promoter.[59] Other regions of DNA known as *activators* or *coactivators* may interact with the preinitiation complex to stimulate or repress transcription.

Once transcription is activated, RNA polymerase II moves along and unwinds the DNA double helix. The growing RNA transcript pairs with one of the DNA strands, called the *template*, where RNA polymerase II adds complementary ribonucleotide triphosphates in a 5′ to 3′ direction. It is now known that both DNA strands of the double helix can act as the template for RNA transcription.[4] For example, when the growing RNA transcript pairs with the antisense (−) DNA strand, the resultant RNA molecule is a copy of the sense (+) strand of DNA, and vice versa. Natural antisense transcripts (i.e., RNA transcripts that are copies of the antisense DNA strand) have been better known only in recent years.[45] Both protein-coding and non–protein-coding RNAs have been reported to be natural antisense RNAs.[14]

RNA elongation continues until chain termination occurs. The precise signaling mechanism for chain termination still is not well understood. The RNA transcript quickly detaches from the template DNA because restoration of the DNA-DNA duplex is energetically more favorable than is retention of the DNA-RNA hybrid or a segment of single-stranded DNA. The newly synthesized RNA molecule then undergoes further

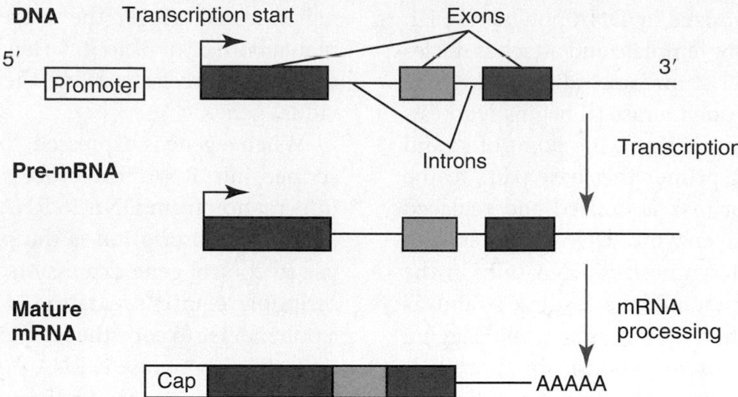

Figure 37-6 DNA transcription and mRNA processing. A gene that encodes for a protein contains a promoter region with variable numbers of introns and exons. Transcription commences at the transcription start site. Pre-mRNA is processed by capping, polyadenylation, and intron splicing and becomes a mature mRNA.

modification depending on its functional class. We shall discuss the fate of the ncRNAs in a later section of this chapter. Here we focus on describing subsequent processing of the protein coding RNAs, which are referred to as mRNA. First, the 5′ end of the RNA molecule is modified by the addition of 7-methylguanosine residues to form a structure called a *cap* (Figure 37-6). The 3′ end is modified by the addition of multiple adenine bases, called the *poly(A) tail* (see Figure 37-6). Both the cap and the tail are necessary for translation of mRNA into protein, and they protect the mRNA molecule from degradation by exonucleases. The coding region of a gene (i.e., segments that will contribute to the amino acid sequence of the protein) is divided into segments called *exons* interspersed with noncoding regions termed *introns* (see Figure 37-6). The number and size of introns and exons differ among genes. Excision or splicing of the noncoding introns is carried out by a molecular complex termed a *spliceosome.* These complexes are composed of multiple small nuclear ribonucleoprotein particles. Spliceosomes mediate the cleavage and ligation of RNA at specific recognition sequences, termed *splicing donor and acceptor sequences.* After the introns have been removed, the exons are juxtaposed to each other, forming a mature mRNA molecule (see Figure 37-6) that is transported into the cytoplasm, where protein translation takes place.

Translation

Translation is the process whereby the mRNA sequence directs the amino acid sequence during protein synthesis. Amino acids are the building blocks of a polypeptide chain. To date, 22 amino acids have been reported in nature. Each amino acid is specified by a three-nucleotide sequence known as a *codon.* Because 64 possible codons are known, most amino acids are specified by more than one codon. One codon, UAA, does not code for amino acids but always signals termination of protein synthesis (a stop codon). UGA codes for a stop or for selenocysteine, and UAG codes for a stop or for pyrrolysine, depending on adjacent sequences or RNA-binding proteins. With the exception of pyrrolysine, which is the most recently identified amino acid and so far has been found in proteins of bacteria and archaea only, all other amino acids are involved in human protein synthesis.[38] The full menu of codon sequences forms the genetic code, which is shown in Table 37-1.

Translation takes place on ribosomes, which are ribonucleoprotein complexes that function as protein synthesis factories. A ribosome binds to the initiation site on mRNA to form an initiation complex. Protein synthesis begins at the translation initiation codon, AUG, which codes for the amino acid, methionine. The region of the mRNA molecule preceding the initiation codon is termed the *5′ untranslated region (5′UTR).* The initiation codon and each subsequent codon are "read" by tRNA, short RNA molecules that have a sequence complementary to an amino acid codon (anticodon) and are bound to the amino acid molecule specified by the codon.[3] As synthesis proceeds, the appropriate tRNA anticodon base pairs with the next mRNA codon and thus brings this amino acid bound to it into close proximity of the growing peptide chain. An enzyme on the ribosome then catalyzes the formation of a peptide bond between the amino acid and the growing peptide chain. The previous tRNA is released and the next tRNA is added. The ribosome moves along the mRNA until a stop codon is reached and synthesis is complete. The ribosome and the protein product are then dissociated from the mRNA. More than one ribosome can move along an mRNA molecule at a time, forming a polyribosome. The rest of the mRNA molecule downstream to the stop codon is termed the *3′ untranslated region (3′UTR).*

Genetics and Epigenetics

Genetic and epigenetic phenomena are intimately related and work in concert to bring about the normal development and functioning of each cell and the whole organism. In general, genetic events are related to the sequence information of DNA, and thus include the consequences of transmission of a particular DNA sequence (e.g., inheritance of DNA

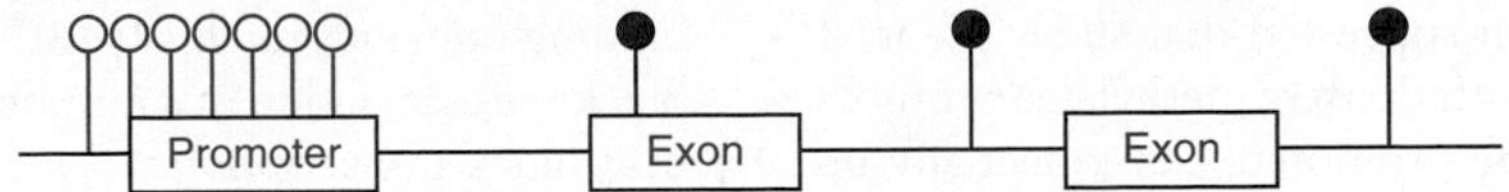

Figure 37-7 Normal DNA methylation pattern in the human genome. Sites of CpG dinucleotides are indicated by *circles*. CpG islands in association with gene promoters are generally unmethylated, but isolated CpG dinucleoctides are methylated. *Filled circles*, methylated; *open circles*, unmethylated.

TABLE 37-1 The Genetic Code (Translation of mRNA to Amino Acids During Protein Synthesis)

		Nucleotide Position in the Codon			
1st	**2nd**	**3rd**			
		U	**C**	**A**	**G**
U	U	Phenylalanine	Phenylalanine	Leucine	Leucine
	C	Serine	Serine	Serine	Serine
	A	Tyrosine	Tyrosine	Stop	Pyrrolysine*
	G	Cysteine	Cysteine	Selenocysteine*	Tryptophan
C	U	Leucine	Leucine	Leucine	Leucine
	C	Proline	Proline	Proline	Proline
	A	Histidine	Histidine	Glutamine	Glutamine
	G	Arginine	Arginine	Arginine	Arginine
A	U	Isoleucine	Isoleucine	Isoleucine	Methionine
	C	Threonine	Threonine	Threonine	Threonine
	A	Asparagine	Asparagine	Lysine	Lysine
	G	Serine	Serine	Arginine	Arginine
G	U	Valine	Valine	Valine	Valine
	C	Alanine	Alanine	Alanine	Alanine
	A	Aspartic acid	Aspartic acid	Glutamic acid	Glutamic acid
	G	Glycine	Glycine	Glycine	Glycine

*The codon UGA can code for selenocysteine or stop, and the codon UAG can code for pyrrolysine or stop.

mutations or polymorphisms) or of acquisition of DNA sequence variations (e.g., accumulation of somatic mutations in aging or cancer development). These pathologies are discussed in some of the subsequent chapters. On the other hand, a broad definition of epigenetics encompasses processes that alter gene function or its interpretation by mechanisms other than those that rely on DNA sequence change.[44] Practically, epigenetics has evolved to include the study of DNA methylation, genomic imprinting, histone modifications, chromatin remodeling, ncRNA regulation, and others. Most of these processes add another dimension to gene expression control and thus play a role in all fundamental cellular events, including cell differentiation, cell growth, cell death, and DNA repair.

DNA Methylation

DNA methylation is possibly the most widely studied epigenetic phenomenon. It refers to the addition of a methyl group to the fifth carbon position of cytosine residues in CpG dinucleotides. CpG dinucleotides are present throughout the genome and may exist singly as an isolated CpG site or in clusters, termed *CpG islands* (Figure 37-7). Most CpG dinucleotides in the human genome are methylated; these include CpG sites within gene bodies, within intergenic regions, and in DNA repeat elements (see Figure 37-7).[57] Unmethylated regions of the human genome are mostly found at CpG islands located at the 5′ ends, in promoters or first exons of genes, and occasionally in some intergenic CpG islands.[12,22,57] However, it is noteworthy that not all gene promoters are associated with CpG islands, and not all promoter-associated CpG islands are unmethylated. About 56% of human genes have promoters with CpG islands.[57] Some 10% of promoter CpG islands are methylated.[12,22]

It has been well accepted that DNA methylation mediates the silencing of gene transcription. The methylation of gene promoters has been shown to hinder the association of methylation-sensitive transcription factors, thus preventing gene activation. Consequently, the promoters of actively transcribed genes are generally unmethylated, while silenced genes are associated with methylated promoters. Because gene expression varies between cell types, the profile of DNA methylation differs between cell and tissue types. Furthermore, a CpG island may be composed of varying arrangements of methylated and unmethylated CpG sites. Hence, a genomic region can be further described in relative degree of methylation using the term *hypomethylated* or *hypermethylated*.[12] It has been suggested that stably silenced genes tend to be associated with densely methylated promoters, and hypomethylated gene promoters can potentially be activated.[57] Methylation of the nonpromoter regions of genes, on the other hand, is thought to suppress inadvertent transcription.[57] Furthermore, methylation of repeat elements in the genome helps to maintain chromosome stability by preventing translocations and insertions of transposons, which are repeat sequences that could randomly insert into the genome, causing gene disruptions.[13]

Because DNA methylation has implications for gene expression, aberrant changes in DNA methylation profiles may cause pathologies. For example, aberrant hypermethylation of gene promoters, particularly those of tumor suppressor genes, contributes to cancer development.[13] Hence, it is important that the DNA methylation pattern of a cell should be faithfully propagated to its daughter cells upon cell division. This process is executed by maintenance DNA methyltransferases (DNMT1).[25] DNMT1 is said to perform a "maintenance" role because the DNA methylation patterns inherited by somatic cells were originally laid down by other de novo DNA methyltransferases (DNMT3a and DNMT3b) in the early embryo.

After embryo fertilization, the genome becomes demethylated (except imprinted loci; see discussion later in this chapter) to pave the way for the establishment of developmentally related patterns of DNA methylation by de novo DNA methyltransferases. Genomic imprinting and gene dosage compensation of X-linked genes in females, termed *X-inactivation* or *lyonization*, are also mediated by DNA methylation. *Genomic imprinting* refers to the phenomenon whereby the function of each of the two alleles of a gene is determined by its parental origin. Differential methylation of the imprinted locus from the time of germ cell development allows recognition of the parental origin of imprinted alleles by cellular processes. The human insulin-like growth factor-2 H19 (IGF2-H19) locus on chromosome 15 is an example of an imprinted locus whereby the maternal allele is unmethylated and the paternal allele is methylated. Disomic inheritance of the paternal or maternal allele results in significantly different clinical outcomes, namely, Prader-Willi and Angelman syndromes, respectively (see Chapter 40).

X chromosome inactivation is an epigenetic phenomenon that occurs in female cells. Each female cell has two X chromosomes, and each male cell has only one X chromosome. The function of one of the X chromosomes in female cells is epigenetically silenced, so that the dosage of X chromosome genes in female and male cells is the same. Gene silencing on the inactive X chromosome is maintained by dense methylation of CpG island promoters. Within each female cell, either of the X chromosomes could be chosen for inactivation.

Histone Modifications

Hypermethylated CpG dinucleotides are also known to attract the binding of methyl-CpG binding proteins, such as methyl-CpG binding protein 2 (MECP2) and methyl-CpG binding domain proteins (MBD1 and MBD2), which further block the association of a number of transcription factors and thus block transcription.[24,34] It is now appreciated that these methyl-CpG binding proteins have the ability to recruit histone deacetylases, a phenomenon that leads to deacetylation of histones and ultimately represses transcription.

As discussed, histones are an integral part of nucleosomes, the basic repeating structural unit of chromatin. The amino termini of histone proteins can be modified posttranslationally by processes that include acetylation, methylation, phosphorylation, and ubiquitination (see Figure 37-4).[29,34] Acetylation of the lysines on amino termini of histones H3 and H4 by histone acetyltransferases decreases histone-DNA interaction and improves accessibility of DNA to transcriptional activation. On the contrary, histone deacetylation by histone deacetylases promotes the formation of compact nucleosomes, leading to repression of transcription. Histone deacetylation is in fact a key component of the assembly of heterochromatin, the transcriptionally inactive chromatin.[19] Methylation of the ninth amino acid residue, lysine, on histone H3 generates a binding site for heterochromatin protein (HP1) and thus is another key event in heterochromatin formation. Phosphorylation of the tenth amino acid, serine, on histone H3 is important for chromosome condensation and mitosis.

Nucleosome Positioning and Remodeling

Besides histone modifications, the position of nucleosomes is known to affect the transcriptional activity of the corresponding region of DNA. It is now known that the positioning of histones is not an entirely random process. It has been demonstrated that nucleosome-free regions are present at the 5′ and 3′ ends of genes. The 5′ nucleosome-free region is thought to be the assembly point of the preinitiation complex for transcription, and the 3′ one is the location of transcription termination.[23] A nucleosome unit is located just upstream to the 5′ nucleosome-free region, and another nucleosome is located just downstream to it, close to the transcription start site. It has been observed that the location of the nucleosome nearest to the transcription start site is predictable and consistent.[23] Positioning of the nucleosomes farther downstream through the gene, however, is shown to be more random. In summary, it seems that mechanisms control the positioning of nucleosomes, so that their presence will not be inhibitory to the initiation of transcription.

During transcription, the nucleosomes along a gene undergo a series of changes successively. First, histones H2A and H3 are replaced by the histone variants, H2A.Z and H3.3. The histone tails would be acetylated and methylated. The nucleosome would then be repositioned laterally and ultimately evicted to clear the DNA for access by the transcription machinery.[23] The nucleosome may then return to the DNA after RNA polymerase II has passed through. Consequently, nucleosomes are dynamic structures that can be remodeled according to the transcriptional demands of the cell.

Noncoding RNAs

It was once thought that much of the transcriptional activity of the human genome was directed toward the production of proteins. Exons of protein-coding genes occupy only 1 to 2% of base pairs in the human genome.[28] Thus, the rest of the genome was previously thought to be "junk" DNA, serving no function, and was merely a fossil of our evolutionary past. The availability of innovative technologies in recent years has enabled researchers to study transcriptional activity or RNA expression on a genome-wide scale.[27] On the contrary, studies have revealed that almost the entire genome was transcribed.[4] Transcription takes place in both sense and antisense directions.[14,28] The same genomic region could serve as the template for many nonoverlapping or overlapping transcription units.[28] Most transcription units do not result in the production of a protein product. Researchers became aware that some of the transcribed RNA molecules serve a direct biological function. An increasing number of classes of such functional RNA molecules have been described; they are collectively termed *ncRNAs*.[58] In retrospect, rRNA and tRNA are the earliest classes of ncRNAs described. Most recently, a class of short ncRNAs, miRNAs, has become the focus of much research interest.

MicroRNA

Mature (i.e., functional) miRNAs are 21 to 24 nucleotides long. The first step in the miRNA biogenesis pathway involves the initial transcription of an RNA molecule in the nucleus by RNA polymerase II. The first transcript, termed the *primary miRNA*, may be derived from short introns or a longer primary transcript that subsequently gives rise to multiple mature miRNAs.[47] Regions of the primary miRNA that would ultimately contribute to sequences of the mature miRNA are typified by their adoption of a stem loop, also known as hairpin, configuration with imperfect base pairing between sequences on both sides of the stem. The primary miRNA is cleaved by an RNase III–like enzyme, Drosha. The resultant RNA molecule, which is approximately 70 nucleotides long, is termed the *precursor miRNA*. The precursor miRNA is exported to the cytoplasm of the cell, where another RNase III–like enzyme, Dicer, cleaves at the loop end of the molecule, thus generating a double-stranded RNA product. The double-stranded product of Dicer is 21 to 24 nucleotides long, consisting of a mature miRNA paired with its imperfect complementary strand, termed *miRNA*. Some evidence suggests that miRNA may serve some biological function, and the conclusion awaits further investigation.[11]

The mature miRNA detaches from its partner and is incorporated into the RNA-silencing complex (RISC), which includes one or more Argonaute proteins. The biological function of miRNA is effected through RISC. The miRNA pairs with the 3′ untranslated region of mRNAs, leading to repression of protein translation or mRNA degradation. The actual biological consequence is determined by the degree of complementarity (i.e., the degree of base pairing) between the miRNA and the target mRNA. mRNAs that can be influenced by a particular miRNA are referred to as the target mRNAs of the corresponding miRNA. More than 850 human mature miRNAs have now been discovered.[16] Because miRNAs can function via imperfect base pairing to mRNA, each miRNA can have an effect on multiple target mRNAs.

miRNAs modulate gene expression at the post-transcriptional level. Therefore, they are involved in many biological processes, including development and cell differentiation.[16] They regulate cell proliferation, apoptosis, and maturation. Because of their important regulatory role, aberrant expression of miRNAs has been reported for a myriad of diseases involving, for example, the cardiovascular, neurologic, musculoskeletal, endocrinologic, and immunologic systems and others.[16] More important, aberrant miRNA expression has been implicated in carcinogenesis.[16] Their association with pathologies, coupled with realization of the presence of miRNAs in plasma and serum, makes them attractive candidate biomarkers for disease diagnosis and monitoring.[6,10]

Other ncRNAs

Besides miRNA, several other novel classes of ncRNAs have been discovered. In general, the ncRNA classes are subdivided into two groups—short and long ncRNAs—based on their nucleotide lengths, using an arbitrary cutoff of 200 bases.[58] Other than miRNAs, short ncRNAs that have been described include small interfering RNAs (siRNAs), which are 21 to 22 nucleotides long and are produced by Dicer cleavage of perfectly complementary double-stranded RNA molecules. siRNAs complex with certain Argonaute proteins and are involved in gene regulation, transposon control, and viral defense.[58] Piwi-interacting RNAs (piRNAs) are 26 to 30 nucleotides long and function in the germline to regulate transposon activity and the chromatin state.[58] piRNAs are derived not from Dicer cleavage but from successive Argonaute cleavage of long ncRNAs. Promoter-associated RNAs (PASRs) and transcription initiation RNAs (tiRNAs) are 20 to 200 nucleotides and 18 nucleotides long, respectively.[58] They are transcribed from promoters and transcription start sites and may be involved in regulating gene expression.

Long ncRNAs include a broad range of transcripts longer than 200 nucleotides and may be as long as 100 kb.[42,58] Some of these long ncRNAs could be 5′ capped, 3′ polyadenylated, and spliced like mRNAs. Because this is a heterogeneous group of transcripts, their reported functions are wide ranging and include modulation of chromatin architecture, regulation of gene expression, and others.[42,58] Long ncRNAs have been shown to regulate expression of protein-coding genes by modulating histone methylation and chromatin accessibility.[58] Long ncRNAs may exert biological effects directly or as an intermediary by acting as the precursor of multiple small ncRNAs. For example, the better known long ncRNA, *XIST*, is a transcript that is expressed exclusively from the inactive X chromosome with a key role in initiating the process of X chromosome inactivation. *XIST* literally coats the X chromosome that is destined to be inactivated and suppresses transcriptional activity.[36] However, besides acting directly, the corresponding transcript in mice, *Xist*, has been shown to anneal with its antisense partner, *Tsix*, another long ncRNA. The *Xist-Tsix* duplex is further cleaved by Dicer to produce siRNAs, which, in turn, are involved in epigenetic modifications that maintain gene silencing on the inactive X chromosome.[46] In summary, much remains to be learned about the roles of ncRNAs in physiology and pathology.

BEYOND THE NUCLEAR GENOME

The Mitochondrial Genome

Up to this point, we have focused our attention on the nuclear genome only. Yet, in fact, it is not the only genome in the cell; the mitochondrial genome is the other important genetic component of eukaryotic cells. The human mitochondrial genome is a circular piece of DNA 16.5 kb in length. Mitochondrial DNA is transmitted between generations by maternal inheritance, with the mitochondria coming from the oocytes and not (usually) from sperm. Multiple copies of mitochondrial DNA are present within each mitochondrion, and each cell contains a variable number of mitochondria, depending on the energy requirements of the particular cell type. Thus certain cell types may contain up to several thousand copies of mitochondrial DNA. This greater abundance, compared with that of nuclear DNA, makes mitochondrial DNA attractive for tests for which sample DNA is limited (e.g., crime scenes, pathogen detection, paleontology). Mitochondrial DNA is double-stranded for most of its length, except at the replication and transcription control region (the D-loop). Unlike the nuclear genome, the mitochondrial genome is not packaged into nucleosomal units. Instead, it has a unique structural organization. It encodes for 13 polypeptides, all involved in the oxidative phosphorylation pathway; two ribosomal RNAs (rRNAs); and all of the 22 tRNAs required for mitochondrial protein synthesis. Several other proteins are also required for normal mitochondrial function and are encoded by nuclear genes.

The mutation rate of mitochondrial DNA is 10 to 20 times higher than that of nuclear DNA. This high rate has been viewed as resulting from the poor fidelity of mitochondrial DNA polymerase. Germline mutations in the mitochondrial genome generally lead to neurodegenerative and/or myopathic disease, such as MELAS (myopathy, encephalopathy, lactic acidosis, and strokelike episodes) and Leber's hereditary optic neuropathy. Somatic mutations, on the other hand, are associated with aging and cancer development.[61] Consequent to the accumulation of sequence variations, more than one population of mitochondrial DNA sequences may be present in a cell. This state is termed *heteroplasmy* as opposed to *homoplasmy*, in which the cell contains a homogeneous population of mitochondrial genomes. When genetic analysis is performed for mitochondrial DNA, a note of caution is warranted on potential problems related to the presence of nuclear pseudogenes, which are DNA segments in the nuclear genome with significant homology to the mitochondrial genome.[64] The close resemblance of the nuclear and mitochondrial DNA segments may result in false-positive detection of mitochondrial DNA sequences; thus the specificity of polymerase chain reaction (PCR) systems for mitochondrial DNA detection needs to be carefully evaluated. Disorders associated with mitochondrial DNA and tests for the disorders are discussed in Chapter 40.

Circulating Nucleic Acids

Besides being confined within cellular boundaries, nucleic acid molecules are present in the blood circulation. It is now known that cell-free DNA and RNA molecules exist in human plasma. DNA, RNA, miRNA, and methylated DNA sequences derived from tumors, the unborn fetus, transplant donors, and traumatized tissues have been found in the plasma of cancer patients, pregnant women, transplant recipients, and patients suffering acute pathologies, respectively. Because cell-free nucleic acid molecules could be sampled simply through collection of a peripheral blood sample, the potential for developing molecular diagnostic applications based on their detection is vast. For details, the reader is referred to Chapter 45.

UNDERSTANDING OUR GENOME

Evident from the discussion so far, our understanding of the structure and function of the human genome has vastly expanded over the past decade. This is a consequence of the availability of high-throughput technologies that allow scientists to study almost every aspect of the human genome on a genome-wide scale. For example, both sequencing and hybridization techniques that allow the interrogation of nucleic acid pools from the entire genome have been extensively employed in research. In terms of sequencing, the so-called next-generation sequencers decode millions to billions of nucleotide fragments in a massively parallel fashion and are capable of producing giga bases of sequence output in a matter of days.[43] Regarding hybridization techniques, high-density microarrays with probes carpeting the entire genome, referred to as *tiling arrays*, are readily available.[18] Both sequencing and hybridization techniques can be coupled with various sample preparation protocols for analysis of pools of DNA, RNA, or complementary DNA (DNA generated by reverse-transcribing RNA) from the entire genome or subsets enriched with exon sequences, transcription factor–binding sites, methylated CpG sites, short RNAs, polyadenylated RNAs, and so on. Each of these experiments generates vast quantities of data. Basic management and analysis and further interpretation of such large data sets require the use of high-throughput computing. Hence, the field of bioinformatics has flourished and become an essential and fundamental component of life science research.[48]

The first of the whole genome scale project tackled by humankind was the Human Genome Project. It is the biggest biological project completed to date. Apart from its ambitious goal of deciphering the 3 billion base pairs that make up the human genetic code, it also represents a model for the planning, organization, and execution of large-scale biological projects.[7,8] The first serious discussion of the feasibility of such a project can be traced back to the mid-1980s. It was visionary of early proponents to conceive of the project before the advent of high-throughput sequencing technologies. In fact, the proposal was suggested just years after the invention of DNA sequencing in 1977. Based on technology available at the time, sequencing of the human genome would be a mammoth task, requiring a multinational effort. In 1988, a special committee of the U.S. National Research Council of the U.S. National Academy of Sciences formulated a 15-year human genome project, costing some $200 million a year. A genetic map with 1cM resolution was accomplished in September 1994. A physical map involving 52,000 sequence-tagged sites (STSs) was completed in October 1998. The final journey to completion of this project was marked by a highly publicized race between a publicly funded group of investigators and a private effort. The public effort, undertaken by the International Human Genome Sequencing Consortium, consisted of investigators from 20 centers located in six countries: the United States, the United Kingdom, Japan, China, France, and Germany. Completion of a draft sequence was announced on June 26, 2000, and it was published in two landmark papers, one from the public team and one from the private team, in February 2001.[33,60] The final sequence was accomplished in April 2003, with 99.99% sequencing accuracy.

The Human Genome Project has far reaching implications. Technologically, it accelerated the pace of development of sequencing technologies, computational tools for alignment of stretches of DNA reads, and organization of the data. Biologically, the human race has produced a copy of its genetic code. However, many more questions stem from having the reference human genome sequence. For example, how different is the genome between individuals? With the reduction in the cost of genome sequencing and a reduction in its technical complexity, sequencing of the genomes of a handful of individuals, including that performed by Watson[63] and Venter,[37] the pioneers of the Human Genome Project, has been completed recently.[37,50,62,63] Cross-comparisons have been made between the sequences of these genomes.

To enhance understanding of human genomic diversity on a broader scale, two large-scale projects were launched. The first one, the International HapMap Project, was launched to study heritable variations (i.e., polymorphisms, patterns of linkage disequilibrium, and haplotypes) across the human genome.[15,55] The HapMap Project primarily focuses on one class of genome variations, namely, single-nucleotide polymorphisms (SNPs). Cataloguing genetic variations between different ethnic populations would help one to understand the ancestral relationships between those populations. Once identified, a catalog of SNPs is also useful in providing landmarks of genomic locations for identification of disease-causing genes.[31] If an SNP allele is found to be associated with a particular disease, the SNP allele could further serve as a marker for assessment of an individual's susceptibility (statistical probability) of developing said disease.

The second project, the 1000 Genomes Project, also aims to study genomic diversity and disease-causing genes in humans.[56] The approach is based on whole genome sequencing of 1000 individuals, and the analysis is not limited to SNPs. Most recently, researchers have embarked on another approach to identify disease-causing genes through whole genome sequencing of families.[40,54] This approach entails the comparison of genomic sequences between affected and unaffected relatives within families known to propagate a hereditary disease under investigation.

After the alphabets of the human genome have been spelled out, another obvious follow-up would be to decode the meaning of the 3 billion nucleotides (i.e., the functional aspects of the human genome). This led to the launch of the Encyclopedia of DNA Elements (ENCODE) Project (http://www.genome.gov/ENCODE/), which aims to identify all functional elements within the human genome. A feasibility study targeting 1% of the human genome has been done.[4] Data from just this 1% of the genome have already led to many surprises that overturned many of our earlier simplistic views of the genome. Just to name a few of these surprises, as discussed earlier, other than the 1 to 2% of the genome that was previously annotated as protein-coding, we have come to realize that much of the entire genome is transcribed. Promoters that activate transcription are not limited to the 5′ ends of genes but instead are distributed at various locations of the transcription unit. Transcription takes place on both sense and antisense strands with highly overlapping units. Such new information redefines many previously established concepts including very fundamental ones, for example, what is a gene?[17,49] Our renewed understanding has brought about our appreciation of the highly sophisticated and complex nature of the workings of the human genome. All this new information is facilitated by the advent of high-throughput technologies, as discussed earlier. Our macroscopic view of some functional aspects of the human genome is now improving. However, a long journey lies ahead until we can attain a full understanding of each of the specific cellular and molecular mechanisms. Although our current understanding of the wonders of the genome is very limited, it is hoped that ultimately, humankind will have a better grasp of the causative mechanisms of pathologies to facilitate our efforts in predicting, diagnosing, monitoring, and treating disease.

Other large-scale projects that researchers are currently tackling include the Human Epigenome Project, which aims to identify, catalog, and interpret genome-wide DNA methylation patterns of all human genes in all major tissues.[12] This would represent yet another major challenge because only one reference human genome is known and many methylomes are present, given the different DNA methylation profiles between cells.[35] Besides genetic polymorphisms such as SNPs, it is now known that structural variations between individuals are characterized by comparatively large regions of gains and losses in DNA and are known as *copy number variations*. Hence, a copy number variation project aims to catalog and interpret the functional implications of copy number varations.[52]

In conclusion, our understanding of the human genome will continue to expand at an unimaginable rate. This will continue to drive changes in the way we practice medicine and diagnostics. An emerging theme shows that each individual is a unique being, and much heterogeneity is seen even within the same disease entity. Thus, it is possible that personalized medicine with individualized therapies will be the standard of the future.[20]

REFERENCES

1. Aleman EA, Lamichhane R, Rueda D. Exploring RNA folding one molecule at a time. Curr Opin Chem Biol 2008;12:647-54.
2. Allshire RC, Karpen GH. Epigenetic regulation of centromeric chromatin: old dogs, new tricks? Nat Rev Genet 2008;9:923-37.
3. Banerjee R, Chen S, Dare K, Gilreath M, Praetorius-Ibba M, Raina M, et al. tRNAs: cellular barcodes for amino acids. FEBS Lett 2010;584: 387-95.
4. Birney E, Stamatoyannopoulos JA, Dutta A, Guigo R, Gingeras TR, Margulies EH, et al. Identification and analysis of functional elements in 1% of the human genome by the ENCODE pilot project. Nature 2007;447:799-816.
5. Blasco MA. Telomeres and human disease: ageing, cancer and beyond. Nat Rev Genet 2005;6:611-22.
6. Chim SS, Shing TK, Hung EC, Leung TY, Lau TK, Chiu RW, et al. Detection and characterization of placental microRNAs in maternal plasma. Clin Chem 2008;54:482-90.
7. Collins FS, Green ED, Guttmacher AE, Guyer MS. A vision for the future of genomics research. Nature 2003;422:835-47.
8. Collins FS, Morgan M, Patrinos A. The human genome project: lessons from large-scale biology. Science 2003;300:286-90.
9. Corpet A, Almouzni G. Making copies of chromatin: the challenge of nucleosomal organization and epigenetic information. Trends Cell Biol 2009;19:29-41.
10. Cortez MA, Calin GA. MicroRNA identification in plasma and serum: a new tool to diagnose and monitor diseases. Expert Opin Biol Ther 2009;9:703-11.
11. Czech B, Zhou R, Erlich Y, Brennecke J, Binari R, Villalta C, et al. Hierarchical rules for Argonaute loading in Drosophila. Mol Cell 2009;36:445-56.
12. Eckhardt F, Lewin J, Cortese R, Rakyan VK, Attwood J, Burger M, et al. DNA methylation profiling of human chromosomes 6, 20 and 22. Nat Genet 2006;38:1378-85.
13. Esteller M. Cancer epigenomics: DNA methylomes and histone-modification maps. Nat Rev Genet 2007;8:286-98.
14. Faghihi MA, Wahlestedt C. Regulatory roles of natural antisense transcripts. Nat Rev Mol Cell Biol 2009;10:637-43.
15. Frazer KA, Ballinger DG, Cox DR, Hinds DA, Stuve LL, Gibbs RA, et al. A second generation human haplotype map of over 3.1 million SNPs. Nature 2007;449:851-61.
16. Friedman JM, Jones PA. MicroRNAs: critical mediators of differentiation, development and disease. Swiss Med Wkly 2009;139: 466-72.
17. Gerstein MB, Bruce C, Rozowsky JS, Zheng D, Du J, Korbel JO, et al. What is a gene, post-ENCODE? History and updated definition. Genome Res 2007;17:669-81.
18. Gregory BD, Belostotsky DA. Whole-genome microarrays: applications and technical issues. Methods Mol Biol 2009;553:39-56.
19. Grewal SI, Jia S. Heterochromatin revisited. Nat Rev Genet 2007;8:35-46.
20. Guttmacher AE, McGuire AL, Ponder B, Stefansson K. Personalized genomic information: preparing for the future of genetic medicine. Nat Rev Genet 2010;11:161-5.
21. Hall PA, Reis-Filho JS, Tomlinson IP, Poulsom R. An introduction to genes, genomes and disease. J Pathol 2010;220:109-13.
22. Illingworth R, Kerr A, Desousa D, Jorgensen H, Ellis P, Stalker J, et al. A novel CpG island set identifies tissue-specific methylation at developmental gene loci. PLoS Biol 2008;6:e22.
23. Jiang C, Pugh BF. Nucleosome positioning and gene regulation: advances through genomics. Nat Rev Genet 2009;10:161-72.
24. Jones PA, Baylin SB. The fundamental role of epigenetic events in cancer. Nat Rev Genet 2002;3:415-28.
25. Jones PA, Liang G. Rethinking how DNA methylation patterns are maintained. Nat Rev Genet 2009;10:805-11.
26. Juven-Gershon T, Hsu JY, Theisen JW, Kadonaga JT. The RNA polymerase II core promoter—the gateway to transcription. Curr Opin Cell Biol 2008;20:253-9.
27. Kapranov P, Cheng J, Dike S, Nix DA, Duttagupta R, Willingham AT, et al. RNA maps reveal new RNA classes and a possible function for pervasive transcription. Science 2007;316:1484-8.
28. Kapranov P, Willingham AT, Gingeras TR. Genome-wide transcription and the implications for genomic organization. Nat Rev Genet 2007;8: 413-23.
29. Khorasanizadeh S. The nucleosome: from genomic organization to genomic regulation. Cell 2004;116:259-72.
30. Kloc A, Martienssen R. RNAi, heterochromatin and the cell cycle. Trends Genet 2008;24:511-7.
31. Ku CS, Loy EY, Pawitan Y, Chia KS. The pursuit of genome-wide association studies: where are we now? J Hum Genet 2010;55: 195-206.
32. Kumar D. Genomic medicine: a new frontier of medicine in the twenty first century. Genomic Med 2007;1:3-7.
33. Lander ES, Linton LM, Birren B, Nusbaum C, Zody MC, Baldwin J, et al. Initial sequencing and analysis of the human genome. Nature 2001;409:860-921.
34. Latham JA, Dent SY. Cross-regulation of histone modifications. Nat Struct Mol Biol 2007;14:1017-24.
35. Laurent L, Wong E, Li G, Huynh T, Tsirigos A, Ong CT, et al. Dynamic changes in the human methylome during differentiation. Genome Res 2010;20:320-31.
36. Leeb M, Steffen PA, Wutz A. X chromosome inactivation sparked by non-coding RNAs. RNA Biol 2009;6:94-9.
37. Levy S, Sutton G, Ng PC, Feuk L, Halpern AL, Walenz BP, et al. The diploid genome sequence of an individual human. PLoS Biol 2007;5: e254.
38. Lobanov AV, Kryukov GV, Hatfield DL, Gladyshev VN. Is there a twenty third amino acid in the genetic code? Trends Genet 2006;22: 357-60.
39. Loeb LA, Monnat RJ Jr. DNA polymerases and human disease. Nat Rev Genet 2008;9:594-604.
40. Lupski JR, Reid JG, Gonzaga-Jauregui C, Rio Deiros D, Chen DC, Nazareth L, et al. Whole-genome sequencing in a patient with Charcot-Marie-Tooth neuropathy. N Engl J Med 2010;362:1181-91.
41. Margulies M, Egholm M, Altman WE, Attiya S, Bader JS, Bemben LA, et al. Genome sequencing in microfabricated high-density picolitre reactors. Nature 2005;437:376-80.
42. Mercer TR, Dinger ME, Mattick JS. Long non-coding RNAs: insights into functions. Nat Rev Genet 2009;10:155-9.
43. Metzker ML. Sequencing technologies—the next generation. Nat Rev Genet 2010;11:31-46.
44. Mohn F, Schubeler D. Genetics and epigenetics: stability and plasticity during cellular differentiation. Trends Genet 2009;25:129-36.
45. Munroe SH, Zhu J. Overlapping transcripts, double-stranded RNA and antisense regulation: a genomic perspective. Cell Mol Life Sci 2006;63: 2102-18.
46. Ogawa Y, Sun BK, Lee JT. Intersection of the RNA interference and X-inactivation pathways. Science 2008;320:1336-41.
47. Olena AF, Patton JG. Genomic organization of microRNAs. J Cell Physiol 2010;222:540-5.
48. Ostrowski J, Wyrwicz LS. Integrating genomics, proteomics and bioinformatics in translational studies of molecular medicine. Expert Rev Mol Diagn 2009;9:623-30.
49. Pesole G. What is a gene? An updated operational definition. Gene 2008;417:1-4.
50. Pushkarev D, Neff NF, Quake SR. Single-molecule sequencing of an individual human genome. Nat Biotechnol 2009;27:847-52.
51. Rando OJ, Chang HY. Genome-wide views of chromatin structure. Annu Rev Biochem 2009;78:245-71.

52. Redon R, Ishikawa S, Fitch KR, Feuk L, Perry GH, Andrews TD, et al. Global variation in copy number in the human genome. Nature 2006;444:444-54.
53. Reymond C, Beaudoin JD, Perreault JP. Modulating RNA structure and catalysis: lessons from small cleaving ribozymes. Cell Mol Life Sci 2009;66:3937-50.
54. Roach JC, Glusman G, Smit AF, Huff CD, Hubley R, Shannon PT, et al. Analysis of genetic inheritance in a family quartet by whole-genome sequencing. Science 2010;328:636-9.
55. Sabeti PC, Varilly P, Fry B, Lohmueller J, Hostetter E, Cotsapas C, et al. Genome-wide detection and characterization of positive selection in human populations. Nature 2007;449:913-8.
56. Siva N. 1000 Genomes Project. Nat Biotechnol 2008;26:256.
57. Suzuki MM, Bird A. DNA methylation landscapes: provocative insights from epigenomics. Nat Rev Genet 2008;9:465-76.
58. Taft RJ, Pang KC, Mercer TR, Dinger M, Mattick JS. Non-coding RNAs: regulators of disease. J Pathol 2010;220:126-39.
59. Thomas MC, Chiang CM. The general transcription machinery and general cofactors. Crit Rev Biochem Mol Biol 2006;41:105-78.
60. Venter JC, Adams MD, Myers EW, Li PW, Mural RJ, Sutton GG, et al. The sequence of the human genome. Science 2001;291:1304-51.
61. Wallace DC, Fan W, Procaccio V. Mitochondrial energetics and therapeutics. Annu Rev Pathol 2010;5:297-348.
62. Wang J, Wang W, Li R, Li Y, Tian G, Goodman L, et al. The diploid genome sequence of an Asian individual. Nature 2008;456:60-5.
63. Wheeler DA, Srinivasan M, Egholm M, Shen Y, Chen L, McGuire A, et al. The complete genome of an individual by massively parallel DNA sequencing. Nature 2008;452:872-6.
64. Woischnik M, Moraes CT. Pattern of organization of human mitochondrial pseudogenes in the nuclear genome. Genome Res 2002;12:885-93.

CHAPTER 38

Genomes and Nucleic Acid Alterations

Carl T. Wittwer, M.D., Ph.D., and Noriko Kusukawa, Ph.D.

Molecular diagnostics focuses on medically important sequence variations within a background of complex genomic structure. This chapter reviews the organization of human, bacterial, viral, and fungal genomes and the spectrum of variations in nucleic acids that are of medical concern.

HUMAN GENOME

Each human cell contains two copies of a 3 billion member sequence code of nucleic acids on 46 chromosomes.[4,5,12] Box 38-1 lists statistics for the human genome and the types of variations that are important in clinical diagnostics.

Three quarters of human DNA is intergenic, or between genes. More than 60% of this intergenic sequence consists of "parasitic" DNA regions of transposable elements 100 to 11,000 bases in length. Between 2 million and 3 million of these elements are present in each copy of the genome. They contribute to genetic recombination and chromosome structure and provide an evolutionary record of sequence variation and selection.

Segmental duplications constitute 5.3% of the human genome. They are over 1 kilobase (a thousand bases, or kb) in length and have a sequence identity of at least 90%; they are not transposable. Segmental duplications are common in the human genome and are prone to deletion and/or rearrangement, often with medical consequences.

Intergenic DNA carries most of the simple sequence repeats (SSRs) present in the genome. These repeats are known as *microsatellites* or *short tandem repeats (STRs)* when the repeat unit is 1 to 13 bases, and *minisatellites* or *variable number of tandem repeats (VNTRs)* when the repeat unit is 14 to 500 bases. SSRs are critical markers in genetic linkage studies and in forensic or medical identity testing. They are formed by slippage during replication and are highly polymorphic between individuals. The most common SSRs are dinucleotide repeats, such as ACACAC and ATATAT. On average, approximately one SSR occurs every 2000 bases.

Approximately 2% of DNA is required to maintain the structure of chromosomes and is located at chromosome centers (centromeres) and ends (telomeres). Centromeric DNA consists of many tandem copies of nearly identical 171 base pair (bp) repeats encompassing 0.24 to 5.0 Mb per chromosome. Each chromosome end is capped with several kb of the telomeric 6 base repeat TTAGGG.

Although intergenic DNA does not code for protein and was originally considered "junk," much of this DNA is transcribed to RNA, producing a complex "transcriptome" network of RNA control elements whose function and mechanics are active areas of investigation.[1]

One quarter of the human genome consists of genes. A total of 20,000 to 25,000 genes are found in the human genome. The average gene covers 27 kb, but only about 1300 of these bases code for amino acid sequences. The primary RNA transcript is processed by splicing to retain exons that are interspersed throughout the gene and have a higher GC content than noncoding regions. On average, 95% of a gene is spliced out as introns, retaining a mean of 10.4 exons, of which 9.1 are translated into proteins. Exons make up only 1.9% of the total genome, with 1.1% of the genome coding for proteins. Some important genes are present in many copies, so that overall protein expression is not affected if a chance variation occurs in one copy. If extra copies of genes lose their function, they are known as *pseudogenes*. At least as many pseudogenes as functional genes are present in the human genome. It is important to distinguish pseudogenes from functional genes because sequence variations in pseudogenes are seldom of clinical importance.

Even though 99% of the genome does not code for protein, most of it is transcribed into noncoding RNA. At least 93% of the genome is transcribed,[1] producing more than 10 times the amount of RNA that is produced from the coding segments of genes.[2] Both strands of DNA may be transcribed, and long noncoding transcripts may overlap coding regions, producing a complex transcriptome of functional RNA molecules that may variably regulate transcription of coding regions, RNA processing, mRNA stability, translation, protein stability, and secretion. In addition to long noncoding RNA, ribosomal RNA, and transfer RNA, specific classes of noncoding RNAs include small nuclear RNAs critical for splicing,

BOX 38-1 The Human Genome and Its Sequence Variation

- The human genome
  - 3.08 billion base pairs in 24 chromosomes
  - 23 chromosome pairs (46 to 244 million base pairs per chromosome)

75% Intergenic Sequences

Transposable elements	45%
Segmental duplications	5%
Simple sequence repeats [SSRs, short tandem repeats (STRs)]	3%
Structural (centromeres, telomeres)	2%
Other	20%

25% Genes That Code for Proteins

Introns	23%
Exons	1.9%
• Coding segments	1.2%
• Untranslated regions	0.7%
Number of genes	20,000 to 25,000
Average gene	27,000 base pairs 10.4 exons with 9.1 that are transcribed 1340 bases coding for 446 amino acids

- Sequence variants
  - 99.9% identity (1 difference every 1250 bases between randomly selected haploid genomes)

Single-nucleotide polymorphisms (SNPs): identified every 100 to 300 bases

Noncoding	97%
Average number within a gene	126
Average number within the coding region of a gene	5

Copy number variants (CNVs): involve 5 to 12% of the genome

Disease-causing variants

SNPs	68%
• Missense (amino acid substitution)	45%
• Nonsense (termination)	11%
• Splicing	10%
• Regulatory	2%
Small insertions and/or deletions	24%
Structural variants (copy number variations, inversions, translocations, rearrangements, repeats)	8%

- Epigenetic alterations
  - Variable initiation and alternative splicing
  - Cytosine methylation
- Histone phosphorylation, methylation, acetylation

Data compiled from the Human Gene Mutation Database[11] and the International Human Genome Sequencing Consortium.[4,12]

small nucleolar RNAs that modify rRNA, telomerase RNAs for maintenance of telomeres, small interfering RNAs, and microRNAs that regulate gene expression.[8,9]

MicroRNAs (or miRNAs) are noncoding but functional single-stranded RNAs that are about 22 bases long and are expressed in a tissue-specific manner. They are initially transcribed as longer precursors that undergo two rounds of truncations as they are transported from nucleus to cytoplasm in the cell. The mature miRNA is then integrated into a protein complex called the *RNA-induced silencing complex*, which regulates translation of mRNA. MicroRNAs hybridize to a 6 to 8 base sequence in the 3′ untranslated region of a target mRNA and inhibit mRNA expression, by mRNA degradation if the remaining bases are perfectly complementary, or by blocking of translation if they are imperfectly complementary. More than 700 different miRNAs have been reported,[3] and sequences encoding for miRNA have been found on every chromosome except the Y chromosome.

Variation Within the Human Genome

Consider the genome as a book. Nucleotides are the individual letters, and three bases make up each word as an amino acid codon. The words are organized into sentences or exons that are separated by periods or introns. Each sentence is further organized into paragraphs or genes. Many paragraphs constitute a chapter or chromosome, and several chapters make up a book or genome. If the DNA of any two individuals is compared, on average one spelling difference is noted every 1250 bases (i.e., approximately 99.9% of the sequence is identical between randomly chosen copies of the genome). However, different individuals (copies of the same book) vary in a subtler way. Some of the pages are copied more than once and may be scattered throughout the book. Such copy number variants involve a greater amount of text than the spelling differences, with 0.5% of the genome differing on average between two individuals when 50 kb pages are considered,[7] that is, between individuals, at least five times as many bases are affected by copy number changes than by small sequence differences.

Any sequence change (compared with a reference sequence) is called a *sequence variant* or *alteration.* If a sequence variant or alteration is present in at least 1% of a population, it is a *polymorphism.* Many sequence variants, alterations, and polymorphisms in the genome do not affect human health and are benign or silent. For example, most copy number variations do not cause disease. Furthermore, most single-base changes [also known as *single-nucleotide polymorphisms (SNPs)*] and SSRs found between genes are seldom associated with disease. Similarly, most of the SNPs within introns, except for splicing and regulatory variants, are not known to affect gene function. In addition, some of the SNPs within exons are silent alterations that do not code for a change in amino acid sequence because of the redundancy in the genetic code. Still other SNPs in exons code for amino acid changes that do not affect protein function. Even such silent SNPs nonetheless may be of considerable interest as genetic markers.

The most commonly observed sequence variations are SNPs. Millions of SNPs have been described, and many new SNPs continue to be reported. Some SNPs are common in the population, with allele frequencies of 0.1 to 0.5 (i.e., present in 10 to 50 of every 100 haploid copies studied), although other single-base changes are very rare. Although single-base variants have been identified every 100 to 300 bases, many of these are not found frequently in the population. A vast majority of SNPs (97%) occur in noncoding regions; only 3% of SNPs are within coding sequences.

Although SNPs are the most common sequence variant, copy number variants cover more of the genome than SNPs. These copy number variants (CNVs) occur in stretches of DNA that may range from 100 bases up to several Mb (megabases, or million bases) in size. CNVs may be duplicated in tandem or may involve complex gains or losses of homologous sequences at multiple sites in the genome. CNV regions exist in every chromosome and involve 5 to 12% of the human genome.[7,10] Most CNVs are inherited and biallelic, similar to SNPs.[7] More than 6000 CNV loci have been reported, and many of them overlap with genes. Individuals differ on average at more than 200 CNV loci, and these overlap the transcribed regions of more than 100 genes.[7]

Variations That Cause Human Disease

Sequence alterations that are known to cause disease are often called *mutations*, although the more cumbersome term, *disease-causing variant*, is more politically correct and precise. About 68% of known disease-causing variants are SNPs (see Box 38-1). Most of the remaining disease-causing variants (24%) are small insertions and/or deletions. However, 8% involve more complex sequence changes, including copy number variants, inversions, balanced translocations, repeat expansions, and rearrangements.

Single-Nucleotide Polymorphisms

Most SNPs that cause disease are missense and result in an amino acid substitution, whereas significantly fewer are nonsense variants that result in premature polypeptide chain termination. Approximately 10% of disease-causing variants are SNPs that affect splicing sites and result in altered concatenation of coding sequences. Finally, less than 2% of known disease-causing variants are SNPs that affect the regulatory efficiency of transcription by altering promoter and/or enhancer regions in introns or the stability of the RNA transcript.

Small Insertions and/or Deletions

Small insertion and/or deletion variants account for about 24% of nucleic acid sequence alterations that cause disease. An *insertion* refers to the presence of extra bases, whereas *deletion* implies the absence of certain bases in comparison with a reference sequence. Insertions and deletions often cause a shift in the codon reading frame, resulting in an altered amino acid sequence downstream of the variation; this is commonly followed by chain termination from a nonsense codon. A small *indel* is an insertion and a deletion at the same locus (for instance, TG is deleted and is replaced by AGGTC).

Structural Variants

The remaining 8% of variants that cause disease are mostly large structural anomalies, including copy number variations, inversions, balanced translocations, gene rearrangements (e.g., B- and T-cell gene rearrangements), and complex polymorphic loci related to health and disease [e.g., human leukocyte antigen (HLA)]. SSR expansions (e.g., increased numbers of STRs such as trinucleotide repeats) can also cause disease.

Interest in CNV in relation to disease has increased recently as the extent of variation has become clear.[13] CNVs can involve genes or contiguous sets of genes. When the normal dosage of the gene is two, but more than two functional copies of a gene are present, then the gene is "amplified." If a dosage-sensitive gene, such as HER-2-neu *(ERBB2)*, is amplified, this usually leads to overexpression of mRNA and protein, resulting in cellular abnormalities and possible progression to disease such as cancer. When the normal gene dosage is two, and loss of one of the functional copies of the gene occurs, disorders such as mental retardation and developmental delay may result. Structural variants can be determined by cytogenetic techniques, including karyotyping, fluorescent in situ hybridization, comparative genomic hybridization, and virtual karyotyping by SNP microarrays.

Haplotypes

Often, sequence variants are inherited together in a contiguous block, or haplotype. A schematic representation of alleles arranged as haplotypes is shown in Figure 38-1. Disease associations may depend not on any particular sequence variant but on the overall effect of several linked alleles that define the haplotype. For example, enzyme function depends on the haplotype that defines the amino acid sequence in the protein. When the haplotype linkage of alleles is strong, genotype determination at a single locus may identify the haplotype (and disease association) with high confidence. However, methods for determining the *cis* or *trans* phase of alleles are necessary when the haplotype linkage is weak and when the disease association and/or haplotype linkage is first being established. Haplotypes may be defined by the phases of many polymorphic loci.

Alterations in Hemizygous Genes and Mitochondrial DNA

Most human genetic material is present in two copies (on paired chromosomes), with the exception of the unpaired sex chromosome in males and genes on mitochondrial DNA. When mutations occur in single-copy *(hemizygous)* genes on the X or Y chromosomes in males, they lead to sex-linked

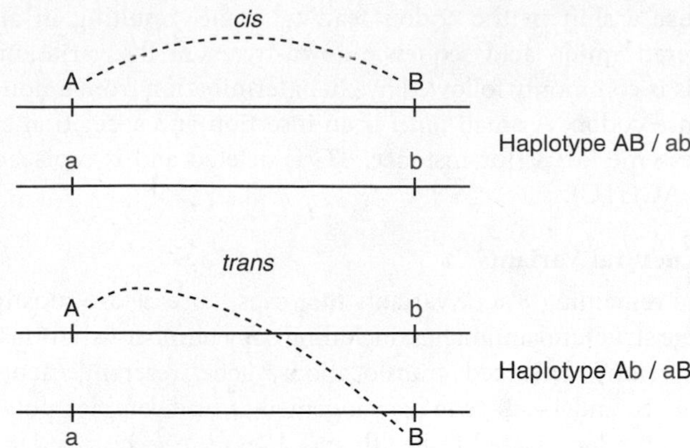

Figure 38-1 Schematic diagram of alleles arranged in haplotypes. Consider two polymorphic sites: one site is allele "A" or "a," the other is "B" or "b." Given a doubly heterozygous genotype *(A/a, B/b)* in a diploid organism, possible haplotypes are as follows: *AB/ab*, in which *A* and *B* are on the same chromosome (*cis* configuration shown on top), or *Ab/aB*, in which *A* and *B* are on different chromosomes (*trans* configuration shown on bottom).

disorders. In contrast, the 16,500 bp mitochondrial genome is present in more than 1000 copies per cell, constituting about 0.3% of human DNA. Allele fractions may vary over a wide range when all mitochondria in a cell are considered, that is, sequence variations in mitochondrial DNA are *heteroplasmic*, meaning that the ratio of wild-type to variant alleles within a cell can vary almost continuously, sometimes resulting in a wide range of symptoms even when only one sequence variant is involved.

Human Epigenetic Alterations

In addition to the sequence alterations considered previously, epigenetic alterations, including alternative splicing and methylation, may affect gene expression. Even though the number of genes may be limited to 20,000 to 25,000, variable transcription initiation and exon splicing are estimated to produce about 90,000 mRNA transcripts and protein products.

Methylation of cytosine to form 5-methylcytosine occurs frequently; about 70% of CpG dinucleotides in the human genome are methylated. Although not inherited, interest in this "5th base" has increased as correlations with cancer have been reported.[6] CpG islands are about 1000 bases in length and often are found near the 5′ ends of genes. These regions consist of clusters of CG dinucleotides that usually are not methylated in normal cells. However, CpG methylation correlates with condensed chromatin structure and promoter inactivation; an important example is seen in tumor suppressor genes.

DNA is associated with proteins in nucleosomes. Gene expression can be altered by histone phosphorylation, acetylation, and methylation. Our understanding of epigenetic alterations and their relation to disease is rapidly developing.

BACTERIAL GENOMES

Bacterial genomes are considerably less complex than human or other eukaryotic genomes. Common bacteria have only one chromosome, usually a circular DNA double helix of 4 million to 5 million bp—about 1000 times less than the amount of DNA in a human cell. About 90% of the DNA in bacteria codes for protein. No introns are present, but multiple small intergenic regions of repetitive sequences are dispersed throughout the genome. The common bacterium *Escherichia coli* contains about 4300 genes.

In addition to the large circular chromosome that carries essential genes, bacteria carry accessory genes in smaller circles of double-stranded DNA (dsDNA) known as *plasmids*. Plasmids range in size from 1000 to more than 1 million bp. Plasmids are important in molecular diagnostics because they often encode pathogenic factors and antibiotic resistance.

The bacterial repertoire of DNA can be altered by (1) gain or loss of plasmids; (2) single-base changes, small insertions, and/or deletions, as in eukaryotic genomes; and (3) larger segmental rearrangements, including inversions, deletions, and duplications. Some genes, such as those for ribosomal RNA, are present in many copies and have been used to identify different species of bacteria. In addition, the intergenic repetitive sequences serve as multiple targets for oligonucleotide probes, enabling the generation of unique DNA profiles or fingerprints for individual bacterial strains.

VIRAL GENOMES

Viral genomes are considerably less complex than bacterial genomes. Common viruses that infect humans vary in genome size from about 5000 to 250,000 bases, or from 20 to 1000 times less than the amount of nucleic acid in *E. coli*. Because viruses use the cellular machinery of the host, they do not need as many genes. Small viruses may encode only several genes, but larger viruses can encode hundreds. The viral genome consists of DNA or RNA, and the nucleic acid may be single stranded or double stranded, linear, or circular, with one or multiple fragments and/or copies per viral particle. As in bacteria, no introns are present. In fact, in some viruses, the exons overlap with different reading frames coding different products from the same nucleic acid sequence. Noncoding regions are usually present at the terminal ends of linear genomes. Repeat segments are often found as terminal or internal repeats and may be inverted.

Sequence alterations in viruses are common. Areas of high sequence variation may be interspersed between conserved domains. Higher frequencies of variation have been correlated with lower polymerase fidelity and may allow escape from antibody recognition and from antiviral drugs. Common sequence variants in viruses include single-base changes, insertions, and deletions. Sequence diversity within a viral species may be so great that consensus sequences for molecular typing are difficult to find.

FUNGAL GENOMES

Fungi are eukaryotes, and their genomes are more complex than the genomes of bacteria or viruses. Common fungi that cause human disease have genome sizes of 7.5 to 30 million bases and 8 to 14 chromosomes, as well as mitochondrial genomes. Some fungi have diploid genomes, and others have haploid genomes. Many of their genes have introns. For instance, *Aspergillus fumigatus* (a fungus that causes allergic reactions and systemic disease with a high mortality rate) has a haploid genome of about 30 million bases with more than 9900 predicted genes on eight chromosomes. Its genes are smaller than human genes, with an average length of 1400 bp and 2.8 exons per gene.[6] Some fungi such as *Pneumocystis jiroveci* (a yeastlike fungus that causes pneumonia) cannot be cultured, and the use of nucleic acid tests is helpful in detecting them.

REFERENCES

1. Amaral PP, Dinger ME, Mercer TR, Mattick JS. The eukaryotic genome as an RNA machine. Science 2008;319:1787-9.
2. Carninci P, Kasukawa T, Katayama S, Gough J, Frith MC, Maeda N, et al. The transcriptional landscape of the mammalian genome. Science 2005;309:1559-63.
3. Griffiths-Jones S, Saini HK, van Dongen S, Enright AJ. miRBase: tools for microRNA genomics. Nucleic Acids Res 2008;36:D154-8.
4. International Human Genome Consortium. Finishing the euchromatic sequence of the human genome. Nature 2004;431:931-45.
5. Lander ES, Linton LM, Birren B, Nusbaum C, Zody MC, Baldwin J, et al. Initial sequencing and analysis of the human genome. Nature 2001;409:860-921.
6. Lopez J, Percharde M, Coley HM, Webb A, Crook T. The context and potential of epigenetics in oncology. Br J Cancer 2009;100:571-7.
7. McCarroll SA, Kuruvilla FG, Korn JM, Cawley S, Nemesh J, Wysoker A, et al. Integrated detection and population-genetic analysis of SNPs and copy number variation. Nat Genet 2008;40: 1166-74.
8. Mendes Soares LM, Valcarcel J. The expanding transcriptome: the genome as the "Book of Sand." EMBO J 2006;25:923-31.
9. Mercer TR, Dinger ME, Mattick JS. Long non-coding RNAs: insights into functions. Nat Rev Genet 2009;10:155-9.
10. Redon R, Ishikawa S, Fitch KR, Feuk L, Perry GH, Andrews TD, et al. Global variation in copy number in the human genome. Nature 2006; 444:444-54.
11. Stenson PD, Mort M, Ball EV, Howells K, Phillips AD, Thomas NS, et al. The Human Gene Mutation database: 2008 update. Genome Med 2009;1:13.
12. Venter JC, Adams MD, Myers EW, Li PW, Mural RJ, Sutton GG, et al. The sequence of the human genome. Science 2001;291:1304-51.
13. Wain LV, Armour JA, Tobin MD. Genomic copy number variation, human health, and disease. Lancet 2009;15:15.

Genome Databases

NCBI
http://www.ncbi.nlm.nih.gov/sites/entrez?db=genome
Ensembl: http://www.ensembl.org/index.html
UCSC
http://genome.ucsc.edu/

Human Genes and Disease

OMIM
http://www.ncbi.nlm.nih.gov/omim

Sequence Databanks

NCBI GenBank
http://www.ncbi.nlm.nih.gov/Genbank/
EMBL-Bank
http://www.ebi.ac.uk/embl/
DDBJ
http://www.ddbj.nig.ac.jp/
MicroRNAs
http://microrna.sanger.ac.uk/sequences/index.shtml

Human Variation Databases

Mutation Database
http://www.hgmd.cf.ac.uk/ac/index.php
Structural Variants
http://projects.tcag.ca/variation/
Chromosome Imbalance
https://decipher.sanger.ac.uk/application/
SNPs
http://www.ncbi.nlm.nih.gov/SNP/index.html
Transposons
http://dbrip.brocku.ca/
Haplotypes (HapMap)
http://www.hapmap.org/

Nomenclature

HUGO Genes
http://www.genenames.org/
NGVS Mutations
http://www.hgvs.org/mutnomen/

CHAPTER 39

Nucleic Acid Isolation

*Rossa W. K. Chiu, M.B.B.S., Ph.D., F.H.K.A.M.(Pathology), F.R.C.P.A. and Y. M. Dennis Lo, M.A., D.M., D.Phil., F.R.C.P.,(Lond. & Edin.), F.R.C.Path., F.R.S.**

Many of the key advances in our understanding of DNA and RNA have been achieved by the study of purified nucleic acids. In a molecular diagnostic laboratory, some tests can be performed directly on biological fluids, but techniques for *isolation* of nucleic acids often are critical. Nucleic acid *isolation* refers to the process of separating DNA or RNA from its surrounding materials; nucleic acid *extraction* is the technique of removing DNA or RNA from surrounding materials. With the advent of the polymerase chain reaction (PCR), molecular analyses could be performed on a variety of specimens, including whole blood, plasma, serum, tissue biopsies, cultured cells, buccal swabs, cerebrospinal fluids, amniotic fluids, and paraffin-embedded tissues. Isolation of DNA and/or RNA is usually a key preliminary step in molecular analysis.[43]

SPECIMEN PRESERVATION

DNA- and RNA-specific nucleases (DNases and RNases, respectively) can degrade DNA and RNA molecules in biological specimens. Hence, specimens should be properly preserved before molecular analyses. DNA molecules are generally stable in specimens when stored at −80 °C. However, RNA molecules are much more fragile than DNA. This is because, unlike DNA, RNA is not protected by a stable double-helical conformation, and RNA is subject to alkaline hydrolysis via the 2′ hydroxyl group of its ribose moiety. In addition, RNases are ubiquitous and difficult to inactivate or denature. Hence, special attention should be paid when one undertakes operations on RNA.[12] Tissue specimens intended for RNA analysis should be processed promptly upon collection. One preservation method is to snap-freeze the specimens by liquid nitrogen. However, snap-frozen tissues are laborious to handle in the subsequent homogenization step (see later). For example, to minimize the exposure of RNA to RNases, the frozen tissues should be ground to a fine powder before denaturants are added. Moreover, to prevent the release of RNases from thawing cells, the tissues should be kept frozen during the grinding process; thus liquid nitrogen has to be added at intervals. Alternatively, RNA can be protected by incubating tissue specimens in preservation agents such as RNA*later* (Ambion/Applied Biosystems, Austin, Tex) and PrepProtect Stabilization Buffer (Miltenyi Biotec Inc., Auburn, Calif).[33] RNA molecules in such preserved tissues are stable at room temperature for up to a week.[22] Specimen handling and transportation procedures are thereby facilitated. The preserved tissues can be directly homogenized (see later) without further processing.

Blood is the most common specimen type in a diagnostic laboratory because it is more readily available than a biopsy specimen. During peripheral blood collection and processing, ex vivo changes in gene expression and RNA degradation continue to occur, and can affect subsequent analyses.[38] To overcome such problems, vacutainer tubes prefilled with preservation agents, such as those in the PAXgene Blood RNA System (PreAnalytiX GmbH, Hombrechtikon, Switzerland), are available for immediate stabilization of RNA profiles during blood collection.[50]

Plasma and serum are routinely used for circulating nucleic acid studies (see Chapter 45). Plasma DNA has been shown to be stable in unprocessed whole blood for up to 24 hours at room temperature.[45] Plasma RNA has also been shown to be stable in unprocessed whole blood when collected in tubes containing ethylenediaminetetraacetic acid (EDTA) for up to 24 hours at 4 °C.[45] However, in contrast to short-term storage, the concentration of circulating DNA in harvested serum specimens has been reported to decrease by 0.66 copies per milliliter for each month of storage.[25] More marked degradation upon long-term storage was observed for plasma RNA.[49] To protect RNA in plasma and serum during storage, several investigators have suggested mixing RNase-inhibitory agents, such as TRIzol LS (Invitrogen, Life Technologies, Carlsbad, Calif), with specimens before storage at −80 °C.[45,49]

In urine specimens, bacterial and fungal contamination as well as calcium oxalate crystal formation can influence the yield of downstream nucleic acid isolation. Hence, long-term storage of urine specimens with EDTA at −80 °C has been recommended to resolve contamination problems and to inhibit any possible nuclease activity in urine.[20,31,42]

*The authors thank Nancy B.Y. Tsui for assistance in the preparation of this chapter.

TISSUE HOMOGENIZATION AND CELL LYSIS

Homogenization refers to the breakdown of tissue into small fragments by mechanical or enzymatic means. Complete homogenization is essential for isolating nucleic acids with high quality and yield. For DNA isolation from soft tissues, homogenization is usually performed by incubating the specimens with digestion enzymes such as protease K at 56 °C overnight.[51] On the other hand, the roto/stator method is preferred for RNA isolation. This method involves mechanical disruption of tissues in lysis buffer, composed of phenol, sodium dodecyl sulfate, or guanidine salts (e.g., TRIzol from Invitrogen). The buffers not only lyse cells directly, they also inhibit RNase effectively during homogenization.[9]

DNA Isolation

Although various commercial protocols are available for DNA extraction, most protocols can be classified into one of a few categories that involve liquid- or solid-phase extraction. In general, solid-phase extraction methods are more commonly used because of the relative ease of operation, the ability to process large batches of specimens simultaneously, freedom from toxic chemicals, high reproducibility, and adaptability to automation. However, solution-based methods are still favored when large quantities of DNA or large sample volumes are involved.

For solution-based protocols, cellular debris and proteins are separated from the DNA fraction by solvent extraction through the use of solvents with different solubility constants. The well-known phenol-chloroform protocols are based on this principle. After centrifugation of the mixture of phenol-chloroform and sample lysate, proteins, lipids, carbohydrates, and cellular debris are separated from the DNA fraction and are settled in the bottom organic phase. DNA molecules contained in the upper aqueous phase are precipitated by ethanol and rehydrated with sterile distilled water or Tris-EDTA buffer (TE buffer). Because of the number of manual steps involved, the sample throughput of these solution-based methods is limited.

Solid-phase extraction methods are more robust and generally are based on the principle of DNA adsorption onto silica in the presence of chaotropic salts, such as guanidine thiocyanate, and ethanol.[3,37] The silica is typically coated onto membrane filters or magnetic particles. Silica-impregnated filters that are housed in plastic columns are the most commonly adopted format. DNA binds reversibly with silica, depending on the ionic strength of the environment.[41] After cell lysis and protein denaturation, DNA is precipitated by the addition of ethanol. The solution is then passed through the silica-impregnated filter, which binds and purifies DNA from other debris present in the ethanol solution. Centrifugation or vacuum manifolds can be used for the filtration step. The bound DNA is washed and subsequently eluted using nuclease-free water or low ionic strength buffers. Similarly, methods based on the use of silica-coated magnetic particles allow the isolation of ethanol-precipitated DNA by placing the solution under a magnetic field whereby DNA molecules adsorbed to the magnetic beads are retained. The DNA is subsequently eluted from the beads in low ionic strength buffer or water.

RNA Isolation

RNA analysis and therefore RNA extraction are required for studies on gene expression. Utmost care is needed to prevent RNase contamination during the process; this effort is aided by the use of RNase-free reagents, RNase-free plastic-ware, and decontamination of working surfaces and equipment with RNase-free detergents. Water treated with diethylpyrocarbonate (DEPC) for the inactivation of RNase is widely used. During the process of RNA purification, DNA digestion by DNase I is commonly incorporated as an additional step to avoid DNA contamination.

The underlying principles of RNA extraction are essentially identical to those of DNA isolation. Both solution- and solid-phase extraction protocols are available. The most commonly used solution-based method is guanidine thiocyanate-phenol-chloroform extraction.[9,10] Guanidine isothiocynate is a chaotropic agent used for protein denaturation while RNase activity is inhibited. In a mixture of guanidine isothiocynate, phenol (e.g., TRIzol from Invitrogen), sodium acetate, and chloroform in an acidic condition, total RNA is partitioned into the aqueous phase, and DNA molecules and proteins remain in the interphase and the organic phase, respectively. Total RNA in the aqueous phase is next precipitated by the addition of isopropanol. For solid-phase RNA extraction protocols, lysis/binding buffer includes chaotropic salts, such as guanidine isothiocyanate, to protect RNA. The ionic strength of the buffer is optimized to promote the binding of RNA molecules onto the silica matrix.

For specimens with high protein and lipid contents, such as plasma and serum, agglutination of lysed samples with the silica matrix can occur. In addition, genomic DNA present in the specimens competes with the RNA for binding to the silica matrix. These factors can adversely affect the isolation of RNA species that exist at trace amounts in the specimens. One such example is the extraction of cell-free fetal RNA in maternal plasma. To overcome these limitations, several investigators have developed a combined solution- and solid-phase RNA extraction protocol.[34,49] As an initial step, RNA molecules are separated from contaminants such as protein, lipid, and DNA by the TRIzol protocol. RNA molecules contained in the aqueous phase are then isolated by the silica-column method.

The guanidine thiocyanate-phenol-chloroform protocols are relevant to the isolation of total RNA, which comprises messenger RNA (mRNA), ribosomal RNA (rRNA), transfer RNA (tRNA), and small nuclear RNA. Protocols have been developed for the specific isolation of mRNA; these are based on capture of polyadenylated tails on the 3′ ends of mRNA by hybridization to cellulose-bound oligo(dT) molecules.[12] It is worth noting that most of the commercial silica-based kits are inefficient in extracting small nucleic acid species, such as microRNA. Because the binding efficiency of nucleic acids to the silica matrix is dependent on salt concentrations, pH, and the ethanol content of the washing buffer in a size-dependent manner, most commercial kits have optimized these parameters to isolate nucleic acids larger than 150 nucleotides. Hence, microRNA extraction should be performed by using the solution-based method (e.g., TRIzol protocol) or with a silica-column protocol that has been optimized for binding microRNA molecules (e.g., mirVana from Ambion).[32]

ASSESSMENT OF NUCLEIC ACID YIELD AND QUALITY

Nucleic acid molecules absorb ultraviolet light maximally at a wavelength of 260 nm owing almost entirely to the constituent bases. Thus, DNA or RNA yield can be quantified by spectrophotometric measurement of absorbance at 260 nm, with higher absorbance values indicating higher yield. For example, a solution containing 50 mg/L of pure double-stranded DNA has an absorbance of 1.0 at 260 nm. Purity can be evaluated by assessing the ratio of spectrophotometric absorbances at 260 nm and 280 nm (A260/A280). Absorbance ratios greater than 1.8 indicate minimal contamination with proteins. The sizes of the isolated genomic DNA can be estimated by gel electrophoresis. Good quality DNA extractions are generally associated with higher molecular weight fragments (Figure 39-1). Similarly, total RNA integrity can be assessed by estimating the size distribution of the extracted RNA and the appearances of the 18S and 28S rRNA peaks (Figure 39-2). Total RNA preparations of high quality generally have a 28S/18S peak ratio greater than 2.0. With RNase degradation, the RNA size distribution is shifted toward the smaller fragments with a reduction in the 28S/18S rRNA ratio (see Figure 39-2).

In assessment of the yield and quality of DNA/RNA extracts, electrophoretic methods provide better precision and more information regarding quality, for instance, the size distribution of the isolated DNA or RNA. Modern improvements in instrumentation have led to the development of spectrophotometric and electrophoretic systems that require only the input of microvolumes of extracted DNA/RNA for assessment. One spectrophotometer for this purpose uses only 1 μL of sample for the measurement of DNA or RNA concentrations ranging from 2 ng/μL to 3700 ng/μL (ND-1000 Spectrophotometer, NanoDrop Technologies, Wilmington, Del). Automated analyzers that use prefabricated chips with microfluidic channels and are designed for capillary electrophoresis of microvolumes of DNA and RNA have become available; one example is the Agilent 2100 Bioanalyzer (Agilent Technologies Inc., Santa Clara, Calif).[36] This system allows better estimation of sizes, qualities, and concentrations of DNA and RNA when compared with the conventional slab-gel electrophoresis method. For example, the RNA integrity number (RIN) is an RNA integrity score that is calculated based on the entire electropherogram generated by the Bioanalyzer rather than only the 18S and 28S rRNA peaks.[39] The RIN has been shown to be a better estimation of RNA quality when compared with the 28S/18S ratio method.[21] The RNA integrity score has been widely adopted in studies in which RNA quality is critical for the reliability of the experiment, such as for gene expression microarray analysis.[30]

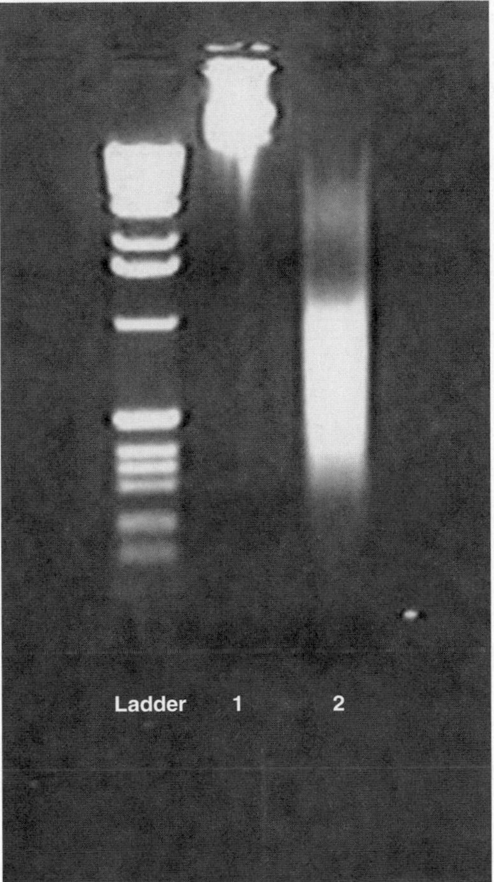

Figure 39-1 Assessment of DNA quality by gel electrophoresis. DNA extracted from two whole blood specimens was resolved on 1% agarose gel and compared with a molecular weight size marker *(ladder)*. High-quality DNA extractions are associated with high molecular weight fragments, as shown in *lane 1*. *Lane 2* illustrates DNA extracted from a degraded whole blood sample wherein the molecular weights of DNA fragments are much reduced.

STORAGE OF PURIFIED NUCLEIC ACIDS

Isolated DNA can be stored temporarily at 4 °C or at −20 °C, but gradual degradation occurs over time. For prolonged storage, DNA should be stored at −80 °C or as a precipitate in ethanol at −20 °C. Similarly, RNA should be stored as aqueous form or ethanol precipitate at −80 °C. If RNA samples are intended for repeated usage, they should be stored as small aliquots to avoid repeated freeze-thaw cycles for maintaining nucleic acid integrity.

AUTOMATED NUCLEIC ACID ISOLATION

Many molecular diagnostic protocols that were originally developed by research laboratories have now been adopted by clinical laboratories. For such adoption, additional

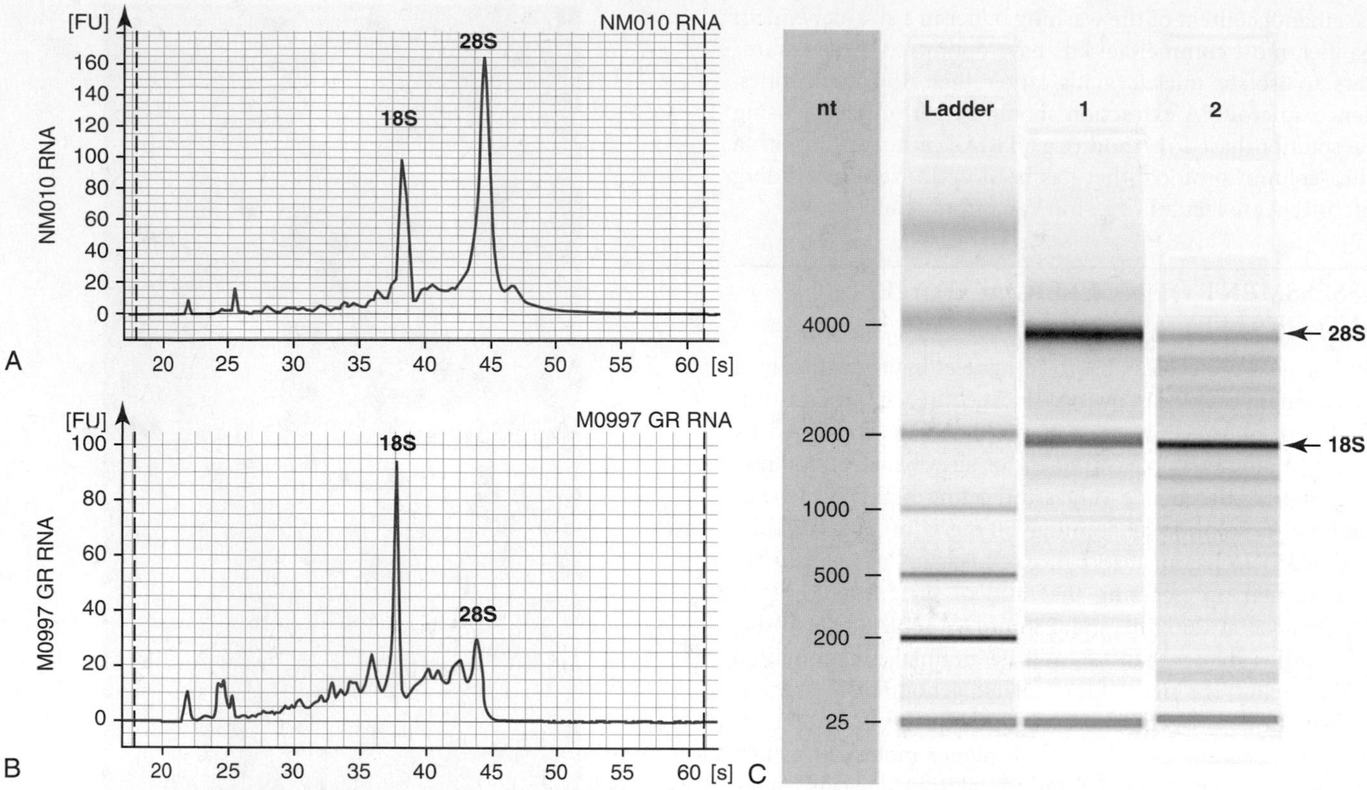

Figure 39-2 Assessment of total RNA quality by gel electrophoresis and densitometry. Total RNA extracted from two whole blood specimens was analyzed on the Agilent 2100 Bioanalyzer using the RNA 6000 Nano LabChip (Agilent Technologies Inc., Santa Clara, Calif) and was compared with a molecular weight size marker *(ladder)*. The gel electropherogram (C) is a simulated image based on the densitometry results shown in A and B. Extracted total RNA appears as a smear with two prominent bands corresponding to 18S and 28S ribosomal RNA (rRNA), respectively. A specimen with a high-quality total RNA extraction is shown in (A) and in lane 1 in (C), and is characterized by a high 28S/18S rRNA ratio with a broad size distribution of other RNA species. A second specimen demonstrating RNase degradation is shown in (B) and in lane 2 in (C), with a reduction in the 28S/18S rRNA ratio and the overall RNA signal. A shift is noted toward shorter fragments of RNA. *nt*, Nucleotides.

protocol requirements need to be considered. These requirements include the need to improve analytical throughput as well as the need to minimize manual handling, to ensure the reliability of assay performance, and to comply with regulatory or accreditation specifications. Automation of molecular diagnostic procedures is often considered and is particularly relevant to the process of nucleic acid isolation, as it involves many manual steps. Many commercial systems address the automation of this process. In general, automated nucleic acid isolation systems are based on the solid-phase extraction principles discussed previously. For example, MagNA Pure instruments from Roche Diagnostics (Branchburg, NJ)[23] adopt the use of silica-coated magnetic bead separation. The BioRobot Universal system (Qiagen, Hilden, Germany), on the other hand, is based on the use of silica-impregnated filter columns. These systems can be utilized as stand-alone instruments or can be integrated with downstream applications. For example, the MagNA Pure LC instrument (Roche Diagnostics) can be integrated with the LightCycler (Roche Diagnostics) for the performance of real-time PCR.[13] Besides the dedicated instruments described previously, open systems are available and are amenable to the setup of liquid handling steps according to end-users' specifications. Examples of such systems include those from Tecan (Durham, NC)[19] and the Biomek series from Beckman Coulter (Fullerton, Calif).[16]

A detailed evaluation of the analytical performance of an automatic nucleic acid protocol is usually required before high-throughput implementation. A number of studies have revealed that certain automated protocols may be less sensitive than manual methods of nucleic acid isolation.[5,7,40] Another relevant issue is the possibility of cross-contamination of specimens. Most systems evaluated to date have been shown to be free from the problem of cross-contamination.[5,13] These analytical factors have to be carefully considered before automatic protocols are adopted.

POINT-OF-CARE NUCLEIC ACID ANALYSIS

The automatic nucleic acid isolation systems described previously are generally designed for high-throughput usage. In contrast, another trend toward the development of compact, low-cost, and small-scale instruments for point-of-care services has been noted.[47] These instruments should be simple to operate by medical personnel or technical assistants with interventional steps reduced to a minimum. A lab-on-a-chip nucleic acid extraction platform has been developed for such a purpose.[37] This prefabricated chip contains networks of microfluidic pipelines for automatic sample and reagent flow control, as well as reservoirs containing reagents necessary for extraction procedures.[1] The only manual operation step is the injection of samples into the chip by a conventional syringe. On-chip nucleic acid isolation procedures are then automatically carried out by passing the sample through a solid-phase extraction filter.[1] To further automate the whole genetic analysis process, a nucleic acid detection module, such as those capable of preparing the reaction mixture and performing PCR amplification, can be integrated in the same microfluidic chip.[14,15]

ISOLATION OF CIRCULATING NUCLEIC ACIDS

In selecting the most appropriate protocol for one's laboratory, some of the issues worth considering include the specimen type and its available volume; the necessary yield, purity, and size of isolated nucleic acids; ease of operation; throughput and cost; whether the protocol involves the use of hazardous reagents; and whether it is amenable to automation. We are devoting this section to discuss these issues by using as an example the extraction of circulating nucleic acids in plasma.

For most applications of circulating nucleic acid analysis, the molecules of interest are those released from a tumor, fetus, or transplanted organ. However, these molecules are present in the circulation among a high background of other DNA and RNA species contributed by the blood cells.[29] As a result, the molecules of interest represent the minority population. Because a low fractional concentration of the DNA/RNA of interest would affect the reliability of their detection, special sample preservation measures are taken to minimize the number of background nucleic acid concentrations. In this regard, plasma is a preferred specimen type over serum because excessive background nucleic acids from blood cells might be released into the serum during the clotting process.[29] In addition, delays in the separation of plasma from whole blood should be avoided to minimize the release of DNA from blood cells.[24] EDTA is the anticoagulant of choice because cellular integrity is better maintained and hence the release of DNA from blood cells is less than when citrate or heparin is used.[24] Circulating cell-free DNA and RNA remain stable in unprocessed EDTA in whole blood for up to 24 hours at room temperature and at 4 °C, respectively.[45] Appropriate blood processing protocols are required to efficiently remove blood cells from the plasma.[8,18]

Concentrations of circulating nucleic acids are several orders of magnitude lower than those in a tissue biopsy specimen or in a whole blood sample.[24,35] Hence, an important factor affecting the successful adoption of plasma-based molecular diagnostics involves maximizing the yield of circulating nucleic acids during the isolation procedure. For example, the volume of sample to be used can be scaled up in each extraction.[6,44,46] When commercial nucleic acid extraction kits are to be used, the types and brands of kits that yield the best extraction efficiency should be assessed. For example, it has been demonstrated that when compared with the widely utilized QIAamp DNA Blood Mini Kit (Qiagen), the QIAamp DSP Virus Kit (Qiagen) showed an improved circulating fetal DNA yield from maternal plasma.[11,27] Studies have also revealed that the automated system of MagNa Pure LC (Roche) performed better than manual column-based procedures for DNA isolation[2] but not for RNA extraction.[7]

Apart from the isolation of *total* nucleic acids from plasma, investigators have studied the possibility of selectively isolating or enriching specific nucleic acid subpopulations. One example is the detection of the fetal-derived rhesus-D gene in the plasma of rhesus-D–negative mothers. Magnetic beads coated with oligonucleotides that specifically capture rhesus-D gene sequences have been used to enrich fetal rhesus-D gene fragments from maternal plasma.[26] Another relevant consideration is the size of circulating DNA or RNA fragments in the plasma. Both DNA and RNA exist in circulation as short fragments. Approximately 80% of DNA molecules in plasma, whether they are derived from a tumor, a fetus, or background blood cells, are 180 or fewer base pairs (bp) in length.[4] Similarly, plasma RNA molecules that are associated with a tumor, a fetus, or background blood cells are found to be fragments of the corresponding full-length transcript.[48] Hence, protocols selected for the isolation of circulating DNA and RNA should favor the isolation of low molecular weight fragments.[17,28]

Standardization of preanalytical and analytical parameters is an important consideration when diagnostic testing is offered. To standardize maternal plasma fetal DNA extraction protocols for noninvasive prenatal diagnosis, an International Workshop was conducted to evaluate the performance of fetal DNA detection across 13 different laboratories.[27] The Workshop reported that analytical and diagnostic sensitivities for fetal rhesus-D gene detection in maternal plasma were variable among different laboratories. These observations highlighted the need to standardize nucleic acid extraction procedures, as well as subsequent analytical steps, to achieve reliable diagnostic performance in clinical laboratories.

REFERENCES

1. Baier T, Hansen-Hagge TE, Gransee R, Crombe A, Schmahl S, Paulus C, et al. Hands-free sample preparation platform for nucleic acid analysis. Lab Chip 2009;9:3399-405.
2. Banzola I, Kaufmann I, Lapaire O, Hahn S, Holzgreve W, Rusterholz C. Isolation of serum nucleic acids for fetal DNA analysis: comparison of manual and automated extraction methods. Prenat Diagn 2008;28: 1227-31.

3. Carter MJ, Milton ID. An inexpensive and simple method for DNA purifications on silica particles. Nucleic Acids Res 1993;21:1044.
4. Chan KCA, Zhang J, Hui AB, Wong N, Lau TK, Leung TN, et al. Size distributions of maternal and fetal DNA in maternal plasma. Clin Chem 2004;50:88-92.
5. Chiu RWK, Jin Y, Chung GTY, Lui WB, Chan ATC, Lim W, et al. Automated extraction protocol for quantification of SARS-coronavirus RNA in serum: an evaluation study. BMC Infect Dis 2006;6:20.
6. Chiu RW, Lo YM. Noninvasive prenatal diagnosis by analysis of fetal DNA in maternal plasma. In: Lo YM, Chiu RW, Chan KC, eds. Clinical applications of PCR, volume 336, 2nd edition. New York, NY: Humana Press, 2006:101-19.
7. Chiu RW, Lui WB, El-Sheikhah A, Chan AT, Lau TK, Nicolaides KH, et al. Comparison of protocols for extracting circulating DNA and RNA from maternal plasma. Clin Chem 2005;51:2209-10.
8. Chiu RW, Poon LL, Lau TK, Leung TN, Wong EM, Lo YM. Effects of blood-processing protocols on fetal and total DNA quantification in maternal plasma. Clin Chem 2001;47:1607-13.
9. Chomczynski P, Sacchi N. Single-step method of RNA isolation by acid guanidinium thiocyanate-phenol-chloroform extraction. Anal Biochem 1987;162:156-9.
10. Chomczynski P, Sacchi N. The single-step method of RNA isolation by acid guanidinium thiocyanate-phenol-chloroform extraction: twenty-something years on. Nat Protoc 2006;1:581-5.
11. Clausen FB, Krog GR, Rieneck K, Dziegiel MH. Improvement in fetal DNA extraction from maternal plasma: evaluation of the NucliSens Magnetic Extraction system and the QIAamp DSP Virus Kit in comparison with the QIAamp DNA Blood Mini Kit. Prenat Diagn 2007;27:6-10.
12. Connolly MA, Clausen PA, Lazar JG. RNA purification. In: Dieffenbach CW, Dveksler GS, eds. PCR primer: a laboratory manual, 2nd edition. New York, NY: Cold Spring Harbor Laboratory Press, 2003:117-33.
13. Costa JM, Ernault P. Automated assay for fetal DNA analysis in maternal serum. Clin Chem 2002;48:679-80.
14. Dimov IK, Garcia-Cordero JL, O'Grady J, Poulsen CR, Viguier C, Kent L, et al. Integrated microfluidic tmRNA purification and real-time NASBA device for molecular diagnostics. Lab Chip 2008;8:2071-8.
15. Easley CJ, Karlinsey JM, Bienvenue JM, Legendre LA, Roper MG, Feldman SH, et al. A fully integrated microfluidic genetic analysis system with sample-in-answer-out capability. Proc Natl Acad Sci U S A 2006;103:19272-7.
16. Greenspoon SA, Ban JD, Sykes K, Ballard EJ, Edler SS, Baisden M, et al. Application of the BioMek 2000 Laboratory Automation Workstation and the DNA IQ System to the extraction of forensic casework samples. J Forensic Sci 2004;49:29-39.
17. Hahn T, Drese KS, O'Sullivan CK. Microsystem for isolation of fetal DNA from maternal plasma by preparative size separation. Clin Chem 2009;55:2144-52.
18. Heung MM, Tsui NB, Leung TY, Lau TK, Lo YMD, Chiu RWK. Development of extraction protocols to improve the yield for fetal RNA in maternal plasma. Prenat Diagn 2009;29:277-9.
19. Hourfar MK, Michelsen U, Schmidt M, Berger A, Seifried E, Roth WK. High-throughput purification of viral RNA based on novel aqueous chemistry for nucleic acid isolation. Clin Chem 2005;51:1217-22.
20. Hung EC, Shing TK, Chim SS, Yeung PC, Chan RW, Chik KW, et al. Presence of donor-derived DNA and cells in the urine of sex-mismatched hematopoietic stem cell transplant recipients: implication for the transrenal hypothesis. Clin Chem 2009;55:715-22.
21. Imbeaud S, Graudens E, Boulanger V, Barlet X, Zaborski P, Eveno E, et al. Toward standardization of RNA quality assessment using user-independent classifiers of microcapillary electrophoresis traces. Nucleic Acids Res 2005;33:e56.
22. Kasahara T, Miyazaki T, Nitta H, Ono A, Miyagishima T, Nagao T, et al. Evaluation of methods for duration of preservation of RNA quality in rat liver used for transcriptome analysis. J Toxicol Sci 2006;31:509-19.
23. Kessler HH, Muhlbauer G, Stelzl E, Daghofer E, Santner BI, Marth E. Fully automated nucleic acid extraction: MagNA Pure LC. Clin Chem 2001;47:1124-6.
24. Lam NY, Rainer TH, Chiu RW, Lo YM. EDTA is a better anticoagulant than heparin or citrate for delayed blood processing for plasma DNA analysis. Clin Chem 2004;50:256-7.
25. Lee T, LeShane ES, Messerlian GM, Canick JA, Farina A, Heber WW, et al. Down syndrome and cell-free fetal DNA in archived maternal serum. Am J Obstet Gynecol 2002;187:1217-21.
26. Legler TJ, Liu Z, Heermann KH, Hempel M, Gutensohn K, Kiesewetter H, et al. Specific magnetic bead-based capture of free fetal DNA from maternal plasma. Transfus Apher Sci 2009;40:153-7.
27. Legler TJ, Liu Z, Mavrou A, Finning K, Hromadnikova I, Galbiati S, et al. Workshop report on the extraction of foetal DNA from maternal plasma. Prenat Diagn 2007;27:824-9.
28. Li Y, Zimmermann B, Rusterholz C, Kang A, Holzgreve W, Hahn S. Size separation of circulatory DNA in maternal plasma permits ready detection of fetal DNA polymorphisms. Clin Chem 2004;50:1002-11.
29. Lui YY, Chik KW, Chiu RW, Ho CY, Lam CW, Lo YM. Predominant hematopoietic origin of cell-free DNA in plasma and serum after sex-mismatched bone marrow transplantation. Clin Chem 2002;48:421-7.
30. Madabusi LV, Latham GJ, Andruss BF. RNA extraction for arrays. Methods Enzymol 2006;411:1-14.
31. Milde A, Haas-Rochholz H, Kaatsch HJ. Improved DNA typing of human urine by adding EDTA. Int J Legal Med 1999;112:209-10.
32. Mraz M, Malinova K, Mayer J, Pospisilova S. MicroRNA isolation and stability in stored RNA samples. Biochem Biophys Res Commun 2009;390:1-4.
33. Mutter GL, Zahrieh D, Liu C, Neuberg D, Finkelstein D, Baker HE, et al. Comparison of frozen and RNALater solid tissue storage methods for use in RNA expression microarrays. BMC Genomics 2004;5:88.
34. Ng EK, Tsui NB, Lam NY, Chiu RW, Yu SC, Wong SC, et al. Presence of filterable and nonfilterable mRNA in the plasma of cancer patients and healthy individuals. Clin Chem 2002;48:1212-7.
35. Ng EK, Tsui NB, Lau TK, Leung TN, Chiu RW, Panesar NS, et al. mRNA of placental origin is readily detectable in maternal plasma. Proc Natl Acad Sci U S A 2003;100:4748-53.
36. Panaro NJ, Yuen PK, Sakazume T, Fortina P, Kricka LJ, Wilding P. Evaluation of DNA fragment sizing and quantification by the Agilent 2100 Bioanalyzer. Clin Chem 2000;46:1851-3.
37. Price CW, Leslie DC, Landers JP. Nucleic acid extraction techniques and application to the microchip. Lab Chip 2009;9:2484-94.
38. Rainen L, Oelmueller U, Jurgensen S, Wyrich R, Ballas C, Schram J, et al. Stabilization of mRNA expression in whole blood samples. Clin Chem 2002;48:1883-90.
39. Schroeder A, Mueller O, Stocker S, Salowsky R, Leiber M, Gassmann M, et al. The RIN: an RNA integrity number for assigning integrity values to RNA measurements. BMC Mol Biol 2006;7:3.
40. Schuurman T, van Breda A, de Boer R, Kooistra-Smid M, Beld M, Savelkoul P, et al. Reduced PCR sensitivity due to impaired DNA recovery with the MagNA Pure LC total nucleic acid isolation kit. J Clin Microbiol 2005;43:4616-22.
41. Smith C, Otto P, Bitner R, Shiels G. DNA purification. In: Dieffenbach CW, Dveksler GS, eds. PCR primer: a laboratory manual, 2nd edition. New York, NY: Cold Spring Harbor Laboratory Press, 2003:87-115.
42. Su YH, Wang M, Brenner DE, Ng A, Melkonyan H, Umansky S, et al. Human urine contains small, 150 to 250 nucleotide-sized, soluble DNA derived from the circulation and may be useful in the detection of colorectal cancer. J Mol Diagn 2004;6:101-7.
43. Tan SC, Yiap BC. DNA, RNA, and protein extraction: the past and the present. J Biomed Biotechnol 2009;2009:574398.
44. Tsui NB, Ng EK, Lo YM. Molecular analysis of circulating RNA in plasma. In: Lo YM, Chiu RW, Chan KC, eds. Clinical applications of PCR, 2nd edition. New York, NY: Humana Press, 2006.
45. Tsui NB, Ng EK, Lo YM. Stability of endogenous and added RNA in blood specimens, serum, and plasma. Clin Chem 2002;48:1647-53.

46. Tsui NB, Wong BC, Leung TY, Lau TK, Chiu RW, Lo YM. Noninvasive prenatal detection of fetal trisomy 18 by RNA-SNP allelic ratio analysis using maternal plasma SERPINB2 mRNA: a feasibility study. Prenat Diagn 2009;29:1031-7.
47. Tudos AJ, Besselink GJ, Schasfoort RB. Trends in miniaturized total analysis systems for point-of-care testing in Clin Chem. Lab Chip 2001;1:83-95.
48. Wong BC, Chiu RW, Tsui NB, Chan KC, Chan LW, Lau TK, et al. Circulating placental RNA in maternal plasma is associated with a preponderance of 5′ mRNA fragments: implications for noninvasive prenatal diagnosis and monitoring. Clin Chem 2005;51:1786-95.
49. Wong SC, Lo ES, Cheung MT. An optimised protocol for the extraction of non-viral mRNA from human plasma frozen for three years. J Clin Pathol 2004;57:766-8.
50. Yamamoto T, Sekiyama A, Sekiguchi H, Yoshida T, Miyagi Y. Examination of stability of bone marrow blood RNA in the PAXgene tube. Lab Hematol 2006;12:143-7.
51. Yu C, Penn LD, Hollembaek J, Li W, Cohen LH. Enzymatic tissue digestion as an alternative sample preparation approach for quantitative analysis using liquid chromatography-tandem mass spectrometry. Anal Chem 2004;76:1761-7.

CHAPTER 40

Inherited Diseases

Cindy L. Vnencak-Jones, Ph.D., F.A.C.M.G.

Since the first description of the use of the polymerase chain reaction (PCR) for the diagnosis of sickle cell anemia in 1985, numerous applications of PCR have been described.[558] The invention of PCR combined with advances in bioinformatics, the chemistry of fluorescent molecules, and the development of DNA chip and next-generation sequencing technology has revolutionized the field of human genetics. In addition, the establishment of public databases and rapid and unrestricted communication among investigators around the world via the Internet have enabled the phenomenal growth of this medical specialty. Upon completion of the Human Genome Project in 2003, the post-genomic era spawned *personalized medicine,* or a tailored approach to healthcare based on an individual's genotype. The relevance of genetic variation has been explored in the areas of nutrigenomics—modulation of nutrition and nutritional requirements; vaccinomics—determination of disease susceptibility and efficacy and response to vaccines; and pharmacogenomics—evaluation of the drug response. A personalized genetic approach to medicine is most important in the area of targeted gene therapy for both inherited and acquired somatic diseases.

This chapter will review deoxyribonucleic acid (DNA) testing for some of the more common inherited autosomal recessive, autosomal dominant, and X-linked genetic diseases, and will discuss testing of several mitochondrial, imprinting, and complex diseases. Because molecular testing for inherited diseases has influenced virtually every discipline of clinical medicine, the reader should refer to other chapters within this textbook for discipline-specific diseases, including inherited disorders of erythrocyte enzymes (see Chapter 23) and inborn errors of carbohydrate metabolism (see Chapter 26). In this rapidly evolving area of diagnostic testing, multiple methods can be used to achieve the same sensitivity and specificity. Similar to other areas of laboratory medicine, the method chosen by the DNA laboratory is determined by the expected volume for the test, the availability of personnel to perform the assay, and the current instrumentation within the laboratory.

In conjunction with scientific discoveries that have been made in the area of human genetics, public awareness of DNA and genetic diseases has been enhanced by the media, the Internet, the judicial system, and direct-to-consumer marketing of personal genetic information services. The Genetic Information Nondiscrimination Act was passed in 2008, thereby protecting an individual from discrimination by employers and health insurance companies based on their genotype; however, many concerns and unanswered questions remain for us as scientists and for our society. Who has a right to know the results of genetic testing—the insurance company or the employer? Once we begin to unravel the interaction between genetic and environmental factors, can insurance or healthcare coverage be denied to the person who engages in a lifestyle likely to cause disease based on his or her genetic predisposition? To what extent will personalized healthcare be conducted? In this time of healthcare reform, which genetic tests will be used for routine carrier or diagnostic screening? What will be the economic impact of these tests, and how will the healthcare system absorb these costs? Can the healthcare community be trained to understand complex principles of genetics and provide comprehensive counseling? Can a person's genetic makeup predisposing him or her to aberrant behavior provide a defense in a court of law? To what extent will manipulation of genetic material be tolerated in our society? Will most couples undergo in vitro fertilization and preimplantation genetic screening to choose the embryo with the most desirable genes? What will be the fate of frozen embryos created for these services? Will cloning be allowed? Although it is difficult to predict what the future will bring, one thing is clear: the future will be both scientifically and intellectually stimulating, yet no doubt controversial.

DISEASES WITH MENDELIAN INHERITANCE

Autosomal Recessive Diseases

An individual with an autosomal recessive disease has inherited two abnormal alleles at a given locus by receiving one mutant allele from each carrier parent; the disease-causing gene is on one of the autosomes (1 to 22) and not on a sex chromosome (X or Y). Typically, the carrier parent with one abnormal allele has no clinical features of the disease, yet possesses a 50% risk of donating the mutant allele to his or her offspring. Matings in which both partners are carriers of an abnormal allele have a 25% chance of producing a child with both normal alleles, a 50% chance of having a child that has received only one abnormal allele, and a 25% chance of having an affected child. The affected patient may be homozygous for a specific mutation by receiving the same mutation from each parent or may be a compound heterozygote by having received a different mutation within the gene from each parent. Regardless of the mechanism, the end result is the same: the patient has no normal allele. The specific mutations present in the patient largely affect the clinical severity of the disease; however, modifier genes and environmental factors also play a role in the phenotypic expression of the disease. Among pedigrees illustrating autosomal recessive disorders, males and females are equally affected, and for rare diseases, consanguinity is likely to be observed.

Cystic Fibrosis

Cystic fibrosis (CF) (Online Mendelian Inheritance in Man [OMIM #602421]) is one of the most common autosomal recessive diseases in people of Northern European ancestry with an estimated incidence in the United States of about 1 in 2500 and a carrier frequency of about 1 in 25.[5] Within other ethnic populations, the disease has an estimated incidence of 1 in 2300 Ashkenazi Jews, 1 in 8500 Hispanics, 1 in 17,000 African Americans, and 1 in 35,000 Asian Americans.[5] CF is a multisystem disorder that primarily affects the pulmonary, gastrointestinal, and reproductive organs.[455] However, the phenotypic expression of the disease is heterogeneous, ranging from meconium ileus and severe respiratory disease in infants to mild pulmonary symptoms and no evidence of gastrointestinal problems even in adulthood. Morbidity and mortality of the disease are most related to mucous accumulation; recurrent infection with pathogens, such as *Pseudomonas aeruginosa, Burkholderia cepacia, Staphylococcus aureus,* and *Haemophilus influenzae;* and excessive inflammation in the lung.[553,559] Although it was previously considered a fatal childhood disease, the U.S. Cystic Fibrosis Foundation reported that in 2008, the median survival age among ≈23,000 patients with CF who received care through 1 of 115 care centers nationwide was 37.4 years.[132] In addition, more than 45% of patients were over the age of 18.[132] The increase in survival age is due to organ transplantation, improved nutrition, and new therapies.[31,160,250,478,661] This success will continue with the likelihood of targeting infectious agents, mucous accumulation, and inflammation with pharmacotherapy and gene therapy to the lung.[16] Further, because of the complexity and frequency of the disease, most patients receive treatment from specialized care centers.[132,256] This approach provides widespread communication between healthcare providers and enables monitoring of a large population of patients with respect to treatment outcome, healthcare, and disease-specific variables.

The severity and frequency of the disease led to an intensive search for the gene. The gene was mapped to 7q31 in 1985 and was subsequently cloned in 1989.[365,374,536,545,633] The CF gene is large, containing 27 exons and producing a transcript of approximately 6.5 kb. It codes for the CF transmembrane conductance regulator protein (CFTR) of 1480 amino acids and a member of the ATP-binding cassette (ABC) transporter superfamily. CFTR consists of two repeated motifs, each containing six hydrophobic transmembrane domains and one hydrophilic intracellular nucleotide-binding fold connected by a highly charged regulatory domain site.[536] The molecule serves as a chloride ion channel and is located within the lipid bilayer, predominantly at the apical membrane of secretory epithelial cells, where it is dependent on phosphorylation by protein kinases through activation by cyclic adenosine monophosphate (cAMP).[259] In addition to epithelial chloride conductance, the molecule is involved in transport of sodium, potassium, and adenosine triphosphate (ATP) from the intracellular compartment to the extracellular surface.[556,571,609] An abnormal sweat chloride concentration is considered the gold standard for the diagnosis of CF (≥60 mmol/L in childhood).[223] However, some patients with *CFTR* mutations may have borderline (30 to 59 mmol/L) or even normal (<30 mmol/L) results.[112,290] Atypical or nonclassic CF patients may have involvement of only one organ, as in congenital bilateral absence of the vas deferens (CBAVD), pancreatitis, pulmonary disease, or nasal polyps.[498,685] Measuring the nasal potential difference is part of the algorithm to distinguish patients with a questionable diagnosis of CF from true CF patients.[142,162,333] Thus although the diagnosis of CF can be made easily in patients with characteristic clinical features and abnormal sweat chloride concentrations, in patients with atypical presentation, mutations in the *CFTR* gene cannot be excluded without complete sequence analysis of the gene.[434] The wide clinical diversity among patients with CF in part is the result of varying effects on the CFTR protein caused by more than 1600 mutations identified thus far in the *CFTR* gene.[133] However, it is possible that the "nonclassic" CF phenotype is caused by factors other than mutations in the *CFTR* gene.[255,579]

Because CF is an autosomal recessive disorder, the CF patient must have two mutant *CFTR* alleles to develop the disease. Some mutations are "private" and unique to a family; others may be common among CF patients. Patients will be homozygous with two copies of the same mutation or will represent a compound heterozygote with one copy of one mutation and one copy of a second mutation. Predictably, the type and location of the mutation have varying effects on CFTR and affect the phenotype of the patient.[6,99,455] The *CFTR* genotype and the clinical phenotype are most closely related for pancreatic involvement rather than for pulmonary manifestations of the disease, which appear to be more dependent on environmental factors and genetic modifiers.[92,121,168,563,722] Environmental modulating factors of lung disease include second-hand smoke and varying exposure to pathogens.[122,559] It is interesting to note that patients with idiopathic chronic pancreatitis have a higher incidence of *CFTR* mutations than the expected carrier frequency and have more severe disease.[8] Pancreatitis in these patients may result from CF with a second *CFTR* gene mutation not detected, or could represent a complex disease resulting from a predisposing mutation in several genes.[358] *CFTR* genotypes in infertile males with only the genital form of CF—CBAVD—usually have a mutation associated with a severe phenotype on one allele and a mutation associated with a mild phenotype on the second allele. The most frequently reported *CFTR* genotype in this population is the 5T polymorphism in intron 8 (corresponding to a sequence of five thymidines).[112,524] The 7T and 9T alleles are more common than the 5T variant, which is observed in only ≈5% of *CFTR* alleles. The 5T variant affects mRNA splicing and can cause exon 9 to be deleted; without it, the chloride channel is not functional.[115,144,608] An adjacent polymorphic TG dinucleotide sequence [(TG)9 to (TG)13] regulates the efficiency of mRNA splicing, with the higher number of TG repeats [(TG)13] associated with decreased efficiency of splicing.[254] Thus, the 5T-(TG)12 or (TG)13 allele is more commonly associated with an abnormal phenotype than is the 5T-(TG)11 allele.

The types of mutations in *CFTR* can illustrate the association of the genotype with the phenotype. More than half of all mutations are missense or frameshift mutations, and more than 9% occur in exon 13.[133] Mutations can be divided into five classes.[455] Patients with class 1 mutations have defects in protein production, and class 2 mutations are associated with defective processing of CFTR. In both cases, CFTR trafficking to the cell membrane does not occur, and both class 1 and class 2 mutations are typically associated with a severe phenotype. Class 3 and 4 mutations have CFTR expression at the cell membrane, but channel activity is reduced. Class 3 mutations can be associated with a more severe phenotype and result from defective regulation; class 4 mutations can be mild and result in diminished conduction of ion flow. Class 5 mutations are associated with abnormal splicing and thus reduced amounts of normal *CFTR* messenger RNA (mRNA). These mutations may be associated with a severe phenotype (621+1G>T) or a mild phenotype (2789+5G>A). The most common mutation, deltaF508, seen in about 70% of CF chromosomes in Caucasians of Northern European descent, affects processing of CFTR and prevents its trafficking to the apical membrane.[111] Prevalent mutations G542X and W1282X cause premature translation termination and thus truncation of the protein.[270] The frequently observed mutation G551D results in CFTR that reaches the apical membrane but improperly regulates the chloride channel.[688]

DNA testing for the identification of *CFTR* mutations is performed for a variety of reasons (Box 40-1). It is performed to confirm the diagnosis of disease in patients with equivocal sweat chloride results, or in instances when insufficient material is collected. A diagnosis of CF can be considered in the patient with only the presenting symptom of chronic pancreatitis. Alternatively, in the known CF patient, mutation analysis can be requested to help predict the prognosis because some genotype-phenotype correlations exist. At the same time, identifying the mutations segregating within a family enables preimplantation diagnosis or prenatal testing for subsequent pregnancies and carrier or diagnostic testing for other at-risk family members. Similarly, state-sponsored newborn screening programs have detected infants with CF and at the same time have identified at-risk family members and have enabled genetic testing. Most important, newborn screening allows for early diagnosis and intervention through treatment to prevent malabsorption of nutrients and to minimize lung damage from infection.[578] Neonatal screening for CF is based on the immunoreactive trypsinogen (IRT) assay and is used to detect elevated levels of this pancreatic enzyme from dried blood spots. States vary in their newborn screening algorithms. In some, a positive result is followed by IRT retesting; in others, blood from the newborn is submitted for *CFTR* mutation analysis.[497,597] A sweat chloride test is ultimately performed for confirmation of CF but may not always be effective in infants younger than 2 weeks.[497] Some families referred for prenatal CF testing have no family history of CF. Rather, in these families, hyperechoic (hyperechogenic) bowel may be diagnosed in the fetus on routine ultrasonography. In one study of 209 fetuses, 7 were subsequently given the diagnosis of CF, which is about 84 times the estimated risk of CF in the general population.[457]

The most challenging and controversial DNA testing for CF is carrier screening for preconception and expectant couples. Carrier screening in these circumstances was recommended in October 2001 by the American College of Obstetricians and Gynecologists (ACOG) in conjunction with the American College of Medical Genetics (ACMG).[14] With the heterogeneity of *CFTR* mutations, testing for more than 1600 mutations in this population would be a daunting task. For this reason, a core panel of 25 mutations was proposed as a minimum standard for CF carrier screening. The mutations initially proposed included those with an estimated prevalence of at least 0.1% of CF mutant alleles and a CF carrier detection rate of about 88% for non-Hispanic Caucasians.[14] However, in 2004, the core panel was revised to 23 mutations with the removal of mutations 1078delT and I148T-3199del6, which are not present at a frequency representing 0.1% of all CF alleles (Table 40-1).[451,607,682] The intent of the screening panel is to identify individuals at risk for classical CF, not CBAVD; thus it is recommended that 5T/7T/9T status be evaluated only in the presence of mutation R117H. In this case, the panel would allow distinction between R117H-5T and R117-7T individuals. This in turn would enable proper genetic counseling and prenatal testing options for individuals who are R117H-5T and at risk of having an offspring with CF if their reproductive partner is also a carrier of CF. Although CF is more common in the Caucasian and

BOX 40-1 Referrals for *CFTR* Mutation Analysis

- Confirm diagnosis of cystic fibrosis (CF)
- Determine prognosis
- Screen patient with pancreatitis
- Family member testing
- Newborn screening
- Preconception couples
- Expectant couples
- Prenatal testing—at-risk fetus
- Prenatal testing—hyperechogenic bowel
- Preimplantation genetic diagnosis
- Infertile male with congenital bilateral absence of the vas deferens (CBAVD)
- Semen and oocyte donors

TABLE 40-1 ACOG/ACMG Mutation Panel

	MUTATION FREQUENCY AMONG PATIENTS WITH CLINICALLY DIAGNOSED CF, %				
***CFTR* Mutation**	**Ashkenazi Jewish**	**Non-Hispanic Caucasian**	**Hispanic Caucasian**	**African American**	**Asian American**
ΔF508	31.41	72.42	54.38	44.07	38.95
G542X	7.55	2.28	5.10	1.45	0.00
W1282X	45.92	1.50	0.63	0.24	0.00
G551D	0.22	2.25	0.56	1.21	3.15
621+1G>T	0.00	1.57	0.26	1.11	0.00
N1303K	2.78	1.27	1.66	0.35	0.76
R553X	0.00	0.87	2.81	2.32	0.76
delI507	0.22	0.88	0.68	1.87	0.00
3489+10kbC>T	4.77	0.58	1.57	0.17	5.31
3120+1G>T	0.10	0.08	0.16	9.57	0.00
R117H	0.00	0.70	0.11	0.06	0.00
1717-1G>T	0.67	0.48	0.27	0.37	0.00
2789+5G>A	0.10	0.48	0.16	0.00	0.00
R347P	0.00	0.45	0.16	0.06	0.00
711+1G>T	0.10	0.43	0.23	0.00	0.00
R334W	0.00	0.14	1.78	0.49	0.00
R560T	0.00	0.38	0.00	0.17	0.00
R1162X	0.00	0.23	0.58	0.66	0.00
3569delC	0.00	0.34	0.13	0.06	0.00
A455E	0.00	0.34	0.05	0.00	0.00
G85E	0.00	0.29	0.23	0.12	0.00
2184delA	0.10	0.17	0.16	0.05	0.00
1898+1G>A	0.10	0.16	0.05	0.06	0.00
Total	**94.04**	**88.29**	**71.72**	**64.46**	**48.93**

ACMG, American College of Medical Genetics; *ACOG,* American College of Obstetricians and Gynecologists; *CF,* cystic fibrosis.
Adapted from Watson et al.[682]

Ashkenzai Jewish population, the standard of care recommended by the ACOG is to make CF testing available to all preconception or expectant couples, especially because it is becoming more difficult to assign a single ethnicity to a patient to best determine her carrier risk.

For *CFTR* mutation testing, a variety of assay platforms are commercially available and varying numbers of mutations are detected.[147] Further, because the detection rate of the panel is lower in some ethnicities, laboratories serving those populations should consider supplementing this screening panel with additional mutation analysis.[611]

Social issues associated with population screening for this genetic disease are in part rather specific to this program (such as the enormous number of mutations in this huge gene), but many others are illustrative of issues that surround genetic testing in general. Issues surrounding this program include (1) the inability to detect CF carriers with *CFTR* mutations other than the 23 included in the screening panel, (2) the need for appropriate genetic counseling of patients before they consent to the analysis, (3) the need for proper understanding of the possibility of a false-negative result, (4) stigmatization of being a "carrier" of a genetic disease, (5) threats to confidentiality of results, (6) effects on health insurability, and (7) a possible increase in the number of abortions following the identification of previously unknown affected fetuses. In addition to these social and/or ethical issues, opposition to this screening panel has arisen over the set of mutations included in the panel, because those currently selected under-represent the mutations found in minorities.[191,224,282,287,288] It is likely that mutations in the *CFTR* screening panel will continue to change as carrier screening evolves and the program is critically evaluated.

It is the standard of care for all prenatal cases that DNA extracted from the fetus is tested for the presence of maternal contamination, because the presence of maternal DNA could interfere with interpretation of the results. This is best performed by using PCR amplification for highly polymorphic short tandem repeat loci coupled with capillary electrophoresis (Figure 40-1). As important as the accuracy of the laboratory results is the interpretation of these results. For carrier screening, with no family history of CF and no mutation detected, it is important for the patient to understand that a residual risk of being a carrier remains (Table 40-2).[5] This is especially important for patients in ethnic groups for which the *CFTR* mutation detection level is reduced. Further, it is very important to know relevant family history when interpreting and reporting rest results to provide accurate genetic risk assessments regarding a residual carrier risk for

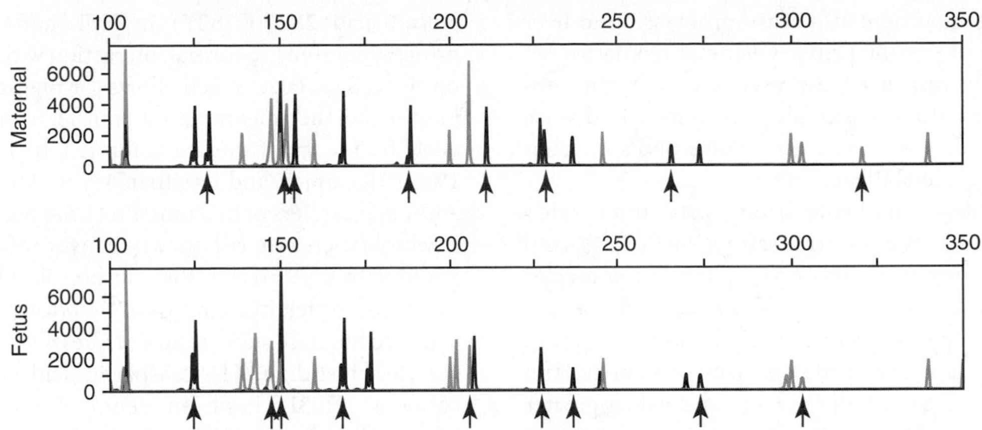

Figure 40-1 Electropherograms obtained following polymerase chain reaction (PCR) amplification of maternal and fetal DNA at nine independently segregating loci and one gender-specific marker. Extracted maternal and fetal DNA was amplified by PCR using a multiplex PCR assay with fluorescent labeled primers (AmpFLSTR Profiler Plus ID PCR Amplification Kit, Applied Biosystems, Foster City, Calif). Amplicons were detected following capillary electrophoresis on an ABI 3130*xl* Genetic Analyzer and were analyzed using GeneMapper version 3.7 software (Applied Biosystems). *Arrows* in the *upper panel* denote maternal alleles absent in the fetal DNA specimen. *Arrows* in the *bottom panel* indicate maternal alleles inherited by the fetus.

TABLE 40-2 Cystic Fibrosis Mutation Carrier Risk

	Ashkenazi Jewish	Non-Hispanic Caucasian	Hispanic Caucasian	African American	Asian American
Detection rate of ACOG/ACMG 23 mutation panel	94%	88%	72%	65%	49%
Estimated carrier risk in population	1/24	1/25	1/46	1/65	1/94
Estimated carrier risk after no mutation detected on screening panel	1/400	1/208	1/164	1/186	1/184

ACMG, American College of Medical Genetics; *ACOG*, American College of Obstetricians and Gynecologists.
Adapted from ACOG Committee Opinion 2005.[5]

a negative result, because the mutation segregating within the family could be one not detected by the test panel, and a false-negative result could occur.[486]

Hereditary Hemochromatosis

Hereditary hemochromatosis (HH) (OMIM #235200) is an autosomal recessive disorder of iron regulation that can result in excess iron deposition in otherwise healthy tissue primarily of the liver, heart, joints, pituitary gland, and pancreas. Affected individuals can absorb approximately 3 to 4 mg of iron per day compared with the normal rate of 1 to 2 mg per day, and although the average male has body iron storage of about 5 g, affected individuals can accumulate as much as 30 g. Symptoms associated with this disease occur during mid to late adulthood, but the diagnosis of HH is often delayed because early symptoms of weakness, lethargy, joint pain, and abdominal pain are nonspecific. Complications of the disease include hepatic cirrhosis, diabetes mellitus, hypopituitarism, hypogonadism, arthritis, and cardiomyopathy.[615] Moreover, patients are at increased risk for hepatocellular carcinoma.[366] The disease is more common in men than in women presumably because of physiologic iron loss during menstruation and pregnancy. However, other sex-related differences may be involved. The phenotypic expression of the disease appears to be dependent on both genetic and environmental factors. Although regular blood donation may be protective against HH, infection with hepatitis C, obesity-related steatosis, increased consumption of dietary iron or vitamin C (an enhancer of iron uptake), and, most notably, excessive alcohol intake can increase the likelihood of symptoms in the presence of an affected genotype.[519,704] Management of the disease may include therapeutic phlebotomy, chelation therapy or erythrocytopheresis to reduce iron stores, and dietary avoidance of red meats, iron supplements, and excess vitamin C, as well as uncooked seafood (to avoid *Vibrio vulnificus* infection); alcohol intake should be minimal.[43,80] Single-nucleotide polymorphisms (SNPs) in transforming growth factor-β_1 and myeloperoxidase have been implicated as modifiers of disease progression to liver fibrosis and cirrhosis, yet the primary genetic risk factor for *HFE*-related disease remains the presence of a Y chromosome.[704] The identification of modifier genes for this disease is an area of active interest and may involve SNPs in genes associated with iron metabolism.[127]

Laboratory testing for hemochromatosis most often includes determination of transferrin saturation (TS) [(serum iron/total iron binding capacity) × 100]; saturation greater than 55 to 60% is considered abnormal for men, and saturation greater than 45 to 50% is abnormal for women. Serum ferritin (SF) levels are also ordered, with serum ferritin greater than 300 μg/L abnormal for men, and values greater than 200 μg/L abnormal for women. Elevated levels of transferrin saturation and serum ferritin often lead to genetic testing. If genetic testing is positive, a liver biopsy follows to determine the amount of stainable iron and the degree of injury.[332]

In 1976, Simon and associates reported an association of human leukocyte antigen (HLA)-A3 and HLA-B14 antigens with idiopathic hemochromatosis, which suggested that the HH gene was located near the major histocompatibility complex (MHC) on chromosome 6p.[590] Classic genetic studies confirmed linkage of the HH gene to the HLA locus, and in 1996, Feder and colleagues cloned the HH gene, *HFE*.[196,335,389] Although *HFE* (6p21.3) remains the primary gene associated with abnormal iron regulation, other autosomal recessive disorders involving the genes *TfR2* (transferrin receptor 2), *HJV* (hemojuvelin), and *HAMP* (hepcidin), as well as an autosomal dominant disorder involving ferroportin 1, have been reported.[32] Additional genes may be associated with inherited forms of abnormal iron metabolism.

The *HFE* gene protein, HFE, encodes a β_2-microglobulin–associated protein with structural resemblance to MHC class I proteins. The *HFE* gene contains seven exons spanning about 10 kb, with a 2.7 kb mRNA that is highly expressed in the hepatocyte. The 40 kDa HFE protein is composed of 348 amino acids and is involved in the highly regulated hepcidin-ferroportin pathway for iron homeostasis.[496] As such, when bound to transferrin receptor 1 (TfR1), HFE is silenced. However, when plasma transferrin is saturated, HFE dissociates from TfR1, making TfR1 available for binding and cellular uptake of iron. Once no longer bound to TfR1, HFE binds to TfR2 and other proteins, possibly HJV, and various bone morphogenetic proteins (BMPs) and their receptors to form an *iron-sensing complex*. This complex signals for the expression of hepcidin, a 25 amino acid liver hormone, using the SMAD signaling pathway. Hepcidin, now upregulated from the iron overload, binds to ferroportin, causing it to be internalized and degraded, thereby maintaining iron within the enterocytes and macrophages.[496]

A founder effect, suggested by linkage disequilibrium between HLA haplotypes and the *HFE* gene, was confirmed in two studies by the identification of homozygosity for a common mutation, G-to-A base pair substitution, in 148 of 178 (83%) and 121 of 147 (82.3%) HH patients.[60,196] This mutation results in a cysteine-to-tyrosine substitution at amino acid 282 (C282Y) in HFE and disrupts disulfide bridges required for normal interaction with β_2-microglobulin on the cell surface, which allows for high-affinity transferrin binding to the uncomplexed transferrin receptor.[196-198] The allele frequency of this mutation is 5 to 10% in Caucasians, 1% in Hispanics, and less than 1% in African Americans.[513] Although carriers of this mutation have been reported to have a twofold increased risk for acute myocardial infarction compared with noncarriers, they do not have higher transferrin saturation or ferritin than C282Y noncarriers.[450,635]

A second base substitution of C-to-G in exon 2 and resulting in a histidine (H)-to-aspartic acid (D) substitution at codon 63 (H63D) has been identified in a higher percentage of C282Y-negative HH patients than would be expected based on the frequency of this mutation in the population.[196] This mutation is observed in 89% of HH chromosomes that do not have mutation C282Y compared with an allele frequency of 15 to 17% in Caucasian control *HFE* genes.[196,513] HFE, with this alteration, is expressed at the cell surface, but its interaction with the transferrin receptor is altered, resulting in increased iron deposition within the cell.[196,669] The frequency of mutation H63D is less in African Americans (0.026) and Hispanics (0.10).[513] Mutation H63D is associated with increased risk of developing a mild form of hemochromatosis, but appears to have little effect in causing iron overload when inherited by itself (wild-type and/or H63D), which represents 2.5% of HH chromosomes, or when two copies of the mutation are inherited (H63D/H63D), which is seen in 1.4% of HH patients.[419] Although many compound heterozygotes (C282Y/H63D) in the general population are asymptomatic, H63D may contribute to disease when inherited with mutation C282Y because 1 to 5% of HH patients have this genotype, although these patients display variability in liver histologic findings and iron indices.[58,334,347,419,566]

A third mutation in the *HFE* gene is associated with a mild form of hemochromatosis.[30,299,461] This A-to-T mutation results in a serine-to-cysteine substitution at codon 65 (S65C) in exon 2 and is in close proximity within the gene to the previously described *H63D* mutation. In one study, mutation S65C was detected in 2.49% of normal controls yet was identified in 10 of 128 (7.8%) HH chromosomes that had neither C282Y nor H63D.[461] Although C282Y is the primary mutation in *HFE*-associated HH, compound heterozygotes C282Y-H63D and C282Y-S65C have an increased risk of developing HH, thus suggesting their role in the development of HH.

DNA analysis of the *HFE* gene is done using a variety of methods and in most laboratories includes testing only for mutations C282Y and H63D (Figure 40-2). Once *HFE* mutation analysis has confirmed the cause of HH in the patient, transferrin saturation (TS), serum ferritin, and DNA testing of at-risk family members can identify those who may benefit from earlier treatment and dietary restrictions.[89] This is especially important because morbidity among first-degree relatives of *HFE*-related hemochromatosis patients is greater than in the general population.[329]

Because HH is a common disorder with clinical symptoms that can be prevented with easy and inexpensive early

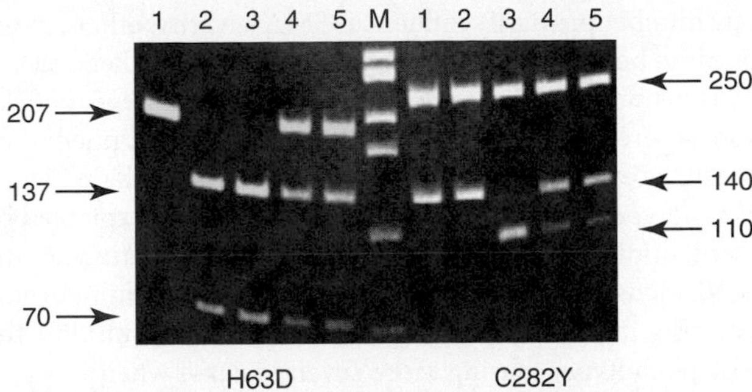

Figure 40-2 Detection of mutations H63D and C282Y in the *HFE* gene. Patient DNA is amplified by polymerase chain reaction (PCR) using oligonucleotide primer pairs that flank mutation H63D or C282Y, respectively. For detection of mutation H63D, 207 base pair (bp) PCR products are digested with restriction endonuclease *BclI* and are subjected to electrophoresis on a 5% polyacrylamide gel *(left)*. Mutation H63D results from a C-to-G base substitution and destroys a *BclI* site, thereby preventing digestion of 207 bp fragments into 137 bp and 70 bp fragments. Detection of mutation C282Y uses digestion of 390 bp amplified products with restriction endonuclease *RsaI* and electrophoresis on a 5% polyacrylamide gel *(right)*. Mutation C282Y results from a G-to-A base substitution and creates an *RsaI* site within the amplicons cleaving 140 bp fragments to 110 bp and 30 bp fragments. In patient 1 *(lane 1)*, the H63D-specific 207 bp amplification products are not digested with *BclI* to yield wild-type bands of 137 bp and 70 bp, thereby indicating that the restriction site has been lost in both alleles. Conversely, the C282Y-specific amplicons from patient 1 yield exclusively wild-type bands of 250 bp and 140 bp fragments. Genotype for patient 1 is interpreted as mutation H63D, wild-type C282Y on both alleles. Genotype for patient 2 *(lane 2)* is wild-type H63D, wild-type C282Y on both alleles. Genotype for patient 3 *(lane 3)* is wild-type H63D, mutant (m) C282Y on both alleles. Patient 4 *(lane 4)* is a compound heterozygote with mH63D, wild-type *C282Y* on one allele and wild-type H63D, mC282Y on the second allele. *Lane 5* represents control DNA heterozygous for mutations H63D and C282Y.

intervention, population-based DNA screening for HH may be appropriate and has been considered.[93,120] Yet, although homozygosity for the *HFE* mutation C282Y is close to 1 in 250 in the general population, making hemochromatosis one of the most common inherited genetic disorders, significant clinical heterogeneity is observed and varies from severe disease to an asymptomatic phenotype with only abnormal iron indices. In one study of 41,000+ patients attending a health clinic in the United States, only 1% of C282Y homozygotes developed clinical hemochromatosis. However, the penetrance of C282Y homozygotes displaying iron overload–related disease in a large study of more than 31,000 people between 40 and 69 years of age was reported to be 28% in males compared with only 1% in females by the age of 65.[10] Further, this study showed that patients with serum ferritin levels greater than 1000 μg/L are at increased risk for developing *HFE* gene-related disease compared with subjects with less than 1000 μg/L. Although clinical expression of the disease is reduced, more than 50% of homozygotes of both sexes will have elevated TS and SF levels. However, these two studies indicate wide variability of true penetrance of this disease. Thus, because of incomplete penetrance, many people with mutations will not have and will never develop iron overload.[59] Inability to predict who will develop disease is the primary reason why population-based genetic screening is not done routinely in the United States. This is a topic of much debate.[9] Targeted screening to adult Caucasian men of Northern European ancestry combined with TS and SF has been proposed.[512] Targeted screening for family members of C282Y homozygotes has been suggested.[330] In the United Kingdom, genetic testing for C282Y and H63D was determined to result in significant cost savings when incorporated into the diagnostic strategy of potentially affected patients and in testing of their offspring.[128] Phenotypic measurements of transferrin saturation or serum ferritin could be more appropriate than genotype studies for population-based screening for HH, but these results can also be misleading in that iron overload can occur from a host of other conditions unrelated to hemochromatosis and mutations in *HFE*.[699]

Spinal Muscular Atrophy

Spinal muscular atrophy (SMA) is an autosomal recessive neurodegenerative disorder with an estimated incidence of 1 in 10,000 births and a carrier frequency of 1 in 40 to 1 in 50. The disease is characterized by progressive symmetric degeneration of spinal cord motor neurons of the anterior horn region and results in skeletal muscle weakness and atrophy.[415] Wide variability in age of onset and motor function impairment has been noted in SMA, and four clinical phenotypes have been identified. Type I (OMIM #253300) is the most severe and the most common (50%); it is associated with age of onset younger than 6 months and death in early childhood. These children have profound hypotonia and no control of head movement, and they are unable to sit. Intercostal muscle weakness leads to respiratory failure and tongue fasciculation, dysphagia, and fatigue, making feeding difficult, worsening the condition, and increasing the risk of aspiration pneumonia. SMA type II (OMIM #253550) is intermediate in its severity and has an age of onset between 7 and 18 months. These children can sit and some can stand, although none can walk independently. Death typically ensues in adolescence. SMA type III (OMIM #253400) has onset of disease after 18 months and a mild phenotype with gradually progressive disease and a normal life expectancy. SMA type IV (OMIM #271150) is the mildest of all forms and is characterized by muscle weakness initially in the second or third decade of life and a normal life span.

The gene for SMA, survival motor neuron I *(SMN1)*, was mapped to 5q11.2-13.3 in 1990 and cloned in 1995.[86,393,438] This gene contains 9 exons (numbered 1, 2a, 2b to 8) spanning about 28,000 bases and encodes a 1.7 kb mRNA transcript producing a 38 kDa protein composed of 294 amino acids that is widely expressed in the nucleus and cytoplasm.[404] The SMN protein forms a multiprotein complex with other proteins, some of which are referred to as Gemins, and is enriched in the nucleus in size and number to form Gems.[46,589] The SMN complex is essential for the biogenesis of small ribonucleoproteins into the spliceosome, a structure that is required in the nucleus for the removal of noncoding sequences during pre-mRNA splicing.[505] In addition, SMN interacts with a whole host of other proteins, indicating that it plays an important role in a variety of cellular functions, including transcription and apoptosis. SMN is essential during embryogenesis in that its absence results in embryonic lethality in *SMN1* knockout mice.[567] It is not understood why it plays such an important role in the cell and is expressed in many tissues, yet deficiency of SMN almost exclusively affects the lower motor neurons. This would suggest that SMN may function in a role unique to motor neurons.[189,717] In most cases, SMA results from homozygous deletions of *SMN1*. Some cases result from gene conversion of *SMN1,* and in less than 5% of cases, patients are compound heterozygotes with an *SMN1* deletion on one allele and loss of function or point mutation on the second allele. In rare cases, a point mutation in *SMN1* is present on both alleles. Reduced amounts of functional SMN in SMA patients limit the formation of the SMN complex, thereby affecting snRNP assembly and ultimately normal mRNA splicing.[201,697,720] *SMN1* is contained within a large inverted repeat sequence that contains the highly homologous *SMN2* gene. *SMN2* differs from *SMN1* by only five bases; it lies in the opposite orientation and is centromeric to *SMN1*.[415,500] It is believed that *SMN2* arose by gene duplication, and that the *SMN2-SMN1* configuration is unique only to primates.[544] Although the five bases that differ between *SMN1* and *SMN2* do not affect the amino acid sequence of the protein; a C-to-T transition in exon 7 of *SMN2* corresponding to codon 280 causes alternative splicing and the deletion of exon 7 in 80 to 90% of *SMN2* transcripts.[408] The C-to-T transition enables the binding of heterogeneous ribonucleoproteins, thereby acting as a splicing silencer element and causing the exclusion of exon 7 from the transcript.[354] In addition, an *SMN2*-specific nucleotide in intron 7 contributes to excision of exon 7 in *SMN2* transcripts.[355] Thus despite the fact that most SMA patients have intact *SMN2* genes, they still have disease, because most *SMN2* transcripts do not contain exon 7; thus they produce negligible functional SMN protein. Without the amino acids encoded by exon 7, SMN is unstable and is unable to efficiently oligomerize to form the SMN complex.[409]

The *SMN2* gene is in part a modifier of the severity of SMA, and its affect is based on the *SMN2* gene copy number.[423,622,681] Some *SMN1* deletion alleles also contain an *SMN2* deletion, whereas other *SMN1* deletion alleles may have two or even three copies of *SMN2*. In patients with milder forms of the disease, three or four copies of *SMN2* may be present. Increased gene copy numbers are therefore producing more *SMN2* transcript, some of which will translate to functional SMN protein, thereby providing some normal SMN protein for required cellular functions. Although *SMN2* copy number primarily influences SMA severity, other factors appear to be contributory. Males with identical biallelic *SMN1* deletions and identical *SMN2* copy numbers appear to be more severely affected than females, and the SMA phenotype is variable even within families whose members share identical genotypes.[337] Phenotypic variability could be explained by recent findings of differences in DNA methylation at the *SMN2* locus.[278] In addition, absence of the adjacent neuronal apoptosis inhibitory protein (NAIP) gene may modify the SMA phenotype, causing more severe disease when it is also deleted.[180,554,681] NAIP is deleted in 1.8% of SMA carriers, yet is homozygously deleted in 67% of SMA patients with type I disease.

Treatment for SMA is mostly supportive for the management of respiratory insufficiency, nutritional deficiency, and orthopedic needs.[95] Because *SMN2* serves to modify the SMA phenotype, it can also provide a therapeutic target for future treatment. One approach is to reduce aberrant splicing of *SMN2*.[367] This was successfully performed in the mouse model of SMA to increase normal SMN levels using bifunctional RNA.[47,443] An alternative strategy would be to increase the expression level of *SMN2* using histone deacetylation inhibitors.[140] Because of the frequency and severity of the disease, therapeutic research is ongoing and many clinical trials are in progress.[95]

DNA testing for SMA is performed at multiple laboratories using a variety of techniques.[218] Establishing diagnostic or carrier testing can be complicated by (1) the polymorphic nature of the *SMN* locus, with alleles containing varying copy numbers of both *SMN1* and *SMN2* genes; (2) the degree of homology between *SMN1* and *SMN2*; (3) a small percentage of affected alleles with point mutations rather than deletions within *SMN1*; and (4) a 2% rate of de novo cases, which most frequently occur during paternal meiosis. A common diagnostic assay for SMA includes PCR amplification coupled with restriction endonuclease digestion with *DraI* and gel electrophoresis.[646] Only amplicons derived from *SMN2* will contain the restriction site; those generated from *SMN1* will not. Because most SMA affected patients have *SMN1* deletions involving exon 7, no bands corresponding to *SMN1* are observed. Although this assay is simple and robust, it is not quantitative and cannot determine the *SMN2* copy number, nor can it identify patients with point mutations within the gene. *SMN2* copy number is important for prognosis and for interpretation of at-risk pregnancies. Further, this assay cannot distinguish SMA carriers from controls—a task that is important for determining recurrence risk and for distinguishing an inherited mutation from a de novo mutation. Thus in some scenarios, quantitative methods such as real-time PCR, multiplex ligation-dependent probe amplification, denaturing high-pressure liquid chromatography, fluorescent PCR coupled with capillary electrophoresis, or DNA sequencing must be used.[238,312,610,674,713] Population-based carrier screening for SMA has been proposed but is not currently the standard of care.[521] With prospects of therapeutic treatment for SMA and early age of onset for the disease, newborn screening for SMA has also been proposed.[523] This testing would allow early identification of patients and would enable timely treatment intervention, thereby minimizing the severity of the disease. Although it is theoretically sound, widespread newborn screening for SMA is not widely available.

Autosomal Dominant Diseases

In autosomal dominant conditions, a single abnormal allele is sufficient to cause disease despite the presence of a normal allele. An individual with an autosomal dominant disease may have inherited an abnormal allele from an affected parent, or alternatively, the mutant allele may have risen de novo as a new mutation during gametogenesis in an unaffected parent. The disease-causing gene is on one of the autosomes (1 to 22) and is not on a sex chromosome (X or Y). An affected individual possesses a 50% risk of donating the mutant allele to an offspring. Different mutations within the gene have varying effects on the protein, so that affected patients can have variability in clinical expression of the disease. In some instances, known mutant gene carriers have no clinical symptoms of the disease in a phenomenon referred to as *reduced penetrance,* yet they possess a 50% chance of having an affected child. Differences in phenotypic expression of the disease despite an identical mutation are most likely explained by the effects of other genes (modifier genes) and/or environmental influences. Among pedigrees illustrating autosomal dominant inheritance, both males and females are affected and male-to-male transmission is observed.

Achondroplasia

Achondroplasia (ACH) (OMIM #100800) is the most common nonlethal form of human genetic dwarfism with a worldwide incidence of 1 in 10,000 to 1 in 30,000.[308] ACH is inherited as an autosomal dominant disorder with 100% penetrance and is characterized by short-limbed dwarfism (rhizomelic form), macrocephaly, frontal and biparietal bossing, bowing of the lower extremities, and normal intelligence. The mean adult height is 131 cm for men and 124 cm for women, with a standard deviation of 5.6 and 5.9 cm, respectively. Close monitoring of patients is essential to prevent morbidity and mortality arising from complications of the disease.[48] Infants with this disease can die within the first year of life from central apnea caused by compression at the craniocervical junction; two copies of the mutant allele are often lethal.[241,473,502] Children undergoing surgical decompression of the craniocervical junction have decreased mortality and demonstrate improvement in neurologic function. During the first 5 years of life, affected children are at risk of death from compression of the brainstem and/or the upper cervical spinal cord. In adult patients, the leading cause of death is heart disease, and life expectancy is about 10 years less than for the general population.[707]

More than 90% of patients are born to parents of normal height. These patients represent sporadic cases arising as de novo mutations—a phenomenon associated with the "paternal effect" and advanced paternal age (older than 35 years).[137,229] Moreover, the estimated germline frequency of the common de novo disease causing mutation may be the highest observed in human beings.[692] The observed paternal effect associated with ACH has been thought to occur as the result of lifelong spermatogonial stem cell divisions, and thus an increase in production of mutant sperm as the male grows older.[131] Analysis of DNA extracted from testicular biopsy samples from older subjects supports this conclusion.[137] Alternatively, it has been proposed that sperm bearing ACH gene mutations may have a selective advantage in spermatogonial cells.[242] With both the paternal effect and a high mutation rate, when two affected siblings born to normal-sized parents shared a 4p haplotype derived from their unaffected father, Sobetzko and coworkers suggested that two de novo, independent, sporadic events had occurred, or that paternal gonadal mosaicism was present.[596] In a second reported family, recurrent affected siblings were shown to arise from paternal germline mosaicism rather than recurrent de novo mutations.[469] In one unusual report, it was concluded that siblings with achondroplasia born to unaffected parents were a result of germline mosaicism from the mother.[286] Although the mother had no clinical features of achondroplasia, a mutant allele was detected in the DNA extracted from her peripheral blood.

In 1994, the gene for achondroplasia was mapped to the telomeric region of chromosome 4p (4p16.3) using linkage studies on multigenerational families.[209,657] The fibroblast growth factor receptor 3 gene *(FGFR3),* mapped to this region and previously considered as a candidate gene for Huntington's disease (HD), was evaluated as a candidate gene for achondroplasia and was reported to contain mutations in patients with achondroplasia.[586,626] The *FGFR3* gene consists of 17 exons and encodes an mRNA of 4000 base pairs (bp). A different set of mutations in the *FGFR3* gene, causing varying effects on the function of *FGFR3,* have been associated with related forms of dwarfism, including thanatophoric dysplasia type I (OMIM #187601) and type II (OMIM #187601), hypochondroplasia (OMIM #146000), and a severe form of achondroplasia with developmental delay and acanthosis nigricans.[274,307]

The *FGFR3* protein product, FGFR3, is one of four human fibroblast growth factor (FGF) receptors and contains three extracellular immunoglobulin-like domains, a single transmembrane domain, and a split intracellular tyrosine kinase domain.[342] FGFR3 is a tyrosine kinase receptor that, when bound to 1 of 22 possible FGFs and heparan sulfate–bearing proteoglycans on the cell surface, induces dimerization of receptor monomers, activates tyrosine kinase activity, and promotes phosphorylation of tyrosine residues in the cytoplasmic domain, which in turn induces multiple signaling pathways, including STAT, MAPK, PLC-γ, and PI3K-AKT.[308,617] Signaling through FGFR3 is complex and is not completely characterized, but FGFR3 is thought to negatively regulate chondrocyte proliferation through apoptosis and differentiation.[124,145,533] Precisely which FGFs serve as ligands for FGFR3 is not known. Different proteoglycans on the cell surface, various isoforms due to alternative splicing, and different FGFs at different stages of development and at different locations of the growth plate give rise to added diversity of FGFR3 ligand binding and subsequent effects.

The primary mutation in achondroplasia results in a defect in normal internalization and ubiquitination and lyosomal degradation of the mutant receptor. Thus it is retained on the cell surface and has uncontrolled and prolonged phosphorylation of FGFR3 signaling in chondrocytes.[274,453] Hence, chondrocyte maturation and terminal differentiation are inhibited. As such, therapies are directed toward the increase in short stature. New therapies can be directed toward the molecular bases of disease, including (1) chemical inhibitors of FGFR3 tyrosine kinase activity, (2) antibodies that prevent binding of FGF ligands to FGFR3, and (3) targeting of regulators of various FGF-induced signaling pathways.[143,263,307]

In the original report identifying the *FGFR3* gene as the cause of achondroplasia, 15 of 16 patients had a G-to-A transition mutation at nucleotide 1138 (c.1138G>A), and the only patient who did not have this mutation instead had a G-to-C transversion mutation at the same position (c.1138G>C).[586] Both mutations result in a glycine-to-arginine substitution in the transmembrane domain of FGFR3 at codon 380. The frequency of the G-to-A transition mutation at codon 380 in achondroplasia patients is well documented and represents more than 95% of the mutation detected in this population.[55,551] This base pair may be prone to mutation because a cytosine residue in a CpG dinucleotide is known to be a hot spot for transition mutations.[41,64,166] If the cytosine residue is methylated (i.e., as 5-methylcytosine), it can spontaneously deaminate to thymine to introduce the change from a G:C base pair to an A:T base pair in subsequent replications of DNA. Because most *FGFR3* mutations causing achondroplasia are c.1138G>A or c.1138G>C, DNA testing includes targeted mutation analysis for both mutations using a variety of techniques.[218] Testing can be performed postnatally to confirm the diagnosis of achondroplasia. Prenatal DNA testing may be requested by couples in which one is affected with ACH and the risk of an affected child is 50%. Alternatively, preimplantation genetic diagnosis can be performed for ACH.[12] In addition, prenatal testing can be requested by unaffected parents with a previous affected child, who may be concerned about germline mosaicism, although the risk of recurrence in these cases would be considered low. Pregnancies involving mating between two affected individuals are not uncommon. Prenatal DNA testing can be requested by these couples because they have a 25% chance of having a child homozygous for an *FGFR3* gene mutation—a potentially lethal condition. This situation presents difficult choices for the couple. In one study, attitudes of affected individuals and their relatives toward termination of the pregnancy based on prenatal findings indicated that if the fetus was homozygous mutant for ACH, 40% would consider termination compared with 41% who would not; 19% were unsure of what they would do.[240] In this same study, if the fetus was heterozygous for a mutation causing achondroplasia, 5% would consider termination and 86% would not; 8% were unsure what they would do. Last, if the fetus was determined to be normal, having not received a mutation from either parent to cause this disease, 90% responded that they would not consider termination of the pregnancy, but 3% would; 6% were unsure of what their decision might be.

Huntington's Disease

Huntington's disease (HD) (OMIM#143100) is an autosomal dominant, late-onset neurodegenerative disorder with an incidence of about 3 to 10 per 100,000 in most populations of European origin. First described by George Huntington in 1872, the disease is progressive and is characterized by frequent involuntary, rapid movements (chorea) and dementia.[320] The mean age of onset is between 35 and 44 years, but approximately 25% of patients first display symptoms after the age of 50, and about 10% of patients have juvenile HD with age of onset before 20 years.[279,465] The median survival time is 15 to 20 years after onset of symptoms. In the first few years of the disease, symptoms include mood disturbances, cognitive deficits, clumsiness, and impairment of voluntary movement.[279] The next stage of the disease is associated with slurred speech (dysarthria), hyperreflexia, chorea, gait abnormalities, and behavioral disturbances such as intermittent explosiveness, apathy, aggression, alcohol abuse, sexual dysfunction and deviations, and increased appetite.[207] As the disease advances, bradykinesia, rigidity, dementia, dystonia, and dysphagia are present. In the late stages of HD, weight loss, sleep disturbances, and incontinence occur.

In 1983, Gusella and associates reported linkage between DNA marker D4S10, on the short arm of chromosome 4, and HD, based on studies from a large kindred in Venezuela.[261] Subsequently, more DNA markers were identified, and the region of the genome containing the HD gene was narrowed to 4p16.3.[50,126,225,420,680] Through an international collaborative effort, and 10 years after its initial localization, the HD gene, *IT15,* was cloned.[321] The molecular basis for HD was determined to be expansion of a glutamine-encoding CAG trinucleotide repeat; this was subsequently confirmed in a worldwide study by the identification of expanded CAG-repeat alleles in HD patients from 565 families, representing 43 national or ethnic groups.[377] In this initial international study, the median CAG-repeat length was reported to be 44 in affected patients and 18 in controls. Normal CAG repeats range from 10 to 26, repeats of 27 to 35 are considered intermediate or "mutable," repeats of 36 to 39 are associated with reduced penetrance of the disease, and repeats of 40 or greater are associated with HD (Figure 40-3). HD is one of about 20 inherited neurologic diseases associated with trinucleotide repeat instability.[83,491] In HD, the number of CAG repeats is inversely correlated with age at onset of the disease. Patients with onset as early as 2 years of life have a repeat number approaching 100 or greater, and late-onset-disease patients have repeat numbers of 36 to 39.[19,81,169,321,377,594] However, an autopsy confirmed that the diagnosis of HD was reported in a 65-year-old male with as few as 29 CAG repeats.[364] Although the CAG-repeat number accounts for the majority of variance in age of onset for HD (≈70%), the remainder of the variance is due to modifier genes or environmental factors. Analysis of the large Venezuelan HD kindreds encompassing 18,149

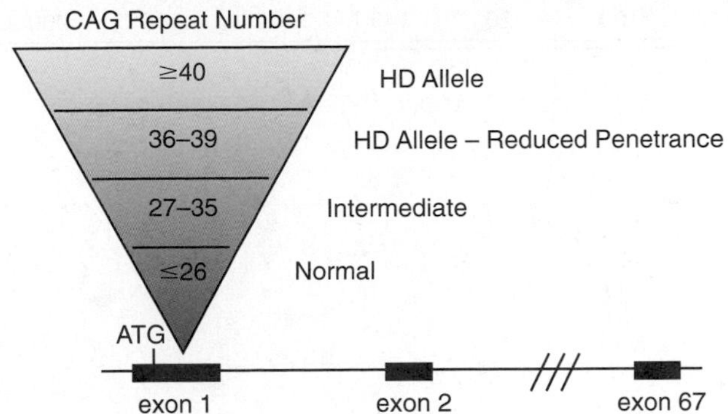

Figure 40-3 Schematic representation of the polyglutamine-encoding CAG repeat in exon 1 of the HD gene and associated alleles. A CAG-repeat number ≤26 is considered normal. CAG-repeat numbers of 27 to 35 are intermediate, and although they are not associated with an abnormal phenotype, these alleles are prone to meiotic expansion to an HD allele. CAG repeats of 36 to 39 are considered HD alleles but with reduced penetrance, indicating that both unaffected and affected patients have been reported with alleles of this size. CAG repeats ≥40 are associated with HD with complete penetrance.

individuals spanning 10 generations indicated that 40% of the remainder of the variance is due to modifier genes, and 60% to environmental factors.[643] The largest genome-wide scan to identify modifying loci was performed on these Venezuelean kindreds.[216] Most significant LOD scores (logarithm of the odds ratio) were identified at chromosomal regions 2p25, 2q35, 5p14, and 5q32, suggesting the physical location of candidate modifying genes.

New mutations for HD (the presence of an affected individual in the absence of a family history) occur from expansion of CAG-intermediate alleles and occur almost exclusively through expansion during paternal transmission.[233] Although intermediate alleles are present in about 1% of the population, it appears that flanking DNA sequences may influence the instability of these alleles by enhancing the formation of hairpin loop structures and causing replication slippage.[114,234] Single sperm analysis studies have demonstrated 11% instability (9% expansions and 2.5% contractions) in CAG repeats of 30 compared with 0.6% instability (contractions only) seen in average-sized alleles of 15 to 18 repeats.[392] These studies indicate that an increase in instability occurs as the repeat number increases. This concept is further supported by observations that CAG repeats of 36 showed 53% instability, and CAG repeats from 38 to 51 had instability ranging from 92 to 99%. In addition, *cis*-elements may play a role in CAG-repeat instability in *IT15*.[678] Warby and colleagues identified a common haplotype (A) of 22 tagged single-nucleotide polymorphisms (tSNPs) that was more common on HD (95%) and intermediate (83%) alleles in patients of European origin than on normal (53%) alleles from the same population. Onset of symptoms occurs at progressively younger ages in successive generations of affected families, a pattern called *anticipation.* Anticipation is explained by meiotic expansion of the unstable CAG repeat during transmission by the affected parent, resulting in an even higher CAG-repeat number in the offspring and an earlier age of onset. In addition, although 69% of affected father-child pairs show expansion, only 32% of affected mother-child pairs demonstrate expansion. Further, <2% of maternal expansions result in a change of >5 repeats, whereas up to 21% of paternal transmissions increase by >7 repeats.[376] The affected parent in most cases of juvenile-onset HD is the father. However, the largest reported CAG-repeat number of ≈130 occurred via maternal expansion of 70 CAG repeats.[467] An increase in the CAG-repeat number is also associated with more rapid progression of disease and greater neuropathologic severity in the striatum.[213,508] However, it is interesting to note that homozygotes with two expanded CAG-repeat alleles do not have more severe disease than heterozygotes.[377,464,690]

The HD gene protein, huntingtin (htt), consists of 3144 amino acids with a molecular mass of ≈349 kDa, is ubiquitously expressed in all tissue, and predominantly resides in the cytoplasm with lesser amounts in the nucleus.[148,262,302,627,655] With universal distribution, it is not known how and/or why the primary phenotype is neuronal loss. In neurons, htt is associated with synaptic vesicles and microtubules and is abundant in dendrites and nerve terminals. Huntingtin interacts with multiple proteins, indicating its function in intracellular trafficking and cytoskeletal organization, as well as in endocytosis, apoptosis, and transcription regulation.* Mutant HD alleles are effectively transcribed and translated, but as a result of the increase in glutamine residues, the protein is misfolded.[564] Thus, abnormal folding may result in aberrant protein-protein interaction of mutant htt with any of its protein partners and could contribute to the pathogenesis of HD. In addition, neuronal mitochondrial dysfunction may play a role in the disease process.[85,675] Further, aggregates of fragmented mutant htt form neuronal nuclear inclusion bodies (IBs), which may be toxic to the cells.[156] Recent data, however, suggest that IBs may result from a normal cellular process to handle abnormal and toxic proteins, and that their formation is facilitated by proteasomal chaperones.[448,550] HD remains an incurable disease; however, various therapeutic strategies have been proposed and/or attempted in animal models. Such strategies include allele-specific silencing of mutant *IT15* mRNA; small molecules targeted toward mutant htt; and cell transplantation therapy.[360,620,719]

DNA testing for HD is performed with the use of PCR so that the exact CAG-repeat number can be determined.[321] Soon after the initial report, it was discovered that the accuracy of determining the CAG-repeat number by PCR was compromised by inclusion of a polymorphic CGG repeat immediately downstream from the CAG repeat. Because the CGG repeat was contained within the amplified sequence, the length of the amplicon could be altered and overestimated.[20,555] Upon this discovery, a new primer pair was identified that flanked the CAG repeat, yet excluded the problematic polymorphic CGG repeat and provided accurate assessment of

*References 39, 178, 353, 395-397, 442, 591, 668, 677, and 725.

BOX 40-2 Ethical Issues Associated With Presymptomatic DNA Testing for HD

Patients must be 18 years of age.
The decision to proceed with testing must be voluntary and informed.
Genetic counseling regarding benefits/pitfalls of testing is required.
A support partner is needed for the patient for counseling and the testing process.
Diagnosis of Huntington's disease (HD) in the family should be confirmed by DNA testing before presymptomatic testing.
Psychiatric assessment of patient is necessary before testing.
Follow-up genetic counseling is recommended after delivery of results.
Discrimination by insurance carriers or employers may occur following completion of testing.
Prenatal testing of fetus is controversial; preimplantation diagnosis is available.

the CAG-repeat number.[679] However, in contrast to earlier years, when PCR involved the use of ^{32}P-labeled primers for this and similar assays, currently the most common method involves the use of PCR with fluorescently labeled primers and capillary electrophoresis[664] (Figure 40-4). Guidelines for diagnostic testing by clinical laboratories with reference to standardization and interpretation have been developed.[518]

Besides the technical and interpretive difficulties associated with HD testing, many ethical issues exist as well, primarily as they relate to presymptomatic testing (Box 40-2). The first policy statement on ethical issues related to genetic testing for HD was adopted in 1989 at a joint meeting with representatives from the International Huntington Association and the World Federation of Neurology.[325] At that time, the gene had not yet been cloned, and predictive testing was performed using linkage studies; the at-risk patient was quoted the likelihood of inheriting the mutant allele. These tests were less than perfect and provided, at best, results in only 60 to 75% of families. Moreover, the possibility of recombination allowed erroneous predictions to occur.[280,463] In other families, living affected members were not available, or markers were not informative. Once the gene had been cloned and direct mutation analysis was possible, risk assessments were reversed in a small percentage of patients.[11]

Following cloning of the gene and the availability of direct mutation analysis, guidelines for predictive testing were re-evaluated, and changes were proposed by the International Huntington Association and the World Federation of Neurology Research Group on Huntington's Chorea.[326] Direct predictive testing was preferred over linkage studies and was readily accepted by the HD community.[33] The approach used for HD has become the model for predictive testing for late-onset single-gene disorders, and similar formats have been applied to other late-onset inherited diseases, including the autosomal dominant cerebellar ataxias and less common, dominantly inherited, fatal familial insomnia.[232,640] If an HD-causing expanded CAG-repeat allele is identified in the

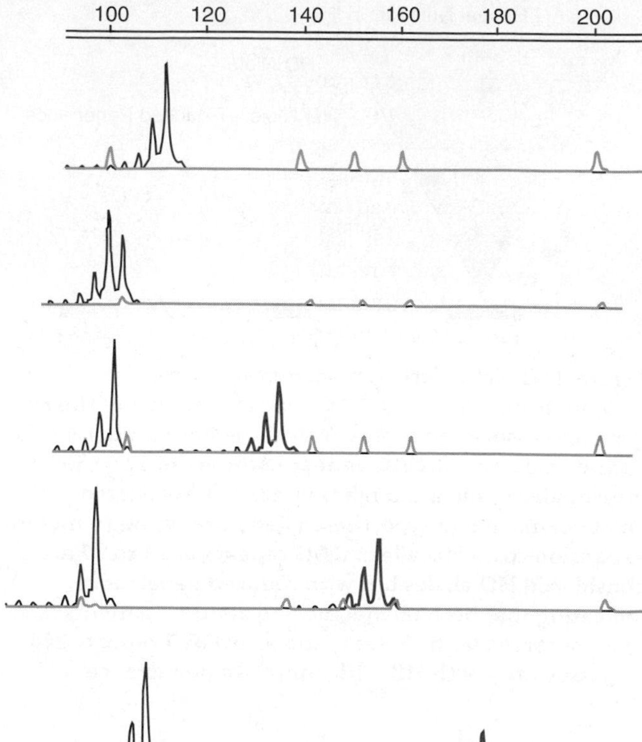

Figure 40-4 Electropherograms representing various patterns observed in patients referred for Huntington's disease (HD) testing. The polyglutamine-encoding CAG repeat in exon 1 is amplified by polymerase chain reaction (PCR) using flanking oligonucleotide primers, one of which is labeled with a fluorescent dye. Amplicons are subjected to electrophoresis on a 5% denaturing polyacrylamide gel on an ABI 377 DNA sequencer and are analyzed using GeneScan software, version 3.1 b3 (Applied Biosystems, Foster City, Calif). Amplicons 100 base pairs (bp) in length contain 18 CAG repeats and flanking DNA. Patient 1 *(row 1, top)* has amplicons 112 bp in length and has 22 CAG repeats on both HD alleles. Patient 2 *(row 2)* has 97 bp and 100 bp amplicons, corresponding to CAG repeats of 17 and 18. The diagnosis of HD can be ruled out in these two patients. Patient 3 *(row 3)* has 97 bp and 133 bp amplicons corresponding to CAG repeats of 17 and 29. The results would not support a diagnosis of HD. However, a CAG repeat of 29 is considered intermediate and can undergo meiotic expansion to an HD allele. Patient 4 *(row 4)* has CAG repeats of 19 and 38, as depicted by amplicons 103 bp and 160 bp in length. In the symptomatic patient, these results would support the diagnosis of HD. However, in the presymptomatic patient, the phenotype of this HD allele with reduced penetrance cannot be predicted with certainty. Patient 5 *(row 5)* has CAG repeats of 21 and 44 because amplicons 109 bp and 178 bp in length were detected. These results would confirm the diagnosis of HD. Genetic counseling regarding the implications of DNA findings in patients 3, 4, and 5 is indicated.

asymptomatic patient (≥40 years), the median age of onset in HD patients with the patient's corresponding CAG-repeat number can be quoted to the patient.[81] Predictive testing should be performed only on adults and only with informed consent. Informed consent implies that the patient has been thoroughly counseled and clearly understands both the advantages and the disadvantages of knowing the results. Advantages of having this test include but are not limited to removal of uncertainty regarding whether patients have or have not inherited the mutant allele and the feeling of relief for those who have not inherited a mutant HD allele. This information can help patients appropriately plan their personal and career paths. Disadvantages of knowing this information include but are not limited to (1) the feeling of "survivor's guilt" in those who learn that they have not inherited a mutant allele and other family members have; (2) fear from learning that they have inherited a mutant HD allele and will develop this incurable disease; (3) risk of discrimination in employment or health insurance coverage if the results are disclosed; (4) worry about a 50% chance of passing this gene on to their offspring; and (5) uncertainty of developing disease if they have inherited a mutant HD allele containing 36 to 39 CAG repeats.

It is important to note that the guidelines indicate that the patient should be accompanied by a trusted friend or loved one throughout the counseling and testing procedure. This person can provide stability to the patient by being able to intimately speak to the patient about the situation and discuss the information shared at the counseling sessions. Most important, as a part of this process, the partner will be present when the results of testing are revealed and can provide comfort and support as needed both then and in the following days, weeks, or months. Ultimately, however, it is the patient's decision to proceed with this testing and to accept both the benefits and pitfalls of knowing this information. The patient's decision to proceed must be his or hers, without coercion from family members, clinicians, friends, or employers.

For at-risk individuals requesting mutation studies, it is important that their mental stability is considered for the safety of the patient; a psychiatric assessment is often part of the testing protocol because HD test results can precipitate depression. Results of the psychiatric evaluation can influence the timing of the DNA test, postponing it until such time when the patient is considered mentally able to deal with the possibly devastating news. Suicidal tendencies associated with HD range from 9.1% in at-risk individuals displaying a normal neurologic examination to as high as 23.5% in at-risk individuals with neurologic findings consistent with "possible Huntington's disease."[503] Suicidal thoughts in patients with confirmed HD range from 16.7% in the early stage of disease to 21.6% later in the disease, when independence diminishes.[503]

If possible before presymptomatic mutation testing, the diagnosis of HD should be confirmed in an affected member of the family to be certain that the disease in the family is indeed HD. Excluding HD cannot rule out a different, dominantly inherited neurodegenerative disease in the family for which the patient likely retains a risk of development. Because HD is a delayed-onset disease, as the asymptomatic at-risk patient ages, the risk of testing positive with an expanded CAG repeat decreases.[276] Thus should the patient elect not to have predictive testing, the genetic counselor can provide information regarding the probability that an HD mutation exists, which, based on the individual's age, may provide some comfort to the patient. Most individuals who seek presymptomatic testing have a mean age of ≈40 years and are more often female.[631] It is also not uncommon for one to begin this multistep counseling process and withdrawal from the study without receiving test results.[631] Counseling in families with no prior family history of HD can be complicated. In these cases, the expanded CAG repeat appears to be de novo. Multiple factors can explain this phenomenon, including (1) expansion of an intermediate (27 to 35) or reduced penetrance allele (36 to 39); (2) premature death of an adult asymptomatic individual; (3) misdiagnosis in other family members; (4) alternative paternity; and (5) undisclosed adoption. For appropriate at-risk assessment of individuals with these pedigrees, it is important to try to determine the likely explanation; however, in some cases, it may not be known, and thus counseling for the risk of HD should be prudent.

Prenatal testing for HD, another complicated issue associated with this disease, may not be provided in all laboratories that perform routine HD testing. If a molecular genetics laboratory chooses not to provide prenatal testing (e.g., because of the possibility of termination of a pregnancy for a late-onset disorder, or because it constitutes presymptomatic testing of the child should the parents choose not to terminate), it is the responsibility of the laboratory to identify an alternative laboratory for testing to which the patient can be referred. Before cloning of the HD gene, prenatal testing was performed using linkage studies, and the likelihood that the child would develop HD was "excluded" if the child had inherited an HD haplotype from an unaffected grandparent.[447,638] The concept of exclusion testing was difficult to understand, however, and not all families were heterozygous for the DNA markers, thereby making the test inconclusive. In some instances, the status of the parent at risk for developing the disease was also revealed. Moreover, testing could in theory lead to abortion of 50% of fetuses who had not inherited HD but rather had inherited the normal HD allele from the affected grandparent. To eliminate some of the controversy of prenatal testing for HD, preimplantation genetic diagnosis (PGD) can be performed. In PGD, in vitro fertilization is used to produce embryos that then undergo a single cell biopsy for analysis of their HD genes. Once PCR has been used to determine the HD CAG-repeat numbers, embryos with normal HD alleles are implanted. This method, which combines direct mutation analysis and PGD, eliminates the necessity for prenatal testing to determine the HD status of the fetus, because the HD alleles of the fetus are known to be normal, and the need for termination of a pregnancy is eradicated. Further, this method can be performed without disclosing the HD status of the asymptomatic, yet at-risk parent. However, this approach of nondisclosure PGD can pose ethical problems for testing personnel.[76] In some testing centers, PGD may be performed by direct mutation analysis in families in which the at-risk parent is knowledgeable regarding his or her carrier status, and embryos with only normal HD alleles are implanted. Alternatively, in families in which the parent is unaware of his or her HD status, PGD can be performed using exclusion testing, whereby only embryos who have not inherited an affected allele are implanted, and information regarding the HD CAG repeat numbers in all tested embryos is not disclosed to the parents.[76,575,576]

Marfan Syndrome

Marfan syndrome (MFS) (OMIM #154700) is an autosomal dominant multisystem connective tissue disorder with primary manifestations involving the ocular, musculoskeletal, and cardiovascular systems and an estimated worldwide incidence of 1 in 5000.[146,155,348] Common ocular features of MFS include myopia, bilateral ectopia lentis, and retinal detachment. In addition, patients with MFS are at increased risk for cataracts at a younger age. Skeletal abnormalities arise from bone overgrowth and joint hypermobility. MFS patients are tall with frequent clinical findings including pectus excavatum or pectus carinatum, arm span-to-height ratio greater than 1.05, and a reduced upper body-to-lower extremity ratio. Scoliosis is present and can be mild to severe and is progressive. Morbidity and early mortality of the disease are linked to cardiovascular manifestations of the disorder, which are characterized by progressive dilation of the aortic root, predisposition to aortic dissection, mitral valve prolapse with or without regurgitation, and dilation of the pulmonary artery. Wide phenotypic variability is observed, with some patients presenting as neonates and others remaining undiagnosed until adulthood. An early diagnosis is associated with an improved long-term outcome.[694] Unfortunately, it is not uncommon to first diagnose MFS in a patient at autopsy when associated with sudden premature death due to aortic dissection and/or rupture.[372,539]

The diagnosis of MFS is based on family history of the disease, although as many as 25% of cases of MFS can arise from a new mutation and thus a negative family history of disease.[154] In the absence of a documented family history of MFS, the clinical diagnosis of MFS is made using the Ghent nosology in adults.[141,146] The MFS diagnosis relies on specific significant clinical manifestations involving two organ systems and minor involvement of a third organ system.[146] Because most clinical manifestations increase with age, these criteria may be less applicable to diagnosis in the pediatric community.[188]

Classic MFS is associated with mutations in the fibrillin gene *(FBN1)* mapped to 15q21.1.[154,298,351] The gene spans 237,414 bp, is composed of 65 exons, and encodes a 10 kb mRNA, prefibrillin-1.[62] *FBN1* is ubiquitously expressed in connective tissue.[62] The ≈350 kDa, 2871 amino acid extracellular glycoprotein, fibrillin-1, self-assembles into macroaggregates to serve as the primary structural component of 10 to 12 nm diameter microfibrils in elastic and nonelastic tissue.[62,313] In elastic tissue, microfibrils make up the scaffold for elastin assembly within the extracellular matrix. In nonelastic tissue, including the ciliary zonule of the eye and of basement membranes, they have an anchoring function and provide tensile strength.[526] Fibrillin-1 contains several motifs, including cysteine-rich calcium binding epidermal growth factor-like domains interspersed with eight cysteine motifs. These motifs are interspersed by transforming growth factor-β (TGF-β) binding protein (LTBP) domains. LTBPs interact with fibrillin-1 and together bind TGF-β to inactivate and thereby prevent signaling through the SMAD 2/3 pathway.[243,314,526] Studies on the MFS mouse deficient in fibrillin-1 demonstrated that reduced LTBP–fibrillin-1 complexes led to the inability to sequester latent TGF-β and resulted in increased activity and dysregulation of TGF-β.[474]

Mutations in *FBN1* are heterogeneous, with more than 600 reported throughout the gene. Phenotype-genotype studies have shown that neonatal MFS and severe MFS, with an earlier age of diagnosis, have an increased likelihood of ectopia lentis, ascending aortic dilation, aortic surgery, mitral valve anomalies, and scoliosis, and a reduced life expectancy, and are associated with mutations spanning exons 24 to 32.[186,187,636] This region of the protein contains the longest stretch of epidermal growth factor (EGF)-like domains and is thought to be important for microfibril biogenesis. More specifically, one study suggested that neonatal MFS is most frequently associated with exon 25 mutations.[186] In this study, in-frame missense mutations were often associated with more severe complications of MFS than were mutations predicted to cause premature truncation of the protein.[186] Further, many of the missense mutations affected highly conserved cysteine residues within the EGF-like domains. It is interesting to note that wide phenotypic variability is observed even for individuals harboring the same recurrent mutation, suggesting the role of modifier genes in the MFS phenotype.[186] The likely effect of yet to be identified modifier genes on the MFS phenotype explains the lack of consistent genotype-phenotype correlations. Further, the lack of consistent genotype-phenotype correlations provides little prognostic value for individual patient management.

Management of patients with MFS is similar to that of patients with other inherited multisystem disorders, involving a team approach with specialists in many areas of medicine. It is now believed that the pathogenesis of MFS is due to the increased availability of TGF-β; therefore, treatment for MFS includes the use of TGF-β antagonists. Studies using this approach on the MFS mouse model have been reported not only to stop the progression of disease but also to reverse the cardiovascular consequences of FBN1 deficiency.[264] As a result, the antihypertensive drug losartan is being used clinically for MFS patients; it acts as an angiotensin II type 1 receptor inhibitor to inhibit excessive TGF-β signaling.[82]

TGF-β signaling also requires the action of matrix metalloproteases to allow for proper release and interaction of TGF-β with its receptor complexes. Thus, targeted treatment through inhibition of matrix metalloproteinase-2 and -9 has also been successfully employed.[116]

FBN1 is one of the largest human genes, and although it is labor intensive and costly, DNA sequencing is the gold standard for DNA testing for Marfan syndrome. Thus, many laboratories invoke a prescreening approach to identify the region of interest within the gene that may harbor a mutation. If an area of interest is detected, DNA sequencing is performed for mutation identification.[318] Using this method, full *FBN1* gene sequencing can be reserved for those patients for whom no mutations are identified by gene scanning approaches to prevent a false-negative result from gene scanning techniques. It is important to note that the presence of an *FBN1* mutation does not imply a clinical diagnosis of MFS because mutations in this gene can be associated with isolated ocular, skeletal, or cardiovascular features also seen in MFS patients.[214] These patients do not meet the clinical criteria of MFS but rather are collectively referred to as having *type I fibrillinopathies. FBN1* mutation detection in this patient population is variable.[605] Despite extensive *FBN1* analysis, as many as 30% of MFS patients will have no mutation detected. These cases could reflect patients with *FBN1* mutations that are contained within regions of the gene that cannot be detected by current screening techniques; patients who do not meet the strict Ghent diagnostic criteria; or patients with genetic heterogeneity whereby mutations in other genes cause the MFS phenotype.[260,407] Once an *FBN1* mutation has been identified within a family, predictive testing for at-risk family members as well as prenatal or preimplantation genetic diagnosis can be performed.

X-Linked Diseases

In X-linked diseases, the mutant allele resides on the X chromosome. In X-linked recessive diseases, females are carriers of the disease with one normal and one mutant allele but typically are not affected. Males receiving the mutant allele from their mothers and having only one X chromosome have no normal allele and thus are affected. All daughters of affected males are carriers of a mutant allele. The carrier female has a 25% chance of transmitting her normal allele to a son, a 25% chance of having an affected son, a 25% chance of having a daughter who carries the mutant allele, and a 25% chance of having a daughter who receives her normal allele. In the absence of a family history, an affected male can have a mutant allele that arose de novo as a new mutation during formation of the egg. Roughly one third of all cases of X-linked disorders represent new mutations, indicating that the mother is not a carrier of a mutant allele and is not at risk for subsequent affected children. In pedigrees associated with X-linked recessive conditions, typically only males are affected, and male-to-male transmission of the disease is not seen. In less frequent, X-linked dominant diseases, one copy of the mutant allele is sufficient to cause disease despite the presence of a normal allele. Further, in males with only a mutant allele, these diseases are often lethal.

Hemophilia A

Hemophilia A (HA) (OMIM #306700) is an X-linked recessive bleeding disorder caused by a deficiency of coagulation factor VIII (FVIII); it affects approximately 1 in 5000 males worldwide.[245] The disease is characterized by prolonged bleeding after injury or surgery, renewed bleeding after the initial bleeding has ceased, and, in severe cases, spontaneous bleeding into the joints. The severity of the disease is classified according to the amount of FVIII coagulant activity present in the plasma; severe, moderate, or mild disease corresponds to FVIII activity levels of <1%, 1 to 5%, or 5 to 30%, respectively. Severe disease is seen in 50% of patients; 10% have moderate disease and 40% have mild disease.[22] In the patient with severe or moderate hemophilia A disease, the activated partial thromboplastin time (aPTT) will be prolonged, while all other routine coagulation tests will be normal. In patients with mild hemophilia A disease, however, aPTT is often normal. Age at diagnosis is typically younger in cases of severe disease and in cases with a family history of disease.[106] Most patients with severe disease are diagnosed in the first year of life; patients with mild disease may not be diagnosed until several years later. Diagnosis may also be delayed because about 30% of cases arise as a new mutation in the absence of a family history. As an X-linked disease, HA typically presents in males; however, females with the disease have been reported. Carrier females can present with severe disease caused by (1) skewed X-chromosome inactivation, in which the X chromosome with the mutant *FVIII* gene is not inactivated because of its involvement in an X-autosome translocation; (2) an X inactive transcript gene, *XIST*, mutation; or (3) the presence of a mutant *FVIII* gene on each of the X chromosomes.[61,454,572,644,696]

The clinical phenotype of HA is variable for both frequency and type of bleeding and is most often associated with the baseline plasma FVIII level for the patient. Treatment for bleeding episodes consists of intravenous infusions of FVIII concentrate given as quickly as possible to prevent pain, disability, and chronic joint disease. For children with severe hemophilia, the standard of care is to provide prophylactic infusions of FVIII concentrate within the first 2 years of life to maintain their clotting activity above 1% and to decrease the number of spontaneous bleeding episodes.[416] As a result, clotting factor consumption has increased dramatically over the years and is quite costly, but this regime has significantly decreased hemophiliac arthropathy and has extended the life span to near normal.[206] Management of 30% of patients with severe disease is complicated by immunoglobulin (Ig)G antibody formation, termed *inhibitors*, to exogenous FVIII that is caused by repeated infusions. These antibodies can rapidly neutralize infused FVIII. Inhibitor formation generally occurs early in treatment, usually before the 15th infusion, and is suspected when a poor response to FVIII infusion therapy is observed.[362,623] The formation of inhibitors is dependent on the type of FVIII mutation, as well as on other genetic and environmental factors.[623] A risk stratification score was recently devised to assist with identification of patients at high risk for inhibitor formation, thereby enabling individualized treatment strategies to minimize inhibitor formation.[623] Before the use of recombinant FVIII, management of the disease was further complicated in patients who had contracted bloodborne pathogens, human immunodeficiency virus, and/or hepatitis C virus from contaminated plasma-derived FVIII concentrates. Great interest in gene therapy for hemophilia A remains, despite limited success thus far.[310,662] However, Margaritis and associates reported promising results using in vivo adeno-associated viral vector delivery of continuously expressed recombinant FVIIa in the canine model of HA, thus bypassing FVIII-FIX and avoiding the risk of FVIII inhibitor formation.[427]

The *FVIII* gene is found on Xq28 and was cloned in 1984.[228] This gene spans more than 186,000 base pairs and includes 26 exons.[21] The *FVIII* gene is predominantly expressed in the liver and encodes a 9 kb mRNA transcript.[652] The mature 2332 amino acid FVIII protein is produced after cleavage of a 19 amino acid N-terminal leader peptide. The protein is divided into several domains, referred to as A1, A2, B (heavy chain), A3, and C1 and C2 (light chain).[652] FVIII circulates in the plasma, and is protected and stabilized through noncovalent binding to the complex multimeric glycoprotein von Willebrand factor (vWF) through binding at the C2 domain. In the intrinsic coagulation pathway, proteolytic activation of FVIII occurs following cleavage by thrombin at multiple sites, where it participates as a cofactor with activated factor IX to catalyze the conversion of factor X to factor Xa.[193] The B domain of the protein is removed in the activated form, and the other components are held in a complex with Cu^{2+}.[245] Factor Xa hydrolyzes and activates prothrombin to thrombin. As the concentration of thrombin increases, FVIIIa is ultimately cleaved by thrombin and inactivated. This dual action of thrombin on FVIII regulates the formation of the FVIIIa, IXa, and X complex, thus regulating the clotting cascade. A deficiency of coagulation FVIII then leads to uncontrolled bleeding.

A plethora of nucleotide substitutions and gene deletions, insertions, and rearrangements throughout the *FVIII* gene account for more than 1000 mutations reported in patients with hemophilia.[285] The type of mutation, its location within the gene, and ultimately its effect on the functional activity of the FVIII protein account for much of the clinical heterogeneity that is observed with this disease.[239,246,634] Gross rearrangements of the *FVIII* gene, including intrachromosomal inversions or large deletions and duplications, are typically associated with severe disease.[239] Small deletions and insertions are also common in severe HA. Missense mutations are most frequently observed (95%) in patients with moderate and mild disease.[239] Further, patients with null mutations, large deletions, nonsense mutations, and common intron 22 inversions are most susceptible to inhibitor formation and have more complicated disease management issues.[362] Patients with nonsense mutations in the 5′ region of the gene have a lower risk of inhibitor formation than those with mutations involving the 3′ region of the gene.

Before the early 1990s, routine screening of coding, splice junctions, the promoter region, and the polyadenylation site of the gene could detect the mutation in most patients with mild to moderate disease, yet the disease-causing mutation in about half of those with severe disease remained elusive.[291] In 1993, a common inversion mutation was identified in approximately 45% of patients with severe disease.[386,472] The *int22h*-related inversions arose from genetic recombination between a small intronless gene within intron 22, gene A, and one of two additional copies of gene A located approximately 500 kb upstream from the *FVIII* gene. The mechanism for the inversion involves flipping of the tip of the X chromosome, allowing pairing between homologous sequences and genetic recombination between one of the upstream copies of gene A and the copy of gene A within intron 22. Consequently, the *FVIII* gene is divided into two parts, with exons 1 to 22 widely separated and in an opposite orientation and thus inverted from exons 23 to 26. Most (>75%) inversion mutations involve the distal copy of gene A upstream from the *FVIII* gene as compared with the adjacent proximal copy of gene A.[386] Rossiter and colleagues showed that this genetic recombination between homologous intragenic and extragenic copies of gene A occurred as a new mutation predominantly during male meiosis with a male-to-female ratio of 302 : 1.[549] Because Xq is unpaired with a homolog during male meiosis, it is able to flip on itself for an intrachromosomal recombination event. The role of this mutation as a primary cause of severe hemophilia A disease was subsequently confirmed by analysis of DNA from patients with hemophilia from around the world.[23] Additionally, this mutation has been identified in the Chapel Hill dog colony with hemophilia A disease and presumably arose from the same mechanism of genetic recombination between homologous sequences.[412] Subsequently, a second, less common inversion mutation resulting in about 1% of cases with severe disease was identified.[34] This inversion results from homologous recombination between a segment in intron 1 *(int1h1)* and a 1041 bp repeat that is 140 kb telomeric to *FVIII*.

In the mid-1980s, after the discovery of the *FVIII* gene and before our current DNA technologies were developed, DNA testing for hemophilia A primarily involved the use of linkage studies and restriction fragment length polymorphisms to determine the carrier status of at-risk females in the family and to perform prenatal testing.[24,698] Although accurate, these studies could be complicated by (1) the large number of family members required for participation in the analysis, (2) a limited number of alleles for each marker [limiting the chance that key members of the family would be informative (i.e., heterozygous) for a given marker], and (3) genetic recombination between the informative marker and the *FVIII* gene mutation, which could affect the accuracy of the results. Moreover, in the absence of a family history, the carrier status of the mother of a sporadic case was uncertain (although as many as two thirds of these mothers might be carriers). PCR and analysis of polymorphic microsatellite repeats within the

FVIII gene increased the number of families in which linkage studies could be performed and significantly improved turnaround times.[388]

The most significant improvements in DNA testing included the identification of the inversion mutation in families with severe disease and the ability to offer direct mutation analysis as opposed to linkage studies.[339,665] As a result, the carrier status of the mother of a sporadic case with a detectable inversion mutation could now be determined with certainty, and her risk for carrying another affected son could be precisely predicted to be 25% (Figure 40-5). In addition, prenatal and carrier testing results would be completely informative and accurate and would not be subjected to the inaccuracy of linkage studies caused by the possibility of genetic recombination. Subsequently, a PCR assay was developed for detection of the inversion mutation. It eliminated the necessity for labor-intensive and expensive Southern blot analysis and significantly improved turnaround times.[405,406,548]

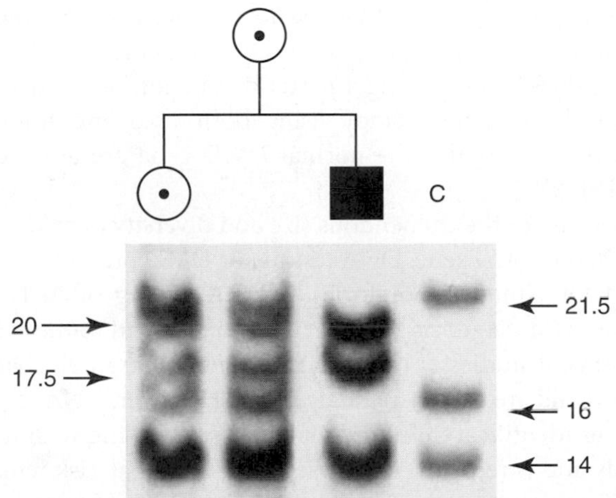

Figure 40-5 Southern blot analysis for the detection of a common inversion mutation present in the DNA of about 50% of patients with severe hemophilia A disease. Patient DNA is digested with restriction endonuclease *BclI*, blotted to a nylon membrane, and is hybridized with a ^{32}P-labeled probe corresponding to sequences in intron 22 of the factor VIII gene. Autoradiography was performed at −70 °C for 24 hours. Normal control DNA *(lane C)* yields bands 21.5 kb, 16 kb, and 14 kb in length. The pattern observed for the affected male *(shaded box)* in this family yields an altered banding pattern with bands of 20 kb, 17.5 kb, and 14 kb. Bands of these sizes confirm the presence of an inversion mutation resulting from homologous recombination between a copy of gene A within intron 22 of the factor VIII gene and the distal copy of gene A 5′ to the factor VIII gene. DNA analysis of the patient's mother and sister indicates that they are carriers of the inversion mutation with bands at 21.5 kb, 16 kb, and 14 kb generated from their wild-type allele and bands at 20 kb, 17.5 kb, and 14 kb generated from their mutant allele. Identification of the inversion mutation in this family will facilitate accurate carrier screening in other at-risk females in this family.

DNA testing for HA involves the use of a variety of techniques, including PCR to detect common inversion mutations, multiplex ligation-dependent probe amplification (MLPA) to identify deletions and duplications, and DNA sequencing to uncover the abundant numbers of missense, nonsense, and splice-site disease-causing mutations in this gene.[239] The testing algorithm for the proband is initially based on the clinical presentation of the patient.[522] For patients with severe disease, screening begins for inversion mutations involving introns 22 and 1. If negative, the *FVIII* gene is screened for the disease-causing mutation. In contrast, if the patient has moderate or mild disease, testing for common inversion mutations would not be necessary. Identification of the mutation in the affected male confirms the diagnosis, detects patients at high risk for inhibitor formation, and identifies the mutation segregating within the family. The ability to perform direct mutation analysis enables future prenatal or preimplantation genetic diagnosis studies or carrier studies for at-risk females in the family. Although the causative mutation in most patients can be identified through a combination of various screening techniques, in as many as 5% of patients the causative *FVIII* gene mutation is not identified.[373] In these situations, linkage studies may be required for prenatal, preimplantation, or carrier studies. These patients may have mutations buried in *FVIII* gene introns, or in 5′ upstream sequences, or perhaps at other gene loci whose proteins interact with the FVIII molecule.

Duchenne Muscular Dystrophy

Duchenne muscular dystrophy (DMD) (OMIM #310200) is a fatal X-linked recessive disorder characterized by progressive skeletal muscle wasting. The incidence of DMD is about 1 in 3500 male births, making it the most common severe neuromuscular disease in man. Classic DMD presents in early childhood, most often with motor delay or an abnormal gait. This is followed by progressive myopathic weakness with pseudohypertrophy of calves, and grossly elevated serum creatine kinase (>10× normal) as a result of degenerating muscle fibers. A muscle biopsy can confirm the diagnosis and shows variation in fiber size, necrosis, inflammation, fibrosis, and fiber regeneration. Immunohistochemistry staining using antibodies directed against different epitopes of dystrophin shows complete or almost complete absence of carboxy-terminal antibodies in the majority of DMD patients. Progressive weakness first affects the lower extremities such that most DMD patients are wheelchair bound between 10 and 15 years of age. Continual degeneration and regeneration of muscle eventually lead to the replacement of muscle tissue by adipose and connective tissue, causing progressive disease. Scoliosis is common and affects respiratory function. Chronic respiratory insufficiency develops in all patients, and cardiac disease can include dilated cardiomyopathy due to cardiac fibrosis and/or rhythm and conduction abnormalities. Death usually occurs in the third decade of life as the result of respiratory and cardiac failure. In some patients, however, only the heart is affected, causing DMD-associated dilated cardiomyopathy. In addition, one third of DMD patients have an IQ below 70. The primary treatment for DMD patients consists of corticosteroids to combat muscle weakness, angiotensin-converting enzyme inhibitors and β-blockers for cardiac disease, and noninvasive ventilation for respiratory care. A national newborn screening program requiring informed parental consent is ongoing in Wales and is performed by measuring plasma creatine kinase from dried blood spots.[499] This approach has been used to identify affected males before the onset of clinical signs, to prevent delay in the diagnosis, and to offer immediate medical intervention and genetic services to the patient and family. In the United States, although DMD is a candidate condition for which newborn screening could be considered, insufficient data are available regarding the cost-effectiveness of screening, as well as the possible risks and potential benefits, and such screening is not being performed.[361] Because DMD is an X-linked recessive disorder, most carrier females are asymptomatic. However, some may have muscle weakness and elevated serum creatine kinase levels (2 to 10× normal). Varying degrees of clinical symptoms in females depend on the degree of inactivation of the X chromosome harboring the mutant *DMD* gene in various tissues where the DMD protein is expressed.[301] Females with severe disease most often result from a carrier female with skewed lyonization or an X-autosome translocation involving the *DMD* gene.*

Cytogenetic abnormalities in DMD patients and DNA linkage studies localized the DMD locus to Xp21.† By mixing DNA enhanced for X-linked genes from a 49,XXXXY cell line with DNA from a patient with DMD and a cytogenetic deletion in Xp21, Kunkel and colleagues cleverly used subtraction hybridization to clone the DNA corresponding to the patient's deletion.[382] During hybridization, Xp21 sequences from the cell line had no complementary sequences with which to anneal in the patient's DNA, thus they were available for cloning. The *DMD* gene (Xp21.2) is complex and is the largest gene in the human genome, spanning 2.4 megabases. It is interesting to note that it contains 79 exons, representing less than 1% of the gene, it encodes a 14 kb mRNA, and it has multiple tissue-specific promoters.[67,293] The full-length protein product, dystrophin, contains 3685 amino acids, has a molecular weight of 427 kDa, and contains four distinct domains, including actin-binding, central rod, cysteine-rich, and the unique COOH-terminal domain. Dystrophin is expressed predominantly in skeletal and cardiac muscle but is also expressed in neuronal tissue.[670] However, various dystrophin isoforms and splice variants are found in nonmuscle organs throughout the body.[67] Dystrophin is a cytoskeletal protein and a critical component of the dystrophin-glycoprotein complex (DGC), which also includes dystroglycans, sarcoglycans, sarcospan, dystrobrevins, and syntrophins.[138,182,670]

The DGC interacts with a host of cytoskeletal, transmembrane, extracellular, and trafficking proteins, as well as with cell signaling proteins.[181,184,670] In skeletal muscle, DGC plays a structural role by connecting the actin cytoskeleton to the extracellular matrix, stabilizing the sarcolemma during repeated cycles of contraction and relaxation, and transmitting force generated in the muscle sarcomeres to the extracellular matrix.[172] The DGC is also important for Ca^{2+} homeostasis.[45] In the absence of normal dystrophin and the DGC, the sarcolemmal integrity is compromised, and an influx of extracellular calcium triggers calcium-activated proteases and fiber necrosis and abnormal intracellular signaling.[38,184,304,606] The *DMD* animal models, including canine *(cxmd)* and mouse models *(mdx),* are an important resource for understanding the pathogenesis of DMD disease and for developing treatments.[38,167] Cerletti and coworkers described the use of mouse skeletal muscle progenitor cells to restore muscle fibers and regain normal dystrophin expression in the *mdx* mouse.[69,104] In addition to stem cell therapy for muscle growth and regeneration, other forms of treatment are being investigated. One method is the use of drugs to enable read-through of stop codons arising from nonsense mutations to prevent premature truncation of the protein.[402] Another promising molecular approach is the use of synthetic antisense oligonucleotides designed to redirect mRNA splicing and induce exon skipping of a specific mutation containing exons, thereby producing a partially functioning dystrophin protein.[244,449] Gene therapy using both viral and nonviral vectors to introduce the normal *DMD* gene are also being studied.[77,309,673]

Because of the tremendous size and diversity of mutations within the *DMD* gene, DNA testing for DMD presents a challenge for clinical laboratories.[394] DNA testing often is not required for diagnosis because morphologic and immunohistochemical studies of biopsied muscle tissue are well characterized and are considered diagnostic. However, DNA testing enables identification of the mutation segregating within the family and is required for carrier detection of at-risk females and for prenatal testing. Intragenic deletions, often encompassing multiple exons, represent 65% of mutations, affect the translational reading frame of the protein, and lead to a truncated and nonfunctional protein.[2] Duplications of the gene are observed in about 5% of patients. Deletions and duplications can be rapidly detected using multiplex PCR or fluorescence in situ hybridization.[53,105,458,654] More recently, the multiplex ligation-dependent probe amplification assay has been developed to screen for all 79 exons.[387] This method is simple and rapid and reliably determines whether the exon is present, deleted, or doubled when compared to control DNA. This technique is particularly useful for carrier detection in at-risk females by providing an accurate method for quantification of exon copy number. Alternatively, quantitative real-time PCR can be used to identify carrier females.[343] Direct sequence analysis is required for detection of the remaining 30% of mutations. Because of the sheer size of the gene, laboratories may first employ a screening technique to localize the likely area of the gene containing the disease-causing mutation prior to sequencing.[295]

Becker muscular dystrophy (BMD) (OMIM #300376) is a milder and less common form of muscular dystrophy with an

*References 75, 249, 532, 659, 710, and 714.

†References 35, 139, 208, 249, 659, and 714.

estimated incidence of 1 in 18,500 births. BMD is an allelic variation of DMD that is caused by different mutations within the *DMD* gene and is associated with a milder phenotype with a mean age of death in the mid-40s.* About 85% of BMD patients have deletions within *DMD,* 5 to 10% have a duplication, and 5 to 10% have a small insertion, deletion, or point mutation. Patients with deletions involving the distal rod domain of dystrophin (exons 45 to 60) show the mild BMD phenotype and in some cases remain free of symptoms until their 50s. However, BMD patients with deletions involving the amino-terminal domain of dystrophin (exons 1 to 9) have a more severe BMD phenotype with an earlier age of onset and more rapid progression of disease.

Patients with X-linked dilated cardiomyopathy have mutations at the dystrophin locus and *DMD*-associated dilated cardiomyopathy (DCM).[200,203,446,460,490] DCM is a rapidly progressive, fatal disease with an onset of symptoms early in the third decade of life.[205] Mutations associated with DCM are varied and involve the promoter region and exon 1, or splice sites, as well as exonic duplications and deletions.[205]

For families in which no mutation is detected, carrier and prenatal testing can be offered using DNA linkage studies. However, because the intragenic recombination frequency for this gene is estimated to be about 12%, these studies require the use of multiple intragenic, as well as 5′ and 3′, flanking markers for accurate carrier or prenatal results.[4] Particularly difficult are sporadic cases of DMD or BMD in which no other family member with DMD or BMD is known, and no mutation in the affected individual is detected. Generally, one third of sporadic cases are thought to represent a new mutation in the mother's gamete from which that individual was derived. Thus neither the mother nor female siblings would be carriers, and the risk to the mother for a second affected son would be considered minimal. In addition, in mutation-negative families, carrier assessment involves measurement of serum CK activity and linkage studies.[323] Linkage studies are complex, require participation of multiple family members, and are confounded by inaccuracy caused by meiotic recombination or germline mosaicism. Serum CK is, by definition, above the reference interval (defined as the 95th percentile of a healthy reference group of age-matched women) in ≈1 of 20 noncarrier women. Moreover, serum CK decreases in DMD carrier women as they age.

In 1987, Bakker and associates first described the phenomenon of germline mosaicism, in which no *DMD* gene mutation is present in lymphocyte DNA, but a *DMD* gene mutation is present in germline tissue.[36] Presumably these mutations occur during mitosis in germline proliferation, which explains the report of multiple affected children of women whose lymphocyte DNA contains no *DMD* mutation.

Fragile X Syndrome

Fragile X syndrome (OMIM #309550) is one of the most commonly inherited forms of mental retardation, with an estimated incidence of ≈1 in 4000 males and ≈1 in 4000 to 8000 females.[580] The name of the condition reflects the cytogenetic abnormality of a breakpoint or fragile site in the X chromosome. The clinical syndrome was first described by Martin and Bell in 1943 in a family with sex-linked mental retardation in both males and females who had no dysmorphic features.[428] The disease was later redefined by Lubs, who noted the presence of a marker X chromosome in the leukocytes of some mentally retarded males following incubation of cells in cell culture media depleted of folate and thymidine; the marker segregated with mental retardation within the family.[414] The chromosomal locus for this fragile site would later be localized to Xq27.3.[277] Common clinical features associated with fragile X syndrome are mental retardation, delayed motor and speech development, macro-orchidism, long face, prominent forehead and jaw, large ears, flat feet, and abnormal behavioral characteristics such as hyperactivity, hand flapping, temper tantrums, persevering speech patterns, poor eye contact, and occasionally autism.[151] These features often are less frequent and milder in affected females than in affected males because of random X inactivation of their abnormal fragile X gene and expression of their normal gene in half of their tissue.

As a sex-linked disease, fragile X syndrome has a complicated inheritance pattern. Affected females are heterozygous for the mutation, and unaffected males can transmit the mutation through the family. For this reason, Sherman and colleagues proposed that fragile X syndrome was an X-linked dominant disorder with reduced penetrance (79% for males and 35% for females), but the penetrance of the disease appeared to increase in subsequent generations within a family.[582,584] The mechanism of this "Sherman paradox" was resolved when the gene causing fragile X syndrome, *FMR1* (*F*ragile X *M*ental *R*etardation 1), was cloned in 1991.[54,378,484,660,711] *FMR1* was the first gene discovered to cause disease through expansion of an unstable trinucleotide repeat sequence. The unstable CGG repeat is located in the 5′ untranslated region (5′UTR) of the *FMR1* gene in exon 1. The gene spans 38 kb, with 17 exons, encodes a 4.4 kb mRNA transcript, that contains 190 bp of the 5′UTR.[176] *FMR1* mRNA is expressed in neural and non-neural tissues during both embryonic and postnatal development.[401] The FMR1 protein, FMRP, is a 71 kDa RNA-binding protein (RBP) with three RNA-binding domains, KH1 and KH2 and an RGG box; it is associated with polyribosomes as part of a messenger ribonucleoprotein complex, where it serves to suppress the translation of specific mRNAs.[40,202,384,398,592] Binding about 4% of total mRNA, it is primarily observed in the cytoplasm but shuttles between the cytoplasm and the nucleus. It is suggested that FMRP binds specific RNA ligands then recruits the RNA-induced silencing complex to selectively repress translation of targeted mRNA.[103,328,432]

In addition, FMRP is involved in synaptic plasticity through regulation of mRNA transport into dendrites to regulate local protein synthesis of specific RNAs in response to synaptic stimulation signals; most notable is its ability to inhibit the effects of metabotrophic glutamate receptor 5 (mGluR5).[44,152,676] Thus, loss of function of FMRP in fragile X

*References 2, 52, 96, 125, 294, and 709.

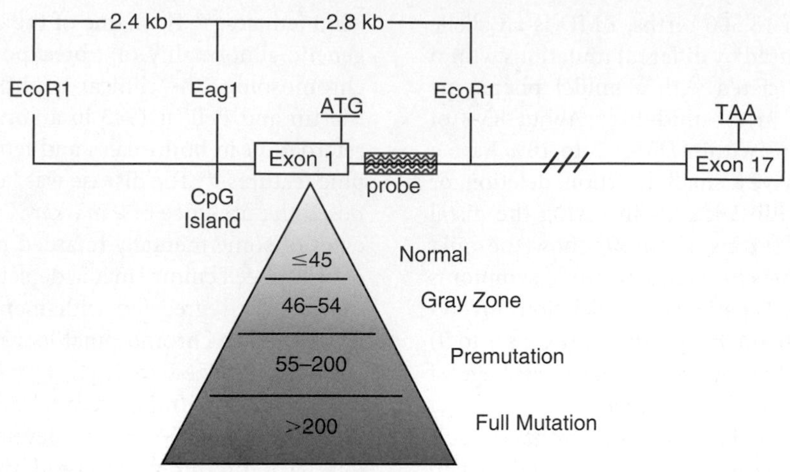

Figure 40-6 Schematic representation of the CGG repeat in exon 1 of *FMR1* and associated alleles. A CGG-repeat number less than or equal to 45 is normal. A CGG-repeat number of 46 to 54 is in the gray zone and has been reported to expand to a full mutation in some families. A CGG-repeat number of 55 to 200 is considered a premutation allele and is prone to expansion to a full mutation during female meiosis. A CGG-repeat number in excess of 200 is considered a full mutation and is diagnostic of fragile X syndrome.

patients results in abnormal translation profiles and altered synapse structure and signaling.[66,531]

FMR1 alleles contain blocks of CGG repeats usually 7 to 13 repeats in length, which can be interspersed with single AGG repeats.[383,595] Allelic diversity results from the variable numbers and lengths of these CGG-repeat blocks. No distinct boundaries separate the repeat number categories; however, normal alleles have 5 to 45 repeats; gray zone alleles have 46 to 54; premutation alleles have 55 to 200; and full mutation expansion alleles contain more than 200 repeats[422] (Figure 40-6). Individuals with a normal number of CGG repeats do not have fragile X syndrome, nor are they at risk of having an affected child. Individuals with 46 to 54 repeats represent alleles in the upper range of normal or a smaller than average premutation allele. These individuals do not have fragile X syndrome, yet may have a slightly increased risk of repeat instability and expansion to a full mutation in their offspring in some families. Premutation alleles are unstable and can expand to a larger allele in the premutation range when transmitted or can expand to a full mutation allele and an offspring with fragile X syndrome.[481] Although rare, premutation alleles have been reported to undergo rather drastic contractions (82 to 33, 95 to 35, 145 to 43, 130 to 10, and 70 to 54).[84,481] The risk of CGG expansion from a premutation to a full mutation allele is dependent on several factors, including the number of pure uninterrupted CGG repeats, the number and position of interspersed AGG repeats, haplotype background, and less well-characterized heritable factors.*

In a large collaborative study among 13 laboratories in 8 countries and involving more than 1500 premutation carrier females, the smallest premutation alleles shown to expand contained 59 repeats with no AGG interruptions.[481] Most data from humans suggest that expansion occurs before zygote formation, but the possibility that CGG expansion will occur very early in embryogenesis cannot be excluded.[424,456] CGG expansions of premutations to full mutations are largely confined to maternal transmissions to the offspring, and the sex of the fetus has no apparent effect on this process.[481] Expansion occurs during DNA replication and results from hairpin formation and slippage within the expanded CGG-repeat sequence corresponding to the lagging strand, but it likely involves other factors and processes as well.[237,687] Premutation repeat alleles transmitted in males remained stable in 16% of cases, decreased in size in 22% of transmissions, and expanded to a larger premutation allele in 62% of transmissions.[482]

Premutation carriers do not have fragile X syndrome. However, although *FMR1* is overexpressed in these individuals, FMRP appears to be significantly diminished, suggesting reduced translation efficiency.[363] Diminished FMRP levels in premutation carriers are negatively correlated with the repeat number, and overexpression of *FMR1* has a positive correlation with the repeat number. It is interesting to note that ≈20% of premutation carrier females have primary ovarian insufficiency with cessation of menstrual periods before 40 years of age.[612,700] However, this clinical finding is not observed in full mutation carrier females, nor in their nonpremutation carrier sisters.[581] Further, a positive association of ovarian insufficiency and CGG repeat size indicates that *FMR1* RNA toxicity may mediate these clinical symptoms.

Premutation carrier males exhibit fragile X–associated tremor/ataxia syndrome (FXTAS), a neurodegenerative syndrome characterized by progressive intention tremor, cerebellar gait ataxia, parkinsonism, neuropathy, cognitive decline, psychiatric features, and generalized brain atrophy.[74,266,268]

*References 94, 173-175, 179, 284, 482, and 583.

FXTAS occurs in about one third of premutation carrier males over the age of 50; also, 17% of males between the ages of 50 and 59 and as many as 75% of males older than 80 years are affected.[331] FXTAS can be seen in premutation carrier females but is observed at a lower percentage.[266,267] The lower incidence of FXTAS in females may be explained by the presence of a second X chromosome and a normal *FMR1* gene in approximately half of all cells. Although patients with FXTAS may demonstrate a neuropsychiatric illness, the existence of a distinct neuropsychologic phenotype in premutation carriers without FXTAS remains controversial. Most recently however, Hunter and coworkers showed that premutation males and females younger than 50 years appear to have no significant difference in their neuropsychologic profile compared with nonpremutation carriers,[319] although this study showed that premutation carrier females may have an increased number of symptoms associated with attention-deficit hyperactivity disorder (ADHD). Thus, although FMRP is decreased, increased concentrations of *FMR1* transcript may be toxic to the cell and may have a gain-of-function affect.[266]

The molecular basis of fragile X syndrome includes expansion of the 5′UTR CGG repeat and hypermethylation coupled with histone deacetylation of this region and the adjacent CpG island in the promoter region of the *FMR1* gene, resulting in transcriptional silencing of the gene and no production of FMRP.[54,119,515,516,614] Males with full expansion alleles but incomplete methylation—"mosaic males"—may have severe mental retardation or a milder phenotype.[433,552] One report describes two males from unrelated fragile X syndrome families who although they had the full mutation allele did not have the fragile X phenotype.[618] In vitro analysis indicated that their alleles lacked the complete specific epigenetic methylation-deacetylation patterns observed in abnormal *FMR1* genes. These results are interesting because expanded repeats may trigger chromatin remodeling and may recruit cellular mechanisms to cause epigenetic changes.[381] Although in vitro reactivation of the *FMR1* gene has been reported to occur by inducing DNA demethylation and the reassociation of acetylated histones, reactivation of *FMR1* may not be sufficient to restore FMRP concentrations because transcripts with large repeats may not be efficiently translated.[113,363]

DNA testing for fragile X syndrome using Southern blot analysis of peripheral blood enables detection of the majority of cases of fragile X syndrome (Figure 40-7). PCR analysis with capillary electrophoresis is used to complement the testing by providing the precise CGG-repeat number. However, because of the CG-rich sequence, large full mutation alleles are difficult to amplify by PCR. As the CGG-repeat length increases, the risk of expansion from a premutation to a full mutation in premutation carrier females increases. Thus PCR testing to determine the exact CGG-repeat number is most useful for determining the risk of an affected offspring during genetic counseling of a premutation carrier female. Although a woman with a premutation CGG repeat of 55 to 59 is given about a 5% risk of expansion to a full mutation, a woman with a repeat length of 70 to 79 is given a 31% risk of expansion, and a woman with a CGG-repeat length greater than 100 is given close to a 100% chance of expansion.[481] Chorionic villus samples or amniotic fluid can be tested, but the methylation pattern expected in adult tissue may be absent. Although expansion of the CGG repeat in 5′UTR of *FMR1* accounts for more than 99% of all cases of fragile X syndrome, CGG deletions and point mutations have also been described.[686] The American College of Human Genetics has published guidelines for testing in the laboratory.[422]

DNA testing for *FMR1* is requested for children with (1) the fragile X phenotype, (2) developmental delay, (3) mental retardation, or (4) autism. Fragile X DNA testing is performed for carrier testing in at-risk pregnant or preconception females with a family history of fragile X or mental retardation of unknown cause. Carrier testing is performed on patients with clinical suspicion of FXTAS. In addition, a pilot newborn screening test for fragile X syndrome was conducted to determine the feasibility of this testing.[561] In this study, two families were identified, and the incidence of disease was 1 in 730 births. Because of the carrier frequency of FXS, a population-based carrier screening program has been considered but would require significant planning, educational resources, and counseling programs to be established before such testing could be implemented. [441]

Treatment of patients with FXS includes therapies for behaviors related to ADHD, anxiety, aggression, and seizures.[265] A better understanding of the molecular function of FMRP may lead to targeted treatment options in the future.

DISEASES WITH NONMENDELIAN INHERITANCE

Mitochondrial DNA Diseases

Mitochondria are organelles ubiquitous to the cytoplasm of all eukaryotic cells of animals, higher plants, and some microorganisms. Mitochondria generate energy for the cellular processes by producing ATP through oxidative phosphorylation (OXPHOS); they are important in maintaining both calcium homeostasis and various intracellular signaling cascades, including apoptosis.[199,511,598] The matrix of the mitochondrion is surrounded by a cardiolipin-rich inner membrane, and both are enclosed by a second outer membrane. Within the matrix are copies of mitochondrial deoxyribonucleic acid (mtDNA). Each mitochondria contains between about 2 and 10 copies of mtDNA, so with hundreds of mitochondria per cell, an estimated 10^3 to 10^4 copies of mtDNA exist within each cell, with brain, skeletal, and cardiac muscle having particularly high concentrations. Alterations in mtDNA copy number or mutations in mtDNA are associated with both inherited and acquired diseases.[117,153,577] The mtDNA is a double-stranded, circular molecule containing 16,569 base pairs that encodes 37 genes, including two ribosomal RNAs (rRNA), 22 transfer RNAs (tRNA), and 13 subunits required for the OXPHOS system, with seven belonging to complex I, one to complex III, three to complex IV, and two to complex V.[17] Most subunits involved in the OXPHOS system are nuclear-encoded, as are several nuclear gene products that regulate mitochondrial gene

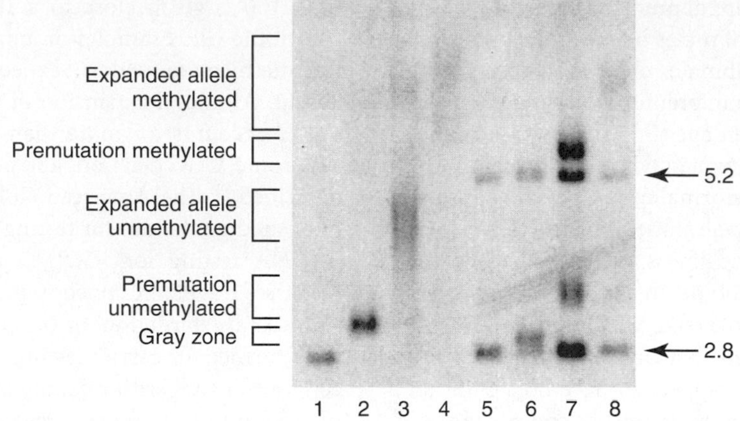

Figure 40-7 Southern blot analysis for the diagnosis of fragile X syndrome. Patient DNA is simultaneously digested with restriction endonucleases *EcoR*I and *Eag*I, is blotted to a nylon membrane, and is hybridized with a ^{32}P-labeled probe adjacent to exon 1 of *FMR1* (see Figure 40-6). *Eag*I is a methylation-sensitive restriction endonuclease that will not cleave the recognition sequence if the cytosine in the sequence is methylated. Normal male control DNA with a CGG-repeat number of 22 on his single X chromosome *(lane 1)* generates a band about 2.8 kb in length, corresponding to *Eag*I-*EcoR*I fragments (see Figure 40-6). Normal female control DNA with a CGG-repeat number of 20 on one X chromosome and a CGG-repeat number of 25 on the second X chromosome *(lane 5)* generates two bands: one at about 2.8 kb and a second at 5.2 kb. *EcoR*I-*EcoR*I fragments approximately 5.2 kb in length represent methylated DNA sequences characteristic of the lyonized chromosome in each cell that is not digested with restriction endonuclease *Eag*I. DNA in *lane 2* contains an *FMR1* CGG-repeat number of 90 and is characteristic of a normal transmitting male. The banding pattern observed in lane 3 is representative of a mosaic male with a single X chromosome with a full mutation (>200 repeats). However, the full mutation in some cells is unmethylated; in other cells, the full mutation is fully methylated, hence the term *mosaic*. In those cells in which the full mutation is unmethylated, digestion by both *Eag*I and *EcoR*I occurs, and in those cells in which the full mutation is fully methylated, digestion of the DNA by *Eag*I is inhibited. The banding pattern observed in *lane 4* is diagnostic of a male with fragile X syndrome, illustrating the typical expanded allele fully methylated in all cells. *Lane 6* is characteristic of a female with a normal allele and a CGG-repeat number of 29 and a larger gray zone allele with a CGG-repeat number of 54. *Lane 7* is the banding pattern observed from a premutation carrier female with one normal allele having a CGG-repeat number of 23 (band at about 2.8 kb) and a second premutation allele with CGG repeats of 120 to about 200 (band at about 3.1 kb). In premutation carrier females, in cells in which the X chromosome with the premutation allele is lyonized, the normal 5.2 kb *EcoR*I-*EcoR*I band is larger because of the increased CGG-repeat number and is about 5.5 kb in length. *Lane 8* is diagnostic of a female with fragile X syndrome with one full expansion mutation allele that is completely methylated and transcriptionally silenced on one X chromosome but with a second normal allele with a CGG-repeat number of 33.

expression. It is interesting to note that the mitochondrial genetic code is slightly different from the universal code. For example, in mtDNA, TGA codes for tryptophan, rather than a termination codon, and all mitochondrial-encoded polypeptides contain codons requiring only 22 mitochondrial-encoded tRNA molecules for translation, rather than the 31 predicted by Crick's wobble hypothesis.[42] The high copy number of mtDNA per cell coupled with a small genome and highly polymorphic sequence variations between individuals makes mtDNA sequence analysis an ideal tool for forensic studies.[439,639]

Mitochondria-related diseases have an incidence of 1 : 1000 to 1 : 5000 and can result from mutations in nuclear DNA (85 to 90%) or, as first reported in 1988, can result from mutations in the mitochondrial genome (10 to 15%).[300,671,716] Mutations in mtDNA occur at a higher rate than nuclear DNA, probably because of differences in chromatin structure, lack of DNA repair machinery, and the continual generation of reactive oxygen species. Mitochondrial genetics is different from mendelian genetics in several aspects. First, all mtDNA is maternally inherited, with mature oocytes having the highest mtDNA copy number per cell at 10^5 and with sperm having the lowest mtDNA copy number per cell at 10^2. After fertilization, sperm mtDNA is selectively degraded so that only maternal mtDNA remains. Thus if a mother is carrying an mtDNA mutation, it will be transmitted to all of her children, but only her daughters can transmit the disease to their offspring. Although this is considered the rule, paternal mtDNA inheritance has been reported and may result from incomplete degradation of sperm mtDNA in early embryogenesis.[569,570] If an mtDNA mutation arises, it will exist among a population of normal mtDNA. This coexistence of normal and mutant mtDNA copies within the same cell is referred to as *heteroplasmy* and is the second unique feature of mitochondrial genetics. Third, during cell division, the proportions of normal and mutant mtDNA can shift as mitochondria, and their accompanying genomes are partitioned into daughter cells. Thus in development and differentiation, the proportions of normal and mutant mtDNA can vary among cells and tissues within the body. Last, the percentage of mutant mtDNA required within a cell, tissue, or organ system to produce a deleterious phenotype is referred to as the *threshold effect.* The threshold for disease varies between people, energetic requirements for tissue, and the mtDNA mutation. As is evident, genetic counseling for families with mtDNA disorders is complicated by an inability to accurately predict phenotype caused by the phenomena of heteroplasmy and the threshold effect.

Two types of mtDNA mutations exist: those that affect mitochondrial protein synthesis (tRNA and rRNA genes) and those within the protein-encoding genes themselves.[153,702] Direct sequencing of mtDNA is considered the gold standard for mutation detection, but this method may be unable to detect a low percentage of mutant mtDNA in a heteroplasmic state. Alternatively, a simple and effective method referred to as *temporal temperature-gradient gel electrophoresis,* coupled with PCR and DNA sequencing, can detect heteroplasmic mutations as low as 4%.[703] Although mtDNA mutations are now associated with a significant number of inherited diseases, acquired mtDNA deletions are associated with the aging process, and mitochondrial dysfunction is associated with neurodegenerative diseases and cancer.[231,527] Many somatic mtDNA mutations occur via damage by oxygen free radicals produced as byproducts of aerobic metabolism.[15,534]

Leber Hereditary Optic Neuropathy

Leber hereditary optic neuropathy (LHON) (OMIN #53500), the most common mitochondrial disease, is the first linked to maternal inheritance through a mutation in the mtDNA.[671] LHON is characterized by acute or subacute bilateral loss of central vision caused by focal degeneration of the retinal ganglion cell (RGC) layer and, in some individuals, impairment of optic nerve function.[712] The specific nature of the disease in terms of RGC degeneration is unknown, but it could be due to differences in superoxide regulation.[292] Age of onset is typically in the second to fourth decade of life, and after initial symptoms, both eyes are usually affected within 6 months. Approximately 50% of males and only 10% of females who possess the mtDNA mutation will develop disease.[712] In addition, yet to be defined environmental factors, nuclear-encoded modifier genes that affect mtDNA expression, mtDNA products, or mitochondrial metabolism may modify the phenotypic expression of LHON. The explanation for differences in rates between genders has not been determined but could be related to genes on the X chromosome.[315] Genetic counseling in LHON is complicated in that the amount of mutant mtDNA transmitted by heteroplasmic females cannot be predicted, and testing cannot predict which individuals will develop visual symptoms.[322] LHON can be confused with autosomal dominant optic atrophy (OMIN #165500), which shares a similar ocular phenotype but results from mutations primarily in the gene *OPA1* (3q28-29). It is interesting to note that OPA1 is a nuclear-encoded mitochondrial protein required for mitochondrial fusion, maintenance of cristae architecture, and regulation of apoptosis.[598]

LHON is a disorder caused by OXPHOS deficiency. Although many mutations have been associated with this disease, mtDNA mutations G3460A, G11778A, and T14484C represent 95% of those identified.[421] Mutation G11778A was the first described, is the most common, and accounts for at least 50% of cases. In most affected individuals, LHON mutations appear to be homoplasmic, with only mutant mtDNA detected, but in 15% of cases, the mutations are heteroplasmic, with a mixture of both normal and mutant mtDNA detected.[593,663] Each of the common mutations affects a subunit of the nicotinamide adenine dinucleotide : ubiquinone oxidoreductase in complex I of the OXPHOS pathway. The mechanism by which these mutations cause the LHON phenotype is not well understood.[476]

Clinical DNA testing for LHON-associated mutations is widely available and utilizes an array of techniques.[18,218,462] If the patient's mtDNA is negative for the three common mutations, testing for other mtDNA mutations associated with LHON should be considered.[462,712] DNA sequencing of the entire mitochondrial genome may be required but is labor intensive and costly, so it should be pursued only when clinical suspicion for LHON is high.[18,476]

Leigh Syndrome

Leigh syndrome (LS) (OMIM #256000), or subacute necrotizing encephalopathy, is a progressive neurodegenerative disorder that most often leads to death before the age of 5. In contrast to LHON, most patients present within the first year of life with hypotonia, failure to thrive, psychomotor regression, ocular movement abnormalities, ataxia, and brainstem and basal ganglia dysfunction caused by severe dysfunction of mitochondrial energy metabolism. The clinical phenotype for LS is variable in patients with the same pathogenic mtDNA mutation and largely results from differences in the percentages of mutant mtDNA among organs and tissues within an individual (Figure 40-8).[632]

LS exhibits extensive genetic heterogeneity, with disease-causing mutations identified in both nuclear-encoded genes and mtDNA, making both mendelian and maternal patterns of inheritance possible for this syndrome.[157] Mutations in mitochondrial-encoded genes affecting complexes I, IV, and

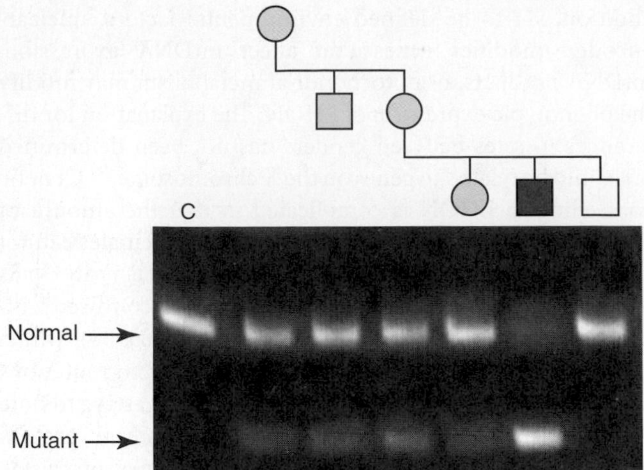

Figure 40-8 Detection of varying degrees of heteroplasmy for mitochondrial deoxyribonucleic acid (mtDNA) mutation A8344G in a family with Leigh syndrome. Mitochondrial DNA was extracted from a peripheral blood specimen from an affected male with Leigh syndrome and from family members. Mitochondrial DNA was amplified using an oligonucleotide primer pair that flanks mitochondrial mutation A8344G. The A-to-G base substitution creates an *Nae*I recognition site (GCCGGC) that is not present in normal control mtDNA (C). Amplicons from each member of the family and from the control were digested with *Nae*I and subjected to gel electrophoresis. The virtual absence of undigested amplicons in the affected male *(red box in pedigree)* indicates the presence of almost 100% mutant mtDNA in the cells from this specimen and coincides with the severe phenotype of Leigh syndrome in this patient. In contrast, his sister, mother, and grandmother with 30%, 40%, and 20% mutant mtDNA suffer only from migraine headaches. His uncle, with 30% mutant mtDNA present, suffers from attention-deficit hyperactivity disorder and learning disabilities. Heteroplasmy, or variation in the percentages of normal and mutant mitochondria, largely explains observed phenotypic differences in this family.
(Courtesy Thomas W. Prior, PhD, Departments of Pathology and Neurology, Ohio State University, Columbus, Ohio.)

V, as well as several tRNA genes, or nuclear-encoded genes affecting the pyruvate dehydrogenase complex, the respiratory chain complexes I, II, and IV, or coenzyme Q have been reported.[204] The most common mitochondrial-encoded mutation associated with Leigh is seen in the *ATPase 6* gene (complex V) with a common T>G transversion mutation at nucleotide 8993. The most common nuclear-encoded mutation associated with Leigh syndrome is in the *SURF1* gene, which encodes a cytochrome oxidase assembly factor. Regardless of which gene is involved, the overall prognosis of these patients is generally poor, and treatment of mitochondrial disease is in its infancy.[375] Because of the lethality of Leigh syndrome, preimplantation genetic diagnosis can be considered and has been successfully performed with the implantation of a disease-free embryo.[642]

Clinical DNA testing for mitochondrially inherited LS includes targeted mutation analysis for a common mutation or DNA sequencing of the mitochondrial genome.[218] Because of the heterogeneity of nuclear-encoded genes associated with LS, testing is limited to a few locations within the United States and most frequently involves DNA sequence analysis of the entire coding region of multiple genes.[218]

Imprinting

Imprinting refers to the differential marking or "imprinting" of specific paternally and maternally inherited alleles during gametogenesis, resulting in differential expression of those genes. Such imprints on the DNA during gametogenesis must be maintained through DNA replication in the somatic cells of the offspring, must be reversible from generation to generation, and must influence transcription. DNA methylation is the primary mechanism for genomic imprinting. The number of imprinted genes in the human genome is estimated to be fewer than 200, and most are clustered around imprinting control centers. Alterations in normal imprinting patterns can result in disease.

Prader-Willi and Angelman Syndromes

Prader-Willi syndrome (PWS) is a complex multisystem, neurogenetic disorder with an incidence of 1 in 15,000 to 30,000.[98] Prenatally, the affected fetus exhibits diminished movement, peculiar fetal position, and often polyhydramnios.[63] At birth, dysmorphic features, small hands and feet, and hypogonadism are observed. The affected child is lethargic with persistent hypotonia that results in poor feeding and failure to thrive. Development is delayed for both motor skills and language, and this delay continues throughout life, with a mean IQ of 60 to 70. Early in childhood, a unique and characteristic insatiable appetite that is hypothalamic in origin presents. Obesity soon ensues with associated complications and is the major cause of morbidity, mortality, and sleep disorders. In addition, patients have short stature and abnormal body composition characteristic of growth hormone deficiency. This aspect of the disorder can be treated with exogenous growth hormone, although many other aspects of this disease are difficult to manage and require a multidisciplinary approach.[235,403] The syndrome is associated with specific behavioral characteristics, and some patients can have psychiatric disorders; both of these situations present challenging management issues.

Angelman syndrome (AS) is another neurogenetic disorder with a similar incidence in the population as PWS; it is characterized by severe mental retardation (IQ<40), inappropriate bouts of laughter, absence of speech, gait ataxia, progressive microcephaly, dysmorphic facial features, and epilepsy.[336] Unique electroencephalographic (EEG) patterns are seen in most AS patients at younger than 2 years of life and can be helpful in diagnosing the condition. As many as 6% of patients with both mental retardation and epilepsy may have AS. Some of the phenotypic features associated with AS can be nonspecific or can occur separately in other syndromes or nonsyndromic conditions; thus, it is the combination of many of these and the associated laughter, unique smiling, and happy demeanor of the AS patient that aids in making the diagnosis. Feeding problems and/or truncal hypotonia may be present at birth, and sleep disturbances and abnormal food-related behaviors can be displayed in older children. Apparent from the characteristic physical findings, PWS and AS are clinically distinct syndromes; yet each results from genetic changes involving a 4 Mb region on chromosome 15q11-q13.[306] Within this region are multiple genes that are imprinted with gene expression dependent on parental origin. PWS results when the paternal allele on 15q11-q13 is missing, defective, or epigenetically silenced through DNA methylation, and only the inactive maternal allele remains. In contrast, AS results from loss of function of the maternally expressed allele in this region.

Multiple paternally expressed genes for PWS exist in 15q11-q13. Most notable is the *SNURF-SNRPN* locus and >70 C/D box small nucleolar RNA (snoRNA) genes.[306,493] Extensive DNA methylation and histone H3 Ly59 demethylation at the CpG island regulate the single transcriptional unit encoding these genes on the maternal allele, leading to transcriptional silencing of this allele. The *cis*-acting regulatory region referred to as the *imprinting center (IC)* controls resetting of parental imprints in the 15q11-13 region during gametogenesis. SNRPN is involved in mRNA splicing in the brain, and SNURF (*SNRPN* Upstream Reading Frame) is found in the nucleus, contains 71 amino acids, may bind RNA, and has a C-terminal motif similar to ubiquitin. SnoRNAs are noncoding RNA molecules that modify both rRNA and snRNA by methylation of the ribose 2′ hydroxyl group of specific nucleotides, which may vary between them.[371] Sahoo and associates described a patient with a Prader-Willi phenotype and de novo deletion of 174,584 bp comprising all 29 snoRNAs of the HBII-85 snoRNA cluster and the proximal 23 of the 42 snoRNAs of the HBII-52 cluster on his paternal allele.[557] This finding provided convincing evidence that deficiency of HBII-85 snoRNAs causes the main features of PWS. This finding is significant in that it is also the first disorder associated with a deficiency of snoRNA.[509] Perhaps other paternal-only expressed genes in this region, such as *NDN,* which encodes necdin, a protein important for neuronal differentiation and a suppressor for cell proliferation; *IPW,* which encodes a 2.2 kb RNA but is not translated into a polypeptide; *MKRN3,* which encodes makorin ring zinc-finger protein 3; and *MAGEL2,* which encodes melanoma antigen-like gene 2, could have additive roles in the phenotype of PWS.[346,391,468,477,689]

Loss of normally expressed paternal genes in 15q11-q13 resulting in PWS can occur by several mechanisms. Most commonly, PWS (70%) results from a de novo deletion following unequal homologous recombination involving one of the three common breakpoints on the paternal allele. This would render the zygote monosomic for these genes, and the zygote would possess only the maternal copy of this region. Alternatively, 25 to 30% of cases of PWS are caused by uniparental disomy (UPD). In the case of PWS, although two copies of the genes located in 15q11-q13 exist, both are maternal in origin, arising in most cases from meiosis I nondisjunction followed by postzygotic mitotic loss of the third, paternally derived chromosome 15 via a process referred to as *trisomy rescue.* This mechanism rescues the zygote from trisomy 15, a condition that is incompatible with life.[541] Although the fetus is genetically complete with two chromosome 15's (disomy), both chromosomes are received from the same parent (uniparental), and no normal expression of paternally expressed genes occurs in this imprinted region. In about 1% of cases, PWS results from microdeletions encompassing the paternal IC. Or, in some cases, no DNA mutation is detectable, but rather, an abnormal imprint occurs.[87,88] A mutation involving the IC prevents this *cis*-acting control center from resetting the imprint in the germline. These mutations will result in PWS, because if they are present on the maternal chromosome of phenotypically normal fathers, they will be transmitted to offspring, as now the paternal chromosome will maintain the maternal imprint and will be silenced. Finally, less than 1% of PWS cases are caused by chromosomal rearrangements disrupting the genes in the 15q11-q13 region.[613] Some genotype correlations have been noted. It is interesting to note that PWS patients with uniparental disomy are more likely to have psychotic episodes, compulsive behaviors (e.g., skin-picking), and autism spectrum disorders than are PWS patients with deletions.[170,658,683]

The genes *UBE3A* and *ATP10A* are located downstream and in the opposite orientation to *SNURF-SNRPN* in 15q11-q13; both are predominantly maternally expressed in brain.[370,440] The *UBE3A* gene contains 16 exons and encodes E6-AP (E6-associated protein), a member of the E3 ubiquitin ligase family, which is involved in the ubiquitin proteasome pathway for degradation of a diverse range of yet unidentified protein substances.[431] Three protein isoforms that differ at the N-termini result from alternative splicing.[708] It is interesting to note that even though the paternal *UBE3A* allele is imprinted in some parts of the brain, it is expressed in other tissues throughout the body.[667] Studies on mice suggest that E6-AP may localize to the dendritic spines and may function to regulate spinal development or synaptic plasticity.[158] Deregulation of ubiquitination from lack of E6-AP could result in an inability to degrade or functionally alter targeted proteins. Similar to PWS, most AS patients (70%) have a deletion of the critical 15q11-q13 region. However, unlike PWS, in which a deletion occurs on the paternal allele, in AS, a deletion occurs on the maternally derived chromosome 15. Inversion mutations involving this region have been identified in a subset of mothers of AS patients with a deletion.[226] It is likely that the presence of these inverted DNA sequences in these women predisposed this region to deletions in their offspring by interfering with normal homologous synapses, or by pairing homologous chromosomes, during meiosis.

In 7% of AS patients, the syndrome is attributed to uniparental disomy from the inheritance of two paternally derived chromosome 15's. As a consequence, with two paternal *UBE3A* genes silenced, no functional UBE3A protein is present. In 3% of AS patients, an imprinting defected has been described.[87,305] A cytogenetic rearrangement has been detected in about 1% of AS cases, and in 11% of cases, a mutation in the *UBE3A* gene itself has been reported.[190] It is odd that a small number of AS cases and of another imprinting disorder at chromosome 11p15, Beckwith-Wiedemann syndrome, have been associated with assisted reproductive technologies, but the exact mechanism by which this occurs is not known.[425] Although mutations causing AS can arise de novo, they can be silently transmitted through several generations. For example, if a *UBE3A* mutation arose de novo on a paternal allele transmitted to a son, the son could transmit the mutation to a son or daughter to produce a normal phenotype. However, although this son could transmit the silenced *UBE3A* mutation to his offspring, his sister could donate her mutated *UBE3A* and her paternally derived allele to her offspring, and the child would have AS. In about 10 to 15% of patients with a firm diagnosis of AS, the cause of the disease has not been established. Clinical presentation does correlate with the underlying genetic cause for some features of the disease. AS patients with deletions are more likely to have hypopigmentation of skin, eye, and hair or microcephaly and are more likely to be severely affected.[410] A more severe phenotype may arise because of haploinsufficiency of nonimprinted *UBE3A* adjacent and co-deleted genes. In contrast, AS patients arising from UPD have normal head circumference and are mildly affected.

Diagnostic testing for individuals suspected of having AS or PWS can involve a variety of techniques. Determining the genetic mechanism for the cause of the disease is important in determining recurrence risks for the family.[91] Under most circumstances, initiation of testing with methylation-specific PCR (mPCR) is one scenario that can be used and may be the most cost-effective approach[452] (Figure 40-9). In methylation-specific PCR, genomic DNA is treated with sodium bisulfite before PCR to convert unmethylated cytosine residues to uracil without altering the methylated cytosine residues (those silenced in the 15q11-13 region). Subsequent PCR reactions use oligonucleotide primers specific to DNA strands that contain uracil (unmethylated) or cytosine (methylated).[379,656] Methylation-specific PCR provides a rapid and reliable diagnostic test to rule out PWS or AS. If the result is negative, more than 99% of those with PWS and about 80% of AS patients can be ruled out. Alternatively, aberrant CpG methylation can be commonly detected with the use of methylation-specific MLPA.[483] PWS patients with a chromosomal rearrangement disrupting the genes in this area will not be identified by this test. Similarly, AS patients with a *UBE3A* mutation, a chromosome rearrangement disrupting the genes in this region, and those with AS resulting from an unknown cause will not be diagnosed with this method. However, if the result is positive, fluorescent in situ hybridization (FISH) studies can be performed to detect a deletion within 15q11-13, and/or uniparental disomy DNA testing should be done to determine the genetic mechanism of disease for appropriate genetic counseling of the family. Alternatively, real-time PCR can be used to identify and characterize the deletion, and PCR analysis of short tandem repeats coupled with capillary electrophoresis can be used to detect uniparental disomy.[222,459] Mechanisms and tests for PWS and AS are summarized and contrasted in Table 40-3.

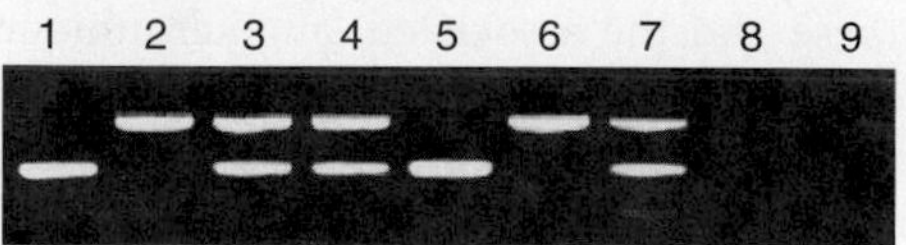

Figure 40-9 Methylation-specific polymerase chain reaction (PCR) assay for the diagnosis of Prader-Willi syndrome (PWS) and Angelman syndrome (AS). Extracted DNA is treated with sodium bisulfate before amplification using multiplex PCR and oligonucleotide primers specific for modified DNA. Normal individuals show amplicons representing their methylated maternal allele and amplicons from their unmethylated paternal allele. PWS patients show only the maternal allele, and AS patients show only the paternal allele. Results observed following PCR amplification and gel electrophoresis of patients referred for PWS and AS testing. Patient DNA with patterns diagnostic of AS *(lanes 1 and 5)* and PWS *(lanes 2 and 6)* and patients referred for AS or PWS but who have normal methylation patterns *(lanes 3 and 4)* are shown. Normal control DNA patterns and a negative control reaction in which no template DNA was added are indicated in *lanes 7 and 8*, respectively. No amplification products are observed in unmodified normal control DNA *(lane 9)*, illustrating the specificity of PCR primers prepared specifically for sodium bisulfate–modified DNA. *(Courtesy Jack Tarleton, PhD, Director of Genetics Laboratory, Fullerton Genetics Center, Mission Hospitals, Asheville, NC.)*

Complex Diseases

A complex or multifactorial inheritance pattern indicates interaction of one or more genes with one or more environmental factors. Multifactorial diseases can be more prevalent in some families with several affected family members, but the disease does not follow typical mendelian inheritance patterns. Disease may present in multiple family members because of sharing of similar disease-predisposing alleles and often sharing of similar daily habits, routines, and diet. The degree of genetic and environmental contribution to a disease process varies among complex diseases, and identification of causative genetic and environmental factors is challenging. Further, it is difficult to assess the relative importance of genetic and environmental influences in the development of a disease, although twin studies are often used. Among twins who were raised together, a greater concordance of disease among monozygotic (MZ) twins—who share all of their genes—than in dizygotic (DZ) twins, who share 50% of their genes, provides strong evidence of a genetic component of the disease. Conversely, disease concordance less than 100% in MZ twins is strong evidence that nongenetic factors play a role in the disease. Large genome-wide association (GWA) studies are being used to identify common genetic variants that play a role in the pathogenesis of common complex

TABLE 40-3 Molecular Mechanisms and Tests for Prader-Willi and Angelman Syndromes

Molecular Mechanism	Angelman Syndrome (Frequency)	Prader-Willi Syndrome (Frequency)	Methylation-Specific PCR Result	Possible Detection Methods
Deletion (≈4 Mb) of chromosome 15q11-13	70% (maternal)	70% (paternal)	Abnormal	High-resolution cytogenetics or FISH
Uniparental disomy	7% (paternal)	25 to 30% (maternal)	Abnormal	PCR for microsatellite analysis
Imprinting center defect	3%	1 to 2%	Abnormal	IC sequencing
UBE3A mutation (specific to AS)	11%	N/A	Normal	*UBE3A* sequencing
Chromosomal rearrangement in chromosome 15q11-13 region	<1% (maternal)	<1% (paternal)	Normal	High-resolution cytogenetics or FISH
No detectable abnormality	10 to 15%	Very few cases	Normal	N/A

AS, Angelman syndrome; *FISH,* fluorescent in situ hybridization; *IC,* imprinting center; *N/A,* not applicable; *PCR,* polymerase chain reaction.
Modified from a table prepared by Allison Presley, MD, University of Virginia.

diseases.[275] Examples of largely adult-onset complex diseases include type 1 diabetes, rheumatoid arthritis, Parkinson disease, hypertension, alcoholism, and thrombophilia.

Thrombophilia

Deep vein thrombosis (DVT) occurs in about 1 per 1000 individuals, and associated complications, including pulmonary embolism, account for about 50,000 deaths per year.[588] Venous thrombosis results from disruption of normal hemostasis. As a complex or multifactorial disease, thrombophilia is caused by the interaction of genetic and environmental factors and/or acquired conditions, including the use of oral contraceptives, trauma, obesity, immobility, pregnancy, advancing age, or surgery.[283,400] Protein products of many genes are involved in the anticoagulation and coagulation pathway to regulate hemostasis. Yet it is sequence variants in the factor V (FV) (lq23) and prothrombin (PT) (11p11-q12) genes that are associated with DVT, represent the most frequent lifelong genetic cause of thrombophilia, and are common in the Caucasian population.[57,517] Patients with mutations in both genes have increased risk of a recurrent DVT and may require different management than patients with a mutation in only one of these two genes.[149] Despite the known presence of these mutations and some environmental and/or acquired factors, it is impossible to predict a patient's clinical course even within members of the same family. This illustrates our lack of understanding of the interaction between known and uncharacterized risk factors in predisposition to a complex disease. Activated protein C in conjunction with its cofactor, protein S, plays a key role in the anticoagulant system by inactivating membrane-bound factors Va and VIIIa. The inability to inactivate procoagulant factors Va or VIIIa can disturb hemostasis, heighten the coagulation pathway, increase the generation of thrombin, and promote clot formation.[135] In 1993, Dahlbäck reported that familial thrombophilia caused resistance to activated protein C (APC).[136] In 1994, Bertina and colleagues observed linkage of the FV gene with the APC resistance phenotype and reported a G-to-A base substitution at nucleotide 1691 (c.1691G>A) in exon 10 of the FV gene (OMIM #188055).[57] This nucleotide change results in an arginine-to-glutamine substitution at codon 506 (R506Q) in the FV protein and is commonly referred to as FV Leiden, named for the Dutch city in which it was discovered.[57]

The c.1691G>A substitution is common in the Caucasian population of Northern European descent, with a frequency of 3 to 5%, but it is rare in Asian, African, or indigenous Australian populations.[57,303,528,535] Because c.1691G>A occurs on the same FV gene haplotype, it is speculated that the G-to-A substitution occurred as a single event approximately 21,000 to 34,000 years ago, after the evolutionary divergence of non-Africans from Africans and of Caucasians from Mongoloids.[723]

The arginine residue at codon 506 is one of three peptide bonds (Arg306, Arg506, and Arg679) cleaved by APC to inhibit factor Va activity to decrease affinity for factor Xa and reduce efficiency in catalyzing the conversion of prothrombin to thrombin.[134,352,426] Substitution of a glutamine residue at this site prolongs APC inactivation of factor Va by approximately 10-fold, thereby shifting the balance of hemostasis to favor coagulation and increasing thrombin production.[281] In addition, R506Q prolongs APC-mediated protein S inactivation of FVIII.[648]

Heterozygous c.1691G>A carriers have a lifelong 7.9-fold increased relative risk of venous thrombosis compared with increased risk for homozygotes as high as 80-fold.[400,546] However, the FV Leiden does not confer increased risk for arterial thrombosis.[350] The mean age of onset of symptoms associated with thrombosis is 44 years for heterozygotes and 31 years for homozygotes.[546] Further, although it is transmitted as a dominant trait because thrombophilia is a complex disease resulting from the interaction of genetic and environmental and/or acquired factors, many heterozygote carriers can remain asymptomatic.[248,546]

Also in Leiden, Poort and coworkers in 1996 described a genetic variant (c.20210G>A) in the 3′ untranslated region of the PT gene (OMIM #176930) in 18% of patients with a documented family history of venous thrombosis.[517] In this population-based case-controlled study, the presence of c.20210G>A resulted in a hypercoagulable state with increased levels of plasma prothrombin (>1.15 kU/L) and a 2.8-fold lifelong increased risk of venous thrombosis. Similar to FV Leiden, this allele is largely confined to Caucasian populations and is rare in Asians, Africans, and indigenous populations of Australia.[724] Likewise, it is hypothesized that c.20210G>A represents a founder mutation after the divergence of Africans from non-Africans and of Caucasians from Mongoloid subpopulations approximately 24,000 years ago.[724]

Prothrombin, also referred to as factor II, is the precursor of thrombin and plays a primary role in fibrin production and clot formation. The G-to-A substitution does not change the coding region of the protein, rather it enhances processing of the 3′ end of pre-mRNA and thus functions as a gain-of-function mutation, culminating in increased mRNA accumulation and increased synthesis of protein.[217] This aberration of RNA metabolism results in increased synthesis of prothrombin and can enhance clot formation. The risk of venous thrombosis is increased 16-fold in c.20210G>A carriers using oral contraceptives, and the risk of cerebral vein thrombosis increases 149-fold in c.20210G>A carriers using oral contraceptives.[429,430] In the Caucasian population, this base substitution is present in 6.2% of patients with venous thrombosis compared with 2.3% of controls.

Inherited together, c.1691G>A and c.20210G>A convey at least a 20-fold increased risk for a venous thromboembolic event (VTE). They are commonly seen together in thrombophilia patients, thus supporting the additive genetic effects associated with complex diseases.[49,101,149,177,628] In addition, the presence of both mutations is associated with a sixfold increased risk of ischemic heart disease.[684] Further, women with one or both of these mutations are at increased risk of preeclampsia and have a higher rate of recurrent preeclampsia in subsequent pregnancies.[165,185] Treatment of the patient with a VTE typically involves the initial use of both heparin and vitamin K antagonists.[135] After several days, heparin is discontinued and vitamin K antagonist (warfarin) therapy is continued for 3 to 6 months or longer, depending on the type of thrombotic event, the precipitating factors, and the combination of genetic and other risk factors. Treatment is regularly monitored to avoid overdosing and possible bleeding complications using prothrombin time, and results are reported as the international normalized ratio (INR).

DNA testing for c.1691G>A and c.20210G>A in clinical laboratories is most often performed by any one of several common methods, including the Invader assay, PCR coupled with restriction-endonuclease digestion and gel electrophoresis, and real-time PCR.[57,273,390,517,691] However, many other techniques have been described.[37,68,164,289,501] Any testing platform is acceptable for clinical use as long as the procedure has been properly validated in the laboratory and follows appropriate quality assurance guidelines.[252]

DNA-based testing for factor V may be requested on a patient following the factor V Leiden-specific functional assay (Coatest APC resistance, Chromogenix AB, Mölndal, Sweden) to confirm the diagnosis and to distinguish between heterozygotes and homozygotes. Similarly, DNA testing can be ordered in place of the functional assay, especially for patients with lupus anticoagulant and a markedly prolonged baseline aPTT (which may interfere with the assay).[715] The clinical utility of knowing the FV or PT genotype is debated because it may not affect the clinical management of patients.[444] However, most experts believe that testing is appropriate for targeted patients such as those with (1) venous thrombosis or pulmonary embolism before 50 years of age; (2) venous thrombosis at an unusual site (hepatic, mesenteric, portal, or cerebral veins); (3) recurrent VTE; (4) VTE and a strong family history of thrombotic disease; or (5) VTE in pregnancy or associated with contraceptive use.[252,435,520] Routine screening before hormone use is not routinely performed, nor is it cost-effective.[647] Modifications to patient management after knowledge of this information may involve length of treatment with anticoagulants and management of other procoagulation risk factors. Use of DNA testing for these two common mutations in the pediatric thrombosis patient is less well defined because often multiple coexisting risk factors exist, and patient management is not currently provided on the basis of test results.[525]

Benefits from DNA testing in the adult include identification of individuals at risk for recurrent events, especially in situations that predispose to thrombosis, such as oral contraceptive use, management of pregnancy complications, or hormone replacement therapy, and in identification of at-risk family members,[150,520] although it is not clear whether this knowledge improves VTE-related outcomes of these individuals or the management of family members who have been genotyped.[573] Screening is not recommended for the general population or for newborns, nor is prenatal screening advised. Although factor V mutation is present in more than 50% of families with thrombosis, inherited defects in protein C, protein S, and antithrombin are detectable in approximately 10 to 15% of families with venous thrombosis. These latter, less common deficiencies can be diagnosed through laboratory assays and do not typically involve DNA testing because of the heterogeneity of mutations in these genes.[51,72,530] Mutations at two other factor V arginine-cleavage sites have been reported, but these mutations are rare and are not part of routine FV DNA testing.[107,693]

Inherited Breast Cancer

Mutations in *BRCA1* (OMIM #113705) or *BRCA2* (OMIM #600185) predispose patients to breast and ovarian cancer. In addition, *BRCA2* mutation carriers are at increased risk for pancreas cancer, and males are at increased risk for prostate and male breast cancer. The incidence of mutations in these genes within the population is estimated to be about 1 in 500. The combined frequency of two founder mutations in *BRCA1* (185delAG, 5382InsC) and one in *BRCA2* (6174delT) in the Ashkenazi Jewish population is as high as almost 3%.[540] Breast carcinoma is second only to lung carcinoma as a cause of cancer-related death among women in the Western hemisphere. Although most cases are sporadic (average lifetime risk, 12%), about 15% show familial clustering, and only about 5% demonstrate a distinct inheritance pattern. *BRCA1* mutations are associated with younger age at onset (average age, 43); they have a higher histologic grade with a high mitotic index, show a syncytial growth pattern, along with pushing margins, foci of necrosis, a high degree of aneuploidy, and lymphocytic infiltrate, and are usually negative for the expression of estrogen (ER), progestin (PR), and HER-2.[385] *BRCA2* mutation carriers have a slightly later age of onset (average age, 48) and exhibit higher overall grade, but these tumors are less distinct from sporadic breast cancer and more often are ER and PR positive.[385] In families in which breast cancer is segregating, but in which no *BRCA1* or *BRCA2* gene mutation has been detected, other genes that predispose to breast cancer are likely to be involved but have not yet been identified.[653]

The inability to identify breast cancer susceptibility genes in these families may reflect (1) genetic heterogeneity in the family with mutations in several genes; (2) low penetrance of these mutations, making it difficult to distinguish family members without mutation from asymptomatic carriers in the studies; (3) an autosomal recessive mode of inheritance; or (4) breast cancer acting as a complex disease that results from the interaction of several genes and lifestyle/environmental factors, thereby making it difficult to tease out the genetic component of the disease. Lifestyle/environmental factors that have been shown to affect breast cancer susceptibility include smoking, age at menarche and menopause, childbearing, breast feeding, hormonal contraception, and hormone replacement therapy. A candidate gene approach looking at genetic variation in DNA repair genes and large genome-wide association studies have identified multiple possible breast cancer susceptibility loci.[7,171,215,272,625] The significance of these findings requires additional studies, but the results of these and other studies begin to provide potential insight into the pathogenesis of this complex disease.

Offspring of *BRCA1* and *BRCA2* carriers possess a 50% chance of inheriting the predisposing cancer gene mutation. However, inheritance of the mutation does not convey certainty of developing cancer. *BRCA1* and *BRCA2* gene mutations are highly penetrant with a lifetime risk of breast cancer of about 65% and about 45% for *BRCA1* and *BRCA2*, respectively.[25] For the development of ovarian cancer, *BRCA1* mutation carriers have about a 39% risk, and *BRCA2* mutation carriers have an 11% chance.[25] Penetrance of disease is determined by both environmental and genetic factors. However, little is known regarding the identity of genetic modifiers; thus an intense, multicenter effort is under way for their characterization.[110,316] It is interesting to note that some susceptibility loci identified in sporadic breast cancer have been linked to *BRCA1* and *BRCA2* mutation carriers.[28] Homozygosity for a single-nucleotide polymorphism (SNP) c.-98G>C that affects splicing within the 5′UTR of *RAD51* was identified as increasing the risk of disease among *BRCA2* heterozygotes and homozygotes with hazard ratios of 1.17 and 3.18, respectively.[27] RAD51 interacts with BRCA1 and BRCA2 in the repair of double-stranded DNA. Although *BRCA1* and *BRCA2* genes are associated with the most common cause of hereditary breast cancer, much less common yet other highly penetrant genes and associated syndromes include *TP53*, Li-Fraumeni syndrome; *STK11*, Peutz-Jeghers syndrome; *PTEN*, Cowden syndrome; and *CDH1*, causing hereditary diffuse gastric cancer and familial lobular breast cancer.[538] Mutations in other genes involved in DNA repair such as *ATM*, *CHEK2*, *BRIP1*, *PALB2*, and *RAD50* also convey moderate susceptibility to breast cancer with odds ratios of between 2 and 4.[538]

Using DNA linkage studies, Hall and coworkers mapped the gene for early-onset familial breast cancer to 17q21.[269] In 1994, *BRCA1* was cloned; it was later confirmed by several other investigators as the susceptibility gene in breast and ovarian cancer kindreds.[100,212,445] The *BRCA1* gene spans 80 kb and is composed of 24 exons; 22 encode the 7.8-kb mRNA that is translated into a protein of 1863 amino acids. The large exon 11 (3427 bp) accounts for 63% of the coding portion of the gene. It is interesting to note that exon 11 is alternatively spliced in a number of tissues. In families in whom linkage to *BRCA1* was excluded, a second susceptibility locus at 13q12-13, *BRCA2*, was proposed and subsequently cloned.[621,705,706] The *BRCA2* gene, unrelated in sequence to *BRCA1*, spans 70 kb, contains 26 exons, encodes an 11.5-kb mRNA, and is translated into a protein of 3418 amino acids.

BRCA1 and *BRCA2* are considered tumor suppressor genes that require inactivation of both alleles for progression to neoplasm. In a patient with familial breast cancer, a mutant allele is inherited, and the second allele (the patient's wild-type allele) is inactivated through loss of the second allele (i.e., LOH). It is interesting to note that somatic mutations in these genes are not common in tumor DNA from sporadic breast cancer cases. However, LOH and epigenetic changes have been documented in a subset of sporadic breast and ovarian tumors, and RNA-binding protein HuR, which is commonly overexpressed in sporadic breast cancer, has been shown to post-transcriptionally regulate *BRCA1* expression.[102,562,603] BRCA1 and BRCA2 are large multifunctional proteins, expressed in a wide variety of tissues, where they are localized to the nucleus.[258] Each interacts with numerous proteins in complex and separate systems involved in DNA repair, transcriptional regulation of the response to DNA damage, protein ubiquitination, and chromatin remodeling.

Mutations in *BRCA1* and *BRCA2* are heterogeneous and are located throughout each gene.[78] The range of mutations varies greatly among different populations, with founder mutations observed in many ethnic groups.[399,471,616] In Ashkenazi Jewish breast and ovarian cancer families, the mutations 185delAG and 5382insC are primarily observed in *BRCA1*, and in families in whom these mutations are not present, identification of other *BRCA1* mutations is rare.[514] *BRCA2* mutation 6174delT has been observed in 6 of 80 (8%) Ashkenazi Jewish women diagnosed with breast cancer before age 42 as compared with 0 of 93 non-Jewish women diagnosed with breast cancer at the same age.[475] *BRCA1* mutation 943ins10 is a founder mutation of West African origin, and mutation 2804delAA, estimated to have occurred about 32 generations ago, is seen in Dutch and Belgian families.[436,487,504] The *BRCA2* mutation 999del5 is common in the Icelandic population, whereas the founder *BRCA2* mutations S2835X and 5802del4 are common in Japanese breast cancer families.[324,341] In contrast, *BRCA1* and *BRCA2* mutations are less commonly associated with familial breast cancer in Taiwanese and Chinese populations.[109,721]

Testing for disease-associated mutations is made more difficult by the heterogeneity of disease-causing mutations and the complexity of the *BRCA1* and *BRCA2* genes. Moreover, some gene variations may be family specific and may not result in an obvious biological functional change to the protein. Further, small families or unavailable DNA specimens from multiple family members may prevent additional studies to support segregation analysis of the DNA variant with disease, to confirm it as the disease-causing mutation in the family. Variants of uncertain significance (VUS) have been reported for *BRCA1* and *BRCA2*, and various mathematical and histologic models have been proposed to assist in the classification of VUS.[296,601] The development of functional assays and the maintenance of locus-specific databases will assist in determining the pathogenicity of variants and in disseminating their clinical significance throughout the clinical and research community.[129,247] Most *BRCA1* and *BRCA2* disease-associated mutations result in premature truncation of the protein and thus loss of function. Genotype-phenotype correlations indicate that *BRCA1* mutation carriers, with truncating mutations 3′ to codon 1358 and 5′ to codon 800, have a decreased ovarian-to-breast cancer ratio, and those with mutations between these 5′ and 3′ regions have a higher ovarian-to-breast cancer ratio.[297] Similarly, in *BRCA2*, mutations centrally located between nucleotides 4075 and 6503 of exon 11 cause an increased risk for ovarian cancer.[600] About 10% of patients with epithelial ovarian carcinoma (EOC) have a *BRCA1* or *BRCA2* germline mutation. These tumors tend to have serous histology, high response rates to chemotherapy, longer treatment-free intervals between each line of therapy, and improved overall survival compared with nonhereditary EOC.[619] It is interesting to note that some rare biallelic mutations in *BRCA2* can be associated with a Fanconi anemia (FA-D1) phenotype, while heterozygosity for a *BRCA2* mutation results in breast and/or ovarian cancer.[311] Other groups of FA patients have germline mutations in genes whose protein products interact with BRCA2.[529] Further, the type of *BRCA1* or *BRAC2* mutation in the affected patient may be used to determine the most appropriate drug and treatment plan.[488,637]

DNA sequencing of *BRCA1* and *BRCA2* genes is both laborious and costly. To minimize time and expense, some laboratories may use one or more of a variety of techniques to rapidly screen these genes for alterations, while maintaining maximum sensitivity in mutation detection and achieving a high throughput of specimens.[90,219] Once a region of the gene has been identified as containing a possible DNA perturbation, DNA sequence analysis of that particular region is performed to precisely identify the base or bases involved. Some testing algorithms may begin with mutation-specific screening assays that look specifically for common founder mutations when information regarding the ethnicity of the patient is provided. Alternatively, some laboratories prefer no prior gene screening technique and choose to perform DNA sequence analysis of the entire gene to maximize mutation detection and prevent a possible false-negative result caused by the presence of a mutation not detected by screening techniques. When a mutation has been identified as the disease-causing mutation within the family, at-risk family members will be tested specifically for that mutation, and complete *BRCA1* and/or *BRCA2* gene analysis is not required.

Clinical testing for *BRCA1* and *BRCA2* gene mutations should be considered for a woman if (1) multiple cases of breast cancer (<50 years of age) and/or ovarian cancer (any age) are present in her family, in more than one generation; (2) she has breast or ovarian cancer and is younger than 40 years; (3) both breast and ovarian cancers are present in her or in a family member; (4) she has breast and/or ovarian cancer and is of Ashkenazi Jewish descent; (5) she has a male relative with breast cancer; (6) she has a family member with a known *BRCA1* or *BRCA2* mutation, or (7) she has breast cancer and a family history of *BRCA1*- or *BRCA2*-related tumors.[568] *BRCA1* and *BRCA2* testing should also be performed on any man with breast cancer.[568] However, it is important to note that some mutations have been found in families who do not meet these criteria. Further, clinical testing for *BRCA1* and *BRCA2* mutations within the United States is currently available only at a single location within the United States because of exclusive licensing of patented genes. Absolute control of diagnostic testing at one location for these genes is an issue of much debate.[56]

In presymptomatic cases, extensive genetic counseling that addresses both positive and negative aspects of genetic testing must be provided to the patient before genetic testing is undertaken. Counseling often involves the participation of family members, usually spouses. Based on the family history, the genetic counselor should inform the patient of the likelihood that a *BRCA1* or *BRCA2* mutation could be segregating within the family, and that the risk of disease(s) may be associated with various mutations; an overview of prevention and surveillance options available for mutation carriers should be presented.[543] Mathematical models are available to determine the likelihood that a *BRCA1* or *BRCA2* mutation will be found that is based on the pedigree; these models should be used to assist in counseling.[26,192,495] In addition, counseling may be needed for psychologic issues, including fear of cancer or medical procedures, past experiences involving loved ones with cancer, and feelings of guilt about possibly transmitting a cancer-causing gene to children.[73] Continued anxiety and uncertainty regarding some test results should be discussed as well. For example, in some instances, when DNA from an affected family member is not available for testing, the presymptomatic patient must clearly understand that a negative result could imply a false negative because of the inability to detect the specific *BRCA1* or *BRCA2* gene mutation segregating within the family or the possibility of a mutation in another breast cancer susceptibility gene that may be present in the family. As previously discussed, there exists the possibility of identifying a DNA variant of uncertain significance.

As important as pretest counseling is post-test counseling to explain the test results, answer additional questions, and provide referral to various follow-up services as needed. In addition, the genetic counselor should always be available for further future questions that may arise after the patient has had time to synthesize the results of the disclosure counseling.

Management of the mutation-positive woman is complex and often involves a multidisciplinary approach. The woman may wish to undergo risk reduction surgery, including some type of prophylactic mastectomy and/or salpingo-oophorectomy. Alternatively, she may choose to utilize increased surveillance and prevention strategies for the early detection of breast and ovarian cancer. Surveillance for breast cancer should include annual mammography and breast magnetic resonance imaging and biannual clinical breast examinations.[512,547] Surveillance for ovarian cancer should include transvaginal ultrasound and CA125 measurement every 6 months.[542] Although surveillance may be the choice of some patients, prophylactic surgeries have proved more effective in cancer prevention.[161,437] In addition to facing increased risk of cancer for themselves, most *BRCA1* and *BRCA2* mutation carriers are concerned about transmitting a gene mutation to their offspring. However, one survey showed that only a minority of *BRCA1* or *BRCA2* carriers would be interested in assisted reproductive technologies to minimize the risk of passing a mutant allele on to their children.[604] Although preimplantation genetic diagnosis is available for inherited breast and ovarian cancers, the ethical use of this technology for these adults with late-onset disease is debated.[480]

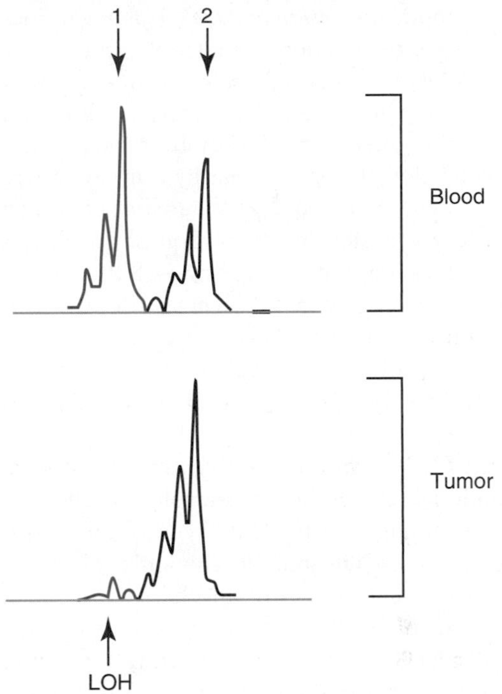

Figure 40-10 Electropherograms illustrating loss of heterozygosity (LOH) in tumor DNA. Patient DNA is extracted from peripheral blood and tumor tissue and is amplified by polymerase chain reaction (PCR) using an oligonucleotide primer pair specific for a polymorphic, microsatellite repeat locus contained within the chromosomal region and thought to be deleted during tumorigenesis. One of the primers within the pair is labeled with a fluorescent dye. Amplicons are subjected to electrophoresis on a 5% denaturing polyacrylamide gel in an ABI DNA sequencer and are analyzed using GeneScan software 3.1 b3 (Applied Biosystems, Foster City, Calif). Constitutive DNA from the patient's blood illustrates heterozygosity for this marker with amplicons represented by alleles 1 and 2. In DNA from the tumor, a single peak representing a typical homozygous pattern is observed. Thus LOH is present in tumor DNA. This loss signifies loss of the second allele and indicates loss of this region on the chromosome.

Inherited Colon Cancer

Colorectal cancer (CRC) is the third leading cause of cancer death in the United States with approximately 150,000 new cases each year. About 3 to 5% of CRC cases are associated with inherited mutations linked to highly penetrant colon cancer syndromes. In as many as one third of cases, familial clustering is observed, thereby suggesting the involvement of less penetrant susceptibility genes and environmental factors. The molecular basis of sporadic and inherited CRC involves two major and distinct pathways: one of chromosomal instability and one associated with microsatellite instability. The original model of chromosome instability proposed in 1990 to explain the pathogenesis of most sporadic tumors (>85%) has been further characterized to reveal a complex chain of events whereby normal colon lining (mucosa) is transformed into adenomatous and then into malignant mucosa via the inactivation of tumor suppressor genes and the activation of genes involved in tumor cell proliferation.[195]

The *chromosomal instability (CIN) pathway* begins with loss of function of the adenomatous polyposis coli *(APC)* tumor suppressor gene product, most often caused by a somatic inactivating gene mutation on one allele followed by a second inactivating mutation such as a chromosomal deletion encompassing the second *APC* allele and adjacent flanking DNA on chromosome 5q (Figure 40-10).[195] Because *APC* is involved early in the tumorigenic process, it has been referred to as the "gatekeeper."[369] The cascade of events proceeds with continued activation of the *KRAS* (Kirsten rat sarcoma virus) proto-oncogene on 12p12.1 through somatic gene mutations (most frequently occurring in codon 12, 13, or 61), which, in the presence of *APC* inactivation, increase growth and proliferation of the cell. Subsequent inactivation of the tumor suppressor gene *DCC* (deleted in colon cancer), frequent loss of adjacent tumor suppressor genes on 18q, including *SMAD4* and *SMAD2,* and inactivation of tumor suppressor gene *TP53* on 17p are identified in late adenoma and carcinoma.

The *microsatellite instability (MSI) pathway* in sporadic CRC arises from mutations or altered expression of genes involved in DNA mismatch repair (MMR). MMR is a ubiquitous DNA repair process that occurs in all dividing cells. As a result of an altered and thus dysfunctional MMR system, DNA replication errors, primarily within microsatellite repeats or repetitive sequences, remain uncorrected and accumulate. Expansion or contraction of the microsatellite-repeat number in noncoding areas of the genome is of little significance. However, if changes occur within coding microsatellites of the genome and specifically within targeted genes whose protein products are involved in cell growth (TGFβR2), apoptosis (*BAX*), and DNA repair *(MSH6)* then CRC may result.[701]

Inherited CRC syndromes occur as the result of an inherited mutation in one of the genes involved in the CIN or MSI pathway. Although several CRC syndromes exist, the two most common are autosomal dominantly inherited familial adenomatous polyposis (FAP) and hereditary nonpolyposis colorectal cancer (HNPCC).[108] Tumors in FAP kindreds and tumors displaying CIN more frequently are found in the distal part of the colon (left-sided), whereas tumors in HNPCC families and tumors displaying MSI more commonly occur in the proximal part of the colon (right-sided).

FAP (OMIM #175100) is characterized by hundreds to thousands of adenomatous polyps throughout the large bowel and has an estimated incidence of 1 in 8000.[65] FAP accounts for less than 1% of CRC observed in the United States. In about 25% of cases, no family history exists, indicating that these cases arise as the result of a new mutation; however, there is no tendency for paternal versus maternal origin of the mutated allele.[65,537] Polyps first appear during the second decade of life.[510] CRC ultimately develops approximately 10 to 15 years after the onset of polyposis, with the median age of CRC in untreated FAP patients being about 40.[65,510] It is the sheer number of polyps in these patients that increases the likelihood that one will progress to cancer. Further, patients with FAP have about a 1 to 2% risk of developing malignant extraintestinal manifestations of disease, including papillary thyroid carcinoma, hepatoblastoma, brain tumor, and pancreatic cancer.[253] In addition, these patients have a 7 to 20% lifetime risk of developing benign extraintestinal manifestations of the disease, including adrenal or desmoid tumors, osteomas, and dental abnormalities.[253] Desmoids have been reported as a cause of death in as many as 21% of patients with FAP.[344] It is important to note that close clinical surveillance of FAP patients and at-risk family members is critical to reducing CRC, CRC-associated mortality, and mutant APC-associated complications.[650] The gene responsible for FAP, adenomatous polyposis coli *(APC)*, was ultimately cloned in 1991, following linkage to chromosome 5q21 in FAP kindreds in 1987.[70,251,368,479] The *APC* gene spans 8535 base pairs, contains 15 exons, and encodes a protein of 2843 amino acids with a molecular weight of about 312 kDa. The APC protein is a multidomain, multifunctional protein that plays a key role in regulating the β-catenin level in the Wnt signaling pathway.[666] This tumor suppressor protein is also involved in other cellular processes, including cell adhesion and migration, signal transduction, microtubule assembly, and chromosome segregation.[29] However, the main tumor suppressor function of *APC* appears to be its regulation of β-catenin. Many *APC* truncation germline mutations affect the glycogen synthase kinase-3β, APC, and axin complex, which is unable to phophorylate cytoplasmic β-catenin for ubiquitin-dependent degradation. This, in turn, results in lack of β-catenin regulation and constitutive Wnt signaling, promoting cell proliferation and suppression of apoptosis.[29,357]

Studies on FAP families indicate that more than 700 germline mutations exist; more than 95% result in truncated proteins because of a nonsense mutation (30%) or a frameshift mutation, and most are contained within the 5′ half of the gene.[317] The penetrance of most mutations is 80 to 90% of the lifetime risk of colon cancer. Two hot spots for mutations occur at codons 1061 and 1309 representing 11% and 13% of all mutations, respectively. Genotype-phenotype correlations exist for some *APC* mutations. The AAAAG deletion at codon 1309 is associated with a younger age of onset.[97] Approximately 10% of patients who have truncating mutations at the extreme 5′ end of the gene (codons 1 to 163) or mutations at the carboxyl-terminal end of the gene (codons 1860 to 1987) have the attenuated form of the disease—attenuated FAP (AFAP). These patients develop a smaller number of polyps (5-100) and have a 10-year delay in the development of both polyps and cancer.* FAP patients with mutations between codons 1250 and 1464, or truncating mutations between codons 1403 and 1578, have a severe phenotype and are at increased risk for extracolonic disease.[159,466] Intra- and interfamilial phenotypic variability exists even in the presence of an identical mutation and may be explained by a modifier gene or genes.[130,221]

In 2002, *APC* mutation-negative FAP patients were found to have biallelic mutations in the base excision repair gene *MUTYH* or *MAP* (OMIM #604933).[13,560] This gene is located on 1p34.3-p32.1 and encodes an adenine-specific DNA glycosylase, which removes adenine when it is inappropriately paired with guanine, cytosine, or oxidatively damaged DNA containing 8-oxo-7,8-dihydroguanine. This results in G : C to T : A transversion mutations in the *APC* and *KRAS* genes.[13,345] Most patients with these mutations have fewer than 100 polyps. Following screening for common mutations in this gene, data from a multicenter case-controlled study showed that compared with *MUTYH*-negative CRC patients, an increased proportion of *MUTYH* homozygous or compound heterozygous patients tended to have a greater proportion of right-sided, synchronous tumors with an earlier age of onset (mean, 51.7 ± 9.5 years).[118] Although this is an autosomal recessive condition, this study showed that *MUTYH* heterozygous carriers are at increased for CRC, thus indicating that early clinical surveillance may be indicated in this population as well.[118,489] Clinical care of these patients should be similar to that provided for those with FAP or AFAP.

*References 79, 194, 211, 587, 599, 645, and 672.

The protein truncation test can be used to test for *APC* mutations because most mutations cause a frameshift in the protein and result in a truncated product.[227] However, most DNA laboratories use sequence analysis of the entire coding region of the gene coupled with multiplex ligation-dependent probe amplification for the detection of exonic insertions or deletions. Sensitivity of about 80 to 90% can be achieved for patients with classic FAP, but it may be as low as 20% in patients with AFAP.[210] If the mutation within the family can be identified, it is recommended that the family be referred for genetic counseling. Many studies have reviewed genetic testing associated with FAP.[163] Most of these studies found that a majority of individuals choose to have presymptomatic testing, yet clinically relevant levels of anxiety and depression can be observed after positive results are received.[163] DNA testing is recommended in at-risk family members as young as 10 to 12 years of age.[220] Genetic testing can significantly alter the 50% pretest risk for disease to a risk of 0% or 100%. Although DNA testing on an asymptomatic minor typically is not endorsed by the genetic community, in this scenario, early identification of the mutation in these patients will clearly affect their clinical management because intense screening programs and possible prophylactic colectomy can be initiated in that decade of life. Family members who test negative for the mutation do not have increased risk of CRC and can avoid intensive screening programs. Further, in some FAP mutation–positive families, preimplantation genetic diagnosis can be used to prevent the birth of a child with an inherited predisposition to FAP or another cancer syndrome.[602] If the mutation in the family cannot be identified, DNA linkage studies may be useful for presymptomatic identification of at-risk family members. If the mutation in the family cannot be identified, and if DNA linkage studies are not informative or available, screening with sigmoidoscopy is recommended every 1 to 2 years, starting as early as age 12. Further, when repeatedly negative sigmoidoscopy results are obtained, the frequency of such examinations can be reduced in each subsequent decade of life. It is important to distinguish AFAP from MAP families because at-risk individuals within the pedigree may shift. In AFAP, the risk to offspring is 50% a priori, whereas in the MAP family, the patient's children have a much lower risk of developing CRC because in most cases, a second mutation in their alternate *MUTYH* allele must be inherited from the other parent.

The most common inherited CRC susceptibility syndrome is HNPCC (OMIM #120435), which represents about 2 to 3% of all CRC cases. In contrast to FAP, HNPCC is characterized by a few polyps that possess an accelerated transformation potential to carcinoma in as little as 1 to 2 years. HNPCC is inherited as an autosomal dominant disorder with a penetrance of 80 to 85%. HNPCC is sometimes referred to as *Lynch syndrome* because of Dr. Lynch's observation of an autosomal dominant predisposition to early-onset CRC with proximal involvement and cancers of other organs in two large Midwestern kindreds.[418] HNPCC patients have a lifetime risk of 70 to 80% of developing CRC, thereby suggesting a role for other factors in this disease process.[257] To assist clinicians in identifying patients in HNPCC kindreds, and to help standardize the ascertainment and study of these families, the International Collaborative Group on HNPCC developed the Amsterdam criteria (AC) in 1991.[649] Basically, criteria for inclusion as an HNPCC family included at least three affected members spanning two successive generations with the diagnosis of colon cancer before the age of 50. In addition, one affected individual must be a first-degree relative of two other individuals, and because this mode of inheritance is consistent with autosomal dominant, the diagnosis of FAP must be excluded.

Because some HNPCC families were excluded by these stringent criteria, and because these criteria did not account for the risk to these patients for cancers of other organs as well, an expanded, more inclusive set of criteria was subsequently developed in Bethesda in 1998, as the Amsterdam criteria II in 1999, and as the Revised Bethesda Criteria (RBC) in 2004.[71,641,651] According to the RBC, tumors from individuals should be tested for microsatellite instability to identify a member of an HNPCC family under the following circumstances: (1) the patient is younger than 50; (2) regardless of age, synchronous, metachronous colorectal, or other HNPCC-associated tumor, including endometrium, ovary, stomach, hepatobiliary system, small bowel, ureter, renal, pelvis, and brain, is present; (3) CRC in someone younger than 60 shows a histology of tumor-infiltrating lymphocytes, Crohn's-like lymphocytic reaction, mucinous/signet ring differentiation, or a medullary growth pattern; (4) CRC occurs in one or more first-degree relatives with an HNPCC-associated tumor, and one is diagnosed before age 50; or (5) CRC occurs in two or more first- or second-degree relatives with HNPCC-related tumors, regardless of their age.[641] Use of the RBG for MSI testing has enhanced the detection of microsatellite instability and the potential to identify HNPCC cases.[236] Although these guidelines reflect improvement, some index cases are still missed, causing some investigators to propose a molecular approach to identifying these patients.[349]

The first MMR gene was mapped to 2p15-16 using large HNPCC kindreds.[506] Simultaneously, MSI was noted in a subset of sporadic CRC.[327,624] MMR genes associated with HNPCC include *MSH2* (2p15-16), *MSH6* (2p15-16), *MLH1* (3p21), *hPMS1* (2q31), *hPMS2* (7p22), and *hMLH3* (14q24.3); however, more than 90% of HNPCC mutations are observed in *hMSH2* and *hMLH1*.[417] In addition, *MLH1* and *MSH2* mutations have been identified in families with Muir-Torre syndrome (MTS), which is characterized by sebaceous gland neoplasia, other skin tumors, and other HNPCC-associated tumors, and is considered a variant of Lynch syndrome.[3] Patients with biallelic germline mutations in an MMR gene resulting in constitutional mismatch repair deficiency syndrome have childhood hematologic or brain tumors, early-onset CRC, and light-brown café au lait spots on the skin.[695]

HNPCC-related MMR gene mutations are diverse and are located throughout these genes.[507] Almost all errors made during DNA replication are repaired through the proofreading 3′-to-5′ exonuclease activity of DNA polymerase.

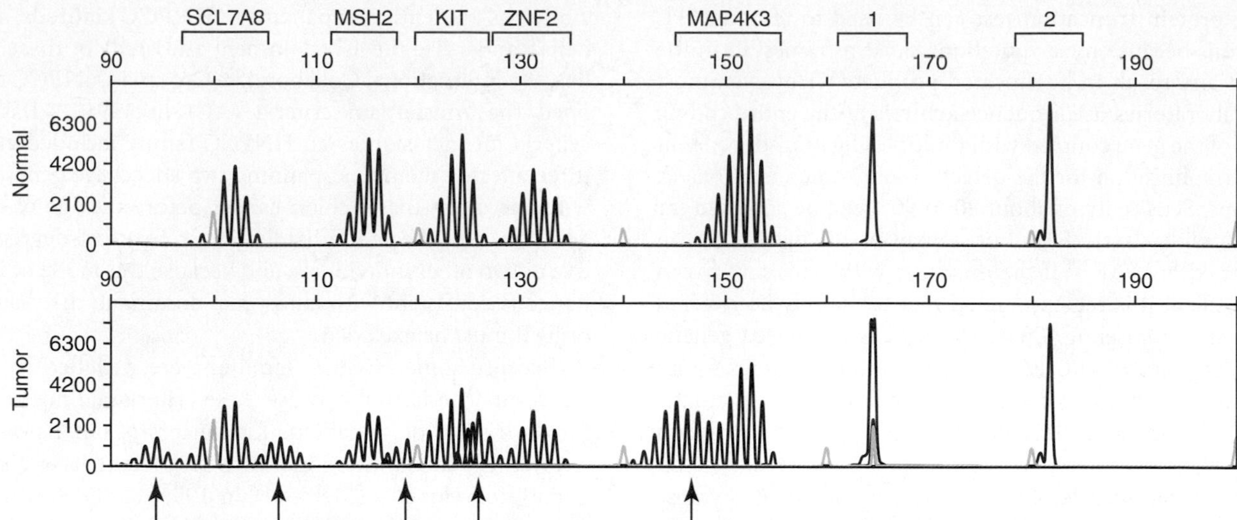

Figure 40-11 Electropherograms illustrating microsatellite instability (MSI) in tumor DNA. Patient DNA is extracted from peripheral blood or normal tissue and is compared with DNA extracted from tumor tissue. DNA is amplified in a multiplex polymerase chain reaction (PCR) assay using fluorescent labeled primers corresponding to 5 mononucleotide loci *(SCL7A8, MSH2, KIT, ZNF2, MAP4K3)* and two pentanucleotide loci (1 and 2) (Promega Corporation, Madison, Wis). Amplicons were detected following capillary electrophoresis on an ABI 3130*xl* Genetic Analyzer (Applied Biosystems, Foster City, Calif) and were analyzed using Gene Mapper v.3.7 software (Applied Biosystems). *Arrows* denote a shift in polymerase chain reaction (PCR) products at 5/5 mononucleotide loci, indicating microsatellite instability. Identical patterns between normal and tumor DNA at the polymorphic pentanucleotide markers suggest that normal and tumor DNA is derived from the same individual.

Uncorrected errors of mismatched bases between the two strands are repaired before cell division by the MMR proteins.[340] In addition to providing the repair of a mismatched base pair, the MMR system repairs "loop outs" from unmatched bases that can occur during replication of a microsatellite or small repetitive sequences. When the normal function of MMR proteins is altered through DNA mutations, mismatched bases generated through DNA replication are not fixed, leading to strands of DNA of different lengths. In the case of HNPCC, a germline mutation in one of the six known MMR genes is inherited, causing one allele to be nonfunctional. In the tumor tissue of these patients, the second allele has been rendered inactive through a somatic mutation or LOH. Uncorrected somatic replication errors thus accumulate in noncoding and insignificant locations throughout the genome, but significantly in coding regions of genes involved in cell growth and signaling and in the DNA of genes involved in DNA repair.

Although MSI is identified in ≈90% of cases of HNPCC-related CRC, it is observed in approximately 15 to 20% of cases of sporadic CRC.[1] MSI in sporadic CRC is attributed to epigenetic silencing of *MLH1* expression through biallelic methylation.[380,630] Thus a category of CRC consisting of the CpG island methylator phenotype (CIMP) has been recognized.

Testing of tumor tissue for MSI is often the first laboratory step in the investigation of HNPCC patients, because MSI is a measure of MMR deficiency that indicates probable defects in MMR genes through germline and somatic changes. Because mononucleotide microsatellite repeats are more susceptible to errors resulting from MMR enzyme deficiencies, testing for MSI most often includes multiplex analysis at multiple mononucleotide loci (Figure 40-11). MSI is characterized by the expansion or contraction of DNA sequences through the insertion or deletion of repeated sequences. If MSI is detected at two or more of the five loci, or more than 30%, the tumor has a "high" frequency of MSI. If MSI is detected at one locus, or less than 30%, the tumor has a "low" frequency of MSI. If MSI is not detected at any locus, the tumor is considered to be microsatellite stable. If MSI is detected, it is necessary to determine whether the MSI results from an inherited MMR germline mutation, or from somatic CpG methylation and inactivation of an MMR gene. Because somatic CpG methylation is frequently associated with mutation V600E in the *BRAF* proto-oncogene, V600E mutation analysis is often performed (Figure 40-12).[411,485] If MSI is present but a *BRAF* mutation is not detected, MMR gene mutation analysis is considered, requiring the submission of a peripheral blood specimen to screen for germline mutations in *MLH1, MSH2, PMS2,* and *MSH6*. To minimize the cost of screening all four genes for mutations, immunohistochemistry (IHC) testing can be performed on tumor tissue to identify the likely defective protein, thereby indicating which gene should be screened for using DNA sequence analysis. However, the best laboratory method for the identification of

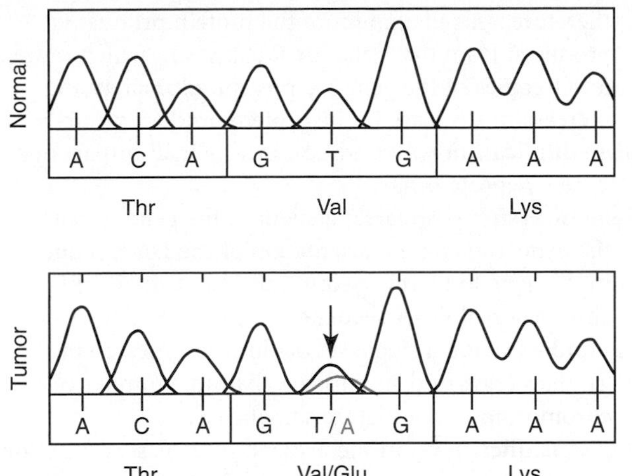

Figure 40-12 DNA sequencing results for *BRAF* mutation c.1799T>A. DNA extracted from normal tissue and paraffin-embedded colon tumor tissue was amplified for exon 15 of the *BRAF* gene by polymerase chain reaction (PCR) and was sequenced using the BigDye Terminator v3.1 cycle sequencing kit (Applied Biosystems, Foster City, Calif). Amplicons were subjected to capillary electrophoresis on an ABI 3030*xl* Genetic Analyzer (Applied Biosystems). The *arrow* indicates the presence of mutation c.1799T>A, resulting in substitution of glutamic acid for valine at codon 600 in the tumor tissue.

HNPCC patients and their families, MSI versus IHC, is still debated.[183,271,494,585,718] It is important for patient care that a systematic and comprehensive approach be developed and followed.

HNPCC-associated gene mutations are heterogeneous, consisting predominantly of point mutations, which impair the activity of the protein, or deletions, which result in premature truncation of the protein and loss of function.[317] An inherent problem with DNA sequence analysis is the identification of sequence variants without obvious biological significance. Thus, it is difficult to assign a pathologic role to these variants without functional assays to confirm their relevance in the disease process. Studies have shown that most of these variants are associated with splicing defects.[629] Further, a database has been developed to assist clinicians in interpreting these variants and to facilitate communication between investigators.[492]

Genotype-phenotype correlations for *MLH1* and *MSH2* from two large European and U.S. studies representing 236 *MLH1* and 330 *MSH2* mutations led to similar conclusions.[230,356] These studies showed that (1) CRC is more prevalent with *MLH1* mutations and is diagnosed at a younger age in males; (2) endometrial cancer is equally present in *MLH1* and *MSH2* families; and (3) extracolonic tumors, excluding endometrial tumors, are more prevalent with *MSH2* mutations. It is interesting to note that a study of *PMS2* mutation carriers reported a lower penetrance of disease with highly variable clinical characteristics, including a wide range of HNPCC-related tumors and a wide age of onset ranging from 23 to 77 years.[574]

If a mutation is identified, at-risk adult family members can pursue presymptomatic testing. Genetic counseling is important to reduce distress associated with test results.[359] Similar to presymptomatic testing for other adult-onset disorders, the counseling session should include verification of the family history and discussion of the clinical course of the disease, including risk of developing the disease and issues associated with disease management. Discussions should be incorporated into the session, including how the patient will act upon both positive and negative results, feelings of survivor guilt or stigmatization, and the possibility of discrimination for insurance and employment. If a germline mutation is detected, a colonoscopy should be performed every 1 or 2 years, or at 5 years younger than the youngest age of diagnosis in the family.[470] Because the risk of endometrial cancer is 40 to 60% for at-risk women with Lynch syndrome, screening for endometrial cancer annually with endometrial aspiration biopsy and transvaginal ultrasound beginning at 30 to 35 years of age is recommended.[565] Further, prophylactic hysterectomy and bilateral salpingo-oophorectomy can be considered. Alternatively, if genetic testing is not pursued, relatives should begin an intensive screening program with a colonoscopy every 1 to 2 years, starting at between 20 and 30 years of age, and then annually after age 40. If no mutation is detected in the proband, presymptomatic DNA testing for family members is not recommended. Some testing strategies may result in false-negative results caused by the inability of the assays employed to identify all mutations at these loci. However, some mutation-negative families may have germline mutations in other, yet unknown MMR genes.[338] Although detection of a mutation in a family that meets HNPCC criteria is not always possible, careful surveillance of at-risk family members in mutation-negative families is considered critical.

REPORTING OF TEST RESULTS

As the preceding pages make clear, DNA testing for inherited diseases is complex, and it is most important to convey the results of a genetic test thoroughly. Results must be presented in a manner that can be easily and accurately understood by a professional whose expertise is not genetics, because in many instances, primary care providers will be communicating test results to the patient. Unfortunately, however, with the increasing clinical demand for genetic testing and the increasing numbers of laboratories performing such tests, uniformity in communicating these complex results to referring clinicians does not exist. However, efforts are ongoing to develop standardized and comprehensive, yet "clinician-friendly," reports.[413] The Molecular Pathology Laboratory Inspection Checklist of the College of American Pathologists (CAP) indicates that failure to include pertinent information within the patient report constitutes a deficiency.[123]

A comprehensive genetic report should include the patient's name; medical record number and/or birth date; sex of the patient; ethnicity of the patient (if relevant); type of specimen and date received; specimen's laboratory identification number; laboratory test requested; name and address of laboratory performing the test; name and address of referring physician, hospital, or genetic counselor; date of report; brief interpretation of the results; and a descriptive comments section explaining the test results. Although preparation of the comments can be labor-intensive, the comments section is vital to a genetic report and should include the following: (1) brief clinical history of patient (indicating the reason for referral); (2) detailed explanation of the method (citing literature if possible); (3) description of the patient's results using standard nomenclature; (4) sensitivity and specificity of the assay (e.g., number of mutations analyzed, percentage of mutations not detected, possibility of genetic heterogeneity, chance of genetic recombination); (5) clinical significance of the results (e.g., recurrence risk, genotype-phenotype correlation or penetrance, with citations of literature if possible); and (6) a statement that genetic counseling for the patient is recommended to discuss the implications of the results for the health and management of the patient, and when mutations are identified, to inform the patient of the potential risk of disease for other family members.

Because many assays performed in clinical DNA laboratories have been developed by the laboratory and are not approved by the U.S. Food and Drug Administration (FDA), reports must include a disclaimer that states, "This test was developed and its performance characteristics determined by [laboratory name]. It has not been cleared or approved by the U.S. Food and Drug Administration." In addition, the CAP recommends inclusion of these additional statements: "The FDA has determined that such clearance or approval is not necessary. This test is used for clinical purposes. It should not be regarded as investigational or for research. This laboratory is certified under the Clinical Laboratory Improvement Amendments of 1988 (CLIA 88) as qualified to perform high complexity clinical laboratory testing." Last, the report should be reviewed and signed by the laboratory director.

Glossary

Allele—An alternative form of a gene found at a specific location on a chromosome.

Crossover—*See* "Recombination."

Diploid—Having a full set of (paired) chromosomes (46 chromosomes in humans, half from each parent).

DNA marker—A polymorphic locus that is easily assayed, yielding reproducible results.

DNA methylation—The addition of a methyl residue to the 5′ position of the pyrimidine ring of a cytosine base to form 5-methylcytosine; this most often occurs at CpG DNA sequences. DNA methylation can serve as a mode of gene regulation by preventing gene transcription.

Downstream—A DNA sequence located 3′ to another DNA sequence.

Gene deletion—A circumstance in which all or part of a gene is lost.

Gene dosage—The number of copies of a particular gene. In most cases, there are two copies of each gene; therefore, a fixed amount of the protein product is produced from that gene. In situations in which more or fewer copies of the gene are present, ultimately an increase or decrease in the protein product occurs.

Gene duplication—A condition in which all or part of a gene is repeated.

Gene inversion—A rearrangement of the gene or part of the gene, causing the orientation of the DNA sequences in the gene to be reversed in relation to the flanking chromosomal DNA sequences.

Haploid—Having a single set of chromosomes, as in gametes (eggs and sperm) (i.e., half the number of chromosomes in a mature somatic cell).

Haploinsufficiency—In the presence of a loss-of-function DNA mutation, the remaining normal allele is unable to produce sufficient quantities of the protein product of the specific gene, and disease results.

Homologous sequences—DNA sequences that share a similar order of DNA bases. If two sequences are 95% homologous, 95% of their bases are identical at a particular location.

Linkage disequilibrium—The occurrence of two alleles from two loci inherited together on a chromosome more frequently than would be predicted by chance.

Linkage studies—A method using DNA markers physically adjacent (i.e., "linked") to a disease gene. Through this "indirect" analysis, the disease gene can be tracked through a family to determine the disease status of at-risk individuals without the need for knowledge of the disease-causing mutation segregating within the family.

Meiosis—Two-step process of cell division that produces gametes (ova in females and sperm in males) with one half the number of chromosomes of the parent cell. Contrast with mitosis.

Microsatellite repeat markers—Highly polymorphic DNA sequences of short repeats generally comprising <6 bases. These repeats are widely prevalent in both coding and noncoding regions of the human genome.

Mitosis—Process of cell division that produces daughter cells that are genetically identical to the parent cell with the same number of chromosomes as the parent cell. Contrast with meiosis.

Nondisjunction—Failure of chromosomes to separate during cell division.

Penetrance—Percentage of individuals who carry the disease genotype and have symptoms of the disease. *Complete penetrance* implies that all individuals who possess the abnormal allele will develop the disease, whereas *incomplete or reduced penetrance* indicates that not all individuals who have the disease allele will become symptomatic. Incomplete penetrance of a disease suggests that other genetic loci and/or environmental factors can influence or modify the pathogenesis of the disease.

Primer—A short oligonucleotide designed to anneal to single-stranded DNA and from which DNA polymerase can add deoxynucleotide triphosphate (dNTP) in a complementary fashion to the template DNA. A primer pair flanks the target DNA to be amplified in PCR and creates the specificity of the reaction.

Recombination—Crossing over between DNA sequences that results in an exchange of information between two alleles. This process occurs in meiosis between homologous chromosomes and during mitosis between sister chromatids. *Homologous recombination* refers to this process when it occurs between similar sequences in corresponding regions. Crossing over between misaligned yet similar sequences is called *unequal homologous recombination* and results in a duplication on one allele and the reciprocal deletion on the alternate allele.

Restriction fragment length polymorphism—A polymorphism in the DNA sequence that creates or destroys a restriction endonuclease recognition site, thereby enabling detection by altered base-pair lengths of digested DNA fragments.

Skewed X-inactivation (lyonization) —A process by which inactivation of the X chromosome is not random.

REFERENCES

1. Aaltonen LA, Salovaara R, Kristo P, Canzian F, Hemminki A, Peltomaki P, et al. Incidence of hereditary nonpolyposis colorectal cancer and the feasibility of molecular screening for the disease. N Engl J Med 1998;338:1481-7.
2. Aartsma-rus A, Van Deutekom JC, Fokkema IF, Van Ommen GJ, Den Dunnen JT. Entries in the Leiden Duchenne muscular dystrophy mutation database: an overview of mutation types and paradoxical cases that confirm the reading frame rule. Muscle Nerve 2006;34:135-44.
3. Abbas O, Nahalingam M. Cutaneous sebaceous neoplasms as markers of Muir-Torre syndrome: a diagnostic algorithm. J Cutan Pathol 2009;36:613-9.
4. Abbs S, Roberts RG, Mathew CG, Bentley DR, Bobrow M. Accurate assessment of intragenic recombination frequency within the Duchenne muscular dystrophy gene. Genomics 1990;7:602-6.
5. ACOG Committee Opinion. Update on carrier screening for cystic fibrosis. Obstet Gynecol 2005;106:1465-8.
6. Acton JD, Wilmott RW. Phenotype of CF and the effects of possible modifier genes. Paediatr Respir Rev 2001;2:332-9.
7. Ahmed S, Thomas G, Ghoussaini M, Healey CS, Humphreys MK, Platte R, et al. Newly discovered breast cancer susceptibility loci on 3p24 and 17q23.2. Nat Genet 2009;41:585-9.
8. Alazmi WM, Fogel EL, Schmidt S, Watkins JL, McHenry L, Sherman S, et al. ERCP findings in idiopathic pancreatitis: patients who are cystic fibrosis gene positive and negative. Gastrointest Endosc 2006;63:234-9.
9. Allen KJ. Population genetic screening for hereditary haemochromatosis: are we a step closer? Med J Aust 2008;189:300-1.
10. Allen KJ, Gurrin LC, Constantine CC, Osborne NJ, Delatycki MB, Nicoll AJ, et al. Iron-overload-related disease in HFE hereditary hemochromatosis. N Engl J Med 2008;358:221-30.
11. Almqvist E, Adam S, Bloch M, Fuller A, Welch P, Eisenberg D, et al. Risk reversals in predictive testing for Huntington disease. Am J Hum Genet 1997;61:945-52.
12. Altarescu G, Renbaum P, Brooks BP, Margalioth EJ, Chetrit AB, Munter G, et al. Successful polar body-based preimplantation genetic diagnosis for achondroplasia. Reprod Biomed Online 2008;16:276-82.
13. Al-Tassan N, Chmiel NH, Maynard J, Fleming N, Livingston AL, Williams GT, et al. Inherited variants of MYH associated with somatic G:C→T:A mutations in colorectal tumors. Nat Genet 2002;30:227-32.
14. American College of Obstetricians and Gynecologists, American College of Medical Genetics. Preconception and prenatal carrier screening for CF: clinical and laboratory guidelines. Washington, DC: American College of Obstetricians and Gynecologists, 2001.
15. Ames BN, Shigenaga MK, Hagen TM. Oxidants, antioxidants, and the degenerative diseases of aging. Proc Natl Acad Sci U S A 1993;90:7915-22.
16. Amin R, Ratjen F. Cystic fibrosis: a review of pulmonary and nutritional therapies. Adv Pediatr 2008;55:99-121.
17. Anderson S, Bankier AT, Barrell BG, de Bruijn MH, Coulson AR, Drouin J, et al. Sequence and organization of the human mitochondrial genome. Nature 1981;290:457-65.
18. Andreu AL, Marti R, Hirano M. Analysis of human mitochondrial DNA mutations. Methods Mol Biol 2003;217:185-97.
19. Andrew SE, Goldberg YP, Kremer B, Telenius H, Theilmann J, Adam S, et al. The relationship between trinucleotide (CAG) repeat length and clinical features of Huntington's disease. Nat Genet 1993;4:398-403.
20. Andrew SE, Goldberg YP, Theilmann J, Zeisier J, Hayden MR. A CGG repeat polymorphism adjacent to the CAG repeat in the Huntington disease gene: implications for diagnostic accuracy and predictive testing. Hum Mol Genet 1994;3:65-7.
21. Antonarakis S. Molecular genetics of coagulation factor VIII gene and hemophilia A. Thromb Haemost 1995;74:322-8.
22. Antonarakis SE, Kazazian HH, Tuddenham, EG. Molecular etiology of factor VIII deficiency in hemophilia A. Hum Mutat 1995;5:1-22.
23. Antonarakis SE, Rossiter JP, Young M, Horst J, de Moerloose P, Sommer SS, et al. Factor VIII inversions in severe hemophilia A: results from an international consortium. Blood 1995;86:2206-12.
24. Antonarakis SE, Waber PG, Kittur SD, Patel AS, Kazazian HH, Mellis MA, et al. Hemophilia A: detection of molecular defects and of carriers by DNA analysis. N Engl J Med 1985;313:842-8.
25. Antoniou A, Pharoah PDP, Narod S, Risch HA, Eyfjord JE, Hopper JL, et al. Average risks of breast and ovarian cancer associated with *BRCA1* or *BRCA2* mutations detected in case series unselected for family history: a combined analysis of 22 studies. Am J Hum Genet 2003;72:1117-30.
26. Antoniou AC, Hardy R, Walker L, Evans DG, Shenton A, Eeles R, et al. Predicting the likelihood of carrying a *BRCA1* or *BRCA2* mutation: validation of BOADICEA, BRCAPRO, IBIS, Myriad and the Manchester scoring system using data from UK genetics clinics. J Med Genet 2008;45:425-31.
27. Antoniou AC, Sinilnikova OM, Simard J, Léoné M, Dumont M, Neuhausen SL, et al. *RAD51* 135G→C modifies breast cancer risk among *BRCA2* mutation carriers: results from a combined analysis of 19 studies. Am J Hum Genet 2007;81:1186-200.
28. Antoniou AC, Spurdle AB, Sinilnikova OM, Healey S, Pooley KA, Schmutzler RK, et al. Common breast cancer-predisposition alleles are associated with breast cancer risk in *BRCA1* and *BRCA2* mutation carriers. Am J Hum Genet 2008;82:937-48.
29. Aoki K, Taketo MM. Adenomatous polyposis coli (APC): a multi-functional tumor suppressor gene. J Cell Sci 2007;120:3327-35.
30. Asberg A, Thorstensen K, Hveem K, Bjerve KS. Hereditary hemochromatosis: the clinical significance of the S65C mutation. Genet Testing 2002;6:59-62.
31. Aurora P, Carby M, Sweet S. Selection of cystic fibrosis patients for lung transplantation. Curr Opin Pulm Med 2008;14:589-94.
32. Ayondrinde OT, Milward EA, Chua AC, Trinder D, Olynyk JK. Clinical perspectives on hereditary hemochromatosis. Crit Rev Clin Lab Sci 2008;45:451-84.
33. Babul R, Adam S, Kremer B, Dufrasne S, Wiggins S, Huggins M, et al. Attitudes toward direct predictive testing for the Huntington disease gene. JAMA 1993;270:2321-5.
34. Bagnall RD, Waseem N, Green PM, Giannelli F. Recurrent inversion breaking intron 1 of the factor VIII gene is a frequent cause of severe hemophilia A. Blood 2002;99:168-74.
35. Bakker E, Hofker MH, Goor N, Mandel JL, Wrogemann K, Davies KE, et al. Prenatal diagnosis and carrier detection of Duchenne muscular dystrophy with closely linked RFLPs. Lancet 1985;1:655-8.

36. Bakker E, Van Broeckhoven C, Bonten EJ, van de Vooren MJ, Veenema H, Van Hul W, et al. Germline mosaicism and Duchenne muscular dystrophy mutations. Nature 1987;329:554-6.
37. Ballering LA, Bon MA, Steffens-Nakken HM, Van den Bergh FA. Chemiluminescent detection of factor V Leiden in a routine laboratory. Ann Clin Biochem 1996;33:259-62.
38. Banks GB, Chamberlain JS. The value of mammalian models for Duchenne muscular dystrophy in developing therapeutic strategies. Curr Topics Dev Biol 2008;84:431-53.
39. Bao J, Sharp AH, Wagster MV, Becher M, Schilling G, Ross CA, et al. Expansion of polyglutamine repeat in huntingtin leads to abnormal protein interactions involving calmodulin. Proc Natl Acad Sci U S A 1996;93:5037-42.
40. Bardoni B, Mandel J-L. Advances in understanding of fragile X pathogenesis and FMRP function, and in identification of X linked mental retardation genes. Curr Opin Genet Dev 2002;12:284-93.
41. Barker D, Schafer M, White R. Restriction sites containing CpG show a higher frequency of polymorphisms in human DNA. Cell 1984;36:131-8.
42. Barrell BG, Bankier AT, Drouin J. A different genetic code in human mitochondria. Nature 1979;282:189-94.
43. Barton JC, McDonnell SM, Adams PC, Brissot P, Powell LW, Edwards CQ, et al. Management of hemochromatosis. Ann Intern Med 1998;129:932-9.
44. Bassell GJ, Warren ST. Fragile X syndrome: loss of local mRNA regulation alters synaptic development and function. Neuron 2008;60:201-14.
45. Batchelor CL, Winder SJ. Sparks, signals and shock absorbers: how dystrophin loss causes muscular dystrophy. Trends Cell Biol 2006;16:198-205.
46. Battle DJ, Kasim M, Yong J, Lotti F, Lau CK, Mouaikel J. The SMN complex: an assembly machine for RNPs. Cold Spring Harb Symp Quant Biol 2006;71:313-20.
47. Baughan TD, Dickson A, Osman EY, Lorson CL. Delivery of bifunctional RNAs that target an intronic repressor and increase SMN levels in an animal model of spinal muscular atrophy. Hum Mol Genet 2009;18:1600-11.
48. Baujat G, Legeai-Mallet L, Finidori G, Cormier-Daire V, Le Merrer M. Achondroplasia. Best Pract Res Clin Rheumatol 2008;22:3-18.
49. Bavikatty NR, Killeen AA, Akel N, Normolle D, Schmaier AH. Association of the prothrombin G20210A mutation with factor V Leiden in a Midwestern American population. Am J Clin Pathol 2000;114:272-5.
50. Baxendale S, MacDonald ME, Mott R, Francis F, Lin C, Kirby SF, et al. A cosmid contig and high resolution restriction map of the 2 megabase region containing the Huntington's disease gene. Nat Genet 1993;4:181-6.
51. Bayston TA, Lane DA. Antithrombin: molecular basis of deficiency. Thromb Haemost 1997;78:339-43.
52. Beggs AH, Hoffman EP, Snyder JR, Arahata K, Speecht L, Shapiro F, et al. Exploring the molecular basis for variability among patients with Becker muscular dystrophy: dystrophin gene and protein studies. Am J Hum Genet 1991;49:54-67.
53. Beggs AH, Koenig M, Boyce FM, Kunkel LM. Detection of 98% of DMD/BMD gene deletions by polymerase chain reaction. Hum Genet 1990;86:45-8.
54. Bell MV, Hirst MC, Nakahori Y, MacKinnin RN, Roche A, Flint TJ, et al. Physical mapping across the fragile X: hypermethylation and clinical expression of the fragile X syndrome. Cell 1991;64:861-6.
55. Bellus GA, Hefferon TW, Ortiz de Luna RI, Hecht JT, Horton WA, Machado M, et al. Achondroplasia is defined by recurrent G380R mutations of FGFR3. Am J Hum Genet 1995;56:368-73.
56. Benowitz S. European groups oppose Myriad's latest patent on *BRCA1*. J Natl Cancer Inst 2003;95:8-9.
57. Bertina RM, Koeleman BPC, Koster T, Rosendaal FR, Dirven RJ, de Ronde H, et al. Mutation in blood coagulation factor V associated with resistance to activated protein C. Nature 1994;369:64-7.
58. Beutler E. The significance of the 187G (H63D) mutation in hemochromatosis. Am J Hum Genet 1997;61:762-4.
59. Beutler E, Felitti VJ, Koziol JA, Ho NJ, Gelbart T. Penetrance of 845G-A (C282Y) *HFE* hereditary haemochromatosis mutation in the USA. Lancet 2002;359:211-8.
60. Beutler E, Gelbart T, West C, Lee P, Adams M, Blackstone R, et al. Mutation analysis in hereditary hemochromatosis. Blood Cells Mol Dis 1996;22:187-94.
61. Bicocchi MP, Migeon BR, Pasino M, Lanza T, Bottini F, Boeri E, et al. Familial nonrandom inactivation linked to the X inactivation centre in heterozygotes manifesting haemophilia A. Eur J Hum Genet 2005;13:635-40.
62. Biery NJ, Eldadah ZA, Moore CS, Stetten G, Spencer F, Dietz HC. Revised genomic organization of *FBN1* and significance for regulated gene expression. Genomics 1999;56:70-7.
63. Bigi N, Faure JM, Coubes C, Puechberty J, Lefort G, Sarda P, et al. Prader-Willi syndrome: is there a recognizable fetal phenotype? Prenat Diagn 2008;28:796-9.
64. Bird AP. DNA methylation and the frequency of CpG in animal DNA. Nucleic Acids Res 1980;8:1499-04.
65. Bisgaard ML, Fenger K, Bulow S, Niebuhr E, Mohr J. Familial adenomatous polyposis (FAP): frequency, penetrance, and mutation rate. Hum Mutat 1994;3:121-5.
66. Bittel DC, Kibiryeva N, Butler MG. Whole genome microarray analysis of gene expression in subjects with fragile X syndrome. Genet Med 2007;9:464-72.
67. Blake DJ, Weir A, Newey SE, Davies KE. Function and genetics of dystrophin and dystrophin-related proteins in muscle. Physiol Rev 2002;82:291-329.
68. Blasczyk R, Ritter M, Thiede C, Wehling J, Hintz G, Neubauer A, et al. Simple and rapid detection of factor V Leiden by allele specific PCR amplification. Thromb Haemost 1996;75:757-9.
69. Blau HM. Cell therapies for muscular dystrophy. N Engl J Med 2008;359:1403-5.
70. Bodmer WF, Bailey CJ, Bodmer J, Bussey HJ, Ellis A, Gorman P, et al. Localization of the gene for familial adenomatous polyposis on chromosome 5q. Nature 1987;328:614-6.
71. Boland CR, Thibodeau SN, Hamilton SR, Sidransky D, Eshleman JR, Burt RW, et al. A National Cancer Institute workshop on microsatellite instability for cancer detection and familial predisposition: development of international criteria for the determination of microsatellite instability in colorectal cancer. Cancer Res 1998;58:5248-57.
72. Borgel D, Grandrille S, Aiach M. Protein S deficiency. Thromb Haemost 1997;78:351-6.
73. Botkin JR, Croyle RT, Smith KR, Baty BJ, Lerman C, Goldgar DE, et al. A model protocol for evaluating the behavioral and psychosocial effects of *BRCA1* testing. J Natl Cancer Inst 1996;88:872-82.
74. Bourgeois JA, Coffey SM, Rivera SM, Hessl D, Gane LW, Tassone F, et al. A review of fragile X premutation disorders: expanding the psychiatric perspective. J Clin Psychiatry 2009;70:852-62.
75. Boyd Y, Buckle V, Holt S, Munro E, Hunter D, Craig I. Muscular dystrophy in girls with X: autosome translocations. J Med Genet 1986;23:484-90.
76. Braude PR, De Wert GM, Evers-Kiebooms E, Pettigrew RA, Geraedts JP. Non-disclosure preimplantation genetic diagnosis for Huntington's disease: practical and ethical dilemmas. Prenat Diagn 1998;18:1422-6.
77. Braun S. Muscular gene transfer using nonviral vectors. Curr Gene Ther 2008;8:391-405.
78. Breast Cancer Information Core. Available at: http://research.nhgri.nih.gov/bic/ (accessed July 2009).
79. Brensinger JD, Laken SJ, Luce MC, Powell SM, Vance GH, Ahnen DJ, et al. Variable phenotype of familial adenomatous polyposis in pedigrees with 3′ mutation in the *APC* gene. Gut 1998;43:548-52.
80. Bring P, Partovi N, Ford JA, Yoshida EM. Iron overload disorders: treatment options for patients refractory to or intolerant of phlebotomy. Pharmacotherapy 2008;28:331-42.

81. Brinkman RR, Mezei MM, Theilmann J, Almqvist E, Hayden MR. The likelihood of being affected with Huntington disease by a particular age, for a specific CAG size. Am J Hum Genet 1997;60:1202-10.
82. Brooke BS, Habashi JP, Judge DP, Patel N, Loeys B, Dietz HC III. Angiotensin II blockade and aortic-root dilation in Marfan's syndrome. N Engl J Med 2008;358:2787-95.
83. Brouwer JR, Willemsen R, Oostra BA. Microsatellite repeat instability and neurological disease. BioEssays 2009;31:71-83.
84. Brown WT, Houck GE, Ding X, Zhong N, Nolin S, Glicksman A, et al. Reverse mutations in the fragile X syndrome. Am J Med Genet 1996;64:287-92.
85. Browne SE. Mitochondria and Huntington's disease pathogenesis: insight from genetic and chemical models. Ann N Y Acad Sci 2008; 1147:358-82.
86. Brzustowicz LM, Lehner T, Castilla LH, Penchaszadeh GK, Wilhelmsen KC, Daniels R, et al. Genetic mapping of chronic childhood-onset spinal muscular atrophy to chromosome 5q11.2-13.3. Nature 1990;344:540-1.
87. Buiting K, Dittrich B, Gross S, Lich C, Farber C, Buchholz T, et al. Sporadic imprinting defects in Prader-Willi syndrome and Angelman syndrome: implications for imprint-switch models, genetic counseling and prenatal diagnosis. Am J Hum Genet 1998;63:170-80.
88. Buiting K, Saitoh S, Gross S, Dittrich B, Schwartz S, Nicholls RD, et al. Inherited microdeletions in the Angelman and Prader-Willi syndromes define an imprinting centre on human chromosome 15. Nat Genet 1995;9:395-400.
89. Bulaj ZJ, Ajioka RS, Phillips JD, LaSalle BA, Jorde LB, Griffen LM, et al. Disease-related conditions in relatives of patients with hemochromatosis. N Engl J Med 2000;343:1529-35.
90. Bunyan DJ, Eccles DM, Sillibourne J, Wilkins E, Thomas N, Shea-Simonds J, et al. Dosage analysis of cancer predisposition genes by multiplex ligation-dependent probe amplification. Br J Cancer 2004;91:1155-9.
91. Burger J, Buiting K, Dittrich B, Gross S, Lich C, Sperling K, et al. Different mechanisms and recurrence risks for imprinting defects in Angelman syndrome. Am J Hum Genet 1997;61:88-93.
92. Burke W, Aitken ML, Chen SH, Scott CR. Variable severity of pulmonary disease in adults with identical cystic fibrosis mutations. Chest 1992;102:506-9.
93. Burke W, Thomson E, Khoury MJ, McDonnell SM, Press N, Adams PC, et al. Hereditary hemochromatosis: gene discovery and its implications for population-based screening. JAMA 1998;280:172-8.
94. Burman RW, Anoe KS, Popovich BW. Fragile X full mutations are more similar in siblings than in unrelated patients: further evidence for a familial factor in CGG repeat dynamics. Genet Med 2000;2: 242-8.
95. Burnett BG, Crawford TO, Sumner CJ. Emerging treatment options for spinal muscular atrophy. Curr Treat Options Neurol 2009;11:90-101.
96. Bushby KMD, Gardner-Medwin D. The clinical, genetic and dystrophin characteristics of Becker muscular dystrophy. I. Natural history. J Neurol 1993;240:98-104.
97. Caspari R, Friedl W, Mandl M, Moselein G, Kadmon M, Knapp M, et al. Familial adenomatous polyposis: mutation at codon 1309 and early onset of colon cancer. Lancet 1994;343:629-32.
98. Cassidy SB, Driscoll DJ. Prader-Willi syndrome. Eur J Hum Genet 2009;17:3-13.
99. Castellani C, Cuppens H, Macek M, Cassiman JJ, Kerem E, Durie P, et al. Consensus on the use and interpretation of cystic fibrosis mutation analysis in clinical practice. J Cyst Fibros 2008;7:179-96.
100. Castilla LH, Couch FJ, Erdos MR, Hoskins KF, Calzone K, Garber JE, et al. Mutations in the BRCA1 gene in families with early-onset breast and ovarian cancer. Nat Genet 1994;8:387-91.
101. Cattaneo M, Chantarangkul V, Tailoi E, Santos JH, Tagliabue L. The G20210A mutation of the prothrombin gene in patients with previous first episodes of deep-vein thrombosis: prevalence and association with factor V G1691A, methylenetetrahydrofolate reductase C677T and plasma prothrombin levels. Thromb Res 1999;93:1-8.
102. Catteau A, Harris WH, Xu CF, Solomon E. Methylation of the BRCA1 promoter region in sporadic breast and ovarian cancer: correlation with disease characteristics. Oncogene 1999;18:1957-65.
103. Caudy AA, Myers M, Hannon GJ, Hammond SM. Fragile X-related protein and VIG associated with the RNA interference machinery. Genes Dev 2002;16:2491-6.
104. Cerletti M, Jurga S, Witczak C, Hirshman HF, Shadrach JL, Goodyear LJ, et al. Highly efficient, functional engraftment of skeletal muscle stem cells in dystrophic muscles. Cell 2008;134:37-47.
105. Chamberlain JS, Gibbs RA, Ranier JE, Caskey CT. Multiplex PCR for the diagnosis of Duchenne muscular dystrophy. In: Innis MA, Gelfand DH, Sninsky JJ, White TJ, eds. PCR protocols: a guide to methods and applications. San Francisco: Academic Press, 1990:272-81.
106. Chambost H, Gaboulud V, Coatmelec B, Rafowicz A, Schneider P, Calvez T, et al. What factors influence the age at diagnosis of hemophilia? Results of the French hemophilia cohort. J Pediatr 2002;141:548-52.
107. Chan WP, Lee CK, Kwong YL, Lam CK, Liang R. A novel mutation of Arg 306 of factor V gene in Hong Kong Chinese. Blood 1998;91:1135-9.
108. Chea PY. Recent advances in colorectal cancer genetics and diagnostics. Crit Rev Oncol Hematol 2009;69:45-55.
109. Chen ST, Chen RA, Kuo SJ, Chien YC. Mutational screening of breast cancer susceptibility gene 1 from early onset, bi-lateral, and familial breast cancer patients in Taiwan. Breast Cancer Res Treat 2003;77: 133-43.
110. Chenevix-Trench G, Milne RL, Antoniou AC, Couch FJ, Easton DF, Goldgar DE. An international initiative to identify genetic modifiers of cancer risk in *BRCA1* and *BRCA2* mutation carriers: the Consortium of Modifiers of *BRCA1* and *BRCA2* (CIMBA). Breast Cancer Res 2007;9:104-7.
111. Cheng SH, Gregory RJ, Marshall J, Paul S, Souza DW, White GA, et al. Defective intracellular transport and processing of CFTR is the molecular basis of most cystic fibrosis. Cell 1990;63:827-34.
112. Chillon M, Casals T, Mercier B, Bassas L, Lissens W, Silber S, et al. Mutations in the cystic fibrosis gene in patients with congenital absence of the vas deferens. N Engl J Med 1995;332:1475-80.
113. Chiurazzi P, Pomponi MG, Willemsen R, Oostra BA, Neri G. In vitro reactivation of the FMR1 gene involved in fragile X syndrome. Hum Mol Genet 1998;7:109-13.
114. Chong SS, Almqvist E, Telenius H, LaTray L, Nichol K, Bourdelat-Parks B, et al. Contribution of DNA sequence and CAG size to mutation frequencies of intermediate alleles for Huntington disease: evidence from single sperm analyses. Hum Mol Genet 1997;6:301-9.
115. Chu CS, Trapnell BC, Curristin S, Cutting GR, Crystal RG. Genetic basis of variable exon 9 skipping in cystic fibrosis transmembrane conductance regulator mRNA. Nat Genet 1993;3:151-6.
116. Chung AW, Yang HH, Radomski MW, van Breeman C. Long-term doxycycline is more effective than atenolol to prevent thoracic aortic aneurysm in Marfan syndrome through the inhibition of matrix metalloproteinase-2 and -9. Circ Res 2008;102:e73-85.
117. Clay Montier LL, Deng JJ, Bai Y. Number matters: control of mammalian mitochondrial DNA copy number. J Genet Genomics 2009;36:125-31.
118. Cleary SP, Cotterchio M, Jenkins MA, Kim H, Bristow R, Green R, et al. Germline MutY human homologue mutations and colorectal cancer: a multisite case-control study. Gastroenterology 2009;136:1251-60.
119. Coffee B, Zhang F, Warren ST, Reines D. Acetylated histones are associated with FMR1 in normal but not fragile X-syndrome cells. Nat Genet 1999;22:98-101.
120. Cogswell ME, Burke W, McDonnell SM, Franks AL. Screening for hemochromatosis: a public health perspective. Am J Prev Med 1999; 16:134-40.
121. Collaco JM, Cutting GR. Update on gene modifiers in cystic fibrosis. Curr Opin Pulm Med 2008;14:559-66.
122. Collaco JM, Vanscoy L, Bremer L, McDougal K, Blackman SM, Bowers A, et al. Interactions between secondhand smoke and genes that affect cystic fibrosis lung disease. JAMA 2008;299:417-24.

123. College of American Pathologists. Molecular pathology checklist. Available at: http://www.cap.org (accessed July 2009).
124. Colvin JS, Bohne BA, Harding GW, McEwen DG, Ornitz DM. Skeletal overgrowth and deafness in mice lacking fibroblast growth factor receptor 3. Nat Genet 1996;12:390-7.
125. Comi GP, Prelle A, Bresolin N, Moggio M, Bardoni A, Gallanti A, et al. Clinical variability in Becker muscular dystrophy: genetic, biochemical and immunhistochemical correlates. Brain 1994;117:1-14.
126. Conneally PM, Haines JL, Tanzi RE, Wexler NS, Penchaszadeh GK, Harper PS, et al. Huntington's disease: no evidence for heterogeneity. Genomics 1989;5:304-8.
127. Constantine CC, Gurrin LC, McLaren CE, Bahlo M, Anderson GJ, Vulpe CD, et al. SNP selection for genes of iron metabolism in a study of genetic modifiers of hemochromatosis. BMC Med Genet 2008;9:18.
128. Cooper K, Bryant J, Picot J, Clegg A, Roderick PR, Rosenberg WM, et al. A decision analysis model for diagnostic strategies using DNA testing for hereditary haemochromatosis in at risk populations. QJM 2008;101:631-41.
129. Couch FJ, Rasmussen LJ, Hofstra R, Monteiro ANA, Greenblatt MS, de Wind N. Assessment of functional effects of unclassified genetic variants. Hum Mutat 2008;29:1314-26.
130. Crabtree MD, Tomlinson IPM, Hodgson SV, Neale K, Phillips RKS, Houlston RS. Explaining variation in familial adenomatous polyposis: relationship between genotype and phenotype and evidence for modifier genes. Gut 2002;51:420-3.
131. Crow JF. The origins, patterns and implications of human spontaneous mutation. Nat Rev Genet 2000;1:40-7.
132. Cystic Fibrosis Foundation Website. Available at: http://www.cff.org (accessed July 2009).
133. Cystic Fibrosis Mutation database. Available at: www.genet.sickkids.on.ca/cftr/ (accessed July 2009).
134. Dahlbäck B. Inherited thrombophilia: resistance to activated protein C as a pathogenic factor of venous thromboembolism. Blood 1995;85: 607-14.
135. Dahlbäck B. Advances in understanding pathogenic mechanisms of thrombophilic disorders. Blood 2008;112:19-27.
136. Dahlbäck B, Carlsson M, Svensson PJ. Familial thrombophilia due to a previously unrecognized mechanism by poor anticoagulant response to activated protein C: prediction of a cofactor to activated protein C. Proc Natl Acad Sci U S A 1993;90:1004-8.
137. Dakouane Giudicelli M, Serazin V, Le Sciellour CR, Albert M, Selva J, Giudicelli Y. Increased achondroplasia mutation frequency with advanced age and evidence for G1138A mosaicism in human testis biopsies. Fertil Steril 2008;89:1651-6.
138. Davies KE, Nowak KJ. Molecular mechanisms of muscular dystrophies: old and new players. Nat Rev Mol Cell Biol 2006;7: 762-72.
139. Davies KE, Pearson PL, Harper PS, Murray JM, O'Brien T, Sarfarazi M, et al. Linkage analysis of two cloned DNA sequences flanking the Duchenne muscular dystrophy locus on the short arm of the human X chromosome. Nucleic Acids Res 1983;11:2303-12.
140. Dayangaç-Erden D, Bora G, Ayhan P, Kocaefe Ç, Dalkara S, Yelkçi K, et al. Histone deacetylase inhibition activity and molecular docking of (E)-resveratrol: its therapeutic potential in spinal muscular atrophy. Chem Biol Drug Des 2009;73:355-64.
141. Dean JCS. Marfan syndrome: clinical diagnosis and management. Eur J Hum Genet 2007;15:724-33.
142. De Boeck K, Wilschanksi M, Castellani C, Taylor C, Cuppens H, Dodge J, et al. Cystic fibrosis: terminology and diagnostic algorithms. Thorax 2006;61:627-35.
143. de Frutos CA, Vega S, Manzanares M, Flores JM, Huertas H, Martínez-Frías ML, et al. Snail1 is a transcriptional effector of FGFR3 signaling during chondrogenesis and achondroplasias. Dev Cell 2007;13:872-83.
144. Delaney SJ, Rich DP, Thomson SA, Hargrave MR, Lovelock PK, Welsh MJ, et al. Cystic fibrosis transmembrane conductance regulator splice variants are not conserved and fail to produce chloride channels. Nat Genet 1993;4:426-31.
145. Deng C, Wynshaw-Boris A, Zhou F, Kuo A, Leder P. Fibroblast growth factor receptor 3 is a negative regulator of bone growth. Cell 1996;84:911-21.
146. De Paepe A, Devereux RB, Dietz HC, Hennekam RC, Pyeritz RE. Revised diagnostic criteria for the Marfan syndrome. Am J Med Genet 1996;62:417-26.
147. Dequeker E, Stuhrmann M, Morris MA, Casals T, Castellani C, Claustres M, et al. Best practice guidelines for molecular genetic diagnosis of cystic fibrosis and CFTR-related disorders: updated European recommendations. Eur J Hum Genet 2009;17:51-65.
148. De Rooij KE, Dorsman JC, Smoor MA, Den Dunnen JT, van Ommen GJ. Subcellular localization of the Huntington's disease gene product in cell lines by immunofluorescence and biochemical subcellular fractionation. Hum Mol Genet 1996;5:1093-9.
149. De Stefano V, Martinelli I, Mannucci PM, Paciaroni K, Chiusolo P, Casorelli I, et al. The risk of recurrent deep venous thrombosis among heterozygous carriers of both factor V Leiden and the G20210A prothrombin mutation. N Engl J Med 1999;341:801-6.
150. De Stefano V, Rossi E, Paciaroni K, Leone G. Screening for inherited thrombophilia: indications and therapeutic implications. Haematologica 2002;87:1095-108.
151. de Vries BBA, Halley DJJ, Oostra BA, Niermeijer MF. The fragile X syndrome. J Med Genet 1998;35:579-89.
152. Dictenberg JB, Swanger SA, Antar LN, Singer RH, Bassell GJ. A direct role for FMRP in activity-dependent dendritic mRNA transport links filopodial-spine morphogenesis to fragile X syndrome. Dev Cell 2008; 14:926-39.
153. Di Donato S. Multisystem manifestations of mitochondrial disorders. J Neurol 2009;256:693-10.
154. Dietz HC, Cutting GR, Pyeritz RE, Maslen CL, Sakai LY, Corson GM, et al. Marfan syndrome caused by a recurrent de novo missense mutation in the fibrillin gene. Nature 1991;352:337-9.
155. Dietz HC, Loeys B, Carta L, Ramirez F. Recent progress towards a molecular understanding of Marfan syndrome. Am J Med Genet C Semin Med Genet 2005;139C:4-9.
156. Difiglia M, Sapp E, Chase KO, Davies SW, Bates GP, Vonsattel JP, et al. Aggregation of huntingtin in neuronal intranuclear inclusions and dystrophic neuritis in brain. Science 1997;277:1990-3.
157. DiMauro S, De Vivo DC. Genetic heterogeneity in Leigh syndrome. Ann Neurol 1996;40:5-7.
158. Dindot SV, Antalffy BA, Bhattacharjee MB, Beaudet AL. The Angelman syndrome ubiquitin ligase localizes to the synapse and nucleus, and maternal deficiency results in abnormal dendritic spine morphology. Hum Mol Genet 2008;17:111-8.
159. Dobbie Z, Spycher M, Mary JL, Haner M, Guldenschuh I, Hurliman R, et al. Correlation between the development of extracolonic manifestations in FAP patients and mutations beyond codon 1403 of the APC gene. J Med Genet 1996;33:274-80.
160. Dodge JA, Turck D. Cystic fibrosis: nutritional consequences and management. Best Pract Res Clin Gastroenterol 2006;20:531-46.
161. Domchek SM, Friebel TM, Neuhausen SL, Wagner T, Evans G, Isaacs C, et al. Mortality after bilateral salpingo-oophorectomy in *BRCA1* and *BRCA2* mutations carriers: a prospective cohort study. Lancet Oncol 2006;7:223-9.
162. Domingo-Ribas C, Bosque-Garcia M. Nasal potential difference test to diagnose cystic fibrosis. Arch Bronconeumol 2006;42: 33-8.
163. Douma KF, Aaronson NK, Vasen HFA, Bleiker EMA. Psychosocial issues in genetic testing for familial adenomatous polyposis: a review of the literature. Psychooncology 2008;17:737-45.
164. Dubreuil Lastrucci RM, Dawson DA, Bowden JH, Munster M. Development of a simple multiplex polymerase chain reaction for the simultaneous detection of factor V Leiden and prothrombin 20210A mutations. Mol Diagn 1999;4:247-50.
165. Dudding T, Heron J, Thakkinstian A, Nurk E, Golding J, Pembrey M, et al. Factor V Leiden is associated with pre-eclampsia but not with fetal growth restriction: a genetic association study and meta-analysis. J Thromb Haemost 2008;6:1869-75.

166. Duncan B, Miller J. Mutagenic deamination of cytosine residues in DNA. Nature 1980;287:560-1.
167. Durbeej M, Campbell KP. Muscular dystrophies involving the dystrophin-glycoprotein complex: an overview of current mouse models. Curr Opin Genet Dev 2002;12:349-61.
168. Durno C, Corey M, Zielenski J, Tullis E, Tsui LC, Durie P. Genotype and phenotype correlations in patients with cystic fibrosis and pancreatitis. Gastroenterology 2002;123:1857-64.
169. Duyao M, Ambrose C, Myers R, Novelletto A, Persichetti F, Frontali M, et al. Trinucleotide repeat length instability and age of onset in Huntington's disease. Nat Genet 1993;4:387-92.
170. Dykens EM, Roof E. Behavior in Prader-Willi syndrome: relationship to genetic subtypes and age. J Child Psychol Psychiatry 2008;49:1001-8.
171. Easton DF, Pooley KA, Dunning AM, Pharoah PDP, Thompson D, Ballinger DG, et al. Genome-wide association study identifies novel breast cancer susceptibility loci. Nature 2007;447:1087-93.
172. Ehmsen J, Poon E, Davies K. The dystrophin-associated protein complex. J Cell Sci 2002;115:2801-3.
173. Eichler EE, Hammond HA, Macpherson JN, Ward PA, Nelson DL. Population survey of the human FMR1 CGG repeat substructure suggests biased polarity for the loss of AGG interruptions. Hum Mol Genet 1995;4:2199-208.
174. Eichler EE, Holden JJA, Popovich BW, Reiss AL, Snow K, Thibodeau SN, et al. Length of uninterrupted CGG repeats determines instability in the FMR1 gene. Nat Genet 1994;8:88-94.
175. Eichler EE, Macpherson JN, Murray A, Jacobs PA, Chakravarti A, Nelson DL. Haplotype and interspersion analysis of the FMR1 CGG repeat identifies two different mutational pathways for the origin of the fragile X syndrome. Hum Mol Genet 1996;5:319-30.
176. Eichler EE, Richards S, Gibbs RJ, Nelson DL. Fine structure of the human FMR1 gene. Hum Mol Genet 1993;2:1147-53.
177. Emmerich J, Rosendaal FR, Cattaneo M, Margaglione M, DeStefano V, Cumming T, et al. Combined effect of Factor V Leiden and prothrombin 20210A on the risk of venous thromboembolism. Thromb Haemost 2001;86:809-16.
178. Engelender S, Sharp AH, Colomer V, Tokito MK, Lanahan A, Worley P, et al. Huntingtin-associated protein 1 (HAP1) interacts with the $p150^{Glued}$ subunit of dynactin. Hum Mol Genet 1997;6:2205-12.
179. Ennis S, Murray A, Brightwell G, Morton NE, Jacobs PA. Closely linked cis-acting modifier of expansion of the CGG repeat in high risk FMR1 haplotypes. Hum Mutat 2007;28:1216-24.
180. Erdem H, Pehlivan S, Topaloglu H, Ozguc M. Deletion analysis in Turkish patients with spinal muscular atrophy. Brain Dev 1999;21:86-9.
181. Ervasti JM. Dystrophin, its interactions with other proteins, and implications for muscular dystrophy. Biochim Biophys Acta 2007;1772:108-17.
182. Ervasti JM, Sonnemann KJ. Biology of the striated muscle dystrophin-glycoprotein complex. Int Rev Cytol 2008;265:191-225.
183. Evaluation of Genomic Applications in Practice and Prevention (EGAPP) Working Group. Recommendations from the EGAPP Working Group: genetic testing strategies in newly diagnosed individuals with colorectal cancer aimed at reducing morbidity and mortality from Lynch syndrome in relatives. Genet Med 2009;11:35-41.
184. Evans NP, Misyak SA, Robertson JL, Bassaganya-Riera J, Grange RW. Dysregulated intracellular signaling and inflammatory gene expression during initial disease onset in Duchenne muscular dystrophy. Am J Phys Med Rehabil 2009;88:502-22.
185. Facchinetti F, Marozio L, Frusca T, Grandone E, Venturini P, Tiscia GL, et al. Maternal thrombophilia and the risk of recurrence of preeclampsia. Am J Obstet Gynecol 2009;200:46e1-5.
186. Faivre L, Collod-Béroud G, Callewaert B, Child A, Binquet C, Gautier E, et al. Clinical and mutation-type analysis from an international series of 198 probands with a pathogenic FBN1 exons 24-32 mutation. Eur J Hum Genet 2009;17:491-501.
187. Faivre L, Collod-Béroud G, Loeys BL, Child A, Binquet C, Gautier E, et al. Effect of mutation type and location on clinical outcome in 1,013 probands with Marfan syndrome or related phenotypes and FBN1 mutations: an international study. Am J Hum Genet 2007;81:454-66.
188. Faivre L, Masurel-Paulet A, Collod-Béroud G, Callewaert BL, Child AH, Stheneur C, et al. Clinical and molecular study of 320 children with Marfan syndrome and related type I fibrillinopathies in a series of 1009 probands with pathogenic FBN1 mutations. Pediatrics 2009;123:391-8.
189. Fan L, Simard LR. Survival motor neuron (SMN) protein: role in neurite outgrowth and neuromuscular maturation during neuronal differentiation and development. Hum Mol Genet 2002;11:1605-14.
190. Fang P, Lev-Lehman E, Tsai TF, Matsuura T, Benton CS, Sutcliffe JS, et al. The spectrum of mutations in *UBE3A* causing Angelman syndrome. Hum Mol Genet 1999;8:129-135.
191. Farrell PM, Fost N. Prenatal screening for cystic fibrosis: where are we now? J Pediatr 2002;141:758-63.
192. Fasching PA, Bani MR, Nestle-Kramling C, Goecke TO, Niederacher D, Beckmann MW, et al. Evaluation of mathematical models for breast cancer risk assessment in routine clinical use. Eur J Cancer Prev 2007;15:216-24.
193. Fay PJ. Factor VIII structure and function. Thromb Haemost 1993;70:63-7.
194. Fearnhead NS, Britton MP, Bodmer WF. The ABC of APC. Hum Mol Genet 2001;10:721-33.
195. Fearon ER, Vogelstein B. A genetic model for colorectal tumorigenesis. Cell 1990;61:759-67.
196. Feder JN, Gnirke A, Thomas W, Tsuchihashi Z, Ruddy DA, Basava A, et al. A novel MHC class I-like gene is mutated in patients with hereditary haemochromatosis. Nat Genet 1996;13:399-408.
197. Feder JN, Penny DM, Irrinki A, Lee VK, Lebron JA, Watson N, et al. The hemochromatosis gene product complexes with the transferrin receptor and lowers its affinity for ligand binding. Proc Natl Acad Sci U S A 1998;95:1472-7.
198. Feder JN, Tsuchihashi Z, Irrinki A, Lee VK, Mapa FA, Morikang E, et al. The hemochromatosis founder mutation in HLA-H disrupts beta2-microglobulin interaction and cell surface expression. J Biol Chem 1997;272:14025-8.
199. Feissner RF, Skalska J, Gaum WE, Sheu SS. Crosstalk signaling between mitochondrial Ca^{2+} and ROS. Front Biosci 2009;14:1197-218.
200. Feng J, Yan J, Buzin CH, Sommer SS, Towbin JA. Comprehensive mutation scanning of the dystrophin gene in patients with nonsyndromic X-linked dilated cardiomyopathy. J Am Coll Cardiol 2002;40:1120-4.
201. Feng W, Gubitz AK, Wan L, Battle DJ, Dostie J, Golembe TJ, et al. Gemins modulate the expression and activity of the SMN complex. Hum Mol Genet 2005;14:1605-11.
202. Feng Y, Absher D, Eberhart DE, Brown V, Malter HE, Warren ST. FMRP associates with polyribosomes as an mRNP and the I304N mutation of severe fragile X syndrome abolishes this association. Mol Cell 1997;1:109-18.
203. Ferlini A, Sewry C, Melis MA, Matteddu A, Muntoni F. X-linked dilated cardiomyopathy and the dystrophin gene. Neuromuscul Disord 1999;9:339-46.
204. Finsterer J. Leigh and Leigh-like syndrome in children and adults. Pediatr Neurol 2008;39:223-35.
205. Finsterer J, Stollberger C. The heart in human dystrophinopathies. Cardiology 2003;99;1-19.
206. Fischer K, Van der bom JG, Mauser-Bunschoten EP, Roosendaal G, Prejs R, Grobbee DE, et al. Changes in treatment strategies for severe haemophilia over the last 3 decades: effects on clotting factor consumption and arthropathy. Haemophilia 2001;7:446-52.
207. Folstein SE. The psychopathology of Huntington's disease. Res Publ Assoc Res Nerv Ment Dis 1991;69:181-91.
208. Francke U, Ochs HD, de Martinville B, Giacalone J, Lindgren V, Disteche C, et al. Minor Xp21 chromosome deletion in a male associated with expression of Duchenne muscular dystrophy, chronic granulomatous disease, retinitis pigmentosa and McLeod syndrome. Am J Hum Genet 1985;37:250-67.

209. Francomano CA, Ortiz de Luna RI, Hefferon TW, Bellus GA, Turner CE, Taylor E, et al. Localization of the achondroplasia gene to the distal 2.5 Mb of human chromosome 4p. Hum Mol Genet 1994;3:787-92.
210. Friedl W, Caspari R, Sengteller M, Uhlhaas S, Lamberti C, Jungck M, et al. Can APC mutation analysis contribute to therapeutic decisions in familial adenomatous polyposis? Experience from 680 FAP families. Gut 2001;48:515-21.
211. Friedl W, Meuschel S, Caspari R, Lamberti C, Krieger S, Sengteller M, et al. Attenuated familial adenomatous polyposis due to a mutation in the 3′ part of the *APC* gene: a clue for understanding the function of the APC protein. Hum Genet 1996;97:579-84.
212. Friedman LS, Ostermeyer EA, Szabo CI, Dowd P, Lynch ED, Rowell SE, et al. Confirmation of BRCA1 by analysis of germline mutations linked to breast and ovarian cancer in ten families. Nat Genet 1994;8: 399-404.
213. Furtado S, Suchowersky O, Rewcastle B, Graham L, Klimek M, Garber A. Relationship between trinucleotide repeats and neuropathological changes in Huntington's disease. Ann Neurol 1996;39:132-6.
214. Furthmayer H, Francke U. Ascending aortic aneurysm with or without features of Marfan syndrome and other fibrillinopathies: new insights. Semin Thorac Cardiovasc Surg 1997;9:191-5.
215. Gaudet MM, Milne RL, Cox A, Camp NJ, Goode EL, Humphreys MK, et al. Five polymorphisms and breast cancer risk: results from the Breast Cancer Association Consortium. Cancer Epidemiol Biomarkers Prev 2009;18:1610-6.
216. Gayan J, Brocklebank D, Andresen JM, Alkorta-Aranburu G, The US Venezuela Collaborative Research Group, Cader MZ, et al. Genomewide linkage scan reveals novel loci modifying age of onset of Huntington's disease in the Venezuelan HD kindreds. Genet Epidemiol 2008;32:445-53.
217. Gehring NH, Frede U, Neu-Yilik G, Hundsdoerfer P, Vetter B, Hentze MW, et al. Increased efficiency of mRNA 3′ end formation: a new genetic mechanism contributing to hereditary thrombophilia. Nat Genet 2001;28:389-92.
218. GeneTests: Medical Genetics Information Resource (database online). A listing of research and clinical labs for disease specific referrals. Available at: www.genetests.org (accessed July 2009).
219. Gerhardus A, Schleberger H, Schlegelberger B, Gadzicki D. Diagnostic accuracy of methods for the detection of *BRCA1* and *BRCA2* mutations: a systematic review. Eur J Hum Genet 2007;15:619-27.
220. Giardiello FM, Brensinger JD, Peterson G. American Gastroenterological Association technical review on hereditary colorectal cancer and genetic testing. Gastroenterology 2001;121: 198-213.
221. Giardiello FM, Krush AJ, Peterson GM, Booker SV, Kerr M, Tong LL, et al. Phenotypic variability of familial adenomatous polyposis in 11 unrelated families with identical *APC* gene mutation. Gastroenterology 1994;106:1542-7.
222. Giardina E, Peconi C, Cascella R, Sinibaldi C, Nardone AM, Novelli G. A multiplex assay for the detection of uniparental disomy for human chromosome 15. Electrophoresis 2008;29:4775-9.
223. Gibson LE, Cooke RE. A test for the concentration of electrolytes in sweat in cystic fibrosis of the pancreas utilizing pilocarpine by iontophoresis. Pediatrics 1959;23:545-9.
224. Gilbert F. Cystic fibrosis carrier screening: steps in the development of a mutation panel. Genet Testing 2001;5:223-7.
225. Gilliam TC, Tanzi RE, Haines JL, Bonner TI, Faryniarz AG, Hobbs WJ, et al. Localization of the Huntington's disease gene to a small segment of chromosome 4 flanked by D4S10 and the telomere. Cell 1987;50:565-71.
226. Gimelli G, Pujana MA, Patricelli MG, Russo S, Giardino D, Larizza L, et al. Genomic inversions of human chromosome 15q11-q13 in mothers of Angelman syndrome patients with class II (BP2/3) deletions. Hum Mol Genet 2003;12:849-58.
227. Gite S, Lim M, Carlson R, Olejnik J, Zehnbauer B, Rothschild K. A high throughput nonisotopic protein truncation test. Nat Biotech 2003;21:194-7.
228. Gitschier J, Wood WI, Goralka JM, Wion KL, Chen EY, Eaton DH, et al. Characterization of the human factor VIII gene. Nature 1984; 312:326-30.
229. Glaser RL, Jabs EW. Dear old dad. Sci Aging Knowledge Environ 2004;3:re1.
230. Goecke T, Schulmann K, Engel C, Holinski-Feder E, Pagenstecher C, Schackert HK, et al. Genotype-phenotype comparison of German MLH1 and MSH2 mutation carriers clinically affected with Lynch syndrome: a report by the German HNPCC Consortium. J Clin Oncol 2006;24:4285-92.
231. Gogvadze V, Orrenius S, Zhivotovsky B. Mitochondria as targets for chemotherapy. Apoptosis 2009;14:624-40.
232. Goizet C, Lesca G, Durr A. Presymptomatic testing in Huntington's disease and autosomal dominant cerebellar ataxias. Neurology 2002;59:1330-6.
233. Goldberg YP, Kremer B, Andrew SE, Theilmann J, Graham RK, Squitieri F, et al. Molecular analysis of new mutations for Huntington's disease: intermediate alleles and sex of origin effects. Nat Genet 1993;5:174-9.
234. Goldberg YP, McMurray CT, Zeisler CT, Almqvist E, Sillence D, Richards F, et al. Increased instability of intermediate alleles in families with sporadic Huntington disease compared to similar sized intermediate alleles in the general population. Hum Mol Genet 1995;4:1911-8.
235. Goldstone AP, Holland AJ, Hauffa BP, Hokken-Koelega AC, Tauber M. Recommendations for the diagnosis and management of Prader-Willi syndrome. J Clin Endocrinol Metab 2008;93:4183-97.
236. Gologan A, Krasinskas A, Hunt Jennifer, Thull DL, Farkas L, Sepulveda AR. Performance of the revised Bethesda guidelines for identification of colorectal carcinomas with a high level of microsatellite instability. Arch Pathol Lab Med 2005;129:1390-7.
237. Gomes-Pereira M, Fortune MT, Ingram L, McAbney JP, Monckton DG. Pms2 is a genetic enhancer of trinucleotide CAG.CTG repeat somatic mosaicism: implications for the mechanism of triplet repeat expansion. Hum Mol Genet 2004;13:1815-25.
238. Gómez-Curet I, Robinson KG, Funanage VL, Crawford TO, Scavina M, Wang W. Robust quantification of the SMN gene copy number by real-time TaqMan PCR. Neurogenetics 2007;8:271-8.
239. Goodeve A. Molecular genetic testing of hemophilia A. Semin Thromb Hemost 2008;34:491-501.
240. Gooding HC, Boehm K, Thompson RE, Hadley D, Francomano CA, Biesecker BB. Issues surrounding prenatal genetic testing for achondroplasia. Prenat Diagn 2002;22:933-40.
241. Gordon N. The neurological complications of achondroplasia. Brain Dev 2000;22:3-7.
242. Goriely A, McVean GA, Röjmyr M, Ingemarsson B, Wilkie AO. Evidence for selective advantage of pathogenic FGFR2 mutations in the male germ line. Science 2003;301:643-6.
243. Goumans MJ, Liu Z, ten Dijke P. TGF-β signaling in vascular biology and dysfunction. Cell Res 2009;19:116-27.
244. Goyenvalle A, Babbs A, van Ommen GJ, Garcia L, Davies KE. Enhanced exon-skipping induced by U7 snRNA carrying a splicing silencer sequence: promising tool for DMD therapy. Mol Ther 2009;17:1234-40.
245. Graw J, Brackmann HH, Oldenburg J, Schneppenheim R, Spannagl M, Schwaab R. Haemophilia A: from mutation analysis to new therapies. Nat Rev Genet 2005;6:488-501.
246. Green PM, Bagnall RD, Waseem NH, Giannelli F. Haemophilia A mutations in the UK: results of screening one-third of the population. Br J Haematol 2008;143:115-28.
247. Greenblatt MS, Brody LC, Foulkes WD, Genuardi M, Hofstra RMW, Olivier M, et al. Locus-specific databases and recommendations to strengthen their contribution to the classification of variants in cancer susceptibility genes. Hum Mutat 2008;29:1273-81.
248. Greengard JS, Eichinger S, Griffin JH, Bauer KA. Variability of thrombosis among homozygous siblings with resistance to activated protein C due to an Arg-Gln mutation in the gene for factor V. N Engl J Med 1994;331:1559-62.

249. Greenstein RM, Reardon MP, Chan TS. An X-autosome translocation in a girl with Duchenne muscular dystrophy: evidence for DMD gene localization. Pediatr Res 1977;11:475A.
250. Griesenbach U, Alton EW. Gene transfer to the lung: lessons learned from more than 2 decades of CF gene therapy. Adv Drug Deliv Rev 2009;61:128-39.
251. Groden J, Thliveris A, Samowitz W, Carlson M, Gelbert L, Albertsen H, et al. Identification and characterization of the familial adenomatous polyposis coli gene. Cell 1991;66:589-600.
252. Grody WW, Griffin JH, Taylor AK, Korf BR, Heit JA. American College of Medical Genetics consensus statement on factor V Leiden mutation testing. Genet Med 2001;3:139-48.
253. Groen EJ, Roos A, Muntinghe FL, Enting RH, de Vries J, Kleibeuker JH, et al. Extraintestinal manifestations of familial adenomatous polyposis. Ann Surg Oncol 2008;15:2439-50.
254. Groman JD, Hefferon TW, Casals T, Bassas L, Estivill X, Des Georges M, et al. Variation in a repeat sequence determines whether a common variant of the cystic fibrosis transmembrane conductance regulator gene is pathogenic or benign. Am J Hum Genet 2004;74:176-9.
255. Groman JD, Meyer ME, Wilmott RW, Zeitlin PL, Cutting GR. Variant cystic fibrosis phenotypes in the absence of CFTR mutations. N Engl J Med 2002;347:401-7.
256. Grosse SD, Schechter MS, Kulkarni R, Lloyd-Puryear, MA, Strickland B, Trevathan E. Models of comprehensive multidisciplinary care for individuals in the United States with genetic disorders. Pediatrics 2009;123:407-12.
257. Gryfe R, Kim H, Hsieh ETK, Aronson MD, Holowaty EJ, Bull SB, et al. Tumor microsatellite instability and clinical outcome in young patients with colorectal cancer. N Engl J Med 2000;342:69-77.
258. Gudmundsdottir K, Ashworth A. The roles of BRCA1 and BRCA2 and associated proteins in the maintenance of genomic stability. Oncogene 2006;25:5864-74.
259. Guggino WB, Stanton BA. New insights into cystic fibrosis: molecular switches that regulate CFTR. Nat Rev Mol Cell Biol 2006;7:426-36.
260. Guo DC, Gupta P, Tran-Fadulu V, Guuidry TV, Leduc MS, Schaefer FV, et al. An FBN1 pseudoexon mutation in a patient with Marfan syndrome: confirmation of cryptic mutations leading to disease. J Hum Genet 2008;53:1007-11.
261. Gusella JA, Wexler NS, Conneally PM, Naylor S, Anderson MA, Tanzi RE, et al. A polymorphic DNA marker genetically linked to Huntington's disease. Nature 1983;306:234-8.
262. Gutekunst CA, Levey A, Heilman C, Waley W, Yi H, Nash N, et al. Identification and localization of huntingtin in brain and human lymphoblastoid cell lines with anti-fusion protein antibodies. Proc Natl Acad Sci U S A 1995;92:8710-4.
263. Guzmán-Aránguez A, Crooke A, Yayon A, Pintor J. Effect of PPADS on achondroplastic chondrocytes: inhibition of FGF receptor type 3 over-activity. Eur J Pharmacol 2008;584:72-7.
264. Habashi JP, Judge DP, Holm TM, Cohn RD, Loeys BL, Cooper TK, et al. Losartan, an AT1 antagonist, prevents aortic aneurysm in a mouse model of Marfan syndrome. Science 2006;312:117-21.
265. Hagerman RJ, Berry-Kravis E, Kaufmann WE, Ono MY, Tartaglia N, Lachiewicz A, et al. Advances in the treatment of fragile X syndrome. Pediatrics 2009;123:378-90.
266. Hagerman PJ, Hagerman RJ. The fragile-X premutation: a maturing perspective. Am J Hum Genet 2004;74:805-16.
267. Hagerman RJ, Leavitt BR, Farzin F, Jacquemont S, Greco CM, Brunberg JA, et al. Fragile-X-associated tremor/ataxia syndrome (FXTAS) in females with the FMR1 premutation. Am J Hum Genet 2004;74:1051-6.
268. Hagerman RJ, Leehey M, Heinrichs W, Tassone F, Wilson R, Wills J, et al. Intention tremor, parkinsonism, and generalized brain atrophy in male carriers of fragile X. Neurology 2001;57:127-30.
269. Hall JM, Lee MK, Newman B, Morrow JE, Anderson LA, Huey B, et al. Linkage of early-onset familial breast cancer to 17q21. Science 1990;250:1684-9.
270. Hamosh A, Rosenstein BJ, Cutting GR. CFTR nonsense mutations G542X and W1282X associated with severe reduction of CFTR mRNA in nasal epithelial cells. Hum Mol Genet 1992;1:542-4.
271. Hampel H, Frankel WL, Martin E, Arnold M, Khanduja K, Kuebler P, et al. Feasibility of screening for Lynch syndrome among patients with colorectal cancer. J Clin Oncol 2008;26:5783-8.
272. Han J, Haiman C, Niu T, Guo Q, Cox DG, Willett WC, et al. Genetic variation in DNA repair pathway genes and premenopausal breast cancer risk. Breast Cancer Res Treat 2009;115:613-22.
273. Happich D, Schwaab R, Hanfland P, Hoernschemeyer D. Allelic discrimination of factor V Leiden using a 5′ nuclease assay. Thromb Haemost 1999;82:1294-6.
274. Harada D, Yamanaka Y, Ueda K, Nishimura R, Morishima T, Seino Y, et al. Sustained phosphorylation of mutated FGFR3 is a crucial feature of genetic dwarfism and induces apoptosis in the ATDC5 chondrogenic cell line via PLCγ-activated STAT1. Bone 2007;41:273-81.
275. Hardy J, Singleton A. Genome wide association studies and human disease. N Engl J Med 2009;360:1759-68.
276. Harper PS, Newcombe RG. Age at onset and life table risks in genetic counseling for Huntington's disease. J Med Genet 1992;29:239-42.
277. Harrison CJ, Jack EM, Allen TD, Harris R. The fragile X: a scanning electron microscopic study. J Med Genet 1983;20:280-5.
278. Hauke J, Riessland M, Lunke S, Eyüpoglu I, Blümcke I, El-Osta A, et al. Survival motor neuron gene 2 silencing by DNA methylation correlates with spinal muscular atrophy disease severity and can be bypassed by histone deacetylase inhibition. Hum Mol Genet 2009;18:304-17.
279. Hayden MR. Huntington's chorea. London, Berlin, Heidelberg: Springer, 1981.
280. Hayden MR, Bloch M, Fahy M. Predictive testing for Huntington's disease using linked DNA markers. N Engl J Med 1988;319:583.
281. Heeb MJ, Kojima Y, Greengard JS, Griffin JH. Activated protein C resistance: molecular mechanisms based on studies using purified Gln506—factor V. Blood 1995;85:3405-11.
282. Heim RA, Sugarman EA, Allitto BA. Improved detection of cystic fibrosis mutations in the heterogeneous U.S. population using an expanded, pan-ethnic mutation panel. Genet Med 2001;3:168-76.
283. Heit JA, Silverstein MD, Mohr DN, Petterson TM, O'Fallon WM, Melton LJ. Risk factors for deep vein thrombosis and pulmonary embolism: a population-based case-control study. Arch Intern Med 2000;160:809-15.
284. Heitz D, Devus D, Imbert G, Kretz C, Mandel JL. Inheritance of the fragile X syndrome: size of the fragile X premutation is a major determinant of the transition to full mutation. J Med Genet 1992;29:794-801.
285. Hemophilia A mutation database. Available at: http://europium.csc.mrk.ac.uk (accessed July 2009).
286. Henderson S, Sillence D, Loughlin J, Bennetts B, Sykes B. Germline and somatic mosaicism in achondroplasia. J Med Genet 2000;37:956-8.
287. Henneman L, Bramsen I, Van Der Ploeg HM, Ten Kate LP. Preconception cystic fibrosis carrier couple screening: impact, understanding, and satisfaction. Genet Testing 2002;3:195-202.
288. Henneman L, Poppelaars FAM, Ten Kate LP. Evaluation of cystic fibrosis carrier screening programs according to genetic screening criteria. Genet Med 2002;4:241-9.
289. Hessner MJ, Budish MA, Friedman KD. Genotyping of factor V G1691A (Leiden) without the use of PCR by invasive cleavage of oligonucleotide probe. Clin Chem 2000;46:1051-6.
290. Highsmith WE, Burch LH, Zhou Z, Olsen JC, Boat TE, Spock A, et al. A novel mutation in the cystic fibrosis gene in patients with pulmonary disease but normal sweat chloride concentrations. N Engl J Med 1996;331:974-80.
291. Higuchi M, Kazazian HH, Kasch L, Warren TC, McGinniss MJ, Phillips JA, et al. Molecular characterization of severe hemophilia A suggests that about half the mutations are not within the coding regions and splice junctions of the factor VIII gene. Proc Natl Acad Sci U S A 1991;88:7405-9.

292. Hoegger MJ, Lieven CJ, Levin LA. Differential production of superoxide by neuronal mitochondria. BMC Neurosci 2008;9:4.
293. Hoffman EP, Brown RH, Kunkel LM. Dystrophin: the protein product of the Duchenne muscular dystrophy locus. Cell 1987;51:919-28.
294. Hoffman EP, Kunkel LM. Dystrophin abnormalities in Duchenne/ Becker muscular dystrophy. Neuron 1989;2:1019-29.
295. Hofstra RMW, Mulder IM, Vossen R, de Koning-Gans PAM, Kraak M, Ginjaar IB, et al. DGGE-based whole-gene mutation scanning of the dystrophin gene in Duchenne and Becker muscular dystrophy patients. Hum Mutat 2004;23:57-66.
296. Hofstra RMW, Spurdle AB, Eccles D, Foulkes WD, de Wind N, Hoogeerbrugge N, et al. Tumor characteristics as an analytic tool for classifying genetic variants of uncertain clinical significance. Hum Mutat 2008;29:1292-3.
297. Hohenstein P, Fodde R. Of mice and (wo)men: genotype-phenotype correlations in BRCA1. Hum Mol Genet 2003;12:R271-7.
298. Hollister DW, Godfrey M, Sakai LY, Pyeritz RE. Immunohistologic abnormalities of the microfibrillar-fiber system in the Marfan syndrome. N Engl J Med 1990;323:152-9.
299. Holmstrom P, Marmur J, Eggertsen G, Gafvels M, Stal P. Mild iron overload in patients carrying the *HFE* S65C gene mutation: a retrospective study in patient with suspected iron overload and healthy controls. Gut 2002;51:723-30.
300. Holt IJ, Harding AE, Morgan-Hughes JA. Deletions of muscle mitochondrial DNA in patients with mitochondrial myopathies. Nature 1988;331:717-9.
301. Hoogerwaard EM, Bakker E, Ippel PF, Oosterwijk JC, Majoor-Krakauer DF, Leschot NJ, et al. Signs and symptoms of Duchenne muscular dystrophy and Becker muscular dystrophy among carriers in the Netherlands: a cohort study. Lancet 1999;353:2116-9.
302. Hoogeveen AT, Willemsen R, Meyer R, De Rooij K, van Ommen G, Galjaard H. Characterization and localization of the Huntington disease gene product. Hum Mol Genet 1993;2:2069-73.
303. Hooper WC, Dilley A, Ribeiro MJA, Benson J, Austin H, Silva V, et al. A racial difference in the prevalence of the Arg506-Gln mutation. Thromb Res 1996;81:577-81.
304. Hopf FW, Turner PR, Steinhardt RA. Calcium misregulation and the pathogenesis of muscular dystrophy. Subcell Biochem 2007;45:429-64.
305. Horsthemke B, Dittrich B, Buiting K. Imprinting mutations on human chromosome 15. Hum Mutat 1997;10:329-37.
306. Horsthemke B, Wagstaff J. Mechanisms of imprinting of the Prader-Willi/Angelman region. Am J Med Genet A 2008;146A:2041-52.
307. Horton WA. Recent milestones in achondroplasia research. Am J Med Genet A 2006;140A:166-9.
308. Horton WA, Hall JG, Hecht JT. Achondroplasia. Lancet 2007;370: 162-72.
309. Hoshiya H, Kazuki Y, Abe S, Takiguchi M, Kajitani N, Watanabe Y, et al. A highly stable and nonintegrated human artificial chromosome (HAC) containing the 2.4 Mb entire human dystrophin gene. Mol Ther 2009;17:309-17.
310. Hough C, Lillicrap D. Gene therapy for hemophilia: an imperative to succeed. J Thromb Haemost 2005;3:1195-205.
311. Howlett NG, Taniguchi T, Olson S, Cox B, Waisfisz Q, de Die-Smulders C, et al. Biallelic inactivation of *BRCA2* in Fanconi anemia. Science 2002;297:606-9.
312. Huang CH, Chang YY, Chen CH, Kuo YS, Hwu WL, Gerdes T, et al. Copy number analysis of survival motor neuron genes by multiplex ligation-dependent probe amplification. Genet Med 2007;9:241-8.
313. Hubmacher D, El-Hallous EI, Nelea V, Kaartinen MT, Lee ER, Reinhardt DP. Biogenesis of extracellular microfibrils: multimerization of the fibrillin-1 C terminus into bead-like structures enables self-assembly. Proc Natl Acad Sci U S A 2008;105:6548-53.
314. Hubmacher D, Tiedemann K, Reinhardt D. Fibrillins: from biogenesis of microfibrils to signaling functions. Curr Top Dev Biol 2006;75: 93-123.
315. Hudson G, Keers S, Yu Wai Man P, Griffiths P, Huoponen K, Savontaus ML, et al. Identification of an X-chromosomal locus and haplotype modulating the phenotype of a mitochondrial DNA disorder. Am J Hum Genet 2005;77:1086-91.
316. Hughes DJ. Use of association studies to define genetic modifiers of breast cancer risk in *BRCA1* and *BRCA2* mutation carriers. Fam Cancer 2008;7:233-44.
317. Human Gene Mutation Database. Available at: www.hgmd.org (accessed July 2009).
318. Hung CC, Lin SY, Lee CN, Cheng HY, Lin CY, Chang CH, et al. Identification of fibrillin-1 gene mutations in Marfan syndrome by high-resolution melting analysis. Anal Biochem 2009;389:102-6.
319. Hunter JE, Allen EG, Abramowitz A, Rusin M, Leslie M, Novak G, et al. No evidence for a difference in neuropsychological profile among carriers and noncarriers of the FMR1 premutation in adults under the age of 50. Am J Hum Genet 2008;83:692-702.
320. Huntington G. On chorea. Medical and Surgical Reporter 1872;26:320-21.
321. Huntington's Disease Collaborative Research Group. A novel gene containing a trinucleotide repeat that is expanded and unstable on Huntington's disease chromosomes. Cell 1993;72:971-83.
322. Huoponen K, Puomila A, Savontaus ML, Mustonen E, Kronqvist E, Nikoskelainen E. Genetic counseling in Leber hereditary optic neuropathy (LHON). Acta Ophthalmol Scand 2002;80:38-43.
323. Hyser CL, Doherty RA, Griggs RC, Mendell JR, Polakowska R, Quirk S, et al. Carrier assessment for mothers and sisters of isolated Duchenne dystrophy cases: the importance of serum enzyme determinations. Neurology 1987;37:1476-80.
324. Ikeda N, Miyoshi Y, Yoneda K, Shiba E, Sekihara Y, Moritoshi K, et al. Frequency of *BRCA1* and *BRCA2* germline mutations in Japanese breast cancer families. Int J Cancer 2001;91:83-8.
325. International Huntington Association/World Federation of Neurology. Ethical issues: policy statement on Huntington's disease molecular genetics predictive test. J Med Genet 1990;27:34-8.
326. International Huntington Association (IHA) and the World Federation of Neurology (WFN) Research Group on Huntington's Chorea. Guidelines for the molecular genetics predictive test in Huntington's disease. Neurology 1994;44:1533-6.
327. Ionov Y, Peinado MA, Malkhosyan S, Shibata D, Perucho M. Ubiquitous somatic mutations in simple repeated sequences reveal a new mechanism for colonic carcinogenesis. Nature 1993;363: 558-61.
328. Ishizuka A, Siomi MC, Siomi H. A Drosophila fragile X protein interacts with components of RNAi and ribosomal proteins. Genes Dev 2002;16:2497-508.
329. Jacobs EM, Hendriks JC, Marx JJ, van Deursen CT, Kreeftenberg HG, de Vries RA, et al. Morbidity and mortality in first-degree relatives of C282Y homozygous probands with clinically detected haemochromatosis compared with the general population: the HEmochromatosis FAmily Study (HEFAS). Neth J Med 2007;65: 425-33.
330. Jacobs EM, Hendriks JC, van Deursen CT, Kreeftenberg HG, de Vries RA, Marx JJ, et al. Severity of iron overload of proband determines serum ferritin levels in families with HFE-related hemochromatosis: the HEmochromatosis FAmily Study. J Hepatol 2009;50:174-83.
331. Jacquemont S, Hagerman RJ, Leehey MA, Hall DA, Levine RA, Brunberg JA, et al. Penetrance of the fragile X-associated tremor/ ataxia syndrome in a permutation carrier population. JAMA 2004;291: 460-9.
332. Janssen MC, Swinkels DW. Hereditary haemochromatosis. Best Pract Res Clin Gastroenterol 2009;23:171-83.
333. Jaron R, Yaakov Y, Rivlin J, Blau H, Bentur L, Yahav Y, et al. Nasal potential difference in non-classic cystic fibrosis—long term follow up. Pediatr Pulmonol 2008;43:545-9.
334. Jazwinska EC, Cullen LM, Busfield F, Pyper WR, Webb SI, Powell LW, et al. Haemochromatosis and HLA-H (Letter). Nat Genet 1996;14: 249-51.
335. Jazwinska EC, Lee SC, Webb SI, Halliday JW, Powell LW. Localization of the hemochromatosis gene close to D6S105. Am J Hum Genet 1993;53:347-52.

336. Jedele KB. The overlapping spectrum of Rett and Angelman syndromes: a clinical review. Semin Pediatr Neurol 2007;14:108-17.
337. Jędrezjowska M, Borkowska J, Zimowski J, Kostera-Pruszczyk A, Milewski M, Jurek M, et al. Unaffected patients with a homozygous absence of the SMN1 gene. Eur J Hum Genet 2008;16:930-4.
338. Jenkins Ma, Baglietto L, Dite GS, Jolley DJ, Southey MC, Whitty J, et al. After *hMSH2* and *hMLH1*—What next? Analysis of three-generational, population-based, early-onset colorectal cancer families. Int J Cancer 2002;102:166-71.
339. Jenkins PV, Collins PW, Goldman E, McCraw A, Riddell A, Lee CA, et al. Analysis of intron 22 inversions of the factor VIII gene in severe hemophilia A: implications for genetic counseling. Blood 1994;84:2197-201.
340. Jiricny J, Nystrom-Lahti M. Mismatch repair defects in cancer. Curr Opin Genet Dev 2000;10:157-61.
341. Johannesdottir G, Gudmundsson J, Bergthorsson JT, Arason A, Agnarsson BA, Eiriksdottier G, et al. High prevalence of the 999del5 mutation in Icelandic breast and ovarian cancer patients. Cancer Res 1996;56:3663-5.
342. Johnson DE, Lu J, Chen H, Werner S, Williams LT. Human fibroblast growth factor receptor genes: a common structural arrangement underlies the mechanisms for generating receptor forms that differ in their third immunoglobulin domain. Mol Cell Biol 1991;11:4627-34.
343. Joncourt F, Neuhaus B, Jostarndt-Foegen K, Kleinle S, Steiner B, Gallati S. Rapid identification of female carriers of DMD/BMD by quantitative real-time PCR. Hum Mutat 2004;23:385-91.
344. Jones IT, Jagelman DG, Fazio VW, Lavery IC, Weakley FL, McGannon E. Desmoid tumors in familial polyposis coli. Ann Surg 1986;204:94-7.
345. Jones S, Lambert S, Williams GT, Best JM, Sampson JR, Cheadle JP. Increased frequency of the k-ras G12C mutation in MYH polyposis colorectal adenomas. Br J Cancer 2004;90:1591-3.
346. Jong MT, Gray TA, Ji Y, Glenn CC, Saitoh S, Driscoll DJ, et al. A novel imprinted gene, encoding a RING zinc-finger protein, and overlapping antisense transcript in Prader-Willi syndrome critical region. Hum Mol Genet 1999;8:783-93.
347. Jouanolle AM, Fergelot P, Gandon G, Yaouanq J, Le Gall JY, David V. A candidate gene for hemochromatosis: frequency of the C282Y and H63D mutations. Hum Genet 1997;100:544-7.
348. Judge DP, Dietz HC. Marfan's syndrome. Lancet 2005;366:1965-76.
349. Julié C, Trésallet C, Brouquet A, Vallot C, Zimmerman U, Mitry E, et al. Identification in daily practice of patients with Lynch syndrome (hereditary nonpolyposis colorectal cancer): revised Bethesda guidelines-based approach versus molecular screening. Am J Gastroenterol 2008;103:2825-35.
350. Juul K, Tybjærg-Hansen A, Steffensen R, Kofoed S, Jensen G, Nordestgaard BG. Factor V Leiden: the Copenhagen City Heart Study and 2 meta-analyses. Blood 2002;100:3-10.
351. Kainulainen K, Pulkkinen L, Savolainen A, Kaitila I, Peltonen L. Location on chromosome 15 of the gene defect causing Marfan syndrome. N Engl J Med 1990;323:935-9.
352. Kalafatis M, Bertina RM, Rand MD, Mann KG. Characterization of the molecular defect in factor V^{R506Q}. J Biol Chem 1995;270:4053-7.
353. Kaltenback LS, Romero E, Becklin RR, Chettier R, Bell R, Phansalkar A, et al. Huntington interacting proteins are genetic modifiers of neurodegeneration. PLoS Genet 2007;3:e82.
354. Kashima T, Rao N, David CJ, Manley JL. hnRNP A1 functions with specificity in repression of SMN2 exon 7 splicing. Hum Mol Genet 2007;16:3149-59.
355. Kashima T, Rao N, Manley JL. An intronic element contributes to splicing repression in spinal muscular atrophy. Proc Natl Acad Sci U S A 2007;104:3426-31.
356. Kastrinos F, Stoffel EM, Balmana J, Steyerberg EW, Mercado R, Syngal S. Phenotype comparison of MLH1 and MSH2 mutation carriers in a cohort of 1,914 individuals undergoing clinical genetic testing in the United States. Cancer Epidemiol Biomarkers Prev 2008;17:2044-51.
357. Katoh M, Katoh M. WNT signaling pathway and stem cell signaling network. Clin Cancer Res 2007;13:4042-5.
358. Keiles S, Kammesheidt A. Identification of *CFTR, PRSS1,* and *SPINK1* mutations in 381 patients with pancreatitis. Pancreas 2006;33:221-7.
359. Keller M, Jost R, Haunstetter CM, Sattel H, Schroeter C, Bertsch U, et al. Psychosocial outcome following genetic risk counselling for familial colorectal cancer: a comparison of affected patients and family members. Clin Genet 2008;74:414-24.
360. Kelly CM, Dunnett SB, Rosser AE. Medium spiny neurons for transplantation in Huntington's disease. Biochem Soc Trans 2009;37:323-8.
361. Kemper AR, Wake MA. Duchenne muscular dystrophy: issues in expanding newborn screening. Curr Opin Pediatr 2007;19:700-4.
362. Kempton CL, White GC II. How we treat a hemophilia A patient with a factor VIII inhibitor. Blood 2009;113:11-7.
363. Kenneson A, Zhang F, Hagedorn CH, Warren ST. Reduced FMRP and increased FMR1 transcription is proportionally associated with CGG repeat number in intermediate-length and premutation carriers. Hum Mol Genet 2001;10:1449-54.
364. Kenney C, Powell S, Jankovic J. Autopsy-proven Huntington's disease with 29 trinucleotide repeats. Mov Disord 2007;22:127-30.
365. Kerem BS, Rommens JM, Buchanan JA, Markiewicz D, Cox TK, Chakravarti A, et al. Identification of the cystic fibrosis gene: genetic analysis. Science 1989;245:1073-80.
366. Kew MC. Hepatic iron overload and hepatocellular carcinoma. Cancer Lett 2009;286:38-43.
367. Khoo B, Krainer AR. Splicing therapeutics in SMN2 and APOB. Curr Opin Mol Ther 2009;11:108-15.
368. Kinzler KW, Nilbert MC, Su LK, Vogelstein B, Bryan TM, Levy DB, et al. Identification of FAP locus genes from chromosome 5q21. Science 1991;253:661-5.
369. Kinzler KW, Vogelstein B. Landscaping the cancer terrain. Science 1998;280:1036-7.
370. Kishino T, Lalande M, Wagstaff J. UBE3A/E6AP mutations cause Angelman syndrome. Nat Genet 1997;15:70-3.
371. Kiss T. Small nucleolar RNAs: an abundant group of noncoding RNAs with diverse cellular functions. Cell 2002;109:145-8.
372. Klintschar M, Bilkenroth U, Arslan-Kirchner M, Schmidtke J, Stiller D. Marfan syndrome: clinical consequences resulting from a medicolegal autopsy of a case of sudden death due to aortic rupture. Int J Legal Med 2009;123:55-8.
373. Klopp N, Oldenburg J, Uen C, Schneppenheim R, Graw J. 11 hemophilia A patients without mutations in the factor VIII encoding gene. Thromb Haemost 2002;88:357-60.
374. Knowlton RG, Cohen-Haguenauer O, Van Cong N, Grezal J, Brown VA, Barker D, et al. A polymorphic DNA marker linked to cystic fibrosis is located on chromosome 7. Nature 1985;318:380-2.
375. Koene S, Smeitink J. Mitochondrial medicine: entering the era of treatment. J Intern Med 2009;265:193-9.
376. Kremer B, Almqvist E, Theilmann J, Spence N, Telenius H, Goldberg YP, et al. Sex-dependent mechanisms for expansions and contractions of the CAG repeat on affected Huntington disease chromosomes. Am J Hum Genet 1995;57:343-50.
377. Kremer B, Goldberg P, Andrew SE, Theilmann J, Telenius H, Ziesler J, et al. A worldwide study of the Huntington's disease mutation: the sensitivity and specificity of measuring CAG repeats. N Engl J Med 1994;330:1401-6.
378. Kremer EJ, Pritchard M, Lynch M, Yu S, Holman K, Baker E, et al. Mapping of DNA instability at the fragile X to a trinucleotide repeat sequence p(CGG)n. Science 1991;252:1711-4.
379. Kubota T, Das S, Christian SL, Baylin SB, Herman JG, Ledbetter DH. Methylation-specific PCR simplifies imprinting analysis. Nat Genet 1997;16:16-7.
380. Kuismanen SA, Holmberg MT, Salovaara R, de la Chapelle A, Peltomaki P. Genetic and epigenetic modification of *MLH1* accounts for a major share of microsatellite-unstable colorectal cancers. Am J Pathol 2000;156:1773-9.
381. Kumari D, Usdin K. Chromatin remodeling in the noncoding repeat expansion diseases. J Biol Chem 2009;284:7413-7.

382. Kunkel LM, Monaco AP, Middlesworth W, Ochs H, Latt SA. Specific cloning of DNA fragments absent from the DNA of a male patient with an X-chromosome deletion. Proc Natl Acad Sci U S A 1985;82:4778-82.
383. Kunst CB, Warren ST. Cryptic and polar variation of the fragile X repeat could result in predisposing normal alleles. Cell 1994;77:853-61.
384. Laggerbauer B, Ostareck D, Keidel EM, Ostareck-Lederer A, Fischer U. Evidence that fragile X mental retardation protein is a negative regulator of translation. Hum Mol Genet 2001;10:329-38.
385. Lakhani SR, van de Vijver MJ, Jacquemier J, Anderson TJ, Osin PP, McGuffog L, et al. The pathology of familial breast cancer: predictive value of immunohistochemical markers estrogen receptor, progesterone receptor, HER-2, and p53 in patients with mutations in *BRCA1* and *BRCA2*. J Clin Oncol 2002;20:2310-8.
386. Lakich D, Kazazian HH, Antonarakis SE, Gitschier J. Inversions disrupting the factor VIII gene are a common cause of severe hemophilia A. Nat Genet 1993;5:236-41.
387. Lalic T, Vossen RH, Coffa J, Schouten JP, Guc-Scekic M, Radivojevic D, et al. Deletion and duplication screening in the DMD gene using MLPA. Eur J Hum Genet 2005;13:1231-4.
388. Lalloz MR, McVey JH, Pattinson JK, Tuddenham EGD. Haemophilia A diagnosis by analysis of a hypervariable dinucleotide repeat within the factor VIII gene. Lancet 1991;338:207-11.
389. Lalouel JM, Le Mignon L, Simon M, Fauchet R, Bourel M, Rao DC, et al. Genetic analysis of idiopathic hemochromatosis using both qualitative (disease status) and quantitative (serum iron) information. Am J Hum Genet 1985;37:700-18.
390. Ledford M, Friedman KD, Hessner MJ, Moehlenkamp C, Williams TM, Larson RS. A multi-site study for detection of the factor V (Leiden) mutation from genomic DNA using a homogeneous invader microtiter plate fluorescence resonance energy transfer (FRET) assay. J Mol Diagn 2000;2:97-104.
391. Lee S, Kozlov S, Hernandez L, Chamberlain SJ, Brannan CI, Stewart CL, et al. Expression and imprinting of MAGEL2 suggest a role in Prader-Willi syndrome and the homologous murine imprinting phenotype. Hum Mol Genet 2000;9:1813-9.
392. Leeflang EP, Zhang L, Tavare S, Hubert R, Srinidhi J, MacDonald ME, et al. Single sperm analysis of the trinucleotide repeats in the Huntington's disease gene: quantification of the mutation frequency spectrum. Hum Mol Genet 1995;4:1519-26.
393. Lefebvre S, Bürglen L, Reboullet S, Clermont O, Burlet P, Viollet L, et al. Identification and characterization of a spinal muscular atrophy-determining gene. Cell 1995;80:155-65.
394. Leiden muscular dystrophy pages (database online). Dystrophin (DMD) sequence variations. Available at: http://www.dmd.nl/database.html (accessed July 2009).
395. Li SH, Gutekunst CA, Hersch SM, Li XJ. Association of HAP1 isoforms with a unique cytoplasmic structure. J Neurochem 1998;71:2178-85.
396. Li XJ, Li SH, Sharp AH, Nucifora FC, Schilling G, Lanahan A, et al. A huntingtin-associated protein enriched in brain with implications for pathology. Nature 1995;378:398-402.
397. Li Y, Chin LS, Levey AI, Li L. Huntingtin-associated protein-1 interacts with Hrs and functions in endosomal trafficking. J Biol Chem 2002;277:28212-21.
398. Li Z, Zhang Y, Ku L, Wilkinson KD, Warren ST, Feng Y. The fragile X mental retardation protein inhibits translation via interacting with mRNA. Nucleic Acids Res 2001;29:2276-83.
399. Liede A, Narod SA. Hereditary breast and ovarian cancer in Asia: genetic epidemiology of *BRCA1* and *BRCA2*. Hum Mutat 2002;20:413-24.
400. Liem TK, DeLoughery TG. First episode and recurrent venous thromboembolism: who is identifiably at risk? Semin Vasc Surg 2008;21:132-8.
401. Lim JH, Booker AB, Fallon JR. Regulating fragile X gene transcription in the brain and beyond. J Cell Physiol 2005;205:170-5.
402. Linde L, Kerem B. Introducing sense into nonsense in treatments of human genetic diseases. Trends Genet 2008;24:552-63.
403. Lindgren AC, Lindberg A. Growth hormone treatment completely normalizes adult height and improves body composition in Prader-Willi syndrome: experience from KIGS (Pfizer International Growth Database). Horm Res 2008;70:182-7.
404. Liu Q, Dreyfuss G. A novel nuclear structure containing the survival of motor neurons protein. EMBO J 1996;15:3555-65.
405. Liu Q, Nozari G, Sommer SS. Single tube polymerase chain reaction for rapid diagnosis of the inversion hotspot of mutation in hemophilia A. Blood 1998;92:1458-9.
406. Liu Q, Sommer SS. Subcycling-PCR for multiplex long-distance amplification of regions with high and low GC content: application to the inversion hotspot in the factor VIII gene. Biotechniques 1998;25:1022-8.
407. Loeys B, De Backer J, Van Acker P, Wettinck K, Pals G, Nuytinck L, et al. Comprehensive molecular screening of the FBN1 gene favors locus homogeneity of classical Marfan syndrome. Hum Mutat 2004;24:140-6.
408. Lorson CL, Hahnen E, Androphy EJ, Wirth B. A single nucleotide in the SMN gene regulates splicing and is responsible for spinal muscular atrophy. Proc Natl Acad Sci U S A 1999;96:6307-11.
409. Lorson CL, Strasswinner J, Yao JM, Baleja JD, Hahnen E, Wirth B, et al. SMN oligomerization defect correlates with spinal muscular atrophy severity. Nat Genet 1998;19:63-6.
410. Lossie AC, Whitney MM, Amidon D, Dong HJ, Chen P, Theriaque D, et al. Distinct phenotypes distinguish the molecular classes of Angelman syndrome. J Med Genet 2001;38:834-45.
411. Loughrey MB, Waring PM, Tan A, Trivett M, Kovalenko S, Beshay V, et al. Incorporation of somatic BRAF mutation testing into an algorithm for the investigation of hereditary non-polyposis colorectal cancer. Fam Cancer 2007;6:301-10.
412. Lozier JN, Dutra A, Pak E, Zhou N, Zheng Z, Nichols TC, et al. The Chapel Hill hemophilia A dog colony exhibits a factor VIII gene inversion. Proc Natl Acad Sci U S A 2002;99:12991-6.
413. Lubin IM, McGovern MM, Gibson Z, Gross SJ, Lyon E, Pagon RA, et al. Clinician perspectives about molecular genetic testing for heritable conditions and development of a clinician-friendly laboratory report. J Mol Diagn 2009;11:162-71.
414. Lubs H. A marker X chromosome. Am J Hum Genet 1969;21:231-44.
415. Lunn MR, Wang CH. Spinal muscular atrophy. Lancet 2008;371:2120-33.
416. Lusher JM. Considerations for current and future management of haemophilia and its complications. Haemophilia 1995;1:2-10.
417. Lynch HT, de la Chapelle A. Hereditary colorectal cancer. N Engl J Med 2003;348:919-32.
418. Lynch HT, Shaw MW, Magnuson CW, Larsen AL, Krush AJ. Hereditary factors in two large Midwestern kindreds. Arch Intern Med 1966;117:206-12.
419. Lyon E, Frank EL. Hereditary hemochromatosis since discovery of the HFE gene. Clin Chem 2001;47:1147-56.
420. MacDonald ME, Anderson MA, Gilliam TC, Tranebjaerg L, Carpenter NJ, Magenis E, et al. A somatic cell hybrid panel for localizing DNA segments near the Huntington's disease gene. Genomics 1987;1:29-34.
421. Mackey DA, Costra RJ, Rosenberg T, Nikoskelainen E, Bronte-Stewart J, Poulton J, et al. Primary pathogenic mtDNA mutations in multigeneration pedigrees with Leber hereditary optic neuropathy. Am J Hum Genet 1996;59:481-5.
422. Maddalena A, Richards CS, McGinniss MJ, Brothman A, Desnick RJ, Grier RE, et al. Technical standards and guidelines for fragile X: the first of a series of disease-specific supplements to the standards and guidelines for clinical genetics laboratories of the American College of Medical Genetics. Genet Med 2001;3:200-5.
423. Mailman MD, Heinz JW, Papp AC, Snyder PJ, Sedra MS, Wirth B, et al. Molecular analysis of spinal muscular atrophy and modification of the phenotype by SMN2. Genet Med 2002;4:20-6.
424. Malter HE, Iber JC, Willemsen R, deGraaff E, Tarleton JC, Leisti J, et al. Characterization of the full fragile X syndrome mutation in fetal gametes. Nat Genet 1997;15:165-9.

425. Manipalviratn S, DeCherney A, Segars J. Imprinting disorders and assisted reproductive technology. Fertil Steril 2009;91:305-15.
426. Mann KG, Kalafatis M. Factor V: a combination of Dr Jekyll and Mr Hyde. Blood 2003;101:20-30.
427. Margaritis P, Roy E, Aljamali MN, Downey HD, Giger U, Zhou S, et al. Successful treatment of canine hemophilia by continuous expression of canine FVIIa. Blood 2009;113:3682-9.
428. Martin JP, Bell J. A pedigree of mental defect showing sex-linkage. J Neurol Psych 1943;6:154-7.
429. Martinelli I, Sacchi E, Landi G, Taili E, Duca F, Mannucci PM. High risk of cerebral-vein thrombosis in carriers of a prothrombin-gene mutation and in users of oral contraceptives. N Engl J Med 1998;338: 1840-1.
430. Martinelli I, Taioli E, Bucciarelli P, Akhavan S, Mannucci PM. Interaction between the G20210A mutation of the prothrombin gene and oral contraceptive use in deep vein thrombosis. Arterioscler Thromb Vasc Biol 1999;19:700-3.
431. Matentzoglu K, Scheffner M. Ubiquitin ligase E6-AP and its role in human disease. Biochem Soc Trans 2008;36:797-01.
432. Mazroul R, Huot ME, Tremblay S, Filion C, Labelle Y, Khandjian EW. Trapping of messenger RNA by fragile X mental retardation protein into cytoplasmic granules induces translation repression. Hum Mol Genet 2002;11:3007-17.
433. McConie-Rosell A, Lachiewicz AM, Spiridigliozzi GA, Tarleton J, Schoenwald S, Phelan MC, et al. Evidence that methylation of the FMR-1 locus is responsible for variable phenotypic expression of the fragile X syndrome. Am J Hum Genet 1993;53:800-9.
434. McGinniss MJ, Chen C, Redman JB, Buller A, Quan F, Peng M, et al. Extensive sequencing of the CFTR gene: lessons learned from the first 157 patient samples. Hum Genet 2005;118:31-8.
435. McGlennen RC, Key NS. Clinical and laboratory management of the prothrombin G20210A mutation. Arch Pathol Lab Med 2002;126: 1319-25.
436. Mefford HC, Baumbach L, Panguluri RC, Whitfield-Broome C, Szabo C, Smith S, et al. Evidence for a *BRCA1* founder mutation in families of West African ancestry. Am J Hum Genet 1999;65:575-8.
437. Meijers-Heijboer H, van Geel B, van Putten WLJ, Henzen-Logmans SC, Seynaeve C, Menke-Pluymers MBE, et al. Breast cancer after prophylactic bilateral mastectomy in women with a *BRCA1* or *BRCA2* mutation. N Engl J Med 2001;345:159-64.
438. Melki J, Abdelhak S, Sheth P, Bachelot MF, Burlet P, Marcadet A, et al. Gene for chronic proximal spinal muscular atrophies maps to chromosome 5q. Nature 1990;344:767-8.
439. Melton T, Clifford S, Kayser M, Nasidze I, Batzer M, Stoneking M. Diversity and heterogeneity in mitochondrial DNA of North American populations. J Forensic Sci 2001;46:46-52.
440. Mequro M, Kashiwagi A, Mitsuya K, Nakao M, Kondo I, Saitoh S, et al. A novel maternally expressed gene, ATPIOC, encodes a putative aminophospholipid translocase associated with Angelman syndrome. Nat Genet 2001;28:19-20.
441. Metcalfe S, Jacques A, Archibald A, Burgess T, Collins V, Henry A, et al. A model for offering carrier screening for fragile X syndrome to nonpregnant women: results from a pilot study. Genet Med 2008;10: 525-35.
442. Metzler M, Legendre-Guillemin V, Gan L, Chopra V, Kwok A, McPherson PS, et al. HIP1 functions in clathrin-mediated endocytosis through binding to clathrin and adaptor protein 2. J Biol Chem 2001;276:39271-6.
443. Meyer K, Marquis J, Trüb J, Nlend Nlend R, Verp S, Ruepp MD, et al. Rescue of a severe mouse model for spinal muscular atrophy by U7 snRNA-mediated splicing modulation. Hum Mol Genet 2009;18: 546-55.
444. Middeldorp S, van Hylckama Vlieg A. Does thrombophilia testing help in the clinical management of patients? Br J Haematol 2008; 143:321-35.
445. Miki Y, Swensen J, Shattuck-Eidens D, Futreal PA, Harshman K, Tavtigian S, et al. A strong candidate for the breast and ovarian cancer susceptibility gene *BRCA1*. Science 1994;266:66-71.
446. Milasin J, Muntoni F, Severini GM, Bartoloni L, Vatta M, Krajinovic M, et al. A point mutation in the 5′ splice site of the dystrophin gene first intron responsible for X-linked dilate cardiomyopathy. Hum Mol Genet 1996;5:73-9.
447. Millan FA, Curtis A, Mennie M, Holloway S, Boxer M, Faed MJW, et al. Prenatal exclusion testing for Huntington's disease: a problem of too much information. J Med Genet 1989;26:83-5.
448. Mitra S, Tsvetkov AS, Finkbeiner S. Single neuron ubiquitin-proteasome dynamics accompanying inclusion body formation in Huntington disease. J Biol Chem 2009;284:4398-403.
449. Mitrpant C, Adams AM, Meloni PL, Muntoni F, Fletcher S, Wilton SD. Rational design of antisense oligomers to induce dystrophin exon skipping. Mol Ther 2009;17:1418-26.
450. Moirand R, Guyader D, Mendler MH, Jouanolle AM, Le Gall JY, David V, et al. HFE based re-evaluation of heterozygous hemochromatosis. Am J Med Genet 2002;111:356-61.
451. Monaghan KG, Highsmith WE, Amos J, Pratt VM, Roa B, Friez M, et al. Genotype-phenotype correlation and frequency of the 3199del6 cystic fibrosis mutation among I148T carriers: results from a collaborative study. Genet Med 2004;6:421-6.
452. Monaghan KG, Wiktor A, Van Dyke DL. Diagnostic testing for Prader-Willi syndrome and Angelman syndrome: a cost comparison. Genet Med 2002;4:448-50.
453. Monsonego-Ornan E, Adar R, Feferman T, Segev O, Yayon A. The transmembrane mutation G380R in fibroblast growth factor receptor 3 uncouples ligand-mediated receptor activation from down-regulation. Mol Cell Biol 2000;20:516-22.
454. Mori PG, Pasino M, Vadala CR, Bisogni MC, Tonini GP, Scarabicchi S. Haemophilia A in a 46,X, i(Xq) female. Br J Haematol 1979;43: 143-7.
455. Moskowitz SM, Chmiel JF, Sternen DL, Cheng E, Gibson RL, Marshall SG, et al. Clinical practice and genetic counseling for cystic fibrosis and CFTR-related disorders. Genet Med 2008;10:851-68.
456. Moutou C, Vincent MC, Biancalana V, Mandel JL. Transition from premutation to full mutation in fragile X syndrome is likely to be prezygotic. Hum Mol Genet 1997;6:971-9.
457. Muller F, Dommergues M, Simon-Bouy B, Ferec C, Oury JF, Aubry MC, et al. Cystic fibrosis screening: a fetus with hyperechogenic bowel may be the index case. J Med Genet 1998;35:657-60.
458. Multicenter Study Group. Diagnosis of Duchenne and Becker muscular dystrophies by polymerase chain reaction. JAMA 1992;267:2609-15.
459. Munce T, Simpson R, Bowling F. Molecular characterization of Prader-Willi syndrome by real-time PCR. Genet Test 2008;12: 319-24.
460. Muntoni F, Cau M, Ganau A, Congiu R, Arvedi G, Mateddu A, et al. Brief report: deletion of the dystrophin muscle-promoter region associated with X-linked dilated cardiomyopathy. N Engl J Med 1993;329:921-5.
461. Mura C, Raguenes O, Ferec C. *HFE* mutation analysis in 711 hemochromatosis probands: evidence for S65C implication in mild form of hemochromatosis. Blood 1999;93:2502-5.
462. Muralidharan K. Detection of mitochondrial DNA mutations associated with Leber hereditary optic neuropathy. Methods Mol Biol 2003;217:199-205.
463. Myers RH, Farber LA, Busella JF, Martin JB. Predictive testing for Huntington's disease using linked DNA markers. N Engl J Med 1988;319:583-4.
464. Myers RH, Leavitt J, Farrer LA, Jagadeesh J, McFarlane H, Mastromauro CA, et al. Homozygote for Huntington disease. Am J Hum Genet 1989;45:615-8.
465. Myers RH, Sax DS, Schoenfeld M, Bird ED, Wolf PA, Vonsattrel JP, et al. Late onset of Huntington's disease. J Neurol Neurosurg Psychiatry 1985;48:530-4.
466. Nagase H, Miyoshi Y, Horii A, Aoki T, Agawa M, Utsunomiya J, et al. Correlation between the location of germ-line mutations in the *APC* gene and the number of colorectal polyps in familial adenomatous polyposis patients. Cancer Res 1992;52:4055-7.

467. Nahhas FA, Garbern J, Krajewski KM, Roa BB, Geldman GL. A juvenile onset Huntington disease resulting from a very large maternal expansion. Am J Med Genet 2005;137A:328-31.
468. Nakada Y, Taniura H, Uetsuki T, Inazawa J, Yoshikawa K. The human chromosomal gene for necdin, a neuronal growth suppressor, in the Prader-Willi syndrome deletion region. Gene 1998;213:65-72.
469. Natacci F, Baffico M, Cavallari U, Bedeschi MF, Mura I, Paffoni A, Setti PL, et al. Germline mosaicism in achondroplasia detected in sperm DNA of the father of three affected sibs. Am J Med Genet A 2008;146A:784-6.
470. National Comprehensive Cancer Network. NCCN colorectal cancer screening practice guidelines. Oncology 1999;13:152-79.
471. Nauhausen S. Founder populations and their uses for breast cancer genetics. Breast Cancer Res 2000;2:77-81.
472. Naylor J, Brinke A, Hassock S, Green PM, Giannelli F. Characteristic mRNA abnormality found in half the patients with severe haemophilia A is due to large DNA inversions. Hum Mol Genet 1993;2:1773-8.
473. Nelson FW, Hecht JT, Horton WA, Butler IJ, Goldie WD, Miner M. Neurological basis of respiratory complications in achondroplasia. Ann Neurol 1988;24:89-93.
474. Neptune ER, Frischmeyer PA, Arking DE, Myers L, Bunton TE, Gayraud B, et al. Dysregulation of TGF-β activation contributes to pathogenesis in Marfan syndrome. Nat Genet 2003;33:407-11.
475. Neuhausen S, Gilewski T, Norton L, Tran T, McGuire P, Swensen J, et al. Recurrent *BRCA2* 6174delT mutations in Ashkenazi Jewish women affected by breast cancer. Nat Genet 1996;13:126-8.
476. Newman NJ. From genotype to phenotype in Leber hereditary optic neuropathy: still more questions than answers. J Neuroophthalmol 2002;22:257-61.
477. Nicholls RD, Saitoh S, Horsthemke B. Imprinting in Prader-Willi and Angelman syndromes. Trends Genet 1998;14:194-200.
478. Nichols DP, Konstan MW, Chmiel JF. Anti-inflammatory therapies for cystic fibrosis-related lung disease. Clin Rev Allergy Immunol 2008;35:135-53.
479. Nishisho I, Nakamura Y, Miyoshi Y, Miki Y, Ando H, Horii A, et al. Mutations of chromosome 5q21 genes in FAP and colorectal cancer patients. Science 1991;253:665-9.
480. Noble R, Bahadur G, Iqbal M, Sanyal A. Pandora's box: ethics of PGD for inherited risk of late-onset disorders. Reprod Biomed Online 2008;17S:55-60.
481. Nolin SL, Brown WT, Glicksman A, Houck GE, Gargano AD, Sullivan A, et al. Expansion of the fragile X CGG repeat in females with premutation or intermediate alleles. Am J Hum Genet 2003;72:454-64.
482. Nolin SL, Lewis FA, Ye LL, Houck GEJ, Glicksman AE, Limprasert P, et al. Familial transmission of the FMR1 CGG repeat. Am J Hum Genet 1996;59:1252-61.
483. Nygren AO, Ameziane N, Duarte HM, Vijzelaar RN, Waisfisz Q, Hess CJ, et al. Methylation-specific MPLA (MS-MLPA): simultaneous detection of CpG methylation and copy number changes of up to 40 sequences. Nucleic Acids Res 2005;33:e128.
484. Oberle I, Rousseau F, Heitz D, Kretz C, Devys D, Hanauer A, et al. Instability of a 550-base pair DNA segment and abnormal methylation in fragile X syndrome. Science 1991;252:1097-102.
485. Ogino S, Kawasaki T, Kirkner GJ, Kraft P, Loda M, Fuchs CS. Evaluation of markers for CpG island methylator phenotype (CIMP) in colorectal cancer by a large population-based sample. J Mol Diagn 2007;9:305-14.
486. Ogino S, Wilson RB, Gold B, Hawley P, Grody WW. Bayesian analysis for cystic fibrosis risks in prenatal and carrier screening. Genet Med 2004;6:439-49.
487. Olopade OI, Fackenthal JD, Dunston G, Tainsky MA, Collins F, Whitfield-Broome C. Breast cancer genetics in African Americans. Cancer 2003;97:236-45.
488. Olopade OI, Grushko TA, Nanda R, Huo D. Advances in breast cancer: pathways to personalized medicine. Clin Cancer Res 2008;14:7988-99.
489. Olschwang S, Blanché H, De Moncuit C, Thomas G. Similar colorectal cancer risk in patients with monoallelic and biallelic mutations in the MYH gene identified in a population with adenomatous polyposis. Genet Test 2007;11:315-20.
490. Oritz-Lopez R, Li H, Su J, Goytia V, Towbin J. Evidence for a dystrophin missense mutation as a cause of X-linked dilated cardiomyopathy. Circulation 1997;95:2434-40.
491. Orr HT, Zoghbi HY. Trinucleotide repeat disorders. Annu Rev Neurosci 2007;30:575-621.
492. Ou J, Niessen RC, Vonk J, Westers H, Hofstra RMW, Sijmons RH. A database to support the interpretation of human mismatch repair gene variants. Hum Mutat 2008;29:1337-41.
493. Ozcelik T, Leff S, Robinson W, Donlon T, Lalande M, Sanjines E, et al. Small nuclear ribonucleoprotein polypeptide N (SNRPN), an expressed gene in the Prader-Willi syndrome critical region. Nat Genet 1992;2:265-9.
494. Palomaki GE, McClain MR, Mclillo S, Hampel HL, Thibodeau SN. EGAPP supplementary evidence review: DNA testing strategies aimed at reducing morbidity and mortality from Lynch syndrome. Genet Med 2009;11:42-65.
495. Panchal SM, Ennis M, Canon S, Bordeleau LJ. Selecting a *BRCA* risk assessment model for use in a familiar cancer clinic. BMC Med Genet 2008;9:116-24.
496. Pantopoulos K. Function of the hemochromatosis protein HFE: lessons from animal models. World J Gastroenterol 2008;14:6893-901.
497. Parad RB, Comeau AM, Dorkin HL, Dovey M, Gerstle R, Martin T, et al. Sweat testing infants detected by cystic fibrosis newborn screening. J Pediatr 2005;147:S69-72.
498. Paranjape SM, Zeitlin PL. Atypical cystic fibrosis and CFTR-related diseases. Clin Rev Allergy Immunol 2008;35:116-23.
499. Parsons EP, Clarke AJ, Bradley DM. Newborn screening for Duchenne muscular dystrophy, a psychosocial study. Arch Dis Child 2002;86:F91-5.
500. Parsons DW, McAndrew PE, Iannaccone T, Mendell JR, Burghes AH, Prior TW. Intragenic telSMN mutations: frequency, distribution, evidence of a founder effect, and modification of the spinal muscular atrophy phenotype by cenSMN copy number. Am J Hum Genet 1998;63:1712-23.
501. Patrushev LI, Zykiva ES, Kayushin AL, Korosteleva MD, Miroshnikov AI, Bokarew IN, et al. New DNA diagnostic system for detection of factor V Leiden. Thromb Res 1998;92:251-9.
502. Pauli RM, Horton VK, Glinski LP, Reiser CA. Prospective assessment of risks for cervicomedullary-junction compression in infants with achondroplasia. Am J Hum Genet 1995;56:732-44.
503. Paulsen JS, Ferneyhough Hoth, K, Nehl C, Stierman L, The Huntington Study Group. Critical periods of suicide risk in Huntington's disease. Am J Psychiatry 2005;162:725-31.
504. Peelen T, van Vliet M, Petrij-Bosch A, Mieremet R, Szabo C, von den Ouweland AMW, et al. A high proportion of novel mutations in *BRCA1* with strong founder effects among Dutch and Belgian hereditary breast and ovarian cancer families. Am J Hum Genet 1997;60:1041-9.
505. Pellizzoni L, Yong J, Dreyfuss G. Essential role for the SMN complex in the specificity of snRNP assembly. Science 2002;298:1775-9.
506. Peltomaki P, Aaltonen LA, Sistonen P, Pylkkanen L, Mecklin JP, Jarvinen H, et al. Genetic mapping of a locus predisposing to human colorectal cancer. Science 1993;260:810-2.
507. Peltomaki P, Vasen H. Mutations associated with HNPCC predisposition—update of ICG-HNPCC/INSIGHT mutation database. Dis Markers 2004;20:269-76.
508. Penney JB, Vonsattel JP, MacDonald M, Gusella J, Myers R. CAG repeat number governs the development rate of pathology in Huntington's disease. Ann Neurol 1997;41:689-92.
509. Peters J. Prader-Willi and snoRNAs. Nat Genet 2008;40:688-9.
510. Petersen GM, Slack J, Nakamura Y. Screening guidelines and premorbid diagnosis of familial adenomatous polyposis using linkage. Gastroenterology 1991;100:1658-64.

511. Petit E, Oliver L, Vallette FM. The mitochondrial outer membrane protein import machinery: a new player in apoptosis? Front Biosci 2009;14:3563-70.
512. Phatak PD, Bonkovsky HL, Kowdley KV. Hereditary hemochromatosis: time for targeted screening. Ann Intern Med 2008;149:270-2.
513. Phatak PD, Ryan DH, Cappuccio J, Oakes D, Braggins C, Provenzano K, et al. Prevalence and penetrance of *HFE* mutations in 4865 unselected primary care patients. Blood Cells Mol Dis 2002;29:41-7.
514. Phelan CM, Kwan E, Jack E, Li S, Morgan C, Aube J, et al. A low frequency of non-founder *BRCA1* mutations in Ashkenazi Jewish breast-ovarian cancer families. Hum Mutat 2002;20:352-7.
515. Pieretti M, Zhang F, Fu YH, Warren ST, Oostra BA, Caskey CT, et al. Absence of expression of the *FMR1* gene in fragile X syndrome. Cell 1991;66:817-22.
516. Pietrobono R, Tabolacci E, Zalfa F, Zito I, Terracciano A, Moscato U, et al. Molecular dissection of the events leading to inactivation of the *FMR1* gene. Hum Mol Genet 2005;14:267-77.
517. Poort SR, Rosendaal FR, Reitsma PH, Bertina RM. A common genetic variation in the 3′-untranslated region of the prothrombin gene is associated with elevated plasma prothrombin levels and an increase in venous thrombosis. Blood 1996;88:3698-703.
518. Potter NT, Spector EB, Prior TW. Technical standards and guidelines for Huntington disease testing. Genet Med 2004;6:61-5.
519. Powell LW, Burt MJ, Halliday JW, Jazwinska EC. Hemochromatosis: genetics and pathogenesis. Semin Liver Dis 1996;16:55-63.
520. Press RD, Bauer KA, Kujovich JL, Heit JA. Clinical utility of factor V Leiden (R506Q) testing for the diagnosis and management of thromboembolic disorders. Arch Pathol Lab Med 2002;126:1304-18.
521. Prior TW. Carrier screening for spinal muscular atrophy. Genet Med 2008;10:840-2.
522. Pruthi RK. Hemophilia: a practical approach to genetic testing. Mayo Clin Proc 2005;80:1485-99.
523. Pyatt RE, Prior TW. A feasibility study for the newborn screening of spinal muscular atrophy. Genet Med 2006;8:428-37.
524. Radpou R, Gourabi H, Dizaj AV, Holzgreve W, Zhong XY. Genetic investigations of CFTR mutations in congenital absence of vas deferens, uterus, and vagina as a cause of infertility. J Androl 2008;29:506-13.
525. Raffini L. Thrombophilia in children: who to test, how, when, and why? Hematology Am Soc Hematol Educ Program 2008;228-35.
526. Ramirez F, Dietz HC. Fibrillin-rich microfibrils: structural determinants of morphogenetic and homeostatic events. J Cell Physiol 2007;213:326-30.
527. Reddy PH. Mitochondrial medicine for aging and neurodegenerative diseases. Neuromol Med 2008;10:291-315.
528. Rees DC, Cox M, Clegg JB. World distribution of factor V Leiden. Lancet 1995;346:1133-4.
529. Reid S, Schindler D, Hanenberg H, Barker K, Hanks S, Kalb R, et al. Biallelic mutations in *PALB2* cause Fanconi anemia subtype FA-N and predispose to childhood cancer. Nat Genet 2007;39:162-4.
530. Reitsma PH, Bernardi F, Doig RG, Gandrille S, Greengard JS, Ireland H, et al. Protein C deficiency: a database of mutations, 1995 update. Thromb Haemost 1995;73:876-89.
531. Repicky S, Broadie K. Metabotropic glutamate receptor-mediated-use-dependent down-regulation of synaptic excitability involves the fragile X mental retardation protein. J Neurophysiol 2009;101:672-87.
532. Richards CS, Watkins SC, Hoffman EP, Schneider NR, Milsark IW, Katz KS, et al. Skewed X inactivation in a female MZ twin results in Duchenne muscular dystrophy. Am J Hum Genet 1990;46:672-81.
533. Richette P, Bardin T, Stheneur C. Achondroplasia: from genotype to phenotype. Joint Bone Spine 2008;75:125-30.
534. Richter C, Park JW, Ames BN. Normal oxidative damage to mitochondrial and nuclear DNA is extensive. Proc Natl Acad Sci U S A 1988;85:6465-7.
535. Ridker PM, Miletich JP, Hennekens CH, Buring JE. Ethnic distribution of factor V Leiden in 4047 men and women. JAMA 1997;277:1305-7.
536. Riordan JR, Rommens JM, Kerem BS, Alon N, Rozmahel R, Grzelczak Z, et al. Identification of the cystic fibrosis gene: cloning and characterization of complementary DNA. Science 1989;245:1066-73.
537. Ripa R, Bisgaard ML, Bulow S, Nielsen FC. De novo mutations in familial adenomatous polyposis (FAP). Eur J Hum Genet 2002;10: 631-7.
538. Ripperger T, Gadzicki D, Meindl A, Schlegelberger B. Breast cancer susceptibility: current knowledge and implications for genetic counseling. Eur J Hum Genet 2008;17:1-10.
539. Ripperger T, Tröger HD, Schmidtke J. The genetic message of a sudden, unexpected death due to thoracic aortic dissection. Forensic Sci Int 2009;187:1-5.
540. Roa BB, Boyd AA, Volcik K, Richards CS. Ashkenazi Jewish population frequencies for common mutations in *BRCA1* and *BRCA2*. Nat Genet 1996;14:185-7.
541. Robinson WP, Christian SL, Kuchinka BD, Penaherrera MS, Das S, Schuffenhauer S, et al. Somatic segregation errors predominantly contribute to the gain or loss of a paternal chromosome leading to uniparental disomy for chromosome 15. Clin Genet 2000;57:349-58.
542. Robson M, Offit K. Management of an inherited predisposition to breast cancer. N Engl J Med 2007;357:154-62.
543. Robson ME. Clinical considerations in the management of individuals at risk for hereditary breast and ovarian cancer. Cancer Control 2002; 9:457-65.
544. Rochette CF, Gilbert N, Simard LR. SMN gene duplication and the emergence of the SMN2 gene occurred in distinct hominids: SMN2 is unique to *Homo sapiens*. Hum Genet 2001;108:255-66.
545. Rommens JM, Iannuzzi MC, Kerem BS, Drumm ML, Melmer G, Dean M, et al. Identification of the cystic fibrosis gene: chromosome walking and jumping. Science 1989;245:1059-65.
546. Rosendaal FR, Koster T, Vandenbroucke JP, Reitsma PH. High risk of thrombosis in patients homozygous for factor V Leiden (activated protein C resistance). Blood 1995;85:1504-8.
547. Rosman DS, Kaklamani V, Pashe B. New insights into breast cancer genetics and impact on patient management. Curr Treat Options Oncol 2007;8:61-73.
548. Rossetti LC, Radic CP, Larripa IB, De Brasi CD. Genotyping the hemophilia inversion hotspot by use of inverse PCR. Clin Chem 2005;51:1154-8.
549. Rossiter JP, Young M, Kimberland ML, Hutter P, Ketterling RP, Gitschier J, et al. Factor VIII gene inversions causing severe hemophilia A originate almost exclusively in male germ cells. Hum Mol Genet 1994;3:1035-9.
550. Rousseau E, Kojima R, Hoffner G, Djian P, Bertolotti A. Misfording of proteins with a polyglutamine expansion is facilitated by proteasomal chaperones. J Biol Chem 2009;284:1917-29.
551. Rousseau F, Bonaventure J, Legeai-Mallet L, Pelet A, Rozet JM, Maroteaux P, et al. Mutations in the gene encoding fibroblast growth factor receptor-3 in achondroplasia. Nature 1994;371:252-4.
552. Rousseau F, Heitz D, Tarleton J, MacPherson J, Malmgren H, Dahl N, et al. A multicenter study on genotype-phenotype correlations in the fragile X syndrome, using direct diagnosis with probe StB12.3: the first 2,253 cases. Am J Hum Genet 1994;55:225-37.
553. Rowe SM, Miller S, Sorscher EJ. Cystic fibrosis. N Engl J Med 2005; 352:1992-2001.
554. Roy N, Mahadevan MS, Mclean M, Shutler G, Yaraghi Z, Farahana R, et al. The gene for neuronal apoptosis inhibitory protein is partially deleted in individuals with spinal muscular atrophy. Cell 1995;80: 167-78.
555. Rubinsztein DC, Leggo J, Barton DE, Ferguson-Smith MA. Site of (CGG) polymorphism in the HD gene. Nat Genet 1993;5:214-5.
556. Sabirov RZ, Okada Y. ATP release via anion channels. Purinergic Signal 2005;1:311-28.
557. Sahoo T, del Gaudio D, German JR, Shinawi M, Peters SU, Person RE, et al. Prader-Willi phenotype caused by paternal deficiency for the HBII-85 C/D box small nucleolar RNA cluster. Nat Genet 2008;40: 719-21.

558. Saiki RK, Scharf S, Faloona F, Mullis KB, Horn GT, Erlich HA, et al. Enzymatic amplification of beta-globin genomic sequences and restriction site analysis for diagnosis of sickle cell anemia. Science 1985;230:1350-4.
559. Saiman L, Siegel J. Infection control in cystic fibrosis. Clin Microbiol Rev 2004;17:57-71.
560. Sampson JR, Jones S, Dolwani S, Cheadle JP. MutYH (MYH) and colorectal cancer. Biochem Soc Trans 2005;33:679-83.
561. Saul RA, Friez M, Eaves K, Stapleton GA, Collins JS, Schwartz CE, et al. Fragile X syndrome detection in newborns—pilot study. Genet Med 2008;10:714-9.
562. Saunus JM, French JD, Edwards SL, Beveridge DJ, Hatchell EC, Wagner SA, et al. Posttransciptional regulation of the breast cancer susceptibility gene *BRCA1* by the RNA binding protein Hur. Cancer Res 2008;68:9469-78.
563. Schechter MS, Shelton BJ, Margois PA, Fitzsimmons SC. The association of socioeconomic status with outcomes in cystic fibrosis patients in the United States. Am J Respir Crit Care Med 2001;163: 1331-7.
564. Schilling G, Sharp AH, Love SJ, Wagster MV, Li SH, Stine OC, et al. Expression of the Huntington's disease (IT15) protein product in HD patients. Hum Mol Genet 1995;4:1365-71.
565. Schmeler KM, Lu KH. Gynecologic cancers associated with Lynch syndrome/HNPCC. Clin Transl Oncol 2008;10:313-7.
566. Schoniger-Hekele M, Muller C, Polli C, Wrba F, Penner E, Ferenci P. Liver pathology in compound heterozygous patients for hemochromatosis mutations. Liver 2002;22:295-301.
567. Schrank B, Götz R, Gunnersen JM, Ure JM, Toyka KV, Smith AG, et al. Inactivation of the survival motor neuron gene, a candidate gene for human spinal muscular atrophy, leads to massive cell death in early mouse embryos. Proc Natl Acad Sci U S A 1997;94:9920-5.
568. Schwartz GF, Hughes KS, Lynch HT, Fabian CJ, Fentiman IS, Robson ME, et al. Proceedings of the International Consensus Conference on Breast Cancer Risk, Genetics, & Risk Management, April 2007. Cancer 2008;113:2627-37.
569. Schwartz M, Vissing J. Paternal inheritance of mitochondrial DNA. N Engl J Med 2002;347:576-80.
570. Schwartz M, Vissing J. New patterns of inheritance in mitochondrial disease. Biochem Biophys Res Commun 2003;310:247-51.
571. Schwiebert EM, Egan ME, Hwang TH, Fulmer SB, Allen SS, Cutting WB, et al. CFTR regulates outwardly rectifying chloride channels through an autocrine mechanism involving ATP. Cell 1995;82:1063-73.
572. Seeler RA, Vnencak-Jones CL, Bassett LM, Gilbert JB, Michaelis RC. Severe hemophilia A in a female: a compound heterozygote with nonrandom X-inactivation. Haemophilia 1999;5:445-9.
573. Segal JB, Brotman DJ, Necochea AJ, Emadi A, Samal L, Wilson LM, et al. Predictive value of factor V Leiden and prothrombin G20210A in adults with venous thromboembolism and in family members of those with a mutation: a systematic review. JAMA 2009;301:2472-85.
574. Senter L, Clendenning M, Sotamaa K, Hampel H, Green J, Potter JD, et al. The clinical phenotype of Lynch syndrome due to germ-line PMS2 mutations. Gastroenterology 2008;135:419-28.
575. Sermon K, De Rijcke M, Lissens W, De Vos A, Platteau P, Bonduelle M, et al. Preimplantation genetic diagnosis for Huntington's disease with exclusion testing. Eur J Hum Genet 2002;10:591-8.
576. Sermon K, Goossens V, Seneca S, Lissens W, De Vos A, Vanderborst M, et al. Preimplantation diagnosis for Huntington's disease (HD): clinical application and analysis of the HD expansion in affected embryos. Prenat Diagn 1998;18:1427-36.
577. Shapira AH. Mitochondrial disease. Lancet 2006;368:70-82.
578. Sharp JK, Rock MJ. Newborn screening for cystic fibrosis. Clin Rev Allergy Immunol 2008;35:107-15.
579. Sheridan MB, Fong P, Groman JD, Conrad C, Flume P, Diaz R, et al. Mutations in the beta-subunit of the epithelial Na^+ channel in patients with a cystic fibrosis-like syndrome. Hum Mol Genet 2005;14:3493-8.
580. Sherman S. Epidemiology. In: Hagerman RJ, Hagerman PJ, eds. Fragile X syndrome: diagnosis, treatment, and research. Baltimore: Johns Hopkins University Press, 2002:136-68.
581. Sherman SL. Premature ovarian failure among fragile X premutation carriers: parent of origin effect? Am J Hum Genet 2000;67:11-3.
582. Sherman SL, Jacobs PA, Morton NE, Froster-Iskenius U, Howard-Peebles PN, Nielsen KB, et al. Further segregation analysis of the fragile X syndrome with special reference to transmitting males. Hum Genet 1985;69:289-99.
583. Sherman SL, Meadows KL, Ashley AE. Examination of factors that influence the expansion of the fragile X mutation in a sample of conceptuses from known carrier females. Am J Med Genet 1996; 64:256-60.
584. Sherman SL, Morton NE, Jacobs PA, Turner G. The marker (X) syndrome: a cytogenetic and genetic analysis. Ann Hum Genet 1984;48:21-37.
585. Shia J. Immunohistochemistry versus microsatellite instability testing for screening colorectal cancer patients at risk for hereditary nonpolyposis colorectal cancer syndrome. Part I. The utility of immunohistochemistry. J Mol Diagn 2008;10:293-300.
586. Shiang R, Thompson LM, Zhu YZ, Church DM, Fielder TJ, Bocian M, et al. Mutations in the transmembrane domain of FGFR3 cause the most common genetic form of dwarfism, achondroplasia. Cell 1994; 78:335-42.
587. Shirio L, Otterud B, Stauffer D, Lynch H, Lynch P, Watson P, et al. Alleles of the APC gene: an attenuated form of familial polyposis. Cell 1993;75:951-7.
588. Silverstein MD, Heit JA, Mohr DN, Petterson TM, O'Fallon WM, Melton LJ. Trends in the incidence of deep vein thrombosis and pulmonary embolism: a 25-year population based cohort study. Arch Intern Med 1998;158:585-93.
589. Simic G. Pathogenesis of proximal autosomal recessive spinal muscular atrophy. Acta Neuropathol 2008;116:223-34.
590. Simon M, Bourel M, Fauchet R, Genete B. Association of HLA-A3 and HLA-B14 antigens with idiopathic haemochromatosis. Gut 1976;17:332-4.
591. Singaraja RR, Hadano S, Metzler M, Givan S, Wellington CL, Warby S, et al. HIP14, a novel ankyrin domain-containing protein, links huntingtin to intracellular trafficking and endocytosis. Hum Mol Genet 2002;11:2815-28.
592. Siomi H, Siomi MC, Nussbaum RL, Dreyfuss G. The protein product of the fragile X gene, *FMR1,* has characteristics of an RNA-binding protein. Cell 1993;74:291-8.
593. Smith KH, Johns DR, Heher KL, Miller NR. Heteroplasmy in Leber's hereditary optic neuropathy. Arch Ophthalmol 1993;111:1486-90.
594. Snell RG, MacMillan JC, Cheadle JP, Fenton I, Lazarou LP, Davies P, et al. Relationship between trinucleotide repeat expansion and phenotypic variation in Huntington's disease. Nat Genet 1993;4: 393-7.
595. Snow K, Doud LK, Hagerman R, Pergolizzi RG, Erster SH, Thibodeau SN. Analysis of CGG sequence at the FMR1 locus in fragile X families and in the general population. Am J Hum Genet 1993;53:1217-28.
596. Sobetzko D, Braga S, Rudeberg A, Superti-Furga A. Achondroplasia with the FGFR3 1138-g to a (G380R) mutation in two sibs sharing a 4p haplotype derived from their unaffected father. J Med Genet 2000; 37:958-9.
597. Sontag MK, Hammond KB, Zielenski J, Wagener JS, Accurso FJ. Two-tiered immunoreactive trypsinogen-based newborn screening for cystic fibrosis in Colorado: screening efficacy and diagnostic outcomes. J Pediatr 2005;147:S83-8.
598. Soubannier V, McBride HM. Positioning mitochondrial plasticity within cellular signaling cascades. Biochim Biophys Acta 2009;1793: 154-70.
599. Sovavia C, Berk T, Madlensky L, Mitri A, Cheng H, Gallinger S, et al. Genotype-phenotype correlations in attenuated adenomatous polyposis coli. Am J Hum Genet 1998;62:1290-301.
600. Sowter HM, Ashworth A. *BRCA1* and *BRCA2* as ovarian cancer susceptibility genes. Carcinogenesis 2005;26:1651-6.
601. Spearman AD, Sweet K, Zhou XP, McLennan J, Couch FJ, Toland AE. Clinically applicable models to characterize *BRCA1* and *BRCA2* variants of uncertain significance. J Clin Oncol 2008;26:5393-400.

602. Spits C, De Rycke M, Van Ranst N, Verpoest W, Lissens W, Van Steirteghem A, et al. Preimplantation genetic diagnosis for cancer predisposition syndromes. Prenat Diagn 2007;27:447-56.
603. Staff S, Isola J, Tanner M. Haplo-insufficiency of *BRCA1* in sporadic breast cancer. Cancer Res 2003;63:4978-83.
604. Staton AD, Kurian AW, Cobb K, Mills MA, Ford JM. Cancer risk reduction and reproductive concerns in female *BRCA1/2* mutation carriers. Fam Cancer 2008;7:179-86.
605. Stheneur C, Collod-Béroud G, Faivre L, Buyck JF, Gouya L, Le Parc JM, et al. Identification of the minimal combination of clinical features in probands for efficient mutation detection in the *FBN1* gene. Eur J Hum Genet 2009;17:1121-8.
606. Straub V, Campbell KP. Muscular dystrophies and the dystrophin-glycoprotein complex. Curr Opin Neurol 1997;10:168-75.
607. Strom CM, Crossley B, Redman JB, Buller A, Quan F, Peng M, et al. Cystic fibrosis screening: lessons learned from the first 320,000 patients. Genet Med 2004;6:136-40.
608. Strong TV, Wilkinson DJ, Mansoura MK, Devor DC, Henze K, Yang Y, et al. Expression of an abundant alternatively spliced form of the cystic fibrosis transmembrane conductance regulator *(CFTR)* gene is not associated with cAMP-activated chloride conductance. Hum Mol Genet 1993;2:225-30.
609. Stutts MJ, Canessa CM, Olsen JC, Hamrick M, Cohn JA, Rossier BC, et al. CFTR as a cAMP-dependent regulator of sodium channels. Science 1995;269:847-50.
610. Su YN, Hung CC, Li H, Cheng WF, Tsai PN, Chang MC, et al. Quantitative analysis of *SMN1* and *SMN2* genes based on DHPLC: a highly efficient and reliable carrier-screening test. Hum Mutat 2005;25:460-7.
611. Sugarman EA, Rohlfs EM, Silverman LM, Allitto BA. *CFTR* mutation distribution among U.S. Hispanic and African American individuals: evaluation in cystic fibrosis patient and carrier screening populations. Genet Med 2004;6:392-9.
612. Sullivan AK, Marcus M, Epstein MP, Allen EG, Anido AE, Paquin JJ, et al. Association of FMR1 repeat size with ovarian dysfunction. Hum Reprod 2005;20:402-12.
613. Sun Y, Nicholls RD, Butler MG, Saitoh S, Hainline BE, Palmer CG. Breakage in the SNRPN locus in a balanced 46,XY,t(15;19) Prader-Willi syndrome patient. Hum Mol Genet 1996;5:517-24.
614. Sutcliffe JS, Nelson DL, Zhang F, Pieretti M, Caskey CT, Saxe D, et al. DNA methylation represses FMR-1 transcription in fragile X syndrome. Hum Mol Genet 1992;1:397-400.
615. Swinkels DW, Janssen MC, Bergmans J, Marx JJ. Hereditary hemochromatosis: genetic complexity and new diagnostic approaches. Clin Chem 2006;52:950-68.
616. Szabo CI, King MC. Population genetics of *BRCA1* and *BRCA2*. Am J Hum Genet 1997;60:1013-20.
617. Szebenyi G, Fallon JF. Fibroblast growth factors as multifunctional signaling factors. Int Rev Cytol 1999;185:45-106.
618. Tabolacci E, Moscato U, Zalfa F, Bagni C, Chiurazzi P, Neri G. Epigenetic analysis reveals a euchromatic configuration in the *FMR1* unmethylated full mutations. Eur J Hum Genet 2008;16: 1487-98.
619. Tan DSP, Rothermundt C, Thomas K, Bancroft E, Eeles R, Shanley S, et al. "BRCAness" syndrome in ovarian cancer: a case-control study describing the clinical features and outcome of patients with epithelial ovarian cancer associated with *BRCA1* and *BRCA2* mutations. J Clin Oncol 2008;26:5530-6.
620. Tanaka M, Machida Y, Nukina N. A novel therapeutic strategy for polyglutamine diseases by stabilizing aggregation-prone proteins with small molecules. J Mol Med 2005;83:343-52.
621. Tavtigian SV, Simard J, Rommens J, Couch F, Shattuck-Eidens D, Neuhausen S, et al. The complete *BRCA2* gene and mutations in chromosome 13q-linked kindreds. Nat Genet 1996;12:333-7.
622. Taylor JE, Thomas NH, Lewis CM, Abbs SJ, Rodrigues NR, Davies KE, et al. Correlation of SMNt and SMNc gene copy number with age of onset and survival in spinal muscular atrophy. Eur J Hum Genet 1998;6:467-74.
623. ter Avest PC, Fischer K, Mancuso ME, Santagostino E, Yuste VJ, van den Berg HM, et al. Risk stratification for inhibitor development at first treatment for severe hemophilia A: a tool for clinical practice. J Thromb Haemost 2008;6:2048-54.
624. Thibodeau SN, Bren G, Schaid D. Microsatellite instability in cancer of the proximal colon. Science 1993;260:816-9.
625. Thomas G, Jacobs KB, Kraft P, Yeager M, Wacholder S, Cox DG, et al. A multistage genome-wide association study in breast cancer identifies two new risk alleles at 1p11.2 and 14q24.1 *(RAD51L1)*. Nat Genet 2009;41:579-84.
626. Thompson LM, Plummer S, Schalling M, Altherr MR, Gusella JF, Housman DE, et al. A gene encoding a fibroblast growth factor receptor isolated from the Huntington disease gene region of human chromosome 4. Genomics 1991;11:1133-42.
627. Tolttier Y, Devys D, Imbert G, Saudou G, An I, Lutz Y, et al. Protein cellular localization of the Huntington's disease protein and discrimination of the normal and mutated form. Nat Genet 1995;10: 104-10.
628. Tosetto A, Rodeghiero F, Martinelli I, De Stefano V, Missiaglia E, Chiusolo P, et al. Additional genetic risk factors for venous thromboembolism in carriers of the factor V Leiden mutation. Br J Haematol 1998;103:871-6.
629. Tournier I, Vezain M, Martins A, Charbonnier F, Baert-Desurmont S, Olschwang S, et al. A large fraction of unclassified variants of the mismatch repair genes *MLH1* and *MSH2* is associated with splicing defects. Hum Mutat 2008;29:1412-24.
630. Toyota M, Ahuja N, Ohe-Toyota M, Herman JG, Baylin SB, Issa JP. CpG island methylator phenotype in colorectal cancer. Proc Natl Acad Sci U S A 1999;96:8681-6.
631. Trembath MK, Tassicker RJ, Collins V, Mansie S, Sheffield LJ, Delatycki MB. Fifteen years of experience in predictive testing for Huntington disease at a single testing center in Victoria, Australia. Genet Med 2006;8:673-80.
632. Tsao CY, Herman G, Boue DR, Prior TW, Lo WD, Atkin JR, et al. Leigh disease with mitochondrial DNA A8344G mutation: case report and brief review. J Child Neurol 2003;18:62-4.
633. Tsui LC, Buchwald M, Barker D, Braman JC, Knowlton R, Schumm JW, et al. Cystic fibrosis locus defined by a genetically linked polymorphic DNA marker. Science 1985;230:1954-7.
634. Tuddenham EGD, Schwaab R, Seehafer J, Miller DS, Gitschiver J, Higuchi M, et al. Haemophilia A: database of nucleotide substitutions, deletions, insertions and rearrangements of the factor VIII gene, 2nd ed. Nucleic Acids Res 1994;22:3511-33.
635. Tuomainen TP, Kontula K, Nyyssonen K, Lakka TA, Helio T, Salonen JT. Increased risk of acute myocardial infarction in carriers of the hemochromatosis gene cyc282tyr mutation. Circulation 1999;100: 1274-9.
636. Turner CL, Emery H, Collins AL, Howarth RJ, Yearwood CM, Cross E, et al. Detection of 53 FBN1 mutations (41 novel and 12 recurrent) and genotype-phenotype correlations in 113 unrelated probands referred with Marfan syndrome, or a related fibrillinopathy. Am J Med Genet A 2009;149A:161-70.
637. Tutt A, Ashworth A. Can genetic testing guide treatment in breast cancer? Eur J Cancer 2008;44:2774-80.
638. Tyler A, Quarrell OWJ, Lazarou LP, Meredith AL, Harper PS. Exclusion testing in pregnancy for Huntington's disease. J Med Genet 1990;27:488-95.
639. Tzen CY, Wu TY, Liu HF. Sequence polymorphism in the coding region of mitochondrial genome encompassing position 8389-8865. Forensic Sci Int 2001;120:204-9.
640. Ulm J, Vnencak-Jones CL, Bosque P. Research on familial Creutzfeldt-Jacob disease (FCJD) resulting in presymptomatic testing: implications for the Human Genome Project. J Genet Counseling 1993;2:9-15.
641. Umar A, Boland CR, Terdiman JP, Syngal S, de la Chapelle A, Rüschoff J, et al. Revised Bethesda Guidelines for hereditary nonpolyposis colorectal cancer (Lynch syndrome) and microsatellite instability. J Natl Cancer Inst 2004;96:261-8.

642. Ünsal E, Aktaş Y, Üner Ö, Baltaci A, Özcan S, Turhan F, et al. Successful application of preimplantation genetic diagnosis for Leigh syndrome. Fertil Steril 2008;90:2017e11-3.
643. The U.S.-Venezuela Collaborative Research Project, Wexler NS. Venezuelan kindreds reveal that genetic and environmental factors modulate Huntington's disease age of onset. Proc Natl Acad Sci U S A 2004;101:3498-503.
644. Valleix S, Vinciguerra C, Lavergne JM, Leuer M, Delpech M, Negrier C. Skewed X-chromosome inactivation in monochorionic diamniotic twin sisters results in severe and mild hemophilia A. Blood 2002;100: 3034-6.
645. van der Luijt R, Meera Khan P, Vasen HFA, Breukel C, Tops CM, Scott RJ, et al. Germline mutations in the 3′ part of APC exon 15 do not result in truncated proteins and are associated with attenuated adenomatous polyposis coli. Hum Genet 1996;98: 727-34.
646. van der Steege G, Grootscholten PM, van der Vlies P, Draaijers TG, Osinga J, Cobben JM, et al. PCR-based DNA test to confirm clinical diagnosis of autosomal recessive spinal muscular atrophy. Lancet 1995;345:985-6.
647. Vandenbroucke JP, Koster T, Briet E, Reitsma PH, Bertina RM, Rosendaal FR. Increased risk of venous thrombosis in oral-contraceptive users who are carriers of factor V Leiden mutation. Lancet 1994;344:1453-7.
648. Váradi K, Rosing J, Tans G, Pabinger I, Keil B, Schwarz HP. Factor V enhances the cofactor function of protein S in the APC-mediated inactivation of factor VIII: influence of the factor VR506Q mutation. Thromb Haemost 1996;76:208-14.
649. Vasen HF, Mecklin JP, Khan PM, Lynch HT. The International Collaborative Group on Hereditary Non-Polyposis CRC (ICG-HNPCC). Dis Colon Rectum 1991;34:424-5.
650. Vasen HFA, Moslein G, Alonso A, Aretz S, Bernstein I, Bertario L, et al. Guidelines for the clinical management of familial adenomatous polyposis (FAP). Gut 2008;57:704-13.
651. Vasen HFA, Watson P, Mecklin JP, Lynch HT, The International Collaborative Group on HNPCC. New clinical criteria for hereditary nonpolyposis colorectal cancer (Lynch syndrome) proposed by the International Collaborative Group on HNPCC. Gastroenterology 1999;116:1453-6.
652. Vehar GA, Keyt B, Eaton D, Rodriguez H, O'Brien DP, Rotblat F, et al. Structure of human factor VIII. Nature 1984;312:337-42.
653. Vehmanen P, Friedman LS, Eerola H, McClure M, Ward B, Sarantaus L, et al. Low proportion of *BRCA1* and *BRCA2* mutations in Finnish breast cancer families: evidence for additional susceptibility genes. Hum Mol Genet 1997;6:2309-15.
654. Velázquez-Wong AC, Hernández-Huerta C, Márquez-Calixto A, Hernández-Aguilar FO, Rodríguez-Cruz M, Salamanca-Gómez F, et al. Identification of Duchenne muscular dystrophy female carriers by fluorescence in situ hybridization and RT-PCR. Genet Testing 2008;12:221-3.
655. Velier J, Kim M, Schwarz C, Kim TW, Sapp E, Chase K, et al. Wild-type and mutant huntingtins function in vesicle trafficking in the secretory and endocytic pathways. Exp Neurol 1998;152: 34-40.
656. Velinov M, Jenkins EC. PCR-based strategies for the diagnosis of Prader-Willi/Angelman syndromes. Methods Mol Biol 2003;217: 209-16.
657. Velinov M, Slaugenhaupt SA, Stoilov I, Scott CI, Gusella JF, Tsipouras P. The gene for achondroplasia maps to the telomeric region of chromosome 4p. Nat Genet 1994;6:314-7.
658. Veltman MWM, Craig EE, Bolton PF. Autism spectrum disorders in Prader-Willi and Angelman syndromes: a systematic review. Psychiatr Genet 2005;15:243-54.
659. Verellen-Domoulin C, Freund M, de Meyer T, Laterre C, Frederic J, Thompson MW, et al. Expression of an X-linked muscular dystrophy in a female due to translocation involving Xp21 and non random X-inactivation. Hum Genet 1984;67:115-9.
660. Verkerk AJ, Pieretti M, Sutcliffe JS, Fu YH, Kuhl DP, Pizzuti A, et al. Identification of a gene *(FMR-1)* containing a CGG repeat coincident with a breakpoint cluster region exhibiting length variation in fragile X syndrome. Cell 1991;65:905-14.
661. Verkman AS, Galietta LJ. Chloride channels as drug targets. Nat Rev Drug Discov 2009;8:153-171.
662. Viiala NO, Larsen SR, Rasko JE. Gene therapy for hemophilia: clinical trials and technical tribulations. Semin Thromb Hemost 2009;35: 81-92.
663. Vilkki J, Savontaus ML, Nikoskelainen EK. Segregation of mitochondrial genomes in a heteroplasmic lineage with Leber hereditary optic neuroretinopathy. Am J Hum Genet 1990;47:95-100.
664. Vnencak-Jones CL. Fluorescence PCR and GeneScan analysis for the detection of CAG repeat expansions associated with Huntington's disease. Methods Mol Biol 2003;217:101-10.
665. Vnencak-Jones CL, Phillips JA, Janco RL, Cohen MP, Dupont WD, Kazazian HH, et al. Analysis of factor VIII gene inversion mutations in 166 unrelated haemophilia A families: frequency and utility in genetic counseling. Haemophilia 1996;2:18-23.
666. Vogelstein B, Kinzler KW. Cancer genes and the pathways they control. Nat Med 2004;10:789-99.
667. Vu TH, Hoffman AR. Imprinting of the Angelman syndrome gene, *UBE3A,* is restricted to brain. Nat Genet 1997;17:12-3.
668. Waelter S, Scherzinger E, Hasenbank R, Nordhoff E, Lurz R, Goehler H, et al. The huntingtin interacting protein HIP1 is a clathrin and alpha-adaptin-binding protein involved in receptor-mediated endocytosis. Hum Mol Genet 2001;10:1807-17.
669. Waheed A, Parkkila S, Zhou XY, Tomatsu S, Tsuchihashi Z, Feder JN. Hereditary hemochromatosis: effects of C282Y and H63D mutations on association with B2-microglobulin, intracellular processing, and cell surface expression of the HFE protein in COS-cells. Proc Natl Acad Sci U S A 1997;94:12384-9.
670. Waite A, Tinsley CL, Locke M, Blake DJ. The neurobiology of the dystrophin-associated glycoprotein complex. Ann Med 2009;41: 344-59.
671. Wallace DC, Singh G, Lott MT, Hodge JA, Schurr TG, Lezza AMS, et al. Mitochondrial DNA mutation associated with Leber's hereditary optic neuropathy. Science 1988;242:1427-30.
672. Walon C, Kartheuser A, Michils G, Smaers M, Lannoy N, Ngounou P, et al. Novel germline mutations in the *APC* gene and their phenotypic spectrum in familial adenomatous polyposis kindreds. Hum Genet 1997;100:601-5.
673. Wang B, Li J, Xiao X. Adeno-associated virus vector carrying human minidystrophin genes effectively ameliorates muscular dystrophy in mdx mouse model. Proc Natl Acad Sci U S A 2000;97:13714-9.
674. Wang CC, Chang JG, Jong YJ, Wu SM. Universal multiplex PCR and CE for quantification of *SMN1/SMN2* genes in spinal muscular atrophy. Electrophoresis 2009;30:1102-10.
675. Wang H, Lim PJ, Karbowski M, Monteiro MJ. Effects of overexpression of Huntingtin proteins on mitochondrial integrity. Hum Mol Genet 2009;18:737-52.
676. Wang H, Wu LJ, Kim SS, Lee FJS, Gong B, Toyoda H, et al. FMRP acts as a key messenger of dopamine modulation in the forebrain. Neuron 2008;59:634-47.
677. Wanker EE, Rovira C, Scherzinger E, Hasenbank R, Walter S, Tait D, et al. HIP-I: a huntingtin interacting protein isolated by the yeast two-hybrid system. Hum Mol Genet 1997;6:487-95.
678. Warby SC, Montpetit A, Hayden AR, Carroll JB, Butland SL, Visscher H, et al. CAG expansion in the Huntington disease gene is associated with a specific and targetable predisposing haplogroup. Am J Hum Genet 2009;84:351-66.
679. Warner JP, Barron LH, Brock DJH. A new polymerase chain reaction (PCR) assay for the trinucleotide repeat that is unstable and expanded on Huntington's disease chromosomes. Mol Cell Probes 1993;7:235-9.
680. Wasmuth JJ, Hewitt J, Smith B, Allard D, Haines JL, Skarecky D, et al. A highly polymorphic locus very tightly linked to the Huntington's disease gene. Nature 1988;332:734-6.

681. Watihayati MS, Fatemeh H, Marini M, Atif AB, Zahiruddin WM, Sasongko TH, et al. Combination of SMN2 copy number and NAIP deletion predicts disease severity in spinal muscular atrophy. Brain Dev 2009;31:42-5.
682. Watson MS, Cutting GR, Desnick RJ, Driscoll DA, Klinger K, Mennuti M, et al. Cystic fibrosis population carrier screening: 2004 revision of American College of Medical Genetics mutation panel. Genet Med 2004;6:387-91.
683. Webb T, Maina EN, Soni S, Whittington J, Boer H, Clarke D, et al. In search of the psychosis gene in people with Prader-Willi syndrome. Am J Med Genet A 2008;146A:843-53.
684. Weischer M, Juul K, Zacho J, Jensen GB, Steffensen R, Schroeder TV, et al. Prothrombin and risk of venous thromboembolism, ischemic heart disease and ischemic cerebrovascular disease in the general population. Atherosclerosis 2010;208:480-3.
685. Weiss FU, Simon P, Bogdanova N, Mayerle J, Dworniczak B, Horst J, et al. Complete cystic fibrosis transmembrane conductance regulator gene sequencing in patients with idiopathic chronic pancreatitis and controls. Gut 2005;54:1456-60.
686. Wells RD. Mutation spectra in fragile X syndrome induced by deletions of CGG.CCG repeats. J Biol Chem 2009;284:7407-11.
687. Wells RD, Dere R, Hebert ML, Napierala M, Son LS. Advances in mechanisms of genetic instability related to hereditary neurological diseases. Nucleic Acids Res 2005;33:3785-98.
688. Welsh MJ, Smith AE. Molecular mechanisms of CFTR chloride channel dysfunction in cystic fibrosis. Cell 1993;73:1251-4.
689. Wevrick R, Kerns JA, Francke U. Identification of a novel paternally expressed gene in the Prader-Willi syndrome region. Hum Mol Genet 1994;3:1877-82.
690. Wexler NS, Young AB, Tanzi RE, Travers H, Starosta-Rubinstein SS, Penney JB, et al. Homozygotes for Huntington's disease. Nature 1987;326:194-7.
691. Whitcombe D, Brownie J, Gillard HL, McKechnie D, Theaker J, Newton CR, et al. A homogeneous fluorescence assay for PCR amplicons: its application to real-time, single-tube genotyping. Clin Chem 1998;44:918-23.
692. Wilkin DJ, Szabo JK, Cameron R, Henderson S, Bellus GA, Mack ML, et al. Mutations in fibroblast growth-factor receptor 3 in sporadic cases of achondroplasia occur exclusively on the paternally derived chromosome. Am J Hum Genet 1998;63:711-6.
693. Williamson D, Brown K, Luddington R, Baglin C, Baglin T. Factor V Cambridge: a new mutation (Arg306-Thr) associated with resistance to activated protein C. Blood 1998;91:1140-4.
694. Willis L, Roosevelt GE, Yetman AT. Comparison of clinical characteristics and frequency of adverse outcomes in patients with Marfan syndrome diagnosed in adulthood versus childhood. Pediatr Cardiol 2009;30:289-92.
695. Wimmer, K, Etzler J. Constitutional mismatch repair-deficiency syndrome: have we so far seen only the tip of an iceberg? Hum Genet 2008;124:105-22.
696. Windsor S, Lyng A, Taylor SAM, Ewenstein BM, Neufeld EJ, Lillicrap D. Severe haemophilia A in a female resulting from two de novo factor VIII mutations. Br J Haematol 1995;90:906-9.
697. Winkler C, Eggert C, Gradl D, Meister G, Giegerich M, Wedlich D, et al. Reduced U snRNP assembly causes motor axon degeneration in an animal model for spinal muscular atrophy. Genes Dev 2005;19: 2320-30.
698. Wion KL, Tuddenham EGD, Lawn RM. A new polymorphism in the factor VIII gene for prenatal diagnosis of hemophilia A. Nucleic Acid Res 1986;14:4535-42.
699. Witte DL, Crosby WH, Edwards CQ, Fairbanks VF, Mitros FA. Practice guideline development task force of the College of American Pathologists: hereditary hemochromatosis. Clin Chim Acta 1996;245: 139-200.
700. Wittenberger MD, Hagerman RJ, Sherman SL, McConkie-Rosell A, Welt CK, Rebar RW, et al. The FMR1 premutation and reproduction. Fertil Steril 2007;87:456-65.
701. Woerner SM, Kloor M, Mueller A, Rueschoff J, Friedrichs N, Buetnner R, et al. Microsatellite instability of selective target genes in HNPCC-associated colon adenomas. Oncogene 2005;24:2525-35.
702. Wong LJ. Pathogenic mitochondrial DNA mutations in protein-coding genes. Muscle Nerve 2007;36:279-93.
703. Wong LJC, Liang MH, Kwon H, Park J, Bai RK, Tan DJ. Comprehensive scanning of the entire mitochondrial genome for mutations. Clin Chem 2002;48:1901-2.
704. Wood MJ, Powell LW, Ramm GA. Environmental and genetic modifiers of the progression to fibrosis and cirrhosis in hemochromatosis. Blood 2008;111:4456-62.
705. Wooster R, Bignell G, Lancaster J, Swift S, Seal S, Mangion J, et al. Identification of the breast cancer susceptibility gene *BRCA2*. Nature 1995;378:789-92.
706. Wooster R, Neuhausen SL, Mangion J, Quirk Y, Ford D, Collins N, et al. Localization of a breast cancer susceptibility gene, *BRCA2*, to chromosome 13q12-13. Science 1994;265:2088-90.
707. Wynn J, King TM, Bambello MJ, Waller DK, Hecht JT. Mortality in achondroplasia study: a 42-year follow-up. Am J Med Genet A 2007;143A:2502-11.
708. Yamamoto Y, Huibregtse JM, Howley PM. The human E6-AP gene *(UBE3A)* encodes three potential protein isoforms generated by differential splicing. Genomics 1997;41:263-6.
709. Yazaki M, Yoshida K, Nakamura A, Koyama J, Nanba T, Ohori N, et al. Clinical characteristics of aged Becker muscular dystrophy patients with onset after 30 years. Eur Neurol 1999;42:145-9.
710. Yoshioka M, Yorifuji T, Mituyoshi I. Skewed X inactivation in manifesting carriers of Duchenne muscular dystrophy. Clin Genet 1998;52:102-7.
711. Yu S, Pritchard M, Kremer E, Lynch M, Nancarrow J, Baker E, et al. Fragile X genotype characterized by an unstable region of DNA. Science 1991;252:1179-81.
712. Yu-Wai-Man P, Griffiths PG, Hudson G, Chinnery PF. Inherited mitochondrial optic neuropathies. J Med Genet 2009;46:145-58.
713. Zapletalová E, Hedvičáková P, Kozák L, Vondráček P, Gaillyová R, Maříková T, et al. Analysis of point mutations in the SMN1 gene in SMA patients bearing a single SMN1 copy. Neuromuscul Disord 2007;17:476-81.
714. Zatz M, Vianna-Morgante AM, Campos P, Diament AJ. Translocation (X;6) in a female with Duchenne muscular dystrophy, implications for the localization of the DMD locus. J Med Genet 1981;18:442-7.
715. Zehnder JL, Benson RC. Sensitivity and specificity of the APC resistance assay in detection of individuals with factor V Leiden. Am J Clin Pathol 1996;106:107-11.
716. Zeviani M, Moraes CT, DiMauro S, Nakase H, Bonilla E, Schon EA, et al. Deletions of mitochondrial DNA in Kearns-Sayre syndrome. Neurology 1988;38:1339-46.
717. Zhang H, Xing L, Rossoll W, Wichterle H, Singer RH, Bassell GJ. Multiprotein complexes of the survival of motor neuron protein SMN with Gemins traffic to neuronal processes and growth cones of motor neurons. J Neurosci 2006;26:8622-32.
718. Zhang L. Immunohistochemistry versus microsatellite instability testing for screening colorectal cancer patients at risk for hereditary nonpolyposis colorectal cancer syndrome. Part II. The utility of microsatellite instability testing. J Mol Diagn 2008;10:301-7.
719. Zhang Y, Engelman J, Friedlander RM. Allele-specific silencing of mutant Huntington's disease gene. J Neurochem 2009;108: 82-90.
720. Zhang Z, Lotti F, Dittmar K, Younis I, Wan L, Kasim M, et al. SMN deficiency causes tissue-specific perturbations in the repertoire of snRNAs and widespread defects in splicing. Cell 2008;133: 585-600.
721. Zhi X, Szabo C, Chopin S, Suter N, Wang QS, Ostrander EA, et al. *BRCA1* and *BRCA2* sequence variants in Chinese breast cancer families. Hum Mutat 2002;20:474.
722. Zielenski J. Genotype and phenotype in cystic fibrosis. Respiration 2000;67:117-33.

723. Zivelin A, Griffin JH, Xiao X, Pabinger I, Samama M, Conard J, et al. A single origin for a common Caucasian risk factor for venous thrombosis. Blood 1997;89:397-402.
724. Zivelin A, Mor-Cohen R, Kovalsky V, Kornbrot N, Conard J, Peyvandi F, et al. Prothrombin 20210G>A is an ancestral prothrombotic mutation that occurred in whites approximately 24,000 years ago. Blood 2006;107:4666-8.
725. Zuccato C, Tartari M, Crotti A, Goffredo D, Valenza M, Conti L, et al. Huntingtin interacts with REST/NRSF to modulate the transcript of NRSE-controlled neuronal genes. Nat Genet 2003;35:76-83.

CHAPTER 41

Identity Assessment

Thomas M. Williams, M.D., Howard J. Baum, Ph.D., Victor W. Weedn, M.D., J.D., and Malek Kamoun, M.D., Ph.D.

Identity testing exploits variations present within the human genome to distinguish among individuals. Identity assessment has six basic uses: (1) to confirm or refute that a sample is from a specific person in forensic testing; (2) to identify unknown human remains or victims of a mass disaster; (3) to resolve questions regarding the identity of a clinical specimen; (4) to select donors for a planned transplant recipient to minimize rejection and improve graft survival via histocompatibility testing; (5) to assess whether hematopoietic cells are donor- or recipient-derived following stem cell transplantation; and (6) to identify the parents of a child.

VARIATION IN THE HUMAN GENOME

Identity testing began with the use of serologic methods to identify variations in proteins that differ among individuals. The discovery of the genetic basis for these protein differences and of genetic variability at loci not encoding proteins, coupled with technical advances, allowed the field to move to direct analysis of DNA. Genetic variation among individuals is extensive, with about one sequence difference for every 400 to 1250 nucleotides on autosomal chromosomes. Variants of a genetic locus in a population are referred to as *alleles.* A locus is said to be polymorphic when the least common allele has a frequency ≥0.01 in a population. Although several alleles may be found in a population for an autosomal locus, an individual may have at most two alleles at that locus. Individuals may have one or two alleles for X-linked loci.

Genetic Variation Useful in Identity Testing

Several classes of genetic variants are found in the genome; some are more useful than others for identity testing. Most of the variants used occur in the noncoding genetic regions, such as introns, regulatory domains, and regions between genes, whereas some variants occur in gene domains transcribed into RNA, that is, the exons. Highly repetitive sequence elements that contribute to the structure of centromeres and telomeres and hundreds of thousands of copies of transposable elements that move about the genome over time may vary among individuals. However, these repetitive sequence elements generally are not useful for identity testing.

Several million single-nucleotide polymorphisms (SNPs) have been identified in the genome (see Chapter 38). A subset of SNPs can be identified based on the ability of a restriction endonuclease to digest double-stranded DNA at the site of the variation. These SNPs are referred to as restriction fragment length polymorphisms (RFLPs). SNPs and most RFLPs are not very useful for identity testing because they usually have only two alleles.

Variable numbers of tandem repeat loci (VNTRs) or minisatellite loci consist of repeated sequences of DNA. The core sequence is from 8 to 80 nucleotides long. The core is repeated from 4 to 40 times, thus forming 4 to 40 alleles. The allele size difference can be detected as an RFLP if the locus containing the VNTR is digested with a restriction endonuclease, which cuts the DNA outside of the VNTR, and the resulting restriction fragments are hybridized to a labeled DNA probe in Southern hybridization assays. VNTRs are attractive for identity testing, because the loci usually have a number of different alleles with relatively high allele frequencies. Minisatellite regions are commonly near the telomeric end of the chromosome and have core repeats of 8 to 80 base pair lengths, resulting in DNA fragment lengths of 0.5 to >20 kilobases.

Short tandem repeat (STR) or microsatellite loci consist of DNA sequence motifs that have core repeats of two to seven base pairs.[6,15] Examples include the dinucleotide 5′ CACACACA 3′ and the tetranucleotide 5′ TTTATTTATTTA 3′. Thousands of STRs are scattered throughout the genome. Because they are flanked by unique sequences, each can be specifically amplified with the polymerase chain reaction (PCR) for analysis. In populations of individuals, multiple alleles may be present based on differences in the numbers of repeated motifs at the locus. STRs have many characteristics that make them ideal for identity testing: (1) they can be analyzed in fluorescent automated systems; (2) alleles can be assigned in a definitive manner following analysis; (3) STR loci are almost always transmitted in families in a Mendelian fashion; (4) the loci may have 10 or more alleles, often with substantial allele frequencies, making them highly informative and making it easier to resolve mixtures of DNA; and (5) extensive information is available about allele frequencies in many human populations for STRs commonly used in identity testing.[7]

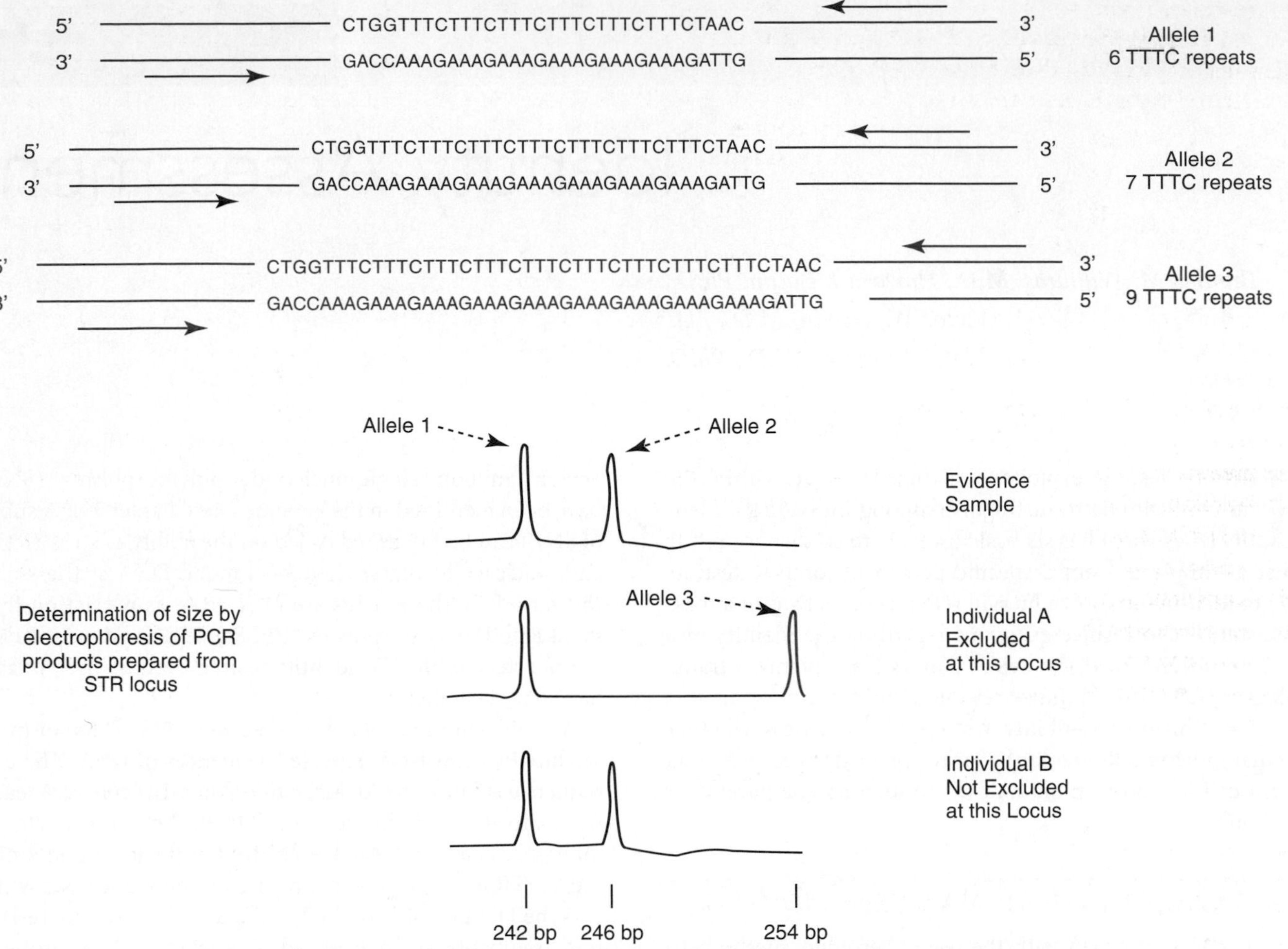

Figure 41-1 Identity testing via short tandem repeat (STR) analysis. An STR locus can be specifically amplified with the polymerase chain reaction (PCR) using primers binding to unique sequences adjacent to the repeat motif in the genome. In the example shown, the polymorphic repeat is the tetramer TTTC. Three example alleles with 6, 7, and 9 repeats at this locus are shown. The genotype for an individual or for an evidence sample can be determined by performing PCR with a fluorescently labeled primer and sizing the products on a high-resolution gel with laser detection. PCR products should differ in size from each other by multiples of 4 nucleotides (nt). Use of several fluorescent dyes and PCR products of different sizes allows multiplexing for simultaneous assessment of a number of independently segregating STR loci.

Commercially available STR systems employ tetrameric and pentameric repeat loci, which produce fewer artifactual bands and are characterized by roughly equal amplification of both alleles within an individual (Figure 41-1). Fragments can be labeled during PCR amplification with fluorescently tagged primers that facilitate multiplexing.

Apart from STRs distributed across the whole genome, two special genetic regions with sufficient sequence variability for identity testing include the human leukocyte antigen (HLA) loci within the major histocompatibility complex (MHC) and mitochondrial DNA. The HLA loci described in the "Transplantation Testing" section later in this chapter are interesting in that the polymorphisms are densely packed and are preferentially located in the exons rather than the introns of these genes on chromosome 6. Mitochondrial genome variation is also useful in forensic identity testing and is described in that section.

Exclusion of Tested Individuals

Identity testing frequently excludes the tested person with almost absolute reliability. Exclusion results can indicate that a suspect did not commit a murder or rape, or that an alleged man did not father a child. The exclusion is based on the presence of alleles at a locus that make it impossible for him or her to be a contributor to the tested sample. For example, if the person has the alleles j and k at the autosomal locus L, then, in the absence of mutations, it is not possible for him to be the major contributor to an evidence sample with the alleles m and n at L, or to be the father of a child with the alleles m and p at L. In practice, laboratory protocols require that exclusion be based on incompatible results for at least two loci to rule out mutation events or other sources of error. In this context, "impossible" implies a situation in which samples have been collected correctly and have not been mislabeled, testing has been performed accurately, and results have been interpreted and reported appropriately.

Likelihood of Inclusion of Tested Individuals

If a tested individual has genotypes at several loci that are identical to the genotypes found in an evidence sample, then that person is not excluded as the contributor to the sample. Inclusion of a tested individual in identity testing is based on a probability calculation that relies on knowledge of the allele frequencies in human populations for the tested loci. For each locus, the likelihood that a random person of relevant ethnicity would have a genotype identical to that found in the evidence sample can be calculated. If the tested loci independently segregate during meiosis, the overall probability that a random person rather than the accused is responsible can be calculated by multiplying the likelihoods for each locus. When several loci are tested and each has many possible alleles, it becomes extremely likely that an individual whose genotypes match those found in the evidence sample is the person who contributed the DNA to the sample. For genetically linked systems such as mitochondrial DNA testing or Y chromosome STRs, inclusion statistics are calculated using the upper bound confidence level of the database frequency of the entire haplotype. In these systems, the loci do not independently segregate during meiosis.

Discriminatory power is the ability of an identity testing system to distinguish an individual or group from the rest of the population. The power of discrimination of a locus or testing system should not be confused with accuracy. ABO blood group typing is accurate but poorly discriminating, in that this locus results in only a few phenotypes of generally high frequency in populations. Current identity test systems that employ a number of highly polymorphic loci may have powers of discrimination that exceed 1×10^{-14}, making it very unlikely that any unrelated individual on earth other than a nonexcluded suspect or his identical twin could be the source of an evidence sample. However, likelihoods of this magnitude should be viewed with knowledge that a variety of potential problems extraneous to the testing technology, involving sample collection and labeling and test interpretation and reporting, may lead to an erroneous result.

Parentage calculations are often performed using Bayesian methods that consider the prior probability that an individual is the father of a child. It is obvious, for example, that the prior probability of a man living in Boston is the father of a coworker's child is much greater than that of a Beijing inhabitant with no overt connection to the mother. Most crime laboratories in the United States do not report calculations using Bayesian analyses, but instead report population phenotypic frequencies for Caucasian, African American, and Hispanic populations, and sometimes a likelihood ratio that an individual is the source of a DNA specimen. Many times, forensic evidence samples contain a mixture of DNA because they are collected in the real world and not under controlled laboratory conditions. In a mixed sample, if the individual constituents of the mixture cannot be separated, a forensic laboratory will calculate a likelihood ratio or a probability of exclusion, which determines the percentage of the population who could not contribute to the mixture. When questions arise regarding assumptions that must be made during the calculation of inclusion probabilities, laboratories generally choose the conservative option that favors the accused individual.

Samples Employed for Identity Testing

A sample for identity testing can be any specimen that contains DNA. Samples obtained from an individual for parentage testing or as a reference sample to be compared with DNA prepared from evidence are usually peripheral blood or buccal mucosa or objects contaminated with human cellular remains or body fluids. Samples useful for forensic testing, engraftment assays, and the identification of clinical samples may range from plucked hairs to dried biological fluid stains to bone marrow aspirates to paraffin-embedded tissue. Although subject to degradation over time in the presence of enzymes, acidic or basic conditions, or high temperature, DNA is a remarkably stable molecule that can be recovered and successfully analyzed from solutions, surfaces, and cells, sometimes decades or centuries after it was deposited.

FORENSIC DNA TYPING

DNA testing has revolutionized criminalistics.[19,33] Only fingerprint evidence can sometimes rival the ability of DNA as trace evidence left at a scene to identify a perpetrator. As a general rule, other trace evidence merely links an article, instrument, or material to a scene. The origin of DNA-based identity testing is generally traced to a 1985 article in *Nature* by Alec Jeffreys.[18] He coined the term "DNA fingerprint" and suggested that the hybridization of DNA probes to polymorphic genetic loci could be exploited for forensic purposes. Jeffreys first applied his techniques to civil and criminal cases in England. In the United States, DNA-based identity testing was introduced via commercial laboratories and later the Federal Bureau of Investigation (FBI). Today approximately 200 forensic DNA typing laboratories have been established in the United States, along with many other DNA laboratories around the globe. Forensic DNA testing is also used to identify decomposed unknown human remains through kinship analysis and can be used to identify victims of a mass disaster.[4]

Forensic Applications

Forensic testing differs from clinical laboratory testing in several ways: (1) the forensic question is usually one of identity rather than one of presence or absence of a trait or analyte quantification, as is done in most clinical laboratory analyses; (2) specimens received by forensic laboratories are much

TABLE 41-1 DNA Typing Systems and Their Characteristics

Genetic Systems	Time Frame	PCR-Based	Discrimination	Comments
RFLP analysis of VNTRs	1980s-1990s	–	++++	Labor intensive
PCR dot-blots	1980s-1990s	+	+	Limited discrimination
STRs	Mid-1990s to present	+	++++	Current mainstay
mtDNA	Mid-1990s to present	+	++	Used in hairs, skeletons
Y-markers	1998 to present	+	++	Male DNA
Alu repeats	Not yet in use	+	++	Population marker
SNPs	Not yet in use	+	+++	Useful for samples with highly degraded DNA

mtDNA, Mitochondrial DNA; *PCR,* polymerase chain reaction; *RFLP,* restriction fragment length polymorphism; *SNPs,* single-nucleotide polymorphisms; *STRs,* short tandem repeats; *VNTRs,* variable numbers of tandem repeat loci.

more diverse than the typical blood, fluid, and tissue samples handled by clinical laboratories; (3) clinical samples are collected under controlled circumstances, while evidence from which DNA must be isolated may be exposed to the environment in a variety of ways. This can lead to degradation of the sample. Experiments may be necessary to validate testing for a particular case; (4) forensic samples may include a mixture of DNA such as a vaginal swab containing female epithelial cells and sperm from one or more donors. In addition, a surface may contain more than one biological fluid such as blood from a victim and saliva from someone else; (5) evidentiary material cannot be replenished and may be present in only trace amounts. Testing may consume the sample, and thus complete or repeat testing may be impossible; and (6) forensic identity testing is scrutinized in a judicial environment, requiring complete accounting for chain of custody following its collection and strict validation of procedures.

Most other laboratories perform routine analyses of samples collected in defined ways. Forensic identity testing must contend with much greater variability in samples and testing conditions.

Genetic Systems Used in Forensic Identification

Numerous genetic systems that are employed by forensic laboratories are summarized in Table 41-1.[3,24]

VNTR Analysis by RFLP

Jeffreys described a method to create a barcode-like DNA fingerprint based on VNTRs. Because the probes used bind to several loci in Southern hybridization experiments and produce numerous bands per probe, they are termed *multilocus probes.* In the United States, laboratories have preferred single-locus probe (SLP) systems that hybridize only to a single genetic locus. However, Southern hybridization–based RFLP analysis is expensive, labor intensive, difficult to automate, and less sensitive than PCR-based methods. Finally, RFLP is sensitive to DNA degradation—an important issue with environmentally exposed forensic specimens. RFLP tests have been largely abandoned in favor of the more efficient PCR-based assays discussed later.[5]

Short Tandem Repeats

Most identity testing performed today relies on the PCR. PCR testing is inherently sensitive, allowing routine analysis of nanogram quantities of genomic DNA and often successful testing of picogram quantities (one cell contains 5 to 10 pg of DNA). Low copy number (LCN) STR analysis[8] detects quantities of DNA down to the single cell level PCR, which underlies the characterization of STR and other loci for forensic identity testing loci described in this and later sections.

STR testing is quick, less expensive, more forgiving with respect to technical skills needed, less sensitive to DNA degradation, and more amenable to automation in comparison with the Southern hybridization methods described earlier. Although less discriminating than RFLP genetic markers, STR analysis can be made as powerful as Southern RFLP analysis through the use of large numbers of informative loci.

The National Institute of Justice provided funding for the initial application of STRs in forensics. STRs were used in forensic casework during the first Persian Gulf War and were widely adopted for testing by forensic laboratories in the United Kingdom and the United States in the mid to late 1990s.

The FBI laboratory's combined DNA index system (CODIS) blends forensic science and computer technology into an effective tool for investigating violent crimes. CODIS enables federal, state, and local crime laboratories to exchange and compare DNA profiles electronically, thereby linking crimes to each other and to convicted offenders. The FBI convened a panel of forensic scientists in 1998 that chose a panel of 13 STR loci for use in the National DNA Index System. These 13 core loci have become the standard for casework and databanking for most forensic laboratories around the world (Table 41-2). They have been commercialized as kits in a variety of formats. STRs are now routinely used in crime laboratories globally and typically yield discriminatory values of one in trillions to sextillions.

Low copy number STR testing is currently being used in the United Kingdom, Australia, New Zealand, and the United States. Its extreme sensitivity is both an advantage and a disadvantage. Very small samples can be detected, but because of the small amounts of DNA analyzed, the system suffers

TABLE 41-2 List of Short Tandem Repeat (STR) Core Loci

Core Loci	Currently Available Commercial STR Kits		
	MiniFiler	**Identifiler**	**Powerplex 16**
D3S1358		D3S1358	D3S1358
D5S818		D5S818	D5S818
D7S820	D7S820	D7S820	D7S820
D8S1170		D8S1170	D8S1170
D13S317	D13S317	D13S317	D13S317
D16S539	D16S539	D16S539	D16S539
D18S51	D18S51	D18S51	D18S51
D21S11	D21S11	D21S11	D21S11
CSF1PO	CSF1PO	CSF1PO	CSF1PO
FGA	FGA	FGA	FGA
THO1		THO1	THO1
TPOX		TPOX	TPOX
vWA		vWA	vWA
	D2S1338	D2S1338	Penta D
		D19S433	Penta E
	Amelogenin	Amelogenin	Amelogenin

The 13 STR core loci are listed against the STR systems present in currently available commercial STR kits. Identifiler and MiniFiler are available from Applied Biosystems, Inc. (Foster City, Calif), and Powerplex 16 is available from Promega Corporation (Madison, Wis).

from stochastic effects. Contamination and secondary transfer are potential problems with this system. Another approach to increase the sensitivity of degraded DNA samples is the use of mini STRs, which essentially are the same tandem repeats used in the commercial kits described previously, but the flanking PCR primers are moved closer to the tandem repeats. This results in amplification of smaller fragments, which decreases the likelihood that degradation will affect an STR. Greater sensitivity has been seen with mini STRs.

Gender Markers and Y Chromosome Markers

Amelogenin is a low molecular weight protein found in tooth enamel. The amelogenin gene is useful as a gender marker. The X chromosome amelogenin gene differs from its homolog on chromosome Y by a six–base pair polymorphism, allowing the distinction between individuals with 46,XY and 46,XX karyotypes. Males will display amelogenin locus heterozygosity; females will exhibit homozygosity. Reagents for assessing the amelogenin locus are incorporated into commercially available STR kits.

Y chromosome polymorphic loci can be used as identifying loci found only in males. In this way, male-specific DNA obtained from a vaginal swab can be typed without the usual *differential extraction,* in which the DNA from spermatozoa is released after the female fraction has been isolated from epithelial cells. Y chromosome loci useful for identity testing include STRs or SNPs (described later in this chapter). Laboratories typically employ commercially available panels of 12

TABLE 41-3 Y Chromosome Markers*

European Minimal Haplotype	European Extended Haplotype	U.S. Minimal Haplotype	U.S. Extended Haplotype
DYS19	DYS19	DYS19	DYS19
DYS385a/b	DYS385a/b	DYS385a/b	DYS385a/b
DYS389 I/II	DYS389 I/II	DYS389 I/II	DYS389 I/I
DYS390	DYS390	DYS390	DYS390
DYS391	DYS391	DYS391	DYS391
DYS392	DYS392	DYS392	DYS392
DYS393	DYS393	DYS393	DYS393
	YCAIIa/b	DYS437	DYS437
		DYS438	DYS438
		DYS439	DYS439
			DYS448
			DYS456
			DYS458
			DYS635
			Y GATA H4

*Y chromosome markers are listed in their major haplotype groups.

to 17 Y chromosome STRs for analyses (Table 41-3). Y chromosome SNPs are in development.

Y chromosome polymorphic loci are linked, resulting in discriminatory power that is significantly less than that of a panel of independently segregating somatic STR loci. Discriminatory values can be increased by using a large panel of Y chromosome markers in conjunction with a large database of typed individuals.

Mitochondrial DNA

Mitochondrial genomes are circular double-stranded DNA molecules that are 16,569 bp long and are present as one or more copies within the mitochondria of a cell. Thus mitochondrial DNA (mtDNA) is present in hundreds to thousands of copies per cell. mtDNA, unlike chromosomal DNA, does not undergo meiosis and does not participate in genetic recombination events. mtDNA remains stable over generations, except for the acquisition of mutations at a rate 10 to 20 times that of nuclear DNA.

mtDNA is transmitted to children via oocytes. Although it is generally thought that mitochondrial DNA is exclusively derived from the mother, a minor contribution from the father is occasionally present, particularly in disease states. The normal state of mitochondria is generally thought to be one of *homoplasmy,* in which all the mtDNA has the same sequence. However, because of mutational events, a state of *heteroplasmy,* in which more than one mtDNA sequence is present in the same tissue, may exist. High-level heteroplasmy is generally on the order of 30% of the mtDNA sequence before it is reported. Unrecognized low-level heteroplasmy is common. Heteroplasmy appears to be somewhat tissue-specific rather than uniform throughout the body. Thus two shed hairs may show discrepant mtDNA sequences. Because of heteroplasmy, one or two nucleotide mismatches between two individuals are not an absolute basis for exclusion of a tested individual.

In the human mitochondrial genome, only approximately 1200 bases in the region of transcription origin (15971-579), known as the *displacement loop (D-loop)* or the *control region,* are noncoding. This D-loop consists of two hypervariable regions that contain the majority of polymorphisms useful for identity (HVI: 16024-16365; HVII: 73-340). Polymorphisms outside this region can also be employed for testing. mtDNA polymorphisms are typically identified for forensic testing via DNA sequencing of hypervariable regions.[15] This method is expensive, labor intensive, and highly sensitive to contamination.

The mtDNA sequence obtained from a specimen is compared with a reference sequence (revised Cambridge sequence, www.mitomap.org/MITOMAP, accessed May 24, 2010). As in the case with Y chromosome STRs, because mtDNA polymorphisms are linked, individual polymorphism frequencies cannot be multiplied together to generate a likelihood of identity such as by independently segregating chromosomal locus allele frequencies. Instead the mtDNA haplotype identified in a sample is compared with those deposited in a database to derive a frequency statistic. Many mitochondrial haplotypes in the database are unique. Because the database has more than 6000 entries, it can be fairly stated that many mitochondrial haplotypes have a discriminatory value greater than 1 in 6000. However, 18 common haplotypes have population frequencies greater than 0.5%, including a haplotype present in 7% of the population. In aggregate, these common haplotypes account for 20% of all haplotypes.

mtDNA is useful primarily for identity testing in four contexts. First, a sample may be available that contains mitochondrial but not nuclear DNA. For example, shed hairs that do not have roots generally contain only mtDNA. Second, when the DNA within a specimen, such as skeletal remains, is substantially degraded, the high copy number and small size of mtDNA make it more likely to yield a result than nuclear DNA. Third, mtDNA analysis may become essential when only a distant relative is available for a reference specimen. In this example, nuclear DNA requires samples from multiple close kindred, but mtDNA matching would require only a distant maternal relative. Fourth, in database searches of unidentified human remains or missing person relatives, the algorithms for the search often produce several matches, and mitochondrial DNA analysis is needed to identify the true match.

Single-Nucleotide Polymorphisms

A DNA locus whose polymorphism extends over a short region can be preferable for identity testing because it may remain intact and available for analysis in the face of extensive levels of DNA degradation. These loci are particularly amenable to automation and chip technology using hybridization, polymerase extension, or ligation reaction assays. Despite a four-base possibility, most are biallelic with a dominant and a nondominant allele. A large set of SNPs must be used to obtain significant discriminatory values. SNPs are not used in forensic laboratories at this time but are likely to be used in the near future. Unfortunately, because of its biallelic nature, SNPs are not able to discriminate mixtures of DNA. As mentioned previously, many forensic samples contain mixtures, sometimes of more than two individuals, because they are collected under real-world conditions.

Other Systems

Other systems are being pursued for forensic identity testing, generally for phenotypic information. The Alu family of mobile elements constitutes 5% of the human genome. These elements repeatedly insert themselves into the human genome. Polymorphisms occur within these elements, so that the age of the element can be inferred. In Alu systems that are inherited, recent polymorphisms become markers of descent, and older elements (without the Alu insertion site) are markers of root ancestry. Similarly, the L1 family of long interspersed elements (LINEs) can be used to trace evolutionary ancestry. In combination with other genetic systems, Alu and LINE markers will provide some statistical inference about human evolution and race and ethnicity that may be helpful to investigators.

Instrumentation Used in Forensic Laboratories

Most forensic DNA testing is performed with the use of capillary electrophoretic (CE) systems. These systems have a substantially faster run time and higher resolution than slab gels. Several genetic analyzers are commercially available through various vendors.

Instrumentation under development for forensic testing generally focuses on a goal of miniaturization, yielding ultrafast and portable assays that would be useful for field testing. These technologies use miniaturized capillary arrays by etching microchannels into large chips, resulting in an ultrafast CE array that has run times of seconds and produces sharper bands than conventional CE instruments.

Currently being validated by the FBI and its regional mitochondrial laboratories is an electrospray ionization time-of-flight mass spectrometer, which can detect STRs and any SNPs within the STR region. At this time, SNPs within the STR are not detected and are not used for identity testing. This instrument will be used first for mitochondrial sequencing, which is essentially SNP detection, and later will be used for STRs.

Quality Assurance and Accreditation in Forensic DNA Analysis

Crime laboratories are regulated only because they receive federal grants or submit DNA results to the National DNA Index System (NDIS) through the Combined DNA Index System software. Therefore every state or local governmental DNA laboratory in the United States is regulated, but not every general crime laboratory. The DNA Identification Act of 1994 gave the FBI regulatory oversight of DNA profiles entered into the national database. The legislation called for a DNA Advisory Board that produced recommended standards, based largely on guidelines of the FBI's Technical Working Group on DNA Analysis Methods (TWGDAM). The Scientific Working Group on DNA Analysis Methods (SWGDAM), which has replaced the TWGDAM, now advises the FBI Director to create standard revisions. These standards are now called FBI Quality Assurance Standards, and every forensic DNA laboratory must comply with them.

One aspect of the FBI Quality Assurance Standards is a requirement for accreditation. Forensic Quality Systems Inc. and the American Society of Crime Laboratory Directors/ Laboratory Accreditation Board (ASCLD/LAB) accredit crime laboratories to International Organization for Standardization (ISO) 17025 standards. Each laboratory must meet more than 500 separate standards, in addition to the FBI Quality Assurance Standards, to be accredited. ASCLD/LAB requirements include minimal educational credits and experience, proficiency testing twice a year per analyst, and annual audits. All testing requires a technical and an administrative review. Judicial scrutiny provides another layer of critical review of those cases heard in court. Defense review and challenge, however, vary greatly.

Proficiency test providers for forensic laboratories in the United States include the Collaborative Testing Service, the College of American Pathologists, and Orchid Cellmark.

Standard reference materials from the National Institute of Standards and Technology (NIST) are available for PCR-Based Profiling DNA Standard (SRM 2391b), Mitochondrial DNA Sequencing (SRM 2392, 2392-I, and 2394), Human DNA Quantitation (SRM 2372), and Y chromosome testing (SRM 2395). Standards require annual NIST-traceable comparisons.

Statistical Interpretation

In the early days of DNA-based identity testing, significant challenges were launched regarding the interpretation of DNA typing results.[9,13,20,34] Questions included whether loci exhibit Hardy-Weinberg equilibrium, and whether allele frequencies vary significantly among ethnic groups. Current forensic genetic systems have not demonstrated significant deviation from Hardy-Weinberg equilibrium. These systems show greater intragroup allelic diversity than between-group diversity. A National Research Council panel was created to address these issues.[22] The resultant report (so-called NRC I) introduced a *ceiling principle* to ensure the conservativism of the frequency estimates, which itself generated considerable controversy. This led to NRC II, which articulated the current standards of statistical analysis.[23] Statistical formulas are routinely applied to Caucasian, Black, and Hispanic population databases. Specialized databases also exist for Native American Indian and for Pacific and African populations. Current statistical formulas assume that populations are substructured or inbred and correct for this occurrence. In a substructured population, mates are not chosen randomly from the population. Instead, a person will choose a mate of similar religious, ethnic, or geographic origin, such as by marrying within his or her own religion. In a substructured population, an individual is more likely to marry a distant relative such as a second, third, or fourth cousin, because selection of a mate is limited, leading to an inbred population.

Convicted Offender Databases

In the United States, all 50 states now have convicted offender databases. Initially, most databases exclusively contained sexual offenders, but the recent trend is to expand the databases to include all felons and some misdemeanors. States have begun to consider collecting DNA evidence in connection with lesser crimes, such as burglaries, to help solve these cases, to potentially interdict the progression to more serious future offenses, and to identify "hits" in the databases linked to past serious crimes. Twenty-one states and the federal government have recently adopted legislation allowing collection of DNA specimens on arrest or detention. Several states are allowing the release of names of convicted offenders who do not exactly match a crime scene sample (low stringency searches) on the premise that if there is a near database match, then a relative of the convicted offender may have left the sample. This approach has solved several crimes in the United States and in the United Kingdom.

DNA profiles are placed in the NDIS. If a "hit" is determined, the local crime laboratories of the involved states are contacted to discuss details. Identifying information other than the DNA profile is not entered into the system. Uploading of DNA profiles triggers quality assurance requirements and legal constraints on the use of DNA specimens and profiles.

The use of identity testing and linked databases in crime investigation has been aggressively pursued in the United Kingdom. U.K. forensic scientists maintain that approximately 50% of biological specimens from crime scenes result in hits in their databases, suggesting that a relatively small group of professional criminals perpetrate most crimes. They believe that DNA-based testing may be a more efficient tool for investigating crimes than traditional methods, such as canvassing neighborhoods.

Legal Issues

Early challenges to the practice and interpretation of DNA-based forensic identification have faded as the public, attorneys, and judges have become more knowledgeable about this technology. The most common challenges today involve issues regarding sample collection, preservation of the evidence, chain-of-custody documentation, and validation studies. New applications of DNA-based testing to assess ethnicity, to infer phenotypic features from evidence, to release the names of arrestees or potential family members of convicted offenders, or to identify an assailant from very small samples, such as fingerprints,[32] are likely to cause controversy in the future.

USE OF DNA TESTING FOR THE IDENTIFICATION OF CLINICAL SPECIMENS

Identity testing can also be used to confirm the identity of a clinical or anatomic pathology laboratory patient specimen.[27,29] Occasionally, questions arise regarding the identity of specimens in the clinical laboratory. DNA prepared from a peripheral blood or buccal mucosa specimen can be compared with the pathology specimen to confirm that it is derived from the same patient. The authors have encountered a variety of scenarios resulting in requests for this specialized identity service. (1) A patient lost confidence that her breast biopsy results were hers following a series of reporting errors involving the spelling of her name and her birth date. (2) A biopsy of a colonic lesion revealed adenocarcinoma. The subsequent colectomy specimen was devoid of a tumor. (3) A gastrectomy was performed after a biopsy diagnosis of adenocarcinoma. No tumor was seen in the gastrectomy specimen. (4) Multiple blocks from two breast lumpectomy procedures were processed. Because of labeling errors, it was unclear to which patient the various paraffin-embedded blocks belonged. (5) A young male fractured his femur and developed osteomyelitis. Curettings from the fracture site demonstrated acute inflammation as well as a fragment of tissue that appeared to be a squamous cell carcinoma.

In cases 1 to 4, identity testing with STRs demonstrated that all specimens in question truly belonged to the involved patients. In case 5, testing after microdissection of tissue fragments revealed that the squamous carcinoma "floater" had been derived from another individual. The availability of identity testing in situations such as these can be a significant benefit for involved patients and healthcare providers.

In prenatal testing for inherited disorders, chorionic villus sampling (CVS) performed early in pregnancy is sometimes employed as a source of fetal DNA for testing. Testing for a disorder such as cystic fibrosis may reveal that the genotypes for the mother and the fetus are identical, for example, that they are both heterozygous carriers of a cystic fibrosis mutation. This result is entirely consistent with the usual segregation of chromosomes during meiosis. However, it is possible that the CVS material was not derived largely from the fetus but consists of decidual cells primarily from the mother. If the father is a carrier of a cystic fibrosis mutation, this may result in failure to diagnose cystic fibrosis in a fetus. Identity testing can be employed to confirm that tested cells have a genotype distinct from that of the mother and are a valid sample from the fetus. Some advocate that identity testing should be performed to detect maternal contamination on all prenatal specimens.

TRANSPLANTATION TESTING

Obtaining well-matched tissue enhances transplanted organ and bone marrow survival. Human leukocyte antigen (HLA) alleles determine the tissue compatibility for acceptance of transplanted graft donated from another person (allograft). HLA genes encode highly polymorphic cell surface molecules that are strong alloantigens. An allograft is rejected as the result of an immune response directed against HLA alloantigens, which are expressed on the graft but are absent from the host.

Genetic Features of HLA Genes

The HLA genes are located within a genetic complex designated as the major histocompatibility complex (MHC). The extended MHC includes about 7.6 Mb on the short arm of chromosome 6 (6p21.3). Of the 421 loci, 252 (60%) are classified as expressed genes on the basis of complementary DNA (cDNA) and/or expressed sequence tag evidence.[16,17] The MHC is divided into three subregions containing different types of genes (Figure 41-2). With 58 (23%) of the expressed genes, the class III region is the most gene-dense subregion of the extended MHC and of the human genome.[17] Many of the MHC genes are involved in regulation of the immune response.[17] HLA variation is a critical determinant of susceptibility to a large number of infectious and autoimmune diseases.[10,17] The genes encoding the HLA class I (A, B, and C) and class II (DR, DQ, and DP) molecules are the most polymorphic loci in the human genome (see Figure 41-2 and Table 41-4). This polymorphism made the HLA loci an attractive and powerful early resource for identity testing.

HLA genes are codominantly expressed, and most individuals are heterozygous at HLA class I and class II loci. Most of the sequence diversity for HLA class I loci is seen in the second and third exons, and for the class II loci, in the second exon. These domains encode the peptide-binding regions of HLA molecules. The pattern of allelic sequence diversity noted in class I and class II loci is unusual; most alleles differ from their closest neighbor by multiple substitutions, with some alleles differing in the second and third exons by as much as 15%. This pattern is suggestive of segmental exchange of nucleotide motifs between alleles of the same locus. As a result, different HLA alleles are mosaic-like combinations of subsets of all polymorphisms.[12,21,28]

Although a very large number of alleles (e.g., >785 for HLA-DRB1) can be found in the worldwide population, a much smaller number (e.g., 30 to 50 for HLA-DRB1) is present with allele frequencies greater than 0.5% in most individual populations. Different populations tend to have different frequency distributions of alleles and exhibit different patterns of linkage disequilibrium. This variability exists among both racial and ethnic groups.

The HLA genes exist in linkage disequilibrium, also referred to as *gametic association*. Gametic associations are regularly found between certain HLA alleles of A and B, C and B, B and DRB1, and DRB1 and DQB1 loci. HLA genes are transmitted in families as haplotypes. The number of possible haplotypes is vast. However, because of linkage disequilibrium, the number of haplotypes found in a population is limited.[21] Genetic recombination or crossing over in the HLA region is a relatively rare event, occurring for the most part at a rate not greater than 1% per meiosis between A and B, and between B and DRB1. Recombination can also occur

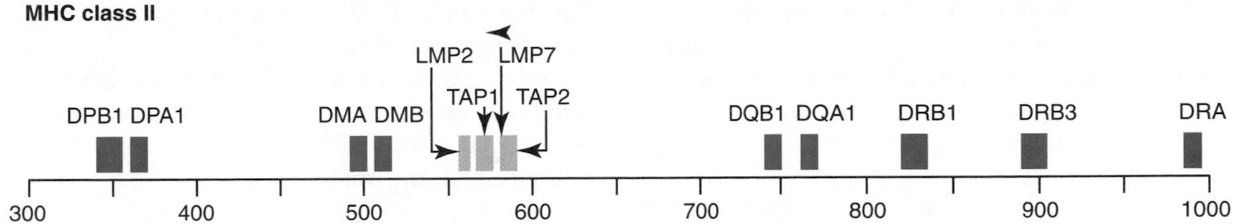

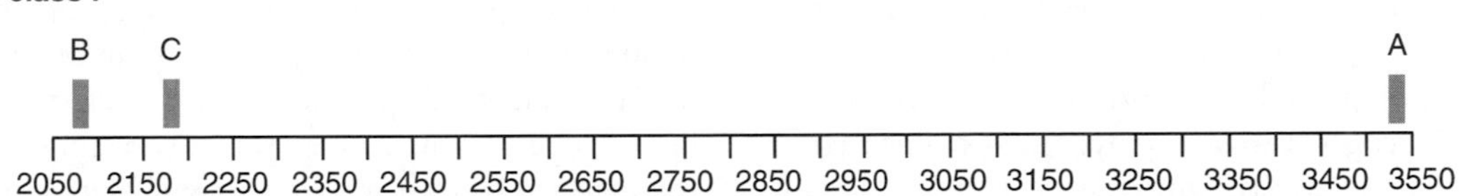

Figure 41-2 Map of the human major histocompatibility complex (MHC) region. The organization of the most important class I and class II genes of the MHC is shown, with approximate genetic distances given in thousands of base pairs (kb). Genes are ordered from telomere *(right)* to centromere *(left)*. The human leukocyte antigen (HLA) class I supercluster comprises the classical class I genes (HLA-A, -B, and -C). Not shown in this class I region are the nonclassical class I genes (HLA-E, -F, -G, HFE, and 12 pseudogenes) and the class I–like genes (MICA, MICB, and five pseudogenes). At the centromeric end of the MHC region is the class II region, which contains all expressed class II genes and several nonfunctional genes. Separating the class I and class II regions is a 1 megabase region of DNA containing the class III genes *(not shown)*.

TABLE 41-4 Names of the Most Important HLA Class I and Class II Genes and Their Encoded Polypeptides Ordered from Telomere to Centromere

Name	Previous Equivalents	Encoded Polypeptide
HLA-A		Class I α-chain
HLA-C		Class I α-chain
HLA-B		Class I α-chain
MICA	MICA, PERB11.1	Class I chain-related gene
MICB	MICB, PERB11.2	Class I chain-related gene
HLA-DRA	DR α	DR α-chain
HLA-DRB3	DRβIII	DR β3-chain determining DR52 specificities
HLA-DRB1	DRβI	DR β1-chain determining specificities DR1, DR2, DR3, DR4, DR5, etc.
HLA-DQA1	DQα1, DQ1A	DQ α-chain
HLA-DQB1	DQβ1, DQ1B	DQ β-chain
TAP2	RING11, Y1, PSF2	ABC (ATP-binding cassette) transporter (associated with antigen presentation)
PSMB8	LMP7, RING10	Proteasome-related sequence (role in loading class I molecules with peptides)
TAP1	RING4, Y3, PSF1	ABC (ATP-binding cassette) transporter (associated with antigen presentation)
PSMB9	LMP2, RING12	Proteasome-related sequence (role in loading class I molecules with peptides)
HLA-DMB	RING7	DM β-chain (control peptide loading by class II molecules)
HLA-DMA	RING6	DM α-chain (control peptide loading by class II molecules)
HLA-DPA1	DP1A	DP α-chain
HLA-DPB1	DP1B	DP β-chain

between A and C, and between B and C (0.6% and 0.2%, respectively).

Historical Applications of HLA Typing

HLA allele identification has been used for transplantation and for forensic, parentage, and chimerism testing. The latter three are of historical interest and are discussed in this section.

Forensic DNA Testing

The first case in the United States in which DNA-based identity testing was used, *Pestinikas v. Pennsylvania* (1986), involved HLA-DQA1 oligonucleotide, dot-blot hybridization analysis for forensic identification. This commercially available DQA1 system was later modified with five additional non-HLA genetic loci, resulting in discriminatory power of approximately 1 in 2000. The relatively low discriminatory power and problems with interpreting mixtures resulted in the migration of forensic laboratories to other methods and genetic loci as described previously.

Parentage Testing

Use of HLA loci for parentage testing has been replaced by methods described later in this chapter. The polymorphism of the loci was first inferred from antisera that distinguished among antigenic specificities. These specificities were especially numerous within the Class I loci, and it was recognized that they could be exploited in identity testing. Typically, a panel of serologic reagents was employed that defined HLA loci and red cell antigens. The emergence of many highly informative non-HLA polymorphic loci that could be conveniently genotyped led to reduced utility of HLA loci for parentage testing in the 1990s.

Chimerism

Chimerism is defined as mosaicism with coexistence of cells derived from two different individuals. Although HLA loci can be used to study the engraftment of transplanted hematopoietic stem cells (see later in this chapter), other more convenient loci are genotyped for this purpose. These other loci are essential when the transplant donor/recipient pair consists of HLA-identical siblings or allele-matched unrelated individuals.

Transplantation

Matching the HLA alleles of donors and recipients for renal transplantation improves long-term graft survival of kidneys from living related and unrelated donors and from deceased donors. For example, the half-life survival for a graft from an HLA-identical sibling is 23 years compared with a one haplotype–related donor with a half-life of 12.8 years.[12,30] It is important to note that the effect of HLA matching remains significant even with the most recent forms of immunosuppression. The effect of HLA matching on the survival of heart and lung transplants is statistically significant. In contrast, the effect of HLA matching for liver transplants is uncertain.

Hematopoietic cell transplantation (HCT) is employed to treat several classes of disorders, such as leukemia and hereditary immune deficiencies. HLA compatibility between donor and recipient in HCT affects not only the ability to achieve sustained engraftment of donor HCT, but also the risk of developing acute and chronic graft-versus-host disease (GVHD). Post-transplant risk of graft failure, GVHD, and mortality can be affected by quantitative and qualitative characteristics of donor-recipient HLA allele mismatching. In allogeneic stem cell transplantation, the donor is an individual who is genetically nonidentical and either related or unrelated to the recipient. Three different categories of donors are usually considered in the following order of preference: HLA genotypically identical siblings, HLA mismatched relatives, and unrelated donors, matched or mismatched. The goal when screening for an HLA-matched sibling donor is to identify which of any siblings have inherited the same HLA haplotypes from their parents.

When a matched sibling donor does not exist for a patient requiring allogeneic HCT (70% of cases), searching for extended family members or donors from an unrelated bone marrow registry would be the next option. Identifying a patient's haplotypes by testing the immediate family can help predict the probability of finding matching donors and can assist in developing a search strategy, because some alleles and haplotypes are more common than others, and they are distributed at different frequencies in different racial and ethnic groups. When searching for a donor, for some alleles, an allele-level match is more likely to be found among persons of a particular ethnicity. The National Marrow Donor Program (NMDP) matching algorithm, HapLogic, is based on this principle. The NMDP recommends that when possible, patients and adult donors (marrow or peripheral blood stem cells) should be fully matched (8 of 8 loci) at high resolution for HLA-A, -B, -C, and -DRB1. Matching for cord blood units is less stringent.

Registries of volunteer bone marrow donors and cord blood exist in most developed countries (http://www.marrow.org). Currently, approximately 65% of patients can find an acceptable donor among the more than 7 million individuals registered in the United States–based NMDP. However, patients belonging to racial groups that are not well represented in these registries have a considerably decreased probability of finding a donor (http://www.marrow.org).[3]

DNA-Based HLA Allele Identification

Most of the common molecular diagnostic methods have been used to identify HLA alleles. Strategies based on oligonucleotide probe hybridization, DNA sequencing, and allele-specific DNA amplification have become the most commonly used for HLA typing. Each of these methods relies on amplification with PCR of genomic DNA of relevant regions of an HLA gene from the tested individual.[12] Samples for testing usually consist of peripheral blood but may include any tissue containing nucleated cells.

Typing methods involve the design of primer pairs that are able to amplify all alleles at the target HLA locus with the polymorphic sequence motifs situated between the primer sites. Laboratories usually amplify at least exons 2 and 3 of class I genes and exon 2 of class II genes. Some prepare larger amplification products that include exon 1 and/or exon 4 of class I genes. Amplification primers may be located within exons or introns. Primers positioned in introns allow complete analysis of exons and inspection of exon/intron junctions for splice-site polymorphisms. Primers must be carefully chosen to attain locus-specific amplification because HLA loci are the products of gene duplication and divergence and retain substantial homology. Further, many HLA loci have closely related pseudogenes that do not encode functional polypeptides but may result in nonspecific PCR products.[12]

The PCR products prepared are subsequently analyzed by a variety of methods. They can be hybridized to oligonucleotide probes in reverse or forward dot-blot assays. The panel of probes is chosen to cover critical polymorphic positions in the HLA gene tested. A typical format for this method today is a multiplexed series of fluorescent microspheres coated with oligonucleotide probes that are hybridized to amplicons prepared from the HLA loci and detected in a flow cytometer. The pattern of reactivity of the panel can then be analyzed to assign allele identities.[12]

Alternatively, amplicons can be directly sequenced via dideoxynucleotide chain termination methods. This approach is increasingly attractive for allele level typing because of the large numbers of alleles known to exist at the HLA loci. The homozygous or heterozygous sequence obtained can be compared with a library of known sequences of alleles for allele assignment.[35]

A third commonly employed method, sequence-specific primer PCR (SSP-PCR) employs pairs of PCR primers chosen so that their 3′-most nucleotide or nucleotides are complementary to a polymorphic position that distinguishes an allele or an allele group from other alleles. If the individual possesses the allele(s) of interest, the PCR will lead to a product whose size and presence are typically identified by agarose gel electrophoresis or can be detected with real-time methods. Typing can be performed by choosing many pairs of primers in independent reactions to cover all allele groups.[12]

Commercial reagents and software for analysis of results are available for each of these three methods. Laboratories tailor HLA typing assays to the specific applications discussed previously. Choice of methods depends on typing volume, turnaround requirements, and the resolution needed.

Interpretation of HLA Test Results

An international nomenclature committee assigns each HLA allele an identifying number of at least four digits, with additional digits used if required to uniquely specify an allele. Fields in the identifying number are separated by colons, with each field providing a different form of information. For example, HLA-DRB1*13:01 is an allele found at the DRB1 locus in which the first two digits "13" describe the serologic antigen carried by an allotype, and the third and fourth digits "01" identify a specific subtype based on nucleotide sequence. Allele names are assigned in the order in which DNA sequences are first discovered and determined. Alleles whose names differ in the first four digits must differ in one or more nucleotide substitutions that change the amino acid sequence of the encoded protein. Alleles that differ only by synonymous nucleotide substitutions (also called *silent* or *noncoding substitutions*) within the coding sequence are distinguished by the digits in a third field. For example, HLA-A*02:171:01 and A*02:171:02 encode identical proteins but differ in sequence. Alleles that differ only by sequence polymorphisms in the introns or in the 5′ or 3′ untranslated regions that flank the exons and introns are distinguished by the use of a fourth field. In addition to the unique allele number, optional suffixes may be added to an allele to indicate its expression status. Alleles that have been shown not to be expressed—Null alleles—have been given the suffix "N."

The number of alleles at the HLA class I and class II loci and a listing of serologically defined specificities and their allele equivalents are shown in Table 41-5; updates of the numbers of these alleles are available online at http://www.ebi.ac.uk/imgt/hla (accessed May 11, 2009). The alleles of each of the HLA antigens are numbered according to the original serologic nomenclature. HLA alleles are now designated by a superscripted asterisk after the locus of origin and a number corresponding to the particular allele (e.g., HLA-A*0201). Parallel testing using serologic and DNA genotyping of HLA alleles has led to the use of one nomenclature for the description of low-resolution typing in which the HLA assignment might include more than one possible related allele (e.g., HLA-A A*02) and a nomenclature reflecting the high-resolution allelic typing. Thus different HLA allele subtypes (e.g., for A*02) can appear indistinguishable when

TABLE 41-5 HLA Allele Numbers

HLA Class I

Gene	*A*	*B*	*C*
Alleles	965	1543	626
Proteins	718	1230	464
Nulls	53	43	11

HLA Class II

Gene	*DRA*	*DRB1*	*DRB3*	*DRB4*	*DRB5*	*DQA1*	*DQB1*	*DPA1*	*DPB1*	*DMA*	*DMB*
Alleles	3	855	50	13	18	34	96	27	133	4	7
Proteins	2	657	40	7	15	25	70	16	116	4	7
Nulls	0	10	0	3	2	1	1	0	3	0	0

Other Non-HLA Genes

Gene	*MICA*	*MICB*	*TAP1*	*TAP2*
Alleles	68	30	7	4
Proteins	57	19	5	4
Nulls	0	2	1	0

tested by serology or with a limited panel of nucleic acid probes so a generic or low-resolution typing is obtained. New HLA alleles are named by an international nomenclature committee. Annual HLA nomenclature reports with frequent updates are available at the Website given in this paragraph.

Quality Assurance and Quality Control Issues

Quality control and assurance programs for HLA testing should be similar to those for other types of PCR-based testing. The NMDP and the American Society for Histocompatibility and Immunogenetics (ASHI) maintain a cell repository of a subset of known alleles (http://www.ashi-hla.org/; accessed April 20, 2009). As in other PCR-based testing, strict measures to prevent contamination of pre-PCR areas with genomic DNA and PCR products are essential. Testing for contamination arising from products prepared in SSP-PCR can be challenging because the many PCR reactions necessary to type an individual often result in products varying in size and composition. Measures to prevent contamination in PCR-based testing have been widely described; such information is available online at the ASHI Website.

Proficiency Testing

Several proficiency testing programs are available in the United States. These include the College of American Pathologists (CAP), ASHI, and the Southeastern Organ Procurement Foundation. Each offers comprehensive programs to assess the ability of laboratories to correctly identify HLA alleles. The University of California at Los Angeles has offered an international cell exchange program for many years. Laboratories are challenged to correctly type samples that often include unusual or recently described alleles.

Accreditation and Certification of Laboratories and Professionals

Clinical histocompatibility laboratories are high-complexity laboratories that in the United States must have a Clinical Laboratory Improvement Amendments (CLIA) license. Laboratories may be inspected and accredited by CAP or ASHI. The United Network for Organ Sharing, NMDP, and CLIA all have designated ASHI with deemed status for purposes of accreditation of HLA laboratories. Laboratories are generally directed by individuals with a PhD, an MD, or both degrees. ASHI administers a program to assess the qualifications of doctoral level individuals to direct ASHI-accredited laboratories. Directors can take a certifying examination administered by the American Board of Histocompatibility and Immunogenetics (ABHI). The ABHI also certifies laboratory staff as histocompatibility technologists and specialists. Information is available on the ASHI Website.

CHIMERISM AND HEMATOPOIETIC CELL ENGRAFTMENT ANALYSIS

Successful HCT effectively results in chimerism with the recipient's hematopoietic cells derived from the donor. With the exception of monozygotic twins, it is virtually always possible to use polymorphic loci on chromosomes to distinguish between DNA prepared from cells derived from the recipient and DNA obtained from donor cells. This is true even for siblings if enough loci are studied. Suppose the father and the mother of two siblings have alleles j and k and s and t, respectively, at a locus. The likelihood that the two siblings will inherit an identical genotype at this locus is 1 in 4. The likelihood that the siblings will be identical for other studied loci for which the parents are similarly heterozygous is also 1 in 4. In this particular example of complete parental heterozygosity, the risk that no locus will be found at which the two siblings can be distinguished is $\frac{1}{4}^N$, where N is the number of independently segregating loci tested. Commercial engraftment testing reagents that include 9 to 16 independently segregating loci will virtually always reveal at least a single locus at which donor and recipient cells can be distinguished.

Methods for Performing Engraftment Analysis

Sources of DNA for engraftment testing are typically peripheral white blood cells or bone marrow aspirates. It is crucial to obtain genomic DNA samples from the recipient before the transplant to determine his or her native genotypes at the tested loci. Then post-transplant samples can be compared with "pure" specimens from the donor and from the pretransplant recipient. If a pretransplant sample from the recipient is not available, another sample such as buccal cells may be obtained. Care should be taken in interpreting results from these alternate sources, however, because donor-derived inflammatory cells may be present.

Testing can be performed on genomic DNA isolated from the entire cell population of the specimen. Alternatively, the sample can be sorted by flow cytometry or immunorosetting to assess engraftment of specific cell lineages.[14] For example, engraftment of T-cell versus non–T-cell components can be assessed after flow cytometry sorting based on expression of the CD3 surface molecule, a T-cell marker.

DNA typing methods used in engraftment analysis are summarized in Table 41-6. These methods have evolved similarly to those used for identity testing in general. Initial methods relied on Southern blotting to detect RFLPs or VNTRs. These labor-intensive hybridization assays have been largely replaced by PCR-based methods.

One PCR-based strategy is to amplify a series of VNTR loci with subsequent separation of the DNA fragments on polyacrylamide gels.[26] Alleles can be assigned via comparison with size standards after staining with ethidium bromide. The sensitivity of this method for detecting a small admixture of donor or recipient DNA is roughly 10%. Sensitivity can be increased to the <1% to 1% range with silver staining of the amplification products.

As described earlier in this chapter for forensic identification, fluorescent detection of PCR products derived from STR, or microsatellite loci, has been adopted by many laboratories for engraftment assays.[25] This method is attractive because of the ability to automate the assay, the extensive characterization of these loci in a variety of populations, and their high degree of polymorphism. Surveys from the

TABLE 41-6 DNA Typing Methods Used in Engraftment Testing

Method	Description	Comment
RFLP analysis of VNTR loci	Digest genomic DNA with restriction endonuclease and detect polymorphic VNTR loci by Southern blotting	Highly informative identity testing method also used in early forensics, now discarded because of its labor-intensive nature
PCR analysis of VNTR loci	Amplify VNTR loci and size by gel electrophoresis	This assay can be quite sensitive when bands are detected by silver staining.
STR analysis	Multiplex amplification of several STR loci with sizing by fluorescent detection	Becoming the standard method in the field because of its efficiency and partial automation
Cytogenetics	Interphase analysis of X and Y chromosomes with fluorescent in situ hybridization	May be useful when donor and recipient are of different genders

PCR, Polymerase chain reaction; *RFLP,* restriction fragment length polymorphism; *STRs,* short tandem repeats; *VNTRs,* variable numbers of tandem repeat loci.

proficiency testing programs described later indicate that most laboratories providing clinical engraftment testing currently analyze STR loci.

When the donor and the recipient are of different genders, analysis of sex chromosomes in post-transplant hematopoietic cells can be useful in engraftment testing. Cytogenetic analysis of chromosomes in interphase cells with X- and Y-specific probes may be performed with fluorescent in situ hybridization assays. The percent donor or recipient cells can be determined by assessing the ratio of cells with XX signals to those with XY signals. Alternatively, PCR-based analysis of X and Y chromosome loci can be carried out. For example, the reappearance of Y-specific amplification products in a male whose donor was his sister may indicate relapse of a malignancy. Polymorphic loci on chromosome X can be studied similarly to the autosomal STR previously discussed.

Selection and Interpretation of Short Tandem Repeat Loci

Engraftment testing is accomplished by preparing genomic DNA from donor and pretransplant and post-transplant recipient specimens and performing PCR amplification of selected STR loci. Amplification reactions are typically multiplexed using fluorescently labeled commercially available reagents as described for forensic identity testing. Products are then separated via high-resolution slab or capillary electrophoresis on an automated genetic analyzer. Comparison of DNA fragment sizes with a reference ladder allows software to assign alleles for each locus.

Analysis of a donor sample and a pretransplant recipient sample allows the laboratory to identify which STR loci are informative (nonidentical genotypes) for the pair. A post-transplant sample can then be studied. If only fluorescent peaks from the donor are observed, the cells studied are donor in origin. Rarely, only recipient peaks will be seen, consistent with a recipient origin of the cells. These assays can detect admixtures of cell populations down to approximately 3%. Therefore, results indicating that a sample has been obtained exclusively from the donor are often reported as ≥97% donor. If fluorescent peaks derived from both the donor and the recipient are seen, the sample must be a mixture of cells from the two individuals.

The percent recipient in a mixed sample can be calculated by summing the intensities of the informative recipient peaks and dividing by the sum of the intensities of the informative recipient and donor peaks. Many laboratories then average the percent recipient for each locus to arrive at a final result. Some laboratories run a calibration curve of artificial mixtures of donor and recipient DNA for each tested pair. Other laboratories validate the assay with calibration curves for a number of control "donor" and "recipient" mixtures, and do not run new calibration curves for each new donor-recipient pair.

Applications of Microsatellite Locus Testing to Engraftment Analysis

Several clinical questions can be answered with engraftment testing.[31] Is engraftment of donor cells proceeding well in the weeks following a stem cell transplant? In the setting of a history of successful engraftment, do subsequent studies demonstrate a resurgence of recipient-derived hematopoietic cells indicating a relapse? Has stable chimerism developed following transplantation with the production of hematopoietic cells derived from both the donor and the recipient?

Correlation of engraftment testing results with the clinical history is crucial for interpretation of results. Thus appropriate communication between the engraftment testing laboratory and the transplantation team is essential. Consultation with a hematopathologist may be helpful in interpreting results in complex cases.

A result indicating 85% donor cells and 15% recipient cells might be equally consistent with an engrafting marrow 3 weeks after transplantation or with relapse 6 months following transplantation. The date of the transplant in relation to sample collection, the conditioning regimen used before transplant, and evidence from peripheral smear or bone marrow aspirate examination may be helpful in interpreting results. Unusual history, if unknown, can cause considerable confusion. For example, some recipients may have received more than one stem cell transplant or may have had a donor who is an identical twin.

Interpretation of an engraftment result from a single sample can be difficult. Multiple samples collected at intervals after transplantation may reveal changes in the fractions of donor and recipient over time that can be correlated with the evolving clinical picture.

Proficiency Testing

Proficiency testing programs for engraftment testing are offered by CAP and ASHI. Challenge specimens are typically artificial mixtures of genomic DNA from two related or unrelated individuals. In both surveys, participant laboratories have demonstrated a high degree of agreement for challenge samples. The standard deviation from the mean of participant results in a 50 50 mixture of "donor" and "recipient" cells is typically ±2 to 4%. For mixtures that approach the sensitivity threshold of the assay (e.g., 6% recipient, 94% donor), somewhat broader standard deviations may be seen.

Quality Assurance and Quality Control

Quality control and assurance programs for engraftment testing should be similar to those for other types of identity testing. Assays may require as little as 1 ng of genomic DNA. Thus strict measures to prevent contamination of pre-PCR areas with genomic DNA and PCR products are important.

Accreditation

Accreditation of programs may be provided through ASHI or CAP. Because engraftment testing is a variant of identity testing, the standards used are often those written for paternity and other forms of identity testing. However, because engraftment testing deals with subpopulations of cells and the relative proportions of cells, organizations such as ASHI have developed accreditation standards specifically for engraftment testing.

PARENTAGE TESTING

Questions regarding the parentage of minor and adult children arise frequently in modern society. Generally at issue is whether a particular man is the father of a child. As discussed in the chapter introduction, parentage testing allows an individual to be excluded or not excluded as the parent of a child. If not excluded, the likelihood that he is the father can be calculated. The same methods can be applied to the search for a mother, a situation that sometimes arises when an adopted person is trying to find his or her biological parents. Court-ordered or privately sought parentage testing is usually performed to facilitate decisions regarding responsibility for the financial support of a child. However, individuals may wish to establish parentage for other reasons; an example is the settlement of an estate. Laboratories that perform other types of identification tests for purposes unrelated to parentage (e.g., HLA typing for transplantation) should be aware of the possibility of inadvertently uncovering "false paternity."

Methods, Instrumentation, and Sample Requirements

Methods for parentage testing have evolved considerably over time, similar to other human identification applications. Early methods relied on serologic techniques to identify red cell antigens, such as ABO and MNS groups and the highly polymorphic HLA antigens found on most cells. Since 1990, a substantial migration of parentage laboratories to DNA-based methods has occurred, especially to those based on analysis of STR alleles. The significant advantages of these PCR-based assays with detection of fluorescently labeled DNA fragments on automated genetic analyzers have been discussed in the section on forensic identification. SNPs have also been introduced in commercial parentage laboratories.

Selection and validation of testing methods are key issues in parentage testing. Specific requirements for paternity testing may be mandated by local laws and agreements. Thus the choice of methods and genetic systems should be based on an agreement between the client(s) and the laboratory.

Nonstandardized methods should not be used as the sole methods within a paternity testing laboratory. Also, a nonstandard method should be used only if it can be documented that the method is used in at least one other laboratory, thus making it possible to obtain a second opinion based on repeated testing.

Similar to other forms of identity testing, a sample for parentage testing may be any specimen containing chromosomal DNA. In practice, programs generally perform testing on peripheral blood samples or buccal smears. Buccal smears are increasingly preferred as they offer a noninvasive means of sample collection, which is especially convenient when testing minors.

Reporting of Test Results

In addition to the usual parentage test reports, laboratories are occasionally asked to provide interpretative reports when less than complete information is available. The usual report is discussed next, and interpretive reports are discussed afterward.

Test Reports

Results should include all information requested by the client and necessary for the interpretation of test results and all information required by the method used. If the weight of evidence is calculated, this must be based on likelihood ratio principles, such as the paternity index.[2,11]

Exclusion of a Tested Man

Standard parentage testing involves genotyping of several polymorphic loci in samples from a trio consisting of the mother, child, and presumed father. Inspection of the alleles found in the mother and child at the genetic loci analyzed reveals alleles that must have been contributed by the child's biological father. If the accused father does not have an obligatory allele at one of the tested loci, he is excluded as the biological father. Laboratories require the absence of an obligatory allele for at least *two* loci in a tested man to exclude him as the father. The requirement of multiple loci reduces the possibility of an error caused by a technical problem or by a rare mutation at one of the examined loci.

The power of an analyzed locus to exclude a tested man depends on the number of alleles found at the locus and allele frequencies in human populations. ABO typing can exclude a tested man but has a relatively poor probability of exclusion of about 15%. HLA and VNTR loci have many alleles, and a single locus may have a greater than 90% probability of excluding a falsely accused man. The STR loci have an intermediate number of alleles. A single STR locus typically has a 30 to 60% likelihood of excluding a wrongly accused man. The ease of STR analysis makes these loci attractive for parentage testing even with their lower exclusion power. If several STRs that independently segregate during meiosis are studied, a cumulative probability of exclusion can be calculated that is based on the product of exclusion power for each tested locus. The use of 9 to 16 unlinked, and therefore independent, STRs provided in commercially available human identity reagents generally results in at least a 99% probability of exclusion of a falsely accused man.

Inclusion of a Tested Man

The alleles found at the analyzed loci may be entirely consistent with the accused man being the biological father of the child. In this case, the likelihood that he is truly the father rather than a random individual who is not excluded can be calculated. A number of assumptions underlie accurate calculations of the likeliness of paternity. Tested individuals must be properly identified, testing must be accurate, and allele frequencies in relevant populations must be well characterized.

The probability of paternity (W) and the paternity index (PI) are two closely related values that express the likelihood that the tested man is truly the father, rather than another man who by chance shares alleles at a tested locus. Calculation of the PI takes into account allele frequencies at the locus in relevant populations. If multiple independent loci are analyzed, a cumulative PI based on the products of individual loci can be calculated. Government entities typically require that the PI be greater than 100:1 and that the probability of paternity be greater than 99% for inclusion of a man. Other evidence bearing on the probability that a man is the father before testing is performed can be integrated with test results using Bayesian analysis to calculate a posterior probability of paternity. The prior probability that an accused man is the father is typically set at 50%, but a range of likelihoods given different prior probabilities (e.g., 10 to 50%) can be calculated for comparison.

Opinions, Interpretations, and Problems

Standard parentage testing requires samples from the trio previously described. However, in many cases, the mother, child, and putative father may not all be available for testing. If a sample cannot be obtained from the mother, it may still be possible to exclude a tested man or to calculate his probability of paternity. For example, the finding of locus L genotypes 1,3 for the child and 4,5 for the tested man is inconsistent with the hypothesis that he is the father, whether or not we know the mother's genotype. Similarly, when the accused man is not available, testing performed for individuals related to him may be used to calculate the likelihood that he is the biological father of the child in question.

Although STRs and VNTRs are usually transmitted in a faithful mendelian fashion, mutations can occur. A child and a tested man may be encountered who share an allele at all but one of the tested loci. The possibility that the man is truly the father and that a mutation has occurred at the mismatched locus should then be entertained. If additional loci are tested and no additional genetic inconsistencies are discovered, the likelihood of paternity can be calculated by considering the frequency of mutations at the mismatched locus. Alternatively, additional genotyping may reveal more exclusions, making it unlikely that the tested man is truly the father. Laboratories should apply procedures for estimating the uncertainty of measurement. The measurement of uncertainty of tests should be known and should be included in the interpretation of test results.

Quality Assurance and Quality Control

Quality control and assurance measures for parentage testing are similar to those for other types of human identity testing. Positive identification of samples, prevention of DNA contamination, use of control alleles of known size, and validation of software employed for genetic analysis and calculation are among measures common to identity testing programs. Population distribution data for the systems used must be documented. In addition, mutation frequencies of the systems used must be documented and used appropriately.

Policy and Procedures for Resolution of Complaints

The laboratory should have a policy and a procedure for the resolution of complaints received from clients or other parties. Paternity testing programs involving knowledge of sensitive family information results may be employed in legal proceedings. Samples and records, including information stored electronically, must be handled carefully to ensure their privacy, confidentiality, and security. Laboratory procedures for documenting the identity of individuals who contribute samples for study and the chain of custody of specimens should be very detailed.

Accreditation

Recommendations and standards for paternity testing are formulated by government agencies or professional organizations [e.g., the Standards for Parentage Testing Laboratories of the American Association of Blood Banks (AABB)]. The AABB administers a laboratory inspection and accreditation program.[1] ASHI and CAP also publish relevant standards. CAP and AABB jointly offer a proficiency testing survey.

REFERENCES

1. American Association of Blood Banks (AABB). Standards for parentage testing laboratories, 6th edition. Bethesda, Md: AABB; 2004:1-57.
2. Baur MP, Elston RC, Gurtler H, Henningsen K, Hummel K, Matsumoto H, et al. No fallacies in the formulation of the paternity index. Am J Hum Genet 1986;39:528-36.
3. Beatty PG, Mori M, Milford E. Impact of racial genetic polymorphism on the probability of finding an HLA-matched donor. Transplantation 1995;60:778-83.
4. Biesecker L, Bailey-Wilson J, Ballantyne J, Baum H, Bieber F, Brenner C, et al. DNA identifications after the 9/11 World Trade Center attack. Science 2005;310:1122-3.
5. Budowle B, Smith J, Moretti T, DiZinno J. DNA typing protocols: molecular biology and forensic analysis. Natick, Mass: Eaton Publishing Co., 2000.
6. Butler JM. Forensic DNA typing: biology and technology behind STR markers. London, UK: Academic Press, 2005.
7. Butler JM, Reeder DJ. STR DNA Internet database. Available at: http://www.cstl.nist.gov/div831/strbase (accessed on June 29, 2009).
8. Caragine T, Mikulasovich R, Tamariz J, Bajda E, Sebestyen J, Baum H, et al. Validation of testing and interpretation protocols for low template DNA samples suing AmpFLSTR® Identifiler®. Croatian Med J 2009;50: 250-67.
9. Chakraborty R, Kidd KK. The utility of DNA typing in forensic casework. Science 1991;254:1735-9.
10. de Bakker PI, McVean G, Sabeti PC, Miretti MM, Green T, Marchini J, et al. A high-resolution HLA and SNP haplotype map for disease association studies in the extended human MHC. Nat Genet 2006;38: 1166-72.
11. Elston RC. Probability and paternity testing. Am J Hum Genet 1986;39: 112-22.
12. Erlich HA, Opelz G, Hansen J. HLA DNA typing and transplantation. Immunity 2001;14:347-56.
13. Evett IW, Weir B. Interpreting DNA evidence: statistical genetics for forensic scientists. Sunderland, Mass: Sinauer Associates Inc., 1998.
14. Fernandez-Aviles F, Urbano-Ispizua A, Aymerich M, Colomer D, Rovira M, Martinez C, et al. Serial quantification of lymphoid and myeloid mixed chimerism using multiplex PCR amplification of short tandem repeat-markers predicts graft rejection and relapse, respectively, after allogeneic transplantation of CD34+ selected cells from peripheral blood. Leukemia 2003;17:613-20.
15. Holland MM, Parsons TJ. Mitochondrial DNA sequence analysis—validation and use for forensic casework. Forensic Sci Rev 1999;11: 21-50.
16. Horton R, Gibson R, Coggill P, Miretti M, Allcock RJ, Almeida J, et al. Variation analysis and gene annotation of eight MHC haplotypes: the MHC Haplotype Project. Immunogenetics 2008;60:1-18.
17. Horton R, Wilming L, Rand V, Lovering RC, Bruford EA, Khodiyar VK, et al. Gene map of the extended human MHC. Nat Rev Genet 2004;5:889-99.
18. Jeffreys AJ, Wilson V, Thein SL. Hypervariable "minisatellite" regions in human DNA. Nature 1985;314:67-73.
19. Jeffreys AJ, Wilson V, Thein SL. Individual specific "fingerprints" of human DNA. Nature 1985;316:76-9.
20. Lander ES, Budowle B. DNA fingerprinting dispute laid to rest. Nature 1994;371:735-8.
21. Little AM, Parham P. Polymorphism and evolution of HLA class I and II genes and molecules. Rev Immunogenet 1999;1:105-23.
22. National Research Council. DNA technology in forensic science. Washington, DC: National Academy Press, 1992.
23. National Research Council. The evaluation of forensic DNA evidence. Washington, DC: National Academy Press, 1996.
24. Rudin N, Inman K. An introduction to forensic DNA analysis, 2nd edition. Boca Raton, Fla: CRC Press, 2001.
25. Scharf SJ, Smith AG, Hansen JA, McFarland C, Erlich HA. Quantitative determination of bone marrow transplant engraftment using fluorescent polymerase chain reaction primers for human identity markers. Blood 1995;85:1954-63.
26. Schichman SA, Suess P, Vertino AM, Gray PS. Comparison of short tandem repeat and variable number tandem repeat genetic markers for quantitative determination of allogeneic bone marrow transplant engraftment. Bone Marrow Transplant 2002;29:243-8.
27. Shibata D. Identification of mismatched fixed specimens with a commercially available kit based on the polymerase chain reaction. Am J Clin Pathol 1993;100:666-70.
28. Traherne JA, Horton R, Roberts AN, Miretti MM, Hurles ME, Stewart CA, et al. Genetic analysis of completely sequenced disease-associated MHC haplotypes identifies shuffling of segments in recent human history. PLoS Genet 2006;2:82-96.
29. Tsongalis GJ, Wu AH, Silver H, Ricci A Jr. Applications of forensic identity testing in the clinical laboratory. Am J Clin Pathol 1999;112(1 Suppl 1):S93-103.
30. United Network for Organ Sharing (UNOS). 2007 annual report, the U.S. Scientific Registry of Transplant Recipients and the Organ Procurement and Transplantation Network, Transplant data 1997-2006. Washington, DC: Department of Health and Human Services, Health Resources and Services Administration, 2007.
31. Van Deerlin VM, Leonard DG. Bone marrow engraftment analysis after allogeneic bone marrow transplantation. Clin Lab Med 2000;20: 197-225.
32. Van Oorschot RAH, Jones MK. DNA fingerprints from fingerprints. Nature 1997;387:767.
33. Weedn VW, Hicks JW. The unrealized potential of DNA testing: research in action. Washington, DC: National Institute of Justice, 1998.
34. Wooley J, Harmon RP. The forensic brouhaha: science or debate? Am J Hum Genet 1992;51:1164-5.
35. Wu J, Bassinger S, Griffith BB, Williams TM. Analysis of HLA Class I alleles via direct sequencing of PCR products: ASHI laboratory manual, 4. 2 edition. Lenexa, Ks: ASHI, 2006.

World Wide Web Sites

The Anthony Nolan Trust, HLA Informatics Page

www.anthonynolan.org/Healthcare-professionals/Research-at-Anthony-Nolan/HLA-Informatics-Group.aspx

American Society for Histocompatibility and Immunogenetics

www.ashi-hla.org

National Institute of Standards and Technology, Short Tandem Repeat DNA Internet DataBase

www.cstl.nist.gov/div831/strbase

European Bioinformatics Institute, IMGT/HLA Sequence Database

www.ebi.ac.uk/imgt/hla

National Marrow Donor Program

www.marrow.org

CHAPTER 42

Molecular Methods in Diagnosis and Monitoring of Infectious Diseases

Aaron D. Bossler, M.D., Ph.D., and Angela M. Caliendo, M.D., Ph.D.

In the short time since their introduction, nucleic acid tests have profoundly impacted the management of infectious diseases. In contrast to microbial culture methods, molecular methods are rapid, allowing early decisions about treatment to be based on data about the pathogen(s) in an individual patient. Molecular methods have provided a means to detect pathogens that could not be easily detected by traditional methods using culture, antigen detection, or serology. By providing rapid identification and in some cases quantification of pathogen nucleic acids, these methods have transformed the clinical practice of assessing the risk of disease development, determining disease prognosis, and predicting and monitoring response to therapy.

Interpretation of the results of molecular assays for infectious diseases requires an understanding of the biology of the target organism, the pathogenesis of related infectious disease(s), and the advantages and limitations of the technology used. An advantage of molecular methods is their exquisite sensitivity for the detection of pathogen nucleic acids whether from viable or nonviable organisms. The nucleic acids of the organism may persist for varying lengths of time after adequate treatment of an infection. Therefore, one of the challenges can be interpreting the significance of a positive molecular test result. For example, *Chlamydia trachomatis* DNA can be detected in the urine of patients for as long as 3 weeks after initiation of appropriate therapy.[48] Similarly, herpes simplex virus (HSV) DNA can be detected in the cerebrospinal fluid (CSF) of patients with encephalitis for 2 weeks or longer after initiation of acyclovir therapy.[84] Thus, in this case and most others, monitoring response to therapy with qualitative assays has limited clinical utility and is best done using quantitative methods. Detection of the nucleic acid of a pathogen does not ensure that the organism is the cause of the disease. The organism may be part of the normal flora, colonizing a specific area or causing infection but not disease. For example, interpretation of molecular tests for the detection and quantification of herpesviruses after primary infection is complicated by the fact that these viruses establish a life-long latent infection. Early studies evaluating the clinical utility of cytomegalovirus (CMV) DNA assays used very sensitive qualitative methods and peripheral blood mononuclear cells as the specimen of choice. As a result, CMV DNA was detected in immunocompromised patients with disease, as well as in those without CMV disease. Studies are needed to establish viral load values that distinguish between latent infection, asymptomatic disease, and active disease.

A common application for quantitative molecular assays involves monitoring of disease progression or response to therapy over time. To determine whether changes in quantitative values are clinically significant or are due to expected variability of the measurement, one must consider the analytical variability of the test and biological variability of the pathogen. For example, for the current human immunodeficiency virus (HIV)-1 viral load assays, to allow for both assay and biological variability, a change in the viral load must exceed 0.5 $\log_{10}$ (or a threefold change in concentration) to represent a biologically significant change in viral replication.

Interpretation of a negative result requires consideration of assay sensitivity and efficiencies of nucleic acid extraction and amplification. A false-negative result may be due to inhibition of or decreased efficiency of amplification, and proper controls are important. Insufficient sample, inappropriate specimen type, inappropriate timing of sample collection, and degradation of nucleic acid during transport and handling are other sources of false-negative results.

Factors that need to be considered when a positive result is interpreted include assay specificity and contamination. Specificity of molecular infectious disease assays is related to the primers and probes used during amplification and detection/quantification steps. If primers allow amplification of nucleic acids from other pathogens normally present in a patient specimen, false-positive results are possible. Although uncommon, problems with primer specificity have been reported; primers designed to amplify the 5′ untranslated region of the enterovirus genome have also been shown to amplify rhinovirus RNA.[129] This will not be an issue if the assay is used only for cerebrospinal fluid, but it will likely cause false-positive results if respiratory specimens are tested.

False-positive results can also occur as the result of carryover contamination of amplified products. This is not a problem with signal amplification methods, but it can be of significant concern for target amplification methods, such as polymerase chain reaction (PCR), nucleic acid sequence-based amplification (NASBA), transcription-mediated amplification (TMA), and strand displacement amplification (SDA). The use of real-time assays, which do not require postamplification handling of the product, greatly reduces the risk of carryover contamination. Cross-contamination of clinical specimens with target DNA during specimen collection, transport, and processing can occur with any method. Strict attention to good laboratory practices is needed to minimize the risk of cross-contamination.

Molecular infectious disease tests are used in a variety of ways including identification of pathogens, particularly those that do not grow using conventional methods or that grow very slowly; monitoring of response to therapy; assessment of risk of disease development; and determination of disease prognosis. The balance of this chapter will review nucleic acid testing as it applies to specific pathogens, with a focus on those pathogens for which nucleic acid testing is considered the standard of care.

CHLAMYDIA TRACHOMATIS AND *NEISSERIA GONORRHOEAE*

Chlamydia trachomatis (CT) and *Neisseria gonorrhoeae* (GC, for gonococcus) will be discussed together because several of the available nucleic acid tests for these pathogens are multiplex assays. Although both CT and GC can cause a variety of clinical infections, here we will focus on genital infections.

Detection of CT is a challenging and important public health issue. CT is a major cause of genital infections, with an estimated 1 million cases occurring annually among sexually active adolescents and young adults in the United States.[53] More than half of the infections are asymptomatic.[144] Even when symptomatic, the diagnosis can be missed as the manifestations are protean. In males, CT infection may present as urethritis, epididymitis, prostatitis, or proctitis[17,105] and as cervicitis, endometritis, and urethritis in women, with 10 to 40% of infections in women progressing to pelvic inflammatory disease (PID) if untreated.[122,145] Related complications include chronic pelvic pain, ectopic pregnancy, and infertility. In the United States, CT infection is a likely cause of most secondary infertility in females. In pregnant women, there is the additional risk of transmitting the infection to the newborn during labor and delivery, leading to pneumonia or conjunctivitis in the newborn.

GC, too, may present in various ways, and the clinical presentations overlap those of CT. Males may have acute urethritis with discharge, epididymitis, prostatitis, and urethral strictures. In women, GC infection can produce cervicitis, which if left untreated can lead to PID, abscesses, or salpingitis.

Traditional methods for the diagnosis of CT infection include cell culture, antigen detection by immunofluorescence-based techniques, enzyme immunoassay, and, more recently, nonamplified nucleic acid detection. These traditional methods have been replaced in many laboratories by amplified nucleic acid tests, which provide greater sensitivity in detecting CT from genital specimens. For GC, which was traditionally diagnosed based on culture methods that relied on selective culture media, nucleic acid testing does not offer significant improvement in sensitivity compared with culture when culture is performed under ideal conditions. GC is a fastidious organism, however, and is highly susceptible to extreme temperatures and desiccation, which can lead to decreased sensitivity of detection by culture, particularly when specimen transport is required prior to culturing.[76] Nucleic acid testing for GC offers a sensitive and reliable alternative to culture.

Nucleic Acid Testing for CT and GC

In addition to high diagnostic and analytical sensitivity and specificity, nucleic acid testing offers several advantages over conventional culture and antigen detection methods for the diagnosis of CT and GC. Testing for both pathogens can be done on a single specimen, and for some multiplex assays, testing is performed in a single reaction. Unlike the infectious organism itself, the DNA and RNA of GC and CT are quite stable in commercial transport devices, thus accounting for some of the increased diagnostic sensitivity of these assays compared with culture. The stability of nucleic acid avoids the necessity of immediate transport to the laboratory, and specimens may be stored refrigerated or at room temperature prior to transport. Transport and storage requirements vary among tests, so it is important to refer to the package insert for specific details. An additional advantage of nucleic acid testing is the use of urine specimens, which for women allows testing to be done without the need for a pelvic examination. In males, urine offers a convenient and diagnostically sensitive alternative to collection with a urethral swab and increases the likelihood that asymptomatic males will agree to be tested.

Tests for the detection of CT and GC from clinical specimens (Table 42-1) use a variety of specimens, including cervical and vaginal swabs, urethral swabs, and urine from both asymptomatic and symptomatic individuals. Not all assays are cleared by the U.S. Food and Drug Administration (FDA) for use in the United States for all conditions, and the current assays are not FDA-cleared for oral, rectal, respiratory, or conjunctival specimens. Performance characteristics vary among assays (details are available in the package inserts), but some general comments can be made. The diagnostic sensitivity of the tests varies according to the specimen type and whether the patient is asymptomatic or symptomatic. Interpretation of the results of nucleic acid testing for CT can be challenging because many studies have shown these assays to be more diagnostically sensitive than culture, which was

TABLE 42-1 Summary of FDA-Cleared Testing for *Chlamydia trachomatis* (CT) and *Neisseria gonorrhoeae* (NG)[a]

Test	Assay Method	Gene Target	Comments
AMPLICOR CT[b]/NG[c] COBAS AMPLICOR CT/NG (Roche Diagnostics, Indianapolis, Ind)	PCR[d]	CT: cryptic plasmid NG: M-Ngo PII[e]	Internal control, multiplex assays
BD ProbeTec ET, *C. trachomatis* and *N. gonorrhoeae* amplified DNA assay (Becton-Dickinson, Franklin Lakes, NJ)	SDA[f]	CT: cryptic plasmid NG: Piv_{Ng} gene	Internal control
APTIMA Combo 2 Assay[g] (Gen-Probe, San Diego, Calif)	TMA[h]	CT: 23S rRNA NG: 16S rRNA	Multiplex assay Target capture nucleic acid extraction
Abbott RealTime CT/NG (Abbott Molecular Inc., Des Plaines, Ill)	Real-time PCR	CT: cryptic plasmid NG: *Opa* gene	Multiplex assay, nucleic acid extraction, internal control
HC 2 CT ID HC 2 GC ID HC 2 CT/GC Combo test (Digene Corporation, Gaithersburg, Md)	Hybrid capture	CT: Cryptic plasmid and GC[c]: genomic DNA	Signal amplification

[a]For FDA listings of these and any newer tests, see http://www.accessdata.fda.gov/scripts/cdrh/cfdocs/cfRL/listing.cfm. Use test codes LSK and LSL for *C. trachomatis* and *N. gonorrhoeae*, respectively.
[b]*Chlamydia trachomatis.*
[c]*Neisseria gonorrhoeae.*
[d]Polymerase chain reaction.
[e]Cytosine DNA methyltransferase.
[f]Strand displacement assay.
[g]Confirmatory assays for CT and NG are also available.
[h]Transcription mediated amplification.

previously used as the gold standard for clinical trials. For males, the diagnostic sensitivity of testing urine specimens is nearly equivalent to that of testing urethral swabs.[16,29,36,72,155] A limited volume (20 to 50 mL) of first-passed urine is preferred because larger volumes will lead to a decreased concentration of the organism in the sample and thus reduced diagnostic sensitivity. With proper specimen collection, male urethral swabs and urine specimens have a sensitivity of nearly 100% for the detection of GC or CT infection. For women, cervical swab specimens provide the highest sensitivity for the detection of GC and CT infection, with many studies showing a sensitivity of 90 to 95%.[29,36,86,115] Urine specimens can be used, but they generally result in a lower diagnostic sensitivity than cervical swabs (75 to 85%).[29,36,86,115] An alternative to urine testing in women is the use of self-collected vaginal swabs, which have been shown in some studies to have a diagnostic sensitivity that is equal to that obtained with cervical swabs; several of the tests have been cleared for use with vaginal swabs.[65,134]

Decisions regarding the selection of a specific amplification test for the detection of CT and GC should not be based solely on the cost of reagents. Other key factors to consider include test performance characteristics, such as diagnostic sensitivity and specificity, and applicability for urine and swab specimens in both symptomatic and asymptomatic individuals. (In the United States, FDA clearance for various specimen types and individuals varies among methods.) Ideally the test should include an internal control, particularly if a crude lysate is used in the assay. Other factors to consider are degree of automation, ease of use, work flow issues, and space and equipment needs.

False-Positive Test Results

For several of the GC assays, reduced specificity is due to cross-hybridization of primers with nongonococcal *Neisseria* species.[56,104] The ProbeTec test (Becton-Dickinson, Franklin Lakes, NJ) has been reported to produce false-positive results with *N. flavescens, N. lactamica, N. subflava,* and *N. cinerea,* and the AMPLICOR assay (Roche Diagnostics, Indianapolis, Ind) can produce false-positive results with *N. flavescens, N. lactamica,* and *N. sicca.* There is concern about generating false-positive results with pharyngeal specimens that may contain these nongonococcal species of *Neisseria.* However, *N. cinerea, N. lactamica, N. subflava,* and *N. sicca* have also been isolated from genital mucosa, so it is possible to generate false-positive results from genital specimens.

Other sources of false-positive results include carryover contamination of amplified product and cross-contamination during specimen collection, transport, or processing. Concerns over these issues have led to discussion of confirmatory testing for CT and GC, because false-positive results can have psychosocial or medicolegal ramifications. False-positive results in a low-prevalence population can significantly reduce the predictive value of a positive result. For example, although the specificity of nucleic acid testing for GC or CT generally ranges from 98 to 99%, the positive predictive value may be as low as 60 to 70% in a population with a low prevalence.

Nucleic acid testing for the detection of CT or GC should not be used as a test of cure. Because DNA can persist in urine samples for up to 3 weeks after completion of therapy,[48] test of cure using nucleic acid testing is discouraged. If this must be done, then testing should be delayed for at least 3 weeks after therapy is begun to allow time for clearance of the DNA of the pathogen.

False-Negative Test Results

False-negative results from inhibition of amplification are a consideration for both GC and CT testing and have been reported for both cervical swabs and urine specimens.[30,89,127] Inhibition rates may vary considerably depending on the amplification method used and are related, in part, to the method used for nucleic acid extraction.[89] For tests that use a crude lysate in testing (such as the AMPLICOR and ProbeTec tests), inhibition rates tend to be higher than those seen with the APTIMA Combo test (Gen-Probe Inc., San Diego, Calif), which uses a target capture method to purify nucleic acid. For assays that test a crude lysate, it is useful to amplify another nucleic acid sequence as an internal control (or "amplification control") to assess for inhibition of amplification. Results are reported as negative for GC or CT only when amplification of the internal control is documented.

A variant strain of CT has been identified in Sweden with a 377-base-pair deletion in the cryptic plasmid, which is the target for several of the CT tests. This deletion leads to false-negative results with some but not all of the tests that target the cryptic plasmid. Tests that target other regions of the organism are not affected. The ability of a test to detect this variant is important when a test is chosen, particularly if this variant is commonly found in the geographic area where the test will be used.[91,124]

Liquid Cytology Specimens

Performing CT and GC testing for liquid cytology specimens is a matter of interest because a single specimen can be used for cervical cytology (PAP smear) and for CT and GC testing.[8] The latter two tests would be performed on the liquid specimen that remained after completion of the PAP and human papillomavirus testing. However, several drawbacks to this approach must be considered. The instruments used to prepare liquid PAP smears were not designed to control for cross-contamination during processing, and this may lead to false-positive results. CT and GC testing would not be performed until after the PAP smear and human papillomavirus testing were completed, which could delay diagnosis and treatment of CT or GC infection. Moreover, the remaining specimen may be inadequate to complete CT and GC testing, thus requiring the patient to make a return visit for collection of an additional sample. Removing an aliquot for CT and GC testing before PAP testing is performed may be helpful in overcoming some of these issues, provided adequate volume of sample remains for PAP testing. This approach does not completely remove the risk of cross-contamination, so specimens must be handled in a manner consistent with procedures used in molecular laboratories, such as uncapping and aliquoting one specimen at a time.

Recommendations on Laboratory Testing for CT and GC

In January of 2009, an expert panel was convened by the Association of Public Health Laboratories in cooperation with the Centers for Disease Control and Prevention to update recommendations on laboratory diagnostic testing for CT and GC (document available at www.aphl.org; Laboratory Diagnostic Testing for *Chlamydia trachomatis* and *Neisseria gonorrhoeae*). Several of the new and updated recommendations are as follows:

1. Urine is the preferred specimen in males. Vaginal swabs are the preferred specimen for screening females, because the sensitivity of tests with vaginal specimens is equal to or superior to that with cervical swabs.
2. Nucleic acid testing (NAT) is recommended for the detection of rectal and oropharyngeal infections caused by CT and GC. Because currently available CT and GC tests are not cleared for this specimen type, laboratories must perform a validation study to establish the performance characteristics of the test. A NAT test with minimal cross-reactivity with commensal *Neisseria* species should be used.
3. Routine repeat testing of NAT-positive screening tests is not recommended.
4. NAT testing is superior to culture for the detection of CT in cases of adult rape or abuse. For GC, positive results of tests that have significant cross-reactivity with nongonococcal *Neisseria* species should be retested with a different NAT.
5. In cases of pediatric sexual abuse, NAT for CT has been shown to be superior to culture. For GC, positive results of tests that have significant cross-reactivity with nongonococcal *Neisseria* species should be retested with a different NAT.

HUMAN PAPILLOMAVIRUS

Human papillomaviruses (HPVs) are small, double-stranded DNA viruses that infect squamous epithelium, subverting normal cell growth and potentially leading to squamous cell carcinoma.[98] Anogenital HPV infections are common in both men and women. It is estimated that more than 24 million men and women in the United States are currently infected with HPV. HPV is a sexually transmitted infection; it is most common among sexually active young women ages 15 through 25 years. In one study, cervicovaginal HPV was found in up to 43% of sexually active college women during a 3-year period.[63] Infections, however, are usually transient, and progression to cancer requires persistence of viral infection over several years. The types of HPV that are spread through sexual contact are classified as low risk or high risk for progression to malignancy, and there are multiple types. Infections with low-risk HPV such as types 6 and 11 can lead to benign genital warts or condyloma acuminata and have a low likelihood of progressing to malignancy. In contrast, high-risk types such as types 16, 18, and 45 are associated with development of squamous cell carcinoma of the anogenital region and oropharynx. The cervix is particularly affected, and worldwide cervical squamous cell carcinoma continues to cause significant morbidity and mortality (5% of cancer deaths).

Productive infections usually result in cytologic and histologic changes including cellular and nuclear enlargement, nuclear hyperchromasia, and perinuclear halos (koilocytosis). These changes can be identified on a stained smear of cells collected from the cervix (the "Pap smear," developed by Dr. George Papanicolaou in the 1940s) or in a biopsy taken during colposcopy or a loop electrosurgical excision procedure (LEEP). The Pap smear has been used very successfully to identify women with cervical cancer and, more important, for the detection of precursor lesions, so that biopsy or excision can be performed to remove the lesion earlier in the disease process, before metastasis can occur.

The histologic types of squamous precursor lesions are divided into three categories: (1) mild dysplasia, or cervical intraepithelial neoplasia (CIN)1; (2) moderate dysplasia, or CIN2; and (3) severe dysplasia, or carcinoma in situ, or CIN3. In the Bethesda System for Cytologic Classification, squamous precursor lesions are divided into low-grade and high-grade squamous intraepithelial lesions (LSIL and HSIL). LSIL corresponds with CIN1, and HSIL corresponds to CIN2 and CIN3. Frequently, the cytologic evaluation demonstrates mildly atypical cells that do not meet these criteria and are referred to as *atypical squamous cells of undetermined significance (ASCUS);* these cells may correspond to an early HPV infection. The prevalence of ASCUS on Pap smears is approximately 5 to 10%, with rates as high as 20% reported in sexually active women. Not all women with a cytology result of ASCUS progress to cervical cancer.

Primarily as a result of the ALTS trial (ASCUS and LSIL Triage Study), performed in the late 1990s, HPV testing now plays an important role in assessing which women with ASCUS are at highest risk of developing cervical cancer. The 2006 Guidelines recommend that women 20 years or older in whom ASCUS is found on Pap testing should be tested for the presence of high-risk HPV.[167] Those women testing positive for high-risk HPV DNA should undergo further clinical and pathologic examination (colposcopy), and those testing negative for HPV DNA can be followed according to routine practice. The Guidelines also recommended that women 30 years or older with a normal Pap and a negative HPV test result could have less-frequent examinations (every 3 years), and those with an HPV-positive test result could have (1) repeat Pap or HPV testing in a year, or (2) HPV genotyping performed; if found to be positive for type 16 or 18, they should be referred for immediate colposcopy.

Nucleic Acid Testing for HPV

Three tests for the detection of HPV DNA and one for genotype identification of HPV 16 and 18 have been cleared by the FDA for use in the United States: Hybrid Capture 2 (Qiagen Inc., Valencia, Calif), Cervista HPV HR (Hologic Inc., Danbury, Conn), cobas® HPV Test (Roche Diagnostics) and Cervista HPV-16 and -18 Genotyping test. All four tests have been cleared by the FDA for use with ThinPrep PreservCyt liquid-based cytology media (Hologic Inc.), but not with the other commonly used SurePath media (Becton-Dickinson). The Hybrid Capture 2 (HC2) test relies on hybridization of an RNA probe to the HPV DNA, followed by use of an antibody for capture of the duplex (RNA-DNA) hybrids, and then detection with chemiluminescent signal amplification. The test uses a pool of RNA probes spanning the entire genome that are specific for 13 high-risk HPV types (16, 18, 31, 33, 35, 39, 45, 51, 52, 56, 58, 59, and 68). The specific type is not identified. The test uses a 96-well microtiter plate format and can be performed manually or with the semiautomated Rapid Capture system (Qiagen) for reagent and plate handling. It is also cleared for use on Digene specimen transport media (STM). The HC2 test has been used in several large studies and reproducibly demonstrates high sensitivity of 93 to 96%, but false-positive results occur as a result of cross-reaction with low-risk HPV types.[23]

The Cervista HPV HR assay also uses a signal amplification method that is based on Invader technology (Hologic Inc.) and detects the same 13 high-risk types, along with HPV 66. A combination of DNA probes and invader oligonucleotides targeting the late gene (L)1 sequence and secondary fluorescently labeled probes are divided into three phylogenetically related reactions that are performed on 96-well microtiter plates. Unlike the HC2 assay, this assay includes an internal control with each reaction. Both assays have low limits of detection of around 3000 to 5000 genome copies per milliliter. The Cervista HPV HR assay appears to have less frequent cross-reactivity with low-risk types. Studies comparing the two assays demonstrate concordance of 82 to 88%. The Cervista HPV-16 and -18 Genotyping test is the first assay cleared by the FDA for HPV genotyping; it uses the same Invader technology.

The cobas HPV Test is the first real-time PCR method FDA-approved for cervical cancer screening. It utilizes a multiplexed primer and hydrolysis probe (TaqMan-based chemistry) assay to individually detect both HPV types 16 and 18 simultaneously with the 12 other high-risk HPV types using different fluorescently labeled probes. The assay includes detection of the human beta-globin gene as an internal control for extraction and amplification adequacy. The cobas 4800 system utilizes automated bead-based nucleic acid extraction and PCR reaction assembly. The sensitivity and specificity have been reported similar to the HC2 and Cervista HPV HR assays.

Other manufacturers that are developing HPV tests or performing clinical trials for FDA submission include Abbott, AutoGenomics, and Gen-Probe. Several of these tests are already available outside the United States. The assays use various methods such as real-time PCR, transcription-mediated amplification, and array hybridization for detection and genotyping.

HUMAN IMMUNODEFICIENCY VIRUS TYPE 1

Human immunodeficiency virus type 1 (HIV-1), the causative agent of the acquired immunodeficiency syndrome (AIDS), is an RNA virus belonging to the genus *Lentivirus* of the family Retroviridae. Replication of the virus is complex and involves reverse transcription of the RNA genome into a double-stranded DNA molecule or provirus, which is integrated into the host genome. HIV-1 enters the cell using CD4 as a receptor and CXCR4 or CCR5 as a coreceptor. In general, CCR5 coreceptors are found on macrophages, and CXCR4 coreceptors are found on T cells. Determining the cellular tropism of the virus has become important, now that a new antiretroviral drug targets the CCR5 coreceptor. The HIV-1 reverse transcriptase enzyme does not have proofreading capabilities, leading to the marked genetic diversity of HIV-1. Several distinct genetic subtypes or clades have been identified and are categorized into three groups: major (M), outlier (O), and N (nonmajor and nonoutlier). The major group is divided into nine clades (A, B, C, D, F, G, H, J, and K) and circulating recombinant forms (CRFs), which are determined on the basis of sequence diversity within the HIV-1 *gag* and *env* genes.[42] Group M virus is found worldwide, with clade B predominating in Europe and North America, clade C in Africa and India, and clade E in much of Southeast Asia. Complex replication cycles and genetic diversity are two factors that influence the design and interpretation of HIV-1 molecular assays.

The management of HIV-1 infection has been revolutionized by tests performed to measure the concentrations of HIV-1 RNA in blood (viral load testing) and tests for resistance to antiviral drugs. With these tools, it is possible to maximize the effectiveness of antiretroviral therapy for an individual.

HIV-1 Viral Load Testing

Viral load testing became the standard of care around 1996, followed by resistance testing. The clinical utility of viral load testing (usually using blood plasma) has been well established. Testing is used (1) to determine when to initiate antiretroviral therapy, (2) to monitor response to therapy, and (3) to predict time to progression to AIDS. Higher viral loads are associated with more rapid progression to AIDS and death.[99,100,111] Viral load testing is used routinely in decisions regarding when to initiate antiretroviral therapy and in monitoring response to therapy. Current treatment guidelines [U.S. Department of Health and Human Services (DHHS) Panel on Antiretroviral Guidelines, http://AIDSinfo.nih.gov] recommend initiating therapy for individuals on the basis of several factors, including concentrations of CD4-positive cells in blood (CD4 cell counts), viral loads, and symptoms.

The current standard for treating HIV-1–infected individuals is to use combinations of highly active antiretroviral drugs. Multiple classes of drugs are used, including nucleoside reverse transcriptase inhibitors (NRTIs), non-nucleoside reverse transcriptase inhibitors (NNRTIs), protease inhibitors (PIs), fusion inhibitors, integrase inhibitors, and CCR5 entry inhibitors. Current guidelines (DHHS Panel on Antiretroviral Guidelines, http://AIDSinfo.nih.gov) recommend an initial regimen of two NRTIs and either an NNRTI or a PI. This combination therapy is often referred to as *highly active antiretroviral therapy,* or *HAART.* Initial use of these effective drug combinations in individuals who have not been treated with them before ("naive" individuals) is expected to decrease viral loads by at least 100-fold, or 2 $\log_{10}$ copies/mL. The goal of therapy is to achieve viral loads below the limit of detection of currently available assays (50 copies/mL), although this is not always possible in all individuals, particularly in those with very high pretreatment viral load values, or in those who have failed prior therapeutic regimens. Guidelines for the use of HIV-1 RNA viral load values in clinical practice have been published[131] and are frequently updated (http://www.aidsinfo.nih.gov/, http://www.iasusa.org). In general, a plasma HIV-1 viral load should be measured before therapy is begun (baseline), and then again at 2 to 8 weeks after initiation of therapy to determine the response to therapy. Testing is then repeated at 3- to 4-month intervals to evaluate continued effectiveness of the regimen. Any increase in viral load should be confirmed with repeat testing because a variety of other illnesses can transiently increase viral load. When a significant increase in viral load has been documented, HIV-1 resistance testing should be considered (see later).

The use of HIV-1 viral load testing for *diagnosing* acute HIV-1 infection in adults is more controversial. Currently available viral load assays are approved by the FDA for use only in patients known to be infected with HIV-1, but they have clear utility in the diagnosis of acute infection, which is defined as the period after exposure to the virus but before seroconversion, that is, while the enzyme-linked immunosorbent assay (ELISA) and Western blot assays for antibodies to HIV-1 are negative or indeterminate. In this "window period," additional testing is required and viral load assays are often used. Individuals with acute infection are often symptomatic with a mononucleosis-type syndrome, which may include fever, fatigue, rash, lymphadenopathy, and oral ulcers.[77] During this acute infection, the plasma concentration of viral RNA is very high, usually 10^5 to 10^7 copies/mL, and viral load measurements are a useful diagnostic tool. Acute HIV-1 infection should be suspected in an individual presenting with appropriate symptoms and risk factors. In these individuals, testing for acute HIV-1 infection would include an ELISA and a viral load assay. Care must be taken to correctly interpret these test results, because individuals with acute HIV-1 infection would be expected to have a negative or indeterminate ELISA and/or Western blot, and a very high viral load (>100,000 copies/mL). The concern with using viral load testing to diagnose acute HIV infection is that false-positive results have been reported.[37] In one study, false-positive results (usually lower than 2000 copies/mL) were found when the VERSANT bDNA test (Siemens Healthcare Diagnostics, Deerfield, Ill) was used.[37] Before acute HIV infection is diagnosed, individuals must be educated regarding the limitations of these tests and must give informed consent prior to testing. To minimize the likelihood of reporting a false-positive result, repeat testing should be done on all specimens with a detectable viral load, and an HIV-1/-2 ELISA should be obtained at the time of viral load testing. It is critical to remember that patients with acute retroviral syndrome should have very high concentrations of HIV-1 RNA.

Available HIV-1 Viral Load Assays

HIV-1 viral load assays that are currently approved by the FDA are listed in Table 42-2. (FDA-approved devices have been found by the FDA to be safe and effective for a defined clinical use. Many of the other tests described in this chapter are FDA-cleared devices; they have been deemed substantially equivalent to an existing "predicate" device.) In addition to conventional molecular tests [AMPLICOR MONITOR, and VERSANT], two real-time HIV-1 viral load tests have been approved by the FDA. The lower limit of quantification differs among the assays, although most tests reach levels of 40 to 50 copies/mL. The reportable concentration range of each of the conventional AMPLICOR assays is limited, so both an ultrasensitive and a standard version of the test are needed to cover the clinically important range of viral load values. Viral load assays must be able to accurately quantify the various viral subtypes. In the United States and Europe, subtype B predominates, although infections with non-B subtypes are becoming more common and are certainly an important cause of HIV-1 infection globally. The VERSANT bDNA assay will accurately quantify HIV-1 subtypes A through G,[71] and the AMPLICOR reverse transcriptase polymerase chain reaction (RT-PCR), version 1.5 (Roche Diagnostics), will perform accurate quantification of subtypes A through H.[71,109,113,114] The real-time RT-PCR tests have been designed to detect genetically diverse types and subtypes of HIV-1. The COBAS TaqMan test (Roche Diagnostics) quantifies all subtypes of group M and group N viruses and many CRFs.[137] Version 2 of the COBAS TaqMan test is now available and has a lower limit of quantification of 20 copies/mL and accurately quantifies Group O virus and a broader range of CRFs compared to the version 1 test. The RealTime TaqMan test quantifies all group M and N viruses, CRFs, and group O virus.[54,149] Real-time viral load tests have several other important advantages compared with conventional viral load tests, including broader linear range, greater automation, and decreased risk of carryover contamination. Viral load values obtained with the different assays may not always agree, so it is recommended that one assay is chosen when patients are monitored over time.

Analytical characteristics of viral load assays have been examined in several studies.[14] The intra-assay imprecision (SD) of the assays is approximately 0.12 to 0.2 $\log_{10}$, with the VERSANT bDNA assay showing the best precision. The biological variation (as SD) of the virus in patients not receiving therapy is approximately 0.3 $\log_{10}$ copies/mL.[88,131] For the AMPLICOR (version 1.0) assay, the total variation was approximately 0.26 $\log_{10}$, including intra-assay, interassay, and biological variation, with biological variation accounting for 56 to 80% of the total variation.[15] Changes in viral load must exceed 0.5 $\log_{10}$ (a fivefold change) or more to suggest a change in viral replication rather than a change in viral load attributable to analytical and day-to-day biological variation. Reporting viral load results as $\log_{10}$ copies/mL is recommended[33] and will assist in preventing clinicians from

TABLE 42-2 Quantitative HIV (Viral Load) Assays Approved by the FDA*

Test	Amplification Method	Linear Range
AMPLICOR HIV MONITOR v. 1.5 test (Roche Diagnostics, Indianapolis, Ind)	RT-PCR†	Ultrasensitive: 50 to 100,000 copies/mL Standard: 400 to 750,000 copies/mL
COBAS AMPLICOR HIV-1 MONITOR v. 1.5	RT-PCR RT-PCR	Ultrasensitive: 50 to 100,000 copies/mL Standard: 400 to 750,000 copies/mL
COBAS AmpliPrep/ COBAS Amplicor HIV-1 MONITOR v. 1.5	RT-PCR	Ultrasensitive: 50 to 100,000 copies/mL Standard: 500 to 1,000,000 copies/mL
COBAS AmpliPrep/ COBAS TaqMan HIV-1 version 1	Real time RT-PCR	48 to 10,000,000 copies/mL
COBAS AmpliPrep/ COBAS TaqMan HIV-1 version 2	Real time RT-PCR	20 to 10,000,000 copies/mL
VERSANT HIV-1 RNA 3.0 Assay (Siemens Healthcare Diagnostics, Tarrytown, NY)	bDNA‡	75 to 500,000 copies/mL
RealTime TaqMan HIV-1 (Abbott Molecular, Des Plaines, Ill)	Real-time RT-PCR	40 to 10,000,000 copies/mL

*For FDA listings of these and any newer tests, visit http://www.accessdata.fda.gov/scripts/cdrh/cfdocs/cfRL/listing.cfm and use test code MTL.
†Reverse transcriptase polymerase chain reaction.
‡Branched DNA.

overinterpreting small changes in viral load. This is particularly important for values near the limit of quantification, where assay variability is the greatest. A variety of acute and opportunistic infections and vaccinations can transiently increase HIV-1 RNA in plasma,[39,111,147] so it is recommended not to measure viral load for monitoring of individuals who are acutely ill and those who have been recently vaccinated.

Viral load testing is routinely performed on plasma specimens, and ethylenediaminetetraacetic acid (EDTA) is the anticoagulant of choice. Acid-citrate-dextrose is also an acceptable anticoagulant, but blood anticoagulated in heparin is unacceptable for most tests. Viral load testing can be done on specimens other than plasma, including serum, dried blood (or plasma) spots on filter paper, CSF, and genital secretions. The assays have not been approved by the FDA for all of these specimen types, and testing of these specimens is usually reserved for research studies. It is critical to handle clinical specimens properly to minimize the risk of RNA degradation during specimen collection and transport. Plasma should be separated within 6 hours of collection and ideally stored at −20 °C, although plasma viral RNA is stable at 4 °C for several days. For laboratories performing testing from specimens collected at remote sites, sample handling can require careful attention. Special blood collection containers, or tubes, are available that contain a gel that provides a physical barrier between the plasma and cells after centrifugation. The tubes can be shipped without the need to transfer the plasma into a separate tube.[64] Vacutainer brand plasma preparation tubes (PPTs) (Becton-Dickinson), similar to plasma separation tubes (PSTs), are an example of such a container. Tubes should not be frozen prior to pouring off of the plasma, as this may lead to a false increase in results of viral load assays.[47,52]

Qualitative and Proviral HIV-1 RNA Testing

Both qualitative RNA and proviral DNA tests are useful for the diagnosis of HIV-1 infection in newborns (Guidelines for the Use of Antiretroviral Agents in Pediatric HIV Infection, http://AIDSinfo.nih.gov). Because maternal immunoglobulin (Ig)G crosses the placenta, an uninfected child of an HIV-positive mother may be seropositive into the second year of life. The diagnosis or exclusion of HIV-1 infection requires use of testing at several different time points, usually (1) shortly after birth (14 to 21 days), (2) at 1 to 2 months, and (3) at 4 to 6 months after birth. The diagnosis of HIV-1 infection requires two positive RNA or DNA tests performed on separate blood samples regardless of age. RNA and DNA tests have different strengths and weaknesses. HIV-1 DNA tests may be less sensitive for the detection of non-B subtype infections than are HIV-1 RNA tests, particularly the FDA-approved APTIMA HIV-1 RNA Qualitative Assay (Gen-Probe), which is the first qualitative NAT approved by the FDA for the diagnosis of acute HIV-1 infection. Proviral DNA tests are also useful for the diagnosis of neonatal infection because they remain positive when the infant is receiving antiretroviral therapy. Currently, no proviral DNA tests have been approved by the FDA; the AMPLICOR HIV-1 DNA PCR assay (Roche Diagnostics) is available as a research-use-only (RUO) test.

The APTIMA test has also been approved for the diagnosis of acute HIV-1 infection in adults, for confirming a repeatedly positive antibody screen, or for resolving indeterminate Western blots. This test targets both the 5′ long terminal repeat (LTR) and the *pol* gene of the HIV-1 genome, and it detects all HIV-1 group M, N, and O viruses. The test is analytically sensitive with a limit of detection of 30 copies/mL. One reason this test has not been widely adopted in clinical laboratories is that it is a manual test, and the volume of testing in any given laboratory is very low, so this type of testing is often sent to referral laboratories.

HIV-1 Resistance Testing

Six general classes of antiretroviral drugs are used in clinical care: nucleoside reverse transcriptase inhibitors (NRTIs), non-nucleoside reverse transcriptase inhibitors (NNRTIs), protease inhibitors (PIs), fusion inhibitors, integrase inhibitors, and CCR5 entry inhibitors. Viral resistance can occur with each of these classes of drug, particularly when viral replication is not maximally suppressed during therapy. The current standard of care is to use regimens that contain a combination of drugs because resistance is less likely to occur on the complex regimens than on monotherapy.

A variety of studies have evaluated the clinical utility of antiviral resistance testing in HIV-1–infected individuals. Several early prospective randomized clinical trials of genotypic resistance testing were conducted with persons who had failed therapy with multidrug regimens including PIs and NRTIs. In both the VIRADAPT[32,40] and GART[6] studies, selection of the salvage regimen was determined by using genotypic resistance testing (genotype arm) or by considering which antiretroviral drugs had been used in prior treatment regimens (control arm). Response rates in the genotype arms were higher than in the control arm. For example, in the VIRADAPT study, patients in the genotype arm had a greater decrease in viral load 6 months after salvage therapy was initiated, and more of them (32% vs. 14 %) had plasma viral loads <200 copies/mL.[32,40] The HAVANA trial helped establish the utility of expert advice in interpreting genotypic resistance data by comparing genotype resistance testing, expert advice, or both with the standard of care for selecting a regimen in patients failing therapy.[154] Although either genotyping or expert advice improved response compared with the control group, the best response was seen in the group receiving both genotyping and expert advice. The VIRA3001 study, a prospective randomized trial that compared standard of care versus phenotypic resistance testing in patients who failed a PI-containing regimen, found a better virologic outcome for patients in the phenotypic arm.[34] Although some trials of resistance testing have not shown improved clinical outcomes compared with standard of care,[59,101,103] the results of randomized trials favor use of resistance testing.

Guidelines for the appropriate use of HIV-1 resistance testing in adults have been established and are regularly updated (DHHS Panel on Antiretroviral Guidelines, http://

AIDSinfo.nih.gov). Resistance testing is recommended in the following situations: (1) when changing antiretroviral regimens, (2) before initiating therapy in patients who have never received therapy, (3) during management of patients who have not obtained an optimal decrease in viral load values, and (4) before initiating therapy in all pregnant women.

HIV-1 resistance testing can be done by genotypic or phenotypic methods. Genotypic assays identify specific mutations or nucleotide changes that are associated with decreased susceptibility to an antiviral drug. The effective use of genotypic resistance testing requires an extensive understanding of the genetics of antiretroviral resistance. This discussion will be limited to automated sequencing methods, because this is the method used in the overwhelming majority of genotypic resistance testing performed for management of patients. Currently available FDA-cleared assays will detect mutations in the reverse transcriptase and protease gene; modifications of existing assays will be needed to detect resistance mutations associated with other classes of drugs such as fusion inhibitors.

The first step in genotypic assays is the isolation of HIV-1 RNA from plasma, followed by RT-PCR amplification and sequencing of reverse transcriptase and protease genes. Analysis of the results involves sequence alignment and editing, mutation identification by comparison with wild-type sequence, and interpretation of the clinical significance of the mutations identified. Most clinical laboratories performing genotypic resistance testing rely on commercial assays that provide reagents and software programs to assist with interpretation of the results. Two assays have been cleared by the FDA: the Trugene HIV-1 Genotyping Kit and OpenGene DNA Sequencing System (Siemens Healthcare Diagnostics) and the ViroSeq HIV-1 Genotyping System (Abbott Molecular, Des Plaines, Ill).

Interpretation of genotypic resistance testing is complex. Interpretation of resistance mutations uses "rules-based" software that takes into account cross-resistance and interactions of mutations. The commercially available systems generate a summary report that lists the various mutations that have been identified in the reverse transcriptase and protease genes, and each drug is reported as resistant, possibly resistant, no evidence of resistance, or insufficient evidence. A comprehensive discussion of the specific mutations associated with each antiretroviral drug and the interactions of mutations is beyond the scope of this chapter, but is available from a variety of sources (http://www.iasusa.org, http://hivdb.stanford.edu/).

Phenotypic resistance assays measure viral replication in the presence of antiretroviral drugs. Results of phenotypic assays are typically reported as the inhibitory concentration of a drug that reduces in vitro HIV-1 replication by 50% (IC_{50}). The IC_{50} is usually reported as the fold change in IC_{50} relative to a wild-type strain. Initially, phenotypic assays required the isolation of infectious HIV-1 from a blood specimen. Newer phenotypic assays use high-throughput automated assays based on recombinant DNA technology. For these assays, HIV-1 RNA is amplified from a plasma specimen, eliminating the need for a viral isolate. This testing is not performed in clinical laboratories, and the technology is available from only two commercial laboratories. For the PhenoSense assay (Monogram Biosciences, South San Francisco, Calif), the protease and reverse transcriptase genes are amplified using RT-PCR and are inserted into a modified HIV-1 vector that has a luciferase reporter gene in place of the viral envelope gene.[117] Drug resistance is assessed by quantification of luciferase expression in the presence of various concentrations of antiretroviral drugs. The reproducibility of the assay is such that increases in IC_{50} greater than 2.5-fold can be reliably detected in the assay. The other assay (Antivirogram, VIRCO Lab Inc., Bridgewater, NJ) combines patient and HIV-1 vector sequences using in vitro recombination.[34] Viral replication is measured using a reporter gene system. Based on replicate studies performed by the company, reduced susceptibility is defined as a greater than fourfold increase in IC_{50} compared with wild-type virus. This technical cutoff often differs from the cutoff that is associated with clinical resistance to a drug, which is referred to as the *clinical cutoff.* The change in IC_{50} associated with clinical failure may differ for each drug tested. For example, with the protease inhibitor lopinavir, the IC_{50} that correlates with clinical resistance may be in the range of a 10-fold or greater increase in IC_{50},[156] compared with twofold for the NRTI didanosine (ddI). It is likely that IC_{50} cutoffs will continue to be modified as more clinical outcomes data become available. Results of phenotypic assays include not only the change in IC_{50} value, but an interpretation of whether there is an increase or decrease in susceptibility compared with wild-type virus. Phenotypic tests are available to measure susceptibility to NRTIs, NNRTIs, PIs, fusion inhibitors, and integrase inhibitors.

A "virtual phenotype" is also available commercially for assessing HIV-1 drug resistance. With a virtual phenotype, rather than performing a phenotypic assay directly, the information is inferred from the genotypic assay. Results of the genotypic assay are entered into a database containing matching genotypic and phenotypic results from thousands of clinical specimens, and the closest matching phenotypic results are averaged and reported as the virtual phenotype.

Both phenotypic and genotypic assays are used in clinical care. Some clinicians prefer phenotypic testing because it is a direct measure of viral susceptibility; others prefer genotypic testing because the development of a mutation may precede phenotypic expression of resistance.[62] Other advantages of genotypic testing include relatively rapid turnaround time (a few days), easier availability, and lower cost compared with phenotypic testing. Providers often use genotypic testing routinely and rely on phenotypic testing for patients who have failed multiple regimens and have very complex genotypic results. If both assays are used, it is important to remember that the results of the two assays may not agree, as the presence of a resistance mutation does not ensure its expression in a phenotypic assay.

A limitation of currently used genotypic and phenotypic assays is that they can detect only those mutants that make up at least 20% of the total viral population. Regimens chosen based on resistance testing may not always be effective because the minority populations will quickly predominate in the presence of drug. Drug selection pressure is also needed for some resistance mutations to persist at detectable concentrations in the viral population; when drug therapy is discontinued, the wild-type virus may quickly predominate. For this reason, it is recommended that specimens for resistance testing be obtained while the patient is on antiretroviral therapy.

The minimum viral load required for reliable resistance testing is approximately 1000 copies/mL. Because genotyping assays are especially sensitive to RNA degradation, care must be taken to properly handle the specimen after collection. Guidelines outlined for collection and transport of specimens for testing in viral load assays should be followed for resistance testing.

HIV-1 Tropism Testing

Maraviroc, the new CCR5 inhibitor, is effective only against HIV-1 that uses CCR5 as a coreceptor for entry into the cell. Virus may use CCR5 (R5-tropic) or CXCR4 (X4-tropic) of both (dual/mixed-tropic) coreceptors. The tropism test must be performed before therapy with maraviroc is initiated, as the drug is not effective against virus that is X4-tropic or dual/mixed tropic. Two tropism assays are commercially available: Trofile (Monogram Biosciences) and Sensitrop II HIV Co-Receptor Tropism Assay (Pathway Diagnostics, Malibu, Calif). The Trofile test is a cell-based assay in which pseudoviruses are constructed using the *env* gene sequence amplified from the patient's plasma. This pseudovirus is then used to infect cells that express CXCR4 or CCR5. The tropism is determined according to which cell populations the pseudovirus infects.[160] The Sensitrop assay uses a heteroduplex tracking assay (HTA) along with sequencing to identify minor viral populations that may be CXCR-4 tropic. HTA is performed using labeled probes with coreceptor-specific sequence combinations that are annealed to denatured PCR products derived from the total viral population and separated by gel electrophoresis. Mismatches with the probe result in altered migration of the heteroduplex and reveal distinct subpopulations of coreceptor-specific viral genomes.

HERPES SIMPLEX VIRUS

Herpes simplex virus (HSV), a member of the herpesvirus family, is a double-stranded DNA virus. Following primary infection, the virus remains latent in sensory neurons and can be reactivated under a variety of situations, including stress, trauma, sun exposure, and various immunocompromised states. HSV types 1 and 2 produce various clinical syndromes involving the skin, eye, central nervous system (CNS), and genital tract. Although nucleic acid testing has been used to detect HSV DNA in all of these clinical manifestations, this discussion will focus on the use of HSV PCR for the diagnosis of CNS infections, because nucleic acid amplification testing is widely viewed as the standard of care for their diagnosis.

HSV causes both encephalitis and meningitis. In adults, HSV encephalitis is usually attributable to infection with HSV type 1, while HSV meningitis is most commonly caused by HSV type 2. HSV encephalitis is a severe infection with high morbidity and mortality; treatment with acyclovir reduces mortality from approximately 70% in untreated infection to 19 to 28%. Neurologic impairment is common (about 50%) in those who survive.[161,162] HSV encephalitis may reflect primary infection or reactivation of latent infection. HSV meningitis is usually a self-limited disease that resolves over the course of several days without therapy. In some patients the disease may recur as a lymphocytic meningitis over a period of years.[150,161]

Neonatal HSV infection occurs in 1 : 3500 to 1 : 5000 deliveries in the United States.[161] It is most commonly acquired by intrapartum contact with infected maternal genital secretions and is usually due to HSV type 2. In the newborn, three general presentations of the disease are known: (1) skin, eye, and mouth disease, which accounts for approximately 45% of infections; (2) encephalitis, which accounts for 35%; and (3) disseminated disease, 20%. Because disseminated disease is often associated with neurologic disease, CNS disease occurs in about 50% of newborns with neonatal HSV infection.

HSV encephalitis cannot be distinguished clinically from encephalitis caused by other viruses such as West Nile Virus, St. Louis encephalitis virus, and Eastern equine encephalitis virus. Historically, the gold standard for the diagnosis of HSV encephalitis required brain biopsy with identification of HSV by cell culture or immunohistochemical staining. This approach provided high sensitivity (99%) and specificity (100%), but it required an invasive procedure, and several days elapsed before results were available. Cell culture of CSF has a sensitivity of less than 10% for the diagnosis of HSV encephalitis in adults. Tests that measure HSV antigen or antibody in CSF have diagnostic sensitivities of 75 to 85%, and diagnostic specificities of 60 to 90%.[161] Because of the limitations of conventional methods, there was interest in assessing the clinical utility of PCR for the detection of HSV DNA from CSF of patients with encephalitis.

Nucleic Acid Testing for HSV

The two largest studies compared HSV PCR on CSF specimens versus brain biopsy[4,84] in patients with suspected HSV encephalitis. The sensitivity and specificity of PCR were greater than 95%, and the sensitivity of HSV PCR did not decrease significantly until 5 to 7 days after the start of therapy. PCR is positive early in the course of illness, usually within the first 24 hours of symptoms, and in some individuals, HSV DNA can persist in the CSF for weeks after therapy is initiated.[4,84,163]

The clinical utility of HSV PCR has also been established for the diagnosis of neonatal HSV infection. In one study,[79] HSV DNA was detected in the CSF of 76% (26 of 34) of infants with CNS disease; 94% (13 of 14) of those with disseminated infection; and 24% (7 of 29) of infants with skin, eye, or mouth disease. The persistence of HSV DNA in the CSF of newborns for longer than 1 week after therapy is initiated is associated with a poor outcome.[90] Based on these findings, detection of HSV DNA in CSF by PCR has become the standard of care for the diagnosis of HSV encephalitis and neonatal HSV infection. In newborns with disseminated disease, HSV DNA may be detected in serum or plasma specimens, and it can be a useful diagnostic tool in newborns if it is not possible to do a lumbar puncture. Although the sensitivity of HSV PCR is high, it is not 100%, so a negative PCR test may not rule out neurologic disease due to HSV, particularly if the pretest probability is high. In this situation, it is important to consider repeat testing.

As with HSV encephalitis, HSV meningitis cannot be distinguished clinically from other viral meningitides, although recurrence of viral meningitis is a strong clue that HSV may be the etiologic agent. Unlike HSV encephalitis, HSV meningitis has not been the subject of large studies evaluating the clinical utility of PCR for diagnosis. Nonetheless, because the sensitivity of cell culture of CSF specimens is only 50%, HSV PCR of CSF is commonly used in the evaluation of meningitis and has been described as accurate in anecdotal reports.[135,150]

Molecular tests for the detection of HSV DNA from genital specimens have been cleared by the FDA, importantly none of these tests have been cleared for use with CSF specimens. Several companies provide primers and probes as analyte-specific reagents (ASRs), which can be used as components in laboratory-developed tests (LDTs).

Molecular tests are often designed to detect HSV types 1 and 2 with equal sensitivity. Distinguishing between HSV types 1 and 2 may not be necessary because the clinical management of CNS disease is the same for both infections. Primers used for the detection of HSV DNA commonly target the polymerase, glycoprotein B, glycoprotein D, or thymidine kinase genes. It is important that the primers not amplify DNA from other herpesviruses that are associated with neurologic disease; these include cytomegalovirus, varicella zoster virus, human herpes virus type 6, and Epstein-Barr virus.

HSV PCR assays need low detection limits (several hundred copies/mL of specimen) to be useful in evaluating neurologic disease. This is particularly true for the diagnosis of meningitis, where CSF concentrations of DNA tend to be lower than those seen with encephalitis. HSV neurologic disease rarely occurs in individuals without an increased CSF white blood cell count or protein concentration.[140] Caution should be exercised in applying this generalization to immunocompromised individuals, as they may not mount a typical inflammatory response to HSV infection. Although HSV PCR of CSF specimens is clearly the gold standard for the diagnosis of neurologic disease, results should be interpreted with caution because neither sensitivity nor specificity is 100%. Test results should always be interpreted within the context of the clinical presentation of the patient. If results do not correlate with the clinical impression, repeat testing should be performed.

ENTEROVIRUS 2

Enteroviruses are a diverse group of single-stranded RNA viruses belonging to the Picornavirus family. This group includes polioviruses, enterovirus types A through D, and parechovirus (human echovirus). Numerous clinical presentations are seen with the nonpolioviruses, including acute aseptic meningitis, encephalitis, exanthems, conjunctivitis, acute respiratory disease, gastrointestinal disease, myopericarditis, and sepsis-like syndrome in neonates. Diagnoses typically are based on clinical presentation and/or culture methods. Cell culture methods have several drawbacks, including the requirement to inoculate multiple cell lines because no single cell line is optimal for all enterovirus types, the inability to grow some enterovirus types in cell culture, the limited diagnostic sensitivity of cell culture (65 to 75%), and the long turnaround time of 3 to 8 days for those enteroviruses that do grow in cell culture.[31] The long turnaround time for culture means that results are rarely available in a time frame to influence clinical management. Nucleic acid testing offers several important advantages over cell culture, including improved sensitivity and turnaround time. As a result, nucleic acid testing is considered the new gold standard for the diagnosis of aseptic meningitis and neonatal sepsis syndrome due to enterovirus.

Nucleic Acid Testing for Enteroviruses

Two methods are used for the detection of enteroviral RNA from clinical specimens: reverse transcriptase PCR (RT-PCR) and nucleic acid sequence-based amplification (NASBA). The primers used in clinical testing most commonly target the highly conserved 5′ untranslated region of the gene (5′ UTR)[128,130] and will detect polioviruses and enteroviruses. These primers will not detect parechoviruses (formerly echovirus types 22 and 23), although these viruses can cause aseptic meningitis. In general, molecular assays have good detection limits ranging from 0.1 to 50 tissue culture infectious doses 50 (TCID50) per assay.* The assays are quite specific, but sequence similarities may allow amplification of some types of rhinoviruses.[11,158] Currently, two tests for the detection of enteroviruses from CSF specimens have been cleared by the FDA: the NucliSENS EasyQ Enterovirus (bioMérieux) and Xpert EV (Cepheid, Sunnyvale, Calif). A clinical evaluation of the NASBA assay showed it to be more sensitive than CSF viral culture for the detection of enterovirus, and it had a specificity of 100%.[169] Likewise, the Gene Xpert enterovirus test has been shown to have a sensitivity of 97% and a specificity of 100% for the diagnosis of enteroviral meningitis.[81] The Gene Xpert test has the advantage of being very simple to perform: the specimen and reagents are added to a cartridge, which is inserted into the instrument. Nucleic acid extraction, amplification, and detection are fully automated, and results are available within about 2½ hours. The system permits random access, which allows for on-demand testing.

*References 11, 46, 112, 120, 128, 148, 158, 169, and 170.

Nucleic acid testing for the diagnosis of enteroviral infection has been evaluated in a variety of clinical studies,[1,2,78] with testing showing a sensitivity equal to or greater than that of cell culture, a high specificity, and faster turnaround times than cell culture. Several studies have suggested that the use of molecular methods for the diagnosis of enteroviral infection in infants and pediatric patients can lead to an overall cost savings by reducing the use of antibiotics and of imaging studies.[57,92,107,120] To maximize the benefits for patient care and cost savings, testing should be available on a daily basis.

As mentioned earlier, many molecular assays detect rhinoviruses, and most detect polioviruses. These two factors can lead to unexpected and misleading positive results when respiratory or stool specimens are tested. The diagnosis of enterovirus meningitis should be based on testing of CSF specimens, and sepsis syndrome is best diagnosed in the neonate by testing serum, plasma, or CSF samples.

PERINATAL GROUP B STREPTOCOCCAL DISEASE

In the 1970s, group B streptococcal (GBS) disease was the leading infectious cause of neonatal morbidity and mortality, with case rates of two to three per 1000 live births and case-fatality rates as high as 50%.[24] In 1996, consensus guidelines from the Centers for Disease Control and Prevention, the American Academy of Pediatrics, and the American College of Obstetrics and Gynecology were issued in an effort to reduce the rate of GBS disease in newborns.[24] The guidelines called for administration of intrapartum prophylactic antibiotics for GBS using a risk-based or screening-based approach. In the risk-based approach, antibiotics were administered based on identification of one of the following risk factors: intrapartum fever, prolonged rupture of membranes, or imminent preterm delivery. For the screening-based approach, vaginal/rectal cultures were collected at 35 to 37 weeks' gestation, and those women with positive cultures received intrapartum antibiotics. Since the widespread implementation of these guidelines, the number of cases of GBS disease has decreased, but GBS remains a serious cause of neonatal infection. GBS disease in the newborn may be classified as early disease, which occurs within 1 week of life and usually presents as a sepsis syndrome or pneumonia, or late disease, which is defined as that presenting at greater than 1 week of life, and which presents most commonly as sepsis or meningitis.

GBS colonization of pregnant women is common, with a prevalence of 10 to 30%; colonization may be transient, chronic, or intermittent.[123] Those women who are colonized are 25 times more likely to deliver infants with early-onset GBS disease.[12] The effectiveness of the 1996 guidelines for the prevention of neonatal GBS was re-evaluated, and it was determined that the screening approach to GBS prevention was greater than 50% more effective than the risk-based approach.[136] Based on these findings, the Centers for Disease Control and Prevention (CDC) in 2002 issued updated guidelines recommending that vaginal/rectal GBS screening cultures be done on all pregnant women. Exceptions included women with a previous infant who had GBS disease and those with GBS bacteriuria during pregnancy, because these women require intrapartum antibiotics. The risk-based approach is to be used only for women with unknown GBS status at the time of labor and delivery. See the CDC guidelines[24] for a more detailed description, and refer to the CDC Website for; updated guidelines that were published in 2010.

Methods for GBS screening of cultures have been standardized and include collection of a vaginal/rectal swab and transport to the laboratory in Amies or Stuart media. The specimen is then inoculated into an enrichment broth (LIM broth), incubated for 18 to 24 hours, and subcultured onto a sheep-blood agar plate. GBS is identified according to colony morphology, hemolysis, and latex agglutination testing. This two-step method ensures maximal sensitivity for GBS detection. GBS cultures usually require 2 to 3 days to complete. Because GBS is universally susceptible to penicillin and ampicillin, antimicrobial susceptibility testing is not routinely performed, but it is needed for women with a serious allergy to penicillin.

Nucleic Acid Testing for GBS

The clinical utility of a real-time PCR assay (Light Cycler assay, Roche Diagnostics) for the detection of GBS in pregnant women[7] was compared with culture in 112 pregnant women and was found to have a sensitivity of 97%, a specificity of 100%, and negative and positive predictive values of 98.8% and 100%, respectively. Testing results were available within 45 minutes of the time the specimen arrived in the laboratory, which raised the possibility of offering real-time testing to women who present in labor. This could be especially useful for women who present with an unknown GBS status; based on current guidelines, these women would receive intrapartum antibiotics based on risk factors. Because women without risk factors are still at risk of delivering newborns with GBS disease,[136] PCR testing would undoubtedly offer a more sensitive method for GBS detection than one based on risk factors alone. In addition, intrapartum testing would be useful in identifying women whose GBS status changes in the interval between screening-culture (weeks 35 to 37 of gestation) and the time of delivery.

Currently, several real-time PCR tests for the detection of GBS directly from rectal/vaginal swabs from pregnant women have been cleared by the FDA: the IDI-Strept B Assay (BD Diagnostics-GeneOhm, San Diego, Calif), the BD Max™ GBS Assay (BD Diagnostics-GeneOhm, San Diego, Calif), Smart GBS (Cepheid), and Xpert GBS (Cepheid). In a multicenter clinical trial, the IDI-Strept B test demonstrated a sensitivity of 94% and a specificity of 96% compared with intrapartum culture (IDI-Strept B package insert). The assay requires a few simple hands-on steps to prepare the specimen, the testing cartridge is inserted into the Smart Cycler, and testing is complete within an hour. The test also includes an internal control to monitor for inhibition of amplification. The Xpert GBS test has a sensitivity of 92% and a specificity of 96% for intrapartum testing. The test is rapid, with results available within an hour; it is easy to use and is designed for use in the clinical laboratory, as well as by nonlaboratory professionals such as labor and delivery nurses. These real-time GBS tests offer a rapid and sensitive alternative to GBS culture. Advantages need to be balanced with the challenge of providing intrapartum test results to clinicians within 1 to 2 hours at any time of day or night; also, the cost of nucleic acid testing must be compared with the cost of culture. If intrapartum testing is done at the time of labor and delivery, there will not be adequate time for erythromycin and clindamycin susceptibility testing, so women with severe penicillin allergies will require therapy with vancomycin. An alternative approach is to replace antepartum culture at 35 to 37 weeks' gestation with the real-time PCR assay. With the availability of an FDA-cleared test, there will be more discussion on the use of GBS PCR testing of pregnant women. Readers are referred to the CDC Website for updated recommendations, which are in preparation (http://www.cdc.gov/groupbstrep/hospitals/hospitals_guidelines.htm).

CYTOMEGALOVIRUS

CMV, a member of the herpesvirus family, is a double-stranded enveloped DNA virus. CMV causes a clinically minor infection in immunocompetent individuals but remains an important pathogen in immunocompromised individuals, including persons with AIDS, transplant recipients, and those on immune-modulating drugs. Primary infection is usually asymptomatic in immunocompetent persons, although a small percentage of individuals with CMV infection may develop a mononucleosis type of syndrome. Following primary infection, a life-long latent infection is established that does not cause clinical symptoms. However, if an infected individual becomes immunocompromised, the virus can reactivate, leading to a wide variety of clinical syndromes.

The most severe CMV infections are seen in those individuals who acquire their primary infection while immunocompromised. In persons with AIDS, CMV disease rarely occurs when the CD4+ cell count is above 100 cells/mm^3; the most common clinical presentations are retinitis, esophagitis, and colitis. In transplant recipients, the occurrence and severity of CMV disease are related to the CMV serostatus of the organ donor and recipient, the type of organ transplanted, and the overall degree of immunosuppression. For example, CMV disease tends to be more severe in lung transplant recipients than in renal transplant recipients. For all types of organ recipients, the most severe disease occurs when CMV-seronegative recipients receive an organ from a CMV-seropositive donor, and the primary CMV infection occurs while the person is immunosuppressed. CMV disease can also occur in seropositive individuals, whether they receive an organ from a seropositive or seronegative donor. Clinical findings associated with CMV disease in transplant recipients are diverse and include interstitial pneumonitis, esophagitis and colitis, fever, leukopenia, and, less commonly, retinitis and encephalitis.

The diagnosis of CMV disease represents a challenge because of the presence of latent infection. Immunocompromised individuals can have an asymptomatic, clinically insignificant, low-level, persistent infection that must be distinguished from clinically important active CMV disease. The distinction can be challenging when sensitive molecular assays are used that can detect small amounts of CMV DNA in clinical specimens.

Traditionally, the diagnosis of CMV disease relied on the detection of CMV from clinical specimens by the use of cell culture techniques in human diploid fibroblasts. Although considered the gold standard, these conventional culture methods are labor-intensive and have a long turnaround time of 1 to 3 weeks.[94] In addition, the assays lack adequate sensitivity for detecting CMV present in blood specimens. The (relatively) rapid shell-vial culture method can provide results in 1 to 2 days and is useful for detection of CMV in tissue, respiratory, and urine specimens. However, this assay may also fail to detect CMV in blood. Many laboratories rely on the antigenemia assay, which detects the matrix protein pp65 in polymorphonuclear cells. This semiquantitative assay is rapid, and the number of CMV antigen-positive cells correlates with the likelihood of CMV disease, but the assay is labor-intensive, and CMV antigen is not stable in whole blood specimens for periods greater than 24 hours.

Nucleic Acid Testing for CMV

In light of the limitations of culture and antigen detection methods, there has been great interest in using nucleic acid testing for the detection and quantification of CMV DNA from plasma and blood specimens. Few assays have been cleared by the FDA, and those that were have been withdrawn from the market. Many commercially available analyte specific reagents (ASRs) were removed from the market in 2008 to fulfill FDA ASR regulations. Some of these assays may become available after obtaining clearance from the FDA. Quantitative molecular CMV assays that remain commercially available include the AMPLICOR CMV MONITOR test (Roche Diagnostics), a DNA PCR assay that is an RUO test, and the artus CMV ASR (owned and distributed by Qiagen, with a distribution agreement with Abbott Molecular). Many studies have reported on performance of these assays. These LDTs use various specimen types, nucleic acid extraction methods, target genes, calibrators, and detection methods. As a result, viral load values obtained with the different assays may be inconsistent. This makes it difficult to compare results among clinical studies that use these assays and to establish concentrations of CMV DNA that correlate with clinical disease.

The analytical performance of the AMPLICOR CMV MONITOR RUO and that of the Artus CMV ASR tests have been evaluated.[18,19] The PCR-based AMPLICOR CMV MONITOR was shown to have a limited range of quantification of approximately 2.7 to 4.7 $\log_{10}$ and a limit of detection of 3.0 $\log_{10}$ copies/mL,[19] while the Artus-based real-time PCR assay is linear from 2.0 to 6.0 $\log_{10}$ copies/mL, with a limit of detection of 2.3 $\log_{10}$ copies/mL. Comparison of quantitative results between the two assays showed a mean difference of 0.012 log_{10}, varying from −0.869 to 0.845 log_{10} copies/mL.[18] The reproducibility of the Artus-based assay is such that changes in viral load (copies/mL) less than fivefold to sevenfold may represent assay variability rather than clinically relevant changes in viral replication.

An unsettled issue for CMV molecular assays is the appropriate specimen type for testing. Almost all assays use plasma or whole blood, with concentrations of CMV DNA measured in whole blood higher than those measured in plasma.[121] The AMPLICOR PCR assay and the Artus real-time PCR assay can accommodate blood or plasma specimens. CMV DNA may be detected in whole blood or leukocytes of individuals without active CMV disease. Some studies have shown a good association between high CMV DNA concentrations in plasma and active CMV disease[22] and suggest that detecting CMV DNA in plasma rather than in leukocytes may provide a better correlation with clinical disease, because the detection of CMV DNA in plasma suggests active viral replication.[121] However, it is clear that CMV DNA can also be detected in the plasma in patients without active CMV disease.[21,22] Others prefer to test whole blood because CMV DNA can be detected more frequently in blood samples than in plasma. With either sample type, the key requirement is to establish a concentration of CMV DNA that correlates with the likelihood of disease. The concentration of DNA that predicts disease will be higher in assays that use whole blood specimens than in those that test plasma specimens.

The clinical uses of CMV molecular assays are diverse and include assisting in decisions regarding (1) initiation of preemptive therapy, (2) diagnosis of active CMV disease, and (3) monitoring of response to therapy. *Preemptive therapy* refers to the use of a laboratory test to identify a group of individuals at higher risk for developing CMV disease. For example, all members of the group would be tested for the presence of CMV DNA in their blood or plasma, and only those testing positive would be treated. Therapy is administered before development of symptoms in an attempt to prevent the onset of active disease. By contrast, with *prophylactic therapy*, all patients in the group are treated, without further stratification of risk, thus involving treatment of a greater number of patients.

Molecular assays have utility for the diagnosis of active CMV disease, because CMV DNA concentrations are higher in patients with active CMV disease than in those with asymptomatic infection.[35,67] A study in liver transplant recipients using the AMPLICOR PCR assay showed that the median peak viral load in patients with asymptomatic infection was 1850 copies/mL compared with 55,000 copies/mL for those with active disease.[67] The viral load cutoff that was most predictive of the development of active disease was between 2000 and 5000 copies/mL of plasma. It is important to note that viral load cutoffs will differ in studies using different assays and different specimen types (plasma vs. whole blood).

Once active CMV disease has been diagnosed, molecular assays are useful in monitoring response to therapy. Viral load values decrease rapidly after appropriate antiviral therapy is begun, and several studies have reported that CMV DNA is cleared from the plasma within several weeks of initiation of therapy.[21,22,68] Failure of viral loads to decrease promptly should raise concerns of possible treatment failure, because persistently elevated concentrations of CMV DNA during therapy have been seen in patients with documented resistance of CMV to the therapy.[21] Molecular assays also have clinical utility in identifying patients at risk for relapsing CMV infection. In solid organ transplant recipients, patients with a detectable viral load after completing 14 days of ganciclovir therapy for CMV infection are at increased risk of relapse. Similarly, an increased risk of relapse has been shown for patients with persistent pp67 mRNA after completion of a course of therapy. The rate of decline in CMV DNA after initiation of therapy can be used to predict risk of relapse of CMV infection. In one study, CMV DNA was cleared from the plasma in 17 days for patients without recurrent CMV disease compared with 34 days for those with evidence of recurrent disease.[68] By following viral load concentrations weekly after initiating antiviral therapy, it may be possible to identify those at risk of recurrent disease and thus intensify therapy and possibly prevent recurrent disease.

CMV DNA concentrations are also useful in assessing the risk of developing CMV disease in persons with AIDS. Detection of CMV DNA in plasma has been associated with increased risk of developing CMV disease and increased risk of death. In addition, each log_{10} increase in viral load (i.e., each 10-fold increase in concentration) has been associated with a threefold increase in the risk of developing CMV disease.[143] The clinical importance of CMV viral load in patients was further established in patients with advanced AIDS, in whom the CMV DNA load was found to be more predictive of developing CMV disease or death than was HIV-1 viral load. Individuals with a CD4+ cell count lower than 50 cells/μL (50 cells/mm^3) and an HIV-1 viral load greater than 10,000 copies/mL of plasma are at greatest risk of developing end-organ CMV disease. In this group of individuals, an increase in CMV DNA to above the limit of detection of the AMPLICOR PCR assay was associated with the development of CMV end-organ disease. This study identifies a group of HIV-1–infected individuals who may benefit from monitoring of CMV viral load and preemptive therapy for the prevention of CMV end-organ disease.

A major challenge that remains for laboratories offering these assays is the difference in results among assays. The available international standard for CMV, should improve the agreement of viral load values between the different tests; this was certainly seen for hepatitis C virus (HCV) viral load testing once that international standard became available. The availability of commutable calibrators has also been shown to improve agreement between two viral load tests.[20] These types of well-characterized standards and calibrators will assist in achieving better agreement of viral load values among different tests and will facilitate the determination of CMV concentrations that predict or correspond to clinical events.

MYCOBACTERIUM TUBERCULOSIS

Mycobacterium tuberculosis (MTb) causes a wide range of clinical infections, including pulmonary disease, miliary tuberculosis, meningitis, pleurisy/pericarditis/peritonitis, gastrointestinal disease, genitourinary disease, and lymphadenitis. MTb infection was in steady decline in the United States until the late 1980s into the early 1990s. The infection rate had declined to an all-time low by the late 1990s,[26] when the number of reported cases began to increase. This resurgence in the number of infections was related to the AIDS epidemic, homelessness, and a decreased focus on tuberculosis control programs. The infection rate continues to rise in foreign-born persons as the result of immigration from countries with a high prevalence of MTb infection.[26] This increase in MTb infection has focused considerable attention on the development of assays for its rapid diagnosis; molecular methods were at the center of this effort. The goal was to design very sensitive assays that would enable the direct detection of MTb from clinical specimens. However, this goal has proved to be more difficult to reach than was originally anticipated.

Standard methods for detection of MTb include acid-fast bacilli (AFB) smear and conventional and liquid culture methods. The AFB smear is rapid but has poor sensitivity of 20 to 80%.[13] Another challenge with AFB smear is that it cannot distinguish MTb from nontuberculous mycobacteria (NTM), such as *Mycobacterium avium*-complex (MAC). This distinction is important because both disseminated MAC and MTb are common infections in persons with AIDS. Culture methods for the detection of MTb are sensitive, but growth detectable by standard methods may require 6 to 8 weeks in culture. Growth often occurs more quickly in liquid culture than with conventional methods but can still require weeks. With these limitations of culture methods, there was great enthusiasm for nucleic acid testing as a rapid, sensitive method for detection of MTb, especially given the need to rapidly isolate patients with active, untreated disease and to initiate prompt therapy, particularly in immunocompromised hosts.

Nucleic Acid Testing for MTb

The Amplified *Mycobacterium tuberculosis* Direct test [MTD test (Gen-Probe) is the only available FDA approved amplification test for the detection of MTb from clinical samples. The MTD test is based on transcription-mediated amplification of ribosomal RNA and can be used to test both AFB smear-positive and smear-negative respiratory specimens. The MTD test has not been approved for nonrespiratory specimens; this limits its clinical utility for diagnosis of extrapulmonary MTb infection. This is unfortunate because diagnosis of some of these infections is often difficult. In addition to these commercially available assays, LDTs are widely used, and a key advantage of these assays is their ability to test respiratory as well as nonrespiratory specimens.

The MTD test has a sensitivity of 95 to 98% when AFB smear-positive respiratory specimens are used, and the specificity ranges from 99 to 100%. However, early studies showed that sensitivity for AFB smear-negative specimens was ≈50%.[25] Based on these data, it was clear that the test could not be used to rule out MTb infection on smear-negative respiratory specimens. This further limited the clinical utility of these tests because it became clear that nucleic acid testing would be used to supplement AFB smear and culture, rather than replace these testing modalities. Another limitation of currently available nucleic acid assays is that they can be used only on specimens from patients who have not received antituberculosis therapy in the previous 12 months. This limitation was included because DNA can persist in respiratory secretions (and other body fluids) for months after the mycobacteria are no longer viable. The MTD test was subsequently reformulated and evaluated in a clinical trial that compared this test versus culture and versus the probability of MTb infection as determined by a panel of experts.[75] The sensitivity and specificity of the test were 86% and 98%, respectively. Positive and negative predictive values were 91% and 97%, respectively. Based on this study, the reformulated MTD test was approved by the FDA for use on both AFB smear-positive and AFB smear-negative specimens.

In spite of the limitations discussed previously, nucleic acid amplification tests do provide added value in managing patients with tuberculosis. Advantages include rapid turnaround time, greater positive predictive value (>95%) with AFB smear-positive specimens in settings where nontuberculous mycobacteria are common, and rapid confirmation of MTb in 50 to 80% of AFB smear-negative, culture-positive specimens.[27] Because of increasing use of nucleic acid amplification tests, the CDC has provided updated guidelines for the use of nucleic acid amplification tests in the diagnosis of tuberculosis.[27] It is now recommended that nucleic acid amplification testing be performed on at least one respiratory specimen from each patient with signs and symptoms of pulmonary MTb for whom a diagnosis of MTb is being considered but has not yet been established, and for whom the test result would alter case management or MTb control activities. Patients with a positive AFB smear and a positive nucleic acid testing result should be presumed to have MTb infection, and there is no need for additional nucleic acid testing. If the sputum smear is AFB-positive and two or three specimens are negative by nucleic acid testing, and inhibition of amplification has been ruled out, then the patient can be presumed to have nontuberculous mycobacterial infection. If the sputum specimen is AFB smear-negative and repeatedly positive by the MTD test, then the patient can be presumed to have MTb infection. For patients with an AFB-negative smear, a negative nucleic acid test does not rule out MTb infection.

A key consideration with molecular assays is controlling for inhibition of amplification. This is particularly critical for the detection of MTb nucleic acid from respiratory specimens, as these specimen types often contain blood or glycoprotein, which can inhibit amplification. The MTD test does not contain an inhibition control, although many laboratories include such a control by adding a positive control material to a second aliquot of the clinical specimen.

An important role for molecular assays is in the diagnosis of extrapulmonary MTb infection, such as meningitis, pleuritis, pericarditis, or peritonitis, as these infections can be very difficult to diagnose using traditional methods. Amplification assays have been used on CSF specimens for the diagnosis of MTb meningitis,[5,10,85] although the tests have not been approved by the FDA for this indication. In addition, LDTs have been developed with the flexibility needed to test a variety of clinical specimens. As mentioned for respiratory specimens, it is critical to remember that a negative nucleic acid test result does not rule out extrapulmonary MTb infection, and molecular assays using these complex body fluids should include an inhibition control.

Updated guidelines on the use of nucleic acid amplification tests have expanded their role in the diagnosis of MTb infection. However, culture remains the gold standard for laboratory confirmation of MTb infection, and an isolate of the organism is needed for susceptibility testing. Although nucleic acid testing is recommended, a portion of the clinical specimen should always be reserved for culture.

HEPATITIS C VIRUS

HCV, an RNA virus, is a major cause of chronic liver disease. According to the National Health and Nutrition Examination Survey (NHANES) of 1988-1994, approximately 4 million Americans were infected with HCV, and 2.7 million were estimated to have chronic infection. After acute infection, 80 to 85% of individuals develop a chronic infection, and 2 to 4% of these individuals develop cirrhosis and end-stage liver disease, making end-stage liver disease secondary to HCV the most common indication for liver transplantation in the United States. The development of molecular testing for HCV infection has been a major advance in the clinical care of infected individuals.

Detection and Quantification of HCV

Applications of HCV RNA testing include (1) assisting in the diagnosis of HCV infection, (2) excluding HCV infection as the etiologic agent of symptoms, (3) screening the blood supply, (4) monitoring response to therapy, and (5) determining the duration of therapy. Qualitative molecular assays can be used to confirm the diagnosis of HCV infection, although improvements in quantitative assays have made them just as sensitive. A low detection limit is particularly important in distinguishing seropositive individuals who have cleared the infection (undetectable HCV RNA) from seropositive persons who have chronic infection (persistent HCV RNA).

Data from the CDC have shown that 95% of positive results of screening ELISA that have a high signal-to-cutoff ratio can be confirmed as true positives. For these specimens, confirmation testing is not routinely needed. For specimens with a low signal-to-cutoff ratio, confirmation testing should be done with a recombinant immunoblot assay (RIBA) or by detection of HCV RNA. If HCV RNA detection is used as the confirmatory test, then RNA-negative specimens should be tested in the RIBA. This is done to distinguish a false-positive ELISA result from true infection. Alternatively, repeat testing for HCV RNA should be conducted, because viremia may be intermittent and HCV infection should not be ruled out on the basis of one negative HCV RNA test.

Qualitative molecular assays are also used to diagnose HCV infection in infants born to HCV-infected mothers. Because maternal IgG antibody can cross the placenta, these infants can be seropositive into the second year of life. Detection of HCV RNA in the plasma or serum of the newborn shortly after birth would be diagnostic of infection.

Detection of HCV RNA in plasma or serum can be a useful diagnostic test in immunocompromised individuals, such as those with end-stage HIV-1 infection, because they may not mount a normal immune response to the virus and may not be seropositive.

Qualitative HCV RNA testing is also used to define a treatment response to therapy for HCV infection because these assays are very sensitive, with lower limits of detection between 5 and 50 copies/mL plasma. Response to therapy is defined as an undetectable HCV RNA after completion of therapy; a sustained virologic response (SVR) is defined as an undetectable viral load 24 weeks after completion of therapy.

More recently, qualitative HCV RNA assays have been developed for screening the blood supply. HCV RNA is detectable in serum during the "window period" (when tests for HCV antibodies are negative) between infection and seroconversion. Because most individuals with recently acquired HCV infection are asymptomatic, testing of blood donors for HCV RNA allows identification of individuals at risk for transmitting HCV infection that would have been missed if testing were done with only serologic assays. Nucleic acid testing for HCV RNA has reduced the window period by an average of 26 days.[80] By screening the blood supply with HCV antibody testing alone, it was estimated that 1 in 100,000 transfused units contained HCV RNA, but with the addition of testing by nucleic acid amplification technology (often called NAT) for HCV, the risk is projected to be reduced to 1 in 367,000 units.[80]

Several large clinical trials have established the benefit of treatment of chronic HCV infection with ribavirin and pegylated interferon-α [interferon-α with addition of polyethylene glycol (PEG)].[44,55] Overall SVRs of approximately 55% are obtained; patients who have the common genotype 1 have SVRs of only 42 to 46%, compared with 76 to 82% for those with genotype 2 or 3 infection. In addition, no additional benefit was derived from treating genotype 2 and 3 infection for 48 weeks compared with 24 weeks, thus allowing for a shorter course of therapy for genotype 2 and 3 infections. New, specific antiviral agents offer additional therapeutic choices; the HCV NS3/4A protease inhibitor, telaprevir, is one that has shown significant improvement in SVR as high as 25% over standard of care using ribavirin and pegylated interferon-α.[61,97] Both telaprevir and boceprevir have been approved by the FDA for use in combination with ribavirin and peginterferon to treat chronic HCV infection, both drugs have shown substantial increases in the rate of SVR compared to with ribavirin and peginterferon alone. Although genotype is a strong predictor of response to therapy, studies have shown the utility of determining the viral load during the course of therapy. Patients who fail to have a 2 $\log_{10}$ drop in HCV RNA concentrations at 12 weeks [defined as an early virologic response (EVR)] after initiating interferon and ribavirin have a 3% likelihood of responding to therapy compared with 65% for patients who do achieve a 2 $\log_{10}$ drop in viral load. More recently, achieving an undetectable HCV RNA result at 4 weeks [defined as a rapid virologic response (RVR)] has been associated with an 89% likelihood of responding to just 24 weeks of therapy with ribavirin and pegylated interferon-α and achieving an SVR.[73,118,168] By determining HCV viral load at baseline, at 4 weeks, and again after 12 weeks of therapy, patients who are unlikely to respond to therapy can be identified earlier in the course of therapy. This will allow for (a) discontinuation of potentially toxic drugs and a reduction in the cost of therapy, or (b) increasing doses of these drugs, or (c) the addition of new antiviral medications. On the other hand, individuals who attain an RVR or EVR will likely have a good response to treatment and will have therapy continued for 24 to 48 weeks, depending on the HCV genotype, other risk factors, and drug side effects.

Available Assays for Detection and Quantification

Several qualitative assays have been approved by the FDA for the detection of HCV RNA in plasma or serum specimens (Table 42-3). The AMPLICOR HCV test, the COBAS AMPLICOR HCV test, and the COBAS Ampliprep/COBAS AMPLICOR HCV test (Roche Diagnostics) are based on RT-PCR technology; the COBAS AMPLICOR test allows for automation of the amplification and detection steps, and the COBAS Ampliprep adds automation for the nucleic acid extraction step. The first two versions of the AMPLICOR test have a lower limit of detection of 50 international units (IU)/mL, and the COBAS Ampliprep/COBAS AMPLICOR is lower at 13.9 or 18.8 IU/L for plasma because of the larger specimen volume that is extracted. The VERSANT HCV RNA Qualitative Assay (Siemens Healthcare Diagnostics) uses transcription-mediated amplification (TMA) and can detect as few as 5 IU/mL. In addition to these tests, laboratories have developed their own reverse transcription PCR and real-time PCR assays. Two additional qualitative assays are available only for screening the blood supply: the Procleix HIV-1/HCV Assay (Novartis Vaccines and Diagnostics Inc., Emeryville, Calif, in partnership with Gen-Probe) based on TMA technology,[70] and the AMPLISCREEN HCV test (Roche Diagnostics), which uses the reverse transcription PCR method. Both assays report a lower limit of detection of less than 50 IU/mL. Next generation blood screening instruments are currently in development.

Various tests are available for the quantification of HCV RNA. The VERSANT HCV RNA assay (Siemens Healthcare Diagnostics) was the first FDA-approved assay for HCV viral load testing (see Table 42-3). The assay is based on bDNA

TABLE 42-3 HCV RNA Tests in Clinical Use[a]

Test	Assay Method	Comments
RealTime HCV assay ASR[b]	RT-PCR[c]	Qualitative, LOD[d] defined by the individual laboratory
RealTime HCV assay ASR (Abbott Molecular, Des Plaines, Ill)	RT-PCR	Quantitative, range defined by the individual laboratory
AMPLICOR HCV Test v. 2.0	RT-PCR	Qualitative, LOD 50 IU/mL
COBAS AMPLICOR HCV test v. 2.0	RT-PCR	Qualitative, LOD 50 IU/mL
COBAS AmpliPrep/ COBAS AMPLICOR v. 2.0	RT-PCR	Qualitative, LOD 50 IU/mL
COBAS AMPLICOR HCV MONITOR Test v. 2.0	RT-PCR	Quantitative, range 600 to 500,000 IU/mL
COBAS TaqMan HCV v. 2.0 (for use with high pure system)	Real-time RT-PCR	Quantitative, range 43 to 69 million IU/mL
COBAS AmpliPrep/ COBAS TaqMan HCV test (Roche Diagnostics, Indianapolis, Ind)	Real-time RT-PCR	Quantitative, range 43 to 69 million IU/mL
Abbott Real-time HCV (Abbott Molecular, Inc. Des Plaines, IL)	Real-time RT-PCR	Quantitative range 12 to 100 million IU/mL
Versant HCV RNA assay	TMA[e]	Qualitative, limit of detection 5 IU/mL
Versant HCV RNA v. 3.0 Assay Systems 340 and 440 (Siemens Healthcare Diagnostics, Tarrytown, NY)	bDNA[f]	Quantitative, range 615 to 7.69 million IU/mL

[a]Excluding molecular testing for the blood supply.
[b]Analyte-specific reagent.
[c]Reverse transcriptase-polymerase chain reaction.
[d]Limit of detection.
[e]Transcription-mediated amplification.
[f]Branched DNA.

signal amplification technology and has a reasonably broad dynamic range and a lower limit of quantification of 615 IU/mL. The COBAS AMPLICOR HCV MONITOR test (Roche Diagnostics) uses RT-PCR and has a similar limit of quantification (600 IU/mL), but a more limited linear range requiring dilution of the clinical specimen to measure viral loads greater than 500,000 IU/mL. The first FDA-approved real-time PCR assay, the COBAS Ampliprep/COBAS TaqMan HCV test (CAP/CTM; Roche Diagnostics), has a lower limit of quantification of 43 IU/mL with a broad linear range across 6 $\log_{10}$ and uses the Ampliprep nucleic acid extraction automation. A real-time PCR assay from Abbott Molecular is also FDA-approved and has a linear range of 12 IU/ml to 100 million IU/ml. With their improved sensitivity and broad linear range, real-time tests are now widely used for monitoring response to antiviral therapy.

Several studies have evaluated and compared the FDA-cleared assays and the laboratory-developed assays; most have demonstrated good correlation.[45,102,119,133,165] Genotype-specific variability in quantification for particular HCV assays has been reported. Earlier versions of the AMPLICOR RT-PCR and bDNA assays did not accurately quantify all genotypes of HCV and usually underestimated the concentrations of genotypes 2 and 3. However, current versions of the AMPLICOR RT-PCR (version 2.0) and the VERSANT bDNA (version 3.0) quantify all HCV genotypes. The CAP/CTM assay may overquantify genotype 1 and underquantify genotype 4 specimens in comparison with the other assays.[132,157] However, all assays appear to perform well in determining SVR in patients.[93] The availability of an established World Health Organization (WHO) international standard has allowed standardization of HCV assays with reporting of results as IU per milliliter.

The intra-assay imprecision (SDs) of the HCV VERSANT bDNA, the AMPLICOR RT-PCR, and the CAP/CTM real-time PCR assays ranges from 0.05 to 0.3 $\log_{10}$; the VERSANT bDNA assay is most precise. The biological variation of HCV viral load (as SD) ranges from 0.5 $\log_{10}$ to 0.75 $\log_{10}$. Changes in HCV viral load need to exceed 1 $\log_{10}$ (i.e., a 10-fold change in concentration) or more to represent statistically significant changes beyond those explained by analytical and biological variation.

HCV Genotyping

A hallmark of HCV infection is genetic heterogeneity resulting from the low fidelity of the RNA-dependent RNA polymerase, which frequently introduces random nucleotide errors during viral replication. These replication errors could yield 10 to 100 nucleotide changes per position per year, giving rise to many genetic variants (quasispecies) of the virus in a single patient. Based on identification of these genomic differences, HCV has been classified into six major genotypes and multiple subtypes within each genotype. Geographic differences in the distribution of HCV types have been noted. In the United States, approximately two thirds of the infections are type 1, with the remaining being predominantly types 2 and 3.

The HCV genome contains well-defined 5′ and 3′ untranslated regions (5′UTR and 3′UTR). The 5′UTR is the most conserved portion of the genome and is frequently used as the target for molecular assays, including genotyping assays. The HCV genome is divided into seven areas: the core region that encodes the capsid C protein, the E1 and E2 regions that encode the envelope proteins (gp33 and gp72), and several nonstructural protein regions (NS2, NS3, NS4, and NS5). The NS5B region shows less sequence conservation than the 5′UTR, and sequencing of NS5B has been successfully used for genotyping HCV.

HCV genotyping, along with pretreatment viral load, age, gender, and the presence of hepatic fibrosis, can be used to determine the duration of antiviral therapy, with genotype being a strong predictor of a sustained virologic response. Several methods have been developed for genotyping and/or subtyping HCV, but most clinical laboratories use the reverse hybridization-based line probe assay (INNO-LiPA HCV II, Siemens Healthcare Diagnostics) or direct DNA sequencing. The INNO-LiPA assay is based on reverse hybridization of 5′UTR and core amplified products with genotype-specific probes. The INNO-LiPA HCV II discriminates and identifies the 6 HCV genotypes and subtypes.

Automated sequencing assays, developed both commercially and in-laboratory, are available to genotype HCV; the genomic regions commonly used include 5′UTR, NS5B, and core. Sequencing methods require sequence alignment and comparison with reference sequences to determine the genotype and subtype. An HCV genotyping kit based on automated sequencing (Trugene HCV 5′NC, Siemens Healthcare Diagnostics) targets the 5′UTR region. Although this assay can accurately type HCV, sequence variation in this region is not adequate to accurately subtype the virus.[110] When more variable regions of the virus are sequenced, such as NS5B, it is possible to determine both viral type and subtype. Several methods using real-time PCR technology, with or without melting curve analysis, are in limited use, and others are under development.

CLOSTRIDIUM DIFFICILE

Clostridium difficile is a gram-positive spore-forming anaerobic bacillus that is frequently found in the stool flora of healthy infants, but is rarely found in the stool flora of healthy adults and children older than 12 months. The organism is acquired by ingesting spores, which survive the gastric acid barrier and germinate in the colon. Alteration of the intestinal flora with the use of antibiotics facilitates colonization of the intestinal tract. Once colonized, patients may develop symptoms of diarrhea and/or colitis. Most strains of *C. difficile* make two toxins: toxin A and toxin B; the regulatory protein TcdC represses expression of the toxin A and B genes. These toxins are responsible for symptomatic disease; strains that lack these toxins do not cause diarrhea or colitis. Detection of these toxins or of their activity is essential in diagnostic tests for *C. difficile*–associated disease. An additional toxin, the binary toxin, has been described in some strains of

C. difficile, and recent reports have suggested that strains encoding the binary toxin have a deletion in the *tcdC* gene, leading to overexpression of toxins A and B (BI/NAP1/027), and are causing outbreaks of more severe disease.[95,96]

C. difficile is a frequent cause of antibiotic-associated diarrhea and colitis. In hospitals, the risk of infection increases with the length of hospital stay, and use of antimicrobial therapy greatly increases the likelihood of acquiring *C. difficile* colitis. *C. difficile* causes a spectrum of disease ranging from asymptomatic carrier state, to fulminant, relapsing, and fatal colitis. Diarrhea may be mild to severe. Pseudomembranous colitis is a classic presentation of *C. difficile* disease, and toxic megacolon may also be seen. Although clindamycin, penicillins, and cephalosporins have commonly been associated with disease, almost all antibiotics have been associated with disease.

Various non–nucleic acid tests are available for the diagnosis of *C. difficile* infection. Culture of the organism alone is not helpful in the diagnosis, as there needs to be confirmation that the organism is producing toxin. The cell culture cytotoxicity test neutralization assay (CCNA), which detects the cytopathic effect of toxin B, is considered the gold standard for the diagnosis of clinically important *C. difficile* infection. The test is highly sensitive and specific but is labor-intensive and technically demanding. The turnaround time of 1 to 3 days limits its clinical utility.[164] The most commonly used tests are enzyme immunoassays (EIAs) and lateral flow devices that detect toxin A and/or toxin B. Overall these tests have lower sensitivities (45 to 95%) and specificities (75 to 100%) than the cytotoxicity test.[116,141] In general, EIAs that detect both toxins A and B are preferred because some strains may not produce toxin A.[3,164] An alternative testing approach is detection of the common antigen glutamate dehydrogenase (GDH). The test does not distinguish between toxigenic and nontoxigenic strains and cannot be used alone for the diagnosis of *C. difficile* disease. A positive result needs to be confirmed with the cytotoxicity test, an EIA, or PCR for the detection of toxin. The GDH test is a useful screening test because it has a high negative predictive value. One study evaluated a two-step approach using the GDH test as the initial screen followed by a CCNA for antigen-positive specimens to confirm the presence of toxin. A negative antigen test was more than 99% predictive of a negative CCNA.[153] A limitation of this approach is the delay in obtaining a result because of the long turnaround time of the CCNA test.

Nucleic Acid Tests for *C. difficile*

In view of the limitations of traditional methods, molecular tests have recently been investigated as an alternative for the diagnosis of *C. difficile* infection. Four tests have been cleared by the FDA for the detection of *C. difficile* directly from stool specimens: GeneOhm Cdiff Assay (BD Diagnostics-GeneOhm), ProGastro Cd Assay (Gen-Probe), and the Xpert *C. difficile* test (Cepheid), and the Illumigene™ *C. difficile* (Meridian Bioscience Cincinnati, OH). These tests are designed to detect the toxin B gene *(tcdB)* or toxin A and B. The Xpert™ *C. difficile/Epi* Test also detects the binary toxin and the deletion of *tcdC,* thus allowing specific identification of the hypervirulent strain of *C. difficile* (027/NAP1/BI), although this test is cleared for epidemiologic studies only. A study comparing the GeneOhm test versus a CCNA test using anaerobic toxigenic culture as the gold standard found the CCNA test to have a sensitivity of 67.2% and a specificity of 99.1% [positive predictive value (PPV) 93.2%, negative predictive value (NPV) 94.4%], while the GeneOhm test had a sensitivity of 83.6% and a specificity of 98.2% (PPV 89.5%, NPV 97.1%).[146] Peterson and associates[116] evaluated an EIA that detects toxins A and B, a laboratory-developed real-time PCR test targeting a conserved region of *tcdB,* a CCNA, and anaerobic toxigenic culture. Culture test results and clinical criteria were used to assess the performance of the four tests. The sensitivities of the EIA, PCR, CCNA, and toxigenic culture were 73.3%, 93.3%, 76.7%, and 100%, respectively. The PCR test had a turnaround time of less than 4 hours, which was equivalent to the EIA, and it had a much greater sensitivity. Overall, PCR tests appear to be more sensitive than EIAs that detect toxin and more sensitive than CCNA tests. Concerns have arisen about the possibility of *C. difficile* with variant *tcdB* and the emergence of *tcdB*-negative *C. difficile* strains, which will not be detected by some of these PCR tests.

METHICILLIN-RESISTANT *STAPHYLOCOCCUS AUREUS* (MRSA)

Staphylococcus aureus is an important human pathogen and a leading cause of hospital-acquired infection (HAI). Colonization of the nares and skin is common. Transmission occurs primarily through contact with those who are infected or are carriers of the organism. This gram-positive coccus is responsible for a wide clinical spectrum of infections from minor skin infections such as folliculitis (furuncles) or carbuncles (boils), to more severe sepsis and CNS infection, to death. HAIs have become a significant problem affecting the health of millions of patients, extending their stay in the hospital and contributing to mortality. The National Healthcare Safety Network estimates a rate of 2 million HAIs per year in the United States, with 90,000 deaths per year[41]; *S. aureus* contributes to a significant number of these cases.

Treatment of *S. aureus* infection has become more difficult with its acquisition of resistance to the antibiotics oxacillin and methicillin. These organisms, referred to as methicillin-resistant *S. aureus* (MRSA), most often are acquired in the hospital and then are termed *hospital-acquired (HA) MRSA.* MRSA infections of individuals who have not been hospitalized within the previous year and have not undergone an invasive medical procedure including catheterization are termed *community-acquired (CA) MRSA.* These two types of MRSA have been shown to be genetically and biologically different. In the past few years, the number of cases of CA-MRSA has dramatically increased; it often occurs in otherwise healthy individuals. MRSA is usually resistant to all β-lactam agents, including cephalosporins and carbapenems. Unlike CA-MRSA, HA-MRSA is usually multidrug resistant and is resistant to erythromycin and clindamycin. Vancomycin has been the mainstay in the treatment of MRSA, and the emergence of vancomycin-intermediate MRSA (VISA) and vancomycin-resistant MRSA (VRSA) is particularly disturbing. Additionally, when patients with MRSA have been compared with patients with methicillin-susceptible *S. aureus* (MSSA), MRSA-colonized patients more frequently developed symptomatic infection and had a higher case fatality rate for certain MRSA infections, including bacteremia and surgical site infection.[38]

Prevention of nosocomial transmission has become an important concern for healthcare facilities. Use of rapid molecular diagnostic tests for the detection of MRSA has been studied as a component of an approach to decrease the rate of nosocomial transmission of MRSA. One observational study evaluated clinical disease during hospitalization before and after implementing a universal surveillance program. The program used (1) rapid PCR-based MRSA detection for all hospital admissions, (2) decolonization procedures, and (3) contact isolation of patients who tested positive. The interventions reduced MSRA by almost 70% [confidence interval (CI), 89.2 to 19.6%].[125] Other studies, however, found no decrease in hospital acquisition of MRSA infection, although some demonstrated a reduction in the time patients spent in preemptive contact isolation because molecular surveillance testing was more rapid than conventional culture-based MRSA detection.[58,74,108] Recommendations for MRSA surveillance testing have been published.[106,139]

Resistance to methicillin is conferred by activity of the *mecA* gene product, penicillin-binding protein (PBP) 2a. It has a lower affinity for binding by methicillin, allowing it to evade inhibition by methicillin and to complete the transglycosidation step in cell wall synthesis in the bacteria. The *mecA* gene is carried on a mobile genetic element 21 to 67 kilobase pairs in length, and is referred to as a staphylococcal chromosomal cassette *mec* (SCC*mec*). The SCC*mec* contains several other antibiotic resistance determinants: the gene complex that encodes the recombinases for excision and integration from the staphylococcal chromosome and terminal repeat sequences necessary for mobilizing the cassette. At least six identified types of SCC*mec* cassettes based on the DNA sequence and the combination of *mecA* and recombinase gene complexes have been identified: types I, II, III, IV, V, and VI. SCC*mec* types I, II, and III are associated with HA-MRSA, and types IV and V have been associated with CA-MRSA. Some coagulase-negative staphylococci (CoNS) also carry the SCC elements with the *mecA* gene, and it is clinically important to differentiate them from MRSA. The SCC*mec* insertion into *S. aureus* is seen at the 3′ end of the open reading frame *(orf) X attB* gene sequence, which is an *S. aureus*–specific sequence. This provides one means of differentiating MRSA from *mecA*-containing CoNS by targeting PCR primers to this junction so that amplification occurs only if MRSA is present. The limitation of this method is that a separate amplification is required to detect the *mecA* gene.

Traditional methods of culture and antibiotic susceptibility testing have been important in the detection and identification of MRSA, and in distinguishing it from CoNS, but the requirement for 48 to 72 hours of culture to obtain a definitive result is a major disadvantage. Test results often are available too late to inform treatment decisions. The development of selective media with chromogenic indicators has decreased the time to detection, but at least overnight incubation is still required. Because methicillin resistance is almost always induced in the presence of β-lactam antibiotics when the *mecA* gene is present, detection using molecular methods is considered indicative of the presence of the organism with antibiotic resistance. The move toward reducing nosocomial transmission has further propelled the development of molecular assays for detection of the *mecA* gene to reduce the time to obtaining a result.

Nucleic Acid Testing for MRSA

Molecular tests can identify MRSA in a few hours or in a day, rather than the 3 to 4 days currently needed for culture methods. Timeliness not only reduces healthcare costs for the patient but also reduces the risk of transmitting the MRSA to healthcare workers and to other patients—a crucial step for infection control. Molecular tests are also sensitive and thus can increase the detection rate of MRSA. The high sensitivity of molecular assays permits direct detection of MRSA from clinical samples such as nasal swabs without the need for culture. Molecular assays are also highly specific and thus are able to distinguish, for example, *mecA*-carrying CoNS from true MRSA. Finally, on rare occasions, phenotypic tests for *S. aureus* give equivocal results, creating the need for alternative methods. Testing for susceptibility to oxacillin also sometimes gives equivocal results, again highlighting the need for alternative methods.

Four manufacturers have molecular assays for the detection of MRSA from nasal swab specimens cleared by the FDA: the GeneOhm MRSA assay (Becton-Dickinson; previously IDI-MRSA from Infectio Diagnostic Inc.) for the Smartcycler (Cepheid), the Xpert MRSA assays for the GeneXpert (Cepheid), the LightCycler MRSA Advanced Test (Roche), and the NucliSENS EasyQ MRSA (bioMérieux). The GeneOhm, Xpert MRSA, and LightCycler MRSA Advanced assays are designed for the detection of unique sequences at the junction of the SCC*mec* cassette in *S. aureus* but not for *mecA* gene detection. Another version of the Xpert MRSA assay, the Cepheid Xpert MRSA/SA Blood Culture Assay, has been cleared for MRSA determination from positive blood cultures using BD BACTEC Plus Aerobic/F blood culture bottles; it detects the *mecA* gene and the *S. aureus* protein A *(spa)* gene, along with the SCC*mec*. The NucliSENS EasyQ MRSA detects the SCCmec cassette junction *(orf X)* and the *mecA* gene. All the assays except the LightCycler MRSA Advanced Test demonstrate detection of the six primary SCC*mec*. Reports of loss of the *mecA* gene from the SCC element have been described, and the assays that lack direct *mecA* detection demonstrate false-positive results in these instances, requiring subsequent evaluation specifically for the *mecA* gene or antibiotic susceptibility.[66]

The BD GeneOhm MRSA Assay was the first assay cleared by the FDA for direct detection of nasal colonization by MRSA. It applies a manual lysis step before assembly of the real-time PCR reaction using fluorescently labeled hybridization probes in the Smartcycler reaction tube. In the clinical trial, it demonstrated sensitivity of 93% and specificity of 96% compared with culture-based methods, although analysis of the culture-negative/MRSA assay–positive discrepant results showed that most cases were true positives [FDA 510(k) number k033415]. The limit of detection is reported as 15 genome copies per reaction, or approximately 325 colony-forming units (cfu) per swab.

The Cepheid Xpert MRSA Assays (Xpert MRSA, Xpert MRSA/SA Blood Culture, Xpert MRSA/SA Nasal, and Xpert MRSA/SA SSTI [from skin and soft tissue] assays) are unique among FDA-cleared molecular-based diagnostics because of the rating as "moderate complexity" assays according to Clinical Laboratory Improvement Amendments (CLIA) categorization. This is because the assays are performed on the GeneXpert Dx System, which utilizes automated nucleic acid extraction and real-time PCR amplification in a self-contained cartridge. This advance in test design allows for use with the "moderate complexity" designation. The single-use cartridge contains chambers for holding the specimen and the extraction and real-time PCR reagents, a pump and valve system for controlling the movement of fluids between chambers, and an integrated PCR reaction tube with a high surface area for rapid amplification. The Xpert MRSA assay detects the presence of the SCC*mec* cassette at the *orfX attB* site, along with an internal control for amplification. The Xpert MRSA/SA Blood Culture, Nasal, and SSTI assays are similar in design to the Xpert MRSA assay, except for modification of the nucleic acid extraction procedure and inclusion of detection of the *mecA* and the *S. aureus* protein A *(spa)* genes.

The LightCycler® MRSA Advanced is another real-time PCR method for the detection of the presence of the SCC*mec* cassette at the *orfX attB* site, and includes an internal control for amplification. The NucliSENS EasyQ MRSA test uses nucleic acid sequence based amplification (NASBA), to detect two DNA targets for the presence of MRSA; the SCCmec cassette junction *(orfX)* and the *mecA* gene. Unlike the GeneXpert system, both require separate nucleic acid preparation before performing.

In a multisite study[166] involving nasal specimens with MRSA prevalence ranging from 5 to 44%, the Cepheid Xpert MRSA assay was compared with chromogenic agar with or without preceding broth enrichment. The assay showed (1) 100% sensitivity and specificity (after clerical errors were removed), (2) a limit of detection of approximately 80 cfu per reaction, and (3) linearity across six logs from 68 cfu to 6.8×10^7. Other ASRs for MRSA detection are commercially available from several other vendors.

RESPIRATORY VIRUSES

The viruses that infect the respiratory tract consist of diverse groups that cause disease in humans, and new ones continue to be discovered. The more common viruses that infect humans include influenza A and B, parainfluenza virus (PIV) types 1 to 4, respiratory syncytial virus (RSV), metapneumovirus, adenovirus (more than 50 different types), rhinovirus (more than 100 different types), and coronavirus. All of these viruses can be associated with symptoms of the common cold, including fever, myalgia, malaise, headache, pharyngitis, cough, and sore throat. Some virus types are associated with typical presentations in distinct populations, for instance, tracheolaryngobronchitis or croup in a 4- to 6-year-old is most frequently associated with PIV 1 infection, but bronchiolitis (infection and inflammation of the medium- to small-caliber airways) in toddlers is associated with RSV infection and can suffocate the child through closure of the airway from inflammation. The disease spectrum ranges from the common cold to severe life-threatening pneumonia. It can be difficult to differentiate the viral origin based on signs and symptoms alone, and treatment options vary depending on the viral etiology. Infection with these viruses has demonstrated the potential for a public health threat of epidemic and pandemic proportions. The history of pandemic influenza is well known, starting with the 1918 influenza A. More recently, presentations of the deadly avian influenza A [hemagglutinin (H) type 5 and neuraminidase (N) type 1 H5N1] in 1997[142] and the severe acute respiratory syndrome (SARS) coronavirus in 2003 have been reminders of the potential for human infection by new or reassorted viruses.[43] Neither of these viruses seemed to acquire significant human-to-human transmission. In 2009, however, a multiply reassorted novel (swine-like) influenza A H1N1 was easily transmitted between humans and was declared a pandemic, although it appeared to be less deadly than seasonal influenza infection. Detection of emerging respiratory viruses will require multiple modalities, and molecular methods will be critical in evaluating these new viruses.

Acute respiratory viral infection (1) is a leading cause of hospitalization and death in infants and young children[60,126,138]; (2) contributes to problems of asthma exacerbation, otitis media, and lower respiratory tract infection[9]; and (3) contributes to acute disease in immunocompromised and elderly patients. Rapid diagnosis aids in effective treatment (e.g., with antiviral medications such as oseltamivir for influenza A infection) and management (e.g., reduction in inappropriately prescribed antibiotics for viral infection). Rapid antigen-based EIAs provide short turnaround times (minutes) but are hampered by poor diagnostic sensitivity compared with culture methods or molecular assays, and low positive predictive values, especially when the prevalence is low.[28,50,51,69] Direct fluorescent antibody (DFA) detection assays for viral antigens on centrifuged cellular material (cytospun) from nasopharyngeal swabs, aspirates, or wash specimens demonstrate greater rates of detection than the rapid antigen assays, and provide results in a relatively short time frame of 2 to 4 hours. Rates of detection, however, are lower for antigen detection methods than for PCR methods.[49,51,87]

Cell culture methods, although slower than antigen detection methods, have been considered the gold standard for detection of a wide range of viral pathogens. In recent years, culture methods have been optimized for detection by combining multiple cell lines and improving turnaround time from weeks to days through the use of shell-vial spin amplification cultures. Here, the patient's specimen is concentrated onto cells grown on a coverslip, and fluorescent antibody detection is performed after 16 to 24 hours of incubation, instead of waiting for the development of a cytopathic effect. Although this has hastened the time to detection, 1 to 2 days is still required for results, along with significant technologist labor, and this method is not quite as sensitive as molecular methods of detection.

Nucleic Acid Testing for Respiratory Viruses

Molecular detection of respiratory viruses offers several advantages over traditional virologic culture or antigen detection. Most important, analytical sensitivity of molecular assays, primarily using PCR or real-time PCR, is consistently found to be better than that of traditional methods.* Results from molecular testing are more accurate and thus the patient benefits from the most appropriate treatment decision; also, infection control practitioners can more effectively implement strategies to prevent or reduce nosocomial transmission. Molecular assays can be designed to detect a wide range of viral pathogens, including for detection of new viruses. Multianalyte testing in a single or a small number of reaction tubes decreases the cost of reagents and technologist time and allows robotic implementation of specimen handling and testing.

Two important considerations in the design of a molecular-based detection method are whether the genetic material is DNA or RNA, and which method is appropriate for detection. For PCR, which is used most commonly, a DNA template is required, so RNA viruses must be reverse transcribed into a complementary DNA product (cDNA) before PCR amplification can be performed. Furthermore, it must be determined which viruses should be included in the detection process. Many different laboratory-developed assays have been designed specifically for particular needs with any number of organisms detected, and several commercial vendors have developed analyte specific reagents (ASRs). PCR-based assays that have been cleared by the FDA, include the ProFlu+, ProFast+, ProParaFlu+, Pro hMPV+, PROAdeno+ from Gen-Probe, the xTAG Respiratory Viral Panel from Luminex Corporation (Austin, Tex), the Verigene Respiratory Virus and Respiratory Virus Plus Nucleic Acid tests from NanoSphere Inc. (Northbrook, Ill), the Simplexa FluA/B and RSV test from Focus Diagnostics, Inc. (Cypress, California), the Xpert Flu Assay (Cepheid), and the FilmArray Respiratory Panel from Idaho Technologies (Salt Lake City, UT) (Table 42-4). All assays are cleared for

*References 49, 83, 87, 151, 152, and 159.

TABLE 42-4 In Vitro Diagnostic Kits for Respiratory Virus Detection

Test	Method	Extraction Method	Viruses Detected	Sensitivity/ Specificity, %
xTAG Respiratory Viral Panel (Luminex Corp., Austin, Tex)	RT-PCR and xMAP bead array	NucliSENS miniMAG or NucliSENS easyMAG (bioMérieux Inc., Durham, NC), or QIAamp MiniElute Virus Spin Kit (Qiagen Inc., Valencia, Calif)	Influenza A nonsubtype H1 (seasonal) H3 Influenza B RSV A RSV B PIV 1 PIV 2 PIV 3 Metapneumovirus Rhinovirus Adenovirus	 96.4/95.9* 100/100 91.7/98.7 91.5/96.0 100/98.4 100/97.4 100/99.0 100/99.0 84.2/99.0 100/91.3 78.3/100
ProFlu+ (Gen-Probe Inc., San Diego, Calif)	RT-PCR for real-time PCR instruments, including Lightcycler (LC, Roche Diagnostics, Indianapolis, Ind), or SmartCycler (Cepheid Inc., Sunnyvale, Calif)	MagNA Pure LC Total Nucleic Acid Isolation (TNAI) (Roche Diagnostics)	Influenza A Influenza B RSV*	100/92.6*,† 97.8/98.6 89.5/94.9

TABLE 42-4 In Vitro Diagnostic Kits for Respiratory Virus Detection—cont'd

Test	Method	Extraction Method	Viruses Detected	Sensitivity/ Specificity, %
ProhMPV+ (Gen-Probe)		MagNA Pure LC TNAI or NucliSENS easyMAG	hMPV*	94.1/99.3‡
ProParaFlu+ (Gen-Probe)	SmartCycler II (Cepheid)	MagNA Pure LC TNAI or NucliSENS easyMAG	PIV 1*	88.9/99.9*
			PIV 2	96.3/99.8
			PIV 3	97.3/99.2
ProFast+ (Gen-Probe)		MagNA Pure LC TNAI or NucliSENS easyMAG	Influenza A	
			H1	93.2/98.0§
			H3	86.7/98.9
			H1N1(2009)	87.3/99.5
ProAdeno+ Assay		MagNA Pure LC TNAI or NucliSENS easyMAG	Adenovirus	97.5/95.6
Verigene Respiratory Virus Nucleic Acid test (Nanosphere Inc., Northbrook, Ill)	Multiplex RT-PCR and hybridization detection using a microfluidics cartridge system	NucliSENS easyMAG	Influenza A	99.2*,‡
			Influenza B	96.8
			RSV	89.9
Verigene Respiratory Virus Plus Nucleic Acid test (Nanosphere)	Multiplex RT-PCR and hybridization detection using a microfluidics cartridge system	NucliSENS easyMAG	Influenza A	98.7/93.2*
			H1	100/99.9
			H3	100/100
			H1N1(2009)	99.5/100
			Influenza B	100/99.7
			RSV A	100/100
			RSV B	100/99.9
Simplexa FluA/ B&RSV (Focus Diagnostics, Cypress, Calif)	RT-PCR for 3M Integrated Cycler real-time PCR instrument		Influenza A	100/99[4]
			Influenza B	100/100
			RSV	100/99.4
Xpert Flu Assay (Cepheid)	Multiplex RT-PCR for GeneXpert real-time PCR instrument (Cepheid)	Sample preparation integrated into GeneXpert cartridge	Influenza A	99.4/100§
			H1N1(2009)	98.4/99.7
			Influenza B	97.5/100
FilmArray RP (Idaho Technologies, Salt Lake City, UT	Multiplex real-time RT-PCR for FilmArray Instrument	Sample preparation integrated into FilmArray pouch	Adenovirus,	88.9/98.3
			Coronavirus HKU 1	95.8/99.8
			Coronavirus NL63	95.8/100
			hMPV	94.6/99.2
			Influenza A	90.0/99.8
			Subtype H1	100/100
			Subtype H3	100/100
			Subtype H1 2009	88.9/99.6
			Influenza B	100/100
			PIV 1	100/99.9
			PIV 2	87.4/99.8
			PIV 3	95.8/98.8
			PIV 4	100/99.9
			Rhinovirus/enterovirus	92.7/94.6
			RSV	100/89.1

hMPV, Human metapneumovirus; *PIV,* parainfluenza virus; *RSV,* respiratory syncytial virus; *RT-PCR,* reverse transcriptase polymerase chain reaction.
*Compared with direct fluorescent antibody (DFA) and shell-vial culture as the gold standard.
†Compared with xTAG Respiratory Viral Panel as the predicate device.
‡hMPV comparator assays are two-step RT-PCR assays that target conserved regions of the hMPV nucleocapsid or fusion gene.
§Compared with ProFlu+ as the predicate device.

use on nasopharyngeal swabs, and all use internal controls for amplification. The ProFlu+, the Verigene Respiratory Virus Nucleic Acid, and the Simplexa FluA/B & RSV tests detect influenza A and B and respiratory syncytial viruses while the Verigene Respiratory Virus Plus Nucleic Acid test includes influenza A subtyping. The ProFast+ is only performed for influenza A subtyping. The xTAG Respiratory Viral Panel and the FilmArray Respiratory Panel detect the influenza types and subtypes, RSV, and many more viruses. The ProParaFlu+ assay detects parainfluenza types 1, 2, and 3 and the ProAdeno+ detects adenoviruses. All influenza assays are reported to be capable of detecting the 2009 H1N1 influenza A.[51]

ProFlu+, ProFast+, ProParaFlu+, ProhMPV+, and ProAdeno+ from Gen-Probe use real-time PCR with reverse transcription followed by multiplex amplification and then detection through the use of fluorescently labeled TaqMan probes. All four kits include an internal control added to the specimen before extraction of the nucleic acids to monitor extraction and amplification efficiencies. The limit of detection, defined as the lowest concentration at which 95% or more of replicates tested positive, ranged from 10^2 to 10^{-1} tissue culture infective dose $(TCID)_{50}/mL$, depending on the specific virus detected.

The Verigene Respiratory Virus and Respiratory Virus Plus Nucleic Acid tests from Nanosphere use a unique single-use microfluidics cartridge in which products of the multiplex RT-PCR are captured to a microarray format and are detected with the use of gold nanoparticle probes. The nanoprobes are illuminated using a fixed wavelength light source and are detected with a single-image sensor in the dedicated detection instrument, the Verigene System. The assays include two internal controls: a process control for sample isolation, and an inhibition control for amplification. The Verigene Respiratory Virus Nucleic Acid test has been cleared by the FDA for the detection of influenza A, influenza B, and RSV, and for nucleic acid extraction performed with the NucliSENS easyMAG System (bioMérieux). Sensitivity ranges from 89 to 99% in comparison with culture and DFA detection, and depending on the virus tested. The limit of detection is reported to range from 0.05 to 50.0 $TCID_{50}/mL$, depending on the viral strain.

The xTAG Respiratory Viral Panel (RVP) assay is a multiplexed RT-PCR–based assay with fluorescently color-coded microsphere (bead) hybridization for simultaneous detection and identification of 12 respiratory viruses and subtypes (see Table 42-4). The multiplexed RT-PCR primers amplify conserved regions of the viruses, and the products are labeled with biotin-containing deoxynucleotides (dNTPs) in a second target-specific primer extension reaction. The extension product has a proprietary tag sequence incorporated for hybridization to the virus-specific probe on the color-coded bead. After hybridization, phycoerythrin-conjugated streptavidin is bound by the biotin-labeled primer extension products, and the fluorescent signal is quantified on the Luminex xMAP instrument. The instrument contains two lasers: one for identification of the color-coded bead, and the other for detection of the phycoerythrin signal attached to the primer extension product. The data are recorded as mean fluorescent intensities, and the software analyzes the data and reports the positive results. The assay includes a separate lambda phage amplification control and an MS-2 bacteriophage internal control for extraction and amplification.

Clinical trials with the Luminex xMAP for FDA submission demonstrated sensitivities ranging from 78.3 to 100%, depending on the virus (see Table 42-4). The manufacturer reports that the assay cannot adequately detect adenovirus species C, or serotypes 7a and 41, and that the RVP primers for detection of rhinovirus cross-react with enterovirus. Analyses by investigators prior to FDA approval (when the assay existed with detection for 20 viruses and subtypes) demonstrated a detection rate for influenza 5 to 10% more sensitive than that of DFA and culture.[82] Specificity is also high, ranging from 91.3 to 100%.

The Film Array Respiratory Panel combines multiplex testing with ease of use. Nucleic acid extraction, a multiplex amplification, and second round of target specific amplifcation and detection occurs within a single pouch. Test set up is simple and requires two pipetting steps one to add buffer to the pouch to hydrate the reagents and another to add sample. The test includes an internal control and detects the adenoviruses, coronaviruses HKU1 and NL63, hMPV, human rhinovirus/enterovirus, influenza A (subtypes H1, H3, H1 2009), influenza B, PIV 1-4, and RSV. Results are completed in an hour, currently the instrumentis designed to test a single sample per run, though multiple instruments can be linked.

Molecular testing for respiratory viruses will likely continue to include tests designed to detect the most common pathogens (influenza A and B and RSV), as well as tests that detect a broad array of viruses, as there are clinical needs for both types of tests. Other assays will likely be cleared by the FDA in the coming years, as several other commercial analyte-specific reagents are available, and reports of laboratory-developed assays are abundant.

REFERENCES

1. Abzug MJ, Loeffelholz M, Rotbart HA. Diagnosis of neonatal enterovirus infection by polymerase chain reaction. J Pediatr 1995;126:447-50.
2. Ahmed A, Brito F, Goto C, Hickey SM, Olsen KD, Trujillo M, et al. Clinical utility of the polymerase chain reaction for diagnosis of enteroviral meningitis in infancy. J Pediatr 1997;131:393-7.
3. Alfa MJ, Kabani A, Lyerly D, Moncrief S, Neville LM, Al-Barrak A, et al. Characterization of a toxin A-negative, toxin B-positive strain of *Clostridium difficile* responsible for a nosocomial outbreak of *Clostridium difficile*-associated diarrhea. J Clin Microbiol 2000;38:2706-14.
4. Aurelius E, Johansson B, Skoldenberg B, Staland A, Forsgren M. Rapid diagnosis of herpes simplex encephalitis by nested polymerase chain reaction assay of cerebrospinal fluid. Lancet 1991;337:189-92.
5. Baker CA, Cartwright CP, Williams DN, Nelson SM, Peterson PK. Early detection of central nervous system tuberculosis with the Gen-Probe nucleic acid amplification assay: utility in an inner city hospital. Clin Infect Dis 2002;35:339-42.
6. Baxter JD, Mayers DL, Wentworth DN, Neaton JB, Hoover ML, Winters MA, et al. A randomized study of antiretroviral management

based on plasma genotypic antiretroviral resistance testing in patients failing therapy. AIDS 2000;14:F83-F93.

7. Bergeron MG, Ke D, Menard C, Picard FJ, Gagnon M, Bernier M, et al. Rapid detection of group B streptococci in pregnant women at delivery. N Engl J Med 2000;343:175-9.
8. Bianchi A, Moret F, Desrues JM, Champenois T, Dervaux Y, Desvouas O, et al. PreservCyt transport medium used for the ThinPrep Pap test is a suitable medium for detection of *Chlamydia trachomatis* by the COBAS Amplicor CT/NG test: results of a preliminary study and future implications. J Clin Microbiol 2002;40:1749-54.
9. Bloom B, Cohen RA, Freeman G. Summary health statistics for U.S. children: National Health Interview Survey, 2007. Vital and Health Statistics 2009:1-80.
10. Bonington A, Strang JI, Klapper PE, Hood SV, Rubombora W, Penny M, et al. Use of Roche AMPLICOR *Mycobacterium tuberculosis* PCR in early diagnosis of tuberculous meningitis. J Clin Microbiol 1998;36:1251-4.
11. Bourlet T, Caro V, Minjolle S, Jusselin I, Pozzetto B, Crainic R, Colimon R. New PCR test that recognizes all human prototypes of enterovirus: application for clinical diagnosis. J Clin Microbiol 2003; 41:1750-2.
12. Boyer KM, Gotoff SP. Strategies for chemoprophylaxis of GBS early-onset infections. Antibiot Chemother 1985;35:267-80.
13. Bradley SP, Reed SL, Catanzaro A. Clinical efficacy of the amplified *Mycobacterium tuberculosis* direct test for the diagnosis of pulmonary tuberculosis. Am J Respir Crit Care Med 1996;153:1606-10.
14. Brambilla D, Leung S, Lew J, Todd J, Herman S, Cronin M, et al. Absolute copy number and relative change in determinations of human immunodeficiency virus type 1 RNA in plasma: effect of an external standard on kit comparisons. J Clin Microbiol 1998;36: 311-4.
15. Brambilla D, Reichelderfer P, Bremer J, Shapiro DE, Hershow RC, Katzenstein DA, et al. The contribution of assay variation and biological variation to the total variability of plasma HIV-1 RNA measurements. AIDS 1999;13:2269-79.
16. Buimer M, van Doornum GJ, Ching S, Peerbooms PG, Plier PK, Ram D, et al. Detection of *Chlamydia trachomatis* and *Neisseria gonorrhoeae* by ligase chain reaction-based assays with clinical specimens from various sites: implications for diagnostic testing and screening. J Clin Microbiol 1996;34:2395-400.
17. Burstein GR, Zenilman JM. Nongonococcal urethritis—a new paradigm. Clin Infect Dis 1999;28:S66-73.
18. Caliendo AM, Ingersoll J, Fox-Canale AM, Pargman S, Bythwood T, Hayden MK, et al. Evaluation of real-time PCR laboratory-developed tests using analyte-specific reagents for cytomegalovirus quantification. J Clin Microbiol 2007;45:1723-7.
19. Caliendo AM, Schuurman R, Yen-Lieberman B, Spector SA, Andersen J, Manjiry R, et al. Comparison of quantitative and qualitative PCR assays for cytomegalovirus DNA in plasma. J Clin Microbiol 2001;39:1334-8.
20. Caliendo AM, Shahbazian MD, Schaper C, Ingersoll J, Abdul-Ali D, Boonyaratanakornkit J, et al. A commutable cytomegalovirus calibrator is required to improve the agreement of viral load values between laboratories. Clin Chem 2009;55:1701-10.
21. Caliendo AM, St George K, Kao SY, Allega J, Tan BH, LaFontaine R, et al. Comparison of quantitative cytomegalovirus (CMV) PCR in plasma and CMV antigenemia assay: clinical utility of the prototype AMPLICOR CMV MONITOR test in transplant recipients. J Clin Microbiol 2000;38:2122-7.
22. Caliendo AM, St. George K, Allega J, Bullotta AC, Gilbane L, Rinaldo CR. Distinguishing cytomegalovirus (CMV) infection and disease with CMV nucleic acid assays. J Clin Microbiol 2002;40:1581-6.
23. Castle PE, Solomon D, Wheeler CM, Gravitt PE, Wacholder S, Schiffman M. Human papillomavirus genotype specificity of hybrid capture 2. J Clin Microbiol 2008;46:2595-604.
24. Centers for Disease Control and Prevention. Prevention of perinatal group B streptococcal disease. MMWR Morb Mortal Wkly Rep 2002; 51:1-26.
25. Centers for Disease Control and Prevention. Rapid diagnostic tests for tuberculosis: what is the appropriate use? American Thoracic Society Workshop. Am J Respir Crit Care Med 1997;155:1804-14.
26. Centers for Disease Control and Prevention. Tuberculosis morbidity—United States, 1997. MMWR Morb Mortal Wkly Rep 1998;47:253-7.
27. Centers for Disease Control and Prevention. Updated guidelines for the use of nucleic acid amplification tests in the diagnosis of tuberculosis. MMWR Morb Mortal Wkly Rep 2009;58:7-10.
28. Chan KH, Peiris JS, Lim W, Nicholls JM, Chiu SS. Comparison of nasopharyngeal flocked swabs and aspirates for rapid diagnosis of respiratory viruses in children. J Clin Virol 2008;42:65-9.
29. Chernesky MA, Jang D, Lee H, Burczak JD, Hu H, Sellors J, et al. Diagnosis of *Chlamydia trachomatis* infections in men and women by testing first-void urine by ligase chain reaction. J Clin Microbiol 1994;32:2682-5.
30. Chong S, Jang D, Song X, Mahony J, Petrich A, Barriga P, et al. Specimen processing and concentration of *Chlamydia trachomatis* added can influence false-negative rates in the LCx assay but not in the APTIMA Combo 2 assay when testing for inhibitors. J Clin Microbiol 2003;41:778-82.
31. Chonmaitree T, Menegus MA, Powell KR. The clinical relevance of "CSF viral culture": a two-year experience with aseptic meningitis in Rochester, NY. JAMA 1982;247:1843-7.
32. Clevenbergh P, Durant J, Halfon P, Giudice PD, Mondain V, Montagne N, et al. Persisting long-term benefit of genotype-guided treatment for HIV-infected patients failing HAART. The VIRADAPT study: week 48 follow-up. Antivir Ther 2000;5:65-70.
33. Clinical and Laboratory Standards Institute (CLSI). MM6: quantitative molecular methods for infectious diseases; approved guideline. CLSI 2003;23:1-55.
34. Cohen CJ, Hunt S, Sension M, Farthing C, Conant M, Jacobson S, et al. A randomized trial assessing the impact of phenotypic resistance testing on antiretroviral therapy. AIDS 2002;16:579-88.
35. Cope AV, Sabin C, Burroughs A, Rolles K, Griffiths PD, Emery VC. Interrelationships among quantity of human cytomegalovirus (HCMV) DNA in blood, donor-recipient serostatus, and administration of methylprednisolone as risk factors for HCMV disease following liver transplantation. J Infect Dis 1997;176:1484-90.
36. Crotchfelt KA, Pare B, Gaydos C, Quinn TC. Detection of *Chlamydia trachomatis* by the Gen-Probe AMPLIFIED *Chlamydia trachomatis* Assay (AMP CT) in urine specimens from men and women and endocervical specimens from women. J Clin Microbiol 1998;36:391-4.
37. Daar ES, Little S, Pitt J, Santangelo J, Ho P, Harawa N, et al. Diagnosis of primary HIV-1 infection. Los Angeles County Primary HIV Infection Recruitment Network. Ann Intern Med 2001;134:25-9.
38. Davis KA, Stewart JJ, Crouch HK, Florez CE, Hospenthal DR. Methicillin-resistant *Staphylococcus aureus* (MRSA): nares colonization at hospital admission and its effect on subsequent MRSA infection. Clin Infect Dis 2004;39:776-82.
39. Donovan RM, Bush CE, Markowitz NP, Baxa DM, Saravolatz LD. Changes in virus load markers during AIDS-associated opportunistic diseases in human immunodeficiency virus-infected persons. J Infect Dis 1996;174:401-3.
40. Durant J, Clevenbergh P, Halfon P, Delgiudice P, Porsin S, Simonet P, et al. Drug-resistance genotyping in HIV-1 therapy: the VIRADAPT randomised controlled trial. Lancet 1999;353:2195-9.
41. Edwards JR, Peterson KD, Andrus ML, Dudeck MA, Pollock DA, Horan TC. National Healthcare Safety Network (NHSN) Report: data summary for 2006 through 2007, issued November 2008. Am J Infect Control 2008;36:609-26.
42. Eshleman SH, Hackett J Jr, Swanson P, Cunningham SP, Drews B, Brennan C, et al. Performance of the Celera Diagnostics ViroSeq HIV-1 Genotyping System for sequence-based analysis of diverse human immunodeficiency virus type 1 strains. J Clin Microbiol 2004;42:2711-7.
43. Falsey AR, Walsh EE. Novel coronavirus and severe acute respiratory syndrome. Lancet 2003;361:1312-3.

44. Ferenci P, Fried MW, Shiffman ML, Smith CI, Marinos G, Goncales FL Jr, et al. Predicting sustained virological responses in chronic hepatitis C patients treated with peginterferon alfa-2a (40 KD)/ribavirin. J Hepatol 2005;43:425-33.
45. Forman MS, Valsamakis A. Performance characteristics of a quantitative hepatitis C virus RNA assay using COBAS AmpliPrep total nucleic acid isolation and COBAS TaqMan hepatitis C virus analyte-specific reagent. J Mol Diagn 2008;10:147-53.
46. Fox JD, Han S, Samuelson A, Zhang Y, Neale ML, Westmoreland D. Development and evaluation of nucleic acid sequence based amplification (NASBA) for diagnosis of enterovirus infections using the NucliSens Basic Kit. J Clin Virol 2002;24:117-30.
47. Garcia-Bujalance S, Ladron de Guevara C, Gonzalez-Garcia J, Arribas JR, Zamora F, Gutierrez A. Elevation of viral load by PCR and use of plasma preparation tubes for quantification of human immunodeficiency virus type 1. J Microbiol Methods 2007;69:384-6.
48. Gaydos CA, Crotchfelt KA, Howell MR, Kralian S, Hauptman P, Quinn TC. Molecular amplification assays to detect chlamydial infections in urine specimens from high school female students and to monitor the persistence of chlamydial DNA after therapy. J Infect Dis 1998;177:417-24.
49. Gharabaghi F, Tellier R, Cheung R, Collins C, Broukhanski G, Drews SJ, et al. Comparison of a commercial qualitative real-time RT-PCR kit with direct immunofluorescence assay (DFA) and cell culture for detection of influenza A and B in children. J Clin Virol 2008;42:190-3.
50. Ghebremedhin B, Engelmann I, Konig W, Konig B. Comparison of the performance of the rapid antigen detection Actim Influenza A&B test and RT-PCR in different respiratory specimens. J Med Microbiol 2009;58:365-70.
51. Ginocchio CC, Zhang F, Manji R, Arora S, Bornfreund M, Falk L, et al. Evaluation of multiple test methods for the detection of the novel 2009 influenza A (H1N1) during the New York City outbreak. J Clin Virol 2009;45:191-5.
52. Griffith BP, Mayo DR. Increased levels of HIV RNA detected in samples with viral loads close to the detection limit collected in plasma preparation tubes (PPT). J Clin Virol 2006;35:197-200.
53. Groseclose SL, Zaidi AA, DeLisle SJ, Levine WC, St Louis ME. Estimated incidence and prevalence of genital *Chlamydia trachomatis* infections in the United States, 1996. Sex Transm Dis 1999;26:339-44.
54. Gueudin M, Plantier JC, Damond F, Roques P, Mauclere P, Simon F. Plasma viral RNA assay in HIV-1 group O infection by real-time PCR. J Virol Methods 2003;113:43-9.
55. Hadziyannis SJ, Sette H Jr, Morgan TR, Balan V, Diago M, Marcellin P, et al. Peginterferon-alpha2a and ribavirin combination therapy in chronic hepatitis C: a randomized study of treatment duration and ribavirin dose. Ann Intern Med 2004;140:346-55.
56. Hagblom P, Korch C, Jonsson AB, Normark S. Intragenic variation by site-specific recombination in the cryptic plasmid of *Neisseria gonorrhoeae*. J Bacteriol 1986;167:231-7.
57. Hamilton MS, Jackson MA, Abel D. Clinical utility of polymerase chain reaction testing for enteroviral meningitis. Pediatr Infect Dis J 1999;18:533-8.
58. Harbarth S, Fankhauser C, Schrenzel J, Christenson J, Gervaz P, Bandiera-Clerc C, et al. Universal screening for methicillin-resistant *Staphylococcus aureus* at hospital admission and nosocomial infection in surgical patients. JAMA 2008;299:1149-57.
59. Haubrich R, Keiser P, Kemper C, Witt M, Leedom J, Forthal D, et al. CCTG 575: a randomized, prospective study of phenotype testing versus standard of care for patients failing antiretroviral therapy. Abstract 80. In: 5th International Workshop on HIV Drug Resistance and Treatment Strategies, vol 6. San Diego, Calif: International Medical Press Ltd., 2001:63.
60. Henrickson KJ, Hoover S, Kehl KS, Hua W. National disease burden of respiratory viruses detected in children by polymerase chain reaction. Pediatr Infect Dis J 2004;23:S11-8.
61. Hezode C, Forestier N, Dusheiko G, Ferenci P, Pol S, Goeser T, et al. Telaprevir and peginterferon with or without ribavirin for chronic HCV infection. N Engl J Med 2009;360:1839-50.
62. Hirsch MS, Conway B, D'Aquila RT, Johnson VA, Brun-Vezinet F, Clotet B, et al. Antiretroviral drug resistance testing in adults with HIV infection: implications for clinical management. International AIDS Society—USA Panel. JAMA 1998;279:1984-91.
63. Ho G, Bierman R, Beardsley L, Chang C, Burk R. Natural history of cervicovaginal papillomavirus infection in young women. N Engl J Med 1998;338:423-8.
64. Holodniy M, Rainen L, Herman S, Yen-Lieberman B. Stability of plasma human immunodeficiency virus load in VACUTAINER PPT plasma preparation tubes during overnight shipment. J Clin Microbiol 2000;38:323-6.
65. Hook EW 3rd, Smith K, Mullen C, Stephens J, Rinehardt L, Pate MS, et al. Diagnosis of genitourinary *Chlamydia trachomatis* infections by using the ligase chain reaction on patient-obtained vaginal swabs. J Clin Microbiol 1997;35:2133-5.
66. Huletsky A, Giroux R, Rossbach V, Gagnon M, Vaillancourt M, Bernier M, et al. New real-time PCR assay for rapid detection of methicillin-resistant *Staphylococcus aureus* directly from specimens containing a mixture of staphylococci. J Clin Microbiol 2004;42: 1875-84.
67. Humar A, Gregson D, Caliendo AM, McGeer A, Malkan G, Krajden M, et al. Clinical utility of quantitative cytomegalovirus viral load determination for predicting cytomegalovirus disease in liver transplant recipients. Transplantation 1999;68:1305-11.
68. Humar A, Kumar D, Boivin G, Caliendo AM. Cytomegalovirus (CMV) viral load kinetics to predict recurrent disease in solid organ transplant patients with CMV disease. J Infect Dis 2002;186: 829-33.
69. Hurt AC, Alexander R, Hibbert J, Deed N, Barr IG. Performance of six influenza rapid tests in detecting human influenza in clinical specimens. J Clin Virol 2007;39:132-5.
70. Jackson JB, Smith K, Knott C, Korpela A, Simmons A, Piwowar-Manning E, et al. Sensitivity of the Procleix HIV-1/HCV assay for detection of human immunodeficiency virus type 1 and hepatitis C virus RNA in a high-risk population. J Clin Microbiol 2002;40:2387-91.
71. Jagodzinski LL, Wiggins DL, McManis JL, Emery S, Overbaugh J, Robb M, et al. Use of calibrated viral load standards for group M subtypes of human immunodeficiency virus type 1 to assess the performance of viral RNA quantitation tests. J Clin Microbiol 2000; 38:1247-9.
72. Jaschek G, Gaydos CA, Welsh LE, Quinn TC. Direct detection of *Chlamydia trachomatis* in urine specimens from symptomatic and asymptomatic men by using a rapid polymerase chain reaction assay. J Clin Microbiol 1993;31:1209-12.
73. Jensen DM, Morgan TR, Marcellin P, Pockros PJ, Reddy KR, Hadziyannis SJ, et al. Early identification of HCV genotype 1 patients responding to 24 weeks peginterferon alpha-2a (40 kd)/ribavirin therapy. Hepatology 2006;43:954-60.
74. Jeyaratnam D, Whitty CJ, Phillips K, Liu D, Orezzi C, Ajoku U, et al. Impact of rapid screening tests on acquisition of methicillin resistant *Staphylococcus aureus:* cluster randomised crossover trial. BMJ 2008; 336:927-30.
75. Jonas V, Acedo M, Clarridge JE, et al. A multi-center evaluation of MTD and culture compared to clinical diagnosis. Abstract L-31. Presented at: 98th General Meeting of the American Society for Microbiology, May 17-21, 1998, Atlanta, Ga.
76. Judson FN. Gonorrhea. Med Clin North Am 1990;74:1353-66.
77. Kahn JO, Walker BD. Acute human immunodeficiency virus type 1 infection. N Engl J Med 1998;339:32-9.
78. Kessler HH, Santner B, Rabenau H, Berger A, Vince A, Lewinski C, et al. Rapid diagnosis of enterovirus infection by a new one-step reverse transcription-PCR assay. J Clin Microbiol 1997;35:976-7.
79. Kimberlin DW, Lakeman FD, Arvin AM, Prober CG, Corey L, Powell DA, et al. Application of the polymerase chain reaction to the diagnosis and management of neonatal herpes simplex virus disease. National Institute of Allergy and Infectious Diseases Collaborative Antiviral Study Group. J Infect Dis 1996;174:1162-7.

80. Kolk DP, Dockter J, Linnen J, Ho-Sing-Loy M, Gillotte-Taylor K, McDonough SH, et al. Significant closure of the human immunodeficiency virus type 1 and hepatitis C virus preseroconversion detection windows with a transcription-mediated amplification-driven assay. J Clin Microbiol 2002;40:1761-6.
81. Kost CB, Rogers B, Oberste MS, Robinson C, Eaves BL, Leos K, et al. Multicenter beta trial of the GeneXpert enterovirus assay. J Clin Microbiol 2007;45:1081-6.
82. Krunic N, Yager TD, Himsworth D, Merante F, Yaghoubian S, Janeczko R. xTAG RVP assay: analytical and clinical performance. J Clin Virol 2007;40(Suppl 1):S39-46.
83. Kuypers J, Wright N, Ferrenberg J, Huang ML, Cent A, Corey L, et al. Comparison of real-time PCR assays with fluorescent-antibody assays for diagnosis of respiratory virus infections in children. J Clin Microbiol 2006;44:2382-8.
84. Lakeman F, Whitley RJ. Diagnosis of herpes simplex encephalitis: application of polymerase chain reaction to cerebrospinal fluid from brain-biopsied patients and correlation with disease. National Institute of Allergy and Infectious Diseases Collaborative Antiviral Study Group. J Infect Dis 1995;171:857.
85. Lang AM, Feris-Iglesias J, Pena C, Sanchez JF, Stockman L, Rys P, et al. Clinical evaluation of the Gen-Probe Amplified Direct Test for detection of *Mycobacterium tuberculosis* complex organisms in cerebrospinal fluid. J Clin Microbiol 1998;36:2191-4.
86. Lee HH, Chernesky MA, Schachter J, Burczak JD, Andrews WW, Muldoon S, et al. Diagnosis of *Chlamydia trachomatis* genitourinary infection in women by ligase chain reaction assay of urine. Lancet 1995;345:213-6.
87. Legoff J, Kara R, Moulin F, Si-Mohamed A, Krivine A, Belec L, et al. Evaluation of the one-step multiplex real-time reverse transcription-PCR ProFlu-1 assay for detection of influenza A and influenza B viruses and respiratory syncytial viruses in children. J Clin Microbiol 2008;46:789-91.
88. Lew J, Reichelderfer P, Fowler M, Bremer J, Carrol R, Cassol S, et al. Determinations of levels of human immunodeficiency virus type 1 RNA in plasma: reassessment of parameters affecting assay outcome. TUBE Meeting Workshop Attendees. Technology Utilization for HIV-1 Blood Evaluation and Standardization in Pediatrics. J Clin Microbiol 1998;36:1471-9.
89. Mahony J, Chong S, Jang D, Luinstra K, Faught M, Dalby D, et al. Urine specimens from pregnant and nonpregnant women inhibitory to amplification of *Chlamydia trachomatis* nucleic acid by PCR, ligase chain reaction, and transcription-mediated amplification: identification of urinary substances associated with inhibition and removal of inhibitory activity. J Clin Microbiol 1998;36:3122-6.
90. Malm G, Forsgren M. Neonatal herpes simplex virus infections: HSV DNA in cerebrospinal fluid and serum. Arch Dis Child Fetal Neonatal Ed 1999;81:F24-9.
91. Marions L, Rotzen-Ostlund M, Grillner L, Edgardh K, Tiveljung-Lindell A, Wikstrom A, et al. High occurrence of a new variant of *Chlamydia trachomatis* escaping diagnostic tests among STI clinic patients in Stockholm, Sweden. Sex Transm Dis 2008;35:61-4.
92. Marshall GS, Hauck MA, Buck G, Rabalais GP. Potential cost savings through rapid diagnosis of enteroviral meningitis. Pediatr Infect Dis J 1997;16:1086-7.
93. Matsuura K, Tanaka Y, Hasegawa I, Ohno T, Tokuda H, Kurbanov F, et al. Abbott RealTime hepatitis C virus (HCV) and Roche Cobas AmpliPrep/Cobas TaqMan HCV assays for prediction of sustained virological response to pegylated interferon and ribavirin in chronic hepatitis C patients. J Clin Microbiol 2009;47:385-9.
94. Mazzulli T, Drew L, Yen-Lieberman B, Jekic-McMullen D, Kohn DJ, Isada CM, et al. Multicenter comparison of the Digene Hybrid Capture CMV DNA assay (version 2.0), the pp65 antigenemia assay, and cell culture for detection of cytomegalovirus viremia. J Clin Microbiol 1999;37:958-63.
95. McDonald LC, Killgore GE, Thompson A, Owens RC Jr, Kazakova SV, Sambol SP, et al. An epidemic, toxin gene-variant strain of *Clostridium difficile*. N Engl J Med 2005;353:2433-41.
96. McEllistrem MC, Carman RJ, Gerding DN, Genheimer CW, Zheng L. A hospital outbreak of *Clostridium difficile* disease associated with isolates carrying binary toxin genes. Clin Infect Dis 2005;40:265-72.
97. McHutchison JG, Everson GT, Gordon SC, Jacobson IM, Sulkowski M, Kauffman R, et al. Telaprevir with peginterferon and ribavirin for chronic HCV genotype 1 infection. N Engl J Med 2009;360:1827-38.
98. McMurray HR, Nguyen D, Westbrook TF, McAnce DJ. Biology of human papillomaviruses. Int J Exp Pathol 2001;82:15-33.
99. Mellors JW, Kingsley LA, Rinaldo CR Jr, Todd JA, Hoo BS, Kokka RP, et al. Quantitation of HIV-1 RNA in plasma predicts outcome after seroconversion. Ann Intern Med 1995;122:573-9.
100. Mellors JW, Rinaldo CR Jr, Gupta P, White RM, Todd JA, Kingsley LA. Prognosis in HIV-1 infection predicted by the quantity of virus in plasma. Science 1996;272:1167-70.
101. Meynard J-L, Vray M, Morand-Joubert L, Race E, Descamps D, Peytavin G, et al. Phenotypic or genotypic resistance testing for choosing antiretroviral therapy after treatment failure: a randomized trial. AIDS 2002;16:727-36.
102. Michelin BD, Muller Z, Stelzl E, Marth E, Kessler HH. Evaluation of the Abbott RealTime HCV assay for quantitative detection of hepatitis C virus RNA. J Clin Virol 2007;38:96-100.
103. Miller V. HIV drug resistance: overview of clinical data. J HIV Ther 2001;6:68-72.
104. Miyada CG, Born TL. A DNA sequence for the discrimination of *Neisseria gonorrhoeae* from other *Neisseria* species. Mol Cell Probes 1991;5:327-35.
105. Moss T. International handbook of *Chlamydia*. Exeter, UK: Polestar Wheatons Ltd., 2001.
106. Muto CA, Jernigan JA, Ostrowsky BE, Richet HM, Jarvis WR, Boyce JM, et al. SHEA guideline for preventing nosocomial transmission of multidrug-resistant strains of *Staphylococcus aureus* and *Enterococcus*. Infect Control Hosp Epidemiol 2003;24:362-86.
107. Nigrovic LE, Chiang VW. Cost analysis of enteroviral polymerase chain reaction in infants with fever and cerebrospinal fluid pleocytosis. Arch Pediatr Adolesc Med 2000;154:817-21.
108. Nijssen S, Bonten MJ, Weinstein RA. Are active microbiological surveillance and subsequent isolation needed to prevent the spread of methicillin-resistant *Staphylococcus aureus*? Clin Infect Dis 2005;40:405-9.
109. Nkengasong JN, Bile C, Kalou M, Maurice C, Boating E, Sassan-Morokro M, et al. Quantification of RNA in HIV type 1 subtypes D and G by NucliSens and Amplicor assays in Abidjan, Ivory Coast. AIDS Res Hum Retroviruses 1999;15:495-8.
110. Nolte FS, Green AM, Fiebelkorn KR, Caliendo AM, Sturchio C, Grunwald A, et al. Clinical evaluation of two methods for genotyping hepatitis C virus based on analysis of the 5′ noncoding region. J Clin Microbiol 2003;41:1558-64.
111. O'Brien WA, Grovit-Ferbas K, Namazi A, Ovcak-Derzic S, Wang HJ, Park J, et al. Human immunodeficiency virus-type 1 replication can be increased in peripheral blood of seropositive patients after influenza vaccination. Blood 1995;86:1082-9.
112. Oberste MS, Maher K, Flemister MR, Marchetti G, Kilpatrick DR, Pallansch MA. Comparison of classic and molecular approaches for the identification of untypeable enteroviruses. J Clin Microbiol 2000;38:1170-4.
113. Parekh B, Phillips S, Granade TC, Baggs J, Hu DJ, Respess R. Impact of HIV type 1 subtype variation on viral RNA quantitation. AIDS Res Hum Retroviruses 1999;15:133-42.
114. Pasquier C, Sandres K, Salama G, Puel J, Izopet J. Using RT-PCR and bDNA assays to measure non-clade B HIV-1 subtype RNA. J Virol Methods 1999;81:123-9.
115. Pasternack R, Vuorinen P, Miettinen A. Evaluation of the Gen-Probe *Chlamydia trachomatis* transcription-mediated amplification assay with urine specimens from women. J Clin Microbiol 1997;35:676-8.
116. Peterson LR, Manson RU, Paule SM, Hacek DM, Robicsek A, Thomson RB Jr, et al. Detection of toxigenic *Clostridium difficile* in stool samples by real-time polymerase chain reaction for the diagnosis of *C. difficile*-associated diarrhea. Clin Infect Dis 2007;45:1152-60.

117. Petropoulos CJ, Parkin NT, Limoli KL, Lie YS, Wrin T, Huang W, et al. A novel phenotypic drug susceptibility assay for human immunodeficiency virus type 1. Antimicrob Agents Chemother 2000;44:920-8.
118. Poordad F, Reddy KR, Martin P. Rapid virologic response: a new milestone in the management of chronic hepatitis C. Clin Infect Dis 2008;46:78-84.
119. Pyne MT, Konnick EQ, Phansalkar A, Hillyard DR. Evaluation of the Abbott investigational use only RealTime hepatitis C virus (HCV) assay and comparison to the Roche TaqMan HCV analyte-specific reagent assay. J Clin Microbiol 2009;47:2872-8.
120. Ramers C, Billman G, Hartin M, Ho S, Sawyer MH. Impact of a diagnostic cerebrospinal fluid enterovirus polymerase chain reaction test on patient management. JAMA 2000;283:2680-5.
121. Razonable RR, Brown RA, Wilson JA, Groettum CM, Kremers W, Espy MJ, et al. The clinical use of various blood compartments for cytomegalovirus (CMV) DNA quantitation in transplant recipients with CMV disease. Transplantation 2002;73:968-73.
122. Rees E. The treatment of pelvic inflammatory disease. Am J Obstet Gynecol 1980;138:1042-7.
123. Regan JA, Klebanoff MA, Nugent RP. The epidemiology of group B streptococcal colonization in pregnancy. Vaginal Infections and Prematurity Study Group. Obstet Gynecol 1991;77:604-10.
124. Ripa T, Nilsson PA. A *Chlamydia trachomatis* strain with a 377-bp deletion in the cryptic plasmid causing false-negative nucleic acid amplification tests. Sex Transm Dis 2007;34:255-6.
125. Robicsek A, Beaumont JL, Peterson LR. Duration of colonization with methicillin-resistant *Staphylococcus aureus*. Clin Infect Dis 2009;48: 910-3.
126. Robinson CC. The value of RVP in children's hospitals. J Clin Virol 2007;40(Suppl 1):S51-2.
127. Rosenstraus M, Wang Z, Chang SY, DeBonville D, Spadoro JP. An internal control for routine diagnostic PCR: design, properties, and effect on clinical performance. J Clin Microbiol 1998;36:191-7.
128. Rotbart HA. Diagnosis of enteroviral meningitis with the polymerase chain reaction. J Pediatr 1990;117:85-9.
129. Rotbart HA. Nucleic acid detection systems for enteroviruses. Clin Microbiol Rev 1991;4:156-68.
130. Rotbart HA, Sawyer MH, Fast S, Lewinski C, Murphy N, Keyser EF, et al. Diagnosis of enteroviral meningitis by using PCR with a colorimetric microwell detection assay. J Clin Microbiol 1994;32: 2590-2.
131. Saag MS, Holodniy M, Kuritzkes DR, O'Brien WA, Coombs R, Poscher ME, et al. HIV viral load markers in clinical practice. Nat Med 1996;2:625-9.
132. Sarrazin C, Dragan A, Gartner BC, Forman MS, Traver S, Zeuzem S, et al. Evaluation of an automated, highly sensitive, real-time PCR-based assay (COBAS Ampliprep/COBAS TaqMan) for quantification of HCV RNA. J Clin Virol 2008;43:162-8.
133. Sarrazin C, Gartner BC, Sizmann D, Babiel R, Mihm U, Hofmann WP, et al. Comparison of conventional PCR with real-time PCR and branched DNA-based assays for hepatitis C virus RNA quantification and clinical significance for genotypes 1 to 5. J Clin Microbiol 2006; 44:729-37.
134. Schachter J, Chernesky MA, Willis DE, Fine PM, Martin DH, Fuller D, et al. Vaginal swabs are the specimens of choice when screening for *Chlamydia trachomatis* and *Neisseria gonorrhoeae*: results from a multicenter evaluation of the APTIMA assays for both infections. Sex Transm Dis 2005;32:725-8.
135. Schlesinger Y, Tebas P, Gaudreault-Keener M, Buller RS, Storch GA. Herpes simplex virus type 2 meningitis in the absence of genital lesions: improved recognition with use of the polymerase chain reaction. Clin Infect Dis 1995;20:842-8.
136. Schrag SJ, Zell ER, Lynfield R, Roome A, Arnold KE, Craig AS, et al. A population-based comparison of strategies to prevent early-onset group B streptococcal disease in neonates. N Engl J Med 2002;347: 233-9.
137. Schumacher W, Frick E, Kauselmann M, Maier-Hoyle V, van der Vliet R, Babiel R. Fully automated quantification of human immunodeficiency virus (HIV) type 1 RNA in human plasma by the COBAS AmpliPrep/COBAS TaqMan system. J Clin Virol 2007;38: 304-12.
138. Shay DK, Holman RC, Newman RD, Liu LL, Stout JW, Anderson LJ. Bronchiolitis-associated hospitalizations among US children, 1980-1996. JAMA 1999;282:1440-6.
139. Siegel JD, Rhinehart E, Jackson M, Chiarello L. 2007 guideline for isolation precautions: preventing transmission of infectious agents in health care settings. Am J Infect Control 2007;35:S65-164.
140. Simko JP, Caliendo AM, Hogle K, Versalovic J. Differences in laboratory findings for cerebrospinal fluid specimens obtained from patients with meningitis or encephalitis due to herpes simplex virus (HSV) documented by detection of HSV DNA. Clin Infect Dis 2002;35:414-9.
141. Sloan LM, Duresko BJ, Gustafson DR, Rosenblatt JE. Comparison of real-time PCR for detection of the tcdC gene with four toxin immunoassays and culture in diagnosis of *Clostridium difficile* infection. J Clin Microbiol 2008;46:1996-2001.
142. Snacken R, Kendal AP, Haaheim LR, Wood JM. The next influenza pandemic: lessons from Hong Kong, 1997. Emerg Infect Dis 1999;5: 195-203.
143. Spector SA, Wong R, Hsia K, Pilcher M, Stempien MJ. Plasma cytomegalovirus (CMV) DNA load predicts CMV disease and survival in AIDS patients. J Clin Invest 1998;101:497-502.
144. Stamm WE. *Chlamydia trachomatis* infections of the adult. In: Holmes KK, Sparling PF, Mardh P-A, et al, eds. Sexually transmitted diseases, 3rd edition. New York: McGraw-Hill, 1999:407-22.
145. Stamm WE, Guinan ME, Johnson C, Starcher T, Holmes KK, McCormack WM. Effect of treatment regimens for *Neisseria gonorrhoeae* on simultaneous infection with *Chlamydia trachomatis*. N Engl J Med 1984;310:545-9.
146. Stamper PD, Alcabasa R, Aird D, Babiker W, Wehrlin J, Ikpeama I, et al. Comparison of a commercial real-time PCR assay for tcdB detection to a cell culture cytotoxicity assay and toxigenic culture for direct detection of toxin-producing *Clostridium difficile* in clinical samples. J Clin Microbiol 2009;47:373-8.
147. Staprans SI, Hamilton BL, Follansbee SE, Elbeik T, Barbosa P, Grant RM, et al. Activation of virus replication after vaccination of HIV-1-infected individuals. J Exp Med 1995;182:1727-37.
148. Stellrecht KA, Harding I, Hussain FM, Mishrik NG, Czap RT, Lepow ML, et al. A one-step RT-PCR assay using an enzyme-linked detection system for the diagnosis of enterovirus meningitis. J Clin Virol 2000; 17:143-9.
149. Swanson P, Holzmayer V, Huang S, Hay P, Adebiyi A, Rice P, et al. Performance of the automated Abbott RealTime HIV-1 assay on a genetically diverse panel of specimens from London: comparison to VERSANT HIV-1 RNA 3.0, AMPLICOR HIV-1 MONITOR v1.5, and LCx HIV RNA quantitative assays. J Virol Methods 2006;137: 184-92.
150. Tedder D, Ashley R, Tyler K, Levin M. Herpes simplex virus infection as a cause of benign recurrent lymphocytic meningitis. Ann Intern Med 1994;121:334-8.
151. Templeton KE, Scheltinga SA, Beersma MF, Kroes AC, Claas EC. Rapid and sensitive method using multiplex real-time PCR for diagnosis of infections by influenza and influenza B viruses, respiratory syncytial virus, and parainfluenza viruses 1, 2, 3, and 4. J Clin Microbiol 2004;42:1564-9.
152. Templeton KE, Scheltinga SA, van den Eeden WC, Graffelman AW, van den Broek PJ, Claas EC. Improved diagnosis of the etiology of community-acquired pneumonia with real-time polymerase chain reaction. Clin Infect Dis 2005;41:345-51.
153. Ticehurst JR, Aird DZ, Dam LM, Borek AP, Hargrove JT, Carroll KC. Effective detection of toxigenic *Clostridium difficile* by a two-step algorithm including tests for antigen and cytotoxin. J Clin Microbiol 2006;44:1145-9.

154. Tural C, Ruiz L, Holtzer C, Schapiro J, Viciana P, Gonzalez J, et al. Clinical utility of HIV-1 genotyping and expert advice: the Havana trial. AIDS 2002;16:209-18.
155. Van Der Pol B, Ferrero DV, Buck-Barrington L, Hook E 3rd, Lenderman C, Quinn T, et al. Multicenter evaluation of the BDProbeTec ET System for detection of *Chlamydia trachomatis* and *Neisseria gonorrhoeae* in urine specimens, female endocervical swabs, and male urethral swabs. J Clin Microbiol 2001;39:1008-16.
156. Van Houtte M. Update on resistance testing. J HIV Ther 2001;6:61-4.
157. Vermehren J, Kau A, Gartner BC, Gobel R, Zeuzem S, Sarrazin C. Differences between two real-time PCR-based hepatitis C virus (HCV) assays (RealTime HCV and Cobas AmpliPrep/Cobas TaqMan) and one signal amplification assay (VERSANT HCV RNA 3.0) for RNA detection and quantification. J Clin Microbiol 2008;46:3880-91.
158. Verstrepen WA, Bruynseels P, Mertens AH. Evaluation of a rapid real-time RT-PCR assay for detection of enterovirus RNA in cerebrospinal fluid specimens. J Clin Virol 2002;25:S39-43.
159. Weinberg GA, Erdman DD, Edwards KM, Hall CB, Walker FJ, Griffin MR, et al. Superiority of reverse-transcription polymerase chain reaction to conventional viral culture in the diagnosis of acute respiratory tract infections in children. J Infect Dis 2004;189:706-10.
160. Whitcomb JM, Huang W, Fransen S, Limoli K, Toma J, Wrin T, et al. Development and characterization of a novel single-cycle recombinant-virus assay to determine human immunodeficiency virus type 1 coreceptor tropism. Antimicrob Agents Chemother 2007;51: 566-75.
161. Whitley R, Lakeman F. Herpes simplex virus infections of the central nervous system: therapeutic and diagnostic considerations. Clin Infect Dis 1995;20:414-20.
162. Whitley RJ, Alford CA, Hirsch MS, Schooley RT, Luby JP, Aoki FY, et al. Vidarabine versus acyclovir therapy in herpes simplex encephalitis. N Engl J Med 1986;314:144-9.
163. Wildemann B, Ehrhart K, Storch-Hagenlocher B, Meyding-Lamade U, Steinvorth S, Hacke W, et al. Quantitation of herpes simplex virus type 1 DNA in cells of cerebrospinal fluid of patients with herpes simplex virus encephalitis. Neurology 1997;48:1341-6.
164. Wilkins TD, Lyerly DM. *Clostridium difficile* testing: after 20 years, still challenging. J Clin Microbiol 2003;41:531-4.
165. Wolff D, Gerritzen A. Comparison of the Roche COBAS Amplicor MONITOR, Roche COBAS Ampliprep/COBAS TaqMan and Abbott RealTime test assays for quantification of hepatitis C virus and HIV RNA. Clin Chem Lab Med 2007;45:917-22.
166. Wolk DM, Picton E, Johnson D, Davis T, Pancholi P, Ginocchio CC, et al. Multicenter evaluation of the Cepheid Xpert methicillin-resistant *Staphylococcus aureus* (MRSA) test as a rapid screening method for detection of MRSA in nares. J Clin Microbiol 2009;47:758-64.
167. Wright TC Jr, Massad LS, Dunton CJ, Spitzer M, Wilkinson EJ, Solomon D. 2006 consensus guidelines for the management of women with abnormal cervical cancer screening tests. Am J Obstet Gynecol 2007;197:346-55.
168. Zeuzem S, Buti M, Ferenci P, Sperl J, Horsmans Y, Cianciara J, et al. Efficacy of 24 weeks treatment with peginterferon alfa-2b plus ribavirin in patients with chronic hepatitis C infected with genotype 1 and low pretreatment viremia. J Hepatol 2006;44:97-103.
169. Zhang F, Ginocchio CC, Malhotra A, et al. Clinical performance and financial impact of rapid enterovirus detection in cerebrospinal fluid (CSF) using the NucliSens Basic kit and nucleic acid sequence based amplification. Abstract T5. Presented at: 18th Annual Meeting of the PanAmerican Society for Clinical Virology, 2002, Clearwater, Fla.
170. Zoll GJ, Melchers WJ, Kopecka H, Jambroes G, van der Poel HJ, Galama JM. General primer-mediated polymerase chain reaction for detection of enteroviruses: application for diagnostic routine and persistent infections. J Clin Microbiol 1992;30:160-5.

CHAPTER 43

Pharmacogenetics

*Gwendolyn A. McMillin, Ph.D., D.A.B.C.C.(C.C., T.C.)**

The term *pharmacogenetics* comes from merging the names of *pharmacology* (the study of drugs, particularly drug handling and drug response) and *genetics* (the study of how traits are inherited). Pharmacogenetic testing is intended to predict or explain how people will respond to medicines and other pharmacologically or toxicologically active compounds, based on discrete genetic characteristics. Pharmacogenetics is a rapidly evolving and expanding field and a critical component of personalized medicine. Related work associating drug handling and response with the entire genome is known as *pharmacogenomics,* although some use the terms interchangeably. Pharmacogenetics and pharmacogenomics could include human germline mutations, somatic mutations such as those observed in a malignant tumor, gene copy number, or nonhuman (e.g., viral genome) mutations. Pharmacogenetic or pharmacogenomic profiles hold the potential to improve prescribing practices for most if not all drugs.[64,213]

The goal of pharmacogenetics today is to relate a discrete aspect of a patient's genetic inheritance (genotype) to phenotype, specifically, one or more aspects of pharmacokinetics (drug handling) and/or pharmacodynamics (drug action). Pretreatment pharmacogenetic testing has the potential to predict a phenotype before a drug is ever administered. Predicted phenotype information can be used to select a specific drug(s) that a patient is likely to respond to or select the optimal dosing interval for that patient, while at the same time avoiding or minimizing the incidence of adverse drug reactions (ADRs), including drug hypersensitivity. ADRs are a leading cause of morbidity and mortality in the United States, and the likelihood of response for many drug classes is less than 50%.[26,76,97,165,170] Approximately 10% of all drug labels now include references to pharmacogenetic findings, and several pharmacogenetic tests are available clinically that are designed to identify patients that may be genetically predisposed to ADRs or therapeutic failure.[39] However, clinical use of pharmacogenetics in prescribing most drugs requires more specific dosing guidelines and algorithms based on pharmacogenetic information. Such tools are being considered, developed, and/or evaluated to assist with the use of pharmacogenetic data to inform drug and dose selection, and are likely to improve uptake and utility of pharmacogenetic testing in the coming years.

The goal of this chapter is to familiarize the clinical laboratorian with concepts and examples of pharmacogenetic testing involving human germline variants. The chapter includes descriptions of several polymorphic genes and their applications to drugs used in major areas of medicine in which pharmacogenetic testing is currently applied. For a more in-depth discussion of pharmacogenetics or pharmacogenomics, or regarding specific clinical applications, the reader is encouraged to consult the excellent review articles and websites cited here, as well as the contemporary peer-reviewed literature.

DEFINING PHARMACOGENETIC TARGETS

For simplicity, the term *drug(s)* will be used throughout this chapter to reflect any xenobiotic (foreign compound absorbed by the human body) that is capable of evoking a physiologic or behavioral response, whether desirable (therapeutic) or undesirable (toxic). Responses to drugs and drug handling depend on many variables such as drug formulation, route of administration, clinical status (e.g., kidney function, liver function, protein status), age, gender, comedications, and genetics. Many of the variables surrounding drug handling and drug response are measurable and could be considered relative to optimizing drug therapy choices. However, most drugs are historically dosed according to population-based dosage and dose frequency recommendations. Dosing is typically optimized through trial and error, based on how a patient handles and responds to a drug or combination of drugs. Minimizing this process of trial and error is one of several strategies proposed to reduce the incidence of ADRs and improve rates of efficacy. Pharmacogenetic testing can be used to understand and predict specific aspects of the two major processes upon which pharmacology is based: pharmacokinetics and pharmacodynamics.

Pharmacokinetics describes the processes through which the body acts on a drug: absorption, distribution, metabolism, and elimination. Pharmacokinetic targets may therefore represent genes that code for transport proteins, metabolic

The author gratefully acknowledges the original contributions of Drs. Mark W. Linder and Bonny Lewis Bukaveckas on which portions of this chapter are based.

enzymes, or drug-binding proteins. Pharmacokinetics is often evaluated by measuring drugs and/or drug metabolites in biological fluids that are collected at specific times relative to the time of last drug administration. From these results, time-versus-concentration curves can be generated, and parameters such as clearance calculated.

Pharmacodynamics deals with responses to drugs and describes the processes that mediate those responses, whether the response is desirable or undesirable. Pharmacodynamic targets may represent genes that code for enzymes, receptors, ion channels, or other signaling proteins. Response to a drug may or may not show a relationship to drug dose or to the concentration of drug in blood. Pharmacodynamics can be measured for some drugs based on biomarkers [e.g., the international normalized ratio (INR) for warfarin] or based on clinical measurements [e.g., blood pressure, for antihypertensive drugs].

Pharmacogenetic testing provides information about the predicted pharmacokinetics and pharmacodynamics of an individual patient that otherwise are not readily measured. Testing can be used to predict unique characteristics of drug handling and drug response that could minimize the traditional trial and error style of dose optimization, particularly when used in combination with biochemical and clinical (measurable) factors. See Chapter 34 of this book for further discussion of pharmacokinetic and pharmacodynamic processes.

The first recognized pharmacogenetic targets largely described variation in drug metabolism. The early focus on drug metabolism reflects the fact that measurements of drug and drug metabolite concentrations in biological fluids predate detailed understanding of genetics and development of most biomarkers that describe pharmacodynamics. Distinct metabolic phenotypes were characterized and were subsequently found to cluster within families. For example, the metabolic phenotype for *N*-acetyltransferase (NAT), attributed to an enzyme originally called *isoniazid transacetylase,* was recognized in the 1950s with isoniazid (L-isonicotinyl hydrazide), a drug used to treat tuberculosis.[11,199] Population studies revealed a bimodal distribution in plasma and urine concentrations of the *N*-acetylated isoniazid metabolite. The concentration of the parent drug was highly correlated with the prevalence of toxic symptoms, including hepatotoxicity and a painful and progressive peripheral neuropathy that affected up to one third of Caucasian and African American patients. From this initial work, patients were phenotypically described as "fast acetylators" or "slow acetylators." Slow acetylators excrete large amounts of the parent drug relative to the acetylated metabolite when compared with fast acetylators. Family studies identified a strong genetic linkage of this phenotype and suggested that the phenotype was inherited as an autosomal recessive trait. However, details of the genetics, which are described later in this chapter, were not elucidated until several years later.

Clinical use of pharmacogenetic testing requires an understanding of how genetic variation of a metabolic enzyme affects drug response or drug dosing. Drug metabolism can effectively inactivate a substrate or increase water solubility of the substrate to promote its excretion. Conversely, metabolism can activate a substrate or prodrug (e.g., codeine, clopidogrel, tamoxifen). Less commonly, metabolism serves to extend the elimination half-life of a pharmacologically active or potentially toxic metabolite.[131]

Reactions catalyzed by metabolic enzymes are often categorized as Phase I and Phase II. Phase I reactions convert the parent compound into a more polar metabolite by introducing or removing a single functional group. Examples include (1) oxidation, (2) reduction, and (3) hydrolysis. The metabolites may or may not be pharmacologically or toxicologically active. Most Phase I reactions are oxidative and are mediated by cytochrome P450 isoenzymes (CYPs). Genetic variants of CYPs have been associated with changes in enzyme activity, stability, and/or substrate affinity that can lead to clinically significant phenotypes. In addition to genetic variability, many CYP isoenzymes are susceptible to dramatic differences in expression (>1000-fold) and drug-drug interactions that can change the phenotype from that which might be predicted based on genetics alone. This concept is known as *phenocopying.* A drug that can inhibit its own metabolism is known to exhibit autophenocopying.[134,144]

A relatively common fate of Phase I metabolic products is additional modification, such as through Phase II reactions. Phase II reactions may also occur independent of, or before, Phase I reactions. Phase II enzymes are generally transferases that conjugate drugs with acetyl, glucuronyl, amino acyl, or sulfate groups. Many Phase II enzymes exhibit genetic variation that has been associated with clinically significant phenotypical differences caused by changes in enzyme activity, stability, and/or substrate affinity.[187] For example, thiopurine *S*-methyl transferase (TPMT), *N*-acetyltransferase (NAT1, NAT2), and uridine diphosphate glucuronosyl transferase (UGT1A1) exhibit genetic variation and are discussed later in this chapter primarily relative to metabolism of drugs used in oncology and infectious disease.

Through genome-wide association studies and improved definition of response phenotypes, pharmacogenetic targets associated with several aspects of pharmacokinetics and pharmacodynamics are frequently proposed and described in the peer-reviewed literature, considerably increasing the breadth and complexity of drug-gene relationships. Thus far, most drug-gene associations are not sufficiently well studied clinically to be used to direct therapy. Therefore, it is not now practical, medically indicated, nor cost-effective to provide pharmacogenetic profiles for every drug. Based on successful applications to date, pharmacogenetic targets are most likely to be successful clinically when they:

1. Define a major pathway for metabolism of, or response to, a specific drug, thereby providing clear guidance for drug selection or avoidance.
2. Are associated with a clinically significant and actionable effect on the relationship between dose and plasma drug concentration or a measurable biomarker.
3. Predict dosing for a drug that has a narrow therapeutic index or limited temporal opportunity to exert efficacy, or

TABLE 43-1 Overview of Drugs for Which Revised Labeling Includes Pharmacogenetic Information

Drug	Relevant Area of Medicine	Year FDA Approved Revised Labeling	Approximate Rate of ADRs or Resistance	Gene or Allele	Other Drugs With Pharmacogenetic Relationship to Gene or Allele
6-Mercaptopurine	Oncology	2003	1 to 10% ADRs	*TPMT*	Azathioprine, 6-thioguanine
Irinotecan	Oncology	2004	30 to 40% ADRs	*UGT1A1*	Topotecan, nilotinib, protease inhibitors
Tamoxifen	Oncology	Proposed 2006	30% resistant	*CYP2D6*	Codeine
5-Fluorouracil	Oncology	2003	20% ADRs	*DYPD*	Capecitabine
Atomoxetine	Psychiatry	2004	5 to 10% ADRs	*CYP2D6*	Antidepressants, amphetamine
Carbamazepine	Psychiatry, Neurology	2007	10% ADRs	*HLA-B*1502*	Phenytoin, lamotrigine
Abacavir	Infectious Disease	2007	5 to 8% ADRs	*HLA-B*5701*	
Isoniazid	Infectious Disease	Not Available		*NAT*	Rifampin, hydralazine
Warfarin	Cardiology	2007	5 to 40% ADRs	*CYP2C9, VKORC1*	
Clopidogrel	Cardiology	2009	30% resistant	*CYP2C19*	Voriconazole, omeprazole, diazepam, nelfinavir, antidepressants, tamoxifen

ADRs, Adverse drug reactions.

for a drug that requires a long period of time to establish efficacy.

The utility of pharmacogenetic testing may be compromised when (1) no alternative drugs are available for an indication, (2) incorporation of pharmacogenetic testing does not clearly improve patient care, (3) less sophisticated or less expensive tools or tests are sufficient for making prescribing decisions, or (4) accommodations to specific dose or dosing strategies are not available. Some specific gene-drug relationships for which the labeling has been revised to include pharmacogenetic information are shown in Table 43-1. Although these gene-drug examples apply primarily to oncology, psychiatry, neurology, infectious disease, and cardiology, other areas of medicine are likely to benefit from pharmacogenetic testing as well. The examples are intended to provide a foundation of concepts that the reader can translate to future applications as they emerge and develop.

APPROACHES TO PHARMACOGENETIC TESTING

Pharmacogenetic testing can predict that a patient is likely to (1) fail therapy, (2) suffer an ADR, or (3) exhibit altered pharmacokinetics. This knowledge then assists in selection of drug, drug dosage, and dosing frequency, thus promoting successful therapy and avoiding undesirable outcomes such as an ADR. Pharmacogenetic testing is designed to detect a phenotype (phenotyping) or a genetic sequence that has been associated with a phenotype (genotyping). Examples of both approaches (phenotyping and genotyping) will be provided; however, more emphasis is given to the genetic approaches, which are currently more common. Neither phenotyping nor genotyping is intended to replace the need for clinical assessments of drug response, or to replace the need for therapeutic drug monitoring. Several considerations of these two testing approaches are summarized in Table 43-2 and are described in greater detail later.

Phenotyping defines the "state" rather than the "trait." Phenotyping has been applied most frequently to detecting pharmacokinetic variation, particularly in drug metabolism and clearance. Measurement of the drug metabolism phenotype, under highly controlled circumstances, can provide extremely meaningful information.

A common approach to phenotyping is to administer a probe drug, that is, a drug that is known to be metabolized by the same enzyme or pathway as the intended therapeutic drug. Biological fluid, typically urine and/or blood, is collected at specific times after administration of the probe drug. The concentrations of parent drug and one or more drug metabolites are then determined. The ratios of parent to metabolite or of two metabolite concentrations (e.g., metabolite A/metabolite B) are compared, and a metabolic ratio is calculated. The phenotype associated with *CYP2D6* has historically been determined through the use of probe drugs. For this particular enzyme, a continuum of metabolic phenotypes is described, varying from poor (little to no activity) to intermediate, to extensive (normal), to ultra-rapid. Urine collected at a specified time after administration of the probe drug (e.g., 8 hours) is analyzed for the parent drug and a metabolite that is generated primarily via CYP2D6. Example

TABLE 43-2 Comparing Phenotype and Genotype Testing Strategies

	Phenotype	Genotype
Represents	"State" represents current response; may not represent inheritance	"Trait" represents inheritance; may not be consistent with the phenotype
Sensitive to gene expression	Yes	No
Sensitive to protein function	Yes	No
Requires collection of multiple specimens	Commonly	No
Requires administration of a probe drug	Possibly	No
Other limitations	• Specimen instability for enzyme or other protein of interest may lead to inaccurate results • May have to be repeated for patients who recently received a blood transfusion • May be influenced by comedications (drug-drug interactions)	• May not include all clinically relevant genes and/or alleles • Genotype-phenotype relationship (interpretation) may not be known

parent-metabolite pairs used to calculate a metabolic ratio for phenotyping of CYP2D6 include dextromethorphan/dextrorphan, debrisoquine/4-hydroxydebrisoquine, sparteine/dehydrosparteine, and nortriptyline/10-hydroxynortriptyline.[38] An example of phenotype results generated with the probe drug debrisoquine is shown in Figure 43-1. A "cutoff" metabolic ratio is used to distinguish a normal, extensive metabolizer (EM) from a poor metabolizer (PM). Although the metabolic ratio is theoretically a good indicator of enzyme expression and function at the time of the test, marked variation in metabolic ratio has been demonstrated among the phenotypes.[20] Similar variation in metabolic ratio is commonly observed with other probe drugs as well.

Another example of a probe drug is caffeine, which is used to determine acetylator phenotype mediated by NAT.[21,72,121] To determine the NAT phenotype with this probe drug, the patient is given 200 mg caffeine after an overnight fast. Urine is collected 4 and 5 hours later. The 4-hour specimen is discarded, and the 5-hour specimen is analyzed for caffeine metabolites 5-acetylamino-6-formylamino-3-methyluracil (AFMU) and 1-methylxanthine (1X). See Figure 43-2 for sample data. Cutoffs for acetylator phenotypes are based on the ratio of AFMU/1X. Considering a bimodal distribution of acetylators, a ratio of less than 0.66 is used to define slow acetylators. Because a trimodal distribution has now been described and may be of interest, a ratio higher than 3.0 could define "ultrarapid" acetylators; a ratio between 0.66 and 3.0 would define an "intermediate" acetylator phenotype.[57]

Phenotype testing based on probe drug administration requires that the probe compound be (1) safe, (2) easy to administer in the target population, (3) relatively inexpensive, and (4) it must exhibit pharmacokinetics that support convenient collection of specimens from the patient. The need to administer a probe drug and to collect urine over several hours has always limited the practical utility of patient phenotyping with a probe drug. Even with the logistics managed,

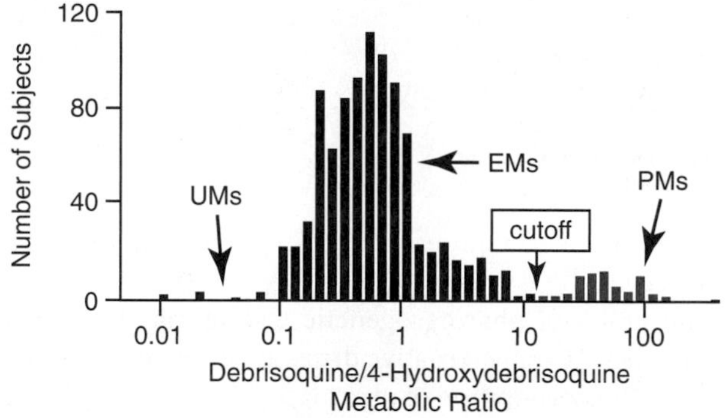

Figure 43-1 Histogram of the "debrisoquine metabolic ratio" in a typical Caucasian population. Metabolic ratios were determined from the concentrations of debrisoquine and 4-hydroxydebrisoquine (metabolite) in a urine specimen collected 8 hours after a 10 mg dose of debrisoquine was given. The data demonstrate a clear distinction between poor metabolizer (PM), extensive metabolizer (EM), and ultra-rapid metabolizer (UM) phenotypes. *(From Caldwell J. Pharmacogenetics and individual variation in the range of amino acid adequacy: the biological aspects. J Nutr 2004;134:1600S-4S; discussion 30S-2S, 67S-72S. Reproduced by permission from the American Society for Nutritional Sciences.)*

phenotyping may be difficult to accomplish because of limited availability and appreciable costs of laboratory testing. Phenotype results based on a probe drug may be difficult to interpret as a result of potentially unrecognized or unrecorded confounding factors, such as diet, comedications, consumption of alcohol or over-the-counter medications, disease status, gender, and age.

Phenotyping is also performed in vitro by measuring the activity of a particular metabolic enzyme using peripheral blood cells as a surrogate to metabolism by the whole patient. For example, a common method of phenotyping TPMT activity is to isolate red blood cells, lyse the cells, and incubate

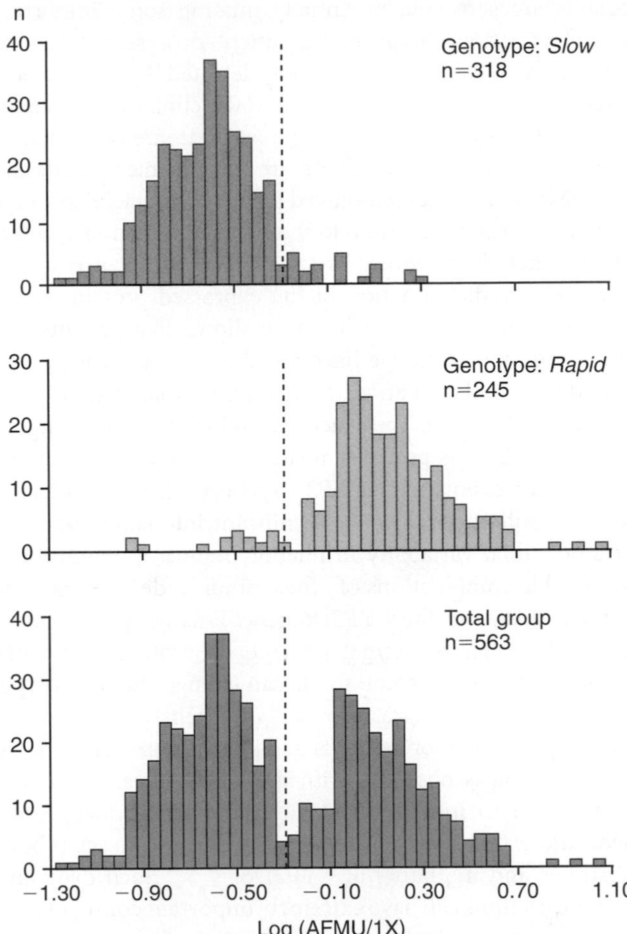

Figure 43-2 Histogram of *N*-acetyltransferase (NAT2) phenotypical activities as obtained by the caffeine test: 5 hour urine collection obtained after administration of caffeine and analyzed for caffeine metabolite concentrations. Values represent the logarithmically transformed ratio of metabolites 5-acetylamino-6-formylamino-3-methyl-uracil (AFMU) and 1-methylxanthine (1X). From the distinct bimodal distribution, an antimode of log(0.50) = −0.30 was obtained *(dotted line)*. *(From Cascorbi I, Drakoulis N, Brockmoller J, Maurer A, Sperling K, Roots I. Arylamine N-acetyltransferase (NAT2) mutations and their allelic linkage in unrelated Caucasian individuals: correlation with phenotypical activity. Am J Hum Genet 1995;57:581-92. Reproduced by permission from the University of Chicago Press.)*

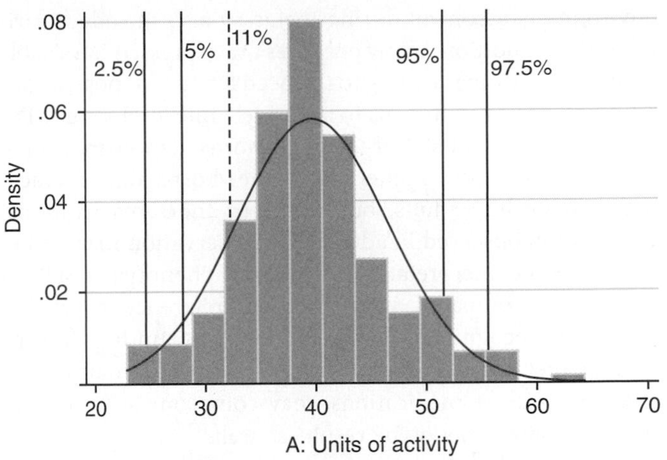

Figure 43-3 Histogram of thiopurine *S*-methyltransferase (TPMT) phenotypical activity obtained with blood samples from 199 healthy Caucasian adult volunteers. Blood lysate was incubated with *S*-adenosyl-L-methionine and 6-mercaptopurine at 37 °C for 60 minutes. The reaction was stopped, and concentrations of 6-methyl-mercaptopurine were determined by ultraviolet high-performance liquid chromatography (HPLC-UV). Data indicate that the activity of TPMT is variable, and that the definition of enzyme impairment is challenging based on phenotype studies alone. Percentiles could be used to phenotype patients, with the 11% mark (corresponding to published incidence of TPMT impairment in Caucasians) used as a cutoff to identify patients who might require a dose adjustment.

the lysate with substrate 6-mercaptopurine (6-MP) and a methyl donor such as *S*-adenosyl-L-methionine for 1.5 hours at 37 °C.[74,201] The concentration of methylated product, 6-methyl mercaptopurine (6-MMP), is measured and compared with a reference interval. An example of TPMT phenotype data generated in a healthy adult population is shown in Figure 43-3. Reduced or deficient TPMT activity is detected when low 6-MMP concentrations are measured. The clinical significance of low TPMT activity is high risk of myelosuppression due to an accumulation of 6-thioguanines (6-TGNs) when patients are treated with 6-MP or azathioprine (AZA), a related prodrug that is metabolized to 6-MP. Patients with impaired TPMT activity require lower doses of these drugs and close clinical monitoring to minimize the risk of toxicity and ensure efficacy of the drug.[7,36] This application is discussed in greater detail in the following section on TPMT genetics. Other examples of enzymes that have been successfully evaluated for in vitro phenotypes include (1) pseudocholinesterase, for detecting individuals with susceptibility to prolonged apnea when treated with succinylcholine or other similar medications; (2) glucose-6-phosphate dehydrogenase (G6PD), for detecting susceptibility to hemolysis in response to drugs such as primaquine, sulfonamides, chloramphenicol, and vitamin K; and (3) NAT, for detecting poor metabolism of drugs such as sulfonamides, isoniazid, and clonazepam.[33,50] With each, a substrate for the enzyme is incubated with the isolated cells under conditions (temperature, time, cofactors, pH, etc.) optimal for the enzyme of interest. The reaction is stopped and the product is measured with an analytical technique such as spectrophotometry or liquid chromatography with ultraviolet or mass spectrometric detection.

The in vitro phenotype approach has several limitations, for example, data are not valid if the patient from whom cells are collected is receiving the same drug used by the laboratory as a substrate in the phenotyping assay for that drug, at the time of specimen collection. Factors such as (1) recent blood transfusions, (2) hormonal fluctuations, (3) handling of the blood before and after isolation of cells, and (4) inadequate environmental control during the assay also introduce variability.[81] In addition, many enzymes are expressed in variable quantities with age, leading to the need for age- or population-specific reference intervals to accurately interpret results. For example, a study of 60 full-term newborns demonstrated that TPMT activity was higher in the newborns than in race-matched healthy adults, but displayed the same tri-modal distribution observed in adults. This observation may lead to inappropriate interpretation of newborn phenotype results, if results are compared with an adult reference interval.[118] Finally, unrecognized or unrecorded confounding factors, such as diet, comedications, and consumption of alcohol or over-the-counter medications, may compromise interpretation of in vitro phenotype results as well.[165]

The second major approach to detecting and evaluating pharmacogenetic variability is through genotyping. Genetic testing may be useful for predicting specific pharmacokinetic and/or pharmacodynamic variables that are well characterized. The value of genotyping depends very much on a strong genotype-phenotype correlation. In the simplest scenario, a genotype result will account for 100% of the anticipated phenotype. Completely definitive genotype-phenotype relationships (100% certainty) are rare—a fact that creates controversy surrounding the value of a single-gene association. It is estimated, for example, that genotyping of *TPMT* can reliably predict the phenotype 80 to 90% of the time.[151] However, the complexity of the metabolism surrounding thiopurine drugs (see TPMT discussion later) raises questions regarding other potentially important genes that contribute to the overall pharmacokinetics of these drugs. For example, variants in three other genes have recently been demonstrated to influence metabolism of azathioprine, and a polymorphism in the inosine trisphosphatase gene *(ITPA)* appears to be responsible for ADRs experienced by some patients treated with AZA.[168,193]

When a good genotype-phenotype relationship exists, genotyping assays have advantages over phenotyping because they (1) can be less expensive than phenotyping, (2) are more reproducible between laboratories, and (3) are not subject to intraindividual variability caused by a specific set of clinical conditions or expected biological variations that complicate phenotyping assays. Genotyping assays are also less invasive and less time-consuming for the patient. Thus, the single sample required for genotyping may be collected anytime, anywhere. Saliva-based testing, which generates an adequate quantity and quality of DNA for most genetic testing, would make at-home collections particularly convenient.[66]

Despite advantages of genotyping over phenotyping, genotyping has limitations that must be recognized. For example, some of the assays using target amplification are prone to false negatives because they rely on the presence or absence of a polymerase chain reaction (PCR) product. The specific allelic variants detected by a given analytical method vary, and, short of sequencing the entire gene, currently available genotyping techniques cannot detect all possible variants. Because of the large amount of variation in many genes, suites of variants are screened, potentially missing some important genetic variations because the patient possesses a rare or novel polymorphism that is not detected by the screen. Further, polymorphisms with unknown clinical significance may be identified by some techniques. Extreme care must be taken to ensure that these data are not misinterpreted, and that the laboratory test employed provides sufficient coverage of genetic variants common to the ethnic population of interest. Another disadvantage of genotyping is that it may not accurately predict function of the expressed protein. Using *CYP2D6* as an example, it has been shown that patients of a single common genotype have metabolic ratios (with probe drug dextromethorphan or debrisoquine) that span a 1000- to 10,000-fold range. The exact reason for this broad range is unknown, but it is probably related to (1) individual differences in expression of the *CYP2D6* gene, (2) inherent alternative metabolic pathways, (3) significant interlaboratory and intraindividual variability in phenotype measurements, and (4) possible combinations of other minor undetected genetic polymorphisms in the *CYP2D6* gene. Finally, specific interactions between the target enzyme or protein and other drugs, chemicals, or some foods can change the phenotype, such as by converting a "normal" or extensive metabolizer phenotype to a poor metabolizer phenotype. This type of phenocopying is observed with grapefruit juice, which has been shown to inhibit CYP3A4, and many antidepressant medications (e.g., fluoxetine), which are known to act as both substrates and inhibitors of CYP2D6.[63,135,144] Such drug and food interactions can have extremely important consequences for the phenotype and can be difficult to both recognize and monitor.

CLINICAL APPLICATION OF PHARMACOGENETIC TESTING

Pharmacogenetic testing is clinically useful only when information is sufficient to allow interpretation of the results. This information must be derived from in vivo human studies. Many examples of this type of information can be found in the peer-reviewed literature. One limitation of existing literature, however, is that most data are based on retrospective studies, and there is no single printed source in which all of this information has been collated. The Pharmacogenetics and Pharmacogenomics Knowledge Base is a publicly available Internet research tool developed by Stanford University with funding from the National Institutes of Health (NIH) and is part of the NIH Pharmacogenetics Research Network (PGRN), a nationwide collaborative research consortium. Its aim is to aid researchers in understanding how genetic variation among individuals contributes to differences in reactions to drugs. This regularly updated database is an excellent source of genetic and clinical information derived from research studies at various medical centers in the PGRN (www.pharmgkb.org, accessed June 28, 2011). Several of the figures illustrating pharmacogenetically important drug metabolism pathways are found in this chapter, with permission from PharmGKB and Stanford University.[91]

Many ongoing clinical trials designed to study the efficacy and toxicity of new pharmaceutical products or new indications for previously developed pharmaceuticals have employed pharmacogenetic testing, or have incorporated pharmacogenetic testing into the study protocol (for a current listing, see www.clinicaltrials.gov, accessed June 28, 2011). Thus it is anticipated that pharmacogenetic guidelines, and possibly new companion diagnostics that would be simultaneously released to market with the pharmaceutical, will be available in the coming years. In addition, drugs that were previously removed from development because of ADRs may be reconsidered if a genetic test can be demonstrated to identify individuals at high risk for ADRs, that would then avoid use of that drug. A discussion of pharmacogenetic testing of clinical relevance to the areas of oncology, psychiatry and neurology, cardiology, and infectious disease is provided in the next section. For each of the major genes discussed in this chapter, Table 43-1 provides a list of common drugs for which pharmacogenetic associations with these genes have been made and drug labels revised. Because many other drug-gene combinations are recognized that may lead to additional drug label revisions, the discussion provided here is in no way comprehensive. In addition, many of the specific genes discussed later have applications to other areas of medicine, some of which are mentioned briefly. The purpose of the discussion in this chapter is to provide examples against which additional pharmacogenetic tests and applications can be compared, critiqued, and understood, and to guide involvement of the clinical laboratorian in this emerging new field of laboratory medicine.

Pharmacogenetics in Oncology

Oncology is an area of medicine in which correct or incorrect choice of therapy can lead to a life or death situation. The temporal opportunity for a therapy to exert effect is narrow, the incidence of ADRs with many available drugs is high, and the overall rates of efficacy are low. It is estimated that as many as 40% of oncology patients receive the wrong drug.[27,198] Many of the tests routinely used to characterize tumor tissue are based on detecting overexpression of specific proteins (e.g., HER2/neu) or the presence of somatic gene variants in a tumor (e.g., *K-ras*). Tumor profiling tests, which evaluate the expression of many genes (e.g., Oncotype DX), can be used to assess the prognosis of certain cancers. Results of these tests certainly guide therapeutic decisions but are not discussed here. The germline pharmacogenetics that is the focus of this chapter is complementary to these tumor-based tests. Some pharmacogenetic tests that predict metabolism are potentially applicable to cancer chemotherapy because metabolic enzymes are required to activate many drugs used in oncology (e.g., tamoxifen, cyclophosphamide). Metabolic enzymes are also required to inactivate some drugs commonly used in oncology (e.g., irinotecan, 6-MP, 5-fluorouracil). Impairment or altered expression of a key metabolic enzyme could make the difference between therapeutic success and ADRs.[70] In theory, optimal dose could be determined for these and all other drugs, based on understanding and coordinated application of pretherapeutic pharmacogenetics with post-therapeutic pharmacokinetic and pharmacodynamic monitoring. Table 43-3 lists examples of genes that are potentially important in selecting and dosing cancer therapies.

Pharmacogenetics has also been applied to risk stratification; this is particularly relevant for cancers that could be triggered by environmental or dietary exposure to a wide variety of xenobiotics.[15,164] Also shown in Table 43-3 are some of the genetic targets and known substrates that have been studied with regard to risk of various cancers. Genes that encode drug-metabolizing enzymes are of greatest interest for this application because it is through these enzymes that xenobiotics become activated or inactivated. For example, several substrates of NAT1 and NAT2 are potentially cancer-causing. In addition to NAT1 and NAT2, the glutathione *S*-transferases (GSTs) are important contributors in establishing the risk of cancer triggered by xenobiotic exposures. At least 16 GSTs have been identified, and these are divided into eight classes. The key members are listed in Table 43-3: alpha (GSTA1, GSTA2), mu (GSTM1), pi (GSTP1) and theta (GSTT1). Additional classes are called kappa, sigma, zeta, and omega. The *GSTM1*-deficient trait has, for example, been associated with higher risks of lung and bladder cancer, although the specific trigger or substrate is not known.[60] With additional study and validation of these and other genetic markers, testing to identify individuals with high susceptibility to chemicals may become important, particularly in high-risk occupational settings such as agriculture and manufacturing.

Three thoroughly-characterized gene-drug associations used to direct therapy in oncology are discussed in detail later in this chapter: *TPMT* for 6-mercaptopurine (6-MP), *UGT1A1* for irinotecan, and *CYP2D6* for tamoxifen.

Pharmacogenetics in Psychiatry and Neurology

Pharmacogenetics testing has shown promise in selecting or optimizing drug therapy for depression, schizophrenia, pain, and addictive behaviors. Many drugs used in psychiatry and neurology have low (<50%) efficacy rates, high interindividual variation in pharmacokinetics, and life-threatening ADRs. In addition, the response to drugs used for depression and schizophrenia cannot be adequately assessed for weeks to months after initiation. Standard-of-care practices today are based on the traditional trial-and-error approach. Pharmacogenetic tests could contribute to drug and dose selection by evaluating patient candidacy for specific drugs, and by allowing pretherapeutic identification of individual differences in pharmacokinetics or pharmacodynamics, particularly for drugs with a narrow therapeutic index.[28,112] It is no surprise that initial applications of pharmacogenetics in these clinical areas were related to thoroughly-characterized metabolic phenotypes. Of particular interest have been drug substrates of CYP2D6, CYP2C19, and CYP2C9. Dosing guidelines for many antidepressant and antipsychotic medications based on predicted metabolic phenotypes have been published.[88,89] A more conservative recommended strategy is to avoid drugs

TABLE 43-3 Pharmacogenetic Targets Potentially Important to Risk of Cancer, Selection of Therapeutic Cancer Drugs, and Optimization of Drug Dose

Gene or Protein Target	Chemotherapeutic Drug	Carcinogen Substrates
CD117 (C-KIT)	Imatinib	
CYP2B6	Cyclophosphamide, ifosfamide	
CYP2C9	Cyclophosphamide, ifosfamide	
CYP2C19	Tamoxifen	
CYP2D6	Tamoxifen	
CYP3A4	Cyclophosphamide, etoposide Ifosfamide, teniposide, vindesine, vinblastine, vincristine	Aflatoxin B1 6-Aminochrysene
DPYD	5-Fluorouracil, capecitabine	
EGFR	Erlotinib, cetuximab, gefitinib	
GSTA1, GSTA2	Cyclophosphamide	Cumene hydroperoxides
GSTM1		Aflatoxin B1 epoxides Benzo(a)pyrene 4,5 oxide Trans-stilbene oxide
GSTP1	Thiotepa, cyclophosphamide, ethacrynic acid	4-Nitrochinolone 1-oxide
GSTT1		Ethylene oxide, methyl chloride, dichloromethane
Her2/neu	Trastuzumab, lapatinib	
KRAS	Cetuximab, panitumumab	
MTHFR	Methotrexate, 5-fluorouracil	
NAT2	Amonafide	*p*-Aminobenzoic acid, 4-aminobiphenyl, 2-aminofluorene, *p*-aminosalicylic acid, benzidine, toluidine
Philadelphia chromosome	Busulfan, dasatinib, nilotinib	
PML/RAR (alpha) fusion	Tretinoin, arsenic oxide	
TPMT	6-Mercaptopurine, azathioprine, 6-thioguanine	
TYMS	5-Fluorouracil, capecitabine	
UGT1A1	Irinotecan, nilotinib	
UGT2B15	Tamoxifen	

that are associated with extreme phenotypes (e.g., UM, PM) or high risk of ADRs, unless alternative therapies are not available.[29]

Risk of ADRs may be associated with inappropriate drug concentrations, as a result of impaired metabolism, or may be unrelated to concentration and dose. For example, severe cutaneous reaction syndromes (SCARS), such as Stevens-Johnson syndrome and toxic epidermal necrolysis, lead to life-threatening and extremely painful rashes. Approximately one third of all drug-induced SCARS are associated with the antiepileptic drug carbamazepine. The occurrence of SCARS in patients treated with carbamazepine has been associated with a specific allele of human leukocyte antigen (HLA), *HLA-B*1502*.[207] This allele occurs most commonly in patients of Asian ancestry. In the Han Chinese population, the odds ratio for carbamazepine-induced SCARS is 2504 when the *IILA-B*1502* allele is present. Associations of this allele with SCARS induced by phenytoin and lamotrigine have also been reported.[111] Detection of HLA alleles associated with drug-induced SCARS before therapy is initiated could allow drug avoidance and substantially reduced risk of the associated ADR.

Resistance to drugs used in psychiatry and neurology is common and is not necessarily related to drug concentration or dose of drug. Genes related to pharmacodynamics of these drugs primarily code for various components within the neurotransmitter systems on which the drugs act. Genes associated with the serotoninergic (e.g., *SLC6A4*), noradrenergic *(SLC6A2)*, and dopaminergic (e.g., *DRD2*) neurotransmitter systems are best characterized. Serotonin-receptor variants have been correlated with response to antidepressants such as escitalopram, fluoxetine, and paroxetine. In addition, the S allele of the serotonin transporter gene *(SLC6A4)*, also known as the short form of the long/short polymorphism, predicts poor response and increased risk of ADRs with fluvoxamine, mirtazapine, and paroxetine. Variants in the glucocorticoid receptor gene *(NR3C1)* have also been proposed to predict response to nortriptyline and escitalopram. Time to response to the antipsychotics risperidone and olanzapine has been associated with variants in the promoter region of the dopamine D2 receptor gene *(DRD2)*. Genes associated with the biosynthesis and disposition of neurotransmitters *(MAOA, TPH)* may be important as well.[100,129,159,189]

Optimal dosing of the anticonvulsant drug phenytoin can be predicted by testing for variation in *CYP2C9, CYP2C19,* and *MDR1;* the latter encodes the p-glycoprotein. CYP2C9 is estimated to contribute to 90% of phenytoin metabolism, and CYP2C19 is thought to contribute to 10% of phenytoin metabolism, in persons with EM phenotypes for both enzymes. In patients who are CYP2C9 PM (poor metabolizers), CYP2C19 is the primary route of phenytoin elimination, and hence the importance of testing for CYP2C19 increases.[46,84,110] However, pharmacogenetics has not been helpful in elucidating resistance mechanisms in epilepsy.[82,166]

Three thoroughly-characterized gene-drug associations used to direct therapy in psychiatry and neurology are discussed in detail here: *CYP2D6* and *CYP2C19* for antidepressants, *CYP2D6* for codeine, and *HLA-B*1501* for carbamazepine.

Pharmacogenetics in Cardiology

Clinical management of acute cardiovascular events, such as myocardial infarction, pulmonary embolism, and a major bleed, cannot wait for genetic testing results to guide therapeutic decisions, at least based on the technologies and methods for genetic testing that are used today. However, preventive cardiovascular medicines are among the most widely prescribed of all drugs. Prominent examples include (1) prophylactic warfarin to prevent thromboses, (2) statins and antiplatelet therapies to minimize the risk of future coronary events, and (3) therapies used to treat hypertension. Each provides opportunities for pharmacogenetics to improve therapy in cardiology.

Procainamide is a classic antiarrhythmic, the metabolism of which is primarily mediated by *N*-acetylation. The rate of acetylation is genetically determined, based on NAT, and shows a bimodal (possibly trimodal) distribution of slow and fast acetylators that correlates to genetic variants in *NAT1* or *NAT2*. The *N*-acetylated metabolite, known commonly as NAPA, is routinely monitored with parent drug to optimize dose. Many CYP substrates have cardiovascular applications as well. For example, clopidogrel is a commonly prescribed CYP2C19 substrate. Clopidogrel is a prodrug and, much like tamoxifen and codeine, will exert little to no benefit unless metabolically activated. Indeed, approximately one third of patients are classified as resistant to clopidogrel, in part because of this pharmacokinetic variation. Pharmacodynamic variability can also explain drug resistance and toxicity. For example, drug transporters that facilitate uptake and elimination of statins may have pharmacogenetic implications. Variants of the OATP1B1, encoded by *SLCO1B1,* and the ABCB1, encoded by the *ABCB1,* are associated with pharmacokinetic variability and statin-induced myopathy.[103,138] In the PROSPER study, Iakoubova and colleagues[73] have reported that elderly carriers of the *KIF6 719Arg* variant with prior vascular disease receive significant benefit from pravastatin therapy; however, no benefit was observed in noncarriers with prior disease or in those without prior disease (carriers or noncarriers).

Ideally, pharmacogenetic testing predicts key aspects of pharmacokinetic and pharmacodynamic variability to guide therapeutic decisions. Combining testing for a key pharmacokinetic gene and a key pharmacodynamic gene is best exemplified by the association of warfarin dose with variants in *CYP2C9,* which is responsible for inactivation of warfarin, and *VKORC1,* the gene that codes for the primary target for the anticoagulant action of warfarin. Another gene, *CYP4F2,* is associated with increased dose requirements of warfarin.

Three thoroughly-characterized gene-drug associations used to direct therapy in cardiology are discussed in detail here: *CYP2C19* for clopidogrel, *CYP2C9* for warfarin, and *VKORC1* for warfarin.

Pharmacogenetics in Infectious Disease

Pharmacogenomics has been applied to infectious disease, primarily to understand organism susceptibility, to study comparative genomics, and to target drug development efforts. This growing area of research will be complementary to host pharmacogenetics, the focus of this chapter. In patients treated with interferon, overlap in the relationship between organism and host has been exemplified by the association of clearance of hepatitis C virus and variants of the gene for interleukin 28B *(IL28B)*.[44]

Regarding more traditional host pharmacogenetics of infectious disease, several targets related to pharmacokinetics are substrates of NAT: isoniazid, dapsone, and the sulfonamides. Although pharmacogenetic testing for *NAT1* and *NAT2* is not routine, variation in these genes has the potential to influence metabolism and steady-state concentrations of these drugs. Concentrations of proguanil are affected by variant *CYP2C19,* and *CYP2C8* is associated with risk of toxicity from amodiaquine. Other pharmacogenetic associations include (1) *CYP2B6* alleles and risk of central nervous system ADRs from efavirenz,[19] (2) *UGT1A* gene variants and severe hyperbilirubinemia associated with protease inhibitors,[95] and (3) variants of the CYP3A family and rates of clarithromycin clearance.[140]

Pharmacodynamic targets that are unrelated to the desirable response of the drug represent a unique opportunity for pharmacogenetic testing. An example of a very successful pharmacogenetic test for predicting risk of ADRs is detection of *HLA-B*5701,* which predicts abacavir-induced hypersensitivity reaction. Genotyping for *HLA-B*5701* before an abacavir-containing regimen is prescribed was recommended in the 2008 guidelines on the use of antiretroviral agents in HIV-1–infected adults and adolescents, which were developed through the Office of AIDS Research Advisory Council and have now become routine clinical practice.[109,147,188]

Three thoroughly-characterized gene-drug associations used to direct infectious disease therapies are discussed in detail here: *CYP2C19* for omeprazole and proguanil, *HLA-B*5701* for abacavir, and *UGT1A1* for protease inhibitors.

The following sections of this chapter provide information on selected key pharmacogenetic targets, the relationship between genotype and phenotype for each, and clinical applications of testing.

PHASE I METABOLIC ENZYMES: CYTOCHROME P450 ISOZYMES

As stated earlier, most Phase I reactions are oxidative and are mediated by cytochrome P450 enzymes (CYPs). CYPs are heme-containing enzymes that are synthesized from a superfamily of CYP genes and are classified into families, and further into subfamilies, based on amino acid homology. The major CYPs that are believed to contribute to drug metabolism are CYP1A2, CYP2B6, CYP2C9, CYP2C19, CYP2D6, CYP2E1, and the CYP3A family. Examples of drug substrates, inhibitors, and inducers are shown in Table 43-4. Although the pharmacogenetics of only CYP2C9, CYP2C19, and CYP2D6 are specifically discussed here, all the CYP families exhibit genetic variation that could influence optimal prescribing practices for drug substrates.[187] Alleles for all CYP genes are described according to international consensus.[77] In brief, the *1 ("star 1") allele is the normal (EM) allele that codes for a protein predicted to function with full enzymatic activity and to be expressed in typical quantities. Often *1 describes a scenario wherein no variant alleles are detected. Therefore, the true accuracy of a *1 allele designation is dependent on whether the assay used to make that call is comprehensive. All alleles are described with a star followed by a number, and possibly a letter to describe an allele subtype. Subtypes have not been shown to influence the phenotype, and identification of them probably is not important clinically but could be important for haplotype assignment or to support research studies. Numerical assignments of other alleles are based largely on chronology of identification, wherein alleles identified earliest in time have the lowest numbers. Some alleles are associated with normal protein function and expression, others with impaired function, altered expression, or no predicted enzyme activity at all (e.g., truncated protein, complete gene deletion). Common alleles for *CYP2C9, CYP2C19,* and *CYP2D6* are shown in Table 43-5. A common single-nucleotide polymorphism (SNP) used to detect each allele is bolded, but in many cases detection of other SNPs is required to accurately classify a genotype. The assignment of phenotype predictions from genotype is described in detail for CYP2D6 (Figure 43-4) but applies generally to other CYPs as well.

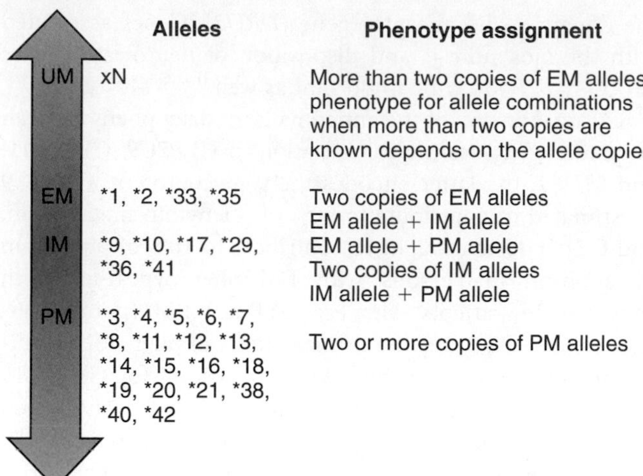

Alleles
Phenotype assignment
UM
xN
More than two copies of EM alleles phenotype for allele combinations when more than two copies are known depends on the allele copied
EM
*1, *2, *33, *35
Two copies of EM alleles
EM allele + IM allele
IM
*9, *10, *17, *29, *36, *41
EM allele + PM allele
Two copies of IM alleles
IM allele + PM allele
PM
*3, *4, *5, *6, *7, *8, *11, *12, *13, *14, *15, *16, *18, *19, *20, *21, *38, *40, *42
Two or more copies of PM alleles

Figure 43-4 CYP2D6 phenotype can be estimated based on the combination of alleles detected. Shown here is a continuum of metabolic phenotypes: poor (PM), extensive (normal, EM), intermediate (IM), and ultra-rapid (UM). The alleles that correspond to enzyme activity are also listed, adjacent to the formulas for establishing a clinical phenotype, based on the combination of two or more alleles.

CYTOCHROME P450 2D6 (CYP2D6)

Cytochrome P450 2D6 (CYP2D6), originally named debrisoquine hydroxylase, is a Phase I enzyme known to metabolize more than 100 drugs and environmental toxins.[8,51,144] As shown in Table 43-4, CYP2D6 is inhibited by several compounds, some of which are substrates. When a CYP2D6 inhibitor is administered along with a CYP2D6 substrate, the phenotype for the patient may appear impaired. This concept, known as *phenocopying,* is of significant concern with CYP2D6. Also, CYP2D6 is frequently implicated in ADRs and has been the subject of many U.S. Food and Drug Administration (FDA)-issued public health advisories. Metabolic phenotypes of CYP2D6 are best described as a continuum that varies from no activity to very high activity. For ease of characterization, a tetra-modal distribution of CYP2D6 activity is described containing the four groups of people called ultra-rapid metabolizers (UMs), extensive (normal) metabolizers (EMs), intermediate metabolizers (IMs), and poor metabolizers (PMs). Translation of a phenotype to a clinical application can be somewhat difficult, as the actual phenotype is dependent not only on the genetic makeup of CYP2D6, but also on (1) expression of CYP2D6, (2) whether drug-drug interactions affect the phenotype, and (3) whether CYP2D6 activates or inactivates the drug of interest.[34] The pharmacogenetics of CYP2D6 and/or phenotype testing can potentially be applied to improve prescribing of any medications known to be transformed by this enzyme. Two clinical applications for CYP2D6 pharmacogenetics include tamoxifen (described later), neuroleptics (some described in the psychiatry section of this chapter), and codeine.

Genotype to Phenotype

The relationship between the CYP2D6 enzyme metabolic rate (phenotype) and the *CYP2D6* genotype has been extensively characterized.[3,98,127,132,149] The *CYP2D6* gene contains 4408 bases and is located on chromosome 22q13.2, near two pseudogenes with greater than 90% homology. More than 90 allelic variants have been described in the *CYP2D6* gene. Alleles, listed with associated nucleotide changes and known effects on enzyme activity for *CYP2D6,* are shown in Table 43-5. Effects on enzyme activity are used to group the alleles according to the predicted phenotype, assuming that two

TABLE 43-4 Examples of Drug Substrates, Inhibitors, and Inducers of Cytochrome P450 Subfamilies

1A2	2B6	2C9	2C19	2D6	2E1	3A4/5/7
Substrates						
Amitriptyline	Buproprion	Celecoxib	Amitriptyline	Amitriptyline	Acetaminophen	Alprazolam
Caffeine	Cyclophosphamide	Diclofenac	Carisoprodol	Amphetamine	Aniline	Clarithromycin
Clomipramine	Efavirenz	Fluvastatin	Citalopram	Aripiprazole	Benzene	Cyclosporine
Clozapine	Ifosfamide	Glipizide	Chloramphenicol	Clomipramine	Chlorzoxazone	Diazepam
Cyclobenzaprine	Methadone	Ibuprofen	Clomipramine	Codeine	Enflurane	Erythromycin
Fluvoxamine	Sorafenib	Irbesartan	Clopidogrel	Desipramine	Ethanol	Gleevac
Haloperidol		Losartan	Cyclophosphamide	Dextromethorphan	Formamide	Haloperidol
Imipramine		Naproxen	Diazepam	Flecainide	Halothane	Lovastatin
Mexiletine		Nateglinide	Imipramine	Fluoxetine	Isoflurane	Methadone
Naproxen		Phenytoin	Indomethacin	Haloperidol	Methoxyflurane	Nitrendipine
Olanzapine		Piroxicam	Nelfinavir	Imipramine	Sevoflurane	Quinine
Propranolol		Rosiglitazone	Omeprazole	Methylphenidate	Theophylline	Sildenafil
Tacrine		Sulfamethoxazole	Primadone	Risperidone		Tamoxifen
Theophylline		Tamoxifen	Progesterone	Tamoxifen		Trazodone
Verapamil		Tolbutamide	Propranolol	Tramadol		Verapamil
R-Warfarin		*S*-Warfarin	*R*-Warfarin	Venlafaxine		Vincristine
Inhibitors						
Cimetidine	Thiotepa	Amiodarone	Fluoxetine	Bupropion	Disulfiram	Clarithromycin
Fluoroquinolones	Ticlopidine	Fluconazole	Fluvoxamine	Fluoxetine		Grapefruit juice
Fluvoxamine		Isoniazid	Ketoconazole	Paroxetine		Itraconazole
Ticlopidine			Omeprazole	Quinidine		Indinavir
Inducers						
Tobacco	Phenobarbital	Rifampin	N/A	N/A	Ethanol	Carbamazepine
	Phenytoin	Secobarbital			Isoniazid	Phenobarbital
	Rifampin					Phenytoin
						St. John Wort

Modified from http://medicine.iupui.edu/flockhart/table.htm (accessed on November 28, 2009), with the permission of David A. Flockhart, MD, PhD.
NA, Not applicable.

TABLE 43-5 Common *CYP2D6*, *CYP2C9*, and *CYP2C19* Alleles*

Allele	Nucleotide Changes (cDNA)	Effect	ENZYME ACTIVITY	
			In Vivo	**In Vitro**
*CYP2D6*1A*	None		Normal	Normal
*CYP2D6*1XN*		N active genes	Increased	
*CYP2D6*2A*	**−1584C→G**; −1235A→G; −740C→T; −678G→A; CYP2D7 conversion in intron 1; 1661G→C; 2850C→T; 4180G→C	R296C; S486T	Normal	Normal
*CYP2D6*3A*	**2549delA**	Frame shift	None	None
*CYP2D6*4A*	**100C→T**; 974C→A; 984A→G; 997C→G; 1661G→C; **1846G→A**; 4180G→C	P34S; L91M; H94R; splicing defect; S486T	None	None
*CYP2D6*5*	Gene deletion		None	
*CYP2D6*6A*	**1707delT**	Frame shift	None	
*CYP2D6*7*	**2935A→C**	H324P	None	
*CYP2D6*8*	1661G→C; **1758G→T**; 2850C→T; 4180G→C	G169X	None	
*CYP2D6*9*	**2615_2617delAAG**	K281del	Decreased	Decreased
*CYP2D6*10A*	**100C→T**; 1661G→C; 4180G→C	P34S; S486T	Decreased	Decreased
*CYP2D6*17*	**1023C→T**; 1661G→C; 2850C→>T; 4180G→C	T1071; R296C; S486T	Decreased	Decreased
*CYP2D6*29*	**1659G→A**; 1661G→C; 2850C→T; 3183G→A; 4180G→C	V136M; R296C; V338M; S486T	Decreased	Decreased
*CYP2D6*35*	−1584C→G; **31G→A**; 1661G→C; 2850C→T; 4180G→C	V136M; R296C; V338M; S486T	Normal	Normal
*CYP2D6*41*	1075A→C −1235A→G; −740C→T; −678G→A; CYP2D7 conversion in intron 1; 1661G→C; 2850C→T **2988G→A**; 4180G→C	R296C; splicing defect; S486T	Decreased	Decreased
*CYP2C9*1A*	None		Normal	Normal
*CYP2C9*2*	**430C→T**	R144C		Decreased
*CYP2C9*3*	**1075A→C**	I359L	Decreased	Decreased
*CYP2C9*4*	**1076T→C**	I359T		
*CYP2C9*6*	**818delA**	Frame shift	None	
*CYP2C9*8*	**449G→A**	R150H	Decreased	Increased
*CYP2C19*1A*	None		Normal	Normal
*CYP2C19*2A*	99C→T; **681G→A**; 990C→T; 991A→G	Splicing defect; I331V	None	
*CYP2C19*3A*	**636G→A**; 991A→G; 1251A→C	W212X; I331V	None	
*CYP2C19*4A*	**1A→G;** 99C→T; 991A→G	GTG initiation codon; I331V	None	
*CYP2C19*17*	**-806C>T** (promoter, not c.DNA)	Expression	Increased	Increased

*Commonly used analytical target for genotyping is bolded.

Modified from the Human Cytochrome P450 (CYP) Allele Nomenclature Committee. Available at: http://www.imm.ki.se/CYPalleles (accessed on June 28, 2011). Reproduced with permission of Sarah C. Sim, Webmaster. No information regarding enzyme activity is listed in the above table when none was present at this reference.

copies of that allele were inherited: PM, IM, EM, and UM. However, the actual phenotype will reflect a sum of the alleles. A summary of *CYP2D6* alleles and assignment of phenotypes are shown in Figure 43-4. Among Caucasians, approximately 1 to 10% are genetically UM, and 5 to 10% are PM. Only 1 to 3% of African Americans and Asians are PM, but many are IM.[75]

The CYP2D6 phenotype that is most simple to characterize is the PM phenotype, for which essentially no CYP2D6 activity is anticipated. The PM phenotype is expected when two or more copies of PM alleles are inherited. The sensitivity and specificity of the genotype to predict the PM phenotype are estimated to be 100%, but are far less for the other phenotypes. Other phenotype assignments are based largely on the highest functioning phenotype prediction. For example, at least one functional EM allele is thought to generate a phenotype that falls within the limits of normal. The UM phenotype is assigned when more than two copies of functional EM alleles are identified; this is often referred to as a *gene duplication*. Duplication of PM alleles has no effect on the phenotype, and duplication of IM alleles may or may not affect the phenotype.[210] An *activity score* has been proposed to help translate genotype to phenotype.[41]

Based on the AmpliChip CYP2D6 test (Roche Molecular Diagnostics, Pleasanton, California), which is an FDA-cleared in vitro diagnostic test that detects 33 allelic variants, the EM genotype predicts an EM phenotype with 95% sensitivity and 47% specificity. For the IM phenotype, the sensitivity of genotyping is estimated at 42% and specificity at 97%. For the UM phenotype, the sensitivity of genotyping is estimated at 6% and specificity at 99%.[142] These results illustrate that difficulties exist in detection and in incorporation of nongenetic factors when CYP2D6 phenotypes are assigned for all but the PM, based on genotype data alone.

Testing

The *CYP2D6* gene is challenging to genotype because of (1) the presence of the pseudogenes, (2) the sheer number of genetic variants, (3) the complexity of the genetic variants, and (4) the need for identification of gene dose, specifically, duplications and deletions of the gene. *CYP2D6* pharmacogenetic screening protocols vary tremendously in ability to accurately detect gene dose and to detect many versus only a few of the most common variants.

To separate *CYP2D6* from structurally similar pseudogenes, *CYP2D6* genotyping protocols often employ long PCR or nested PCR strategies with a first PCR step designed to amplify a large *CYP2D6*-specific region.[61] Small nucleotide changes within this region, including SNPs and smaller insertions/deletions of one or a few bases, are then detected in a second amplification step designed as a PCR restriction fragment length polymorphism (RFLP) assay or as an allele-specific PCR without subsequent digestion. By evaluating the entire gene, such as through use of the single-strand conformation polymorphism technique described by Broly and colleagues, both known and unknown variants in the *CYP2D6* gene can be detected.[16] Other technologies used for genotyping *CYP2D6* include real-time PCR methods and microarrays.[22,62,130,142] It is important that an assay identify a sufficient number of variants to accurately classify an allele. For example, both the *CYP2D6*10* and *CYP2D6*4* alleles contain the 100C→T variant. Because the phenotype predictions differ for the two, it is clinically relevant to determine which allele is present. The pattern of additional SNPs unique to each allele helps distinguish the two and suggests the likelihood that both alleles could be present. Because complete gene deletion *(CYP2D6*5)* and duplication events *(CYP2D6*1XN)* occur relatively commonly and have significant effect on the phenotype, analytical techniques that can detect and quantify these events are preferred. Successful published methods have utilized RFLP, long-product PCR assays, microarrays, or real-time quantitative PCR of *CYP2D6*, sometimes in relation to an internal reference gene.[69,104,152]

Tamoxifen Application

Tamoxifen is an antiestrogenic prodrug widely used to treat and prevent breast cancer; it is a good example of a drug for which pharmacogenetic testing of CYP2D6 is applied clinically.[67] Tamoxifen mediates its therapeutic effects through modulation of estrogen receptors (ERs), leading to suppression of estrogen-mediated cell proliferation. Therefore, hormone-sensitive breast tumors (ER-positive) are most likely to respond to tamoxifen. A meta-analysis of the Early Breast Cancer Trialist Collaborative Group (EBCTCG) study at the 15-year follow-up period for ER-positive breast cancer showed that 5 years of tamoxifen reduced the recurrence rate by 50% and the mortality rate by a third.[1] However, the success of tamoxifen therapy is variable, and 30 to 45% of patients on tamoxifen relapse or die from recurrent cancer.[133]

Tamoxifen is extensively metabolized by many Phase I and Phase II enzymes (Figure 43-5). The lack of efficacy with tamoxifen can be explained, in part, by interindividual differences in the metabolic activation of tamoxifen. Tamoxifen is a prodrug and must be metabolized to the active principles to elicit the desired therapeutic effect. The most potent antiestrogenic metabolites are 4-hydroxy tamoxifen and endoxifen, each shown to exhibit approximately 100-fold greater affinity for the ER than the parent drug tamoxifen. The concentrations of these metabolites compared with the concentrations of *N*-desmethyl tamoxifen, an inactive metabolite, and tamoxifen itself, are shown in Table 43-6. Because the amounts of endoxifen are greater than the amounts of 4-hydroxy tamoxifen, endoxifen is largely credited with producing antiestrogenic effects of tamoxifen.[14] Considerable

TABLE 43-6 Involvement of CYP2D6 in Steady-State Concentrations of Tamoxifen and Major Tamoxifen Metabolites

	Expected Plasma Concentration Range, nmol/L	Involvement of CYP2D6	Estrogen Receptor Effect
Tamoxifen	190 to 420		Weak antagonist
N-Desmethyltamoxifen	280 to 800	Minor	Weak antagonist
N,N-Didesmethyltamoxifen	90 to 120	Minor	Weak antagonist
Endoxifen	14 to 130	Major	Strong antagonist
4-Hydroxytamoxifen	3 to 17	Among others	Strong antagonist

Modified from Brauch H, Mürdter TE, Eichelbaum M, Schwab M. Pharmacogenomics of tamoxifen therapy. Clin Chem 2009;55:1770-82.

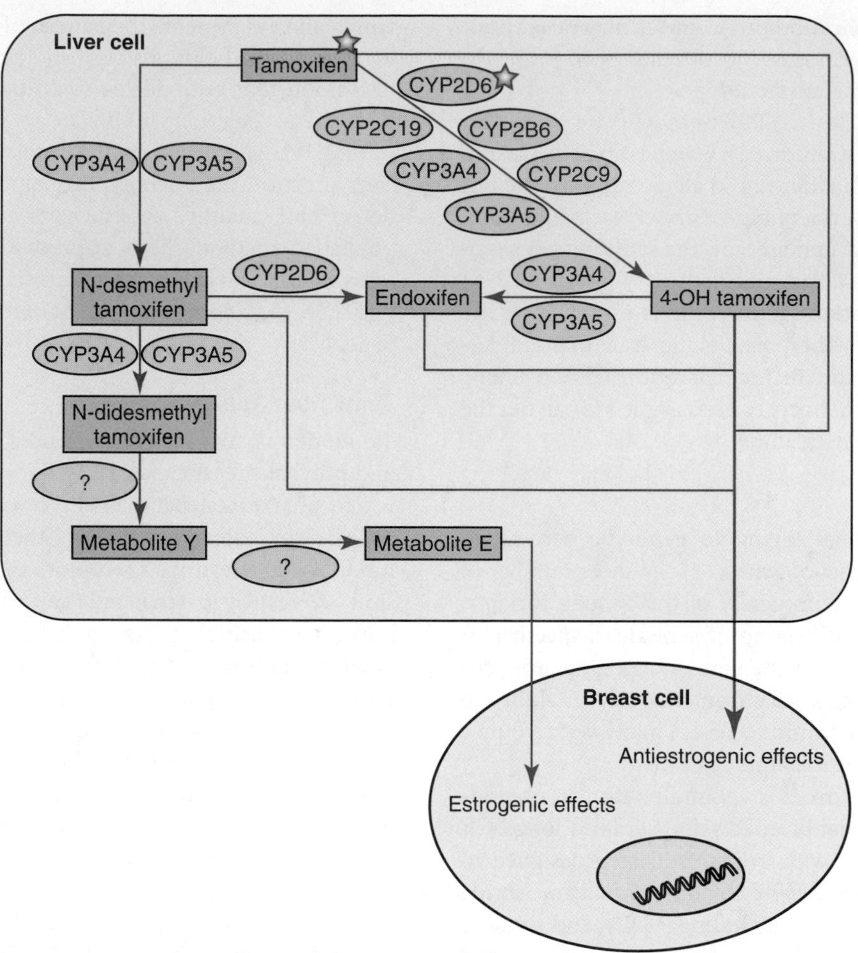

Figure 43-5 Illustrated pharmacokinetic and pharmacodynamic pathways for tamoxifen. Cytochrome P450 (CYP) isozymes are involved in the activation and inactivation of tamoxifen, and CYP2D6 is key to production of the active metabolite endoxifen. Most of the antiestrogenic effects of tamoxifen are attributed to endoxifen. Many additional factors in the pharmacokinetics and pharmacodynamics of tamoxifen are not known. *(Reproduced by permission from PharmGKB and Stanford University.[91])*

evidence suggests that CYP2D6 is a major route for production of endoxifen. Thus, patients with impaired CYP2D6 have been shown to produce less endoxifen than patients with a CYP2D6 EM phenotype. In addition, a PM phenotype and lower endoxifen concentrations are observed in patients with EM genotype, who are coprescribed known strong inhibitors of CYP2D6, such as fluoxetine or paroxetine. It is interesting to note that patients treated with CYP2D6 strong inhibitors and patients who are known CYP2D6 PMs have been shown to exhibit fewer of the common antiestrogenic ADRs such as hot flashes.[14,49,128]

One way in which pharmacogenetic testing of CYP2D6 is used clinically is to qualify patients as good metabolic candidates for tamoxifen pretherapeutically. In this scenario, patients with a PM genotype are not expected to respond appropriately to standard doses of tamoxifen and might be considered for alternative antiestrogenic therapy, such as an aromatase inhibitor. Thus a CYP2D6 PM may be best served clinically by selecting a different agent. An IM is likely to require higher doses of tamoxifen than an EM, and a UM may require lower doses of tamoxifen than an EM. However, appropriate dose optimization studies and determination of a target therapeutic range for tamoxifen are currently lacking. In any case, the best drug must be considered relative to side effect profiles, cost to the patient, and the specific clinical scenario. If tamoxifen is prescribed, the patient should be counseled regarding the phenocopying effects that occur through drug-drug interactions, particularly with the use of CYP2D6 strong inhibitors that are likely to compromise the efficacy of tamoxifen by inhibiting tamoxifen activation.

Other genes are likely to play an important role in the pharmacogenetics of tamoxifen. For example, the *CYP2C19*17* allele, which confers a rapid metabolizer phenotype, is associated with improved response to tamoxifen. The roles of CYP3A4 and CYP3A5 have not been clearly defined.[31,200] The active metabolites endoxifen and 4-hydroxy tamoxifen are inactivated by several enzyme-mediated Phase II (conjugation) reactions (see Figure 43-5). In theory, impairment in Phase II enzymes would lead to accumulation of endoxifen and exaggerated response. The sulfotransferase isoform 1A1 *(SULT1A1)* and UDP-glucuronosyltransferase isoform 2B15 *(UGT2B15)* genes encode for the most common conjugative enzymes associated with inactivation and elimination of the active tamoxifen metabolites. The *SULT1A1*2* allele (reduced activity) has been associated with improved response to tamoxifen.[47,200] However, the distinct role of these and other genes is not well studied or understood. Also of interest would be genes associated with the pharmacodynamics of tamoxifen, such as estrogen receptors and genes associated with estrogen-mediated cell proliferation. Correlation of metabolites with ADRs, particularly risk of endometrial cancer, a rare but significant ADR of tamoxifen, would be useful as well.

Codeine Application

Codeine, an alkaloid obtained from opium or prepared from morphine by methylation, is a widely used analgesic medication. Codeine must be activated by conversion to morphine, through a demethylation reaction mediated primarily by CYP2D6, to produce analgesia. Therefore, a CYP2D6 PM would not be predicted to activate codeine as an EM would, and analgesia may not be experienced with standard doses. A PM may be best served clinically by selecting a different analgesic agent. An IM is likely to require higher doses of codeine than an EM, and a UM may require lower doses of codeine than an EM. In a typical EM scenario, only about 10% of the codeine is converted to morphine. Administration of codeine to a person with the UM phenotype is a significant safety concern because higher than expected concentrations of morphine can be produced, leading to risk of unintentional overdose and opioid toxicity. In an example case report, respiratory depression and coma were observed in a 62-year-old man with the UM phenotype who was given a moderate dose of codeine. Concentrations of morphine were 80 times higher than expected.[43] Of particular concern clinically is administration of codeine to a woman who exhibits a CYP2D6 UM phenotype and is breast-feeding.[108,202] After clinical reports of opioid toxicity in breast-fed newborns of UM mothers, the FDA issued a public health advisory in 2007 warning that codeine administration to mothers with a CYP2D6 UM phenotype could lead to higher than expected morphine concentrations in the breast milk.

Antidepressant Application

Antidepressant dosing is challenging because several weeks is required to assess efficacy, and optimizing dose may require many months of trial and error.[112] Most of the antidepressants available today are substrates of CYP2D6, and many are also inhibitors. Case reports of CYP2D6-related toxicity and death have been published. The first of these involved a child with a PM genotype who was prescribed the antidepressant fluoxetine.[150] Fluoxetine is a selective serotonin reuptake inhibitor (SSRI) that is demethylated to form the only active metabolite, norfluoxetine. Fluoxetine is a racemic mixture of two enantiomers, S and R. S-fluoxetine and S-norfluoxetine are much more potent in the inhibition of serotonin reuptake than the R-enantiomers. Although several CYP isozymes are involved in the metabolism of fluoxetine, metabolism by CYP2D6 is considered the major route. CYP2D6 is also inhibited by both fluoxetine and norfluoxetine, leading to prolongation in the half-life of the drug and the metabolite within the first weeks of therapy. A CYP2D6 PM would require lower doses of fluoxetine and might be best managed with another drug, one that does not require CYP2D6.[29,89]

Tricyclic antidepressants such as nortriptyline are also metabolized by CYP2D6. The relationship between drug concentrations and toxicity for CYP2D6 phenotypes and genotypes has been extensively characterized for nortriptyline. As shown in Figure 43-6, a CYP2D6 PM requires lower doses of nortriptyline than an EM to produce similar serum concentrations of active drug. Nortriptyline, which is also an active metabolite of amitriptyline, is hydroxylated by CYP2D6 to form an inactive metabolite (10-hydroxynortriptyline). Clearance of amitriptyline, nortriptyline, and other tricyclic antidepressants is reduced by at least 50% in PMs of CYP2D6.[107] Tricyclic antidepressants have a narrow

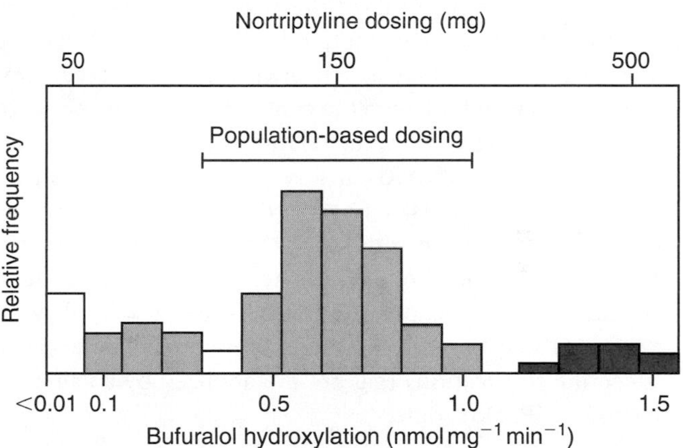

Figure 43-6 Variation in drug metabolism and nortriptyline dosing in the European population, based on cytochrome P450 CYP2D6 activity (hydroxylation of bufuralol). Within the population, four phenotypes can be identified: poor metabolizers (PMs), who lack the functional enzyme; intermediary metabolizers (IMs), who are heterozygous for one functional allele or have two partially defective alleles encoding the enzyme; extensive metabolizers (EMs), who have two normal alleles; and ultra-rapid metabolizers (UMs), who carry duplicated or multiduplicated functional *CYP2D6* genes. The relative frequency of these phenotypes refers to the European population as a whole. The doses of nortriptyline that are required to achieve therapeutic concentrations in all phenotypes are given. Despite this variation in metabolizing capability, population-based dosing is used today and is based on the average plasma concentrations obtained in a given population for a given dose. *(From Ingelman-Sundberg M. Pharmacogenetics of cytochrome P450 and its applications in drug therapy: the past, present and future. Trends Pharmacol Sci 2004;25:193-200. Reproduced by permission from Elsevier.)*

therapeutic index and are associated with severe anticholinergic ADRs that may be life-threatening. Despite these concerns, the drugs are attractive because response rates are higher than for many other classes of antidepressants, and they are available in generic (cost-effective) formulations. The *CYP2D6* genotype has been used to pretherapeutically triage patients as high-risk or low-risk relative to ADRs and response to amitriptyline and nortriptyline. For example, the proportion of patients with ADRs during treatment with these drugs was 12.1% in carriers of two functioning CYP2D6 alleles versus 76.5% in carriers of only one functional allele, in one study.[171,172] Such predictions of pharmacokinetics can be clinically useful and may include multiple relevant genes. The only in vitro diagnostic test currently cleared by the FDA for CYP2D6, the Roche Amplichip, also includes CYP2C19.[142]

Average recommended adjustments for these and other antidepressants vary from 20% of the usual dose for the CYP2D6 PM phenotype to 300% of the usual dose for the CYP2D6 UM. However, some studies have shown no relationship between drugs and CYP2D6 genotype, and the Evaluation of Genomic Applications in Practice and Prevention (EGAPP) Working Group recommends against genetic testing for SSRIs in particular.[2] This may be a result of the fact that most drugs can be metabolized through alternative minor pathways and may act through multiple mechanisms that may or may not relate to the concentration of parent and/or metabolites. In addition, the relationship between circulating concentrations of SSRIs and response is poor. This may reflect unrecognized risks associated with drug metabolites generated by routes considered to be minor. For example, potentially toxic metabolites may accumulate as a result of UM status, possibly leading to ADRs. Thus individuals with the PM or the UM genotype-phenotype may be best served by selecting medications that are metabolized by an alternative (non-CYP2D6) route.[29]

Cytochrome P450 2C9 (CYP2C9)

CYP2C9 is a member of the CYP2C family, which includes CYP2C8, CYP2C9, CYP2C18, and CYP2C19. CYP2C9 is primarily expressed in the liver, at substantially higher quantities than the other CYP isozymes. Concentrations of CYP2C9 are exceeded only by those of CYP3A4.[145,169] CYP2C9 is associated with the metabolism of 15 to 20% of all drugs. Examples of drugs metabolized by CYP2C9 include warfarin, anticonvulsants, nonsteroidal anti-inflammatory drugs (NSAIDs), antidiabetic agents, cholesterol-lowering drugs, and drugs used to treat infection (see Table 43-4). Genotype-based dosing guidelines have been proposed for CYP2C9 substrates and are the subject of intense clinical study for the anticoagulant drug warfarin.[144,154] Similar to CYP2D6, CYP2C9 is subject to induction and inhibition through drug-drug interactions, which will affect the phenotype. For example, CYP2C9 is induced by rifampicin, which will significantly increase the clearance of drugs eliminated by CYP2C9. Common inhibitors of CYP2C9 that reduce clearance of drugs include amiodarone and fluconazole.[80,126,194] Coadministration of CYP2C9 substrates and inducers or inhibitors can lead to life-threatening ADRs, based on whether CYP2C9 activates or inactivates a drug.[105,161]

Genotype to Phenotype

The *CYP2C9* gene is clustered in a 500 kb region on chromosome 10q24 containing CYP genes in the order *CYP2C8-CYP2C9-CYP2C19-CYP2C18*. At least 34 allelic variants have been described in this gene.[55,91] However, two variant alleles, *CYP2C9*2* and *CYP2C9*3*, account for most impaired CYP2C9 PM phenotypes.[127] These alleles are defined by nonsynonymous variants that are relatively common in Caucasians, but have significantly lower allele frequencies in African and Asian populations.[99,167] The *2 allele is identified by R144C (430C→T), and the *3 allele is identified by I359L (1075A→C). The allelic frequency of *CYP2C9*2* has been reported as 8 to 19% in Caucasians, and as 1 to 4% in African Americans and Canadian Native Indians. This allele has not been detected in Asians. The allelic frequency of *CYP2C9*3* has been reported as 6 to 10% in Caucasians, 1.7 to 5% in Asians, and 0.5 to 1.5% in African Americans. Homozygosity for the *CYP2C9*3* allele is relatively rare in Caucasians (1 to 2%).[157] Studies in vitro have shown that the protein produced by the *CYP2C9*3* variant is less than 5% as efficient as the *CYP2C9*1*; *CYP2C9*2* shows about 12% of *CYP2C9*1* activity in most assays. Both variant alleles result in PM in the homozygous state and IM phenotypes when heterozygous. However, the clinical impact of a *CYP2C9*3* variant is more significant than that of a *CYP2C9*2* variant. Additional alleles of interest include *CYP2C9*4, CYP2C9*6,* and *CYP2C9*8.* The *CYP2C9*4* (I359T, 1076T→C) is also more common in Caucasians (6%) than in African Americans (0.5%).[86,175] In contrast, *CYP2C9*6* (frame shift, 818delA), a null allele with lack of activity due to a splicing mutation that causes a frame shift resulting in a truncated protein, has a high prevalence in African Americans. The *CYP2C9*6* in a homozygous individual was shown to contribute to an extremely long phenytoin elimination, with a half-life approximately 5.8 times longer than that of *CYP2C9* extensive metabolizers.[85] The *CYP2C9*8* allele (R150H, 449G→A) has been shown in vitro to have greater activity than the wild-type enzyme, demonstrating 175% tolbutamide hydroxylase activity of recombinant wild type, suggesting that a UM phenotype for CYP2C9 may exist.[9] Many promoter variants are known as well, but their clinical significance has yet to be determined.[92]

Testing

Several protocols have been published for detecting variants in this gene. Most focus on detection of only the *2 and *3 alleles, although multiplexed assays have been described that screen the entire gene for variants.[139,174] Genetic tests have been cleared by the FDA as in vitro diagnostic tests and are available clinically with intent to identify patients at risk for impaired S-warfarin metabolism. These tests include genotyping of *CYP2C9, VKORC1,* and, in at least one test, *CYP4F2*.[87,106]

Warfarin Application

Warfarin is the most widely used anticoagulant drug in the world. Individual response to warfarin is highly variable, and the drug is implicated in life-threatening adverse events, especially when dosed inappropriately. Too much warfarin leads to bleeding, and too little warfarin fails to prevent blood clots. The dose for individual patients is routinely adjusted to achieve a target therapeutic INR (international normalized ratio), usually between 2 and 3. INR is calculated from the prothrombin (clotting) time (PT) of blood samples (see Chapter 59). Factors known to affect warfarin dose requirements include age, gender, clinical status, body size, dietary factors, concomitant medications, and the presence of genetic variation in genes associated with drug metabolism (primarily *CYP2C9*) and response (primarily *VKORC1*). CYP2C9 is the enzyme responsible for inactivating the S-isomer of warfarin that is principally responsible for the anticoagulant effect of the drug. As illustrated in Figure 43-7, standard 5 mg/d maintenance dosing of warfarin in subjects with *CYP2C9* genetic variants can lead to excessive warfarin exposure, resulting in an exaggerated anticoagulant response. Some drug-drug interactions produce a similar result. The clinical impact of a *CYP2C9* polymorphism includes increased risk of ADRs and increased time to achieve a stable INR. Individuals with these variants are at risk of prolonged bleeding time and increased incidence of severe bleeding in warfarin therapy. It is now known that CYP2C9 genotype accounts for only part of the variability in warfarin sensitivity because VKORC1 genotype, age, and weight are also key factors in predicting the therapeutic dose for warfarin.[4,177,179,180] The *VKORC1* gene is discussed in greater detail below.

Cytochrome P450 2C19 (CYP2C19)

CYP2C19 is a member of the CYP2C family, which includes CYP2C8, CYP2C9, CYP2C18, and CYP2C19, of which *CYP2C9* and *CYP2C19* exhibit substantial genetic and clinically significant variability. CYP2C19 is involved in the metabolism of a number of other therapeutic drugs, including citalopram, diazepam, omeprazole, propranolol, and proguanil (see Table 43-4).[144] Of particular relevance to defining phenotypes of CYP2C19 metabolism is the anticonvulsant mephenytoin. CYP2C19 specifically mediates 4-hydroxylation of the S-enantiomer of mephenytoin, and variation in this reaction led to the characterization of CYP2C19, which was originally called *mephenytoin hydroxylase.*[25] Poor, intermediate, extensive, and ultra-rapid metabolizer phenotypes (PM, IM, EM, UM) are described.

Genotype to Phenotype

Genetic variation in CYP2C19 correlates with the IM and PM phenotype. Although at least 25 allelic variants of *CYP2C19* have been described, CYP2C19*2 and CYP2C19*3 account for 99% of PM in Asians and approximately 87% in Caucasians.[17,30,37,91] The PM phenotype occurs in 2 to 5% of Caucasian and Black Zimbabwean Shona populations, and 10 to 23% of Asian populations.[212] The *CYP2C19*2* arises from a 681G→A, which results in a splicing defect and essentially

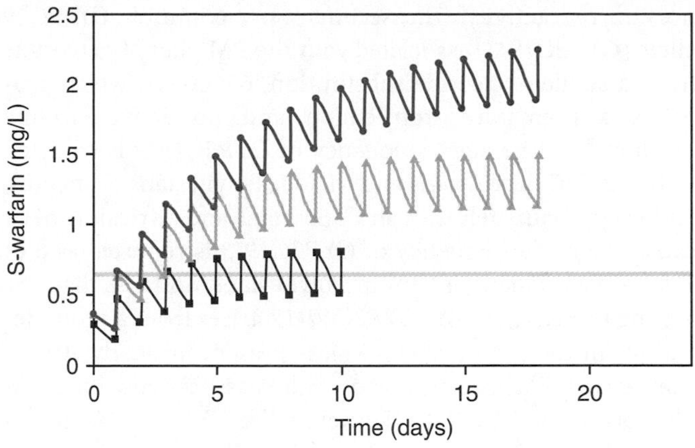

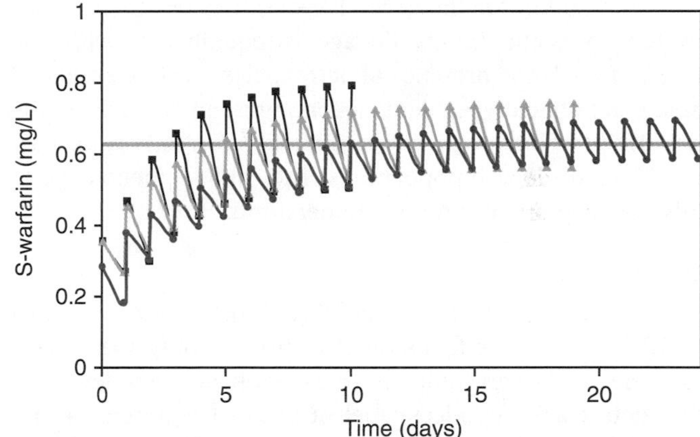

Figure 43-7 Model of warfarin dosing based on *CYP2C9* genetics. In both panels, the conventional therapeutic *S*-warfarin target concentration is shown *(horizontal line)* for reference. The *top panel* depicts a model for warfarin therapy in patients using the standard 5 mg/d dose with all genotypes. *CYP2C9*1/*1* individuals (■) on 5 mg twice per day would attain stable and therapeutic serum *S*-warfarin concentrations (0.68 µg/mL) in approximately 4 days. *CYP2C9*1/*2* (▲) and *CYP2C9*1/*3* (•) individuals on the same 5 mg dose are modeled to attain *S*-warfarin serum concentrations that are too high by the second day and if not adjusted would lead to overanticoagulation. *CYP2C9*1/*2* patients would stabilize at twice therapeutic serum concentrations after 10 to 12 days, but *CYP2C9*1/*3,* if not adjusted, would continue to rise. The *bottom panel* depicts serum *S*-warfarin concentration outcomes for a dosing regimen modified for genotype. All patients would be given the standard 5 mg dose twice, then would be switched to a *CYP2C9* genotype adjusted dose for maintenance, with *CYP2C9*1/*2* receiving 3 mg and *CYP2C9*1/*3* receiving 1.5 mg. This genotype adjusted dosing could result in *CYP2C9*1/*2* and *CYP2C9*1/*3* achieving stable, therapeutic *S*-warfarin concentrations in 10 days, thereby avoiding overanticoagulation in these individuals. *(Adapted from Linder MW, Looney S, Adams JE III, Johnson N, Antonino-Green D, Lacefield N, et al. Warfarin dose adjustments based on CYP2C9 genetic polymorphisms. J Thromb Thrombolysis 2002;14:227-32. Reproduced by permission from Springer.)*

no enzyme activity. The second most common *CYP2C19* allele *(CYP2C19*3)* associated with the PM phenotype results from a single nucleotide substitution, 636G→A, which produces a premature stop codon and no active enzyme product.[30,127] The allele frequency of *CYP2C19*2* is reported to be 32% in East Asians and 71% in Polynesians (Vanuatu), and is approximately 15% in Caucasians and African Americans. The allele frequency of *CYP2C19*3* is reported as 6 to 10% in East Asians, 13.3% in Polynesians, and less than 1% among Caucasians. The *CYP2C19*17* arises from a promoter variant in the gene (-806C→T), is present in nearly 40% of Caucasians, Blacks, and Asians, and is associated with a UM phenotype for CYP2C19. However, the *CYP2C19*4* allele, a relatively rare loss of function (PM) allele, that affects the initiation codon for the gene (1A→G), has been demononstrated to occur in cis linkage disequilibrium with the *CYP2C19*17*. The presence of both alleles must be evaluated based on haplotype, and when present, is called the *CYP2C19*4B* haplotype, observed thus far in only Ashkenazi and Sephardi Jewish populations. The clinical phenotoype of this new haplotype is not yet understood.[157A]

Testing

Several protocols have been published for detecting variants in CYP2C19. Most focus on detection of only the *2 and *3 alleles, although multiplexed assays have been described that detect an expanded panel of alleles (including *4 and *17 alleles), and/or screen the entire gene for variants. The only genetic test for *CYP2C19* that is currently cleared by the FDA as an in vitro diagnostic test is the Roche Amplichip, which also includes *CYP2D6*.[142] Other assay reagents are sold in the United States through research-use-only (RUO) labeling.

Clopidogrel Application

Clopidogrel is a second-generation thienopyridine that inhibits platelet aggregation. This drug is widely used in combination with aspirin to reduce the incidence of thrombotic and ischemic events in patients with coronary artery disease, with acute coronary syndrome (ACS), and/or after percutaneous coronary intervention (PCI) with stenting. Yet, a significant proportion of patients realize insufficient clopidogrel-induced platelet inhibition, and rates of drug resistance are estimated at 30%.[59] One explanation for drug resistance is based on the fact that clopidogrel is an inactive prodrug that requires metabolism to generate the active metabolite. The active metabolite irreversibly inhibits the platelet adenosine diphosphate (ADP) receptor, P2Y12. Carriers of the *CYP2C19*2 and *3* alleles have reduced formation of the active metabolite of clopidogrel, demonstrate reduction in clopidogrel-induced platelet inhibition, and have a higher incidence of major thrombotic events.[13,120,163] Two potential treatment strategies for carriers of *CYP2C19*2 and *3* are to use higher doses of clopidogrel or alternative P2Y12 inhibitors. Higher loading and maintenance doses (e.g., 1200 mg loading and 150 mg maintenance) appear, in part, to overcome the genetic deficiency of the *2 allele, although maintenance doses of up to 300 mg/d might be required to achieve adequate platelet inhibition.[48,136] For carriers of two impaired alleles (e.g., homozygous for *2), an alternative therapy may be preferred, such as the newly approved prasugrel, which does not require CYP-mediated activation.[13,120] The impact of the *CYP2C19*17* genotype, other variant genotypes, and *CYP2C19*4B* haploytpe remain to be defined.

Antidepressant Application

A common reason for genotyping *CYP2C19* is to explain inappropriate response to antidepressant medications. For example, CYP2C19 is the primary enzyme responsible for converting amitriptyline to its active metabolite nortriptyline. Monitoring serum or plasma concentrations of both amitriptyline and nortriptyline as a sum is used to guide amitriptyline therapy.[102,137] The utility of *CYP2C19* genotyping is somewhat controversial. Using a quantitative gene-dose model, it was found that *CYP2D6* but not *CYP2C19* genotyping is most useful in amitriptyline therapy based on the fact that *CYP2C19* polymorphisms alter the ratio of amitriptyline to nortriptyline, but not the sum of the two.[171] The model was derived in a Caucasian population, whereas *CYP2C19* PMs are much more common in Asian populations.[160] CYP2D6 is also thought to be more important than CYP2C19 for newer antidepressants.[54] However, CYP2C19 becomes very important for a drug that is a substrate of both CYP2D6 and CYP2C19 when CYP2D6 is impaired or deficient.

Omeprazole and Proguanil Applications

Omeprazole, a proton pump inhibitor, is primarily inactivated by the CYP2C19 enzyme. It has been reported that homozygous variant subjects had 100% cure of upper gastrointestinal (GI) ulcers after omeprazole-based therapy versus 65% and 25% for heterozygous and homozygous wild-type patients, respectively. Studies have also demonstrated greater effectiveness of single-dose omeprazole for management of *Helicobacter pylori* infection and peptic ulcer in subjects with one or more *CYP2C19* PM alleles. This is thought to be the result of greater exposure to a therapeutic compound in PMs and IMs. This difference in exposure is illustrated in Figure 43-8, wherein the area under the time-versus-concentration curve after a single dose of omeprazole was dramatically larger for *CYP2C219* PMs. However, using triple therapy with rabeprazole, amoxicillin, and clarithromycin, *H. pylori* antimicrobial susceptibility was shown to be a more important factor than *CYP2C19* genotype.[123] No dose adjustments have been proposed to adjust for *CYP2C19* genotype. Gene-gene interactions may indicate a need to test for genetic variation in more than one gene to guide therapy. Multigene studies have shown that interleukin-1β genetic polymorphisms *(IL-1B),* although not an independent factor in treatment outcome, influence the impact of the *CYP2C19* genotype on the cure rate of 1-week triple therapy for *H. pylori* infection.[181]

The antimalarial prodrugs proguanil and chlorproguanil require CYP2C19-dependent bioactivation for therapeutic

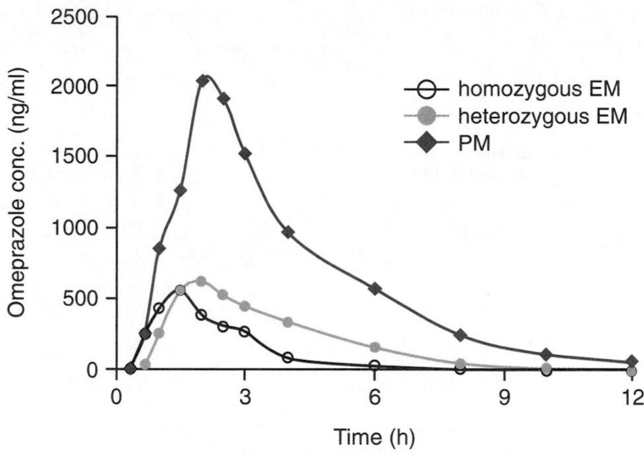

Figure 43-8 Mean plasma concentration-time profile of omeprazole after oral administration of 40 mg omeprazole (in the form of 2 × 20 mg Losec capsules) to 27 male Chinese subjects phenotyped for CYP2C19 activity with mephenytoin. Plasma concentrations of omeprazole were significantly higher in poor metabolizers (PMs) (♦) than in homozygous extensive metabolizers (EMs) (•) or heterozygous EMs (○). In addition, the elimination half-life for omeprazole was 2.3-fold greater in PMs than in EMs (*P* < 0.001). *(From Yin OQ, Tomlinson B, Chow AH, Waye MM, Chow MS. Omeprazole as a CYP2C19 marker in Chinese subjects: assessment of its gene-dose effect and intrasubject variability. J Clin Pharmacol 2004;44:582-9. Reproduced by permission from Sage Publications Inc.)*

efficacy. A clear gene-dose effect has been observed for the oxidation of proguanil to cycloguanil and 4-chlorophenylbiguanide. Clinical response has been shown to be affected in CYP2C19 PM individuals.[68,205]

Other Cytochrome P450 Genes

Additional CYPs including *CYP2B6, CYP3A4,* and *CYP3A5* have been proposed as important pharmacogenetic targets. CYP3A4 and CYP3A5 have been the subject of extensive study, as they are believed to be the predominant CYP expressed in adult human liver and are responsible for the metabolism of at least 50% of all currently used drugs, as well as many endogenous steroid hormones. Linkage results from a Japanese population demonstrate that CYP3A4 and CYP3A5 are closely linked, and that the two genes are in close proximity, so some effects originally thought to be due to a *CYP3A4* allele are probably actually due to a *CYP3A5* allele in linkage disequilibrium.[40] The most common and clinically significant nonfunctional variant of *CYP3A5* is an A→G change at position 6986 that leads to mis-splicing, and is known as *CYP3A5*3*.[93] CYP3A5 is expressed in about 50% of African Americans and only 10 to 30% of Caucasians and Asians. This expression level correlates with allele frequencies of the *3 allele of approximately 50% in African Americans, and 70 to 90% in Caucasians. Because of the allele frequency of the *3, *CYP3A4* is most common in Caucasians, and *CYP3A5* in African Americans. As in the CYP3A subfamily, high interindividual variation is seen in CYP2B6 expression, estimated at 20- to 250-fold, which may be due to differences in transcriptional regulation, as well as genetic variation.[94,186] Many alleles have been reported that correlate with increased or decreased expression, and are present in high frequencies, yet their clinical significance is not well defined. Like for CYP2D6, defining the phenotype is complicated by the fact that many of the drugs that are metabolized by CYP2B6 are also inducers or inhibitors of this enzyme; examples of such drugs include cyclophosphamide, phenobarbital, rifampicin, phenytoin, artemisinin, carbamazepine, efavirenz, and nevirapine.[209]

PHASE II METABOLIC ENZYMES

As described earlier, Phase II enzymes are generally transferases that conjugate drugs with acetyl, glucuronyl, amino acyl, or sulfate groups. Phase II reactions may occur before or after Phase I reactions or independent of them. The enzymes are not typically induced or inhibited to the same degree as CYPs. However, exhausting the substrates or cofactors for transfer, such as glutathione or acetyl-CoA, will prevent the corresponding transferase reactions from occurring. Similar to Phase I enzymes, Phase II enzymes are synthesized from genes that are classified into families and further into subfamilies based on homology.

N-Acetyltransferases (NAT1 and NAT2)

The *N*-acetyltransferase (NAT) polymorphism is one of the earliest pharmacogenetic targets recognized and characterized. NATs are Phase II enzymes that catalyze the transfer of an acetyl moiety from acetyl-CoA to homocyclic and heterocyclic arylamines and hydrazines. Substrates include drugs, carcinogens, toxicants, and possibly endogenous compounds. Slow metabolizer phenotypes, which may affect up to 90% of some populations, are manifested by changes in protein expression, protein stability, and/or enzyme kinetics.

Genotype to Phenotype

Studies with additional substrates for NAT have demonstrated that the phenotype was not relevant to all substrates. For example, the NAT phenotype was clearly recognized for arylamines such as isoniazid, some sulfonamides, amrinone, dapsone, procainamide, caffeine, and clonazepam. The phenotype was not observed with other arylamine substrates such as *p*-aminobenzoate (PABA) and *p*-aminosalicylate (PAS). A folate catabolite, *p*-aminobenzoylglutamate, is the only endogenous NAT substrate proposed.[125] However, *NAT2* knock-out and *NAT1* and *NAT2* double knock-out mice do not express phenotypical abnormalities, suggesting that these enzymes are not required for development or function.[176]

In 1965 it was proposed that two isoforms of NAT, later named *NAT1* and *NAT2,* were responsible for the differences in phenotypes observed previously. Of the two proposed isoforms, NAT2 correlated best with the isoniazid (polymorphic) phenotype.[78] It was also suggested that the fast and slow acetylator phenotypes were caused by differences in expression rather than in enzyme kinetics. Subsequently, it was found that although most substrates exhibit higher specificity for NAT1 or NAT2, most substrates have affinity for both NAT1 and NAT2. Nonetheless, substrates were commonly classified as monomorphic (substrates of NAT1) or polymorphic (substrates of NAT2) until the mid 1990s.

NAT1, which is now recognized to be polymorphic, is extremely unstable and therefore more difficult to study than NAT2. Because of stability differences and overlapping substrate specificity, tissue localization studies for the NATs have been challenging. It is now recognized that both NAT1 and NAT2 are expressed throughout the GI tract, and in the lung, bladder, ureter, and liver.[52,203]

Three human NAT genes are mapped to chromosome 8p22 and were first cloned in 1990. The *NAT1* and *NAT2* genes share 87% nucleotide sequence identity and 81% amino acid sequence identity. The third gene, *NATP,* is thought to be a noncoding pseudogene. Each of the NAT genes has an intronless open reading frame exon of 870 bp and codes for 290 amino acids. Many variant alleles have been described for both NAT1 and NAT2. A consensus nomenclature was published in 1995 and updated in 2000.[10,12,191] *NAT1*3* and *NAT2*4* are considered the wild-type alleles, although the designation is somewhat arbitrary in view of the high frequencies of multiple alleles in the population. For *NAT2,* the former common nomenclature included M1 for *NAT2*5A,* M2 for *NAT2*6A,* and M3 for *NAT2*7A.* The *NAT2*5, *6, *7, *13,* and **14* alleles are thought to account for more than 99% of slow acetylator phenotypes. The *NAT1*10* is the most common variant *NAT1* allele in many human populations, but the phenotype-genotype relationship is not well defined. Other *NAT1* alleles that are rare in humans and produce enzymes with definitively reduced activity and potential clinical implications include *NAT1*14, *15, *17, *19,* and **22.*

The three-dimensional crystal structures of the two NAT isoenzymes have been determined. Structural studies suggest that the active catalytic site of the NATs involves three amino acids: a cysteine residue juxtaposed with histidine, and aspartate residues. The C-terminus is responsible for substrate specificity.[162] The acetylation reaction occurs through a classical two-step mechanism, whereby an acetyl moiety is transferred from acetyl CoA to NAT, and then from NAT to the arylamine to form an arylamide. As shown in Figure 43-9, *N*-acetylation, thought to primarily generate nontoxic stable products, is mediated by both NAT1 and NAT2. *O*-Acetylation of cytochrome P450 *N*-hydroxylated products is also mediated by both NAT1 and NAT2 and is thought to generate reactive products that may spontaneously decompose to form nitrenium ions. Nitrenium ions are electrophiles that may subsequently bind covalently to intracellular nucleophiles such as DNA or proteins and be responsible for cell death, mutagenesis, or other toxicities. An intramolecular *N,O*-acetyltransfer reaction is mediated primarily by NAT1 and may lead to reactive products. Other enzymes that may interrupt or contribute to these reactions include CYP1A2, prostaglandin H synthase, UDP-glucuronosyltransferase, and sulfotransferase.[53,204]

N-Acetylation
NAT1 & NAT2
N-Oxidation
(cytochrome P450)
N-Oxidation
(cytochrome P450)
O-Acetylation
NAT1 & NAT2
Intramolecular
N,O-acetyltransfer
NAT1
Reaction with DNA
Detoxification
(e.g. glutathione
S-transferases)

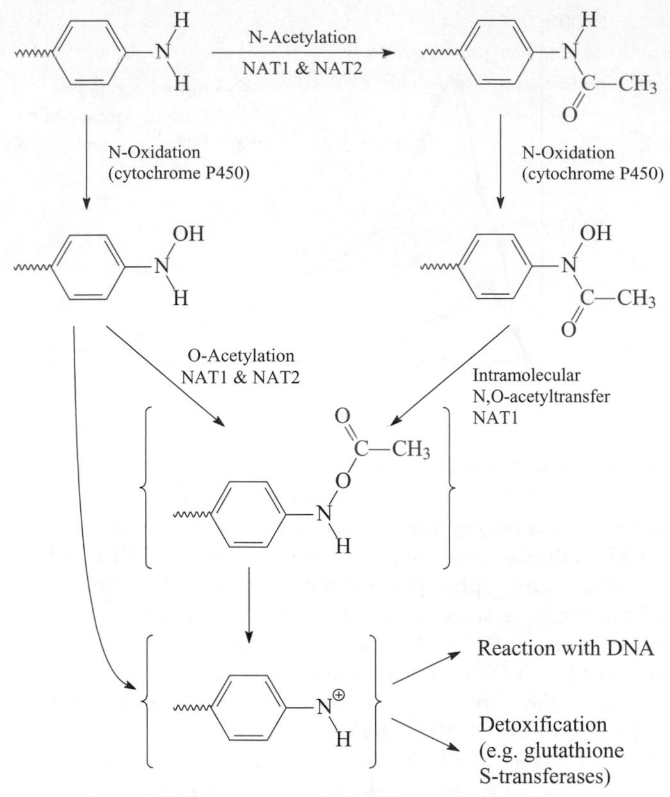

Figure 43-9 Schematic view of the role of *N*-acetyltransferase (NAT) enzymes in the metabolism of aromatic amines. *N*-acetylation might be a detoxification reaction in a number of cases; however, after *N*-hydroxylation of aromatic amines [e.g., by cytochrome P450 (CYP) enzymes], NAT enzymes can bioactivate these intermediates by O-acetylation or by intramolecular *N,O*-acetyltransfer, leading to the formation of nitrenium ions, which might react with DNA or alternatively be detoxified by, for example, GST enzymes. It is shown that a number of other biotransformation enzymes are involved in the metabolism of aromatic amines as well. *(Redrawn from Wormhoudt LW, Commandeur JNM, Vermeulen NPE. Genetic polymorphisms of human N-acetyltransferase, cytochrome P450, glutathione-S-transferase, and epoxide hydrolase enzymes: relevance to xenobiotic metabolism and toxicity. Crit Rev Toxicol 1999;29:59-124. Reproduced by permission from Taylor and Francis, Inc.)*

Testing

NAT2 slow acetylators are common in many populations, including approximately 83% of Egyptians; 40 to 60% of Caucasians, Europeans, and African Americans; 10 to 30% of Asians; and 5% of Canadian Eskimos.[57,122] *NAT1*10* allele frequency is reported to be high in a Japanese population (62.3%) compared with a European population (29%), but additional efforts are required to fully elucidate the population frequencies of the various *NAT1* alleles currently identified.[83] Variables that affect NAT phenotyping include the substrate or probe drug used, the age and disease status of the individual, medications, dietary factors such as ingestion of well-cooked meat, and lifestyle factors such as cigarette smoking or occupational exposure to NAT substrates.

Genotyping can predict NAT phenotype quite well, with concordance of 90 to 100% for *NAT2*. Methods have primarily employed PCR-RFLP, but real-time PCR and other allele-specific detection methods have been described.

Clinical Applications

NAT status has been implicated in propensity for experiencing ADRs and, unlike the CYPs and TPMT, has been associated with risk of disease, including immunologic disorders, such as rheumatoid arthritis and systemic lupus erythematosus, and several cancers, particularly bladder, lung, gastric, and colorectal. NAT substrate exposure can be related to cigarette smoking, some medications, occupational exposure (cooking, dye, and rubber industries), and several environmental toxicants (see Table 43-3). NAT testing may be important for individuals at high risk of exposure to NAT substrates or in whom adverse reactions to probable NAT substrates have been experienced.

Neither genotyping nor phenotyping methods are widely available for clinical testing. However, research involving the genotyping or phenotyping of NAT polymorphisms has significantly impacted pharmacotherapy with NAT substrates and drug development. With isoniazid, recognition of distinct phenotypical differences that led to ADRs resulted in further research into the pathologic mechanisms. For example, the neuropathic consequences are linked to pyridoxine deficiency, which can be avoided by coadministration of pyridoxine to all patients. Because rapid acetylators are less likely to respond to the conventionally administered dose, isoniazid dosing intervals are changed from once a week to twice per week. For procainamide, determining the acetylator status is accomplished through routine therapeutic drug monitoring of the parent and the metabolite, *N*-acetylprocainamide (NAPA). The dose of procainamide is adjusted based on the parent/metabolite ratio. In the development of amonafide, a chemotherapeutic agent inactivated by NAT conjugation, acetylator-based dosing was defined through clinical trials. Although the drug is no longer in development, it is an example of how pharmacogenetic phenomena can support individualized therapy.

Thiopurine S-Methyltransferase

TPMT is a Phase II metabolic enzyme that catalyzes the inactivation of 6-MP by S-methylation, thus preventing it from forming thioguanine nucleotides (TGNs). TPMT also affects AZA, which is another prodrug that is metabolized to 6-MP, as illustrated in Figure 43-10. Endogenous substrates for TPMT are currently unknown. AZA and 6-MP are used in the therapeutic management of leukemias, particularly acute lymphoblastic leukemia (ALL) in children, but are also used to treat a diverse range of conditions, including rheumatic disease, inflammatory bowel disease, and solid organ transplantation. These agents are cytotoxic, acting via incorporation of TGN into DNA. Outside the bone marrow, these agents can be oxidatively inactivated by xanthine oxidase or methylated by TPMT. In hematopoietic tissue, however, the effect of xanthine oxidase is negligible, leaving TPMT as the only significant inactivation pathway. Thus hematopoietic tissues are susceptible to damage in cases in which TPMT activity is very low. TPMT activity is highly variable in all large populations studied to date; approximately 90% of individuals have high activity, 10% have immediate activity, and 0.3% have low or undetectable enzyme activity. This trimodal activity is a direct result of enhanced proteasomal degradation of TPMT.[178] Numerous studies have shown that TPMT-deficient patients are at high risk for severe, and sometimes fatal, hematologic toxicity.

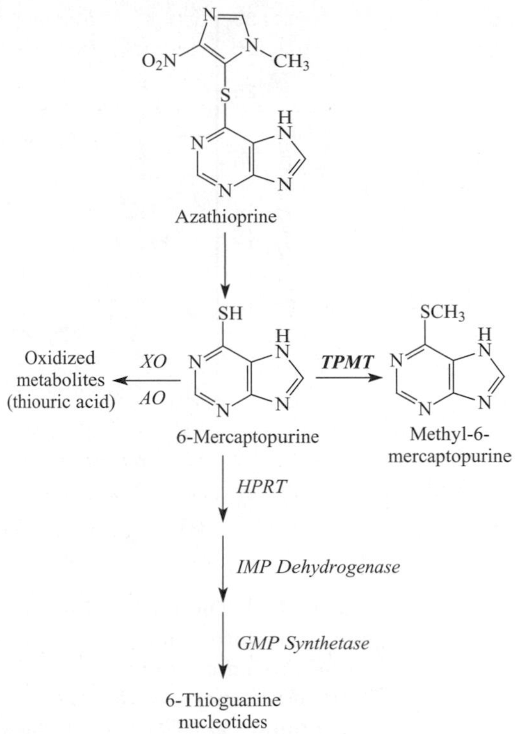

O_2N N CH$_3$ S H N N N N
Azathioprine
SH H SCH$_3$ H
Oxidized metabolites (thiouric acid) ← *XO* *AO* 6-Mercaptopurine → *TPMT* Methyl-6-mercaptopurine
HPRT
IMP Dehydrogenase
GMP Synthetase
6-Thioguanine nucleotides

Figure 43-10 Simplified metabolic pathway for prodrug thiopurines azathioprine and 6-mercaptopurine. *AO,* Aldehyde oxidase; *GMP,* guanine monophosphate; *HPRT,* hypoxanthine phosphoribosyltransferase; *IMP,* inositol monophosphate; *TPMT,* thiopurine *S*-methyltransferase; *XO,* xanthine oxidase.

Genotype to Phenotype

TPMT was the first widely used pharmacogenetic marker for individualizing drug therapy based on a patient's biochemical phenotype (erythrocyte enzyme activity) or genotype. Patients with a "low methylator" status are at significantly greater risk of toxicity, often necessitating a lower dose of these medications (as low as 5% of standard doses) because of accumulation of active drug. Prospective determination of functional TPMT status is useful for preventing mercaptopurine toxicity.[24,158] Whether TPMT testing is based on

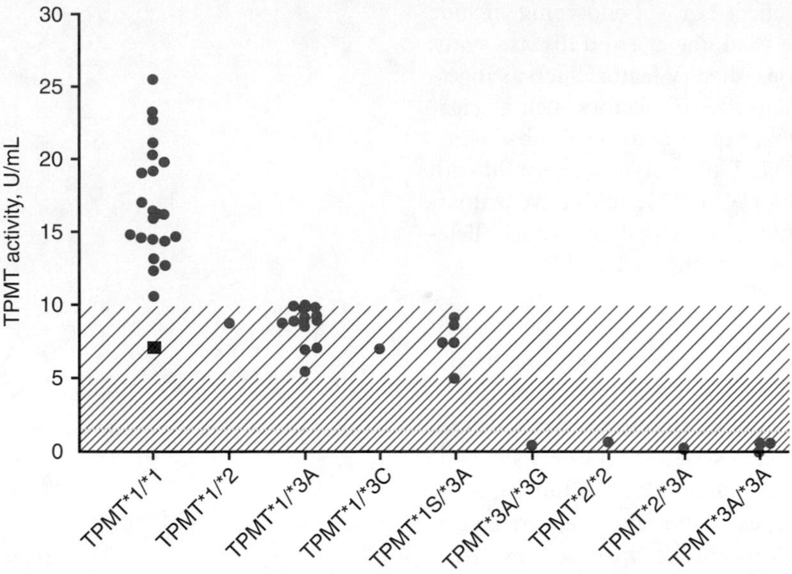

Figure 43-11 Thiopurine *S*-methyltransferase (TPMT) activity as related to genotypes determined by mutation-specific polymerase chain reaction methods. The *heavily shaded area* depicts the range of TPMT activity in erythrocytes that defines TPMT deficiency (<5 U/mL of packed red blood cells); the *lightly shaded area* depicts intermediate activity that defines TPMT heterozygous phenotypes (5 to 10 U/mL of packed red blood cells); and the *nonshaded area* depicts the range of TPMT activity in patients who have homozygous wild-type phenotypes. *Black circles* indicate patients with concordant genotype and phenotype; the *black square* indicates one patient with discordant genotype and phenotype (*TPMT*1/*1*). *(From Yates CR, Krynetski EY, Loennechen T, Fessing MY, Tai HL, Pui CH, et al. Molecular diagnosis of thiopurine* **S***-methyltransferase deficiency: genetic basis for azathioprine and mercaptopurine intolerance. Ann Intern Med 1997;126:608-14. Reproduced by permission from the American College of Physicians.)*

phenotype or genotype, the goal is individualized dosing with controlled systemic exposure.[35]

The molecular basis for variable TPMT activity has now been defined for the majority of patients.[119] The *TPMT* gene is located on chromosome 6p22.3 and is 26,833 bases long, exhibiting genetic polymorphism in all populations studied to date. At least 28 *TPMT* alleles have been identified, including single-nucleotide polymorphisms (SNPs) that lead to amino acid substitutions, formation of a stop codon, or a change that destroys a splice site. Four alleles, *TPMT*2, *3A, *3B,* and **3C,* account for 80 to 95% of intermediate or low enzyme activity cases in most ethnic groups. The **3A* allele is most common in Caucasians, whereas **3C* is most common in African American and Asian populations. The *TPMT *2* and **3B* alleles are rare in comparison with *TPMT*3A* or **3C. TPMT*3A* contains two nonsynonymous SNPs, one in exon 7 and another in exon 10, that result in Ala154Thr and Tyr240Cys alterations in encoded amino acids. *TPMT*3B* occurs rarely and contains only the exon 7 SNP; *TPMT*3C* contains only the exon 10 SNP. Thus a heterozygote **3B/*3C* could be mistaken for a **3A,* which would adversely impact assignment of phenotype. *TPMT*3C* is the most common variant allele in East Asian and African American populations (frequency approximately 2%). Patients with one wild-type allele and one of these variant alleles (i.e., heterozygous) have intermediate activity, and patients inheriting two variant alleles are TPMT deficient.[151] The relationship between phenotype and genotype is very good for most patients, as illustrated in Figure 43-11.

Trinucleotide repeat variants in the promoter region have been described that may explain the 1 to 2% of Caucasians who demonstrate ultra-metabolizer phenotype. A promoter region VNTR (variable number tandem repeat) that may have functional significance has also been investigated.

Testing

TPMT testing may occur via at least three routes: (1) biochemical phenotyping by determination of TPMT activity within erythrocytes from the patient; (2) metabolic phenotyping by determination of concentrations of 6-MP and thioguanine in the patient; or (3) genotyping. Biochemical phenotyping depends on stable enzyme activity between the times of blood collection and analytical testing. This approach therefore is challenged by storage and stability concerns and is limited to patients who have not received a blood transfusion over the weeks previous to TPMT testing, and who have healthy red blood cells at the time of testing (often not the case at the time ALL is diagnosed). When these or other limitations of biochemical phenotyping apply, *TPMT* genotyping is the preferred pretherapeutic testing approach. Metabolic phenotyping requires that AZA or 6-MP be administered before testing. This approach is therefore most useful for optimizing dose once steady-state concentrations have been achieved, or for troubleshooting for patients who have experienced toxicity or an ADR. *TPMT* genotype correlates well with TPMT activity in leukemia cells, as would be expected for germline mutations. By using PCR-based assays to detect the three signature mutations in these alleles, a rapid and relatively inexpensive assay identifies ≈90% of all variant alleles. In Caucasian populations, *TPMT*3A* is the most common variant *TPMT* allele (3.2 to 5.7% of *TPMT* alleles), although *TPMT*3C* has an allele frequency of 0.2 to 0.8%, and *TPMT*2* represents 0.2 to 0.5% of *TPMT* alleles.[2,24,104] Studies in Caucasian, African, and Asian populations have revealed that the frequency of these variant *TPMT* alleles differs among various ethnic populations. East and West African populations have a frequency of variant alleles similar to Caucasians, but the variant alleles in the African populations were predominantly *TPMT*3C*.[5] Among African Americans, *TPMT*3C* is the most prevalent allele, but *TPMT*2* and *TPMT*3A* are also found, reflecting the integration of Caucasian and African American genes in the U.S. population.[65] In Japanese and Chinese populations, *TPMT*3C* is almost exclusively the causative variant allele. In other Asian populations, *TPMT*3C* is also predominant.[115]

Many common genotyping tests do not detect TPMT deficiency in all patients, particularly those with a rare or unknown but clinically significant variant. Compound heterozygotes also present a challenge to PCR-based genetic testing in this gene. For example, patients with the heterozygous genotype *TPMT*1/*3A* have a 35% risk of hematopoietic toxicity versus a 7% risk for patients with a homozygous wild-type genotype. Alternatively, patients with the *TPMT*3B/*3C* genotype are TPMT-deficient and are at very high risk for thiopurine toxicity. These two genotypes are impossible to distinguish when conventional PCR genotyping is used.[18,115] The *TPMT*3B* allele is rare (≈1% of variant alleles), but its presence can have grave clinical consequences. A haplotyping method and a matrix-assisted laser desorption/ionization–time-of-flight (MALDI-TOF) mass spectrometric method, both using genomic DNA, discriminate *TPMT*1/*3A* from *TPMT*3B/*3C*.[151,153]

6-Mercaptopurine and Azathioprine Applications

An analysis of mercaptopurine therapy for childhood ALL found that TPMT-deficient patients tolerated full doses of mercaptopurines for only a brief period (7% of the scheduled weeks of therapy), whereas heterozygous and homozygous wild-type patients tolerated full doses for 65% and 84% of scheduled weeks of therapy during the 2½ years of treatment, respectively. The percentage of weeks in which mercaptopurine dosage had to be decreased to prevent toxicity was 2%, 16%, and 76% in wild-type, heterozygous, and homozygous variant individuals. Collectively, these studies demonstrate that the influence of *TPMT* genotype on hematopoietic toxicity is most dramatic for homozygous variant patients, but is also of clinical relevance for heterozygous individuals, who represent about 10% of patients treated with these medications. The labeling for 6-MP was revised in 2004 to include TPMT testing options. It is advised that patients who are TPMT PMs seek alternative therapies. In the absence of alternative therapy, 5 to 10% of the conventional dose, with careful monitoring, has been recommended. For patients who are predicted to be TPMT IMs, a dose reduction of 30 to 70% has been recommended, based on the specific clinical scenario. This testing is routinely performed pretherapeutically at many children's oncology centers for ALL patients.[70]

A growing and potentially valuable use of TPMT status testing is before intravenous AZA loading, a strategy used in the management of Crohn's disease. Dose-related toxicities resulted in AZA discontinuation in 10 to 20% of cases, and it has been estimated that over 6 months, 20% of patients would need TPMT analysis to avoid one serious ADR. TPMT status testing before taking AZA has been modeled to be cost-effective in a variety of theoretical situations. Analysis of some recent studies suggests that by optimizing the maximum AZA dose between 0.75 and 3 mg/kg/d, depending on TPMT status testing (with a drastic reduction in dosage for patients homozygous for variant *TPMT* alleles), considerable cost savings can be made by avoiding hospitalization and rescue therapy for leukopenic events.[116,184,192] Furthermore, one study reported that the median dose reduction required for TPMT-deficient patients was 90.8% (range, 50 to 94%) and the median dose reduction in *TPMT* for heterozygotes was 67% (range, 0 to 93%).[36] This study included only patients referred for hematopoietic toxicity. However, previous studies have reported that heterozygous patients needed only 15 to 30% dose reduction to avoid ADRs. TPMT phenotyping or genotyping is performed by approximately half of gastroenterologists surveyed.[208]

Although detection of *TPMT* polymorphisms is thought to prospectively identify approximately 10% of patients likely to experience dose-limiting toxicity from AZA and 6-MP therapy, toxicity is estimated to occur in 15 to 28% of patients. Thus, toxicity related to thiopurine therapeutics cannot be explained by known *TPMT* polymorphisms alone. Cao and Hegele described an inosine triphosphatase (ITPA)-deficient phenotype that may provide an additional mechanism for thiopurine-related toxicity.[143] This phenotype, similar to TPMT deficiency, is clinically benign until a patient is exposed to a thiopurine therapeutic such as 6-MP or AZA. The ITPA deficiency phenotype is associated with a 94C→A polymorphism of *ITPA* and approximately 25% residual red cell ITPA activity. Consequently, the metabolite 6-thio-ITP accumulates and may contribute to toxicities previously associated only with TPMT deficiency. Variants in xanthine oxidase/dehydrogenase (XDH) and aldehyde oxidase (AO) and molybdenum cofactor sulfurase (MOCOS) have also been reported to affect treatment outcome with azathioprine.[208] Therefore, other indicators of 6-MP and AZA phenotype may become important for predicting risk of ADRs in the future.

UDP-Glucuronosyltransferase 1A1 (UGT1A1)

The mammalian uridine diphosphate (UDP) glucuronosyl transferase (UGT) family comprises 117 members that can be divided among UGT1, UGT2, UGT3, and UGT4. The

UGT1 and UGT2 families are most efficient at glucuronidation in humans, and the UGT1 family is of most interest clinically. Hepatic isoforms include UGT1A1, 1A3, 1A4, 1A6, and 1A9; UGT1A7, 1A8, and 1A10 have been localized to extrahepatic tissues such as mouth, esophagus, intestine, pancreas, and colon. Of these, the clinical consequences of genetic and clinical variations have been best studied for UGT1A1. The primary goal of glucuronidation is to increase the water solubility of a compound, which typically inactivates that compound and promotes its elimination. An important endogenous substrate for UGT1A1 is bilirubin. Impairment of UGT1A1 leads to accumulation of bilirubin. UGT1A1 is also involved in the glucuronidation of drugs. Impairment of UGT1A1-mediated glucuronidation of drugs was first recognized in patients with Gilbert disease (also known as Gilbert-Meulengracht disease) who were administered irinotecan. An inverse relationship between expression of UGT1A1 and bilirubin concentration was recognized in patients with Gilbert disease and ultimately led to recognition of variation in the promoter region of the gene. These Gilbert patients experienced grade 4 neutropenia when irinotecan was administered—a consequence of reduced glucuronidation of the active irinotecan metabolite, a UGT1A1 substrate.[107,114,141,173]

Genotype to Phenotype

The *UGT1A1* gene is located on chromosome 2q37.1, along with other *UGT* genes, and is 155,596 bases long. The 5-exon genes of the UGT1 family each contain a unique first exon plus four exons that are shared between the genes; the exons may have evolved by a process of duplication, leading to the synthesis of proteins with identical carboxyl-terminal and variable amino-terminal domains. UGT1A1 is the most 3′ of the UGT1A isoform genes. More than 30 SNPs that lead to nonfunctional UGT1A1 have been identified in the promoter and unique exon 1 for this gene. Mutations in the *UGT1A1* gene that lead to complete absence of UGT1A1 activity have been associated with the severe hyperbilirubinemia seen with Crigler-Najjar syndrome. Variations in the number of TA repeats within the TATA box region of the UGT1A1 promoter have been associated with Gilbert disease, a clinically benign, mild hyperbilirubinemia.[15]

The most common number of TA repeats found in the TATA sequence of the *UGT1A1* promoter region in Caucasians is 6. This allele is known as $(TA)_6$ or *UGT1A1*1*. The most common variant of this sequence is the presence of seven repeats, known as $(TA)_7$ or *UGT1A1*28*, and leads to a 30% reduction in promoter activity of the UGT1A1and a reduction in transcription.[96] Tests for detection of *UGT1A1*28* are commercially available. Both $(TA)_5$ and $(TA)_8$ variants of this sequence, although relatively rare, are recognized to exist and correlate with higher and lower expression than the $(TA)_6$, respectively, thus preserving the anticipated inverse relationship between *UGT1A1* expression and the number of dinucleotide repeats. Genotypes are typically referred to as 6/6 for no variants, or 7/7 for homozygosity of *UGT1A1*28*. A nonsynonymous coding variant G71R *(UGT1A1*6)* is also known. The *UGT1A1*28* allele is common in Caucasian populations and populations of African origin (0.26 to 0.56). The *UGT1A1*6* variant is found almost exclusively in Asian populations, with a frequency of 0.13 to 0.25, and is also associated with hyperbilirubinemia.

Irinotecan Application

A well studied example of a pharmacogenetic application for *UGT1A1*28* genotyping is seen with irinotecan. Irinotecan is widely used in metastatic colorectal cancer and in other tumors such as lung and liver. Irinotecan is a prodrug, converted by carboxylesterases to produce the active, cytotoxic metabolite SN-38. This metabolite is a topoisomerase 1 inhibitor and the active agent against malignant cells. Approximately 20 to 35% of patients experience dose-limiting and potentially life-threatening (grade 3 or 4) diarrhea and/or neutropenia when treated with irinotecan.

The toxicity of irinotecan (and of the similar camptothecin analog, topotecan) is related to the accumulation of SN-38. A major route for inactivation of SN-38 is formation of the glucuronide conjugate (SN-38G), a reaction mediated by UGT1A1. Individuals possessing variant TA repeats in UGT1A1 are susceptible to dose-limiting toxicity with irinotecan. It is proposed that the risk of toxicity is near 0% for patients with the TA6/6 genotype, approximately 12.5% for patients with the TA6/7 genotype, and approximately 50% for patients with the TA7/7 genotype. It is generally recommended that patients with the TA7/7 genotype receive a reduced dose of irinotecan as compared with the dose given to patients with a TA6/6 genotype, although specific dosing guidelines are lacking, and the effect is probably most relevant only in "high dose" irinotecan regimens.

UGTs are known to be induced by aryl hydrocarbons and phenobarbital. The flavonoid chrysin has been studied for its ability to induce UGT1A1 specifically in the gastrointestinal tract, because it is not well absorbed and therefore would stay within the gastrointestinal tract, potentially minimizing the opportunity for drug-induced diarrhea. Coadministration of other drugs, such as loperamide, may prevent or alleviate the diarrhea associated with irinotecan. Similarly, coadministration of erythropoietin, granulocyte-colony stimulating factor, or other agents may minimize or shorten the duration of the neutropenic effects of irinotecan.[21] Because the disposition of irinotecan involves other UGTs, as well as the CYP3A family and drug transporters such as ABCB1, ABCC2, and ABCG2, additional study will be required to determine the most effective strategy for identification and management of individuals susceptible to the toxicity of irinotecan. As data accumulate, the utility of genotype-based dose optimization versus coadministration of compounds that counteract or relieve the associated toxicities will be better characterized.

Protease Inhibitors Application

Hyperbilirubinemia with clinically apparent jaundice is frequently observed in patients with human immunodeficiency virus (HIV) who are receiving protease inhibitors such as indinavir and atazanavir. Both of these drugs are glucuronidated by and are potent inhibitors of UGT1A1.[211] Thus patients who are carriers for *UGT1A1*28* would be at high risk of jaundice, because the consequences of indinavir inhibition would be more pronounced in people with *UGT1A1*28,* who are predisposed to reduced bilirubin glucuronidation activity. Indeed, the presence of *UGT1A1*28* is highly predictive of elevated post-therapeutic bilirubin concentrations in patients treated with indinavir.[214] Case reports of grade 4 hyperbilirubinemia related to *UGT1A1*28* resulting in hepatotoxicity have been published.[58] In addition, a genotype-phenotype association study of *UGT1A1, UGT1A3,* and *UGT1A7* genotypes and hyperbilirubinemia have identified combinations of four *UGT1A* SNPs spanning these three different genes and have associated these variants with grades 3 and 4 hyperbilirubinemia after treatment with atazanavir.[95,96] Patients who were homozygous for all four SNPs expressed the highest incidence of severe hyperbilirubinemia, suggesting a strong association between genetics and response. Genotyping for the combination of these SNPs may be useful in predicting susceptibility to severe hyperbilirubinemia and, in view of the high allele frequency of *UGT1A1*28,* could theoretically reduce drug-induced jaundice by 75%.[148]

Other Phase II Metabolism Enzymes

Other Phase II enzymes that exhibit marked genetic variability among individuals may be clinically important. For example, genetic variations in glutathione *S*-transferases, alcohol dehydrogenase, catechol-*O*-methyltransferase, and dihydropyrimidine dehydrogenase have been studied. Dihydropyrimidine dehydrogenase (coded from *DPYD*) is the initial and rate-limiting enzyme in the three-step pathway of uracil and thymidine catabolism and in the pathway leading to formation of β-alanine. It is also responsible for degrading fluoropyrimidines, such as the commonly used cancer chemotherapeutic drugs 5-fluorouracil and capecitabine. Decreased enzyme activity is associated with a higher risk of severe or fatal toxicity from standard doses of 5-fluorouracil.[117,182,190]

PHARMACODYNAMIC GENES

Vitamin K Epoxide Reductase Complex 1 *(VKORC1)*

Vitamin K epoxide reductase (VKOR), a 163 amino acid protein encoded by the subunit complex 1 gene *(VKORC1),* is a key enzyme in the vitamin K cycle, and is the primary site of action for the commonly used oral anticoagulant warfarin. VKOR converts vitamin K epoxide to vitamin K, which is the rate-limiting step in vitamin K recycling. Several coagulation factors are vitamin K dependent. Impairment of VKOR therefore limits activation of the vitamin K–dependent coagulation factors and explains the anticoagulation effect of warfarin.[42] Further, the amount of VKOR expressed, which may be genetically controlled, will dictate a person's sensitivity to warfarin. Although the activity of VKOR has been recognized since the 1970s, the gene was not cloned and characterized until 2004-2005.[101,197]

Genotype to Phenotype

The *VKORC1* gene is located on chromosome 16 and contains 5126 base pairs arranged in three exons. More than 30 variants have been described that originally were grouped and defined on the basis of haplotypes. *VKORC1* variants are associated most commonly with warfarin sensitivity, but also with warfarin resistance, and are implicated in multiple coagulation factor deficiency disorders. In 2005, two independent laboratories defined a haplotype indicative of warfarin sensitivity (*2 and Group A), based on low dose requirements. The allele frequency of the low-dose or "sensitive" haplotypes was approximately 15% for African Americans, 40% for Caucasians, and 90% for Asian populations.[45,146] It was later recognized that a promoter variant is in very strong linkage disequilibrium with the warfarin-sensitive haplotypes. Because this variant was shown to directly affect expression of the VKOR protein, it is thought to be causative for the warfarin sensitivity phenotype.[79] Most clinical testing currently available detects only the promoter variant of *VKORC1* (−1639G→A). Typically, this variant is tested along with the two common variants of CYP2C9: *CYP2C9*2* (430C→T) and *CYP2C9*3* (1075A→C). Other variants in these and other genes that have been studied to date would appear to have little importance for warfarin dosing.[155,196]

Warfarin Sensitivity Application

As discussed previously, warfarin is a commonly prescribed oral anticoagulant used to prevent thromboembolic disease after surgery and on a long-term basis for patients with deep vein thrombosis, atrial fibrillation, recurrent stroke, or heart valve prosthesis. Warfarin acts through inhibition of Vitamin K epoxide reductase (VKOR), which leads to a reduced amount of vitamin K available to serve as a cofactor for active clotting proteins. Warfarin is a very difficult drug to dose correctly because it has a narrow therapeutic range and wide interindividual and intraindividual variability in response. The dose of warfarin is typically adjusted based on a target range for the INR, for example, 2.0 to 3.0. Inappropriate dosing of warfarin has been associated with substantial risk of major and minor hemorrhage or thomboemboli. Genetic variants of *VKORC1,* representing sensitivity in response to warfarin, and of *CYP2C9,* representing pharmacokinetics of warfarin, are thought to account for approximately one third of the variability among patients. When the genetic variants are combined with common clinical factors and early INR data, up to 70% of the variability seen among patients is thought to be explained. These sources of variability are discussed in detail in the 2008 practice guidelines published by the American College of Chest Physicians, as well as in the product labeling for the popular formulation of warfarin sold as Coumadin.[6]

Among the many mathematical algorithms published for predicting warfarin dose, consistently included covariates include age, gender, an index of body size, and the three common genetic variants: *CYP2C9*2, CYP2C9*3,* and a promoter variant of *VKORC1* (−1639G→A). Some algorithms account for factors such as smoking status, interfering

TABLE 43-7 Example Doses of Warfarin Predicted by the Scone Algorithm[156] for a 6 Foot Tall, 55-Year-Old Person

	CALCULATED DAILY MAINTENANCE DOSE (MG) OF WARFARIN PER GENOTYPE AND PERCENT DIFFERENCE FROM THE NO VARIANT DETECTED DOSE PREDICTION		
***CYP2C9* Variants**	***VKORC1* GG (No Variants)**	***VKORC1* AG**	***VKORC1* AA**
*1/*1 (no variants)	6.8 mg/d	5.6 (−18%)	4.5 (−34%)
*1/*2	5.6 (−18%)	4.5 (−34%)	3.6 (−47%)
*1/*3	5.0 (−26%)	4.0 (−41%)	3.1 (−54%)
*2/*2	4.5 (−34%)	3.6 (−47%)	2.7 (−60%)
*2/*3	4.0 (−41%)	3.0 (−56%)	2.3 (−66%)
*3/*3	3.5 (−49%)	2.6 (−62%)	1.9 (−72%)

concomitant medications (e.g., amiodarone), liver disease, and existing INR data.[124] An example of doses predicted with one of the first published algorithms[156] for a patient that is 6 feet tall and 55 years of age is shown in Table 43-7. Comparisons of several published algorithms demonstrate good agreement in predicting maintenance dose requirements for populations studied.[56,206] The overall goals of algorithm-guided dosing include reducing the risk of bleeding events, achieving a stable and therapeutic dose sooner, and maintaining therapeutic INRs more consistently. The International Warfarin Pharmacogenetics Consortium has demonstrated some improvement in pharmacogenetics-guided management over fixed dose or clinical monitoring alone, particularly for people who require low doses.[90] However, specific guidelines for application of pharmacogenetic data and related dosing algorithms to clinical practice are lacking, and prospective clinical studies are few in number. Moreover, clinical studies have not consistently demonstrated improved outcomes for patients who receive gene-based dosing of warfarin. Several multisite international studies are currently under way to gather more information as to how and whether pharmacogenetic testing should be routinely applied to warfarin initiation.[32,113,185,195]

Human Leukocyte Antigen (HLA) Complex, Class I, B

The human leukocyte antigen (HLA) complex is a cornerstone for the immune system because of its involvement in identification of foreign proteins. HLA is the human version of the major histocompatibility complex (MHC), a gene family common to many species. The HLA proteins produced from these genes are expressed on the surface of nearly all cells, where they bind to peptides that are exported from the cell. These peptides are thereby captured and displayed to the circulating cells of the immune system. If the immune system recognizes the peptides as foreign (e.g., viral or bacterial peptides), it responds by triggering the infected cell to self-destruct.

Genotype to Phenotype

The MHC in humans consists of more than 200 genes, clustered on chromosome 6. Genes in this complex are categorized into three groups: class I, class II, and class III. Humans have three major class I genes, known as *HLA-A, HLA-B,* and *HLA-C.* It is the *HLA-B* gene that has been best characterized from the perspective of pharmacogenetics, based on a high degree of polymorphism and association of variants with drug hypersensitivity reactions. Some HLA genes have hundreds of variant alleles, classified by a number (such as *HLA-B27*); closely related alleles are categorized together. For example, more than 40 very similar alleles are subtypes of *HLA-B27.* These subtypes are designated as *HLA-B*2701* to *HLA-B*2743. HLA-B* gene variants are also associated with risk of disease, particularly immune-mediated inflammatory disease.

Risk of SCARS and Related Drug Hypersensitivity Applications

Severe cutaneous reaction syndromes (SCARS), such as Stevens-Johnson syndrome and toxic epidermal necrolysis, lead to extremely painful rashes that sometimes are life-threatening. The diagnosis of Stevens-Johnson syndrome versus toxic epidermal necrolysis is based on the amount of skin affected, whereas toxic epidermal necrolysis affects more than 30% of the body surface area and therefore is more serious. Overall, drug-induced SCARS occur rarely (1 to 6 per 10,000), but the incidence is approximately 10-fold greater in Asian populations, and reactions are characteristically observed with certain drugs. For example, drug-induced hypersensitivity reactions like SCARS are associated with the antiepileptic drugs carbamazepine, phenytoin, and lamotrigine; drugs used in the management of infectious disease, including abacavir, nevirapine, and sulfamethoxazole; the antiplatelet drug ticlopidine; and the antigout agent allopurinol. The best characterized HLA-drug associations today are *HLA-B*1502* and carbamazepine, *HLA-B*5801* and allopurinol, and *HLA-B*5701* with abacavir. Although not common in most populations, the mortality rates are 5 to 10% for Stevens-Johnson syndrome and up to 40% for toxic epidermal necrolysis.[23,183] Therefore, detection of a high-risk allele before therapy is initiated could allow drug avoidance and substantially reduced risk of the associated ADR.

Genetic testing for HLA variants is highly variable among laboratories, ranging from complete gene sequencing, to identification of single SNPs that are in linkage disequilibrium with high-risk haplotypes. Phenotyping for abacavir is also available. Pretherapeutic testing to identify patients at risk for abacavir hypersensitivity was incorporated into the 2008 guidelines for the use of antiretroviral agents in HIV-1–infected adults and adolescents, published by the Office of AIDS Research Advisory Council, and has been shown to be cost-effective.[71,109]

FUTURE DIRECTIONS

As discussed previously in this chapter, any protein for which the related gene exhibits polymorphism has potential pharmacogenetic implications. The future success of pharmacogenetics depends on understanding (1) the interrelationship of the various proteins involved in pharmacokinetics and pharmacodynamics, (2) the balance between major versus minor pathways, and (3) the mechanisms of action of specific drugs. Also important is an understanding of haplotype relationships, the possible implications of heterozygote variants, and gene dose, for single genes and for combinations of genes. Genome-wide association studies are anticipated to increase the complexity of pharmacogenetics, but they also improve our understanding and utility of genotype-phenotype relationships. Additional clinical studies, particularly prospective and outcome-related studies, are needed to guide implementation of pharmacogenetic findings in the clinic. Finally, closer integration of pharmacy professionals with clinical laboratories and clinicians and increased availability of cost-effective commercial testing will improve the success of pharmacogenetic applications.

REFERENCES

1. Effects of chemotherapy and hormonal therapy for early breast cancer on recurrence and 15-year survival: an overview of the randomised trials. Lancet 2005;365:1687-717.
2. Recommendations from the EGAPP Working Group. Testing for cytochrome P450 polymorphisms in adults with nonpsychotic depression treated with selective serotonin reuptake inhibitors. Genet Med 2007;9:819-25.
3. Agundez JA, Ledesma MC, Ladero JM, Benitez J. Prevalence of CYP2D6 gene duplication and its repercussion on the oxidative phenotype in a white population. Clin Pharmacol Ther 1995;57:265-9.
4. Aithal GP, Day CP, Kesteven PJ, Daly AK. Association of polymorphisms in the cytochrome P450 CYP2C9 with warfarin dose requirement and risk of bleeding complications. Lancet 1999;353:717-9.
5. Ameyaw MM, Collie-Duguid ES, Powrie RH, Ofori-Adjei D, McLeod HL. Thiopurine methyltransferase alleles in British and Ghanaian populations. Hum Mol Genet 1999;8:367-70.
6. Ansell J, Hirsh J, Hylek E, Jacobson A, Crowther M, Palareti G. Pharmacology and management of the vitamin K antagonists: American College of Chest Physicians evidence-based clinical practice guidelines, 8th edition. Chest 2008;133:160S-198S.
7. Balis FM, Adamson PC. Application of pharmacogenetics to optimization of mercaptopurine dosing. J Natl Cancer Inst 1999;91: 1983-5.
8. Bertilsson L, Dahl ML, Dalen P, Al-Shurbaji A. Molecular genetics of CYP2D6: clinical relevance with focus on psychotropic drugs. Br J Clin Pharmacol 2002;53:111-22.
9. Blaisdell J, Jorge-Nebert LF, Coulter S, Ferguson SS, Lee SJ, Chanas B, et al. Discovery of new potentially defective alleles of human CYP2C9. Pharmacogenetics 2004;14:527-37.
10. Blum M, Grant DM, McBride W, Heim M, Meyer UA. Human arylamine *N*-acetyltransferase genes: isolation, chromosomal localization, and functional expression. DNA Cell Biol 1990;9:193-203.
11. Bonicke R, Reif W. Enzymatic inactivation of isonicotinic acid hydrazide in humans and animals. Arch Exp Pathol Pharmacol 1953;220:321-33.
12. Boukouvala S, Price N, Plant KE, Sim E. Structure and transcriptional regulation of the Nat2 gene encoding for the drug-metabolizing enzyme arylamine *N*-acetyltransferase type 2 in mice. Biochem J 2003;375:593-602.
13. Brandt JT, Close SL, Iturria SJ, Payne CD, Farid NA, Ernest CS 2nd, et al. Common polymorphisms of CYP2C19 and CYP2C9 affect the pharmacokinetic and pharmacodynamic response to clopidogrel but not prasugrel. J Thromb Haemost 2007;5:2429-36.
14. Brauch H, Murdter TE, Eichelbaum M, Schwab M. Pharmacogenomics of tamoxifen therapy. Clin Chem 2009;55: 1770-82.
15. Brockmoller J, Cascorbi I, Henning S, Meisel C, Roots I. Molecular genetics of cancer susceptibility. Pharmacology 2000;61:212-27.
16. Broly F, Marez D, Sabbagh N, Legrand M, Millecamps S, Lo Guidice JM, et al. An efficient strategy for detection of known and new mutations of the CYP2D6 gene using single strand conformation polymorphism analysis. Pharmacogenetics 1995;5:373-84.
17. Brosen K, de Morais SM, Meyer UA, Goldstein JA. A multifamily study on the relationship between CYP2C19 genotype and S-mephenytoin oxidation phenotype. Pharmacogenetics 1995;5:312-7.
18. Brouwer C, Marinaki AM, Lambooy LH, Duley JA, Shobowale-Bakre M, De Abreu RA. Pitfalls in the determination of mutant alleles of the thiopurine methyltransferase gene. Leukemia 2001;15:1792-3.
19. Cabrera SE, Santos D, Valverde MP, Dominguez-Gil A, Gonzalez F, Luna G, et al. Influence of the cytochrome P450 2B6 genotype on population pharmacokinetics of efavirenz in human immunodeficiency virus patients. Antimicrob Agents Chemother 2009;53:2791-8.
20. Caldwell J. Pharmacogenetics and individual variation in the range of amino acid adequacy: the biological aspects. J Nutr 2004;134: 1600S-4S; discussion 30S-2S, 67S-72S.
21. Cascorbi I, Drakoulis N, Brockmoller J, Maurer A, Sperling K, Roots I. Arylamine *N*-acetyltransferase (NAT2) mutations and their allelic linkage in unrelated Caucasian individuals: correlation with phenotypic activity. Am J Hum Genet 1995;57:581-92.
22. Chou WH, Yan FX, Robbins-Weilert DK, Ryder TB, Liu WW, Perbost C, et al. Comparison of two CYP2D6 genotyping methods and assessment of genotype-phenotype relationships. Clin Chem 2003;49: 542-51.
23. Chung WH, Hung SI, Chen YT. Human leukocyte antigens and drug hypersensitivity. Curr Opin Allergy Clin Immunol 2007;7:317-23.
24. Clunie GP, Lennard L. Relevance of thiopurine methyltransferase status in rheumatology patients receiving azathioprine. Rheumatology (Oxford) 2004;43:13-8.
25. Daniel HI, Edeki TI. Genetic polymorphism of S-mephenytoin 4′-hydroxylation. Psychopharmacol Bull 1996;32:219-30.
26. Davies EC, Green CF, Mottram DR, Pirmohamed M. Adverse drug reactions in hospitals: a narrative review. Curr Drug Saf 2007;2:79-87.
27. Dawood S, Leyland-Jones B. Pharmacology and pharmacogenetics of chemotherapeutic agents. Cancer Invest 2009;27:482-8.
28. de Leon J. The future (or lack of future) of personalized prescription in psychiatry. Pharmacol Res 2009;59:81-9.
29. de Leon J, Armstrong SC, Cozza KL. Clinical guidelines for psychiatrists for the use of pharmacogenetic testing for CYP450 2D6 and CYP450 2C19. Psychosomatics 2006;47:75-85.
30. de Morais SM, Wilkinson GR, Blaisdell J, Nakamura K, Meyer UA, Goldstein JA. The major genetic defect responsible for the polymorphism of S-mephenytoin metabolism in humans. J Biol Chem 1994;269:15419-22.
31. Desta Z, Ward BA, Soukhova NV, Flockhart DA. Comprehensive evaluation of tamoxifen sequential biotransformation by the human cytochrome P450 system in vitro: prominent roles for CYP3A and CYP2D6. J Pharmacol Exp Ther 2004;310:1062-75.
32. Eby CS. Counterpoint: pharmacogenetic-based initial dosing of warfarin: not ready for prime time. Clin Chem 2009;55:712-4.
33. Eichelbaum M, Evert B. Influence of pharmacogenetics on drug disposition and response. Clin Exp Pharmacol Physiol 1996;23:983-5.
34. Ereshefsky L. Drug-drug interactions involving antidepressants: focus on venlafaxine. J Clin Psychopharmacol 1996;16:37S-50S; discussion 53S.
35. Evans WE. Pharmacogenetics of thiopurine S-methyltransferase and thiopurine therapy. Ther Drug Monit 2004;26:186-91.

36. Evans WE, Hon YY, Bomgaars L, Coutre S, Holdsworth M, Janco R, et al. Preponderance of thiopurine S-methyltransferase deficiency and heterozygosity among patients intolerant to mercaptopurine or azathioprine. J Clin Oncol 2001;19:2293-301.
37. Ferguson RJ, De Morais SM, Benhamou S, Bouchardy C, Blaisdell J, Ibeanu G, et al. A new genetic defect in human *CYP2C19*: mutation of the initiation codon is responsible for poor metabolism of S-mephenytoin. J Pharmacol Exp Ther 1998;284:356-61.
38. Frank D, Jaehde U, Fuhr U. Evaluation of probe drugs and pharmacokinetic metrics for *CYP2D6* phenotyping. Eur J Clin Pharmacol 2007;63:321-33.
39. Frueh FW, Amur S, Mummaneni P, Epstein RS, Aubert RE, DeLuca TM, et al. Pharmacogenomic biomarker information in drug labels approved by the United States Food and Drug Administration: prevalence of related drug use. Pharmacotherapy 2008;28:992-8.
40. Fukushima-Uesaka H, Saito Y, Watanabe H, Shiseki K, Saeki M, Nakamura T, et al. Haplotypes of *CYP3A4* and their close linkage with *CYP3A5* haplotypes in a Japanese population. Hum Mutat 2004;23:100.
41. Gaedigk A, Simon SD, Pearce RE, Bradford LD, Kennedy MJ, Leeder JS. The *CYP2D6* activity score: translating genotype information into a qualitative measure of phenotype. Clin Pharmacol Ther 2008;83:234-42.
42. Garcia AA, Reitsma PH. VKORC1 and the vitamin K cycle. Vitam Horm 2008;78:23-33.
43. Gasche Y, Daali Y, Fathi M, Chiappe A, Cottini S, Dayer P, et al. Codeine intoxication associated with ultrarapid CYP2D6 metabolism. N Engl J Med 2004;351:2827-31.
44. Ge D, Fellay J, Thompson AJ, Simon JS, Shianna KV, Urban TJ, et al. Genetic variation in IL28B predicts hepatitis C treatment-induced viral clearance. Nature 2009;461:399-401.
45. Geisen C, Watzka M, Sittinger K, Steffens M, Daugela L, Seifried E, et al. *VKORC1* haplotypes and their impact on the inter-individual and inter-ethnical variability of oral anticoagulation. Thromb Haemost 2005;94:773-9.
46. Giancarlo GM, Venkatakrishnan K, Granda BW, von Moltke LL, Greenblatt DJ. Relative contributions of CYP2C9 and 2C19 to phenytoin 4-hydroxylation in vitro: inhibition by sulfaphenazole, omeprazole, and ticlopidine. Eur J Clin Pharmacol 2001;57:31-6.
47. Gjerde J, Hauglid M, Breilid H, Lundgren S, Varhaug JE, Kisanga ER, et al. Effects of *CYP2D6* and *SULT1A1* genotypes including *SULT1A1* gene copy number on tamoxifen metabolism. Ann Oncol 2008;19:56-61.
48. Gladding P, Webster M, Zeng I, Farrell H, Stewart J, Ruygrok P, et al. The antiplatelet effect of higher loading and maintenance dose regimens of clopidogrel: the PRINC (Plavix Response In Coronary Intervention) trial. JACC Cardiovasc Interv 2008;1:612-9.
49. Goetz MP, Rae JM, Suman VJ, Safgren SL, Ames MM, Visscher DW, et al. Pharmacogenetics of tamoxifen biotransformation is associated with clinical outcomes of efficacy and hot flashes. J Clin Oncol 2005;23:9312-8.
50. Goodall R. Cholinesterase: phenotyping and genotyping. Ann Clin Biochem 2004;41:98-110.
51. Gough AC, Miles JS, Spurr NK, Moss JE, Gaedigk A, Eichelbaum M, et al. Identification of the primary gene defect at the cytochrome *P450 CYP2*D locus. Nature 1990;347:773-6.
52. Grant DM, Blum M, Beer M, Meyer UA. Monomorphic and polymorphic human arylamine *N*-acetyltransferases: a comparison of liver isozymes and expressed products of two cloned genes. Mol Pharmacol 1991;39:184-91.
53. Grant DM, Hughes NC, Janezic SA, Goodfellow GH, Chen HJ, Gaedigk A, et al. Human acetyltransferase polymorphisms. Mutat Res 1997;376:61-70.
54. Grasmader K, Verwohlt PL, Rietschel M, Dragicevic A, Muller M, Hiemke C, et al. Impact of polymorphisms of cytochrome-P450 isoenzymes 2C9, 2C19 and 2D6 on plasma concentrations and clinical effects of antidepressants in a naturalistic clinical setting. Eur J Clin Pharmacol 2004;60:329-36.
55. Gray IC, Nobile C, Muresu R, Ford S, Spurr NK. A 2.4-megabase physical map spanning the *CYP2C* gene cluster on chromosome 10q24. Genomics 1995;28:328-32.
56. Grice GR. Periprocedural anticoagulation management in orthopedic patients: overview and description of a program utilizing pharmacogenetics. J Clin Outcome Manag 2008;15:183-90.
57. Gross M, Kruisselbrink T, Anderson K, Lang N, McGovern P, Delongchamp R, et al. Distribution and concordance of *N*-acetyltransferase genotype and phenotype in an American population. Cancer Epidemiol Biomarkers Prev 1999;8:683-92.
58. Gupta B, LeVea C, Litwin A, Fakih MG. Reversible grade 4 hyperbilirubinemia in a patient with *UGT1A1 7/7* genotype treated with irinotecan and cetuximab. Clin Colorectal Cancer 2007;6:447-9.
59. Gurbel PA, Bliden KP, Hiatt BL, O'Connor CM. Clopidogrel for coronary stenting: response variability, drug resistance, and the effect of pretreatment platelet reactivity. Circulation 2003;107:2908-13.
60. Hayes JD, Strange RC. Glutathione S-transferase polymorphisms and their biological consequences. Pharmacology 2000;61:154-66.
61. Heim MH, Meyer UA. Genetic polymorphism of debrisoquine oxidation: restriction fragment analysis and allele-specific amplification of mutant alleles of *CYP2D6*. Methods Enzymol 1991;206:173-83.
62. Heller T, Kirchheiner J, Armstrong VW, Luthe H, Tzvetkov M, Brockmoller J, et al. AmpliChip CYP450 GeneChip: a new gene chip that allows rapid and accurate *CYP2D6* genotyping. Ther Drug Monit 2006;28:673-7.
63. Ho PC, Saville DJ, Wanwimolruk S. Inhibition of human CYP3A4 activity by grapefruit flavonoids, furanocoumarins and related compounds. J Pharm Sci 2001;4:217-27.
64. Holmes MV, Shah T, Vickery C, Smeeth L, Hingorani AD, Casas JP. Fulfilling the promise of personalized medicine? Systematic review and field synopsis of pharmacogenetic studies. PLoS One 2009;4:e7960.
65. Hon YY, Fessing MY, Pui CH, Relling MV, Krynetski EY, Evans WE. Polymorphism of the thiopurine S-methyltransferase gene in African-Americans. Hum Mol Genet 1999;8:371-6.
66. Hong J, Leung E, Fraser A, Krissansen GW. Nucleic acid from saliva and salivary cells for noninvasive genotyping of Crohn's disease patients. Genet Test 2008;12:587-9.
67. Hoskins JM, Carey LA, McLeod HL. CYP2D6 and tamoxifen: DNA matters in breast cancer. Nat Rev Cancer 2009;9:576-86.
68. Hoskins JM, Shenfield GM, Gross AS. Concordance between proguanil phenotype and *CYP2C19* genotype in Chinese. Eur J Clin Pharmacol 2003;59:611-4.
69. Hosono N, Kato M, Kiyotani K, Mushiroda T, Takata S, Sato H, et al. *CYP2D6* genotyping for functional-gene dosage analysis by allele copy number detection. Clin Chem 2009;55:1546-54.
70. Huang RS, Ratain MJ. Pharmacogenetics and pharmacogenomics of anticancer agents. CA Cancer J Clin 2009;59:42-55.
71. Hughes DA, Vilar FJ, Ward CC, Alfirevic A, Park BK, Pirmohamed M. Cost-effectiveness analysis of *HLA B*5701* genotyping in preventing abacavir hypersensitivity. Pharmacogenetics 2004;14:335-42.
72. Hughes NC, Janezic SA, McQueen KL, Jewett MAS, Castranio T, Bell DA, et al. Identification and characterization of variant alleles of human acetyltransferase NAT1 with defective function using p-aminosalicylate as an in-vivo and in-vitro probe. Pharmacogenetics 1998;8:55-66.
73. Iakoubova OA, Robertson M, Tong CH, Rowland CM, Catanese JJ, Blauw GJ, et al. KIF6 Trp719Arg polymorphism and the effect of statin therapy in elderly patients: results from the PROSPER study. Eur J Cardiovasc Prev Rehabil. 2010;17:455-61.
74. Indjova D, Shipkova M, Atanasova S, Niedmann PD, Armstrong VW, Svinarov D, et al. Determination of thiopurine methyltransferase phenotype in isolated human erythrocytes using a new simple nonradioactive HPLC method. Ther Drug Monit 2003;25:637-44.
75. Ingelman-Sundberg M. Pharmacogenetics: an opportunity for a safer and more efficient pharmacotherapy. J Intern Med 2001;250:186-200.

76. Ingelman-Sundberg M. Pharmacogenomic biomarkers for prediction of severe adverse drug reactions. N Engl J Med 2008;358:637-9.
77. Ingelman-Sundberg M, Oscarson M, Daly AK, Garte S, Nebert DW. Human cytochrome *P-450 (CYP)* genes: a web page for the nomenclature of alleles. Cancer Epidemiol Biomarkers Prev 2001;10:1307-8.
78. Jenne JW. Partial purification and properties of the isoniazid transacetylase in human liver: its relationship to the acetylation of p-aminosalicylic acid. J Clin Invest 1965;44:1992-2002.
79. Johnson AD, Zhang Y, Papp AC, Pinsonneault JK, Lim JE, Saffen D, et al. Polymorphisms affecting gene transcription and mRNA processing in pharmacogenetic candidate genes: detection through allelic expression imbalance in human target tissues. Pharmacogenet Genomics 2008;18:781-91.
80. Kanebratt KP, Diczfalusy U, Backstrom T, Sparve E, Bredberg E, Bottiger Y, et al. Cytochrome P450 induction by rifampicin in healthy subjects: determination using the Karolinska cocktail and the endogenous CYP3A4 marker 4beta-hydroxycholesterol. Clin Pharmacol Ther 2008;84:589-94.
81. Kashuba AD, Nafziger AN, Kearns GL, Leeder JS, Shirey CS, Gotschall R, et al. Quantification of intraindividual variability and the influence of menstrual cycle phase on CYP2D6 activity as measured by dextromethorphan phenotyping. Pharmacogenetics 1998;8:403-10.
82. Kasperaviciute D, Sisodiya SM. Epilepsy pharmacogenetics. Pharmacogenomics 2009;10:817-36.
83. Katoh T, Boissy R, Nagata N, Kitagawa K, Kuroda Y, Itoh H, et al. Inherited polymorphism in the *N*-acetyltransferase 1 *(NAT1)* and 2 *(NAT2)* genes and susceptibility to gastric and colorectal adenocarcinoma. Int J Cancer 2000;85:46-9.
84. Kerb R, Aynacioglu AS, Brockmoller J, Schlagenhaufer R, Bauer S, Szekeres T, et al. The predictive value of *MDR1, CYP2C9*, and *CYP2C19* polymorphisms for phenytoin plasma levels. Pharmacogenomics J 2001;1:204-10.
85. Kidd RS, Curry TB, Gallagher S, Edeki T, Blaisdell J, Goldstein JA. Identification of a null allele of *CYP2C9* in an African-American exhibiting toxicity to phenytoin. Pharmacogenetics 2001;11:803-8.
86. Kimura M, Ieiri I, Mamiya K, Urae A, Higuchi S. Genetic polymorphism of cytochrome *P450s, CYP2C19*, and *CYP2C9* in a Japanese population. Ther Drug Monit 1998;20:243-7.
87. King CR, Porche-Sorbet RM, Gage BF, Ridker PM, Renaud Y, Phillips MS, et al. Performance of commercial platforms for rapid genotyping of polymorphisms affecting warfarin dose. Am J Clin Pathol 2008;129:876-83.
88. Kirchheiner J, Brosen K, Dahl ML, Gram LF, Kasper S, Roots I, et al. *CYP2D6* and *CYP2C19* genotype-based dose recommendations for antidepressants: a first step toward subpopulation-specific dosages. Acta Psychiatr Scand 2001;104:173-92.
89. Kirchheiner J, Nickchen K, Bauer M, Wong ML, Licinio J, Roots I, et al. Pharmacogenetics of antidepressants and antipsychotics: the contribution of allelic variations to the phenotype of drug response. Mol Psychiatry 2004;9:442-73.
90. Klein TE, Altman RB, Eriksson N, Gage BF, Kimmel SE, Lee MT, et al. Estimation of the warfarin dose with clinical and pharmacogenetic data. N Engl J Med 2009;360:753-64.
91. Klein TE, Chang JT, Cho MK, Easton KL, Fergerson R, Hewett M, et al. Integrating genotype and phenotype information: an overview of the PharmGKB project. Pharmacogenetics Research Network and Knowledge Base. Pharmacogenomics J 2001;1:167-70.
92. Kramer MA, Rettie AE, Rieder MJ, Cabacungan ET, Hines RN. Novel CYP2C9 promoter variants and assessment of their impact on gene expression. Mol Pharmacol 2008;73:1751-60.
93. Kuehl P, Zhang J, Lin Y, Lamba J, Assem M, Schuetz J, et al. Sequence diversity in CYP3A promoters and characterization of the genetic basis of polymorphic *CYP3A5* expression. Nat Genet 2001;27:383-91.
94. Lamba JK, Lin YS, Schuetz EG, Thummel KE. Genetic contribution to variable human CYP3A-mediated metabolism. Adv Drug Deliv Rev 2002;54:1271-94.
95. Lankisch TO, Behrens G, Ehmer U, Mobius U, Rockstroh J, Wehmeier M, et al. Gilbert's syndrome and hyperbilirubinemia in protease inhibitor therapy—an extended haplotype of genetic variants increases risk in indinavir treatment. J Hepatol 2009;50:1010-8.
96. Lankisch TO, Moebius U, Wehmeier M, Behrens G, Manns MP, Schmidt RE, et al. Gilbert's disease and atazanavir: from phenotype to UDP-glucuronosyltransferase haplotype. Hepatology 2006;44: 1324-32.
97. Lazarou J, Pomeranz BH, Corey PN. Incidence of adverse drug reactions in hospitalized patients: a meta-analysis of prospective studies. JAMA 1998;279:1200-5.
98. Leathart JB, London SJ, Steward A, Adams JD, Idle JR, Daly AK. *CYP2D6* phenotype-genotype relationships in African-Americans and Caucasians in Los Angeles. Pharmacogenetics 1998;8:529-41.
99. Lee CR, Goldstein JA, Pieper JA. Cytochrome *P450 2C9* polymorphisms: a comprehensive review of the in-vitro and human data. Pharmacogenetics 2002;12:251-63.
100. Lencz T, Robinson DG, Xu K, Ekholm J, Sevy S, Gunduz-Bruce H, et al. DRD2 promoter region variation as a predictor of sustained response to antipsychotic medication in first-episode schizophrenia patients. Am J Psychiatry 2006;163:529-31.
101. Li T, Chang CY, Jin DY, Lin PJ, Khvorova A, Stafford DW. Identification of the gene for vitamin K epoxide reductase. Nature 2004;427:541-4.
102. Linder MW, Keck PE Jr. Standards of laboratory practice: antidepressant drug monitoring. National Academy of Clinical Biochemistry. Clin Chem 1998;44:1073-84.
103. Link E, Parish S, Armitage J, Bowman L, Heath S, Matsuda F, et al. *SLCO1B1* variants and statin-induced myopathy—a genomewide study. N Engl J Med 2008;359:789-99.
104. Lovlie R, Daly AK, Molven A, Idle JR, Steen VM. Ultrarapid metabolizers of debrisoquine: characterization and PCR-based detection of alleles with duplication of the *CYP2D6* gene. FEBS Lett 1996;392:30-4.
105. Lu Y, Won KA, Nelson BJ, Qi D, Rausch DJ, Asinger RW. Characteristics of the amiodarone-warfarin interaction during long-term follow-up. Am J Health Syst Pharm 2008;65:947-52.
106. Lyon E, McMillin G, Melis R. Pharmacogenetic testing for warfarin sensitivity. In: Reynolds KK, Valdes R, Wells A, eds. Clinics in laboratory medicine: pharmacogenetics, vol 28. Philadelphia: WB Saunders, 2009:525-37.
107. Mackenzie PI, Bock KW, Burchell B, Guillemette C, Ikushiro S, Iyanagi T, et al. Nomenclature update for the mammalian UDP glycosyltransferase (UGT) gene superfamily. Pharmacogenet Genomics 2005;15:677-85.
108. Madadi P, Shirazi F, Walter FG, Koren G. Establishing causality of CNS depression in breastfed infants following maternal codeine use. Paediatr Drugs 2008;10:399-404.
109. Mallal S, Phillips E, Carosi G, Molina JM, Workman C, Tomazic J, et al. HLA-B*5701 screening for hypersensitivity to abacavir. N Engl J Med 2008;358:568-79.
110. Mamiya K, Ieiri I, Shimamoto J, Yukawa E, Imai J, Ninomiya H, et al. The effects of genetic polymorphisms of *CYP2C9* and *CYP2C19* on phenytoin metabolism in Japanese adult patients with epilepsy: studies in stereoselective hydroxylation and population pharmacokinetics. Epilepsia 1998;39:1317-23.
111. Man CB, Kwan P, Baum L, Yu E, Lau KM, Cheng AS, et al. Association between *HLA-B*1502* allele and antiepileptic drug-induced cutaneous reactions in Han Chinese. Epilepsia 2007;48: 1015-8.
112. Mann JJ. The medical management of depression. N Engl J Med 2005; 353:1819-34.
113. Mannucci PM, Spreafico M, Peyvandi F. Dosing anticoagulant therapy with coumarin drugs: is genotyping clinically useful? No. J Thromb Haemost 2008;6:1450-2.
114. Marcuello E, Altes A, Menoyo A, Del Rio E, Gomez-Pardo M, Baiget M. *UGT1A1* gene variations and irinotecan treatment in patients with metastatic colorectal cancer. Br J Cancer 2004;91:678-82.

115. Marez D, Legrand M, Sabbagh N, Guidice JM, Spire C, Lafitte JJ, et al. Polymorphism of the cytochrome P450 *CYP2D6* gene in a European population: characterization of 48 mutations and 53 alleles, their frequencies and evolution. Pharmacogenetics 1997;7:193-202.
116. Marra CA, Esdaile JM, Anis AH. Practical pharmacogenetics: the cost effectiveness of screening for thiopurine S-methyltransferase polymorphisms in patients with rheumatological conditions treated with azathioprine. J Rheumatol 2002;29:2507-12.
117. Mattison LK, Soong R, Diasio RB. Implications of dihydropyrimidine dehydrogenase on 5-fluorouracil pharmacogenetics and pharmacogenomics. Pharmacogenomics 2002;3:485-92.
118. McLeod HL, Krynetski EY, Wilimas JA, Evans WE. Higher activity of polymorphic thiopurine S-methyltransferase in erythrocytes from neonates compared to adults. Pharmacogenetics 1995;5:281-6.
119. McLeod HL, Siva C. The thiopurine S-methyltransferase gene locus—implications for clinical pharmacogenomics. Pharmacogenomics 2002;3:89-98.
120. Mega JL, Close SL, Wiviott SD, Shen L, Hockett RD, Brandt JT, et al. Cytochrome p-450 polymorphisms and response to clopidogrel. N Engl J Med 2009;360:354-62.
121. Meisler MH, Reinke C. A sensitive fluorescent assay for *N*-acetyltransferase activity in human lymphocytes from newborns and adults. Clin Chim Acta 1979;1979:91-6.
122. Meyer UA, Zanger UM. Molecular mechanisms of genetic polymorphisms of drug metabolism. Annu Rev Pharmacol Toxicol 1997;37:269-96.
123. Miki I, Aoyama N, Sakai T, Shirasaka D, Wambura CM, Maekawa S, et al. Impact of clarithromycin resistance and *CYP2C19* genetic polymorphism on treatment efficacy of *Helicobacter pylori* infection with lansoprazole- or rabeprazole-based triple therapy in Japan. Eur J Gastroenterol Hepatol 2003;15:27-33.
124. Millican EA, Lenzini PA, Milligan PE, Grosso L, Eby C, Deych E, et al. Genetic-based dosing in orthopedic patients beginning warfarin therapy. Blood 2007;110:1511-5.
125. Minchin RF. Acetylation of p-amino benzoylglutamate, a folic acid catabolite, by recombinant arylamine *N*-acetyltransferase and U937 cells. Biochem J 1995;307:1-3.
126. Miners JO, Birkett DJ. Cytochrome P4502C9: an enzyme of major importance in human drug metabolism. Br J Clin Pharmacol 1998;45:525-38.
127. Mizutani T. PM frequencies of major CYPs in Asians and Caucasians. Drug Metab Rev 2003;35:99-106.
128. Mortimer JE, Flatt SW, Parker BA, Gold EB, Wasserman L, Natarajan L, et al. Tamoxifen, hot flashes and recurrence in breast cancer. Breast Cancer Res Treat 2008;108:421-6.
129. Murphy GM Jr, Hollander SB, Rodrigues HE, Kremer C, Schatzberg AF. Effects of the serotonin transporter gene promoter polymorphism on mirtazapine and paroxetine efficacy and adverse events in geriatric major depression. Arch Gen Psychiatry 2004;61:1163-9.
130. Murphy GM Jr, Pollock BG, Kirshner MA, Pascoe N, Cheuk W, Mulsant BH, et al. *CYP2D6* genotyping with oligonucleotide microarrays and nortriptyline concentrations in geriatric depression. Neuropsychopharmacology 2001;25:737-43.
131. Nebert DW, Dieter MZ. The evolution of drug metabolism. Pharmacology 2000;61:124-35.
132. Nelson DR, Kamataki T, Waxman DJ, Guengerich FP, Estabrook RW, Feyereisen R, et al. The P450 superfamily: update on new sequences, gene mapping, accession numbers, early trivial names of enzymes, and nomenclature. DNA Cell Biol 1993;12:1-51.
133. Osborne CK. Tamoxifen in the treatment of breast cancer. N Engl J Med 1998;339:1609-18.
134. Owen RP, Sangkuhl K, Klein TE, Altman RB. Cytochrome P450 2D6. Pharmacogenet Genomics 2009;19:559-62.
135. Paine MF, Criss AB, Watkins PB. Two major grapefruit juice components differ in intestinal CYP3a4 inhibition kinetic and binding properties. Drug Metab Dispos 2004;32:1146-53.
136. Pena A, Collet JP, Hulot JS, Silvain J, Barthelemy O, Beygui F, et al. Can we override clopidogrel resistance? Circulation 2009;119:2854-7.
137. Perry PJ, Pfohl BM, Holstad SG. The relationship between antidepressant response and tricyclic antidepressant plasma concentrations: a retrospective analysis of the literature using logistic regression analysis. Clin Pharmacokinet 1987;13:381-92.
138. Peters BJ, Klungel OH, Visseren FL, de Boer A, Maitland-van der Zee AH. Pharmacogenomic insights into treatment and management of statin-induced myopathy. Genome Med 2009;1:120.
139. Pickering JW, McMillin GA, Gedge F, Hill HR, Lyon E. Flow cytometric assay for genotyping cytochrome *p450 2C9* and *2C19*: comparison with a microelectronic DNA array. Am J Pharmacogenomics 2004;4:199-207.
140. Pinto AG, Wang YH, Chalasani N, Skaar T, Kolwankar D, Gorski JC, et al. Inhibition of human intestinal wall metabolism by macrolide antibiotics: effect of clarithromycin on cytochrome P450 3A4/5 activity and expression. Clin Pharmacol Ther 2005;77:178-88.
141. Rantner B, Kollerits B, Anderwald-Stadler M, Klein-Weigel P, Gruber I, Gehringer A, et al. Association between the *UGT1A1 TA*-repeat polymorphism and bilirubin concentration in patients with intermittent claudication: results from the CAVASIC study. Clin Chem 2008;54:851-7.
142. Rebsamen MC, Desmeules J, Daali Y, Chiappe A, Diemand A, Rey C, et al. The AmpliChip CYP450 test: cytochrome P450 2D6 genotype assessment and phenotype prediction. Pharmacogenomics J 2009;9:34-41.
143. Relling MV, Hancock ML, Rivera GK, Sandlund JT, Ribeiro RC, Krynetski EY, et al. Mercaptopurine therapy intolerance and heterozygosity at the thiopurine S-methyltransferase gene locus. J Natl Cancer Inst 1999;91:2001-8.
144. Rendic S, Di Carlo FJ. Human cytochrome P450 enzymes: a status report summarizing their reactions, substrates, inducers, and inhibitors. Drug Metab Rev 1997;29:413-580.
145. Rettie AE, Jones JP. Clinical and toxicological relevance of CYP2C9: drug-drug interactions and pharmacogenetics. Annu Rev Pharmacol Toxicol 2005;45:477-94.
146. Rieder MJ, Reiner AP, Gage BF, Nickerson DA, Eby CS, McLeod HL, et al. Effect of *VKORC1* haplotypes on transcriptional regulation and warfarin dose. N Engl J Med 2005;352:2285-93.
147. Roca B. Pharmacogenomics of antiretrovirals. Recent Pat Antiinfect Drug Discov 2008;3:132-5.
148. Rotger M, Taffe P, Bleiber G, Gunthard HF, Furrer H, Vernazza P, et al. Gilbert syndrome and the development of antiretroviral therapy-associated hyperbilirubinemia. J Infect Dis 2005;192:1381-6.
149. Sachse C, Brockmoller J, Bauer S, Roots I. Cytochrome *P450 2D6* variants in a Caucasian population: allele frequencies and phenotypic consequences. Am J Hum Genet 1997;60:284-95.
150. Sallee FR, DeVane CL, Ferrell RE. Fluoxetine-related death in a child with cytochrome *P-450 2D6* genetic deficiency. J Child Adolesc Psychopharmacol 2000;10:27-34.
151. Schaeffeler E, Fischer C, Brockmeier D, Wernet D, Moerike K, Eichelbaum M, et al. Comprehensive analysis of thiopurine S-methyltransferase phenotype-genotype correlation in a large population of German-Caucasians and identification of novel TPMT variants. Pharmacogenetics 2004;14:407-17.
152. Schaeffeler E, Schwab M, Eichelbaum M, Zanger UM. *CYP2D6* genotyping strategy based on gene copy number determination by TaqMan real-time PCR. Hum Mutat 2003;22:476-85.
153. Schaeffeler E, Zanger UM, Eichelbaum M, Asante-Poku S, Shin JG, Schwab M. Highly multiplexed genotyping of thiopurine S-methyltransferase variants using MALD-TOF mass spectrometry: reliable genotyping in different ethnic groups. Clin Chem 2008;54: 1637-47.
154. Schwarz UI. Clinical relevance of genetic polymorphisms in the human *CYP2C9* gene. Eur J Clin Invest 2003;33(Suppl 2):23-30.
155. Schwarz UI, Ritchie MD, Bradford Y, Li C, Dudek SM, Frye-Anderson A, et al. Genetic determinants of response to warfarin during initial anticoagulation. N Engl J Med 2008;358:999-1008.
156. Sconce EA, Khan TI, Wynne HA, Avery P, Monkhouse L, King BP, et al. The impact of *CYP2C9* and *VKORC1* genetic polymorphism and

patient characteristics upon warfarin dose requirements: proposal for a new dosing regimen. Blood 2005;106:2329-33.

157. Scordo MG, Aklillu E, Yasar U, Dahl ML, Spina E, Ingelman-Sundberg M. Genetic polymorphism of cytochrome P450 2C9 in a Caucasian and a black African population. Br J Clin Pharmacol 2001;52:447-50.

157A. Scott SA, Martis S, Peter I, Kasai Y, Kornreich R, Desnick RJ. "Identification of CYP2C19*4B: pharmacogenetic implications for drug metabolism including clopidogrel responsiveness." Pharmacogenomics J 2011; Epub March 1, doi:10.1038

158. Seidman EG, Furst DE. Pharmacogenetics for the individualization of treatment of rheumatic disorders using azathioprine. J Rheumatol 2002;29:2484-7.

159. Serretti A, Artioli P. The pharmacogenomics of selective serotonin reuptake inhibitors. Pharmacogenomics J 2004;4:233-44.

160. Shimoda K, Someya T, Yokono A, Morita S, Hirokane G, Takahashi S, et al. The impact of *CYP2C19* and *CYP2D6* genotypes on metabolism of amitriptyline in Japanese psychiatric patients. J Clin Psychopharmacol 2002;22:371-8.

161. Siddoway LA. Amiodarone: guidelines for use and monitoring. Am Fam Physician 2003;68:2189-96.

162. Sim E, Pinter K, Mushtaq A, Upton A, Sandy J, Bhakta S, et al. Arylamine *N*-acetyltransferases: a pharmacogenomic approach to drug metabolism and endogenous function. Biochem Soc Trans 2003;31:615-9.

163. Simon T, Verstuyft C, Mary-Krause M, Quteineh L, Drouet E, Meneveau N, et al. Genetic determinants of response to clopidogrel and cardiovascular events. N Engl J Med 2009;360:363-75.

164. Singh MS, Michael M. Role of xenobiotic metabolic enzymes in cancer epidemiology. Methods Mol Biol 2009;472:243-64.

165. Singh SS. Preclinical pharmacokinetics: an approach towards safer and efficacious drugs. Curr Drug Metab 2006;7:165-82.

166. Sisodiya SM, Marini C. Genetics of antiepileptic drug resistance. Curr Opin Neurol 2009;22:150-6.

167. Sistonen J, Fuselli S, Palo JU, Chauhan N, Padh H, Sajantila A. Pharmacogenetic variation at *CYP2C9, CYP2C19*, and *CYP2D6* at global and microgeographic scales. Pharmacogenet Genomics 2009; 19:170-9.

168. Smith MA, Marinaki AM, Arenas M, Shobowale-Bakre M, Lewis CM, Ansari A, et al. Novel pharmacogenetic markers for treatment outcome in azathioprine-treated inflammatory bowel disease. Aliment Pharmacol Ther 2009;30:375-84.

169. Soars MG, Gelboin HV, Krausz KW, Riley RJ. A comparison of relative abundance, activity factor and inhibitory monoclonal antibody approaches in the characterization of human CYP enzymology. Br J Clin Pharmacol 2003;55:175-81.

170. Spear BB, Heath-Chiozzi M, Huff J. Clinical application of pharmacogenetics. Trends Mol Med 2001;7:201-4.

171. Steimer W, Zopf K, Von Amelunxen S, Pfeiffer H, Bachofer J, Popp J, et al. Allele-specific change of concentration and functional gene dose for the prediction of steady-state serum concentrations of amitriptyline and nortriptyline in CYP2C19 and CYP2D6 extensive and intermediate metabolizers. Clin Chem 2004;50:1623-33.

172. Steimer W, Zopf K, von Amelunxen S, Pfeiffer H, Bachofer J, Popp J, et al. Amitriptyline or not, that is the question: pharmacogenetic testing of CYP2D6 and CYP2C19 identifies patients with low or high risk for side effects in amitriptyline therapy. Clin Chem 2005;51: 376-85.

173. Strassburg CP. Pharmacogenetics of Gilbert's syndrome. Pharmacogenomics 2008;9:703-15.

174. Stubbins MJ, Harries LW, Smith G, Tarbit MH, Wolf CR. Genetic analysis of the human cytochrome P450 *CYP2C9* locus. Pharmacogenetics 1996;6:429-39.

175. Sullivan-Klose TH, Ghanayem BI, Bell DA, Zhang ZY, Kaminsky LS, Shenfield GM, et al. The role of the *CYP2C9-Leu359* allelic variant in the tolbutamide polymorphism. Pharmacogenetics 1996;6:341-9.

176. Summerscales JE, Josephy PD. Human acetyl CoA:arylamine N-acetyltransferase variants generated by random mutagenesis. Mol Pharmacol 2004;65:220-6.

177. Tabrizi AR, Zehnbauer BA, Borecki IB, McGrath SD, Buchman TG, Freeman BD. The frequency and effects of cytochrome P450 *(CYP) 2C9* polymorphisms in patients receiving warfarin. J Am Coll Surg 2002;194:267-73.

178. Tai HL, Fessing MY, Bonten EJ, Yanishevsky Y, d'Azzo A, Krynetski EY, et al. Enhanced proteasomal degradation of mutant human thiopurine S-methyltransferase (TPMT) in mammalian cells: mechanism for TPMT protein deficiency inherited by TPMT*2, TPMT*3A, TPMT*3B or TPMT*3C. Pharmacogenetics 1999;9:641-50.

179. Takahashi H, Wilkinson GR, Caraco Y, Muszkat M, Kim RB, Kashima T, et al. Population differences in S-warfarin metabolism between *CYP2C9* genotype-matched Caucasian and Japanese patients. Clin Pharmacol Ther 2003;73:253-63.

180. Takahashi H, Wilkinson GR, Nutescu EA, Morita T, Ritchie MD, Scordo MG, et al. Different contributions of polymorphisms in *VKORC1* and *CYP2C9* to intra- and inter-population differences in maintenance dose of warfarin in Japanese, Caucasians and African-Americans. Pharmacogenet Genomics 2006;16:101-10.

181. Take S, Mizuno M, Ishiki K, Nagahara Y, Yoshida T, Inaba T, et al. Interleukin-1beta genetic polymorphism influences the effect of cytochrome P 2C19 genotype on the cure rate of 1-week triple therapy for *Helicobacter pylori* infection. Am J Gastroenterol 2003;98:2403-8.

182. Takechi T, Okabe H, Ikeda K, Fujioka A, Nakagawa F, Ohshimo H, et al. Correlations between antitumor activities of fluoropyrimidines and DPD activity in lung tumor xenografts. Oncol Rep 2005;14:33-9.

183. Tassaneeyakul W, Jantararoungtong T, Chen P, Lin PY, Tiamkao S, Khunarkornsiri U, et al. Strong association between HLA-B*5801 and allopurinol-induced Stevens-Johnson syndrome and toxic epidermal necrolysis in a Thai population. Pharmacogenet Genomics 2009;19: 704-9.

184. Tavadia SM, Mydlarski PR, Reis MD, Mittmann N, Pinkerton PH, Shear N, Sauder DN. Screening for azathioprine toxicity: a pharmacoeconomic analysis based on a target case. J Am Acad Dermatol 2000;42:628-32.

185. Thacker SM, Grice GR, Milligan PE, Gage BF. Dosing anticoagulant therapy with coumarin drugs: is genotyping clinically useful? Yes. J Thromb Haemost 2008;6:1445-9.

186. Thummel KE. Does the *CYP3A5*3* polymorphism affect in vivo drug elimination? Pharmacogenetics 2003;13:585-7.

187. Tomalik-Scharte D, Lazar A, Fuhr U, Kirchheiner J. The clinical role of genetic polymorphisms in drug-metabolizing enzymes. Pharmacogenomics J 2008;8:4-15.

188. Tozzi V. Pharmacogenetics of antiretrovirals. Antiviral Res 2010;85: 190-200.

189. Uher R, Huezo-Diaz P, Perroud N, Smith R, Rietschel M, Mors O, et al. Genetic predictors of response to antidepressants in the GENDEP project. Pharmacogenomics J 2009;9:225-33.

190. Van Kuilenburg AB, Vreken P, Abeling NG, Bakker HD, Meinsma R, Van Lenthe H, et al. Genotype and phenotype in patients with dihydropyrimidine dehydrogenase deficiency. Hum Genet 1999; 104:1-9.

191. Vatsis KP, Weber WW, Bell DA, Dupret JM, Evans DAP, Grant DM, et al. Nomenclature for *N*-acetyltransferases. Pharmacogenetics 1995;5:1-17.

192. Veenstra DL, Higashi MK, Phillips KA. Assessing the cost-effectiveness of pharmacogenomics. AAPS Pharm Sci 2000;2:E29.

193. von Ahsen N, Armstrong VW, Behrens C, von Tirpitz C, Stallmach A, Herfarth H, et al. Association of inosine triphosphatase 94C→A and thiopurine S-methyltransferase deficiency with adverse events and study drop-outs under azathioprine therapy in a prospective Crohn disease study. Clin Chem 2005;51:2282-8.

194. Vormfelde SV, Brockmoller J, Bauer S, Herchenhein P, Kuon J, Meineke I, et al. Relative impact of genotype and enzyme induction on the metabolic capacity of CYP2C9 in healthy volunteers. Clin Pharmacol Ther 2009;86:54-61.

195. Wadelius M. Point: use of pharmacogenetics in guiding treatment with warfarin. Clin Chem 2009;55:709-11.

196. Wadelius M, Pirmohamed M. Pharmacogenetics of warfarin: current status and future challenges. Pharmacogenomics J 2007;7: 99-111.
197. Wajih N, Sane DC, Hutson SM, Wallin R. Engineering of a recombinant vitamin K-dependent gamma-carboxylation system with enhanced gamma-carboxyglutamic acid forming capacity: evidence for a functional CXXC redox center in the system. J Biol Chem 2005; 280:10540-7.
198. Walko CM, McLeod H. Pharmacogenomic progress in individualized dosing of key drugs for cancer patients. Nat Clin Pract Oncol 2009;6: 153-62.
199. Weber WW, Hein DW. Clinical pharmacokinetics of isoniazid. Clin Pharmacokinet 1979;4:401-22.
200. Wegman P, Elingarami S, Carstensen J, Stal O, Nordenskjold B, Wingren S. Genetic variants of CYP3A5, CYP2D6, SULT1A1, UGT2B15 and tamoxifen response in postmenopausal patients with breast cancer. Breast Cancer Res 2007;9:R7.
201. Weinshilboum RM, Raymond FA, Pazmino PA. Human erythrocyte thiopurine methyltransferase: radiochemical microassay and biochemical properties. Clin Chim Acta 1978;85:323-33.
202. Willmann S, Edginton AN, Coboeken K, Ahr G, Lippert J. Risk to the breast-fed neonate from codeine treatment to the mother: a quantitative mechanistic modeling study. Clin Pharmacol Ther 2009; 86:634-43.
203. Windmill KF, Gaedigk A, Hall PM, Samaratunga H, Grant DM, McManus ME. Localization of *N*-acetyltransferases NAT1 and NAT2 in human tissues. Toxicol Sci 2000;54:19-29.
204. Wormhoudt LW, Commandeur JNM, Vermeulen NPE. Genetic polymorphisms of human *N*-acetyltransferase, cytochrome P450, glutathione-S-transferase, and epoxide hydrolase enzymes: relevance to xenobiotic metabolism and toxicity. Crit Rev Toxicol 1999;29: 59-124.
205. Wright JD, Helsby NA, Ward SA. The role of S-mephenytoin hydroxylase (CYP2C19) in the metabolism of the antimalarial biguanides. Br J Clin Pharmacol 1995;39:441-4.
206. Wu AH. Use of genetic and nongenetic factors in warfarin dosing algorithms. Pharmacogenomics 2007;8:851-61.
207. Yang CW, Hung SI, Juo CG, Lin YP, Fang WH, Lu IH, et al. HLA-B*1502-bound peptides: implications for the pathogenesis of carbamazepine-induced Stevens-Johnson syndrome. J Allergy Clin Immunol 2007;120:870-7.
208. Yip JS, Woodward M, Abreu MT, Sparrow MP. How are azathioprine and 6-mercaptopurine dosed by gastroenterologists? Results of a survey of clinical practice. Inflamm Bowel Dis 2008;14:514-8.
209. Zanger UM, Klein K, Saussele T, Blievernicht J, Hofmann MH, Schwab M. Polymorphic *CYP2B6*: molecular mechanisms and emerging clinical significance. Pharmacogenomics 2007;8:743-59.
210. Zanger UM, Raimundo S, Eichelbaum M. Cytochrome P450 2D6: overview and update on pharmacology, genetics, biochemistry. Naunyn Schmiedebergs Arch Pharmacol 2004;369:23-37.
211. Zhang D, Chando TJ, Everett DW, Patten CJ, Dehal SS, Humphreys WG. In vitro inhibition of UDP glucuronosyltransferases by atazanavir and other HIV protease inhibitors and the relationship of this property to in vivo bilirubin glucuronidation. Drug Metab Dispos 2005;33:1729-39.
212. Zhou HH. *CYP2C19* genotype determines enzyme activity and inducibility of S-mephenytoin hydroxylase. Clin Chim Acta 2001;313: 203-8.
213. Zhou SF, Di YM, Chan E, Du YM, Chow VD, Xue CC, et al. Clinical pharmacogenetics and potential application in personalized medicine. Curr Drug Metab 2008;9:738-84.
214. Zucker SD, Qin X, Rouster SD, Yu F, Green RM, Keshavan P, et al. Mechanism of indinavir-induced hyperbilirubinemia. Proc Natl Acad Sci U S A 2001;98:12671-6.

CHAPTER 44

Hematopoietic Malignancies

Kojo S. J. Elenitoba-Johnson, M.D.

The hematologic malignancies include leukemias, lymphomas, myeloproliferative disorders, and plasma cell neoplasia. The leukemias are primarily bone marrow and peripheral blood–based processes, whereas the lymphomas are tissue based. The plasma cell dyscrasias are predominantly bone marrow–based diseases. The genetic aberrations that occur in hematopoietic neoplasia may be point mutations, deletions or amplifications of genetic material, chromosomal gains or losses, or translocations. These genetic abnormalities generally lead to deregulation of the function of proto-oncogenes, tumor suppressor genes, or genes involved in the regulation of apoptosis. Identification of genetic abnormalities that underlie the pathogenesis of various hematopoietic malignancies has permitted the development of tumor classification schemes based on nonrandom genetic alterations, the creation of tumor-specific therapeutic interventions, and the use of molecular tests that serve as important adjuncts in the monitoring, prognostics, and overall management of patients with hematopoietic malignancies.

This chapter reviews the molecular basis for the development of human hematopoietic malignancies and includes a discussion of the diagnostic techniques that are used routinely in molecular diagnostic laboratories for the detection and quantification of the distinctive molecular genetic abnormalities that are characteristic of different human leukemias and lymphomas. Where relevant, some detail is provided on the pathogenesis of specific neoplasms that provide insights into the molecular basis for the particular assay design. Additionally, somatic mutations in "karyotypically normal" leukemias that carry important prognostic implications are discussed. Finally, the ability to profile mutations that confer resistance to tyrosine kinase inhibitors ushers in the era of personalized medicine such that specific treatment options can be offered, depending on the known resistance properties conferred by specific mutations.

ANTIGEN RECEPTOR REARRANGEMENTS FOR DETERMINATION OF CLONALITY

The histologic features that distinguish benign reactive lymphocytic proliferations from malignant populations can be subtle and somewhat subjective. The introduction of molecular biological techniques into diagnostic pathology has refined lymphoma diagnostics and classification. B and T lymphocytes exhibit the unique property of rearrangement of the immunoglobulin (Ig) and T-cell receptor (TCR) genes, respectively. Immunoglobulin and T-cell receptor genes encode the amino acid sequences of polypeptides that constitute the corresponding antigen receptor. Antigen receptor molecules mediate antigen recognition and are responsible for the specificity of the normal immune response. B lymphocytes are the mediators of humoral response and produce immunoglobulins, and T lymphocytes mediate the cellular response. Each reactive lymphocyte carries a unique antigen receptor gene sequence; therefore, identification of clonal populations arising from a parent malignant lymphocyte becomes feasible because the malignant population is characteristically monoclonal. Tests for monoclonality were originally developed using the Southern blotting hybridization (SBH) method, which remains the gold standard for specificity for detection of clonality throughout a broad range of lymphoid malignancies (Table 44-1). More recently, SBH has been complemented by polymerase chain reaction (PCR)-based strategies.

Molecular Genetic Basis for Immunoglobulin Gene Rearrangements

Humoral immunity is achieved by the cognitive and effector functions provided by B lymphocytes. Immunoglobulins are produced exclusively by B lymphocytes and constitute the hallmark of the humoral response. Ig molecules are heterodimeric polypeptides composed of two identical 50 to 70 kDa

TABLE 44-1 Detection Frequency of Antigen Receptor Gene Rearrangements by Southern Blot Analysis

	Cases With Antigen Receptor Gene Rearrangement, %					
	Immunoglobulin Genes			T-Cell Receptor Genes		
	IgH	Igκ	Igλ	TCRβ	TCRγ	TCRδ
B-Cell Neoplasms						
Precursor B-cell acute lymphoblastic leukemia/ lymphoma	100	40-50	20-25	20-30	50-60	70-80
Chronic lymphocytic leukemia/small lymphocytic lymphoma	100	100	30	<10	<10	<10
Prolymphocytic leukemia	100	100	30	Rare	Rare	NA
Hairy cell leukemia/variant	100	100	30-50	Rare	NA	NA
Lymphoplasmacytic lymphoma/immunocytoma	100	100	30	Rare	NA	NA
Marginal Zone B-Cell Lymphoma						
Low-grade, B-cell lymphoma of mucosa-associated lymphoid tissue	100	100	30	<10	Rare	NA
Splenic marginal zone lymphoma	100	100	30	0	NA	NA
Mantle cell lymphoma	100	100	50	Rare	NA	NA
Follicular lymphoma	100	100	30	<10	<10	<10
Diffuse large B-cell lymphoma	100	100	30	<10	<10	NA
Burkitt lymphoma	100	100	30-40	Rare	Rare	NA
Plasma cell myeloma	90	90	30	10	10	NA
T-Cell Neoplasms						
Precursor T-cell acute lymphoblastic leukemia/ lymphoma	20	Rare	Rare	90-95	90-95	>95
Chronic lymphocytic leukemia/prolymphocytic leukemia	<10	0	0	100	100	>90
Large Granular Lymphocytic Leukemia						
T cell	Rare	0	0	>90	>90	>90
Natural killer cell	0	0	0	0	0	0
Peripheral T-cell lymphoma, unspecified	<10	Rare	0	>90	>90	>90
Peripheral T-Cell Lymphoma, Specific Variants						
Adult T-cell leukemia/lymphoma	<10	0	0	100	>90	>90
Nasal-T/NK lymphoma	0	0	0	<10	0	Rare
Angioimmunoblastic T-cell lymphoma	20	10-20	10-20	90	90	90
Intestinal T-cell lymphoma	0	0	0	100	NA	NA
Anaplastic large cell lymphoma	10	Rare	0	60-70	60-70	90
Hepatosplenic T-cell lymphoma	0	0	0	70-80	70-80	80-90
Subcutaneous panniculitis-like T-cell lymphoma	0	0	0	>90	>90	50
Mycosis fungoides/Sézary syndrome	0	0	0	70-80	70-80	>90

Ig, Immunoglobulin; *NA,* not applicable; *NK,* natural killer cell; *TCR,* T-cell receptor.

heavy chains, associated with two identical light chains, kappa (κ) or lambda (λ) of approximately 23 kDa. The Ig chains are linked by noncovalent forces and interchain disulfide bridges, and together form a bilaterally symmetric structure. The heavy and light chain proteins encoded by their corresponding genes are composed of a tandem series of homologous segments consisting of approximately 110 amino acid residues. These segments undergo folding into 12 kDa domains with single intrachain disulfide bridges. Heavy chains contain one variable (V) and three constant (C) domains; light chains contain one N-terminal V and one C domain. In both heavy and light chains, the V domain consists of four relatively invariable framework regions of 15 to 30 amino acids separated by three 9 to 12 amino acid–long hypervariable or complementarity determining regions (CDRs). In both heavy and light chains, the CDR3 region is the farthest away from the N-terminus, and it exhibits the greatest sequence variability among the three CDRs. The

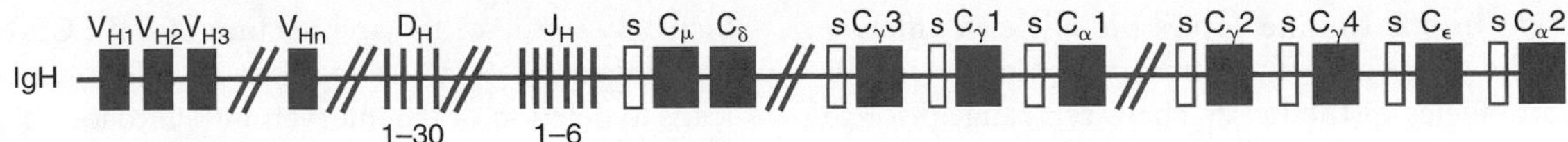

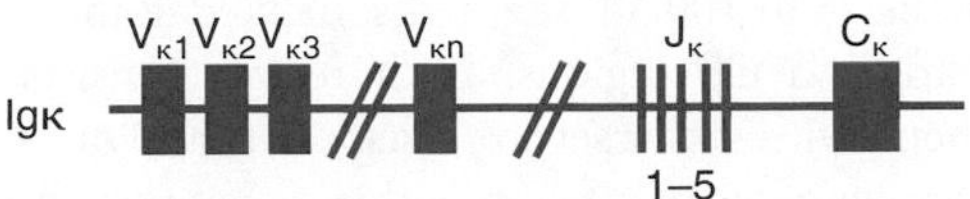

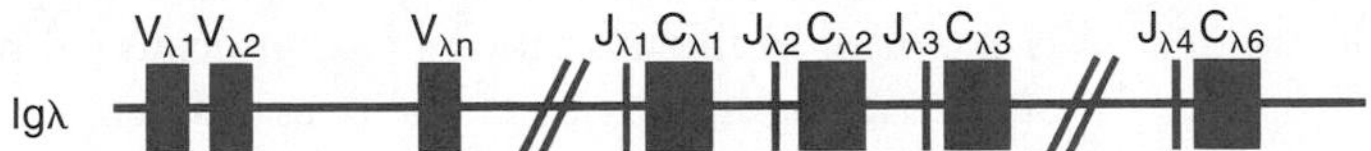

Figure 44-1 Schematic representation of germline configurations of the antigen receptor gene loci. Immunoglobulin heavy chain (IgH), immunoglobulin kappa (Igκ), and immunoglobulin lambda (Igλ) light chains. Each gene comprises several variable (V), joining (J), and constant (C) segments. Note that the IgH gene contains diversity (D) gene segments. Switch regions are indicated by *S*.

C-terminal region of secreted Ig molecules binds to complement components and Fc receptors. The genes encoding the Ig proteins are the target of DNA-based studies for clonality assessment.

The organization of Ig genes in the germline is fundamentally similar in all species studied. Genes encoding the two light chains, (κ and λ), and the single locus containing the various heavy chain genes are located on different chromosomes. To generate the large number of antibody molecules needed, B cells have evolved a unique strategy that involves recombination of germline-encoded immunoglobulin gene segments and a somatic hypermutation mechanism that further diversifies the reactivities of the rearranged antigen receptor molecules.[140] The immunoglobulin heavy and light chain gene loci—IgH, Igκ, and Igλ—are located at chromosomes 14q32, 2p12, and 22q11, respectively. In the germline configuration, all antigen receptor genes are composed of discontinuous DNA segments that are referred to as variable (V), diversity (D), joining (J), and constant (C) regions. Although both Ig heavy and light chain genes contain V, J, and C regions, only the IgH genes contain D regions (Figure 44-1). The IgH gene contains approximately 87 VH, 30 DH, and 6 JH segments. The IgH VH segment genes can be categorized into seven families, based on relatedness of the DNA sequences. The ability of Ig genes to undergo recombination in a manner analogous to shuffling of cards affords the capacity to generate an enormous primary repertoire of 10^9 Ig molecules (Figure 44-2). The human Ig C region contains 11 C region segments, which define nine functional immunoglobulin classes and subclasses (IgM, IgD, IgG1, IgG2, IgG3, IgG4, IgA1, IgA2, and IgE). The C region genes are initially uninvolved in the rearrangement process, but are subsequently juxtaposed to the VDJ complex during RNA splicing. Incorporation of C regions into the rearranged VDJ recombination permits class switching. Thus, the specific V(D)J rearrangement can be expressed as IgG, IgA, or other Ig classes. Following the formation of a productive IgH rearrangement, the light chain loci undergo a similar recombination process involving the joining of V to J segments, because no D segments are present in the light chain loci.[28]

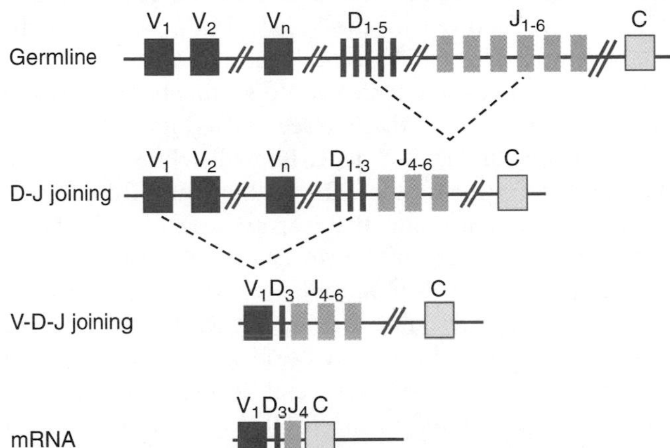

Figure 44-2 Schematic representation of antigen receptor gene rearrangement mechanism using the immunoglobulin heavy chain (IgH) locus as a model. An initial DJ joins in a partial/incomplete recombination, followed by a VDJ joining to complete the rearrangement. The C regions are included at the mRNA level via RNA splicing to form a V(D)JC transcript.

The Igκ light chain gene is located on chromosome 2p11-13 and contains up to 1000 Vκ genes, five Jκ segments, and one Cκ gene. A κ-deleting sequence (element) is present 3′ to the Cκ region. In Igλ-expressing B cells in which the Igκ genes are not productively rearranged, the κ-deleting element undergoes rearrangement such that the Cκ locus is deleted. The Igλ light chain is situated on chromosome 22q11 and is composed of several Vλ segments with Jλ and Cλ segments arranged in tandem. The Cλ locus is polymorphic and may be present in one to nine copies per allele in different individuals. The hierarchy of the rearrangement events is such that both alleles of the heavy chain rearrange prior to the light chain genes, and the kappa (κ) light chain locus is productively rearranged before (in most cases, but not always) the λ light chain genes. Thus, the immunoglobulin lambda (λ) light chain gene is not favored for clonality analysis because it frequently rearranges after the κ light chain gene. In addition, because most clonal rearrangements of the immunoglobulin heavy chain gene can be detected in up to 95% of clonal processes, it has become customary to perform only Southern blot analysis for the IgH locus in many laboratories.

Molecular Genetic Basis for T-Cell Receptor Gene Rearrangements

A similar process as described for the Ig genes occurs in the T-cell receptor (TCR) genes, with the notable exception of the absence of a somatic hypermutation mechanism in T-cell receptor gene rearrangements. The developmental hierarchy of T-cell receptor genes is such that the TCR-δ gene is the first to rearrange, followed by the TCRγ, TCRβ, and then the TCRα genes.[26] The TCR-δ gene is located on chromosome 14q11 and contains six or fewer Vδ segments, only two or three Dδ segments, and three Jδ segments (Figure 44-3). It is located within the TCR-α gene, immediately 3′ to the last TCR-Vα gene and 5′ to the TCR-Jα segments. This location is important in that productive rearrangements of the TCRδ gene lead to expression of the γ/δ TCR. In the event that the TCRδ rearrangement is nonproductive, Vα to Jα rearrangements obligatorily require that the TCRδ be deleted. The TCRα gene is located on band 14q11 and flanks the TCRδ gene on either side; it contains several Vα segments, an extensive J region composed of up to 50 Jα genes, and one Cα locus. By virtue of the architecture of the TCRα and δ loci, rearrangement of a Vα segment to a Jα segment typically leads to deletion of the intervening TCRδ loci. T cells undergoing such rearrangements may go on to express the TCR-α/β protein. The TCRβ gene is located on band 7q34 and contains 75 to 100 Vβ segments, flanked at the 3′ end by two Dβ, Jβ, and Cβ regions. Each region consists of one Dβ segment, with six or seven Jβ segments and one Cβ segment. Rearrangements may occur within or between segments (e.g., Vβ1 to Jβ1, Vβ2 to Jβ1). Extensive sequence homology is noted between the Cβ1 and Cβ2 segments. This phenomenon is exploited in the utilization of a consensus Cβ probe in the Southern blotting–based clonality assessment of TCR genes. The TCRγ gene is located on band 7q15 and contains about 11 Vγ segments and two Jγ genes.[24] The simple structure of the architecture of this gene favors its utilization as a target for TCR receptor PCR, where consensus primers are designed to encompass the relatively few Vγ and the Jγ genes.

Southern Blot Hybridization Analysis for Antigen Receptor Gene Rearrangements

In this procedure, high-quality total cellular DNA extracted from a fresh or fresh-frozen specimen is subjected to digestion using different bacterial restriction endonucleases, which produce DNA fragments of different sizes encompassing the Ig or TCR gene region segments to be interrogated (Figures 44-4 and 44-5). Enzyme-restricted DNA from each enzyme is subjected to gel electrophoresis and is transferred by blotting and immobilized on a membrane. A labeled probe complementary to the Ig J region segment is hybridized to the membrane. Clonal rearrangements are recognized by the identification of one or two novel rearranged bands that are distinct from the germline pattern obtained with a benign sample or placental DNA. One or two novel rearranged

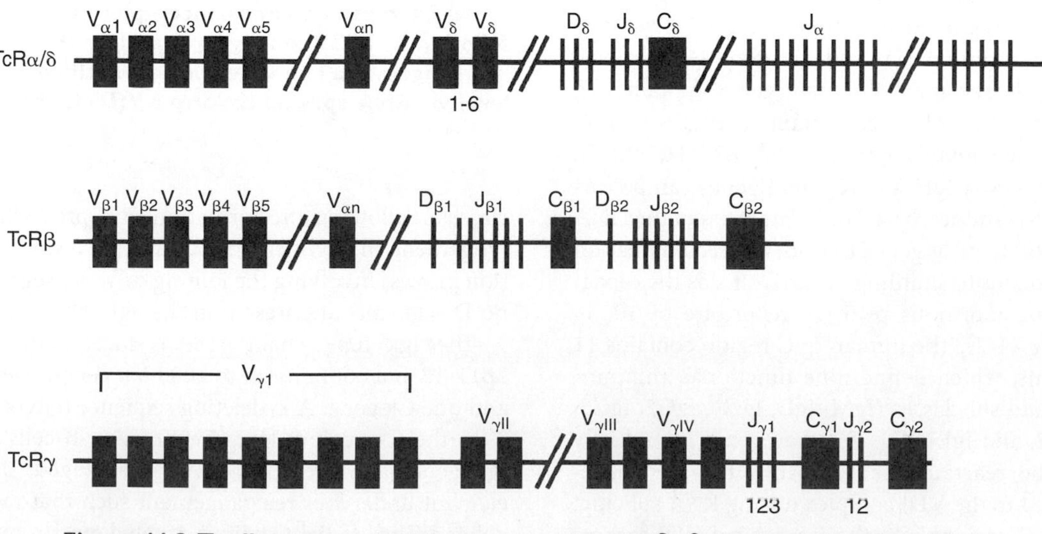

Figure 44-3 T-cell receptor (TCR) genes consist of α/δ-, β-, and γ-chain genes. The architectural configurations are similar to those of the immunoglobulin (Ig) loci. Note that only the TCRβ- and δ-chain genes contain diversity (D) regions.

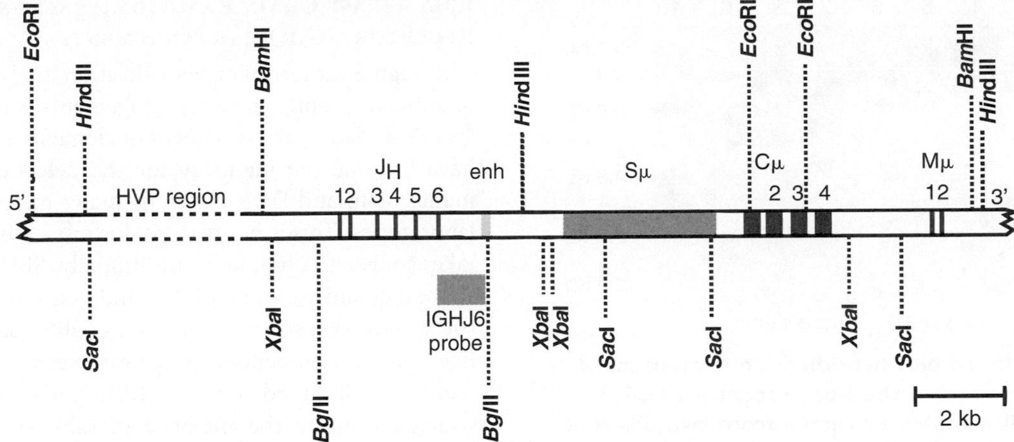

Figure 44-4 Restriction map of the immunoglobulin heavy chain (IgH) locus. The sites of the enzyme restriction sites determine the sizes of the fragments that are visualized using the IgH J6 probe as illustrated (e.g., BamHI, XbaI, and BglII enzymes yield 16 kb, 6.2 kb, and 3.8 kb fragments, respectively). Restriction patterns different from the germline patterns are indicative of a novel rearrangement event.

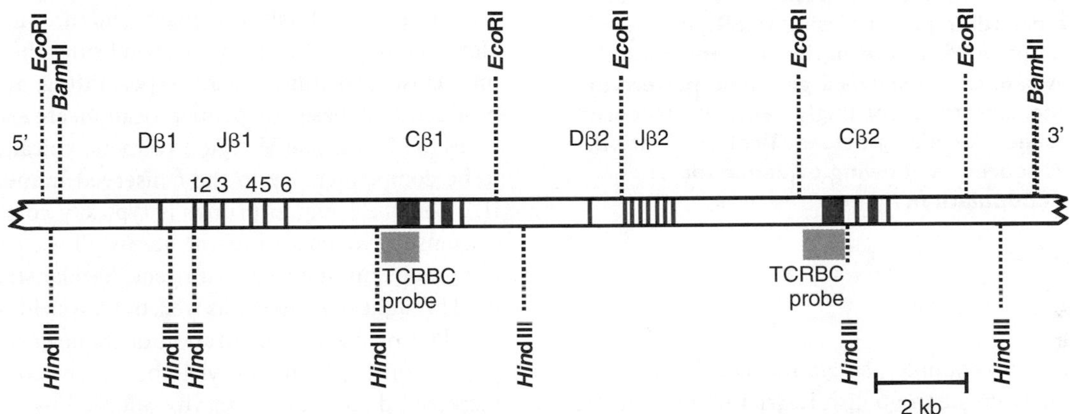

Figure 44-5 Restriction map of the T-cell receptor (TCR)β chain locus. The probe is complementary to the TCRβ constant region. Extensive sequence homology is noted between the Cβ1 and Cβ2 segments. Thus the Cβ probe hybridizes to both the Cβ1 and Cβ2 segments, thereby resulting in two germline band signals for all enzymes depicted, except BamHI. The EcoRI site located between the Cβ1 and Jβ2 segments is notoriously resistant to digestion and may yield a partial digest with a band of 8.0 kb.

(nongermline) bands may be identifiable, depending on whether a clonal monoallelic or biallelic rearrangement is present (Figure 44-6).

Material suitable for Southern blot analysis includes fresh tissue or aspiration biopsy material, as long as sufficient cellular material can be obtained from the specimen of interest. Ethanol-fixed tissue can also be successfully utilized. However, formalin-fixed tissue yields DNA of insufficient quality to permit reliable Southern blotting because of cross-linking of proteins to DNA. A Southern blot hybridization assay using three enzymes requires approximately 1.5×10^7 cells (approximately 15 μg of intact total cellular DNA). Hypothetically, all of the antigen receptor genes could be utilized as potential targets for assessment of clonality status. However, only the immunoglobulin heavy and light chains and the T-cell receptor β-chain loci have gained widespread use for clonality testing. With regard to the other T-cell loci, the TCR-α locus is impractical because it is composed of several J segments that are distributed widely apart, and it would pose practical challenges in the optimization of assays for multiple probes. Evaluation of TCRγ and δ loci is not favored because they have only a limited number of V segments, such that even reactive T-cell populations may yield confusing nongermline bands.

The diagnostic hallmark of a clonal population is the presence a nongermline novel rearranged band (see Figure 44-6). However, it is important to recognize that under certain circumstances, nongermline bands do not indicate

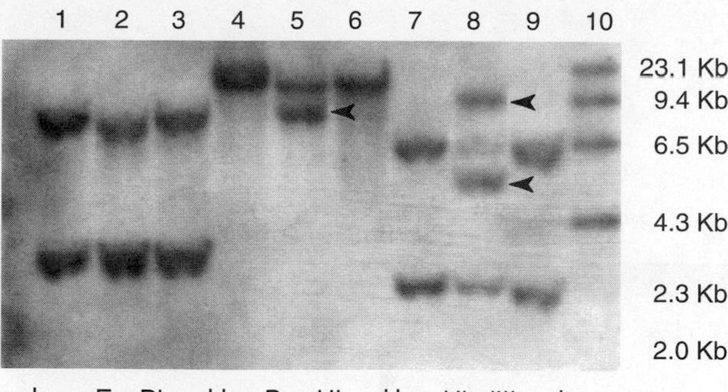

Figure 44-6 Southern blot hybridization analysis for clonal rearrangements of the T-cell receptor (TCR)β chain locus. DNA samples extracted from two different patients with a suspected diagnosis of T-cell lymphoma are assessed. *Lanes 1 to 3* represent the EcoRI digests. *Lanes 4 to 6* show the BamHI digests, and *lanes 7 to 9* demonstrate the HindIII digests from both samples run side by side. *Lane 10* shows the DNA size marker. *Lanes 1, 4,* and *7* show the restriction patterns in the germline control (placenta) using the EcoRI, BamHI, and HindIII enzymes, respectively. DNA from patient 1 *(lanes 2, 5,* and *8)* shows a germline pattern using EcoRI, but novel rearrangements *(arrowheads)* using BamHI and HindIII. Patient 2 *(lanes 3, 6,* and *9)* shows a germline pattern in all three enzyme digests. Accordingly, sample 1 is scored as showing evidence for a monoclonal T-cell population, and sample 2 is scored as showing evidence for a polyclonal T-cell population.

monoclonality. For example, single-nucleotide polymorphisms (SNPs) may create or abolish restriction enzyme recognition sites, thus yielding fragments with novel restriction banding patterns. In this scenario, utilization of a different enzyme would yield a germline configuration. The potential of these SNPs to confound the interpretation of Southern blot studies justifies the utilization of up to three or more enzymes for the unequivocal assignment of monoclonality. A second situation in which a nongermline band may occur and yet not indicate monoclonality is partial digestion. This is typically evident in the control sample (placental DNA) and invalidates the significance of any such band in the test sample. Clonal rearrangements of the Ig or TCR genes have been used to ascertain the lineage of hematologic neoplasms that do not express B- or T-cell specific markers. Intuitively, clonal rearrangements of Ig genes would indicate B-cell processes, and clonal rearrangements of TCR genes would indicate T-cell processes. However, some malignant lymphomas and leukemias may demonstrate both Ig and TCR rearrangements. In particular, acute leukemias and lymphoblastic lymphomas may demonstrate both Ig and TCR gene rearrangements. Further, up to 20% of acute myeloid leukemias may demonstrate rearrangements of Ig or TCR genes.[20,59,73] Hence, lineage is best assigned using a combination of immunophenotypical and molecular studies.

Polymerase Chain Reaction Analysis of Antigen Receptor Gene Rearrangements

Although Southern blot hybridization analysis for detection of antigen receptor gene rearrangements is recognized as the "gold standard" for assessment of clonality, PCR-based assays have become the mainstay for the detection of rearrangements of Ig and TCR genes in many molecular diagnostic laboratories. This is because SBH is more labor-intensive and takes longer to complete. Additionally, SBH requires a substantial quantity of intact DNA and hence is less amenable to specimens with suboptimal DNA quality (as is the case with fixed paraffin-embedded tissue samples). PCR on the other hand is well suited for the utilization of such specimens, which constitute the majority of samples analyzed in the clinical laboratory.

Application of PCR for the identification of clonality entails the utilization of consensus V region and J region primers and in vitro amplification of DNA across the V(D)J junction, followed by gel electrophoresis or other methods to determine the size distribution of PCR-generated fragments. In the germline configuration, V and J region segments are located several kilobases apart and are not amplifiable. However, the V(D)J recombination brings the VDJ segments into close proximity, thereby permitting amplification of products that, based on primer location, are usually 80 to 350 bases in length. The V region primers typically are designed to be complementary to the conserved framework (I, II, or III), and the J region primer is typically complementary to consensus sequences present across all six J regions in the immunoglobulin heavy chain gene. Similar strategies may be used for light chain genes as well, but the yield is lower; hence, IgH-PCR is favored. Utilization of framework III consensus primers offers the highest yield but can be complemented by increased diagnostic sensitivity afforded by the inclusion of framework II and/or framework I primer-mediated IgH-PCR for clonality. With regard to T-cell assays, the TCRγ-PCR is the most informative. In these assays, monoclonal populations yield one or two dominant bands (Figure 44-7), while polyclonal cells, each of which carries a unique rearrangement with slightly different band sizes, demonstrate a ladder or smear pattern on gel electrophoresis.[81,130] Thus the specificity of each rearrangement identified by PCR is determined by the junctional sequence; hence the marker of clonality in PCR differs from that in SBH analysis, wherein the marker is the configuration of rearranged antigen receptor genes.

Following PCR, the amplification products are analyzed by agarose or polyacrylamide gel electrophoresis and are visualized by ethidium bromide staining.[38,138] Agarose gels, although less expensive, do not provide resolution of polyacrylamide, which can be configured to reliably discriminate bands differing in size by as few as three bases. This is often very useful in the assessment of PCR products for antigen receptor gene rearrangement assays. Further resolution may be achieved by evaluating sequence-specific and melting characteristics of double-stranded DNA using denaturation gradient gel electrophoresis or temperature gradient gel electrophoresis.[55] More recently, capillary gel electrophoresis has

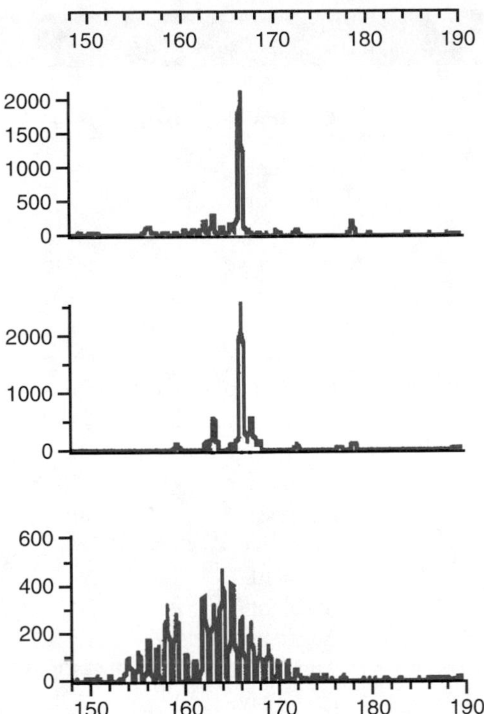

Figure 44-7 Polymerase chain reaction (PCR) analysis for clonal rearrangements of the antigen receptor gene loci. PCR analysis of the T-cell receptor (TCR) γ-chain locus is shown. The *upper and middle panels* show duplicate assays with monoclonal capillary electrophoretic peaks of identical size (≈166 bp) in the two replicates. The *bottom panel* shows a polyclonal pattern.

become a preferred method for analysis of antigen receptor gene rearrangement. A successful study would exhibit PCR products in the expected size range, appropriate results in positive and negative controls, and absence of bands in the template-free (H_2O) control.

PCR-based clonality assays are less sensitive in detecting all possible clonal rearrangements when compared with SBH analysis, which approaches 100% if sufficient restriction enzymes and a variety of probes are used. Depending on the assay and the lymphoid neoplasm tested, PCR-based clonality studies may show false-negative rates from 10 to 40% when compared with SBH. False negatives occur for several reasons. First, in contrast to SBH, PCR does not detect partial DJ rearrangements, wherein V and J region genes are not approximated to one another and are too distant for conventional PCR to generate an amplification product. Second, the consensus primers are incapable of hybridizing to all of the different V regions, any one of which could be potentially present in any single neoplasm. Of particular importance to the Ig genes, somatic mutations occurring within the Ig V region genes result in decreased ability for the consensus V region primers to anneal optimally to the V region genes in the template DNA. Thus lymphoid neoplasias with a high somatic hypermutation rate, such as follicular lymphoma, yield lower positive rates by PCR-based Ig clonality tests.[125,126] Most of the difficulties described previously can be overcome by the utilization of multiple primer sets. In the event of a negative PCR result, SBH analysis may be performed if sufficient high-quality genomic DNA is available. The main drawback for PCR is the propensity for contamination. Various strategies for contamination control such as maintaining separate DNA extraction and amplification rooms, utilization of laminar flow hoods, and incorporation of uracil DNA glycosylase into PCR should be employed as a rule to prevent contamination problems.

The ability to detect rare DNA species carrying a specific molecular aberration (sensitivity) of PCR is dependent on the particular application. For antigen receptor gene rearrangement studies, PCR can detect a monoclonal population in a background of 10^2 to 10^3 polyclonal cells of the same phenotype (B or T cells). By comparison, PCR can detect one cell harboring a chromosomal translocation within a background of 10^5 to 10^6cells negative for the translocation.[92]

MOLECULAR GENETICS OF MALIGNANT LYMPHOMAS

Antigen receptor gene rearrangements, which are integral to normal B- and T-cell development, and the elaboration of an appropriate immune response are fraught with susceptibility for abnormal translocation of foreign genes, deregulation of which contributes to the development of lymphoid neoplasia. A translocation typically involves the transfer of chromosomal material from one chromosome to a different chromosome. Indeed, nonrandom chromosomal translocations are frequently observed in hematologic neoplasia, and in many cases are characteristic of specific types of tumors. Translocations typically occur in one of two structural configurations, each with distinctive genetic consequences. In the first scenario, the translocation results in the juxtaposition of the intact coding sequence of an oncogene in close proximity with an antigen receptor gene, leading to dysregulated expression and increased production of the structurally normal oncoprotein. This mechanism is most frequently seen in malignant lymphomas, as exemplified by the t(14;18)(q32;q21) characteristic of follicular lymphoma. This translocation juxtaposes the *BCL2* gene on 18q21 adjacent to the IgH gene on 14q32, leading to overexpression of BCL2 mRNA and protein.[142] In the second scenario, chromosomal translocation leads to an in-frame juxtaposition of two different genes, with resultant creation of a novel chimeric gene. This mechanism is most commonly observed in the leukemias, and less commonly in malignant lymphomas. The t(2;5)(2p23;q35) seen in anaplastic large cell lymphoma is one example wherein an abnormal fusion gene *(NPM-ALK)* is formed and is central to pathogenesis.[96] As another example, the t(11;18)(q21;q21) seen in a subset of extranodal marginal zone B-cell lymphomas of mucosa-associated lymphoid tissue leads to formation of an abnormal *API-MALT1* chimeric gene fusion.[29] Reverse transcription PCR is a well-suited strategy for the diagnostic detection of such chimeric fusions, because the fusion product is often within the size range of amplifiability of conventional PCR. Many of the translocation

TABLE 44-2 Common Recurrent Genetic Alterations in Human Malignant Lymphoma

Aberration	Genes (@) Involved Loci*	Disease	Clinical Features	Frequency, %
t(14;18)(q32;q21)	*BCL2/IGH@*	FL	Indolent	≈90
t(2;18)(p12;q21)	*IGK@/BCL2*	FL	Indolent	<5
t(3;14)(q27;q32)	*BCL6/IGH@*	FL	Indolent	≈10
t(11;14)(q13;q32)	*BCL1/IGH@*	MCL	Aggressive	>90
Trisomy 3	Unknown	MZBCL-MALT	Indolent	Variable
t(11;18)(p21;q21)	*BIRC3*/MALT1	MZBCL	Antibiotic resistant	50
t(1;14)(p22;q32)	*BCL10/IGH@*	MZBCL	Indolent	†
t(8;14)(q24;q32)	*CMYC/IGH@*	Burkitt lymphoma	Highly aggressive	75
t(2;8)(p12;q24)	*CMYC/IGK@*	Burkitt lymphoma	Highly aggressive	15
t(8;22)(q24;q11)	*CMYC/IGL@*	Burkitt lymphoma	Highly aggressive	10
t(3;14)(q27;q32)	*BCL6/IGH@*	DLBCL	Aggressive	≈30
t(14;18)(q32;q21)	*BCL2/IGH@*	DLBCL	Aggressive	30
Amplification 9p	*REL*	PMLBCL	Agressive	†
Del 13q14	Unknown	B-CLL	Indolent	25-50
Trisomy 12	Unknown	B-CLL	Indolent	30
t(11;14)(q13;q32)	*CCND1/IGH@*	B-PLL	Aggressive	†
t(2;5)(p23;q35)	*NPM/ALK*	ALCL,T/NK	Aggressive	≈40
Inv 14(q11;q32) or complex translocations involving both chromosomes 14	Unknown	T-PLL	Aggressive	75
Isochromosome 7q	Unknown	Hepatosplenic γ/δ	Aggressive	†
Trisomy 8	Unknown	Hepatosplenic γ/δ	Aggressive	†
Del 6q23.3-q24	*A20/TNFAIP3* mutations	DLBCL	Aggressive	38
		MZBCL	Indolent	21
		cHL (NS)	Good prognosis	33

*Note that IGK and IGL are symbols for genes Igκ and Igλ, respectively.
†An insufficient number of patients were studied to permit accurate assessment of percentage of tumors with the cytogenetic aberration indicated.
ALCL, Anaplastic large-cell lymphoma; *ALL,* acute lymphoblastic leukemia; *B-CLL,* B-chronic lymphocytic leukemia; *cHL(NS),* classical Hodgkin lymphoma, nodular sclerosis subtype; *DLBCL,* diffuse large B-cell lymphoma; *FL,* follicular lymphoma; *LPL,* lymphoplasmacytic lymphoma; *MALT,* mucosa-associated lymphoid tissue; *MCL,* mantle-cell lymphoma; *MZBCL,* marginal-zone B-cell lymphoma; *NK,* natural killer; *PLL,* prolymphocytic leukemia; *PMLBCL,* primary mediastinal large B-cell lymphoma.

breakpoints are widely dispersed and are not clustered. If DNA were to be considered as the template for such PCR, it would best be performed as a long-distance (LD) PCR protocol. However, LD PCR protocols are not applicable to many clinical sample types. A list of common chromosomal translocations, participating genes, and associated lymphomas is provided in Table 44-2.

Southern Blot Hybridization Analysis for the Detection of Chromosomal Translocations

Southern blot hybridization analysis is an excellent method for the detection of chromosomal translocations. A sequence-specific probe to the gene of interest is utilized for SBH analysis, as described for the antigen receptor genes. Detection of a pattern of bands of different sizes from those seen in the germline configuration of the gene suggests the presence of a translocation. This approach method does not, however, identify the translocation partner of the gene of interest. As with the antigen receptor gene rearrangement studies by SBH, SNPs at enzyme restriction sites may result in nongermline patterns that may be misinterpreted as translocations. In this scenario, utilization of a different restriction enzyme will correctly show the gene locus to be of germline size. The labor-intensive nature of SBH and the requirement for high-quality DNA have diminished its popularity for routine detection of chromosomal translocations in the clinical laboratory. In this regard, PCR continues to gain in utilization for detection of recurrent chromosomal translocations.

Polymerase Chain Reaction Analysis for Detection of Chromosomal Translocations

PCR is well suited for analysis of chromosomal translocations, particularly when the translocation breakpoints are clustered and the sequences flanking the translocation breakpoints are well characterized.

t(14;18)(q32;21)—*BCL2/JH* Aberration

The translocation t(14;18)(q32;21), characteristic of follicular lymphoma, exemplifies the utility of PCR in the detection of a chromosomal translocation characteristic of a specific form

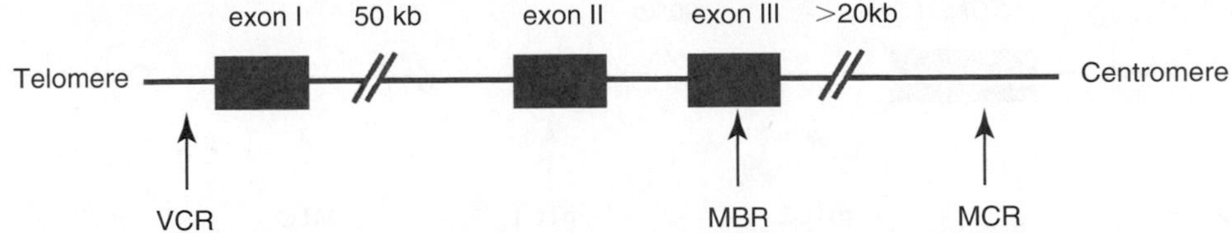

Figure 44-8 Schematic representation of the organization of the *BCL2 gene* and the most frequent breakpoints on chromosome 18q21 involved in the t(14;18). The *BCL2*exons are represented as rectangles. MBR represents the major breakpoint cluster region, where approximately 50 to 60% of breakpoints occur. MCR represents the minor breakpoint cluster region, where 20 to 25% of breakpoints may be found. VCR represents the variant cluster region, where 5 to 20% of breakpoints may be found.

of non-Hodgkin lymphoma. The t(14;18) is a balanced reciprocal translocation involving the *BCL2 gene* (18q21) and the IgH locus (14q32) (Figure 44-8). The *BCL2* gene is composed of three exons and two introns.[128] At up to four different regions on 18q21, breakpoints are frequently found. The 18q21 breakpoints in most translocations are clustered in the *major breakpoint cluster* region (MBR). The MBR is a 150 bp sequence located within the 3′ untranslated region of exon 3 of the *BCL2 gene,* and harbors approximately 60% of the breakpoints found in follicular lymphoma.[141,152] Another 20% of follicular lymphomas harbor t(14;18) aberrations in which the breakpoint is located at the *minor cluster* region, which is located 30 kb further 3′ to the *BCL2 gene.* An additional cluster of breakpoints occur within the *variant cluster region* located 5′ upstream to the *BCL2* gene, accounting for approximately 5% of the breakpoints found in follicular lymphoma (see Figure 44-8).[112] More recently, an intermediate cluster region (ICR) has been described with additional 18q21 breakpoints associated with follicular lymphoma.[1] Although initial studies comparing conventional cytogenetics, Southern blot, and PCR-based methods for detection of the t(14;18) (not including the ICR) showed that 86% of cases were identified by Southern blotting and 75% by PCR,[66] the inclusion of PCR assays targeting the ICR improves the PCR detection rate for the t(14;18).[1] Figure 44-9 shows fluorescence in situ hybridization (FISH) analysis demonstrating the t(14;18) in a sample that tested negative by PCR. An important caveat to note is that the t(14;18) has been detected in benign tonsils and reactive lymph nodes,[4,87] and in the peripheral blood of normal blood donors.

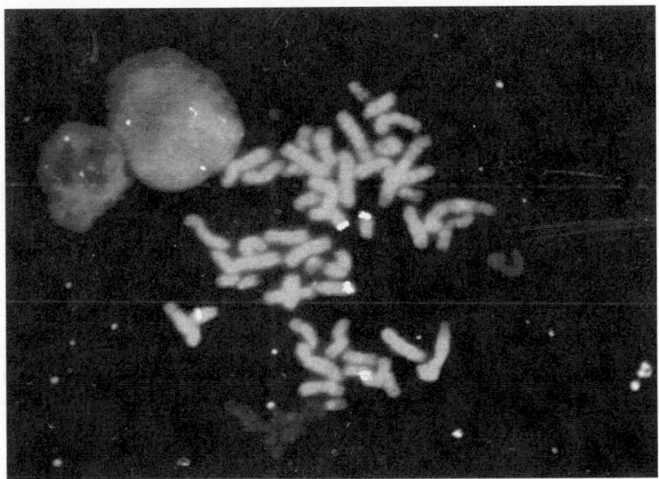

Figure 44-9 Fluorescence in situ hybridization for the t(14;18) anomaly on metaphase spreads of a case of follicular lymphoma. The immunoglobulin heavy chain sequences on 14q32 when juxtaposed to the *BCL2* sequences on 18q21 yield a fusion signal indicative of the presence of the t(14;18).

t(11;14)(q13;32)—*CCND1/JH* Aberration*

The t(11;14)(q13;32) abnormality is characteristic of mantle cell lymphoma,[85,151] but is rare in other types of malignant lymphoma. This translocation juxtaposes the *CCND1* locus on 11q13 with the immunoglobulin heavy chain gene enhancer locus at 14q32.[143] This leads to deregulation of the cyclin D1 gene with a quantitative increase in the production of normal cyclin D1 transcripts. Structurally, multiple breakpoints are found on chromosome 11. The most frequently involved location on 11q13 is the major translocation cluster (MTC) region, located 110 kb 5′ to the *CCND1* locus.[143] Other breakpoints occurring within minor translocation cluster regions have been described 3′ to the major translocation cluster but 5′ to the *CCND1* locus (Figure 44-10).[111] The *CCND1* gene is composed of five exons covering a genomic distance of approximately 15 kb.[97] The gene encodes cyclin D1, which regulates cellular transition from G1 to S phase. Despite the diversity of breakpoints flanking the *CCND1* gene, the t(11;14) does not lead to disruption of the coding region of the *CCND1* gene. Consequently, the expression of cyclin D1 is qualitatively normal but quantitatively increased. One of the practical consequences of the multiple breakpoints in mantle cell lymphoma is that approximately 70% of cases of mantle cell lymphoma can be demonstrated to harbor the t(11;14) by Southern blotting analysis using multiple probes for detection of the various breakpoints.[155] By comparison,

*Accepted gene names and symbols can be found at http://www.genenames.org/accessed July 15, 2011.

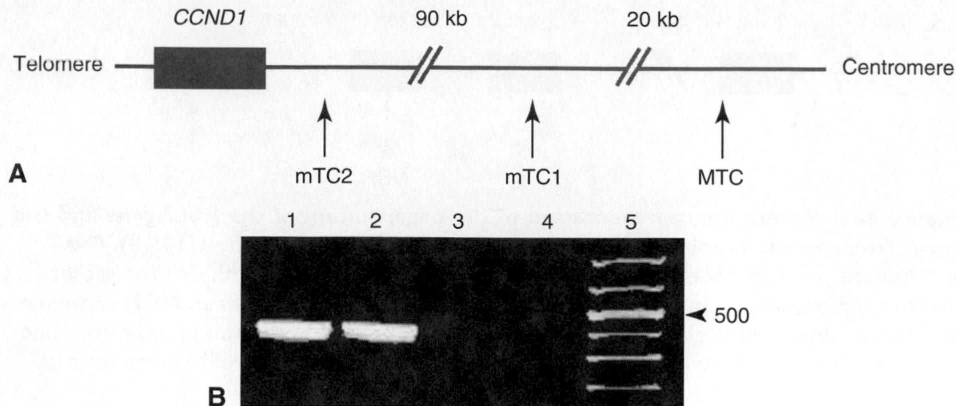

Figure 44-10 A, Schematic representation of the organization of the *CCND1* gene on chromosome 11q13 and the breakpoint regions associated with the t(11;14). The *CCND1* gene is represented as a *red rectangle*. The relative locations of the major translocation cluster (MTC), where up to 40% of the breakpoints are clustered and the minor translocation cluster regions (mTC1 and mTC2) are indicated. The size of the amplified polymerase chain reaction (PCR) product may vary, depending on the location of the breakpoints. B, PCR analysis and agarose gel electrophoresis for the detection of t(11;14). The primers were directed against the MTC of *CCND1*. *Lane 1* represents a positive control with a band at ≈450 bp. *Lane 2* is the patient sample with a positive band also at ≈450 bp. *Lane 3* contains a negative control (reactive tonsil). *Lane 4* represents a no-template (H_2O) control. *Lane 5* shows the size marker.

most published PCR protocols detect only approximately 40% of the t(11;14) anomalies in mantle cell lymphoma, and most of these are clustered in the MTC.[155] This is in marked contrast to DNA fiber FISH, which reportedly may detect up to 95% of the t(11;14) aberrations, making FISH the most sensitive method for detection of this abnormality.[145]

MOLECULAR GENETICS OF LEUKEMIAS

Human leukemias are characterized by recurrent genetic abnormalities that can be utilized as genetic markers of the specific leukemia. The genetic abnormalities are most often recurrent chromosomal translocations that result in chimeric fusions with dysregulated cellular functions, leading to differentiation block or enhancement of proliferation. The chronic leukemias of myeloid-derived cells are characterized by constitutive activation of tyrosine kinases, which primarily confer an excessive proliferative signal and an increased survival advantage. An example of this is the t(9;22), which results in the *BCR-ABL* chimeric fusion characteristic of chronic myelogenous leukemia (CML). Inhibition of activated tyrosine kinases is a bonafide therapeutic option, as in the case of imatinib mesylate (Gleevec) in CML. By comparison, the chromosomal translocations in acute myeloid leukemias typically result in loss-of-function aberrations within transcription factors that lead to maturational arrest or differentiation blocks at early stages of hematopoietic development. The preponderance of evidence suggests that genetic aberrations leading to maturational arrest in the acute myeloid leukemias are by themselves insufficient to cause leukemia. The concomitant occurrence of cooperating mutations in the *RAS* and tyrosine kinase genes *FLT3* and *C-KIT* permits progression to a frank leukemia. In either case, the presence of genetic aberrations provides a target for disease detection and monitoring, and for potential gene-specific therapy. A comprehensive list of translocations and fusions thereby arising in acute leukemias is provided in Table 44-3. The most frequently employed technique for the detection of chimeric transcripts in the molecular laboratory is reverse transcriptase–polymerase chain reaction (RT-PCR). Although it is recognized that the definitive method for detection of point mutations is sequencing, a variety of techniques may be used to screen for the presence of point mutations (e.g., single-strand conformation polymorphism analysis,[102,134] denaturation gradient gel electrophoresis,[12] fluorescence real-time PCR-based melting curve analysis).[39]

Recurrent Chromosomal Translocations in Acute Myeloid Leukemias

The translocations that occur in the acute myeloid leukemias target transcription factors or transcriptional coactivators. The transcription factors are involved in the differentiation of hematopoietic cells, and disruption of their normal function by the translocation leads to developmental arrest and maturational block at immature stages of differentiation. Targeted transcription factors include the retinoic acid receptor alpha (RARα) in acute promyelocytic leukemia (APL) and several members of the core binding factor (CBF) complex. Core binding factor is a transcription factor composed of heterodimers including a DNA-binding component known as *AML1 (RUNX1/CBFA2/PEBP2A)* and a subunit CBFβ that activates the transcription of *AML1*. CBF is targeted in the t(8;21)[43] aberration, which results in the AML/*ETO* fusion characteristic of acute myelogenous

TABLE 44-3 Common Recurrent Genetic Alterations in Human Leukemia

Aberration or Locus	Genes (@) Involved Loci	Disease	Clinical Features	Frequency, %*
t(9;22)(q34;q11)	*BCR/ABL (p210)*	CML	Good prognosis	95
9p24	*JAK2 V617F*	PV	Fair prognosis	95
9p24	*JAK2 V617F*	ET	Fair prognosis	50
9p24	*JAK2 V617F*	IMF	Poor prognosis	35
1p34	*MPL S505N*	IMF	Poor prognosis	9
1p34	*MPL W515X*	IMF	Poor prognosis	5
t(12;21) cryptic	*TEL/AML1*	Precursor B-cell ALL	Good prognosis	20-25
t(9;22)(q34;q11)	*BCR/ABL (p190)*	Precursor B-cell ALL	Poor prognosis	5-20
t(1;19)(q23;p13)	*E2A/PBX*	Precursor B-cell ALL	Pre-B phenotype (cytoplasmic μ), poor response to antimetabolites	3-6
t(4;11)(q21;q23)	*MLL/AF4*	Precursor B-cell ALL	Mixed lineage, infants, poor prognosis, leukocytosis	3
t(11;19)(q23;p13)	*MLL/ENL*	Precursor B-cell ALL	Leukocytosis	<1
t(8;14)(q24;q32)	*CMYC/IGH@*	B-ALL	FAB L3, mature B-cell phenotype, extramedullary disease	85
t(2;8)(p12;q24)	*CMYC/IGK@*	B-ALL	FAB L3, mature B-cell phenotype, extramedullary disease	10
t(8;22)(q24;q11)	*CMYC/IGL@*	B-ALL	FAB L3, mature B-cell phenotype, extramedullary disease	5
None	*TAL1* deletion	Precursor T-cell ALL	Extramedullary disease, CD2+, CD10+	25
t(1;14)(p32;q11)	*TRD@/TAL1*	Precursor T-cell ALL	Extramedullary disease, CD2+, CD10+	3
t(1;7)(p32;q35)	*TRB@/TAL1*	Precursor T-cell ALL	Extramedullary disease, CD2+, CD10+	<1
t(8;14)(q24;q11)	*TRA@/CMYC*	Precursor T-cell ALL	Extramedullary disease	2
t(11;14)(p15;q11)	*TRD@/RBTN1*	Precursor T-cell ALL	Extramedullary disease	<1
t(11;14)(p13;q11)	*TRD@/RBTN2*	Precursor T-cell ALL	Extramedullary disease	7
t(10;14)(q24;q11)	*TRD@/HOX11*	Precursor T-cell ALL	Extramedullary disease	4
t(1;7)(p34;q34)	*TRB@/LCK*	Precursor T-cell ALL	Extramedullary disease	1
t(8;13)(p11;q11-12)	*FGFRI/ZNF198*	Precursor T-cell ALL	Extramedullary disease	<1
t(8;21)(q22;q22)	*AML1/ETO*	AML	AML-FAB M2	10-15
inv(16)(p13;q22)	*CBFβ/MYH11*	AML	FAB M4EO	10
t(6;9)(p23;q34)	*DEK/CAN*	AML	Basophilia	2
t(9;11)(p22;q23)	*MLL/AF9*	AML	FAB M4-M5, infants	5
t(8;16)(p11;p13)	*MOZ/CBP*	AML	FAB M4, M5	<1
t(7;11)(p15;p15)	*NUP98/HOXA9*	AML	FAB M2, M4	1
t(3;5)(q25;q34)	*NPM/MLF 1*	AML	Myelodysplastic syndrome	1
t(15;17)(q22;q21)	*PML/RARA*	AML	FAB M3, coagulopathy, good retinoic acid response	7
t(11;17)(q23;q21)	*PLZF/RARA*	AML	FAB M3, coagulopathy, poor retinoic acid response	<1
t(5;17)(q32;q21)	*NPM/RARA*	AML	FAB M3, coagulopathy, poor retinoic acid response	<1

*Estimated frequency per clinical disease category.

ALL, Acute lymphoblastic leukemia; *AML*, acute myelogenous leukemia; *CML*, chronic myelogenous leukemia; *ET*, essential thrombocythemia; *FAB* (with L3, M3, M4EO, etc.), French-American-British classifications; *IMF*, idiopathic myelofibrosis; *LOH*, loss of heterozygosity; *p210* and *p190*, chimeric proteins (see text); *MPL*, myeloproliferative leukemia virus oncogene homology; *PV*, polycythemia vera; *TRB@*, *TRD@*, T-cell receptor β and δ loci.

leukemia (AML) with differentiation (AML FAB-M2). CBF is similarly targeted in the inv(16), which leads to generation of a fusion gene *(CBFβ/SMMHC)* comprised of *CBFβ* and the smooth muscle myosin heavy chain gene *(SMMHC)* found in a subset of AML4Eo.[88] The multilineage importance of CBF is manifest in a subset of precursor B-cell acute lymphoblastic leukemias, where it is targeted in the t(12;21), which leads to the TEL/*AML1* fusion.[54] All chimeric proteins that result from chimeric fusions are dominant negative inhibitors of CBF-mediated transcription.[49,62] The transcriptional repression of CBF target genes caused by CBF-chimeric proteins partially involves recruitment of the histone deacetylase complex.

By comparison, APL is characterized by translocations involving the RARα gene (see Table 44-3). These translocations result in a block of myeloid differentiation at the promyelocytic stage. It has been shown that maturational arrest is due in part to recruitment of the nuclear corepressor–histone deacetylase complex. The ability of all-*trans* retinoic acid (ATRA) to bind to *PML/RARα*, resulting in release of the nuclear corepressor complex, explains in part the ability of ATRA to relieve the maturational block in promyelocytes central to the development of APL.

t(8;21)(q22;q22)—AML1-ETO

The t(8;21)(q22;q22) was originally described in a case of acute leukemia by Janet Rowley in 1973.[113] The translocation is found in approximately 7% of cases of de novo AML and is more common in young individuals. The translocation is found in 20 to 40% of AMLs of the FAB-M2 subtype.[3] It has been reported infrequently in AML FAB-M1, AML FAB-M4, and rare cases of therapy-associated AML. The translocation leads to fusion of the *AML1* gene (acute myeloid leukemia 1 gene), also known as *CBFA2* (core binding factor subunit A2) or *PEBP2α* (polyoma enhancer binding protein 2 subunit α), to the *ETO* gene (8;21), also known as *MTG8* (myeloid translocation gene on chromosome 8).

The t(8;21) portends a good prognosis in cases of de novo AML, with a favorable response to treatment with cytosine arabinoside.[98] The *AML1-ETO* chimeric fusion is detectable by RT-PCR in the vast majority of t(8;21)-positive AMLs, thus making RT-PCR a good choice for detection of the t(8;21) in clinical samples. The *AML1-ETO* fusions join exon 5 of *AML1* to exon 2 of *ETO* (Figure 44-11), and the fusion transcript can be detected in complex translocations in a significant proportion of cases that are t(8;21) negative by conventional cytogenetics.[3,94] Specifically, RT-PCR has been reported to detect *AML1-ETO* fusions in 8 to 12% of AML.[3,79,94] It is interesting to note that the *AML1-ETO* fusion transcript may be detected using sensitive end point PCR assays several years after chemotherapy or bone marrow transplant (BMT), thus limiting its predictive value for relapse in affected patients.[70] Quantitative studies using recently developed real-time PCR protocols (Figure 44-12) provide a better indication of increasing transcript copies and hence disease recurrence.

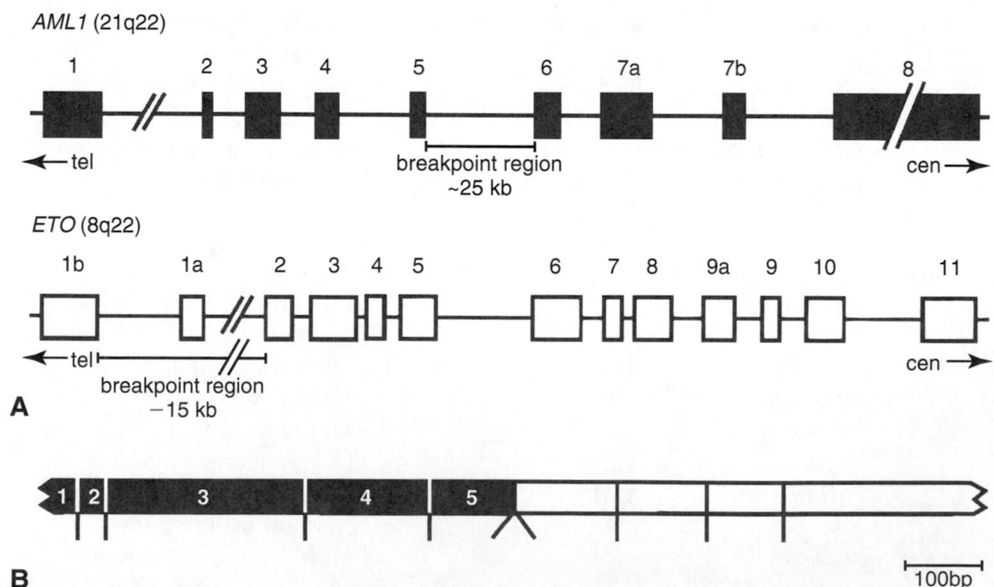

Figure 44-11 Schematic representation of the organization of the *AML1* (21q22) and *ETO* genes (8q22) involved in the t(8;21) anomaly that is characteristic of FAB AML-M2. The centromeric *(cen)* and telomeric (tel) directions are indicated. In A, the exons of the *AML1* gene are depicted in *red rectangles;* the exons of the *ETO* gene are depicted in *white rectangles.* In B, the configuration of the AML1/ETO chimeric fusion is shown. The numbers below the fusion transcript indicate the position of the first nucleotide in the exon involved, or the last nucleotide of the exon immediately 5′ to the fusion.

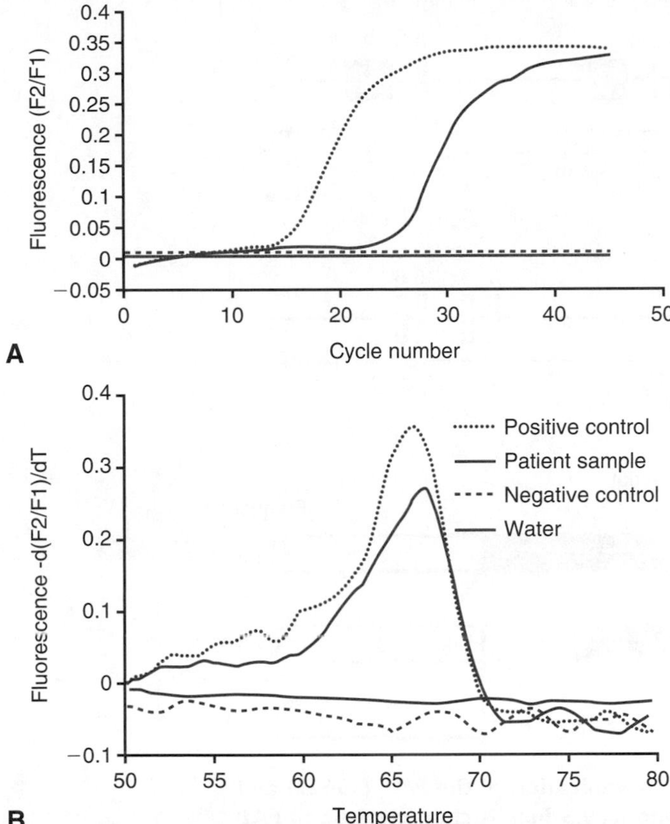

Figure 44-12 Real-time polymerase chain reaction (PCR) detection of *AML1/ETO* fusion transcript. Real-time PCR detection was performed using a sequence-specific hybridization probe format with oligonucleotide probes labeled with fluorescein as the donor fluorophore and LCRed640 as the acceptor. Postamplification melting analysis was performed to provide confirmation of amplicon identity through the probe melting temperature. A shows the fluorescence (F) versus cycle number (C) on the LightCycler (Roche Diagnostics, Indianapolis, Ind). The characteristic three-phase profiles of amplification curves are recognizable (i.e., initial lag, exponential or log/linear, and the final plateau phase). The *red dotted curve* represents the positive amplification signal for the t(8;21) in the Kasumi cell line positive control. The *red solid curve* represents the patient sample, also showing the presence of the *AML1/ETO* fusion. The *red dashed line* represents a negative control (placental cDNA), and the *red flat line* is the no-template (H_2O) control. B shows the derivative melting curves with positive melting peaks at ≈65 °C in both the Kasumi cell line positive control and the patient sample. Both negative and water controls show flat lines indicating the absence of the t(8;21) *AML1/ETO* product.

t(15;17)(q22;q21)—*PRAM1* (also known as PML-RARA)

The t(15;17) is the characteristic molecular abnormality in APL, which is classified as AML FAB-M3. This abnormality is present in virtually all cases of APL, which accounts for 5 to 10% of all AMLs. The t(15;17) results in juxtaposition of the putative transcription factor *PML* on 15q22[13,90] to the retinoic acid receptor-α gene on 17q21.[107] The breakpoints on chromosome 17 are confined to a 15 kB fragment within intron 2 of the *RARα* locus. The breakpoints on chromosome 15 are more varied with involvement of three or more distinct regions (Figure 44-13, *A*). These include intron 6 *(BCR 1)*, which is involved in approximately 55% of cases, exon 6 *(BCR 2)*, which is involved in 5% of cases, and intron 3 *(BCR 3)*, which is involved in 40% of cases. Similar to the scenario seen in the t(9;22) leading to *BCR-ABL* fusion, the different breakpoints on *PML*, the alternatively spliced transcripts, and usage of two different polyadenylation sites further give rise to a greater variety of *PML-RARα* fusion transcripts of different sizes (Figure 44-13, *B*).[10] Recognition of these varied transcripts is important in the design of diagnostic RT-PCR assays that are capable of detecting the majority of t(15;17) fusions. In this regard, most assays have been directed at the *PML-RARAα* fusion, because the reciprocal *(RARα-PML)* fusion is not detectable in some cases of APL. The PML-RARA chimeric protein contributes to leukemogenesis by blocking the differentiation of myeloid cells at the level of promyelocytes. The persistent detection of *PML-RARA* transcripts in treated patients is an ominous indicator of a tendency for relapse. Quantitative real-time PCR provides an opportunity for sensitive and specific monitoring of consecutive samples at appropriate intervals.

Recurrent Chromosomal Translocations in Chronic Leukemias of Myeloid/Monocytic Lineage

The chronic myeloid leukemias are characterized by translocations that lead to constitutive activation of tyrosine kinases. The most frequent is the t(9;22)(q34;q11), resulting in the *BCR/ABL* fusion characteristic of CML. Up to seven different chromosomal translocations are associated with the chronic leukemias of myeloid/monocytic lineage, and all are characterized by the formation of a chimeric fusion with a carboxy-terminal tyrosine kinase domain and an oligomerization motif in the amino-terminus of the fusion protein. The oligomerization motif is important for the constitutive activation of tyrosine kinase, which transforms hematopoietic cells and confers them with ligand-independent growth potential.

t(9;22)(q34;q11)—*BCR-ABL* Aberration

The t(9;22) Philadelphia chromosome is the diagnostic hallmark of CML and is found in virtually 100% of cases. The translocation is also found in up to 20 to 50% of acute lymphoblastic leukemias (ALLs) in adults, in 2 to 10% of childhood ALLs, and in rare cases of malignant lymphoma and myeloma.[11,75-77,91] The t(9;22) results in the juxtaposition of 3′ sequences on the *c-ABL* tyrosine kinase proto-oncogene (9q34) to the 5′ sequences of the breakpoint cluster region *BCR* gene (22q11). The t(9;22) results in the formation of two hybrid genes: *BCR-ABL* on the derivative chromosome 22, and *ABL-BCR* on the derivative chromosome 9.[27] The *BCR-ABL* fusion encodes a chimeric protein with constitutively activated tyrosine kinase activity. Although the breakpoints on chromosome 9 are relatively constant and 5′ to exon 2 of

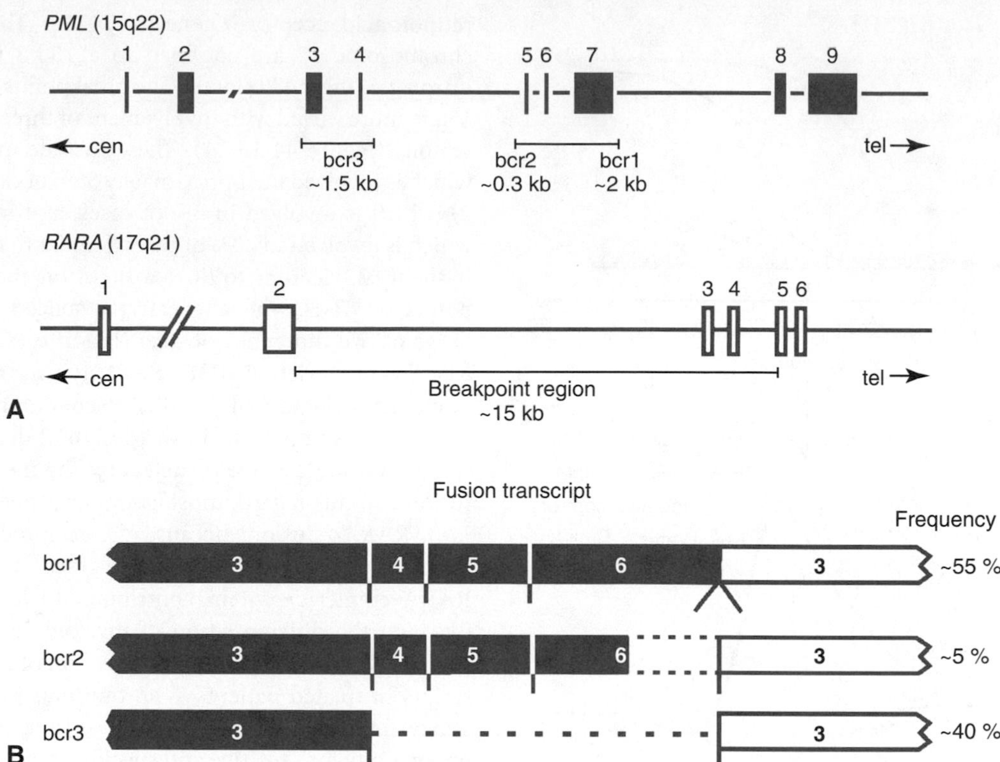

Figure 44-13 Schematic representation of the organization of the *PML* (15q22) and *RARα* (17q11) genes involved in the t(15;17) anomaly, which is characteristic of FAB AML-M3. The centromeric *(cen)* and telomeric (tel) directions are indicated. In A, the exons of the *PML* gene are depicted in *red rectangles,* and the exons of the *RARα* gene are depicted in *white rectangles.* In *B,* the configuration of the *PML-RARα* chimeric fusions is shown.

c-*ABL*, the breakpoints on chromosome 22 are quite variable and within the *BCR* gene (Figure 44-14).[61,75] Depending on the location of the breakpoint, the fusion protein resulting from *BCR-ABL* fusion can vary in size from 190 to 230 kDa. Up to 95% of CMLs, 30 to 50% of adult t(9;22)-positive ALLs, and 20 to 30% of childhood t(9;22)-positive ALLs harbor breakpoints in the M-*BCR* region of the *BCR* gene.[56,104,109,119] The *BCR* breakpoints in virtually all CML cases occur in the 9.0 kb region between exons 13 and 15 (also known as b2 and b4, respectively). Fusion occurs to a breakpoint located in the large intron between exons 1b and 2 of the *ABL* gene.[21] The resulting *BCR-ABL* transcript measures 8.5 kb and contains *BCR* exon b2 or b3 and ABL exon 2 (exon a2). This transcript encodes the 210 kDa BCR-ABL chimeric protein (p210$^{BCR/ABL}$). The most frequent fusions found in CML are b3-a2 fusions, which account for 55% of *BCR-ABL* junctions, and the b2-a2 transcript (40%).[129] Less frequently (5%), both b3-a2 and b2-a2 fusions may occur as a result of alternative splicing.[129] Thus far, no significant prognostic differences between p210-positive CMLs with different transcripts are apparent.[129]

In rare cases of CML, the breakpoint in the *BCR* gene occurs at the ALL-associated m-*BCR*, which leads to generation of the p190$^{BCR/ABL}$ fusion protein.[127] p190-positive CML patients characteristically exhibit relative and absolute monocytosis in peripheral blood reminiscent of chronic myelomonocytic leukemia.[93] Another distinct but rare fusion that has been described in t(9;22)-positive CML is one that results in the formation of a large 230 kDa fusion protein as a consequence of a fusion between exon 19 (c3) of *BCR* and exon 2 (a2) or ABL. The *BCR* breakpoints for this fusion are located in the micro breakpoint cluster region (μ-*BCR*) located between exons 19 and 20 (see Figure 44-14). The p230 fusion is characteristic of a peculiar form of chronic myelogenous leukemia with prominent neutrophilic proliferation. The clinical course of p230-positive CML is reportedly indolent in most cases.[105]

Another distinct breakpoint cluster region in the *BCR* gene has been uniquely associated with t(9;22)-positive ALLs.[61] Up to 60% of t(9;22)-positive ALLs carry translocations in which the *BCR* breakpoint genes are located in a distinct region known as the *minor breakpoint cluster region* (m-*BCR*). m-*BCR* is located between the two alternative exons and exon 2. The ABL breakpoints are located in the large intron between exon 1b and exon 2 of the ABL gene. The resulting e1-a2 fusion encodes a 190 kDa *BCR-ABL* chimeric protein[22] that is expressed mostly in ALLs, and rather infrequently as the exclusive *BCR-ABL* transcript in CML.[114,127] On the other hand, the remaining 40% of t(9;22)-positive ALLs may express the p210 *BCR-ABL* fusion, thus indicating

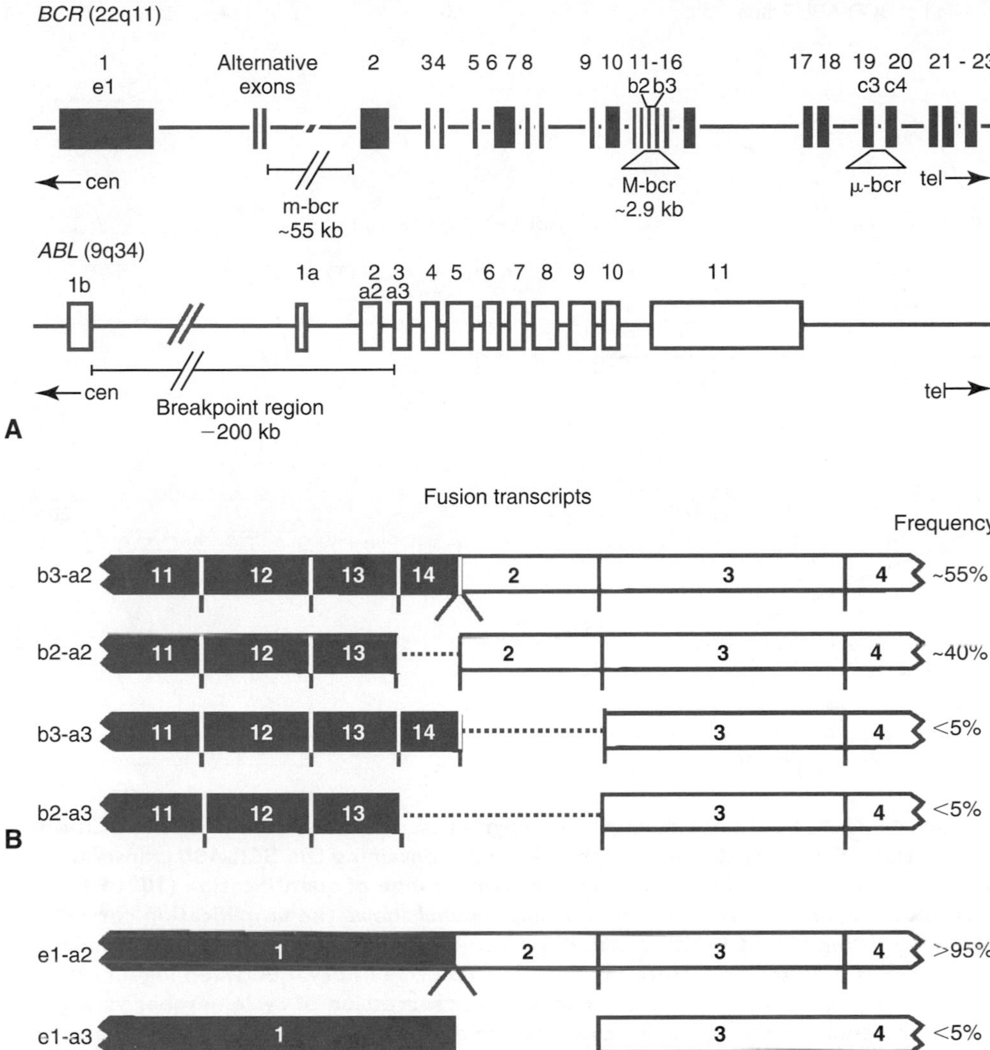

Figure 44-14 Schematic representation of the *BCR* (22q11) and *ABL* (9q34) genes involved in the t(9;22), which is characteristic of all chronic myelogenous leukemias (CMLs) and a subset of acute lymphoblastic leukemias (ALLs). The centromeric (cen) and telomeric (tel) directions are indicated. The relative positions of the major breakpoint cluster (M-*BCR*), the minor breakpoint cluster (m-*BCR*), and the micro breakpoint cluster regions (μ-*BCR*) are shown. The previously used alternative nomenclature for the *BCR* and *ABL* exons is included where relevant. In A, the exons of the *BCR* genes are depicted in *red rectangles,* and those of the *ABL* genes are depicted in *white rectangles.* In B, the configuration and varieties of the *BCR-ABL* chimeric fusions seen in CML are shown. In the *lower part* of B, the configuration and varieties of the *BCR-ABL* fusions seen in *ALL* are shown. The e1-a2 transcript is most commonly detected in t(9;22)-positive *ALL,* but the b3-a2 and b2-a2 fusions are most commonly detected in CML.

its relative lack of specificity. A significant number of CML cases express the low levels of e1-a2 transcripts, in addition to p210, via an alternative splicing mechanism.[25,64,114,146]

Conventional cytogenetics, FISH, and RT-PCR have been reliably utilized for the laboratory detection of the t(9;22). RT-PCR detection is possible in up to 95% of cases and may detect up to 10% of cases missed by conventional cytogenetics[25]; it is an important modality for minimal residual disease detection. Quantitative real-time PCR-based approaches have improved our ability to detect and quantitate *BCR-ABL* transcripts in CML patients[37,74] (Figure 44-15, *A*). The availability of the tyrosine kinase inhibitor imatinib mesylate for CML is an important development in the treatment of CML[36-37]; it underscores the importance of methods for sensitive and specific identification and quantification of *BCR-ABL* fusions in patients with a clinical suspicion for CML.

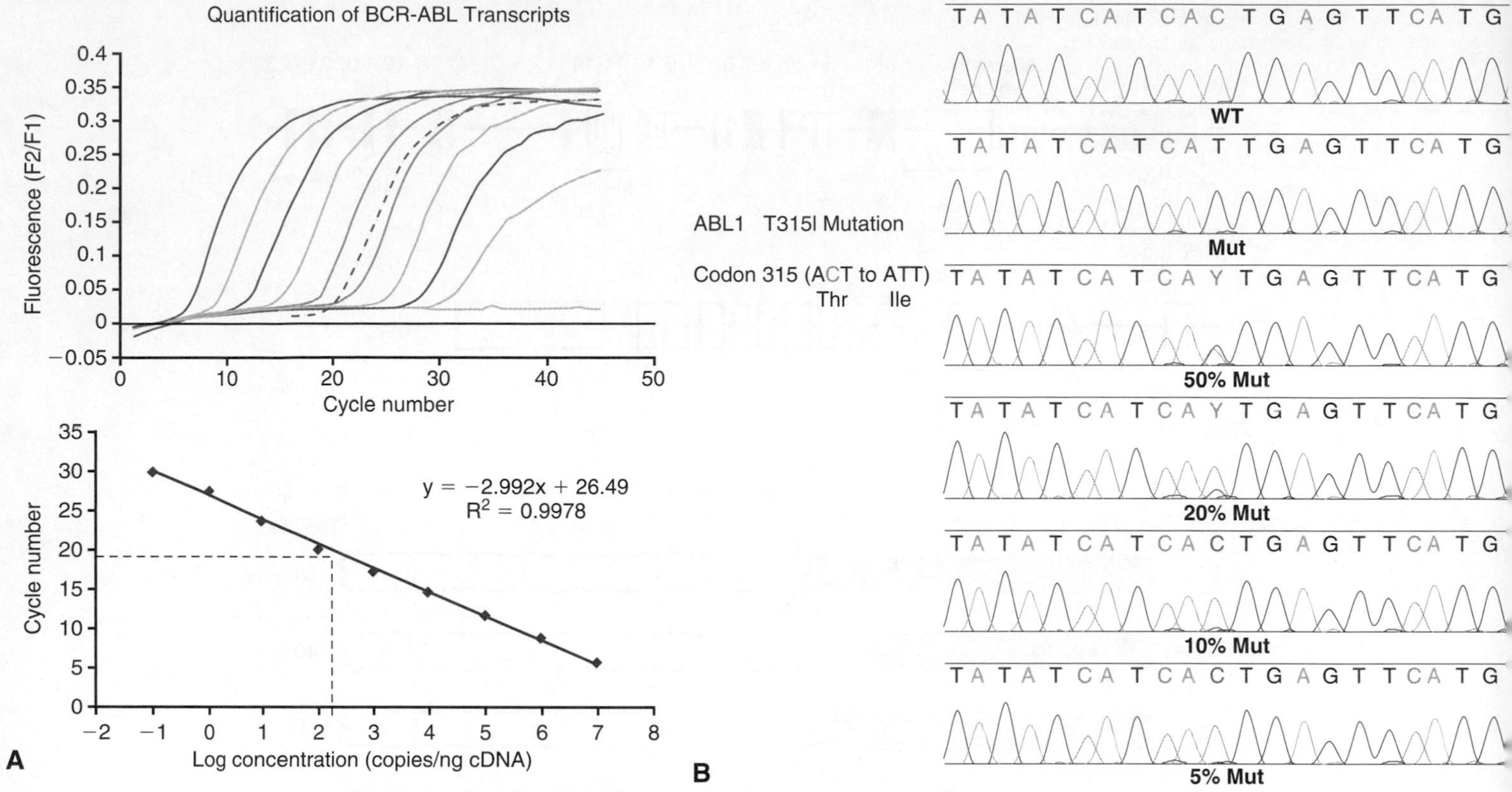

Figure 44-15 A, Real-time quantitative polymerase chain reaction (PCR) of *BCR-ABL* transcripts. Serial log dilutions of the plasmids containing the *BCR-ABL* transcripts. Real-time PCR provides a remarkable dynamic range of quantification (10^9 to 10^0 template copies) in this example. The *upper panel* shows the amplification curves obtained using the *BCR-ABL*–containing plasmids and an unknown patient sample depicted as a *dotted line.* Note the regular ≈3.3-cycle interval between log dilutions. The *lower panel* shows a standard curve (linear regression of cycle number vs. log template concentration). As indicated by the *dotted line* in the *lower panel,* the cycle threshold (onset of the log-linear phase of the amplification curve) can be used to quantitate the copy number of the target in the tested sample. B, Detection of *ABL1* kinase mutation by direct sequencing. The ACT→ATT transition at codon 315 results in a threonine→isoleucine substitution at the amino acid level: the *T315I* mutation. The *T315I* mutation confers resistance to imatinib, nilotinib, and dasatinib and is an important cause of resistance to tyrosine kinase inhibitors in Ph+ leukemias (CML and ALL). The mutated peak is clearly visible even to a dilution of tumor concentration of 10%.

t(9:22) in ALL

The t(9;22) has emerged as a sine qua non for the diagnosis of CML, and the recent development of novel tyrosine kinase inhibitor therapy portends a favorable prognosis. By contrast, the presence of the t(9;22) is an independent poor prognostic factor in ALLs.[45,124,154]

Reverse Transcription Polymerase Chain Reaction

Reverse transcription polymerase chain reaction (RT-PCR) involves the initial synthesis of complementary DNA (cDNA) from messenger RNA (mRNA) using a reverse transcriptase enzyme. Reverse transcription can be performed using oligo-dT priming, random hexamers, or gene-specific primers. The cDNA generated is utilized as the template for PCR. This strategy is indicated for the detection of chromosomal translocations wherein breakpoints are widely separated by large intervening introns between juxtaposed fragments that limit the practicality of conventional PCR.

Real-Time Polymerase Chain Reaction

PCR assays have traditionally entailed a two-step procedure comprising an initial amplification reaction, followed by analysis of PCR products in a separate process. PCR product analysis has generally entailed size fractionation by gel electrophoresis and product visualization by ultraviolet (UV) transillumination of ethidium bromide–stained gels or chemiluminescent or radioisotopic detection. The advent of real-time PCR techniques led to PCR amplification with simultaneous monitoring of product accumulation.[63]

Real-time PCR methods employ variations of three fundamental fluorescence chemistries to monitor product accumulation. Higuchi and associates introduced the incorporation of a double-stranded DNA (dsDNA) binding dye (ethidium bromide) into amplification reactions, with fluorescence monitoring at each cycle for quantitative analysis.[63] Real-time PCR using dsDNA-binding dyes such as ethidium bromide and SYBR Green I (Invitrogen Ltd, Paisley, United Kingdom) is relatively inexpensive and easy to use, but does not offer specificity beyond that inherent within the PCR. In poorly optimized reactions, nonspecific dsDNA binding dye- or intercalator-based assays may be prone to yielding false-positive results. It is thus important to carefully optimize primer design to minimize primer dimer and nonspecific product formation.[17] By comparison, sequence-specific fluorescence probe-based systems provide definitive identification of the sequence of interest by virtue of hybridization of fluorescently labeled internal probes to the amplified target sequence.[156]

The most commonly utilized sequence-specific chemistries include exonuclease (TaqMan, Applied Biosystems, Carlsbad, Calif), linear hybridization probe, and hairpin-based (molecular beacon) systems. The TaqMan chemistry takes advantage of the 5→3 exonucleolytic activity of the *Taq* polymerase. In this system, an oligonucleotide probe is dually labeled with a donor fluorophore at the 5′ end, and then with a fluorescence quencher at the 3′ end. The proximity of the quencher to the fluorescent effectively quenches the fluorescence of the donor fluorophore. The labeled probe hybridizes to the amplicon during PCR, but the exonuclease activity of Taq leads to probe hydrolysis and release of the donor fluorophore from the effect of the quencher. Hence, the generation of signals using the TaqMan system requires both hybridization and cleavage of the probe to separate the donor fluorophore and the quencher. The ensuing increase in fluorescence is indicative of new strand synthesis and can be used to monitor PCR progress. Another variation on the dual-labeled sequence-specific probe theme is the hairpin (molecular beacon) system.[144] In this system, a single-stranded molecule is configured in such a way that it possesses a stem-and-loop structure. The sequence of the loop segment of the molecule is complementary to a specific sequence within the target of interest. The stem is composed of two complementary arm sequences that flank the loop sequence. The arm sequences when annealed form the stem and are dissimilar to those of the target sequences. The 5′ end of the probe is labeled with a fluorescent donor (e.g., EDANS), and the 3′ end is labeled with a quencher (e.g., DABCYL). Hybridization of the probe to the target leads to the formation of a hybrid that is longer and more stable than that formed with the arm sequences in the stem configuration (in the absence of target). In a nonhybridized state, the molecular beacon fluorescence is quenched. When linearized by hybridized to target, quenching is removed and fluorescence emission occurs.

The adjacent hybridization probe-based systems employ two oligonucleotide probes. One of the probes is labeled at its 3′ end with fluorescein, and the other is labeled at its 5′ end with a fluorescent acceptor (e.g., Cy5). Hybridization of both probes to the template leads to juxtaposition of the fluorophores to within a distance of one nucleotide base. An accompanying increase in fluorescence is the result of fluorescence resonance energy transfer (FRET) between the excited donor fluorophore and the acceptor. The specificity of oligonucleotide probe hybridization–based schemes ensures that no signal is generated when a nonspecific product is amplified. In sequence-specific probe formats, the probes are included in the amplification reaction in marked excess compared with the template.

Quantification

Real-time PCR is particularly advantageous for the quantitative analysis of nucleic acid sequences. Previously, quantitative PCR was based on end point or competitive assays, which measured band intensities in ethidium bromide–stained gels or via radioisotopic labeling.[148] Fluorescence-based real-time PCR assays characteristically demonstrate three time succession phases: an initial background phase, an exponential or logarithmic phase, and a plateau phase. Onset of the exponential phase is inversely related to the abundance of the target of interest at the beginning of the PCR. By using controls with known quantities of a specific target, a standard curve can be plotted with a crossing threshold (*y*-axis) against log concentration (*x*-axis) for the target of interest. The crossing threshold for a control and specific gene targets in unknown samples can be derived from their PCRs and read off the standard curve to yield a copy number for the target transcript.

ABL-1 Drug Resistance Mutations in Ph+ Chromosome–Positive Leukemias

Philadelphia choromosome–positive chronic myeloid leukemia represents a prototypical disease for targeted cancer therapeutics with the advent of tyrosine kinase inhibitors (TKIs) such as imatinib mesylate (Gleevec). Although imatinib is associated with durable responses in most patients, TKI-resistant clones carrying mutations in the ABL kinase domain have emerged as a frequent mechanism for disease recurrence. Disease remission may be achieved by changing to a different TKI with different kinase inhibitory characteristics, which retains activity against the particular ABL-1 kinase mutation. In this regard, molecular diagnostics testing involving sequencing of the ABL-1 kinase gene plays a role in the selection of appropriate TKIs and the identification of resistance mutations (Figure 44-15, *B*).[16,68]

Mutations of Oncogenes and Tumor Suppressor Genes in Hematopoietic Malignancies

Malignant Lymphomas

Mutations involving several oncogenes and tumor suppressor genes have been identified as important in the pathogenesis of malignant lymphomas. These include mutations targeting *p53* and *p16* tumor suppressor genes.[40,116] It is significant that mutations occurring in genes encoding components of the nuclear factor–kappaB (NF-κB) signaling pathway have been identified in several histologic subtypes of lymphoma. These include *CARD11,*[82] *A20/TNFAIP3, TRAF2,* and *TRAF5* genes.[23] *A20/TNFAIP3* is targeted most frequently across diverse histologic subtypes of malignant lymphoma[71] and is discussed briefly in the following section.

A20/TNFAIP3

Tumor necrosis factor-α–induced protein 3 *(TNFAIP3)* is induced by TNF-α and is a negative regulator of NF-κB. TNFAIP3 is a ubiquitin ligase with deubiquitinating activity,[153] and is capable of inhibiting TNF-induced apoptosis. The gene that encodes TNFAIP3/A20 maps to chromosome 6q23, a locus that is frequently deleted in non-Hodgkin lymphoma. Studies have demonstrated that TNFAIP3/A20 is frequently inactivated by deletions involving 6q23, or by mutations[23,71] or by promoter hypermethylation[65] in diverse forms of malignant lymphoma.

Acute Myeloid Leukemias

Various somatic mutations occur in AMLs and have been demonstrated to carry important implications for prognosis. Among these are mutations involving *RAS, FLT3, NPM1, CEBP-α,* and *c-KIT.* Many of these are routinely tested in molecular diagnostics reference laboratories and are discussed in the sections that follow here.

RAS Mutations

The concomitant occurrence of genetic aberrations and chromosomal translocations is common in hematologic malignancies. The *RAS* oncogene, one of the most frequently mutated genes in cancer,[14] is mutated in up to 25 to 44% of hematopoietic malignancies and myelodysplastic syndromes (MDSs).[7] The presence of *RAS* mutations has been reported to confer a worse prognosis on patients with AML and MDS.[100,101] The mutations are clustered in "hot spots" that occur in codon 12, 13, or 61, rendering them fairly straightforward to detect with the use of different technical strategies.

FMS-like Tyrosine Kinase 3

Mutations of the tyrosine kinase gene, *FLT3,* have been described in acute myeloid leukemias.[99,157] Most mutations are internal tandem duplications (ITDs) within the juxtamembrane domain (JMD) of the gene, and are present in up to 24% of AML cases. ITDs have been identified in all FAB subtypes of AML, most frequently in acute promyelocytic leukemia (AML FAB-M3). Figure 44-16 shows an example of an *FLT3* ITD detected by PCR and capillary electrophoresis in a case of acute myeloid leukemia, which also demonstrated the presence of the *PML-RARα* fusion transcript. The presence of the ITD was inferred by the larger PCR product size and was subsequently confirmed by sequencing. Additional mutations distinct from ITDs occurring in the JMD have been described in a subset of AMLs. The most frequent of these is a base substitution occurring at aspartic acid residue 835 in the activation loop of *FLT3. D835* mutations have been identified in 7% of AML, 3% of MDS, and 3% of ALL.[157] In considering *FLT3* ITDs and activation mutations combined, *FLT3* may be the most frequently mutated gene in acute myeloid leukemia. Mutations in the activation loop of another receptor tyrosine kinase, *c-KIT,* have been reported in mast cell proliferations[89] and in a small proportion of AMLs.[18]

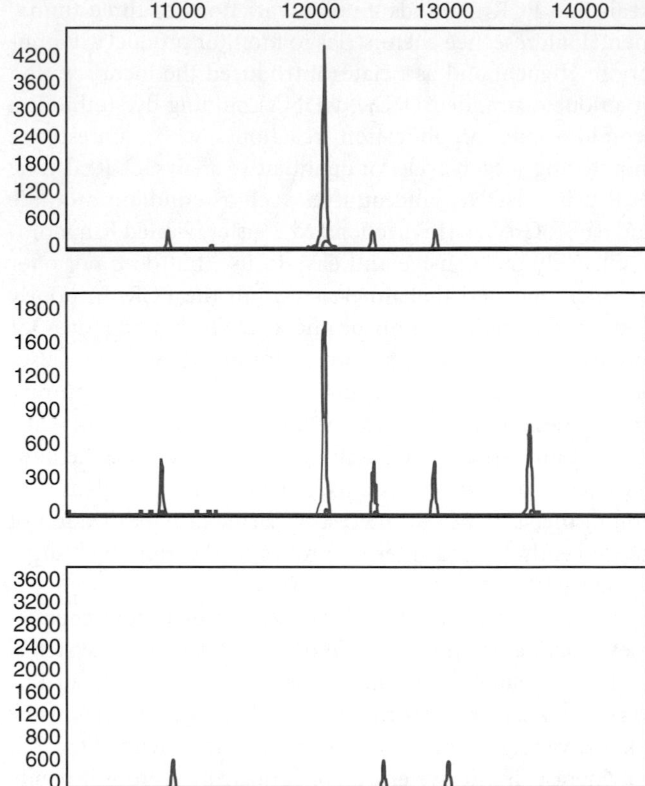

Figure 44-16 Detection of internal tandem duplications of the *FLT3* gene by polymerase chain reaction (PCR) and capillary gel electrophoresis of PCR products. Capillary electropherograms show clear resolution of PCR products. The *x*-axis represents the sizes of PCR products, and the *y*-axis shows the fluorescence intensity, which correlates with the abundance of the PCR product. The *upper panel* shows a wild type of pattern *(red peak).* The *middle panel* shows an additional peak of greater size than the wild-type peak *(red peak on the left).* The *red peak on the right* represents an *FLT3* internal tandem duplication. The *lower panel* shows the size markers *(red peaks)* also present in the upper and middle panels.

Nucleophosmin 1 *(NPM1)* Gene Mutations

The nucleophosmin *(NPM1)* gene encodes a nucleolar phosphoprotein that shuttles between the nucleus and the cytoplasm. Mutations in exon 12 of the gene were found to result in abnormal cytoplasmic localization of *NPM1.*[46] The most common of these is a four-base pair insertion, TCTG, which leads to the loss of critical tryptophan residues required for *NPM1* nucleolar localization, and to the generation of an additional nuclear export signal in the C-terminus of *NPM1.*[47] *NPM1* gene mutations are the most prevalent genetic aberration in AML in adults, and are detectable in 24 to 35% of all cases.[46,133,139] The prevalence of *NPM1* mutations is even greater in karyotypically normal AMLs with detection in 43 to 62% of cases. By comparison, *NPM1* mutations are found at much lower frequencies in AMLs occurring in children (8% of childhood AML).[24] *NPM1* mutations appear to associate with distinct clinical features such as female sex, high total white blood cell count (WBC) and bone marrow blast counts, high CD33, and low to absent CD34 expression. *NPM1* mutations are preferentially associated with the AMLs with monocytic differentiation. It is important to note that *NPM1* mutations are associated with a favorable prognosis after intensive induction therapy.[52,117,122] However, this association with a favorable prognosis is lost when *NPM1* mutations are detected concomitantly with ITDs of the *FLT3* gene,[33,139] or with partial tandem duplications of the *MLL* gene.[118]

CCAAT Enhancer–Binding Protein Alpha (CEBPα) Gene Mutations

The CCAAT enhancer–binding protein alpha (CEBPα) is an important transcriptional regulator of differentiation of pluripotent myeloid progenitors into mature granulocytes.[50,103] As with *NPM1,* CEBPα mutations are found predominantly in AMLs with normal karyotype. CEBPα mutations can be divided into two major categories. The first category of mutations consists of nonsense mutations located in the N-terminal region of the protein that result in a truncated protein with dominant negative properties. In the second variety, the mutations are distributed mainly in the leucine zipper domain in the C-terminal basic region, resulting in CEBPα proteins with decreased DNA binding and dimerization activity. It is interesting to note that N- and C-terminal mutations may be detectable in the same AML case, and mutations may coexist on the same (monoallelic) or on different alleles (biallelic). Clinically, karyotypically normal AMLs with CEBPα mutations exhibit distinct clinical features such as high peripheral blood blast counts, lower platelets, and lower likelihood of extramedullary disease.[118]

Partial Tandem Duplications (PTDs) of the Myeloid/Lymphoid or Mixed Lineage Leukemia *(MLL)* Gene

MLL-PTD is detectable in 5 to 11% of karyotypically normal AMLs. In comparison with *NPM1*-mutation positive AMLs, the clinical features of MLL-PTD–positive AMLs are not distinctive. Although concurrent existence of *NPM1* and CEBPα mutations is infrequent in cases with MLL-PTD, MLL-PTD–positive AMLs may harbor *FLT3* ITD mutations in up to 40% of cases.[50,103] MLL-PTD is associated with inferior relapse-free survival in some studies, without significant effect on overall survival.[34,118,132]

Wilms' Tumor Suppressor 1 Gene *(WT1)*

The Wilms' tumor suppressor gene, *WT1,* located on chromosome 11p13, encodes a 45 kDa protein that appears to function in transcriptional regulation by suppressing the expression of growth-inducing genes, such as early growth response, insulin-like growth factor 2, and platelet-derived growth factor A chain genes.[84] Other chromosomal changes in Wilms' tumors indicate that mutations of *WT1* may be only one step in the process of carcinogenesis. Mutations involving the *WT1* gene are detectable in up to 12.6% of karyotypically normal AMLs.[51,72] Although initial studies indicated that *WT1* mutations by themselves conferred an adverse impact on AML prognosis, these findings have not been confirmed by other studies.[51] More recent studies show data to support that it is the *WT1*^{mut}/*FLT*-ITD–positive genotype that confers a worse clinical outcome.

The *p53* gene is a tumor suppressor gene that encodes a nuclear phosphoprotein/transcription factor, which regulates diverse cellular processes, including DNA repair, cell cycle arrest, and apoptosis. *p53* inactivation is associated with genomic instability and deregulated cell cycle entry and progression. The *p53* gene is the most commonly mutated tumor suppressor gene in cancer, and *p53* mutations are commonly present in a variety of hematologic disorders, including blast crisis in CML, AML, MDS,[83,150] and adult T-cell leukemia/lymphoma.[115] *p53* mutations are implicated in the histologic transformation of follicular lymphoma into diffuse large B-cell lymphoma,[116] and have been described in a small subset of cases of Hodgkin disease.[41] *p53* mutations correlate with resistance to chemotherapy and portend a worse prognosis.[150] The *p53* mutations are localized mainly to mutational "hot spots" in exons 5 through 8, and may be single base substitutions, deletions, or insertions. Dominant negative inactivation of critical p53 protein function can be achieved by a mutation on one allele, because the wild-type protein can dimerize with mutated proteins and consequent functional impairment.[53] denaturing gradient gel electrophoresis (DGGE),[57] constant gradient gel electrophoresis,[12] and single strand confirmation polymorphism (SSCP)[41] have been used with success in screening for *p53* mutations.

Myeloproliferative Disorders

Janus Kinase (JAK) 2 Gene Mutations

The myeloproliferaative disorders include polycythemia vera (PV), essential thrombocythemia (ET), and primary myelofibrosis (PMF). In 2005, an activating mutation in exon 14 of the Janus kinase 2 gene was discovered in patients with PV, ET, and PMF by independent researchers.[6,69,86] This mutation, *JAK2V617F,* occurs as a result of a nucleotide change at position 1849, leading to the substitution of a phenyl alanine for a valine at codon 617. *JAK2V617F* is detectable in approximately 95% of cases of PV, 50% of ET, and 30% of PMF. It is interesting to note that the burden of the mutant allele in patients with PV and PMF is higher than that seen in patients with ET.[136] In PV, the higher mutant allele burden is attributed to *JAK2V617F* homozygosity, which occurs by mitotic recombination.[6,86] This mutation develops in an early-stage hematopoietic progenitor with stem cell characteristics. Aside from the *JAK2V617F* mutation, other mutations have been reported in exon 14 of JAK2 and include *D620E* (PV, unclassifiable myeloproliferative neoplasm) and *E627E* (unclassifiable myeloproliferative neoplasm). Other exon 14 mutations have been described in rare AMLs *(K607N)*. The importance of detection of the *JAK2* mutation is underscored by the fact that it is considered a major criterion for the diagnosis of PV in the 2008 revision of the World Health Organization (WHO) classification of myeloid neoplasms and acute leukemia.[137,147]

Rare patients with PV with a dominant clinical picture of erythrocytosis have been shown to carry mutations in exon 12 of the *JAK2* gene [N542-E543del (most common), F537-K539delinsL, and K539L]. These mutant alleles have been demonstrated to induce cytokine-independent proliferation and constitutive activation of JAK-STAT signaling, as is the case with the *V617F* allele.[123]

Myeloproliferative Leukemia Virus Oncogene Homology (MPL) Gene Mutations

The hematopoietic receptor superfamily includes the myeloproliferative leukemia virus oncogene, which encodes the thrombopoietin (TPO) receptor. The *MPL* gene maps to band 1p34.[80] Codon 515 is affected in a number of somatic mutations associated with *MPL (W515L, W515K, W515S, W515A, W515R)*.[120,121] Additionally, a subset of patients with familial thrombocytosis have been demonstrated to harbor germline *MPL* mutations *(MPLS505N)*.[30] Somatic *S505N* mutations have been identified in cases of sporadic ET and PMF.[106] Mutations involving the *MPL* gene are estimated to be present in as many as 4% of cases of ET (9% of *JAK2V17F*-negative cases) and in 10% of cases of PMF.[121]

MINIMAL RESIDUAL DISEASE DETECTION AND MONITORING

The occurrence of characteristic genetic aberrations and the uniqueness of antigen receptor gene rearrangements in lymphoid neoplasia provide an attractive opportunity for the exploitation of the high sensitivity and specificity of molecular techniques for the detection of minimal residual disease and for therapeutic monitoring. The sensitivity and specificity of molecular techniques capable of detecting one aberrant cell in a background of 10^3 to 10^6 are superior to those provided solely by clinical or microscopic examination. In this regard, PCR-based studies have enjoyed the greatest usefulness for the detection of clonal antigen receptor rearrangements and recurrent chromosomal translocations. With regard to antigen receptor gene rearrangements, clonal identity may be established by designing sequence-specific primers for the unique antigen receptor rearrangement, or by sequencing the PCR product. The ideal scenario for analysis of antigen receptor rearrangements for monitoring of minimal residual disease (MRD) requires previous identification of the specific clonal antigen receptor gene rearrangement in the tumor of interest by PCR and DNA sequencing, followed by clonality analysis and sequencing of initial and subsequent samples. The antigen receptor gene rearrangement sequences of initial and subsequent biopsies are compared for sequence homology. Alternatively, tumor-specific antigen receptor primers may be designed for amplification of the subsequent sample, with successful amplification considered evidence of clonal identity.

Minimal residual disease monitoring using antigen receptor PCR based–monitoring is especially significant in the pediatric population among patients with acute lymphoblastic leukemia/lymphoma.[95] Detection of clonal rearrangements of the antigen receptor genes at the end of induction therapy has been shown to be predictive of patients with high relapse potential.[44,149] In addition, the demonstration of persistent positivity in successive analyses is an indicator of future clinical relapse, although persistent negativity is indicative of a durable remission.[131]

The detection of chromosomal aberrations by PCR-based methods continues to evolve as a tool for MRD detection. Indeed, the clinical significance of the qualitative detection of chromosomal translocations has been the subject of intense study with varying implications, depending on the natural biology of the hematologic disorder (if present), the specific clinical context, the translocation detected, or the method employed. For instance, the t(14;18) has been detected in the peripheral blood and reactive lymphoid tissues of healthy individuals, leading to uncertainty about the significance of qualitative detection of the t(14;18).[35,87] Similarly, highly sensitive PCR assays have detected the t(9;22) in the peripheral blood of otherwise healthy elderly individuals.[9,15]

The implications of qualitative detection of translocations vary with the translocation detected. For instance, a very high risk of relapse is associated with the detection of residual *PML-RARα* transcripts after therapy.[31,32] By contrast, the t(8;21) *AML1-ETO* fusion may be detected in patients who have sustained and durable clinical remissions following treatment. The *AML1-ETO* fusion may also be detected in patients who have undergone chemotherapy or bone marrow transplantation.[70,78] On the other hand, detection of the t(9;22) *BCR-ABL* fusion transcript is prognostically significant for relapse, if conversion to positivity occurs within 6 to 12 months of treatment. The predictive value of the presence of chimeric transcripts can be affected by therapy-associated factors such as graft-versus-host disease or the type of transplant.[110] Nevertheless, persistent molecular negativity for the *BCR-ABL* transcript is indicative of good response to therapy and favors a durable remission.

The recent availability of quantitative real-time PCR-based assays for the quantitative detection of specific genetic alterations holds great promise in the quantification of tumor burden, response to therapy, and relapse potential. Appropriately done, the tests should be performed at a series of regular and successive time points during management of the disease. This approach is more apt to identify increasing, decreasing, or stabilizing trends in the abundance of the translocation product in tested samples. Figure 44-15 shows a quantitative RT-PCR study for the *BCR-ABL* transcript that incorporates several quantification standards for determination of the number of copies of the fusion transcript present in the sample. An alternative approach involves expression of the ratio of expression levels of the fusion transcript being tested against those of a stably expressed housekeeping gene, and monitoring the changes that ensue over time.

DETECTION OF VIRAL GENOMES

Viruses involved in the pathogenesis of abnormal proliferations of hematopoietic cells include the human T-cell leukemia virus type I, found in adult T-cell leukemia/lymphoma, and Kaposi sarcoma herpesvirus/human herpesvirus-8 (KSHV/HHV8), seen in primary effusion lymphoma and multicentric Castleman disease.[19] These viruses can be detected using the standard molecular biology techniques described in this chapter. Primer design should take into consideration the propensity for shared sequences within related viruses. Optimal specificity can be obtained by assigning primers to unique portions of the genome of the virus of interest. Because of its well-established role in the pathogenesis of a variety of lymphoproliferative disorders, Epstein-Barr virus (EBV) and its detection are discussed in the following section as an example of a virus that may be detected by in situ hybridization.

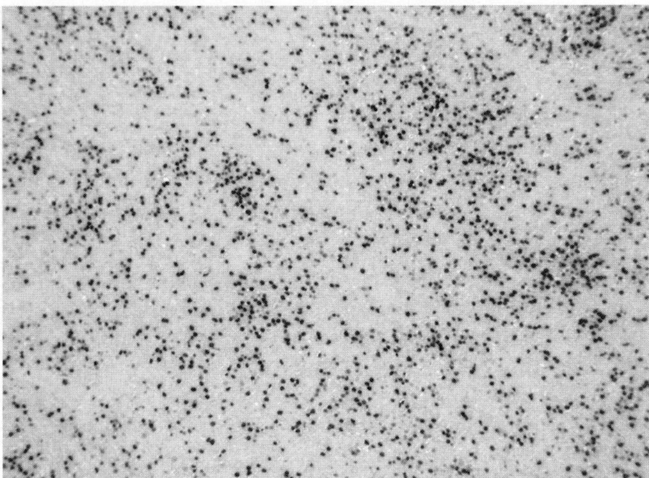

Figure 44-17 In situ hybridization (ISH) for the Epstein-Barr virus (EBV). ISH hybridization for EBV shows numerous positive signals *(dark-black spots)* for EBV using the EBER-1 probe. The tissue sample was obtained from a solid organ transplant patient who developed widespread nodal and extranodal masses. The positive reaction for EBV in this assay supports a diagnosis of post-transplant lymphoproliferative disease.

Epstein-Barr Virus

Epstein-Barr virus (EBV) was identified in 1964 by Epstein, Achong, and Barr in cultured cells obtained from a malignant lymphoma described by Dennis Burkitt.[42] EBV was subsequently identified by Werner Henle and colleagues as the cause of infectious mononucleosis.[60] EBV is a lymphotropic virus that has been associated with different malignant neoplasms, including endemic Burkitt lymphoma, nasopharyngeal carcinoma, nasal natural killer cell (NK)/T cell or NK-/T- type lymphoma, and some subtypes of Hodgkin lymphoma. EBV is also implicated in the pathogenesis of most post-transplant lymphoproliferative disorders.[67] Figure 44-17 shows an example of positive EBV signals (EBER in situ hybridization) in a case of post-transplant lymphoproliferative disease.

EBV is an enveloped icosahedral virus containing a double-stranded DNA genome of 172 kb with more than 100 open reading frames, potentially encoding an equivalent number of proteins.[5] The precise size of each virion varies from particle to particle because of the presence of tandemly repeated sequences, each 500 bp long and present in the virus termini. Viral tropism is mediated via attachment of the gp350/220 viral envelope protein to the complement receptor type 2 C3d (CR2) or CD21.[48,135] The virus exhibits tropism for B cells, some T cells, dendritic cells, and epithelial cells. After infection, typically via the oropharyngeal mucosa, EBV undergoes lytic replication in vivo. In the lytic replication, the linear genome is duplicated and assembled into viral capsid, and it exits the cell by budding or lysis. By contrast, B cells are efficiently immortalized by EBV in vitro. In immortalized cells, the viral genome is circularized by fusion of the termini (episomal), and the viral infection is latent with lack of production of viral particles. In the latent phase, viral replication occurs coordinately with host cell division. During latent infection, 11 genes are actively transcribed, including six nuclear antigens (EBNA-1, -2, -3A, -3B, -3C, and -LP), 3 membrane proteins (latent membrane proteins LMP-1, -2A, and -2B), and 2 EBV-encoded, small, nonpolyadenylated RNAs (EBER-1/-2).[2] The EBERs are present at very high copy numbers in the nuclei of latently infected cells.[84] The abundance of this transcript makes it very attractive for detection of latent EBV infection in cells and tissue specimens by in situ hybridization (see Figure 44-17).

Three latency patterns of expression have been described that relate to the expression of latency gene products. In latency pattern I, exemplified by Burkitt lymphoma cells, EBNA-1 is the only antigen that is expressed. In latency pattern II (exemplified by Hodgkin lymphoma), EBNA-1 and LMP-1 are expressed, and in latency pattern III (exemplified by post-transplant lymphoproliferative disease), all nuclear and latent membrane antigens are expressed. Based on the premise that one virion infects one host cell, and each virion has a unique number of terminal repeats with each episome being exactly replicated in all of its progeny, the clonality status of different cell populations has been assessed using probes complementary to the EBV termini by Southern blotting hybridization analysis.[58] Genomic probes that are complementary to sequences adjacent to the EBV termini, so-called terminal repeat region probes, are utilized. In this assay, a specimen yielding a single size of episomal EBV DNA is considered monoclonal. This is based on the premise that all cells arose from a parent cell containing the same EBV DNA episome that was replicated in the progeny. By contrast, a sample yielding episomes of various sizes, with a ladder pattern in which fragments differ by 500 bp, is indicative of a polyclonal population wherein each different progenitor cell harbored a different EBV DNA episome.[108]

An obvious advantage of using EBV terminal repeat probes for assessment of clonality is that they can also be used for assessment of clonality in EBV-positive nonhematopoietic neoplasms (e.g., nasopharyngeal carcinoma) in which antigen receptor gene rearrangements are not informative.[108] EBV in situ hybridization using probes targeting the EBER-1 transcript has contributed significantly to the identification of EBV in several hematopoietic and nonhematopoietic disorders.

IN SITU HYBRIDIZATION

The ability to visualize the cellular localization of different gene products is an important aspect of molecular biology and pathology. In situ hybridization (ISH) is a method that permits identification of the exact cellular location of target DNA or RNA in cytologic preparations or microscopic sections. In situ hybridization entails the synthesis of a nucleic acid (DNA or RNA) probe that is complementary to the gene sequence of interest. The probe may be labeled by nonisotopic or radioisotopic methods. ISH hybridization of fixed paraffin-embedded tissue sections entails initial dissolution of paraffin in xylene and serial dehydration in graded ethanols. For DNA targets, the tissue section is subjected to denaturation, followed by application of the probe for hybridization. Several washing steps with modulation of stringency (temperature, ionic/salt concentration) are necessary to ensure specificity of the hybridization. Development of signals indicative of specific hybridization depends on the system used. Colorimetric detection using avidin-biotin and peroxidase chemistry with a substrate yielding a visible precipitate (e.g., diaminobenzidine) is currently favored for light microscopic applications. In situ hybridization is versatile and is not limited to the detection of viral targets; it has found utility in a number of diagnostic settings, including the assessment of B-cell clonality by light chain restriction. Developments that have led to widespread utility of ISH include nonfluorescent chromophore in situ hybridization protocols that permit ISH analysis of a variety of targets using the light microscope.[8]

CONCLUSIONS

Hematopoietic neoplasms are associated with distinctive molecular aberrations that are amenable to diagnostic detection. In addition, identification of the molecular abnormality in many cases also carries important prognostic and disease-specific treatment implications. The method chosen depends on the nature of the aberration being evaluated, the nature of available samples, and the level of sensitivity afforded by available methods. Technical issues aside, the clinical significance of each test has to be determined on an individual basis. Most important, molecular tests should be utilized as adjunctive parameters in evaluation of the patient, and they should never be used in isolation without consideration of clinical findings. Ideally, the management of a patient should incorporate the entire complement of clinical and diagnostic information pertinent to the individual and his or her disorder.

REFERENCES

1. Albinger-Hegyi A, Hochreutener B, Abdou MT, Hegyi I, Dours-Zimmermann MT, Kurrer MO, et al. High frequency of t(14;18)-translocation breakpoints outside of major breakpoint and minor cluster regions in follicular lymphomas: improved polymerase chain reaction protocols for their detection. Am J Pathol 2002;160:823-32.
2. Anagnostopoulos I, Hummel M. Epstein-Barr virus in tumours. Histopathology 1996;29:297-315.
3. Andrieu V, Radford-Weiss I, Troussard X, Chane C, Valensi F, Guesnu M, et al. Molecular detection of t(8;21)/AML1-ETO in AML M1/M2: correlation with cytogenetics, morphology and immunophenotype. Br J Haematol 1996;92:855-65.
4. Aster JC, Kobayashi Y, Shiota M, Mori S, Sklar J. Detection of the t(14;18) at similar frequencies in hyperplastic lymphoid tissues from American and Japanese patients. Am J Pathol 1992;141:291-9.
5. Baer R, Bankier AT, Biggin MD, Deininger PL, Farrell PJ, Gibson TJ, et al. DNA sequence and expression of the B95-8 Epstein-Barr virus genome. Nature 1984;310:207-11.
6. Baxter EJ, Scott LM, Campbell PJ, East C, Fourouclas N, Swanton S, et al. Acquired mutation of the tyrosine kinase JAK2 in human myeloproliferative disorders. Lancet 2005;365:1054-61.
7. Beaupre DM, Kurzrock R. RAS and leukemia: from basic mechanisms to gene-directed therapy. J Clin Oncol 1999;17:1071-9.
8. Beck RC, Tubbs RR, Hussein M, Pettay J, Hsi ED. Automated colorimetric in situ hybridization (CISH) detection of immunoglobulin (Ig) light chain mRNA expression in plasma cell (PC) dyscrasias and non-Hodgkin lymphoma. Diagn Mol Pathol 2003;12:14-20.
9. Biernaux C, Loos M, Sels A, Huez G, Stryckmans P. Detection of major bcr-abl gene expression at a very low level in blood cells of some healthy individuals. Blood 1995;86:3118-22.
10. Biondi A, Rambaldi A, Pandolfi PP, Rossi V, Giudici G, Alcalay M, et al. Molecular monitoring of the myl/retinoic acid receptor-alpha fusion gene in acute promyelocytic leukemia by polymerase chain reaction. Blood 1992;80:492-7.
11. Bloomfield CD, Goldman AI, Alimena G, Berger R, Borgstrom GH, Brandt L, et al. Chromosomal abnormalities identify high-risk and low-risk patients with acute lymphoblastic leukemia. Blood 1986;67:415-20.
12. Borresen AL, Hovig E, Smith-Sorensen B, Malkin D, Lystad S, Andersen TI, et al. Constant denaturant gel electrophoresis as a rapid screening technique for p53 mutations. Proc Natl Acad Sci U S A 1991;88:8405-9.
13. Borrow J, Goddard AD, Sheer D, Solomon E. Molecular analysis of acute promyelocytic leukemia breakpoint cluster region on chromosome 17. Science 1990;249:1577-80.
14. Bos JL. Ras oncogenes in human cancer: a review. Cancer Res 1989;49:4682-9.
15. Bose S, Deininger M, Gora-Tybor J, Goldman JM, Melo JV. The presence of typical and atypical BCR-ABL fusion genes in leukocytes of normal individuals: biologic significance and implications for the assessment of minimal residual disease. Blood 1998;92:3362-7.
16. Branford S, Rudzki Z, Walsh S, Parkinson I, Grigg A, Szer J, et al. Detection of BCR-ABL mutations in patients with CML treated with imatinib is virtually always accompanied by clinical resistance, and mutations in the ATP phosphate-binding loop (P-loop) are associated with a poor prognosis. Blood 2003;102:276-83.
17. Brownie J, Shawcross S, Theaker J, Whitcombe D, Ferrie R, Newton C, et al. The elimination of primer-dimer accumulation in PCR. Nucleic Acids Res 1997;25:3235-41.
18. Care RS, Valk PJ, Goodeve AC, Abu-Duhier FM, Geertsma-Kleinekoort WM, Wilson GA, et al. Incidence and prognosis of c-KIT and FLT3 mutations in core binding factor (CBF) acute myeloid leukaemias. Br J Haematol 2003;121:775-7.

19. Cesarman E, Knowles DM. Kaposi's sarcoma-associated herpesvirus: a lymphotropic human herpesvirus associated with Kaposi's sarcoma, primary effusion lymphoma, and multicentric Castleman's disease. Semin Diagn Pathol 1997;14:54-66.
20. Cheng GY, Minden MD, Toyonaga B, Mak TW, McCulloch EA. T cell receptor and immunoglobulin gene rearrangements in acute myeloblastic leukemia. J Exp Med 1986;163:414-24.
21. Chissoe SL, Bodenteich A, Wang YF, Wang YP, Burian D, Clifton SW, et al. Sequence and analysis of the human ABL gene, the BCR gene, and regions involved in the Philadelphia chromosomal translocation. Genomics 1995;27:67-82.
22. Clark SS, McLaughlin J, Crist WM, Champlin R, Witte ON. Unique forms of the abl tyrosine kinase distinguish Ph1-positive CML from Ph1-positive ALL. Science 1987;235:85-8.
23. Compagno M, Lim WK, Grunn A, Nandula SV, Brahmachary M, Shen Q, et al. Mutations of multiple genes cause deregulation of NF-kappaB in diffuse large B-cell lymphoma. Nature 2009;459: 717-21.
24. Cossman J, Uppenkamp M, Sundeen J, Coupland R, Raffeld M. Molecular genetics and the diagnosis of lymphoma. Arch Pathol Lab Med 1988;112:117-27.
25. Costello R, Lafage M, Toiron Y, Brunel V, Sainty D, Arnoulet C, et al. Philadelphia chromosome-negative chronic myeloid leukaemia: a report of 14 new cases. Br J Haematol 1995;90:346-52.
26. Davey MP, Bongiovanni KF, Kaulfersch W, Quertermous T, Seidman JG, Hershfield MS, et al. Immunoglobulin and T-cell receptor gene rearrangement and expression in human lymphoid leukemia cells at different stages of maturation. Proc Natl Acad Sci U S A 1986;83: 8759-63.
27. de Klein A, van Kessel AG, Grosveld G, Bartram CR, Hagemeijer A, Bootsma D, et al. A cellular oncogene is translocated to the Philadelphia chromosome in chronic myelocytic leukaemia. Nature 1982;300:765-7.
28. de Villartay JP, Hockett RD, Coran D, Korsmeyer SJ, Cohen DI. Deletion of the human T-cell receptor delta-gene by a site-specific recombination. Nature 1988;335:170-4.
29. Dierlamm J, Baens M, Wlodarska I, Stefanova-Ouzounova M, Hernandez JM, Hossfeld DK, et al. The apoptosis inhibitor gene API2 and a novel 18q gene, MLT, are recurrently rearranged in the t(11;18)(q21;q21) associated with mucosa-associated lymphoid tissue lymphomas. Blood 1999;93:3601-9.
30. Ding J, Komatsu H, Wakita A, Kato-Uranishi M, Ito M, Satoh A, et al. Familial essential thrombocythemia associated with a dominant-positive activating mutation of the c-MPL gene, which encodes for the receptor for thrombopoietin. Blood 2004;103: 4198-200.
31. Diverio D, Pandolfi PP, Rossi V, Biondi A, Pelicci PG, Lo Coco F. Monitoring of treatment outcome in acute promyelocytic leukemia by RT-PCR. Leukemia 1994;8(Suppl 2):S63-5.
32. Diverio D, Rossi V, Avvisati G, De Santis S, Pistilli A, Pane F, et al. Early detection of relapse by prospective reverse transcriptase-polymerase chain reaction analysis of the PML/RARalpha fusion gene in patients with acute promyelocytic leukemia enrolled in the GIMEMA-AIEOP multicenter "AIDA" trial. GIMEMA-AIEOP Multicenter "AIDA" Trial. Blood 1998;92:784-9.
33. Dohner K, Schlenk RF, Habdank M, Scholl C, Rucker FG, Corbacioglu A, et al. Mutant nucleophosmin (NPM1) predicts favorable prognosis in younger adults with acute myeloid leukemia and normal cytogenetics: interaction with other gene mutations. Blood 2005;106:3740-6.
34. Dohner K, Tobis K, Ulrich R, Frohling S, Benner A, Schlenk RF, et al. Prognostic significance of partial tandem duplications of the MLL gene in adult patients 16 to 60 years old with acute myeloid leukemia and normal cytogenetics: a study of the Acute Myeloid Leukemia Study Group Ulm. J Clin Oncol 2002;20:3254-61.
35. Dolken G, Illerhaus G, Hirt C, Mertelsmann R. BCL-2/JH rearrangements in circulating B cells of healthy blood donors and patients with nonmalignant diseases. J Clin Oncol 1996;14:1333-44.
36. Druker BJ, Talpaz M, Resta DJ, Peng B, Buchdunger E, Ford JM, et al. Efficacy and safety of a specific inhibitor of the BCR-ABL tyrosine kinase in chronic myeloid leukemia. N Engl J Med 2001;344:1031-7.
37. Druker BJ, Tamura S, Buchdunger E, Ohno S, Segal GM, Fanning S, et al. Effects of a selective inhibitor of the Abl tyrosine kinase on the growth of Bcr-Abl positive cells. Nat Med 1996;2:561-6.
38. Eisenstein BI. The polymerase chain reaction: a new method of using molecular genetics for medical diagnosis. N Engl J Med 1990;322: 178-83.
39. Elenitoba-Johnson KS, Bohling SD, Wittwer CT, King TC. Multiplex PCR by multicolor fluorimetry and fluorescence melting curve analysis. Nat Med 2001;7:249-53.
40. Elenitoba-Johnson KS, Gascoyne RD, Lim MS, Chhanabai M, Jaffe ES, Raffeld M. Homozygous deletions at chromosome 9p21 involving p16 and p15 are associated with histologic progression in follicle center lymphoma. Blood 1998;91:4677-85.
41. Elenitoba-Johnson KS, Medeiros LJ, Khorsand J, King TC. P53 expression in Reed-Sternberg cells does not correlate with gene mutations in Hodgkin's disease. Am J Clin Pathol 1996;106:728-38.
42. Epstein MA, Achong BG, Barr YM. Virus particles in cultured lymphoblasts from Burkitt's lymphoma. Lancet 1964;1:702-3.
43. Erickson P, Gao J, Chang KS, Look T, Whisenant E, Raimondi S, et al. Identification of breakpoints in t(8;21) acute myelogenous leukemia and isolation of a fusion transcript, AML1/ETO, with similarity to *Drosophila* segmentation gene, *runt*. Blood 1992;80:1825-31.
44. Evans PA, Short MA, Owen RG, Jack AS, Forsyth PD, Shiach CR, et al. Residual disease detection using fluorescent polymerase chain reaction at 20 weeks of therapy predicts clinical outcome in childhood acute lymphoblastic leukemia. J Clin Oncol 1998;16:3616-27.
45. Faderl S, Kantarjian HM, Talpaz M, Estrov Z. Clinical significance of cytogenetic abnormalities in adult acute lymphoblastic leukemia. Blood 1998;91:3995-4019.
46. Falini B, Mecucci C, Tiacci E, Alcalay M, Rosati R, Pasqualucci L, et al. Cytoplasmic nucleophosmin in acute myelogenous leukemia with a normal karyotype. N Engl J Med 2005;352:254-66.
47. Falini B, Nicoletti I, Martelli MF, Mecucci C. Acute myeloid leukemia carrying cytoplasmic/mutated nucleophosmin (NPMc+ AML): biologic and clinical features. Blood 2007;109:874-85.
48. Fingeroth JD, Weis JJ, Tedder TF, Strominger JL, Biro PA, Fearon DT. Epstein-Barr virus receptor of human B lymphocytes is the C3d receptor CR2. Proc Natl Acad Sci U S A 1984;81:4510-4.
49. Frank R, Zhang J, Uchida H, Meyers S, Hiebert SW, Nimer SD. The AML1/ETO fusion protein blocks transactivation of the GM-CSF promoter by AML1B. Oncogene 1995;11:2667-74.
50. Frohling S, Schlenk RF, Stolze I, Bihlmayr J, Benner A, Kreitmeier S, et al. CEBPA mutations in younger adults with acute myeloid leukemia and normal cytogenetics: prognostic relevance and analysis of cooperating mutations. J Clin Oncol 2004;22:624-33.
51. Gaidzik VI, Schlenk RF, Moschny S, Becker A, Bullinger L, Corbacioglu A, et al. Prognostic impact of WT1 mutations in cytogenetically normal acute myeloid leukemia: a study of the German-Austrian AML Study Group. Blood 2009;113:4505-11.
52. Gale RE, Green C, Allen C, Mead AJ, Burnett AK, Hills RK, et al. The impact of FLT3 internal tandem duplication mutant level, number, size, and interaction with NPM1 mutations in a large cohort of young adult patients with acute myeloid leukemia. Blood 2008;111: 2776-84.
53. Galmarini CM, Falette N, Tabone E, Levrat C, Britten R, Voorzanger-Rousselot N, et al. Inactivation of wild-type p53 by a dominant negative mutant renders MCF-7 cells resistant to tubulin-binding agent cytotoxicity. Br J Cancer 2001;85:902-8.
54. Golub TR, Barker GF, Bohlander SK, Hiebert SW, Ward DC, Bray-Ward P, et al. Fusion of the TEL gene on 12p13 to the AML1 gene on 21q22 in acute lymphoblastic leukemia. Proc Natl Acad Sci U S A 1995;92:4917-21.
55. Greiner TC, Raffeld M, Lutz C, Dick F, Jaffe ES. Analysis of T cell receptor-gamma gene rearrangements by denaturing gradient gel electrophoresis of GC-clamped polymerase chain reaction products:

correlation with tumor-specific sequences. Am J Pathol 1995;146: 46-55.
56. Groffen J, Stephenson JR, Heisterkamp N, de Klein A, Bartram CR, Grosveld G. Philadelphia chromosomal breakpoints are clustered within a limited region, bcr, on chromosome 22. Cell 1984;36:93-9.
57. Guldberg P, Nedergaard T, Nielsen HJ, Olsen AC, Ahrenkiel V, Zeuthen J. Single-step DGGE-based mutation scanning of the p53 gene: application to genetic diagnosis of colorectal cancer. Hum Mutat 1997;9:348-55.
58. Gulley ML, Raphael M, Lutz CT, Ross DW, Raab-Traub N. Epstein-Barr virus integration in human lymphomas and lymphoid cell lines. Cancer 1992;70:185-91.
59. Ha K, Minden M, Hozumi N, Gelfand EW. Immunoglobulin gene rearrangement in acute myelogenous leukemia. Cancer Res 1984;44: 4658-60.
60. Henle G, Henle W, Diehl V. Relation of Burkitt's tumor-associated herpes-type virus to infectious mononucleosis. Proc Natl Acad Sci U S A 1968;59:94-101.
61. Hermans A, Heisterkamp N, von Linden M, van Baal S, Meijer D, van der Plas D, et al. Unique fusion of bcr and c-abl genes in Philadelphia chromosome positive acute lymphoblastic leukemia. Cell 1987;51:33-40.
62. Hiebert SW, Sun W, Davis JN, Golub T, Shurtleff S, Buijs A, et al. The t(12;21) translocation converts AML-1B from an activator to a repressor of transcription. Mol Cell Biol 1996;16:1349-55.
63. Higuchi R, Fockler C, Dollinger G, Watson R. Kinetic PCR analysis: real-time monitoring of DNA amplification reactions. Biotechnology 1993;11:1026-30.
64. Hochhaus A, Lin F, Reiter A, Skladny H, Mason PJ, van Rhee F, et al. Quantification of residual disease in chronic myelogenous leukemia patients on interferon-alpha therapy by competitive polymerase chain reaction. Blood 1996;87:1549-55.
65. Honma K, Tsuzuki S, Nakagawa M, Tagawa H, Nakamura S, Morishima Y, et al. TNFAIP3/A20 functions as a novel tumor suppressor gene in several subtypes of non-Hodgkin lymphomas. Blood 2009;114:2467-75.
66. Horsman DE, Gascoyne RD, Coupland RW, Coldman AJ, Adomat SA. Comparison of cytogenetic analysis, southern analysis, and polymerase chain reaction for the detection of t(14;18) in follicular lymphoma. Am J Clin Pathol 1995;103:472-8.
67. Hsieh WS, Lemas MV, Ambinder RF. The biology of Epstein-Barr virus in post-transplant lymphoproliferative disease. Transpl Infect Dis 1999;1:204-12.
68. Jabbour E, Kantarjian H, Jones D, Talpaz M, Bekele N, O'Brien S, et al. Frequency and clinical significance of BCR-ABL mutations in patients with chronic myeloid leukemia treated with imatinib mesylate. Leukemia 2006;20:1767-73.
69. James C, Ugo V, Le Couedic JP, Staerk J, Delhommeau F, Lacout C, et al. A unique clonal JAK2 mutation leading to constitutive signalling causes polycythaemia vera. Nature 2005;434:1144-8.
70. Jurlander J, Caligiuri MA, Ruutu T, Baer MR, Strout MP, Oberkircher AR, et al. Persistence of the AML1/ETO fusion transcript in patients treated with allogeneic bone marrow transplantation for t(8;21) leukemia. Blood 1996;88:2183-91.
71. Kato M, Sanada M, Kato I, Sato Y, Takita J, Takeuchi K, et al. Frequent inactivation of A20 in B-cell lymphomas. Nature 2009;459: 712-6.
72. King-Underwood L, Renshaw J, Pritchard-Jones K. Mutations in the Wilms' tumor gene WT1 in leukemias. Blood 1996;87:2171-9.
73. Kitchingman GR, Rovigatti U, Mauer AM, Melvin S, Murphy SB, Stass S. Rearrangement of immunoglobulin heavy chain genes in T cell acute lymphoblastic leukemia. Blood 1985;65:725-9.
74. Kreuzer KA, Lass U, Bohn A, Landt O, Schmidt CA. LightCycler technology for the quantitation of bcr/abl fusion transcripts. Cancer Res 1999;59:3171-4.
75. Kurzrock R, Gutterman JU, Talpaz M. The molecular genetics of Philadelphia chromosome-positive leukemias. N Engl J Med 1988;319: 990-8.
76. Kurzrock R, Kloetzer WS, Talpaz M, Blick M, Walters R, Arlinghaus RB, et al. Identification of molecular variants of p210bcr-abl in chronic myelogenous leukemia. Blood 1987;70:233-6.
77. Kurzrock R, Shtalrid M, Gutterman JU, Koller CA, Walters R, Trujillo JM, et al. Molecular analysis of chromosome 22 breakpoints in adult Philadelphia-positive acute lymphoblastic leukaemia. Br J Haematol 1987;67:55-9.
78. Kusec R, Laczika K, Knobl P, Friedl J, Greinix H, Kahls P, et al. AML1/ ETO fusion mRNA can be detected in remission blood samples of all patients with t(8;21) acute myeloid leukemia after chemotherapy or autologous bone marrow transplantation. Leukemia 1994;8:735-9.
79. Langabeer SE, Walker H, Rogers JR, Burnett AK, Wheatley K, Swirsky D, et al. Incidence of AML1/ETO fusion transcripts in patients entered into the MRC AML trials. MRC Adult Leukaemia Working Party. Br J Haematol 1997;99:925-8.
80. Le Coniat M, Souyri M, Vigon I, Wendling F, Tambourin P, Berger R. The human homolog of the myeloproliferative virus maps to chromosome band 1p34. Hum Genet 1989;83:194-6.
81. Lehman CM, Sarago C, Nasim S, Comerford J, Karcher DS, Garrett CT. Comparison of PCR with Southern hybridization for the routine detection of immunoglobulin heavy chain gene rearrangements. Am J Clin Pathol 1995;103:171-6.
82. Lenz G, Davis RE, Ngo VN, Lam L, George TC, Wright GW, et al. Oncogenic CARD11 mutations in human diffuse large B cell lymphoma. Science 2008;319:1676-9.
83. Lepelley P, Preudhomme C, Vanrumbeke M, Quesnel B, Cosson A, Fenaux P. Detection of p53 mutations in hematological malignancies: comparison between immunocytochemistry and DNA analysis. Leukemia 1994;8:1342-9.
84. Lerner MR, Andrews NC, Miller G, Steitz JA. Two small RNAs encoded by Epstein-Barr virus and complexed with protein are precipitated by antibodies from patients with systemic lupus erythematosus. Proc Natl Acad Sci U S A 1981;78:805-9.
85. Leroux D, Le Marc'Hadour F, Gressin R, Jacob MC, Keddari E, Monteil M, et al. Non-Hodgkin's lymphomas with t(11;14)(q13;q32): a subset of mantle zone/intermediate lymphocytic lymphoma? Br J Haematol 1991;77:346-53.
86. Levine RL, Wadleigh M, Cools J, Ebert BL, Wernig G, Huntly BJ, et al. Activating mutation in the tyrosine kinase JAK2 in polycythemia vera, essential thrombocythemia, and myeloid metaplasia with myelofibrosis. Cancer Cell 2005;7:387-97.
87. Limpens J, de Jong D, van Krieken JH, Price CG, Young BD, van Ommen GJ, et al. Bcl-2/JH rearrangements in benign lymphoid tissues with follicular hyperplasia. Oncogene 1991;6:2271-6.
88. Liu P, Tarle SA, Hajra A, Claxton DF, Marlton P, Freedman M, et al. Fusion between transcription factor CBF beta/PEBP2 beta and a myosin heavy chain in acute myeloid leukemia. Science 1993;261: 1041-4.
89. Longley BJ Jr, Metcalfe DD, Tharp M, Wang X, Tyrrell L, Lu SZ, et al. Activating and dominant inactivating c-KIT catalytic domain mutations in distinct clinical forms of human mastocytosis. Proc Natl Acad Sci U S A 1999;96:1609-14.
90. Longo L, Pandolfi PP, Biondi A, Rambaldi A, Mencarelli A, Lo Coco F, et al. Rearrangements and aberrant expression of the retinoic acid receptor alpha gene in acute promyelocytic leukemias. J Exp Med 1990;172:1571-5.
91. Maurer J, Janssen JW, Thiel E, van Denderen J, Ludwig WD, Aydemir U, et al. Detection of chimeric BCR-ABL genes in acute lymphoblastic leukaemia by the polymerase chain reaction. Lancet 1991;337:1055-8.
92. Medeiros LJ, Carr J. Overview of the role of molecular methods in the diagnosis of malignant lymphomas. Arch Pathol Lab Med 1999;123: 1189-207.
93. Melo JV, Myint H, Galton DA, Goldman JM. P190BCR-ABL chronic myeloid leukaemia: the missing link with chronic myelomonocytic leukaemia? Leukemia 1994;8:208-11.
94. Mitterbauer M, Kusec R, Schwarzinger I, Haas OA, Lechner K, Jaeger U. Comparison of karyotype analysis and RT-PCR for AML1/ETO in 204 unselected patients with AML. Ann Hematol 1998;76:139-43.

95. Moppett J, Burke GA, Steward CG, Oakhill A, Goulden NJ. The clinical relevance of detection of minimal residual disease in childhood acute lymphoblastic leukaemia. J Clin Pathol 2003;56:249-53.
96. Morris SW, Kirstein MN, Valentine MB, Dittmer KG, Shapiro DN, Saltman DL, et al. Fusion of a kinase gene, ALK, to a nucleolar protein gene, NPM, in non-Hodgkin's lymphoma. Science 1994;263:1281-4.
97. Motokura T, Arnold A. PRAD1/cyclin D1 proto-oncogene: genomic organization, 5′ DNA sequence, and sequence of a tumor-specific rearrangement breakpoint. Genes Chromosomes Cancer 1993;7:89-95.
98. Mrozek K, Heinonen K, de la Chapelle A, Bloomfield CD. Clinical significance of cytogenetics in acute myeloid leukemia. Semin Oncol 1997;24:17-31.
99. Nakao M, Yokota S, Iwai T, Kaneko H, Horiike S, Kashima K, et al. Internal tandem duplication of the flt3 gene found in acute myeloid leukemia. Leukemia 1996;10:1911-8.
100. Neubauer A, Dodge RK, George SL, Davey FR, Silver RT, Schiffer CA, et al. Prognostic importance of mutations in the ras proto-oncogenes in de novo acute myeloid leukemia. Blood 1994;83:1603-11.
101. Neubauer A, Greenberg P, Negrin R, Ginzton N, Liu E. Mutations in the ras proto-oncogenes in patients with myelodysplastic syndromes. Leukemia 1994;8:638-41.
102. Orita M, Iwahana H, Kanazawa H, Hayashi K, Sekiya T. Detection of polymorphisms of human DNA by gel electrophoresis as single-strand conformation polymorphisms. Proc Natl Acad Sci U S A 1989;86:2766-70.
103. Pabst T, Mueller BU, Zhang P, Radomska HS, Narravula S, Schnittger S, et al. Dominant-negative mutations of CEBPA, encoding CCAAT/enhancer binding protein-alpha (C/EBPalpha), in acute myeloid leukemia. Nat Genet 2001;27:263-70.
104. Paietta E, Racevskis J, Neuberg D, Rowe JM, Goldstone AH, Wiernik PH. Expression of CD25 (interleukin-2 receptor alpha chain) in adult acute lymphoblastic leukemia predicts for the presence of BCR/ABL fusion transcripts: results of a preliminary laboratory analysis of ECOG/MRC Intergroup Study E2993. Eastern Cooperative Oncology Group/Medical Research Council. Leukemia 1997;11:1887-90.
105. Pane F, Frigeri F, Sindona M, Luciano L, Ferrara F, Cimino R, et al. Neutrophilic-chronic myeloid leukemia: a distinct disease with a specific molecular marker (BCR/ABL with C3/A2 junction). Blood 1996;88:2410-4.
106. Pardanani AD, Levine RL, Lasho T, Pikman Y, Mesa RA, Wadleigh M, et al. MPL515 mutations in myeloproliferative and other myeloid disorders: a study of 1182 patients. Blood 2006;108:3472-6.
107. Petkovich M, Brand NJ, Krust A, Chambon P. A human retinoic acid receptor which belongs to the family of nuclear receptors. Nature 1987;330:444-50.
108. Raab-Traub N, Flynn K. The structure of the termini of the Epstein-Barr virus as a marker of clonal cellular proliferation. Cell 1986;47:883-9.
109. Radich J, Gehly G, Lee A, Avery R, Bryant E, Edmands S, et al. Detection of bcr-abl transcripts in Philadelphia chromosome-positive acute lymphoblastic leukemia after marrow transplantation. Blood 1997;89:2602-9.
110. Radich JP, Gehly G, Gooley T, Bryant E, Clift RA, Collins S, et al. Polymerase chain reaction detection of the BCR-ABL fusion transcript after allogeneic marrow transplantation for chronic myeloid leukemia: results and implications in 346 patients. Blood 1995;85:2632-8.
111. Rimokh R, Berger F, Delsol G, Charrin C, Bertheas MF, French M, et al. Rearrangement and overexpression of the BCL-1/PRAD-1 gene in intermediate lymphocytic lymphomas and in t(11q13)-bearing leukemias. Blood 1993;81:3063-7.
112. Rimokh R, Gadoux M, Bertheas MF, Berger F, Garoscio M, Deleage G, et al. FVT-1, a novel human transcription unit affected by variant translocation t(2;18)(p11;q21) of follicular lymphoma. Blood 1993;81:136-42.
113. Rowley J. Identification of a translocation with quinicrine fluorescence in a patient with acute leukemia. Ann Genet 1973;16:109-12.
114. Saglio G, Pane F, Gottardi E, Frigeri F, Buonaiuto MR, Guerrasio A, et al. Consistent amounts of acute leukemia-associated P190BCR/ABL transcripts are expressed by chronic myelogenous leukemia patients at diagnosis. Blood 1996;87:1075-80.
115. Sakashita A, Hattori T, Miller CW, Suzushima H, Asou N, Takatsuki K, et al. Mutations of the p53 gene in adult T-cell leukemia. Blood 1992;79:477-80.
116. Sander CA, Yano T, Clark HM, Harris C, Longo DL, Jaffe ES, et al. p53 mutation is associated with progression in follicular lymphomas. Blood 1993;82:1994-2004.
117. Schlenk RF, Dohner K, Kneba M, Gotze K, Hartmann F, Del Valle F, et al. Gene mutations and response to treatment with all-trans retinoic acid in elderly patients with acute myeloid leukemia. Results from the AMLSG Trial AML HD98B. Haematologica 2009;94:54-60.
118. Schlenk RF, Dohner K, Krauter J, Frohling S, Corbacioglu A, Bullinger L, et al. Mutations and treatment outcome in cytogenetically normal acute myeloid leukemia. N Engl J Med 2008;358:1909-18.
119. Schlieben S, Borkhardt A, Reinisch I, Ritterbach J, Janssen JW, Ratei R, et al. Incidence and clinical outcome of children with BCR/ABL-positive acute lymphoblastic leukemia (ALL): a prospective RT-PCR study based on 673 patients enrolled in the German pediatric multicenter therapy trials ALL-BFM-90 and CoALL-05-92. Leukemia 1996;10:957-63.
120. Schnittger S, Bacher U, Haferlach C, Beelen D, Bojko P, Burkle D, et al. Characterization of 35 new cases with four different MPLW515 mutations and essential thrombocytosis or primary myelofibrosis. Haematologica 2009;94:141-4.
121. Schnittger S, Bacher U, Haferlach C, Dengler R, Krober A, Kern W, et al. Detection of an MPLW515 mutation in a case with features of both essential thrombocythemia and refractory anemia with ringed sideroblasts and thrombocytosis. Leukemia 2008;22:453-5.
122. Schnittger S, Schoch C, Kern W, Mecucci C, Tschulik C, Martelli MF, et al. Nucleophosmin gene mutations are predictors of favorable prognosis in acute myelogenous leukemia with a normal karyotype. Blood 2005;106:3733-9.
123. Scott LM, Tong W, Levine RL, Scott MA, Beer PA, Stratton MR, et al. JAK2 exon 12 mutations in polycythemia vera and idiopathic erythrocytosis. N Engl J Med 2007;356:459-68.
124. Secker-Walker LM, Craig JM, Hawkins JM, Hoffbrand AV. Philadelphia positive acute lymphoblastic leukemia in adults: age distribution, BCR breakpoint and prognostic significance. Leukemia 1991;5:196-9.
125. Segal GH, Jorgensen T, Masih AS, Braylan RC. Optimal primer selection for clonality assessment by polymerase chain reaction analysis. I. Low grade B-cell lymphoproliferative disorders of nonfollicular center cell type. Hum Pathol 1994;25:1269-75.
126. Segal GH, Jorgensen T, Scott M, Braylan RC. Optimal primer selection for clonality assessment by polymerase chain reaction analysis. II. Follicular lymphomas. Hum Pathol 1994;25:1276-82.
127. Selleri L, von Lindern M, Hermans A, Meijer D, Torelli G, Grosveld G. Chronic myeloid leukemia may be associated with several bcr-abl transcripts including the acute lymphoid leukemia-type 7 kb transcript. Blood 1990;75:1146-53.
128. Seto M, Jaeger U, Hockett RD, Graninger W, Bennett S, Goldman P, et al. Alternative promoters and exons, somatic mutation and deregulation of the Bcl-2-Ig fusion gene in lymphoma. EMBO J 1988;7:123-31.
129. Shepherd P, Suffolk R, Halsey J, Allan N. Analysis of molecular breakpoint and m-RNA transcripts in a prospective randomized trial of interferon in chronic myeloid leukaemia: no correlation with clinical features, cytogenetic response, duration of chronic phase, or survival. Br J Haematol 1995;89:546-54.
130. Sioutos N, Bagg A, Michaud GY, Irving SG, Hartmann DP, Siragy H, et al. Polymerase chain reaction versus Southern blot hybridization: detection of immunoglobulin heavy-chain gene rearrangements. Diagn Mol Pathol 1995;4:8-13.
131. Steenbergen EJ, Verhagen OJ, van Leeuwen EF, van den Berg H, Behrendt H, Slater RM, et al. Prolonged persistence of PCR-detectable

minimal residual disease after diagnosis or first relapse predicts poor outcome in childhood B-precursor acute lymphoblastic leukemia. Leukemia 1995;9:1726-34.

132. Stirewalt DL, Kopecky KJ, Meshinchi S, Appelbaum FR, Slovak ML, Willman CL, et al. FLT3, RAS, and TP53 mutations in elderly patients with acute myeloid leukemia. Blood 2001;97:3589-95.
133. Suzuki T, Kiyoi H, Ozeki K, Tomita A, Yamaji S, Suzuki R, et al. Clinical characteristics and prognostic implications of NPM1 mutations in acute myeloid leukemia. Blood 2005;106:2854-61.
134. Suzuki Y, Orita M, Shiraishi M, Hayashi K, Sekiya T. Detection of ras gene mutations in human lung cancers by single-strand conformation polymorphism analysis of polymerase chain reaction products. Oncogene 1990;5:1037-43.
135. Tanner J, Weis J, Fearon D, Whang Y, Kieff E. Epstein-Barr virus gp350/220 binding to the B lymphocyte C3d receptor mediates adsorption, capping, and endocytosis. Cell 1987;50:203-13.
136. Tefferi A, Strand JJ, Lasho TL, Knudson RA, Finke CM, Gangat N, et al. Bone marrow JAK2V617F allele burden and clinical correlates in polycythemia vera. Leukemia 2007;21:2074-5.
137. Tefferi A, Thiele J, Orazi A, Kvasnicka HM, Barbui T, Hanson CA, et al. Proposals and rationale for revision of the World Health Organization diagnostic criteria for polycythemia vera, essential thrombocythemia, and primary myelofibrosis: recommendations from an ad hoc international expert panel. Blood 2007;110:1092-7.
138. Templeton NS. The polymerase chain reaction: history, methods, and applications. Diagn Mol Pathol 1992;1:58-72.
139. Thiede C, Koch S, Creutzig E, Steudel C, Illmer T, Schaich M, et al. Prevalence and prognostic impact of NPM1 mutations in 1485 adult patients with acute myeloid leukemia (AML). Blood 2006;107: 4011-20.
140. Tonegawa S. Somatic generation of antibody diversity. Nature 1983;302:575-81.
141. Tsujimoto Y, Cossman J, Jaffe E, Croce CM. Involvement of the BCL2gene in human follicular lymphoma. Science 1985;228: 1440-3.
142. Tsujimoto Y, Gorham J, Cossman J, Jaffe E, Croce CM. The t(14;18) chromosome translocations involved in B-cell neoplasms result from mistakes in VDJ joining. Science 1985;229:1390-3.
143. Tsujimoto Y, Yunis J, Onorato-Showe L, Erikson J, Nowell PC, Croce CM. Molecular cloning of the chromosomal breakpoint of B-cell lymphomas and leukemias with the t(11;14) chromosome translocation. Science 1984;224:1403-6.
144. Tyagi S, Kramer FR. Molecular beacons: probes that fluoresce upon hybridization. Nat Biotechnol 1996;14:303-8.
145. Vaandrager JW, Schuuring E, Zwikstra E, de Boer CJ, Kleiverda KK, van Krieken JH, et al. Direct visualization of dispersed 11q13 chromosomal translocations in mantle cell lymphoma by multicolor DNA fiber fluorescence in situ hybridization. Blood 1996;88:1177-82.
146. van Rhee F, Marks DI, Lin F, Szydlo RM, Hochhaus A, Treleaven J, et al. Quantification of residual disease in Philadelphia-positive acute lymphoblastic leukemia: comparison of blood and bone marrow. Leukemia 1995;9:329-35.
147. Vardiman JW, Thiele J, Arber DA, Brunning RD, Borowitz MJ, Porwit A, et al. The 2008 revision of the World Health Organization (WHO) classification of myeloid neoplasms and acute leukemia: rationale and important changes. Blood 2009;114:937-51.
148. Wang AM, Doyle MV, Mark DF. Quantitation of mRNA by the polymerase chain reaction. Proc Natl Acad Sci U S A 1989;86:9717-21.
149. Wasserman R, Galili N, Ito Y, Silber JH, Reichard BA, Shane S, et al. Residual disease at the end of induction therapy as a predictor of relapse during therapy in childhood B-lineage acute lymphoblastic leukemia. J Clin Oncol 1992;10:1879-88.
150. Wattel E, Preudhomme C, Hecquet B, Vanrumbeke M, Quesnel B, Dervite I, et al. p53 mutations are associated with resistance to chemotherapy and short survival in hematologic malignancies. Blood 1994;84:3148-57.
151. Weisenburger DD, Sanger WG, Armitage JO, Purtilo DT. Intermediate lymphocytic lymphoma: immunophenotypic and cytogenetic findings. Blood 1987;69:1617-21.
152. Weiss LM, Warnke RA, Sklar J, Cleary ML. Molecular analysis of the t(14;18) chromosomal translocation in malignant lymphomas. N Engl J Med 1987;317:1185-9.
153. Wertz IE, O'Rourke KM, Zhou H, Eby M, Aravind L, Seshagiri S, et al. De-ubiquitination and ubiquitin ligase domains of A20 downregulate NF-kappaB signalling. Nature 2004;430:694-9.
154. Westbrook CA, Hooberman AL, Spino C, Dodge RK, Larson RA, Davey F, et al. Clinical significance of the BCR-ABL fusion gene in adult acute lymphoblastic leukemia: a Cancer and Leukemia Group B Study (8762). Blood 1992;80:2983-90.
155. Williams ME, Swerdlow SH, Rosenberg CL, Arnold A. Chromosome 11 translocation breakpoints at the PRAD1/cyclin D1 gene locus in centrocytic lymphoma. Leukemia 1993;7:241-5.
156. Wittwer CT, Herrmann MG, Moss AA, Rasmussen RP. Continuous fluorescence monitoring of rapid cycle DNA amplification. Biotechniques 1997;22:130-1, 4-8.
157. Yamamoto Y, Kiyoi H, Nakano Y, Suzuki R, Kodera Y, Miyawaki S, et al. Activating mutation of D835 within the activation loop of FLT3 in human hematologic malignancies. Blood 2001;97:2434-9.

CHAPTER 45

Plasma Nucleic Acids

Y. M. Dennis Lo, M.A., D.M., D.Phil., F.R.C.P.(Lond. & Edin.), F.R.C.Path., F.R.S.,, and Rossa W. K. Chiu, M.B.B.S., Ph.D., F.H.K.A.M.(Pathology), F.R.C.P.A.

With the notable exception of virology, much of molecular diagnostics has been built on the detection of nucleic acids from cellular materials. However, over the past 15 years or so, much interest has developed in the molecular diagnostic applications of cell-free nucleic acids in plasma and serum. This chapter reviews the remarkable developments in this emerging area.

DISCOVERY AND EARLY WORK

It is generally agreed that cell-free nucleic acids in plasma were first discovered by Mandel and Metais in 1948.[136] It was especially remarkable that this work preceded the discovery of the double-helical structure of DNA in 1953.[204] However, the significance of the work by Mandel and Métais was not recognized for many years. It was not until 1966 that interest in the area re-emerged with the finding of DNA in the serum of patients with systemic lupus erythematosus.[187] Similar findings in other autoimmune diseases were subsequently reported.[101] In the 1970s, it was reported that increased concentrations of cell-free DNA were found in the serum of cancer patients, when compared with controls.[102] Furthermore, it was shown that the reduction in concentrations of serum DNA correlated with treatment response. However, the origin of such serum DNA remained unclear.

CIRCULATING DNA AS A TUMOR MARKER

In 1989, Stroun and associates proposed that such DNA might have originated from cancer cells.[182] However, definitive proof of this hypothesis had to wait until 1994, when two groups used polymerase chain reaction (PCR)-based technologies to show that oncogene mutations were indeed detectable in the plasma of patients with pancreatic cancer,[179] myelodysplastic syndrome, and acute myelogenous leukemia.[197] Two years later, two groups confirmed these observations by showing that tumor-derived microsatellite alterations could be found in the plasma and serum of patients with small cell lung cancer[25] and head and neck cancer,[146] respectively. These results laid the foundation for rapid developments in the field over the following decade (Table 45-1).

Measurement of Total Plasma DNA Concentrations

Several groups have replicated the previously mentioned pioneering work on plasma and serum DNA. On the simplest level, the total concentrations of DNA in plasma are measured. Thus, some groups have demonstrated that the total concentrations of DNA in the plasma of cancer patients are generally higher than those in controls.[5,8,171,174,180] For example, Sozzi and colleagues showed that the median concentration of plasma DNA in lung cancer patients is almost eight times higher than that in controls.[180] Similar results have been reported by Paci and coworkers.[154] However, it is important to note that the total concentration of plasma/serum DNA is relatively nonspecific and could be influenced by pathologies other than cancer (e.g., tissue injury, as discussed later). Thus, most workers in the field have focused on a variety of tumor-derived genetic and other molecular alterations.

Plasma DNA Size as a Tumor Marker

Circulating DNA in plasma consists of short fragments of DNA.[87] In 2003, it was shown that the DNA molecules in the plasma of gynecologic and breast cancer patients were shorter than those in the plasma of control subjects.[200] In this study, the length of plasma DNA molecules was assessed by measuring the relative abundance of a longer versus a shorter fragment of DNA using quantitative PCR.[200] Results were expressed as a *DNA integrity index.* This approach was similar to the method used to analyze the length of Epstein-Barr virus (EBV) DNA in the plasma of patients with nasopharyngeal carcinoma (NPC).[20] Wang and associates attributed the success of plasma DNA size as a tumor marker to the fact that necrosis might be a relatively commonly phenomenon in tumor tissues and might be associated with the liberation of relatively longer fragments of DNA into the plasma. It was also suggested that cell death in normal tissues might be more related to apoptosis, which might be associated with the release of shorter DNA fragments into the circulation. Various groups have confirmed the potential usefulness of plasma DNA integrity analysis for cancer patients.[18,73,89,196] For example, Chan and colleagues reported that the plasma DNA integrity of NPC patients was higher than that of controls.[18] Furthermore, radiotherapy was associated with a reduction

TABLE 45-1 Plasma Nucleic Acid Features Associated With Tumors

Features	Examples
Total plasma DNA concentration	Elevated in cancer patients over controls
Plasma DNA size	Plasma DNA molecules are longer (higher integrity) in cancer patients than in controls
Loss of heterozygosity	Microsatellite and single-nucleotide polymorphism analysis
Gene mutations	*KRAS, APC, TP53, EGFR*
Aberrant DNA methylation	P16, *SEPT9* (septin 9), *APC, GSTP1, RASSF1, rarB2*
Tumor-associated viral DNA	HBV, HPV, EBV
Plasma RNA	Tyrosinase, VEGF, thymidylate synthase, *BMI1,* laminin B1
Plasma RNA integrity	Plasma RNA molecules are more fragmented (reduced integrity) in cancer patients than in controls
Plasma microRNA	Aberrant concentrations of certain microRNA species in a number of malignancies

EBV, Epstein-Barr virus; *HBV,* hepatitis B virus; *HPV,* human papillomavirus; *VEGF,* vascular endothelial growth factor.

in the plasma DNA integrity index in 70% of patients. Most important, patients who did not demonstrate this reduction had a worse prognosis than those who had normalization in the DNA integrity index. However, Holdenrieder and coworkers and Boddy and associates were unable to reproduce the value of DNA integrity analysis for the plasma and serum of cancer patients.[9,77] Chan and colleagues studied preanalytical factors associated with the measurement of DNA integrity.[19] These workers showed that clotting and delayed separation of plasma from blood cells for 24 hours would significantly increase the concentration and observed size of cell-free DNA in blood samples. They also showed that repeated freezing and thawing of plasma samples, but not extracted DNA, leads to fragmentation of DNA. These factors should be taken into consideration if DNA integrity should become a clinical molecular test.

Detection of Loss of Heterozygosity in Plasma

Numerous groups have reported the detection of tumor-associated loss of heterozygosity (LOH) in the plasma/serum of cancer patients. As examples, this has been reported in lung cancer,[68] prostate cancer,[143,172] breast cancer,[173] melanoma,[185,186] renal cancer,[69] and transitional cell carcinoma of the urinary bladder.[199] Most workers have used microsatellites as the targets for such analysis. However, debate regarding the robustness of this approach is ongoing, as it has been demonstrated that PCR artifacts might occasionally result in the false identification of LOH when in fact none is present.[40] It has been suggested that fractionation of plasma DNA and specific targeting of lower-molecular-weight DNA might improve the detection of LOH in plasma.[143] Targeting of single-nucleotide polymorphisms (SNPs), instead of microsatellites, is an alternative method for the detection of LOH.[22]

Detection of Somatic Gene Mutations in Plasma

Another approach for the detection of tumor-derived DNA in plasma is to target mutant gene sequences. Examples of genes that have been studied in this fashion include the *KRAS* oncogene in colorectal carcinoma[94,166,167,183] and pancreatic carcinoma,[12,58,210] the adenomatosis polyposis coli *(APC)* gene in colorectal carcinoma,[97] and the *TP53* gene (coding for the p53 protein) in lung cancer,[72] ovarian cancer,[152] and hepatocellular carcinoma (HCC).[79,90,92] Much interest has been expressed in mutations in the epidermal growth factor receptor *(EGFR)* gene in non–small-cell lung cancer and its relation to response to tyrosine kinase inhibitors.[133,155] It has been shown that the mutational status of the *EGFR* gene can be predicted from plasma/serum DNA analysis and is strongly correlated with response to tyrosine kinase inhibitor treatment.[91,134,213]

The main challenge faced by investigators working with the detection of tumor-derived gene mutations is that the minority mutant DNA molecules are surrounded by a "sea" of nonmutant molecules. Thus, detection methods should allow the sensitive and specific detection of such mutant sequences from the background. Many workers initially used allele-specific PCR amplification.[40,91]

Much promise has been shown with the use of techniques that allow analysis of single DNA molecules. One such method is single-molecule PCR or digital PCR (see Chapter 17), in which the DNA template is diluted and then amplified in a series of PCRs.[198] The degree of dilution is such that each PCR will contain approximately 0.5 copy of the template. In such a situation, distribution of the template DNA molecule among the PCRs will follow the Poisson distribution,[125] with some reactions containing no target molecule and other reactions containing a single target molecule. The Poisson distribution also predicts that some reactions will contain more than a single target molecule. However, the latter will be the minority at the template concentration of 0.5 copy of target per reaction. Reactions containing a single target molecule, mutant or wild-type, can be analyzed without the interference of closely related sequences. Another advantage of the digital PCR approach lies in its quantitative applications. In this regard, the number of positive reactions will reflect the number of starting template molecules. The number of reactions containing more than one template molecule can be mathematically "corrected" by using the Poisson distribution.[125] The main disadvantage of digital PCR is the need to carry out numerous parallel PCRs. However, the development of several platforms for high-throughput implementation of digital PCR has offered the hope that this method might eventually be used in routine molecular diagnostics. One such method employs microfluidics to distribute the reaction mixture to hundreds or thousands of nanoliter chambers.[203] This method has been used for the detection and measurement of the concentration of *EGFR* mutations in the plasma of non–small-cell lung cancer patients.[213] Another method involves the performance of PCR in emulsions, following the capture of PCR products on beads.[48] This method, which is referred to as *BEAMing (beads, emulsion, amplification, and magnetics)*, has been used to detect and measure the concentration of mutant DNA molecules in the plasma of colorectal cancer patients.[44,45]

Detection of Aberrant DNA Methylation in Plasma

Much interest has arisen in the study of epigenetic alterations in tumors. *Epigenetics* is the study of molecular changes that influence gene expression, but that do not involve a change in DNA sequence.[175] One of the best studied epigenetic mechanisms is DNA methylation, which typically involves the methylation of the cytosine residue of the CpG dinucleotide. DNA methylation in the promoter region of genes is associated with gene silencing.[85] This is one of the mechanisms for the inactivation of tumor suppressor genes in cancer.[139] In 1999, two groups first demonstrated the presence of tumor-associated DNA methylation in the plasma and serum of cancer patients.[51,208] Both groups used a method known as methylation-specific PCR (MSP).[75] DNA for MSP analysis is first treated with bisulfite, a process that converts unmethylated cytosine to uracil, while leaving methylated cytosine unchanged.[62] Hence, methylated and unmethylated sequences can then be amplified using different primers. The versatility of MSP has since been enhanced by the development of quantitative MSP, in which the concentration of targets with different methylation status can be measured.[49,117]

Tumor-associated DNA methylation changes have since been detected for many tumor suppressor genes and for many types of cancer. Examples include the gene for p16 in non–small-cell lung cancer,[51] colorectal cancer,[145] and HCC[208] patients; the *SEPT9* gene (septin 9) in colorectal cancer[71]; the *APC* and several other genes in breast cancer[78]; and the *GSTP1* gene in prostate cancer.[4] The main advantage of the methylation-based approach is that one methylation assay can typically be used for several tumor types. This is different from the previously mentioned approach of targeting tumor-specific gene mutations in which multiple assays are often needed to target the many possible mutations of a gene.

The main disadvantage of the MSP-based approach is that the bisulfite conversion step is known to degrade the input of DNA significantly, with certain workers estimating that in some cases, the degree of degradation might be greater than 90%.[70] In addition, many workers have reported that the sensitivity of detecting a single aberrantly methylated marker might be quite low. Possible explanations for this observation include the fact that a particular tumor suppressor gene may be aberrantly methylated in only a proportion of tumors, and the fact that bisulfite-related DNA degradation might reduce the target DNA available for analysis. Thus, many researchers have used a combination of methylated markers for cancer detection purposes.[78]

In an attempt to bypass the use of the bisulfite conversion step, Chan and associates investigated the use of methylation-sensitive restriction enzyme digestion followed by real-time PCR detection of the *RASSF1 (RASSF1A)* gene, which is hypermethylated in a significant proportion of HCC.[17] The methylation-sensitive restriction enzyme will not cleave the hypermethylated, tumor-derived *RASSF1* sequences while digesting the background nonmethylated sequences of non-tumoral origin. This assay shows that hypermethylated *RASSF1* sequences are detectable in 93% of the plasma of patients with HCC, in only 58% of chronic carriers of the hepatitis B virus (HBV), and in 8% of healthy controls. Furthermore, for the former two groups, the median plasma concentration of hypermethylated *RASSF1A* sequences in the cancer group is some 6.5 times higher than that in the HBV carrier group. A possible disadvantage of this approach is the possibility that incomplete digestion by the restriction enzyme will lead to false-positive results. In this regard, quality control steps for assessing the enzyme digestion step are essential. Future studies are needed to investigate the robustness of this approach in a large-scale clinical setting.

Another exciting development in plasma-based methylation analysis is the use of BEAMing for methylation analysis, so-called methyl-BEAMing.[108] This technology allows the digital analysis of individual bisulfite-converted DNA molecules through emulsion PCR, bead capture, and magnetic separation. This technology allows the detection of one methylated DNA molecule in a background of approximately 5000 unmethylated molecules. Clinical utility of this approach has been demonstrated through detection of the hypermethylated vimentin gene in the plasma of colorectal cancer patients.

Viral DNA in Plasma

Several tumor types are associated with viral infection. Examples include the association of HBV infection with HCC, human papillomavirus (HPV) with cervical carcinoma, and EBV infection with NPC. Numerous workers have looked for tumor-associated viral sequences in the plasma or serum of cancer patients. The most convincing data have been reported for detection of EBV DNA in the plasma or serum of NPC patients.[119,144] With the use of real-time PCR technology, EBV DNA has been detected in NPC patients with a sensitivity of 96% and a specificity of 93%.[119] The plasma concentrations appear to be positively correlated with tumor load and stage, and can serve as a prognosticator.[15,104,113,118] Furthermore, measurement of circulating EBV DNA concentrations can allow one to monitor treatment response and to predict tumor relapse.[14,115] Preliminary data suggest that detection of circulating EBV DNA is a marker for the screening of NPC.[103] It has been shown that circulating EBV DNA in NPC patients consists of short DNA fragments, instead of complete virions.[20] EBV has also been associated with certain lymphomas and a small proportion of gastric carcinomas; plasma/

serum EBV DNA has been detected in the plasma of a proportion of such patients.[99,100,120]

A similar approach has been applied to the detection of HPV DNA in the plasma/serum of patients with cervical cancer.* However, the sensitivity of this approach varies greatly from group to group, with several groups reporting very low values. For example, Dong and colleagues reported that only 6.9% of plasma samples obtained from patients with invasive cervical cancer were HPV DNA positive.[47] Similarly, Sathish and coworkers reported a plasma positivity rate of only 11.8% in cervical cancer patients.[169] Thus, the clinical role, if any, of detecting HPV DNA in the plasma of cervical cancer patients remains unclear at the present time.

CIRCULATING RNA AS A TUMOR MARKER

With the success of detecting tumor-derived DNA molecules in the plasma of cancer patients, some workers have started to explore the detection of tumor-derived RNA in plasma. This was first achieved in 1999 by two groups: through the detection of tyrosinase mRNA in the serum of melanoma patients, and through EBV RNA in the plasma of NPC patients.[93,114] These observations were initially rather intriguing, because RNA has been generally regarded as a highly unstable class of molecules. Subsequent work has demonstrated that plasma RNA is particle associated—a configuration that might protect the RNA molecules from degradation in plasma.[64,74,149] Indeed, endogenous plasma RNA has been demonstrated to be stable enough to be processed with several hours' delay from sample collection to preparation. Consistent with its particle-associated nature, plasma RNA has been shown to be degraded rapidly if subjected to detergent treatment (which would disrupt the particles),[50] filtration with submicron-size filters,[50,149] and high-speed centrifugation.[149] Although plasma RNA is stable enough to be detectable by sensitive molecular techniques such as PCR, such molecules nonetheless are fragmented and partially degraded, instead of existing as intact mRNA molecules.[13] Indeed, many species of tumor-derived mRNA have now been successfully detected in the plasma and serum of cancer patients. Examples include vascular endothelial growth factor (VEGF) and thymidylate synthase mRNA in the plasma of patients with colorectal carcinoma,[65,66] Bmi-1 mRNA and RNA subunits of the telomerase complex in the plasma of breast cancer patients,[24,178] and lamin B1 mRNA in the plasma of HCC patients.[184]

Analogous to plasma DNA, investigators have studied the integrity of plasma RNA in cancer patients. However, the observation is reversed, namely, that cancer patients appear to have lower plasma RNA integrity than do controls.[207] A possible explanation of this observation is that the concentration of RNase in the plasma/serum of cancer patients is increased.[163,176]

Much interest has been focused on micro RNAs (miRNAs), a class of short (19 to 25 nucleotides), single-stranded, non–protein-coding RNA that plays an important role in the regulation of gene expression.[86] Chim and associates first reported that cell-free miRNA is detectable in human plasma, using placental miRNA in the plasma of pregnant women as a model system.[26] Following this publication, a flurry of reports were published confirming the presence of miRNA in plasma and serum.* These reports further show that plasma/serum miRNA can be used as a biomarker for various types of cancer, including lymphoma,[98] prostate cancer,[141] ovarian cancer,[164] lung cancer,[23] and colorectal cancer.[147] Chim and colleagues showed that miRNA appeared to be very stable in plasma, indeed even more stable than mRNA in plasma.[26] Furthermore, it was shown by these workers that most of the detected plasma miRNA passed through a 0.22 μm filter. This finding suggests that plasma miRNAs are predominantly non–particle associated, or that they are associated with particles smaller than 0.22 μm. This issue requires continued investigation because other workers have reported the presence of miRNA in plasma in microparticles referred to as *exosomes* or *microvesicles.*[81,160]

FETAL NUCLEIC ACIDS IN MATERNAL PLASMA

Demonstration of the presence of tumor-derived DNA in the plasma of cancer patients prompted Lo and coworkers in 1997 to explore whether an analogous phenomenon might also be present in pregnancy (i.e., whether the fetus would release its DNA into the plasma of its mother).[122] This analogy is particularly intriguing because there are similarities between the placenta of the fetus and a tumor, with the former being referred to as a *pseudomalignant tissue.*[181]

Discovery and Basic Biology of Fetal DNA in Maternal Plasma

Using a sequence on the Y chromosome as a marker for a male fetus, Lo and associates demonstrated that this DNA was detectable in the plasma and serum of a woman bearing a male fetus, thus demonstrating the existence of fetal DNA in maternal plasma.[122] This group of investigators went on to develop a real-time PCR-based assay for measuring the fractional and absolute concentrations of fetal DNA in maternal plasma.[126] It has since been reported that fetal DNA represents a mean of 3 to 6% of the DNA that is present in maternal plasma, as measured by PCR-based techniques. With the use of more precise digital PCR-based techniques, the median fractional concentration of fetal DNA in maternal plasma has been found to be some two times higher, with a median value around 10% in the first and second trimesters, and 20% during the third trimester.[131] The absolute concentration of circulating fetal DNA increases with gestational age, probably as a consequence of the increase in fetal tissue mass. Following delivery, fetal DNA is cleared very rapidly, with a half-life on the order of 16 minutes.[129]

*References 47, 169, 205, 206, 211, and 212.

*References 23, 81, 98, 141, 160, and 164.

The tissue of origin of fetal DNA in maternal plasma has been generally agreed to be the placenta. This conclusion is supported by various findings. First, fetal DNA has been found in maternal plasma even in anembryonic pregnancies, in which no embryo was found, but in which the placenta was present.[2] Second, it has been shown that fetal DNA in maternal serum carries the placental karyotype in cases in which the fetus proper and the placenta contain different cytogenetic signatures.[60] Finally, fetal DNA in maternal plasma has been shown to carry the DNA methylation signature of the placenta.[16,27,28,151]

Through the use of a series of quantitative PCR assays with different amplicon lengths, Chan and colleagues showed that circulating fetal DNA in maternal plasma consisted of short DNA fragments.[21] These observations are consistent with the suggestion that fetal DNA is released from the placenta into the maternal plasma as a result of apoptosis or necrosis.[188] Furthermore, it was shown that circulating fetal DNA was generally shorter in length than the maternally derived DNA in maternal plasma.[21] This observation has opened up the possibility of preferentially enriching for fetal DNA by targeting short DNA fragments. One way of doing this is by electrophoresis of plasma DNA fragments.[109,112] Another method consists of digital PCR analysis of plasma DNA from maternal plasma using a nested set of PCR primers.[132] The nested set of primers would produce amplicons of different sizes. A digital PCR well containing a long (e.g., maternal) template DNA molecule would be predicted to produce both a long and a short amplicon. Conversely, a digital PCR well containing a short (e.g., fetal) DNA molecule would produce only the short amplicon. This has been referred to as *digital size selection.*[132] One advantage of this system is that the size cutoff can be readily changed by designing PCR primers with different amplicon sizes.

Rapid clearance of circulating fetal DNA following delivery has prompted some investigators to study the mechanisms of clearance. Botezatu and associates postulated that a proportion of fetal DNA in maternal plasma might be cleared via the urinary system, with some fetal DNA still detectable in maternal urine.[10] However, several other groups have been unable to detect fetal DNA in maternal urine, or they did so only at a relatively low proportion, even during the third trimester, or in pathologies associated with increased concentrations of fetal DNA in maternal plasma (e.g., preeclampsia).[83,111,135] One possible explanation for the difficulties experienced by these latter groups is that fetal DNA in maternal urine, if present, would be even more fragmented than its counterpart in maternal plasma. Thus, very short amplicons or special methods for urine DNA extraction might be required for such analysis.[177]

Applications to Sex-Linked Diseases, RhD Genotyping, and Monogenic Disease

The first diagnostic applications of cell-free fetal DNA in maternal plasma have centered on those that could be achieved through the detection of fetal-derived paternally inherited sequences that are not present in the genome of the pregnant woman (Figure 45-1). One example of such an application is fetal sex determination by the detection of Y chromosomal sequences from a male fetus in maternal plasma. This strategy is useful for the noninvasive prenatal diagnosis of sex-linked disorders.[38,82] This approach is also useful for the prenatal investigation of congenital adrenal hyperplasia, because if the fetus can be shown to be male, then prenatal steroid treatment to avoid virilization could be avoided.[82,165] Another example of such an application is the prenatal determination of fetal RhD status in pregnancies involving an RhD-negative pregnant woman.[52,59,123] The robustness of the fetal sex and RhD applications is high, and these applications have been utilized for clinical purposes in a number of centers in Europe and the United States.

Several groups have reported the detection of paternally inherited fetal gene mutations in maternal plasma. Examples include mutations causing achondroplasia,[110,168] myotonic dystrophy,[3] α-thalassemia,[34] β-thalassemia,[76] and cystic fibrosis.[11,67] For autosomal dominant disorders, such as achondroplasia, the detection of a fetal-derived mutation from the plasma of a woman who does not carry the mutation is indicative of an at-risk fetus (see Figure 45-1). However, for autosomal recessive disorders, early work in this area was focused on families in which the father and mother carried different mutations (see Figure 45-1). Thus, detection of the mutation that the father has passed on to the fetus would only increase the fetal risk of being a compound heterozygous victim of the disease from 25 to 50%. Conversely, if the paternal mutation is shown to be undetectable in maternal plasma, an affected fetus can be excluded (see Figure 45-1).[34] Diagnostically, the latter scenario is more useful for patient management than the former scenario. An alternative way is to examine genetic polymorphisms linked to the wild-type (i.e., nonmutant) gene in the father and demonstrate that the fetus has inherited the wild-type paternal marker combination.[31,46]

A technical challenge for these applications is the need to detect a minority sequence (i.e., the fetal target) that might differ from the majority background (i.e., the maternal background) by as little as a single base pair (e.g., for the detection of a single point mutation, or an SNP allele). Examples of methods that have been developed for this purpose include single-allele base extension[46] or allele-specific base extension,[191] followed by mass spectrometry or peptide nucleic acid clamping.[109] Investigators have combined (1) the previously mentioned size selection strategy for enriching shorter fetal DNA molecules, and (2) such assays for detecting fetal-derived gene mutations or polymorphisms in maternal plasma.[109] Another very promising approach for the sensitive and specific detection of fetal-derived gene mutations and polymorphisms is through the use of digital PCR.[125,131,132] Thus, by the use of highly diluted DNA samples and multiple digital PCRs, in which each reaction contains a mean of some 0.5 target molecule, most reactions would contain just a single target template molecule or no target molecule. In other words, fetal and maternal DNA molecules derived from the same locus would be distributed into separate PCR wells, and thus would not interfere with each other during the

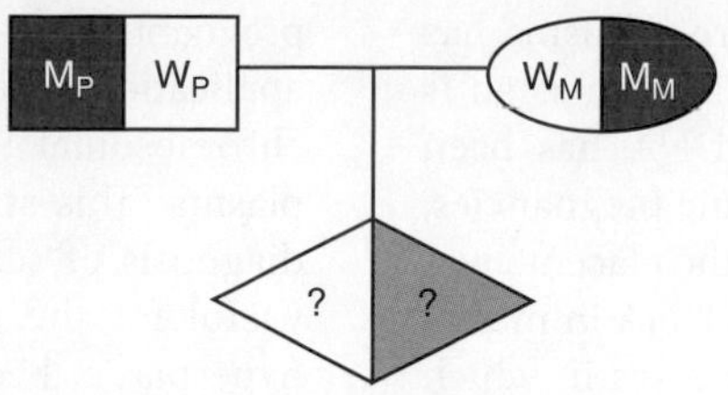

Condition	Approach
Autosomal dominant traits or mutations	
Paternally inherited	Qualitative detection of M_P
Maternally inherited	Quantitative comparison between M_M and W. **If M_M = W, fetus has inherlted M_M.** If M_M < W, fetus has not inherited M_M.
Autosomal recessive conditions or diseases	
When M_P and M_M are identical	Quantitative comparison between M and W. If M = W, fetus is heterozygous. If M > W, fetus is homozygous for the mutation. If M < W, fetus has not inherited the mutation.
When M_P and M_M are different	Assess which paternal allele has been transmitted to the fetus by qualitative detection of M_P or W_P by a polymorphism that distinguishes W_P from M_P, M_M and W_M. Assess which maternal allele has been transmitted to the fetus by quantitative comparison between M_M and W. If M_M = W, fetus has inherited M_M. If M_M < W, fetus has not inherited M_M.

Figure 45-1 Approaches to the noninvasive prenatal diagnosis of monogenic disease by maternal plasma DNA analysis. *M,* Mutant allele; *MM,* maternally inherited mutant allele; *MP,* paternally inherited mutant allele; *W,* wild-type allele; *WM,* maternally inherited wild-type allele; *WP,* paternally inherited wild-type allele.

amplification process. This is analogous to the detection of tumor-derived gene mutations using the digital PCR-based approach described earlier in this chapter. The advent of refinements to the digital PCR process, including microfluidics[131] and BEAMing,[44,45,48] potentially makes this approach more suited to routine clinical application.

Another challenge in this field is to extend the application of plasma DNA-based fetal diagnostics beyond the detection of paternally inherited gene mutations or polymorphic alleles that are absent in the maternal genome. For autosomal recessive disease, such a development would allow a complete diagnosis to be made, instead of just limiting the approach to the exclusion of an affected compound heterozygous fetus.[31,34] This goal has been achieved through the development of the concept of relative mutation detection (RMD) (see Figure 45-1).[132] Thus, for an autosomal recessive disease in which the mother and the father are carriers of the same mutation, the ratio of mutant and wild-type alleles in the parental genomes would be 1 : 1. If the fetus has inherited a mutant allele from both of its parents, then the ratio of the mutant to the wild-type allele in its genome would be 2 : 0. When this fetus then releases its DNA into the maternal plasma, a slight excess of mutant over wild-type alleles in the mixture of genomes is seen in the maternal circulation. This allelic imbalance will be small and correlated with the fractional fetal DNA concentration in maternal plasma. With the use of the superior quantitative precision of digital PCR techniques, such an allele imbalance has been detected successfully in maternal plasma.[132] Conversely, if the fetus has inherited one mutant allele from one of its parents and a wild-type allele from the other parent, then the ratio of mutant to wild-type alleles in its genome would also be 1 : 1. Thus, when this fetus then releases its DNA into the maternal plasma, no allelic imbalance would be observed. With future developments in digital PCR technologies and other digital counting techniques (e.g., massively parallel DNA sequencing described later), it is hoped that this approach will enter clinical practice.

Detection of Chromosomal Aneuploidies

The detection of fetal chromosomal aneuploidies, such as trisomy 21, using cell-free fetal nucleic acids in maternal plasma is challenging because the cell-free nature of such nucleic acids obviates the use of cell-based methods such as fluorescence in situ hybridization (FISH) for counting the number of the target chromosome in a fetal cell. The second

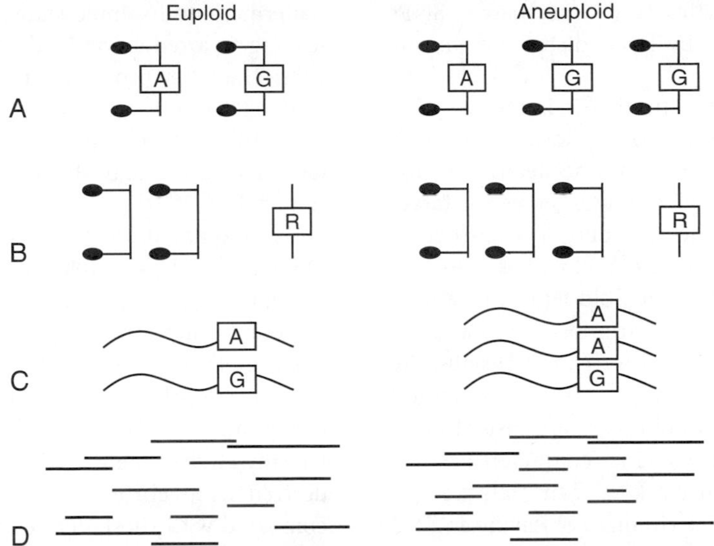

Figure 45-2 Approaches to the noninvasive prenatal diagnosis of fetal aneuploidy by maternal plasma DNA analysis. *A,* Epigenetic allelic ratio approach. Fetal DNA molecules derived from the potentially aneuploid chromosome are distinguished from the maternal counterpart by differential DNA methylation. Chromosome dosage assessment is achieved by comparing the ratio of polymorphic alleles within the locus. *Filled lollipops* denote CpG sites. *Box A* and *Box G* denote different alleles at a single-nucleotide polymorphism (SNP) site. *B,* Epigenetic genetic approach. Fetal DNA molecules derived from the potentially aneuploid chromosome are distinguished from the maternal counterpart by differential DNA methylation. Chromosome dosage assessment is achieved by comparing the relative amounts of aneuploid chromosome against a paternally inherited genetic marker on a reference chromosome. *Box R* denotes a marker on a reference chromosome. *C,* RNA-SNP approach. Chromosome dosage assessment is based on comparing the ratio of heterozygous alleles within fetal-specific RNA molecules derived from the aneuploid chromosome. *Box A* and *Box G* denote different alleles at an SNP site. *D,* Chromosome dosage imbalance approach. Total (maternal + fetal) amount or proportion of plasma DNA molecules derived from the potentially aneuploid chromosome is increased in pregnancies involving an aneuploid fetus rather than a euploid fetus. *Red lines* represent fetal DNA molecules from the aneuploid chromosome. *Black lines* represent maternal DNA molecules from the aneuploid chromosome.

challenge reflects the fact that fetal DNA represents only a small fraction of the total DNA in maternal plasma.[126,131]

Several approaches have been developed to address the challenges of detecting aneuploidies (Figure 45-2). One approach is to target a fetal-specific subset of plasma nucleic acids. One family of such markers consists of loci that demonstrate different DNA methylation patterns between fetal and maternal DNA in maternal plasma.[158] The *SERPINB5* gene, coding for maspin, is the first fetal DNA methylation marker that can be used as a generic indicator of the presence of fetal DNA in maternal plasma.[28] The fetal-derived subset of *SERPINB5* promoter sequences in maternal plasma is characterized by a hypomethylated nature, when compared with maternally derived ones. In other words, when one analyzes hypomethylated *SERPINB5* promoter sequences in maternal plasma, one is essentially just analyzing the fetal-derived sequences. This feature allows one to overcome the challenge concerning low fractional concentrations of fetal DNA in maternal plasma. It is therefore fortunate that the *SERPINB5* gene is present on chromosome 18, the chromosome that is involved in trisomy 18. One would still have to develop a technology to measure the dosage of chromosome 18 through analysis of hypomethylated *SERPINB5* sequences in maternal plasma.

In 2006, Tong and associates achieved this goal through development of the epigenetic allelic ratio (EAR) approach (see Figure 45-2).[189] With this method, one targets fetuses that are heterozygous for an SNP within the region of the *SERPINB5* gene that is hypomethylated in the placenta when compared with maternal blood cells. The latter requirement exists because most of the fetal DNA in maternal plasma is released by the placenta,[2,7,60] while the background maternal DNA has been postulated to be derived from maternal blood cells.[130] For a fetus that has two copies of chromosome 18, the ratio of the two SNP alleles should be 1:1. However, for a fetus that has three copies of chromosome 18, the ratio would be changed to 2:1 or 1:2. The main limitation of the EAR approach is that it requires markers with both usable

DNA methylation characteristics and informative SNPs within a close (e.g., amplifiable by PCR) distance from one another.

Another variant of the epigenetic theme is the so-called epigenetic-genetic (EGG) chromosome dosage approach (see Figure 45-2).[190] With this method, one determines the ratio between a fetal DNA methylation marker on the target chromosome (e.g., chromosome 21) and a fetal-specific genetic marker (e.g., a marker on the Y chromosome for a male fetus). As an illustration, for a euploid fetus, the ratio of a fetal DNA methylation marker on chromosome 21 and a Y chromosomal marker will be 2:1. For a trisomy 21 fetus, the ratio will be 3:1. The main advantage of the EGG method over the EAR method is that it would be much easier to find markers with the required epigenetic characteristics for the EGG approach than to find markers with both the epigenetic characteristics and the requirement of having an SNP marker in the same region for the EAR approach. In this regard, many groups have reported candidate fetal DNA methylation markers on the chromosomes commonly involved in chromosomal aneuploidies of importance for prenatal diagnosis.[27,151,156,190]

Another family of fetal-specific nucleic acid markers in maternal plasma is the group of mRNA molecules produced in placenta.[150] For fetal trisomy detection, one has to identify placental mRNA transcribed from genes located on the target chromosomes (e.g., chromosome 21).[153] The discovery of such markers has been facilitated by the development of a microarray-based approach in which thousands of such genes could be interrogated in a single experiment.[195] One of the most promising of such genes is the *PLAC4* gene (placenta-specific 4) located on chromosome 21.[128,193] The mRNA coded by *PLAC4* is detectable in maternal plasma from the first trimester onward and is cleared rapidly following delivery.[128] For the detection of trisomy 21, one could use the RNA-SNP allelic ratio approach,[128] which is analogous to the EAR approach for fetal DNA methylation markers (see Figure 45-2). Thus, one would be detecting a 2:1 or 1:2 ratio for a trisomy 21 fetus versus the 1:1 ratio for a euploid fetus. The RNA-SNP allelic ratio approach has also been demonstrated for the prenatal detection of trisomy 18.[194] The main limitation of the RNA-SNP allelic ratio approach is that one could cover only a proportion of the population (i.e., individuals informative for the SNP marker) with a single RNA-SNP marker. Thus, to obtain high population coverage, one would require multiple RNA-SNP markers, and this would increase the complexity of development and eventual applications. Apart from the use of placental mRNA for RNA-SNP allelic ratio analysis, the absolute concentration of *PLAC4* can be used as a risk indicator for trisomy 21.[193] Although this approach is not as sensitive and specific as the RNA-SNP allelic ratio approach, it does offer the advantage of having broad population coverage.

Another approach reported in the literature and using fetal DNA in maternal plasma for aneuploidy detection is the use of formaldehyde treatment.[42,43] It has been postulated by Dhallan and associates that treatment by formaldehyde of a maternal blood sample stabilizes maternal blood cells, thus leading to a reduction in the liberation of DNA from these cells. The latter process, if not prevented, would potentially lead to the dilution of fetal DNA in maternal plasma.[42] Unfortunately, several groups have not been able to replicate these data, and the diagnostic impact of this approach remains uncertain.[29,37,80,121]

Yet another alternative strategy for detecting fetal-specific DNA and RNA aneuploidy involves the detection of fetal chromosomal aneuploidy, despite the fact that fetal DNA represents only a minor fraction of DNA in maternal plasma. Such methods attempt to detect the slight quantitative sequence imbalance that would exist in maternal plasma if an aneuploid fetus were present. For example, if the fetus has trisomy 21, then there should be a slight increase in sequences derived from chromosome 21 in maternal plasma, when compared with those derived from the other chromosomes. In other words, one is attempting to measure the relative chromosome dosage (RCD) (see Figure 45-2). For a maternal plasma sample containing 10% fetal DNA, one would need to detect a 5% increase in the sequences derived from chromosome 21 if one wishes to detect the presence of a trisomy 21 fetus.[54,125] Two groups have outlined strategies for using digital PCR for RCD analysis.[54,125] Indeed, this concept can be generalized to other single-molecule counting methods.[30] The discrimination power of such methods increases with the increase in the number of molecules analyzed. With the advent of massively parallel DNA sequencing,[6,137,170] millions or even billions of molecules are readily analyzed in a single run. Thus, it has been shown that fetal trisomy 21 can be detected with high accuracy using the sequencing-by-synthesis[33,53] and sequencing-by-ligation[32] platforms. With the rapid reduction in the costs of sequencing and the increase in throughput and in the amount of sequencing per run, this technology is expected to impact clinical practice in the near future, subject to large-scale validation trials.

Pregnancy-Associated Disorders

Several groups have shown that the concentration of fetal DNA in maternal plasma is increased in a variety of pregnancy-associated disorders, including preeclampsia[124,215] and preterm labor.[56,106] In particular, the relationship between circulating fetal DNA concentrations and preeclampsia has been studied by a number of groups.[124,215] Following the onset of preeclampsia, both fetal and total cell-free DNA concentrations are increased in maternal plasma,[215] and fetal DNA clearance appears to be impaired in preeclamptic pregnancies.[96] In addition, several workers have reported that circulating cell-free fetal DNA is already elevated before the onset of clinical features of preeclampsia.[39,84,105,107,214] These latter observations thus open up the possibility that circulating fetal DNA measurement might identify pregnant women at increased risk of developing preeclampsia.

Most of the previously mentioned data on preeclampsia were generated using Y chromosomal markers that could be used only in pregnancies involving male fetuses. Two approaches have been used to generate fetal sex-independent and genetic polymorphism-independent nucleic acid markers. The first involves the use of fetal DNA methylation markers. Hypomethylated *SERPINB5* and hypermethylated *RASSF1* sequences, both markers for fetal DNA in maternal plasma, have been shown to be elevated in the plasma of pregnant women with preeclampsia.[28,192] Hypermethylated *RASSF1*, in particular, has the advantage that it is detected with relatively simple methylation-sensitive restriction enzyme digestion, followed by real-time PCR.[16]

The second approach involves the detection of placental mRNA in maternal plasma.[150] Various groups have demonstrated that a number of such mRNA markers are increased in the plasma of women suffering from preeclampsia.[55,148,159]

The final word has not been said concerning the relative merit of using fetal DNA versus RNA in the prediction, detection, and monitoring of preeclamptic pregnancies. Both approaches require extra steps specific to the marker chosen. For example, when one uses DNA methylation markers, one has to use steps that allow analysis of DNA methylation status (e.g., methylation-sensitive restriction enzyme digestion,[16] methylation-specific PCR).[28,75] Plasma RNA analysis, however, has the disadvantage that a number of groups have advocated the use of potentially hazardous reagents (e.g., Trizol) in preserving the integrity of RNA.[149,209] Plasma RNA markers, on the other hand, offer the advantage that each copy of a fetal gene can theoretically transcribe multiple copies of mRNA, thus providing a biological amplification system.

An emerging class of plasma RNA markers for pregnancy-associated disorders consists of plasma miRNA. In 2008, it was first demonstrated that placental miRNA could be detected in the plasma of pregnant women.[26] Plasma miRNA appears to be more stable than plasma mRNA. Because miRNA expression has been reported to be aberrant in preeclampsia,[157,216] it is possible that some of such plasma miRNA markers might be used to detect and monitor pregnancy-associated disorders.

OTHER APPLICATIONS OF PLASMA NUCLEIC ACIDS

The finding of circulating tumor-derived and fetal-derived DNA in the plasma of cancer patients and pregnant women has prompted researchers to look for other nonhost nucleic acid species in plasma. In 1998, Lo and colleagues reported that donor-derived DNA can be detected in the plasma of patients who have received liver and kidney transplantation.[127] This phenomenon was first observed using sex-mismatched transplantations in which the donor was a male subject and the recipient was a female subject. This observation has been replicated by a number of independent groups in both human subjects[63,140,142] and a rat model.[138] Cell death has generally been regarded as the mechanism through which DNA is released by cells into the plasma. Because graft rejection is a cause of cell death following transplantation, it has been proposed that the measurement of donor-derived DNA concentration in the plasma of transplant recipients might serve as a marker for graft rejection.[127] This hypothesis has been shown to be correct.[63,142] Furthermore, it has been shown that the total concentration of plasma DNA can serve as a rejection marker.[142] This would significantly facilitate the ease with which this technology could be used clinically, as one does not have to use genetic polymorphisms that are informative for only a proportion of donor-recipient pairs.

Plasma nucleic acid technology has been studied as a tool to detect a variety of pathologies associated with tissue damage. Examples include trauma,[116] stroke,[162] myocardial infarction,[41,161] exercise-induced injury,[57] and burns.[36] Furthermore, persistent elevation of plasma DNA has been associated with poor prognosis in trauma patients.[95]

Plasma RNA markers have also been used in monitoring tissue damage. Plasma RNA markers offer the advantage that different tissues have their own RNA expression profiles. For example, plasma albumin mRNA is increased in multiple liver pathologies, including liver cancer, cirrhosis, and chronic hepatitis B.[35] When used in this fashion, plasma albumin mRNA appears to be more sensitive than conventional markers such as alanine aminotransferase. As another example, plasma endothelial specific mRNA has been shown to be elevated in patients with burn injuries and to correlate with the severity of the injury.[61] With the emergence of plasma miRNA markers, these molecules have also been used for assessment of tissue injury. One example is the use of plasma miR-122 and miR-192 in assessment of drug-induced liver injury.[202] Another example is the use of miR-208[88,201] and miR-1[1] in the detection of acute myocardial infarction.

CONCLUDING REMARKS

Over the past 15 years or so, the field of circulating nucleic acids has developed very rapidly. This development has coincided with a number of important technological advances in nucleic acid detection, such as real-time PCR, mass spectrometry, and massively parallel DNA sequencing. It is likely that some of these developments will have a significant impact on the clinical practice of molecular diagnostics in the near future.

REFERENCES

1. Ai J, Zhang R, Li Y, Pu J, Lu Y, Jiao J, et al. Circulating microRNA-1 as a potential novel biomarker for myocardial infarction. Biochem Biophys Res Commun 2010;391:73-7.
2. Alberry M, Maddocks D, Jones M, Abdel Hadi M, Abdel-Fattah S, Avent N, et al. Free fetal DNA in maternal plasma in anembryonic pregnancies: confirmation that the origin is the trophoblast. Prenat Diagn 2007;27:415-8.
3. Amicucci P, Gennarelli M, Novelli G, Dallapiccola B. Prenatal diagnosis of myotonic dystrophy using fetal DNA obtained from maternal plasma. Clin Chem 2000;46:301-2.
4. Bastian PJ, Palapattu GS, Lin X, Yegnasubramanian S, Mangold LA, Trock B, et al. Preoperative serum DNA GSTP1 CpG island hypermethylation and the risk of early prostate-specific antigen recurrence following radical prostatectomy. Clin Cancer Res 2005;11:4037-43.
5. Bastian PJ, Palapattu GS, Yegnasubramanian S, Lin X, Rogers CG, Mangold LA, et al. Prognostic value of preoperative serum cell-free circulating DNA in men with prostate cancer undergoing radical prostatectomy. Clin Cancer Res 2007;13:5361-7.

6. Bentley DR, Balasubramanian S, Swerdlow HP, Smith GP, Milton J, Brown CG, et al. Accurate whole human genome sequencing using reversible terminator chemistry. Nature 2008;456:53-9.
7. Bianchi DW. Fetal DNA in maternal plasma: the plot thickens and the placental barrier thins. Am J Hum Genet 1998;62:763-4.
8. Boddy JL, Gal S, Malone PR, Harris AL, Wainscoat JS. Prospective study of quantitation of plasma DNA levels in the diagnosis of malignant versus benign prostate disease. Clin Cancer Res 2005;11: 1394-9.
9. Boddy JL, Gal S, Malone PR, Shaida N, Wainscoat JS, Harris AL. The role of cell-free DNA size distribution in the management of prostate cancer. Oncol Res 2006;16:35-41.
10. Botezatu I, Serdyuk O, Potapova G, Shelepov V, Alechina R, Molyaka Y, et al. Genetic analysis of DNA excreted in urine: a new approach for detecting specific genomic DNA sequences from cells dying in an organism. Clin Chem 2000;46:1078-84.
11. Bustamante-Aragones A, Gallego-Merlo J, Trujillo-Tiebas MJ, de Alba MR, Gonzalez-Gonzalez C, Glover G, et al. New strategy for the prenatal detection/exclusion of paternal cystic fibrosis mutations in maternal plasma. J Cyst Fibros 2008;7:505-10.
12. Castells A, Puig P, Mora J, Boadas J, Boix L, Urgell E, et al. K-ras mutations in DNA extracted from the plasma of patients with pancreatic carcinoma: diagnostic utility and prognostic significance. J Clin Oncol 1999;17:578-84.
13. Cerkovnik P, Perhavec A, Zgajnar J, Novakovic S. Optimization of an RNA isolation procedure from plasma samples. Int J Mol Med 2007; 20:293-300.
14. Chan AT, Lo YM, Zee B, Chan LY, Ma BB, Leung SF, et al. Plasma Epstein-Barr virus DNA and residual disease after radiotherapy for undifferentiated nasopharyngeal carcinoma. J Natl Cancer Inst 2002; 94:1614-9.
15. Chan KC, Chan AT, Leung SF, Pang JC, Wang AY, Tong JH, et al. Investigation into the origin and tumoral mass correlation of plasma Epstein-Barr virus DNA in nasopharyngeal carcinoma. Clin Chem 2005;51:2192-5.
16. Chan KC, Ding C, Gerovassili A, Yeung SW, Chiu RW, Leung TN, et al. Hypermethylated RASSF1A in maternal plasma: a universal fetal DNA marker that improves the reliability of noninvasive prenatal diagnosis. Clin Chem 2006;52:2211-8.
17. Chan KC, Lai PB, Mok TS, Chan HL, Ding C, Yeung SW, et al. Quantitative analysis of circulating methylated DNA as a biomarker for hepatocellular carcinoma. Clin Chem 2008;54:1528-36.
18. Chan KC, Leung SF, Yeung SW, Chan AT, Lo YM. Persistent aberrations in circulating DNA integrity after radiotherapy are associated with poor prognosis in nasopharyngeal carcinoma patients. Clin Cancer Res 2008;14:4141-5.
19. Chan KC, Yeung SW, Lui WB, Rainer TH, Lo YM. Effects of preanalytical factors on the molecular size of cell-free DNA in blood. Clin Chem 2005;51:781-4.
20. Chan KC, Zhang J, Chan AT, Lei KI, Leung SF, Chan LY, et al. Molecular characterization of circulating EBV DNA in the plasma of nasopharyngeal carcinoma and lymphoma patients. Cancer Res 2003;63:2028-32.
21. Chan KCA, Zhang J, Hui AB, Wong N, Lau TK, Leung TN, et al. Size distributions of maternal and fetal DNA in maternal plasma. Clin Chem 2004;50:88-92.
22. Chang HW, Lee SM, Goodman SN, Singer G, Cho SK, Sokoll LJ, et al. Assessment of plasma DNA levels, allelic imbalance, and CA 125 as diagnostic tests for cancer. J Natl Cancer Inst 2002;94:1697-703.
23. Chen X, Ba Y, Ma L, Cai X, Yin Y, Wang K, et al. Characterization of microRNAs in serum: a novel class of biomarkers for diagnosis of cancer and other diseases. Cell Res 2008;18:997-1006.
24. Chen XQ, Bonnefoi H, Pelte MF, Lyautey J, Lederrey C, Movarekhi S, et al. Telomerase RNA as a detection marker in the serum of breast cancer patients. Clin Cancer Res 2000;6:3823-6.
25. Chen XQ, Stroun M, Magnenat JL, Nicod LP, Kurt AM, Lyautey J, et al. Microsatellite alterations in plasma DNA of small cell lung cancer patients. Nat Med 1996;2:1033-5.
26. Chim SS, Shing TK, Hung EC, Leung TY, Lau TK, Chiu RW, et al. Detection and characterization of placental microRNAs in maternal plasma. Clin Chem 2008;54:482-90.
27. Chim SSC, Jin S, Lee TYH, Lun FMF, Lee WS, Chan LYS, et al. Systematic search for placental epigenetic markers on chromosome 21: towards noninvasive prenatal diagnosis of fetal trisomy 21. Clin Chem 2008;54:500-11.
28. Chim SSC, Tong YK, Chiu RWK, Lau TK, Leung TN, Chan LYS, et al. Detection of the placental epigenetic signature of the maspin gene in maternal plasma. Proc Natl Acad Sci U S A 2005;102:14753-8.
29. Chinnapapagari SK, Holzgreve W, Lapaire O, Zimmermann B, Hahn S. Treatment of maternal blood samples with formaldehyde does not alter the proportion of circulatory fetal nucleic acids (DNA and mRNA) in maternal plasma. Clin Chem 2005;51:652-5.
30. Chiu RW, Cantor CR, Lo YM. Non-invasive prenatal diagnosis by single molecule counting technologies. Trends Genet 2009;25:324-31.
31. Chiu RW, Lau TK, Cheung PT, Gong ZQ, Leung TN, Lo YMD. Noninvasive prenatal exclusion of congenital adrenal hyperplasia by maternal plasma analysis: a feasibility study. Clin Chem 2002;48: 778-80.
32. Chiu RW, Sun H, Akolekar R, Clouser C, Lee C, McKernan K, et al. Maternal plasma DNA analysis with massively parallel sequencing by ligation for noninvasive prenatal diagnosis of trisomy 21. Clin Chem 2010;56:459-63.
33. Chiu RWK, Chan KCA, Gao Y, Lau VYM, Zheng W, Leung TY, et al. Noninvasive prenatal diagnosis of fetal chromosomal aneuploidy by massively parallel genomic sequencing of DNA in maternal plasma. Proc Natl Acad Sci U S A 2008;105:20458-63.
34. Chiu RWK, Lau TK, Leung TN, Chow KCK, Chui DHK, Lo YMD. Prenatal exclusion of beta-thalassaemia major by examination of maternal plasma. Lancet 2002;360:998-1000.
35. Chiu RWK, Wong J, Chan HL, Mok TS, Lo WY, Lee V, et al. Aberrant concentrations of liver-derived plasma albumin in liver pathologies. Clin Chem 2010;56:82-9.
36. Chiu TW, Young R, Chan LYS, Burd A, Lo DYM. Plasma cell-free DNA as an indicator of severity of injury in burn patients. Clin Chem Lab Med 2006;44:13-7.
37. Chung GT, Chiu RWK, Chan KCA, Lau TK, Leung TN, Lo YMD. Lack of dramatic enrichment of fetal DNA in maternal plasma by formaldehyde treatment. Clin Chem 2005;51:655-8.
38. Costa JM, Benachi A, Gautier E. New strategy for prenatal diagnosis of X-linked disorders. N Engl J Med 2002;346:1502.
39. Cotter AM, Martin CM, O'Leary JJ, Daly SF. Increased fetal RhD gene in the maternal circulation in early pregnancy is associated with an increased risk of pre-eclampsia. BJOG 2005;112:584-7.
40. Coulet F, Blons H, Cabelguenne A, Lecomte T, Lacourreye O, Brasnu D, et al. Detection of plasma tumor DNA in head and neck squamous cell carcinoma by microsatellite typing and p53 mutation analysis. Cancer Res 2000;60:707-11.
41. Destouni A, Vrettou C, Antonatos D, Chouliaras G, Traeger-Synodinos J, Patsilinakos S, et al. Cell-free DNA levels in acute myocardial infarction patients during hospitalization. Acta Cardiol 2009;64:51-7.
42. Dhallan R, Au WC, Mattagajasingh S, Emche S, Bayliss P, Damewood M, et al. Methods to increase the percentage of free fetal DNA recovered from the maternal circulation. JAMA 2004;291:1114-9.
43. Dhallan R, Guo X, Emche S, Damewood M, Bayliss P, Cronin M, et al. A non-invasive test for prenatal diagnosis based on fetal DNA present in maternal blood: a preliminary study. Lancet 2007;369: 474-81.
44. Diehl F, Li M, Dressman D, He Y, Shen D, Szabo S, et al. Detection and quantification of mutations in the plasma of patients with colorectal tumors. Proc Natl Acad Sci U S A 2005;102:16368-73.
45. Diehl F, Schmidt K, Choti MA, Romans K, Goodman S, Li M, et al. Circulating mutant DNA to assess tumor dynamics. Nat Med 2008;14: 985-90.
46. Ding C, Chiu RWK, Lau TK, Leung TN, Chan LC, Chan AY, et al. MS analysis of single-nucleotide differences in circulating nucleic acids:

application to noninvasive prenatal diagnosis. Proc Natl Acad Sci U S A 2004;101:10762-7.
47. Dong SM, Pai SI, Rha SH, Hildesheim A, Kurman RJ, Schwartz PE, et al. Detection and quantitation of human papillomavirus DNA in the plasma of patients with cervical carcinoma. Cancer Epidemiol Biomarkers Prev 2002;11:3-6.
48. Dressman D, Yan H, Traverso G, Kinzler KW, Vogelstein B. Transforming single DNA molecules into fluorescent magnetic particles for detection and enumeration of genetic variations. Proc Natl Acad Sci U S A 2003;100:8817-22.
49. Eads CA, Danenberg KD, Kawakami K, Saltz LB, Blake C, Shibata D, et al. MethyLight: a high-throughput assay to measure DNA methylation. Nucleic Acids Res 2000;28:E32.
50. El-Hefnawy T, Raja S, Kelly L, Bigbee WL, Kirkwood JM, Luketich JD, et al. Characterization of amplifiable, circulating RNA in plasma and its potential as a tool for cancer diagnostics. Clin Chem 2004;50: 564-73.
51. Esteller M, Sanchez-Cespedes M, Rosell R, Sidransky D, Baylin SB, Herman JG. Detection of aberrant promoter hypermethylation of tumor suppressor genes in serum DNA from non-small cell lung cancer patients. Cancer Res 1999;59:67-70.
52. Faas BH, Beuling EA, Christiaens GC, von dem Borne AE, van der Schoot CE. Detection of fetal RHD-specific sequences in maternal plasma. Lancet 1998;352:1196.
53. Fan HC, Blumenfeld YJ, Chitkara U, Hudgins L, Quake SR. Noninvasive diagnosis of fetal aneuploidy by shotgun sequencing DNA from maternal blood. Proc Natl Acad Sci U S A 2008;105: 16266-71.
54. Fan HC, Quake SR. Detection of aneuploidy with digital polymerase chain reaction. Anal Chem 2007;79:7576-9.
55. Farina A, Chan CW, Chiu RW, Tsui NB, Carinci P, Concu M, et al. Circulating corticotropin-releasing hormone mRNA in maternal plasma: relationship with gestational age and severity of preeclampsia. Clin Chem 2004;50:1851-4.
56. Farina A, LeShane ES, Romero R, Gomez R, Chaiworapongsa T, Rizzo N, et al. High levels of fetal cell-free DNA in maternal serum: a risk factor for spontaneous preterm delivery. Am J Obstet Gynecol 2005; 193:421-5.
57. Fatouros IG, Destouni A, Margonis K, Jamurtas AZ, Vrettou C, Kouretas D, et al. Cell-free plasma DNA as a novel marker of aseptic inflammation severity related to exercise overtraining. Clin Chem 2006;52:1820-4.
58. Feng DX, Zhang SD, Han TQ, Jiang Y, Lei RQ, Yuan ZR, et al. A prospective study of detection of pancreatic carcinoma by combined plasma K-ras mutations and serum CA19-9 analysis. Pancreas 2002; 25:336-41.
59. Finning K, Martin P, Summers J, Massey E, Poole G, Daniels G. Effect of high throughput RHD typing of fetal DNA in maternal plasma on use of anti-RhD immunoglobulin in RhD negative pregnant women: prospective feasibility study. BMJ 2008;336:816-8.
60. Flori E, Doray B, Gautier E, Kohler M, Ernault P, Flori J, et al. Circulating cell-free fetal DNA in maternal serum appears to originate from cyto- and syncytio-trophoblastic cells: case report. Hum Reprod 2004;19:723-4.
61. Fox A, Gal S, Fisher N, Smythe J, Wainscoat JS, Tyler MPH, et al. Quantification of circulating cell-free plasma DNA and endothelial gene RNA in patients with burns and relation to acute thermal injury. Burns 2008;34:809-16.
62. Frommer M, McDonald LE, Millar DS, Collis CM, Watt F, Grigg GW, et al. A genomic sequencing protocol that yields a positive display of 5-methylcytosine residues in individual DNA strands. Proc Natl Acad Sci U S A 1992;89:1827-31.
63. Gadi VK, Nelson JL, Boespflug ND, Guthrie KA, Kuhr CS. Soluble donor DNA concentrations in recipient serum correlate with pancreas-kidney rejection. Clin Chem 2006;52:379-82.
64. Garcia JM, Garcia V, Pena C, Dominguez G, Silva J, Diaz R, et al. Extracellular plasma RNA from colon cancer patients is confined in a vesicle-like structure and is mRNA-enriched. RNA 2008;14:1424-32.
65. Garcia V, Garcia JM, Pena C, Silva J, Dominguez G, Hurtado A, et al. Thymidylate synthase messenger RNA expression in plasma from patients with colon cancer: prognostic potential. Clin Cancer Res 2006;12:2095-100.
66. Garcia V, Garcia JM, Silva J, Pena C, Dominguez G, Lorenzo Y, et al. Levels of VEGF-A mRNA in plasma from patients with colorectal carcinoma as possible surrogate marker of angiogenesis. J Cancer Res Clin Oncol 2008;134:1165-71.
67. Gonzalez-Gonzalez MC, Garcia-Hoyos M, Trujillo MJ, Rodriguez de Alba M, Lorda-Sanchez I, Diaz-Recasens J, et al. Prenatal detection of a cystic fibrosis mutation in fetal DNA from maternal plasma. Prenat Diagn 2002;22:946-8.
68. Gonzalez R, Silva JM, Sanchez A, Dominguez G, Garcia JM, Chen XQ, et al. Microsatellite alterations and TP53 mutations in plasma DNA of small-cell lung cancer patients: follow-up study and prognostic significance. Ann Oncol 2000;11:1097-104.
69. Gonzalgo ML, Eisenberger CF, Lee SM, Trock BJ, Marshall FF, Hortopan S, et al. Prognostic significance of preoperative molecular serum analysis in renal cancer. Clin Cancer Res 2002;8:1878-81.
70. Grunau C, Clark SJ, Rosenthal A. Bisulfite genomic sequencing: systematic investigation of critical experimental parameters. Nucleic Acids Res 2001;29:E65-75.
71. Grutzmann R, Molnar B, Pilarsky C, Habermann JK, Schlag PM, Saeger HD, et al. Sensitive detection of colorectal cancer in peripheral blood by septin 9 DNA methylation assay. PLoS One 2008;3:e3759.
72. Hagiwara N, Mechanic LE, Trivers GE, Cawley HL, Taga M, Bowman ED, et al. Quantitative detection of p53 mutations in plasma DNA from tobacco smokers. Cancer Res 2006;66:8309-17.
73. Hanley R, Rieger-Christ KM, Canes D, Emara NR, Shuber AP, Boynton KA, et al. DNA integrity assay: a plasma-based screening tool for the detection of prostate cancer. Clin Cancer Res 2006;12: 4569-74.
74. Hasselmann DO, Rappl G, Tilgen W, Reinhold U. Extracellular tyrosinase mRNA within apoptotic bodies is protected from degradation in human serum. Clin Chem 2001;47:1488-9.
75. Herman JG, Graff JR, Myohanen S, Nelkin BD, Baylin SB. Methylation-specific PCR: a novel PCR assay for methylation status of CpG islands. Proc Natl Acad Sci U S A 1996;93:9821-6.
76. Ho SS, Chong SS, Koay ES, Ponnusamy S, Chiu L, Chan YH, et al. Noninvasive prenatal exclusion of haemoglobin Bart's using foetal DNA from maternal plasma. Prenat Diagn 2010;30:65-73.
77. Holdenrieder S, Burges A, Reich O, Spelsberg FW, Stieber P. DNA integrity in plasma and serum of patients with malignant and benign diseases. Ann N Y Acad Sci 2008;1137:162-70.
78. Hoque MO, Feng Q, Toure P, Dem A, Critchlow CW, Hawes SE, et al. Detection of aberrant methylation of four genes in plasma DNA for the detection of breast cancer. J Clin Oncol 2006;24:4262-9.
79. Huang XH, Sun LH, Lu DD, Sun Y, Ma LJ, Zhang XR, et al. Codon 249 mutation in exon 7 of p53 gene in plasma DNA: maybe a new early diagnostic marker of hepatocellular carcinoma in Qidong risk area, China. World J Gastroenterol 2003;9:692-5.
80. Hulten MA, Old RW. Non-invasive prenatal diagnosis of Down's syndrome. Lancet 2007;369:1997; author reply 8-9.
81. Hunter MP, Ismail N, Zhang X, Aguda BD, Lee EJ, Yu L, et al. Detection of microRNA expression in human peripheral blood microvesicles. PLoS One 2008;3:e3694.
82. Hyett JA, Gardener G, Stojilkovic-Mikic T, Finning KM, Martin PG, Rodeck CH, et al. Reduction in diagnostic and therapeutic interventions by non-invasive determination of fetal sex in early pregnancy. Prenat Diagn 2005;25:1111-6.
83. Illanes S, Denbow ML, Smith RP, Overton TG, Soothill PW, Finning K. Detection of cell-free fetal DNA in maternal urine. Prenat Diagn 2006;26:1216-8.
84. Illanes S, Parra M, Serra R, Pino K, Figueroa-Diesel H, Romero C, et al. Increased free fetal DNA levels in early pregnancy plasma of women who subsequently develop preeclampsia and intrauterine growth restriction. Prenat Diagn 2009;29:1118-22.

85. Illingworth RS, Bird AP. CpG islands—'a rough guide.' FEBS Lett 2009;583:1713-20.
86. Iorio MV, Croce CM. MicroRNAs in cancer: small molecules with a huge impact. J Clin Oncol 2009;27:5848-56.
87. Jahr S, Hentze H, Englisch S, Hardt D, Fackelmayer FO, Hesch RD, et al. DNA fragments in the blood plasma of cancer patients: quantitations and evidence for their origin from apoptotic and necrotic cells. Cancer Res 2001;61:1659-65.
88. Ji X, Takahashi R, Hiura Y, Hirokawa G, Fukushima Y, Iwai N. Plasma miR-208 as a biomarker of myocardial injury. Clin Chem 2009;55: 1944-9.
89. Jiang WW, Zahurak M, Goldenberg D, Milman Y, Park HL, Westra WH, et al. Increased plasma DNA integrity index in head and neck cancer patients. Int J Cancer 2006;119:2673-6.
90. Kimbi GC, Kew MC, Yu MC, Arakawa K, Hodkinson J. 249ser p53 mutation in the serum of black Southern African patients with hepatocellular carcinoma. J Gastroenterol Hepatol 2005;20: 1185-90.
91. Kimura H, Suminoe M, Kasahara K, Sone T, Araya T, Tamori S, et al. Evaluation of epidermal growth factor receptor mutation status in serum DNA as a predictor of response to gefitinib (IRESSA). Br J Cancer 2007;97:778-84.
92. Kirk GD, Camus-Randon AM, Mendy M, Goedert JJ, Merle P, Trepo C, et al. Ser-249 p53 mutations in plasma DNA of patients with hepatocellular carcinoma from The Gambia. J Natl Cancer Inst 2000;92:148-53.
93. Kopreski M, Benko FA, Kwak LW, Gocke CD. Detection of tumor messenger RNA in the serum of patients with malignant melanoma. Clin Cancer Res 1999;5:1961-5.
94. Kopreski MS, Benko FA, Borys DJ, Khan A, McGarrity TJ, Gocke CD. Somatic mutation screening: identification of individuals harboring K-ras mutations with the use of plasma DNA. J Natl Cancer Inst 2000;92:918-23.
95. Lam NY, Rainer TH, Chan LY, Joynt GM, Lo YM. Time course of early and late changes in plasma DNA in trauma patients. Clin Chem 2003;49:1286-91.
96. Lau TW, Leung TN, Chan LY, Lau TK, Chan KC, Tam WH, et al. Fetal DNA clearance from maternal plasma is impaired in preeclampsia. Clin Chem 2002;48:2141-6.
97. Lauschke H, Caspari R, Friedl W, Schwarz B, Mathiak M, Propping P, et al. Detection of APC and k-ras mutations in the serum of patients with colorectal cancer. Cancer Detect Prev 2001;25:55-61.
98. Lawrie CH, Gal S, Dunlop HM, Pushkaran B, Liggins AP, Pulford K, et al. Detection of elevated levels of tumour-associated microRNAs in serum of patients with diffuse large B-cell lymphoma. Br J Haematol 2008;141:672-5.
99. Lei KI, Chan LY, Chan WY, Johnson PJ, Lo YM. Diagnostic and prognostic implications of circulating cell-free Epstein-Barr virus DNA in natural killer/T-cell lymphoma. Clin Cancer Res 2002;8: 29-34.
100. Lei KI, Chan LY, Chan WY, Johnson PJ, Lo YMD. Quantitative analysis of circulating cell-free Epstein-Barr virus (EBV) DNA levels in patients with EBV-associated lymphoid malignancies. Br J Haematol 2000;111:239-46.
101. Leon SA, Ehrlich GE, Shapiro B, Labbate VA. Free DNA in the serum of rheumatoid arthritis patients. J Rheumatol 1977;4:139-43.
102. Leon SA, Shapiro B, Sklaroff DM, Yaros MJ. Free DNA in the serum of cancer patients and the effect of therapy. Cancer Res 1977;37: 646-50.
103. Leung SF, Tam JS, Chan AT, Zee B, Chan LY, Huang DP, et al. Improved accuracy of detection of nasopharyngeal carcinoma by combined application of circulating Epstein-Barr virus DNA and anti-Epstein-Barr viral capsid antigen IgA antibody. Clin Chem 2004;50:339-45.
104. Leung SF, Zee B, Ma BB, Hui EP, Mo F, Lai M, et al. Plasma Epstein-Barr viral deoxyribonucleic acid quantitation complements tumor-node-metastasis staging prognostication in nasopharyngeal carcinoma. J Clin Oncol 2006;24:5414-8.
105. Leung TN, Zhang J, Lau TK, Chan LY, Lo YM. Increased maternal plasma fetal DNA concentrations in women who eventually develop preeclampsia. Clin Chem 2001;47:137-9.
106. Leung TN, Zhang J, Lau TK, Hjelm NM, Lo YMD. Maternal plasma fetal DNA as a marker for preterm labour. Lancet 1998;352:1904-5.
107. Levine RJ, Qian C, Leshane ES, Yu KF, England LJ, Schisterman EF, et al. Two-stage elevation of cell-free fetal DNA in maternal sera before onset of preeclampsia. Am J Obstet Gynecol 2004;190:707-13.
108. Li M, Chen WD, Papadopoulos N, Goodman SN, Bjerregaard NC, Laurberg S, et al. Sensitive digital quantification of DNA methylation in clinical samples. Nat Biotechnol 2009;27:858-63.
109. Li Y, Di Naro E, Vitucci A, Zimmermann B, Holzgreve W, Hahn S. Detection of paternally inherited fetal point mutations for beta-thalassemia using size-fractionated cell-free DNA in maternal plasma. JAMA 2005;293:843-9.
110. Li Y, Page-Christiaens GC, Gille JJ, Holzgreve W, Hahn S. Non-invasive prenatal detection of achondroplasia in size-fractionated cell-free DNA by MALDI-TOF MS assay. Prenat Diagn 2007;27:11-7.
111. Li Y, Zhong XY, Kang A, Troeger C, Holzgreve W, Hahn S. Inability to detect cell free fetal DNA in the urine of normal pregnant women nor in those affected by preeclampsia associated HELLP syndrome. J Soc Gynecol Investig 2003;10:503-8.
112. Li Y, Zimmermann B, Rusterholz C, Kang A, Holzgreve W, Hahn S. Size separation of circulatory DNA in maternal plasma permits ready detection of fetal DNA polymorphisms. Clin Chem 2004;50:1002-11.
113. Lin JC, Wang WY, Chen KY, Wei YH, Liang WM, Jan JS, et al. Quantification of plasma Epstein-Barr virus DNA in patients with advanced nasopharyngeal carcinoma. N Engl J Med 2004;350:2461-70.
114. Lo KW, Lo YM, Leung SF, Tsang YS, Chan LY, Johnson PJ, et al. Analysis of cell-free Epstein-Barr virus associated RNA in the plasma of patients with nasopharyngeal carcinoma. Clin Chem 1999;45: 1292-4.
115. Lo YM, Chan LY, Chan AT, Leung SF, Lo KW, Zhang J, et al. Quantitative and temporal correlation between circulating cell-free Epstein-Barr virus DNA and tumor recurrence in nasopharyngeal carcinoma. Cancer Res 1999;59:5452-5.
116. Lo YM, Rainer TH, Chan LY, Hjelm NM, Cocks RA. Plasma DNA as a prognostic marker in trauma patients. Clin Chem 2000;46:319-23.
117. Lo YM, Wong IH, Zhang J, Tein MS, Ng MH, Hjelm NM. Quantitative analysis of aberrant p16 methylation using real-time quantitative methylation-specific polymerase chain reaction. Cancer Res 1999;59:3899-903.
118. Lo YMD, Chan ATC, Chan LYS, Leung SF, Lam CW, Huang DP, et al. Molecular prognostication of nasopharyngeal carcinoma by quantitative analysis of circulating Epstein-Barr virus DNA. Cancer Res 2000;60:6878-81.
119. Lo YMD, Chan LY, Lo KW, Leung SF, Zhang J, Chan AT, et al. Quantitative analysis of cell-free Epstein-Barr virus DNA in plasma of patients with nasopharyngeal carcinoma. Cancer Res 1999;59: 1188-91.
120. Lo YMD, Chan WY, Ng EKW, Chan LYS, Lai PBS, Tam JS, et al. Circulating Epstein-Barr virus DNA in the serum of patients with gastric carcinoma. Clin Cancer Res 2001;7:1856-9.
121. Lo YMD, Chiu RWK, Chan KCA, Chung GT. Free fetal DNA in maternal circulation. JAMA 2004;292:2835.
122. Lo YMD, Corbetta N, Chamberlain PF, Rai V, Sargent IL, Redman CW, et al. Presence of fetal DNA in maternal plasma and serum. Lancet 1997;350:485-7.
123. Lo YMD, Hjelm NM, Fidler C, Sargent IL, Murphy MF, Chamberlain PF, et al. Prenatal diagnosis of fetal RhD status by molecular analysis of maternal plasma. N Engl J Med 1998;339:1734-8.
124. Lo YMD, Leung TN, Tein MS, Sargent IL, Zhang J, Lau TK, et al. Quantitative abnormalities of fetal DNA in maternal serum in preeclampsia. Clin Chem 1999;45:184-8.
125. Lo YMD, Lun FMF, Chan KCA, Tsui NBY, Chong KC, Lau TK, et al. Digital PCR for the molecular detection of fetal chromosomal aneuploidy. Proc Natl Acad Sci U S A 2007;104:13116-21.

126. Lo YMD, Tein MS, Lau TK, Haines CJ, Leung TN, Poon PM, et al. Quantitative analysis of fetal DNA in maternal plasma and serum: implications for noninvasive prenatal diagnosis. Am J Hum Genet 1998;62:768-75.
127. Lo YMD, Tein MSC, Pang CCP, Yeung CK, Tong KL, Hjelm NM. Presence of donor-specific DNA in plasma of kidney and liver-transplant recipients. Lancet 1998;351:1329-30.
128. Lo YMD, Tsui NB, Chiu RWK, Lau TK, Leung TN, Heung MM, et al. Plasma placental RNA allelic ratio permits noninvasive prenatal chromosomal aneuploidy detection. Nat Med 2007;13:218-23.
129. Lo YMD, Zhang J, Leung TN, Lau TK, Chang AM, Hjelm NM. Rapid clearance of fetal DNA from maternal plasma. Am J Hum Genet 1999;64:218-24.
130. Lui YY, Chik KW, Chiu RW, Ho CY, Lam CW, Lo YM. Predominant hematopoietic origin of cell-free DNA in plasma and serum after sex-mismatched bone marrow transplantation. Clin Chem 2002;48: 421-7.
131. Lun FMF, Chiu RWK, Chan KCA, Leung TY, Lau TK, Lo YMD. Microfluidics digital PCR reveals a higher than expected fraction of fetal DNA in maternal plasma. Clin Chem 2008;54:1664-72.
132. Lun FMF, Tsui NBY, Chan KCA, Leung TY, Lau TK, Charoenkwan P, et al. Noninvasive prenatal diagnosis of monogenic diseases by digital size selection and relative mutation dosage on DNA in maternal plasma. Proc Natl Acad Sci U S A 2008;105:19920-5.
133. Lynch TJ, Bell DW, Sordella R, Gurubhagavatula S, Okimoto RA, Brannigan BW, et al. Activating mutations in the epidermal growth factor receptor underlying responsiveness of non-small-cell lung cancer to gefitinib. N Engl J Med 2004;350:2129-39.
134. Mack PC, Holland WS, Burich RA, Sangha R, Solis LJ, Li Y, et al. EGFR mutations detected in plasma are associated with patient outcomes in erlotinib plus docetaxel-treated non-small cell lung cancer. J Thorac Oncol 2009;4:1466-72.
135. Majer S, Bauer M, Magnet E, Strele A, Giegerl E, Eder M, et al. Maternal urine for prenatal diagnosis—an analysis of cell-free fetal DNA in maternal urine and plasma in the third trimester. Prenat Diagn 2007;27:1219-23.
136. Mandel P, Métais P. Les acides nucléiques du plasma sanguin chez l'homme. C R Acad Sci Paris 1948;142:241-3.
137. Margulies M, Egholm M, Altman WE, Attiya S, Bader JS, Bemben LA, et al. Genome sequencing in microfabricated high-density picolitre reactors. Nature 2005;437:376-80.
138. Martins PN, Mashreghi MF, Reutzel-Selke A, Neuhaus P, Volk HD, Tullius SG, et al. Quantification of donor-derived DNA in serum: a new approach of acute rejection diagnosis in a rat kidney transplantation model. Transplant Proc 2005;37:87-8.
139. Merlo A, Herman JG, Mao L, Lee DJ, Gabrielson E, Burger PC, et al. 5′ CpG island methylation is associated with transcriptional silencing of the tumour suppressor p16/CDKN2/MTS1 in human cancers Nat Med 1995;1:686-92.
140. Minon JM, Senterre JM, Schaaps JP, Foidart JM. An unusual false-positive fetal RHD typing result using DNA derived from maternal plasma from a solid organ transplant recipient. Transfusion 2006;46:1454-5.
141. Mitchell PS, Parkin RK, Kroh EM, Fritz BR, Wyman SK, Pogosova-Agadjanyan EL, et al. Circulating microRNAs as stable blood-based markers for cancer detection. Proc Natl Acad Sci U S A 2008;105: 10513-8.
142. Moreira VG, Garcia BP, Martin JMD, Suarez FO, Alvarez FV. Cell-free DNA as a noninvasive acute rejection marker in renal transplantation. Clin Chem 2009;55:1958-66.
143. Muller I, Beeger C, Alix-Panabieres C, Rebillard X, Pantel K, Schwarzenbach H. Identification of loss of heterozygosity on circulating free DNA in peripheral blood of prostate cancer patients: potential and technical improvements. Clin Chem 2008;54:688-96.
144. Mutirangura A, Pornthanakasem W, Theamboonlers A, Sriuranpong V, Lertsanguansinchi P, Yenrudi S, et al. Epstein-Barr viral DNA in serum of patients with nasopharyngeal carcinoma. Clin Cancer Res 1998;4:665-9.
145. Nakayama H, Hibi K, Taguchi M, Takase T, Yamazaki T, Kasai Y, et al. Molecular detection of p16 promoter methylation in the serum of colorectal cancer patients. Cancer Lett 2002;188:115-9.
146. Nawroz H, Koch W, Anker P, Stroun M, Sidransky D. Microsatellite alterations in serum DNA of head and neck cancer patients. Nat Med 1996;2:1035-7.
147. Ng EK, Chong WW, Jin H, Lam EK, Shin VY, Yu J, et al. Differential expression of microRNAs in plasma of patients with colorectal cancer: a potential marker for colorectal cancer screening. Gut 2009;58: 1375-81.
148. Ng EK, Leung TN, Tsui NB, Lau TK, Panesar NS, Chiu RW, et al. The concentration of circulating corticotropin-releasing hormone mRNA in maternal plasma is increased in preeclampsia. Clin Chem 2003;49: 727-31.
149. Ng EK, Tsui NB, Lam NY, Chiu RW, Yu SC, Wong SC, et al. Presence of filterable and nonfilterable mRNA in the plasma of cancer patients and healthy individuals. Clin Chem 2002;48:1212-7.
150. Ng EKO, Tsui NBY, Lau TK, Leung TN, Chiu RWK, Panesar NS, et al. mRNA of placental origin is readily detectable in maternal plasma. Proc Natl Acad Sci U S A 2003;100:4748-53.
151. Old RW, Crea F, Puszyk W, Hulten MA. Candidate epigenetic biomarkers for non-invasive prenatal diagnosis of Down syndrome. Reprod Biomed Online 2007;15:227-35.
152. Otsuka J, Okuda T, Sekizawa A, Amemiya S, Saito H, Okai T, et al. Detection of p53 mutations in the plasma DNA of patients with ovarian cancer. Int J Gynecol Cancer 2004;14:459-64.
153. Oudejans CB, Go AT, Visser A, Mulders MA, Westerman BA, Blankenstein MA, et al. Detection of chromosome 21-encoded mRNA of placental origin in maternal plasma. Clin Chem 2003;49:1445-9.
154. Paci M, Maramotti S, Bellesia E, Formisano D, Albertazzi L, Ricchetti T, et al. Circulating plasma DNA as diagnostic biomarker in non-small cell lung cancer. Lung Cancer 2009;64:92-7.
155. Paez JG, Janne PA, Lee JC, Tracy S, Greulich H, Gabriel S, et al. EGFR mutations in lung cancer: correlation with clinical response to gefitinib therapy. Science 2004;304:1497-500.
156. Papageorgiou EA, Fiegler H, Rakyan V, Beck S, Hulten M, Lamnissou K, et al. Sites of differential DNA methylation between placenta and peripheral blood: molecular markers for noninvasive prenatal diagnosis of aneuploidies. Am J Pathol 2009;174:1609-18.
157. Pineles BL, Romero R, Montenegro D, Tarca AL, Han YM, Kim YM, et al. Distinct subsets of microRNAs are expressed differentially in the human placentas of patients with preeclampsia. Am J Obstet Gynecol 2007;196:261.e1-6.
158. Poon LLM, Leung TN, Lau TK, Chow KC, Lo YMD. Differential DNA methylation between fetus and mother as a strategy for detecting fetal DNA in maternal plasma. Clin Chem 2002;48:35-41.
159. Purwosunu Y, Sekizawa A, Koide K, Farina A, Wibowo N, Wiknjosastro GH, et al. Cell-free mRNA concentrations of plasminogen activator inhibitor-1 and tissue-type plasminogen activator are increased in the plasma of pregnant women with preeclampsia. Clin Chem 2007;53:399-404.
160. Rabinowits G, Gercel-Taylor C, Day JM, Taylor DD, Kloecker GH. Exosomal microRNA: a diagnostic marker for lung cancer. Clin Lung Cancer 2009;10:42-6.
161. Rainer TH, Lam NY, Man CY, Chiu RW, Woo KS, Lo YM. Plasma beta-globin DNA as a prognostic marker in chest pain patients. Clin Chim Acta 2006;368:110-3.
162. Rainer TH, Wong LK, Lam W, Yuen E, Lam NY, Metreweli C, et al. Prognostic use of circulating plasma nucleic acid concentrations in patients with acute stroke. Clin Chem 2003;49:562-9.
163. Reddi KK, Holland JF. Elevated serum ribonuclease in patients with pancreatic cancer. Proc Natl Acad Sci U S A 1976;73:2308-10.
164. Resnick KE, Alder H, Hagan JP, Richardson DL, Croce CM, Cohn DE. The detection of differentially expressed microRNAs from the serum of ovarian cancer patients using a novel real-time PCR platform. Gynecol Oncol 2009;112:55-9.
165. Rijnders RJ, van der Schoot CE, Bossers B, de Vroede MA, Christiaens GC. Fetal sex determination from maternal plasma in

pregnancies at risk for congenital adrenal hyperplasia. Obstet Gynecol 2001;98:374-8.
166. Ryan BM, Lefort F, McManus R, Daly J, Keeling PW, Weir DG, et al. A prospective study of circulating mutant KRAS2 in the serum of patients with colorectal neoplasia: strong prognostic indicator in postoperative follow up. Gut 2003;52:101-8.
167. Ryan BM, McManus RO, Daly JS, Keeling PW, Weir DG, Lefort F, et al. Serum mutant K-ras in the colorectal adenoma-to-carcinoma sequence: implications for diagnosis, postoperative follow-up, and early detection of recurrent disease. Ann N Y Acad Sci 2000;906:29-30.
168. Saito H, Sekizawa A, Morimoto T, Suzuki M, Yanaihara T. Prenatal DNA diagnosis of a single-gene disorder from maternal plasma. Lancet 2000;356:1170.
169. Sathish N, Abraham P, Peedicayil A, Sridharan G, John S, Shaji RV, et al. HPV DNA in plasma of patients with cervical carcinoma. J Clin Virol 2004;31:204-9.
170. Schuster SC. Next-generation sequencing transforms today's biology. Nat Methods 2008;5:16-8.
171. Schwarz AK, Stanulla M, Cario G, Flohr T, Sutton R, Moricke A, et al. Quantification of free total plasma DNA and minimal residual disease detection in the plasma of children with acute lymphoblastic leukemia. Ann Hematol 2009;88:897-905.
172. Schwarzenbach H, Chun FK, Muller I, Seidel C, Urban K, Erbersdobler A, et al. Microsatellite analysis of allelic imbalance in tumour and blood from patients with prostate cancer. BJU Int 2008; 102:253-8.
173. Schwarzenbach H, Muller V, Beeger C, Gottberg M, Stahmann N, Pantel K. A critical evaluation of loss of heterozygosity detected in tumor tissues, blood serum and bone marrow plasma from patients with breast cancer. Breast Cancer Res 2007;9:R66.
174. Schwarzenbach H, Stoehlmacher J, Pantel K, Goekkurt E. Detection and monitoring of cell-free DNA in blood of patients with colorectal cancer. Ann N Y Acad Sci 2008;1137:190-6.
175. Sharma S, Kelly TK, Jones PA. Epigenetics in cancer. Carcinogenesis 2010;31:27-36.
176. Sheid B, Lu T, Pedrinan L, Nelson JH Jr. Plasma ribonuclease: a marker for the detection of ovarian cancer. Cancer 1977;39:2204-8.
177. Shekhtman EM, Anne K, Melkonyan HS, Robbins DJ, Warsof SL, Umansky SR. Optimization of transrenal DNA analysis: detection of fetal DNA in maternal urine. Clin Chem 2009;55:723-9.
178. Silva J, Garcia V, Garcia JM, Pena C, Dominguez G, Diaz R, et al. Circulating BMI-1 mRNA as a possible prognostic factor for advanced breast cancer patients. Breast Cancer Res 2007;9:R55.
179. Sorenson GD, Pribish DM, Valone FH, Memoli VA, Bzik DJ, Yao SL. Soluble normal and mutated DNA sequences from single-copy genes in human blood. Cancer Epidemiol Biomarkers Prev 1994;3:67-71.
180. Sozzi G, Conte D, Leon M, Ciricione R, Roz L, Ratcliffe C, et al. Quantification of free circulating DNA as a diagnostic marker in lung cancer. J Clin Oncol 2003;21:3902-8.
181. Strickland S, Richards WG. Invasion of the trophoblasts. Cell 1992;71:355-7.
182. Stroun M, Anker P, Maurice P, Lyautey J, Lederrey C, Beljanski M. Neoplastic characteristics of the DNA found in the plasma of cancer patients. Oncology 1989;46:318-22.
183. Su YH, Wang M, Brenner DE, Norton PA, Block TM. Detection of mutated K-ras DNA in urine, plasma, and serum of patients with colorectal carcinoma or adenomatous polyps. Ann N Y Acad Sci 2008;1137:197-206.
184. Sun S, Xu MZ, Poon RT, Day PJ, Luk JM. Circulating Lamin B1 (LMNB1) biomarker detects early stages of liver cancer in patients. J Proteome Res 2010;9:70-8.
185. Taback B, Fujiwara Y, Wang HJ, Foshag LJ, Morton DL, Hoon DS. Prognostic significance of circulating microsatellite markers in the plasma of melanoma patients. Cancer Res 2001;61:5723-6.
186. Taback B, O'Day SJ, Boasberg PD, Shu S, Fournier P, Elashoff R, et al. Circulating DNA microsatellites: molecular determinants of response to biochemotherapy in patients with metastatic melanoma. J Natl Cancer Inst 2004;96:152-6.
187. Tan EM, Schur PH, Carr RI, Kunkel HG. Deoxyribonucleic acid (DNA) and antibodies to DNA in the serum of patients with systemic lupus erythematosus. J Clin Invest 1966;45:1732-40.
188. Tjoa ML, Cindrova-Davies T, Spasic-Boskovic O, Bianchi DW, Burton GJ. Trophoblastic oxidative stress and the release of cell-free feto-placental DNA. Am J Pathol 2006;169:400-4.
189. Tong YK, Ding C, Chiu RWK, Gerovassili A, Chim SSC, Leung TY, et al. Noninvasive prenatal detection of fetal trisomy 18 by epigenetic allelic ratio analysis in maternal plasma: theoretical and empirical considerations. Clin Chem 2006;52:2194-202.
190. Tong YK, Jin S, Chiu RW, Ding C, Chan KC, Leung TY, et al. Noninvasive prenatal detection of trisomy 21 by an epigenetic-genetic chromosome-dosage approach. Clin Chem 2010;56:90-8.
191. Tsang JC, Charoenkwan P, Chow KC, Jin Y, Wanapirak C, Sanguansermsri T, et al. Mass spectrometry-based detection of hemoglobin E mutation by allele-specific base extension reaction. Clin Chem 2007;53:2205-9.
192. Tsui DW, Chan KC, Chim SS, Chan LW, Leung TY, Lau TK, et al. Quantitative aberrations of hypermethylated RASSF1A gene sequences in maternal plasma in pre-eclampsia. Prenat Diagn 2007; 27:1212-8.
193. Tsui NB, Akolekar R, Chiu RW, Chow KC, Leung TY, Lau TK, et al. Synergy of total PLAC4 RNA concentration and measurement of the RNA single-nucleotide polymorphism allelic ratio for the noninvasive prenatal detection of trisomy 21. Clin Chem 2010;56: 73-81.
194. Tsui NB, Wong BC, Leung TY, Lau TK, Chiu RW, Lo YM. Non-invasive prenatal detection of fetal trisomy 18 by RNA-SNP allelic ratio analysis using maternal plasma SERPINB2 mRNA: a feasibility study. Prenat Diagn 2009;29:1031-7.
195. Tsui NBY, Chim SSC, Chiu RWK, Lau TK, Ng EKO, Leung TN, et al. Systematic microarray-based identification of placental mRNA in maternal plasma: towards non-invasive prenatal gene expression profiling. J Med Genet 2004;41:461-7.
196. Umetani N, Kim J, Hiramatsu S, Reber HA, Hines OJ, Bilchik AJ, et al. Increased integrity of free circulating DNA in sera of patients with colorectal or periampullary cancer: direct quantitative PCR for ALU repeats. Clin Chem 2006;52:1062-9.
197. Vasioukhin V, Anker P, Maurice P, Lyautey J, Lederrey C, Stroun M. Point mutations of the N-Ras gene in the blood plasma DNA of patients with myelodysplastic syndrome or acute myelogenous leukemia. Br J Haematol 1994;86:774-9.
198. Vogelstein B, Kinzler KW. Digital PCR. Proc Natl Acad Sci U S A 1999;96:9236-41.
199. von Knobloch R, Hegele A, Brandt H, Olbert P, Heidenreich A, Hofmann R. Serum DNA and urine DNA alterations of urinary transitional cell bladder carcinoma detected by fluorescent microsatellite analysis. Int J Cancer 2001;94:67-72.
200. Wang BG, Huang HY, Chen YC, Bristow RE, Kassauei K, Cheng CC, et al. Increased plasma DNA integrity in cancer patients. Cancer Res 2003;63:3966-8.
201. Wang GK, Zhu JQ, Zhang JT, Li Q, Li Y, He J, et al. Circulating microRNA: a novel potential biomarker for early diagnosis of acute myocardial infarction in humans. Eur Heart J 2010;31:659-66.
202. Wang K, Zhang SD, Marzolf B, Troisch P, Brightman A, Hu Z, et al. Circulating microRNAs, potential biomarkers for drug-induced liver injury. Proc Natl Acad Sci U S A 2009;106:4402-7.
203. Warren L, Bryder D, Weissman IL, Quake SR. Transcription factor profiling in individual hematopoietic progenitors by digital RT-PCR. Proc Natl Acad Sci U S A 2006;103:17807-12.
204. Watson JD, Crick FHC. A structure of deoxyribose nucleic acid. Nature 1953;171:737-8.
205. Wei YC, Chou YS, Chu TY. Detection and typing of minimal human papillomavirus DNA in plasma. Int J Gynaecol Obstet 2007;96:112-6.
206. Widschwendter A, Blassnig A, Wiedemair A, Muller-Holzner E, Muller HM, Marth C. Human papillomavirus DNA in sera of cervical cancer patients as tumor marker. Cancer Lett 2003;202:231-9.

207. Wong BC, Chan KC, Chan AT, Leung SF, Chan LY, Chow KC, et al. Reduced plasma RNA integrity in nasopharyngeal carcinoma patients. Clin Cancer Res 2006;12:2512-6.
208. Wong IH, Lo YM, Zhang J, Liew CT, Ng MH, Wong N, et al. Detection of aberrant p16 methylation in the plasma and serum of liver cancer patients. Cancer Res 1999;59:71-3.
209. Wong SC, Lo ES, Cheung MT. An optimised protocol for the extraction of non-viral mRNA from human plasma frozen for three years. J Clin Pathol 2004;57:766-8.
210. Yamada T, Nakamori S, Ohzato H, Oshima S, Aoki T, Higaki N, et al. Detection of K-ras gene mutations in plasma DNA of patients with pancreatic adenocarcinoma: correlation with clinicopathological features. Clin Cancer Res 1998;4:1527-32.
211. Yang H, Yang K, Khafagi A, Tang Y, Carey TE, Opipari AW, et al. Sensitive detection of human papillomavirus in cervical, head/neck, and schistosomiasis-associated bladder malignancies. Proc Natl Acad Sci U S A 2005;102:7683-8.
212. Yang HJ, Liu VW, Tsang PC, Yip AM, Tam KF, Wong LC, et al. Quantification of human papillomavirus DNA in the plasma of patients with cervical cancer. Int J Gynecol Cancer 2004;14:903-10.
213. Yung TK, Chan KC, Mok TS, Tong J, To KF, Lo YM. Single-molecule detection of epidermal growth factor receptor mutations in plasma by microfluidics digital PCR in non-small cell lung cancer patients. Clin Cancer Res 2009;15:2076-84.
214. Zhong XY, Holzgreve W, Hahn S. The levels of circulatory cell free fetal DNA in maternal plasma are elevated prior to the onset of preeclampsia. Hypertens Pregnancy 2002;21:77-83.
215. Zhong XY, Laivuori H, Livingston JC, Ylikorkala O, Sibai BM, Holzgreve W, et al. Elevation of both maternal and fetal extracellular circulating deoxyribonucleic acid concentrations in the plasma of pregnant women with preeclampsia. Am J Obstet Gynecol 2001;184:414-9.
216. Zhu XM, Han TQ, Sargent IL, Yin GW, Yao YQ. Differential expression profile of microRNAs in human placentas from preeclamptic pregnancies vs normal pregnancies. Am J Obstet Gynecol 2009;200:661.e1-7.

SECTION V

Pathophysiology

CHAPTER 46

Diabetes Mellitus

David B. Sacks, M.B., Ch.B., F.R.C.Path.

Diabetes mellitus is a group of metabolic disorders of carbohydrate metabolism in which glucose is underused, producing hyperglycemia. Some patients may experience acute life-threatening hyperglycemic episodes, such as ketoacidosis or hyperosmolar coma. As the disease progresses, patients are at increased risk for the development of specific complications, including *retinopathy* leading to blindness, *nephropathy* leading to renal failure, and *neuropathy* (nerve damage), collectively known as microvascular complications, as well as *atherosclerosis,* which is considered a *macrovascular complication.*[169,218] The last may result in stroke, gangrene, or coronary artery disease.

Diabetes is a common disease, although the exact prevalence is unknown. It is estimated that ≈250 million people currently have diabetes, and by 2025 this number will reach 280 million, 80% of whom will live in developing countries. In the United States, the number of people with diabetes has increased dramatically. The prevalence in 1999-2002 was 9.3%, 30% of whom were undiagnosed.[57] Analysis of the 2005-2006 National Health and Nutritional Examination Survey (NHANES) using both fasting glucose and oral glucose tolerance testing (OGTT) shows a prevalence of diabetes in the United States in persons 20 years of age and older of 12.9% (equivalent to ≈40 million people).[58] Of these, ≈40% are undiagnosed. Similarly, the prevalence of diabetes in Asian populations has increased rapidly in recent decades, reaching more than 110 million in 2007.[50] These statistics led to a description of diabetes as "one of the main threats to human health in the twenty-first century."[267] The prevalence of diabetes mellitus increases with age, and approximately half of all cases occur in people older than 55 years. In the United States, more than 20% of the population older than 65 years have diabetes.[99] A racial predilection has been noted, and by the age of 65, 33%, 25%, and 17% of Hispanics, blacks, and whites, respectively, in the United States have diabetes. In 2007, diabetes mellitus was estimated to be responsible for $174 billion in healthcare expenditures in the United States.[17] The direct costs were $116 billion, with 56% of that total incurred by those 65 years and older. An estimated 3.8 million people worldwide died from diabetes-related causes in 2007.[115] Diabetes is the fourth most common cause of death in the developed world.

CLASSIFICATION

Diabetes was initially diagnosed by OGTT. Values greater than two standard deviations above the mean of the value found in a selected population of healthy volunteers without a family history of diabetes mellitus were accepted as diagnostic. This criterion led to the identification of large numbers of asymptomatic people with abnormally high 1 to 2 hour postload glucose values, but normal fasting blood glucose. They were presumed to have early or mild diabetes mellitus. In 1975 it was estimated that more than half the population older than 60 years was abnormal. Follow-up on these individuals indicated that most of them with lesser degrees of glucose intolerance did not manifest definite evidence of diabetes mellitus in the next 10 years, and a large percentage returned to normal glucose tolerance.

Most populations have plasma glucose values that exhibit a unimodal, log-normal distribution (a distribution curve that is skewed to the high end but becomes bell shaped on a logarithmic axis). Ethnic groups with a high prevalence of diabetes, such as the Pima Indians and Nauruans, exhibit bimodal blood glucose distributions.[80] Optimal distinction between normal and diabetic individuals in these groups occurs at a fasting glucose around 140 mg/dL and glucose concentrations greater than 200 mg/dL 2 hours after an oral glucose load. Furthermore, the specific microvascular complications of diabetes were believed to be rare in patients with fasting or 2 hour postprandial glucose concentrations less than 140 or 200 mg/dL, respectively. These observations formed the basis for the criteria proposed in 1979 by a workgroup of the National Diabetes Data Group[174] and later endorsed by the World Health Organization (WHO) Committee on Diabetes.

The 1979 classification scheme recognized two major forms of diabetes: type I (insulin-dependent) diabetes mellitus (IDDM) and type II (non–insulin-dependent) diabetes mellitus (NIDDM).[174] The terms *juvenile-onset* and *adult-onset diabetes* were abolished. To base the classification on cause rather than on treatment, the American Diabetes Association (ADA) established a workgroup in 1995 to re-examine the classification and diagnosis of diabetes mellitus. The revised classification, published in 1997,[9] eliminates the terms *insulin-dependent diabetes mellitus* and *non–insulin-dependent diabetes mellitus,* which now are termed *type 1*

BOX 46-1 Classification of Diabetes Mellitus

Type 1 diabetes
- Immune-mediated
- Idiopathic

Type 2 diabetes

Other specific types of diabetes
- Gestational diabetes mellitus (GDM)
- Impaired glucose tolerance (IGT)
- Impaired fasting glucose (IFG)

From the American Diabetes Association. Report of the expert committee on the diagnosis and classification of diabetes mellitus. Diabetes Care 1997; 20:1183-201.

and *type 2 diabetes,* respectively (Box 46-1). Furthermore, the categories of previous abnormality of glucose tolerance and potential abnormality of glucose tolerance have been eliminated.

Type 1 Diabetes Mellitus

Approximately 5 to 10% of all cases of diabetes mellitus are included in this category. Patients usually have abrupt onset of symptoms (e.g., polyuria, polydipsia, rapid weight loss). They have insulinopenia (a deficiency of insulin) caused by loss of pancreatic islet β-cells and are dependent on insulin to sustain life and prevent ketosis. Most patients have antibodies that identify an autoimmune process (see later discussion); some have no evidence of autoimmunity and are classified as type 1 idiopathic. The peak incidence occurs in childhood and adolescence. Approximately 75% acquire the disease before the age of 18, but onset in the remainder may occur at any age. Age at presentation is not a criterion for classification.

Type 2 Diabetes Mellitus

This group accounts for approximately 90% of all cases of diabetes. Patients have minimal symptoms, are not prone to ketosis, and *are not dependent on insulin* to prevent ketonuria. *Insulin concentrations may be normal, decreased, or increased,* and most people with this form of diabetes have impaired insulin action. *Obesity* is commonly associated, and weight loss alone usually improves hyperglycemia in these persons. However, many individuals with type 2 diabetes may require dietary manipulation, oral hypoglycemic agents, or insulin to control hyperglycemia. Most patients acquire the disease after age 40, but it may occur in younger people. Type 2 diabetes in children and adolescents is an emerging, significant problem.[12,59,267] Among children in Japan, type 2 diabetes is now more common than type 1.[267]

Other Specific Types of Diabetes Mellitus

This subclass includes uncommon patients in whom hyperglycemia is due to a specific underlying disorder, such as genetic defects of β-cell function; genetic defects in insulin action; disease of the exocrine pancreas; endocrinopathies (e.g., Cushing's syndrome, acromegaly, glucagonoma); administration of hormones or drugs known to induce β-cell dysfunction (e.g., dilantin, pentamidine) or to impair insulin action (e.g., glucocorticoids, thiazides, β-adrenergics); infection; uncommon forms of immune-mediated diabetes; or other genetic conditions (e.g., Down syndrome, Klinefelter syndrome, porphyria; see Reference 18 for a detailed list). This was formerly termed *secondary diabetes.*

Gestational Diabetes Mellitus

This is defined as any degree of glucose intolerance *with onset or first recognition during pregnancy*[157] (i.e., diabetic women who become pregnant are not included in this category). Estimates of the frequency of abnormal glucose tolerance during pregnancy range from 1 to 14%, depending on the population studied and the diagnostic tests employed.[131] In the United States, gestational diabetes mellitus (GDM) occurs in 6 to 8% of pregnancies (≈200,000 cases annually). Women with GDM are at significantly increased risk for the subsequent development of type 2 diabetes mellitus, which occurs in 6 to 62%.[130] The risk is particularly high in women who have marked hyperglycemia during or soon after pregnancy, women who are obese, and those whose GDM was diagnosed before 24 weeks' gestation.[135] At 6 to 12 weeks postpartum, all patients who had GDM should be evaluated for diabetes using nonpregnant OGTT criteria. If diabetes is not present, patients should be re-evaluated for diabetes at least every 3 years.[19]

Impaired Glucose Tolerance

Impaired glucose tolerance (IGT) is diagnosed in people who have fasting blood glucose concentrations less than those required for a diagnosis of diabetes mellitus, but have a plasma glucose response during the OGTT between normal and diabetic states. The 2 hour postload plasma glucose following an OGTT is 140 to 199 mg/dL for this classification. An OGTT is required to assign a patient to this class. Development of overt diabetes occurs at a rate of 1 to 5% per year, but a large proportion of cases spontaneously revert to normal glucose tolerance. Microvascular disease is rare in this group, and patients usually do not experience the renal or retinal complications of diabetes. Patients have an increased prevalence of atherosclerosis and mortality from cardiovascular disease.[65]

Impaired Fasting Glucose

This category is analogous to IGT, but it is diagnosed by a *fasting* glucose value between those of normal and diabetic individuals, namely, fasting plasma glucose (FPG) between 100 and 125 mg/dL. It is a metabolic stage between normal glucose homeostasis and diabetes. As with IGT, persons with impaired fasting glucose (IFG) are at increased risk for the development of diabetes and cardiovascular disease. IFG and IGT are not clinical entities, but rather are risk factors for diabetes and cardiovascular disease.

HORMONES THAT REGULATE BLOOD GLUCOSE CONCENTRATION

During a brief fast, a precipitous decline in the concentration of blood glucose is prevented by breakdown of glycogen stored in the liver and synthesis of glucose in the liver. Some glucose is derived from gluconeogenesis in the kidneys.[84] These organs contain glucose-6-phosphatase, which is necessary to convert glucose-6-phosphate (derived from gluconeogenesis or glycogenolysis) to glucose. Skeletal muscle lacks this enzyme; muscle glycogen therefore cannot contribute directly to blood glucose. With more prolonged fasting (>42 hours), gluconeogenesis accounts for essentially all glucose production. In contrast, after a meal, the absorbed glucose is converted to glycogen (for storage in the liver and skeletal muscle) or fat (for storage in adipose tissue). Despite large fluctuations in the supply and demand of carbohydrates, the concentration of glucose in the blood is normally maintained within a fairly narrow range by hormones that modulate the movement of glucose into and out of the circulation. These include insulin, which decreases blood glucose, and the counter-regulatory hormones (glucagon, epinephrine, cortisol, and growth hormone), which increase blood glucose concentrations (Figure 46-1).[84] Normal glucose disposal depends on (1) the ability of the pancreas to secrete insulin, (2) the ability of insulin to promote uptake of glucose into peripheral tissue, and (3) the ability of insulin to suppress hepatic glucose production. The major insulin target organs are liver, skeletal muscle, and adipose tissue. These organs exhibit some differences in their responses to insulin. For example, the hormone stimulates glucose uptake through a specific glucose transporter—GLUT4—into muscle and fat cells, but not into liver cells.

Insulin

Insulin is a protein hormone produced by the β-cells of the islets of Langerhans in the pancreas. Insulin was the first protein hormone to be sequenced, the first substance to be measured by radioimmunoassay (RIA), and the first compound produced by recombinant DNA technology for clinical use. It is an anabolic hormone that stimulates the uptake of glucose into fat and muscle, promotes the conversion of glucose to glycogen or fat for storage, inhibits glucose production by the liver, stimulates protein synthesis, and inhibits protein breakdown.

Chemistry

Human insulin [molecular weight (MW) 5808 Da] consists of 51 amino acids in two chains (A and B) joined by two disulfide bridges, with a third disulfide bridge within the A chain. The amino acid sequence of human insulin differs slightly from insulin of other species, but the carboxyl terminal region of the B chain (B23 to B26), which appears crucial for the biological actions of insulin, is highly conserved among species. Insulin from most animals is immunologically and biologically similar to human insulin, and in the past, patients were treated with insulin purified from beef or pig pancreas. The most commonly used forms now are recombinant human insulins.

Synthesis

Preproinsulin, a protein of about 100 amino acids (MW 12,000 Da), is formed by ribosomes in the rough endoplasmic reticulum of the pancreatic β-cells (Figure 46-2). Preproinsulin is not detectable in the circulation under normal conditions because it is rapidly converted by cleaving enzymes to proinsulin (MW 9000 Da), an 86 amino acid polypeptide. This is stored in secretory granules in the Golgi complex of the β-cells, where *proteolytic cleavage to insulin and connecting peptide (C-peptide) occurs.*[179] Cleavage of proinsulin is catalyzed by two Ca^{2+}-regulated endopeptidases: prohormone convertases 1 and 2 (PC1 and PC2).[195] PC1 (sometimes designated PC3) hydrolyzes the molecule on the *C*-terminal

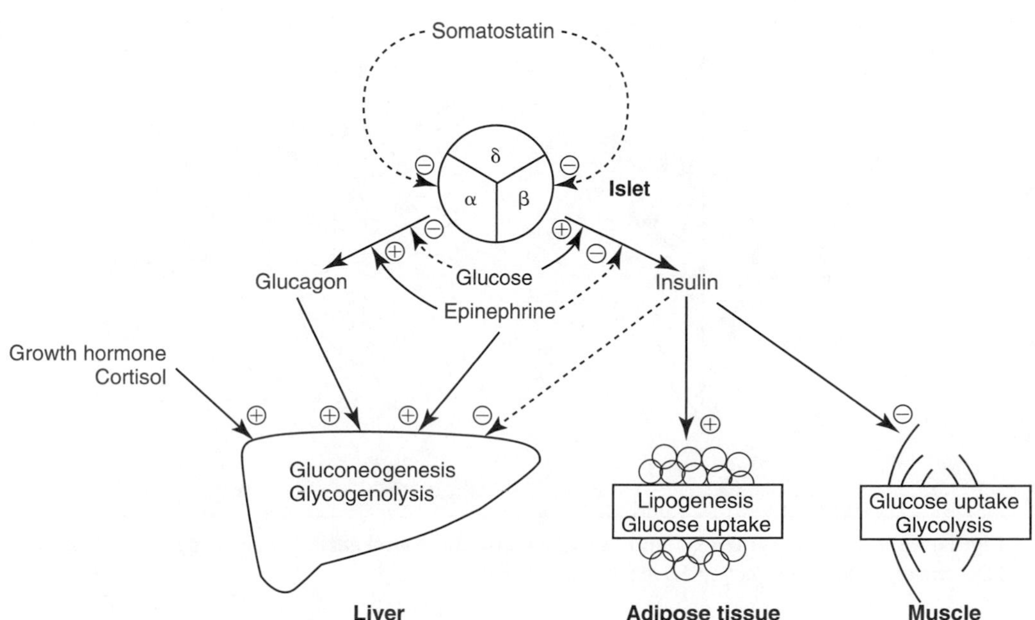

Figure 46-1 Hormonal regulation of blood glucose. Key: +, stimulation; –, inhibition. Cortisol, growth hormone, and epinephrine antagonize the effects of insulin.

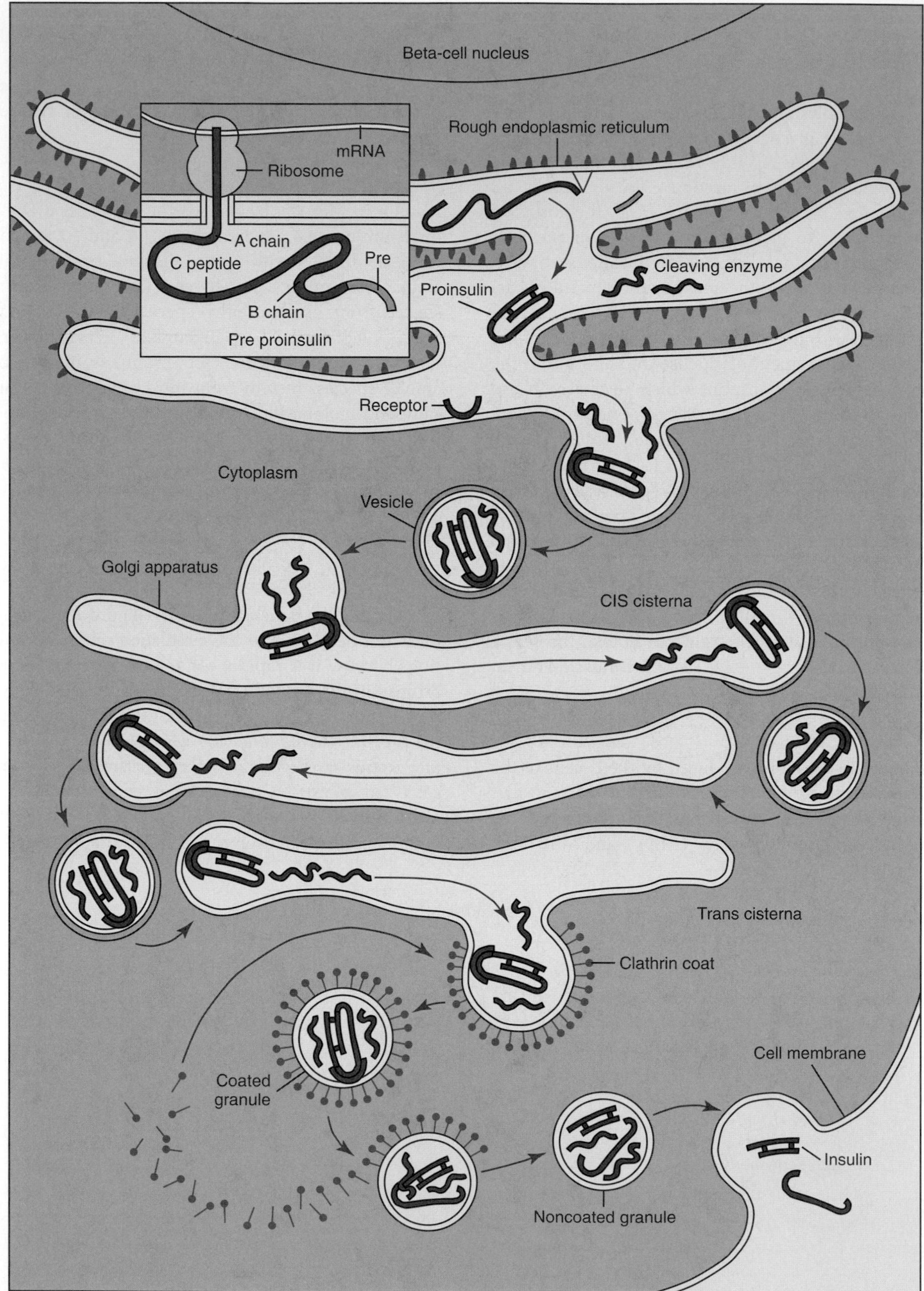

Figure 46-2 Insulin synthesis and release from the pancreatic β-cell. *(From Orci L, Vassalli J-D, Perrelet A. The insulin factory. Sci Am 1988;259:85-94.)*

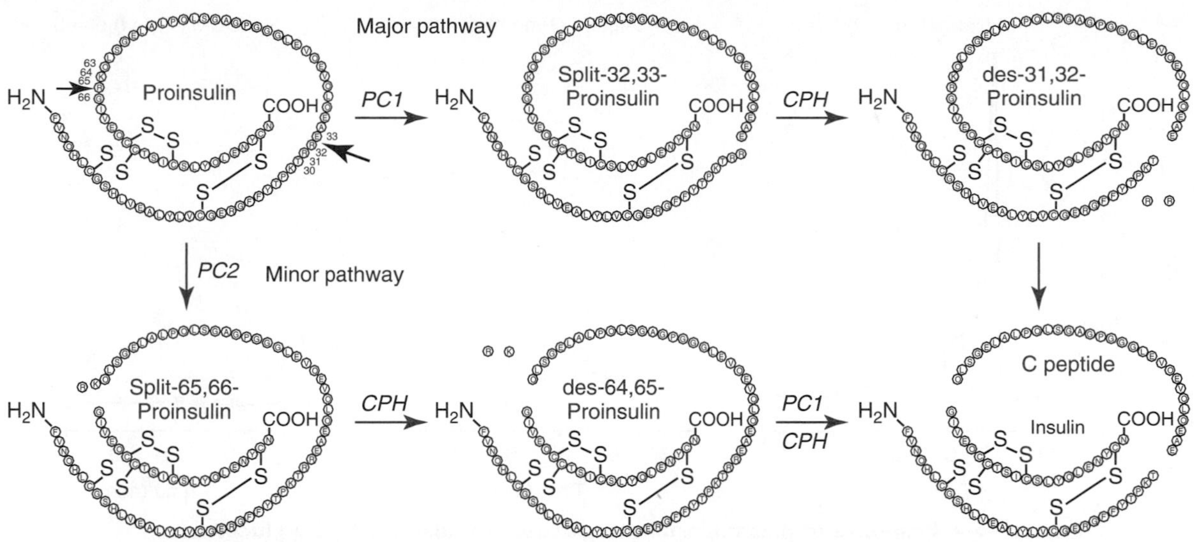

Figure 46-3 Processing of proinsulin. The enzymes prohormone convertase 1 and 2 (PC1 and PC2) act on proinsulin to form the appropriate split proinsulins. Carboxypeptidase-H (CPH) removes the two exposed basic amino acid residues *(circles)*.

end of Arg-31 and Arg-32 (at the BC junction) to yield split-32, 33-proinsulin (Figure 46-3). PC2 cleaves proinsulin on the *C*-terminal side of dibasic residues Lys-64 and Arg-65 (at the AC junction) to generate split-65,66-proinsulin. Each enzymatic hydrolysis is rapidly followed by the removal of two newly exposed *C*-terminal basic amino acids by carboxypeptidase-H to produce insulin and C-peptide.

The split proinsulin intermediates are rarely detected in patient samples because of the relatively high quantity of carboxypeptidase-H. This enzyme produces the more commonly observed proinsulin intermediates, des-31,32-proinsulin and des-64,65-proinsulin (see Figure 46-3). Most proinsulin processing is sequential. Intact proinsulin is initially hydrolyzed by PC1 or carboxypeptidase-H. The resultant des-31,32-proinsulin is converted by PC2 and carboxypeptidase-H to insulin and C-peptide. Less than 10% of proinsulin is metabolized via des-(64-65)-proinsulin, which is present in negligible amounts in humans. Des-31,32-proinsulin is the major proinsulin conversion intermediate.[223] Glucose regulates biosynthesis of both proinsulin and PC1, but has no effect on PC2 or carboxypeptidase-H. At the cell membrane, insulin and C-peptide are released into the portal circulation in equimolar amounts. In addition, small amounts of proinsulin and intermediate cleavage forms enter the circulation.

Release

Glucose, amino acids, pancreatic and gastrointestinal hormones (e.g., glucagon, gastrin, secretin, pancreozymin, gastrointestinal polypeptide), and some medications (e.g., sulfonylureas, β-adrenergic agonists) stimulate insulin secretion. Insulin release is inhibited by hypoglycemia, somatostatin (produced in the pancreatic δ-cells), and various drugs (e.g., α-adrenergic agonists, β-adrenergic blockers, diazoxide, phenytoin, phenothiazines, nicotinic acid).[184] In healthy individuals, insulin is secreted in a pulsatile fashion, with glucose and insulin the main signals in the feedback loop. Glucose elicits the release of insulin from the pancreas in two phases. The first phase begins 1 to 2 minutes after intravenous injection of glucose and ends within 10 minutes. This phase, illustrated by the sharp spike in Figure 46-4, *A*, represents the rapid release of stored insulin. The second phase, beginning at the point where the first phase ends, depends on continuing insulin synthesis and release and lasts until normoglycemia has been restored, usually within 60 to 120 minutes. With progressive failure of β-cell function, the first-phase insulin response to glucose is lost, but other stimuli such as glucagon or amino acids may be able to elicit this response. Although the second-phase insulin response is preserved in most patients with type 2 diabetes mellitus, both the first-phase response (Figure 46-4, *B*) and normal pulsatile insulin secretion[174] are lost. In contrast, patients with type 1 diabetes mellitus exhibit minimal or no insulin response (Figure 46-4, *C*).

Degradation

On the first pass through the portal circulation, approximately 50% of insulin is extracted by the liver, where it is degraded. Because the amount extracted is variable, plasma insulin concentrations may not accurately reflect the rate of insulin secretion. Additional insulin degradation occurs in the kidneys. Insulin is filtered through the glomeruli, reabsorbed, and degraded in the proximal tubule. The basal insulin secretory rate is about 1 U (43 μg)/h, with total daily secretion of about 40 U. The half-life of insulin in the circulation is between 4 and 5 minutes.

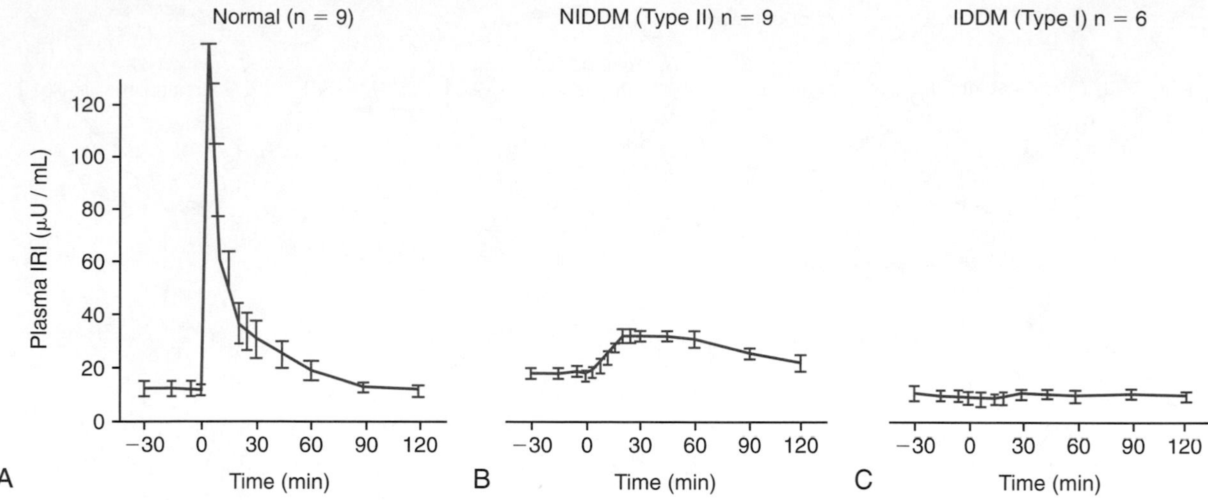

Figure 46-4 Response of plasma insulin to glucose stimulation. A 20 g glucose pulse is given intravenously at time 0. A, Healthy subjects. B, Patients with type 2 diabetes mellitus (NIDDM). C, Patients with type 1 diabetes mellitus (IDDM). *IRI*, Immunoreactive insulin. Values before time 0 represent baseline. *(From Pfeifer MA, Halter JB, Porte D Jr. Insulin secretion in diabetes mellitus. Am J Med 1981;70:579-88.)*

Proinsulin

Proinsulin, which has relatively low biological activity (approximately 10% of insulin potency), is the major storage form of insulin.[198] Normally, only small amounts (about 3% of the amount of insulin, on a molar basis) of proinsulin enter the circulation. However, the hepatic clearance rate for proinsulin is only 25% of that for insulin, and the half-life of proinsulin is ≈30 minutes. Therefore in the fasting state, circulating proinsulin concentrations are approximately 10 to 15% of insulin concentrations.

C-Peptide

Proinsulin is cleaved to a 31 amino acid connecting (C) peptide (MW 3600 Da) and insulin (see Figure 46-3). C-peptide is devoid of biological activity but appears necessary to ensure the correct structure of insulin.[104] Although insulin and C-peptide are secreted into the portal circulation in equimolar amounts, fasting C-peptide concentrations are fivefold to 10-fold higher than those of insulin owing to the longer half-life of C-peptide (≈35 minutes). The liver does not extract C-peptide, which is removed from the circulation by the kidneys and degraded, with a fraction excreted unchanged in the urine.

Antibodies to Insulin

Antibodies to insulin develop in almost all patients who are treated with exogenous insulin.[197] These antibodies are usually present at low titer and produce no adverse effects. On rare occasions (usually in patients with type 2 diabetes), high titers of insulin antibodies may cause insulin resistance. Improvement in the purity of animal insulins and the widespread use of human insulin have reduced, but not totally eliminated, antibody production. Recent advances in insulin delivery systems, namely, continuous subcutaneous insulin infusion and inhaled insulin, have significantly increased concentrations of insulin antibodies.[189] Antibodies to insulin rarely develop in patients who have not received exogenous insulin.

Although rare, patients with antibodies to the insulin receptor have been described.[79] On binding the receptor, these antibodies act as antagonists, producing hyperglycemia (e.g., in patients with acanthosis nigricans), or agonists, resulting in hypoglycemia.

The Mechanism of Insulin Action

Although the metabolic effects produced by insulin are well known, the molecular mechanism of insulin action remains incompletely understood.[40,231] It is generally accepted that the initial event is the binding of insulin to specific receptors in the plasma membrane (Figure 46-5). The human insulin receptor, which is well characterized, is a heterotetramer, comprising two α- and two β-subunits. The α-subunit (MW 135,000 Da) is located on the outer surface of the plasma membrane and contains the site where insulin binds. The β-subunit (MW 95,000 Da) extends intracellularly through the plasma membrane and contains an intrinsic tyrosine kinase. Binding of insulin to the α-subunits induces a conformational change in the receptor, resulting in activation of tyrosine kinase, which catalyzes the phosphorylation of tyrosine residues on several proteins. One of the major substrates for this tyrosine kinase is the receptor itself.

In addition to phosphorylating itself, the insulin receptor catalyzes the tyrosine phosphorylation of various specific intracellular proteins (see Figure 46-5). These include the four members of the family of insulin-receptor substrate (IRS) proteins (termed IRS-1, IRS-2, IRS-3, and IRS-4), Shc, and Gab-1. The phosphorylated tyrosines on these target proteins act as docking sites for selected intracellular signal transducer

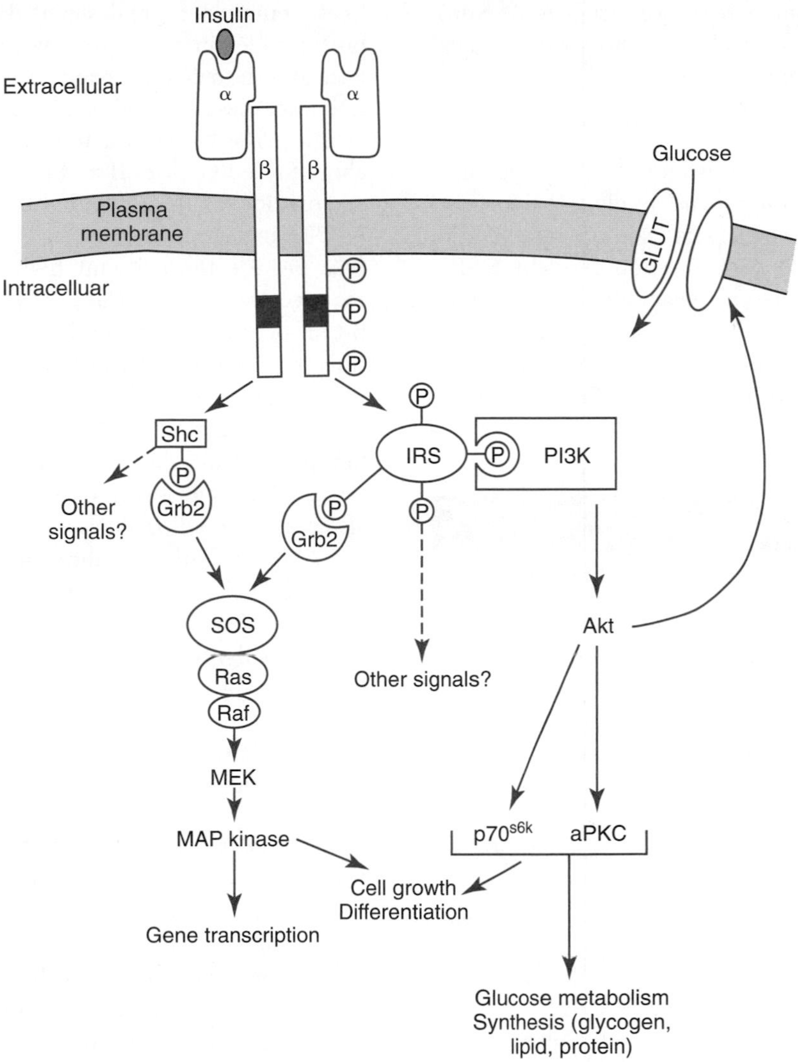

Figure 46-5 Mechanism of insulin action. Binding of insulin to the extracellular α-subunit of the insulin receptor induces autophosphorylation of the β-subunit of the receptor and phosphorylation of selected intracellular proteins, such as Shc and the insulin-receptor substrate (IRS) family. These latter phosphoproteins interact with other targets, thereby activating phosphorylation cascades, which result in glucose uptake (in adipose tissue and skeletal muscle), glucose metabolism, synthesis (of glycogen, lipid, and proteins), enhanced gene expression, cell growth, and differentiation. *aPKC*, Atypical protein kinase C; *p*, protein phosphorylation. See text for details.

proteins.[231] Most of these transducer proteins contain one or more Src homology 2 (SH2) domains. The SH2 domain is a sequence of approximately 100 amino acids that recognizes phosphotyrosine.[183] Sequence differences in the SH2 domain dictate the specificity of binding. SH2-containing proteins depicted in Figure 46-5 include those labeled phosphatidylinositol 3-kinase (PI3K) and growth factor receptor–bound protein 2 (Grb2), both of which mediate downstream signal transduction events. Similar to other growth factors, insulin stimulates the mitogen-activated protein (MAP) kinase cascade via Ras. In addition, phosphatidylinositol 3′-kinase activates atypical protein kinase C (aPKC) via Akt. The latter enzymes regulate glucose transport by modulating translocation of GLUT4 (the insulin-sensitive glucose transporter) to the plasma membrane. Akt also phosphorylates and inactivates GSK-3, thereby enhancing glycogen synthesis. Some of these events are listed in Figure 46-5. The pathways are elaborate, and although several components have been identified, there remain considerable gaps in our knowledge and understanding. Recent studies have clarified a fundamental concept—that insulin-mediated signaling events are highly redundant. For example, when two key insulin-signaling molecules, IRS-1 and GLUT4, were knocked out in transgenic mouse experiments, the resulting animals had minor metabolic defects rather than overt diabetes.[196] Similarly, mice with knockout of insulin receptors from skeletal muscle or liver do not develop diabetes.

Glucose Transport

The transport of glucose into cells is modulated by two families of proteins.[263] The sodium-dependent glucose transporters (SGLTs) use the electrochemical sodium gradient to transport glucose against its concentration gradient. SGLTs promote the uptake of glucose and galactose from the lumen of the small bowel and their reabsorption from urine in the kidney. Members of the second family of glucose carriers are called *facilitative glucose transporters* (GLUT) (Table 46-1).

TABLE 46-1 Facilitative Human Glucose Transporters

Name	Class	Tissue	Function
GLUT1	I	Wide distribution, especially brain, kidney, colon, and fetal tissues	Basal glucose transport
GLUT2	I	Liver, β-cells of pancreas, small intestine, and kidney	Non–rate-limiting glucose transport
GLUT3	I	Wide distribution, especially neurons, placenta, and testis	Glucose transport in neurons
GLUT4	I	Skeletal muscle, cardiac muscle, adipose tissue	Insulin-stimulated glucose transport
GLUT5	II	Small intestine, kidney, skeletal muscle, brain, and adipose tissue	Transports fructose (not glucose)
GLUT6	III	Brain, spleen, leukocytes	
GLUT7	II	Intestine, testis, prostate	
GLUT8	III	Testis, heart, brain	
GLUT9	II	Kidney, liver	
GLUT10	III	Liver, pancreas	
GLUT11	II	Pancreas, kidney, placenta, skeletal muscle	
GLUT12	III	Heart, prostate	
HMIT		Brain	Transports *myo*-inositol (not glucose)
GLUT14	III	Testis	

These transporters are designated GLUT1 to GLUT14, based on the order in which they were identified.[209] Eleven have been shown to catalyze sugar transport. They can be divided into three classes, based on sequence similarities and characteristics. The best characterized are class I. Less is known about those in classes II and III. GLUT1 is widely expressed and provides many cells with their basal glucose requirement. GLUT1 in the blood-brain barrier and GLUT3 in neuronal cells provide the constant high concentrations of glucose required by the brain. GLUT2 is expressed in hepatocytes, β-cells of the pancreas, and basolateral membranes of intestinal and renal epithelial cells. It is a low-affinity, high-capacity transport system that allows non–rate-limiting movement of glucose into and out of these cells. GLUT4 catalyzes the rate-limiting step for glucose uptake and metabolism in skeletal muscle, the major organ of glucose consumption. GLUT4 is also present in adipose tissue.

When circulating insulin concentrations are low, most of the GLUT4 is localized in intracellular compartments and is inactive. After eating, the pancreas releases insulin, which stimulates the translocation of GLUT4 to the plasma membrane, thereby promoting glucose uptake into skeletal muscle and fat. Insulin-stimulated glucose transport into skeletal muscle is defective in type 2 diabetes mellitus, but the mechanism has not been established.

Insulin-like Growth Factors

Insulin-like growth factors 1 and 2 (IGF-1 and IGF-2) are polypeptides structurally related to insulin.[190] These hormones (previously referred to as *nonsuppressible insulin-like activity* or *somatomedin*) exhibit metabolic and growth-promoting effects similar to those of insulin. Accumulating evidence implicates the IGF axis in the development of several common cancers.[207] IGF-1 (previously known as somatomedin C) is an important mediator of growth hormone action and is one of the major regulators of cell growth and differentiation. The physiologic role of IGF-2 is not known. Synthesis of IGF-1 depends on growth hormone and occurs predominantly in the liver. In addition, many other cells produce IGF-1 that does not enter the circulation but acts locally. Circulating IGF concentrations are approximately 1000-fold higher than insulin concentrations, and the hormone is kept inactive by binding to a family of at least six specific binding proteins.[113] These proteins regulate IGF by protecting the ligands in the circulation and delivering them to their target tissue. In contrast to insulin, which is unbound in the circulation, less than 10% of total serum IGF-1 is free. The biological actions of IGF are exerted through specific IGF receptors or the insulin receptor. The IGF-1 receptor is closely related to the insulin receptor in structure and biochemical properties. In contrast, the IGF-2 receptor is quite different; it lacks tyrosine kinase activity, and its physiologic relevance is not understood. The IGF-1 receptor has a high affinity for both IGF-1 and IGF-2, but a low affinity for insulin. The IGF-2 receptor has high, low, and no affinity for IGF-2, IGF-1, and insulin, respectively. The insulin receptor binds insulin with high affinity and IGF-1 and IGF-2 with low affinity.

The significance of IGFs in normal carbohydrate metabolism is not known. Exogenous administration produces hypoglycemia, whereas a deficiency of IGF-1 results in dwarfism (pygmies and Laron dwarfs). IGFs, particularly IGF-2, may be produced in excess by extrapancreatic neoplasms, and patients may have fasting hypoglycemia.[60] The high concentrations of both IGF-2 protein in the blood and IGF-2 messenger RNA (mRNA) in tumor extracts have led to the proposal that IGF-2 is the humoral mediator of non–islet cell tumor–induced hypoglycemia.[217] Measurement of plasma IGF-1 concentration may be useful in evaluating growth hormone deficiency and excess (acromegaly), and in monitoring response to nutritional support.

Counter-Regulatory Hormones

Several hormones have actions opposite to those of insulin. These counter-regulatory hormones are catabolic and increase hepatic glucose production initially by enhancing the breakdown of glycogen to glucose (glycogenolysis), and later by stimulating the synthesis of glucose (gluconeogenesis).[83,84] The initial response (within minutes) to low blood glucose is an increase in glucose production, stimulated by glucagon and epinephrine. Over time (3 to 4 hours), growth hormone and cortisol increase glucose mobilization and decrease glucose use (see Figure 46-1). Evidence also suggests that glucose production by the liver is an inverse function of ambient glucose concentration, independent of hormonal factors *(glucose autoregulation)*. The role of other hormones or neurotransmitters is not clear but appears relatively unimportant. Multiple counter-regulatory hormones exhibit both redundancy and hierarchy. Glucagon is the most important, and epinephrine becomes critical when glucagon is deficient. The other factors have lesser roles. These hormones, briefly described here, are discussed further in Chapters 30, 51, 53, and 54.

Glucagon

Glucagon is a 29 amino acid polypeptide secreted by α-cells of the pancreas. The major target organ for glucagon is the liver, where it binds to specific receptors and increases both intracellular adenosine-5′-monophosphate and calcium. Glucagon stimulates the production of glucose in the liver by glycogenolysis and gluconeogenesis.[144] In addition, glucagon enhances ketogenesis in the liver. A minor target organ for glucagon is adipose tissue, where the hormone increases lipolysis. Glucagon secretion is regulated primarily by plasma glucose concentrations, with low and high plasma glucose being stimulatory and inhibitory, respectively. Long-standing diabetes mellitus impairs the glucagon response to hypoglycemia, resulting in an increased incidence of hypoglycemic episodes. Stress, exercise, and amino acids induce glucagon release. Insulin inhibits glucagon release from the pancreas and decreases glucagon gene expression, thereby attenuating its biosynthesis. Increased glucagon concentrations, secondary to insulin deficiency, are believed to contribute to the hyperglycemia and ketosis of diabetes.

Proglucagon is also produced in the distal gut by L-cells, which process it into glucagon, glucagon-like peptide-1 (GLP-1), and GLP-2. Food ingestion stimulates release of GLP-1, which acts on β-cells of the pancreas to stimulate insulin gene transcription and potentiate glucose-induced insulin secretion. GLP-1 and glucose-dependent insulinotropic polypeptide (GIP) are incretin hormones that are responsible for 70% of postprandial insulin secretion.[55] GLP-1 reduces hyperglycemia by regulating insulin and glucagon secretion, thus providing gastric emptying and satiety. For these reasons, GLP-1 analogs are generating interest in the treatment of type 2 diabetes,[55] and two (exenatide and liraglutide) have received Food and Drug Administration (FDA) approval.

Epinephrine

Epinephrine, a catecholamine secreted by the adrenal medulla, stimulates glucose production (glycogenolysis) and decreases glucose use, thereby increasing blood glucose concentrations. It also stimulates glucagon secretion and inhibits insulin secretion by the pancreas (see Figure 46-1). Epinephrine appears to have *a key role in glucose counter-regulation when glucagon secretion is impaired* (e.g., in type 1 diabetes mellitus). Physical or emotional stress increases epinephrine production, releasing glucose for energy. Tumors of the adrenal medulla, known as *pheochromocytomas,* secrete excess epinephrine or norepinephrine and produce moderate hyperglycemia as long as glycogen stores are available in the liver.

Growth Hormone

Growth hormone is a polypeptide secreted by the anterior pituitary gland. It stimulates gluconeogenesis, enhances lipolysis, and antagonizes insulin-stimulated glucose uptake.

Cortisol

Cortisol, secreted by the adrenal cortex in response to adrenocorticotropic hormone (ACTH), stimulates gluconeogenesis and increases the breakdown of protein and fat. Patients with Cushing's syndrome have *increased cortisol* owing to tumor or hyperplasia of the adrenal cortex and may become hyperglycemic. In contrast, people with Addison's disease have *adrenocortical insufficiency* caused by destruction or atrophy of the adrenal cortex and may exhibit hypoglycemia.

Other Hormones Influencing Glucose Metabolism

Thyroxine

Thyroxine, secreted by the thyroid gland, is not directly involved in glucose homeostasis, but it stimulates glycogenolysis and increases the rates of gastric emptying and intestinal glucose absorption. These factors may produce glucose intolerance in thyrotoxic individuals, but patients usually have a fasting plasma glucose concentration in the reference interval.

Somatostatin

Somatostatin, also called *growth hormone–inhibiting hormone,* is a 14 amino acid peptide found in the gastrointestinal tract, the hypothalamus, and the δ-cells of the pancreatic islets.

Although somatostatin does not appear to have a direct effect on carbohydrate metabolism, it inhibits the release of growth hormone from the pituitary. In addition, *somatostatin inhibits secretion of glucagon and insulin by the pancreas,* thus modulating the reciprocal relationship between these two hormones.

CLINICAL UTILITY OF MEASURING INSULIN, PROINSULIN, C-PEPTIDE, AND GLUCAGON

Box 46-2 lists the clinical conditions in which hormones that regulate glucose, namely, insulin, proinsulin, C-peptide, and glucagon, have been measured. Although there is interest in the possible clinical value of measurement of the concentrations of insulin and its precursors, the assays are useful primarily for research purposes. There is no role for routine testing for insulin, proinsulin, or C-peptide in most patients with diabetes mellitus.[204] Measurement of C-peptide is sometimes necessary in the United States for patients to obtain insurance coverage for continuous subcutaneous insulin infusion pumps. It must be emphasized that the diagnostic criteria for diabetes mellitus do not include measurements of hormones, which remain predominantly research tools.

BOX 46-2 Clinical Utility of Insulin, Proinsulin, C-Peptide, and Glucagon Assays

Insulin
- Evaluation of fasting hypoglycemia
- Evaluation of the polycystic ovary syndrome
- Classification of diabetes mellitus
- Prediction of diabetes mellitus
- Assessment of β-cell activity
- Selection of optimal therapy for diabetes
- Investigation of insulin resistance
- Prediction of the development of coronary artery disease

Proinsulin
- Diagnosis of β-cell tumors
- Familial hyperproinsulinemia
- Cross-reactivity of insulin assays

C-Peptide
- Evaluation of fasting hypoglycemia
  - β-Cell tumors
  - Factitious
- Classification of diabetes mellitus
- Assessment of β-cell activity
- Obtaining insurance coverage for insulin pump
- Monitoring therapy
  - Pancreatectomy
  - Transplant (pancreas-islet cell)
  - Immunomodulation of type 1 diabetes

Glucagon
- Diagnosis of α-cell tumors

Insulin

The primary clinical application of insulin measurement is in the evaluation of patients with fasting hypoglycemia (discussed in more detail in Chapter 26). Measurement of circulating insulin could be helpful in evaluating insulin resistance and insulin secretion. Insulin determination has also been proposed to be of value in selecting the optimal initial therapy for patients with type 2 diabetes mellitus. In theory, the lower the pretreatment insulin concentration, the more appropriate might be insulin or an insulin secretagogue as the treatment of choice. Although intellectually appealing, no evidence suggests that knowledge of the insulin concentration leads to more efficacious treatment. Evidence indicates that increased concentrations of insulin in nondiabetic individuals predict the development of coronary artery disease.[96] Nevertheless, it is not clear whether the increased insulin is responsible for the risk of coronary disease, and the clinical value is questionable.[204] In the past, measurement of insulin was advocated in the evaluation and management of patients with polycystic ovary syndrome.[204] Women with this condition have insulin resistance and abnormal carbohydrate metabolism that may respond to oral hypoglycemic agents. However, it is not clear whether assessing insulin resistance by measuring insulin concentrations affords any advantage over clinical signs of insulin resistance (body mass index, acanthosis nigricans), and the American College of Obstetrics and Gynecology does not recommend routine measurements of insulin.[5] Although a few investigators have recommended measuring insulin along with glucose during an OGTT as an aid to the early diagnosis of diabetes mellitus, this approach is not recommended.[204]

Proinsulin

High proinsulin concentrations are usually noted in patients with benign or malignant β-cell tumors of the pancreas. Most patients with β-cell tumors have increased insulin, C-peptide, and proinsulin concentrations, but occasionally only proinsulin is increased[82] because the tumors have defective conversion of proinsulin to insulin. Despite its low biological activity, proinsulin production may be adequate to produce hypoglycemia. In addition, a rare form of familial hyperproinsulinemia, produced by impaired conversion to insulin, has been described. Measurement of proinsulin can be useful to determine the amount of proinsulin-like material that cross-reacts in an insulin assay. Patients with type 2 diabetes have increased proportions of proinsulin and proinsulin conversion intermediates,[143] high concentrations of which are associated with cardiovascular risk factors.[167] Even relatively mild hyperglycemia produces hyperproinsulinemia, with values greater than 40% of insulin concentration in type 2 diabetes.[143] Similarly, women with GDM have higher concentrations of proinsulin and split-32,33-proinsulin than pregnant normoglycemic control subjects. An increased ratio of proinsulin-like molecules to insulin-like molecules at screening may be a better predictor of GDM than age, obesity, or hyperglycemia.[226] Increased proinsulin concentrations may also be detected in patients with chronic renal failure, cirrhosis, or hyperthyroidism.

Accurate measurement of proinsulin has been difficult for several reasons: the blood concentrations are low; antibody production is difficult; most antisera cross-react with insulin and C-peptide, which are present in much higher concentrations; the assays measure intermediate cleavage forms of proinsulin; and reference preparations of pure proinsulin are not readily available. However, a more sensitive nonequilibrium RIA method for measuring proinsulin was developed by adsorbing the initial antiserum with biosynthetic human C-peptide coupled with agarose to eliminate cross-reactivity with C-peptide.[42,101] An enzyme-linked immunosorbent assay (ELISA) has been described that employs an antibody to C-peptide as the coating antibody and anti-insulin antibody for detection.[85] The detection limit is 0.25 pmol/L.[134]

C-Peptide

Measurement of C-peptide has a number of advantages over insulin measurement. Because hepatic metabolism is negligible, C-peptide concentrations are better indicators of β-cell function than is peripheral insulin concentration.[186] Furthermore, C-peptide assays do not measure exogenous insulin and do not cross-react with insulin antibodies, which interfere with the insulin immunoassay.

Fasting Hypoglycemia

The primary indication for measuring C-peptide is for the evaluation of fasting hypoglycemia. Some patients with insulin-producing β-cell tumors, particularly if hyperinsulinism is intermittent, may exhibit increased C-peptide concentrations with normal insulin concentrations. When hypoglycemia is due to surreptitious insulin injection, *insulin* concentrations will be high but C-peptide values will be low[108]; this occurs because C-peptide is not found in commercial insulin preparations and exogenous insulin suppresses β-cell function.

Insulin Secretion

Basal or stimulated (by glucagon or glucose) C-peptide concentrations provides estimates of a patient's insulin secretory capacity and rate. For example, diabetic patients with C-peptide concentrations greater than 1.8 μg/L (1.8 ng/mL) after stimulation with glucagon behave clinically like patients with type 2 diabetes, and those with low peak C-peptide values (<0.5 μg/L) behave like patients with type 1 diabetes.[105] In rare cases, this strategy may be helpful before discontinuation of insulin treatment (e.g., in an obese adolescent). Urinary and fasting serum C-peptide concentrations appear to be of some value in differentiating patients with type 1 diabetes from those with type 2 diabetes.[124] In addition, patients who have type 1 diabetes but who have no C-peptide response are usually more labile than those with some residual β-cell function. Despite these observations, C-peptide measurement has a negligible role in the routine management of patients with diabetes. A relatively new indication for C-peptide analysis is the recent requirement that Medicare patients in the United States must have low C-peptide concentrations to be eligible for coverage of insulin pumps.[204]

Monitoring Therapy

Measurement of C-peptide is used to monitor patients' response to pancreatic surgery. C-peptide should be undetectable after a radical pancreatectomy and should increase after a successful pancreas or islet cell transplant. In addition, a stable C-peptide concentration is used as an endpoint in immunomodulatory trials for the prevention of type 1 diabetes.[1]

Measurements of urine C-peptide are useful when continuous assessment of β-cell function is desired, or when frequent blood sampling is not practical. The 24-hour urine C-peptide content (in the absence of renal failure, which produces increased concentrations) correlates well with fasting serum C-peptide concentration or with the sum of C-peptide concentrations in sequential specimens after a glucose load. However, the fraction of secreted C-peptide that is excreted in the urine exhibits high intersubject and intrasubject variability, limiting the value of urine C-peptide as a measure of insulin secretion.[237]

Glucagon

Very high concentrations of glucagon are seen in patients with α-cell tumors of the pancreas called *glucagonomas*. Patients with this tumor frequently have weight loss, necrolytic migratory erythema, diabetes mellitus, stomatitis, and diarrhea.[252] Skin lesions often occur first and are frequently overlooked. Most tumors have metastasized when finally diagnosed. Low glucagon concentrations are associated with chronic pancreatitis and long-term sulfonylurea therapy.

METHODS FOR THE MEASUREMENT OF SPECIFIC HORMONES

Insulin

Although insulin has been assayed for over 50 years, no highly accurate, precise, and reliable procedure is available to measure the amount of insulin in a patient sample. Many insulin assays are commercially available.[52,150,160] The techniques most widely used are immunometric.[150,160] Bioassays, although of greater physiologic relevance because they measure biological activity, are labor intensive and are not widely used. A stable isotope dilution mass spectrometry assay yields lower values than an immunoassay.[132]

Patients treated with exogenous insulin may develop circulating anti-insulin antibodies, which compete with antibodies in the RIA. Endogenous antibodies and their bound insulin can be precipitated from serum with polyethylene glycol (PEG), and free insulin measured by RIA. Total insulin can be determined by eluting antibody-bound insulin with hydrochloric acid (HCl), precipitating the antibody with PEG, and performing RIA. The bound insulin is the difference between total and free insulin. Unless a patient's insulin requirements change dramatically, total insulin concentrations are usually constant in patients with type 1 diabetes, and repeated assays are not necessary.

Principle

In a typical RIA procedure for measuring insulin, ^{125}I-labeled insulin competes with insulin in a patient sample for binding to an insulin-specific antibody immobilized on the walls of a polypropylene tube. The supernatant is decanted, and the bound ^{125}I determined in a gamma counter. The amount of insulin in the sample is established by comparison with a calibration curve obtained by plotting on logit-log graph paper the percent of total radioactivity bound (B/T%) against the concentration of the calibrators. Various commercial kits for insulin measurement are now available.

Comments

General comments on the measurement of insulin include the following:

1. The term *immunoreactive insulin* is used in reference to assays that may recognize, in addition to insulin, substrates that share antigenic epitopes with insulin. Examples include proinsulin, proinsulin conversion intermediates, and insulin derivatives, produced by glycation or dimerization.
2. Various insulin preparations, including human insulin, are used as insulin calibrators. For ease of comparison of results among laboratories, the insulin calibrator is expressed in terms of international units (IU). One international unit of insulin is equal to approximately 43 µg of the World Health Organization (WHO) first International Reference Preparation (1st IRP) Code 66/304 (National Institute of Biological Standards and Control, South Mimms, Potters Bar, Hertfordshire, United Kingdom), which is 100% human insulin.
3. *Antisera raised against insulin show some cross-reactivity with proinsulin but not with C-peptide.* Specificity is not a problem in healthy individuals because the low proinsulin concentrations do not appreciably affect the absolute values of insulin. In certain situations (e.g., islet cell tumors and diabetic individuals), proinsulin is present at higher concentrations, and direct assay of plasma may falsely overestimate the true insulin concentration. Because proinsulin has very low activity, incorrect conclusions regarding the availability of biologically active insulin may be reached in patients with diabetes. The magnitude of the error depends on the concentration of proinsulin and the extent of cross-reactivity of the antiserum with proinsulin. Monoclonal antibody-based assays that are specific for insulin and do not measure proinsulin,[234] although theoretically advantageous, are not superior to nonspecific assays.[197]
4. A stable isotope dilution mass spectrometry (IDMS) assay has been developed to measure insulin, proinsulin, and C-peptide.[132] The difference in mass among the three analytes allows specific measurement of each protein. Comparison of patient samples revealed that most, but not all, results were higher by immunoassay than by mass spectrometry.[132] Thus immunoassays may overestimate insulin, particularly at low concentrations. The high protein concentration in the serum requires extraction of proteins (e.g., by immunoaffinity) and purification by high-performance liquid chromatography (HPLC) before quantification by mass spectrometry. This method is not suitable for routine laboratory analysis, but is the best higher-order measurement procedure available and can be used as a candidate reference measurement procedure.
5. The American Diabetes Association (ADA) appointed a task force to standardize the insulin assay.[197] Evaluation of unknown samples by 17 different laboratories revealed a wide range in insulin values, with interlaboratory variation up to threefold.[197] Large differences were observed even among laboratories using the same assays. Use of a common calibrator did not improve agreement among laboratories. Assay coefficients of variation (CVs) ranged from less than 2% to greater than 30%, with ELISAs exhibiting the lowest imprecision. Certain characteristics of some assays, including commercial kits, were unacceptable. The task force judged available proficiency and certification programs for insulin to be inadequate, and recommended the establishment of a central laboratory to provide certification for insulin assays. Complete interlaboratory standardization was deemed to be neither practical nor universally acceptable. ADA recommendations for analysis of insulin[197] are as follows:
   a. Each laboratory should carefully evaluate its insulin assay to ensure acceptable assay performance.
   b. Each laboratory should compare the performance of its assay with others using common calibrators and unknown samples.
   c. Because assay performance may change with time or with new reagents or equipment, performance characteristics must be remeasured periodically.
6. In 2004 the ADA convened an international workgroup to establish guidelines for acceptability of insulin assays and to develop a standardization program that can be used to achieve uniform accuracy-based values.[152] Evaluation of 10 commercial insulin methods from 9 manufacturers revealed within-assay CVs ranging from 3.7 to 39%, and 7 assays had a CV ≤10.6%.[152] Among-assay CVs ranged from 12 to 66%. Results from six assays agreed within a total error of 32%.[152] Cross-reactivity with proinsulin and split-32,33-proinsulin was <2% for nine methods and <3% for eight methods, respectively. A common insulin reference preparation failed to improve harmonization of results. The workgroup concluded that not all commercial insulin assays have acceptable performance characteristics. A study in the United Kingdom published at the same time[150] compared 11 commercially available insulin assays and made analogous observations. Insulin values among the different assays varied up to twofold.

The ADA workgroup subsequently compared results of 10 commercial insulin assays against IDMS. Four methods were within 32% of the IDMS concentration.[160] Most methods had bias greater than 15.5%. Bias was reduced by calibration with serum pools, but remained high for many methods at low insulin concentrations (<60 pmol/L) (10 μIU/mL).

7. Based on biological variability, desirable measurement bias of ±15%, imprecision of 10.6% CV, and total analytical error of 32.0% have been proposed for a single insulin measurement.[152]
8. Patient samples with high values should be diluted with the zero calibrator.
9. The presence of antibodies to insulin produces spuriously increased or decreased (depending on the method used) insulin values.

Reference Intervals

Reference intervals vary among assays, and each laboratory should establish its own reference intervals. After an overnight fast, insulin concentrations in healthy, normal, nonobese people vary from 12 to 150 pmol/L (2 to 25 μIU/mL).* More specific assays that have minimal cross-reactivity with proinsulin reveal a fasting plasma insulin concentration of less than 60 pmol/L (10 μIU/mL). Concentrations up to 1200 pmol/L (200 μIU/mL) can be reached during a glucose tolerance test. Representative values for insulin concentrations after glucose are shown in Figure 46-4. Fasting insulin values are higher in obese, nondiabetic people and lower in trained athletes.

Insulin Antibodies

Assays for insulin antibodies fall into three categories: (1) quantitative radioimmunoelectrophoresis, which measures the binding of immunoglobulin (Ig)G antibody to radiolabeled insulin by rocket immunoelectrophoresis into anti–IgG-containing agarose; (2) RIAs with separation of bound and free insulin by precipitation with PEG or a second antibody; and (3) solid-phase immobilization of insulin to test tubes or Sepharose. These are discussed in greater detail in Reeves.[194]

Proinsulin

Principle

Accurate measurement of proinsulin has been difficult for several reasons: the blood concentrations are low; antibody production is difficult; most antisera cross-react with insulin and C-peptide, which are present in much higher concentrations; the assays measure intermediate cleavage forms of proinsulin; and reference preparations of pure proinsulin were not readily available.[247] Therefore few accurate data are available in the literature on plasma proinsulin. These problems have, to a large extent, been overcome by the availability of biosynthetic proinsulin, which has allowed the production of monoclonal antibodies to proinsulin[67,223] and has provided reliable proinsulin calibrators and reference preparations. An International Reference Preparation for human proinsulin (code 84/611) is available from the National Institute of Biological Standards and Controls (Potters Bar, United Kingdom). Earlier assays may have overestimated proinsulin concentrations.[180]

Reference Intervals

Reference intervals for proinsulin are highly dependent on the method of analysis, the degree of cross-reactivity of the antisera, and the purity of proinsulin calibrators. Each laboratory should establish its own reference intervals.

Reference intervals in healthy, fasting individuals reported in the literature vary from 1.1 to 6.9 pmol/L to 2.1 to 12.6 pmol/L (see Reference 109 and references therein).

C-Peptide

Principle

C-peptide undergoes minimal liver metabolism, and, in contrast to proinsulin assays, assays are not affected by anti-insulin antibodies. However, several methodologic problems produce large between-method variation. These difficulties include variable specificity among different antisera, variable cross-reactivity with proinsulin, and various types of C-peptide preparation used as a calibrator. A 2008 comparison of 40 serum samples using nine commercial C-peptide assay methods showed within- and between-run CVs varying from less than 2% to greater than 10%, and from less than 2% to greater than 18%, respectively.[146] Some methods had high imprecision, with between-run CVs exceeding 15%. Two isotope-dilution liquid chromatography–mass spectrometry methods for measuring C-peptide have been developed.[48,199] Calibrating C-peptide measurements to a reference method using mass spectrometry increased comparability among laboratories.[146]

Reference Intervals

Each laboratory should establish its own reference interval for C-peptide. Fasting serum concentrations of C-peptide in healthy people range from 0.78 to 1.89 ng/mL (0.25 to 0.6 nmol/L). After stimulation with glucose or glucagon, values range from 2.73 to 5.64 ng/mL (0.9 to 1.87 nmol/L), or three to five times the prestimulation value. Urinary C-peptide is usually in the range of 74 ± 26 μg/L (25 ± 8.8 μmol/L). C-peptide is excreted primarily by the kidney, and concentrations in the serum are increased in renal disease.

Glucagon

Principle

A competitive RIA is available for measuring glucagon (Siemens Medical Solutions Diagnostics, Malvern, Pa). ^{125}I-labeled glucagon competes with glucagon in the patient specimen for binding to the polyclonal glucagon antibody.

*The conversion factor of 6.0 used to convert μIU/mL (or mIU/L) of insulin to pmol/L is based on an MW of insulin of 5807.58 and specific activity of 30 IU/mg.

Bound glucagon is separated from free glucagon by the use of PEG and a second antibody. Bound radioactivity for the patient specimen is compared with that of glucagon calibrators. Calibrator values are assigned at the manufacturer using the WHO glucagon international standard (69/194).

Reference Intervals

Fasting plasma concentrations of glucagon vary from 70 to 180 ng/L (20 to 52 pmol/L). Values up to 500 times the upper reference limit may be found in patients with autonomously secreting α-cell neoplasms.

PATHOGENESIS OF TYPE 1 DIABETES MELLITUS

Type 1 diabetes mellitus results from cellular-mediated autoimmune destruction of the insulin-secreting cells of pancreatic β-cells.[22,100] In the vast majority of patients, destruction is mediated by T cells. This is termed type 1A or immune-mediated diabetes (see Box 46-1). The α-, δ-, and other islet cells are preserved. The islet cells have a chronic mononuclear cell infiltrate, called *insulitis.* The autoimmune process leading to type 1 diabetes begins months or years before the clinical presentation, and an 80 to 90% reduction in the volume of β-cells is required to induce symptomatic type 1 diabetes. The rate of islet cell destruction is variable and is usually more rapid in children than in adults.

Antibodies

The most practical markers of β-cell autoimmunity are circulating antibodies, which have been detected in the serum years before the onset of hyperglycemia. The best characterized antibodies are as follows[22,100,204,251]:

1. *Islet cell cytoplasmic antibodies* (ICAs) react with a sialoglycoconjugate antigen present in the cytoplasm of all endocrine cells of the pancreatic islets. These antibodies are detected in the serum of 0.5% of normal subjects and 75 to 85% of patients with newly diagnosed type 1 diabetes. The antibodies are detected by immunofluorescence microscopy on frozen sections of human pancreatic tails. Results are compared with standard serum of the Immunology of Diabetes Workgroup[162] and are expressed in Juvenile Diabetes Foundation (JDF) units. Although not universal, many laboratories use 10 JDF units on two separate occasions or a single result of greater than or equal to 20 JDF units as a significant titer. The ICA assay is labor intensive and difficult to standardize. Few clinical laboratories are likely to implement this assay, which has marked interlaboratory variability in sensitivity and specificity.[204]
2. *Insulin autoantibodies* (IAAs) are present in more than 90% of children who develop type 1 diabetes before age 5, but in less than 40% of individuals who develop diabetes after age 12. Their frequency in healthy people is similar to that of ICA. A radioisotopic method that calculates the displaceable insulin radio ligand binding after the addition of excess nonradiolabeled insulin is recommended for IAA. Results are positive when concentrations exceed the 99th percentile or the mean + 2 (or 3) standard deviations (SDs) in healthy controls. Proficiency evaluation revealed poor concordance for IAA among laboratories.[35] An important caveat is that insulin antibodies develop after insulin therapy, even in those persons who use human insulin.
3. *Antibodies to the 65 kDa isoform of glutamic acid decarboxylase* (GAD_{65})[24] have been found up to 10 years before the onset of clinical type 1 diabetes and are present in ≈60% of patients with newly diagnosed diabetes. GAD_{65} antibodies may be used to identify patients with apparent type 2 diabetes who will subsequently progress to type 1 diabetes. Several different assay formats have been used for the measurement of anti-GAD_{65} antibodies, including enzymatic immunoprecipitation assay, radiobinding assay, ELISA, immunofluorescence, and Western blotting.[214] Considerable variability among laboratories has been significantly reduced by the Second International GADAb Workshop.[214] A monoclonal antibody, MICA 3, was suggested as a reference standard. A dual micromethod and RIA performed with ^{3}H-labeled human recombinant GAD_{65} in a rabbit reticulocyte expression system is used by many laboratories. Methods for measurement of GAD_{65} are now commercially available.
4. *Insulinoma-associated antigens* (IA-2A and IA-2βA), directed against two tyrosine phosphatases, have been detected in more than 50% of newly diagnosed type 1 diabetes patients. A widely used method to measure IA-2A uses ^{35}S-labeled recombinant IA-2 in a dual micromethod and RIA. Concurrent analysis of IA-2 and GAD_{65} in a single assay has been reported.[205]
5. *Zinc transporter ZnT8* was identified recently as a major autoantigen in type 1 diabetes.[251] Initial analysis identified ZnT8 in 60 to 80% of patients with new-onset type 1 diabetes compared with less than 2% of controls and less than 3% of individuals with type 2 diabetes.

Although antibodies to bovine serum albumin have been reported in patients with newly diagnosed type 1 diabetes,[123] this model is contentious, and conflicting data exist.[21,23,149]

The Centers for Disease Control and Prevention (CDC) and the Immunology of Diabetes Society have developed the Diabetes Autoantibody Standardization Program (DASP). The major goals of DASP are (1) to assist laboratories in improving methods, (2) to organize workshops for harmonization of antibody testing for type 1 diabetes, and (3) to provide reference materials.[35,239] DASP provides serum from 50 patients with newly diagnosed type 1 diabetes and from 50 to 100 control patients. A WHO standard for GAD_{65} and IA-2A (97-550) has been established and allows laboratories to express results in common units.[239] Several workshops have been held. The first assay proficiency evaluation revealed poor performance for IAA among 23 laboratories.[35] Good concordance among laboratories was observed for GAD_{65} and IA-2A, with the latter improving with successive comparisons.[239] Ongoing harmonization is likely to enhance assay performance.

Autoantibody markers of immune destruction are present in 85 to 90% of individuals with immune-mediated diabetes when fasting hyperglycemia is initially detected.[9] Approximately 5 to 10% of white adult patients who have the type 2 diabetes phenotype also have islet cell autoantibodies, particularly to GAD_{65}. This condition has been termed *latent autoimmune diabetes of adulthood (LADA).*[188] Up to 1 to 2% of healthy individuals have a single autoantibody and are at low risk of developing immune-mediated diabetes. Because the prevalence of immune-mediated diabetes is low (approximately 0.3% in the general population), the positive predictive value of a single autoantibody will be low. The presence of multiple islet autoantibodies (IAA, GAD_{65}, and IA-2A and/or IA-2βA) is associated with a greater than 90% risk of immune-mediated diabetes. However, no acceptable therapy has been documented to prevent the clinical onset of diabetes in islet cell autoantibody–positive individuals.[22] New strategies under development for treatment of type 1 diabetes focus on immunosuppressive therapy to attenuate the autoimmune response, replacement of insulin-producing β-cells by transplantation, or restoration of insulin with gene therapy.[86,176] Hyperglycemia in diabetic mice was completely reversed by gene therapy that induced the development of β-cells of the pancreas in the liver.[138] Although type 1 diabetes can be prevented in animal models,[41] the possible role of immune intervention in humans remains unresolved.

Genetics

Susceptibility to type 1 diabetes is inherited,[238] but the mode of inheritance is complex and has not been defined. It is a multigenic trait, and the major locus is the major histocompatibility complex on chromosome 6. At least 11 other loci on 9 chromosomes also contribute, with the regulatory region of the insulin gene *INS* on chromosome 11p15 being an important locus. The human leukocyte antigen (HLA)-DQ and -DR genetic factors are by far the most important determinants for risk of type 1 diabetes.[56] The concordance rate between identical twins is approximately 30%, and approximately 95% of whites with type 1 diabetes express HLA-DR3 or HLA-DR4 histocompatibility antigens. However, up to 40% of the nondiabetic population also express these alleles. In contrast, the *HLA-DQB1*0602* allele significantly decreases the risk of type 1 diabetes. HLA typing can indicate absolute risk of diabetes.[204] The risk of a sibling developing diabetes is 1%, 5%, and 10 to 20% if the number of haplotypes shared is none, one, and two, respectively. However, only 10% of patients with type 1 diabetes have an affected first-degree relative. Genome-wide association studies have also identified non-HLA genetic factors that increase risk, including the insulin gene variable number tandem repeat (*INS* VNTR, *CTLA4,* and *PTPN22*).[56] The multiplicity of independent chromosomal regions associated with a predisposition to type 1 diabetes suggests that other susceptibility genes will be identified. Routine measurement of genetic markers is not of value at this time for the diagnosis or management of patients with type 1 diabetes.[204]

Environment

Reports describe that environmental factors are involved in initiating diabetes. Viruses, such as rubella, mumps, and coxsackievirus B, have been implicated.[114] It seems likely that autoimmunity to β-cells is initiated by a viral protein (that shares amino acid sequence with a β-cell protein) or some other environmental insult. Genetic susceptibility and other host factors (e.g., HLA type) determine the progression of the β-cell destruction.

PATHOGENESIS OF TYPE 2 DIABETES MELLITUS

At least two major identifiable pathological defects have been reported in patients with type 2 diabetes.[66,121,206] One is a decreased ability of insulin to act on peripheral tissue. This is called *insulin resistance* and is thought by many to be the primary underlying pathologic process. The other is *β-cell dysfunction,* which is an inability of the pancreas to produce sufficient insulin to compensate for the insulin resistance. Thus a relative deficiency of insulin occurs early in the disease and absolute insulin deficiency late in the disease. The debate over whether type 2 diabetes is due primarily to a defect in β-cell secretion or to peripheral resistance to insulin, or to both, has been raging for decades. However, data are available to support the concept that insulin resistance is the primary defect, preceding the derangement in insulin secretion and clinical diabetes by as much as 20 years.[121,206] Despite the lack of consensus, it is clear that type 2 diabetes mellitus is an extremely heterogeneous disease, and no single cause is adequate to explain the progression from normal glucose tolerance to diabetes. The fundamental molecular defects in insulin resistance and insulin secretion result from a combination of environmental and genetic factors.

Loss of β-Cell Function

Increased β-cell demand induced by insulin resistance is ultimately associated with progressive loss of β-cell function that is necessary for the development of fasting hyperglycemia. The major defect is a *loss of glucose-induced insulin release* (see Figure 46-4), which is termed *selective glucose unresponsiveness.* Hyperglycemia appears to render the β-cells increasingly unresponsive to glucose (called *glucotoxicity*), and the degree of dysfunction correlates with both glucose concentration and duration of hyperglycemia. Restoration of euglycemia rapidly resolves the defect. Increased free fatty acids in serum have also been implicated in β-cell failure.[29] Other insulin secretory abnormalities in type 2 diabetes include disruption of the normal pulsatile release of insulin and an increased ratio of plasma proinsulin to insulin.[143] More recently, evidence obtained from knockout mice reveals that insulin resistance in the β-cells may contribute to alterations in insulin secretion, as occur in type 2 diabetes.[140]

Insulin Resistance

Insulin resistance is defined as "a decreased biological response to normal concentrations of circulating insulin"[78]; it is found in obese, nondiabetic individuals and in patients with type 2 diabetes. The underlying pathophysiologic defect(s) has (have) not been identified, but insulin resistance is usually attributed to a defect in insulin action. Measurement of insulin resistance in a routine clinical setting is difficult, and surrogate measures, namely, fasting insulin concentration or the euglycemic insulin clamp,[10] are used to provide an indirect assessment of insulin function. The euglycemic clamp is performed in hospital under close supervision. The subject receives a constant intravenous infusion of insulin in one arm with concurrent intravenous infusion of variable amounts of glucose in the other arm to maintain blood glucose at a normal fasting concentration. A broad clinical spectrum of insulin resistance varies from euglycemia (with marked increase in endogenous insulin) to hyperglycemia (despite large doses of exogenous insulin). Several rare clinical syndromes are also associated with insulin resistance. The prototype is the type A insulin resistance syndrome, which is characterized by hyperinsulinemia, acanthosis nigricans, and ovarian hyperandrogenism.

The insulin resistance syndrome (also known as *syndrome X*, or *the metabolic syndrome*) is a constellation of associated clinical and laboratory findings, consisting of insulin resistance, hyperinsulinemia, obesity, dyslipidemia [high triglyceride and low high-density lipoprotein (HDL) cholesterol], and hypertension.[191] Individuals with this syndrome are at increased risk for cardiovascular disease. The metabolic syndrome is diagnosed if an individual meets three or more of the following criteria[76]:

- Abdominal obesity: waist circumference greater than 35 inches (women) or 40 inches (men)
- Triglycerides greater than 150 mg/dL
- HDL cholesterol less than 50 mg/dL (women) or less than 40 mg/dL (men)
- Blood pressure greater than or equal to 130/85 mm Hg
- Fasting plasma glucose greater than or equal to 110 mg/dL

The diagnostic criteria proposed by the WHO differ from those listed here.[264] The concept of the "metabolic syndrome" has been questioned by several experts, including the person who first described it,[192] and major clinical diabetes organizations.[122]

Environment

Environmental factors, such as diet and exercise, are important determinants in the pathogenesis of type 2 diabetes. Convincing evidence links obesity to the development of type 2 diabetes, but the association is complex. Although 60 to 80% of patients with type 2 diabetes are obese, diabetes develops in less than 15% of obese individuals. In contrast, virtually all obese subjects, even those with normal carbohydrate tolerance, have hyperinsulinemia and are insulin resistant. Other factors, such as family history of type 2 diabetes (genetic predisposition), the duration of obesity, and the distribution of fat are important. Nevertheless, the rising prevalence of diabetes is believed to be a consequence of the increase in obesity (defined as a body mass index ≥30 kg/m^2), which was reported to be 25.6% in U.S. adults in 2007.[2] Evaluation of 84,941 healthy women after 16 years in the Nurses' Health Study revealed that obesity was the most important predictor of type 2 diabetes.[110] Compared with women with a body mass indices less than 23, the relative risks of developing diabetes were 38.8 and 20.1 with body mass indexes greater than or equal to 35 and 30 to 34.9, respectively. It is important to note that intervention can delay or prevent the onset of type 2 diabetes. Two randomized studies documented that life-style changes (weight reduction and exercise) in individuals with IGT reduced the incidence of type 2 diabetes.[136,241] Although the weight loss was modest (5 to 7%), the rate of progression to type 2 diabetes was reduced by 58% in both studies.

An inverse relationship has been noted between the degree of physical activity and the prevalence of type 2 diabetes. For every 500 kcal increase in daily energy expenditure, a 6% decrease in age-adjusted risk of type 2 diabetes occurs. This effect is independent of both body weight and a parental history of diabetes. The mechanism of the protective effect of exercise is thought to be increased sensitivity to insulin in skeletal muscle and adipose tissue.

Diabetogenes

It is widely acknowledged that genetic factors contribute to the development of type 2 diabetes.[121] For example, the concordance rate for type 2 diabetes in identical twins approaches 100%. Type 2 diabetes is 10 times more likely to occur in an obese person with a diabetic parent than in an equally obese person without a diabetic family history. However, the mode of inheritance is unknown, and type 2 diabetes has been described as a "geneticist's nightmare."[175] Many less common diseases (e.g., cystic fibrosis, Duchenne muscular dystrophy) are caused by mutations at a single locus. More common diseases, such as diabetes mellitus, schizophrenia, atherosclerosis, hypertension, and osteoporosis, are not inherited according to simple mendelian rules. These conditions are genetically more complex, and multiple genetic factors interact with exogenous influences (such as environmental factors) to produce the phenotype.

Numerous mutations of the insulin receptor gene, *INSR*, have been identified.[78] Many patients with these defects have extreme insulin resistance, but the mutations are exceptionally rare and usually are found in only one patient or a single family. Mutations of substrates for the insulin receptor that causes diabetes are not known. Few mutations have been described in other potential candidate genes, including those coding for GLUT4 and glycogen synthase.

Initial success in the search for diabetogenes was seen in maturity-onset diabetes of the young (MODY), a rare group of disorders characterized by nonketotic diabetes.[29,204] The clinical spectrum of MODY is broad, ranging from asymptomatic hyperglycemia to an acute presentation. Several types of MODY may result from mutations in the genes that encode glucokinase (an enzyme that phosphorylates glucose in the β-cell) or several transcription factors. These can be diagnosed by molecular diagnostic testing. Although MODY is not a form of type 2 diabetes, interest in the genetics of MODY offers hope of insight into type 2 diabetes.

Multiple factors complicate the search for diabetogenes in type 2 diabetes.[206] A variety of approaches have produced several genes that are associated with type 2 diabetes. Recent genome-wide association studies (GWAS) have substantially contributed to our understanding of the genetic architecture of type 2 diabetes, with 17 genetic loci identified.[94,224] Most of these genetic loci are associated with the insulin secretion pathway, rather than with insulin resistance. Despite considerable effort to identify the genetic basis of type 2 diabetes mellitus, *genetic defects identified to date account for only ≈5% of patients with type 2 diabetes.* Therefore, the gene or genes causing common forms of type 2 diabetes remain unknown. Moreover, the risk alleles in these loci all have relatively small effects (odds ratios, 1.1 to 13). Incorporation of 18 different risk loci to construct a genotype score did not significantly improve clinical prediction based on current phenotype risk factors.[156]

DIAGNOSIS

For many years the diagnosis of diabetes mellitus was dependent solely on the *demonstration of hyperglycemia* (Box 46-3). In 2009, an International Expert Committee recommended that diabetes be diagnosed by measurement of hemoglobin A1c (HbA_{1c}), which reflects long-term blood glucose concentrations[235] (for additional information, see "Glycated Hemoglobin" section, later in this chapter). For type 1 diabetes, the diagnosis is usually easy because hyperglycemia appears abruptly, is severe, and is accompanied by serious metabolic derangements. Diagnosis of type 2 diabetes may be difficult because hyperglycemia often is not severe enough for the patient to notice symptoms of diabetes. Nevertheless, the risk of complications makes it important to identify people with the disease.

BOX 46-3 Criteria for the Diagnosis of Diabetes Mellitus

Any one of the following is diagnostic:

A. Glucose
   1. Fasting plasma glucose (FPG) ≥7.0 mmol/L (126 mg/dL)*
   OR
   2. Symptoms of hyperglycemia and casual plasma glucose ≥11.1 mmol/L (200 mg/dL)†
   OR
   3. 2 hour plasma glucose ≥11.1 mmol/L (200 mg/dL) during an oral glucose tolerance test (OGTT)‡
B. Hemoglobin A1c (HbA_{1c})§
   $HbA_{1c} \geq 6.5\%$

In the absence of unequivocal hyperglycemia, these criteria should be confirmed by repeating the same test on a different day. Mixing different methods to diagnose diabetes should be avoided.

*Fasting is defined as no calorie intake for at least 8 hours.
†Casual is defined as any time of day without regard to time since last meal. The classic symptoms of hyperglycemia include polyuria, polydipsia, and unexplained weight loss.
‡The OGTT should be performed as described by the World Health Organization (WHO), using a glucose load containing the equivalent of 75 g of anhydrous glucose dissolved in water.
§The test should be performed in a laboratory that is NGSP-certified and standardized to the DCCT assay. Point-of-care assays should not be used for diagnosis.
From the American Diabetes Association. Standards of medical care in diabetes—2010. Diabetes Care 2010;33(Suppl 1):S11-61.

The diagnostic criteria recommended in 1979 were (1) classic symptoms of diabetes with unequivocal increase in plasma glucose, (2) FPG greater than or equal to 140 mg/dL on more than one occasion, or (3) a 2 hour and one other postload glucose concentration greater than or equal to 200 mg/dL during an OGTT.[174] These criteria were widely adopted but are imperfect. The OGTT is more sensitive than fasting glucose early in the course of type 2 diabetes, resulting in lack of equivalence between fasting and 2 hour glucose values. Virtually all persons with an FPG concentration greater than or equal to 140 mg/dL have 2 hour glucose greater than or equal to 200 mg/dL in an OGTT. In contrast, in persons without previously identified diabetes, fasting glucose greater than or equal to 140 mg/dL is present in only 25% of those who have 2 hour glucose greater than or equal to 200 mg/dL. To address these and other discrepancies, the diagnostic criteria were revised in 1997 (see Box 46-3).[9,201] The major modification was lowering the diagnostic threshold for fasting glucose from 140 to 126 mg/dL (7 mmol/L) to better identify individuals at risk of retinopathy and nephropathy. The lower cutoff was suggested to provide earlier diagnosis of diabetes, with consequent earlier therapeutic intervention.[201]

Fasting Plasma Glucose Concentrations

FPG concentrations of 126 mg/dL (7.0 mmol/L) or greater on more than one occasion are diagnostic of diabetes mellitus (see Box 46-3). The diagnosis of most cases of diabetes mellitus can be established with this criterion. However, some investigators believe that fasting hyperglycemia may be a relatively late development in the course of type 2 diabetes, delaying the diagnosis and leading to underestimation of the prevalence of diabetes mellitus in the population.[233] Complications of diabetes, such as retinopathy, proteinuria, and neuromuscular disease, are present in approximately 30% of patients at clinical diagnosis of type 2 diabetes, and onset of type 2 diabetes probably occurs at least 4 to 7 years before clinical diagnosis. Screening of high-risk individuals for diabetes is now recommended.[9,19,95] Fasting glucose should be measured in all asymptomatic persons at age 45 (or younger in subjects at increased risk), with follow-up testing every 3 years (see discussion later in this chapter). However, no published evidence indicates that treatment based on screening is efficacious.

Oral Glucose Tolerance Test

Serial measurement of plasma glucose before and after a specific amount of glucose given orally should provide a standard

BOX 46-4 Factors Other Than Diabetes That Influence the Oral Glucose Tolerance Test

Patient Preparation
- Duration of fast
- Prior carbohydrate intake
- Medications (e.g., thiazides, oral contraceptives, corticosteroids)
- Trauma
- Intercurrent illness
- Age
- Activity
- Weight

Administration of Glucose
- Form of glucose (anhydrous or monohydrate)
- Quantity of glucose ingested
- Volume in which administered
- Rate of ingestion

During the Test
- Posture
- Anxiety
- Caffeine
- Smoking
- Activity
- Time of day
- Sample preservation

method by which to evaluate individuals and establish values for healthy and diseased subjects. Although more sensitive than FPG determinations, glucose tolerance testing is affected by multiple factors that result in *poor reproducibility* (Box 46-4).[6] Moreover, approximately 20% of OGTTs fall into the nondiagnostic category (e.g., only one blood sample exhibits increased glucose concentration). Unless results are grossly abnormal initially, *the OGTT should be performed on two separate occasions* to establish the diagnosis of diabetes.

The following conditions should be met before an OGTT is performed: discontinue, when possible, medications known to affect glucose tolerance; perform in the morning after 3 days of unrestricted diet (containing at least 150 g of carbohydrate per day) and activity; and perform the test after a 10 to 16 hour fast only in ambulatory outpatients (bed rest impairs glucose tolerance), who should remain seated during the test without smoking cigarettes. Glucose tolerance testing should not be performed on hospitalized, acutely ill, or inactive patients. The test should begin between 7 AM and 9 AM. Venous plasma glucose should be measured fasting, then 2 hours after an oral glucose load. For nonpregnant adults, the recommended load is 75 g, which may not be a maximum stimulus[174]; for children, 1.75 g/kg, up to 75 g maximum is given. The glucose should be dissolved in 300 mL of water and ingested over 5 minutes. A commercial, more palatable form of glucose may be ingested, but whether the anhydrous or monohydrate form of glucose should be used is still in question.[255]

An OGTT is rarely necessary for the diagnosis of diabetes mellitus. It continues to be recommended in a limited fashion by the WHO.[204,265] The sensitivity of FPG concentrations is lower than the OGTT for diagnosing diabetes, and some authors claim that the OGTT better identifies patients at risk for developing complications of diabetes. An FPG value less than 100 mg/dL or a random glucose concentration less than 140 mg/dL is sufficient to rule out the diagnosis of diabetes mellitus. An OGTT is indicated in the following situations:

1. Diagnosis of GDM (discussed later).
2. Diagnosis of IGT. This remains controversial. Individuals with IGT have increased risk of cardiovascular disease, but many of them do not have IFG by ADA criteria.[204]
3. Evaluation of a patient with unexplained nephropathy, neuropathy, or retinopathy, with random glucose concentration less than 140 mg/dL. Abnormal results in this setting do not necessarily denote a cause-and-effect relationship, and other diseases must be ruled out.
4. Population studies for epidemiologic data.

As mentioned earlier, 2009 guidelines advocate the use of HbA_{1c} for diagnosis of diabetes in nonpregnant individuals.[235]

Intravenous Glucose Tolerance Test

Poor absorption of orally administered glucose may result in a "flat" tolerance curve. Some patients are unable to tolerate a large oral carbohydrate load or may have altered gastric physiology (e.g., after gastric resection). In these patients, an intravenous glucose tolerance test may be performed to eliminate factors related to the rate of glucose absorption. In addition, measurement of the first-phase insulin response can identify the subgroup of individuals with increased concentrations of multiple autoantibodies who are at greatest risk of progression to type 1 diabetes.[36]

Preparation of patients is the same as for the OGTT. The dose of glucose is 0.5 g/kg of body weight (maximum 35 g), given as a 25 g/dL solution. The dose is administered intravenously over 3 minutes ± 15 seconds, and blood is collected every 10 minutes after the midinjection time for 1 hour. A single forearm vein cannula may be used for infusion and sampling, but it should be flushed with saline after the glucose is infused, and dead space should be cleared with several volumes of blood before each sample is drawn. If insulin assays are performed, a specimen is also obtained 5 minutes after the start of the injection. Blood glucose concentrations decrease in an exponential manner, and the rate of glucose disappearance can be calculated from the formula $K = 70/t_{1/2}$, where $t_{1/2}$ is the number of minutes required for the blood glucose value to decrease to one half of the 10 minute value, and K is the rate of disappearance of blood glucose, expressed as percent per minute. The glucose values are plotted on the log scale of semilog paper versus time on the abscissa. The best-fitting straight line is drawn through the points, and the time (in minutes) for the glucose concentration to decrease by 50% ($t_{1/2}$) is read. In healthy individuals, K usually exceeds 1.5%; values less than 1.0% are considered diagnostic of diabetes. A poor correlation is found between the results of intravenous and oral glucose tolerance tests.[81] Similar to oral glucose tolerance, intravenous glucose tolerance deteriorates with age.

In the formula $K = 70/t_{1/2}$, the value of 70 is derived from the logarithmic nature of the decrease in glucose concentration over time. The concentration of glucose at 10 minutes will be twice that of the value obtained from the plot $t_{1/2}$. Using natural logarithms, the rate of decrease in glucose concentration, expressed as percent per minute *(K)*, is given by

$$K = 100\,(\ln 2 - \ln 1)/t_{1/2} = 69.3/t_{1/2} \cong 70/t_{1/2}$$

The main indication for the intravenous glucose tolerance test is in clinical research to evaluate the first-phase insulin response to glucose (see Figure 46-4).[37] The test is performed as described earlier, but samples are drawn as follows: two baseline samples 5 minutes apart (the latter immediately before infusion) and samples 1, 3, 5, and 10 minutes after the end of the glucose infusion. The first-phase insulin release is usually measured by the sum of the insulin concentrations 1 and 3 minutes after the glucose bolus. Alternatively, the 0 to 10 minute incremental insulin area may be used. Analogous to the OGTT, the intravenous glucose tolerance test has poor reproducibility.

GESTATIONAL DIABETES MELLITUS

Normal pregnancy is associated with increased insulin resistance, especially in the late second and third trimesters. Euglycemia is maintained by increased insulin secretion, with GDM developing in those women who fail to augment insulin sufficiently. Risk factors for GDM include a family history of diabetes in a first-degree relative, obesity, advanced maternal age, glycosuria, and selected adverse outcomes in a previous pregnancy (e.g., stillbirth, macrosomia). Recommendations for screening and diagnosis were formulated in 1984 at the Second International Workshop-Conference on Gestational Diabetes Mellitus,[225] and were refined at the Third, Fourth, and Fifth International Workshop-Conferences in 1990, 1998, and 2007,[157] respectively. Based on the Fourth Workshop-Conference, the ADA modified its recommendations for laboratory diagnosis of GDM by adopting 5 to 10% lower glucose values.[11] These modified guidelines are as follows[14,19]:

1. Low-risk patients require no testing. Low-risk status is limited to women who meet all of the following:
   - Age younger than 25 years
   - Weight normal before pregnancy
   - Member of an ethnic group with a low prevalence of diabetes
   - No known diabetes in first-degree relatives
   - No history of abnormal glucose tolerance
   - No history of poor obstetric outcome
2. Average-risk patients (all patients who fall between low and high risk) should be tested at 24 to 28 weeks' gestation (see below for testing strategy).
3. Very high-risk patients should undergo immediate testing. They are defined as having any of the following:
   - Severe obesity
   - Prior history of GDM or delivery of large-for-gestational age infant
   - Glycosuria
   - Strong family history of type 2 diabetes
   - Diagnosis of polycystic ovarian syndrome

Average- and high-risk patients receive a glucose challenge test given by one of two methods (Table 46-2):

1. One step: Perform a diagnostic 100 g OGTT without prior plasma or serum glucose screening. This one-step approach may be cost-effective in high-risk patients or populations (e.g., some Native American groups).
   - A 75 g OGTT is deemed acceptable by some, but it is not as well validated as the 100 g test.
2. Two step (see Table 46-2): The first step is a 50 g oral glucose load (the patient does not need to be fasting), followed by a plasma or serum glucose determination at 1 hour. A plasma glucose value greater than or equal to 140 mg/dL (7.7 mmol/L) indicates the necessity for definitive testing. Approximately 15% of patients have a 1 hour venous plasma glucose concentration of 140 mg/dL (7.7 mmol/L) or greater, and require a full diagnostic glucose tolerance test. That subgroup includes ≈80% of all women with GDM. Some experts have recommended a

TABLE 46-2 Screening and Diagnosis of Gestational Diabetes Mellitus

Screening

1. Perform at between 24 and 28 weeks' gestation on all average and very high-risk pregnant women not identified as having glucose intolerance.
2. Give 50 g oral glucose load without regard to time of day or time of last meal.
3. Measure venous plasma glucose at 1 hour.
4. If glucose is ≥140 mg/dL,* perform glucose tolerance test.

Diagnosis

1. Perform in the morning after an overnight fast of at least 8 hours.
2. Measure fasting venous plasma glucose.
3. Give 75 or 100 g of glucose orally.
4. Measure plasma glucose hourly for 3 hours (or for 2 hours if 75 g of glucose is given)
5. At least two values must meet or exceed the following:

	100 g Load	75 g Load
Fasting	95 mg/dL	95 mg/dL
1 hour	180 mg/dL	180 mg/dL
2 hour	155 mg/dL	155 mg/dL
3 hour	140 mg/dL	—

6. If results are normal in a clinically suspect situation, repeat during the third trimester.

*Some experts recommend a cutoff of 130 mg/dL.

value of greater than or equal to 130 mg/dL. This cutoff will increase the sensitivity for GDM to greater than 90%, but will include ≈25% of all pregnant women. Women who exceed the chosen threshold on 50 g screening should have a diagnostic 100 g OGTT performed on a different day.

The criteria for diagnosis are different from those for nonpregnant patients (see Table 46-2).[181] The WHO recommends a one-step 75 g OGTT in the developing world.[3] In the 75 g test, diagnostic criteria for plasma glucose values are the same as for the 100 g test, except that there is no 3 hour measurement (see Table 46-2). Although the 75 g OGTT appears practical and acceptable, more data are obtained with the 100 g OGTT.

Screening and diagnostic criteria for GDM will almost certainly be modified extensively in the near future. Changes will be motivated by results of the HAPO (Hyperglycemia and Adverse Pregnancy Outcome) study, which was a prospective, randomized, multinational study of ≈25,000 women. Initial published results[159] show that risk of adverse maternal, fetal, and neonatal outcomes increased continuously as a function of maternal glycemia at 24 to 28 weeks, even within ranges previously considered normal for pregnancy. Based on outcomes in the HAPO study, an international group of experts representing both obstetric and diabetic organizations developed new diagnostic criteria that were published in 2010.[114A] The panel recommended that all pregnant women not previously known to have diabetes should be evaluated for GDM at 24-28 weeks of gestation by a 75 g OGTT. Diagnostic cut points were established for FPG (92 mg/dL), 1-hour (180 mg/dL) and 2-hour (153 mg/dL) plasma glucose concentrations. If one or more of these values is equaled or exceeded, a diagnosis of GDM is made. Using these criteria will result in a considerable increase in the prevalence of GDM because only one increased glucose value (as opposed to two increased glucose concentrations with prior recommendations) is required to diagnose GDM.

Although GDM is usually asymptomatic and not life-threatening to the mother, it is associated with an increased incidence of neonatal mortality and morbidity, including hypocalcemia, hypoglycemia, and macrosomia.[135,158] Maternal hyperglycemia causes the fetus to secrete more insulin, resulting in stimulation of fetal growth and macrosomia. Recognition is important because therapy can reduce perinatal morbidity and mortality.[172] Maternal complications include a high rate of cesarean delivery and hypertension. In addition, mothers with GDM are at significantly increased risk of subsequent diabetes, predominantly type 2. A 2009 meta-analysis and systematic review indicated that women with GDM have a sevenfold increased risk of developing type 2 diabetes compared with those who had a normoglycemic pregnancy.[30] The largest single study observed a 12.6-fold increased risk. The cumulative incidence of type 2 diabetes varies among populations, ranging from about 40 to 70%.[130] It rises markedly in the first 5 years and reaches a plateau after 10 years.

Distinct from GDM is pregnancy in a patient with preexisting diabetes (≈19,000 per annum in the United States). This is associated with an increased incidence of congenital malformation, but meticulous glycemic control during the first 8 weeks of pregnancy can significantly decrease the risk of congenital malformation.[133] Tight control results in an increased incidence of maternal hypoglycemia, which is teratogenic in animals but does not cause malformation in humans.[161]

Women with GDM should be screened for diabetes 6 to 12 weeks postpartum using nonpregnant OGTT criteria (see Box 46-3). If glucose values are normal, glycemia should be reassessed at least every 3 years.

CHRONIC COMPLICATIONS OF DIABETES MELLITUS

Pathogenesis

Patients with both type 1 and type 2 diabetes are at high risk for the development of chronic complications.[44,169] Diabetes-specific microvascular pathology in the retina, renal glomerulus, and peripheral nerve produces retinopathy, nephropathy, and neuropathy. As a result of these microvascular complications, diabetes is the most frequent cause of new cases of blindness in the industrialized world in persons between 25 and 74 years and the leading cause of end-stage renal disease. Diabetes is also associated with a marked increase in atherosclerotic macrovascular disease involving cardiac, cerebral, and peripheral large vessels. The consequence is that patients with diabetes have a high rate of myocardial infarction (the major cause of mortality in diabetes), stroke, and limb amputation. Prospective clinical studies document a strong relationship between hyperglycemia and the development of microvascular complications.[62,242] Both hyperglycemia and insulin resistance appear to be important in the pathogenesis of macrovascular complications.[44,88,242]

Progress has been made in our understanding of the molecular mechanisms underlying derangements produced by hyperglycemia.[44,218] Four main hypotheses have been proposed to explain how hyperglycemia causes the neural and vascular pathology. These include increased aldose reductase (or polyol pathway) flux; enhanced formation of advanced glycation end products (AGE); activation of protein kinase C; and increased hexosamine pathway flux. Inhibitors of each of these have been shown to ameliorate diabetes-induced abnormalities in cell culture and animal models.[44] Overproduction of superoxide by the mitochondrial electron transport chain integrates these four apparently disparate mechanisms. Clinical trials are under way using novel therapies specifically directed at the signaling molecules (such as protein kinase C) or employing antioxidants to neutralize the effects of the oxidants.

Effects of Intensive Therapy

Type 1 Diabetes

Although it had been theorized for many years that better glycemic control would decrease rates of long-term complications of diabetes mellitus, it was not until the publication of the Diabetes Control and Complications Trial (DCCT) in 1993[62] that this hypothesis was verified. The DCCT was a multicenter, randomized trial that compared the effects of intensive and conventional insulin therapy on the development and progression of complications in 1441 patients with type 1 diabetes. During the study period, which averaged 6.5 years, intensively managed patients maintained significantly lower mean blood glucose concentrations. Compared with conventional therapy, intensive therapy reduced the risk of retinopathy, nephropathy, and neuropathy by 40 to 75%.[62] Intensive therapy delayed the onset and slowed the progression of these three complications, regardless of age, gender, or duration of diabetes. The absolute risks of retinopathy and nephropathy were proportional to the mean glycated hemoglobin (GHb) (discussed later in the chapter). Although intensive therapy also reduced the development of hypercholesterolemia, major cardiovascular and peripheral vascular diseases were not significantly decreased in the initial assessment. However, analysis after 17 years of follow-up showed that the incidence of cardiovascular disease was 42% lower in the intensively treated group.[170] This landmark study has had a considerable impact on therapeutic goals and comprehension of the pathogenesis of complications of diabetes.

At the conclusion of the DCCT, 95% of participants enrolled in the long-term follow-up study, termed the Epidemiology of Diabetes Interventions and Complications (EDIC). Five years after the end of the DCCT, no difference in metabolic control (assessed by HbA_{1c} measurements) was noted between the former conventional and intensively treated groups. Nevertheless, further progression of retinopathy and neuropathy was significantly lower in the former intensive group, demonstrating that the beneficial effects of intensive treatment persisted for at least several years beyond the period of strictest intervention.[64,154]

Type 2 Diabetes

The role of hyperglycemia in the development of complications in individuals with type 2 diabetes was established in the United Kingdom Prospective Diabetes Study (UKPDS).[242] The UKPDS was a major randomized, multicenter clinical study that included 5102 patients with newly diagnosed type 2 diabetes who were followed for an average of 10 years. Analogous to the findings of the DCCT, the UKPDS demonstrated in patients with type 2 diabetes that intensive treatment diminishes by approximately 10 to 40% the development of microvascular complications.[242] Intensive treatment decreased the rate of occurrence of macrovascular complications. Although the reduction was not statistically significant initially, follow-up 10 years after the study ended showed a significant reduction in myocardial infarction among patients who had received intensive therapy.[107] Analogous to the EDIC findings, long-term benefits for microvascular complications were observed with follow-up of patients in the UKPDS despite loss of glycemic separation between intensive and standard cohorts after the study ended.[107] An important caveat of both the DCCT and the UKPDS was that intensive therapy produced a threefold increase in the incidence of severe hypoglycemia.[62,242]

ROLE OF THE CLINICAL LABORATORY IN DIABETES MELLITUS

The clinical laboratory has a vital role in both the diagnosis and management of diabetes mellitus.[203A] Some of the important variables assayed are outlined in Table 46-3. In 2002 the National Academy of Clinical Biochemistry (referred to as the NACB) published evidence-based guidelines for laboratory analysis in diabetes mellitus.[204] These guidelines were reviewed by the Professional Practice Committee of the ADA and were consistent in those areas where the ADA also published recommendations. Specific recommendations for laboratory testing based on published data or derived from expert consensus are presented.[204] An updated version of these guidelines was published in 2011.[203A] The revised guidelines were also published as a Position Statement by the ADA.[203B,203C] A brief overview is presented here.

Diagnosis

Preclinical (Screening)

Type 1 Diabetes

Evidence from animal studies suggests that immune intervention therapy before the appearance of clinical symptoms can delay or prevent type 1 diabetes. Results from human studies have been disappointing. Nevertheless, several large clinical trials are under way to assess a variety of therapeutic strategies designed to delay or prevent the onset of type 1 diabetes.[39,219] The Diabetes Prevention Trial-Type 1 (DPT-1) screened 84,228 relatives of patients with diabetes for islet cell antibodies.[68] Half of the 339 individuals deemed to be at high (greater than 50%) risk for disease were randomly assigned to low-dose insulin therapy. Unfortunately, neither insulin injections nor oral insulin delayed the development of type 1 diabetes.[68,221] Despite the negative results, the ADA encourages screening of first-degree relatives of patients with type 1 diabetes by measuring immune-related markers (autoantibodies), provided that individuals who have positive screening results are referred to defined research studies.[15] Until effective intervention therapy becomes available and cost-effective screening strategies are developed for young children, screening for antibodies is not recommended outside of clinical studies.[204]

Some experts have proposed that testing for islet cell autoantibodies may be useful in the following situations: (1) to identify a subset of adults initially thought to have type 2 diabetes but who have islet cell autoantibody markers of type 1 diabetes and progress to insulin dependency; (2) to screen nondiabetic family members who wish to donate a kidney or part of their pancreas for transplantation; (3) to screen women with GDM to identify those at high risk of progression to type 1 diabetes; and (4) to distinguish type 1 from type 2 diabetes in children to institute insulin therapy at the time of diagnosis.[204] Wide variability in clinical practice has been noted regarding the use of islet cell autoantibodies. Proponents argue that the results of autoantibody assays are clinically useful, whereas others point to lack of evidence. Although some clinicians, particularly those who treat

TABLE 46-3 Role of the Laboratory in Diabetes Mellitus

Diagnosis		
Preclinical (Screening)	Immunologic markers	
		ICA
		IAA
		GAD antibodies
		Protein tyrosine phosphatase antibodies (IA-2)
		Zinc transporter ZnT8 antibodies
	Genetic markers [e.g., human leukocyte antigen (HLA)]	
	Insulin secretion	
		Fasting
		Pulses
		In response to a glucose challenge
	Blood glucose	
	Hemoglobin A1c (HbA_{1c})	
Clinical	Blood glucose	
	Oral glucose tolerance test (OGTT)	
	HbA_{1c}	
	Ketones (urine and blood)	
	Other (e.g., insulin, C-peptide, stimulation tests)	
Management		
Acute	Glucose	
		Blood
		Urine
	Ketones	
		Blood
		Urine
	Acid-base status (pH, bicarbonate)	
	Lactate	
	Other abnormalities related to cellular dehydration or therapy (e.g., potassium, sodium, phosphate, osmolality)	
Chronic	Glucose	
		Blood (fasting-random)
		Urine
	Glycated proteins	
		Glycated hemoglobin (GHb) (HbA_{1c})
		Fructosamine
		Glycated serum albumin
	Urinary protein	
		Urinary albumin excretion (UAE) ("microalbuminuria")
		Proteinuria
	Evaluation of complications (e.g., creatinine, cholesterol, triglycerides)	
	Evaluation of pancreas transplant (C-peptide, insulin)	
	Eligibility for insulin pump (C-peptide)	

pediatric patients, use autoantibody assays, clinical studies are necessary to provide outcome data to validate the clinical use of autoantibody assays.

Screening by determining HLA type is not currently warranted, except in research studies.[204] A decrease in glucose-stimulated insulin secretion is the first functional abnormality in both type 1 and type 2 diabetes. Nevertheless, tests of insulin secretion are not currently recommended for routine clinical use.

Type 2 Diabetes

Screening of asymptomatic individuals for type 2 diabetes has been the subject of much controversy.[95] The ADA, which previously did not support screening, now advocates screening in all asymptomatic individuals over the age of 45 years.[13,75] Prior screening recommendations were that FPG or the 2 hour OGTT could be used.[19] The new guidelines include the use of HbA_{1c} for screening.[235] If the HbA_{1c} is less than 5.7% or the FPG is less than 100 mg/dL, testing should be repeated at 3 year intervals. Testing may be considered at a younger age or may be carried out more frequently in individuals at increased risk of diabetes (e.g., family history, members of certain ethnic groups).[13] The rising incidence of type 2 diabetes in adolescents has led to the recommendation for screening overweight youths with any two of the following risk factors: (1) they have a family history of type 2 diabetes in first- and second-degree relatives; (2) they belong to a certain race and/or ethnic group; (3) they have signs of insulin resistance or conditions associated with insulin resistance; or (4) there is a maternal history of diabetes or GDM during the child's gestation.[13,19,204] Testing should be done every 3 years starting at 10 years of age. Rationales for screening are that at least 33% of individuals with type 2 diabetes are undiagnosed, complications are often present by the time of diagnosis, and treatment delays the onset of complications.[95] Notwithstanding these recommendations, no published evidence indicates that treatment based on screening has value.

Clinical

The laboratory diagnosis of diabetes is made exclusively by the demonstration of hyperglycemia, by measuring venous plasma glucose or HbA_{1c}. Although other tests (e.g., C-peptide, insulin analysis) have been proposed to assist in the diagnosis and classification of the disease, these do not at present have a role outside of research studies.[204]

Management

Acute

In diabetic ketoacidosis, hyperosmolar nonketotic coma, and hypoglycemia, the clinical laboratory has an essential role in both diagnosis and monitoring of therapy. Several analytes are frequently measured to guide clinicians in treatment regimens to restore euglycemia and correct other metabolic disturbances. The metabolic abnormalities of these conditions are beyond the scope of this book, and interested readers are referred to a standard textbook of medicine. The NACB guidelines also provide information on the tests that are used.

Chronic

The DCCT[62] and UKPDS[242] studies documented a correlation between blood glucose concentrations and the development of long-term complications of diabetes. Measurement of glucose and glycated proteins provides an index of short- and long-term glycemic control, respectively (see section on glycated proteins later in the chapter). Detection and monitoring of complications are achieved by assaying creatinine, urinary albumin excretion, and serum lipids. The success of newer therapies, such as islet cell or pancreas transplantation, can be monitored by measuring serum C-peptide or insulin concentrations.

SELF-MONITORING OF BLOOD GLUCOSE

Diabetic patients, especially those who need insulin therapy, require careful monitoring to maintain control of blood glucose. This has become particularly important with the results of the DCCT[62] and the recommendation that patients use intensive insulin therapy to achieve nearly normal glycemia. These regimens include multiple daily insulin injections, insulin pumps, and continuous subcutaneous insulin injections. Estimating blood glucose concentrations by monitoring urine glucose concentrations—a simple and convenient method—is undesirable for the following reasons:

1. The renal threshold (the blood glucose concentration above which glucose appears in the urine) averages 160 to 180 mg/dL but varies widely among individuals. It may increase in long-standing diabetes or with age and may be lower in pregnancy or childhood. A decreased threshold (±100 mg/dL) is known as *renal glycosuria.*
2. Monitoring of urine glucose concentrations lacks sensitivity and specificity. For example, one study demonstrated that patients with plasma glucose concentrations between 150 and 199 mg/dL exhibited normal urine test results 75% of the time. Furthermore, 9% of patients with plasma glucose concentrations below 149 mg/dL had glycosuria.[165]
3. A negative test result does not distinguish between hypoglycemia, euglycemia, and mild or moderate hyperglycemia.
4. Urine testing, which uses a color chart, is not accurate.
5. Other factors (e.g., fluid intake, urine concentration, ingestion of salicylates or ascorbic acid, urinary tract infections) may influence testing.

Testing urine for glucose is therefore not adequate for monitoring patients on insulin therapy.[8] Although some evidence suggests that it may be effective for monitoring type 2 diabetes,[4] the ADA states that limitations of urine testing make blood glucose measurements the preferred method of assessing glycemic control.[91]

Glucose Meters

Portable meters for measurement of blood glucose concentrations are used in three major settings: (1) in acute and chronic care facilities (at the patient's bedside and in clinics or hospitals); (2) in physicians' offices; and (3) by patients at home, work, and school. The last, self-monitoring of blood glucose (SMBG), used by approximately 1 million diabetic patients, is performed in the United States at least once a day by 40% and 26% of individuals with type 1 and 2 diabetes, respectively.[204] The worldwide market for SMBG is $2.7 billion per year, with annual growth estimated at 10 to 12%.[204]

Patients measure their own blood glucose concentration and modify their insulin dose based on this glucose value. It is impractical for patients themselves to perform glucose determinations by the methods described earlier, but a large number of simple test strips that are available permit rapid measurements on a drop of whole blood.[8] These use the same methodology as described earlier for glucose analysis—predominantly glucose oxidase or glucose dehydrogenase. In many strips, a dye is colored by the glucose oxidase-peroxidase chromogenic reaction. The reagents are combined in dry form on a small surface area of a test strip, and the colors that develop may be evaluated visually by comparison with a color chart (rarely used any more) or quantified in a specially designed meter. *Visual reading with a color chart is not accurate enough* for most clinical circumstances. More than 30 different blood glucose meters are commercially available; these vary in size, weight, calibration method, and other features. They are reviewed annually in the ADA's *Resource Guide.*[16]

To perform the measurement, a sample of blood [usually from a fingerstick, but anticoagulated whole blood collected in ethylenediaminetetraacetic acid (EDTA) or heparin may be used] is placed on the test pad, which is attached to a plastic support. The test strip is then inserted into the meter. (In some devices, the strip is inserted into the meter before the sample is applied.) After a fixed period of time, the result appears on a digital display screen. These meters use reflectance photometry or electrochemistry to measure the rate of the reaction or the final concentration of the products. Reflectance photometry measures the amount of light reflected from a test pad containing reagent. In electrochemical systems, the enzymatic reaction in an electrode incorporated on the test strip produces a flow of electrons. The current, which is directly proportional to the amount of glucose in the sample, is converted to a digital readout. Large variability has been noted among meters as to the test time (5 to 45 seconds) and the claimed reading range (30 to 500 mg/dL to 0 to 600 mg/dL). Calibration is automatic on some devices, whereas others use lot-specific code chips or strips. All manufacturers supply control solutions. Strict adherence to the instructions is necessary to obtain accurate results. Some meters have a porous membrane that separates erythrocytes, and analysis is performed on the resultant plasma. *Whole blood glucose concentrations are approximately 10 to 15% lower than plasma or serum concentrations, but meters can be calibrated to report plasma glucose values, even when the sample is whole blood.* An International Federation of Clinical Chemistry (IFCC) working group recommended that glucose meters be harmonized using a factor of 1.11× to report the concentration of glucose in plasma, irrespective of the sample type or technology.[70]

Analytical Goals

Multiple analytical goals have been proposed for the performance of glucose meters. The rationale for these is not always clear. In 1987 the ADA recommended a goal of total error (in the hands of users) of less than 10% at glucose concentrations of 30 to 400 mg/dL 100% of the time.[7] This recommendation was modified in response to the significant reduction in complications by tight glucose control in the DCCT. The revised performance goal, published in 1996,[8] is for analytical error to be less than 5%. No published studies of glucose meters have achieved this goal. The recommendations promulgated by the Clinical and Laboratory Standards Institute (CLSI) [previously called the National Committee for Clinical Laboratory Standards (NCCLS)] and the International Organization for Standardization (ISO)[173] are that 95% of results should fall within 20% of laboratory-measured glucose concentrations when greater than 75 mg/dL, and within 15 mg/dL of laboratory glucose if the glucose concentration is less than or equal to 75 mg/dL. Several experts believe these acceptance criteria to be too wide. The CLSI and ISO documents are undergoing revision at the time of this writing, with publication anticipated in 2012.

A different method was proposed by Clarke,[53] who developed an error grid that attempts to define clinically important errors by identifying fairly broad target ranges. In addition, a novel approach using simulation modeling reached the conclusion that meters that achieve both a CV and a bias less than 5% rarely lead to major errors in insulin dose.[43] Lack of consensus on quality goals for glucose meters reflects the absence of agreed-upon objective criteria. When biological variation criteria are used, a goal for total error (including both bias and imprecision) of less than or equal to 6.9% has been proposed.[203A]

Glucose meters are also used to calculate insulin dose in patients without diabetes on tight glucose control protocols in intensive care units (ICUs). Evidence in 2001[245] showed that intensive insulin therapy significantly reduced mortality and morbidity of critically ill patients in the surgical ICU. Although some subsequent studies were unable to replicate these findings,[77,257] tight glucose is used extensively in hospital ICUs. Many factors, such as hypoxia, shock, and low hematocrit, are common in these patients and can compromise glucose analysis in capillary blood samples.[72] The use of glucose meters in these settings has been questioned by some experts.[216]

Performance of Glucose Meters

The most common errors in SMBG, such as proper application, timing, and removal of excess blood, have been reduced by advances in technology but can still occur. Additional innovations that reduce operator error include (1) systems that abort testing if the sample volume is inadequate, (2) built-in programs that simplify quality control, and (3) increased memory that allows the instrument to store up to several hundred glucose readings that can be downloaded into a computer.

Several factors affect the accuracy and reproducibility of SMBG. These include (1) user variability—up to 50% of values may vary by more than 20% from reference values[8]; (2) hematocrit—the presence of anemia (false increase) or polycythemia (false depression) may result in up to 30% variability; and (3) defective reagent strips or instrument malfunction (rare). Other variables include changes in altitude, environmental temperature, or humidity; hypotension; hypoxia; and high triglyceride concentrations. In addition, *these assays are unreliable at very high and very low glucose concentrations* (<60 and >500 mg/dL). Because dehydration, a common feature of diabetic ketoacidosis, greatly increases blood viscosity, inaccurately low blood glucose results may be obtained. Several drugs interfere, but not with all meters.[230] Another important factor is the lack of correlation among meters, even from a single manufacturer, caused by different assay methods and architecture. Moreover, results from two meters of the same brand have been observed to differ substantially.[232] The analytical performance characteristics of several meters have been published.[118,244] Patient factors are also important, particularly adequacy of training. Recurrent education at clinic visits and comparison of SMBG with concurrent laboratory glucose analysis improved the accuracy of patients' blood glucose readings.[120] In addition, it is important to evaluate the patient's technique at regular intervals.

The performance of different meters varies widely. Although current meters, as predicted, exhibit performance superior to prior generations of meters,[249] imprecision remains high. Under carefully controlled conditions in which all assays were performed by a single medical technologist, ≈50% of analyses met the ADA criterion of less than 5% deviation from reference values.[249] Performance of older meters was substantially worse. Note that the performance of glucose meters achieved by medical technologists is better than that achieved by patients. Another study that evaluated meter performance in 226 hospitals by split samples analyzed simultaneously on meters and laboratory glucose analyzers revealed that 45.6%, 25%, and 14% differed from each other by greater than 10%, greater than 15%, and greater than 20%, respectively.[177] Comparison with laboratory values of almost 22,000 measurements of capillary glucose by patients using meters revealed no significant improvement in meter performance between 1989 and 1999.[38] The imprecision of meters precludes their use in the diagnosis of diabetes.[204]

Indications and Frequency of SMBG

The indications and frequency of self-monitoring vary among patients. *SMBG should be performed by all patients treated with insulin.* The role of SMBG in patients with type 2 diabetes not treated with insulin has not been defined.[204] A consensus statement by the ADA[8] recommended the following specific indications for SMBG: (1) patients undergoing intensive insulin treatment programs (in this group, glucose should be measured at least four times a day to achieve glycemic control); (2) prevention and detection of hypoglycemia, especially in people who are asymptomatic or unable to recognize the early warning signs; (3) avoidance of severe hyperglycemia, particularly in situations of increased risk (e.g., medications that alter insulin secretion or action, intercurrent illness, elderly people); (4) adjusted pharmacologic therapy in response to changes in life-style, such as exercise or altering food intake; and (5) determination of the necessity for initiating insulin therapy in GDM. *Glucose meters should not be used to diagnose diabetes mellitus,* and their role in screening remains uncertain.[204]

Current ADA recommendations[19] are that SMBG should be performed three or more times per day in patients using multiple insulin injections or insulin pump therapy. Monitoring less frequently results in deterioration of glycemic control.[8,168,210] Published studies reveal that self-monitoring is performed by patients much less frequently than recommended: at least once a day by 39% of patients using insulin and by 5 to 6% of those treated with oral agents or diet alone.[98] Moreover, 29% and 65% of patients treated with insulin and oral agents, respectively, monitored their blood glucose less than once per month. More recent evidence shows a gradual increase, with 63.4% of patients with diabetes now reported to monitor blood glucose at least once daily.[103] Guidelines on the recommended frequency and timing of SMBG vary among international diabetes associations.[34] Recent recommendations suggest that the frequency and timing of SMBG should be dictated by the particular needs and goals of the individual patient.[19,34]

The value of SMBG for patients with type 2 diabetes not on insulin therapy is controversial owing, in part, to the lack of well-designed studies. A meta-analysis of SMBG in non–insulin-treated patients with type 2 diabetes showed that SMBG improved glycemic control.[250] However, many studies in this analysis included patient education, and the contribution of SMBG to glucose control in non–insulin-treated patients remains contentious.[103] Despite controversy in the literature, a survey conducted in 14 countries in 2007 revealed unexpectedly high SMBG use in non–insulin-treated patients, with up to 75% of patients performing SMBG.[222]

MINIMALLY INVASIVE MONITORING OF BLOOD GLUCOSE

A major limitation to performing SMBG is that it is painful and inconvenient. Since the 1960s, attempts have been made to develop a painless method for monitoring blood glucose concentrations. Three general approaches have been used, namely, implanted sensors, minimally invasive monitoring, and noninvasive monitoring.

Implanted Sensors

Several implanted biosensors have been developed and evaluated in both animals and humans. Detection systems are based on enzymes, electrodes, or fluorescence.[89,126] The most widely studied method is an electrochemical sensor that is usually implanted subcutaneously. The first device approved for patient use was the CGMS (Medtronic, Minneapolis, Minn); several others are now available.[89] All monitoring devices use glucose oxidase to measure glucose every 1 to 5 minutes. The values are sent to a monitor. Results are recorded and, depending on the system, may be downloaded later in the physician's office or are available to the patient in real-time. These devices are subject to some limitations. Implantation of a needle type of sensor into the subcutaneous tissue induces inflammatory responses in the host that alter the sensitivity of the device. Therefore, the devices can be worn for only 3 to 7 days. These sensors require calibration by the user several times per day with a glucose meter and are subject to the imprecision of the meter. In addition, changes in glucose concentration in the interstitial fluid occur 4 to 20 minutes later than in the blood. A 2008 randomized study of 322 patients with type 1 diabetes showed that adults age 25 and older using intensive insulin treatment and real-time continuous glucose monitoring had better long-term glycemic control than patients using intensive insulin therapy and SMBG.[229]

Another available strategy is the Glucoday (A. Menarini Diagnostics, Florence, Italy), which uses microdialysis and measures glucose outside the body. Fluid is pumped from a storage bag through a microfiber under the skin. The solution carries the glucose sample back to a biosensor, which displays the glucose result every second. This device, which is available in parts of Europe but not in the United States, can be worn for 48 hours.

Minimally Invasive Glucose Monitoring

The concept underlying these methods is that the concentration of glucose in the interstitial fluid correlates with the blood glucose concentration. The principle of the FDA-approved Gluco Watch Biographer (Animas Corporation, West Chester, Pa) involves the application of a low-level electric current to the skin. This induces movement by electro-osmosis of glucose across the skin, where it is measured by a glucose oxidase detector.[228] Glucose concentrations in transdermal fluid and plasma are highly correlated. The clearest application of the Gluco Watch, which is designed to measure glucose three times per hour for up to 12 hours, appears to be in the detection of unsuspected hypoglycemia. Calibration with reference plasma glucose is required. Initial clinical studies reveal reasonable correlation of the Gluco Watch with SMBG.[228] This device has been withdrawn from the market, but it is likely to stimulate enhanced efforts to bring other technologies into clinical use.

Noninvasive Glucose Monitoring

Noninvasive in vivo monitoring of glucose has been an area of active investigation for many years. Near-infrared spectroscopic devices measure the absorption or the reflection of light from subcutaneous tissue. Although glucose has a specific absorption at 1035 nm, many substances interfere. A computer, individually calibrated, screens out interfering information to obtain the glucose result. Alternative approaches include Raman scattering spectroscopy and photoacoustic spectroscopy. Notwithstanding the investment of considerable resources, no noninvasive sensing technology is approved for glucose measurement in patients.

KETONE BODIES

The development of ketosis requires changes in both adipose tissue and the liver. *The primary substrates for ketone body formation are free fatty acids* from adipose stores. Normally, long-chain fatty acids are taken up by the liver, re-esterified to triglycerides, and stored in the liver or incorporated in very low-density lipoproteins and returned to the plasma. In contrast to other tissue, the brain cannot use free fatty acids for energy. When glucose is unavailable, ketone bodies supply the vast majority of the brain's energy. After a 3 day fast, ketone bodies provide 30 to 40% of the body's energy requirements.[142] In uncontrolled diabetes, the low insulin concentrations result in increased lipolysis and decreased re-esterification, thereby increasing plasma free fatty acids. In addition, the increased glucagon/insulin ratio enhances fatty acid oxidation in the liver. Increased counter-regulatory hormones also augment lipolysis and ketogenesis in fat and liver, respectively. Thus increased hepatic ketone production and decreased peripheral tissue metabolism lead to acetoacetate accumulation in the blood. A small fraction undergoes spontaneous decarboxylation to form acetone, but most of it is converted to β-hydroxybutyrate.

Acetoacetate
β-Hydroxybutyrate dehydrogenase (in liver)
NADH + $H^{\oplus}$ $NAD^{\oplus}$
β-Hydroxybutyrate
$H^{\oplus}$
Spontaneous
CO_2
Acetone

The relative proportions in which the three ketone bodies are present in blood vary, depending on the redox state of the cell. In healthy people, β-hydroxybutyrate and acetoacetate—which are present at approximately equimolar concentrations[142,187,258]—constitute virtually all the serum ketones. Acetone is a minor component. In severe diabetes, the ratio of β-hydroxybutyrate to acetoacetate may increase to 6 : 1 owing to the presence of a large concentration of nicotinamide adenine dinucleotide (NADH), which favors β-hydroxybutyrate production.

None of the commonly used methods for the detection and determination of ketone bodies in serum or urine reacts with all three ketone bodies. Gerhardt's ferric chloride test reacts with acetoacetate only. Tests using nitroprusside are at least 10 times more sensitive to acetoacetate than to acetone, and give no reaction at all with β-hydroxybutyrate.

Most of the tests for ketosis essentially detect or measure acetoacetate only. This may produce a paradoxical situation. When a patient initially presents in ketoacidosis, the test results for ketones may be only weakly positive. With therapy, *β-hydroxybutyrate is converted to acetoacetate, and the ketosis appears to worsen.*

Traditional tests for β-hydroxybutyrate are indirect; they require brief boiling of the urine to remove acetone and acetoacetate by evaporation (acetoacetate first breaks down spontaneously to acetone), followed by gentle oxidation of β-hydroxybutyrate to acetoacetate and acetone with peroxide, ferric ions, or dichromate. The acetoacetate thus formed may be detected with Gerhardt's test or by one of the procedures in which nitroprusside is used.

Specific determination of β-hydroxybutyrate in urine is not considered to be a routine procedure. A paper strip for semiquantitative measurement of β-hydroxybutyrate in serum and urine has been described[97] but has not gained general acceptance. Quantitative enzymatic assays for β-hydroxybutyrate that can be performed directly on blood or serum have become commercially available. Originally available commercially as a bench-top analyzer (KetoSite, GDS Diagnostics, Elkhart, Ind), hand-held devices are also available now (Precision Xtra, Abbot and KetoSite, Stanbio Laboratory, Boeme, Tex).[47]

Clinical Significance

Excessive formation of ketone bodies results in increased blood concentrations *(ketonemia)* and increased excretion in the urine *(ketonuria)*. This process is observed in conditions associated with decreased availability of carbohydrates (such as starvation or frequent vomiting) or decreased use of carbohydrates [such as diabetes mellitus, glycogen storage disease (von Gierke's disease), and alkalosis]. The popular high-fat, low-carbohydrate diets are ketogenic and increase ketone bodies in the circulation. Diabetes mellitus and alcohol consumption are the most common causes of ketoacidosis in adults. (Hyperglycemia is not usually present in the latter condition.) Ingestion of isopropyl alcohol and salicylate poisoning can also produce ketoacidosis. Urine ketone test results are positive in ≈30% of first morning void specimens from pregnant women. Semiquantitative determination of ketone bodies in blood is more accurate than determination of these compounds in urine in the treatment of diabetic ketoacidosis. Although not always excreted in proportion to blood ketone concentrations, because of convenience, urine ketones are widely used for monitoring control in patients with type 1 diabetes. The ADA states that *urine ketone testing is an important part of monitoring by patients with diabetes,* particularly those with type 1 diabetes, pregnancy with preexisting diabetes, and GDM.[91] Patients with type 1 diabetes should test for ketones during acute illness or stress, with consistent increases in blood glucose (greater than 300 mg/dL), during pregnancy, or when symptoms of ketoacidosis are present.[91] Measurement of ketones in urine and blood is widely performed in patients with diabetes for both diagnosis and monitoring of diabetic ketoacidosis.[204]

Determination of Ketone Bodies in Body Fluids

Although quantitative determination of individual ketone bodies is possible, these methods are not used as routine tests. The semiquantitative Acetest, Ketostix (Bayer Health Care, Pine Brook, NJ), and DiaScreen 1K (Arkray, Edina, MN) are frequently used but are insensitive to β-hydroxybutyrate.[236] It is important to bear in mind, therefore, that a *negative nitroprusside test result does not rule out ketoacidosis.*

Detection of Ketone Bodies by Acetest

The Acetest tablets contain a mixture of glycine, sodium nitroprusside, disodium phosphate, and lactose. Acetoacetate or acetone (to a lesser extent) in the presence of glycine forms a lavender-purple complex with nitroprusside. β-Hydroxybutyrate does not react with nitroprusside. The disodium phosphate provides an optimum pH for the reaction, and lactose enhances the color.[116]

Detection of Ketone Bodies by Ketostix

Ketostix is a modification of the nitroprusside test in which a reagent strip is used instead of a tablet. The Ketostix test gives a positive reaction within 15 seconds with a specimen containing at least 50 mg of acetoacetate per liter. The accompanying color chart gives readings for ketone concentrations of 50, 150, 400, 800, and 1600 mg/L. Acetone also reacts, but the test is less sensitive to it.

Determination of β-Hydroxybutyrate

A 1995 short report on patients with diabetic ketoacidosis indicated that β-hydroxybutyrate correlated better than acetoacetate with changes in acid-base status.[243]

In this test, β-hydroxybutyrate in the presence of nicotinamide adenine dinucleotide (NAD^+) is converted by β-hydroxybutyrate dehydrogenase to acetoacetate, producing nicotinamide adenine dinucleotide phosphate (NADH). Diaphorase catalyzes the reduction of nitroblue tetrazolium (NBT) by NADH to produce a purple compound, and its absorbance is read in a special meter that provides a digital readout.

$$\beta\text{-Hydroxybutyrate} \xrightleftharpoons[\text{NAD}^{\oplus} \;\to\; \text{NADH} + \text{H}^{\oplus}]{\beta\text{-Hydroxybutyrate dehydrogenase}} \text{Acetoacetate}$$

$$\text{NADH} + \text{NBT} \xrightleftharpoons{\text{Diaphorase}} \text{NAD}^{\oplus} + \text{Reduced NBT}$$

Determination of Ketone Bodies in Urine

Acetest and Ketostix are also suitable for detecting ketone bodies in urine. The sensitivity and specificity of these tests are the same as outlined for serum.

Reference Interval

Serum β-hydroxybutyrate values vary from 0.02 to 0.27 mmol/L (0.21 to 2.81 mg/dL) in healthy people after an overnight fast. Ketone bodies in the blood can reach 2 mmol/L (20 mg/dL) with prolonged exercise.[142] Patients with diabetic ketoacidosis usually have β-hydroxybutyrate concentrations greater than 2 mmol/L (20 mg/dL).

GLYCATED PROTEINS

Measurement of glycated proteins, primarily GHb, is effective in monitoring long-term glucose control in people with diabetes mellitus. It provides a retrospective index of integrated plasma glucose values over an extended period of time and is not subject to the wide fluctuations observed when blood glucose concentrations are assayed. GHb concentrations therefore are a valuable and widely used adjunct to blood glucose determinations for monitoring long-term glycemic control. In addition, GHb has recently been recommended for the diagnosis of diabetes and is a measure of risk for the development of microvascular complications of diabetes.

Glycated Hemoglobin*

Glycation is the nonenzymatic addition of a sugar residue to amino groups of proteins. Human adult hemoglobin (Hb) usually consists of HbA (97% of the total), HbA_2 (2.5%), and HbF (0.5%). HbA is made up of four polypeptide chains, two α- and two β-chains. Chromatographic analysis of HbA identifies several minor hemoglobins, namely, HbA_{1a}, HbA_{1b}, and HbA_{1c},which are collectively referred to as HbA_1, *fast hemoglobins* (because they migrate more rapidly than HbA in an electrical field), *glycohemoglobins,* or *glycated hemoglobins* (Table 46-4). The Joint Commission on Biochemical Nomenclature of the International Union of Pure and Applied Chemistry recommends the term *neoglycoprotein* for such derivatives and the term *glycation* to describe this process. Therefore although *glycosylated* and *glucosylated* have been widely used in the literature, the term *glycated* is preferred. HbA_{1c} is formed by the condensation of glucose with the *N*-terminal valine residue of each β-chain of HbA to form an unstable Schiff base (aldimine, pre-HbA_{1c}; see Figure 46-6). The Schiff base may dissociate or may undergo an Amadori rearrangement to form a stable ketoamine, HbA_{1c}. HbA_{1a1} and HbA_{1a2}, which make up HbA_{1a}, have fructose-1,6-diphosphate and glucose-6-phosphate, respectively, attached to the amino terminal of the β-chain (see Table 46-4). The structure of HbA_{1b}, identified by mass spectrometry, contains pyruvic acid linked to the amino terminal valine of the β-chain, probably by a ketamine or enamine bond. *HbA_{1c} is the major fraction,* constituting approximately 80% of HbA_1.

Glycation may also occur at sites other than the end of the β-chain, such as lysine residues, or the α-chain. These GHbs,

*A note on terminology: In this chapter, the term glycated hemoglobin is used to refer to the set of all glycated hemoglobins, and hemoglobin A1c is used to refer to a specific molecular form as described in text.

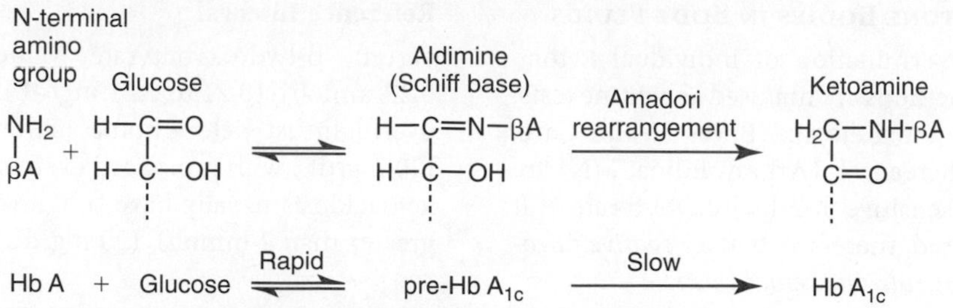

N-terminal amino group, Glucose, Aldimine (Schiff base), Amadori rearrangement, Ketoamine

NH_2–βA + H–C=O / H–C–OH ⇌ H–C=N–βA / H–C–OH → H_2C–NH-βA / C=O

Hb A + Glucose $\underset{\text{Rapid}}{\rightleftharpoons}$ pre-Hb A_{1c} $\xrightarrow{\text{Slow}}$ Hb A_{1c}

Figure 46-6 Formation of hemoglobin A_{1c}.

TABLE 46-4 Nomenclature of Selected Hemoglobins

Name	Component(s)
HbA	Constitutes ≈97% adult hemoglobin
HbA_0	Synonymous with HbA
HbA_{1a1}	HbA with fructose-1,6-diphosphate attached to the *N*-terminal of the β-chain
HbA_{1a2}	HbA with glucose-6-phosphate attached to the *N*-terminal of the β-chain
HbA_{1a}	Comprises HbA_{1a1} and HbA_{1a2}
HbA_{1b}	HbA with pyruvic acid attached to the *N*-terminal of the β-chain
HbA_{1c}	HbA with glucose attached to the *N*-terminal valine of the β-chain
Pre-HbA_{1c}	Unstable Schiff base (aldimine); a labile intermediary component in the formation of HbA_{1c}
HbA_1	Consists of HbA_{1a}, HbA_{1b}, and HbA_{1c}
Total glycated hemoglobin*	Consists of HbA_{1c} and other hemoglobin-carbohydrate adducts

*Also termed *glycated hemoglobin* or *glycohemoglobin.*
Hb, Hemoglobin.

referred to as glycated HbA_0 or total glycated hemoglobin (see Table 46-4), cannot be separated from nonglycated hemoglobin by methods based on charge, but are measured by boronate affinity chromatography.

Formation of GHb is essentially irreversible, and the concentration in the blood depends on both the lifespan of the red blood cell (RBC; average lifespan is 120 days) and the blood glucose concentration. Because the rate of formation of GHb is directly proportional to the concentration of glucose in the blood, *the GHb concentration represents integrated values for glucose over the preceding 8 to 12 weeks.* This provides an additional criterion for assessing glucose control because GHb values are free of day-to-day glucose fluctuations and are unaffected by recent exercise or food ingestion. It is important to realize that the contribution of the plasma glucose concentration to GHb depends on the time interval, with more recent values providing a larger contribution than earlier values. The plasma glucose in the preceding 1 month determines 50% of the HbA_{1c}, whereas days 60 to 120 determine only 25%.[227] After a sudden alteration in blood glucose concentrations, the rate of change of HbA_{1c} is rapid during the initial 2 months, followed by a more gradual change approaching steady state 3 months later.

Interpretation of GHb depends on red blood cells having a normal lifespan. Patients with hemolytic disease or other conditions with shortened red blood cell survival exhibit a substantial reduction in GHb.[46] Similarly, individuals with recent significant blood loss have falsely low values owing to a higher fraction of young erythrocytes. GHb concentrations can still be used to monitor these patients, but values must be compared with previous values from the same patient—not with published reference intervals. High GHb concentrations have been reported in iron deficiency anemia, probably because of the high proportion of old erythrocytes. The effects of hemoglobin variants (such as HbF, HbS, and HbC) depend on the specific method of analysis used (discussed later).[46] Depending on the particular hemoglobinopathy and assay, results may be spuriously increased or decreased. Most manufacturers of HbA_{1c} assays have modified their assays to eliminate interference from many of the common hemoglobin variants. Therefore, accurate measurement of HbA_{1c} is possible by selecting an appropriate instrument, provided the erythrocyte lifespan is not altered (see www.NGSP.org for additional information). Another source of error in selected methods is *carbamylated hemoglobin.* This is formed by attachment of urea and is present in large amounts in renal failure, which is common in diabetic patients. Most of the interferents produce relatively small effects, and for the vast majority of patients with diabetes, HbA_{1c} can be measured accurately.

Labile intermediates (pre-HbA_{1c}, Schiff base) may be included in measurements of HbA_{1c}, especially in the common ion-exchange methods,[166] and produce misleadingly high results. The *labile fraction changes rapidly with acute changes in blood glucose concentration and thus is not an indicator of long-term glycemic control.* Pre-HbA_{1c} amounts to 5 to 8% of total HbA_1 in healthy individuals and ranges from 8 to 30% in patients with diabetes, depending on the degree of control of blood glucose concentration at or near the time of blood sampling.[112] If the analytical method measures both fractions, the labile pre-HbA_{1c} should be removed first, to prevent falsely increased results. In the absence of glucose, pre-HbA_{1c} reverts to glucose and HbA (see Figure 46-6). This provides the basis for some procedures to eliminate the labile fraction by incubating washed red blood cells in saline. In some boronate affinity methods, the assay conditions favor rapid dissociation of the Schiff base.

Clinical Utility

Diagnosis of Diabetes

A major change in the diagnosis of diabetes was recommended in 2009.[203,235] An International Expert Committee advised that HbA_{1c} could be used for the diagnosis of diabetes (see Box 46-3). An HbA_{1c} value ≥6.5% was selected as the decision point, based on the prevalence of retinopathy.[235] This recommendation has been endorsed by both the ADA[19A] and the WHO. HbA_{1c} concentrations 5.7 to 6.4% indicate subjects at high risk of developing diabetes. HbA_{1c} was also recommended as an alternative to glucose for screening for diabetes. This last recommendation has also been accepted by the ADA.[19A]

Monitoring Diabetes

GHb has been firmly established as an index of long-term blood glucose concentrations and as a measure of the risk for development of microvascular complications in patients with diabetes mellitus.[91] GHb was a cornerstone of the DCCT.[62] [To prevent assay variability (see section on assay standardization later in this chapter), all GHb assays in the DCCT were done in a single laboratory that measured HbA_{1c} by HPLC.] The DCCT documented a direct relationship between blood glucose concentrations (assessed by HbA_{1c}) and the risk of microvascular complications.[62] The absolute risks of retinopathy and nephropathy were directly proportional to the mean HbA_{1c} concentration. The risk of retinopathy increased continuously with increasing HbA_{1c}, and a single measure of HbA_{1c} predicted the progression of retinopathy 4 years later. Subsequent analysis revealed that the mean HbA_{1c} was the dominant predictor of retinopathy progression, and a 10% lower HbA_{1c} concentration was associated with a 45% lower risk.[63] The risk of microvascular complications varies continuously with HbA_{1c}, and there is no HbA_{1c} concentration below which the risk is eliminated.

Analogous correlations between HbA_{1c} and complications were observed in patients with type 2 diabetes in the UKPDS trial.[242] To ensure that HbA_{1c} results in the UKPDS were comparable with DCCT findings, an ion-exchange HPLC method calibrated to the DCCT was used. Mean HbA_{1c} values for the intensively treated and conventionally treated groups were 7.0% and 7.9%, respectively.[242] Despite the small difference in HbA_{1c}, microvascular complications were reduced by ≈25%. Each 1% reduction in HbA_{1c} (e.g., from 8 to 7%) was associated with risk reductions of 37% for microvascular disease, 21% for death related to diabetes, and 14% for myocardial infarction.[242] In patients without diabetes, HbA_{1c} is directly related to cardiovascular disease. In the European Prospective Investigation into Cancer and Nutrition (EPIC-Norfolk), an increase of 1% in HbA_{1c} was associated with a 28% increase in the risk of death.[127] Based on the DCCT and the UKPDS, major clinical diabetes organizations recommend that the goal for most patients with diabetes should be HbA_{1c} less than 6.5 to 7%.[33] The more frequent use of this test in the management of patients is reflected in the increased number of laboratories participating in College of American Pathologists (CAP) GHb surveys. In 1985, 1990, 2003, and 2009, approximately 300, 700, 2000, and 3250 laboratories, respectively, were enrolled in the GHb surveys.

Methods for the Determination of Glycated Hemoglobins

More than 100 different methods may be used for the determination of GHbs. These methods separate GHb from nonglycated hemoglobin using techniques based on *charge differences* (ion-exchange chromatography, HPLC, electrophoresis, and isoelectric focusing), *structural differences* (affinity chromatography and immunoassay), or *chemical analysis* (photometry and spectrophotometry).[92] Regardless of the method used, the result is expressed as a percentage of total hemoglobin. Analysis by electrophoresis, isoelectric focusing, or chemical techniques is rarely used and is not addressed further here. (Interested readers are referred to earlier editions of this book.) The selection of method by a laboratory is influenced by several factors, including sample volume, patient population, and cost. It is advisable to consult clinicians in this process. The ADA recommends that laboratories use only HbA_{1c} assays that are certified by the National Glycohemoglobin Standardization Program (now known as the NGSP) as traceable to the DCCT reference.[91] These assays are listed on the NGSP Website (www.NGSP.org/accessed July 28, 2011) and are updated at least annually.

The GHb assays most widely used in the United States are depicted in Table 46-5. These data are based on results from 1947 laboratories participating in a 1995 quality control survey and 2398 laboratories participating in a 2009 quality control survey conducted by the CAP. The results demonstrate that in 2009, virtually all laboratories used immunoassay or ion-exchange chromatography. HbA_{1c} was measured by more than 99% of laboratories (see Table 46-5). Total GHb and HbA_1 measurements had essentially disappeared. These results reflect significant changes from the methods used in 1995, when affinity chromatography was the most common analytical method (see Table 46-5). Also, only 60% of laboratories reported HbA_{1c} in 1995. In addition, variation among mean values—both between and within methods—and imprecision were substantially lower in 2009. It should be borne in mind that these data refer only to these CAP surveys and are weighted to laboratories that participate. All of the methods described are commercially available from several different manufacturers.

Ion-Exchange Minicolumns

Ion-exchange chromatography separates hemoglobin variants on the basis of charge. The cation-exchange resin (negatively charged), packed in a disposable minicolumn, has an affinity for hemoglobin, which is positively charged. The patient's sample is hemolyzed, and an aliquot of the hemolysate is applied to the column. A buffer is applied and the eluent collected. The ionic strength and pH of the eluent buffer are selected so that GHbs are less positively charged than HbA, do not bind as well to the negatively charged resin, and therefore are eluted first. The GHbs—A_{1a} + A_{1b} + A_{1c},

TABLE 46-5 Methods of Glycated Hemoglobin Analysis[a]

Method	Component	Year: 1995 (N = 1947)[b] Number[c]	% of Total	Mean, %[d]	CV, %[d]	2009 (N = 2396) Number[c]	% of Total	Mean, %[e]	CV, %[d]
Charge Reported									
Ion exchange			15				35		
	HbA_{1c}	279		4.9-5.7	4.4-13.8	832		6.0-6.3	1.3-3
	HbA_1	22		6.5	15.2	—[f]			
Electrophoresis			12						
	HbA_{1c}	138		4.9	16.5	0		—	—
	HbA_1	99		6.4-7.8	9.6-12.7	—			
Structure									
Affinity			66				<1		
	HbA_{1c}	642		6.5	8.1	12		5.9	2.3
	Total GHb	638		5.9-7.9	6.9-9.3	0		—	—
Immunoassay			7				65		
	HbA_{1c}	129		5.7	3.5	1552		5.7-6.2	2.7-8

[a]Results are based on 1995 CAP Survey, Set EC-B, Specimen GH-03 and 2009 CAP Survey, Set GH2-A, Specimen GH2-02 (Copyright, 1995 and 2009 College of American Pathologists; data used with permission). See text for discussion of methods.
[b]*n* is the number of laboratories that participated in the survey.
[c]Indicates how many laboratories use the indicated method.
[d]Where more than one value is listed, the data vary among commercial assays. The range is presented.
[e]The NGSP value in 2009 was 6.0%.
[f]Number of participants was too low to permit statistical analysis.
CV, Coefficient of variation; *GHb*, glycated hemoglobin; *Hb*, hemoglobin.

expressed collectively as HbA_1—are measured in a spectrophotometer. A second buffer of different ionic strength can be added to the column to elute the more positively charged main hemoglobin fraction. This is read in the spectrophotometer, and GHb is expressed as a percentage of total hemoglobin. Alternatively, only the HbA_1 is eluted and a separate dilution of the original hemolysate is made, against which the HbA_1 is compared. Numerous commercial modifications have been developed. Simple agitation of resins with hemolysates (batch technique) to adsorb HbA has also been described. In this approach, the supernatant solution containing the HbA_1 fraction is removed by filtration or centrifugation. Methods that separate HbA_{1a+b} from HbA_{1c} by using two different buffers have also been described.[151] Most of the current commercial ion-exchange methods use HPLC.

In all ion-exchange column methods, it is important to *control the temperature of the reagents and columns* to obtain accurate and reproducible results. This is best done by thermostatting the columns. Alternatively, a temperature correction factor can be applied if the room temperature differs from the specified optimum. In addition, rigid control of pH and ionic strength must be maintained. Sample storage conditions are also important.

The labile pre-HbA_1 fractions elute with the stable ketoamine and produce spuriously high values unless destroyed by pretreatment of the red blood cells. Spuriously increased values are also obtained when the charge on hemoglobin is altered by the attachment of noncarbohydrate moieties, which may co-chromatograph with GHbs, as in uremia (carbamylated hemoglobin), alcoholism, lead poisoning, or chronic treatment with large doses of aspirin (acetylated hemoglobin). Hemoglobin variants or chemically modified hemoglobins that elute separately from HbA and HbA_{1c} have little effect on HbA_{1c} measurements. If the modified hemoglobin (or its glycated derivative) cannot be separated from HbA or HbA_{1c}, spuriously increased or reduced results will be obtained.[46] A variant that elutes with HbA_{1c} will yield a gross overestimation of HbA_{1c}, and a variant that coelutes with HbA will underestimate HbA_{1c}. Note that a single variant may falsely increase or decrease HbA_{1c}, depending on the method used.[46]

High-Performance Liquid Chromatography

HbA_{1c} and other hemoglobin fractions can be separated by HPLC, which employs cation-exchange chromatography.[61] Several fully automated systems are commercially available. Assays require only 5 µL of whole blood, and fingerstick samples can be collected in a capillary tube for analysis. Anticoagulated blood is diluted with a hemolysis reagent containing borate. Samples are incubated at 37 °C for 30 minutes to remove the Schiff base and are inserted into the autosampler. [Some instruments have a shorter preincubation step, and others (e.g., Tosoh A_{1c}2.2) separate labile A_{1c} chromatographically, eliminating the step to remove the Schiff base.[87]] A step gradient using three phosphate buffers of increasing ionic strength is passed through the column. Detection is performed at both 415 and 690 nm, and results are quantified by integrating the area under the peaks. Analysis time is as short as 3 to 5 minutes. All HPLC methods had CVs less than or equal to 3.0% in a 2009 CAP survey (see Table 46-5). HbA_{1c} by HPLC was used for analysis of all patient samples in the DCCT.[61]

Immunoassay

Assays for HbA_{1c} have been developed using antibodies raised against the Amadori product of glucose (ketoamine linkage) plus the first few (four to eight) amino acids at the *N*-terminal end of the β-chain of hemoglobin.[74,117] A widely used assay measures HbA_{1c} in whole blood by inhibition of latex agglutination. The agglutinator, a synthetic polymer containing multiple copies of the immunoreactive portion of HbA_{1c}, binds the anti-HbA_{1c} monoclonal antibody that is attached to latex beads. This agglutination produces light scattering, measured as an increase in absorbance. HbA_{1c} in the patient's sample competes for the antibody on the latex, inhibiting agglutination, thereby decreasing light scattering. Enzyme immunoassays using monoclonal antibodies are commercially available, and most exhibit reasonable imprecision (see Table 46-5). These assays are generally calibrated to give values that match and correlate with HPLC values. The antibodies do not recognize labile intermediates or other GHbs (such as HbA_{1a} or HbA_{1b}) because both ketoamine with glucose and specific amino acid sequences are required for binding. Similarly, several hemoglobin variants, such as HbF, HbA_2, HbS, and carbamylated hemoglobin, are not detected.[46] The procedure has been adapted for capillary blood samples using a bench-top analyzer with reagent cartridges designed for use in physicians' office laboratories.

Affinity Chromatography

Affinity gel columns are used to separate GHb, which binds to the column, from the nonglycated fraction. *m*-Aminophenylboronic acid is immobilized by cross-linking to beaded agarose or another matrix (e.g., glass fiber). The boronic acid reacts with the *cis*-diol groups of glucose bound to hemoglobin to form a reversible five-member ring complex, thus selectively holding the GHb on the column (Figure 46-7). The nonglycated hemoglobin does not bind. Sorbitol is then added to elute the GHb. Absorbance of bound and nonbound fractions, measured at 415 nm, is used to calculate the percentage of GHb.

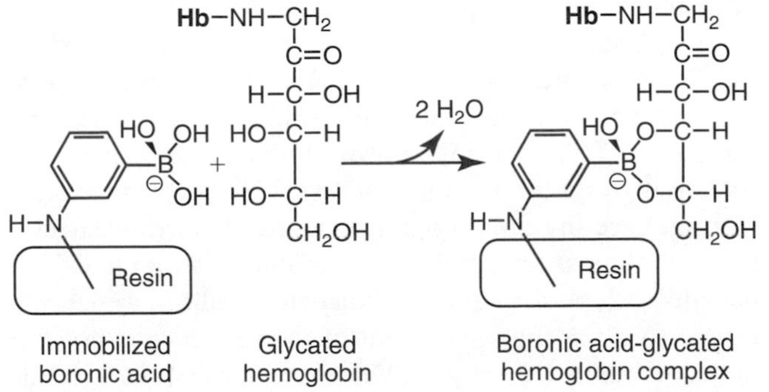

Figure 46-7 Reaction of glycated hemoglobin (GHb) with immobilized boronic acid.

A commercial assay is performed on an automated analyzer that uses a soluble reagent consisting of dihydroxyboronate coupled with high molecular weight polyacrylic acid.[259] GHb binds to the boronate. The polyanionic-glycated hemoglobin affinity complex attaches by electrostatic interactions to the cationic surface of the solid-phase matrix (ion capture). Nonglycated hemoglobin does not bind and is removed in a wash step. GHb is quantified by measuring quenching by hemoglobin of the fluorescence of an added fluorophore, 4-methyl-umbelliferone. Total hemoglobin is determined by fluorescence quenching of a second sample containing sorbitol. The sorbitol competes for boronate binding sites, and both nonglycated hemoglobin and GHb contribute to inhibition of the quenching. The fluorescence measurements are converted to glycated and total hemoglobin concentrations from separate stored calibration curves.

The major advantages of affinity chromatography are as follows: there is no interference from nonglycated hemoglobins and negligible interference from the labile intermediate form of HbA_{1c}. It is unaffected by variations in temperature and has reasonably good precision. Hemoglobin variants such as HbS, HbC, HbD, or HbE produce little effect. Affinity methods measure total GHb. This includes components other than HbA_{1c} because the assay detects ketoamine structures on lysine and valine residues on both α- and β-chains of hemoglobin.

Although the method detects all GHbs, most commercially available systems are calibrated to report a standardized HbA_{1c} value. The value is derived from an equation obtained from linear regression between total GHb and HbA_{1c} analysis by HPLC.[259] A linear relationship has been demonstrated, and standardized HbA_{1c} values are thus comparable to values obtained by methods specific for HbA_{1c}. Columns and reagents are commercially available.

Removal of Labile Glycated Hemoglobin from Red Blood Cells

The concentration of the labile form of HbA_{1c} (Schiff base) fluctuates rapidly in response to acute changes in plasma glucose concentrations and should be removed before analysis by charge-based assays. This may be accomplished by incubating red blood cells in saline[93] or in buffer solutions at pH 5 to 6,[28] or by dialysis or ultrafiltration of hemolysates. Most kits for column assays contain reagents to remove this labile component.

Assay Standardization

Clinical laboratories measure GHb with diverse assays that use multiple methods and quantify different components. The DCCT results accentuated the need for accurate GHb measurement and provided a strong impetus for standardization of GHb assays. At the end of the DCCT, it was noted that absence of both a reference method and a single GHb standard had generated confusion.[208] Interlaboratory comparisons were not possible, and even a single quality control sample analyzed by a single method exhibited interlaboratory CVs as high as 16.5%. Similar large variability among laboratories was observed in Europe.[254] Committees were established under the auspices of the American Association for Clinical Chemistry (AACC) in 1993 and the IFCC in 1995 to standardize GHb assays.[146A]

The NGSP was established in 1996 to implement the protocol developed by the AACC to calibrate GHb results to DCCT-equivalent values. Employing a network of reference laboratories, the NGSP interacts with manufacturers of GHb methods to help them calibrate their methods and trace values to the DCCT.[147] Manufacturers apply for certification by performing precision testing according to CLSI EP5-A guidelines and report results in DCCT-equivalent HbA_{1c} values. This calibration effort has markedly improved harmonization of results and has reduced imprecision.[146A,147] Results obtained using NGSP-certified assays can be compared with results of the DCCT and UKPDS, allowing alignment with clinical outcomes data. The ADA recommends that clinical laboratories use only assays certified by the NGSP and participate in proficiency testing offered by the CAP. The CAP-GH2 survey uses pooled whole blood specimens at three HbA_{1c} concentrations. Target values are assigned by the NGSP network. Thus individual laboratories can directly compare their HbA_{1c} results with those of the DCCT (and UKPDS).

A different approach was adopted by the IFCC. A working group was established to devise a reference system for standardization based on HbA_{1c}. The IFCC group developed a mixture of purified HbA_{1c} and HbA_0 as primary reference material.[137] Two candidate reference methods, namely, electrospray ionization mass spectrometry (ESI-MS) and capillary electrophoresis, were proposed.[137] These specifically measure the glycated *N*-terminal valine of the β-chain of hemoglobin. Analysis is performed by digesting the hemoglobin molecule with endoproteinase Glu-C, which cleaves the β-chain between Glu-6 and Glu-7, releasing the *N*-terminal hexapeptide. Glycated and nonglycated hexapeptides are separated and quantified by HPLC-ESI-MS or by HPLC-capillary electrophoresis.[137] HbA_{1c} is measured as the ratio between glycated and nonglycated *N*-terminal hexapeptides. The IFCC Working Group has established a network of laboratories to implement and maintain the reference system.[253] Comparisons between IFCC and NGSP reference methods (and reference systems from Japan and Sweden) indicate a close and stable relationship and allow manufacturers to calibrate their instruments to a higher-level reference method.[253] However, HbA_{1c} results obtained using IFCC reference methods are 1.5 to 2% absolute HbA_{1c} units lower than those of the NGSP (and lower than other reference systems). The difference is possibly due to measurement of glycated components other than HbA_{1c} by HPLC. The IFCC method is time-consuming and technically complex, thus it is not designed to be used for routine analysis of patient samples.

Reporting HbA_{1c}

HbA_{1c} typically is reported as a percentage of total hemoglobin in the NGSP system. These values, which are equivalent to those reported in the DCCT and the UKPDS, represent the most widely used reporting system in patient care and the published literature. The IFCC method reports HbA_{1c} as mmol/mol (HbA_{1c}/total Hb).[168] Comparison between the IFCC and NGSP networks produced a master equation that permits conversion between the two reference systems.[106] For example, an HbA_{1c} result of 7% (in NGSP/DCCT/UKPDS units) is equivalent to 53 mmol/mol (in IFCC units). A 2008 multinational, prospective study [termed A_{1c} Derived Average Glucose (ADAG)] evaluated the relationship between HbA_{1c} concentrations and long-term glucose values.[171] A linear correlation was observed, permitting estimated average glucose (eAG) to be calculated from the HbA_{1c} measurement. The regression equations are as follows: eAG mg/dL $= 28.7 \times HbA_{1c} - 46.7$, and eAG mmol/L $= 1.59 \times HbA_{1c} - 2.59$. For example, an HbA_{1c} value of 7% translates into an eAG of 140 mg/dL. Some clinicians and many diabetes educators believe that the eAG will facilitate communication with patients.[202] The ADA and the AACC recommend that laboratories report both HbA_{1c} and eAG. Nevertheless, the concept of expressing HbA_{1c} in terms of average glucose is not accepted by all.[128,148]

Specimen Collection and Storage

Patients need not be fasting. Venous blood should be collected in tubes containing EDTA, oxalate, or fluoride. Sample stability depends on the assay method used.[204] Whole blood may be stored at 4 °C for up to 1 week. Above 4 °C, HbA_{1a+b} increases in a time- and temperature-dependent manner, but HbA_{1c} is only slightly affected.[220] Storage of samples at −20 °C is not recommended. For most methods, whole blood samples stored at −70 °C or colder are stable for at least 18 months.[71] Heparinized samples should be assayed within 2 days and may not be suitable for some methods of analysis (e.g., electrophoresis).

Reference Intervals

Values for GHbs are expressed as a percentage of total blood hemoglobin. One of three major GHb species, namely, HbA_1, HbA_{1c}, or total GHb, is usually measured. The United States and several other countries, including Canada, Australia, New Zealand, and the United Kingdom, now report virtually all results as HbA_{1c}. Reference intervals vary, depending on the GHb component measured. The reference interval for HbA_{1c} (using an NGSP-certified method) is 4 to 6% (20 to 42 mmol/mol).

The effects of age on reference intervals are controversial.[204] Some studies show age-related increases (≈0.1% per decade after age 30), and other reports show no increase.[129,182,256] It is not known whether these small, but statistically significant, increases in HbA_{1c} concentrations with age have any clinical significance. Results are not affected by acute illness. Intraindividual variability is minimal.[200] In patients with poorly controlled diabetes mellitus, values may extend to twice the upper limit of the reference interval or more, but rarely exceed 15%. Values greater than 15% should prompt additional studies to determine the possible presence of variant hemoglobin.[46] Note that ADA target values derived from DCCT and UKPDS, not the reference values, are used to evaluate metabolic control in diabetic patients.

There is no specific value of HbA_{1c} below which the risk of diabetic complications is eliminated completely. The ADA states that the goal of treatment should be to maintain HbA_{1c} at less than 7%.[19] (Some organizations recommend an HbA_{1c} target of less than 6.5%.) These goal values are applicable only if the assay method is certified as traceable to the DCCT reference. Each laboratory should establish its own nondiabetic reference interval. Assay precision is important because each 1% change in HbA_{1c} represents an approximate 30 mg/dL change in average blood glucose.

No consensus has been reached on optimum frequency of testing. The ADA recommends that *HbA_{1c} should be routinely monitored at least every 6 months in patients meeting treatment goals (and who have stable glycemic control).*[19] These recommendations are for patients with type 1 or type 2 diabetes.

Fructosamine

Clinical Significance

In selected patients with diabetes mellitus (e.g., GDM, change in therapy), assays may be needed that are more sensitive than GHb to shorter-term alterations in average blood glucose concentrations. Nonenzymatic attachment of glucose to amino groups of proteins other than hemoglobin (e.g., serum proteins, membrane proteins, lens crystallins) to form ketoamines also occurs. Because serum proteins turn over more rapidly than erythrocytes (the circulating half-life for albumin is about 20 days), *the concentration of glycated serum albumin reflects glucose control over a period of 2 to 3 weeks.* Therefore, both deterioration of control and improvement with therapy are evident earlier than with GHb.

Fructosamine is the generic name for plasma protein ketoamines (for reviews, see Armbruster[20] and Hill and associates[102]). The name refers to the structure of the ketoamine rearrangement product formed by the interaction of glucose with the ε-amino group on lysine residues of albumin. Analogous to GHb, measurement of fructosamine may be used as an index of the average concentration of blood glucose over an extended period of time, but one that is about ¼ as long as the time examined with GHb.

Because all glycated serum proteins are fructosamines and albumin is the most abundant serum protein, measurement of fructosamine is thought to be largely a measure of glycated albumin, but this has been questioned by some investigators.[212] Although the fructosamine assay can be automated and is cheaper and faster than GHb, *there is a lack of consensus on its clinical utility.* For example, evaluation of 65 studies led the authors to conclude that fructosamine determination is not a reliable test, and it has not been evaluated sufficiently for routine clinical use.[260] In contrast, a review of essentially the same data concluded that fructosamine could provide information useful in the management of diabetes.[20] Early work using the original assay, introduced in 1983,[25,119] indicated that fructosamine concentrations were significantly higher in diabetic individuals than in healthy subjects. Over the succeeding decade, the assay underwent numerous modifications because several artifacts were identified that rendered data from the first-generation fructosamine assay difficult to interpret. These include apparent lack of specificity for glycated proteins (up to 60% of the value was due to nonfructosamine reducing substances), lack of standardization among laboratories, difficulty in calibrating the assay, and interference by urates and hyperlipidemia.[31] Substantial modifications produced second-generation assays that contain uricase and higher detergent concentrations and are calibrated with glycated lysine.[213] In addition, an industry standard was adopted. These improvements resulted in average fructosamine values in nondiabetic individuals that are approximately 10% of those obtained with the first-generation assay. Some clinical evidence suggests that fructosamine may be useful in the elderly[49] and in those with gestational diabetes.[125] The potential role of the second-generation fructosamine assay in providing rapid, reliable, inexpensive, and technically easy monitoring of glycemic control requires evaluation. The clinical value of fructosamine has not been firmly established, and no convincing evidence relates its concentration to the chronic complications of diabetes.[204]

Because fructosamine determination monitors short-term glycemic changes different from GHb, it may have a role in conjunction with GHb rather than instead of it. In addition, fructosamine may be useful in patients with hemoglobin variants, such as HbS or HbC, that are associated with decreased erythrocyte lifespan, where GHb is of little value. Gross changes in protein concentration and half-life may have large effects on the proportion of protein that is glycated. Thus fructosamine results may be invalid in patients with nephrotic syndrome, cirrhosis of the liver, or dysproteinemias, or after rapid changes in acute-phase reactants. Initial reports indicated that, in the absence of significant alterations in serum protein concentrations, fructosamine results were independent of protein concentrations.[26] However, this observation has been questioned by other investigators, who recommend that fructosamine values be corrected for protein concentrations. This issue remains to be resolved. It is generally accepted that the test should not be performed when serum albumin is less than 30 g/L. Although it was initially postulated that the fructosamine assay would replace the OGTT, *there is no role for the fructosamine assay in the diagnosis of diabetes mellitus.* The second-generation fructosamine assay has been reported to have sensitivity and specificity close to 80% in screening patients for GDM,[111] but this study requires verification.

Determination of Fructosamine

Methods for measuring glycated proteins include (1) affinity chromatography using immobilized phenylboronic acid (similar to the GHb assay)[266]; (2) HPLC of glycated lysine residues after hydrolysis of the glycated proteins[211]; (3) a photometric procedure in which mild acid hydrolysis releases 5-hydroxymethylfurfural—proteins are precipitated with trichloroacetic acid and the supernatant is reacted with 2-thiobarbituric acid[69]; and (4) other procedures using phenylhydrazine and ε-*N*-(2-furoylmethyl)-L-lysine (furosine). None of these assays is popular because they are not suitable for routine clinical laboratories. The development of monoclonal antibodies to glycated albumin,[54] although theoretically advantageous, has not yet resulted in the widespread availability of commercial glycated albumin assays. It should be noted that prolonged storage at ultra-low temperatures (−96 °C) prevents in vitro glycation of serum proteins.[27]

An alternative method for the measurement of fructosamine is a modification[145,213] of the original method of Johnson and colleagues.[119] This method is conducted under alkaline conditions and results in fructosamine undergoing an Amadori rearrangement with the resultant compounds having reducing activity that can be differentiated from other reducing substances. In the presence of carbonate buffer, fructosamine rearranges to the eneaminol form, which reduces NBT to a formazan (Figure 46-8). Absorbance at 530 nm is measured at two time points, and the absorbance change is proportional to the fructosamine concentration. A 10 minute preincubation is necessary to allow fast-reacting interfering reducing substances to react. It is unnecessary to remove endogenous glucose from patients' samples because a pH greater than 11 is required for glucose to reduce NBT. The assay is easily automated and has excellent between-batch analytical precision. Hemoglobin (>100 mg/dL) and bilirubin (>4 mg/dL) may interfere; therefore moderate to grossly hemolyzed and icteric samples should not be used. Ascorbic acid concentrations greater than 5 mg/dL may cause negative interference. Kits are commercially available (Roche Diagnostics, Indianapolis, Ind). An assay that measures fructosamine by oxidizing the ketoamine bond using ketoamine oxidase, with release of H_2O_2 that is quantified by a photometric reaction, is available (Randox, Oceanside, Calif). An alternative approach has been described.[246] Samples are incubated with proteases, followed by the enzyme fructosaminase, resulting in the release of H_2O_2, which is quantified. The assay, which can be run on an automated analyzer, is commercially available (Diazyme, San Diego, Calif).

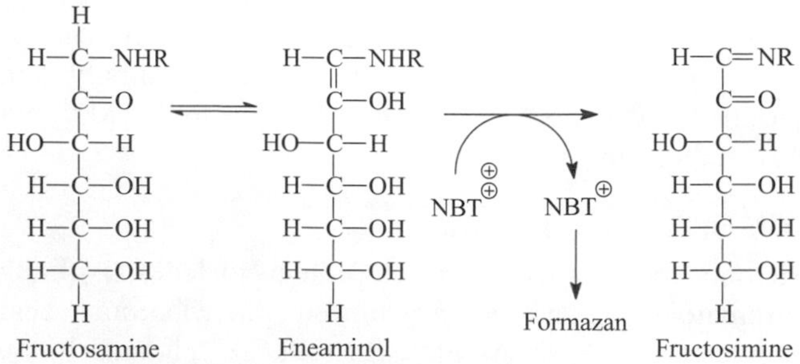

A different way to measure glycated albumin is used in Japan. Glycated albumin is hydrolyzed by proteinases to glycated amino acids, which are oxidized by ketoamine oxidase, producing H_2O_2.[139] The H_2O_2 is quantified and glycated albumin is expressed as a percentage of total albumin. This assay is not available in the United States at the time of this writing, but the manufacturer has applied to the FDA for approval.

Reference Intervals

Values in a nondiabetic population vary from 205 to 285 μmol/L. The reference interval corrected for albumin is 191 to 265 μmol/L.

Advanced Glycation End Products

The molecular mechanism by which hyperglycemia produces toxic effects is unknown, but glycation of tissue proteins may be important. Nonenzymatic attachment of glucose to long-lived proteins, lipids, or nucleic acids produces stable Amadori early-glycated products. These undergo a series of additional rearrangements, dehydration, and fragmentation reactions, resulting in stable *advanced glycation end products* (AGEs). The amounts of these products do not return to normal when hyperglycemia is corrected, and they accumulate continuously over the lifespan of the protein. Hyperglycemia accelerates the formation of protein-bound AGE, and patients with diabetes mellitus thus have more AGE than healthy subjects. Through effects on the functional properties of protein and extracellular matrix, AGE may contribute to the microvascular and macrovascular complications of diabetes mellitus.[45,90] AGEs can also activate the receptor for AGE (RAGE) to induce intracellular signaling that leads to enhanced oxidative stress and the production of proinflammatory cytokines.[90] Moreover, inhibitors of AGE formation, such as aminoguanidine, have been shown to prevent several of the complications of diabetes in experimental animal models and are undergoing clinical trials in patients.

Fructosamine ⇌ Eneaminol → Fructosimine (NBT⊕ → Formazan)

Figure 46-8 Reaction of fructosamine with nitroblue tetrazolium (NBT).

URINARY ALBUMIN EXCRETION

Clinical Significance

Patients with diabetes mellitus are at high risk of suffering renal damage. End-stage renal disease requiring dialysis or transplantation develops in approximately one third of patients with type 1 diabetes,[193] and diabetes is the most common cause of end-stage renal disease in the United States and Europe.[164] Although nephropathy is less common in patients with type 2 diabetes, approximately 60% of all cases of diabetic nephropathy occur in these patients because of the higher incidence of this form of diabetes. Early detection of diabetic nephropathy relies on tests of urinary excretion of albumin. Persistent proteinuria detectable by routine screening tests [equivalent to a urinary albumin excretion (UAE) rate ≥200 μg/min] indicates overt diabetic nephropathy. This is usually associated with long-standing disease and is unusual less than 5 years after the onset of type 1 diabetes. Once diabetic nephropathy occurs, renal function deteriorates rapidly and renal insufficiency evolves. Treatment at this stage can retard the rate of progression without stopping or reversing the renal damage. Preceding this stage is a period of increased UAE not detected by routine dipstick methods. This range of 20 to 200 μg/min (or 30 to 300 mg/24 h) of increased UAE has been called *microalbuminuria.* Note that it is not defined in terms of urinary albumin concentration, although the ratio of the urinary albumin concentration to the urinary creatatinine concententration (albumin-to-creatinine ratio) in an untimed urine specimen can be used as a substitute for albumin measurements in a timed collection of urine, as described later. The term *microalbuminuria,* although widely used, is misleading. It implies a small version of the albumin molecule rather than an excretion rate of albumin greater than normal but less than that detectable by routine methods. Use of the term is discouraged.

The presence of increased UAE denotes an increase in the transcapillary escape rate of albumin and therefore is a marker of microvascular disease. Persistent UAE greater than 20 μg/min represents a 20-fold greater risk for the development of clinically overt renal disease in patients with type 1 and type 2 diabetes. Prospective studies have demonstrated that increased UAE precedes and is highly predictive of diabetic nephropathy, end-stage renal disease, cardiovascular mortality, and total mortality in patients with diabetes mellitus.[163,164] The DCCT and the UKPDS showed that intensive diabetes therapy can significantly reduce the risk of development of increased UAE and overt nephropathy in individuals with diabetes.[62,242] In addition, increased UAE identifies a group of nondiabetic subjects at increased risk for coronary artery disease.[85,141] Interventions, such as control of blood glucose concentrations and blood pressure, particularly with angiotensin-converting enzyme (ACE) inhibitors, slow the rate of decline in renal function.[164]

Methods for Measuring Urinary Albumin Excretion

No consensus has been reached about how a urine sample should be collected for measuring UAE. Variations in urine flow rate in a person may be corrected by expressing albumin as a ratio to creatinine (i.e., albumin:creatinine). *UAE is increased by physiologic factors* (e.g., exercise, posture, diuresis), and the method of urine collection must be standardized. Samples should not be collected after exertion, in the presence of urinary tract infection, during acute illness, immediately after surgery, or after an acute fluid load. All the following urine samples are currently acceptable: (1) 24 hour collection; (2) overnight (8 to 12 hours, timed) collection; (3) 1 to 2 hour timed collection (in laboratory or clinic); and (4) first morning sample for simultaneous albumin and creatinine measurement. Only results for timed specimens can be reported as mg albumin excreted per hour, but the albumin-to-creatinine ratio is more practical and convenient for the patient and is the recommended method. A first morning void sample is recommended because it has lower within-person variation for the albumin-to-creatinine ratio than a random urine sample.[204,261] *At least three separate specimens, collected on different days, should be assayed* because of high intraindividual variation (CV of 30 to 50%) and diurnal variation (50 to 100% higher during the day). Urine should be stored at 4 °C after collection. Alternatively, 2 mL of 50 g/L sodium azide can be added per 500 mL of urine, but preservatives are not recommended for some assays. Bacterial contamination and glucose have no effect. Specimens are stable for 2 weeks at 4 °C and for at least 5 months at −80 °C. Freezing samples has been reported to decrease albumin,[73] but mixing immediately before assay eliminates this effect.

Semiquantitative Assays

Several semiquantitative assays are available for screening for increased UAE. These test strips, most of which are optimized to read "positive" at a predetermined albumin concentration, have been recommended for screening programs. In view of the wide variability in UAE, it must be borne in mind that a "normal" value does not rule out renal disease. *Because these assays measure albumin concentration, dilute urine may yield a false-negative test result.* Refrigerated urine samples should be allowed to reach at least 10 °C before analysis. Albu Screen and Albu Sure (Cambridge Life Sciences, Cambridge, United Kingdom) detect urinary albumin concentrations exceeding 20 and 30 mg/L, respectively. The assay is a latex agglutination inhibition test. Briefly, one drop of urine is mixed with one drop of goat antihuman albumin, the titer of which is adjusted so that all antibody-binding sites are occupied at urinary albumin concentrations of 30 mg/L or greater. Excess albumin-binding sites are detected by adding one drop of albumin-coated latex microspheres and rocking for 2 minutes. Albumin concentrations less than 20 mg/L produce agglutination. Microbumintest (Bayer Diagnostics Tarrytown, NY) uses bromophenol blue in an alkaline matrix to detect albumin concentrations exceeding 40 mg/L. The assay sensitivity for increased urinary albumin as measured by quantitative assays is approximately 95%, but because other proteins are also detected, the specificity is approximately 80%.

Micral (Roche Diagnostics Indianapolis, IN) uses a monoclonal antialbumin IgG complexed to β-galactosidase. The albumin in the urine binds to the antibody-enzyme conjugate in the test strip. Excess conjugate is retained in a separation zone containing immobilized albumin, and only albumin bound to the antibody-enzyme immunocomplex diffuses to the reaction zone. Here it reacts with a buffered substrate (chlorophenol red galactoside) to produce a red color when the β-galactosidase hydrolyzes galactose. The test strip is dipped into the urine for 5 seconds, and the intensity of the color after 5 minutes is proportional to the urinary albumin concentration. Direct visual comparison is made with printed color blocks, with yellow, light brown, medium brown, brick red, and burgundy representing 0, 10, 20, 50, and 100 mg/L, respectively. No interference is observed with drugs, glucose, urea, or other proteins. Comparison with a reference method demonstrates a sensitivity and specificity for albumin concentrations greater than 20 mg/L (not for microalbuminuria defined by UAE rate) of approximately 100% and 91%, respectively.[153] The *time that the stick is in contact with the urine and the time of reading are critical.* A modification (Micral II) uses a gold-labeled, instead of an enzyme-labeled, antibody. This enhances the stability, allowing the strip to be read at any time from 1 to at least 60 minutes. Urine samples with albumin concentrations greater than 100 to 300 mg/L may be diluted and reassayed. The assigned concentration of the color block is multiplied by the dilution factor to obtain the concentration in the sample. These semiquantitative assays have been *recommended for screening only.* However, published studies reveal sensitivities for detection of increased UAE from 67 to 91%.[204] These low sensitivities limit the value of semiquantitative tests even for screening, and additional studies are necessary before dipstick tests can be recommended as replacements for quantitative tests.[204]

Quantitative Assays

All sensitive, specific assays for urine albumin use immunochemistry with antibodies to human albumin. Four methods are available: RIA, ELISA, radial immunodiffusion, and immunoturbidimetry.[155] Each method has advantages and disadvantages, and the choice depends on local experience and technical support. In general, these *methods have similar imprecisions, detection limits, and reference intervals.* A comparison of these methods has been performed.[248] Although dye-binding[215] and protein-precipitation[185] assays have been described, these are insensitive and nonspecific and should not be used.

Radial Immunodiffusion

Radial immunodiffusion has not gained wide acceptance because it requires long incubation and a high level of technical skill and cannot be automated. The antibody is incorporated into an agar gel. Aliquots of samples and calibrators are added to wells and are allowed to diffuse into the agar. The antigen-antibody complexes precipitate at equilibrium, and after staining, the distance of migration is measured.

Radioimmunoassay

Standard RIA methods have been described[262] with ^{125}I-labeled albumin and antialbumin antiserum, but reagents are radioactive and have a short shelf life. Commercial kits are available.

Enzyme-Linked Immunosorbent Assay

Both competitive and "sandwich" ELISAs are available.[51,240] Although the competitive ELISA is faster because it uses only one incubation with an antibody, it is reported to be less sensitive and exhibits large imprecision. ELISA can be performed on a microplate reader, allowing semiautomation. In the sandwich assay, the primary antibody (antialbumin antiserum) is fixed on the plastic plate, which is then washed. Samples, controls, and calibrators are added, and the complexes are detected and quantified by a second antibody conjugated to an enzyme label.

Immunoturbidimetry

Albumin in the urine sample forms an insoluble complex with antibodies to human albumin. PEG accelerates complex formation. The turbidity caused by these complexes is measured by a spectrophotometer at 340 nm and is a measure of albumin concentration. The background absorbance of the initial urine sample is subtracted automatically. This method is simple and less expensive than RIA, and rapid analysis of large numbers of samples is possible. Assays may be performed as kinetic or equilibrium reactions. Kits are commercially available for use with automated analyzers (Roche Diagnostics).

Reference Intervals

URINARY ALBUMIN EXCRETION

	μg/min	mg/24 h	Corrected (mg/g Urine Creatinine)
Normal	<20	<30	<30
Increased UAE	20-200	30-300	30-300
Clinical albuminuria*	>200	>300	>300

*Also termed *overt nephropathy.*

The ADA position statement[19] recommends initial UAE measurement in patients with type 1 diabetes who have had diabetes for 5 years or longer, and in all type 2 diabetic patients. Because of the difficulty involved in dating the onset of type 2 diabetes, screening should commence at diagnosis. Analysis should be performed annually in all patients who have a negative screening result. Screening may be performed with a semiquantitative assay. If the screening result is positive, UAE should be evaluated by a quantitative assay. Diagnosis requires the demonstration of increased UAE in at least two of three tests measured within a 3 to 6 month period.

If the confirmatory test result is positive, treatment with an ACE inhibitor or an angiotensin-receptor blocker should be initiated. ACE inhibitors delay progression to overt nephropathy, and the National Kidney Foundation recommends their use in both normotensive and hypertensive type 1 and 2 diabetic patients.[32] The role of monitoring UAE in patients on ACE inhibitor therapy is less clear, although many experts recommend continued surveillance. Untreated, the UAE would increase by 10 to 30% per year, whereas the albumin-to-creatinine ratio in patients on ACE inhibitors should stabilize or decrease by up to 50%.

REFERENCES

1. Anonymous. Effects of insulin in relatives of patients with type 1 diabetes mellitus. N Engl J Med 2002;346:1685-91.
2. Anonymous. State-specific prevalence of obesity among adults—United States, 2007. MMWR Morb Mortal Wkly Rep 2008;57:765-8.
3. Alberti KG, Zimmet PZ. Definition, diagnosis and classification of diabetes mellitus and its complications. Part 1. Diagnosis and classification of diabetes mellitus provisional report of a WHO consultation. Diabet Med 1998;15:539-53.
4. Allen BT, DeLong ER, Feussner JR. Impact of glucose self-monitoring on non-insulin-treated patients with type II diabetes mellitus: randomized controlled trial comparing blood and urine testing. Diabetes Care 1990;13:1044-50.
5. American College of Obstetrics and Gynecology. ACOG practice bulletin. Polycystic ovary syndrome, Number 41, December 2002. Int J Gynaecol Obstet 2003;80:335-48.
6. American Diabetes Association. Standardization of the oral glucose tolerance test. Report of the Committee on Statistics of the American Diabetes Association, June 14, 1968. Diabetes 1969;18:299-307.
7. American Diabetes Association. Consensus statement on self-monitoring of blood glucose. Diabetes Care 1987;10:93-9.
8. American Diabetes Association. Self-monitoring of blood glucose. Diabetes Care 1996;19(suppl 1):S62-6.
9. American Diabetes Association. Report of the Expert Committee on the Diagnosis and Classification of Diabetes Mellitus. Diabetes Care 1997;20:1183-97.
10. American Diabetes Association. Consensus Development Conference on Insulin Resistance, 5-6 November 1997. Diabetes Care 1998;21: 310-4.
11. American Diabetes Association. Gestational diabetes mellitus. Diabetes Care 2000;23:S77-9.
12. American Diabetes Association. Type 2 diabetes in children and adolescents. Diabetes Care 2000;23:381-9.
13. American Diabetes Association. Screening for type 2 diabetes. Diabetes Care 2003;26(suppl 1):S21-4.
14. American Diabetes Association. Gestational diabetes mellitus. Diabetes Care 2004;27(suppl 1):S88-90.
15. American Diabetes Association. Prevention of type 1 diabetes. Diabetes Care 2004;27(suppl 1):S133.
16. American Diabetes Association. 2008 resource guide. Diabetes Forecast 2008;61:RG31-2, RG34-48.
17. American Diabetes Association. Economic costs of diabetes in the U.S. in 2007. Diabetes Care 2008;31:596-615.
18. American Diabetes Association. Diagnosis and classification of diabetes mellitus. Diabetes Care 2009;32(suppl 1):S62-7.
19. American Diabetes Association. Standards of medical care in diabetes—2009. Diabetes Care 2009;32(suppl 1):S13-61.

19A. American Diabetes Association. Standards of medical care in diabetes—2010. Diabetes Care 2010;33(Suppl 1):S11-61

20. Armbruster DA. Fructosamine: structure, analysis, and clinical usefulness. Clin Chem 1987;33:2153-63.
21. Atkinson MA, Bowman MA, Kao KJ, Campbell L, Dush PJ, Shah SC, et al. Lack of immune responsiveness to bovine serum albumin in insulin-dependent diabetes. N Engl J Med 1993;329:1853-8.
22. Atkinson MA, Eisenbarth GS. Type 1 diabetes: new perspectives on disease pathogenesis and treatment. Lancet 2001;358:221-9.
23. Atkinson MA, Maclaren NK. The pathogenesis of insulin-dependent diabetes mellitus. N Engl J Med 1994;331:1428-36.
24. Baekkeskov S, Aanstoot HJ, Christgau S, Reetz A, Solimena M, Cascalho M, et al. Identification of the 64K autoantigen in insulin-dependent diabetes as the GABA-synthesizing enzyme glutamic acid decarboxylase [published erratum appears in Nature 1990 Oct 25;347(6295):782]. Nature 1990;347:151-6.
25. Baker J, Metcalf P, Tatnell M, Lever M, Johnson R. Quality assessment of determinations of serum fructosamine in 33 clinical chemistry laboratories. Clin Chem 1986;32:2133-6.
26. Baker JR, O'Connor JP, Metcalf PA, Lawson MR, Johnson RN. Clinical usefulness of estimation of serum fructosamine concentration as a screening test for diabetes mellitus. BMJ (Clin Res Ed) 1983;287: 863-7.
27. Balland M, Schiele F, Henny J. Effect of a 6-month storage on human serum fructosamine concentration. Clin Chim Acta 1994;230:105-7.
28. Bannon P. Effect of pH on the elimination of the labile fraction of glycosylated hemoglobin. Clin Chem 1982;28:2183.
29. Bell GI, Polonsky KS. Diabetes mellitus and genetically programmed defects in beta-cell function. Nature 2001;414:788-91.
30. Bellamy L, Casas JP, Hingorani AD, Williams D. Type 2 diabetes mellitus after gestational diabetes: a systematic review and meta-analysis. Lancet 2009;373:1773-9.
31. Benjamin RJ, Sacks DB. Glycated protein update: implications of recent studies, including the diabetes control and complications trial. Clin Chem 1994;40:683-7.
32. Bennett PH, Haffner S, Kasiske BL, Keane WF, Mogensen CE, Parving HH, et al. Screening and management of microalbuminuria in patients with diabetes mellitus: recommendations to the Scientific Advisory Board of the National Kidney Foundation from an ad hoc committee of the Council on Diabetes Mellitus of the National Kidney Foundation. Am J Kidney Dis 1995;25:107-12.
33. Berg AH, Sacks DB. Haemoglobin A1c analysis in the management of patients with diabetes: from chaos to harmony. J Clin Pathol 2008;61: 983-7.
34. Bergenstal RM, Gavin JR 3rd. The role of self-monitoring of blood glucose in the care of people with diabetes: report of a global consensus conference. Am J Med 2005;118:1S-6S.
35. Bingley PJ, Bonifacio E, Mueller PW. Diabetes antibody standardization program: first assay proficiency evaluation. Diabetes 2003;52:1128-36.
36. Bingley PJ, Bonifacio E, Ziegler AG, Schatz DA, Atkinson MA, Eisenbarth GS. Proposed guidelines on screening for risk of type 1 diabetes. Diabetes Care 2001;24:398.
37. Bingley PJ, Colman P, Eisenbarth GS, Jackson RA, McCulloch DK, Riley WJ, et al. Standardization of IVGTT to predict IDDM. Diabetes Care 1992;15:1313-6.
38. Bohme P, Floriot M, Sirveaux MA, Durain D, Ziegler O, Drouin P, et al. Evolution of analytical performance in portable glucose meters in the last decade. Diabetes Care 2003;26:1170-5.
39. Bollyky J, Sanda S, Greenbaum CJ. Type 1 diabetes mellitus: primary, secondary, and tertiary prevention. Mt Sinai J Med 2008;75:385-97.
40. Boura-Halfon S, Zick Y. Phosphorylation of IRS proteins, insulin action, and insulin resistance. Am J Physiol Endocrinol Metab 2009;296:E581-91.
41. Bowman MA, Leiter EH, Atkinson MA. Prevention of diabetes in the NOD mouse: implications for therapeutic intervention in human disease. Immunol Today 1994;15:115-20.
42. Bowsher RR, Wolny JD, Frank BH. A rapid and sensitive radioimmunoassay for the measurement of proinsulin in human serum. Diabetes 1992;41:1084-90.
43. Boyd JC, Bruns DE. Quality specifications for glucose meters: assessment by simulation modeling of errors in insulin dose. Clin Chem 2001;47:209-14.
44. Brownlee M. Biochemistry and molecular cell biology of diabetic complications. Nature 2001;414:813-20.
45. Brownlee M, Cerami A, Vlassara H. Advanced glycosylation end products in tissue and the biochemical basis of diabetic complications. N Engl J Med 1988;318:1315-21.
46. Bry L, Chen PC, Sacks DB. Effects of hemoglobin variants and chemically modified derivatives on assays for glycohemoglobin [Review]. Clin Chem 2001;47:153-63.
47. Byrne HA, Tieszen KL, Hollis S, Dornan TL, New JP. Evaluation of an electrochemical sensor for measuring blood ketones. Diabetes Care 2000;23:500-3.
48. Cabaleiro DR, Stockl D, Kaufman JM, Fiers T, Thienpont LM. Feasibility of standardization of serum C-peptide immunoassays with

isotope-dilution liquid chromatography-tandem mass spectrometry. Clin Chem 2006;52:1193-6.
49. Cefalu WT, Ettinger WH, Bell-Farrow AD, Rushing JT. Serum fructosamine as a screening test for diabetes in the elderly: a pilot study. J Am Geriatr Soc 1993;41:1090-4.
50. Chan JC, Malik V, Jia W, Kadowaki T, Yajnik CS, Yoon KH, et al. Diabetes in Asia: epidemiology, risk factors, and pathophysiology. JAMA 2009;301:2129-40.
51. Chesham J, Anderton SW, Kingdon CF. Rapid, competitive enzymoimmunoassay for albumin in urine. Clin Chem 1986;32:669-71.
52. Clark PM. Assays for insulin, proinsulin(s) and C-peptide. Ann Clin Biochem 1999;36(Pt 5):541-64.
53. Clarke WL, Cox D, Gonder-Frederick LA, Carter W, Pohl SL. Evaluating clinical accuracy of systems for self-monitoring of blood glucose. Diabetes Care 1987;10:622-8.
54. Cohen MP, Hud E. Production and characterization of monoclonal antibodies against human glycoalbumin. J Immunol Methods 1989;117:121-9.
55. Combettes MM. GLP-1 and type 2 diabetes: physiology and new clinical advances. Curr Opin Pharmacol 2006;6:598-605.
56. Concannon P, Rich SS, Nepom GT. Genetics of type 1A diabetes. N Engl J Med 2009;360:1646-54.
57. Cowie CC, Rust KF, Byrd-Holt DD, Eberhardt MS, Flegal KM, Engelgau MM, et al. Prevalence of diabetes and impaired fasting glucose in adults in the U.S. population: National Health and Nutrition Examination Survey 1999-2002. Diabetes Care 2006;29: 1263-8.
58. Cowie CC, Rust KF, Ford ES, Eberhardt MS, Byrd-Holt DD, Li C, et al. Full accounting of diabetes and pre-diabetes in the U.S. population in 1988-1994 and 2005-2006. Diabetes Care 2009;32: 287-94.
59. Dabelea D, Bell RA, D'Agostino RB Jr, Imperatore G, Johansen JM, Linder B, et al. Incidence of diabetes in youth in the United States. JAMA 2007;297:2716-24.
60. Daughaday WH. The possible autocrine/paracrine and endocrine roles of insulin-like growth factors of human tumors. Endocrinology 1990;127:1-4.
61. DCCT. Feasibility of centralized measurements of glycated hemoglobin in the Diabetes Control and Complications Trial: a multicenter study. Clin Chem 1987;33:2267-71.
62. DCCT. The effect of intensive treatment of diabetes on the development and progression of long-term complications in insulin-dependent diabetes mellitus. N Engl J Med 1993;329:977-86.
63. DCCT. The relationship of glycemic exposure (HbA1c) to the risk of development and progression of retinopathy in the Diabetes Control and Complications Trial. Diabetes 1995;44:968-83.
64. DCCT. Effect of intensive therapy on the microvascular complications of type 1 diabetes mellitus. The Diabetes Control and Complications Trial Research Group. JAMA 2002;287:2563-9.
65. DECODE Study Group. Is the current definition for diabetes relevant to mortality risk from all causes and cardiovascular and noncardiovascular diseases? Diabetes Care 2003;26:688-96.
66. DeFronzo RA, Bonadonna RC, Ferrannini E. Pathogenesis of NIDDM: a balanced overview. Diabetes Care 1992;15:318-68.
67. Dhahir FJ, Cook DB, Self CH. Amplified enzyme-linked immunoassay of human proinsulin in serum (detection limit: 0.1 pmol/L). Clin Chem 1992;38:227-32.
68. Diabetes Prevention Trial, Type 1 Study Group. Effects of insulin in relatives of patients with type 1 diabetes mellitus. N Engl J Med 2002;346:1685-91.
69. Dolhofer R, Wieland OH. Increased glycosylation of serum albumin in diabetes mellitus. Diabetes 1980;29:417-22.
70. D'Orazio P, Burnett RW, Fogh-Andersen N, Jacobs E, Kuwa K, Kulpmann WR, et al. Approved IFCC recommendation on reporting results for blood glucose (abbreviated). Clin Chem 2005;51:1573-6.
71. Duck SC, Lee M, D'Alessio D. 24-42 month stability of internal blood standards for glycated hemoglobin analysis. Diabetes Res Clin Pract 1990;9:195-9.
72. Dungan K, Chapman J, Braithwaite SS, Buse J. Glucose measurement: confounding issues in setting targets for inpatient management. Diabetes Care 2007;30:403-9.
73. Elving LD, Bakkeren JA, Jansen MJ, de Kat Angelino CM, de Nobel E, van Munster PJ. Screening for microalbuminuria in patients with diabetes mellitus: frozen storage of urine samples decreases their albumin content. Clin Chem 1989;35:308-10.
74. Engbaek F, Christensen SE, Jespersen B. Enzyme immunoassay of hemoglobin A1c: analytical characteristics and clinical performance for patients with diabetes mellitus, with and without uremia. Clin Chem 1989;35:93-7.
75. Engelgau MM, Narayan KM, Herman WH. Screening for type 2 diabetes. Diabetes Care 2000;23:1563-80.
76. Expert Panel. Executive summary of the third report of the National Cholesterol Education Program (NCEP) Expert Panel on Detection, Evaluation, and Treatment of High Blood Cholesterol in Adults (Adult Treatment Panel III). JAMA 2001;285:2486-97.
77. Finfer S, Chittock DR, Su SY, Blair D, Foster D, Dhingra V, et al. Intensive versus conventional glucose control in critically ill patients. N Engl J Med 2009;360:1283-97.
78. Flier JS. Lilly Lecture. Syndromes of insulin resistance: from patient to gene and back again. Diabetes 1992;41:1207-19.
79. Flier JS, Kahn CR, Roth J, Bar RS. Antibodies that impair insulin receptor binding in an unusual diabetic syndrome with severe insulin resistance. Science 1975;190:63-5.
80. Flock EV, Bennett PH, Savage PJ, Webner CJ, Howard BV, Rushforth NB, et al. Bimodality of glycosylated hemoglobin distribution in Pima Indians: relationship to fasting hyperglycemia. Diabetes 1979;28: 984-9.
81. Ganda OP, Day JL, Soeldner JS, Connon JJ, Gleason RE. Reproducibility and comparative analysis of repeated intravenous and oral glucose tolerance tests. Diabetes 1978;27:715-25.
82. Gerbitz KD, Spelsberg F. Pancreatic B-cell peptides as parameters for diagnosis and localisation of hormone secreting tumours. J Clin Chem Clin Biochem 1985;23:377-80.
83. Gerich JE. Lilly Lecture 1988. Glucose counterregulation and its impact on diabetes mellitus. Diabetes 1988;37:1608-17.
84. Gerich JE. Physiology of glucose homeostasis. Diabetes Obes Metab 2000;2:345-50.
85. Gerstein HC, Mann JF, Yi Q, Zinman B, Dinneen SF, Hoogwerf B, et al. Albuminuria and risk of cardiovascular events, death, and heart failure in diabetic and nondiabetic individuals. JAMA 2001; 286:421-6.
86. Giannoukakis N, Rudert WA, Robbins PD, Trucco M. Targeting autoimmune diabetes with gene therapy. Diabetes 1999;48:2107-21.
87. Gibb I, Parnham A, Fonfrede M, Lecock F. Multicenter evaluation of Tosoh glycohemoglobin analyzer. Clin Chem 1999;45:1833-41.
88. Ginsberg HN. Insulin resistance and cardiovascular disease. J Clin Invest 2000;106:453-8.
89. Girardin CM, Huot C, Gonthier M, Delvin E. Continuous glucose monitoring: a review of biochemical perspectives and clinical use in type 1 diabetes. Clin Biochem 2009;42:136-42.
90. Goh SY, Cooper ME. Clinical review: the role of advanced glycation end products in progression and complications of diabetes. J Clin Endocrinol Metab 2008;93:1143-52.
91. Goldstein DE, Little RR, Lorenz RA, Malone JI, Nathan D, Peterson CM, et al. Tests of glycemia in diabetes. Diabetes Care 2004;27: 1761-73.
92. Goldstein DE, Little RR, Wiedmeyer H-M, England JD, Rohlfing CG. Glycated haemoglobin estimation in the 1990s: a review of assay methods and clinical interpretation. In Marshall SM, Home PD, eds. The diabetes annual. New York, NY: Elsevier Science BV, 1994:193-212.
93. Goldstein DE, Peth SB, England JD, Hess RL, Da Costa J. Effects of acute changes in blood glucose on HbA1c. Diabetes 1980;29:623-8.
94. Grant RW, Moore AF, Florez JC. Genetic architecture of type 2 diabetes: recent progress and clinical implications. Diabetes Care 2009;32:1107-14.

95. Greenberg RA, Sacks DB. Screening for diabetes: is it warranted? Clin Chim Acta 2002;315:61-9.
96. Grundy SM. Hypertriglyceridemia, insulin resistance, and the metabolic syndrome. Am J Cardiol 1999;83:25F-9F.
97. Harano Y, Kosugi K, Hyosu T, Suzuki M, Hidaka H, Kashiwagi A, et al. Ketone bodies as markers for type 1 (insulin-dependent) diabetes and their value in the monitoring of diabetic control. Diabetologia 1984;26:343-8.
98. Harris MI. Frequency of blood glucose monitoring in relation to glycemic control in patients with type 2 diabetes. Diabetes Care 2001;24:979-82.
99. Harris MI, Flegal KM, Cowie CC, Eberhardt MS, Goldstein DE, Little RR, et al. Prevalence of diabetes, impaired fasting glucose, and impaired glucose tolerance in U.S. adults. The Third National Health and Nutrition Examination Survey, 1988-1994. Diabetes Care 1998;21:518-24.
100. Harrison LC. Risk assessment, prediction and prevention of type 1 diabetes. Pediatr Diabetes 2001;2:71-82.
101. Heding LG. Specific and direct radioimmunoassay for human proinsulin in serum. Diabetologia 1977;13:467-74.
102. Hill RP, Hindle EJ, Howey JE, Lemon M, Lloyd DR. Recommendations for adopting standard conditions and analytical procedures in the measurement of serum fructosamine concentration. Ann Clin Biochem 1990;27(Pt 5):413-24.
103. Hirsch IB, Bode BW, Childs BP, Close KL, Fisher WA, Gavin JR, et al. Self-monitoring of blood glucose (SMBG) in insulin- and non-insulin-using adults with diabetes: consensus recommendations for improving SMBG accuracy, utilization, and research. Diabetes Technol Ther 2008;10:419-39.
104. Hoekstra JB, van Rijn HJ, Erkelens DW, Thijssen JH. C-peptide. Diabetes Care 1982;5:438-46.
105. Hoekstra JB, Van Rijn HJ, Thijssen JH, Erkelens DW. C-peptide reactivity as a measure of insulin dependency in obese diabetic patients treated with insulin. Diabetes Care 1982;5:585-91.
106. Hoelzel W, Weykamp C, Jeppsson JO, Miedema K, Barr JR, Goodall I, et al. IFCC reference system for measurement of hemoglobin A1c in human blood and the national standardization schemes in the United States, Japan, and Sweden: a method-comparison study. Clin Chem 2004;50:166-74.
107. Holman RR, Paul SK, Bethel MA, Matthews DR, Neil HA. 10-year follow-up of intensive glucose control in type 2 diabetes. N Engl J Med 2008;359:1577-89.
108. Horwitz DL, Kuzuya H, Rubenstein AH. Circulating serum C-peptide: a brief review of diagnostic implications. N Engl J Med 1976;295: 207-9.
109. Houssa P, Dinesen B, Deberg M, Frank BH, Van Schravendijk C, Sodoyez-Goffaux F, et al. First direct assay for intact human proinsulin. Clin Chem 1998;44:1514-9.
110. Hu FB, Manson JE, Stampfer MJ, Colditz G, Liu S, Solomon CG, et al. Diet, lifestyle, and the risk of type 2 diabetes mellitus in women. N Engl J Med 2001;345:790-7.
111. Hughes PF, Agarwal M, Newman P, Morrison J. An evaluation of fructosamine estimation in screening for gestational diabetes mellitus. Diabet Med 1995;12:708-12.
112. Huisman W, Kuijken JP, Tan-Tjiong HL, Duurkoop EP, Leijnse B. Unstable glycosylated hemoglobin in patients with diabetes mellitus. Clin Chim Acta 1982;118:303-9.
113. Hwa V, Oh Y, Rosenfeld RG. The insulin-like growth factor-binding protein (IGFBP) superfamily. Endocr Rev 1999;20:761-87.
114. Hyoty H, Taylor KW. The role of viruses in human diabetes. Diabetologia 2002;45:1353-61.
114A. International Association of Diabetes and Pregnancy Study Groups. International Association of Diabetes and Pregnancy Study Groups recommendations on the diagnosis and classification of hyperglycemia in pregnancy. Diabetes Care 2010;33:676-682.
115. International Diabetes Federation. Diabetes atlas, 3rd edition. Brussels, Belgium: International Diabetes Federation, 2008.
116. James RC, Chase GR. Evaluation of some commonly used semiquantitative methods for urinary glucose and ketone determinations. Diabetes 1974;23:474-9.
117. John WG, Gray MR, Bates DL, Beacham JL. Enzyme immunoassay—a new technique for estimating hemoglobin A1c. Clin Chem 1993;39: 663-6.
118. Johnson RN, Baker JR. Error detection and measurement in glucose monitors. Clin Chim Acta 2001;307:61-7.
119. Johnson RN, Metcalf PA, Baker JR. Fructosamine: a new approach to the estimation of serum glycosylprotein. An index of diabetic control. Clin Chim Acta 1983;127:87-95.
120. Kabadi UM, O'Connell KM, Johnson J, Kabadi M. The effect of recurrent practice at home on the acceptability of capillary blood glucose readings: accuracy of self blood glucose testing. Diabetes Care 1994;17:1110-23.
121. Kahn CR. Banting Lecture. Insulin action, diabetogenes, and the cause of type II diabetes. Diabetes 1994;43:1066-84.
122. Kahn R, Buse J, Ferrannini E, Stern M. The metabolic syndrome: time for a critical appraisal. Joint statement from the American Diabetes Association and the European Association for the Study of Diabetes. Diabetes Care 2005;28:2289-304.
123. Karjalainen J, Martin JM, Knip M, Ilonen J, Robinson BH, Savilahti E, et al. A bovine albumin peptide as a possible trigger of insulin-dependent diabetes mellitus. N Engl J Med 1992;327:302-7.
124. Katzeff HL, Savage PJ, Barclay-White B, Nagulesparan M, Bennett PH. C-peptide measurement in the differentiation of type 1 (insulin-dependent) and type 2 (non-insulin-dependent) diabetes mellitus. Diabetologia 1985;28:264-8.
125. Kennedy DM, Johnson AB, Hill PG. A comparison of automated fructosamine and HbA1c methods for monitoring diabetes in pregnancy. Ann Clin Biochem 1998;35(Pt 2):283-9.
126. Khalil OS. Spectroscopic and clinical aspects of noninvasive glucose measurements. Clin Chem 1999;45:165-77.
127. Khaw KT, Wareham N, Luben R, Bingham S, Oakes S, Welch A, et al. Glycated haemoglobin, diabetes, and mortality in men in Norfolk cohort of European prospective investigation of cancer and nutrition (EPIC-Norfolk). BMJ 2001;322:15-8.
128. Kilpatrick ES. Haemoglobin A1c in the diagnosis and monitoring of diabetes mellitus. J Clin Pathol 2008;61:977-82.
129. Kilpatrick ES, Dominiczak MH, Small M. The effects of ageing on glycation and the interpretation of glycaemic control in Type 2 diabetes. Q J Med 1996;89:307-12.
130. Kim C, Newton KM, Knopp RH. Gestational diabetes and the incidence of type 2 diabetes: a systematic review. Diabetes Care 2002;25:1862-8.
131. King H, Aubert RE, Herman WH. Global burden of diabetes, 1995-2025: prevalence, numerical estimates, and projections. Diabetes Care 1998;21:1414-31.
132. Kippen AD, Cerini F, Vadas L, Stocklin R, Vu L, Offord RE, et al. Development of an isotope dilution assay for precise determination of insulin, C-peptide, and proinsulin levels in non-diabetic and type II diabetic individuals with comparison to immunoassay. J Biol Chem 1997;272:12513-22.
133. Kitzmiller JL, Gavin LA, Gin GD, Jovanovic-Peterson L, Main EK, Zigrang WD. Preconception care of diabetes: glycemic control prevents congenital anomalies. JAMA 1991;265:731-6.
134. Kjems LL, Roder ME, Dinesen B, Hartling SG, Jorgensen PN, Binder C. Highly sensitive enzyme immunoassay of proinsulin immunoreactivity with use of two monoclonal antibodies. Clin Chem 1993;39:2146-50.
135. Kjos SL, Buchanan TA. Gestational diabetes mellitus. N Engl J Med 1999;341:1749-56.
136. Knowler WC, Barrett-Connor E, Fowler SE, Hamman RF, Lachin JM, Walker EA, et al. Reduction in the incidence of type 2 diabetes with lifestyle intervention or metformin. N Engl J Med 2002;346:393-403.
137. Kobold U, Jeppsson JO, Dulffer T, Finke A, Hoelzel W, Miedema K. Candidate reference methods for hemoglobin A1c based on peptide mapping. Clin Chem 1997;43:1944-51.

138. Kojima H, Fujimiya M, Matsumura K, Younan P, Imaeda H, Maeda M, et al. NeuroD-betacellulin gene therapy induces islet neogenesis in the liver and reverses diabetes in mice. Nat Med 2003;9:596-603.
139. Kouzuma T, Uemastu Y, Usami T, Imamura S. Study of glycated amino acid elimination reaction for an improved enzymatic glycated albumin measurement method. Clin Chim Acta 2004;346:135-43.
140. Kulkarni RN, Bruning JC, Winnay JN, Postic C, Magnuson MA, Kahn CR. Tissue-specific knockout of the insulin receptor in pancreatic beta cells creates an insulin secretory defect similar to that in type 2 diabetes. Cell 1999;96:329-39.
141. Kuusisto J, Mykkanen L, Pyorala K, Laakso M. Hyperinsulinemic microalbuminuria: a new risk indicator for coronary heart disease. Circulation 1995;91:831-7.
142. Laffel L. Ketone bodies: a review of physiology, pathophysiology and application of monitoring to diabetes. Diabetes Metab Res Rev 1999; 15:412-26.
143. Leahy JL. Natural history of beta-cell dysfunction in NIDDM. Diabetes Care 1990;13:992-1010.
144. Lefebvre PJ. Glucagon and its family revisited. Diabetes Care 1995;18: 715-30.
145. Lin MJ, Hoke C, Ettinger B, Coyne RV. Technical performance evaluation of BM/Hitachi 747-200 serum fructosamine assay. Clin Chem 1996;42:244-8.
146. Little RR, Rohlfing CL, Tennill AL, Madsen RW, Polonsky KS, Myers GL, et al. Standardization of C-peptide measurements. Clin Chem 2008;54:1023-6.
146A. Little RR, Rohlfing CL, Sacks DB; National Glycohemoglobin Standardization Program (NGSP) Steering Committee. Status of hemoglobin A1c measurement and goals for improvement: from chaos to order for improving diabetes care. Clin Chem 2011;57:205-14.
147. Little RR, Rohlfing CL, Wiedmeyer HM, Myers GL, Sacks DB, Goldstein DE. The national glycohemoglobin standardization program: a five-year progress report. Clin Chem 2001;47:1985-92.
148. Little RR, Sacks DB. HbA1c: how do we measure it and what does it mean? Curr Opin Endocrinol Diabetes Obes 2009;16:113-8.
149. Luopajarvi K, Savilahti E, Virtanen SM, Ilonen J, Knip M, Akerblom HK, et al. Enhanced levels of cow's milk antibodies in infancy in children who develop type 1 diabetes later in childhood. Pediatr Diabetes 2008;9:434-41.
150. Manley SE, Stratton IM, Clark PM, Luzio SD. Comparison of 11 human insulin assays: implications for clinical investigation and research. Clin Chem 2007;53:922-32.
151. Maquart FX, Gillery P, Bernard JF, Mante JP, Borel JP. A method for specifically measuring haemoglobin AIC with a disposable commercial ion-exchange column. Clin Chim Acta 1980;108:329-32.
152. Marcovina S, Bowsher RR, Miller WG, Staten M, Myers G, Caudill SP, et al. Standardization of insulin immunoassays: report of the American Diabetes Association Workgroup. Clin Chem 2007;53:711-6.
153. Marshall SM, Shearing PA, Alberti KG. Micral-test strips evaluated for screening for albuminuria. Clin Chem 1992;38:588-91.
154. Martin CL, Albers J, Herman WH, Cleary P, Waberski B, Greene DA, et al. Neuropathy among the Diabetes Control and Complications Trial cohort 8 years after trial completion. Diabetes Care 2006;29: 340-4.
155. Medcalf E, Newman DJ, Gorman EG. Rapid latex-enhanced turbidimetric assay for urine albumin. Ann Clin Biochem 1988;25(suppl):1645-55.
156. Meigs JB, Shrader P, Sullivan LM, McAteer JB, Fox CS, Dupuis J, et al. Genotype score in addition to common risk factors for prediction of type 2 diabetes. N Engl J Med 2008;359:2208-19.
157. Metzger BE, Buchanan TA, Coustan DR, de Leiva A, Dunger DB, Hadden DR, et al. Summary and recommendations of the Fifth International Workshop Conference on Gestational Diabetes Mellitus. Diabetes Care 2007;30(suppl 2):S251-60.
158. Metzger BE, Coustan DR. Summary and recommendations of the Fourth International Workshop–Conference on Gestational Diabetes Mellitus. The Organizing Committee. Diabetes Care 1998;21:B161-7.
159. Metzger BE, Lowe LP, Dyer AR, Trimble ER, Chaovarindr U, Coustan DR, et al. Hyperglycemia and adverse pregnancy outcomes. N Engl J Med 2008;358:1991-2002.
160. Miller WG, Thienpont LM, Van Uytfanghe K, Clark PM, Lindstedt P, Nilsson G, et al. Toward standardization of insulin immunoassays. Clin Chem 2009;55:1011-8.
161. Mills JL, Knopp RH, Simpson JL, Jovanovic-Peterson L, Metzger BE, Holmes LB, et al. Lack of relation of increased malformation rates in infants of diabetic mothers to glycemic control during organogenesis. N Engl J Med 1988;318:671-6.
162. Mire-Sluis AR, Gaines Das R, Lernmark A. The World Health Organization International Collaborative Study for islet cell antibodies. Diabetologia 2000;43:1282-92.
163. Mogensen CE. Microalbuminuria, blood pressure and diabetic renal disease: origin and development of ideas. Diabetologia 1999;42:263-85.
164. Molitch ME, DeFronzo RA, Franz MJ, Keane WF, Mogensen CE, Parving HH. Diabetic nephropathy. Diabetes Care 2003;26(suppl 1): S94-8.
165. Morris LR, McGee JA, Kitabchi AE. Correlation between plasma and urine glucose in diabetes. Ann Intern Med 1981;94:469-71.
166. Mullins RE, Austin GE. Sensitivity of isoelectric focusing, ion exchange, and affinity chromatography to labile glycated hemoglobin. Clin Chem 1986;32:1460-3.
167. Nagi DK, Hendra TJ, Ryle AJ, Cooper TM, Temple RC, Clark PM, et al. The relationships of concentrations of insulin, intact proinsulin and 32-33 split proinsulin with cardiovascular risk factors in type 2 (non-insulin-dependent) diabetic subjects. Diabetologia 1990;33:532-7.
168. Nathan D. The importance of intensive supervision in determining the efficacy of insulin pump therapy. Diabetes Care 1983;6:295-7.
169. Nathan DM. Long-term complications of diabetes mellitus. N Engl J Med 1993;328:1676-85.
170. Nathan DM, Cleary PA, Backlund JY, Genuth SM, Lachin JM, Orchard TJ, et al. Intensive diabetes treatment and cardiovascular disease in patients with type 1 diabetes. N Engl J Med 2005;353: 2643-53.
171. Nathan DM, Kuenen J, Borg R, Zheng H, Schoenfeld D, Heine RJ. Translating the hemoglobin A1c assay into estimated average glucose values. Diabetes Care 2008;31:1473-8.
172. Naylor CD, Sermer M, Chen E, Sykora K. Cesarean delivery in relation to birth weight and gestational glucose tolerance: pathophysiology or practice style? Toronto Trihospital Gestational Diabetes Investigators. JAMA 1996;275:1165-70.
173. NCCLS. Point-of-care blood testing in acute and chronic care facilities: approved guideline, 2nd edition. CLSI document C30-A2. Wayne, Pa: NCCLS, 2002.
174. NCCLS. Classification and diagnosis of diabetes mellitus and other categories of glucose intolerance. National Diabetes Data Group. Diabetes 1979;28:1039-57.
175. Neel JV. Diabetes mellitus: a geneticist's nightmare. In Creutzfeldt W, Kobberling J, Neel JV, eds. The genetics of diabetes. New York, NY: Springer Verlag, 1976:1-11.
176. Notkins AL. Immunologic and genetic factors in type 1 diabetes. J Biol Chem 2002;277:43545-8.
177. Novis DA, Jones BA. Interinstitutional comparison of bedside blood glucose monitoring program characteristics, accuracy performance, and quality control documentation: a College of American Pathologists Q-Probes study of bedside blood glucose monitoring performed in 226 small hospitals. Arch Pathol Lab Med 1998;122: 495-502.
178. O'Rahilly S, Turner RC, Matthews DR. Impaired pulsatile secretion of insulin in relatives of patients with non-insulin-dependent diabetes. N Engl J Med 1988;318:1225-30.
179. Orci L, Vassalli JD, Perrelet A. The insulin factory. Sci Am 1988;259: 85-94.
180. Ostrega D, Polonsky K, Nagi D, Yudkin J, Cox LJ, Clark PM, et al. Measurement of proinsulin and intermediates: validation of immunoassay methods by high-performance liquid chromatography. Diabetes 1995;44:437-40.

181. O'Sullivan JB, Mahan CM. Criteria for the oral glucose tolerance test in pregnancy. Diabetes 1964;13:278-85.
182. Pani LN, Korenda L, Meigs JB, Driver C, Chamany S, Fox CS, et al. Effect of aging on A1C levels in individuals without diabetes: evidence from the Framingham Offspring Study and the National Health and Nutrition Examination Survey 2001-2004. Diabetes Care 2008;31: 1991-6.
183. Pawson T. Specificity in signal transduction: from phosphotyrosine-SH2 domain interactions to complex cellular systems. Cell 2004;116:191-203.
184. Pfeifer MA, Halter JB, Porte D Jr. Insulin secretion in diabetes mellitus. Am J Med 1981;70:579-88.
185. Phillipou G, James SK, Seaborn CJ, Phillips PJ. Screening for microalbuminuria by use of a rapid, low-cost colorimetric assay. Clin Chem 1989;35:456-8.
186. Polonsky K, Frank B, Pugh W, Addis A, Karrison T, Meier P, et al. The limitations to and valid use of C-peptide as a marker of the secretion of insulin. Diabetes 1986;35:379-86.
187. Porter WH, Yao HH, Karounos DG. Laboratory and clinical evaluation of assays for beta-hydroxybutyrate. Am J Clin Pathol 1997;107:353-8.
188. Pozzilli P, Di Mario U. Autoimmune diabetes not requiring insulin at diagnosis (latent autoimmune diabetes of the adult): definition, characterization, and potential prevention. Diabetes Care 2001;24: 1460-7.
189. Radermecker RP, Renard E, Scheen AJ. Circulating insulin antibodies: influence of continuous subcutaneous or intraperitoneal insulin infusion, and impact on glucose control. Diabetes Metab Res Rev 2009;25:409-501.
190. Rajpathak SN, Gunter MJ, Wylie-Rosett J, Ho GY, Kaplan RC, Muzumdar R, et al. The role of insulin-like growth factor-I and its binding proteins in glucose homeostasis and type 2 diabetes. Diabetes Metab Res Rev 2009;25:3-12.
191. Reaven GM. Banting Lecture 1988. Role of insulin resistance in human disease. Diabetes 1988;37:1595-607.
192. Reaven GM. The metabolic syndrome: requiescat in pace. Clin Chem 2005;51:931-8.
193. Reddi AS, Camerini-Davalos RA. Diabetic nephropathy: an update. Arch Intern Med 1990;150:31-43.
194. Reeves WG. Insulin antibody determination: theoretical and practical considerations. Diabetologia 1983;24:399-403.
195. Rhodes CJ, Alarcon C. What beta-cell defect could lead to hyperproinsulinemia in NIDDM? Some clues from recent advances made in understanding the proinsulin-processing mechanism. Diabetes 1994;43:511-7.
196. Rhodes CJ, White MF. Molecular insights into insulin action and secretion. Eur J Clin Invest 2002;32(suppl 3):3-13.
197. Robbins DC, Andersen L, Bowsher R, Chance R, Dinesen B, Frank B, et al. Report of the American Diabetes Association's Task Force on standardization of the insulin assay. Diabetes 1996;45:242-56.
198. Robbins DC, Tager HS, Rubenstein AH. Biologic and clinical importance of proinsulin. N Engl J Med 1984;310:1165-75.
199. Rogatsky E, Balent B, Goswami G, Tomuta V, Jayatillake H, Cruikshank G, et al. Sensitive quantitative analysis of C-peptide in human plasma by 2-dimensional liquid chromatography-mass spectrometry isotope-dilution assay. Clin Chem 2006;52:872-9.
200. Rohlfing C, Wiedmeyer HM, Little R, Grotz VL, Tennill A, England J, et al. Biological variation of glycohemoglobin. Clin Chem 2002;48:1116-8.
201. Sacks DB. Implications of the revised criteria for diagnosis and classification of diabetes mellitus. Clin Chem 1997;43:2230-2.
202. Sacks DB. Translating hemoglobin A1c into average blood glucose: implications for clinical chemistry. Clin Chem 2008;54:1756-8.
203. Sacks DB. The diagnosis of diabetes is changing: how implementation of hemoglobin A1c will impact clinical laboratories. Clin Chem 2009;55:1612-4.
203A. Sacks DB, Arnold M, Bakris GL, Bruns DE, Horvath AR, Kirkman MS, et al.Guidelines and recommendations for laboratory analysis in the diagnosis and management of diabetes mellitus. Clin Chem. 2011;57(6):e1-e47. Epub 2011 May 26.
203B. Sacks DB, Arnold M, Bakris GL, Bruns DE, Horvath AR, Kirkman MS, et al. Position statement executive summary: guidelines and recommendations for laboratory analysis in the diagnosis and management of diabetes mellitus. Diabetes Care. 2011 ;34(6):1419-23.
203C. Sacks DB, Arnold M, Bakris GL, Bruns DE, Horvath AR, Kirkman MS, et al. Guidelines and recommendations for laboratory analysis in the diagnosis and management of diabetes mellitus. Diabetes Care. 2011;34(6):e61-99.
204. Sacks DB, Bruns DE, Goldstein DE, Maclaren NK, McDonald JM, Parrott M. Guidelines and recommendations for laboratory analysis in the diagnosis and management of diabetes mellitus. Clin Chem 2002;48:436-72.
205. Sacks DB, Lernmark A. Molecular manipulation of autoantibody testing in type 1 diabetes: two for one. Clin Chem 2001;47:803-4.
206. Sacks DB, McDonald JM. The pathogenesis of type II diabetes mellitus: a polygenic disease. Am J Clin Pathol 1996;105:149-56.
207. Samani AA, Yakar S, LeRoith D, Brodt P. The role of the IGF system in cancer growth and metastasis: overview and recent insights. Endocr Rev 2007;28:20-47.
208. Santiago JV. Lessons from the Diabetes Control and Complications Trial. Diabetes 1993;42:1549-54.
209. Scheepers A, Joost HG, Schurmann A. The glucose transporter families SGLT and GLUT: molecular basis of normal and aberrant function. JPEN J Parenter Enteral Nutr 2004;28:364-71.
210. Schiffrin A, Belmonte M. Multiple daily self-glucose monitoring: its essential role in long-term glucose control in insulin-dependent diabetic patients treated with pump and multiple subcutaneous injections. Diabetes Care 1982;5:479-84.
211. Schleicher E, Wieland OH. Specific quantitation by HPLC of protein (lysine) bound glucose in human serum albumin and other glycosylated proteins. J Clin Chem Clin Biochem 1981;19:81-7.
212. Schleicher ED, Mayer R, Wagner EM, Gerbitz KD. Is serum fructosamine assay specific for determination of glycated serum protein? Clin Chem 1988;34:320-3.
213. Schleicher ED, Vogt BW. Standardization of serum fructosamine assays. Clin Chem 1990;36:136-9.
214. Schmidli RS, Colman PG, Bonifacio E. Disease sensitivity and specificity of 52 assays for glutamic acid decarboxylase antibodies. The Second International GADAB Workshop. Diabetes 1995;44: 636-40.
215. Schosinsky KH, Vargas M, Luz Esquivel A, Chavarria MA. Simple spectrophotometric determination of urinary albumin by dye-binding with use of bromphenol blue. Clin Chem 1987;33:223-6.
216. Scott MG, Bruns DE, Boyd JC, Sacks DB. Tight glucose control in the intensive care unit: are glucose meters up to the task? Clin Chem 2009;55:18-20.
217. Shapiro ET, Bell GI, Polonsky KS, Rubenstein AH, Kew MC, Tager HS. Tumor hypoglycemia: relationship to high molecular weight insulin-like growth factor-II. J Clin Invest 1990;85:1672-9.
218. Sheetz MJ, King GL. Molecular understanding of hyperglycemia's adverse effects for diabetic complications. JAMA 2002;288:2579-88.
219. Sherr J, Sosenko J, Skyler JS, Herold KC. Prevention of type 1 diabetes: the time has come. Nat Clin Pract Endocrinol Metab 2008;4:334-43.
220. Simon M, Hoover JD. Effect of sample instability on glycohemoglobin (HbA1) measured by cation-exchange chromatography. Clin Chem 1982;28:195-8.
221. Skyler JS, Krischer JP, Wolfsdorf J, Cowie C, Palmer JP, Greenbaum C, et al. Effects of oral insulin in relatives of patients with type 1 diabetes: the Diabetes Prevention Trial—type 1. Diabetes Care 2005;28:1068-76.
222. SMBG International Working Group. Self-monitoring of blood glucose in type 2 diabetes: an inter-country comparison. Diabetes Res Clin Pract 2008;82:e15-8.
223. Sobey WJ, Beer SF, Carrington CA, Clark PM, Frank BH, Gray IP, et al. Sensitive and specific two-site immunoradiometric assays for

human insulin, proinsulin, 65-66 split and 32-33 split proinsulins. Biochem J 1989;260:535-41.
224. Stolerman ES, Florez JC. Genomics of type 2 diabetes mellitus: implications for the clinician. Nat Rev Endocrinol 2009;5:429-36.
225. Summary and recommendations of the Second International Workshop-Conference on Gestational Diabetes Mellitus. Diabetes 1985;34(suppl 2):123-6.
226. Swinn RA, Wareham NJ, Gregory R, Curling V, Clark PM, Dalton KJ, et al. Excessive secretion of insulin precursors characterizes and predicts gestational diabetes. Diabetes 1995;44:911-5.
227. Tahara Y, Shima K. Kinetics of HbA1c, glycated albumin, and fructosamine and analysis of their weight functions against preceding plasma glucose level. Diabetes Care 1995;18:440-7.
228. Tamada JA, Garg S, Jovanovic L, Pitzer KR, Fermi S, Potts RO. Noninvasive glucose monitoring: comprehensive clinical results. Cygnus Research Team. JAMA 1999;282:1839-44.
229. Tamborlane WV, Beck RW, Bode BW, Buckingham B, Chase HP, Clemons R, et al. Continuous glucose monitoring and intensive treatment of type 1 diabetes. N Engl J Med 2008;359:1464-76.
230. Tang Z, Du X, Louie RF, Kost GJ. Effects of drugs on glucose measurements with handheld glucose meters and a portable glucose analyzer. Am J Clin Pathol 2000;113:75-86.
231. Taniguchi CM, Emanuelli B, Kahn CR. Critical nodes in signalling pathways: insights into insulin action. Nat Rev Mol Cell Biol 2006;7: 85-96.
232. Tate PF, Clements CA, Walters JE. Accuracy of home blood glucose monitors. Diabetes Care 1992;15:536-8.
233. Taylor R, Zimmet P. Limitation of fasting plasma glucose for the diagnosis of diabetes mellitus. Diabetes Care 1981;4:556-8.
234. Temple RC, Carrington CA, Luzio SD, Owens DR, Schneider AE, Sobey WJ, et al. Insulin deficiency in non-insulin-dependent diabetes. Lancet 1989;1:293-5.
235. The International Expert Committee. International Expert Committee report on the role of the A1c assay in the diagnosis of diabetes. Diabetes Care 2009;32:1327-34.
236. Thomas GH, Howell RR. Selected screening tests for genetic metabolic diseases. Chicago: Year Book Medical Publishers, 1973.
237. Tillil H, Shapiro ET, Given BD, Rue P, Rubenstein AH, Galloway JA, et al. Reevaluation of urine C-peptide as measure of insulin secretion. Diabetes 1988;37:1195-201.
238. Todd JA. Genetic analysis of type 1 diabetes using whole genome approaches. Proc Natl Acad Sci U S A 1995;92:8560-5.
239. Torn C, Mueller PW, Schlosser M, Bonifacio E, Bingley PJ. Diabetes antibody standardization program: evaluation of assays for autoantibodies to glutamic acid decarboxylase and islet antigen-2. Diabetologia 2008;51:846-52.
240. Townsend JC. A competitive immunoenzymometric assay for albumin in urine. Clin Chem 1986;32:1372-4.
241. Tuomilehto J, Lindstrom J, Eriksson JG, Valle TT, Hamalainen H, Ilanne-Parikka P, et al. Prevention of type 2 diabetes mellitus by changes in lifestyle among subjects with impaired glucose tolerance. N Engl J Med 2001;344:1343-50.
242. U.K. Prospective Diabetes Study (UKPDS) Group. Intensive blood-glucose control with sulphonylureas or insulin compared with conventional treatment and risk of complications in patients with type 2 diabetes (UKPDS 33). U.K. Prospective Diabetes Study (UKPDS) Group. Lancet 1998;352:837-53.
243. Umpierrez GE, Watts NB, Phillips LS. Clinical utility of beta-hydroxybutyrate determined by reflectance meter in the management of diabetic ketoacidosis. Diabetes Care 1995;18:137-8.
244. Urdang M, Ansede-Luna G, Muller B, Newson R, Lacy-Pettit A, O'Shea D. An independent pilot study into the accuracy and reliability of home blood glucose monitors. Lancet 1999;353: 1065-6.
245. van den Berghe G, Wouters P, Weekers F, Verwaest C, Bruyninckx F, Schetz M, et al. Intensive insulin therapy in the critically ill patients. N Engl J Med 2001;345:1359-67.
246. Wang Y, Dou C, Yuan C, Datta A. Development of an automated enzymatic assay for the determination of glycated serum protein in human serum. Clin Chem 2005;51:1991-2.
247. Ward WK, Paquette TL, Frank BH, Porte D Jr. A sensitive radioimmunoassay for human proinsulin, with sequential use of antisera to C-peptide and insulin. Clin Chem 1986;32:728-33.
248. Watts GF, Bennett JE, Rowe DJ, Morris RW, Gatling W, Shaw KM, et al. Assessment of immunochemical methods for determining low concentrations of albumin in urine. Clin Chem 1986;32:1544-8.
249. Weitgasser R, Gappmayer B, Pichler M. Newer portable glucose meters—analytical improvement compared with previous generation devices? Clin Chem 1999;45:1821-5.
250. Welschen LM, Bloemendal E, Nijpels G, Dekker JM, Heine RJ, Stalman WA, et al. Self-monitoring of blood glucose in patients with type 2 diabetes who are not using insulin: a systematic review. Diabetes Care 2005;28:1510-7.
251. Wenzlau JM, Juhl K, Yu L, Moua O, Sarkar SA, Gottlieb P, et al. The cation efflux transporter ZnT8 (Slc30A8) is a major autoantigen in human type 1 diabetes. Proc Natl Acad Sci U S A 2007;104:17040-5.
252. Wermers RA, Fatourechi V, Wynne AG, Kvols LK, Lloyd RV. The glucagonoma syndrome: clinical and pathologic features in 21 patients. Medicine (Baltimore) 1996;75:53-63.
253. Weykamp C, John WG, Mosca A, Hoshino T, Little R, Jeppsson J, et al. The IFCC reference measurement system for HbA1c: a 6-year progress report. Clin Chem 2008;54:240-8.
254. Weykamp CW, Penders TJ, Miedema K, Muskiet FA, van der Slik W. Standardization of glycohemoglobin results and reference values in whole blood studied in 103 laboratories using 20 methods. Clin Chem 1995;41:82-6.
255. Wiener K. What is 75g of glucose? Ann Clin Biochem 1990;27(Pt 4): 283-4.
256. Wiener K, Roberts NB. Age does not influence levels of HbA1c in normal subject. Q J Med 1999;92:169-73.
257. Wiener RS, Wiener DC, Larson RJ. Benefits and risks of tight glucose control in critically ill adults: a meta-analysis. JAMA 2008;300:933-44.
258. Wiggam MI, O'Kane MJ, Harper R, Atkinson AB, Hadden DR, Trimble ER, et al. Treatment of diabetic ketoacidosis using normalization of blood 3-hydroxybutyrate concentration as the endpoint of emergency management: a randomized controlled study. Diabetes Care 1997;20:1347-52.
259. Wilson DH, Bogacz JP, Forsythe CM, Turk PJ, Lane TL, Gates RC, et al. Fully automated assay of glycohemoglobin with the Abbott IMx analyzer: novel approaches for separation and detection. Clin Chem 1993;39:2090-7.
260. Windeler J, Kobberling J. The fructosamine assay in diagnosis and control of diabetes mellitus scientific evidence for its clinical usefulness? J Clin Chem Clin Biochem 1990;28:129-38.
261. Witte EC, Lambers Heerspink HJ, de Zeeuw D, Bakker SJ, de Jong PE, Gansevoort R. First morning voids are more reliable than spot urine samples to assess microalbuminuria. J Am Soc Nephrol 2009;20: 436-43.
262. Woo J, Floyd M, Cannon DC, Kahan B. Radioimmunoassay for urinary albumin. Clin Chem 1978;24:1464-7.
263. Wood IS, Trayhurn P. Glucose transporters (GLUT and SGLT): expanded families of sugar transport proteins. Br J Nutr 2003;89:3-9.
264. World Health Organization. Definition, diagnosis and classification of diabetes mellitus and its complications: report of a WHO consultation. Part 1. Diagnosis and classification of diabetes mellitus. Geneva, Switzerland: World Health Organization, 1999.
265. World Health Organization. Definition and diagnosis of diabetes mellitus and intermediate hyperglycemia: report of a WHO/IDF consultation. Geneva, Switzerland: World Health Organization, 2006.
266. Yatscoff RW, Tevaarwerk GJ, MacDonald JC. Quantification of nonenzymically glycated albumin and total serum protein by affinity chromatography. Clin Chem 1984;30:446-9.
267. Zimmet P, Alberti KG, Shaw J. Global and societal implications of the diabetes epidemic. Nature 2001;414:782-7.

CHAPTER 47

Cardiac Function

Fred S. Apple, Ph.D., Jens Peter Goetze, M.D., D.M.Sc., and Allan S. Jaffe, M.D.

Although the heart is an efficient and durable pump, a variety of pathologies are known to diminish cardiac function, possibly leading to a multiplicity of dysfunctional clinical states. Heart failure, which is increasing as we improve the treatment of acute ischemic heart disease, and acute ischemic heart disease itself are the most common cardiac diseases that rely on a biochemical diagnosis and thus will be the focus of this chapter.[41]

The term *acute myocardial infarction (AMI)* refers to a situation in which death of myocytes is due to an imbalance between myocardial oxygen supply and demand. When the blood supply to the heart is interrupted, "gross necrosis" of the myocardium results. In addition, a substantial number of cells die as the result of apoptosis. Such extensive damage is most often associated with a thrombotic occlusion superimposed on coronary atherosclerosis. Initially, it was thought that the population of myocytes was fixed; however, it is now believed that the migration of a variety of precursor stem cells has the potential at least to replace some of the damaged myocytes. It is now thought that the process of plaque rupture or erosion and thrombosis is one of the ways in which coronary atherosclerosis progresses, and that we recognize only more severe events.[283,284] Total loss of coronary blood flow results in a clinical syndrome associated with what is known as ST segment elevation AMI (STE AMI). Partial loss of coronary perfusion if severe can lead to necrosis as well, which is generally less severe and is known as NSTEMI (non–ST elevation myocardial infarction). Other events of still lesser severity may be missed entirely or may be called *angina,* which can range from stable to unstable.

In the United States, approximately 700,000 patients suffer from an initial AMI annually and another 500,000 from recurrent AMI. Coronary heart disease causes 20% of all deaths in the United States, and cardiovascular disease causes up to 38.5% of all mortality in the United States. About 1.7 million patients are hospitalized each year in the United States with acute coronary syndrome (ACS). Historically, most deaths caused by ischemic heart disease were acute, but as our therapeutic abilities have increased, the disease is becoming more chronic. Deaths that occur acutely result from ventricular arrhythmias or pump dysfunction and congestive heart failure with or without cardiogenic shock. Death rates are sharply age dependent, both during hospitalization and in the year following infarction. In the United States, the yearly economic burden of coronary artery disease (CAD) is in excess of $133.2 billion—more than a third of the total of $503.2 billion attributed to cardiovascular disease overall.

Before the advent of coronary care units, treatment of AMI was directed toward allowing healing of the infarcted area. The concept that infarctions evolve over time and that their size can be moderated led to rethinking of this passive philosophy.[319] We now know that re-establishment of perfusion reduces the extent of myocardial injury and is an important determinant of prognosis.[330] Today the management of AMI suggested by most guidelines is aggressive and invasively oriented in the hope of reducing the extent of myocardial damage and thus improving prognosis.[63A,67] In addition, prevention is finally being recognized as a key element in the long-term treatment of patients with atherosclerosis.

BASIC ANATOMY

The average human adult heart weighs approximately 325 g in men and 275 g in women and is 12 cm in length. The heart is a hollow muscular organ, shaped like a blunt cone, and is about the size of a human fist. It is located in the mediastinum, between the lower lobes of each lung, and rests upon the diaphragm. It is enclosed in a sac called the *pericardium.* The cardiac wall is composed of three layers: the *epicardium,* which is the outermost layer; a middle layer; and an inner layer, called the *endocardium.* The heart has four chambers. The two upper chambers are termed the *right* and *left atria,* and the two lower chambers are termed the *right* and *left ventricles* (Figure 47-1). Under normal circumstances, the atria are compliant structures, so that intracavitary pressure is low. When anatomy is normal, each atrium is connected to its ventricle through an atrioventricular (AV) valve, which opens and closes (see discussion later in this chapter). The valve on the left side is called the *mitral valve* and the one on the right side, the *tricuspid valve.* The right ventricle is banana shaped and pumps blood into the *pulmonary artery* through a tri-leaflet *pulmonic valve.* The left ventricle pumps blood into the *aorta* through a tri-leaflet *aortic valve.* The ventricles, especially the left ventricle, are thicker and less compliant in keeping with the need to generate higher pressures than the right ventricle, and intercavitary pressures are much higher

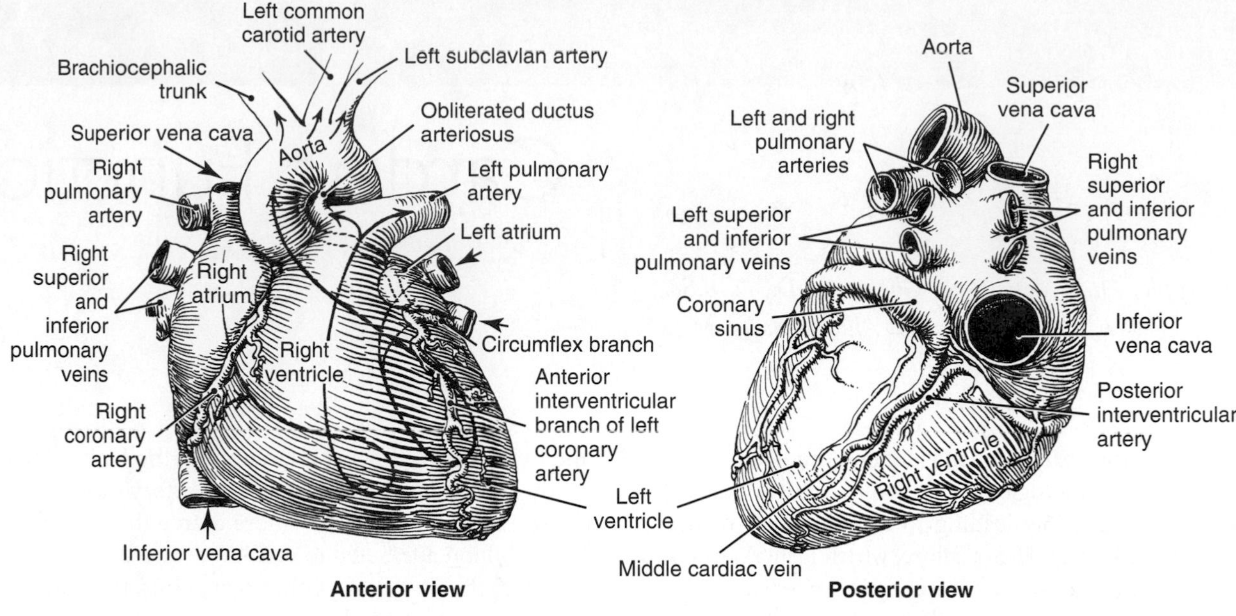

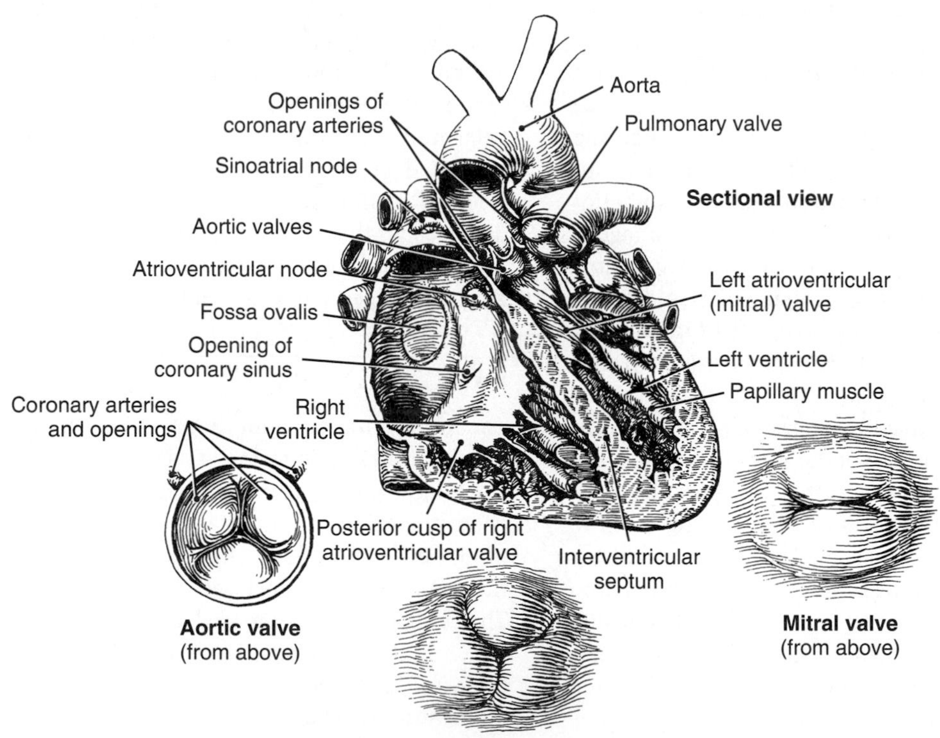

Figure 47-1 Anatomy of the heart. *(From Dorland's illustrated medical dictionary, 30th edition. Philadelphia, Pa: WB Saunders, 2003:Panel 20.)*

than in the atria. Under normal conditions, the conduction or electrical system of the heart coordinates the sequential contraction of first the atria and then the ventricles. Given that they are connected, each side can affect the other. Under normal circumstances, the sequence of activation optimizes this interaction and thus the efficiency of cardiac function. The right and left coronary arteries originate from two of three cusps of the aortic valve. They provide blood flow and thus nutritive perfusion to the heart. The largest vessels are on the epicardium, and these can be accessed therapeutically fairly easily. Subsequent smaller branches divide to supply the remaining myocardium. The endocardium is the layer most susceptible to ischemia because its perfusion relies on the smallest vessels.

The myocardium contains bundles of striated muscle fibers, each of which is typically 10 to 15 mm in diameter and

30 to 60 mm in length. Work of the heart is generated by the alternating of contraction and relaxation of these fibers. The fibers are composed of the cardiac-specific contractile proteins actin and myosin, and regulatory proteins called *troponins*. They also contain a variety of enzymes and proteins that are vital for energy use, such as myoglobin, creatine kinase (CK), and lactate dehydrogenase (LD), some of which can be used as markers of cardiac injury.

PHYSIOLOGY

Cardiac Cycle

A typical cardiac cycle consists of two intervals known as *systole* and *diastole* (Figure 47-2). During diastole, oxygenated blood returns from the lungs to the left atrium via the pulmonary veins, and deoxygenated blood returns from other parts of the body to fill the right atrium. During this period, the AV valves are open, allowing passive filling of the ventricle. At the end of diastole, the atria contract, forcing additional blood through the AV valves and into the respective ventricles. During systole, the ventricles contract. This closes the AV valves when ventricular pressure exceeds atrial pressure, and the pulmonary and aortic valves are opened when ventricular pressure exceeds pressure in the pulmonary arteries and/or the aorta, and blood flows into those conduits. During systole, a normal blood pressure in the aorta is typically 120 mm Hg; during diastole, it falls to about 70 mm Hg. At rest, the heart pumps between 60 and 80 times per minute. Stroke volume (i.e., the amount of blood expelled with each contraction) is roughly 50 mL, so cardiac output per minute is roughly 3 L. Typically, values are corrected for body surface area and are usually in the range of 2.5 to 3.6 L/min/m^2. Measurements of cardiac output and ventricular filling pressures are the standards for assessing cardiac performance and function. Furthermore, therapeutic intervention in patients with heart disease often includes assessment of cardiac output and ventricular pressures.

Cardiac Conducting System

The cardiac cycle is tightly controlled by the cardiac conducting system, which initiates electrical impulses and carries them, via a specialized conducting system, to the myocardium. The surface electrocardiogram (ECG) records changes in potential and is a graphic tracing of the variations in electrical potential caused by excitation of the heart muscle and detected at the body surface.[264] Clinically, the ECG is used to identify (1) anatomic, (2) metabolic, (3) ionic, and (4) hemodynamic changes in the heart. The clinical sensitivity and specificity of ECG abnormalities are influenced by a wide spectrum of physiologic and anatomic changes and by the clinical situation.

Under normal circumstances, cardiac cycles are similar and each includes three major components (Figure 47-3): atrial depolarization (the P wave), ventricular depolarization (the QRS complex), and repolarization (the ST segment and T wave). Atrial depolarization, which is depicted by the P wave, produces atrial contraction. Ventricular depolarization, marked by the QRS complex, produces contraction of the ventricles. It is composed of as many as three deflections: (1) the Q wave, which when present is the first negative deflection; (2) the R wave, which is the first positive deflection; and (3) the S wave, which is a negative deflection following the R wave. On occasion, there is an R prime, which is a second positive deflection. Whether each of these occurs depends on the path of depolarization of the ventricles, as does the significance. Thus not every QRS complex will have discrete Q, R, and S waves. The ST segment and the T wave are produced by electrical recovery of the ventricles, and their mean electrical vector is under normal circumstances concordant (i.e., in roughly the same direction) with the mean QRS vector.

A routine ECG is composed of 12 leads. Six are called limb leads (I, II, III, aVR, aVL, and aVF), because they are recorded between arm and leg electrodes; six are called precordial or chest leads (V_1, V_2, V_3, V_4, V_5, and V_6) and are recorded across the sternum and left precordium. Each lead records the same electrical impulse but in a different position relative to the heart. Areas of pathology shown on the ECG can be localized by analyzing differences between the tracing in question and what is known to be normal in the 12 different leads.

CARDIAC DISEASE

Cardiac disease occurs in many forms. This chapter briefly covers congestive heart failure (CHF) and acute coronary syndromes, such as AMI. The vast number of other cardiac diseases is not discussed in depth here because of the smaller role of clinical laboratory tests in these disorders.

Congestive Heart Failure

CHF is a syndrome characterized by ineffective pumping of the heart leading to an accumulation of fluid in the lungs. Typically, it results from loss of cardiac tissue and subsequent function.[88] Medically, it is defined as the pathophysiologic condition in which an abnormality of cardiac function is responsible for failure of the heart to pump sufficient blood to satisfy the requirements of metabolizing tissues. Encompassed in this definition are a wide spectrum of clinical conditions, ranging from (1) a primary impairment in pump function, such as might occur after a large AMI; (2) increased cardiac stiffness, which causes increased pressure in the heart, restricts filling, and increases hydrostatic pressures behind the area of reduced compliance; and (3) situations in which peripheral demand is excessive, resulting in what is known as high-output heart failure, which is defined as the inability of the heart to increase pumping sufficiently to meet the peripheral demands for blood.

Epidemiology

In the United States, CHF is the only cardiovascular disease with an increasing incidence. The National Heart, Lung, and Blood Institute estimates current prevalence at 4.9 million Americans with CHF, with an incidence of approximately 400,000 new cases each year.[171] CHF is the leading cause of

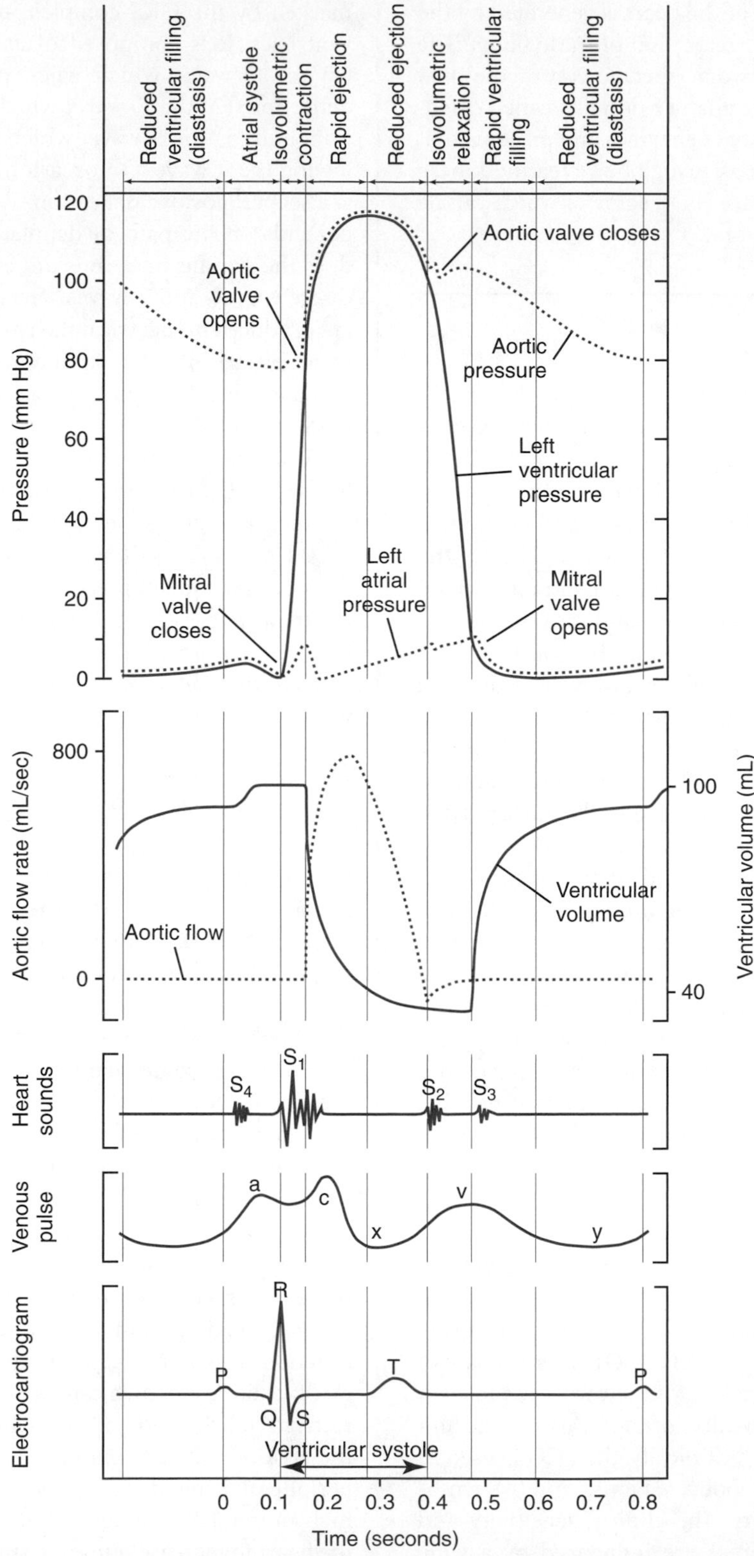

Figure 47-2 The cardiac cycle. *(From Dorland's illustrated medical dictionary, 30th edition. Philadelphia, Pa: WB Saunders, 2003, with permission from the National Kidney Foundation.)*

hospitalization in individuals 65 years of age and older. It has become clear that a larger component of heart failure is attributable to what has been called diastolic dysfunction, or heart failure (HF) with preserved ejection fraction (HFPEF). Therapeutic options for such patients are more limited than for those who have systolic abnormalities.[313] Current prognosis is dependent on disease severity, but overall it is poor. Five-year mortality is approximately 10% in mild CHF, 20 to 30% in moderate CHF, and up to 80% in end-stage disease.[205] These poor outcomes are not without substantial cost, estimated at $18.8 billion per year in the United States.

Currently, CHF patients are staged with the New York Heart Association (NYHA) functional classifications I to IV. Class I patients are generally considered asymptomatic, with no restrictions on physical activity; class IV patients are often symptomatic at rest, with severe limitations on physical activity. The problem with this classification system is that much of it is based on subjective criteria. Thus patients with comorbidities that reduce their activities are hard to classify. In addition, dyspnea, which is the primary symptom in many of these individuals, has many causes. Finally, many patients with ventricular dysfunction modify their activities to accomplish activities of daily living and thus lack overt symptoms until late in their disease. Thus patients with CHF often go

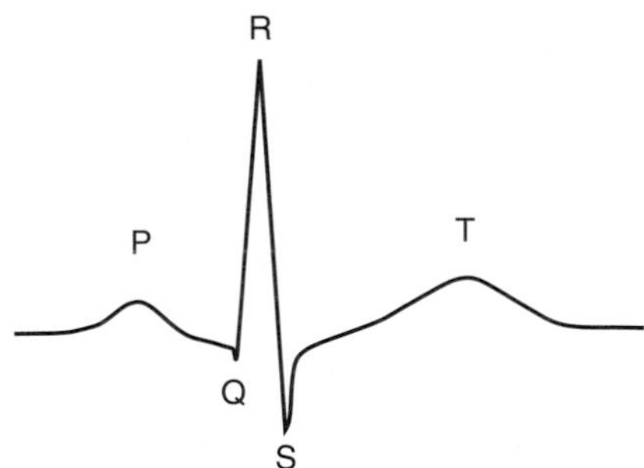

Figure 47-3 Electrocardiogram, serial tracing of a normal single heartbeat. Each beat manifests as five major waves: P, Q, R, S, and T. The QRS complex represents the ventricular contraction.

undiagnosed and untreated early in their disease or are misdiagnosed because of conditions such as pulmonary disease. Initiating treatment in the more advanced disease state (higher degree of irreversible cardiac function and patient deconditioning) is challenging and more expensive (often requiring extended inpatient stay) and leaves patients with considerable morbidity on a daily basis. Obviously, misdiagnoses often lead to patient morbidity.

Acute Coronary Syndrome

The term *acute coronary syndrome (ACS)* encompasses patients who present with unstable ischemic heart disease.[67] If they have ST segment elevation, they are called STEMI (Figure 47-4). Usually, but not always, these individuals will develop Q waves on their ECGs, hence the term *Q-wave MI*. If patients do not have STE but have biochemical criteria for cardiac injury, they are called NSTEMI, and most do not develop ECG Q waves. Those who have unstable ischemia and do not manifest necrosis are designated patients with unstable angina (UA). Most of these syndromes occur in response to an acute event in the coronary artery, when circulation to a region of the heart is obstructed for some reason. If the obstruction is high grade and persists, then necrosis usually ensues. Because necrosis is known to take some time to develop, it is apparent that opening the blocked coronary artery in a timely fashion can often prevent some of the death of myocardial tissue. This is clearly the case with STEMI. With non-STEMI [American Heart Association (AHA)/American College of Cardiology (ACC) guidelines], early but not immediate intervention is advocated, because most often the infarct-related coronary artery is not totally occluded, and thus immediate intervention is less necessary. These syndromes are usually but not always associated with chest discomfort (see discussion later in this chapter).[286]

The major cause of ACS is atherosclerosis, which contributes to significant narrowing of the artery lumen and a tendency for plaque disruption and thrombus formation.[67,283,284] Myocardial ischemia and infarction are usually segmental diseases. In up to 90% of patients with these diseases, focal

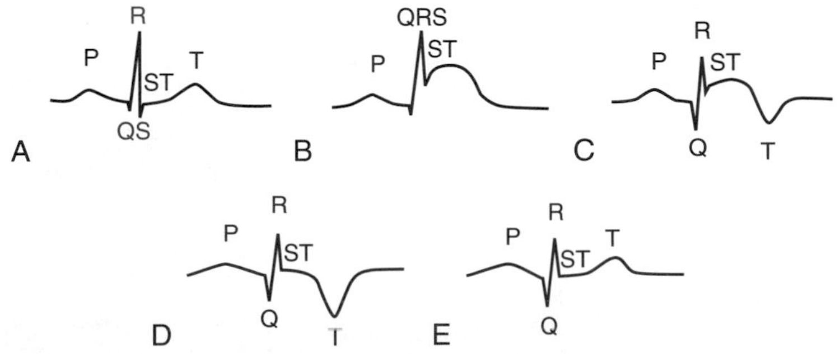

Figure 47-4 Electrocardiogram, serial tracing of a patient with an acute myocardial infarction. The sequence is (A) normal; (B) hours after infarction, the ST segment becomes elevated; (C) hours to days later, the T wave inverts and the Q wave becomes larger; (D) days to weeks later, the ST segment returns to near normal; and (E) weeks to months later, the T wave becomes upright again, but the large Q wave may remain.

occlusion of only one of the three large coronary vessels or branches occurs. The resulting impaired contractile performance of that segment occurs within seconds and is initially restricted to the affected segment(s). Myocardial ischemia and subsequent infarction usually begin in the endocardium and spread toward the epicardium.[319] The extent of myocardial injury reflects (1) the extent of occlusion, (2) the needs of the area deprived of perfusion, and (3) the duration of the imbalance in coronary supply. Irreversible cardiac injury consistently occurs in animals when the occlusion is complete for at least 15 to 20 minutes. Most damage occurs within the first 2 to 3 hours. Restoration of flow within the first 60 to 90 minutes evokes maximal salvage of tissue, but benefits of increased survival are possible up to 4 to 6 hours. In some situations, the restoration of coronary perfusion even later is of benefit.[330] The percentage of tissue at risk of necrosis (infarct size) depends on the amount of antegrade flow, the existing collateral flow, which is highly variable and difficult to predict, and the metabolic needs of the tissue.[246,328,366]

In almost all instances, the left ventricle is affected by AMI. However, with right coronary and/or circumflex occlusion, the right ventricle can also be involved, and there is a clinical syndrome in which damage to the right ventricle predominates and is the major determinant of hemodynamics. Coronary thrombi will undergo spontaneous lysis, even if untreated, in about 50% of cases within 10 days. However, for patients with STE AMI, opening the vessel earlier with clot-dissolving agents (thrombolysis) and/or percutaneous intervention can often save myocardium and lives (Figure 47-5). At present, immediate percutaneous intervention (PCI) with

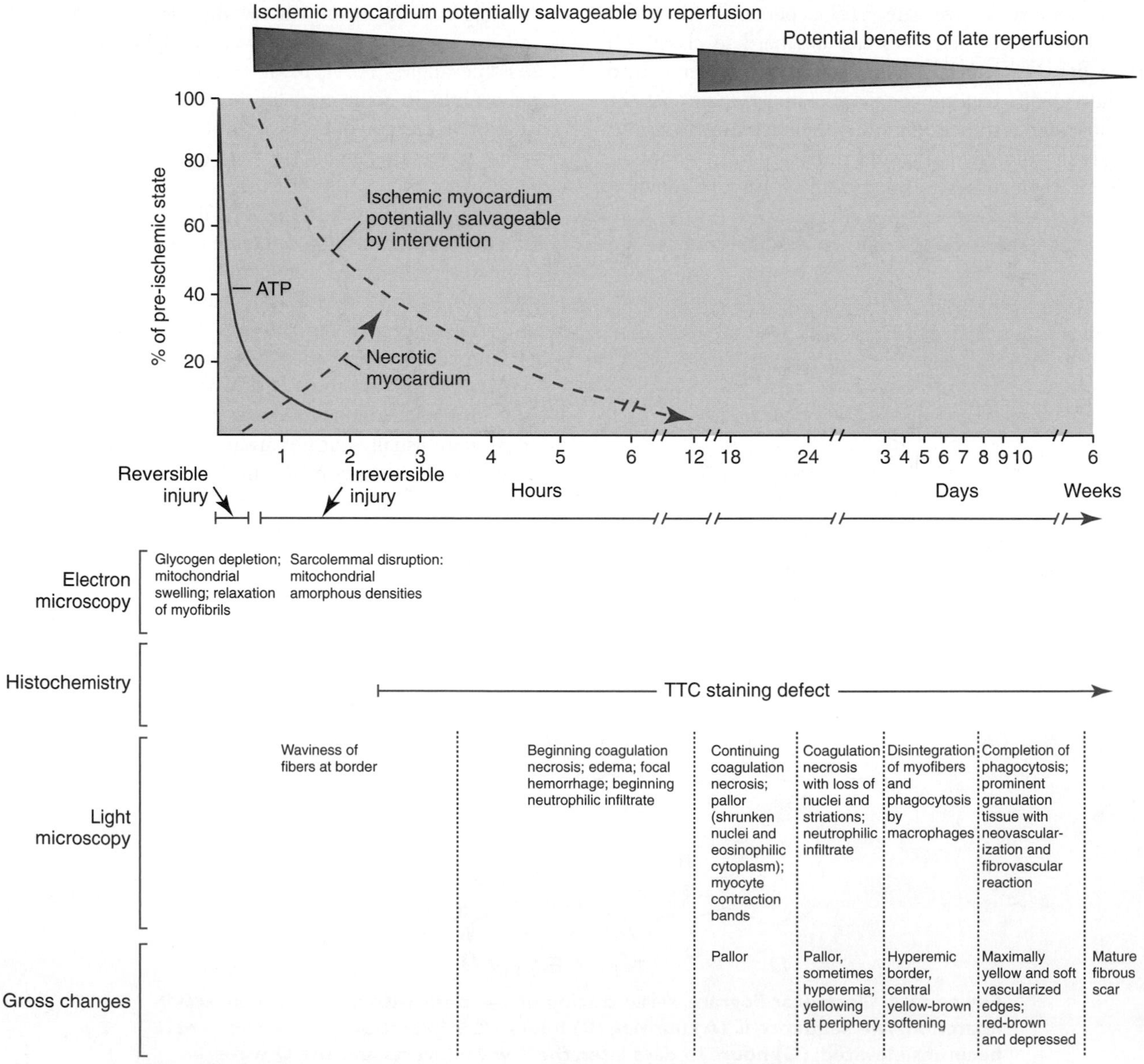

Figure 47-5 Temporal sequence of myocardial infarction. *(From Antman EM, Braunwald E. Acute myocardial infarction. In: Braunwald E, ed. Heart disease: a textbook of cardiovascular medicine, 5th edition. Philadelphia, Pa: WB Saunders, 1997:1189.)*

stenting is the preferred therapy for STE AMI. However, many hospitals cannot or do not offer urgent PCI 24 hours a day, 365 days per year. Thus clot-dissolving medications still play a major role in the treatment of these patients. In addition, it is now apparent that urgent but not necessarily immediate invasive revascularization benefits those with NSTEMI.[67] These individuals usually have only partial coronary occlusion and smaller amounts of cardiac damage acutely. However, untreated, repetitive episodes often eventually damage larger amounts of myocardium, leading to increased morbidity and mortality over time. Treatments such as newer anticoagulants and antiplatelet and anti-inflammatory agents, in conjunction with coronary revascularization, save lives in this group.

The prognosis for patients with ischemia but without necrosis is far better. Some studies based on biomarkers would suggest that in patients with no troponin elevation, interventional therapies may be harmful.[395] A major determinant of mortality and morbidity is the amount of myocardial damage that occurs. With STE AMI, most damage is acute, whereas with NSTEMI, damage may evolve as the result of repetitive events over many months; thus, interrupting the process improves survival.

Precipitating Factors

In many patients with AMI, no precipitating factor can be identified. Studies have noted the following patient activities at the onset of AMI: (1) heavy physical exertion, 13%; (2) modest or usual exertion, 18%; (3) surgical procedure, 6%; (4) rest, 51%; and (5) sleep, 8%. Exertion before infarction is somewhat more common among patients without preexisting angina than in those who have a history of angina.[342]

Causes of infarction other than acute atherothrombotic coronary occlusion have been identified. For example, prolonged vasospasm can induce infarction, and spontaneous dissection is becoming more commonly appreciated, especially in pregnant females.[67] In addition, it is now clear that some patients, particularly women, can have acute infarction with normal-appearing angiographic coronary arteries.[247] Other conditions (Box 47-1) can also cause the death of cardiomyocytes, leading to a biochemical signal (such as increased circulating concentrations of cardiac troponins) of myocyte damage, but these conditions should not be confused with myocardial infarction.[176] Pulmonary embolism (PE) is another common cause of biochemical elevations that is caused by right ventricular damage related to acute increases in wall stress and reduced subendocardial perfusion.[132,170,216]

Chronobiology

There is a pronounced periodicity for the time of onset of STE AMI.[68,115,342] Often an AMI occurs in the morning hours soon after arising; this is a period of (1) increasing adrenergic activity, (2) increased plasma fibrinogen levels, (3) increased inhibition of fibrinolysis, and (4) increased platelet adhesiveness. Studies have demonstrated that the early morning peak in MI parallels the peak incidence of death from ischemic heart disease, which occurs at about 8 AM to 9 AM. A second peak has been noted at approximately 5 PM. Diurnal differences affect many physiologic and biochemical parameters; the early morning hours are associated with rises in plasma catecholamines and cortisol and increases in platelet aggregability. Tissue plasminogen activator activity is low and plasminogen activator inhibitor activity is high during the early morning hours. Thus it is possible that some cyclic aspects of combined vasospastic, prothrombotic, and fibrinolytic factors, in the setting of preexisting atherosclerosis, lead to AMI. NSTEMI does not exhibit this diurnal pattern.

BOX 47-1 Elevation of Troponins Without Overt Ischemic Heart Disease

Trauma (including contusion, ablation, pacing, and cardioversion)
Congestive heart failure—acute and chronic*
Aortic valve disease and HOCM with significant LVH*
Hypertension
Hypotension, often with arrhythmias
Postoperative noncardiac surgery patients who seem to do well*
Renal failure*
Critically ill patients, especially those with diabetes, respiratory failure*
Drug toxicity (e.g., Adriamycin, 5-FU, herceptin, snake venoms)*
Hypothyroidism
Coronary vasospasm, including apical ballooning syndrome
Inflammatory disease (e.g., myocarditis, parvovirus B19, Kawasaki disease, sarcoid, smallpox vaccination)
Post-PCI patients whose condition appears to be uncomplicated*
Pulmonary embolism, severe pulmonary hypertension*
Sepsis*
Burns, especially if TBSA > 30%*
Infiltrative disease, including amyloidosis, hemochromatosis, sarcoidosis, and scleroderma*
Acute neurologic disease, including CVA, subarachnoid bleeds*
Rhabdomyolysis with cardiac injury
Transplant vasculopathy
Vital exhaustion

*Designation implies that prognostic information has been reported.
CVA, cerebrovascular accident; *5-FU,* 5-fluorouracil; *HOCM,* hypertrophic cardiomyopathy; *LVH,* left ventricular hypertrophy; *PCI,* percutaneous intervention; *TBSA,* total body surface area.

Prognosis

STE and non-STE infarctions have distinctly different short-term prognoses. STE AMI is associated with higher early and in-hospital mortality. It is said that mortality associated with STE AMI can occur up to 6 months post event, but the vast majority (at least two thirds) occur during the first 30 or 40 days. It is this risk that coronary recanalization seems to benefit. NSTE AMI is associated with lower acute mortality and complication rates but a longer period of vulnerability to reinfarction and death. As a result, 1- to 2-year survival rates are similar to those for STEMI.[67] This is why intervention has been so effective in this group.

Clinical History

The clinical history remains of substantial value in establishing a diagnosis.[330] A prodromal history of angina can be elicited in 40 to 50% of patients with AMI. Among patients with AMI who present with prodromal symptoms, approximately one third have had symptoms from 1 to 4 weeks before hospitalization; in the remaining two thirds, symptoms predate admission by a week or less, with one third of patients having had symptoms for 24 hours or less.

In most patients the pain of AMI is severe, but it is rarely intolerable. The pain may be prolonged, lasting up to 30 minutes. The discomfort is described as constricting, crushing, oppressing, or compressing; often the patient complains of something sitting on or squeezing the chest. Although usually described as a squeezing, choking, viselike, or heavy pain, it may be characterized as a stabbing, knifelike, boring, or burning discomfort. The pain is usually retrosternal in location, spreading frequently to both sides of the chest, favoring the left side. Often the pain radiates down the left arm. Some patients note only a dull ache or numbness in the wrists in association with severe substernal discomfort. In some instances, the pain of AMI may begin in the epigastrium, simulating a variety of abdominal disorders; this often causes MI to be misdiagnosed as indigestion. In other patients, the discomfort of AMI radiates to the shoulders, upper extremities, neck, and jaw, again usually favoring the left side. In patients with preexisting angina, the pain of infarction usually resembles that of the angina pain with respect to features and location. However, it is generally much more severe, lasts longer, and/or is not relieved by rest and nitroglycerin.

Older individuals, patients with diabetes, and women often present atypically. For example, among individuals older than 80 years, less than 50% of those with AMI will have chest discomfort at the time of AMI. Sometimes these patients will present with shortness of breath, fatigue, or even confusion. The pain of AMI may have disappeared by the time physicians first encounter the patient (or the patient reaches the hospital), or it may persist for a few hours.

Myocardial Changes Following Acute Myocardial Infarction

Figure 47-5 shows the temporal sequence of early biochemical, histochemical, and histologic findings after the onset of AMI. On gross pathologic examination, AMI can be divided into subendocardial (nontransmural) infarctions and transmural infarctions.[11] In the former, necrosis involves the endocardium, the intramural myocardium, or both without extending all the way through the ventricular wall to the epicardium. In the latter, myocardial necrosis involves the full thickness of the ventricular wall. The histologic pattern of necrosis may differ: contraction band injury occurs almost twice as often in nontransmural infarctions as in transmural infarctions. Unfortunately, the pathologic changes correlate poorly with clinical, ECG, and biochemical markers of necrosis, which is why those terms are no longer used clinically. Statistically, patients are more apt to have STE MI Q waves on the ECG and larger biochemical signals when the infarction is transmural pathologically.

Ultrastructural (Electron Microscopic) Changes in Myocardium

In experimental infarction, the earliest ultrastructural changes in cardiac muscle following occlusion of a coronary artery, noted within 20 minutes by electron microscopy, consist of reduction in the size and number of glycogen granules, intracellular edema, and swelling and distortion of the transverse tubular system, the sarcoplasmic reticulum, and the mitochondria. These early changes are partially reversible. Changes after 60 minutes of occlusion include myocardial cell swelling; mitochondrial abnormalities, such as swelling and internal disruption; development of amorphous, flocculent aggregation and margination of nuclear chromatin; and relaxation of myofibrils. After 20 minutes to 2 hours of ischemia, changes in some cells become irreversible, and progression of these alterations occurs; additional changes include swollen sacs of the sarcoplasmic reticulum at the level of the A band, greatly enlarged mitochondria with few cristae, thinning and fractionation of myofilaments, disorientation of myofibrils, and clumping of mitochondria. Cells irreversibly damaged by ischemia are usually swollen, with an enlarged sarcoplasmic reticulum. Defects in the plasma membrane may appear, and the mitochondria are fragmented. Many of these changes become more intense when blood flow is restored.

Histologic (Light Microscopic) Changes in Myocardium

Although it was previously believed that no light microscopic changes could be seen in infarcted myocardium until 8 hours after interruption of blood flow, in some infarcts a pattern of wavy myocardial fibers may be seen 1 to 3 hours after onset, especially at the periphery of the infarct.[11] After 8 hours, edema of the interstitium becomes evident, as do increased fatty deposits in the muscle fibers, along with infiltration of neutrophilic polymorphonuclear leukocytes and red blood cells.

By 24 hours, clumping of the cytoplasm and loss of cross-striations are seen, with the appearance of irregular cross-bands in the involved myocardial fibers. The nuclei sometimes even disappear. Myocardial capillaries in the involved region dilate, and polymorphonuclear leukocytes accumulate, first at the periphery and then in the center of the infarct. During the first 3 days, the interstitial tissue becomes edematous. Generally, on about day 4 after infarction, removal of necrotic fibers by macrophages begins, again commencing at the periphery. By day 8, the necrotic muscle fibers have become dissolved; by about 10 days, the number of polymorphonuclear leukocytes is reduced, and granulation tissue first appears at the periphery. Removal of necrotic muscle cells continues until the fourth to sixth week following infarction, by which time much of the necrotic myocardium has been removed. This process continues, along with increasing collagenization of the infarcted area. By the sixth week, the infarcted area usually has been converted to a firm connective tissue scar with interspersed intact muscle fibers.

Gross Changes in Myocardium

Gross alterations of the myocardium are difficult to identify until at least 6 to 12 hours following the onset of necrosis.[11] However, several histochemical approaches have been used to identify zones of necrosis that can be observed after only 2 to 3 hours. Initially, the myocardium in the affected region may appear pale and slightly swollen. By 18 to 36 hours after onset of the infarct, the myocardium is tan or reddish purple (because of trapped erythrocytes). These changes persist for approximately 48 hours; the infarct then turns gray, and fine yellow lines, secondary to neutrophilic infiltration, appear at its periphery. This zone gradually widens and during the next few days extends throughout the infarct.

Eight to 10 days following infarction, the thickness of the cardiac wall in the area of the infarct is reduced as necrotic muscle is removed by mononuclear cells. The cut surface of an infarct of this age is yellow and is surrounded by a reddish purple band of granulation tissue that extends through the necrotic tissue by 3 to 4 weeks. Over the next 2 to 3 months, the infarcted area gradually acquires a gelatinous, gray appearance, eventually converting into a shrunken, thin, firm scar that whitens and firms progressively with time. This process begins at the periphery of the infarct and gradually moves centrally. In addition, more hemorrhage is seen in the area of damage because of the use of potent thrombolytic and anticoagulant agents.

Development and Progression of Atherosclerosis[229]

Intrinsic to modern day understanding of ischemic heart disease and to the intense interest in the development of markers of inflammation is the concept that atherosclerosis is a chronic inflammatory disease. The concept is that some event damages the endothelium of blood vessels, which facilitates the egress of lipid into the subendothelial space. Putative injurious stimuli include turbulent flow in a blood vessel, which could occur for example because of hypertension or a noxious metabolite from a lipid fraction. This damage tends to occur at branch points of blood vessels. Regardless of the initial stimulus, once damaged, low-density lipoprotein (LDL) can cross into the vessel wall more easily in a nicotinamide adenine dinucleotide phosphate (NADPH) oxidase–mediated fashion. Whether minimal oxidation facilitates that egress or whether it occurs once the LDL is within the vessel wall is unclear, but a minimal degree of oxidation once in the vessel wall facilitates the egress of smooth muscle cells from the media of the vessel and macrophages that ingest cholesterol, hence the rationale for the measurement of oxidized lipids in blood. The process of atherosclerosis progresses slowly with involvement of lymphocytes, monocytes, macrophages, and smooth muscle cells. The dynamic within a given plaque may vary, but there clearly is an inflammatory milieu, in part mediated by substances such as CD40 ligand, which can be measured directly or indirectly as C-reactive protein (CRP). Interleukins-1, -6, -8, and -18 also participate to various extents as part of this chronic inflammatory process. This process involves adherence of white blood cells to the damaged endothelial surface with subsequent degranulation and elaboration of myeloperoxidase. A procoagulant component is due predominantly to the presence of tissue factor, which is localized immediately under the cap of the plaque. Intermittent instability is noted because of inflammatory products within the plaque that release chemicals, such as metalloproteinases. Initially the plaque expands by stretching the adventitia through a process of small ruptures with release of procoagulant and proinflammatory materials and then remodeling over time as anti-inflammatory and anticoagulant and thrombolytic substances are elaborated. This process of stretching the adventitia preserves the lumen such that by the time luminal encroachment occurs, there is a very large plaque burden.[136]

A categorization of plaques has been proposed to facilitate identification of those at risk of rupture that could lead to an acute event. It is acknowledged that the propensity for a plaque to rupture probably reflects a systemic predilection rather than a local one. Thus for a given patient at risk, there likely are many plaques that are metabolically at risk of rupture at any given time.[283,284] High-risk plaques have

1. An active inflammatory environment that not only may be intrinsic but may be stimulated additionally by systemic infection.
2. A thin fibrous cap on the endothelial surface with a large lipid core that is filled with procoagulant substances, predominantly tissue factor.
3. Endothelial denudation and fissuring caused by the elaboration of metalloproteinases.
4. Local high shear stress, usually because they are severe, at branch points in the vessel.

Events likely occur because of superimposed thrombosis. This can be the result of erosions on the surface of the plaque or more often rupture of the plaque at its edges, where the cap is thinnest and most of the metalloproteinases reside. If rupture induces total thrombotic occlusion, the event is usually an STE AMI. If lesser degrees of occlusion occur, an NSTE AMI or UA may ensue. One of the causes that may participate in subtotal occlusive plaque rupture involves platelets and abnormal coronary vasomotion. It is known that diseased coronary arteries respond atypically to many stimuli, often constricting rather than dilating. Because the cross-sectional area of a vessel is related to the square of the radius, even modest amounts of constriction can markedly increase the extent of occlusion. Whether constriction occurs first, leading to changes of coronary flow and platelet aggregation on the plaque, or whether platelets stick and cause the aggregation, is not certain, but these processes reinforce one another. Platelets secrete vasoconstricting substances in response to a denuded area, which expresses cell adhesion molecule (CAM) receptors. This, in addition to stagnant blood flow, will cause platelets and white blood cells to adhere to the surfaces of vessels. It appears likely that platelets adhere and enhance vasoconstriction and then break off, causing small vessel emboli, sometimes in association with plaque debris and sometimes without. These processes, in addition to a reduction in flow, can lead to necrosis or at least recurrent ischemia. It is apparent that the process that eventually leads to acute events involves a systemic propensity to platelet aggregation and inflammation, because effluent flowing from the nonculprit vessel (distant from the putative coronary lesion causing the acute event) elaborates inflammatory mediators (e.g., myeloperoxidase) similar to those observed from the affected vessel. Finally, necrosis when present stimulates an acute-phase reaction and inflammation. Given this pathophysiology, many therapies are now oriented toward inhibition of thrombosis, fibrinolysis, platelet aggregation, and inflammation. Many inflammatory markers are used diagnostically and for assessment of therapeutic efficiency.

Diagnosis of Acute Myocardial Infarction

The diagnosis of AMI established by the World Health Organization in 1986 included biomarkers as an integral part of the disorder and required that at least two of the following criteria be met: (1) a history of chest pain, (2) evolutionary changes on the ECG, and/or (3) elevations of serial cardiac markers to a level two times the normal value. However, over time, it became rare for a diagnosis of AMI to be made in the absence of biochemical evidence of myocardial injury. A 2000 European Society of Cardiology/American College of Cardiology (ESC/ACC) consensus conference[66] updated in 2007 (Global Task Force)[372] codified the role of markers by advocating that the diagnosis should be regarded as evidence of myocardial injury based on markers of cardiac damage in the appropriate clinical situation (Box 47-2).[372] The criteria for diagnosis of an established MI are listed in Box 47-3. The guidelines thus recognized the reality that neither the clinical presentation nor the ECG had adequate sensitivity and specificity. This guideline does not suggest that all elevations of these biomarkers should elicit a diagnosis of AMI—only those associated with appropriate clinical and ECG findings (see discussion later in this chapter). When elevations that are not caused by acute ischemia occur, the clinician is obligated to search for another cause for the elevation.[176,181,401,406] The criteria suggested for use with these markers by the Biochemistry Panel of the ESC/ACC Committee are listed in Box 47-4.[181] In the 2007 revision of the guidelines, several types of AMI were recognized, including the spontaneous type, which is associated with plaque rupture or erosion, and the type associated with fixed or transient coronary abnormalities but not thrombotic occlusion. These are discussed in greater detail in the following paragraphs. It is also recognized that one can have a classic AMI and succumb before markers are obtained or become elevated, and cardiac injury can occur in association with cardiac procedures.[372] In addition, criteria for use with coronary interventions and bypass surgery were suggested.

ECG Findings

At one time, the initial ECG was thought to be diagnostic of AMI in about 50% of patients.[179] As the frequency of STE AMI has diminished and the diagnosis has been made with greater and greater sensitivity, this percentage has been greatly reduced. Serial tracings are helpful for STE AMI but not for what is now almost 70% of AMIs that are known as non-STE (NSTE) AMIs. The classic ECG changes of an STE AMI are ST segment elevation, which often evolves to the

BOX 47-2 Criteria for the Definition of Acute Myocardial Infarction

1. Detection of rise and/or fall of cardiac biomarkers (preferably troponin) above the 99th percentile of the upper reference limit, together with evidence of ischemia with at least one of the following:
   a. Ischemic symptoms
   b. Electrocardiogram (ECG) changes of new ischemia [new ST-T changes or new left bundle branch block (LBBB)]
   c. Development of pathologic Q waves on the ECG
   d. Imaging evidence of new loss of viable myocardium or new regional wall motion abnormality

From reference 372.

BOX 47-3 Diagnosis of Established Myocardial Infarction

Any one of the following criteria satisfies the diagnosis for established MI:

1. Development of new pathologic Q waves on serial electrocardiograms (ECGs). The patient may or may not remember previous symptoms. Biochemical markers of myocardial necrosis may have normalized, depending on the length of time that has passed since the infarct developed.
2. Pathologic findings of a healed or healing myocardial infarction (MI).

BOX 47-4 Clinical Classification of Different Types of Myocardial Infarction

Type 1: spontaneous myocardial infarction related to ischemia due to a primary coronary event, such as plaque fissuring or rupture

Type 2: myocardial infarction secondary to ischemia due to imbalance between oxygen demand and supplies (e.g., coronary spasm)

Type 3: sudden cardiac death with symptoms of myocardial ischemia, accompanied by new ST elevation or left bundle branch block (LBBB), or verified coronary thrombus by angiography, but with death occurring before blood samples could be obtained

Type 4: myocardial infarction associated with percutaneous innervation (PCI)

Type 5: myocardial infarction associated with coronary artery bypass grafting (CABG)

From reference 372.

development of Q waves if intervention is not provided (see Figure 47-4). Pericarditis, some normal variants, and transient causes that may result in myocardial injury such as myocarditis are well described and on occasion can mimic the changes of AMI. Most NSTE AMIs present as ST segment depression, with or without T-wave changes; as T-wave changes alone; or on occasion in the absence of any ECG findings. Those with ST segment change have a substantially worse prognosis.[372]

In some patients, the clinical history and ECG may be definitive. In others, they may not be as clear. Many other clinical aspects might suggest acute ischemia as the origin of a given biomarker elevation. For example, the finding of significant coronary obstructive lesions, especially in a pattern suggestive of recent plaque rupture, is highly suggestive. At times, a positive stress test with or without imaging may be what helps in making the diagnosis. However, if the clinical situation is not suggestive, other sources for cardiac injury should be sought.

BIOMARKERS IN ACUTE CORONARY SYNDROME

Analytical Considerations

Myocardial damage detected by elevations of cardiac troponin (cTn) are almost invariably associated with impaired clinical outcomes for patients. This statement summarizes more than 20 years of analytical and clinical investigations pertaining to the clinical utility of cTnI and cTnT. This section of the chapter will focus on cTn biochemistry; the analytical aspects of assays used to measure cTn in whole blood, serum, and plasma; preanalytical and analytical specifications that manufacturers of assays need to strive to optimize; reference (normal) limit determinations; and point-of-care (POC) testing strategies.

Biochemistry

The contractile proteins of the myofibril include the three troponin regulatory proteins (Figure 47-6).[85,196,244] The troponins are a complex of three protein subunits: troponin C (the calcium-binding component), troponin I (the inhibitory component), and troponin T (the tropomyosin-binding component). The subunits exist in a number of isoforms. The distribution of these isoforms varies between cardiac muscle and slow and fast twitch skeletal muscle. Only two major isoforms of troponin C are found in human heart and skeletal muscle. These are characteristic of slow and fast twitch skeletal muscle. The heart isoform is identical to the slow twitch skeletal muscle isoform, thus the reason why cTnC was never developed as a cardiac specific biomarker. Isoforms of cardiac-specific troponin T (cTnT) and cardiac-specific troponin I (cTnI) also have been identified and are the products of unique genes.[62,63,94,194] Troponin is localized primarily in the myofibrils (94 to 97%), with a smaller cytoplasmic fraction

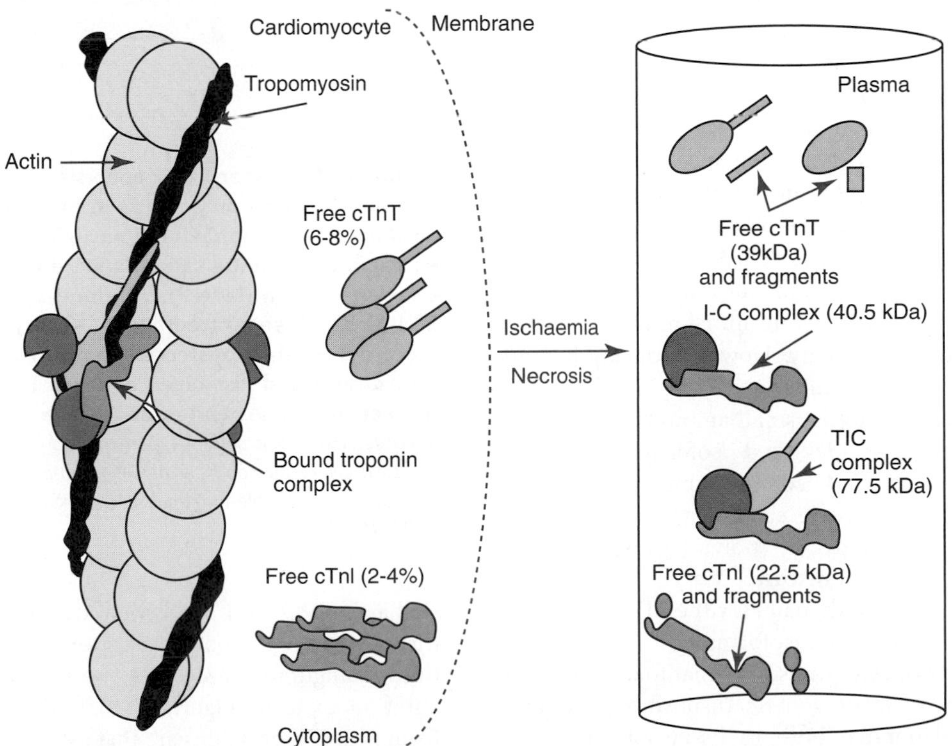

Figure 47-6 Structure of cardiac troponin complex and troponin forms released following myofibril necrosis. *(From Gaze DC, Collinson PO. Multiple molecular forms of circulating cardiac troponin: analytical and clinical significance. Ann Clin Biochem 2008;45:349-59. Figure courtesy Paul Collinson.)*

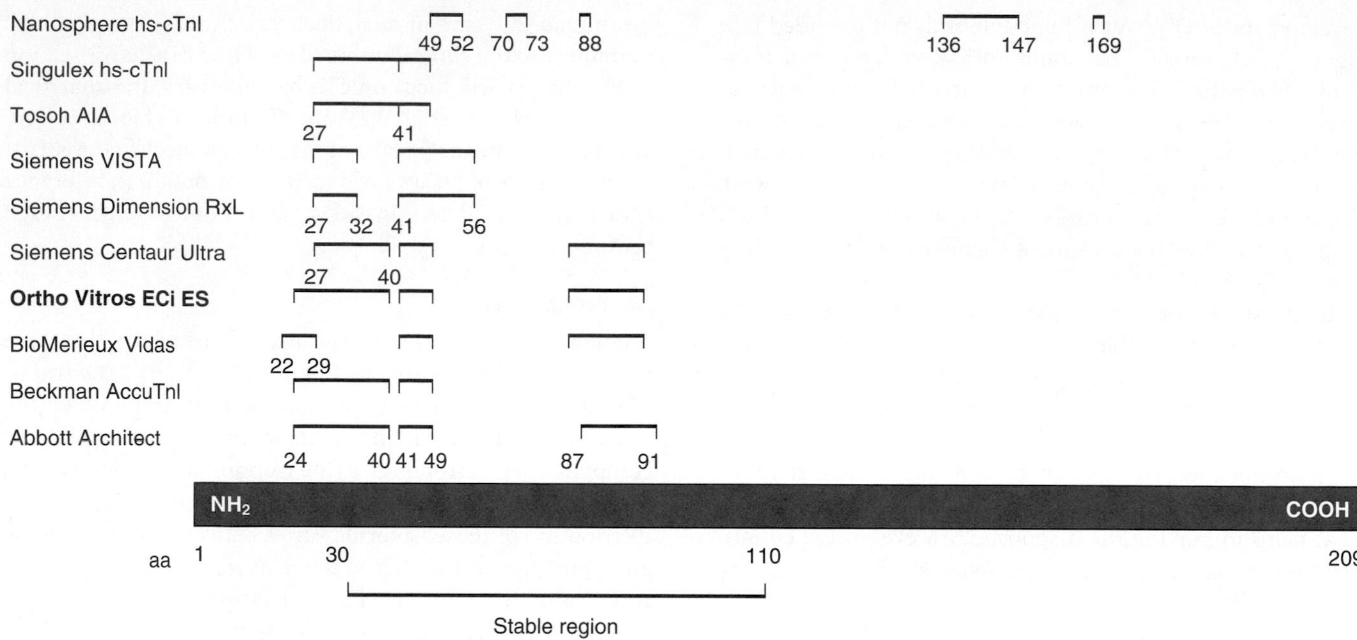

Figure 47-7 Amino acid sequence of cardiac troponin I (cTnI), with identification of epitopes used by antibodies in cTnI assays. Antibodies are named in the boxes that have attached arrows. *(Figure courtesy David Gaze and Paul Collinson.)*

(3 to 6%).[122] Some experts in the field think that 100% of cTn is myofibril bound and that the "cytoplasmic fraction" represents a more easily mobilizable fraction, rather than representing a different cellular localization.

cTnI and cTnT have different amino acid sequences from the skeletal isoforms and are encoded by unique genes. Human cTnI has an additional 31-amino-acid residue on the amino terminal end compared with skeletal muscle TnI, giving it complete cardiac specificity (Figure 47-7). Only one isoform of cTnI has been identified. cTnI has never been shown to be expressed in normal, regenerating, or diseased human or animal skeletal muscle.[62] cTnT is encoded for by a different gene than the one that encodes for skeletal muscle isoforms. An 11 amino acid amino-terminal residue gives this marker unique cardiac specificity. However, during human fetal development, in regenerating rat skeletal muscle, and in diseased human skeletal muscle, small amounts of cTnT are expressed as one of four identified isoforms in skeletal muscle.[10,63,335] In humans, cTnT isoform expression has been demonstrated in skeletal muscle specimens obtained from patients with muscular dystrophy, polymyositis, dermatomyositis, and end-stage renal disease.[63,255,298,320,371] Thus, care is necessary to choose antibody pairs for the cTnT assay that do not detect these re-expressed isoforms.[130,217]

A substantial body of evidence shows that following myocardial injury or because of genetic disposition, multiple forms of cTn are elaborated both in tissue and in blood (Figure 47-8).[193,194,406] These include the following: T-I-C ternary complex, IC binary complex, and free I; multiple modification of these three forms can occur, involving oxidation, reduction, phosphorylation, and dephosphorylation, as well as both C- and N-terminal degradation. Depending on the selection of antibodies used to detect cTnI, different antibody configurations can lead to a substantially different recognition pattern (Figure 47-9).[85] The conclusions derived from these observations are that assays need to be developed in which the antibodies recognize epitopes in the stable region of cTnI and, ideally, demonstrate an equimolar response to the different cTnI forms that circulate in the blood.

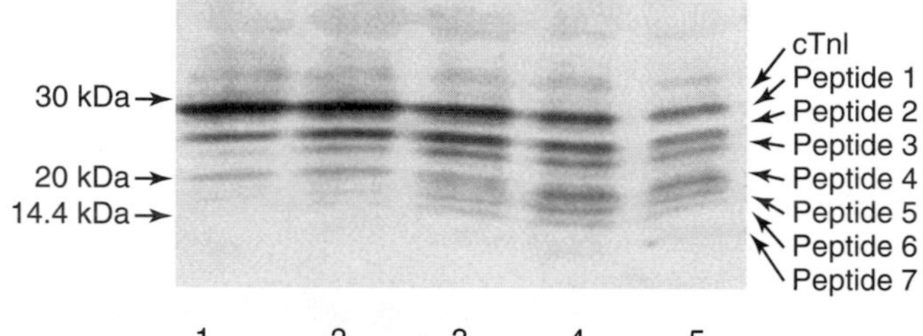

Figure 47-8 Western blot analysis of endogenous cardiac troponin I (cTnI) proteolysis in human heart tissue visualized with monoclonal anti-cTnI antibody. Protein extracts from tissue samples were incubated at 37 °C for 0 h (lane 1), 2 h (lane 2), 5 h (lane 3), 8 h (lane 4), and 20 h (lane 5), separated by 10%–20% gradient SDS-gel electrophoresis, transferred to a nitrocellulose membrane, and visualized by MAb 19C7. The apparent molecular masses and peptides are marked by arrows. *(From Katrukha AG, Bereznikova AV, Filtaov VL, Esakova TV, Kolosova OV, Pettersson K, et al. Degradation of cardiac troponin I: implication for reliable immunodetection. Clin Chem 1998;44: 2433-40.)*

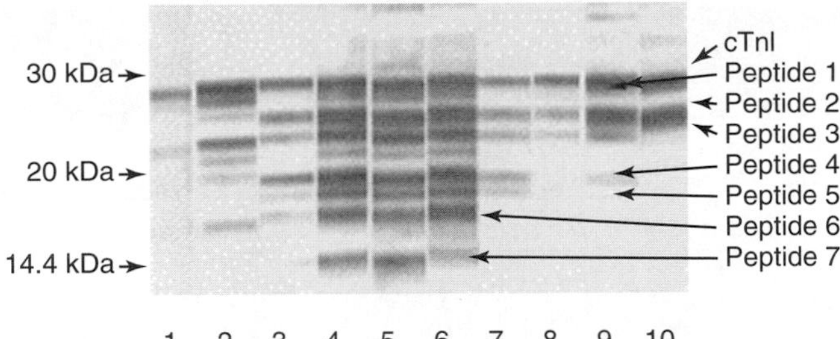

Figure 47-9 Western blot analysis of endogenous proteolytic fragments of cardiac troponin I (cTnI) antibodies. Human cardiac tissue was incubated for 8 h at 37 °C. Proteins were extracted and separated using 10–20% gradient SDS-gel electrophoresis, and then transferred to a nitrocellulose membrane. Bands corresponding to cTnI proteolytic peptides were visualized by different MAbs: lane 1, 10B11; lane 2, 4G6; lane 3, 10F4; lane 4, 19C7; lane 5, 414; lane 6, 16A11; lane 7, 18H7; lane 8, 10B7; lane 9, 6F9; lane 10, 7F4. The apparent molecular masses and peptides are marked by arrows. *(From Katrukha AG, Bereznikova AV, Filtaov VL, Esakova TV, Kolosova OV, Pettersson K, et al. Degradation of cardiac troponin I: implication for reliable immunodetection. Clin Chem 1998;44: 2433-40.)*

Immunoassays

Cummins and coworkers were the first to develop an RIA to measure cTnI, using polyclonal anti-cTnI antibodies.[94] The first monoclonal enzyme-linked immunosorbent assay (ELISA), an anti-cTnI antibody–based immunoassay, was described by Bodor and Ladenson.[61] Numerous manufacturers have now described the development of monoclonal antibody–based diagnostic immunoassays for the measurement of cTnI in serum.[14,17,18,22,28,29,34,37,85,87,90,161,195] As shown in Table 47-1, numerous assays have been approved by the U.S. Food and Drug Administration (FDA) for patient testing within the United States on central laboratory and POC testing platforms. In addition to these quantitative assays, several assays have been cleared by the FDA for the qualitative determination of cTnI. Further development has led to the design of research (prototype) high-sensitivity cTn (hs-cTn) I and T assays. In practice, two obstacles limit the ease of switching from one assay to another in clinical practice or research. First, no primary reference cTnI material is currently available for manufacturers to use in standardizing cTnI assays. Second, assay concentrations fail to be consistent because cTnI circulate in its various forms and the different antibodies use in the available assays recognize different epitopes of cTnI.

The cTnI standardization subcommittee of the American Association for Clinical Chemistry (AACC) in collaboration with the National Institute of Standards and Technology (NIST) developed a cTnI reference material (SRM #2921) that is a TnC-cTnI-cTnT complex purified from human heart under nondenaturing conditions.[74] A cTnI value was assigned by a combination of reversed-phase liquid chromatography with ultraviolet detection and amino acid analysis. However, because this material demonstrated commutability with only 50% of current cTnI assays, it is of limited value for assay harmonization of current assays and cannot be used as a common calibrator. Although standardization of assays remains elusive, differences of cTnI concentrations reported by studied assays has been narrowed from a 20-fold difference to a twofold to threefold difference using the SRM 2921. Further, this material allows for traceability to a common reference material. It appears that the only way to achieve complete standardization for cTnI would be for manufacturers to agree to use the same antibodies showing similar specificity for the cTnI molecule; this would also overcome matrix effects with a serum-based common reference material for calibration.

Several adaptations of the Roche cTnT immunoassay have been described over the years.[383,405] The current FDA-cleared assay available worldwide involves two monoclonal, anti–cardiac troponin T antibodies. Skeletal muscle TnT is no longer a potential interferant, as was found in the first-generation ELISA cTnT assay. In contrast to cTnI, no standardization bias exists for cTnT, because the same antibodies (M11, M7) are used in the central laboratory and in POC assay systems.

Assay Specifications

In 2001 and 2004, the International Federation of Clinical Chemistry and Laboratory Medicine (IFCC) Committee on Standardization of Markers of Cardiac Damage (C-SMCD) recommended quality specifications for cTn assays.[300,301] These specifications were intended for use by the manufacturers of commercial assays and by clinical laboratories utilizing cTn assays. The overall goal was to attempt to establish uniform criteria so that all assays could be evaluated objectively for their analytical qualities and clinical performance. Both analytical and preanalytical factors were addressed and are in the process of being updated with an expected publication date of 2012. An adequate description of the analytical principles, method design, and assay components should include the following: (1) antibody specificity and epitope locations identified need to be delineated; (2) epitopes located on the stable part of the cTnI molecule should be a priority; (3) assays need to clarify whether different cTnI forms (e.g., binary vs. ternary complex) are recognized in an equimolar fashion by the antibodies used; (4) specific relative responses need to be described for each of the cTnI forms (free cTnI, the 1-C binary complex, the T-I-C ternary complex, and oxidized, reduced, and phosphorylated isoforms of the three cTnI forms); (5) the effects of different anticoagulants on binding of cTnI need to be addressed; and (6) the source of material used to calibrate cTn assays, specifically for cTnI, should be reported (Box 47-5).

Defining Normal Reference Limits for Cardiac Troponin

Advancements in cTn assay technology have created a conundrum for clinicians and laboratory scientists, who must determine which assays are best for optimal patient care.

TABLE 47-1 Analytical Characteristics of Commercial and Research High Sensitive Cardiac Troponin I and T Assays as Stated by Manufacturer

Company/ Platform/Assay	LoD μg/L	99th% μg/L	%CV 99th%	10% CV μg/L	Risk Stratification†	Epitopes Recognized by Antibodies	Detection Antibody Tag
Abbott AxSYM ADV	0.02	0.04	15.0	0.16	Yes	C: 87-91, 41-49; D: 24-40	ALP
Abbott ARCHITECT	<0.01	0.028	15.0	0.032	No	C: 87-91, 24-40: D: 41-49	Acridinium
Abbott i-STAT*	0.02	0.08	16.5	0.10	Yes	C: 41-49, 88-91; D: 28-39, 62-78	ALP
Beckman Coulter Access Accu	0.01	0.04	14.0	0.06	Yes	C: 41-49; D: 24-40	ALP
bioMerieux Vidas Ultra	0.01	0.01	27.7	0.11	No	C: 41-49, 22-29; D: 87-91, 7B9	ALP
Inverness Biosite Triage*	0.05	<0.05	NA	NA	No	C: NA; D: 27-40	Fluorophor
Inverness Biosite Triage (r)*	0.01	0.056	17.0	NA	No	NA	Fluorophor
Mitsubishi Chemical PATHFAST*	0.008	0.029	5.0	0014	No	C: 41-49; D: 71-116, 163-209	ALP
Ortho Vitros ECi ES	0.012	0.034	10.0	0.034	Yes	C: 24-40, 41-49; D: 87-91	HRP
Radiometer AQT90*	0.0095	0.023	17.7	0.039	NA	C: 41-49, 190-196; D: 137-149	Europium
Response Biomedical RAMP*	0.03	<0.1	18.5	0.21	No	C: 85-92; D: 26-38	Flourophor
Roche E170	0.01	<0.01	18.0	0.03	Yes	C: 125-131; D: 136-147	Ruthenium
Roche Elecsys 2010	0.01	<0.01	18.0	0.030	Yes	C: 125-131; D: 136-147	Ruthenium
Roche Cardiac Reader	<0.05	<0.05	NA	NA	No	C: 125-131; D: 136-147	Gold particules
Siemens Centaur Ultra	0.006	0.04	10.0	0.03	Yes	C: 41-49, 87-91; D: 27-40	Acridinium
Siemens Dimension RxL	0.04	0.07	20.0	0.14	Yes	C: 27-32; D: 41-56	ALP
Siemens Immulite 2500 STAT	0.1	0.2	NA	0.42	No	C: 87-91; D: 27-40	ALP
Siemens Immulite 1000 Turbo	0.15	NA	NA	0.64	No	C: 87-91; D: 27-40	ALP
Siemens Stratus CS*	0.03	0.07	10.0	0.06	Yes	C: 27-32; D: 41-56	ALP
Siemens VISTA	0.015	0.045	10.0	0.04	Yes	C: 27-32; D: 41-56	Chemiluminescent
Tosoh AIA II	0.06	<0.06	8.5	0.09	No	C: 41-49; D: 87-91	ALP
High Sensitive cTnIAssays hs-cTnI Assays							
Abbott Architect	0.009	0.16	5.6	0.003	No	C: 24-40; D: 41-49	
Beckman Coulter Access	0.002	0.0086	10.0	0.0086	No	C: 41-49; D: 24-40	ALP
Nanosphere	0.002	0.0028	9.5	0.0005	No	C: 136-147; D: Ab PA1010	
Singulex Errena	0.0009	0.0101	9.0	0.0008	No	C: 41-49; D: 27-41	
Siemens VISTA	0.15	0.009	5.0	0.003	No	C: 27-32; D: 41-56	

TABLE 47-1 Analytical Characteristics of Commercial and Research High Sensitive Cardiac Troponin I and T Assays as Stated by Manufacturer—cont'd

Company/ Platform/Assay	LoD µg/L	99th% µg/L	%CV 99th%	10% CV µg/L	Risk Stratification+	Epitopes Recognized by Antibodies	Detection Antibody Tag
hs-cTnT Assays							
Roche Elecsys	0.001	0.013	8.0	0.012	No	C: 125-131; D: 136-147	Ruthenium Gold-nanoparticles Capillary flow fluorescence

*POC testing assay.
LoD, Limit of detection; *99th%,* 99th percentile concentrations; *NA,* not available; + designates FDA clearance; *(r),* revised assay under review by FDA.

BOX 47-5 Quality Specifications—Cardiac Troponin Assays

Analytical Factors
1. Antibody specificity—recognize epitopes as part of molecule and equimolar for all forms
2. Influence of anticoagulants
3. Calibration against natural form of molecule
4. Defined type of material useful for dilutions
5. Demonstrated recovery and linearity of method
6. Described detection limit and imprecision (10% CV)
7. Addressing interferants (i.e., RF, heterophile antibodies)

Preanalytical Factors
1. Storage time and temperature conditions
2. Centrifugation effects—gel separators
3. Serum-plasma—WB correlations

CV, Coefficient of variation; *RF,* rheumatoid factor; *WB,* whole blood.
Adapted from Panteghini M, Gerhardt W, Apple FS, Dati F, Ravkilde J, Wu AH. Quality specifications for cardiac troponin assays. Clin Chem Lab Med 2001;39:174-8.

Unfortunately, few resources are available to guide the medical and scientific communities in this regard. International guidelines have defined an increased cTn above the 99th percentile limit as an abnormal result, as described in the clinical section.[17,273,372] What is lacking, unfortunately, is an approach to define the 99th percentile limit across the heterogeneity of assays. In spite of evidence-based literature demonstrating that cTn concentrations tend to increase in individuals older than 60 years, likely because of unrecognized comorbidities, 99th percentile reference limits are often determined across wide age ranges using subjects as old as 80 years (convenience samples).[14,21,116] Further frustrating the problem of selecting relevant reference subjects is the fact that in clinically defined normal individuals without known cardiovascular disease, increased cTn concentrations are indicative of a significantly higher risk of death. Given such problems, most laboratories (1) accept the manufacturer's reference limit from the FDA-cleared package insert; (2) perform an underpowered normal range study to establish a reference limit; or (3) accept a cutoff value published in the literature.

Consensus guidelines from the Global Task Force for the Universal Definition of Myocardial Infarction and the National Academy of Clinical Biochemistry (NACB) plus the updated American College of Cardiology/American Heart Association and Epidemiology[133,240] guidelines have recommended that, in patients who present with ischemic symptoms, at least 1 cTn concentration higher than the 99th percentile value during the first 24 hours after onset of symptoms indicates myocardial necrosis. If this elevation occurs in a clinical situation consistent with myocardial infarction (MI), that diagnosis should be made (see Box 47-2). It is recommended that cTn assays with appropriate quality control and optimal total imprecision [coefficient of variation (CV) ≤10%] at the 99th percentile limit are preferred.[86,301] Better imprecision at low cTn concentrations appears to improve the value of cTn as a diagnostic and risk indicator. Use of cTn assays with intermediate imprecision (10 to 20% CV) at the 99th percentile, however, does not lead to significant patient misclassification when serial cTn results are interpreted.

A challenge that arises as the FDA clears improved cTn assays with higher analytical sensitivity for use in laboratory practice is determining how these new assays compare with the older assays. Diagnostic sensitivities using specimens collected at presentation for detection of myocardial infarction (MI) have improved from 15 to 35% for early cTn assays to 50 to 75% for contemporary assays (Table 47-2). Unfortunately, definitive data about how long it takes to totally exclude AMI are still lacking. Over the past 10 years, the science of reagent and technology formulation of cTn assays has allowed measurement of this biomarker with greatly improved precision at concentrations approaching the 99th percentile limit of an assay. The goal is to better define the clinical playing field for assays used to assist the diagnosis of MI and to better stratify patients by risk of adverse events. To summarize these discussions, the optimal goals that the FDA would like to achieve include the following: (1) to transition from the current practice of approving assays based on

TABLE 47-2 Diagnostic Accuracy of Current cTn Assays 99th Percentile at Presentation of Patient to Hospital

	Sensitivity	Specificity
2003 Collinson, Roche Elecsys cTnT	82%	60%
2004 Eggers, Siemens Dimension cTnI	78%	NA
2006 Apple, Siemens Stratus CS cTnI	68%	82%
2007 Apple, Ortho-Clinical Diagnostics ECi cTnI ES	83%	79%
2007 Apple, bioMerieux VIDAS cTnI	88%	79%
2008 Apple, Siemens Centaur Ultra cTnI	74%	83%
2009 Reichlin, Abbott ARCHITECT cTnI	86%	92%
2009 Reichlin, Roche Elecsys cTnI	84%	94%
2009 Reichlin, Roche Elecsys hs-cTnT	95%	80%
2011 Apple, Mitsubishi PATHFAST	73%	92.7%

Diagnostic accuracy values may vary based on patient populations and prevalence of disease in each study.
cTn, Cardiac troponin; *NA,* not published.

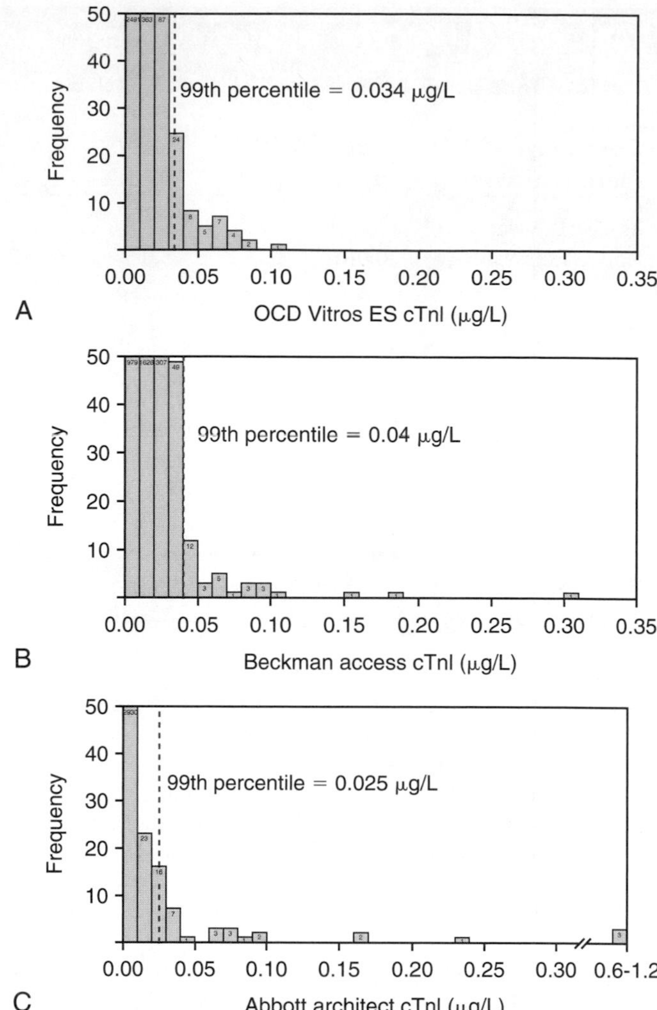

Figure 47-10 Histograms of serum specimens from apparently healthy individuals measured for cardiac troponin I (cTnI) by the (A) OCD, (B) Beckman, and (C) Abbott assays. *(From Apple FS, Murakami MM. Serum and plasma cardiac troponin I 99th percentile reference values for 3 2nd-generation assays. Clin Chem 2007;53:1558-60.)*

receiver operating characteristic (ROC)-optimized cutoffs to using the 99th percentile value; (2) to ensure that cTn assays are accurate enough at the 99th percentile values for clinical use; and (3) to define the effects of implementing the 99th percentile value in clinical practice on minimizing false-negative and false-positive findings. Understanding what is truly normal for cTn, once high-sensitivity assays are incorporated into clinical practice, will be a major step forward in the cardiac biomarker field. The authors advocate for worldwide acceptance of the 99th percentile cTn value as the MI diagnostic cutoff—not ROC curve–derived cTn cutoff values.

To solve the conundrum of assay-to-assay differences, head-to-head comparison of leading market share assays used in clinical practice, as well as hs-cTn assays that will enter the marketplace within 2 years, is needed. One rational approach would be to use a common normal reference population within a focused, young, healthy age group to establish 99th percentile limits. Multiple studies using first-generation, contemporary, and prototype hs-cTn assays have demonstrated that the cTn 99th percentile limit strongly depends on selection of individuals to be included in the reference population. In one study examining four contemporary assays, measurable concentrations below the 99th percentile concentration ranged from 1 to 67% across assays (Figure 47-10). Studies using high-sensitivity assays detect cTn in almost 100% of normal samples, with results appearing to have a near-Gaussian distribution* (Figure 47-11). Some manufacturers report gender differences at these very low levels, but others do not.

To overcome the barrier for accurate interpretation of cTn values in clinical practice, a two-tiered system of analysis using both 99th percentiles and imprecision values at the 99th percentile, based on a young, healthy reference population that is diversified by sex, race, and ethnicity, has been proposed. This approach has been challenged because it does not provide an age-matched normal cohort matching the ACS patient population that typically presents to rule out an AMI. This approach establishes a scorecard (1) to capture the essence of which assays are acceptable for use in clinical practice; (2) to assist the FDA in assay clearance criteria; and (3) to facilitate the transition to future generations of hs-cTn assays. The proposed assay-dependent scorecard shown in

*References 57, 199, 215, 263, 332, 394, 399, and 400.

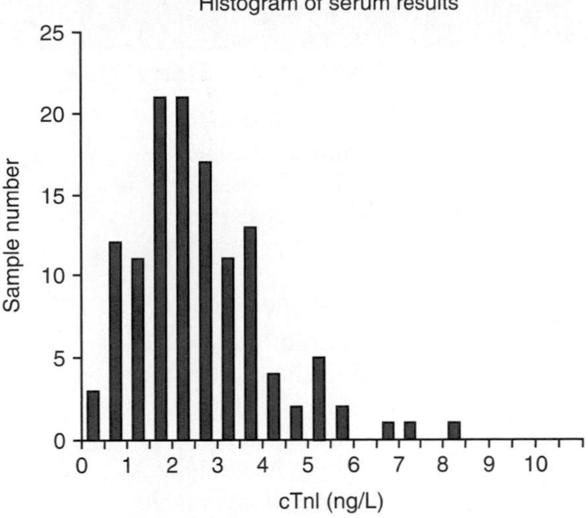

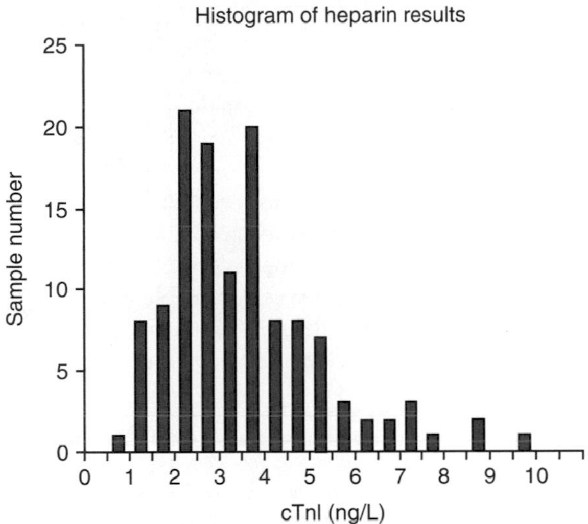

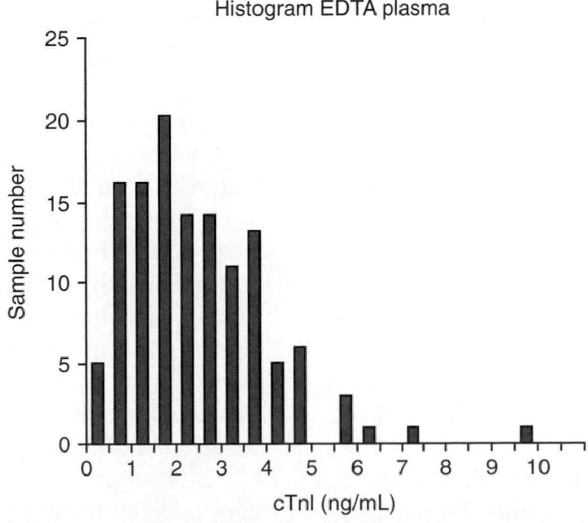

Figure 47-11 Distribution of high-sensitivity cardiac troponin I (hs-cTnI) (Beckman Coulter) concentrations in serum *(top panel)*, heparin plasma *(middle panel)*, and EDTA plasma *(bottom panel)* from 125 healthy individuals. The hs-cTnI was measured by the Beckman Coulter assay. *(From Kavsak PA, MacRae AR, Yerna MJ, Jaffe AS. Analytic and clinical utility of a next-generation, highly sensitive cardiac troponin I assay for early detection of myocardial injury. Clin Chem 2009;53:573-7. Figure courtesy Allan Jaffe.)*

TABLE 47-3 Cardiac Troponin Assay Scorecard Designations

Company/Platform/Assay[a]	Acceptance Designation	Assay Designation
Abbott AxSYM ADV	Clinically usable	Level 1
Abbott Architect	Clinically usable	Level 1
Abbott i-STAT	Clinically usable	Level 1
Beckman Access Accu	Clinically usable	Level 2
bioMerieux Vidas Ultra	Not acceptable	Level 1
Inverness Biosite Triage	NA	Level 1
Inverness Biosite Triage (r)	Clinically usable	Level 1
Mitsubishi PATHFAST	Guideline acceptable	Level 1
Ortho-Clinical Diag Vitros ES	Guideline acceptable	Level 1
Radiometer AQT90	Clinically usable	Level 1
Response Biomedical RAMP	Clinically usable	Level 1
Roche Elecsys 2010	Clinically usable	Level 1
Siemens Centaur Ultra	Guideline acceptable	Level 1
Siemens Dimension RxL	Clinically usable	Level 1
Siemens Immulite 2500 STAT	Not acceptable	Level 1
Siemens Stratus CS	Guideline acceptable	Level 1
Siemens VISTA	Guideline acceptable	Level 1
Tosoh AIA II	Clinically usable	Level 1
High Sensitivity Assay		
Abbott ARCHITECT	Guideline acceptable	Level 3
Beckman Access hs-cTnI	Guideline acceptable	Level 4
Roche Elecsys hs-cTnT	Guideline acceptable	Level 4
Nanosphere hs-cTnI	Guideline acceptable	Level 3
Siemens VISTA	Guideline acceptable	Level 4
Singulex hs-cTnI	Guideline acceptable	Level 4

[a]Per manufacturer's package insert; NA, insufficient information to designate.
Adapted from Apple FS. A new season for cardiac troponin assays: it's time to keep a scorecard. Clin Chem 2009;55:1303-6.
Acceptance criteria based on CV at 99th percentile: "Guideline acceptable", CV ≤ 10%; "Clinically useable", CV >10 to ≤ 20%; "Not acceptable", CV > 20%.
Assay designations based on % of normal subjects in whom cardiac troponin is measureable: Level 4, ≥95% of subjects have measurable concentrations; Level 3, 75 to <95% measurable; Level 2, 50 to <75% measurable; Level 1, <50% measurable.

Table 47-3 is based on designations of the total imprecision (CV%) of each assay at the 99th percentile and how many specimens from normal individuals have cTn concentrations that are actually measurable below the 99th percentile.[14] The ultimate goal is to have all assays be level 4 (third-generation) guideline acceptable.

The likely clinical effects of using assays rated by the scorecard as guideline acceptable or clinically usable include the following: (1) emergency medicine physicians will achieve improvements in triage through earlier ruling out (improved specificity) and ruling in (improved sensitivity) of patients with MI; (2) cardiology and internal medicine physicians will see improved outcomes for both inpatients (hospitalized, short-term risk) and outpatients (post hospitalization, long-term risk); (3) other medical specialty physicians will be better able to identify patients, often without clinical symptoms, who may be at risk of cardiac-related adverse outcomes; and (4) clinical trial investigators will be able to identify appropriate and optimal patient re-enrollment and outcome measures.

Optimal discrimination between a small amount of myocardial injury and analytical noise requires assays that have low limits of quantitation (LoQ) and detection (LoD), both of which require high precision at low cTn concentrations. Efforts to improve the precision of cTn assays are warranted. Irrespective of how the testing is performed, whether in the central laboratory or at the bedside using POC assays, manufacturers need to define the imprecision profile [i.e., the scattergraph showing the %CV vs. increasing cTn concentrations obtained using the Clinical and Laboratory Standards Institute (CLSI) EP5-A2 protocol] by assessing pools of human samples containing different cTn concentrations (Figure 47-12).[301] In particular, at least two cTn concentrations that cover the range between the LoD and the 99th percentile decision limit of the assay are recommended to be included. Imprecision characteristics, including the 10% CV concentration, the LoD, and 99th percentile data from currently commercially available assays, are shown in Table 47-1. It is a matter of concern that in clinical practice, different cTn concentrations are obtained with the same manufacturer's assay by independent users of the assay. Such discrepancies highlight the need for local analytical validation whenever feasible. Laboratories at a minimum should determine total imprecision and should continue to monitor

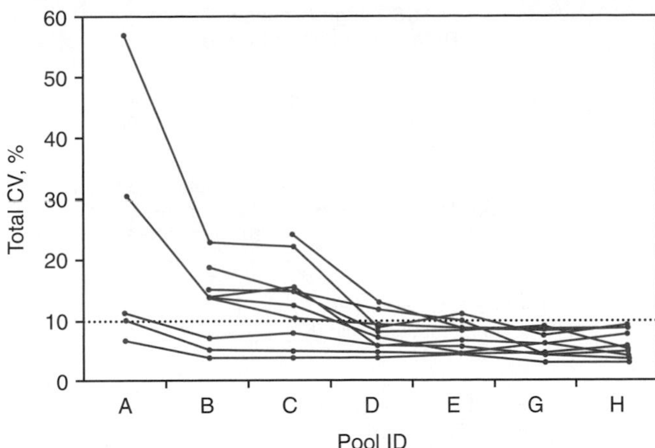

Figure 47-12 Cardiac troponin I imprecision profiles for human serum pools using different cardiac troponin I (cTnI) assays, with 10% coefficient of variation (CV) concentration indicated by the *dashed line*. *(From Panteghini M, Pagani F, Yeo KT, Apple FS, Christenson RH, Dati F, et al. Evaluation of the imprecision at low range concentrations of the assays for cardiac troponin determination. Clin Chem 2004;50:327 32.)*

assay performance over time using internal quality control materials that include the lowest concentration corresponding to the 10% CV, as well as at the 99th percentile value if different from the 10% CV concentration. Patient specimen comparisons such as regression analysis and bias assessment should be performed according to CLSI guidelines.

The 2007 NACB and IFCC C-SMCD laboratory medicine practice guidelines outlined the following analytical recommendations for cTn and other biomarkers of ACS. Objectives were to recommend the appropriate implementation and utilization of cardiac biomarkers, specifically, cTn, to aid in the diagnosis of MI, complementing the quality specifications for the cTn assay previously published. It should be noted that these recommendations build on and, in many cases, are identical to the previously established 1999 IFCC C-SMCD guidelines and the 2007 Global Task Force for the Universal Definition of MI guidelines.[372,398]

1. Reference decision limits should be established for each cardiac biomarker based on a population of normal, healthy individuals without a known history of heart disease (reference population). For cardiac troponin I (cTnI) and T (cTnT), as well as for CK-MB mass, the 99th percentile of the reference population should be the decision limit for myocardial injury. The CLSI (formerly, the NCCLS) recommends a minimum of 120 individuals per group of healthy individuals for appropriate statistical determination of a normal reference limit cutoff. [This number was suggested as a minimum number of subjects for estimating endpoints of a central 95% reference interval (with limits at the 2.5 and 97.5 percentile) by use of the nonparametric estimation method. This number of subjects is not adequate for determination of a 99th percentile for which *N* s of 300 to 500 individuals have been recommended.[161A]] Sex-specific reference limits should be used in clinical practice for CK-MB mass.
2. One decision limit, the 99th percentile, is recommended as the optimum cutoff for cTnI, cTnT, and CK-MB mass. Patients with ACS with cTnI and cTnT results above the decision limit should be labeled as having myocardial injury and at high risk.
3. Assays for cardiac biomarkers should strive for total imprecision (%CV) of less than 10% at the 99th percentile reference limit. Before introduction into clinical practice, cardiac biomarker assays must be characterized with respect to potential interferences, including rheumatoid factors, human antimouse antibodies, and heterophile antibodies. Preanalytical and analytical assay characteristics should include biomarker stability (over time and across temperature ranges) for each acceptable specimen type used in clinical practice and identification of antibody/epitope recognition sites for each biomarker. Analytical and preanalytical specifications developed by professional groups such as the IFCC should be followed.
4. Serum, plasma, and anticoagulated whole blood are acceptable specimens for the analysis of cardiac biomarkers. Choice of specimen must be based on sufficient evidence and the known characteristics of individual biomarker assays.

Point-of-Care Testing

The NACB has developed Laboratory Medicine Practice Guidelines for point-of-care testing for the use of cardiac biomarkers in ACS.[10A] These guidelines address administrative issues, cost-effective utilization, and clinical and technical performance of cardiac biomarkers in the emergency medicine department (ED). Eleven proposed elements of the guidelines are:

1. Members of EDs, primary care physicians, cardiologists, hospital administrators, and clinical laboratory staff should work collectively to develop an accelerated protocol for the use of biomarkers in the evaluation of patients with possible ACS.
2. This protocol should be applied to facilitate the diagnosis of MI in the ED, or to continue the diagnosis at other locations in the hospital.
3. Quality assurance measures should be used with monitoring to reduce medical errors and improve patient treatment.
4. Blood collection should be referenced to the time of presentation in the ED and, if available, to the reported time of symptom onset.
5. The interdisciplinary team should include personnel who are knowledgeable about local reimbursement.
6. The laboratory should perform biomarker testing with a maximum turnaround time (TAT) of 1 hour, optimally 30 minutes. The TAT is defined as the time from blood collection to reporting of results to the provider.
7. Institutions that cannot consistently provide a 1 hour TAT should implement POC testing assays.
8. Performance specifications and characteristics for central laboratory and POC testing assays should not differ.

9. Laboratory personnel must be involved in selection of POC assays, training of individuals to perform the analysis (whether laboratory or nonlaboratory personnel), maintenance of POC equipment, oversight of proficiency and competency of operators, and compliance with requirements of regulatory agencies.
10. POC assays should provide quantitative results.
11. Manufacturers are encouraged to work closely with professional organizations to develop structured committees and to establish quality performance specifications for new biomarkers.

For both point-of-care and central laboratory testing, and for practical considerations, anticoagulated whole blood or plasma appears to be the optimal specimen for rapid emergent processing. This eliminates the extra time needed for clotting and additional sample handling. However, differences have been described between plasma, whole blood, and serum specimens for cTnI concentration measurement by an individual assay. Both ethylenediaminetetraacetic acid (EDTA) and heparin are known to interfere with cTnI and cTnT antibody-binding affinity, as well as produce some matrix effect differences.[131] It is not recommended that different sample types are mixed during an individual's workup when serial, timed samples are being drawn to rule in or out an MI. Although clinicians and laboratorians continue to publish guidelines supporting TATs of less than 60 minutes for cardiac biomarkers, the largest TAT study (published in 2005) demonstrated that TAT expectations are not being met in a large proportion of hospitals. A College of Pathologists (CAP) Q-probe survey study[293] of 7020 cardiac troponin and 4368 CK-MB determinations in 159 hospitals demonstrated that median and 90th percentile TATs for troponin and CK-MB were as follows: 74.5 minutes, 129 minutes; and 82 minutes, 131 minutes, respectively. Less than 25% of hospitals were able to meet the less than 60 minute TAT, representing the biomarker order-to-report time. However, data have shown that implementation of POC cardiac troponin testing can decrease TATs to less than 30 minutes in cardiology critical care and short stay units.[10A,15,16,224,249,287,352]

The following example demonstrates how an institution that addressed a poor TAT problem for cTn improved laboratory services through cross-department cooperation.[16,281] Based at a 400 bed county hospital with 120,000 patient presentations a year through the emergency department, approximately 30,000 cTn orders per year were tested for both outpatients and the 1800 to 2000 patients admitted for short- or long-term care. A 2 month survey of the TAT for cTn showed a 90% TAT of 118 minutes. To better meet the published guideline of 60 minutes 100% of the time, the laboratory medical director, the emergency medicine staff whose primary responsibility involved ACS MI presentations, and the cardiology medical director who was responsible for the 11 bed cardiac 24 to 48 hour observation unit [cardiac short stay unit (CSSU)], 28 bed telemetry unit, and 8 bed cardiac care unit (CCU) met and designed an ACS triage protocol, outlined in Figure 47-13. Two point-of-care cTnI assay systems were placed in the small ED laboratory, staffed by

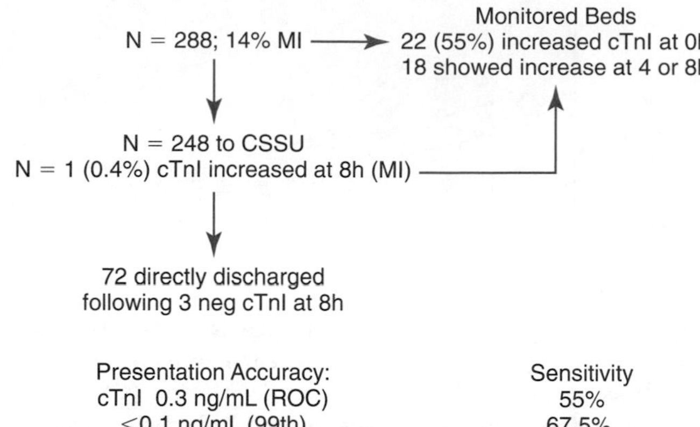

Figure 47-13 Role of cardiac troponin testing correlated with patient flow in the triage process from the emergency room, cardiac short stay unit, and coronary care unit. *(From Betti I, Castelli G, Barchielli A, Beligni C, Boscherini V, De Luca L, et al. The role of N-terminal PRO-brain natriuretic peptide and echocardiography for screening asymptomatic left ventricular dysfunction in a population at high risk for heart failure. The PROBE-HF study. J Card Fail 2009;15:377-84.)*

the clinical laboratory around the clock, in support of the hospital's level 1 trauma center. Two additional POC assays were placed in the CSSU, in which 42 nurses were trained by the laboratories' POC coordinators. The flow of specimens was such that initial presentation cTnI requests ordered through the ER were analyzed in the ED laboratory—about 6000 to 8000 per year. TAT from the time of blood draw to the provider result report was less than 18 minutes, 100% of the time. Patients admitted to the hospital to rule in/out MI who were at low risk were admitted to the CSSU, where staff nurses provided less than 20-minute TAT 100% of the time from blood draw to results to provider. In the CSSU, in compliance with the hospital protocol that at least a 6-hour postpresentation sample had to remain normal for cTnI, two blood specimens, in addition to the ED presentation sample, were measured at 4 and 8 hours. The uniform timed ordering protocol for ruling out MI included four timed draws at 0, 4, 8, and 12 hours. In patients admitted to the telemetry unit or the coronary care unit, a dedicated blood draw was tubed to the central laboratory, where specimens were given priority testing status, and thus met a TAT of less than 60 minutes 98% of the time.

During this process, it was recognized that POC testing was not cost-effective for patients in telemetry or CCU units; these were mostly patients at moderate to high risk in whom a clinical diagnosis had already been made; thus urgent cTn values were less necessary. The CSSU was successful in decreasing the length of stay in the unit by 0.8 day through implementation of POC testing, allowing triage to lower levels of care and/or discharge on a 24/7 basis. Although the

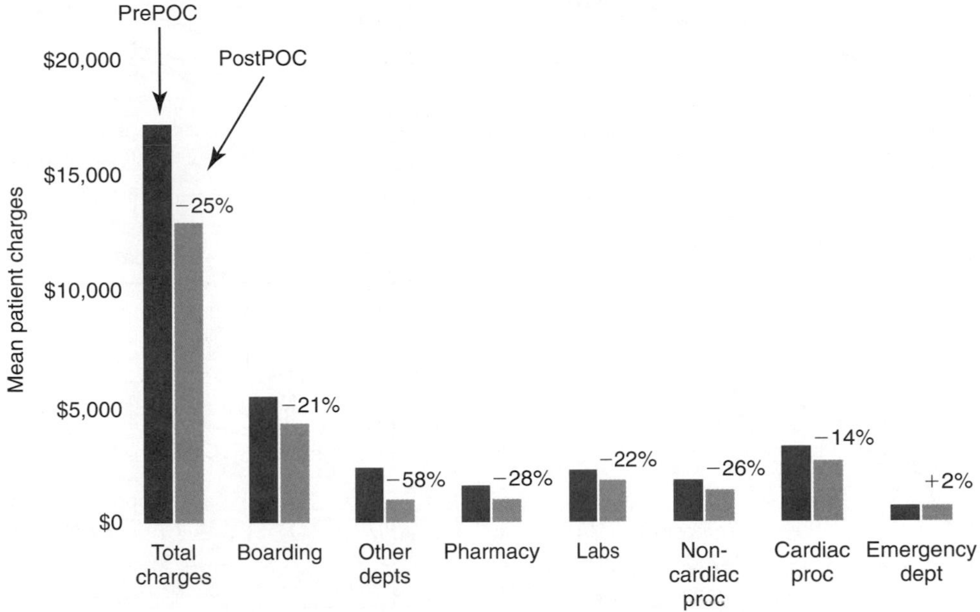

Figure 47-14 Financial impact of incorporating point-of-care (POC) cardiac troponin I (cTnI) testing into a cardiology service compared with central laboratory cTnI testing. In each pair of bars, the left and right bars indicate the costs before and after introduction of POC testing, respectively. *(From Betti I, Castelli G, Barchielli A, Beligni C, Boscherini V, De Luca L, et al. The role of N-terminal PRO-brain natriuretic peptide and echocardiography for screening asymptomatic left ventricular dysfunction in a population at high risk for heart failure. The PROBE-HF study. J Card Fail 2009;15:377-84.)*

direct cost per assay reagent increased from $3.83 (central laboratory) to $10.51 (POC testing), the overall cost to the patient decreased by more than $4000 per admission (Figure 47-14), primarily based on decreased bed charges from a more costly cardiac bed to a less expensive general medicine bed or to discharge. These data highlight the continued need for laboratory services and healthcare providers to work together to develop better processes to meet a less than 60 minute TAT, as requested by physicians. It is important to indicate that the POC testing assay used in the previous study example (Siemens Stratus CS; Siemens Healthcare Diagnostics, Inc., Deerfield, Ill) appears to be the only POC cTn assay with adequate analytical sensitivity, similar to central laboratory contemporary assays, and that other POC assays that are not as analytically sensitive will need to be independently validated. Further, it has been shown that a less sensitive POC assay may miss a positive cTn value that would be detected as increased by a more sensitive contemporary assay, as noted in Figure 47-15.

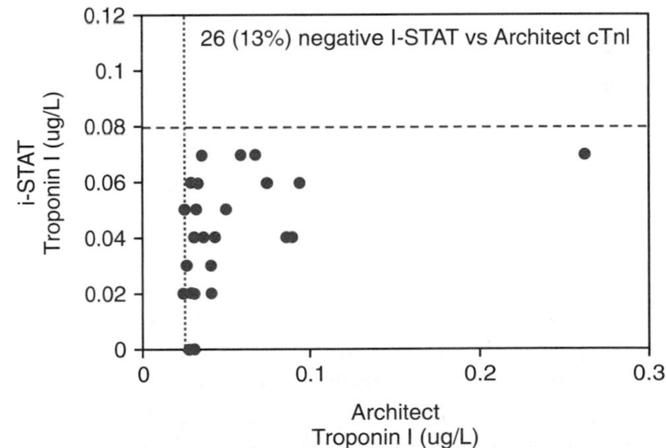

Figure 47-15 Scatterplot of i-STAT-negative and Architect-positive samples. The *dotted line* represents the 99th percentile cutoff for each instrument. *(From Singh J, Akbar MS, Adabag S. Discordance of cardiac troponin I assays on the point-of-care i-STAT and Architect assays from Abbott Diagnostics. Clin Chim Acta 2009;403:59-260. Figure courtesy Jasbir Singh.)*

Clinical Use of Cardiac Troponin

cTns have been available for clinical use since 1995, when the first cTn T (cTnT) assay was approved. Since that time, it has become clear that enhanced cardiac specificity and particularly improved sensitivity lead to more frequent and more accurate diagnosis of cardiovascular abnormalities (see Table 47-2, Figure 47-16).[178] Initial use of these assays was influenced in large part by the previous use of markers such as CK-MB. CK-MB is substantially less sensitive and less cardiac specific than cTn, but because of its long use, it had become entrenched in the thinking of clinicians and laboratorians. For this reason perhaps, the first set of guidelines by the NACB attempted to compromise between the use of these two markers in setting guidelines for clinical use.[398] These guidelines suggested that there should be two cutoffs.

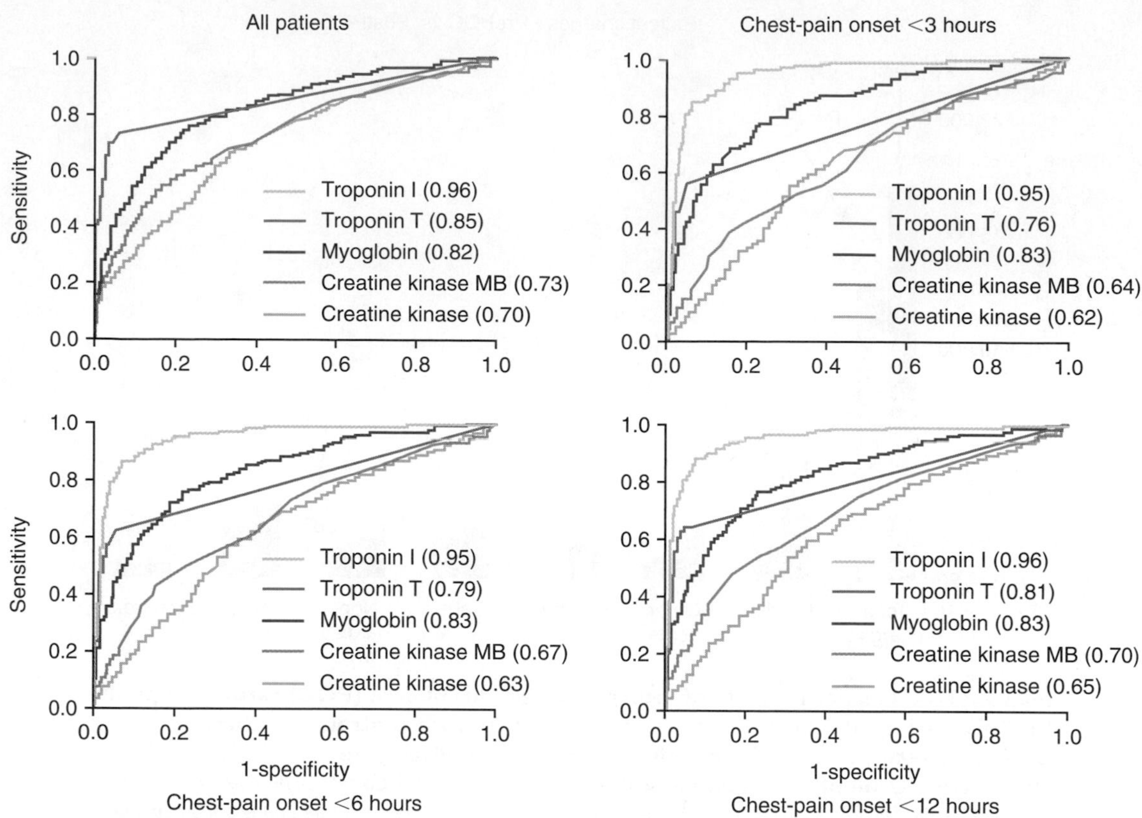

Figure 47-16 Receiver operating characteristic (ROC) curve analysis of troponin, myoglobin, and CK-MB by time from onset of symptoms to presentation.

One cutoff was selected to be equivalent to values of CK-MB in the clinical identification of patients. This cutoff, known as the ROC curve–derived cutoff value, considered CK-MB as the gold standard, as it had been for years. However, this cutoff did not take advantage of the increased sensitivity of cTn values.[299] A second cutoff was recommended for use at a lower level (the 97.5th percentile of a normal patient population), which was poorly clinically defined, above which patients were considered to have cardiac injury. But even patients with a classic history of AMI were designated as having "unstable angina with minimal myocardial necrosis." The guidelines followed extensive research demonstrating large numbers of patients with chest pain (roughly an additional 33%) whose prognoses in terms of subsequent frequency and timing of events were identical, and who had increased cTn values but normal CK-MB values.[299] These findings were documented despite the fact that the initial version of cTn assays was relatively insensitive compared with contemporary assays.

This concept of using prognosis to confirm diagnosis rapidly became the paradigm not only for cTn but for the validation of most other markers as well. It was not until 1999, when a task force empaneled by the American College of Cardiology (ACC) and the European Society of Cardiology (ESC) took issue with these guidelines, that the concept of using only one cutoff value was initiated.[6] ESC/ACC guidelines suggested the use, not of the 97.5th percentile of a reference population but, in recognition of increased sensitivity of the marker that led to many elevations that were difficult to explain, of the 99th percentile. This had the potential benefit of reducing the overlap to 1% between those with disease and normal individuals.[181] It was conceptually important because even by this time, it was clear that enhanced sensitivity of cTn was leading to the identification of a substantial number of patients in whom the cause of cardiac injury (see later sections) could not be determined. This is often the case when one moves from a relatively insensitive measure to one that has substantially greater sensitivity (i.e., when one uncovers new diagnostically and prognostically important increases).[148,233,234] Nonetheless, clinicians had difficulty understanding this because such elevations had not been described previously, and the pathophysiology was obscure. This problem continues today as newer assays become more and more sensitive. The ESC/ACC biochemical group at that time also recommended that the 99th percentile should be measurable with excellent precision and suggested, not mandated, a criterion of 10% CV or less at the 99th percentile. The group did not, however, recommend that if assays did not reach that level of precision, the values should be raised. Unfortunately, this was the extrapolation of some, and it led to even greater heterogeneity in how cTn values were interpreted.

Some individuals persisted in using the NACB recommendations, some utilized the ESC/ACC recommendations, and some because of fear of false positives caused by imprecision employed a value higher than the 99th percentile, usually at the level of the 10% CV value. Add to this the fact that local laboratories often felt the need (appropriately) to validate the assays in their own hands and came up with different values, and one can see how the use of cTn values became fragmented and idiosyncratic. This problem also led to tremendous heterogeneity in the published literature and attendant confusion on the part of clinicians.[128,172,392]

It is now very clear that normal cTn values are substantially lower than concentrations that are being reported for healthy individuals by contemporary assays (see Table 47-1). (The reported concentrations in healthy individuals often represent "noise" in the contemporary assays.) Research assays are beginning to have the ability to measure healthy individuals' low concentrations accurately, but only one (the high-sensitivity cTnT assay) has been released for clinical use and, as of this time, it is unavailable in the United States.[197,394,399] Nonetheless, this documentation and a wealth of clinical information has made it clear that for contemporary assays, the 99th percentile value is the key value to use when measuring cardiac cTn.[33,184,274] Any value above the 99th percentile should be considered abnormal. Concerns about false positives induced by such criteria should be minimal because assuming adequate quality assurance of the assays, even reduced precision should not lead to false-positive results.[26] Usually, reduced precision simply impairs the sensitivity of the assay. Statistical modeling of this issue suggests that as long as one does not look at a huge number of consecutive samples, the clinical impact of utilizing even an imprecise assay is negligible with regard to false-positive results. For this reason, along with the clinical data, the criteria in all guidelines now include use of the 99th percentile.[273,372] Once one recognizes that the 99th percentile is the criterion for abnormality, and therefore is the criterion that one should at least keep in mind, one can progress to understanding how to use cTn in a variety of clinical situations. The recent publication of several papers has clearly demonstrated this point, which will be discussed in the following section.

Use of cTn for the Diagnosis of Acute Myocardial Infarction

Acute myocardial infarction is a state characterized by abnormalities between nutrient perfusion and myocardial oxygen consumption. It is usually diagnosed when abnormalities in coronary flow at least in part contribute to the pathogenesis of cardiac injury. Because of the high sensitivity and specificity of cTn, it has become the cornerstone of the diagnosis of myocardial infarction (see Box 47-2, Figure 47-17). Accordingly, one needs an increased value of cardiac cTn in the appropriate clinical setting with values that manifest a rising pattern for the diagnosis of acute myocardial infarction. Some clarification concerning the specifics of that definition are necessary:

1. The clinical substrate (usually risk factors for AMI in the patient) is key. An increased cTn value is not synonymous with the diagnosis of myocardial infarction.[178] First, both the substrate (such as risk factors) and the presentation (most often chest discomfort) must be compatible with the diagnosis. At times, imaging, whether performed at the time of intervention by angiography or thereafter, may provide proof of the substrate.[273,372]
2. Many clinical situations can mimic acute myocardial infarction, the most common of which is myocarditis. Apical ballooning is another.[119,354,363]
3. Because of the increased sensitivity of cardiac cTn, clinicians need to be astute to the possibility that a given elevation in cTn even with a rising pattern suggesting that it is acute may not be due to ischemic heart disease (see Box 47-1).[178] This is conceptually difficult for many clinicians because with CK-MB, which was reasonably insensitive, most substantive elevations were associated with coronary heart disease, albeit not all.
4. Acute events leading to cardiac injury usually will manifest a changing pattern of values.[175] The rationale for this is that as assays have become more sensitive, it has become clear that elevations of cTn can exist chronically.[24,95,189,386,417] The

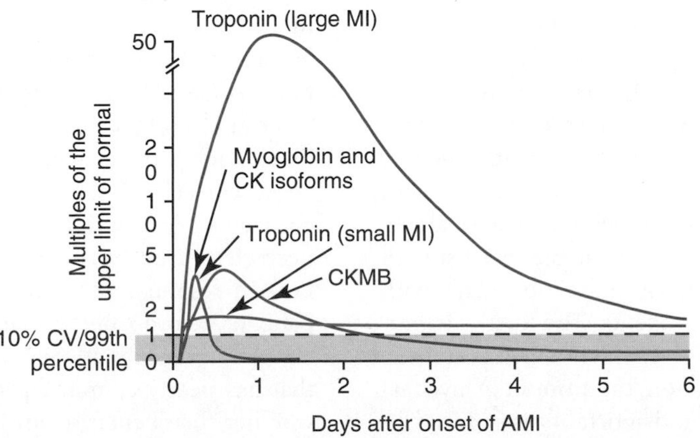

Figure 47-17 Kinetics of myoglobin, troponin, and CK-MB. With contemporary assays, cardiac troponin (cTn) rises more rapidly than do other markers. With small myocardial infarctions (MT), two types of time courses are possible, as indicated by the two arrows.

most overt case of this is seen in patients with renal failure,[29] but as indicated later, in a large number of clinical circumstances, elevations of cTn exist and are maintained over time. This is also the pattern manifest when artifactual increases occur as the result of analytical problems caused by interferences from substances in the blood of some patients.[123,210] Although patients with chronic elevations (not those with artifactual causes) are at high risk over time, they are not necessarily at high risk short term. For this reason, the guidelines groups have advocated the need for a rising pattern of cTn values in patients who present early after the onset of symptoms, because such increases usually are indicative of an acute process. However, the acute process may not be acute myocardial infarction. Whether acute myocardial infarction is present is a clinical decision, but if the values are not rising, one might seriously question whether acute disease of any kind is present, or whether the elevations are of a more chronic nature. Care is necessary to ensure that one does not miss individuals who come in late, after the onset of symptoms, whose cTn values may be near peak values, or whose values are on the long persistent tail of the time-concentration curve (see Figure 47-17). They may appear not to have a changing pattern of values because they are near the peak of the time-concentration curve or on the gradual down slope.
5. With contemporary assays, values should exceed the 99% value of the reference population. Use of such a value maximizes the sum of sensitivity and specificity.[33,184,273,274,372]

The guidelines distinguish five different types of acute myocardial infarction (see Box 47-4); two will be considered here because they both present with chest discomfort and increased biomarkers. One is the so-called spontaneous, or what some would call "wild type", in which acute plaque rupture leads to some degree of thrombosis, or an episode wherein platelet accretion occurs on a plaque, leading to thrombosis.[273] The second type includes coronary abnormalities with possible supply-demand imbalance, vasospasm, or endothelial dysfunction, which provides evidence of myocardial injury. For example, supply-demand imbalance with fixed coronary artery disease is thought to be the cause of most perioperative myocardial infarctions,[218] and these patients do not require the same care as those with a spontaneous AMI.[273]

Individuals with spontaneous AMI can have STEMI or non-STEMI as indicated by the ECG pattern that they manifest.[9,273] Data indicate that immediate treatment aimed at opening the occluded artery is mandatory for patients with STEMI; this should be done based on the ECG pattern alone, even before biomarker values become available to assist with diagnosis. Opening of the artery is done nowadays with primary PCI and/or thrombolytic agents. The former is preferred whenever the two are available in similar timeframes. With prompt coronary recanalization, the amount of myocardium that is lost is minimized, and mortality is reduced. It should be noted that coronary recanalization increases the rapidity of cTn release, and thus the rate of rise of the time-concentration curve is increased, and the time to peak values is shortened.[178]

A non-STEMI is less often associated with total coronary occlusion and usually is identified by ECG changes, which show not ST segment elevation, but rather ST segment depression or T-wave changes. Given the sensitivity of cTn for this diagnosis, the ECG is even at times totally normal. Patients who present with chest pain due to coronary artery disease should have risk factors, an appropriate presentation, or imaging evidence of this syndrome; patients with an increased cTn, using contemporary assays and recommended cutoff values, are known to have more severe coronary heart disease than individuals without increased cTns. Likely for this reason, they also have more procoagulant activity; multiple intervention studies have shown that these patients benefit from aggressive anticoagulation, including heparin (the data for low molecular weight heparin are much stronger than the data for unfractionated heparin), glycoprotein IIb/IIIa antiplatelet agents, and an early invasive strategy consisting of PCI or coronary artery bypass grafting (CABG). Use of these strategies in patients without increased cTn values has been shown to be of no benefit and, in some trials, has actually proved detrimental.[14]

However, not all patients have easily identifiable culprit lesions[42,81,247,297] upon which to intervene, and this explains some apparent spontaneous AMIs without severe coronary artery disease. These patients, often women, may have endothelial dysfunction, coronary vasospasm, or some other transient process that has resolved prior to investigation. These patients might be designated as having type 2 myocardial infarction according to the guidelines. This group might also include those individuals who have fixed but stable coronary artery disease but have some degree of damage due to excessive myocardial oxygen consumption, such as that caused by severe tachycardia or by hypotension or hypertension. Coronary arteries that are diseased tend to vasoconstrict rather than dilating in response to stimuli that would normally evoke vasodilation and increases in coronary flow.[218] This can be identified by special studies utilizing provocative stimuli and documenting these paradoxical responses; these paradoxical responses occur in response to cold, to changes in catecholamines, and to changes in potassium that probably induce a degree of vasoconstriction on top of coronary lesions.[362] Because the cross-sectional area of a tube is related to the square of the radius, small degrees of vasoconstriction can cause marked changes in blood flow through the artery. Thus, some patients, whether with vasoconstriction or simply because fixed coronary disease inhibits the ability to increase coronary perfusion, have increased cTns and myocardial necrosis caused by an inability to improve coronary blood flow in response to increased oxygen consumption. These patients are probably fundamentally different from individuals who have spontaneous MIs and likely are not a subgroup that has nearly as much procoagulant activity; it is unclear whether they benefit from interventional therapy. This may be one of the reasons why women who tend to have more severe endothelial dysfunction seem to have a different profile.[81,247] Nonetheless, depending on the specific study reviewed, substantial numbers—10 to 15% of patients at least, and perhaps as high as 30% of patients—may not have an identifiable lesion that has caused the event, leading to consideration of this alternative pathophysiology.[297] From the perspective of diagnosis, however, the cTn criteria are identical. Distinctions between types has to be made on the basis of clinical characteristics and other diagnostic studies.

Three other types of MIs are recognized.[372] One does not use biomarkers at all. This case includes patients who may present classically with both chest pain and ECG changes but succumb either (1) before blood tests can be obtained, or (2) before enough time has elapsed for the circulating concentration of cTn to exceed the 99th percentile. Two other types of myocardial infarctions have been designated; these are related to PCI and CABG and will be covered later under "Special Situations."

Operationalization of a Changing Pattern of cTn Values

This is a challenging area. Minor changes in values may be due to analytical causes. In general, two values are different if they differ by more than 2.77 standard deviations (SDs) (assuming the variances are comparable at the two concentrations).[400] Ideally, one would like to include both analytical and biological variation in calculation of the SDs.[402] Unfortunately, analysis of biological variation requires studies of stable subjects, and only the developing high-sensitivity assays can provide data on healthy people. Thus, at present, the analysis has focused on the use of data on analytical imprecision alone. At high concentrations of troponins, the analytical coefficient of variation (CV) is 5 to 7%, so a difference of 20% is unlikely to be attributable to measurement imprecision.[273] But as values begin to approach the low concentrations corresponding to the 99th percentile value, analytical CV increases, making the relative difference between two consecutive values prone to increases by chance alone.[400] To calculate percent changes, one might need the values to be reported with more than the number of decimal points usually reported for clinical use of troponin assays. Local analysis of imprecision should be used to guide interpretation of differences in results for consecutive samples, with larger percentage changes necessary to suggest real change at very low levels of troponin. Obviously, defining a consistent period of time for analysis is also key to an accurate approach to this analysis. High-sensitivity assays will help with this problem because they make it possible to calculate a reference change value, i.e., the value that must be exceeded before a change in consecutive test results is statistically significant.[126,274]

Special Situations With Acute Myocardial Infarction

Post Percutaneous Coronary Intervention

It has long been appreciated that interventions done on the coronary arteries can result in the release, from heart muscle, of biomarkers indicative of cardiac injury.[58] For this reason, a variety of criteria have been promulgated, starting years ago with CK-MB. It was shown initially that elevations of CK-MB that occurred post procedure were highly predictive of adverse events over the long term. These findings were difficult to explain because the amount of injury involved often was very minor but was nonetheless easy to document with sophisticated techniques such as cardiac magnetic resonance (cMR) imaging. However, controversy about the mechanisms continued, and a large number are being hypothesized. The advent of cTn markers has rendered this issue far less complex. Patients who have elevations of circulating cTn and who present with acute coronary problems have much more severe abnormalities in coronary anatomy than those who do not have elevations of cTn.[9] In recent studies, the baseline cTn value has been added to the analysis of these post-PCI elevations.[260,309] This was done for many years by others, but not with assays that measured cTn concentrations even close to the 99th percentile. Accordingly, it is only recently that the data have confirmed several important conceptual issues.

The first concept is that a vast majority of patients with significant elevations (threefold to fivefold increase in CK-MB or cTn) that in the past were associated with an adverse prognosis are those with increased cTn values at baseline. This usually (although not always) is indicative of an acute presentation and therefore a rising pattern of values. In the setting with a rising pattern of values, it is hard know whether one should attribute the increases to the PCI or to the initial insult. Nonetheless, when one incorporates the baseline value into the analysis, most of the prognostic significance of the cTn values post procedure is ablated.[260,309] Indeed, those data suggest that it is only when one has an elevation of cTn at baseline that one is apt to frequently find marked elevations in cTn post procedure, suggesting that in most instances, at least a blend of the two processes occurs. These issues have been confounded not only by failure to use appropriate cutoffs for cTn, but by the use of insensitive assays. More recent guidelines clarify this circumstance substantially by indicating that if one has an increased cTn at baseline prior to PCI, the diagnosis of post-PCI injury is confounded and cannot be made.[273] Thus, one requires a normal baseline cTn in almost all instances to identify procedure-related myocardial injury. If the baseline cTn is increased, then subsequent increases may not be attributable to the procedure itself, and a diagnosis of post-PCI injury cannot be made.

Marked elevations as indicated previously are uncommon but can occur. When they do occur, they are rarely of cardiovascular importance in the sense that the more marked elevations are easily presaged by clinical information at the time of the procedure. Thus, cTn adds very little that is new. In addition, it is unclear whether patients have an adverse cardiovascular prognosis over time. In the most recent analysis done by using the most appropriate cutoff values and contemporary cTn assays, borderline statistical significance was attributed to elevations post PCI.[309] However, most events that did occur were noted during procedures in patients who had severe underlying noncardiac comorbidities and therefore underwent palliative procedures. The event rate if one excluded patients with non–cardiac-related subsequent complications would not have been of statistical importance and even with their inclusion was of only borderline significance. Thus, it

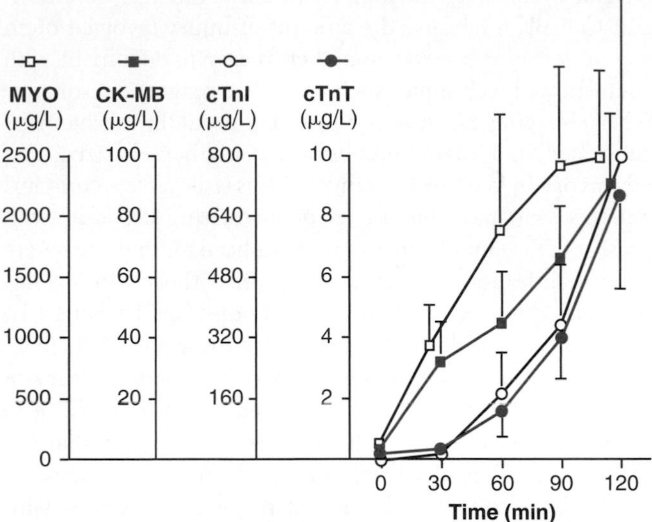

Figure 47-18 Time course (mean and standard error) of serum cardiac troponin I (cTnI), cardiac troponin T (cTnT), creatine kinase-2 (CK-MB), and myoglobin (MYO) concentrations after initiation of thrombolytic therapy in patients with thrombolysis in myocardial infarction (TIMI) grade 3 reperfusion flow. *(From Apple FS, Sharkey SW, Henry TD. Early serum cardiac troponin I and T concentrations following successful thrombolysis for acute myocardial infarction. Clin Chem 1995;41:1197-8.)*

now appears that collection of this information post PCI is not necessary. Nonetheless, criteria still exist for these occasional patients who may have post-PCI injury. The appropriate cutoff value is unclear, but it is clear that very few patients will reach the marked threefold to fivefold elevations previously advocated if the baseline cTn is not increased.[260] Thus, if cTn is increased post-PCI more than threefold, with a normal baseline cTn value assumed, they can be diagnosed as having had a periprocedural myocardial infarction. No specific therapy is mandated. Regarding biomarker changes that occur following reperfusion of an occluded vessel after PCI or thrombolytic therapy[1] in AMI patients, greater than twofold increases in biomarkers occur within 90 minutes of reperfusion, the rate of increase of biomarkers within the first 4 hours separates reperfused from nonreperfused patients, and after myocardial reperfusion in AMI patients, washouts of all biomarkers parallel each other (Figure 47-18).[12,36,390,414] However, increased washout does not define the level of reperfusion; this is what clinicians need to know diagnostically, so this approach has not become clinically widespread.

One unique subset needs to be taken into account, and that is the small group of patients who may have chronic preprocedure elevations in cTn. These individuals will manifest a rising pattern, albeit from an increased baseline, when they have events including post-PCI events. Accordingly, what has been suggested is that the criteria used for reinfarction of an increased value of 20% or more should be used to define post-PCI infarction in this group.[273] This, as with other values that utilize changing patterns, must be done over a constrained period of time.

Post-CABG Myocardial Infarction

Abundant data indicate that patients post cardiac surgery have elevations in cardiac cTn. Indeed in the vast majority of studies, such elevations are of prognostic importance: the higher the elevation, the worse the prognosis.[267,336,369] However, the underlying propensity for elevation is moderated in part by the details of the procedure. Thus, for example, procedures that are done off cardiopulmonary bypass evoke less cTn release,[267] as one might expect, because they cause less direct cardiac injury. In addition, a relationship has been noted between the duration of cross-clamp time and the amount of marker that is elaborated, the temperature of the cardioplegia, and the duration of the procedure. Most of the injury as assessed from cMR studies is subendocardial and often apical. Higher biomarker values post CABG are associated with transmural injury.[340,359] Thus procedures that are longer, such as those that include valve replacement, are very likely to evoke more cardiac damage than those that are shorter. Accordingly, finding a single value that separates all of these different subsets is impossible. Accordingly, most recent guidelines have elected not to try to define separate criteria for subsets of these procedures, but instead have preferred to define a single cutoff that can be used for all the situations already described for which ancillary criteria need to be employed. The decision of most of the most recent guidelines has been that one should employ a fivefold increase in cTn post procedure and add to that additional criteria such as ECG changes, changes with imaging, and the development of new regional wall-motion abnormalities.

The value of such an approach is that it allows one to use a single cutoff. The downside of the approach is that this cutoff lacks some precision when it comes to the types of procedures performed. Thus, one might well do better if one could devise specific criteria for each subset of the procedures. This is an extensive task because of multiple variations in the way in which cardiac surgery is done, but it is a task that at some point in time might be worthwhile. Nonetheless, the key concept is that the prognostic impact of increased cTn concentrations is related to the magnitude of the increase. Unfortunately, because of the complexity of these considerations, no one has been able to define a value at which one can attribute increases in cTn to a specific coronary-related event such as graft or native vessel occlusion.[370] Thus, although the aggregate amount of marker that is released is prognostic (for both CK-MB and cTn), it does not distinguish the mechanism of injury.

Patients Who Have Increased cTns at Baseline

As indicated previously, some patients may have cardiovascular comorbidities such as heart failure, left ventricular hypertrophy, renal failure, and diabetes, along with elevations in cTn that are stable and chronic. In these circumstances, it is known that dialysis patients, to take but one example, increase their values from the increased baseline after AMI and the values come back down over time to the original baseline, suggesting that a changing pattern can be used despite increased baseline. This is likely the case for these other entities and is what has been incorporated into most of the guideline documents.

Evaluating Possible Acute Myocardial Infarction

Between 5 and 6 million individuals present to emergency departments yearly with complaints that could be compatible with acute myocardial infarction. The screening done in emergency room settings takes a very broad approach because many patients have atypical symptoms. For example, patients with diabetes and hypertension often have what has been termed *silent,* or perhaps a better term would be *unrecognized,* acute myocardial infarction.[9,227] In addition, patients who are older (e.g., over the age of 80) often present with myocardial infarction in the absence of chest discomfort. Thus, a very broad screen in the emergency department is appropriate. Accordingly, the diagnosis of AMI often relies heavily on abnormalities in cardiac biomarkers such as cTn. The criteria for ruling in myocardial infarction are listed in Box 47-2 and often can be accomplished in a fairly short time.[29,201,242,317] Recent data suggest that use of a changing pattern can identify 80% of patients with acute myocardial infarction within 2 to 3 hours of presentation.[242] Although at times not adequately emphasized, this of course implies the use of more sensitive rather than less sensitive assays and use of appropriate cutoff values.[177] Of course, these data take advantage of the fact that often patients with chest discomfort do not immediately come to the hospital; thus, often it is many hours since their initial chest discomfort.

Exclusion of myocardial infarction is far more problematic. In the United States,[9] at most 20% of patients who are evaluated with ischemic symptoms suggestive of ACS (it is somewhat higher in Europe,[201,317] where selection seems to be done in a different manner) rule in for AMI or have increased cTn values. Thus, in the United States, one must identify the relatively small proportion of the patients who have ACS. Data suggest that patients sent home with a missed diagnosis do poorly; it is perhaps not surprising that they are a common source of litigation. A variety of protocols have been advocated for the early evaluation of patients with possible acute myocardial infarction. These have often presumed that cTn rises late because the initial assays were relatively insensitive, causing that to occur. Thus, there has been advocacy for myoglobin, heart fatty acid–binding protein, or even CK-MB as early markers. Recent data utilizing contemporary assays and contemporary cutoffs suggest that use of other markers is rarely necessary because cTn, as measured with current assays, increases rapidly (see Figure 47-17).[118,197,201] With criteria of the 99th percentile and a rising pattern, 80% of rule-ins are detected within 2 to 3 hours.[201,242,317]

It appears from the most recent literature that the cumulative value of additional markers is small, if not totally negated, by the use of the 99th percentile and criteria for interpreting changes of concentration of cTns. In fact, it appears that with contemporary (i.e., those in use today) assays, cTn rises more rapidly than the other so-called early rising markers. How long it takes to rule out AMI, however, is less clear. This is a difficult issue to study because one needs longer periods of observation to see who eventually will be determined to have AMI at a time when protocols are attempting to move people more rapidly through systems. Thus, present standards suggest that 6 hours is the length of time that should be designated for cTn monitoring to occur. Some data suggest that one should make sure that the patient is at least 6 hours from the onset of chest pain to completely ensure that infarction has not occurred.[147] Others, because of relative insecurity of the timing of onset of chest symptoms, believe that the clock for this timing should be started at the time the patient presents to the emergency room. This at present is an unadjudicated issue, but 6 hours appears to be the preferred time. It would be ideal if this time could be cut substantially in the interest of more rapid discharge. Additional research is needed.

Other Causes of Acute cTn Elevation in the Absence of Acute Ischemic Heart Disease

Many acute diseases are associated with elevated cTns (see Box 47-1). This can occur for many reasons,[78,112,208,257,358] including direct trauma to the heart; we know that contemporary cTn assays are sufficiently sensitive to detect implantable cardioverter-defibrillator (ICD) firings, biopsies, cardioversions, and so forth. Also, some patients may have type 2 myocardial infarction, as indicated previously. Critically ill patients often have tachycardia, hypertension, or hypotension with or without drugs that may be given therapeutically such as catecholamines, which in and of themselves can directly damage myocardium. Thus in some instances, these individuals have what could be called type 2 AMI. On the other hand, in the absence of at least some coronary artery abnormality to negatively affect perfusion, these episodes would not be designated as type 2 AMIs. Patients in the absence of coronary artery disease who have very severe supply/demand imbalance may have elevated cTn; these individuals probably do not have AMI. Finally, direct toxic effects of circulating cytokines and catecholamines can end up causing severe myocardial toxicity. Such is the case in sepsis. Thus, consideration of each mechanism for a given elevation is important. A short, brief tabulation is provided here:

1. *Trauma:* Contusion, slow potential (S/P) cardiac ablation, pacing, ICD firings, cardioversion, myocardial biopsy, and closure following a variety of interventional procedures commonly cause elevations in cTn and should be expected. These elevations are usually modest. More marked elevations should engender suspicion of additional processes.
2. *Congestive heart failure:* Heart failure can cause acute elevations,[302] and elevations have been noted during long-term monitoring of patients as well.[261] In both circumstances, they are markedly adverse prognostic signals and indicate more severe heart failure and an increased proximate likelihood of mortality. Such patterns can be rising but need not be, especially with more chronic heart failure. The prognostic significance of cTn is additive to that of the natriuretic peptides. Elevations are usually modest.

3. *Severe valvular heart disease* with volume or pressure overload can be associated with elevations in cTn. Elevations may be more apt to occur with cTnI for volume overload via a calpain-mediated mechanism and may be more common with cTnT with left ventricular hypertrophy (LVH).
4. *Hypertension:* Hypertension in and of itself can cause LVH or cardiac enlargement, which increases wall stress and reduces nutritive perfusion, causing increases in cTn. LVH is associated with reduced subendocardial perfusion caused by increased wall stress; therefore, subendocardial injury may occur in response to severe hypertension.[149] Obviously, because hypertension is a risk factor for coronary artery disease, these processes may be exacerbated by each other, but this is not necessary for elevations to be observed. Elevations most often are modest.
5. *Hypotension and tachycardia:* These can be synergistic with underlying coronary abnormalities or may occur independently.[48] Nonetheless, at some point, their severity can be sufficient to cause some degree of cTn release, usually modest.
6. *Postoperative noncardiac surgery patients:* Data suggest that most of these events are similar if not identical to type 2 MI, that is to say, most often among vascular surgery patients who have been best studied, these cTn elevations seem to be related to underlying coronary heart disease in association with an abnormality in acute myocardial oxygen consumption, usually hypertension or hypotension and/or tachycardia, anemia, and the like.[204] This is an area of expanding interest as it has become clear that more and more noncardiac surgery patients suffer events in the hospital, and it is likely that a more diverse group of patients will soon be elucidated. Data have already been gathered from some orthopedic surgery patients.[100] Causes of observed elevations may differ among the groups involved and may include, for example, pulmonary embolism, which is common in postoperative patients.
7. *Patients with renal failure*[43]: Patients with renal failure often have elevations in cTn that are highly prognostic. Elevations occur more frequently with cTnT than with cTnI, perhaps because processing of the two proteins is different in the renal failure circumstance. Nonetheless, elevations are highly prognostic in this group, but not necessarily for coronary artery disease.[162] A large percentage of renal failure patients die of sudden cardiac death. One should not presume that all cTn elevations occur in such groups, although this group does have an increased prevalence of coronary artery disease.
8. *Critically ill patients:* These individuals may or may not have underlying coronary heart disease, which is negatively synergistic with their acute illness, but they often have reasons for very substantial increases in myocardial oxygen consumption.[46,144] Elevations in cTn are common and usually modest but nonetheless are highly negative prognostically in the short and long term. An understanding of various subsets of patients in the large group should in the long run provide better ideas about how to treat such patients. Unfortunately, these data are missing at present.
9. *Drug toxicity:* Carbon monoxide poisoning is an archetypical example.[159] Elevations in response to drug toxicity have prognostic significance. Recent data show that one can detect[77] and with early treatment obviate the effects of some toxic chemotherapies by monitoring cTn and, when elevations occur, by using angiotensin-converting enzyme (ACE) inhibitors.[76] Snake bite venom can be another cause. It is very likely that over time, a far larger number of drug toxicities will be documented.
10. *Inflammatory heart disease:* Myocarditis, when acute, commonly causes elevations of cTn.[125] Myocarditis can also cause coronary vasospasm and is a common mimicker of acute coronary syndromes.[413] Elevation in this circumstance can be very high, even higher than that associated with acute infarction, or very modest, depending on whether patients have acute or chronic conditions.
11. *Pulmonary embolism*[132,216]: In general, the degree of cTn elevation is related to the degree of right ventricular (RV) dysfunction, and therefore to the severity of pulmonary hypertension induced. Increased cTn defines a patient who is at high risk; some have advocated that it should be used as an indication for the use of thrombolytic therapy of PE. This recommendation is premature at the present time. Elevations that occur with PE usually resolve within 40 hours. If they do not, one should consider recurrent emboli or another cause, along with or independent of pulmonary embolism.
12. *Sepsis*[7,46,384]: Severe septicemia with hypotension probably has multifactorial causes for increases in cTn. Such increases are often related to elaboration of toxic cytokines such as tumor necrosis factor (TNF) alpha and heat shock proteins; a relationship has also been noted between the magnitude of cTn elevation and the extent of myocardial depression associated with cTn elevation. Nonetheless, the extent of myocardial suppression is over and above that associated with a modest increase in cTn. In addition, catecholamines often used to treat these patients may contribute to the supply-demand imbalance associated with type 2 AMI.
13. *Burns:* Only when they are severe are elevations observed; this probably reflects the marked hemodynamic changes associated with severe burns.[282]
14. *Acute neurologic disease*[183,285,377]: Increases probably represent reflex stimulation from the central nervous system. A very substantial literature suggests that such is the case, and that such increases seem to be related to insults in the midbrain[44]; they are particularly prominent with subarachnoid bleeds. Such elevations are highly prognostic but not necessarily for coronary heart disease.
15. *Rhabdomyolysis:* Rhabdomyolysis can occur systemically with associated cardiac injury.[37]
16. *Transplant vasculopathy:* Monitoring of cTn has not been useful as an early marker, but elevations do occur with both transplant vasculopathy and rejection.[259]

17. *Vital exhaustion*[80,99,263,327]: Severe exercise has been shown to cause release of cTn. Whether this implies an element of minor myocardial injury or whether this could be release of cTn from the "cytosolic" pool is a difficult issue. Nonetheless, studies suggest that patients, despite some having cMR evidence of cardiac injury, do well and do not require emergency hospitalization.[70]
18. *Chronic elevations of cTn:* Any chronic cardiac comorbidity, whether it is coronary artery disease, LVH, heart failure, or diabetes, can be associated with elevations in cTn. In general, these patients are the ones who have the most severe disease and poorest prognosis. Recent data suggest that one can identify patients with chronic heart disease at risk for subsequent events by looking simply at whether a cTn is detectable or not. This suggests that with more sensitive assays, we may be able to identify patients who are at greater versus lesser risk from chronic heart disease. In addition, left ventricular hypertrophy and heart failure, both of which can cause increased wall stress and reduced subendocardial myocardial perfusion, are known to be associated with elevations in cTn. The prognostic significance of such elevations in older individuals is clear.
19. *Hypothyroidism:* This is a rare cause of cTn elevation.[349] Usually, hypothyroidism in the modern era is detected fairly early and treated, and it seems to take fairly severe hypothyroidism for elevations in cTn to occur. This is in contrast to previous literature, which suggested a high frequency of elevated CK-MB. Given the cTn data, it is likely that CK-MB elevations were due to skeletal muscle abnormalities, rather than to cardiac problems, as some might have initially surmised.
20. *Infiltrative disease such as amyloid*[113,114] and cardiomyopathies such as hemochromatosis are capable of causing increased cTns. In general, elevations are modest but very negatively prognostic.

In addition, one should always consider the possibility that chronic elevations are artifactual. Heterophilic antibodies can interfere in cTn assays (though less commonly than in the past) by binding to antibodies in the reagent. Some patients have antibodies that bind cTn, creating immunoglobulin-cTn complexes that are poorly cleared from the circulation, leading to increased concentrations of cTn in blood that do not indicate cardiac injury. Unexpected cTn results should be evaluated by the laboratory. Usually, when an interferant is present, dilution studies fail to give a linear pattern. Heterophile-blocking reagents can be used to minimize the effects of heterophilic antibodies. On occasion, even more sophisticated methods may be necessary to document false positives. Nonetheless, false-positive elevations appear to be relatively uncommon with present day cTn assays.

The Future

High-sensitivity cTn assays are being developed (see Table 47-1).* They have the ability to define normal values in most, if not all, individuals (see Figure 47-11). Present data indicate that these assays have the ability to allow for much more rapid diagnosis of acute myocardial infarction, and that values have prognostic significance (Figure 47-19). Perhaps with this approach, patients previously thought to have unstable angina (no cTn elevations) will be detected as having elevations. In addition, recent information suggests that positive stress tests might be predicted by increases of cTn measured by hs-cTn assays, although this result is controversial.[215,332] If so, a very rapid rule-out strategy might be possible that involves eliminating an acute coronary syndrome by finding the absence of an increasing pattern of cTn, precluding the need for stress testing. This would allow for the very rapid triage of patients with chest discomfort. In addition, recent data suggest that cTn increases may be useful in monitoring patients with more chronic heart disease, as indicated by data showing an adverse prognosis related to cTn levels in the Prevention of Events with Angiotensin Converting Enzyme Inhibition (PEACE) trial. Essential to the ability to use these assays properly will be the need to eliminate the use of large numbers of zeros. Thus, values will need to be reported as pg/mL or ng/L.

*References 57, 197, 198, 280, 382, 394, and 399.

Clinical Use of Creatine Kinase-MB (CK-MB)

Considering CK-MB an obsolete test has met with considerable resistance,[60,67,134,334] in part because of difficulty clinicians have had in understanding how to utilize cTn measurements. This has been fueled in part by heterogeneity in the cTn assays available, diversity in the cutoffs intermittently advocated, and difficulty in understanding how to respond to elevations in cTn that are seen with cTns but not with CK-MB because troponin is so much more diagnostically sensitive than CK-MB. Nonetheless, several groups have advocated that CK-MB assays should be eliminated. The major push for this comes from the thought that not only do they add expense while not adding value, but because clinicians who continue to rely on CK-MB often do patients a disservice. In addition, these assays retard clinicians' ability to learn how to use cTn measurements properly, which would be more efficacious in almost every situation. Accordingly, serious consideration should be given by laboratories to discontinuing the use of CKMB. Testing is not essential even for skeletal muscle disease in which total CK is appropriate, but it does eliminate a source of what some would argue is confusion for clinicians. This position has been well articulated in a recent editorial.[334]

Those who advocate continued use of CK-MB point to a small number of instances that are worthy of consideration. The first includes the most controversial, which is the area of recurrent infarction after an index AMI. When initial guidelines for the use of cTn were developed, how well one would do in diagnosing recurrent injury with cTn was called into question because cTn elevations persist for so long. Recent data suggest that cTn values detect acute recurrent injury very well (Figure 47-20), and that re-elevations occur with sufficient robustness that they can be detected promptly.[20] From first principles related to both sensitivity and specificity (see earlier), some would argue that cTn would be clearly superior

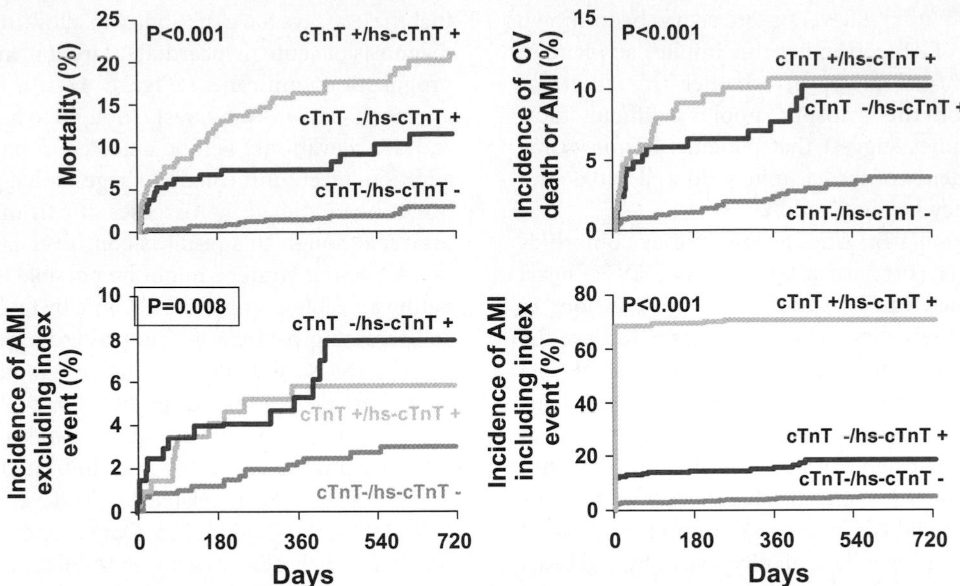

Figure 47-19 Kaplan-Meier analyses according to cutoffs of troponin T assays. Result above the cutoff is indicated by +; result equal to or below the cutoff is indicated by −. The cTnT assay used a cutoff of 0.010 μg/L (i.e., the lower limit of detection) because the 99th percentile was below this cutoff). The hs-cTnT used a cutoff of 0.014 μg/L (99th percentile). *P* value by log-rank test. *(From Hochholzer W, Reichlin T, Twerenbold R, Stelzig C, Hochholzer K, Meissner J, et al. Incremental value of high-sensitivity cardiac tropinin T for risk prediction in patients with suspected acute myocardial infarction. Clin Chem 2011;57:1318-26.)*

in this area. Nonetheless, the diagnosis of reinfarction is common after non–Q-wave myocardial infarction, and because CK-MB was initially used to unmask this, people have retained some enthusiasm for its use. This occurred in part because in the past, if individuals had had chest pain, this did not trigger a rapid evaluation. Thus, because CK-MB returns to normal earlier, its elevation was helpful. In modern practice, most patients with ACS are seen when chest pain is present and serial values are obtained. Thus, in the series by Apple,[20] every patient identified had normal values of CK-MB, which subsequently increased to reach an abnormal threshold (see Figure 47-20). Accordingly, serial samples are required for both analytes; if this is done, CK-MB possesses no characteristics that would make it superior to cTn. This early surveillance is needed in part because non-STEMI in the modern era is optimally treated by an invasive strategy, meaning that almost all patients go for cardiac catheterization and often undergo percutaneous intervention.

When such patients have recurrent chest discomfort, most immediately go back for coronary angiography to evaluate whether the chest pain is indicative of a problem with the area that has undergone intervention (e.g., stent thrombosis), or whether severe diminution in flow is present in that vessel. Thus, the only patients who are really held for evaluation are those in whom there is uncertainty about the diagnosis, and for this group, one needs to wait for serial samples. Indeed, this is the recommendation of the ACC/AHA committee on the management of patients with unstable angina and non–Q-wave myocardial infarction. Despite this recommendation, the committee does suggest in its guidelines that CK-MB may be useful. As indicated earlier, a substantial number of individuals would disagree.

Other uses for which CK-MB is often talked about have to do with patients with renal failure. Such an advocacy is misplaced because prior data suggest that as many as 20% of renal failure patients have increased CK-MB, probably as the result of concurrent skeletal muscle myopathy.[182] Similar claims have been made for the evaluation of patients after extreme or severe exercise, because it is well known that cTn elevations occur in these individuals. However, this advocacy does not take into account the very extensive literature documenting marked elevations in serum CK-MB in almost all individuals after extreme exercise; these elevations are due predominantly to the release of skeletal muscle CK and re-expression of the B chain of CK, which increases the percentage of CK-MB with respect to total CK in skeletal muscle.[5,350]

Very few other indications exist for the use of CK-MB, except when cTn measurements are unavailable. This is a rare circumstance in the United States and in most of western Europe but probably does occur elsewhere in the world, perhaps in countries with a much lower incidence of myocardial infarction, or countries that are resource poor and cannot afford the equipment needed to measure cTn. In this circumstance, most countries would rely on total CK moving back even another step. In addition, immunoassays for cTn and CK-MB are reasonably comparably priced and use similar types of equipment. Nonetheless, if CK-MB is to be used, mass assays are considered far preferable. This is due to the fact that they are more sensitive and less prone to artifactual

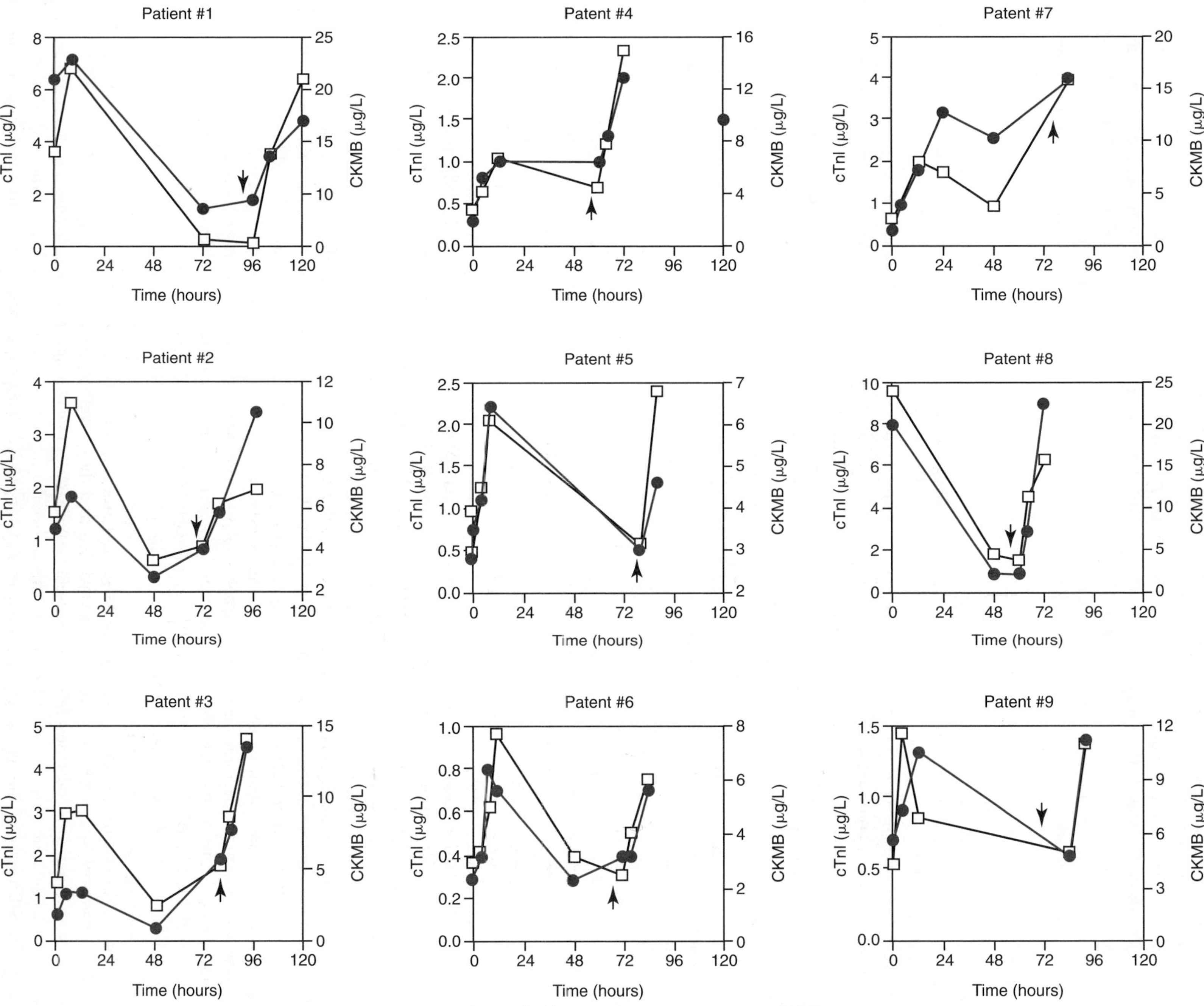

Figure 47-20 Time course of changes in biomarker concentrations in nine myocardial infarction patients who experienced reinfarction during hospitalization. *Red closed circles,* CTnI; *black open squares,* CKMB. *(From Apple FS, Murakami MM. Cardiac troponin and creatine kinase MB monitoring during in-hospital myocardial reinfarction. Clin Chem 2005;51:460-3.)*

elevations. However, increases in CK-MB from skeletal muscle injury clearly confound this measure and need to be taken into account. Use of the relative index (CK-MB divided by total CK), which used to be advocated by some because the percentage of CK-MB in cardiac muscle is so much higher than that in skeletal muscle, was discredited during the initial evaluation of cTn assays. The specificity of diagnosis is clearly improved when the index is used, but because so much CK is present in skeletal muscle, modest concurrent cardiac injury does not provide an adequate signal, so that sensitivity is lost.

Differences between males and females in reference values for CK-MB are likely related to differences in body mass.[30] Thus, if one is using CK-MB, one is obligated to use gender-specific reference intervals, which improve the sensitivity.[209,230,396] This will correct in part for the relative lack of sensitivity of CK-MB, particularly in women. When used, the same criteria as with cTn should be employed (i.e., a rising and/or falling pattern of results with at least one value above the 99th percentile of a normal reference population). However, very clear data indicate that elevations of CK-MB when cTn is normal identify patients who have skeletal muscle injury and not cardiac injury, as suggested strongly by the fact that these individuals do extremely well prognostically and do not appear to have an increased incidence of subsequent cardiovascular events.[141]

Early studies involving animal hearts or specimens obtained at autopsy from human hearts suggested a uniform distribution of CK-MB ranging from 5 to 50% of total CK activity.[220] However, it has been shown that the proportion of CK-MB was 6 to 15% lower in surrounding normal areas of tissue than in infarcted myocardium in humans. Further, in response to acute and chronic coronary artery occlusion in a dog model, myocardium showed twofold to threefold increases in CK-MB in both ischemic and nonischemic myocardium.[343,344] When studied more completely in humans, CK-MB concentrations in heart tissue were found to be variable, ranging from 15 to 24% of total CK in myocardial tissue obtained from patients with LVH caused by aortic stenosis, from patients with CAD without LVH, and from patients with CAD and LVH due to aortic stenosis. In contrast, patients with normal left ventricular tissue had a low percentage of CK-MB (<2%).[173] These data suggest that changes in CK isoenzyme distribution are dynamic and occur in hypertrophied and diseased human myocardium. Diseased cells also have less total CK per cell.

Normal skeletal muscle, depending on its location, contains very little CK-MB.[220] Percentages as high as 5% to 7% have been reported, but values less than 2% are much more common. Some differences are related to slow versus fast twitch muscle, and thus also to race. Severe skeletal muscle injury following trauma or surgery can lead to absolute elevations of CK-MB to above the upper reference limit of CK-MB in serum. However, the percent CK-MB in serum would be low (percentages advocated vary, but in comparisons of activity versus activity, a percentage less than 5% is often used, and when one compares CK activity with CK-MB mass, a percentage less than 2.5% is usually advocated).[220] Increases in serum total CK and CK-MB in several patient groups present a diagnostic challenge to the clinician. Persistent elevations of serum CK-MB resulting from chronic muscle disease occur in patients with muscular dystrophy, end-stage renal disease, or polymyositis, and in healthy subjects who undergo extreme exercise or physical activity. The increase in serum CK-MB in runners, for example, may be related to adaptation by skeletal muscle during regular training and after acute exercise, resulting in increased CK-MB tissue concentrations.[32]

Biomarkers No Longer of Clinical Use

Creatine Kinase (CK) Isoenzyme Electrophoresis and CK Isoforms

Three cytosolic isoenzymes (CK-3, CK-2, CK-1) and one mitochondrial isoenzyme (CK-Mt) of creatine kinase (CK) (MW 80,000 Da for all four isoenzymes) have been identified and are easily separated on agarose and cellulose acetate by electrophoresis.[13,311] Three different genes have been identified that encode for and are specific for CK-M, CK-B, and mitochondrial CK subunits.[306,329] Although CK-3 (CK-MM) is predominant in both heart and skeletal muscle, CK-2 (CK-MB) has been shown to be more specific for the myocardium, which contains 10 to 20% of its total CK activity as CK-MB, compared with amounts varying from 2% to 5% in skeletal muscle.

Numerous investigators have shown that electrophoresis of CK isoenzymes, with extended electrophoresis times or electrophoresis at higher voltages, further separates the bands of CK-MM and CK-MB.[391] At least three CK-MM isoforms and at least four CK-MB isoforms (subtypes of individual isoenzymes) exist. The tissue isoform (gene product) of CK-MM is designated CK-MM_3. When this protein/enzyme is released into the circulation, a time-mediated carboxypeptidase hydrolysis of C-terminal lysine residues occurs, giving rise to at least two post-translational products: CK-MM_2 and CK-MM_1.[305] Similarly, following release of the CK-MB tissue isoform into the circulation, carboxypeptidase cleavage of the CK-B carboxy-terminal lysine residue gives rise to a B-chain–negative product, and then a product devoid of lysines on both chains. Only tiny amounts of the M-chain–negative, B-chain–positive form are reproduced. Because only two forms are separated by electrophoresis (the B-chain–negative, M-chain–positive form comigrates with the tissue form and a small amount of the M-chain–negative, B-chain–positive form migrates with the ultimate conversion product), only two forms have been used diagnostically, and they have been labeled CK-MB_2 and CK-MB_1.[1,2,59] The clearance rate of total CK activity from blood is a composite of the clearance rates of the individual isoforms.[3] More prolonged half-lives are associated with the post-translational degradation isoforms. Thus the orders of half-lives are CK-MM_1>CK-MM_2>CK-MM_3, and CK-MB_1>CK-MB_2. Studies in an experimental animal model and in humans have shown that post-translational modifications of isoforms occur in blood, are unidirectional, and do not occur in the lymphatic system or in necrotic tissue.[4]

Myoglobin

Myoglobin is an oxygen-binding protein of cardiac and skeletal muscle with a molecular mass of 17,800 Da. The low molecular weight and cytoplasmic location of the protein probably account for its early appearance in the circulation following muscle (heart or skeletal) injury. No difference in myoglobin protein localization has been noted in the heart versus skeletal muscle. Increases in serum myoglobin occur after trauma to skeletal or cardiac muscle, as is seen in crush injury or MI.[378] Serum myoglobin methods are unable to distinguish the tissue of origin because the proteins are identical.[351] Even minor injury to skeletal muscle may result in elevated concentrations of serum myoglobin, which may lead to misinterpretation of myocardial injury.[376] Because myoglobin is cleared renally, changes in the glomerular filtration rate (GFR) will cause increases. It has a very short half-life of 10 minutes in blood.

Lactate Dehydrogenase Isoenzymes

Lactate dehydrogenase (LD) (MW 180,000 Da) is localized in the cytoplasm of tissue.[231] Even though LD isoenzymes are rarely used in clinical practice anymore, for historical purposes their biochemistry will be described here, and readers are referred to previous versions of this chapter. The highest activities of LD are found in skeletal muscle, liver, heart, kidney, and red blood cells. Electrophoresis on a variety of gels and buffer media, combined with kinetic and immunologic studies, has provided convincing evidence of the existence of at least five isoenzymes, composed of four subunit peptides of two distinct types, designated M (for muscle) and H (for heart). LD-1 (H_4) moves fastest toward the anode, while LD-5 (M_4) is closest to the cathode on an electrophoretic gel. LD-1 is found in highest concentrations in the heart, kidney (cortex), and red blood cells. LD-5 is found in highest concentrations in liver and skeletal muscle. The hybrid LD isoenzymes LD-2 (H_3M), LD-3 (H_2M_2), and LD-4 (HM_3) are also found in these and several other tissues.

Because LD is not a tissue-specific enzyme, it is not surprising that serum total LD is increased in a wide variety of diseases. Studies have demonstrated that activities of total LD and LD-1 increase from right to left ventricles, with H subunit activity varying twofold between different locations of the heart. As with CK-2 in skeletal muscle, the heart-specific LD-1 isoenzyme in skeletal muscle can increase twofold (from 10 to 20% of total LD activity) during a 9 week period of exercise training, with parallel decreases in LD-5.[19] Thus one must be aware that acute and chronic injury incurred during exercise training and racing increases total LD in serum, especially LD-1 and the ratio of LD-1 to LD-2. The tissue source of these increases is likely skeletal muscle as opposed to myocardium.[19,31,180]

CONGESTIVE HEART FAILURE

Natriuretic Peptides—Analytical Considerations

Biochemistry

An endocrine phenotype of the heart muscle was suggested by anatomic findings half a century after the discovery of endocrine substances by Drs. Starling and Bayliss.[51] In the 1960s, electron microscopy revealed granules in the cytoplasm of atrial myocytes, which structurally resemble secretory granules in known peptide hormone–producing cells.[186,206] In 1981, the Canadian physiologist Adolfo de Bold and his colleagues reported that infusion of atrial tissue extracts elicits renal excretion of sodium and water.[102] Moreover, a rapid decrease in blood pressure and increase in blood hematocrit were observed, and the substance was named *atrial natriuretic factor.* Soon after, this factor was purified and identified as a peptide comprising 28 amino acid residues; it was renamed *atrial natriuretic peptide (ANP).*[103,124] This discovery paved the way for identification of two structurally related peptides in the porcine brain: brain natriuretic peptide (BNP) and C-type natriuretic peptide (CNP).[288,360,361] However, BNP is mainly expressed in the heart, and the name *brain natriuretic peptide* is now often replaced with B-type natriuretic peptide (Figure 47-21).[360,361] CNP is expressed in the invertebrate heart and can be considered the ancestor gene for the natriuretic peptide family.[174] Nevertheless, the CNP gene is not expressed to the same extent in mammalian hearts and should not be considered as a cardiac-derived peptide in humans, where the gene is expressed dominantly in other tissues, including the vasculature and the male reproductive glands.[291,338]

The endocrine heart gained clinical interest when it was reported that patients with cardiac disease displayed increased concentrations of ANP in plasma.[72,75] In parallel, BNP circulates in highly increased concentrations in patients suffering from congestive heart failure.[277,278] The concept of a quantitative plasma marker of the heart failure syndrome was thereby introduced and has been intensely pursued with a dominant focus on clinical applications. In addition to the bioactive end products, N-terminal fragments from the precursors of ANP and BNP, proANP and proBNP, were shown to circulate in heart failure plasma and provided new molecular targets for biochemical detection.[65,72,169,228] As of today, proBNP-derived peptides have become the preferred routine markers in heart failure diagnosis and prognosis because of the available automated assays; the clinical relevance of peptide measurement is frequently and extensively reviewed.[84,91,92,96]

In contrast to the clinical focus on the diagnostic possibilities, much less is known concerning the biosynthesis of proBNP-derived peptides.[137] The post-translational phase of gene expression and the cellular secretion still remain incompletely characterized. The first data on molecular composition in tissue and plasma suggested an overall simple cellular maturation with only one endoproteolytic cleavage of proBNP prior to secretion of BNP. However, cardiac myocytes possess

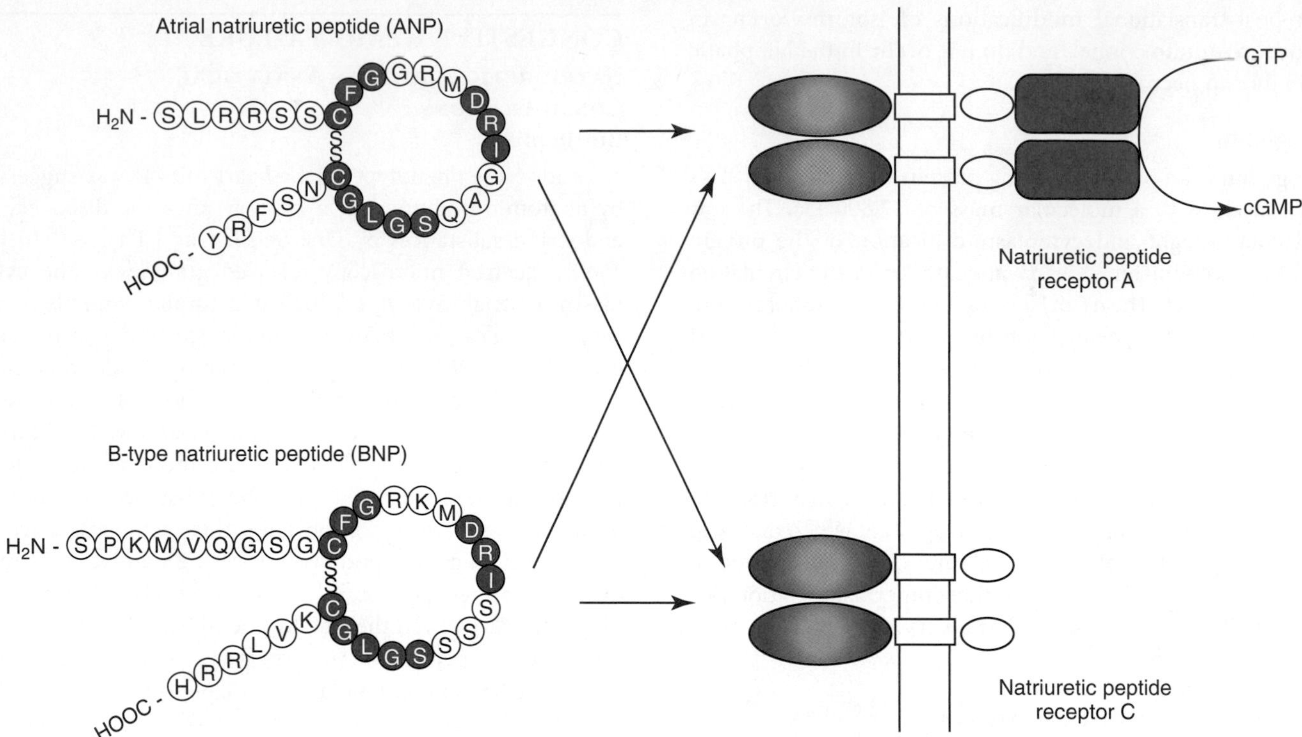

Figure 47-21 Schematic presentation of human atrial and B-type natriuretic peptides with their principal receptors. Homolog amino acid residues between the natriuretic peptides are marked in *bold circles*. The natriuretic peptide receptor (NPR)-A mediates atrial natriuretic peptide (ANP) and brain natriuretic peptide (BNP) signal transduction through induction of cyclic guanosine monophosphate (cGMP); the NPR-C receptor lacks the intracellular domain and has been classed primarily as a clearance receptor.

a biosynthetic apparatus, including several enzymes for propeptide processing, and cardiac prohormone maturation has proved to be much more complex than was initially assumed. Clinical studies have also revealed that plasma concentrations of the different proBNP-derived peptides vary greatly, which suggests that cardiac myocytes may not always release different biosynthetic products on a simple equimolar basis.[137,167]

Peptide Nomenclature and Biosynthesis

Some confusion has arisen as the result of an incoherent nomenclature for cardiac natriuretic peptides. In some ways, this confusion reflects underlying lack of knowledge of biosynthetic products, which has led researchers to apply nonspecific terms for the measured substances. However, a stringent nomenclature is essential for an understanding of peptide structure and function.[315] If the measured peptide is not readily distinguishable by its name, simple comparisons of reported concentrations may confuse and at worst may lead to incorrect decisions. For instance, some of the abbreviations used do not identify the measured peptide(s), which should be the primary goal of a name. A common abbreviation "NT-proBNP" is used for one particular analytical method; this refers to the measurement of nonglycosylated proBNP 1-76, against which the immunoanalysis is calibrated. However, the abbreviation does not provide specific information on the primary structure that is actually measured, which includes the intact precursor (proBNP 1-108) with some cross-reactivity to the glycosylated forms (see later). Other investigators have used broader terms for plasma measurement, as for instance "N-BNP," which refers to measurement of intact proBNP 1-108, as well as its N-terminal fragment(s). However, this abbreviation leaves the less astute user with the impression that it is the N-terminus of BNP that is measured. The use of abbreviations such as "BNP 77-108" is simply incorrect (BNP includes only 32 amino acid residues). Thus, BNP-32 is synonymous with proBNP 77-108. A rational nomenclature needs to be structurally informative and should see the name in relation to its origin (i.e., with insight into and reference to biosynthesis of the precursor). If this information is not available, then that should be stated. In the following section, a nomenclature based on these premises will be attempted.

Pretranslational Phase of B-Type Natriuretic Peptide Gene Expression

Human atrial natriuretic peptide (ANP) is encoded by the gene natriuretic peptide A (symbol *NPPA*), and B-type natriuretic peptiede (BNP) is encoded by the gene natriuretic peptide B (gene symbol *NPPB*). Both are located on chromosome 1.[40,411] In rodents, these genes are located on chromosome 4 (mouse) or chromosome 5 (rat). The overall gene structure is simple and resembles that of other peptide hormone genes in size and composition, with three exons separated by two introns. For both ANP and BNP, the major part of the coding sequence resides in exon 2. Genetic polymorphisms and mutations have been reported in both genes, as well as in the natriuretic peptide receptor genes.[219] Although the impact of genetic variation on the ANP and BNP systems remains to be fully established, it seems reasonable to suspect that it may affect the plasma concentrations in a heritable manner, which in fact has been reported in the general population.[387] A common polymorphism in the BNP promoter region has been associated with the prevalence of type 2 diabetes.[256] Genetic variation in cardiac natriuretic peptides may thus be involved in the pathophysiology of a common metabolic disorder. To complicate matters, diabetes mellitus induces increased risk for development of cardiovascular disease with concomitant changes in cardiac natriuretic peptide expression.[83] In addition to the promoter polymorphism, a frameshift mutation in the ANP gene has been reported in heritable atrial fibrillation. The frameshift introduces a C-terminally extended ANP peptide.[164] The "mutant" ANP exerts an exaggerated effect on potassium current in a cultured cell line.[4A]

Mature ANP and BNP transcripts consist of approximately 500 to 700 base pairs. Although intracellular regulation of natriuretic gene transcription is extensive as has been reviewed elsewhere,[129,221,253,254] both genes seem regulated by the same transcriptional factors, including p38 mitogen-activated protein kinase (MAPK). p38 MAPK activates the transcription factor nuclear factor-kappaB (NF-κB) and subsequently ANP and BNP gene transcription.[228A,371A] Vasoactive substances such as catecholamines and angiotensin II increase natriuretic gene transcription in a p38 MAPK–dependent manner. Myocyte stretching increases the intracellular calcium concentration and modulates calcium-binding proteins that regulate downstream modulators, including calcineurin, which stimulates myocyte natriuretic gene expression.[214A] Thus, cardiac natriuretic gene expression can be modulated by blocking p38 MAPK and calcineurin pathways. Finally, the hypoxia-inducible transcription factor (HIF) 1-alpha activates both ANP and BNP transcription, which is of importance in ischemic heart disease.[83A,389A] One scenario in which ANP and BNP genes seem not to be coregulated is inflammation driven by specific cytokines, where BNP gene expression is increased and ANP gene expression is unaffected.[241A] This differential gene expression has led to the suggestion that concurrent measurements of ANP and BNP and their related peptides might be clinically useful in conditions with both hemodynamic changes and a proinflammatory drive on the cardiac myocytes, as seen after cardiac transplantation.[101]

One feature of ANP and BNP messenger RNA (mRNA) regulation should be recapitulated. Although gene expression is regulated at the transcriptional level, another relevant mechanism involves changes in mRNA stability and the half-life of transcripts. This RNA regulatory mechanism has been demonstrated for BNP mRNA through stimulation of alpha-adrenergic receptors.[149A,149B] BNP mRNA stabilization is thought to be mediated through AU-rich elements in the 3′-untranslated region, which is not present in the ANP gene. Consequently, mRNA stabilization seems to involve only BNP, not ANP, mRNA.

Primary Structure of proBNP

Human proBNP comprises 108 amino acid residues (Figure 47-22). The primary structure is slightly shorter in mouse but with a similar C-terminal region, including the bioactive receptor-binding motif. Mammalian precursor sequences have been deduced from complementary DNA (cDNA) sequences that encode the entire preprostructure.[41A,236A,359A,360A] Amino acid homology between species is largely confined to the amino- and carboxy-terminal regions, whereas the remaining prostructure varies considerably between animals. Moreover, the principal motifs for amino acid modifications and enzymatic prohormone processing are not well conserved between species.

Human preproBNP contains an N-terminal hydrophobic signal peptide of 26 amino acid residues (see Figure 47-22). As with most regulatory peptides, this sequence is removed

cDNA-deduced proBNP sequences in 4 mammals

```
Cat    HPLGGPGPAS--EASAIQELLDGLRDTVSELQEAQMALGPLQQGHSPAESWEAQEEPPAR 58
Dog    HPLGGPGPAS--EASAIQELLDGLRDTVSELQEAQMALGPLQQGHSPAESWEAQEEPPAR 58
Man    HPLGSPGSASDLETSGLQEQRNHLQGKLSELQVEQTSLEPLQESPRPTGVWKSREVATEG 60
Mouse  YPLGSPSQSP--EQFKMQKLLELIREKSEEMAQRQLLKD---QG--------LTKEHPKR 47

Cat    VLAPHDNVLRALRRLGSSKMMRDSRCFGRRLDRIGSLSGLGCNVLRRH 106
Dog    VLAPHDNVLRALRRLGSSKMMRDSRCFGRRLDRIGSLSGLGCNVLRRH 106
Man    IRGHRKMVLYTLRAPRSPKMVQGSGCFGRKMDRISSSSGLGCKVLRRH 108
Mouse  VLRSQGSTLRVQQRPQNSKVTHISSCFGHKIDRIGSVSRLGCNALKLL 95
```

Figure 47-22 The primary structure of proBNP (pro-brain natriuretic peptide) in four mammals. The human proBNP sequence comprises 108 amino acid residues. The precursor sequence is evolutionary and is conserved in the C-terminal region that makes up the bioactive natriuretic peptide. In contrast, the cleavage site corresponding to position 73-76 in the human sequence is not well conserved. Amino acids are indicated by their single-letter codes.

during translation before synthesis of the C-terminal portion of the precursor is completed. Therefore, preproBNP does not exist as a separate entity but is only a theoretical structure. On the other hand, proBNP is likely to be an existing polypeptide; this has been indicated by chromatographic profiling and sequence-specific immunoassays.[135,169,338A,339A] The precursor molecule remains to be purified together with the processing intermediates there of—apart from the C-terminal 32 amino acid cleavage product (i.e., BNP-32) and the N-terminal region of the precursor.[4B,124A,163A,192A,262A] Thus, whenever the primary proBNP structure is mentioned, it still refers to the cDNA-deduced preprosequence combined with antibody-based data derived from chromatographic elution, Western blotting, or immunoassays.

Post-Translational Phase of B-Type Natriuretic Peptide Gene Expression

Post-translational BNP processing has only recently become a subject of interest. One contributing factor to this may relate to the troublesome lack of useful in vitro cellular models. Although neonatal atrial myocytes can be cultured for short periods of time, they do not anatomically or functionally resemble differentiated atrial or, for that matter, ventricular myocytes. Moreover, only a few immunoassays have been available for characterizing the molecular heterogeneity of the processing intermediates. Recent advances through mass spectrometry combined with the development of sequence-specific antibodies nevertheless have revealed a complex cardiac biosynthesis of cardiac natriuretic peptides.

Disulfide Bond Formation

The proBNP structure appears simple (see Figures 47-21 and 47-22). In humans, it is divided into two principal regions by a cleavage site in position 73-76 (Arg-Ala-Pro-Arg). The first region is the N-terminal fragment proBNP 1-76, and the second region is the C-terminal BNP-32 (proBNP 77-108). In contrast to other prohormones, proBNP does not contain a C-terminal flanking region. The C-terminal region contains a ring structure formed by a disulfide bond between the cystyl residues in positions 86 and 102, respectively (see Figure 47-21). The ring formation is essential for receptor binding and biological activity.[265] This crucial modification in ANP and BNP synthesis takes place in the endoplasmic reticulum and may be considered the first step in post-translational processing. The protein disulfide isomerase family and thiol-disulfide oxidoreductases are likely candidate enzymes involved in cardiac myocyte disulfide bond formation. Cardiac expression of the protein disulfide isomerase transcript was recently reported to be upregulated in cardiac disease.[341A] Cellular in vitro experiments further suggest a direct cardioprotective effect of this regulation. It may even be that not all cardiac natriuretic peptides are activated through this enzymatic process, which introduces the earliest possible regulatory step in natriuretic peptide biosynthesis and hormone activation. Regulation of protein disulfide isomerase has been classified as *endoplasmic reticulum stress,* which is a hallmark of several pathologic disorders, including diabetes mellitus, neurodegenerative disorders, and ischemic heart disease.

Glycosylation

Larger forms of BNP than the purified BNP-32 were first suspected from gel filtration studies of cardiac tissue extracts and plasma from patients with severe cardiac disease.[136A,169,338A,347,348] Some data even suggested molecular forms larger than the predicted precursor. Independently, several groups observed immunoreactive forms with molecular masses of 25 to 45 kDa in cardiac tissue and plasma (Figure 44-23). Intact proBNP, however, has an expected mass of ≈11 kDa based on the primary structure. Whether the peculiar elution patterns were in vitro artifacts or represented peptide binding to other molecules was put aside when it was shown that human proBNP exists as an O-linked glycoprotein.[337A] In the precursor structure, the midregion (proBNP 36-71) contains seven seryl and threonyl residues, where O-linked glycosylation occurs fully or partially (see Figure 47-23). This major modification of a polypeptide apparently does not affect the overall structure of the precursor.[93] On the other hand, the presence of carbohydrate groups clearly affects immunodetection if the epitope recognition resides within this region.[339] No specific immunoassay has yet been developed against the glycosylated forms, and the ratio between glycosylated versus nonglycosylated proBNP products can be deduced only from assays that specifically measure the nonglycosylated forms or cross-react with both forms. Whether O-linked glycosylation is an "unlimited" post-translational modification or is affected by increased BNP gene expression, as in heart disease, will be an important question for future studies. It should also be noted that the ANP precursor may be subject to glycosylation. In addition, the proBNP sequence varies considerably between species in the midregion (see Figure 47-22), which probably makes glycosylation a species-specific modification. Finally, it is not known whether atrial and ventricular myocytes possess the same capacity to glycosylate natriuretic precursor peptides.

Glycosylation could perhaps be a biochemical target for diagnostic applications, if the modification is affected by cardiac disease and/or reflects changes in BNP gene expression. Most captivating, however, is the potential impact of early biosynthetic glycosylation on cellular sorting and subsequent precursor processing. Because O-linked glycosylation can occur close to the principal maturation site in position 74-76 (on the threonyl residue in position 71), it should be suspected that the presence of carbohydrate groups can affect processing and hormonal maturation. In turn, this modification could regulate prohormone cleavage by blocking or guiding endoproteolytic enzymes, which may leave the propeptide with reduced or no biological activity. Such post-translational regulation has been shown for other regulatory peptides, as for instance insulin-like growth factor (IGF)-2.[98] Conceptually, immunoreactive BNP with little or no biological activity has been nicknamed "junk-BNP." This "junk" may nevertheless prove to be the most useful peptide forms for diagnostic measurement.

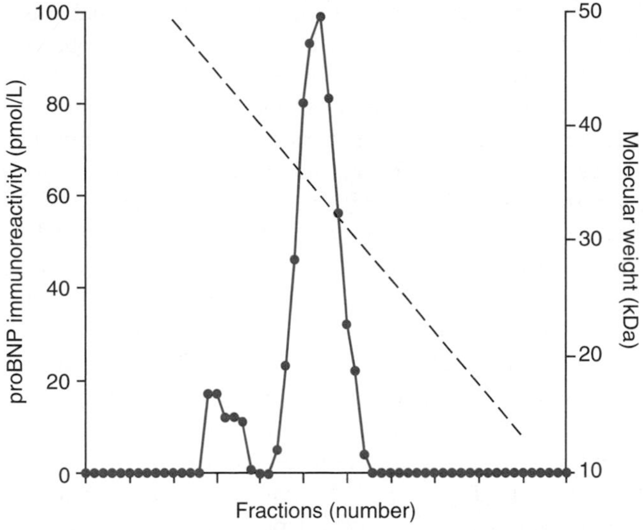

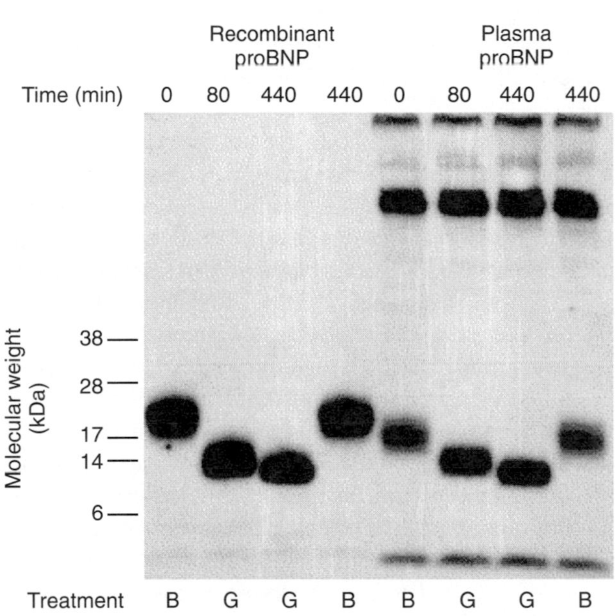

Figure 47-23 The *upper panel* shows a chromatographic profile of proBNP (pro-brain natriuretic peptide) immunoreactivity in human atrial tissue. Cardiac tissue extract was subjected to size exclusion high-performance liquid chromatography (HPLC). Molecular size calibrators, eluted in a separate run, were used in determining molecular sizes *(dashed line)*. The proBNP immunoreactivity eluted in positions approximately three times higher than the theoretical molecular weight of intact proBNP. The *lower panel* displays Western blotting of recombinant *(left)* and patient *(right)* proBNP in buffer *(B)* or after deglycosylation *(G)*. The incubation time is also listed. *(Modified with permission from Schellenberger U, O'Rear J, Guzzetta A, Jue RA, Protter AA, Pollitt NS. The precursor to B-type natriuretic peptide is an O-linked glycoprotein. Arch Biochem Biophys 2006;451:160-6.)*

Endoproteolysis

Human proBNP was first suggested to be cleaved by the ubiquitous endoprotease furin, because furin and the BNP gene are coexpressed in cardiac myocytes.[336A,336B] The Arg-Ala-Pro-Arg motif in position 73-76 in human proBNP has been shown to be a target for furin-mediated cleavage. In fact, endoproteolytic processing can be blocked in vitro by inhibition of furin, and furin has been shown to be essential for maturation of the structurally related CNP.[407] A novel protease named *corin* has been identified from human heart cDNA.[129,408,409] Corin is a serine protease that can cleave both proANP and proBNP in vitro, presumably at a similar cleavage site.[408,409] Corin contains a transmembrane domain anchored in the cell membrane and is thought to cleave the precursors upon secretion. The enzymatic activity, however, does not require the transmembrane domain because a mutant soluble form also is capable of processing proANP.[206A] A role of corin in the processing of cardiac natriuretic peptides in vivo has been further substantiated by genetic coupling of corin mutations to clinical phenotypes that can be explained by reduced ANP and BNP bioactivity in circulation such as hypertension.[114B,388A] Corin thus seems to be a relevant candidate for cardiac processing of natriuretic peptides generating the N-terminal processing fragments and C-terminal bioactive peptides.[408,410] Of note, no study has yet demonstrated exactly where corin cleaves the proBNP structure. Moreover, atrial post-translational processing of proANP and proBNP is likely to differ from ventricular processing, because isolated atrial granules have been reported to contain both unprocessed proANP and mature BNP-32.[413A] Corin activity alone therefore cannot fully explain the endoproteolytic maturation of cardiac natriuretic propeptides. It should be mentioned that the putative corin site in the BNP precursor is not conserved between mammals, and accordingly, it would be interesting to examine whether human corin can cleave precursor peptides from other mammalian species.

A well-established family of intracellular processing enzymes deeply involved in prohormone maturation is the proprotein/prohormone convertases, or the PCs. In addition to the already mentioned furin, the subtilisin-like endoproteases PC1/3 and PC2 are expressed in the mammalian heart,[51A,60A] and PC1/3 expression has been demonstrated in both normal and pathologic human cardiac tissue.[114C] Atrial myocytes transfected with an adenoviral vector expressing PC1/3 process proANP both to mature ANP and to a truncated form.[248] Although the precise cleavage site was not established and the processing capacity was somewhat inefficient, this singular report does underscore the possibility that other proteases than furin and corin may be involved in the post-translational endoproteolysis of proANP and proBNP. PC1/3 is active in secretory granules and therefore could be an important regulator of atrial proBNP processing. Cardiac PC1/3 expression has been reported to be upregulated at the transcriptional level in heart disease.[190A] Unfortunately, no data are available on other proBNP-derived fragments stemming from endoproteolytic processing. This may reflect the lack of specific tools for identifying such peptide fragments, which requires antibodies directed at epitopes other than the ones used so far for biochemical identification. Sandwich-based immunoassays usually are not ideal for this type of experiment. The precursor sequence contains several basic amino acid residues that potentially could represent cleavage sites for the PCs, and molecular characterization may not be complete when it comes to identifying processing intermediates from the natriuretic peptide precursors.

Exoproteolysis

N-terminal trimming of proBNP-derived peptides seems to be a biological feature, as both the N-terminus of the biosynthetic precursor and the C-terminal bioactive BNP product contain an amino acid motif for aminopeptidase recognition and cleavage. The N-terminus of both proBNP and BNP-32 (proBNP 77-108) contains a prolyl residue in position 2 (His-Pro and Ser-Pro, respectively). Although prolyl residues are important for peptide structure and folding, they can also be involved in exoproteolytic trimming when located near the N-terminus.[379] N-terminal trimming has in fact been demonstrated for BNP in vitro.[65] When synthetic BNP-32 (proBNP 77-108) is incubated in its presence, dipeptidyl peptidase (DPP)-IV removes the N-terminal Ser-Pro residues. DPP-IV is an enzyme located mainly on endothelial cells and in the circulation, with a preference for cleaving N-termini with prolyl or alanyl residues in the second position.[5A] Thus, this DPP-IV cleavage in BNP-32 cannot per se be considered part of the biosynthetic maturation, but rather is related to the elimination phase. An N-terminally trimmed form of proBNP lacking the His-Pro residues in position 1-2 has been reported in heart failure patients.[217A] This report disclosed that a truncated proBNP 3-108 form circulates in increased concentrations in heart failure patients. In this context, it is noteworthy that the initial report on glycosylated proBNP in a recombinant expression system (CHO cells) also identified a truncated proBNP 3-108 form in cell extracts.[337A] Although this finding may be explained by experimental handling of extracts and medium, it could also imply that N-terminal exoproteolysis is a biosynthetic event. N-terminal trimming as a part of peptide biosynthesis has for instance been demonstrated for melittin, which is a secretory peptide produced in honey bee venom glands.[209A,209B] In mammalian cells, intracellular aminopeptidase has been reported in compartments different from the lysosomes, suggesting N-terminal trimming as a possible part of the biosynthetic peptide maturation.[80A,377A] Whether the trimming of BNP and its molecular precursor serves an actual regulatory function in cardiac natriuretic peptide physiology remains an open question for future experimental research. One could speculate that amino-terminal trimming affects the metabolic fate of the peptides and thus their turnover in circulation. However, no data are available on the actual biological relevance of these trimmings.

Cellular Storage and Secretion

BNP gene expression is a feature of both atrial and ventricular myocytes. In the normal heart, the main site of BNP expression is in the atrial regions.[82,238A] Ventricular BNP gene expression increases drastically in cardiac disease that affects the ventricles (i.e., congestive heart failure).[278] The observation of ventricular BNP gene expression in ventricular disease may have given rise to the common statement that BNP is predominantly a ventricular hormone. Atrial and ventricular myocytes, however, differ considerably with respect to their endocrine phenotypes, and it is reasonable to expect major differences in peptide storage and secretion patterns.[114A,140A] For instance, atrial myocytes contain intracellular granules for peptide storage and maturation; this actually contributed to the primary hypothesis of the endocrine heart.[186,206] Atrial granules contain both intact precursors and biosynthetic end products (i.e., bioactive ANP-28 and BNP-32). In contrast, normal ventricular myocytes do not seem to express such granules, and normal ventricular myocytes do not contain proBNP-derived peptides.[82] A few reports have observed granules and proBNP-derived peptides in ventricular myocytes sampled from pathologic hearts.[152,289,364] Thus, ventricular myocytes not only regulate the BNP gene at the transcriptional and post-translational levels but also seem to be able to differentiate with respect to the biosynthetic apparatus per se.

An acidic protein class involved in granule formation is the chromogranins.[368] Chromogranins, or just granins, comprise at least three proteins (A, B, and C) that possess aggregation characteristics suggesting a function in the formation of secretory granules. Cardiac expression of chromogranin A and B has been established.[156,356,374] With cardiac chromogranins, however, the focus has mainly been on the potential biological activity of chromogranin-derived fragments (the vasostatins) or on plasma measurement for diagnostic purposes. Whether cardiac chromogranins are involved in the biosynthesis of ANP and BNP through formation of granules remains an area for future study. It should be recapitulated that chromogranin A–deficient mice do not reveal obvious changes in granule formation in, for instance, adrenal chromaffin cells.[157] Cardiac chromogranin B has also been suggested to be directly involved in BNP gene expression through a Ca^{2+}-dependent induction of the BNP promoter.[156] Future in vitro experiments targeted at proANP and proBNP maturation in cardiac cell systems devoid of chromogranin A and B may thus reveal a specific role for the granins in storage and secretion of natriuretic peptides.

ProBNP-Derived Peptides in Plasma

ProBNP-derived peptides are secreted by cardiac myocytes and circulate in plasma. Their molecular heterogeneity has been characterized primarily by chromatography in combination with sequence-specific immunoassays. Much of our present conception of cellular synthesis in fact is derived from the plasma phase, which represents the sum of secretion and metabolism. The picomolar concentrations in plasma limit the possibilities for full biochemical identification and underscore careful understanding of epitope recognition by the immunoassays. With this in mind, it is established that bioactive BNP is secreted from the heart and circulates without binding to plasma proteins.[154] Synthetic BNP-32 (proBNP

77-108) is trimmed when incubated in whole blood, generating a BNP form lacking the two N-terminal amino acid residues.[153,347] As mentioned earlier, this molecular form can also be generated in vitro by enzymatic trimming by DPP-IV and possibly other aminopeptidases.[65] Further processing of plasma BNP seems to involve degradation with loss of bioactivity through disruption of the ring structure mediated by neutral endopeptidase (NEP 24.11) or by receptor-mediated cellular uptake. This has been known for some time; however, the therapeutic potential of inhibiting neutral endopeptidase with increased plasma concentrations of "beneficial" natriuretic peptides is still an appealing strategy.[89] The metabolic fate of BNP-32 has been reported to be 13 to 20 minutes.[321,353] Immunoreactive BNP is also excreted in urine, but the precise contribution of renal excretion to renal metabolism has not yet been clarified. A minor degree of hepatic clearance has been shown; this is not significantly altered in patients with liver failure.[158]

In addition to bioactive BNP, other proBNP-derived fragments circulate in plasma.[140,243] These fragments are commonly referred to as *N-terminal proBNP,* but molecular heterogeneity also includes the intact precursor, in particular in heart failure patients.[139,167,169] Cardiac secretion of proBNP and its N-terminal fragments has been demonstrated by blood sampling from the coronary sinus. The molar ratio of secreted proBNP 1-76 to intact proBNP is not yet fully clarified but is likely to depend on cardiac status (i.e., more unprocessed precursor compared with biosynthetic cleavage products in severe heart failure) (Figure 47-24). In the metabolic phase, major discrepancies remain in the suggested half-life of N-terminal precursor fragments, which at least partially reflect epitope recognition in the assays. Theoretically, the half-life of proBNP 1-76 in circulation should be around 25 minutes[211] and thus does not differ greatly from the established metabolism of BNP-32 (proBNP 77-108). One report, however, suggested a considerably longer half-life (≈90 minutes after cardiac pacing), which would fit well with the higher plasma concentrations of N-terminal proBNP

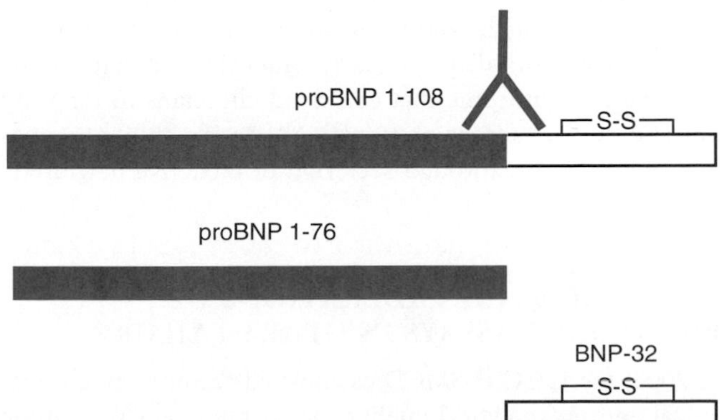

Figure 47-24 Immunoassay for detection of unprocessed human proBNP (pro-brain natriuretic peptide). The assay utilizes antibody recognition of an epitope spanning the Arg-Ala-Pro-Arg site (proBNP74-76) thought to be cleaved by Corin.

fragments compared with bioactive BNP in healthy individuals and in cardiac patients.[304] Our perception of molecular heterogeneity in plasma has changed radically over recent years; therefore, new pharmacokinetic experiments are urgently needed to separate the biosynthetic phase from peripheral elimination. Ideally, experiments should be performed by classical peptide infusion strategies with measurement across organ beds.

Biosynthesis and Assay Calibration

Elucidation of cardiac natriuretic peptide biosynthesis has disclosed a complex post-translational maturation that produces a variety of peptides targeted for cellular secretion (Figure 47-25). The different phases of gene expression not only are region specific but also depend on changes within the secretory apparatus in cardiac myocytes. The main clinical application of the peptides today strongly relates to plasma measurement in cardiovascular diagnosis and prognosis. Immunoassays thus need to be designed with insight into the biosynthesis of the peptides. Another defining aspect of immunoassay measurement is the choice of calibrator. This aspect so far has not been scrutinized by researchers, apart from observations of disturbingly large discrepancies between the different assays.[239] On the other hand, it has not been possible to raise meaningful assay calibration issues before now, because the existence of a complex molecular heterogeneity had not been established. One way of bypassing this lack of information has been introduced as a "processing-independent-assay," which in principle quantifies one in vitro cleavage product that represents all secreted precursor molecules. This assay can then be calibrated with the specific cleavage product and assay measurement performed on a stoichiometricly correct basis.

If one is to choose a proBNP-derived calibrator peptide for plasma measurement, the situation becomes more blurry. As the ratio of bioactive BNP to intact precursor shifts toward fewer processed biosynthetic products, one would perhaps choose the dominant "disease" form over the more prevalent forms in healthy individuals. However, large comparative studies have not revealed major differences between BNP and proBNP measurements in terms of overall clinical performance. One report on assay calibration has shown that assays directed at the C-terminal BNP region do not really cross-react with larger biosynthetic products.[239] However, plasma measurement based on assays directed against the N-terminal proBNP fragment is greatly influenced by the degree of O-linked glycosylation. Clearly, this issue is far from settled, and our present perception of "normal" concentrations of various biosynthetic products may have to be redefined.

Inefficient Prohormone Maturation in Heart Failure

Heart failure patients display highly increased plasma concentrations of bioactive ANP and BNP. With dramatic upregulation of gene expression and concomitant high concentrations of immunoreactive ANP and BNP in plasma, it seems reasonable to expect increased natriuresis. The

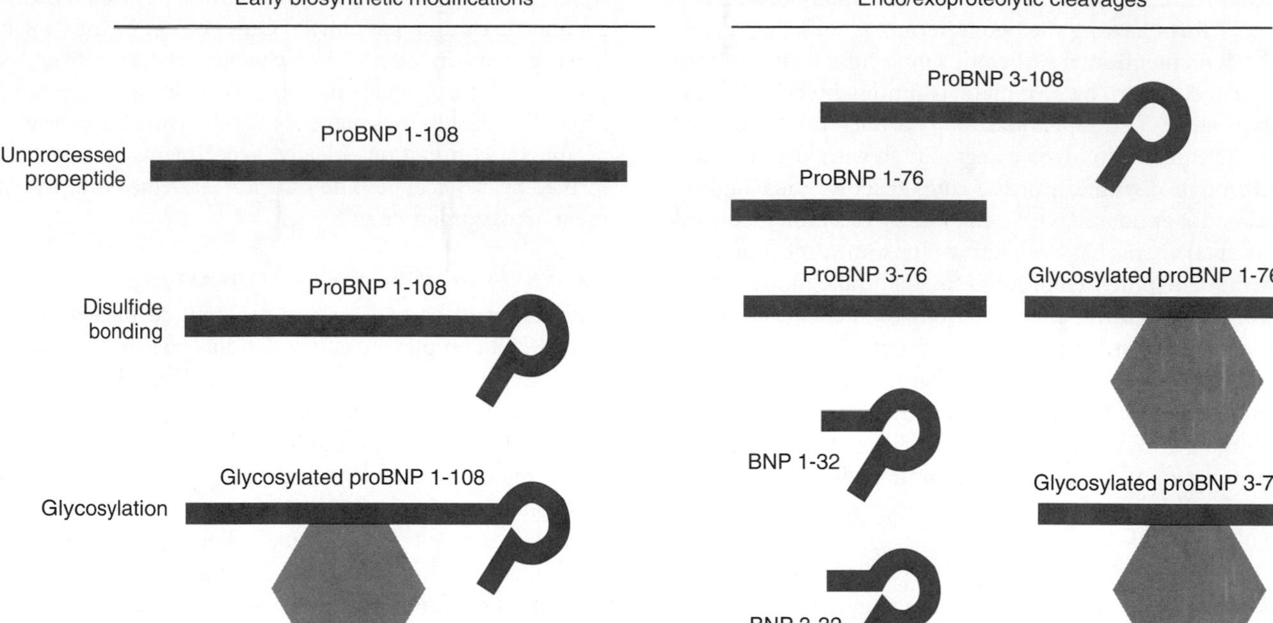

Figure 47-25 Schematic presentation of possible proBNP-derived peptide products. Note that most peptides are not chemically identified but rather are suggested by biochemical methods that rely on antibody recognition. Carbohydrate is indicated by the hexagons.

common presentation of heart failure, however, consists of congestion, sodium retention, and edema. Although heart failure is a complex syndrome with both activation and inhibition of multiple neurohumoral systems, the paradoxical lack of ANP and BNP bioactivity is still compelling. Heart failure patients respond to intravenous administration of chemically synthesized ANP and BNP, which has led to the introduction of a BNP-32 analog: nesiritide.[268] This peptide is a potent drug in heart failure; it has raised serious concerns regarding patient safety by causing unwanted hypotension.[373] Experts have further explored the possibilities of natriuretic peptide drugs by constructing structurally related peptides that possess natriuretic effects but without the undesirable hypotension.[235] Obviously, this research area could prove of major relevance to medical therapy, because all the different physiologic effects of natriuretic peptides could have specific roles in the modern treatment of heart failure and other cardiovascular pathologies.

The endocrine paradox of sodium and water retention in heart failure, where the gold standard biomarkers are the cardiac natriuretic peptides, relates to insufficient post-translational maturation of the biosynthetic precursors.[138] A well-established analogy to this phenomenon is enhanced secretion of proinsulin over mature insulin in patients with type 2 diabetes. In the early stages of the disease, selective proinsulin measurement is therefore a valuable tool in evaluating pancreatic β-cell dysfunction. A shift toward secretion of unprocessed precursors in cardiac disease may represent early involvement of ventricular expression and secretion, as efficient precursor maturation seems to be an endocrine feature of atrial biosynthesis. In support of this explanation, the intracellular processing enzymes involved in ANP and BNP maturation are dominantly expressed in atrial myocytes. Moreover, ventricular myocytes do not, at least in the early stages of disease, contain secretory granules for peptide storage and maturation. The post-translational processing of ventricular precursors may not be efficient in the production of needed natriuretic potency, while immunoassays cross-react to various degrees with the unprocessed biosynthetic products. Although speculative, there may be large individual differences in the ability of the heart to process the precursor peptides; this could help explain the highly variable heart failure phenotypes. The ratio of mature BNP to unprocessed proBNP might be of diagnostic relevance in parallel with the present application of proinsulin to insulin measurement. If specific assays for the various forms are applied in concert, it may be possible to define an early endocrine hallmark of the heart failure syndrome that could aid clinicians in tailoring diuretic therapy according to patient-specific ability to ameliorate congestion through secretion of bioactive natriuretic hormones.

ANALYTICAL CONSIDERATIONS OF BIOMARKER ASSAYS IN HEART FAILURE

In 2005, the IFCC C-SMCD established recommended analytical and preanalytical quality specifications for natriuretic peptide (NP) assays.[25] The objectives were intended for use by the manufacturers of commercial assays and by clinical laboratories utilizing NP assays. The overall goal was to attempt to establish uniform criteria so that all NP assays could be evaluated objectively for their analytical qualities and clinical performance. As BNP and NT-proBNP become more integrated into clinical practice as diagnostic and prognostic biomarkers, understanding differences between individual assay characteristics becomes extremely important. The influence of clinical and analytical and preanalytical factors on increasing numbers of commercially available BNP and NT-proBNP assays (as shown in Table 47-4), shows the need for improved understanding by clinicians of how to interpret findings of different studies predicated on BNP or NT-proBNP concentrations monitored by different assays.[168,365,412] The laboratory community must work closely with in vitro diagnostics companies to assist in defining the numerous assay characteristics.[38] When BNP or NT-proBNP assays are used as biomarkers for diagnosis, therapy decisions, and prognosis, or when they are used in clinical trials or studies, they should be well characterized, as suggested in the list of recommendations that follow. It is further recommended that when designing studies using BNP or NT-proBNP, investigators should review the STARD (Standards for Reporting Diagnostic Accuracy)[64] initiative for assay characterization issues and for clinical and patient enrollment issues when BNP or NT-proBNP levels are monitored.

A growing diversity of BNP and NT-proBNP assays are used worldwide, emphasizing the need for both analytical and clinical validation of all commercial assays to support definitive clinical acceptance of these new biomarkers. At present, four companies have BNP assays that have been cleared by the U.S. Food and Drug Administration (FDA) [Inverness Biosite, Siemens (Bayer), Abbott including POC, and Beckman Coulter using Biosite reagents], and at least seven companies have FDA-cleared NT-proBNP assays [Roche, and six others that use Roche antibodies and calibrators: Siemens (Dade Behring and DPC), bioMérieux, Response Biomedical, Mitsubishi Chemical, Ortho-Clinical Diagnostics, and Nanogen]. POC platforms (Response Biomedical, Mitsubishi Chemical, Inverness Biosite) are suitable for whole blood use. Research and development is under way for commercialization of proBNP assays, with preliminary assays described by BioRad, HyTest, and Biosite Inverness. As the number of assays for all three NP biomarkers grows, it is even more essential that appropriate clinical and analytical assay criteria are uniformly adopted. The accurate clinical performance of each BNP or NT-proBNP assay, and likely proBNP in the future, which may serve as the basis for life and death medical decisions, sets the stage in establishing assay criteria as indispensable.

BNP and NT-proBNP are determined by a number of different immunoassays using antibodies directed to different epitopes located on the antigen molecules (see Table 47-4). For BNP, one antibody binds to the ring structure and the other antibody to the carboxy- or amino-terminal end. Degradation of BNP is known to occur by proteolytic cleavage of serine and proline residues in vivo and in vitro (see Figure 47-25).[25,346,348] This degradation may affect antibody affinities and thus may be responsible for differences in stability of BNP32 monitored by different commercial BNP assays, as discussed earlier. For NT-proBNP (a.a.1-76) monitoring, an improved understanding of potential cross-reactivity with split products of the N-terminal portion of NT-proBNP and proBNP itself is needed. For both assays—BNP and NT-proBNP—minimizing interference from heterophilic antibodies and rheumatoid factor, for example, needs to be optimized. The influence, stabilizing or destabilizing, of anticoagulant additives, as well as the type of collection tube, has been well described.[52,346] For BNP, EDTA-anticoagulated whole blood or plasma appears to be the only acceptable specimen choice. For NT-proBNP, serum, heparin plasma, and EDTA plasma (reads 10% lower) appear acceptable. Plastic blood collection tubes are necessary for BNP; for NT-proBNP, either glass or plastic is acceptable.

In the clinical setting,[35,226,236,238,381] BNP and NT-proBNP assay characteristics need to be better understood or better established for optimal consideration as diagnostic and prognostic biomarkers, as discussed later. Further, proBNP, the precursor peptide that splits into BNP and NT-proBNP, appears to be detected in both BNP and NT-proBNP assays; this may have substantial implications regarding clinical utilization of these assays.[135] The influence of age, gender, ethnicity, and non-HF pathologies has been shown to substantially influence what may otherwise be considered a normal reference concentration.[25,314] Renal impairment has been shown to substantially increase NT-proBNP concentrations and, to a lesser extent, BNP concentrations.*

For BNP, a single cutoff has been designated at 100 pg/mL, likely driven by FDA clearance of this value as the ROC curve value optimized for diagnostic accuracy. However, as shown in Figure 47-26, normal subjects older than 75 years have concentrations above the 100 pg/mL cutoff. For NT-proBNP, the FDA-cleared cutoffs are based on age: for patients younger

*References 23, 25, 79, 108, 191, and 252.

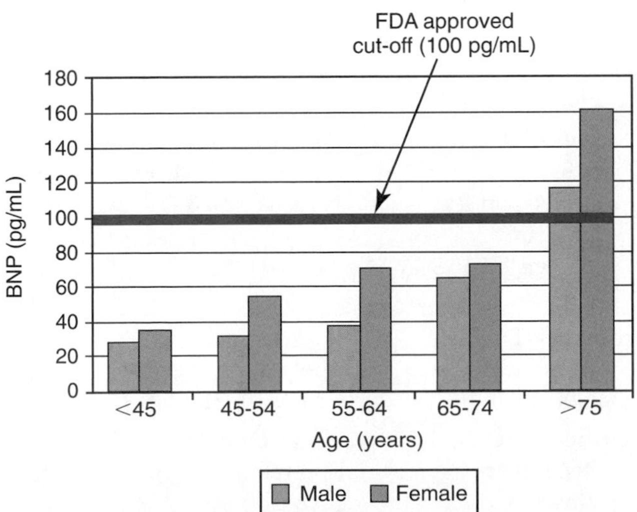

Figure 47-26 Representative brain natriuretic peptide (BNP) concentration distributions in normal males and females by decade (years) with indication of the U.S. Food and Drug Administration (FDA)-cleared 100 pg/mL cutoff value.

TABLE 47-4 Analytical Characteristics of Commercial BNP and NT-proBNP Assays per Manufacturer

Assay	Capture Antibody	Detection Antibody	Standard Material	FDA Claim
BNP				
Inverness (Biosite) Triage	NH_2 terminus and part of the ring structure (Scios), murine monoclonal AB, aa 5-13	BNP (Biosite), murine Omniclonal AB, epitope not characterized	Recombinant BNP	Diagnosis of HF Assess severity of HF Risk of ACS Risk of HF
Beckman Coulter Access, Access 2, DxL	NH_2 terminus and part of the ring structure (Scios), murine monoclonal AB, aa 5-13	BNP (Biosite), murine Omniclonal AB, epitope not characterized	Recombinant BNP	Diagnosis of HF Assess severity of HF Risk of ACS Risk of HF
Abbott Architect, AxSYM, iSTAT	NH_2 terminus and part of the ring structure (Scios), murine monoclonal AB, aa 5-13	COOH terminus, murine monoclonal AB, aa 26-32	Synthetic BNP 32	Assist in diagnosis of HF Assess severity of disease
Siemens (Bayer) ACS 180, Advia Centaur, Advia Centaur CP	COOH terminus (BC-203), murine monoclonal AB, aa 27-32	Ring structure (KY-hBNP-II), murine monoclonal AB, aa 14-21	Synthetic BNP	Aid in diagnosis and assessment of severity of HF Predict survival and likelihood of future HF in ACS patients
Shionogi	Ring structure (KY-hBNP-II), murine monoclonal AB, aa 14-21	COOH terminus (BC-203), murine monoclonal AB, aa 27-32	Synthetic BNP	Not FDA cleared
NT-proBNP				
Roche proBNP I Elecsys, E170	NH_2 terminus polyclonal sheep AB, aa 1-21	Central molecule, polyclonal sheep AB, aa 39-50	Synthetic NT-proBNP 1-76	Diagnosis of HF Assess severity of HF Risk of ACS Risk of HF
proBNP II Elecsys, E170	Murine monoclonal AB, aa 27-31	Sheep monoclonal AB, aa 42-46	Synthetic NT-proBNP 1-76	Treatment monitoring in LVD
Siemens (Dade Behring) Dimension RxL, Stratus CS, Dimension VISTA	NH_2 terminus monoclonal sheep AB, aa 22-28	Central molecule, sheep monoclonal AB, aa 42-46	Synthetic NT-proBNP 1-76	Aid in the diagnosis of CHF and assessment of severity Risk stratification of patients with ACS and HF
Siemens (DPC) Immulite 1000, 2000 2500	NH_2 terminus polyclonal sheep AB, aa 1-21	Central molecule, polyclonal sheep AB, aa 39-50	Synthetic NT-proBNP 1-76	Not FDA cleared
Ortho-Clinical Diagnostics Vitros ECi	NH_2 terminus polyclonal sheep AB, aa 1-21	Central molecule, polyclonal sheep AB, aa 39-50	Synthetic NT-proBNP 1-76	Aid diagnosis of CHF Risk stratification of ACS and CHF Risk assessment of CV events and mortality in patients at risk for HF with stable CAD Assess severity of HF

TABLE 47-4 Analytical Characteristics of Commercial BNP and NT-proBNP Assays per Manufacturer—cont'd

Assay	Capture Antibody	Detection Antibody	Standard Material	FDA Claim
Response Biomedical RAMP	Murine monoclonal AB, aa 27-31	Central molecule, polyclonal sheep AB, aa 39-50	Synthetic NT-proBNP 1-76	Diagnosis of HF Assess severity of HF
bioMérieux VIDAS	NH_2 terminus polyclonal sheep AB, aa 1-21	Central molecule, polyclonal sheep AB, aa 39-50	Synthetic NT-proBNP 1-76	Diagnosis of HF
Mitsubishi Chemical PATHFAST	NH_2 terminus polyclonal sheep AB, aa 1-21	Central molecule, polyclonal sheep AB, aa 39-50	Synthetic NT-proBNP 1-76	Aid diagnosis of CHF Assess severity of CHF Risk stratification in ACS and stable CAD
Nanogen LifeSign DXpress Reader	Monoclonal (mouse) and polyclonal (goat) ABs	Polyclonal sheep AB	Synthetic NT-proBNP 1-76	Diagnosis of HF

AB, Antibody; *ACS*, acute coronary syndrome; *CAD*, coronary artery disease; *CHF*, congestive heart failure; *CV*, cardiovascular; *LVD*, left ventricular dysfunction; *N/A*, not available.

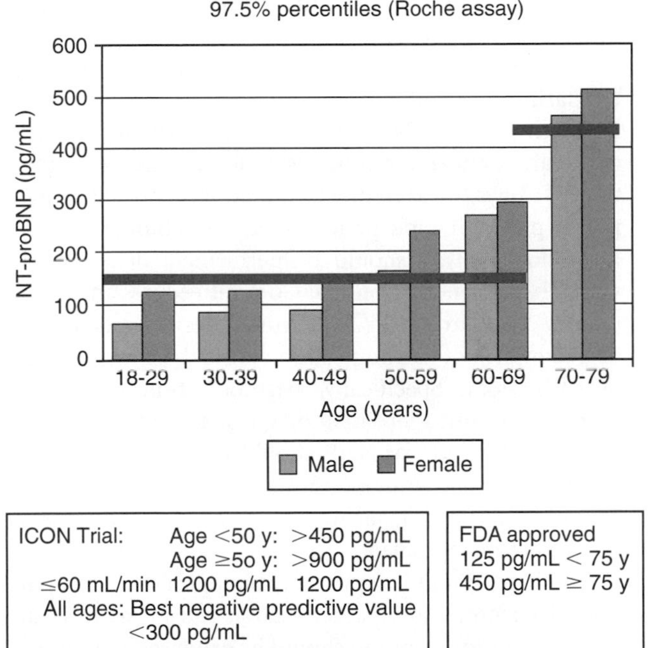

Figure 47-27 Representative N-terminal pro brain natriuretic peptide (NT-proBNP) concentration distributions in normal males and females by decade (years) with indication of the U.S. Food and Drug Administration (FDA)-cleared age-related cutoff values compared with ICON (International Collaborative on NT-proBNP) study) trial recommended values determined by age and renal function.

than 75 years, 125 pg/mL, and for those older than 75 years, 450 pg/mL. Again, these cutoffs appear to misclassify many normal individuals, as shown in Figure 47-27. Clinical studies [ProBNP Investigation of Dyspnea in the Emergency Department (PRIDE) Study] have more appropriately defined cutoffs by sex, age, and renal function, as shown in Figure 47-27, and estimated GRF, with an optimal negative predictive value at less than 300 pg/mL that is independent of age, gender, and eGFR. Obesity has also been shown to have an impact on BNP and NT-proBNP measurements[150,160,203,279]; an inverse relationship has been noted between increased BMI and decreased BNP in CHF patients. HF patients who receive the drug nesiritide (human recombinant BNP) for therapy and management may have confounding BNP results because nesiritide is molecularly identical to endogenous BNP. Thus, if BNP were to be monitored for regulation of nesiritide infusion within a time window before an appropriate decrease in exogenous BNP could occur (half-life ≈22 minutes), the potential for falsely increased concentrations could arise. Nesiritide does not directly confound NT-proBNP measurements. Finally, lack of understanding of the physiologic and biological variability of BNP and NT-proBNP in HF patients may cause clinicians to misinterpret changing (increasing or decreasing) BNP and NT-proBNP concentrations in the context of establishing the success or failure of therapy.

BNP and NT-proBNP exhibit intraindividual biological variability (CV) of 33 to about 50%.[404] The authors of this study [404] suggested that changes of 130% for B-type natiuretic peptide (BNP) and 90% for N-terminal (NT)-proBNP are necessary before results of serially collected data can be considered statistically different. A small study has shown that in HF patients monitored for BNP over at least 2 time periods during a 2 week period, less than 50% of concentrations were found to be outside the expected biological variability (Figure 47-28).[403] This implies that results of BNP or NT-proBNP monitoring may be overinterpreted and re-emphasizes the role of these tests as confirmatory biomarkers, not as a tests that clinicians should rely upon solely when managing HF patients.

Presently, no available data have established a correlation between BNP and NT-proBNP concentrations using commercially available technology. In addition, the literature is

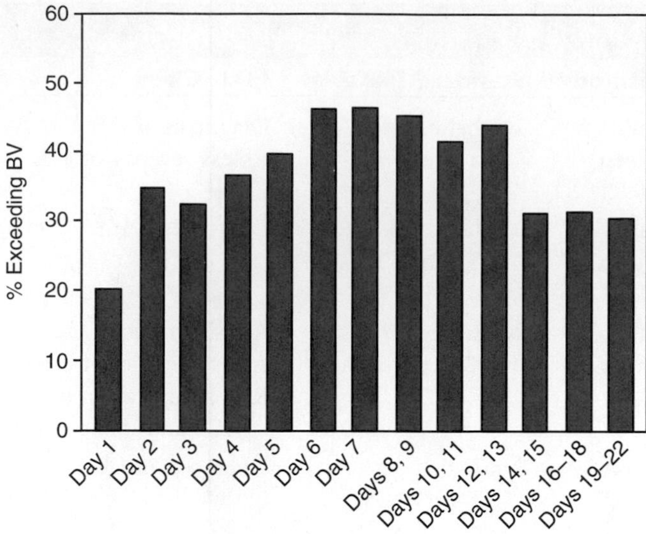

Figure 47-28 Variability of brain natriuretic peptide (BNP) concentrations by day from initial admission order, with demonstration that more than 50% exceed biological variability (100% change) over a 2 week time period. *(From Reference 403 with permission from Excerpta Medica.)*

scattered with BNP and NT-proBNP assays that were developed and standardized in individual laboratories. All of these factors add to the confusion of clinicians when interpreting and comparing data from different studies, whether for diagnosing or ruling out HF, managing HF, screening for asymptomatic left ventricular dysfunction, or determining risk stratification and prognostication for patients with HF, ACS, or other pathologies. One must consider the assay used, the available clinical evidence based on the individual assay, and the aim of the biomarker-based studies. No peer-reviewed studies have demonstrated that the two tests (BNP and NT-proBNP) are equivalent. Thus until large studies become available that include proBNP measurements as well, caution is suggested before conclusions based on one particular BNP or NT-proBNP assay are translated to another assay.

The following practice guidelines pertaining to analytical issues for biomarkers of heart failure have been recommended by the NACB and the IFCC Committee for Standardization of Markers of Cardiac Damage:

1. Normal reference limits (95th or 97.5th percentile) should be established independently for both BNP and NT-proBNP based on age (by decade) and by gender. Each commercial assay should be validated separately. The effects of ethnicity and renal function need to be evaluated as possible independent variables.
2. ROC curves should be established to evaluate clinical effectiveness and to establish optimal medical decision cutoffs for BNP and NT-proBNP assays for diagnostic usefulness.
3. Assays for BNP and NT-proBNP should have total imprecision (%CV) ≤15% at their age- and gender defined upper reference limits, as well as at the New York State Heart Association (NYSHA)-defined medical decision concentrations.
4. Before introduction into clinical practice, BNP and NT-proBNP assays must be characterized with respect to the following preanalytical and analytical issues:

   Preanalytical:
   a) Effects of storage time and temperature
   b) Influence of different anticoagulants
   c) Influence of gel separator tubes
   d) Need for plastic blood collection tubes for BNP; for NT-proBNP, either glass or plastic is acceptable

   Analytical:
   a) Identification of both antibody recognition epitopes
   b) Cross-reactivity characteristics with related natriuretic peptides, including NT-proANP, ANP, CNP, BNP, and glycosylated and nonglycosylated NT-proBNP and proBNP
   c) Identification of interference from heterophile antibodies, rheumatoid factors, human antimouse antibodies
   d) Description of calibration material used, how the material was defined, and the concentration value assigned
   e) Clarification of dilution response
5. For both BNP and NT-proBNP, until a primary reference material is defined for either assay for appropriate calibration of assays, measurements should be reported in ng/L, not in pmol/mL; and patient specimen comparisons and regression analysis should be performed, in accordance with CLSI [formerly National Committee for Clinical Laboratory Standards (NCCLS)] guidelines, to establish the degree or lack of harmonization across the dynamic range of each assay. Specifically, harmonization around the current presumed optimal diagnostic medical decision cutoff of 100 ng/L for BNP should be validated. Because there is only one source of antibodies and calibrators for NT-proBNP (Roche), harmonization of NT-proBNP assays should not be a problem.
6. For both BNP and NT-proBNP, biological variability has been determined to be at least 50%, and in many studies higher. Therefore, caution should be exercised in interpreting concentration changes of less than 50 to 80% as reflective of medical therapy. However, consistent trends should be followed as clinically important.

In summary, laboratorians and clinicians must be cognizant of numerous considerations inherent in NPs as markers for management of cardiology patients, including (1) the form of the biomarker itself (BNP or NT-proBNP); (2) lack of standardization of immunoassays; (3) that reference and medical decision limits are dependent on age and gender; (4) that biological variation among NPs in individuals is inherently high; (5) the diagnostic time window (admission or monitoring of trends over time); (6) the clinical setting in which NPs are used (e.g., general practice, emergency room, coronary care unit); (7) the patient subset being tested (e.g., renal failure, sepsis); and (8) whether application is for diagnostic use, for prognostic use, or for a future potential application of therapeutic guidance. All of these aspects must be taken into consideration with the implementation of biomarkers such as NPs, to avoid the possibility of misinterpretation of a result for patient care.

Clinical Use of Natriuretic Peptides

BNP, NT-proBNP, and novel assays that are being developed have been shown to be of assistance to clinicians in the evaluation of patients with impaired left ventricular function, with or without congestive heart failure, and with coronary heart disease.* On the other hand, the more we have learned about natriuretic peptides, the more complicated the biology of these biomarkers has become (see earlier).

Use in the Diagnosis of Congestive Heart Failure

Natriuretic peptides were initially validated on the basis of their ability to facilitate the diagnosis of congestive heart failure. The situations chosen to test this hypothesis did not occur in sophisticated cardiology offices, but in the emergency department and in primary care practices.[187,245] The emergency setting is an extremely busy environment where there is often a severe press for time, making cautious and careful evaluation difficult. In addition, emergency department physicians are generalists who must triage problems related to trauma, infectious disease, and a variety of other complaints related to almost any organ system. Some are very sophisticated with regard to cardiovascular issues and the presenting symptoms and cardiovascular examination associated with heart failure; others are not. Accordingly, some have objected to the use of this setting as the primary testing ground for the use of natriuretic peptides in the diagnosis of heart failure. General internists are in a similar position, especially in the outpatient setting where these evaluations were done, where physicians have limited resources and a heterogeneity of expertise related to this particular diagnosis. Thus, the relatively marginal improvement in diagnostic yield [74 to 81% in the Breathing Not Properly (BNP) trial and 92 to 96% in the PRIDE trial] is not terribly impressive in one sense. However, in parsing the data, it is clear that most of the benefit derived from the use of natriuretic peptides for diagnosis resides in the triage of patients about whom clinicians are ambivalent, as was recently elegantly documented.[357]

When patients have a very low risk of heart failure, it is not clear whether natriuretic peptides help at all; similarly, with a classic presentation, patients have such a high frequency of heart failure and such a high pretest probability that natriuretic peptides are unlikely to be helpful. However, in the group of patients with dyspnea about whom the clinician is ambivalent, natriuretic peptides are helpful. Of importance in the interpretation of natriuretic peptides in this situation is that marginal values often are not helpful. The Breathing Not Properly Trial suggested the use of one cutoff value at 100 ng/mL in making the diagnosis of heart failure. This value could have been altered to increase sensitivity or specificity (Figure 47-29).[251] However, 26% of the population had values between 100 and 500 ng/mL. One third of this group did not have congestive heart failure according to subsequent adjudication, and two thirds did, but unfortunately, no cutoff value distinguished these groups. For this reason, a group of investigators [ICON (International Collaborative on NT-proBNP) study] have analyzed their data with NT-proBNP, looking to generate values that will help to both include and exclude disease.[188] This is an extremely valuable approach. Investigators have reported that a value for NT-proBNP less than 300 ng/mL effectively excludes congestive heart failure. Values greater than 450 ng/mL in individuals younger than 50 rule in heart failure, and values greater than 900 ng/mL permit diagnosis of heart failure in patients over the age of 50.

As is clear, gaps between these values describe the fact that clinical judgment is still importantly necessary in the use of natriuretic peptides. It is for this reason that most guideline groups have not suggested the routine use of natriuretic peptides for diagnosis in every patient who presents with dyspnea.[111,170,367] Instead, group members recommend their judicious use in patients in whom the diagnosis is not clear. It is axiomatic to suggest that consideration of gender, age, and weight (see earlier) in interpreting such values is advised. In addition, it is clear that the worse the clinical class of heart failure is, the higher are the natriuretic peptide levels (Figure 47-30). The diagnosis may be problematic, especially in patients who have other comorbidities.[212,310,401] Chronic obstructive pulmonary disease and cardiovascular disease frequently overlap, and it is in these types of patients that the optimal use of natriuretic peptides for diagnosis likely can be applied. Other disease processes (Box 47-6) can cause elevations and must be taken into account by including the clinical situation in interpretation of natriuretic peptide values.

Special Situations

Several additional caveats are necessary clinically. The epidemic of heart failure with preserved ventricular function is increasing (Box 47-7). Controversy continues concerning the mechanisms involved in this clinical entity, and some even question its existence; however, a stiff, noncompliant left

BOX 47-6 Causes of Increased Natriuretic Peptides

1. Acute or chronic systolic or diastolic HF
2. LV hypertrophy
3. Inflammatory cardiac disease
4. Systemic arterial hypertension with LVH
5. Pulmonary hypertension
6. Acute or chronic renal failure
7. Ascitic liver cirrhosis
8. Endocrine disorders (e.g., hyperaldosteronism, Cushing's syndrome)
9. Sepsis

HF, Heart failure; *LV,* left ventriular; *LVH,* left ventricular hypertrophy.

*References 250, 272, 290, 393, 397, and 415.

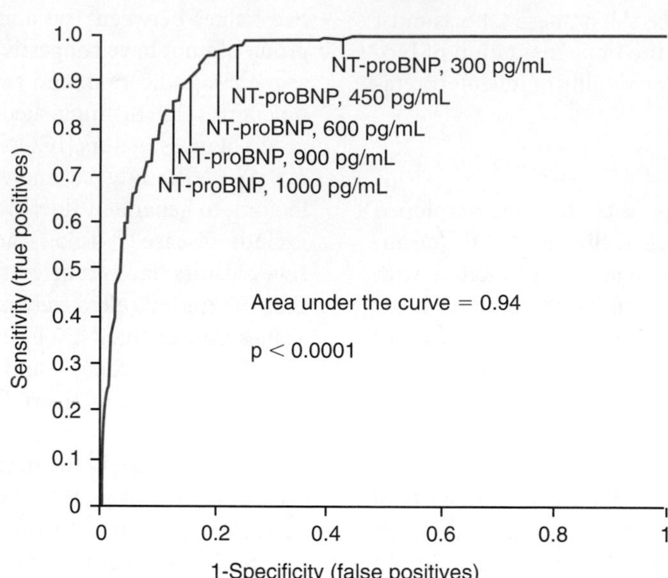

Cut point	Sensitivity	Specificity	Positive predictive value	Negative predictive value	Accuracy
300 pg/mL	99%	68%	62%	99%	79%
450 pg/mL	98%	76%	68%	99%	83%
600 pg/mL	96%	81%	73%	97%	86%
900 pg/mL	90%	85%	76%	94%	87%
1000 pg/mL	87%	86%	78%	91%	87%

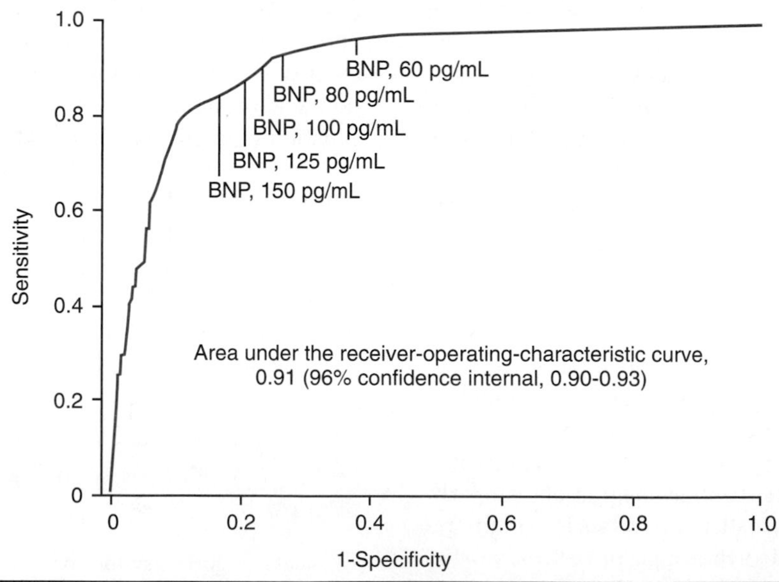

BNP pg//mL	Sensitivity	Specificity	Positive predictive value	Negative predictive value	Accuracy
50	97 (98-98)	62 (60-66)	71 (68-74)	96 (94-97)	79
80	98 (91-96)	74 (70-77)	77 (76-80)	92 (89-94)	83
100	90 (88-92)	76 (73-78)	79 (78-81)	92 (87-91)	83
125	87 (86-90)	79 (78-82)	80 (78-83)	87 (84-89)	83
150	86 (82-88)	83 (80-86)	83 (80-86)	85 (83-88)	84

Figure 47-29 Receiver operating characteristic (ROC) analysis for brain natriuretic peptide (BNP) and N-terminal pro brain natriuretic peptide (NTproBNP) for the diagnosis of acute heart failure. *(With permission, References 245 and 316.)*

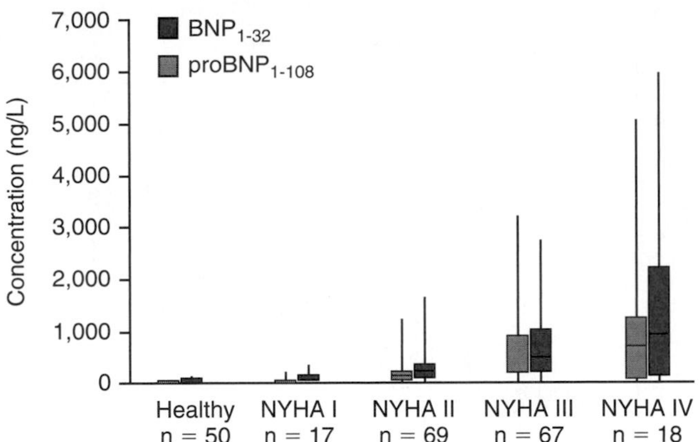

Figure 47-30 Relationship between proBNP$_{1-108}$ and NYHA classifications. *(From Giuliani I, Rieunier F, Larue C, Delagneau JF, Granier C, Pau B. Assay for measurement of intact B-type natriuretic peptide prohormone in blood. Clin Chem 2006;52: 1054-61.)*

BOX 47-7 Special Situations

1. Well HF patients
2. HF due to diastolic dysfunction
3. Acute mitral regurgitation
4. Pulmonary edema <1 hour old
5. Constrictive epicarditis
6. Other cases "upstream" from
   a. Left ventricle
   b. Mitral stenosis
   c. Atrial myoxma

HF, Heart failure.
Modified from Thygesen K, Alpert JS, White HD. Universal definition of myocardial infarction. Eur Heart J 2007;28:2525-38.

ventricle is clearly an important contributor. Unfortunately, the therapeutic modalities used for treatment have been shown to be ineffective.[313] In addition, because natriuretic peptides are predominantly released in response to end-systolic wall stress, values are much lower in this disease state. Thus natriuretic peptides provide aid in the inclusion or exclusion of heart failure due to systolic dysfunction, but they do not provide similarly robust triage in patients with diastolic dysfunction, or so-called heart failure with preserved systolic function. The presence of primary or secondary valvular abnormalities, which increase pressure or volume overload, particularly the latter, will cause increases in natriuretic peptide values because they increase wall stress. Thus, the presence of these abnormalities must be taken into account when natriuretic peptide values are interpreted. Additionally, the presence of atrial fibrillation defines a group of patients with underlying cardiovascular disease. Natriuretic peptides in the presence and the absence of heart failure will be higher in this setting; this needs to be taken into account when values are interpreted for diagnostic purposes.[207] Abnormalities in right ventricular function, even when due to volume overload that will cause increased wall stress, are associated with a blunted natriuretic peptide response, likely due to the smaller mass of myocardium involved. Because the pericardium inhibits increases in wall stress, natriuretic peptide values often are not elevated in constrictive pericarditis despite overt heart failure, unless the constrictive process is superimposed on prior cardiac disease.[45]

Screening for Ventricular Dysfunction

The use of natriuretic peptides in screening to identify patients with impaired ventricular function that has not previously been appreciated has been proposed. The sensitivity and specificity of such an approach are far less than those of the acute circumstance; for this reason, most groups have not advocated use of this analyte in this particular area; however, as the criteria for diagnosis improve, as more specific assays are developed, this is an area where natriuretic peptides may prove to be of value, especially if confined to high-risk groups.[56,120,163,337]

Prognostic Use of Natriuretic Peptides

Some have argued for the ubiquitous use of natriuretic peptides in all patients with dyspnea. The logic for such an approach is related to the fact that individuals with higher natriuretic peptide values have a more adverse prognosis (Figure 47-31) in general than those with lower levels when they present acutely or chronically.* There may be an exception to the idea that higher levels are always more negatively prognostic.[258] (It has been reported that in the extremely ill end-stage patient, lower values are observed, and this could reflect exhaustion of the natriuretic peptide system; however, these observations remain to be confirmed.) One could argue that obtaining a natriuretic peptide value at the time of admission to hospital in a patient who has suspected congestive heart failure is valuable from the perspective of determining eventual risk. Indeed, it is well established that values obtained in this circumstance are highly prognostic, with very high risk ratios and higher values by and large associated with worse disease. Maximal prognostic significance usually is associated with the value at the time of discharge. Thus, a reasonable strategy would be to obtain one level at the time of admission and another at the time of discharge.

Recent data suggest that if natriuretic peptide values are reduced substantially during hospitalization, patients tend to do better. However, most of the reductions that have been reported are modest compared with the biological variability (see earlier). Thus, it is difficult to know how to interpret these changes, especially in individual patients. Recent data in the outpatient setting suggest that the changes needed to overcome biological variability of 80% or greater (Figure 47-32) lead to substantive alterations in prognosis.[71,262] Nonetheless, in the clinical perspective, there probably are differences between those individuals with more chronic disease and those with only acute disease. Those with more chronic disease have a chronically induced natriuretic peptide system that probably responds more slowly than the system in individuals who have simply an acute diathesis and in whom

*References 8, 47, 55, 146, 188, 222, 223, 238, and 294.

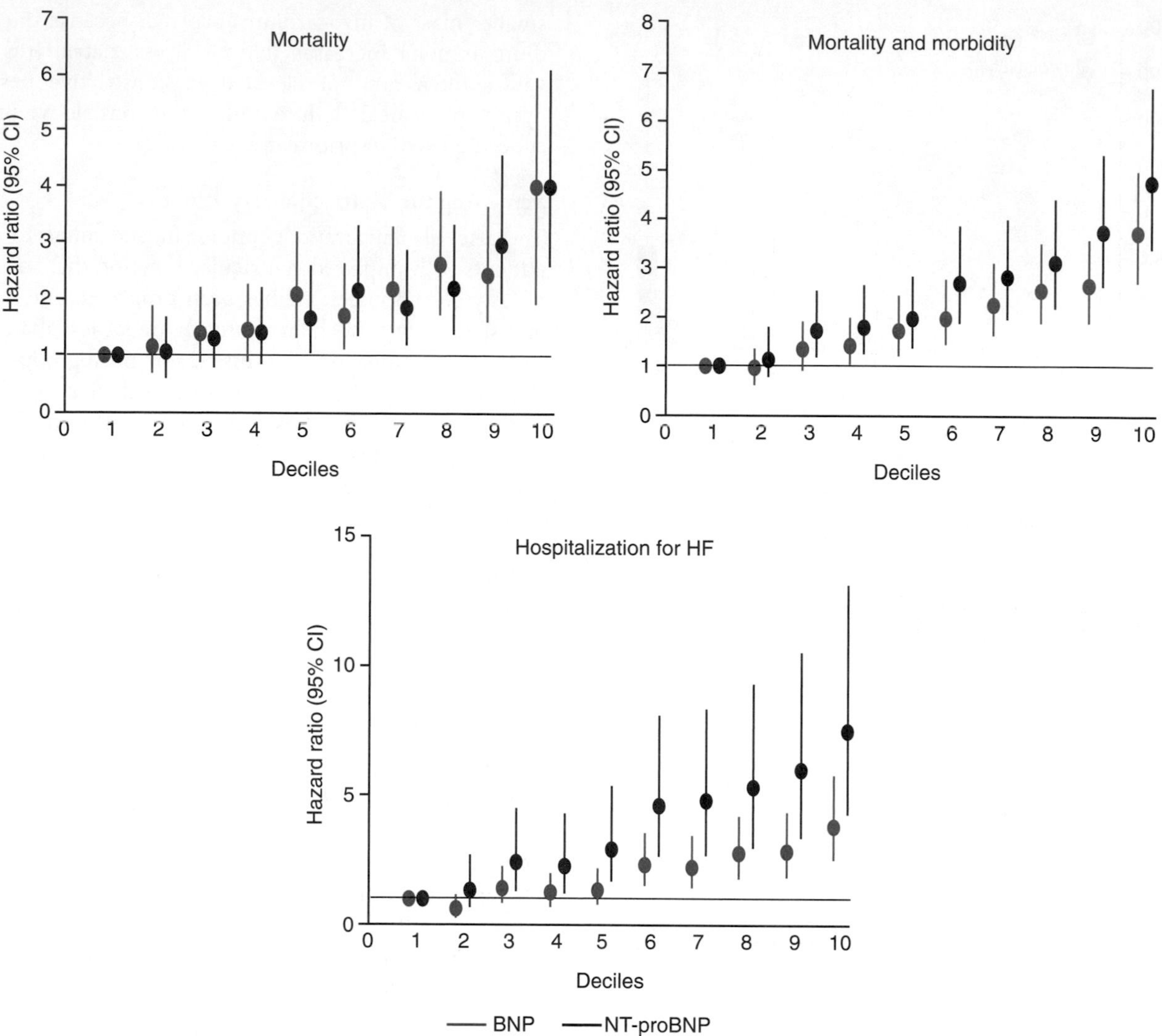

Covariates for adjustment: age, gender, NYHA class, ischemic etiology, LVEF, LVIDd, serum creatinine and bilirubin, randomized treatment, prescription of beta-blockers, digitalis and diuretics, presence of AF or diabetes at study entry.

Figure 47-31 Relationships of brain natriuretic peptide (BNP) and N-terminal pro brain natriuretic peptide (NTproBNP) values and outcomes. *(With permission from Anand IS, Fisher LD, Chiang YT, Latini R, Masson S, Maggioni AP, et al. Changes in brain natriuretic peptide and norepinephrine over time and mortality and morbidity in the Valsartan Heart Failure Trial (Val-HeFT). Circulation 2003;107:1278-83.)*

natriuretic peptide levels may respond somewhat more rapidly. Accordingly, some effort in subclassifying these patients with regard to these parameters is essential.

Unfortunately, studies have not defined what should be done if natriuretic peptide levels do not respond rapidly. It would be important if one could show that keeping patients in the hospital, for example, would mitigate some of these problems, but this information simply is not available at present. Some studies have actually claimed benefit in reducing costs, but at times those studies have included very long hospital stays.[276] Thus, management decisions cannot be made solely on the basis of the natriuretic peptide concentrations. In addition, one needs to be extremely careful because of the subset of patients who may have low levels if they are chronically ill, and because of the heterogeneity of values associated with differences in body physiognomy likely related to clearance of the natriuretic peptides.

Use of Natriuretic Peptides to Guide Therapy

Perhaps the most interesting use of these markers is seen in the patient with heart failure, in whom they are used in the hope of titering therapy more efficaciously.[151,200,322,324] The logic of this approach suggests that many individuals are not as astute as they could be regarding their symptoms, and that having an objective measure may be helpful. This theory has been tested in several randomized controlled trials. The first, STARS-BNP, suggested benefit of such an approach, but subsequent trials have not confirmed those findings.[192] Two other studies have been presented, but not published, at this time. It has been argued that negative results may be due to the fact

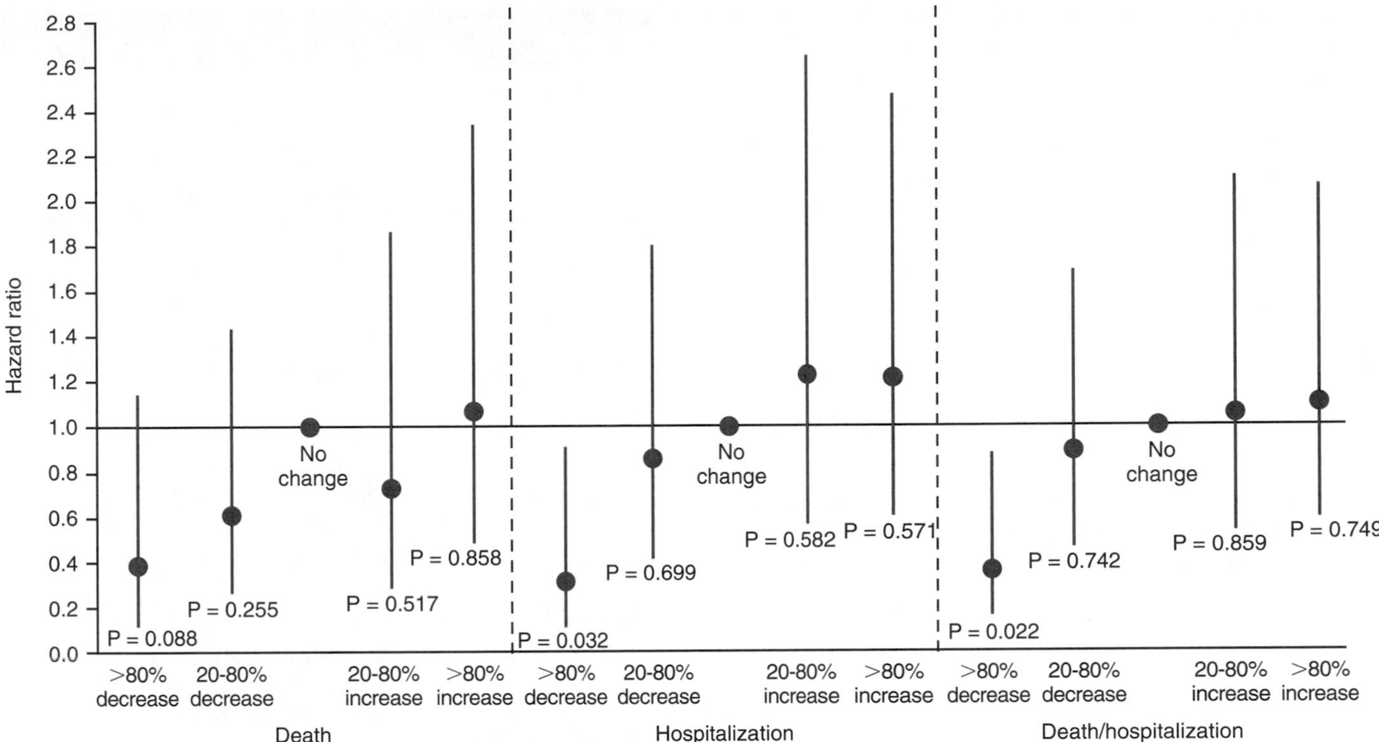

Figure 47-32 Relationship of the change in brain natriuretic peptide (BNP) values over time to outcomes. *(With permission from Jeremias A, Kleiman NS, Nassif D, Hsieh WH, Pencina M, Maresh K, et al; Evaluation of Drug Eluting Stents and Ischemic Events [EVENT] Registry Investigators. Prevalence and prognostic significance of preprocedural cardiac troponin elevation among patients with stable coronary artery disease undergoing percutaneous coronary intervention: results from the evaluation of drug eluting stents and ischemic events registry. Circulation 2008;118:632-8.)*

that, in many of the trials, a large percentage of patients have been elderly (>75 years), and the thought is that elderly patients may not tolerate the increased doses of therapeutic agents used in the management protocols predicated on natriuretic peptides. Indeed, if one excludes those older than 75 years, substantial benefit is associated with this strategy.[307] If this were a finding in only one trial, one might be highly cynical; this is why reports of the other studies are awaited anxiously. If confirmed, the idea of utilizing natriuretic peptides to adjust therapy so as to reduce values toward normal or to attain a change from baseline greater than 80% has the possibility of markedly improving prognosis. Time will tell.

Other Situations

Several investigations have suggested that one can use natriuretic peptides to determine when to intervene in patients with aortic stenosis and mitral regurgitation.[54,110,308,389] Unfortunately, usually only one value has been used, and that value (corrected for differences in the assays) tends to be quite low. Thus, how to distinguish these values from those of normal or less severely affected individuals is unclear. However, it is possible that using changes in natriuretic peptides over time might provide a better paradigm. Several situations can be associated with severe congestive heart failure in the absence of increased concentrations of natriuretic peptides. These include very acute heart failure that manifests before the stimulus to produce increased levels of natriuretic peptides has had time to occur. In addition, patients in situations where the abnormality is above the ventricle, such as atrial myxoma or mitral stenosis, can present with heart failure and normal natriuretic peptide values. Finally, constrictive pericarditis is associated with low values because increases in wall stress are precluded by the constricting pericardium.

Other situations in which natriuretic peptide concentrations are increased in blood include any disease that increases blood volume and thus wall stress, such as sepsis, anemia, renal dysfunction, Cushing's syndrome and/or hyperaldosteronism, hypertension with LVH, and cirrhosis. Some have suggested that values can be used to assess prognosis in patients with renal failure, albeit using higher cutoff values, and it does appear that the mechanisms for release are the same.[289] However, mixing values between GFR groups is likely to lead to confusion. Using values within groups (e.g., those with severe disease on or off long-term dialysis) appears much more salutary.[109,292]

Ischemic Heart Disease

Several investigations have suggested that natriuretic peptides can be used to assess prognosis in patients who present with acute coronary syndromes and normal cardiac troponin values.* Most of these studies have used relatively insensitive cardiac troponin assays or higher cutoff values, but such

*References 104-106, 190, 275, 284, 295, 296, 323, 333, and 388.

assays and cutoff values are still in common use. If so, the finding of an elevated natriuretic peptide level may be helpful. In one study, such patients benefited from an invasive strategy.[395] The subgroup involved was mostly female, and it appears that women may have lower cardiac troponin levels than men. However, if this strategy is to be used, a relatively low cutoff value has been advocated (80 ng/L with the Biosite BNP assay). Whether these low values will allow adequate discrimination in large groups of patients is unclear. However, it is clear that use of natriuretic peptides may be helpful after the acute episode in predicting the subsequent risk of events. Indeed, over time in some studies, they appear to be even more prognostic than troponin.[117] Thus, eventually, it is likely that natriuretic peptides may become part of a long-term risk stratification panel. Natriuretic peptides are also elaborated, albeit to a modest extent, in those with positive treadmill stress tests.[332] Some of this release comes directly from the coronary arteries. Elevations also occur in those with diastolic abnormalities.[269] The changes appear too small to be used diagnostically.

The Future

The potential future use of natriuretic peptides, as indicated in the analytical sections, is growing as we understand more about the biochemistry and mechanisms of natriuretic peptide release. It appears that congestive heart failure is in part a clinical syndrome characterized by abnormalities in how the natriuretic peptide system works. The system synthesizes and releases large amounts of protein, but much of the protein is poorly functional. Whether this is because it is inadequately cleaved or whether it is due to glycosylation[93,339] or to other biochemical processes has yet to be determined. However, what is clear is that very little circulating active BNP is present in patients with heart failure.[341] Most of what appears to circulate is proBNP,[153] which is uncleaved, suggesting probable abnormalities in corin and furin that are indigenous to the pathophysiology of congestive heart failure. If one could manipulate these systems to facilitate the presence of active BNP or of other fragments that might have biological importance, one might substantially improve congestive heart failure. These are some of the approaches currently being pursued in the hope of improving therapy for this very large group of patients.

In addition, novel biomarkers (Tables 47-5 and 47-6) have the potential to contribute substantially to this work. Recent data suggest that one can measure intact proBNP directly, which may lead to better understanding of underlying pathophysiology. As with other natriuretic peptides, its circulating concentration tracks with the clinical class of heart failure (see Figure 47-29).[135] In addition, a new test for ANP has been developed (MR-proANP) that may have some advantages.[271] Preliminary data suggest that it is equivalent to other natriuretic peptides in its ability to diagnose acute heart failure.[266] Such testing might allow the more rapidly responding atrial peptide and the more slow to respond B-type natriuretic peptide to be used synergistically. Again, additional research is necessary.

TABLE 47-5 Biomarkers in Heart Failure

Inflammation*†‡	C-reactive protein Tumor necrosis factor-α Fas (APO-1) Interleukins-1, -6, and -18
Oxidative stress*†§	Oxidized low-density lipoproteins Myeloperoxidase Urinary biopyrrins Urinary and plasma isoprostanes Plasma malondialdehyde
Myocyte injury*†§	Cardiac-specific troponins I and T Myosin light-chain kinase I Heart-type fatty acid protein Creatine kinase MB fraction
Myocyte stress†§¶	BNP NT-proBNP MR-proANP ST2
Extracellular matrix remodeling*†§	Matrix metalloproteinases Tissue inhibitors of metalloproteinases Collagen propeptides
New biomarkers†	Chromogranin Galectin 3 Osteoprotegerin Adiponectin Growth differentiation factor 15
Neurohormones*†§	Norepinephrine Renin Angiotensin II Arginine vasopressin Endothelin

*Biomarkers in this category aid in elucidating the pathogenesis of heart failure.
†Biomarkers in this category provide prognostic information and enhance risk stratification.
‡Biomarkers in this category can be used to identify subjects at risk for heart failure.
§Biomarkers in this category are potential targets of therapy.
¶Biomarkers in this category are useful in the diagnosis of heart failure and in monitoring therapy.
Adapted from Braunwald E. Biomarkers in heart failure. N Engl J Med 2008;358:2148-59.

Natriuretic peptides may be of additional value in several different intriguing areas that are being explored. One is sudden cardiac death. Several studies have associated elevated natriuretic peptide values with mortality and/or ICD discharges.[53,385] A second area involves the follow-up of patients who received cardiac resynchronization therapy (CRT) devices. It appears that higher values help define a group apt to benefit, and although it takes some time for natriuretic peptides to fall, their reduction is associated with clinical benefit over time.[127,225] Finally, several suggestions have indicated that BNP may be useful in helping to diagnose pulmonary emboli when they occur and to determine prognosis. Unfortunately, levels often are not markedly elevated,

TABLE 47-6 Biomarkers in ACS

Type	Markers
Serologic biomarkers of arterial vulnerability	Lipid profile
	Apo B
	Lp(a)
	LDL particle number
	CETP
	Lp-PLA_2
	Inflammation
	hsCRP
	sICAM-1
	IL-6
	IL-18
	SAA
	MPO
	sCD40
	Oxidized LDL
	GPX1 activity
	Nitrotyrosine
	Homocysteine
	Cystatin-C
	Natriuretic peptides
	ADMA
	MMP-9
	TIMP-1
Structural markers of arterial vulnerability	Carotid IMT
	Coronary artery calcium
Functional markers of arterial vulnerability	Blood pressure
	Endothelial dysfunction
	Arterial stiffness
	Ankle-brachial index
	Urine albumin excretion
Serologic markers of blood vulnerability	Fibrinogen
	D-Dimer
Decreased fibrinolysis	TPA/PAI-1
Increased coagulation	von Willebrand factor
Structural markers of myocardial vulnerability	Exercise stress echo
	PET
Serologic markers of myocardial injury	Cardiac troponins

ADMA, Asymmetric dimethylarginine; *Apo,* apolipoprotein; *CETP,* cholesterol ester transfer protein; *hsCRP,* high-sensitivity C-reactive protein; *IL,* interleukin; *IMT,* Intimal-medial thickness; *LDL,* low-density lipoprotein; *Lp(a),* lipoprotein a; *Lp-PLA₂,* phospholipase A2; *MMP,* matrix metalloproteinase; *MPO,* myeloperoxidase; *PET,* positron emission tomography; *SAA,* ribonucleoprotein; *sCD40,* soluble CD40 ligand; *sICAM,* soluble intracellular adhesion molecule; *TIMP,* tissue inhibitor of metalloproteinase; *TPA/PAI,* tissue plasminogen activator, plasminogen activator inhibitor-1.

Adapted from Vasan RS. Biomarkers of cardiovascular disease: molecular basis and practical considerations. Circulation 2006;113:2335-62.

but with time this indication may be developed more fully.[213,214]

Two other major areas need to be discussed: multimarker testing and ST2. First, it is clear that for ischemic heart disease, the addition of natriuretic peptides to other markers in a multimarker strategy improves risk stratification, especially over the long term.[331,416,419] It also appears that benefit may be derived from the prediction of events in older, less acutely ill individuals. Recently, the group from Upsalla reported a rather striking improvement in the prediction of events (changes in the kappa c statistic from 0.644 to 0.766) with the use of a multimarker panel that included natriuretic peptides. The panel included cTn, NT-proBNP, cystatin C, and CRP. If confirmed, this approach may become more widely used for risk prediction. Second, markers have been found that may be synergistic with the natriuretic peptides. One such marker, ST2, a "decoy receptor for IL33," has substantially better predictive ability for mortality than the natriuretic peptides.[316] Other "death markers" such as GDF-15 may also provide benefit in this area.[202]

BIOMARKERS OF INTEREST, ALTHOUGH THEY ARE NOT CURRENTLY USED ROUTINELY

Figure 47-33 portrays a biochemical profile in coronary vascular disease that correlates staging of biomarker release into the circulation with various pathophysiologic mechanisms of acute coronary syndrome and heart failure. As shown in Tables 47-5 and 47-6, numerous biomarkers have been studied and used for different clinical reasons, and other promising novel biomarkers are trying to establish themselves alongside cTn and NPs as routine clinical tools. We highlight some characteristics of several of these here. This list is not meant to be all inclusive.

C-Reactive Protein

CRP is an acute-phase reactant that was initially developed to evaluate patients with infection.[73,185,303,325] It now appears that concentrations below those seen in infection but above healthy values (as measured by so-called high-sensitivity CRP, or hsCRP, assays) can be a marker of the atherosclerotic process, because both chronic and acute atherosclerotic processes involve an inflammatory component (see Chapter 27). Among the ligands that can stimulate CRP are tissue necrosis factor (TNF) and interleukin 1 (IL-1), which are thought to stimulate IL-6, which then causes the elaboration of CRP from the liver (see Chapters 21 and 27). It is now clear that CRP itself can enhance the inflammatory and prothrombotic response. A large number of assays for hsCRP are available, as is a standard protocol for their reporting.

For primary prevention, values greater than 3 mg/L are considered high risk. Recent data suggest that using hsCRP data with the calculated low-density lipoprotein (LDL) is a potent way to predict risk. For risk stratification in primary prevention, the use of routine hsCRP is not recommended by the AHA/CDC panel. When used, less than 1 mg/L is

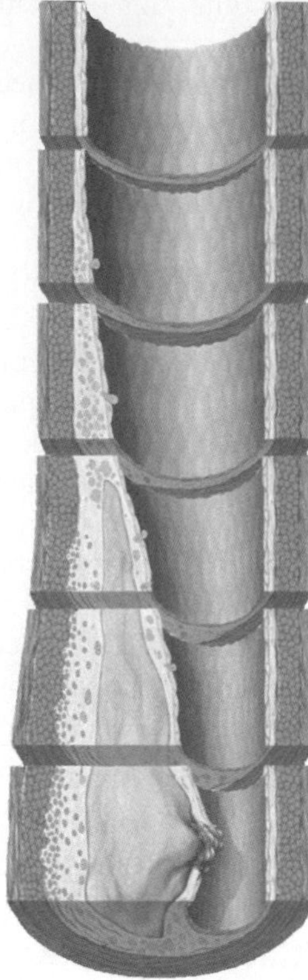
• Proinflammatory Cytokines
• IL-6, TNFa
• Plaque Destabilization
• MPO, MMPs, CAMs
• Plaque Rupture
• sCD40L, PIGF, PAPP-A
• Acute Phase Reactants
• hs-CRP, serum amyloid
• Ischemia
• Choline, FFAu, copeptin, GPBB
• Necrosis
• cTnT, cTnI, CKMB, myoglobin, FABP
• Myocardial Dysfunction/CHF
• BNP, NT-proBNP, MR-proANP, proBNP, ST2, GDF-15, galactin

Figure 47-33 Complete spectrum of acute coronary pathophysiologic process from initiation of atherosclerosis to cell death to myocardial dysfunction. *(Modified from Apple F. Cardiac ischemia: where no biomarker has gone before. Clin Lab News 2009;35:8-10.)*

considered low risk, 1 to 3 mg/L intermediate risk, and more than 3 mg/L high risk.

In patients who present with ACS, the initial value for hsCRP has prognostic significance. Whether it is short or long term depends on the study. In most studies, the influence of cardiac troponin measurements is the predominant short-term prognostic factor, and hsCRP adds to long-term prognosis. However, this is not always the case. Of interest, hsCRP measurements, similar to BNP, seem to predict death, but not recurrent infarction. This could be true because of the effect of mortality, which can confound multivariable models, but it is different from the data related to cardiac troponin (see discussion in this chapter).[184] It should be appreciated that once necrosis has occurred, hsCRP values rise and the ability to use them prognostically is attenuated.

Serum Amyloid Protein A

Serum amyloid protein A, an acute-phase protein and an apolipoprotein, has been used with hsCRP in cross-sectional studies. It can be synergistic with hsCRP[326] but is much less commonly used. At present, no standardized assays, reference interval studies, nor consistent assay validations are available.

sCD40 Ligand

CD40 ligand is a transmembrane protein related to TNF. It has multiple prothrombotic and proatherogenic effects. What is usually measured is the soluble form of the receptor, sCD40 ligand, which has been shown to be a predictor of events after acute presentation.[380] At present, standardized assays, reference interval studies, nor consistent assay validations are not available.

Cytokines

A variety of stimulatory and inhibitory interleukins (TNF, IL-1, IL-6, IL-8, IL-12, IL-18) are thought to help mediate the elaboration of CRP and the development of atherosclerosis and acute events.[121] These cytokines may stimulate or inhibit leukocytes, often through T cell–mediated processes and effects on monocytes, which are indigenous to atherogenesis.[237] In some studies, IL-6 is more prognostic than hsCRP. These cytokines often have inhibitors and/or binding proteins that modulate their effects. At present, standardized assays, reference intervals studies, and consistent assay validations are not available.

Myeloperoxidase

Myeloperoxidase (MPO) is released when neutrophils aggregate; this may indicate an active inflammatory response in blood vessels. It has been shown to be elevated chronically when chronic CAD is present.[418] It is increased when patients present with ACS.[39A,69] Initial prognostic studies were encouraging but were done without adequate consideration of other analytes and specifically cardiac troponin. A multi-biomarker study has shown that myeloperoxidase as a prognostic tool was dependent on the outcomes studied (cardiac death) and the demographics of the patient population enrolled.[27] Accordingly, additional studies are needed. At present, no standardized assays, reference interval studies, nor consistent assay validations are available. Further, it has been demonstrated that the type of specimen collected is critical for the stability and accurate measurement of myeloperoxidase.[345] For further information on this enzyme, see Chapter 22.

Lipoprotein-Associated Phospholipase A_2

Phospholipase A2 (Lp-PLA_2) is a phospholipase associated with LDL that is thought to be an inflammatory marker. It was previously known as platelet-activating factor (PAF) acetyl hydrolase. It is synthesized by monocytes and lymphocytes and is thought to cleave oxidized lipids to produce lipid fragments that are more atherogenic and that increase endothelial adhesion. An FDA-approved assay for this analyte includes obligatory reference intervals. It has been shown to be predictive of events in a primary prevention cohort, even when hsCRP is present in the model, suggesting that it measures something different from what is measured by the acute-phase reactants associated with hsCRP.[49] For more information on Lp-PLA_2, see Chapter 22.

Pregnancy-Associated Plasma Protein A

Pregnancy-associated plasma protein A (PAPP-A) is a metalloproteinase that is thought to be expressed in plaques that may be prone to rupture. The literature in this regard is mixed at present concerning its use.[50,241,312] At present, standardized assays, reference interval studies, and consistent assay validations are not available. Recent data suggest that heparin administration in MI patients is associated with increased PAPP-A concentrations; this may limit its prognostic role. For further information on this enzyme, see Chapter 22.

Oxidized LDL

Oxidized LDL has been attributed a key role in the development of atherosclerosis (see Chapter 27). Several methods have been used to measure it, but they yield potentially different data. Some have correlated malondialdehyde LDL with the development of atherosclerosis and short-term events.[165] Direct identification with antibodies suggests that oxidized LDL may be released from vessels and may colocalize with lipoprotein a [Lp(a)] after acute events.[375]

Placental Growth Factor

Placental growth factor is an angiogenic factor related to vascular endothelial growth factor (VEGF), which stimulates smooth muscle cells and macrophages.[135A,155] It also increases TNF and MCP-1. A novel assay for this analyte is thought to provide additional prognostic information on patients who present with ACS.[39] At present, standardized assays, reference interval studies, and consistent assay validations are not available.

Matrix Metalloproteinases

Matrix metalloproteinases (MMPs) can degrade the collagen matrix in coronary artery or myocardium. They are integral to remodeling of the coronary artery and/or the heart after acute events. Elaboration of MMP-9, a gelatinase, is thought to be important in plaque destabilization; thus some have tried to measure it as a prognostic index.[39] Other MMPs participate in the elaboration of extracellular matrix in the heart. Many MMPs also have inhibitors [tissue inhibitors of metalloproteinase (TIMPs)] that modulate their effects. At present, standardized assays, reference intervals studies, and consistent assay validations are not available.

Monocyte Chemotactic Protein

Monocyte chemotactic protein (MCP-1) is a chemokine that is thought to be responsible for the recruitment of monocytes into atherosclerotic plaque (see Chapter 22). It has been reported to be elevated in patients with ACS and to have long-term predictive value.[107] However, at present, standardized assays, reference interval studies, and consistent assay validations are not available.

Tissue Plasminogen Activator Antigen (t-PA) and Plasminogen Activator Inhibitor 1 (PAI-1)

t-PA is the body's physiologic fibrinolytic activator. PAI-1, its endogenous inhibitor, binds to t-PA (see Chapter 59). Inhibition of fibrinolysis has been suggested to be a reason for recurrent infarction; the fact that maximal inhibition usually occurs in the early morning hours provides a potential explanation for the circadian variability of AMI.[166] It may also be the reason why persons with diabetes have such unstable disease; the growth factor properties of insulin stimulate increases in PAI-1.[355] An accurate assessment of this system includes both t-PA and PAI-1, along with some assessment of bound versus free levels.

Secreted Platelet Granular Substances

Both platelet factor 4 (PF4) and beta thromboglobulin (BTG) are secreted when platelets aggregate. PF4 has a short half-life and is released by heparin (see Chapter 59). BTG is not released by heparin and has a longer half-life. Both markers have been used to assess platelet aggregation.[145] BTG is by far the more reliable. At present, standardized assays, reference interval studies, and consistent assay validations are not available.

Isoprostanes

Isoprostanes are the end breakdown products of lipid peroxidation, and urinary levels have been used to assess the level of oxidative stress.[142,143] It is thought that oxidation of LDL is essential for the development of atherosclerosis, and that HDL and other antioxidants work by antagonizing this oxidative stress. Urinary isoprostanes give some assessment of this critical process. The most commonly measured are F_2-isoprostanes, but a large number of others are available for measurement. It does appear that they will eventually be helpful in assessing oxidative stress.

Urinary Thromboxane

Urinary thromboxane is the end metabolite of thromboxane A2, which is a measure of platelet aggregation. Urinary levels are elevated in patients with unstable coronary disease, in keeping with the known participation of platelets in the pathogenesis of CAD. This level is difficult to ascertain, and collecting urine in the acute situation is at times problematic.

Adhesion Molecules

Adhesion molecules are a wide variety of molecules that can potentially be measured as a way of assessing the adherence of leukocytes and/or platelets or other adhesive proteins to the endothelial matrix.[232] Some are receptors. Examples include PECAM-1 (platelet-endothelial adhesion molecule 1), P-selectin, e-selectin, and VCAM-1 (vascular cell adhesion molecule 1). At times, the receptor itself is measured, but often it is a soluble portion that circulates that is measured. At present, standardized assays, reference interval studies, and consistent assay validations are not available.

Choline

Choline is released after stimulation by phospholipase D and has been touted as a test of prognosis in patients with chest discomfort.[97] At present, standardized assays, reference interval studies, and consistent assay validations are not available.

Unbound Free Fatty Acid

Unbound free fatty acid (uFFA)[39] has also been touted as a marker of ischemia. Most fatty acid is bound, and ischemia is thought to increase the small unbound fraction. Initial studies have reported mixed results. At present, standardized assays, reference interval studies, and consistent assay validations are not available.

Nourin

Nourin I is a small protein released rapidly by "stressed myocytes." It induces changes in a variety of inflammatory cytokines and attracts neutrophils. Preliminary studies have been done to attempt to validate its use. At present, standardized assays, reference interval studies, and consistent assay validations are not available.

Copeptin

Copeptin, a 30 amino acid glycoprotein constituting the C-terminal portion of arginine vasopressin, has been shown to be a prognostic biomarker in hemorrhagic and septic sepsis. More recently, data have shown that measurement of copeptin serves as a rapid and early rule-out biomarker for AMI at presentation in patients with symptoms suggestive of ACS with a normal cTn value.[256A,318] An assay measuring copeptin (CT-proAVP) has been described using the Brahms Kryptor Immunology Analyzer, Diamond Diagnostics Holliston, MA.[270] Additional clinical and analytical validation studies will be necessary, especially head-to-head comparisons of copeptin versus the new hs-cTn assays.

REFERENCES

1. Abendschein DR, Fontanet HL, Nohara R. Optimized preservation of isoforms of creatine kinase MM isoenzyme in plasma specimens and their rapid quantification by semi-automated chromatofocusing. Clin Chem 1990;36:723-7.
2. Abendschein DR. Rapid diagnosis of myocardial infarction and reperfusion by assay of plasma isoforms of creatine kinase isoenzymes. Clin Biochem 1990;23:399-407.
3. Abendschein D, Seacord LM, Nohara R, Sobel BE, Jaffe AS. Prompt detection of myocardial injury by assay of creatine kinase isoforms in initial plasma samples. Clin Cardiol 1988;11:661-4.
4. Abendschein DR, Morelli RL, Carlson CJ, Emilson B, Rapaport E. Creatine kinase MM isoenzyme subforms in myocardium, cardiac lymph and blood after coronary artery occlusion in dogs. Cardiovasc Res 1984;18:690-6.

4A. Abraham RL, Yang T, Blair M, Roden DM, Darbar D. Augmented potassium current is a shared phenotype for two genetic defects associated with familial atrial fibrillation. J Mol Cell Cardiol 2010;48: 181–90.

4B. Aburaya M, Hino J, Minamino N, Kangawa K, Matsuo H. Isolation and identification of rat brain natriuretic peptides in cardiac atrium. Biochem Biophys Res Commun 1989;163:226-32.

5. Adams JE 3rd, Bodor GS, Davila-Roman VG, Delmez JA, Apple FS, Ladenson JH, et al. Cardiac troponin I. A marker with high specificity for cardiac injury. Circulation 1993;88:101-6.

5A. Ahrén B. DPP-4 inhibitors. Best Pract Res Clin Endocrinol Metab 2007;21:517-33.

6. Alpert JS, Thygesen K, Antman E, Bassand JP. Myocardial infarction redefined—a consensus document of The Joint European Society of Cardiology/American College of Cardiology Committee for the redefinition of myocardial infarction. J Am Coll Cardiol 2000;36: 959-69.
7. Ammann P, Fehr T, Minder EI, Gunter C, Bertel O. Elevation of troponin I in sepsis and septic shock. Intensive Care Med 2001;27: 965-9.
8. Anand IS, Fisher LD, Chiang YT, Latini R, Masson S, Maggioni AP, et al. Changes in brain natriuretic peptide and norepinephrine over time and mortality and morbidity in the Valsartan Heart Failure Trial (Val-HeFT). Circulation 2003;107:1278-83.
9. Anderson JL, Adams CD, Antman EM, Bridges CR, Califf RM, Casey DE Jr, et al. ACC/AHA 2007 guidelines for the management of patients with unstable angina/non ST-elevation myocardial infarction: a report of the American College of Cardiology/American Heart Association Task Force on Practice Guidelines (Writing Committee to Revise the 2002 Guidelines for the Management of Patients With Unstable Angina/Non ST-Elevation Myocardial Infarction): developed in collaboration with the American College of Emergency Physicians, the Society for Cardiovascular Angiography and Interventions, and the Society of Thoracic Surgeons: endorsed by the American Association of Cardiovascular and Pulmonary Rehabilitation and the Society for Academic Emergency Medicine. Circulation 2007;116:e148-304.
10. Anderson PA, Malouf NN, Oakeley AE, Pagani ED, Allen PD. Troponin T isoform expression in humans: a comparison among normal and failing adult heart, fetal heart, and adult and fetal skeletal muscle. Circ Res 1991;69:1226-33.

10A. Anonymous. The National Academy of Clinical Biochemistry. Laboratory Medicine Practice Guidelines. Evidence-based practice for point-of-care testing http://www.aacc.org/members/nacb/LMPG/OnlineGuide/PublishedGuidelines/poct/Pages/default.aspx/accessed July 20, 2011.

11. Antman EM, Braunwald E. Acute myocardial infarction. In: Braunwald E, ed. Heart disease: a textbook of cardiovascular medicine, 6th edition. Philadelphia, Pa: WB Saunders, 2001:1114-231.
12. Apple FS. Acute myocardial infarction and coronary reperfusion: serum cardiac markers for the 1990s. Am J Clin Pathol 1992;97: 217-26.
13. Apple FS. Diagnostic use of CK-MM and CK-MB isoforms for detecting myocardial infarction. Clin Lab Med 1989;9:643-54.

14. Apple FS. A new season for cardiac troponin assays: it's time to keep a scorecard. Clin Chem 2009;55:1303-6.
15. Apple FS. Point-of-care cardiac troponin testing: process improvements for detection of acute myocardial infarction. Point Care 2006;5:25-7.
16. Apple FS, Chung AY, Kogut ME, Bubany S, Murakami MM. Decreased patient charges following implementation of point-of-care cardiac troponin monitoring in acute coronary syndrome patients in a community hospital cardiology unit. Clin Chim Acta 2006;370:191-5.
17. Apple FS, Jesse RL, Newby LK, Wu AH, Christenson RH, Cannon CP, et al. National Academy of Clinical Biochemistry and IFCC Committee for Standardization of Markers of Cardiac Damage Laboratory Medicine Practice Guidelines: analytical issues for biochemical markers of acute coronary syndromes. Clin Chem 2007;53:547-51.
18. Apple FS, Ler R, Chung AY, Berger MJ, Murakami MM. Point-of-care i-STAT cardiac troponin I for assessment of patients with symptoms suggestive of acute coronary syndrome. Clin Chem 2006;52:322-5.
19. Apple FS, McGue MK. Serum enzyme changes during marathon training. Am J Clin Pathol 1983;79:716-9.
20. Apple FS, Murakami MM. Cardiac troponin and creatine kinase MB monitoring during in-hospital myocardial reinfarction. Clin Chem 2005;51:460-3.
21. Apple FS, Murakami MM. Serum and plasma cardiac troponin I 99th percentile reference values for 3 2nd-generation assays. Clin Chem 2007;53:1558-60.
22. Apple FS, Murakami MM, Ler R, Walker D, York M. Analytical characteristics of commercial cardiac troponin I and T immunoassays in serum from rats, dogs, and monkeys with induced acute myocardial injury. Clin Chem 2008;54:1982-9.
23. Apple FS, Murakami MM, Pearce LA, Herzog CA. Multi-biomarker risk stratification of N-terminal pro-B-type natriuretic peptide, high-sensitivity C-reactive protein, and cardiac troponin T and I in end-stage renal disease for all-cause death. Clin Chem 2004;50: 2279-85.
24. Apple FS, Murakami MM, Pearce LA, Herzog CA. Predictive value of cardiac troponin I and T for subsequent death in end-stage renal disease. Circulation 2002;106:2941-5.
25. Apple FS, Panteghini M, Ravkilde J, Mair J, Wu AH, Tate J, et al. Quality specifications for B-type natriuretic peptide assays. Clin Chem 2005;51:486-93.
26. Apple FS, Parvin CA, Buechler KF, Christenson RH, Wu AH, Jaffe AS. Validation of the 99th percentile cutoff independent of assay imprecision (CV) for cardiac troponin monitoring for ruling out myocardial infarction. Clin Chem 2005;51:2198-200.
27. Apple FS, Pearce LA, Chung A, Ler R, Murakami MM. Multiple biomarker use for detection of adverse events in patients presenting with symptoms suggestive of acute coronary syndrome. Clin Chem 2007;53:874-81.
28. Apple FS, Pearce LA, Doyle PJ, Otto AP, Murakami MM. Cardiac troponin risk stratification based on 99th percentile reference cutoffs in patients with ischemic symptoms suggestive of acute coronary syndrome: influence of estimated glomerular filtration rates. Am J Clin Pathol 2007;127:598-603.
29. Apple FS, Pearce LA, Smith SW, Kaczmarek JM, Murakami MM. Role of monitoring changes in sensitive cardiac troponin I assay results for early diagnosis of myocardial infarction and prediction of risk of adverse events. Clin Chem 2009;55:930-7.
30. Apple FS, Quist HE, Doyle PJ, Otto AP, Murakami MM. Plasma 99th percentile reference limits for cardiac troponin and creatine kinase MB mass for use with European Society of Cardiology/American College of Cardiology consensus recommendations. Clin Chem 2003;49:1331-6.
31. Apple FS, Rogers MA. Skeletal muscle lactate dehydrogenase isozyme alterations in men and women marathon runners. J Appl Physiol 1986;61:477-81.
32. Apple FS, Rogers MA, Casal DC, Lewis L, Ivy JL, Lampe JW. Skeletal muscle creatine kinase MB alterations in women marathon runners. Eur J Appl Physiol Occup Physiol 1987;56:49-52.
33. Apple FS, Smith SW, Pearce LA, Ler R, Murakami MM. Use of the Centaur TnI-Ultra assay for detection of myocardial infarction and adverse events in patients presenting with symptoms suggestive of acute coronary syndrome. Clin Chem 2008;54:723-8.
34. Apple FS, Smith SW, Pearce LA, Ler R, Murakami MM, Benoit MO, et al. Use of the bioMerieux VIDAS troponin I ultra assay for the diagnosis of myocardial infarction and detection of adverse events in patients presenting with symptoms suggestive of acute coronary syndrome. Clin Chim Acta 2008;390:72-5.
35. Apple FS, Trinity E, Steen J, Prawer S, Wu AH. BNP test utilization for CHF in community hospital practice. Clin Chim Acta 2003;328: 191-3.
36. Apple FS, Voss E, Lund L, Preese L, Berger CR, Henry TD. Cardiac troponin, CK-MB and myoglobin for the early detection of acute myocardial infarction and monitoring of reperfusion following thrombolytic therapy. Clin Chim Acta 1995;237:59-66.
37. Apple FS, Wu AH, Jaffe AS. European Society of Cardiology and American College of Cardiology guidelines for redefinition of myocardial infarction: how to use existing assays clinically and for clinical trials. Am Heart J 2002;144:981-6.
38. Apple FS, Wu AH, Jaffe AS, Panteghini M, Christenson RH, Cannon CP, et al. National Academy of Clinical Biochemistry and IFCC Committee for Standardization of Markers of Cardiac Damage Laboratory Medicine practice guidelines: analytical issues for biomarkers of heart failure. Circulation 2007;116: e95-8.
39. Apple FS, Wu AH, Mair J, Ravkilde J, Panteghini M, Tate J, et al. Future biomarkers for detection of ischemia and risk stratification in acute coronary syndrome. Clin Chem 2005;51:810-24.
39A. Apple FS, Smith SW, Pearce LA, Schulz KM, Ler R, Murakami MM. Myeloperoxidase improves risk stratification in patients with ischemia and normal cardiac troponin I concentrations. Clin Chem 2011;57: 603-8.
40. Arden KC, Viars CS, Weiss S, Argentin S, Nemer M. Localization of the human B-type natriuretic peptide precursor (NPPB) gene to chromosome 1p36. Genomics 1995;26:385-9.
41. American Heart Association. Heart disease and stroke statistics, 2004 update. Dallas, Tex: AHA, 2004.
41A. Asano K, Murakami M, Endo D, Kimura T, Fujinaga T. Complementary DNA cloning, tissue distribution, and synthesis of canine brain natriuretic peptide. Am J Vet Res 1999;60:860-4.
42. Assomull RG, Lyne JC, Keenan N, Gulati A, Bunce NH, Davies SW, et al. The role of cardiovascular magnetic resonance in patients presenting with chest pain, raised troponin, and unobstructed coronary arteries. Eur Heart J 2007;28:1242-9.
43. Aviles RJ, Askari AT, Lindahl B, Wallentin L, Jia G, Ohman EM, et al. Troponin T levels in patients with acute coronary syndromes, with or without renal dysfunction. N Engl J Med 2002;346:2047-52.
44. Ay H, Koroshetz WJ, Benner T, Vangel MG, Melinosky C, Arsava EM, et al. Neuroanatomic correlates of stroke-related myocardial injury. Neurology 2006;66:1325-9.
45. Babuin L, Alegria JR, Oh JK, Nishimura RA, Jaffe AS. Brain natriuretic peptide levels in constrictive pericarditis and restrictive cardiomyopathy. J Am Coll Cardiol 2006;47:1489-91.
46. Babuin L, Vasile VC, Rio Perez JA, Alegria JR, Chai HS, Afessa B, et al. Elevated cardiac troponin is an independent risk factor for short- and long-term mortality in medical intensive care unit patients. Crit Care Med 2008;36:759-65.
47. Baggish AL, van Kimmenade RR, Januzzi JL Jr. Amino-terminal pro-B-type natriuretic peptide testing and prognosis in patients with acute dyspnea, including those with acute heart failure. Am J Cardiol 2008;101:49-55.
48. Bakshi TK, Choo MK, Edwards CC, Scott AG, Hart HH, Armstrong GP. Causes of elevated troponin I with a normal coronary angiogram. Intern Med J 2002;32:520-5.
49. Ballantyne CM, Hoogeveen RC, Bang H, Coresh J, Folsom AR, Heiss G, et al. Lipoprotein-associated phospholipase A2, high-sensitivity C-reactive protein, and risk for incident coronary heart disease in

middle-aged men and women in the Atherosclerosis Risk in Communities (ARIC) study. Circulation 2004;109:837-42.

50. Bayes-Genis A, Conover CA, Overgaard MT, Bailey KR, Christiansen M, Holmes DR Jr, et al. Pregnancy-associated plasma protein A as a marker of acute coronary syndromes. N Engl J Med 2001;345:1022-9.
51. Bayliss WM, Starling EH. The mechanism of pancreatic secretion. J Physiol 1902;28:325-53.
51A. Beaubien G, Schafer MK, Weihe E, Dong W, Chretien M, Seidah NG, Day R. The distinct gene expression of the pro-hormone convertases in the rat heart suggests potential substrates. Cell Tissue Res 1995;279:539-49.
52. Belenky A, Smith A, Zhang B, Lin S, Despres N, Wu AH, et al. The effect of class-specific protease inhibitors on the stabilization of B-type natriuretic peptide in human plasma. Clin Chim Acta 2004; 340:163-72.
53. Berger R, Huelsman M, Strecker K, Bojic A, Moser P, Stanek B, et al. B-type natriuretic peptide predicts sudden death in patients with chronic heart failure. Circulation 2002;105:2392-7.
54. Bergler-Klein J, Klaar U, Heger M, Rosenhek R, Mundigler G, Gabriel H, et al. Natriuretic peptides predict symptom-free survival and postoperative outcome in severe aortic stenosis. Circulation 2004;109: 2302-8.
55. Bettencourt P, Ferreira A, Dias P, Pimenta J, Frioes F, Martins L, et al. Predictors of prognosis in patients with stable mild to moderate heart failure. J Card Fail 2000;6:306-13.
56. Betti I, Castelli G, Barchielli A, Beligni C, Boscherini V, De Luca L, et al. The role of N-terminal PRO-brain natriuretic peptide and echocardiography for screening asymptomatic left ventricular dysfunction in a population at high risk for heart failure. The PROBE-HF study. J Card Fail 2009;15:377-84.
57. Beyrau R, Braun S, Dolci A, Freidank H, Giannitsis E, Handy B, et al. Multicentre evaluation of a high sensitive Elecsys troponin T assay. Clin Chem 2009;55:A71.
58. Bhatt DL, Topol EJ. Does creatinine kinase-MB elevation after percutaneous coronary intervention predict outcomes in 2005? Periprocedural cardiac enzyme elevation predicts adverse outcomes. Circulation 2005;112:906-15; discussion 923.
59. Billadello JJ, Fontanet HL, Strauss AW, Abendschein DR. Characterization of MB creatine kinase isoform conversion in vitro and in vivo in dogs. J Clin Invest 1989;83:1637-43.
60. Bilodeau L, Preese LM, Apple FS. Does low total creatine kinase rule out myocardial infarction? Ann Intern Med 1992;116:523-4.
60A. Bloomquist BT, Eipper BA, Mains RE. Prohormone-converting enzymes: regulation and evaluation of function using antisense RNA. Mol Endocrinol 1991;5:2014-24.
61. Bodor GS, Porter S, Landt Y, Ladenson JH. Development of monoclonal antibodies for an assay of cardiac troponin-I and preliminary results in suspected cases of myocardial infarction. Clin Chem 1992;38:2203-14.
62. Bodor GS, Porterfield D, Voss EM, Smith S, Apple FS. Cardiac troponin-I is not expressed in fetal and healthy or diseased adult human skeletal muscle tissue. Clin Chem 1995;41:1710-5.
63. Bodor GS, Survant L, Voss EM, Smith S, Porterfield D, Apple FS. Cardiac troponin T composition in normal and regenerating human skeletal muscle. Clin Chem 1997;43:476-84.
63A. Bonow RO, Mann DL, Zipes DP, Libby P. Braunwald's Heart Disease: a Textbook of Cardiovascular Medicine. 9th ed. Saunders Philadelphia; 2011.
64. Bossuyt PM, Reitsma JB, Bruns DE, Gatsonis CA, Glasziou PP, Irwig LM, et al. The STARD statement for reporting studies of diagnostic accuracy: explanation and elaboration. Clin Chem 2003;49:7-18.
65. Brandt I, Lambeir AM, Ketelslegers JM, Vanderheyden M, Scharpe S, De Meester I. Dipeptidyl-peptidase IV converts intact B-type natriuretic peptide into its des-SerPro form. Clin Chem 2006;52:82-7.
66. Braunwald E, Antman EM, Beasley JW, Califf RM, Cheitlin MD, Hochman JS, et al. ACC/AHA guidelines for the management of patients with unstable angina and non-ST-segment elevation myocardial infarction: executive summary and recommendations: a report of the American College of Cardiology/American Heart Association Task Force on Practice Guidelines (Committee on the Management of Patients With Unstable Angina). Circulation 2000;102:1193-209.
67. Braunwald E, Antman EM, Beasley JW, Califf RM, Cheitlin MD, Hochman JS, et al. ACC/AHA guideline update for the management of patients with unstable angina and non-ST-segment elevation myocardial infarction—2002. Summary article: a report of the American College of Cardiology/American Heart Association Task Force on Practice Guidelines (Committee on the Management of Patients With Unstable Angina). Circulation 2002;106:1893-900.
68. Bray MS, Shaw CA, Moore MW, Garcia RA, Zanquetta MM, Durgan DJ, et al. Disruption of the circadian clock within the cardiomyocyte influences myocardial contractile function, metabolism, and gene expression. Am J Physiol Heart Circ Physiol 2008;294:H1036-47.
69. Brennan ML, Penn MS, Van Lente F, Nambi V, Shishehbor MH, Aviles RJ, et al. Prognostic value of myeloperoxidase in patients with chest pain. N Engl J Med 2003;349:1595-604.
70. Breuckmann F, Mohlenkamp S, Nassenstein K, Lehmann N, Ladd S, Schmermund A, et al. Myocardial late gadolinium enhancement: prevalence, pattern, and prognostic relevance in marathon runners. Radiology 2009;251:50-7.
71. Bruins S, Fokkema MR, Romer JW, Dejongste MJ, van der Dijs FP, van den Ouweland JM, Muskiet FA. High intraindividual variation of B-type natriuretic peptide (BNP) and amino-terminal proBNP in patients with stable chronic heart failure. Clin Chem 2004;50:2052-8.
72. Buckley MG, Sagnella GA, Markandu ND, Singer DR, MacGregor GA. Concentrations of N-terminal ProANP in human plasma: evidence for ProANP (1-98) as the circulating form. Clin Chim Acta 1990;191:1-14.
73. Buffon A, Biasucci LM, Liuzzo G, D'Onofrio G, Crea F, Maseri A. Widespread coronary inflammation in unstable angina. N Engl J Med 2002;347:5-12.
74. Bunk DM, Welch MJ. Characterization of a new certified reference material for human cardiac troponin I. Clin Chem 2006;52:212-9.
75. Burnett JC Jr, Kao PC, Hu DC, Heser DW, Heublein D, Granger JP, et al. Atrial natriuretic peptide elevation in congestive heart failure in the human. Science 1986;231:1145-7.
76. Cardinale D, Colombo A, Sandri MT, Lamantia G, Colombo N, Civelli M, et al. Prevention of high-dose chemotherapy-induced cardiotoxicity in high-risk patients by angiotensin-converting enzyme inhibition. Circulation 2006;114:2474-81.
77. Cardinale D, Sandri MT, Martinoni A, Tricca A, Civelli M, Lamantia G, et al. Left ventricular dysfunction predicted by early troponin I release after high-dose chemotherapy. J Am Coll Cardiol 2000;36: 517-22.
78. Carson JL, Terrin ML, Magaziner J, Chaitman BR, Apple FS, Heck DA, et al. Transfusion trigger trial for functional outcomes in cardiovascular patients undergoing surgical hip fracture repair (FOCUS). Transfusion 2006;46:2192-206.
79. Cataliotti A, Malatino LS, Jougasaki M, Zoccali C, Castellino P, Giacone G, et al. Circulating natriuretic peptide concentrations in patients with end-stage renal disease: role of brain natriuretic peptide as a biomarker for ventricular remodeling. Mayo Clin Proc 2001;76:1111-9.
80. Chen Y, Serfass RC, Mackey-Bojack SM, Kelly KL, Titus JL, Apple FS. Cardiac troponin T alterations in myocardium and serum of rats after stressful, prolonged intense exercise. J Appl Physiol 2000;88: 1749-55.
80A. Chiravuri M, Agarraberes F, Mathieu SL, Lee H, Huber BT. Vesicular localization and characterization of a novel post-proline-cleaving aminodipeptidase, quiescent cell proline dipeptidase. J Immunol 2000;165:5695-702.
81. Christiansen JP, Edwards C, Sinclair T, Armstrong G, Scott A, Patel H, et al. Detection of myocardial scar by contrast-enhanced cardiac magnetic resonance imaging in patients with troponin-positive chest pain and minimal angiographic coronary artery disease. Am J Cardiol 2006;97:768-71.

82. Christoffersen C, Goetze JP, Bartels ED, Larsen MO, Ribel U, Rehfeld JF, et al. Chamber-dependent expression of brain natriuretic peptide and its mRNA in normal and diabetic pig heart. Hypertension 2002;40:54-60.
83. Christoffersen C, Hunter I, Jensen AL, Goetze JP. Diabetes and the endocrine heart. Eur Heart J 2007;28:2427-9.
83A. Chun YS, Hyun JY, Kwak YG, Kim IS, Kim CH, Choi E, Kim MS, Park JW. Hypoxic activation of the atrial natriuretic peptide gene promoter through direct and indirect actions of hypoxia-inducible factor-1. Biochem J 2003;370:149-57.
84. Clerico A, Emdin M. Diagnostic accuracy and prognostic relevance of the measurement of cardiac natriuretic peptides: a review. Clin Chem 2004;50:33-50.
85. Collinson PO, Boa FG, Gaze DC. Measurement of cardiac troponins. Ann Clin Biochem 2001;38:423-49.
86. Collinson PO, Clifford-Mobley O, Gaze D, Boa F, Senior R. Assay imprecision and 99th-percentile reference value of a high-sensitivity cardiac troponin I assay. Clin Chem 2009;55:1433-4.
87. Collinson PO, Stubbs PJ, Kessler AC. Multicentre evaluation of the diagnostic value of cardiac troponin T, CK-MB mass, and myoglobin for assessing patients with suspected acute coronary syndromes in routine clinical practice. Heart 2003;89:280-6.
88. Colucci WS, Braunwald E. Pathophysiology of heart failure. In: Braunwald E, ed. Heart disease: a textbook of cardiovascular medicine. Philadelphia: WB Saunders, 2001:503-614.
89. Corti R, Burnett JC Jr, Rouleau JL, Ruschitzka F, Luscher TF. Vasopeptidase inhibitors: a new therapeutic concept in cardiovascular disease? Circulation 2001;104:1856-62.
90. Cortina MAQ, Pituley AJ, Shin H, Liu J, Kadijevic L, Bilandzic LM, et al. Comparison of Spectral's enhanced point-of-care test for markers troponin I and myoglobin with clinical analyzers. Clin Chem 2003;49(suppl 6):A71.
91. Costello-Boerrigter LC, Burnett JC Jr. The prognostic value of N-terminal proB-type natriuretic peptide. Nat Clin Pract Cardiovasc Med 2005;2:194-201.
92. Cowie MR, Jourdain P, Maisel A, Dahlstrom U, Follath F, Isnard R, et al. Clinical applications of B-type natriuretic peptide (BNP) testing. Eur Heart J 2003;24:1710-8.
93. Crimmins DL, Kao JL. A glycosylated form of the human cardiac hormone pro B-type natriuretic peptide is an intrinsically unstructured monomeric protein. Arch Biochem Biophys 2008;475:36-41.
94. Cummins B, Auckland ML, Cummins P. Cardiac-specific troponin-I radioimmunoassay in the diagnosis of acute myocardial infarction. Am Heart J 1987;113:1333-44.
95. Daniels LB, Laughlin GA, Clopton P, Maisel AS, Barrett-Connor E. Minimally elevated cardiac troponin T and elevated N-terminal pro-B-type natriuretic peptide predict mortality in older adults: results from the Rancho Bernardo Study. J Am Coll Cardiol 2008;52:450-9.
96. Daniels LB, Maisel AS. Natriuretic peptides. J Am Coll Cardiol 2007;50:2357-68.
97. Danne O, Mockel M, Lueders C, Mugge C, Zschunke GA, Lufft H, et al. Prognostic implications of elevated whole blood choline levels in acute coronary syndromes. Am J Cardiol 2003;91:1060-7.
98. Daughaday WH, Trivedi B, Baxter RC. Serum "big insulin-like growth factor II" from patients with tumor hypoglycemia lacks normal E-domain O-linked glycosylation, a possible determinant of normal propeptide processing. Proc Natl Acad Sci U S A 1993;90:5823-7.
99. Davila-Roman VG, Guest TM, Tuteur PG, Rowe WJ, Ladenson JH, Jaffe AS. Transient right but not left ventricular dysfunction after strenuous exercise at high altitude. J Am Coll Cardiol 1997;30:468-73.
100. Dawson-Bowling S, Chettiar K, Cottam H, Worth R, Forder J, Fitzgerald-O'Connor I, et al. Troponin T as a predictive marker of morbidity in patients with fractured neck of femur. Injury 2008;39: 775-80.
101. de Bold AJ. Determinants of brain natriuretic peptide gene expression and secretion in acute cardiac allograft rejection. Curr Opin Cardiol 2007;22:146-50.
102. de Bold AJ, Borenstein HB, Veress AT, Sonnenberg H. A rapid and potent natriuretic response to intravenous injection of atrial myocardial extract in rats. Life Sci 1981;28:89-94.
103. de Bold AJ, Flynn TG. Cardionatrin I: a novel heart peptide with potent diuretic and natriuretic properties. Life Sci 1983;33:297-302.
104. de Lemos JA, McGuire DK, Drazner MH. B-type natriuretic peptide in cardiovascular disease. Lancet 2003;362:316-22.
105. de Lemos JA, Morrow DA. Combining natriuretic peptides and necrosis markers in the assessment of acute coronary syndromes. Rev Cardiovasc Med 2003;4(suppl 4):S37-46.
106. de Lemos JA, Morrow DA, Bentley JH, Omland T, Sabatine MS, McCabe CH, et al. The prognostic value of B-type natriuretic peptide in patients with acute coronary syndromes. N Engl J Med 2001;345: 1014-21.
107. de Lemos JA, Morrow DA, Sabatine MS, Murphy SA, Gibson CM, Antman EM, et al. Association between plasma levels of monocyte chemoattractant protein-1 and long-term clinical outcomes in patients with acute coronary syndromes. Circulation 2003;107:690-5.
108. deFilippi C, Wasserman S, Rosanio S, Tiblier E, Sperger H, Tocchi M, et al. Cardiac troponin T and C-reactive protein for predicting prognosis, coronary atherosclerosis, and cardiomyopathy in patients undergoing long-term hemodialysis. JAMA 2003;290:353-9.
109. DeFilippi CR, Fink JC, Nass CM, Chen H, Christenson R. N-terminal pro-B-type natriuretic peptide for predicting coronary disease and left ventricular hypertrophy in asymptomatic CKD not requiring dialysis. Am J Kidney Dis 2005;46:35-44.
110. Detaint D, Messika-Zeitoun D, Avierinos JF, Scott C, Chen H, Burnett JC Jr, Enriquez-Sarano M. B-type natriuretic peptide in organic mitral regurgitation: determinants and impact on outcome. Circulation 2005; 111:2391-7.
111. Dickstein K, Cohen-Solal A, Filippatos G, McMurray JJ, Ponikowski P, Poole-Wilson PA, et al. ESC guidelines for the diagnosis and treatment of acute and chronic heart failure 2008: the Task Force for the Diagnosis and Treatment of Acute and Chronic Heart Failure 2008 of the European Society of Cardiology; developed in collaboration with the Heart Failure Association of the ESC (HFA) and endorsed by the European Society of Intensive Care Medicine (ESICM). Eur Heart J 2008;29:2388-442.
112. Diris JH, Hackeng CM, Kooman JP, Pinto YM, Hermens WT, van Dieijen-Visser MP. Impaired renal clearance explains elevated troponin T fragments in hemodialysis patients. Circulation 2004;109: 23-5.
113. Dispenzieri A, Gertz MA, Kyle RA, Lacy MQ, Burritt MF, Therneau TM, et al. Serum cardiac troponins and N-terminal pro-brain natriuretic peptide: a staging system for primary systemic amyloidosis. J Clin Oncol 2004;22:3751-7.
114. Dispenzieri A, Kyle RA, Gertz MA, Therneau TM, Miller WL, Chandrasekaran K, et al. Survival in patients with primary systemic amyloidosis and raised serum cardiac troponins. Lancet 2003;361: 1787-9.
114A. Doyama K, Fukumoto M, Takemura G, Tanaka M, Oda T, Hasegawa K, Inada T, Ohtani S, Fujiwara T, Itoh H, Nakao K, Sasayama S, Fujiwara H. Expression and distribution of brain natriuretic peptide in human right atria. J Am Coll Cardiol 1998;32:1832-8.
114B. Dries DL, Victor RG, Rame JE, Cooper RS, Wu X, Zhu X, Leonard D, Ho SI, Wu Q, Post W, Drazner MH. Corin gene minor allele defined by 2 missense mutations is common in blacks and associated with high blood pressure and hypertension. Circulation 2005;112:2403-10.
114C. Dschietzig T, Richter C, Bartsch C, Laule M, Armbruster FP, Baumann G, Stangl K. The pregnancy hormone relaxin is a player in human heart failure. FASEB J 2001;15:2187-95.
115. Durgan DJ, Hotze MA, Tomlin TM, Egbejimi O, Graveleau C, Abel ED, et al. The intrinsic circadian clock within the cardiomyocyte. Am J Physiol Heart Circ Physiol 2005;289:H1530-41.
116. Eggers KM, Jaffe AS, Lind L, Venge P, Lindahl B. Value of cardiac troponin I cutoff concentrations below the 99th percentile for clinical decision-making. Clin Chem 2009;55:85-92.

117. Eggers KM, Lagerqvist B, Venge P, Wallentin L, Lindahl B. Prognostic value of biomarkers during and after non-ST-segment elevation acute coronary syndrome. J Am Coll Cardiol 2009;54:357-64.
118. Eggers KM, Oldgren J, Nordenskjold A, Lindahl B. Diagnostic value of serial measurement of cardiac markers in patients with chest pain: limited value of adding myoglobin to troponin I for exclusion of myocardial infarction. Am Heart J 2004;148:574-81.
119. Eitel I, Behrendt F, Schindler K, Kivelitz D, Gutberlet M, Schuler G, et al. Differential diagnosis of suspected apical ballooning syndrome using contrast-enhanced magnetic resonance imaging. Eur Heart J 2008;29:2651-9.
120. Ewald B, Ewald D, Thakkinstian A, Attia J. Meta-analysis of B type natriuretic peptide and N-terminal pro B natriuretic peptide in the diagnosis of clinical heart failure and population screening for left ventricular systolic dysfunction. Intern Med J 2008;38:101-13.
121. Feldman AM, Kadokami T, Higuichi Y, Ramani R, McTiernan CF. The role of anticytokine therapy in heart failure: recent lessons from preclinical and clinical trials? Med Clin North Am 2003;87:419-40.
122. Fishbein MC, Wang T, Matijasevic M, Hong L, Apple FS. Myocardial tissue troponins T and I: an immunohistochemical study in experimental models of myocardial ischemia. Cardiovasc Pathol 2003;12:65-71.
123. Fitzmaurice TF, Brown C, Rifai N, Wu AH, Yeo KT. False increase of cardiac troponin I with heterophilic antibodies. Clin Chem 1998;44: 2212-4.
124. Flynn TG, de Bold ML, de Bold AJ. The amino acid sequence of an atrial peptide with potent diuretic and natriuretic properties. Biochem Biophys Res Commun 1983;117:859-65.
124A. Flynn TG, Brar A, Tremblay L, Sarda I, Lyons C, Jennings DB. Isolation and characterization of iso-rANP, a new natriuretic peptide from rat atria. Biochem Biophys Res Commun 1989;161:830-7.
125. Franz WM, Remppis A, Kandolf R, Kubler W, Katus HA. Serum troponin T: diagnostic marker for acute myocarditis. Clin Chem 1996;42:340-1.
126. Fraser CG. Reference change values: the way forward in monitoring. Ann Clin Biochem 2009;46:264-5.
127. Fruhwald FM, Fahrleitner-Pammer A, Berger R, Leyva F, Freemantle N, Erdmann E, et al. Early and sustained effects of cardiac resynchronization therapy on N-terminal pro-B-type natriuretic peptide in patients with moderate to severe heart failure and cardiac dyssynchrony. Eur Heart J 2007;28:1592-7.
128. Galvani M, Panteghini M, Ottani F, Cappelletti P, Chiarella F, Chiariello M, et al. The new definition of myocardial infarction: analysis of the ESC/ACC Consensus Document and reflections on its applicability to the Italian Health System. Ital Heart J 2002;3: 543-57.
129. Gardner DG, Chen S, Glenn DJ, Grigsby CL. Molecular biology of the natriuretic peptide system: implications for physiology and hypertension. Hypertension 2007;49:419-26.
130. Gaze DC, Collinson PO. Multiple molecular forms of circulating cardiac troponin: analytical and clinical significance. Ann Clin Biochem 2008;45:349-55.
131. Gerhardt W, Nordin G, Herbert AK, Burzell BL, Isaksson A, Gustavsson E, et al. Troponin T and I assays show decreased concentrations in heparin plasma compared with serum: lower recoveries in early than in late phases of myocardial injury. Clin Chem 2000;46:817-21.
132. Giannitsis E, Muller-Bardorff M, Kurowski V, Weidtmann B, Wiegand U, Kampmann M, et al. Independent prognostic value of cardiac troponin T in patients with confirmed pulmonary embolism. Circulation 2000;102:211-7.
133. Gibler WB, Cannon CP, Blomkalns AL, Char DM, Drew BJ, Hollander JE, et al. Practical implementation of the Guidelines for Unstable Angina/Non-ST-Segment Elevation Myocardial Infarction in the emergency department. Ann Emerg Med 2005;46:185-97.
134. Gibler WB, Runyon JP, Levy RC, Sayre MR, Kacich R, Hattemer CR, et al. A rapid diagnostic and treatment center for patients with chest pain in the emergency department. Ann Emerg Med 1995;25:1-8.
135. Giuliani I, Rieunier F, Larue C, Delagneau JF, Granier C, Pau B, et al. Assay for measurement of intact B-type natriuretic peptide prohormone in blood. Clin Chem 2006;52:1054-61.
135A. Glaser R, Peacock WF, Wu AHB, Muller R, Möckel M, Apple FS. Placental growth factor and B type natriuretic peptide: independent predictors of risk from a multi-biomarker panel in suspected acute coronary syndrome ARROW (Acute Risk and Related Outcomes assessed With cardiac biomarkers) Study. Am J Cardiol 2011:107: 821-6
136. Glagov S, Weisenberg E, Zarins CK, Stankunavicius R, Kolettis GJ. Compensatory enlargement of human atherosclerotic coronary arteries. N Engl J Med 1987;316:1371-5.
136A. Goetze JP, Kastrup J, Pedersen F, Rehfeld JF. Quantification of pro-B-type natriuretic peptide and its products in human plasma by use of an analysis independent of precursor processing. Clin Chem 2002;48:1035-42.
137. Goetze JP. Biochemistry of pro-B-type natriuretic peptide-derived peptides: the endocrine heart revisited. Clin Chem 2004;50:1503-10.
138. Goetze JP, Kastrup J, Rehfeld JF. The paradox of increased natriuretic hormones in congestive heart failure patients: does the endocrine heart also fail in heart failure? Eur Heart J 2003;24:1471-2.
139. Goetze JP, Rehfeld JF, Videbaek R, Friis-Hansen L, Kastrup J. B-type natriuretic peptide and its precursor in cardiac venous blood from failing hearts. Eur J Heart Fail 2005;7:69-74.
140. Goetze JP, Yongzhong W, Rehfeld JF, Jorgensen E, Kastrup J. Coronary angiography transiently increases plasma pro-B-type natriuretic peptide. Eur Heart J 2004;25:759-64.
140A. Goetze JP, Friis-Hansen L, Rehfeld JF, Nilsson B, Svendsen JH. Atrial secretion of B-type natriuretic peptide. Eur Heart J 2006;27: 1648-50.
141. Goodman SG, Steg PG, Eagle KA, Fox KA, Lopez-Sendon J, Montalescot G, et al. The diagnostic and prognostic impact of the redefinition of acute myocardial infarction: lessons from the Global Registry of Acute Coronary Events (GRACE). Am Heart J 2006;151:654-60.
142. Griendling KK, FitzGerald GA. Oxidative stress and cardiovascular injury. Part I. Basic mechanisms and in vivo monitoring of ROS. Circulation 2003;108:1912-6.
143. Griendling KK, FitzGerald GA. Oxidative stress and cardiovascular injury. Part II. Animal and human studies. Circulation 2003;108:2034-40.
144. Guest TM, Ramanathan AV, Tuteur PG, Schechtman KB, Ladenson JH, Jaffe AS. Myocardial injury in critically ill patients: a frequently unrecognized complication. JAMA 1995;273:1945-9.
145. Gurney D, Lip GY, Blann AD. A reliable plasma marker of platelet activation: does it exist? Am J Hematol 2002;70:139-44.
146. Gustafsson F, Steensgaard-Hansen F, Badskjaer J, Poulsen AH, Corell P, Hildebrandt P. Diagnostic and prognostic performance of N-terminal ProBNP in primary care patients with suspected heart failure. J Card Fail 2005;11:S15-20.
147. Hamm CW, Goldmann BU, Heeschen C, Kreymann G, Berger J, Meinertz T. Emergency room triage of patients with acute chest pain by means of rapid testing for cardiac troponin T or troponin I. N Engl J Med 1997;337:1648-53.
148. Hamm CW, Heeschen C, Goldmann B, Vahanian A, Adgey J, Miguel CM, et al. Benefit of abciximab in patients with refractory unstable angina in relation to serum troponin T levels. c7E3 Fab Antiplatelet Therapy in Unstable Refractory Angina (CAPTURE) Study Investigators. N Engl J Med 1999;340:1623-9.
149. Hamwi SM, Sharma AK, Weissman NJ, Goldstein SA, Apple S, Canos DA, et al. Troponin-I elevation in patients with increased left ventricular mass. Am J Cardiol 2003;92:88-90.
149A. Hanford DS, Thuerauf DJ, Murray SF, Glembotski CC. Brain natriuretic peptide is induced by alpha 1 adrenergic agonists as a primary response gene in cultured rat cardiac myocytes. J Biol Chem 1994;269:26227-33.
149B. Hanford DS, Glembotski CC. Stabilization of the B-type natriuretic peptide mRNA in cardiac myocytes by alpha-adrenergic receptor

activation: potential roles for protein kinase C and mitogen-activated protein kinase. Mol Endocrinol 1996;10:1719-27.
150. Hanusch-Enserer U, Hermann KM, Cauza E, Spak M, Mahr B, Dunky A, et al. Effect of gastric banding on aminoterminal pro-brain natriuretic peptide in the morbidly obese. Obes Res 2003;11:695-8.
151. Hara Y, Hamada M, Shigematsu Y, Suzuki M, Kodama K, Kuwahara T, et al. Effect of beta-blocker on left ventricular function and natriuretic peptides in patients with chronic heart failure treated with angiotensin-converting enzyme inhibitor. Jpn Circ J 2000;64:365-9.
152. Hasegawa K, Fujiwara H, Doyama K, Mukoyama M, Nakao K, Fujiwara T, et al. Ventricular expression of atrial and brain natriuretic peptides in dilated cardiomyopathy: an immunohistocytochemical study of the endomyocardial biopsy specimens using specific monoclonal antibodies. Am J Pathol 1993;142:107-16.
153. Hawkridge AM, Heublein DM, Bergen HR 3rd, Cataliotti A, Burnett JC Jr, Muddiman DC. Quantitative mass spectral evidence for the absence of circulating brain natriuretic peptide (BNP-32) in severe human heart failure. Proc Natl Acad Sci U S A 2005;102:17442-7.
154. Hawkridge AM, Muddiman DC, Hebulein DM, Cataliotti A, Burnett JC Jr. Effect of plasma protein depletion on BNP-32 recovery. Clin Chem 2008;54:933-4.
155. Heeschen C, Dimmeler S, Fichtlscherer S, Hamm CW, Berger J, Simoons ML, et al. Prognostic value of placental growth factor in patients with acute chest pain. JAMA 2004;291:435-41.
156. Heidrich FM, Zhang K, Estrada M, Huang Y, Giordano FJ, Ehrlich BE. Chromogranin B regulates calcium signaling, nuclear factor kappaB activity, and brain natriuretic peptide production in cardiomyocytes. Circ Res 2008;102:1230-8.
157. Hendy GN, Li T, Girard M, Feldstein RC, Mulay S, Desjardins R, et al. Targeted ablation of the chromogranin a (Chga) gene: normal neuroendocrine dense-core secretory granules and increased expression of other granins. Mol Endocrinol 2006;20:1935-47.
158. Henriksen JH, Gotze JP, Fuglsang S, Christensen E, Bendtsen F, Moller S. Increased circulating pro-brain natriuretic peptide (proBNP) and brain natriuretic peptide (BNP) in patients with cirrhosis: relation to cardiovascular dysfunction and severity of disease. Gut 2003;52: 1511-7.
159. Henry CR, Satran D, Lindgren B, Adkinson C, Nicholson CI, Henry TD. Myocardial injury and long-term mortality following moderate to severe carbon monoxide poisoning. JAMA 2006;295:398-402.
160. Hermann-Arnhof KM, Hanusch-Enserer U, Kaestenbauer T, Publig T, Dunky A, Rosen HR, et al. N-terminal pro-B-type natriuretic peptide as an indicator of possible cardiovascular disease in severely obese individuals: comparison with patients in different stages of heart failure. Clin Chem 2005;51:138-43.
161. Hermsen D, Apple F, Garcia-Beltran L, Jaffe A, Karon B, Lewandrowski E, et al. Results from a multicenter evaluation of the 4th generation Elecsys Troponin T assay. Clin Lab 2007;53:1-9.
161A. Hickman PE, Badrick T, Wilson SR, McGill D. Reporting of cardiac troponin—problems with the 99th population percentile. Clin Chim Acta 2007;381:182-3.
162. Hickson LJ, Cosio FG, El-Zoghby ZM, Gloor JM, Kremers WK, Stegall MD, et al. Survival of patients on the kidney transplant wait list: relationship to cardiac troponin T. Am J Transplant 2008;8:2352-9.
163. Hill SA, Balion CM, Santaguida P, McQueen MJ, Ismaila AS, Reichert SM, et al. Evidence for the use of B-type natriuretic peptides for screening asymptomatic populations and for diagnosis in primary care. Clin Biochem 2008;41:240-9.
163A. Hino J, Tateyama H, Minamino N, Kangawa K, Matsuo H. Isolation and identification of human brain natriuretic peptides in cardiac atrium. Biochem Biophys Res Commun 1990;167:693-700.
164. Hodgson-Zingman DM, Karst ML, Zingman LV, Heublein DM, Darbar D, Herron KJ, et al. Atrial natriuretic peptide frameshift mutation in familial atrial fibrillation. N Engl J Med 2008;359:158-65.
165. Holvoet P, Mertens A, Verhamme P, Bogaerts K, Beyens G, Verhaeghe R, et al. Circulating oxidized LDL is a useful marker for identifying patients with coronary artery disease. Arterioscler Thromb Vasc Biol 2001;21:844-8.
166. Huber K, Christ G, Wojta J, Gulba D. Plasminogen activator inhibitor type-1 in cardiovascular disease: status report 2001. Thromb Res 2001;103(suppl 1):S7-19.
167. Hunt PJ, Espiner EA, Nicholls MG, Richards AM, Yandle TG. The role of the circulation in processing pro-brain natriuretic peptide (proBNP) to amino-terminal BNP and BNP-32. Peptides 1997;18:1475-81.
168. Hunt PJ, Richards AM, Nicholls MG, Yandle TG, Doughty RN, Espiner EA. Immunoreactive amino-terminal pro-brain natriuretic peptide (NT-PROBNP): a new marker of cardiac impairment. Clin Endocrinol (Oxf) 1997;47:287-96.
169. Hunt PJ, Yandle TG, Nicholls MG, Richards AM, Espiner EA. The amino-terminal portion of pro-brain natriuretic peptide (Pro-BNP) circulates in human plasma. Biochem Biophys Res Commun 1995;214:1175-83.
170. Hunt SA, Abraham WT, Chin MH, Feldman AM, Francis GS, Ganiats TG, et al. ACC/AHA 2005 guideline update for the diagnosis and management of chronic heart failure in the adult: a report of the American College of Cardiology/American Heart Association Task Force on Practice Guidelines (Writing Committee to Update the 2001 Guidelines for the Evaluation and Management of Heart Failure): developed in collaboration with the American College of Chest Physicians and the International Society for Heart and Lung Transplantation: endorsed by the Heart Rhythm Society. Circulation 2005;112:e154-235.
171. Hunt SA, Baker DW, Chin MH, Cinquegrani MP, Feldman AM, Francis GS, et al. ACC/AHA guidelines for the evaluation and management of chronic heart failure in the adult: executive summary. A report of the American College of Cardiology/American Heart Association Task Force on Practice Guidelines (Committee to Revise the 1995 Guidelines for the Evaluation and Management of Heart Failure): developed in collaboration with the International Society for Heart and Lung Transplantation: endorsed by the Heart Failure Society of America. Circulation 2001;104:2996-3007.
172. Hutter AM Jr, Amsterdam EA, Jaffe AS. 31st Bethesda Conference. Emergency cardiac care. Task force 2: acute coronary syndromes. Section 2B: chest discomfort evaluation in the hospital. J Am Coll Cardiol 2000;35:853-62.
173. Ingwall JS, Kramer MF, Fifer MA, Lorell BH, Shemin R, Grossman W, et al. The creatine kinase system in normal and diseased human myocardium. N Engl J Med 1985;313:1050-4.
174. Inoue K, Naruse K, Yamagami S, Mitani H, Suzuki N, Takei Y. Four functionally distinct C-type natriuretic peptides found in fish reveal evolutionary history of the natriuretic peptide system. Proc Natl Acad Sci U S A 2003;100:10079-84.
175. Jaffe AS. Chasing troponin: how low can you go if you can see the rise? J Am Coll Cardiol 2006;48:1763-4.
176. Jaffe AS. Elevations in cardiac troponin measurements: false false-positives: the real truth. Cardiovasc Toxicol 2001;1:87-92.
177. Jaffe AS, Apple FS. High-sensitivity cardiac troponin: hype, help, and reality. Clin Chem 2010;56:342-4.
178. Jaffe AS, Babuin L, Apple FS. Biomarkers in acute cardiac disease: the present and the future. J Am Coll Cardiol 2006;48:1-11.
179. Jaffe AS, Davidenko J, Clements I. Diagnosis of acute coronary syndromes including myocardial infarction. In: Crawford MH, DiMarco JP, Paulus WJ, eds. Cardiology, 2nd edition. St Louis: Mosby, 2004:311-28.
180. Jaffe AS, Landt Y, Parvin CA, Abendschein DR, Geltman EM, Ladenson JH. Comparative sensitivity of cardiac troponin I and lactate dehydrogenase isoenzymes for diagnosing acute myocardial infarction. Clin Chem 1996;42:1770-6.
181. Jaffe AS, Ravkilde J, Roberts R, Naslund U, Apple FS, Galvani M, Katus H. It's time for a change to a troponin standard. Circulation 2000;102:1216-20.
182. Jaffe AS, Ritter C, Meltzer V, Harter H, Roberts R. Unmasking artifactual increases in creatine kinase isoenzymes in patients with renal failure. J Lab Clin Med 1984;104:193-202.
183. James P, Ellis CJ, Whitlock RM, McNeil AR, Henley J, Anderson NE. Relation between troponin T concentration and mortality in patients

presenting with an acute stroke: observational study. BMJ 2000;320: 1502-4.

184. James S, Armstrong P, Califf R, Simoons ML, Venge P, Wallentin L, Lindahl B. Troponin T levels and risk of 30-day outcomes in patients with the acute coronary syndrome: prospective verification in the GUSTO-IV trial. Am J Med 2003;115:178-84.
185. James SK, Lindahl B, Siegbahn A, Stridsberg M, Venge P, Armstrong P, et al. N-terminal pro-brain natriuretic peptide and other risk markers for the separate prediction of mortality and subsequent myocardial infarction in patients with unstable coronary artery disease: a Global Utilization of Strategies To Open occluded arteries (GUSTO)-IV substudy. Circulation 2003;108:275-81.
186. Jamieson JD, Palade GE. Specific granules in atrial muscle cells. J Cell Biol 1964;23:151-72.
187. Januzzi JL Jr, Camargo CA, Anwaruddin S, Baggish AL, Chen AA, Krauser DG, et al. The N-terminal Pro-BNP investigation of dyspnea in the emergency department (PRIDE) study. Am J Cardiol 2005;95: 948-54.
188. Januzzi JL, van Kimmenade R, Lainchbury J, Bayes-Genis A, Ordonez-Llanos J, Santalo-Bel M, et al. NT-proBNP testing for diagnosis and short-term prognosis in acute destabilized heart failure: an international pooled analysis of 1256 patients: the International Collaborative of NT-proBNP Study. Eur Heart J 2006;27:330-7.
189. Jeremias A, Kleiman NS, Nassif D, Hsieh WH, Pencina M, Maresh K, et al. Prevalence and prognostic significance of preprocedural cardiac troponin elevation among patients with stable coronary artery disease undergoing percutaneous coronary intervention: results from the evaluation of drug eluting stents and ischemic events registry. Circulation 2008;118:632-8.
190. Jernberg T, Lindahl B, Siegbahn A, Andren B, Frostfeldt G, Lagerqvist B, et al. N-terminal pro-brain natriuretic peptide in relation to inflammation, myocardial necrosis, and the effect of an invasive strategy in unstable coronary artery disease. J Am Coll Cardiol 2003;42:1909-16.

190A. Jin H, Fedorowicz G, Yang R, Ogasawara A, Peale F, Pham T, Paoni NF. Thyrotropin-releasing hormone is induced in the left ventricle of rats with heart failure and can provide inotropic support to the failing heart. Circulation 2004;109:2240-5.

191. Johnston N, Jernberg T, Lindahl B, Lindback J, Stridsberg M, Larsson A, et al. Biochemical indicators of cardiac and renal function in a healthy elderly population. Clin Biochem 2004;37:210-6.
192. Jones CB, Sane DC, Herrington DM. Matrix metalloproteinases: a review of their structure and role in acute coronary syndrome. Cardiovasc Res 2003;59:812-23.

192A. Kambayashi Y, Nakao K, Mukoyama M, Saito Y, Ogawa Y, Shiono S, Inouye K, Yoshida N, Imura H. Isolation and sequence determination of human brain natriuretic peptide in human atrium. FEBS Lett 1990; 259:341-5.

193. Katrukha AG, Bereznikova AV, Esakova TV, Pettersson K, Lovgren T, Severina ME, et al. Troponin I is released in bloodstream of patients with acute myocardial infarction not in free form but as complex. Clin Chem 1997;43:1379-85.
194. Katrukha AG, Bereznikova AV, Filatov VL, Esakova TV, Kolosova OV, Pettersson K, et al. Degradation of cardiac troponin I: implication for reliable immunodetection. Clin Chem 1998;44:2433-40.
195. Katus HA, Looser S, Hallermayer K, Remppis A, Scheffold T, Borgya A, et al. Development and in vitro characterization of a new immunoassay of cardiac troponin T. Clin Chem 1992;38:386-93.
196. Katus HA, Remppis A, Scheffold T, Diederich KW, Kuebler W. Intracellular compartmentation of cardiac troponin T and its release kinetics in patients with reperfused and nonreperfused myocardial infarction. Am J Cardiol 1991;67:1360-7.
197. Kavsak PA, MacRae AR, Newman AM, Lustig V, Palomaki GE, Ko DT, et al. Effects of contemporary troponin assay sensitivity on the utility of the early markers myoglobin and CKMB isoforms in evaluating patients with possible acute myocardial infarction. Clin Chim Acta 2007;380:213-6.
198. Kavsak PA, MacRae AR, Yerna MJ, Jaffe AS. Analytic and clinical utility of a next-generation, highly sensitive cardiac troponin I assay for early detection of myocardial injury. Clin Chem 2009;55:573-7.
199. Kavsak PA, Wang X, Ko DT, MacRae AR, Jaffe AS. Short- and long-term risk stratification using a next-generation, high-sensitivity research cardiac troponin I (hs-cTnI) assay in an emergency department chest pain population. Clin Chem 2009;55:1809-15.
200. Kawai K, Hata K, Takaoka H, Kawai H, Yokoyama M. Plasma brain natriuretic peptide as a novel therapeutic indicator in idiopathic dilated cardiomyopathy during beta-blocker therapy: a potential of hormone-guided treatment. Am Heart J 2001;141:925-32.
201. Keller T, Zeller T, Peetz D, Tzikas S, Roth A, Czyz E, et al. Sensitive troponin I assay in early diagnosis of acute myocardial infarction. N Engl J Med 2009;361:868-77.
202. Kempf T, von Haehling S, Peter T, Allhoff T, Cicoira M, Doehner W, et al. Prognostic utility of growth differentiation factor-15 in patients with chronic heart failure. J Am Coll Cardiol 2007;50:1054-60.
203. Kenchaiah S, Evans JC, Levy D, Wilson PW, Benjamin EJ, Larson MG, et al. Obesity and the risk of heart failure. N Engl J Med 2002;347:305-13.
204. Kim LJ, Martinez EA, Faraday N, Dorman T, Fleisher LA, Perler BA, et al. Cardiac troponin I predicts short-term mortality in vascular surgery patients. Circulation 2002;106:2366-71.
205. Kinugawa T, Kato M, Ogino K, Osaki S, Igawa O, Hisatome I, Shigemasa C. Plasma endothelin-1 levels and clinical correlates in patients with chronic heart failure. J Card Fail 2003;9:318-24.
206. Kisch B. A significant electron microscopic difference between the atria and the ventricles of the mammalian heart. Exp Med Surg 1963;21:193-221.

206A. Knappe S, Wu F, Masikat MR, Morser J, Wu Q. Functional analysis of the transmembrane domain and activation cleavage of human corin: design and characterization of a soluble corin. J Biol Chem 2003;278:52363-70.

207. Knudsen CW, Omland T, Clopton P, Westheim A, Wu AH, Duc P, et al. Impact of atrial fibrillation on the diagnostic performance of B-type natriuretic peptide concentration in dyspneic patients: an analysis from the breathing not properly multinational study. J Am Coll Cardiol 2005;46:838-44.
208. Konstantinides S, Geibel A, Olschewski M, Kasper W, Hruska N, Jackle S, Binder L. Importance of cardiac troponins I and T in risk stratification of patients with acute pulmonary embolism. Circulation 2002;106:1263-8.
209. Kontos MC, Fritz LM, Anderson FP, Tatum JL, Ornato JP, Jesse RL. Impact of the troponin standard on the prevalence of acute myocardial infarction. Am Heart J 2003;146:446-52.

209A. Kreil G. Processing of precursors by dipeptidylaminopeptidases: a case of molecular ticketing. Trends Biochem Sci 1990;15:23-6.

209B. Kreil G, Haiml L, Suchanek G. Stepwise cleavage of the pro part of promelittin by dipeptidylpeptidase IV. Evidence for a new type of precursor–product conversion. Eur J Biochem 1980;111:49-58.

210. Kricka LJ. Human anti-animal antibody interferences in immunological assays. Clin Chem 1999;45:942-56.
211. Kroll MH, Twomey PJ, Srisawasdi P. Using the single-compartment ratio model to calculate half-life, NT-proBNP as an example. Clin Chim Acta 2007;380:197-202.
212. Kruger S, Graf J, Merx MW, Koch KC, Kunz D, Hanrath P, et al. Brain natriuretic peptide predicts right heart failure in patients with acute pulmonary embolism. Am Heart J 2004;147:60-5.
213. Kucher N, Printzen G, Doernhoefer T, Windecker S, Meier B, Hess OM. Low pro-brain natriuretic peptide levels predict benign clinical outcome in acute pulmonary embolism. Circulation 2003;107:1576-8.
214. Kucher N, Printzen G, Goldhaber SZ. Prognostic role of brain natriuretic peptide in acute pulmonary embolism. Circulation 2003;107:2545-7.

214A. Kudoh S, Akazawa H, Takano H, Zou Y, Toko H, Nagai T, Komuro I. Stretch-modulation of second messengers: effects on cardiomyocyte ion transport. Prog Biophys Mol Biol 2003;82:57-66.

215. Kurz K, Giannitsis E, Zehelein J, Katus HA. Highly sensitive cardiac troponin T values remain constant after brief exercise- or pharmacologic-induced reversible myocardial ischemia. Clin Chem 2008;54:1234-8.
216. La Vecchia L, Ottani F, Favero L, Spadaro GL, Rubboli A, Boanno C, et al. Increased cardiac troponin I on admission predicts in-hospital mortality in acute pulmonary embolism. Heart 2004;90:633-7.
217. Labugger R, Organ L, Collier C, Atar D, Van Eyk JE. Extensive troponin I and T modification detected in serum from patients with acute myocardial infarction. Circulation 2000;102:1221-6.
217A. Lam CS, Burnett JC Jr, Costello-Boerrigter L, Rodeheffer RJ, Redfield MM. Alternate circulating pro-B-type natriuretic peptide and B-type natriuretic peptide forms in the general population. J Am Coll Cardiol 2007;49:1193-1202.
218. Landesberg G, Beattie WS, Mosseri M, Jaffe AS, Alpert JS. Perioperative myocardial infarction. Circulation 2009;119:2936-44.
219. Lanfear DE. Genetic variation in the natriuretic peptide system and heart failure. Heart Fail Rev 2010;15:219-28.
220. Lang H. Creatine kinase isoenzymes. New York: Springer-Verlag, 1981.
221. LaPointe MC. Molecular regulation of the brain natriuretic peptide gene. Peptides 2005;26:944-56.
222. Latini R, Masson S, Anand I, Judd D, Maggioni AP, Chiang YT, et al. Effects of valsartan on circulating brain natriuretic peptide and norepinephrine in symptomatic chronic heart failure: the Valsartan Heart Failure Trial (Val-HeFT). Circulation 2002;106:2454-8.
223. Latini R, Masson S, Anand I, Salio M, Hester A, Judd D, et al. The comparative prognostic value of plasma neurohormones at baseline in patients with heart failure enrolled in Val-HeFT. Eur Heart J 2004;25: 292-9.
224. Lee-Lewandrowski E, Januzzi JL, Green SM, Tannous B, Wu AH, Smith A, et al. Multi-center validation of the Response Biomedical Corporation RAMP NT-proBNP assay with comparison to the Roche Diagnostics GmbH Elecsys proBNP assay. Clin Chim Acta 2007;386: 20-4.
225. Lellouche N, De Diego C, Cesario DA, Vaseghi M, Horowitz BN, Mahajan A, et al. Usefulness of preimplantation B-type natriuretic peptide level for predicting response to cardiac resynchronization therapy. Am J Cardiol 2007;99:242-6.
226. Levin ER, Gardner DG, Samson WK. Natriuretic peptides. N Engl J Med 1998;339:321-8.
227. Li G, Lau JT, McCarthy ML, Schull MJ, Vermeulen M, Kelen GD. Emergency department utilization in the United States and Ontario, Canada. Acad Emerg Med 2007;14:582-4.
228. Liang F, O'Rear J, Schellenberger U, Tai L, Lasecki M, Schreiner GF, et al. Evidence for functional heterogeneity of circulating B-type natriuretic peptide. J Am Coll Cardiol 2007;49:1071-8.
228A. Liang F, Gardner DG. Mechanical strain activates BNP gene transcription through a p38/NF-kappa B-dependent mechanism. J Clin Invest 1999;104:1603-12.
229. Libby P. Vascular biology of atherosclerosis: overview and state of the art. Am J Cardiol 2003;91:3A-6A.
230. Lin JC, Apple FS, Murakami MM, Luepker RV. Rates of positive cardiac troponin I and creatine kinase MB mass among patients hospitalized for suspected acute coronary syndromes. Clin Chem 2004;50:333-8.
231. Lin L, Sylven C, Sotonyi P, Somogyi E, Kaijser L, Jansson E. Lactate dehydrogenase and its isoenzyme activities in different parts of the normal human heart. Cardiovasc Res 1989;23:601-6.
232. Lind L. Circulating markers of inflammation and atherosclerosis. Atherosclerosis 2003;169:203-14.
233. Lindahl B, Andren B, Ohlsson J, Venge P, Wallentin L. Noninvasive risk stratification in unstable coronary artery disease: exercise test and biochemical markers. FRISC Study Group. Am J Cardiol 1997;80: 40E-4E.
234. Lindahl B, Diderholm E, Lagerqvist B, Venge P, Wallentin L. Mechanisms behind the prognostic value of troponin T in unstable coronary artery disease: a FRISC II substudy. J Am Coll Cardiol 2001;38:979-86.
235. Lisy O, Huntley BK, McCormick DJ, Kurlansky PA, Burnett JC Jr. Design, synthesis, and actions of a novel chimeric natriuretic peptide: CD-NP. J Am Coll Cardiol 2008;52:60-8.
236. Little WC. Assessment of cardiac function. In: Braunwald E, ed. Heart disease: a textbook of cardiovascular medicine, 6th edition. Philadelphia, Pa: WB Saunders, 2001:98.
236A. Liu ZL, Wiedmeyer CE, Sisson DD, Solter PF. Cloning and characterization of feline brain natriuretic peptide. Gene 2002;292: 183-90.
237. Liuzzo G, Biasucci LM, Rebuzzi AG, Gallimore JR, Caligiuri G, Lanza GA, et al. Plasma protein acute-phase response in unstable angina is not induced by ischemic injury. Circulation 1996;94:2373-80.
238. Luchner A, Burnett JC Jr, Jougasaki M, Hense HW, Heid IM, Muders F, et al. Evaluation of brain natriuretic peptide as marker of left ventricular dysfunction and hypertrophy in the population. J Hypertens 2000;18:1121-8.
238A. Luchner A, Stevens TL, Borgeson DD, Redfield M, Wei CM, Porter JG, Burnett JC, Jr. Differential atrial and ventricular expression of myocardial BNP during evolution of heart failure. Am J Physiol 1998;274:H1684-9.
239. Luckenbill KN, Christenson RH, Jaffe AS, Mair J, Ordonez-Llanos J, Pagani F, et al. Cross-reactivity of BNP, NT-proBNP, and proBNP in commercial BNP and NT-proBNP assays: preliminary observations from the IFCC Committee for Standardization of Markers of Cardiac Damage. Clin Chem 2008;54:619-21.
240. Luepker RV, Apple FS, Christenson RH, Crow RS, Fortmann SP, Goff D, et al. Case definitions for acute coronary heart disease in epidemiology and clinical research studies: a statement from the AHA Council on Epidemiology and Prevention; AHA Statistics Committee; World Heart Federation Council on Epidemiology and Prevention; the European Society of Cardiology Working Group on Epidemiology and Prevention; Centers for Disease Control and Prevention; and the National Heart, Lung, and Blood Institute. Circulation 2003;108: 2543-9.
241. Lund J, Qin QP, Ilva T, Pettersson K, Voipio-Pulkki LM, Porela P, et al. Circulating pregnancy-associated plasma protein A predicts outcome in patients with acute coronary syndrome but no troponin I elevation. Circulation 2003;108:1924-6.
241A. Ma KK, Ogawa T, de Bold AJ. Selective upregulation of cardiac brain natriuretic peptide at the transcriptional and translational levels by pro-inflammatory cytokines and by conditioned medium derived from mixed lymphocyte reactions via p38 MAP kinase. J Mol Cell Cardiol 2004;36:505-13.
242. Macrae AR, Kavsak PA, Lustig V, Bhargava R, Vandersluis R, Palomaki GE, et al. Assessing the requirement for the 6-hour interval between specimens in the American Heart Association Classification of Myocardial Infarction in Epidemiology and Clinical Research Studies. Clin Chem 2006;52:812-8.
243. Mair J. Biochemistry of B-type natriuretic peptide—where are we now? Clin Chem Lab Med 2008;46:1507-14.
244. Mair J, Dienstl F, Puschendorf B. Cardiac troponin T in the diagnosis of myocardial injury. Crit Rev Clin Lab Sci 1992;29:31-57.
245. Maisel AS, Krishnaswamy P, Nowak RM, McCord J, Hollander JE, Duc P, et al. Rapid measurement of B-type natriuretic peptide in the emergency diagnosis of heart failure. N Engl J Med 2002;347: 161-7.
246. Maroko PR, Kjekshus JK, Sobel BE, Watanabe T, Covell JW, Ross J Jr, et al. Factors influencing infarct size following experimental coronary artery occlusions. Circulation 1971;43:67-82.
247. Martinez MW, Babuin L, Syed IS, Feng DL, Miller WL, Mathew V, et al. Myocardial infarction with normal coronary arteries: a role for MRI? Clin Chem 2007;53:995-6.
248. Marx R, Mains RE. Adenovirally encoded prohormone convertase-1 functions in atrial myocyte large dense core vesicles. Endocrinology 1997;138:5108-18.

249. McCord J, Nowak RM, McCullough PA, Foreback C, Borzak S, Tokarski G, et al. Ninety-minute exclusion of acute myocardial infarction by use of quantitative point-of-care testing of myoglobin and troponin I. Circulation 2001;104:1483-8.
250. McCullough PA, Hollander JE, Nowak RM, Storrow AB, Duc P, Omland T, et al. Uncovering heart failure in patients with a history of pulmonary disease: rationale for the early use of B-type natriuretic peptide in the emergency department. Acad Emerg Med 2003;10: 198-204.
251. McCullough PA, Nowak RM, McCord J, Hollander JE, Herrmann HC, Steg PG, et al. B-type natriuretic peptide and clinical judgment in emergency diagnosis of heart failure: analysis from Breathing Not Properly (BNP) Multinational Study. Circulation 2002;106:416-22.
252. McCullough PA, Sandberg KR. B-type natriuretic peptide and renal disease. Heart Fail Rev 2003;8:355-8.
253. McGrath MF, de Bold AJ. Determinants of natriuretic peptide gene expression. Peptides 2005;26:933-43.
254. McGrath MF, de Bold ML, de Bold AJ. The endocrine function of the heart. Trends Endocrinol Metab 2005;16:469-77.
255. McLaurin MD, Apple FS, Voss EM, Herzog CA, Sharkey SW. Cardiac troponin I, cardiac troponin T, and creatine kinase MB in dialysis patients without ischemic heart disease: evidence of cardiac troponin T expression in skeletal muscle. Clin Chem 1997;43:976-82.
256. Meirhaeghe A, Sandhu MS, McCarthy MI, de Groote P, Cottel D, Arveiler D, et al. Association between the T-381C polymorphism of the brain natriuretic peptide gene and risk of type 2 diabetes in human populations. Hum Mol Genet 2007;16:1343-50.
256A. Meune C, Zuily S, Wahbi K, Claessens YE, Wever S, Chenevier-Gobeaux C. Combination of copeptin and high-sensitivity cardiac troponin T assay in unstable angina and non-ST-segment elevation myocardial infarction: a pilot study. Arch Cardiovasc Dis 2011;104: 4-10.
257. Miller R, Callas DD, Kahn SE, Ricchiuti V, Apple FS. Evidence of myocardial infarction in mummified human tissue. JAMA 2000;284: 831-2.
258. Miller WL, Burnett JC Jr, Hartman KA, Henle MP, Burritt MF, Jaffe AS. Lower rather than higher levels of B-type natriuretic peptides (NT-pro-BNP and BNP) predict short-term mortality in end-stage heart failure patients treated with nesiritide. Am J Cardiol 2005;96: 837-41.
259. Miller WL, Edwards BS, Kremers WK, Kushwaha SS, McGregor CG, Daly RC, et al. Elevated donor troponin levels are associated with a lower frequency of allograft vasculopathy. J Heart Lung Transplant 2005;24:2075-8.
260. Miller WL, Garratt KN, Burritt MF, Lennon RJ, Reeder GS, Jaffe AS. Baseline troponin level: key to understanding the importance of post-PCI troponin elevations. Eur Heart J 2006;27:1061-9.
261. Miller WL, Hartman KA, Burritt MF, Grill DE, Rodeheffer RJ, Burnett JC Jr, et al. Serial biomarker measurements in ambulatory patients with chronic heart failure: the importance of change over time. Circulation 2007;116:249-57.
262. Miller WL, Hartman KA, Grill DE, Burnett JC Jr, Jaffe AS. Only large reductions in concentrations of natriuretic peptides (BNP and NT-proBNP) are associated with improved outcome in ambulatory patients with chronic heart failure. Clin Chem 2009;55:78-84.
262A. Minamino N, Aburaya M, Ueda S, Kangawa K, Matsuo H. The presence of brain natriuretic peptide of 12,000 daltons in porcine heart. Biochem Biophys Res Commun 1988;155:740-6.
263. Mingels A, Jacobs L, Michielsen E, Swaanenburg J, Wodzig W, van Dieijen-Visser M. Reference population and marathon runner sera assessed by highly sensitive cardiac troponin T and commercial cardiac troponin T and I assays. Clin Chem 2009;55:101-8.
264. Mirvis DM, Goldberger AL. Electrocardiography. In: Braunwald E, ed. Heart disease: a textbook of cardiovascular medicine. 6th edition. Philadelphia, Pa: WB Saunders, 2001:744-61.
265. Misono KS, Fukumi H, Grammer RT, Inagami T. Rat atrial natriuretic factor: complete amino acid sequence and disulfide linkage essential for biological activity. Biochem Biophys Res Commun 1984;119:524-9.
266. Moertl D, Berger R, Struck J, Gleiss A, Hammer A, Morgenthaler NG, et al. Comparison of midregional pro-atrial and B-type natriuretic peptides in chronic heart failure: influencing factors, detection of left ventricular systolic dysfunction, and prediction of death. J Am Coll Cardiol 2009;53:1783-90.
267. Mohammed AA, Agnihotri AK, van Kimmenade RR, Martinez-Rumayor A, Green SM, Quiroz R, et al. Prospective, comprehensive assessment of cardiac troponin T testing after coronary artery bypass graft surgery. Circulation 2009;120:843-50.
268. Mohammed SF, Korinek J, Chen HH, Burnett JC, Redfield MM. Nesiritide in acute decompensated heart failure: current status and future perspectives. Rev Cardiovasc Med 2008;9:151-8.
269. Moller JE, Bergeron S, Jaffe A, Pellikka PA. Influence of left ventricular filling pattern on exercise-induced changes of natriuretic peptides in patients with suspected coronary artery disease. Int J Cardiol 2008;124:204-10.
270. Morgenthaler NG, Struck J, Alonso C, Bergmann A. Assay for the measurement of copeptin, a stable peptide derived from the precursor of vasopressin. Clin Chem 2006;52:112-9.
271. Morgenthaler NG, Struck J, Thomas B, Bergmann A. Immunoluminometric assay for the midregion of pro-atrial natriuretic peptide in human plasma. Clin Chem 2004;50:234-6.
272. Morrison LK, Harrison A, Krishnaswamy P, Kazanegra R, Clopton P, Maisel A. Utility of a rapid B-natriuretic peptide assay in differentiating congestive heart failure from lung disease in patients presenting with dyspnea. J Am Coll Cardiol 2002;39:202-9.
273. Morrow DA, Cannon CP, Jesse RL, Newby LK, Ravkilde J, Storrow AB, et al. National Academy of Clinical Biochemistry Laboratory Medicine practice guidelines: clinical characteristics and utilization of biochemical markers in acute coronary syndromes. Clin Chem 2007;53:552-74.
274. Morrow DA, Cannon CP, Rifai N, Frey MJ, Vicari R, Lakkis N, et al. Ability of minor elevations of troponins I and T to predict benefit from an early invasive strategy in patients with unstable angina and non-ST elevation myocardial infarction: results from a randomized trial. JAMA 2001;286:2405-12.
275. Morrow DA, de Lemos JA, Sabatine MS, Murphy SA, Demopoulos LA, DiBattiste PM, et al. Evaluation of B-type natriuretic peptide for risk assessment in unstable angina/non-ST-elevation myocardial infarction: B-type natriuretic peptide and prognosis in TACTICS-TIMI 18. J Am Coll Cardiol 2003;41:1264-72.
276. Mueller C, Scholer A, Laule-Kilian K, Martina B, Schindler C, Buser P, et al. Use of B-type natriuretic peptide in the evaluation and management of acute dyspnea. N Engl J Med 2004;350:647-54.
277. Mukoyama M, Nakao K, Saito Y, Ogawa Y, Hosoda K, Suga S, et al. Human brain natriuretic peptide, a novel cardiac hormone. Lancet 1990;335:801-2.
278. Mukoyama M, Nakao K, Saito Y, Ogawa Y, Hosoda K, Suga S, et al. Increased human brain natriuretic peptide in congestive heart failure. N Engl J Med 1990;323:757-8.
279. Mundy BJ, McCord J, Nowak RM. B-type natriuretic peptide levels are inversely related to body mass index in patients with heart failure. J Am Coll Cardiol 2003;41(suppl):158A.
280. Murakami MM, Apple FS, Hollander JER, Shipp GW. Preliminary performance of a research high sensitive gold nanoparticle-based cardiac troponin I assay: proof of concept study of the Nanosphere Verigene system. Clin Chem 2009;55(suppl):A64-5.
281. Murakami MM, Chung AY, Kogut ME, Apple FS. Cost effective implementation of the Stratus CS point of care cardiac troponin I testing in coronary care units. Clin Chem 2004;50:A21.
282. Murphy JT, Horton JW, Purdue GF, Hunt JL. Evaluation of troponin-I as an indicator of cardiac dysfunction after thermal injury. J Trauma 1998;45:700-4.
283. Naghavi M, Libby P, Falk E, Casscells SW, Litovsky S, Rumberger J, et al. From vulnerable plaque to vulnerable patient: a call for new definitions and risk assessment strategies: part II. Circulation 2003;108:1772-8.
284. Naghavi M, Libby P, Falk E, Casscells SW, Litovsky S, Rumberger J, et al. From vulnerable plaque to vulnerable patient: a call for new

definitions and risk assessment strategies: part I. Circulation 2003; 108:1664-72.
285. Naidech AM, Kreiter KT, Janjua N, Ostapkovich ND, Parra A, Commichau C, et al. Cardiac troponin elevation, cardiovascular morbidity, and outcome after subarachnoid hemorrhage. Circulation 2005;112:2851-6.
286. Newby LK, Alpert JS, Ohman EM, Thygesen K, Califf RM. Changing the diagnosis of acute myocardial infarction: implications for practice and clinical investigations. Am Heart J 2002;144:957-80.
287. Newby LK, Storrow AB, Gibler WB, Garvey JL, Tucker JF, Kaplan AL, et al. Bedside multimarker testing for risk stratification in chest pain units: the chest pain evaluation by creatine kinase-MB, myoglobin, and troponin I (CHECKMATE) study. Circulation 2001;103:1832-7.
288. Ng LL, Loke I, O'Brien RJ, Squire IB, Davies JE. Plasma urotensin in human systolic heart failure. Circulation 2002;106:2877-80.
289. Nicolau N, Butur G, Laky D. Electronmicroscopic observations regarding the presence of natriuretic granules in the ventricle of patients with cardiopathies. Rom J Morphol Embryol 1997;43: 119-37.
290. Nielsen OW, McDonagh TA, Robb SD, Dargie HJ. Retrospective analysis of the cost-effectiveness of using plasma brain natriuretic peptide in screening for left ventricular systolic dysfunction in the general population. J Am Coll Cardiol 2003;41:113-20.
291. Nielsen SJ, Gotze JP, Jensen HL, Rehfeld JF. ProCNP and CNP are expressed primarily in male genital organs. Regul Pept 2008;146: 204-12.
292. Niizuma S, Iwanaga Y, Yahata T, Tamaki Y, Goto Y, Nakahama H, et al. Impact of left ventricular end-diastolic wall stress on plasma B-type natriuretic peptide in heart failure with chronic kidney disease and end-stage renal disease. Clin Chem 2009;55:1347-53.
293. Novis DA, Jones BA, Dale JC, Walsh MK. Biochemical markers of myocardial injury test turnaround time: a College of American Pathologists Q-Probes study of 7020 troponin and 4368 creatine kinase-MB determinations in 159 institutions. Arch Pathol Lab Med 2004;128:158-64.
294. Omland T, Aakvaag A, Bonarjee VV, Caidahl K, Lie RT, Nilsen DW, et al. Plasma brain natriuretic peptide as an indicator of left ventricular systolic function and long-term survival after acute myocardial infarction: comparison with plasma atrial natriuretic peptide and N-terminal proatrial natriuretic peptide. Circulation 1996;93:1963-9.
295. Omland T, Persson A, Ng L, O'Brien R, Karlsson T, Herlitz J, et al. N-terminal pro-B-type natriuretic peptide and long-term mortality in acute coronary syndromes. Circulation 2002;106:2913-8.
296. Omland T, Richards AM, Wergeland R, Vik-Mo H. B-type natriuretic peptide and long-term survival in patients with stable coronary artery disease. Am J Cardiol 2005;95:24-8.
297. Ong P, Athanasiadis A, Hill S, Vogelsberg H, Voehringer M, Sechtem U. Coronary artery spasm as a frequent cause of acute coronary syndrome: the CASPAR (Coronary Artery Spasm in Patients With Acute Coronary Syndrome) study. J Am Coll Cardiol 2008;52:523-7.
298. Ooi DS, Isotalo PA, Veinot JP. Correlation of antemortem serum creatine kinase, creatine kinase-MB, troponin I, and troponin T with cardiac pathology. Clin Chem 2000;46:338-44.
299. Ottani F, Galvani M, Nicolini FA, Ferrini D, Pozzati A, Di Pasquale G, et al. Elevated cardiac troponin levels predict the risk of adverse outcome in patients with acute coronary syndromes. Am Heart J 2000;140:917-27.
300. Panteghini M, Gerhardt W, Apple FS, Dati F, Ravkilde J, Wu AH. Quality specifications for cardiac troponin assays. Clin Chem Lab Med 2001;39:175-9.
301. Panteghini M, Pagani F, Yeo KT, Apple FS, Christenson RH, Dati F, et al. Evaluation of imprecision for cardiac troponin assays at low-range concentrations. Clin Chem 2004;50:327-32.
302. Peacock WF, De Marco T, Fonarow GC, Diercks D, Wynne J, Apple FS, et al. Cardiac troponin and outcome in acute heart failure. N Engl J Med 2008;358:2117-26.
303. Pearson TA, Mensah GA, Alexander RW, Anderson JL, Cannon RO 3rd, Criqui M, et al. Markers of inflammation and cardiovascular disease: application to clinical and public health practice: a statement for healthcare professionals from the Centers for Disease Control and Prevention and the American Heart Association. Circulation 2003;107:499-511.
304. Pemberton CJ, Johnson ML, Yandle TG, Espiner EA. Deconvolution analysis of cardiac natriuretic peptides during acute volume overload. Hypertension 2000;36:355-9.
305. Perryman MB, Knell JD, Roberts R. Carboxypeptidase-catalyzed hydrolysis of C-terminal lysine: mechanism for in vivo production of multiple forms of creatine kinase in plasma. Clin Chem 1984;30: 662-4.
306. Perryman MB, Strauss AW, Olson J, Roberts R. In vitro translation of canine mitochondrial creatine kinase messenger RNA. Biochem Biophys Res Commun 1983;110:967-72.
307. Pfisterer M, Buser P, Rickli H, Gutmann M, Erne P, Rickenbacher P, et al. BNP-guided vs symptom-guided heart failure therapy: the Trial of Intensified vs Standard Medical Therapy in Elderly Patients with Congestive Heart Failure (TIME-CHF) randomized trial. JAMA 2009;301:383-92.
308. Pizarro R, Bazzino OO, Oberti PF, Falconi M, Achilli F, Arias A, et al. Prospective validation of the prognostic usefulness of brain natriuretic peptide in asymptomatic patients with chronic severe mitral regurgitation. J Am Coll Cardiol 2009;54:1099-106.
309. Prasad A, Rihal CS, Lennon RJ, Singh M, Jaffe AS, Holmes DR Jr. Significance of periprocedural myonecrosis on outcomes after percutaneous coronary intervention: an analysis of preintervention and postintervention troponin T levels in 5487 patients. Circ Cardiovasc Interv 2008;1:10-9.
310. Pruszczyk P, Kostrubiec M, Bochowicz A, Styczynski G, Szulc M, Kurzyna M, et al. N-terminal pro-brain natriuretic peptide in patients with acute pulmonary embolism. Eur Respir J 2003;22:649-53.
311. Puleo PR, Guadagno PA, Roberts R, Perryman MB. Sensitive, rapid assay of subforms of creatine kinase MB in plasma. Clin Chem 1989;35:1452-5.
312. Qin QP, Laitinen P, Majamaa-Voltti K, Eriksson S, Kumpula EK, Pettersson K. Release patterns of pregnancy associated plasma protein A (PAPP-A) in patients with acute coronary syndromes. Scand Cardiovasc J 2002;36:358-61.
313. Redfield MM. Treating diastolic heart failure with AGE crosslink breakers: thinking outside the heart failure box. J Card Fail 2005;11: 196-9.
314. Redfield MM, Rodeheffer RJ, Jacobsen SJ, Mahoney DW, Bailey KR, Burnett JC Jr. Plasma brain natriuretic peptide concentration: impact of age and gender. J Am Coll Cardiol 2002;40:976-82.
315. Rehfeld JF, Bundgaard JR, Goetze JP, Friis-Hansen L, Hilsted L, Johnsen AH. Naming progastrin-derived peptides. Regul Pept 2004;120:177-83.
316. Rehman SU, Martinez-Rumayor A, Mueller T, Januzzi JL Jr. Independent and incremental prognostic value of multimarker testing in acute dyspnea: results from the ProBNP Investigation of Dyspnea in the Emergency Department (PRIDE) study. Clin Chim Acta 2008;392:41-5.
317. Reichlin T, Hochholzer W, Bassetti S, Steuer S, Stelzig C, Hartwiger S, et al. Early diagnosis of myocardial infarction with sensitive cardiac troponin assays. N Engl J Med 2009;361:858-67.
318. Reichlin T, Hochholzer W, Stelzig C, Laule K, Freidank H, Morgenthaler NG, et al. Incremental value of copeptin for rapid rule out of acute myocardial infarction. J Am Coll Cardiol 2009;54:60-8.
319. Reimer KA, Lowe JE, Rasmussen MM, Jennings RB. The wavefront phenomenon of ischemic cell death. 1. Myocardial infarct size vs duration of coronary occlusion in dogs. Circulation 1977;56:786-94.
320. Ricchiuti V, Apple FS. RNA expression of cardiac troponin T isoforms in diseased human skeletal muscle. Clin Chem 1999;45:2129-35.
321. Richards AM, Crozier IG, Holmes SJ, Espiner EA, Yandle TG, Frampton C. Brain natriuretic peptide: natriuretic and endocrine effects in essential hypertension. J Hypertens 1993;11:163-70.

322. Richards AM, Doughty R, Nicholls MG, MacMahon S, Sharpe N, Murphy J, et al. Plasma N-terminal pro-brain natriuretic peptide and adrenomedullin: prognostic utility and prediction of benefit from carvedilol in chronic ischemic left ventricular dysfunction. Australia-New Zealand Heart Failure Group. J Am Coll Cardiol 2001;37:1781-7.
323. Richards AM, Nicholls MG, Espiner EA, Lainchbury JG, Troughton RW, Elliott J, et al. B-type natriuretic peptides and ejection fraction for prognosis after myocardial infarction. Circulation 2003;107:2786-92.
324. Richards AM, Nicholls MG, Lainchbury JG, Fisher S, Yandle TG. Plasma urotensin II in heart failure. Lancet 2002;360:545-6.
325. Ridker PM. Clinical application of C-reactive protein for cardiovascular disease detection and prevention. Circulation 2003;107: 363-9.
326. Ridker PM, Rifai N, Pfeffer MA, Sacks FM, Moye LA, Goldman S, et al. Inflammation, pravastatin, and the risk of coronary events after myocardial infarction in patients with average cholesterol levels. Cholesterol and Recurrent Events (CARE) Investigators. Circulation 1998;98:839-44.
327. Rifai N, Douglas PS, O'Toole M, Rimm E, Ginsburg GS. Cardiac troponin T and I, echocardiographic [correction of electrocardiographic] wall motion analyses, and ejection fractions in athletes participating in the Hawaii Ironman Triathlon. Am J Cardiol 1999;83:1085-9.
328. Roberts R, Henry PD, Sobel BE. An improved basis for enzymatic estimation of infarct size. Circulation 1975;52:743-54.
329. Roman D, Billadello J, Gordon J, Grace A, Sobel B, Strauss A. Complete nucleotide sequence of dog heart creatine kinase mRNA: conservation of amino acid sequence within and among species. Proc Natl Acad Sci U S A 1985;82:8394-8.
330. Ryan TJ, Antman EM, Brooks NH, Califf RM, Hillis LD, Hiratzka LF, et al. 1999 update: ACC/AHA guidelines for the management of patients with acute myocardial infarction: executive summary and recommendations: a report of the American College of Cardiology/ American Heart Association Task Force on Practice Guidelines (Committee on Management of Acute Myocardial Infarction). Circulation 1999;100:1016-30.
331. Sabatine MS, Morrow DA, de Lemos JA, Gibson CM, Murphy SA, Rifai N, et al. Multimarker approach to risk stratification in non-ST elevation acute coronary syndromes: simultaneous assessment of troponin I, C-reactive protein, and B-type natriuretic peptide. Circulation 2002;105:1760-3.
332. Sabatine MS, Morrow DA, de Lemos JA, Jarolim P, Braunwald E. Detection of acute changes in circulating troponin in the setting of transient stress test-induced myocardial ischaemia using an ultrasensitive assay: results from TIMI 35. Eur Heart J 2009;30:162-9.
333. Sabatine MS, Morrow DA, de Lemos JA, Omland T, Desai MY, Tanasijevic M, et al. Acute changes in circulating natriuretic peptide levels in relation to myocardial ischemia. J Am Coll Cardiol 2004;44:1988-95.
334. Saenger AK, Jaffe AS. Requiem for a heavyweight: the demise of creatine kinase-MB. Circulation 2008;118:2200-6.
335. Saggin L, Gorza L, Ausoni S, Schiaffino S. Cardiac troponin T in developing, regenerating and denervated rat skeletal muscle. Development 1990;110:547-54.
336. Salamonsen RF, Schneider HG, Bailey M, Taylor AJ. Cardiac troponin I concentrations, but not electrocardiographic results, predict an extended hospital stay after coronary artery bypass graft surgery. Clin Chem 2005;51:40-6.
336A. Sawada Y, Inoue M, Kanda T, Sakamaki T, Tanaka S, Minamino N, Nagai R, Takeuchi T. Co-elevation of brain natriuretic peptide and proprotein-processing endoprotease furin after myocardial infarction in rats. FEBS Lett 1997;400:177-82.
336B. Sawada Y, Suda M, Yokoyama H, Kanda T, Sakamaki T, Tanaka S, Nagai R, Abe S, Takeuchi T. Stretch-induced hypertrophic growth of cardiocytes and processing of brain-type natriuretic peptide are controlled by proprotein-processing endoprotease furin. J Biol Chem 1997;272:20545-54.
337. Schaufelberger M, Bergh CH, Caidahl K, Eggertsen R, Furenas E, Lindstedt G, et al. Can brain natriuretic peptide (BNP) be used as a screening tool in general practice? Scand J Prim Health Care 2004;22:187-90.
337A. Schellenberger U, O'Rear J, Guzzetta A, Jue RA, Protter AA, Pollitt NS. The precursor to B-type natriuretic peptide is an O-linked glycoprotein. Arch Biochem Biophys 2006;451:160-6.
338. Schulz S. C-type natriuretic peptide and guanylyl cyclase B receptor. Peptides 2005;26:1024-34.
338A. Schulz H, Langvik TA, Lund SE, Smith J, Ahmadi N, Hall C. Radioimmunoassay for N-terminal probrain natriuretic peptide in human plasma. Scand J Clin Lab Invest 2001;61:33-42.
339. Seferian KR, Tamm NN, Semenov AG, Tolstaya AA, Koshkina EV, Krasnoselsky MI, et al. Immunodetection of glycosylated NT-proBNP circulating in human blood. Clin Chem 2008; 54:866-73.
339A. Seferian KR, Tamm NN, Semenov AG, Mukharyamova KS, Tolstaya AA, Koshkina EV, Kara AN, Krasnoselsky MI, Apple FS, Esakova TV, Filatov VL, Katrukha AG. The brain natriuretic peptide (BNP) precursor is the major immunoreactive form of BNP in patients with heart failure. Clin Chem 2007;53:866-73.
340. Selvanayagam JB, Pigott D, Balacumaraswami L, Petersen SE, Neubauer S, Taggart DP. Relationship of irreversible myocardial injury to troponin I and creatine kinase-MB elevation after coronary artery bypass surgery: insights from cardiovascular magnetic resonance imaging. J Am Coll Cardiol 2005;45:629-31.
341. Semenov AG, Postnikov AB, Tamm NN, Seferian KR, Karpova NS, Bloshchitsyna MN, et al. Processing of pro-brain natriuretic peptide is suppressed by O-glycosylation in the region close to the cleavage site. Clin Chem 2009;55:489-98.
341A. Severino A, Campioni M, Straino S, Salloum FN, Schmidt N, Herbrand U, et al. Identification of protein disulfide isomerase as a cardiomyocyte survival factor in ischemic cardiomyopathy. J Am Coll Cardiol 2007;50:1029-37.
342. Servoss SJ, Januzzi JL, Muller JE. Triggers of acute coronary syndromes. Prog Cardiovasc Dis 2002;44:369-80.
343. Sharkey SW, Elsperger KJ, Murakami M, Apple FS. Canine myocardial creatine kinase isoenzyme response to coronary artery occlusion. Am J Physiol 1989;256:H508-14.
344. Sharkey SW, Murakami MM, Smith SA, Apple FS. Canine myocardial creatine kinase isoenzymes after chronic coronary artery occlusion. Circulation 1991;84:333-40.
345. Shih J, Datwyler SA, Hsu SC, Matias MS, Pacenti DP, Lueders C, et al. Effect of collection tube type and preanalytical handling on myeloperoxidase concentrations. Clin Chem 2008;54:1076-9.
346. Shimizu H, Aono K, Masuta K, Asada H, Misaki A, Teraoka H. Degradation of human brain natriuretic peptide (BNP) by contact activation of blood coagulation system. Clin Chim Acta 2001;305: 181-6.
347. Shimizu H, Masuta K, Aono K, Asada H, Sasakura K, Tamaki M, et al. Molecular forms of human brain natriuretic peptide in plasma. Clin Chim Acta 2002;316:129-35.
348. Shimizu H, Masuta K, Asada H, Sugita K, Sairenji T. Characterization of molecular forms of probrain natriuretic peptide in human plasma. Clin Chim Acta 2003;334:233-9.
349. Shuvy M, Shifman OE, Nusair S, Pappo O, Lotan C. Hypothyroidism-induced myocardial damage and heart failure: an overlooked entity. Cardiovasc Pathol 2009;18:183-6.
350. Siegel RJ, Said JW, Shell WE, Corson G, Fishbein MC. Identification and localization of creatine kinase B and M in normal, ischemic and necrotic myocardium: an immunohistochemical study. J Mol Cell Cardiol 1984;16:95-103.
351. Silva DP Jr, Landt Y, Porter SE, Ladenson JH. Development and application of monoclonal antibodies to human cardiac myoglobin in a rapid fluorescence immunoassay. Clin Chem 1991;37:1356-64.
352. Singh J, Akbar MS, Adabag S. Discordance of cardiac troponin I assays on the point-of-care i-STAT and Architect assays from Abbott Diagnostics. Clin Chim Acta 2009;403:259-60.

353. Smith MW, Espiner EA, Yandle TG, Charles CJ, Richards AM. Delayed metabolism of human brain natriuretic peptide reflects resistance to neutral endopeptidase. J Endocrinol 2000;167: 239-46.
354. Smith SC, Ladenson JH, Mason JW, Jaffe AS. Elevations of cardiac troponin I associated with myocarditis: experimental and clinical correlates. Circulation 1997;95:163-8.
355. Sobel BE. Increased plasminogen activator inhibitor-1 and vasculopathy: a reconcilable paradox. Circulation 1999;99: 2496-8.
356. Steiner HJ, Weiler R, Ludescher C, Schmid KW, Winkler H. Chromogranins A and B are co-localized with atrial natriuretic peptides in secretory granules of rat heart. J Histochem Cytochem 1990;38:845-50.
357. Steinhart B, Thorpe KE, Bayoumi AM, Moe G, Januzzi JL Jr, Mazer CD. Improving the diagnosis of acute heart failure using a validated prediction model. J Am Coll Cardiol 2009;54:1515-21.
358. Stelow EB, Johari VP, Smith SA, Crosson JT, Apple FS. Propofol-associated rhabdomyolysis with cardiac involvement in adults: chemical and anatomic findings. Clin Chem 2000;46:577-81.
359. Steuer J, Bjerner T, Duvernoy O, Jideus L, Johansson L, Ahlstrom H, et al. Visualisation and quantification of peri-operative myocardial infarction after coronary artery bypass surgery with contrast-enhanced magnetic resonance imaging. Eur Heart J 2004;25:1293-9.
359A. Steinhelper ME. Structure, expression, and genomic mapping of the mouse natriuretic peptide type-B gene. Circ Res 1993;72:984-92.
360. Sudoh T, Kangawa K, Minamino N, Matsuo H. A new natriuretic peptide in porcine brain. Nature 1988;332:78-81.
360A. Sudoh T, Maekawa K, Kojima M, Minamino N, Kangawa K, Matsuo H. Cloning and sequence analysis of cDNA encoding a precursor for human brain natriuretic peptide. Biochem Biophys Res Commun 1989;159:1427-34.
361. Sudoh T, Minamino N, Kangawa K, Matsuo H. C-type natriuretic peptide (CNP): a new member of natriuretic peptide family identified in porcine brain. Biochem Biophys Res Commun 1990;168:863-70.
362. Suwaidi JA, Hamasaki S, Higano ST, Nishimura RA, Holmes DR Jr, Lerman A. Long-term follow-up of patients with mild coronary artery disease and endothelial dysfunction. Circulation 2000;101: 948-54.
363. Syed IS, Prasad A, Oh JK, Martinez MW, Feng D, Motiei A, et al. Apical ballooning syndrome or aborted acute myocardial infarction? Insights from cardiovascular magnetic resonance imaging. Int J Cardiovasc Imaging 2008;24:875-82.
364. Takemura G, Takatsu Y, Doyama K, Itoh H, Saito Y, Koshiji M, et al. Expression of atrial and brain natriuretic peptides and their genes in hearts of patients with cardiac amyloidosis. J Am Coll Cardiol 1998;31:754-65.
365. Tamm NN, Seferian KR, Semenov AG, Mukharyamova KS, Koshkina EV, Krasnoselsky MI, et al. Novel immunoassay for quantification of brain natriuretic peptide and its precursor in human blood. Clin Chem 2008;54:1511-8.
366. Tanaka H, Abe S, Yamashita T, Arima S, Saigo M, Nakao S, et al. Serum levels of cardiac troponin I and troponin T in estimating myocardial infarct size soon after reperfusion. Coron Artery Dis 1997;8:433-9.
367. Tang WH, Francis GS, Morrow DA, Newby LK, Cannon CP, Jesse RL, et al. National Academy of Clinical Biochemistry Laboratory Medicine practice guidelines: clinical utilization of cardiac biomarker testing in heart failure. Circulation 2007;116:e99-109.
368. Taupenot L, Harper KL, O'Connor DT. The chromogranin-secretogranin family. N Engl J Med 2003;348:1134-49.
369. Thielmann M, Massoudy P, Neuhauser M, Tsagakis K, Marggraf G, Kamler M, et al. Prognostic value of preoperative cardiac troponin I in patients undergoing emergency coronary artery bypass surgery with non-ST-elevation or ST-elevation acute coronary syndromes. Circulation 2006;114:I448-53.
370. Thielmann M, Massoudy P, Schmermund A, Neuhauser M, Marggraf G, Kamler M, et al. Diagnostic discrimination between graft-related and non-graft-related perioperative myocardial infarction with cardiac troponin I after coronary artery bypass surgery. Eur Heart J 2005;26: 2440-7.
371. Thompson PD, Apple FS, Wu A. Marathoner's heart? Circulation 2006;114:2306-8.
371A. Thuerauf DJ, Glembotski CC. Differential effects of protein kinase C, Ras, and Raf-1 kinase on the induction of the cardiac B-type natriuretic peptide gene through a critical promoter-proximal M-CAT element. J Biol Chem 1997;272:7464-72.
372. Thygesen K, Alpert JS, White HD. Universal definition of myocardial infarction. Eur Heart J 2007;28:2525-38.
373. Topol EJ. Nesiritide—not verified. N Engl J Med 2005;353:113-6.
374. Tota B, Angelone T, Mazza R, Cerra MC. The chromogranin A-derived vasostatins: new players in the endocrine heart. Curr Med Chem 2008;15:1444-51.
375. Tsimikas S, Bergmark C, Beyer RW, Patel R, Pattison J, Miller E, et al. Temporal increases in plasma markers of oxidized low-density lipoprotein strongly reflect the presence of acute coronary syndromes. J Am Coll Cardiol 2003;41:360-70.
376. Tucker JF, Collins RA, Anderson AJ, Hauser J, Kalas J, Apple FS. Early diagnostic efficiency of cardiac troponin I and troponin T for acute myocardial infarction. Acad Emerg Med 1997;4:13-21.
377. Tung P, Kopelnik A, Banki N, Ong K, Ko N, Lawton MT, et al. Predictors of neurocardiogenic injury after subarachnoid hemorrhage. Stroke 2004;35:548-51.
377A. Underwood R, Chiravuri M, Lee H, Schmitz T, Kabcenell AK, Yardley K, Huber BT. Sequence, purification, and cloning of an intracellular serine protease, quiescent cell proline dipeptidase. J Biol Chem 1999;274:34053-8.
378. Vaananen HK, Syrjala H, Rahkila P, Vuori J, Melamies LM, Myllyla V, et al. Serum carbonic anhydrase III and myoglobin concentrations in acute myocardial infarction. Clin Chem 1990;36: 635-8.
379. Vanhoof G, Goossens F, De Meester I, Hendriks D, Scharpe S. Proline motifs in peptides and their biological processing. FASEB J 1995;9: 736-44.
380. Varo N, de Lemos JA, Libby P, Morrow DA, Murphy SA, Nuzzo R, et al. Soluble CD40L: risk prediction after acute coronary syndromes. Circulation 2003;108:1049-52.
381. Vasan RS, Benjamin EJ, Larson MG, Leip EP, Wang TJ, Wilson PW, et al. Plasma natriuretic peptides for community screening for left ventricular hypertrophy and systolic dysfunction: the Framingham heart study. JAMA 2002;288:1252-9.
382. Venge P, Johnston N, Lindahl B, James S. Normal plasma levels of cardiac troponin I measured by the high-sensitivity cardiac troponin I access prototype assay and the impact on the diagnosis of myocardial ischemia. J Am Coll Cardiol 2009;54:1165-72.
383. Venge P, Lagerqvist B, Diderholm E, Lindahl B, Wallentin L. Clinical performance of three cardiac troponin assays in patients with unstable coronary artery disease (a FRISC II substudy). Am J Cardiol 2002;89: 1035-41.
384. ver Elst KM, Spapen HD, Nguyen DN, Garbar C, Huyghens LP, Gorus FK. Cardiac troponins I and T are biological markers of left ventricular dysfunction in septic shock. Clin Chem 2000;46: 650-7.
385. Verma A, Kilicaslan F, Martin DO, Minor S, Starling R, Marrouche NF, et al. Preimplantation B-type natriuretic peptide concentration is an independent predictor of future appropriate implantable defibrillator therapies. Heart 2006;92:190-5.
386. Wallace TW, Abdullah SM, Drazner MH, Das SR, Khera A, McGuire DK, et al. Prevalence and determinants of troponin T elevation in the general population. Circulation 2006;113:1958-65.
387. Wang TJ, Larson MG, Levy D, Benjamin EJ, Corey D, Leip EP, et al. Heritability and genetic linkage of plasma natriuretic peptide levels. Circulation 2003;108:13-6.
388. Wang TJ, Larson MG, Levy D, Benjamin EJ, Leip EP, Omland T, et al. Plasma natriuretic peptide levels and the risk of cardiovascular events and death. N Engl J Med 2004;350:655-63.

388A. Wang W, Liao X, Fukuda K, Knappe S, Wu F, Dries DL, Qin J, Wu Q. Corin variant associated with hypertension and cardiac hypertrophy exhibits impaired zymogen activation and natriuretic peptide processing activity. Circ Res 2008;103:502-8.
389. Weber M, Hausen M, Arnold R, Nef H, Moellman H, Berkowitsch A, et al. Prognostic value of N-terminal pro-B-type natriuretic peptide for conservatively and surgically treated patients with aortic valve stenosis. Heart 2006;92:1639-44.
389A. Weidemann A, Klanke B, Wagner M, Volk T, Willam C, Wiesener MS, Eckardt KU, Warnecke C. Hypoxia, via stabilization of the hypoxia-inducible factor HIF-1alpha, is a direct and sufficient stimulus for brain-type natriuretic peptide induction. Biochem J 2008;409:233-42.
390. Weisfeldt ML. Reperfusion and reperfusion injury. Clin Res 1987;35: 13-20.
391. Wevers RA, Olthuis HP, Van Niel JC, Van Wilgenburg MG, Soons JB. A study on the dimeric structure of creatine kinase (EC 2.7.3.2). Clin Chim Acta 1977;75:377-85.
392. White HD. Things ain't what they used to be: impact of a new definition of myocardial infarction. Am Heart J 2002;144:933-7.
393. Wieczorek SJ, Wu AH, Christenson R, Krishnaswamy P, Gottlieb S, Rosano T, et al. A rapid B-type natriuretic peptide assay accurately diagnoses left ventricular dysfunction and heart failure: a multicenter evaluation. Am Heart J 2002;144:834-9.
394. Wilson SR, Sabatine MS, Braunwald E, Sloan S, Murphy SA, Morrow DA. Detection of myocardial injury in patients with unstable angina using a novel nanoparticle cardiac troponin I assay: observations from the PROTECT-TIMI 30 Trial. Am Heart J 2009;158:386-91.
395. Wiviott SD, Cannon CP, Morrow DA, Murphy SA, Gibson CM, McCabe CH, et al. Differential expression of cardiac biomarkers by gender in patients with unstable angina/non-ST-elevation myocardial infarction: a TACTICS-TIMI 18 (Treat Angina with Aggrastat and determine Cost of Therapy with an Invasive or Conservative Strategy-Thrombolysis In Myocardial Infarction 18) substudy. Circulation 2004;109:580-6.
396. Wong ET, Cobb C, Umehara MK, Wolff GA, Haywood LJ, Greenberg T, et al. Heterogeneity of serum creatine kinase activity among racial and gender groups of the population. Am J Clin Pathol 1983;79: 582-6.
397. Wright SP, Doughty RN, Pearl A, Gamble GD, Whalley GA, Walsh HJ, et al. Plasma amino-terminal pro-brain natriuretic peptide and accuracy of heart-failure diagnosis in primary care: a randomized, controlled trial. J Am Coll Cardiol 2003;42:1793-800.
398. Wu AH, Apple FS, Gibler WB, Jesse RL, Warshaw MM, Valdes R Jr. National Academy of Clinical Biochemistry standards of laboratory practice: recommendations for the use of cardiac markers in coronary artery diseases. Clin Chem 1999;45:1104-21.
399. Wu AH, Fukushima N, Puskas R, Todd J, Goix P. Development and preliminary clinical validation of a high sensitivity assay for cardiac troponin using a capillary flow (single molecule) fluorescence detector. Clin Chem 2006;52:2157-9.
400. Wu AH, Jaffe AS. The clinical need for high-sensitivity cardiac troponin assays for acute coronary syndromes and the role for serial testing. Am Heart J 2008;155:208-14.
401. Wu AH, Jaffe AS, Apple FS, Jesse RL, Francis GL, Morrow DA, et al. National Academy of Clinical Biochemistry laboratory medicine practice guidelines: use of cardiac troponin and B-type natriuretic peptide or N-terminal proB-type natriuretic peptide for etiologies other than acute coronary syndromes and heart failure. Clin Chem 2007;53:2086-96.
402. Wu AH, Lu QA, Todd J, Moecks J, Wians F. Short- and long-term biological variation in cardiac troponin I measured with a high-sensitivity assay: implications for clinical practice. Clin Chem 2009;55:52-8.
403. Wu AH, Smith A, Apple FS. Optimum blood collection intervals for B-type natriuretic peptide testing in patients with heart failure. Am J Cardiol 2004;93:1562-3.
404. Wu AH, Smith A, Wieczorek S, Mather JF, Duncan B, White CM, et al. Biological variation for N-terminal pro- and B-type natriuretic peptides and implications for therapeutic monitoring of patients with congestive heart failure. Am J Cardiol 2003;92:628-31.
405. Wu AH, Valdes R Jr, Apple FS, Gornet T, Stone MA, Mayfield-Stokes S, et al. Cardiac troponin-T immunoassay for diagnosis of acute myocardial infarction. Clin Chem 1994;40:900-7.
406. Wu AHB. Cardiac markers: pathology and laboratory medicine, 2nd edition. Totowa, NJ: Humana Press, 2003.
407. Wu C, Wu F, Pan J, Morser J, Wu Q. Furin-mediated processing of Pro-C-type natriuretic peptide. J Biol Chem 2003;278:25847-52.
408. Wu Q. The serine protease corin in cardiovascular biology and disease. Front Biosci 2007;12:4179-90.
409. Yan W, Sheng N, Seto M, Morser J, Wu Q. Corin, a mosaic transmembrane serine protease encoded by a novel cDNA from human heart. J Biol Chem 1999;274:14926-35.
410. Yan W, Wu F, Morser J, Wu Q. Corin, a transmembrane cardiac serine protease, acts as a pro-atrial natriuretic peptide-converting enzyme. Proc Natl Acad Sci U S A 2000;97:8525-9.
411. Yang-Feng TL, Floyd-Smith G, Nemer M, Drouin J, Francke U. The pronatriodilatin gene is located on the distal short arm of human chromosome 1 and on mouse chromosome 4. Am J Hum Genet 1985;37:1117-28.
412. Yeo KT, Wu AH, Apple FS, Kroll MH, Christenson RH, Lewandrowski KB, et al. Multicenter evaluation of the Roche NT-proBNP assay and comparison to the Biosite Triage BNP assay. Clin Chim Acta 2003;338:107-15.
413. Yilmaz A, Mahrholdt H, Athanasiadis A, Vogelsberg H, Meinhardt G, Voehringer M, et al. Coronary vasospasm as the underlying cause for chest pain in patients with PVB19 myocarditis. Heart 2008;94:1456-63.
413A. Yokota N, Bruneau BG, Fernandez BE, de Bold ML, Piazza LA, Eid H, de Bold AJ. Dissociation of cardiac hypertrophy, myosin heavy chain isoform expression, and natriuretic peptide production in DOCA-salt rats. Am J Hypertens 1995;8:301-10.
414. Zabel M, Hohnloser SH, Koster W, Prinz M, Kasper W, Just H. Analysis of creatine kinase, CK-MB, myoglobin, and troponin T time-activity curves for early assessment of coronary artery reperfusion after intravenous thrombolysis. Circulation 1993;87:1542-50.
415. Zaphiriou A, Robb S, Murray-Thomas T, Mendez G, Fox K, McDonagh T, et al. The diagnostic accuracy of plasma BNP and NTproBNP in patients referred from primary care with suspected heart failure: results of the UK natriuretic peptide study. Eur J Heart Fail 2005;7:537-41.
416. Zethelius B, Berglund L, Sundstrom J, Ingelsson E, Basu S, Larsson A, et al. Use of multiple biomarkers to improve the prediction of death from cardiovascular causes. N Engl J Med 2008;358:2107-16.
417. Zethelius B, Johnston N, Venge P. Troponin I as a predictor of coronary heart disease and mortality in 70-year-old men: a community-based cohort study. Circulation 2006;113:1071-8.
418. Zhang R, Brennan ML, Fu X, Aviles RJ, Pearce GL, Penn MS, et al. Association between myeloperoxidase levels and risk of coronary artery disease. JAMA 2001;286:2136-42.
419. Zimmerman J, Fromm R, Meyer D, Boudreaux A, Wun CC, Smalling R, et al. Diagnostic marker cooperative study for the diagnosis of myocardial infarction. Circulation 1999;99:1671-7.

ADDITIONAL READING

Apple FS, Blankenburg S, Morrow D. Impact of clinical markers, proteomics and genomics in cardiovascular disease. Clin Chem; Special Issue January 2012.

CHAPTER 48

Kidney Disease

*Michael P. Delaney, B.Sc., M.D., F.R.C.P., Christopher P. Price, Ph.D., F.R.S.C., F.R.C.Path., and Edmund J. Lamb, Ph.D., F.R.C.Path.**

The kidneys play a central role in the homeostatic mechanisms of the human body, and reduced renal function strongly correlates with increasing morbidity and mortality. Biochemical investigations, both routine and specialized, are an important part of the clinician's diagnostic armamentarium, and investigations of kidney function constitute a significant element of the workload of most laboratories. The aim of this chapter is to ensure that the clinical chemist/biochemist understands the perspective of the nephrologist when dealing with laboratory investigations for patients with kidney disease. The basic anatomy and physiology of the kidneys are described as a foundation for understanding the pathophysiology of disease and the rationale for diagnostic and management strategies in kidney disease. Key analytical methods employed during the investigation of kidney disease are discussed in Chapter 25.

ANATOMY

The kidneys form a paired organ system located in the retroperitoneal space. They extend from the the lower part of the eleventh thoracic vertebra to the upper portion of the third lumbar vertebra, with the right kidney situated slightly lower than the left. The adult kidney is about 12 cm long and weighs about 150 g (Figure 48-1). The kidneys have both sympathetic and parasympathetic nerve supplies, whose function appears to be predominantly associated with vasomotor activity. The renal lymphatic drainage includes fine lymphatics in the glomerulus, some in close proximity to the juxtaglomerular apparatus (JGA; see Box 48-1 for a list of abbreviations), which are associated with removal of material from the glomerular mesangial cells.

Blood Supply

In most cases, each kidney receives its blood supply from a single renal artery derived from the abdominal aorta. However, multiple renal arteries occur commonly. The renal artery divides into posterior and anterior elements, and ultimately into the afferent arterioles, which expand into the highly specialized capillary beds that form the glomerulus (Figure 48-2). These capillaries then rejoin to form the efferent arteriole that forms the capillary plexuses and the elongated vessels (the *vasa recta*) that pass around the remaining parts of the nephron, the proximal and distal tubules, the loop of Henle, and the collecting duct, providing oxygen and nutrients and removing ions, molecules, and water, which have been reabsorbed by the nephron. The efferent arteriole then merges with renal venules to form the renal veins, which merge into the inferior vena cava.

In adults, the kidneys receive approximately 25% of the cardiac output, about 90% of which supplies the renal cortex, maintaining the highly active tubular cells. Maintenance of renal blood flow is essential to kidney function, and a complex array of intrarenal regulatory mechanisms ensure that it is maintained across a wide range of systemic blood pressures (see discussion later in this chapter). The renal glomerular perfusion pressure is maintained at a constant 45 mm Hg across systemic pressures between 90 and 200 mm Hg.

Nephron

The functional unit of the kidney is the *nephron*. Each kidney has been reported to contain between 600,000 and 1.5 million nephrons.[323] The number of nephrons that an individual is born with (the "nephron dose") may determine that individual's susceptibility to renal injury. The nephron consists of a glomerulus, proximal tubule, loop of Henle, distal tubule, and collecting duct (see Figure 48-2). The collecting ducts ultimately combine to develop into the renal calyces, where the urine collects before passing along the ureter and into the bladder. The kidney is divided into several lobes. The outer, darker region of each lobe, the cortex, consists of most of the glomeruli and the proximal and distal tubules. The cortex surrounds a paler inner region, the medulla, which is further divided into a number of conical areas known as the renal

**We are grateful for data supplied by the U.S. Renal Data System (USRDS). Interpretation and reporting of these data are the responsibility of the authors and in no way should be seen as an official policy or interpretation of the U.S. government. We are also grateful for data supplied by the U.K. Renal Registry. Interpretation and reporting of these data are the responsibility of the authors and in no way should be seen as an official policy or interpretation of the U.K. Renal Registry.*

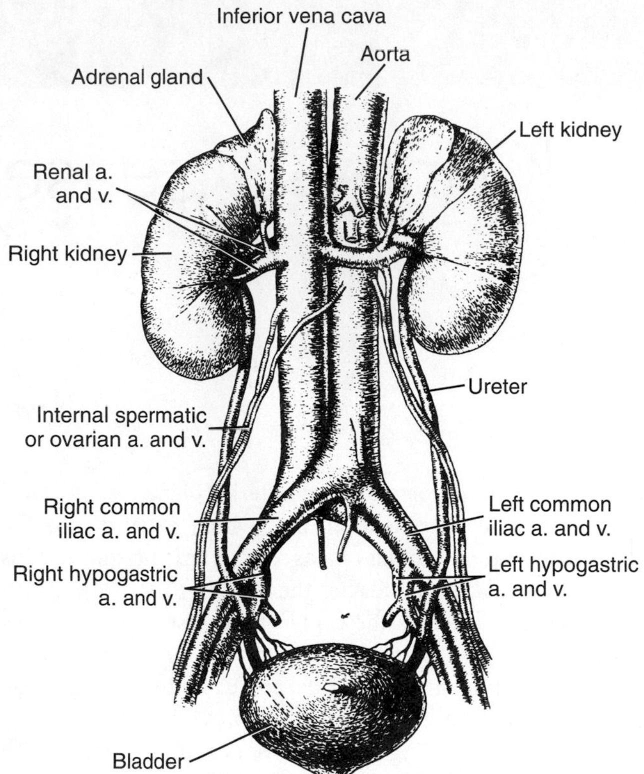

Figure 48-1 Vascular and anatomic relationships of the kidneys in man. *(From Leaf A, Cotran RS. Renal pathophysiology, 3rd edition. Oxford: Oxford University Press, 1985. Reproduced by permission of Oxford University Press.)*

pyramids, the apex of which extends toward the renal pelvis, forming papillae. Medullary rays are visible striations in the renal pyramids that connect the kidney cortex with the medulla. They are composed of descending (straight proximal) and ascending (straight distal) thick limbs of Henle and collecting ducts and associated blood vessels (the vasa recta). The central hilus is where blood vessels, lymphatics, and the renal pelvis (containing the ureter) join the kidney.

Glomerulus

The glomerulus is formed from a specialized capillary network. Each capillary develops into approximately 40 glomerular loops around 200 μm in size and consisting of a variety of different cell types supported on a specialized basement membrane (Figure 48-3, *top*). Some endothelial and epithelial cells act in concert with the specialized glomerular basement membrane (GBM) to form the glomerular filtration barrier, in addition to mesangial cells.

The *capillary endothelial* cells are about 40 nm thick and are in contact with each other. However, in contrast to the continuous endothelial linings seen elsewhere in the body, circular fenestrations (pores) with diameters of approximately 60 nm collectively constitute 20 to 50% of the glomerular endothelial surface.[170] The endothelium permits virtually free access of plasma and small solutes to the basement membrane. However, although the fenestrations are far larger than the diameter of albumin (3.5 nm), it is thought that perm selectivity to such larger molecules begins at the

BOX 48-1 List of Abbreviations

$1,25(OH_2)D_3$	calcitriol	ATG	antithymocyte globulin
11β-HSD	11β-hydroxysteroid dehydrogenase	ATN	acute tubular necrosis
^{99m}Tc-DMSA	technetium-99 m-dimercaptosuccinic acid	AVF	arteriovenous fistula
^{99m}Tc-DTPA	^{99m}Tc-diethylenetriaminepentaacetic acid	AZT	azathioprine
^{99m}Tc-MAG3	^{99m}Tc-mercaptoacetyltriglycerine	BJP	Bence Jones protein
AII	angiotensin II	BP	blood pressure
ACE	angiotensin-converting enzyme	BPH	benign prostatic hyperplasia
ADH	antidiuretic hormone	BSA	body surface area
ADPKD	autosomal dominant polycystic kidney disease	CA II	carbonic anhydrase II
		CA IV	carbonic anhydrase IV
ADQI	Acute Dialysis Quality Initiative	CAN	chronic allograft nephropathy
AE1	anion exchanger 1	CAPD	continuous ambulatory peritoneal dialysis
AGE	advanced glycation end products	CFU	colony-forming units
AIN	acute interstitial nephritis	CHD	coronary heart disease
AKI	acute kidney injury	CKD	chronic kidney disease
AKIN	Acute Kidney Injury Network	CMV	cytomegalovirus
ALG	antilymphocyte globulin	CNI	calcineurin inhibitor
ANA	antinuclear antibody	CO_2	carbon dioxide
ANCA	antineutrophil cytoplasmic antibody	COL4A5	A5 chain of type IV collagen
ANP	atrial natriuretic peptide	COX	cyclooxygenase
anti-GBM	anti–glomerular basement membrane	CRF	chronic renal failure
APD	automated peritoneal dialysis	CRP	C-reactive protein
AQP	aquaporin	CT	computed tomography
ARAS	atheromatous renal artery stenosis	CVP	central venous pressure
ARB	angiotensin receptor blocker	DCCT	Diabetes Control and Complications Trial
ARF	acute renal failure	dRTA	distal renal tubular acidosis

BOX 48-1 List of Abbreviations—cont'd

DTPA	^{99m}Tc-diethylenetriaminepentaacetic acid
DVT	deep vein thrombosis
EDTA	ethylenediaminetetraacetic acid
EM	electron microscopy
EMT	epithelial-mesenchymal transition
EMU	early morning urine
ENaC	apical sodium channel
EPO	erythropoietin
ERF	established renal failure
ESA	erythropoiesis-stimulating agent
ESRD	end-stage renal disease
ESWL	extracorporeal shock wave lithotripsy
FENa	fractional excretion of sodium
FGF-23	fibroblast growth factor-23
FSGS	focal segmental glomerulosclerosis
GBM	glomerular basement membrane
GFR	glomerular filtration rate
GN	glomerulonephritis
GSC	glomerular sieving coefficient
H_2CO_3	carbonic acid
HD	hemodialysis
HDF	hemodiafiltration
HDL	high-density lipoprotein
HF	hemofiltration
HIV	human immunodeficiency virus
HLA	human leukocyte antigen
HOT	Hypertension Optimal Treatment
HPLC	high-performance liquid chromatography
IDL	intermediate-density lipoprotein
ID-MS	isotope dilution mass spectrometry
Ig	immunoglobulin
IL-6	interleukin-6
IM	immunoperoxidase
IVP	intravenous pyelography
IVU	intravenous urography
JGA	juxtaglomerular apparatus
JNC 7	Joint National Committee on Prevention, Detection, Evaluation, and Treatment of High Blood Pressure
KDIGO	Kidney Disease Improving Global Outcomes
LDL	low-density lipoprotein
LM	light microscopy
LVH	left ventricular hypertrophy
LVMI	left ventricular mass index
MCD	minimal change disease
MCGN	mesangiocapillary glomerulonephritis
MCP-1	monocyte chemoattractant protein-1
MDRD	Modification of Diet in Renal Disease
MHC	major histocompatibility complex
MMF	mycophenolate mofetil
6-MP	6-mercaptopurine
MPA	mycophenolic acid
MR	mineralocorticoid receptor
MRA	magnetic resonance angiography
MRI	magnetic resonance imaging
Na^+-K^+-ATPase	sodium-potassium adenosine triphosphatase
NAG	*N*-acetyl-β-D-glucosaminidase
NBC-1	Na^+-HCO_3^- cotransporter
NCCT	Na^+-Cl^- cotransporter
NCX1	sodium calcium exchanger
NHANES III	Third National Health and Nutrition Examination Survey
NHE-3	Na^+-H^+ exchanger
NHS	National Health Service
NICE	National Institute for Health and Clinical Excellence
NKCC2	Na^+-K^+-$2Cl^-$ cotransporter
NKF-K/DOQI	National Kidney Foundation–Kidney Disease Outcomes Quality Initiative
NO	nitric oxide
NOS	nitric oxide synthase
NSAID	nonsteroidal anti-inflammatory drug
PD	peritoneal dialysis
PET	peritoneal equilibration test
pIgA	polymeric IgA
PKC-β1	protein kinase C-β1
pmp	per million population
PR3	proteinase 3
PRA	panel-reactive antibody
pRTA	proximal renal tubular acidosis
PTH	parathyroid hormone
QOF	Quality and Outcomes Framework
RAAS	renin-angiotensin-aldosterone system
RBP	retinol-binding protein
rhEPO	recombinant human erythropoietin
RIFLE	Risk, Injury, Failure, Loss, End-stage kidney disease
RPGN	rapidly progressive glomerulonephritis
RRF	residual renal function
RRT	renal replacement therapy
RTA	renal tubular acidosis
RVT	renal vein thrombosis
SAP	serum amyloid protein
SIGN	Scottish Intercollegiate Guideline Network
SLE	systemic lupus erythematosus
SPK	simultaneous pancreas and kidney
TGF-β	transforming growth factor-β
THG	Tamm Horsfall glycoprotein
TIN	tubulointerstitial nephritis
Tm	tubular maximal uptake
TMB	tetramethyl benzidine
TNF-α	tissue necrosis factor-α
TPMT	thiopurine methyltransferase
UF	ultrafiltration
UK	United Kingdom
UKM	urea kinetic modeling
UKNEQAS	United Kingdom National External Quality Assessment Scheme
UKPDS	United Kingdom Prospective Diabetes Study
UKT	United Kingdom transplant
UNOS	United Network for Organ Sharing
URR	urea reduction ratio
US	United States
USRDS	United States Renal Data System
UTI	urinary tract infection
VDR	vitamin D receptor
VLDL	very low-density lipoprotein

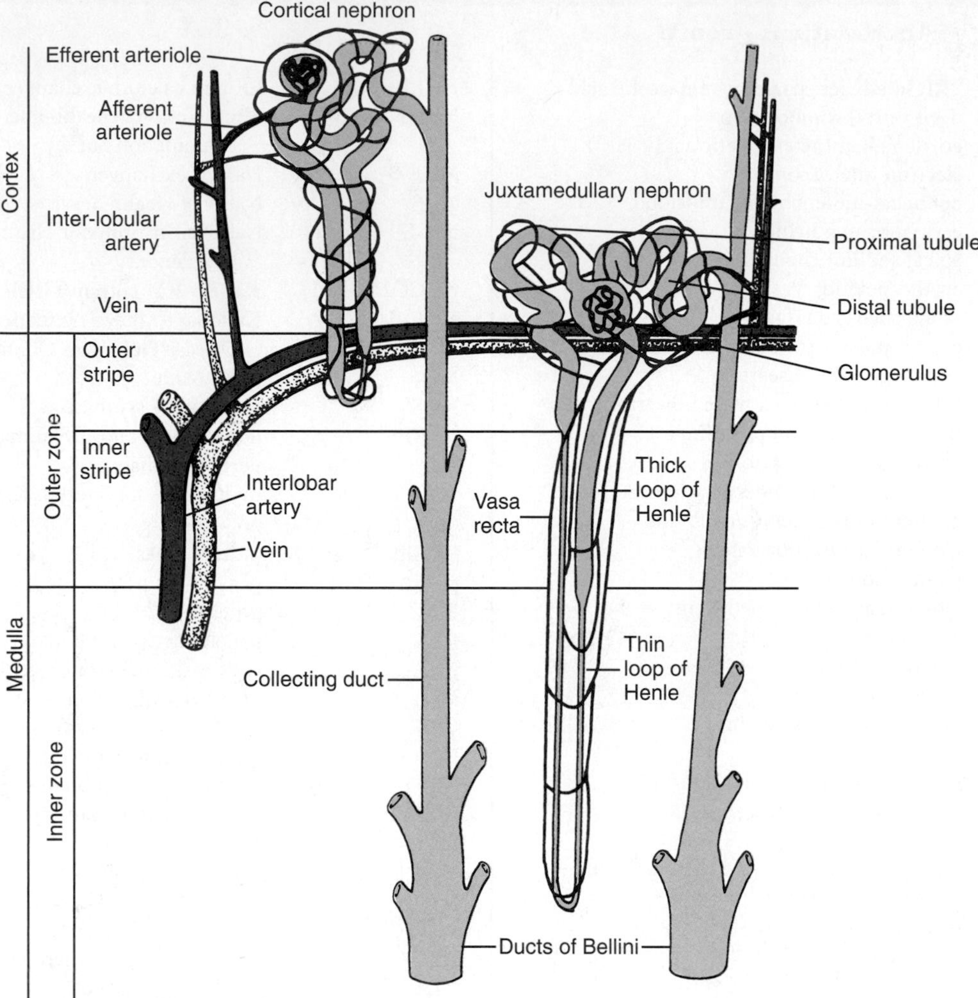

Figure 48-2 Diagrammatic representation of the nephron, the functional unit of the kidney, illustrating anatomic and vascular arrangements. *(From Pitts RF: Physiology of the kidney and body fluids, 3rd edition. Chicago, Ill: Year Book Medical Publishers, 1974.)*

endothelium because of the endothelial surface lining—a glycocalyx coating of negatively charged glycoproteins, glycosaminoglycans, proteoglycans, and absorbed plasma proteins, including orosomucoid and albumin. Estimates of the thickness of this layer vary depending on the visualization and preparation techniques used, but it may be between 200 and 400 nm thick.[170]

The *basement membrane* (Figure 48-3, *bottom*) of the glomerular capillaries is much thicker (approximately 300 nm) than that of other vascular beds and consists of three distinct electron-dense layers: the *lamina rara interna,* the *lamina densa,* and the *lamina rara externa.* The lamina densa consists of a close feltwork of fine, mainly type IV, collagen fibrils (each 3 to 5 nm thick) embedded in a gel-like matrix of laminin, nidogen/entactin, glycoproteins, and proteoglycans such as agrin and perlecan. The lamina densa forms the main size discriminant barrier to protein passage into the tubular lumen. The other two layers of the basement membrane are rich in negatively charged polyanionic glycoproteins, such as heparan sulfate; these may form a charge discriminant barrier to the passage of proteins, although the importance of the GBM in charge discrimination is still uncertain.[170]

The *epithelial cells* of the glomerulus line the outside of the glomerular capillaries, thus facing Bowman's capsule and the primary urine (see Figure 48-3, *top*). These cells are called *podocytes* and have an unusual octopus-like structure in that they have a large number of cytoplasmic extensions or foot processes that are embedded in the basement membrane. Foot processes are anchored to the GBM via integrin molecules and dystroglycans and are divided into primary and secondary. The secondary processes between adjacent cells interdigitate to form filtration slits, which are 25 to 60 nm wide.[170] The podocytes are covered by a complex diaphragm ("slit diaphragm"), some of the molecular components of which (e.g., nephrin) appear crucial for the maintenance of larger proteins within the circulation. The resulting structure is relatively impermeable to most proteins above 60 kDa, but passage of proteins is modulated by their charge and shape.

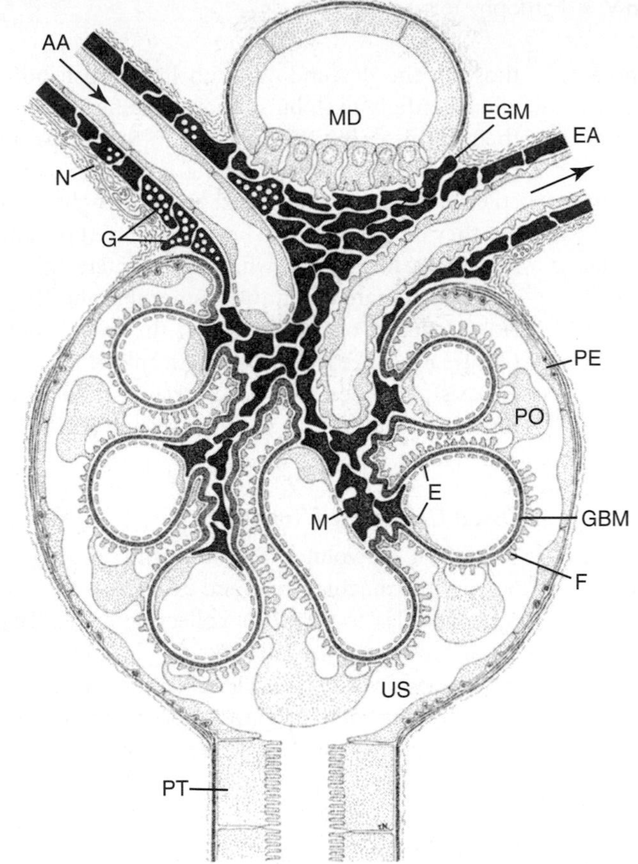

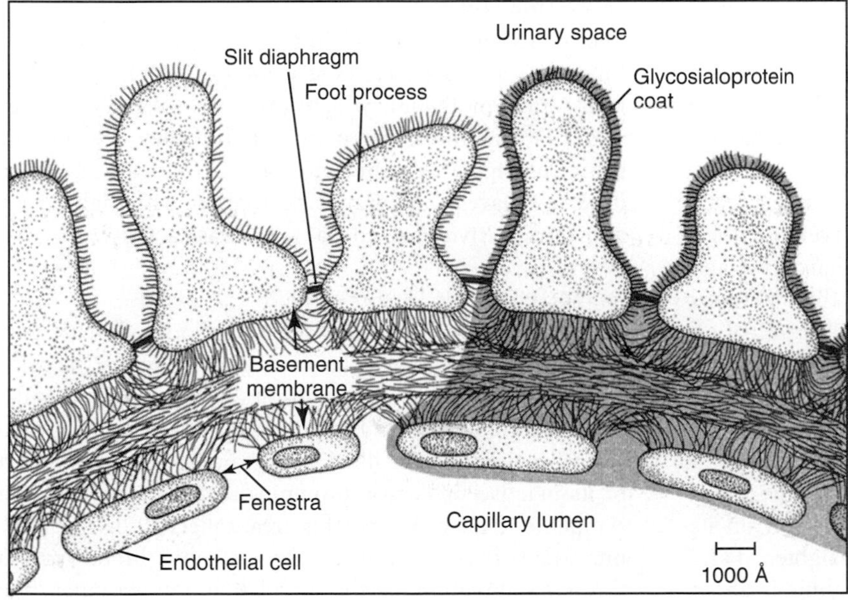

Figure 48-3 The glomerular cells and the glomerular filtration barrier. A, Longitudinal section through a glomerulus and its juxtaglomerular apparatus. The capillary tuft consists of a network of specialized capillaries, which are outlined by a fenestrated endothelium *(E)*. At the vascular pole, the afferent arteriole *(AA)* enters, branching into capillaries immediately after its entrance; the efferent arteriole *(EA)* is established inside the tuft and passes through the glomerular stalk before leaving at the vascular pole. The capillary network and the mesangium are enclosed in a common compartment bounded by the glomerular basement membrane *(GBM)*. Note that there is no basement membrane at the interface between the capillary endothelium and the mesangium. The glomerular visceral epithelium consists of highly branched podocytes *(POs)*, which, in a typical interdigitating pattern, cover the outer aspect of the GBM. At the vascular pole, the visceral epithelium and the GBM are reflected into the parietal epithelium *(PE)* of Bowman's capsule, which passes over into the epithelium of the proximal tubule *(PT)* at the urinary pole. At the vascular pole, the glomerular mesangium is continuous with the extraglomerular mesangium *(EGM)*, which consists of extraglomerular mesangial cells and an extraglomerular mesangial matrix. The EGM and the granular cells *(G)* of the afferent arteriole, along with the macula densa *(MD)*, establish the juxtaglomerular apparatus. All cells that are suggested to be of smooth muscle origin are shown in black. *US*, Urinary space; *F*, foot processes; *N*, sympathetic nerve terminals; *M*, messenger cells. B, Glomerular capillary wall. In glomerular filtration, filtered fluid is believed to traverse the capillary wall via an extracellular route, that is, through endothelial fenestrae, basement membrane, and slit diaphragms. Circulating polyanions (e.g., albumin) are thought to be retarded by the rich distribution in inner barriers of negatively charged sialylated glycoproteins (*shaded area* in schematic diagram). (**A** *From Elger M, Kriz W. The renal glomerulus—the structural basis of ultrafiltration. In: Cameron JS, Davison AM, Grunfeld JP, Kerr D, Ritz E, eds. Oxford textbook of clinical nephrology, volume 1, 2nd edition. Oxford: Oxford University Press, 1998:Chapter 3.1. Reproduced by permission of Oxford University Press;* **B** *From Brenner BM, Beeuwkes R III. The kidney in health and disease: III. The renal circulations. Hosp Pract 1978;13:35-46.)*

Podocytes are also covered by a glycocalyx of sulfated molecules, including glycosaminoglycans and glycoconjugates (e.g., podocalyxin). The surface anionic charge helps to maintain the foot process structure and the distance between the parietal and visceral epithelial cells constituting Bowman's space.[170]

The final cellular components of the glomerulus are the *mesangial cells,* which are found in the central part ("stalk") of the glomerulus between and within the capillary loops suspended in a matrix that they synthesize. They are in direct contact with glomerular endothelial cells and the inner layer of the GBM (lamina rara interna), and also with the extraglomerular mesangium and the JGA (see Figure 48-3, *top*). Mesangial cells have the characteristics of smooth muscle cells (pericytes), in that they are rich in microfilaments and respond to and produce a variety of stimuli [e.g., angiotensin II (AII) and antidiuretic hormone (ADH) or arginine vasopressin].[391] Mesangial matrix is rich in collagens and proteoglycans but is different in composition from the matrix of the GBM. Its composition and volume are tightly regulated in health but can be markedly altered during certain diseases [e.g., diabetic nephropathy, immunoglobulin (Ig)A nephropathy]. Mesangial cells have both structural and housekeeping functions. They have anchoring filaments to GBM opposite the podocytes, and their contractile properties enable them to alter intraglomerular capillary flow and glomerular ultrafiltration surface area, and thereby single nephron glomerular filtration rate (GFR). The cells appear to respond to capillary stretch by generating soluble factors such as vascular endothelial growth factor and transforming growth factor-β (TGF-β), and by activating intracellular signaling pathways. Mesangial cells also have specific and nonspecific mechanisms for removing macromolecules that reach the mesangial and subendothelial space, preventing their accumulation. These mechanisms include phagocytosis and degradation by the cells and trafficking along the mesangial stalk to the juxtaglomerular region, followed by elimination via the renal lymphatics, or by regurgitation into the glomerular capillary.

Proximal Tubule

Bowman's capsule forms the beginning of the tightly coiled, proximal convoluted tubule *(pars convoluta),* which on its progress toward the renal medulla becomes straightened and is then called the *pars recta.* The proximal tubule is about 15 mm long. Epithelial cells lining the convoluted section are cuboidal/columnar cells with a luminal brush border consisting of millions of microvilli, which expand the surface area for absorption of tubular fluid. The proximal tubule is the most metabolically active part of the nephron (Table 48-1).

Loop of Henle

The pars recta drains into the descending thin loop of Henle, which, after passing through a hairpin loop, becomes first the thin ascending limb, and then the thick ascending limb. The cells of the thin ascending limb are very similar to those in the descending (with little brush border, flattened and interdigitated), but important differences are evident in their permeability to water and in their capability for active transport. The thick ascending limb is lined with cuboidal/columnar cells similar in size to those in the proximal tubule, but they do not possess a brush border. At the end of the thick ascending limb, near where it re-enters the cortex and is closely associated with the glomerulus and the efferent arteriole, a cluster of cells known as the *macula densa* is present (Figure 48-4; see later). The main role of the loop of Henle is to assist in generating concentrated urine, hypertonic with respect to plasma; it also has several other functions (see Table 48-1).

Distal Convoluted Tubule

The distal convoluted tubule begins at a variable distance beyond the macula densa and extends to the first fusion with other tubules to form the collecting ducts. The cells of the distal convoluted are tall and cuboidal and contain numerous mitochondria. Na^+,K^+-ATPase activity is higher than in any other segment of the nephron, being located in the basolateral membrane and providing the main driving force for ion transport. Reabsorption of sodium and chloride, with passive reabsorption of water, is the main function of the distal convoluted tubule (see later).

Collecting Duct

The collecting ducts are formed from approximately six distal tubules. These are successively joined by other tubules to form ducts of Bellini, which ultimately drain into a renal calyx. Two main cell types are found in the collecting duct: principal (light) cells and intercalated (dark) cells. Intercalated cells have a dark granular cytoplasm with high carbonic anhydrase activity but no Na^+,K^+-ATPase activity.

Juxtaglomerular Apparatus

Where the thick ascending limb of the loop of Henle passes very close to the glomerulus of its own nephron, the cells of the tubule and the afferent arteriole show regional specialization (see Figure 48-4). The tubule forms the macula densa; the arteriolar cells are filled with granules (containing renin or its inactive precursor, prorenin) and are innervated with sympathetic nerve fibers. This area, called the *JGA,* plays an important part in maintaining systemic blood pressure through regulation of the circulating intravascular blood volume and sodium concentration via the renin-angiotensin-aldosterone system (RAAS). The proteolytic enzyme renin is released primarily in response to decreased afferent arteriolar pressure and decreased intraluminal sodium delivery to the macula densa. Renin is an enzyme of the hydrolase class that catalyzes cleavage of the leucine-leucine bond in angiotensinogen to generate angiotensin I. Renin release from the macula densa is also influenced by nitric oxide, renal cortical prostaglandins (predominantly PGI_2), and the sympathetic nervous system. Angiotensin I is converted in the lungs by angiotensin-converting enzyme (ACE) to the potent vasoconstrictor and stimulator of aldosterone

TABLE 48-1 Metabolic Functions of the Different Parts of the Nephron

	Proximal		Loop of Henle		Distal Tubule		Collecting Duct	
Molecule	**R**	**S**	**R**	**S**	**R**	**S**	**R**	**S**
Urea	+			(+)			+	
Proteins	+							
Peptides	+							
Phosphate	+							
Sulfate	+							
Organic anions			+					
Urate	+	+						
Sodium	+		+		+		+	
Chloride	+		+		+		+	
Water	+		+				+	
Potassium	+		+	(+)		+	+	
Hydrogen ion		+		+		+	+	+
Bicarbonate	+		+		+		+	+
Ammonium		+	+					+
Calcium	+		+		+		+	

R, Reabsorption; *S*, secretion; + indicates function; (+) indicates partial function.

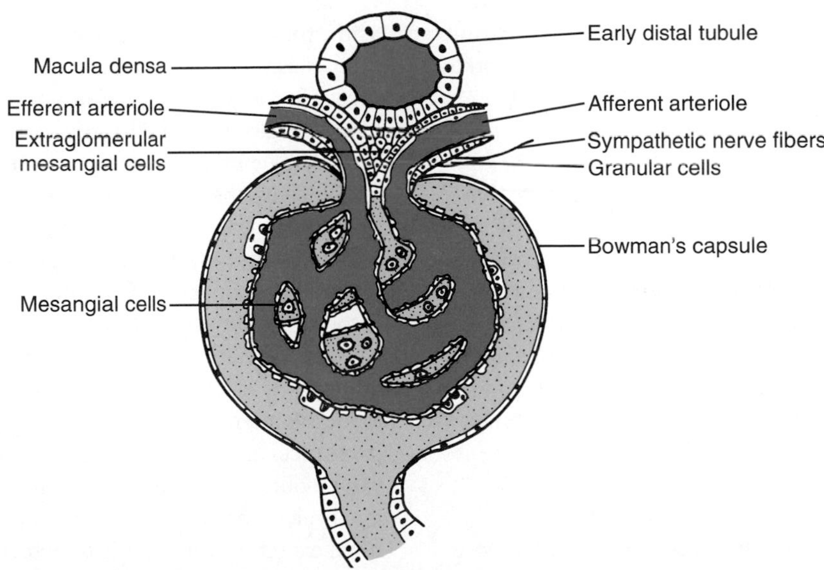

Figure 48-4 The juxtaglomerular apparatus. The beginning of the distal tubule (i.e., where the loop of Henle re-enters the cortex) lies very close to the afferent and efferent arterioles, and the cells of both the afferent arteriole and the tubule show specialization. The cells of the afferent arteriole are thickened, granular (juxtaglomerular) cells that are innervated by sympathetic nerve fibers. The mesangial cells are irregularly shaped and contain filaments of contractile proteins. Identical cells are found just outside the glomerulus and are termed *extraglomerular mesangial cells* or *Goormaghtigh cells*. *(From Lote CJ. Principles of renal physiology, 4th edition. London: Kluwer Academic Publishers, 2000:Chapter 2.)*

release, AII. Vasoconstriction and aldosterone release (with increased distal tubular sodium retention) act in concert with the other action of AII to increase the release of the nonapeptide ADH, and to increase proximal tubular sodium reabsorption, intravascular volume, and pressure. AII also has an inhibitory effect on renin release as part of a negative feedback loop.

Renal Interstitium

In a normal renal cortex, the interstitium is sparse (7 to 9% by volume) because the tubules lie very close together; however, a large proportion of the reabsorbed tubular fluid has to traverse a true interstitial space before entering the capillaries. The interstitium contains a variety of cell types, including lymphocytes and fibroblast-like cells.[361]

The medullary interstitium contains a further specialized cell, lipid-laden interstitial cells, which are arranged in a characteristic ladder-like pattern across the loops of Henle and the capillaries. The extracellular space is rich in glycosaminoglycans, resulting in a gelatinous matrix that contains various poorly characterized osmolytes, osmotically active molecules that help stabilize the high osmotic gradient essential to the countercurrent mechanism involved in the generation of hyperosmotic urine. The interstitium becomes very important in a variety of kidney diseases, and its expansion, as a consequence or cause of nephron loss, plays an important part in progressive kidney disease. Interstitial expansion includes cellular infiltration and increased interstitial matrix synthesis and interstitial fibrosis.

TABLE 48-2 Important Components of Kidney Function

Filtration	Preparation of an ultrafiltrate
Reabsorptive	Glucose, amino acids, electrolytes, proteins
Homeostatic	Extracellular volume, acid-base status, blood pressure, electrolytes
Metabolic	Synthetic: glutathione, glyconeogenesis, ammonia Catabolic: hormones, cytokines
Endocrine	Erythropoietin synthesis, activation of vitamin D, renin release

KIDNEY FUNCTION AND PHYSIOLOGY

The kidneys regulate and maintain the constant optimal chemical composition of the blood and interstitial and intracellular fluids throughout the body—the internal milieu—through integration of the major renal functions, namely, filtration, reabsorption, and excretion. Mechanisms of differential reabsorption and secretion, located in the tubule of a nephron, are the effectors of regulation (Table 48-2).

Excretory and Reabsorptive Functions

The *excretory function* of the kidneys serves to rid the body of many end products of metabolism and of excessive inorganic substances ingested in the diet. Waste products include the nonprotein nitrogenous compounds urea, creatinine, and uric acid; a number of other organic acids, including amino acids, are excreted in small quantities. Dietary intake contains a variable and usually excessive supply of sodium, potassium, chloride, calcium, phosphate, magnesium, sulfate, and bicarbonate. The efficiency of the homeostatic role of kidney function is illustrated by the way the sodium content of the body is maintained essentially constant, regardless of whether daily sodium intake is 1 or 150 mmol or more. Daily intake of water is also variable and may, on occasion, greatly exceed the requirements of the body. Under such circumstances, water becomes additional waste material requiring excretion. To achieve excretion of metabolic wastes and ingested surpluses without disrupting homeostasis, the kidneys must exercise both their *excretory* and *reabsorptive* functions.

Mechanisms for the regulation of electrolytes, nitrogenous wastes, and organic acids are similar, although not identical. For all, except potassium and hydrogen ions and a few organic acids, the maximal excretory rate is limited or established by their plasma concentrations and the rate of their filtration through the glomeruli. Bulk transfer of substances from blood to glomerular filtrate determines the initial mass on which the nephron must operate to produce and excrete urine. Thus the maximal amount of substance excreted in urine does not exceed the amount transferred through the glomeruli by ultrafiltration except in the case of those substances capable of being secreted by tubular cells. Depending on the activity of the renal tubular epithelial cells and their several reabsorptive capacities, excreted amounts of urinary constituents are in general less than the amounts filtered. Because of this general behavior, for many substances an estimate of the excretory capacity of the kidneys can be obtained by measuring the GFR or some variable that is closely related to it. The primary objective in evaluating renal excretory function is to detect quantitatively the degradation of normal capacities or the improvement of impaired ones.

Definitions

Urine is defined as a fluid excreted by the kidneys, passed through the ureters, stored in the bladder, and discharged through the urethra. In health, it is sterile and clear and has an amber color, a slightly acid pH (≈5.0 to 6.0), and a characteristic odor. In addition to dissolved compounds, it contains a number of cellular fragments and complete cells, derived from normal turnover of tubular cells, casts, and crystals (formed elements). Urinary casts are cylindrical proteinaceous structures formed in the distal convoluted tubule and collecting ducts, which dislodge and pass into the urine, where they can be detected by microscopy.

Urination, also termed *micturition,* is the discharge of urine. In normal adults, adequate homeostasis is maintained with a urine output of 400 to 2000 mL/d. Alterations in urinary output are described as *anuria* (<100 mL/d), *oliguria* (<400 mL/d), and *polyuria* (>3 L/d or 50 mL/kg body weight/d). The most common disorder of urination is altered frequency, which may be associated with increased urinary volume or with partial urinary tract obstruction (e.g., in prostatic hypertrophy).

Formation of Urine—An Overview

The first step in urine formation is filtration of plasma water at the glomeruli. A net filtration pressure of about 17 mm Hg in the capillary bed of the tuft drives the filtrate through the glomerular membrane. The filtrate is called an *ultrafiltrate* because its composition is essentially the same as that of plasma, but with a notable reduction in molecules of molecular weight exceeding 15 kDa. Each nephron produces about 100 μL of ultrafiltrate per day. Overall, approximately 170 to 200 L of ultrafiltrate passes through the glomeruli daily. In the passage of ultrafiltrate through the tubules, reabsorption of solutes and water in various regions of the tubules reduces the total urine volume.

Transport of solutes and water occurs both across and between the epithelial cells that line the renal tubules. Transport is both active requiring energy and passive, but many of the so-called passive transport processes are dependent upon or secondary to active transport processes, particularly those involving sodium transport. All known transport processes involve receptor or mediator molecules, the activity of many of which is regulated by phosphorylation facilitated by protein kinase C or A. Their renal distribution has been shown to correlate with known regional functional activities, but the same transporters, or isoforms of them, can be found in other tissues, particularly the digestive tract. For instance, at least five independent proximal tubular transport processes may be noted for amino acids, including those for (1) basic amino acids plus cystine, (2) glutamic and aspartic acid, (3) neutral amino acids, (4) imino amino acids, and (5) glycine.[489] Inherited disorders of tubular transporters, discussed later in this chapter, may occur, as well as a well-known generalized disorder affecting all of the transport processes, causing Fanconi syndrome and resulting in decreased reabsorption of electrolytes and nutrients (e.g., glucose, amino acids).

Direct coupling of adenosine triphosphate (ATP) hydrolysis is an example of an active transport process. The most important enzymatic transporter in the nephron is Na^+ K^+-ATPase, which is located on the basolateral membranes of the tubuloepithelial cells, accounts for much of the renal oxygen consumption, and drives more than 99% of renal sodium reabsorption (Figure 48-5). Other examples of primary active transport mechanisms include a calcium-ATPase, an H^+-ATPase, and an H^+,K^+-ATPase. These enzymes establish ionic gradients, polarizing cell membranes and thus driving secondary transport processes.

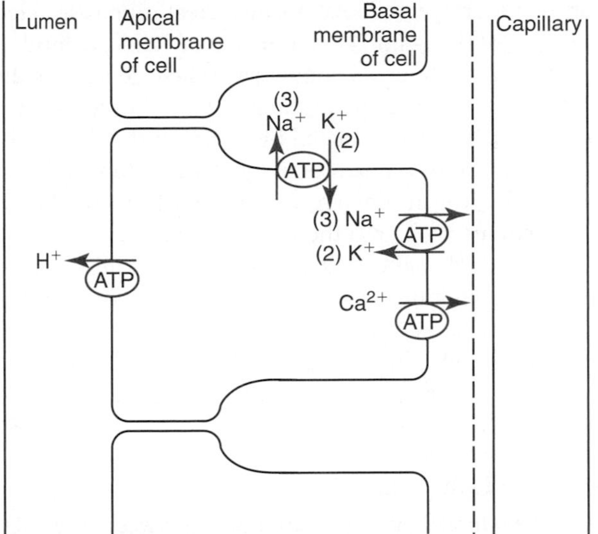

Figure 48-5 Tubular reabsorptive mechanisms: the major primary active transport processes in the proximal nephron. The renal tubular epithelium consists of a single layer of cells. At the luminal side, adjacent cells are in contact (the tight junction), whereas toward the basal side of the cells, there are gaps between adjacent cells (lateral intercellular spaces). *(From Lote CJ. Principles of renal physiology, 4th edition. London: Kluwer Academic Publishers, 2000:Chapter 4.)*

Many renal epithelial cell membranes also contain proteins that act as ion channels. For example, there is one for sodium that is closed by amiloride and modulated by hormones such as atrial natriuretic peptide (ANP). Ion channels enable much faster rates of transport than ATPases but are relatively fewer in number (e.g., ≈100 sodium and chloride channels vs. 10^7 Na^+,K^+-ATPase molecules per cell).

Different regions of the tubule have been shown to specialize in certain functions. The proximal tubule facilitates the reabsorption of 60 to 80% of the glomerular filtrate volume, including 70% of the filtered load of sodium and chloride, and most of the potassium, glucose, bicarbonate, calcium, phosphate, sulfate, and other ions—secreting 90% of the hydrogen ion excreted by the kidney (see Table 48-1). Glucose is virtually completely reabsorbed, predominantly in the proximal tubule, by a passive but sodium-dependent process that is saturated at a blood glucose concentration of about 180 mg/dL (10 mmol/L). Uric acid is also reabsorbed in the proximal tubule by a passive sodium-dependent mechanism, but an active secretory mechanism is present. Creatinine is secreted but only to a small extent—approximately 2.5 μmol/min.

Certain nonbiological compounds, such as phenolsulfonphthalein and *p*-aminohippurate, are secreted by the proximal tubule and have been used for the evaluation of renal tubular secretory capacity. When blood concentrations of creatinine increase to above normal, creatinine is secreted in this region of the nephron. In the loop of Henle, chloride and more sodium without water are reabsorbed, generating dilute urine. Water reabsorption in the more distal tubules and collecting ducts is then regulated by ADH. In the distal tubule, secretion is the prominent activity; organic ions, potassium ions, and hydrogen ions are transported from the blood in the efferent arteriole into the tubular fluid.

Tubular epithelial cells synthesize a vast range of growth factors and cytokines in response to a variety of stimuli that can have both autocrine and paracrine effects. All cells secrete a variety of cell adhesion molecules that are essential for cellular attachment to the tubular basement membrane.

Regulatory Function

Electrolyte Homeostasis

A complex interplay has been noted between the tubular transport systems regulating individual electrolytes. For simplicity, we have considered each electrolyte individually and have restricted our discussion to the systems of major physiological, pharmacologic, and pathologic significance.

Sodium

Sodium reabsorption is required for the reabsorption of water and many solutes. The proximal tubule is highly permeable to sodium, and the net flux of reabsorption from the tubular lumen is achieved against a high backflux, particularly from paracellular* movement. Approximately 60% of filtered sodium is reabsorbed in the proximal tubule in an energy-dependent manner, driven by basolateral Na^+,K^+-ATPase pumps. Approximately 80% of sodium entering proximal tubular cells does so in exchange for hydrogen ion secretion, facilitated by apical Na-H exchangers. This process in turn permits bicarbonate reabsorption via carbonic anhydrases that are present in both the brush border and the intracellular compartment. A variety of apical sodium cotransporters also allow for reabsorption of other organic and inorganic solutes (e.g., chloride, calcium, phosphates, bicarbonate, sulfates,[406] glucose, urea, amino acids). Sodium transport activity is regulated by many factors, including protein kinase–dependent phosphorylation, which can increase both activity and channel numbers.

A further 30% of filtered sodium is reabsorbed in the thick ascending limb of the loop of Henle, where it is achieved by an apical, bumetanide-sensitive, 130 kDa, electroneutral, Na-K-2Cl cotransporter (NKCC2), itself driven by a favorable inward gradient generated by the basolateral Na^+,K^+-ATPase pump (Figure 48-6). NKCC2 is a kidney-specific member of a class of such channels found throughout secretory epithelia. Activation of these cotransporters appears, in part, to be a result of cell shrinkage. The distal tubule reabsorbs 5 to 8% of sodium via the apical thiazide-sensitive Na-Cl cotransporter (NCCT). Final sodium balance is achieved in the

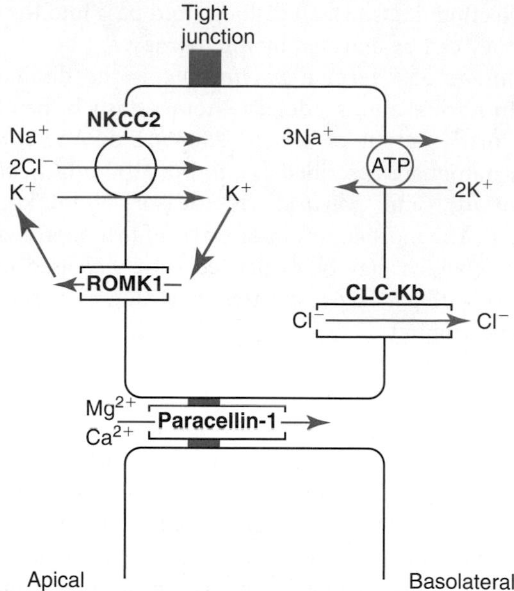

Figure 48-6 Schematic diagram showing the major pathways of solute reabsorption in the thick ascending limb of the loop of Henle. Sodium chloride is reabsorbed by the apical NKCC2 transporter. This electroneutral transport is driven by the low intracellular sodium and chloride concentrations generated by the basolateral Na^+,Ka^+-ATPase and the basolateral chloride channel CLC-Kb. The availability of potassium is rate-limiting for NKCC2, so potassium entering the cell is recycled back to the lumen via the ROMKI potassium channel. This potassium movement is electrogenic and drives paracellular resorption of Mg^{2+} and Ca^{2+} via paracellin-1. Mutations in NKCC2, ROMK1, or CLC-Kb cause Bartter's syndrome. Mutations in paracellin-1 lead to disruption of this paracellular pathway and the tubular disease known as *hypomagnesemic hypercalciuric nephrolithiasis*.[3] *(From Sayer JA, Pearce SHS. Diagnosis and clinical biochemistry of inherited tubulopathies. Ann Clin Biochem 2001;38: 459-70.)*

collecting duct via selective amiloride-sensitive, apical sodium channels (ENaCs) in exchange for potassium. ENaCs are controlled in part by the effects of aldosterone on the mineralocorticoid receptor (Figure 48-7).

Potassium

Approximately 90% of daily potassium loss occurs via renal elimination. Potassium is freely filtered across the glomerulus and normally is almost completely reabsorbed in the proximal tubule. However, most regulatory mechanisms affect the loop of Henle, the distal tubule, and the collecting duct. Indeed, urinary losses can exceed filtered load, indicating the importance of distal secretion. Determinants of urinary potassium loss are dietary intake of potassium and plasma potassium concentration, acid-base disturbances (acidosis reduces potassium secretion and vice versa), circulating ADH concentration (ADH increases potassium loss[119]), tubular flow rate (increased flow rate increases potassium loss[240]), and aldosterone secretion (enhances potassium loss and increases

*Paracellular transport is that occurring between tubular epithelial cells and occurs by passive diffusion or by solvent drag.

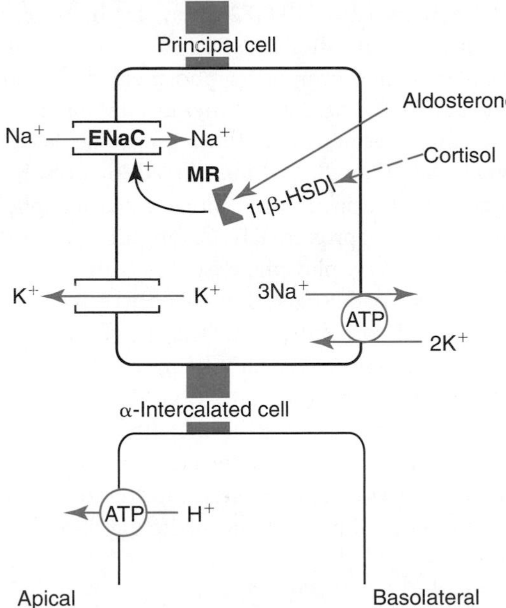

Figure 48-7 Schematic diagram showing the major pathways of solute reabsorption in the collecting duct. In principal cells, sodium reabsorption occurs through the amiloride-sensitive epithelial sodium channel (ENaC). Sodium reabsorption is influenced by the actions of aldosterone on the mineralocorticoid receptor (MR), with hyperaldosteronism producing an increase in channel activity. Cortisol, if permitted, will also bind to the MR, but a degree of specificity is maintained by 11β-hydroxysteroid dehydrogenase (11β-HSD), which inactivates cortisol to cortisone. Sodium uptake drives potassium secretion from principal cells and proton secretion from α-intercalated cells. In Liddle's syndrome, mutations lead to an increase in ENaC activity, with increased Na^+ reabsorption and consequent potassium and proton loss. In pseudohypoaldosteronism type Ia, loss-of-function mutations inactivate ENaC, whereas in pseudohypoaldosteronism type Ib, there are MR abnormalities. Both lead to reduced sodium entry via ENaC, causing salt wasting and decreased secretion of potassium and protons. Licorice causes hypertension and a hypokalemic metabolic alkalosis by inactivating 11β-HSD, allowing cortisol to act as a mineralocorticoid. *(From Sayer JA, Pearce SHS. Diagnosis and clinical biochemistry of inherited tubulopathies. Ann Clin Biochem 2001;38:459-70.)*

sodium retention).[153] Potassium ions are actively accumulated within tubular cells as a result of basolateral Na^+,K^+-ATPase activity, resulting in elevation of intracellular potassium concentration to above its electrochemical equilibrium. Several types of potassium channels exist that have a number of functions: (1) maintenance of a negative resting cell membrane potential, (2) regulation of intracellular volume, (3) recycling of potassium across apical and basolateral membranes to supply NKCC2 and enable sodium reabsorption, and (4) potassium secretion in the cortical collecting tubule.[32] As mentioned previously, potassium is reabsorbed with sodium by NKCC2 in the thick ascending limb of the loop of Henle, but it is recycled back into the lumen by the potassium-secreting channel, ROMK1, thus generating an electrical gradient that drives passive paracellular reabsorption of calcium and magnesium down their electrochemical gradient[3] (see Figure 48-6). ROMK1 is a pH-sensitive, membrane-spanning protein with several serine residues. At least two of these residues require phosphorylation by protein kinase A for the channel to be active.[32]

In the principal cells of the collecting duct, sodium reabsorption via ENaC is accompanied by movement of potassium into the lumen through potassium channels or through a K-Cl symporter* (see Figure 48-7).

Chloride

Approximately 60% of chloride is reabsorbed in the proximal tubule. In the early part of the proximal tubule, avid reabsorption of sodium in combination with glucose and amino acids occurs, creating a lumen-negative potential difference. The negative potential difference drives chloride reabsorption by diffusion through the paracellular pathway. Preferential reabsorption of glucose, amino acids, and bicarbonate in association with sodium in the early proximal tubule causes an increase in the luminal chloride concentration. This high chloride composition heralds the second phase of proximal chloride (and sodium) reabsorption: passive diffusion of sodium chloride via the paracellular pathway, and active reabsorption involving several antiporter† systems, by which chloride is exchanged for secretion of other anions (e.g., bicarbonate, formate, oxalate). In the thick ascending limb of the loop of Henle, further chloride reabsorption occurs in association with sodium via NKCC2. The concentration gradient is maintained by a basolateral chloride pump, CLC-Kb (see Figure 48-6).[239]

Calcium

Approximately 98% of filtered calcium is reabsorbed: 65 to 75% in the proximal tubule (via a paracellular pathway), 20 to 25% in the thick ascending limb of the loop of Henle, 10% in the distal tubule, and, finally, small amounts in the collecting ducts. Calcium reabsorption is predominantly a passive process linked to active sodium reabsorption. For example, in the thick ascending limb of the loop of Henle, paracellular calcium transport is driven by the potential difference created by ROMK1. Active processes, particularly in the distal tubule, tightly regulate the final amount of calcium excreted. Here, calcium reabsorption is transcellular, occurring against the existing electrochemical gradient, and is stimulated by parathyroid hormone (PTH). Following entry into the cell from

*A symporter is an integral membrane protein that is involved in movement of two or more different molecules or ions across a phospholipid membrane such as the plasma membrane in the same direction, and is therefore a type of cotransporter.

†An antiporter (also called exchanger or counter-transporter) is an integral membrane protein which is involved in secondary active transport of two or more different molecules or ions (i.e., solutes) across a phospholipid membrane such as the plasma membrane in opposite directions.

the lumen via an apical epithelial active transport mechanism (ECaC1), calcium binds to calbindin-D and is delivered to the basolateral membrane. Here it is extruded by a calcium-ATPase (PMCA1b) and an Na-Ca exchanger (NCX1). Transcription of messenger RNA coding for both ECaC1 and calbindin is stimulated by calcitriol [1,25(OH_2)D_3], possibly synthesized locally in the distal nephron and acting in a paracrine and autocrine fashion. A functional vitamin D response element has been identified in the promoter region of the calbindin-D gene, along with a putative site in the ECaC1 gene. ECaC1 is a pH-sensitive, 83 kDa protein with six transmembrane-spanning domains. Activation of the ion channel probably involves protein kinase C phosphorylation. Evidence indicates that stimulation of the renal calcium-sensing receptor by calcium in the tubular lumen can directly affect tubular reabsorption of calcium, independent of the effects of calciotropic hormones.[187]

Phosphate

Reabsorption of phosphate occurs predominantly in the proximal tubule and is mediated by a secondary active transport mechanism. Three families (types I, II, and III) of sodium-dependent, phosphate cotransporters have been identified, of which type IIa (NPT2a, SLC34A1), a 640 amino acid protein located in the apical plasma membrane, is thought to be the most physiologically important. NPT2a sodium-phosphate transporter is electrogenic (i.e., involves the inward flux of a positive charge), with three sodium ions and one phosphate ion (preferentially divalent) being transferred. Acute regulation of transport is achieved primarily by an alteration in the amount of NPT2a protein present in the apical membrane, with longer-term changes also involving increased transcription of the protein [e.g., in response to 1,25(OH_2)D_3]. Tonic amounts of NPT2a in the apical membrane are thought to be high, with regulation predominantly involving internalization of the protein. Increased intracellular movement of the channel from the plasma membrane to the lysosomes is believed to follow both protein kinase A and C phosphorylation initiated by PTH receptor binding.[429,430] Fibroblast growth factor 23 (FGF-23), is a 32 kDa phosphate-regulating peptide, largely produced by bone cells. It was discovered during the 1990s following studies of severe hereditary osteomalacia characterized by severe hypophosphatemia and inappropriate phosphaturia.[56] Its major action is the inhibition of sodium-coupled reabsorption of inorganic phosphate in the renal proximal tubule. Autosomal dominant hypophosphatemic rickets is due to a mutation in the *FGF-23* gene that results in a hyperstable form of this protein.[26] The current paradigm suggests that phosphate ingestion and/or hyperphosphatemia causes FGF-23 release into the circulation from skeletal osteocytes and osteoblasts and interacts with receptors within the kidney via a transmembrane protein, klotho, thereby inhibiting the sodium-coupled phosphate cotransporter in the proximal tubule (Na-Pi type IIa, or NPt2a) and causing phosphaturia. FGF-23 also inhibits 1α-vitamin D hydroxylase, leading to reduced calcitriolproduction. These effects will reduce plasma phosphate concentrations. FGF23 may act in concert with PTH by reducing expression of NPT2a at the proximal tubule brush border, hence promoting phosphaturia.[196] Efflux of phosphate across the basolateral membrane may involve an anion-exchange mechanism and/or a phosphate leak.

Normally, less than 20% of the filtered load of phosphate is excreted into the urine, but above a plasma phosphate concentration of approximately 3.6 mg/dL (1.2 mmol/L), increments in urinary phosphate excretion increase linearly with the filtered load, suggesting that there is T_m (tubular maximal uptake) for phosphate. The T_m for phosphate is decreased by increases in the circulating PTH concentration and the ratio of T_m for phosphate to GFR (T_mP/GFR). T_mP/GFR has been used as a test in the differential diagnosis of hypercalcemia. Although superseded in this context by modern PTH assays, it may be useful in the investigation of inherited disorders of tubular phosphate handling.[340]

Bicarbonate and Hydrogen Ion

The kidney plays a central role in the maintenance of acid-base homeostasis through reabsorption of filtered bicarbonate and secretion of ammonium and acid. The tubular mechanisms underlying these processes are discussed in Chapter 49.

Water Homeostasis

Approximately 180 L glomerular filtrate is formed each day. The unique physiology of the kidney enables approximately 99% of this to be reabsorbed in the production of urine with variable osmolality (between 50 and 1400 mOsmol/kg H_2O at extremes of water intake). Plasma membranes of all mammalian cells are water permeable but to variable degrees. In the kidney, different segments of the nephron show differing permeability to water, enabling the body to both retain water and produce urine of variable concentration. Water reabsorption occurs both isosmotically, in association with electrolyte reabsorption in the proximal tubule, and differentially, in the loop of Henle, distal tubule, and collecting duct in response to the action of ADH. Absorption of water depends on the driving force for water reabsorption (predominantly active sodium transport) and the osmotic equilibration of water across the tubular epithelium. The generation of concentrated urine depends upon medullary hyperosmolality; this in turn requires low water permeability in some kidney segments (ascending limb of the loop of Henle), whereas in other kidney segments (e.g., proximal tubule), there is a requirement for high water permeability. Differing permeability and enaction of hormonal control appear to be largely caused by differential expression along the nephron of a family of proteins known as the aquaporins (AQPs), which act as water channels.

At least 11 different mammalian AQPs have been identified, of which seven (AQP1, -2, -3, -4, -6, -7, -8) are expressed in the kidney.[320,321] Many of these have extrarenal expression sites as well (e.g., AQP1 may be important in fluid removal across the peritoneal membrane). Two asparagine-proline-alanine sequences in the molecule are thought to interact in the membrane to form a pathway for water translocation. AQP1, which is found in the proximal tubule and the descending thin limb of the loop of Henle, constitutes almost 3% of total membrane protein in the kidney. It appears to be constitutively expressed and is present in both the apical and basolateral plasma membranes, representing entry and exit ports for water transport across the cell, respectively. Approximately 70% of water reabsorption occurs at this site, predominantly via a transcellular (e.g., AQP1) rather than a paracellular route. Water reabsorption in the proximal tubule passively follows sodium reabsorption, so that fluid entering the loop of Henle is almost isosmotic with plasma.

Urinary concentration is predominantly achieved by countercurrent multiplication in the loop of Henle (Figure 48-8).[364,383] The descending thin limb is very permeable to water, but the ascending limb and the collecting duct are not (the collecting ducts are also poorly permeable to urea). Fluid entering the loop of Henle is isotonic to plasma but is hypotonic on leaving it. The ascending limb has active sodium reabsorption driven by Na^+,K^+-ATPase with electroneutralizing transport of chloride—a combined process that can be inhibited by the so-called loop diuretics (e.g., furosemide; see discussion later in this chapter). In this section of the nephron, sodium reabsorption is not accompanied by water, creating a hypertonic medullary interstitium and facilitating water reabsorption from the anatomically adjacent descending limb. The descending limb cells are permeable to sodium chloride, which is cycled from the descending limb back to the ascending limb. Continuous flow along the loop generates an osmotic gradient at the tip of the loop that can reach 1400 mOsmol/kg H_2O. Approximately 5% of water is reabsorbed in the loop of Henle.

A further 10% of water reabsorption occurs in the distal tubule, with the remainder (>20 L/d) reabsorbed in the collecting ducts. Entry of water into the collecting duct cells occurs via apical AQP2 channels, with exit probably occurring via basolateral AQP3 (cortical and outer medullary collecting ducts) and AQP4 (inner medullary collecting ducts). AQP2 appears to be the primary target for ADH regulation of water reabsorption. AQP2 is stored in subapical vesicles in the collecting duct cells. In response to ADH stimulation, these vesicles are cycled through, and inserted into, the plasma membrane by a cytoskeletal, dynein-mediated transport process. Stimulation occurs following binding of ADH

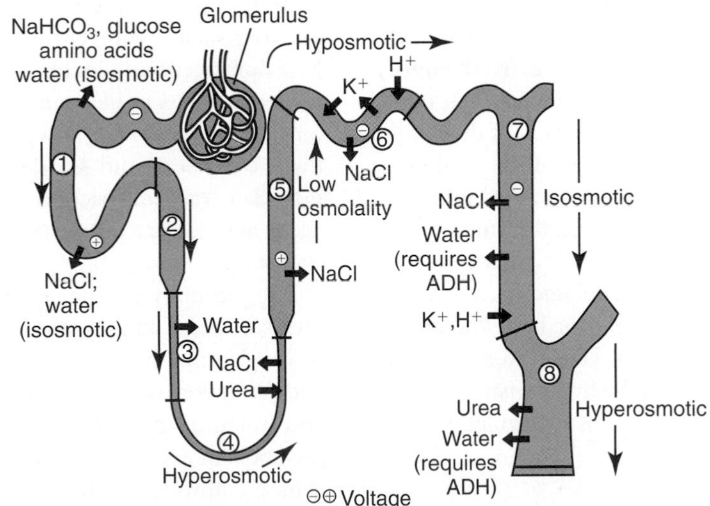

Figure 48-8 Countercurrent multiplication mechanism: schematic representation of the principal processes of transport in the nephron. In the convoluted portion of the proximal tubule *(1)*, salts and water are reabsorbed at high rates in isotonic proportions. Bulk reabsorption of most of the filtrate (65 to 70%) and virtually complete reabsorption of glucose, amino acids, and bicarbonate take place in this segment. In the pars recta *(2)*, organic acids are secreted and continuous reabsorption of sodium chloride takes place. The loop of Henle comprises three segments: the thin descending *(3)* and ascending *(4)* limbs and the thick ascending limb *(5)*. The fluid becomes hyperosmotic, because of water abstraction, as it flows toward the bend of the loop, and hyposmotic, because of sodium chloride reabsorption, as it flows toward the distal convoluted tubule *(6)*. Active sodium reabsorption occurs in the distal convoluted tubule and in the cortical collecting tubule *(7)*. This latter segment is water impermeable in the absence of antidiuretic hormone (ADH), and reabsorption of sodium in this segment is increased by aldosterone. The collecting duct *(8)* allows equilibration of water with the hyperosmotic interstitium when ADH is present. For additional details, see text.
(From Burg MB. The nephron in transport of sodium, amino acids, and glucose. Hosp Pract 1978;13:100. Adapted from a drawing by A. Iselin.)

to a V_2 receptor in the basolateral plasma membrane of the principal cells of the collecting duct, which promotes a cyclic adenosine monophosphate (cAMP)/protein kinase A cascade, resulting in phosphorylation and activation of AQP2. ADH regulates the acute cellular water-retaining response (AQP2 trafficking) and its longer-term regulation via a conditioning effect on AQP2 gene transcription. The AQP2 gene has a cAMP response element that is involved in the long-term upregulation of AQP2 expression by ADH. It is likely that there are also ADH-independent regulatory pathways of AQP2 expression. Membrane insertion of AQP2 allows water to pass into the collecting duct cells under the influence of medullary hyperosmolality. Maintenance of medullary hyperosmolality depends upon efficient fluid removal, which is the function of the ascending vasa recta, a specialized medullary vasculature, and the close anatomic relations of all medullary constituents (see Figure 48-2). AQP2 expression is decreased in a variety of polyuric conditions (e.g., diabetes insipidus, lithium treatment, hypokalemia, hypercalcemia, urinary obstruction) and is increased in some water-retaining states (e.g., heart failure, cirrhosis, pregnancy).[321,396] A variety of V_2 receptor antagonists have been designed that block the actions of ADH. In contrast to diuretics, these agents promote the excretion of electrolyte-free water and have exciting therapeutic potential in water-retaining states.[396]

ADH also increases the permeability of collecting duct cells to urea, which is the major osmotically active component of luminal fluid in the distal tubule. Fluid of high urea concentration therefore enters the deepest layers of the medullary interstitium, passing down its concentration gradient, contributing to medullary hyperosmolality. Regulation of ADH excretion is of vital importance to fluid homeostasis. Normal plasma osmolality is maintained very tightly between 280 and 290 mOsmol/kg H_2O and is regulated by means of specific osmoreceptors found in the anterior hypothalamus. These receptors modulate the release of ADH and also affect thirst. ADH release may be stimulated by hypotension, hypovolemia, and vomiting independently of osmoregulation.

Endocrine Function

The *endocrine functions* of the kidneys may be regarded as primary, because the kidneys are endocrine organs producing hormones, or as secondary, because the kidneys are a site of action for hormones produced or activated elsewhere. In addition, the kidneys are a site of degradation for hormones such as insulin and aldosterone. In their primary endocrine function, the kidneys produce erythropoietin (EPO), prostaglandins and thromboxanes, $1,25(OH_2)D_3$, and renin. The importance of renin in the maintenance of systemic blood pressure was discussed previously (see earlier, "Juxtaglomerular Apparatus").

Erythropoietin

EPO is a large glycoprotein hormone (MW 34 kDa) containing 165 amino acids and is responsible for stimulating erythroid progenitor cells within the bone marrow to produce red blood cells. It is secreted chiefly by renal peritubular capillary endothelial cells in the adult and by the liver in the fetus. Physiologically, the kidneys sense a reduction in oxygen delivery to tissues by blood and release EPO, thereby stimulating erythropoiesis. Conversely, with a surplus of oxygen in blood traversing the kidneys, as in some forms of polycythemia, the release of EPO into blood is diminished. The use of recombinant human erythropoietin (rhEPO, epoetin) in the management of anemia of kidney disease is discussed later.

Prostaglandins and Thromboxanes

Prostaglandins and thromboxanes are synthesized from arachidonic acid by the cyclooxygenase (COX) enzyme system (see Chapter 27 for further details). The COX system is present in many parts of the kidney and has an important role in regulating the physiologic action of other hormones on renal vascular tone, mesangial contractility, and tubular processing of salt and water. Prostaglandins have a critical role in renal hemodynamics, control of tubular function, and renin release. The major renal vasodilatory prostaglandin is PGE_2, which is synthesized predominantly in the medulla. The major vasoconstrictor prostaglandin is thromboxane A_2, which is produced primarily within the renal cortex.[101] PGE_2 increases renal blood flow rate, inhibits sodium reabsorption in the distal nephron and collecting duct, and stimulates renin release.[101] These actions promote natriuresis and diuresis. In patients with chronic kidney disease (CKD), renal PGE_2 production is increased, representing a compensatory response to loss of nephron mass.[438] Vasodilatory prostaglandins are synthesized following stimulation with renal sympathetic adrenergic and AII-dependent mechanisms to offset or modulate vasoconstriction.[295] In the tubule, prostaglandins act as autocoids, exerting their effects locally, near the site of synthesis.

In pathophysiologic circumstances, including various forms of acute kidney injury, thromboxane A_2 and various prostaglandins may have a significant role in inflammation and alteration of vascular tone. The effects of nonsteroidal anti-inflammatory drugs (NSAIDs) on renal prostaglandin metabolism are considered later in this chapter. The lipoxygenase pathway, which leads to formation of leukotrienes, is also present within the kidneys, although the major source of leukotrienes in inflammatory disease of the kidneys is infiltrating white cells and macrophages.

$1,25(OH_2)D_3$

The kidneys are primarily responsible for producing $1,25(OH_2)D_3$ from 25-hydroxycholecalciferol as a result of the action of the enzyme 25-hydroxycholecalciferol 1α-hydroxylase found in proximal tubular epithelial cells. Regulation of this system is discussed in Chapter 52. The management of renal osteodystrophy is considered later in this chapter.

Glomerular Filtration Rate

The GFR is considered to be the most reliable measure of the functional capacity of the kidneys and is often thought of as indicative of the number of functioning nephrons. As a physiological measurement, it has proved to be the most sensitive and specific marker of changes in overall renal function. Measurement of GFR is discussed in Chapter 25.

The rate of formation of the glomerular filtrate depends on the balance between hydrostatic and oncotic forces along the afferent arteriole and across the glomerular filter. The net pressure difference must be sufficient not only to drive filtration across the glomerular filtration barrier but also to drive the ultrafiltrate along the tubules against their inherent resistance to flow. In the absence of sufficient pressure, the lumina of the tubules will collapse. This balance of forces can be expressed as follows:

$$\text{Rate of Filtration} = K_f\left(\left(P_{GCap} + \Pi_{BC}\right) - \left(P_{BG} + \Pi_{GCap}\right)\right)$$

where

K_f = (hydraulic permeability × surface area)
P_{GCap} = glomerular-capillary hydrostatic pressure
Π_{BC} = oncotic pressure in Bowman's capsule
P_{BC} = hydrostatic pressure in Bowman's capsule
Π_{GCap} = oncotic pressure in the glomerular capillary

Because the oncotic pressure in Bowman's capsule (Π_{BC}) can be considered to be negligible (protein concentration is usually 10 to 100 mg/L), this equation becomes

$$\text{Rate of Filtration} = K_f\left(P_{GCap} - P_{BC} - \Pi_{GCap}\right)$$

Changes in K_f are caused by drugs and by glomerular disease, but it is also physiologically regulated. Mesangial cell contraction, which is thought to be the main mechanism, causes a reduction in K_f, tending to reduce GFR. Net P_{GCap} represents a balance between renal arterial pressure and afferent and efferent arteriolar resistance. Although an increase in arterial pressure will tend to increase P_{GCap}, the magnitude of the change is modulated by differential manipulation of afferent and efferent tone, which can result in minimal change to the P_{GCap}. When the renal blood flow is low, oncotic pressure can change as the plasma passes along the renal capillaries. As filtrate is removed, the oncotic pressure rises, and by the end of the capillary, the net filtration rate may become zero; thus GFR falls, and this limits the amount of filtrate that can be obtained from a given volume of plasma. The average ($P_{GCap} - P_{BC} - \Pi_{GCap}$) or net filtration pressure is only about 17 mm Hg. This pressure is sufficient to drive the filtration of 180 L of fluid per day, only because the K_f for glomerular capillaries is several orders of magnitude greater than for nonrenal capillaries.

Regulation of GFR

The factors involved in regulation of GFR are listed in Table 48-3. Autoregulation of renal blood flow and GFR is widely thought to be explained by the *myogenic theory.* This theory is based on the principle that an increase in wall tension of the afferent arterioles, brought about by an increase in perfusion pressure, causes automatic contraction of arteriolar smooth muscle, thus increasing resistance and keeping the flow constant despite the increase in perfusion pressure.

The *tubuloglomerular feedback mechanism,* involving the macula densa and release of the vasodilator adenosine, must also be considered. Although not fully understood, this mechanism appears to regulate GFR, with changes in renal blood flow as a secondary consequence. For individual nephrons, evidence indicates that each single nephron GFR (SNGFR) is influenced by the composition of the tubular fluid in the distal tubule, which in turn is influenced by the filtration rate. The macula densa is thought to sense the distal tubular sodium chloride content, its osmolality, or the rate at which sodium chloride is transported. The macula densa then signals the JGA via an uncertain mechanism to cause the release of adenosine and possibly AII and prostaglandins, which in turn affects vascular resistance.*

TABLE 48-3 Summary of Factors That Influence the Glomerular Filtration Rate (see text for explanation of terminology)

	Major Influencing Factors	Effect on GFR
Kf	Increased glomerular surface area due to relaxation of mesangial cells	Increase
	Decreased glomerular surface area due to contraction of mesangial cells	Decrease
P_{GCap}	Altered renal arterial pressure	
	Afferent dilation	Increase
	Afferent constriction	Decrease
	Efferent constriction	Increase
	Efferent dilation	Decrease
P_{BC}	Increased intratubular pressure (e.g., tubular obstruction)	Decrease
Π_{GCap}	Altered plasma oncotic pressure: increased	Decrease
	Altered renal blood flow: decreased	Decrease

The result of the combination of myogenic mechanisms and tubuloglomerular feedback is that the net filtration pressure or P_{GCap} is kept reasonably constant over a wide variety of systemic arterial pressures. It should be noted that renal blood flow and GFR change across this variety of systemic pressures but to a significantly smaller extent than would be predicted if these autoregulatory mechanisms were not in place.

Other factors influencing renal blood flow are indicated in Table 48-4. The afferent and efferent arterioles are richly supplied with renal sympathetic nerves. Epinephrine acts via α-adrenergic receptors, leading to constriction of both arterioles and causing a decrease in renal blood flow.

Nitric oxide (NO) has been identified as an important vasodilator produced by vascular endothelial cells. NO is synthesized from L-arginine and oxygen by nitric oxide synthetase (NOS), of which three isoenzymes are differentially located and regulated. Within the kidney are eNOS

*Vascular resistance is the resistance to flow that must be overcome to push blood through the circulatory system.

TABLE 48-4 Factors Altering Renal Artery Tone and Renal Blood Flow

	Effect On		Effect On	
Factor	**Afferent Arteriole**	**Efferent Arteriole**	**RBF**	**GFR**
Adenosine	Constriction	Dilation	N	N→NE
Angiotensin II	Constriction	Constriction	N	N
Epinephrine/norepinephrine	Constriction	Constriction	N	N→NE
Antidiuretic hormone (ADH)	Constriction	Constriction	NE	N→NE
Endothelin	Constriction	Constriction	NE	N→NE
Leukotrienes	Constriction	Constriction	NE	N→NE
Thromboxane A_2	Constriction	Constriction	NE	N→NE
Prostaglandins (PGE_2, PGI_2)	Dilation	Dilation	NE	NE
Nitric oxide	Dilation	Dilation	N	N
Atrial natriuretic factor	Dilation	Constriction	N	N→P
Dopamine	–	Dilation	N	N

GFR, Glomerular filtration rate; *N,* negative; *NE,* negligible; *P,* positive; *RBF,* renal blood flow.

(endothelial) and iNOS (inducible) isoenzymes. Activation of NOS has been shown to occur as a result of shear stress (e.g., increased arteriolar tone). A variety of physiologic vasoconstrictors are present, including acetylcholine, bradykinin, endothelin, and serotonin; a rise in intracellular ionized calcium is required for the vasoconstrictors. NO synthesis is now known to play an important role in the regulation of human vascular tone and has a crucial role in control of blood pressure and kidney function.[102,160,359] It has also been found in the macula densa and has been implicated in the regulation of renin release.

Age and the Kidney

Kidney function is not constant throughout life. In utero, urine is produced by the developing fetus from about the ninth week of gestation. Nephrogenesis is complete by approximately 35 weeks' gestation, although kidney function remains immature during the first 2 years of life. The kidney of the term infant receives approximately 6% of the cardiac output, compared with 25% in adults. Renal vascular resistance is relatively high, and the low renal blood flow is particularly directed to the medulla and inner cortex. The gradual increase in renal blood flow that occurs with increasing age is directed mainly to the outer cortex and is mediated by local neurohormonal mechanisms.[216] The GFR at birth is approximately 30 mL/min/1.73 m^2.[72] It increases rapidly during the first weeks of life to reach approximately 70 mL/min/1.73 m^2 by age 16 days.[72] Normal adult values are achieved by age 14 years. Tubular functions, including salt and water conservation, are also immature at birth. Birth is associated with rapid changes in kidney function, with a switch to salt and water conservation mediated by catecholamines, the renin-angiotensin system, ADH, glucocorticoids, and thyroid hormone.[72] The immaturity of the neonatal kidney contributes to the relatively common problems of water and electrolyte disturbances in infants. These disturbances are more likely to occur in premature infants, particularly those born before 35 weeks' gestation.

Aging is associated with a variety of structural changes in the kidney, which begin in early middle age, including decreasing kidney weight and number of glomeruli, with the cortical glomeruli being particularly affected.[110,222] Changes in the afferent and efferent arteriolar systems are evident, with formation of direct channels (shunts) between afferent and efferent arterioles in the medulla. Aging is also associated with the development of tubulointerstitial fibrosis, loss of tubular mass, and decreasing length of the proximal tubule.

Structural change is accompanied by functional changes, which in many respects are the reverse of those seen in early life. On average, GFR declines with age by approximately 1 mL/min/1.73 m^2/y over the age of 40 years.[11,92,375,459] Renal blood flow, particularly to the cortical area, also decreases with age, while the filtration fraction (i.e., GFR/renal plasma flow)[11] and renal vascular resistance[123,124] increase. Tubular function, such as the ability to concentrate urine and excrete a water and salt load, is decreased, and nocturnal polyuria is common. Renal salt conservation is impaired,[110] and the prevalence of albuminuria rises over the age of approximately 40 years.[95,213]

It is not known whether these changes are the result of a normal aging process (i.e., involutional) or whether they are caused by the interplay of pathology and age. Cumulative exposure to common causes of CKD such as (1) atherosclerosis, (2) hypertension, (3) heart failure, (4) diabetes,[65] (5) obstructive nephropathy, (6) infection, (7) immune insult, (8) nephrotoxins such as lead,[262] and (9) dietary protein[5,47] increases with age, and it is difficult to separate these effects from those of "healthy" aging. The decline in GFR with increasing age may be largely attributable to hypertension,[265,266] atherosclerosis,[222] or heart failure.[122] In the absence of these and other identifiable causes of kidney disease, many individuals have stable GFR as they age.

Loss of kidney function with aging appears to be heterogeneous and is not inevitable.[123,264] Kidney function may be well preserved in healthy older people, and assumptions with respect to GFR based solely on age could be erroneous.

Conversely, attention to the common causes of CKD could preserve function in older people.[395] Kidney disease is more common among older people. Studies from England,[116] France,[217] and Iceland[281] have demonstrated a near exponential rise in CKD with age. Data from the United States on CKD prevalence show the prevalence of a GFR between 30 and 60 mL/min/1.73 m^2 to be 4.3% of the total noninstitutionalized population overall, but this rises to 25% among those over 70 years.[83] The prevalence may be even higher among institutionalized older people (e.g., 82% of a residential home population were identified as having a GFR <60 mL/min/1.73 m^2).[61] The incidence of acute kidney injury also increases with age.[230]

Glomerular and Tubular Protein Handling

Glomerular permselectivity to proteins is a function of the integrated actions of endothelial cells, the GBM, and the podocytes, although the exact contribution and importance of each is still a matter of some debate. A variety of methods have been used to study the permeability of the glomerular barrier, including urinalysis in vivo, micropuncture of single nephrons, isolated perfused kidneys, isolated glomeruli, isolated GBMs, and artificial membranes. All of these techniques have contributed to knowledge of glomerular permeability characteristics, and all have advantages and disadvantages. For example, micropuncture techniques may damage the barrier. These issues have been reviewed by Haraldsson and associates.[170] Additionally, a number of different markers, including endogenous and modified proteins, dextran, and Ficoll polymers, have been used to study glomerular permeability.[170]

Glomerular Sieving

The glomerular permeability of a molecule is expressed in terms of its glomerular sieving coefficient (GSC). Molecules smaller than approximately the molecular weight of inulin (5 kDa) are freely filtered. Therefore, inulin, urea, creatinine, glucose, and electrolytes all have a GSC = 1.0. Classic experiments in the 1970s used linear dextran chains of varying molecular weight and charge to study glomerular filtration characteristics. However, linear carbohydrate chains do not necessarily behave in the same manner as a globular protein of equal molecular weight or charge. For example, neutral dextran chains of 15 kDa (diameter 2.4 nm) have GSC = 1.0, whereas the smaller β_2-microglobulin (11.8 kDa, diameter 1.6 nm) has GSC = 0.7.[24] Linear molecules have higher GSC than globular proteins, hence theoretical glomerular pore dimensions based on dextran studies were overestimated. More recently, Ficoll polymers have been used. These are neutral, heavily cross-linked, sucrose-epichlorohydrin copolymers that behave as rigid hydrated spheres and are thought to behave more like globular proteins in their sieving behavior.[170]

As a result of such studies, some general conclusions can be drawn with respect to glomerular protein handling. The glomerulus acts as a selective filter of the blood passing through its capillaries, restricting the passage of macromolecules in a size-, charge-, and shape/configuration-dependent manner. Sieving coefficients (1) decrease as molecular size increases, (2) are lower for anionic proteins than for neutral proteins of equivalent size, and (3) are lower for globular rather than elongated proteins. Examples of the GSC for major urinary proteins are listed in Table 25-2.

The protein concentration in the glomerular filtrate has been measured in several animal models by direct glomerular puncture. The concentration of total protein found is in the range of several hundred mg/L (≈1% of plasma), with albumin concentrations varying from less than 40 to a few hundred mg/L. The filtered load of protein depends on the product of the GSC and the free plasma concentration; therefore the albumin load per nephron is much greater than that of the other filtered proteins.[24,275] In general, proteins larger than albumin (66 kDa, diameter 3.5 nm, charge −23) are retained by the healthy glomerulus and are termed high molecular weight proteins. However, lower molecular weight proteins are also retained to a significant extent.

Tubular Reabsorption

The final urinary concentration of proteins depends on the filtered load, but also on the efficiency of the proximal tubular reabsorptive process, in addition to any contribution of tubular secretion. Proteins are reabsorbed by receptor-mediated, low-affinity, high-capacity processes. Megalin (MW 600 kDa) and cubulin (MW 460 kDa) are endocytic, multiligand receptors that are important in protein reabsorption.[455] Megalin belongs to the low-density lipoprotein (LDL) receptor family, whereas cubulin is identical to the intestinal intrinsic factor–vitamin B_{12} receptor. In the kidney, both are localized in clathrin-coated pits in the apical brush border of renal proximal tubular cells and bind filtered proteins in a calcium-dependent process. Megalin appears capable of both binding and internalizing its ligands, whereas the cubulin-ligand complex requires megalin to be internalized. Some proteins such as albumin will bind to either receptor, whereas others are specific [e.g., transferrin binds to cubulin only, retinol-binding protein (RBP) and α_1-microglobulin to megalin only]. Once proteins have been internalized, they are transported by the endocytic vesicle and fuse with lysosomes. Proteolysis occurs, and the resultant amino acids are released into the tubulointerstitial space across the basolateral surface of the tubular epithelial cell. The membrane vesicles are then recycled to the brush border to complete the reabsorption cycle. In health, the reabsorptive mechanism removes 99% of the filtered protein, thus retaining most of the essential amino acid constituents for reuse.[24,162,275] Capture of filtered transport proteins is also important in conserving vitamin status (e.g., vitamin A associated with RBP).

The tubular reabsorptive process is saturable. Any increase in the filtered load [caused by glomerular damage, increased glomerular vascular permeability (e.g., inflammatory response), or increased circulating concentration of low molecular weight proteins] or decrease in reabsorptive capacity (caused by tubular damage) can result in increased urinary protein loss *(proteinuria)*.

Tubular secretion of proteins also contributes to urinary total protein concentration; in particular, in health, Tamm Horsfall glycoprotein (THG) accounts for ≈50% of urinary total protein. THG (MW 200 kDa), a highly glycosylated acidic protein, is secreted into the tubular fluid only by the thick ascending limb and the early distal convoluted tubule and is thought to play a role in inhibiting kidney stone formation.[190,373] It is a major constituent of renal tubular casts, along with albumin and traces of other proteins. Investigation for increased urinary protein loss is mandatory in any patient with suspected kidney disease and was considered in Chapter 25.

Consequences of Proteinuria

It is increasingly accepted that proteinuria is not just a marker of, but contributes directly to, progression of kidney disease.[52,54] The accumulation of proteins in abnormal amounts in the tubular lumen may trigger an inflammatory reaction, which in turn may contribute to interstitial structural damage and expansion, and progression of kidney disease.[51] Increasing evidence suggests that megalin may not just be a scavenger receptor for albumin, but that it may have signaling functions that regulate cell survival. Excessive quantities of albumin in the tubular lumen may downregulate proximal tubular megalin expression, increasing cell sensitivity to apoptosis.[13] Evidence gathered from in vitro studies suggests that glomerular filtration of abnormal amounts or types of protein induces mesangial cell injury, leading to glomerulosclerosis, and that these same proteins can have adverse effects on proximal tubular cell function.[105] Numerous studies have demonstrated that proteinuria is a potent risk marker for progression of renal disease in both nondiabetic[202,346,377] and diabetic[48,189] kidney disease. Furthermore, reducing proteinuria slows the rate of progression of proteinuric kidney disease. This effect has been observed in clinical trials in patients treated with ACE inhibitors and angiotensin II receptor blockers (ARBs), given alone or in combination.[337,376] These drugs reduce protein excretion by reducing intraglomerular filtration pressure and possibly by stabilizing the glomerular epithelial cell slit diaphragm proteins.[6,276] Consequently, reduction of proteinuria is an important therapeutic target.[185,203,225]

PATHOPHYSIOLOGY OF KIDNEY DISEASE

Despite the diverse initial causes of injury to the kidney, progression of kidney disease leading to loss of function and ultimately to kidney failure is a remarkably monotonous process characterized by (1) early inflammation, followed by (2) accumulation and deposition of extracellular matrix, (3) tubulointerstitial fibrosis, (4) tubular atrophy, and (5) glomerulosclerosis. Proteinuria is thought to be one of the most important risk factors for progression of kidney disease (see earlier). Nephrons are also lost via toxic, anoxic, or immunologic injury that initially may occur in the glomerulus, the tubule, or both. Glomerular damage can involve endothelial, epithelial, or mesangial cells and/or the basement membrane.

The RAAS plays a pivotal role in many of the pathophysiologic changes that cause kidney injury and is an important therapeutic target (Figure 48-9).[380] Renal cells are able to produce AII in a concentration that is much higher than in the systemic circulation, and AII generates potentially toxic reactive oxygen species within renal cells affecting signal transduction. In addition, many profibrogenic and proinflammatory mediators are induced within the kidney by AII. Aldosterone has been reported to enhance profibrogenic processes. Inflammatory mediators released include cytokines, chemokines, and growth factors, such as TGF-β, monocyte chemoattractant protein-1 (MCP-1), interleukin-6 (IL-6), interferon-γ, or tissue necrosis factor-α (TNF-α); these inflammatory factors activate resident lymphocytes and macrophages and recruit additional cells from the peripheral circulation. Thus, cellular infiltration is a common but not

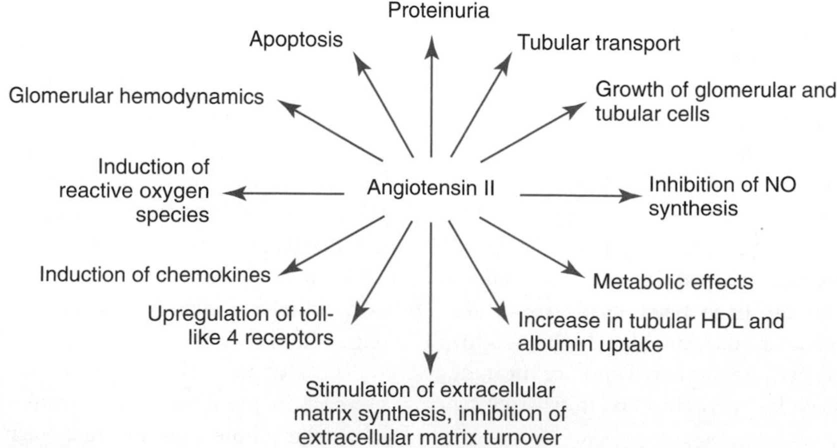

Figure 48-9 Role of angiotensin II in renal pathology. Angiotensin II is a cytokine with many effects on the kidney, clearly beyond its classical function as a hemodynamic mediator. *(From Ruster C, Wolf G: Renin-angiotensin-aldosterone system and progression of renal disease. J Am Soc Nephrol 2006;17:2985-91.)*

universal finding in renal biopsy specimens. These activated cells can cause T cell–mediated cell lysis, activation, and proliferation of interstitial fibroblasts. Fibroblast activity results in increased extracellular matrix synthesis and eventually in glomerular and tubular fibrosis. Extracellular matrix expansion causes disruption of local blood flow, exaggerating regional ischemia, and a vicious cycle of inflammation, fibrosis, and cell death is propagated.

Elucidation of this common pathway is incomplete but is the focus of considerable research interest because novel therapies are required to reduce progression and ideally to reverse fibrosis. A strong relationship has been described for proteinuria and MCP-1–mediated interstitial damage in a prospective study of patients undergoing kidney biopsy for CKD.[104] In rodent models, anti–MCP-1 gene therapy reduced interstitial inflammation and fibrosis.[404] Increased production and activity of TGF-β have also been demonstrated in glomerular disease; this acts as a key mediator, along with AII, of fibrogenesis.[267] Data support the hypothesis that during tubulointerstitial fibrosis, α-smooth muscle actin-expressing mesenchymal cells might derive from the tubular epithelium via epithelial-mesenchymal transition (EMT) under the influence of TGF-β.[199] Strategies to block the process of EMT are being explored for future therapeutic targets in CKD. For example, an endogenous antagonist of TGF-β–induced EMT has been identified as bone morphogenic protein-7, a member of the TGF-β superfamily. Systemic administration of bone morphogenic protein-7 repaired severely damaged tubular cells in mice and reversed renal injury.[488]

The kidneys have considerable ability to increase their functional capacity in response to injury. Thus, a significant reduction in functioning renal mass (50 to 60%) may occur before the onset of any significant symptoms, or even before any major biochemical alterations appear. The most sensitive and specific measure of functional change, the GFR, can be reduced to less than 60 mL/min/1.73 m^2 before signs and symptoms of kidney failure will be observed. This increase in workload per nephron is thought to be an important cause of progressive renal injury.[486] A well-recognized hypothesis suggests that independent of primary renal injury, a point is reached in the decline in nephron number when further loss becomes inevitable and progressive as a consequence of a common pathway leading to interstitial fibrosis.[366]

Overview of Kidney Disease and Its Clinical Manifestations

Most often, kidney disease is detected opportunistically by measurement of blood pressure and urine testing and blood tests in asymptomatic individuals. Such testing can occur in the primary care setting or for health clearance purposes for insurance. Typical findings include isolated hematuria and isolated proteinuria. Kidney disease may also present with macroscopic hematuria, swollen ankles, headaches, and visual disturbances due to severe hypertension, or as a manifestation of systemic disease, such as in the vasculitides and systemic lupus erythematosus (SLE) (kidney diseases are discussed in greater detail later). Symptoms suggestive of advanced kidney disease include fatigue, nausea, vomiting, poor appetite, shortness of breath, fluid retention, poor memory, loss of libido, and itching. Unfortunately, as many as 30% of individuals present very late in their disease and may require urgent dialysis with no previous experience with the specialist nephrology service. These patients have a poor prognosis compared with patients who have been cared for in a multidisciplinary specialist environment for at least 1 year. Therefore, early recognition of kidney disease is of paramount importance to outcome.

Detection and diagnosis of kidney disease requires a detailed history to include current symptoms, past medical and family history, social history, and a full drug history. A focused examination may identify potential causes of kidney disease such as obstructive uropathy in which the bladder is easily palpable, or may indicate vascular disease associated with narrowing of the arteries supplying the kidneys (renal artery stenosis), systemic disease, or de novo kidney disease. Blood pressure measurement and urinalysis (see Chapter 25) are crucial baseline assessments. Examination of the skin may reveal evidence of advanced kidney disease with excoriations due to the intense itch that can occur. Signs of fluid overload can be seen in the ankles, or effusions may be noted in the chest. Abdominal examination may detect a palpable bladder, renal bruits, or enlarged kidneys. Fundoscopic examination is performed in hypertensive and diabetic patients to identify microvascular damage to the retina.

Kidney disease may present with heavy blood and protein detected in a sample of the urine—a so-called active urinary sediment. An acute "nephritic" syndrome may occur as the result of postinfectious glomerulonephritis, for example, following a streptococcal throat or skin infection. The patient presents with poor urine output, edema, hypertension and acute kidney failure, and brown discolored urine. This pattern of acute nephritis is commonly seen in the developing world and is relatively unusual in developed countries.

Proteinuria may be the only indicator of kidney disease in many people. Proteinuria, particularly if in excess of 1 g/d, is indicative of glomerular disease. Most cases of glomerular disease are chronic, and patients may be followed for many years with monitoring of GFR and quantification of proteinuria.

Kidney disease presenting as nephrotic syndrome is characterized by the triad of heavy proteinuria (typically defined as exceeding an arbitrary threshold of 3 g/d), hypoalbuminemia, and edema. It is almost always caused by glomerular disease as opposed to tubular proteinuria. Several distinct pathologic entities may cause nephrotic syndrome (and are discussed in detail later in the present chapter), including minimal change nephropathy, focal segmental glomerular sclerosis, and membranous nephropathy. Nephrotic syndrome can also be a manifestation of diabetic kidney disease (diabetic nephropathy). Amyloid light chain amyloidosis (AL-amyloid) is a relatively common cause of nephrotic syndrome in older people.

Kidney disease often accompanies systemic diseases such as diabetes mellitus, vasculitis, SLE, and disorders of immunoglobulin light chains. The whole spectrum of kidney involvement may be seen, including an active urinary sediment, isolated proteinuria or hematuria, nephrotic syndrome, and rapidly progressive kidney failure.

Imaging of the renal tract to include kidneys, ureters, bladder, and prostate gland is very important in many kidney diseases and provides useful information. It is mandatory in all cases of new acute kidney injury (AKI; see later) to identify size and symmetry of kidneys and to exclude obstruction to urine flow anywhere within the tract. Renal ultrasound, the imaging technique of choice in most cases, gives reliable data on the size of kidneys and evidence of obstruction where present. Additionally, underlying structural abnormalities such as polycystic kidneys, renal cysts and tumors, and anatomic and congenital malformations may be demonstrated. Renal ultrasonography is easy, cheap, noninvasive, and without risk. Intravenous urography/pyelography (IVU/IVP) is utilized in urologic practice mainly to identify kidney stone disease and to investigate structural disease of the urinary tract such as a transitional cell carcinoma of the ureter or bladder. Imaging of soft tissues with computed tomography (CT) scanning or magnetic resonance imaging (MRI) may also be necessary to identify structural abnormalities. Invasive investigations of the urinary tract, particularly in patients with obstruction and hematuria, include cystoscopic examination of the bladder lining under direct vision, which allows for selective cannulation of each ureteric orifice and imaging with x-rays following injection of radiocontrast medium (retrograde study). The location of the lesion in an obstructed kidney can be ascertained by percutaneous insertion of a catheter into the kidney via a nephrostomy and subsequent injection of contrast via the nephrostomy tube, with x-rays taken as the contrast is drained from the kidney into the ureter and bladder (antegrade study).

Nuclear medicine scintigraphy is used to identify scars or cortical defects within kidneys and to assess the differential function of each kidney relative to the other. In addition, patients with well-preserved kidney function who are suspected of having renal artery stenosis can be challenged with an ACE inhibitor, such as captopril. This investigation assesses whether the flow of the radioisotope alters significantly following captopril administration. Radioisotopes are also utilized in some cases when obstruction is suspected but cannot be reliably demonstrated on ultrasound scanning, or when the collecting system with the kidney is dilated to assess whether there is a functional obstruction. Excretion of the radioisotope is tested following administration of the loop diuretic furosemide.

In patients with suspected renal artery disease, direct examination of the blood supply is undertaken. This can be performed by direct selective renal angiography following x-ray screening of a fine-bore catheter inserted into the aorta via the femoral artery in the groin or the brachial artery approach at the elbow. Magnetic resonance angiography is proving a valuable tool in the noninvasive testing of patients for renovascular disease.

Despite all these investigations, it is occasionally necessary to perform a kidney biopsy. Biopsy typically is indicated in patients with (1) nephrotic syndrome, (2) moderate proteinuria in the presence of hematuria, (3) rapidly progressive disease, (4) AKI, and in patients with (5) CKD (see below) that is progressive despite attention to treatments targeted to preserve kidney function. A biopsy is taken from one kidney only following injection of local anesthetic. To minimize the risk of bleeding, the lower pole of the kidney is chosen, because the lower pole is away from the hilum, where the major blood vessels are present. The lower pole is identified using ultrasound scanning, and a semiautomatic needle device is placed on the capsule of the kidney and is released into the cortex and medulla. A sample of tissue is obtained, and light microscopy, immunofluorescence, or immunoperoxidase staining is performed, as well as electron microscopy. It should be emphasized that although approximately 13% of the adult population is estimated to have CKD,[84] only a minority of patients undergo a kidney biopsy. A kidney biopsy should be undertaken only for nonmalignant disease in a specialist nephrology setting. Histopathologic examination of the specimen confirms the diagnosis and gives some indication of prognosis and the need for specific treatment.

Classification of Kidney Disease

The terminology associated with kidney disease has been amended and is clarified here. Previously, renal failure was divided into (1) *acute renal failure* (ARF) and (2) *chronic renal failure* (CRF). These terms indicate the rate at which damage occurs, rather than the mechanism by which it occurs. Landmark guidelines developed in the United States by the National Kidney Foundation-Kidney Disease Outcomes Quality Initiative (NKF-K/DOQI)[315] attempted to evaluate, classify, and stratify CKD. These guidelines have been revised and updated by the Kidney Disease: Improving Global Outcomes (KDIGO) working group initiative[255] and the National Institute for Health and Clinical Excellence (NICE) in the United Kingdom[311] (Table 48-5).

The term *renal* has largely been replaced by *kidney* in reference to *chronic* disease, because it is more easily understood by patients and nonspecialists. The commonly used term, *acute renal failure (ARF),* has been replaced by *acute kidney injury (AKI). End-stage renal disease (ESRD)* is a U.S. federal government–defined term that indicates the need for long-term treatment by dialysis or transplantation. Each patient with ESRD is registered through the Medical Evidence form (2728), submitted by all dialysis and transplant providers. The term now includes both Medicare and non-Medicare populations. Kidney failure is defined by NKF-K/DOQI as a GFR of less than 15 mL/min/1.73 m^2. In the National Service Framework for Renal Services in the United Kingdom, the term *kidney failure* in the NKF-K/DOQI classification has been replaced by *established renal failure (ERF),* defined as "chronic kidney disease that has progressed so far that renal replacement therapy (RRT; i.e., dialysis and transplantation) is required to maintain life."[99]

TABLE 48-5 Stages of Chronic Kidney Disease (CKD): Metabolic and Management Consequences

Stage*	Description	GFR, mL/min/1.73 m²	Population Prevalence in the U.S., %[84]	Population Prevalence in the U.K., %[421]	Metabolic Consequences	Management
1†	Kidney damage with normal or increased GFR	>90	1.78	—	Hypertension more frequent than among patients without CKD	Diagnosis and treatment Treatment of comorbid conditions Slowing progression CVD risk reduction
2†	Kidney damage with mildly decreased GFR	60-89	3.24	—	• Hypertension frequent • Concentration of PTH starts to rise (GFR, 60-80)	Estimating progression
3‡	Moderately decreased GFR	30-59	7.69	9.19	• Hypertension frequent • Decrease in calcium absorption (GFR < 50) • More markedly increased PTH concentration • Reduced phosphate excretion • Malnutrition (reduced spontaneous protein intake) • Onset of left ventricular hypertrophy • Onset of anemia (erythropoietin deficiency)	Evaluating and treating complications
4	Severely reduced GFR	15-29	0.35	0.35	• As above but more pronounced, plus: • Triglyceride concentrations start to rise • Hyperphosphatemia • Metabolic acidosis • Tendency to hyperkalemia • Decreased libido	Preparation for RRT
5§	Kidney failure	<15	—	0.06	• As above but more pronounced, plus: • Saline retention causing apparent heart failure • Anorexia • Vomiting • Pruritus (itching without skin disease)	RRT, if uremia present

CVD, Cardiovascular disease; *GFR,* glomerular filtration rate; *PTH,* parathyroid hormone; *RRT,* renal replacement therapy.

*The National Institute of Health and Clinical Excellence (NICE) has recommended that the suffix (p) should be used to denote the presence of proteinuria.[311]

†The diagnosis of stage 1 and 2 CKD requires additional evidence of kidney damage or disease (e.g., proteinuria).

‡NICE has recommended that stage 3 CKD should be subdivided into two subcategories defined by a GFR of 45 to 59 mL/min/1.73 m² (stage 3A) and a GFR of 30 to 44 mL/min/1.73 m² (stage 3B).[311]

§In the U.K. National Service Framework for Renal Services, the term *kidney failure* has been replaced by *established renal failure,* defined as "chronic kidney disease which has progressed so far that renal replacement therapy is needed to maintain life."[99]

Adapted from National Kidney Foundation. K/DOQI clinical practice guidelines for chronic kidney disease: evaluation, classification, and stratification. Am J Kidney Dis 2002;39:S1-266; Parmar MS. Chronic renal disease. BMJ 2002;325:85-90.

Chronic Kidney Disease

Studies established to identify the incidence, causes, and complications of CKD have largely focused on advanced disease and kidney failure. Because the numbers of patients with ESRD continue to rise, with associated poor prognosis despite modern replacement therapies (e.g., 33% 5-year survival on dialysis) and an enormous healthcare cost (e.g., $23 billion total Medicare spending on ESRD in the United States in 2006),[79] it has been recognized that CKD is an important public health problem, emphasizing the need for early identification and treatment.[336] Historically, data obtained from epidemiologic surveys had been compromised by lack of consistent surrogate markers of kidney function to identify established disease. For example, serum creatinine, calculated creatinine clearance, and measured creatinine clearance were variously used. The NKF-K/DOQI published a definition of CKD partly in an effort to identify its early stages.[315] The guidelines have been widely distributed and have facilitated the undertaking of comparative studies and analysis. Criteria for the definition of CKD include the following: "kidney damage or GFR <60 mL/min/1.73 m^2 for at least 3 months." Kidney damage is defined as "pathologic abnormalities or markers of damage, including abnormalities in blood or urine tests or imaging studies."

The NKF-K/DOQI guidelines stratify CKD from stage 1 at the milder end of the spectrum to stage 5, with kidney failure or GFR less than 15 mL/min/1.73 m^2. Although the cutoff values between stages are somewhat arbitrary, the process may allow for consistency in prevalence reporting for epidemiologic studies, as well as focused treatment schedules for individual patients (see Table 48-5). In addition, it has been recognized that risk of cardiovascular disease and death associated with moderate kidney disease is increased, and therefore CKD alerts the physician to the need to modify relevant risk factors.[149] One of the concerns regarding classification is the high prevalence of CKD imposed by the classification system itself. In the United States, it is estimated that 27 million individuals have CKD, representing almost 1 in 7 adults.[84] Population samples from elsewhere indicate similar prevalence rates. Most individuals with CKD do not progress to ESRD, with prevalence rates of stage 3 CKD 10 to 20 times greater than the prevalence rates of stages 4 and 5.[207,474] In the NICE guideline, the classification system has been revised to include the presence or absence of albuminuria/proteinuria, and stage 3 has been subdivided into 3A (GFR 45 to 59 mL/min/1.73 m^2) and 3B (GFR 30 to 44 mL/min/1.73 m^2), on the basis of their differing epidemiologic and prognostic significance.[311] The prognostic value of proteinuria has been established in CKD and reveals a much higher probability of progression to ESRD (see earlier).[163] Since the introduction of the classification system, the documented prevalence of CKD has increased sharply, and recognition of the importance of CKD led to the introduction of new diagnostic codes during 2006 (ICD-9-CM diagnosis codes). The importance of early diagnosis of CKD is highlighted by the recognition that 40% of patients commenced on dialysis (so-called "incident" patients) in the United States during 2006 had not previously seen a nephrologist, and most individuals had not had a serum creatinine measurement within the previous year.[79]

The incidence and major causes of CKD in the United States, the United Kingdom, and Australasia were previously identified from community-based studies and registry databases, such as the U.S. Renal Data System (USRDS), the U.K. Renal Registry Report, and the Australia and New Zealand Dialysis and Transplant Registry (ANZDATA). As indicated, registry databases tend to highlight those patients who develop advanced CKD or ESRD requiring treatment with dialysis or transplantation. The incidence of less advanced stages of CKD and of ESRD among patients not accepted for RRT is less clear.

The annual acceptance rate for RRT is increasing worldwide and has done so for the past 2 decades. The annual acceptance rate in the United States during 2006 was 360 per million population (pmp), although much higher among African Americans and Native Americans (Figure 48-10),[79] and in the United Kingdom in 2007 was 109 pmp.[7] The age of patients accepted for RRT is increasing, with most new patients undergoing RRT within the ages varying from 66 to 74 years.[7] It should be noted that the incidence of ESRD increases with age. The prevalence rates of patients with ESRD are also increasing and reached 1600 pmp in 2006 in the United States.[79]

The main causes of CKD leading to kidney failure from 1990 to 2006 in the United States are indicated in Figure 48-11. As indicated, diabetes mellitus is the largest single cause of advanced CKD and accounts for almost 50% of new dialysis patients in the United States. Hypertension is the underlying diagnosis in around 25% of new dialysis patients and is particularly prevalent among African Americans. The myriad of kidney diseases, including glomerulonephritis, infection, and hereditary, systemic, interstitial, and obstructive conditions, as well as those of unknown origin, account for the remainder. In the United Kingdom, diabetic nephropathy as a cause of kidney failure is seen in approximately 20% of new patients.[7]

Ethnic origin also modifies risk of kidney disease.[115] The lifetime risk of developing ESRD in 20-year-old African American men and women respectively has been estimated to be 7.3% and 7.8%, compared with 2.5% in white men and 1.8% in white women.[231] Family history of kidney disease is also a risk factor for developing ESRD. For example, a ninefold increased risk for ESRD has been noted in the African American community for those individuals with a first-degree relative with ESRD.[135] Therefore, genetic influences may be involved in the development of kidney disease and in the rate of progression to ESRD.

In summary, the presence of kidney disease is easily identified through simple blood and urine testing. Subsequent diagnosis of the cause of kidney disease relies on medical history, examination, and laboratory and radiologic investigations and will be discussed in the relevant disease sections later in this chapter.

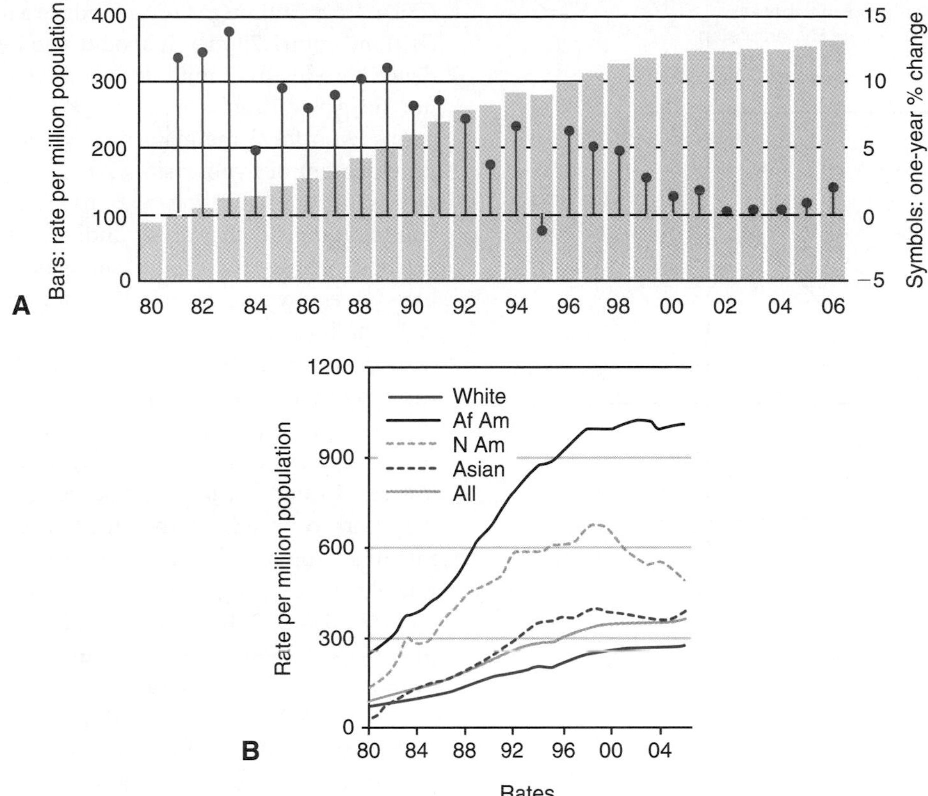

Figure 48-10 Changes in annual acceptance rate for renal replacement therapy (RRT) in the United States. The annual acceptance rate for incident end-stage renal disease (ESRD) patients reached 360 pmp up until 2006 (A: *bars*), although much higher rates for incident patients of approximately 1000 pmp (B) were recorded in African Americans. The percentage change in annual acceptance rate, shown in A, confirms a rise in 2006, compared with leveling of the incident rate during the early part of the decade. *(Reproduced from U.S. Renal Data System. USRDS 2008 annual data report: atlas of chronic kidney disease and end-stage renal disease in the United States. Bethesda, Md: National Institutes of Health, National Institute of Diabetes and Digestive and Kidney Diseases, 2008.[79])*

General Management of CKD

Complications of CKD that develop before the need for RRT are numerous (see Table 48-5) and include cardiovascular disease, metabolic acidosis, bone disease, and anemia. GFR cutoff values in the NKF-K/DOQI guidelines have been selected on the basis of limited data with respect to the relationship between complications and value of GFR. Additional studies may refine these values. Nevertheless, there is often a causal relationship between the burden of illness and the severity of CKD.

Rate of progression of CKD, irrespective of underlying cause, is dependent on both nonmodifiable factors, such as age, gender, race, and level of kidney function at diagnosis, and modifiable characteristics, including proteinuria, blood pressure control, and smoking. Progression and specific treatment options for diabetic and hypertensive nephropathy are discussed separately later in the chapter. The current discussion focuses on optimal treatment for nondiabetic CKD.

Lowering blood pressure and reducing proteinuria have been shown to ameliorate the progression of CKD. The Modification of Diet in Renal Disease (MDRD) study compared the rates of decline in GFR in 840 patients with various causes of CKD versus a "usual" or "low" blood pressure goal.[234] Patients with type 1 diabetes were excluded. Outcome data suggest that a low blood pressure goal had some beneficial effect in those patients with higher amounts of proteinuria.[194,234] The study supported the concept that proteinuria is an independent risk factor for progression of kidney disease. For patients with proteinuria greater than 1 g/d, the suggested target for mean blood pressure was 92 mm Hg (125/75 mm Hg).[346] The target blood pressure recommended by the seventh report of the Joint National Committee on Prevention, Detection, Evaluation, and Treatment of High Blood Pressure (JNC 7) is 130/80 mm Hg for patients with diabetes or kidney disease.[73] Strong consensus among national and international renal, hypertension, and diabetes organizations has led to the recommendation of a target systolic blood pressure of less than 140 mm Hg (range 120-139 mm Hg) and diastolic blood pressure less than 90 mm Hg for most patients with CKD.[446] Whereas some evidence supports a

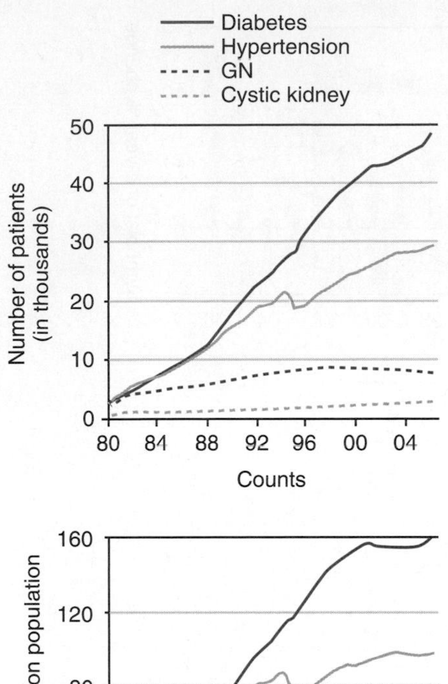

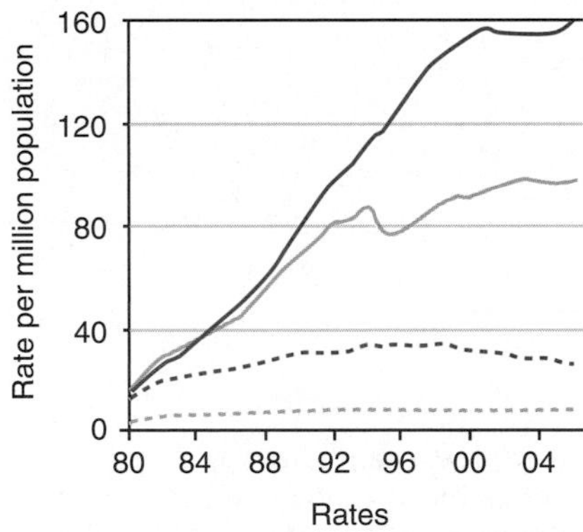

Figure 48-11 Trends in incident rates of end-stage renal disease (ESRD) by primary diagnosis in the United States. The number of patients with diabetes as the primary cause of ESRD reached 48,157 in 2006, 4.6% higher than the previous year, and 17.2% higher than in 2000. Incident rates for these patients have grown by 3.7% since 2000. The incidence of ESRD due to glomerulonephritis, in contrast, continues to fall—by 15.6% since 2000, to reach 26 pmp. In the *lower panel*, rates have been adjusted for age, gender, and race. *(Reproduced from U.S. Renal Data System. USRDS 2008 annual data report: atlas of chronic kidney disease and end-stage renal disease in the United States. Bethesda, Md: National Institutes of Health, National Institute of Diabetes and Digestive and Kidney Diseases, 2008.[79])*

lower target of less than 125/75 mm Hg in patients with more than 1 g/d of proteinuria, the concern is that lower blood pressure may be associated with adverse outcomes in some patients.

Data from the Third National Health and Nutrition Examination Survey (NHANES III) (1988-1994) reveal that among hypertensive individuals with an increased serum creatinine concentration, 75% were on antihypertensive treatment, and only 11% had their blood pressure reduced to lower than 130/85 mm Hg.[85]

ACE inhibitors are more effective than other antihypertensive drugs in slowing the rate of progression of proteinuric CKD,[146,289,376] although they do induce a mild decrease in GFR (<10 mL/min/1.73 m^2). It should also be noted that the evidence base for ACE inhibitor use in the setting of CKD may not be generalizable to older (>70 years), nonproteinuric adults, who form the majority of patients with CKD.[324] The development of hypotension, AKI, or hyperkalemia (plasma potassium concentration >5.5 mmol/L) should prompt discontinuation of the drug until other causes have been excluded. Short-term studies show that ARBs have effects on blood pressure and proteinuria that are similar to those of ACE inhibitors.

Low-nitrogen (protein) diets have been advocated from the early years of treatment of severe chronic uremia.[145] The very low protein diets tested in the MDRD study were of marginal benefit in these well-supervised patients with very low renal function, but are not well adhered to in practice, may lead to negative nitrogen balance, and are not recommended. Protein intake is restricted spontaneously to approximately 0.6 to 0.8 g/kg/d by uremic patients not receiving dietary advice.[195] To prevent malnutrition, patients receive professional dietary advice, with diets containing an increased proportion of protein and a total calorie content of up to 35 kcal/kg/d. The NHANES III has confirmed an association with reduced GFR and malnutrition in noninstitutionalized individuals studied in a cross-sectional survey of more than 5000 participants stratified according to GFR.[143]

In 2009, a relatively small trial demonstrated that bicarbonate supplementation slows the rate of progression of CKD.[94] General health measures, including cessation of cigarette smoking, should be encouraged.

Cardiovascular Complications of CKD

The spectrum of cardiovascular pathology predominant among patients with CKD (hypertensive cardiomyopathy, arrhythmias, heart failure, valvular disease, and peripheral vascular disease) differs from that predominant in the general population (atheromatous coronary artery disease).[12] The incidence of cardiovascular disease is seven- to tenfold greater in patients with CKD than in non-CKD age- and gender-matched controls.[467] By the time patients develop the need for RRT, there is an approximately 17 times greater risk of cardiovascular death or nonfatal myocardial infarction than among age- and sex-matched individuals without kidney disease.[12,126] Among patients treated by dialysis, the prevalence of coronary artery disease is approximately 40% and the prevalence of left ventricular hypertrophy (LVH) is approximately 75%.[127,405] Cardiovascular mortality, defined as death caused by (1) arrhythmias, (2) cardiomyopathy, (3) cardiac arrest, (4) myocardial infarction, (5) atherosclerotic heart disease, and (6) pulmonary edema, has been estimated to be approximately 9% per year in dialysis patients, accounting for 50% of deaths of all patients with ESRD. Even after stratification by age, gender, race, and the presence or absence of diabetes, cardiovascular mortality in dialysis patients is 10 to 20 times higher than in the general population (Figure 48-12).[130,384] Patients with ESRD should be considered in the highest risk group for subsequent cardiovascular events.

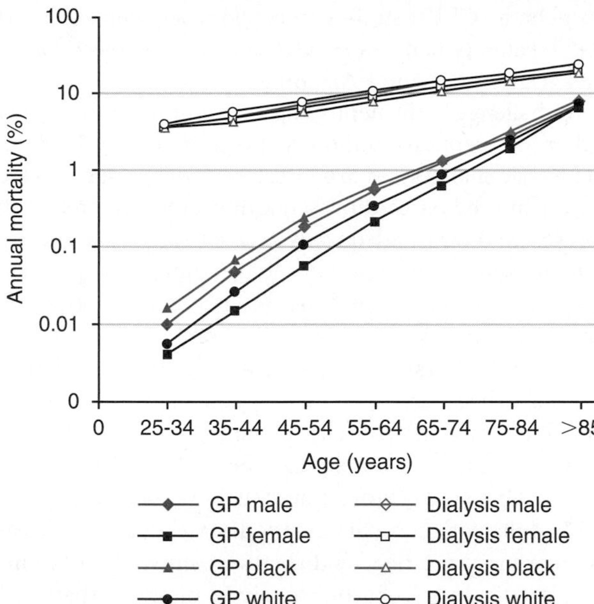

Figure 48-12 Cardiovascular disease mortality defined by death caused by arrhythmias, cardiomyopathy, cardiac arrest, myocardial infarction, atherosclerotic heart disease, and pulmonary edema in the general population (GP). Data from NCHS multiple cause of mortality data files compared with end-stage renal disease (ESRD) treated by dialysis. Data are stratified by age, race, and gender. *[From Foley RN, Parfrey PS, Sarnak MJ. Clinical epidemiology of cardiovascular disease in chronic renal disease. Am J Kidney Dis 1998;32(suppl 3):S112-19, with permission from the National Kidney Foundation.]*

TABLE 48-6 Traditional and Chronic Kidney Disease (CKD)-Related Risk Factors for Cardiovascular Disease in CKD

Traditional risk factors for cardiovascular disease	Older age Male gender White race Hypertension Elevated LDL cholesterol Decreased HDL cholesterol Smoking Diabetes mellitus Menopause Sedentary lifestyle Family history
CKD-related risk factors for cardiovascular disease	Extracellular fluid overload Left ventricular hypertrophy Proteinuria Anemia Abnormal calcium and phosphate metabolism (vascular calcification) Dyslipidemia MIA syndrome Infection Thrombogenic factors Oxidative stress Elevated homocysteine Uremic toxins

LDL, Low-density lipoprotein; *HDL,* high-density lipoprotein; *MIA,* malnutrition inflammation atherosclerosis.

Risk factors for cardiovascular disease in CKD consist of a mixture of traditional and CKD-specific factors. Traditional risk factors such as diabetes, hypertension, and dyslipidemia are more likely in CKD patients.[467] In addition, many other risk factors are CKD related (Table 48-6).

Observational studies indicate that cardiovascular disease occurs at an early stage in CKD.[457] Thus among middle-aged men, a moderate increase in serum creatinine concentration [>1.5 mg/dL (>130 μmol/L)] was associated with an age-adjusted relative risk (RR) of 1.5 for coronary disease and 3.0 for stroke. Reduction of GFR is associated with increased risk of composite end points of cardiovascular death, myocardial infarction, and stroke.[286] Microalbuminuria and proteinuria have also been shown to be associated with increased risk of cardiovascular disease, cardiovascular mortality, and all-cause mortality.[2,45,88] These associations may arise because (1) CKD causes an elevated level of cardiovascular disease, (2) cardiovascular disease causes CKD, or (3) some other factor, such as diabetes and hypertension, causes both CKD and cardiovascular disease. Significantly, there are many more patients with stage 3 than stage 5 CKD (see Table 48-5). A longitudinal population study of 40,000 patients with stage 3 to 4 CKD in Northern California reported after a mean follow-up period of almost 4 years that the age-adjusted rate for development of ESRD in the white population was 0.67 per 100 person-years, whereas the rate for any cardiovascular event and death from any cause was 10.94 and 5.25 per 100 person-years, respectively.[345]

Two large prospective randomized controlled studies reported significant reductions in cardiovascular morbidity and mortality associated with ACE inhibitor treatment among patients at high risk for future cardiovascular events.[132,485] A secondary analysis of the Prevention of Events with ACE Inhibition (PEACE) trial data revealed a higher risk of death among patients with an estimated GFR of less than 60 mL/min/1.73 m^2 at baseline, and a significant reduction in all-cause mortality associated with ACE inhibitor treatment in this subgroup.[416] Whereas none of the studies already mentioned specifically included patients with CKD, and all excluded patients with severe renal impairment, these data do provide support for the notion that ACE inhibitor treatment reduces cardiovascular risk in high-risk patients. Because cardiovascular disease remains the most important cause of death among CKD patients, it seems reasonable to recommend ACE inhibitor or ARB treatment for reduction of cardiovascular risk and for slowing of CKD progression.

Left Ventricular Hypertrophy

Among dialysis patients, the prevalence of congestive heart failure is approximately 40%. Both coronary artery disease and LVH are risk factors for the development of heart failure. In practice, it is difficult to determine whether cardiac failure reflects left ventricular dysfunction or extracellular fluid volume overload. LVH is demonstrable early in the course of CKD, with the proportion of patients with LVH increasing as kidney function declines. Univariate analysis of a single-center cohort of CKD patients in Canada revealed that age, systolic blood pressure, and hemoglobin were significantly different between the groups with or without LVH.[258] For each 5 mm Hg increase in systolic BP, the risk of LVH increased by 3%. A fall in blood hemoglobin concentration of 1 g/dL increased the risk of LVH by 6%. A large prospective multi-center study confirmed progressive increases in left ventricular mass index (LVMI) over a 12-month period, with the incidence of new LVH at 10% per year.[259] Again, lower hemoglobin concentrations and higher systolic blood pressures were associated with left ventricular growth. Anemia has both direct and indirect effects on left ventricular function and growth. Cardiac output increases because of a combination of increased cardiac preload and a reduction in afterload. Such changes lead to ventricular remodeling, with initial left ventricular dilation followed by subsequent hypertrophy. In ESRD, other factors contribute to LVH, including hypertension, volume expansion, and the metabolic consequences of uremia, to which may be added the effects of diabetes.[125]

Dyslipidemia in CKD

Various dyslipidemias are associated with CKD.[291,362,467] The pattern of dyslipidemia in CKD differs from that seen in non-CKD. It is characterized by an accumulation of partially metabolized triglyceride-rich particles [predominantly very low-density lipoprotein (VLDL) and intermediate-density lipoprotein (IDL) remnants], due mainly to abnormal lipase function.[325] This causes hypertriglyceridemia and low high-density lipoprotein (HDL) cholesterol. Although total cholesterol concentration may be normal, there is often a highly abnormal lipid subfraction profile with a predominance of atherogenic small, dense LDL particles.[12] In a large cross-sectional analysis of 1047 hemodialysis patients in the Dialysis Morbidity and Mortality Study, only 20% of patients had low-risk lipid concentrations [i.e., LDL <130 mg/dL (3.36 mmol/L), HDL >40 mg/dL (1.03 mmol/L), and triglycerides <150 mg/dL (1.69 mmol/L)] (see http://www.kidney.org/professionals/KDOQI/guidelines_lipids/ii.htm#Table16, accessed on July 12, 2011). Low cholesterol was found to be associated with increased mortality, but this is probably a reflection of other conditions that lower cholesterol, such as inflammation and malnutrition ("reverse causality"). It is possible that other, nontraditional atherogenic lipoprotein abnormalities [e.g., lipoprotein (a) and oxidized LDL] are present in hemodialysis patients.[136,280] Similar profiles are seen in peritoneal dialysis patients.

Lipoprotein (a) concentrations are also increased in CKD. Baseline data from the Chronic Renal Impairment in Birmingham (CRIB) study confirmed dyslipidemia in early CKD.[467] Patients had lower HDL and LDL cholesterol and higher triglyceride concentrations.

The challenge to the nephrology community is to establish whether interventions to modify the pattern of dyslipidemia with lifestyle changes and drug treatment will preserve kidney function and reduce cardiovascular morbidity and mortality. At present, no large, adequately controlled trials are testing the hypotheses that treatment of dyslipidemia preserves kidney function. The major trials of intervention with statins [3-hydroxy-3-methylglutaryl-Co-enzyme A (HMG-CoA) reductase inhibitors] in the general population and those with established cardiovascular disease have been limited with reference to CKD, because patients with CKD have been excluded from trials as perceived to be too high risk for inclusion.[76,349] The Heart Protection Study randomly allocated 20,536 adults with coronary artery disease, occlusive disease of noncoronary arteries, or diabetes to simvastatin (40 mg) or placebo.[297] In a subgroup analysis of more than 1300 patients with serum creatinine concentration between 1.2 and 2.3 mg/dL (110 and 200 μmol/L), fewer major vascular events were reported in the simvastatin group.

Guidelines from the U.K. Renal Association[446] and NICE[311] recommend that statins should be considered for primary prevention in all patients with CKD, including dialysis patients, if their 10-year risk of cardiovascular disease is calculated as greater than 20% according to the guidelines of the Joint British Societies.[211] However, these risk calculations have not been validated in patients with kidney disease. The target total cholesterol should be less than 156 mg/dL (<4 mmol/L) or a 25% reduction from baseline; also, a fasting LDL cholesterol of less than 78 mg/dL (<2 mmol/L), or a 30% reduction from baseline, should be achieved, whichever is the greatest reduction in all patients. However, this guidance remains controversial.[82] At present there is no data to suggest that statins are of benefit in patients receiving dialysis. A major study, known as the 4D Study, investigated the use of atorvastatin in more than 1200 patients with type 2 diabetes mellitus undergoing hemodialysis and followed for a median period of 4 years. The study group concluded that atorvastatin had no statistically significant effect on the composite primary end point of cardiovascular death, nonfatal myocardial infarction, and stroke.[458] A 2009 study, called AURORA, evaluated the use of rosuvastatin in subjects on hemodialysis and failed to demonstrate any beneficial effects of statins on cardiovascular outcomes despite markedly reduced lipid concentrations.[117] Although these studies have limitations, the most likely explanation for the lack of benefit associated with statins is that patients on dialysis have a different type of cardiovascular disease than individuals with earlier stages of CKD.

The Study of Heart and Renal Protection (SHARP), evaluated the use of cholesterol lowering with simvastatin and ezetimibe in a broad variety of patients with CKD for benefit in terms of cardiovascular risk, but also amelioration of progression of CKD. This randomized double-blind placebo-controlled study of more than 9000 patients (including 3000 dialysis patients) has been reported.[12A] There were significant reductions in atherosclerotic endpoints including non-hemorrhagic stroke and arterial revascularization in the treated patients followed for a median of 4.9 years. In addition, a randomized controlled trial of proteinuric CKD patients receiving ACE inhibitors and ARBs reported additional benefit from treatment with atorvastatin in terms of reduction in proteinuria and progression of disease.[33]

Vascular Calcification

It has been known for many years that patients with kidney failure have vascular calcification. Serial x-ray studies and ultrasound imaging of large arteries confirm increased calcification in patients on dialysis over many years.[150] Studies from France have linked the presence of vascular calcification with reduced survival on dialysis.[35,36,158] Calcification of the major arteries occurs along the intimal lining of blood vessels in association with atheroma. However in CKD, medial and adventitial calcification also occurs, reducing the compliance of the vessel. Reductions in vessel compliance can be observed by measuring pulse wave velocities along major arteries such as the aorta. The pulse wave velocity is increased in stiff (less compliant) vessels, causing the rebound pulse wave to return more quickly to the heart during the cardiac cycle. Early rebound of the pulse wave places extra strain on the heart, leading to LVH.[35] Vascular calcification has been studied in both CKD and non-CKD populations using modern sophisticated imaging. Electron beam CT acquires serial sections of the aortic arch, the coronary vessels, and the aorta. Areas of calcification can be identified and allocated a calcium score (Agatston score).[1] This approach cannot distinguish between intimal and medial calcification, but in non-CKD patients, the higher the calcium score, the more predictive it is of stenotic vascular disease.[224,379] Dialysis patients as young as 20 years exhibit vascular calcification,[151] and calcium scores increased rapidly within several months when the scans were repeated.

The pathophysiology of vascular calcification in CKD patients is an exciting area of study, with many new developments and hypotheses. Vascular calcification was previously thought to be a passive process caused by precipitation of mineral from the circulation. However, it is increasingly recognized that vascular calcification is a tightly regulated process with true bone marrow, osteo/chondrocytic cells, cytokines, matrix proteins, and matrix vesicles characteristic of mature bone-forming cells (osteoblasts) within calcified vascular lesions.[394,401,442] Mineralization-regulating proteins are deposited at sites of vascular calcification. The generation of a matrix gamma-carboxyglutamic acid (Gla) protein knockout mouse, which exhibits extensive and lethal calcification and cartilaginous metaplasia of the media of all elastic arteries, has refocused attention on the role of Gla-containing proteins in vascular calcification.[401] A number of proteins, including matrix Gla protein, osteonectin, and osteoprotegerin, are constitutively expressed by vascular smooth muscle cells in normal media but are downregulated in calcified arteries. In calcified plaques, vascular smooth muscle cells express osteoblast-like gene expression profiles, as demonstrated by in situ hybridization,[442] and are able to transdifferentiate into osteo/chondrocytic cells in the arterial wall and to orchestrate bone formation and calcification in response to multiple factors such as hypertension, reactive oxygen species, advanced glycation end products, lipids, and inflammatory proteins. Identification of natural inhibitors of calcification in plasma, such as human fetuin-A [α_2-Heremans Schmid glycoprotein (AHSG)] and matrix-Gla protein, suggests that the vascular endothelium may be continually subjected to calcification stresses, and that regulatory systems break down in uremia. A cross-sectional study in hemodialysis patients demonstrated that AHSG concentrations were significantly lower in plasma of patients on hemodialysis than in healthy controls.[229]

The use of calcium-containing oral phosphate binders (see later) may be associated with increased risk of calcification.[151] The Treat to Goal study explored the use of a noncalcium, nonaluminum-containing phosphate binder, sevelamer hydrochloride, in 200 hemodialysis patients from Europe and North America.[68] This study demonstrated significant attenuation in the rate of calcification of vessels with sevelamer hydrochloride at 12 months. Patients were less likely to develop hypercalcemia and had lower plasma LDL cholesterol concentrations, but a tendency toward worsening acidosis was noted. Still other studies have identified a potential survival benefit for new ("incident") hemodialysis patients derived from treatment with sevelamer hydrochloride compared with calcium-based oral phosphate binders when treatment was provided for at least 18 months.[38] However, a study comparing sevelamer hydrochloride versus calcium-based binders in more than 2000 prevalent hemodialysis patients failed to show a significant difference between therapies in terms of all-cause mortality and cause-specific mortality.[424]

Disturbances in Calcium and Phosphate Metabolism

CKD is associated with complex metabolic disturbances in divalent ion and phosphate metabolism. Although this is commonly referred to as *renal osteodystrophy,* there has been a paradigm shift in terms of calcium, phosphate, and PTH management in patients receiving dialysis. The impetus for this change in approach has been recognition of the importance of the previously unheralded phosphate moiety in terms of increased risk of death in ESRD and the almost universal development of *cardiovascular calcification* (see earlier) that is seen in dialysis patients. It is likely that treatment of hyperphosphatemia in dialysis patients with calcium-based therapies may be contributing to vascular calcification; therefore these two problems are intricately linked. In an effort to clarify the terminology of renal metabolic bone disease, KDIGO proposed that the term *CKD-mineral and bone disorder* (CKD-MBD) should be used to describe the syndrome of biochemical, bone, and extraskeletal calcification abnormalities that occur in patients with CKD, and the term *renal osteodystrophy* should be used exclusively to define alterations in bone morphology, following bone biopsy, associated with CKD.[232]

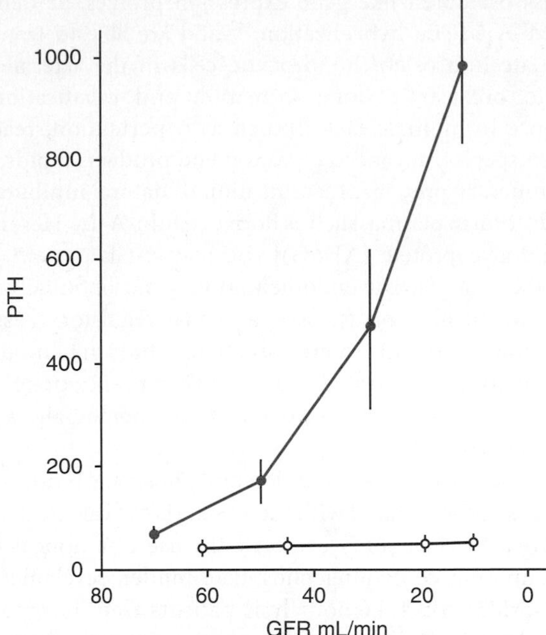

Figure 48-13 The relationship between parathyroid hormone (PTH) concentration and glomerular filtration rate (GFR) in two groups of dogs: those maintained on a normal phosphate diet *(closed circles)* and those maintained on a diet containing <100 mg of phosphate per day *(open circles)*. The vertical lines represent ±1 SEM. PTH is expressed in μEq/mL. *(From Slatopolsky E, Caglar S, Pennell JP, Taggart DD, Canterbury JM, Reiss E, et al. On the pathogenesis of hyperparathyroidism in chronic experimental renal insufficiency in the dog. J Clin Invest 1971;50:492-9.)*

As GFR declines, plasma phosphate concentration rises, resulting in reduced ionized calcium. The consequence of this is increased production of PTH by the parathyroid glands. PTH-producing cells are regulated tightly through complex feedback mechanisms to maintain normocalcemia (see Chapter 52). The calcium-sensing receptor (CaSR) is stimulated by calcium and has an inhibitory effect on PTH production.[50] In addition, phosphate has been reported to directly stimulate the production of PTH in vitro.[413] Elegant experiments on dogs with varying levels of induced kidney failure have confirmed the increase in PTH as GFR fell, with attenuation noted in animals fed a modified diet with very low concentrations of phosphate (Figure 48-13).[411] FGF-23 may stimulate PTH production. FGF-23 concentrations increase markedly in CKD (between 10 and 600 times higher than the normal range) and are correlated with predialysis phosphate concentrations, but not with bone mineral density.[448] Ongoing studies are evaluating the importance of this peptide in terms of skeletal resistance to PTH as seen in CKD patients.

In addition to hyperphosphatemia contributing to hypocalcemia, reduced 1α-hydroxylation of 25-hydroxycholecalciferol by the renal proximal tubular cells may lead to reduced production of calcitriol, the active form of vitamin D and a vitamin D receptor activator. Vitamin D is required in health to increase calcium absorption from the gut; it also increases phosphate absorption from the gut. PTH-producing cells in the parathyroid gland have receptors for vitamin D (VDRs). The VDR is a 427 amino acid peptide that is widely found in tissues, including parathyroid glands, intestine, and osteoblast-like cells. Binding of vitamin D to the VDR inhibits its PTH production. The result of these complex metabolic disturbances is secondary hyperparathyroidism. Increased secretion of PTH stimulates resorption of calcium and phosphate from the major calcium reservoir, the bone. Problems can develop early, and patients with a GFR of less than 60 mL/min/1.73 m^2 should be evaluated for these metabolic disturbances.[315] Secondary hyperparathyroidism classically causes bone changes consistent with osteitis fibrosa cystica. Bony erosions and intramedullary cysts are seen because of direct effects of PTH on osteoclasts and osteoblasts. Unchecked, this can lead to bone pain and fracture. Eventually, PTH secretion can become unhinged completely from feedback control; this autonomous production is called *tertiary hyperparathyroidism*. Severe secondary hyperparathyroidism is associated with hyperplasia of the glands and ultimately with nodular hyperplasia. These grossly enlarged glands tend to be resistant to medical therapies of secondary hyperparathyroidism, as they have significantly reduced expression of both the CaSR and VDR. In this setting, medical treatment has failed and parathyroidectomy is required. A severe and often terminal manifestation of long-standing ESRD is calcemic uremic arteriolopathy *(calciphylaxis)*. Calciphylaxis is characterized by calcium deposition within the arterioles of the microcirculation, leading to destruction of the vessel, and in turn causing necrosis of tissues, particularly the skin and adipose tissue on the legs and torso.

Adynamic bone in patients with CKD is characterized by low turnover and poor bone formation and is highly prevalent in CKD. It is much more common in older people and those with diabetes and malnutrition. Adynamic bone is associated with a low PTH concentration and abnormal calcium balance, hyperphosphatemia, and acidosis. Progression of CKD adds to the risk profile for adynamic bone, because 1,25-dihydroxyvitamin D becomes markedly reduced in advanced CKD.[257] The diagnosis of adynamic bone is ultimately made on bone biopsy, but patients are reluctant to undertake this procedure. Unfortunately, PTH alone does not correlate with bone biopsy findings. However, serum bone-specific alkaline phosphatase measured using an immunoassay technique has very good predictive value in separating high from low bone turnover, particularly in combination with PTH measurements. For example, low bone formation has been associated with bone-specific alkaline phosphatase activity less than 20 U/L and PTH less than 100 ng/L.[78] Although it has not proved to be associated with increased fracture risk in ESRD patients, dialysis patients with adynamic bone are less able to incorporate calcium into bone and are at increased risk of vascular calcification.[272] Excessive use of vitamin D analogs (e.g., alfacalcidol [1α-hydroxyvitamin D3]) is implicated in the high prevalence of adynamic bone in dialysis patients. However, recent data have revealed that this is less likely to occur with the synthetic vitamin D

TABLE 48-7 K/DOQI Target Guidelines for Serum Calcium, Phosphate, Calcium × Phosphate Product and Plasma PTH Concentrations in CKD Stages 4 and 5

Stage of CKD	Phosphate	Calcium (Corrected for Albumin)	PTH	Calcium × Phosphate Product
4	2.7 mg/dL-4.6* mg/dL (0.87 mmol/L-1.49* mmol/L)	Normal laboratory range	70-110* ng/L (7.7-12.1 pmol/L)	<55 mg^2/dL^2 (<4.51 $mmol^2/L^2$)
5	3.5 mg/dL-5.5 mg/dL (1.13 mmol/L-1.78 mmol/L)	8.4-9.5 mg/dL (2.10*-2.38* mmol/L)	150-300 ng/L (15-30 pmol/L)	<55 mg^2/dL^2 (<4.51 $mmol^2/L^2$)

Conversion to SI units:
Phosphate: mg/dL to mmol/L × 0.323.
Calcium: mg/dL to mmol/L × 0.25.
Calcium phosphate product: mg^2/dL^2 to $mmol^2/L^2$ × 0.0807.
PTH: ng/L to pmol/L × 0.1 (approx).
CKD, Chronic kidney disease; *K/DOQI,* Kidney Disease Outcomes Quality Initiative; *PTH,* parathyroid hormone.

receptor activator, paricalcitol (19-nor-1,25-dihydroxyvitamin D_2), which reduces bone resorption and intestinal calcium reabsorption, than with calcitriol or alfacalcidol.[412]

Bone disease in CKD is also complicated by the relatively high prevalence of hypogonadism in men on dialysis and the high prevalence of osteoporosis in postmenopausal women.

High concentrations of plasma phosphate are associated with increased mortality in hemodialysis patients.[37] In at least 50% of hemodialysis patients, the serum phosphate is greater than 6.0 mg/dL (1.9 mmol/L), and in 25% of patients, it is greater than 7.2 mg/dL (2.3 mmol/L). Higher corrected calcium and PTH concentrations are associated with death in hemodialysis patients. Patients with low phosphate concentrations are also at increased risk of death (RR of death increased by approximately 50% with phosphate <3 mg/dL) because low phosphate is associated with intercurrent illness and malnutrition. The U.K. Renal Association standard for midweek predialysis serum phosphate concentration is 3.3 to 5.6 mg/dL (1.1 to 1.8 mmol/L).[446] National guidelines were published in the United States by NKF-K/DOQI during 2003 (Table 48-7).[108] Achievement of these targets is variable between dialysis providers, with approximately 60% of patients within the phosphate target and 25% within the PTH target. As few as 8% of patients simultaneously achieve all four targets.[7]

Strategies to reduce phosphate concentrations are employed routinely in the treatment of patients on dialysis. Inorganic phosphate within the blood accounts for less than 0.1% of total body phosphate. Clearance of phosphate on intermittent hemodialysis is approximately one third of that seen with urea and is subject to postdialysis rebound because of efflux from the intracellular to the extracellular space. Phosphate is present in many foods and is linearly associated with protein ingestion. The recommended allowance of phosphate is reduced for patients on dialysis to around 800 mg/d. Treatment with vitamin D analogs increases gut absorption of phosphate from approximately 65 to almost 85%. The use of phosphate binders, taken with meals, is almost universal in dialysis patients; treatment may include calcium-containing and non–calcium-containing binders (Table 48-8). Prescribing of phosphate binders should be individualized for each patient because each binder has pros and cons. Recent interest has focused on the increased propensity to vascular calcification noted in those dialysis patients receiving calcium-containing phosphate binders. These binders reduce phosphate absorption to 30 to 40% and decrease serum phosphate concentrations. However, a 2009 systematic review of randomized controlled trials concluded that no evidence suggests that phosphate binders reduce all-cause or cardiovascular mortality compared with placebo.[318] Further, no survival advantages of newer phosphate-binding agents (sevelamer, lanthanum carbonate) over traditional calcium-based therapies were found.[318] In summary, patients on conventional three times weekly dialysis are in a net positive phosphate balance. It has been possible to normalize phosphate balance in patients treated by daily hemodialysis.[307]

Medical treatment strategies are designed to limit phosphate intake and normalize calcium. With the advent of vitamin D analogs, it has been possible to supplement vitamin D, resulting in increased plasma calcium concentrations and switching off of PTH production. Unfortunately, commonly used analogs, such as 1α-hydroxyvitamin D3, also lead to increased reabsorption of calcium and phosphate from the gut. In the setting of aggressive treatment with vitamin D analogs, hypercalcemia may develop that is associated with low, suppressed concentrations of PTH. Alternative vitamin D receptor activators, such as paricalcitol, are associated with improved survival in U.S. dialysis patients and have a lower incidence of treatment-related hyperphosphatemia and hypercalcemia than calcitriol.[288,431] The vitamin D receptor is ubiquitous, and its stimulation has wide-ranging effects on the cardiovascular and immune systems; this may explain the benefits of treatment in CKD patients over and above the effects on reducing PTH.[238]

A further development in the management of CKD-MBD has been the generation of calcimimetic agents such as cinacalcet.[8,263] Calcimimetics mimic calcium by directly stimulating the CaSR and can affect the molecular configuration of

TABLE 48-8 Summary of Currently Available Oral Phosphate Binders

Phosphate Binder	Advantages	Disadvantages
Aluminum salts	Calcium free High binder efficiency regardless of pH Cheap Moderate tablet burden	Risk of aluminum toxicity Requires frequent monitoring—extra cost
Calcium carbonate	Aluminum free Moderate binding efficacy Relatively low cost Moderate tablet burden Chewable	Calcium containing—potential risk of hypercalcemia and ectopic calcification Parathyroid hormone oversuppression Gastrointestinal side effects Efficacy pH dependent
Calcium acetate	Aluminum free Higher efficacy than calcichew/sevelamer Moderately cheap Lower calcium load than calcium carbonate	Calcium containing—potential risk of hypercalcemia and ectopic calcification, PTH oversuppression Gastrointestinal side effects Large tablets, nonchewable formulation
Sevelamer hydrochloride	Aluminum and calcium free No gastrointestinal absorption Moderate efficacy Reduces total and low-density lipoprotein cholesterol	Relatively costly High pill burden Large tablets, nonchewable formulation Gastrointestinal side effects Binds fat-soluble vitamins
Lanthanum carbonate	Aluminum and calcium free Minimal gastrointestinal absorption High efficacy across full pH range Chewable formulation Palatable Low tablet burden	Relatively costly Gastrointestinal side effects

PTH, Parathyroid hormone.

the CaSR to enhance its sensitivity to extracellular calcium.[263] Stimulation of the CaSR switches off PTH production selectively with no risk of increased phosphate absorption. Use of cinacalcet has increased the proportion of patients who reach the K/DOQI targets for CKD-MBD and has reduced the need for parathyroidectomy in patients with secondary hyperparathyroidism.[89] Prospective randomized controlled trials evaluating the effects of adding calcimimetics to standard therapy on cardiovascular outcomes and mortality are ongoing and include the Evaluation of Cinacalcet HCL Therapy to Lower CardioVascular Events (EVOLVE).

Aluminum Toxicity

A causative factor for renal bone disease, historically, has been aluminum intoxication (see Chapter 36). Aluminum concentrations in dialysis fluids were previously high, but with modern dialysis facilities, this is no longer such a problem. However, some dialysis patients are treated intermittently with aluminum-containing phosphate binders; therefore regular monitoring of blood aluminum concentration is recommended in such patients.[446] Aluminum accumulation has been associated with deposition along the mineralization surface of the osteoid and a low-turnover form of bone disease. Aluminum accumulation may be treated by infusions of the chelating agent desferrioxamine. Aluminum intoxication may be associated with neurologic disturbances characterized by dementia (dialysis dementia) and with a hypochromic microcytic anemia.

Anemia

The World Health Organization defines anemia, when the patient is at sea level, as a blood hemoglobin concentration of less than 13 g/dL in adult men and less than 12 g/dL in adult, nonpregnant women.[478] It is clearly established that anemia is inevitable as CKD progresses. Therapies are available to correct anemia; therefore it is mandatory that a patient with CKD should be assessed for anemia. The NKF-K/DOQI recommends that an estimated GFR of less than 60 mL/min/1.73 m^2 should be the cutoff value for determining the presence or absence of anemia.[314] The U.K. Renal Association recommends that anemia should be investigated in CKD when hemoglobin is less than 13 g/dL in adult males and postmenopausal females and less than 12 g/dL in premenopausal females.[446] In addition, CKD should be considered as a possible cause of anemia when the GFR is less than 60 mL/min/1.73 m^2. It is more likely to be the cause if the GFR is less than 30 mL/min/1.73 m^2 (<45 mL/min/1.73 m^2 in patients with diabetes) and no other cause (e.g., blood loss, folic acid or vitamin B_{12} deficiency) is identified. The prevalence of anemia increases as GFR declines. In the NHANES

III data set, the prevalence of anemia (defined as Hb <12.0 g/dL in men, Hb <11.0 g/dL in women) was 33% at a GFR of 15 mL/min/1.73 m^2 and 9% at a GFR of 30 mL/min/1.73 m^2.[83] CKD-related anemia occurs earlier in patients with diabetes and is highly prevalent among such patients.[109]

Detection is important because if left untreated, anemia causes many of the side effects of CKD, such as fatigue, breathlessness on exertion, intolerance to cold, and decreased exercise capacity. As indicated earlier, it is also a major factor in the high prevalence of cardiovascular disease in patients with CKD and contributes to the development of LVH. In patients on dialysis, large observational studies have clearly shown that anemia is associated with increased mortality rates and increased hospitalization.[81,269,274,482] In hemodialysis patients, hematocrit percentages of 33 to 36% (corresponding to hemoglobin concentrations of 11 to 12 g/dL) were associated with the lowest risk for all-cause and cardiac mortality[274]; these patients also had the lowest risk of hospitalization.[326,482]

Etiology of Anemia in CKD

The etiology of anemia in CKD is multifactorial. A major cause, however, is the loss of peritubular fibroblasts within the renal cortex that synthesize EPO. Failure of EPO production in the kidney leads to inappropriately low concentrations within the blood for the concomitant hemoglobin concentration. Other causes of anemia include absolute or functional iron deficiency, folic acid and vitamin B_{12} deficiencies, and chronic inflammation. Red cell survival may also be reduced. Hemodialysis patients tend to have more severe anemia than peritoneal dialysis patients because of greater blood losses and hemolysis.

Several national and international organizations such as NKF-K/DOQI,[317] the European Renal Association,[112] and NICE,[310] have published algorithms for the treatment of anemia in CKD and dialysis patients. The NICE guideline recommends that treatment should aim to maintain hemoglobin concentration between 10.5 and 12.5 g/dL in adults.[310] The NKF-K/DOQI Work Group recommends a slightly different target reference interval for hemoglobin of 11 to 12 g/dL, and that hemoglobin concentration should not exceed 13 g/dL.[317] The mainstays of treatment are iron supplementation and the use of erythropoiesis-stimulating agents (ESAs). Warnings, indications, precautions, and instructions for dosing and administration of ESAs are available from national regulatory agencies, including the U.S. Food and Drug Administration (FDA), and from product package inserts.

Assessment of Iron and Iron Supplementation

Iron status is assessed by measurement of serum ferritin and transferrin saturation. Transferrin saturation gives an indication of iron "delivery." Ferritin is used to represent iron stores. In patients with CKD, a serum ferritin concentration less than 100 μg/L is considered to suggest iron deficiency, and a serum ferritin of 100 to 200 μg/L in association with transferrin saturation less than 20% represents "functional" iron deficiency. Treatment of anemia in CKD requires adequate iron stores. A very high concentration of ferritin (>800 μg/L) may suggest iron overload (see Chapter 32). However, these indices have limitations (e.g., a high ferritin concentration is also generated by an inflammatory process; transferrin varies with nutritional state and is also influenced by inflammation). Clinical hematology laboratories may offer an automated estimate of the percentage of hypochromic red blood cells. A value above 10% is indicative of functional iron deficiency, and the target is less than 2.5%.[112]

Iron deficiency (absolute or functional) was the main cause of ESA resistance in the United Kingdom, but this has been resolved by iron replacement strategies. In hemodialysis patient populations, the inverse relationship between ESA dose and iron stores continues to maintain a linear relationship up to a mean ferritin of 500 μg/L. Parenteral iron is the treatment of choice for absolute and functional iron deficiency because oral iron has low efficacy in CKD. Parenteral iron can easily be administered during dialysis in patients receiving hemodialysis. Hemodialysis patients have additional iron losses from gastrointestinal bleeding, blood tests, and losses in dialysis lines that result in iron supplementation requirements that outstrip the capacity of the gut to absorb iron. Maintenance intravenous iron in hemodialysis patients greatly reduces ESA requirements and costs.[29] Maintaining iron stores at steady state in a hemodialysis population requires 50 to 60 mg/wk of intravenous iron.

In non–dialysis-treated CKD, a randomized study of intravenous iron versus oral iron in predialysis patients demonstrated a greater improvement in hemoglobin outcome in those on intravenous iron, but no difference in the proportion of patients who had to commence ESA after the start of the study.[450]

Nevertheless, oral iron is easy and cheap to prescribe and can be used as first-line iron supplementation in nondialysis patients. It is appropriate to treat patients who have not responded to, or have been intolerant of, oral iron with intravenous iron every 6 to 8 weeks to maintain serum ferritin greater than 100 μg/L.

Use of Erythropoiesis-Stimulating Agents

ESAs are synthetic versions of human EPO (rhEPO or epoetin) that are used to treat anemia. Following replenished iron stores and exclusion of other causes of anemia, the addition of ESAs is indicated for the treatment of CKD-related anemia. Measurement of serum EPO concentration is rarely indicated in the setting of renal anemia. The gene for human EPO was cloned in 1985, and epoetin was introduced into clinical practice shortly afterward.[200,475] ESAs are effective in correcting the anemia of CKD in 90 to 95% of patients. The most common side effect is hypertension; therefore blood pressure should be well controlled before treatment is introduced. Hypertension may develop or worsen in a quarter of patients. Failure to respond to treatment requires thorough investigation for many potential causes (Box 48-2). It is estimated that 3 million patients worldwide have received treatment with ESAs. A rare complication of ESA treatment is the generation of neutralizing antibodies to the ESA. These

BOX 48-2 Causes of Failure to Respond to Erythropoiesis-Stimulating Agents (ESAs)

Iron status
Occult blood loss
Vitamin B_{12} or folate deficiency
Infection and inflammation
Inadequate dialysis
Hyperparathyroidism
Aluminum toxicity
Patient adherence
Hypothyroidism
Primary disease activity
Transplant rejection
Malignancy
Pure red cell aplasia

antibodies stop bone marrow erythroid cells from producing mature red blood cells, so-called pure red cell aplasia.[62] If a case of pure red cell aplasia is proven, then no additional recombinant ESAs are administered.

Many clinical benefits are derived from correcting anemia with ESAs, including (1) improved exercise capacity,[294] (2) improved cognitive function,[287] (3) better quality of life,[306,367] and (4) increased libido. Much of the evidence has been taken from studies in dialysis patients. In patients with advanced CKD not yet on dialysis, small nonrandomized studies have suggested that regression of LVH is possible with partial correction of anemia with epoetin.[175,353] Patients who receive an ESA consistently over the 2 years before commencement of dialysis may have improved survival,[483] although larger prospective randomized trials have not confirmed these observations. Two important studies focused on patients not yet on dialysis. The Correction of Hemoglobin and Outcomes in Renal Insufficiency (CHOIR) study showed no benefit of higher hemoglobin concentration (13.5 g/dL vs. 11.3 g/dL) in CKD patients. Higher outcome target hemoglobin concentrations showed increased risk (using composite end points of death, myocardial infarction, and hospitalization for congestive cardiac failure) and no incremental improvement in quality of life.[407] The Cardiovascular Risk Reduction in Early Anaemia Treatment with Epoetin Beta (CREATE) study reported early correction of anemia to normal hemoglobin concentration (13 to 15 g/dL vs. 10.5 to 11.5 g/dL) but did not reduce the risk of cardiovascular events in patients followed for 3 years.[103] Indeed the hazards ratio for primary end points of death from any cause or death from cardiovascular disease consistently (but not significantly) favored the lower hemoglobin target group. LVH remained stable in both groups, and quality of life was significantly better in the higher hemoglobin outcome group.

A large randomized controlled trial has tested the hypothesis that normalization of anemia would have benefits in terms of morbidity and mortality for hemodialysis patients with New York Heart Association (NYHA) heart disease stage I to III.[30] Patients were randomized to normalization of anemia (618 patients and target hemoglobin concentration of 14 g/dL) or to the control group (615 patients and target hemoglobin concentration of 10 g/dL).

The study was terminated early because of a nonsignificant higher risk of death in the normalization group [RR 1.3, confidence interval (CI) 0.9 to 1.9]. These studies have been instructive in setting the current hemoglobin target of 10.0 to 12.0 g/dL and in recommending ESA dose adjustments when hemoglobin is less than 10.5 or greater than 11.5 g/dL, to balance benefit versus safety to patients.[446A]

The Uremic Syndrome

Uremia is defined as the excess within the blood of urea, creatinine, and other nitrogenous end products of amino acid and protein metabolism that are normally excreted in the urine. The *uremic syndrome,* the terminal clinical manifestation of kidney failure, is the group of symptoms, physical signs, and abnormal findings on diagnostic studies that result from failure of the kidneys to maintain adequate excretory, regulatory, and endocrine function.

Classic signs of uremia include (1) progressive weakness and easy fatigue, (2) loss of appetite followed by nausea and vomiting, (3) muscle wasting, (4) tremors, (5) abnormal mental function, (6) frequent but shallow respirations, and (7) metabolic acidosis. The syndrome evolves to produce stupor, coma, and ultimately death unless support is provided by dialysis or successful kidney transplantation. Regulation of body fluids is impaired in patients with uremia because of failure to excrete excess ingested fluid or to cope with fluid losses caused by vomiting or diarrhea. Patients also have difficulty excreting a salt load or retaining sodium when intake is low or vascular volume inadequate. Acid excretion is impaired, as is the ability to excrete nitrogenous metabolites from dietary sources. In relation to the stages of kidney disease defined by NKF-K/DOQI (see Table 48-5), kidney failure is present at a GFR $\leq$ 15 mL/min/1.73 m^2 (stage 5).[315] At this rate, signs and symptoms of uremia or the need for RRT is generally present. Biochemical characteristics of the uremic syndrome are summarized in Box 48-3. In addition to the consequences of reduced excretory, regulatory, and endocrine function of the kidneys, the uremic syndrome has several systemic manifestations—among them (1) pericarditis, (2) pleuritis, (3) disordered platelet and granulocyte function, and (4) encephalopathy—that have been difficult to explain.

For longer than 200 years, scientists have been studying the nature of uremia, but no single retained molecule has yet qualified for the title "uremic toxin," and many now agree that a variety of compounds are potential uremic toxins (Table 48-9). At least 90 organic compounds are known to be retained in uremia.[14,451] Many more still unidentified solutes are possibly retained and might exert systemic toxicity. Although urea was the first metabolite to be identified at increased concentrations in uremia, this does not appear to be responsible for the systemic manifestations of uremia. Urea is a 60 Da water-soluble compound that has the highest

BOX 48-3 Biochemical Characteristics of the Uremic Syndrome

Retained Nitrogenous Metabolites
- Urea
- Cyanate
- Creatinine
- Guanidine compounds
- "Middle molecules"
- Uric acid

Fluid, Acid-Base, and Electrolyte Disturbances
- Fixed urine osmolality
- Metabolic acidosis (decreased blood pH, bicarbonate)
- Hyponatremia or hypernatremia or hyperkalemia
- Hyperchloremia
- Hypocalcemia
- Hyperphosphatemia
- Hypermagnesemia

Carbohydrate Intolerance
- Insulin resistance (hypoglycemia may also occur)
- Plasma insulin normal or increased
- Delayed response to carbohydrate loading
- Hyperglucagonemia

Abnormal Lipid Metabolism
- Hypertriglyceridemia
- Decreased high-density lipoprotein cholesterol
- Hyperlipoproteinemia

Altered Endocrine Function
- Secondary hyperparathyroidism
- Osteomalacia (secondary to abnormal vitamin D metabolism)
- Hyperreninemia and hyperaldosteronism
- Hyporeninemia
- Hypoaldosteronism
- Decreased erythropoietin production
- Altered thyroxine metabolism
- Gonadal dysfunction (increased prolactin and luteinizing hormone, decreased testosterone)

concentrations of presently known uremic retention solutes in uremic plasma. Although its removal by dialysis is directly related to patient survival, the effects of urea on biological systems are not clear. Urea removal by dialysis is not necessarily representative of other molecules retained in the uremic syndrome, particularly protein-bound solutes such as *p*-cresol, or higher molecular weight molecules such as PTH and cystatin C.[319] Urea may be the source of other, more toxic moieties.[452] However, it is more likely that the syndrome is a result of the cumulative effect of many retained compounds, which may act as toxins and may have an effect on metabolism in general, for example, through enzyme inhibition or derangement in membrane transport. The decreased ability of the kidneys to degrade or eliminate hormones may also have a role.

TABLE 48-9 Potential Uremic Toxins

Toxin	Effect
Urea	At very high concentrations [>300 mg/dL (>50 mmol/L)] can cause headache, vomiting, and fatigue, carbamylation of proteins
Creatinine	Possibly affects glucose tolerance and erythrocyte survival
Cyanate	Causes drowsiness, hyperglycemia; a breakdown product of urea, it can cause carbamylation of proteins, altering protein function
Polyols (e.g., myoinositol)	Can cause peripheral neuropathy
Phenols	Can be highly toxic as they are lipid soluble and therefore can cross cell membranes easily
Middle molecules (e.g., atrial natriuretic peptide, cystatin C, delta sleep-inducing protein, IL-6, TNF-α, PTH)	Peritoneal dialysis patients clear middle molecules more efficiently than HD patients and show fewer signs of neuropathy than hemodialysis patients (many candidate molecules but none paramount)
β_2-Microglobulin	Causative agent in renal amyloid

HD, Hemodialysis; *IL-6,* interleukin-6; *PTH,* parathyroid hormone; *TNF-α,* tumor necrosis factor-alpha.

Acute Kidney Injury

AKI has largely replaced the older term *acute renal failure* and describes a sudden decline in kidney function over hours and days. AKI is an increasingly common and potentially catastrophic complication of systemic illness. Identifying the true incidence and prevalence of AKI has been difficult because of wide variation in the accepted definition of AKI. Several studies have reported multicenter experience with AKI in the intensive care unit setting and note wide variation in practice and outcomes.[69,299]

In 2003, a new classification of AKI was proposed that was based on the combination of susceptibility, nature and timing of insult, biomarker response, urine output, and end-organ consequences.[298] In recognition of the potential clinical importance of small changes in kidney function and the need to standardize definitions of AKI for clinical and research purposes, the RIFLE criteria were adopted by the Acute Dialysis Quality Initiative (ADQI), providing a graded definition of AKI severity.[226] The acronym RIFLE defines three grades of increasing severity of AKI (risk, injury, and failure) and two outcome variables (loss and end-stage renal disease). Grades of severity are established on the basis of change in serum creatinine concentration and decline in urine output

TABLE 48-10 Acute Kidney Injury Network (AKIN) Criteria for Acute Kidney Injury (AKI)*

AKIN Stage	Serum Creatinine Criteria	Urine Output Criteria
1	↑ SCr ≥ 0.3 mg/dL (26 μmol/L) *or* ↑ SCr ≥ 150-200% from baseline	<0.5 mL/kg/h for >6 h
2	↑ SCr > 200-300% from baseline	<0.5 mL/kg/h for >12 h
3	↑ SCr > 300% (>3-fold) from baseline *or* SCr ≥ 4 mg/dL (354 μmol/L) with an acute rise of ≥0.5 mg/dL (44 μmol/L) in ≤24 h *or* Initiation of renal replacement therapy (irrespective of stage at time of initiation)	<0.3 mL/kg/h for >24 h *or* Anuria for 12 h

*Only one criterion needs to be fulfilled to qualify for a stage.
SCr, Serum creatinine concentration.

from baseline. The most powerful tool to improve outcome in AKI is prevention, and the advantage of the RIFLE criteria is the definition of "risk," where it is envisaged that intervention may prevent injury and failure. In 2007, the Acute Kidney Injury Network (AKIN) proposed three stages of increasing disease severity (Table 48-10).[303] This expert working group, from all aspects of nephrology and critical care, modified the RIFLE criteria slightly to incorporate smaller changes in serum creatinine concentration into the definition of risk, because it was appreciated that small changes in kidney function can affect outcome. In essence, the AKIN has provided the following diagnostic criteria for AKI: (1) an abrupt (within 48 hours) reduction in kidney function, currently defined as an increase in serum creatinine concentration of 0.3 mg/dL (26 μmol/L); (2) an increase of 50% or greater (1.5-fold from baseline); or (3) a reduction in urine output (documented oliguria <0.5 mL/kg/h for >6 hours).

A prospective study of the initial hospital management of AKI confirmed that in almost 40% of cases, AKI was iatrogenic or preventable.[422] Early identification of intravascular volume depletion, use of nephrotoxic drugs, and early diagnosis of causative conditions can prevent AKI. Therefore, prompt administration of intravenous crystalloid solutions such as 0.9% sodium chloride may prevent further deterioration of AKI in many cases. Patients at risk for AKI include older persons; those with preexisting CKD, sepsis, diabetes, and heart disease; and those taking nephrotoxic drugs, particularly in the setting of hypovolemia. Fluid replacement requirements need careful monitoring and review of the patient, with emphasis on restoring an optimal circulatory volume without developing signs of fluid overload such as pulmonary edema. Additional monitoring may include use of a central venous pressure (CVP) line. Insertion of a CVP line is a specialist skill that requires cannulation of the internal jugular vein, ideally utilizing ultrasonic guidance facilities. However, where hypovolemia is clinically apparent, the priority is to resuscitate the patient with fluid, rather than delay treatment, by establishing invasive monitoring. The target CVP is 8 to 12 cm H_2O. A series of CVP measurements are useful for check response to fluids.

Clinical assessment of AKI should consider whether the precipitant is prerenal, intrarenal (intrinsic), or postrenal. The most common causes are listed in Box 48-4. Intrinsic AKI can be caused by primary vascular, glomerular, or interstitial disorders. It is therefore important that all patients presenting with AKI undergo urinalysis to test for infection, hematuria, and proteinuria. In most cases, the kidney lesion seen on histology is referred to as acute tubular necrosis (ATN). ATN is caused by ischemic or nephrotoxic injury to the kidney. In 50% of cases of hospital-acquired AKI, the cause is multifactorial. (The term *ATN* is somewhat misleading, insofar as necrosis per se is seldom seen, rather tubular *damage* occurs.) Although the pathogenesis is uncertain, a well-recognized clinical pattern is associated with the development of ATN, with anuria or oliguria and abnormalities indicating tubular dysfunction (Figure 48-14).[40] Necrosis of tubular cells need not be extensive, but obstruction by tubular casts, back-leak of glomerular filtrate through gaps in the tubular epithelium caused by cellular denudation, and primary reductions in GFR caused by altered intrarenal hemodynamics, known as tubuloglomerular feedback, may occur.[248] Direct vasoconstriction of glomerular capillaries in response to ischemic insults can also occur and may be mediated by AII, endothelin,[144,471] and serotonin.[453]

Urinary electrolyte measurements are seldom required or useful in the investigation of AKI. In practice, the treatment of prerenal AKI and ATN requires prompt and continued correction of hypovolemia, so urinary findings generally are not helpful.

Laboratory testing of blood is crucial in the management of AKI. Blood tests also assist in establishing the underlying diagnosis, and specific investigations are requested if kidney function has not improved following volume correction. An *acute renal screen* should clearly focus on most likely diagnoses and include the tests shown in Table 48-11.

The role of imaging in kidney disease is mentioned in Table 48-11, and exclusion of obstruction is important in AKI. Kidney biopsy is generally reserved for cases of AKI wherein an ultrasound scan has excluded obstructed kidneys, kidney sizes are maintained and the cause of AKI is otherwise unexplained, and an intrinsic pathology is suspected.

Metabolic acidosis is the most common acid-base disorder in patients with AKI. Reduced renal excretion of potassium and the effects of acidosis on the generation of extracellular

BOX 48-4 Causes of Acute Kidney Injury

Prerenal AKI
- Hemorrhage
- Diarrhea
- Postoperative fluid and blood losses
- Sepsis
- Acute cardiac failure

Intrinsic renal disease
- Tubular
- Glomerular
- Vascular

Any of the prerenal causes that are severe or that are not corrected promptly leading to ATN

Other causes of ATN
- Drug nephrotoxicity
- NSAIDs, ACE inhibitors
- Aminoglycoside antibiotics
- Amphotericin

TIN
- Allergic TIN associated with antibiotics and NSAIDs
- Sarcoidosis
- Pyelonephritis

Renal parenchymal disease
- RPGN (ANCA-associated vasculitides, Goodpasture's disease, SLE, other crescentic glomerulonephritides)
- Thrombotic microangiopathies
- Cryoglobulinemia

Myeloma

Miscellaneous
- Contrast nephropathy
- Poisoning
- Rhabdomyolysis
- Atheroembolism
- Urate nephropathy
- Hepatorenal syndrome

Vascular causes
- Aortic dissection
- Renal vein thrombosis

Postrenal AKI

Bladder outflow obstruction
- Benign and malignant prostate disease
- Invasive bladder carcinoma

Bilateral renal calculi or calculi within a single kidney

Retroperitoneal fibrosis

ACE, Angiotensin-converting enzyme; *AKI,* acute kidney injury; *ANCA,* antineutrophil cytoplasmic antibody; *ATN,* acute tubular necrosis; *NSAIDs,* nonsteroidal anti-inflammatory drugs; *RPGN,* rapidly progressive glomerulonephritis; *SLE,* systemic lupus erythematosus; *TIN,* tubulointerstitial nephritis.

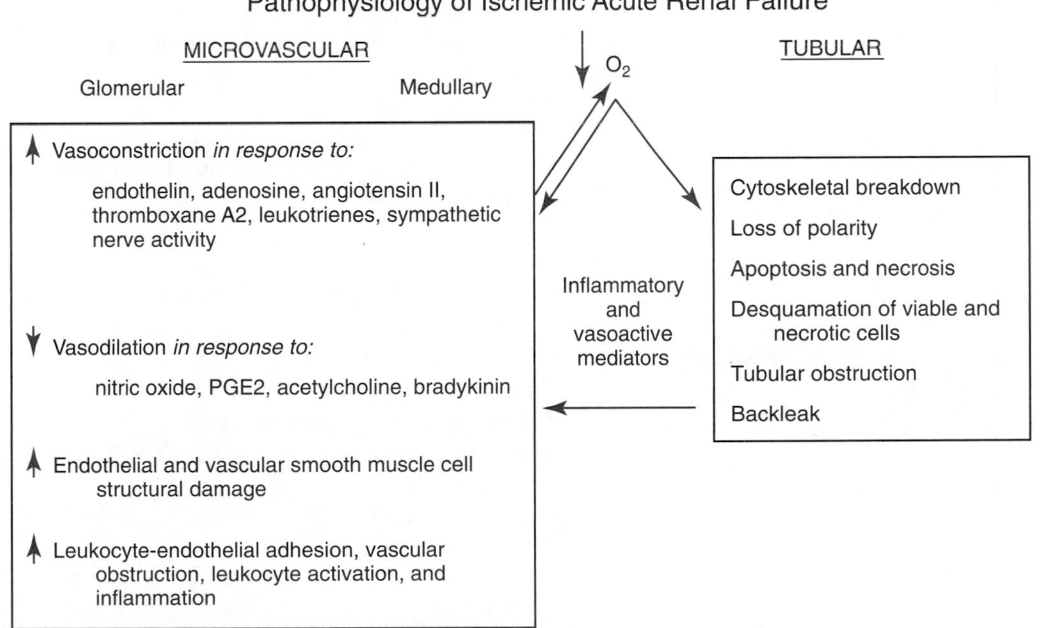

Figure 48-14 Pathogenesis of ischemic acute kidney injury. Hypoxic insults cause vascular responses and tubular damage. *(From Bonventre JV, Weinberg JM. Recent advances in the pathophysiology of ischemic acute renal failure. J Am Soc Nephrol 2003;14:2199-210.)*

TABLE 48-11 Investigation of Acute Kidney Injury (AKI)

Test	Indication/Comments
Urine Testing	
Urine reagent strip ("dipstick")	Hematuria and proteinuria may indicate glomerular origin
Red cell casts on microscopy	Not available universally: may need bedside microscope
Urine microscopy and culture	Identify urinary tract infection
Urine protein electrophoresis and immunofixation	
Blood Tests	
Baseline Studies	
Urea, electrolytes, creatinine, and calcium, phosphate, albumin	Check previous laboratory reports: AKI or AKI with preexisting CKD
Liver function tests	
Acid-base studies	Suspected multiorgan involvement or abnormal coagulation
Full blood count	Arterial blood gas or venous plasma bicarbonate concentration
Coagulation studies	Anemia, hemolysis, thrombocytopenia
	Evidence of intravascular coagulation; need to normalize if considering kidney biopsy and central line insertion
Selected Additional Investigations	
Blood culture	Any infection but especially endocarditis, severe pneumonia, or urinary tract sepsis
Creatine kinase	Very high in cases of muscle inflammation and necrosis (rhabdomyolysis)
Lactate dehydrogenase	If high, suspect renal infarction and consider hemolysis
Antineutrophil cytoplasmic antibodies	Vasculitides
Anti–glomerular basement membrane antibody	Anti–glomerular basement membrane disease
Antinuclear antibodies	Systemic lupus erythematosus
Anti-dsDNA antibodies, extractable nuclear antigens	Systemic lupus erythematosus
Low C4 complement	Systemic lupus erythematosus, atheroembolism, cryoglobulinemia
Cryoglobulin	Cryoglobulinemia
Urate	Urate nephropathy
Serum protein electrophoresis	Myeloma
Virology studies	Hepatitis serology, antistreptolysin O titer, human immunodeficiency virus
Imaging	
Chest x-ray	Pulmonary edema, pneumonia, effusions, malignancy, and granulomas
Abdominal x-ray (kidney, ureter, and bladder)	Renal stones
Renal tract ultrasound scan	Identify size and symmetry of kidneys
	Evidence of an obstructed system
	Small shrunken kidneys in advanced CKD
Computed tomography scan	Anatomy and perfusion
Magnetic resonance imaging	Angiography to identify renovascular lesions
Formal angiography	Critical renal artery stenosis
Kidney Biopsy	Reserved for patients with unexplained AKI in whom acute tubular necrosis is not suspected. It is anticipated that additional therapy such as steroids, cytotoxic drugs, and plasma exchange may be required.

CKD, Chronic kidney disease; *dsDNA,* double-stranded DNA.

potassium may lead to a very high concentration of potassium in the plasma. Severe hyperkalemia (serum potassium concentration >6.5 mmol/L) is associated with life-threatening cardiac arrhythmias. Emergency treatment of hyperkalemia should be instituted as necessary. Patients who have an abnormal electrocardiogram in the setting of high plasma potassium concentration, or a potassium concentration of 6.5 mmol/L or greater, should receive 10% calcium gluconate intravenously over 2 to 3 minutes through a large-bore peripheral venous cannula or a central line. This treatment stabilizes myocardial cells. However, calcium gluconate will not lower the potassium concentration. Infusion of high concentrations of glucose stimulates insulin secretion from the pancreas and uptake of potassium into the intracellular space. A fall in potassium concentration should be expected within 60 minutes. In addition, low-dose rapid-acting insulin can be administered with the glucose bolus. Serum potassium concentration should be monitored hourly until risk of a life-threatening cardiac event has passed and no evidence of potassium rebound is found. Blood glucose concentration should be monitored because hypoglycemia may occur following exogenous insulin. Again, care should be taken with 50% glucose infusions that good venous access is established, because extravasation can cause severe tissue necrosis.

When hyperkalemia persists despite appropriate medical measures, then RRT should be considered. Options for RRT include intermittent hemodialysis, peritoneal dialysis, and continuous renal replacement therapies (hemofiltration and hemodiafiltration) (see later). Continuous modalities are particularly appropriate for the intensive care unit setting in cases of multiple-organ failure. Continuous therapies are useful in the treatment of septic shock, cardiac failure, pancreatitis, and acute respiratory distress syndrome. They also allow the use of supplementary feeding, which is important in the oliguric patient with established AKI, in whom fluid is restricted to avoid overload.

If the patient survives, recovery usually will occur within days or weeks following removal of the initiating event. Uncomplicated AKI has a mortality rate of 5 to 10%,[186] although AKI complicating nonrenal organ system failure in the intensive care unit setting is associated with mortality rates approaching 50 to 70%, despite advances in dialysis treatment.[298]

The role of the clinical laboratory in assessment and monitoring of AKI is limited to assessment of electrolyte disturbance and fluid status, because during the recovery period, an initial polyuric phase occurs, as glomerular function recovers before tubular function recovers. This polyuric phase recedes after a few days to weeks, but careful monitoring is required to enable suitable fluid and electrolyte replacement.

Serum creatinine is the most widely used parameter for everyday assessment of GFR, but it has poor sensitivity and specificity in AKI because it lags behind both kidney injury and recovery. Several urinary and serum biomarkers of early tubular injury are being studied to assess whether injury can be detected before GFR is decreased.[77] These include urinary kidney injury molecule-1 (KIM-1), urinary neutrophil gelatinase-associated lipocalin (NGAL), urine IL-18, and serum cystatin C (see Chapter 25).

AKI Associated With Radiocontrast Media

Many procedures and tests that are undertaken within the hospital environment may contribute to the burden of AKI. In particular, intravascular administration of radiocontrast media during enhanced CT scanning and angiographic procedures accounts for many cases of AKI.[186] This is important as preventative strategies should be employed in patients with preexisting kidney disease, in patients with diabetes mellitus, and in those who are dehydrated and at increased risk of developing AKI when undergoing imaging. In 2003, 80 million doses of contrast media were administered worldwide.[223] Radiocontrast media are iodinated and may be ionic or nonionic. At concentrations required for angiography or CT scanning, the various agents used have differing osmolality. First-generation agents were ionic monomers with a very high osmolality with respect to plasma (e.g., 1500 to 1800 mOsmol/kg). Second-generation agents such as iohexol are nonionic monomers with a lower osmolality, although still higher than that of plasma (e.g., 600 to 850 mOsmol/kg). An iso-osmolal agent, iodixanol, has been introduced in 2003 (osmolality 290 mOsmol/kg). The use of iso-osmolar agents may lower the risk of AKI in high-risk diabetic patients undergoing angiography.[10] Preventative measures should be considered before a radiocontrast load is administered, regardless of the agent used. If possible, alternative investigations should be performed. However, when radiocontrast is required, the patient should be adequately hydrated with normal saline or isotonic sodium bicarbonate. An antioxidant, *N*-acetylcysteine, is commonly used to prevent contrast nephropathy following a reported benefit in reducing the incidence of AKI.[432] Reports of efficacy have been conflicting, but *N*-acetylcysteine is well tolerated and safe.[309] NSAIDs should be avoided because they interfere with vasodilator prostaglandins, causing increased renal vasoconstriction. The drug metformin should be discontinued at the time of the exposure to contrast in patients with diabetes.

DISEASES OF THE KIDNEY

Diabetic Nephropathy

Diabetes mellitus is a state of chronic hyperglycemia sufficient to cause long-term damage to specific tissues, notably the retina, kidney, nerves, and arteries (see Chapter 46). In 2000, the World Health Organization (WHO) estimated that 171 million people worldwide were affected by diabetes, with the prevalence set to reach 366 million by 2030.[479] In the United Kingdom, approximately 3% (1.9 million adults) of the population have diabetes. The WHO and national diabetes agencies have approved diagnostic criteria for diabetes based on venous plasma glucose concentrations.[479] In 2007, the Centers for Disease Control and Prevention in the United States took the unusual step for a noninfectious disease of classifying the increase in the incidence of diabetes as an epidemic.

Type 1 diabetes is due to autoimmune destruction of pancreatic islet β-cells, causing loss of insulin secretion. Type 2 diabetes is due to the combination of cellular resistance to insulin and β-cell failure. Tissue lesions are common to both types of diabetes, and chronic hyperglycemia (or a closely related metabolic abnormality) is responsible for diabetic complications including diabetic nephropathy.

Background

Diabetic nephropathy is a clinical diagnosis based on the finding of proteinuria in a patient with diabetes in whom there is no evidence of urinary tract infection. Overt nephropathy is characterized by protein loss greater than 0.5 g/d, approximately equivalent to albumin loss of greater than 300 mg/d. It is preferable to assess proteinuria as albuminuria because it is a more sensitive marker for CKD due to diabetes.[312,315] Albumin has been uniformly adopted as the "criterion standard" in evaluating diabetes-related kidney damage. The NKF-K/DOQI Work Group concluded that albumin should be measured to detect and monitor kidney damage in adults. Patients with urinary albumin loss of between 30 and 300 mg/d have so-called microalbuminuria (see Chapter 25).

Diabetic nephropathy is the most common cause of ESRD in the United States: the number of incident patients with diabetes as the cause of ESRD exceeded 48,000 during 2006—17.2% higher than in 2000 (see Figure 48-11).[79] Almost 200,000 people receiving RRT in the United States have diabetes as the cause of their ESRD, and this continues to rise steadily at around 2.5% per year.[79] Among patients who require dialysis, those with diabetes have a 22% higher mortality at 1 year and a 15% higher mortality at 5 years than patients without diabetes. Diabetic nephropathy as a cause of ESRD in the United Kingdom is seen in approximately 20% of new patients—a lower percentage than that of the United States and Europe.[7] In the United States, a number of objectives were developed for reducing threats to the health of the nation in the *Healthy People 2010* report. One of the objectives (HP 2010 Objective 4.7) is to reduce the incidence rate of ESRD caused by diabetes from 145 per million population to 78 per million people by 2010.[447] However, the overall rate for new cases of ESRD caused by diabetes was 153 pmp in 2008.[79,447A]

Diabetic nephropathy is clinically a very slowly developing condition, but ultrastructural evidence of glomerular damage has been found in renal biopsies taken from type 1 diabetic patients within a few years of their diagnosis.[18,65,120] In type 1 diabetes, early macroscopic changes include kidney enlargement and pallor. With disease progression, the kidneys become smaller. Type 2 diabetes is typified by variable kidney contraction caused by associated ischemia. On histologic examination, glomerular changes include diffuse mesangial sclerosis with accentuation of matrix and irregularly thickened basement membranes; sclerotic, acellular mesangial nodules (so-called Kimmelstiel-Wilson lesions); hyaline fibrin cap lesions around peripheral capillary loops; capsular drop lesions located within Bowman's capsule; and hyalinosis of arterioles.

Clinical progression is defined in terms of changes in rate of urinary albumin loss and decline in GFR and blood pressure changes (Table 48-12). In type 1 diabetes, it is unusual to develop microalbuminuria within the first 5 years of diagnosis, but it can occur anytime thereafter, and even after 40 years. Patients with type 1 diabetes and microalbuminuria will progress to overt nephropathy at an average rate of 20% over 5 years.[131] Long-term follow-up data on microalbuminuric patients confirm that 30% become normoalbuminuric (i.e., disease regression) and the rest remain microalbuminuric at 10 years.[59] Because the onset of type 2 diabetes is difficult to define, it is difficult to estimate the incidence of microalbuminuria, although 1% of patients in the United Kingdom have overt nephropathy at diagnosis. As albuminuria worsens and blood pressure increases, a relentless decline in GFR occurs.

Family studies of patients with type 1 diabetes have shown that diabetic siblings of patients with nephropathy have a fourfold risk of nephropathy compared with siblings without nephropathy. A family history of hypertension

TABLE 48-12 Development of Diabetic Nephropathy

Stage	Designation	Characteristics	Structural Changes	Glomerular Filtration Rate, mL/min/1.73 m²	Blood Pressure, mm Hg
I	Hyperfunction	Hyperfiltration	Glomerular hypertrophy	>150	Normal
II	Normoalbuminuria	Normal albumin loss	Basement membrane thickening	150	Normal
III	Incipient diabetic nephropathy (microalbuminuria)	Increased albumin loss	Albumin loss correlates with structural damage and hypertrophy of remaining glomeruli	125	Increased
IV	Overt diabetic nephropathy	Clinical proteinuria	Advanced structural damage	<100	Hypertension
V	Uremia	Kidney failure	Glomerular closure	0-10	High

and cardiovascular disease may increase nephropathy rates.[41] However, the best available predictor for development of nephropathy is microalbuminuria, although cellular markers are being investigated—such as increased erythrocyte Na^+/Li^+ countertransporter and overactivity of the Na^+/H^+ antiporter.[23] Considerable work has been undertaken to look for genetic linkages with the development of nephropathy in diabetes.[393]

Pathophysiology

Observational studies have shown that sustained poor glycemic control is associated with a greater risk for development of nephropathy in both type 1 and type 2 diabetes.[100,235,362,444] The exact mechanism for hyperglycemic tissue damage probably includes (1) glycation of proteins, leading to the formation of advanced glycation end products (AGEs); (2) overactivity of the polyol pathway; and (3) generation of reactive oxygen species.[220] Polyols are sugar alcohols formed from their respective sugars under the action of aldose reductase. Glucose is preferentially shunted through the polyol pathway under hyperglycemic conditions, generating sorbitol that accumulates within cells. A key step linking glucotoxicity to cell dysfunction in diabetic nephropathy is the excess of extracellular matrix within the glomerulus and interstitium. A number of genes encoding matrix proteins in hyperglycemic conditions have been identified.[290] For example, transcription of the gene for TGF-β is stimulated by hyperglycemia, AGE, AII, and reactive oxygen species.[182,334,463]

One important consequence of glucose-stimulated TGF-β transcription is upregulation of the insulin-independent GLUT-1 transporter in mesangial cells. Glucose is transported to the cells through GLUT-1 and is metabolized mainly by the glycolytic pathway. Increased de novo synthesis of diacylglycerol results in the activation of protein kinase C and mitogen-activated kinases. Activation of these enzymes can lead to stimulation of certain genes, including TGF-β. Activation of TGF-β can induce the expression of GLUT-1, and these signaling pathways induce the expression of extracellular matrix proteins. The formation of AGE also generates reactive oxygen species, which can activate latent TGF-β.[290] Studies employing neutralizing anti–TGF-β antibodies have provided evidence that the prosclerotic and hypertrophic effects of high ambient glucose in cultured renal cells are largely mediated by autocrine production and activation of TGF-β.[198,491] These antibodies can reverse established nephropathy in animal models.[67,490] Furthermore, glomerular TGF-β mRNA is markedly increased in kidney biopsy specimens from patients with proven diabetic kidney disease, and blood and urine sampling across the renal vascular bed confirms net renal production of TGF-β in diabetic patients.[403] Treatment with the ACE inhibitor captopril lowers circulating TGF-β concentrations in patients with diabetic nephropathy.[402]

The receptor for AGE (RAGE) has been identified.[392] RAGE is selectively expressed in the glomerular epithelial cells (podocytes) and not in the mesangial cell or the glomerular endothelium.[427] Increased accumulation of AGE in diabetes engages podocyte RAGE and may lead to increased glomerular permeability.[466] Vascular hyperpermeability, a hallmark feature of diabetes, can be suppressed by inhibiting RAGE in the animal model of diabetes, the streptozotocin-treated rat.[461]

Studies of experimental diabetes in the rat suggest that hyperfiltration alone could cause glomerular changes; conflicting reports have described the effects in humans. Increased GFR could be a predictor of progression to microalbuminuria but is also a reflection of poor metabolic control. In the Diabetes Control and Complications Trial (DCCT),[100] no association was noted between hyperfiltration and subsequent development of microalbuminuria.[23] Systemic blood pressure is higher in patients with diabetes who subsequently develop microalbuminuria, although it is not clear which comes first. Tubulointerstitial fibrosis occurs in diabetic nephropathy, in addition to glomerulosclerosis. Decreased GFR correlates with interstitial and glomerular expansion.[469]

Treatment Strategies

The cornerstones of treatment for diabetic nephropathy consist of glycemic control, blood pressure control, particularly with drugs that block the RAAS, and management of cardiovascular risk.[100,140,327,444] Guidelines published by NICE in 2008 recommend negotiation and individual target setting of glycated hemoglobin (HbA_{1c}) of around 6.5%, while specifically avoiding highly intensive management to values less than 6.5%.[312] High blood pressure accelerates the progressive increase in albuminuria in patients with initially normal urinary albumin loss and accelerates loss of kidney function in those with overt nephropathy in type 2 diabetes.[15,169] The NKF Task Force on Cardiovascular Disease has recommended a target blood pressure of less than 125/75 mm Hg in diabetic kidney disease.[256] ACE inhibitors and ARBs slow the progression of diabetic kidney disease.[46,260,302,337] A trial that was reported in 2000 confirmed that even normoalbuminuric patients with type 2 diabetes should be managed with ACE inhibitors or ARBs to prevent cardiovascular events.[485] In addition to lowered systemic blood pressure, such patients have lowered glomerular capillary blood pressure and protein filtration.[176,487] ACE inhibitors and ARBs also reduce AII-mediated effects on glomerular permeability and cell proliferation and fibrosis[276,308] and should be incorporated into the treatment schedules of all patients with type 2 diabetes and those with type 1 diabetes and microalbuminuria. ACE inhibitors may exacerbate hyperkalemia in patients with advanced kidney disease and/or hyporeninemic hypoaldosteronism. In older patients with renal artery stenosis, they may cause a rapid decline in kidney function. A low sodium diet potentiates the antihypertensive and antiproteinuric effects of AII blockade in type 2 diabetes.[188] Patients should be encouraged to stop smoking cigarettes because smoking increases the risk of microalbuminuria.[329] Dyslipidemias should be managed as outlined for nondiabetic proteinuric CKD. For many years, the Steno Diabetes Center in Copenhagen, Denmark, has advocated multifactorial interventions in the management of type 2 diabetes. For example, intensified interventions including tight glucose regulation, use of RAAS blockers, aspirin, lipid-lowering agents and lifestyle changes, were shown to reduce nonfatal cardiovascular disease among patients with type 2 diabetes[139] and subsequently beneficial effects with respect to vascular complications and on all-cause mortality.[138]

Hypertensive Nephropathy

Hypertension is second only to diabetes as a primary diagnosis of ESRD for incident patients commencing dialysis in the United States (see Figure 48-11).[79] The incidence is higher in older people and especially among the black population in the United States. Hypertension often develops as a consequence of CKD because of alterations in salt and water metabolism and activation of the sympathetic nervous and renin-angiotensin systems.[134,261] Hypertension can act as an accelerating force in the development of ESRD. As described earlier, treatment of hypertension to predefined target blood pressure values is critical in preventing progression to ESRD.[212,234,346] Various national and international guidelines on the treatment of hypertension have been published, although variability is evident among these recommendations. The JNC 7 report suggests that the risk of cardiovascular disease doubles for each increment in BP of 20/10 mm Hg, beginning at 115/75 mm Hg. The report identifies 120/80 mm Hg as normotension. All patients with hypertension (>140/90 mm Hg) should receive life-style change advice and antihypertensive medication if necessary.[73]

Hypertension is grouped with large vessel *renovascular disease* in the USRDS Annual Data Report database. Primary diseases of the renal arteries usually involve the origin of the renal arteries at the aorta (ostial lesions). Secondary diseases with hypertension and CKD with small vessel and intrarenal disease are referred to as *ischemic nephropathy.* A complex interplay occurs between renal artery stenosis and ischemic nephropathy. Atherosclerosis accounts for more than 90% of renal artery stenosis. The disease is progressive and may cause renal artery occlusion.[58] Prevalence increases with age and is associated with refractory hypertension, low body mass index, smoking, diabetes, and established vascular disease elsewhere. In general, as a marker of established cardiovascular disease, atheromatous renal artery stenosis is associated with a poor prognosis.[283] Diagnosis requires a high index of suspicion and is guided by radiologic examination of the renal arterial anatomy. Patients who receive ACE inhibitors and ARBs may develop AKI in the setting of severe bilateral renovascular disease or severe disease to a single functioning kidney. Kidney function should be carefully monitored following the introduction of these drugs, and a fall of GFR in excess of 15 to 20% should raise the suspicion of renovascular disease. The diagnosis is important to make because radiologic placement of intraluminal stents[39] is possible, and surgical repair can be performed to prolong vessel patency.[168] Patients are at risk, however, of atheroembolism following intervention.[398] A correctable atherosclerotic renal artery stenosis (ARAS) lesion is found in less than 1% of all hypertensive patients, so investigation has to be targeted to high-risk groups.

Renal artery stenosis in younger patients is characteristically due to fibromuscular dysplasia. The medial part of the artery is most commonly affected and presents radiologically as alternate bands of narrowing and dilatation, giving rise to a "string of beads" appearance. If the diagnosis is made, then hypertension can be cured following balloon angioplasty to the artery in at least 50% of cases.

Noninvasive imaging is readily available and includes CT angiogram and MRI angiography with gadolinium-based contrast media. A rare but potentially fatal disease, nephrogenic systemic fibrosis, has been described in patients with advanced kidney disease receiving gadolinium-based contrast media during MRI. Because many patients who are investigated for ARAS will have CKD, the approach to investigation has changed. Nephrogenic systemic fibrosis was first described in 2000 as a cutaneous scleromyxedema-like disorder in patients with ESRD.[87] Gadolinium-based contrast media are not recommended for patients with advanced renal impairment, particularly those on dialysis.[426]

Glomerular Disease

Glomerular disease is suggested clinically by the finding of blood and protein in the urine on urine reagent strip testing. Proteinuria greater than 1 g/d (≈0.88 g/g creatinine; ≈100 mg/mmol creatinine) in the absence of an overflow-type proteinuria such as myoglobinuria or light chain–related disease is invariably glomerular in origin. Although a detailed discussion of each glomerular disease is beyond the scope of this book, the most important diseases will be discussed to illustrate the spectrum of disease. Whereas the incidence of kidney failure in the Western world has increased dramatically over recent years, in the United States, the incidence rate due to glomerulonephritis has fallen (see Figure 48-11).[79] In the United Kingdom, glomerulonephritis accounts for 10% of new cases of established renal failure.[7]

Primary Glomerular Disease

Glomerulonephritis can be primary (affecting only the kidneys) or secondary (in which the kidneys are involved as part of a systemic process). Histopathologic classification of glomerulonephritis may appear slightly cumbersome but is readily simplified by consideration of the glomerular structures and cells that may be involved, and the presence or absence of immune complexes (Table 48-13). In essence, only three cell types are involved (endothelial, epithelial, and mesangial) plus the acellular GBM. The glomerular cells and the GBM have a limited range of response to injury, namely, proliferation, scarring (sclerosis), and GBM thickening. The term *focal* is used if less than half of the glomeruli are involved in the disease process as seen on light microscopy, whereas *diffuse glomerulonephritis* refers to cases in which all glomeruli are involved. Immune deposits identified following immunofluorescence or immunoperoxidase staining do not define whether a disease is focal or diffuse. Primary glomerular diseases that will not be considered further

TABLE 48-13 Overview of Some Primary Glomerular Diseases

Disease	Histologic Findings	Clinical Spectrum	Treatment	Prognosis
IgA nephropathy	• Focal mesangial cell proliferation on LM • IgA deposited within mesangial cells on IM	• Variable: incidental finding; episodes of macroscopic hematuria; proteinuria and declining GFR • Male preponderance • Peak incidence occurs in second and third decades of life • May be associated with systemic vasculitis in HSP	• Generic treatment targeting blood pressure and RAAS blockade • Selected cases receive corticosteroids and cytotoxic drugs	• Variable, but 30-40% progress to kidney failure over 20 years
Minimal change disease (MCD)	• Little evidence of cellular involvement on LM • Podocyte foot process effacement demonstrated on EM • No immune deposits	• Most common cause of nephrotic syndrome in children • Usually idiopathic • Relapsing and remitting course	• Oral corticosteroids and cytotoxic drugs	• Does not cause kidney failure • Significant side effects of immunosuppressant drugs
Focal segmental glomerulosclerosis (FSGS)	• Glomerular scarring and nonspecific trapping of immune complexes in scarred areas	• Common cause of nephrotic syndrome in adults • Congenital forms described • Secondary causes include collapsing variety seen in HIVAN	• Idiopathic disease requires corticosteroids and cytotoxic drugs in selected cases	• Nephrotic syndrome commonly refractory to treatment • 30-40% develop kidney failure at 10 years
Membranous nephropathy	• Thickened GBM with immune deposits in subepithelial GBM • Classically, "spikes" are seen along the GBM and represent new GBM squeezed between deposits	• Common cause of nephrotic syndrome • Secondary causes in 20% of cases	• Treat underlying condition • Idiopathic membranous • Treat generically and if progressive add immunosuppressive drugs	• Variable outcome: "rule of thirds" (see text)

EM, Electron microscopy; *ESRD*, end-stage renal disease; *FSGS*, focal segmental glomerulosclerosis; *GBM*, glomerular basement membrane; *GFR*, glomerular filtration rate; *HIVAN*, human immunodeficiency virus–associated nephropathy; *HSP*, Henoch-Schönlein purpura; *IM*, immunofluorescence or imunoperoxidase microscopy; *LM*, light microscopy; *RAAS*, renin-angiotensin-aldosterone system.

include mesangiocapillary glomerulonephritis and hereditary nephritis (Alport's syndrome).

IgA Nephropathy

IgA nephropathy is an example of a focal glomerulonephritis with focal mesangial cell proliferation demonstrated by light microscopy. However, diffuse and global deposition of the immunoglobulin, IgA, can be demonstrated following immunostaining. It is the most common type of glomerulonephritis worldwide and has a particularly high prevalence around the Pacific rim, where it is commonly reported as an incidental finding in kidney biopsy specimens from potential kidney donors.[22] The disease tends to be slowly progressive (in terms of loss of kidney function) depending, as with most kidney diseases, on the degree of proteinuria, kidney function at the time of diagnosis, and degree of interstitial fibrosis on kidney biopsy. Up to 50% of patients exhibit elevated concentrations of serum IgA, although diagnosis depends on kidney biopsy findings. Clinical presentation varies considerably from asymptomatic microscopic hematuria to macroscopic hematuria; proteinuria including nephrotic syndrome; and crescentic glomerulonephritis with kidney failure. Episodic macroscopic hematuria is seen in some patients at the same time as an upper respiratory tract infection. IgA nephropathy may also present with established proteinuria, renal impairment, and hypertension. Variation in clinical and histologic features leads to difficulty in reaching conclusions regarding treatment protocols that have been tested in clinical trials.

No treatment is available that specifically modifies mesangial deposition of IgA, and available options are limited to downstream immune and inflammatory events that may lead to scarring. Treatment options vary from tonsillectomy in patients with macroscopic hematuria associated with respiratory infection to no treatment in those with isolated microscopic hematuria or those with proteinuria of less than 1 g/d. In progressive disease, all patients are treated in a similar generic fashion as for most kidney diseases, including targeting blood pressure to less than 125/75 mm Hg and using comprehensive RAAS blockade to minimize proteinuria. Assessment of the impact of immunosuppressive therapy is compromised by the heterogeneity of the disease and the duration of a randomized controlled study with sufficient numbers to allow a conclusion. Nevertheless, a large Italian study with more than 10 years of follow-up data demonstrated benefit from oral corticosteroids in high doses for 6 months.[354,423] Cytotoxic therapy can be considered for rapidly progressing or vasculitic IgA.[17]

Nephrotic Syndrome

Nephrotic syndrome is defined as (1) heavy proteinuria (>3 g/d), (2) reduced serum albumin concentration, and (3) edema. In comparison with nephritic syndrome, nephrotic patients may exhibit an otherwise bland urinary sediment with little hematuria. Nephrotic syndrome can occur at any age from neonate to elderly. Although the underlying kidney disease tends to vary with age, in all cases the lesion is within the glomerulus and is associated with damage to the specialized visceral epithelial cells, the podocytes (see earlier). Proteinuria is a consequence of a reduction in the charge-selective properties of the filtration barrier, particularly the GBM, and of alterations in the slit diaphragms of interdigitating foot processes of adjacent podocytes (Figure 48-15).[91,365] Following the discovery of numerous genes and podocyte proteins that make up the slit diaphragm, the pathophysiology of glomerular proteinuria is beginning to be elucidated. The primary glomerular diseases that cause nephrotic syndrome have recently been termed *podocytopathies,* and a new

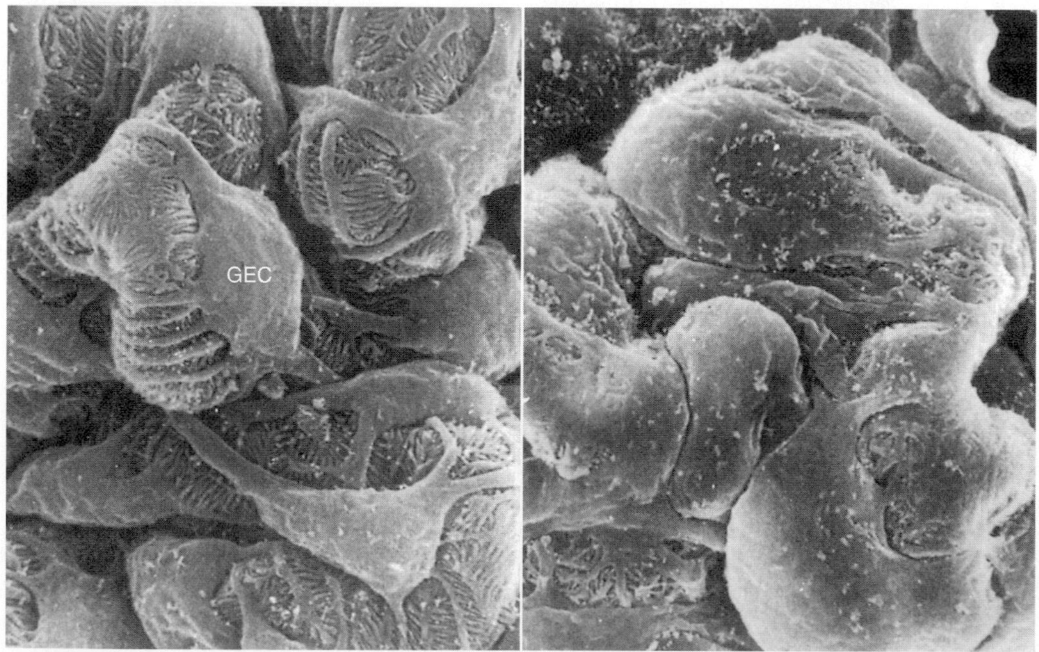

Figure 48-15 Graphic example of glomerular changes in nephrotic syndrome. Scanning electron microscopic view of glomerular epithelial podocytes from a vehicle-treated rat *(left)* and a puromycin aminonucleoside (PAN)-treated (180 mg/kg body wt) rat *(right)*. Note the extensive loss of podocyte foot processes, which occurs in response to PAN-induced nephrotic syndrome and illustrates the major cellular changes that can occur in nephrotic syndrome. *GEC,* Glomerular epithelial cell. *(From Ricardo SD, Bertram JF, Ryan GB: Antioxidants protect podocyte foot processes in puromycin aminonucleoside–treated rats. J Am Soc Nephrol 1994;4:1974-86.)*

classification scheme has been proposed that will identify diseases based on both morphology and etiology.[20]

The most common causes of nephrotic syndrome are minimal change disease (MCD), focal segmental glomerulosclerosis (FSGS), and membranous nephropathy (see later). Secondary causes are discussed separately and include diabetic nephropathy, amyloidosis, and SLE. A kidney biopsy is generally undertaken in all adult patients who present with nephrotic syndrome. Diagnosis is made only on kidney biopsy, and a biopsy is generally undertaken in all adult patients who present with nephrotic syndrome. Nephrotic syndrome is associated with significant morbidity regardless of cause, and patients with the disease have increased cardiovascular disease as the result of marked hyperlipidemia and increased risk of infection and thromboembolic disease. Between 10 and 40% of patients with nephrotic syndrome develop evidence of arterial and venous thromboemboli, particularly deep vein and renal vein thrombosis. Renal vein thrombosis may be unilateral or bilateral and may extend into the inferior vena cava. However, most cases of renal vein thrombosis have an insidious onset and produce no symptoms. Infrequently, patients develop acute renal vein thrombosis and present with signs of renal infarction, including flank pain and microscopic or gross hematuria. In addition, AKI may supervene in cases of nephrotic syndrome (Box 48-5), and prolonged proteinuria with a poor response to treatment may lead to kidney failure.

The management of nephrotic syndrome depends on the underlying glomerular lesion, although general principles apply in all cases (Box 48-6). In addition to general measures, specific treatment targeted at inducing remission from proteinuria usually requires a combination of immunosuppressive drugs, including corticosteroids and cytotoxic drugs.

MCD is the most common cause of nephrotic syndrome in children and young adults. The incidence of MCD is estimated at 1 to 5 cases per 100,000 children per year. It typically presents with severe edema and hypoalbuminemia, and urine testing confirms heavy proteinuria. Kidney function is normal, with little evidence of a reduced GFR. MCD does not progress to kidney failure, except in some cases of severe refractory disease that may be complicated by glomerular scarring lesions. Nephrotic syndrome in a noninfant child is assumed to be caused by MCD, and a kidney biopsy generally is not performed, because the condition typically is responsive to a trial of corticosteroids with remission within 2 weeks. Following the disappearance of proteinuria, or 1 week after remission is induced, the corticosteroid dose can be reduced and tapered slowly. An attempt to stop treatment may be indicated after 8 weeks. Longer duration of corticosteroid therapy significantly reduces the risk of relapse, and many centers will treat for a minimum of 12 weeks, particularly with a first episode of steroid-responsive nephrotic syndrome. Around 60% of steroid-responsive patients experience multiple relapses. Some of these patients can be managed with low-dose corticosteroids given daily or on alternate days, but relapses do occur, especially if intercurrent infection is present. In addition to the comorbidity associated with nephrotic syndrome, the burden of long-term exposure to corticosteroids and cytotoxic drugs has to be considered. Cyclophosphamide, azathioprine, and cyclosporine are reserved for refractory cases and can be used as corticosteroid-sparing agents with the aim of reducing relapse rates. Treatment with cyclophosphamide is limited to 8 to 12 weeks to reduce risk of gonadal toxicity, and the cumulative dose threshold whereby this risk increases significantly is 200 mg/kg in children.

The histologic lesion is by definition "minimal" when viewed on light microscopy. However, electron microscopy confirms disruption to the epithelial surface of the glomerular capillary. Podocyte foot processes are detached (effaced) from the GBM, conferring absence of the slit diaphragm, and therefore the final barrier to filtration fails (see Figure 48-15). The glomerular architecture is restored following prompt treatment with high-dose corticosteroids. In MCD, the onset of nephrotic syndrome is often preceded by an infection or allergic reaction, and it has been proposed that nephrotic syndrome may be the result of an exaggerated response to normal physiologic and immune mechanisms that increase proteinuria during infection. MCD does occur in adults who present with nephrotic syndrome. MCD occasionally complicates NSAID ingestion, and secondary MCD has been

BOX 48-5 Causes of AKI in Nephrotic Syndrome

- Acute tubular necrosis, usually in MCD and patients >50 years of age
- Minimal change disease with acute interstitial nephritis induced by NSAIDs
- Tubular injury in collapsing FSGS idiopathic or associated with HIV infection
- Crescentic glomerulonephritis superimposed upon membranous nephropathy

FSGS, Focal segmental glomerulosclerosis; *HIV,* human immunodeficiency virus; *MCD,* minimal change disease; *NSAIDs,* nonsteroidal anti-inflammatory drugs.

BOX 48-6 Management of Nephrotic Syndrome

- Low-sodium diet
- Protein intake of 1.0 g/kg/d
- Fluid management: usually includes loop diuretics
- Thromboembolism prophylaxis: may include formal anticoagulation in high-risk patients (serum albumin <20 g/L or in nephrotic syndrome due to membranous nephropathy or mesangiocapillary glomerulonephritis)
- Vigilance for infection
- Treatment of hyperlipidemia with 3-hydroxy-3-methylglutaryl-Co-enzyme A (HMG)-CoA-reductase inhibitors (statins)
- Treatment of hypertension, primarily with RAAS blockade
- Supportive treatment of AKI
- Education and psychologic support for patients and relatives

AKI, Acute kidney injury; *RAAS,* renin-angiotensin-aldosterone system.

described in patients with malignancy (particularly Hodgkin's lymphoma).

Focal segmental glomerulosclerosis (FSGS) is the most important cause of the nephrotic syndrome in adults and remains a frequent cause in children and adolescents, particularly in the United States, Brazil, and many other countries.[161] Genetic studies in children with familial nephrotic syndrome have identified mutations in genes that encode important podocyte proteins.[44,228] Nephrin was the first slit diaphragm protein identified, and mutations in this transmembrane protein cause congenital (Finnish-type) nephrotic syndrome, which occurs with a frequency of 1/8200 live births in Finland. Among children with inherited nephrotic syndrome, other podocyte proteins (podocin, α-actinin 4, CD2-AP) have been described; all proteins are crucial to the interaction of the slit diaphragm with the podocyte cytoskeleton. Compelling evidence advocating a soluble permeability factor has been proposed as causing nephrotic syndrome in FSGS. Evidence includes experience in kidney transplantation, whereby FSGS may recur within hours of transplantation of a normal kidney into a recipient with FSGS.[387] The nature of the permeability factor remains unknown, but it can be removed by immunoabsorption to protein A and plasma exchange prior to transplantation.

Several disease processes lead to the description of FSGS on kidney biopsy and are shown in Box 48-7. Proteinuria in secondary FSGS, as in primary FSGS, reflects epithelial injury, although the mechanism is different. Following nephron loss, the remaining glomeruli undergo hypertrophy. Because podocytes are usually in a state of terminal differentiation and unable to replicate, the density of available foot processes to cover the enlarged glomerular surface is decreased. Focal areas of denudation from the GBM ensue, leading to proteinuria. Corticosteroids and other immunosuppressant drugs are not recommended for secondary forms of FSGS or for congenital forms. The treatment of primary disease causing nephrotic syndrome is typically a course of high-dose corticosteroids given for at least 6 months as tolerated. Remission of nephrotic syndrome is characterized by absence of proteinuria, loss of edema, and normalization of serum albumin concentration.

BOX 48-7 Causes of Secondary Focal Segmental Glomerulosclerosis

- Glomerular hypertrophy/hyperfiltration
  - Unilateral renal agenesis
  - Massive obesity
- Scarring due to previous injury
  - Focal proliferative glomerulonephritis
  - Vasculitis
  - Lupus
- Toxins (pamidronate)
- Human immunodeficiency virus–associated nephropathy (HIVAN)
- Heroin nephropathy

Membranous Nephropathy

The term *membranous nephropathy* reflects the primary histologic change noted on light microscopy: basement membrane thickening with little or no cellular proliferation or infiltration. Electron microscopy (EM) reveals electron-dense deposits across the glomerular basement membrane. The immune nature of these deposits is confirmed by immunostaining with immunoglobulins, and complement components are readily demonstrated. Idiopathic membranous nephropathy is a common cause of nephrotic syndrome, accounting for approximately 30% of adult cases. The clinical features are variable and are classically described as follows ("rule of thirds"): (1) a third of cases undergo spontaneous remission of proteinuria and recovery of kidney function; (2) a third of cases have nonprogressive disease but evidence of ongoing proteinuria; and (3) a third of cases continue to exhibit nephrotic syndrome and are at high risk of progressive kidney failure.

The clinical course therefore is difficult to predict at the onset of the disease, although 40% of patients develop kidney failure after 10 years. Patients generally are observed for 6 months to assess the likely natural history of the condition and are treated generically. In progressive cases and in those who have evidence of nephrotic syndrome for at least 6 months, a course of immunosuppressive drugs is indicated. Typical immunosuppressive schedules include high-dose corticosteroids, calcineurin inhibitors such as cyclosporine, and cytotoxic drugs (chlorambucil and cyclophosphamide).[350]

Secondary causes of membranous nephropathy are associated with a wide spectrum of diseases, including SLE, hepatitis B, falciparum malariae, malignancy, and drugs (e.g., gold, penicillamine, captopril). In comparison with idiopathic disease, the clinical outcome depends on the underlying disease process. Underlying malignancy has been thought to be responsible for up to 5 to 10% of cases of membranous nephropathy in adults; the risk is highest in patients older than 60 years of age. A solid tumor (such as carcinoma of the lung, colon, or prostate) is most often involved and usually is clinically obvious.[253]

Rapidly Progressive Glomerulonephritis

Rapidly progressive glomerulonephritis (RPGN) is a heterogeneous group of disorders characterized by a fulminant clinical course that leads to kidney failure in only weeks or a few months. The clinical picture of RPGN is often preceded by a systemic illness for several months associated with general malaise, weight loss, breathlessness, upper respiratory tract abnormalities, and skin changes. Clinical examination may reveal nailfold infarcts affecting the fingernails and toenails and palpable purple lesions on the skin of the legs. In severe cases, a renal-pulmonary syndrome supervenes with kidney failure and alveolitis with associated pulmonary hemorrhage. In some cases, the condition may be limited to the kidneys (renal-limited vasculitis).

These syndromes are often characterized by focal glomerulonephritis with glomerular ischemia, infarction, and tissue death (necrosis). Following release of inflammatory cytokines and chemokines from the necrotic capillaries the epithelial cells of Bowman's capsule proliferate. These cells lie on top of adjacent cells and form a partial circle around the inner rim of Bowman's capsule that is referred to as a *crescent*. Proliferating epithelial cells and macrophages eventually compress the glomeruli and obstruct the proximal convoluted tubules, thus severely compromising nephron function.

RPGN may be classified as idiopathic kidney disease or as a disease secondary to other conditions, such as infectious disease, multisystem disease, and occasionally an adverse reaction to medication. Anti-GBM antibodies may be present along the GBM in anti-GBM disease. Most commonly, however, there is no immunoglobulin deposition within the glomerulus (pauci-immune). Approximately 80% of patients with active pauci-immune necrotizing and crescentic glomerulonephritis have been shown to possess antineutrophil cytoplasmic antibodies (ANCAs), irrespective of the presence or absence of a concomitant systemic vasculitis. This strong association has allowed serologic discrimination of this type of glomerulonephritis from other types of RPGN. Wegener's granulomatosis, microscopic polyangiitis, and Churg-Strauss syndrome are small-vessel vasculitides characterized by an association with ANCAs.

ANCAs were first reported in 1982 in patients with pauci-immune serologic glomerulonephritis.[93] Three years later, ANCAs were detected by indirect immunofluorescence on human neutrophils in patients with active Wegener's granulomatosis.[449] Since 1989, two subtypes of ANCA have been described: cytoplasmic (C-ANCA) and perinuclear (P-ANCA), reflecting the patterns observed by indirect immunofluorescence microscopy using alcohol-fixed neutrophils as a substrate.[470] C-ANCAs are directed toward a plasma proteinase (PR3) in neutrophil primary granules and are associated with Wegener's granulomatosis, whereas the P-ANCA target antigen is usually myeloperoxidase (MPO) and is associated with microscopic polyangiitis.[113,322] Immunoassays have been used to measure anti-PR3 and anti-MPO antibody titers. Vasculitis or angiitis is an inflammatory reaction in the wall of any blood vessel that can have diverse clinical presentations. The exact sequence of events that triggers perivascular inflammation leading to injury is unclear, but ANCAs have been identified that have at least diagnostic and prognostic usefulness. ANCAs appear in the plasma of almost all patients with active and generalized disease and are useful in diagnosis of the disease and in monitoring response to therapy, because a falling titer of ANCA suggests response. Autoantibodies of other specificities in rheumatoid arthritis, SLE, and inflammatory bowel disease may mimic the P-ANCA pattern, and in isolation, the finding of P-ANCA has a low specificity for vasculitis. The International Consensus Statement on Testing and Reporting of Antineutrophil Cytoplasmic Antibodies (ANCA) was developed to optimize ANCA testing.[386] It requires that all sera are tested by indirect immunofluorescence examination of peripheral blood neutrophils and, where there is positive fluorescence, by immunoassays for antibodies against PR3 and MPO. Following this protocol, false-positive rates of less than 1% can be achieved. Testing will be further improved by standardization and use of common immunoassay methods.

Rapidly progressive glomerulonephritis accounts for 15% of patients presenting to specialist nephrology units for renal replacement therapy and therefore is an important disease category to be aware of, because if treatment is initiated early, independent kidney function can be restored, particularly if active lesions are seen on biopsy.[173] In addition to measurement of ANCA, C-reactive protein (CRP) is extremely helpful in assessment of the acute-phase reaction in active disease processes and is critical in helping to define disease remission. In patients in whom the CRP has returned to normal, disease remission is indicated; this prompts the clinician to reduce immunosuppressant treatment doses.[385]

Highly intensive immunosuppressive schedules are commenced in patients who present with RPGN. This *induction* phase of treatment is continued until the disease has remitted. Once remission is attained, a longer maintenance phase of treatment with less intensive schedules is commenced. In cases with a high index of suspicion on clinical grounds, treatment should begin empirically. Usually the diagnosis is made following a kidney biopsy and an ANCA or anti-GBM antibody test. High-dose oral prednisolone and oral or intravenous cyclophosphamide are given as standard baseline treatment. Adjunctive treatments that may be used routinely in severe cases include pulses of intravenous methylprednisolone (1 g/d for 3 days) or a series of plasma exchanges.[204] The rationale for these approaches is to switch off production of the antibody and attenuate the proinflammatory response to tissue damage. Patients are closely followed for many months for evidence of disease activity and signs of treatment-related toxicity. This involves monitoring of kidney function, full blood count, ANCA serology, and anti-MPO/PR3 titer, as well as CRP. Following remission of active disease, drug doses are tapered, and cyclophosphamide may be exchanged for azathioprine. Serologic testing for ANCA and measurement of CRP are performed prior to immunosuppressant dose reduction to ensure that the disease activity has abated. Plans for long-term follow-up are made, and treatment is expected to be ongoing for at least 3 to 5 years. Relapses may occur as immunosuppression is reduced or withdrawn. The untreated mortality of ANCA-associated vasculitis is 90% at 1 year. With current management strategies, the mortality rate has fallen to 20 to 30%. The elderly are most susceptible both to the disease and to treatment-related morbidities, particularly infection. Patients who require dialysis or ventilatory support for pulmonary involvement have a higher mortality rate.

Anti-GBM disease (Goodpasture's disease) affects 0.5 to 1 per million population per year in the United Kingdom. Serologic detection of anti-GBM antibodies is helpful for assisting diagnosis in cases of RPGN. In this process, the antigens are well characterized and the antibody is directed at the $\alpha 3$ chain of type IV collagen. The disease is characterized by a relative lack of prodromal illness; a very rapid deterioration in kidney function; and a poor prognosis if oliguria or anuria should develop. The kidney biopsy typically demonstrates crescents in all the glomeruli ("100% crescents"), and each crescent is at a similar stage of development. The GBM stains positively with anti-GBM antibodies upon immunostaining in a linear pattern. In addition to renal involvement, lung basement membrane can be affected, leading to pulmonary hemorrhage (Goodpasture's syndrome). The environment plays a critical role in determining whether anti-GBM antibodies cause lung injury, because pulmonary hemorrhage occurs only in current cigarette smokers.

Systemic Lupus Erythematosus (SLE)

SLE is a chronic inflammatory disease of unknown cause that can affect the (1) skin, (2) joints, (3) kidneys, (4) lungs, (5) nervous system, (6) serous membranes, and/or (7) other organs of the body. The clinical course of SLE is variable and may be characterized by periods of remissions and chronic or acute relapses. Women, especially in their 20s and 30s, are affected more frequently than men. Renal involvement, termed *lupus nephritis,* occurs in up to 60% of adults with SLE. Lupus nephritis is especially common in African American and Hispanic patients in the United States.[21] Lupus nephritis may present variably from incidental hematuria and proteinuria, nephrotic syndrome, or a fulminating RPGN. Most patients with SLE (≈75%) develop an abnormal urinalysis or impaired kidney function during the course of the disease. A pathologic description is required to stage the disease process in lupus nephritis. The classification of lupus nephritis has been revised, and treatment is targeted depending on the stage of disease.[462] In general terms, pathologic findings include a spectrum from focal mesangial proliferation to diffuse global necrotizing glomerulonephritis. Membranous nephropathy may also be present. Detection of lupus nephritis involves urine testing for blood and protein and tests of kidney function. In addition, serologic testing for autoantibodies to nuclear antigens and measurement of complement components C3 and C4 are undertaken (Table 48-14). Significant hypocomplementemia and elevated anti-DNA titers suggest active disease. Combined use of corticosteroids and intravenous or oral cyclophosphamide has been the conventional treatment for diffuse proliferative lupus nephritis since the 1970s.[419] Treatment duration with cyclophosphamide is limited because of severe toxicity, including gonadal toxicity, hemorrhagic cystitis, bone marrow suppression, and carcinogenicity. Data from a 2009 study suggest that mycophenolate mofetil and corticosteroids can be as effective, but not superior to, intravenous cyclophosphamide for induction treatment for lupus nephritis.[9]

TABLE 48-14 Laboratory Investigation of Vasculitic Syndromes

Disease	Serologic Test	Antigens	Associated Laboratory Features
SLE	ANA including antibodies to dsDNA and ENA [including SM, Ro (SSA), La (SSB), and RNP]	Nuclear antigens	Leukopenia, thrombocytopenia, Coombs' test Complement activation: low serum concentrations of C3 and C4 Positive immunofluorescence using *Crithidia luciliae* as substrate Antiphospholipid antibodies (i.e., anticardiolipin, lupus anticoagulant, false-positive VDRL)
Goodpasture's disease	Anti-GBM antibody	Epitope on noncollagen domain of type IV collagen	
Small Vessel Vasculitis			
Microscopic polyangiitis	P-ANCA	MPO	↑ CRP
Wegener's granulomatosis	C-ANCA	Proteinase 3 (PR3)	↑ CRP
Churg-Strauss syndrome	P-ANCA in some cases	MPO	↑ CRP and eosinophilia
Henoch-Schönlein purpura	None		
Cryoglobulinemia			Cryoglobulins, rheumatoid factor, complement components, hepatitis C
Medium Vessel Vasculitis			
Classical PAN	None		↑ CRP and eosinophilia

ANA, Antinuclear antibodies; *ANCA,* antineutrophil cytoplasmic antibody; *C-ANCA,* cytoplasmic ANCA; *CRP,* C-reactive protein; *dsDNA,* double-stranded DNA; *ENA,* extractable nuclear antigens; *GBM,* glomerular basement membrane; *MPO,* myeloperoxidase; *P-ANCA,* perinuclear ANCA; *PAN,* polyarteritis nodosa; *RNP,* ribonucleoproteins; *SLE,* systemic lupus erythematosus; *VDRL,* Venereal Disease Research Laboratory.

Acute Nephritic Syndrome

This disorder is characterized by rapid onset of hematuria, proteinuria, reduced GFR, and sodium and water retention, with resulting hypertension and localized peripheral edema. Congestive heart failure and oliguria may also develop. In a number of patients with the acute nephritic syndrome, the pathologic process is related to recent group A α-hemolytic streptococcal infection of the pharynx or, less commonly, the skin. Only certain strains of streptococci are capable of inducing acute nephritis. A latent period averaging about 2 weeks exists between the time of streptococcal infection and clinical evidence of nephritis. In patients suspected of having acute poststreptococcal glomerulonephritis, evidence of recent infection may be found in increased titers of antibodies to streptococcal extracellular products: antistreptolysin O, anti-hyaluronidase, and anti–deoxyribonuclease-B. Serial measurements that document rising antibody titers against streptococcal antigens provide stronger evidence of recent infection than is provided by a single determination. Most patients have moderate reductions in total hemolytic complement activity (CH_{50}) and in the C3 component of the complement cascade. Typical poststreptococcal glomerulonephritis is now rare in developed countries, and a kidney biopsy may be performed in adult cases to establish the diagnosis pending serologic test results. A kidney biopsy of patients with post-streptococcal glomerulonephritis reveals diffuse involvement with enlarged hypercellular glomeruli infiltrated by polymorphonuclear leukocytes and monocytes. Electron microscopy reveals deposits, presumably immune complexes, on the epithelial side of the basement membrane. Abnormal laboratory results are usually present early in the course of acute nephritis. Hematuria, which may be gross ("cola-colored" urine) or microscopic, and proteinuria, usually <3 g/d, are almost always present. Red blood cell casts are highly suggestive of glomerulonephritis. These casts are commonly present in urine but are observed only if the specimen is fresh and acidic, centrifugation is light, and sediment (after decantation) is resuspended gently. Large numbers of hyaline and granular casts are common; waxy casts suggest a chronic process and should raise the possibility of acute exacerbation of a preexisting disease. Persistent and severe depression of C3 concentrations should suggest membranoproliferative glomerulonephritis, SLE, endocarditis, or other forms of sepsis. Although depressed concentrations of complement imply disease activity, they are not useful for grading the severity or determining the prognosis of the illness.

Other causes of acute nephritis include reactions to drugs, acute infection of the kidneys, systemic disease with immune complexes such as SLE, bacterial endocarditis, and finally disease in which the antigen is unknown but is possibly related to antecedent viral infection.

Interstitial Nephritis

A variety of chemical, bacterial, and immunologic injuries to the kidney may cause generalized or localized changes that primarily affect the tubulointerstitium rather than the glomerulus. This group of disorders is characterized by alterations in tubular function that, in advanced cases, may cause secondary vascular and glomerular damage. Interstitial nephritis, including chronic pyelonephritis, is the primary diagnosis, accounting for 3.8% of patients admitted onto dialysis programs in the United States[447] and 6.4% in the United Kingdom.[7] *Pyelonephritis,* the term associated with a bacterial infection that causes this kind of damage, is the most common of the interstitial nephritides.[435] Both acute and chronic types of pyelonephritis may occur; the acute type is most commonly associated with urinary tract infection (UTI). Acute pyelonephritis may develop into chronic pyelonephritis, usually as a result of a renal tract abnormality such as abnormal urethral valves. Interstitial nephritis is also associated with proteinuria that is less severe than in glomerular disease. In addition to conventional pyelonephritis, interstitial nephritis may present in acute and chronic forms and has many causes. Acute allergic interstitial nephritis presents with AKI and marked inflammation of the interstitium. Lymphocytes, polymorphonuclear cells, and eosinophils are prominent. The incidence is variable and depends on kidney biopsy practice. It may account for up to 7% of cases of AKI when an intrinsic kidney disease is diagnosed as opposed to purely toxic and/or ischemic acute tubular damage.[355] Higher values are likely in older people because of the increased incidence of drug reactions. A drug hypersensitivity reaction is the most common form of acute interstitial nephritis. Urinary findings may be normal, or decreased proteinuria and eosinophils may be seen on light microscopy. More than 100 different drugs have been implicated, but NSAIDs and β-lactam antibiotics are the drugs most commonly identified.[141] Nephrotic syndrome may accompany an acute interstitial nephritis associated with NSAIDs. Treatment is directed at removing any causative agent. Steroids are used to promote early resolution of the clinical course, although patients can develop chronic interstitial fibrosis.[397]

Sarcoidosis is a multisystem disorder associated with chronic granulomatous interstitial nephritis. Biochemical abnormalities include hypercalcemia, hypercalciuria, and increased serum ACE activity.[372] The condition may be effectively treated with steroids.

Prostaglandins and NSAIDs in Kidney Disease

NSAIDs block synthesis of prostaglandins by cyclooxygenase (COX) enzymes. Two isoforms of COX synthesize prostaglandins. COX-1 is a resident or constitutive form, and COX-2 is an inducible form that increases with disorders of inflammation.[399] NSAIDs are nonspecific inhibitors of both COX isoforms. Analgesic nephropathy is a common cause of kidney failure in many countries, causing 10% of such failures in Switzerland and Australia, but it is essentially a preventable condition for which monitoring of kidney function has proved useful. The incidence of this disease has decreased over the past decade as awareness has improved, and phenacetin was withdrawn from over-the-counter analgesic mixtures. In the United States, 1 in 5 citizens (50 million) report that they use an NSAID for an acute complaint.[468] Although most healthy individuals tolerate NSAIDs well, a study of the very old (mean age, 88 years) demonstrated significant reduction of GFR within 1 week of ingestion of NSAIDs.[159] Renal blood flow, particularly within the medulla, is dependent on systemic and local production of vasodilatory prostaglandins, and analgesic-related kidney damage is seen mostly within the medulla, with late changes causing papillary necrosis and interstitial fibrosis. Hyperkalemia can develop as a consequence of reduced GFR or secondary to hyporeninemic hypoaldosteronism. In addition, NSAIDs can rarely cause nephrotic syndrome and drug-related acute allergic interstitial nephritis.

Monoclonal Light Chains and Kidney Disease

Immunoglobulin (Ig) molecules are formed in secretory B cells. The heavy chains α, β, γ, δ, and ε identify the antibody isotype, and light chains include peptide molecules that are called kappa (κ) and lambda (λ). A complete Ig molecule will contain either κ or λ. The proportion of Ig containing κ versus λ is 3:2 in humans. The molecular weight of light chains is approximately 23 kDa. Excess production of light over heavy chains appears to be required for efficient Ig synthesis, resulting in the release of free light chains into the circulation. In normal individuals, the small quantity of circulating polyclonal light chains is filtered by the glomerulus, and ≈90% is reabsorbed in the proximal tubule and degraded by proteases. Increased concentrations of filtered light chains lead to alteration in the proximal tubule cells, including prominent cytoplasmic vacuolation, loss of the microvillous border, and epithelial cell exfoliation.[382]

Light chains can deposit in the kidney as casts, fibrils, and precipitates or crystals, giving rise to a spectrum of disease including cast nephropathy, amyloid, light chain deposition disease, and the Fanconi syndrome. However, not all patients with excessive production of monoclonal light chains develop disease. Other promoters include dehydration, hypercalcemia, contrast medium, and NSAIDs. Evidence suggests that light chains are directly pathogenic.[415] The pattern of human renal injury associated with monoclonal light chains can be reproduced in mice injected intraperitoneally with large quantities of light chains isolated from patients with myeloma or light chain–associated amyloid (AL-amyloid).[237]

Myeloma or multiple myeloma is a neoplastic proliferation of secretory B cells (plasma cells) that produce excessive amounts of a monoclonal Ig (paraprotein)—so-called M protein, because of the characteristic peaks obtained from serum protein electrophoresis on agarose gel. A serum IgG greater than 2 g/dL (often much higher), or IgA or IgM greater than 10 g/dL, or the finding of an IgD or IgE paraprotein at any concentration suggests a malignant paraproteinemia. The clonal production of immunoglobulin is associated with excess or pure light chain production. In multiple myeloma, complete monoclonal Igs (usually IgG or IgA) are accompanied in the plasma by variable concentrations of free light chains that appear in the urine as Bence Jones proteins, named after Henry Bence Jones, who first described these in 1848. M proteins and light chains can be identified in the blood and/or the urine in 98% of patients with myeloma using protein electrophoresis and immunofixation. Immunoparesis, with reduction in nonparaprotein Ig, is characteristic of myeloma. The incidence of myeloma is 40 new cases per million population per year.[473] Myeloma is more common in men than in women, and the median age at presentation is 65 years.[242] It is the second most commonly diagnosed hematologic malignancy, with an annual incidence of 15,000 and a prevalence of 45,000 in the United States.[408]

Impairment of kidney function at presentation occurs in almost 50% of myeloma patients.[98,473] Although most recover following treatment for other factors contributing to renal impairment (e.g., dehydration, hypercalcemia, infection, nephrotoxic drugs), about 10% have severe renal involvement caused by the effects of light chains on the kidney. Severe kidney failure may occur in myeloma following deposition of light chains within tubules—so-called cast nephropathy (myeloma kidney). Cast nephropathy can present acutely, again precipitated by dehydration, hypercalcemia, or NSAIDs, or de novo in the absence of these factors. It occurs when the reabsorptive capacity of proximal tubule cells is exceeded by overproduction of light chains. In myeloma, light chain excretion can exceed 20 g/d. Casts are large and numerous and are found predominantly in the distal convoluted tubule and collecting ducts, causing obstruction to urine flow. They have a hard and fractured appearance with lamination visible on histologic examination of kidney biopsy specimens. Immunofluorescence confirms that casts are composed of monoclonal light chains and THG. Casts usually are stained exclusively with anti-κ or anti-λ antibodies. At biopsy, there is often an interstitial inflammatory infiltrate, and fibrosis and tubular atrophy can be extensive. Not all light chains induce cast formation. The ability of light chains to form casts is based on binding to THG.[373] Light chains interfere with proximal tubule cell function, and this promotes delivery to the distal tubule. A specific binding site for light chains has been identified on THG, and light chains with high affinity appear to be more likely to produce obstructing intratubular casts.[191]

Physicochemical determinants of binding of light chains to THG include the isoelectric point (pI) of the light chain. Those molecules with a pI above 5.1 (above the tubular fluid pH in the distal nephron) will have a net positive charge that may promote binding via charge interaction to anionic THG (pI, 3.2). Urinary alkalinization reduces binding of light chains to THG in animal models.[183] Nephrotoxicity may be determined by the ability of light chains to self-associate, leading to the formation of high molecular weight aggregates that are more likely to deposit in tissues, particularly in the setting of volume depletion.

The clinical features of myeloma include a normochromic normocytic anemia, bone pain with pathologic fractures (back or chest rather than extremities), and hypercalcemia in 20% of patients. Severe kidney failure may dominate the clinical picture, and 84% of patients studied retrospectively with severe renal impairment required dialysis.[197] Only 15% of these patients regained independent kidney function. Treatment has two main objectives: therapy is targeted at predisposing factors for cast nephropathy as indicated, and chemotherapy is used to reduce the production of monoclonal antibodies and light chains from monoclonal plasma cells. Supportive therapy includes increased fluid intake where permissible to 3 L/d, treatment of hypercalcemia, treatment of infection, and withdrawal of NSAIDs. Anemia can be addressed by replacement with blood products or the use of ESAs. Skeletal complications are common in myeloma, and pathologic fractures occur in the setting of apparently trivial injury. Increased osteoclastic activity is mediated by IL-1, IL-6, TNF, and macrophage inflammatory protein-1α.[167] Bisphosphonates, which are specific inhibitors of osteoclastic activity, have beneficial effects in myeloma.[25] Bisphosphonates may exert direct antitumor effects on myeloma because they induce significant expansion of γδ-T cells in peripheral blood mononuclear cells, which exhibit specific cytotoxicity against myeloma cell lines in vitro.[241]

Chemotherapy can be considered as part of urgent treatment for patients with kidney involvement in myeloma. The aim is to reduce the concentration of free light chains. Chemotherapy with alkylating agents, such as melphalan, and combination treatment with cytotoxic agents and dexamethasone are the preferred initial treatment regimens, and doses and schedules are adjusted depending on the lrate of GFR. Combination chemotherapy results in partial responses but only rarely in complete remission.[4,155,277]

The disease is incurable and eventually relapses. Poor prognostic features in myeloma include increased serum concentrations of β_2-microglobulin, CRP, and lactate dehydrogenase, and abnormal cytogenetics (especially deletion of 13q). With modern, intensive therapy, including autologous hematopoietic stem cell transplantation, the median survival is 5 years. Refractory disease is associated with a short survival and requires salvage therapy. Development of the newer agents bortezomib and lenalidomide, in addition to the antiangiogenesis compound thalidomide,[328,409] has improved the outlook for relapsed disease. The rationale for use of thalidomide comes from observations that prominent bone marrow vascularization occurs in myeloma and correlates with markers of poor prognosis, and that plasma concentrations of angiogenic cytokines are elevated in myeloma. Clinical trials of thalidomide in myeloma were first described in 1965, and reduction in the paraprotein load and improved 1-year survival have been reported.[409,484] Significant side effects include thromboembolic disease and peripheral neuropathy, and the agent is highly teratogenic. Bortezomib is an inhibitor of the 26S proteosome (an intracellular organelle responsible for protein degradation). It causes rapid clonal cell reduction by inducing apoptosis, reversing drug resistance in myeloma cells, and blocking angiogenesis in vitro,[181] and has been demonstrated to be superior to dexamethasone for relapsed disease.[368]

In addition to chemotherapy, plasma exchange is often used in the treatment of myeloma cast nephropathy to acutely reduce free light chain load. There is a paucity of trial data,[209,492] but one prospective study of 29 patients demonstrated increased 1-year survival following plasma exchange treatment. Several early deaths in the control group render the data difficult to interpret.[492] Further study of 21 patients with myeloma and AKI demonstrated advantages of plasma exchange in patients with kidney failure severe enough to require dialysis.[209] The U.K. Renal Association and the U.K. Myeloma Forum are currently recruiting almost 300 patients to a national study of plasma exchange in myeloma cast nephropathy (Myeloma Renal Impairment Trial-MERIT). However, a study from Canada of 104 patients presenting with myeloma and AKI, randomized to five to seven plasma exchange treatments in addition to conventional treatment, showed no significant difference in the composite outcome of death, dialysis dependence, and GFR less than 30 mL/min/1.73 m^2 at 6 months.[75]

In cast nephropathy, glomerular filtration of *intact* light chains may occur. Excess production of monoclonal light chains (or rarely heavy chains) causes disorders in which *fragments* are deposited in the kidney and other tissues. Amyloidosis is a condition characterized by extracellular deposition of fibrils in an antiparallel β-pleated sheet arrangement. The type of amyloid is defined by the abnormal protein deposited. For example, in "primary amyloid" or "AL-amyloid," fibrils derived from the variable region of light chains are deposited in the tissue. Seventy-five percent are derived from the λ-light chain. Because it is the variable region that is deposited, it is often difficult to assess with immune reactants. Only 50% of AL-amyloid cases are stainable with commercially available antisera to κ and λ. The deposits are fibrillar in nature and bind to Congo red. Amyloid fibrils also bind to the serum amyloid P component, allowing noninvasive evaluation by radiolabeled serum amyloid P scanning.[174] The diagnosis of AL-amyloid can be suspected from the clinical findings of nephrotic proteinuria (>3.5 g/d) and serum or urinary paraprotein. However, 10 to 15% of patients with primary amyloid do not have a detectable serum or urinary paraprotein. Demonstration of a clonal excess of plasma cells on bone marrow biopsy may help with the diagnosis in those without detectable paraprotein. AL-amyloid has a poor prognosis, and mean survival is 18 months, with 50% of patients dying from cardiac failure. Treatment options are unsatisfactory, although prednisolone and melphalan may be tried.[243,244,410] Circulating free light chains can be detected by a nephelometric immunoassay in most patients with AL-amyloid, and patient outcome following treatment is improved if the concentration of free light chains can be reduced by 50%.[245]

The French Myeloma Group has published results of bone marrow or stem cell transplantation in AL-amyloid.[305] In a retrospective analysis of 21 patients treated with melphalan and stem cell transplantation, 43% died within 1 month, and the remainder had a favorable outcome.

Light chains may cause tubular dysfunction, especially of the proximal tubular cells. Characteristically, the light chain variable domain is resistant to degradation by proteases in lysosomes in the tubular cells. The variable domain fragments accumulate in proximal tubular cells, and clinical features include renal tubular acidosis and phosphate wasting.

Polycystic Kidney Disease

Autosomal dominant polycystic kidney disease (ADPKD) is the second most common inherited monogenic disease (after familial hypercholesterolemia), with an estimated incidence of 1 : 1000. It is by far the most common inherited kidney disease; ≈12.5 million people worldwide are affected.[254] In the United Kingdom, ADPKD is responsible for 10% of new ESRD in patients younger than 65 years and 2.5% of incident patients over age 65 years.[7] The prevalence of the disease varies from 1 in 200 to 1 in 1000 of the population, but many cases, possibly up to 50%, remain clinically undiagnosed during life. Approximately 50% of ADPKD patients develop kidney failure by age 55 years.[137] It is therefore important to make the diagnosis in affected families and to monitor kidney function regularly. The intervals between estimations of GFR will depend on the stage of CKD, as with other progressive kidney diseases. An important clinical observation is the highly variable phenotype within families. The disease causes the development of multiple kidney cysts and extrarenal cysts occurring in the liver and pancreas. About 10% of ADPKD families have a strong family history of intracranial arterial aneurysm rupture. Hypertension is an early and frequent manifestation, and gross hematuria is a common presenting symptom. On the basis of effectiveness, cost, and safety, ultrasound is the imaging modality most commonly used to make the diagnosis. Screening for polycystic kidney disease is controversial, and age-dependent ultrasound diagnostic criteria for ADPKD have been developed. According to recent criteria, the presence of fewer than two renal cysts has a negative predictive value of 100% and is enough to exclude the disease in at-risk individuals who are 40 years of age and older.[342]

ADPKD is caused by mutations in the genes (*PKD1* and *PKD2*) that encode polycystin 1 and 2, which are located in primary cilia.[192,233,363] Mutations affecting *PKD1* are more prevalent than those of *PKD2* and tend to have a worse prognosis, with larger kidneys and earlier development of kidney failure. Genetic testing is not used routinely as a screening tool because current techniques identify only 70% of the hundreds of different *PKD1* and *PKD2* mutations.[152] The function of primary cilia is to act as flow sensors in the tubules, with flow-induced deformation resulting in calcium influx that leads to a proliferative cellular response mediated by intracellular cAMP. Animal model studies have demonstrated abnormalities in vasopressin and vasopressin receptors in ADPKD and these receptors may be therapeutic targets in the future. Other mutations include the *PKD2* mutation on chromosome 4 (110 kDa) and *APKD3*, for which the gene product and the chromosomal location remain unknown.[339] *PKD2* appears to be a more slowly progressive form of the disease.[172] The median age of onset of ESRD with *PKD2* is 15 years later than with *PKD1*. Also, a rare (incidence 1/20,000) autosomal recessive form of the disease may present in childhood.

Specific treatments for ADPKD in clinical practice are currently lacking. Generic treatment should include treatment of hypertension with ACE inhibitors and/or ARBs and maintaining a fluid intake of 2 to 3 L/d to reduce risk of kidney stone disease. Specific therapies, in development, are targeted at reducing cyst development and enlargement. Estimates of cyst volume can be determined using MRI techniques and changes documented over a relatively short period of time.[64] This has allowed the performance of clinical trials of novel drugs such as vasopressin receptor antagonists and other antiproliferative drugs such as sirolimus.[86]

Obstructive Uropathy

Benign prostatic hyperplasia (BPH) is one of the most common types of obstructive uropathy and is an almost universal finding in aging men.[296] For example, for men aged 50 years, the reported prevalence of BPH is 40%, and for men aged over 70 years, it is at least 75%.[27] No close relationship between the degree of enlargement and the symptoms experienced has been observed.[66] Among the most common symptoms are disorders of micturition, in particular increased frequency, and in many cases this progresses to bladder outflow obstruction. Between 10 and 40% of men with bladder outflow obstruction caused by BPH present in acute retention.[296] Approximately 5% of this group have high-pressure chronic retention of urine, which can result in upper urinary tract obstruction, and consequently CKD as a result of glomerular and tubular damage. Although medical treatments are available to decrease the rate of enlargement of the prostate, resection of the enlarged gland remains the most common surgical procedure performed on men. Urinary retention can be a chronic disorder, with acute exacerbations requiring bladder decompression by catheterization. If the obstruction is not removed by surgery, progressive kidney injury can occur as a result of backpressure along the urinary tract. It is important to identify those patients at risk of developing CKD, because failure to remove their enlarged gland can cause kidney failure. Obstruction can also occur because of kidney stones, which can cause bilateral or unilateral damage. In children, severe kidney damage can be caused by vesicoureteric reflux. One of the main complications of reflux, whether caused by obstruction or by an inherited defect, is the increased incidence of urinary tract infection. When the obstruction is relieved, the kidney often regains some independent function. A tendency toward slower progression to kidney failure has been noted in obstructive uropathy compared with other kidney diseases.

Tubular Disease

Types of tubular disease discussed in this section include renal tubular acidoses (RTAs) and inherited tubulopathies.

Renal Tubular Acidoses

The RTAs constitute a diverse group of inherited and acquired disorders affecting the proximal or distal tubule. They are characterized by a hyperchloremic, normal anion gap; metabolic acidosis; and urinary bicarbonate or hydrogen ion excretion inappropriate for the plasma pH. They may result from failure to retain bicarbonate or from inability of the renal tubules to secrete hydrogen ion. Typically, the GFRs in RTAs are normal or slightly reduced, and there is no retention of anions, such as phosphate and sulfate (as opposed to the acidosis of kidney failure). Before attempting to understand the pathology of these conditions, the reader should ensure a good comprehension of normal renal acid-base (and ammonia) regulation (see Chapter 49).

Classification of RTAs is based on the biochemical expression and region of the defect, rather than on an understanding of the exact molecular defect. The three categories of RTA are distal (dRTA, type I); proximal (pRTA, type II); and type IV, which occurs secondary to aldosterone deficiency or resistance. [The term "type III RTA" (mixed proximal/distal defect) has been abandoned by some authors because it is not considered a separate entity.[343] It may arise as the result of a mutation in the gene coding for carbonic anhydrase type 2.[369]]

Distal RTA (Type I)

Type I dRTA occurs most often in infants (sometimes transiently) and young children, but it may also be encountered in adults, in whom it is more common than pRTA. Clinical features generally include metabolic acidosis, muscle weakness, nephrocalcinosis (i.e., diffuse, fine, renal parenchymal calcification), and urolithiasis (i.e., the formation of calculi in the urinary tract). The defect is an inability to secrete hydrogen ions in the distal tubule in the presence of a systemic acidosis. Several subtypes may be seen: urinary pH greater than 5.5 is a common feature.[343] Biochemical features typically include hypokalemia, hypocitraturia, and low urinary ammonium ion.

Classic (Hypokalemic, Secretory) dRTA. The molecular basis is not known but may include defects in the H-ATPase or H,K-ATPase transporters. dRTA may occur in association with a wide variety of conditions, including (1) an autosomal dominant condition (more common in females); (2) a sporadic, nonfamilial disease; (3) other genetic disorders (e.g., Wilson's disease); (4) dysproteinemias (e.g., hypergammaglobulinemia, cryoglobulinemia, amyloidosis); (5) disorders of calcium metabolism (e.g., primary hyperparathyroidism); and (6) a variety of autoimmune disorders (e.g., SLE, Sjögren's syndrome, primary biliary cirrhosis, thyroiditis). The pathogenesis of nephrocalcinosis and urolithiasis may be the result of decreased urinary citrate excretion secondary to cellular acidosis.

Back-leak dRTA. Although the kidney tubule retains the ability to secrete hydrogen ions, the gradient is not maintained because of back-diffusion. Typically, this occurs in association with specific drug treatments (e.g., amphotericin B).

Voltage-Dependent (Hyperkalemic) dRTA. This is due to failure to maintain an intraluminal negative potential that restricts hydrogen (and potassium) ion secretion; it may be seen with urinary tract obstruction, sickle cell disease, and treatment with amiloride or triamterene. Voltage-dependent (hyperkalemic) dRTA has many features in common with type IV RTA (see discussion later in this chapter). It is frequently associated with mild to moderate CKD, and hyperkalemia is caused in part by decreased GFR, in addition to decreased potassium excretion relative to the filtered load. In contrast to classic dRTA, potassium excretion cannot be increased in response to sodium sulfate (Na_2SO_4) administration, suggesting an isolated defect in hydrogen ion secretion. However, because hydrogen ion secretion is dependent on sodium reabsorption in the distal tubules, the primary defect could be impairment of distal tubular sodium reabsorption.

Incomplete dRTA. This is a less severe, normokalemic form, which may represent an early stage of overt dRTA. Some patients acidify urine at a submaximal rate, but at a rate that is generally sufficient to maintain acid-base balance. Potassium wasting, hypokalemia, and hyperchloremia generally are not present. However, when patients are stressed or are given an acid load test, their ability to excrete acid and to lower urine pH is suboptimal, and urinary pH may exceed 5.5.

Proximal RTA (Type II)

In pRTA the primary defect is failure of proximal tubular bicarbonate reabsorption. Proximal RTA may occur as an isolated defect (primary or sporadic type II pRTA) that occurs chiefly in infant males and is commonly associated with growth retardation, or that produces a generalized proximal tubular disorder (Fanconi syndrome). Proximal tubular bicarbonate reabsorption is still incompletely understood at the molecular level, but some candidate transporters associated with hereditary forms of pRTA are discussed by Ring and associates.[369] Most cases of pRTA are secondary to genetic disorders that affect the proximal tubule (e.g., cystinosis, fructose intolerance) or to acquired diseases including multiple myeloma, Sjögren's syndrome, and amyloidosis; heavy metal poisoning (lead, mercury, cadmium); drugs (e.g., ifosfamide); and renal transplant rejection. Drugs that act as carbonic anhydrase inhibitors (e.g., acetazolamide, topiramate) have also produced a pRTA condition. (Note that several of these disorders and agents also cause dRTA.) In pRTA the threshold for bicarbonate reabsorption is lowered (from a plasma concentration of 22 mmol/L to 15 mmol/L).[343] Once plasma bicarbonate falls below this threshold, filtered bicarbonate is reclaimed, and urinary pH generally will be less than 5.5. In pRTA, contrary to dRTA, nephrocalcinosis and nephrolithiasis are rarely observed, but metabolic bone disease is common. Other features of the Fanconi syndrome (e.g., glycosuria, aminoaciduria, hypophosphatemia, hypouricemia) are commonly present.

Selective Aldosterone Deficiency (Type IV RTA)

In type IV RTA failure of distal potassium and hydrogen ion secretion results from aldosterone deficiency or resistance due to a number of steroid or steroid receptor synthetic defects or from hyporeninemic hypoaldosteronism (e.g., due to diabetic nephropathy, tubulointerstitial disease, urinary obstruction, renal transplantation, or SLE). Hyperkalemia, although mild, is a usual manifestation. Type IV RTA associated with pseudohypoaldosteronism type 2 is thought to be due to a mutation in the *WNK* gene, which encodes a protein that interacts with several renal electrolyte transport systems (Table 48-15).[369]

TABLE 48-15 Characteristics of Some Inherited Tubulopathies*

Disorder [OMIM Number]	Protein Defect	Chromosome Localization	Inheritance	Clinical Features/Notes	Biochemical Features
Proximal Tubule					
Lowe's syndrome (oculocerebral dystrophy) [309000]	OCRL1	Xq26.1	XR	Hydrophthalmia, cataract, mental retardation, hyporeflexia, hypotonia, and progressive kidney failure; normotensive	Plasma: ↓K, ↓CO_2 Urine: ↑LMWP, ↑AA, ↑PO_4, ↑K
Wilson's disease [277900]	ATP7B	13q14.3-q21.1	AR	Liver disease or neurologic symptoms, or both, Kayser-Fleischer rings, normotensive	Plasma: ↑free copper, abnormal LFTs Urine: ↑copper excretion, ↑LMWP, ↑AA, ↑PO_4, ↑Glycosuria
Dent's disease (X-linked recessive hypophosphatemic rickets) [300009]	CLCN5	Xp11.22	XR	Nephrocalcinosis, nephrolithiasis, rachitic and osteomalacic bone disease, progressive kidney failure, normotensive	Plasma: ↓PO_4, N/↓K Urine: ↑LMWP, ↑AA, ↑K, ↑Ca, ↑PO_4, ↑Glycosuria
X-linked dominant hypophosphatemic rickets [307800]	PHEX	Xp22.2-p22.1	XD	Growth retardation, rachitic and osteomalacic bone disease, hypophosphatemia, and renal defects in phosphate reabsorption and vitamin D metabolism	Plasma: ↓PO_4, ↑ALP Urine: ↑PO_4
Loop of Henle					
Bartter's syndrome [601678] [241200] [607364] [602522]	NKCC2 (type I) ROMK (type II) ClC-Kb (type III, "classic") Barttin (type IV)	15q15-q21.1 11q24 1p36 1p31	AR AR AR AR	Polyuria, polydipsia, muscle weakness, hypovolemia, normotensive or hypotensive (all types). Maternal polyhydramnios, premature birth, perinatal salt wasting, nephrocalcinosis and kidney stones (types I and II), milder phenotype with normocalciuria (type III), sensorineural deafness, motor retardation, renal failure (type IV)	Plasma: ↑renin, ↓K, ↑CO_2, mild ↓Mg in some patients Urine: ↑Ca
Hypomagnesemic hypercalciuric nephrocalcinosis (magnesium-losing kidney) [248250]	PCLN1	3q27	AR	Nephrocalcinosis, renal failure, ocular/hearing defects, polyuria, polydipsia, recurrent urinary tract infections, recurrent renal colic, normotensive	Plasma: ↓Mg, ↑PTH Urine: ↑Ca, ↑Mg

Distal Tubule/Collecting Duct					
Liddle's syndrome [177200][†]	ENaC (activating)	16p13-p12	AD	Early, and frequently severe, hypertension, stroke	Plasma: ↓renin, ↓K, ↓Mg, ↑CO_2 Urine: ↑K
Pseudohypoaldosteronism type Ia [264350][†]	ENaC (inactivating)	12p13, 16p13-p12	AR	Presents in infancy with salt-wasting and hypotension. Cough, respiratory infections	Plasma: ↑renin, ↓Na, ↑K, ↓CO_2 Urine: ↑K
Pseudohypoaldosteronism type Ib [177735][†]	Mineralocorticoid receptor	4q31.1	AD	Presents in infancy with salt-wasting and hypotension. Milder than type 1a and remits with age	Plasma: ↑renin, ↓Na, ↑K, ↓CO_2 Urine: ↑K
Pseudohypoaldosteronism type II (Gordon's syndrome) [145260]	Unknown (?WNK)	1q31-q42 12p13 17q21-q22	AD	Hypertension (±muscle weakness, short stature, intellectual impairment). Correction of physiologic abnormalities by thiazide diuretics	Plasma: ↓renin, ↑K, ↓CO_2, ↑Cl Urine: ↓K
Gitelman's syndrome [263800]	NCCT	16q13	AR	Hypotension, weakness, paresthesias, tetany, fatigue, and salt craving. Presentation generally much later in life than in Bartter's, and hypocalciuria is typical	Plasma: ↑renin, ↓K, ↓Mg, ↑CO_2 Urine: ↓calcium:creatinine excretion ratio (useful in distinguishing Gitelman's and Bartter's) (*Note:* biochemically can mimic thiazide use)
X-linked nephrogenic diabetes insipidus type I [304800]	V2 receptor	Xq28	XR	Hyperthermia, polyuria, polydipsia, dehydration, inability to form concentrated urine, mental retardation if diagnosis delayed. Symptoms in infancy	Hyperosmolar plasma, dilute urine
Autosomal dominant nephrogenic diabetes insipidus type II [192340]	AQP2	12q13	AD and AR	Polyuria, polydipsia, dehydration, inability to form concentrated urine. Symptoms after first year of life	Hyperosmolar plasma, dilute urine

*Note: This list is not exhaustive. Some of the material in this table has been adapted from Sayer JA, Pearce SHS.[388] A useful resource for further information is the Online Mendelian Inheritance in Man (OMIM) Website, which may be searched using the OMIM numbers given in the table (http://www.ncbi.nlm.nih.gov/entrez/query.fcgi?db=OMIM).

[†]See Figure 48-7.

AA, Aminoaciduria; *AD,* autosomal dominant; *AR,* autosomal recessive; *LFTs,* liver function tests; *LMWP,* low molecular weight proteinuria; *XD,* X-linked dominant; *XR,* X-linked recessive.

Diagnosis of RTA

The finding of a hyperchloremic metabolic acidosis in a patient without obvious gastrointestinal bicarbonate losses (e.g., due to excessive diarrhea or small intestinal fistulas) and with no obvious pharmacologic cause should prompt suspicion of an RTA. The presence of suggestive clinical (e.g., nephrocalcinosis in dRTA) or biochemical (e.g., hypophosphatemia and hypouricemia as a result of proximal tubular wasting in pRTA) features should also be considered.

In addition to plasma electrolyte (including potassium) measurement, preliminary investigation should include measurement of urinary pH in a fresh, early morning urine sample. The finding of urine pH greater than 5.5 in the presence of systemic acidosis supports the diagnosis of dRTA, although it is not specific and will also be seen in types II and IV RTAs. If appropriate urinary acidification cannot be demonstrated, further investigation may involve assessing the ability of the kidneys to excrete an acid load (ammonium chloride load test) and to reabsorb filtered bicarbonate (fractional bicarbonate excretion). Additional details on the conduct and interpretation of these tests may be found in a review article.[343]

Treatment of RTA

Treatment of the RTAs is aimed at (1) correcting the biochemical disturbance and, where possible, underlying disorder; (2) improving growth in children; and (3) avoiding the development and progression of CKD. In both type I and II RTAs, bicarbonate is administered to correct the metabolic acidosis. Fludrocortisone and loop diuretics (see "Diuretics" section later) may be used to treat type IV RTA.

Inherited Tubulopathies

The inherited tubulopathies make up a heterogeneous set of disorders often characterized by electrolyte disturbances (see Table 48-15). Most are eponymous and have been described clinically for many years. However, enhanced understanding of the molecular biology of the tubular ion channel and transport pumps has delineated the mechanism of disease in many of these disorders. In addition to electrolyte disturbances (particularly of potassium), general reasons to suspect a tubulopathy include a familial disease pattern, renal impairment, nephrocalcinosis, and stone formation, especially if these should present at an early age. In cases in which a diuretic-sensitive channel is affected, these disorders will clearly mimic the effects of diuretic use (see discussion later in this chapter), and exclusion of covert use of diuretics is important. Although they are individually uncommon or rare, an awareness of these disorders is critical for the clinical biochemist when considering the potential differential diagnoses in patients presenting with electrolyte imbalances. A brief description of these disorders follows; for more detailed information, the reader is referred to the citation list, including several reviews on this subject.[341,388,389] This section should be considered in conjunction with the aforegoing description of tubular electrolyte handling (see "Electrolyte Homeostasis").

Bartter's Syndrome

This group of autosomal recessive disorders is characterized by (1) renal salt wasting; (2) polyuria; (3) polydipsia; (4) impaired urinary concentrating ability; (5) a hyperreninemic, hypokalemic metabolic alkalosis; and (6) a mild hypomagnesemia in some patients. Biochemically, the effects resemble those of loop diuretic use, but clinically, the phenotype is highly variable. This variability arises because of the fact that the syndrome encompasses defects of three different transporters/channels in the loop of Henle. The biochemical effects are predictable from knowledge of the function of these transporters and channels (see Figure 48-6).

Mutations in the genes encoding for NKCC2 (type I) or ROMK1 (type II) are associated with the more severe phenotype, including polyhydramnios, premature birth, life-threatening salt wasting in the perinatal period, and hypercalciuria. Patients with ROMK1 defects tend to have less severe hypokalemia.

The milder ("classic," type III) Bartter's syndrome is due to defects in the basolateral pump, CLC-Kb. Although the phenotype is extremely variable (neonatal, life-threatening presentations do occur), patients typically present in the first year of life with weakness and hypovolemia and normal urinary calcium excretion. Nephrocalcinosis and kidney stone formation usually are not features.

A fourth variant of Bartter's syndrome (type IV) has been described as due to a mutation in the gene coding for Barttin. Barttin is an essential subunit of CLC-Kb that influences its function and expression in the cell membrane. Bartter's syndrome type IV is characterized by severe, early-onset salt wasting, leading to polydramnios, premature birth, and inner-ear deafness.[239]

Gitelman's Syndrome

This autosomal recessive disorder is characterized by a hypokalemic, hyperreninemic, hypomagnesemic, metabolic alkalosis, but presentation is generally much later in life than with Bartter's syndrome, and hypocalciuria is typical. Clinical features include reduced blood pressure, weakness, paresthesia, tetany, fatigue, and salt craving.[19] The molar urinary calcium/creatinine excretion ratio can be useful in distinguishing between Gitelman's ($\leq$0.20) and Bartter's (>0.20) syndromes.[31] The molecular defect is seen in the thiazide-sensitive NCCT transporter (see Figure 48-6), and the biochemistry can therefore mimic the effects of thiazide use (see "Diuretics" section later).

Liddle's Syndrome

This autosomal dominant disorder is characterized by a hypokalemic, hypomagnesemic metabolic alkalosis but, in contrast to Bartter's and Gitelman's syndromes, hypertension and hyperreninism also occur. The disease is due to activating mutations, which increase sodium transport through the ENaC channel with consequent enhanced kaliuresis (see Figure 48-7).

Pseudohypoaldosteronism Type I

This condition presents in infancy with salt wasting, hypotension, hyperkalemia, and significant hyperreninism and aldosteronism. Two different molecular mechanisms are causative. Type Ia (autosomal recessive) is caused by inactivating mutations of the *ENaC* gene, and type Ib (autosomal dominant) is caused by mutations in the mineralocorticoid gene. In both cases, sodium loss in the collecting duct is increased with consequent retention of potassium.

Dent's Disease

Dent's disease is an X-linked condition characterized by hypercalciuria and kidney stone formation, low molecular weight proteinuria, aminoaciduria, hypophosphatemia, and rickets.[481] The disease arises from single-base change mutations, of which approximately 60 have been described, in the gene coding for the tubular endosomal chloride channel CLC-5. The exact relationship between loss of function of this protein and the resulting Fanconi syndrome remains unclear, but CLC-5 appears to have an important role in proximal tubular endocytosis.[205] Although X-linked, a mild form of the disease can be seen in females because of lyonization. The related syndromes (1) X-linked recessive nephrolithiasis, (2) X-linked recessive hypophosphatemic rickets, and (3) Japanese idiopathic low molecular weight proteinuria are also all related to defects in CLC-5.[434]

Phosphate Disorders

Several disorders of tubular phosphate handling have been described, including X-linked dominant hypophosphatemic rickets (XLH; previously known as vitamin D–resistant rickets), autosomal dominant hypophosphatemic rickets, and acquired oncogenic hypophosphatemic osteomalacia. Our understanding of the molecular biology of these and other renal phosphate transport disorders has advanced greatly in recent years.[429]

Many other tubulopathies exist[341,388,389] and the features of some of these are described in Table 48-15.

Treatment With Diuretics

Diuretics are among the most widely prescribed drugs. They are used predominantly to treat hypertension and/or disorders associated with fluid overload. All diuretics act by interfering with tubular reabsorption of sodium and/or chloride, thereby promoting water loss from the peripheral circulation. Diuretics are taken up by tubular cells across the basolateral membrane by specific anion- (e.g., furosemide, thiazides) or cation- (e.g., amiloride, triamterene) exchangers and then are secreted into the lumen through a process that has not been fully elucidated.[389] Different classes of diuretics act at different sites along the nephron. A basic understanding of these processes is helpful in understanding both the potency of different diuretic classes and their importance in the investigation of electrolyte disorders, in particular hypokalemia. Many diuretics will cause hypokalemia to some degree, depending on potency, dose, duration of treatment, and the patient's underlying potassium balance.

Loop Diuretics

Loop diuretics act largely by blocking sodium and chloride reabsorption in the ascending limb of the loop of Henle. Because this is a site at which 30% of sodium reabsorption normally occurs, these are considered potent diuretics. Loop diuretics specifically inhibit NKCC2; therefore, they also have an effect on potassium handling in the ascending limb. Consequent changes in transepithelial potential result in a direct kaliuretic effect in this region,[153] causing hypercalciuria (see Figure 48-6). Loop diuretics also paralyze the macula densa segment, stimulating renin secretion and subsequent aldosterone release, promoting sodium reabsorption and potassium loss in the distal tubule, and so further exacerbating the kaliuresis. Most significantly, blockage of loop sodium reabsorption results in enhanced delivery of sodium ions to the distal tubule, where sodium is reabsorbed in exchange for potassium secretion.[153] The affinity of loop diuretics for NKCC2 is bumetanide>torasemide>piretanide>furosemide>azosemide.[154] The net effect of loop diuretics is that increased sodium chloride with associated water is lost from the body: potassium loss as a result of the various mechanisms described here means that hypokalemia is a common side effect.

Thiazide Diuretics

The benzothiadiazine group of compounds inhibits NCCT in the distal tubule. Because only 5 to 10% of sodium reabsorption occurs at this site, these agents are less potent than the loop diuretics, but hypokalemia is still common as a result of increased sodium delivery to the collecting duct. Thiazide diuretics also have secondary effects, resulting in increased calcium reabsorption, which may lead to hypercalcemia.[154]

"Potassium-Sparing" Diuretics

These diuretics act by reducing sodium reabsorption in the collecting duct, hence increasing potassium retention. Spironolactone acts as a competitive antagonist of aldosterone, blocking its stimulatory effects on sodium reabsorption via the mineralocorticoid receptor. Both amiloride and triamterene inhibit ENaC. The danger associated with this group of diuretics is that they can induce hyperkalemia; this is particularly likely to occur in patients with kidney disease.

Diabetes Insipidus

Primary functions of the kidney include conservation of water and production of a concentrated urine. A number of conditions are associated with disturbances of the renal concentrating mechanism, resulting in polyuria and an inability to produce hypertonic urine. General conditions giving rise to this picture include hypercalcemia, hypokalemia, and CKD. Specifically, diabetes insipidus is due to the absence of an ADH effect, caused by impaired or failed secretion (cranial or central diabetes insipidus) or lack of end-organ response to ADH (nephrogenic diabetes insipidus). A further disorder, psychogenic polydipsia, or compulsive water drinking can also present as diabetes insipidus. Polyuria is common to both diabetes insipidus and diabetes mellitus, but in diabetes insipidus, no hyperglycemia and no glycosuria are present. These individuals may fail to concentrate urine even in response to fluid restriction or synthetic ADH as a result of medullary "washout"; sustained fluid ingestion destroys the hyperosmolality of the medulla, which may take some time to recover. Differentiation and the pathology of these three conditions are discussed in Chapter 53. It should be noted that a vast diuresis can be induced by consumption of excessive fluid volumes (e.g., among heavy beer drinkers).

Congenital nephrogenic diabetes insipidus is associated with defects that have been characterized at the molecular level (see Table 48-15).[34] Most (>90%) congenital nephrogenic diabetes insipidus patients have mutations in the *AVPR2* gene, which codes for the ADH V2 receptor. This results in an X-linked form of diabetes insipidus, with an estimated prevalence of 4 per 1 million males.[34] In less than 10% of cases, an autosomal recessive inheritance pattern is caused by mutations in the *AQP2* gene. It has been suggested that measurement of the urinary excretion of AQP may be useful diagnostically.[97,321] Downregulation of AQP2 has been observed in a variety of acquired forms of diabetes insipidus, including lithium treatment, hypokalemia, hypercalcemia, ureteric obstruction, and, in animal models, chronic kidney failure.[321] Acquired forms of diabetes insipidus are more common than congenital forms.

Assessment of Renal Concentrating Ability: Urinary Osmolality

Urinary concentration can be quantified by measuring specific gravity (see Chapter 25) or by measuring urinary osmolality. For most clinical purposes, measuring specific gravity is probably sufficient,[344] but urinary osmolality measurement is critical in the diagnosis of diabetes insipidus using the water deprivation test (see Chapter 53).

Urinary osmolality may vary widely, depending on the state of hydration. After excessive intake of fluids, for example, the osmotic concentration may fall to as low as 50 mOsm/kg H_2O, whereas in individuals with severely restricted fluid intake, concentrations of up to 1400 mOsm/kg H_2O can be observed. In individuals on an average fluid intake, values of 300 to 900 mOsm/kg H_2O are typically seen. If a random urine specimen has an osmolality greater than 600 mOsm/kg H_2O (or >850 mOsm/kg H_2O after 12 hours of fluid restriction), it generally can be assumed that the renal concentrating ability is normal.

In chronic progressive kidney disease, the concentrating ability of the tubules is diminished, and in ATN, the urinary osmolality, if there is urine output at all, approaches that of plasma. For a discussion on measurement of urinary and plasma osmolality, readers are referred to Chapter 28.

Renal Calculi

Nephrolithiasis is the disease condition associated with the presence of renal calculi. Renal calculi, commonly termed *kidney stones,* occur in the renal pelvis, the ureter, or the bladder. Calcification also occurs scattered throughout the parenchyma (nephrocalcinosis). Kidney stone formation is often considered to be a nutritional or environmental disease, linked to affluence, but genetic or anatomical abnormalities are significant. Approximately 5 to 10% of the population of the Western world are thought to have formed at least one kidney stone by the age of 70 years,[201,381] and the prevalence of kidney stones is increasing.[418] For most stone types, there is a male preponderance. The passage of a stone is associated with severe pain called *renal colic,* which may last for 15 minutes to several hours and is commonly associated with nausea and vomiting.[472] Kidney stone formation contributes to the development of CKD.[142,378]

Background

Chemically, urine contains many mineral salts that are present in concentrations that approach their solubility products at body temperature. Anyone who has seen a urine sample before and after refrigeration has witnessed the consequences of this in the massive crystal deposits that can form on cooling. Crystals are able to form spontaneously if the salt concentrations are high enough or, alternatively, may bind to organic material, acting as a "seed": hyaluronic acid, a large glycosaminoglycan, has been suggested as one such promoter of crystal formation.[454] Human urine contains a number of promoters of stone formation and a variety of inhibitors, the concentrations of which can be influenced by dietary and metabolic factors (Figure 48-16).

Initial diagnosis and investigation of stones require radiologic investigation to explore the degree of intrarenal calcification and papillary damage. Plain x-rays are undertaken at initial presentation, although it should be noted that urate and other purine stones and some cystine stones are radiolucent. An intravenous urogram or spiral CT scan may be performed to establish the presence and extent of urinary tract obstruction, intrarenal reflux, and ureteric dilation. Further investigation of the patient with kidney stones or suspected of being a stone former involves analysis of blood, urine, and the stone itself, should one be obtained.[177]

Small stones (<5 mm in diameter) pass spontaneously in the urine as "gravel."[472] Although surgical treatment to remove large staghorn calculi may still be necessary, the most common form of treatment is ultrasonic extracorporeal shock wave lithotripsy (ESWL),[358] which can be applied to stones between 5 mm and 2 cm in diameter. Although this allows noninvasive destruction of stones, the long-term sequelae of exposing the kidney to high-intensity sound waves have not been fully established.[142] Additionally, evidence is mounting that ESWL may be associated with higher recurrence rates than invasive treatment.[425] Percutaneous nephrolithotomy may be required if ESWL fails and also in the removal of cystine stones.

After treatment and successful removal of a stone, follow-up monitoring is required, as many patients will have recurrent disease: in the absence of medical treatment, the recurrence rate may be as high as 50% at 10 years.[268] The mechanisms responsible for multiple recurrences of kidney stones in only certain individuals are not completely understood. Factors involved include (1) urine flow (fluid intake); (2) excretion of excess quantities of stone components; (3) the

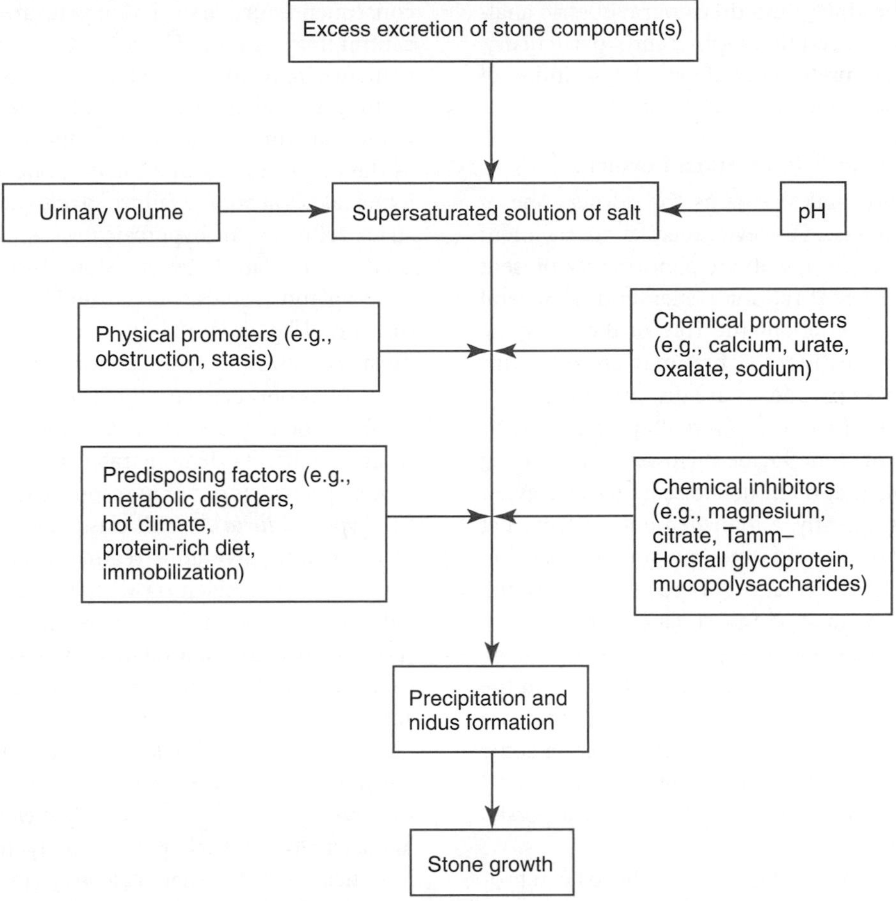

Figure 48-16 Diagrammatic representation of the interplay of factors involved in kidney stone formation. High or low pH may act as a promoter or inhibitor of stone formation depending on the stone type in question (e.g., calcium stone formation is favored by inadequate acidification, while urate is less soluble in acidic urine). Controversy exists as to whether formed stones become trapped as they pass through the nephron ("free particle theory"), or whether stone formation occurs at damaged sites on the tubule wall ("fixed particle theory").

relative absence of a substance, or substances, in the urine that inhibit stone formation; and (4) urinary pH (see Figure 48-16). The predominant risk factor is poor hydration, with concentrated urine further increasing the concentrations of the mineral salts, predisposing to crystallization. Urinary concentration at least partially explains the increased incidence of kidney stone disease in hot climates, for example, in the Gulf States.

Kidney Stone Analysis

A majority of kidney stones found in the Western world are composed of one or more of the following substances: (1) calcium oxalate with or without phosphate (frequency 67%); (2) magnesium ammonium phosphate (12%); (3) calcium phosphate (8%); (4) urate (8%); (5) cystine (1 to 2%); and (6) complex mixtures of these substances (2 to 3%).[381] These poorly soluble substances crystallize within an organic matrix, the nature of which is not well understood.

When available, analysis of the chemical constituents of stones may be useful in establishing the cause and in planning rational therapy. It complements and guides metabolic investigation of patients and may be particularly useful in identifying rare stone types (e.g., xanthine, dihydroxyadenine), artifacts (e.g., Munchausen syndrome), or drugs precipitating in the urinary tract, such as triamterene[417] and indinavir.[236] Conversely, it has been argued that stone analysis is not useful clinically,[178] because the stone material that is passed often does not represent the initial metabolic derangement. This is a result of the phenomenon known as *epitaxy,* whereby nonspecific stone material, typically arising as a result of urinary tract infection (e.g., struvite), may accumulate on a preexisting "metabolic" nidus, the latter of which may not be detected during stone analysis. Clearly, for stone analysis to be useful, it must be accurate. A variety of techniques have been used over the years. Traditionally, stones were crushed and solubilized, and the resulting solution analyzed (at several dilutions when appropriate) with the use of conventional qualitative or semiquantitative chemical methods. Such techniques require relatively large amounts of stone, may miss rare and artifactual material, and analytically often perform poorly.[381] More sophisticated approaches including thermogravimetric analysis,[374] x-ray diffraction crystallography, and, particularly, infrared spectroscopy are preferred, a detailed description of the which is beyond the scope of this chapter.[28,180,221]

Metabolic Investigation of Kidney Stone Formers

Ensuring adequate fluid intake remains the cornerstone of management of stone disease. However, specific management of disease depending on the metabolic abnormality present is important, and a treatment rationale is emerging. Several misconceptions have arisen about the role of diet in stone formation, and optimal treatment at first may appear counterintuitive; some of these paradoxes are discussed here.

Further investigation of stone formers may be guided by knowledge of the type of stone formed. However, increasing use of lithotripsy means that often no stone material is available for analysis. Consequently, a management strategy that focuses on the cause of stone formation and is based on knowledge of blood and urinary composition is useful. Although historically, metabolic investigations have often been targeted at recurrent stone formers only, the increasing availability of simple assays for chemical risk factors and the health economic burden of renal colic suggest that they are likely to become more widespread.[178,357,428] However, in some instances, it is not possible to demonstrate a biochemical abnormality in stone-forming individuals beyond a persistently small urine volume.

A variety of metabolic screening strategies have been proposed in stone-forming patients.[177,179,381,437] The chosen strategy should balance convenience for the patient and the laboratory against ability to intervene therapeutically. For example, although THG is known to inhibit stone formation, in the absence of a specific treatment, there is little merit in measuring it. A reasonable approach would probably include measurement of plasma sodium, potassium, chloride, bicarbonate, creatinine, calcium, phosphate, and urate, together with 24-hour urinary volume, calcium, magnesium, phosphate, oxalate, urate, creatinine, sodium, citrate, and microbiology (to exclude infection). Additionally, urinary pH and cystine should be measured on a fresh, early morning urine sample. Some investigators have proposed complex "supersaturation indices" that combine the information obtained from these studies in a numeric index.[335,371,436] Metabolic evaluation should be undertaken at least 6 weeks after the episode of renal colic and ideally should be done on several occasions.[179] Evaluation is most informative when undertaken on an outpatient basis with patients pursuing their normal diet and lifestyle. A brief description of the role and measurement of these risk factors is given here, with focus predominantly on the investigation of calcium stone formers.

Calcium

Most of the stones formed in the Western world are composed of calcium, most commonly in association with oxalate, although calcium phosphate and urate may also be present, alone or in combination with calcium oxalate. As a consequence, urinary calcium measurement has served as the central investigation. However, the significant role of oxalate is increasingly appreciated, and this has resulted in changes to the optimal management of hypercalciuria. As a rough guide, calcium oxalate stones tend to suggest hyperoxaluria as the main cause, while calcium phosphate stones implicate hypercalciuria and/or failure to adequately acidify urine.[381] A strict definition of hypercalciuria is difficult because of significant overlap between stone-forming and non–stone-forming individuals, but a cutoff of 4 mg/kg body weight (0.1 mmol/kg) is useful.[55,477] Excretion in excess of this, the most common metabolic abnormality seen in calcium stone formers, is observed in up to 50% of patients.

Traditionally, some investigation strategies focused on whether patients demonstrated hypercalciuria while fasting *(renal hypercalciuria)* or in response to a calcium load *(absorptive hypercalciuria)*.[472] This classification was used as the basis of an investigative and treatment strategy in patients with absorptive hypercalciuria who have abnormally high intestinal calcium absorption compared with non–stone formers (possibly because of a relative increase in $1,25[OH]_2D_3$ concentration and/or changes in intestinal vitamin D receptor activity). Treatment in these patients focused on dietary modification of calcium intake. Patients with renal hypercalciuria are now thought not to have a renal transport defect, but to have increased turnover of skeletal calcium, although management of such patients may involve pharmacologic modification of renal calcium handling (e.g., thiazide diuretics).[472]

However, convincing evidence questions the usefulness of this classification and these therapeutic approaches. Dietary restriction of calcium now is generally regarded as ineffective, and actually counterproductive, as it results in an increase in intestinal oxalate absorption and increased risk of stone formation.[63,90] Further, patients with hypercalciuria are known to have reduced bone mineral density, and dietary calcium restriction may exacerbate a tendency toward osteopenia and/or osteoporosis.[439,465]

A more useful approach is to classify hypercalciuric patients into hypercalcemic or nonhypercalcemic causes. The former is most commonly due to primary hyperparathyroidism, which is seen in approximately 5% of stone formers. Treatment involves neck exploration and removal of the adenoma, although the risk of a stone recurring remains high for several years after parathyroidectomy.[304]

Nonhypercalcemic causes of hypercalciuria account for the majority of patients and generally are classified as idiopathic (although causes such as RTA, high sodium intake, and prolonged immobilization should be excluded). Most patients with idiopathic hypercalciuria appear to have a generalized acceleration of calcium transport, with increased absorption from the gut, increased mobilization from bone, and abnormal renal calcium conservation, all contributing to hypercalciuria.[477] In addition to increasing fluid consumption, idiopathic hypercalciuric patients appear to benefit from a diet that is low in animal protein and sodium.[42,370] Animal protein consumption increases the production of metabolic acids, increasing urinary calcium and uric acid excretion and decreasing urinary citrate (see discussion later in this chapter).[55] High sodium excretion as a result of high consumption inhibits tubular reabsorption of calcium, with a consequent increase in risk of calcium stone formation. Sodium is easily measured in urine and represents a modifiable risk factor. Other therapeutic maneuvers that may be useful include using thiazide diuretics or alkaline citrate, reducing oxalate, and increasing fiber intake.[437] Some of these factors are discussed in greater detail in the following sections.

Magnesium

With calcium stone disease, magnesium is an inhibitor of stone growth. Magnesium forms complexes with oxalate that are more soluble than calcium oxalate. Increased urinary magnesium therefore inhibits stone formation.[165] Administration of magnesium has been shown to reduce enteral calcium absorption and has been proposed as a treatment for idiopathic hypercalciuric stone formers.[96] However, oral magnesium supplementation may have unpleasant side effects, and a positive benefit in terms of reducing stone recurrence has not been demonstrated.[437]

Urate

Some investigators believe that urate may potentiate calcium stone formation, although this perception is not universally accepted.[381] However, hyperuricosuria is common in calcium stone–forming patients, and treatment with allopurinol, by decreasing urate synthesis, reduces the rate of stone recurrence. Allopurinol treatment therefore is recommended for hyperuricosuric patients with calcium stone disease.[437] The formation and management of pure urate stones are discussed in Chapter 25.

Oxalate

Oxalate is an end product of metabolism, predominantly derived from breakdown of glyoxylate and glycine. The plasma concentration of oxalate is 1.0 to 2.4 mg/L (11 to 27 μmol/L), and it is excreted in the urine at a rate of 17.5 to 35.1 mg/d (200 to 400 μmol/d).[476] Only 10 to 15% of urinary oxalate is derived directly from dietary sources.[437] Intestinal oxalate absorption is increased when the availability of calcium in the intestine is reduced. Hyperoxaluria is a powerful promoter of calcium oxalate stone formation; indeed, it is more significant in this respect than calcium itself.[381]

Hyperoxaluria may occur as a result of excessive dietary intake, because of malabsorption and/or steatorrhea (enteric hyperoxaluria), or because of an inborn error of metabolism (primary hyperoxaluria). Enteric hyperoxaluria commonly occurs in association with inflammatory bowel disease and may contribute to an increased incidence of stone formation in such patients.[476] Fat malabsorption contributes to the formation of calcium–fatty acid complexes ("soaps") in the intestine, increasing the enteric concentration of unbound oxalate that is absorbed through the damaged bowel wall. Primary hyperoxaluria may be type 1 (glycolic aciduria) or type 2 (L-glyceric aciduria). Patients with type 1 disease present in the first decade of life with recurrent calcium oxalate nephrolithiasis. Inheritance is autosomal recessive and survival is poor. Type 2 disease is rarer and has been claimed to run a milder course, despite the passage of similarly high concentrations of urinary oxalate. The urinary excretion of oxalate may increase to approximately 60 mg/d (700 μmol/d) when a diet containing an excess of oxalate-rich foods is taken, and to as much as 260 mg/d (3 mmol/d) in patients with primary hyperoxaluria.

Ideally, urine for oxalate analysis should be collected into acid to prevent the crystallization of calcium oxalate crystals. Acidification also prevents ex vivo formation of oxalate from ascorbate—a cause of factitious hyperoxaluria in individuals ingesting excessive amounts of vitamin C.[171] A number of approaches to the measurement of urinary oxalate have been employed, including high-performance liquid chromatography (HPLC), enzymatic assays, and capillary electrophoretic methods.[184,251,347] The enzymatic methods employ the enzyme oxalate oxidase (EC 1.2.3.4. oxalate:oxygen oxidoreductase). With this method, the sample of urine is initially acidified to pH 1.8 (typically with 2 mmol/L HCl) to ensure complete solubilization of any calcium oxalate crystals. The oxalate is oxidized to carbon dioxide and hydrogen peroxide by oxalate oxidase, and the hydrogen peroxide is detected with horseradish peroxidase and is coupled with an oxygen acceptor reagent such as 3-dimethyl aminobenzoic acid and 3-methyl-2-benzothiazolinone hydrazone to yield an indamine dye that absorbs at 590 nm. A charcoal column pretreatment step to remove interferents from the urine has been used,[246] although this may not be necessary.[347] An alternative approach to the detection of hydrogen peroxide using catalase has been described. The oxalate oxidase is specific for oxalate; however, the peroxide detection reaction may suffer from interferences (e.g., turbidity in the catalase-mediated reaction, ascorbic acid, other reducing agents in the peroxidase-mediated reaction). The choice of oxygen acceptor will determine the potential for interference from compounds such as ascorbic acid.

A dietary history is important in the evaluation of calcium oxalate stone formers. Patients who are excreting large amounts of oxalate may be offered dietary advice to modify their risk of future stone formation. Foods rich in oxalate include beets, tea, spinach, sorrel, wheat bran, strawberries, rhubarb, blackcurrants, peanuts, and chocolate.[381,437,472] Paradoxically, epidemiologic evidence has actually demonstrated a protective effect of high tea consumption.[90] This has been attributed to the low bioavailability of oxalate in tea and the inhibition of tubular ADH action by caffeine. Patients may be treated with calcium carbonate, which binds oxalate in the gut, rendering it unavailable for absorption. Alternatively, pyridoxine (vitamin B_6) may be used; this increases the catabolism of oxalate to more soluble products.[472] It should be remembered that the use of calcium-lowering diets, once favored in the treatment of calcium stone formers, increases intestinal absorption of oxalate.

Citrate

Urinary citrate inhibits stone formation by forming soluble complexes with calcium. It is present in the diet in many fruits. Excretion [typically between 120 and 930 mg/d (0.6 and 4.8 mmol/d) for adult males and between 250 and 1160 mg/d (1.3 and 6.0 mmol/d) for adult females][381] is reduced in the calcium stone–forming population.[436] Urinary citrate measurement may be of value in the assessment of stone-forming risk, particularly in the setting of distal RTA, where the reduction in filtered bicarbonate appears to increase tubular reabsorption of citrate with consequent hypocitraturia.[166] Inadequate urinary acidification compounds the increased risk of calcium stone formation. Treatment with carbonic anhydrase inhibitors (e.g., acetazolamide,[332] topiramate[215,247]) mimics distal RTA with a consequent increase in stone risk. Hypocitraturia may also be seen in malabsorption and urinary tract infection. Administration of oral alkaline citrate increases urinary citrate concentration by increasing the pH of tubular cells. It has been shown to be effective in the treatment of nephrolithiasis,[333,437] although side effects are reported and compliance is poor.

Citrate is measured by gas chromatography, capillary electrophoresis,[184] or an enzyme-mediated reaction. Although methods using aconitase (EC 4.2.1.3) and isocitrate dehydrogenase (EC 1.1.1.42), or citrate lyase (EC 4.1.3.6) and oxaloacetate decarboxylase (EC 4.1.1.3), have been described, a method using the lyase together with malate dehydrogenase (EC 1.1.1.37) and lactate dehydrogenase (EC 1.1.1.27) is preferred. The combination of the two dehydrogenase pathways has been proposed to ensure that any oxaloacetate ion enzymatically decarboxylated is also measured. The enzyme-mediated decarboxylase pathway is less favored because of the poor stability of the enzyme. Using a reaction sequence that involves incubation of the sample with all constituents except the citrate lyase ensures that all endogenous oxaloacetate and pyruvate are removed. Analysis of serum involves a deproteinization step, and urine should be titrated to pH 8.0 before analysis. A typical incubation period is 10 to 15 minutes, and the citrate can be quantitated from the decrease in absorbance at 340 nm. A cheap, rapid, automated adaptation of this procedure, which does not require a deproteinizing step, has been described.[43]

Struvite Stones

Struvite stones (also called *triple phosphate* or *infection stones*) are composed of magnesium ammonium phosphate hexahydrate. The formation of such stones requires urinary tract infection with urea-splitting organisms; such stones therefore are more common in females and in certain patient populations (e.g., paraplegic individuals).[381] The risk of progression to CKD appears higher in patients who develop infection stones than in those with other forms of stone disease.[142]

Cystinuria

Cystinuria is an autosomal recessive condition in which excessive urinary excretion of cystine results from a defect in proximal renal tubular reabsorption. In the most common form of the disease, there is also excess excretion of the dibasic amino acids (lysine, ornithine, and arginine). These share the same renal tubular transporter, although their presence in excess in urine appears benign. More rarely, isolated cystinuria is seen. The reader should note that cystinuria should not be confused with cystinosis, which is a condition associated with intracellular accumulation of cystine but not with excess urinary excretion of cystine.

The normal urinary excretion of cystine has been reported to be 5 to 48 mg/d (40 to 400 μmol/d).[381] Its relatively low limit of solubility, 18 mg/dL (1500 μmol/L),[472] is exceeded in many patients with cystinuria,[381] resulting in the formation of hexagonal crystals and, ultimately, cystine stones. Cystine stones usually are seen only in homozygotes, although some evidence suggests that heterozygotes are at increased risk of stone formation.[147] Cystinuria may present at any age from infancy to old age, although presentation is most common in the second and third decades.

The finding of a cystine stone should prompt confirmation of cystinuria by urinary analysis.[381] It could be argued, however, that all stone formers should be screened for cystinuria; at least 10% of cystinuric individuals form stones in which cystine cannot be detected, presumably because of epistaxis.[301] The index of suspicion should be increased in patients who are relatively young stone formers and in those with a positive family history. Once a cystinuric patient is diagnosed, it is important to screen all members of the family, particularly to detect affected siblings.

Cystine can be measured in urine by using the cyanide-nitroprusside test, thin-layer chromatography, quantitative amino acid analysis with ion-exchange or liquid chromatographic techniques, or mass spectrometry. In the cyanide-nitroprusside test, cystine is split into two molecules of cysteine by cyanide. Sodium nitroprusside reacts with the free sulfide groups to give a magenta color. This test is hazardous and will give false-negative results in patients with acidified or infected urine, in those receiving penicillamine therapy, and in patients for whom the sodium nitroprusside solution is not fresh. Further, it cannot distinguish between cystine and homocystine or between heterozygote and homozygote cystinuric individuals. It is not useful when treatment is monitored for known cystinuric patients, who require quantitation of their urinary cystine output or concentration. In practice, amino acid analysis allows simultaneous quantitation of the dibasic amino acids, which may be helpful for characterizing the clinical phenotype. Quantitative amino acid analysis is described in Chapter 21.

Treatment of cystinuria is aimed at keeping cystine below its saturation point by maintaining high fluid intake, particularly at night. Other treatments include urinary alkalinization (cystine is more soluble in alkaline urine) and chelation with D-penicillamine. Quantitative analysis is an important adjunct for monitoring penicillamine therapy, which can be optimized on the basis of free cystine versus cystine/penicillamine disulfide. Penicillamine itself may cause glomerular damage; thus regular monitoring of urinary protein excretion is recommended.

Toxic Nephropathy

A wide variety of nephrotoxins exist in the environment, in some cases associated with particular occupations (e.g., heavy metals, such as cadmium and lead; see Chapter 36). Both glomerular and tubulointerstitial damage may result from exposure to toxins; detection of both requires biochemical monitoring of GFR/serum creatinine concentration and tubular and glomerular proteinuria. Anatomic, physiologic, and biochemical features make the kidney susceptible to insult from a variety of medicinal and environmental agents. Factors contributing to the sensitivity of the kidney include its large blood flow, the concentration of filtered solutes during urine production, and the presence of a variety of xenobiotic transporters and metabolizing enzymes. Toxic nephropathy commonly occurs as a result of decreased renal perfusion, because of precipitation within the tubule, or because of direct toxic effects at the proximal tubule. In some cases the conjugation of environmental chemicals (e.g., mercury, cadmium) to glutathione and/or cysteine targets these chemicals to the kidney, where inhibition of renal function occurs through a variety of mechanisms that are not completely understood. Although some drugs can cause kidney damage in the presence of normal renal function, a far greater variety of drugs can cause problems in patients with kidney disease, predominantly because of accumulation resulting from decreased renal elimination. The British National Formulary (www.bnf.org) has an appendix devoted to prescribing issues in the presence of renal impairment. A list of drugs and environmental toxins commonly known to cause kidney damage is given in Table 48-16.

RENAL REPLACEMENT THERAPY

Renal replacement therapy (RRT) includes dialysis procedures such as hemodialysis (HD), peritoneal dialysis (PD), continuous hemofiltration (HF), and continuous hemodiafiltration (HDF). These techniques are used to temporarily or permanently remove toxic substances from the blood when the kidneys cannot satisfactorily remove them from the circulation. In addition, kidney transplantation has become an effective form of RRT. Extensive laboratory support is required by an RRT program (Table 48-17).

Background

In 1861, Thomas Graham Bell in Glasgow, Scotland, carried out the first dialysis experiments (and coined the term *dialysis*), separating crystalloids and colloids in a solution. Bell predicted that this technique could have medical application, but this was not realized until nearly 100 years later in the work of Willem Kolff and then Belding Scribner, who made HD a feasible treatment in the early 1960s. Since that time, HD and more recently PD have extended the lives of many people, sometimes for up to 20 or 30 years.

Dialysis

Dialysis is the process of separating macromolecules from ions and low molecular weight compounds in solution based on the difference in their rates of diffusion through a semipermeable membrane, through which crystalloids can pass readily but colloids pass very slowly or not at all. Two distinct physical processes are involved: diffusion and ultrafiltration.

The timing of initiation of dialysis treatment is controversial and requires judgment, taking into account the treatment of metabolic consequences of advanced CKD, the comorbidities of the patient, and the accepted impact of dialysis treatment on quality of life. No absolute recommendation of commencement of dialysis based on GFR alone can be made, although commencement of dialysis is considered as GFR falls below 15 mL/min/1.73 m^2.[316] The USRDS reports the mean GFR on initiation of dialysis is 10 mL/min/1.73 m^2.[80]

Hemodialysis and Hemofiltration

HD is the technique most commonly used to treat advanced and permanent kidney failure. Clinically, it is considered the default therapy that is utilized in patients unsuitable for other modalities of PD and kidney transplantation. Operationally, it involves connecting the patient to a hemodialyzer, into which his or her blood flows. After filtration to remove wastes and extra fluids, the cleansed blood is returned to the patient. This is a complicated and inconvenient therapy requiring a coordinated effort from a healthcare team that includes the patient, nephrologist, dialysis nurse, dialysis technician, dietitian, and others.

Description

HD utilizes diffusive and convective mass transfer across a semipermeable membrane. The driving force for diffusion is the concentration gradient between blood and dialysate. Smaller solutes with larger concentration gradients give increased diffusion. The concentration gradient is maintained by using countercurrent flows and high flow rates. Heparinized blood is pumped in one direction across the membrane, and the recipient fluid, the dialysate, flows at a rate of 500 to 800 mL/min in the opposite direction, as shown in Figure 48-17. Water molecules and small molecular weight molecules are able to cross the membrane, while larger proteins and cellular elements are retained in the vascular space. Convection is the bulk movement of solvent and dissolved solute across the membrane, down a transmembrane hydrostatic pressure gradient. The most important functional part is the dialyzer membrane. Biocompatibility of the dialyzer membrane is an essential requirement because of high surface areas and long contact times. Patients are dialyzed in home-based or hospital-based units, with dialysis usually performed three times a week for sessions lasting between 3 and 5 hours. This dialysis schedule is largely empirical, insofar as it reconciles adequate treatment with breaks between treatments to provide the patient with a reasonable quality of life. Approaches to increase the dose of dialysis have been explored. These include short daily HD that entails a 2- to 3-hour dialysis on 6 days per week.[292] Alternatively, slow overnight dialysis for 5 to 7 nights has been employed. These regimens have been reported to improve outcome.[292,360,443]

TABLE 48-16 Toxic Nephropathy: Causes, Pattern, and Markers

Compound Category	Drug/Toxin	Type of Renal Injury/Pathology	Biomarkers/Notes
Antibacterial agents	Aminoglycosides (e.g., neomycin, gentamicin, tobramycin, amikacin)	Acute tubular necrosis and interstitial nephritis Nonoliguric AKI	Plasma: ↓K, ↓Mg, ↓Ca Urine: ↑LMWP, ↑glycosuria Nephrotoxicity major and common side effect
	Amphotericin	Initially distal tubular injury followed by medullary injury	Plasma: ↓K, ↑creatinine, dRTA
Antiviral/antiprotozoal agents	Acyclovir	Nonoliguric AKI due to tubular obstruction and interstitial inflammation	Crystalluria and hematuria
	Pentamidine	Tubular toxicity	Plasma: ↓Mg, ↓Ca Urine: ↑Mg, ↑Ca
	Indinavir	Nephrolithiasis, irreversible kidney failure in some patients	Crystalluria and hematuria
Radiocontrast agents	(e.g., iothalamate, iodixanol)	Oliguric or nonoliguric AKI, generally reversible. Proximal tubular damage	↑plasma creatinine after contrast administration
Antitumor drugs	Cisplatin	Irreversible dose-related and cumulative kidney failure. TIN with heavy proteinuria. Often AKI	Urine: ↑Mg, ↑PO_4, tubular casts and ↑LMWP in early stages
	Methotrexate	Nonoliguric AKI. Tubular atrophy and interstitial fibrosis	Seen only in association with high-dose therapy
	Interleukin-2	Reversible AKI due to ↓RBF	Observed in up to 90% of cases of high-dose therapy
Other drugs	ACE inhibitors	Dramatic ↓GFR due to ↓efferent arteriolar tone	Especially in the setting of bilateral renal artery stenosis. ↑plasma creatinine and K
	5-Aminosalicylic acid (e.g., mesalazine, olsalazine)	Occasional ATN and irreversible kidney damage	Tubular proteinuria
	Cyclooxygenase (COX)-2 inhibitors	Probably a similar pattern of renal injury to NSAIDs (see below)	
	Lithium	Distal tubular damage with nephrogenic diabetes insipidus ± dRTA	
	Penicillamine	Membranous glomerulopathy with NS, occasionally AKI	Proteinuria
	NSAIDs	Several forms of nephropathy identified, including (1) hemodynamically mediated AKI, (2) TIN ± NS, (3) salt and/or water retention, (4) hyperkalemia, (5) CKD/ESRD ("analgesic nephropathy")	Depends on type of effect
Heavy metals	Cadmium	Subtle but irreversible TIN	Fanconi syndrome with RTA. ↑urinary metallothionein
	Gold	Membranous glomerulopathy but normal GFR maintained	Proteinuria <3.5 g/24 h
	Lead	Proximal tubular atrophy with interstitial fibrosis	Reversible Fanconi syndrome in children with acute poisoning. In lead workers, urinary proteinuria <2 g/24 h in association with ↑plasma urate, hypertension ± gouty arthritis
	Mercury	Proximal tubular damage with ATN	Urine: ↑LMWP

TABLE 48-16 Toxic Nephropathy: Causes, Pattern, and Markers—cont'd

Compound Category	Drug/Toxin	Type of Renal Injury/Pathology	Biomarkers/Notes
Other environmental agents	Hydrocarbons (e.g., paints, dry cleaning solvents)	ATN, chronic TIN, glomerulonephritis. Caused by renal cytochrome P450 metabolism of chloroform to toxic metabolites	Tubular proteinuria ± ↑plasma creatinine
	Paraquat, diquat	ATN secondary to ↓RBF due to shock and direct toxic effects of paraquat. Intrinsic kidney damage due to production of reactive oxygen species	↑plasma creatinine
Drugs used in transplantation	See Table 48-19.		

ACE, Angiotensin-converting enzyme; *AKI,* acute kidney injury; *ATN,* acute tubular necrosis; *CKD,* chronic kidney disease; *dRTA,* distal renal tubular acidosis; *ESRD,* end-stage renal disease; *LMWP,* low molecular weight proteinuria; *NS,* nephrotic syndrome; *NSAIDs,* nonsteroidal anti-inflammatory drugs; *RBF,* renal blood flow; *TIN,* tubulointerstitial nephropathy.

TABLE 48-17 Laboratory Support for Dialysis Programs

Clinical Condition	Laboratory Tests
Acute Dialysis	
Dialysis disequilibrium	Urea and electrolyes, bicarbonate, calcium
Pyrexia	C-reactive protein, white cell count, blood cultures
Bleeding	Clotting screen, platelets
Chronic Dialysis Programs	
Anemia	Ferritin, transferrin saturation, B_{12}, folate
	Blood film, PTH, C-reactive protein
Sepsis	C-reactive protein, blood, urine specimens for microscopy, culture and sensitivity
Nutrition	Albumin, phosphate
Cardiovascular disease risk	Lipid profile
Dialysis-related amyloid	β_2-Microglobulin (not routinely measured)
CKD-MBD	Predialysis plasma calcium, phosphate (monthly in hemodialysis patients; 3-monthly in peritoneal dialysis patients)
	Alkaline phosphatase
	PTH (at least every 3 months)
	Aluminum in patients receiving aluminum-based phosphate binders (3-monthly)
Adequacy of hemodialysis as assessed by urea clearance	Predialysis and postdialysis urea
Sepsis, abdominal pain in peritoneal dialysis	Microscopy and culture of peritoneal dialysate
Adequacy of peritoneal dialysis as assessed by weekly small solute clearance	Dialysate creatinine, urea
Peritoneal membrane characteristics assessed by peritoneal equilibration test (PET)	Plasma and dialysate glucose and creatinine

CKD, Chronic kidney disease; *MBD,* mineral and bone disorder; *PTH,* parathyroid hormone.

HD relies on good vascular access to the circulation of the patient to enable blood to be pumped around the extracorporeal circuit at a rate in excess of 300 mL/min. Suitable vascular access was not achieved until the 1960s. Although Kolff at Groningen Hospital in the Netherlands performed the first dialysis experiments in humans in 1943, the problem of dialysis support with long-term vascular access was not solved until Scribner developed the arteriovenous cannula in 1960. This advance was followed by the development of the surgically created arteriovenous fistula (AVF), introduced by Brescia and coworkers in 1966, which provided permanent vascular access. The Dialysis Outcomes Practice Patterns

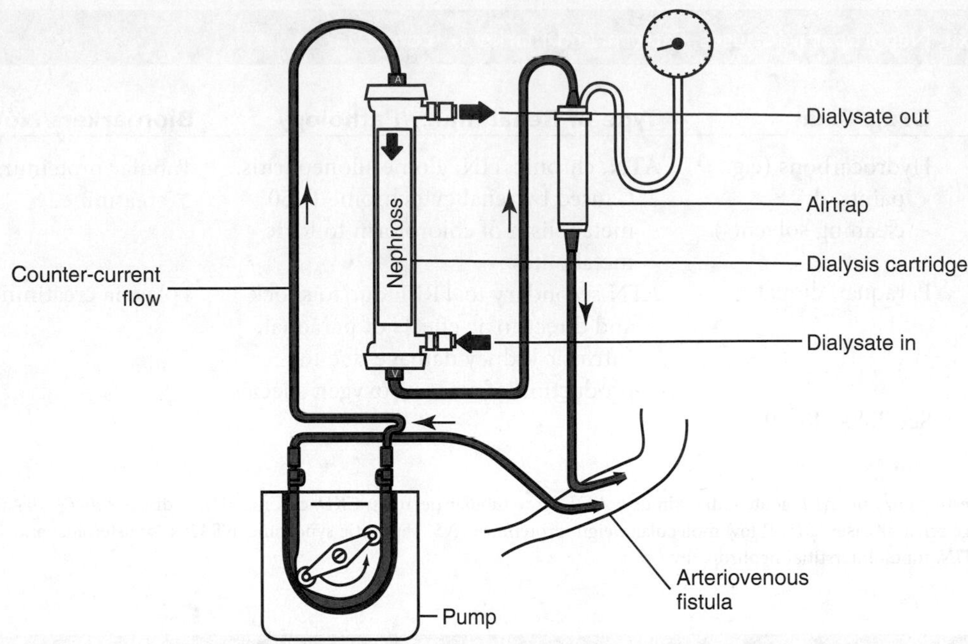

Figure 48-17 A hemodialyzer setup with inset flow diagram.

Study (DOPPS) confirmed a wide variation in how dialysis is achieved throughout the world. For example, most patients in Germany have an AVF as their main access, whereas in the United States, a fistula was used for access in only 13% of patients for their first dialysis in 2006,[79] reflecting suboptimal pre-ESRD care. AVF survival is longer in Europe than in the United States. However, coalition initiatives in 2011 exemplified by the "Fistula First" campaign and the K/DOQI Work Group have delivered service improvements with national AVF rates reported at 58.3% during April 2011.[120A] When used as a patient's first access, AVF survival is considered superior to arteriovenous grafts regarding time to first failure.

Conventional HD uses low-flux dialyzers, allowing diffusive but little convective solute removal. Middle molecule clearance is poor. HF is a convective treatment. Although middle molecule clearances are improved, small molecule clearance is poor. HF is used for continuous treatment in intensive care units in the management of AKI. High-flux HD using biocompatible membranes allows convective and diffusive solute removal. The use of very pure water is crucial in high-flux modes, because dialysis fluid is infused directly into the bloodstream by back-filtration. The Hemodialysis (HEMO) Study, a randomized clinical trial designed to determine whether increasing the dose of dialysis or using a high-flux dialyzer membrane alters major outcomes, concluded that patients undergoing HD three times weekly derived no major benefit from a higher dialysis dose than that recommended by current U.S. guidelines, or from the use of a high-flux membrane.[107] However, subgroup analysis suggested benefit in patients maintained on dialysis for longer than 3.7 years and in those with diabetes.[70] The Membrane Permeability Outcome (MPO) study group reported similar results,[271] and the K/DOQI recommends the use of high-flux membranes.[316]

HDF is HD in which fluid removal exceeds the desired weight loss, and fluid balance is maintained by the infusion of a sterile pyrogen-free solution. HDF offers the advantages of both HD and HF in a single therapy. The replacement fluid, previously supplied in autoclaved bags, is now generated "online" from concentrated bicarbonate, and 20 to 30 L of water is used per session.[252] The result is that HDF provides a 10 to 15% increase in urea clearance compared with HD along with increased middle molecule clearances. Water for online preparation of substitution solution should meet common standards for dialysis water regarding chemical contaminants, but should be of higher quality regarding microbiological contaminants. Online HDF has been used extensively in continental Europe over the past 20 years or so.

After several years of HD, patients may develop carpal tunnel syndrome and evidence of amyloid deposition. The main constituent of dialysis-related amyloid is β_2-microglobulin. Circulating concentrations of β_2-microglobulin can be as high as 30 to 40 mg/dL. Although no correlation is noted between β_2-microglobulin circulating concentration and risk of amyloidosis, evidence from the HEMO study indicates that concentrations are correlated with survival.[71] Retrospective data from Lombardy in Italy indicate that there is a 5% risk that carpal tunnel decompression surgery will be required after 8 years of extracorporeal therapy, and that a reduction in risk of 42% is seen in those patients treated by HDF and HF compared with conventional HD.[270] It is suggested that patients on PD are less prone to developing amyloidosis.

Fluid management on HD is crucial for patient well-being and survival. Because conventional dialysis is based on a thrice weekly schedule, fluid is accumulated by the patient between dialysis sessions. Many patients are anuric or at least oliguric; therefore unrestricted fluid intake would result in fluid overload and complications of pulmonary edema and hypertension. Patients receiving HD are advised to restrict fluid intake to 1 L/d or so. This allowance is recommended to the individual patient by the dialysis nursing staff and the dietitian to ensure that adequate nutrition is maintained. Nevertheless many patients find the fluid restriction very difficult to maintain; therefore large weight gains between dialysis sessions are a common occurrence. During the dialysis session, the patient's "dry" or "target" weight is achieved. At dry weight, the fluid compartments are normal; this value is determined by gradually reducing weight until the patient is edema-free and reaches the point below which hypotension occurs on further fluid removal. The dry weight is difficult to reach in patients with abnormal cardiovascular responses, who may become hypotensive despite being relatively fluid replete.

When HD is begun, most patients have a small amount of residual renal function (RRF). This value of RRF may persist for many months and years; the volume of urine produced each day allows greater fluid intake and provides the benefit of reducing large fluctuations in body fluid volumes. RRF should be taken into consideration when dialysis prescriptions are adjusted. The K/DOQI Work Group 2006 updates include recommendations, as opposed to guidelines (opinion-based rather than evidence-based), for preserving RRF in patients receiving HD.[316]

Assessment of Adequacy of Hemodialysis

Assessment of adequacy of dialysis treatment for individual patients in the clinical setting includes consideration of the patient's well-being, cardiovascular risk, nutritional status, and degree of achievable ultrafiltration. It also includes estimates of a number of laboratory parameters, such as hemoglobin, phosphate, and albumin and clearance of the small solutes urea and creatinine. Although a full description of adequacy is beyond the scope of this text, a brief outline will be provided. Clearance of urea during a dialysis session (Kt/V) is calculated following determination of predialysis and postdialysis plasma urea concentrations, the time of the dialysis session, RRF, total clearance predicted from the dialyzer, and blood and dialysate flow rates. These variables are processed using computerized mathematical formulas. The Kt/V effectively describes the *power* of the dialysis session and continues to be valued as the most precise and accurate measure of dialysis.[316] A retrospective analysis of the National Cooperative Dialysis Study (NCDS) was the first study to identify a threshold in the value of Kt/V and survival in HD.[273] In practice, a simple calculation may be performed to obtain an estimate of dialysis adequacy: the urea reduction ratio (URR). The URR is the percentage fall in plasma urea attained during a dialysis session and is measured as follows:

$$[(\text{Predialysis}\ \{\text{urea}\} - \text{Postdialysis}\ \{\text{urea}\})/(\text{predialysis}\ \{\text{urea}\})] \times 100\%$$

Observational studies in populations of dialysis patients have shown that variations in URR are associated with major differences in mortality.[330]

Following publication of the HEMO study,[107] in 2006 the K/DOQI Work Group recommended that the target dose of delivered dialysis as calculated by Kt/V urea kinetic modeling was 1.4 per dialysis session. This dose is consistent with the target single pool Kt/V of approximately 1.4 set by the European Standards Group[111] and is roughly equivalent to a urea reduction ratio of 70% per dialysis for a patient receiving hemodialysis three times weekly.

Peritoneal Dialysis

Peritoneal dialysis (PD) is a type of dialysis in which dialysate is passed into the patient's peritoneal cavity, with the peritoneum employed as the dialysis membrane. It was first explored by Ganter in 1923 and initially showed poor results. The modern era of PD started in 1953, with intermittent irrigation of the peritoneal cavity with commercially prepared solutions and access achieved through a single disposable catheter (Figure 48-18). Popovich and coworkers in 1976 introduced the concept of portable equipment; this approach led to the use of continuous ambulatory peritoneal dialysis (CAPD),[351] a type of PD performed in ambulatory patients during normal activities. Peritoneal dialysis now accounts for 6.2% and 7.4% of the incident and prevalent dialysis populations in the United States—proportions that have continued to decline over the past decade from peaks of 13% and 11%, primarily as the result of an increase in HD capacity.[79] Use of PD varies between countries depending on access to HD. For example, in the United Kingdom, 21% of prevalent patients receive PD,

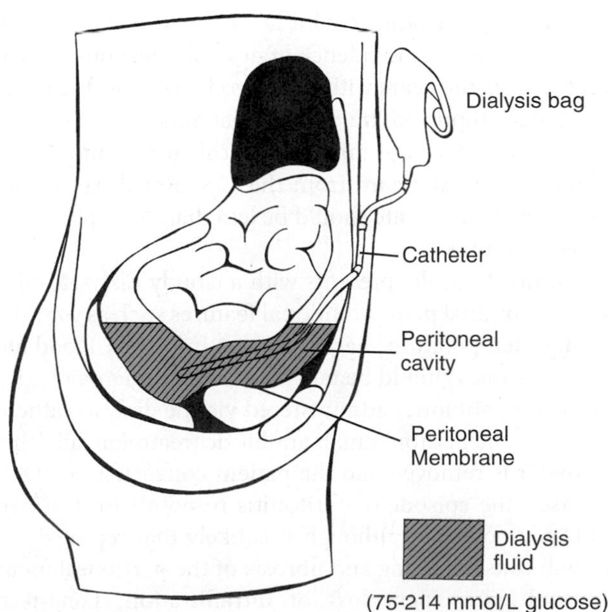

Figure 48-18 Diagrammatic sketch of peritoneal dialysis. *(Redrawn from Nolph KD. Peritoneal anatomy and transport physiology. In: Maher JF, ed. Replacement of renal function by dialysis, 3rd edition. Dordrecht, The Netherlands: Kluwer Academic Publishers/ Springer, 1989:Chapter 23.)* **To convert glucose concentration in mmol/L to mg/dL, multiply by 18.**

reflecting a percentage fall of 10% over 10 years, whereas in Mexico, 90% of patients receive PD.[338]

Description

Operationally, CAPD uses the patient's own peritoneal membrane (surface area ≈2 m^2), across which fluid and solutes are exchanged between the peritoneal capillary blood and the dialysis solution placed in the peritoneal cavity. Fluid removal (ultrafiltration) is achieved by using dialysis fluids containing high concentrations of dextrose acting as an osmotic agent; as dextrose passes across the peritoneal membrane, the rate of fluid removal decreases. Conventional therapies use four daily exchanges of approximately 2 L of fluid with approximately 10 L of spent dialysate generated, including ultrafiltration. RRF is critical to the success of PD because only a few milliliters per minute can contribute substantially to urea clearance and creatinine clearance (C_{Cr}), with each additional milliliter resulting in an extra 10 L of clearance per week. Practical reasons for opting for PD include (1) preservation of RRF and vascular access sites, (2) increased patient autonomy, (3) flexibility as to where the treatment can be administered, and (4) ease of self-treatment, with lower capital costs involved. The higher permeability of the peritoneal membrane provides good removal of β_2-microglobulin and may help to protect patients from the development of dialysis-related amyloid. Blood pressure control and extremes of fluid shifts are not as problematic as those that occur on conventional HD.

Automated PD is now widely available. It requires a programmable machine to regulate flow, dwell time, and drainage, and it may be performed at night. Solute clearance can be increased by leaving fluid in the peritoneum during the day and by performing an additional daytime exchange.

The main disadvantage of PD is the risk of infection causing peritonitis. Incidence rates of peritonitis have decreased over the years with the introduction of disconnect PD systems, improved training of patients with regard to meticulous hygiene, and microbiological surveillance protocols. The current standard from the U.K. Renal Association is that the peritonitis rate should be less than one episode per 18 patient months.[446]

Peritonitis typically presents with a cloudy dialysate effluent and abdominal pain. Additional features such as vomiting and a high temperature suggest serious infection. Blood and dialysate samples should be taken for urgent microbiological analysis and antibiotics administered via the dialysis catheter directly into the peritoneum. If antibiotic treatment fails, then the catheter is removed and the patient converted to HD. In most cases, the episode of peritonitis responds to treatment and PD can continue, although it is likely that repeated episodes will cause scarring and fibrosis of the peritoneal membrane with permanent loss of ultrafiltration. Long-term serious complications may occur, such as sclerosing encapsulating peritonitis caused by adhesions and peritoneal thickening encasing the peritoneal contents and causing bowel obstruction. This unusual condition is associated with increased frequency of peritonitis episodes and longer duration of PD.[16]

Assessment of Adequacy in PD

A series of clinical outcome reports have demonstrated that measures of PD solute removal (urea and creatinine) correlate with patient status and outcome.[249,284,400] In particular, a multicenter prospective cohort study of 680 incident CAPD patients [Canada-United States (CANUSA) Study] showed that a decrease of 0.1 in weekly urea clearance (defined by Kt/V_{urea}) was associated with a 5% increase in the RR of death.[74] Similarly, a decrease of 5 L/wk/1.73 m^2 of total C_{Cr} was associated with a 7% increase in the RR of death. As a consequence of these studies, national guidelines from the United Kingdom,[446] Australia,[60] and the United States[313] have set standards of dialysis adequacy in terms of small solute removal. An estimate of adequacy is performed in all patients within 6 to 8 weeks of commencement of dialysis. Additional studies should be performed at least every 6 months.[446]

Obtaining the weekly Kt/V_{urea} requires measurement of the volume of spent dialysate and urine for a complete 24-hour period. The concentration of urea in dialysate (D) compared with plasma (P) is calculated (the D/P ratio), and this value is then multiplied by the volume of the drained effluent to obtain an estimate of Kt. The calculation of "V," or the volume of distribution of urea, is derived from an estimate of total body water.[193,460] An estimate of weekly Kt/V_{urea} is simply the daily clearance multiplied by a factor of seven. These equations are used for both peritoneal and renal clearance, and the total weekly clearance is obtained by addition. Calculation of C_{Cr} is based on the following clearance (C) formula:

$$C = \frac{U\,(\text{or } D) \times V}{P}$$

where *U* is the concentration of creatinine in urine or dialysate, *V* is the mean daily drain volume or urine volume (measured in liters), and *P* is the concentration of creatinine in the plasma. The daily clearances obtained for both urine and dialysate are added together and multiplied by seven for the total weekly C_{Cr}. Current recommendations from the U.K. Renal Association include a combined urinary and peritoneal Kt/V_{urea} greater than 1.7/wk or a creatinine clearance greater than 50 L/week/1.73 m^2, which should be considered as reflecting minimal treatment doses. The dose should be increased in patients experiencing uremic symptoms.[446]

Compliance with complete collections is mandatory. To avoid sampling errors in patients who void infrequently, urine is collected over a 48 hour period. Dialysate sampling requires that all effluent bags obtained over a 24 hour period should be brought to the center renal unit; this can be difficult because the bags are heavy and bulky. Glucose concentrations in peritoneal dialysis bags may reach 3852 mg/dL (214 mmol/L): it is important that glucose interference in the dialysate creatinine measurement is corrected for when Jaffe assays are used[114] or minimized by the use of an enzymatic creatinine method.[250] An adjunct to assessment of adequacy in PD patients is the peritoneal equilibration test (PET),[441] which assesses peritoneal membrane transport characteristics in terms of creatinine clearance, glucose absorption, and ultrafiltration. The results are used to select dialysis schedules appropriate to the transport characteristics of the patient.

Measurement of adequacy is burdensome, labor intensive, and prone to multiple measurement errors, particularly from volume measurements of urine and dialysate samples; laboratory errors in measurements of urea and creatinine in blood, urine, and dialysate; and finally adjustment of results to predict weekly clearance. Although dialysis center nursing staff and patients may collect the samples required for adequacy testing with the utmost diligence, the very complexity and number of measurements taken will lead to an accumulation of measurement errors. In the opinion of the authors of the NKF-K/DOQI Clinical Practice Guidelines for PD Adequacy, when properly performed, these measures are reproducible enough to be useful in routine clinical practice.[313] However, an alternative, simpler method for defining dialysis adequacy would be very useful in practice.

Malnutrition in Dialysis Patients

Dialysis patients with ESRD tend to have a poor appetite. In addition, protein metabolism is altered in the setting of chronic acidosis and low-grade inflammation. These factors in combination place patients at risk of protein and energy malnourishment. Nutritional screening is recommended in dialysis patients. Such screening may involve subjective global assessment, measurement of the body mass index, a recent history of weight loss, and the measurement of albumin. Serum albumin is often used as a marker of malnutrition, even though it is a relatively poor nutritional marker.[214] However, good evidence indicates that the lower the albumin concentration, the worse is the long-term prognosis.[128,129,330] An albumin concentration less than 3.5 g/dL (measured by a bromocresol green method) or less than 3.0 g/dL (bromocresol purple method) is indicative of undernutrition. Hypoalbuminemia is associated with increased markers of the acute-phase response, such as CRP.[331,420] Persistent elevation of CRP is common in dialysis patients and may occur in the absence of detectable infection. Episodes of peritonitis in PD patients cause significant albumin losses as the result of membrane leakage.

Kidney Transplantation

Kidney transplantation is the most effective form of renal replacement therapy, in terms of long-term survival and quality of life.[352] Data provided by the Organ Procurement and Transplantation Network reveal that 305,000 kidney transplants were performed in the United States between 1988 and June 2011. During 2010, 16,898 kidney transplants were performed in the United States, and more than 89,000 patients are on the waiting list for a kidney transplant.[328A] The median waiting time for a listed patient depends on his or her age. For example, for patients listed between 2003 and 2004, the median waiting time for a child aged 1 to 5 years was 361 days, and for an adult aged 35 to 49 years, 1807 days. Although patients with kidney failure should have equitable access to kidney transplantation, currently only 23% of adult patients on dialysis in the United Kingdom are on the active renal transplant waiting list. Waiting time spent on dialysis has been shown to be an important factor in determining mortality. In England and Wales, 45% of patients younger than 65 years were activated on the transplant list within 1 year of starting dialysis, and 66% were activated within 5 years. Evidence suggests that the very best outcomes are achieved following preemptive (i.e., before dialysis has become necessary) live donor transplants[285]; this has led to increased emphasis on preemptive transplantation, particularly in the United Kingdom following the National Service Framework for Renal Services, published in 2004.[99]

Since Joseph Murray in Boston performed the first successful transplant in 1954 from one twin to the other, progressive developments have occurred in this field of medicine. In 1959, Dameshek and Schwartz used 6-mercaptopurine (6-MP) in place of irradiation to precondition patients for bone marrow transplantation. Calne developed this work with the introduction of a safer derivative of 6-MP called azathioprine (AZA). By 1963, maintenance AZA and corticosteroids had become the standard regimen for kidney transplantation. Kidney transplant or "allograft" survival with these treatment protocols was approximately 40% at 12 months. In the late 1970s to early 1980s, cyclosporine was introduced and has since been the mainstay immunosuppressive regimen in combination with AZA and corticosteroids. Cyclosporine-based protocols led to fewer episodes of acute rejection and improved graft survival at 12 months to 80 to 90%. Tacrolimus, mycophenolate mofetil (MMF), sirolimus (Rapamycin), and everolimus (Ever) were developed for use in kidney transplantation in the mid- to late 1990s (see Chapter 35 for details on the individual drugs). Also, marked progress has been noted in the development and use of biological agents (monoclonal or polyclonal antibodies directed against immune response cellular targets) to suppress the immune response to a graft in human transplant recipients. All these advancements have led to increases in graft and patient survival, with 1-year graft survival of approximately 90% being the norm.[121,157] By contrast, long-term graft survival remains a major problem, with half of transplants failing within 14 years, usually as a result of chronic allograft injury or death with a functioning graft. Transplantation medicine provides a constant challenge to balance the immunologic risk of damage to the allograft (rejection) versus the well-being of the recipient, while avoiding excess immunosuppression that increases the likelihood of opportunistic infection and malignancy. In addition, many of the powerful immunosuppressive drugs have idiosyncratic side effect profiles.

Preoperative Assessment

The criteria for acceptance into a transplant program differ slightly from center to center, and it is easier to consider reasons for exclusion (Box 48-8). Two important psychologic issues remain to be considered: (1) the concept of organ receipt, and (2) the potential difficulty in complying with immunosuppressive therapies. Age is no longer a primary issue in an otherwise healthy individual; however, only 6% of

BOX 48-8 Exclusion Criteria for Consideration for a Kidney Transplant

Serious concomitant illness (particularly if likely to shorten life expectancy or to be exacerbated by immunosuppressive treatment)
- Active malignancy*
- Inoperable ischemic heart disease
- Severe chronic lung disease
- Active systemic infection (e.g., tuberculosis)
- Active immunologic disease
- Severe irreversible hepatic disease
- Severe peripheral vascular disease

Severe obesity [body mass index (BMI) >40 kg/m^2)

Lower urinary tract dysfunction not amenable to surgical repair

Substance abuse

Significant psychiatric disturbance

*Malignancy that has been treated with no evidence of recurrence is not an exclusion, provided the predefined remission period has elapsed.

transplant recipients in the United Kingdom are over the age of 65.[445]

Laboratory assessment includes indicators of general operative health [e.g., electrolytes, acid-base status, clotting profile, full blood cell count, cross-matching (Boxes 48-9 and 48-10)]. In addition, a full screen for infectious diseases, particularly cytomegalovirus (CMV), Epstein-Barr virus, hepatitis B and C, varicella-zoster virus, and human immunodeficiency virus (HIV) status, is undertaken; these infections can be activated by immunosuppressive therapy.

The Operation

The donor kidney is usually placed extraperitoneally in the right or left iliac fossa. Anastomoses are constructed joining the transplant renal artery and vein to the recipient's respective iliac vessels. The ureter is joined to the bladder. The recipient native kidneys are left in situ in most cases. Living donor kidneys can be retrieved through open surgery or with the aid of laparoscopic techniques.

Postoperative Assessment

During the initial postoperative phase of 1 to 2 weeks, careful monitoring of serum creatinine and urine output is required to monitor graft function. Most grafts produce measurable amounts of urine within a matter of hours, and this is a clear sign of a functioning graft; however, in a certain proportion, perhaps 5 to 10% of cases, primary nonfunction is apparent. In this subgroup, continuing dialysis support is necessary. In some patients the condition resolves without treatment, but in others a percutaneous kidney biopsy may be necessary to establish whether the graft is still viable and what form of therapy should be initiated. In otherwise uncomplicated cases, the serum creatinine concentration falls rapidly postoperatively (Figure 48-19). Early allograft rejection episodes are suspected if the creatinine does not fall to the expected concentration, or if there is a rise of 10% in creatinine concentration. The differential diagnoses of graft dysfunction and complications that may ensue following transplant are summarized in Table 48-18. In the very early postoperative phase, in addition to rejection, graft dysfunction may be a consequence of delayed graft function, immunosuppressive drug toxicity, and acute tubular damage. Relative hypotension and dehydration may also contribute. Renal artery and venous thromboses are rare complications, and ureteric obstruction can be readily diagnosed using ultrasonography. Histologic examination of a transplant biopsy is necessary to aid diagnosis and treatment adjustment. Regular monitoring of kidney function, drug concentrations, and viral assay—particularly for CMV viremia and polyoma viruses such as BK virus— is mandated following kidney transplantation in many centers.

BOX 48-9 Immunologic Aspects of Transplantation

Although a detailed description of the immunologic aspects of transplantation is beyond the scope of this chapter, a brief discussion follows to highlight the close collaboration between clinicians and the tissue typing laboratory, and to explore some of the recent advances in transplantation. The tissue type identifies an individual based on human leukocyte antigens (HLAs) expressed on cells. These antigens are coded by genes of the major (and minor) histo- (tissue) compatibility complex (MHC). Individuals who have received blood transfusions or previous transplants of nonidentical tissue and females who have had pregnancies develop antibodies to nonself HLA. These antibodies can be detected by analyzing the recipient serum against a panel of cells containing various HLA types. If a reaction is noted between donor cells and recipient serum in vitro, this is indicative of a potential positive cross-match between donor organ and recipient at the time of transplantation. All recipients are tested regularly by the tissue typing service. Highly sensitive individuals have a number of antibodies or an antibody to a common HLA type and typically have a longer waiting time for a suitable donor kidney. The definition of high sensitization varies, for example, panel-reactive antibody (PRA) >50%. PRA refers to the percentage of typical donors against which the patient has in vitro evidence of potentially toxic alloantibody. Highly sensitized patients form about 30% of those on the waiting list in the United States.[278]

ABO blood group incompatibility and HLA cross-match reactivity between donor organs and recipients result in an accelerated or "hyperacute" rejection of the nonself organ (allograft) and have been traditional barriers to transplantation. Recent developments have led to desensitization protocols to remove pre-formed antibodies from the plasma of potential recipients and have permitted transplantation across ABO and HLA barriers. This has permitted previously unsuitable potential live donors to donate. The outcome for recipients of desensitization programs is very encouraging, with 89% of allografts surviving at 22 months' follow-up in a single center.[279] Following transplantation, clinicians and the tissue typing laboratory must remain vigilant for the persistence or reappearance of antibodies that may mediate rejection of the allograft.

BOX 48-10 Laboratory Assessment of Potential Kidney Transplant Recipient*

Electrolytes, liver function tests, glucose, C-reactive protein
Acid-base status
Full blood cell count
Clotting profile
Cytomegalovirus (CMV)
Hepatitis B and C
Varicella-zoster virus (VZV)
Epstein-Barr virus (EBV)
Human immunodeficiency virus (HIV) 1 and 2
Toxoplasma
Syphilis serology
Blood group: ABO compatibility
Tissue typing: human leukocyte antigen (HLA)
Panel reactive antibodies (PRAs) (see Box 48-9)

*Tests of cardiac disease, vascular disease, and bladder function are also required in most cases.

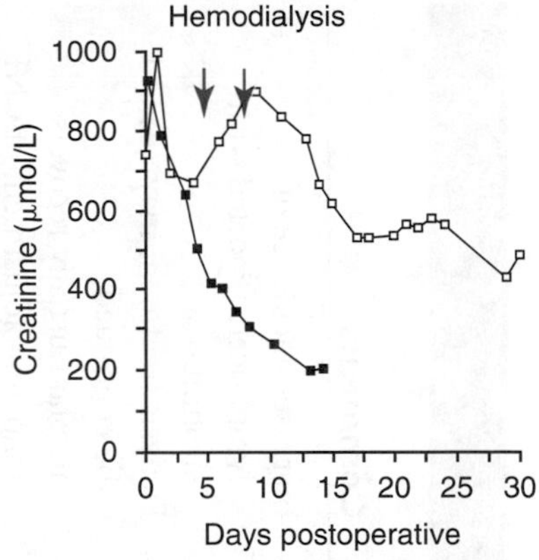

Figure 48-19 Post-transplantation biochemical profile. *Open squares* represent the course of a patient who experienced an early rejection episode (confirmed by biopsy, ↓) and requires initial hemodialysis support. *Solid squares* represent the typical profile of an uncomplicated transplant recipient. To convert creatinine concentration in μmol/L to mg/dL, multiply by 0.011.

Primary glomerular disease may recur following kidney transplantation, resulting in loss of the graft. An Australian study has confirmed the 10 year incidence of graft loss caused by recurrent glomerulonephritis as 8.4%.[49] Recurrence was the third most frequent cause of graft loss (chronic allograft nephropathy and death with a functioning graft were most common). As compared with the average for all recipients with a primary diagnosis of glomerulonephritis, FSGS (11.8%) and mesangiocapillary glomerulonephritis type 1 (10.2%) were most likely to recur, causing graft loss. In contrast, graft loss due to recurrent IgA and pauci-immune crescentic glomerulonephritis occurred in only 2% of patients at 10 years' follow-up.

Allograft Rejection

The immune response to the foreign graft (allograft) is very rapid, and allograft rejection may occur in response to nonidentical HLA molecules. A subtle rise in creatinine of approximately 10% in the first 3 months of a transplant may indicate a rejection episode. However, biopsy of the kidney transplant is necessary to confirm the cause of graft dysfunction and to identify the type of rejection that is occurring. A systematic classification system is employed ("Banff classification") to report transplant biopsy specimens.[414] The latest updates from the Banff report have increasingly recognized the importance of humoral (antibody-mediated) rejection as a cause of allograft failure during the whole life of the transplant. Rejection has classically been divided into cellular and vascular types, and typically has been qualified by the speed of onset of graft dysfunction and the time since transplant. This classification builds on this but incorporates antibody-mediated rejection (acute or chronic) and T cell–mediated rejection (again, acute or chronic). Advances in the diagnoses of humoral rejection have included identification of complement-fixing alloantibody along capillary walls within the transplant following the development of a stain for C4d product.[118] In addition, donor-specific anti-HLA antibodies can often be detected in the serum of the recipient during the course of the transplant and may predict graft dysfunction in some cases.[433,480] It is accepted that antibody- and T cell–mediated rejection may coexist as causes of immunologic damage to the allograft. Allograft rejection typically is treated by escalating immunosuppression schedules, and treatment may include antithymocyte globulin and/or high-dose corticosteroids.

Immunosuppression and Therapeutic Drug Monitoring

As mentioned earlier, the introduction of immunosuppressive drugs in the 1970s led to vast improvement in the success rate of kidney transplantation (see Chapter 35). However, currently used drugs have potentially numerous and serious side effects that are summarized in Table 48-19.

Following the introduction of cyclosporine in the 1980s, a dramatic increase in 1 year graft survival resulted from the reduction in the number of acute rejection episodes.[300] However, a number of important side effects have been observed. Nephrotoxicity was soon apparent in early clinical trials[57] and remains a major clinical problem. During the 1990s, tacrolimus was introduced and 1 year graft and patient survival rates were equivalent to those achieved with cyclosporine therapy, although rates of acute rejection episodes were lower.[148,293,348,440] Five-year follow-up data suggest improved graft survival with tacrolimus compared with cyclosporine.[456]

Sirolimus, in contrast to cyclosporine, does not cause nephrotoxicity, gingival hyperplasia, or tremor. However, patients treated with sirolimus have a higher incidence of thrombocytopenia, hyperlipidemia, and lymphocele formation.[218] Sirolimus and mycophenolate mofetil (MMF), both introduced during the late 1990s, have been studied in the

TABLE 48-18 Complications Following Kidney Transplantation

	Immediate Post Transplant	Early Post Transplant Period Until 3 Months	3-12 Months	After 1 Year	Comments
Surgical complications	Renal venous thrombosis, arterial thrombosis Pelvic lymphocele adjacent to the transplanted kidney Ureteric obstruction			Ureteric obstruction, renal artery stenosis	Increased incidence of lymphocele reported with sirolimus
Kidney	Acute tubular necrosis with delayed graft function				Dialysis treatment may need to be continued Transplant usually recovers following adjustment of CNI doses Electrolytes and creatinine should be measured daily
(a) Immunologic	Hyperacute rejection: occurs as a consequence of pre-formed antibodies in recipient serum to donor blood group or HLA antigens, resulting in graft failure. Plasma exchange may be initiated but transplant nephrectomy likely	Acute rejection in 20-60% of patients Associated with rise in serum creatinine concentration Confirmed on biopsy Pathologic description includes vascular and cellular infiltration by immune reactive cells Requires urgent treatment with high-dose corticosteroids	(i) Chronic allograft injury. Heralded by rising serum creatinine, proteinuria, and hypertension. Common cause of graft failure in the long term. Complex pathogenesis with a combination of donor-specific and recipient influences. Humoral (antibody-mediated) rejection increasingly recognized as contributing to immunologic injury. Transplant biopsy may show peritubular capillary stain for complement degradation product C4d (ii) Subclinical rejection not suspected from serum creatinine concentration. This is a pathologic diagnosis from transplant biopsy and is treated with high-dose corticosteroids		Transplant centers may perform biopsy protocols at 3, 6, and 12 months to guide therapy Clinical episode of rejection considered if serum creatinine concentration increases from baseline Monitor recipient serum for anti-HLA antibodies, particularly donor-specific antibodies Reduction in immunosuppression during maintenance phase of stable transplants
(b) Recurrent disease	Glomerular disease such as FSGS and MCGN may occur early and lead to graft failure		Risk of anti-GBM disease in patients with Alport's syndrome Familial hemolytic-uremic syndrome		Low risk of recurrent disease causing graft failure in diabetes and IgA nephropathy

Infection	Chest infection Urinary tract infection Septicemia	Opportunistic infections: PCP, CMV infection and reactivation. High-risk cases include donor-positive and recipient-negative for prior exposure to CMV (D+/D–) Prophylactic antiviral drugs recommended in high-risk patients Varicella-zoster virus, polyoma virus (BK virus nephropathy), candidiasis	CMV viremia in high-risk cases following discontinuation of prophylactic antiviral medication		Increased risk of infection in all patients receiving immunosuppression Patients advised to receive influenza vaccine annually and vaccination against pneumococcus Regular screening for viremia by PCR methods Routine staining of transplant biopsy specimens for SV40 to identify BK virus nephropathy C-reactive protein, urine microscopy, cultures performed Blood cultures Chest x-ray
Drug-related toxicity	See Table 48-19.				
Lymphoproliferative		PTLD Typically associated with EBV expression in patients exposed to highly potent immunosuppressive protocols	PTLD Includes non–EBV-related lymphoma	PTLD Includes non–EBV-related lymphoma	EBV-PCR CT/MRI scans of chest, abdomen, and pelvis Tissue diagnosis mandatory from lymph node and bone marrow Serum lactate dehydrogenase activity increased
Malignancy	Increased risk of nonmelanotic skin malignancy and solid organ malignancy in all patients				
Cardiovascular disease	Increased incidence of cardiovascular disease following transplantation. Death with a functioning graft is a common cause of "graft failure" Most transplant patients require treatment for hypertension and dyslipidemias				

CMV, Cytomegalovirus; *CNI,* calcineurin inhibitor; *CT,* computed tomography; *EBV,* Epstein-Barr virus; *FSGS,* focal segmental glomerulosclerosis; *GBM,* glomerular basement membrane; *HLA,* human leukocyte antigen; *Ig,* immunoglobulin; *MCGN,* mesangiocapillary glomerulonephritis; *MRI,* magnetic resonance imaging; *PCP, Pneumocystis carinii* pneumonia; *PCR,* polymerase chain reaction; *PTLD,* post-transplant lymphoproliferative disease; *SV40,* simian virus 40 (cross-reacts with BK virus).

TABLE 48-19 Noninfectious Complications of Immunosuppressant Drugs

Drug	Drug Dose	Target Therapeutic Range*	Toxicity Profile
Corticosteroids (e.g., prednisone)	Dose depends on weight of patient and time since transplant. Typically, 40 mg daily during first week and tapering to 5 mg at 6 months and withdrawal at 12 months	Not appropriate	Increased risk of developing diabetes mellitus Deterioration in diabetes control Osteopenia Osteoporosis Psychosis Fat redistribution Hypertension Dyslipidemia Cataracts Weight gain
Calcineurin Inhibitors			
Cyclosporine	Variable Depends on weight, time since transplant, and achieved drug concentration. Given in two divided doses and predose trough level measured in morning blood sample	200-300 μg/L for first 3-12 months. Thereafter aim for 100 μg/L	Nephrotoxicity Hypertension Neurotoxicity Hemolytic-uremic syndrome Tubular electrolyte abnormalities (hypophosphatemia, hypomagnesemia, hyperkalemia) Hirsutism Gingival hyperplasia Bone pain Dyslipidemia
Tacrolimus			As for cyclosporine, except no hirsutism or gingival hyperplasia Increased risk of diabetes mellitus Cardiomyopathy (children) Alopecia
Mycophenolate mofetil	Aim for 2 g daily in divided doses	Not routinely measured	Abdominal pain Diarrhea Myelosuppression
Sirolimus	Dose depends on weight and achieved drug level. The drug is administered once daily	Level depends on time since transplant. Typical early (<3 months) targets are 8-12 μg/L and thereafter 4-8 μg/L	Lymphocele (a fluid-filled collection near to transplanted kidney) Thrombocytopenia Hyperlipidemia
Azathioprine	Usual starting dose of 2 mg/kg body weight in a single daily dose	Levels not measured. Because the enzyme thiopurine methyltransferase (TPMT) metabolizes azathioprine, the risk of myelosuppression is increased in patients with low activity of the enzyme (although the enzyme level is not measured routinely: weekly monitoring of full blood counts is performed for several weeks following commencement of drug)	Myelosuppression Severe interaction if used with allopurinol (treatment for gout)

TABLE 48-19 Noninfectious Complications of Immunosuppressant Drugs—cont'd

Drug	Drug Dose	Target Therapeutic Range*	Toxicity Profile
Biological Agents			
Anti-CD25 monoclonal antibodies	Given at time of transplant and once thereafter		Very well tolerated
Basiliximab and daclizumab			
Polyclonal antithymocyte globulin (ATG) and antilymphocyte globulin (ALG), and monoclonal OKT3	Given in response to refractory rejection episodes in selected patients		Increased risk of malignancy, post-transplant lymphoproliferative disease Hypersensitivity reactions

*These are not recommendations but are illustrative and will vary between centers.

setting of cyclosporine withdrawal and cyclosporine-free strategies in kidney transplantation,* the hypothesis being that withdrawal or avoidance of cyclosporine would improve long-term outcomes because there is no nephrotoxic stimulus. It has been shown in a multinational study that withdrawal of cyclosporine within 3 months of transplantation is feasible.[208] Studies have also shown that sirolimus in combination with MMF is safe and is associated with low rates of acute transplant rejection at 12 months.[121]

These patients also received basiliximab, a monoclonal antibody to a specific target (CD 25) of T-cell activation that occurred in response to a nonidentical graft. However, the CEASAR study (Cyclosporin Sparing with Mycophenolate mofetil, daclizamab and Corticosteroids in Renal Allograft Recipients) found that use of MMF, corticosteroids, and daclizumab induction was associated with increased risk of rejection if cyclosporine was withdrawn by month 6 following the transplant, compared with continuation of low-dose cyclosporine.[106]

Cyclosporine is insoluble and is presented for clinical use as a microemulsion. It has a narrow therapeutic window, and in clinical transplantation it is important to monitor the blood concentration frequently. The most widely accepted practice is to monitor the "trough" blood concentration just before the next dose. Accepted trough concentrations vary from 100 to 300 μg/L (see Table 48-19). The highest concentrations are targeted during the induction phase of treatment for 2 to 3 months; subsequently, lower maintenance concentrations are desirable. The trough concentration within the blood may not provide a truly accurate guide to total drug exposure, because wide variation in absorption is seen over the first 2 to 4 hours following dosing.[210] This is important in that most of the pharmacodynamic effects of cyclosporine occur within 2 hours.[164] Studies from Canada suggest that trough concentrations do not reflect clinical outcomes in terms of acute rejection rates,[282] although high trough concentrations were associated with increased nephrotoxicity. A 2 hour drug (C-2) concentration correlated well with formal area under the curve measurements and is predictive of nephrotoxicity and acute rejection episodes. Among kidney transplant patients, the trough concentration of tacrolimus is well correlated with acute rejection episodes and nephrotoxicity.[227] Trough concentrations also guide sirolimus therapy (see Table 48-19).[219]

MMF is morpholinoethyl ester of mycophenolic acid (MPA), a potent and reversible inhibitor of inosine monophosphate dehydrogenase isoform 2 (IMPDH), and has become the single most used immunosuppressant in solid organ transplantation. Excellent results have been obtained with a fixed-dose regimen. IMPDH is a target for immunosuppression because lymphocytes depend on the de novo guanosine nucleotide synthesis pathway for DNA synthesis and cell division.[206] MMF, because it is a prodrug of MPA, is rapidly absorbed following an oral dose and is de-esterified to MPA, which is highly protein bound. Free MPA concentrations determine the amount of immunosuppressive activity, and this can be affected by hypoalbuminemia and renal insufficiency. Toxicity of MPA is manifested by bone marrow failure. Therapeutic drug monitoring of MPA is possible using HPLC and immunoassay techniques. However, it has not been established whether the extra effort of measuring MPA concentrations would improve clinical end points. Studies have been commenced to compare fixed dosing versus concentration-controlled MMF therapy; until these findings are reported, therapeutic drug monitoring of MPA has not been established in routine clinical practice.[356]

In summary, long-term graft failure is a major problem, and graft loss accounts for the return of increasing numbers of patients to dialysis. The most common cause of graft loss is death with a functioning graft. Kidney failure carries a considerable burden of cardiovascular morbidity. Although some risk factors, such as volume overload and anemia, are improved following transplantation, others, including dyslipidemia and hypertension, persist. The drugs used to prevent rejection can exacerbate these. Challenges to the nephrology

*References 106, 121, 133, 208, 390, and 464.

community are complex and include improving access to transplantation, reducing side effects of the powerful drugs used to prevent rejection, and reducing cardiovascular risk profiles for individual patients.

Simultaneous Pancreas-Kidney Transplantation

Patients with type 1 diabetes and stage 5 CKD with limited secondary complications of diabetes may be considered for simultaneous pancreas and kidney (SPK) transplantation. Patients (aged between 20 and 40 years) tend to be younger than kidney only recipients. Graft and patient survival rates were calculated for more than 3500 recipients of an SPK transplant in the United States from 1994 to 1997, based on data reported to the United Network for Organ Sharing (UNOS) renal registry database.[53] The 1 year graft survival rate was 90%, and patient survival was around 93%. At 5 years, graft survival was in excess of 70%, and patient survival 85%. These results compare favorably with those of cadaveric kidney only transplantation in diabetes. The main reason for the survival advantage of SPK over kidney only is the fact that younger donors and recipients are selected. A separate prospective observational study examined the impact of SPK transplant in terms of quality of life.[156] At 3 years, SPK patients report greater improvements than kidney only recipients in physical functioning, bodily pain, general health, and perception of improvements to secondary complications of diabetes.

The surgical technique for SPK involves whole organ pancreas transplantation with the duodenal segment draining into the urinary bladder through a duodenocystostomy. The kidney is attached as usual to the iliac vessels, and the donor ureter is inserted into the bladder separately. Alternatively, the pancreas can be drained enterically. This distinction is important because of the metabolic consequences outlined below. Postoperatively, blood glucose concentrations are monitored closely and intravenous insulin is given as necessary. Exocrine pancreatic secretion can be measured in the urine. The major fear is rejection and a number of parameters are monitored, including plasma glucose, amylase, lipase, and 12 or 24 hour urinary amylase. Because of high fluid, bicarbonate, and electrolyte losses into the urine, the need for supplementation is increased in SPK recipients. There is a long-term need for high-dose oral sodium bicarbonate supplementation in bladder-drained pancreatic transplantation because of exocrine secretory losses. Hyperamylasemia is common postoperatively and may or may not signify allograft rejection. Immunosuppressive schedules vary between centers and include induction therapy with monoclonal or polyclonal anti–T cell agents and a combination of the drugs outlined previously. Diagnosis of pancreatic rejection in the absence of a simultaneous kidney transplant is very difficult. Signs of rejection include fever, pain, hematuria, reduction of urinary amylase, and unexplained hyperglycemia. Organ scanning and biopsy are also used. However, the function of the kidney in SPK mirrors the pancreas; therefore immunosuppression can be tailored to the requirements of the kidney.

For patients with bladder drainage, enteric conversion may be required for refractory problems, such as dehydration, metabolic acidosis, chronic urethritis caused by trypsinogen activation, urinary tract infection, and recurrent reflux pancreatitis. Enteric conversion involves an anastomosis between the graft duodenal segment and the recipient small bowel.

REFERENCES

1. Agatston AS, Janowitz WR, Hildner FJ, Zusmer NR, Viamonte M Jr, Detrano R. Quantification of coronary artery calcium using ultrafast computed tomography. J Am Coll Cardiol 1990;15:827-32.
2. Agewall S, Wikstrand J, Ljungman S, Fagerberg B. Usefulness of microalbuminuria in predicting cardiovascular mortality in treated hypertensive men with and without diabetes mellitus. Risk Factor Intervention Study Group. Am J Cardiol 1997;80:164-9.
3. Alexander RT, Hoenderop JG, Bindels RJ. Molecular determinants of magnesium homeostasis: insights from human disease. J Am Soc Nephrol 2008;19:1451-8.
4. Alexanian R, Dimopoulos M. The treatment of multiple myeloma. N Engl J Med 1994;330:484-9.
5. Anderson S, Brenner BM. Effects of aging on the renal glomerulus. Am J Med 1986;80:435-42.
6. Anderson S, Meyer TW, Rennke HG, Brenner BM. Control of glomerular hypertension limits glomerular injury in rats with reduced renal mass. J Clin Invest 1985;76:612-9.
7. Ansell D, Feehally J, Fogarty D, Tomson C, Williams AJ, Warwick G. The eleventh annual report of the UK renal registry 2008. Available at: www.renalreg.org/ accessed July 14, 2011.
8. Antonsen JE, Sherrard DJ, Andress DL. A calcimimetic agent acutely suppresses parathyroid hormone levels in patients with chronic renal failure: rapid communication. Kidney Int 1998;53:223-7.
9. Appel GB, Contreras G, Dooley MA, Ginzler EM, Isenberg D, Jayne D, et al. Mycophenolate mofetil versus cyclophosphamide for induction treatment of lupus nephritis. J Am Soc Nephrol 2009;20: 1103-12.
10. Aspelin P, Aubry P, Fransson SG, Strasser R, Willenbrock R, Berg KJ. Nephrotoxic effects in high-risk patients undergoing angiography. N Engl J Med 2003;348:491-9.
11. Back SE, Ljungberg B, Nilsson-Ehle I, Borga O, Nilsson-Ehle P. Age dependence of renal function: clearance of iohexol and p-amino hippurate in healthy males. Scand J Clin Lab Invest 1989;49:641-6.
12. Baigent C, Burbury K, Wheeler D. Premature cardiovascular disease in chronic renal failure. Lancet 2000;356:147-52.

12A. Baigent C, Landray MJ, Reith C. et al., on behalf of the of the SHARP investigators. The effects of lowering LDL cholesterol with simvastatin plus ezetimibe in patients with chronic kidney disease (Study of Heart and Renal Protection): a randomised placebo-controlled trial. Lancet 2011;377:2181-2192.

13. Baines RJ, Brunskill NJ. The molecular interactions between filtered proteins and proximal tubular cells in proteinuria. Nephron Exp Nephrol 2008;110:e67-71.
14. Bakir A, Williams RH, Shaykh M, Dunea G, Dubin A. Biochemistry of the uremic syndrome. Adv Clin Chem 1992;29:61-120.
15. Bakris GL, Williams M, Dworkin L, Elliott WJ, Epstein M, Toto R, et al. Preserving renal function in adults with hypertension and diabetes: a consensus approach. National Kidney Foundation Hypertension and Diabetes Executive Committees Working Group. Am J Kidney Dis 2000;36:646-61.
16. Balasubramaniam G, Brown EA, Davenport A, Cairns H, Cooper B, Fan SL, et al. The Pan-Thames EPS study: treatment and outcomes of encapsulating peritoneal sclerosis. Nephrol Dial Transplant 2009;24: 3209-15.
17. Ballardie FW, Roberts IS. Controlled prospective trial of prednisolone and cytotoxics in progressive IgA nephropathy. J Am Soc Nephrol 2002;13:142-8.
18. Bangstad HJ, Osterby R, Dahl-Jorgensen K, Berg KJ, Hartmann A, Nyberg G, et al. Early glomerulopathy is present in young, type 1 (insulin-dependent) diabetic patients with microalbuminuria. Diabetologia 1993;36:523-9.

19. Barakat AJ, Rennert OM. Gitelman's syndrome (familial hypokalemia-hypomagnesemia). J Nephrol 2001;14:43-7.
20. Barisoni L, Schnaper HW, Kopp JB. A proposed taxonomy for the podocytopathies: a reassessment of the primary nephrotic diseases. Clin J Am Soc Nephrol 2007;2:529-42.
21. Barr RG, Seliger S, Appel GB, Zuniga R, D'Agati V, Salmon J, et al. Prognosis in proliferative lupus nephritis: the role of socio-economic status and race/ethnicity. Nephrol Dial Transplant 2003;18:2039-46.
22. Barratt J, Feehally J. IgA nephropathy. J Am Soc Nephrol 2005;16: 2088-97.
23. Batlle D. Clinical and cellular markers of diabetic nephropathy. Kidney Int 2003;63:2319-30.
24. Beetham R, Cattell WR. Proteinuria: pathophysiology, significance and recommendations for measurement in clinical practice. Ann Clin Biochem 1993;30:425-34.
25. Berenson JR, Lichtenstein A, Porter L, Dimopoulos MA, Bordoni R, George S, et al. Efficacy of pamidronate in reducing skeletal events in patients with advanced multiple myeloma. Myeloma Aredia Study Group. N Engl J Med 1996;334:488-93.
26. Berndt T, Kumar R. Phosphatonins and the regulation of phosphate homeostasis. Annu Rev Physiol 2007;69:341-59.
27. Berry SJ, Coffey DS, Walsh PC, Ewing LL. The development of human benign prostatic hyperplasia with age. J Urol 1984;132:474-9.
28. Berthelot M, Cornu G, Daudon M, Helbert M, Laurence C. Diffuse reflectance technique for infrared analysis of urinary calculi. Clin Chem 1987;33:780-3.
29. Besarab A, Amin N, Ahsan M, Vogel SE, Zazuwa G, Frinak S, et al. Optimization of epoetin therapy with intravenous iron therapy in hemodialysis patients. J Am Soc Nephrol 2000;11:530-8.
30. Besarab A, Bolton WK, Browne JK, Egrie JC, Nissenson AR, Okamoto DM, et al. The effects of normal as compared with low hematocrit values in patients with cardiac disease who are receiving hemodialysis and epoetin. N Engl J Med 1998;339:584-90.
31. Bettinelli A, Bianchetti MG, Girardin E, Caringella A, Cecconi M, Appiani AC, et al. Use of calcium excretion values to distinguish two forms of primary renal tubular hypokalemic alkalosis: Bartter and Gitelman syndromes. J Pediatr 1992;120:38-43.
32. Bhandari S, Hunter M. Inward rectifier renal potassium channel (ROMK), the low-conductance channels for potassium secretion. Nephrol Dial Transplant 1998;13:3019-23.
33. Bianchi S, Bigazzi R, Caiazza A, Campese VM. A controlled, prospective study of the effects of atorvastatin on proteinuria and progression of kidney disease. Am J Kidney Dis 2003;41:565-70.
34. Bichet DG. Nephrogenic diabetes insipidus. Am J Med 1998;105: 431-42.
35. Blacher J, Guerin AP, Pannier B, Marchais SJ, London GM. Arterial calcifications, arterial stiffness, and cardiovascular risk in end-stage renal disease. Hypertension 2001;38:938-42.
36. Blacher J, Safar ME, Guerin AP, Pannier B, Marchais SJ, London GM. Aortic pulse wave velocity index and mortality in end-stage renal disease. Kidney Int 2003;63:1852-60.
37. Block GA, Hulbert-Shearon TE, Levin NW, Port FK. Association of serum phosphorus and calcium × phosphate product with mortality risk in chronic hemodialysis patients: a national study. Am J Kidney Dis 1998;31:607-17.
38. Block GA, Raggi P, Bellasi A, Kooienga L, Spiegel DM. Mortality effect of coronary calcification and phosphate binder choice in incident hemodialysis patients. Kidney Int 2007;71:438-41.
39. Blum U, Krumme B, Flugel P, Gabelmann A, Lehnert T, Buitrago-Tellez C, et al. Treatment of ostial renal-artery stenoses with vascular endoprostheses after unsuccessful balloon angioplasty. N Engl J Med 1997;336:459-65.
40. Bonventre JV, Weinberg JM. Recent advances in the pathophysiology of ischemic acute renal failure. J Am Soc Nephrol 2003;14:2199-210.
41. Borch-Johnsen K, Norgaard K, Hommel E, Mathiesen ER, Jensen JS, Deckert T, et al. Is diabetic nephropathy an inherited complication? Kidney Int 1992;41:719-22.
42. Borghi L, Schianchi T, Meschi T, Guerra A, Allegri F, Maggiore U, et al. Comparison of two diets for the prevention of recurrent stones in idiopathic hypercalciuria. N Engl J Med 2002;346:77-84.
43. Borland WW, Fergusson JC, Dryburgh FJ. A fast automated method for measuring serum and urine citrate. Ann Clin Biochem 1989;26: 286-8.
44. Boute N, Gribouval O, Roselli S, Benessy F, Lee H, Fuchshuber A, et al. NPHS2, encoding the glomerular protein podocin, is mutated in autosomal recessive steroid-resistant nephrotic syndrome. Nat Genet 2000;24:349-54.
45. Brantsma AH, Bakker SJ, de Zeeuw D, de Jong PE, Gansevoort RT. Extended prognostic value of urinary albumin excretion for cardiovascular events. J Am Soc Nephrol 2008;19:1785-91.
46. Brenner BM, Cooper ME, de Zeeuw D, Keane WF, Mitch WE, Parving HH, et al. Effects of losartan on renal and cardiovascular outcomes in patients with type 2 diabetes and nephropathy. N Engl J Med 2001;345:861-9.
47. Brenner BM, Meyer TW, Hostetter TH. Dietary protein intake and the progressive nature of kidney disease: the role of hemodynamically mediated glomerular injury in the pathogenesis of progressive glomerular sclerosis in aging, renal ablation, and intrinsic renal disease. N Engl J Med 1982;307:652-9.
48. Breyer JA, Bain RP, Evans JK, Nahman NS Jr, Lewis EJ, Cooper M, et al. Predictors of the progression of renal insufficiency in patients with insulin dependent diabetes and overt diabetic nephropathy. The Collaborative Study Group. Kidney Int 1996;50:1651-8.
49. Briganti EM, Russ GR, McNeil JJ, Atkins RC, Chadban SJ. Risk of renal allograft loss from recurrent glomerulonephritis. N Engl J Med 2002;347:103-9.
50. Brown EM, Gamba G, Riccardi D, Lombardi M, Butters R, Kifor O, et al. Cloning and characterization of an extracellular Ca(2+)-sensing receptor from bovine parathyroid. Nature 1993;366:575-80.
51. Brunskill NJ. Albumin handling by proximal tubular cells: mechanisms and mediators. Nephrol Dial Transplant 2000;15(suppl 6):39-40.
52. Bruzzi I, Benigni A, Remuzzi G. Role of increased glomerular protein traffic in the progression of renal failure. Kidney Int Suppl 1997;62:S29-31.
53. Bunnapradist S, Cho YW, Cecka JM, Wilkinson A, Danovitch GM. Kidney allograft and patient survival in type I diabetic recipients of cadaveric kidney alone versus simultaneous pancreas kidney transplants: a multivariate analysis of the UNOS database. J Am Soc Nephrol 2003;14:208-13.
54. Burton C, Harris KP. The role of proteinuria in the progression of chronic renal failure. Am J Kidney Dis 1996;27:765-75.
55. Bushinsky DA. Recurrent hypercalciuric nephrolithiasis—does diet help? N Engl J Med 2002;346:124-5.
56. Cai Q, Hodgson SF, Kao PC, Lennon VA, Klee GG, Zinsmiester AR, et al. Brief report: inhibition of renal phosphate transport by a tumor product in a patient with oncogenic osteomalacia. N Engl J Med 1994;330:1645-9.
57. Calne RY, White DJ, Thiru S, Evans DB, McMaster P, Dunn DC, et al. Cyclosporin A in patients receiving renal allografts from cadaver donors. Lancet 1978;2:1323-7.
58. Caps MT, Perissinotto C, Zierler RE, Polissar NL, Bergelin RO, Tullis MJ, et al. Prospective study of atherosclerotic disease progression in the renal artery. Circulation 1998;98:2866-72.
59. Caramori ML, Fioretto P, Mauer M. The need for early predictors of diabetic nephropathy risk: is albumin excretion rate sufficient? Diabetes 2000;49:1399-408.
60. Caring for Australasians with renal impairment (CARI). Available at: www.cari.org.au/ accessed July 14, 2011
61. Carter JL, O'Riordan SE, Eaglestone GL, Delaney MP, Lamb EJ. Chronic kidney disease prevalence in a UK residential care home population. Nephrol Dial Transplant 2008;23:1257-64.
62. Casadevall N, Nataf J, Viron B, Kolta A, Kiladjian JJ, Martin-Dupont P, et al. Pure red-cell aplasia and antierythropoietin antibodies in patients treated with recombinant erythropoietin. N Engl J Med 2002;346:469-75.

63. Caudarella R, Rizzoli E, Buffa A, Bottura A, Stefoni S. Comparative study of the influence of 3 types of mineral water in patients with idiopathic calcium lithiasis. J Urol 1998;159:658-63.
64. Chapman AB. Approaches to testing new treatments in autosomal dominant polycystic kidney disease: insights from the CRISP and HALT-PKD studies. Clin J Am Soc Nephrol 2008;3:1197-204.
65. Chavers BM, Bilous RW, Ellis EN, Steffes MW, Mauer SM. Glomerular lesions and urinary albumin excretion in type I diabetes without overt proteinuria. N Engl J Med 1989;320:966-70.
66. Chen JH, Pu YS, Liu SP, Chiu TY. Renal hemodynamics in patients with obstructive uropathy evaluated by duplex Doppler sonography. J Urol 1993;150:18-21.
67. Chen S, Iglesias-de la Cruz MC, Jim B, Hong SW, Isono M, Ziyadeh FN. Reversibility of established diabetic glomerulopathy by anti-TGF-beta antibodies in db/db mice. Biochem Biophys Res Commun 2003; 300:16-22.
68. Chertow GM, Burke SK, Raggi P. Sevelamer attenuates the progression of coronary and aortic calcification in hemodialysis patients. Kidney Int 2002;62:245-52.
69. Chertow GM, Soroko SH, Paganini EP, Cho KC, Himmelfarb J, Ikizler TA, et al. Mortality after acute renal failure: models for prognostic stratification and risk adjustment. Kidney Int 2006;70:1120-6.
70. Cheung AK, Levin NW, Greene T, Agodoa L, Bailey J, Beck G, et al. Effects of high-flux hemodialysis on clinical outcomes: results of the HEMO study. J Am Soc Nephrol 2003;14:3251-63.
71. Cheung AK, Rocco MV, Yan G, Leypoldt JK, Levin NW, Greene T, et al. Serum beta-2 microglobulin levels predict mortality in dialysis patients: results of the HEMO study. J Am Soc Nephrol 2006;17: 546-55.
72. Chevalier RL. The moth and the aspen tree: sodium in early postnatal development. Kidney Int 2001;59:1617-25.
73. Chobanian AV, Bakris GL, Black HR, Cushman WC, Green LA, Izzo JL Jr, et al. Seventh report of the Joint National Committee on Prevention, Detection, Evaluation, and Treatment of High Blood Pressure. Hypertension 2003;42:1206-52.
74. Churchill DN, Taylor DW, Keshaviah PR. Adequacy of dialysis and nutrition in continuous peritoneal dialysis: association with clinical outcomes. Canada-USA (CANUSA) Peritoneal Dialysis Study Group. J Am Soc Nephrol 1996;7:198-207.
75. Clark WF, Stewart AK, Rock GA, Sternbach M, Sutton DM, Barrett BJ, et al. Plasma exchange when myeloma presents as acute renal failure: a randomized, controlled trial. Ann Intern Med 2005;143: 777-84.
76. Coca SG, Krumholz HM, Garg AX, Parikh CR. Underrepresentation of renal disease in randomized controlled trials of cardiovascular disease. JAMA 2006;296:1377-84.
77. Coca SG, Yalavarthy R, Concato J, Parikh CR. Biomarkers for the diagnosis and risk stratification of acute kidney injury: a systematic review. Kidney Int 2008;73:1008-16.
78. Coen G, Ballanti P, Bonucci E, Calabria S, Centorrino M, Fassino V, et al. Bone markers in the diagnosis of low turnover osteodystrophy in haemodialysis patients. Nephrol Dial Transplant 1998;13:2294-302.
79. Healthy People 2010. U.S. Renal Data System, USRDS 2010 Annual Data Report: Atlas of Chronic Kidney Disease and End-Stage Renal Disease in the United States, National Institutes of Health, National Institute of Diabetes and Digestive and Kidney Diseases, Bethesda, MD, 2010/accessed 2011-06-28.
80. Collins AJ, Kasiske B, Herzog C, Chavers B, Foley R, Gilbertson D, et al. Excerpts from the United States Renal Data System, 2004 annual data report: atlas of end-stage renal disease in the United States. Am J Kidney Dis 2005;45:A5-7, S1-280.
81. Collins AJ, Li S, St Peter W, Ebben J, Roberts T, Ma JZ, et al. Death, hospitalization, and economic associations among incident hemodialysis patients with hematocrit values of 36 to 39%. J Am Soc Nephrol 2001;12:2465-73.
82. Connor A, Tomson C. Should statins be prescribed for primary prevention of cardiovascular disease in patients with chronic kidney disease? BMJ 2009;339:b2949.
83. Coresh J, Astor BC, Greene T, Eknoyan G, Levey AS. Prevalence of chronic kidney disease and decreased kidney function in the adult US population: Third National Health and Nutrition Examination Survey. Am J Kidney Dis 2003;41:1-12.
84. Coresh J, Selvin E, Stevens LA, Manzi J, Kusek JW, Eggers P, et al. Prevalence of chronic kidney disease in the United States. JAMA 2007;298:2038-47.
85. Coresh J, Wei GL, McQuillan G, Brancati FL, Levey AS, Jones C, et al. Prevalence of high blood pressure and elevated serum creatinine level in the United States: findings from the third National Health and Nutrition Examination Survey (1988-1994). Arch Intern Med 2001; 161:1207-16.
86. Cowley BD Jr. Introduction: new insights, treatments, and management strategies for ADPKD. Clin J Am Soc Nephrol 2008; 3:1195-6.
87. Cowper SE, Robin HS, Steinberg SM, Su LD, Gupta S, LeBoit PE. Scleromyxoedema-like cutaneous diseases in renal-dialysis patients. Lancet 2000;356:1000-1.
88. Culleton BF, Larson MG, Parfrey PS, Kannel WB, Levy D. Proteinuria as a risk factor for cardiovascular disease and mortality in older people: a prospective study. Am J Med 2000;109:1-8.
89. Cunningham J, Danese M, Olson K, Klassen P, Chertow GM. Effects of the calcimimetic cinacalcet HCl on cardiovascular disease, fracture, and health-related quality of life in secondary hyperparathyroidism. Kidney Int 2005;68:1793-800.
90. Curhan GC, Willett WC, Rimm EB, Stampfer MJ. A prospective study of dietary calcium and other nutrients and the risk of symptomatic kidney stones. N Engl J Med 1993;328:833-8.
91. D'Amico G, Bazzi C. Pathophysiology of proteinuria. Kidney Int 2003;63:809-25.
92. Davies DF, Shock NW. Age changes in glomerular filtration rate, effective renal plasma flow, and tubular excretory capacity in adult males. J Clin Invest 1950;29:496-507.
93. Davies DJ, Moran JE, Niall JF, Ryan GB. Segmental necrotising glomerulonephritis with antineutrophil antibody: possible arbovirus aetiology? Br Med J (Clin Res Ed) 1982;285:606.
94. de Brito-Ashurst I, Varagunam M, Raftery MJ, Yaqoob MM. Bicarbonate supplementation slows progression of CKD and improves nutritional status. J Am Soc Nephrol 2009;20:2075-84.
95. de Jong PE, Hillege HL, Pinto-Sietsma SJ, de Zeeuw D. Screening for microalbuminuria in the general population: a tool to detect subjects at risk for progressive renal failure in an early phase? Nephrol Dial Transplant 2003;18:10-3.
96. de Swart PM, Sokole EB, Wilmink JM. The interrelationship of calcium and magnesium absorption in idiopathic hypercalciuria and renal calcium stone disease. J Urol 1998;159:669-72.
97. Deen PM, van Aubel RA, van Lieburg AF, van Os CH. Urinary content of aquaporin 1 and 2 in nephrogenic diabetes insipidus. J Am Soc Nephrol 1996;7:836-41.
98. Defronzo RA, Humphrey RL, Wright JR, Cooke CR. Acute renal failure in multiple myeloma. Medicine (Baltimore) 1975;54:209-23.
99. Department of Health. National Service Framework for Renal Services. Part 1: dialysis and transplantation, 2004. www.dh.gov.uk/PolicyAndGuidance/HealthAndSocialCareTopics/Renal/fs/en/ accessed July 14, 2011.
100. Diabetes Control and Complications Trial Research Group. The effect of intensive treatment of diabetes on the development and progression of long-term complications in insulin-dependent diabetes mellitus. N Engl J Med 1993;329:977-86.
101. DiBona GF. Prostaglandins and nonsteroidal anti-inflammatory drugs: effects on renal hemodynamics. Am J Med 1986;80:12-21.
102. Dominiczak AF, Bohr DF. Nitric oxide and hypertension in 1995. Curr Opin Nephrol Hypertens 1996;5:174-80.
103. Drueke TB, Locatelli F, Clyne N, Eckardt KU, Macdougall IC, Tsakiris D, et al. Normalization of hemoglobin level in patients with chronic kidney disease and anemia. N Engl J Med 2006;355:2071-84.
104. Eardley KS, Zehnder D, Quinkler M, Lepenies J, Bates RL, Savage CO, et al. The relationship between albuminuria, MCP-1/CCL2, and

interstitial macrophages in chronic kidney disease. Kidney Int 2006;69:1189-97.
105. Eddy AA, Giachelli CM. Renal expression of genes that promote interstitial inflammation and fibrosis in rats with protein-overload proteinuria. Kidney Int 1995;47:1546-57.
106. Ekberg H, Grinyo J, Nashan B, Vanrenterghem Y, Vincenti F, Voulgari A, et al. Cyclosporine sparing with mycophenolate mofetil, daclizumab and corticosteroids in renal allograft recipients: the CAESAR Study. Am J Transplant 2007;7:560-70.
107. Eknoyan G, Beck GJ, Cheung AK, Daugirdas JT, Greene T, Kusek JW, et al. Effect of dialysis dose and membrane flux in maintenance hemodialysis. N Engl J Med 2002;347:2010-9.
108. Eknoyan G, Levin A, Levin NW. K/DOQI clinical practice guidelines for bone metabolism and disease in chronic kidney disease. Am J Kidney Dis 2003;42(suppl 3):1-201.
109. El-Achkar TM, Ohmit SE, McCullough PA, Crook ED, Brown WW, Grimm R, et al. Higher prevalence of anemia with diabetes mellitus in moderate kidney insufficiency: the Kidney Early Evaluation Program. Kidney Int 2005;67:1483-8.
110. Epstein M. Aging and the kidney. J Am Soc Nephrol 1996;7:1106-22.
111. European Renal Association. Section II. Haemodialysis adequacy. Nephrol Dial Transplant 2002;17(suppl 7):16-31.
112. European Renal Association. European best practice guidelines for the management of anaemia in patients with chronic renal failure. Working Party for European Best Practice Guidelines for the Management of Anaemia in Patients with Chronic Renal Failure. Nephrol Dial Transplant 1999;14(suppl 5):1-50.
113. Falk RJ, Jennette JC. Anti-neutrophil cytoplasmic autoantibodies with specificity for myeloperoxidase in patients with systemic vasculitis and idiopathic necrotizing and crescentic glomerulonephritis. N Engl J Med 1988;318:1651-7.
114. Farrell SC, Bailey MP. Measurement of creatinine in peritoneal dialysis fluid. Ann Clin Biochem 1991;28:624-5.
115. Feehally J. Ethnicity and renal disease. Kidney Int 2005;68:414-24.
116. Feest TG, Mistry CD, Grimes DS, Mallick NP. Incidence of advanced chronic renal failure and the need for end stage renal replacement treatment. BMJ 1990;301:897-900.
117. Fellstrom BC, Jardine AG, Schmieder RE, Holdaas H, Bannister K, Beutler J, et al. Rosuvastatin and cardiovascular events in patients undergoing hemodialysis. N Engl J Med 2009;360:1395-407.
118. Feucht HE, Schneeberger H, Hillebrand G, Burkhardt K, Weiss M, Riethmuller G, et al. Capillary deposition of C4d complement fragment and early renal graft loss. Kidney Int 1993;43:1333-8.
119. Field MJ, Stanton BA, Giebisch GH. Influence of ADH on renal potassium handling: a micropuncture and microperfusion study. Kidney Int 1984;25:502-11.
120. Fioretto P, Steffes MW, Mauer M. Glomerular structure in nonproteinuric IDDM patients with various levels of albuminuria. Diabetes 1994;43:1358-64.
120A. FistulaFirst.org. http://www.fistulafirst.org/, accessed June 30, 2011
121. Flechner SM, Goldfarb D, Modlin C, Feng J, Krishnamurthi V, Mastroianni B, et al. Kidney transplantation without calcineurin inhibitor drugs: a prospective, randomized trial of sirolimus versus cyclosporine. Transplantation 2002;74:1070-6.
122. Fliser D, Franek E, Joest M, Block S, Mutschler E, Ritz E. Renal function in the elderly: impact of hypertension and cardiac function. Kidney Int 1997;51:1196-204.
123. Fliser D, Franek E, Ritz E. Renal function in the elderly—is the dogma of an inexorable decline of renal function correct? Nephrol Dial Transplant 1997;12:1553-5.
124. Fliser D, Zeier M, Nowack R, Ritz E. Renal functional reserve in healthy elderly subjects. J Am Soc Nephrol 1993;3:1371-7.
125. Foley RN, Culleton BF, Parfrey PS, Harnett JD, Kent GM, Murray DC, et al. Cardiac disease in diabetic end-stage renal disease. Diabetologia 1997;40:1307-12.
126. Foley RN, Parfrey PS. Cardiovascular disease and mortality in ESRD. J Nephrol 1998;11:239-45.
127. Foley RN, Parfrey PS, Harnett JD, Kent GM, Martin CJ, Murray DC, et al. Clinical and echocardiographic disease in patients starting end-stage renal disease therapy. Kidney Int 1995;47:186-92.
128. Foley RN, Parfrey PS, Harnett JD, Kent GM, Murray DC, Barre PE. Hypoalbuminemia, cardiac morbidity, and mortality in end-stage renal disease. J Am Soc Nephrol 1996;7:728-36.
129. Foley RN, Parfrey PS, Harnett JD, Kent GM, Murray DC, Barre PE. The impact of anemia on cardiomyopathy, morbidity, and and mortality in end-stage renal disease. Am J Kidney Dis 1996;28:53-61.
130. Foley RN, Parfrey PS, Sarnak MJ. Epidemiology of cardiovascular disease in chronic renal disease. J Am Soc Nephrol 1998;9:S16-23.
131. Forsblom CM, Groop PH, Ekstrand A, Groop LC. Predictive value of microalbuminuria in patients with insulin-dependent diabetes of long duration. BMJ 1992;305:1051-3.
132. Fox KM. Efficacy of perindopril in reduction of cardiovascular events among patients with stable coronary artery disease: randomised, double-blind, placebo-controlled, multicentre trial (the EUROPA study). Lancet 2003;362:782-8.
133. Francois H, Durrbach A, Amor M, Djeffal R, Kriaa F, Paradis V, et al. The long-term effect of switching from cyclosporin A to mycophenolate mofetil in chronic renal graft dysfunction compared with conventional management. Nephrol Dial Transplant 2003;18:1909-16.
134. Freedman BI, Iskandar SS, Appel RG. The link between hypertension and nephrosclerosis. Am J Kidney Dis 1995;25:207-21.
135. Freedman BI, Spray BJ, Tuttle AB, Buckalew VM Jr. The familial risk of end-stage renal disease in African Americans. Am J Kidney Dis 1993;21:387-93.
136. Fujisawa M, Haramaki R, Miyazaki H, Imaizumi T, Okuda S. Role of lipoprotein (a) and TGF-beta 1 in atherosclerosis of hemodialysis patients. J Am Soc Nephrol 2000;11:1889-95.
137. Gabow PA. Autosomal dominant polycystic kidney disease—more than a renal disease. Am J Kidney Dis 1990;16:403-13.
138. Gaede P, Lund-Andersen H, Parving HH, Pedersen O. Effect of a multifactorial intervention on mortality in type 2 diabetes. N Engl J Med 2008;358:580-91.
139. Gaede P, Vedel P, Larsen N, Jensen GV, Parving HH, Pedersen O. Multifactorial intervention and cardiovascular disease in patients with type 2 diabetes. N Engl J Med 2003;348:383-93.
140. Gaede P, Vedel P, Parving HH, Pedersen O. Intensified multifactorial intervention in patients with type 2 diabetes mellitus and microalbuminuria: the Steno type 2 randomised study. Lancet 1999;353:617-22.
141. Galpin JE, Shinaberger JH, Stanley TM, Blumenkrantz MJ, Bayer AS, Friedman GS, et al. Acute interstitial nephritis due to methicillin. Am J Med 1978;65:756-65.
142. Gambaro G, Favaro S, D'Angelo A. Risk for renal failure in nephrolithiasis. Am J Kidney Dis 2001;37:233-43.
143. Garg AX, Blake PG, Clark WF, Clase CM, Haynes RB, Moist LM. Association between renal insufficiency and malnutrition in older adults: results from the NHANES III. Kidney Int 2001;60:1867-74.
144. Gellai M, Jugus M, Fletcher T, Nambi P, Ohlstein EH, Elliott JD, et al. Nonpeptide endothelin receptor antagonists: V. Prevention and reversal of acute renal failure in the rat by SB 209670. J Pharmacol Exp Ther 1995;275:200-6.
145. Giovannetti S, Maggiore Q. A low-nitrogen diet with proteins of high biological value for severe chronic uraemia. Lancet 1964;1:1000-3.
146. GISEN. Randomised placebo-controlled trial of effect of ramipril on decline in glomerular filtration rate and risk of terminal renal failure in proteinuric, non-diabetic nephropathy. The GISEN Group (Gruppo Italiano di Studi Epidemiologici in Nefrologia). Lancet 1997;349:1857-63.
147. Giugliani R, Ferrari I, Greene LJ. Heterozygous cystinuria and urinary lithiasis. Am J Med Genet 1985;22:703-15.
148. Gjertson DW, Cecka JM, Terasaki PI. The relative effects of FK506 and cyclosporine on short- and long-term kidney graft survival. Transplantation 1995;60:1384-8.

149. Go AS, Chertow GM, Fan D, McCulloch CE, Hsu CY. Chronic kidney disease and the risks of death, cardiovascular events, and hospitalization. N Engl J Med 2004;351:1296-305.
150. Goldsmith DJ, Covic A, Sambrook PA, Ackrill P. Vascular calcification in long-term haemodialysis patients in a single unit: a retrospective analysis. Nephron 1997;77:37-43.
151. Goodman WG, Goldin J, Kuizon BD, Yoon C, Gales B, Sider D, et al. Coronary-artery calcification in young adults with end-stage renal disease who are undergoing dialysis. N Engl J Med 2000;342:1478-83.
152. Grantham JJ. Clinical practice: autosomal dominant polycystic kidney disease. N Engl J Med 2008;359:1477-85.
153. Greger R. Why do loop diuretics cause hypokalaemia? Nephrol Dial Transplant 1997;12:1799-801.
154. Greger R. New insights into the molecular mechanism of the action of diuretics. Nephrol Dial Transplant 1999;14:536-40.
155. Gregory WM, Richards MA, Malpas JS. Combination chemotherapy versus melphalan and prednisolone in the treatment of multiple myeloma: an overview of published trials. J Clin Oncol 1992;10:334-42.
156. Gross CR, Limwattananon C, Matthees B, Zehrer JL, Savik K. Impact of transplantation on quality of life in patients with diabetes and renal dysfunction. Transplantation 2000;70:1736-46.
157. Groth CG, Backman L, Morales JM, Calne R, Kreis H, Lang P, et al. Sirolimus (rapamycin)-based therapy in human renal transplantation: similar efficacy and different toxicity compared with cyclosporine. Sirolimus European Renal Transplant Study Group. Transplantation 1999;67:1036-42.
158. Guerin AP, London GM, Marchais SJ, Metivier F. Arterial stiffening and vascular calcifications in end-stage renal disease. Nephrol Dial Transplant 2000;15:1014-21.
159. Gurwitz JH, Avorn J, Ross-Degnan D, Lipsitz LA. Nonsteroidal anti-inflammatory drug-associated azotemia in the very old. JAMA 1990;264:471-5.
160. Guyton AC. Blood pressure control—special role of the kidneys and body fluids. Science 1991;252:1813-6.
161. Haas M, Meehan SM, Karrison TG, Spargo BH. Changing etiologies of unexplained adult nephrotic syndrome: a comparison of renal biopsy findings from 1976-1979 and 1995-1997. Am J Kidney Dis 1997;30:621-31.
162. Hackbarth H, Alt JM, Gartner K, Sindermann H. Renal handling of albumin: clearance studies with bovine and rat serum albumin in conscious rats. Contrib Nephrol 1980;19:225-30.
163. Hallan SI, Ritz E, Lydersen S, Romundstad S, Kvenild K, Orth SR. Combining GFR and albuminuria to classify CKD improves prediction of ESRD. J Am Soc Nephrol 2009;20:1069-77.
164. Halloran PF, Helms LM, Kung L, Noujaim J. The temporal profile of calcineurin inhibition by cyclosporine in vivo. Transplantation 1999;68:1356-61.
165. Hallson PC, Rose GA, Sulaiman S. Magnesium reduces calcium oxalate crystal formation in human whole urine. Clin Sci (Lond) 1982;62:17-9.
166. Hamm LL. Renal handling of citrate. Kidney Int 1990;38:728-35.
167. Han JH, Choi SJ, Kurihara N, Koide M, Oba Y, Roodman GD. Macrophage inflammatory protein-1alpha is an osteoclastogenic factor in myeloma that is independent of receptor activator of nuclear factor kappaB ligand. Blood 2001;97:3349-53.
168. Hansen KJ, O'Neil EA, Reavis SW, Craven TE, Plonk GW Jr, Dean RH. Intraoperative duplex sonography during renal artery reconstruction. J Vasc Surg 1991;14:364-74.
169. Hansson L, Zanchetti A, Carruthers SG, Dahlof B, Elmfeldt D, Julius S, et al. Effects of intensive blood-pressure lowering and low-dose aspirin in patients with hypertension: principal results of the Hypertension Optimal Treatment (HOT) randomised trial. HOT Study Group. Lancet 1998;351:1755-62.
170. Haraldsson B, Nystrom J, Deen WM. Properties of the glomerular barrier and mechanisms of proteinuria. Physiol Rev 2008;88:451-87.
171. Harris AB. Letter: vitamin-C-induced hyperoxaluria. Lancet 1976;1:366.
172. Hateboer N, van Dijk MA, Bogdanova N, Coto E, Saggar-Malik AK, San Millan JL, et al. Comparison of phenotypes of polycystic kidney disease types 1 and 2. European PKD1-PKD2 Study Group. Lancet 1999;353:103-7.
173. Hauer HA, Bajema IM, Van Houwelingen HC, Ferrario F, Noel LH, Waldherr R, et al. Determinants of outcome in ANCA-associated glomerulonephritis: a prospective clinico-histopathological analysis of 96 patients. Kidney Int 2002;62:1732-42.
174. Hawkins PN. Serum amyloid P component scintigraphy for diagnosis and monitoring amyloidosis. Curr Opin Nephrol Hypertens 2002;11:649-55.
175. Hayashi T, Suzuki A, Shoji T, Togawa M, Okada N, Tsubakihara Y, et al. Cardiovascular effect of normalizing the hematocrit level during erythropoietin therapy in predialysis patients with chronic renal failure. Am J Kidney Dis 2000;35:250-6.
176. Heeg JE, de Jong PE, van der Hem GK, de Zeeuw D. Reduction of proteinuria by angiotensin converting enzyme inhibition. Kidney Int 1987;32:78-83.
177. Henderson MJ. Renal stone disease—investigative aspects. Arch Dis Child 1993;68:160-2.
178. Henderson MJ. Stone analysis is not useful in the routine investigation of renal stone disease. Ann Clin Biochem 1995;32:109-11.
179. Hess B, Hasler-Strub U, Ackermann D, Jaeger P. Metabolic evaluation of patients with recurrent idiopathic calcium nephrolithiasis. Nephrol Dial Transplant 1997;12:1362-8.
180. Hesse A, Gergeleit M, Schuller P, Moller K. Analysis of urinary stones by computerized infrared spectroscopy. J Clin Chem Clin Biochem 1989;27:639-42.
181. Hideshima T, Richardson P, Chauhan D, Palombella VJ, Elliott PJ, Adams J, et al. The proteasome inhibitor PS-341 inhibits growth, induces apoptosis, and overcomes drug resistance in human multiple myeloma cells. Cancer Res 2001;61:3071-6.
182. Hoffman BB, Sharma K, Zhu Y, Ziyadeh FN. Transcriptional activation of transforming growth factor-beta1 in mesangial cell culture by high glucose concentration. Kidney Int 1998;54:1107-16.
183. Holland MD, Galla JH, Sanders PW, Luke RG. Effect of urinary pH and diatrizoate on Bence Jones protein nephrotoxicity in the rat. Kidney Int 1985;27:46-50.
184. Holmes RP. Measurement of urinary oxalate and citrate by capillary electrophoresis and indirect ultraviolet absorbance. Clin Chem 1995;41:1297-301.
185. Hou FF, Xie D, Zhang X, Chen PY, Zhang WR, Liang M, et al. Renoprotection of Optimal Antiproteinuric Doses (ROAD) study: a randomized controlled study of benazepril and losartan in chronic renal insufficiency. J Am Soc Nephrol 2007;18:1889-98.
186. Hou SH, Bushinsky DA, Wish JB, Cohen JJ, Harrington JT. Hospital-acquired renal insufficiency: a prospective study. Am J Med 1983;74:243-8.
187. Houillier P, Paillard M. Calcium-sensing receptor and renal cation handling. Nephrol Dial Transplant 2003;18:2467-70.
188. Houlihan CA, Allen TJ, Baxter AL, Panangiotopoulos S, Casley DJ, Cooper ME, et al. A low-sodium diet potentiates the effects of losartan in type 2 diabetes. Diabetes Care 2002;25:663-71.
189. Hovind P, Rossing P, Tarnow L, Smidt UM, Parving HH. Progression of diabetic nephropathy. Kidney Int 2001;59:702-9.
190. Hoyer JR, Seiler MW. Pathophysiology of Tamm-Horsfall protein. Kidney Int 1979;16:279-89.
191. Huang ZQ, Sanders PW. Localization of a single binding site for immunoglobulin light chains on human Tamm-Horsfall glycoprotein. J Clin Invest 1997;99:732-6.
192. Hughes J, Ward CJ, Peral B, Aspinwall R, Clark K, San Millan JL, et al. The polycystic kidney disease 1 (PKD1) gene encodes a novel protein with multiple cell recognition domains. Nat Genet 1995;10:151-60.
193. Hume R, Weyers E. Relationship between total body water and surface area in normal and obese subjects. J Clin Pathol 1971;24:234-8.
194. Hunsicker LG, Adler S, Caggiula A, England BK, Greene T, Kusek JW, et al. Predictors of the progression of renal disease in the Modification of Diet in Renal Disease Study. Kidney Int 1997;51:1908-19.

195. Ikizler TA, Greene JH, Wingard RL, Parker RA, Hakim RM. Spontaneous dietary protein intake during progression of chronic renal failure. J Am Soc Nephrol 1995;6:1386-91.
196. Imel EA, Econs MJ. Fibroblast growth factor 23: roles in health and disease. J Am Soc Nephrol 2005;16:2565-75.
197. Irish AB, Winearls CG, Littlewood T. Presentation and survival of patients with severe renal failure and myeloma. QJM 1997;90:773-80.
198. Isono M, Mogyorosi A, Han DC, Hoffman BB, Ziyadeh FN. Stimulation of TGF-beta type II receptor by high glucose in mouse mesangial cells and in diabetic kidney. Am J Physiol Renal Physiol 2000;278:F830-8.
199. Iwano M, Plieth D, Danoff TM, Xue C, Okada H, Neilson EG. Evidence that fibroblasts derive from epithelium during tissue fibrosis. J Clin Invest 2002;110:341-50.
200. Jacobs K, Shoemaker C, Rudersdorf R, Neill SD, Kaufman RJ, Mufson A, et al. Isolation and characterization of genomic and cDNA clones of human erythropoietin. Nature 1985;313:806-10.
201. Jaeger P. Genetic versus environmental factors in renal stone disease. Curr Opin Nephrol Hypertens 1996;5:342-6.
202. Jafar TH, Stark PC, Schmid CH, Landa M, Maschio G, de Jong PE, et al. Progression of chronic kidney disease: the role of blood pressure control, proteinuria, and angiotensin-converting enzyme inhibition: a patient-level meta-analysis. Ann Intern Med 2003;139:244-52.
203. Jafar TH, Stark PC, Schmid CH, Landa M, Maschio G, Marcantoni C, et al. Proteinuria as a modifiable risk factor for the progression of non-diabetic renal disease. Kidney Int 2001;60:1131-40.
204. Jayne DR, Gaskin G, Rasmussen N, Abramowicz D, Ferrario F, Guillevin L, et al. Randomized trial of plasma exchange or high-dosage methylprednisolone as adjunctive therapy for severe renal vasculitis. J Am Soc Nephrol 2007;18:2180-8.
205. Jentsch TJ. Chloride transport in the kidney: lessons from human disease and knockout mice. J Am Soc Nephrol 2005;16:1549-61.
206. Jeong H, Kaplan B. Therapeutic monitoring of mycophenolate mofetil. Clin J Am Soc Nephrol 2007;2:184-91.
207. John R, Webb M, Young A, Stevens PE. Unreferred chronic kidney disease: a longitudinal study. Am J Kidney Dis 2004;43:825-35.
208. Johnson RW, Kreis H, Oberbauer R, Brattstrom C, Claesson K, Eris J. Sirolimus allows early cyclosporine withdrawal in renal transplantation resulting in improved renal function and lower blood pressure. Transplantation 2001;72:777-86.
209. Johnson WJ, Kyle RA, Pineda AA, O'Brien PC, Holley KE. Treatment of renal failure associated with multiple myeloma: plasmapheresis, hemodialysis, and chemotherapy. Arch Intern Med 1990;150:863-9.
210. Johnston A, David OJ, Cooney GF. Pharmacokinetic validation of neoral absorption profiling. Transplant Proc 2000;32:53S-56S.
211. Joint British Societies. JBS 2: Joint British Societies' guidelines on prevention of cardiovascular disease in clinical practice. Heart 2005;91(suppl 5):v1-52.
212. Joint National Committee. The sixth report of the Joint National Committee on Prevention, Detection, Evaluation, and Treatment of High Blood Pressure. Arch Intern Med 1997;157:2413-46.
213. Jones CA, Francis ME, Eberhardt MS, Chavers B, Coresh J, Engelgau M, et al. Microalbuminuria in the US population: Third National Health and Nutrition Examination Survey. Am J Kidney Dis 2002;39:445-59.
214. Jones CH, Newstead CG, Will EJ, Smye SW, Davison AM. Assessment of nutritional status in CAPD patients: serum albumin is not a useful measure. Nephrol Dial Transplant 1997;12:1406-13.
215. Jones MW. Topiramate—safety and tolerability. Can J Neurol Sci 1998;25:S13-5.
216. Jose PA, Fildes RD, Gomez RA, Chevalier RL, Robillard JE. Neonatal renal function and physiology. Curr Opin Pediatr 1994;6:172-7.
217. Jungers P, Chauveau P, Descamps-Latscha B, Labrunie M, Giraud E, Man NK, et al. Age and gender-related incidence of chronic renal failure in a French urban area: a prospective epidemiologic study. Nephrol Dial Transplant 1996;11:1542-6.
218. Kahan BD. Efficacy of sirolimus compared with azathioprine for reduction of acute renal allograft rejection: a randomised multicentre study. The Rapamune US Study Group. Lancet 2000;356:194-202.
219. Kahan BD, Murgia MG, Slaton J, Napoli K. Potential applications of therapeutic drug monitoring of sirolimus immunosuppression in clinical renal transplantation. Ther Drug Monit 1995;17:672-5.
220. Kanwar YS, Wada J, Sun L, Xie P, Wallner EI, Chen S, et al. Diabetic nephropathy: mechanisms of renal disease progression. Exp Biol Med (Maywood) 2008;233:4-11.
221. Kasidas GP, Samuell CT, Weir TB. Renal stone analysis: why and how? Ann Clin Biochem 2004;41:91-7.
222. Kasiske BL. Relationship between vascular disease and age-associated changes in the human kidney. Kidney Int 1987;31:1153-9.
223. Katzberg RW, Haller C. Contrast-induced nephrotoxicity: clinical landscape. Kidney Int Suppl 2006;S3-7.
224. Kaufmann RB, Sheedy PF 2nd, Maher JE, Bielak LF, Breen JF, Schwartz RS, et al. Quantity of coronary artery calcium detected by electron beam computed tomography in asymptomatic subjects and angiographically studied patients. Mayo Clin Proc 1995;70:223-32.
225. Keane WF, Eknoyan G. Proteinuria, albuminuria, risk assessment, detection, elimination (PARADE): a position paper of the National Kidney Foundation. Am J Kidney Dis 1999;33:1004-10.
226. Kellum JA, Bellomo R, Ronco C, Mehta R, Clark W, Levin NW. The 3rd International Consensus Conference of the Acute Dialysis Quality Initiative (ADQI). Int J Artif Organs 2005;28:441-4.
227. Kershner RP, Fitzsimmons WE. Relationship of FK506 whole blood concentrations and efficacy and toxicity after liver and kidney transplantation. Transplantation 1996;62:920-6.
228. Kestila M, Lenkkeri U, Mannikko M, Lamerdin J, McCready P, Putaala H, et al. Positionally cloned gene for a novel glomerular protein—nephrin—is mutated in congenital nephrotic syndrome. Mol Cell 1998;1:575-82.
229. Ketteler M, Bongartz P, Westenfeld R, Wildberger JE, Mahnken AH, Bohm R, et al. Association of low fetuin-A (AHSG) concentrations in serum with cardiovascular mortality in patients on dialysis: a cross-sectional study. Lancet 2003;361:827-33.
230. Khan IH, Catto GR, Edward N, Macleod AM. Acute renal failure: factors influencing nephrology referral and outcome. QJM 1997;90: 781-5.
231. Kiberd BA, Clase CM. Cumulative risk for developing end-stage renal disease in the US population. J Am Soc Nephrol 2002;13:1635-44.
232. Kidney Disease Improving Global Outcomes (KDIGO). KDIGO clinical practice guideline for the diagnosis, evaluation, prevention, and treatment of chronic kidney disease–mineral and bone disorder (CKD-MBD). Kidney Int Suppl 2009;S1-130.
233. Kimberling WJ, Kumar S, Gabow PA, Kenyon JB, Connolly CJ, Somlo S. Autosomal dominant polycystic kidney disease: localization of the second gene to chromosome 4q13-q23. Genomics 1993;18:467-72.
234. Klahr S, Levey AS, Beck GJ, Caggiula AW, Hunsicker L, Kusek JW, et al. The effects of dietary protein restriction and blood-pressure control on the progression of chronic renal disease. Modification of Diet in Renal Disease Study Group. N Engl J Med 1994;330:877-84.
235. Klein R, Klein BE, Moss SE, Cruickshanks KJ, Brazy PC. The 10-year incidence of renal insufficiency in people with type 1 diabetes. Diabetes Care 1999;22:743-51.
236. Kohan AD, Armenakas NA, Fracchia JA. Indinavir urolithiasis: an emerging cause of renal colic in patients with human immunodeficiency virus. J Urol 1999;161:1765-8.
237. Koss MN, Pirani CL, Osserman EF. Experimental Bence Jones cast nephropathy. Lab Invest 1976;34:579-91.
238. Kovesdy CP, Kalantar-Zadeh K. Vitamin D receptor activation and survival in chronic kidney disease. Kidney Int 2008;73:1355-63.
239. Kramer BK, Bergler T, Stoelcker B, Waldegger S. Mechanisms of disease: the kidney-specific chloride channels ClCKA and ClCKB, the Barttin subunit, and their clinical relevance. Nat Clin Pract Nephrol 2008;4:38-46.
240. Kunau RT Jr, Webb HL, Borman SC. Characteristics of the relationship between the flow rate of tubular fluid and potassium transport in the distal tubule of the rat. J Clin Invest 1974;54:1488-95.
241. Kunzmann V, Bauer E, Feurle J, Weissinger F, Tony HP, Wilhelm M. Stimulation of gammadelta T cells by aminobisphosphonates and

induction of antiplasma cell activity in multiple myeloma. Blood 2000;96:384-92.

242. Kyle RA. Multiple myeloma: review of 869 cases. Mayo Clin Proc 1975;50:29-40.

243. Kyle RA, Gertz MA, Greipp PR, Witzig TE, Lust JA, Lacy MQ, et al. A trial of three regimens for primary amyloidosis: colchicine alone, melphalan and prednisone, and melphalan, prednisone, and colchicine. N Engl J Med 1997;336:1202-7.

244. Kyle RA, Greipp PR. Primary systemic amyloidosis: comparison of melphalan and prednisone versus placebo. Blood 1978;52:818-27.

245. Lachmann HJ, Gallimore R, Gillmore JD, Carr-Smith HD, Bradwell AR, Pepys MB, et al. Outcome in systemic AL amyloidosis in relation to changes in concentration of circulating free immunoglobulin light chains following chemotherapy. Br J Haematol 2003;122:78-84.

246. Laker MF, Hofmann AF, Meeuse BJ. Spectrophotometric determination of urinary oxalate with oxalate oxidase prepared from moss. Clin Chem 1980;26:827-30.

247. Lamb EJ, Stevens PE, Nashef L. Topiramate increases biochemical risk of nephrolithiasis. Ann Clin Biochem 2004;41:166-9.

248. Lameire N, Vanholder R. Pathophysiologic features and prevention of human and experimental acute tubular necrosis. J Am Soc Nephrol 2001;12(suppl 17):S20-32.

249. Lameire NH, Vanholder R, Veyt D, Lambert MC, Ringoir S. A longitudinal, five year survey of urea kinetic parameters in CAPD patients. Kidney Int 1992;42:426-32.

250. Larpent L, Verger C. The need for using an enzymatic colorimetric assay in creatinine determination of peritoneal dialysis solutions. Perit Dial Int 1990;10:89-92.

251. Larsson L, Libert B, Asperud M. Determination of urinary oxalate by reversed-phase ion-pair "high-performance" liquid chromatography. Clin Chem 1982;28:2272-4.

252. Ledebo I. On-line hemodiafiltration: technique and therapy. Adv Ren Replace Ther 1999;6:195-208.

253. Lefaucheur C, Stengel B, Nochy D, Martel P, Hill GS, Jacquot C, et al. Membranous nephropathy and cancer: epidemiologic evidence and determinants of high-risk cancer association. Kidney Int 2006;70: 1510-7.

254. Leuenroth SJ, Crews CM. Targeting cyst initiation in ADPKD. J Am Soc Nephrol 2009;20:1-3.

255. Levey AS, Atkins R, Coresh J, Cohen EP, Collins AJ, Eckardt KU, et al. Chronic kidney disease as a global public health problem: approaches and initiatives—a position statement from Kidney Disease Improving Global Outcomes. Kidney Int 2007;72:247-59.

256. Levey AS, Beto JA, Coronado BE, Eknoyan G, Foley RN, Kasiske BL, et al. Controlling the epidemic of cardiovascular disease in chronic renal disease: what do we know? What do we need to learn? Where do we go from here? National Kidney Foundation Task Force on Cardiovascular Disease. Am J Kidney Dis 1998;32:853-906.

257. Levin A, Bakris GL, Molitch M, Smulders M, Tian J, Williams LA, et al. Prevalence of abnormal serum vitamin D, PTH, calcium, and phosphorus in patients with chronic kidney disease: results of the study to evaluate early kidney disease. Kidney Int 2007;71:31-8.

258. Levin A, Singer J, Thompson CR, Ross H, Lewis M. Prevalent left ventricular hypertrophy in the predialysis population: identifying opportunities for intervention. Am J Kidney Dis 1996;27:347-54.

259. Levin A, Thompson CR, Ethier J, Carlisle EJ, Tobe S, Mendelssohn D, et al. Left ventricular mass index increase in early renal disease: impact of decline in hemoglobin. Am J Kidney Dis 1999;34:125-34.

260. Lewis EJ, Hunsicker LG, Clarke WR, Berl T, Pohl MA, Lewis JB, et al. Renoprotective effect of the angiotensin-receptor antagonist irbesartan in patients with nephropathy due to type 2 diabetes. N Engl J Med 2001;345:851-60.

261. Ligtenberg G, Blankestijn PJ, Oey PL, Klein IH, Dijkhorst-Oei LT, Boomsma F, et al. Reduction of sympathetic hyperactivity by enalapril in patients with chronic renal failure. N Engl J Med 1999;340:1321-8.

262. Lin JL, Lin-Tan DT, Hsu KH, Yu CC. Environmental lead exposure and progression of chronic renal diseases in patients without diabetes. N Engl J Med 2003;348:277-86.

263. Lindberg JS, Moe SM, Goodman WG, Coburn JW, Sprague SM, Liu W, et al. The calcimimetic AMG 073 reduces parathyroid hormone and calcium × phosphorus in secondary hyperparathyroidism. Kidney Int 2003;63:248-54.

264. Lindeman RD. Is the decline in renal function with normal aging inevitable? Geriatr Nephrol Urol 1998;8:7-9.

265. Lindeman RD, Tobin J, Shock NW. Longitudinal studies on the rate of decline in renal function with age. J Am Geriatr Soc 1985;33:278-85.

266. Lindeman RD, Tobin JD, Shock NW. Association between blood pressure and the rate of decline in renal function with age. Kidney Int 1984;26:861-8.

267. Liu Y. Renal fibrosis: new insights into the pathogenesis and therapeutics. Kidney Int 2006;69:213-7.

268. Ljunghall S, Danielson BG. A prospective study of renal stone recurrences. Br J Urol 1984;56:122-4.

269. Locatelli F, Conte F, Marcelli D. The impact of haematocrit levels and erythropoietin treatment on overall and cardiovascular mortality and morbidity—the experience of the Lombardy Dialysis Registry. Nephrol Dial Transplant 1998;13:1642-4.

270. Locatelli F, Marcelli D, Conte F, Limido A, Malberti F, Spotti D. Comparison of mortality in ESRD patients on convective and diffusive extracorporeal treatments. The Registro Lombardo Dialisi E Trapianto. Kidney Int 1999;55:286-93.

271. Locatelli F, Martin-Malo A, Hannedouche T, Loureiro A, Papadimitriou M, Wizemann V, et al. Effect of membrane permeability on survival of hemodialysis patients. J Am Soc Nephrol 2009;20:645-54.

272. London GM, Marty C, Marchais SJ, Guerin AP, Metivier F, de Vernejoul MC. Arterial calcifications and bone histomorphometry in end-stage renal disease. J Am Soc Nephrol 2004;15:1943-51.

273. Lowrie EG, Laird NM, Parker TF, Sargent JA. Effect of the hemodialysis prescription of patient morbidity: report from the National Cooperative Dialysis Study. N Engl J Med 1981;305:1176-81.

274. Ma JZ, Ebben J, Xia H, Collins AJ. Hematocrit level and associated mortality in hemodialysis patients. J Am Soc Nephrol 1999;10:610-9.

275. Maack T, Johnson V, Kau ST, Figueiredo J, Sigulem D. Renal filtration, transport, and metabolism of low-molecular-weight proteins: a review. Kidney Int 1979;16:251-70.

276. Macconi D, Ghilardi M, Bonassi ME, Mohamed EI, Abbate M, Colombi F, et al. Effect of angiotensin-converting enzyme inhibition on glomerular basement membrane permeability and distribution of zonula occludens-1 in MWF rats. J Am Soc Nephrol 2000;11:477-89.

277. MacLennan IC, Chapman C, Dunn J, Kelly K. Combined chemotherapy with ABCM versus melphalan for treatment of myelomatosis. The Medical Research Council Working Party for Leukaemia in Adults. Lancet 1992;339:200-5.

278. Magee C, Clarkson M, Rennke H. A case of desensitization, transplantation, and allograft dysfunction. Clin J Am Soc Nephrol 2008;3:1573-81.

279. Magee CC, Felgueiras J, Tinckam K, Malek S, Mah H, Tullius S. Renal transplantation in patients with positive lymphocytotoxicity crossmatches: one center's experience. Transplantation 2008;86: 96-103.

280. Maggi E, Bellazzi R, Falaschi F, Frattoni A, Perani G, Finardi G, et al. Enhanced LDL oxidation in uremic patients: an additional mechanism for accelerated atherosclerosis? Kidney Int 1994;45:876-83.

281. Magnason RL, Indridason OS, Sigvaldason H, Sigfusson N, Palsson R. Prevalence and progression of CRF in Iceland: a population-based study. Am J Kidney Dis 2002;40:955-63.

282. Mahalati K, Belitsky P, Sketris I, West K, Panek R. Neoral monitoring by simplified sparse sampling area under the concentration-time curve: its relationship to acute rejection and cyclosporine nephrotoxicity early after kidney transplantation. Transplantation 1999;68:55-62.

283. Mailloux LU, Napolitano B, Bellucci AG, Vernace M, Wilkes BM, Mossey RT. Renal vascular disease causing end-stage renal disease, incidence, clinical correlates, and outcomes: a 20-year clinical experience. Am J Kidney Dis 1994;24:622-9.

284. Maiorca R, Brunori G, Zubani R, Cancarini GC, Manili L, Camerini C, et al. Predictive value of dialysis adequacy and nutritional indices for mortality and morbidity in CAPD and HD patients: a longitudinal study. Nephrol Dial Transplant 1995;10:2295-305.
285. Mange KC, Joffe MM, Feldman HI. Effect of the use or nonuse of long-term dialysis on the subsequent survival of renal transplants from living donors. N Engl J Med 2001;344:726-31.
286. Mann JF, Gerstein HC, Pogue J, Bosch J, Yusuf S. Renal insufficiency as a predictor of cardiovascular outcomes and the impact of ramipril: the HOPE randomized trial. Ann Intern Med 2001;134:629-36.
287. Marsh JT, Brown WS, Wolcott D, Carr CR, Harper R, Schweitzer SV, et al. rHuEPO treatment improves brain and cognitive function of anemic dialysis patients. Kidney Int 1991;39:155-63.
288. Martin KJ, Gonzalez EA, Gellens M, Hamm LL, Abboud H, Lindberg J. 19-Nor-1-alpha-25-dihydroxyvitamin D2 (paricalcitol) safely and effectively reduces the levels of intact parathyroid hormone in patients on hemodialysis. J Am Soc Nephrol 1998;9:1427-32.
289. Maschio G, Alberti D, Janin G, Locatelli F, Mann JF, Motolese M, et al. Effect of the angiotensin-converting-enzyme inhibitor benazepril on the progression of chronic renal insufficiency. The Angiotensin-Converting-Enzyme Inhibition in Progressive Renal Insufficiency Study Group. N Engl J Med 1996;334:939-45.
290. Mason RM, Wahab NA. Extracellular matrix metabolism in diabetic nephropathy. J Am Soc Nephrol 2003;14:1358-73.
291. Massy ZA, Nguyen Khoa T, Lacour B, Descamps-Latscha B, Man NK, Jungers P. Dyslipidaemia and the progression of renal disease in chronic renal failure patients. Nephrol Dial Transplant 1999;14:2392-7.
292. Mastrangelo F, Alfonso L, Napoli M, DeBlasi V, Russo F, Patruno P. Dialysis with increased frequency of sessions (Lecce dialysis). Nephrol Dial Transplant 1998;13(suppl 6):139-47.
293. Mayer AD, Dmitrewski J, Squifflet JP, Besse T, Grabensee B, Klein B, et al. Multicenter randomized trial comparing tacrolimus (FK506) and cyclosporine in the prevention of renal allograft rejection: a report of the European Tacrolimus Multicenter Renal Study Group. Transplantation 1997;64:436-43.
294. Mayer G, Thum J, Cada EM, Stummvoll HK, Graf H. Working capacity is increased following recombinant human erythropoietin treatment. Kidney Int 1988;34:525-8.
295. McGiff JC, Crowshaw K, Terragno NA, Lonigro AJ. Renal prostaglandins: possible regulators of the renal actions of pressor hormones. Nature 1970;227:1255-7.
296. McKelvie GB, Collins GN, Hehir M, Rogers AC. A study of benign prostatic hyperplasia—a challenge to British urology. Br J Urol 1993;71:38-42.
297. Medical Research Board. MRC/BHF Heart Protection Study of cholesterol lowering with simvastatin in 20,536 high-risk individuals: a randomised placebo-controlled trial. Lancet 2002;360:7-22.
298. Mehta RL, Chertow GM. Acute renal failure definitions and classification: time for change? J Am Soc Nephrol 2003;14:2178-87.
299. Mehta RL, Pascual MT, Soroko S, Savage BR, Himmelfarb J, Ikizler TA, et al. Spectrum of acute renal failure in the intensive care unit: the PICARD experience. Kidney Int 2004;66:1613-21.
300. Merion RM, White DJ, Thiru S, Evans DB, Calne RY. Cyclosporine: five years' experience in cadaveric renal transplantation. N Engl J Med 1984;310:148-54.
301. Milliner DS. Cystinuria. Endocrinol Metab Clin North Am 1990;19:889-907.
302. Mogensen CE, Neldam S, Tikkanen I, Oren S, Viskoper R, Watts RW, et al. Randomised controlled trial of dual blockade of renin-angiotensin system in patients with hypertension, microalbuminuria, and non-insulin dependent diabetes: the candesartan and lisinopril microalbuminuria (CALM) study. BMJ 2000;321:1440-4.
303. Molitoris BA, Levin A, Warnock DG, Joannidis M, Mehta RL, Kellum JA, et al. Improving outcomes of acute kidney injury: report of an initiative. Nat Clin Pract Nephrol 2007;3:439-42.
304. Mollerup CL, Vestergaard P, Frokjaer VG, Mosekilde L, Christiansen P, Blichert-Toft M. Risk of renal stone events in primary hyperparathyroidism before and after parathyroid surgery: controlled retrospective follow up study. BMJ 2002;325:807.
305. Moreau P, Leblond V, Bourquelot P, Facon T, Huynh A, Caillot D, et al. Prognostic factors for survival and response after high-dose therapy and autologous stem cell transplantation in systemic AL amyloidosis: a report on 21 patients. Br J Haematol 1998;101:766-9.
306. Moreno F, Aracil FJ, Perez R, Valderrabano F. Controlled study on the improvement of quality of life in elderly hemodialysis patients after correcting end-stage renal disease-related anemia with erythropoietin. Am J Kidney Dis 1996;27:548-56.
307. Mucsi I, Hercz G, Uldall R, Ouwendyk M, Francoeur R, Pierratos A. Control of serum phosphate without any phosphate binders in patients treated with nocturnal hemodialysis. Kidney Int 1998;53:1399-404.
308. Nakamura T, Obata J, Kimura H, Ohno S, Yoshida Y, Kawachi H, et al. Blocking angiotensin II ameliorates proteinuria and glomerular lesions in progressive mesangioproliferative glomerulonephritis. Kidney Int 1999;55:877-89.
309. Nallamothu BK, Shojania KG, Saint S, Hofer TP, Humes HD, Moscucci M, et al. Is acetylcysteine effective in preventing contrast-related nephropathy? A meta-analysis. Am J Med 2004;117:938-47.
310. National Institute for Health and Clinical Excellence (NICE). Anaemia management in people with chronic kidney disease. *NICE Clinical Guidelines, No. 39.* National Collaborating Centre for Chronic Conditions (UK). London: Royal College of Physicians (UK); 2006. (http://guidance.nice.org.uk/CG39, accessed July 14, 2011.)
311. National Institute for Health and Clinical Excellence (NICE). Chronic kidney disease: national clinical guideline for early identification and management in adults in primary and secondary care. *NICE Clinical Guidelines, No. 73.* National Collaborating Centre for Chronic Conditions (UK). London: Royal College of Physicians (UK); 2008. (http://guidance.nice.org.uk/CG73, accessed July 14, 2011.)
312. National Institute for Health and Clinical Excellence (NICE). Type 2 diabetes: the management of type 2 diabetes. *NICE Clinical Guidelines, No. 66.* National Collaborating Centre for Chronic Conditions (UK). London: Royal College of Physicians (UK); 2008. (http://www.nice.org.uk/guidance/index.jsp?action=download&o=40803, accessed July 14, 2011.)
313. National Kidney Foundation. II. NKF-K/DOQI clinical practice guidelines for peritoneal dialysis adequacy: update 2000. Am J Kidney Dis 2001;37:S65-S136.
314. National Kidney Foundation. IV. NKF-K/DOQI clinical practice guidelines for anemia of chronic kidney disease: update 2000. Am J Kidney Dis 2001;37:S182-238.
315. National Kidney Foundation. K/DOQI clinical practice guidelines for chronic kidney disease: evaluation, classification, and stratification. Am J Kidney Dis 2002;39:S1-266.
316. National Kidney Foundation. Clinical practice guidelines for hemodialysis adequacy, update 2006. Am J Kidney Dis 2006;48(suppl 1):S2-90.
317. National Kidney Foundation. KDOQI clinical practice guideline and clinical practice recommendations for anemia in chronic kidney disease: 2007 update of hemoglobin target. Am J Kidney Dis 2007;50:471-530.
318. Navaneethan SD, Palmer SC, Craig JC, Elder GJ, Strippoli GF. Benefits and harms of phosphate binders in CKD: a systematic review of randomized controlled trials. Am J Kidney Dis 2009;54:619-37.
319. Newman DJ. Cystatin C. Ann Clin Biochem 2002;39:89-104.
320. Nielsen S, Frokiaer J, Marples D, Kwon TH, Agre P, Knepper MA. Aquaporins in the kidney: from molecules to medicine. Physiol Rev 2002;82:205-44.
321. Nielsen S, Kwon TH, Christensen BM, Promeneur D, Frokiaer J, Marples D. Physiology and pathophysiology of renal aquaporins. J Am Soc Nephrol 1999;10:647-63.
322. Niles JL, McCluskey RT, Ahmad MF, Arnaout MA. Wegener's granulomatosis autoantigen is a novel neutrophil serine proteinase. Blood 1989;74:1888-93.

323. Nyengaard JR, Bendtsen TF. Glomerular number and size in relation to age, kidney weight, and body surface in normal man. Anat Rec 1992;232:194-201.
324. O'Hare AM, Kaufman JS, Covinsky KE, Landefeld CS, McFarland LV, Larson EB. Current guidelines for using angiotensin-converting enzyme inhibitors and angiotensin II-receptor antagonists in chronic kidney disease: is the evidence base relevant to older adults? Ann Intern Med 2009;150:717-24.
325. Oda H, Keane WF. Lipid abnormalities in end stage renal disease. Nephrol Dial Transplant 1998;13(suppl 1):45-9.
326. Ofsthun N, Labrecque J, Lacson E, Keen M, Lazarus JM. The effects of higher hemoglobin levels on mortality and hospitalization in hemodialysis patients. Kidney Int 2003;63:1908-14.
327. Ohkubo Y, Kishikawa H, Araki E, Miyata T, Isami S, Motoyoshi S, et al. Intensive insulin therapy prevents the progression of diabetic microvascular complications in Japanese patients with non-insulin-dependent diabetes mellitus: a randomized prospective 6-year study. Diabetes Res Clin Pract 1995;28:103-17.
328. Olson KB, Hall TC, Horton J, Khung CL, Hosley HF. Thalidomide (N-phthaloylglutamimide) in the treatment of advanced cancer. Clin Pharmacol Ther 1965;6:292-7.
328A. Organ Procurement and Transplantation network (OPTN). http://optn.transplant.hrsa.gov/latestData/rptData.asp, accessed June 30, 2011.
329. Orth SR, Ritz E, Schrier RW. The renal risks of smoking. Kidney Int 1997;51:1669-77.
330. Owen WF Jr, Lew NL, Liu Y, Lowrie EG, Lazarus JM. The urea reduction ratio and serum albumin concentration as predictors of mortality in patients undergoing hemodialysis. N Engl J Med 1993; 329:1001-6.
331. Owen WF, Lowrie EG. C-reactive protein as an outcome predictor for maintenance hemodialysis patients. Kidney Int 1998;54:627-36.
332. Paisley KE, Tomson CR. Calcium phosphate stones during long-term acetazolamide treatment for epilepsy. Postgrad Med J 1999;75:427-8.
333. Pak CY. Citrate and renal calculi. Miner Electrolyte Metab 1987;13: 257-66.
334. Park IS, Kiyomoto H, Abboud SL, Abboud HE. Expression of transforming growth factor-beta and type IV collagen in early streptozotocin-induced diabetes. Diabetes 1997;46:473-80.
335. Parks JH, Coward M, Coe FL. Correspondence between stone composition and urine supersaturation in nephrolithiasis. Kidney Int 1997;51:894-900.
336. Parmar MS. Chronic renal disease. BMJ 2002;325:85-90.
337. Parving HH, Lehnert H, Brochner-Mortensen J, Gomis R, Andersen S, Arner P. The effect of irbesartan on the development of diabetic nephropathy in patients with type 2 diabetes. N Engl J Med 2001;345:870-8.
338. Pastan S, Bailey J. Dialysis therapy. N Engl J Med 1998;338:1428-37.
339. Paterson AD, Pei Y. Is there a third gene for autosomal dominant polycystic kidney disease? Kidney Int 1998;54:1759-61.
340. Payne RB. Renal tubular reabsorption of phosphate (TmP/GFR): indications and interpretation. Ann Clin Biochem 1998;35:201-6.
341. Pearce SH. Straightening out the renal tubule: advances in the molecular basis of the inherited tubulopathies. QJM 1998;91:5-12.
342. Pei Y, Obaji J, Dupuis A, Paterson AD, Magistroni R, Dicks E, et al. Unified criteria for ultrasonographic diagnosis of ADPKD. J Am Soc Nephrol 2009;20:205-12.
343. Penney MD, Oleesky DA. Renal tubular acidosis. Ann Clin Biochem 1999;36:408-22.
344. Penney MD, Walters G. Are osmolality measurements clinically useful? Ann Clin Biochem 1987;24:566-71.
345. Peralta CA, Shlipak MG, Fan D, Ordonez J, Lash JP, Chertow GM, et al. Risks for end-stage renal disease, cardiovascular events, and death in Hispanic versus non-Hispanic white adults with chronic kidney disease. J Am Soc Nephrol 2006;17:2892-9.
346. Peterson JC, Adler S, Burkart JM, Greene T, Hebert LA, Hunsicker LG, et al. Blood pressure control, proteinuria, and the progression of renal disease. The Modification of Diet in Renal Disease Study. Ann Intern Med 1995;123:754-62.
347. Petrarulo M, Cerelli E, Marangella M, Cosseddu D, Vitale C, Linari F. Assay of plasma oxalate with soluble oxalate oxidase. Clin Chem 1994; 40:2030-4.
348. Pirsch JD, Miller J, Deierhoi MH, Vincenti F, Filo RS. A comparison of tacrolimus (FK506) and cyclosporine for immunosuppression after cadaveric renal transplantation. FK506 Kidney Transplant Study Group. Transplantation 1997;63:977-83.
349. Plehn JF, Davis BR, Sacks FM, Rouleau JL, Pfeffer MA, Bernstein V, et al. Reduction of stroke incidence after myocardial infarction with pravastatin: the Cholesterol and Recurrent Events (CARE) study. The Care Investigators. Circulation 1999;99:216-23.
350. Ponticelli C, Altieri P, Scolari F, Passerini P, Roccatello D, Cesana B, et al. A randomized study comparing methylprednisolone plus chlorambucil versus methylprednisolone plus cyclophosphamide in idiopathic membranous nephropathy. J Am Soc Nephrol 1998;9: 444-50.
351. Popovich RP, Moncrief JW, Nolph KD, Ghods AJ, Twardowski ZJ, Pyle WK. Continuous ambulatory peritoneal dialysis. Ann Intern Med 1978;88:449-56.
352. Port FK, Wolfe RA, Mauger EA, Berling DP, Jiang K. Comparison of survival probabilities for dialysis patients vs cadaveric renal transplant recipients. JAMA 1993;270:1339-43.
353. Portoles J, Torralbo A, Martin P, Rodrigo J, Herrero JA, Barrientos A. Cardiovascular effects of recombinant human erythropoietin in predialysis patients. Am J Kidney Dis 1997;29:541-8.
354. Pozzi C, Bolasco PG, Fogazzi GB, Andrulli S, Altieri P, Ponticelli C, et al. Corticosteroids in IgA nephropathy: a randomised controlled trial. Lancet 1999;353:883-7.
355. Prakash J, Sen D, Kumar NS, Kumar H, Tripathi LK, Saxena RK. Acute renal failure due to intrinsic renal diseases: review of 1122 cases. Ren Fail 2003;25:225-33.
356. Premaud A, Le Meur Y, Debord J, Szelag JC, Rousseau A, Hoizey G, et al. Maximum a posteriori bayesian estimation of mycophenolic acid pharmacokinetics in renal transplant recipients at different postgrafting periods. Ther Drug Monit 2005;27:354-61.
357. Preminger GM. The metabolic evaluation of patients with recurrent nephrolithiasis: a review of comprehensive and simplified approaches. J Urol 1989;141:760-3.
358. Preminger GM. Is there a need for medical evaluation and treatment of nephrolithiasis in the "age of lithotripsy"? Semin Urol 1994;12: 51-64.
359. Raij L, Baylis C. Glomerular actions of nitric oxide. Kidney Int 1995; 48:20-32.
360. Raj DS, Charra B, Pierratos A, Work J. In search of ideal hemodialysis: is prolonged frequent dialysis the answer? Am J Kidney Dis 1999;34:597-610.
361. Rastegar A, Kashgarian M. The clinical spectrum of tubulointerstitial nephritis. Kidney Int 1998;54:313-27.
362. Ravid M, Brosh D, Ravid-Safran D, Levy Z, Rachmani R. Main risk factors for nephropathy in type 2 diabetes mellitus are plasma cholesterol levels, mean blood pressure, and hyperglycemia. Arch Intern Med 1998;158:998-1004.
363. Reeders ST, Breuning MH, Davies KE, Nicholls RD, Jarman AP, Higgs DR, et al. A highly polymorphic DNA marker linked to adult polycystic kidney disease on chromosome 16. Nature 1985; 317:542-4.
364. Reeves WB, Winters CJ, Zimniak L, Andreoli TE. Medullary thick limbs: renal concentrating segments. Kidney Int Suppl 1996;57: S154-64.
365. Reiser J, von Gersdorff G, Simons M, Schwarz K, Faul C, Giardino L, et al. Novel concepts in understanding and management of glomerular proteinuria. Nephrol Dial Transplant 2002;17:951-5.
366. Remuzzi G, Ruggenenti P, Benigni A. Understanding the nature of renal disease progression. Kidney Int 1997;51:2-15.
367. Revicki DA, Brown RE, Feeny DH, Henry D, Teehan BP, Rudnick MR, et al. Health-related quality of life associated with recombinant human erythropoietin therapy for predialysis chronic renal disease patients. Am J Kidney Dis 1995;25:548-54.

368. Richardson PG, Sonneveld P, Schuster MW, Irwin D, Stadtmauer EA, Facon T, et al. Bortezomib or high-dose dexamethasone for relapsed multiple myeloma. N Engl J Med 2005;352:2487-98.
369. Ring T, Frische S, Nielsen S. Clinical review: renal tubular acidosis—a physicochemical approach. Crit Care 2005;9:573-80.
370. Robertson WG, Peacock M, Heyburn PJ, Hanes FA, Rutherford A, Clementson E, et al. Should recurrent calcium oxalate stone formers become vegetarians? Br J Urol 1979;51:427-31.
371. Robertson WG, Peacock M, Heyburn PJ, Marshall DH, Clark PB. Risk factors in calcium stone disease of the urinary tract. Br J Urol 1978;50:449-54.
372. Robson MG, Banerjee D, Hopster D, Cairns HS. Seven cases of granulomatous interstitial nephritis in the absence of extrarenal sarcoid. Nephrol Dial Transplant 2003;18:280-4.
373. Ronco P, Brunisholz M, Geniteau-Legendre M, Chatelet F, Verroust P, Richet G. Physiopathologic aspects of Tamm-Horsfall protein: a phylogenetically conserved marker of the thick ascending limb of Henle's loop. Adv Nephrol Necker Hosp 1987;16:231-49.
374. Rose GA, Woodfine C. The thermogravimetric analysis of renal stones (in clinical practice). Br J Urol 1976;48:403-12.
375. Rowe JW, Andres R, Tobin JD, Norris AH, Shock NW. The effect of age on creatinine clearance in men: a cross-sectional and longitudinal study. J Gerontol 1976;31:155-63.
376. Ruggenenti P, Perna A, Gherardi G, Gaspari F, Benini R, Remuzzi G. Renal function and requirement for dialysis in chronic nephropathy patients on long-term ramipril: REIN follow-up trial. Gruppo Italiano di Studi Epidemiologici in Nefrologia (GISEN). Ramipril Efficacy in Nephropathy. Lancet 1998;352:1252-6.
377. Ruggenenti P, Perna A, Mosconi L, Pisoni R, Remuzzi G. Urinary protein excretion rate is the best independent predictor of ESRF in non-diabetic proteinuric chronic nephropathies. Gruppo Italiano di Studi Epidemiologici in Nefrologia (GISEN). Kidney Int 1998;53: 1209-16.
378. Rule AD, Bergstralh EJ, Melton LJ 3rd, Li X, Weaver AL, Lieske JC. Kidney stones and the risk for chronic kidney disease. Clin J Am Soc Nephrol 2009;4:804-11.
379. Rumberger JA, Simons DB, Fitzpatrick LA, Sheedy PF, Schwartz RS. Coronary artery calcium area by electron-beam computed tomography and coronary atherosclerotic plaque area: a histopathologic correlative study. Circulation 1995;92:2157-62.
380. Ruster C, Wolf G. Renin-angiotensin-aldosterone system and progression of renal disease. J Am Soc Nephrol 2006;17:2985-91.
381. Samuell CT, Kasidas GP. Biochemical investigations in renal stone formers. Ann Clin Biochem 1995;32:112-22.
382. Sanders PW, Herrera GA, Galla JH. Human Bence Jones protein toxicity in rat proximal tubule epithelium in vivo. Kidney Int 1987;32: 851-61.
383. Sands JM, Kokko JP. Current concepts of the countercurrent multiplication system. Kidney Int Suppl 1996;57:S93-9.
384. Sarnak MJ, Levey AS, Schoolwerth AC, Coresh J, Culleton B, Hamm LL, et al. Kidney disease as a risk factor for development of cardiovascular disease: a statement from the American Heart Association Councils on Kidney in Cardiovascular Disease, High Blood Pressure Research, Clinical Cardiology, and Epidemiology and Prevention. Circulation 2003;108:2154-69.
385. Savage CO. ANCA-associated renal vasculitis. Kidney Int 2001;60: 1614-27.
386. Savige J, Gillis D, Benson E, Davies D, Esnault V, Falk RJ, et al. International Consensus Statement on Testing and Reporting of Antineutrophil Cytoplasmic Antibodies (ANCA). Am J Clin Pathol 1999;111:507-13.
387. Savin VJ, Sharma R, Sharma M, McCarthy ET, Swan SK, Ellis E, et al. Circulating factor associated with increased glomerular permeability to albumin in recurrent focal segmental glomerulosclerosis. N Engl J Med 1996;334:878-83.
388. Sayer JA, Pearce SH. Diagnosis and clinical biochemistry of inherited tubulopathies. Ann Clin Biochem 2001;38:459-70.
389. Scheinman SJ, Guay-Woodford LM, Thakker RV, Warnock DG. Genetic disorders of renal electrolyte transport. N Engl J Med 1999;340:1177-87.
390. Schena FP, Pascoe MD, Alberu J, del Carmen Rial M, Oberbauer R, Brennan DC, et al. Conversion from calcineurin inhibitors to sirolimus maintenance therapy in renal allograft recipients: 24-month efficacy and safety results from the CONVERT trial. Transplantation 2009;87:233-42.
391. Schlondorff D, Banas B. The mesangial cell revisited: no cell is an island. J Am Soc Nephrol 2009;20:1179-87.
392. Schmidt AM, Vianna M, Gerlach M, Brett J, Ryan J, Kao J, et al. Isolation and characterization of two binding proteins for advanced glycosylation end products from bovine lung which are present on the endothelial cell surface. J Biol Chem 1992;267:14987-97.
393. Schmidt S, Ritz E. The role of angiotensin I-converting enzyme gene polymorphism in renal disease. Curr Opin Nephrol Hypertens 1996;5: 552-5.
394. Schoppet M, Shroff RC, Hofbauer LC, Shanahan CM. Exploring the biology of vascular calcification in chronic kidney disease: what's circulating? Kidney Int 2008;73:384-90.
395. Schreiner GE. Prevention of renal disease and conservation of renal function. Am J Kidney Dis 1990;16:360-6.
396. Schrier RW. Vasopressin and aquaporin 2 in clinical disorders of water homeostasis. Semin Nephrol 2008;28:289-96.
397. Schwarz A, Krause PH, Kunzendorf U, Keller F, Distler A. The outcome of acute interstitial nephritis: risk factors for the transition from acute to chronic interstitial nephritis. Clin Nephrol 2000;54:179-90.
398. Scoble JE. Do protection devices have a role in renal angioplasty and stent placement? Nephrol Dial Transplant 2003;18:1700-3.
399. Seibert K, Zhang Y, Leahy K, Hauser S, Masferrer J, Perkins W, et al. Pharmacological and biochemical demonstration of the role of cyclooxygenase 2 in inflammation and pain. Proc Natl Acad Sci U S A 1994;91:12013-7.
400. Selgas R, Bajo MA, Fernandez-Reyes MJ, Bosque E, Lopez-Revuelta K, Jimenez C, et al. An analysis of adequacy of dialysis in a selected population on CAPD for over 3 years: the influence of urea and creatinine kinetics. Nephrol Dial Transplant 1993;8:1244-53.
401. Shanahan CM, Proudfoot D, Farzaneh-Far A, Weissberg PL. The role of Gla proteins in vascular calcification. Crit Rev Eukaryot Gene Expr 1998;8:357-75.
402. Sharma K, Eltayeb BO, McGowan TA, Dunn SR, Alzahabi B, Rohde R, et al. Captopril-induced reduction of serum levels of transforming growth factor-beta1 correlates with long-term renoprotection in insulin-dependent diabetic patients. Am J Kidney Dis 1999;34:818-23.
403. Sharma K, Ziyadeh FN, Alzahabi B, McGowan TA, Kapoor S, Kurnik BR, et al. Increased renal production of transforming growth factor-beta1 in patients with type II diabetes. Diabetes 1997;46:854-9.
404. Shimizu H, Maruyama S, Yuzawa Y, Kato T, Miki Y, Suzuki S, et al. Anti-monocyte chemoattractant protein-1 gene therapy attenuates renal injury induced by protein-overload proteinuria. J Am Soc Nephrol 2003;14:1496-505.
405. Silberberg JS, Barre PE, Prichard SS, Sniderman AD. Impact of left ventricular hypertrophy on survival in end-stage renal disease. Kidney Int 1989;36:286-90.
406. Silve C. Tubular handling and regulation of sulphate. Nephrol Dial Transplant 2000;15(suppl 6):34-5.
407. Singh AK, Szczech L, Tang KL, Barnhart H, Sapp S, Wolfson M, et al. Correction of anemia with epoetin alfa in chronic kidney disease. N Engl J Med 2006;355:2085-98.
408. Singhal S, Mehta J. Multiple myeloma. Clin J Am Soc Nephrol 2006;1: 1322-30.
409. Singhal S, Mehta J, Desikan R, Ayers D, Roberson P, Eddlemon P, et al. Antitumor activity of thalidomide in refractory multiple myeloma. N Engl J Med 1999;341:1565-71.
410. Skinner M, Anderson J, Simms R, Falk R, Wang M, Libbey C, et al. Treatment of 100 patients with primary amyloidosis: a randomized trial of melphalan, prednisone, and colchicine versus colchicine only. Am J Med 1996;100:290-8.

411. Slatopolsky E, Caglar S, Pennell JP, Taggart DD, Canterbury JM, Reiss E, et al. On the pathogenesis of hyperparathyroidism in chronic experimental renal insufficiency in the dog. J Clin Invest 1971;50:492-9.
412. Slatopolsky E, Cozzolino M, Finch JL. Differential effects of 19-nor-1,25-(OH)(2)D(2) and 1alpha-hydroxyvitamin D(2) on calcium and phosphorus in normal and uremic rats. Kidney Int 2002;62:1277-84.
413. Slatopolsky E, Finch J, Denda M, Ritter C, Zhong M, Dusso A, et al. Phosphorus restriction prevents parathyroid gland growth: high phosphorus directly stimulates PTH secretion in vitro. J Clin Invest 1996;97:2534-40.
414. Solez K, Colvin RB, Racusen LC, Sis B, Halloran PF, Birk PE, et al. Banff '05 meeting report: differential diagnosis of chronic allograft injury and elimination of chronic allograft nephropathy ('CAN'). Am J Transplant 2007;7:518-26.
415. Solomon A, Weiss DT, Kattine AA. Nephrotoxic potential of Bence Jones proteins. N Engl J Med 1991;324:1845-51.
416. Solomon SD, Rice MM, A Jablonski K, Jose P, Domanski M, Sabatine M, et al. Renal function and effectiveness of angiotensin-converting enzyme inhibitor therapy in patients with chronic stable coronary disease in the Prevention of Events with ACE Inhibition (PEACE) trial. Circulation 2006;114:26-31.
417. Sorgel F, Ettinger B, Benet LZ. The true composition of kidney stones passed during triamterene therapy. J Urol 1985;134:871-3.
418. Stamatelou KK, Francis ME, Jones CA, Nyberg LM, Curhan GC. Time trends in reported prevalence of kidney stones in the United States: 1976-1994. Kidney Int 2003;63:1817-23.
419. Steinberg AD, Decker JL. A double-blind controlled trial comparing cyclophosphamide, azathioprine and placebo in the treatment of lupus glomerulonephritis. Arthritis Rheum 1974;17:923-37.
420. Stenvinkel P, Heimburger O, Paultre F, Diczfalusy U, Wang T, Berglund L, et al. Strong association between malnutrition, inflammation, and atherosclerosis in chronic renal failure. Kidney Int 1999;55:1899-911.
421. Stevens PE, O'Donoghue DJ, de Lusignan S, Van Vlymen J, Klebe B, Middleton R, et al. Chronic kidney disease management in the United Kingdom: NEOERICA project results. Kidney Int 2007;72:92-9.
422. Stevens PE, Tamimi NA, Al-Hasani MK, Mikhail AI, Kearney E, Lapworth R, et al. Non-specialist management of acute renal failure. QJM 2001;94:533-40.
423. Strippoli GF, Manno C, Schena FP. An "evidence-based" survey of therapeutic options for IgA nephropathy: assessment and criticism. Am J Kidney Dis 2003;41:1129-39.
424. Suki WN, Zabaneh R, Cangiano JL, Reed J, Fischer D, Garrett L, et al. Effects of sevelamer and calcium-based phosphate binders on mortality in hemodialysis patients. Kidney Int 2007;72:1130-7.
425. Sun BY, Lee YH, Jiaan BP, Chen KK, Chang LS, Chen KT. Recurrence rate and risk factors for urinary calculi after extracorporeal shock wave lithotripsy. J Urol 1996;156:903-5; discussion 906.
426. Swaminathan S, Shah SV. New insights into nephrogenic systemic fibrosis. J Am Soc Nephrol 2007;18:2636-43.
427. Tanji N, Markowitz GS, Fu C, Kislinger T, Taguchi A, Pischetsrieder M, et al. Expression of advanced glycation end products and their cellular receptor RAGE in diabetic nephropathy and nondiabetic renal disease. J Am Soc Nephrol 2000;11:1656-66.
428. Taylor EN, Curhan GC. Diet and fluid prescription in stone disease. Kidney Int 2006;70:835-9.
429. Tenenhouse HS. Phosphate transport: molecular basis, regulation and pathophysiology. J Steroid Biochem Mol Biol 2007;103:572-7.
430. Tenenhouse HS, Murer H. Disorders of renal tubular phosphate transport. J Am Soc Nephrol 2003;14:240-8.
431. Teng M, Wolf M, Lowrie E, Ofsthun N, Lazarus JM, Thadhani R. Survival of patients undergoing hemodialysis with paricalcitol or calcitriol therapy. N Engl J Med 2003;349:446-56.
432. Tepel M, van der Giet M, Schwarzfeld C, Laufer U, Liermann D, Zidek W. Prevention of radiographic-contrast-agent-induced reductions in renal function by acetylcysteine. N Engl J Med 2000;343:180-4.
433. Terasaki PI, Ozawa M. Predicting kidney graft failure by HLA antibodies: a prospective trial. Am J Transplant 2004;4:438-43.
434. Thakker RV. Pathogenesis of Dent's disease and related syndromes of X-linked nephrolithiasis. Kidney Int 2000;57:787-93.
435. Thomsen OF, Ladefoged J. Pyelonephritis and interstitial nephritis—clinical-pathological correlations. Clin Nephrol 2002;58:275-81.
436. Tiselius HG. Metabolic evaluation of patients with stone disease. Urol Int 1997;59:131-41.
437. Tiselius HG. Possibilities for preventing recurrent calcium stone formation: principles for the metabolic evaluation of patients with calcium stone disease. BJU Int 2001;88:158-68.
438. Toto RD. The role of prostaglandins in NSAID induced renal dysfunction. J Rheumatol Suppl 1991;28:22-5.
439. Trinchieri A, Nespoli R, Ostini F, Rovera F, Zanetti G, Pisani E. A study of dietary calcium and other nutrients in idiopathic renal calcium stone formers with low bone mineral content. J Urol 1998;159:654-7.
440. Trompeter R, Filler G, Webb NJ, Watson AR, Milford DV, Tyden G, et al. Randomized trial of tacrolimus versus cyclosporin microemulsion in renal transplantation. Pediatr Nephrol 2002;17:141-9.
441. Twardowski ZJ, Nolph KD, Khanna R. Peritoneal equilibration test. Perit Dial Bull 1987;7:138-147.
442. Tyson KL, Reynolds JL, McNair R, Zhang Q, Weissberg PL, Shanahan CM. Osteo/chondrocytic transcription factors and their target genes exhibit distinct patterns of expression in human arterial calcification. Arterioscler Thromb Vasc Biol 2003;23:489-94.
443. Uldall R, Ouwendyk M, Francoeur R, Wallace L, Sit W, Vas S, et al. Slow nocturnal home hemodialysis at the Wellesley Hospital. Adv Ren Replace Ther 1996;3:133-6.
444. United Kingdom Prospective Diabetes Study Group. Intensive blood-glucose control with sulphonylureas or insulin compared with conventional treatment and risk of complications in patients with type 2 diabetes (UKPDS 33). UK Prospective Diabetes Study (UKPDS) Group. Lancet 1998;352:837-53.
445. United Kingdom Renal Association, Renal Association Standards Committee. Treatment of adults and children with renal failure: standards and audit measures, 3rd edition. London: Royal College of Physicians, 2002.
446. United Kingdom Renal Association. Clinical practice guidelines, http://www.renal.org/Clinical/GuidelinesSection/Guidelines.aspx/ accessed July 14, 2011.
446A. United KingdomRenal Association. Clinical practice guidelines. Anaemia in CKD. http://www.renal.org/Clinical/GuidelinesSection/AnaemiaInCKD.aspx, accessed June 30, 2011.
447. United States Renal Data Systems. Excerpts from the USRDS 2002 annual data report: atlas of end-stage renal disease in the United States. Am J Kidney Dis 2003;41(suppl 2):S1-260.
447A. U.S. Renal Data System, USRDS 2010 Annual Data Report: Atlas of Chronic Kidney Disease and End-Stage Renal Disease in the United States, National Institutes of Health, National Institute of Diabetes and Digestive and Kidney Diseases, Bethesda, MD, 2010, Healthy People 2010. http://www.usrds.org/2010/pdf/v2_00hp.pdf, accessed 2011-06-28.
448. Urena Torres P, Friedlander G, de Vernejoul MC, Silve C, Prie D. Bone mass does not correlate with the serum fibroblast growth factor 23 in hemodialysis patients. Kidney Int 2008;73:102-7.
449. van der Woude FJ. Anticytoplasmic antibodies in Wegener's granulomatosis. Lancet 1985;2:48.
450. Van Wyck DB, Roppolo M, Martinez CO, Mazey RM, McMurray S. A randomized, controlled trial comparing IV iron sucrose to oral iron in anemic patients with nondialysis-dependent CKD. Kidney Int 2005;68:2846-56.
451. Vanholder R, De Smet R, Glorieux G, Argiles A, Baurmeister U, Brunet P, et al. Review on uremic toxins: classification, concentration, and interindividual variability. Kidney Int 2003;63:1934-43.

452. Vanholder R, Glorieux G, De Smet R, Lameire N. New insights in uremic toxins. Kidney Int Suppl 2003;S6-10.
453. Verbeke M, Smollich B, van de Voorde J, de Ridder L, Lameire N. Beneficial influence of ketanserin on autoregulation of blood flow in post-ischemic kidneys. J Am Soc Nephrol 1996;7:621-7.
454. Verkoelen CF. Crystal retention in renal stone disease: a crucial role for the glycosaminoglycan hyaluronan? J Am Soc Nephrol 2006;17: 1673-87.
455. Verroust PJ, Christensen EI. Megalin and cubilin—the story of two multipurpose receptors unfolds. Nephrol Dial Transplant 2002;17: 1867-71.
456. Vincenti F, Jensik SC, Filo RS, Miller J, Pirsch J. A long-term comparison of tacrolimus (FK506) and cyclosporine in kidney transplantation: evidence for improved allograft survival at five years. Transplantation 2002;73:775-82.
457. Wannamethee SG, Shaper AG, Perry IJ. Serum creatinine concentration and risk of cardiovascular disease: a possible marker for increased risk of stroke. Stroke 1997;28:557-63.
458. Wanner C, Krane V, Marz W, Olschewski M, Mann JF, Ruf G, et al. Atorvastatin in patients with type 2 diabetes mellitus undergoing hemodialysis. N Engl J Med 2005;353:238-48.
459. Watkin DM, Shock NW. Agewise standard values for C_{In}, C_{PAH}, and Tm_{PAH} in adult males. J Clin Invest 1955;34:969.
460. Watson PE, Watson ID, Batt RD. Total body water volumes for adult males and females estimated from simple anthropometric measurements. Am J Clin Nutr 1980;33:27-39.
461. Wautier JL, Zoukourian C, Chappey O, Wautier MP, Guillausseau PJ, Cao R, et al. Receptor-mediated endothelial cell dysfunction in diabetic vasculopathy: soluble receptor for advanced glycation end products blocks hyperpermeability in diabetic rats. J Clin Invest 1996;97:238-43.
462. Weening JJ, D'Agati VD, Schwartz MM, Seshan SV, Alpers CE, Appel GB, et al. The classification of glomerulonephritis in systemic lupus erythematosus revisited. J Am Soc Nephrol 2004;15:241-50.
463. Weigert C, Brodbeck K, Klopfer K, Haring HU, Schleicher ED. Angiotensin II induces human TGF-beta 1 promoter activation: similarity to hyperglycaemia. Diabetologia 2002;45:890-8.
464. Weir MR, Anderson L, Fink JC, Gabregiorgish K, Schweitzer EJ, Hoehn-Saric E, et al. A novel approach to the treatment of chronic allograft nephropathy. Transplantation 1997;64:1706-10.
465. Weisinger JR. New insights into the pathogenesis of idiopathic hypercalciuria: the role of bone. Kidney Int 1996;49:1507-18.
466. Wendt T, Tanji N, Guo J, Hudson BI, Bierhaus A, Ramasamy R, et al. Glucose, glycation, and RAGE: implications for amplification of cellular dysfunction in diabetic nephropathy. J Am Soc Nephrol 2003;14:1383-95.
467. Wheeler DC, Townend JN, Landray MJ. Cardiovascular risk factors in predialysis patients: baseline data from the Chronic Renal Impairment in Birmingham (CRIB) study. Kidney Int Suppl 2003;S201-3.
468. Whelton A. Nephrotoxicity of nonsteroidal anti-inflammatory drugs: physiologic foundations and clinical implications. Am J Med 1999; 106:13S-24S.
469. White KE, Bilous RW. Type 2 diabetic patients with nephropathy show structural-functional relationships that are similar to type 1 disease. J Am Soc Nephrol 2000;11:1667-73.
470. Wiik A. Delineation of a standard procedure for indirect immunofluorescence detection of ANCA. APMIS Suppl 1989;6:12-3.
471. Wilhelm SM, Simonson MS, Robinson AV, Stowe NT, Schulak JA. Endothelin up-regulation and localization following renal ischemia and reperfusion. Kidney Int 1999;55:1011-8.
472. Wilkinson H. Clinical investigation and management of patients with renal stones. Ann Clin Biochem 2001;38:180-7.
473. Winearls CG. Acute myeloma kidney. Kidney Int 1995;48:1347-61.
474. Winearls CG, Glassock RJ. Dissecting and refining the staging of chronic kidney disease. Kidney Int 2009;75:1009-14.
475. Winearls CG, Oliver DO, Pippard MJ, Reid C, Downing MR, Cotes PM. Effect of human erythropoietin derived from recombinant DNA on the anaemia of patients maintained by chronic haemodialysis. Lancet 1986;2:1175-8.
476. Woolfson RG, Mansell MA. Hyperoxaluria and renal calculi. Postgrad Med J 1994;70:695-8.
477. Worcester EM, Coe FL. New insights into the pathogenesis of idiopathic hypercalciuria. Semin Nephrol 2008;28:120-32.
478. World Health Organisation. Nutritional anemia: report of a WHO scientific group. Geneva, Switzerland: WHO, 1968.
479. World Health Organisation. Definition and diagnosis of diabetes mellitus and intermediate hyperglycaemia. Available at: http://www.who.int/diabetes/publications/Definition%20and%20diagnosis%20of%20diabetes_new.pdf 2006 (accessed on July 14, 2011).
480. Worthington JE, Martin S, Al-Husseini DM, Dyer PA, Johnson RW. Posttransplantation production of donor HLA-specific antibodies as a predictor of renal transplant outcome. Transplantation 2003;75: 1034-40.
481. Wrong OM, Norden AG, Feest TG. Dent's disease; a familial proximal renal tubular syndrome with low-molecular-weight proteinuria, hypercalciuria, nephrocalcinosis, metabolic bone disease, progressive renal failure and a marked male predominance. QJM 1994;87:473-93.
482. Xia H, Ebben J, Ma JZ, Collins AJ. Hematocrit levels and hospitalization risks in hemodialysis patients. J Am Soc Nephrol 1999;10:1309-16.
483. Xue JL, St Peter WL, Ebben JP, Everson SE, Collins AJ. Anemia treatment in the pre-ESRD period and associated mortality in elderly patients. Am J Kidney Dis 2002;40:1153-61.
484. Yakoub-Agha I, Attal M, Dumontet C, Delannoy V, Moreau P, Berthou C, et al. Thalidomide in patients with advanced multiple myeloma: a study of 83 patients—report of the Intergroupe Francophone du Myelome (IFM). Hematol J 2002;3:185-92.
485. Yusuf S, Sleight P, Pogue J, Bosch J, Davies R, Dagenais G. Effects of an angiotensin-converting-enzyme inhibitor, ramipril, on cardiovascular events in high-risk patients. The Heart Outcomes Prevention Evaluation Study Investigators. N Engl J Med 2000;342: 145-53.
486. Zatz R. Haemodynamically mediated glomerular injury: the end of a 15-year-old controversy? Curr Opin Nephrol Hypertens 1996;5: 468-75.
487. Zatz R, Dunn BR, Meyer TW, Anderson S, Rennke HG, Brenner BM. Prevention of diabetic glomerulopathy by pharmacological amelioration of glomerular capillary hypertension. J Clin Invest 1986;77:1925-30.
488. Zeisberg M, Hanai J, Sugimoto H, Mammoto T, Charytan D, Strutz F, et al. BMP-7 counteracts TGF-beta1-induced epithelial-to-mesenchymal transition and reverses chronic renal injury. Nat Med 2003;9:964-8.
489. Zelikovic I, Chesney RW. Sodium-coupled amino acid transport in renal tubule. Kidney Int 1989;36:351-9.
490. Ziyadeh FN, Hoffman BB, Han DC, Iglesias-De La Cruz MC, Hong SW, Isono M, et al. Long-term prevention of renal insufficiency, excess matrix gene expression, and glomerular mesangial matrix expansion by treatment with monoclonal antitransforming growth factor-beta antibody in db/db diabetic mice. Proc Natl Acad Sci U S A 2000;97: 8015-20.
491. Ziyadeh FN, Sharma K, Ericksen M, Wolf G. Stimulation of collagen gene expression and protein synthesis in murine mesangial cells by high glucose is mediated by autocrine activation of transforming growth factor-beta. J Clin Invest 1994;93:536-42.
492. Zucchelli P, Pasquali S, Cagnoli L, Ferrari G. Controlled plasma exchange trial in acute renal failure due to multiple myeloma. Kidney Int 1988;33:1175-80.

CHAPTER 49

Physiology and Disorders of Water, Electrolyte, and Acid-Base Metabolism

Joshua L. Hood, M.D., Ph.D., and Mitchell G. Scott, Ph.D.

Adaptation to terrestrial life led to the evolution of physiologic systems to maintain the composition of the internal milieu of animals, including humans. These systems include a variety of chemical buffers and highly specialized mechanisms of the lungs and kidneys that work together to regulate water, electrolytes, and pH between intracellular and extracellular compartments. Perturbations in the dynamic equilibria that exist for water, electrolytes, and pH may arise from external (e.g., trauma, changes in altitude, ingestion of toxic substances) or internal (e.g., normal metabolism, disease state) sources. Endogenous correction of these imbalances may not always be adequate; at these times, the clinical laboratory can provide valuable information for guiding therapy.

TOTAL BODY WATER—VOLUME AND DISTRIBUTION

During gestation, ≈90% of fetal body weight is water.[22] Water is 80% of body weight for preterm infants and 70% for full-term infants. Water gradually decreases as percent of body weight, so that it accounts for 65% of body weight in older children, 60% in adolescents and adult males,[22] and ≈55% for adult females. After middle age, the percentage of body water falls to ≈50%. As depicted in Figure 49-1, approximately two thirds of total body water (TBW) is distributed into the intracellular fluid (ICF) compartment, and one third exists in the extracellular fluid (ECF) compartment. The ICF and ECF compartments are physically separated by the cellular plasma membrane. The ECF may be subdivided into interstitial (≈75% of ECF) and intravascular (≈25% of ECF) fluid compartments, which are separated by the capillary endothelium. The average adult has ≈5 L blood volume (intravascular compartment) and a plasma volume of ≈3.0 L when the hematocrit is ≈40%. Although other clinically relevant ECF compartments (e.g., cerebrospinal fluid,[31] urine) may be analyzed in the clinical laboratory, most laboratory tests used to determine hydration status and electrolyte and acid-base status are performed on samples from the *intravascular* compartment.

The minimum daily requirement for water can be estimated from renal (1200 to 1500 mL in urine) and "insensible" losses (≈400 to 700 mL due to evaporation from the skin and respiratory tract). Activity, environmental conditions, and disease all have dramatic effects on daily water (and electrolyte) requirements. However, on average, an adult must take in ≈1.5 to 2.0 L of water daily to maintain fluid balance. Because primary regulatory mechanisms are designed to first maintain *intracellular* hydration status, imbalances in TBW are initially reflected in the ECF compartment. Table 49-1 lists common causes and clinical manifestations of expansion and contraction of the ECF compartment.

WATER AND ELECTROLYTES—COMPOSITION OF BODY FLUIDS

The primary cationic (positively charged) electrolytes are sodium (Na^+), potassium (K^+), calcium (Ca^{2+}), and magnesium (Mg^{2+}), whereas the anions (negatively charged) include chloride (Cl^-), bicarbonate (HCO_3^-), phosphate (HPO_4^{2-}, $H_2PO_4^-$), sulfate (SO_4^{2-}), organic ions such as lactate, and negatively charged proteins. Electrolyte concentrations of the body fluid compartments are shown in Table 49-2. Na^+, K^+, Cl^-, and HCO_3^- in the plasma or serum are commonly analyzed in an *electrolyte profile,* because their concentrations provide the most relevant information about the osmotic, hydration, and acid-base status of the body. Although hydrogen ion (H^+) is a cation, its concentration is approximately 1 million–fold lower in plasma than the major electrolytes listed in Table 49-2 (10^{-9} mol/L vs. 10^{-3} mol/L) and thus is negligible in terms of osmotic activity.

Any increase in the concentration of one anion is accompanied by a corresponding decrease in other anions, or by an increase in one or more cations or both, as total electrical

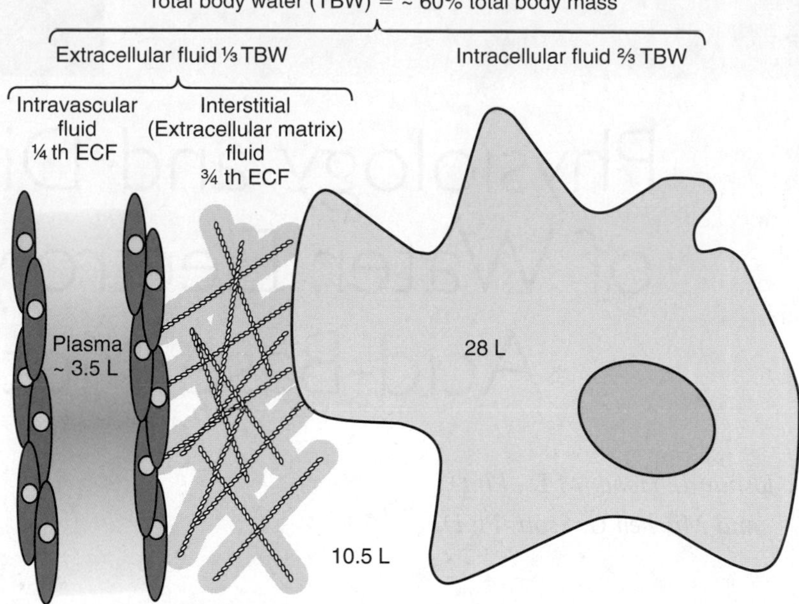

Figure 49-1 Volume and distribution of total body water. Note that the intracellular and extracellular fluid compartments (ICF and ECF, respectively) are separated by cellular plasma membranes, and within the ECF, interstitial and intravascular fluids are separated by the capillary endothelium (red cells). The volumes indicated represent water and not total volume. Endothelial cells = red; interstitial cell = gray; collagen matrix fibers = black cables.

TABLE 49-1 Causes and Clinical Manifestations of Changes in Extracellular Fluid (ECF) Volume

	Clinical Manifestations	Causes
ECF loss	Thirst, anorexia, nausea, lightheadedness, orthostatic hypotension, syncope, tachycardia, oliguria, decreased skin turgor and "sunken eyes," shock, coma, death	Trauma (and other causes of acute blood loss), "third-spacing" of fluid (e.g., burns, pancreatitis, peritonitis), vomiting, diarrhea, diuretics, renal or adrenal (i.e., sodium wasting) disease
ECF gain	Weight gain, edema, dyspnea (due to pulmonary edema), tachycardia, jugular venous distention, portal hypertension (ascites), esophageal varices	Heart failure, cirrhosis, nephrotic syndrome, iatrogenic (intravenous fluid overload)

TABLE 49-2 Electrolyte and Water Composition of Body Fluid Compartments*

Component	Plasma	Interstitial Fluid	Intracellular Fluid†
Volume, H_2O (TBW = 42 L)	3.5 L	10.5 L	28 L
Na^+	142	145	12
K^+	4	4	156
Ca^{2+}	2.4	2-3	0.3
Mg^{2+}	2	1-2	26
Trace elements	1	–	–
Total cations	155	–	–
Cl^-	103	114	4
HCO_3^-	27	31	12
$Protein^-$	16	–	55
Organic $acids^-$	5	–	–
HPO_4^{2-}	2	–	–
SO_4^{2-}	1	–	–
Total anions	154	–	–

*All electrolyte values are expressed in mEq/L of *fluid*. Because the H_2O content of plasma is ≈93% by volume, the corresponding electrolyte concentrations in plasma water are ≈10% higher. Note that the *molar concentration* of divalent ions is one half the depicted value.

†These values are derived from skeletal muscle.

TBW, Total body water.

neutrality must be maintained. Similarly, any decrease in the concentration of anions involves a corresponding increase in other anions or a decrease in cations, or both. In the case of polyvalent ions (e.g., Ca^{2+}, Mg^{2+}), it is important to distinguish between the substance concentration of the ion itself and the concentration of the ion charge. Thus although the concentration of total calcium ions in normal plasma is ≈2.5 mmol/L, the concentration of the total calcium ion *charge* is 5.0 mmol/L [also called 5 milliequivalents per liter (mEq/L)]. This law of *electrical neutrality* should not be confused with acid-base neutrality (pH = 7.0), where the activity of H^+ equals the activity of OH^-.

Extracellular and Intracellular Compartments

The extracellular compartment is composed of plasma and interstitial fluid.

Plasma

Plasma generally has a volume of 1300 to 1800 mL/m² of body surface and constitutes approximately 5% of the body volume (≈3.5 L for a 66 kg subject). Generally, total body volume is derived from body mass by using an estimated body density of 1.06 kg/L. Table 49-2 describes the electrolyte composition of plasma. The mass concentration of water in normal plasma is about 0.933 kg/L, depending on the protein and lipid content (see "Electrolyte Exclusion Effect" in Chapter 28). Thus a concentration of sodium in the plasma of 140 mmol/L would correspond to a molality of sodium in plasma water of 150 mmol/kg H_2O (140 mmol/L divided by 0.933 kg/L). The concentration of net protein ions in plasma is ≈12 mmol/L, with the charge mainly due to albumin, as the charge of globulins is negligible.[8]

Interstitial Fluid

Interstitial fluid is essentially an ultrafiltrate of blood plasma (see Figure 49-1). When all extracellular spaces except plasma are included, the volume accounts for about 26% (10.5 L) of the total body volume. Plasma is separated from the interstitial fluid by the endothelial lining of the capillaries, which acts as a semipermeable membrane and allows passage of water and diffusible solutes but not compounds of high molecular mass, such as proteins. The exchange of water between the interstitial and intravascular compartments is governed by Starling forces.[22] The Starling formula demonstrates that the net movement of fluid across a capillary membrane is a function of membrane permeability and differences in hydrostatic and oncotic pressures on the two sides of the membrane. The "impermeability" to proteins is not absolute, and in some pathologic conditions causing "shock," such as bacterial sepsis, the permeability of the vascular endothelium increases dramatically, resulting in leakage of albumin, a reduction in the effective circulating volume, and hypotension. If not aggressively treated with intravenous fluids and/or vasopressors, this condition can result in death as the result of decreased cerebral perfusion.

Intracellular Fluid

The exact composition of ICF is extremely difficult to measure because of the relative unavailability of cells free of contamination. Although erythrocytes are easily accessible, it would be incorrect to make any generalizations based on the composition of these highly specialized cells. Data for ICF (see Table 49-2), therefore, are considered only approximations. The ICF constitutes ≈66% of the total body volume (see Figure 49-1).

Reasons for Composition Differences of Body Fluids

The composition of ICF can differ markedly from that of ECF because of separation of these compartments by the cell membrane. The composition differences are a consequence of both the Gibbs-Donnan equilibrium and active and passive transport of ions.

Gibbs-Donnan Equilibrium

Two solutions separated by a semipermeable membrane will establish an equilibrium, so that all ions are equally distributed in both compartments, provided that the solutes can move freely through the membrane. At the state of equilibrium, the total ion concentration and therefore the total concentration of osmotically active particles are equal on both sides of the membrane.

If solutions on two sides of a membrane contain different concentrations of ions that cannot freely move through the membrane (e.g., proteins), distribution of diffusible ions (e.g., electrolytes) at the steady state will be unequal, but the sum of the concentrations of ions in one compartment is equal to the sum of ions in the other compartment (Gibbs-Donnan law). Also, the law of electrical neutrality is obeyed for both compartments. An example of the uneven distribution of an ion in two compartments with different protein content (nondiffusible ions) is the concentration of chloride ions in plasma and cerebrospinal fluid (CSF). As a result of increased selectivity of the blood-brain barrier against proteins, Cl^- ions are ≈15% higher in CSF to establish electrical and osmotic equilibrium.[31] Calculations that demonstrate these principles can be found in the first edition of this textbook.[27]

Cells that contain nondiffusible protein anions can withstand only a limited and temporary difference in osmotic pressure across the cell membrane. To some extent, cells adjust osmolality by producing "idiogenic osmoles" from the breakdown of macromolecules; this enhances resistance to cellular dehydration. Osmotic pressure is normally identical inside and outside the cells because the cell membrane can correct concentration differences by excluding some small ions through active, energy-requiring transport processes. If these processes cease, the cells will swell and eventually will burst (osmotic lysis).

Distribution of Ions by Active and Passive Transport

Examination of Table 49-2 reveals that the electrolyte compositions of blood plasma and interstitial fluid (both ECFs) are similar, but their compositions differ markedly from that of ICF. The major ECF ions are Na^+, Cl^-, and HCO_3^-, but in ICF, the main ions are K^+, Mg^{2+}, organic phosphates, and protein. This unequal distribution of ions is due to active transport of Na^+ from inside to outside the cell against an electrochemical gradient. This process requires energy supplied by metabolic processes in the cell (e.g., glycolysis). An active sodium pump deriving its energy from adenosine triphosphate (ATP) is present in most cell membranes and frequently is coupled with transport of K^+ into the cell. The Na^+/K^+ pump is a heterodimer consisting of a catalytic transmembrane α-subunit that is about 1000 amino acid residues long, and an associated, smaller β-subunit.[13] The internal surface has a catalytic binding site for ATP and a binding site for Na^+. The external surface has a binding site for K^+.

In addition to the Na^+/K^+-ATPase, a ubiquitous Na^+-H^+ exchanger (often referred to as an *antiporter*) actively pumps H^+ out of the ICF in exchange for Na^+.[20] This exchanger is critical for maintaining intracellular pH homeostasis in many cell types. At least six different isoforms of this transmembrane protein have been identified, and regulation and tissue distribution of these differ.[20] Of particular importance is the role of this exchanger for acid-base regulation in renal tubular cells, as discussed later in this chapter.

ELECTROLYTES

Disorders of Na^+, K^+, Cl^-, and HCO_3^- will now be separately considered, even though disorders of electrolyte and water homeostasis need a systematic evaluation.[18]

Sodium

Disorders of Na^+ homeostasis can occur because of excessive loss, gain, or retention of Na^+, or as the result of excessive loss, gain, or retention of H_2O. It is difficult to separate disorders of Na^+ and H_2O balance because of their close relationship in establishing normal osmolality in all body water compartments. As described in detail in Chapter 48, the primary organ for regulating body water and extracellular Na^+ is the kidney. As a brief introduction to this section, it is important to remind the reader of the functions of healthy kidneys.

In the proximal tubules, 70 to 80% of filtered Na^+ is actively reabsorbed, with H_2O and Cl^- following passively to maintain electrical neutrality and osmotic equivalence. In the descending loop of Henle, H_2O, but not electrolytes, is passively reabsorbed because of the high osmotic strength of interstitial fluid in the renal medulla. In the ascending loop of Henle, Cl^- is reabsorbed actively, with Na^+ following. At the level of the distal tubule, the first of the two primary Na^+/H_2O regulating processes occurs. Here, aldosterone stimulates the cortical collecting ducts to reabsorb Na^+ (with water following passively) and secrete K^+ (and to a lesser extent, H^+) to maintain electrical neutrality. Aldosterone is produced by the adrenal cortex in response to angiotensin II derived via the action of renin. The secretion of renin by renal juxtaglomerular cells is stimulated by low chloride, by β-adrenergic activity, and by low arteriolar pressure.[26] Thus when the kidneys are hypoperfused (as occurs when blood volume decreases, or when the renal arteries are obstructed), the distal tubules, under the influence of aldosterone, reclaim Na^+.

Further water regulation in the kidney occurs from the distal tubule through the collecting duct, where tubular permeability to H_2O is under the influence of antidiuretic hormone (ADH) (see Chapters 48 and 53). ADH (also called vasopressin) is released by the posterior pituitary under the influence of baroreceptors in the aortic arch and of hypothalamic chemoreceptors that are responsive to circulating osmolality, which is primarily a reflection of Na^+ concentration. When blood volume is decreased, or when plasma osmolality is increased, ADH is secreted, tubular permeability to H_2O increases via aquaporins, and H_2O is reabsorbed in an attempt to restore blood volume or to decrease osmolality. In contrast, when blood volume is increased or osmolality decreased, ADH secretion is inhibited, and more H_2O is excreted in the urine (diuresis).

Besides the kidney, the body's only other mechanism for restoring Na^+/H_2O homeostasis is ingestion of H_2O. Thirst is stimulated by decreased blood volume or by a hyperosmotic condition. It is important to remember that receptors that influence renal handling of Na^+ and H_2O, and thirst, sense changes only in the intravascular blood volume and not the total ECF. Furthermore, laboratory assessment of water and electrolyte disorders is made primarily from the blood volume (plasma). As discussed in subsequent sections, the clinician must assess the status of TBW and blood volume before interpreting laboratory values in the diagnosis of water and electrolyte disorders. The physical findings of these disorders are every bit as important as the laboratory values (see Table 49-1).

Hyponatremia

Hyponatremia is defined as a decreased plasma Na^+ concentration (<130 to 135 mmol/L). Hyponatremia typically manifests clinically as nausea, generalized weakness, and mental confusion at values <120 mmol/L, ocular palsy at <110 mmol/L, and severe mental impairment at between 90 and 105 mmol/L.[25] The rapidity of development of hyponatremia influences the Na^+ concentrations at which symptoms develop [i.e., clinically apparent symptoms may manifest at higher Na^+ concentrations (≈125 mmol/L) when hyponatremia develops rapidly].[25] It is important to note that symptoms are due to changes in osmolality rather than to the Na^+ concentration per se. Central nervous system (CNS) symptoms are due primarily to movement of H_2O into cells to maintain osmotic balance and subsequent swelling of CNS cells.

Hyponatremia can be hypo-osmotic, hyperosmotic, or isosmotic. Thus, measurement of plasma osmolality is an important initial step in the assessment of hyponatremia. Of these, the most common form is hypo-osmotic hyponatremia. Figure 49-2 describes an algorithm for laboratory measurements and physical examination findings in the differential diagnosis of plasma Na^+ <135 mmol/L.

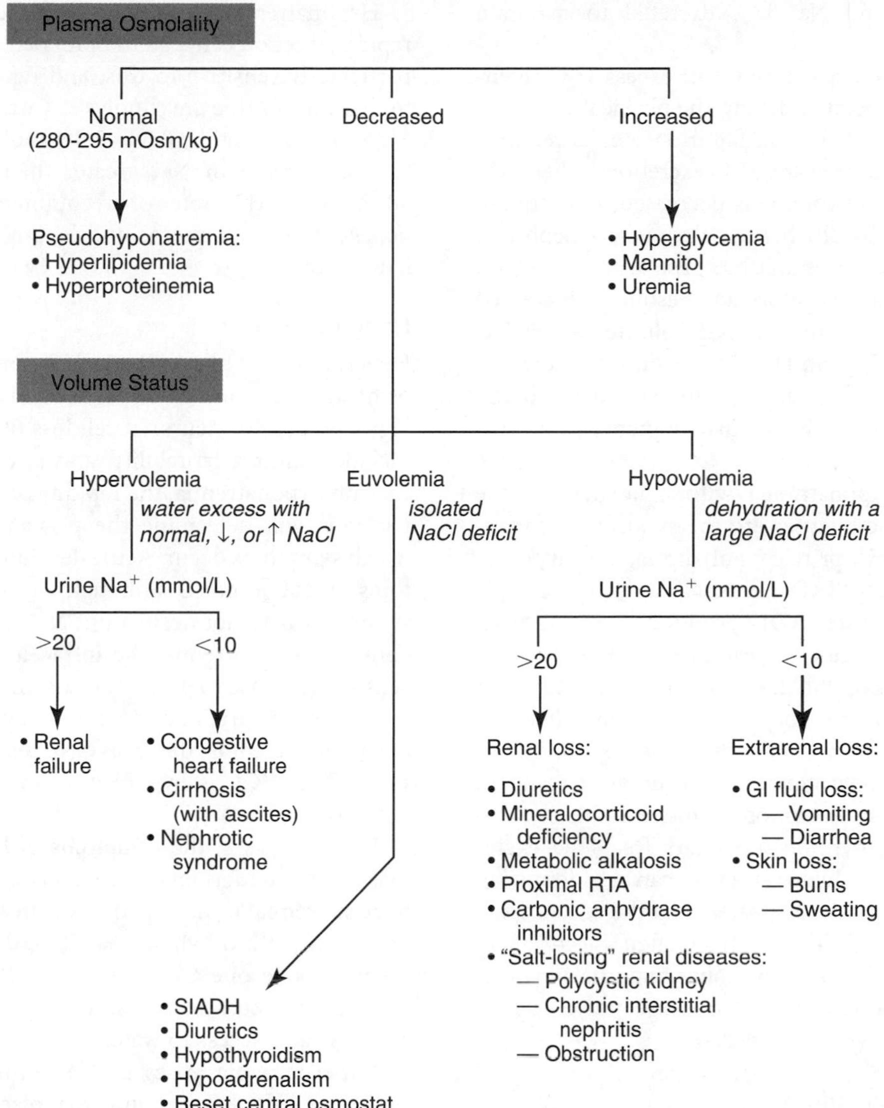

Figure 49-2 Algorithm for the differential diagnosis of hyponatremia. *(Modified from Kirkpatrick W, Kreisberg R. Acid-base and electrolyte disorders. In: Liu P, ed. Blue book of diagnostic tests. Philadelphia: WB Saunders, 1986:239-54.)*

Hypo-Osmotic Hyponatremia

Typically, when plasma Na^+ concentration is low, calculated or measured osmolality will also be low. This type of hyponatremia can be due to excess loss of Na^+ *(depletional hyponatremia)* or increased ECF volume *(dilutional hyponatremia)*. Differentiating these initially requires clinical assessment of TBW and ECF volume by history and physical examination.

Depletional hyponatremia (excess loss of Na^+) is almost always accompanied by loss of ECF water, but to a lesser extent than Na^+ loss. This occurs because thirst leads to ingestion of water, which obviously is more hypotonic than the lost fluids. Hypovolemia is apparent in the physical examination (orthostatic hypotension, tachycardia, decreased skin turgor). If urine Na^+ is low (generally <10 mmol/L), the loss is extrarenal (see Figure 49-2), as the kidneys are properly retaining filtered Na^+ in response to aldosterone, which is stimulated by hypovolemia. Causes of extrarenal loss of Na^+ in excess of H_2O include losses from the gastrointestinal tract or skin (see Figure 49-2).

Alternatively, if urine Na^+ is elevated in this setting (generally >20 mmol/L), renal loss of Na^+ is likely. Renal loss of Na^+ occurs with (1) osmotic diuresis, (2) use of diuretics (inhibit reabsorption of Cl^- and Na^+ in the ascending loop), (3) adrenal insufficiency (no aldosterone or cortisone prevents distal tubule reabsorption of Na^+), or (4) salt wasting nephropathies, as can occur with interstitial nephritis and tubular recovery after acute tubular necrosis or obstructive nephropathy. Renal loss of Na^+ in excess of H_2O can also occur in metabolic alkalosis from prolonged vomiting, because increased renal HCO_3^- excretion is accompanied by Na^+ ions. In this case, urine sodium is elevated (>20 mmol/L), but urine chloride remains low. In proximal renal tubular acidosis (RTA), bicarbonate is lost because of a defect in

HCO_3^- reabsorption, and Na^+ is coexcreted to maintain electrical neutrality.

Dilutional hyponatremia is a result of excess H_2O retention and often can be detected during the physical examination as edema. In advanced renal failure, water is retained because of decreased filtration and H_2O excretion. When ECF is increased but the blood volume is decreased, as occurs in congestive heart failure (CHF), hepatic cirrhosis, or nephrotic syndrome, a vicious cycle is established. The decreased blood volume is sensed by baroreceptors and results in increased aldosterone and ADH, even though ECF volume is excessive. The kidneys reabsorb Na^+ and H_2O in response to increased aldosterone and ADH in an attempt to restore the blood volume, but this simply results in further increases in ECF and further dilution of Na^+.

In hypo-osmotic hyponatremia with a normal volume status, the most common causes are the syndrome of inappropriate ADH (SIADH), primary polydipsia, and hypothyroidism (see Figure 49-2). SIADH is usually a result of ectopic or otherwise "inappropriate" ADH production arising from a variety of conditions[6] (see Chapters 48 and 53) and results in excessive H_2O retention. SIADH is often diagnosed when urine osmolality is greater than plasma osmolality, *but only when renal, adrenal, and thyroid function are normal.* In cortisol insufficiency, hyponatremia can occur as a result of increased cortisol-releasing hormone, which stimulates vasopressin release.[29] Hypothyroidism impairs free H_2O excretion. Finally, euvolemic hyponatremia can be found in polydipsia when water intake is greater than the renal capacity to excrete excess H_2O. This is most often the result of psychiatric illness, but diseases that cause hypothalamic disorders, such as sarcoidosis, may also cause polydipsia by altering the thirst reflex (see Figure 49-2).

Hyperosmotic Hyponatremia

Hyponatremia that occurs in the presence of increased quantities of other solutes in the ECF is the result of an extracellular shift of water or an intracellular shift of Na^+ to maintain osmotic balance between ECF and ICF compartments. The most common cause of this type of hyponatremia is severe hyperglycemia (see Figure 49-2). As a general rule, Na^+ is decreased by ≈1.6 to 2.4 mmol/L for every 100 mg/dL increase in glucose above 100 mg/dL.[30] Correction of hyperglycemia will restore normal blood Na^+.

Isosmotic Hyponatremia

If the measured Na^+ concentration in plasma is decreased, but measured plasma osmolality, glucose, and urea are normal, the most likely explanation is pseudohyponatremia caused by the *electrolyte exclusion effect* (see Chapter 28). This occurs when Na^+ is measured by an indirect ion-selective electrode (and flame photometry in the past) in patients with severe hyperlipidemia. It can also occur when osmotically active agents such as mannitol and glycine are used in irrigation fluids for transurethral resection of the prostate (TURP) and endometrial ablation.

Hyponatremia must be corrected cautiously because too rapid correction can lead to brain demyelination. The pons is particularly sensitive to this, and rapid correction can lead to central pontine myelinolysis. Current recommendations are to increase Na^+ by 0.5 to 2.0 mmol/L/h and not to exceed a total increase in Na^+ greater than 18 to 25 mmol over 48 hours.[30] The rate of recommended Na^+ increase is dependent on symptoms and length of time the patient is hyponatremic.

Hypernatremia[1]

Hypernatremia (plasma Na^+ >150 mmol/L) is always hyperosmolar. Symptoms of hypernatremia are primarily neurologic (because of neuronal cell loss of H_2O to the ECF) and include tremors, irritability, ataxia, confusion, and coma.[25] As with hyponatremia, the rapidity of development of hypernatremia will determine the plasma Na^+ concentration at which symptoms occur. Acute development may cause symptoms at 160 mmol/L, although in chronic hypernatremia, symptoms may not occur until Na^+ exceeds 175 mmol/L. In chronic hypernatremia, the intracellular osmolality of CNS cells will increase to protect against intracellular dehydration. Because of this, rapid correction of hypernatremia can cause dangerous cerebral edema, as CNS cells will take up too much water if the ICF is hyperosmotic when normonatremia is achieved.[25]

In many cases, the symptoms of hypernatremia may be masked by underlying conditions. Indeed, most cases of hypernatremia occur in patients with altered mental status or in infants, both of whom may have difficulty in rehydrating themselves despite a normal thirst reflex. Thus, hypernatremia rarely occurs in an alert patient with a normal thirst response and access to water.

Hypernatremia arises in the setting of (1) hypovolemia (excessive water loss or failure to replace normal water losses), (2) hypervolemia (a net Na^+ gain in excess of water gain), or (3) normovolemia. Again, assessment of TBW status by physical examination and measurement of urine Na^+ and osmolality are important steps in establishing a diagnosis (Figure 49-3).

Hypovolemic Hypernatremia

Hypernatremia in the setting of decreased ECF is caused by renal or extrarenal loss of hypo-osmotic fluid, leading to dehydration. Thus once hypovolemia is established by physical examination, measurement of urine Na^+ and osmolality is used to determine the source of fluid loss. Patients who have large extrarenal losses will have concentrated urine (often >800 mOsmol/L) with low urine Na^+ (<20 mmol/L), reflecting a proper renal response to conserve Na^+ and water to restore ECF volume. Extrarenal causes include diarrhea, skin losses (burns, fever, or excessive sweating), and respiratory losses coupled with failure to replace the water. When gastrointestinal loss is excluded, and the patient has normal mental status and access to H_2O, a hypothalamic disorder (tumor or granuloma) should be suspected, because the

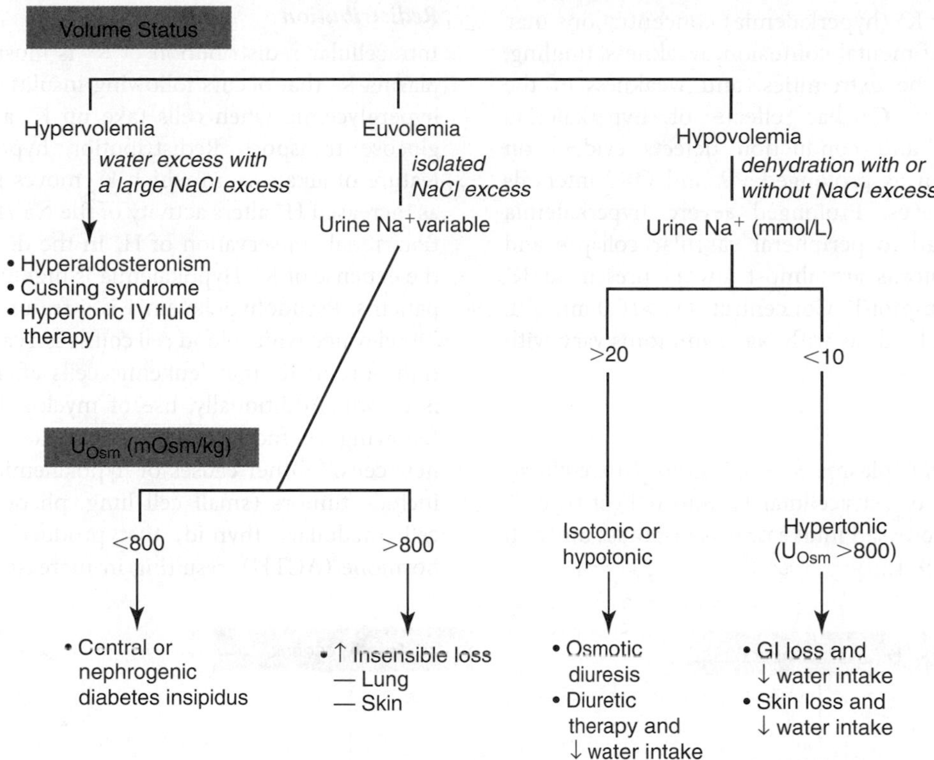

Figure 49-3 Algorithm for the differential diagnosis of hypernatremia. *(Modified from Kirkpatrick W, Kreisberg R. Acid-base and electrolyte disorders. In: Liu P, ed. Blue book of diagnostic tests. Philadelphia: WB Saunders, 1986:239-54.)*

normal thirst response should always replace insensible water losses.[25]

Normovolemic Hypernatremia

Hypernatremia in the presence of normal ECF volume is often a prelude to hypovolemic hypernatremia. Insensible losses through the lung or skin again must be suspected and are characterized by concentrated urine as the kidneys conserve water. Another cause of normovolemic hypernatremia is water diuresis, which is manifested by polyuria (see Figure 49-3). The differential for polyuria (generally defined as >3 L urine output/d) is a water or solute diuresis. Solute diuresis is exemplified by the osmotic diuresis of diabetes mellitus and generally is characterized by urine osmolality >300 mOsmol/L and hyponatremia (see previous discussion in this chapter). Water diuresis, a manifestation of diabetes insipidus (DI), is characterized by dilute urine (osmolality <250 mOsmol/L) and slight hypernatremia.[25] DI can be central or nephrogenic.[21] Central DI is due to decreased or absent ADH secretion resulting from head trauma, hypophysectomy, pituitary tumor, or granulomatous disease. Nephrogenic DI is due to renal resistance to ADH as a result of drugs (e.g., lithium, demeclocycline, amphotericin, propoxyphene); sickle cell anemia and Sjögren syndrome, which affect collecting duct responsiveness to ADH; or, more rarely, mutant ADH receptors.[2] Central DI usually is treated with vasopressin, whereas nephrogenic DI is treated by discontinuing the drug or providing easy access to water, which will maintain normonatremia.

Hypervolemic Hypernatremia

The presence of excess TBW and hypernatremia indicates a net gain of water and Na^+, with Na^+ gain in excess of water (see Figure 49-3). This rare condition is observed most commonly in hospital patients receiving hypertonic saline or sodium bicarbonate.

Potassium

The total body potassium of a 70 kg subject is ≈3.5 mol (40 to 59 mmol/kg), of which only 1.5 to 2% is present in the ECF. Nevertheless, plasma K^+ is often a good indicator of total K^+ stores, unless abnormal K^+ is due to abnormal cellular shifts. Disturbance of K^+ homeostasis has serious consequences. For example, a decrease in extracellular K^+ (hypokalemia) is characterized by muscle weakness, irritability, and paralysis. Plasma K^+ concentrations less than 3.0 mmol/L are often associated with marked neuromuscular symptoms and indicate a critical degree of intracellular depletion. At lower concentrations, tachycardia and cardiac conduction defects are apparent by electrocardiogram (flattened T waves) and can lead to cardiac arrest.[25]

High extracellular K^+ (hyperkalemia) concentrations may produce symptoms of mental confusion, weakness, tingling, flaccid paralysis of the extremities, and weakness of the respiratory muscles.[25] Cardiac effects of hyperkalemia include bradycardia and conduction defects evident on the electrocardiogram as prolonged PR and QRS intervals and "peaked" T waves. Prolonged severe hyperkalemia >7.0 mmol/L can lead to peripheral vascular collapse and cardiac arrest. Symptoms are almost always present at K^+ concentrations >6.5 mmol/L. Concentrations >10.0 mmol/L in most cases are fatal, but as with Na^+, symptoms vary with the rapidity of onset.

Hypokalemia

Causes of *hypokalemia* (plasma K^+ <3.5 mmol/L) are classified as redistribution of extracellular K^+ into ICF, or true K^+ deficits, caused by decreased intake or loss of potassium-rich body fluids (Figure 49-4).

Redistribution

Intracellular redistribution of K^+ is illustrated by the fall in plasma K^+ that occurs following insulin therapy for diabetic hyperglycemia when cells take up K^+ as a consequence of glucose transport. Redistribution hypokalemia is also a feature of alkalosis, in which K^+ moves from ECF into cells as increased H^+ alters activity of the Na^+/K^+-ATPase. In addition, renal conservation of H^+ in the distal tubule occurs at the expense of K^+. Hypokalemia is highly prevalent in cancer patients. Pseudohypokalemia is a feature of acute leukemia. The elevated white blood cell count can cause time-dependent transport of K^+ into leukemic cells after the blood sample is drawn. Additionally, use of myelopoietic growth factors following chemotherapy can lead to rapid K^+ uptake by new cells.[17] Other causes of hypokalemia in cancer patients include tumors (small cell lung, pheochromocytoma, islet cell, medullary thyroid) that produce adrenocorticotropic hormone (ACTH), resulting in increased cortisol and renal

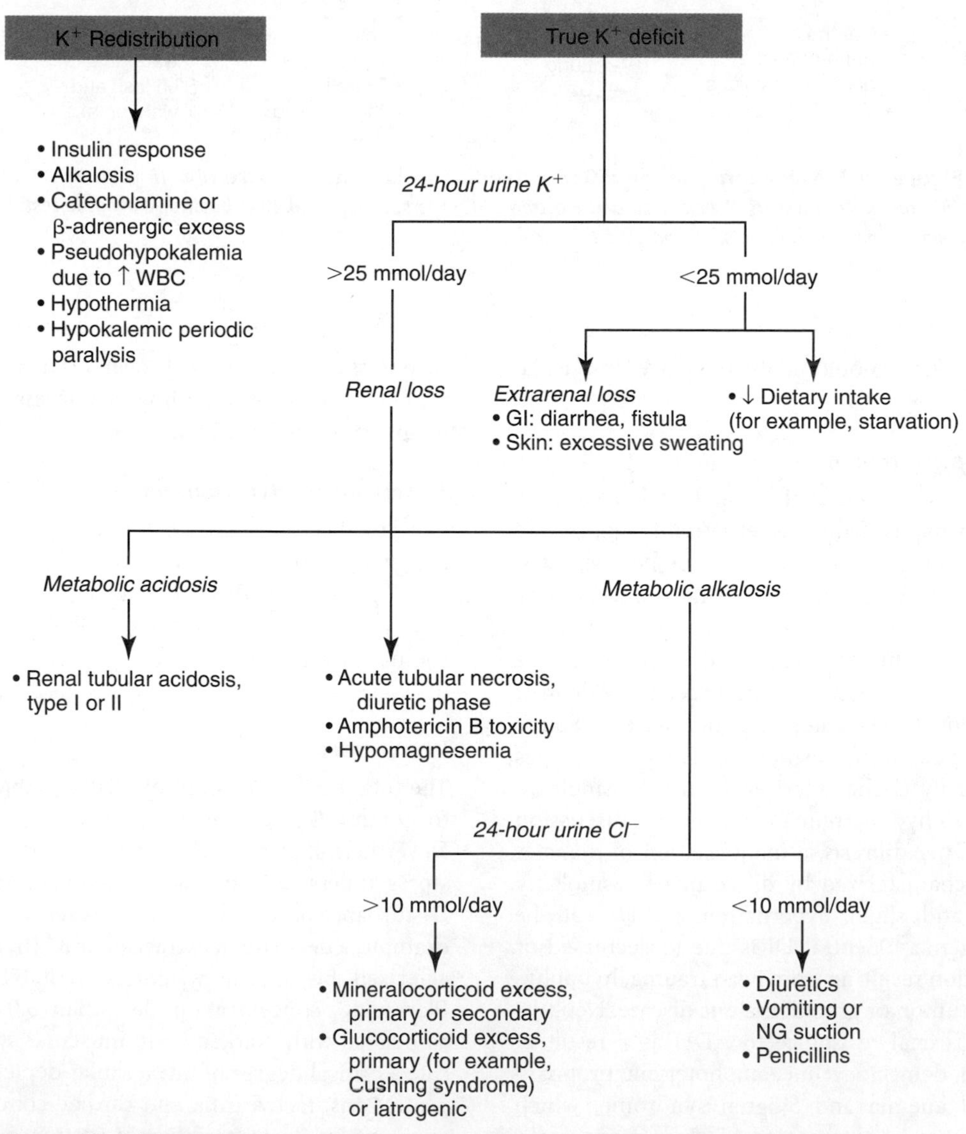

Figure 49-4 Algorithm for the differential diagnosis of hypokalemia. *(Modified from Kirkpatrick W, Kreisberg R. Acid-base and electrolyte disorders. In: Liu P, ed. Blue book of diagnostic tests. Philadelphia: WB Saunders, 1986:239-54.)*

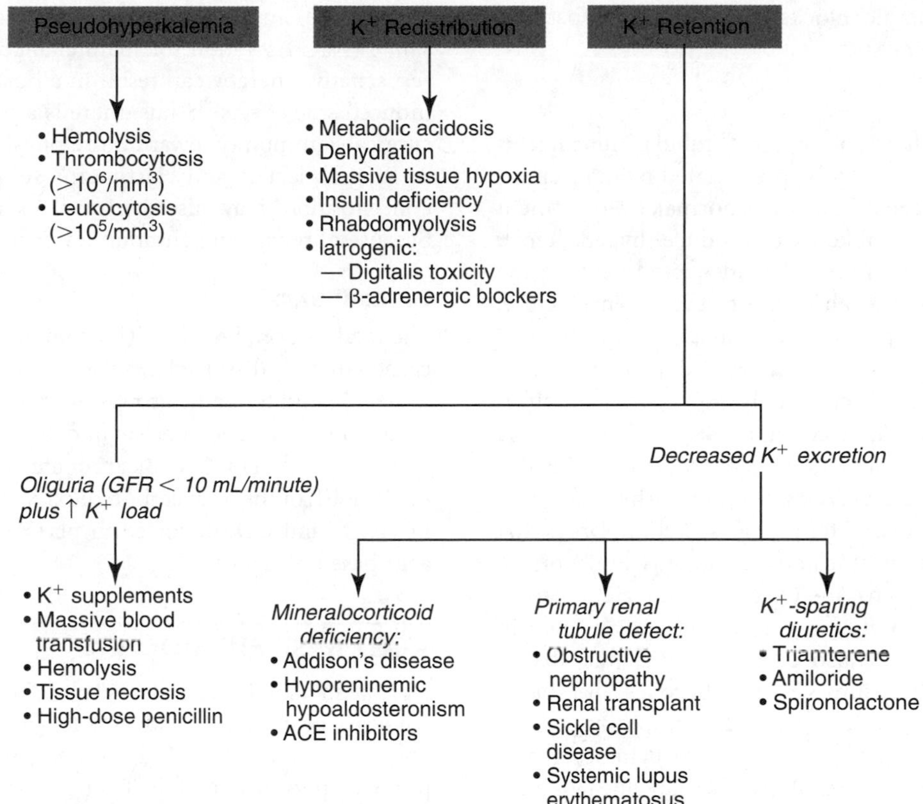

Figure 49-5 Algorithm for the differential diagnosis of hyperkalemia. *(Modified from Kirkpatrick W, Kreisberg R. Acid-base and electrolyte disorders. In: Liu P, ed. Blue book of diagnostic tests. Philadelphia: WB Saunders, 1986:239-54.)*

loss of K^+. Other causes of intracellular redistribution are listed in Figure 49-4.

True Potassium Deficit

Hypokalemia reflecting true total body deficits of K^+ can be classified into renal and nonrenal losses, based on daily excretion of K^+ in the urine (see Figure 49-4). If urine excretion of K^+ is <30 mmol/d, it can be concluded that the kidneys are properly functioning and are attempting to reabsorb K^+ as appropriate in a hypokalemic setting. The cause may be decreased K^+ intake or extrarenal loss of K^+-rich fluid. Situations of decreased intake include chronic starvation and postoperative intravenous fluid therapy with K^+-poor solutions. Gastrointestinal loss of K^+ occurs most commonly with diarrhea and loss of gastric fluid through vomiting or prolonged nasogastric suction.

Urine excretion exceeding 25 to 30 mmol/d in a hypokalemic setting is inappropriate and indicates that the kidneys are the primary source of lost K^+. Renal losses of K^+ may occur during the diuretic (recovery) phase of acute tubular necrosis and during states of excess mineralocorticoid (primary or secondary aldosteronism) or glucocorticoid (Cushing syndrome) when the distal tubules increase Na^+ reabsorption and K^+ excretion. Renal loss of K^+ is also caused by thiazide and loop diuretics.[16] In addition to redistribution of K^+ into cells in an alkalotic setting, K^+ can be lost from the kidneys in exchange for reclaimed H^+ ions. This cause of true hypokalemia will be evident in low urine Cl^- and an alkaline urine. In cancer patients, increased renal K^+ loss is due to chemotherapy (e.g., cisplatin)-induced nephron and tubular damage.[17]

Hyperkalemia

Hyperkalemia (plasma K^+ >5.0 mmol/L) is a result of (singly or in combination) (1) redistribution, (2) increased intake, or (3) increased retention. In addition, preanalytical conditions—such as hemolysis, thrombocytosis (>10^6/μL), and leukocytosis (>10^5/μL)—have been known to cause marked pseudohyperkalemia, as described in detail in Chapter 28 (Figure 49-5).

Redistribution

The transfer of intracellular K^+ into ECF invariably occurs in acidosis as K^+ shifts outward as the result of pH-induced changes in Na^+/K^+-ATPase activity. As a general rule, K^+ concentrations can be expected to rise 0.2 to 0.7 mmol/L for every 0.1 unit drop in pH. When acidosis is corrected, normokalemia will be restored rapidly. Extracellular redistribution of K^+ may also occur in (1) tissue hypoxia; (2) insulin deficiency (e.g., diabetic ketoacidosis); (3) massive intravascular hemolysis; (4) severe burns; (5) violent muscular activity, as in status epilepticus; (6) rhabdomyolysis; and (7) tumor lysis syndrome. Finally, important iatrogenic causes of redistribution hyperkalemia include digoxin toxicity and β-adrenergic blockade, especially in patients with diabetes or on dialysis.[25]

Potassium Retention

When glomerular filtration or renal tubular function is decreased, hyperkalemia may be precipitated by intravenous infusion of K^+. When renal function is normal, overtreatment with K^+ solutions is unlikely to produce hyperkalemia, because renal capacity is more than adequate to excrete the excess K^+. Indeed, in the absence of severe renal failure, hyperkalemia is seldom prolonged. Decreased excretion of K^+ in moderate and acute renal disease and end-stage renal failure (with oliguria or anuria) are the most common causes of prolonged hyperkalemia (see Figure 49-5). Hyperkalemia occurs along with Na^+ depletion in adrenocortical insufficiency (e.g., Addison disease) because diminished Na^+ reabsorption results in decreased tubular K^+ secretion. Drugs that block the production of aldosterone, such as inhibitors of angiotensin-converting enzyme (ACE inhibitors; e.g., lisinopril), nonsteroidal anti-inflammatory drugs, and angiotensin II receptor blockers, may also cause hyperkalemia. Excess administration of potassium-sparing diuretics that block distal tubular K^+ secretion (e.g., triamterene, spironolactone) commonly causes hyperkalemia.[11] In cancer patients, hyperkalemia can be caused by adrenal insufficiency due to metastases to the adrenal glands, nephrotoxic chemotherapy agents (e.g., mitomycin-C, methotrexate, platinum compounds), postrenal obstruction, or tumor lysis syndrome.[17] Treatment of hyperkalemia includes agents that increase cellular uptake of K^+ such as calcium gluconate, glucose and insulin, sodium bicarbonate, and β_2-adrenergic agonists. Potassium can be removed from the circulation with the use of K^+-losing diuretics, cation-exchange resins, and finally hemodialysis.[17]

Chloride

In the absence of acid-base disturbances, Cl^- concentrations in plasma generally will follow those of Na^+. However, determination of plasma Cl^- concentration is useful in the differential diagnosis of acid-base disturbances and is essential for calculating the anion gap. Fluctuations in serum or plasma Cl^- have little clinical consequence, but do serve as signs of an underlying disturbance in fluid or acid-base homeostasis.

Hypochloremia

In general, causes of hypochloremia will parallel causes of hyponatremia. Persistent gastric secretion and prolonged vomiting result in significant loss of Cl^- and ultimately in hypochloremic alkalosis and depletion of total body Cl^- with retention of HCO_3^-. Respiratory acidosis, which is accompanied by increased HCO_3^-, is another common cause of decreased Cl^- with normal Na^+.

Hyperchloremia

Increased plasma Cl^- concentration, similar to increased Na^+ concentration, occurs with dehydration, prolonged diarrhea with loss of sodium bicarbonate, DI, and overtreatment with normal saline solutions, which have a Cl^- content of 154 mmol/L. In fact, mounting evidence suggests that use of saline (NaCl) solution for maintenance, intraoperative, and resuscitative therapy can result in a host of hyperchloremia-induced side effects.[10] Thus, there is a movement among the surgical community toward more physiologic solutions such as Ringer's lactate and Hartmann's solution.[10] A rise in Cl^- concentration may also be seen in respiratory alkalosis because of renal compensation for excreting HCO_3^-.

Bicarbonate

The total carbon dioxide (CO_2) content of plasma consists of carbon dioxide dissolved in an aqueous solution (dCO_2), CO_3 loosely bound to amine groups in proteins (carbamino compounds), HCO_3^-, and very small quantities of CO_3^{2-} ions and carbonic acid (H_2CO_3). Bicarbonate ions make up all but ≈2 mmol/L of the total carbon dioxide of plasma. Alterations in HCO_3^- and CO_2 dissolved in plasma are characteristic of acid-base imbalances.

ACID-BASE PHYSIOLOGY

Normal metabolic processes result in the production of large amounts of carbonic acid and lesser amounts of sulfuric, phosphoric, and other acids. For example, during a 24 hour period, a person weighing 70 kg disposes of about 20 mol of carbon dioxide (the volatile form of carbonic acid) through the lungs, and about 70 to 100 mmol (or ≈1 mmol/kg) of nonvolatile acids (mainly sulfuric and phosphoric acids) through the kidneys. These products of metabolism are transported to the lungs and kidneys via the ECF and blood with no appreciable change in the ECF pH, and with only a minimal difference between arterial (pH 7.35 to 7.45) and venous (pH 7.32 to 7.38) blood. This is accomplished by the buffering capacity of blood and by respiratory and renal regulatory mechanisms.

Acid-Base Balance and Acid-Base Status

A description of acid-base balance involves an accounting of the carbonic (H_2CO_3, HCO_3^-, CO_3^{2-}, and CO_2) and noncarbonic acids and conjugate bases in terms of input (intake plus metabolic production) and output (excretion plus metabolic conversion) over a given time interval. The acid-base status of body fluids is typically assessed by measurements of total CO_2, plasma pH, and PCO_2, because the bicarbonate/carbonic acid system is the most important mammalian buffering system.

The following clinical terms are used to describe acid-base status. *Acidemia* is defined as an arterial blood pH <7.35, and *alkalemia* indicates an arterial blood pH >7.45. *Acidosis* and *alkalosis* refer to pathologic states that often lead to acidemia or alkalemia. For example, in common acid-base disorders such as lactic acidosis and diabetic ketoacidosis, intermediate organic acids (lactic acid and β hydroxybutyric acid, respectively), which normally are metabolized to carbon dioxide and water, may accumulate to a significant extent, resulting in acidemia. Additionally, more than one type of pathologic process can occur simultaneously, giving rise to a mixed acid-base disturbance, in which the blood pH may be low, high, or within the reference interval. To understand how these and other perturbations of acid-base metabolism affect human physiology, it will be necessary to examine briefly the concepts of acids, bases, pH, and buffers in relation to the relevant systems that function to maintain normal acid-base balance in the human body.

Acid-Base Parameters—Definitions and Abbreviations

Acids are chemical substances that can donate protons (H^+ ions) in solution, and *bases* are substances that accept protons. Strong acids readily give up H^+, whereas strong bases readily accept H^+. Thus the conjugate base of a strong acid is a weak base and vice versa.

pH and pK

The pH of a solution is defined as the negative logarithm of the hydrogen ion activity (pH = $-\log aH^+$). Thus *pH is a dimensionless quantity,* such that a decrease in one pH unit represents a tenfold increase in H^+ activity. Potentiometric determinations of blood pH measure H^+ activity and not H^+ concentration, although the activity is assumed to equal the concentration. The average pH of blood (7.40) corresponds to a hydrogen ion concentration of 40 nmol/L, but this assumes an activity coefficient of 1. The relationship between hydrogen ion activity and pH is illustrated in Figure 49-6. This relationship is inverse and is obviously nonlinear. Expressing the acidity of blood in terms of its hydrogen ion concentration in nanomoles per liter (nmol/L) has the advantage of avoiding logarithmic transformations when acid-base calculations are performed. Even though it would be consistent with how other ion concentrations are expressed, this method has not gained widespread use in the United States.

The pK (also, pK' and pK_a) represents the negative logarithm of the ionization constant of a weak acid (K_a), that is, the pK is the pH at which an acid is half dissociated, existing as equal proportions of acid and conjugate base. Thus acids have pK values <7.0, whereas bases have pK values >7.0. The lower the pK, the stronger the acid, and the higher the pK, the stronger the conjugate base. For example, the pK of lactic acid is 3.86, and that of ammonium ion NH_4^+ is 9.5. The high pK for the ammonium ion indicates that this species prefers to hold onto its proton, rather than dissociating into NH_3 and H^+.

The pH of plasma may be considered to be a function of two independent variables: (1) the PCO_2, which is regulated by the lungs and represents the acid component of the carbonic acid/bicarbonate buffer system, and (2) the concentration of titratable base (base excess or deficit, which is defined later), which is regulated by the kidneys. The plasma total CO_2 (bicarbonate) concentration generally is taken as a measure of the base excess or deficit in plasma and ECF, although conditions exist in which it may not accurately reflect the true base excess or deficit.

Bicarbonate and Dissolved CO_2

Bicarbonate is the second largest fraction (behind Cl^-) of plasma anions (≈25 mmol/L). Conventionally, it is defined to include (1) plasma bicarbonate ion (HCO_3^-), (2) carbonate ion (CO_3^{2-}), and (3) CO_2 bound in plasma carbamino compounds (Figure 49-7). At the pH of blood, the plasma carbonate concentration is ≈25 µmol/L, which is ≈ $\frac{1}{700}$ to $\frac{1}{1000}$ of the total bicarbonate fraction. CO_2-bound carbamino compounds (RCNHCOOH) are 0.2 mmol/L in plasma and 1.5 mmol/L in erythrocytes. Actual bicarbonate ion concentration is not measured, but rather is calculated from the

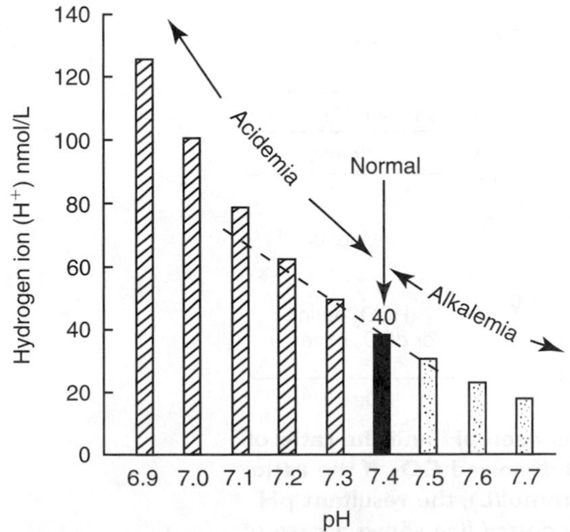

Figure 49-6 Relationship of pH to hydrogen ion concentration. A *broken line* is drawn to emphasize the (approximate) linear relationship between hydrogen ion concentration and pH over the pH range of 7.2 to 7.5. *(From Narins RG, Emmett M. Simple and mixed acid-base disorders: a practical approach. Medicine 1980;59:161-87.)*

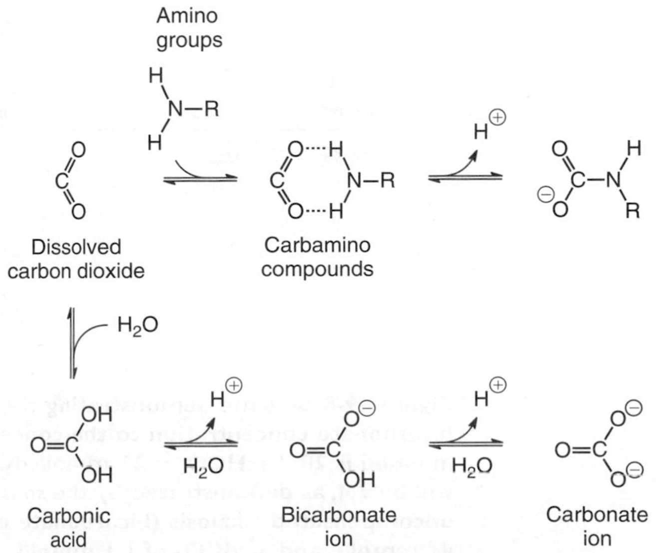

Figure 49-7 Reactions of CO_2 with water and amino groups. Hydrogen bonding is indicated by a *dotted line.* The carbamino acid is fairly strong (—R—NH—COOH → H^+ + R—NH—COO^-).

Henderson-Hasselbalch equation as described later (and discussed in detail in Chapter 28). Also as described in Chapter 28, the analyte usually measured in plasma is total CO_2, which includes bicarbonate and dissolved CO_2 (dCO_2). At the pH of the blood, the amount of dissolved CO_2 is 700 to 1000 times greater than the amount of carbonic acid (H_2CO_3); therefore $cdCO_2$ is the term used to express their combined concentration. It is calculated from the solubility coefficient of CO_2 in blood at 37 °C ($\alpha = 0.0306$ mmol/L per mm Hg) multiplied by the measured PCO_2 in mm Hg. Thus at a PCO_2 of 40 mm Hg, $cdCO_2$ is 1.224 mmol/L (0.0306 mmol/L × 40 mm Hg). This $cdCO_2$ value can then be used, in the Henderson-Hasselbalch equation, to calculate the total bicarbonate concentration.

Henderson-Hasselbalch Equation

The Henderson-Hasselbalch equation is described in detail in Chapter 28. However, it is important to review this equation here because it enhances understanding of pH regulation of body fluids as it relates to compensatory mechanisms of the body in acid-base disturbances. The equation derived in Chapter 28 can also be written as follows:

$$\text{pH} = 6.1 + \log \frac{cHCO_3^-}{cdCO_2}$$

where $cdCO_2$ is equal to α (0.0306 mmol/L per mm Hg) PCO_2 and 6.1 is the pK' for the carbonic acid/bicarbonate system. An alternative expression useful for approximating cH^+ in blood is as follows:

$$cH^+ = K \times \frac{PCO_2}{cHCO_3^-}$$

where $K = 24$ (nmol/L)(mmol/L)(mm Hg^{-1}).

The average normal ratio of the concentrations of bicarbonate and dissolved carbon dioxide in plasma is 25 (mmol/L)/1.25 (mmol/L) = 20/1. It follows then that any change in the concentration of bicarbonate or dissolved CO_2 relative to each other must be accompanied by a change in pH. Such changes in this important ratio can occur through a change in $cHCO_3^-$ (the renal component) or in PCO_2 (the respiratory component). Clinical conditions characterized as *metabolic* disturbances of acid-base balance are classified as primary disturbances in $cHCO_3^-$. Those characterized as *respiratory* disturbances are classified as primary disturbances in $cdCO_2$ (PCO_2). Various compensatory mechanisms attempting to re-establish the normal ratio of $cHCO_3^-/cdCO_2$ may result in changes in bicarbonate concentration, dissolved CO_2 concentration, or both. Application of the Henderson-Hasselbalch equation to human acid-base physiology can be illustrated by a lever-fulcrum (teeter-totter) diagram (Figure 49-8).

Buffer Systems and Their Role in Regulating the pH of Body Fluids

A buffer is a mixture of a weak acid and a salt of its conjugate base that resists changes in pH when a strong acid or base is added to the solution. If concentrations of the acid and base components of a buffer are equal, the pH will equal the pK.

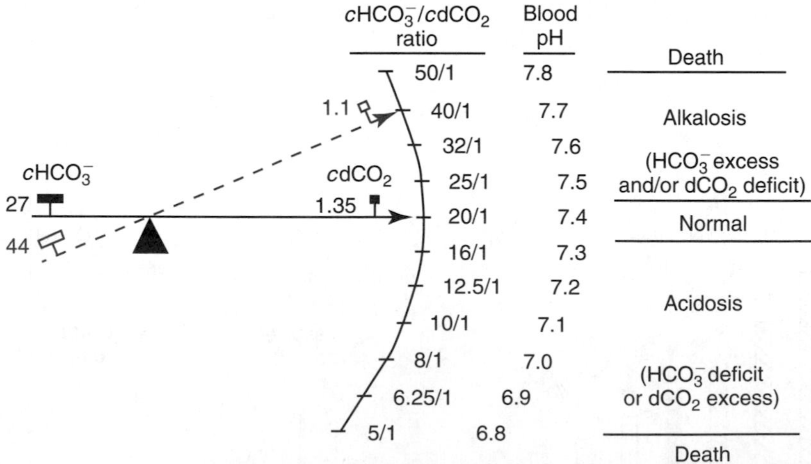

Figure 49-8 Scheme demonstrating the relation between pH and the ratio of bicarbonate concentration to the concentration of dissolved CO_2. If the ratio in blood is 20:1 ($cHCO_3^-$ = 27 mmol/$cdCO_2$ = 1.35 mmol/L), the resultant pH will be 7.4, as demonstrated by the *solid beam*. The *dotted line* shows a case of uncompensated alkalosis (bicarbonate excess) with a bicarbonate concentration of 44 mmol/L and a $cdCO_2$ of 1.1 mmol/L. The ratio therefore is 40:1, and the resultant pH is 7.7. In a case of uncompensated acidosis, the pointer of the balance would point to a pH between 6.8 and 7.35, depending on the $cHCO_3^-/cdCO_2$ ratio. *[From Weisberg HF. A better understanding of anion-cation ("acid-base") balance. Surg Clin North Am 1959;39:93-120.]*

Generally, buffers work best at resisting pH changes in the interval ±1 pH unit of its p*K*, that is, buffers work best when the ratio of acid/base is within the range of 10:1 to 1:10. Buffers are also more effective at higher concentrations, so that a 10 mmol/L buffer solution is more effective than a 1.0 mmol/L solution.

The action of buffers in the regulation of body pH can be explained by using the bicarbonate buffer system as an example. If a strong acid is added to a solution containing HCO_3^- and H_2CO_3, the H^+ will react with HCO_3^- to form more H_2CO_3, and subsequently CO_2 and H_2O. The hydrogen ions are thereby bound, and the increase in the H^+ concentration will be minimal.

$$H^+ + HCO_3^- \rightleftharpoons H_2CO_3 \rightleftharpoons CO_2 + H_2O$$

Bicarbonate/Carbonic Acid Buffer System

The most important buffer of plasma is the bicarbonate/carbonic acid pair. Initially, one might not think that this buffer would be very effective because its p*K* is 6.1, whereas normal plasma pH is 7.4, which is outside the general limits for good buffering capacity. Also note that the normal bicarbonate/dCO_2 ratio is 20:1, which is outside the 10:1 or 1:10 ratio at which buffers work best. However, the effectiveness of the bicarbonate buffer is based on the fact that the lungs can readily dispose of or retain CO_2, and that other than hemoglobin and other serum proteins, it is present at higher concentrations than other buffers. In addition, the renal tubules can increase or decrease the rate of reclamation of bicarbonate from the glomerular filtrate (see Chapter 48). The importance of the relatively high concentration of bicarbonate (relative to H^+) becomes apparent when one considers that at normal plasma pH, 5 mmol/L of lactate (p*K* ≈3.86) generates ≈5 mmol/L of H^+ ion, which is remarkable given that a normal H^+ ion concentration is only 40 nmol/L. The buffer value (β) is defined as the amount of base required to cause a change in pH of one unit. The buffer value of the bicarbonate buffer in plasma is 55.6 mmol/L. Derivation of this value is attained by taking partial differentials of the Henderson-Hasselbalch equation, which is presented in detail in the second edition of this textbook.[28]

Phosphate Buffer System

At a plasma pH of 7.4, the ratio $cHPO_4^{2-}/cH_2PO_4^-$ is 4:1 (pK′ = 6.8). The total concentration of this buffer in both erythrocytes and plasma accounts for about 5% of the nonbicarbonate buffer value of plasma. Organic phosphate, however, in the form of 2,3-diphosphoglycerate (present in erythrocytes in a concentration of about 4.5 mmol/L), accounts for about 16% of the nonbicarbonate buffer value of erythrocytes.

The phosphate buffer reacts with acids and with bases as follows:

$$HPO_4^{\oplus\oplus} + H^{\oplus} \rightarrow H_2PO_4^{\oplus}$$
$$H_2PO_4^{\oplus} + OH^{\ominus} \rightarrow HPO_4^{\oplus\oplus} + H_2O$$

This system is most important in the titration and excretion of acids in urine.

Plasma Protein Buffer System and Plasma Base Excess

The buffer value (β) of the nonbicarbonate buffers of plasma totals about 7.7 mmol/L at pH 7.40 and a normal plasma protein concentration of 72 g/L. Proteins, especially albumin, account for the greatest portion (>90%) of the nonbicarbonate buffer value of plasma. The most important buffer groups of proteins in the physiologic pH range are the imidazole groups of histidines (p*K* ≈7.3). Each albumin molecule contains 16 histidines.

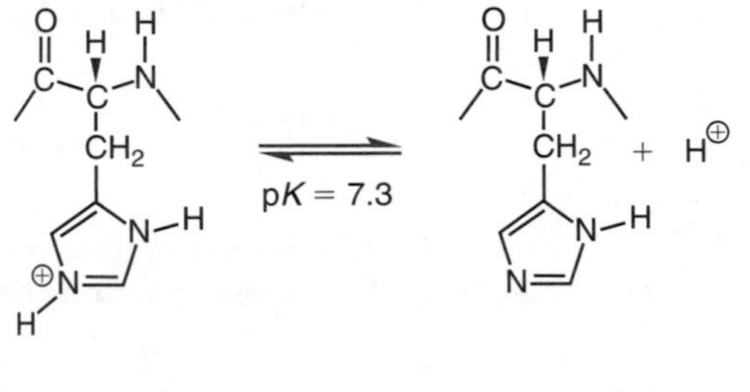

The significance of nonbicarbonate buffers of plasma can be illustrated by the chemical reactions during CO_2 equilibration:

$$CO_2 + H_2O \rightarrow H_2CO_3 \rightarrow HCO_3^{\ominus} + H^{\oplus}$$
$$HPr \rightarrow H^{\oplus} + Pr^{\ominus}$$

where the HPr/Pr^- system represents all nonbicarbonate buffers. Because the purpose of this buffer system is to maintain cH^+ constant, for each molecule of HCO_3^- that is generated, one molecule of nonbicarbonate buffer base disappears. Thus in alkalosis, the cH^+ from CO_2 equilibration falls, and an excess of nonbicarbonate buffer base is the result. As follows, there is a consumption or negative excess of this buffer base in acidosis.

Plasma base excess is defined as the initial concentration of titratable base when the plasma with strong acid or base is titrated to pH (Std) = 7.4 at PCO_2 = 40 mm Hg and 37 °C. The equation for the CO_2 equilibration curve of plasma and for calculation of *plasma base excess* can be written as follows:

$$\Delta cHCO_3^-(P) = [-\beta Pr \times \Delta pH(P)] + \Delta cB'(P)$$

where $\Delta cHCO_3^-$ = actual HCO_3^- minus the standard HCO_3^- of 24.5 mmol/L, ΔpH = measured pH minus 7.40, and $\Delta cB'(P)$ is the plasma base excess.

Hemoglobin Buffer System and Whole Blood Base Excess

The buffer value (β) of the nonbicarbonate buffers of erythrocyte fluid is about 63 mmol/L at pH 7.20, for an erythrocyte hemoglobin concentration of 21 mmol/L (33.8 g/dL). Hemoglobin accounts for the major part (53 mmol/L), with the remainder being caused mainly by 2,3-diphosphoglycerate (2,3-DPG). The imidazole groups of hemoglobin are quantitatively the most important buffer groups.

As in plasma, CO_2 equilibration of whole blood depends on the buffer value of nonbicarbonate buffers. Thus CO_2 equilibration in whole blood is dependent on hemoglobin concentration and also on pH and oxygenation status. It is

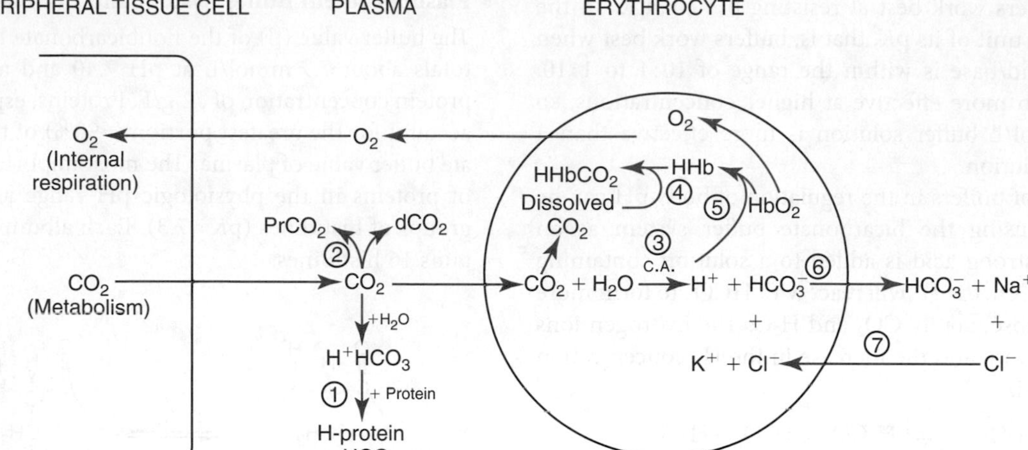

Figure 49-9 Scheme demonstrating the isohydric and chloride shift. The *encircled numbers* refer to the reactions described in the text. For details, see text.

possible to derive an approximate equation for whole blood CO_2 equilibration and calculation of *whole blood base excess* as follows:

$$\Delta c\text{HCO}_3^-(\text{P}) = -\beta \times \Delta\text{pH}(\text{P}) + \frac{\Delta c\text{B}'(\text{B})}{\zeta}$$

where

$\Delta c\text{HCO}_3^-$ = measured plasma $c\text{HCO}_3^-$ (P) − 24.5 mmol/L HCO_3^-

ΔpH = measured pH − the standard pH of 7.40

$\Delta c\text{B}'(\text{B})$ = the *whole blood base excess* [i.e., the concentration of titratable base when the blood is titrated with strong acid or base to pH = 7.40 at PCO_2 (Std) and 37 °C]

$\beta = \beta_m\text{Hb} \times c\text{Hb(B)} + \beta\text{Pr}$, where β_mHb is the molar buffer value of hemoglobin (2.3 mol/mol), *c*Hb(B) is the substance concentration of hemoglobin (Fe) in the blood (unit: mmol/L), and βPr is the buffer value of the plasma proteins (7.7 mmol/L)

$\zeta = 1 - c\text{Hb(B)}/c_{ref}$, where c_{ref} is an empirical parameter (43 mmol/L).

This equation for *whole blood base excess* (known as the Van Slyke equation[23,24]), together with the Henderson-Hasselbalch equation, provides the simplest algorithm for calculation of various acid-base variables. The buffer value of HHb is slightly lower than that for O_2Hb at pH ≈6.5 but higher at pH ≈7.8. This is due to a decrease in the p*K* value of the "oxygen-linked" acid-base groups of Hb (C-terminal histidine and N-terminal valine) when HHb is oxygenated. When oxygenated, H^+ ions are liberated from Hb—a phenomenon called the *Haldane effect.* For additional details on the Haldane effect, see Chapter 31 of the second edition of this textbook.[28]

Isohydric and Chloride Shift

Because of continuous production of carbon dioxide within tissue cells, there is a concentration gradient for carbon dioxide from cells to plasma and thus to erythrocytes. Despite this, all buffer systems discussed previously interact together through a phenomenon known as the *isohydric Cl– shift,* which keeps the $cdCO_2$ and cH^+ (pH) essentially constant between arterial and venous blood. A small portion of the carbon dioxide entering the plasma stays as dissolved carbon dioxide, thus the slightly higher PCO_2 of venous blood. Most reacts with water to form carbonic acid that dissociates into H^+ and HCO_3^-. The increased amount of H^+ is buffered by plasma buffers (Figure 49-9, reaction 1). Another small portion combines with the amino groups of proteins and forms carbamino compounds (Figure 49-9, reaction 2). The normal concentration of carbamino compounds in the plasma is about 0.2 mmol/L. Most of the carbon dioxide enters the erythrocytes and reacts with water to form carbonic acid. This reaction is catalyzed by the enzyme carbonic anhydrase (CA) and proceeds at a relatively high rate (Figure 49-9, reaction 3). Some CO_2 remains as dissolved CO_2, and some combines with Hb to form $HbCO_2$ (Figure 49-9, reaction 4).

The carbonic acid formed in reaction 3 initially increases the H^+ concentration. The pH change, however, is fully or partially compensated by the release of oxygen from O_2Hb, which involves the conversion of stronger acid (O_2Hb) into weaker acid (HHb) that then readily accepts the H^+. For each mole of O_2 released, the hemoglobin binds about 0.5 mol of H^+ ion. Furthermore, the HHb binds significantly more CO_2 in the form of carbamino-CO_2 than does oxyhemoglobin; thus an additional fraction of CO_2 is transported in this form. The oxygen released from O_2Hb moves from the erythrocytes through the plasma into the peripheral tissue cells.

Remaining hydrogen ions formed in reaction 3 are buffered by the nonbicarbonate buffers of the erythrocyte fluid, whereas the concentration of HCO_3^- increases to the same extent that the concentration of Hb anion falls. The transformations described so far (Figure 49-9, reactions 1 through 5) are referred to as the *isohydric shift* (i.e., a shift in which the hydrogen ion concentration remains unchanged).

However, the equilibrium between plasma and red cells has been disturbed by this isohydric shift. The concentration of HCO_3^- has increased relatively more in the erythrocytes than in the plasma; the pH of plasma has fallen relatively more than the pH of erythrocytes; and the nondiffusible ion concentration in the erythrocytes has fallen because of the increase in protonation of hemoglobin. The membrane potential of the erythrocytes therefore becomes less negative, and the distribution of all diffusible ions must change with the new membrane potential. The ion shifts that occur rapidly include movement of HCO_3^- out of the erythrocytes and movement of Cl^- into the erythrocytes to provide electrochemical balance. This shift of chloride ions is referred to as the *chloride shift* (Figure 49-9, reactions 6 and 7). As a result of these ion fluxes, the concentration of chloride in venous plasma is about 1 mmol/L lower than that in arterial plasma.

In the alveoli, low PCO_2 and high PO_2 cause a reversal of reactions 1 through 7, as shown in Figure 49-9.

Respiratory Mechanism in the Regulation of Acid-Base Balance

In addition to supplying O_2 to tissue cells for normal metabolism, the respiratory mechanism contributes to maintenance of normal body pH through elimination or retention of CO_2 in metabolic acidosis and alkalosis, respectively.

Respiration

Exchange of O_2 and CO_2 in the lungs between alveolar air and blood is called *external respiration,* in contrast to internal respiration, which occurs at the tissue level. At inspiration, muscular contraction expands intrathoracic volume and creates a fall in intrapulmonary pressure. Atmospheric air is drawn into the bronchial tree, which terminates at the alveoli, where the exchange of gases between alveolar air and pulmonary blood occurs. Expiration takes place passively as the elastic tissues of the lungs and chest wall rebound and the intrathoracic volume is decreased. Loss of elasticity of the lungs and destruction of the alveolar membranes are basic pathologic mechanisms underlying many pulmonary diseases.

Peripheral venous blood reaches the pulmonary circulation from the right ventricle of the heart and is *arterialized* in the capillaries of the lungs by uptake of O_2 and loss of CO_2. Pulmonary venous blood then returns to the left ventricle by way of the left atrium and is pumped through the aorta to the peripheral tissues. In the capillaries of peripheral tissues, the arterial blood releases O_2 to the tissue cells and takes up CO_2.

In a resting state, the respiration rate is normally 12 to 15 breaths/min. For an average-sized adult with a tidal volume of about 0.5 L, 6 to 8 L of air is moved per minute in either direction. Physical activity increases ventilation. Involuntary increases in rate and depth of respiration are regulated by the medullary respiratory center in the brainstem, which is stimulated by central chemoreceptors located on the anterior surface of the medulla oblongata and by peripheral chemoreceptors located in the carotid arteries and aorta. Peripheral chemoreceptors are stimulated by a fall in pH caused by accumulation of CO_2 or by a decrease in PO_2. Central chemoreceptors are stimulated only by a decrease in pH of the CSF.

The normal response to these chemical receptors that drive respiration can be perturbed by a pathologic condition in the circulatory or respiratory system. Such patients may require assisted ventilation that uses a mechanical device to provide gas mixtures via an endotracheal tube. Adjustments of gas mixtures and rates of mechanical ventilation depend greatly on the results of laboratory blood gas and pH determinations.

Exchange of Gases in the Lungs and Peripheral Tissues

Diffusion of O_2 and CO_2 across alveolar and cell membranes is governed by gradients in the partial pressure of each gas (Figure 49-10). Dry air inspired at a pressure of 1 atm (760 mm Hg) consists of 21% O_2 (PO_2 ≈160 mm Hg), 0.03% CO_2 (PCO_2 ≈0.25 mm Hg), 78% nitrogen, and ≈0.1% other inert gases. As inspired air passes over the moist mucous membranes of the upper respiratory tract, it is warmed to 37 °C, becomes saturated with water vapor, and mixes with air in the respiratory tree, resulting in partial pressures of ≈150 mm Hg for O_2, ≈0.3 mm Hg for CO_2, ≈47 mm Hg for H_2O, and ≈563 mm Hg for nitrogen. Further mixing with alveolar air results in partial pressures at the alveolar membrane of ≈105 mm Hg for O_2, ≈40 mm Hg for CO_2, and ≈47 mm Hg for H_2O. Venous blood on the opposite side of the alveolar membrane has PO_2 ≈40 mm Hg and PCO_2 ≈46 mm Hg. Thus the gradient for O_2 is inward, toward the blood, and for CO_2, it is outward, toward the alveoli. CO_2 removal is so efficient that the PCO_2 in expired air is more than 100 times the PCO_2 in inspired air (see Figure 49-10). In arterial blood, the PO_2 is slightly lower than in alveolar air (90 to 100 vs. 105 mm Hg) as the result of shunting of about 5% of blood that does not equilibrate.

At the arterial end of capillaries of peripheral tissues, the PO_2 at 95 mm Hg is substantially higher than the average PO_2 at the surface of tissue cells (20 mm Hg), and the PCO_2 at 40 mm Hg is substantially lower than that in the cells (50 to 70 mm Hg). Thus in the tissue capillary, the gradient for O_2 is inward to the cell; for CO_2, it is outward to the capillary blood. The arteriovenous difference in partial pressures is approximately 60 mm Hg for O_2 and 6 mm Hg or less for CO_2. This difference in arteriovenous PO_2 is one indicator of the efficiency of O_2 extraction in the passage of blood through the capillaries. During passage through the tissues, the concentration of total oxygen falls on average 2.3 mmol/L, whereas the concentration of total CO_2 of blood rises about 2.0 mmol/L.

Respiratory Response to Acid-Base Perturbations

Most metabolic acid-base disorders develop slowly, within hours in diabetic ketoacidosis and months in chronic renal disease. The respiratory system responds immediately to a change in acid-base status, but several hours may be required

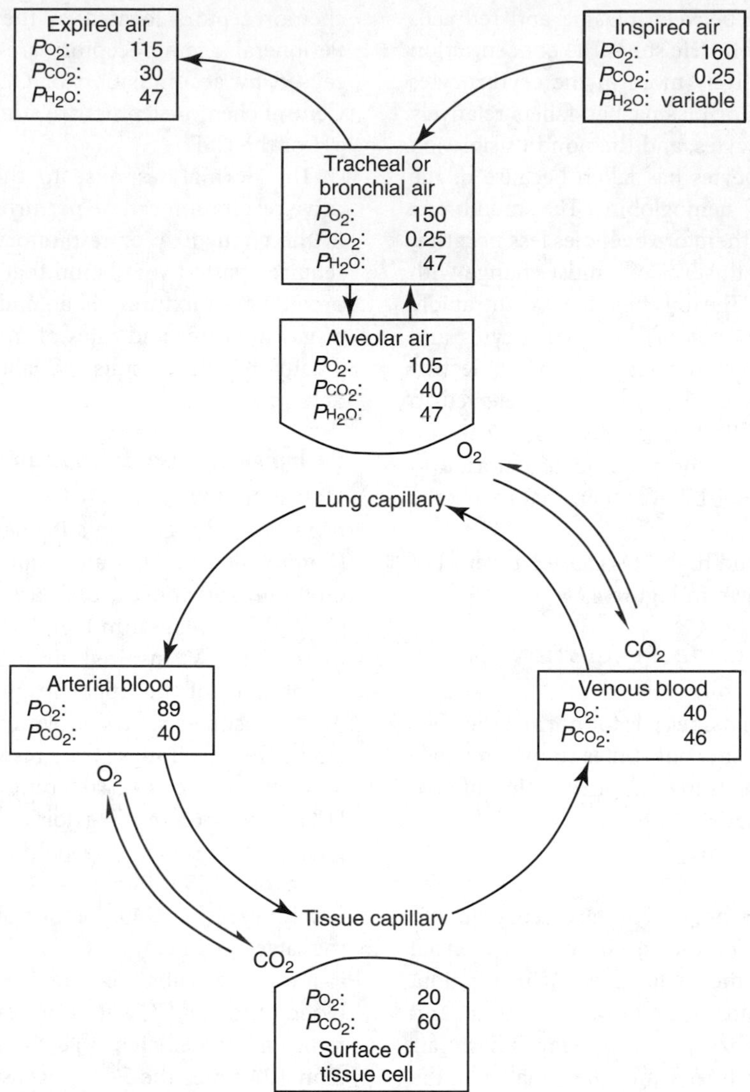

Figure 49-10 Partial pressures of oxygen and carbon dioxide in air, blood, and tissue. Values shown are approximations in mm Hg and are calculated assuming a 5% shunt. *Red arrows* show directions of gradients. *(Modified from Tietz NW. Fundamentals of clinical chemistry, 3rd edition. Philadelphia: WB Saunders, 1987.)*

for the response to become maximal. The maximum response is not attained until both central and peripheral chemoreceptors are fully stimulated. For example, in the early stages of metabolic acidosis, plasma pH decreases, but because H^+ ions equilibrate rather slowly across the blood-brain barrier, the pH in CSF remains nearly normal. However, because peripheral chemoreceptors are stimulated by decreased plasma pH, hyperventilation occurs, and plasma PCO_2 is decreased. When this occurs, the PCO_2 of the CSF decreases immediately because CO_2 equilibrates rapidly across the blood-brain barrier, leading to a rise in pH of the CSF that inhibits the central chemoreceptors. As plasma bicarbonate gradually falls because of acidosis, bicarbonate concentration and pH in the CSF will also eventually fall. At this point, stimulation of respiration becomes maximal from both central and peripheral chemoreceptors.

The reverse is true when a patient with metabolic acidosis is treated with HCO_3^-. When the pH in plasma increases as the result of HCO_3^- administration, stimulation of the peripheral chemoreceptors returns to normal. However, because of slow equilibration of HCO_3^- between plasma and CSF, the central chemoreceptors continue to be stimulated and the patient continues to hyperventilate. Respiration does not return to normal until normal acid-base balance in the CSF is restored.

Renal Mechanisms in the Regulation of Acid-Base Balance

The average pH of plasma and of the glomerular filtrate is ≈7.4, whereas the average urinary pH is ≈6.0, reflecting the renal excretion of nonvolatile acids. Various functions of the kidneys respond to different alterations in acid-base status. In the case of acidosis, excretion of acids is increased and that of base is conserved; in alkalosis, the opposite occurs. The pH of the urine changes correspondingly and may vary in *random* specimens from pH 4.5 to 8.0. This ability to excrete variable amounts of acid or base makes the kidney the final defense mechanism against changes in body pH.

The various acids produced during metabolic processes are buffered in the ECF at the expense of HCO_3^-. Renal excretion of acid and conservation of HCO_3^- occur through several mechanisms, including (1) Na^+-H^+ exchange, (2) production of ammonia and excretion of NH_4^+, and (3) reclamation of HCO_3^-.

Na^+-H^+ Exchange

Nearly all mammalian cells contain a plasma membrane ATP-hydrolyzing protein capable of exchanging sodium ions for protons—the so-called Na^+-H^+ exchanger (Figure 49-11). In 2002 it was reported that at least six isoforms of the Na^+-H^+ exchanger (NHE-1 through NHE-6) are differentially expressed in a wide variety of tissues.[20] In the renal tubules, NHE-1 and NHE-3 appear to be the predominant isoforms that extrude H^+ ions into the tubular fluid in exchange for Na^+ ions.

Na^+-H^+ exchange is enhanced in states of acidosis and is inhibited in alkalosis. Both NHE-1 and NHE-3 are transcriptionally upregulated in response to acidotic states.[20] The proximal tubules, however, cannot maintain an H^+ gradient of more than ≈1 pH unit, whereas the distal tubules cannot maintain 1 of more than ≈3 pH units. Thus maximum urine acidity is reached at ≈pH 4.4. In type I and type IV RTA, this exchange process is defective and may lead to a decrease in blood pH. In type I RTA, an increase in urinary pH is often noted.

Potassium ions compete with H^+ in the renal tubular Na^+-H^+ exchanger. If the intracellular K^+ level of renal tubular cells is high, more K^+ and less H^+ are exchanged for Na^+. As a result, the urine becomes less acidic, thereby increasing the acidity of body fluids. If K^+ is depleted, more H^+ ions are exchanged for Na^+; the urine becomes more acidic and the body fluids more alkaline. Thus hyperkalemia contributes to acidosis and hypokalemia to alkalosis. Because the body's compensatory mechanism against metabolic alkalosis is relatively ineffective, K^+ depletion alone can result in a metabolic alkalosis.

Renal Production of Ammonia and Excretion of Ammonium Ions

Renal tubular cells are able to generate ammonia from glutamine and other amino acids derived from muscle and liver cells according to the following reaction:

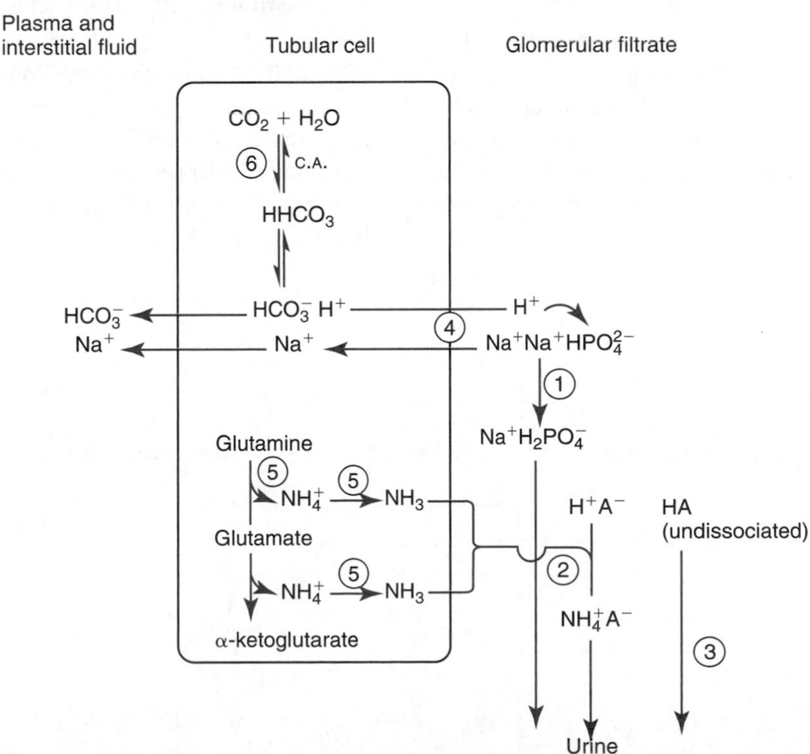

Figure 49-11 Hydrogen ion excretion, sodium hydrogen ion exchange, and ammonia production in the renal tubules. Key: *1*, conversion of HPO_4^{2-} to $H_2PO_4^-$; *2*, reaction of hydrogen ions with NH_3; *3*, excretion of undissociated acids; *4*, Na^+-H^+ exchange; *5*, NH_3 production; and *6*, synthesis of carbonic acid from CO_2.

$$\text{Glutamine} + H_2O \xrightarrow{\text{Glutaminase}} \text{Glutamate} + NH_3$$

$$\text{Glutamate} + NAD^+ \xrightarrow{\text{Glutamate dehydrogenase}} \text{2-Oxoglutarate} + NADH + NH_4^+$$

$$NH_4^+ \rightleftharpoons NH_3 + H^+$$

The ammonium ion produced dissociates into ammonia and hydrogen ions to a degree dependent on the pH (see Figure 49-11). At normal blood pH, the ratio of NH_4^+ to NH_3 is about 100 to 1. Ammonia is a gas that diffuses readily across the cell membrane into the tubular lumen, where it combines with hydrogen ions to form ammonium ions (see Figure 49-11). At the acid pH of urine, the equilibrium between NH_4^+ and NH_3 shifts markedly to the left (≈10,000 to 1), strongly favoring formation of NH_4^+. The NH_4^+ formed in the tubular lumen cannot easily cross cell membranes and thus is trapped in the tubular urine and excreted with anions such as phosphate, chloride, or sulfate. In normal individuals, NH_4^+ production in the tubular lumen accounts for the excretion of ≈60% (30 to 60 mmol) of the hydrogen ions. Finally, the α-oxoglutarate produced in this reaction is converted to bicarbonate (up to 270 mmol/d) that helps to replenish bicarbonate neutralized by metabolic acid production. The amount of H^+ excreted bound to NH_3 can be measured as NH_4^+. The H^+ required for NH_4^+ formation may be present in the glomerular filtrate or may be generated within tubular cells by carbonic anhydrase synthesis of carbonic acid from CO_2 (see Figures 49-11 and 49-12). These hydrogen ions are secreted into the tubular lumen through the Na^+-H^+ exchangers (see Figure 49-11).

Excretion of H^+ as $H_2PO_4^-$

H^+ secreted into the tubular lumen by the Na^+-H^+ exchanger may also react with HPO_4^- to form $H_2PO_4^{2-}$ (see Figure 49-11). This process depends on the amount of phosphate filtered by the glomeruli and the pH of urine. Under normal physiologic conditions, ≈30 mmol of H^+ is excreted per day as $H_2PO_4^-$. Acidemia increases phosphate excretion and thus provides additional buffer for reaction with H^+. A decrease in the glomerular filtration rate (GFR), as observed in renal disease, results in a decrease in $H_2PO_4^-$ excretion. The secretion of H^+ and the subsequent reaction with $H_2PO_4^-$ allow the removal of one H^+ with no significant decrease in urinary pH. As a result, the pH gradient is not greatly affected and more H^+ can be secreted into the tubules, whereas more Na^+ is reabsorbed and conserved.

Reclamation of Filtered Bicarbonate

The unmodified glomerular filtrate has the same concentration of HCO_3^- as does plasma; however, with increasing acidification of proximal tubular urine, the HCO_3^- concentration is decreased. Excreted H^+ reacts with HCO_3^- (catalyzed by carbonic anhydrase, in the brush border of the proximal tubular cells) to form H_2CO_3 and subsequently CO_2 and H_2O (see Figure 49-12).

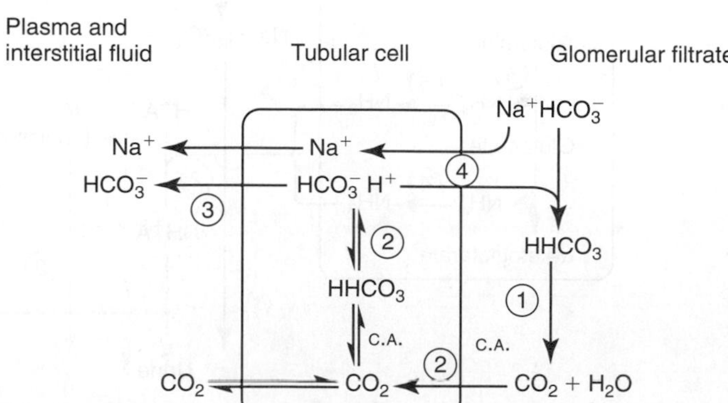

Figure 49-12 Key: *1*, Formation of CO_2 from bicarbonate in the tubular fluid; *2*, formation of H^+ and HCO_3^- from CO_2 in the tubular cell; *3*, new generation of HCO_3^-; and *4*, Na^+-H^+ exchange.

This increase in urinary CO_2 causes carbon dioxide to diffuse across the tubular cell membrane into the tubular cell, where it reacts with H_2O in the presence of *cytoplasmic* carbonic anhydrase to form H_2CO_3 and subsequently H^+ and HCO_3^- (see Figure 49-12). Thus reclamation of bicarbonate consists in fact of diffusion of CO_2 into tubular cells and its subsequent conversion to HCO_3^-. The increase in HCO_3^- helps to maintain or restore a normal pH in the circulation. Normally, ≈90% of filtered HCO_3^- (or about 4500 mmol/d) is reclaimed in the proximal tubule, which parallels Na^+ reabsorption. Thus for each mmol H^+ secreted into the tubular fluid, 1 mmol Na^+ and 1 mmol HCO_3^- enter the tubular cell and return to the general circulation. When plasma HCO_3^- concentration increases above ≈28 mmol/L, the capacity of the proximal and distal tubules to reclaim HCO_3^- is exceeded, and HCO_3^- is excreted in the urine. Type II RTA is caused by a decreased ability to reabsorb HCO_3^- in the proximal tubules, leading to a decrease in blood pH.

CONDITIONS ASSOCIATED WITH ABNORMAL ACID-BASE STATUS AND ABNORMAL ELECTROLYTE COMPOSITION OF THE BLOOD[5,19,25]

Many pathologic conditions are accompanied by acid-base and electrolyte disturbances in the blood. Abnormalities in acid-base status of the blood are always accompanied by characteristic changes in electrolyte concentrations in the plasma. Hydrogen ions cannot accumulate without concomitant accumulation of anions, such as Cl^- or lactate, or without exchange for cations, such as K^+ or Na^+. Consequently, the electrolyte composition of blood serum or plasma is often determined along with measurements of blood gases and pH to assess acid-base disturbances.

Acid-base disturbances are traditionally classified as (1) metabolic acidosis, (2) metabolic alkalosis, (3) respiratory acidosis, or (4) respiratory alkalosis. In simple, straightforward acid-base disorders, the laboratory parameters observed for these groups are shown in Table 49-3. However, interpretation of laboratory values to classify these disorders is rarely straightforward because of compensatory responses by the respiratory and renal systems in attempting to correct the imbalance.

Causes of acid-base disorders, resulting laboratory values, and compensatory responses are discussed here in the traditional categorization of these disorders. However, it is often difficult to remember which disorders fall into which categories, so it is common for mnemonic devices or tables to be used to facilitate description of these disorders. A useful and more logical approach is to realize that an acidosis can only occur as the result of one (or a combination) of three mechanisms: (1) increased addition of acid, (2) decreased elimination of acid, and (3) increased loss of base. Similarly, alkalosis occurs only by (1) increased addition of base, (2) decreased

TABLE 49-3 Classification and Characteristics of Simple Acid-Base Disorders

	Primary Change	Compensatory Response	Expected Compensation
Metabolic			
Acidosis	↓$cHCO_3^-$	↓PCO_2	$PCO_2 = 1.5\,(cHCO_3^-) + 8 \pm 2$ PCO_2 falls by 1 to 1.3 mm Hg for each mmol/L fall in $cHCO_3^-$ Last 2 digits of pH = PCO_2 (e.g., if $PCO_2 = 28$, pH = 7.28) $cHCO_3^- + 15$ = last 2 digits of pH ($cHCO_3^- = 15$, pH = 7.30)
Alkalosis	↑$cHCO_3^-$	↑PCO_2	PCO_2 increases 6 mm Hg for each 10 mmol/L rise in $cHCO_3^-$ $cHCO_3^- + 15$ = last 2 digits of pH ($cHCO_3^- = 35$, pH = 7.50)
Respiratory			
Acidosis			
Acute	↑PCO_2	↑$cHCO_3^-$	$cHCO_3^-$ increases by 1 mmol/L for each 10 mm Hg rise in PCO_2
Chronic	↑PCO_2	↑$cHCO_3^-$	$cHCO_3^-$ increases by 3.5 mmol/L for each 10 mm Hg rise in PCO_2
Alkalosis			
Acute	↓PCO_2	↓$cHCO_3^-$	$cHCO_3^-$ falls by 2 mmol/L for each 10 mm Hg fall in PCO_2
Chronic	↓PCO_2	↓$cHCO_3^-$	$cHCO_3^-$ falls by 5 mmol/L for each 10 mm Hg fall in PCO_2

Modified from Narins RG, Gardner LB. Simple acid-base disturbances. Med Clin North Am 1981;65:321-46.

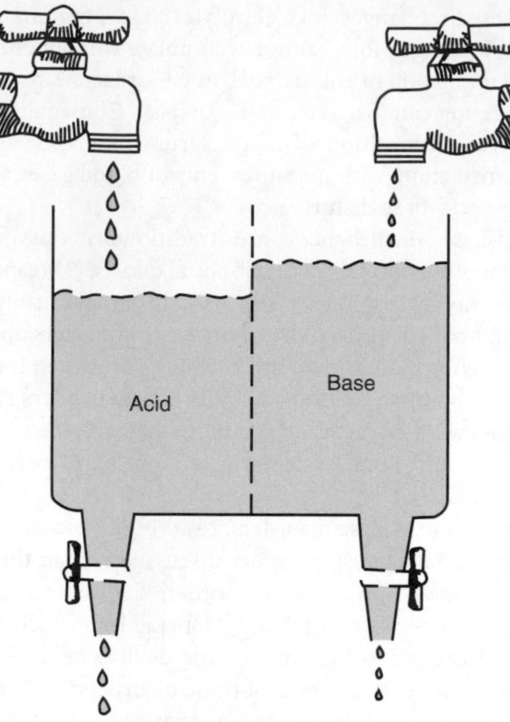

Figure 49-13 Simple depiction of the body as a two-vat system of acid and base. At equilibrium, input and output from each "vat" are equal. *(From Dufour DR. Acid-base disorders. In: Dufour DR, Christenson RH, eds: Professional practice in clinical chemistry: a review. Washington, DC: AACC Press, 1995:604-35.)*

elimination of base, and (3) increased loss of acid. Dufour has illustrated this simple concept by depicting the body as a two-tank vat, one of acid and one of base, with inputs and outputs for each vat (Figure 49-13).[5] In the normal setting, these inputs and outputs are balanced; an acid-base disorder then involves a perturbation in the input or output of these body reservoirs, as is discussed in the next section.

Metabolic Acidosis (Primary Bicarbonate Deficit)

Metabolic acidosis is readily detected by decreased plasma bicarbonate (or a negative extracellular base excess)—the primary perturbation in this acid-base disorder. Causes include the following:

1. Production of organic acids that exceeds the rate of elimination (e.g., production of acetoacetic acid and β-hydroxybutyric acid in diabetic ketoacidosis and of lactic acid in lactic acidosis). Bicarbonate is "lost" in the buffering of excess acid.
2. Reduced excretion of acids (H^+) as occurs in renal failure and some RTAs, resulting in an accumulation of acid that consumes bicarbonate.
3. Excessive loss of bicarbonate due to increased renal excretion (decreased tubular reclamation) or excessive loss of duodenal fluid (as in diarrhea). Plasma $cHCO_3^-$ falls; the fall is associated with a rise in the concentration of inorganic anions (mostly chloride) or, rarely, a concomitant fall in the sodium concentration.

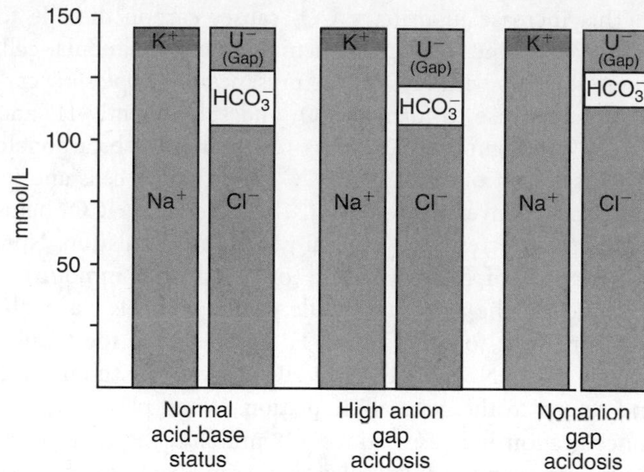

Figure 49-14 Simple "Gambelgram" depiction of normal gap, anion gap acidosis, and nonanion gap acidosis. Cations, Na^+ and K^+, are in left bar for each condition, whereas measured (Cl^- and HCO_3^-) and unmeasured (U^-) anions are in right bar for each condition.

When any of these conditions exists, the ratio of $cHCO_3^-/cCO_2$ is decreased because of the primary decrease in bicarbonate. The resulting drop in pH stimulates respiratory compensation via hyperventilation, which lowers PCO_2 and thereby raises the pH.

Increased Anion Gap Acidosis (Organic Acidosis)

Metabolic acidoses are classified as those associated with an increased anion gap or a normal anion gap (Table 49-4). The concept of the *anion gap* was originally devised as a quality control rule when it was noted that if the sum of Cl^- and HCO_3^- values was subtracted from the Na^+ values [$Na^+ - (Cl^- + HCO_3^-)$], the difference, or "gap," averaged 12 mmol/L in healthy subjects.[14] This *apparent* gap is due to unmeasured anions (e.g., proteins, SO_4^{2-}, $H_2PO_4^{2-}$) that are present in plasma. In reality, unmeasured cations (calcium, magnesium, organic cations) should be included in the equation with sodium and potassium, but their concentration in the blood is relatively small compared with circulating sodium levels. It is important to note that infrequently, low serum anion gaps (<2 mEq/L) can occur. Laboratory error is the most common cause, but bromide, lithium, or iodide intoxication or use of polymyxin B can also lead to a low anion gap, as can low albumin/increased immunoglobulin in cirrhosis and monoclonal gammopathies.[14] The anion gap is increased in many patients with a metabolic acidosis. Indeed, the presence of an elevated anion gap is often the first indication of a metabolic acidosis and should be assessed in the electrolyte profiles of all patients.[14] The gap is also slightly increased in the absence of acidosis by very low calcium, magnesium, or potassium levels, because lower levels of these "unmeasured" cations will result in lower levels of anions (Figure 49-14).

TABLE 49-4 Conditions of Metabolic Acidoses With High and Normal Anion Gaps

Etiology	Retained Acids	Other Laboratory Findings
High AG*		
Methanol toxicity	Formate	↑Osmolal gap (>15 mOsmol/kg)
Uremia of renal failure	Sulfuric, phosphoric, organic	↑BUN† and serum creatinine
Ketoacidoses		
Diabetes mellitus	Acetoacetate and β-hydroxybutyrate	↑Plasma and urine glucose
Ethyl alcohol toxicity		†Osmolal gap (>15 mOsmol/kg)
Starvation		
Paraldehyde toxicity		
Isoniazid or iron toxicity, also ischemia	Organic, mainly lactate	Isoniazid and iron act as mitochondrial poisons
Lactic acidosis	Lactate	
Ethylene glycol toxicity	Hippurate, glycolate, oxalate	↑Osmolal gap (>15 mOsmol/kg), urine oxalate crystals
Salicylate toxicity	Salicylate, organic	Respiratory alkalosis
Normal AG		
Gastrointestinal fluid loss	Primary loss of bicarbonate	
Severe diarrhea		Hypokalemia
Pancreatitis		K^+ variable
Intestinal fistula		
Renal tubular acidoses (RTAs)		
Proximal (type II) RTA		Urine pH <5.5, with K^+ normal or low
Distal (type I) RTA		Urine pH >5.5 with hypokalemia (usually)
Type IV RTA		Urine pH <5.5 with hyperkalemia

*Although there is considerable variability, the anion gap is often >25 mmol/L in these conditions, with the exception of uremic renal failure.
†Blood urea nitrogen (reference interval: 8 to 25 mg/dL, or ≈3.0 to 9.0 mmol/L).

All anion gap metabolic acidoses, besides inborn errors of metabolism, can be explained by one (or a combination) of eight underlying mechanisms listed here according to the common mnemonic device MUDPILES (see Table 49-4). The physiologic basis for the anion gap in these conditions is the consumption of bicarbonate in buffering excess acid. Cl^- values remain normal when the excess acid is any other than HCl, because lost bicarbonate is replaced by unmeasured anions.

Methanol

Although nontoxic itself, methanol is metabolized by the liver to formaldehyde and formic acid. Accumulation of this acid leads to metabolic acidosis with a high anion gap and to clinical symptoms of optic papillitis ("snowfield" blindness), retinal edema, and ultimately blindness caused by optic nerve atrophy and neurologic defects that may lead to coma. Methanol and other ingested alcohols such as ethylene glycol, ethanol, and isopropanol will increase the osmolality of plasma. Thus in the presence of a high anion gap acidosis, determination of the osmolal gap (see Chapter 28) will help determine the source of the unmeasured anion[4] and will suggest specific toxicologic analyses.[4]

Uremia of Renal Failure

Loss of functional renal tubular mass results in decreased ammonia formation, decreased Na^+-H^+ exchange, and decreased GFR. All lead to decreased acid excretion (see Chapter 48). Acidosis usually develops if GFR falls below 20 mL/min. Serum creatinine and blood urea nitrogen levels usually are elevated and are used as an estimate of the degree of renal damage or, more appropriately, as an estimate of remaining functional renal capacity.

Diabetes or Ketoacidosis

The pathogenesis of ketoacidosis is discussed in detail in Chapter 46. Ketoacids such as β-hydroxybutyrate and 2-oxoglutarate accumulate and represent the unmeasured anions. Accumulation of these "ketone bodies" causes a decrease in HCO_3^-, a normal serum chloride, and a high anion gap. Ketoacids also accumulate in states of starvation and alcoholic malnutrition.

Paraldehyde Toxicity

Paraldehyde toxicity may develop after chronic paraldehyde ingestion. The pathogenesis is poorly defined, but the acidosis may actually be a ketosis (nitroprusside negative)

with β-hydroxybutyric acid as the main acidic product. Patients with paraldehyde toxicity have a pungent, apple-like odor to their breath.

Isoniazid, Iron, or Ischemia

These seemingly unrelated causes of high anion gap acidosis share a common feature: the accumulation of organic acids, with a predominance of lactic acid. Thus the "three I's" actually represent special cases in the general category of lactic acidosis, which is described next. Both isoniazid, an antimycobacterial agent commonly used in the treatment or prophylaxis of tuberculosis, and iron toxicity involve the production of toxic peroxides that act as mitochondrial poisons and interfere with normal cellular respiration. In addition, isoniazid may be hepatotoxic, leading to significant liver damage and impairment of lactate clearance.[16]

Tissue ischemia may result from many causes; in general, hypoperfusion leads to hypoxia of cells, resulting in anaerobic metabolism with accumulation of organic (mainly lactic) acids.

Lactic Acidosis

Lactic acid, present in blood entirely as the lactate ion ($pK = 3.86$), is an intermediate of carbohydrate metabolism that is derived mainly from muscle cells and erythrocytes (see Chapter 26). It represents the end product of anaerobic metabolism and is normally metabolized by the liver. Therefore, the blood lactate concentration is affected by the rate of production and the rate of metabolism, both of which are dependent on adequate tissue perfusion. An increase in the concentration of lactate to >3 mmol/L with the associated increase in H^+ is considered lactic acidosis.

Lactic acidosis caused by severe tissue hypoxia is seen in severe anemia, shock, cardiac arrest, and pulmonary insufficiency. Severe oxygen deprivation of tissue blocks aerobic oxidation of pyruvic acid in the tricarboxylic acid cycle, resulting in the reduction of pyruvate to form lactate. Extreme deterioration of the cellular oxidative process is associated with marked tachypnea, weakness, fatigue, stupor, and finally coma. Conditions at these later stages are frequently irreversible, even when treatment for acidosis and hypoxia is instituted. A short-lived lactic acidosis is often observed following grand mal seizures. If the origin of lactate (e.g., seizure, hypoxic tissue) can be rectified, lactate is rapidly metabolized to CO_2, which then is eliminated by an intact respiratory system.

Lactic acidosis is also caused by (1) drugs and toxins such as ethanol, methanol, or isoniazid (see previous discussion); (2) acquired and hereditary defects in enzymes involved in gluconeogenesis; (3) disorders such as uremia, liver failure, tumors, and seizures; (4) anesthesia; and (5) abnormal intestinal bacteria producing D-lactate. Most common methods for lactate do not detect D-lactate acidosis; this form of lactic acidosis should be considered in patients with "short-bowel" syndromes or following other GI surgeries resulting in "blind loops."[12]

Alcohol taken in excess tends to prevent the metabolism of lactate in the liver, because oxidation of ethanol to acetaldehyde competes for the NAD^+ necessary for conversion of lactate to pyruvate.

During exercise, lactate levels may increase significantly, from an average normal concentration of ≈0.9 mmol/L to ≈12 mmol/L. However, under normal conditions, the lactate is rapidly metabolized to CO_2, so the "acidosis" is only transient as hyperventilation eliminates the CO_2.

Lactate in spinal fluid normally parallels blood levels. In cases of biochemical alterations in the central nervous system, however, CSF lactate values change independently of blood values. Increased CSF lactate levels may be seen in intracranial hemorrhage, bacterial meningitis, epilepsy, and other CNS disorders.[31]

Ethylene Glycol

Ingested ethylene glycol is metabolized primarily to glycolic and oxalic acids. Its metabolism leads to an acidosis with high anion and osmolal gaps. Accumulation of toxic metabolites may also contribute to lactic acid production that further contributes to the acidosis. Precipitation of calcium oxalate and hippurate crystals in the urinary tract may lead to acute renal failure. Clinically, patients develop a variety of neurologic symptoms that may lead to coma. The minimal lethal dose of ethylene glycol is ≈100 mL for an average 70 kg adult.

Salicylate Intoxication

Acidosis generally occurs with blood salicylate concentrations above 30 mg/dL. Salicylate, itself an unmeasured anion, alters peripheral metabolism, leading to the production of various organic acids without dominance of any specific acid. These processes eventually result in a metabolic acidosis with a high anion gap. Salicylate also stimulates the respiratory center to increase the rate and depth of respiration, resulting in a low PCO_2 and mixed respiratory alkalosis and metabolic acidosis.

Normal Anion Gap Acidosis (Inorganic Acidosis)

In contrast to high anion gap acidoses, in which bicarbonate is consumed from buffering excess H^+, the cause of acidosis in the presence of a normal anion gap is the loss of bicarbonate-rich fluid from the kidney or the gastrointestinal tract. As bicarbonate is lost, more Cl^- ions are reabsorbed with Na^+ or K^+ to maintain electrical neutrality, so that hyperchloremia ensues (see Figure 49-14). Normal anion gap acidosis can be divided into *hypokalemic, normokalemic,* and *hyperkalemic* acidoses, which can be helpful in the differential diagnosis of this type of disorder (see Table 49-4 and subsequent section on type IV RTA).

GI Losses

Diarrhea may cause acidosis as a result of loss of Na^+, K^+, and HCO_3^-. One of the primary exocrine functions of the pancreas is production of HCO_3^- to neutralize gastric contents on entry into the duodenum. If the water, K^+, and HCO_3^- in the intestine are not reabsorbed, a hypokalemic, normal anion gap metabolic acidosis will develop. The resulting hyperchloremia is due to replacement of lost bicarbonate with Cl^- to maintain electrical balance.

Renal Tubular Acidoses, Types I and II

These syndromes are characterized predominantly by loss of bicarbonate due to decreased tubular secretion of H^+ (distal or type I RTA) or decreased reabsorption of HCO_3^- (proximal or type II RTA).[15] Because the major urine-acidifying power of the kidneys rests in the distal tubules, proximal and distal RTAs may be differentiated by measurement of urine pH after administration of acid. In proximal RTA, urine pH becomes <5.5, whereas in distal RTA, the distal tubules are compromised and urine pH is >5.5.[15]

Carbonic Anhydrase Inhibitors

Acetazolamide is the most commonly used drug in this class of therapeutic agents. It is rarely used as a mild diuretic. More often, it is used for urine alkalinization and in patients suffering from open-angle glaucoma or acute mountain (altitude) sickness.[11] Inhibition of carbonic anhydrase causes wasting of Na^+, K^+, and HCO_3^- in the proximal tubules and represents a pharmacologically induced proximal RTA.

Hyperkalemic Normal Anion Gap Acidosis (RTA Type IV)

Failure of the kidneys to synthesize renin, failure of the adrenal cortex to secrete aldosterone, and renal tubular resistance to aldosterone are the most common causes of this type of acidosis (often called type IV RTA). It inhibits Na^+ reabsorption, and both K^+ and H^+ are thus abnormally retained. The result is decreased renal ammonia formation and therefore decreased elimination of H^+. Hyperkalemia is also usually present.

Compensatory Mechanisms in Metabolic Acidosis

The buffer systems of the blood (mainly the bicarbonate/carbonic acid buffer) minimize changes in pH. In acidoses, the bicarbonate concentration decreases to yield a ratio of $cHCO_3^-/cdCO_2$ of less than 20:1. The respiratory compensatory mechanism responds to correct the ratio with increased rate and depth of respiration to eliminate CO_2. Table 49-3 depicts expected compensation in acidoses and alkaloses and corresponding laboratory values.

Respiratory Compensatory Mechanism

The decrease in pH in metabolic acidosis stimulates hyperventilation (Kussmaul respiration), which results in the elimination of carbonic acid as CO_2, a decrease in PCO_2 (hypocapnia), and thus a decrease in $cdCO_2$. There is also a decrease in $cHCO_3^-$ that is smaller than that in $cdCO_2$. For example, the ratio of $cHCO_3^-/cdCO_2$ might be 16:1.28 (12.5:1) for a pH of 7.2 before compensation, and 14.5:0.9 (16:1) for a pH of 7.30 after compensation (see Figure 49-8).

Renal Compensatory Mechanism

If possible, the kidneys respond to restore the normal pH through increased excretion of acid and preservation of base (increased rate of Na^+-H^+ exchange, increased ammonia formation, and increased reabsorption of bicarbonate). When the renal compensating mechanisms are functioning, urine acidity and ammonia are increased. The total amount of H^+ excreted may be as great as 500 mmol/d. As a result, $cHCO_3^-/cdCO_2$ will increase, for example, to 22:1.1 (20:1) for a pH of 7.40. *This is a fully compensated metabolic acidosis*, because the pH has returned to normal; however, acidosis still exists because a process that consumes HCO_3^- persists. Physiologically, a normal pH suggests that the acidosis is overcompensated.

Laboratory Findings in Metabolic Acidosis

Bicarbonate concentrations have been used to empirically estimate pH and PCO_2. For pH, 15 is added to the determined bicarbonate concentration for an estimate of the decimal digits of pH. For example, a patient who has been acidotic for at least 12 to 24 hours and has a bicarbonate of 10 mmol/L (10 + 15 = 25) will have an estimated pH of 7.25. Another common estimator of proper compensation is that the PCO_2 will equal the last two digits of the pH. If a respiratory acidosis was superimposed on a preexisting metabolic acidosis, the PCO_2 would be higher than expected by this estimate.

Electrolytes are also altered depending on the cause of metabolic acidosis. In diabetic ketoacidosis, the increase in the fraction of organic acids caused by increased ketone body production is reflected by a decrease in plasma bicarbonate and sometimes in chloride. Plasma Na^+ and K^+ are also decreased because of the associated polyuria and coexcretion of these cations with acetoacetate and β-hydroxybutyrate. Furthermore, because of the high glucose, a dilutional effect occurs as a result of the osmotically induced increase in vascular volume. When glucose concentration is decreased following insulin treatment, water leaves the vascular compartment, and Na^+ concentration is increased. Serum potassium concentrations, however, may be normal or even high, despite severe total body depletion of K^+; the serum concentration represents a balance struck between the amount of K^+ lost in the urine, the amount of K^+ shifted from cells into ECF, and the degree of dehydration.

Metabolic Alkalosis (Primary Bicarbonate Excess)

Alkalosis occurs when excess base is added to the system, base elimination is decreased, or acid-rich fluids are lost (Box 49-1). Any of these can lead to a primary bicarbonate excess, such that the ratio of $cHCO_3^-/cdCO_2$ becomes greater than 20:1. For instance, a primary increase in bicarbonate to 48 mmol/L will alter the $cHCO_3^-/cdCO_2$ to 48:1.5 (32:1) for a pH of 7.6 (see Figure 49-8). The patient will hypoventilate to raise PCO_2, thereby lowering the pH toward normal. However, hypoxia usually prevents the patient from achieving a PCO_2 greater than 55 mm Hg. Above pH 7.55, tetany may

BOX 49-1 Conditions Leading to Metabolic Alkalosis

Chloride-Responsive (Urine Cl^- <10 mmol/L)
Contraction alkaloses
- Prolonged vomiting or nasogastric suction
- Pyloric or upper duodenal obstruction
- Prolonged or abusive diuretic therapy (loop diuretics)
- Dehydration

Posthypercapnic state
Cystic fibrosis (systemic ineffective reabsorption of Cl^-)

Chloride-Resistant (Urine Cl^- >20 mmol/L)
Mineralocorticoid excess
- Primary hyperaldosteronism (adrenal adenoma or, rarely, carcinoma)
- Bilateral adrenal hyperplasia
- Secondary hyperaldosteronism
- Congenital adrenal hyperplasia [due to adrenal enzyme deficiencies in cortisol production (11β- or 17α-hydroxylase)]

Glucocorticoid excess
- Primary adrenal adenoma (Cushing syndrome)
- Pituitary adenoma secreting ACTH (Cushing disease)
- Exogenous cortisol therapy
- Excessive licorice ingestion

Bartter syndrome (defective renal Cl^- reabsorption)

Exogenous Base
Iatrogenic
- Bicarbonate-containing intravenous fluid therapy
- Massive blood transfusion (sodium citrate overload)
- Antacids and cation-exchange resins in dialysis patients
- High-dose carbenicillin or penicillin (associated with hypokalemia)

Milk-alkali syndrome

develop, even in the presence of a normal serum total calcium concentration. The cause of the tetany is a decreased concentration of ionized calcium due to increased binding of calcium ions by albumin. Measurement of urine Cl^- can be helpful, as causes of metabolic alkalosis fall into Cl^- responsive, Cl^- resistant, and exogenous base categories (see Box 49-1 and Figure 49-4).

Cl^- Responsive Metabolic Alkalosis

Most causes of Cl^- responsive metabolic alkalosis occur as a result of *hypovolemia* (see Box 49-1). When the ECF is severely depleted, the resulting acid-base disorder is often referred to as *contraction alkalosis.* Hypovolemia will result in increased reabsorption of Na^+, along with increased HCO_3^- absorption and excretion of K^+ and H^+. Urine Cl^- will be less than 10 mmol/L, as both the available Cl^- and HCO_3^- are reabsorbed with Na^+. Urine Na^+ is not useful for classifying metabolic alkalosis because an obligatory loss of Na^+ will occur when filtered HCO_3^- exceeds reclamation. Common causes of contraction alkalosis include prolonged vomiting or nasogastric suction, pyloric or upper duodenal obstruction, and the use of certain diuretics. Following prolonged vomiting or gastric suction, excessive loss of hydrochloric acid from the stomach and *hypovolemia* may occur. In this hypochloremic, hypovolemic setting, the kidneys preferentially reabsorb Na^+ to restore volume, and excess bicarbonate is reabsorbed in the absence of sufficient Cl^- to maintain electrical neutrality. In addition, H^+ and K^+ are secreted in exchange for Na^+. Urine Cl^- will be less than 10 mmol/L in this setting (see Figure 49-4). Treatment consists of replacing TBW with water and NaCl tablets or saline infusion.

Diuretic Therapy

Prolonged administration of certain diuretics has been known to cause an alkalosis similar to that observed in a hypovolemic setting. Most common are those acting on the ascending limb of the loop of Henle [e.g., furosemide (Lasix)] that block sodium, potassium, and chloride reabsorption.[11] The resulting increase in Na^+ concentration reaching the distal convoluted tubule, particularly when combined with activation of the renin-angiotensin-aldosterone axis, leads to increased urinary excretion of K^+ and H^+. Loss of K^+ with furosemide is much greater than with thiazides. Continued abuse or unmonitored use of loop diuretics can lead to volume contraction and a contraction alkalosis. This is commonly seen among patients using diuretics for the purpose of weight loss.

Cl^- Resistant Metabolic Alkalosis

This condition is far less common than Cl^- responsive metabolic alkalosis and is almost always associated with an underlying disease (primary hyperaldosteronism, Cushing syndrome, or Bartter syndrome) or with excess addition of exogenous base. In these conditions, urine Cl^- will usually be greater than 20 mmol/L.

In states of adrenocortical excess (endogenous or pharmacologic, primary or secondary), K^+ and H^+ are "wasted" by the kidneys as a consequence of increased Na^+ reabsorption stimulated by elevated aldosterone or cortisol. The attendant hypokalemia often further contributes to the alkalosis and should be treated with K^+ replacement therapy. The decreased tubular K^+ concentration stimulates NH_3 production and thus renal H^+ excretion as NH_4^+. This is accompanied by enhanced HCO_3^- reabsorption (see Figures 49-3 and 49-12). Diseases in which endogenous mineralocorticoids, glucocorticoids, or both are elevated include primary and secondary hyperaldosteronism, bilateral adrenal hyperplasia, pituitary ACTH-producing adenoma (Cushing disease), and primary adrenal adenomas producing glucocorticoids (Cushing syndrome) or aldosterone.

Excessive licorice ingestion may cause a form of Cl^- resistant alkalosis. Black licorice contains glycyrrhizic acid, which inhibits the enzyme 11-β hydroxysteroid dehydrogenase, which catalyzes the conversion of cortisol to cortisone.[7] The excess cortisol exerts a mineralocorticoid effect on the distal tubule aldosterone receptors.

Finally, a rare cause of Cl^- resistant metabolic alkalosis is a genetic (autosomal recessive) defect in Cl^- reabsorption within the thick ascending limb of the loop of Henle—a condition known as Bartter syndrome.[3]

Exogenous Base

Examples in this category include citrate toxicity following massive blood transfusion, aggressive intravenous therapy with bicarbonate solutions, and ingestion of large quantities of antacids in the treatment of gastritis or peptic ulcer *(milk-alkali syndrome)*.[9] The latter is far less commonly seen since the introduction and now widespread use of H_2-receptor antagonists and proton pump inhibitors.

Compensatory Mechanisms in Metabolic Alkalosis

The compensatory mechanisms for metabolic alkalosis include both respiratory compensation and, if physiologically possible, renal compensation. The increase in pH depresses the respiratory center, causing retention of carbon dioxide (hypercapnia), which in turn causes an increase in cH_2CO_3 and $cdCO_2$. Thus the ratio of $cHCO_3^-/cdCO_2$, which was originally increased, approaches its normal value, although the actual concentrations of both $cHCO_3^-$ and $cdCO_2$ remain increased. The kidneys respond to the state of alkalosis by decreased Na^+-H^+ exchange, decreased formation of ammonia, and decreased reclamation of bicarbonate. This response is blunted, however, in conditions of hypokalemia and hypovolemia.

Laboratory Findings in Metabolic Alkalosis

Plasma values for $cHCO_3^-$, $cdCO_2$, and PCO_2, and therefore the plasma total CO_2 concentration, are increased, and the ratio of $cHCO_3^-/cdCO_2$ is high. In uncomplicated metabolic alkalosis, the PCO_2 is increased by ≈6 mm Hg for each 10 mmol/L rise in $cHCO_3^-$. A higher than expected PCO_2 may indicate superimposed respiratory acidosis. The extent of increase in pH in uncompensated metabolic alkalosis can be estimated by adding 15 to the $cHCO_3^-$ to give the last two digits of the pH. If the $cHCO_3^-$ is 35 mmol/L, the estimated pH would be 7.50 (35 + 15 = 50). In cases of prolonged vomiting, Cl^- (and sometimes K^+) concentrations are low because of loss of these ions through the vomitus. Protein values may be increased owing to dehydration, and if food intake is inadequate, formation of ketoacids may increase the organic acid fraction. In cases of excessive administration of $NaHCO_3$, Na^+ levels are increased.

In patients with adequate renal function, urinary pH values are usually increased as the result of decreased excretion of acid and increased excretion of bicarbonate. Urinary ammonium values are decreased because of decreased formation of ammonium in the tubules. In K^+ depletion, H^+ is preferentially exchanged for Na^+ and the pH of the urine may be low. This is called *paradoxical aciduria*.

Respiratory Acidosis

Any condition that decreases elimination of carbon dioxide through the lungs results in an increase in PCO_2 (hypercapnia) and dCO_2 (respiratory acidosis). Thus respiratory acidosis occurs only through decreased elimination of CO_2. Causes of decreased CO_2 elimination (Box 49-2) are classified as acute or chronic. Alternatively, these conditions may be separated into those caused by factors that directly depress the respiratory center (such as centrally acting drugs, CNS trauma, or infection) and those that affect the respiratory apparatus or cause mechanical obstruction of the airways. Chronic obstructive pulmonary disease is the most common cause. Rebreathing, or breathing air high in CO_2 content, may also cause a high PCO_2. An increase in PCO_2 results in an increase in $cdCO_2$ (and thus H_2CO_3, which dissociates to H^+ and HCO_3^-), which in turn causes a decrease in the $cHCO_3^-/cdCO_2$ ratio [e.g., the ratio may be 28:1.7 (16:1) for a pH of ≈7.30; see Figure 49-8]. Doubling of PCO_2 will cause a fall in pH of about 0.23 when other factors remain constant.

BOX 49-2 Conditions Leading to Respiratory Acidosis

Factors That Directly Depress the Respiratory Center
Drugs such as narcotics and barbiturates
Central nervous system (CNS) trauma, tumors, and degenerative disorders
Infections of the CNS such as encephalitis and meningitis
Comatose states such as cerebrovascular accident due to intracranial hemorrhage
Primary central hypoventilation

Conditions That Affect the Respiratory Apparatus
Chronic obstructive pulmonary disease (most common cause)
Severe pulmonary fibrosis
Status asthmaticus (severe)
Disease of the upper airways such as laryngospasm or tumor
Pulmonary infection (severe)
Impaired lung motion due to pleural effusion or pneumothorax
Adult respiratory distress syndrome
Chest wall disease and chest wall deformity
Neurologic disorders affecting the muscles of respiration

Others
Abdominal distention, as in peritonitis and ascites
Extreme obesity (pickwickian syndrome)
Sleep disorders such as sleep apnea

Compensatory Mechanisms in Respiratory Acidosis

Compensation for respiratory acidosis occurs immediately via buffers, and over time via the kidneys and, if possible, the lungs. Excess carbonic acid present in blood is buffered to a great extent by the hemoglobin and protein buffer systems[8] (see Figure 49-9). Buffering of CO_2 causes a slight rise in $cHCO_3^-$. Thus in the immediate posthypercapnic state, this compensation may appear as a metabolic alkalosis (see Box 49-1). The kidneys respond to respiratory acidosis similarly to the way that they respond to metabolic acidosis, namely, with (1) increased Na^+-H^+ exchange, (2) increased ammonia formation, and (3) increased reclamation of bicarbonate. In a partially compensated chronic respiratory acidosis at steady state, the plasma pH is returned about halfway toward normal as compared with the acute (uncompensated) situation. Renal compensation is not effective before 6 to 12 hours and is not optimal until 2 to 3 days. In chronic respiratory acidosis, such as occurs in patients with chronic obstructive pulmonary disease (COPD), full renal compensation may be seen even in those patients with very high PCO_2 (>50 mm Hg). However, patients with severe COPD often present with a superimposed metabolic alkalosis arising from a variety of causes, such as prolonged administration of diuretics.

The increase in PCO_2 stimulates the respiratory center, resulting in an increased pulmonary rate and depth of respiration, provided that the primary defect is not in the respiratory center. Elimination of carbon dioxide through the lungs results in a decrease in $cdCO_2$; thus the ratio of $cHCO_3^-/cdCO_2$ and pH approach normal.

Laboratory Findings in Respiratory Acidosis

Plasma $cdCO_2$, PCO_2, $cHCO_3^-$, and therefore $ctCO_2$ are elevated in respiratory acidoses. Because of an increase in $cdCO_2$, the ratio of $cHCO_3^-/cdCO_2$ is decreased, resulting in a decreased pH. In the acute phase, $cHCO_3^-$ will increase by ≈1 mmol/L for each 10 mm Hg rise in PCO_2. If respiratory acidosis persists, the change will be ≈3.5 mmol/L, mainly as a result of renal compensation. For every 15 mm Hg increase in PCO_2, pH decreases in the *acute* phase by ≈0.10 pH unit, and in *chronic* conditions by slightly less than 0.05 pH unit. For example, if the PCO_2 increases acutely by 30 mm Hg, the pH drops to ≈7.20. The same PCO_2 increase in a chronic condition results in a pH of ≈7.31. The plasma chloride decreases as plasma bicarbonate increases. Hyperkalemia may occur but is not as predictable as in some forms of metabolic acidosis. For every 0.1 unit decrease in pH, there is generally an inverse change of 0.6 mmol/L in K^+. Urinary acidity and ammonium content are increased as the kidney attempts to compensate.

Respiratory Alkalosis

A decrease in PCO_2 (hypocapnia) and the resulting primary deficit in $cdCO_2$ (respiratory alkalosis) are caused by an increased rate and/or depth of respiration. Therefore, the basic cause of respiratory alkalosis is excess elimination of acid via the respiratory route. Excessive elimination of carbon dioxide reduces the PCO_2 and causes an increase in the $cHCO_3^-/cdCO_2$ ratio. The latter shifts the normal equilibrium of the bicarbonate/carbonic acid buffer system, reducing the hydrogen ion concentration and increasing the pH. This shift also results in a decrease in $cHCO_3^-$, which somewhat ameliorates the change in pH. Analogous to causes of respiratory acidosis, causes of respiratory alkalosis can be classified as those with a direct stimulatory effect on the respiratory center and those due to effects on the pulmonary system. These and some additional conditions underlying respiratory alkaloses are listed in Box 49-3.

BOX 49-3 Factors Causing Respiratory Alkalosis

Nonpulmonary Stimulation of Respiratory Center
Anxiety, hysteria
Febrile state
Gram-negative septicemia
Metabolic encephalopathy (e.g., due to liver disease)
Central nervous system infection such as meningitis, encephalitis
Cerebrovascular accident
Intracranial surgery
Hypoxia [e.g., severe anemia, high altitudes (acute condition)]
Drugs and agents such as salicylates, catecholamines, and progesterone
Pregnancy, mainly third trimester (↑ progesterone?)
Hyperthyroidism

Pulmonary Disorders*
Pneumonia
Pulmonary emboli
Interstitial lung disease
Large right-to-left shunt (PCO_2 <50 mm Hg)
Congestive heart failure
Respiratory compensation after correction of metabolic acidosis

Others
Ventilator-induced hyperventilation

*The severe stages of some of these disorders may be associated with respiratory acidosis if elimination of CO_2 is severely impaired.

Compensatory Mechanisms in Respiratory Alkalosis

The compensatory mechanisms respond to respiratory alkalosis in two stages. In the first stage, erythrocyte and tissue buffers provide H^+ ions that consume a small amount of HCO_3^-. The second stage becomes operational in prolonged respiratory alkalosis and depends on renal compensation as described for metabolic alkalosis (decreased reclamation of bicarbonate).

Laboratory Findings in Respiratory Alkalosis

In this condition, $cdCO_2$, PCO_2, $cHCO_3^-$, and thus total CO_2 concentration all decrease. The ratio of $cHCO_3^-/cdCO_2$ is increased, causing an increase in pH. During the acute phase, $cHCO_3^-$ falls by 2 mmol/L for each 10 mm Hg decrease in PCO_2 (i.e., if the PCO_2 falls by 20 mm Hg, $cHCO_3^-$ is decreased by 4 mmol/L). For the same 20 mm Hg decrease in PCO_2, the (H^+) will decrease by 16 nmol/L.

If the original cH^+ was 40 nmol/L, it would now be 24 nmol/L (40 − 16 = 24), which corresponds to a pH of 7.61 (see Figure 49-6). Finally, individuals living at high altitudes chronically hyperventilate owing to hypoxia and have PCO_2 values lower than those seen at sea level.

REFERENCES

1. Adrogué HJ, Madias NE. Hypernatremia. N Engl J Med 2002;342: 1493-9.

2. Birnbaumer M. The V2 vasopressin receptor mutations and fluid homeostasis. Cardiovasc Res 2001;51:409-15.
3. Chesney R. Specific renal tubular disorders. In: Goldman L, Bennett J, eds. Cecil textbook of medicine, 21st edition. Philadelphia: WB Saunders, 2000:605-10.
4. Dorwart WV, Chalmers L. Comparison of methods for calculating serum osmolality form chemical concentrations, and the prognostic value of such calculations. Clin Chem 1975;21:190-4.
5. Dufour DR. Acid-base disorders. In: Dufour R, Christenson RH, eds. Professional practice in clinical chemistry: a review. Washington, DC: AACC Press, 1995:604-35.
6. Ellison DH, Berl T. The syndrome of inappropriate antidiuresis. N Engl J Med 2007;356:2064-72.
7. Farese RV Jr, Biglieri EG, Shackleton CH, Irony I, Gomez-Fontes R. Licorice-induced hypermineralocorticoidism. N Engl J Med 1991;325: 1223-7.
8. Figge J, Rossing TH, Fencl V. The role of serum proteins in acid-base equilibria. J Lab Clin Med 1991;117:453-67.
9. Gabriely I, Leu JP, Barzel US. Clinical problem-solving: back to basics. N Engl J Med 2008;358:1952-6.
10. Handy JM, Soni N. Physiological effects of hyperchloraemia and acidosis. Br J Anaesth 2008;101:141-50.
11. Jackson E. Diuretics. In: Hardman JG, Linbird LE, eds. Goodman and Gilman's the pharmacological basis of therapeutics, 10th edition. New York: McGraw-Hill, 2001:763-7.
12. Kadakia SC. D-Lactic acidosis in a patient with jejunoileal bypass. J Clin Gastroenterol 1995;20:154-6.
13. Kaplan JH. Biochemistry of Na,K-ATPase. Annu Rev Biochem 2002;71: 511-35.
14. Kraut JA, Madias NE. Serum anion gap: its uses and limitations in clinical medicine. Clin J Am Soc Nephrol 2007;2:162-74.
15. Lash JP, Arruda JA. Laboratory evaluation of renal tubular acidosis. Clin Lab Med 1993;13:117-29.
16. MandPetri WA. Antimicrobial agents. In: Hardman JG, Linbird LE, eds. Goodman and Gilman's the pharmacological basis of therapeutics, 10th edition. New York: McGraw-Hill, 2001:1276-7.
17. Miltiadous G, Christidis D, Kalogirou M, Elisaf M. Causes and mechanisms of acid-base and electrolyte abnormalities in cancer patients. Eur J Intern Med 2008;19:1-7.
18. Palmer BF. Approach to fluid and electrolyte disorders and acid-base problems. Prim Care 2008;35:195-213.
19. Preuss HG. Fundamentals of clinical acid-base evaluation. Clin Lab Med 1993;13:103-16.
20. Putney LK, Denker SP, Barber DL. The changing face of the Na^+/H^+ exchanger, NHE1: structure, regulation, and cellular actions. Annu Rev Pharmacol Toxicol 2002;42:527-52.
21. Robertson GL. Diabetes insipidus. Endocrinol Metab Clin North Am 1995;24:549-72.
22. Ruth JL, Wassner SJ. Body composition: salt and water. Pediatr Rev 2006;27:181-7; quiz 8.
23. Siggaard-Andersen O. An acid-base chart for arterial blood with normal and pathophysiological reference areas. Scand J Clin Lab Invest 1971;27:239-45.
24. Siggaard-Andersen O. The van Slyke equation. Scand J Clin Lab Invest Suppl 1977;37:15-20.
25. Singer G. Fluid and electrode management. In: Ahya SL, Flood K, Paranjothi S, Schaiff R, eds. The Washington manual of medical therapeutics, 30th edition. Philadelphia: Lippincott, Williams and Wilkins, 2001:3-75.
26. Skott O. Renin. Am J Physiol Regul Integr Comp Physiol 2002;282: R937-9.
27. Tietz NW, ed. Textbook of clinical chemistry, 1st edition. Philadelphia: WB Saunders, 1986.
28. Tietz textbook of clinical chemistry, 2nd edition. Philadelphia: WB Saunders, 1994.
29. van der Hoek J, Hoorn EJ, de Jong GM, Janssens EN, de Herder WW. Severe hyponatremia with high urine sodium and osmolality. Clin Chem 2009;55:1905-8.
30. Verbalis JG. Hyponatremia and hypoosmolar disorders. In: Greenberg A, Cheung AK, eds. Primer on kidney diseases, Philadelphia: Elsevier Saunders, 2005:55-65.
31. Watson MA, Scott MG. Clinical utility of biochemical analysis of cerebrospinal fluid. Clin Chem 1995;41:343-60.

ADDITIONAL READING

Adrogué HJ, Madias NE. Management of life-threatening acid-base disorders, first of two parts (review). N Engl J Med 1998;338:26-34. Erratum in: N Engl J Med 1998;340:247.

Adrogué HJ, Madias NE. Management of life-threatening acid-base disorders, second of two parts (review). N Engl J Med 1998;338: 107-11.

Adrogué HJ, Madias NE. Hyponatremia (review). N Engl J Med 2000;342: 1581-9.

CHAPTER 50

Liver Disease

D. Robert Dufour, M.D., F.C.A.P., F.A.C.B.*

The liver has a central and critical biochemical role in the (1) metabolism, (2) digestion, (3) detoxification, and (4) elimination of substances from the body. All blood from the intestinal tract initially passes through the liver, where products derived from digestion of food are processed, transformed, and stored. These include amino acids, carbohydrates, fatty acids, cholesterol, lipids, vitamins, and minerals (see Chapters 21, 26, 27, and 31 respetcively). Most major plasma proteins (with the exception of immunoglobulins and von Willebrand factor) are mainly or exclusively synthesized in the liver. The liver responds to multiple hormonal and neural stimuli to regulate the blood glucose concentration. Not only does it extract glucose from blood for use in generating energy, it also stores dietary glucose as glycogen for later use. The liver is also the major site for gluconeogenesis, which is critical for maintaining blood glucose in the fasting state. The liver is central in lipid metabolism; it extracts and processes dietary lipids, and it is the principal site of cholesterol, triglyceride, and lipoprotein synthesis. Another major liver function is the synthesis of bile acids from cholesterol with secretion of these compounds into the bile, facilitating the absorption of dietary fat and fat-soluble vitamins. The liver is also the primary site of metabolism of both endogenous substances and exogenous compounds, such as drugs and toxins. This process, known as *biotransformation,* converts lipophilic substances to hydrophilic ones for subsequent elimination. The liver is a major site of catabolism of hormones, and thus participates in regulation of plasma hormone concentrations. The liver is also involved in hormone synthesis, producing such hormones as insulin-like growth factor 1, angiotensinogen, hepcidin, thrombopoietin, erythropoietin, and the prohormone 25-OH vitamin D. Many of these hepatic functions may be assessed by laboratory procedures to gain insight into the integrity of the liver.

As a large organ, the liver shares with many other organs the ability to perform its functions with extensive reserve capacity. In many cases, individuals with liver disease maintain normal function despite extensive liver damage. In such cases, liver disease may be recognized only by using tests that detect injury. Most commonly, this is accomplished by measuring plasma activities of enzymes found within liver cells, released in somewhat specific patterns with different forms of injury. Chronic liver injury often involves fibrosis in the liver; markers of the fibrotic process might be indicators of degree of injury. Chronic damage is often due to chronic inflammation; cytokines alter the pattern of liver protein production, allowing detection of inflammation (although not necessarily that involving the liver). Some proteins are produced in increased amounts with liver regeneration and neoplasm; such markers may be useful in detecting liver cell proliferation.

The chapter begins with a discussion of the anatomy and biochemical functions of the liver. Various disease states that involve the liver are then discussed. The chapter concludes with a discussion of the use of laboratory test results in recognizing and characterizing patterns of liver injury.

ANATOMY OF THE LIVER

The adult liver weighs approximately 1.2 to 1.5 kg. It is located beneath the diaphragm in the right upper quadrant of the abdomen and is protected by the ribs and held in place by ligamentous attachments.

Gross Anatomy

The liver is divided into left and right anatomic lobes by the falciform ligament, an anterior extension of the peritoneal folds that connects the liver to the diaphragm and the anterior abdominal wall (Figure 50-1). Two smaller lobes are found on the posterior surface (caudate lobe) and the inferior surface (quadrate lobe) of the right lobe. Riedel's lobe, an anatomic extension of the right lobe of the liver, consists of a projection that may feel like a mobile tumor in the right abdomen.

The liver has a dual blood supply. The portal vein, which carries blood from the spleen and nutrient-enriched blood from the gastrointestinal (GI) tract, supplies approximately 70% of the blood supply; the hepatic artery, a branch of the celiac axis, provides oxygen-enriched arterial blood. Each supplies approximately half of the oxygen reaching the liver, making it highly resistant to infarction. Ultimately, these two blood supplies merge and flow into the sinusoids that course

*The author gratefully acknowledges the original contributions by Drs. Keith G. Tolman and Robert Rej upon which portions of this chapter are based.

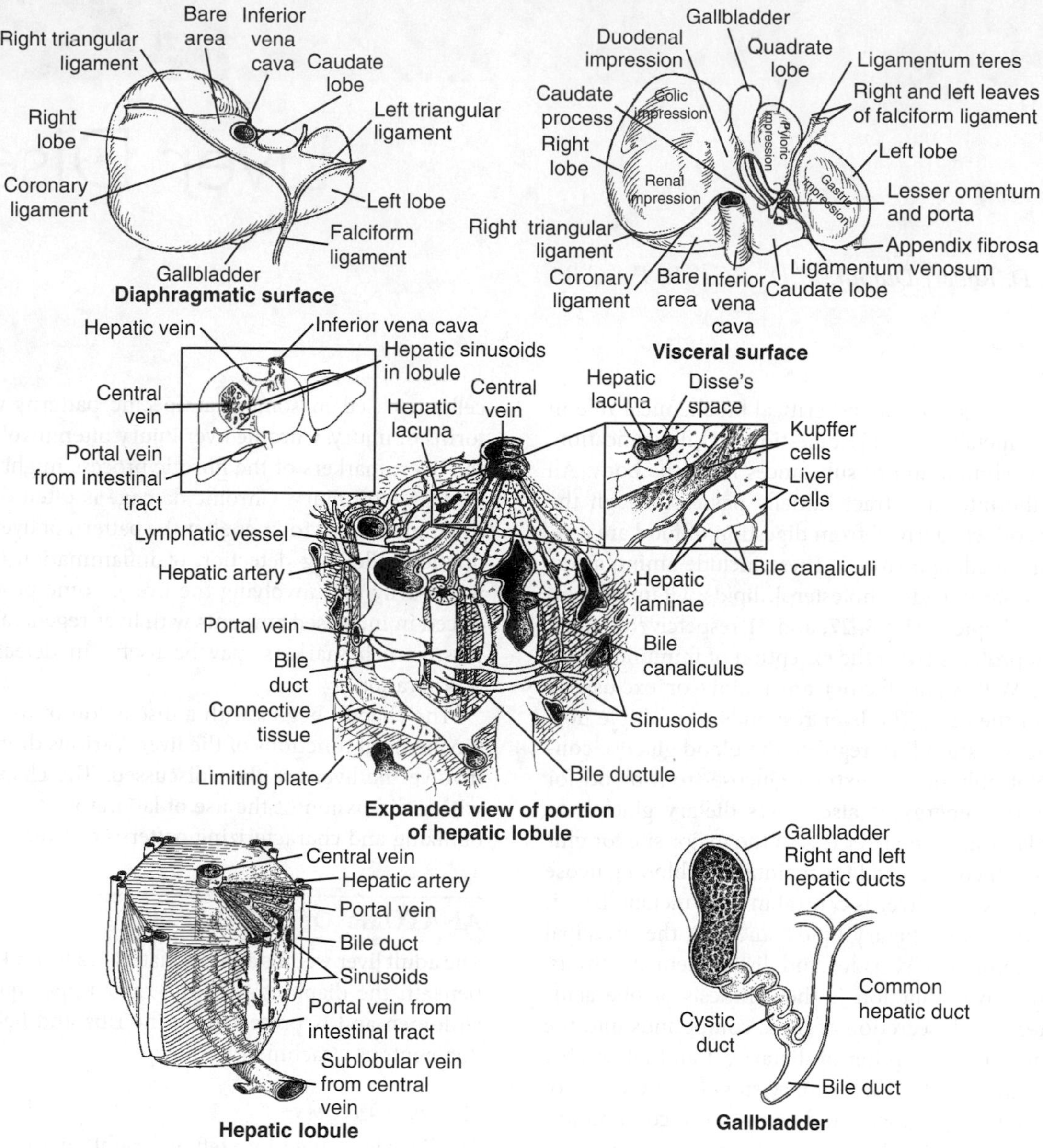

Figure 50-1 Structure of the liver. *(From Dorland's illustrated medical dictionary, 30th edition. Philadelphia, Pa: WB Saunders, 2003, plate 26.)*

between individual hepatocytes. Venous drainage from the liver ultimately converges into the right and left hepatic veins, which exit on the posterior surface of the liver and join the inferior vena cava near its entry into the right atrium.

The liver is covered by an anterior reflection of the peritoneum known as *Glisson's capsule.* Other extensions of the peritoneum form ligaments that hold the liver in place. Internal extensions of the capsule provide an internal supporting framework that divides the liver into lobules and ultimately surrounds blood vessels and nerves. One of the ligaments, the ligamentum teres, is the vestigial remnant of the umbilical vein; it connects the umbilicus to the inferior border of the liver. When portal hypertension occurs, the umbilical veins may reopen, leading to venous dilation around the umbilicus (termed *caput medusae*).

The nerve supply to the liver comes from the vagus and phrenic nerves and the sympathetic ganglia originating from cell bodies in the spinal cord that are located between the seventh and tenth thoracic vertebrae. These merge to accompany the hepatic artery and bile ducts throughout the liver.

Biliary drainage originates at the bile canaliculi; these grooves between adjacent hepatocytes form ductules that merge to create the intrahepatic bile ducts, which ultimately join to form the right and left hepatic bile ducts, which exit from the liver at the porta hepatis and combine to form the common hepatic duct. The hepatic duct is joined by the cystic duct draining the gallbladder to form the common bile duct (see Figure 50-1). The common bile duct then enters the duodenum (usually with the pancreatic duct) at the ampulla of Vater. The duodenal portion of the common bile duct is surrounded by longitudinal and circular muscle fibers that form the sphincter of Oddi. This musculature relaxes when the gallbladder contracts, allowing bile to enter the duodenum; in its normally contracted state, the sphincter prevents reflux of acidic duodenal contents into the bile duct. The gallbladder, located on the undersurface of the right lobe of the liver, is the site for storage and concentration of bile, a complex mixture of bile salts and waste products. In the adult, it averages about 10 cm in length and has a capacity of 30 to 50 mL of bile. Hormonal stimuli initiated by food ingestion cause contraction of the muscular wall of the gallbladder, releasing bile salts into the intestine to facilitate digestion of fat.

Microscopic Anatomy

The functional anatomical unit of the liver is the acinus, adjacent to the portal triad (which consists of a branch of the portal vein, hepatic artery, and bile duct). Each acinus is a diamond-shaped mass of liver parenchyma that is supplied by a terminal branch of the portal vein and of the hepatic artery and is drained by a terminal branch of the bile duct. The blood vessels radiate toward the periphery, forming sinusoids, which perfuse the liver and ultimately drain into the central (terminal) hepatic vein (Figure 50-2). The sinusoids are lined by fenestrated endothelial cells (allowing free filtration of blood) and phagocytic Kupffer cells (see Figure 50-1). The Kupffer cells are derived from blood monocytes. They contain lysosomes with hydrolytic enzymes that break down phagocytized foreign particles, such as bacteria. They also have immunoglobulin and complement receptors and are the main site for clearance of antigen-antibody complexes from blood. Kupffer cells secrete interleukins, tumor necrosis factor, collagenase, prostaglandins, and other factors involved in the inflammatory response.

Hepatocytes are the major functioning cells in the liver and are responsible for about 70% of liver mass and perform most of the metabolic and synthetic functions of the liver. Two other cell types are found in small numbers within the liver. The *stellate cells* (sometimes referred to as *Ito cells*) are located between the endothelial lining of the sinusoids and the hepatocytes within a small cleft referred to as the *space of Disse.* In their normal, quiescent state, stellate cells serve as a site of storage for fat-soluble vitamins, particularly vitamin A. When stimulated, stellate cells are morphologically and functionally transformed. They synthesize collagen and are the cells responsible for fibrosis and, eventually, cirrhosis. They also synthesize nitric oxide, which helps to regulate intrahepatic blood flow. *Oval cells,* found near the portal areas around small bile passages, are believed to be liver stem cells involved in regeneration of hepatocytes and bile ducts after liver injury.[268]

The blood supply to each acinus consists of three zones (Figure 50-3). Zone 1, the area immediately adjacent to the portal tract, is enriched with lysosomes and mitochondria.

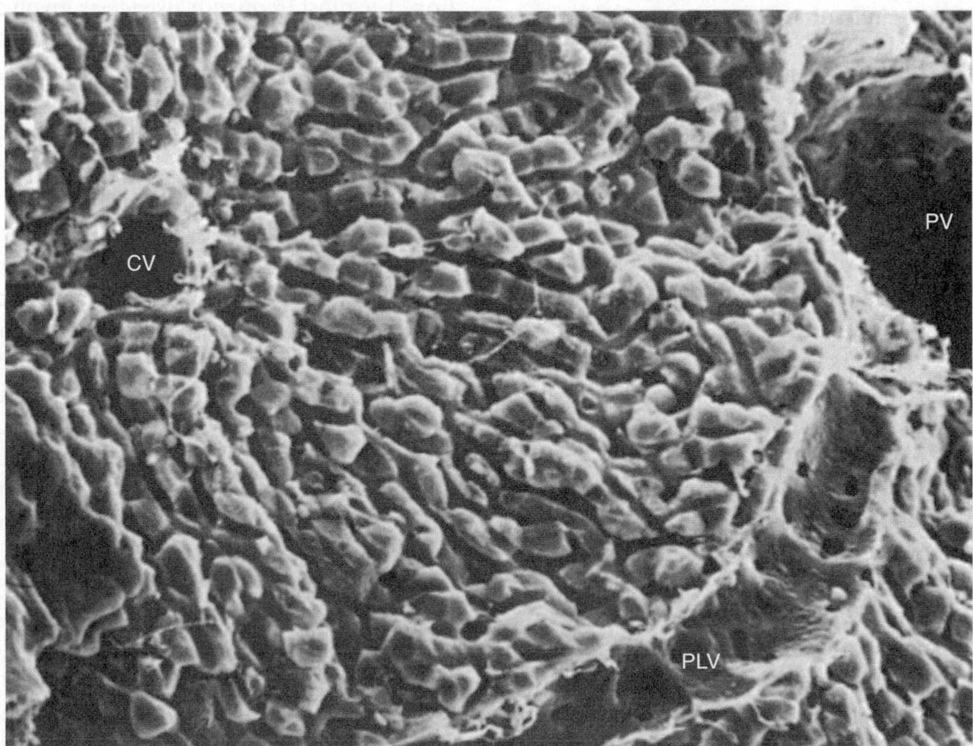

Figure 50-2 A low-magnification scanning electron micrograph depicting a portion of a liver lobule from a rat liver. *CV,* Central vein; *PLV,* perilobular venules; *PV,* portal vein. *(From Zakim O, Boyer TD. Hepatology: a textbook of liver disease, 3rd edition. Philadelphia, Pa: WB Saunders, 1996:9.)*

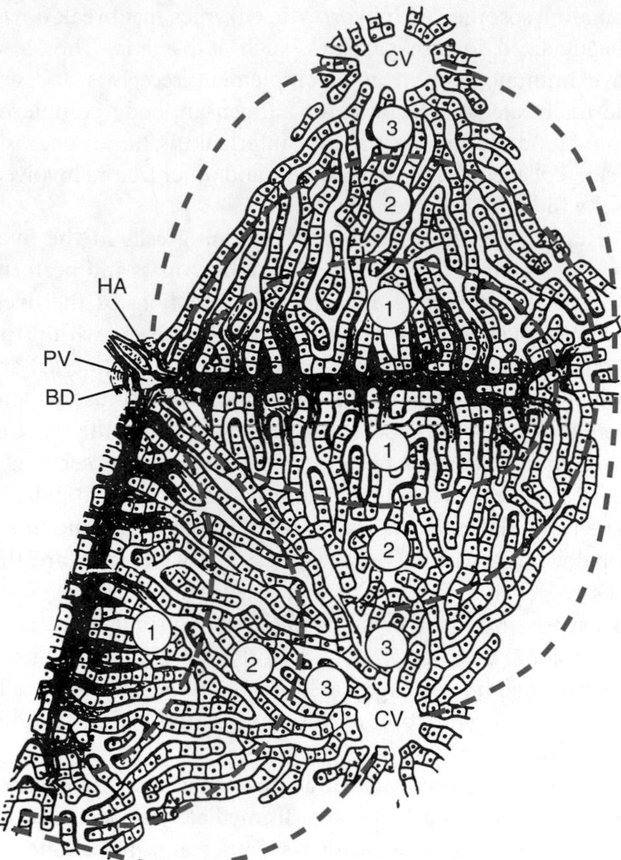

Figure 50-3 Blood supply of the simple liver acinus. *Zones 1, 2,* and *3* indicate corresponding volumes in a portion of an adjacent acinar unit. Oxygen tension and the nutrient level in the blood in sinusoids decrease from zone 1 through zone 3. *BD,* Bile duct; *CV,* central vein; *HA,* hepatic artery; *PV,* portal vein. *(From Zakim O, Boyer TD. Hepatology: a textbook of liver disease, 3rd edition. Philadelphia, Pa: WB Saunders, 1996:10.)*

The periphery of the acinus, zone 3, is enriched with endoplasmic reticulum, is very active metabolically, and has relatively low oxygen tension. This area is most susceptible to injury, although zone 1 appears to be involved in protecting the liver from external injury and providing a base for hepatic regeneration.

Ultrastructure of the Hepatocyte

Hepatocytes contain a well-developed organelle substructure (Figure 50-4). Mitochondria, which constitute approximately 18% of hepatocyte volume, are the sites of oxidative phosphorylation and energy production. They contain enzymes involved in the citric acid cycle and in β-oxidation of fatty acids. The rough endoplasmic reticulum is the site of synthesis of many proteins, including albumin, coagulation factors, enzymes (e.g., glucose-6-phosphatase), and triglycerides. The smooth endoplasmic reticulum contains microsomes that are involved in bilirubin conjugation, detoxification (cytochrome P450–dependent isoenzymes), steroid synthesis, cholesterol synthesis, and bile acid synthesis. Several microsomal enzymes, including γ-glutamyltransferase, are induced by many drugs and inhibited by others. This is the site of most drug metabolism and many important drug interactions.

Peroxisomes are found near the smooth endoplasmic reticulum and contain oxidases that use molecular oxygen to modify a variety of substrates, leading to the production of hydrogen peroxide. They also contain catalase, which decomposes hydrogen peroxide. Peroxisomes catalyze the β-oxidation of fatty acids with chain lengths from 7 to 18. Approximately 5 to 20% of the metabolism of ethanol also occurs in the peroxisomes. Lysosomes are dense organelles that contain hydrolytic enzymes that act as scavengers. Deposition of iron, lipofucsin, bile pigments, and copper occurs in the lysosomes. The Golgi apparatus lies near the canaliculus and is involved in the secretion of various substances, including bile acids and albumin.

BIOCHEMICAL FUNCTIONS OF THE LIVER

The liver is involved in various excretory, synthetic, and metabolic functions. Clinical laboratories perform numerous tests that are useful in the biochemical assessment of these functions.

Hepatic Excretory Function

Organic compounds of both endogenous and exogenous origin are extracted from the sinusoidal blood, biotransformed, and excreted into the bile or urine. Assessment of this excretory function provides valuable clinical information. The most frequently used tests involve the measurement of plasma concentrations of endogenously produced compounds, such as bilirubin and bile acids, and determination of the rate of clearance of exogenous compounds, such as aminopyrine, lidocaine, and caffeine.

Bilirubin

Bilirubin is the orange-yellow pigment derived from heme, mainly as a product of red blood cell turnover. It is extracted and biotransformed in the liver and excreted in bile and urine. The chemistry, biochemistry, and analytical methodsology for bilirubin and related compounds are discussed in Chapter 32; a brief overview of factors relevant to an understanding of liver disease is included here.

Bilirubin is transported from sites of production (mainly the spleen), loosely bound to albumin, in its native, unconjugated form. Bilirubin is transported across the hepatocyte membrane and is rapidly conjugated with glucuronic acid to produce bilirubin glucuronides, which are then excreted into bile by an energy-dependent process. This process is highly efficient, and bilirubin conjugates are detectable in normal plasma only with the use of highly sensitive techniques. In the presence of bilirubin monoglucuronide, albumin (and other proteins) can be postsynthetically modified by covalent attachment to lysine residues. In the case of albumin, this produces a protein-bound form termed *biliprotein* or *δ-bilirubin.* Increases in conjugated bilirubin or δ-bilirubin are highly specific markers of hepatic dysfunction (except in

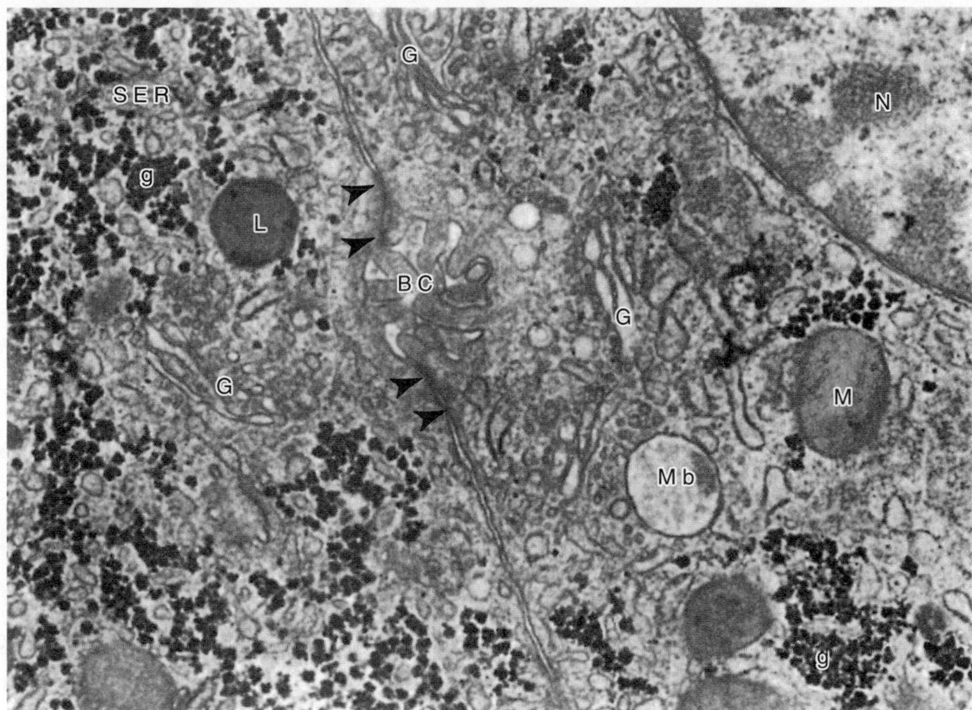

Figure 50-4 Portions of two human liver cells showing the relationship of the organelles and a typical bile canaliculus (BC). ***Arrowheads*** **indicate light junctions.** ***G,*** **Golgi;** ***g,*** **glycogen;** ***L,*** **lysosome;** ***M,*** **mitochondria;** ***Mb,*** **microbody;** ***N,*** **nucleus;** ***SER,*** **smooth endoplasmic reticulum.** *(From Zakim O, Boyer TD. Hepatology: a textbook of liver disease, 3rd edition. Philadelphia, Pa:WB Saunders, 1996:20.)*

the presence of rare inherited disorders that impair excretion of conjugated bilirubin, such as Dubin-Johnson syndrome). In the intestinal tract, bilirubin glucuronides are hydrolyzed and reduced by bacteria to form colorless *urobilinogens,* which undergo an enterohepatic circulation. A small fraction (2 to 5%) escapes the liver and is excreted in urine. In the colon, urobilinogens spontaneously oxidize to stool pigments stercobilin, mesobilin, and urobilin.

Increased plasma bilirubin typically is classified as primarily indirect (an approximation of unconjugated bilirubin) or direct (an approximation of the sum of conjugated bilirubin and biliprotein). Increased indirect bilirubin indicates overproduction of bilirubin, usually caused by hemolysis, or decreased metabolism by the liver [primarily caused by congenital defects involving uridine 5′-phosphate (UDP)-glucuronyl transferase]. With severe liver injury, as occurs with fulminant hepatic failure and end-stage cirrhosis, liver disease may cause primarily unconjugated hyperbilirubinemia. Increased urine urobilinogen occurs when bilirubin delivery to the intestinal tract is increased (as with hemolysis, or following recovery from hepatitis or obstruction), or when liver clearance is decreased, as occurs in portal hypertension.

Increased direct bilirubin generally results from functional or mechanical impairment in bilirubin excretion from the hepatocyte. Increased conjugated bilirubin is found in most cases of acute hepatitis and cholestasis (stoppage or suppression of the flow of bile); the percentage of direct bilirubin is similar in both types of liver disease.[42] Urine bilirubin reflects increased plasma concentrations of conjugated bilirubin. With resolution of liver disease, conjugated bilirubin is rapidly cleared, and biliprotein may become the only form present; urine bilirubin is typically absent in such circumstances. Increased conjugated bilirubin is rarely seen with congenital defects in bilirubin excretion, such as Dubin-Johnson syndrome, and with impaired bilirubin excretion, as occurs in sepsis or other acute illness.

Bile Acids

Regulation of bile acid metabolism is a major function of the liver. Alterations in bile acid metabolism are usually a reflection of liver dysfunction. Cholesterol homeostasis is in large part maintained by the conversion of cholesterol to bile acids and subsequent regulation of bile acid metabolism. Bile acids themselves provide surface-active detergent molecules that facilitate both hepatic excretion of cholesterol and solubilization of lipids for intestinal absorption. Bile acid homeostasis requires normal terminal ileum function to absorb bile acids for recirculation (enterohepatic circulation). Alterations in hepatic bile acid synthesis, intracellular metabolism, excretion, intestinal absorption, or plasma extraction are reflected in derangements of bile acid metabolism.

Chemistry

Four major bile acids are known. Cholic acid and chenodeoxycholic acid, the primary bile acids, are synthesized in the liver. The sequence of reactions involved in the synthesis of

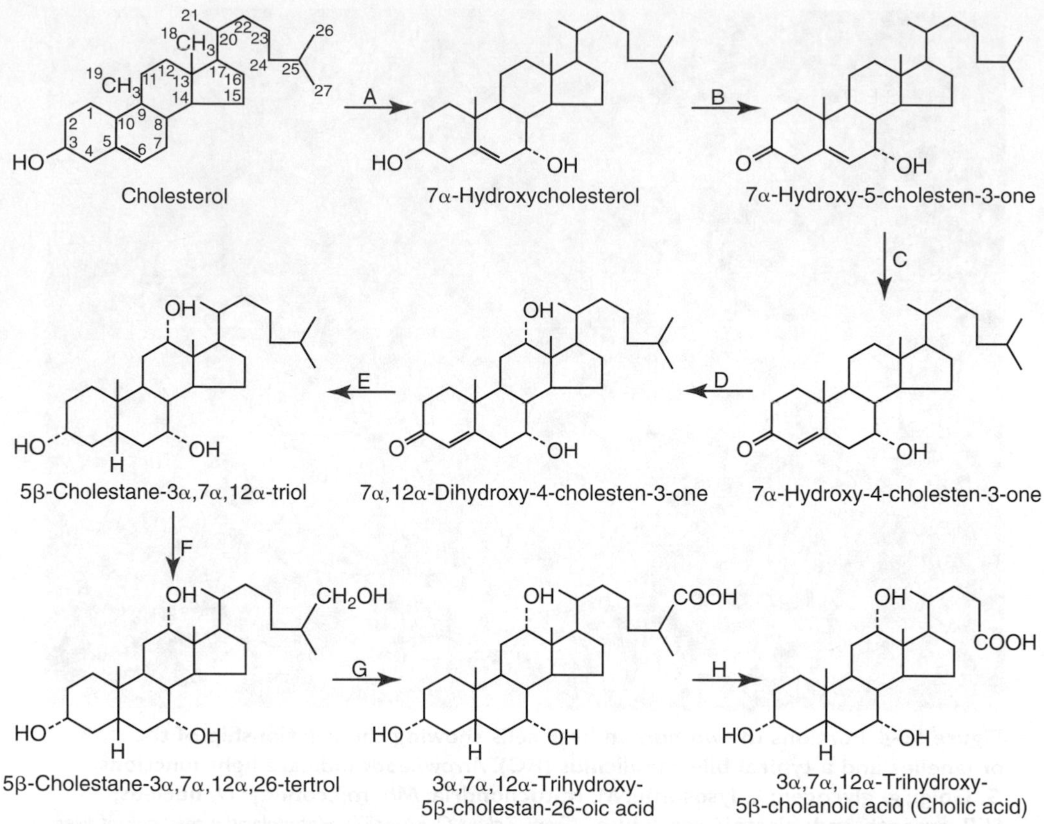

Cholesterol
A
7α-Hydroxycholesterol
B
7α-Hydroxy-5-cholesten-3-one
C
7α-Hydroxy-4-cholesten-3-one
D
7α,12α-Dihydroxy-4-cholesten-3-one
E
5β-Cholestane-3α,7α,12α-triol
F
5β-Cholestane-3α,7α,12α,26-tertrol
G
3α,7α,12α-Trihydroxy-5β-cholestan-26-oic acid
H
3α,7α,12α-Trihydroxy-5β-cholanoic acid (Cholic acid)

Figure 50-5 The biosynthetic pathways of cholesterol conversion to cholic acid. *A,* 7-α-Hydroxylation of cholesterol (addition of —OH group at position 7-α-configuration), the rate-limiting step in the biosynthetic pathway. *B,* Oxidation of the 3-β-hydroxyl group (to form 3-oxo compound). *C,* Isomerization of the 5-ene structure. *D,* 12-α-Hydroxylation (for cholic acid only). *E,* Saturation of the double bond and reduction of the 3-one group. *F,* Hydroxylation of the side chain at C-26 position. *G,* Side chain oxidation to cholestanoic acid. *H,* Hydroxylation at C-24 and β-oxidation to reduce the length of the side chain. *(From Balistreri WF, Setchel KDR. Clinical implications of bile acid metabolism. In: Silverberg M, Daum F, eds. Textbook of pediatric gastroenterology, 2nd edition. Chicago, Ill: Year Book Medical Publishers, 1988:72-89. By permission of Mosby, Inc.)*

cholic acid from cholesterol is shown in Figure 50-5. To date, nine inborn errors of bile acid synthesis have been identified; these can present with neonatal hepatitis, fat malabsorption, or neurologic defects that can progress to chronic liver disease or liver failure and death.[192] The primary bile acids are metabolized (by bacterial 7-α-dehydroxylase) in the intestinal lumen to the secondary bile acids—deoxycholic acid and lithocholic acid. Bile acids (at their carboxylic acid) are conjugated in the liver with the amino acid glycine or taurine. This decreases passive absorption in the biliary tree and proximal small intestine, but permits conservation through active transport in the terminal ileum. Approximately 0.1 to 0.6 g of bile acids is lost in the feces daily.

Because they possess both polar and nonpolar regions, molecules of bile acids are able to solubilize biliary lipids. Such molecules align at water-lipid interfaces and reduce surface tension, acting as detergents. In an aqueous solution, bile acids aggregate to form small polymolecular aggregates ≈5 nm in diameter called *micelles,* which are capable of incorporating cholesterol and phospholipids to form mixed micelles. Micellar solubilization of these water-insoluble constituents maintains cholesterol in solution. In the intestinal lumen, dietary cholesterol and the products of triglyceride digestion (predominantly free fatty acids and monoglycerides) are incorporated into mixed micelles. Micelles deliver lipolytic products to the mucosal surface. To carry out these functions, a critical micellar bile acid concentration of ≈2 mmol/L is necessary. Bile acids are thus important for ensuring the solubility of cholesterol (a major component of most gallstones) in bile and dietary lipids (including fat-soluble vitamins) in the intestinal lumen.

Clinical Significance of Bile Acids

In view of the multiple processes involved in bile acid synthesis, conjugation, and excretion, and in its hepatic and intestinal uptake, several potential sites for primary or secondary disturbances have been identified (Box 50-1). With hepatocyte dysfunction (as occurs in many liver disorders), decreased

BOX 50-1 Disturbances in Bile Acid Metabolism

Defective bile acid synthesis
Inherited defects in bile acid synthesis
Acquired defects in bile acid synthesis secondary to liver disease
Extrahepatic bile duct obstruction
Bile acid malabsorption
Defective uptake or altered intracellular metabolism

bile acid synthesis results in low primary bile acid concentrations and a decreased ratio of primary to secondary bile acids in plasma; in addition, decreased extraction from plasma often leads to increased concentrations of bile acids, particularly in the nonfasting state. With cholestatic disorders, decreased delivery of primary bile acids to the intestine with resulting decreased secondary bile acid production causes an increased ratio of primary to secondary bile acids, as well as increased total bile acid concentrations. With intestinal disease (including bypass operations that may be performed to treat obesity), increased fecal loss of bile acids leads to decreased concentrations of both primary and secondary bile acids and, often, a decrease in cholesterol caused by increased need for bile acid synthesis. Although bile acid concentrations are abnormal in many situations, they add little to standard tests of liver function and are rarely used in clinical medicine.

Analytical Methods

Analytical techniques used to quantify total or individual bile acids in biological fluids include (1) gas-liquid chromatography (GLC), (2) high-performance liquid chromatography (HPLC), (3) enzymatic assay, (4) radioimmunoassay (RIA), (5) enzyme-linked immunosorbent assay (ELISA), and (6) tandem mass spectrometry (MS/MS).

Hepatic Synthetic Function

The liver has extensive synthetic capacity and plays a major role in the regulation of protein, carbohydrate, and lipid metabolism (see Chapters 21, 26, and 27). A bidirectional flux of precursors and products, such as glucose, amino acids, free fatty acids, and other nutrients, occurs across the hepatocyte membrane. Normal blood glucose concentrations are maintained during short fasts by the breakdown of hepatic glycogen and during prolonged fasts by hepatic gluconeogenesis. The primary sources of carbon atoms for gluconeogenesis are amino acids derived from muscle proteins. To a lesser extent, lactate (produced in skeletal muscle and erythrocytes) and glycerol (obtained from hydrolysis of triglycerides) also serve as substrates for gluconeogenesis. In humans, the oxidation of odd-numbered fatty acids yields propionyl-CoA, which can be converted to glucose. However, the formation of glucose in this manner is not quantitatively significant. Protein, triglyceride, fatty acid, cholesterol, and bile acid synthesis also occurs within the liver.

Protein Synthesis

The liver is the primary site of the synthesis of plasma proteins (see Chapter 21). Synthesis occurs in the rough endoplasmic reticulum of hepatocytes, followed by release into the hepatic sinusoids. Although disturbances of protein synthesis occur as a consequence of impaired hepatic function, a variety of other factors may affect plasma protein concentrations. These include (1) decreased availability of amino acids (malnutrition, maldigestion, and malabsorption), (2) catabolic states (hyperthyroidism, Cushing's syndrome, burns, postsurgery recovery), (3) protein-losing states (nephrotic syndrome and protein-losing enteropathy), (4) actions of cytokines (decrease in transport proteins such as albumin, transferrin, and lipoproteins, but increase in inflammatory response modifiers such as α_1-antitrypsin, ceruloplasmin, and α_2-macroglobulin), (5) action of hormones (such as growth hormone, cortisol, estrogen, androgens, and thyroid hormones) to increase or decrease production of specific proteins, and (6) congenital deficiency states (Wilson's disease and α_1-antitrypsin deficiency). In addition, the liver has a significant reserve capacity, preventing protein concentrations from decreasing unless liver damage is extensive. In addition, many liver proteins have relatively long half-lives, such as albumin at approximately 3 weeks. For this reason, the sensitivity and specificity of protein concentrations for diagnosis of liver disease are far from ideal.

The patterns of plasma protein alterations seen in liver disease depend on the type, severity, and duration of liver injury. For example, in acute hepatic dysfunction, usually little change is seen in the plasma protein profile or the total plasma protein concentration; with fulminant hepatic failure or severe liver injury, concentrations of short-lived hepatic proteins (such as transthyretin and prothrombin) fall quickly and become abnormal, whereas proteins with longer half-lives are normal or minimally changed. In cirrhosis, concentrations of liver-synthesized plasma proteins and immunoglobulins decrease and increase, respectively. Serial determination of plasma proteins provides prognostic information, for example, worsening of prothrombin time during acute hepatitis suggests a poor prognosis.

Plasma Proteins

Albumin. Albumin, the most commonly measured serum protein, is synthesized exclusively by the liver. The rate of synthesis varies, depending on hormonal environment, nutritional status, age, and other local factors. In inflammatory conditions, interleukin (IL)-6 inhibits albumin synthesis but induces synthesis of acute-phase response proteins. With liver disease, hypoalbuminemia is noted primarily in cirrhosis, autoimmune hepatitis, and alcoholic hepatitis. The mechanism is multifactorial. In cirrhosis, hepatic synthesis of albumin may be decreased, normal, or increased. Loss of albumin into ascitic fluid seems responsible for the decrease in albumin in many cases. One important consideration in measurement of albumin is the inaccuracy of dye-binding methods in patients with liver disease. Although bromocresol green measurements tend to overestimate albumin concentration at low concentrations,[293] bromocresol purple methods give falsely low values in patients with jaundice because of interference of bilirubin at the site of binding.[207]

Transthyretin. This protein has a short half-life of 24 to 48 hours, making it a sensitive indicator of current synthetic ability. Transthyretin is typically decreased in cirrhosis (among other conditions) as a result of decreased synthesis. It is more commonly used as a measurement of nutritional status.

Immunoglobulins. Immunoglobulins are commonly increased in cirrhosis, autoimmune hepatitis, and primary biliary cirrhosis but are normal in most other types of liver disease. Immunoglobulin (Ig)G is increased in autoimmune hepatitis and cirrhosis; IgM is increased in primary biliary cirrhosis. IgA tends to be increased in all types of cirrhosis. None of these findings are specific, and they are seldom used in the diagnosis of liver disease.

Ceruloplasmin. This protein is decreased in Wilson's disease, cirrhosis, and many causes of chronic hepatitis, but may be increased by inflammation, cholestasis, hemochromatosis, pregnancy, and estrogen therapy. It is discussed in greater detail under Wilson's disease.

α_1-Antitrypsin. This protein, which is the major serine protease inhibitor (serpin) in plasma, is decreased in homozygous deficiency and cirrhosis and is increased by acute inflammation. It is discussed in greater detail later in this chapter under the heading "α_1-Antitrypsin Deficiency."

α-Fetoprotein. This protein, a normal component of fetal blood, falls to adult concentrations by 1 year of age. Mild increases are seen in patients with acute and chronic hepatitis and indicate hepatocellular regeneration. It is present at higher concentrations in hepatocellular carcinoma (HCC) and is discussed in greater detail later and in Chapters 21 and 24.

Coagulation Proteins

The coagulation proteins that are synthesized in the liver are listed in Table 50-1. These proteins interact to produce a fibrin clot (see Chapter 59). Inhibitors of the coagulation system, including antithrombin, protein C, and protein S, are also synthesized in the liver. Some of the coagulation factors (II, VII, IX, and X) require vitamin K for post-translational carboxylation within the hepatocyte. Proteins C and S are also carboxylated by a vitamin K–dependent enzyme. Activated protein C in plasma inhibits coagulation by inactivating factors V and VIII. Parenchymal liver disease of sufficient severity to impair protein synthesis or obstructive liver disease sufficient to impair intestinal absorption of vitamin K is therefore a potential cause of bleeding disorders. Because of the great functional reserve of the liver, failure of hemostasis usually does not occur except in severe or long-standing liver disease.

Prothrombin time (PT) measures the activity of fibrinogen (factor I), prothrombin (factor II), and factors V, VII, and X. Because all of these factors are made in the liver and several are vitamin K dependent, a prolonged PT often indicates the presence of significant liver disease. In cholestasis, vitamin K deficiency may cause an increase in PT. In this case, the coagulation abnormality is corrected within a few days by parenteral injection of 10 mg of vitamin K. In contrast, if PT is prolonged because of hepatocellular disease, factor synthesis is decreased and administration of vitamin K does not typically correct the problem. PT is also prolonged in some patients with liver disease because of the presence of dysfibrinogenemia, an abnormal form of fibrinogen that does not clot normally, and that may predispose to thrombosis.[188]

TABLE 50-1 Blood Coagulation Factors

Number or Acronym	Name
I	Fibrinogen*
II	Prothrombin*†
III	Tissue factor
IV	Calcium (Ca^{2+})
V	Proaccelerin*
VI	–
VII	Proconvertin*†
VIII	Antihemophilic factor
IX	Christmas factor*†
X	Stuart-Prower factor†
XI	Plasma thromboplastin antecedent*
XII	Hageman factor*
XIII	Fibrin-stabilizing factor*
PK	Prekallikrein (Fletcher factor)*
HMWK	High molecular weight kininogen*

*Protein synthesized in liver.
†Synthesis requires vitamin K.

The method for reporting PT in liver disease remains controversial. PT measures the time to clot after exposure of plasma to tissue factor. Reagents differ in the amount of tissue factor present; in patients on warfarin, clotting times are more greatly prolonged when lower amounts of tissue factor and other reagents that stimulate clotting are in the reagents. This makes a reagent more sensitive to clotting factor abnormalities, but makes standardization of results between laboratories difficult. The International Normalized Ratio (INR) was developed by the World Health Organization (WHO) and the International Committee on Thrombosis and Hemostasis (ICTH) for reporting the results of blood coagulation (clotting) tests. All results are standardized using the international sensitivity index (ISI) for the particular thromboplastin reagent and instrument combination used to perform the test. In practice, it requires determination of the ISI based on the slope of the relationship between prothrombin time using the reagent and that using a reference method in patients on warfarin. The INR is then calculated as follows:

$$INR = \left[\frac{\text{PT (patient)}}{\text{PT (geometric mean of normal)}}\right]^{ISI}$$

INR has been found to standardize interpretation of PT measurements between laboratories in those taking warfarin.

Unfortunately, INR does not have the same relationship to impairment of clotting in individuals with liver disease.[216,235] The apparent explanation lies in the mechanism of clotting factor deficiency in liver disease and warfarin administration. Although liver disease inhibits synthesis of clotting factors, warfarin impairs vitamin K–dependent carboxylation, impairing the ability of the factors to bind calcium. These noncarboxylated clotting factors (termed proteins induced by vitamin K antagonists, or PIVKAs) appear to act as inhibitors of coagulation; thus when lower amounts of tissue factor are present, clotting times are more prolonged.[235] In contrast, in liver disease, factor deficiency is due to impaired factor synthesis, and no PIVKAs are present (except in HCC, as discussed later in this chapter). This leads to lesser increases in PT in individuals with liver disease and underestimation of the degree of clotting impairment when reagents with low ISI are used. Studies have shown that calculation of a different ISI using plasma samples from patients with liver disease can standardize PT results with different reagents,[33,454] but to date, such "liver ISI" information is not readily available to laboratories.

Lipid and Lipoprotein Synthesis

The liver plays a key role in the metabolism of lipids and lipoproteins (see Chapter 27). On a daily basis, approximately 33% of the fatty acids originating from adipose tissue enter the liver, where they undergo esterification into triglycerides or are oxidized. Oxidation is favored in the fasting state and esterification is favored in the nonfasting state. Excessive esterification results in "fatty liver," a disorder in which excess triglycerides are deposited in large vacuoles that displace other cellular components. Most cholesterol is endogenously synthesized in the liver. It and cholesterol of dietary origin enter the hepatic pool, where they are converted to bile acids, incorporated into lipoproteins, or used in the synthesis of liver cell membranes. The relative rates of secretion of bile acids, cholesterol, and lecithin are important factors in the pathogenesis of cholesterol gallstones.

Urea Synthesis

Patients with end-stage liver disease may have low concentrations of urea in plasma (see Chapter 48). The rate of urea excretion in urine is lower than in healthy individuals. In addition, plasma concentrations are elevated for the urea precursors—ammonia and amino acids. Lower specific activities of enzymes involved in urea synthesis are also seen. These findings suggest that patients with liver disease have an impaired ability to metabolize protein nitrogen and to synthesize urea. The rate of hepatic urea synthesis also depends on exogenous intake of nitrogen and on endogenous protein catabolism.

Hepatic Metabolic Function

A recurring theme is the central importance of the liver in metabolic and regulatory pathways. The functional expression of the complex, integrated organelle structure includes the metabolism of drugs (activation and detoxification) and the disposal of exogenous and endogenous substances, such as galactose and ammonia. In addition, metabolic abnormalities due to specific, inherited enzyme deficiencies can affect the liver. A classic example is galactosemia. In this condition, congenital absence of galactose-1-phosphate uridyltransferase allows accumulation of the toxic metabolite galactose-1-phosphate, which causes injury to the liver, brain, and kidneys.

Ammonia Metabolism

Biochemistry and Physiology

The major source of circulating ammonia is the GI tract. Plasma ammonia concentration in the hepatic portal vein is typically fivefold to tenfold higher than that in the systemic circulation. It is derived from the action of bacterial proteases, ureases, and amine oxidases on the contents of the colon and from the hydrolysis of glutamine in both the small and large intestines. Under normal circumstances, most of the portal vein ammonia load is metabolized to urea in hepatocytes in the Krebs-Henseleit (urea) cycle during the first pass through the liver; this process includes intramitochondrial and cytosolic enzyme-catalyzed steps (Figure 50-6).

Ammonia enters tissue of the central nervous system by passive diffusion. The rate of entry increases in proportion to the plasma concentration and is dependent on pH. Ammonia crosses the blood-brain barrier membranes more readily than the ammonium ion. As pH increases, the rate of entry of ammonia into the central nervous system tissue increases as the result of an increase in ammonia relative to ammonium. Given that the pK_a of ammonia is 8.9 at 37 °C, approximately 3% of blood ammonia is NH_3 at the normal physiological pH of 7.4. An increase in pH to 7.6 produces an increase in NH_3 to approximately 5% of total blood ammonia—a 67% increase in concentration.

Clinical Significance

Animal and human studies have shown that an elevated concentration of ammonia (hyperammonemia) exerts toxic effects on the central nervous system. Several causes, both inherited and acquired, of hyperammonemia are known. Inherited deficiencies of urea cycle enzymes are the major cause of hyperammonemia in infants.[55] The two major inherited disorders are those involving the metabolism of the dibasic amino acids lysine and ornithine and those involving the metabolism of organic acids, such as propionic acid, methylmalonic acid, isovaleric acid, and others (see Chapter 58).

Acquired causes of hyperammonemia are advanced liver disease and renal failure. Severe or chronic liver failure (as occurs in fulminant hepatitis or cirrhosis, respectively) leads to significant impairment of normal ammonia metabolism. Reye's syndrome, which is primarily a central nervous system disorder with minor hepatic dysfunction, is also associated with hyperammonemia. Hepatic encephalopathy in the cirrhotic patient is often precipitated by GI bleeding, which enhances ammonia production through bacterial metabolism of protein found in blood. Other precipitating causes of encephalopathy include (1) excess dietary protein,

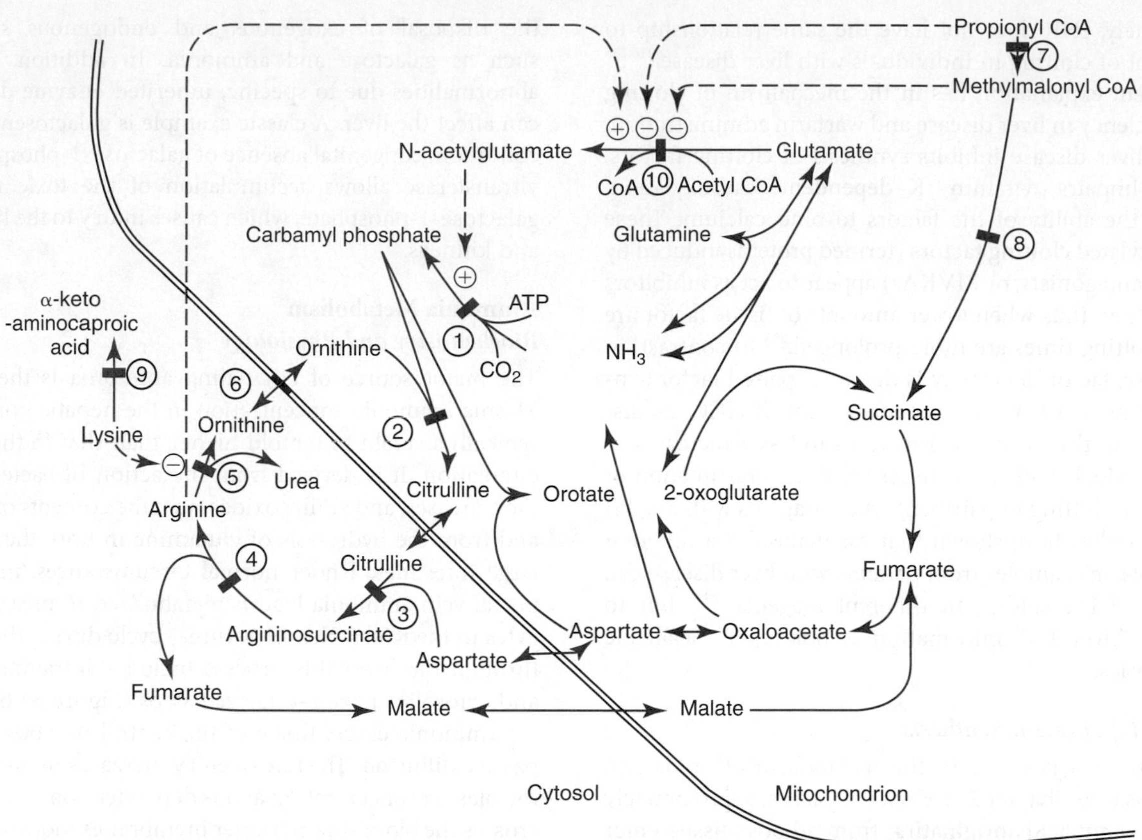

Figure 50-6 Major metabolic pathways for the use of ammonia by the hepatocyte. *Solid bars* indicate the sites of primary enzyme defects in various metabolic disorders associated with hyperammonemia: *(1)* carbamyl phosphate synthetase I, *(2)* ornithine transcarbamylase, *(3)* argininosuccinate synthetase, *(4)* argininosuccinate lyase, *(5)* arginase, *(6)* mitochondrial ornithine transport, *(7)* propionyl CoA carboxylase, *(8)* methylmalonyl CoA mutase, *(9)* L-lysine dehydrogenase, and *(10) N*-acetyl glutamine synthetase. *Dotted lines* indicate the site of pathway activation (+) or inhibition (–). *(From Flannery OB, Hsia YE, Wolf B. Current status of hyperammonemia syndromes. Hepatology 1982;2:495-506.)*

(2) constipation, (3) infection, (4) drugs, and (5) electrolyte and acid-base imbalance. Because cirrhosis is accompanied by portosystemic shunting, ammonia clearance is impaired, leading to increased concentrations of blood ammonia. Impaired renal function also causes hyperammonemia. As blood urea nitrogen (BUN) concentration increases, more diffuses into the GI tract, where is it converted to ammonia.

The fasting venous plasma ammonia concentration is useful in the differential diagnosis of encephalopathy when it is unclear whether encephalopathy is of hepatic origin.[126] It is especially helpful in diagnosing Reye's syndrome and the inherited disorders of urea metabolism, as well as increased ammonia concentrations due to drugs such as salicylates or valproate. In acute liver injury, ammonia concentrations greater than 200 μmol/L are associated with cerebral edema and a poor prognosis,[83] and it has been suggested that ammonia concentrations should be used as part of the evaluation of prognosis in acute liver failure.[37] However, plasma ammonia is not useful in patients with known chronic liver disease.[26] Although ammonia concentrations are higher as the degree of encephalopathy worsens, significant overlap between concentrations is seen in different stages of encephalopathy, and about 70% of those with cirrhosis without encephalopathy have elevated ammonia concentrations.[350] Ammonia concentrations may actually better reflect the presence of shunting blood around the portal veins than the degree of liver dysfunction.[441]

Analytical Methodology

Both enzymatic and chemical methods are used to measure ammonia in body fluids. Enzymatic assay with glutamate dehydrogenase is the most frequently used method. Plasma ammonia measurement is particularly susceptible to contamination, leading to falsely elevated concentrations. Common sampling problems are discussed in the third edition of this textbook.

Reference Intervals

For the enzymatic method, the reference interval is 15 to 45 µg/dL or 11 to 32 µmol/L.

Carbohydrate Metabolism

Because the liver is a major processor of dietary and endogenous carbohydrates, liver disease affects carbohydrate metabolism in a variety of ways (see Chapter 26). However, none of the conventional modes of evaluating carbohydrate metabolism have value in the diagnosis of liver disease. Because the liver is the major site of both glycogen storage and gluconeogenesis, hypoglycemia is a common complication in certain liver diseases, particularly Reye's syndrome, fulminant hepatic failure, advanced cirrhosis, and hepatocellular carcinoma.

Xenobiotic Metabolism and Excretion

Xenobiotics are chemical substances that are foreign to the biological system. Biochemically, they are cleared and/or metabolized by the liver; some have been used as tests of liver function. Rates of metabolism of these compounds are sometimes referred to as *quantitative liver function tests,* to distinguish them from the more commonly used term, *liver function tests,* often used to refer to measurements of liver-associated enzymes. As liver disease progresses, quantitative liver function test results gradually worsen, and their measurement adds slightly to that obtained by widely used tests such as bilirubin, albumin, and INR measurement.[130] Even when these tests are used, significant overlap of values is noted in persons with cirrhosis and less severe degrees of liver scarring, limiting their utility.

Dye Excretion Tests

Dye excretion tests [such as bromsulphthalein (BSP) and indocyanine green (ICG) clearance] were formerly used as indicators of liver disease. With the development of more sensitive and specific indicators of liver disease, dye excretion tests have become obsolete. Until the 1970s, BSP was the most frequently used dye excretion test. Because of reports of fatalities resulting from hypersensitivity and other adverse effects (nausea, syncope, headache, chills, and thrombophlebitis at the site of injection), BSP use has been discontinued. ICG clearance was used for investigating hepatic blood flow and for predicting clearance rates of drugs that undergo first-pass clearance by the liver, such as lidocaine. Typical ICG clearance values in healthy subjects range from 6.5 to 14 mL/min/kg. ICG clearance is still used occasionally.

Drug Clearance Tests

A variety of drugs that are metabolized by the liver have been used to study the action of various P_{450} enzymes. *Aminopyrine* is demethylated to form carbon dioxide and aminoantipyrine. With the use of ^{13}C- or ^{14}C -labeled aminopyrine, the resulting isotopically labeled CO_2 is measured in breath as a reflection of functioning liver mass. Decreases in metabolism are common in persons with cirrhosis,[162] but metabolism is also affected by other factors such as cigarette smoking and use of drugs such as oral contraceptives; significant intraindividual variation in results has been noted.[63] Overall diagnostic sensitivity is similar to that of other more routine laboratory tests.[340] *Caffeine* is rapidly and nearly completely absorbed from the GI tract and then undergoes *N*-demethylation by the hepatic mixed-function oxidase system. Caffeine clearance is altered during hepatic injury, being prolonged in both chronic hepatitis and cirrhosis.[484] A single dose of caffeine (3.5 mg/kg to a maximum dose of 200 mg, dissolved in water, fruit juice, or milk for oral administration) is administered. This caffeine dose is equivalent to that found in one cup of brewed coffee or in one can of commercial soft drink.

Blood (or salivary samples) obtained before and at timed intervals after caffeine ingestion can be analyzed by reversed-phase HPLC or immunoassay. A close correlation is found between plasma and salivary caffeine concentrations. Caffeine half-life is approximately 5.5 hours in healthy adults and 3 hours in healthy children, with clearance of approximately 2 mL/min/kg in healthy adults and 10 mL/min/kg in healthy children. Caffeine clearance correlates with the aminopyrine breath test and has similar limitations, although it is less subject to effects of variables, such as smoking and oral contraceptive use.[63] *Lidocaine* undergoes *N*-de-ethylation in the liver by cytochrome P450 to form monoethylglycinexylidide (MEGX); the rate of appearance of MEGX in plasma reflects hepatic lidocaine clearance. Because lidocaine is highly extracted, its clearance is flow dependent. Thus alterations in hepatic blood flow also influence lidocaine elimination.[502] Lidocaine (1 mg/kg) is given by intravenous bolus; plasma is obtained at baseline and at 15 minutes for MEGX concentration (time of plateau concentration in healthy individuals). MEGX is most commonly measured using immunoassay. Lidocaine clearance has been used to assess liver transplant function, but its use is limited by the effect of hypoperfusion (as occurs in sepsis or volume depletion).[155]

Hepatic Storage Function

Because individual cells are unable to store a sufficient supply of energy-rich carbohydrate substrates, the liver serves as the major site for their storage. For example, hepatic storage of glycogen allows the release of glucose to other tissue when the need exists (e.g., when plasma concentrations of glucose decrease). Other tissues, such as muscle and adipose tissue, store proteins and triglycerides, respectively, and are capable of adaptation. Depending on the availability of oxidizable fuels, these tissues also switch from the storage mode to the synthesis or release mode during periods of decreased carbohydrate intake.

CLINICAL MANIFESTATIONS OF LIVER DISEASE

Various characteristics indicate the presence of liver disease, including (1) jaundice, (2) portal hypertension, (3) abnormal renal function, (4) altered drug metabolism, (5) nutritional and metabolic abnormalities, (6) disordered hemostasis, and (7) release of enzymes into various body fluids.

Jaundice

Jaundice (or icterus) is a physical sign characterized by a yellow appearance of the skin, mucous membranes, and sclera caused by bilirubin deposition. It is the most specific clinical manifestation of hepatic dysfunction, but is not present in many individuals with liver disease (especially chronic liver disease) and may occur in states of bilirubin overproduction (such as hemolysis). Jaundice is seen most easily in the sclera of the eyes, where yellow contrasts sharply with the usual bright white color. Jaundice is usually apparent clinically when the plasma bilirubin concentration reaches 2 to 3 mg/dL (34 to 51 μmol/L), although higher concentrations may be required when fluorescent lighting is used. When bilirubin clearance from the liver to the intestinal tract is impaired (as in acute hepatitis and bile duct obstruction), acholic (gray-colored) stools may be noted. Bilirubin is the source of stercobilin, which produces the brown color of normal stool. Increases in plasma conjugated bilirubin lead to tea-colored urine, because conjugated bilirubin is water soluble. Jaundice may also be due to disorders of bilirubin metabolism. Bilirubin metabolism is discussed more fully in Chapter 32. Classification of jaundice, based on the site of altered bilirubin metabolism, is shown in Box 32-1 of that chapter.

Portal Hypertension

The portal circulation handles all venous outflow of the GI tract, the spleen, the pancreas, and the gallbladder (Figure 50-7). The portal vein is formed by the union of the splenic vein and the superior mesenteric vein. Portal flow is normally 1000 to 1200 mL/min with pressure of 5 to 7 mm Hg. Portal hypertension occurs when portal flow is obstructed anywhere along its course. Causes of obstruction leading to portal hypertension are classified by site: (1) presinusoidal, (2) sinusoidal, and (3) postsinusoidal. Presinusoidal portal hypertension is most commonly caused by portal vein thrombosis or schistosomiasis but may also occur with increased portal flow, such as occurs with Felty syndrome (a combination of chronic rheumatoid arthritis, splenomegaly, leukopenia, pigmented spots on the lower extremities, and sometimes other evidence of hypersplenism, such as anemia and thrombocytopenia). Sinusoidal hypertension is most commonly caused by cirrhosis but may occur transiently with acute and chronic hepatitis or acute fatty liver. The most important cause of postsinusoidal hypertension is hepatic vein occlusion or Budd-Chiari syndrome,[149A] in which sudden obstruction or occlusion of the hepatic veins (associated with myeloproliferative disorders in half of cases) causes hepatomegaly, abdominal pain, severe ascites, mild jaundice, and eventually portal hypertension and liver failure.[364] The most common cause of postsinusoidal hypertension is cardiac disease, most commonly congestive heart failure. Chronic congestive heart failure is usually associated with portal hypertension and ascites, and may even lead to increased activities of aminotransferases.[323] Other causes include abscesses, membranous obstruction of the vena cava, and veno-occlusive disease (as may be seen in patients following

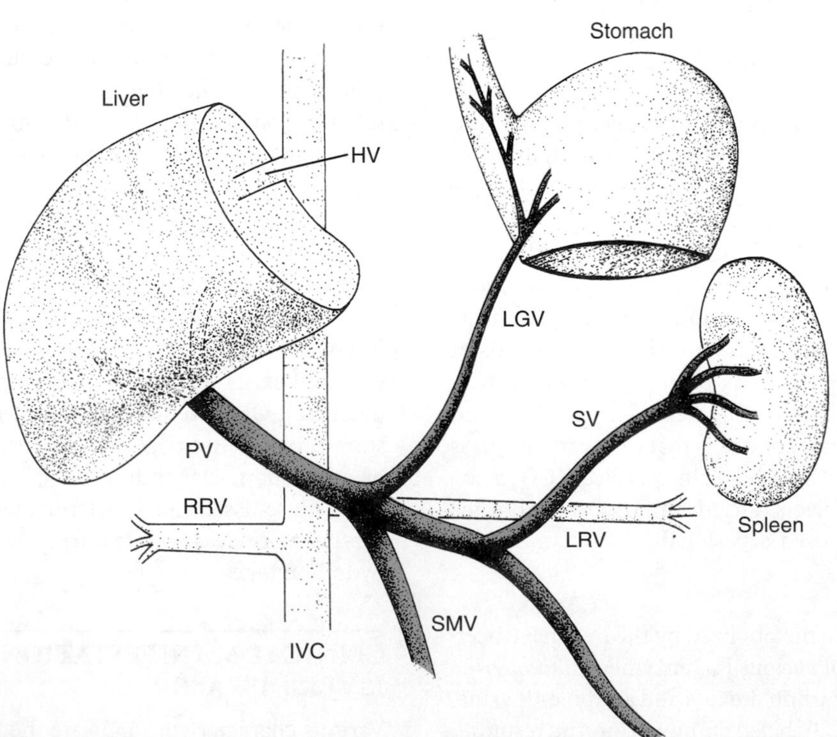

Figure 50-7 The portal-venous system. *HV*, Hepatic vein; *IMV*, inferior mesenteric vein; *IVC*, inferior vena cava; *LGV*, left gastric vein; *LRV*, left renal vein; *PV*, portal vein; *RRV*, right renal vein; *SMV*, superior mesenteric vein; *SV*, splenic vein. *(From Zakim O, Boyer TD. Hepatology: a textbook of liver disease, 3rd edition. Philadelphia, Pa: WB Saunders, 1996:721.)*

bone marrow transplantation). Although increased portal resistance is the major factor causing portal hypertension, it is often accompanied by decreased resistance to blood flow through other blood vessels, which enhances blood flow through the portal veins.

When portal pressure increases, the portal venous system becomes dilated and forms collateral connections to the systemic venous flow (Figure 50-8), leading to portosystemic shunting. Initially, this is clinically silent, but as portal hypertension worsens, it compromises many of the metabolic functions of the liver. One such abnormality is altered estrogen metabolism, which increases the ratio of estrogen to testosterone. Clinical consequences include spider telangiectasias and palmar erythema, gynecomastia in men, and abnormal vaginal bleeding and irregular menstrual periods in women. Impaired protein metabolic functions cause the accumulation of ammonia and abnormal neurotransmitters, ultimately leading to hepatic encephalopathy.[60A] Because most nutrients arrive through the portal vein, synthetic functions are also impaired, leading to hypoalbuminemia (contributing to ascites), decreased clotting factors (predisposing to bleeding), and reduced thrombolytic factors, such as antithrombin (predisposing to venous thrombosis).

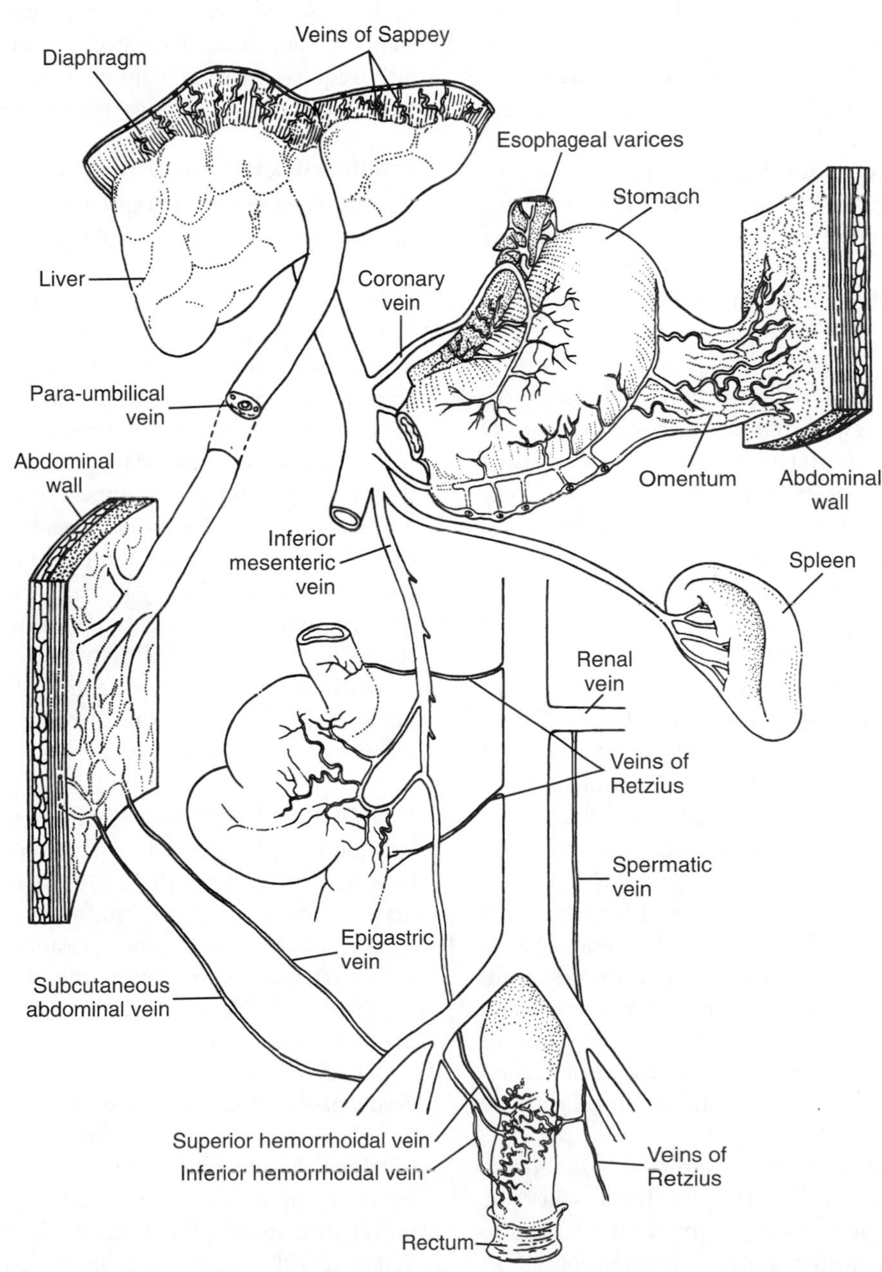

Figure 50-8 Sites of portosystemic collateral circulation in cirrhosis of the liver. *(From Sherlock S, Dooley J, eds. Diseases of the liver and biliary system, 9th edition. London, United Kingdom: Blackwell Scientific Publications, 1993:134.)*

Bleeding Esophageal Varices

The most life-threatening consequence of portosystemic shunting is the development of varices (enlarged and tortuous veins), which can occur throughout the GI tract but are most common in the esophagus and stomach. Bleeding from varices is one of the leading causes of morbidity and mortality in patients with cirrhosis. Varices are present at the time of diagnosis of cirrhosis in about 40% of patients and occur in an additional 6% per year.[156] In general, the risk of bleeding is low until portal vein pressure exceeds 12 mm Hg. The major consequences of varices are rupture and bleeding, usually presenting as hematemesis. Treatment of portal hypertension and varices is directed at obliterating the dilated blood vessels or reducing portal pressure. Pressure can be reduced by pharmacologic agents, such as nonselective β-adrenergic blockers, but if this is not effective, invasive procedures can be used, most commonly by putting rubber bands around large varices ("banding") or, if not successful, by placing a stent through the jugular and hepatic veins to connect to the portal vein, called transjugular intrahepatic portosystemic shunt (TIPS).[46] Because portal flow is already significantly reduced before shunting, minimal change in liver function is usually seen, but the incidence of hepatic encephalopathy following shunts is markedly increased.

Ascites

Ascites is the effusion and accumulation of fluid in the abdominal cavity. Ascites is the most common clinical finding in patients with portal hypertension. Ascites itself is not life threatening, but it is uncomfortable and may compromise respiration (from upward displacement of the diaphragm and compression of the lungs). It predisposes individuals to spontaneous bacterial peritonitis, which is life threatening.

The pathogenesis of ascites is complex because of a number of simultaneously operating factors. Of these, the most important are (1) increased hydrostatic portal venous pressure, with increased resistance to flow, (2) decreased colloid osmotic (oncotic) pressure due to hypoalbuminemia, and (3) leakage of protein-enriched fluid from the surface of the liver, which increases intraperitoneal colloid pressure. The primary event is probably peripheral vasodilation due to an imbalance of vasoactive factors, including endothelins. The net effect of these forces is shrinkage of the central blood volume, which decreases renal perfusion and leads to sodium retention through activation of the renin-angiotensin system. Sodium retention leads to water retention, but because of increased portal hydrostatic pressure and decreased intravascular colloid pressure, the fluid leaks into the so-called third space, causing ascites and edema.

Ascites has many causes, and it is important to differentiate ascites secondary to portal hypertension from ascites due to other causes. This is done by analyzing ascitic fluid. The feature that best distinguishes portal hypertension is an increase in the serum-ascites albumin gradient (sometimes abbreviated as SAAG). A gradient greater than 1.1 g/dL (11 g/L) is characteristic of ascites caused by portal hypertension,[5] but a high SAAG can also be seen in congestive heart failure or nephrotic syndrome.

Ascites due to portal hypertension is managed by creating a negative sodium balance or by relieving portal hypertension. A negative sodium balance is obtained by reducing sodium intake and enhancing sodium excretion with the use of diuretics. In cirrhosis, activation of the renin-aldosterone axis (caused by a variety of factors) necessitates use of agents that act at the distal nephron as the primary diuretic used, but these can be combined with other diuretics that act more proximally. In patients who require more urgent treatment for relief of symptoms, or who do not respond adequately to diuretics, ascitic fluid may be removed with a catheter placed percutaneously through the abdominal wall. More than 10 L of fluid may be drained to relieve patient discomfort or respiratory compromise. Repeated or large-volume paracentesis also requires plasma volume expansion to prevent renal failure; albumin is effective as an expander.[315]

Spontaneous Bacterial Peritonitis

Ascites predisposes to spontaneous bacterial peritonitis, defined as bacteremia (typically gram negative), in the absence of mechanical disruption of the bowel.[234] The condition usually presents in an individual with known cirrhosis who develops abdominal pain, fever, or leukocytosis. The diagnosis is established by examination of the ascitic fluid; greater than 250 neutrophils per microliter, or more than 500 in the absence of a positive blood culture, is considered diagnostic. In contrast, secondary peritonitis is usually associated with higher neutrophil counts, along with high protein and low glucose in ascitic fluid. Several studies have suggested that dipsticks that detect the presence of leukocyte esterase could be used to identify increased leukocytes and to diagnose spontaneous bacterial peritonitis; however, a recent review found poor sensitivity and frequent false-negative results in asymptomatic patients.[334,387] Unless cell counts are not available (e.g., in an office setting in a remote site), use of dipsticks for leukocyte esterase is not recommended.

Hepatic (Portosystemic) Encephalopathy

Hepatic encephalopathy is a metabolic disorder characterized by a wide spectrum of neuropsychiatric dysfunction.[60A,86] It may occur as an acute syndrome in patients with acute hepatic failure, or as a chronic, relapsing syndrome associated with cirrhosis. As implied by the synonym, chronic hepatic encephalopathy occurs in the setting of portosystemic shunting, usually as a result of cirrhosis.

The clinical syndrome is variable but follows a reasonably predictable course. Disturbed consciousness always occurs. It usually starts as hypersomnia and progresses to sleep reversal, in which the patient tends to sleep through the day and be awake at night. This is followed by decreased spontaneous movement, apathy, and gradually increasing levels of coma. Personality changes may be conspicuous, especially in patients with chronic disease. Irritability and disturbed social behavior may follow. Intellectual deterioration occurs and generally progresses to overt confusion. Neurologic abnormalities include slurred speech, a characteristic flapping tremor called *asterixis,* increased muscle tone, and abnormal reflexes. Disturbed gait may ensue. In chronic encephalopathy, these changes typically fluctuate over time and follow a waxing and waning course. Acute encephalopathy progresses rapidly, often within hours, and is characterized by cerebral edema, which may result in brainstem herniation and death.

The pathophysiology of hepatic encephalopathy is not completely understood but includes an increased sensitivity to dietary proteins. Ammonia concentrations are always increased with acute encephalopathy[476] and are usually increased with chronic encephalopathy. A reduction in plasma ammonia is often associated with symptomatic improvement. However, because plasma ammonia concentrations do not correlate with the severity of the encephalopathy, it has been suggested that other factors are involved.[186] It is recognized that a variety of neurotransmitter systems are dysfunctional in hepatic encephalopathy, but the exact cause of the changes is not known. One important contributor is the endogenous benzodiazepine agonist system.

The diagnosis of chronic hepatic encephalopathy is usually made on clinical grounds. Plasma ammonia concentrations are rarely helpful for diagnosis or for monitoring the patient's disorder; normal ammonia concentrations are helpful in excluding hepatic encephalopathy as a cause of cerebral dysfunction when the clinical picture is not clear. As discussed earlier, ammonia is more helpful in acute encephalopathy in proving a hepatic cause, and is of some prognostic importance in acute liver failure.[37] Elevated ammonia concentrations in that situation suggest acute hepatic failure or Reye's syndrome.

Treatment is largely empirical, based on observations that intestinal bacteria and protein loads in the intestinal tract are important in the symptoms of hepatic encephalopathy. Lactulose has long been known to reduce symptoms in chronic hepatic encephalopathy. Antibiotic treatment with a nonabsorbable antibiotic such as rifaxamin reduces the number of bacteria and is especially helpful in patients with GI bleeding. Patients with acute encephalopathy may require measures to reduce intracranial pressure, such as osmotic diuretics.

Hepatorenal Syndrome

Hepatorenal syndrome (HRS) refers to decreased renal function secondary to hepatic disease; portal hypertension is a common factor in all cases of HRS that develop in chronic liver disease, but HRS may also occur in acute liver failure. Although formerly thought to be a rapidly progressing, terminal event in a person with end-stage liver disease, it is now recognized that HRS falls into two major varieties.[322] Type 2 HRS is more common; it represents a slowly progressive or stable decline in renal function that is due to peripheral vasodilation and renal vasoconstriction. Type 1, or classic, HRS represents rapidly declining renal function, which is usually seen in a person with preexisting type 2 HRS. Type 1 HRS usually develops in the setting of an acute decrease in blood pressure, often due to spontaneous bacterial peritonitis or variceal bleeding.

A common feature in both forms of HRS is activation of the renin-angiotensin-aldosterone axis caused by intravascular volume depletion.[26] As with other forms of prerenal azotemia (elevated concentrations of urea, creatinine, and other compounds rich in nitrogen.), HRS in the untreated patient is generally associated with increased antidiuretic hormone and with profound thirst. This leads to the development of (1) hyponatremia, (2) hypokalemia, (3) metabolic alkalosis, (4) low urine sodium, (5) high urine potassium excretion, and (6) high urine osmolality. BUN, creatinine, and creatinine clearance are not reliable indicators of renal function in HRS.[77] Urea is produced by the liver and is often decreased in advanced liver disease; it is also increased after upper GI bleeding—a common cause of worsening renal function in HRS. Creatinine production by muscle is reduced in cirrhosis, causing falsely low serum creatinine and creatinine clearance. Although cystatin-C has better correlation with measured glomerular filtration rate (GFR),[110,462] it has not been widely adopted for monitoring persons with cirrhosis, and one study has suggested that it may be misleading following liver transplantation.[44]

Despite its limitations, the most widely accepted criterion for diagnosis of HRS is an increase in serum creatinine or a reduction in estimated GFR. Because no specific clinical or laboratory features of HRS have been identified, diagnosis depends on (1) the presence of severe liver disease, (2) a rise in creatinine to greater than 1.5 mg/dL (25.6 µmol/L), (3) no evidence of other renal disease by urinalysis and clinical history, and (4) lack of improvement in renal function with treatments that increase intravascular volume (such as stopping diuretics, or administration of fluids and/or albumin).[322] The latter two criteria are important because laboratory findings are similar to those of volume depletion, with low urine output, low urine sodium concentration, and increased urine osmolality.

Treatment of HRS is best accomplished by increasing systemic vascular resistance, as with the vasopressin analog terlipressin, or by reducing portal venous pressure, which is most commonly accomplished with TIPS. Both approaches have shown promise in improving renal function in HRS.[291]

Altered Drug Metabolism

Because of the central role of the liver in drug metabolism and disposition, alterations in drug metabolism may occur in patients with liver disease. In general, this is reflected in delayed metabolism. Only patients with evidence of liver failure, such as encephalopathy, coagulopathy, or ascites, need alterations in dosing. In general, patients with liver disease are not more susceptible to drug-induced hepatotoxicity. However, those with alcoholic liver disease who continue to consume alcohol are susceptible to liver injury from acetaminophen, even at therapeutic doses.[411]

Nutritional and Metabolic Abnormalities

The intake and disposition of nutrients in patients with chronic liver disease are altered, which subjects them to nutritional imbalance. Severe metabolic and nutritional derangements have been observed in the cirrhotic patient, including alterations in glucose metabolism caused by insulin resistance, and hypokalemia caused by secondary hyperaldosteronism. In addition, hypoalbuminemia is frequently present because of decreased production and sinusoidal leakage of albumin in patients with portal hypertension. Also, in patients with chronic cholestasis, impaired delivery of bile salts to the duodenum results in malabsorption of lipids and fat-soluble vitamins, leading to deficiencies in vitamins A, D, E, and K (see Chapters 31 and 52). Vitamin A deficiency may cause night blindness, but rarely progresses to serious visual impairment. Vitamin D deficiency causes osteopenia and, in severe cases, osteomalacia. In fact, osteopenic bone disease may be one of the most crippling results of chronic cholestatic liver disease, such as primary biliary cirrhosis.[189] Vitamin E deficiency is of little clinical significance. Vitamin K deficiency leads to hypoprothrombinemia, with easy bruising and bleeding.

Disordered Hemostasis in Liver Disease

As was discussed earlier and in Chapter 59, the liver manufactures most of the soluble clotting factors (the major exceptions being factor VIII and von Willebrand factor), as well as a number of inhibitors of clotting (proteins C and S, antithrombin). The liver also clears activated clotting factors from the circulation. Bile acids are necessary for vitamin K absorption and are needed to produce the active forms of several clotting factors, as well as proteins C and S. Disorders of fibrinogen also occur in liver disease. For example, dysfibrinogenemia may be seen in both acute and chronic liver disease and leads to prolongation of the partial thromboplastin time.[150] Patients with autoimmune hepatitis may have anticardiolipin antibodies and antibodies to platelets. The liver is the major source of thrombopoietin, which is needed to produce platelets. Portal hypertension results in splenomegaly, which often leads to thrombocytopenia. In addition, persons with liver disease often have evidence of platelet-associated antibodies,[218] although their contribution to low platelet counts in liver disease is questionable.[164]

Although these facts suggest that hemostatic problems are common in patients with liver disease, discordance is often noted between degree of abnormality of laboratory tests of coagulation and clinical evidence of bleeding.[260,446,455] Even in patients bleeding from esophageal varices and having prolonged clotting times, administration of blood components (including activated factor VII) was not associated with any clinical difference in degree of bleeding or need for blood transfusions.[455]

Enzymes Released from Diseased Liver Tissue

Because hepatic function is often normal in many patients with liver disease, the plasma activities of several cytosolic, mitochondrial, and membrane-associated enzymes are measured, because they are increased in many forms of liver disease. Because plasma enzyme measurements are discussed in greater detail in Chapter 22, only those factors relevant to an understanding of liver disease will be summarized here.

Reference Limits for Alanine Aminotransferase

One area of significant concern is the reference limits for liver-associated enzymes, particularly for alanine aminotransferase (ALT, EC 2.6.1.2). In most laboratories, reference intervals are based on samples of the "apparently healthy" population. For ALT, that upper reference limit is often around 40 to 45 U/L in males, but many laboratories have upper reference limits of 65 to 70 U/L.[332] These differences are greater than can be explained by analytical differences between methods.[332] Although ALT values are approximately 40% lower in females (a difference found even in children[128]), not all laboratories have different reference limits for the two genders.

Population-based reference intervals may not, however, be adequate for identifying persons with liver disease, or for recognizing persons who may be at risk for metabolic syndrome or cardiovascular disease. Because many chronic liver disorders (e.g., hepatitis C, alcoholic liver disease, nonalcoholic fatty liver disease) are prevalent in the population, such reference intervals may include many persons with liver disease. A widely cited Italian study, which excluded persons with known or likely liver disease, suggested lowering reference limits for ALT to about 30 U/L in males and 19 U/L in females.[370] A similar study in the author's laboratory (data unpublished), excluding persons with positive anti–hepatitis C virus (HCV), hepatitis B surface antigen (HBsAg), or obesity, found upper reference limits of 33 U/L in males and 19 U/L in females. A study among dialysis patients [who had 25% lower aspartate aminotransferase (AST) and ALT compared with healthy controls] in Taiwan found that the optimal cutoff value for detecting viral hepatitis was 17 U/L.[201] In Korea, risk of development of liver steatosis increased with serum ALT activity, even among those within its usual reference limits,[69] as was true with risk of death from cardiovascular disease.[230] A study using the Framingham offspring in the United States found that risk of metabolic syndrome and cardiovascular disease increased significantly, starting at ALT, above the lowest quartile of the normal reference limits.[166] The National Academy of Clinical Biochemistry and American Association for the Study of Liver Diseases guidelines on liver-related tests recommend that health-related reference limits should be developed for alanine aminotransferase.[118] These data provide some preliminary information toward that end.

Factors Affecting Plasma Enzyme Quantities

Because the pattern and degree of elevation of enzyme activity vary with the type of liver disease, their measurement is extremely helpful in the recognition and differential diagnosis of liver damage. Several factors govern the ability of liver enzymes to assist in diagnosis, including their (1) tissue specificity, (2) subcellular distribution, (3) relative activity of enzyme activity in liver and plasma, (4) patterns of release, and (5) clearance from plasma.

Tissue Specificity

Five enzymes are used in the diagnosis of liver disease: ALT, AST (EC 2.6.1.1), alkaline phosphatase (ALP; 3.1.3.1), and γ-glutamyltransferase (GGT; EC 2.3.2.2) are commonly used to detect liver injury, and lactate dehydrogenase (LD; EC 1.1.1.27) is occasionally used. ALT and GGT are present in several tissues, but increased plasma activities primarily reflect liver injury. AST is found in liver and muscle (cardiac and skeletal), and to a limited extent in red cells. LD has wide tissue distribution and is thus relatively nonspecific. ALP is found in a number of tissues, but in normal individuals primarily reflects bone and liver sources. Thus based on tissue distribution, ALT and GGT would seem to be the most specific markers for liver injury.

Subcellular Distribution

Enzymes are found at different locations within cells. AST, ALT, and LD are cytosolic enzymes. As such, they can be released with cell injury and appear in plasma relatively rapidly. AST and ALT have both mitochondrial and cytosolic isoenzymes in hepatocytes and other cells containing these enzymes. In the case of ALT, the relative amount of mitochondrial isoenzyme is small, and its plasma half-life is extremely short, making it of no diagnostic significance. In the case of AST, the mitochondrial isoenzyme represents a significant fraction of total AST within hepatocytes. In contrast, ALP and GGT are membrane-bound glycoprotein enzymes. The most important location of both enzymes is on the canalicular membrane of hepatocytes.

Relative Activity in Liver and Plasma

For cytoplasmic enzymes, the relative amount of enzyme in the liver relative to plasma is an important determinant of diagnostic sensitivity. The activity of AST within hepatocytes is about twice that of ALT, although plasma activities are similar. In contrast, hepatocyte activities of LD are much lower (relative to plasma) than those of the other two enzymes, and plasma activities of LD are several times higher than those of AST and ALT. This means that a smaller increase in LD is seen with liver injury than occurs with AST and ALT. The relative amount of enzyme in tissue is not necessarily the same in disease; in cirrhosis and malnutrition, and with alcohol abuse, greater decreases are seen in cytoplasmic ALT than in cytoplasmic AST.[272] In addition, other mechanisms may be responsible for this difference in enzyme activity. The development of immunoassays for measuring ALT has led to the observation of discordance between enzymatic activity and mass in several types of liver disease.[227] In chronic hepatitis and in healthy individuals, ALT activity and mass change in parallel. In acute hepatitis, activity is increased to a much greater degree than is mass; the opposite pattern is seen in cirrhosis and hepatocellular carcinoma. Additional studies are necessary to confirm this finding, but these results suggest that as yet, poorly understood factors affect enzyme activity.

Mechanisms of Release

Several mechanisms appear to be involved in release of enzymes from hepatocytes. Cell injury, the simplest mechanism, appears to allow leakage of cytoplasmic enzymes from cells, but minimal release of other types of enzymes. Thus necroinflammatory disease leads to release of AST and ALT, and to a lesser extent LD, but not of mitochondrial isoenzyme of AST nor ALP or GGT. Alcohol appears to induce expression of mitochondrial AST on the surface of hepatocytes.[501]

The mechanism of release of membrane-bound enzymes such as GGT and ALP into the circulation is less well understood. Synthesis of GGT and ALP appears to be increased in diseased human liver.[318] How this enhanced synthesis of tissue-bound enzymes translates into increased activity in plasma is not clear. However, fragments of hepatocyte membrane rich in GGT and ALP activity have been detected in the plasma of patients with cholestasis; this process may be a result of membrane fragmentation by bile acids. Furthermore, bile acids, which are detergents, could solubilize and release GGT and ALP from plasma membranes. In vitro studies of membranes treated with bile acids show that this possibility exists.[398]

Rate of Clearance of Enzyme from Plasma

Clearance of liver enzymes from plasma occurs at variable rates. The half-life of ALT is 47 hours, and of cytosolic AST, 17 hours; thus although more AST is released from the liver, the much longer half-life of ALT leads to higher activities of ALT than AST in most forms of hepatocellular injury. The half-life of the liver isoenzyme of ALP has been variously reported as from 1 to 10 days; the former figure appears to correspond better to changes seen with removal of gallstones. The half-life of GGT has been reported as 4.1 days. The mechanism by which enzymes are removed from the circulation is not completely known, although receptor-mediated endocytosis by liver macrophages is likely involved.

DISEASES OF THE LIVER

The liver has a limited number of ways of responding to injury.[371A] Acute injury to the liver may be asymptomatic, but often presents as jaundice. The major acute liver diseases are (1) acute hepatitis and (2) cholestasis. Chronic liver injury generally takes the clinical form of chronic hepatitis; its long-term complications include cirrhosis and HCC. The discussion of liver disease will focus mainly on these patterns and on a few diseases that differ from this general pattern.

Mechanisms and Patterns of Injury

Cell death occurs by necrosis (death of cell) or apoptosis (programmed cell death) or both. The target cell determines the pattern of injury, with hepatocyte injury leading to hepatocellular disease and biliary cell injury leading to cholestasis. All cellular injury induces fibrosis as an adaptive or healing response, with the duration of injury and genetic factors

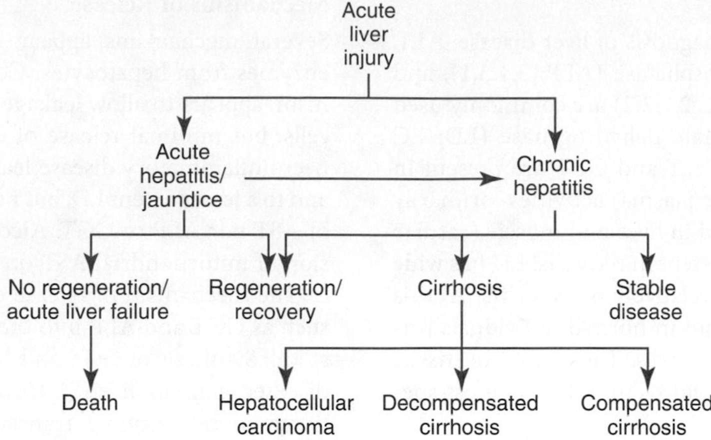

Figure 50-9 Natural history of liver disease. With acute injury to the liver, several outcomes are possible. In many individuals, damage is clinically inapparent and recovery occurs with clearance of the causative agent. In some, clinical acute hepatitis occurs. In the overwhelming majority of these, clearance of the causative agent results in complete recovery; in a very small minority, damage is so severe that acute liver failure (fulminant hepatitis) develops, which is usually fatal without liver transplantation. A variable percentage of persons with acute liver injury (dependent on the cause) progress to chronic hepatitis. In some, recovery eventually occurs naturally or following treatment of the underlying cause. Among those in whom chronic hepatitis persists, many will never progress to cirrhosis. A majority of those who do will remain well for many years, but about 3% per year develop decompensated cirrhosis (bleeding varices, ascites, hepatic encephalopathy) or hepatocellular carcinoma. These are the most common causes of death from liver disease.

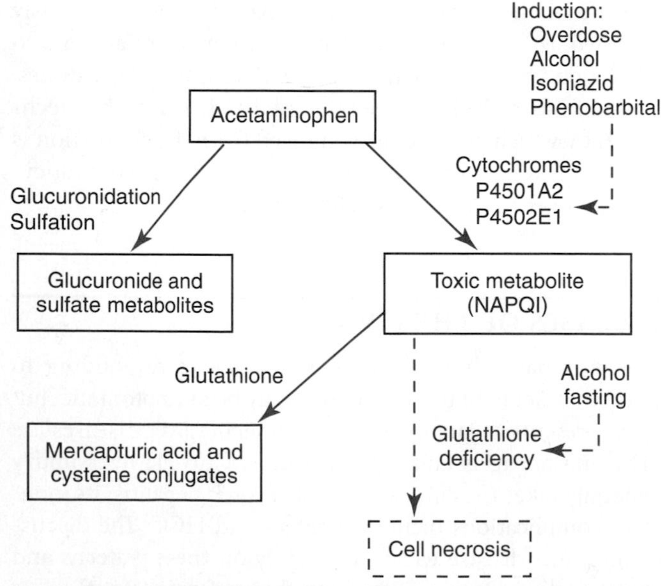

Figure 50-10 Metabolism of acetaminophen by the liver.

determining whether cirrhosis and ultimately carcinoma occur (Figure 50-9).

Cellular necrosis occurs as the result of an injurious environment and has been referred to as "murder." It is characterized by cellular swelling with loss of membrane integrity. Toxic injury from compounds such as carbon tetrachloride, aspirin, and acetaminophen (Figure 50-10) occurs for the most part by necrosis. Apoptosis occurs as the result of accelerated programmed death in which the cell participates in its own demise and thus commits "suicide." It is characterized by cell shrinkage, with nuclear chromatin condensation and fragmentation forming apoptotic bodies. Regardless of the cause, cell death typically leads to leakage of cytoplasmic enzymes. Most forms of hepatitis are associated with apoptosis.

Laboratory tests are helpful in distinguishing (1) the pattern of injury (hepatocellular vs. cholestatic), (2) the chronicity of injury (acute vs. chronic), and (3) the severity of injury (mild vs. severe). In general, the aminotransferase enzymes and ALP are used to distinguish the pattern, the plasma albumin to determine the chronicity, and the PT or factor V concentration to determine the severity. At the present time, the only way to accurately detect fibrosis is by liver biopsy.

Disorders of Bilirubin Metabolism

Defects in bilirubin metabolism resulting in jaundice are known to occur at each step in the metabolic pathway (see Figure 32-22, Chapter 32). Disorders related to these defects are discussed in Chapter 32 (see Box 32-1).

Hepatic Viral Infection

Five viruses have been identified (A, B, C, D, E) as causes of infection that primarily targets the liver. In addition, certain other viruses may infect the liver as part of a more generalized

TABLE 50-2 Types of Viral Hepatitis

	A	B	C	D	E	G
Type	RNA	DNA	RNA	Partial	RNA	RNA
Incubation period, d	45-50	30-150	15-160	30-150	20-40	Unknown
Transmission						
Fecal-oral	Yes	No	Minimal	No	Yes	No
Household	Yes	Min	Min	Yes	Yes	No
Vertical	No	Yes	Min	Yes	No	Yes
Blood	Rare	Yes	Yes	Yes	Unknown	Yes
Sexual	No	Yes	Min	Yes	Unknown	Yes
Diagnosis	Anti-HAV IgM	HBsAg, PCR, anti-HBc IgM	Anti-HCV, PCR	Anti-HDV	Anti-HEV	Anti-HGV
Carrier state	No	Yes	Yes	Yes	Yes	Yes
Chronic hepatitis	No	Depends on age, immune status	50-70%	Yes	Rare†	No
Liver cancer	No	Yes	Yes	No	No	No
Prevention						
Vaccine	Yes	Yes	No	Yes*	No	No
Immunoglobulin	Yes	Yes	No	Yes*	No	No
Response to interferon	Not used	30%	40-80%	Yes	Not used	Yes

*Vaccination and passive immunization against HBV protects against HDV infection.
†Only with severe immunosuppression.
HAV, Hepatitis A virus; *HBc,* hepatitis B core antigen; *HBsAg,* hepatitis B surface antigen; *HCV,* hepatitis C virus; *HDV,* hepatitis D virus; *HEV,* hepatitis E virus; *HGV,* hepatitis G virus; *IgM,* immunoglobulin M; *PCR,* polymerase chain reaction.

infection, among them cytomegalovirus (CMV), Epstein-Barr virus (EBV), and herpes simplex virus (HSV). Several other viruses have been proposed as causes of liver injury; these include hepatitis G virus[1](discussed later), transfusion-transmitted virus (TTV),[194] and the closely related SEN-V virus.[486] Although all three are bloodborne chronic viral infections and, in the case of TTV and SEN-V, have been known to replicate in the liver, none of these viruses appear to cause acute or chronic liver injury.[341,461,494] The various hepatitis viruses are outlined in Table 50-2.

Hepatitis A Virus

Hepatitis A virus (HAV) has historically accounted for about one fourth to one third of cases of clinical acute hepatitis in the United States and 20 to 25% worldwide. Since the mid-1980s, a vaccine has been available for HAV, and incidence has declined to its lowest ever in the United States.[21] Current recommendations are that all children should be immunized for HAV, along with adults at high risk for HAV,[18] as well as persons planning international travel and individuals exposed to HAV.[19] Although most commonly an infection of children and adolescents before immunization, the disease has become more common in adults than children, and most common in young adult men, particularly in injection drug users and in males who have sex with other males.[471] It tends to be most virulent in middle-aged and older people. Epidemics have been associated with waterborne and foodborne contamination. Ingestion of raw shellfish from contaminated waters has caused both sporadic and epidemic cases. Although not as common a cause of liver infection as hepatitis B, it is more frequently associated with jaundice when occurring in adults than hepatitis B or C; an estimated 50 to 70% of infected adults develop jaundice, and mortality is almost 2% with infection in those older than 60.[20] In contrast, hepatitis A infection in children is rarely associated with jaundice, and thus is usually not detected clinically. Hepatitis A may cause severe hepatitis and death in those who have chronic hepatitis, particularly hepatitis C.[465]

Hepatitis A is caused by a 27 nm RNA picornavirus. It has four capsid proteins (VP1-4), but only one serotype has been identified. The virus is not cytopathic to hepatoctyes, but causes liver injury by stimulating both cellular and humoral immune responses. Hepatitis A occurs in sporadic and epidemic forms, with an incubation period of 15 to 50 days. The clinical course of acute hepatitis A is usually that of a mild flulike illness that lasts for a few days to a few weeks. There is no chronic form of hepatitis A, but cholestasis (manifested by several weeks of jaundice and pruritus) may occur in some adults. Although a rare occurrence, relapse has been known to happen 1 to 3 months after the acute illness in up to 5% of patients. It resembles the acute illness and is associated with viremia, but recovery always ensues.

Although tests for HAV RNA are available for research purposes, diagnosis of HAV is based primarily on serologic tests for antibody to HAV. Total anti-HAV is believed to be protective and occurs with natural exposure to HAV and to HAV vaccine. With natural exposure, HAV antibodies appear to persist for life.[424] IgM antibodies to HAV are always present at the time of diagnosis of acute hepatitis A and generally remain present for 3 to 6 months, although they may persist for longer in about 14% of individuals.[221] With the falling prevalence of HAV, the number of cases of "acute" HAV reported to the Centers for Disease Control and Prevention (CDC) that are due to false-positive results exceeds the frequency of actual cases of HAV.[108] For this reason, IgM anti-HAV should be used only in the clinical setting of acute hepatitis.

Hepatitis B Virus

Hepatitis B virus (HBV) is the most common cause of acute hepatitis, and the most common chronic viral infection worldwide. An estimated 350 million individuals are chronically infected with HBV, and several times as many individuals have been exposed to HBV. The frequency of chronic HBV infection varies worldwide and it is highest in most of central and southeast Asia, central Africa, and southern Europe (prevalence >8% of the population), and intermediate (2 to 8%) in most of the rest of Asia, Africa, and South America. It occurs rarely among those born in North America and Europe[5]; one study found that 86% of U.S. residents with chronic HBV were actually born outside the United States.[228] In endemic areas, the incidence of new infection has decreased markedly in those places where HBV vaccine has been introduced. HBV is transmitted through body fluids, primarily by parenteral or sexual contact; it can be transmitted from mother to child, usually at or after delivery (termed *vertical transmission*). In parts of the world with high rates of chronic infection, much of the transmission is vertical. The residual risk from transfusion is estimated to be 1 in 600,000.[56]

Hepatitis B is caused by a 42 nm DNA virus that is a member of the hepadnavirus family. The DNA is partially double stranded and contains 3200 nucleotides with overlapping coding regions, leading to several major open reading frames. The S gene codes for several different length variants of surface protein; the smallest form, HBsAg, is produced independently of and in excess of the amount needed for viral replication; the largest form (S1) makes up the surface coat of circulating viral particles. The C gene encodes the hepatitis B core antigen (HBcAg), which is part of the infectious core of the virus. The X gene codes for a transactivating factor that may be involved with viral replication and the development of malignancy. The precore and basal core promoter regions code for production of hepatitis B e antigen (HBeAg), a protein found only in those with (but separate from) circulating viral particles. The final major viral protein is a polymerase, which has several different enzymatically active sites. Hepadnaviruses are unusual among DNA viruses in that they produce the first strand of DNA from a form of viral messenger RNA, using the reverse transcriptase activity of HBV polymerase. This error-prone reproductive strategy, along with an extremely high rate of viral replication in chronically infected individuals, leads to a very high rate of mutation in HBV. The significance of several mutants is described later.

Hepatitis B was first described in the 1960s by Blumberg and colleagues following discovery of a protein, termed the *Australia antigen,* which was initially believed to be a tumor marker for leukemia.[38] Subsequent studies confirmed it to be a marker for a form of hepatitis initially termed *serum hepatitis.* Later work established that this was hepatitis B surface antigen (HBsAg). The complete HBV virion (Dane particle) consists of a core containing DNA attached to DNA polymerase and core antigen (HBcAg), surrounded by the S1 form of surface protein. HBsAg and other forms of surface protein contain a common determinant, a, and four subdeterminants designated d, y, w, and r. These determinants are responsible for determining HBV genotypes; the eight major genotypes, termed A through H, have less than 92% homology with other types.[80] Geographic differences in genotype distribution have been noted; genotype A predominates among those infected in North America, whereas genotype C is the dominant form in those infected in Asia. Although not routinely determined at present, evidence indicates that genotype is an important predictor of the natural course of HBV and response to certain forms of treatment.[296] For example, genotypes A1 and F1 are associated with hepatocellular carcinoma in young adults and (in Alaska with genotype F1) children.[263] Genotype C has a higher risk of development of cirrhosis and hepatocellular carcinoma than is the case with most other genotypes. Genotype C has a low likelihood of response to interferon treatment.

Several mutants of HBV may have clinical importance.

HBeAg and HBeAg Mutants

Hepatitis B e antigen (HBeAg) is a protein of uncertain function produced by viral messenger RNA. It is released into the circulation by infected hepatocytes and may be involved as a "decoy," preventing the immune system from attacking HBV viral particles. The most common HBV mutations involve the regions that code for production of HBeAg. The highest frequency is for a mutation at nucleotide 1896 that inserts a stop codon in the mRNA, preventing production of HBeAg. Mutations in the precore promoter region, particularly at nucleotides 1762 and 1764, are associated with reduced production of normal HBeAg. Such mutants are associated with undetectable HBeAg, although they are characterized by production of anti-HBe. Precore and core promoter mutants are found in most individuals chronically infected with HBV in areas with high rates of infection, such as Asia and Southern Europe. In North America, it is estimated that 10 to 20% of individuals with chronic HBV infection have such precore mutants.[202] Such mutants may be present at the time of infection or may develop during the course of disease. Although initially it was thought that individuals infected with such mutants are much more likely to have severe acute infection, the high prevalence of such mutants suggests that this is not the case. Infection with these mutant strains is associated with a higher risk of development of hepatocellular carcinoma, and risk is stronger for the basal core promoter mutations.[449]

Polymerase Mutants

Treatment with antiviral agents that inhibit the reverse transcriptase domain of HBV polymerase is now the most widely used therapy for chronic HBV.[112] As is the case with human immunodeficiency virus (HIV), specific amino acid substitutions have been linked to resistance with several of the commonly used agents, particularly lamivudine and adefovir. The longer these agents are used, the greater is the likelihood that resistant mutants will emerge. Testing to detect resistant mutants is becoming more wide performed, particularly from individuals who have been exposed to more than one reverse transcriptase inhibitor (such as those who also are infected with HIV).

HBsAg Mutants

Mutations in the "a" determinant of HBsAg are the most important HBsAg mutants. Antibody to HBsAg, developed by natural exposure or by the HBV vaccine, is primarily directed against the "a" determinant. Exposure to strains that have mutants in this domain can result in infection despite the presence of protective titers of anti-HBs. In areas where HBV is endemic, up to 25% of cases of HBV in immunized infants are due to infection by such mutants.[31,200] In addition, the reagents used to detect HBsAg are antibodies to anti-HBs; therefore, mutant strains can be missed by HBsAg assays.[85,158] In fact, the ability of reagents to identify these mutant strains differs, mainly because of the specific epitopes recognized by the antibody (or antibodies) used in the assay.[312] Use of assays with antibodies to multiple epitopes improves detection of such mutant strains.[125] At present, the importance of such mutant strains is unknown.[117] Data suggest that most individuals infected with mutant strains have such viral particles at low titerss, usually in the presence of larger amounts of wild-type virus. Thus, most infected persons will be detected by the current assays for HBV. However, some infected individuals (perhaps more commonly those immunized for HBV) will be missed by some current assays.

Immunization

Hepatitis B may be prevented by passive [hepatitis B immune globulin (HBIG)] or active (hepatitis B recombinant vaccine) immunization. In the United States, current data suggest that more than 90% of children have been immunized against HBV infection, leading to a historically low incidence of acute HBV infection. Because infants born to HBsAg mothers have a high risk of developing chronic HBV infection, routine prenatal testing for HBsAg is needed to identify infants at risk. Infection occurs in only about 2% of infants before birth[439]; postexposure prophylaxis (typically used in infants of HBsAg-positive mothers) consisting of passive immunization with 0.06 mL/kg of HBIG and the first dose of hepatitis B vaccine within 24 hours of birth is more than 95% effective in preventing infection.[107] A universal immunization program in Taiwan, where vertical transmission of HBV was endemic, has greatly reduced the death rate from HCC in young individuals.[67]

Diagnostic Tests for Hepatitis B

More diagnostic tests exist to measure Hepatitis B than any of the hepatitis viruses; consequently, interpretation of results is complicated. Testing currently involves primarily enzyme-linked immunosorbent assay (ELISA) or related techniques to measure viral antigens or antibodies, but nucleic acid–based tests are becoming more widely used.

Hepatitis B surface antigen, the most widely used marker for detecting current hepatitis B infection, is detected by kits using antibody to HBsAg. Occasionally, false-positive results occur in testing, particularly during pregnancy; a neutralization assay is available. Low-level reactivity [as evaluated by the ratio of the signal from the sample to that of the cutoff for distinguishing positive and negative, termed the *signal/cutoff (S:C) ratio*] is highly predictive of samples that fail to confirm on neutralization.[346] False-negative results can occur with mutants in the surface antigen (see earlier), and they occur more commonly in early HBV infection. Most assays are qualitative; quantitative HBsAg assays have been available in Europe for over a decade. Some studies have shown a direct relationship (in untreated individuals) between quantitative HBV DNA and viral load[507]; others have not.[238] Declines in quantitative HBsAg during treatment have been found predictive of response to treatment for chronic HBV.[52,320]

Antibody to the hepatitis B core antigen (anti-HBc) is the most commonly detected antibody against HBV. Two assays are usually employed: IgM and total anti-HBc. IgM anti-HBc assays typically employ a large dilution of plasma (1:100) before analysis to reduce the likelihood of positivity in individuals with chronic HBV. The total antibody assay measures both IgM and IgG antibodies. Anti-HBc appears to last longer than anti-HBs in natural infection, and is still present in 97% of previously infected individuals more than 30 years after exposure.[410] Isolated anti-HBc is a relatively common finding, particularly in the setting of hepatitis C virus (HCV) coinfection,[472] but also in immunosuppressed individuals.[450] Although this may represent a false-positive result, particularly as a transient phenomenon following influenza vaccination, current guidelines on hepatitis B recommend consideration of individuals with isolated anti-HBc who have been exposed to HBV.[22]

Antibody to the hepatitis B surface antigen (anti-HBs) is considered evidence of immunity to hepatitis B and is the only marker found in those receiving the hepatitis B vaccine. The World Health Organization has developed a reference material that contains 10 IU/mL of anti-HBs. Current guidelines suggest that immunocompetent individuals who ever achieve an anti-HBs of 10 IU/mL or greater have life-long immunity to hepatitis B.

The hepatitis B e antigen (HBeAg) and antibody to the e antigen (anti-HBe) are typically used only in the setting of chronic HBV infection. Although HBeAg typically appears at about the same time as HBsAg in acute hepatitis, it is rarely used as a marker for acute infection. In chronic infection, HBeAg has historically been used as a marker of persistence of infectious virus; its clearance and the appearance of anti-HBe have been used as indicators of conversion to the nonreplicating state and as goals of antiviral treatment. With widespread availability of HBV DNA assays with low detection limits, the discordance between HBeAg and the presence of infectious viral particles has become apparent. Although a vast majority of untreated patients with HBV who are HBeAg positive have very high viral loads (usually >10^6 IU/mL), detectable HBV DNA is also found (usually with lower viral load) in about 70% of those who are HBeAg negative. When HBeAg-positive individuals are treated with reverse transcriptase inhibitors, loss of HBV DNA occurs in the majority, and HBeAg usually remains detectable. Loss of HBeAg during treatment, with development of anti-HBe, indicates a high likelihood that viral suppression will be maintained after discontinuation of treatment.[112] In contrast, in those who were HBeAg negative (and anti-HBe positive) before treatment, discontinuation of treatment almost always leads to recurrence of viremia. Thus, HBeAg remains an important marker for monitoring therapy, but has largely been replaced by HBV DNA for detection of those who harbor infectious virus.

Hepatitis B viral DNA is now routinely measured using amplification techniques (see Chapter 42). The World Health Organization has established an international reference material for HBV DNA, and results are typically reported in IU/mL[391]; conversion from copies/mL differs on the basis of viral load and is different for various assays. Because much older literature and some currently published papers still report HBV DNA in copies/mL, a rough conversion factor is 5 copies/mL = 1 IU/mL. Currently, assays using amplification, particularly polymerase chain reaction (PCR) methods, have detection limits of 100 IU/mL, although nonamplified assays are still available. It is unclear what amount of HBV DNA represents clinically important viremia; however, data (primarily from Taiwan) have shown that risk of progression to cirrhosis or hepatocellular carcinoma increases at viral loads above 10,000 copies/mL (2000 IU/mL).[70] Current treatment guidelines suggest that this number should be used as one criterion in treatment decision making.[265]

Hepatitis B mutants and genotypes are usually determined by direct sequencing or with the use of line probes.

Hepatitis C Virus

The hepatitis C virus (HCV) is the cause of most cases previously known as non-A, non-B hepatitis. It was recognized in 1989[78] and fully characterized 2 years later.[198] It is the most common cause of chronic hepatitis in North America, Europe, and Japan and is estimated to infect approximately 170 million individuals worldwide. Although HBV infection appears to have been present for a long time, evidence suggests that HCV is a more recently developing viral infection, because rates of HCV-related liver disease have been increasing in many parts of the world. Predictions are that HCV-related end-stage chronic liver disease will increase twofold to threefold over the next 20 to 30 years.[102] HCV infection primarily occurs through plasma; major risk factors are injection drug use and transfusion. For example, before the recognition of and availability of tests for HCV, the frequency of

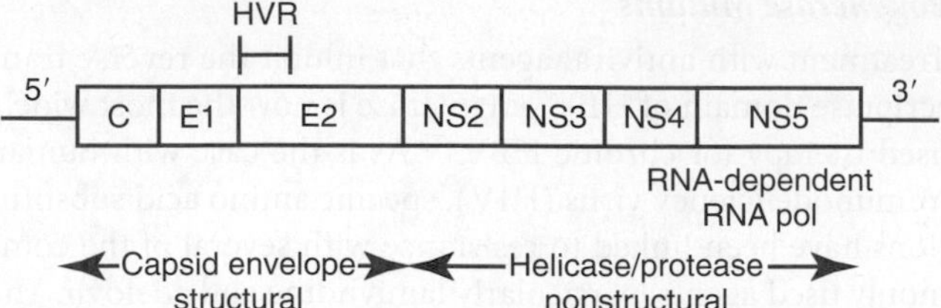

Figure 50-11 Structure of the hepatitis C genome.

post-transfusion hepatitis (mainly due to HCV) was 3.5%[414]; the risk of HCV transmission by transfusion is currently estimated at 1:2,000,000.[56] Because of its mode of spread, HCV infection is rare in children; the only common causes of pediatric infection are vertical transmission from an infected mother (estimated to occur in about 5% of infected women[381]) and, previously, transfusion of infected blood.

HCV is a single-stranded enveloped RNA virus of the flavivirus family, which includes other hepatitis viruses (yellow fever virus) and viruses that cause unrelated disease (such as West Nile virus). HCV RNA contains one reading frame (Figure 50-11). The resulting polypeptide is cleaved to core and envelope antigens and a number of nonstructural (NS) proteins, including a polymerase, a protease, and an interferon-response element. As an RNA virus, HCV is subject to a high rate of spontaneous mutation, giving rise to large numbers of variants. This results in six major genotypes (<70% nucleotide homology), along with a number of subtypes (77 to 80% homology).[53] In a chronically infected individual, numerous quasispecies (>90% homology) develop over time. These quasispecies seem to be important in establishing chronic infection[133] and appear related to the fluctuating nature of chronic inflammation in chronic HCV infection.[134] Quasispecies are unique to the individual infected; those infected from a common source show different patterns of mutation.[258]

Chronic HCV infection is associated with evidence of chronic liver injury in most cases. Elevations in liver-associated enzymes, particularly ALT, are usually mild and fluctuate between normal and abnormal in most infected individuals. In an estimated 15 to 20% of cases, cirrhosis becomes evident an average of 20 to 30 years after exposure. HCC may develop once cirrhosis is present, at an average rate of 1.5 to 3 cases per year. In North America, Europe, and Japan, HCV is the most common risk factor in the development of HCC. Various extrahepatic manifestations of chronic HCV infection may be noted; the most common are cryoglobulinemia and porphyria cutanea tarda. Epidemiologic evidence has linked HCV to increased risk of lymphoma and type 2 diabetes mellitus.

Prevention

Prevention of hepatitis C has proved more difficult than that of HAV and HBV. However, an 80% decrease in the incidence of acute HCV has occurred[6]—similar to what occurred with HAV and HBV; this is thought to be due to testing of blood donors for HCV and to safe injection practices instituted to reduce the risk of HIV infection. Vaccine development has been difficult because of the many subspecies of virus and the presence of many quasispecies with different antigenic determinants. Significant improvement has been noted in the treatment of HCV infection, however. Treatment of acute hepatitis C with α-interferon monotherapy has been found effective in preventing chronic hepatitis in a large majority of patients in nonrandomized trials. The use of pegylated interferon and ribavirin combination therapy leads to viral eradication in about 75% of those infected with genotypes 2, 3, and 4, and in almost half of those infected with genotype 1.

Diagnostic Tests for Hepatitis C

Measurement of the antibody to HCV (anti-HCV) is the principal screening test for HCV exposure. These tests, using ELISA and related microparticle, chemiluminescence formats, detect the presence of antibodies to one or more HCV antigens (derived by recombinant technology from yeast cultures or through production of synthetic peptides). Although the initial assay detected only antibody to a single antigen, subsequent tests have used antigens from four different regions of the HCV genome. Second-generation assays become positive on average 12 weeks after exposure, and third-generation assays become positive on average 9 weeks after exposure. After comparison with a cutoff value, results are interpreted as positive or negative. As is true for HBsAg, samples with a low S:C ratio are often false positive, whereas false-positive results are rare in samples with a high S:C ratio.[120,121] Current CDC recommendations[22] suggest use of an S:C ratio less than 3.8 for both second- and third-generation ELISA assays, and an S:C ratio less than 8.0 for the chemiluminescence assay, to define low-positive results.[22] Samples with a low S:C ratio are recommended to be confirmed, ideally with the use of recombinant immunoblot assay (RIBA).

RIBA is a technique similar in principle to Western blot. HCV antigens used in anti-HCV assays are typically blotted onto a membrane as dots, and reactivity is detected after incubation with serum. Results are interpreted as negative if there is less than 1+ reactivity with any of the four antigens, indeterminate if there is 1+ or greater reactivity to only a single antigen (or to more than one antigen along with the nonspecific yeast marker superoxide dismutase), and positive with 1+ or greater reactivity to multiple antigens. Third-generation RIBA has considerably fewer indeterminate results than second-generation RIBA.

HCV RNA measurement has become the most widely used test to detect current HCV infection. Typical of RNA in general, HCV RNA is labile in whole blood because of the action of RNAses primarily found in blood cells. Rapid separation of serum from clot is critical for accurate measurement of HCV RNA. If serum is separated from the clot by centrifugation within 1 hour, HCV RNA does not show an appreciable decline until 6 hours after collection. If serum is physically separated from cells within 1 hour, samples are stable at room temperature for 3 days, at refrigerator temperatures for 1 week, and indefinitely if frozen.[103] Samples collected in ethylenediaminetetraacetic acid (EDTA), which inhibits enzyme activity, are stable for 24 hours, even if plasma is not separated from red cells.[174]

Assays for HCV RNA historically were divided into qualitative and quantitative variants. An international reference material for quantification of HCV RNA has been developed,[392] and quantitative HCV RNA assay results are calibrated using this material and are reported in international units per milliliter (IU/mL). The relationship between IU/mL and copies/mL differs significantly for different assays. Results expressed in IU/mL agree within 1 log in about 90% of samples, but discrepant results do occur.[419] Until recently, qualitative assays had significantly lower detection limits than quantitative assays, but quantitative assays using real-time PCR have equivalent or lower detection limits compared with qualitative assays; if assays with detection limits of 10 to 20 IU/mL are used (as is the case in many settings), qualitative assays are no longer needed.[161] One of the currently available real-time PCR assays tends to underreport viral load among 15% of individuals infected with genotype 2[73] and may cause falsely negative results with genotype 4.[74]

Hepatitis C core antigen (HCV Ag) is produced by the most constant part of the HCV genome. HCV Ag is one of the major targets of antibody formation, and most HCV Ag circulates bound to antibody. HCV Ag has a similar time course to that of HCV RNA in both acute and chronic HCV infection[438]; the currently available assay for HCV Ag becomes reliably positive when HCV RNA is 20,000 IU/mL or greater.[45] In our experience with several thousand HCV RNA samples, less than 5% of untreated HCV RNA–positive individuals had a viral load lower than 20,000 IU/mL. In contrast to HCV RNA, HCV Ag is stable on storage. Currently, no commercial HCV core antigen assays are available in North America.

Hepatitis C genotype is an important parameter in determining the length and intensity of antiviral therapy. Several methods are currently used to determine the infecting genotype. Although serologic assays to detect antibody to specific genotypes of HCV are available, their correlation with direct tests is approximately 90%,[361] and a significant minority of infected individuals have antibodies to more than one genotype.[451] However, detection of viral RNA of more than one genotype is exceptionally rare. The most reliable method involves direct sequencing of regions of the genome that show characteristic patterns with specific genotypes and subtypes. Commercial assays using the 5′-untranslated region are most widely used,[384] although assays using the NS5b region are now available. All currently available assays show good agreement on genotype, although they differ in their detection limits.[403] Line probe assays are also widely used and show good agreement with direct sequencing assays.[309]

Hepatitis D Virus (Delta Agent)

Hepatitis D virus (HDV) is an incomplete, 36 nm RNA particle that cannot replicate on its own.[425] It is coated with HBsAg and is dependent on HBV for its activation. It is thus a satellite virus similar to that seen in plants. The D virus is a single-stranded antisense RNA virus. It is very infectious and strongly associated with intravenous drug abuse; approximately 10 million persons have been infected worldwide, although the incidence is declining with the fall in incidence of HBV infection.[379] It occurs as simultaneous infection with hepatitis B (coinfection) or as superimposed infection in someone with chronic hepatitis B (superinfection). Coinfection usually runs the same time course as acute hepatitis B, and HDV is spontaneously cleared as the hepatitis B resolves, but the risk of fulminant hepatitis is higher than in HBV infection alone, and mortality is higher. Superinfection typically results in chronic HDV infection, suppression of HBV DNA replication, and more rapid progression to cirrhosis (estimated 4% per year) and hepatocellular carcinoma (estimated 3% per year).[383] It should be suspected in a chronically infected HBV patient whose condition worsens.[488] Although it is traditionally diagnosed serologically by detection of anti-HDV (total or IgM) and/or HDV Ag,[329] HDV RNA measurements are often used as evidence of current infection.[311]

Hepatitis E Virus

Hepatitis E virus (HEV) is a 34 nm, single-stranded, unenveloped RNA virus. It accounts for sporadic and epidemic hepatitis in tropical and semitropical countries and in people returning from these areas.[487] Although considered to be rare in Europe and nontropical areas of North America, HEV RNA is frequently isolated from city sewage treatment plants in such nonendemic areas.[82] A number of small outbreaks have occurred in Europe over the past several years[95]; in one institution in England, HEV was responsible for about 10% of otherwise undiagnosed cases of acute hepatitis.[96] It is enterically transmitted, as is HAV, and viral RNA has been detected in plasma and in stool.[459] There is probably only one species, although four genotypes are known. Tests to detect antibody to HEV have been developed; specificity for HEV is high only for assays detecting antibody to the open reading frame 2 (ORF2) antigen.[285] The prevalence of antibodies to HEV is high in the United States, with 21% of randomly selected individuals having anti-HEV during the period from 1988 to 1994.[240] HEV has been isolated from a number of animals, notably rats[217] and pigs[302]; the significance of this is unclear, although it has been speculated that HEV is a zoonotic disease.[301] In fact, in several countries, HEV has been linked to ingestion of pork,[95] and in the United States, to ingestion of liver (from unclassified species).[240]

As with HAV, IgM anti-HEV, detection of antibodies have been considered diagnostic of acute infection by HEV, but false-positive results have been reported with hepatitis due to cytomegalovirus and Epstein-Barr virus.[143] The clinical course is similar to that of HAV infection in that HEV typically infects young people, has a self-limited course, and was not associated with chronicity. Recently, however, chronic infection with HEV has been documented in organ transplant recipients.[179,219] A peculiar feature of this disease is its virulent course in late pregnancy in India, with mortality generally in the range of 20 to 25%, but rates as high as 50% have been reported[226]; it is interesting to note that mortality during pregnancy is not increased in other parts of the world.[328] Mortality is increased among the elderly and in those with chronic liver disease.[96]

Hepatitis G Virus

Hepatitis G virus (HGV), also known as GBV-C, is an RNA virus of the flavivirus family, closely related to HCV.[7] It is most commonly transmitted by plasma[213]; vertical transmission has been reported.[310] Although it has a very high infectivity rate in recipients of contaminated blood (>90%), HGV infection appears to have no adverse consequences.[473] In fact, although it has been called a hepatitis virus, viral RNA cannot be isolated from the liver in chronic infection.[246] Coinfection with HCV and HGV is common, but coinfection has no effect on prognosis in HCV.[351,491] HGV and HIV coinfection is common; individuals coinfected with HGV and HIV have lower HIV viral loads and a better prognosis than those infected with HIV alone.[251,448,452] The pathogenesis of this presumed viral interaction is still unknown,[27] although stimulation of innate immunity may be involved.[242]

Acute Hepatitis

Acute hepatitis refers to an acute injury directed against the hepatocytes. The injury may be mediated directly, as occurs with certain drugs, such as acetaminophen or with ischemia, or indirectly, as occurs with immunologically mediated injury from most of the hepatitis viruses and most drugs, including ethanol. In direct injury, a typical rapid rise in cytosolic enzymes, such as AST, ALT, and LD, is followed by a rapid fall, with rates of decline similar to known half-lives of the enzymes. With immunologic injury, a gradual rise in cytosolic enzymes occurs, followed by a plateau phase and gradual resolution of enzyme elevation. Although jaundice is a key clinical finding in acute hepatitis, it is often absent (as discussed later under the various forms of viral infection). An increase in AST activity to greater than 200 U/L, or in ALT activity to greater than 300 U/L, has sensitivity and specificity greater than 90% for acute hepatitis.[386]

ALP usually is mildly elevated and is less than three times the upper reference limit in 90% of cases of acute hepatitis.[386] Bilirubin elevation, when present, typically is predominant in direct reacting bilirubin; indirect bilirubin is higher than direct bilirubin in about 15% of cases.[42] The distribution of direct bilirubin percentage is identical in acute hepatitis and bile duct obstruction, making the relative amount of direct bilirubin inconsequential in the differential between hepatitis and obstruction.[42] Liver synthetic function usually is well preserved in most forms of acute hepatitis. These and other features that are helpful in the differential diagnosis of acute hepatitis are summarized in Table 50-3.

The outcome of acute hepatitis is variable. In most cases, complete recovery occurs and liver regeneration leads to normal structure and function. With some viruses, failure to clear infection leads to development of chronic hepatitis. In a small percentage of cases, massive destruction of the liver leads to acute (fulminant) hepatic failure, which is associated with high mortality unless liver transplantation is performed.[2A,25A]

TABLE 50-3 Laboratory Features of Different Forms of Acute Hepatitis

Type	AST/ALT	ALP	Bilirubin	PT	Serology	Other
Viral	8-50× URL	<3× URL	5-15 mg/dL	<15 s	Positive	
HAV					IgM anti-HAV	
HBV					HBsAg, IgM anti-HBc	
HCV					HCV RNA ±anti-HCV	
Alcoholic	<8× URL	>3× URL in 25%	5-15 mg/dL	<15 s	Negative	AST > ALT
Toxic	>50× URL	Normal	<5 mg/dL	>15 s	Negative	Toxin usually detectable; acute renal failure common
Ischemic	>50× URL	Normal	<5 mg/dL	>15 s	Negative	Acute renal failure common
Drug induced	8-50× URL	>3× URL in 50%	5-15 mg/dL	<15 s	Negative	Eosinophilia, skin rash common
Autoimmune	8-50× URL	<3× URL	5-15 mg/dL	<15 s	Positive ANA or ASMA	Low albumin, high globulins
Wilson's	8-50× URL	Low normal or decreased	5-15 mg/dL	<15 s	Negative	Hemolytic anemia, renal failure, low ALP common; low ceruloplasmin often absent

ALP, Alkaline phosphatase; *ALT,* alanine aminotransferase; *ANA,* antinuclear antibody; *ASMA,* anti–smooth muscle (or antiactin) antibody; *AST,* aspartate aminotransferase; *HAV,* hepatitis A virus; *HBc,* hepatitis B core antigen; *HBsAg,* hepatitis B surface antigen; *HBV,* hepatitis B virus; *HCV,* hepatitis C virus; *IgM,* immunoglobulin M; *URL,* upper reference limit.

Acute Viral Hepatitis

All forms of acute viral hepatitis have similar pathology and a similar clinical course. They are all diagnosed on the basis of marked elevations in aminotransferases, usually between 8 and 50 times the upper reference limits, with only slight elevations in ALP and little or no effect on hepatic synthetic function. ALT is typically higher than AST because of slower clearance. Enzyme elevations typically peak before peak bilirubin occurs, and remain increased for an average of 4 to 5 weeks (longer for ALT than AST because of its longer half-life). Bilirubin elevation is variable, as is discussed later. The incidence of acute viral hepatitis due to HAV, HBV, and HCV had reached historically low levels by 2007, the last year for which complete statistics were available at the time of preparation of this chapter.[21]

Acute Hepatitis A

In adults, about 70% of those with acute HAV infection develop jaundice, much more commonly than with HBV or HCV. In children, acute HAV infection typically goes unrecognized and is often considered to be a viral gastroenteritis or other viral disease, because only 10% of children become jaundiced. The disease is more prolonged and serious in individuals over age 60,[4] and can cause liver failure in persons with chronic HCV[465] or cirrhosis,[376] with high mortality. The specific etiologic diagnosis is made with serologic tests. An IgM antibody (anti-HAV IgM) appears early in the course of illness and persists for an average of 2 to 6 months; rarely, IgM antibodies may remain positive for a year or longer. The presence of IgM anti-HAV has therefore been considered diagnostic of recent HAV infection. No antigen tests are available for detection of hepatitis A in plasma. Incubation of stool samples with labeled antibodies to hepatitis A and examination with an electron microscope have been used in the past to detect infectious viral particles. Amplification techniques [usually with reverse transcriptase PCR (rt-PCR)] have been used to detect virus in epidemiologic studies, but are not routinely used to diagnose infection.

Acute Hepatitis B

In most of the world, HBV is the most common cause of acute viral hepatitis. As with HAV, most infections in children are clinically silent. An estimated one third of adolescents and adults with acute HBV infection develop jaundice. The outcome in acute HBV infection is strongly influenced by age and immune status. In healthy adolescents and adults, an estimated 1 to 3% of cases will progress to chronic infection. In a person with immunosuppression, the likelihood of chronic infection increases to 10%. Neonates infected with HBV have a 90% likelihood of chronic infection, and the risk falls gradually over the first 5 years of life.[255]

The serologic course of acute hepatitis B infection is illustrated in Figure 50-12. HBsAg is the first serologic marker to appear, although HBV DNA may be detectable slightly earlier. HBsAg usually appears 1 to 2 months after infection and before the onset of clinical illness, and is the last protein marker to disappear. HBV DNA replication is slower than that of HCV; doubling time averages 2 to 3 days.[477] Persistence of HBsAg for longer than 6 months beyond the onset of acute hepatitis indicates chronic infection. HBeAg appears at about the same time as HBsAg; however, because it is not usually measured except in the setting of chronic HBV infection, it

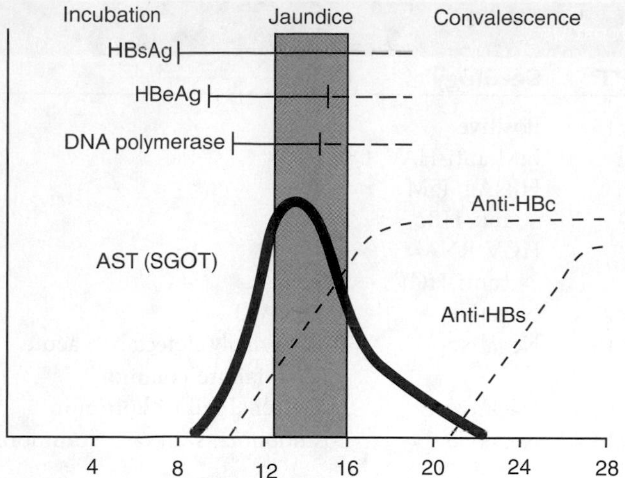

Figure 50-12 Course of acute type B hepatitis with recovery. *1*, Onset of hepatitis with jaundice 3 months after exposure; *2*, detection of hepatitis B surface antigen (HBsAg) 2 to 8 weeks after exposure, followed by appearance of its antibody (anti-HBs) 2 to 4 weeks after HBsAg is no longer detectable; *3*, detection of hepatitis Be antigen (HBeAg) shortly after HBsAg disappears [this is usually followed by the appearance of antibody to HbeAg (anti-HBe), which persists]; *4*, detection of hepatitis B core antibody (anti-HBc) at the time of onset of disease 2 to 3 months after exposure. Anti-HBc immunoglobulin (Ig)M will be detectable in high levels for ≈5 months. *(From Balistreri WF. Viral hepatitis: unique aspects of infection during childhood. Consultant 1984;24:131-53.)*

usually is not helpful as a marker to document acute infection. The first antibody to appear, usually coinciding with the onset of clinical evidence of hepatitis 3 to 6 months after infection, is antibody to the hepatitis B core antigen (anti-HBc). As with hepatitis A, an IgM antibody is the first to appear and usually persists for 3 to 6 months; it is usually considered diagnostic of acute hepatitis B infection. In chronic infection, however, IgM antibody may become detectable with flares of severity of disease and thus is not completely reliable in recognizing a recent infection.[94] The typical pattern at clinical presentation is positive serology for anti-HBc (both total and IgM), HBsAg, HBeAg (when measured), and negative anti-HBs. A small percentage of individuals have negative HBsAg and anti-HBs at the time of initial presentation, leaving IgM anti-HBc as the only commonly measured marker to be positive; this finding has been termed the *core window.* With current, sensitive assays for HBsAg, it is rare to encounter individuals in the core window. Clearance of HBeAg with development of anti-HBe is the first sign of viral clearance and usually predates loss of HBsAg. Clinically, HBsAg clearance from serum is associated with recovery from acute hepatitis and has been thought to confer life-long immunity to HBV.

Accumulating evidence indicates that HBV remains dormant in the body and HBV DNA circulates in many to most individuals who have "recovered" from acute hepatitis. This has been termed *occult* HBV infection.[48] Several studies have demonstrated that HBV DNA is still present in low amounts, in both plasma and liver, in most individuals who had past acute HBV infection and who were HBsAg negative and anti-HBc positive.[450,472,496] Viral loads typically consist of 100 copies/mL or fewer, and it has been estimated that the number of liver cells infected may be as low as 1%. Such individuals have been shown to transmit HBV infection if their organs are used for transplantation (if treatment to prevent this is not given). The significance of circulating HBV DNA for the individual infected or for others (in the absence of transplantation) seems to be minimal, however, in that liver enzymes are usually normal and circulating HBV DNA is found mainly in immune complexes.

In recent years, the problem of reactivation of HBV has been increasingly recognized. *Reactivation* refers to return of viral replication, often accompanied by acute liver injury (and, in a high percentage of cases, liver failure), in a person with occult HBV (sometimes also called *seroreversion*) or, more frequently, in a person with HBsAg but inactive viral replication. Typically, agents that suppress the immune system (chemotherapeutic agents, glucocorticosteroids, anti-lymphoid treatments) allow return of viral replication that had been kept in check by the immune system.[241,267,492] Withdrawal of immune suppression (including immune restoration in persons with HIV[385]) leads to liver injury. Treatment with lamivudine (or other agents that suppress HBV replication) before immune suppression is highly effective in preventing such reactivation, and guidelines have recommended testing all patients who will be receiving immune suppression for HBV before such agents are used.[20,430]

Acute Hepatitis C

Acute HCV infection is responsible for 10 to 15% of cases of acute hepatitis in the United States; an estimated 10 to 30% of those with acute infection develop jaundice. Increased aminotransferases usually develop about 6 to 8 weeks after infection. In those cases in which clinical acute hepatitis develops, jaundice typically begins about 2 to 3 months after exposure. HCV RNA and HCV core antigen are detectable in plasma 2 to 4 weeks after initial exposure. Viremia increases rapidly (average doubling time, 17 hours) and plateaus at high viral loads (often $>10^7$ IU/mL). In acute hepatitis C infection, anti-HCV is present in a little more than half of cases at the time of presentation.[29,176] IgM anti-HCV assays are not commercially available, but in contrast to HAV and HBV, IgM antibodies are encountered in both acute and chronic HCV infection, making the test useless diagnostically.[338] HCV RNA and HCV core antigen usually are both present at the time of diagnosis, and viral load is often significantly elevated compared with values seen in chronic hepatitis. Diagnosis of acute HCV is likely if anti-HCV is absent but HCV RNA is positive. Diagnosis of acute HCV is also likely if HCV RNA viral load is high and anti-HCV titer is low or increases with time.[338,352] Viral load falls with development of antibody to one or more HCV proteins, and may become transiently negative. HCV antibodies never appear, or disappear, in 30 to

50% of those who recover from acute HCV.[412,481] The importance of recognizing acute hepatitis C is that, if virus does not clear spontaneously, treatment is highly effective when given in the first 6 months after diagnosis.[9]

Other Types of Acute Viral Hepatitis

Numerous other viruses can affect the liver, causing acute hepatitis. The most common are the Epstein-Barr virus and cytomegalovirus. Features are otherwise typical of viral hepatitis, although signs of systemic infection are often seen as well. Herpes simplex virus occasionally may cause severe hepatitis in adults.[223] Infection with each of these agents is more commonly associated with hepatitis in the neonatal period, during which it is part of disseminated infection. Diagnosis of infection with these viruses involves serologic and nucleic acid tests; none are specific to the liver.

Sudden flares of activity in individuals with chronic hepatitis B may mimic acute hepatitis. An acute rise in cytoplasmic enzymes commonly occurs, often in association with jaundice and other clinical features, suggesting an acute liver disease. For example, development of an immune response that leads to clearance of HBeAg or HBsAg is often associated with clinical and enzymatic features of acute hepatitis.[296] Recognition of this cause of the clinical picture of acute hepatitis in a person with chronic hepatitis relies on demonstration of antigen loss and antibody development, along with absence of other causes of acute hepatitis.

Toxic Hepatitis

Toxic hepatitis refers to direct damage of hepatocytes by a toxin or toxic metabolite. Toxic reactions are usually predictable and are directly related to the dose of the agent ingested. In North America and Europe, the most common cause of toxic hepatitis (and the most common cause of acute liver failure) is acetaminophen, a widely used nonprescription pain reliever.[249] The metabolism of acetaminophen is affected by dose, induction of metabolic enzymes, and concentrations of glutathione (see Figure 50-10). When a large dose of acetaminophen is ingested (average lethal dose as a single ingestion = 15 g), the metabolic pathways are overwhelmed, glutathione is depleted, and toxic intermediates accumulate, causing liver damage. When metabolic enzymes are induced (such as by ethanol) or glutathione is depleted (as occurs in alcoholism and with starvation), toxicity can occur with relatively small doses of acetaminophen (total doses of 2 to 4 g).[411] Toxicity can also occur with excessive cumulative doses of acetaminophen; such accidental overdoses appear to be responsible for about half of cases of toxicity.[244] Diagnosis is often based on history and increased acetaminophen concentrations; in patients who present later, and for whom history cannot be obtained, measurement of acetaminophen-protein adducts allows diagnosis.[101] The first laboratory abnormality to appear is an increase in PT, followed by increased activity of cytosolic enzymes. Initially, LD is often increased to higher absolute amounts than AST, and AST tends to be higher than ALT.[61] Peak activities (typically more than 100 times the upper reference limits) usually occur by 24 to 48 hours, followed by rapid clearance at rates approximating the known half-lives of the enzymes.[423] PT elevations are typical and are greater than 4 seconds above the control value in most cases.[347] Prognosis is related most closely to the prolonged increase in PT; persistent elevation of PT 4 days after ingestion is associated with a poor prognosis.[184] Other markers of risk include development of acute renal failure and the presence of lactic acidosis, particularly if pH is less than 7.30.

Ischemic Hepatitis ("Shock Liver")

Hepatic hypoperfusion (ischemic hepatitis) is one of the most common causes of elevated cytosolic enzymes; in hospital patients, it is the cause of most cases of acute hepatitis.[193,478] Ischemic hepatitis may follow any cause of shock; the most common causes are septic and cardiogenic shock (sometimes termed *cardiac hepatopathy*[323]). Not all patients with shock develop ischemic hepatitis; in one recent study, only 13.8% of those with septic shock did, but mortality was significantly higher in such patients.[377] Another study found that cardiac dysfunction, especially right heart failure, appeared necessary to cause the clinical picture of ischemic hepatitis.[415] Bilirubin elevations typically are minimal, and they usually peak several days after enzyme activity reaches its greatest point.[122] Laboratory findings are similar to those seen in toxic hepatitis (including high LD), and acute renal failure is a common complicating factor. Prognosis is primarily related to the underlying cause of hypotension[122]; individuals with prolonged elevation of bilirubin appear to have a poor prognosis.[28]

Reye's Syndrome

Acute encephalopathy in combination with fatty degeneration of the viscera was initially described by Reye and associates in Australia in 1963,[378] with nearly simultaneous case descriptions by Johnson and colleagues in the United States.[214] In most of these early cases, the disease was fatal. It most frequently strikes children aged 6 to 11 years and infants, although it may affect other ages. The syndrome is characterized by a prodromal, febrile viral illness (usually influenza B or varicella), followed in about a week by protracted vomiting associated with lethargy and confusion, which may deteriorate rapidly into stupor and coma.[256] At the same time, the liver enlarges, increased aminotransferases and PT develop, and ammonia increases. A prolonged PT greater than 3 seconds above normal and a plasma ammonia concentration greater than 100 μmol/L usually indicate a poor prognosis. Bilirubin typically is normal or only mildly increased. Other laboratory features include hypoglycemia and hyperuricemia.

Only sporadic case descriptions of Reye's syndrome were published until 1974, when 379 cases in the United States were reported to the CDC. The mortality rate in this series was 41%. The number of cases peaked in 1980 at 555.[32] At about the same time, articles began to appear linking Reye's syndrome with aspirin treatment of viral illness[420]; these were followed by a case control study that strongly implicated salicylate in the pathogenesis of Reye's syndrome.[182] Although CDC guidelines recommending avoidance of aspirin in children with febrile illness were not published until 1985,[203] a decline in salicylate use began before this time, and Reye's syndrome has again become a rare disease. A 2008 review suggested that children who present with a clinical picture similar to Reye's syndrome are actually much more likely to have inborn metabolic errors, particularly those involving the urea cycle or mitochondrial enzymes, and should be evaluated for those before a diagnosis of Reye's syndrome is considered.[171]

Other Causes of Acute Hepatitis

Alcoholic hepatitis is discussed more fully in the alcoholic liver disease section later in the chapter. Alcoholic hepatitis is often suspected by the combination of mild elevations in enzymes (peak AST typically <300 U/L), AST-to-ALT ratio greater than 2 : 1, and leukocytosis.[270] Drugs can cause liver injury through a number of mechanisms, but the most common is idiosyncratic, immune-mediated injury to hepatocytes. The most common pattern is similar to that of other types of acute hepatitis; cholestatic hepatitis, with increased aminotransferases and ALP, is more common in drug-induced hepatitis than with other causes of acute hepatitis, but is present only in a minority of cases (40% in a 2008 U.S. study).[65] Criteria used to recognize drug-induced liver injury include a temporal relationship between drug exposure and onset of hepatitis; exclusion of other known causes of hepatitis; the presence of extrahepatic hypersensitivity (especially skin rash, arthralgia, renal injury, and eosinophilia); the development of liver injury on rechallenge; and, ideally, previously published reports of similar reactions.[282] Several standardized approaches to evaluation of possible drug-induced liver disease have been developed.[23,97,147] Hepatic drug reactions represent about 6% of all adverse drug reactions[115] and about 1% of cases of acute hepatitis.[237] Although usually associated with prescription drugs, complementary and alternative products are becoming increasingly recognized as causes of acute hepatitis[99,408] and in a U.S. study were responsible for 9% of all cases.[65] Although drug reactions typically develop soon after that start of treatment, several months may elapse between the time of initial exposure and development of acute hepatitis. Approximately 60% of cases cause severe acute hepatitis with jaundice; fatalities can occur,[145] although often death is not due to liver disease.[65] Serious reactions are more common in individuals who are continued on the medication.[359] In 15 to 30% of cases, liver injury persists and becomes chronic following cessation of the drug.[20,65]

Some of the disorders that usually produce chronic hepatitis (and are discussed more fully later) may occasionally present in an acute fashion. Autoimmune hepatitis has an acute component in up to 40% of cases. Clinically, it differs from other forms of acute hepatitis in having decreased albumin, increased globulins, and a more protracted increase in aminotransferases.[88,185,365] Acute autoimmune hepatitis is diagnosed by the absence of other causes of acute hepatitis and the presence of autoimmune markers (discussed in detail in the section on chronic hepatitis). Wilson's disease is the result of deficiency of an intracellular ATPase[54,362A,440] and typically presents with neuropsychiatric findings, often associated with chronic liver injury. Wilson's disease may also present as acute hepatitis, often associated with fulminant hepatic failure[35]; in one study, 8 of 14 patients who had hepatic injury due to Wilson's disease had an acute presentation.[172] The classic biochemical findings of Wilson's disease are often absent (low ceruloplasmin, low plasma copper, and Kayser-Fleischer rings) or misleading (high urine copper is common to all forms of acute hepatitis) in the setting of acute Wilson's disease.[35,433] Additional features often suggest the diagnosis, including nonimmune hemolytic anemia, acute tubular necrosis, and a low ratio of ALP (in U/L) to bilirubin (in mg/dL); one recent study found that if this ratio was less than 4, sensitivity was 94% and specificity was 96%—far superior to tests such as ceruloplasmin and plasma copper.[233]

Other Disorders With Laboratory Findings Similar to Acute Hepatitis

Several conditions mimic the laboratory picture of acute hepatitis. Hemolytic anemia can cause jaundice, increased LD, and slight increases in AST and ALT. In contrast to hepatitis, the increase in bilirubin is predominantly (often >80%) indirect reacting. LD activity is elevated to several times that of AST, and AST activity usually is several times that of ALT. Acute injury to skeletal or cardiac muscle may cause significant increases in AST and, to a lesser extent, ALT, but the ratio of AST to ALT activity is generally more than 3 : 1 at presentation (although, as with liver injury, the shorter half-life of AST will cause the ratio to become less than 1 with time, usually after 3 days)[327]; bilirubin usually is not elevated, but mild increases in unconjugated bilirubin from metabolism of myoglobin may be seen in severe skeletal muscle injury. Acute bile duct obstruction, particularly when caused by gallstones, can cause a picture that resembles acute hepatitis. In the early stages of obstruction, transient increases in AST and ALT are common,[431] and rarely their activities may exceed 2000 U/L.[15,149] Increases in ALP develop more slowly than those of the aminotransferases, masking the presence of cholestasis early in the course. Increases in bilirubin are typically predominantly direct reacting, creating a presentation similar to that seen in acute hepatitis. Even if obstruction persists, aminotransferase activity falls rapidly, with AST typically returning to normal within 8 days[360] and ALP activity gradually increasing. ALP activities greater than 300 U/L in this setting strongly suggest the presence of obstructive jaundice.[469] Acute biliary obstruction by gallstones is often accompanied by acute pancreatitis; increased amylase and lipase should suggest biliary tract obstruction as the cause of any liver abnormalities noted.

Approach to the Patient With Acute Hepatitis

Once a diagnosis of acute hepatitis has been established, additional laboratory testing is usually required to determine the cause. Although the incidence of acute viral hepatitis has decreased, serologic studies should be performed to rule out infectious causes. A typical panel of tests would include IgM anti-HAV, HBsAg, IgM anti-HBc, anti-HCV, and HCV RNA (or HCV core antigen, if available). Marked elevations (>100 times the upper reference limits) in AST or ALT, particularly if AST is higher than ALT, should suggest the possibility of toxic or ischemic liver injury. Minimal increases (<8 times the reference limit) in AST, with AST greater than ALT, in a patient with jaundice and leukocytosis indicate likely alcoholic hepatitis. Imaging studies of the biliary tract are appropriate to rule out obstruction in those who present with sudden onset of symptoms, especially if accompanied by right upper quadrant pain and tenderness, laboratory evidence of pancreatitis, or a history of gallstones. The presence of increased globulins and decreased albumin, or the presence of hemolytic anemia and acute renal failure, should suggest the possibility of autoimmune hepatitis or Wilson's disease, respectively.

Follow-up of Acute Hepatitis

Important uses of laboratory tests in acute hepatitis are to (1) identify individuals with fulminant hepatic failure, (2) document recovery, and (3) determine clearance of any infectious agents. The most important tests in determining extent of injury are not plasma activities of cytosolic enzymes, but evidence of impaired liver function. The most important indicator of prognosis in acute viral hepatitis is impairment in synthetic function, with PT a widely accepted indicator. In acute viral or alcoholic hepatitis, PT more than 3 seconds above normal is associated with a poor prognosis,[347] whereas in toxic hepatitis, persistent elevation more than 4 days after ingestion has prognostic importance.[184] Low concentrations of other markers of synthetic function, such as transthyretin or actin-free Gc globulin,[397] or of markers of hepatocyte regeneration, such as α-fetoprotein,[197] have been found to predict poor prognosis. In alcoholic hepatitis, bilirubin and INR are the most reliable predictors of prognosis; several indices, discussed later in the section on alcoholic liver disease, have been used to predict risk of death and need for treatment.[270] Cytosolic enzyme activities decrease rapidly in ischemic and toxic hepatitis or obstruction, regardless of outcome, and fall more gradually in viral and alcoholic hepatitis, but are not helpful in evaluating outcome. With hepatitis B and C, cytosolic enzyme activities may return to normal even if viral replication persists[105,211]; serologic tests are the only reliable means to evaluate resolution of infection.

Chronic Hepatitis

Chronic hepatitis is defined as chronic inflammation of the liver that persists for at least 6 months, or signs and symptoms of chronic liver disease in the presence of elevated cytosolic enzymes.[119] It is characterized by ongoing inflammatory damage to hepatocytes, often accompanied by hepatocyte regeneration and scarring. Formerly, chronic hepatitis was subdivided into three forms (chronic persistent, chronic lobular, and chronic active) based on histologic characteristics. It was recognized that individuals often had each of these "diseases" at different points in time, and often in different areas of the liver in the same biopsy. Current classifications describe the cause and evaluate the severity of inflammatory injury (termed *grade*) and the extent of fibrosis (termed *stage*). The importance of these findings will be discussed in detail later. Common causes of chronic hepatitis and tests used to make a specific etiologic diagnosis are listed in Table 50-4.

TABLE 50-4 Causes of Chronic Hepatitis and Diagnostic Strategies

Cause	Diagnosis
Hepatitis B	History, HBsAg, anti-HBs, anti-HBc, HBV DNA
Hepatitis C	Anti-HCV, HCV RNA by PCR
Autoimmune type 1	ANA, anti–smooth muscle antibody
Autoimmune type 2	SLA, anti-LKM_1
Wilson's disease	Ceruloplasmin
Drugs	History
α_1-Antitrypsin deficiency	α_1-AT phenotype
Nonalcoholic fatty liver disease (NAFLD)	Metabolic syndrome, liver ultrasound, liver biopsy
Idiopathic	Liver biopsy, absence of markers

ANA, Antinuclear antibody; *AT*, antitrypsin; *HBc*, hepatitis B core antigen; *HBsAg*, hepatitis B surface antigen; *HBV*, hepatitis B virus; *HCV*, hepatitis C virus; *LKM_1*, liver-kidney microsomal antigen type 1; *PCR*, polymerase chain reaction; *SLA*, soluble liver antigen.

The clinical features of chronic hepatitis are highly variable. Most patients are asymptomatic, but nonspecific features such as fatigue, lack of concentration, and weakness may be present. Most patients are diagnosed because of an unexplained abnormality in aminotransferase activities or detection of positive results on a screening test for a cause of chronic hepatitis. Moderate elevations in aminotransferase activities (an average of about twofold, and in most cases less than fivefold) are characteristic, whereas results of most other tests are normal. Normal aminotransferase activities do not rule out histologic evidence of chronic hepatitis, especially in the presence of chronic viral hepatitis or nonalcoholic steatohepatitis (NASH).[161,180,313] Characteristically, ALT is elevated to a greater degree than AST,[66] although elevations in both are common; reversal of the AST/ALT ratio to greater than 1 suggests coexisting alcohol abuse or development of cirrhosis in patients with a variety of causes of chronic liver disease[16,146,344,345] (as discussed in greater detail later in this chapter). One study found that the AST/ALT ratio was significantly higher in women than in men;[304]however, in most studies in which the AST/ALT ratio is used, separate analyses are not done by gender. Although ALT is relatively specific for the liver, skeletal muscle sources for AST and ALT should always be considered, especially in physically active young individuals.[111,239,327] A finding of persistent elevation of

TABLE 50-5 Patterns of Chronic Hepatitis B Virus Infection

Type	AST/ALT	HBsAg	HBeAg	Anti-HBc	HBV DNA
Occult	Normal	Neg	Neg	Pos	Neg*
Immune control	Normal	Pos	Neg	Pos	Neg*
Immune tolerant	Normal	Pos	Neg/Pos	Pos	Pos
Immune active	Increased	Pos	Pos	Pos	Pos, viral load usually >10^6 IU/mL
HBeAg-negative chronic hepatitis	Increased	Pos	Neg	Pos	Pos, viral load usually <10^6 IU/mL

*May have very low level (usually <10^2 IU/mL) in serum.
ALT, Alanine aminotransferase; *AST,* aspartate aminotransferase; *HBc,* hepatitis B core antigen; *HBeAg,* hepatitis B e antigen; *HBsAg,* hepatitis B surface antigen; *HBV,* hepatitis B virus.

aminotransferase activity should lead to an evaluation for chronic hepatitis using the tests outlined in Table 50-4. A liver biopsy may be helpful in determining the cause, assessing severity, and following treatment. A specific etiologic diagnosis is essential because it dictates the treatment. The most common causes of chronic hepatitis are chronic HBV and HCV and NASH, but a variety of other disease processes may cause chronic hepatitis.

Chronic Hepatitis B

Worldwide, HBV infection is the most important cause of chronic hepatitis.[137] Approximately 350 million individuals worldwide have chronic HBV infection; most cases are found in Asia, Africa, and southern Europe.

In most circumstances, HBV is not cytopathic because the injury results from an immune-mediated inflammatory attack against hepatocytes. Chronic hepatitis results when the immune response is incomplete and the virus is not eliminated from infected cells. This leads to a continuing cycle of viral replication, reinfection of regenerating hepatocytes, and immune damage to newly infected cells that is inadequate to clear infection. The details are not completely understood, but it appears that in the normal circumstance, hepatocytes express surface markers (in this case, HBcAg and HLA class 1 proteins).[316] Primed lymphocytes then attack the infected hepatocytes.[75] Expression of HLA class 1 markers is stimulated by interferon. It appears that many chronic hepatitis B patients are deficient in or have an inadequate response to interferon and, by inference, are unable to express HLA antigens that would attract an appropriate lymphocyte response.[248] The discovery of interferon deficiency led to the successful use of α-interferon (IFN-α) therapy in chronic HBV. The clinical presentation may be complicated by various extrahepatic complications (which occur in 1 to 10% of those with HBV[255]), including (1) polyarteritis, (2) glomerulonephritis, (3) polymyalgia rheumatica, (4) cryoglobulinemia, (5) myocarditis, and (6) Guillain-Barré syndrome. These conditions are associated with circulating immune complexes containing HBsAg.[456] Immunocompromised persons, such as HBV/HIV-coinfected individuals, typically have higher replication markers, less hepatic inflammation, and poorer survival than those with HIV alone.[339,447]

The natural history of chronic hepatitis B (defined by the persistence of HBsAg) varies.[296] Features of the different stages of chronic HBV are given in Table 50-5. It is convenient to divide chronic hepatitis B infection into two basic types—replicative and nonreplicative—although transitions between these stages are common. In the chronic replicative form, viral DNA is found in the cytoplasm of infected hepatocytes, and complete viral particles are produced and released into the circulation. In the replicating form of infection, viral loads in plasma are usually high (>10^5 copies/mL, often >10^8 copies/mL). In those infected later in life who develop chronic hepatitis, evidence of hepatocyte injury (elevated aminotransferase activity and inflammation in liver biopsy sections) is found in most cases (termed *immune active*[296] or *chronic active phase*). In those infected early in life, however, evidence of hepatocyte injury is often minimal; this has been referred to as the *immunotolerant phase of chronic HBV.* Those in the immune tolerant phase may transition to the immune active phase, but do not always do so. In the nonreplicating form, circulating viral load is low or undetectable, and evidence of hepatocyte injury is usually absent. This variant has been termed *HBV carrier state,* although current terminology describes this phase as the *immune control phase.* Traditionally, HBeAg had been used to differentiate replicative and nonreplicative types of chronic hepatitis, with negative HBeAg and positive anti-HBe thought to indicate the nonreplicating stage of infection. As discussed earlier, however, this distinction is inaccurate, and classification is based on HBV DNA concentrations along with ALT activities and histology.[296] All of these three phases of chronic HBV are associated with the presence of HBsAg in serum. As mentioned earlier, occult HBV infection is present in many individuals previously exposed to HBV, but is not associated with inflammation in the liver or elevated aminotransferases.

In general, chronic HBV passes through stages in untreated persons. For those infected early in life, the immune tolerant phase is usually followed by an immune active phase, then often the immune control phase or occult infection. For those affected as older children or adults, the immune active phase usually is seen first, and the immune tolerant phase is never seen or is present for only a short period. About 8 to 10% of persons per year will transition from the immune active to the immune control phase of chronic HBV.[112] A variable, but low, proportion of those in the immune control phase will revert to the immune active phase (mainly dependent on genotype).[296] About 0.5 to 1% of persons per year will convert from HBsAg positive to HBsAg negative, entering the occult phase of infection (or, in a minority, resolved HBV). Each of these transitions can be associated with an acute rise in aminotransferase activities in a clinical picture mimicking acute viral hepatitis, as discussed earlier.

For individuals who have chronic replicating infection, the major risk is development of cirrhosis and HCC. An estimated 20 to 30% of individuals with chronic hepatitis B will develop cirrhosis over a 20-year follow-up period; the risk is directly related to amount of HBV DNA, with risk progressively increasing at viral loads greater than 2000 IU/mL (10,000 copies/mL).[209] Once cirrhosis has developed, a 1.5 to 5% annual risk of development of HCC is noted. Although the risk of HCC is lower in individuals with HBV infection who do not have cirrhosis, risk is directly related to viral load and rises at quantities above 2000 IU/mL.[71] Even a person in the nonreplicating stage of infection has a tenfold higher risk of HCC.[70] On a worldwide basis, hepatitis B infection is the most common cause of liver cancer.

Several agents have been approved for the treatment of chronic HBV infection, including interferon (both standard and pegylated) and several nucleoside/nucleotide inhibitors of HBV polymerase (adefovir, entecavir, lamivudine, telbivudine, and tenofovir).[112] Other polymerase inhibitors (largely used for HIV treatment) have been evaluated in research studies but are not yet approved for use in North America. At present, only single-agent therapy is used, although it has been suggested that combinations of polymerase inhibitors should be used in persons with lack of response to single agents, particularly in those with cirrhosis.[405] Combinations of interferon plus lamivudine show higher rates of response to treatment, but no additional long-term benefit, compared with interferon alone.[444] Major criteria for initiating treatment include HBV viral load and activity of ALT; viral load greater than 20,000 IU/mL (100,000 copies/mL) is currently considered a criterion for treatment, as are ALT at least two times the upper reference limit and detectable HBV DNA.[106] For persons who do not meet these criteria, indications for treatment include active liver disease on biopsy and the presence of cirrhosis. Treatment is about equally effective for persons positive or negative for HBeAg; those who are HBeAg negative have slightly higher response rates on treatment but have a low likelihood of maintaining suppression of viral replication if treatment is stopped.[112]

Efficacy of treatment is typically measured by response of alanine and/or aspartate aminotransferase and HBV DNA; goals of treatment include normalization of ALT and suppression of HBV DNA below the limits of detection of assays, ideally with detection limits of about 20 to 50 IU/mL. With polymerase inhibitors, about 70 to 80% of patients will achieve these goals within 1 year of treatment. Duration of treatment is largely dependent on HBeAg status before the start of therapy and, for those HBeAg positive before treatment, response of HBeAg on therapy. For those who are HBeAg negative, treatment typically is continued indefinitely, as long as treatment is effective. For those who are HBeAg positive before treatment, loss of HBeAg and development of anti-HBe indicate a high likelihood of maintenance of HBV DNA control and normalization of ALT once treatment is stopped (after 6 to 12 months of further treatment once anti-HBe appears). With interferon therapy, response rates to 1 year of treatment are somewhat lower than with polymerase inhibitors, but treatment requires only 6 to 12 months. Loss of HBsAg is uncommon; with most agents, the likelihood of loss of HBsAg usually is not higher than in untreated persons, although it may be higher with interferon and tenofovir.[112]

Chronic Hepatitis C

Approximately 170 million individuals worldwide have been diagnosed with chronic HCV infection; most cases are found in North America, Northern Europe, and Japan.[383A] In contrast to HBV, the risk of chronic hepatitis does not appear related to age at exposure (although perinatal infection is uncommon with HCV), and the likelihood of chronic infection is much higher overall. Many references state about an 80 to 85% likelihood of chronic infection by HCV; this interpretation is based on the frequency of finding HCV RNA on a chronic basis among those who are anti-HCV positive. As mentioned earlier, however, many individuals who clear HCV with acute exposure never develop or lose anti-HCV. Among persons followed prospectively after acute HCV infection, chronic HCV infection actually developed in only about 50 to 70%.[224,413,481] Once viremia becomes established beyond 6 months after initial exposure, it essentially never resolves spontaneously; in one study of 320 patients followed serially for longer than 3 years, only 6 patients with end-stage liver disease lost detectable HCV RNA.[493] HCV viral load fluctuates little over time; in most individuals, viral load differs by less than 0.5 log,[132,181] and gradually increases by an average of 0.2 to 0.3 log/y.[132,333] It is estimated that approximately 20 to 30% of patients with hepatitis C will progress to cirrhosis over a period of 20 years.[409] The frequency of progression appears to be increased by age over 40 at the time of infection, male gender, alcohol abuse,[281] and immunosuppression, but it is less than 5% after 20 years of infection in those infected during the first 20 to 30 years of life.[224,382,413,481] In those who develop recurrent HCV after liver transplantation, the response rate is lower and the rate of progression to cirrhosis is faster than in primary infection. As with HBV, the likelihood of progression to HCC is between 1.5 and 5% per year in those with cirrhosis.[254]

The clinical picture of chronic HCV is similar to that of HBV in producing chronic hepatitis. Infection with HCV is characterized by fluctuating ALT activities over time. Only about one third of those with chronic HCV have continually increased ALT, and many of these individuals show variation in ALT activity.[116] It is common for individuals with fluctuating values to have multiple normal ALT activity values separating elevated values.[211,375] Individuals with normal ALT tend to have milder fibrosis and less severe disease on liver biopsy, but a minority have advanced fibrosis.[161] In contrast to HBV, individuals with continually normal ALT activity have a similar rate of response to antiviral treatment.[161]

TABLE 50-6 Tests for Evaluating Chronic Hepatitis C Virus (HCV) Infection and Its Treatment

Time of Testing	Test	Condition	Use/Interpretation
Pretreatment	HCV viral load	Detectable	Baseline (to compare with 12 wk value)
	Genotype	2 or 3 vs. other	Length of treatment (24 wk genotype if 2 or 3, 48 wk if other genotype)
4 wk on treatment	HCV viral load	Undetectable	Rapid virologic response (RVR)—high likelihood of treatment success
12 wk on treatment	HCV viral load	<2 log drop	Stop treatment (nonresponder)*
		>2 log drop	Continue treatment (on treatment responder)
End of treatment†	Sensitive HCV RNA‡	Detectable	Nonresponder or breakthrough (if was previously undetectable)
24 wk after completion	Sensitive HCV RNA§	Not detectable	Treatment responder
		Detectable	Relapser
		Not detectable	Sustained virologic responder

*Less than 3% chance of sustained virologic response; some continue treatment to 24 weeks and re-evaluate.
†Done at 24 weeks if genotype 2 or 3, done at 48 weeks if other genotypes; not all recommend evaluating end of treatment response.
‡Lower detection limit <50 IU/mL.
§Done only if genotype not 2 or 3.

Treatment of chronic HCV is based predominantly on a combination of pegylated (long-acting) interferon plus ribavirin. New agents, including HCV protease inhibitors, have shown promise in increasing treatment response rates when used along with standard treatment[295]; a high rate of spontaneous mutations to the most widely tested protease inhibitor precludes monotherapy.[157] In contrast to HBV, for which treatment is aimed at inhibiting viral replication, treatment of HCV is often successful in eradicating the virus.

Measurement of HCV RNA at several time points after the start of therapy has been found predictive of the likelihood of the ultimate goal—sustained virologic response (SVR, defined as absent HCV RNA at least 3 to 6 months after completion of treatment). Persons who achieve SVR have a less than 1% likelihood of recurrent viremia, and have no detectable HCV RNA in the liver.[474] Several terms have been used to describe treatment response.[161] Rapid virologic response (RVR) refers to undetectable HCV RNA after 4 weeks of treatment; those who achieve RVR have a 90% likelihood of achieving SVR. Early virologic response (EVR) refers to at least a 2 log decrease in viral load after 12 weeks of treatment. Persons who have undetectable HCV RNA after 12 weeks have a 70% likelihood of SVR; those with reduced, but detectable, HCV RNA have a lower but significant likelihood of SVR. Persons who fail to achieve EVR have a less than 3% likelihood of SVR and usually are not continued on treatment. End of treatment (EOT) response refers to undetectable HCV RNA at the end of therapy. Several factors may influence response to treatment. The most important is genotype; individuals with genotypes 2, 3, and 4 have response rates approximately twice those of other genotypes (SVR 70 to 80% vs. 45%), and those infected by genotypes 2 and 3 require only 6 months of treatment rather than the 12 months needed for other genotypes. Response rates are lower in those of African ancestry with high body mass index (BMI) and with higher viral load. Table 50-6 summarizes laboratory tests used to evaluate and monitor treatment for HCV.

Hepatitis B and C Coinfection

Approximately 2 to 10% of individuals infected with HCV are coinfected with HBV; of those with chronic HBV, 15 to 20% are also HCV positive.[90,500] Clinical and laboratory features of coinfected patients are somewhat contradictory and differ from those in individuals infected with a single hepatitis virus. Coinfected patients have lower viral loads than do those with single infection.[89] In patients with chronic HBV who develop acute HCV infection, the likelihood of progressing to chronic HCV infection is low,[81] and acute infection with HBV can lead to clearance of HCV.[389] These features would suggest a beneficial effect of coinfection. In contrast, patients with chronic HBV/HCV coinfection have more rapid progression to cirrhosis.[388] Patients with acute coinfection more frequently have severe acute hepatitis.[10,500] Some studies suggest a high frequency of HBV DNA viral replication in the liver even in the absence of circulating HBsAg; such subclinically coinfected patients have more severe liver injury and a higher frequency of cirrhosis.[58,232] Despite some favorable findings, the outcome of hepatitis in coinfected patients seems to be worse than for those infected with only a single agent.

Nonalcoholic Fatty Liver Disease[103A] and Nonalcoholic Steatohepatitis

Ludwig first described patients who had histologic features identical to those of alcoholic hepatitis, but who had no history of alcohol abuse and did not have AST higher than ALT.[271] He introduced the term *nonalcoholic steatohepatitis (NASH)* to describe this entity, which was more common in women than in men and usually was associated with diabetes and/or obesity. [Because alcohol ingestion is common in the population, and alcoholic liver disease does not occur with daily ingestion of less than 20 g ethanol, this threshold has been suggested as the maximum alcohol intake compatible with a diagnosis of nonalcoholic fatty liver disease (NAFLD).][84A,331] It is now recognized that NAFLD is associated strongly with the presence of the metabolic syndrome; almost half of individuals who meet the criteria for metabolic syndrome have NAFLD, and as many as 20 to 30% of the population in North America and Europe has NAFLD,[371] making it far and away the most common form of liver disease and an extremely common condition in the population in the developed world. About 10% of those with NAFLD have the more severe form, NASH. The frequency in obese or diabetic individuals is much higher, with NAFLD in 60 to 75% and NASH in 20 to 25%.[331,470] Prospective studies of patients with liver disease have confirmed that NASH is a common cause of elevated liver enzymes in an unselected population of patients referred to gastroenterologists or seen in primary care settings.[57,98,287] The frequency of cirrhosis in NASH is not well established, but it has been suggested that NASH may be a major cause of *cryptogenic* cirrhosis, for which no underlying cause can be determined. As weight loss develops with chronic illness, fat may disappear from the liver, leaving only fibrosis.

Current evidence suggests that accumulation of fat in NAFLD is a consequence of insulin resistance. A variety of mechanisms may lead to insulin resistance, including genetic predisposition, increased concentrations of free fatty acids, and the presence of cytokines such as tumor necrosis factor-alpha (TNF-α). Because TNF-α is produced by fat cells, correlates with body fat, and is critical to development of insulin resistance in obesity, it may be a key factor in the development of NAFLD. The pathogenesis is likely to be more complicated, however, because a variety of other factors lead to increased fat accumulation in the liver, including increased carbohydrate intake, certain drugs, and mutations in lipid synthesis, but they have not been associated with the development of NASH.

Laboratory diagnosis of NASH and NAFLD is currently not possible.[479] Although oxidative stress, inflammation, and abnormal concentrations of adipocyte-produced peptides are believed to be involved in the pathogenesis of NAFLD, laboratory tests evaluating these have not be found to be reliable predictors of histologic changes. A clinical approach typically involves a compatible clinical history and the presence of steatosis on imaging studies, exclusion of other causes of liver injury, and (if indicated) biopsy to confirm the diagnosis and determine the extent of injury. Although increased activities of liver enzymes are often used to distinguish NASH from other forms of NAFLD, the degree of necroinflammatory damage is not related to elevations in AST or ALT activity, and the likelihood of significant liver damage is similar in those with normal or elevated ALT.[313]

To date, major treatments for NAFLD have been aimed at lowering body weight and fat content. Loss of weight is often associated with decreased ALT values; in one study, a 1% decrease in weight was associated with an 8% decrease in ALT activity.[354] The association of NAFLD with insulin resistance has suggested treatment with antidiabetic medications, particularly those that increase insulin responsiveness [such as peroxisome proliferator-activated receptor (PPAR)-γ agonists and metformin]; studies have not been conclusive as to the benefits of such treatment.[426]

Autoimmune Hepatitis

Autoimmune hepatitis (AIH) represents a rapidly progressive form of chronic hepatitis, with up to 40% 6-month mortality in untreated individuals[428] associated with the presence of autoimmune markers. Although typically a chronic disease, it may have an acute presentation in up to 40% of cases, as discussed earlier. It is relatively uncommon, with an annual incidence of 1.9 cases per 100,000 population,[39] but it is responsible for 3 to 6% of all liver transplants[483]; the disease recurs in about 30% of patients after transplantation.[307] As with most autoimmune diseases, there is a strong female predominance. Forms of AIH has been found in individuals of all ages, with no racial or ethnic predilection. It has been associated with specific HLA haplotypes, notably DR3 and DR4, as is true for many other autoimmune diseases. Practice guidelines on autoimmune chronic hepatitis have been developed by the American Association for the Study of Liver Diseases (AASLD).[93]

AIH is associated with the presence of liver and nonliver autoantibodies in plasma. These are helpful in diagnosis, but are not likely to be the cause of liver injury. The most important antibodies for diagnosis include (1) antinuclear antibody (ANA), (2) anti–smooth muscle (or antiactin) antibody (ASMA), (3) anti–liver-kidney microsomal antigen type 1 (LKM_1), and (4) anti–soluble liver antigen (SLA), which is insensitive but highly specific. A variety of other autoantibodies are found frequently in AIH, some of which are found in other disorders. A summary of the most common autoantibodies, their associations, and their molecular targets (when known) is given in Table 50-7. Tests for these autoimmune markers initially used cell or tissue preparations studied by indirect immunofluorescence, but these have largely been replaced by assays that detect antibodies to purified proteins. Individuals who are negative for common autoantibodies, but otherwise meet criteria for diagnosis, have a similar prognosis and response to treatment.[297]

Criteria for the diagnosis of AIH were developed by an international group[215] and subsequently revised[13]; a simplified scoring system has also been developed.[190] The simplified criteria include (1) exclusion of viral hepatitis, (2) increased IgG, (3) positive autoantibodies, and (4) compatible histologic features.

It is controversial whether AIH should be further divided into subtypes; the international group that codified diagnostic criteria does not recommend use of subtypes,[19] but many authorities recognize three different forms (Types 1, 2, and 3). Although differences in epidemiology may be evident among the different forms, there do not seem to be differences in clinical course or response to treatment. Type 1, which is the most common form and the only one seen

TABLE 50-7 Serologic Markers of Autoimmune Liver Disease

Antibody Name	Antigen Target	Associations
Antiactin	Actin	AIH type 1; more specific than ASMA, poor response to corticosteroids, early age of onset
Anti-asialoglycoprotein receptor (ASGPR)	Transmembrane antigen binding protein	AIH, correlate with activity, disappear with successful treatment
Anti–liver-kidney microsome (LKM_1)	Cytochrome P450 2D6	AIH type 2; seen in only 4% of U.S. cases; usually in children
Anti–liver-specific cytosol (LC_1)	Enzyme (possibly formiminotransferase cyclodeaminase or argininosuccinate lyase)	AIH in younger patients, often with anti-LKM_1, primary sclerosing cholangitis; vary with activity of disease
Antimitochondrial antibody (AMA M2 type)	Dihydrolipoamide acyltransferase	Primary biliary cirrhosis
Antineutrophil cytoplasmic antibodies (ANCAs)	Bactericidal/permeability protein, cathepsin G, lactoferrin	Primary sclerosing cholangitis (PSC; 50-70%), ulcerative colitis (50-70%), AIH; nonspecific
Antinuclear antibody (ANA)	Multiple targets (centromere, ribonucleoproteins); may not be detected by ELISA	AIH type 1, some PSC cases
Anti–smooth muscle antigen (ASMA)	Actin, tubulin, vimentin, desmin, skelitin	AIH type 1, seen in other autoimmune diseases in lower titers
Anti–soluble liver antigen/liver pancreas (SLA)	UGA tRNA suppressor–associated transfer protein	AIH type 3; very specific for AIH, correlate with relapse after corticosteroid withdrawal

AIH, Autoimmune hepatitis; *ELISA,* enzyme-linked immunosorbent assay.

frequently in North America, is predominantly a disease of middle-aged women. It is characterized by ASMA or anti-actin (found in 87% of cases) and/or ANA (found in 67% of cases); one or the other is present in nearly 100% of cases. Because of the nonspecific nature of these antibodies, the strength of the antibody reaction (titer or immunoassay signal) is important in determining the likelihood of AIH. In children, the strength of the reaction is typically lower than in adults. Type 2 AIH, which characteristically occurs in children (although 20% occurs in adults), represents up to 20% of cases in Europe. It is associated with antibodies to liver-kidney microsomal antigen 1 (anti-LKM_1) or cytochrome P450 2D6 (CYP2D6).[499] Some cross-reactivity has been noted between this antibody and certain HCV antigens, leading to positive anti-CYP2D6 in individuals with HCV infection. The epitopes recognized by anti-HCV antibodies are different from those in persons with type 2 AIH.[273] Type 3 often lacks other autoimmune markers but is positive for antibody to soluble liver antigen liver-pancreas. This antibody is directed against UGA tRNA suppressor–associated antigenic protein.[466]

Immunosuppressive treatment using prednisone, alone or in combination with azathioprine, is effective in inducing clinical remission of disease in about 80% of cases; other immunosuppressants are now being used to reduce dependence on corticosteroids.[445] Because inherited differences in the activity of thiopurine methyltransferase affect about 10% of the population,[253] it has been recommended that pretreatment determination of enzyme activity should be used to reduce the likelihood of toxicity. Remission typically begins with improvement in symptoms, followed by normalization in laboratory abnormalities, and finally histologic resolution.[93] Laboratory remission generally does not occur until after at least 12 months of treatment, but it almost always occurs within 24 months in responders. Histologic remission is less common and usually requires at least 3 to 6 months longer than laboratory evidence of remission.[428] Sustained remission can persist off treatment in 80% of those with normal histology following therapy, but relapse occurs in 50% within 6 months if inflammation persists in the liver biopsy.[92]

Inherited Liver Disease Presenting as Chronic Hepatitis

Inherited liver diseases that present as chronic hepatitis include (1) hemochromatosis, (2) Wilson's disease, and (3) α_1-antitrypsin (AAT) deficiency.

Hemochromatosis

Hereditary hemochromatosis (HH) is an autosomal recessive disorder of iron metabolism that results in excessive iron absorption and accumulation in tissue (see Chapter 32). The gene for HH has long been linked to chromosome 6, close to the genes for the HLA system; it has been definitively identified and termed the *HFE* gene, which codes for a transmembrane protein similar to the class 1 major histocompatibility complex (MHC) molecule.[140] In North America and Europe, more than 90% of individuals with HH are homozygous for a single point mutation that inserts a tyrosine instead of cysteine at residue 282 (termed the *C282Y* mutation).[442] Although it is a frequent genetic trait (estimated 1 in 8 persons of northern European ancestry are carriers, with about 1 in 250 being homozygous), most individuals who are homozygous for this mutation do not develop evidence of iron overload. A large population-based study showed that only 28% of males and about 1% of females homozygous for the *C282Y* mutation develop HH.[11] Other mutations in the *HFE* gene have been linked to hemochromatosis, and mutations in other proteins that regulate iron absorption have been identified as causes of HH.[363]

Liver disease due to hemochromatosis is rare in younger individuals, but becomes more common after the age of 30. The likelihood of liver disease is related to serum ferritin concentrations. Ferritin greater than 1000 ng/mL is associated with a high likelihood of significant liver disease, and concentrations between 500 and 1000 indicate moderate risk[17]; in those who are not found to have liver disease, serum ferritin less than 300 indicates a low likelihood of progressive rise in ferritin to greater than 1000 during follow-up for an average of 12 years.[178] Treatment consists of phlebotomy to remove iron, or iron chelation therapy for those who cannot tolerate phlebotomy (with the goal of serum ferritin <50 ng/mL).[349]

Wilson's Disease

Wilson's disease is an autosomal recessive disorder of copper metabolism (see Chapters 31 and 40).[362A] It has a gene frequency of 1 in 200 and a disease frequency of 1 in 30,000. It is due to one of more than 200 mutations in a gene on chromosome 13 coding for a copper-transporting ATPase (ATP7B).[54,440] This enzyme, found mainly in the liver, is involved in movement of copper into bile; deficiency leads to accumulation of copper in the liver and, eventually, in other tissues. Guidelines on diagnosis and treatment of Wilson's disease have been updated.[380]

Wilson's disease usually manifests before age 30 and patients in their 70s have rarely been identified.[6] For reasons that are unknown, patients usually have the hepatic or the neuropsychiatric form of the disease. In children, hepatic involvement tends to predominate, whereas in adolescents and adults, the neuropsychiatric form becomes more common. Hepatic manifestations include fulminant hepatitis (as discussed earlier), but more commonly chronic hepatitis, with or without cirrhosis, is the presenting finding.[396,404] Occasionally, the features mimic those of autoimmune hepatitis, with increased globulins and positive ANA.[308]

The classic clinical finding of increased copper deposition in the eye is the Kayser-Fleischer ring, caused by deposition of copper at the edge of the cornea. Although found in about 95% of patients with neurologic or psychiatric manifestations, it is present in only about half of patients with hepatic forms of Wilson's disease[433] and is rarely present in children.[393] As mentioned earlier, hemolytic anemia and renal failure commonly accompany acute forms of Wilson's disease; hemolytic anemia may be episodic even in chronic forms of Wilson's disease.[380]

Several laboratory tests are available for the diagnosis of Wilson's disease; ceruloplasmin measurement is discussed in detail in Chapter 21 and copper measurement in Chapter 31. Test results are often affected by other conditions, sometimes making diagnosis difficult. Classic findings of Wilson's disease include (1) decreased ceruloplasmin, (2) decreased total plasma copper, (3) increased plasma-free (or nonceruloplasmin) copper, (4) increased urine copper excretion, and (5) increased hepatic copper content. Ceruloplasmin is a ferroxidase that typically is measured by enzymatic activity or by immunoassay. Although controversy is ongoing over which assay format is preferable, guidelines have not specified one type.[119,380] Ceruloplasmin is very low in infants, gradually rises to higher than adult concentrations in early childhood, then gradually declines to adult concentrations. Use of age-appropriate reference intervals is critical for diagnosis in children. Ceruloplasmin is an acute-phase protein, and its synthesis is induced by estrogen; concentrations may be falsely normal with acute illness or with high estrogen states. Low concentrations of ceruloplasmin are seen with malnutrition, in protein-losing states, and in cirrhosis of any cause. These preanalytical variables cause ceruloplasmin to have a low predictive value as a single test for Wilson's disease; in one study of patients with chronic hepatitis, the positive predictive value was only 6%.[64] Ceruloplasmin is also decreased in about 20% of heterozygous carriers of the Wilson's disease gene.[165] Because most plasma copper is bound to ceruloplasmin, total plasma copper is affected by factors that affect ceruloplasmin. Some estimate free (nonceruloplasmin) copper as the difference between total copper (μg/dL) and ceruloplasmin (3 × mg/dL); values greater than 25 μg/dL suggest Wilson's disease.[154] Urine copper excretion is the most specific noninvasive test for Wilson's disease; 24 hour urine copper excretion is typically more than 100 μg/d in Wilson's disease. Unfortunately, the clinical sensitivity of copper excretion appears to be only 75 to 85%.[393,433]

Treatment of active, symptomatic Wilson's disease is aimed at increasing urine copper excretion to eliminate excess copper from tissue. The primary therapy for Wilson's disease usually involves chelating agents such as D-penicillamine and trientine, which now is more widely used because of its lower rate of side effects. Zinc (particularly zinc acetate) inhibits copper absorption from the intestinal tract; it is usually used for maintenance after copper chelation and can also be used as initial therapy. Monitoring treatment (particularly with zinc) by measuring yearly urine copper excretion can be helpful in ensuring that excess copper is no longer being excreted.[380]

α_1-Antitrypsin Deficiency

Alpha$_1$-antitrypsin (AAT) is the most important of the serine protease inhibitors (collectively termed *serpins*). As its name implies, AAT inhibits trypsin, but it also inhibits other proteolytic enzymes, including neutrophil-derived elastase, cathepsin G, and proteinase 3. The gene for AAT (originally called *PI*, but now called *SERPINA1*) is located on chromosome 14. Several genetic variants of AAT (differing by a single amino acid) have been classified on the basis of their electrophoretic mobility; the slowest migrating of these was termed the *Z variant.* Some variants, particularly S and Z, form loop sheet polymers,[266] causing impaired release from the endoplasmic reticulum, hepatocytic inclusions of AAT, and reduced plasma concentrations. The most severe forms of disease have been associated with homozygosity for the Z variant, found in 1 in 1000 to 2000 individuals in Europe and North America.[206] However, it is estimated that only about 10% of those with AAT deficiency develop disease manifestations.[422]

The effects of AAT deficiency on the liver are controversial. In neonates, AAT deficiency is often associated with hepatitis; in one study, almost one third of infants with prolonged jaundice were found to be AAT deficient.[497] About 20% of AAT-deficient infants develop hepatitis,[366] with up to 25% 1-year mortality.[205] In those who survive the first year, however, evidence of liver injury diminishes and usually resolves by age 12.[436,468] At age 18, none of 183 individuals with AAT deficiency had clinical evidence of liver disease, none had elevated procollagen III peptide, and less than 20% had increased concentrations of liver-associated enzymes in serum.[437]

Data on association of AAT deficiency with liver disease in adults are somewhat contradictory.[131] In several studies, cirrhosis was present in one third to one half of those with AAT deficiency, and HCC was present in about one third of those with cirrhosis.[129,373] The frequency was similar in those with heterozygous and homozygous presence of the PiZ variant.[373] In two studies of patients with cryptogenic liver disease, the frequency of the PiZ heterozygotes was significantly higher than that found in the general population.[59,175] Two other studies, however, found a similar frequency of liver disease in those with AAT deficiency and controls.[142,317] Some evidence suggests that AAT deficiency may increase risk of liver damage from other factors. In one study, most individuals with AAT deficiency and liver injury were also positive for anti-HCV; only 11% had no other liver risk factors.[372] In those with AAT deficiency and no evidence of liver disease (usually viral related), life expectancy was no different from that in healthy controls. A 2007 research conference found evidence that defects in degradation of AAT underlie differences in protein accumulation, which is necessary for the development of liver disease.[362] It is likely that, as with hemochromatosis, the abnormal form of AAT is necessary, but perhaps not sufficient, to cause liver disease.

AAT is estimated by protein electrophoresis, in which it constitutes most of the α_1-globulin band; this was the original means by which AAT deficiency was recognized.[129] It also is quantified by a variety of other techniques (see Chapter 21). AAT is an acute-phase response protein; falsely normal quantitative concentrations have been reported in about 40% of PiZ heterozygotes,[196] although rarely in PiZZ homozygotes. Determination of phenotype was typically accomplished by isoelectric focusing and had been recommended as the diagnostic test of choice in one guideline,[119] but phenotype cannot distinguish true homozygotes from heterozygotes who have a null phenotype on the other AAT gene. Molecular tests are now available to determine AAT genotype.[41] Because the prognosis may vary between those who are actually homozygous for the Z variant and those with null phenotype, such molecular testing of the *SERPINA1* gene is considered preferable.[422]

Drug-Induced Liver Injury

As discussed earlier, most cases of drug-induced liver injury present as acute hepatitis. Less commonly, drugs have produced chronic liver injury in a pattern mimicking chronic hepatitis or other chronic liver injury (chronic cholestasis and hepatic granulomas).[407] The drugs most commonly linked to chronic hepatitis are nitrofurantoin, methyldopa, and HMG-CoA reductase inhibitors; however, a large number of drugs have been associated with liver injury,[504] and herbal medications have been linked to chronic hepatitis.[76,432] In individuals with increased activities of aminotransferases and no obvious cause, prescription drug use was significantly more likely to be present than in those with a known cause for elevated enzyme activities.[286] As with acute drug reactions, establishing drugs as the cause of chronic hepatitis is difficult; temporal relationships to drug ingestion are not as clear as with acute hepatitis, and reactions can be seen first in those who have been taking the medication for many months.[169,262] Most chronic drug reactions resolve when administration of the drug is discontinued.[4,14]

Significance of Chronic Hepatitis

In many cases, chronic hepatitis is a disease with minimal consequences. As mentioned earlier, an average of 20 to 30% of individuals with chronic HBV or HCV progress to cirrhosis over a 20 year period. However, cirrhosis was the 12th leading cause of death in the United States in 2006 (the most recent year for which full data are available).[191] The frequency of cirrhosis and HCC has been increasing in much of the Western world,[229] mostly caused by the increase in cases related to HCV. The proportions of individuals with HCV with cirrhosis and HCC are expected to double by 2020, and the number of deaths caused by liver disease is expected to almost triple.[102] The ability to predict which patients are at increased risk for such late complications of chronic hepatitis would allow more appropriate treatment.

Fibrosis and necroinflammatory activity are the two major components of chronic hepatitis. The extent of fibrosis (stage) is strongly related to the risk of progression,[208,356,490] whereas necroinflammatory activity (grade) is correlated with progression in some,[160,288,490] but not all,[62,367] studies. Because ALT activity is strongly correlated with necroinflammatory activity,[292] it is also associated with risk of progression to cirrhosis in some, but not all, studies. Clinical variables are associated with risk of progression as well; these include age at infection, male gender, alcohol intake, and the presence of immunosuppression.[62,151,284,369]

The process of scar formation in the liver involves numerous factors and differs in some important ways from that in other sites in the body.[7,402] Increasing evidence suggests that the process of fibrosis is reversible, even when cirrhosis is histologically present.[153] For example, two studies found that successful treatment of HBV[113] and HCV[368] was associated with reversal of cirrhosis in 50 to 75% of cases. Although the principal component of hepatic scars is type III collagen, other components include type I and type IV collagen, laminin, elastin, and fibronectin. Proteoglycans, especially hyaluronate, are also involved in scar formation. Production of scar in the liver is affected by the rate of enzymatic degradation; a variety of matrix metalloproteinases (MPs) are found in areas of scar formation, along with several tissue inhibitors of metalloproteinases (TIMPs). MPs are involved in degradation of the normal connective tissue of the liver (a necessary prequel to fibrosis), but they are also involved in breakdown and remodeling of collagen. Hepatic stellate cells are critical in this process; they produce both MP and TIMP, as well as collagen and other matrix materials.[34,152] Recruitment and activation of stellate cells involve the action of a number of cytokines, particularly transforming growth factor (TGF)-β, platelet-derived growth factor (PDGF), and interleukin-6.[152] Evidence indicates that a variety of other cells also contribute to development of scar tissue within the liver.[475]

The gold standard for evaluation of the extent of liver damage has been liver biopsy. Because the degree of injury is not uniform throughout the liver, the sample taken may not be representative of the extent of damage.[280] This has led to interest in the use of laboratory tests to predict the extent of fibrosis in the liver. Several approaches have been used to identify markers that correlate with the extent of fibrosis. One approach uses routine laboratory tests; among the markers found to correlate with extent of fibrosis are the ratio of activities of AST to ALT and AST to platelet count (sometimes called APRI). A second approach evaluates multiple markers, either direct markers of proteins and other compounds involved in scar formation or indirect markers of liver injury,[280] using multivariate analysis to determine indices that correlate with extent of fibrosis. Although a variety of indices of this type have been proposed, the most widely studied is the FibroTest.[210] A third approach uses proteomic analysis of serum to discern patterns that correlate with disease.[72] Significant overlap in such markers is evident between individuals with cirrhosis and those with varying stages of fibrosis in chronic hepatitis; in analyses of published studies of markers, indeterminate scores were found, on average, in 35% of patients in reported series.[357] Evidence also suggests that marker concentrations change with alteration in necroinflammatory activity and may actually reflect the activity of disease at the time of sampling, rather than cumulative fibrosis.[458] Because criteria for treatment in the most common causes of chronic hepatitis, HBV and HCV, depend on the severity of liver damage, perhaps the greatest use of such markers at present is in identifying patients who have minimal cumulative damage (in whom risk of treatment outweighs possible benefit). Many marker panels have high negative predictive value for significant fibrosis; their use alone or in combination may significantly reduce the need for liver biopsy.[406]

Alcoholic Liver Disease

Alcoholic liver disease differs clinically and biochemically from other forms of hepatitis and liver disease.[431A] It is a common cause of liver disease in the developed world, but the incidence of acute alcoholic hepatitis and death from alcoholic cirrhosis is declining in North America and Europe.[278,279] Risk factors for developing alcoholic liver disease include the following:

1. *Duration and magnitude of alcohol ingestion.* As discussed later in the chapter, alcoholic liver disease does not occur in all individuals with chronic ethanol intake; although there appears to be a threshold intake of 40 g/d in men and 10 g/d in women,[303] meta-analysis of published studies shows that risk increases even at intakes below 25 g/d.[87] Most individuals with alcoholic liver disease ingest more than 80 g of alcohol per day.[252] Daily drinking appears to be riskier than intermittent drinking.
2. *Gender.* In women there is a greater likelihood of progression to cirrhosis.[467] Although some studies have suggested that this is due to lower activities of gastric mucosal alcohol dehydrogenase in women, 2002 data show that this is true only in younger women, and that older women actually have higher activities than older men.[358]
3. *Hepatitis B or C infection.* Both may increase the severity of liver damage in persons who drink heavily, and both correlate with degree of liver damage. For example, antibodies to HCV are several times more common in individuals with alcoholic hepatitis than in alcoholic individuals without hepatitis or in age- and gender-matched controls, suggesting a synergistic role for HCV.[300]
4. *Genetic factors.* As discussed later, an inherited predisposition to alcoholism has been clearly established. *HFE* gene mutations are more common in alcoholic individuals with liver disease than in those with no evidence of liver disease.[277]
5. *Nutritional status.* Protein-calorie malnutrition is extremely common among alcoholic individuals. Malnutrition may be due not only to poor intake but also to abnormal nutrient metabolism. Whereas poor nutrition may contribute to the evolution of alcoholic liver disease, adequate nutrition does not prevent its development. In fact, studies suggest that obesity may be a risk factor (perhaps because of the presence of coexisting nonalcoholic fatty liver disease).

Alcohol is metabolized to acetaldehyde by cytosolic alcohol dehydrogenase and microsomal enzymes (primarily CYP2E1). Acetaldehyde is subsequently metabolized to acetyl-CoA by aldehyde dehydrogenase. This is further broken down to acetate, which may be converted to carbon dioxide and water or enter the citric acid cycle to be converted to fatty acids. The latter is a major mechanism for induction of fatty liver by alcohol, but acetaldehyde is probably the primary toxin. It causes most of the injury to liver cells, as well as the induction of collagen synthesis leading to fibrosis and, ultimately, cirrhosis.

The mechanism for liver injury in alcohol abuse is still unclear. Only a minority of patients (less than one third) who abuse alcohol develop alcoholic liver disease,[173] and only 5%

of the heaviest drinkers develop cirrhosis.[270] Acetylation of a variety of liver proteins occurs with alcohol abuse, leading to loss of function of affected proteins in many cases.[417] Antibodies to acetylated liver proteins have been detected in patients with alcoholic liver disease.[2,443] Alcohol causes damage to intestinal epithelial cells, leading to release of lipopolysaccharide, which can also damage liver cells.[395] Activation of innate immunity, through either or both of these mechanisms, appears central to damage in alcoholic liver disease.[40] A variety of other metabolic changes have been observed in alcoholic liver disease, including changes in methionine metabolism and oxidative stress.[8]

Genetic factors seem to play a role in both alcohol abuse[289,401] and alcoholic liver disease.[104] As much as 40 to 60% of alcohol abuse is due to inherited factors.[289] Much effort has been expended in finding specific genetic markers; some of the more commonly implicated specific genes are those coding for alcohol dehydrogenase and several brain receptors, including those for γ-aminobutyric acid (GABA) and acetylcholine. Genetic variants in alcohol-metabolizing enzymes (including alcohol dehydrogenase, aldehyde dehydrogenase, and microsomal enzymes such as CYP2E1) are linked to alcohol abuse. However, most believe that multiple genes are involved in alcohol abuse. Genetic factors may also be important in determining which persons with alcohol abuse develop liver disease; as with alcohol abuse itself, as much as half of the risk of cirrhosis is due to genetic factors.[435] Similar genes may be involved; a 2009 study showed that alcoholic individuals with cirrhosis were much more likely to have mutations in *CPP2E1* and GABA receptors than alcoholics without cirrhosis.[225]

Acute alcoholic hepatitis clinically is an acute febrile illness,[270] characteristically associated with leukocytosis[299] and increased concentrations of acute-phase response proteins.[177] It causes mild increases in cytosolic enzymes; AST activity is typically more than two times greater than that of ALT,[84] and it is rare for AST to be more than eight times the upper reference limit.[299] Among the factors involved in causing the higher AST/ALT ratio in alcoholic hepatitis are damage to mitochondria, causing release of mitochondrial AST,[276,325] deficiency of pyridoxal-5′-phosphate,[272] and reduction in ALT content within the liver.[272] A cholestatic form of the disease, with increases in ALP activity to greater than three times the upper reference limit, is seen in up to 20% of cases; it is associated with higher mortality.[342] Increases in bilirubin are common, and reduced liver-synthesized protein concentrations are commonly present. Increased bilirubin, decreased albumin, and prolonged PT are poor prognostic markers in alcoholic hepatitis.[167] The Maddrey discriminant function [4.6 × (PT − Control PT)] + Plasma bilirubin (mg/dL)] value greater than 32 indicates individuals with a high mortality rate,[303] and a Model for End-Stage Liver Disease (MELD) score greater than 11 has been found to have similar sensitivity and better specificity.[418]

A large number of biochemical markers have been proposed for the detection of excessive alcohol consumption.[100,183,336] Among routine laboratory tests, the most widely used are γ-glutamyltransferase (GGT) and mean corpuscular volume (MCV). Serum GGT activity is commonly used as a screening test for alcohol abuse. However, GGT is an inducible enzyme that is elevated by many drugs and a variety of other factors such as cigarette smoking and other forms of liver disease.[118] The threshold for positivity is about 2 drinks/d, and elevation is more common in those who drink regularly than in binge drinkers. Although the clinical sensitivity of GGT for alcohol abuse is in the range of 70%, specificity is poor.[195] GGT remains elevated for an average of 25 days after alcohol abstention.[24] MCV has similar clinical sensitivity, and specificity is low.[195]

Alcohol leads to production of isoforms of transferrin with low sialic acid content, termed *carbohydrate-deficient transferrin* (CDT; also called hyposialyl- and asialyltransferrin). The use of CDT for detecting problem drinkers has been reviewed.[231] CDT returns to a normal concentration in a mean of 10 days with abstention from alcohol.[24] In a pilot study, CDT was found to be the only test to reliably distinguish alcoholic hepatitis from nonalcoholic fatty liver disease.[348] It has been suggested that combining markers such as CDT and GGT will enhance accuracy in identifying problem drinkers.[195] CDT is frequently elevated in persons with end-stage liver disease regardless of cause.[114]

Other markers of alcohol abuse have been studied, but with fewer data than for the markers mentioned earlier. Fatty acid ethyl esters are formed with acute and chronic alcohol intake.[243] Similarly, alcohol metabolites combine with glucuronic acid, forming ethyl glucuronides in patients who abuse alcohol.[355] Acetaldehyde adducts with serum proteins[335] and sialic acid[79] have also been evaluated as markers of alcohol abuse. Proteomic techniques have been used to try to identify additional markers,[343] with the suggestion that these will perform better than currently used markers such as GGT and CDT.

Cirrhosis

Cirrhosis, defined anatomically as diffuse fibrosis with nodular regeneration, represents the end stage of scar formation and regeneration in chronic liver injury. This response to injury occurs independently of the etiology and thus it is not possible, in most circumstances, to determine the cause of cirrhosis based on histology. Classically, cirrhosis has been classified as (1) micronodular, (2) macronodular, or (3) mixed, based on the histology and gross appearance of the liver. However, this is considered inadequate for etiologic or prognostic purposes. Consequently, it is more common to classify cirrhosis on the basis of its presumed or known etiology. Common causes of cirrhosis and their therapies are listed in Table 50-8. Virtually all chronic liver diseases are known to lead to cirrhosis (see Figure 50-9), but most cases of cirrhosis occur as a result of chronic hepatitis.

In the early stages of transition from chronic hepatitis to cirrhosis, termed *compensated cirrhosis,* no signs or symptoms of liver damage may be noted. Laboratory abnormalities usually appear before clinical findings such as ascites, gynecomastia, palmar erythema (reddening of palms), and portal hypertension begin to develop. The earliest laboratory abnormalities to develop in cirrhosis are (1) fall in platelet count, (2) increase in PT, (3) decrease in the albumin-to-globulin ratio to less than 1, and (4) increase in the AST/ALT activity ratio to greater than 1.[163,274] In those with documented cirrhosis, decompensation occurs slowly, at a rate of about 3% per year; 10-year survival with compensated cirrhosis is 90%.[136] Once decompensation occurs, however, 10-year survival is only about 20%.[136] Jaundice is a late finding in decompensated cirrhosis. A variety of staging systems have been used to predict prognosis in cirrhosis. For many years, the most common classification system was the Child-Pugh class system, summarized in Table 50-9. Currently, the MELD score [calculated as 3.8 + ln bilirubin (mg/dL) + 11.2 ln international normalized ratio + 9.6 ln creatinine (mg/dL) + 6.4 etiology score (0 if alcohol or obstruction, 1 for all other causes)] is used to identify patients with advanced cirrhosis who may be candidates for liver transplantation; it appears superior to the Child-Pugh scoring system in predicting short-term survival.[43,50,148] Risk of death over 3 months is low in those with MELD scores less than 10, intermediate in those with scores of 10 to 20, and high in those with scores greater than 20.[220]

TABLE 50-8 Causes and Treatment of Cirrhosis

Cause	Treatment
Viral	
Hepatitis B	Administration of α-interferon or reverse transcriptase inhibitors
Hepatitis C	Administration of α-interferon
Toxic	
Alcohol	Abstinence, liver transplantation
Metabolic	
Hemochromatosis	Phlebotomy
Wilson's disease	Penicillamine, zinc trientine
α_1-Antitrypsin deficiency	Gene therapy, protein administration
Nonalcoholic fatty liver disease	Diet, exercise, insulin sensitizers
Biliary	
Primary biliary cirrhosis	Ursodeoxycholic acid
Primary sclerosing cholangitis	Liver transplantation
Autoimmune hepatitis	Corticosteroids, azathioprine, other immunosuppressants
Idiopathic	

Laboratory findings in cirrhosis reflect ongoing liver injury and decreased hepatic function. Activities of aminotransferases are variable in cirrhosis and reflect underlying necroinflammatory activity. If the cause of cirrhosis has been eliminated (as by abstinence from ethanol or successful treatment of viral hepatitis), aminotransferase activity is often within the reference interval. If aminotransferases remain increased, risk of development of HCC is increased.[394] As described earlier, the ratio of AST/ALT activity is often greater than 1 in cirrhosis; this is usually associated with a fall in ALT and minimal change in AST activities. The mechanism for the change in ratio is not clear, but there appears to be a decrease in the production of enzymatically active ALT in cirrhotic individuals,[399] along with a high ratio of immunoreactive to enzymatically active ALT.[227] Increases in α-fetoprotein (AFP) are common in cirrhotic patients, even in the absence of HCC.[168]

Hepatic Glycogenoses

The glycogenoses are a group of disorders that are characterized by excessive and/or aberrant glycogen storage in various tissues.[353] Most of these have deficient glucose production by the liver, leading to hypoglycemia. All are inherited by autosomal recessive transmission except for type IV, which is sex linked. The hepatic glycogen storage diseases and their enzyme defects are listed in Table 50-10. Most of these disorders are associated with growth retardation and hepatosplenomegaly. Mental development is usually normal. Hypoglycemia is a prominent feature in types I, III, and VI and needs to be treated with continuous glucose feeding of uncooked cornstarch, which results in slow release of glucose. The diagnosis is based on the demonstration of excess glycogen in the liver biopsy and in vitro identification of the abnormal enzyme or aberrant glycogen. Prognosis and treatment vary with each entity.

TABLE 50-9 Child-Pugh System for Classifying Severity of Cirrhosis

Feature	1 Point	2 Points	3 Points
Encephalopathy	None	Grade 1-2	Grade 3-4
Ascites	None	Slight	Moderate-severe
Albumin, g/dL	>3.5	2.8-3.5	<2.8
Prothrombin time, s prolonged	<4	4-6	>6
Bilirubin, mg/dL	<4	4-10	>10

Scoring: <7 points—class A; 7 to 9 points—class B; >9 points—class C.

TABLE 50-10 Hepatic Glycogen Storage Diseases

Type	Eponym	Enzyme Defect	Involved Tissues
0		Glycogen synthetase	Liver
I	von Gierke's	Ia glucose-6-phosphatase Ib translocase for glucose 6-phosphatase Ic phosphate/pyrophosphate translocase	Liver, kidney, intestines
II	Pompe's	Lysosomal acid α-1,4 glucosidase	Most tissues
III	Cori's	Amylo-1,6 glucosidase debranching enzyme	Liver, muscle, WBCs
IV	Anderson's	Amylo-1,4,1,6 trans-glucosidase (branching enzyme)	Most tissue
VI	Hers'	Liver phosphorylase	Liver, WBCs
VII		Phosphorylase activation	Liver
IXa		Phosphorylase kinase	Liver, WBCs, RBCs

RBCs, Red blood cells; *WBCs,* white blood cells.

Cholestatic Liver Disease

Cholestasis (stoppage or suppression of the flow of bile) is associated with retention of bile within the excretory system. The term *obstruction* is often used inappropriately, because cholestasis has been known to occur occur without mechanical obstruction to the biliary tract. Although intrahepatic cholestasis may be due to functional or mechanical problems, extrahepatic cholestasis is always due to physical obstruction of the bile ducts by processes such as gallstones (choledocholithiasis), biliary strictures, and tumors. The major cholestatic diseases include (1) mechanical obstruction of the bile ducts, (2) primary biliary cirrhosis (PBC), and (3) primary sclerosing cholangitis (PSC). Other cholestatic disorders consist of (1) post–bone marrow transplant cholangiopathy, (2) post–liver transplant cholangiopathy, (3) drug-induced cholestasis, (4) acquired immunodeficiency syndrome (AIDS) cholangiopathy, and (5) bilirubinostasis of acute illness. Cholestatic hepatitis, which was discussed previously, may also cause cholestasis, but generally presents in a fashion closer to hepatitis.

The clinical consequences of prolonged cholestasis are related to impaired biliary drainage. Deficiency of bile acids in the intestinal tract leads to malabsorption of fat and the fat-soluble vitamins A, D, E, and K (see Chapters 31 and 52). Vitamin A malabsorption results in night blindness. Vitamin D malabsorption leads to calcium and phosphate malabsorption, causing rickets in children and osteomalacia in adults. Vitamin K malabsorption results in deficiency of coagulation factors II, VII, IX, and X, leading to prolonged clotting times and, sometimes, bleeding. Lack of excretion of normal bile contents results in their accumulation in plasma. Bile acid retention leads to increased bile acid concentrations in plasma. Bilirubin retention leads to jaundice, dark urine, and pale stools. Increased bilirubin generally occurs only with complete obstruction and thus is more commonly seen with extrahepatic than intrahepatic cholestasis.

Laboratory features of cholestasis vary, depending on whether the process causes complete or partial impairment of biliary drainage. A common feature of all cholestatic disorders is an increase in plasma activities of canalicular enzymes, such as ALP and GGT. Because this process involves both increased synthesis of enzyme and release of enzyme from its membrane-bound forms, a short lag period is generally seen between the onset of cholestasis and the increase in plasma activities. In the early stages of an acute mechanical obstruction (especially from gallstones), transient increases may be noted in plasma activities of liver cytosolic enzymes, such as AST and ALT. Activities of plasma AST and ALT may exceed 400 U/L, and in 1 to 2% of cases are greater than 2000 U/L.[21] Even in the presence of continued obstruction, AST and ALT activity gradually decreases, and AST is typically within the reference interval within 8 to 10 days. Increases in total bilirubin typically occur only with complete extrahepatic obstruction, although they may be seen with extensive intrahepatic cholestasis. Increases in direct bilirubin are more commonly seen, and direct bilirubin has been reported to be the most sensitive functional test for the presence of cholestasis. Prolonged PT is the most commonly detected coagulation abnormality. It usually is corrected by administration of parenteral vitamin K. Accumulation of cholesterol is associated with the development of an abnormal lipoprotein-X,[305,326] containing phospholipids, cholesterol, fragments of cell membrane (along with ALP),[49] and albumin; the lipid may deposit in connective tissue, producing xanthomas. Although it is often measured as low-density lipoprotein (LDL) cholesterol,[144] lipoprotein-X is actually antiatherogenic.[429]

Mechanical Bile Duct Obstruction

The most common cause of cholestasis is biliary tract obstruction by space-occupying lesions.[416] Extrahepatic bile duct obstruction occurs most commonly as the result of gallstones in the common bile duct or because of tumors in the head of the pancreas or duodenum. Other causes of extrahepatic obstruction include (1) bile duct strictures, (2) extrinsic compression of the bile ducts by enlarged lymph nodes, (3) congenital biliary atresia, and (4) PSC. Extrahepatic obstruction is commonly associated with jaundice, especially when obstruction is complete. Elevation in canalicular enzymes is common, but is not present in all cases[269]; marked increases

(>3 × the upper reference limit) are more common with gallstones as a cause of obstruction.[469] Transient increases in aminotransferases are more common with choledocholithiasis than with other causes of extrahepatic obstruction.[212] Transient increases in CA 19-9 occur with bile duct obstruction[30]; this is an important consideration, because CA 19-9 is often used as a diagnostic test for pancreatic and bile duct carcinoma. A key feature of extrahepatic obstruction is dilation of more proximal and intrahepatic bile ducts, which is visualized by imaging studies.

Intrahepatic cholestasis caused by mechanical obstruction is also common, but is rarely associated with jaundice or with visibly dilated ducts on imaging studies, although it may be associated with increased direct bilirubin. Jaundice typically occurs only with lesions that are very large, or are located near the porta hepatis, where they may obstruct both hepatic ducts. Common causes of intrahepatic obstruction include (1) tumors (particularly metastases), (2) granulomatous diseases (such as sarcoidosis and tuberculosis), and (3) infiltrative processes (such as lymphoma, leukemia, and extramedullary hematopoiesis).

Primary Biliary Cirrhosis

PBC, or nonsuppurative destructive cholangitis, is an uncommon autoimmune disorder targeting intrahepatic bile ducts.[330] Its prevalence is approximately 2 to 8 per 100,000 population in the developed world, but it is much lower in developing areas. The median age at onset is 50 years, and the female-to-male ratio is about 6:1. An association with HLA class II antigen DR8 has been noted in some populations. A family history of PBC is seen in 1 to 4% of cases. In up to 80% of cases, the condition is associated with other autoimmune processes, most commonly Sjögren's syndrome and hypothyroidism (which often develops before onset of PBC).[91]

The pathogenesis of PBC is not well understood. However, it is known that destruction of the bile duct is mediated by T cells in the presence of upregulation of HLA class I antigens on hepatocytes and HLA class II antigens on biliary epithelial cells.[159] Although the target antigens of the T cells have not been identified, at least 95% of patients have antimitochondrial antibodies that react against the dihydrolipoamide acyltransferase component of the pyruvate decarboxylase complex.[463] Part of this complex is found on the apical surface of biliary epithelial cells, suggesting a role for this antigen as an immune target.[319] In individuals with coexisting Sjögren's syndrome, the antigen is also expressed on the surface of salivary gland cells.[457]

PBC typically presents as an asymptomatic elevation of ALP, but may present with features of cholestasis or with fatigue.[290] Metabolic bone disease and xanthomas are common complications of PBC.[259] Occasionally, autoantibodies are detected (usually because of the presence of another autoimmune disease or because of a family history of PBC) before elevation of ALP.[306] Aminotransferase activities are increased in 50% of cases, but are more than twice the upper reference limit in only 20% of cases.[264] Increased bilirubin is a late finding and is important in predicting decompensation.[236] Antibodies to mitochondria or to the recombinant pyruvate decarboxylase complex appear similar in sensitivity, although the latter are more specific.[464] A liver biopsy is not required for diagnosis in most cases, but may be helpful in those with low titer antibodies or with a greater than twofold increase in aminotransferase activity.

The natural history of PBC is one of slow progression to portal hypertension, often without development of cirrhosis; average time from diagnosis to death in untreated patients is 22 years.[290] Development of jaundice is the most important indicator of advanced disease and serves as the most important prognostic test.[259] Medical management of PBC consists of ursodeoxycholic acid therapy; most evidence suggests that survival is improved in treated patients.[259] Although a rare complication, the relative risk of developing HCC is significantly increased in individuals with PBC.[337] Liver transplantation is the only definitive treatment, but even when it is performed, PBC may recur in the transplanted organ.[139]

Primary Sclerosing Cholangitis

PSC is a chronic inflammatory disease of the biliary tree, most commonly affecting extrahepatic bile ducts; involvement of intrahepatic ducts, with extrahepatic involvement or as an isolated finding, is also possible.[170,421] In contrast to PBC, PSC has a male predominance (60 to 70%) and a younger median age at onset (30 years). In 70 to 90% of patients, PSC is associated with ulcerative colitis, which usually (but not always) precedes onset of PSC; conversely, only about 2 to 4% of patients with ulcerative colitis develop PSC.[170] This has led to speculation that bacterial antigens in portal blood might be involved in the pathogenesis of PSC.[17] An autoimmune component is likely, as 97% of patients with PSC have one or more autoantibodies present in their plasma.[199] The prevalence of PSC is similar to that of PBC, but geographic differences in prevalence have been observed; it is most common in Northern Europe, where PSC is the most common indication for liver transplantation.[400] A markedly increased prevalence of HLA antigens B8 and DR3 has been noted.[480]

The clinical presentation of PSC, similar to that of PBC, is typically an asymptomatic patient with elevated ALP activities found during routine laboratory screening. Symptoms are ultimately present in most patients with PSC; the most common are pruritus and intermittent abdominal pain, but fever may also be present.[421] Treatment, whether medical or surgical, may improve laboratory tests and symptoms, but does not improve long-term survival.[250,298] Transplantation, the major treatment available for end-stage PSC, has a high rate of long-term survival. Although PSC recurs after transplantation in about 20 to 35% of cases, it does not appear to affect survival.[245] Transplantation also appears to increase the severity of underlying ulcerative colitis, when present.[124] The major cause of death in individuals with PSC is cholangiocarcinoma, which ultimately develops in up to 40% of patients.[170,421] Transplantation in the presence of cholangiocarcinoma is associated with rapid development of metastatic disease and poor survival.[3] PSC also increases the likelihood of colon carcinoma in individuals with coexisting ulcerative colitis, although the risk is not affected by liver transplantation.[482]

At the time of diagnosis, most patients with PSC have elevated ALP activities and other canalicular enzymes; bilirubin concentration is typically normal, although it may increase with acute exacerbations. The diagnosis of PSC is based on the typical radiographic appearance of beading and irregularity of the bile ducts. Antineutrophil cytoplasmic antibodies (ANCAs) are present in approximately 80% of patients[321] but are not specific for PSC; they are also present in PBC and autoimmune hepatitis. Typically, the antibodies have an atypical perinuclear pattern, being located near the nucleus in formalin- and methanol-fixed preparations. Antigens include lactoferrin, bactericidal/permeability increasing protein, and cathepsin G.[199]

Drug-Induced Cholestasis

Drugs are a common cause of cholestasis, causing about 15% of cases.[505,506] Drug reactions are especially common in older individuals, among whom up to 50% of individuals have increased enzymes because of medications.[505] Nonmedicinal drugs are also increasingly recognized as a cause of cholestasis.[314] Drugs can cause a cholestatic picture by two major mechanisms.[503] In some cases, only conjugated bilirubin is increased, whereas canalicular enzymes are not elevated. This picture, often seen with estrogen and anabolic steroids, appears due to inhibition of production of MRP2,[453] as discussed earlier in other cholestatic disorders. More commonly, drugs induce a cholestatic hepatitis, as discussed earlier.

Gallstones

Gallstones are solid formations in the gallbladder that are composed of cholesterol and bile salts. Although they vary in chemical composition, they generally contain a mixture of cholesterol, bilirubin, calcium, and mucoproteins. In the United States, 70 to 85% of all gallstones are predominantly cholesterol, and more than 10% of the adult population is affected.

Three major types of gallstones are (1) cholesterol gallstones, (2) pigmented gallstones, and, most common, (3) mixed gallstones. These stones form whenever bile is supersaturated with cholesterol or unconjugated bilirubin. Most gallstones are mixed cholesterol and pigment stones. For these stones or cholesterol gallstones to form, bile must be supersaturated with cholesterol. Whenever an increase in cholesterol or a decrease in bile acids or lecithin occurs, bile becomes lithogenic (prone to stone formation), and cholesterol may precipitate. Factors that predispose to cholesterol hypersecretion are (1) obesity, (2) aging, (3) certain drugs such as clofibrate and nicotine, and (4) certain hormones such as estrogen. Factors that decrease bile acid secretion are terminal ileal disease and cholestatic diseases, such as PBC, PSC, and cystic fibrosis. Genetic factors also appear to be involved. Within racial groups, women are more frequently affected than men. Diet may play a role because it appears that people who ingest diets high in polyunsaturated fats have a higher incidence, whereas those with a diet high in fiber have a decreased incidence.

Pigmented gallstones are associated with conditions in which the bilirubin concentration is increased, such as hemolytic anemia, or bilirubin becomes insoluble (i.e., deconjugated), such as occurs in cholestasis or chronic biliary infection.

Rare Causes of Cholestasis

Several other disorders are associated with cholestasis. Because they occur in specific settings, they are often suggested by the clinical picture. Laboratory tests are of little help in establishing the correct diagnosis.

Cholestasis may develop following bone marrow transplantation because of a variety of factors. Acute graft-versus-host disease (GVHD) is a consequence of the infusion of allogeneic immunocompetent T-lymphoid cells into an immunocompromised host that cannot reject these cells.[427] Periductular epithelial cells are the primary targets of injury in both acute and chronic GVHD.[36] Clinical features of GVHD include skin rash, intestinal symptoms (nausea, vomiting, diarrhea, and abdominal pain), and cholestasis. The histologic appearance is characteristic, but a liver biopsy is somewhat hazardous in these patients; thus most cases are diagnosed on clinical grounds.

Although acute liver transplant rejection is associated with necroinflammatory changes and increased aminotransferases, chronic rejection is often associated with cholestasis. The primary targets of immunologic injury are bile ductules and blood vessels.[109] Because of cholestasis, plasma bile acids are often increased early in the process of rejection. Increased numbers of canalicular membranes are often the first evidence of rejection.[109] Although eosinophilia is common in rejection,[324] it is also a common finding in drug-induced cholestasis and thus is not helpful in the differential diagnosis.

AIDS cholangiopathies are caused by organisms not previously known to infect the biliary tree; they have become less common with reduction in the frequency of immunosuppression because of combination antiretroviral treatment. *Cryptosporidium* is the most common organism. *Microsporidium*, cytomegalovirus, *Mycobacterium avium* complex, and *Cyclospora* have also been identified. The clinical presentation usually includes abdominal pain, diarrhea, and cholestasis manifested by threefold to tenfold elevations in plasma ALP, mild elevations in aminotransferases, and rarely jaundice. Papillary stenosis at the ampulla of Vater is present in patients with pain, and the bile ducts have features of PSC. Cholangiography is needed for the diagnosis but is indicated only in patients with pain. Brushings and biopsies at the time of cholangiography will establish the diagnosis. Treatment is primarily endoscopic. Sphincterotomy will give pain relief in approximately 70% of patients.

Hepatic Tumors

The liver is host to a wide variety of benign and malignant primary tumors. It is the second most common site of metastases; metastatic tumors account for 90 to 95% of all hepatic

TABLE 50-11 Classification of Hepatic Tumors

Type	Benign	Malignant
Epithelial	Adenoma Bile duct adenoma Cystadenoma Carcinoid Focal nodular hyperplasia Diffuse nodular hyperplasia	Hepatocellular carcinoma Cholangiocarcinoma Cystadenocarcinoma Squamous carcinoma
Mesenchymal tumors	Cavernous hemangioma Fibroma Leiomyoma Hematoma	Hemangiosarcoma Fibrosarcoma Leiomyosarcoma Hepatoblastoma
Metastatic tumors (most common sources)	Colon Pancreas Stomach Breast Lung Unknown primary	

malignancies. Primary tumors may arise from many cell lines in the liver, but they arise most commonly from parenchymal and biliary epithelial cells and mesenchymal cells (Table 50-11). The two most important primary liver tumors are HCC and cholangiocarcinoma.

Hepatocellular Carcinoma

HCC is the fifth most common cancer worldwide and a leading cause of cancer death; more than 500,000 cases occur annually, with a similar number of deaths.[204] Wide geographic and ethnic variations are noted in the incidence, suggesting that both host and environmental factors are involved in its origin. For example, approximately 75% of HCC cases occur in Asia, with an annual incidence of HCC in China of approximately 30 cases per 100,000 males. Worldwide, the incidence is twofold to threefold higher among men than among women. The incidence of HCC has been increasing in the United States[12,127] and much of Europe because of the increasing frequency of cirrhosis caused by HCV; however, incidence has declined in many parts of the world, owing to success in prevention of infection by HBV.[68,247] Although cirrhosis is present in most patients with HCC, it is absent in about 25 to 30% of cases, often in association with HBV.[47,498] More important, the presence of cirrhosis had been recognized before diagnosis of HCC in only about one third of cases.[495,498] Wide variations in the incidence of HCC are associated with different causes of cirrhosis. For example, HCC occurs commonly in cirrhosis caused by alcohol abuse, hemochromatosis, AAT deficiency, HBV, and HCV, but is rare in that caused by autoimmune hepatitis and Wilson's disease.

In most parts of the world, the major risk factors for development of HCC are infection with HBV or HCV. In Asia, Africa, and Alaska, the major risk factor is HBV infection. The presence of HBsAg and HBeAg is associated with a relative risk of HCC of 60, whereas the presence of HBsAg with negative HBeAg is associated with a relative risk of 10.[489] This is probably due to the lower viral loads in HBeAg-negative chronic HBV; in all forms of chronic HBV, risk of HCC is directly related to viral load.[71] Once cirrhosis has developed, the rate of development of HCC is about 1.5 to 5% per year in both HBV and HCV[137,138]; the relative risk of HCC doubles in those coinfected with these viruses.[135] The risk of HCC is higher in those with cirrhosis who have elevated aminotransferase activities than in those with normal ALT activity.[187,394] The mechanism of increased risk in HBV is thought to be related to integration of HBV DNA into the host genome, possibly caused by the action of the HBV X gene, which may block the activity of p53.[141,460] The mechanism of increased risk of HCC in HCV has not been identified, but may be related to ongoing injury.

Aflatoxin, a product of *Aspergillus flavus* contamination of grain, has been linked to risk of HCC; although it is harmless, it is metabolized to aflatoxin 8,9-epoxide. This reactive intermediate binds to guanosine bases in DNA, leading to mutagenesis. If the formed adduct is not repaired, G-to-T transversion occurs in codon 249 of the *TP53* gene *(p53),* causing an inactivating mutation.[374] Under normal circumstances, the mutagenic aflatoxin 8,9-epoxide is rendered harmless by glutathione-S-transferase, which converts it to a glutathione conjugate, which in turn is metabolized to 1,2-dihydrodiol by epoxide hydrolase.[261] However, both detoxifying enzymes are polymorphic in humans, and the mutant forms are less active. Patients with HCC are more likely to have the mutant forms of epoxide hydrolase and glutathione-S-transferase; this allows accumulation of the epoxide.[294]

The clinical presentation of HCC is variable and usually does not occur until late in the course of disease, when the tumor is large and resection is impossible. In some cases, acute decompensation occurs in a patient with cirrhosis, but clinical presentation may include detection of a right upper quadrant mass, shock due to hemorrhage into the peritoneal cavity, or right upper quadrant pain. Nonspecific signs and symptoms, such as fever, malaise, anorexia, and anemia, are common, and jaundice may occur with central tumors that obstruct biliary drainage. In a small number of cases, paraneoplastic features, such as hypoglycemia, hypercalcemia [due to parathyroid hormone–related peptide (PTHrP) production], or erythrocytosis (due to erythropoietin production), may be the initial presenting findings; such paraneoplastic findings occur in up to 20% of cases, usually in association with poor prognosis.[222,275] Laboratory findings include those of cirrhosis and cholestasis and (except for tumor markers discussed later) are nonspecific.

Because treatment usually is not possible in individuals with clinically diagnosed HCC, much interest has focused on screening high-risk individuals. Most professional societies have not advocated screening for HCC in Europe or North America, although the American Association for the Study of Liver Diseases (AASLD) has endorsed screening of high-risk patients every 6 to 12 months.[51] Although some data have suggested that screening is effective in detecting small, treatable tumors, other data have not been as supportive.

The most common screening programs have used plasma tumor marker concentrations or tumor markers plus imaging studies; the AASLD recommends imaging as the primary screening modality and recommends against using only tumor markers (although tumor markers were noted to be useful as an addition to imaging).[51] Ultrasound is typically used as the imaging modality for screening because of its low cost. The tumor marker most widely used for screening purposes is AFP; it is typically quantified using assays that measure its total concentration. Although it appears to be relatively sensitive,[283] elevation of AFP is common in individuals with chronic hepatitis and cirrhosis—the group at highest risk for HCC. In our experience, AFP above the upper reference limit has a positive predictive value of only 16% for HCC. Use of higher cutoff values than the upper reference limit improves clinical specificity of total AFP, at the expense of clinical sensitivity; for example, at a cutoff of 20 ng/mL, about three times the upper reference limit, sensitivity is only 60%.[51] As discussed in Chapter 24, modified forms of AFP are more specific for tumors, particularly the L3 isoform recognized by lens culinaris (lentil) lectin. The L3 isoform by itself has low sensitivity for HCC,[434] and in only a small number of cases, it is the only positive tumor marker. On the other hand, specificity and positive predictive value are significantly improved when the L3 isoform is combined with the AFP total.[434] An L3 isoform more than 15% of total AFP may be associated with more aggressive and less well-differentiated tumors.[60]

Des-γ-carboxy prothrombin (DCP)—also called PIVKA-2 (factor II protein induced by vitamin K antagonists)—is the inactive form of prothrombin found in individuals taking warfarin or other vitamin K antagonists. It was first found to be increased in HCC in 1984,[257] but was not widely used until the early 1990s. Initial studies found that DCP was increased in some patients who did not have elevated AFP, but was insensitive to small HCC that might be curable. DCP immunoassays with lowered detection limits have been developed and have shown increased sensitivity for small HCC, and DCP seems directly related to tumor size[123] and prognosis.[434] Pretreatment with vitamin K, to eliminate other causes of increased DCP, further improves specificity.[390] DCP is best used as an adjunct to AFP, because tumors often produce one or the other tumor marker.[25]

Treatment of HCC is dependent on the extent of the tumor. Small tumors are often treated by transplantation, which has a low rate of recurrent tumor. Local techniques, such as ethanol injection, chemoembolization, and use of radiofrequency ablation, are increasingly used before transplant or instead of transplantation. Larger tumors generally are not resectable, but may be treated by chemoembolization if a single feeding vessel is identified. A novel approach to identifying micrometastases has been described using rt-PCR to amplify mRNA for AFP to detect recurrence or metastasis.[485]

Tumors of the Gallbladder and Bile Ducts

Benign lesions such as papillomas or adenomas may be seen as an incidental finding at cholecystectomy; malignant disease of the gallbladder is uncommon. Cholelithiasis may be an etiologic factor, because 85% of gallbladder carcinomas occur in patients with gallstones. However, less than 1% of patients with gallstones develop carcinoma. It has been suggested that a calcified gallbladder is especially prone to malignant transformation. Various pathologic forms exist, including papillary adenocarcinoma, squamous cell carcinoma, and anaplastic tumors. These tumors usually arise in the neck of the gallbladder and spread rapidly, causing obstruction and cholestasis. Physical examination reveals a hard, tender mass in the gallbladder fossa. These lesions are particularly difficult to treat, and most cases are inoperable at the time of diagnosis.

Cholangiocarcinoma, or primary carcinoma of the bile ducts, can arise at any point in the biliary tree, including the small intrahepatic bile duct radicals. This lesion is typically associated with underlying liver disease, such as (1) PSC, (2) congenital cystic lesions, or (3) chronic infestation with *Clonorchis sinensis*. The clinical presentation is that of cholestasis, including jaundice, dark urine, tan-colored stool, and pruritus. This condition is differentiated from other cholestatic diseases by visualizing the biliary tree.

DIAGNOSTIC STRATEGY

Liver function tests are useful in detecting and diagnosing liver disease and dysfunction, as well as in evaluating severity, monitoring therapy, and assessing prognosis. They are also useful in directing further diagnostic work-up. The array of tests useful for these purposes (Table 50-12) includes measurement in plasma of total and direct bilirubin, protein, and albumin concentrations and the activity of enzymes such as the aminotransferases (AST and ALT), ALP, LD, and GGT. By using a combination of these tests, it is possible to categorize broad types of liver disease, which can then be more accurately diagnosed through disease-specific tests. An algorithm for this process is presented in Figure 50-13.

Plasma Enzymes

In practice, plasma aminotransferases and ALP are the most useful tests, because they allow differentiation of hepatocellular disease from cholestatic disease in most cases. The importance of this distinction cannot be overstated: failure to recognize cholestatic disease caused by extrahepatic biliary obstruction will result in liver failure if the obstruction is not quickly corrected. It is also important to recognize that there may be a gray zone of mixed hepatocellular and cholestatic

TABLE 50-12 Tests of Hepatic Function and Injury

Test	Utility
Bilirubin	Diagnosing jaundice, modest correlation with severity
Alkaline phosphatase (ALP)	Diagnosing disorders of metabolism and disorders of the newborn
Bilirubin fractionation	Diagnosing cholestasis and space-occupying lesions
Aspartate aminotransferase (AST)	Sensitive test of hepatocellular disease; AST > ALT in alcoholic disease
Alanine aminotransferase (ALT)	Sensitive and more specific test of hepatocellular disease
Albumin	Indicator of chronicity and severity
Prothrombin time (PT)	Indicator of severity of cholestasis

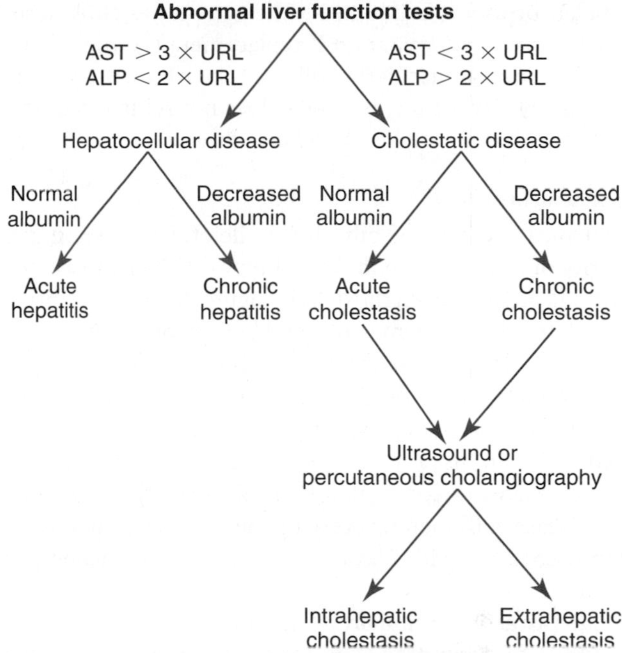

Figure 50-13 Algorithm for using abnormal liver function tests to classify and diagnose various types of liver disease. *ALP,* Alkaline phosphatase; *AST,* aspartate aminotransferase; *URL,* upper reference limit. Initial evaluation is best accomplished by examining the pattern of liver-associated enzymes. If elevation primarily affects one of the aminotransferases, then hepatocellular disease is likely; an increase primarily in ALP suggests a cholestatic disorder. If only ALP is elevated, then it is appropriate to consider nonhepatic sources before further investigation [using measurement of other canalicular enzymes such as γ-glutamyltransferase (GGT) or alkaline phosphatase isoenzymes]. If liver is the source of elevated ALP, then an imaging study to evaluate the ducts is the next test performed; dilated ducts establish a mechanical cause of obstruction, and normal ducts indicate intrahepatic cholestasis requiring further evaluation, as discussed in the text. Predominant increases in aminotransferases suggest hepatocellular injury; values greater than 10× URL usually indicate acute hepatitis, and lower values are typical of chronic hepatitis. If AST > ALT, common causes include very early hepatic injury, nonhepatic injury (such as muscle injury), and, with mildly increased values, cirrhosis.

disease wherein the tests do not distinguish one disease from the other. In this case, it is wise to assume that the problem is cholestatic and rule out biliary obstruction.

Patients are occasionally seen with isolated elevations in ALP or aminotransferase enzyme activities. In practice, an isolated increase in ALP activity is difficult to interpret. In children, *benign transient hyperphosphatasemia* should always be considered. In adults, it is necessary to first confirm that the ALP is of hepatobiliary origin. This can be done by isoenzyme fractionation (see Chapter 22) or by measurement of activity of another canalicular enzyme such as 5′ nucleotidase or GGT, which tends to parallel the activity of ALP in cholestasis. The most important aspect of the work-up is to rule out space-occupying lesions by visualizing the liver with computed tomography (CT), and biliary tract disease by visualizing the biliary tree with ultrasound or cholangiography.

Elevated plasma activities of AST and ALT are common in many disorders (see Chapter 21). To determine whether this elevation is liver related, administration of all drugs and alcohol intake (especially if AST is higher than ALT) should be discontinued. If the elevation persists, ultrasound (looking for nonalcoholic fatty liver) and hepatitis B and C serology should be performed. More than 50% of isolated enzyme elevations of liver origin will be caused by these disorders. A liver biopsy is often needed to allow a more specific diagnosis. No reliable test other than liver biopsy can be used to detect fibrosis.

Plasma Albumin

Plasma albumin measurements are useful in assessing the chronicity and severity of liver disease. For example, the plasma albumin concentration is decreased in advanced chronic liver disease. However, its utility for this purpose is somewhat limited, as the plasma albumin concentration is also decreased in severe acute liver disease and is lowered by many other disorders, and nonspecifically in acute illness. Serial measurements of plasma albumin can be used to assess the severity of liver disease.

Prothrombin Time

Serial PT measurements can be used to differentiate between cholestasis and severe hepatocellular disease. In practice, PT should be measured again after vitamin K injection, because cholestasis will cause a decrease in PT as the result of malabsorption of vitamin K. The patient has cholestasis if the PT corrects after vitamin K replacement (10 mg subcutaneously or intramuscularly, followed by PT measurement 4 hours later). Over time, if the PT does not return to normal, the patient has severe hepatocellular disease.

Serum Bilirubin

Serial measurement of bilirubin is helpful in assessing the severity of liver damage in several types of liver disease (e.g., alcoholic hepatitis, cirrhosis). In acute hepatitis, bilirubin peaks later than enzymes do, and serum bilirubin remains elevated for longer than urine bilirubin because of the presence of biliprotein (δ-bilirubin). Increases in bilirubin in most liver diseases are primarily due to an increase in conjugated bilirubin, usually detected as direct reacting bilirubin. An increase in unconjugated bilirubin usually is not due to liver disease, although severe acute hepatitis and cirrhosis are often associated with elevations primarily of unconjugated bilirubin.

Patients are occasionally seen with isolated elevations in bilirubin concentration and normal quantitess of liver-associated enzymes. Increased unconjugated (indirect reacting) bilirubin in such situations is usually due to increased production of bilirubin (hemolysis, rhabdomyolysis, large hematomas) or to impaired conjugation (inherited decrease in activity of conjugation in Gilbert's syndrome or Crigler-Najjar syndrome, drug-induced inhibition of enzyme activity by atazanavir, immaturity of liver in physiologic jaundice of the newborn). Increases in conjugated (direct reacting) bilirubin are common in seriously ill individuals (bilirubinostasis of sepsis) and are less common with inherited defects in excretion of conjugated bilirubin (Dubin-Johnson syndrome, Rotor syndrome). An algorithm for differentiating the familial causes of hyperbilirubinemia is presented in Figure 50-14.

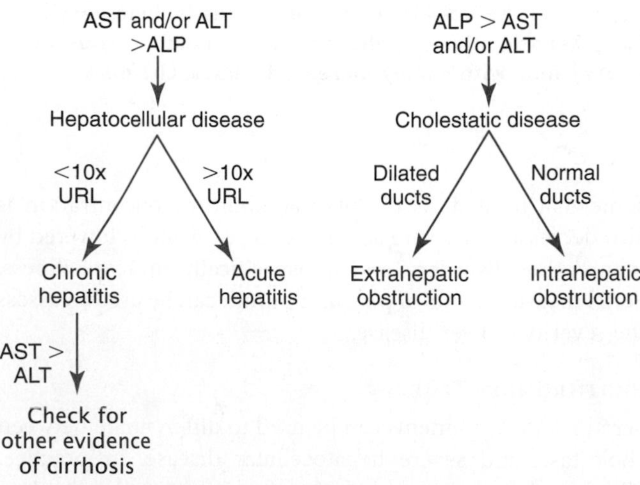

Figure 50-14 Algorithm for differentiating familial causes of hyperbilirubinemia.

REFERENCES

1. Abe K. GB virus-C/hepatitis G virus. Jpn J Infect Dis 2001;54:55-63.
2. Actis G, Ponzetto A, Rizzetto M, Verme G. Cell-mediated immunity to acetaldehyde in alcoholic liver disease demonstrated by leukocyte migration test. Am J Dig Dis 1978;23:883-6.
2A. Åberg F, Isoniemi H, Höckerstedt K. Long-term results of liver transplantation. Scand J Surg 2011;100:14-21.
3. Ahrendt S, Pitt H, Nakeeb A, Klein A, Lillemoe K, Kalloo A, et al. Diagnosis and management of cholangiocarcinoma in primary sclerosing cholangitis. J Gastrointest Surg 1999;3:357-67.
4. Aithal P, Day C. The natural history of histologically proved drug induced liver disease. Gut 1999;44:731-5.
5. Akriviadis E, Kapnias D, Hadjigavriel M, Mitsiou A, Goulis J. Serum/ascites albumin gradient: its value as a rational approach to the differential diagnosis of ascites. Scand J Gastroenterol 1996;31:814-7.
6. Ala A, Borjigin J, Rochwarger A, Schilsky M. Wilson disease in septuagenarian siblings: raising the bar for diagnosis. Hepatology 2005;41:668-70.
7. Albanis E, Friedman S. Hepatic fibrosis: pathogenesis and principles of therapy. Clin Liver Dis 2001;5:315-34, v-vi.
8. Albano E. New concepts in the pathogenesis of alcoholic liver disease. Expert Rev Gastroenterol Hepatol 2008;2:749-59.
9. Alberti A, Boccato S, Vario A, Benvegnu L. Therapy of acute hepatitis C. Hepatology 2002;36:S195-200.
10. Alberti A, Pontisso P, Chemello L, Fattovich G, Benvegnu L, Belussi F, et al. The interaction between hepatitis B virus and hepatitis C virus in acute and chronic liver disease. J Hepatol 1995;22:38-41.
11. Allen K, Gurrin L, Constantine C, Osborne N, Delatycki M, Nicoll A, et al. Iron-overload-related disease in HFE hereditary hemochromatosis. N Engl J Med 2008;358:221-30.
12. Altekruse S, McGlynn K, Reichman M. Hepatocellular carcinoma incidence, mortality, and survival trends in the United States from 1975 to 2005. J Clin Oncol 2009;27:1485-91.
13. Alvarez F, Berg P, Bianchi F, Bianchi L, Burroughs A, Cancado E, et al. International Autoimmune Hepatitis Group Report: review of criteria for diagnosis of autoimmune hepatitis. J Hepatol 1999;31:929-38.
14. Amacher D. Serum transaminase elevations as indicators of hepatic injury following the administration of drugs. Regul Toxicol Pharmacol 1998;27:119-30.
15. Anciaux M, Pelletier G, Attali P, Meduri B, Liguory C, Etienne J. Prospective study of clinical and biochemical features of symptomatic choledocholithiasis. Dig Dis Sci 1986;31:449-53.
16. Angulo P, Hui J, Marchesini G, Bugianesi E, George J, Farrell G, et al. The NAFLD fibrosis score: a noninvasive system that identifies liver fibrosis in patients with NAFLD. Hepatology 2007;45:846-54.
17. Angulo P, Lindor K. Primary sclerosing cholangitis. Hepatology 1999;30:325-32.
18. Anonymous. Centers for Disease Control and Prevention (CDC). Prevention of hepatitis A through active or passive immunization: recommendations of the Advisory Committee on Immunization Practices (ACIP). MMWR Morb Mortal Wkly Rep 2006;55:RR-7.
19. Anonymous. Centers for Disease Control and Prevention (CDC). Update: prevention of hepatitis A after exposure to hepatitis A virus and in international travel. Updated recommendations of the Advisory Committee on Immunization Practices (ACIP). MMWR Morb Mortal Wkly Rep 2007;56:1080-4.
20. Anonymous. Centers for Disease Control and Prevention (CDC). Recommendations for identification and public health management of persons with chronic hepatitis B virus infection. MMWR Morb Mortal Wkly Rep 2008;57:RR08.
21. Anonymous. Centers for Disease Control and Prevention (CDC). Surveillance for acute viral hepatitis—United States, 2007. Surveillance summaries. MMWR Morb Mortal Wkly Rep 2009;58:SS-3.
22. Anonymous. Guidelines for laboratory testing and results reporting of antibody to hepatitis C virus. MMWR Morb Mortal Wkly Rep 2003;52:RR03.

23. Anonymous. Standardization of definitions and criteria of causality assessment of adverse drug reactions. Drug-induced liver disorders: report of an international consensus meeting. Int J Clin Pharmacol Ther Toxicol 1990;28:317-22.
24. Anttila P, Järvi K, Latvala J, Romppanen J, Punnonen K, Niemelä O. Biomarkers of alcohol consumption in patients classified according to the degree of liver disease severity. Scand J Clin Lab Invest 2005;65: 141-51.
25. Aoyagi Y, Oguro M, Yanagi M, Mita Y, Suda T, Suzuki Y, et al. Clinical significance of simultaneous determinations of alpha-fetoprotein and des-gamma-carboxy prothrombin in monitoring recurrence in patients with hepatocellular carcinoma. Cancer 1996;77:1781-6.
25A. Arulraj R, Neuberger J. Liver transplantation: filling the gap between supply and demand. Clin Med 2011;11:194-8.
26. Arroyo V, Fernandez J, Ginès P. Pathogenesis and treatment of hepatorenal syndrome. Semin Liver Dis 2008;28:81-95.
27. Baggio-Zappia G, Hernandes Granato C. HIV-GB virus C co-infection: an overview. Clin Chem Lab Med 2009;47:12-9.
28. Banks J, Foulis A, Ledingham I, Macsween R. Liver function in septic shock. J Clin Pathol 1982;35:1249-52.
29. Barrera J, Bruguera M, Ercilla M, Gil C, Celis R, Gil M, et al. Persistent hepatitis C viremia after acute self-limiting posttransfusion hepatitis C. Hepatology 1995;21:639-44.
30. Basso D, Fabris C, Plebani M, Del FG, Muraca M, Vilei M, et al. Alterations in bilirubin metabolism during extra- and intrahepatic cholestasis. Clin Investig 1992;70:49-54.
31. Basuni A, Butterworth L, Cooksley G, Locarnini S, Carman W. Prevalence of HBsAg mutants and impact of hepatitis B infant immunisation in four Pacific Island countries. Vaccine 2004;22:2791-9.
32. Belay E, Bresee J, Holman R, Khan A, Shahriari A, Schonberger L. Reye's syndrome in the United States from 1981 through 1997. N Engl J Med 1999;340:1377-82.
33. Bellest L, Eschwege V, Poupon R, Chazouilleres O, Robert A. A modified international normalized ratio as an effective way of prothrombin time standardization in hepatology. Hepatology 2007;46:528-34.
34. Benyon R, Arthur M. Extracellular matrix degradation and the role of hepatic stellate cells. Semin Liver Dis 2001;21:373-84.
35. Berman D, Leventhal R, Gavaler J, Cadoff E, Van TD. Clinical differentiation of fulminant Wilsonian hepatitis from other causes of hepatic failure. Gastroenterology 1991;100:1129-34.
36. Berman M, Rabin L, O'Donnell J, Gratwohl A, Graw R, Deisseroth A, et al. The liver in long-term survivors of marrow transplant—chronic graft-versus-host disease. J Clin Gastroenterol 1980;2:53-63.
37. Bernal W, Hall C, Karvellas C, Auzinger G, Sizer E, Wendon J. Arterial ammonia and clinical risk factors for encephalopathy and intracranial hypertension in acute liver failure. Hepatology 2007;46: 1679-81.
38. Blumberg B, Alter H. A "new" antigen in leukemia sera. JAMA 1965; 191:101-6.
39. Boberg K. Prevalence and epidemiology of autoimmune hepatitis. Clin Liver Dis 2002;6:347-59.
40. Bode C, Bode J. Activation of the innate immune system and alcoholic liver disease: effects of ethanol per se or enhanced intestinal translocation of bacterial toxins induced by ethanol? Alcohol Clin Exp Res 2005;29:166S-71S.
41. Bornhorst J, Procter M, Meadows C, Ashwood E, Mao R. Evaluation of an integrative diagnostic algorithm for the identification of people at risk for alpha1-antitrypsin deficiency. Am J Clin Pathol 2007;128: 482-90.
42. Borsch G, Baier J, Glocke M, Nathusius W, Gerhardt W. Graphical analysis of laboratory data in the differential diagnosis of cholestasis: a computer-assisted prospective study. J Clin Chem Clin Biochem 1988; 26:509-19.
43. Botta F, Giannini E, Romagnoli P, Fasoli A, Malfatti F, Chiarbonello B, et al. MELD scoring system is useful for predicting prognosis in patients with liver cirrhosis and is correlated with residual liver function: a European study. Gut 2003;52:134-9.
44. Boudville N, Salama M, Jeffrey G, Ferrari P. The inaccuracy of cystatin C and creatinine-based equations in predicting GFR in orthotopic liver transplant recipients. Nephrol Dial Transplant 2009;24:2926-30.
45. Bouvier-Alias M, Patel K, Dahari H, Beaucourt S, Larderie P, Blatt L, et al. Clinical utility of total HCV core antigen quantification: a new indirect marker of HCV replication. Hepatology 2002;36:211-8.
46. Boyer T, Haskal Z. The role of transjugular intrahepatic portosystemic shunt in the management of portal hypertension. Hepatology 2005;41: 386-400.
47. Bralet M, Regimbeau J, Pineau P, Dubois S, Loas G, Degos F, et al. Hepatocellular carcinoma occurring in nonfibrotic liver: epidemiologic and histopathologic analysis of 80 French cases. Hepatology 2000;32:200-4.
48. Brechot C, Thiers V, Kremsdorf D, Nalpas B, Pol S, Paterlini-Brechot P. Persistent hepatitis B virus infection in subjects without hepatitis B surface antigen: clinically significant or purely "occult"? Hepatology 2001;34:194-206.
49. Brocklehurst D. The alkaline phosphatase-lipoprotein X complex. Clin Chem 1981;27:1317-8.
50. Brown R, Kumar K, Russo M, Kinkhabwala M, Rudow D, Harren P, et al. Model for end-stage liver disease and Child-Turcotte-Pugh score as predictors of pretransplantation disease severity, posttransplantation outcome, and resource utilization in United Network for Organ Sharing status 2A patients. Liver Transpl 2002;8: 278-84.
51. Bruix J, Sherman M: Management of hepatocellular carcinoma. Hepatology 2005;42:1208-36.
52. Brunetto M, Moriconi F, Bonino F, Lau G, Farci P, Yurdaydin C, et al. Hepatitis B virus surface antigen levels: a guide to sustained response to peginterferon alfa-2a in HBeAg-negative chronic hepatitis B. Hepatology 2009;49:1141-50.
53. Bukh J, Miller R, Purcell R. Genetic heterogeneity of hepatitis C virus: quasispecies and genotypes. Semin Liver Dis 1995;15:41-63.
54. Bull P, Thomas G, Rommens J, Forbes J, Cox D. The Wilson disease gene is a putative copper transporting P-type ATPase similar to the Menkes gene. Nat Genet 1993;5:327-37.
55. Burton B. Urea cycle disorders. Clin Liver Dis 2000;4:815-30.
56. Bush M, Kleinman S, Nemo G. Current and emerging infectious risks of blood transfusions. JAMA 2003;289:959-62.
57. Byron D, Minuk G. Clinical hepatology: profile of an urban, hospital-based practice. Hepatology 1996;24:813-5.
58. Cacciola I, Pollicino T, Squadrito G, Cerenzia G, Orlando M, Raimondo G. Occult hepatitis B virus infection in patients with chronic hepatitis C liver disease. N Engl J Med 1999;341:22-6.
59. Carlson J, Eriksson S. Chronic "cryptogenic" liver disease and malignant hepatoma in intermediate $alpha_1$-antitrypsin deficiency identified by a Pi Z-specific monoclonal antibody. Scand J Gastroenterol 1985;20:835-42.
60. Carr B, Kanke F, Wise M, Satomura S. Clinical evaluation of lens culinaris agglutinin-reactive alpha-fetoprotein and des-gamma-carboxy prothrombin in histologically proven hepatocellular carcinoma in the United States. Dig Dis Sci 2007;52:776-82.
60A. Cash WJ, McConville P, McDermott E, McCormick PA, Callender ME, McDougall NI. Current concepts in the assessment and treatment of hepatic encephalopathy. QJM 2010;103:9-16.
61. Cassidy W, Reynolds T. Serum lactic dehydrogenase in the differential diagnosis of acute hepatocellular injury. J Clin Gastroenterol 1994;19: 118-21.
62. Castera L, Hezode C, Roudot-Thoraval F, Bastie A, Zafrani E, Pawlotsky J, et al. Worsening of steatosis is an independent factor of fibrosis progression in untreated patients with chronic hepatitis C and paired liver biopsies. Gut 2003;52:288-92.
63. Caubet M, Laplante A, Caille J, Brazier J. [13C]aminopyrine and [13C]caffeine breath test: influence of gender, cigarette smoking and oral contraceptives intake. Isotopes Environ Health Stud 2002;38:71-7.
64. Cauza E, Maier-Dobersberger T, Polli C, Kaserer K, Kramer L, Ferenci P. Screening for Wilson's disease in patients with liver diseases by serum ceruloplasmin. J Hepatol 1997;27:358-62.

65. Chalasani N, Fontana R, Bonkovsky H, Watkins P, Davern T, Serrano J, et al. Causes, clinical features, and outcomes from a prospective study of drug-induced liver injury in the United States. Gastroenterology 2008;135:1924-34.
66. Chang C, Ko Y, Liu H. Serum alanine aminotransferase levels in relation to hepatitis B and C virus infections among drug abusers in an area hyperendemic for hepatitis B. Dig Dis Sci 2000;45: 1949-52.
67. Chang M, Chen C, Lai M, Hsu H, Wu T, Kong M, et al. Universal hepatitis B vaccination in Taiwan and the incidence of hepatocellular carcinoma in children. Taiwan Childhood Hepatoma Study Group. N Engl J Med 1997;336:1855-9.
68. Chang M, Shau W, Chen C, Wu T, Kong M, Liang D, et al. Hepatitis B vaccination and hepatocellular carcinoma rates in boys and girls. JAMA 2000;284:3040-2.
69. Chang Y, Ryu S, Sung E, Jang Y. Higher concentrations of alanine aminotransferase within the reference interval predict nonalcoholic fatty liver disease. Clin Chem 2007;53:686-92.
70. Chen C, Yang H, Iloeje U. Hepatitis B virus DNA levels and outcomes in chronic hepatitis B. Hepatology 2009;49:S72-S84.
71. Chen C, Yang H, Su J, Jen C, You S, Lu S, et al. Risk of hepatocellular carcinoma across a biological gradient of serum hepatitis B virus DNA level. JAMA 2006;295:65-73.
72. Cheung K, Tilleman K, Deforce D, Colle I, Van Vlierberghe H. Proteomics in liver fibrosis is more than meets the eye. Eur J Gastroenterol Hepatol 2008;20:450-64.
73. Chevaliez S, Bouvier-Alias M, Brillet R, Pawlotsky J. Overestimation and underestimation of hepatitis C virus RNA levels in a widely used real-time polymerase chain reaction-based method. Hepatology 2007;46:22-31.
74. Chevaliez S, Bouvier-Alias M, Castéra L, Pawlotsky J. The Cobas AmpliPrep-Cobas TaqMan real-time polymerase chain reaction assay fails to detect hepatitis C virus RNA in highly viremic genotype 4 clinical samples. Hepatology 2009;49:1397-8.
75. Chisari F, Ferrari C. Hepatitis B virus immunopathology. Springer Semin Immunopathol 1995;17:261-81.
76. Chitturi S, Farrell G. Herbal hepatotoxicity: an expanding but poorly defined problem. J Gastroenterol Hepatol 2000;15:1093-9.
77. Cholongitas E, Shusang V, Marelli L, Nair D, Thomas M, Patch D, et al. Review article: renal function assessment in cirrhosis—difficulties and alternative measurements. Aliment Pharmacol Ther 2007;26:969-78.
78. Choo Q-L, Kuo G, Weiner A, Bradley D, Houghton M. Isolation of a c-DNA clone derived from a blood-borne non-A, non-B viral hepatitis genome. Science 1989;244:359-62.
79. Chrostek L, Cylwik B, Korcz W, Krawiec A, Koput A, Supronowicz Z, et al. Serum free sialic acid as a marker of alcohol abuse. Alcohol Clin Exp Res 2007;31:996-1001.
80. Chu C, Lok A. Clinical significance of hepatitis B virus genotypes. Hepatology 2002;35:1274-6.
81. Chu C, Yeh C, Sheen I, Liaw Y. Acute hepatitis C virus (HCV) infection in chronic carriers of hepatitis B virus (HBV): the impact of underlying active HBV replication on persistence of HCV infection and antibody responses to HCV. Gut 2002;51:95-9.
82. Clemente-Casares P, Pina S, Buti M, Jardi R, Martin M, Bofill-Mas S, et al. Hepatitis E virus epidemiology in industrialized countries. Emerg Infect Dis 2003;9:448-54.
83. Clemmesen J, Larsen F, Kondrup J, Hansen B, Ott P. Cerebral herniation in patients with acute liver failure is correlated with arterial ammonia concentration. Hepatology 1999;29:648-53.
84. Cohen J, Kaplan M. The SGOT/SGPT ratio—an indicator of alcoholic liver disease. Dig Dis Sci 1979;24:835-8.
84A. Cohen JC, Horton JD, Hobbs HH. Human fatty liver disease: old questions and new insights. Science 2011;332:1519-23.
85. Coleman P: Detecting hepatitis B surface antigen mutants. Emerg Infect Dis 2006;12:198-203.
86. Córdoba J, Mínguez B. Hepatic encephalopathy. Semin Liver Dis 2008;28:70-80.
87. Corrao G, Bagnardi V, Zambon A, Torchio P. Meta-analysis of alcohol intake in relation to risk of liver cirrhosis. Alcohol Alcohol 1998;33: 381-92.
88. Crapper R, Bhathal P, Mackay I, Frazer I. "Acute" autoimmune hepatitis. Digestion 1986;34:216-25.
89. Crespo J, Lozano J, Carte B, de las Heras B, de la Cruz F, Pons-Romero F. Viral replication in patients with concomitant hepatitis B and C virus infections. Eur J Clin Microbiol Infect Dis 1997;16:445-51.
90. Crespo J, Lozano J, de la Cruz F, Rodrigo L, Rodriguez M, San Miguel G, et al. Prevalence and significance of hepatitis C viremia in chronic active hepatitis B. Am J Gastroenterol 1994;89:1147-51.
91. Crowe J, Christensen E, Butler J, Wheeler P, Doniach D, Keenan J, et al. Primary biliary cirrhosis: the prevalence of hypothyroidism and its relationship to thyroid autoantibodies and sicca syndrome. Gastroenterology 1980;78:1437-41.
92. Czaja A, Davis G, Ludwig J, Taswell H. Complete resolution of inflammatory activity following corticosteroid treatment of HBsAg-negative chronic active hepatitis. Hepatology 1984;4:622-7.
93. Czaja A, Freese D. Diagnosis and treatment of autoimmune hepatitis. Hepatology 2002;36:479-97.
94. Czaja A, Shiels M, Taswell H, Wood J, Ludwig J, Chase R. Frequency and significance of immunoglobulin M antibody to hepatitis B core antigen in corticosteroid-treated severe chronic active hepatitis B. Mayo Clin Proc 1988;63:119-25.
95. Dalton H, Bendall R, Ijaz S, Banks M. Hepatitis E: an emerging infection in developed countries. Lancet Infect Dis 2008;8:698-709.
96. Dalton H, Stableforth W, Thurairajah P, Hazeldine S, Remnarace R, Usama W, et al. Autochthonous hepatitis E in Southwest England: natural history, complications and seasonal variation, and hepatitis E virus IgG seroprevalence in blood donors, the elderly and patients with chronic liver disease. Eur J Gastroenterol Hepatol 2008;20: 784-90.
97. Danan G: Causality assessment of drug-induced liver injury. Hepatology Working Group. J Hepatol 1988;7:132-6.
98. Daniel S, Ben-Menachem T, Vasudevan G, Ma C, Blumenkehl M. Prospective evaluation of unexplained chronic liver transaminase abnormalities in asymptomatic and symptomatic patients. Am J Gastroenterol 1999;94:3010-4.
99. Dara L, Hewett J, Lim J. Hydroxycut hepatotoxicity: a case series and review of liver toxicity from herbal weight loss supplements. World J Gastroenterol 2008;14:6999-7004.
100. Das S, Dhanya L, Vasudevan D. Biomarkers of alcoholism: an updated review. Scand J Clin Lab Invest 2008;68:81-92.
101. Davern TN, James L, Hinson J, Polson J, Larson A, Fontana R, et al. Measurement of serum acetaminophen-protein adducts in patients with acute liver failure. Gastroenterology 2006;130:687-94.
102. Davis G, Albright JE, Cook SF, Rosenbert DM: Projecting future complications of chronic hepatitis C in the United States. Liver Transpl 2003;9:331-8.
103. Davis G, Lau J, Urdea M, Neuwald P, Wilber J, Lindsay K, et al. Quantitative detection of hepatitis C virus RNA with a solid-phase signal amplification method: definition of optimal conditions for specimen collection and clinical application in interferon-treated patients. Hepatology 1994;19:1337-41.
103A. Day CP. Non-alcoholic fatty liver disease: a massive problem. Clin Med 2011;11:176-8.
104. de Alwis N, Day C. Genetics of alcoholic liver disease and nonalcoholic fatty liver disease. Semin Liver Dis 2007;27:44-54.
105. de Franchis R, Meucci G, Vecchi M, Tatarella M, Colombo M, Del Ninno E, et al. The natural history of asymptomatic hepatitis B surface antigen carriers. Ann Intern Med 1993;118:191-4.
106. Degertekin B, Lok A. Indications for therapy in hepatitis B. Hepatology 2009;49:S129-S37.
107. Delage G, Remy-Prince S, Montplaisir S. Combined active-passive immunization against the hepatitis B virus: five-year follow-up of children born to hepatitis B surface antigen-positive mothers. Pediatr Infect Dis J 1993;12:126-30.

108. Dembek Z, Hadler J, Castrodale L, Funk B, Fiore A, Openo K, et al. Positive test results for acute hepatitis A virus infection among persons with no recent history of acute hepatitis—United States, 2002-2004. MMWR Morb Mortal Wkly Rep 2005;54:453-6.
109. Demetris A, Adams D, Bellamy C, Blakolmer K, Clouston A, Dhillon A, et al. Update of the International Banff Schema for Liver Allograft Rejection: working recommendations for the histopathologic staging and reporting of chronic rejection. An international panel. Hepatology 2000;31:792-9.
110. Demirtas S, Bozbas A, Akbay A, Yavuz Y, Karaca L. Diagnostic value of serum cystatin C for evaluation of hepatorenal syndrome. Clin Chim Acta 2001;311:81-9.
111. Dickerman R, Pertusi R, Zachariah N, Dufour D, McConathy W. Anabolic steroid-induced hepatotoxicity: is it overstated? Clin J Sport Med 1999;9:34-9.
112. Dienstag J. Hepatitis B virus infection. N Engl J Med 2008;359: 1486-500.
113. Dienstag J, Goldin R, Heathcote E, Hann H, Woessner M, Stephenson S, et al. Histological outcome during long-term lamivudine therapy. Gastroenterology 2003;124:105-17.
114. DiMartini A, Day N, Lane T, Beisler A, Dew M, Anton R. Carbohydrate deficient transferrin in abstaining patients with end-stage liver disease. Alcohol Clin Exp Res 2001;25:1729-33.
115. Dossing M, Andreasen P. Drug-induced liver disease in Denmark: an analysis of 572 cases of hepatotoxicity reported to the Danish Board of Adverse Reactions to Drugs. Scand J Gastroenterol 1982;17:205-11.
116. Dufour D. Alanine aminotransferase variation in chronic hepatitis C infection: an analysis of 357 cases. Clin Chem 2001;47:A26-7.
117. Dufour D. Hepatitis B surface antigen (HBsAg) assays: are they good enough for their current uses? Clin Chem 2006;52:1457-9.
118. Dufour D, Lott J, Nolte F, Gretch D, Koff R, Seeff L. Diagnosis and monitoring of hepatic injury. I. Performance characteristics of laboratory tests. Clin Chem 2000;46:2027-49.
119. Dufour D, Lott J, Nolte F, Gretch D, Koff R, Seeff L. Diagnosis and monitoring of hepatic injury. II. Recommendations for use of laboratory tests in screening, diagnosis, and monitoring. Clin Chem 2000;46:2050-68.
120. Dufour D, Talastas M, Fernandez M, Harris B, Strader D, Seeff L. Low positive anti-hepatitis C virus enzyme immunoassay results: an important predictor of low likelihood of hepatitis C infection. Clin Chem 2003;49:479-86.
121. Dufour D, Talastas M, Fernandez M, Harris B. Chemiluminescence assay improves specificity of hepatitis C antibody detection. Clin Chem 2003;49:940-4.
122. Dufour D, Teot L. Laboratory identification of ischemic hepatitis (shock liver). Clin Chem 1988;34:1287.
123. Durazo F, Blatt L, Corey W, Lin J, Han S, Saab S, et al. Des-gamma-carboxyprothrombin, alpha-fetoprotein and AFP-L3 in patients with chronic hepatitis, cirrhosis and hepatocellular carcinoma. J Gastroenterol Hepatol 2008;23:1541-8.
124. Dvorchik I, Subotin M, Demetris A, Fung J, Starzl T, Wieand S, et al. Effect of liver transplantation on inflammatory bowel disease in patients with primary sclerosing cholangitis. Hepatology 2002;35: 380-4.
125. Echevarria J, Avellon A. Improved detection of natural hepatitis B virus surface antigen (HBsAg) mutants by a new version of the VITROS HBsAg assay. J Med Virol 2008;80:598-602.
126. Elgouhari H. What is the utility of measuring the serum ammonia level in patients with altered mental status? Cleveland Clin J Med 2009;76:252-4.
127. El-Serag H, Mason A. Rising incidence of hepatocellular carcinoma in the United States. N Engl J Med 1999;340:745-50.
128. England K, Thorne C, Pembrey L, Tovo P, Newell M. Age- and sex-related reference ranges of alanine aminotransferase levels in children: European paediatric HCV network. J Pediatr Gastroenterol Nutr 2009;49:71-7.
129. Eriksson S. Alpha 1-antitrypsin deficiency and the liver. Acta Paediatr 1994;83:444-7.
130. Everson G, Shiffman M, Morgan T, Hoefs J, Sterling R, Wagner D, et al. The spectrum of hepatic functional impairment in compensated chronic hepatitis C: results from the Hepatitis C Anti-viral Long-term Treatment against Cirrhosis Trial. Aliment Pharmacol Ther 2008;27: 798-809.
131. Fairbanks K, Tavill A. Liver disease in alpha 1-antitrypsin deficiency: a review. Am J Gastroenterol 2008;103:2136-41.
132. Fanning L, Kenny-Walsh E, Levis J, Choudhury K, Cannon B, Sheehan M, et al. Natural fluctuations of hepatitis C viral load in a homogeneous patient population: a prospective study. Hepatology 2000;31:225-9.
133. Farci P, Purcell R. Clinical significance of hepatitis C virus genotypes and quasispecies. Semin Liver Dis 2000;20:103-26.
134. Farci P, Shimoda A, Coiana A, Diaz G, Peddis G, Melpolder J, et al. The outcome of acute hepatitis C predicted by the evolution of the viral quasispecies. Science 2000;288:339-44.
135. Fattovich G. Progression of hepatitis B and C to hepatocellular carcinoma in Western countries. Hepatogastroenterology 1998; 45(Suppl 3):1206-13.
136. Fattovich G, Giustina G, Degos F, Tremolada F, Diodati G, Almasio P, et al. Morbidity and mortality in compensated cirrhosis type C: a restrospective follow-up study of 384 patients. Gastroenterology 1997;112:463-72.
137. Fattovich G, Bortolotti F, Donato F. Natural history of chronic hepatitis B: special emphasis on disease progression and prognostic factors. J Hepatol 2008 Feb;48(2):335-52. Epub 2007 Dec 4.
138. Fattovich G, Giustina G, Schalm S, Hadziyannis S, Sanchez-Tapias J, Almasio P, et al. Occurrence of hepatocellular carcinoma and decompensation in western European patients with cirrhosis type B. The EUROHEP Study Group on Hepatitis B Virus and Cirrhosis. Hepatology 1995;21:77-82.
139. Faust T. Recurrent primary biliary cirrhosis, primary sclerosing cholangitis, and autoimmune hepatitis after transplantation. Liver Transpl 2001;7:S99-108.
140. Feder J, Gnirke A, Thomas W, Tsuchihashi Z, Ruddy D, Basava A, et al. A novel MHC class I-like gene is mutated in patients with hereditary haemochromatosis. Nat Genet 1996;13:399-408.
141. Feitelson M, Zhu M, Duan L, London W. Hepatitis B x antigen and p53 are associated in vitro and in liver tissues from patients with primary hepatocellular carcinoma. Oncogene 1993;8:1109-17.
142. Fisher R, Taylor L, Sherlock S. Alpha-1-antitrypsin deficiency in liver disease: the extent of the problem. Gastroenterology 1976;71:646-51.
143. Fogeda M, de Ory F, Avellón A, Echevarría J. Differential diagnosis of hepatitis E virus, cytomegalovirus and Epstein-Barr virus infection in patients with suspected hepatitis E. J Clin Virol 2009;45:259-61.
144. Foley K, Silveira M, Hornseth J, Lindor K, McConnell J. A patient with primary biliary cirrhosis and elevated LDL cholesterol. Clin Chem 2009;55:187-92.
145. Fontana R. Acute liver failure due to drugs. Semin Liver Dis 2008;28: 175-87.
146. Fontana R, Lok A. Noninvasive monitoring of patients with chronic hepatitis C. Hepatology 2002;36:S57-64.
147. Fontana R, Watkins P, Bonkovsky H, Chalasani N, Davern T, Serrano J, et al. Drug-Induced Liver Injury Network (DILIN) prospective study: rationale, design and conduct. Drug Saf 2009;32:55-68.
148. Forman L, Lucey M. Predicting the prognosis of chronic liver disease: an evolution from child to MELD. Mayo End-stage Liver Disease. Hepatology 2001;33:473-5.
149. Fortson W, Tedesco F, Starnes E, Shaw C. Marked elevation of serum transaminase activity associated with extrahepatic biliary tract disease. J Clin Gastroenterol 1985;7:502-5.
149A. Fox MA, Fox JA, Davies MH Budd-Chiari syndrome–a review of the diagnosis and management. Acute Med 2011;10:5-9.
150. Francis J, Armstrong D. Acquired dysfibrinogenaemia in liver disease. J Clin Pathol 1982;35:667-72.
151. Freeman A, Dore G, Law M, Thorpe M, Von OJ, Lloyd A, et al. Estimating progression to cirrhosis in chronic hepatitis C virus infection. Hepatology 2001;34:809-16.

152. Friedman S. Mechanisms of hepatic fibrogenesis. Gastroenterology 2008;134:1655-69.
153. Friedman S, Bansal M. Reversal of hepatic fibrosis—fact or fantasy? Hepatology 2006;43:S82-8.
154. Gaffney D, Fell G, O'Reilly D. ACP Best Practice No 163. Wilson's disease: acute and presymptomatic laboratory diagnosis and monitoring. J Clin Pathol 2000;53:807-12.
155. Gao L, Ramzan I, Baker A. Potential use of pharmacological markers to quantitatively assess liver function during liver transplantation surgery. Anaesth Intensive Care 2000;28:375-85.
156. Garcia-Tsao G, Sanyal A, Grace N, Carey W. Prevention and management of gastroesophageal varices and variceal hemorrhage in cirrhosis. Hepatology 2007;46:922-38.
157. Gentile I, Viola C, Borgia F, Castaldo G, Borgia G. Telaprevir: a promising protease inhibitor for the treatment of hepatitis C virus infection. Curr Med Chem 2009;16:1115-21.
158. Gerlich W. Diagnostic problems caused by HBsAg mutants—a consensus report of an expert meeting. Intervirology 2004;47:310-3.
159. Gershwin M, Mackay I. Primary biliary cirrhosis: paradigm or paradox for autoimmunity. Gastroenterology 1991;100:822-33.
160. Ghany M, Kleiner D, Alter H, Doo E, Khokar F, Promrat K, et al. Progression of fibrosis in chronic hepatitis C. Gastroenterology 2003;124:97-104.
161. Ghany M, Strader D, Thomas D, Seeff L. Diagnosis, management, and treatment of hepatitis C: an update. Hepatology 2009;49:1335-74.
162. Giannini E, Fasoli A, Borro P, Botta F, Malfatti F, Fumagalli A, et al. 13C-galactose breath test and 13C-aminopyrine breath test for the study of liver function in chronic liver disease. Clin Gastroenterol Hepatol 2005;3:279-85.
163. Giannini E, Risso D, Botta F, Chiarbonello B, Fasoli A, Malfatti F, et al. Validity and clinical utility of the aspartate aminotransferase-alanine aminotransferase ratio in assessing disease severity and prognosis in patients with hepatitis C virus-related chronic liver disease. Arch Intern Med 2003;163:218-24.
164. Giannini E, Savarino V. Thrombocytopenia in liver disease. Curr Opin Hematol 2008;15:473-80.
165. Gibbs K, Walshe J. A study of the caeruloplasmin concentrations found in 75 patients with Wilson's disease, their kinships and various control groups. Q J Med 1979;48:447-63.
166. Goessling W, Massaro J, Vasan R, D'Agostino RS, Ellison R, Fox C. Aminotransferase levels and 20-year risk of metabolic syndrome, diabetes, and cardiovascular disease. Gastroenterology 2008;135:1935-44.
167. Goldberg S, Mendenhall C, Anderson S, Garcia-Pont P, Kiernan T, Seeff L, et al. VA Cooperative Study on Alcoholic Hepatitis. IV. The significance of clinically mild alcoholic hepatitis—describing the population with minimal hyperbilirubinemia. Am J Gastroenterol 1986;81:1029-34.
168. Goldstein N, Blue D, Hankin R, Hunter S, Bayati N, Silverman A, et al. Serum alpha-fetoprotein levels in patients with chronic hepatitis C: relationships with serum alanine aminotransferase values, histologic activity index, and hepatocyte MIB-1 scores. Am J Clin Pathol 1999;111:811-6.
169. Goodman Z. Drug hepatotoxicity. Clin Liver Dis 2002;6:381-97.
170. Gordon F. Primary sclerosing cholangitis. Surg Clin North Am 2008;88:1385-407.
171. Gosalakkal J, Kamoji V. Reye syndrome and Reye-like syndrome. Pediatr Neurol 2008;39:198-200.
172. Gow P, Smallwood R, Angus P, Smith A, Wall A, Sewell R. Diagnosis of Wilson's disease: an experience over three decades. Gut 2000;46:415-9.
173. Grant B, Dufour M, Harford T. Epidemiology of alcoholic liver disease. Semin Liver Dis 1988;8:12-25.
174. Grant P, Kitchen A, Barbara J, Hewitt P, Sims C, Garson J, et al. Effects of handling and storage of blood on the stability of hepatitis C virus RNA: implications for NAT testing in transfusion practice. Vox Sang 2000;78:137-42.
175. Graziadei I, Joseph J, Wiesner R, Therneau T, Batts K, Porayko M. Increased risk of chronic liver failure in adults with heterozygous alpha1-antitrypsin deficiency. Hepatology 1998;28:1058-63.
176. Gretch D. Diagnostic tests for hepatitis C. Hepatology 1997;26:43S-7S.
177. Gupta S, Slaughter S, Akriviadis E, Valenzuela R, Deodhar S. Serial measurement of serum C-reactive protein facilitates evaluation in alcoholic hepatitis. Hepatogastroenterology 1995;42:516-21.
178. Gurrin L, Osborne N, Constantine C, McLaren C, English D, Gertig D, et al. The natural history of serum iron indices for HFE C282Y homozygosity associated with hereditary hemochromatosis. Gastroenterology 2008;135:1945-52.
179. Haagsma E, van den Berg A, Porte R, Benne C, Vennema H, Reimerink J, et al. Chronic hepatitis E virus infection in liver transplant recipients. Liver Transpl 2008;14:547-53.
180. Hadziyannis E, Papatheodoridis G. Hepatitis B e antigen-negative chronic hepatitis B: natural history and treatment. Semin Liver Dis 2006;26:130-41.
181. Halfon P, Bourliere M, Halimi G, Khiri H, Bertezene P, Portal I, et al. Assessment of spontaneous fluctuations of viral load in untreated patients with chronic hepatitis C by two standardized quantitation methods: branched DNA and Amplicor Monitor. J Clin Microbiol 1998;36:2073-5.
182. Halpin T, Holtzhauer F, Campbell R, Hall L, Correa-Villasenor A, Lanese R, et al. Reye's syndrome and medication use. JAMA 1982;248:687-91.
183. Hannuksela M, Liisanantti M, Nissinen A, Savolainen M. Biochemical markers of alcoholism. Clin Chem Lab Med 2007;45:953-61.
184. Harrison P, O'Grady J, Keays R, Alexander G, Williams R. Serial prothrombin time as prognostic indicator in paracetamol induced fulminant hepatic failure. BMJ 1990;301:964-8.
185. Hartleb M, Nowak A, Kajor M, Wlaszczuk P. Autoimmune LKM1 hepatitis presenting in the form of recurrent acute episodes. Am J Gastroenterol 2002;97:1267-8.
186. Häussinger D, Schliess F. Pathogenetic mechanisms of hepatic encephalopathy. Gut 2008;57:1156-65.
187. Hayashi K, Kumada T, Nakano S, Takeda I, Kiriyama S, Sone Y, et al. Incidence of hepatocellular carcinoma in chronic hepatitis C after interferon therapy. Hepatogastroenterology 2002;49:508-12.
188. Hayes T. Dysfibrinogenemia and thrombosis. Arch Pathol Lab Med 2002;126:1387-90.
189. Heathcote E. Management of primary biliary cirrhosis. Hepatology 2000;31:1005-13.
190. Hennes E, Zeniya M, Czaja A, Parés A, Dalekos G, Krawitt E, et al. Simplified criteria for the diagnosis of autoimmune hepatitis. Hepatology 2008;48:169-76.
191. Heron M, Hoyert D, Murphy S, Xu J, Kochanek K, Tejada-Vera B. Deaths: final data for 2006. National Vital Statistics Reports 2009;57:1-136.
192. Heubi J, Setchell K, Bove K. Inborn errors of bile acid metabolism. Semin Liver Dis 2007;27:282-94.
193. Hickman P, Potter J. Mortality associated with ischaemic hepatitis. Aust N Z J Med 1990;20:32-4.
194. Hijikata M, Takahashi K, Mishiro S. Complete circular DNA genome of a TT virus variant (isolate name SANBAN) and 44 partial ORF2 sequences implicating a great degree of diversity beyond genotypes. Virology 1999;260:17-22.
195. Hock B, Schwarz M, Domke I, Grunert V, Wuertemberger M, Schiemann U, et al. Validity of carbohydrate-deficient transferrin (%CDT), gamma-glutamyltransferase (gamma-GT) and mean corpuscular erythrocyte volume (MCV) as biomarkers for chronic alcohol abuse: a study in patients with alcohol dependence and liver disorders of non-alcoholic and alcoholic origin. Addiction 2005;100:1477-86.
196. Hodges J, Millward-Sadler G, Barbatis C, Wright R. Heterozygous MZ alpha 1-antitrypsin deficiency in adults with chronic active hepatitis and cryptogenic cirrhosis. N Engl J Med 1981;304:557-60.

197. Horn K, Wax P, Scheider S, Martin T, Nine J, Moraca M, et al. Biomarkers of liver regeneration allow early prediction of hepatic recovery after acute necrosis. Am J Clin Pathol 1999;112:351-7.
198. Houghton M, Weiner A, Han J, Kuo G, Choo Q. Molecular biology of the hepatitis C viruses: implications for diagnosis, development, and control of viral disease. Hepatology 1991;14:381-8.
199. Hoy J, Boberg K, Karlsen T. Autoantibodies in primary sclerosing cholangitis. World J Gastroenterol 2008;14:3781-91.
200. Hsu H, Chang M, Ni Y, Chen H. Survey of hepatitis B surface variant infection in children 15 years after a nationwide vaccination programme in Taiwan. Gut 2004;53:1499-503.
201. Hung K, Lee K, Yen C, Wu K, Tsai T, Chen W. Revised cutoff values of serum aminotransferase in detecting viral hepatitis among CAPD patients: experience from Taiwan, an endemic area for hepatitis B. Nephrol Dial Transplant 1997;12:180-3.
202. Hunt C, McGill J, Allen M, Condreay L. Clinical relevance of hepatitis B virus mutations. Hepatology 2000;31:1037-44.
203. Hurwitz E, Barrett M, Bregman D, Gunn W, Schonberger L, Fairweather W, et al. Public Health Service study on Reye's syndrome and medications: report of the pilot phase. N Engl J Med 1985;313: 849-57.
204. Hussain K, El-Serag H. Epidemiology, screening, diagnosis and treatment of hepatocellular carcinoma. Minerva Gastroenterol Dietol 2009;55:123-38.
205. Hussain M, Mieli-Vergani G, Mowat A. Alpha 1-antitrypsin deficiency and liver disease: clinical presentation, diagnosis and treatment. J Inherit Metab Dis 1991;14:497-511.
206. Hutchison D. Alpha 1-antitrypsin deficiency in Europe: geographical distribution of Pi types S and Z. Respir Med 1998;92:367-77.
207. Ihara H, Nakamura H, Aoki Y, Aoki T, Yoshida M. Effects of serum-isolated vs synthetic bilirubin-albumin complexes on dye-binding methods for estimating serum albumin. Clin Chem 1991;37:1269-72.
208. Ikeda K, Saitoh S, Suzuki Y, Kobayashi M, Tsubota A, Koida I, et al. Disease progression and hepatocellular carcinogenesis in patients with chronic viral hepatitis: a prospective observation of 2215 patients. J Hepatol 1998;28:930-8.
209. Iloeje U, Yang H, Su J, Jen C, You S, Chen C. Predicting cirrhosis risk based on the level of circulating hepatitis B viral load. Gastroenterology 2006;130:678-86.
210. Imbert-Bismut F, Ratziu V, Pieroni L, Charlotte F, Benhamou Y, Poynard T. Biochemical markers of liver fibrosis in patients with hepatitis C virus infection: a prospective study. Lancet 2001;357:1069-75.
211. Inglesby T, Rai R, Astemborski J, Gruskin L, Nelson K, Vlahov D, et al. A prospective, community-based evaluation of liver enzymes in individuals with hepatitis C after drug use. Hepatology 1999;29:590-6.
212. Isogai M, Hachisuka K, Yamaguchi A, Nakano S. Etiology and pathogenesis of marked elevation of serum transaminase in patients with acute gallstone disease. HPB Surg 1991;4:95-105.
213. Jarvis L, Davidson F, Hanley J, Yap P, Ludlam C, Simmonds P. Infection with hepatitis G virus among recipients of plasma products. Lancet 1996;348:1352-5.
214. Johnson G, Scurletis T, Carroll N. A study of sixteen fatal cases of encephalitis-like disease in North Carolina children. NC Med J 1963;24:464-73.
215. Johnson P, McFarlane I. Meeting report: International Autoimmune Hepatitis Group. Hepatology 1993;18:998-1005.
216. Johnston M, Harrison L, Moffat K, Willan A, Hirsh J. Reliability of the international normalized ratio for monitoring the induction phase of warfarin: comparison with the prothrombin time ratio. J Lab Clin Med 1996;128:214-7.
217. Kabrane-Lazzi Y, Fine J, Elm J, Glass G, Higa H, Diwan A, et al. Evidence for widespread infection of wild rats with hepatitis E virus in the United States. Am J Trop Med Hyg 1999;61:331-5.
218. Kajihara M, Kato S, Okazaki Y, Kawakami Y, Ishii H, Ikeda Y, et al. A role of autoantibody-mediated platelet destruction in thrombocytopenia in patients with cirrhosis. Hepatology 2003;37: 1267-76.
219. Kamar N, Selves J, Mansuy J, Ouezzani L, Péron J, Guitard J, et al. Hepatitis E virus and chronic hepatitis in organ-transplant recipients. N Engl J Med 2008;358:811-7.
220. Kamath P, Wiesner R, Malinchoc M, Kremers W, Therneau T, Kosberg C, et al. A model to predict survival in patients with end-stage liver disease. Hepatology 2001;33:464-70.
221. Kao H, Ashcavai M, Redeker A. The persistence of hepatitis A IgM antibody after acute clinical hepatitis A. Hepatology 1984;4:933-6.
222. Kassianides C, Kew M. The clinical manifestations and natural history of hepatocellular carcinoma. Gastroenterol Clin North Am 1987;16: 553-62.
223. Kaufman B, Gandhi S, Louie E, Rizzi R, Illei P. Herpes simplex virus hepatitis: case report and review. Clin Infect Dis 1997;24:334-8.
224. Kenny-Walsh E. Clinical outcomes after hepatitis C infection from contaminated anti-D immune globulin. N Engl J Med 1999;340: 1228-33.
225. Khan A, Ruwali M, Choudhuri G, Mathur N, Husain Q, Parmar D. Polymorphism in cytochrome P450 2E1 and interaction with other genetic risk factors and susceptibility to alcoholic liver cirrhosis. Mutat Res 2009;664:55-63.
226. Khuroo M, Kamili S. Aetiology, clinical course and outcome of sporadic acute viral hepatitis in pregnancy. J Viral Hepat 2003;20:61-9.
227. Kim H, Oh S, Kin D, Choi E. Abundance of immunologically active alanine aminotransferase in sera of liver cirrhosis and hepatocellular carcinoma patients. Clin Chem 2009;55:1022-5.
228. Kim W, Benson J, Therneau T, Torgerson H, Yawn B, Melton LR. Changing epidemiology of hepatitis B in a U.S. community. Hepatology 2004;39:811-6.
229. Kim W, Brown R, Terrault N, El-Serag H. Burden of liver disease in the United States: summary of a workshop. Hepatology 2002;36: 227-42.
230. Kim W, Flamm S, Di Bisceglie A, Bodenheimer H. Serum activity of alanine aminotransferase (ALT) as an indicator of health and disease. Hepatology 2008;47:1363-70.
231. Koch H, Meerkerk G, Zaat J, Ham M, Scholten R, Assendelft W. Accuracy of carbohydrate-deficient transferrin in the detection of excessive alcohol consumption: a systematic review. Alcohol Alcohol 2004;39:75-85.
232. Koike K, Kobayashi M, Gondo M, Hayashi I, Osuga T, Takada S. Hepatitis B virus DNA is frequently found in liver biopsy samples from hepatitis C virus-infected chronic hepatitis patients. J Med Virol 1998;54:249-55.
233. Korman J, Volenberg I, Balko J, Webster J, Schiodt F, Squires RJ Jr, et al: Screening for Wilson disease in acute liver failure: a comparison of currently available diagnostic tests. Hepatology 2008;48:1167-74.
234. Koulaouzidis A, Bhat S, Saeed A. Spontaneous bacterial peritonitis. World J Gastroenterol 2009;15:1042-9.
235. Kovacs M, Wong A, MacKinnon K, Weir K, Keeney M, Boyle E, et al. Assessment of the validity of the INR system for patients with liver impairment. Thromb Haemost 1994;71:727-30.
236. Krzeski P, Zych W, Kraszewska E, Milewski B, Butruk E, Habior A. Is serum bilirubin concentration the only valid prognostic marker in primary biliary cirrhosis? Hepatology 1999;30:865-9.
237. Kshirsagar N, Karande S, Potkar C. A prospective survey of drug induced hepatotoxicity in a large hospital. Indian J Gastroenterol 1992;11:13-5.
238. Kuhns M, Kleinman S, McNamara A, Rawal B, Glynn S, Busch M. Lack of correlation between HBsAg and HBV DNA levels in blood donors who test positive for HBsAg and anti-HBc: implications for future HBV screening policy. Transfusion 2004;44:1332-9.
239. Kundrotas L, Clement D. Serum alanine aminotransferase (ALT) elevation in asymptomatic US Air Force basic trainee blood donors. Dig Dis Sci 1993;38:2145-50.
240. Kuniholm M, Purcell R, McQuillan G, Engle R, Wasley A, Nelson K. Epidemiology of hepatitis E Virus in the United States: results from

the Third National Health and Nutrition Examination Survey, 1988-1994. J Infect Dis 2009;200:48-56.
241. Lalazar G, Rund D, Shouval D. Screening, prevention and treatment of viral hepatitis B reactivation in patients with haematological malignancies. Br J Haematol 2007;136:699-712.
242. Lalle E, Sacchi A, Abbate I, Vitale A, Martini F, D'Offizi G, et al. Activation of interferon response genes and of plasmacytoid dendritic cells in HIV-1 positive subjects with GB virus C co-infection. Int J Immunopathol Pharmacol 2008;21:161-71.
243. Laposata M. Fatty acid ethyl esters: short-term and long-term serum markers of ethanol intake. Clin Chem 1997;43:1527-34.
244. Larson A, Polson J, Fontana R, Davern T, Lalani E, Hynan L, et al. Acetaminophen-induced acute liver failure: results of a United States multicenter, prospective study. Hepatology 2005;42:1364-72.
245. LaRusso N, Shneider B, Black D, Gores G, James S, Doo E, et al. Primary sclerosing cholangitis: summary of a workshop. Hepatology 2006;44:746-64.
246. Laskus T, Radkowski M, Wang L, Vargas H, Rakela J. Lack of evidence for hepatitis G virus replication in the livers of patients coinfected with hepatitis C and G viruses. J Virol 1997;71:7804-6.
247. Lee C, Ko Y. Hepatitis B vaccination and hepatocellular carcinoma in Taiwan. Pediatrics 1997;99:351-3.
248. Lee W. Hepatitis B virus infection. N Engl J Med 1997;337:1733-45.
249. Lee W. Acetaminophen-related acute liver failure in the United States. Hepatology Research 2008;38:S3-S8.
250. Lee Y, Kaplan M. Treatment of primary biliary cirrhosis and primary sclerosing cholangitis: use of ursodeoxycholic acid. Curr Gastroenterol Rep 1999;1:38-41.
251. Lefrere J, Roudot-Thoraval F, Morand-Joubert L, Petit J, Lerable J, Thauvin M, et al. Carriage of GB virus C/hepatitis G virus RNA is associated with a slower immunologic, virologic, and clinical progression of human immunodeficiency virus disease in coinfected persons. J Infect Dis 1999;179:783-9.
252. Lelbach W. Cirrhosis in the alcoholic and its relation to the volume of alcohol abuse. Ann N Y Acad Sci 1975;252:85-105.
253. Lennard L. Clinical implications of thiopurine methyltransferase—optimization of drug dosage and potential drug interactions. Ther Drug Monit 1998;20:527-31.
254. Leone N, Rizzetto M. Natural history of hepatitis C infection: from chronic hepatitis, to cirrhosis, to hepatocellular carcinoma. Minerva Gastroenterol Dietol 2005;51:31-46.
255. Liang T. Hepatitis B: the virus and disease. Hepatology 2009;49:S13-21.
256. Lichtenstein P, Heubi J, Daugherty C, Farrell M, Sokol R, Rothbaum R, et al. Grade I Reye's syndrome: a frequent cause of vomiting and liver dysfunction after varicella and upper-respiratory-tract infection. N Engl J Med 1983;309:133-9.
257. Liebman H, Furie B, Tong M, Blanchard R, Lo K, Lee S, et al. Des-gamma-carboxy (abnormal) prothrombin as a serum marker of primary hepatocellular carcinoma. N Engl J Med 1984;310:1427-31.
258. Lin HJ, Seeff LB, Barbosa L, Hollinger FB. Occurrence of identical hypervariable region 1 sequences of hepatitis C virus in transfusion recipients and their respective blood donors: divergence over time. Hepatology 2001;34:424-9.
259. Lindor K, Gershwin M, Poupon R, Kaplan M, Bergasa N, Heathcote E. Primary biliary cirrhosis. Hepatology 2009;50:291-308.
260. Lisman T, Leebeek F. Hemostatic alterations in liver disease: a review on pathophysiology, clinical consequences, and treatment. Dig Surg 2007;24:250-8.
261. Liu Y, Taylor J, Linko P, Lucier G, Thompson C. Glutathione S-transferase mu in human lymphocyte and liver: role in modulating formation of carcinogen-derived DNA adducts. Carcinogenesis 1991;12:2269-75.
262. Liu Z, Kaplowitz N. Immune-mediated drug-induced liver disease. Clin Liver Dis 2002;6:467-86.
263. Livingston S, Simonetti J, McMahon B, Bulkow L, Hurlburt K, Homan C, et al. Hepatitis B virus genotypes in Alaska Native people with hepatocellular carcinoma: preponderance of genotype F. J Infect Dis 2007;195:5-11.
264. Lohse A, Zum BK, Franz B, Kanzler S, Gerken G, Dienes H. Characterization of the overlap syndrome of primary biliary cirrhosis (PBC) and autoimmune hepatitis: evidence for it being a hepatic form of PBC in genetically susceptible individuals. Hepatology 1999;29:1078-84.
265. Lok A, McMahon B. Chronic hepatitis B. Hepatology 2007;45:507-39.
266. Lomas D. Loop-sheet polymerization: the mechanism of alpha1-antitrypsin deficiency. Respir Med 2000;94(Suppl C):S3-6.
267. Loomba R, Rowley A, Wesley R, Liang J, Hoofnagle J, Pucino F, et al. Systematic review: the effect of preventive lamivudine on hepatitis B reactivation during chemotherapy. Ann Intern Med 2008;148:519-28.
268. Lowes K, Croager E, Olynyk J, Abraham L, Yeoh G. Oval cell-mediated liver regeneration: role of cytokines and growth factors. J Gastroenterol Hepatol 2003;18:4-12.
269. Lucas W, Chuttani R. Pathophysiology and current concepts in the diagnosis of obstructive jaundice. Gastroenterologist 1995;3:105-18.
270. Lucey M, Marthurin P, Morgan T. Alcoholic hepatitis. N Engl J Med 2009;360:2758-69.
271. Ludwig J, Viggiano T, McGill D, Oh B. Nonalcoholic steatohepatitis: Mayo Clinic experiences with a hitherto unnamed disease. Mayo Clin Proc 1980;55:434-8.
272. Ludwig S, Kaplowitz N. Effect of pyridoxine deficiency on serum and liver transaminases in experimental liver injury in the rat. Gastroenterology 1980;79:545-9.
273. Lunel F, Abuaf N, Frangeul L, Grippon P, Perrin M, Le CY, et al. Liver/kidney microsome antibody type 1 and hepatitis C virus infection. Hepatology 1992;16:630-6.
274. Luo J, Hwang S, Chang F, Chu C, Lai C, Wang Y, et al. Simple blood tests can predict compensated liver cirrhosis in patients with chronic hepatitis C. Hepatogastroenterology 2002;49:478-81.
275. Luo J, Hwang S, Wu J, Lai C, Li C, Chang F, et al. Clinical characteristics and prognosis of hepatocellular carcinoma patients with paraneoplastic syndromes. Hepatogastroenterology 2002;49:1315-9.
276. Macchia T, Mancinelli R, Gentili S, Ceccanti M, Devito R, Attilia M, et al. Mitochondrial aspartate aminotransferase isoenzyme: a biochemical marker for the clinical management of alcoholics? Clin Chim Acta 1997;263:79-96.
277. Machado M, Ravasco P, Martins A, Almeida M, Camilo M, Cortez-Pinto H. Iron homeostasis and H63D mutations in alcoholics with and without liver disease. World J Gastroenterol 2009;15:106-11.
278. Mandayam S, Jamal M, Morgan T. Epidemiology of alcoholic liver disease. Semin Liver Dis 2004;24:217-32.
279. Mann R, Smart R, Govoni R. The epidemiology of alcoholic liver disease. Alcohol Res Health 2003;27:209-19.
280. Manning D, Afdhal N. Diagnosis and quantitation of fibrosis. Gastroenterology 2008;134:1670-81.
281. Marcellin P, Asselah T, Boyer N. Fibrosis and disease progression in hepatitis C. Hepatology 2002;36:S47-56.
282. Maria V, Victorino R. Development and validation of a clinical scale for the diagnosis of drug-induced hepatitis. Hepatology 1997;26:664-9.
283. Marrero J, Feng Z, Wang Y, Nguyen M, Befeler A, Roberts L, et al. Alpha-fetoprotein, des-gamma carboxyprothrombin, and lectin-bound alpha-fetoprotein in early hepatocellular carcinoma. Gastroenterology 2009;137:110-8.
284. Martinez-Sierra C, Arizcorreta A, Diaz F, Roldan R, Martin-Herrera L, Perez-Guzman E, et al. Progression of chronic hepatitis C to liver fibrosis and cirrhosis in patients coinfected with hepatitis C virus and human immunodeficiency virus. Clin Infect Dis 2003;36:491-8.
285. Mast E, Alter M, Holland P, Purcell R. Evaluation of assays for antibody to hepatitis E virus by a serum panel. Hepatitis E Virus Antibody Serum Panel Evaluation Group. Hepatology 1998;27:857-61.
286. Mathiesen U, Franzen L, Fryden A, Foberg U, Bodemar G. The clinical significance of slightly to moderately increased liver transaminase values in asymptomatic patients. Scand J Gastroenterol 1999;34:85-91.
287. Mathiesen U, Franzen L, Fryden A, Fosberg U, Bodemar G. The clinical significance of slightly to moderately increased liver

transaminase values in asymptomatic patients. Scand J Gastroenterol 1999;34:85-91.

288. Mattsson L, Weiland O, Glaumann H. Application of a numerical scoring system for assessment of histological outcome in patients with chronic posttransfusion non-A, non-B hepatitis with or without antibodies to hepatitis C. Liver 1990;10:257-63.
289. Mayfield R, Harris R, Schuckit M. Genetic factors influencing alcohol dependence. Br J Pharmacol 2008;154:275-87.
290. Mayo M. Natural history of primary biliary cirrhosis. Clin Liver Dis 2008;12:277-88.
291. McCormick P, Donnelly C. Management of hepatorenal syndrome. Pharmacol Ther 2008;119:1-6.
292. McCormick S, Goodman Z, Maydonovitch C, Sjogren M. Evaluation of liver histology, ALT elevation, and HCV RNA titer in patients with chronic hepatitis C. Am J Gastroenterol 1996;91:1516-22.
293. McGinlay J, Payne R. Serum albumin by dye-binding: bromocresol green or bromocresol purple? The case for conservatism. Ann Clin Biochem 1988;25:417-21.
294. McGlynn K, Rosvold E, Lustbader E, Hu Y, Clapper M, Zhou T, et al. Susceptibility to hepatocellular carcinoma is associated with genetic variation in the enzymatic detoxification of aflatoxin B1. Proc Natl Acad Sci U S A 1995;92:2384-7.
295. McHutchison J, Everson G, Gordon S, Jacobson I, Sulkowski M, Kauffman R, et al. Telaprevir with peginterferon and ribavirin for chronic HCV genotype 1 infection. N Engl J Med 2009;360:1827-38.
296. McMahon B. The natural history of chronic hepatitis B virus infection. Hepatology 2009;49:S45-55.
297. Mehendiratta V, Mitroo P, Bombonati A, Navarro V, Rossi S, Rubin R, et al. Serologic markers do not predict histologic severity or response to treatment in patients with autoimmune hepatitis. Clin Gastroenterol Hepatol 2009;7:98-103.
298. Meier P, Manns M. Medical and endoscopic treatment in primary sclerosing cholangitis. Best Pract Res Clin Gastroenterol 2001;15: 657-66.
299. Mendenhall C. Alcoholic hepatitis. Clin Gastroenterol 1981;10:417-41.
300. Mendenhall C, Seeff L, Diehl A, Ghosn S, French S, Gartside P, et al. Antibodies to hepatitis B virus and hepatitis C virus in alcoholic hepatitis and cirrhosis: their prevalence and clinical relevance. The VA Cooperative Study Group (No. 119). Hepatology 1991;14:581-9.
301. Meng X. Novel strains of hepatitis E virus identified from humans and other animal species: is hepatitis E a zoonosis? J Hepatol 2000; 33:842-5.
302. Meng X, Dea S, Engle R, Friendship R, Lyoo Y, Sininarumitr T, et al. Prevalence of antibodies to the hepatitis E virus in pigs from countries where hepatitis E is common or is rare in the human population. J Med Virol 1999;59:297-302.
303. Menon K, Gores G, Shah V. Pathogenesis, diagnosis, and treatment of alcoholic liver disease. Mayo Clin Proc 2001;76:1021-9.
304. Mera J, Dickson B, Feldman M. Influence of gender on the ratio of serum aspartate aminotransferase (AST) to alanine aminotransferase (ALT) in patients with and without hyperbilirubinemia. Dig Dis Sci 2008;53:799-802.
305. Meredith J. Lipoprotein-X. Arch Pathol Lab Med 1986;110:1123-7.
306. Metcalf J, Mitchison H, Palmer J, Jones D, Bassendine M, James O. Natural history of early primary biliary cirrhosis. Lancet 1996;348: 1399-402.
307. Milkiewicz P, Hubscher S, Skiba G, Hathaway M, Elias E. Recurrence of autoimmune hepatitis after liver transplantation. Transplantation 1999;68:253-6.
308. Milkiewicz P, Saksena S, Hubscher S, Elias E. Wilson's disease with superimposed autoimmune features: report of two cases and review. J Gastroenterol Hepatol 2000;15:570-4.
309. Mitchell P, Sloan L, Majewski D, Rys P, Heimgartner P, Rosenblatt J, et al. Comparison of line probe assay and DNA sequencing of 5′ untranslated region for genotyping hepatitis C virus: description of novel line probe patterns. Diagn Microbiol Infect Dis 2002;42:175-9.
310. Moaven L, Tennakoon P, Bowden D, Locarnini S. Mother-to-baby transmission of hepatitis G virus. Med J Aust 1996;165:84-5.
311. Modahl L, Lai M. Hepatitis delta virus: the molecular basis of laboratory diagnosis. Crit Rev Clin Lab Sci 2000;37:45-92.
312. Moerman B, Moons V, Sommer H, Schmitt Y, Stetter M. Evaluation of sensitivity for wild type and mutant forms of hepatitis B surface antigen by four commercial HBsAg assays. Clin Lab 2004;50:159-62.
313. Mofrad P, Contos M, Haque M, Sargeant C, Fisher R, Luketic V, et al. Clinical and histologic spectrum of nonalcoholic fatty liver disease associated with normal ALT values. Hepatology 2003;37:1286-92.
314. Mohiuddin R, Lewis J. Drug- and chemical-induced cholestasis. Clin Liver Dis 2004;8:95-132.
315. Moore K, Wong F, Gines P, Bernardi M, Ochs A, Salerno F, et al. The management of ascites in cirrhosis: report on the consensus conference of the International Ascites Club. Hepatology 2003;38:258-66.
316. Moradpour D, Wands J. Understanding hepatitis B virus infection. N Engl J Med 1995;332:1092-3.
317. Morin T, Martin J, Feldmann G, Rueff B, Benhamou J, Ropartz C. Heterozygous alpha 1-antitrypsin deficiency and cirrhosis in adults, a fortuitous association. Lancet 1975;1:250-1.
318. Moss D. Release of membrane-bound enzymes from cells and the generation of isoforms. Clin Chim Acta 1994;226:131-42.
319. Moteki S, Leung P, Dickson E, Van TD, Galperin C, Buch T, et al. Epitope mapping and reactivity of autoantibodies to the E2 component of 2-oxoglutarate dehydrogenase complex in primary biliary cirrhosis using recombinant 2-oxoglutarate dehydrogenase complex. Hepatology 1996;23:436-44.
320. Moucari R, Mackiewicz V, Lada O, Ripault M, Castelnau C, Martinot-Peignoux M, et al. Early serum HBsAg drop: a strong predictor of sustained virological response to pegylated interferon alfa-2a in HBeAg-negative patients. Hepatology 2009;49:1151-7.
321. Mulder A, Horst G, Haagsma E, Limburg P, Kleibeuker J, Kallenberg C. Prevalence and characterization of neutrophil cytoplasmic antibodies in autoimmune liver diseases. Hepatology 1993;17:411-7.
322. Munoz S. The hepatorenal syndrome. Med Clin North Am 2008;92:813-37.
323. Myers R, Cerini R, Sayegh R, Moreau R, Degon C, Lebrec D, et al. Cardiac hepatopathy: clinical, hemodynamic, and histologic characteristics and correlations. Hepatology 2003;37:393-400.
324. Nagral A, Quaglia A, Sabin C, Dhillon A, Bearcroft C, Millar A, et al. Blood and graft eosinophils in acute cellular rejection of liver allografts. Transplant Proc 2001;33:2588-93.
325. Nalpas B, Vassault A, Le GA, Lesgourgues B, Ferry N, Lacour B, et al. Serum activity of mitochondrial aspartate aminotransferase: a sensitive marker of alcoholism with or without alcoholic hepatitis. Hepatology 1984;4:893-6.
326. Narayanan S. Lipoprotein-X. CRC Crit Rev Clin Lab Sci 1979;11: 31-51.
327. Nathwani R, Pais S, Reynolds T, Kaplowitz N. Serum alanine aminotransferase in skeletal muscle diseases. Hepatology 2005;41: 380-2.
328. Navaneethan U, Al Mohajer M, Shata M. Hepatitis E and pregnancy: understanding the pathogenesis. Liver Int 2008;28:1190-9.
329. Negro F, Rizzetto M. Diagnosis of hepatitis delta virus infection. J Hepatol 1995;22:136-9.
330. Neuberger J. Primary biliary cirrhosis. Lancet 1997;350:875-9.
331. Neuschwander-Tetri B, Caldwell S. Nonalcoholic steatohepatitis: summary of an AASLD single topic conference. Hepatology 2003;37: 1202-19.
332. Neuschwander-Tetri B, Unalp A, Creer M. Influence of local reference populations on upper limits of normal for serum alanine aminotransferase levels. Arch Intern Med 2008;168:663-6.
333. Nguyen T, Sedghi-Vaziri A, Wilkes L, Mondala T, Pockros P, Lindsay K, et al. Fluctuations in viral load (HCV RNA) are relatively insignificant in untreated patients with chronic HCV infection. J Viral Hepat 1996;3:75-8.
334. Nguyen-Khac E, Cadranel J, Thevenot T, Nousbaum J. Review article: the utility of reagent strips in the diagnosis of infected ascites in cirrhotic patients. Aliment Pharmacol Ther 2008;28:282-8.

335. Niemelä O. Acetaldehyde adducts in circulation. Novartis Found Symp 2007;285:183-92.
336. Niemelä O. Biomarkers in alcoholism. Clin Chim Acta 2007;377: 39-49.
337. Nijhawan P, Therneau T, Dickson E, Boynton J, Lindor K. Incidence of cancer in primary biliary cirrhosis: the Mayo experience. Hepatology 1999;29:1396-8.
338. Nikolaeva L, Blokhina N, Tsurikova N, Voronkova N, Miminoshvili M, Braginsky D, et al. Virus-specific antibody titres in different phases of hepatitis C virus infection. J Viral Hepat 2002;9:429-37.
339. Nikolopoulos G, Paraskevis D, Hatzitheodorou E, Moschidis Z, Sypsa V, Zavitsanos X, et al. Impact of hepatitis B virus infection on the progression of AIDS and mortality in HIV-infected individuals: a cohort study and meta-analysis. Clin Infect Dis 2009;48:1763-71.
340. Nikopoulos A, Giannoulis E, Doutsos I, Grammaticos P, Tourkantonis A, Arvanitakis C. Evaluation of [14C]aminopyrine breath test, peripheral clearance of [99mTc]EHIDA, and serum bile acid levels in liver function and disease. Dig Dis Sci 1992;37:1655-60.
341. Nishiguchi S, Enomoto M, Shiomi S, Tanaka M, Fukuda K, Tamori A, et al. TT virus infection in patients with chronic liver disease of unknown etiology. J Med Virol 2000;62:392-8.
342. Nissenbaum M, Chedid A, Mendenhall C, Gartside P. Prognostic significance of cholestatic alcoholic hepatitis. VA Cooperative Study Group #119. Dig Dis Sci 1990;35:891-6.
343. Nomura F, Tomonaga T, Sogawa K, Wu D, Ohashi T. Application of proteomic technologies to discover and identify biomarkers for excessive alcohol consumption: a review. J Chromatogr B Analyt Technol Biomed Life Sci 2007;855:35-41.
344. Nyblom H, Björnsson E, Simrén M, Aldenborg F, Almer S, Olsson R. The AST/ALT ratio as an indicator of cirrhosis in patients with PBC. Liver Int 2006;26:840-5.
345. Nyblom H, Nordlinder H, Olsson R. High aspartate to alanine aminotransferase ratio is an indicator of cirrhosis and poor outcome in patients with primary sclerosing cholangitis. Liver Int 2007;27: 694-9.
346. O'Brien J. Hepatitis B surface antigen: decreased need for confirmation of reactive results. Clin Chem 2000;46:582.
347. O'Grady J, Alexander G, Hayllar K, Williams R. Early indicators of prognosis in fulminant hepatic failure. Gastroenterology 1989;97: 439-45.
348. Ohtsuka T, Tsutsumi M, Fukumura A, Tsuchishima M, Takase S. Use of serum carbohydrate-deficient transferrin values to exclude alcoholic hepatitis from non-alcoholic steatohepatitis: a pilot study. Alcohol Clin Exp Res 2005;29:236S-9S.
349. Olynyk J, Trinder D, Ramm G, Britton R, Bacon B. Hereditary hemochromatosis in the post-HFE era. Hepatology 2008;48:991-1001.
350. Ong J, Aggarwal A, Krieger D, Easley K, Karafa M, Van Lente F, et al. Correlation between ammonia levels and the severity of hepatic encephalopathy. Am J Med 2003;114:188-93.
351. Orito E, Mizokami M, Nakano T, Wu R, Cao K, Ohba K, et al. GB virus C/hepatitis G virus infection among Japanese patients with chronic liver diseases and blood donors. Virus Res 1996;46:89-93.
352. Orland J, Wright T, Cooper S. Acute hepatitis C. Hepatology 2001;33:321-7.
353. Ozen H. Glycogen storage diseases: new perspectives. World J Gastroenterol 2007;13:2541-53.
354. Palmer M, Schaffner F. Effect of weight reduction on hepatic abnormalities in overweight patients. Gastroenterology 1990;99: 1408-13.
355. Palmer R. A review of the use of ethyl glucuronide as a marker for ethanol consumption in forensic and clinical medicine. Semin Diagn Pathol 2009;26:18-27.
356. Paradis V, Mathurin P, Laurent A, Charlotte F, Vidaud M, Poynard T, et al. Histological features predictive of liver fibrosis in chronic hepatitis C infection. J Clin Pathol 1996;49:998-1004.
357. Parkes J, Guha I, Roderick P, Rosenberg W. Performance of serum marker panels for liver fibrosis in chronic hepatitis C. J Hepatol 2008;44:2006.
358. Parlesak A, Billinger M, Bode C, Bode J. Gastric alcohol dehydrogenase activity in man: influence of gender, age, alcohol consumption and smoking in a Caucasian population. Alcohol Alcohol 2002;37:388-93.
359. Parrish A, Robson S, Trey C, Kirsch R. Retrospective survey of drug-induced liver disease at Groote Schuur Hospital, Cape Town—1983-1987. S Afr Med J 1990;77:199-202.
360. Patwardhan R, Smith O, Farmelant M. Serum transaminase levels and cholescintigraphic abnormalities in acute biliary tract obstruction. Arch Intern Med 1987;147:1249-53.
361. Pawlotsky J, Prescott L, Simmonds P, Pellet C, Laurent-Puig P, Labonne C, et al. Serological determination of hepatitis C virus genotype: comparison with a standardized genotyping assay. J Clin Microbiol 1997;35:1734-9.
362. Perlmutter D, Brodsky J, Balistreri W, Trapnell B. Molecular pathogenesis of alpha-1-antitrypsin deficiency-associated liver disease: a meeting review. Hepatology 2007;45:1313-23.
362A. Pfeiffer RF. Wilson's disease. Handb Clin Neurol 2011;100:681-709.
363. Pietrangelo A. Hereditary hemochromatosis—a new look at an old disease. N Engl J Med 2004;350:2383-97.
364. Plessier A, Valla D. Budd-Chiari syndrome. Semin Liver Dis 2008;28: 259-69.
365. Porta G, Gayotto L, Alvarez F. Anti-liver-kidney microsome antibody-positive autoimmune hepatitis presenting as fulminant liver failure. J Pediatr Gastroenterol Nutr 1990;11:138-40.
366. Povey S. Genetics of alpha 1-antitrypsin deficiency in relation to neonatal liver disease. Mol Biol Med 1990;7:161-72.
367. Poynard T, Bedossa P, Opolon P. Natural history of liver fibrosis progression in patients with chronic hepatitis C. The OBSVIRC, METAVIR, CLINIVIR, and DOSVIRC Groups. Lancet 1997;349: 825-32.
368. Poynard T, McHutchison J, Manns M, Trepo C, Lindsay K, Goodman Z, et al. Impact of pegylated interferon alfa-2b and ribavirin on liver fibrosis in patients with chronic hepatitis C. Gastroenterology 2002;122:1303-13.
369. Poynard T, Ratziu V, Charlotte F, Goodman Z, McHutchison J, Albrecht J. Rates and risk factors of liver fibrosis progression in patients with chronic hepatitis C. J Hepatol 2001;34:730-9.
370. Prati D, Taioli E, Zanella A, Della Torre E, Butelli S, Del Vecchio E, et al. Updated definitions of healthy ranges for serum alanine aminotransferase levels. Ann Intern Med 2002;137:1-10.
371. Preiss D, Sattar N. Non-alcoholic fatty liver disease: an overview of prevalence, diagnosis, pathogenesis and treatment considerations. Clin Sci (Lond) 2008;115:141-50.
371A. Privette TW Jr, Carlisle MC, Palma JK. Emergencies of the liver, gallbladder, and pancreas. Emerg Med Clin North Am 2011;29: 293-317, viii-ix.
372. Propst T, Propst A, Dietze O, Judmaier G, Braunsteiner H, Vogel W. High prevalence of viral infection in adults with homozygous and heterozygous alpha 1-antitrypsin deficiency and chronic liver disease. Ann Intern Med 1992;117:641-5.
373. Propst T, Propst A, Dietze O, Judmaier G, Braunsteiner H, Vogel W. Alpha-1-antitrypsin deficiency and liver disease. Dig Dis 1994;12: 139-49.
374. Puisieux A, Lim S, Groopman J, Ozturk M. Selective targeting of p53 gene mutational hotspots in human cancers by etiologically defined carcinogens. Cancer Res 1991;51:6185-9.
375. Puoti C, Castellacci R, Montagnese F, Zaltron S, Stornaiuolo G, Bergami N, et al. Histological and virological features and follow-up of hepatitis C virus carriers with normal aminotransferase levels: the Italian prospective study of the asymptomatic C carriers (ISACC). J Hepatol 2002;37:117-23.
376. Radha Krishna Y, Saraswat V, Das K, Himanshu G, Yachha S, Aggarwal R, et al. Clinical features and predictors of outcome in acute hepatitis A and hepatitis E virus hepatitis on cirrhosis. Liver Int 2009;29:392-8.
377. Raurich J, Pérez O, Llompart-Pou J, Ibáñez J, Ayestarán I, Pérez-Bárcena J. Incidence and outcome of ischemic hepatitis complicating septic shock. Hepatol Res 2009;39:700-5.

378. Reye R, Morgan G, Baral J. Encephalopathy and fatty degeneration of the viscera: a disease entity in childhood. Lancet 1963;ii:249-52.
379. Rizzetto M. Hepatitis D: thirty years after. J Hepatol 2009;50:1043-50.
380. Roberts E, Schilsky M. Diagnosis and treatment of Wilson disease: an update. Hepatology 2008;47:2089-111.
381. Roberts E, Yeung L. Maternal-infant transmission of hepatitis C virus infection. Hepatology 2002;36:S106-13.
382. Rodger A, Roberts S, Lanigan A, Bowden S, Brown T, Crofts N. Assessment of long-term outcomes of community-acquired hepatitis C infection in a cohort with sera stored from 1971 to 1975. Hepatology 2000;32:582-7.
383. Romeo R, Del Ninno E, Rumi M, Russo A, Sangiovanni A, de Franchis R, et al. A 28-year study of the course of hepatitis Delta infection: a risk factor for cirrhosis and hepatocellular carcinoma. Gastroenterology 2009;136:1629-38.
383A. Rosen HR. Clinical practice. Chronic hepatitis C infection. N Engl J Med 2011;364:2429-38.
384. Ross R, Viazov S, Hoffmann S, Roggendorf M. Performance characteristics of a transcription-mediated nucleic acid amplification assay for qualitative detection of hepatitis C virus RNA. J Clin Lab Anal 2001;15:308-13.
385. Rouanet I, Peyriere H, Mauboussin J, Terrail N, Vincent D. Acute clinical hepatitis by immune restoration in a human immunodeficiency virus/hepatitis B virus co-infected patient receiving antiretroviral therapy. Eur J Gastroenterol Hepatol 2003;15:95-7.
386. Rozen P, Korn R, Zimmerman H. Computer analysis of liver function tests and their interrelationship in 347 cases of viral hepatitis. Isr J Med Sci 1970;6:67-79.
387. Runyon B. Management of adult patients with ascites due to cirrhosis: an update. Hepatology 2009;49:2087-107.
388. Sagnelli E, Coppola N, Messina V, Di Caprio D, Marrocco C, Marotta A, et al. HBV superinfection in hepatitis C virus chronic carriers, viral interaction, and clinical course. Hepatology 2002;36:1285-91.
389. Sagnelli E, Coppola N, Pisaturo M, Masiello A, Tonziello G, Sagnelli C, et al. HBV superinfection in HCV chronic carriers: a disease that is frequently severe but associated with the eradication of HCV. Hepatology 2009;49:1090-7.
390. Sakon M, Monden M, Gotoh M, Kobayashi K, Kanai T, Umeshita K, et al. The effects of vitamin K on the generation of des-gamma-carboxy prothrombin (PIVKA-II) in patients with hepatocellular carcinoma. Am J Gastroenterol 1991;86:339-45.
391. Saldanha J, Gerlich W, Lelie N, Dawson P, Heermann K, Heath A. An international collaborative study to establish a World Health Organization international standard for hepatitis B virus DNA nucleic acid amplification techniques. Vox Sang 2001;80:63-71.
392. Saldanha J, Lelie N, Heath A. Establishment of the first international standard for nucleic acid amplification technology (NAT) assays for HCV RNA. WHO Collaborative Study Group. Vox Sang 1999;76: 149-58.
393. Sanchez-Albisua I, Garde T, Hierro L, Camarena C, Frauca E, de la Vega A, et al. A high index of suspicion: the key to an early diagnosis of Wilson's disease in childhood. J Pediatr Gastroenterol Nutr 1999;28: 186-90.
394. Sato A, Kato Y, Nakata K, Nakao K, Daikoku M, Ishii N, et al. Relationship between sustained elevation of serum alanine aminotransferase and progression from cirrhosis to hepatocellular carcinoma: comparison in patients with hepatitis B virus- and hepatitis C virus-associated cirrhosis. J Gastroenterol Hepatol 1996;11:944-8.
395. Schaffert C, Duryee M, Hunter C, Hamilton BR, DeVeney A, Huerter M, et al. Alcohol metabolites and lipopolysaccharide: roles in the development and/or progression of alcoholic liver disease. World J Gastroenterol 2009;15:1209-18.
396. Schilsky M, Scheinberg I, Sternlieb I. Prognosis of Wilsonian chronic active hepatitis. Gastroenterology 1991;100:762-7.
397. Schiødt F, Bangert K, Shakil A, McCashland T, Murray N, Hay J, et al. Predictive value of actin-free Gc-globulin in acute liver failure. Liver Transplantation 2007;13:1324-9.
398. Schlaeger R, Haux P, Kattermann R. Studies on the mechanism of the increase in serum alkaline phosphatase activity in cholestasis: significance of the hepatic bile acid concentration for the leakage of alkaline phosphatase from rat liver. Enzyme 1982;28:3-13.
399. Schmidt E, Schmidt F. Progress in the enzyme diagnosis of liver disease: reality or illusion? Clin Biochem 1990;23:375-82.
400. Schrumpf E, Boberg K. Epidemiology of primary sclerosing cholangitis. Best Pract Res Clin Gastroenterol 2001;15:553-62.
401. Schuckit M. An overview of genetic influences in alcoholism. J Subst Abuse Treat 2009;36:S5-14.
402. Schuppan D, Koda M, Bauer M, Hahn E. Fibrosis of liver, pancreas and intestine: common mechanisms and clear targets? Acta Gastroenterol Belg 2000;63:366-70.
403. Schutzbank T, Sefers S, Kahmann N, Li H, Tang Y. Comparative evaluation of three commercially available methodologies for hepatitis C virus genotyping. J Clin Microbiol 2006;44:3797-8.
404. Scott J, Gollan J, Samourian S, Sherlock S. Wilson's disease, presenting as chronic active hepatitis. Gastroenterology 1978;74:645-51.
405. Scott J, McMahon B. Role of combination therapy in chronic hepatitis B. Curr Gastroenterol Rep 2009;11:28-36.
406. Sebastiani G. Non-invasive assessment of liver fibrosis in chronic liver diseases: implementation in clinical practice and decisional algorithms. World J Gastroenterol 2009;15:2190-203.
407. Seeff L. Drug-induced chronic liver disease, with emphasis on chronic active hepatitis. Semin Liver Dis 1981;1:104-15.
408. Seeff L. Herbal hepatotoxicity. Clin Liver Dis 2007;11:577-96.
409. Seeff L. The history of the "natural history" of hepatitis C (1968-2009). Liver Int 2009;29:89-99.
410. Seeff L, Beebe G, Hoofnagle J, Norman J, Buskell-Bales Z, Waggoner J, et al. A serologic follow-up of the 1942 epidemic of post-vaccination hepatitis in the United States Army. N Engl J Med 1987;316:965-70.
411. Seeff L, Cuccherini B, Zimmerman H, Adler E, Benjamin S. Acetaminophen hepatotoxicity in alcoholics: a therapeutic misadventure. Ann Intern Med 1986;104:399-404.
412. Seeff L, Hollinger F, Alter H, Wright E, Cain C, Buskell Z, et al. Long-term mortality and morbidity of transfusion-associated non-A, non-B, and type C hepatitis: a National Heart, Lung, and Blood Institute collaborative study. Hepatology 2001;33:455-63.
413. Seeff L, Miller R, Rabkin C, Buskell-Bales Z, Straley-Eason K, Smoak B, et al. 45-year follow-up of hepatitis C virus infection in healthy young adults. Ann Intern Med 2000;132:105-11.
414. Seeff L, Wright E, Zimmerman H, McCollum R. VA cooperative study of post-transfusion hepatitis, 1969-1974: incidence and characteristics of hepatitis and responsible risk factors. Am J Med Sci 1975;270: 355-62.
415. Seeto R, Fenn B, Rockey D. Ischemic hepatitis: clinical presentation and pathogenesis. Am J Med 2000;109:109-13.
416. Sharma M, Ahuja V. Aetiological spectrum of obstructive jaundice and diagnostic ability of ultrasonography: a clinician's perspective. Trop Gastroenterol 1999;20:167-9.
417. Shepard B, Tuma P. Alcohol-induced protein hyperacetylation: mechanisms and consequences. World J Gastroenterol 2009;15: 1219-30.
418. Sheth M, Riggs M, Patel T. Utility of the Mayo End-Stage Liver Disease (MELD) score in assessing prognosis of patients with alcoholic hepatitis. BMC Gastroenterol 2002;2:2.
419. Shiffman M, Ferreira-Gonzalez A, Reddy K, Sterling R, Luketic V, Stravitz R, et al. International unit standard: implications for management of patients with chronic hepatitis C virus infection in clinical practice. Am J Gastroenterol 2003;98:1159-66.
420. Sillanpaa M, Makela A, Koivikko A. Acute liver failure and encephalopathy (Reye's syndrome?) during salicylate therapy. Acta Paediatr Scand 1975;64:877-80.
421. Silveira M, Lindor K. Primary sclerosing cholangitis. Can J Gastroenterol 2008;22:689-98.
422. Silverman A, Sandhaus R. Alpha1-antitrypsin deficiency. N Engl J Med 2009;360:2749-57.

423. Singer A, Carracio T, Mofenson H. The temporal profile of increased transaminase levels in patients with acetaminophen-induced liver dysfunction. Ann Emerg Med 1995;26:49-53.
424. Skinhoj P, Mikkelsen F, Hollinger F. Hepatitis A in Greenland: importance of specific antibody testing in epidemiologic surveillance. Am J Epidemiol 1977;105:140-7.
425. Smedile A, Rizzetto M, Gerin J. Advances in hepatitis D virus biology and disease. Prog Liver Dis 1994;12:157-75.
426. Socha P, Horvath A, Vajro P, Dziechciarz P, Dhawan A, Szajewska H. Pharmacological interventions for nonalcoholic fatty liver disease in adults and in children: a systematic review. J Pediatr Gastroenterol Nutr 2009;48:587-96.
427. Soiffer R. Immune modulation and chronic graft-versus-host disease. Bone Marrow Transplant 2008;42:S66-9.
428. Soloway R, Summerskill W, Baggenstoss A, Geall M, Gitnick G, Elveback I, et al. Clinical, biochemical, and histological remission of severe chronic active liver disease: a controlled study of treatments and early prognosis. Gastroenterology 1972;63:820-33.
429. Sorokin A, Brown J, Thompson P. Primary biliary cirrhosis, hyperlipidemia, and atherosclerosis risk: a systematic review. Atherosclerosis 2007;194:293-9.
430. Sorrel M, Belongia E, Costa J, Gareen I, Grem J, Inadomi J, et al. National Institutes of Health consensus development conference statement: management of hepatitis B. Ann Intern Med 2009;150: 104-9.
431. Souza M, Castro-e-Silva JO, Picinato M, Franco C, Mazzetto S, Ceneviva R, et al. Serum transaminase levels in the acute phase of chronic extrahepatic cholestasis. Braz J Med Biol Res 1990;23:995-7.
431A. Stubbs MA, Morgan MY. Managing alcohol dependence and alcohol-related liver disease: a problem for the hepatologist, psychiatrist or economist? Clin Med 2011 Apr;11(2):189-93.
432. Stedman C. Herbal hepatotoxicity. Semin Liver Dis 2002;22:195-206.
433. Steindl P, Ferenci P, Dienes H, Grimm G, Pabinger I, Madl C, et al. Wilson's disease in patients presenting with liver disease: a diagnostic challenge. Gastroenterology 1997;113:212-8.
434. Sterling R, Jeffers L, Gordon F, Venook A, Reddy K, Satomura S, et al. Utility of lens culinaris agglutinin-reactive fraction of alpha-fetoprotein and des-gamma-carboxy prothrombin, alone or in combination, as biomarkers for hepatocellular carcinoma. Clin Gastroenterol Hepatol 2009;7:104-13.
435. Stickel F, Osterreicher C. The role of genetic polymorphisms in alcoholic liver disease. Alcohol Alcohol 2006;41:209-24.
436. Sveger T. The natural history of liver disease in alpha 1-antitrypsin deficient children. Acta Paediatr Scand 1988;77:847-51.
437. Sveger T, Eriksson S. The liver in adolescents with alpha 1-antitrypsin deficiency. Hepatology 1995;22:514-7.
438. Tanaka E, Ohue C, Aoyagi K, Yamaguchi K, Yagi S, Kiyosawa K, et al. Evaluation of a new enzyme immunoassay for hepatitis C virus (HCV) core antigen with clinical sensitivity approximating that of genomic amplification of HCV RNA. Hepatology 2000;32:388-93.
439. Tang J, Hsu H, Lin H, Ni Y, Chang M. Hepatitis B surface antigenemia at birth: a long-term follow-up study. J Pediatr 1998;133:374-7.
440. Tanzi R, Petrukhin K, Chernov I, Pellequer J, Wasco W, Ross B, et al. The Wilson disease gene is a copper transporting ATPase with homology to the Menkes disease gene. Nat Genet 1993;5:344-50.
441. Tarantino G, Citro V, Esposito P, Giaquinto S, de Leone A, Milan G, et al. Blood ammonia levels in liver cirrhosis: a clue for the presence of portosystemic collateral veins. BMC Gastroenterol 2009;17:21.
442. Tavill A. Diagnosis and management of hemochromatosis. Hepatology 2001;33:1321-8.
443. Teare J, Carmichael A, Burnett F, Rake M. Detection of antibodies to acetaldehyde-albumin conjugates in alcoholic liver disease. Alcohol Alcohol 1993;28:11-6.
444. Terrault N. Benefits and risks of combination therapy for hepatitis B. Hepatology 2009;49:S122-8.
445. Teufel A, Galle P, Kanzler S. Update on autoimmune hepatitis. World J Gastroenterol 2009;15:1035-41.
446. Thachil J. Relevance of clotting tests in liver disease. Postgrad Med J 2008;84:177-81.
447. Thio C. Hepatitis B and human immunodeficiency virus coinfection. Hepatology 2009;49:S138-45.
448. Tillmann H, Heiken H, Knapik-Botor A, Heringlake S, Ockenga J, Wilber J, et al. Infection with GB virus C and reduced mortality among HIV-infected patients. N Engl J Med 2001;345:715-24.
449. Tong M, Blatt L, Kao J, Cheng J, Corey W. Basal core promoter T1762/A1764 and precore A1896 gene mutations in hepatitis B surface antigen-positive hepatocellular carcinoma: a comparison with chronic carriers. Liver Int 2007;27:1356-63.
450. Torbenson M, Kannangai R, Astemborski J, Strathdee S, Vlahov D, Thomas D. High prevalence of occult hepatitis B in Baltimore injection drug users. Hepatology 2004;39:51-7.
451. Toyoda H, Fukuda Y, Hayakawa T, Kumada T, Nakano S, Takamatsu J, et al. Presence of multiple genotype-specific antibodies in patients with persistent infection with hepatitis C virus (HCV) of a single genotype: evidence for transient or occult superinfection with HCV of different genotypes. Am J Gastroenterol 1999;94:2230-6.
452. Toyoda H, Fukuda Y, Hayakawa T, Takamatsu J, Saito H. Effect of GB virus C/hepatitis G virus coinfection on the course of HIV infection in hemophilia patients in Japan. J Acquir Immune Defic Syndr Hum Retrovirol 1998;17:209-13.
453. Trauner M, Meier P, Boyer J. Molecular pathogenesis of cholestasis. N Engl J Med 1998;339:1217-27.
454. Tripodi A, Chantarangkul V, Primignani M, Fabris F, Dell'era A, Sei C, et al. The international normalized ratio calibrated for cirrhosis [INR(liver)] normalizes prothrombin time results for model for end-stage liver disease calculation. Hepatology 2007;46:520-7.
455. Trotter J. Coagulation abnormalities in patients who have liver disease. Clin Liver Dis 2006;10:665-78.
456. Tsai J, Margolis H, Jeng J, Ho M, Chang W, Hsieh M, et al. Hepatitis B surface antigen- and immunoglobulin-specific circulating immune complexes in acute hepatitis B virus infection. Clin Immunol Immunopathol 1996;80:278-82.
457. Tsuneyama K, Van de Water J, Nakanuma Y, Cha S, Ansari A, Coppel R, et al. Human combinatorial autoantibodies and mouse monoclonal antibodies to PDC-E2 produce abnormal apical staining of salivary glands in patients with coexistent primary biliary cirrhosis and Sjogren's syndrome. Hepatology 1994;20:893-8.
458. Tsutsumi M, Takase S, Urashima S, Ueshima Y, Kawahara H, Takada A. Serum markers for hepatic fibrosis in alcoholic liver disease: which is the best marker, type III procollagen, type IV collagen, laminin, tissue inhibitor of metalloproteinase, or prolyl hydroxylase? Alcohol Clin Exp Res 1996;20:1512-7.
459. Turkoglu S, Lazizi Y, Meng H, Kordosi A, Dubreuil P, Crescenzo B, et al. Detection of hepatitis E virus RNA in stools and serum by reverse transcription-PCR. J Clin Microbiol 1996;34:1568-71.
460. Ueda H, Ullrich S, Gangemi J, Kappel C, Ngo L, Feitelson M, et al. Functional inactivation but not structural mutation of p53 causes liver cancer. Nat Genet 1995;9:41-7.
461. Umemura T, Yeo A, Sottini A, Moratto D, Tanaka Y, Wang R, et al. SEN virus infection and its relationship to transfusion-associated hepatitis. Hepatology 2001;33:1303-11.
462. Ustundag Y, Samsar U, Acikgoz S, Cabuk M, Kiran S, Kulah E, et al. Analysis of glomerular filtration rate, serum cystatin C levels, and renal resistive index values in cirrhosis patients. Clin Chem Lab Med 2007;45:890-4.
463. Van de Water J, Cooper A, Surh C, Coppel R, Danner D, Ansari A, et al. Detection of autoantibodies to recombinant mitochondrial proteins in patients with primary biliary cirrhosis. N Engl J Med 1989;320:1377-80.
464. Van de Water J, Gershwin M, Leung P, Ansari A, Coppel R. The autoepitope of the 74-kD mitochondrial autoantigen of primary biliary cirrhosis corresponds to the functional site of dihydrolipoamide acetyltransferase. J Exp Med 1988;167:1791-9.
465. Vento S, Garofano T, Renzini C, Cainelli F, Casali F, Ghironzi G, et al. Fulminant hepatitis associated with hepatitis A virus superinfection in patients with chronic hepatitis C. N Engl J Med 1998;338:286-90.

466. Volkmann M, Martin L, Bäurle A, Heid H, Strassburg C, Trautwein C, et al. Soluble liver antigen: isolation of a 35-kd recombinant protein (SLA-p35) specifically recognizing sera from patients with autoimmune hepatitis. Hepatology 2001;33:591-6.
467. Wagnerberger S, Schäfer C, Schwarz E, Bode C, Parlesak A. Is nutrient intake a gender-specific cause for enhanced susceptibility to alcohol-induced liver disease in women? Alcohol Alcohol 2008;43: 9-14.
468. Wall M, Moe E, Eisenberg J, Powers M, Buist N, Buist A. Long-term follow-up of a cohort of children with alpha-1-antitrypsin deficiency. J Pediatr 1990;116:248-51.
469. Wang C, Mo L, Lin R, Kuo J, Chang K. Rapid diagnosis of choledocholithiasis using biochemical tests in patients undergoing laparoscopic cholecystectomy. Hepatogastroenterology 2001;48: 619-21.
470. Wanless I, Lentz J. Fatty liver hepatitis (steatohepatitis) and obesity: an autopsy study with analysis of risk factors. Hepatology 1990;12:1106-10.
471. Wasley A, Samandari T, Bell B. Incidence of hepatitis A in the United States in the era of vaccination. JAMA 2005;294:194-201.
472. Weber B, Melchior W, Gehrke R, Doerr H, Berger A, Rabenau H. Hepatitis B virus markers in anti-HBc only positive individuals. J Med Virol 2001;64:312-9.
473. Wejstal R, Norkrans G, Widell A. Chronic non-A, non-B, non-C hepatitis: is hepatitis G/GBV-C involved? Scand J Gastroenterol 1997;32:1046-51.
474. Welker M, Zeuzem S. Occult hepatitis C: how convincing are the current data? Hepatology 2009;49:665-75.
475. Wells R. Cellular sources of extracellular matrix in hepatic fibrosis. Clin Liver Dis 2008;12:759-68.
476. Wendon J, Lee W. Encephalopathy and cerebral edema in the setting of acute liver failure: pathogenesis and management. Neurocrit Care 2008;9:97-102.
477. Whalley S, Murray J, Brown D, Webster G, Emery V, Dusheiko G, et al. Kinetics of acute hepatitis B virus infection in humans. J Exp Med 2001;193:847-54.
478. Whitehead M, Hawkes N, Hainsworth I, Kingham J. A prospective study of the causes of notably raised aspartate aminotransferase of liver origin. Gut 1999;45:129-33.
479. Wieckowska A, Feldstein A. Diagnosis of nonalcoholic fatty liver disease: invasive versus noninvasive. Semin Liver Dis 2008;28: 386-95.
480. Wiencke K, Spurkland A, Schrumpf E, Boberg K. Primary sclerosing cholangitis is associated to an extended B8-DR3 haplotype including particular MICA and MICB alleles. Hepatology 2001;34:625-30.
481. Wiese M, Berr F, Lafrenz M, Porst H, Oesen U. Low frequency of cirrhosis in a hepatitis C (genotype 1b) single-source outbreak in Germany: a 20-year multicenter study. Hepatology 2000;32:91-6.
482. Wiesner R. Liver transplantation for primary sclerosing cholangitis: timing, outcome, impact of inflammatory bowel disease and recurrence of disease. Best Pract Res Clin Gastroenterol 2001;15: 667-80.
483. Wiesner R, Demetris A, Belle S, Seaberg E, Lake J, Zetterman R, et al. Acute hepatic allograft rejection: incidence, risk factors, and impact on outcome. Hepatology 1998;28:638-45.
484. Wittayalertpanya S, Israsena S, Thamaree S, Tongnopnoua P, Komolmit P. Caffeine clearance by two point analysis: a measure of liver function in chronic liver disease. Tokai J Exp Clin Med 1996;21: 195-201.
485. Witzigmann H, Geissler F, Benedix F, Thiery J, Uhlmann D, Tannapfel A, et al. Prospective evaluation of circulating hepatocytes by alpha-fetoprotein messenger RNA in patients with hepatocellular carcinoma. Surgery 2002;131:34-43.
486. Wong S, Primi D, Kojima H, Sottini A, Giulivi A, Zhang M, et al. Insights into SEN virus prevalence, transmission, and treatment in community-based persons and patients with liver disease referred to a liver disease unit. Clin Infect Dis 2002;35:789-95.
487. Worm H, van der Poel C, Brandstatter G. Hepatitis E: an overview. Microbes Infect 2002;4:657-66.
488. Wu J, Chen T, Huang Y, Yen F, Ting L, Sheng W, et al. Natural history of hepatitis D viral superinfection: significance of viremia detected by polymerase chain reaction. Gastroenterology 1995;108:796-802.
489. Yang H, Lu S, Liaw Y, You S, Sun C, Wang L, et al. Hepatitis B e antigen and the risk of hepatocellular carcinoma. N Engl J Med 2002;347:168-74.
490. Yano M, Kumada H, Kage M, Ikeda K, Shimamatsu K, Inoue O, et al. The long-term pathological evolution of chronic hepatitis C. Hepatology 1996;23:1334-40.
491. Yashina T, Favorov M, Khudyakov Y, Fields H, Znoiko O, Shkurko T, et al. Detection of hepatitis G virus (HGV) RNA: clinical characteristics of acute HGV infection. J Infect Dis 1997;175:1302-7.
492. Yeo W, Johnson P. Diagnosis, prevention and management of hepatitis B virus reactivation during anticancer therapy. Hepatology 2006;43: 209-20.
493. Yokosuka O, Kojima H, Imazeki F, Tagawa M, Saisho H, Tamatsukuri S, et al. Spontaneous negativation of serum hepatitis C virus RNA is a rare event in type C chronic liver diseases: analysis of HCV RNA in 320 patients who were followed for more than 3 years. J Hepatol 1999;31:394-9.
494. Yoshida H, Kato N, Shiratori Y, Shao R, Wang Y, Shiina S, et al. Weak association between SEN virus viremia and liver disease. J Clin Microbiol 2002;40:3140-5.
495. Yuen M, Cheng C, Lauder I, Lam S, Ooi C, Lai C. Early detection of hepatocellular carcinoma increases the chance of treatment: Hong Kong experience. Hepatology 2000;31:330-5.
496. Yuki N, Nagaoka T, Yamashiro M, Mochizuki K, Kaneko A, Yamamoto K, et al. Long-term histologic and virologic outcomes of acute self-limited hepatitis B. Hepatology 2003;37:1172-9.
497. Zakiah I, Zaini A, Jamilah B, Zawiah A. Alpha-1-antitrypsin deficiency in babies with prolonged jaundice. Malays J Pathol 1992;14:91-4.
498. Zaman S, Johnson P, Williams R. Silent cirrhosis in patients with hepatocellular carcinoma: implications for screening in high-incidence and low-incidence areas. Cancer 1990;65:1607-10.
499. Zanger U, Hauri H, Loeper J, Homberg J, Meyer U. Antibodies against human cytochrome P-450db1 in autoimmune hepatitis type II. Proc Natl Acad Sci U S A 1988;85:8256-60.
500. Zarski J, Bohn B, Bastie A, Pawlotsky J, Baud M, Bost-Bezeaux F, et al. Characteristics of patients with dual infection by hepatitis B and C viruses. J Hepatol 1998;28:27-33.
501. Zhou S, Gordon R, Bradbury M, Stump D, Kiang C, Berk P. Ethanol up-regulates fatty acid uptake and plasma membrane expression and export of mitochondrial aspartate aminotransferase in HepG2 cells. Hepatology 1998;27:1064-74.
502. Ziebell J, Shaw-Stiffel T. Update on the use of metabolic probes to quantify liver function: caffeine versus lidocaine. Dig Dis 1995;13: 239-50.
503. Zimmerman H. Intrahepatic cholestasis. Arch Intern Med 1979;139: 1038-45.
504. Zimmerman H. Hepatotoxicology: the adverse effects of drugs and other chemicals on the liver, 2nd edition. Philadelphia, Pa: JB Lippincott, 1999.
505. Zimmerman H. Drug-induced liver disease. Clin Liver Dis 2000;4: 73-96.
506. Zimmerman H, Lewis J. Drug-induced cholestasis. Med Toxicol 1987; 2:112-60.
507. Zoulim F, Mimms L, Floreani M, Pichoud C, Chemin I, Kay A, et al. New assays for quantitative determination of viral markers in management of chronic hepatitis B virus infection. J Clin Microbiol 1992;30:1111-9.

CHAPTER 51

Gastric, Pancreatic, and Intestinal Function

Peter G. Hill, B.Sc., Ph.D., F.R.C.Path., Dip.Hlth.Mgt.*

The stomach, intestinal tract, and pancreas are closely related, both anatomically and functionally, and symptoms, such as diarrhea or malabsorption, may be associated with diseases or disorders of any of these organs. It is therefore appropriate to discuss them together. Advances in imaging techniques and improvements in endoscopic procedures have led to enormous changes in the investigation of gastrointestinal (GI) and pancreatic function so that many laboratory tests, once considered important, have now been superseded.

In this chapter, the anatomy and physiology of the GI tract, and the normal processes of digestion and absorption, are briefly reviewed. Disorders of the stomach, pancreas, and intestine associated with malabsorption or diarrhea, in which the laboratory can play a role in diagnosis and monitoring, are discussed. The chapter concludes with an overview of GI regulatory peptides and neuroendocrine tumors in which GI symptoms are prominent, and with two sections that present more integrated approaches to the problems of investigating malabsorption and diarrhea.

INTRODUCTION TO ANATOMY AND PHYSIOLOGY OF THE GASTROINTESTINAL TRACT[176]

The major organs of the GI tract include the stomach, the small and large intestines, the pancreas, and the gallbladder, all of which are involved in the digestive processes that commence with the ingestion of food and water and culminate in the excretion of feces.

Anatomy

The GI tract is a tube, 8 meters in length, beginning with the mouth and ending with the anus. The esophagus, which is about 25 cm in length, is a muscular tube connecting the pharynx to the stomach. For this chapter, the key organs are the stomach, intestines, and pancreas.

Stomach[152]

The stomach consists of three major zones: the cardiac zone, the body, and the pyloric zone (Figure 51-1). The upper cardiac zone, which includes the fundus, contains mucus-secreting surface epithelial cells, which also secrete group II pepsinogens and several types of endocrine secreting cells. The body of the stomach contains cells or cell groups of many different types: (1) surface epithelial cells, which secrete mucus; (2) parietal (oxyntic) cells, which secrete hydrochloric acid and intrinsic factor; (3) the chief, zymogen, or peptic cells, which secrete group I and II pepsinogens; (4) enterochromaffin cells, which secrete serotonin; and (5) several types of endocrine secreting cells. The pyloric zone is subdivided into the antrum (which is approximately the distal third of the stomach), the pyloric canal, and the sphincter. The cells of the pyloric zone secrete mucus, group II pepsinogens, serotonin, gastrin, and several other hormones but no hydrochloric acid.

Small Intestine

In the stomach, food is converted into a semifluid, homogeneous, gruel-like material (chyme) that passes through the pyloric sphincter into the small intestine. The small intestine consists of three parts: the duodenum, jejunum, and ileum. In the adult human, the small intestine is approximately 6 m long and decreases in cross-section as it proceeds distally. The duodenum is about 25 cm long and is the shortest and widest part of the small intestine. The jejunum and ileum make up the remainder of the small intestine. There is no clear demarcation, but the ileum is the distal 3.5 m.

The wall of the small intestine consists of four layers: mucous, submucous, muscular, and serous. The internal surface of the upper small intestine contains valvelike circular folds (valvulae conniventes or plicae circulares) that project 3 to 10 mm into the lumen of the intestine. Covering the entire mucous surface of the small intestine are very small (1 mm) finger-like projections (villi), giving it a "velvety"

*The author gratefully acknowledges the original contributions of Drs. A. Ralph Henderson and Alan D. Rinker, upon which a portion of this chapter is based.

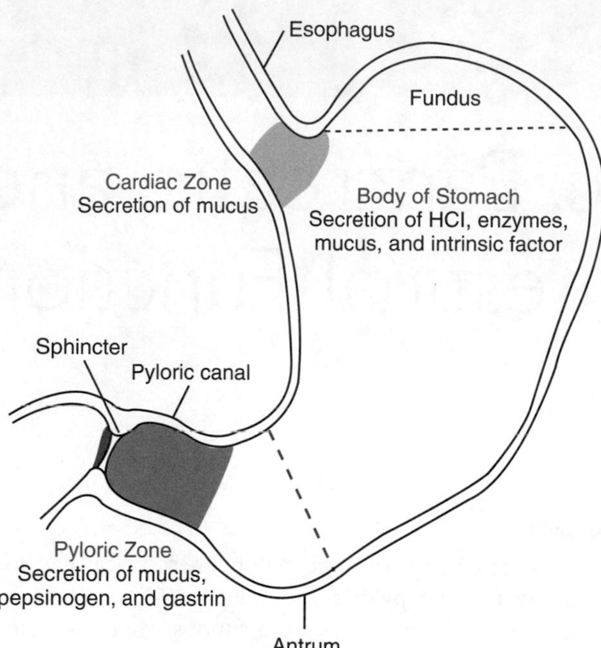

Figure 51-1 Schematic drawing of the stomach, with major zones.

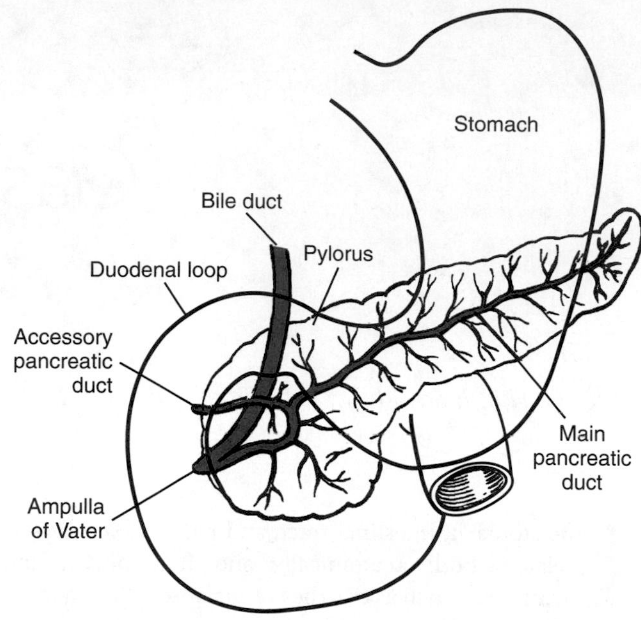

Figure 51-2 Cross-section through the pancreas.

appearance. The luminal surface (brush border) of each epithelial cell consists of some 1700 microvilli projecting about 1 μm from the cell. The folds, villi, and microvilli together present an absorptive surface some 600 times greater than would be inferred from the length and diameter of this portion of the gut. The absorptive surface area of the small intestine is estimated to be about 250 m^2,[73] which is comparable with the area of a doubles tennis court.

Large Intestine

The large intestine is about 1.5 m in length, extending from the ileum to the anus, and includes the cecum, appendix, colon, rectum, and anal canal. The cecum is a blind pouch that begins the large intestine; it is connected to the terminal ileum via the ileocecal sphincter. The appendix is a "worm-shaped" tube connected to the blind end of the cecum. The colon is about 1 m long and is divided into the ascending, transverse, descending, and sigmoid sections. The sigmoid colon connects to the rectum, which is approximately 15 cm long. The rectum in turn connects to the anal canal—the terminal end of the large intestine.

Pancreas

The pancreas is 12 to 15 cm in length and lies across the posterior wall of the abdominal cavity. The head is located in the duodenal curve; the body and tail are directed toward the left, extending to the spleen (Figure 51-2). Pancreatic digestive enzymes, in bicarbonate-rich juice, enter the duodenum through the ampulla of Vater and the sphincter of Oddi and mix with the food bolus as it passes through the small bowel.

Phases of Digestion

The process of digestion can be conveniently subdivided into neurogenic, gastric, and intestinal phases.

Neurogenic Phase

The neurogenic or cephalic phase is initiated by the intake of food into the mouth; the sight, smell, and taste of food stimulate the cerebral cortex and subsequently the vagal nuclei. The process is chemically mediated by acetylcholine from postganglionic parasympathetic nerve endings, which acts on gastric parietal cells. The vagus also stimulates gastric chief and parietal (oxyntic) cells to secrete pepsinogen and hydrochloric acid. [Cutting of the vagus nerve (vagotomy) decreases the volume and acidity of gastric secretion.]

The mechanism of acid secretion is still widely debated; there is, however, significant agreement that acetylcholine, histamine, and gastrin act through their respective neurocrine, paracrine, and endocrine pathways to stimulate the parietal cells, and that specific parietal cell receptors to these transmitters exist. Also, potentiating interactions between the mentioned secretagogues probably occur at the parietal cell itself. Histamine has a role as a mediator or a potentiator of the actions of other secretagogues. Administration of histamine markedly increases the secretion provoked by pentagastrin or by cholinergic agonists. Histamine H_2-receptor antagonists inhibit acid secretion provoked by most types of stimulation, confirming the important role of histamine in acid secretion.

The parietal cell undergoes marked changes when acid secretion is stimulated. The tubulovesicular membranes, prominent in the resting cell, diminish, whereas a marked increase in the apical plasma membrane (the secretory surface of the cell) is noted, together with the appearance of long apical microvilli.

Cimetidine (Tagamet) and other H_2-receptor antagonists [such as ranitidine (Zantac) and famotidine (Pepcid)] block both the morphologic changes of the parietal cell and H^+ secretion. Proton pump inhibitors (PPIs) have a different mechanism of action. Omeprazole (a PPI) is taken up by the parietal cell and is converted to an active metabolite that inactivates the parietal H^+,K^+-ATPase. H^+ secretion is inhibited until new ATPase is synthesized, which takes at least 24 hours.

The secretion of H^+ against a million-fold concentration gradient requires energy from the cell, and this process is coupled to H^+,K^+-ATPase. Histamine-stimulated acid secretion involves cyclic adenosine monophosphate (cAMP); cholinergic stimulation is not associated with increases in intracellular cAMP in isolated parietal cells, and this process may be mediated by changes in permeability of the cell's plasma membrane to Ca^{2+}. The latter activates a chain of events that alter cell function in various ways. In addition to the previously mentioned mechanisms, vagal fibers to the pyloric glandular mucosa cause the release of gastrin, which also stimulates hydrochloric acid and pepsinogen secretion.

Agents that inhibit acid secretion include somatostatin, prostaglandins, gastric inhibitory polypeptide (GIP), secretin, glucagon, vasoactive intestinal polypeptide (VIP), neurotensin, calcitonin gene-related peptide, corticotropin-releasing factor, thyrotropin-releasing hormone, peptide YY, dopamine, and serotonin. Acid secretion is decreased in the presence of decreased quantities of circulating pituitary, adrenal, thyroid, and parathyroid hormones. Pituitary hormones are apparently essential for maintenance of the structural integrity of the gastric mucosa and are necessary for secretory function; human growth hormone may be necessary for growth of the gastric mucosa.

Gastric Phase

When food enters the stomach, the resulting distention initiates the gastric phase of digestion, mediated by local and vagal reflexes. Hydrochloric acid release is caused by (1) direct vagal stimulation of the parietal cells; (2) local distention of the antrum and vagal stimulation of antral cells to secrete gastrin, which causes hydrochloric acid release from parietal cells; and (3) release of gastrin, stimulated by the near neutralization (pH 5 to 7) of gastric hydrochloric acid by ingested food entering the pyloric zone. Gastrin also stimulates antral motility, secretion of pepsinogens and of pancreatic fluid rich in enzymes, and release of a number of GI hormones (secretin, insulin, acetylcholine, somatostatin, and pancreatic polypeptide; for further information on GI hormones, see the later section of this chapter, "GI Regulatory Peptides"). As a result of the acid environment, pepsinogen is rapidly converted to the active proteolytic enzyme, pepsin. Food is mixed by contractions of the stomach and is partially degraded into chyme by the chemical secretions of the stomach. The pylorus plays a role in emptying chyme into the duodenum by virtue of its strong musculature.

Intestinal Phase

The intestinal phase of digestion begins when the weakly acidic digestive products of proteins and lipids enter the duodenum. Many GI hormones and other regulatory peptides are released by both neural and local stimulation and act within the GI tract to regulate digestion and absorption. These are described in greater detail in the section, "GI Regulatory Peptides." Digestion, absorption, and storage functions are stimulated or inhibited by different hormones, creating an intricate hormonal control system that regulates the action of intestinal hormones and provides for secretion of bile acids, bicarbonate, and numerous enzymes involved in the digestion of food. In this system, the intestinal hormones secretin and VIP, for example, inhibit gastrin release and decrease the secretion of hydrochloric acid and pepsinogen; cholecystokinin (CCK; see discussion later in this chapter) binds to gastrin receptors and thus also decreases hydrochloric acid secretion. Somatostatin inhibits gastrin, secretin, CCK, and other hormones.

During the intestinal phase, carbohydrates, proteins, and fats are broken down and absorbed as described in the next section. Most nutrients, including vitamins and minerals, have been absorbed by the time the food passes from the jejunum and ileum into the large bowel. In the large intestine, water is actively absorbed, electrolyte balance is regulated, and bacterial actions take place. These processes result in the formation of feces.

PROCESSES OF DIGESTION AND ABSORPTION[52]

The total quantity of fluid absorbed each day by the gut is estimated to be about 9 L, which is composed of 2 L oral intake, 1.5 L saliva, 2.5 L gastric juice, 0.5 L bile, 1.5 L pancreatic juice, and 1 L intestinal secretions. More than 90% of this fluid is absorbed in the small intestine. The maximal absorptive capacity for fluid is probably at least 20 L. Several hundred grams of carbohydrates, about 100 g of fat, and 50 to 100 g of amino acids are absorbed daily in the small gut, but maximal absorptive capacity is believed to be at least 10 times greater. This considerable reserve capacity may compensate for mild to moderate degrees of dysfunction induced by disease processes, at least in the early phases. The efficiency of absorption is due to the unique features of the absorptive surface of the bowel and the relationship of the epithelial cells to the underlying rich vascular plexus and the lymphatic vessels.

Digestion of ingested food takes place both within the lumen of the small intestine and at the mucosal (brush border) surface. Defects of digestion may occur at one or more stages in the process. The terms *maldigestion* and *malabsorption* refer to different functional abnormalities. *Maldigestion* is a dysfunction of the digestive process that may occur at various sites in the GI tract. For example, hypoacidity in the stomach will reduce peptic digestion of protein; hyperacidity of the duodenum (e.g., due to overproduction of gastrin by tumor in the Zollinger-Ellison syndrome) can inactivate pancreatic enzymes; loss of brush border enzymes in the small intestine, because of any of a variety of processes, can prevent oligosaccharides and disaccharides from being further hydrolyzed; pancreatic insufficiency will reduce intraluminal enzyme activity in the small gut, causing maldigestion of fats and proteins. By contrast, *malabsorption* is strictly a dysfunction of the absorptive process in the small gut due to loss of absorptive epithelial cells caused, for example, by gluten, inflammation, infection, surgical resection, and infiltration. Various transport defects also lead to malabsorption of specific substances (e.g., glucose-galactose malabsorption or zinc deficiency in the congenital disorder acrodermatitis enteropathica). In clinical practice, however, the term *malabsorption* is often used to encompass all aspects of impaired digestion and absorption. As Figure 51-3 shows, absorption of the different nutrients proceeds at different rates and at different sites within the small bowel.

In the following three sections, the digestion and absorption of fats, carbohydrates, and proteins will be discussed separately. It must be remembered, however, that a complex interplay takes place among nutrients, regulatory peptides, enzymes, gallbladder and pancreatic function, and bowel motility, leading to an integrated absorptive process that commences with the ingestion of food and culminates in the excretion of feces.

Digestion and Absorption of Carbohydrates

After the action of salivary and pancreatic α-amylases on dietary starch and glycogen, the carbohydrate content of the small intestine consists of newly formed maltose; ingested monosaccharides; dietary disaccharides, such as lactose, sucrose, maltose, and trehalose; oligosaccharides, such as dextrins and maltotriose; and indigestible oligosaccharides and polysaccharides, such as cellulose, agar, and other oligosaccharide dietary fibers.

The brush border enzymes with disaccharidase and oligosaccharidase activity are listed in Table 51-1. The sucrase-isomaltase complex comprises most of the sucrase, isomaltase, and maltase (80%) activity of the small intestine. It hydrolyzes sucrose to its constituent monosaccharides, cleaves glucose

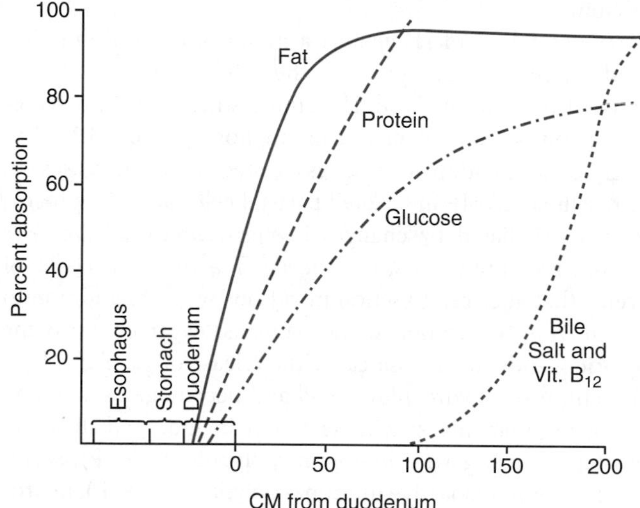

Figure 51-3 The location of small intestinal absorption. *(Modified from Morris JA, Selivanov V, Sheldon GF. Nutritional management of patients with malabsorption syndrome. Clin Gastroenterol 1983;12;463-74, based on Borgstrom B, et al. Studies of intestinal digestion and absorption in the human. J Clin Invest 1957;36:1521-36.)*

TABLE 51-1 Brush Border Oligosaccharidases

Enzyme or Complex	Principal Substrate(s)	Products
β-Glycosidase Complex		
Lactase (EC 3.2.1.23)	Lactose	Glucose + galactose
Glycosylceramidase (EC 3.2.1.45-46) [also called phlorizin hydrolase (EC 3.2.1.62)]	Galactosyl and glucosyl-β-ceramides	Galactose/glucose + ceramides
Sucrase-Isomaltase Complex		
Sucrase-(maltase) (EC 3.2.1.48)	Maltose/sucrose	Glucose/fructose + glucose
Isomaltase-(maltase) (EC 3.2.1.10)	1,6-α-linkages in isomaltose and α-dextrins	Glucose
	Maltose	Glucose
Trehalase (EC 3.2.1.28)	Trehalose	Glucose
Glucoamylase Complex (EC 3.2.1.20)		
Glucoamylase-(maltase)-1 and glucoamylase-(maltase)-2 (have similar substrate specificities)	1,4-α-linkages at nonreducing ends of amylose, amylopectin, glycogen, and straight chain 1,4-α-glucopyranosyl oligomers, including maltose	Glucose

From Semenza G, Auricchio S, Mantei N. Small-intestinal disaccharidases. In: Scriver CR, Beaudet AL, Sly WS, Valle D, eds. The metabolic and molecular bases of inherited disease, 8th edition. New York, NY: McGraw-Hill, 2001:1623-50.

from α-limit dextrins with 1,6 bonds, and hydrolyzes maltose. The activity of the complex is fourfold to fivefold greater in the jejunum than in the ileum. Changes in diet have a marked effect on the expression of the complex; starvation leads to a rapid decline in activity, which is rapidly restored on refeeding. All small intestinal saccharidases may decrease with infection or inflammation of the small bowel to the extent that carbohydrate malabsorption occurs, leading to diarrhea, flatulence, and weight loss. Paradoxically, diabetes mellitus causes a striking increase in sucrase-isomaltase activity; an increase is also observed in monosaccharide and amino acid transport. The lactase–phlorizin hydrolase complex is the only brush border enzyme able to hydrolyze lactose and therefore is essential for the survival of mammals early in life.

This complex also has glycosylceramidase, β-glycosidase, and phlorizin hydrolase activities. Infectious and inflammatory diseases greatly reduce lactase–phlorizin hydrolase activity, leading to symptomatic intolerance to milk. Recovery of enzyme activity following intestinal disease may be slow. The activity of the complex is resistant to starvation. The developmental regulation of lactase is discussed later in the section on disaccharidase deficiencies. Also present in the brush border is the α-glucosidase maltase-glucoamylase, which removes individual glucose molecules from the nonreducing end of α(1,4) oligosaccharides and disaccharides. This enzyme accounts for about 20% of the total maltase activity of the small intestine. Trehalase is also found in the brush border of the small intestine and hydrolyzes trehalose, an α(1,1) disaccharide of glucose found in yeast and mushrooms. The developmental pattern of trehalase appears to follow that of sucrase-isomaltase.

In addition to their actions on disaccharides, the brush border enzymes further hydrolyze the products of amylase action, including maltose, maltotriose, and α-limit dextrins. The brush border enzymes appear to act in an integrated manner in that a flow of substrate occurs from glucoamylase and isomaltase to sucrase producing the monosaccharides glucose, galactose, and fructose. These monosaccharides are transported into the enterocyte by facilitative transport systems, such as the Na^+-dependent glucose (and galactose) transporter (SGLT1) and GLUT5 (one of the GLUT family of monosaccharide transporters), which transports fructose across the apical membrane of the enterocyte. Subsequently, absorbed glucose and fructose are transported across the basolateral membrane and out of the enterocyte and into the portal system by the GLUT2 transporter.

It is increasingly being realized that the limiting factor in carbohydrate digestion and absorption may be diffusion from the intestinal lumen to the membrane surface where the enzymes are localized. Normally, little disaccharidase activity is seen in the luminal contents. For most oligosaccharides (with the exception of lactose), hydrolysis is rapid, and transport is the rate-limiting step in reducing the concentration of monosaccharides and the osmotic load in the gut. When the transport system is operating at its maximum rate but monosaccharide concentration is still high, inhibition of hydrolases by their monosaccharide products (i.e., product inhibition) slows hydrolytic activity, keeping monosaccharide concentrations relatively constant, thereby controlling osmotic load and water concentration in the gut. The importance of this control is evident from the consequences of intestinal disorders in which ingested disaccharide is not split and absorbed, leading to increased fluid secretion into the gut and increased intestinal motility. Enteric bacteria ferment the unabsorbed sugars, producing hydrogen, carbon dioxide, and organic acids causing abdominal discomfort such as bloating, distention and cramping. Absorption of fermentation products may lead to metabolic acidosis. In the large bowel, the presence of CO_2 and organic acids decreases pH and keeps the osmolality high, so that water reabsorption is decreased. The result is an acidic, liquid stool. Normally, however, accumulation of monosaccharide products does not occur, because the transport system is sufficiently fast to remove them. Mucosal lactase activity is the lowest of all the disaccharidases; for lactose, the rate-limiting step in absorption is thought to be hydrolysis. Lactase activity is not increased by feeding large amounts of lactose, as is the case for maltase and sucrase. Lactase, maltase, and sucrase all show circadian rhythms in their activities; minimum and maximum activities may vary by a factor of 2.

Carbohydrate digestion is not always complete in the small intestine. Indeed, it is likely that some starch and sucrose normally pass undigested and unabsorbed into the colon. It has been estimated that colonic bacteria require 70 g of carbohydrate/d. Much of this is derived from endogenous sources, such as from glycoproteins in GI secretions, with the remainder coming from unabsorbed dietary carbohydrate and dietary fiber. Up to 15% of the carbohydrate from white bread reaches the colon, and the effects of indigestible oligosaccharides upon reaching the large bowel are well known. As was pointed out earlier, bacterial action creates short chain fatty acids, which are rapidly absorbed by the colonic mucosa and are thought to provide fuel for the colonocyte. Starch and oligosaccharides are osmotically active and draw water into the gut. The colon, however, can absorb up to four times the normal colonic water load; for this reason, diarrhea is not always present in oligosaccharide malabsorption.

Digestion and Absorption of Lipids

The recommended daily dietary fat intake in Europe and North America is 70 to 95 g. Less than 5 g/24 h is recovered in the feces, indicating the overall efficiency of the normal processes of fat digestion and absorption. Most dietary fat is in the form of long chain triacylglycerols (triglycerides). Pancreatic lipase is quantitatively the most important hydrolytic enzyme, but the contribution of gastric lipase to overall hydrolysis should not be underestimated. Gastric lipase is secreted by the gastric mucosa and normally accounts for up to 17.5% of fatty acids released from triglycerides following a meal.[18] The enzyme has a wide pH optimum and is active in both the stomach and the duodenum. This nonpancreatic lipase may have a significant role in lipid digestion when pancreatic function is impaired and in the neonatal period before pancreatic lipase activity is fully developed. A lingual lipase is also present, secreted by the tongue, but is thought not to be of much significance normally in humans. Fats first are emulsified in the stomach by its churning action and are stabilized by interaction with luminal lecithin and protein fragments. The lingual and gastric lipases do not require bile salts or cofactors to function; they have a pH optimum of 3 to 6, and their action produces 1,2-diacylglycerols and fatty acids. These products further stabilize the surface of the triglyceride emulsion and in the duodenum promote the binding of pancreatic colipase. In addition, the liberated fatty acids stimulate release of CCK from the duodenal mucosa.

Pancreatic lipase, in the presence of bile salts and colipase, acts at the oil-water interface of the triglyceride emulsion to produce fatty acids and 2-monoacylglycerols. Colipase is secreted in pancreatic juice as an inactive proenzyme, which is converted to the active form by trypsin. Other significant enzymes involved in the breakdown of fats within the intestinal lumen are cholesterol ester hydrolase, phospholipase A2, and a nonspecific bile salt–activated lipase.

Only a small proportion of ingested triacylglycerol is completely hydrolyzed to glycerol and fatty acids. These products form micelles with bile salts and lysophosphoglycerides; the micelles convey the nonpolar lipid molecules from the lumen to the epithelial cell surface and dissociate there to produce a high concentration of monoacylglycerols, lysophosphoglycerides, and fatty acids, which are absorbed into the mucosal cell. Absorption involves both passive and active transport processes and is facilitated by a fatty acid–binding protein in the cytosol of the cell that has a high affinity for fatty acids. Within the cell, triacylglycerols are resynthesized from the absorbed 2-monoacylglycerols and fatty acids. The triacylglycerols, together with phospholipids, cholesterol and its esters, fat-soluble vitamins, and a specific apolipoprotein, are formed into chylomicrons, which are then released by exocytosis into the lymphatic system of the small bowel. The absorption of long chain fatty acids is facilitated by transmembrane fatty acid transport proteins.

From the lymphatics, chylomicrons enter the bloodstream via the thoracic duct and are distributed to the liver, adipose tissue, and other organs. Medium and short chain fatty acids (chain length <12 carbon atoms) in mixed triglycerides are preferentially split by lipases and pass into the aqueous phase, from which they are rapidly absorbed. Medium chain triglycerides can be absorbed without complete lipolysis and in the absence of bile. They do not require micellar solubilization and are transported from the intestinal epithelial cells predominantly via the hepatic portal vein. Figure 51-4 summarizes the processes involved in fat absorption and conditions that compromise the efficiency of one or more stages in the process of fat digestion and absorption leading to fat malabsorption.[24]

Digestion and Absorption of Proteins

Average daily dietary intake of protein in North America is about 100 g compared with an estimated requirement for adults of 50 to 70 g. Another 50 to 60 g of protein enters the intestinal tract daily in GI secretions and from desquamated mucosal cells. Normal daily fecal loss of protein is about 10 g.

Protein digestion is initiated in the stomach by the action of pepsin in a highly acid medium. The acidity also denatures the protein, unfolding the polypeptide chains for better access by the gastric, pancreatic, and intestinal proteolytic enzymes. The polypeptides and amino acids produced in the stomach

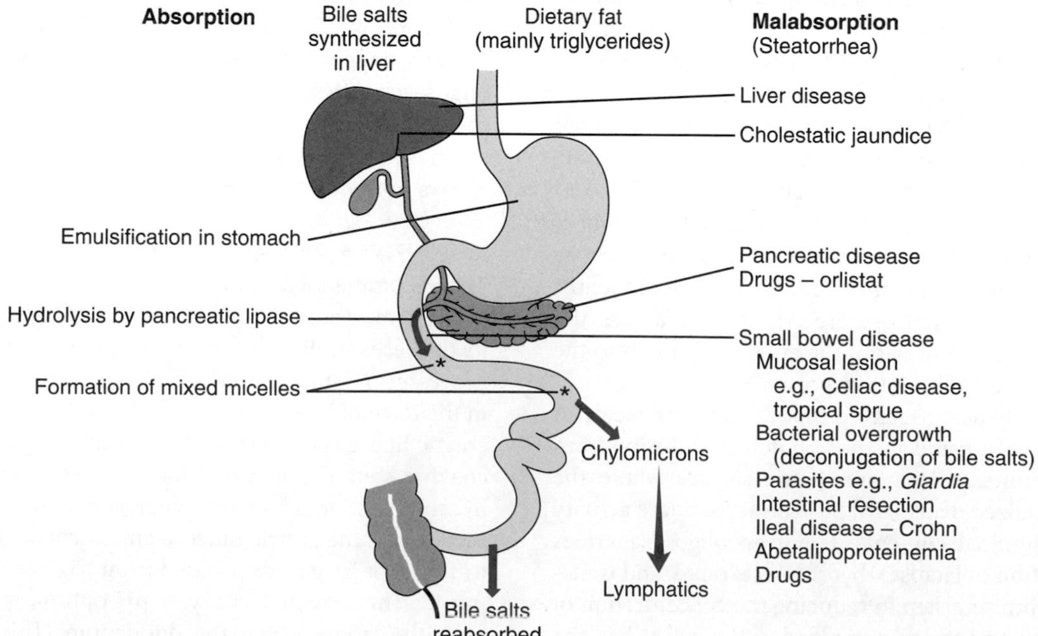

Figure 51-4 Summary of the processes involved in fat absorption and malabsorption. *(From Clark ML, Silk DB. Gastrointestinal disease. In: Kumar P, Clark M, eds. Clinical medicine, 6th edition. Edinburgh: WB Saunders, 2005:265-345.)*

by the action of pepsin are potent secretagogues for hormones that stimulate the pancreas and intestine. Stimulated pancreatic secretion contains proenzyme forms of the proteolytic enzymes trypsin, chymotrypsin, elastase, exopeptidases, and carboxypeptidases. Proteolytic enzymes may be endopeptidases (e.g., pepsin, trypsin, chymotrypsin, elastase), which hydrolyze peptide bonds within the polypeptide chain, or exopeptidases, which hydrolyze peptide bonds of the terminal amino acids (enzymes such as carboxypeptidase and aminopeptidase). Stimulation of the intestine by GI hormones liberates several proteolytic enzymes from the brush border. One of them, enterokinase, selectively cleaves a hexapeptide from the *N*-terminus of trypsinogen to form trypsin. Trypsin then activates more trypsin (autocatalysis) and also converts other pancreatic proenzymes into their active forms. The action of the pancreatic enzymes on partially digested proteins within the lumen produces peptides that are 2 to 6 amino acid residues in length, as well as single amino acids. The peptides are largely hydrolyzed to single amino acids by the aminopeptidases and dipeptidases of the brush border before absorption, although some dipeptides and tripeptides are absorbed and are hydrolyzed to amino acids by cytosolic peptidases within the enterocytes. Multiple carrier systems with overlapping specificities for the 20 amino acids are involved in the transport of amino acids into the cells. Absorption of amino acids by these transport systems is faster in the jejunum than in the ileum. The amino acids pass across the enterocyte basolateral membrane by passive diffusion and by active transport systems, which are distinct from those at the brush border membrane. The underlying rich vascular plexus is drained by the portal circulation, and it is by this route that absorbed amino acids reach the liver and then the systemic circulation.

Individuals with achlorhydria or total gastrectomy have normal protein digestion and absorption because small intestinal function compensates for the lack of pepsin activity. Pancreatic and small intestinal diseases are the major causes of protein maldigestion and malabsorption. However, fecal loss of protein rarely becomes significant in pancreatic insufficiency until trypsin levels fall to about 10% of normal. Two rare disorders, trypsin deficiency and enterokinase deficiency, have far-reaching effects on the efficiency of protein digestion, as would be expected from their roles in the activation of proteolytic proenzymes. Mucosal diseases may affect protein assimilation through a number of mechanisms. Reduction in the number of mucosal cells decreases peptidase activity in the intestine and intestinal absorptive capacity for amino acids. Disease may increase the turnover of intestinal cells and the rate of desquamation. This cell loss, together with increased losses of plasma proteins from the damaged intestinal surface, can cause a negative nitrogen balance. Surgical resection of the intestine not only reduces the total intestinal absorptive surface but also may remove a segment of the gut that is specialized for absorption of certain nutrients (e.g., resection of the distal ileum removes the active transport system for the vitamin B_{12}–intrinsic factor complex). Resection may also alter intestinal motility, leading to stasis and bacterial overgrowth that can intensify a negative nitrogen balance. Also, rare hereditary defects in amino acid transporters (e.g., Hartnup's disease) may produce distinct syndromes.

STOMACH: DISEASES AND LABORATORY INVESTIGATIONS

Growth in endoscopic procedures, with direct visualization of the interior of the stomach, has largely removed the need for the clinical laboratory to carry out analysis of gastric contents. Situations remain, however, in which the laboratory continues to play a significant role in diagnosing gastric diseases and in monitoring the effectiveness of treatment. This section describes peptic ulcer disease, tests for *Helicobacter pylori (H. pylori),* and measurement of basal acid output from the stomach.

Peptic Ulcer Disease and *Helicobacter pylori*[64,123,158,180]

Although the presence of spiral-shaped organisms in the stomach has been acknowledged for many years, it was only in 1985 that the association was described between *H. pylori* (known then as *Campylobacter pylori*) and peptic ulcer disease.[125] Most estimates suggest that the bacterium is present in the mucous layer of the stomach in half the population of the world. In Europe, 30 to 50% of adults, and in the United States, at least 20% of the adult population, are infected with the organism. In all cases, colonization with *H. pylori* causes a chronic inflammatory reaction in the gastric mucosa even when direct endoscopic observation of the mucosa appears normal. Carriers of the organism are at increased risk for gastric cancer (twofold to tenfold) and peptic ulcer (threefold to tenfold).[12] Some of this increased risk is due to infection with strains of the organism that produce the cytotoxic CagA protein. About 90% of gastric cancer patients are infected with *H. pylori,* compared with 40 to 60% of age-matched controls.[141,142] In a European study comparing the prevalence of *H. pylori* versus gastric cancer rates in 13 countries, a significant correlation was observed between infection rate and gastric cancer incidence and mortality.[175] It is, however, important to remember that although a large proportion of gastric cancer can be attributed to infection with *H. pylori,* only in a minority of infected subjects will the inflammatory reaction progress to gastric cancer. Gastric cancer rates in Western countries have declined in recent decades, but the incidence remains high in less developed countries.

At least 95% of patients with duodenal ulcer disease are infected with *H. pylori,* and eradication of the organism leads to healing of the ulcer and a reduction in relapse rates.[147] Eradication of *H. pylori* is now the recommended treatment for patients with duodenal or gastric ulcer who are *H. pylori*–positive. Effective combined antibiotic and acid suppression regimens (using PPIs) are available with eradication rates of up to 90% after first-line treatment.[64] However, increases in the prevalence of antibiotic resistance have led to the development of alternative treatment regimes to maintain high eradication rates.[122A]

H. pylori infection predominantly affects the gastric mucosa, with the antrum usually the most densely colonized area. The reasons why a gastric mucosal infection predisposes to duodenal ulceration are complex and involve several pathways leading to increased acid production. Before there was an awareness of the role of *H. pylori* in the pathogenesis of peptic ulcer disease, vagotomy (surgical sectioning, or cutting, of the vagus nerve) was the mainstay of treatment as a means of reducing gastric acid output, thereby leading to an environment more conducive to healing of the ulcer.

Infection with the organism, with or without duodenal ulceration, leads to increases in both basal and meal-stimulated serum gastrin concentrations, principally due to an increase in gastrin-17.[134] Basal acid output is increased in *H. pylori*–positive subjects (Figure 51-5) and resolves completely after successful eradication of the organism. Hypergastrinemia is believed to be only one of the mechanisms leading to increased acid output. Studies using the neuropeptide gastrin-releasing peptide (GRP) suggest that impairment of inhibitory control mechanisms that regulate acid production may be responsible for the increased acid output associated with *H. pylori* infection.[49] In addition to stimulating G cells of the antrum to release gastrin, which leads to acid secretion by parietal cells, GRP activates neuroendocrine pathways that inhibit gastric acid secretion—an effect that is mediated via peptides (including cholecystokinin and secretin) that stimulate release of the inhibitory peptide somatostatin from the gastric mucosa.

H. pylori produces urease, and hydrolysis of endogenous urea to bicarbonate and ammonia may create a more hospitable microenvironment for survival of the organism in the stomach. Mammalian cells do not hydrolyze urea, and it was only in 1984 that "gastric urease" was associated with the presence of *H. pylori*.[110] The ability of the organism to rapidly hydrolyze urea is the basis of urea breath tests and of direct urease tests on gastric biopsy samples.

Diagnostic Tests for *H. pylori*

Numerous invasive and noninvasive diagnostic tests for *H. pylori* have been described (Box 51-1), and many have been reviewed.[68]

All tests in the "invasive" group necessitate oral gastroduodenoscopy with biopsy of the gastric mucosa; false-negative results may occur as the result of sampling errors, as colonization may be patchy. The antrum is the preferred biopsy site, but multiple biopsies from the anterior and posterior walls of the antrum and the body of the stomach are recommended for maximum diagnostic accuracy of this group of tests. False negatives may also occur when biopsy specimens are taken during treatment with PPIs or within 2 weeks of stopping PPI therapy. These drugs alter the intragastric distribution of *H. pylori* and suppress its activity.[118] During PPI therapy, biopsies

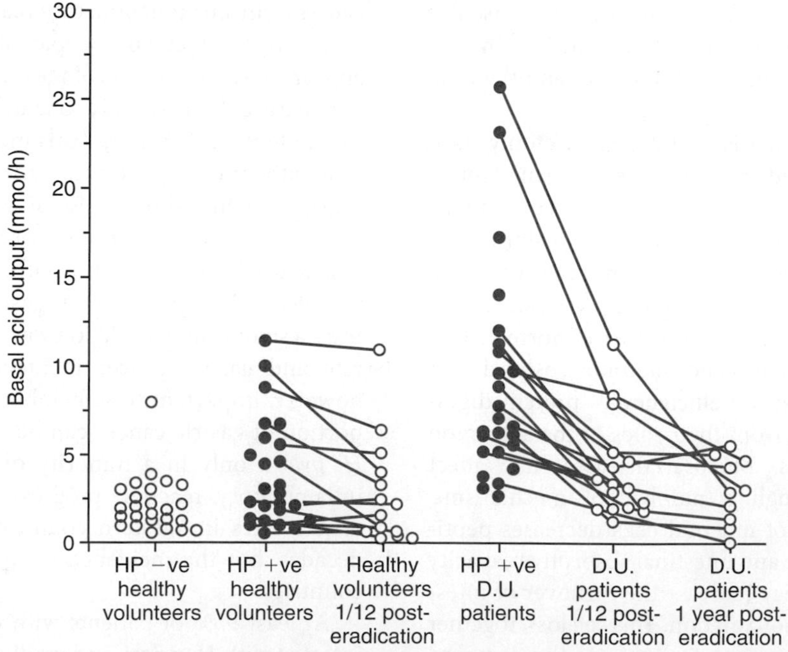

Figure 51-5 Basal acid output in healthy volunteers and patients with duodenal ulcers (DUs) of varying *Helicobacter pylori* status (•, *H. pylori* positive). Compared with *H. pylori*–negative healthy volunteers, basal acid output is increased in *H. pylori*–positive healthy volunteers ($P < 0.05$), *H. pylori*–positive patients with DU ($P < 0.0001$), and patients with DU 1 month after eradication ($P < 0.01$). *(From El-Omar EM, Penman ID, Ardill JES, Chittajallu RS, Howie C, McColl KE.* **H. pylori** *infection and abnormalities of acid secretion in patients with duodenal ulcer disease. Gastroenterology 1995;109:681-91, with permission from the American Gastroenterological Association.)*

BOX 51-1 Diagnostic Tests for *Helicobacter pylori*

Invasive Tests—Using Gastric Mucosal Biopsy Samples
Histology: microscopy after Giemsa or silver staining
Histology: microscopy after immunohistochemical staining
Direct urease test: biopsy incubated in urea/indicator solution; visual end point
Culture: incubation on suitable media for 4 to 10 days
Polymerase chain reaction: amplification of specific DNA sequences

Noninvasive Tests—Using Breath, Blood, Saliva, or Feces
Breath tests: rise in breath $^{14}CO_2$ or $^{13}CO_2$ after ingestion of ^{14}C- or ^{13}C-labeled urea
Serum tests: laboratory measurement of specific immunoglobulin (Ig)G antibody
Whole blood tests: point-of-care tests for specific IgG antibody
Saliva tests: detection of specific IgG antibody
Fecal tests: detection of specific antigen

should be taken from the body and fundus to prevent false negatives. PPIs can also lead to falsely negative urea breath test results. If PPIs cannot be withheld for at least 2 weeks before a breath test, a negative result must be interpreted with caution. Histamine H_2-receptor antagonists should be stopped at least 24 hours before a breath test. Antacids do not affect the test results.

Tests for *H. pylori* are required for the diagnosis of infection and to ascertain, in some situations, whether eradication therapy has been successful. High sensitivity is required to ensure that positives are not missed; similarly, high specificity is essential to prevent inappropriate use of eradication therapy. The Maastricht III Consensus Guidelines[123] recommend a "test and treat" strategy in adults with appropriate dyspeptic symptoms younger than 45 years using a breath test or a stool antigen test. The age limit may vary depending on local prevalence and the age distribution of gastric cancer (e.g., in the United Kingdom, testing and treatment are now an option in any patients with uncomplicated dyspepsia, although for those aged 55 years and older with unexplained and persistent recent-onset dyspepsia alone, referral should be made for urgent endoscopy).[139] Successful eradication of *H. pylori* should be confirmed with the urea breath test or by a monoclonal antibody-based stool antigen test if urea breath tests are not available. Other national guidelines confirm the urea breath test as the preferred procedure, both for initial diagnosis and for confirmation of eradication.[22A,86,139] Testing to confirm eradication should be done at least 4 weeks after completion of the course of treatment.

Urea breath tests are simple to perform, and both sensitivity and specificity are greater than 95%. Urea labeled with ^{14}C or ^{13}C is given orally as a drink or a capsule to be swallowed with water; urease from gastric *H. pylori* rapidly hydrolyzes the ingested urea to produce labeled bicarbonate, which is absorbed into the blood and exhaled as $^{14}CO_2$ or $^{13}CO_2$. The principal advantages of the ^{13}C-urea breath test over the ^{14}C-urea breath test are the simplicity of breath collection and the avoidance of regulations and environmental issues related to the use and disposal of radioisotopes. In the ^{14}C-urea breath test, CO_2 in expired air is trapped in methanolic hyamine hydroxide as the patient exhales through a straw, which should be fitted with a one-way valve to ensure that the patient does not suck the trapping solution into the mouth. A color change of an indicator (thymol blue) in the solution shows that the required quantity of CO_2 has been trapped. Scintillant is then added and $^{14}CO_2$ measured. In the ^{13}C-urea breath test, the patient blows through a straw into an empty 15 mL tube, which is then capped. $^{13}CO_2/^{12}CO_2$ ratios are compared for basal and postdose samples using isotope ratio mass spectrometry or alternative infrared measurement methods.[106,117]

In the stool test, specific *H. pylori* antigens are detected in microtiter plates coated with polyclonal or monoclonal antibodies. Sensitivity and specificity are lower than for the ^{13}C-urea breath test. Monoclonal antibody tests are recommended for posteradication testing if the urea breath test is not available.[123]

Although still widely available, serologic tests are recommended only in specific situations (e.g., when PPI therapy cannot be withheld, when a patient with a bleeding ulcer is investigated).[123] The systemic antibody response is variable, leading to equivocal results in some subjects; in subjects older than 50 years, diagnostic accuracy is unsatisfactory. Serology cannot be used to confirm eradication because of the slow decline in antibody levels after treatment. Laboratory-based enzyme-linked immunosorbent assays (ELISAs) and point-of-care tests are available to measure specific immunoglobulin (Ig)G antibodies in serum or whole blood samples. In younger subjects, laboratory-based tests generally perform well, although some have sensitivity and/or specificity less than 95%. Office-based serology testing has inadequate sensitivity and specificity and currently is not recommended.[123] Calculations based on reported diagnostic accuracy data show that when these tests are used for diagnosis, as many as 28% of those receiving eradication therapy are being treated as a result of false-positive test results.[23]

Determination of Basal Acid Output[35,91]

Documentation of increased basal acid output (BAO) in gastric juice provides strong evidence that a high serum gastrin concentration is caused by Zollinger-Ellison syndrome. Therefore, this test is used in patients with duodenal ulceration and a raised serum gastrin concentration. The test is not appropriate in patients with atrophic gastritis. Pernicious anemia, which also causes hypergastrinemia, should be excluded before BAO is assessed. PPIs must be stopped for at least 14 days, and H_2-receptor antagonists for at least 3 days, before the test. *H. pylori* as a cause of increased serum gastrin should be excluded before BAO is estimated.

A basal condition, in the context of gastric analysis, is one in which the patient is at complete rest and is not exposed to any visual, auditory, or olfactory stimuli. Such a condition is maintained during sleep. It is for this reason that a 12 hour overnight collection of gastric juice has been used traditionally for the determination of BAO. Such an approach has the disadvantage that the patient is exposed to significant discomfort because of the need to retain the tube overnight, while sitting upright and slightly turned to the left to prevent loss of gastric contents into the duodenum. Close supervision throughout the entire night is necessary. A satisfactory alternative is the collection of gastric juice for 60 minutes after the patient has had a restful night's sleep in a quiet separate room. After waking, the patient must remain fasting; smoking and exercise must be avoided before and during the test.

Collection of Gastric Juice

A gastric tube is inserted orally, or nasal intubation may be used if the patient has a hyperactive gag reflex. X-ray or fluoroscopic confirmation that the tip of the radiopaque tube is in the lowest portion of the stomach is necessary. Ten or 15 minutes after the patient has become calm and adjusted to the presence of the tube, the patient is positioned with the trunk upright and inclined slightly to the left. Gastric juice is then aspirated and discarded. After checking that no further juice can be aspirated, note the time, and collect and transfer to plastic bottles all gastric juice that can be aspirated over the next 60 minutes. The patient must be asked to expectorate all saliva during the collection period. The total volume of collected juice is recorded and free acid determined by titration as described in the following section.

Determination of Free Hydrochloric Acid in Gastric Juice

1. Measure and transfer a convenient volume of gastric juice (e.g., 5.0 to 10.0 mL) into a clean titration vessel. If the gastric juice contains food particles or mucus, centrifuge the sample or filter it through gauze.
2. Determine the pH of the gastric specimen with a pH meter. If the pH is above 3.5, no free acid is present. Such a specimen need not be titrated.
3. Titrate the sample with NaOH, 0.10 mol/L, to a pH of 3.5, using a pH meter.

   Calculation:

$$\text{Free HCl (mmol/L)} = \frac{\text{mL of NaOH} \times 100}{\text{mL of gastric juice titrated}}$$

If 5 mL of gastric specimen is titrated, the calculation becomes as follows:

$$\text{Free HCl (mmol/L)} = \text{mL of NaOH} \times 20$$

$$\text{Free HCl (mmol/hr)} = \frac{\text{mL of NaOH} \times 20 \times 60 \text{ min volume of gastric juice in mL}}{1000}$$

Comments and Sources of Error

Titration to a pH of 3 to 3.5 detects essentially all free hydrochloric acid. (Because HCl is the only strongly ionized acid in gastric contents, this test is essentially a test for free HCl.) Titration beyond a pH of 3.5, as recommended by some, will overestimate the HCl concentration to varying degrees, depending on the composition of the gastric residue. On the other hand, titration to pH 3.5 may underestimate the amount of free H^+ secreted if some of these H^+ ions are bound to or have reacted with other constituents of gastric contents. Thus no fully satisfactory procedure is available to measure accurately the true total amount of free acid secreted by the gastric mucosa.

The effectiveness of gastric aspiration may be compromised by both the position of the patient and the position of the tube in the stomach (likened to the position of a straw above or below the fluid level in a glass), by the loss of gastric fluid into the pylorus, and by regurgitation of pyloric contents into the stomach. Some evidence suggests that the exact position of the tube in the stomach does not appear to alter the recovery of gastric juice, because the stomach is not rigid and its walls contract, thus shifting the stomach contents toward the tip of the tube.

Interpretation

Gastric juice pH: if the pH is greater than 2.5, then it is unlikely that the raised gastrin is caused by Zollinger-Ellison syndrome.

BAO: Normal: male 0 to 10.5 mmol/h; female: 0 to 5.6 mmol/h

Zollinger-Ellison syndrome: 15 to 100 mmol/h, or greater than 5 mmol/h if acid-reducing surgery was performed previously.

A level of free acid greater than 15 mmol/h should prompt suspicion of gastrinoma but is not diagnostic; a level greater than 25 mmol/h with high serum gastrin is virtually diagnostic of Zollinger-Ellison syndrome.

Further discussion of the Zollinger-Ellison syndrome can be found in the section of this chapter on neuroendocrine tumors.

INTESTINAL DISORDERS AND THEIR LABORATORY INVESTIGATION

This section includes discussions of celiac disease, disaccharidase deficiency, bacterial overgrowth, bile salt malabsorption, inflammatory bowel disease, and protein-losing enteropathy, and the main laboratory investigations associated with diagnosing or monitoring these disorders.

Celiac Disease (Celiac Sprue, Gluten-Sensitive Enteropathy)[53,54,124,162,181A]

Celiac disease is sometimes called nontropical sprue, celiac sprue, or gluten-sensitive enteropathy.

Pathophysiology of Celiac Disease

Celiac disease occurs in genetically predisposed subjects as a consequence of an inappropriate T cell–mediated immune response to ingestion of gluten from wheat and to similar proteins in barley and rye.

The role of genetic factors in celiac disease has been recognized for many years; a 70% concordance for celiac disease has been reported in identical twins, and typically 10% of first-degree relatives of an affected individual will be found to have the disease. Only recently has the major genetic component been localized to the human leukocyte antigen (HLA) region of chromosome 6. Approximately 95% of subjects with celiac disease express a specific HLA heterodimer (HLA DQ2 α/β heterodimer). Most Caucasian populations have a high frequency (20 to 30%) of DQ2, but only a small minority will develop celiac disease.

The external trigger to the development of celiac disease in genetically susceptible individuals is found in gluten, which is the complex group of proteins present in wheat that form a sticky mass when dough is washed with water and the starch is removed. All proteins (and peptides) that are toxic to the small bowel mucosa in subjects with celiac disease contain large amounts of glutamine. The major toxic proteins of wheat are the gliadins, with homologous proteins (the hordeins and secalins) occurring in barley and rye, respectively. The gliadins are a large family of proteins accounting for about 50% of the wheat protein.

Recent evidence indicates that oats do not lead to an immune-mediated response nor to mucosal damage in subjects with celiac disease.[90] Addition of oats to the list of permitted cereals increases choices and would be welcomed by most subjects with celiac disease. However, if oats are to be introduced into the diet, they must be obtained from a reliable source to ensure no contamination from wheat, barley, or rye proteins at any stage in the process from harvesting to packaging.

The identification in 1997 of small bowel tissue transglutaminase (tTG)-2 as the autoantigen of celiac disease[36] was a major step forward in understanding the pathogenesis of this disorder. The tissue transglutaminases are a family of calcium-dependent cytoplasmic enzymes that are released from cells during wounding. Although their physiologic role is incompletely understood, they are able to catalyze the cross-linking of proteins, leading to stabilization of the wound area. Expression of the enzyme is increased during apoptosis and in active celiac disease. It selectively cross-links or deamidates protein-bound glutamine residues. Deamidation of gliadin peptides by the enzyme enhances their binding to HLA DQ2/DQ8 and increases recognition of these peptides by gut-derived T cells from subjects with celiac disease.[163] The pathogenesis of the disease is therefore believed to involve an interaction between tissue transglutaminase and gliadin peptides in genetically susceptible individuals.

The toxic cereal proteins lead to intestinal epithelial damage, releasing tissue transglutaminase. Cross-linking by the enzyme produces gliadin-gliadin or gliadin-enzyme complexes, unmasking new antigenic epitopes that bind to HLA DQ2 molecules on the antigen-presenting cells, producing an immune response by gut-derived T cells. The characteristic enteropathy is then induced by the release of interferon-γ and other proinflammatory cytokines, as outlined in Figure 51-6.

A 33-mer peptide of gluten appears to be the primary initiator of the inflammatory response.[156] It is resistant to breakdown by all gastric, pancreatic, and intestinal brush border membrane proteases, thus allowing it to reach the small intestine intact. After deamidation by tissue transglutaminase, it is a potent inducer of gut-derived human T-cell lines from patients with celiac disease. Homologs of the peptide are found in food grains that are toxic to patients with celiac disease, but are absent from nontoxic food grains. The peptide could be detoxified by exposure to a bacterial prolyl endopeptidase, suggesting a therapeutic strategy for celiac disease.[156]

Increased intestinal permeability in untreated celiac disease that is reversible on withdrawal of gluten from the diet has been recognized since the early 1980s.[74] Evidence suggests that this may be mediated by increased expression of zonulin,[56] a protein that opens small intestinal tight junctions, or by decreased expression of intercellular epithelial cell adhesion molecules, such as Z0-1, catenin, and cadherin.[144] The zonulin pathway is now thought to play a significant role in the entry of allergens into the cell and hence in the autoimmune response.[54A]

Clinical Considerations

Celiac disease is a common chronic disorder in Caucasian populations, with a prevalence of about 1%.[122,186] It also occurs in northern Indian and North African populations. It is rare among Chinese, Japanese, and African-Caribbean people. It was previously considered to be a rare disorder in North America, but recent serologic and histologic evidence shows that the disease has been underdiagnosed, and that its prevalence is comparable, as might be expected, with that found in Europe.[55,77]

A wide spectrum has been noted in the clinical presentation of celiac disease, with most diagnoses made in adult life. Classical celiac disease, presenting in infancy up to the age of 2 years, with failure to thrive, abdominal distention, and diarrhea, is now an uncommon presentation. The spectrum of presenting symptoms in adults has changed over the past 20 years, and frank malabsorption is now uncommon.[87,185] Most adults present now with nonspecific symptoms; mild iron deficiency is common. A strong association with other autoimmune disease, especially with type 1 diabetes mellitus and autoimmune thyroid disease, has been reported. In type 1 diabetes, the prevalence of celiac disease is about 5%, and serologic screening to detect these cases has been advocated.[84] The initial presentation may be seen by a wide range of clinical specialties, as shown in Table 51-2. To make the diagnosis, there must be a high index of suspicion, along with awareness of the wide range of nonspecific symptoms and easy availability of serologic tests to select those patients in whom endoscopy is indicated to confirm the diagnosis.

Tests for Celiac Disease

Serologic tests have played a significant role in raising awareness of the high prevalence of this disorder, and appropriately standardized tests have high clinical sensitivity and specificity for diagnosis and for monitoring compliance with a gluten-free diet during treatment after diagnosis.

Table 51-3 compares the sensitivity and specificity of the four IgA class antibodies commonly used. Both antireticulin

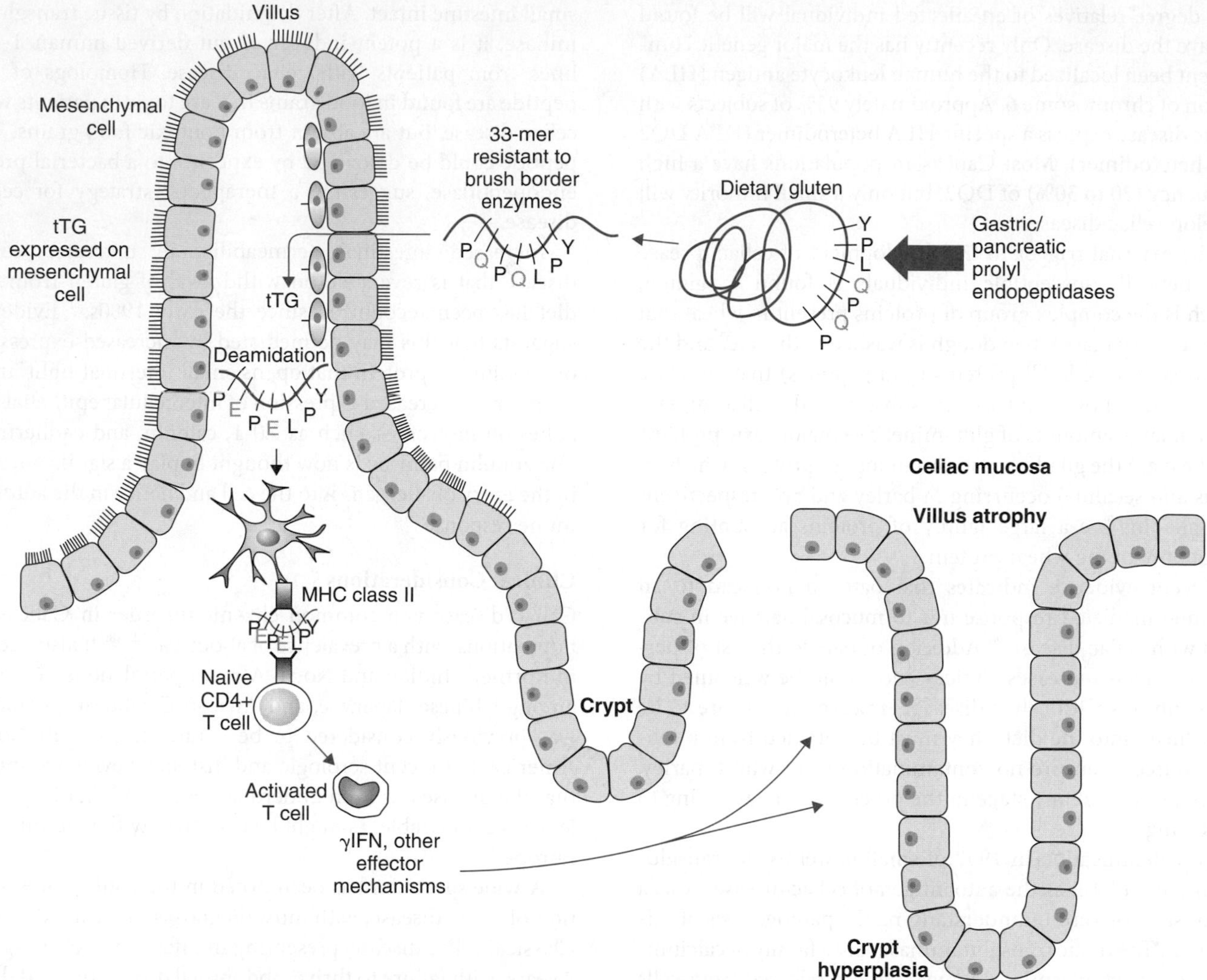

Figure 51-6 Hypothetical scheme for interaction between intestinal protein processing and the specific immune system in celiac disease. Dietary gluten is exposed to intraluminal digestive enzymes (including prolyl endopeptidases), producing stable 33-mer peptide-containing overlapping proline-rich epitopes with the PQPQLPY central motif. 33-mer peptide is absorbed intact by transcellular or paracellular routes into the lamina propria, and exposure to tTG results in deamidation of glutamine residues to glutamic acid. Modified peptide is presented to specific CD4$^+$ T cells in association with HLA DQ2 or DQ8. Activated IFN-γ–producing T-effector cells return to the mucosa and produce characteristic villous atrophy and crypt hyperplasia. *E,* Glutamate; *F,* phenylalanine; *IFN,* interferon; *L,* leucine; *P,* proline; *Q,* glutamine; *tTG,* tissue transglutaminase; and *Y,* tyrosine. *(From Mowat AM. Coeliac disease—a meeting point for genetics, immunology, and protein chemistry. Lancet 2003;361:1290-2.)*

(ARA) and endomysial (EMA) antibodies are measured by indirect immunofluorescence, ARA on rat kidney sections and EMA on monkey esophagus or human umbilical cord sections. The presence of ARA indicates the need to measure antibodies with higher specificity before small bowel histology is recommended for confirmation of the diagnosis. ARA and EMA are tissue type–dependent methods that detect autoantibodies to tissue transglutaminase-2.[107]

Lack of standardization of assays for IgA-antigliadin antibodies (AGA) contributes to the variable diagnostic accuracy of this marker,[81] but the sensitivity and specificity of AGA are poor, and use of this test should be abandoned. The sensitivity and specificity of current deamidated gliadin peptide antibody tests offer no advantages over tissue transglutaminase antibody (TGA) and may give significantly more false positives in subjects with liver disease.[80,136] The sensitivity of EMA in some reports is compromised by selection bias,[115] but most larger series in which patients have not been selected for a biopsy on the basis of positive serology indicate that the true sensitivity for EMA is between 90% and 95% (i.e., 5 to

10% of subjects with celiac disease have a negative EMA at diagnosis). When carried out correctly, the assay has very high specificity (>99%); laboratories should monitor their performance, as small reductions in specificity will lead to a significant increase in the numbers of patients subjected unnecessarily to a small bowel biopsy. Table 51-4 shows the effects of test specificity on the numbers of true and false positives per 1000 subjects tested, and on the positive predictive value at disease prevalence (in the population tested) of 3%, assuming a sensitivity of 95%.

Many commercial kits are now available to measure IgA antibodies against tissue transglutaminase ["transglutaminase antibody" (TGA)] using human recombinant tissue transglutaminase or purified human enzyme as antigen. Their role in the investigation of celiac disease has been reviewed.[80] Lack of standardization and differences in recombinant technology (e.g., the use of eukaryotic or prokaryotic organisms to produce tTG) can lead to variable performance.[11,126] Specificity should be evaluated using a large series of samples representative of those routinely tested, and procedures should be selected on the basis of high specificity (minimum 99%) and high sensitivity (>90%). The use of TGA has advantages over EMA. Unlike EMA, which may be subject to observer bias, TGA is a quantitative procedure that does not require the use of primate tissue. It can be automated and therefore is appropriate for larger numbers of samples. This test has replaced EMA as the antibody of choice for performing serologic testing and for assessing dietary compliance of subjects on a gluten-free diet.[14,79] As with all tests, not all kits perform to the same high standards, and laboratories should ensure that they participate in external quality assessment programs and select a well-validated method.[45,80] In view of the growing public interest in celiac disorder, further standardization of these kits is urgently needed.

For diagnosis, current guidelines require a jejunal biopsy with the characteristic villous atrophy, increased intraepithelial lymphocytes, and hyperplasia of the crypts.[124] Wider use of serology has led to the recognition of more cases with minimal histologic changes and to use of the terms *potential* and *latent* celiac disease.[83] Patients with positive EMA or TGA are described as having *potential celiac disease* when the jejunal biopsy has normal villi but shows subtle changes, such as increased numbers of intraepithelial lymphocytes. It is thought that in time these patients will develop a flat mucosa. The term *latent celiac disease* is used to describe patients who have at some time had positive antibodies and a flat mucosa that recovers on a gluten-free diet, but have also been found to have a normal mucosa while on a normal diet.

Subjects with selective IgA deficiency (IgA <0.05 g/L, incidence about 1:600) are at greater risk of celiac disease. It is therefore important to identify these individuals rather than risk excluding the diagnosis on the basis of a negative test for IgA class antibodies.[22] When EMA is used, total serum IgA should be measured on all samples submitted for celiac serology to identify those patients with IgA deficiency. A TGA method should be used that can distinguish those with a "normal" concentration from the small proportion of subjects with *very* low concentrations, in whom total IgA measurement is indicated to confirm or exclude IgA deficiency.[57] When IgA deficiency is identified, IgG antibodies (IgG-EMA, IgG-TGA, and IgG anti-deamidated gliadin peptide) should be used as serologic screening tests.[21] In view of the increased risk of the disorder in IgA deficiency, a small bowel biopsy should be considered in all IgA-deficient subjects with symptoms of celiac disease.[22]

Strict adherence to a gluten-free diet leads to mucosal recovery in celiac disease and reduces the risk of bowel

TABLE 51-2 An Indication of the Wide Range of Clinical Specialties to Which a Child or Adult With Celiac Disease May Present

Clinical Specialty	Symptoms/Manifestations
General medicine	Tired all the time
Gastroenterology	Diarrhea, flatulence, weight loss
Hematology	Anemia
Obstetrics/gynecology	Infertility
Orthopedics	Fracture, osteopenia
Dermatology	Dermatitis herpetiformis, hyperkeratosis
Neurology	Peripheral neuropathy
Rheumatology	Arthropathy
Endocrinology	Short stature, thyroid disease
Diabetes	Diarrhea, anemia

TABLE 51-3 Comparison of Serologic Tests for Celiac Disease

Antibody	Method	Sensitivity	Specificity
Antireticulin antibody (R1-ARA)	Immunofluorescence on rat or mouse kidney	25-30%	>90%
IgA-endomysial antibody	Immunofluorescence on monkey esophagus or human umbilical cord	80-100%	>99%
IgA-antigliadin antibody	Quantitative ELISA	75-95%	95%
IgA-antitissue transglutaminase antibody (human antigen)	Quantitative ELISA	>90%	>99%
IgA-deamidated gliadin peptide antibody	Quantitative ELISA	90%	90%

ELISA, Enzyme-linked immunosorbent assay; *Ig,* immunoglobulin.

TABLE 51-4 Comparison of True and False Positives and Positive Predictive Values at Different Specificities, Assuming a Prevalence of Celiac Disease of 3% in the Population (n = 1000) Tested (Test Sensitivity of 95%)

Specificity	True Positives	False Positives	Positive Predictive Value
90%	29	97	0.23
95%	29	49	0.38
98%	29	19	0.60
99%	29	10	0.74
99.5%	29	5	0.85

malignancy. TGA can be used as a marker for monitoring dietary compliance, in addition to its diagnostic role.[14] Failure of symptoms to respond to a prescribed gluten-free diet may indicate (1) nonadherence to the diet, (2) other coexisting conditions (such as small bowel bacterial overgrowth, lactose intolerance, and microscopic colitis), or (3) the presence of *refractory celiac disease.* Refractory celiac disease is characterized by persistent villous atrophy with an increase in intraepithelial lymphocytes in the small bowel while the patient is on a long-term gluten-free diet. In both responsive and refractory celiac disease, celiac antibodies typically are decreased with dietary therapy and remain within reference intervals unless individuals are re-exposed to gluten.

Two types of refractory celiac disease may occur and are differentiated by the types of T-cell populations found in the intestinal mucosa—polyclonal in type I disease and clonal in type II disease. Differentiation of the two types is accomplished by immunohistochemical, flow cytometric, or T-cell receptor γ gene rearrangement analysis of intestinal mucosal T cells.[129A] Type II celiac disease has an unfavorable prognosis and typically is viewed as a precursor to enteropathy-associated T-cell lymphoma (EATL).

With the availability now of serologic tests with high diagnostic accuracy, older tests used to investigate celiac disease should be abandoned. For example, there is no place now in routine use for the xylose absorption test. Dual sugar tests (e.g., cellobiose and mannitol) to assess small bowel permeability have a role in research studies but as yet have not established a place in the routine diagnosis or monitoring of celiac disease. Tests of fat malabsorption are also inappropriate in the diagnosis of celiac disease, although appropriate tests of pancreatic function (e.g., fecal elastase) may be indicated in patients diagnosed with celiac disease who fail to respond to a gluten-free diet.

Disaccharidase Deficiencies[155,171]

The presence of the brush border disaccharidases is essential for carbohydrate absorption, and a reduction in their activity leads to carbohydrate malabsorption and intolerance. Carbohydrate malabsorption does not always lead to clinical symptoms, but when symptoms do occur (e.g., abdominal pain, flatulence, diarrhea) as a consequence of malabsorption, the patient is described as having carbohydrate intolerance.

TABLE 51-5 Prevalence of Hypolactasia in Adults

Racial Group	Prevalence, %
Chinese	>90
American blacks	54-81
Asians	60-90
Greeks	60-78
Northern Europeans	5-30

Adult-type hypolactasia is the single most common absorptive defect in adults, with an incidence of 5 to 90% depending on the racial group, as shown in Table 51-5.

Congenital Lactase Deficiency

Intestinal lactase is essential in infancy, and congenital lactase deficiency is a very rare disorder in which lactase activities in the mucosa are low or undetectable at birth. Severe diarrhea occurs as soon as milk is taken; stools have a low pH and contain large amounts of lactose and glucose produced by bacterial action on undigested lactose. A definitive diagnosis must be deferred until after maturation of the lactase synthesis system has occurred. In the interim, relief is dependent on adjustments to dietary composition that appear to reduce the severity of symptoms. An abnormal oral lactose tolerance test obtained a few months after birth could also be caused by congenital glucose-galactose intolerance (see discussion later in this chapter); the differential diagnosis requires performance of an oral glucose tolerance test in conjunction with the lactose tolerance test.

Adult-type Hypolactasia ("Acquired Lactase Deficiency")

In most humans (and in all other mammals), expression of the enzyme decreases during childhood, and by adulthood lactase levels are 10% or less of those seen in infancy. If symptoms of flatulence, abdominal discomfort, bloating, or diarrhea occur after consumption of one or two glasses of milk or of a large portion of ice cream or yogurt, lactose intolerance should be suspected. Suspicion would be increased in a subject from an ethnic group with a high incidence of lactose intolerance (see Table 51-5).

Lactose intolerance may also occur as a result of reduced enzyme activity following diffuse intestinal damage from infection (giardiasis, bacterial overgrowth, or viral gastroenteritis), ulcerative colitis, celiac disease, and tropical sprue. This deficiency is usually reversible following recovery from the disorder.

Diagnostic Tests for Lactase Deficiency

Many methods have been proposed for detecting lactase deficiency (Box 51-2). Disaccharidase activities can be measured in homogenates of an intestinal biopsy.[32] These assays are rarely required for routine diagnostic purposes, but when

BOX 51-2 Methods for Detecting Lactase Deficiency

Lactase in mucosal biopsy
Oral lactose tolerance
- Measure increase in plasma glucose
- Measure increase in plasma galactose
- Measure increase in breath H_2
- Measure increase in breath $^{13}CO_2$

necessary (e.g., in investigations in infancy), they must be carried out by laboratories with expertise in these tests. Breath hydrogen is now the preferred test for diagnosing lactase deficiency. The use of hydrogen breath tests in disorders of carbohydrate absorption and in bacterial overgrowth has been reviewed.[159]

Oral Lactose Tolerance Tests

Oral tolerance tests, measuring the increase in plasma glucose or galactose following ingestion of lactose, have been used to diagnose lactase deficiency. The usual dose of lactose is 50 g in 200 mL water; lower doses should be used in children (2 g/kg, up to a maximum of 50 g). Multiple blood samples are collected over a 2 hour period and the peak increment in glucose (or galactose) noted. To exclude lactase deficiency, the increase above baseline for capillary plasma glucose should be greater than 1.1 mmol/L[138] (20 mg/dL) or greater than 1.4 mmol/L (25 mg/dL) when venous plasma is used.[20] In a survey of laboratory practice in the United Kingdom, widely varying cutoffs were found to be in use (1.0 to 2.7 mmol/L) even with the same lactose dose.[44] The requirement for multiple blood samples and lack of procedural standardization suggest that these tests should be abandoned in favor of noninvasive breath hydrogen testing.

Hydrogen Breath Tests

Hydrogen is not an end product of mammalian metabolism, and breath hydrogen is derived from bacterial metabolism in the intestinal tract.[114] Following lactose ingestion, the disaccharide normally will be split into its constituent monosaccharides and absorbed. With lactase deficiency, unabsorbed disaccharide will pass into the large bowel, and bacterial metabolism will produce hydrogen that is absorbed into the systemic circulation and exhaled in the breath. Breath hydrogen can be measured in end-expiratory breath with the use of laboratory or hand-held direct-reading electrochemical hydrogen monitors.

Patient Preparation. Appropriate patient preparation is essential to ensure stable baseline breath hydrogen levels (Box 51-3). Avoidance of wheat-based foods and fiber for 12 hours before the test minimizes the availability of substrates for bacterial metabolism in the large bowel. Fasting breath hydrogen is typically less than 5 ppm (5 µL/L), and concentrations greater than 20 ppm (20 µL/L) may be an indication of malabsorption or bacterial overgrowth.[143] Oral hygiene

BOX 51-3 Protocol for Lactose Tolerance Test With Measurement of Breath Hydrogen

Meal before 0700 (restriction on wheat and fiber), then fasting until test completed
Brush teeth (night and morning) or use mouthwash
Measure end-expiratory fasting breath H_2
Give lactose solution (50 g in 180 mL water for adults)
Rinse mouth with further 20 mL water and swallow
Measure breath H_2 at 15, 30, 60, 90, and 120 minutes
Test can be stopped if earlier rise of greater than 20 ppm above fasting level

before ingestion of the substrate in hydrogen breath tests minimizes the production of hydrogen by oral bacteria. Brushing of teeth or use of an antibacterial mouthwash (e.g., 1% chlorhexidine) is recommended.[128] Mouthwash containing alcohol should not be used, because this may interfere with the measurement of hydrogen. Cigarette smoke contains high hydrogen levels; smoking therefore is not permitted immediately before or during the test.

After an overnight fast, a baseline breath hydrogen level is recorded and 50 g of lactose in 180 mL water is drunk, followed by a further 20 mL of water to rinse the mouth and further reduce the possibility of an early rise in breath hydrogen from the action of oral bacteria. The dose in children should be 2 g/kg up to a maximum of 50 g. Breath hydrogen is then measured at 15, 30, 60, 90, and 120 minutes.

Interpretation. Most publications indicate that an increase in breath hydrogen greater than 20 ppm (20 µL/L) above the baseline fasting concentration within 2 hours of ingestion of lactose is indicative of lactose malabsorption.[129,138] However, 1999 data suggest that a cutoff of 10 ppm (10 µL/L) improves diagnostic sensitivity without increasing the number of false-positive test results.[98] In most patients with normal lactose absorption, breath hydrogen levels will remain at 2 to 5 ppm throughout the test. Occasionally, high levels may occur within the first 30 minutes after lactose ingestion. This may indicate very rapid transit of lactose to the cecum or bacterial metabolism in the small bowel due to bacterial overgrowth. Repeating the breath test with lactulose or glucose as the substrate or using imaging techniques to confirm transit time will normally clarify the cause of such results.

In lactose malabsorption, breath hydrogen is typically elevated (30 to 100 ppm, 30 to 100 µL/L) at 60 to 120 minutes after lactose ingestion. In a few subjects, the large bowel bacteria do not produce hydrogen; in such patients a normal result does not exclude lactase deficiency. Very low hydrogen when fasting and throughout the test may therefore indicate a false-negative result. Some estimates suggest that up to 10 to 13% of the population have large bowel bacteria that do not produce hydrogen,[105] although others have found the prevalence of hydrogen nonproducers to be less than 2%.[129,168] Such false negatives can be confirmed by failure to produce hydrogen at 45 to 180 minutes after ingestion of lactulose

(10 g), which is a nonabsorbable disaccharide and therefore is available for bacterial metabolism in the large bowel.

A positive breath hydrogen result following ingestion of lactose may also occur in glucose-galactose malabsorption, which may cause intestinal symptoms. When necessary, glucose-galactose malabsorption can be confirmed or excluded by a breath test in which 25 g each of glucose and galactose is substituted for 50 g lactose. An increase in breath hydrogen confirms the diagnosis.

Sucrase-Isomaltase and Trehalase Deficiencies and Monosaccharide Malabsorption

Sucrase-isomaltase deficiency usually presents clinically in infancy when sucrose and fruit are introduced into the diet,[102] but sometimes first presents in adulthood.[133,179] The deficiency is rare in Caucasians and is more common among Eskimo groups. Deficiencies of both lactase and sucrase-isomaltase may occur secondary to other small bowel diseases (e.g., celiac disease, Crohn's disease,[178] acute gastroenteritis). Trehalase deficiency is a rare disorder,[132,135] except in Greenland, where it occurs in 8% of the population.[70] It is manifested by diarrhea following the ingestion of mushrooms.

Malabsorption of monosaccharides can also cause intestinal symptoms more commonly attributed to maldigestion of disaccharides. Glucose-galactose malabsorption is also inherited as an autosomal recessive trait. Symptoms occur in the affected neonate as soon as milk (lactose) is taken, but they also may follow ingestion of glucose- or galactose-containing foods. Symptoms caused by fructose malabsorption occur upon ingestion of fruit. This dietary intolerance is quite a different disorder from hereditary fructose intolerance, in which the hepatic enzyme aldolase is defective.

The breath hydrogen test described previously can be used to diagnose sucrase-isomaltase deficiency. A total of 50 g sucrose is used instead of lactose. An increase in breath hydrogen greater than 20 ppm (20 μL/L) within 2 hours is diagnostic. It is rarely necessary to test for trehalase deficiency, although a breath test using 25 g trehalose has been described.[4]

Bacterial Overgrowth

The proximal small intestine (duodenum and jejunum) normally contains few bacteria. Most ingested bacteria do not survive the acidic environment of the stomach; therefore few live organisms normally enter the small bowel. The motility of the jejunum prevents fecal-type organisms from progressing up into the jejunum from the cecum. The ileum normally contains some fecal-type bacteria. Colonization of the upper small bowel is described as bacterial overgrowth and usually occurs as a consequence of other abnormalities (structural or motility disorders) of the small intestine (Box 51-4). Use of PPIs is associated with an increased risk of bacterial colonization.

BOX 51-4 Abnormalities of the Small Intestine Associated With Bacterial Overgrowth

Jejunal diverticuli
Crohn's disease
Autonomic neuropathy
Scleroderma (systemic sclerosis)
Pseudo-obstruction
Post gastrectomy

Bacteria colonizing the small bowel (such as *Escherichia coli* and *Bacteroides* species) deconjugate and dehydroxylate bile salts, leading to conjugated bile salt deficiency, which causes fat malabsorption. Bacterial metabolism of vitamin B_{12} may also occur, leading to vitamin B_{12} deficiency. The clinical symptoms of bacterial overgrowth include abdominal pain, diarrhea, and steatorrhea.[108]

The diagnostic gold standard requires intubation with aspiration of jejunal contents and demonstration of a bacterial count of more than 10^5 colonic-type organisms/mL.[159] In practice, hydrogen breath tests using lactulose or preferably glucose as the substrate are used more frequently. An alternative diagnostic approach is to use a therapeutic trial of antibiotics.

For hydrogen breath tests, patient preparation is the same as that described in the previous section for the lactose breath hydrogen test. Lactulose (usually given in a dose of 10 g in 200 mL water) is a nonabsorbable disaccharide. In a normal subject, breath hydrogen does not increase until lactulose enters the large intestine; the time from ingestion to a rise in breath hydrogen therefore is normally an indication of small bowel transit time. In bacterial overgrowth, an early rise in breath hydrogen of at least 20 ppm (20 μL/L) is noted within 30 minutes of ingestion of lactulose. The early increase is diagnostic when it can be distinguished clearly from the later colonic rise. Frequent measurements (e.g., at 5-minute intervals) are essential in the first 30 minutes, followed by measurements every 15 minutes thereafter for up to 3 hours.[150]

Glucose is an alternative substrate; the usual adult dose is 50 g (as monohydrate) in 250 mL water.[101,184] An increase in breath hydrogen greater than 12 ppm (12 μL/L) above the fasting concentration indicates bacterial overgrowth. In bacterial overgrowth, breath hydrogen usually increases within 75 minutes of ingestion of glucose and sometimes within 30 minutes. The finding of an increased fasting breath hydrogen has high specificity for bacterial overgrowth but poor sensitivity; however, a fasting breath hydrogen greater than 15 ppm and an increment of at least 12 ppm within 2 hours of a 50 g glucose challenge are diagnostic of bacterial overgrowth.[101,143] The high fasting breath hydrogen levels, even after adequate dietary preparation, are thought to be caused by stasis of gut contents or by intestinal bacteria producing hydrogen from endogenous glycoproteins.[143] Table 51-6 compares some of the published data for diagnostic accuracy of tests using lactulose or glucose.

Variations in gastric emptying rate and in small bowel transit times are problems that limit the diagnostic accuracy

TABLE 51-6 Reported Sensitivity and Specificity of Lactulose and Glucose Hydrogen Breath Tests for the Diagnosis of Bacterial Overgrowth

Substrate	Increment Over Baseline*	Sensitivity	Specificity	Reference
Glucose 50 g	≥12 ppm	93	78	Kerlin and Wong, 1988[101]
Glucose 50 g	>10 ppm	78	89	Flourie et al, 1989[60A]
Glucose 50 g	≥15 ppm	90	—	Stotzer and Kilander, 2000[167]
Glucose 75 g	≥10 ppm	62	83	Corazza et al, 1990[26]
Lactulose 12 g	>10 ppm	68	44	Corazza et al, 1990[26]

*1 ppm = 1 μL/L.

of breath hydrogen tests. In the face of an appropriate clinical picture and a negative breath hydrogen test, an alternative diagnostic approach is a therapeutic trial of appropriate antibiotics.[5]

Other tests for bacterial overgrowth have used ^{14}C-xylose or ^{14}C-glycocholic acid.[105] When bacterial overgrowth occurs, bacteria deconjugate the glycocholic acid to produce ^{14}C-glycine that is absorbed and metabolized with an increase in breath $^{14}CO_2$. As in other tests, an early rise in the marker indicates bacterial overgrowth or rapid transit to the large bowel, where the normal colonic flora releases ^{14}C-glycine. These tests using radioactive isotopes have been superseded by hydrogen breath tests that offer comparable diagnostic performance and methodologic advantages.[167]

Bile Salt Malabsorption[33]

Bile acids are synthesized in the liver and pass into the lumen of the small bowel via the gallbladder. Bile acids are present in bile as taurine or glycine conjugates; because the pH of bile is slightly alkaline and contains significant amounts of sodium and potassium, most of the bile acids and their conjugates exist as salts (i.e., bile salts). In practice, the terms *bile acids* and *bile salts* are frequently used as synonyms. Their major function is to act as surface-active agents, forming micelles and facilitating the digestion of triglycerides and the absorption of cholesterol and fat-soluble vitamins. Little reabsorption of bile acid occurs in the proximal small bowel, but normally more than 90% is reabsorbed in the terminal ileum. It returns to the liver in the portal circulation and is resecreted into the bile. This is known as the *enterohepatic circulation*. Less than 10% of secreted bile acid is lost in the feces, or about 0.2 to 0.6 g/d.

Bile acid malabsorption leading to chronic diarrhea occurs when ileal disease (e.g., Crohn's disease) is present, or after resection of the terminal ileum; it may also occur following cholecystectomy and in some patients with irritable bowel syndrome.[165] Malabsorption of bile salts produces diarrhea by two different mechanisms. When significant bile salt depletion occurs, the deficiency of intraluminal bile salts leads to fat malabsorption and steatorrhea. More commonly, malabsorption of bile salts in the ileum leads to increased concentrations of bile salts in the colon, where they alter water and electrolyte absorption. This leads to net secretion of water into the lumen and diarrhea. Bile salt malabsorption is probably an underdiagnosed condition and should be suspected in patients with unexplained chronic diarrhea.[161,177,188]

Three different procedures have been used to make a diagnosis of bile salt malabsorption: the ^{75}selenohomocholyltaurine test, measurement of serum 7α-hydroxy-4-cholesten-3-one in serum, and a therapeutic trial of bile acid sequestrants such as cholestyramine. The most widely used test involves the oral administration of the synthetic radioactive bile acid ^{75}selenohomocholyltaurine (^{75}SeHCAT). Following the dose, whole body gamma counting is carried out to estimate the basal level at 1 hour (100%). The gamma count is measured again after 7 days, when normally more than 15% of the administered dose is retained. Retention of less than 10% indicates bile salt malabsorption. Patients with less than 5% retention of ^{75}SeHCAT often have a good response to treatment with bile acid sequestrants.

Measurement of 7α-hydroxy-4-cholesten-3-one has been proposed as a simpler alternative to ^{75}SeHCAT. Evidence indicates that the fasting serum level of this intermediary between cholesterol and taurocholic acid reflects the activity of hepatic cholesterol 7α-hydroxylase and therefore the rate of bile acid synthesis. Bile acid malabsorption is associated with increased serum concentrations of 7α-hydroxy-4-cholesten-3-one as hepatic synthesis increases to maintain the pool of circulating bile acids.[6] Good correlation has been demonstrated between serum 7α-hydroxy-4-cholesten-3-one and results of the ^{75}SeHCAT test.[51] Two subsequent publications on patients with chronic diarrhea have documented the high sensitivity of this measurement for identifying those with bile acid–induced diarrhea.[13,153] The test has been compared with ^{75}SeHCAT and with the response to cholestyramine. The latter avoids the problems of assuming 100% sensitivity and specificity for the ^{75}SeHCAT test. With use of the therapeutic response to cholestyramine as the "gold standard," the positive predictive value of serum 7α-hydroxy-4-cholesten-3-one increased to 74% (from 71%), and the negative predictive value increased to 98% (from 94%).

With growing awareness of the likely role of bile salt malabsorption in the chronic diarrhea of a proportion of patients with irritable bowel syndrome and the therapeutic effectiveness of cholestyramine,[161,165] measurement of serum

7α-hydroxy-4-cholesten-3-one, with its high negative predictive value, could be used to exclude bile salt malabsorption. High concentrations would be confirmed at follow-up ^{75}SeHCAT testing or by a therapeutic trial with cholestyramine.

Inflammatory Bowel Disease

Inflammatory bowel disease (IBD) includes Crohn's disease, ulcerative colitis, and a number of microscopic inflammatory bowel disorders. IBD has a high prevalence in the United States and Europe and a much lower, although increasing, prevalence in most Asian countries. Significant overlap in the clinical presentation has been noted, as well as in radiologic and histologic findings in Crohn's disease (which may affect any part of the GI tract) and ulcerative colitis (which is confined to the large bowel). Both conditions present with diarrhea and abdominal pain or discomfort, often associated with fatigue and anemia, and less commonly with inflammation of the joints, skin, and eyes.

Causes of these disorders are unknown; environmental, genetic, and immune factors are believed to be involved in the inflammatory response, which occurs in the mucosa and submucosa as a consequence of activation of innate immune mechanisms. Tissue damage is a consequence of neutrophil activation and the production of proinflammatory mediators. Immunosuppressive drugs and tumor necrosis factor alpha inhibitors are the main medical treatment options, although for many patients, surgery will be required to remove diseased areas of the bowel.

Intestinal symptoms are common to both IBD and irritable bowel syndrome (IBS), although the latter is not an inflammatory disorder and is not associated with organic disease of the bowel. Interest is increasing in the use of markers to differentiate between IBD and IBS when required, and to monitor disease activity or response to anti-inflammatory treatment in patients with IBD.[61,65,113A,170] Interest initially focused on the use of fecal lactoferrin and calprotectin to distinguish organic from functional bowel disorders, but it is now clear that both are markers of the infiltration of neutrophils into the mucosa and are sensitive markers of intestinal inflammation. Negative tests for these proteins therefore exclude significant neutrophilic intestinal inflammation but may not exclude other organic bowel diseases such as celiac disease. Lactoferrin and calprotectin can be used as predictors of relapse in IBD and as markers of mucosal healing following treatment.[160]

Although they have similar diagnostic accuracy, these two markers reflect different aspects of neutrophil function and innate immunity. Lactoferrin (80 kDa) is stored in the granules within neutrophils and is a marker of neutrophil degranulation. Calprotectin is a major cytosolic component of neutrophils and is a complex of two proteins of the S100 family: S100A8 and S100A9. Unlike lactoferrin, which has antibacterial properties and is involved in host defense, the S100 proteins are proinflammatory and are believed to cause tissue damage in IBD. Advances in understanding of the molecular mechanisms surrounding the inflammatory process and of the role of damage-associated molecular pattern proteins suggest that a third member of the S100 family, S100A12, is a strong candidate as a more specific marker of neutrophil activation than calprotectin or lactoferrin.[61,95]

Protein-Losing Enteropathy

Loss of significant quantities of serum proteins into the bowel lumen and their passage into the feces are consequences of a wide range of GI disorders. These may be associated with inflammation or ulceration of a segment of the small or large bowel (as in Crohn's disease and ulcerative colitis) or stomach, with diseases in which the intestinal lymphatics are obstructed or where lymphatic pressure is elevated (e.g., lymphoma, Whipple's disease), or with disorders associated with altered immune status, such as systemic lupus erythematosus and some food allergies.

In the healthy bowel, fecal protein is largely derived from enterocytes shed from the mucosal surface and from intestinal secretions. The normal GI loss of albumin is less than 10% of albumin catabolism, representing a daily loss of less than 1 to 2% of the serum protein pool.[69] Protein loss may be greatly increased in disease. In studies using ^{51}Cr-labeled proteins, 0.1 to 0.7% of an injected dose was excreted in feces over 4 days in healthy subjects; in protein-losing enteropathies this may increase to 40%, leading to hypoalbuminemia and edema.

The diagnosis of protein-losing enteropathy should be considered in the investigation of patients with hypoalbuminemia in whom renal loss, liver disease, and malnutrition have been excluded. The classical test for the diagnosis of protein-losing enteropathy is the measurement of fecal ^{51}Cr-albumin following an intravenous injection, although this test is now rarely available. Imaging techniques that seek to detect the specific site of protein loss by using ^{99m}Tc-human serum albumin or ^{99m}Tc-dextran have been described.

Fecal clearance of alpha-1-antitrypsin (AT) can also be used as a marker of GI protein loss. AT is a glycoprotein (Mw 54,000 Da) that is synthesized in the liver and is normally present in the serum at a concentration of about 1.5 to 2 g/L. It is a protease inhibitor and therefore is resistant to degradation by proteolytic enzymes in the GI tract. The fecal clearance of AT correlates with protein loss measured by ^{51}Cr techniques ($r = 0.96$).[60] The correlation is not influenced by serum AT concentrations or by fecal weight. AT clearance can be used for both small and large bowel disease and is applicable to the evaluation of enteric protein loss in children and adults.[60,82] Work reported in 1990 has confirmed these findings but shown that fecal AT concentration alone does not reliably predict AT clearance (i.e., a timed fecal sample and measurement of serum AT are required).[169] An important observation is that experimentally induced diarrhea in normal subjects leads to increased AT clearance. The mechanism is unclear but may be related to decreased time for degradation of AT if intestinal transit time is shorter. The upper limits of the reference interval [estimated as means ±2 standard deviations (SD)] were found to be 56 mL/d and

24 mL/d in normal subjects with and without diarrhea, respectively. In inflammatory bowel disease, AT clearance may be as high as 200 mL/d; this represents a loss of about 6 g albumin/d.[169] AT clearance must be interpreted with caution in patients with positive fecal occult blood tests, as blood loss might be sufficient to falsely increase AT clearance. Measurement of fecal AT has been suggested as an alternative to fecal occult blood for the detection of colorectal cancer.[131] AT is rapidly destroyed in gastric juice (and in vitro) when the pH is below 3.0; this has meant that the test can be used only to assess protein loss distal to the pylorus.[60] However, administration of PPIs can be used to inhibit gastric acid secretion before collection of the fecal sample, thereby enabling assessment of protein loss from the stomach.[173]

A study evaluating the use of AT clearance as a marker of clinical relapse in patients with Crohn's disease showed a negative predictive value of 94% for predicting relapse in the subsequent 6 months (at a cutoff of 120 mL/d). Sensitivity was only 50% and comparable results were noted when the Bristol Simple Index score was used to predict relapse, so that at present the test appears to have little clinical value in this context.[10]

AT in feces and serum can be measured most conveniently by radial immunodiffusion. Feces should be collected quantitatively, preferably for 3 days, in preweighed containers and kept refrigerated. The AT is extracted into saline before analysis. AT clearance is calculated as follows:

$$\text{AT clearance (mL/day)} = \frac{(\text{fecal weight} \times \text{fecal AT concentration})}{\text{Serum AT}}$$

where fecal weight is expressed in g/d, fecal AT in mg/kg feces, and serum AT in mg/L.

THE PANCREAS: DISEASES AND ASSESSMENT OF EXOCRINE PANCREATIC FUNCTION

It will be evident from the section on digestion and absorption that the pancreas plays a central role in the absorptive process for carbohydrates, fats, and proteins. Disorders of the exocrine pancreas therefore are frequently associated with GI symptoms of malabsorption or diarrhea. In this section, pediatric and adult exocrine pancreatic disorders are briefly discussed, and tests that can be used to assess exocrine pancreatic function are described. Information on exocrine pancreatic tumors can be found in the later section on GI regulatory peptides. Recent textbooks on gastroenterology or medicine provide greater detail on the clinical aspects of exocrine pancreatic disorders.[15,62]

Pediatric Disorders of the Exocrine Pancreas

Pancreatic disorders in childhood have been reviewed[27]; and are summarized in Box 51-5.

BOX 51-5 Spectrum of Pancreatic Disease in Childhood

Disorders of Morphogenesis
Annular pancreas, pancreas divisum, pancreatic hypoplasia and agenesis, heterotopic pancreas

Inherited Syndromes Affecting the Pancreas
Cystic fibrosis
Shwachman-Diamond syndrome, Johnson-Blizzard syndrome, Pearson bone marrow pancreas syndrome

Gene Mutations Leading to Pancreatic Disease
Hereditary pancreatitis; cationic trypsinogen gene mutations, trypsin inhibitor gene mutations

Pancreatic Insufficiency Syndrome
Isolated enzyme deficiencies, lipase, colipase, enterokinase

Pancreatic Insufficiency Secondary to Other Disorders
Celiac disease

Acquired Pancreatitis in Childhood
Idiopathic, traumatic, drugs, viral, metabolic, collagen vascular disease, autoimmune, fibrosing, nutritional (tropical)

Cystic fibrosis (CF) is the most common severe autosomal recessive disease, with an estimated gene frequency in Western Europe and the United States of between 1:25 and 1:35 and a disease incidence of about 1 in 2500 to 1 in 3200. The pathogenesis and diagnosis of CF are described in Chapter 40. Pancreatic insufficiency is present at birth in 65% of infants with CF, and a further 15% develop it during infancy and early childhood. The 20% who do not develop pancreatic insufficiency have a better prognosis and develop fewer complications.

Measurement of pancreatic elastase-1 in feces (see section on noninvasive tests of exocrine pancreatic function) is considered to be a reliable test for pancreatic insufficiency in infants over the age of 2 weeks with CF and in older children at the time of diagnosis of the disorder.[17,113,145] This test can also be used to detect the onset of pancreatic insufficiency in those previously pancreatic sufficient.

Adult Disorders of the Exocrine Pancreas[62]

The major exocrine pancreatic disorders presenting in adult life are acute pancreatitis, chronic pancreatitis,[12A] and carcinoma of the pancreas. The use of enzyme tests in the diagnosis of acute pancreatitis is discussed in Chapter 22. The causes of pancreatitis are given in Box 51-6.

Chronic pancreatitis is defined by irreversible pancreatic damage with histologic evidence of inflammation and fibrosis leading to destruction of endocrine and exocrine function. The major histologic features are similar regardless of the cause. In Western countries, the most common cause is alcohol (60 to 90% of all cases of chronic pancreatitis), although because only 5 to 15% of heavy drinkers develop the disease, clearly other predisposing factors are present (e.g., smoking, diet high in fat and protein).

The role of invasive and noninvasive pancreatic exocrine tests in chronic pancreatitis has been reviewed.[66]

BOX 51-6 Causes of Pancreatitis in Adults

Acute
Gallstones
Alcohol
Infection (e.g., mumps, Coxsackie B)
Pancreatic tumors
Drugs (e.g., azathioprine, estrogens, corticosteroids, didanosine)
Iatrogenic [e.g., postsurgical, endoscopic retrograde cholangiopancreatography (ERCP)]
Hyperlipidemias
Miscellaneous—trauma, scorpion bite, cardiac surgery
Idiopathic

Chronic
Alcohol
Tropical (nutritional)
Hereditary [trypsinogen and inhibitory protein defects, cystic fibrosis]
Idiopathic
Trauma
Hypercalcemia

From Burroughs AK, Westaby D. Liver, biliary tract disease and pancreatic disease. In: Kumar P, Clark M, eds. Clinical medicine, 7th edition. Edinburgh: Elsevier Saunders, 2009:319-85.

Tests of Exocrine Function of the Pancreas

The predominant exocrine functions of the pancreas are the production and secretion of pancreatic juice, which is rich in enzymes and bicarbonate. Normal pancreatic juice is colorless and odorless; it has a pH of 8.0 to 8.3 and a specific gravity of 1.007 to 1.042. The total 24 hour secretion volume may be as high as 3000 mL.[151]

Laboratory tests used to measure exocrine function in the investigation of pancreatic insufficiency (most commonly caused by CF in children and chronic pancreatitis in adults) fall into one of two categories: invasive and noninvasive. Invasive tests require GI intubation to collect pancreatic samples; noninvasive ("tubeless") tests were developed to avoid intubation, which is uncomfortable for the patient, time-consuming, and therefore expensive. Noninvasive tests are simpler and cheaper to perform but in general lack the sensitivity and specificity of invasive tests, particularly for the diagnosis of mild pancreatic insufficiency. It is important to recognize that biochemical tests have a limited clinical application in the diagnosis of pancreatic disease because of the complexity of the invasive tests or the inadequate sensitivity and specificity for mild and moderate pancreatic disease of the noninvasive tests. Of greater importance are the imaging procedures (Box 51-7). These techniques continue to be developed. One study shows that administration of secretin, causing stimulation of fluid and bicarbonate secretion, leads to anatomic changes that can be quantified by magnetic resonance cholangiopancreatography, with significant differences between normal volunteers and patients with pancreatic insufficiency.[31] In the future, it may therefore be possible to confidently diagnose pancreatic insufficiency with the use of imaging techniques alone.

BOX 51-7 Pancreatic Imaging Procedures

Plain abdominal radiograph
- May show pancreatic calcification, particularly when alcohol is the cause

Ultrasound
- Useful screening investigation for inflammation and neoplasia. Views may be limited by overlying bowel gas.

Spiral computed tomography (CT)
- With contrast enhancement and following a specific pancreatic protocol remains the gold standard imaging technique for the investigation of pancreatic disease.

Magnetic resonance imaging (MRI) scanning
- An alternative to CT. Magnetic resonance cholangiopancreatography (MRCP) gives clear definition of the pancreatic duct and the biliary tree. Gallstones (including microcalculi) may also be identified in the biliary tree using MRI/MRCP.

Endoscopic ultrasound
- Very useful for identifying distal common bile duct stones which may be the cause of an episode of acute pancreatitis.
- Can identify early changes of chronic pancreatic before these are evident on other imaging methods.
- Has an increasing role for staging the operability of pancreatic adenocarcinoma, particularly with respect to vascular invasion.
- Considered to be the imaging technique of choice for investigating cystic lesions of the pancreas.
- Is a sensitive means of detecting small pancreatic tumors, particularly those of neuroendocrine origin.

Endoscopic retrograde cholangiopancreatography (ERCP)
- This has been considered the gold standard for diagnosing pancreatic disease. However, with MRCP and endoscopic ultrasound, ERCP is restricted to therapeutic intervention.

From Burroughs AK, Westaby D. Liver, biliary tract disease and pancreatic disease. In: Kumar P, Clark M, eds. Clinical medicine, 7th edition. Edinburgh: Elsevier Saunders, 2009:319-85.

Invasive Tests of Exocrine Pancreatic Function

The main types of invasive tests are summarized in Table 51-7.

Total volume of pancreatic juice, the amount or concentration of bicarbonate, and activities of pancreatic enzymes are measured in duodenal contents. The enzyme most commonly measured is trypsin, but amylase, lipase, chymotrypsin, and elastase may also be evaluated. The *Lundh test* consists of administering a standardized meal consisting of 5% protein, 6% fat, 15% carbohydrate, and 74% non-nutrient fiber, which provides a physiologic stimulus to the pancreas and is simple to administer. However, administration of the meal prevents determination of the total enzyme and bicarbonate or secretory volume, and in the presence of mucosal disease (e.g., celiac disease), in which hormone release from the duodenal mucosa is impaired, it provides inadequate or no stimulation. In view of these limitations, the Lundh test is largely of historical interest.

The *secretin test* is based on the principle that secretion of pancreatic juice and bicarbonate output are related to the functional mass of pancreatic tissue. After an overnight fast, basal samples of fluid are collected from the stomach and duodenum. One clinical unit (CU) of secretin/kg body weight is administered intravenously, and duodenal fluid is collected at 15 minute intervals for at least 1 hour. Purified porcine secretin has traditionally been used for the test, but synthetic porcine secretin (0.2 μg/kg) can also be used.[164]

Secretin stimulates the secretion of pancreatic juice and bicarbonate, but stimulation of the secretion of pancreatic enzymes is inconsistent. Addition of CCK (or a synthetic equivalent) to the secretin test provides a stimulus to the secretion of pancreatic enzymes, allowing a more complete assessment of pancreatic reserve than can be obtained with secretin alone. The functional activity of CCK resides in the C-terminal octapeptide sequence (CCK-8); this octapeptide or ceruletide (a synthetic decapeptide identical to the natural decapeptide cerulein) can be used to stimulate pancreatic enzyme secretion (Figure 51-7).

The procedure for the *secretin-ceruletide test* is similar to that described for the secretin test. Patients are required to fast overnight; a gastroduodenal tube is then placed into the duodenum under x-ray control. After basal fluid is collected for 15 minutes, 1 U secretin/kg body weight/h is given continuously intravenously for 2 hours; 30 mg ceruletide/kg body weight/h is given simultaneously for the second hour. Pancreatic juice is collected during 15 minute intervals, and volume, pH, bicarbonate, and enzymes are measured.[120]

TABLE 51-7 Summary of Invasive Tests of Pancreatic Exocrine Function

Procedure	Pancreatic Stimulant	Analysis of Duodenal Contents
Lundh test	Standardized meal	Enzyme output
Secretin stimulation test	Purified or synthetic porcine secretin	Bicarbonate output
Secretin-cholecystokinin (CCK) test	Secretin as above plus CCK analog (CCK-8 or ceruletide)	Bicarbonate and enzymes

Procedures and reference values are not standardized among laboratories. It is recommended that doses of secretagogues should be high enough to provide maximal pancreatic stimulation and should be given for at least 60 to 90 minutes to ensure better diagnostic accuracy, especially in mild pancreatic insufficiency.[66]

Noninvasive Tests of Exocrine Pancreatic Function

"For many years, gastroenterologists have searched for the holy grail of pancreatic function tests—the tubeless test."[38] It is not surprising that a range of tests have been proposed, but none has adequate sensitivity for reliably detecting early pancreatic disease. When malabsorption is present, such tests are of value in confirming or excluding pancreatic disease. Considerable overlap often occurs between results observed in normal individuals and those found in patients with pancreatic disorders; this is due mainly to the large functional reserve of the pancreas. It has been estimated that pancreatic insufficiency cannot clearly be demonstrated until at least 50% of the acinar cells have been destroyed. Clinical signs of pancreatic insufficiency often do not appear until 90% of acinar tissue has been destroyed. In general, the noninvasive tests may therefore be used when causes of malabsorption are investigated, but they have inadequate sensitivity for the diagnosis of chronic pancreatitis. Comparison between studies and of different markers is difficult because the "gold standard" may be functional tests, which may differ in procedure and reference values,[111,120,166] or morphologic assessment. In some cases, one noninvasive test has been compared with another. Table 51-8 compares the diagnostic performance of noninvasive tests.

The noninvasive tests are based on the reduction in secretion of pancreatic enzymes with measurement of enzymes in feces (chymotrypsin or elastase) or detection of products of their catalytic reactions, after oral administration of synthetic substrates, in urine [*N*-benzoyl-L-tyrosyl-*p*-aminobenzoic acid (NBT-PABA) or pancreolauryl test] or in breath (^{13}C-mixed chain triglyceride breath test).[183] Fecal elastase (measured by the monoclonal antibody method) is currently the noninvasive test of choice for assessing pancreatic insufficiency.

Pancreatic chymotrypsin is almost completely digested during its passage through the gut in adults, but the residual activity of the enzyme in feces is stable for several days at 20 °C. Its output in stool correlates poorly with chymotrypsin

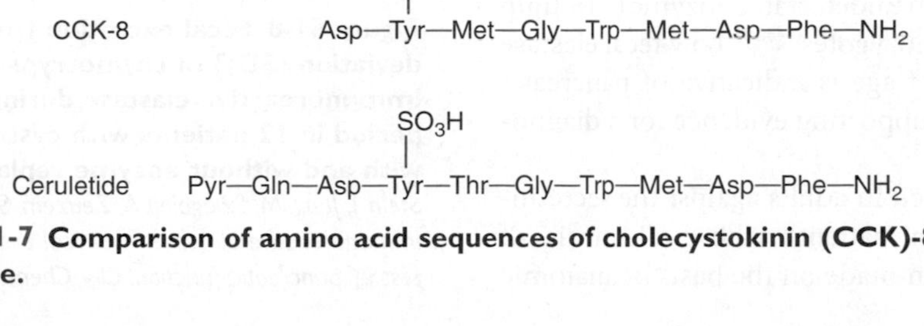

CCK-8: Asp—Tyr(SO_3H)—Met—Gly—Trp—Met—Asp—Phe—NH_2

Ceruletide: Pyr—Gln—Asp—Tyr(SO_3H)—Thr—Gly—Trp—Met—Asp—Phe—NH_2

Figure 51-7 Comparison of amino acid sequences of cholecystokinin (CCK)-8 and ceruletide.

TABLE 51-8 Diagnostic Accuracy of Noninvasive Tests for Mild, Moderate, and Severe Pancreatic Insufficiency, as Assessed by Anatomic or Functional Criteria

Sensitivity for Pancreatic Insufficiency				
Test	**Mild**	**Moderate**	**Severe**	**Specificity**
Fecal chymotrypsin[71]	11%	54%	77%	85%
Fecal elastase-1[71]	22%	77%	100%	96%
NBT-PABA[63,140]	—	50%	70%	72%
Pancreolauryl[38,140]	<50%	50%	85%	50%
^{13}C-MCT absorption[119]	62%	—	100%	85%

MCT, Medium chain triglyceride; *NBT-PABA, N*-benzoyl-L-tyrosyl-*p*-aminobenzoic acid.

secretion in duodenal contents when both are measured after stimulation with secretin-CCK. In patients without pancreatic disease, the incidence of falsely low results is about 10 to 15% and may be due to (a) voluminous stools (>300 g/d) and thus less enzyme per gram of feces; (b) inadequate food intake; (c) partial gastrectomy or mucosal disease (e.g., celiac disease), which causes inadequate stimulation of pancreatic secretion; or (d) obstruction of the bile duct. Falsely normal results in patients with mild pancreatic insufficiency may be as high as 50%.[72] In a collaborative study in children, both fecal chymotrypsin and elastase showed 100% sensitivity for detecting pancreatic insufficiency in CF, but the specificity of chymotrypsin was lower than that of elastase in a control group of children with small intestinal disease.[19] Most recent papers conclude that although chymotrypsin measurement is easier than elastase measurement, the latter test has significant advantages in terms of diagnostic accuracy. The recommended procedure[99] uses a stool pretreatment stage that dissociates particle-bound chymotrypsin.

Pancreatic elastase-1 is a pancreas-specific protease present in pancreatic juice. It is not degraded during passage through the gut, and concentrations in feces are fivefold to sixfold greater than those in pancreatic juice.[172] The enzyme can be identified in feces with a commercial ELISA assay that uses two monoclonal antibodies specific to the human enzyme (Schebo Biotech, Giessen, Germany). Treatment of patients with pancreatic enzyme supplements therefore does not interfere with the test (Figure 51-8). Table 51-9 compares chymotrypsin and elastase, indicating some of the advantages of fecal elastase measurement.

Fecal elastase-1 has been evaluated extensively both in CF and in adult pancreatic insufficiency, and its use is recommended in both children and adults.[30,177] In children with CF, the test discriminates between those with and without pancreatic insufficiency.[71] Very low elastase-1 is seen in a wide range of *CFTR* genotypes with undetectable enzyme (<15 μg/g of stool) in most ΔF508 homozygotes.[145,183] Low fecal elastase (<200 μg/g) after 4 weeks of age is indicative of pancreatic insufficiency and provides supporting evidence for a diagnosis of CF.[17]

The test has been evaluated in adults against the secretin-cerulein test[111,120,166] and in patients whose diagnosis of chronic pancreatitis has been made on the basis of anatomic

TABLE 51-9 Comparison of Fecal Chymotrypsin and Elastase

	Fecal Enzyme	
	Chymotrypsin	**Elastase**
10 day intraindividual variation, mean CV	30%	15%
Loss of activity, 7 days at 4 °C	17%	2.5%
Overall diagnostic sensitivity	64%	93%
Overall diagnostic specificity	89%	93%

CV, Coefficient of variation.
From Loser C, Mollgaard A, Folsch UR. Faecal elastase 1: a novel, highly sensitive, and specific tubeless pancreatic function test. Gut 1996;39:580-6.

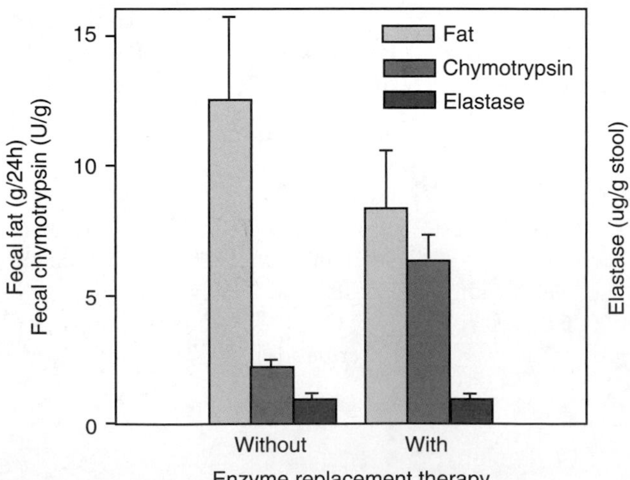

Figure 51-8 Fecal excretion [mean and standard deviation (SD)] of chymotrypsin, fat, and immunoreactive elastase during a 24 hour collection period in 12 patients with cystic fibrosis and steatorrhea, with and without enzyme replacement therapy. *(From Stein J, Jung M, Sziegoleit A, Zeuzem S, Caspary WF, Lembcke B. Immunoreactive elastase I: clinical evaluation of a new non-invasive test of pancreatic function. Clin Chem 1996;42:222-6.)*

and morphologic changes detected by ultrasound and endoscopic retrograde pancreatography or computed tomography.[39,72,127] The test is routinely carried out on a small random fecal sample, thus it might be expected to give inferior diagnostic accuracy compared with those evaluations carried out on portions of 24 hour or 72 hour fecal collections. However, with random fecal samples, specificities of 98% and 100% have been reported in healthy controls, and specificities of 90 to 97% in patients with nonpancreatic GI disease. Positive results (i.e., <200 μg/g) have been reported in patients with clinical or laboratory evidence of malnutrition who also have inflammatory bowel disease or chronic diarrhea (nonpancreatic). These observations may actually be due to impaired pancreatic secretion as a consequence of malnutrition.[127] The authors also suggest that increased bacterial degradation of the enzyme might be the cause of false positives in some patients with bacterial overgrowth. Similar results have been reported in children with nonpancreatic disease; the finding of low fecal elastase in a child with steatorrhea probably indicates coexisting pancreatic insufficiency.[19]

Measurement of pancreatic elastase-1 in feces has high sensitivity for the detection of severe and moderate chronic pancreatitis in adults. It has better sensitivity than other tests for detecting mild chronic pancreatitis, and high sensitivity and high negative predictive value for discriminating between diarrhea of pancreatic and nonpancreatic origin. The test is not specific for pancreatitis and detects moderate to severe impairment of pancreatic exocrine secretion from any cause. It is considered to be the most suitable test to confirm pancreatic insufficiency in screened cystic fibrosis infants older than 2 weeks,[17] and as previously noted, the test result is not influenced by the administration of pancreatic enzyme supplements. A negative test does not exclude mild disease, and false positives in some nonpancreatic diseases and in very watery samples limit its diagnostic accuracy. Measurement of the enzyme in dried feces avoids the problem associated with watery stool samples.[97] An ELISA based on polyclonal antibodies (and also called a test for "elastase 1") appears to have binding characteristics different from those of the monoclonal antibody assay.[75] Quantitative results differ between the polyclonal and monoclonal assays but a comparative study of 68 patient samples showed that both procedures were comparable in categorizing subjects as normal or as having moderately or severe pancreatic insufficiency.[49A]

The *NBT-PABA test* of pancreatic function is not now available but was based on the intestinal hydrolysis, by chymotrypsin, of a synthetic tripeptide—*N*-benzoyl-L-tyrosyl-*p*-aminobenzoic acid. The tripeptide, variously called NBT-PABA, BTP, and bentiromide, was administered orally together with a test meal to stimulate pancreatic secretion. BTP is specifically hydrolyzed by chymotrypsin in the duodenum to release *p*-aminobenzoic acid (PABA). The amount of PABA detected in serum or urine by high-performance liquid chromatography is an indirect measure of chymotrypsin activity in duodenal content. The test had a lower diagnostic sensitivity and specificity for pancreatic insufficiency than fecal elastase (see Table 51-8).

The *pancreolauryl test* (fluorescein dilaurate test) is also obsolete but was similar in its principle to the NBT-PABA test. Fluorescein dilaurate (FDL), which is specifically hydrolyzed to fluorescein by pancreatic cholesterol esterase, was given orally in the middle of a standard "breakfast" (50 g white bread, 20 g butter, and 1 cup of tea) and is specifically hydrolyzed by pancreatic cholesterol esterase, which requires bile salts for its activity. Fluorescein is water-soluble, readily absorbed by the small intestine, conjugated in the liver, and excreted in the urine. Urine was collected for 10 hours; the test was repeated on a second day using free fluorescein to correct for individual variability in intestinal absorption, hepatic conjugation, and urinary excretion. Urinary recovery of fluorescein was measured on a spectrophotometer each day at 492 nm after hydrolysis with 0.1 mol/L sodium hydroxide under standard conditions. The FDL test produces results very similar to those obtained with the PABA test, although sensitivity was higher (see Table 51-8). Analytically, measurement of fluorescein is simple, and good agreement between laboratories was found from external quality assessment (EQA) results for measurements of fluorescein in urine.[44] The test results could also be expressed as peak serum fluorescein concentration; high sensitivity (100%) was reported in moderate and severe chronic pancreatitis; specificity was poor in small bowel disease because of the influence of factors other than pancreatic enzyme hydrolysis on the absorption of fluorescein.[39] Liver diseases are associated with false-positive results because bile salts are necessary for the digestion and absorption of FDL.

Several different ^{13}C breath tests have been proposed for the evaluation of fat absorption[112]; most of them assess the overall ("global") process of fat absorption and are not able to differentiate fat malabsorption from pancreatic and nonpancreatic causes.

The *^{13}C-mixed chain triglyceride test* is designed as a test of intraluminal pancreatic lipase activity.[182] The substrate for the test is 1,3-distearyl,2(carboxyl-^{13}C) octanoyl glycerol, which contains long chain fatty acids in positions 1 and 3 and the ^{13}C-labeled medium chain fatty acid (octanoic acid) in position 2 (Figure 51-9). The labeled substrate is administered orally to fasting patients with a standard meal of toast and butter. Breath samples are collected over a 5 hour period, and exhaled $^{13}CO_2$ is expressed as a percentage of the

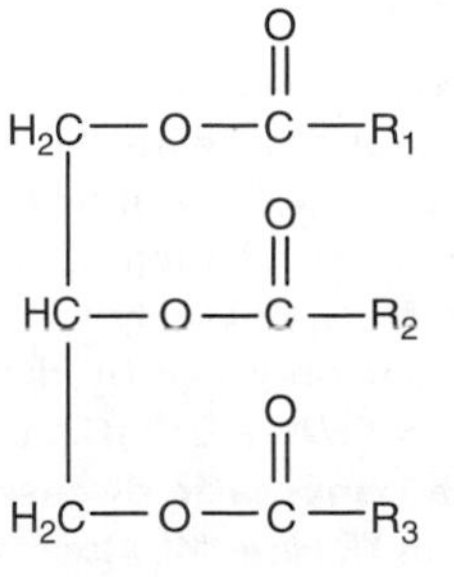

$H_2C-O-C(=O)-R_1$
$HC-O-C(=O)-R_2$
$H_2C-O-C(=O)-R_3$

R_1 and R_3= stearic acid (18:0)

R_2= ^{13}C-octanoic acid

Figure 51-9 The substrate for the ^{13}C-mixed chain triglyceride breath test: 1,3 distearyl,2(carboxyl-^{13}C) octanoyl glycerol.

administered dose. The rationale of the procedure is that before absorption or metabolism of the ^{13}C-octanoate, or ^{13}C-octanoyl monoglyceride, the stearyl groups must be hydrolyzed by the activity of pancreatic lipase. Decreased pancreatic lipase secretion will therefore lead to a reduction in the amount of ^{13}C label absorbed and subsequently metabolized to $^{13}CO_2$.

In an initial assessment, a group of 25 normal control subjects were compared with 29 patients with pancreatic disease. $^{13}CO_2$ in breath (cumulative over 6 hours) was highly correlated with pancreatic lipase output (Figure 51-10).

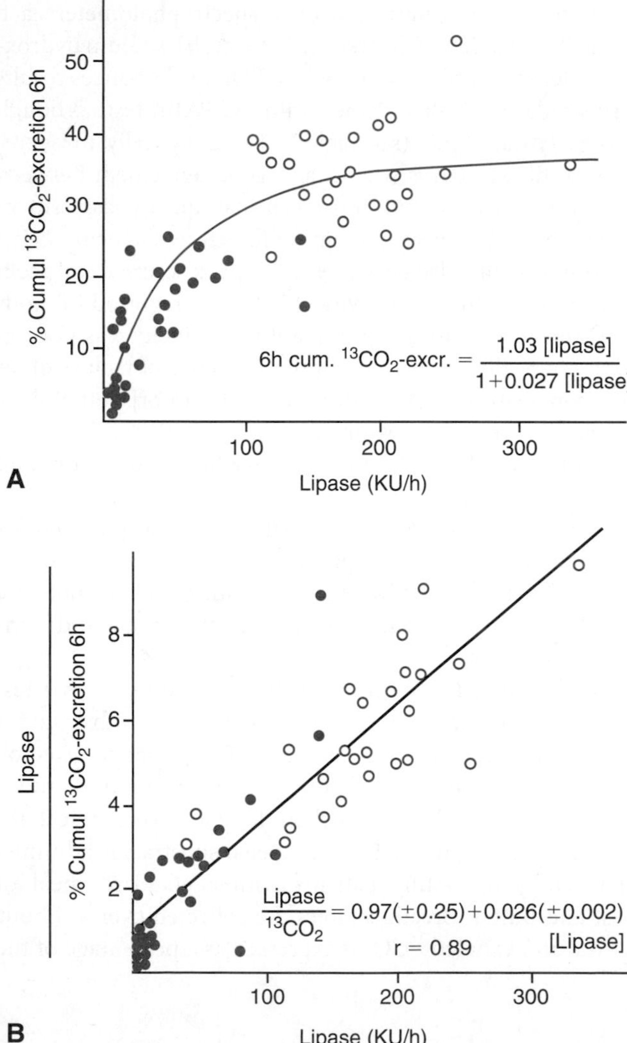

Figure 51-10 A, Cumulative $^{13}CO_2$ excretion (in percentage of ingested dose) 6 hours after intake of the ^{13}C-labeled mixed triglyceride as a function of lipase activity (in kilounits per hour) in normal subjects ○ and patients with pancreatic disease ●. B, Linearly modified saturation curve following the relation given by the following equation: Lipase/$^{13}CO_2$ = (1/A + B/A)(lipase), normal subjects ○, patients with pancreatic disease ●. *(From Vantrappen GR, Rutgeerts PJ, Ghoos YF, Hiele MI. Mixed triglyceride breath test: a noninvasive test of pancreatic lipase activity in the duodenum. Gastroenterology 1989;96:1126-34, with permission from the American Gastroenterological Association.)*

The test was superior to the estimation of fecal fat for detecting impaired pancreatic function. Sensitivity and specificity were 89% and 81%, respectively. In a later evaluation, the test was compared with results from the secretin-cerulein test, with patients categorized as having mild (n = 13) or severe (n = 13) pancreatic insufficiency.[119] Fecal elastase and chymotrypsin were also measured. Fecal elastase and the ^{13}C-mixed chain triglyceride test detected all cases of severe pancreatic insufficiency, but sensitivity was higher for fecal elastase in those with mild disease (see Table 51-8). Similar results were obtained when cholesteryl ^{13}C-octanoate was used as a substrate for a noninvasive test of pancreatic function.[25]

The sensitivity and specificity of these tests are limited by the complexity of the processes of absorption and metabolism. The substrates are specific for pancreatic lipases and the product is absorbed independently of micelle formation, but results of the test are affected by other factors, such as gastric emptying, mucosal absorption, hepatic metabolism, endogenous $^{13}CO_2$, and total CO_2 production.[1,42] These factors may explain the limited diagnostic sensitivity of the test in mild and moderate pancreatic insufficiency and its lack of specificity in nonpancreatic GI disease.

GI REGULATORY PEPTIDES

The gut is the largest endocrine organ in the body[149]; it is also a major target for many hormones, released locally and from other sites. GI regulatory peptides are released from the pancreatic islets (e.g., somatostatin) or from endocrine cells spread throughout the gut mucosa and collectively are referred to as the *diffuse endocrine system.* Many of these peptides (such as VIP and somatostatin) are present in the enteric nerves. They are also found in the central nervous system, and have important roles in the neuroendocrine control of the gut. Although many of them (such as secretin and gastrin) fulfill the classic criteria for a hormone by acting on distant cells (see Chapter 29), others function as neurotransmitters or have local (paracrine) effects on adjacent cells. Collectively, they influence motility, secretion, digestion, and absorption in the gut. They regulate bile flow and secretion of pancreatic hormones and affect the tonicity of vascular walls, blood pressure, and cardiac output.

Understanding of the role of the neuroendocrine system and gut peptides, and of the importance of the gut-hypothalamic pathway, in the normal control of food intake is growing, as is knowledge of the possibility of disorders of these mechanisms as causes of obesity.[154] The gastric peptide ghrelin and cholecystokinin act as short-term regulators of appetite and satiety. The neuropeptide PYY_{3-36}, a member of the neuropeptide Y family, is secreted by endocrine cells in the distal small intestine and colon in response to ingestion of food. Recent evidence shows that infusion of PYY_{3-36} to physiologic plasma concentrations in humans significantly decreases appetite with a 33% reduction in food intake over 24 hours. In mice, the relevant pathway is via the arcuate nucleus of the hypothalamus.[8] PYY_{3-36} therefore is a further

TABLE 51-10 Characteristics of Prominent Forms of Principal Gut Regulatory Peptides

Hormone/ Peptide	Molecular Wt (Da)	No. of Amino Acids	Main Gut Localization	Principal Physiologic Actions
Gastrin Family				
Cholecystokinin	3918	33 (also 385, 59)	Duodenum and jejunum Enteric nerves	Stimulates gallbladder contraction and intestinal motility; stimulates secretion of pancreatic enzymes, insulin, glucagon, and pancreatic polypeptides; has a role in indicating satiety; the C-terminal 8 amino acid peptide cholecystokinin (CCK)-8 retains full activity
Little gastrin Big gastrin	2098 3839	17 34	Both forms of gastrin are found in the gastric antrum and duodenum	Gastrins stimulate the secretion of gastric acid, pepsinogen, intrinsic factor, and secretin; stimulate intestinal mucosal growth; increase gastric and intestinal motility
Secretin-Glucagon Family				
Secretin	3056	27	Duodenum and jejunum	Stimulates pancreatic secretion of HCO_3, enzymes, and insulin; reduces gastric and duodenal motility, inhibits gastrin release and gastric acid secretion
Vasoactive intestinal polypeptide (VIP)	3326	28	Enteric nerves	Relaxes smooth muscle of gut, blood, and genitourinary system; increases water and electrolyte secretion from pancreas and gut; releases hormones from pancreas, gut, and hypothalamus
Glucose-dependent insulinotropic	4976	42	Duodenum and jejunum	Stimulates insulin release; reduces gastric and intestinal motility; increases fluid and electrolyte secretion from small intestine

addition to a growing list of hormones with a role in the regulation of energy balance.

Table 51-10 summarizes basic chemical characteristics of five of the major GI regulatory peptides and indicates their site of origin and major functions. More detailed descriptions of these five peptides are given in the following paragraphs, followed by a listing of other regulatory peptides of the GI tract in Table 51-11.

CHOLECYSTOKININ[130,149]

CCK is a linear polypeptide that exists in multiple molecular forms. The first form to be isolated was the 33 amino acid peptide CCK-33. Other major forms are CCK-8, CCK-39, and CCK-58. In all forms, the five C-terminal amino acids are identical to those of gastrin and are necessary, together with a sulfated tyrosyl residue, for physiologic activity. All forms of CCK are produced by enzymatic cleavage of a single 115 amino acid precursor, preprocholecystokinin.

CCK is found in the I cells of the upper small intestinal mucosa. Mixtures of polypeptides and amino acids (especially tryptophan and phenylalanine) stimulate CCK secretion, whereas pure undigested protein does not elicit a response. Secretion is also stimulated by gastric acid entering the duodenum and by fatty acids with chains of nine or more carbons, especially in the form of micelles. Circulating concentrations of CCK therefore are increased following ingestion of a mixed meal. CCK is rapidly cleared from plasma ($t_{1/2} = <3$ min), predominantly by the kidneys. Secretion of CCK is completely inhibited after somatostatin infusion.

CCK regulates gallbladder contraction and increases small intestinal motility. It possesses the same terminal pentapeptide as gastrin, and therefore also has a mild stimulatory effect on gastric HCl and pepsinogen secretion, antral motility, and pancreatic bicarbonate secretion. Secretion of the less potent CCK results in decreased output of HCl because CCK competes with gastrin for receptor sites on the HCl-secreting cells. Conversely, gastrin and CCK are additive in their stimulation of the pancreas, and both increase the effects of secretin on pancreatic function. CCK also stimulates pancreatic growth, relaxes the sphincter of Oddi, and stimulates secretions from Brunner's (duodenal) glands.

CCK is also present in the brain, with highest concentrations in the cerebral cortex; its function in the CNS is unclear. It is released from the GI tract and acts as a short-term, meal-related satiety signal, thus regulating appetite. CCK is widely

TABLE 51-11 Brief Description of Other GI Regulatory Peptides

Hormone/Peptide	Major Tissue Locations in Gut	Principal Known Actions
Bombesin	Throughout the gut and pancreas	Stimulates release of cholecystokinin (CCK) and gastrin
Calcitonin gene-related peptide	Enteric nerves	Unclear
Chromogranin A	Neuroendocrine cells	Secretory protein
Enkephalins	Stomach, duodenum	Opiate-like actions
Enteroglucagon	Small intestine, pancreas	Inhibits insulin secretion
Galanin	Enteric nerves	
Ghrelin	Stomach	Stimulates appetite, increases gastric emptying
Glucagon-like peptide 1	Pancreas, ileum	Increases insulin secretion
Glucagon-like peptide 2	Ileum, colon	Enterocyte-specific growth hormone
Growth factors	Throughout the gut	Cell proliferation and differentiation
Growth hormone–releasing factor	Small intestine	Unclear
Leptin	Stomach	Appetite control
Motilin	Throughout the gut	Increases gastric emptying and small bowel motility
Neuropeptide Y	Enteric nerves	Regulation of intestinal blood flow
Neurotensin	Ileum	Affects gut motility; increases jejunal and ileal fluid secretion
Pancreastatin	Pancreas	Inhibits pancreatic endocrine and exocrine secretion
Pancreatic polypeptide	Pancreas	Inhibits pancreatic and biliary secretion
$PYY_{3\text{-}36}$	Colon	Inhibits food intake
Somatostatin	Stomach, pancreas	Inhibits secretion and action of many hormones
Substance P	Enteric nerves	Unclear
Trefoil peptides	Stomach, intestine	Mucosal protection and repair

distributed throughout the central and peripheral nervous systems.

Gastrin[130,149]

Three major molecular forms of gastrin occur in blood and tissues: big gastrin (G-34), a linear polypeptide of 34 amino acids; little gastrin (G-17); and mini gastrin (G-14). In addition to these, G-71, G-52, and G-6 are present in small amounts. Gastrins originate from the cleavage of a single precursor, preprogastrin, a peptide consisting of 101 amino acids. The smallest peptide sequence of gastrin possessing biological activity is the carboxy-terminal tetrapeptide (G-4, tetrin); on a molar basis, it is only one sixth to one tenth as potent as G-17. A synthetic pentapeptide (pentagastrin) may be used for stimulation of HCl secretion in gastric function testing.

Gastrin is produced and stored mainly by endocrine cells (G cells) of the antral mucosa and to a lesser extent by G cells of the proximal duodenum and delta cells of the pancreatic islets. After secretion, gastrin is transported by the blood through the liver to the parietal cells of the fundus of the stomach, where it stimulates the secretion of gastric acid. Gastrin also stimulates secretion of gastric pepsinogens and intrinsic factor by the gastric mucosa, release of secretin by the small intestinal mucosa, and secretion of pancreatic bicarbonate and enzymes and hepatic bile; it increases gastric and intestinal motility, mucosal growth, and blood flow to the stomach. It is secreted in response to antral distention meals and by amino acids, peptides, and polypeptides from partially digested proteins in the stomach. Of the free amino acids, glycine, tryptophan, and phenylalanine are the most potent stimulators. Other stimuli of gastrin include alcohol, caffeine, insulin-induced hypoglycemia, and ingestion or intravenous infusion of calcium; vagal stimulation may be initiated by smelling, tasting, chewing, and swallowing food.

Maximal secretion of gastrin occurs at an antral pH of 5 to 7. At pH 2.5, secretion is reduced by about 80%; maximal suppression occurs at pH 1.0. Secretion is inhibited by the direct action of acid on the G cells. This negative feedback safeguards against overacidification by any and all stimulants.

The principal circulating form of gastrin is G-34 in healthy individuals and in patients with hypergastrinemia. Trypsin cleaves G-34 into two fragments, one of which is identical to G-17. On a molar basis, G-17 is six to eight times more potent than G-34 as a stimulant for gastric acid secretion. In the fasting state, the ratio of G-34 to G-17 is about 2 : 1. After meals, the concentration of G-34 doubles but that of G-17 increases four times, so that the ratio of these two forms in the circulation becomes 1 : 1. The half-lives of endogenous human G-17 and G-34 in the circulation are about 6 and 36 minutes, respectively; this difference probably accounts for the higher concentration of G-34 in the peripheral blood of individuals in the fasting state.

Secretin[130]

Secretin, a linear polypeptide containing 27 amino acids, has structural similarities to glucagon, VIP, GIP, peptide histidine-isoleucine (PHI), and growth hormone–releasing hormone. The amino acid residues at 14 positions within the molecule are identical to those found in glucagon; 8 are the same as in GIP, and 9 are the same as in VIP. The intact secretin molecule is required for biological activity.

Secretin is secreted by mucosal granular S cells located in greatest concentration in the duodenum but present throughout the small intestine. It is released primarily on contact of the S cells with gastric HCl; however, as pancreatic juice flows into the duodenum, it neutralizes gastric acid, thereby removing one stimulus for its own secretion. Secretin is not released until the pH is lowered to at least 4.5. Below this pH, secretin release is proportional to the amount of acid entering the duodenum. A pH less than 4.5 normally occurs only in the first few centimeters of the duodenum, causing little increase in plasma secretin after a normal meal. Thus secretin release after exposure of S cells to HCl may not be an important physiologic stimulus. However, plasma secretin concentrations that are too low to be measured by current methods may stimulate the pancreas in the presence of physiologic concentrations of CCK, which is known to strongly potentiate the action of secretin. Undigested fat does not stimulate secretin release, but fatty acids with chains of 10 or more carbons are weak stimulants. Alcohol increases secretin release through stimulation of gastric acid secretion with subsequent lowering of duodenal pH rather than by a direct stimulatory effect. The half-life of secretin is about 4 minutes. The kidney is the major site of its degradation. The only known physiologic inhibitor of secretin release is somatostatin.

The primary physiologic role of secretin is stimulation of the pancreas to secrete an increased volume of juice with high bicarbonate content. Other actions include stimulation of bicarbonate and water secretion from the liver and from Brunner's glands; augmentation of gallbladder contraction and increased hepatic bile flow; weak stimulation of insulin secretion (a pharmacologic effect); stimulation of parathyroid hormone (PTH) secretion; release of pancreatic enzymes and of pepsinogen by the chief cells of the stomach; reduction of gastric and duodenal motility; reduction of lower esophageal sphincter pressure; and promotion of pancreatic growth. Secretin inhibits normal gastrin secretion (but does not decrease serum gastrin in the Zollinger-Ellison syndrome) and therefore gastric acid secretion.

Vasoactive Intestinal Polypeptide[130]

VIP is a linear polypeptide consisting of 28 amino acids; it has structural similarities to secretin, GIP, and glucagon. VIP is present throughout the body and is found in highest concentrations in the nervous system and gut. Unlike secretin and other GI hormones, VIP is not found in the mucosal endocrine cells of the GI tract. VIP is believed to be a neurotransmitter limited to peripheral and central nervous tissue. VIP-containing nerve fibers are found throughout the GI tract from the esophagus to the colon and in all tissue layers of the gut.

Little is known about the conditions that cause VIP to be released into the circulation. No evidence suggests that VIP is released during digestion, but its secretion is increased by vagal stimulation. It has a plasma half-life of about 1 minute, and most of the hormone is inactivated by a single passage through the liver.

VIP has a large number of ill-defined physiologic actions, some of which are shared with other similar polypeptide hormones (secretin and GIP). It acts as a neurotransmitter in the central and autonomic nervous systems and causes vasodilation and relaxation of the smooth muscles of the circulatory and genitourinary systems and the gut. Other actions of VIP include an increase of water and electrolyte secretion from the pancreas and gut; release of hormones from the pancreas, gut, and hypothalamus; stimulation of lipolysis, glycolysis, and bile flow; and inhibition of gastrin and gastric acid secretion. Most of the actions of VIP tend to be of short duration because of its rapid degradation.

Glucose-Dependent Insulinotropic Peptide (GIP, Gastric Inhibitory Polypeptide)[130]

GIP is a linear peptide consisting of 42 amino acids. Its N-terminal end has a close resemblance to glucagon and secretin, but the C-terminal amino acid sequence of 17 residues is not common to any other known intestinal hormone.

GIP is synthesized and released by K cells located in the duodenal and jejunal mucosa. Plasma GIP is increased by oral administration of glucose or triacylglycerols, or intraduodenal infusion of solutions containing a mixture of amino acids; none of these, however, increases GIP concentrations when given intravenously. Protein ingestion does not significantly increase GIP. For food components to stimulate GIP release, they must be absorbed by the intestinal mucosa.

The biological actions of GIP include (1) stimulation of insulin secretion in the presence of hyperglycemia; (2) reduction of intestinal motility with stimulation of small intestinal fluid and electrolyte secretion; and (3) in supraphysiologic concentrations, inhibition of gastric acid, pepsin, and gastrin secretion. The insulinotropic action of GIP appears to be the most important of its biological actions; as a result, this hormone has been called *glucose-dependent insulinotropic peptide* as a more accurate description of its physiologic action.

Other Regulatory Peptides

Table 51-11 provides a brief description of tissue locations and the actions of other gut regulatory peptides, although the function of some of these is unclear. The growth factors belong to several families of peptides and have important roles in the control of a wide range of cell functions in the intestine.[37] The current clinical use of GI hormone/regulatory peptide measurements is in the diagnosis of neuroendocrine tumors of the pancreas and GI tract. It is likely that they will have wider applications as understanding of their functions grows (e.g., in the fields of obesity and appetite modulation).[28,29,137]

GASTROINTESTINAL NEUROENDOCRINE TUMORS AND TUMOR MARKERS

GI neuroendocrine tumors may be endocrine pancreatic tumors or carcinoid tumors arising from enterochromaffin cells that occur throughout the GI tract. Carcinoid tumors are discussed in Chapter 30.

Approximately two thirds of patients with tumors arising from pancreatic islet cells present with clinical syndromes associated with excessive hormone production.[109] This group of tumors includes insulomas, gastrinomas, VIPomas, glucagonomas, and somatostatinomas. Insulinomas and glucagonomas are not usually associated with GI symptoms. Gastrinomas and VIPomas are discussed later. The somatostatinoma syndrome is associated with steatorrhea, gallstones, and diabetes. The remaining one third of patients with endocrine pancreatic tumors have no specific clinical symptoms associated with the tumors, which are described as nonfunctional. Clinical features of these uncommon tumors and measurement of their secretory products have been reviewed.[3]

The pattern of hormone and precursor production by neuroendocrine tumors is complex. Most secrete several tumor markers. Chromogranin A, a member of a family of secretory proteins, has the highest diagnostic sensitivity (94%) for endocrine pancreatic tumors, followed by pancreatic polypeptide (74%).[50] Chromogranin A is elevated in most patients and is an alternative to more specific markers in monitoring the effectiveness of surgery or drug therapy. However, as with other protein and peptide tumor markers, the epitope specificity of antiserum used in the assay has a profound effect on the diagnostic sensitivity of the assay.[109] Although chromogranin A has high sensitivity, false positives have been observed in several nonendocrine tumors, including prostatic cancer.

Gastrinoma and the Zollinger-Ellison Syndrome[7,34,93]

In 1955, Zollinger and Ellison described a syndrome (Zollinger-Ellison, or Z-E, syndrome) consisting of fulminant peptic ulcers, massive gastric hypersecretion, and non-β–islet cell tumors of the pancreas. Hypergastrinemia, diarrhea, steatorrhea, and other endocrinopathies are frequent characteristics of this syndrome. Most cases occur between the ages of 30 and 50 years, although the condition has been described in patients from 7 to 90 years. It is more common in men (60% of cases) than in women. In about 25% of cases, ulcers are found beyond the first portion of the duodenum; such ulcers should always raise suspicion of Z-E syndrome. About 25% of all gastrinomas are part of the multiple endocrine neoplasia 1 syndrome (MEN1), which is characterized by tumors or hyperplasia in the duodenum or pancreatic islets and the parathyroid and pituitary glands. Fasting plasma gastrin usually is greatly increased, ranging from 2 to 2000 times normal. Concentrations more than 10 times the upper limit of normal, in the presence of gastric acid hypersecretion, are virtually diagnostic of gastrinoma. No correlation has been noted between the severity of symptoms and the degree of elevation of the circulating gastrin concentration. However, the fasting plasma gastrin concentration at presentation in sporadic Z-E syndrome is associated with the size and site of the tumor and the presence of hepatic metastases, and therefore has prognostic value.[9] Because management of the patient with Z-E syndrome usually requires surgical intervention, it is important to distinguish hypergastrinemia caused by gastrinoma from other conditions that may lead to similar increases in plasma gastrin.

Increased plasma gastrin occurs in hypochlorhydria or achlorhydria as a consequence of atrophic gastritis or the use of acid-suppressing drugs [e.g., histamine H_2-receptor antagonists, proton pump inhibitors (PPIs)]. Z-E syndrome cannot be diagnosed (or excluded) in patients taking PPIs. These drugs cause a profound reduction in gastric acid secretion and hence a large increase in plasma gastrin. *H. pylori* infection can also lead to increased plasma gastrin and to increased basal acid output, and in some cases to atrophic gastritis and high plasma gastrin.[88] Pernicious anemia and chronic atrophic gastritis associated with parietal cell antibodies are commonly associated with gastrin concentrations that overlap with those found in Z-E syndrome. Increases in plasma gastrin in chronic renal failure appear to be related to the severity of renal failure. A direct correlation has been found between G-cell density and parathyroid function in patients with chronic renal failure, suggesting that secondary hyperparathyroidism may play a role in increasing plasma gastrin. Surgical resection or disease of the kidneys or small intestine can cause hypergastrinemia, possibly because these are important sites of gastrin degradation or excretion.

Increased basal gastrin concentrations may be classified as "appropriate" or "inappropriate" according to their association with decreased or increased gastric acid secretion. In patients with very low or absent acid secretion and a functionally intact gastric antrum, an increase in plasma gastrin is physiologically appropriate and is expected. This increase is caused by hyperplasia of antral G cells as observed in atrophic gastritis, pernicious anemia, previous vagotomy, and renal failure. Inappropriate hypergastrinemia may be caused by gastrinoma, isolated retained antrum after gastric surgery, or primary G-cell hyperfunction.

A secretin stimulation test may assist in the differential diagnosis of Z-E syndrome.[3] The secretin test proved the more useful but is little used now with improved computed tomography scanning and the use of somatostatin-receptor imaging using the somatostatin analog octreotide.[109]

Measurement of Plasma Gastrin

In serum from healthy subjects, the predominant forms of gastrin are amidated G-34 and G-17. In subjects with gastrinomas, the circulating gastrins display unpredictable heterogeneity with a shift toward larger peptides. For the detection of gastrinomas, the assay therefore should be able to detect all secreted forms of gastrin to prevent false negatives.[67]

Gastrin is unstable in serum or plasma, and samples may lose up to 50% of their immunoreactivity during 48 hours at 2 to 8 °C, largely because of the action of proteolytic enzymes. Blood samples should be collected into a tube containing heparin as anticoagulant and aprotinin (e.g., Trasylol, 0.2 mL, 2000 KIU, in a 10 mL tube) to prevent proteolytic degradation. Samples should be mixed by inversion and transported rapidly on ice to the laboratory; the plasma should be separated in a refrigerated centrifuge. The plasma should be frozen at −20 °C within 15 minutes of venipuncture. Samples collected in this way are suitable for analysis of gastrin, VIP, pancreatic polypeptide, somatostatin, neurotensin, and chromogranins A and B.

The Watery Diarrhea Hypokalemia Achlorhydria Syndrome (Werner-Morrison Syndrome, WDHA Syndrome, VIPoma)[92]

The WDHA syndrome may be suspected in a patient who produces large volumes (>1 L/24 h) of secretory diarrhea (see the section on fecal osmolal gap) with dehydration and hypokalemia. The diagnosis is confirmed by the finding of a high plasma VIP concentration and demonstration of the tumor by somatostatin-receptor imaging.

INVESTIGATION OF MALDIGESTION/ MALABSORPTION

This section summarizes causes of malabsorption and suggests the general laboratory approach to these disorders.

Box 51-8 summarizes the main causes of malabsorption under the three categories of (1) intraluminal disorders and malabsorption due to disorders of (2) transport into the mucosal cells, and (3) transport out of the mucosal cells.

BOX 51-8 Summary of Disorders Leading to Malabsorption

Disorders of Intraluminal Digestion	
a. Altered gastric function	Postgastrectomy syndrome Zollinger-Ellison syndrome
b. Pancreatic insufficiency	Chronic pancreatitis Cystic fibrosis Pancreatic cancer
c. Bile acid deficiency	Disease/resection of terminal ileum Small bowel bacterial overgrowth
Disorders of Transport Into the Mucosal Cell	
a. Generalized disorders due to reduction in absorptive surface area	Celiac disease, tropical sprue
b. Specific disorders	Hypolactasia Vitamin B_{12} in pernicious anemia Zn in acrodermatitis enteropathica
Disorders of Transport out of the Mucosal Cell	
a. Blockage of the lymphatics	Abdominal lymphoma Primary lymphangiectasia
b. Inherited disorders	α-β-lipoproteinemia

Clinical presentation of the patient suffering from malabsorption or maldigestion classically includes the following features:

- *Evidence of general ill health.* Anorexia, weight loss, fatigue following minor effort, and dyspnea may be seen. Edema (due to hypoalbuminemia or weakness), tetany, and dehydration due to electrolyte imbalance and water loss may be present. In pancreatic exocrine insufficiency, however, hyperphagia is the rule; patients often report a very high (5000 kcal/d) food intake.
- *Isolated nutritional deficiencies.* Iron, folate, or vitamin B_{12} deficiency may manifest as anemia, which may be mild; vitamin K deficiency as a bleeding tendency; and vitamin D deficiency as bone disease. They are reflected by a variety of signs and symptoms (glossitis, pallor, dermatitis, petechiae, bruising, hematuria, muscle or bone pain, or neurologic abnormalities).
- *Abdominal symptoms,* such as discomfort, distention, flatulence, and borborygmi (rumbling and gurgling sounds due to movement of gas in the intestine).
- *Watery diarrhea and possible steatorrhea.* In severe cases of steatorrhea (excess fat in feces), the stool is typically loose, bulky, offensive, greasy, light-colored, and difficult to flush away. Alternatively, the stools may appear normal but may be more bulky or may be passed with greater frequency.

Early presentation of malabsorption will, however, be more subtle than this list would indicate. The alteration in volume or consistency of the stool may be slight, and only mild symptoms may be attributable to the GI tract. The patient may complain only of anorexia, fatigue, and lack of interest in daily activities. It is in these cases that the physician who suspects malabsorption on clinical grounds will rely on the laboratory to assist in the diagnosis. Initial laboratory investigations consist of routine tests, abnormalities of which may point to the possibility of malabsorption [e.g., blood hemoglobin concentration; mean red cell volume; serum concentrations of folate, ferritin, calcium, albumin, and alkaline phosphatase; tests for antibodies in celiac disease (celiac serology)].

Evaluation of Fat Absorption[78]

The evaluation of fat absorption or malabsorption is required in a small minority of patients undergoing investigation for GI disorders. The guidelines of the British Society of Gastroenterology (BSG)[174] state that gastroenterologists should have access to such tests to "…assess patients with malabsorption who are proving difficult to diagnose."

In a survey in 1997 of 231 hospitals in the United Kingdom,[44] fecal fat was the most widely available of all tests, with an estimated number of fecal fat measurements of 6100 performed annually in the United Kingdom. Fecal fat measurement has many limitations,[85] some of which were highlighted in the 1997 survey, that must be brought to the attention of clinicians to dissuade them from relying on an inherently unreliable test. In addition, dialogue with local gastroenterologists is necessary to reach consensus that the quantitative demonstration of fat malabsorption is of little value for most patients.

Limitations of Fecal Fat Measurement

The case for abandoning fecal fat measurement can be made on the grounds of physiology and of analytical performance. The physiologic problems of sample collection were convincingly demonstrated in a study in which radiopaque pellets were administered orally (8, three times a day) for 5 days (120 total), and feces were collected for days 3 to 5.[187] Radiographic detection of 72 pellets was taken to indicate 100% recovery. In 52 patients studied, recovery ranged from 14 to 125%, and recovery was within the range of 85 to 115% in only 32 of them. In seven patients, fecal fat was normal but became abnormal after adjustment for marker recovery. Despite this evidence, few laboratories attempt to assess the completeness of collection using markers.

Absorption of dietary fat is a remarkably efficient process, so that in normal health, fecal fat is largely (if not entirely) derived from endogenous rather than dietary sources.[40,76,104] Adequate dietary fat intake therefore is essential to minimize false-negative results. The BSG guidelines recommend a diet containing at least 70 g fat for 6 days.[174] In the United Kingdom, only a minority of laboratories try to control (20%) or retrospectively assess (8%) fat intake.[44] Patients with steatorrhea may reduce their fat intake to control their diarrhea and despite laboratory instructions may not increase their dietary fat before and during the 72 hours of fecal collection; this will result in misleadingly low results.[40]

Also, it is often forgotten that diarrhea increases fecal fat excretion. In 58% of subjects with normal fat excretion, experimental induction of severe diarrhea (fecal weight >800 g/d) led to increased fecal fat (values of up to 49 mmol/d).[58] A borderline increase in fecal fat (i.e., two to three times the upper limit of normal, which is 18 mmol/d) therefore is not specific for a primary defect in fat digestion or absorption.

Available analytical performance data for fecal fat measurements in the United Kingdom indicate that the test should now be consigned to history. Eighty-two percent of laboratories use no internal quality control, and EQA is impractical. When the titration step was assessed in an EQA exercise, between-laboratory coefficients of variation for three samples ranged from 31 to 42%.[44] Infrared spectroscopy offers the possibility of improved within- and between-laboratory precision for fecal fat measurements,[89] but does not address the problems of dietary input and sample collection, and is unlikely to be available to most laboratories.

At the end of an extensive survey of hospital laboratories in the United Kingdom, Duncan (unpublished report of the Clinical Resource and Audit Group, Scottish Office, Edinburgh, 1997) concluded that "the current utilization of the test, with no control of dietary fat intake, no correction for incomplete fecal collections and misgivings over analytical reliability, makes it a highly unsatisfactory investigation and probably of little clinical value."

Quantitative Demonstration of Fat Malabsorption Is Rarely Necessary

Many requests for fecal fat can be avoided or rejected by asking the requesting physician how the demonstration of fat malabsorption will help in diagnosis of the disorder or management of the patient (Table 51-12). In most cases, it will become evident that neither fecal fat nor an alternative test for assessing fat absorption is necessary. There is no justification for assessing fat absorption for the diagnosis or management of celiac disease, and fecal elastase is a more appropriate test for the investigation of suspected pancreatic disease. Measuring fecal fat in patients with offensive, floating, putty-colored stools will not provide a diagnosis.

It is essential to encourage clinicians to use appropriate newer tests of GI function directed toward specific clinical situations (Table 51-13). The availability and use of these tests will discourage the inappropriate use of fecal fat measurement.

The question remains: "Which test should be used when the assessment of fat malabsorption really is indicated?" Box 51-9 indicates the range of possible tests. In the 1997 survey, performance of fecal microscopy was very poor (sensitivity 26%, specificity 64%); however, several studies have reported

TABLE 51-12 Common Situations in Which Fecal Fat May Be Requested but Is Unhelpful in Diagnosis and Management

Clinical Picture or Question	Appropriate Laboratory Response
Abdominal pain, weight loss, and diarrhea; possible small bowel problem	Celiac serology: consider small bowel radiology
Offensive, floating, light-colored stools	None (demonstrating fat malabsorption will not provide a diagnosis)
Elderly patient, weight loss, possible malabsorption	Fat intake probably too low for fecal fat measurement; encourage use of appropriate investigations (see Table 51-13)
Pancreatic insufficiency, patient on enzyme supplements	Monitor stool consistency and clinical response (weight gain); may occasionally need to assess fat absorption
Abdominal pain, weight loss, and possible pancreatic insufficiency	Use a specific pancreatic function test
Child, foul stool, possible malabsorption	May sometimes need to confirm presence of fat globules in stool

From Hill PG. Faecal fat: time to give it up. Ann Clin Biochem 2001;38:164-7.

TABLE 51-13 Laboratory Tests to Assess GI Function

Clinical Application	Appropriate Laboratory Investigations
Investigating diarrhea	Possible lactase deficiency: breath hydrogen after oral lactose Possible bacterial overgrowth: breath hydrogen after oral glucose or lactulose Possible laxative abuse: urine laxative screen Possibly induced by bile acid: ^{75}selenohomocholyltaurine whole body retention or serum 7α-hydroxy-4-cholesten-3-one Fecal osmotic gap: fecal Na, K
Assessing pancreatic function	Pancreolauryl test, fecal elastase
Screening for celiac disease	Tissue transglutaminase antibodies
Assessing fat absorption	^{14}C-triolein absorption (breath $^{14}CO_2$) or fecal microscopy
Other tests	Fecal α-1-antitrypsin for protein-losing enteropathy; gut hormones (gastrin)

From Hill PG. Faecal fat: time to give it up. Ann Clin Biochem 2001;38:164-7.

BOX 51-9 Tests for Assessing Fat Absorption and Malabsorption

Measurement of fecal fat
- Problems of poor recovery during sample collection (requires use of markers), inadequate dietary fat (minimum of 70 g/d), inaccurate analysis, and uncertain interpretation

Butter fat test
- Unreliable, poor discrimination

^{14}C-glyceryl trioleate
- Sensitivity 85%, specificity 93%
- Important factors to consider
  - Fat load (20 g) and form of "meal"
  - Effect of fat load on timing of peak of breath CO_2
  - Effect of assuming a constant CO_2 output of 9 mmol/kg/h

  Inappropriate in
  - Liver, thyroid, and severe respiratory disease, diabetes, obesity, pregnancy

Mixed chain triglyceride breath test
- Valid test for pancreatic steatorrhea

Fat globules (fecal microscopy)
- Need for standardized procedure

high sensitivity and specificity figures when compared with those derived from fecal fat measurement.[116,121] Some have argued that fecal microscopy after staining with Sudan III has advantages over fecal fat measurement, because it detects fecal triglycerides and fatty acids, which are principally of dietary origin; fecal fats include phospholipids and cholesteryl esters, which largely originate from the turnover of intestinal epithelial cells and gut bacteria.[103] There is still a need to evaluate a well-defined standardized technique for fat globules by fecal microscopy in a multilaboratory study. Meanwhile, Duncan has made several recommendations (unpublished report as previously noted) to improve current performance related to method, interpretation, quality control, and adequate dietary fat before fecal samples are collected.

In a prospective evaluation of the ^{14}C-triolein test in 57 patients, reported sensitivity was 85%, with specificity of 93% for the detection of fat malabsorption.[181] The procedure used a fat load of 19.3 g prepared as a palatable lemon mousse, containing protein (1.4 g) and carbohydrate (10 g). Peak $^{14}CO_2$ occurred within 6 hours in all subjects studied who had normal fat absorption. The "gold standard" for fat malabsorption was the final diagnosis made on clinical, histologic, and radiologic or laboratory grounds. Various fat loads and procedures have been used,[44] and it is clear that larger fat loads (e.g., 60 g) result in significant delays in peak $^{14}CO_2$ in exhaled breath.[42] When a similar fat load was used without the inclusion of protein and carbohydrates, peak $^{14}CO_2$ occurred later in some patients. In 53 patients in whom $^{14}CO_2$ excretion peaked within 6 hours, the sensitivity and specificity of the tests were 100% and 96%, respectively.[42] An additional source of error is that the usually presumed CO_2 output of 9 mmol/kg/h may lead to significant errors in results because actual output varies from 5 to 12.4 mmol/kg/h.[42]

Breath samples for $^{14}CO_2$ measurement are not easily transportable, and the requirement for a scintillation counter and administrative regulations surrounding the use of radioisotopes deter many laboratories from using the test.

With growing interest in the application of stable isotopes, ^{13}C-substrates may replace the use of ^{14}C-triolein. A breath test using ^{13}C-mixed chain triglycerides [1,3-distearyl, 2(carboxyl-^{13}C) octanoyl glycerol] has been used in children[2] and adults.[182] With a medium chain fatty acid in the 2-position, the test is designed to assess intraluminal pancreatic lipase activity and therefore is not a substitute for fecal fat measurement. The ^{13}C-triolein test, using a uniformly labeled long chain triglyceride, is an alternative to fecal fat measurement.[112]

The van de Kamer method[96] for measuring fecal fat has survived for 5 decades but should now be abandoned as a routine diagnostic test; the wider use of more specific tests for investigating disorders of GI function should be encouraged.[177]

INVESTIGATION OF CHRONIC DIARRHEA

Although diarrhea is a common problem, no clear definition has existed to distinguish it from the range of stool weight, frequency, consistency, or volume that occurs in the normal population. A 2003 proposal, which seeks to encompass these different elements, suggests that for a Western diet, diarrhea may be defined as "the abnormal passage of loose or liquid stools more than three times daily and/or a volume of stool [with a weight] greater than 200 g/day."[177] Guidelines suggest that diarrhea may be defined as chronic when it has continued for 4 weeks; such persistence indicates the likelihood of a noninfectious cause requiring further investigation.

Several quite different mechanisms can lead to diarrhea. In carbohydrate malabsorption, the presence of unabsorbed solutes in the bowel causes an osmotic diarrhea as water enters the bowel from the tissue. By contrast, the diarrhea of most laxative abuse and VIPomas is due to active secretion of water and electrolytes into the bowel, which is described as secretory diarrhea. Inflammatory bowel disease (ulcerative colitis and Crohn's disease) causes diarrhea as a consequence of the inflammatory process with loss of fluid into the bowel.

Many diseases commonly thought to cause "diarrhea" in fact lead to more frequent passage of stools but not usually to an increased stool weight (or volume). Such disorders (e.g., irritable bowel syndrome) generally fall outside the scope of the definition of *chronic diarrhea.* Guidelines for the management of irritable bowel syndrome are available.[40A,94,164A]

Box 51-10 describes the many causes of chronic diarrhea; most chronic diarrhea is due to disease of the colon in which laboratory diagnostic tests are currently of little value. A helpful algorithm for the investigation of chronic diarrhea is given in Figure 51-11.

Investigation of laxative abuse and measurement of fecal osmotic gap are described in the following sections. The other laboratory tests required for the investigation of chronic diarrhea are described in the previous sections on intestinal disease, pancreatic disease, and neuroendocrine tumors.

BOX 51-10 Causes of Chronic Diarrhea

Colonic
- Colonic neoplasia
- Ulcerative and Crohn's colitis
- Microscopic colitis

Small bowel
- Celiac disease
- Crohn's disease
- Other small bowel enteropathies (e.g., Whipple's disease, tropical sprue, amyloid, intestinal lymphangiectasia)
- Bile salt malabsorption
- Disaccharidase deficiency
- Small bowel bacterial overgrowth
- Mesenteric ischemia
- Radiation enteritis
- Lymphoma
- Giardiasis (and other chronic infection)

Pancreatic
- Chronic pancreatitis
- Pancreatic carcinoma
- Cystic fibrosis

Endocrine
- Hyperthyroidism
- Diabetes
- Hypoparathyroidism
- Addison's disease
- Hormone-secreting tumors (VIPoma, gastrinoma, carcinoid)

Other
- Factitious diarrhea
- "Surgical" causes (e.g., small bowel resection, internal fistulas)
- Drugs
- Alcohol
- Autonomic neuropathy

From Thomas PD, Forbes A, Green J, Howdle P, Long R, Playford R, et al. Guidelines for the investigation of chronic diarrhoea, 2nd edition. Gut 2003;52(suppl V):vol 1-15; reproduced with permission from the BMJ Publishing Group.

Laxative Abuse[42,151A]

Surreptitious laxative abuse is an important cause of chronic diarrhea that is often overlooked. It is the final diagnosis for chronic diarrhea in 15 to 26% of patients investigated in secondary or tertiary referral centers[16,46,146,148] and in 4% of a consecutive series of new primary care referrals to a gastroenterology clinic for evaluation of diarrhea.[46] The financial benefits of screening for laxative abuse have been established, and when the diagnosis is not considered early in the investigative pathway, extensive and unnecessary investigations may occur.[16] In Munchausen syndrome by proxy, adults have administered laxatives surreptitiously to young children. A clinical diagnosis can rarely be made; no single clinical feature reliably predicts a positive test, making laboratory support essential.[59,177] The main initial prerequisite for making a diagnosis of surreptitious laxative abuse is a high index of clinical suspicion,[41] followed by a request for appropriate analyses in urine and fecal samples at a time when the patient has diarrhea.

The pattern of laxative abuse has changed following legislation in several countries banning over-the-counter sales of laxatives containing phenolphthalein, traditionally the most widely abused laxative. Abuse of phenolphthalein has therefore decreased, and the laxatives most frequently encountered by clinical laboratories are colonic stimulants containing bisacodyl or anthraquinones (e.g., senna, aloin, cascara). Their absorption, metabolism, and excretion have been reviewed.[41] They can be detected in urine for at least 32 hours after a single dose.[189] Magnesium salts are the active ingredient in some over-the-counter laxatives; these may also be abused. The only reliable diagnostic procedure is the measurement of magnesium in fecal water. Concentrations greater than 30 mmol/L are suggestive of magnesium-induced diarrhea.[43]

A pilot National External Quality Assurance Scheme was set up in the United Kingdom in 1996. In the light of poor overall performance highlighted by the scheme, recommendations were made for a laxative screening service. Subsequently, thin layer chromatography (TLC) methods were extensively evaluated to optimize the detection of

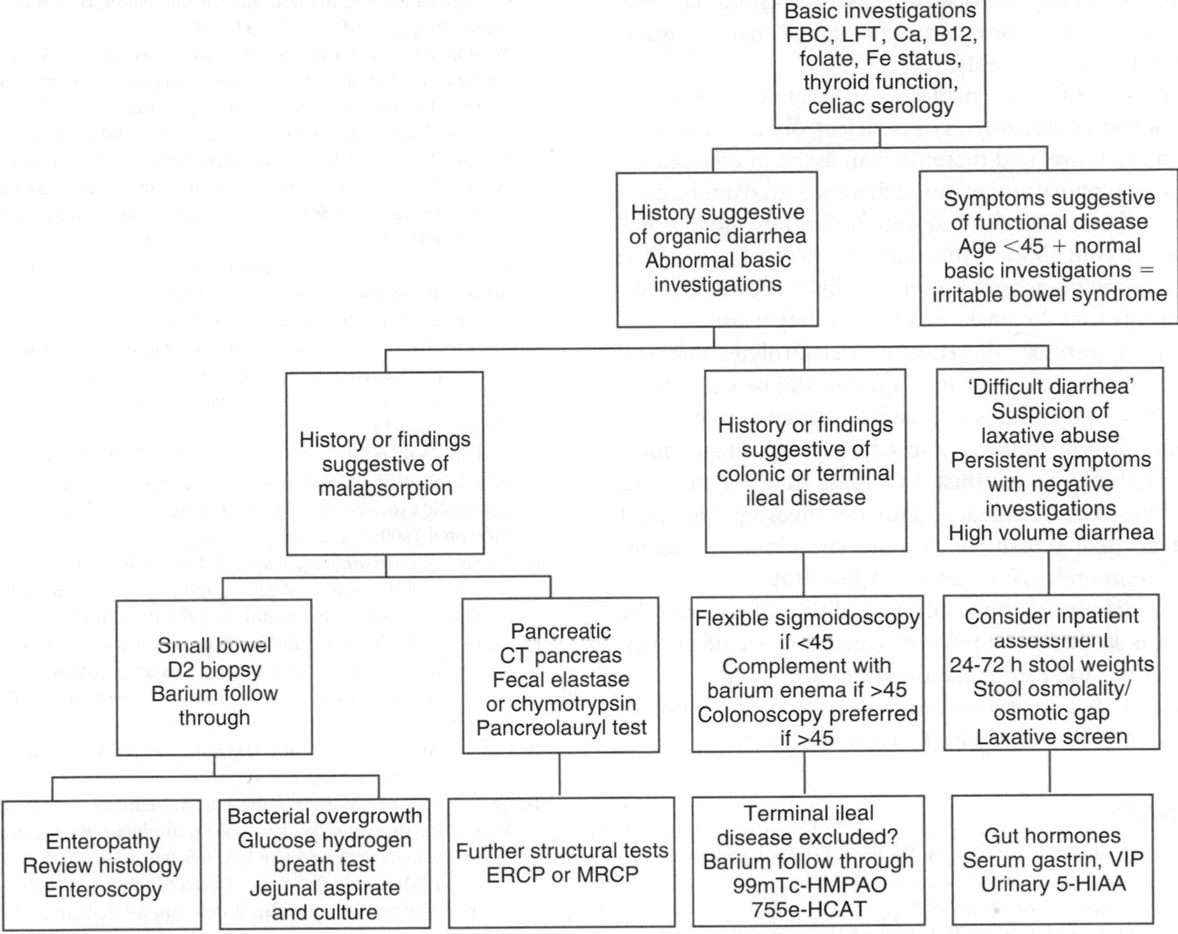

Figure 51-11 An algorithm for the investigation of chronic diarrhea. *CT,* Computed tomography; *ERCP,* endoscopic retrograde cholangiopancreatography; *FBC,* full blood count; *5-HIAA,* 5-hydroxyindoleacetic acid; *LFT,* liver function tests; *MRCP,* magnetic resonance cholangiopancreatography; *75Se-HCAT,* 75Se homotaurocholate; *Tc-HMPAO,* technetium hexa-methyl-propyleneamine oxime. *(From Thomas PD, Forbes A, Green J, Howdle P, Long R, Playford R, et al. Guidelines for the investigation of chronic diarrhoea, 2nd edition. Gut 2003;52(suppl V):v1-15. Used with permission of the BMJ Publishing Group.)*

laxatives.[47] The most important findings for the successful detection of laxatives by TLC were (1) the skill and experience of the operator, (2) the choice of the mobile phase [ethyl acetate:toluene:glacial acetic acid (4:16:1) and hexane:toluene:glacial acetic acid (3:1:1) gave the best results], and (3) use of high-performance TLC plates with a concentrating zone. Increased centralization of laxative analysis led to some improvement in analytical performance, but an assessment of the performance of a reference laboratory in the United States has again highlighted the unreliability of TLC with problems identified for both bisacodyl and senna detection.[157]

For such tests, false positives or false negatives have particularly important implications for the management of the condition, and poor sensitivity and specificity for laxative analysis are unacceptable. The analysis of laxatives should be regarded as part of the toxicology service; the problems identified with TLC suggest that these techniques should be replaced by gas chromatography–mass spectrometry (GC-MS) for all samples requiring laxative analysis.[41] Analyses should be undertaken only by laboratories with appropriate expertise and ability to demonstrate good performance for these tests, so as to ensure that chronic diarrhea is correctly diagnosed and managed.

Fecal Osmotic (Osmolal) Gap

The osmolality of stool "water" normally will be that of serum (i.e., 290 mosm/kg), but the contribution of electrolytes and of nonelectrolytes to the total osmolality will vary, depending on the cause of the diarrhea. Fecal osmotic (osmolal) gap (FOG) expresses the difference between the theoretical normal osmolality (290 mosm/kg) and the contribution of Na^+ and K^+, as follows:

$$\text{Fecal osmotic gap} = 290 - [2(\text{fecal Na}^+ + \text{K}^+)]$$

Fecal sodium and potassium are measured in the fluid obtained by rapid centrifugation of a fecal sample. Total fecal osmolality increases significantly in unrefrigerated samples, and use of the serum osmolality of 290 mosm/kg has been recommended in the above formula, rather than measurement of total fecal osmolality.[48]

Measurement of FOG enables an estimate to be made of the contribution of electrolytes or nonelectrolytes to retention of water in the bowel and therefore can assist in distinguishing between secretory and osmotic diarrhea. In osmotic diarrhea, unabsorbed solutes lead to water retention and thus will make a larger contribution than normal to fecal osmolality; fecal sodium and potassium therefore will be present at lower concentrations than normal, leading to a larger *osmotic gap.* Conversely, in secretory diarrhea, it is electrolytes that lead to water retention, and the FOG therefore will be small. FOG greater than 50 mosm/kg is consistent with an osmotic diarrhea from carbohydrate malabsorption or magnesium-induced diarrhea[43]; by contrast, FOG less than 50 mosm/kg suggests a secretory diarrhea, and further investigation might include a laxative screen for colonic stimulants or, rarely, testing for neuroendocrine tumor.[59] A low FOG will be found in factitious diarrhea because of the addition of water to the stool; if this is suspected and if other causes are excluded, then measurement of total stool osmolality may be helpful.[100]

Measurement of creatinine can be used as an indication of contamination of the fecal sample with urine.

REFERENCES

1. Amarri S, Coward WA, Harding M, Weaver LT. Importance of measuring CO_2 production rate when using ^{13}C-breath tests to measure fat digestion. Br J Nutr 1998;79:541-5.
2. Amarri S, Harding M, Coward WA, Evans TJ, Weaver LT. ^{13}C-mixed triglyceride breath test and pancreatic enzyme supplementation in children with cystic fibrosis. Arch Dis Childhood 1997;76:349-51.
3. Ardill JES. Circulating markers for endocrine tumors of the gastropancreatic tract. Ann Clin Biochem 2008;45:539-59.
4. Arola H, Koivula T, Karvonen AL, Jokela H, Ahola T, Isokoski M. Low trehalase activity is associated with abdominal symptoms caused by edible mushrooms. Scand J Gastroenterol 1999;34:898-903.
5. Attar A, Flourie B, Rambaud JC, Franchisseur C, Ruszniewski P, Bouhnik Y. Antibiotic efficacy in small intestinal bacterial overgrowth-related chronic diarrhoea: a crossover, randomized trial. Gastroenterology 1999;117:794-7.
6. Axelson M, Bjorkhem I, Reihner E, Einarsson K. The plasma level of 7α-hydroxy-4-cholesten-3-one reflects the activity of hepatic cholesterol 7α-hydroxylase in man. FEBS Lett 1991;284:216-8.
7. Barakat MT, Meeran K, Bloom SR. Neuroendocrine tumours. Endocrine-Related Cancer 2004;11:1-18.
8. Batterham RL, Cowley MA, Small CJ, Herzog H, Cohen MA, Dakin CL, et al. Gut hormone PYY_{3-36} physiologically inhibits food intake. Nature 2002;418:650-4.
9. Berger AC, Gibril F, Venzon DJ, Doppman JL, Norton JA, Bartlett DL, et al. Prognostic value of initial fasting serum gastrin levels in patients with Zollinger-Ellison syndrome. J Clin Oncol 2001;19:3051-7.
10. Biancone L, Fantini M, Tosti C, Bozzi R, Vavassori P, Pallone F. Fecal α_1-antitrypsin clearance as a marker of clinical relapse in patients with Crohn's disease of the distal ileum. Eur J Gastroenterol Hepatol 2003;15:261-6.
11. Blackwell PJ, Hill PG, Holmes GK. Autoantibodies to human tissue transglutaminase: superior predictors of coeliac disease. Scand J Gastroenterol 2002;37:1282-5.
12. Blaser MJ. *Helicobacter pylori* and gastric diseases. BMJ 1998;316: 1507-10.

12A. Braganza JM, Lee SH, McCloy RF, McMahon MJ. Chronic pancreatitis. Lancet 2011;377:1184-97.

13. Brydon WG, Nyhlin H, Eastwood MA, Merrick MV. Serum 7α-hydroxy-4-cholesten-3-one and selenohomocholyltaurine (SeHCAT) whole body retention in the assessment of bile acid induced diarrhoea. Eur J Gastroenterol Hepatol 1996;8:117-23.
14. Burgin-Wolff A, Dahlbom I, Hadziselimovic F, Petersson CJ. Antibodies against human tissue transglutaminase and endomysium in diagnosing and monitoring coeliac disease. Scand J Gastroenterol 2002;37:685-91.
15. Burroughs AK, Westaby D. Liver, biliary tract disease and pancreatic disease. In: Kumar P, Clark M, eds. Clinical medicine, 7th edition. Edinburgh: Elsevier Saunders, 2009:319-85.
16. Bytzer P, Stokholm M, Andersen I, Klitgaard NA, de Muckadell OBS. Prevalence of surreptitious laxative abuse in patients with diarrhoea of uncertain origin: a cost benefit analysis of a screening procedure. Gut 1989;30:1379-84.
17. Cade A, Walters MP, McGinley N, Firth J, Brownlee KG, Conway SP, et al. Evaluation of fecal pancreatic elastase-1 as a measure of pancreatic exocrine function in children with cystic fibrosis. Pediatr Pulmonol 2000;29:172-6.
18. Carriere F, Barrowman J, Verger R, Laugier R. Secretion and contribution to lipolysis of gastric and pancreatic lipases during a test meal in humans. Gastroenterology 1993;105:876-88.
19. Carroccio A, Verghi F, Santini B, Lucidi V, Iacono G, Cavataio F, et al. Diagnostic accuracy of fecal elastase 1 assay in patients with pancreatic maldigestion or intestinal malabsorption. Dig Dis Sci 2001;46:1335-42.
20. Caspary WF. Diarrhea associated with carbohydrate malabsorption. Clin Gastroenterol 1986;15:631-55.
21. Cataldo F, Lio D, Marino V, Picarelli A, Venturer A, Corazza GR. IgG_1 antiendomysium and IgG antitissue transglutaminase antibodies in coeliac patients with selective IgA deficiency. Gut 2000;47:366-9.
22. Cataldo F, Marino V, Bottaro G, Greco P, Venture A. Celiac disease and selective immunoglobulin A deficiency. J Pediatr 1997;131: 306-8.

22A. Chey WD, Wong BCY, Practice Parameters Committee of the American College of Gastroenterology. American College of Gastroenterology guidelines on the management of *Helicobacter pylori* infection. Am J Gastroenterol 2007;102:1808-25.

23. Churchill RD, Hill PG, Holmes GK. Breath test is better than near patient blood tests. BMJ 1998;316:1389.
24. Clark ML, Silk DB. Gastrointestinal disease. In: Kumar P, Clark M, eds. Clinical medicine, 6th edition. Edinburgh: Elsevier Saunders, 2005:265-345.
25. Cole SG, Rossi S, Stern A, Hofmann AF. Cholesteryl octanoate breath test—preliminary studies on a new noninvasive test of human pancreatic exocrine function. Gastroenterology 1987;93:1372-80.
26. Corazza GR, Menozzi MG, Strocchi A, Rasciti L, Vaira D, Lecchini R, et al. The diagnosis of small bowel bacterial overgrowth. Gastroenterology 1990;98:302-9.
27. Couper R, Belli D, Durie P, Gaskin K, Sarles J, Werlin S. Pancreatic disorders and cystic fibrosis: working group report of the First World Congress of Pediatric Gastroenterology, Hepatology and Nutrition. J Pediatr Gastroenterol Nutr 2002;35:S213-23.
28. Cummings DE, Foster KE. Ghrelin-Leptin tango in body weight regulation. Gastroenterology 2003;124:1532-5.
29. Cummings DE, Weigle DS, Frayo RS, Breen PA, Ma MK, Dellinger EP, et al. Plasma Ghrelin levels after diet-induced weight loss or gastric bypass surgery. N Engl J Med 2002;346:1623-30.
30. Cystic Fibrosis Trust: Standards for the clinical care of children and adults with cystic fibrosis in the UK, Bromley 2001. Available at: www.cftrust.org.uk/aboutcf/publications/consensusdoc/C_3000Standards_of_Care.pdf (accessed July 2011).
31. Czako L, Endes J, Takacs T, Boda K, Lonovics J. Evaluation of pancreatic exocrine function by secretin-enhanced magnetic resonance cholangiopancreatography. Pancreas 2001;23:323-8.

32. Dahlquist A. Method for assay of intestinal disaccharidases. Anal Biochem 1964;7:18-25.
33. Dawson PA. Bile secretion and the enterohepatic circulation. In: Feldman M, Friedman LS, Brandt LJ, eds. Sleisenger and Fordtran's gastrointestinal and liver disease, 8th edition. Philadelphia, Pa: WB Saunders, 2006:1369-85.
34. Del Valle J. Zollinger-Ellison syndrome. In: Yamada T, ed. Textbook of gastroenterology, 5th edition. Oxford, United Kingdom: Wiley-Blackwell, 2009:982-1004.
35. Deveney CW, Deveney KE. Zollinger Ellison syndrome. In: Clark OH, Weber CA, eds. The surgical clinics of North America. Philadelphia, Pa: WB Saunders, 1987:411-22.
36. Dieterich W, Ehnis T, Bauer M, Donner P, Volta U, Riecken EO, et al. Identification of tissue transglutaminase as the autoantigen of celiac disease. Nat Med 1997;3:797-801.
37. Dignass AU, Sturm A. Peptide growth factors in the intestine. Eur J Gastroenterol Hepatol 2001;13:763-70.
38. Dimagno EP. A perspective on the use of tubeless pancreatic function tests in diagnosis. Gut 1998;43:2-3.
39. Dominguez-Munoz J, Hieronymus C, Sauerbruch T, Malfertheiner P. Fecal elastase test: evaluation of a new non-invasive pancreatic function test. Am J Gastroenterol 1995;90:1834-7.
40. Donowitz M, Kokke FT, Saidi M. Evaluation of patients with chronic diarrhea. N Engl J Med 1995;332:725-9.
40A. Drossman DA, Camilleri M, Mayer EA, Whitehead WE. AGA technical review on irritable bowel syndrome. Gastroenterol 2002;123:2108-31.
41. Duncan A. Screening for surreptitious laxative abuse. Ann Clin Biochem 2000;37:1-8.
42. Duncan A, Cameron A, Stewart MJ, Russell RI. Limitations of the triolein breath test. Clin Chim Acta 1992;205:51-64.
43. Duncan A, Forrest JAH. Surreptitious abuse of magnesium laxatives as a cause of chronic diarrhoea. Eur J Gastroenterol Hepatol 2001;13: 599-601.
44. Duncan A, Hill PG. A UK survey of laboratory-based gastrointestinal investigations. Ann Clin Biochem 1998;35:492-503.
45. Duncan A, Hill PG. A review of the quality of gastrointestinal investigations performed in UK laboratories. Ann Clin Biochem 2007;44:145-58.
46. Duncan A, Morris AJ, Cameron A, Stewart MJ, Brydon WG, Russell RI. Laxative-induced diarrhoea—a neglected diagnosis. J R Soc Med 1992;85:203-5.
47. Duncan A, Phillips IJ. Evaluation of thin-layer chromatography methods for laxative detection. Ann Clin Biochem 2001;38:64-6.
48. Duncan A, Robertson C, Russell RI. The fecal osmotic gap: technical aspects regarding its calculation. J Lab Clin Med 1992;119:359-63.
49. El-Omar EM, Penman ID, Ardill JES, Chittajallu RS, Howie C, McColl KEL. *Helicobacter pylori* infection and abnormalities of acid secretion in patients with duodenal ulcer disease. Gastroenterology 1995;109:681-91.
49A. Erickson JA, Aldeen WE, Grenache DG, Ashwood ER. Evaluation of a fecal pancreatic elastase-1 enzyme-linked immunosorbent assay: assessment versus an established assay and implications in classifying pancreatic function. Clin Chim Acta 2008; 397:87-91.
50. Eriksson B, Oberg K, Stridsberg M. Tumour markers in neuroendocrine tumours. Digestion 2000;62(suppl 1):33-8.
51. Eusufzai S, Axelson M, Angelin B, Einarsson K. Serum 7α-hydroxy-4-cholesten-3-one concentrations in the evaluation of bile acid malabsorption in patients with diarrhoea: correlation to the SeHCAT test. Gut 1993;34:698-701.
52. Farrell JJ. Digestion and absorption of nutrients and vitamins. In: Feldman M, Friedman LS, Brandt LJ, eds. Sleisenger and Fordtran's gastrointestinal and liver disease, 8th edition. Philadelphia, Pa: WB Saunders, 2006:2147-97.
53. Farrell RJ, Kelly CP. Current concepts: celiac sprue. N Engl J Med 2002;346:180-8.
54. Farrell RJ, Kelly CP. Celiac sprue and refractory sprue. In: Feldman M, Friedman LS, Brandt LJ, eds. Sleisenger and Fordtran's gastrointestinal and liver disease, 8th edition. Philadelphia: WB Saunders, 2006: 2277-2306.
54A. Fasano A. Zonulin and its regulation of intestinal barrier function: the biological door to inflammation, autoimmunity and cancer. Physiol Rev 2011;91:151-75.
55. Fasano A, Berti I, Gerarduzzi T, Not T, Colletti RB, Drago S, et al. Prevalence of celiac disease in at-risk and not-at-risk groups in the United States: a large multicenter study. Arch Intern Med 2003;163: 286-92.
56. Fasano A, Not T, Wang W, Uzzau S, Berti I, Tommasini A, et al. Zonulin, a newly discovered modulator of intestinal permeability, and its expression in coeliac disease. Lancet 2000;355:1518-9.
57. Fernandez E, Blanco C, Garcia S, Dieguez A, Riestra S, Rodrigo L. Use of low concentrations of human IgA anti-tissue transglutaminase to rule out selective IgA deficiency in patients with suspected celiac disease. Clin Chem 2005;51:1014-6.
58. Fine KD, Fordtran JS. The effect of diarrhea on fecal fat excretion. Gastroenterology 1992;102:1936-9.
59. Fine KD, Schiller LR. AGA technical review on the evaluation and management of chronic diarrhea. Gastroenterology 1999;116:1464-86.
60. Florent C, L'Hirondel C, Desmazures C, Aymes C, Bernier JJ. Intestinal clearance of α_1-antitrypsin: a sensitive method for the detection of protein-losing enteropathy. Gastroenterology 1981;81:777-80.
60A. Flourie B, Turk J, Lemann M, Florent C, Colimon R, Rambaud JC. Breath hydrogen in bacterial overgrowth. Gastroenterology 1989;96: 1225.
61. Foell, D, Wittkowski H, Roth J. Monitoring disease activity by stool analysis: intestinal inflammation and damage from occult blood to molecular markers of disease activity. Gut 2009;58:859-68.
62. Forsmark CE. Chronic pancreatitis. In: Feldman M, Friedman LS, Brandt LJ, eds. Sleisenger and Fordtran's gastrointestinal and liver disease, 8th edition. Philadelphia, Pa: WB Saunders, 2006:1271-308.
63. Foster PN, Mitchell CJ, Robertson DRC, Hamilton I, Irving H, Kelleher J, et al. Prospective comparison of three non-invasive tests for pancreatic disease. Br Med J 1984;289:13-6.
64. Fuccio L, Laterza L, Zagari RM, Cennamo V, Grillo D, Bazzoli F. Treatment of *Helicobacter pylori* infection. BMJ 2008;337:746-50.
65. Gisbert JP, McNicholl AG, Gomollon F. Questions and answers on the role of fecal lactoferrin as a biological marker in inflammatory bowel disease. Inflamm Bowel Dis 2009;15:1746-54.
66. Glasbrenner B, Kahl S, Malfertheiner P. Modern diagnostics of chronic pancreatitis. Eur J Gastroenterol Hepatol 2002;14:935-41.
67. Goetze JP, Rehfeld JF. Impact of assay epitope specificity in gastrinoma diagnosis. Clin Chem 2003;49:333-4.
68. Granstrom M, Bengtsson C, Megraud F. Diagnosis of *Helicobacter pylori*. Helicobacter 2008;13(suppl 1):7-12.
69. Greenwald DA. Protein losing enteropathy. In: Feldman M, Friedman LS, Brandt LJ, eds. Sleisenger and Fordtran's gastrointestinal and liver disease, 8th edition. Philadelphia, Pa: WB Saunders, 2006:557-64.
70. Gudmund-Hoyer E, Fenger HJ, Skovbjerg H, Kern-Hansen P, Madsen PR. Trehalase deficiency in Greenland. Scand J Gastroenterol 1988;23: 775-8.
71. Gullo L, Graziano L, Babbini S, Battistini A, Lazzari R, Pezzilli R. Fecal elastase 1 in children with cystic fibrosis. Eur J Pediatr 1997;156:770-2.
72. Gullo L, Ventrucci M, Tomassetti P, Migliori M, Pezzilli R. Fecal elastase 1 determination in chronic pancreatitis. Dig Dis Sci 1999;44:210-3.
73. Guyton AC, Hall JE. Human physiology and mechanisms of disease, 6th edition. Philadelphia, Pa: WB Saunders, 1997.
74. Hamilton I, Cobden I, Rothwell J, Axon AT. Intestinal permeability in coeliac disease: the response to gluten withdrawal and single dose gluten challenge. Gut 1982;23:202-10.
75. Hardt PD, Hauenschild A, Nalop J, Marzeion AM, Porsch-Ozcurumez M, Luley C, et al. The commercially available ELISA for pancreatic elastase 1 based on polyclonal antibodies does measure an as yet

unknown antigen different from purified elastase 1. Z Gastroenterol 2003;41:903-6.
76. Hernell O. Assessing fat malabsorption. J Paediatr 1999;135:407-9.
77. Hill I, Fasano A, Schwartz R, Counts D, Glock M, Horvath K. The prevalence of celiac disease in at-risk groups of children in the United States. J Pediatr 2000;136:86-90.
78. Hill PG. Faecal fat: time to give it up. Ann Clin Biochem 2001;38:164-7.
79. Hill PG, Forsyth JM, Semeraro D, Holmes GK. IgA antibodies to human tissue transglutaminase: audit of routine practice confirms high diagnostic accuracy. Scand J Gastroenterol 2004;39:1078-82.
80. Hill PG, McMillan SA. Anti-tissue transglutaminase antibodies and their role in the investigation of coeliac disease. Ann Clin Biochem 2006;43:105-17.
81. Hill PG, Thompson SP, Holmes GKT. IgA anti-gliadin antibodies in adult celiac disease. Clin Chem 1991;37:647-50.
82. Hill RE, Comm B, Herez A, Corey ML, Gilday DL, Eng B, et al. Fecal clearance of alpha-1-antitrypsin: a reliable measure of enteric protein loss in children. J Pediatr 1981;99:416-8.
83. Holmes GKT. Potential and latent coeliac disease. Eur J Gastroenterol Hepatol 2001;13:1057-60.
84. Holmes GKT. Screening for coeliac disease in type 1 diabetes. Arch Dis Child 2002;87:495-9.
85. Holmes GKT, Hill PG. Do we still need to measure faecal fat? BMJ 1988;296:1552-3.
86. Howden CW, Hunt RH. Guidelines for the management of *Helicobacter pylori* infection. Am J Gastroenterol 1998;93:2330-8.
87. Howdle PD, Losowsky MS. Coeliac disease in adults. In: Marsh MN, ed. Coeliac disease. Oxford, United Kingdom: Blackwell, 1992:49-80.
88. Huang SM, Lin HH, Hsu YH. Extreme hypergastrinaemia caused by atrophic gastritis and *Helicobacter pylori* infection—a case report. Hepatogastroenterology 2001;48:1215-6.
89. Jakobs BS, Volmer M, Swinkels DW, Hofs MTW, Donkervoort S, Joostings MMJ, et al. New method for faecal fat determination by mid-infrared spectroscopy, using a transmission cell: an improvement in standardization. Ann Clin Biochem 2000;37:343-9.
90. Janatuinen EK, Kemppainen TA, Julkunen RJ, Kosma VM, Maki M, Heikkinen M, et al. No harm from five year ingestion of oats in coeliac disease. Gut 2002;50:332-5.
91. Jensen RT. Gastrinoma. In: O'Shea D, Bloom SR, eds. Baillieres clinical gastroenterology. London, United Kingdom: Bailliere Tindall, 1996:603-43.
92. Jensen RT. Endocrine neoplasms of the pancreas. In: Yamada T, ed. Textbook of gastroenterology, 5th edition. Oxford, United Kingdom: Wiley-Blackwell, 2009:1875-1920.
93. Jensen RT, Niederle B, Mitry E, Ramage JK, Steinmüller T, Lewington V, et al. Gastrinoma (duodenal and pancreatic). Neuroendocrinology 2006;84:173-82.
94. Jones J, Boorman B, Cann P, Forbes A, Gomborone J, Heaton K, et al. Guidelines for the management of the irritable bowel syndrome, British Society of Gastroenterology, 2000. Available at: http://www.bsg.org.uk/pdf_word_docs/man_ibd.pdf (accessed July2011).
95. Kaiser T, Langhorst J, Wittkowski H, Becker K, Friedrich AW, Rueffer A, et al. Faecal S100A12 as a non-invasive marker distinguishing inflammatory bowel disease from irritable bowel syndrome. Gut 2007;56:1706-13.
96. van de Kamer JH, Ten Huinink BH, Weyers HA. Rapid method for the determination of fat in feces. J Biol Chem 1949;177:347-55.
97. Kampanis P, Ford L, Berg J. Development and validation of an improved test for the measurement of human fecal elastase-1. Ann Clin Biochem 2009;46:33-7.
98. Karcher RE, Truding RM, Stawick LE. Using a cutoff of <10 ppm for breath hydrogen testing: a review of 5 years' experience. Ann Clin Lab Sci 1999;29:1-8.
99. Kaspar P. Chymotrypsin in stool. In: Bergmeyer HU, Bergmeyer J, Grassl M, eds. Methods of enzymatic analysis, volume 5, 3rd edition. Weinheim: Verlag Chemie, 1984:109-18.
100. Katz SL, McGee P, Geist R, Durie P. Factitious diarrhea: a case of watery deception. J Pediatr Gastroenterol Nutr 2001;33:607-9.
101. Kerlin P, Wong L. Breath hydrogen testing in bacterial overgrowth of the small intestine. Gastroenterology 1988;95:982-8.
102. Kerner JA. Formula allergy and intolerance. Gastroenterol Clin North Am 1995;24:1-25.
103. Khouri MK, Huang G, Shiau YF. Sudan stain of fecal fat: new insight into an old test. Gastroenterology 1989;96:421-7.
104. Khouri MK, Huang G, Shiau YF. Dietary fat intake, 72-h excretion and Sudan stain for fecal fat. Gastroenterology 1989;97:550-3.
105. King CE, Toskes PP. Comparison of the 1-gram [^{14}C]xylose, 10-gram lactulose-H_2, and 80-gram glucose-H_2 breath tests in patients with small intestine bacterial overgrowth. Gastroenterology 1986;91: 1447-51.
106. Koletzko S, Haisch M, Seeboth I, Braden B, Hengels K, Koletzko B, et al. Isotope-selective non-dispersive infrared spectrometry for detection of *Helicobacter pylori* infection with ^{13}C-urea breath test. Lancet 1995;345:961-2.
107. Korponay-Szabo IR, Laurila K, Szondy Z, Halttunen T, Szalai Z, Dahlbom I, et al. Missing endomysial and reticulin binding of coeliac antibodies in transglutaminase 2 knockout tissues. Gut 2003;52: 199-204.
108. Kumar PJ, Clark ML. Malabsorption and weight loss. In: Bloom S, ed. Practical gastroenterology. London: Martin Dunitz, 2002:371-82.
109. Lamberts SW, Hofland LJ, Nobels FR. Neuroendocrine tumor markers. Front Neuroendocrinol 2001;22:309-39.
110. Langenberg ML, Tytgat GN, Schipper ME, Rietra PJ, Zanen HC. *Campylobacter*-like organisms in the stomachs of patients and healthy individuals. Lancet 1984;i:1348.
111. Lankisch PG, Schmidt I, Konig H, Lehnick D, Knollman R, Lohr M, et al. Faecal elastase 1: not helpful in diagnosing chronic pancreatitis associated with mild to moderate exocrine pancreatic insufficiency. Gut 1998;42:551-4.
112. Lembcke B, Braden B, Caspary WF. Exocrine pancreatic insufficiency: accuracy and clinical value of the uniformly labelled ^{13}C-Hiolein breath test. Gut 1996;39;668-74.
113. Leus J, Van Biervliet S, Robberecht E. Detection and follow up of exocrine pancreatic insufficiency in cystic fibrosis: a review. Eur J Pediatr 2000;159:563-8.
113A. Lewis JD. The utility of biomarkers in the diagnosis and therapy of inflammatory bowel disease. Gastroenterol 2011;140:1817-26.
114. Levitt MD. Production and excretion of hydrogen gas in man. N Engl J Med 1969;281:122-7.
115. Lijmer J, Bol MW, Heisterkamp S, Bonsel GJ, Prins MH, van der Meulen JH, et al. Empirical evidence of design-related bias in studies of diagnostic tests. JAMA 1999;282:1061-6.
116. Lip-Bin T, Stopard M, Anderson S, Grant A, Quantrill D, Wilkinson RH, et al. Assessment of fat malabsorption. J Clin Pathol 1983;36: 1362-6.
117. Logan RP, Dill S, Bauer FE, Walker MM, Hirschl AM, Gummett PA, et al. The European ^{13}C-urea breath test for the detection of *Helicobacter pylori*. Eur J Gastroenterol Hepatol 1991;3:915-21.
118. Logan RPH, Walker MM, Misiewicz JJ, Gummett PA, Karim QN, Baron JH. Changes in intragastric distribution of *Helicobacter pylori* during treatment with omeprazole. Gut 1995;36:12-6.
119. Loser C, Brauer C, Aygen S, Hennemann O, Folsch UR. Comparative clinical evaluation of the ^{13}C-mixed triglyceride breath test as an indirect test of pancreatic function. Scand J Gastroenterol 1998;33: 327-34.
120. Loser C, Mollgaard A, Folsch UR. Faecal elastase 1: a novel, highly sensitive, and specific tubeless pancreatic function test. Gut 1996;39: 580-6.
121. Luk GD. Screening for steatorrhea. Gastroenterology 1979;77:205-6.
122. Maki M, Mustalahti K, Kokkonen J, Kulmala P, Haapalahti M, Karttunen T, et al. Prevalence of celiac disease among children in Finland. N Engl J Med 2003;348:2517-24.
122A. Malfertheiner P, Bazzoli F, Delchier J-C, Celinski K, Giguere M, Riviere M et al. *Helicobacter pylori* eradication with a capsule containing bismuth subcitrate potassium, metronidazole, and tetracycline given with omeprazole versus clarithromycin-based triple

therapy: a randomized, open-label, non-inferiority, phase 3 trial. Lancet 2011;377:905-913.

123. Malfertheiner P, Megraud F, O'Morain C, Bazzoli F, El-Omar E, Graham D, et al. Current concepts in the management of *Helicobacter pylori* infection—the Maastricht III Consensus Report. Gut 2007;56: 772-81.

124. Marsh MN, ed. Coeliac disease. Oxford, United Kingdom: Blackwell, 1992.

125. Marshall BJ, McGechie DB, Rogers PA, Glancy RJ. Pyloric *Campylobacter* infection and gastroduodenal disease. Med J Aust 1985;142:439-44.

126. Martini S, Mengozzi G, Aimo G, Giorda L, Pagni R, Guidetti CS. Comparative evaluation of serologic tests for celiac disease diagnosis and follow-up. Clin Chem 2002;48:960-3.

127. Masoero G, Zaffino C, Laudi C, Lombardo L, Rocca R, Gallo L, et al. Fecal pancreatic elastase 1 in the work up of patients with chronic diarrhea. Int J Pancreatol 2000;28:175-9.

128. Mastropaolo G, Rees WD. Evaluation of the hydrogen breath test in man: definition and elimination of the early hydrogen peak. Gut 1987;28:721-5.

129. Metz G, Blendis LM, Jenkins DJ. H_2 breath test for lactase deficiency. N Engl J Med 1976;294:730.

129A. Mikesh LM, Crowe SE, Bullock GC, Taylor NE, Bruns DE. Celiac disease refractory to a gluten-free diet? Clin Chem 2008;54:441-5.

130. Miller LJ. Gastrointestinal hormones and receptors. In: Yamada T, ed. Textbook of gastroenterology, 5th edition. Oxford, United Kingdom: Wiley-Blackwell, 2009:56-85.

131. Moran A, Radley S, Neoptolomos J, Jones AF, Asquith P. Detection of colorectal cancer by faecal α_1-antitrypsin. Ann Clin Biochem 1993;30: 28-33.

132. Morris JA, Selivanov V, Sheldon GF. Nutritional management of patients with malabsorption syndrome. Clin Gastroenterol 1983; 12:463-74.

133. Muldoon C, Maguire P, Gleeson F. Onset of sucrase-isomaltase deficiency in late adulthood. Am J Gastroenterol 1999;94:2298-9.

134. Mulholland G, Ardill JES, Fillmore D, Chittajallu RS, Fullarton GM, McColl KE. *Helicobacter pylori*–related hypergastrinaemia is due to a selective increase in gastrin G17. Gut 1993;34:757-61.

135. Murray IA, Coupland K, Smith JA, Ansell ID, Long RG. Intestinal trehalase activity in a UK population: establishing a normal range and the effect of disease. Br J Nutr 2000;83:241-5.

136. Naiyer AJ, Hernandez L, Ciaccio EJ, Papadakis K, Manavalan JS, Bhagat G, et al. Comparison of commercially available serologic kits for the detection of celiac disease. J Clin Gastroenterol 2009;43:225-32.

137. Neary NM, Small CJ, Bloom SR. Gut and mind. Gut 2003;52:918-21.

138. Newcomer AD, McGill DB, Thomas PJ, Hofmann AF. Prospective comparison of indirect methods for detecting lactase deficiency. N Engl J Med 1975;293:1232-5.

139. NICE guideline: dyspepsia, management of dyspepsia in primary care. London, United Kingdom: National Institute for Clinical Excellence, 2004. Available at: www.nice.org.uk/nicemedia/pdf/CG017NICEguideline.pdf (accessed July 2011).

140. Niederau C, Grendell JH. Diagnosis of chronic pancreatitis. Gastroenterology 1985;88:1973-95.

141. Nomura A, Stemmermann GN, Chyou P-H, Kato I, Perez-Perez GI, Blaser MJ. *Helicobacter pylori* infection and gastric carcinoma among Japanese Americans in Hawaii. N Engl J Med 1991;325:1132-6.

142. Parsonnet J, Friedman GD, Vandersteen DP, Chang Y, Vogelman JH, Orentreich N, et al. *Helicobacter pylori* infection and the risk of gastric carcinoma. N Engl J Med 1991;325:1127-31.

143. Perman JA, Modler S, Barr RG, Rosenthal P. Fasting breath hydrogen concentration: normal values and clinical application. Gastroenterology 1984;87:1358-63.

144. Perry I, Iqbal T, Cooper B. Intestinal permeability in coeliac disease. Lancet 2001;358:1729-30.

145. Phillips IJ, Rowe DJ, Dewar P, Connett GJ. Faecal elastase 1: a marker of exocrine pancreatic insufficiency in cystic fibrosis. Ann Clin Biochem 1999;36:739-42.

146. Phillips S, Donaldson L, Geisler K, Pera A, Kochar R. Stool composition in factitial diarrhea: a 6-year experience with stool analysis. Ann Intern Med 1995;123:97-100.

147. Rauws EA, Tytgat GN. Cure of duodenal ulcer associated with eradication of *H. pylori*. Lancet 1990;335:1233-5.

148. Read NW, Kerjs GJ, Read MG, Santa Ana CA, Morawski SG, Fordtran JS. Chronic diarrhea of unknown origin. Gastroenterology 1980;78: 264-71.

149. Rehfeld JF. The new biology of gastrointestinal hormones. Physiol Rev 1998;78:1087-108.

150. Rhodes JM, Middleton P, Jewell DP. The lactulose hydrogen breath test as a diagnostic test for small-bowel bacterial overgrowth. Scand J Gastroenterol 1979;14:333-6.

151. Rinderknecht H, Renner IG, Douglas AP, Adham NF. Profiles of pure pancreatic secretions obtained by direct pancreatic duct cannulation in normal healthy human subjects. Gastroenterology 1978;75:1083-9.

151A. Roerig JL, Steffan KJ, Mitchell JE, Zunker C. Laxative abuse, Epidemiology, Diagnosis and Management. Drugs 2010;12:1487-1503.

152. Russo MA, Redel CA. Anatomy, histology, embryology and developmental anatomy of the stomach and duodenum. In: Feldman M, Friedman LS, Brandt LJ, eds. Sleisenger and Fordtran's gastrointestinal and liver disease, 8th edition. Philadelphia, Pa: WB Saunders, 2006:981-98.

153. Sauter GH, Munzing W, von Ritter C, Paumgartner G. Bile acid malabsorption as a cause of chronic diarrhea: diagnostic value of 7α-hydroxy-4-cholesten-3-one in serum. Dig Dis Sci 1999;44:14-9.

154. Schwartz MW, Morton GJ. Keeping hunger at bay. Nature 2002;418: 595-7.

155. Semenza G, Auricchio S, Mantei N. Small intestinal disaccharidases. In: Scriver CR, Beaudet AL, Sly WS, Valle D, eds. The metabolic and molecular bases of inherited disease, 8th edition. New York, NY: McGraw-Hill, 2001:1623-50.

156. Shan L, Molberg O, Parrot I, Hausch F, Filiz F, Gray GM, et al. Structural basis for gluten intolerance in celiac sprue. Science 2002;297:2275-9.

157. Shelton JH, Santa Ana CA, Thompson DR, Emmett M, Fordtran JS. Factitious diarrhea induced by stimulant laxatives: accuracy of diagnosis by a clinical reference laboratory using thin layer chromatography. Clin Chem 2007;53:85-90.

158. Shiotani A, Graham D. Pathogenesis and therapy of gastric and duodenal ulcer disease. Med Clin N Am 2002;86:1447-66.

159. Simren M, Stotzer PO. Use and abuse of hydrogen breath tests. Gut 2006;55:297-303.

160. Sipponen T, Savilahti E, Karkkainen P, Kolho K-L, Hannu M, Turunen U et al. Fecal calprotectin, lactoferrin, and endoscopic disease activity monitoring with anti-TNF-alpha therapy for Crohn's disease. Inflamm Bowel Dis 2008;14:1392-8.

161. Smith MJ, Cherian P, Raju GS, Dawson BF, Mahon S, Bardhan KD. Bile acid malabsorption in persistent diarrhoea. J R Coll Physicians Lond 2000;34:448-51.

162. Sollid LM. Coeliac disease: dissecting a complex inflammatory disorder. Nat Rev Immunol 2002;2:647-55.

163. Sollid LM, Scott H. New tool to predict celiac disease on its way to the clinics. Gastroenterology 1998;115:1584-94.

164. Somogyi L, Cintron M, Toskes PP. Synthetic porcine secretin is highly accurate in pancreatic function testing in individuals with chronic pancreatitis. Pancreas 2000;21:262-5.

164A. Spiller R, Aziz Q, Creed F, Emmanuel A, Houghton L, Hungin P et al. Guidelines on the irritable bowel syndrome: mechanisms and practical management. Gut 2007;56:1770-98.

165. Spiller RC. Postinfectious irritable bowel syndrome. Gastroenterology 2003;124:1662-71.

166. Stein J, Jung M, Sziegoleit A, Zeuzem S, Caspary WF, Lembcke B. Immunoreactive elastase 1: clinical evaluation of a new non-invasive test of pancreatic function. Clin Chem 1996;42:222-6.

167. Stotzer PO, Kilander AF. Comparison of the 1-gram ^{14}C-D-xylose breath test and the 50-gram hydrogen glucose breath test for diagnosis of small intestinal bacterial overgrowth. Digestion 2000;61:165-71.

168. Strocchi A, Corazza G, Ellis CJ, Gasbarrini G, Levitt MD. Detection of malabsorption of low doses of carbohydrate: accuracy of various breath H_2 criteria. Gastroenterology 1993;105:1404-10.
169. Strygler B, Nicar M, Santangelo WC, Porter JL, Fordtran JS. α_1-Antitrypsin excretion in stool in normal subjects and in patients with gastrointestinal disorders. Gastroenterology 1990;99:1380-7.
170. Sutherland AD, Gearry RB, Frizelle FA. Review of fecal biomarkers in inflammatory bowel disease. Dis Colon Rectum 2008;51:1283-91.
171. Swallow DM, Hollox EJ. Genetic polymorphism of intestinal lactase activity in adult humans. In: Scriver CR, Beaudet AL, Sly WS, Valle D, eds. The metabolic and molecular bases of inherited disease, 8th edition. New York, NY: McGraw-Hill, 2001:1651-63.
172. Sziegoleit A, Linder D. Studies on the sterol-binding capacity of human pancreatic elastase. Gastroenterology 1991;100:768-74.
173. Takeda H, Nishise S, Furukawa M, Nagashima R, Shinzawa H, Takahas T. Fecal clearance of alpha-1-antitrypsin with lansoprazole can detect protein losing gastropathy. Dig Dis Sci 1999;44:2313-8.
174. Tests for malabsorption.British Society of Gastroenterology, 1996. Available at: http:// www.bsg.org.uk/pdf_word_docs/ malabsorbtion.pdf (accessed July 2011).
175. The EUROGAST Study Group. An international association between *Helicobacter pylori* infection and gastric cancer. Lancet 1993;341: 1359-62.
176. Thibodeau GA, Patton KT. Anatomy and physiology, 6th edition. St Louis: Mosby, 2007.
177. Thomas PD, Forbes A, Green J, Howdle P, Long R, Playford R, et al. Guidelines for the investigation of chronic diarrhoea, 2nd edition. Gut 2003;52(suppl V):v1-15.
178. von Tirpitz C, Kohn C, Steinkamp M, Geerling I, Maier V, Möller P, et al. Lactose intolerance in active Crohn's disease: clinical value of duodenal lactase analysis. J Clin Gastroenterol 2002;34:49-53.
179. Treem WR. Congenital sucrase-isomaltase deficiency. J Pediatr Gastroenterol Nutr 1995;21:1-14.
180. Trevisani L, Sartori S. The accuracy of the *Helicobacter pylori* stool antigen test in diagnosing *H. pylori* in treated patients. Eur J Gastroenterol Hepatol 2002;14:89.
181. Turner JM, Lawrence S, Fellows IW, Johnson I, Hill PG, Holmes GK. ^{14}C-Triolein absorption: a useful test in the diagnosis of malabsorption. Gut 1987;28:694-700.
181A. van Heel DA, West J. Recent advances in coeliac disease. Gut 2006;55:1037-46.
182. Vantrappen GR, Rutgeerts PJ, Ghoos YF, Hiele MI. Mixed triglyceride breath test: a noninvasive test of pancreatic lipase activity in the duodenum. Gastroenterology 1989;96:1126-34.
183. Wallis C, Leung T, Cubitt D, Reynolds A. Stool elastase as a diagnostic test for pancreatic function in children with cystic fibrosis. Lancet 1997;350:1001.
184. Watts D, Brydon G, Crichton S, Ghosh S. Glucose hydrogen breath test in the investigation of diarrhoea. Gut 2000;46(suppl II):A23.
185. West J, Palmer BP, Holmes GK, Logan RF. Trends in clinical presentation of adult coeliac disease: a 25-year prospective study. Gut 2001;48(suppl I):A78.
186. West J, Logan RFA, Hill PG, Lloyd A, Lewis S, Hubbard R, et al. Seroprevalence, correlates, and characteristics of undetected coeliac disease in England. Gut 2003;52:960-5.
187. West PS, Levin GS, Griffin GE, Maxwell JD. Comparison of simple screening tests for fat malabsorption. BMJ 1981;282:1501-4.
188. Williams AJ, Merrick MV, Eastwood MA. Idiopathic bile acid malabsorption—a review of clinical presentation, diagnosis and response to treatment. Gut 1991;32:1004-6.
189. de Wolff FA, de Haas EJ, Verweij M. A screening method for establishing laxative abuse. Clin Chem 1981;27:914-7.

CHAPTER 52

Bone and Mineral Metabolism

Juha Risteli, M.D., Ph.D., F.E.B.M.B.,
William E. Winter, M.D.,
Michael Kleerekoper, M.D., F.A.C.B., M.A.C.E.,
*and Leila Risteli, M.D., Ph.D., M.A., F.E.B.M.B.**

The skeletal system is one of the largest organs in the body and the storehouse for 98 to 99% of the body's calcium. Bones are mineralized connective tissue in which type I collagen forms a network of flexible fibers. Mineralization of this network, or matrix, with calcium salts is required to produce the rigid skeleton. Bones are a living tissue that is constantly being remodeled by degradation of old tissue and its replacement with new bone matrix. Two bone cell types, osteoclasts and osteoblasts, are mainly responsible for remodeling. It is now possible to analyze both bone formation and resorption by clinical laboratory methods.

Calcium is required for mineralization of bone and is a key regulator of body processes. Calcium ions play critical roles in intracellular signaling, in regulation of events at the plasma membrane, and in the function of extracellular proteins such as those involved in blood coagulation. The circulating concentration of calcium ions normally is kept constant under the control of parathyroid hormone and metabolites of vitamin D. Deviations of the concentration of free (unbound) calcium outside its very narrow reference interval can be life threatening. The importance of the tight regulation of free calcium is underscored by the recognition that skeletal health is allowed to suffer markedly to allow physiologic processes in other organs to be maintained.

In this chapter, after providing an overview of skeletal metabolism, we discuss (1) the clinical chemistry of several components of free calcium and review other ions, particularly phosphate and magnesium; (2) key hormones regulating these minerals; (3) markers of bone formation and degradation; and (4) major disorders of bone.

OVERVIEW OF SKELETAL METABOLISM

Bone is composed primarily of an extracellular mineralized matrix with a smaller cellular fraction. Bone is a dynamic tissue that is under continuous turnover or *remodeling,* which enables bone to repair damage and adjust strength. *Osteoclasts* and *osteoblasts,* the two main types of bone cells, are located on bone surfaces and are responsible for bone resorption and formation, respectively. Osteoclasts resorb bone, osteoblasts lay down new bone at a site of previous bone resorption, and osteocytes nourish the skeleton (Figure 52-1). Bone remodeling does not occur at random, but occurs instead in discrete packets known as *bone remodeling units.* Bone resorption and bone formation normally are coupled, with synthesis of new bone following the resorption of old. During menopause, the remodeling rate is often increased, but with excess resorption (a negative bone balance). The remodeling cycle can be divided into activation, resorption, reversal, formation, and termination phases.

Circulating mononuclear osteoclast precursors are recruited, proliferate, and fuse to form osteoclasts. These giant multinucleated cells resorb bone by producing hydrogen ions to mobilize minerals and lysosomal enzymes to digest the organic matrix. Deep foldings of their plasma membrane (ruffled border) are in contact with the bone surface, forming the osteoclastic bone-resorbing compartment (Figure 52-2). The resorption lacuna contains degradative enzymes such as cathepsin K and several matrix metalloproteinases (MMPs). After resorption ceases, a cement line is deposited in the resorption cavity, probably by mononucleated cells. Stromal lining cells differentiate to osteoblasts. Osteoblasts form bone by synthesizing the organic matrix, including type I collagen, and participating in the mineralization of newly synthesized matrix. The development of the osteoblast phenotype has been divided into three consecutive phases, each with its typical gene expression patterns (Figure 52-3).[181] Remodeling is followed by a quiescent or termination phase.

The organic matrix of bone is primarily type I collagen (90%) combined with lesser amounts of a large number of

**The authors gratefully acknowledge the contributions to previous editions by Drs. David B. Endres and Robert K. Rude, upon which portions of this chapter are based.*

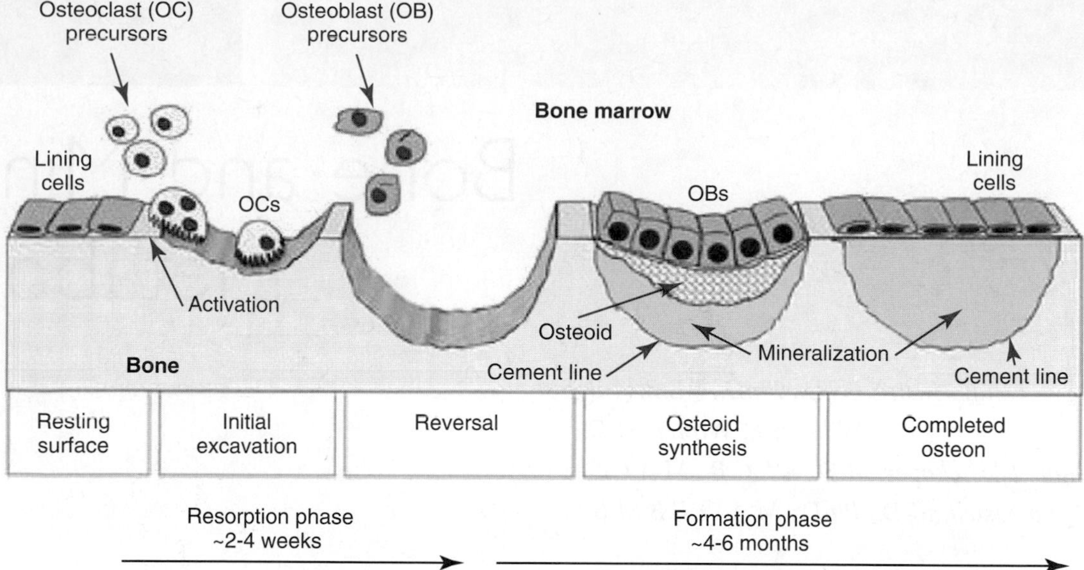

Figure 52-1 Bone remodeling sequence. A cartoon depiction of the sequential action of osteoclasts and osteoblasts in removing old bone and replacing it with new bone. For simplicity of illustration, the cartoon shows remodeling in only two dimensions, whereas in vivo, it occurs in three dimensions, with osteoclasts continuing to enlarge the cavity at one end and osteoblasts beginning to fill it in at the other end. *(From Riggs BL, Parfitt AM. Drugs used to treat osteoporosis: the critical need for a uniform nomenclature based on their action on bone remodeling. J Bone Miner Res 2005;20:177-84.)*

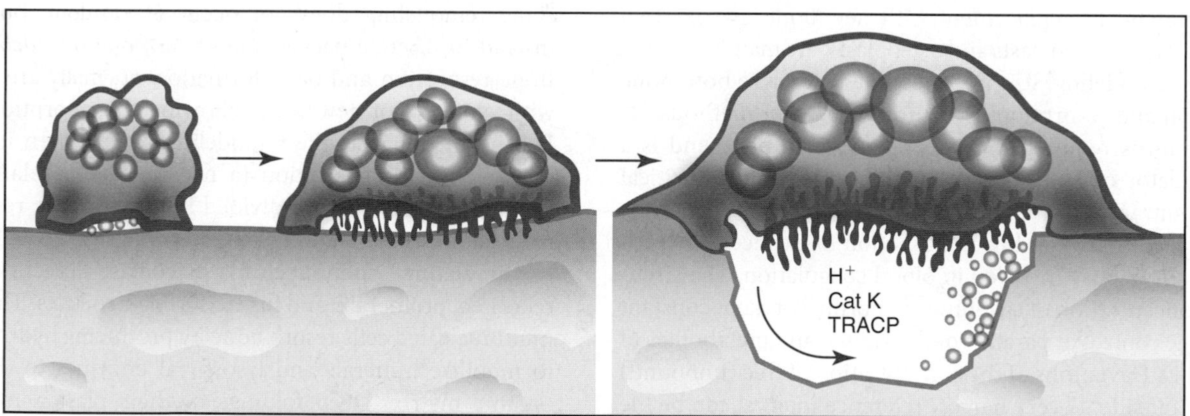

Figure 52-2 Activation of bone resorption. Multinucleated cells are recruited by the action of colony-stimulating factor 1 (CSF-1) and receptor activator for nuclear factor κ B ligand (RANKL) and adhere to bone, undergoing differentiation into mature osteoclasts. RANKL stimulates osteoclast activation by inducing secretion of protons and lytic enzymes into a sealed resorption vacuole formed between the basal surface of the osteoclast and the bone surface. Acidification of the vacuole leads to activation of tartrate-resistant acid phosphatase (TRACP) and cathepsin K (Cat K). *(Modified from Boyle WJ, Simonet WS, Lacey DL. Osteoclast differentiation and activation. Nature 2003;423:337-42.)*

noncollagenous proteins, some of which are found only in bone. Type I collagen is a product of two genes—*COL1A1* on chromosome 17 and *COL1A2* on chromosome 7—that encode two chains of the collagen molecule, called α1(I) and α2(I) chains. The organic matrix is mineralized by the deposition of inorganic calcium and phosphate in small crystals with lesser amounts of carbonate, magnesium, sodium, potassium, and various other ions.

The skeleton is not just a storehouse for ions but is essential for locomotion, protection of vital organs, and production and maturation of major components of the hematopoietic system. Bone contains nearly all of the calcium (≈99%), most of the phosphate (85%), and much of the magnesium (55%) of the body. The structural component of bone required for locomotion and protection of organs is the outer cortical shell, which accounts for 80% of skeletal mass. The less robust

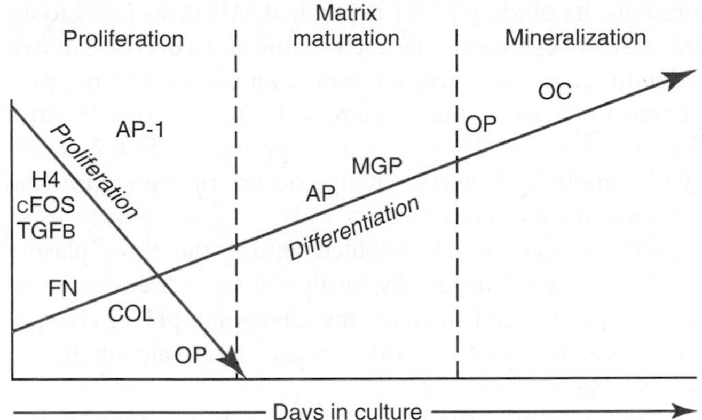

Figure 52-3 Schematic representation of the development of the osteoblast phenotype. The reciprocal relationship between cell growth and differentiation is shown, with *arrows* depicting expression of cell cycle and cell growth–related genes *(proliferation arrow)* and that of genes related to maturation of the osteoblast phenotype and production of the extracellular matrix *(differentiation arrow)*. The three principal periods in the developmental sequence are designated by *vertical broken lines*. *AP*, Alkaline phosphate; *COL*, type I collagen; *MGP*, matrix Gla protein; *OC*, osteocalcin; *OP*, osteopontin. *(Modified from Lian JB, Stein GS. Development of the osteoblast phenotype: molecular mechanisms mediating osteoblast growth and differentiation. Iowa Orthop J 1995;15;118-40.)*

inner cancellous (trabecular) bone also has a role in the mechanical stability of the skeleton, in that disruption of its microarchitecture is the dominant contributor to minimal-trauma fractures.

Cell Signaling in Bone

Over the past few years, much new information about control of the bone remodeling cycle has become available. Understanding of signaling pathways has led to the development of potential new therapies.[157] Two key signaling pathways are known as RANK/RANKL/OPG and Wnt.

RANK (receptor activator of nuclear factor κ B) is a membrane protein expressed on the surface of osteoclasts. Its ligand (RANK ligand, or RANKL) is found on the surface of osteoblasts (also on stromal and T cells). Binding of RANK to RANKL activates osteoclasts (see Figure 52-2). Osteoprotegerin (OPG) is a cytokine [a member of the tumor necrosis factor (TNF) receptor superfamily] and a RANK homolog that can inhibit the production and maturation of osteoclasts by blocking the interaction of RANK with its ligand RANKL. OPG production is stimulated by estrogen, and the marked decrease in estrogen at menopause diminishes OPG production, leaving the way open for increased activation of osteoclasts and the resultant accelerated bone loss that accompanies menopause.

The Wnt signaling pathway is far more complex and is involved in many physiologic systems beyond the skeleton. Key components that have been best studied thus far with respect to skeletal physiology include (1) the Frizzled family of G protein–coupled receptor proteins, (2) low-density lipoprotein receptor–related protein 5 encoded by the *LRP5* gene and associated with high bone mass in affected families, (3) cathepsin K, (4) Dickkopf-related protein 1 (DKK1), and (5) sclerostin.[238]

Bone Remodeling

An estimated 10 to 30% of the skeleton is remodeled each year, with wide variation among individuals. Bone growth and turnover are influenced by the metabolism of calcium, phosphate, and magnesium and several hormones, the primary ones being parathyroid hormone (PTH) and 1,25-dihydroxyvitamin D [$1,25(OH)_2D$]. Bone formation and resorption are affected, however, by a large number of other hormones and factors, including thyroid hormones, estrogens, androgens, cortisol, insulin, growth hormone, insulin-like growth factors (IGF-I and IGF-II), transforming growth factor-β (TGF-β), fibroblast growth factor (FGF), and platelet-derived growth factor (PDGF). Numerous cytokines alter bone remodeling primarily by stimulating resorption; these factors include interleukins (IL)-1, -4, -6 and -11; macrophage and granulocyte/macrophage colony-stimulating factors; and tumor necrosis factor-α (TNF-α). Findings suggest that leptin, which is secreted by adipocytes, can negatively regulate bone formation by osteoblasts.[304,305]

Exercise is a major factor in maintaining bone mass, and immobilization leads to rapid bone loss. Lack of gravity, as occurs during space flight, results in dramatic bone loss.

During childhood and adolescence, bone formation markedly exceeds bone resorption (bone modeling)—a situation that ends with epiphyseal closure at the end of puberty and is followed by a period of consolidation for the next 5 to 10 years, during which time the bone becomes fully mineralized. In healthy individuals, resorption and formation remain in balance for the next several decades. At menopause, the decline in estrogen triggers an increase in bone resorption that exceeds the capacity of the formation process and results in a rapid decrease in bone mass. This imbalance continues at an accelerated rate for approximately 5 years before slowing down to a slower rate of loss of bone, termed *age-related bone loss.* Men do not experience the phase of rapid bone loss unless they develop male hypogonadism, but they do experience age-related loss at a rate similar to that seen in women. The disease resulting from remodeling imbalance is osteoporosis.

Several diseases and medications have adverse effects on bone remodeling and bone balance, in which case the term *secondary osteoporosis* is used. Systemic skeletal disease is also seen in primary and secondary abnormalities in parathyroid hormone regulation. This latter group includes osteomalacia caused by deficiency of active metabolites of the vitamin D endocrine system or metabolic disruption of the vitamin D system, as is seen in patients with chronic renal failure. Nonsystemic skeletal disease also occurs as in skeletal metastases or Paget disease of bone. These diseases will be discussed in a later section of this chapter.

CALCIUM

Calcium is the fifth most common element in the body and the most prevalent cation. An average human body contains about 1 kg, or ≈25 mol, of calcium (Table 52-1). The skeleton contains ≈99% of the body's calcium, predominantly as extracellular crystals of unknown structure and a composition approaching that of hydroxyapatite [$Ca_{10}(PO_4)_6(OH)_2$]. Soft tissues and extracellular fluid contain about 1% of the body's calcium.

BIOCHEMISTRY AND PHYSIOLOGY

In blood, virtually all of the calcium is found in the plasma, which has a mean calcium concentration of ≈9.5 mg/dL (2.38 mmol/L). Calcium exists in three physicochemical states in plasma (Table 52-2): ≈50% is free (ionized), 40% is bound to plasma proteins, and 10% is complexed with small diffusible inorganic and organic anions, including bicarbonate, lactate, phosphate, and citrate.[249]

The free calcium fraction is the biologically active form. Its concentration in plasma is tightly regulated by the calcium-regulating hormones PTH and $1,25(OH)_2D$.

About 80% of protein-bound calcium is associated with albumin,[88,168] with the remaining 20% associated with globulins. Because calcium binds to negatively charged sites on proteins, its binding is pH dependent. Alkalosis leads to an increase in negative charge and binding and a decrease in free calcium; conversely, acidosis leads to a decrease in negative charge and binding and an increase in free calcium. In vitro, for each 0.1 unit change in pH, approximately 0.2 mg/dL (0.05 mmol/L) of inverse change occurs in the serum free calcium concentration.

Calcium can be redistributed among the three plasma pools, acutely or chronically, by alterations in the concentrations of protein and small anions, changes in pH, or changes in the quantities of free calcium and total calcium in the serum (Figure 52-4).

Physiologically, calcium may be classified as intracellular or extracellular. Intracellular calcium has key roles in many important physiologic functions, including muscle contraction, hormone secretion, glycogen metabolism, and cell division.[239] The intracellular concentration of calcium in the cytosol of unstimulated cells is around 0.1 μmol/L, which is less than 1/10,000 of that in extracellular fluid.

Extracellular calcium provides calcium ion for the maintenance of intracellular calcium, bone mineralization, blood coagulation, and plasma membrane potential. Calcium stabilizes the plasma membranes and influences permeability and excitability. A decrease in the serum free calcium concentration causes increased neuromuscular excitability and tetany; an increased concentration reduces neuromuscular excitability.

TABLE 52-1 Distribution of Calcium, Phosphate, and Magnesium in the Body

Tissue	Calcium	Phosphate	Magnesium
Skeleton	99%	85%	55%
Soft tissues	1%	15%	45%
Extracellular fluid	<0.2%	<0.1%	1%
Total	1000 g (25 mol)	600 g (19.4 mol)	25 g (1.0 mol)

Modified from Aurbach GD, Marx SJ, Speigel AM. Parathyroid hormone, calcitonin, and the calciferols. In: Wilson JD, Foster DW, eds. Williams textbook of endocrinology, 8th edition. Philadelphia, Pa: WB Saunders, 1992:1397-476.

TABLE 52-2 Physicochemical States of Calcium, Phosphate, and Magnesium in Human Plasma

	APPROXIMATE PERCENT OF TOTAL		
State	Calcium	Phosphate	Magnesium
Free (ionized)	50	55	55
Protein-bound	40	10	30
Complexed	10	35	15
Total, mg/dL	8.6-10.3	2.5-4.5	1.7-2.4
Total mmol/L	2.15-2.57	0.81-1.45	0.70-0.99

Modified from Marshall RW. Plasma fractions. In: Nordin BEC, ed. Calcium, phosphate and magnesium metabolism. London: Churchill Livingstone, 1976:162-85.

CLINICAL SIGNIFICANCE

Hypocalcemia

Low total serum calcium (hypocalcemia) may be due to a reduction in albumin-bound calcium, the free fraction of calcium, or both (Box 52-1).[272] Hypoalbuminemia is the most common cause of apparent hypocalcemia on a standard biochemical profile, particularly in hospitalized patients, because 1 g/dL of albumin binds approximately 0.8 mg/dL of calcium. Common clinical conditions associated with low serum albumin include chronic liver disease, nephrotic syndrome, congestive heart failure, malnutrition, and postsurgical volume replacement with saline or colloidal solutions. In

BOX 52-1 Differential Diagnosis of Hypocalcemia

- Hypoalbuminemia
- Chronic renal failure
- Magnesium deficiency
- Hypoparathyroidism
- Pseudohypoparathyroidism
- Osteomalacia and rickets due to vitamin D deficiency or resistance
- Acute hemorrhagic and edematous pancreatitis, septic shock
- Malignancy, osteoblastic metastases
- Rhabdomyolysis
- Healing phase of bone disease of treated hyperparathyroidism, hyperthyroidism, and hematologic malignancies (hungry bone syndrome)

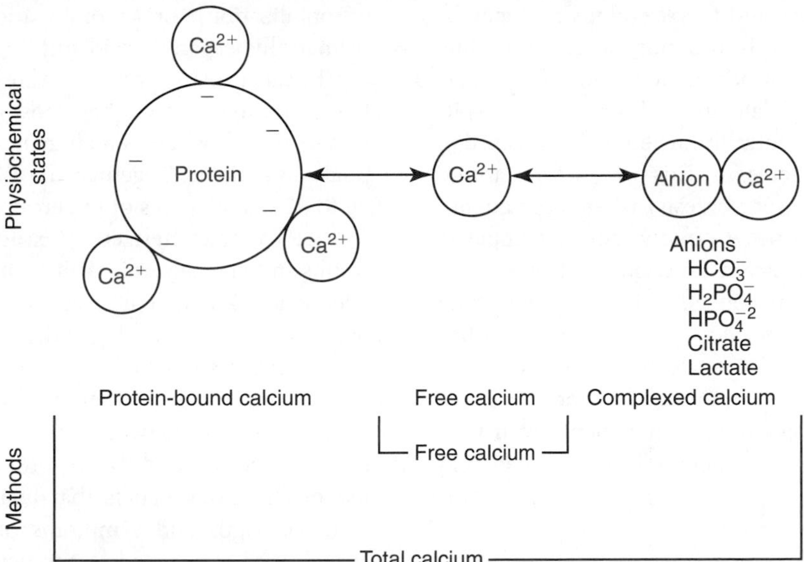

Figure 52-4 Equilibria and determinations of calcium in serum. Calcium can move between three physiochemical pools: (1) free calcium, (2) protein-bound calcium, and (3) calcium complexed with inorganic and organic anions. Methods for determining total calcium measure all three pools, whereas methods for determining free calcium measure only that pool.

these conditions, the concentration of free calcium typically is maintained in its physiologic reference interval. Common causes of true hypocalcemia are chronic renal failure and hypomagnesemia. In chronic renal failure, hypoproteinemia, hyperphosphatemia, low serum $1,25(OH)_2D$ (caused by reduced renal synthesis), and/or skeletal resistance to PTH contribute to hypocalcemia. Magnesium deficiency also can lead to hypocalcemia through several mechanisms, including impairment of PTH secretion and decreased responsiveness of target organs to PTH action (end-organ resistance). Less common causes of hypocalcemia include hypoparathyroidism, pseudohypoparathyroidism, and activating mutations of the calcium-sensing receptor (CaSR). Hypoparathyroidism is due most commonly to parathyroid gland destruction during neck surgery (90%), and less commonly is associated with autoimmune endocrine disorders. Pseudohypoparathyroidism is biochemically similar to hypoparathyroidism, but these patients have (1) an inherited resistance to PTH, and (2) increased concentrations of PTH.[190] The molecular basis for the most common form, pseudohypoparathyroidism type I [Albright's hereditary osteodystrophy (AHO)], is an inactivating mutation in the gene coding for the stimulatory guanine nucleotide-binding protein in the adenylate cyclase complex.

Clinically, hypocalcemia most commonly presents with neuromuscular hyperexcitability, such as tetany, paresthesia, and seizures. A rapid fall in serum calcium may be associated with hypotension and electrocardiographic abnormalities. The severity of symptoms is related to the rate of fall in serum calcium concentration. When symptomatic hypocalcemia is considered, the initial laboratory evaluation must include measurement of ionized calcium and is directed toward assessment of renal function and measurement of serum albumin and magnesium concentrations. Serum intact PTH concentrations are low or inappropriately normal in hypoparathyroidism and elevated in pseudohypoparathyroidism. Vitamin D deficiency is an uncommon cause of symptomatic hypocalcemia and is characterized by low serum 25(OH)D, high PTH (secondary hyperparathyroidism), and high serum alkaline phosphatase (ALP). For symptomatic hypocalcemia, calcium may be administered intravenously, and biochemical response to therapy can be monitored by measurement of total serum calcium. If hypocalcemia is secondary to hypoparathyroidism or pseudohypoparathyroidism, vitamin D and oral calcium supplements are administered.

Activating mutations of the CaSR as a cause of hypocalcemia have been described. Intervention to correct the hypocalcemia may not be needed long term, but in affected neonates, calcium replacement must be provided until genetic confirmation of CaSR status is obtained. Autoimmune destruction of the parathyroid glands may occur in isolation or in combination with other endocrine abnormalities. Postsurgical hypoparathyroidism is uncommon in patients undergoing surgery for primary hyperparathyroidism (PHPT) or secondary hyperparathyroidism (SHPT), but not in patients undergoing extensive neck surgery for treatment of head and neck malignancies. Hypocalcemia in the presence of functional parathyroid glands is a very late manifestation of disease because the interaction of PTH and $1,25(OH)_2D$ will maintain normocalcemia until body stores of 25(OH)D are severely depleted or, in the later stages of chronic renal failure (CRF), $1,25(OH)_2D$ production is inadequate.

Symptoms of hypocalcemia include tingling around the mouth and in the fingers and toes. When more severe, intense, painful spasm of the fingers and toes develops and may be sustained for several minutes. In the most severe cases, life-threatening laryngospasm may occur. These symptoms reflect decreases in the plasma free calcium and may occur despite a normal total calcium concentration when the complexed or protein-bound fraction is increased. This occurs, for example, during massive transfusion (or pheresis) when large quantities of citrated blood are infused rapidly; citrate complexes calcium, leading to lower free calcium concentration without decreasing the total calcium concentration. An important exception to symptomatic hypocalcemia occurs in CRF when marked acidosis is present. Hypocalcemia triggers muscle contraction, but acidosis hampers muscle contraction. Rapid correction of low serum bicarbonate in patients with CRF without assurance that serum calcium is maintained may trigger muscle spasm.

Hypercalcemia

Hypercalcemia is commonly encountered in clinical practice and results when the influx of calcium into the extracellular fluid compartment from the skeleton, intestine, or kidney is greater than the efflux. For example, when excessive resorption of bone mineral occurs in malignancy, hypercalciuria develops. When the capacity of the kidney to excrete filtered calcium is exceeded, hypercalcemia develops. Hypercalcemia can be caused by increased intestinal absorption (as with rare vitamin D intoxication), increased renal retention (e.g., thiazide diuretics), increased skeletal resorption (e.g., immobilization), or a combination of mechanisms (as in primary hyperparathyroidism).

The causes of hypercalcemia are listed in Box 52-2. Primary hyperparathyroidism is the most common pathologic cause in outpatients, whereas malignancy is more common in hospitalized patients. Together, these two disorders account for 90 to 95% of all cases of hypercalcemia.

PHPT is characterized by excessive secretion of PTH that results in hypercalcemia.[282] It is most often due to a solitary adenoma (80 to 85% of cases), less frequently (about 15%) to hyperplasia involving all glands, and infrequently to parathyroid carcinoma (<1%).[207]

More than 80% of hyperparathyroid patients in developed countries are free of overt symptoms on presentation because of early detection of this disorder through the widespread use of chemistry panels that include calcium.[282] The most common signs and symptoms of hypercalcemia are nonspecific and are related to the neuromuscular system. They include fatigue, malaise, and weakness with mild hypercalcemia (calcium <12 mg/dL or <3 mmol/L); depression, apathy, and inability to concentrate may be present at higher calcium concentrations. Hypercalcemia may induce mild nephrogenic diabetes insipidus with thirst, polydipsia, and polyuria. Renal colic caused by kidney stones can result from chronic hypercalcemia and hypercalciuria. Nephrocalcinosis can lead to slowly developing renal failure. Most patients with primary hyperparathyroidism (>60%) are postmenopausal women.

BOX 52-2 Differential Diagnosis of Hypercalcemia

Primary hyperparathyroidism
- Adenoma, hyperplasia, carcinoma
- Familial
    - Multiple endocrine neoplasia type 1 with pituitary and pancreatic tumors
    - Multiple endocrine neoplasia type 2 with medullary thyroid carcinoma and pheochromocytoma

Malignancy
- With skeletal involvement
    - Direct tumor erosion of the bone
    - Local tumor production of bone-resorbing agents
- No skeletal involvement (humoral hypercalcemia of malignancy)
    - Parathyroid hormone–related protein
    - Growth factor(s) (tumor growth factor, epidermal growth factor, platelet-derived growth factor)
- Hematologic malignancy
    - Cytokines (interleukin-1, tumor necrosis factor, lymphotoxin)
    - 1,25-Dihydroxyvitamin D (lymphoma)
- Coexistent primary hyperparathyroidism

Other endocrine disorders
- Hyperthyroidism
- Hypothyroidism
- Acromegaly
- Acute adrenal insufficiency
- Pheochromocytoma

Familial hypocalciuric hypercalcemia

Idiopathic hypercalcemia of infancy
- Loss-of-function mutations in *CYP24A1* (25-hydroxyvitamin D 24-hydoxylase)

Vitamin overdose
- Vitamin D
- Vitamin A

Granulomatous disease
- Sarcoidosis
- Tuberculosis
- Berylliosis
- Coccidioidomycosis

Renal failure
- Chronic renal failure
- Acute renal failure—diuretic phase
- Post renal transplantation

Chlorothiazide diuretics

Lithium therapy

Milk-alkali syndrome

Hyperalimentation regimens

Immobilization

Increased serum proteins
- Hemoconcentration
- Hyperglobulinemia due to multiple myeloma

PHPT is diagnosed by laboratory studies. Hypercalcemia should be documented by measuring total calcium and serum albumin, or by measuring free calcium, on more than one occasion. Measurement of intact PTH (with concomitant measurement of calcium) is the most sensitive and specific test for parathyroid function and is central to the differential diagnosis of hypercalcemia. Serum PTH may not be elevated in some patients, but this should not detract from the diagnosis because, with rare exceptions, nonparathyroid causes of hypercalcemia are associated with suppressed PTH concentrations. Serum $1,25(OH)_2D$ is often in the upper half of the reference interval or is increased in primary hyperparathyroidism, as PTH stimulates its production. By contrast, $1,25(OH)_2D$ (similar to PTH) is low-normal or suppressed in nonparathyroid hypercalcemia, except in sarcoidosis, other granulomatous diseases, and certain lymphomas, in which pathologic tissues contain the 25-hydroxyvitamin D-1α-hydroxylase required to produce $1,25(OH)_2D$.

PTH increases the renal clearance of bicarbonate and phosphate such that in PHPT a mild hyperchloremic metabolic acidosis may be observed, whereas in nonparathyroid hypercalcemia, a mild hypochloremic metabolic alkalosis may be observed. Although hypophosphatemia is often seen in PHPT, measurement of serum phosphate is of limited value because hypophosphatemia is also found in hypercalcemic cancer patients.

Symptomatic patients with PHPT should undergo parathyroid surgery. If the patient is asymptomatic, guidelines have been established recommending surgery over monitoring depending on serum calcium concentration, creatinine clearance, urine calcium, bone mineral density, and age.[282] In the "Guidelines for Management of Asymptomatic Primary Hyperparathyroidism" from the Third International Workshop on the topic,[20A] a serum calcium concentration greater than 1 mg/dL (0.25 mmol/L) above the reference interval was considered an indication for surgical intervention, as was a calculated creatinine clearance less than 60 mL/min. For patients who were to be managed without surgery, annual measurements of serum calcium and creatinine were recommended.

Hypercalcemia occurs in 5 to 30% of individuals with cancer.[188] Solid tissue malignancies commonly produce parathyroid hormone–related peptide (PTHrP), which is secreted into the circulation and stimulates bone resorption. PTHrP binds to the PTH receptor and is the principal mediator of humoral hypercalcemia of malignancy (HHM).[294] Skeletal metastases from cancer also can produce hypercalcemia, but this is a late manifestation, reflecting a large metastatic burden, and less often presents a diagnostic problem. Cytokines such as lymphotoxin, interleukin-1, tumor necrosis factor, and PTHrP appear to be important mediators of hypercalcemia in multiple myeloma and other hematologic malignancies. Some lymphomas associated with acquired immunodeficiency syndrome or human T-lymphotropic virus type 1 (HTLV-1) infection cause hypercalcemia by producing $1,25(OH)_2D$. It is estimated that less than 5% of patients with hypercalcemic cancer have coexisting primary hyperparathyroidism.[188]

Signs and symptoms of hypercalcemia are more evident in patients with hypercalcemia due to malignancy because the serum calcium increases rapidly and often reaches concentrations higher than those usually seen in PHPT. Lethargy, obtundation, nausea, and vomiting are additional symptoms.

Laboratory test selection is similar to that in suspected hyperparathyroidism, with the addition of PTHrP in some individuals with HHM. However, PTHrP is rarely informative if the PTH is not suppressed.[92] In specific instances (e.g., lymphoma, sarcoidosis), measurement of $1,25(OH)_2D$ may be useful.

Therapies are directed toward treating the malignancy, decreasing the serum calcium concentration by saline diuresis, and decreasing osteoclastic resorption (bisphosphonates, calcitonin, etc.). Corticosteroids are useful in reducing intestinal absorption of calcium in $1,25(OH)_2D$-mediated hypercalcemia, particularly in granulomatous disease.

Familial hypocalciuric hypercalcemia (also called *benign familial hypercalcemia*) is characterized, as its name implies, by the presence of hypercalcemia and hypocalciuria. It is due to a mutation in the CaSR found in the parathyroids and the kidney tubules.

Very recent studies of four families with idiopathic hypercalcemia of infancy (see Box 52-2) have identified a genetic basis for this condition.[270A] Sequence analysis of *CYP24A1*, which encodes 25-hydroxyvitamin D 24-hydroxylase, the key enzyme for degrading the active metabolite of vitamin D3, revealed recessive mutations in the affected children. In addition, *CYP24A1* mutations were identified in a group of infants in whom severe hypercalcemia developed after bolus prophylaxis with vitamin D. Functional characterization revealed a complete loss of function in all *CYP24A1* mutations.[270a] The decreased ability to prevent vitamin D actions (see below) appears to explain the hypercalcemia seen in the patients.

Measurement of Calcium

The methods used for quantifying calcium in blood can measure the free Ca^{2+} ion or the total concentration of calcium. The term *ionized calcium*, although widely used, is a misnomer because all calcium in plasma or serum is ionized, irrespective of whether or not it is free or is associated with protein or small anions by ionic binding.

Free calcium is the biologically active fraction of blood calcium; it is tightly regulated by PTH and $1,25(OH)_2D$, and thus is the best indicator of calcium status. Methods for both total and free calcium are currently in use and have their own sources of error. Free calcium measurements have been recommended because of the consequences of delayed treatment and the cost of working-up patients with misleading total calcium results.[30]

Measurement of Total Calcium

Various methods have been described for total calcium measurement. At present, only photometric, ion selective electrode (ISE), and occasionally atomic absorption spectrophotometry methods are used in clinical laboratories for measuring serum and urine total calcium.[272]

ISEs for the measurement of total calcium were introduced more recently than photometric methods. The specimen is acidified to convert protein-bound and complexed calcium to free calcium before calcium is measured by ISE. Calcium ISEs are discussed later in this chapter.

Photometric Methods

Total calcium is most frequently measured by spectrophotometry using metallochromic indicators or dyes. Of the metallochromic indicators that change color on selectively binding calcium (Figure 52-5), *o*-cresolphthalein complexone (CPC) [3′,3″-bis({bis-[carboxymethyl]amino}-methyl)-5′,5″-dimethylphenolphthalein] and arsenazo III are most widely used. These methods, although less accurate and reproducible than atomic absorption spectrometry, have been readily automated on chemistry analyzers.

***o*-Cresolphthalein Complexone Method.** In alkaline solution, the metal-complexing dye CPC forms a red chromophore with calcium; the color is usually measured at a wavelength between 570 and 580 nm. The sample is diluted with acid to release protein-bound and complexed calcium. Organic base, most often diethylamine, 2-amino-2-methyl-1-propanol, or 2-ethylaminoethanol, is added to buffer the reaction and to produce an alkaline pH. Interference by magnesium is reduced: (1) by adding 8-hydroxyquinoline (see Figure 52-5); (2) by buffering the reaction mixture to near pH 12; and (3) by measuring the absorbance near 580 nm. Urea may be added to reduce the turbidity of lipemic specimens and to enhance complex formation. Blank absorbance may be reduced by adding ethanol or other organic solvents. Calcium forms both 1 : 1 and 2 : 1 complexes with CPC, with the former predominating at lower concentrations.[60] Because the 1 : 1 complex has lower molar absorptivity, the calibration curves are nonlinear at low calcium concentrations. Multipoint calibration of CPC methods has been recommended. Linearity may be improved by adding sodium acetate.[61] The temperature must be carefully controlled because the reaction is temperature sensitive.

Arsenazo III Method. Arsenazo III [1,8-dihydroxynaphthalene-3,6-disulfonic acid-2,7-bis(azo-2)-phenylarsonic acid] (see Figure 52-5), at mildly acidic pH, has much higher affinity for calcium than magnesium and binds it to produce an intense, purple complex. A reaction pH of about 6 is commonly used; imidazole has been used to buffer the reaction. The solution must be thoroughly buffered because the spectral properties of arsenazo III are dependent on pH. Binding of calcium to arsenazo III can be influenced by buffer and sodium concentration. Interference from most biological pigments is reduced by measuring the calcium-dye complex near 650 nm. Citrate has been reported to cause negative interference, particularly with dry-slide techniques; in these, the only source of fluid is the sample, and the effective concentration of citrate is much higher than in wet-chemistry methods.[16,106] Clinically significant interference may be noted in patients receiving citrated blood or blood products. Unlike CPC, which has limited stability when used as a single reagent, the arsenazo III reagent is stable.[174]

Many photometric methods should not be used within 24 hours after a magnetic resonance imaging (MRI) examination of the patient in which gadolinium has been used as contrast medium, particularly if the patient has impaired renal function.[220] A predictive model has been described to calculate, in patients who have received gadodiamide, the minimum length of time to wait before blood collection to avoid pseudohypocalcemia when the Roche *o*-cresolphthalein method is used.[156]

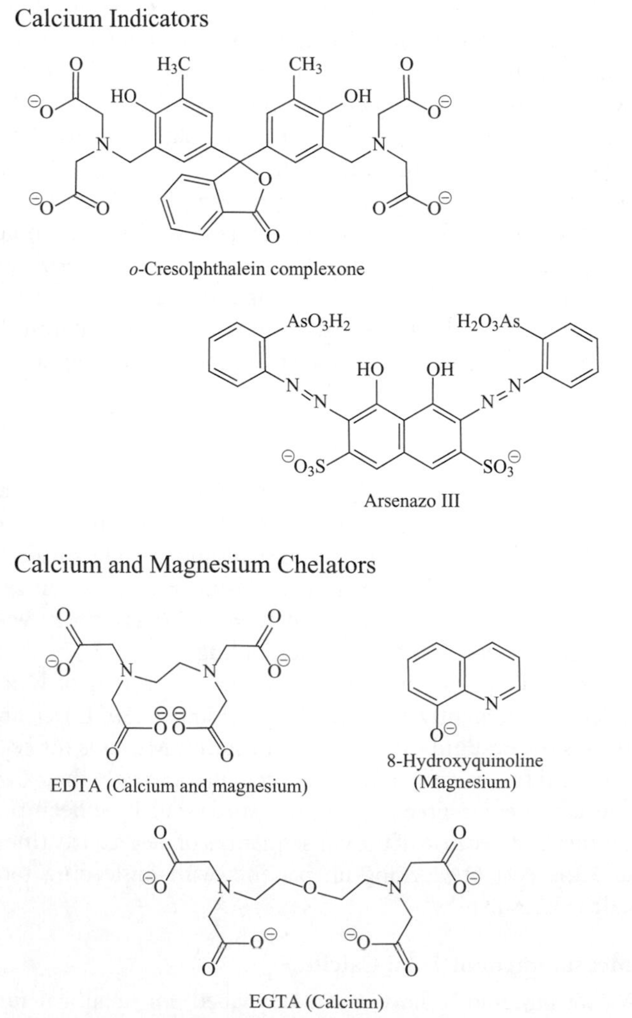

Calcium Indicators

o-Cresolphthalein complexone

Arsenazo III

Calcium and Magnesium Chelators

EDTA (Calcium and magnesium)

8-Hydroxyquinoline (Magnesium)

EGTA (Calcium)

Figure 52-5 Metallochromic indicators for calcium and chelators for calcium and magnesium.

Atomic Absorption Spectrometry Methods

The Clinical Laboratory and Standards Institute (CLSI) has approved a method by which atomic absorption spectrophotometry (AAS) is used as a reference method in measuring total serum calcium.[44,333] This method has been compared with isotope dilution-mass spectrometry (ID-MS), the definitive method for total serum calcium developed by the National Institute of Standards and Technology. The reference method is reported to have an accuracy of 100 ± 2%, compared with 100 ± 0.2% for ID-MS.[44] Although AAS provides better accuracy and precision for total serum calcium than the widely used photometric methods, it is used by only a few laboratories. It should continue to be used for validating new total calcium methods. For further information, see the previous edition of this book and the references.[30,44,47,236,272,333]

Adjusted or Corrected Total Calcium

Wide variation in the concentrations of compounds that bind calcium in blood may be noted; this variation will affect the measured total calcium concentration without changing the free calcium fraction. Several types of calculation have been suggested to "adjust" the measured calcium concentration. The goal is to produce a corrected result that would have been found if the concentrations of all compounds that bind calcium had been within their respective reference intervals. In practice, only adjustments based on albumin are used. The term *adjusted calcium* is preferable to *corrected calcium,* because "corrected" may suggest that the result has been corrected because of an error.[105,150,152]

Adjusted calcium is calculated from total calcium and albumin by first calculating a correction factor by multiplying the deviation of plasma albumin from the mean of its reference interval by the slope of the regression of total calcium against albumin. The following two equations can be found in textbooks for results expressed as mg/dL and mmol/L, respectively:

$$\text{Adjusted total calcium (mg/dL)} = \text{Total calcium (mg/dL)} + 0.8\,[4 - \text{Albumin (g/dL)}]$$

$$\text{Adjusted total calcium (mmol/L)} = \text{Total calcium (mmol/L)} + 0.02\,[40 - \text{Albumin (g/L)}]$$

However, it has proved practically impossible to establish calculation methods that would be suitable for all pathologies and all laboratories. This is consistent with the fact that many factors affect the distribution of calcium among free, complexed, and protein-bound fractions (Box 52-3). The reliability of adjustment for serum albumin deteriorates in patients with very low serum albumin concentrations.[105] Equations that are derived for a specific patient group, such as hemodialysis patients[150] or patients with liver disease, may be better than no adjustment in that group of patients. Direct determination of free calcium by ISE is preferable to adjustments.

Specimen Requirements

Serum and heparinized plasma are the preferred specimens. Citrate, oxalate, and ethylenediaminetetraacetic acid (EDTA) anticoagulants should not be used for the spectrophotometric methods, because they interfere by forming complexes with calcium. Total calcium measurements are little affected by storage, provided that loss of water associated with prolonged refrigerator or freezer storage is prevented (by the use of tightly capped containers designed for such storage), although coprecipitation of calcium with fibrin (e.g., in heparinized plasma) or lipids has been reported with storage or freezing. Plastic and glass may also adsorb calcium from dilute solutions during storage.

BOX 52-3 Factors Altering the Distribution Between Protein-Bound, Complexed, and Free Calcium and Compounding the Interpretation of Total Calcium

Factors Altering Protein Binding of Calcium
Altered concentration of albumin or globulins
Abnormal proteins
Heparin
pH
Free fatty acids
Bilirubin
Drugs
Temperature

Factors Altering Complex Formation
Citrate
Bicarbonate
Lactate
Phosphate
Pyruvate and β-hydroxybutyrate
Sulfate
Anion gap

Interferences

Hemolysis, icterus, lipemia, paraproteins, and magnesium have been reported to interfere positively or negatively with photometric methods. Many methods use bichromatic analysis, multiwavelength corrections, or blanking to reduce interference. Lipemic specimens should be ultracentrifuged before analysis.

Although hemolysis can cause a negative error because red blood cells contain lower concentrations of calcium than does serum, more significant errors may be caused by the spectral interference of hemoglobin. Depending on the method used, hemoglobin has been reported to produce negative or positive interference. In photometric methods, if hemolyzed specimens must be analyzed, blanking with ethylene glycol-*O,O′*-bis(2-aminoethyl)-*N,N,N′,N′*-tetraacetic acid (EGTA)-treated serum is suggested.

Individual instruments and methods should be evaluated for their susceptibility to interference from magnesium, hemoglobin, bilirubin, turbidity, and other interferents. Care should be taken in handling specimens, calibrators, and solutions to prevent contamination with calcium. Any glassware or plastic ware that is reused should be washed with dilute hydrochloric acid (HCl), followed by distilled water, to eliminate calcium contamination. Corks should not be used because they can contaminate specimens with calcium. How the patient is prepared and how the specimen is obtained can have a significant effect on both free and total calcium measurements. For information on these preanalytical effects,

BOX 52-4 Preanalytical Factors Affecting Measurement of Serum Total or Free Calcium

In Vivo
Tourniquet use and venous occlusion
Changes in posture: 10 to 12% increase in total calcium and 5 to 6% increase in free calcium on standing
Exercise
Hyperventilation
Fist clenching
Alimentary status
Alterations in protein binding (see Box 52-3)
Alterations in complex formation (see Box 52-3)

In Vitro
Inappropriate anticoagulants
Dilution with liquid heparin
Interfering levels of heparin
Contamination with calcium
  Corks, glassware, tubes
Specimen handling
  Alterations in pH (free calcium)
  Adsorption or precipitation of calcium
Spectrophotometric interference
  Hemolysis, icterus, lipemia

see a later section in this chapter on the subject as well as Box 52-4.

Measurement of Free (Ionized) Calcium

(See also Chapters 11 and 28.)

Many blood gas analyzers, using ISEs, provide rapid whole blood determinations of plasma free calcium and electrolytes, as well as determinations of blood gases.[30,40,71,272,277] The free calcium analyzer consists of a system of pumps under microprocessor control that transport calibration solutions, samples, and wash solutions through a measuring cell containing calcium ion-selective, reference, and pH electrodes. Sensitive potentiometers measure the voltage difference between the calcium or pH and reference electrodes for calibrating solutions or samples. A microprocessor calibrates the system and calculates calcium concentration and pH. Most instruments simultaneously measure the actual free calcium and pH at 37 °C.

Calcium ISEs contain a calcium-selective membrane, which encloses an inner reference solution of calcium chloride often containing saturated silver chloride (AgCl) and physiologic concentrations of sodium chloride and potassium chloride (KCl) and an internal reference electrode.[30,40,180,222,272] The reference electrode, usually of Ag/AgCl, is immersed in this inner reference solution. Modern calcium ISEs use liquid membranes containing the ion-selective calcium sensor dissolved in an organic liquid trapped in a polymeric matrix. The Ca^{2+} ionophores may be based on a polyvinyl chloride matrix and contain ETH1001 or ETH129 as a carrier. Instead of these two neutral carriers, ion exchangers, such as organophosphate sensors (Figure 52-6), have been used.[30] Neutral carrier membranes contain an uncharged calcium-selective organic molecule, such as ETH1001, dissolved in a plasticizer and trapped in a polyvinyl chloride membrane. These molecules have a favorable steric and electrostatic pocket or site for selectively binding calcium. Ion exchangers or negatively charged carrier membranes are calcium salts, such as calcium bis(di-*n*-octylphenyl) phosphate, dissolved in di-*n*-octylphenyl phosphonate and trapped in a polyvinyl chloride membrane.

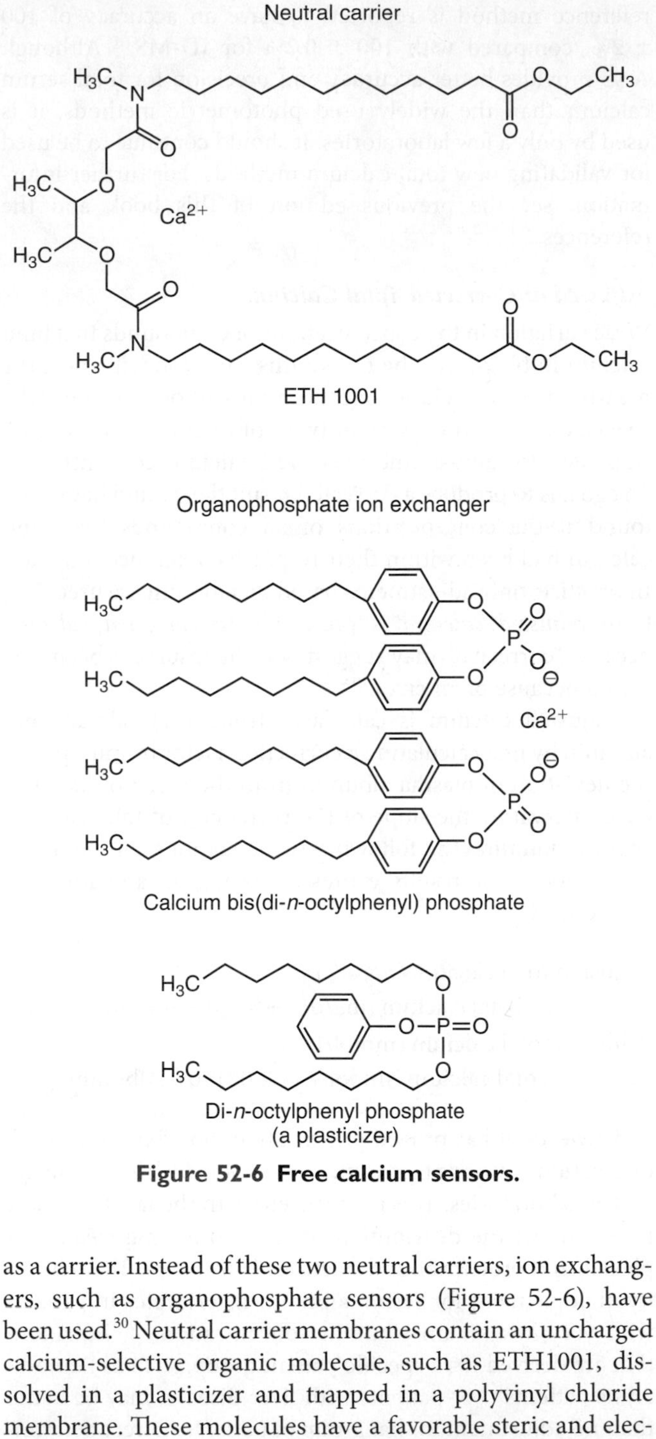

The electrochemical cell is completed by the external reference electrode, an Ag/AgCl or calomel electrode, which is in contact with the specimen by a liquid/liquid junction or a salt bridge of KCl or sodium formate. The potential difference across the cell is logarithmically related to the activity of free calcium ions in the sample by the Nernst equation. By

Figure 52-6 Free calcium sensors.

convention, free calcium is converted from activity to concentration with its activity coefficient, which is itself dependent on ionic strength.

Temperature affects electrode response and the extent of calcium binding by protein and small anions. Most free calcium analyzers adjust and maintain samples at 37 °C, thereby ensuring that results are physiologically relevant for most patients.

Carryover has been minimized by various techniques, including (1) using flush solutions containing 5.0 mg/dL (1.25 mmol/L) of free calcium, (2) using the leading edge of the specimen to clean the fluid path, or (3) purging with air.[40] Significant carryover is noted only at extremely low or high concentrations of free calcium.

The International Federation of Clinical Chemistry and Laboratory Medicine (IFCC) has recommended a reference method for free calcium.[41]

Interferences

Because ISEs measure ion activity, they are affected by the ionic strength of a specimen.[71,272] Free calcium analyzers (and the associated calibrators) are optimized for specimens of serum, plasma, or whole blood. Because the ionic strength of these fluids is primarily a result of Na^+ and Cl^-, calibrators usually are prepared in buffer and NaCl with a final ionic strength of 160 mmol/kg.[40,71,277] Although the range of Na^+ and Cl^+ concentrations usually observed in serum or plasma does not cause a clinically significant error in the measurement of free calcium, significant errors can occur with other specimens unless the matrices and the ionic strength of the calibrators and samples are matched closely.

Modern electrodes have high selectivity for calcium over Na^+, K^+, Mg^{2+}, H^+, and Li^+.[40,71] At normal concentrations, these cations have little effect on the accuracy of free calcium measurements. Wide variations in the concentration of Na^+ and high concentrations of Mg^{2+} and Li^+ may influence the apparent concentration of free calcium. Electrodes are quite insensitive to H^+, with insignificant interference noted between pH 5 and 9.

Many physiologic anions, including protein, phosphate, citrate, lactate, sulfate, and oxalate, form complexes with calcium ions. Although these anions reduce the concentration of free calcium by complex formation, they do not directly interfere with measurement of the calcium that is free. Protein deposits on the electrode may act as a divalent cation exchanger, resulting in positive interference with high concentrations of Mg^{2+}. Older electrodes were sensitive to the concentration of protein in the sample. Newer electrodes use a dialysis membrane or a neutral carrier to reduce or eliminate this protein effect,[40,196,222,229] which typically is less than +0.02 mmol/L for 1 g/dL (10 g/L) of protein. Regular instrument maintenance and protein removal are reported to minimize this interference.

Chemicals may interfere with the measurement of free calcium. Anionic surfactants and ethanol have been reported to affect the calcium-selective membrane.

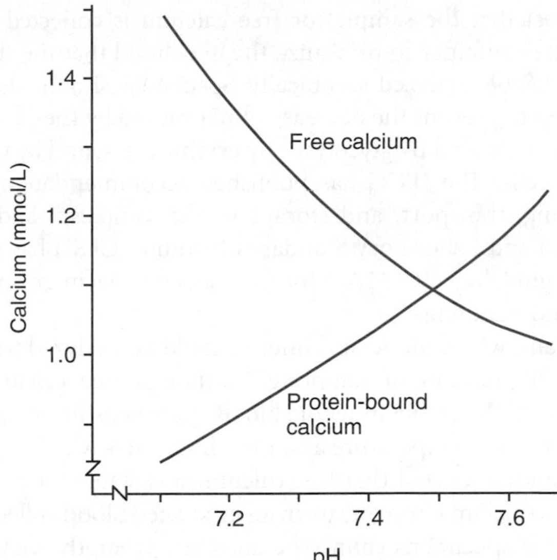

Figure 52-7 Effect of pH on free and protein-bound calcium.

Effect of pH

The binding of calcium by protein and small anions is influenced by pH in vitro and in vivo.[40,71] Albumin, with up to 30 binding sites for calcium,[88,168] accounts for approximately 80% of the protein-bound calcium. Increasing the pH of a specimen in vitro increases the ionization and negative charge on albumin and other proteins, leading to an increase in protein-bound calcium and a decrease in free calcium. Decreasing pH in vitro decreases ionization and negative charge, thereby decreasing protein-bound calcium and increasing free calcium. Free calcium changes by about 5% for each 0.1 unit change in pH (Figure 52-7).

Because of this inverse relationship between free calcium and pH, specimens must be analyzed at the patient's in vivo pH. Usually, this requires that specimens should be handled to prevent alterations in pH.

Specimen Requirements

Preanalytical considerations, including specimen collection and handling, are particularly important for free calcium. Specimens for free calcium must be collected and handled to minimize alterations in pH and free calcium caused by (1) loss of CO_2, and (2) metabolism by blood cells. Free calcium may be measured in heparinized whole blood, heparinized plasma, or serum. For most laboratories in which specimens are analyzed rapidly (within minutes of sampling) by the use of blood gas analyzers, heparinized whole blood is preferable because it reduces processing time and the required specimen volume and avoids the alteration in pH associated with centrifugation. All syringes and evacuated tubes should be filled completely, kept tightly sealed, and handled anaerobically to prevent the loss of CO_2 and the increase in pH that may occur when specimens are exposed to air. If other tests are ordered that are not available on the blood gas analyzer, it is best that the sample for free calcium is collected in a separate container to minimize the likelihood that the specimen may be analyzed aerobically. Specimens should also be handled to prevent the decrease in pH caused by the production of lactic acid by glycolysis, by erythrocytes, and by white blood cells. The IFCC has published recommendations on sampling, transport, and storage of the samples,[25] and the Clinical and Laboratory Standards Institute (CLSI) has published guidelines (C-31A2) for free calcium specimen collection and handling.[214]

Ideally, whole blood specimens should be analyzed within 15 to 30 minutes of sampling,[25] although free calcium is reported to be stable in whole blood specimens for at least 1 hour at room temperature and for 4 hours at 4 °C.[25,40,307,313] A 2009 study reported that free calcium was stable for at least 7 hours at room temperature in an evacuated blood collection tube.[129] If specimens cannot be analyzed promptly, they can be collected in an ice-water slurry to minimize metabolism. If measurements of plasma K^+ are needed on the sample, cooling will not be appropriate; K^+ concentrations will be increased because of the inhibition of ATPase activity at low temperature.[87]

For delayed analysis, serum may be the optimal sample type because of elimination of the anticoagulant and reduction in the occurrence of microclots. Serum specimens can be collected in evacuated gel tubes.[173,313] These tubes should be filled completely and centrifuged to form an effective barrier between the serum and the clot with its cellular elements. Once centrifuged, specimens are stable for hours at 25 °C and for days at 4 °C, provided the tube remains sealed. Free calcium has been reported to be less stable in specimens from both acidotic and nonacidotic patients with uremia.[217]

The practice of using aerobic specimens for the measurement of free calcium with correction of the free calcium to pH 7.4[40,308] has been criticized[40,263,306,330] and is not recommended. The free calcium value at pH 7.4 may be misleading in patients with respiratory and metabolic alkalosis or acidosis.[217] Furthermore, aerobic handling of specimens may lead to irreversible precipitation of calcium-phosphate complexes and a decrease in free calcium in some specimens that have a high total calcium and phosphate content or a high pH (pH > 7.9).

Effects of Anticoagulants

Because citrate, oxalate, and EDTA bind calcium and significantly reduce free calcium, heparin is the only acceptable anticoagulant for free calcium determinations. However, heparin, a polyanion, significantly lowers free calcium at the concentrations (≥30 to 100 U/mL) found in many conventional blood gas syringes (Table 52-3).[42,71] In addition, the use of liquid heparin should be avoided; it can result in errors in free calcium caused by dilution, as well as high and variable concentrations of heparin.

Several commercially available syringes containing lyophilized heparin are suitable for free calcium determinations: (1) electrolyte-balanced or calcium-titrated heparin syringes (final concentration of 40 to 50 U/mL); (2) very low heparin syringes with heparin in an inert filler, providing a final heparin concentration of 2 to 3 U/mL; and (3) lithium-zinc heparin syringes.[314] With electrolyte-balanced or calcium-titrated heparin syringes, the heparin is titrated with calcium so that the free calcium is not significantly altered over most observed concentrations (3.6 to 6.4 mg/dL or 0.9 to 1.6 mmol/L); however, some bias may be apparent at very low and high free calcium concentrations. Electrolyte-balanced heparin may also produce a bias in specimens with pathologically low protein concentrations.[189] In very low heparin syringes that contain 2 to 3 U/mL of heparin dispersed in a puff of inert proprietary material, the puff allows the heparin to be accurately dispensed during manufacturing and to rapidly dissolve with proper mixing, providing effective anticoagulation. A blend of lithium and zinc heparins has been reported to eliminate the heparin interference in free calcium measurements.[171,300,316] In addition, lithium-zinc heparin did not alter total calcium, unlike electrolyte-balanced or calcium-titrated heparin. Three-milliliter syringes containing a total of 50 U of a 1 : 1 blend of lithium and zinc heparins did not alter results of any general chemistry tests except total magnesium, which was increased by 0.19 mg/dL or 0.08 mmol/L. In practice individuals obtaining the blood specimen should not place additional liquid heparin in heparinized syringes.

Most evacuated collection tubes, when filled completely, contain concentrations of heparin (15 U/mL) that only slightly decrease free calcium.[311] Specific brands of syringes, evacuated tubes, and heparin should be carefully evaluated. It is important that all syringes and tubes be filled completely to minimize dilution and/or heparin effects.

TABLE 52-3 Effects of Heparin on Free Calcium

		Free Calcium	
Specimen	**Heparin, U/mL**	**mg/dL**	**mmol/L**
Serum	0	5.00	1.25
Plasma	44 (Ca-heparin)	4.96	1.24
Plasma	29 (Na-heparin)	4.84	1.21
Plasma	100 (Na-heparin)	3.76	0.94
Whole blood	44 (Ca-heparin)	5.08	1.27
Whole blood	19 (Na-heparin)	5.04	1.26
Whole blood	100 (Na-heparin)	3.88	0.97

Modified from Toffaletti J. Ionized calcium. In: Pesce AJ, Kaplan LA, eds. Methods in clinical chemistry. St Louis: CV Mosby, 1987:1010-20.

Calibrators and Quality Controls

Various calibration solutions are used by manufacturers for free calcium analyzers. The buffers in which these calibrators are prepared may have an effect on the liquid junction potential and on calcium binding; however, this is usually corrected for by the instrument software.[40] Until reference solutions are available, it is best to use the calibrators provided by the instrument manufacturer.

Aqueous quality control materials are commercially available for free calcium. Because simple aqueous controls may not reliably detect changes in performance with patient specimens, use of serum-based quality control materials has been recommended.[315] Serum-based controls may be prepared by acidifying serum with 10 μL of 1 mol/L HCl and leaving it exposed in the refrigerator for 1 week to remove carbon dioxide. The pH is then adjusted to 7.4, and the serum is aliquoted and frozen. Alternatively, serum-based controls can be equilibrated with carbon dioxide before undergoing analysis.

Patient Preparation and Sources of Preanalytical Error for Total and Free Calcium Measurements

Patient preparation and the manner of specimen collection can significantly affect the results of total and free calcium determinations (see Box 52-4).[40,115]

A common and important source of preanalytical error in the measurement of calcium is the increase in total, but not free, calcium concentration associated with tourniquet use and venous occlusion during sampling.[245] Errors of 0.5 to 1.0 mg/dL or 0.12 to 0.25 mmol/L in total calcium may result from the increase in protein-bound calcium caused by the efflux of water from the vascular compartment during stasis. Only small and clinically insignificant increases in free calcium have been reported with venous stasis. If a tourniquet is required, it should be applied just before sampling and released as soon as possible.

Fist clenching or other forearm exercise should be avoided before phlebotomy[245] because forearm exercise causes a decrease in pH (lactic acid production) and an increase in free calcium. The NCCLS and the IFCC have published recommendations on blood collection.[42,214]

Changes in posture cause fluid shifts within 10 minutes and thus alter the concentrations of cells and large molecules, including albumin and total calcium (as part of it is protein bound), in the vascular compartment. Standing decreases intravascular water and increases the total calcium concentration by 0.2 to 0.8 mg/dL or 0.05 to 0.20 mmol/L, whereas a much smaller effect has been reported for free calcium.[40,115,245] One partial explanation (along with hypoalbuminemia) for the mild hypocalcemia observed in many hospital patients may be the hemodilution associated with recumbency.

Prolonged immobilization and bed rest[131,295] increase bone resorption, which increases total and free calcium. Hyperventilation and exercise decrease and increase the concentration of free calcium, respectively, because of changes in serum pH.[40,245] Both serum free calcium concentration and calcium excretion are decreased during the night.[45] Food ingestion has been reported to have various effects but usually causes a mild increase in serum calcium. Ingestion of calcium salts may increase serum calcium. Hemolysis can alter free calcium because of dilution and alterations in pH and binding (see previous discussion under "Interferences").

Reference Intervals for Total and Free Calcium in Serum and Plasma

Total Calcium

The reference interval for serum and plasma is usually defined by an upper limit of 10.1 to 10.5 mg/dL (2.52 to 2.62 mmol/L) and a lower limit between 8.5 and 8.8 mg/dL (2.12 to 2.20 mmol/L). The reference interval depends on the method and the reference population chosen.

An analytical goal, or quality specification, for between-day imprecision, expressed as the coefficient of variation (CV), is 0.9% or less based on within-person biological variation.[90] Current methods achieve between-day CVs of 1.5% or less within laboratories.

Free Calcium

For adults, the reference interval of free calcium has been reported as follows:

Adults: 4.6 to 5.3 mg/dL or 1.15 to1.33 mmol/L

Because of the dependence of free calcium on pH, it is recommended that pH be measured and reported with all free calcium determinations. This will assist the laboratory and the physician in identifying specimens in which inappropriate preanalytical handling has led to an in vitro change in pH. Some laboratories report the free calcium corrected to pH 7.4.

Whole blood specimens develop a liquid junction potential different from that of serum or plasma because of the presence of erythrocytes.[40,71,222] A positive bias that is directly proportional to the hematocrit has been reported. In addition, free calcium values have been reported to differ among capillary blood, venous blood, and serum samples because of differences in pH. Therefore, reference intervals should be determined by each laboratory using the local instrument, specimen type, and collection protocol, and reference subjects representative of the patient population served.

Physiologic Variation in Calcium

Calcium has been reported to vary with age, gender, and season and during pregnancy.[166,167,272] Total and free calcium have been reported to decline modestly and to remain unchanged in the elderly.[281] In a healthy ambulatory group of men and women residing in the Southwest of the United States, no age-related decline or gender-related difference could be found in total or free calcium values.[78] During pregnancy, total calcium declines in parallel with serum albumin, whereas free calcium is unchanged.[166,167] The fetal circulation is relatively hypercalcemic,[165,329] as evidenced by higher total and free calcium in cord blood than in maternal serum. Calcium concentrations decline after birth in healthy term neonates during the first few days, but soon rise to concentrations slightly greater than those observed in adults.[166,329]

Interpretation of Total and Free Calcium Results

Calcium status is more accurately determined by measuring free calcium, the tightly regulated, biologically active species.[30,84] Interpretation of total serum calcium value is

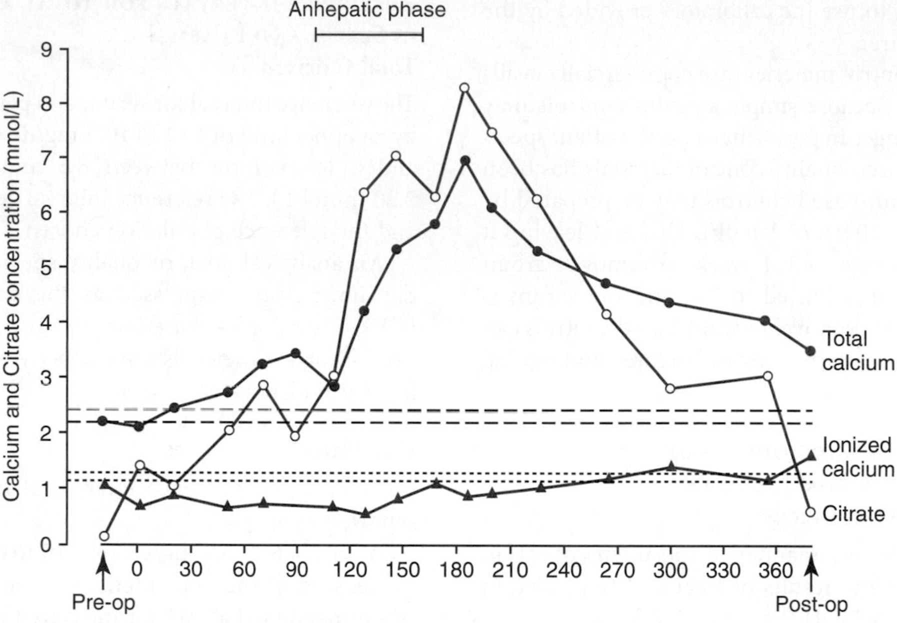

Figure 52-8 Free calcium (▲), total calcium (●), and citrate (○) concentrations in a patient undergoing liver transplantation. Reference intervals are indicated by the *upper* (total calcium) and *lower* (free calcium) sets of *dashed horizontal lines.* The reference interval for citrate is 0.03 to 0.15 mmol/L. *(From Gray TA, Paterson CR. The clinical value of ionized calcium assays. Ann Clin Biochem 1988;25:210-9.)*

complicated by its association with protein and inorganic and organic ions. Interpretation of free calcium concentration is less complicated, provided the specimen has been properly obtained, handled, and analyzed. Disagreement between free and total calcium (abnormal total calcium and normal free calcium, or vice versa) values occurs in a high percentage of specimens. One study of 1213 patients suspected of having calcium disorders found disagreement between free calcium and total calcium or corrected calcium values in 18% and 31% of patients, respectively.[309]

Free calcium is reportedly more useful than total calcium determination in hospital patients, especially those undergoing major surgery (Figure 52-8) who have received citrated blood or platelets, heparin, bicarbonate, intravenous solutions, or calcium.[40] Alterations in blood pH and temperature further reduce the usefulness of total calcium assay in these patients. Rapid measurement of free calcium, blood gases, and potassium permits maintenance of good cardiac function during liver transplant operations and other major operations such as those in which cardiopulmonary bypass is used. Free calcium is more useful than total calcium determination in patients in intensive care because of abnormal protein concentrations and putative circulating factors that alter calcium binding to albumin. Abnormally low free calcium is frequently found in critically ill patients.[12,48,341] A study at one hospital where free calcium has replaced total calcium determinations found that 41% of free calcium concentrations were abnormal among inpatients.[30] Of these cases, 31% were below and 10% were above the reference interval. The recovery room, surgical intensive care unit, renal transplantation ward, medical intensive care unit, and medical oncology unit had the highest percentages of abnormal values.

Another study has questioned the value of frequent measurements of free calcium in hospital patients.[11] In a large academic hospital setting, serial and daily testing was responsible for a large fraction of free calcium analyses. Half of all patients tested had free calcium concentrations below the reference interval. Free calcium was increased by intravenous (IV) administration of calcium, but the increase attributable to administered calcium was small compared with the increase that occurred in patients given no calcium. Retrospective analysis suggested that a total calcium below 8 mg/dL (2 mmol/L) identified most patients with low free calcium (<4 mg/dL, <1.0 mmol/L). Introduction of a reflexive strategy in which free calcium was measured only when total calcium was below that limit reduced free calcium testing by 72 to 76% and reduced IV calcium gluconate therapy by 45 to 81%. An outcomes study showed no evidence of an increase in adverse events.

Bone and mineral disorders are common in patients with renal disease. Therapy and calcium metabolism of these patients is best evaluated by the determination of free calcium because of alterations in protein, pH, protein binding of calcium, and calcium complexes with organic and inorganic anions.

Free calcium may be useful in the diagnosis of hypercalcemia. Patients with subsequently surgically proven primary hyperparathyroidism more often have increases in free calcium than in total calcium (Figure 52-9). Free calcium is more sensitive than total calcium in detecting hypercalcemia

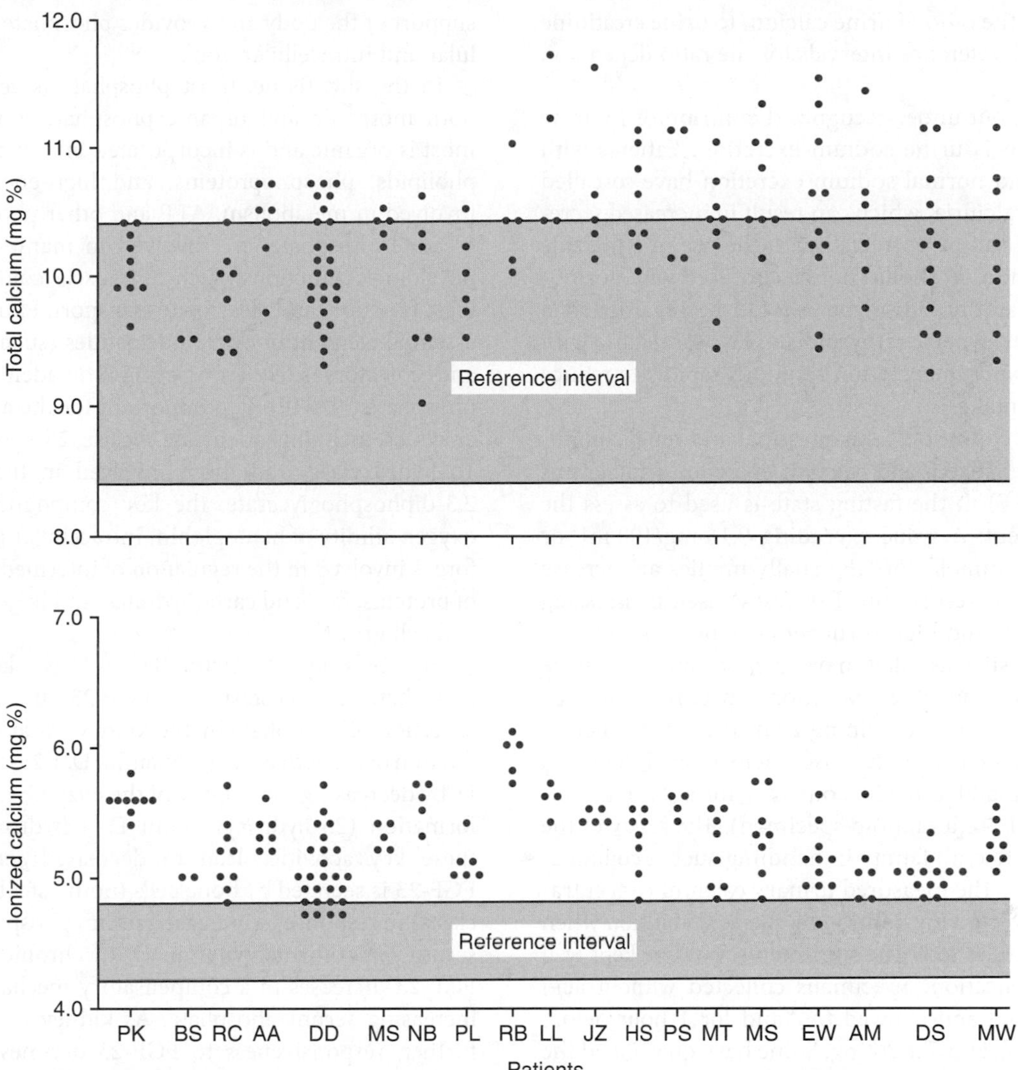

Figure 52-9 Concurrent total and free calcium in patients with primary hyperparathyroidism and intermittent total hypercalcemia. *Shaded areas* represent the reference intervals. *(From McLeod MK, Monchik JM, Martin HF. The role of ionized calcium in the diagnosis of subtle hypercalcemia in symptomatic primary hyperparathyroidism. Surgery 1984;95:667-73.)*

associated with malignancy, as may be expected in patients who frequently have decreased serum albumin. Less commonly, paraproteins produced in myeloma may bind calcium, complicating the interpretation of total or adjusted calcium measurements.

In neonates, assay of free calcium rather than total calcium is recommended because of its speed and the ability to use small skin-puncture specimens, and because of its greater validity in the presence of hyperphosphatemia, with alterations in pH, and with the persistence of α-fetoprotein after birth.[329]

Urinary Calcium

The rate of urinary calcium excretion reflects calcium intake, intestinal absorption, skeletal resorption, and renal tubular filtration and reabsorption.[249] Healthy men and women excrete up to 300 mg or ≈7.5 mmol of calcium per day on a diet with unrestricted calcium content, and up to 200 mg/d or ≈5 mmol/d on a calcium-restricted diet (500 mg or 12.5 mmol dietary calcium per day or less for several days). The reference data for urine calcium are not well established, and it may be preferable to use a value of 4 mg/kg body weight (or 0.1 mmol/kg body weight) as the upper reference limit in an individual patient.

The reference interval for urinary calcium (UCa) for spot fasting or timed specimens collected after an overnight fast is less than 0.16 mg/100 mL or less than 0.04 mmol/L of glomerular filtrate (GF), as calculated by the following equation:

$$\text{UCa (mg/100 mL GF)} = \frac{[\text{UCa (mg/dL)}] \times [\text{Serum creatinine (mg/dL)}]}{\text{Urinary creatinine (mg/dL)}}$$

Alternatively, the ratio of urine calcium to urine creatinine can be calculated; reference intervals for the ratio depend on age and sex.

An important but under-recognized contributor to urine calcium excretion is urine sodium excretion. Patients with hypercalciuria and normal sodium excretion have so-called renal leak hypercalciuria, which can result in increased secretion of PTH and can be corrected with the use of a thiazide diuretic. This condition should not be confused with normocalcemic hyperparathyroidism but should be regarded as a form of secondary hyperparathyroidism. Hypercalciuria with increased urine sodium excretion responds rapidly to reduce dietary sodium intake.

Under fasting conditions, the intestinal and renal components are relatively fixed, and calcium excretion (milligrams per 100 mL of GF) in the fasting state is used to assess the skeletal component. A value exceeding 0.16 mg/100 mL or greater than 0.04 mmol/L of GF usually implies an increase in osteoclastic bone resorption. This test is used in assessing renal stone disease and high-turnover osteoporosis.

Calcium salts, such as calcium oxalate, precipitate in urine specimens during and after collection. Specimens may be collected in a container containing acid to prevent calcium salt precipitation. A commonly used acid is HCl, 6 mol/L, with 20 to 30 mL added to the container for a 24 hour collection (1 to 2 mL for a random specimen). The safety of the patient and the patient's family in handling such a container may be a concern. The measured urinary calcium concentration must be corrected for dilution by the acid solution when the urinary volume is low. The specimen should be kept well mixed during collection. Specimens collected without acid should be acidified and allowed to stand for 1 hour before thorough remixing and aliquoting. Some have questioned the ability of postcollection acidification to redissolve all of the calcium salts with or without heating.[115]

PHOSPHATE

An adult has about 600 g or approximately 20 mol of phosphorus in inorganic and organic phosphates, of which about 85% is in the skeleton, and the rest is principally in soft tissue (see Table 52-1).[249,332]

Biochemistry and Physiology

Plasma contains both inorganic and organic phosphate, but only inorganic phosphate is measured. Inorganic phosphate exists as both monovalent ($H_2PO_4^-$) and divalent (HPO_4^{2-}) phosphate anions. The ratio of $H_2PO_4^-$ to HPO_4^{2-} is pH dependent and varies from approximately 1 : 1 in acidosis to 1 : 4 at pH 7.4 and 1 : 9 in alkalosis. Approximately 10% of the phosphate in serum is protein-bound; 35% is complexed with sodium, calcium, and magnesium; and the remainder, or 55%, is free (see Table 52-1). The organic phosphate esters are located primarily within the cellular elements of blood.

Inorganic phosphate is a major component of hydroxyapatite in bone; thus it plays an important role in the structural support of the body and provides phosphate for the extracellular and intracellular pool.

In the soft tissue, most phosphate is cellular. Although both inorganic and organic phosphate is present in cells, most is organic and is incorporated into nucleic acids, phospholipids, phosphoproteins, and high-energy compounds involved in metabolism. ATP and other phosphates, such as creatine phosphate, are involved in many energy-intensive physiologic functions, such as muscle contractility, neurologic function, and electrolyte transport. Phosphate is also an essential element of cyclic nucleotides (such as cyclic AMP) and cofactors such as nicotinamide-adenine dinucleotide phosphate (NADP). It is important for the activity of several enzymes, including adenylate cyclase, 25-hydroxyvitamin-D-1α-hydroxylase, and those involved in the production of 2,3-diphosphoglycerate, the key compound regulating the oxygen affinity of hemoglobin. Intracellular phosphate therefore is involved in the regulation of intermediary metabolism of proteins, fats, and carbohydrates, and in gene transcription and cell growth.

Fibroblast growth factor (FGF)-23 is a key modulator of phosphate homeostasis.[154A] FGF-23 increases fractional excretion of phosphate by the kidneys. It also decreases production of the active form of vitamin D, 1,25-dihydoxyvitamin D, by decreasing the activity of the enzyme responsible for its formation (25-hydroxyvitamin D, 1-hydroxylase). Both of these key activities lead to decreased serum phosphate. FGF-23 is secreted by bone cells (both osteoblasts and osteoclasts) in response to increased serum phosphate or increased serum 1,25-dihydoxyvitamin D. In chronic kidney disease, FGF-23 increases in a compensatory mechanism to counter increasing serum phosphate. As kidney failure deteriorates further, responsiveness to FGF-23 declines (in association with loss of Klotho, the coreceptor for FGF-23) and thus FGF-23 cannot lower serum phosphate.

Clinical Significance

Disorders of phosphate metabolism are separated into those causing hypophosphatemia and those causing hyperphosphatemia.

Hypophosphatemia

Hypophosphatemia, defined as the concentration of inorganic phosphate in the serum below the reference interval (usually <2.5 mg/dL or <0.81 mmol/L), is relatively common in hospitalized patients (≈2%). Hypophosphatemia is not necessarily associated with intracellular phosphate depletion. Hypophosphatemia may be present when cellular concentrations are normal, and cellular phosphate depletion may exist when serum concentrations are normal or even high.

Hypophosphatemia or phosphate depletion in blood may be caused by (1) a shift of phosphate from extracellular to intracellular spaces, (2) renal phosphate wasting, (3) decreased intestinal absorption, and (4) loss from intracellular phosphate.[249,260,332] Box 52-5 lists the commonly encountered causes of hypophosphatemia and phosphate depletion.

BOX 52-5 Common Causes of Hypophosphatemia and Phosphate Depletion

Intracellular shift
- Glucose
  - Oral or intravenous
  - Hyperalimentation
- Insulin
- Respiratory alkalosis

Lowered renal phosphate threshold
- Primary or secondary hyperparathyroidism
- Renal tubular defects
  - Familial hypophosphatemia
  - Fanconi syndrome

Decreased net intestinal phosphate absorption
- Increased loss
  - Vomiting
  - Diarrhea
  - Phosphate-binding antacids
- Decreased absorption
  - Malabsorption syndrome
  - Vitamin D deficiency

Intracellular phosphate loss
- Acidosis
  - Ketoacidosis
  - Lactic acidosis

A shift of phosphate from extracellular to intracellular fluid is a common cause of hypophosphatemia. A major cause of low serum phosphate is carbohydrate-induced stimulation of insulin secretion, which promotes the transport of glucose and phosphate into insulin-sensitive cells, where phosphate is incorporated into sugar phosphates and ATP. Oral or intravenous carbohydrate and injected insulin decrease serum phosphate. Refeeding of malnourished individuals creates an anabolic state, causing an intracellular shift of phosphate. Respiratory alkalosis leads to an increase in intracellular pH, which activates phosphofructokinase and accelerates glycolysis, causing a shift of phosphate into the cell. Low serum phosphate in these conditions does not indicate a deficiency of phosphate, and hypophosphatemia is self-correcting with stabilization of the patient's condition.

Renal phosphate wasting may also cause hypophosphatemia. Any cause of excessive PTH secretion (primary and secondary hyperparathyroidism) lowers the renal phosphate threshold and may result in hypophosphatemia and phosphate depletion. However, this may not occur if renal failure is the cause of secondary hyperparathyroidism when hyperphosphatemia is more common. The renal phosphate threshold is also lowered in Fanconi syndrome, X-linked hypophosphatemic rickets, and tumor-induced osteomalacia.

Hypophosphatemia and phosphate depletion may result from inadequate intestinal phosphate absorption. Patients taking aluminum- or magnesium-containing antacids may develop hypophosphatemia because these antacids bind phosphate in the intestine, rendering it nonabsorbable. The hypophosphatemia observed in patients with malabsorption may be more closely related to their secondary hyperparathyroidism than to malabsorption of phosphate. Because phosphate is abundant in most foods, dietary deprivation is not usually a cause of phosphate depletion in patients with normal intestinal function and an adequate diet.

Intracellular phosphate may be lost in acidosis as a result of catabolism of organic compounds within the cell. Diabetic ketoacidosis is associated initially with high-normal to increased serum phosphate. Treatment of ketosis and acidosis with insulin and intravenous fluids, however, results in a rapid reduction in the serum phosphate concentration. Consequently, patients being treated for diabetic ketoacidosis may have both intracellular phosphate depletion and hypophosphatemia.

The clinical manifestations of serum phosphate depletion depend on the length and the degree of deficiency. Moderate hypophosphatemia of 1.5 to 2.4 mg/dL, or 0.48 to 0.77 mmol/L, usually is not associated with clinical signs and symptoms (unless chronic, when osteomalacia or rickets develops). Plasma concentrations less than 1.5 mg/dL or 0.48 mmol/L may produce clinical manifestations. Because phosphate is necessary for the formation of ATP, glycolysis and cellular function are impaired by low intracellular phosphate concentrations. Muscle weakness, acute respiratory failure, and decreased cardiac output may occur in phosphate depletion. At very low serum phosphate (<1 mg/dL or <0.32 mmol/L), rhabdomyolysis may be seen. Phosphate depletion in erythrocytes decreases erythrocyte 2,3-diphosphoglycerate, which causes tissue hypoxia as the result of increased affinity of hemoglobin for oxygen. Severe hypophosphatemia (serum phosphate concentration <0.5 mg/dL or <0.16 mmol/L) may result in hemolysis of the red blood cells. Mental confusion and frank coma may be secondary to low ATP and tissue hypoxia. If hypophosphatemia is chronic, impaired mineralization of bone produces rickets in children and osteomalacia in adults.

Treatment of hypophosphatemia depends on the degree of hypophosphatemia and on the presence of symptoms. Patients with moderate hypophosphatemia often require only treatment of the underlying disorder and, possibly, oral phosphate supplementation. In patients with marked symptoms of hypophosphatemia, particularly if respiratory muscle weakness is present, parenteral administration of phosphate may be indicated.

Hyperphosphatemia

Common causes of hyperphosphatemia are listed in Box 52-6.

The most common cause of hyperphosphatemia is inability of the kidneys to excrete phosphate.[260,332] Hyperphosphatemia is a major clinical problem in chronic kidney disease (see Chapter 48). In acute or chronic renal failure, a decrease in glomerular filtration rate (GFR) reduces the renal excretion of phosphate, resulting in hyperphosphatemia. Moderate increases in serum phosphate occur in individuals with low PTH (hypoparathyroidism), PTH resistance (pseudohypoparathyroidism), or acromegaly (increased growth hormone) caused by an increased renal phosphate threshold. Growth

BOX 52-6 Common Causes of Hyperphosphatemia

Decreased renal phosphate excretion
- Decreased glomerular filtration rate
  - Renal failure, chronic and acute
- Increased tubular reabsorption
  - Hypoparathyroidism
  - Pseudohypoparathyroidism
  - Acromegaly
  - Disodium etidronate

Increased phosphate intake
- Oral or intravenous administration
- Phosphate-containing laxatives or enemas

Increased extracellular phosphate load
- Transcellular shift
  - Lactic acidosis
  - Respiratory acidosis
  - Untreated diabetic ketoacidosis
- Cell lysis
  - Rhabdomyolysis
  - Intravascular hemolysis
  - Cytotoxic therapy
  - Leukemia
  - Lymphoma

hormone is responsible for the increased renal phosphate threshold and the higher phosphate concentrations observed in children. EDTA therapy has also been associated with hyperphosphatemia.

Increased intake and a shift of phosphate from the tissues into the extracellular fluid are also causes of hyperphosphatemia. Excessive oral, rectal, or intravenous phosphate administration for the treatment of phosphate depletion is a common cause of hyperphosphatemia. Release of phosphate as the result of cell breakdown in cases of rhabdomyolysis, intravascular hemolysis, or chemotherapy of certain malignancies may cause hyperphosphatemia. Hyperphosphatemia may also be associated with acidosis, a consequence of the hydrolysis of intracellular organic phosphate-containing compounds, with the release of phosphate into the plasma.

The clinical manifestations of hyperphosphatemia depend on its rate of onset. A rapid increase in serum phosphate may be associated with hypocalcemia. Therefore, symptoms may include tetany, seizures, and hypotension. Long-term hyperphosphatemia may be associated with secondary hyperparathyroidism, osteitis fibrosa, and soft tissue calcification of the kidneys, blood vessels, cornea, skin, and periarticular tissue.

Therapy for hyperphosphatemia is directed toward correcting the cause of the increased serum phosphate. In renal failure and in hypoparathyroidism, dietary restriction of phosphate and agents that bind phosphate in the intestine (calcium carbonate and others) are useful in lowering the serum phosphate concentration.[260,332]

Measurement of Phosphate

Most methods used to measure serum inorganic phosphate are based on the reaction of phosphate ions with ammonium molybdate to form a phosphomolybdate complex that is then measured by a spectrophotometer[272]:

$$7H_3PO_4 + 12(NH_4)_6Mo_7O_{24} \bullet 4H_2O \rightarrow 7(NH_4)_3[PO_4(MoO_3)_{12}] + 51NH^{+4} + 51OH^- + 33H_2O$$

The colorless phosphomolybdate complex may be measured directly by ultraviolet absorption (340 nm) or reduced to molybdenum blue and measured at 600 to 700 nm. An acidic pH is necessary for the formation of complexes, but it must be controlled because both complex formation and reduction of molybdate are dependent on pH. A less acidic pH can result in spontaneous reduction of molybdate. The rate of complex formation is also influenced by protein concentration. Solubilizing agents such as Tween 80 are used to prevent protein precipitation.

Measurement of unreduced complexes has several advantages, including simplicity, speed, and reagent stability, and it is the assay that is used in most laboratory analyzers. Disadvantages of the method include greater interference by hemolysis, icterus, and lipemia at 340 nm.

Many reducing agents have been used in producing the blue phosphomolybdate complex, including aminonaphtholsulfonic acid, stannous chloride, methyl-*p*-aminophenol sulfate, ferrous ammonium sulfate, ascorbic acid, and *N*-phenyl-*p*-phenyldiamine (semidine) HCl. Each of these reagents appears to have some individual advantage, such as increased stability, increased color stability, lower detection limit, or reduced hydrolysis of organic esters. Ferrous sulfate and especially ascorbic acid have often been used for biological specimens containing organic esters, because they cause fewer breakdowns of labile phosphate esters. Aminonaphtholsulfonic acid has been used widely but is unstable, tends to precipitate, and requires careful timing because color continues to increase for several hours. With this reagent, color formation is increased with heating. Stannous chloride provides greater color intensity. Hydrazine has been added to stannous chloride to stabilize the reagent and improve the linearity. Methyl-*p*-aminophenol sulfate is acid tolerant, allowing for a one-component acid-molybdate reagent. A method using semidine HCl was published as a "Selected Method" by the American Association for Clinical Chemistry.[97,204]

Phosphate concentrations can also be determined by several other procedures, including the vanadate-molybdate and enzymatic methods. Vanadate and molybdate form a yellow complex with phosphate at acid pH, but the method tends to overestimate inorganic phosphate because of hydrolysis of organic esters. Enzymatic methods are rarely used[272]; for descriptions, see the previous edition of this book.

Specimen Requirements

Serum and heparinized plasma are preferred specimens for the measurement of phosphate. Concentrations of inorganic phosphate are about 0.2 to 0.3 mg/dL or 0.06 to 0.10 mmol/L lower in heparinized plasma than in serum. Other anticoagulants such as citrate, oxalate, and EDTA may interfere with formation of the phosphomolybdate complex and thus are not suitable.[272]

The apparent concentration of inorganic phosphate in whole blood specimens may decrease or increase with time, depending on the type of specimen, the storage temperature, and the duration of storage. Phosphate concentrations in plasma or serum are increased by prolonged storage with cells at room temperature or 37 °C. Hemolyzed specimens are unacceptable because erythrocytes contain high concentrations of organic phosphate esters, which can be hydrolyzed to inorganic phosphate during storage. Inorganic phosphate increases by 4 to 5 mg/dL or 1.29 to 1.61 mmol/L per day in hemolyzed specimens stored at 4 °C, and more rapidly at room temperature or 37 °C. Glucose phosphate, creatine phosphate, and other organic phosphates may also be hydrolyzed by assay conditions, resulting in overestimation of inorganic phosphate concentrations.

Phosphate is considered to be stable in separated serum for days at 4 °C and for months when frozen, provided evaporation and lyophilization are prevented.

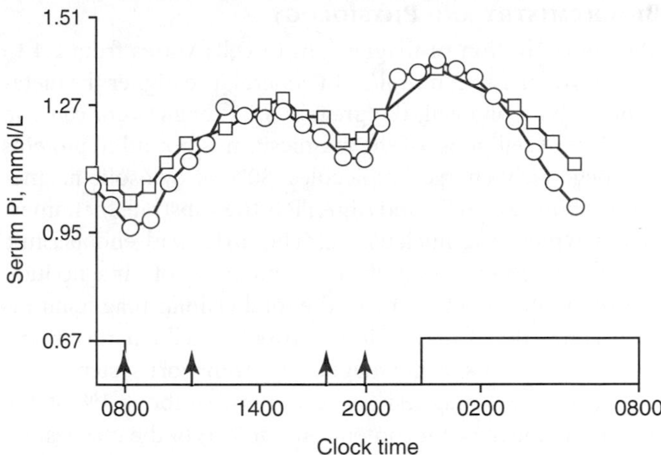

Figure 52-10 Diurnal variation of serum phosphate in men (○) and women (□). Meals and snacks are indicated by *arrows;* the *bar* indicates recumbent posture. *(From Calvo MS, Eastell R, Offord KP, Bergstralh EJ, Burritt MF. Circadian variation in ionized calcium and intact parathyroid hormone: evidence for gender differences in calcium homeostasis. J Clin Endocrinol Metab 1991;72:69-76, © The Endocrine Society.)*

Interferences

Depending on the method used, positive or negative interference has been noted with hemolyzed, icteric, and lipemic specimens.[272] Mannitol,[73] fluoride, and monoclonal immunoglobulins[18,172,231] have also been reported to interfere. Glassware should be properly cleaned and rinsed because phosphate is a common component of many detergents.

Reference Intervals

Phosphate is often referred to as "phosphorus," a practice that is inaccurate and misleading because only phosphate, not elemental phosphorus, circulates in blood and is measured. This practice originated because results were reported as milligrams per deciliter of phosphorus, rather than phosphate. When results are reported in molar units (as in SI), the numeric results and the reference intervals are the same for phosphorus and phosphate, but confusion occurs when results are reported in milligrams per deciliter.

In adults, the reference interval for serum phosphate is 2.5 to 4.5 mg of phosphorus/dL or 0.81 to 1.45 mmol/L. In children, it is 4.0 to 7.0 mg phosphorus/dL or 1.29 to 2.26 mmol/L. Adult plasma reference intervals are about 0.2 mg/dL or 0.06 mmol/L lower than for serum (2.3 to 4.3 mg/dL or 0.75 – 1.39 mmol/l).

Serum phosphate concentrations are about 50% higher in infants than in adults and decline throughout childhood as a consequence of the ability of growth hormone to increase the renal phosphate threshold.[112] The reference interval for serum phosphate in elderly women is similar to that in younger adult women, whereas in elderly men it is lower than in other adult men.[78,281]

Because a diurnal variation in serum phosphate has been reported, fasting morning specimens are recommended (Figure 52-10).[272] Concentrations are higher in the afternoon and evening. Serum phosphate concentrations are influenced by dietary intake and meals and are increased by exercise.

Urinary phosphate excretion varies with age, muscle mass, renal function, PTH, time of day, and other factors. Urinary excretion of phosphate varies widely with diet and is essentially equivalent to dietary intake.[249] On a nonrestricted diet, the reference interval for urinary phosphate is 0.4 to 1.3 g/day or 12.9 to 42.0 mmol/day.

Urine should be collected in 6 mol/L HCl, 20 to 30 mL for a 24 hour specimen, to avoid precipitation of phosphate complexes. Simultaneous measurement of phosphate and creatinine in serum and urine with fasting morning spot or 1 to 2 hour timed collections permits calculation of the renal phosphate threshold ($TmPO_4$/GFR); this calculation is considered the best method for assessing renal tubular reabsorption of phosphate.[272] The clearance of phosphate divided by creatinine clearance can be plotted on a nomogram,[328] and the $TmPO_4$/GFR determined. This index expresses phosphate reabsorption as a function of both serum phosphate concentration and GFR and is more useful than urinary phosphate excretion.

MAGNESIUM

Magnesium is the fourth most abundant cation in the body and the second most prevalent intracellular cation.[258,267] The total body magnesium content is about 25 g or approximately 1 mol, of which about 55% resides in the skeleton (see Table 52-1). One third of skeletal magnesium is exchangeable and is thought to serve as a reservoir for maintaining the extracellular magnesium concentration. About 45% of magnesium is intracellular.

Biochemistry and Physiology

The concentration of magnesium in cells varies from 2.4 to 7.3 mg/dL or 1 to 3 mmol/L. In general, the higher the metabolic activity of a cell, the greater is its magnesium content. Within the cell, most of the magnesium is bound to proteins and negatively charged molecules; 80% of cytosolic magnesium is bound to ATP, and MgATP is the substrate for numerous enzymes. The nucleus, mitochondria, and endoplasmic reticulum contain significant amounts of magnesium. Approximately 0.5 to 5.0% of the total cellular magnesium is free. Transport of magnesium across the cellular membrane is regulated by a specific magnesium transport system.

Extracellular magnesium accounts for about 1% of the total body magnesium content. About 55% of the magnesium in plasma is free, 30% is associated with proteins (primarily albumin), and 15% is complexed with phosphate, citrate, and other anions (see Table 52-2).

Magnesium is a cofactor for more than 300 enzymes in the body.[257,332] It is required for formation of substrates of enzymes (e.g., MgATP is a substrate for numerous enzymes that require ATP). In addition, magnesium is an allosteric activator of many enzyme systems. Examples of enzymes that require magnesium for action include adenylate cyclase, Na^+-K^+-adenosine triphosphatase (ATPase), Ca^{2+}-ATPase, phosphofructokinase, and creatine kinase. The guanine nucleotide containing regulatory proteins Gs and Gi require magnesium for activity. Magnesium is important in oxidative phosphorylation, glycolysis, cell replication, nucleotide metabolism, and protein biosynthesis. A decrease in the serum magnesium concentration lowers the threshold of axonal stimulation and increases nerve conduction velocity. Magnesium also influences neurotransmitter release at the neuromuscular junction by competitively inhibiting the entry of calcium into the presynaptic nerve terminal. Reducing the serum magnesium concentration results in increased neuromuscular excitability. Magnesium deficiency can thus result in a variety of metabolic abnormalities and clinical consequences.[332]

BOX 52-7 Differential Diagnosis of Magnesium Deficiency

Gastrointestinal disorders
- Prolonged nasogastric suction
- Malabsorption syndromes
- Extensive bowel resection
- Acute and chronic diarrhea
- Intestinal and biliary fistulas
- Protein-calorie malnutrition
- Acute hemorrhagic pancreatitis
- Primary hypomagnesemia (neonatal)

Renal loss
- Chronic parenteral fluid therapy
- Osmotic diuresis
  - Glucose (diabetes mellitus)
  - Mannitol
  - Urea
- Hypercalcemia
- Alcohol
- Drugs
  - Diuretics (furosemide, ethacrynic acid)
  - Aminoglycosides
  - Cisplatin
  - Cyclosporine
  - Amphotericin B
  - Cardiac glycosides
  - Pentamidine
- Metabolic acidosis (starvation, ketoacidosis, alcoholism)
- Renal disease
  - Chronic pyelonephritis, interstitial nephritis, and glomerulonephritis
  - Diuretic phase of acute tubular necrosis
  - Postobstructive nephropathy
  - Renal tubular acidosis
  - Post renal transplantation

Primary hypomagnesemia

Phosphate depletion

Clinical Significance

Disorders of magnesium metabolism are separated into those causing hypomagnesemia/magnesium deficiency and hypermagnesemia.

Hypomagnesemia/Magnesium Deficiency

Hypomagnesemia is common in patients in hospitals.[257,258,332] Ten percent of patients admitted to city hospitals and as many as 65% of patients in intensive care units may be hypomagnesemic.[320,332] Moderate or severe magnesium deficiency is usually due to loss of magnesium from the gastrointestinal (GI) tract or kidneys (Box 52-7).

Vomiting and nasogastric suction may deplete body stores of magnesium in that upper GI fluids contain approximately 0.5 mmol/L of magnesium. More commonly, magnesium deficiency is associated with losses from the lower intestine. Diarrhea may result in marked losses of magnesium; therefore, acute diarrheal states, regional enteritis, and ulcerative colitis are frequently complicated by magnesium deficiency. Magnesium is most efficiently absorbed from the distal small bowel.

Excessive urinary losses of magnesium from the kidneys are important causes of magnesium deficiency. Clinically important causes include alcohol, diabetes mellitus (osmotic diuresis), loop diuretics (furosemide), and aminoglycoside antibiotics. Increased sodium excretion (parenteral fluid therapy) and increased calcium excretion (hypercalcemic states) also result in renal magnesium wasting.

Because magnesium deficiency is usually secondary to another disease process or to a therapeutic agent, features of the primary disease process may complicate or mask magnesium deficiency. Neuromuscular hyperexcitability with tetany and seizures may be present. These symptoms and signs may also be due to hypocalcemia, and magnesium deficiency is a common cause of hypocalcemia. Magnesium deficiency impairs PTH secretion and causes resistance to PTH in the kidneys and bone; it has been linked to osteoporosis in epidemiologic studies[257] and in animal experiments.[259]

One of the more serious complications of magnesium deficiency is cardiac arrhythmia. Premature atrial complexes, atrial tachycardia and fibrillation, premature ventricular complexes, ventricular tachycardia, and ventricular fibrillation may be associated with magnesium deficiency. These effects may be caused in part by the hypokalemia, renal wasting, and intracellular depletion of potassium caused by hypomagnesemia.

Although extracellular magnesium accounts for only about 1% of total body magnesium, and plasma magnesium concentrations correlate poorly with total body magnesium, determination of serum magnesium is the most widely used test to assess magnesium deficiency. Hypomagnesemia is often transient and is not an indication of magnesium deficiency. Conversely, intracellular magnesium depletion and magnesium deficiency may exist despite a normal serum magnesium concentration. Consequently, hypocalcemia, hypokalemia, neuromuscular hyperirritability, and cardiac arrhythmias should alert one to the possible presence of magnesium deficiency. Other tests less commonly used include the magnesium loading test (also known as the magnesium tolerance test)[257] and measurements of intracellular magnesium (e.g., in red blood cell, lymphocyte, or skeletal muscle).

Acute symptomatic magnesium deficiency usually is treated with parenteral magnesium; mild depletion may be treated with oral magnesium.[332]

Hypermagnesemia

Magnesium intoxication is not a frequently encountered clinical problem, although a mild to moderate elevation in the serum magnesium concentration may be noted in as many as 12% of hospital patients.[258] Symptomatic hypermagnesemia is almost always caused by excessive intake, resulting from administration of antacids, enemas, and parenteral fluids containing magnesium (Box 52-8). Most of these patients have concomitant renal failure, thereby limiting the ability of the kidneys to excrete excess magnesium. Magnesium used to treat preeclampsia and eclampsia may cause magnesium intoxication in mothers and their neonates.

Depression of the neuromuscular system is the most common manifestation of magnesium intoxication. Deep tendon reflexes disappear at a serum magnesium concentration above 5 to 9 mg/dL or 2.06 to 3.70 mmol/L, whereas depressed respiration and apnea, caused by voluntary muscle paralysis, may occur at serum magnesium concentrations greater than 10 to 12 mg/dL or 4.11 to 4.94 mmol/L. Higher concentrations may result in cardiac arrest. Somnolence, hypotension, nausea, vomiting, and cutaneous flushing may also be seen. Hypermagnesemia induces a decrease in the serum concentration of calcium, presumably because of the inhibition of both PTH secretion and end-organ action of PTH by magnesium.

The possibility of magnesium intoxication should be anticipated in patients receiving magnesium, especially those with renal failure. Replacement therapy should be discontinued in patients with mildly to moderately increased serum magnesium. Higher serum concentrations are used in the treatment of preeclampsia and eclampsia. Because calcium acutely antagonizes the toxic effects of magnesium, patients with severe magnesium intoxication may be treated with intravenous calcium. If necessary, peritoneal dialysis or hemodialysis against a low-magnesium dialysis bath effectively lowers the serum magnesium concentration.[258,332]

BOX 52-8 Causes of Hypermagnesemia

Excessive intake
- Orally (usually in the presence of chronic renal failure)
  - Antacids
  - Cathartic
- Rectally
  - Purgation
- Parenterally
  - Treatment of pregnancy-induced hypertension
  - Treatment of magnesium deficiency

Renal failure
- Chronic (usually with administration of magnesium)
  - Antacid
  - Cathartic
  - Enema
  - Infusion
  - Dialysis
- Acute
  - Rhabdomyolysis

Familial hypocalciuric hypercalcemia

Lithium ingestion

Measurement of Total Magnesium

Serum magnesium has been measured by various techniques including photometry, fluorometry, flame emission spectroscopy, and atomic absorption spectrometry (AAS).[272,327,336] Today, photometric methods are most commonly used by clinical laboratories; although AAS[195,272] is considered the reference method, it is rarely used today.

Photometric Methods

Several metallochromic indicators or dyes change color on selectively binding magnesium and have been used to measure it in biological samples.[272,310,327,336]

Calmagite [1-(1-hydroxy-4-methyl-2-phenylazo)-2-naphthol-4-sulfonic acid] (Figure 52-11), a metallochromic indicator, forms a colored complex with magnesium in alkaline solution, which is measured at 530 to 550 nm.[1,182,270,327] A specific calcium-chelating agent, EGTA (see Figure 52-5), is added to reduce interference by calcium. Reagents may include potassium cyanide (to prevent formation of heavy metal complexes) and polyvinylpyrrolidone and surfactants to reduce interference from protein and lipemia.

Methylthymol blue (see Figure 52-11) forms a blue complex with magnesium, which is measured around 600 nm[310,336]; EGTA is added to reduce interference by calcium.

A formazan dye [1,5-bis(3,5-dichloro-2-hydroxyphenyl)-3-formazan carbonitrile] forms a complex with magnesium

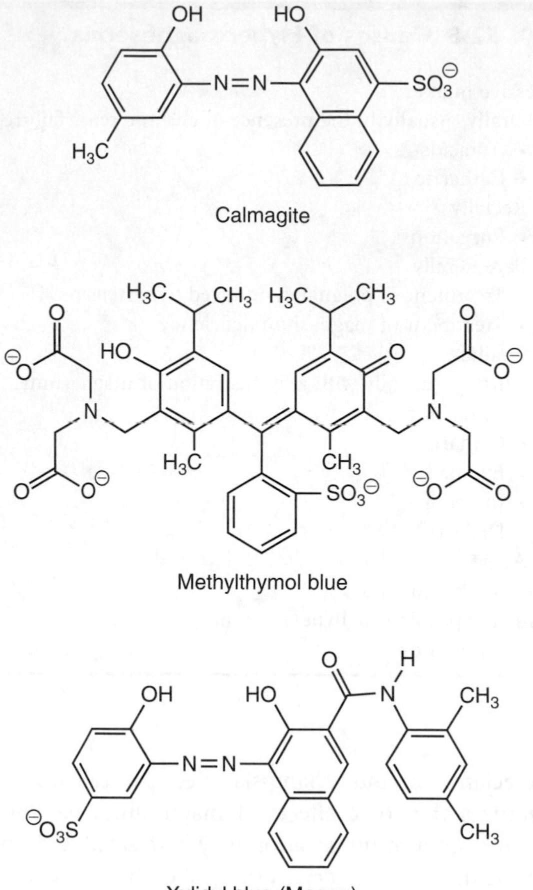

Calmagite

Methylthymol blue

Xylidyl blue (Magon)

Figure 52-11 Metallochromic indicators for magnesium.

at alkaline pH, which has been measured at 630 nm by thin-film reflectance photometry.[312] *N,N′*-[1,2-ethanediylbis(oxy-2,1-phenylene)bis(N-carboxymethyl)] glycine is used to chelate calcium. This thin-film reflectance method shows relatively little interference from icteric, lipemic, and hemolyzed specimens. Elevated calcium concentrations cause a measurable but small overestimation.

Magon, or xylidyl blue [1-azo-2-hydroxy-3-(2,4-dimethylcarboxanilido)-naphthalene-1′-(2-hydroxybenzene)] (see Figure 52-11), binds magnesium in alkaline solution, causing a spectral shift and forming a red complex.[14,65] Absorbance most often has been measured around 600 nm. Calcium and protein interferences are reduced by EGTA and dimethyl sulfoxide, respectively.

All of these methods have been applied to automated analyzers.[272]

Atomic Absorption Spectrometry

As with calcium, AAS methods provide greater accuracy and precision for magnesium measurements than do photometric methods.[272] For furher information,[195,336] refer to previous editions of this book.

Enzymatic methods have been developed with hexokinase or another enzyme that uses Mg^{2+}-ATP as a substrate. The rate of the enzyme-catalyzed reaction is dependent on the concentration of magnesium. When hexokinase is used with glucose-6-phosphate dehydrogenase, the rate of the dehydrogenase reaction is monitored by measuring the formation of NADPH monitored at 340 nm.[302] A simple one-step reaction using stabilized isocitrate dehydrogenase has been reported.[93,296] This enzyme is activated by magnesium and produces NADPH.

Measurement of Free (Ionized) Magnesium

Instruments for the measurement of free magnesium in whole blood, plasma, or serum were developed in the 1990s.[17,71,242] These instruments use ISEs with neutral carrier ionophores, including ETH5220, ETH7025, or a proprietary ionophore. Current ionophores or electrodes have insufficient selectivity for magnesium over calcium. Thus it is necessary to determine the two ions simultaneously in each sample and to correct the result for Ca^{2+} interference. Also pH should be measured simultaneously, as the binding of Mg in plasma is pH dependent.[331]

Comparisons of instruments for free magnesium determinations have been reported.[47,52,144,146,243] Differences in measured free magnesium were apparent among analyzers, mainly because of interference from free calcium.

Decreased total serum magnesium is a common finding in hospital patients. Magnesium salts are frequently administered to patients for antiarrhythmic, vasomotor, and neuronal actions, and to patients with preeclampsia, myocardial infarction, and ischemic heart disease. Monitoring of free magnesium concentrations has been suggested because both low and high concentrations can be life threatening.[257,258,320,332]

Discordance between total and free magnesium measurements has been reported in selected patient populations, including those with cardiovascular disorders, diabetes mellitus, alcoholism, migraine headaches, asthma, renal transplant, and head trauma, and in pregnant women. Interferences, such as that from thiocyanate in smokers,[71] in measurement of free magnesium may explain some of these discrepancies. Free magnesium determinations may be helpful in some of these disorders, in critically ill patients, and during cardiopulmonary bypass, preeclampsia, neonatal distress, and therapy with a number of drugs.[258,266,267]

Specimen Requirements for Total and Free Magnesium

Serum and heparinized plasma are the preferred specimens for measuring free and total magnesium.[17,242] Zinc heparin, lithium-zinc heparin, and some of the newer heparins developed for free calcium determination should be avoided because they significantly increase the apparent free magnesium concentration.[242,316,335] Other anticoagulants, such as citrate, oxalate, and EDTA, are not acceptable because they form complexes with magnesium. Storage of serum for days at 4 °C and for months frozen does not affect measured concentrations of total magnesium, provided evaporation of the specimen is prevented.

Serum or plasma must be separated from the clot or red blood cells as soon as possible to prevent an increase in serum magnesium due to cell leakage. Because erythrocytes contain higher concentrations of magnesium than serum or plasma, hemolyzed specimens are unacceptable. Interference by icterus or lipemia depends on the method and can be decreased by the use of bichromatic analysis or blanking with EDTA. Lipemic specimens should be ultracentrifuged.

Factors that alter free calcium concentration by altering the distribution of calcium between free, protein-bound, and complexed pools can also alter free magnesium concentration. Therefore specimens should be handled anaerobically to prevent loss of CO_2 and analyzed without delay to prevent changes in pH caused by metabolism. As with free calcium, high concentrations of heparin should be avoided. Certain silicones or other tube additives as well as thiocyanate (smokers and diet) interfere with free magnesium determinations.

Magnesium is primarily an intracellular ion. Thus magnesium depletion is not necessarily reflected in decreased concentrations of the metal in serum. The magnesium status of an individual is best measured by a parenteral magnesium load test,[227] also known as a magnesium tolerance test.[257] In this test, the percentage magnesium retention is assessed after an intravenous magnesium load. After baseline collection of 24 hour urine, 0.1 mmol/kg body weight of magnesium is administered intravenously in 5% dextrose and another 24 hour urine collection is carried out. In individuals with adequate magnesium stores, 60 to 80% of the magnesium load is excreted within 24 hours.[227,257]

Urine specimens should be collected in acid (e.g., HCl, 6 mol/L, with 20 to 30 mL added to the container for a 24 hour collection) to prevent precipitation of magnesium complexes. As with calcium, if acid must be added after collection, the entire specimen must be acidified, warmed, and mixed thoroughly before a sample is removed for analysis.

Reference Intervals for Total and Free (Ionized) Magnesium

For adults, reference intervals for total serum magnesium of 1.7 to 2.4 mg/dL or 0.66 to 1.07 mmol/L have been reported. However, the adequate reference interval is somewhat a matter of debate, as concentrations from the lower end may be associated with cardiovascular risk.[272] Magnesium concentrations in erythrocytes are approximately three times those of serum. Conversion factors for the units used to express magnesium concentration are given below:

$$\text{mmol/L} = \text{mEq/L} \times 0.5 = \text{mg/dL} \times 0.41$$
$$\text{mEq/L} = \text{mmol/L} \times 2 = \text{mg/dL} \times 0.82$$
$$\text{mg/dL} = \text{mEq/L} \times 1.22 = \text{mmol/L} \times 2.43$$

The reference interval for free magnesium is instrument dependent[71,272]; a typical interval for the CRT (Nova Biomedical, Waltham, Mass) is 0.45 to 0.60 mmol/L.

Reference intervals for total magnesium in infants, children, and adolescents have been published; they do not differ significantly from those of adults.[272]

HORMONES REGULATING MINERAL METABOLISM

PTH and 1,25-dihydroxyvitamin D are the primary hormones regulating bone and mineral metabolism. Calcitonin has pharmacologic actions, but a physiologic role has not been established in adults. PTHrP is the principal mediator of humoral hypercalcemia of malignancy, but it also has physiologic functions in fetuses and in women during pregnancy and lactation.

Parathyroid Hormone

PTH is synthesized and secreted by the parathyroid glands, usually two superior and two inferior, located bilaterally on or near the thyroid gland capsule. The chief cells of the gland are responsible for synthesizing, storing, and secreting the hormone. The chromosomal location of the gene for PTH is 11p15.3-p15.1.

Biochemistry and Physiology

The concentration of PTH in blood is determined by its synthesis and secretion by the parathyroids and its metabolism and clearance by the liver and kidneys. The primary regulators of PTH secretion are calcium, 1,25-dihydroxyvitamin D, and phosphate. PTH acts directly on bone and kidney, and indirectly on intestine, to increase the plasma concentration of free calcium and decrease the plasma concentration of phosphate.

Synthesis and Secretion

Parathyroid cells have relatively few secretory granules for storage of PTH. Thus PTH must be synthesized as needed for secretion. Control of PTH synthesis by calcium and phosphate occurs largely at the post-transcriptional level. Specific proteins bind to a sequence in the 3′-untranslated region of the PTH mRNA with resultant alteration of the stability of the mRNA.[213]

The primary translation product leading to PTH is the 115 amino acid long pre-pro-PTH (Figure 52-12).[85,219] The amino-terminal hydrophobic "pre" or leader sequence is involved in transporting PTH across the endoplasmic reticulum membrane into the cisternae. Both the pre sequence and the six amino acid long N-terminal "pro" sequence are enzymatically cleaved during intracellular processing and before packaging in the Golgi apparatus. After processing, intact PTH (84 amino acids, molecular mass 9425 Da) is secreted, stored, or degraded intracellularly. Intracellular degradation is increased when plasma calcium concentration is high and secretion of PTH is low. When PTH secretion is high (e.g., with low plasma calcium), intracellular degradation of PTH is low. Unlike proinsulin, pro PTH does not appear to be secreted or to circulate in measurable concentrations. However, together with intact PTH, several C-terminal fragments of the molecule are secreted from the parathyroid.[210]

The classical biological activity of PTH resides in the N-terminal third of the molecule.[136,210] Synthetic PTH(1-34) is at least as potent as intact PTH(1-84) in interacting with

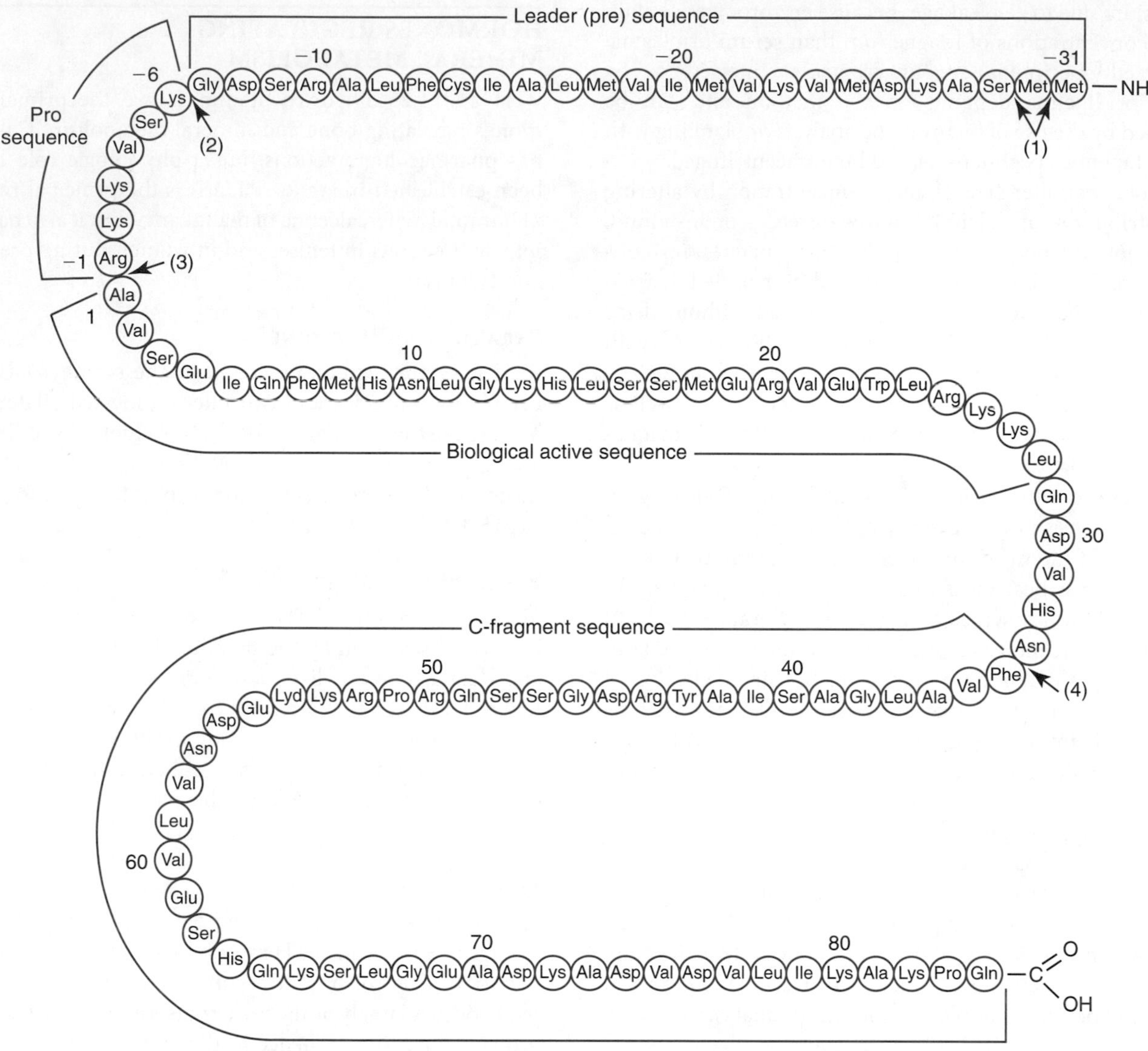

Figure 52-12 Amino acid sequence of human preproparathyroid hormone. ***Arrows*** **indicate the sites of cleavage by proteases to remove the N-terminal methionine and isoleucine** ***(1)*****, the leader (pre) sequence** ***(2)*****, and the pro sequence** ***(3)*****, producing intact PTH(1-84). Cleavage at position 4 produces inactive carboxyl (C)-terminal fragments.** *(From Habener JF, Rosenblatt M, Potts JT Jr. Parathyroid hormone: biochemical aspects of biosynthesis, secretion, action, and metabolism. Physiol Rev 1984;64:985-1053.)*

the PTH/PTHrP receptor (PTH1R, type 1 PTH receptor) and stimulating calcemic, phosphaturic, and other biological responses in kidney and bone. Oxidation of the methionine residues at position 8 or 18 results in loss of biological activity.

The PTH molecule contains a large number of basic amino acids. The middle portion of the molecule is quite immunogenic because of its hydrophobicity and species specificity. The C-terminal part of PTH, PTH(7-84), has some effects that antagonize those of PTH[286] and is involved in some functions of the hormone, having its own receptors in kidney and bone, that are distinct from those mediated by PTH1R.[210]

The concentration of free calcium in blood or extracellular fluid is the primary acute physiologic regulator of PTH synthesis, metabolism, and secretion.[36,85,219] Free calcium is sensed by a G-protein–coupled calcium-sensing receptor (CaSR) in the plasma membrane of parathyroid cells; intracellular signal transduction pathways following activation of the receptor involve release of free calcium from intracellular stores and opening of plasma membrane calcium channels.[35] The 1078 amino acid CaSR (gene symbol *CASR,* gene location chromosome 3q13.3-q21) is a member of subfamily C of the G-protein–coupled receptors. Other subfamily members include gamma-aminobutyric acid type B (GABAB) receptors, metabotropic glutamate receptors (mGluR), and pheromone receptors. The CaSR has a large extracellular domain for the detection of ionized calcium, seven transmembrane domains, and an intracellular domain that couples the receptor to G proteins. An increase in extracellular free calcium concentration inhibits PTH synthesis and secretion and

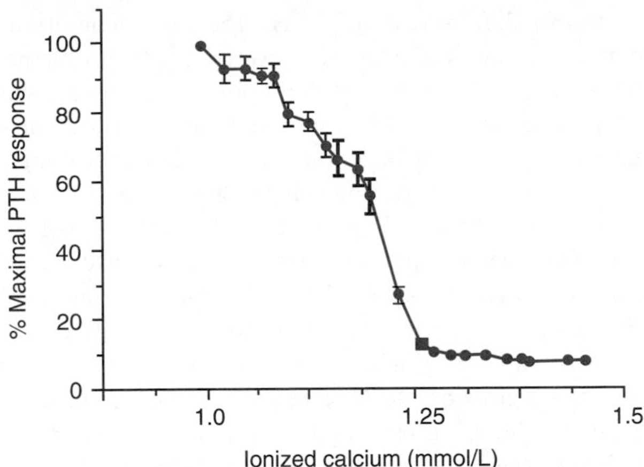

Figure 52-13 Regulation of secretion of intact parathyroid hormone (PTH) by calcium in healthy humans. Calcium and ethylenediaminetetraacetic acid (EDTA) were infused to demonstrate the sigmoidal relationship between PTH secretion and free calcium. *[From Brown EM. Extracellular Ca^{2+} sensing, regulation of parathyroid cell function, and role of Ca^{2+} and other ions as extracellular (first) messengers. Physiol Rev 1991;71:371-411.]*

increases PTH metabolism, whereas a decrease has the opposite effect. An inverse sigmoid relationship exists between PTH secretion and free extracellular calcium (Figure 52-13).[219] Maximal secretion and suppression are attained with mild hypocalcemia and mild hypercalcemia, respectively. The midpoint of this relationship, or the set point, is the calcium concentration at which PTH secretion is half maximal. Set points appear to vary somewhat from individual to individual and may be altered by physiologic or pathologic processes.

$1,25(OH)_2D$, phosphate, and magnesium also influence the synthesis and secretion of PTH.[84,85,219] $1,25(OH)_2D$ interacts with vitamin D receptors in the parathyroid glands to chronically decrease PTH secretion by suppressing PTH gene transcription and subsequent secretion. Hyperphosphatemia and hypophosphatemia increase and decrease PTH synthesis and secretion,[5] respectively, and the hyperphosphatemia of chronic renal failure leads to parathyroid hyperplasia and hyperparathyroidism. Magnesium probably does not play an important role in PTH secretion except at the extremes of magnesium concentration.[84] Chronic severe hypomagnesemia, such as that occurring in alcoholism, has been associated with impaired PTH secretion, whereas acute hypomagnesemia may stimulate secretion. Chronic hypomagnesemia can cause resistance to the effects of PTH.[177] Hypermagnesemia suppresses PTH secretion via the calcium-sensing receptor, although not as effectively as does calcium.[84]

Biological Actions

PTH influences calcium and phosphate homeostasis directly through its actions on both bone and kidney and indirectly through its actions on the intestine through $1,25(OH)_2D$.[85,219] The hormone exerts its actions by interacting with type 1 PTH receptors (PTH/PTHrP receptors) located in the plasma membrane of target cells. This interaction initiates a cascade of intracellular events, including generation of cAMP, activation of kinases, phosphorylation of proteins, increased entry of calcium and intracellular calcium stimulated phospholipase C activity with generation of diacylglycerol and phosphoinositide-activated enzyme and transport systems, and secretion of lysosomal enzymes.[85,228] Two active domains have been identified in the receptor binding region of PTH that activate two separate second messenger pathways upon binding to the receptor[271]; in its classical target cells, PTH normally activates both pathways.

In the kidneys, PTH has several functions: (1) induces 25-hydroxyvitamin D-1α-hydroxylase, increasing the production of $1,25(OH)_2D$, which in turn stimulates intestinal absorption of both calcium and phosphate; (2) increases calcium reabsorption in the distal convoluted tubule of the nephron; (3) decreases reabsorption of phosphate by the proximal tubule; and (4) inhibits Na^+-H^+ antiporter activity, which favors mild hyperchloremic metabolic acidosis in hyperparathyroid states. The effects of PTH on bone are complex, as evidenced by its stimulation of bone resorption or bone formation, depending on the concentration of PTH and the duration of exposure.[85,136] Chronic exposure to high concentrations of PTH leads to increased bone resorption. Bone resorption, a prompt effect, is important for the maintenance of calcium homeostasis, whereas the delayed skeletal effects of PTH are important for extreme systemic needs and skeletal homeostasis.

Despite the extent and rapidity of catabolic effects in bone, it has not been possible to find PTH receptors on osteoclasts, whereas they are found on osteoblasts and adjacent bone marrow stromal cells. These cell types mediate PTH action to osteoclasts via several cytokines.[210] Actions include enhanced differentiation of osteoclast precursors and stimulation of resorbing activity in mature osteoclasts.

PTH also has an anabolic effect on the skeleton. It increases the number of osteoblasts and enhances their differentiation from stromal cells. Different fragments and the intact hormone may have different effects on osteoblast gene expression.[85] Because of its anabolic effect on bone, PTH(1-34) is used as a therapeutic agent for osteoporosis under the name teriparatide (see "Biochemical markers of bone turnover").[136] Osteoblasts, via macrophage-colony stimulating factor (M-CSF), stimulate osteoclast precursor formation from macrophages. Therefore osteoclasts are ultimately derived from the bone marrow and from hematopoietic stem cells located in the bone marrow.

Integration of the direct effects of PTH on bone and kidney, and of the indirect effects on intestine through $1,25(OH)_2D$, results in alterations in calcium and phosphate concentrations in blood and urine. In blood, total and free calcium concentrations are increased, whereas the concentration of phosphate is decreased. In urine, inorganic phosphate and cAMP concentrations are increased. Urinary calcium excretion usually is increased because the larger filtered load of calcium, derived from bone resorption and intestinal calcium absorption, overrides the increased tubular reabsorption of calcium. In the absence of disease, the increase in blood calcium reduces PTH secretion through a negative feedback loop, maintaining homeostasis.

Heterogeneity of Circulating PTH

PTH circulates partially as the biologically active hormone and partially as a series of N-terminally truncated fragments containing the midregion and C-terminal amino acids. Many of these fragments have been identified[33,187] (Figure 52-14). The heterogeneity is due to (1) the secretion of both intact hormone and C-terminal fragments by the parathyroids, (2) peripheral metabolism of intact hormone by liver and kidney to C-terminal fragments, and (3) renal clearance of intact hormone and C-terminal fragments (Figure 52-15). In the parathyroids, secretion of intact PTH is increased by hypocalcemia and is greatly reduced or absent in hypercalcemia, whereas some secretion of C-terminal fragments persists in hypercalcemia. Biologically active intact PTH (amino acids 1-84) is rapidly cleared from plasma (half-life <5 minutes) by Kupffer cells of the liver (60 to 70%) and by glomerular filtration in the kidneys (20 to 30%).[85] Peripheral metabolism appears to inactivate intact hormone without releasing measurable concentrations of biologically active N-terminal fragments.[33,210]

Circulating PTH measured by most immunoassays is composed of "inactive" fragments and intact hormone. Fragments consisting of the middle and carboxyl regions of the molecule (e.g., amino acids 34-84, 36-84) are devoid of the N-terminal region and classical PTH biological activity and were earlier considered to be inactive degradation products. However, reports have identified separate receptors for C-terminal PTH in bone cells and have suggested that such fragments may affect the maturation and biological activity of these cells. C-terminal fragments are cleared by glomerular filtration and normally have a half-life of less than 1 hour. Their half-life and circulating concentration are significantly increased in individuals with impaired renal function. In most current assays, 5 to 25% of the total circulating PTH is intact hormone, and 75 to 95% consists of C-terminal fragments in individuals with normal renal function.[85]

Clinical Significance

Determination of PTH is useful in the differential diagnosis of both hypercalcemia and hypocalcemia, for assessing parathyroid function in renal failure, and for evaluating parathyroid function in bone and mineral disorders (see "Calcium, Clinical Significance," "Hypocalcemia," and "Hypercalcemia"; "Metabolic Bone Diseases"; and "Interpretation of PTH Results").

Measurement of PTH

Radioimmunoassay for PTH was among the first modern immunoassays to be put to clinical use in the 1960s, adding a new dimension to diagnosis and treatment of hypocalcemic and hypercalcemic states. However, it soon became clear that not all immunoreactive substances measured in blood by the assay were active PTH—a finding that led to the identification of C-terminal fragments of PTH. The next generation of immunoassays was developed to overcome this problem. To date, there have been three generations of PTH assay, which have yielded partially different results as the result of the presence of a series of immunologic determinants along the molecule and the physiologic heterogeneity of circulating PTH-related antigens (Figure 52-16).[33,95,194,325,342] Noncompetitive (sandwich) immunoassays generally are used now for the measurement of intact PTH. Radioimmunoassays (RIAs) of the first generation of PTH assays were competitive immunoassays involving a single antibody directed toward epitopes in the midregion or the C-terminal half of the molecules, these being the most immunogenic parts. Today, such assays have been largely discontinued because of their limited specificity and/or sensitivity. Midregion and C-terminal methods (1) measure primarily C-terminal fragments, which are present in much higher concentrations than is the biologically active hormone; (2) often provide poor identification of parathyroid function, as the measured concentration is affected by peripheral metabolism and glomerular filtration of the fragments; (3) are difficult to interpret in patients with impaired renal function, as an apparent high value does not necessarily indicate secondary hyperparathyroidism; and (4) produce results that are not suppressed in nonparathyroid hypercalcemia and are often falsely modestly elevated.[79] Other RIAs were developed to recognize epitopes in the N-terminal part of PTH, but these suffered from inaccuracy.[325,342] Competitive immunoassays lacked the sensitivity required to measure intact PTH in patients with normal or modestly elevated concentrations.

The second generation of PTH assays were designed to detect the intact molecule only and were called *intact assays*. This was accomplished by the use of noncompetitive (sandwich) immunometric assays using two antibodies[33,342]: a solid-phase capture antibody directed against the C-terminus, and a labeled detection antibody raised against the N-terminus (amino acids 1-34), or vice versa. The following advances permitted the development of noncompetitive methods for intact PTH: (1) determination of the amino acid sequence of human (h)PTH; (2) increased understanding of the secretion, metabolism, clearance, and circulating forms of PTH; and (3) synthesis of hPTH, fragments of hPTH, and analogs of fragments for use as immunogens, tracers, and calibrators, for characterization of antiserum and antibody specificity, and for affinity purification of antibodies. The clinical utility of the first generation of so-called intact PTH assays in diagnosing primary hyperparathyroidism and in monitoring secondary hyperparathyroidism is well established.[33] Yet, it has become clear that they overestimate the severity of PTH-related bone disease because they also detect several molecular species of PTH, which can be separated when a serum sample is fractionated on high-performance liquid chromatography (HPLC). Indeed, if PTH concentration in the serum of a patient with end-stage kidney disease was decreased to normal as measured by these assays, adynamic bone disease was a possible outcome.[33,342] Again, blood was found to contain N-terminally truncated PTH fragments that are long

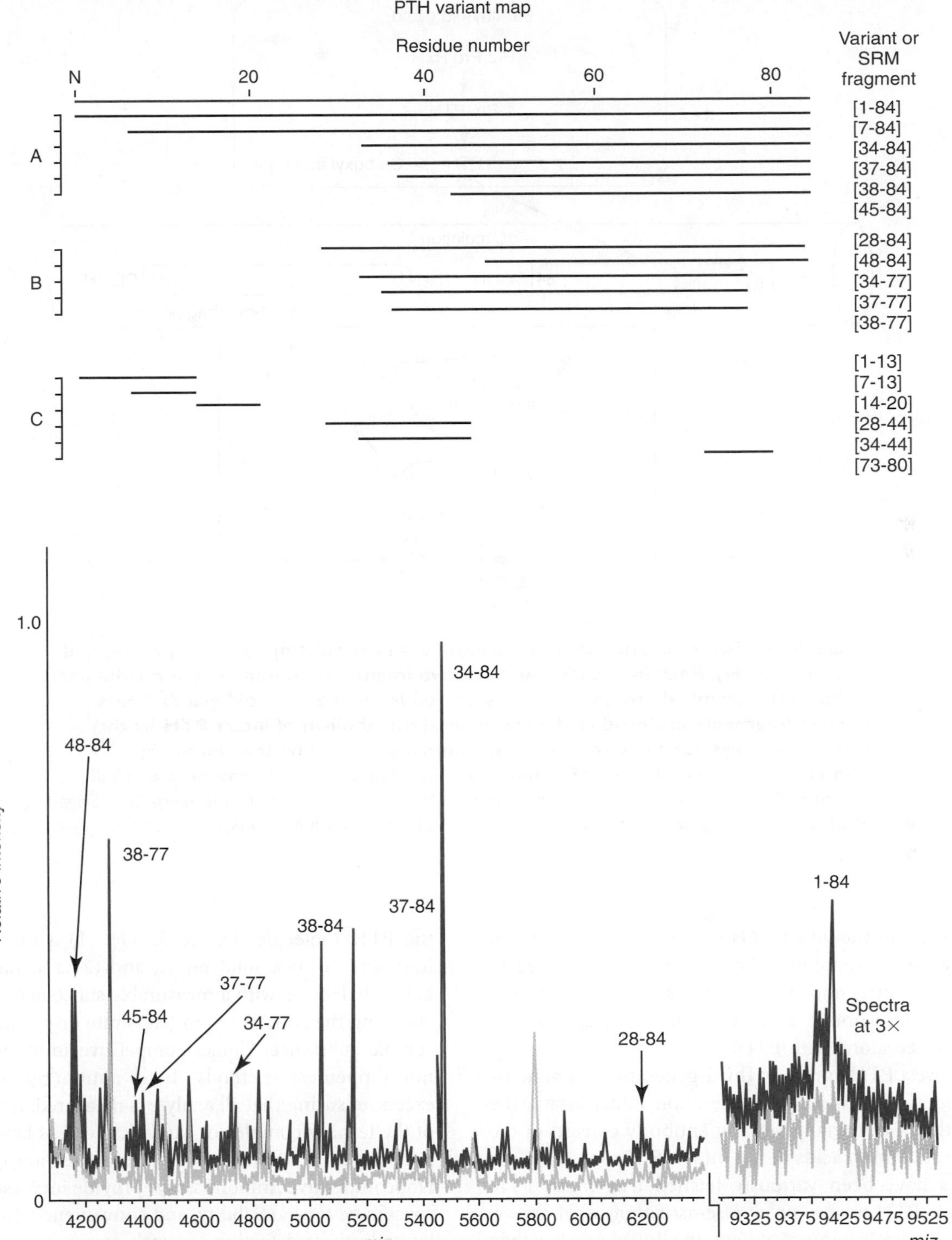

Figure 52-14 Parathyroid hormone (PTH) fragments in plasma. *Upper panel: (A)* N-terminally truncated PTH variants identified before 2010. *(B)* Variants added to map by study of Lopez and associates. *(C)* Conserved and truncated tryptic fragments chosen for study reported in bottom panel. *Bottom panel:* Spectra representative of 12 samples from patients with renal failure *(red/upper tracing)* and 12 from healthy controls *(light red/lower tracing)*. The marked species were consistently found at higher relative abundance in the renal failure cohort. *(From Lopez MF, Rezai T, Sarracino DA, Prakash A, Krastins B, Athanas M, et al. Selected reaction monitoring—mass spectrometric immunoassay responsive to parathyroid hormone and related variants. Clin Chem 2010;56:281-90.)*

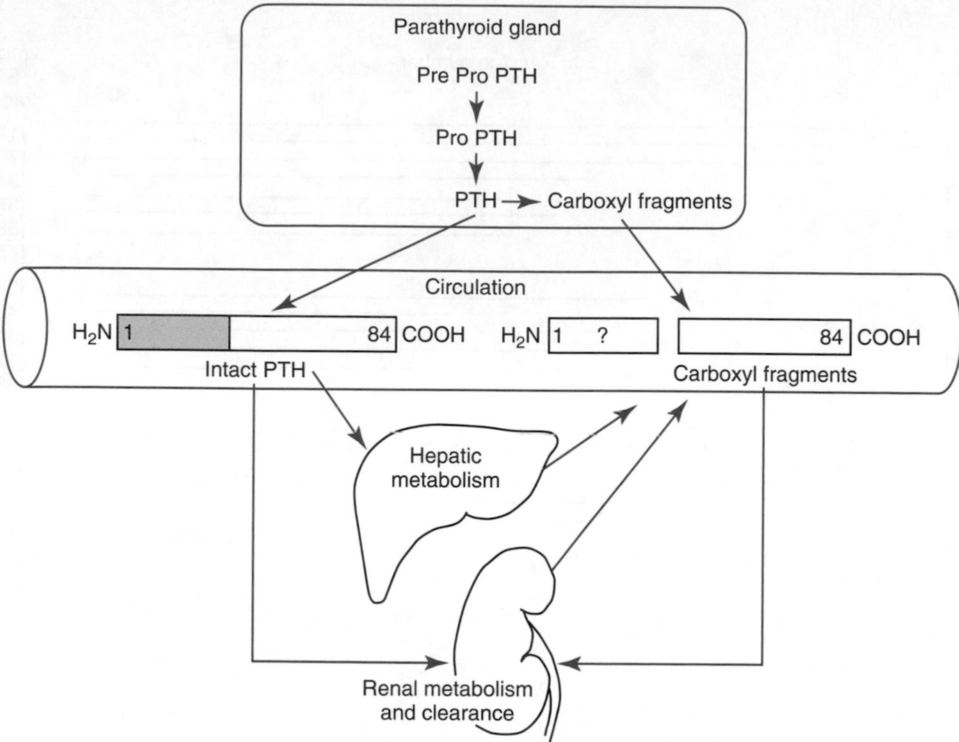

Figure 52-15 Secretion, metabolism, clearance, and circulating forms of parathyroid hormone (PTH). Both intact PTH and inactive fragments containing the middle and carboxyl (C)-terminal amino acids are secreted by the parathyroid glands. These inactive fragments are produced by peripheral metabolism of intact PTH by the liver and kidneys. Carboxy-terminal fragments are cleared by the kidneys by glomerular filtration. The half-life and concentration of intact hormone are small compared with those of inactive fragments. *(From Endres DB, Villanueva R, Sharp CF Jr, Singer FR. Measurement of parathyroid hormone. Endocrinol Metab Clin North Am 1989;18:611-29.)*

enough to react in the intact PTH assays but do not bind to the PTH receptor. Therefore, the term *intact* as applied to these immunometric intact PTH assays is somewhat of a misnomer because non–1-84 PTH fragments [e.g., PTH(7-84)] are detected along with PTH(1-84).

In the newest PTH assays, in third-generation immunoassays in general, and in second-generation intact assays, the epitope of the N-terminally binding antibody consists of the first four to six amino acids of the intact PTH molecule.[292,325] Such assays have been variously termed *true intact* PTH assays, *whole* PTH assays, or *cyclase-activating* PTH assays. Despite the theoretical improvement, in clinical practice they have not shown clear advantages over earlier immunoradiometric assays (IRMAs).[27,33] In addition to intact PTH, these assays have been reported to detect another molecular species in blood, called *amino PTH* by D'Amour and associates,[64] which possibly has its amino-terminal serine residue in a phosphorylated form.

Noncompetitive Methods for Intact PTH

Noncompetitive (also known as two-site, sandwich, or immunometric) methods (see Chapter 16) require two antibodies capable of simultaneously binding two separate epitopes on the PTH molecule (Figure 52-17): (1) a capture antibody immobilized to a solid phase, and (2) a signal or reporter antibody labeled with a measurable substance or an enzyme, changing the concentration (substrate or product) of a measurable substance. Unlike competitive immunoassays, with noncompetitive methods, both antibodies are added in excess, ensuring that all analyte is measured. After formation of the ternary complex or sandwich, excess labeled antibody is removed by washing before quantification of complexes. Noncompetitive immunoassays provide increased sensitivity, specificity, reproducibility, and convenience. In practice, the lower limit of detection for such assays is often lower than that observed in competitive immunoassays, and the upper linear limit is higher than that observed in competitive immunoassays.

For measuring intact PTH, the capture antibody is most often directed against the carboxyl or middle region of the molecule (e.g., amino acid sequences 39-84, 44-84) and the signal antibody against the N-terminal amino acid sequence (1-34).[33] A few methods have reversed this, using capture antibodies against the N-terminal amino acid sequence (e.g., amino acids 26-32) and signal antibodies against the middle or C-terminal amino acid sequence (e.g., 55-64).[292] With the

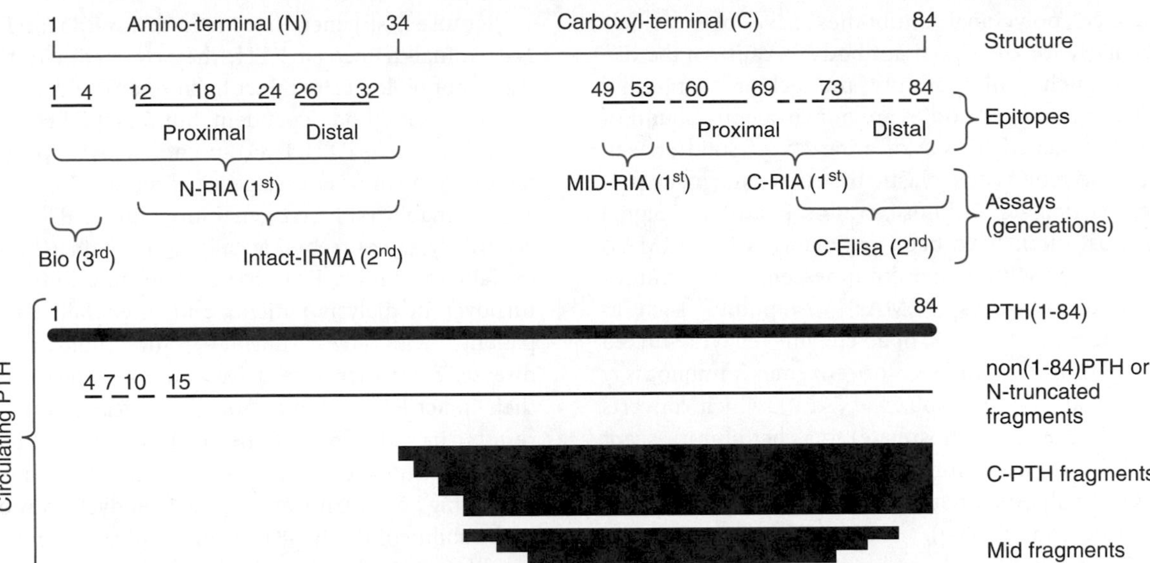

Figure 52-16 Relationship between parathyroid hormone (PTH) assays, PTH assay epitopes, and PTH molecular forms detected in circulation. The *upper panel* depicts the structure of human PTH and epitopes detected by various PTH assays. First-generation PTH assays detect full-length PTH(1-84), in addition to PTH fragments. These assays include radioimmunoassays (RIAs) that use antisera specific for the amino-terminal (N-RIA), middle (MID-RIA), or carboxy-terminal (C-RIA) region of PTH. Second-generation "intact PTH" assays detect full-length PTH(1-84) and non–(1-84)PTH fragments. Third-generation PTH assays (Bio) detect the full-length PTH(1-84). The *bottom panel* depicts the PTH molecular forms present in the circulation. *(Modified from Henrich LM, Rogol AD, D'Amour P, Levine MA, Hanks JB, Bruns DE. Persistent hypercalcemia after parathyroidectomy in an adolescent and effect of treatment with cinacalcet HCl. Clin Chem 2006;52:2286-93.)*

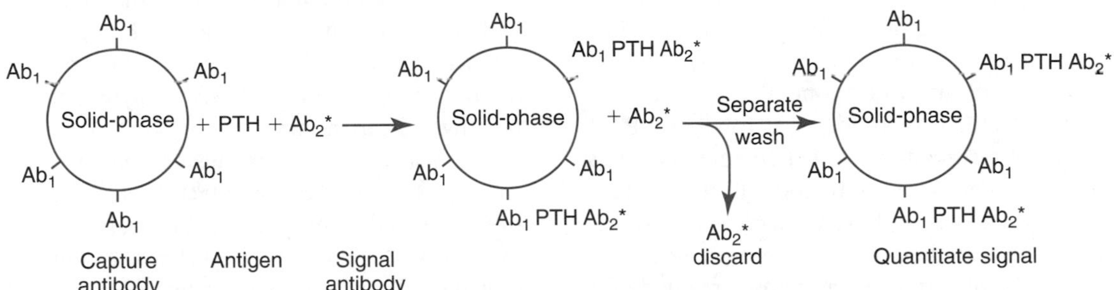

Figure 52-17 Principle of a noncompetitive immunoassay for parathyroid hormone (PTH). PTH is reacted with immobilized capture antibody (Ab_1) against one antigenic determinant and with a labeled signal antibody (Ab_2*) against a second antigenic determinant. PTH forms a bridge between the two antibodies, producing a "sandwich" or ternary complex. Both antibodies are added in excess, ensuring that all PTH reacts and is measured. Free signal antibody is separated, and the solid-phase antibody-PTH-labeled antibody complexes are quantified with an appropriate detection system. The signal increases with increasing concentrations of PTH. *(Modified from Endres DB, Villanueva R, Sharp CF Jr, Singer FR. Measurement of parathyroid hormone. Endocrinol Metab Clin North Am 1989;18:611-29.)*

latter arrangement, a higher concentration of signal antibody is needed because of the high concentration of inactive fragments relative to intact hormone, potentially adversely impacting sensitivity by increasing the blank (signal in the absence of intact PTH). The specificity of these noncompetitive methods depends on the sequence specificity of the antibodies used; they do not measure classical C-terminal fragments that lack the N-terminal amino acid sequence (1-34).

Antibodies used in immunometric assays may be monoclonal or polyclonal antibodies purified by affinity chromatography to produce sequence-specific antibodies.

Affinity-purified polyclonal antibodies have been widely used, particularly for the signal antibody, because of the difficulty of producing high-affinity monoclonal antibodies against PTH. Capture antibodies are noncovalently bound or are covalently attached to one of a variety of solid phases, including polystyrene beads, plastic tubes, paramagnetic particles, microparticulate cellulose, and sepharose.[290] Signal antibodies most often have been radiolabeled (for IRMAs) with ^{125}I, or labeled with a chemiluminescent [for immunochemiluminometric assays (ICMAs)] compound, such as acridinium ester or isoluminol, or an enzyme [enzyme-linked immunosorbent assay (ELISA) or enzyme immunoassay (EIA)], such as alkaline phosphatase (ALP), which converts a substrate (1,2-dioxetane phosphate) to a chemiluminescent product.[290,292] Other assay formats used on fully automated immunoassay analyzers include electrochemiluminescence detection (ruthenium chelate).

Intact PTH assays available commercially have been listed and compared.[244,292]

N-Terminal–Truncated PTH and Second-Generation Intact PTH Methods

The N-terminal–truncated fragment(s) [also called non-(1-84)PTH and PTH(7-84)], containing all but a few of the N-terminal amino acids of PTH,[34,179] account, on average, for 20 and 50% of intact PTH concentrations measured by first-generation intact PTH assays in healthy subjects and patients with chronic renal failure, respectively. Furthermore, the relative concentration of N-terminal–truncated PTH increases with hypercalcemia and decreases with hypocalcemia. Similar to classical C-terminal fragments, N-terminal–truncated PTH originates from both secretion by the parathyroids and peripheral metabolism of intact hormone.[216]

The first noncompetitive methods used for intact PTH cross-reacted with N-terminal–truncated fragment(s), thus overestimating the concentration of biologically active, truly intact PTH. Synthetic PTH(7-84) has shown cross-reactivities of 40 to 160% in these methods.[96,179] These findings stimulated the development of a new generation of methods for intact PTH, using antibodies against the very N-terminal region of PTH that do not cross-react with synthetic PTH(7-84) (see Figure 52-16).

One of the newest-generation methods uses antibodies against PTH(1-4) and even requires the presence of the most N-terminal amino acid, as evidenced by its failure to recognize PTH(2-34).[96,292]

Studies have suggested that N-terminal–truncated PTH [e.g., PTH(7-84)] may be biologically active and antagonistic to the action of PTH. Synthetic PTH(7-84), used as the available representative of N-terminal–truncated PTH, decreased serum calcium; antagonized the calcemic, phosphatemic, and phosphaturic effects of intact PTH in thyroparathyroidectomized animals; and was bound by a C-terminal PTH receptor distinct from the PTH/PTHrP receptor.[72]

Because first-generation methods for intact PTH measure N-terminal–truncated PTH, they overestimate the concentration of biologically intact hormone. The degree of overestimation is method dependent, but intact PTH is 50% higher on average than PTH(1-84) in patients with primary hyperparathyroidism or end-stage renal disease.[96]

The inability of first-generation intact PTH methods to accurately measure biologically active intact hormone may explain why intact PTH is not a reliable indicator of bone turnover in dialysis patients and often fails to distinguish patients with low-, normal-, and high-turnover bone disease.[193] Furthermore, treatment of patients to suppress their intact PTH value to normal or near normal frequently results in adynamic bone disease. The PTH(1-84)/N-terminal–truncated fragment ratio has been proposed for evaluating bone turnover in renal osteodystrophy on the basis of the ability of PTH(7-84) to antagonize the biological activity of intact PTH and preliminary experimental evidence for the predictive value of this ratio.[209] The ratio is calculated after intact PTH and PTH(1-84) are measured and N-terminal–truncated fragments are calculated by subtracting PTH(1-84) from intact PTH. This issue is still unclear, however, because subsequent studies were unable to substantiate the greater clinical utility of measuring both PTH(1-84) and intact PTH and calculating this ratio to assess bone turnover in end-stage kidney disease.[114,193]

Even second-generation intact PTH assays are not absolutely specific for intact PTH, as evidenced by demonstration of an amino-terminal form of PTH distinct from both the intact hormone and the N-truncated fragment. This form represented approximately 20% of the intact PTH measured with a second-generation intact PTH method.[64] The clinical implications of this form have not yet been established, but it has been reported in patients with hyperparathyroidism and parathyroid carcinoma.

Mass spectrometry has been used to characterize PTH fragments and to measure intact PTH.[169,187] In the mass spectrometric method of Kumar and colleagues used for measurement of PTH in serum,[169] PTH was captured on antibody-coated beads and was digested by trypsin. The N-terminal 13 amino acids were then quantified by selected reaction monitoring in a liquid chromatography-tandem mass spectrometry system. As expected, the assay showed no detectable cross-reactivity with PTH fragments, including PTH(7-84), which was captured on the antibody-coated beads.

Specimen Requirements

Specimen requirements may depend on the specific method. Serum or EDTA plasma generally is preferred, and results may vary with sample type. After separation, serum or plasma should be frozen if analysis is delayed. Lower concentrations of PTH are observed in serum incubated at room temperature for longer than a few hours, or after one to several days at 4 °C. PTH has been reported to be more stable in EDTA plasma; this is a probable consequence of reduced proteolytic activity.

Reference Intervals

Reference intervals for PTH vary greatly with the method used.[292,342] Typical reference intervals are as follows:

Intact PTH: 10 to 65 pg/mL or 1.1 to 6.8 pmol/L
PTH(1-84): 6 to 40 pg/mL or 0.6 to 4.2 pmol/L

Interpretation of PTH concentrations should take into account the patient's circulating calcium concentration at the time of sampling.

The upper limit of the reference interval for PTH may be inappropriately high because of the prevalence of vitamin D insufficiency and mild secondary hyperparathyroidism in the reference group. Significantly lower intervals have been established for these methods by excluding individuals with vitamin D insufficiency (see "Vitamin D, Reference Intervals").[292]

Intact PTH concentrations vary with age and are low or normal during pregnancy,[167] lower in fetuses and umbilical cord blood,[165] and increased during the first few days of life, in response to neonatal hypocalcemia. Concentrations in children and adolescents are reportedly similar, if not identical, to those in adults.[264] In healthy adults, circulating concentrations of intact PTH increase with age.[78]

Intact PTH is secreted in a pulsatile fashion with an overall circadian rhythm characterized by a nocturnal rise. Measurement of PTH on more than one occasion should assist in preventing misinterpretation of parathyroid status as the result of episodic secretion.

Interpretation of PTH Results

PTH is the most important test for the differential diagnosis of hypercalcemia. The serum concentration of intact PTH is increased in most patients with primary hyperparathyroidism (Figure 52-18) and is below normal or close to the lower limit of the reference interval in most patients with nonparathyroid hypercalcemia, including hypercalcemia-associated malignancy. In patients with stable hypercalcemia, a PTH value in the upper half of the reference interval is inappropriately high and is suggestive of primary hyperparathyroidism. Whenever possible, PTH specimens should be obtained before therapy is provided for hypercalcemia, because PTH secretion may be stimulated by declining serum calcium.

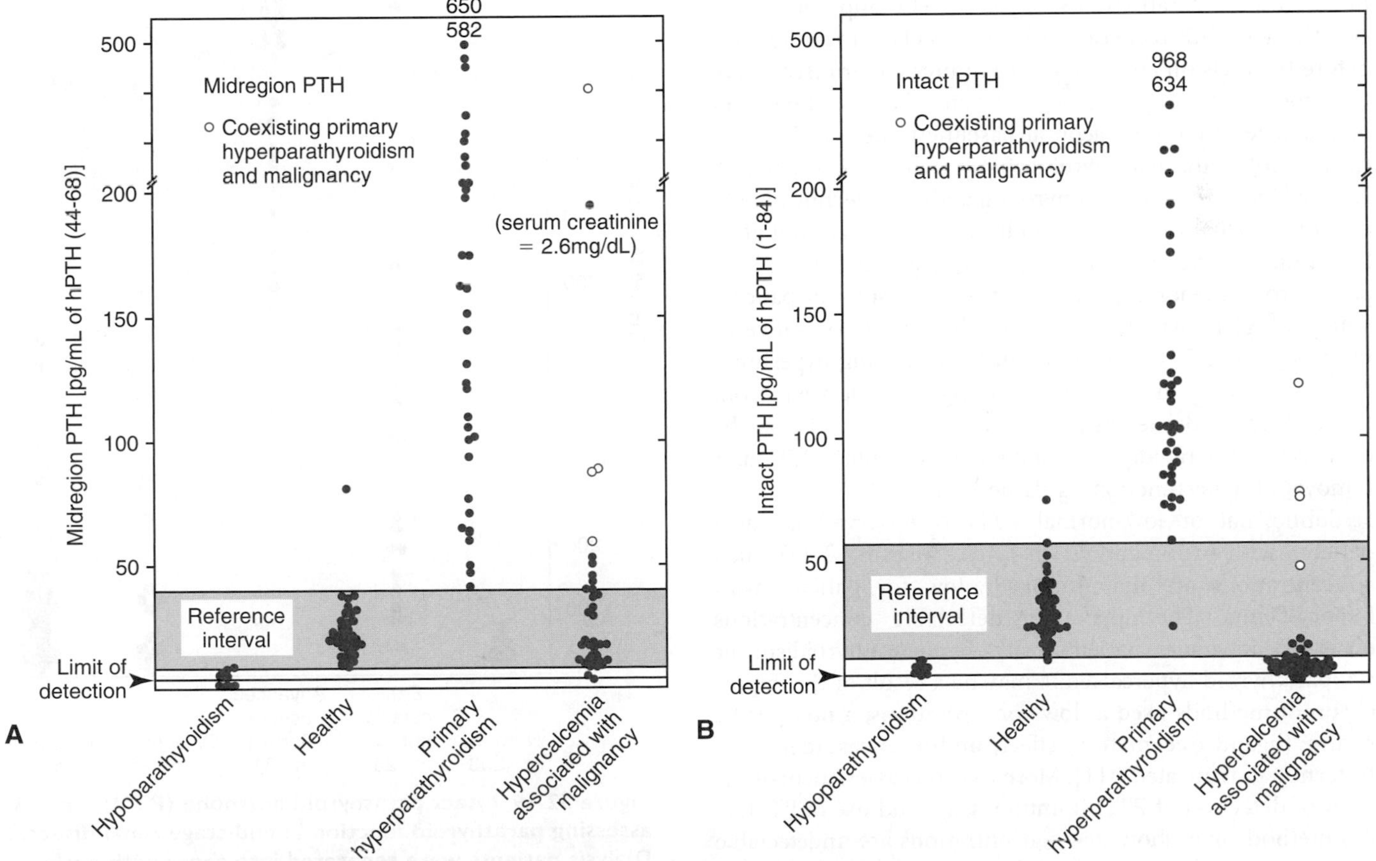

Figure 52-18 Parathyroid hormone (PTH) in healthy individuals and patients with primary hyperparathyroidism, hypercalcemia associated with malignancy, and hypoparathyroidism. PTH was measured with immunoassay for its midregion (A) and for intact PTH (B). *(Modified from Endres DB, Villanueva R, Sharp CF Jr, Singer FR. Measurement of parathyroid hormone. Endocrinol Metab Clin North Am 1989;18:611-29.)*

Increased PTH in patients with hypercalcemia and malignancy suggests coexisting hyperparathyroidism and malignancy, in that ectopic PTH production appears to be extremely rare. Hypercalcemia in malignancy is usually associated with bone metastases (e.g., local osteolytic hypercalcemia) and/or production of PTHrP (e.g., humoral hypercalcemia of malignancy). PTHrP does not cross-react in any of the PTH immunoassays that have been evaluated. According to a 2003 study, PTH(1-84) is more sensitive in diagnosing primary hyperparathyroidism than intact PTH.[283] In this study, PTH(1-84) and intact PTH were elevated in 96% and 73% of 56 patients with primary hyperparathyroidism, respectively.

Measurements of urinary calcium excretion are necessary to confirm hypocalciuria in cases of suspected familial hypocalciuric hypercalcemia. Such patients do not usually display hypercalcemia above 12 mg/dL or above 0.3 mmol/L. Because having this disorder in the heterozygous state leads to no ill effects, parathyroidectomy is not indicated. However, infants with homozygous familial hypocalciuric hypercalcemia can present with life-threatening hypercalcemia, even requiring emergency parathyroidectomy.

Because of the short half-life of PTH (≤5 minutes), intraoperative determination of intact PTH is useful for assessing the completeness of parathyroidectomy and facilitating minimally invasive parathyroid surgery, thereby improving cost-effectiveness and cosmetic outcomes.[50] PTH is measured just before the incision and again at 10 minutes after resection of the hyperfunctioning parathyroid tissue. The neck should not be massaged by the surgeon at baseline (where PTH could rise) or following parathyroidectomy (when PTH could be released from injured parathyroid glands). A decline of 50% or more is usually considered indicative of the removal of all hyperfunctioning tissue. In contrast to patients with solitary parathyroid adenomas, interpretation of results in patients with multiglandular disease is complicated. Preoperative or intraoperative PTH may be useful for localizing hyperfunctioning parathyroid tissue by sampling multiple veins from the cervical and mediastinal regions. PTH(1-84) may be decreased more rapidly and completely than intact PTH after removal of hyperfunctioning tissue.[339]

Subnormal or low-normal PTH is observed in most patients with hypoparathyroidism (see Figure 52-18); such concentrations are inappropriately low for patients with hypocalcemia. The apparently detectable concentrations observed in many patients with hypoparathyroidism or nonparathyroid hypercalcemia may be a result of the imprecision of methods used at low concentrations, a nonspecific serum (ligand-free matrix) effect, and/or measurement of N-terminal–truncated PTH. More rigorous assessment of the limit of detection of PTH immunoassays and use of PTH(1-84) methods may show that concentrations are undetectable in these patients.

In secondary hyperparathyroidism, PTH is increased before total or free calcium becomes abnormally low—a consequence of homeostatic mechanisms for maintenance of serum calcium. Consequently, PTH is more sensitive than calcium in identifying secondary hyperparathyroidism.

In patients with end-stage renal disease, measurement of PTH is helpful in assessing parathyroid function, in estimating bone turnover, and in improving management. Patients with high-turnover bone disease caused by secondary hyperparathyroidism (advanced osteitis fibrosa) have the highest concentrations of PTH, whereas those with low-turnover, adynamic bone disease, including osteomalacia, have the lowest concentrations (Figure 52-19). Intermediate concentrations are seen in low-turnover adynamic (aplastic) disease and early osteitis fibrosa. Considerable overlap in intact PTH concentrations is apparent among the various forms of renal osteodystrophy. In dialysis patients, cut points ("decision levels") of less than 100 or 150 pg/mL and greater than 250 to 300 pg/mL have been suggested for distinguishing patients with low-turnover and high-turnover bone disease, respectively. The Kidney Disease Outcomes Quality Initiative (KDOQI) guidelines of the National Kidney Foundation

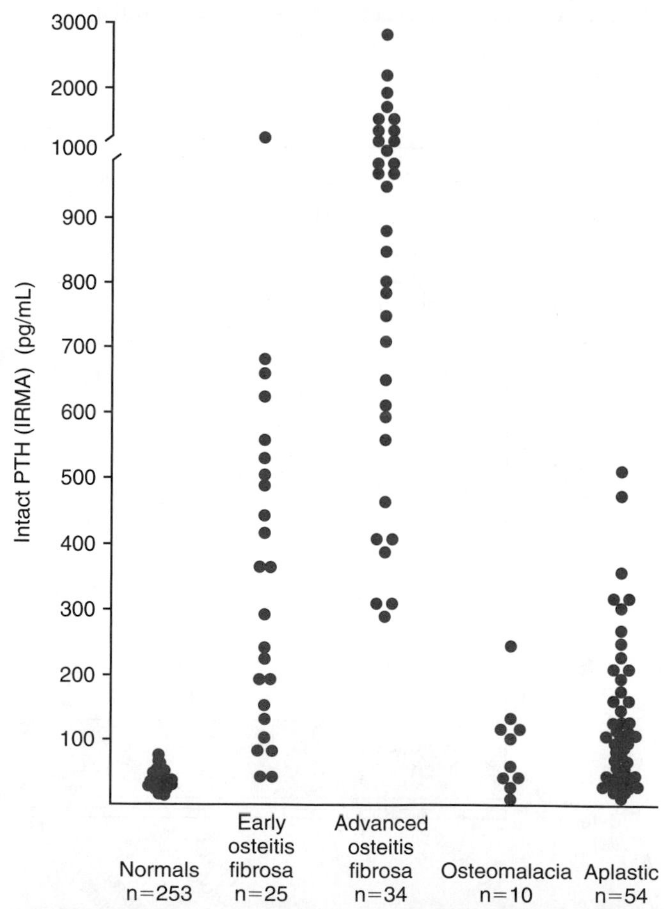

Figure 52-19 Intact parathyroid hormone (PTH) for assessing parathyroid function in end-stage renal disease. Dialysis patients were separated into those with early and advanced osteitis fibrosa, osteomalacia, and aplastic disease by quantitative histomorphometric analysis of undecalcified bone biopsies. *[From Segre GV, Sherrard DJ, Pandian MR, et al. Intact PTH (IRMA) II: New applications to issues in parathyroid hormone and mineral metabolism. San Juan Capistrano, Calif: Nichols Institute, 1989.]*

define reasonable therapeutic goals for intact PTH concentrations (first-generation IRMA or second-generation assay in general) in end-stage kidney disease as two to four times the upper limit of the reference interval to prevent parathyroid-suppressed, adynamic, and hyperparathyroid bone disease.[76]

Parathyroid status is usually determined by measuring PTH on predialysis specimens because various factors, including changes in serum calcium and the type of dialysis membrane, affect PTH secretion and clearance. Comparison of predialysis and postdialysis specimens has been suggested for determining acute parathyroid responsiveness to alterations in serum calcium concentrations.

The PTH(1-84) assay theoretically should more accurately assess parathyroid status and bone turnover and thus better guide therapy in patients with end-stage renal disease compared with the intact PTH assay [see "Noncompetitive Methods for Intact PTH" and "N-Terminal–Truncated PTH and Second-Generation Intact PTH Methods"].[193,209] However, the benefits of the new generation of PTH assays have not been as expected,[321] and it has not been easy to define the therapeutic targets for PTH(1-84).[163] Noncompetitive immunoassays for intact PTH or PTH(1-84) must have high concentrations of the C-terminal antibody to avoid underestimation of PTH in dialysis patients with secondary hyperparathyroidism who have high concentrations of C-terminal fragments. Absence of interference can be assessed by confirming that specimens from dialysis patients with the highest concentrations of PTH dilute in a parallel fashion. Alternatively, recovery can be determined by adding a known amount of intact PTH to these specimens.

PTH concentrations may be altered in hyperthyroidism, in hypothyroidism, and with lithium carbonate treatment. PTH is decreased and is inversely correlated with T3 concentrations in hyperthyroid patients. Serum PTH is increased in patients who become hypothyroid after radioactive iodine treatment, and is decreased with replacement therapy; these changes apparently are mediated by serum calcium. Long-term lithium carbonate therapy has been reported to increase parathyroid gland size and circulating intact PTH. Lithium may produce a state of relative resistance to calcium negative feedback, raising PTH concentrations.

An uncommon use for PTH methods measuring C-terminal fragments involves analysis of fluid from suspected parathyroid cysts. Parathyroid cyst fluid appears to contain primarily inactive fragments of PTH, not intact hormone.[22]

Vitamin D and Its Metabolites

Vitamin D is produced endogenously through exposure of skin to sunlight, and is absorbed from foods containing or supplemented with vitamin D. The vitamin is metabolized to its biologically active form, 1,25-dihydroxyvitamin D [1,25(OH)$_2$D], a hormone that regulates calcium and phosphate metabolism. Deficiency of vitamin D results in impaired formation of bone, producing rickets in children and osteomalacia in adults.

Biochemistry and Physiology

Vitamin D and its metabolites may be categorized as cholecalciferols or ergocalciferols (Figure 52-20). Cholecalciferol (vitamin D_3) is the parent compound of the naturally occurring family and is produced in the skin from 7-dehydrocholesterol on exposure to the ultraviolet B portion of sunlight.[20,178] Latitude, season, aging, sunscreen use, and skin pigmentation influence production of vitamin D_3 by the skin. Vitamin D_2 (ergocalciferol), the parent compound of the other family, is manufactured by irradiation of ergosterol produced by yeasts. Vitamin D_2 differs from vitamin D_3 by the double bond between carbon 22 and carbon 23 and a methyl group on carbon 24. When vitamin D or its metabolites are written without a subscript, both families are included.

Only a few foods, primarily fish liver oils, fatty fish, egg yolks, and liver, naturally contain significant amounts of vitamin D. Consequently, before foods were supplemented with vitamin D_2 or vitamin D_3, most vitamin D in the body was that produced by synthesis in the skin. In North America, a considerable fraction of vitamin D is acquired by ingestion of fortified foods (some cereals, bread products, and milk) or vitamin D supplements. The recommended daily allowance is 400 IU (10 μg). In some European countries, the recommendation for people older than 60 years is 800 IU or 20 μg. However, some clinicians in the United States are prescribing up to 2000 IU of vitamin D daily to treat or prevent osteoporosis and to ensure optimal dietary calcium absorption.[130]

Metabolism, Regulation, and Transport

Vitamin D_2 and vitamin D_3 are metabolized to 25-hydroxyvitamin D [25(OH)D] in the liver by vitamin D 25-hydroxylase, a cytochrome P450 enzyme (Figure 52-21).[70,178] The concentration of 25(OH)D in serum is approximately 10 to 65 ng/mL or 25 to 162 nmol/L (Table 52-4). The half-life of circulating 25(OH)D is 2 to 3 weeks. At 25(OH)D concentrations near 30 ng/mL, dietary calcium absorption is maximal. Therefore any reference interval for 25(OH)D should not be confused with the "optimal" or "healthy" range for 25(OH)D. At physiologic concentrations, 25(OH)D is biologically inactive in affecting dietary calcium absorption.

25(OH)D_2 and 25(OH)D_3 are metabolized to 1,25-dihydroxyvitamin D [1,25(OH)$_2$D], the biologically active hormone, by 25(OH)D 1α-hydroxylase, a cytochrome P450 enzyme, in kidney and placenta (see Figure 52-21). Normal circulating concentrations are approximately 15 to 60 pg/mL or 36 to 144 pmol/L—about $\frac{1}{1000}$ that of 25(OH)D (see Table 52-4). The half-life of 1,25(OH)$_2$D is 4 to 6 hours.

Circulating concentrations of 1,25(OH)$_2$D are tightly regulated, primarily by PTH, phosphate, calcium, and 1,25(OH)$_2$D.[49,70] PTH and hypophosphatemia increase the synthesis of 1,25(OH)$_2$D by increasing 25(OH)D-1α-hydroxylase activity, whereas hypocalcemia acts indirectly by stimulating the secretion of PTH. Hypercalcemia, hyperphosphatemia, and 1,25(OH)$_2$D reduce 25(OH)D 1α-hydroxylase and 1,25(OH)$_2$D. 1,25(OH)$_2$D also induces 25(OH)D 24-hydroxylase, an enzyme producing 24,25-dihydroxyvitamin D [24,25(OH)$_2$D], the most prevalent

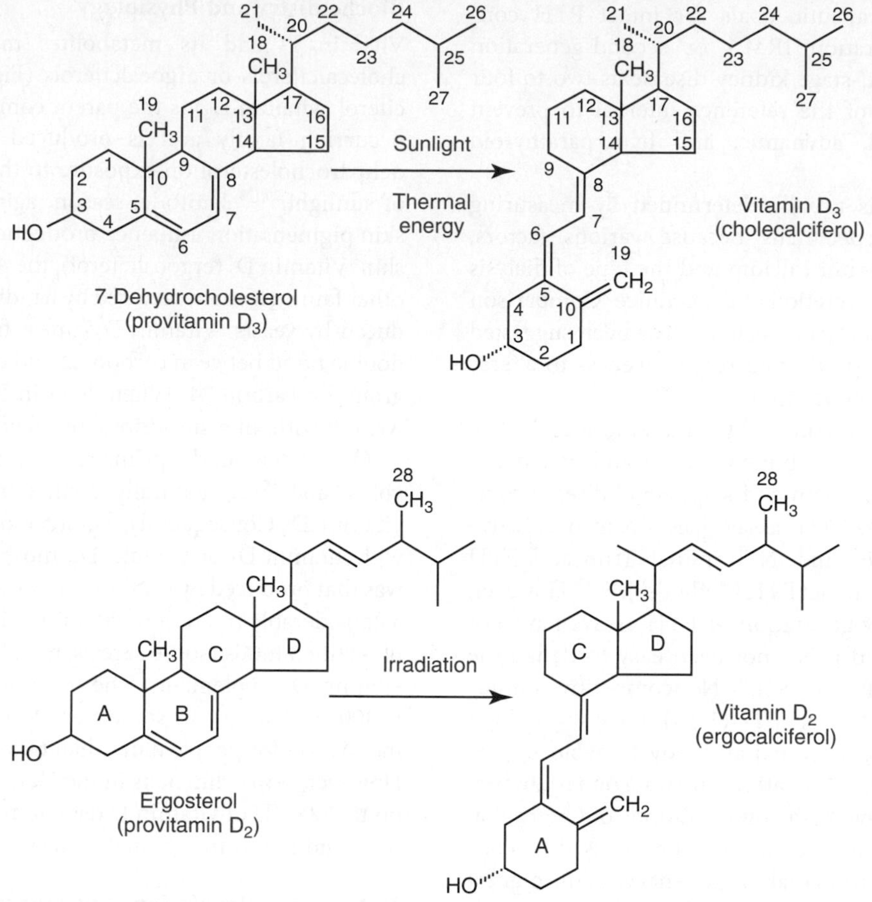

Figure 52-20 Structures of vitamin D_3 (cholecalciferol) and vitamin D_2 (ergocalciferol) and their precursors. 7-Cholecalciferol is produced in the skin from 7-dehydrocholesterol on exposure to sunlight. Ergocalciferol is produced commercially by irradiation of ergosterol. *(Modified from Holick MF, Adams JS. Vitamin D metabolism and biological function. In: Avioli LV, Krane SM, eds. Metabolic bone disease, 2nd edition. Philadelphia, Pa: WB Saunders, 1990:155-95.)*

TABLE 52-4 Vitamin D and Its Metabolites in Plasma

Compound	Concentration	Free, %	Half-life
Vitamin D	<0.2-20 ng/mL <0.5-52 nmol/L	—	1-2 d
25-Hydroxyvitamin D	10-65 ng/mL 25-162 nmol/L	0.03	2-3 wk
1,25-Dihydroxyvitamin D	15-60 pg/mL 36-144 pmol/L	0.4	4-6 h

dihydroxylated vitamin D form in serum. This enzyme is also responsible for inactivating 1,25(OH)vitamin D through the 24-oxidation pathway, leading to formation of calcitroic acid.[270a]

In the circulation, vitamin D, 25(OH)D, and $1,25(OH)_2D$ are bound to vitamin D–binding protein (DBP), a specific, high-affinity transport protein also known as *group-specific component of serum* or *Gc-globulin.*[20,49,119] DBP belongs to the albumin and α-fetoprotein gene family. In humans, DBP contains 458 amino acid residues and has a molecular mass of 51,335 Da. DBP is constitutively synthesized by the liver and circulates in great excess (at about 400 mg/L), with less than 5% of the vitamin D binding sites normally occupied. DBP binds vitamin D and its metabolites, particularly the 25-hydroxylated metabolites 25(OH)D, $24,25(OH)_2D$, and $1,25(OH)_2D$.[20,119] Only 0.03% of 25(OH)D and 0.4% of

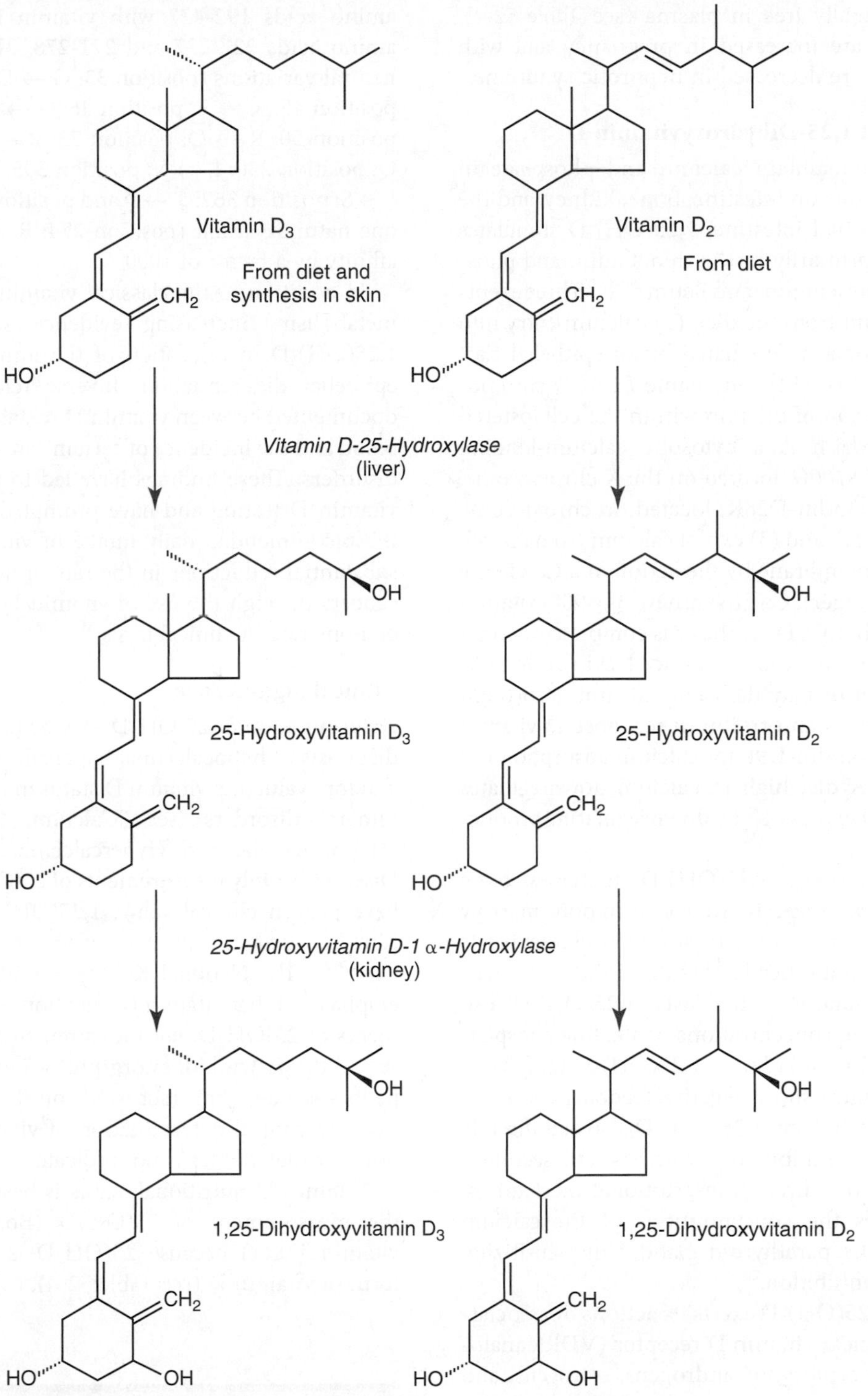

Vitamin D_3

From diet and synthesis in skin

CH_2

HO

Vitamin D_2

From diet

CH_2

HO

Vitamin D-25-Hydroxylase
(liver)

OH

25-Hydroxyvitamin D_3

CH_2

HO

OH

25-Hydroxyvitamin D_2

CH_2

HO

25-Hydroxyvitamin D-1 α-Hydroxylase
(kidney)

OH

1,25-Dihydroxyvitamin D_3

CH_2

HO OH

OH

1,25-Dihydroxyvitamin D_2

CH_2

HO OH

Figure 52-21 Metabolism of vitamin D. Vitamin D_2 and vitamin D_3 are enzymatically hydroxylated to 25-hydroxyvitamin D in the liver and further to 1,25-dihydroxyvitamin D by the kidneys. 1,25-Dihydroxyvitamin D_2 and 1,25-dihydroxyvitamin D_3 are the biologically active forms of vitamin D.

1,25(OH)$_2$D are normally free in plasma (see Table 52-4). DBP concentrations are increased in pregnancy and with estrogen therapy and are decreased in nephrotic syndrome.

Biological Actions of 1,25-Dihydroxyvitamin D

1,25(OH)$_2$D helps to maintain calcium and phosphate in blood through its actions on intestine, bone, kidney, and the parathyroids. In the small intestine, 1,25(OH)$_2$D stimulates calcium absorption, primarily in the duodenum, and phosphate absorption by the jejunum and ileum.[20,49,70] Three events serve to absorb calcium from the diet: (1) calcium entry into the brush border cytoplasm, mediated by an epithelial Ca^{2+} transporter or channel (CaT1; gene name *ECAC2;* chromosome 7q34); (2) diffusion of calcium within the cell fostered by calbindin-D9k, which is a cytosolic calcium-binding protein [gene symbol *S100G*, located on the X chromosome, and distinct from calbindin-D28K, located on chromosome 8 (gene symbol *CALB1*)]; and (3) exit of calcium from the cell across its basolateral membrane by the action of a CaATPase (e.g., a Na^+/Ca^{2+} exchanger). CaT1 synthesis is ≈90% vitamin D dependent, and calbindin D synthesis is completely dependent on vitamin D. Because knockout mice lacking calbindin D_{9k} expression do not display deficient calcium absorption and can increase calcium absorption in response to vitamin D, the necessity of calbindin-D9k for calcium absorption has been questioned.[5,170] A diet high in calcium downregulates CaT1 and calbindin D expression by downregulating production of 1,25(OH)$_2$D.

At high concentrations, 1,25(OH)$_2$D increases bone resorption by inducing monocytic stem cells in bone marrow to differentiate into osteoclasts and by stimulating osteoblasts to produce cytokines and other factors that influence osteoclast activity. By stimulating osteoblasts, 1,25(OH)$_2$D also increases the circulating concentrations of alkaline phosphatase and osteocalcin. In the kidneys, 1,25(OH)$_2$D inhibits its own synthesis in an ultra-short negative feedback loop and stimulates its own metabolism. 1,25(OH)$_2$D also acts directly on the parathyroids to inhibit the synthesis and secretion of PTH. In addition to a direct transcriptional mechanism, 1,25(OH)$_2$D increases the concentrations of the calcium sensing receptor in the parathyroid gland, thus sensitizing the gland to calcium inhibition.[20]

In target tissues, 1,25(OH)$_2$D exerts its actions by associating with a specific nuclear vitamin D receptor (VDR), analogous to the steroid receptors for androgens, estrogens, and corticosteroids (see Chapters 54 and 56). This receptor is expressed widely in tissues, and most cells respond to 1,25(OH)$_2$D.[28] The vitamin D receptor can form heterodimers with members of the retinoid X receptor. The vitamin D receptor is a member of the NR1I family, whose other members include the pregnane X receptor (PXR) and the constitutive androstane receptor (CAR). The gene for the vitamin D receptor is located on chromosome 12q1. The vitamin D_3 receptor is 427 amino acids long and binds to DNA through amino acids 21-96 with NR C4-type zinc fingers at positions 24-44 and 60-84. A hinge region encompasses amino acids 97-191. The ligand-binding region spans amino acids 192-427 with vitamin D–binding regions at amino acids 227-237 and 271-278. The receptor has many natural variations (position 33: G → D; position 35: H → Q; position 45: K → E; position 46: G → D; position 47: F → I; position 50: R → Q; position 73: R → Q; position 80: R → Q; position 230: L → V; position 305: H → Q; position 314: I → S; position 362: T → I; and position 391: R → C). At least one natural variant (position 274: R → L) decreases ligand affinity by a factor of 1000.

In addition to the classical vitamin D effects on calcium metabolism, increasing evidence suggests the role of 1,25(OH)$_2$D in regulation of the immune response and in epithelial differentiation. Inverse relationships have been documented between vitamin D metabolite concentration in blood and the incidence of certain cancers[66] and various other disorders. These findings have led to increased demand for vitamin D testing and have prompted calls for increases in the recommended daily intake of vitamin D. Nevertheless, substantial reductions in the rate of development of various cancers through the use of vitamin D have been difficult to demonstrate in clinical trials.[66]

Clinical Significance

Determination of 25(OH)D may be useful in the differential diagnosis of hypocalcemia, hypercalcemia, or hypercalciuria and for evaluating vitamin D status in health and in bone and mineral disorders (see "Calcium, Clinical Significance," "Hypocalcemia," and "Hypercalcemia"; and "Metabolic Bone Diseases"). Only measurements of 25(OH)D and 1,25(OH)$_2$D have proven clinical value; 1,25(OH)$_2$D measurements are rarely needed in routine or even subspecialty clinical practice.[176,232] The National Kidney Foundation guidelines have emphasized that vitamin D nutrition is assessed by measurements of 25(OH)D, *not* measurements of 1,25(OH)$_2$D [e.g., see http://www.kidney.org/professionals/kdoqi/guidelines_pedbone/index.htm (accessed on September 20, 2011)]. Routine clinical determination of vitamin D, 24,25(OH)$_2$D, or other metabolites is not indicated.

Vitamin D nutritional status is best determined through the measurement of 25(OH)D (Box 52-9), rather than vitamin D, (1) because 25(OH)D is the main circulating form of vitamin D (see Table 52-4), (2) because of its longer

BOX 52-9 Abnormal Circulating Concentrations of 25(OH)D

Decreased 25(OH)D
- Inadequate exposure to sunlight
- Inadequate dietary vitamin D
- Vitamin D malabsorption
- Severe hepatocellular disease
- Increased catabolism (e.g., drugs, such as anticonvulsants)
- Increased loss (nephrotic syndrome)

Increased 25(OH)D (hypercalcemia)
- Vitamin D or 25(OH)D intoxication

half-life [as a result of this, 25(OH)D is less affected by day-to-day variation, exposure to sunlight, or food intake], and (3) because measurement of 25(OH)D is relatively easy compared with the more technically complicated methods used to measure vitamin D.[138,140,178] Groups at higher risk for developing nutritional vitamin D deficiency include breast-fed infants, strict vegetarians who abstain from eggs and milk, individuals with darker skin pigmentation, and the elderly.

Measurement of circulating 25(OH)D is useful in selected patients in evaluating hypocalcemia, vitamin D status, bone disease, and other disorders of mineral metabolism. Circulating concentrations of 25(OH)D may be decreased by (1) reduced availability of vitamin D, (2) inadequate conversion of vitamin D to 25(OH)D, (3) accelerated metabolism of 25(OH)D, and (4) urinary loss of 25(OH)D with its transport protein DBP. Reduced availability of vitamin D occurs with inadequate exposure to sunlight, dietary deficiency, malabsorption syndromes, and gastric or small bowel resection. Severe hepatocellular disease has been associated with inadequate conversion of vitamin D to 25(OH)D. Drugs such as phenytoin, phenobarbital, and rifampin induce drug-metabolizing enzymes that accelerate the metabolism of vitamin D and its metabolites. Serum 25(OH)D concentrations may be reduced in patients with nephrotic syndrome because of the urinary loss of DBP and 25(OH)D.

Serum 25(OH)D concentration is generally accepted as the functional indicator of an individual's vitamin D status.[293] Studies of serum concentrations of 25(OH)D have suggested that a significant proportion of adults in Europe or North America do not get sufficient vitamin D.[3,147,184,273] It has been notoriously difficult to harmonize the reference intervals for 25(OH)D used in various laboratories; this may be related in part to differences of opinion regarding the definition of subclinical vitamin D insufficiency in apparently healthy populations.[51,178] (See below under reference intervals.)

In patients with hypercalcemia, measurement of 25(OH)D has limited value. Its most common use in this situation is in confirming intoxication after ingestion of large amounts of vitamin D or 25(OH)D; in such patients, the 25(OH)D concentration is typically greater than 100 ng/mL or 250 nmol/L.

A 2011 guideline from the Endocrine Society[136A] recommends that routine screening for vitamin D deficiency is not warranted on a population basis, but is warranted in those at risk of deficiency. Candidates for screening are listed as patients with (1) rickets, (2) osteomalacia, (3) osteoporosis, (4) chronic kidney disease, (5) hepatic failure, (6) malabsorption syndromes (cystic fibrosis, inflammatory bowel disease, Crohn disease, bariatric surgery, radiation enteritis), (7) hyperparathyroidism, (8) medications (antiseizure medications, glucocorticoids, AIDS medications, antifungals, e.g., ketoconazole, cholestyramine), (9) African-American and Hispanic children and adults, (10) pregnant and lactating women, (11) older adults with history of falls, (12) older adults with history of nontraumatic fractures, (13) obese children and adults with BMI > 30 kg/m^2), (14) granuloma-forming disorders (sarcoidosis, tuberculosis, histoplasmosis, coccidiomycosis, berylliosis), and (15) some lymphomas.

BOX 52-10 Abnormal Circulating Concentrations of 1,25(OH)$_2$D

Decreased 1,25(OH)$_2$D
- Renal failure
- Hyperphosphatemia
- Hypomagnesemia
- Hypoparathyroidism
- Pseudohypoparathyroidism
- Vitamin D–dependent rickets, type I
- Hypercalcemia of malignancy

Increased 1,25(OH)$_2$D
- Granulomatous disease
- Primary hyperparathyroidism
- Lymphoma
- 1,25(OH)$_2$D intoxication
- Vitamin D–dependent rickets, type II

Measurement of 1,25(OH)$_2$D is diagnostic in vitamin D–dependent rickets types 1 and 2, and in disease states associated with overproduction of 1,25(OH)$_2$D such as sarcoidosis, tuberculosis, Hodgkin's disease, fungal infection, Wegener's granulomatosis, and lymphoma. In the last of these, activated macrophages convert 25(OH)D to 1,25(OH)$_2$D. In other situations, the test result gives confirmatory information in the evaluation of hypercalcemia, hypercalciuria, hypocalcemia, and bone and mineral disorders (Box 52-10). Concentrations of 1,25(OH)$_2$D are increased in vitamin D–dependent rickets type 2 (as the result of nonfunctioning VDR) and in 1,25(OH)$_2$D intoxication, and may be elevated in primary hyperparathyroidism, although the diagnosis of primary hyperparathyroidism does not require measurement of 1,25(OH)$_2$D. Patients with primary hyperparathyroidism and high concentrations of 1,25(OH)$_2$D do appear to be more prone to developing hypercalciuria and renal stones. Reduced concentrations of 1,25(OH)$_2$D can be observed in patients with renal failure, hypercalcemia of malignancy, hyperphosphatemia, hypoparathyroidism, pseudohypoparathyroidism, type 1 vitamin D–dependent rickets, hypomagnesemia, nephrotic syndrome, and severe hepatocellular disease. Other than in cases of suspected vitamin D–resistant rickets, measurement of 1,25(OH)$_2$D in such circumstances is not required for diagnostic purposes.

Diagnosis of vitamin D deficiency is not based on measurement of 1,25(OH)$_2$D, however, because the circulating concentration of this metabolite is often normal because of a compensatory hyperparathyroidism.[183] Nor is the assay useful in confirming intoxication with vitamin D or 25(OH)D, because in this situation, 1,25(OH)$_2$ concentrations may be low, normal, or increased.

Measurement of Vitamin D Metabolites

Specific and sensitive assays have been developed for measuring vitamin D, 25(OH)D, and 1,25(OH)$_2$D.[138,140,178] 25(OH)D and 1,25(OH)$_2$D assays should measure D_2 and D_3 metabolites equally (with "equimolar" reactivity), because both D_2 and D_3 are metabolized to produce biologically active 1,25(OH)$_2$D.

Separate measurement of the D_2 and D_3 forms does not necessarily distinguish between dietary and endogenous sources of vitamin D, as food is supplemented with D_3 and D_2.

The hydrophobic natures and small circulating concentrations of vitamin D metabolites together with the possibility of matrix effects have presented enormous challenges for the development of assays that would be both specific and suitable for high-throughput clinical analysis needs.[138,140] In general, two or three of the following steps are needed in any assay for 25(OH)D or 1,25$(OH)_2$D: (1) deproteinization or extraction, (2) purification, and (3) quantification. The first step frees the metabolites from DBP and may partially purify them. Purification steps, most often column chromatography, separate the various forms of vitamin D, lipids, and interfering substances. The method of quantification depends on the metabolite that is being measured.

Extraction and Deproteinization

Before the advent of commercially available methods, it was common to use two-phase, liquid-liquid partitions with organic solvents and solvent mixtures, including methylene chloride, hexane, diethyl ether, ethanol/chloroform/water, methylene chloride/methanol, hexane/isopropanol, and cyclohexane/ethyl acetate. Ethanol and methanol have also been used to free 25(OH)D from DBP when 25(OH)D is measured.

Today, the most widely used commercially available methods use acetonitrile to deproteinize the specimen and to denature DBP, thereby freeing the vitamin D metabolites.[138,140,178] Another method uses immunoextraction for 1,25$(OH)_2$D.

Column Chromatography

Differences in their polarities, related to their numbers of hydroxyl groups, have been used to separate vitamin D and its metabolites. With three hydroxyl groups, 1,25$(OH)_2$D is more polar than 25(OH)D, with its two hydroxyls, which is more polar than vitamin D, with one hydroxyl group.

Extracts have been purified by chromatography on, for example, minicolumns of silica, silicic acid, Sephadex LH-20, hydroxyalkoxypropyl Sephadex LH-20 (Lipidex 5000), celite, and alumina. Solid-phase extraction using octadecyl (C_{18})-silica was widely used for measuring 1,25$(OH)_2$D. The most popular method used both a reversed-phase C_{18}-silica minicolumn and a normal-phase silica minicolumn to separate vitamin D metabolites. This method was modified by eliminating the silica cartridge and using "phase switching" with a single non–end-capped C_{18}OH cartridge.

Measurement of 25-Hydroxyvitamin D

Acceptance of serum 25(OH)D as an indicator of an individual's vitamin D status has resulted in the development of several commercial assays for it over the past 15 years.[178] The metabolite is measured by competitive protein binding assay (CPBA), competitive or noncompetitive immunoassay (RIA, EIA, ICMA), ultraviolet (UV) absorption after separation by HPLC, or by mass spectrometry after separation by chromatography. Determination by HPLC with UV absorption requires appropriate HPLC equipment (see Chapter 13), specialized training, and a larger sample. Most clinical laboratories that measure 25(OH)D have chosen the more familiar competitive immunoassays or CPBAs. These assays are relatively easy to perform, use widely available reagent sets, and require only a small volume of plasma. In a 2011 CAP survey of 151 laboratories (mostly in the United States), two methods accounted for two-thirds of the results: 54 laboratories reported results by LC-MS/MS assays and 50 used the Diasorin Liaison assay (discussed below). Although assays easily recognize supranormal concentrations of 25(OH)D, measurement of subnormal and low-normal concentrations is more difficult, requiring well-validated methods free from interference.

External quality assurance surveys and proficiency testing programs have identified differences of results among the different 25(OH)D assays—RIA, chemiluminescence immunoassay (CLIA), and the newer liquid chromatography-mass spectrometry (LC-MS/MS) methods.[288] The differences in results reflect, in part, (1) differences in calibration of the assays, (2) nonequimolar responses of some assays to 25(OH) D_2 and 25(OH)D_3, and (3) noncommutable materials used in surveys. Nonequimolar responses are common among the automated methods, but not in LC-MS/MS and HPLC assays.

Care must be taken in interpreting results from external quality assurance surveys and proficiency testing programs. Survey materials that have been processed extensively are noncommutable and lead to overestimation of between-assay variability. Moreover, survey materials that lack 25(OH)D_2 will give no indication of assays that under-recover that form. To address these concerns, a 2011 accuracy-based survey was prepared by the College of American Pathologists. Five pools of minimally processed human serum were prepared to cover a range of 25(OH)D concentrations from about 15 to 60 ng/mL. Two of the pools contained increased concentrations of 25(OH)D_2; these were made from serum of volunteers who had taken 25-hydoxyvitamin D_2 [not made by addition of 25(OH)D_2 to serum)]. Target values were determined by the LC-MS/MS assay in the reference laboratory at the CDC. This survey showed that some assays underestimated the total 25(OH)D in the samples with increased 25(OH)D_2, but the gross errors of 100% or more seen in previous surveys were absent. Importantly, the differences laboratories using LC-MS/MS assays were comparable to differences among laboratories using single commercial assays, despite the differences among LC-MS/MS assays. Despite the improved overall results, even with a generous acceptance criterion that allowed differences from the target value of 25%, the overall pass rate for the five individual pools was only 83 to 92%. It is hoped that efforts at the NIST and elsewhere will lead to improvements of accuracy of these assays.

Radioimmunoassay and Chemiluminescence Immunoassay. Development of a useful antiserum permitted the development of a competitive immunoassay (RIA) for 25(OH) D.[138,140] The antiserum was raised against a bovine serum albumin (BSA) conjugate of a vitamin D analog lacking the side chain [23,24,25,26,27-pentanor vitamin D-C(22)carboxylic acid]. A radioiodinated vitamin D analog [3-aminopropyl derivative of vitamin D-C(22)-amide] was used as the tracer. Samples and calibrators are deproteinized with acetonitrile and analyzed directly without chromatography. Although the antiserum also recognizes 24,25$(OH)_2$D, 25,26$(OH)_2$D, and 25(OH)D-26,23-lactone, the 25(OH)D results obtained are comparable with those obtained by HPLC because of the much lower concentrations of the other metabolites. The RIA has been reported to be less sensitive to interfering substances in serum extracts than is a CPBA that uses DBP.[142] This assay is commercially available as an RIA and as an automated immunoassay based on chemiluminescence (CLIA) detection.[138] The manufacturer replaced the original RIA antiserum in the late 1990s.

Immunoassays for 25(OH)D have appeared from several manufacturers. Some of these assays underestimate the total concentration of 25(OH)D when 25$(OH)D_2$ is present. This is a particular concern in the United States where the available high-dose supplements are vitamin D_2.

Competitive Protein-Binding Assays With Vitamin D–Binding Protein. Before the development of immunoassays, 25(OH)D was measured primarily with CPBA with DBP as the specific binder, and with tritiated 25$(OH)D_3$ (>100 Ci/mmol) as tracer. Assays based on DBP measure both 25(OH)D_2 and 25$(OH)D_3$, but it is important to verify that they respond equally to 25$(OH)D_2$ and 25$(OH)D_3$. If the assay procedure does not involve a chromatographic step for isolating 25(OH)D, other metabolites are also measured, including 25$(OH)D_3$-23,26-lactone, 24,25$(OH)_2$D, 25,26$(OH)_2$D, and, to a lesser extent, vitamin D, thus overestimating the 25(OH)D concentration by about 10% in healthy subjects. 25(OH)D concentrations are reported to be significantly higher when measured by CPBA than when measured by RIA or HPLC.[183,184]

HPLC and Ultraviolet Absorption. HPLC methods for 25(OH)D have used normal-phase chromatography on silica, reversed-phase chromatography on C_{18}-silica, or a combination of the two followed by quantification by UV absorption at 254 or 265 nm. Most methods have required both extraction and preparative chromatography before HPLC. Methods without preparative chromatography also have been developed using gradient or isocratic reversed-phase HPLC with photodiode-array UV detection.[6,323] A specimen of 0.5 to 1.0 mL is required because of the limited sensitivity of UV detection. HPLC methods allow 25$(OH)D_2$ and 25$(OH)D_3$ to be separated. HPLC is useful for validating the accuracy of immunoassays and CPBAs.[138,140]

LC-MS/MS Assays. Liquid chromatography coupled with tandem mass spectrometry is widely used in the measurement of 25(OH)D.[140,198,326] The LC-MS/MS methods are capable of relatively high throughput, with some laboratories producing 1000 results per day. LC-MS/MS has become more attractive for 25(OH)D measurement as the instrumentation has become more widely available in clinical laboratories.

Despite the high selectivity of mass spectrometry, the C-3 epimer of 25(OH)D is not differentiated from 25(OH)D as it has the same mass. Thus, unless the epimer is separated chromatographically prior to the mass-spectrometric quantification, results of LC-MS/MS assays are increased by the C-3 epimer. This is rarely a problem in adults as the epimer is normally present in only low concentrations, but it is a problem in pediatric patients under the age of 1 year.[283A]

In LC-MS/MS assays, samples typically are denatured by the addition of alcohol (such as a methanol-propanol mixture) containing a stable-isotope–labeled internal standard such as $(^2H_6)$25(OH) D_3 (26,26,26,27,27,27-hexadeutero-25-hydroxycholecalciferol). Following extraction, drying, and reconstituting in solvent, the 25(OH)D is chromatographed and analyzed by multiple reaction monitoring. Between-day (total) CVs of 5 to 10% have been reported within individual laboratories, but between-laboratory variability has been a problem, perhaps no worse than for commercially available competitive binding assays.

The 25(OH) metabolites related to D_2 and D_3 are quantified separately by LC-MS/MS. This may have some limited clinical value in some settings,[138] but it is important to report the sum of the two concentrations [25$(OH)D_2$ + 25$(OH)D_3$] because vitamin D status depends on the total concentration, not on the individual concentrations. One approach to reporting is to provide the concentrations of both forms, but to provide a reference interval only for the sum of the two.

Measurement of 1,25-Dihydroxyvitamin D

1,25$(OH)_2$D circulates at approximately $\frac{1}{1000}$ of the concentration of 25(OH)D and at significantly lower concentrations than other dihydroxylated metabolites—facts that together with the extreme hydrophobicity and instability of the compound greatly complicate its determination in serum.[138,178] The most widely used methods require extraction, chromatography, and quantification by radioreceptor assay (RRA) or RIA.

Radioreceptor Assay. Assays using vitamin D receptors from calf thymus or chick intestine have been reported but are rarely used in clinical laboratories. Details are available in the previous edition of this book.

Radioimmunoassay. The first radioimmunoassay for 1,25$(OH)_2$D was introduced in 1978 and required a cumbersome purification.[138] After several assays of similar characteristics, in 1996 another RIA was introduced, with an iodinated reporter and use of an equivalent serum matrix. For this method, sample purification is not needed.[138,141]

The RIA is more convenient than the RRA for 1,25$(OH)_2$D because a radioiodinated tracer eliminates the need for liquid scintillation, and the antiserum eliminates the need to prepare VDR from calf thymus. The RIA uses an antiserum with 1 to 2% cross-reactivity with the more abundant, non-1-hydroxylated vitamin D metabolites and a ^{125}I-labeled tracer prepared from 1,25$(OH)_2$-24,25,26,27,tetranor-C(23)-carboxylic acid and radiolabeled Bolton-Hunter reagent. Before analysis, specimens are deproteinized with acetonitrile, oxidized with sodium metaperiodate, and purified using C_{18}-OH and silica cartridges. Sodium metaperiodate is necessary to eliminate interference by 24,24$(OH)_2$D and

25,26$(OH)_2$D by oxidizing them to their aldehyde and ketone forms, which are easily removed by chromatography. A silica column was added to the single C_{18}-OH cartridge used with the radioreceptor assay, to reduce interference in the RIA. With this RIA, 1,25$(OH)_2$ D_2 is about 70% as potent as 1,25$(OH)_2D_3$. Recovery of individual samples is not determined, although calibrators are prepared in a stripped serum base and are treated identically to samples. The method does cross-react (13 to 25%) with numerous 1-hydroxylated metabolites, including 1,24,25$(OH)_3$D, 1,25,26$(OH)_3$D, and 1,25$(OH)_2$D-26,23-lactone. 1,25$(OH)_2$D-26,23-lactone is a significant metabolite with a concentration of 0 to 30% of that of 1,25$(OH)_2D_3$. A modification of this method using a single C_{18}-OH "extra clean" cartridge is commercially available.

Another commercially available RIA has been developed that uses selective immunoextraction of 1,25$(OH)_2$D.[139] This method is reported to have greater cross-reactivity with the 1-hydroxylated metabolites, including 1,25-dihydroxyvitamin D_3-26,23-lactone[137] and calcipotriol,[148] which is used for treating psoriasis. Apparent concentrations of 1,25$(OH)_2$D are significantly higher with this method than with RRA in patients with hypoparathyroidism receiving vitamin D treatment, patients with biliary atresia, vitamin D–intoxicated subjects, and some normal specimens.

Troubleshooting Vitamin D Assays

Methods requiring extraction and chromatography should be monitored for recovery of the vitamin D metabolites of interest and for solvent or column blanks. Care must be taken to ensure that D_2 and D_3 metabolites are recovered equally, providing a total measurement of 25(OH)D or 1,25(OH)D. Solvents, chromatographic materials, and cartridges may contain substances that interfere with quantification of vitamin D metabolites by CPBA, RIA, and RRA or UV absorption after HPLC, resulting in an overestimation of vitamin D metabolites. Any interference can be monitored by treating a water blank identically to the specimens. Undetectable concentrations of vitamin D in this blank verify the absence of positive interference.

Calibrators for vitamin D assays should be prepared from stock solutions whose concentration and purity are checked by UV spectrophotometry. Stock solutions are suitable if the ratio of absorbance at 264 nm to that at 228 nm is greater than or equal to 1.5. Stock solutions are adjusted using a molar extinction coefficient of 18,200 L/mol/cm for vitamin D_3 metabolites at 264 nm. Tracers used for recovery must be pure to determine recovery accurately. Both calibrators and tracers may be purified by HPLC.

Specimen Requirements

Serum is typically used for measuring vitamin D metabolites, although plasma generally is acceptable for assays using extraction and chromatography. Once separated from the clot, serum is relatively stable at both room temperature and 4 °C; specimens should be frozen if the analysis is delayed. Vitamin D metabolites in serum or plasma do not appear to be sensitive to light and do not require special handling in the laboratory.[140]

Reference Intervals

Reference intervals for vitamin D metabolites are method dependent. A representative one for 1,25$(OH)_2$D is:

1,25$(OH)_2$D: 15 to 60 pg/mL or 36 to 144 pmol/L

Lower limits of the reference interval for 25(OH)D of 10 or 15 ng/mL (25 to 37 nmol/L) have been increasingly criticized as inappropriately low, as even above this limit the vitamin D status of the individual can be insufficient (Table 52-5).[185] Concentrations of less than 20 to 30 ng/mL or 50 to 75 nmol/L can be associated with increased serum PTH concentrations and reduced calcium absorption. In late 2010, the United States Institute of Medicine published a recommendation that the lower limit for vitamin D sufficiency be lowered from 30 to 20 ng/mL and that concentrations above 50 ng/mL be considered as cause for concern.

In 2002 and 2003, the National Health and Nutrition Examination Survey (NHANES) III study reported an unexpectedly high prevalence of vitamin D insufficiency in adults and adolescents in North America.[46,186] For example, vitamin D insufficiency [25(OH)D <20 ng/mL or 50 nmol/L] was exceedingly common during the winter in adult (30 years and older) Caucasian men (15%) and women (30%) living in the South of the United States. Similar findings have been reported from Europe.[147]

The concentrations of 25(OH)D in African Americans are lower than in non-Hispanic whites, but the clinical significance of this is uncertain. Compared with non-Hispanic

TABLE 52-5 Reported Associations of Serum 25-Hydroxyvitamin D Concentrations With Serum PTH and Bone Histology

25(OH)D	1,25$(OH)_2$D	PTH Increase	Bone Histology
<5 ng/mL or <12.5 nmol/L	Normal or low	>30%	Incipient or overt osteomalacia
5-10 ng/mL or 12.5-25 nmol/L	Normal	15-30%	High turnover
10-20 ng/mL or 25-50 nmol/L	Normal	5-15%	Normal or high turnover
>20 ng/mL or >50 nmol/L	Normal	—	Normal

From Lips P, van Schoor NM, Bravenboer N. Vitamin D-related disorders. In: Rosen CJ, Compston JE, Lian JB, eds. Primer on the metabolic bone diseases and disorders of mineral metabolism. Washington, DC: American Society for Bone and Mineral Research, 2008:329-35.

whites, African Americans have higher bone mineral density, higher plasma concentrations of PTH and 1,25$(OH)_2$D, and lower concentrations of biochemical markers of bone remodeling and lower rates of osteoporosis.

Circulating concentrations of 25(OH)D are increased by exposure to sunlight and show seasonal variation, with the highest concentrations in summer or fall and the lowest concentrations in winter or spring.[281] This has led to the recommendation that testing be done at the end of winter; if results are above the chosen cutoff, the patient is likely to have adequate concentrations throughout the year on his or her usual regimen of sun exposure and oral intake of the vitamin. The concentrations are influenced by latitude, sunscreen use, and skin pigmentation. Serum 25(OH)D concentrations of 100 ng/mL (250 nmol/L) are not uncommon in people with extensive sun exposure, such as lifeguards.

Concentrations of vitamin D metabolites vary with age and are increased in pregnancy.[166,167] Concentrations of 1,25$(OH)_2$D are higher in pregnancy and in children than in adults, with the highest concentrations occurring during periods of greatest growth.[205] Although 25(OH)D and 1,25$(OH)_2$D concentrations have been reported to decrease with age, this decline may be a consequence of poor nutrition, reduced exposure to sunlight, and declining health. Concentrations of these metabolites were unchanged with age in studies limited to healthy and active subjects.

CALCITONIN

Release of calcitonin from the parafollicular or C cells of the thyroid gland is stimulated by circulating calcium. The hormone has been used pharmacologically as an inhibitor of bone resorption, but the physiologic role of endogenous calcitonin is less certain. No apparent alterations in bone or mineral metabolism are evident in humans with calcitonin deficiency or excess. However, calcitonin measurements have a role in the diagnosis and follow-up of medullary thyroid carcinoma, a malignant tumor of the C cells, in particular in its familial form.

The C cells of the thyroid arise from the neural crest and are distributed throughout the gland. These cells belong to the APUD (amine precursor uptake and decarboxylation) family, which explains the association of thyroid medullary carcinoma with other tumors such as multiple endocrine neoplasia type 2A and 2B (MEN2A and MEN2B).

Biochemistry and Physiology

Calcitonin is a 32 amino acid peptide, with a molecular mass of 3418 Da, an N-terminal disulfide bond linking the cysteine residues 1 and 7, and a C-terminal proline-amide (Figure 52-22). The hormone interacts with a specific G-protein–coupled receptor that is found on fully differentiated osteoclasts.[2] The structures necessary for biological function are the C-terminal portion of the molecule, with its proline-amide residue, the disulfide bond between residues 1 and 7, and the methionine residue at position 8. The amino-terminal amino acids are highly conserved. In humans, salmon calcitonin is 10 times as potent as the

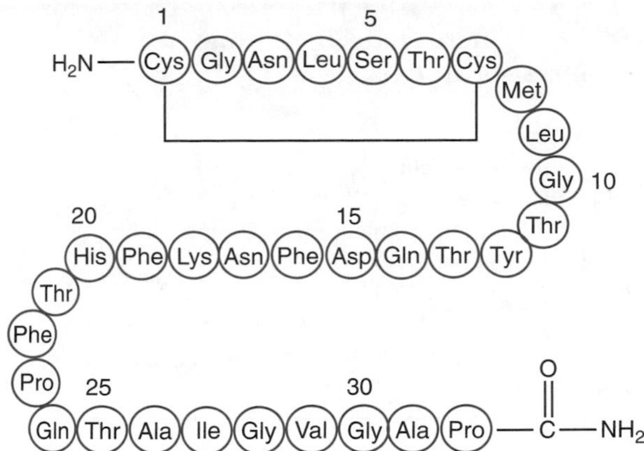

Figure 52-22 Amino acid sequence of human calcitonin.

human hormone and thus is used pharmacologically, usually as nasal spray.[2]

The physiologic regulation of calcitonin secretion is incompletely understood, but the best known secretagogue is the concentration of free calcium in blood. At least in animals, several other peptide hormones (gastrin, cholecystokinin, glucagon, secretin) can stimulate calcitonin secretion, but their physiologic role in humans is uncertain.

Pharmacologic doses of calcitonin reduce serum calcium and phosphate concentrations primarily by inhibiting osteoclastic bone resorption. Salmon calcitonin has been used to treat Paget disease of bone, osteoporosis, and hypercalcemia due to increased bone resorption. Pharmacologic doses of calcitonin also decrease the renal tubular reabsorption of calcium and phosphate. Calcitonin seems to exert an analgesic effect, which is not necessarily solely explained by its effects on bone.[2]

Higher concentrations of circulating calcitonin can be observed in young children[15] and during pregnancy and lactation,[166,167] suggesting that the hormone may be important in protecting the skeleton during periods of calcium stress. Evidence in favor of such a hypothesis has been gained from knockout mice lacking calcitonin.[337]

In serum, multiple forms of calcitonin can be observed both in healthy individuals and in patients with medullary thyroid carcinoma (MTC) or nonthyroidal malignancies. Much of the immunoreactive calcitonin in the circulation is larger than the monomeric hormone.[39] Several reasons for this heterogeneity have been put forward: sulfoxide modification of the monomer, dimerization, glycosylation, presence of biosynthetic precursors of the monomer, and binding to plasma proteins.

During the biosynthesis of calcitonin, the original product is a larger precursor form known as procalcitonin. Procalcitonin has attracted attention as a potential infection marker, in relation to the acute-phase response.[261]

Clinical Significance

Medullary thyroid carcinoma (MTC) occurs as a sporadic disease and as part of the syndromes MEN2A, MEN2B, and familial MTC (FMTC). Together, these account for 5 to 10%

BOX 52-11 Increased Circulating Concentrations of Calcitonin

C-cell hyperplasia
Medullary thyroid carcinoma
Nonthyroidal cancers
- Oat cell carcinoma, small cell carcinoma
- Other malignancies

Acute and chronic renal failure
Hypercalcemia
Hypergastrinemia and other gastrointestinal disorders
Pulmonary disease

of thyroid malignancies, with the sporadic MTC accounting for about 80% of all MTCs. It has been suggested that routine measurement of serum calcitonin in nodular thyroid disease could assist in detecting unsuspected sporadic MTC. After thyroidectomy of MTC patients, calcitonin serves as a tumor marker in the monitoring of treatment response. For more detailed information on the use of calcitonin measurements in oncology, see Chapter 24, "Tumor Markers."

Calcitonin concentrations are increased occasionally in various nonthyroidal cancers (Box 52-11), both in those arising from the neural crest and in others. Increased concentrations or enhanced response to calcitonin secretagogues (calcium, pentagastrin, or both of these) has been reported in cases of nonmalignant disease such as acute and chronic renal failure, hypercalcemia, hypergastrinemia and other gastrointestinal disorders, pulmonary disease, and severe illness.

Assays have been reported also for salmon calcitonin, but it has not been possible to predict the treatment response to this drug by monitoring its circulating concentration. Thus it is advisable to follow the treatment by determining clinical parameters and measuring calcium.

Measurement of Calcitonin

Calcitonin is measured by immunoassay, and interpretation of results in principle can be complicated both by the heterogeneity of the circulating antigen and by the varying characteristics of the different assays.

Historically, the first methods described were RIAs; the different assays showed widely differing reference intervals, sensitivities, and specificities, and they suffered differently from matrix effects. More recently, noncompetitive immunoassays (IRMA, ELISA, EIA, ICMA) have been developed and are available from several diagnostic companies[19]; their results still differ markedly.[318] Some assays may give results that are erroneously low at high concentrations (hook effect); samples with concentrations of 344 ng/L or less (≤344 pg/mL) appear to be unaffected.[318,319]

Reference Intervals

The reference intervals for calcitonin are dependent on the method used. They should be determined for healthy and athyroidal individuals, by gender, in each laboratory for basal and stimulated (calcium and pentagastrin provocation tests) conditions. It is a common finding that men show higher basal and stimulated concentrations than women, but this is not necessarily true for every method.

A typical upper limit for the reference interval for basal calcitonin concentration in adults is about 10 pg/mL or, if the assay gives higher concentrations in men, 5.8 pg/mL (1.7 pmol/L) in women and 8.8 pg/mL (3.8 pmol/L) in men.[15,80] In addition to gender, age, growth, pregnancy, and lactation have been reported to influence[15,159] circulating calcitonin concentrations in healthy people, but reference intervals generally are not given by the assay manufacturer for groups other than healthy adults.

Parathyroid Hormone–Related Protein

Parathyroid hormone–related protein (PTHrP) was discovered as an agent responsible for causing the state known as humoral hypercalcemia of malignancy (HHM) in certain cancers.[43,338] It later proved to be an autocrine/paracrine factor with a multitude of functions in several organ systems.[297,298] Among these are its effects on chondrocyte biology and endochondral bone formation,[110] as well as on calcium metabolism in the fetus[55,206] and during pregnancy and lactation.[338]

Biochemistry and Physiology

PTHrP is derived from a gene on chromosome 12 that is distinct from the *PTH* gene on chromosome 11. Three isoforms of 139, 141, and 173 amino acids are predicted by alternative messenger RNA (mRNA) splicing (Figure 52-23).[110] The N-terminal end of the molecule shows close homology to PTH, with 8 of the first 13 amino acids being identical. The remainder of the PTHrP molecule shows little homology with PTH. The PTH-like activity of PTHrP is contained within the N-terminal amino acids [PTHrP(1-36)].

The primary transcript can undergo a series of post-translational modification reactions, resulting in a series of partially overlapping peptides with biological activities.[55,110,338]

The common N-terminus explains the ability of PTHrP to interact with the PTH/PTHrP receptor, mimicking the biological actions of PTH in classic target tissues, including bone and kidney.[55] Like PTH, PTHrP causes hypercalcemia and hypophosphatemia and increases urinary cyclic AMP. However, when compared with patients with primary hyperparathyroidism, those with PTHrP-induced hypercalcemia have lower concentrations of $1,25(OH)_2D$ and more typically have metabolic alkalosis (instead of hyperchloremic metabolic acidosis), reduced distal tubular calcium reabsorption, and reduced and uncoupled bone formation.

The presence of several basic amino acid residues in PTHrP suggests that it may undergo extensive post-translational processing. Forms of PTHrP containing the following amino acids have been detected in serum[297]: (1) PTHrP(1-36) measured by N-terminal assays; (2) PTHrP containing N-terminal and midregion amino acids measured with noncompetitive immunoassays against PTHrP(1-74 or

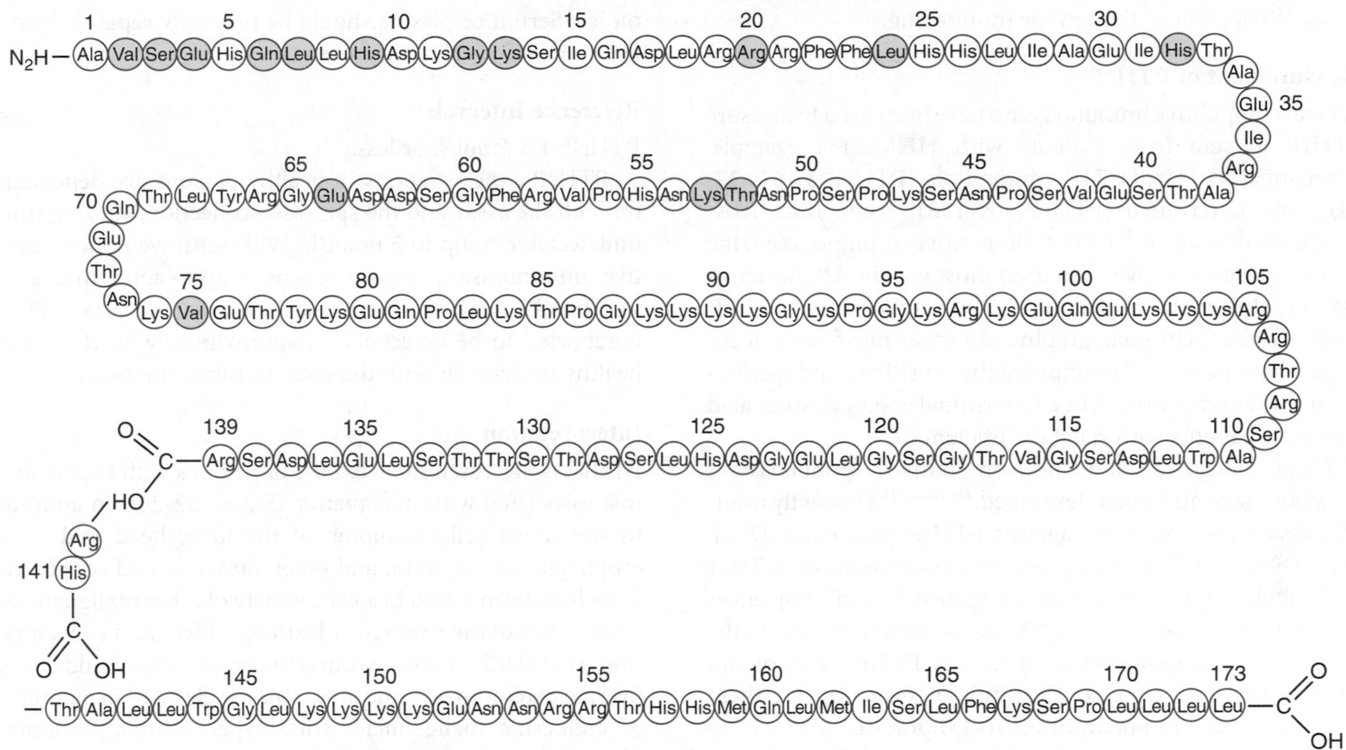

Figure 52-23 Amino acid sequence of human parathyroid hormone–related peptide (PTHrP). Although the exact length of circulating PTHrP is unknown, proteins of 139, 141, and 173 amino acids have been predicted from alternative splicing events. The *shaded circles* show amino acids that are identical in parathyroid hormone (PTH) and PTHrP. *(Modified from Hendy GN, Goltzman D. Parathyroid hormone-like peptide. In: Endocrinology and metabolism inservice, volume 9. Washington, DC: American Association for Clinical Chemistry, 1991:9-24.)*

1-86); (3) midregion fragments, beginning at position 38 and extending 70 to 80 amino acids, measured with midregion assays; and (4) carboxyl fragments, beginning at position 107 or 109, measured with antiserum directed against PTHrP(109 to 138).[338] Midregion and carboxyl forms exert biological actions distinct from the PTH-like actions associated with the N-terminal region.

Besides its endocrine role in the pathophysiology of HHM, PTHrP participates in normal physiology by acting locally on cells or tissues as an autocrine or paracrine factor.[110,298,338] PTHrP is widely expressed in most normal tissues of fetuses and adults. Although it is unlikely that low circulating concentrations of PTHrP have a significant effect on calcium homeostasis in normal adults, PTHrP exerts endocrine effects on skeletal development and calcium homeostasis during fetal life[165,166] and lactation.[167] Breast milk contains extremely high concentrations of PTHrP[338] as does amniotic fluid. Examination of the physiologic effects of PTHrP has identified several themes: (1) PTHrP regulates transepithelial calcium transport; (2) PTHrP is a potent smooth muscle relaxant; and (3) PTHrP regulates growth, differentiation, and development. However, its role of PTHrP in many tissues is unknown.[298]

Clinical Significance

Hypercalcemia associated with malignancy is the second most common cause of hypercalcemia. This frequent paraneoplastic syndrome is believed to occur primarily through two mechanisms: HHM and local osteolysis. HHM is present in approximately 75 to 80% of patients with hypercalcemia associated with malignancy.[143] HHM is common in patients with squamous (lung, head and neck, esophagus, cervix, vulva, and skin), renal, bladder, and ovarian carcinomas. Hypercalcemia due to skeletal metastases and local osteolysis are common in breast cancer and multiple myeloma, lymphoma, and other hematologic malignancies. The hypercalcemia of a subset of lymphomas (human T-cell leukemia virus-1) appears to be caused by HHM. Breast carcinomas may cause hypercalcemia by HHM and/or skeletal metastases with local osteolysis. It is now well established that PTHrP is the principal mediator of HHM, causing dramatic uncoupling of bone resorption from bone formation. After it is secreted by tumors, PTHrP circulates and acts on its target tissues (skeleton and kidney) as an endocrine hormone causing hypercalcemia.

PTHrP determinations usually are considered investigational, because HHM nearly always occurs in advanced disease when the diagnosis is clear. The need for PTHrP determination may increase if it becomes important in prognosis,[322] selection of therapy, or monitoring.

Measurement of PTHrP

Several competitive immunoassays have been used to measure PTHrP in sera from patients with HHM. For example, N-terminal [PTHrP(1-34)], midregion [PTHrP(37-67, 37-74)], and C-terminal [PTHrP(109-138)] competitive RIAs have been developed.[43] Of the competitive immunoassays, the N-terminal assays have been used most widely. Affinity chromatography with immobilized antisera against PTHrP, reversed-phase chromatography, and other purification techniques have been used to improve the sensitivity and specificity of these competitive RIAs. C-terminal assays give elevated results in patients with renal insufficiency.[43]

More sensitive and noncompetitive immunoassays (IRMAs) have also been developed.[43,91,226,240] Currently available assays use antibodies against PTHrP (sequences 37-74, 1-40, 1-40, 1-34, 1-40, and so on) as capture antibodies. Their radiolabeled signal antibodies are against PTHrP (sequences 1-36, 60-72, 57-80, 37-67, 50-83, and so on), respectively; the idea is to measure molecular species of PTHrP that contain large N-terminal regions. The limit of detection for these assays is reported to be from 0.1 to 1.0 pmol/L.

Specimen Requirements

PTHrP is unstable in serum and plasma at 4 °C and at room temperature unless collected in the presence of protease inhibitors. A combination of aprotinin, leupeptin, pepstatin, and EDTA provides the greatest protection. In general, specimens should be collected with protease inhibitors and kept on ice. Serum or plasma should be promptly separated from the clot and/or cells and frozen.

Reference Intervals

PTHrP: 1.3 pmol/L or less.

PTHrP concentrations in healthy persons are dependent on both the assay and the specimen collection, varying from undetectable to up to 5 pmol/L. With sensitive noncompetitive immunoassays, concentrations of up to approximately 1 to 2 pmol/L have been reported in normal subjects. PTHrP is reported to be detectable in approximately 50 to 80% of healthy individuals with the most sensitive methods.

Interpretation

PTHrP is increased in 50 to 90% of patients with hypercalcemia associated with malignancy (Figure 52-24). In addition to squamous cell carcinoma of the lung, head and neck, esophagus, cervix, skin, and other sites, elevated concentrations have been found in a wide variety of other malignancies, irrespective of their source or histology. Increased concentrations of PTHrP have been found in breast, renal, bladder, and ovarian carcinomas. Concentrations are elevated in a number of endocrine malignancies with hypercalcemia, including pheochromocytoma and islet carcinomas. PTHrP is elevated in hypercalcemic patients with adult T-cell lymphoma/leukemia and B-cell lymphoma. PTHrP concentrations have been elevated less frequently in patients with hypercalcemia and other hematologic malignancies (e.g., multiple myeloma).

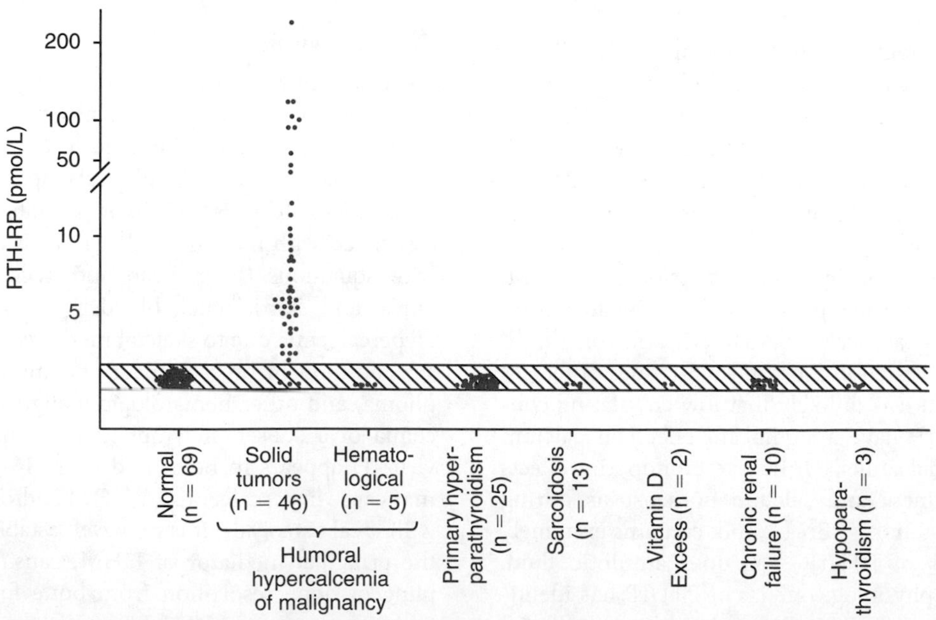

Figure 52-24 Parathyroid hormone–related peptide (PTHrP) in healthy patients and patients with malignancies and other disorders. The *hatched area* indicates the reference interval. *(Adapted from Pandian MR, Morgan CH, Carlton E, Segre GV. Modified immunoradiometric assay of parathyroid hormone-related protein: clinical application in the differential diagnosis of hypercalcemia. Clin Chem 1992;38:282-88.)*

PTHrP is undetectable or normal in most but not all patients with malignancy not associated with hypercalcemia. Increased concentrations of PTHrP have been reported to precede hypercalcemia in some patients with malignancy. Concentrations are normal in patients with primary hyperparathyroidism, hypoparathyroidism, miscellaneous noncancer causes of hypercalcemia, and chronic renal failure (with noncompetitive methods).

SUMMARY OF INTEGRATED CONTROL OF MINERAL METABOLISM

The metabolism of calcium is linked intimately with that of phosphate (Figure 52-25).[84,239,249] The homeostatic mechanisms are directed principally toward the maintenance of normal extracellular calcium and phosphate concentrations, which sustain the extracellular and intracellular processes and provide substrate for skeletal mineralization. The parathyroid gland responds to a decrease in free calcium concentration within seconds. During a time of calcium deprivation, the increase in serum PTH rapidly alters both renal and skeletal metabolism.

Renal Handling of Calcium and Phosphate

Of the about 10 g or approximately 250 mmol of calcium filtered by the kidneys each day, 65% is reabsorbed in the proximal tubule. Calcium reabsorption here is closely linked to sodium and is independent of PTH. Approximately 10 to 20% of calcium is reclaimed in the thick ascending loop of Henle, and 5 to 10% in the distal convoluted tubule. PTH enhances calcium reabsorption at the two latter locations[84] by binding to the PTH receptor.

In contrast to the calcium-conserving effect of PTH on the kidneys, PTH increases renal phosphate excretion at the proximal tubule by directly lowering the renal phosphate threshold. Approximately 6.5 g or 210 mmol of phosphate is filtered by the kidneys each day. Normally, 85 to 90% is reabsorbed by the renal tubules (proximal and distal convoluted tubule). FGF-23 have recently been recognized as a key hormone that lowers serum phosphate.

Intestinal Absorption of Calcium and Phosphate

PTH increases intestinal calcium absorption by increasing $1,25(OH)_2D$ whereas FGF-23 decreases $1,25(OH)_2D$. The effects of PTH and FGF-23 are mediated by opposite effects on renal 25(OH)D 1α-hydroxylase which increases the conversion of 25(OH)D to the active vitamin D metabolite, $1,25(OH)_2D$. About 30 to 40% of a daily calcium intake of 1 g or 25 mmol is absorbed. Approximately 100 to 200 mg (2.5 to 5.0 mmol) of calcium is secreted into the gut lumen by intestinal secretion; therefore, net calcium absorption is 200 mg/d or 5.0 mmol/d. Calcium is absorbed by passive diffusion and by an active transport system. It is estimated that passive diffusion accounts for absorption of about 10% of ingested calcium per day. Active calcium absorption in the duodenum is under the control of $1,25(OH)_2D$.

Dietary phosphate intake is usually 1.2 to 1.4 g/d or 39 to 45 mmol/d, nearly twice the recommended intake, of which approximately 60 to 70% is absorbed, principally in the jejunum. As with calcium, both passive and active transport systems exist; $1,25(OH)_2D$ is the principal regulator of the active transport of phosphate. PTH-stimulated synthesis of $1,25(OH)_2D$ thus offsets the phosphaturic effect of PTH. High serum phosphate concentration stimulates secretion of FGF-23 by bone cells, thus leading to increased phosphate excretion and also decreased $1,25(OH)_2D$. Phosphate depletion or hypophosphatemia stimulates formation of $1,25(OH)_2D$ by the kidneys. At pharmacologic concentrations, calcitonin has the opposite effect to that of PTH. It is unclear, however, whether calcitonin has any physiologic role in mineral homeostasis in adult humans.

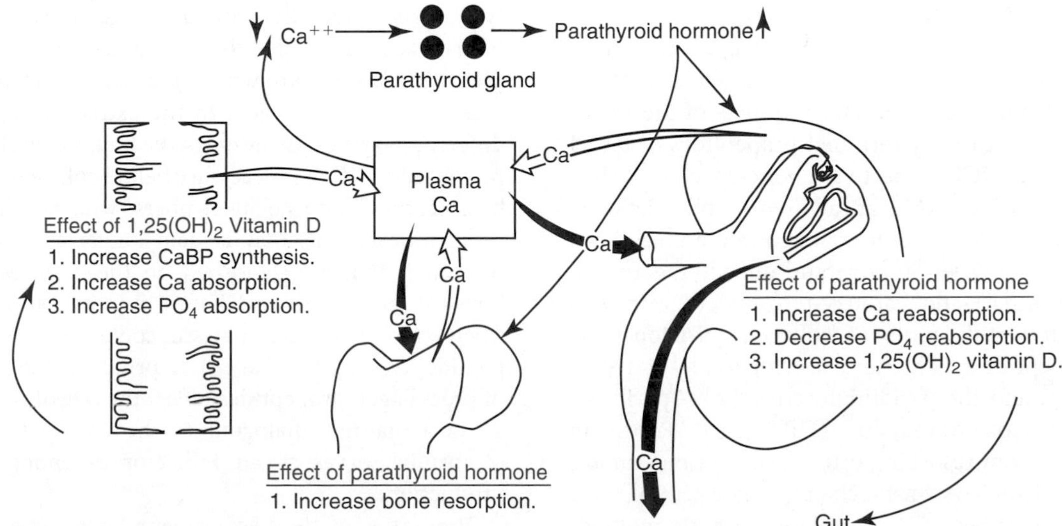

Figure 52-25 **Integrated control of mineral metabolism.** ***CaBP,*** **Calcium-binding protein.**

Bone Metabolism

PTH also has an acute effect on the skeleton. Acutely, PTH decreases collagen synthesis in osteoblasts, but osteoclastic bone resorption is increased, with a net increase in mineral (calcium and phosphate) release from bone into the extracellular fluid. PTH is able to act directly on osteoblasts by interacting with their PTH receptors. The effect of PTH on osteoclasts appears to be indirect, through local mediators produced by the osteoblast (e.g., RANK ligand and OPG) or released from the bone matrix (e.g., TGF-β). Prolonged calcium deprivation results in enhanced recruitment of osteoclasts and an increased number of mature osteoclasts, which continue to resorb bone, releasing calcium, phosphate, and degradation products of the organic matrix. Prolonged exposure to PTH eventually also increases osteoblast activity. This anabolic effect has been the rationale for designing PTH analogs that specifically increase bone formation.[136,215]

Magnesium

Magnesium is efficiently absorbed in the intestinal tract (most efficiently in the distal small bowel). During normal dietary magnesium intake, approximately 30 to 40% of magnesium is absorbed. Magnesium is absorbed by both active and passive transport.

No hormone or factor has been described as primarily regulating magnesium homeostasis. About 25 to 35% of filtered magnesium is passively reabsorbed in the proximal convoluted tubule, where reabsorption is linked closely to sodium and calcium transport. The major site of active reabsorption is the thick ascending loop of Henle, where 60 to 75% of magnesium is reabsorbed. During times of magnesium deprivation, magnesium essentially disappears from the urine (<0.5 mmol/d). The renal threshold for magnesium is close to the filtered load. When magnesium intake is excessive, any amount greater than this maximum is excreted.

BIOCHEMICAL MARKERS OF BONE TURNOVER

In recent years, a large number of specific markers have been developed for measuring both bone formation and degradation. Markers of bone formation are products of the osteoblast: the amino- or carboxy-terminal propeptides of type I collagen, PINP, and PICP, respectively, bone-specific alkaline phosphatase (BAP/BSAP/BALP are all used as abbreviations), and osteocalcin. Markers of bone resorption are breakdown products of type I collagen in bone and include the amino-terminal (N-terminal) and carboxy-terminal (C-terminal) cross-linked telopeptide parts of collagen [N-telopeptide (NTX), C-telopeptide (CTX), and C-telopeptide of type I collagen (ICTP)] and the pyridinium cross-links [pyridinoline (PYD) and deoxypyridinoline (DPD)]. TRAP5b is an enzyme released from resorbing osteoclasts and measurable in blood. Several reviews on biochemical markers of bone metabolism are available.[37,199,247,275,276] More recently, methods have been developed for the measurement of osteoprotegerin and RANK ligand—proteins synthesized by the osteoblast that can influence osteoclast formation, activation, and bone resorption. However, it is unclear whether these newer analytes add information beyond that provided by the markers listed previously. Additional studies are required to determine the roles of RANK ligand and osteoprotegerin as markers of bone turnover.

BOX 52-12 Biochemical Markers of Bone Formation

Propeptides of type I procollagen	PINP and PICP
Bone alkaline phosphatase	BALP
Osteocalcin [bone gla protein (BGP)]	OC

Markers of Bone Formation

Bone formation markers, listed in Box 52-12, can be divided into three families, each of them roughly reflecting a specific phase in development of the osteoblast phenotype. During each remodeling cycle, osteoblasts are formed from undifferentiated mesenchymal cells and pass through the phases of proliferation, matrix maturation, and mineralization (see Figure 52-3).[181] In a steady-state situation without specific disturbances in the production of any of the osteoblast products, the protein products of all three phases should in principle correlate with each other, and their measurements should give the same clinical information on the rate of bone formation. However, marker families can give discordant results if bone formation is affected by a disease state that specifically targets a particular developmental phase of the osteoblast.

Propeptides of Type I Procollagen (PINP and PICP)

Type I collagen accounts for ≈90% of the organic matrix of bone and provides it with tensile strength. The type I collagen molecule, a triple helix of two identical α1(I) chains and a slightly different α2(I) chain, is synthesized as a precursor, type I procollagen that contains large additional domains at both ends of the rodlike collagen molecule (see Figure 52-26). These extensions, known as *propeptides,* are enzymatically cleaved from procollagen in the extracellular space by two different enzymes. Cleavage of the bulky, globular C-terminal propeptide (PICP) is necessary before collagen molecules can be assembled into collagen fibers, whereas the N-terminal propeptide (PINP) may remain longer as a portion of the molecules that are deposited on the surfaces of fibers. In bones, PINP is released before mineralization, but in soft tissues, type I collagen may still contain the N-terminal propeptide (type I pN-collagen). In principle, the concentrations of procollagen propeptides reflect the rate of collagen synthesis in a manner analogous to the way that the C-peptide of insulin serves as an indicator of endogenous insulin production.

Properties of the two propeptides of type I procollagen and the corresponding circulating antigens are summarized in Table 52-6. The serum PICP antigen is homogenous and

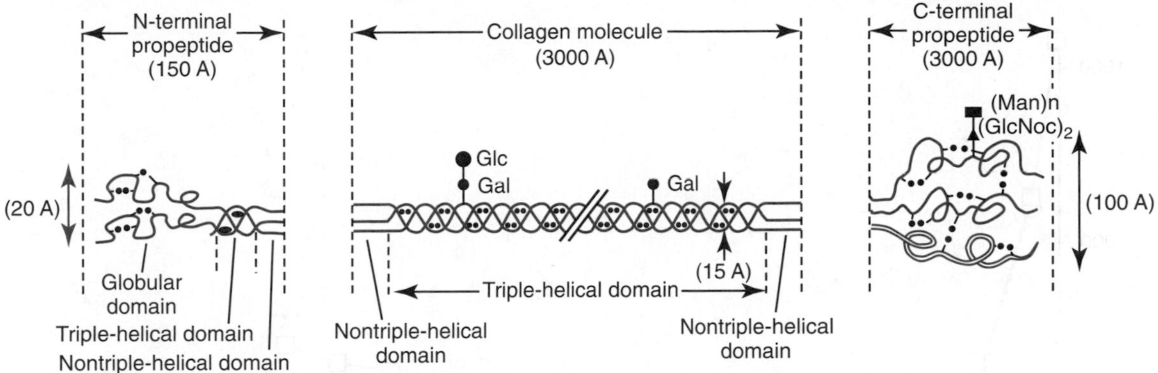

Figure 52-26 Schematic representation of a type I procollagen molecule. The non–triple-helical domains at both ends of the collagen molecule are the telopeptides. The N-terminal propeptide consists of an N-terminal globular domain, a triple-helical domain, and a C-terminal non–triple-helical domain. *(From Prockop DJ, Kivirikko KI, Tuderman L, Guzman NA. The biosynthesis of collagen and its disorders. N Engl J Med 1979;301:13-23, 77-85.)*

TABLE 52-6 Molecular Properties of Propeptides of Type I Procollagen and Corresponding Circulating Antigens

	PINP	PICP
Location	Amino-terminal	Carboxy-terminal
Molecular mass	35,000 Da	100,000 Da
Shape	Elongated	Globular
Chemical nature	Phosphorylated, partially collagenous	Glycoprotein, oligosaccharides of the high-mannose type
Related Serum Antigen		
Homogeneity	One major and one minor form	One form
Size	Same as intact PINP (major) or smaller	Same as PICP
Clearance from blood	Scavenger receptor of liver endothelial cells	Mannose receptor of liver endothelial cells

corresponds in size to the complete propeptide.[202] Also, serum PINP antigen in healthy persons is present mainly in intact, trimeric form.[201] However, in certain situations (e.g., end-stage kidney disease with hemodialysis, bedridden geriatric patients),[163] smaller forms of PINP antigen can be detected in serum. Their exact origin is not known, but in ascitic fluid the molecular mass of a similar antigen (about 10,000 Da) in clearly less than that of a individual monomeric chain of PINP (15,000 Da), suggesting a truncated form such a chain.[193A] In principle this could represent a degradation fragment of tissue type I pN-collagen, an idea strengthened by the finding that the concentration of this smaller antigen correlates with that of the serum marker of type I collagen degradation, ICTP.[163,193A] The PINP assays developed differ with respect to whether they only measure the trimeric form (intact PINP[201]) or both forms (total P1NP[32]) of the serum antigens.

Clearance of Propeptides

For each molecule of type I collagen deposited in the tissues, one molecule of each propeptide is released. For a kilogram of type I collagen synthesized, which is an estimated yearly production rate for adults, about 450 g of propeptide is produced. An efficient recycling mechanism has been noted for this material, which has no known further function once cleaved from procollagen. The intact propeptides are taken up from the circulation via two specific receptor-mediated pathways and are degraded by the endothelial cells of the liver (see Table 52-6).[200,287] PICP and PINP behave differently after exogenous thyroxine treatment, which increases the PINP concentration while PICP is decreased.[317] There are also families with a genetic defect in the uptake mechanism for PICP, which results in an increased concentration of this antigen with no other abnormalities in type I collagen metabolites or other biochemical markers of bone metabolism.[291] When clearance of PINP was studied using an assay that detects both forms of antigens, it was found that renal clearance also occurs for the smaller circulating propeptides.[274]

Clinical Significance

After they are set free from procollagen, the two propeptides behave as two individual proteins, and their fates and metabolism are dependent on their structures. In principle, measurement of either propeptide should give the same information. This is the case when PICP and PINP concentrations are compared in situ (e.g., during the fibroproliferative response in a healing wound, where the concentrations of both propeptides increase up to 1000-fold in 1 week).[201] In children, circulating propeptides closely reflect the somatic

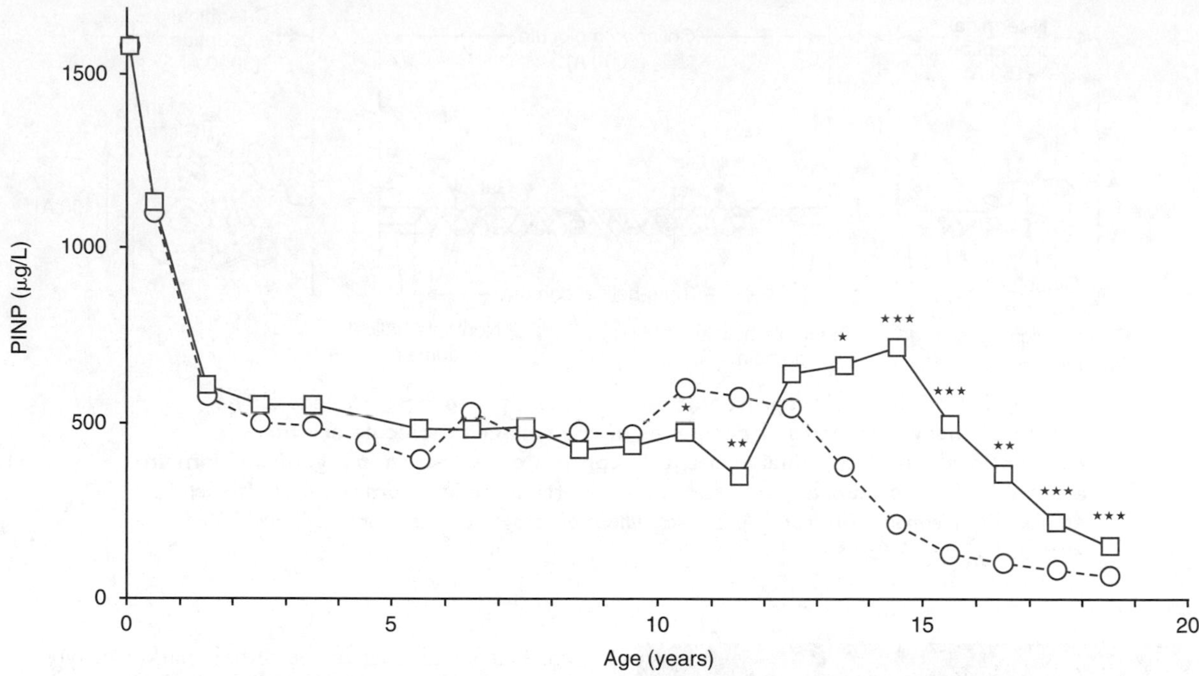

Figure 52-27 Serum concentrations of the amino-terminal propeptide of type I procollagen (PINP) in infants, children, and adolescents in relation to age and gender. Geometric means are shown, defined as the arithmetic mean of log-transformed PINP concentrations, raised to the power of 10. □ ,boys; ○, girls. Geometric means for each age band are plotted at the midpoint of that age band. Unpaired t-tests between age-matched boys and girls: *P *< 0.05;* **P *< 0.01;* ***P *< 0.001.* *(From Crofton PM, Evans N, Taylor MRH, Holland CV. Procollagen type I amino-terminal propeptide: pediatric reference data and relationship with procollagen type I carboxyl-terminal propeptide. Clin Chem 2004;50:2173-6.)*

growth rate, and the peak of PICP and PINP concentrations occurs earlier in girls than in boys (Figure 52-27).[62] During puberty, the increase is larger in boys than in girls.

Various drug therapies affect PINP and PICP concentrations. For example, during the first 2 days of teriparatide [PTH(1-34)] treatment, PINP and PICP increase rapidly and continue to increase until the end of 1 month of treatment to a net increase of 110% (Figure 52-28).[108] By contrast, large doses of intravenous methylprednisolone decrease PICP rapidly, reflecting the inhibition of bone formation by glucocorticoids.[230]

Several studies suggest that the serum concentration of PINP is increased more during active bone growth than is the concentration of PICP.[108,299] The ratio of PICP/PINP in serum is expected to be about 3 when the concentrations are expressed as μg/L. In adults, this ratio is indeed about 3, but in children it is less than 1.[303] In Paget disease of bone, a similar discrepancy is seen between circulating concentrations of the two propeptides.[279] A low PICP/PINP ratio is associated with aggressive breast cancer.[154]

Specimen Requirements

The preferred sample for measuring either of the procollagen propeptides is serum. The antigens are very stable in serum or plasma. Storage of a serum sample at room temperature for 1 week does not decrease measurable concentrations.[202]

Assays for PICP and PINP

The PICP antigen has been purified from the cell culture medium of human fibroblasts and used for establishing a radioimmunoassay.[202] A similar EIA is commercially available (called *CICP*). Assays for PINP can be divided into two families: intact PINP[201] and total P1NP.[32,104,225] So far, only a radioimmunoassay for intact PINP has been approved by the U.S. Food and Drug Administration (FDA). This assay has been used in several clinical studies (e.g., for monitoring the effects of alendronate,[75] denosumab,[63] and teriparatide on bone).[108,208,262]

Reference Intervals

The reported reference intervals for PICP are to be 38 to 202 μg/L in men and 50 to 170 μg/L in women.[202] For intact PINP, the original reference intervals reported in men are 20 to 78 μg/L and in women were 19 to 84 μg/L.[201] The reference interval for total P1NP in young healthy premenopausal women (n = 637; age 30 to 39 years) is 16.3 to 72.2 μg/L in France, Belgium, the United States, and the United Kingdom.[109] Significant differences have been noted between countries; the values being significantly higher in France and Belgium than in the United Kingdom and the United States. The reference interval for total PINP in men is 13.9 to 85.5 μg/L.[104] Children have higher concentrations immediately after birth and later during growth spurts (see Figure 52-27); reference

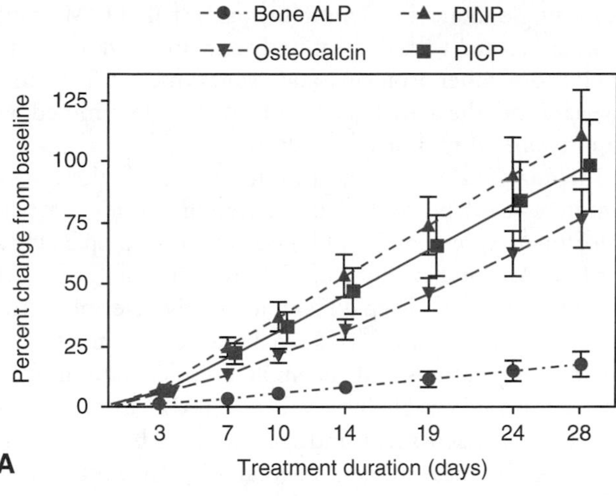

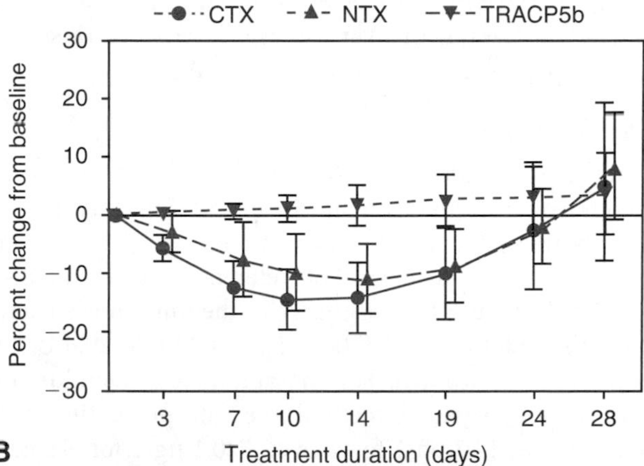

Figure 52-28 Changes in biochemical markers of bone metabolism during 28 days of teriparatide [PTH(1-34)] treatment of osteoporosis. ***Line plots*** **show estimated mean and 90% confidence intervals for percentage change from baseline in (A) markers of bone formation and (B) markers of bone resorption.** ***Bullet points*** **at some time points have been slightly shifted horizontally to increase readability. For bone ALP, osteocalcin, PINP, and PICP, all changes from baseline are statistically significant (P < *0.0001*). For CTX, all changes from baseline until day 19 are statistically significant (P < *0.0004*). For NTX, all changes from baseline to days 7 to 10 are statistically significant (P < *0.03*). For TRACP5b, no changes are statistically significant.** *(From Glover SJ, Eastell R, McCloskey EV, Rogers A, Garnero P, Lowery J, et al. Rapid and robust response of biochemical markers of bone formation to teriparatide therapy. Bone 2009;45:1053-8.)*

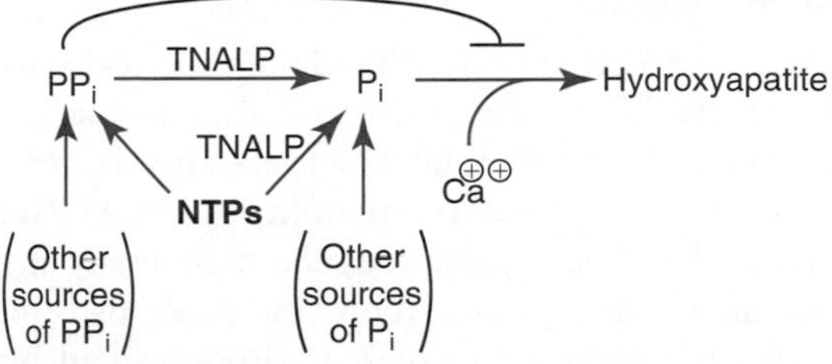

Figure 52-29 Schematic representation of the role of bone alkaline phosphatase in hydroxyapatite formation. Alkaline phosphatase catalyzes the hydrolysis of pyrophosphate (PP_i) produced by the activity of nucleoside triphosphate pyrophosphohydrolase from nucleoside triphosphates (NTPs). Alkaline phosphatase has a positive effect on mineralization primarily by controlling the size of the inhibitory pool of PP_i. The enzyme also generates P_i by using NTPs and PP_i as substrates, but other major sources of P_i (e.g., intestinal absorption) are likely to contribute to the bulk of the P_i needed for hydroxyapatite deposition. *(Modified from Hessle L, Johnson KA, Anderson HC, Narisawa S, Sali A, Goding JW, et al. Tissue-nonspecific alkaline phosphatase and plasma cell membrane glycoprotein-1 are central antagonistic regulators of bone mineralization. Proc Natl Acad Sci U S A 2002;99:9445-9.)*

intervals for children have been reported.[62] In neonates (younger than 1 month of age), the reference interval of intact PINP concentration is very high at 770 to 3202 μg/L.

Bone Alkaline Phosphatase (BAP)

Alkaline phosphatases (ALPs; EC 3.1.3.1) are membrane-bound ectoenzymes that catalyze the hydrolysis of monophosphates from ester linkage under alkaline conditions (pH 8 to 10). Four different genes codes are known for the tissue-nonspecific, intestinal, placental, and germ cell (placental-like) isoenzymes. The alkaline phosphates of liver, bone, and kidney are isoforms of the same gene product, the tissue-nonspecific gene located in chromosome 1 (TNALP). These isoforms are N-glycosylated, and only the liver ALP does not contain O-linked glycans.[221] ALP is attached to the outer surface of the cell membrane by a glycosylphosphatidylinositol (GPI) anchor. Serum ALP is a homodimer in which the anchor has been removed by the action of endogenous or exogenous (e.g., serum) GPI-specific phospholipase D.[8] Bone ALP can be further separated by anion-exchange HPLC or isoelectric focusing into four isoforms—B/I, B1x, B1, and B2—which differ in their sialic acid content.[123,280] Using the same procedure, liver ALP is divided into three isoforms.[280] As glycoproteins, ALPs are cleared by the liver.

During mineralization of bone, the main function of bone ALP is to hydrolyze inorganic pyrophosphate (PPi) to generate phosphate (Pi) (Figure 52-29).[127,135,153] Matrix vesicles are markedly enriched in tissue-nonspecific alkaline phosphatase.[153] The balance between Pi and PPi is thought to be critical for mineralization because PPi inhibits the formation of hydroxyapatite. Studies on TNALP knockout mice, whose condition resembled the human disease hypophosphatasemia (or hypophosphatasia), have suggested that skeletal ALP is necessary for the propagation step but not for the initiation of mineralization.[7,334]

Bone ALP is produced by the osteoblast during the matrix maturation phase (see Figure 52-3),[181] when the newly formed collagenous matrix is prepared for the deposition of mineral. However, because ALP is firmly bound to the cell membrane, its release to plasma can be delayed, and the increase in plasma activity takes time.

Clinical Significance

Total ALP or BALP provides the highest clinical sensitivity and specificity in the diagnosis and monitoring of Paget disease of bone. Although total ALP is used most often, BALP is more sensitive than total ALP in mild disease. ALP is markedly increased in Paget disease and reflects generally increased bone formation in this condition. In severe osteomalacia, BALP may be markedly increased without an increase in bone mineralization because of a mineralizing defect.

BALP is increased in metabolic bone disease, including osteoporosis, osteomalacia and rickets, hyperparathyroidism, renal osteodystrophy, and thyrotoxicosis, and in individuals with acromegaly, bone metastases, and other disorders with increased bone formation.

Because the half-life of ALP is relatively long (≈40 hours), it is less sensitive than procollagen propeptides or osteocalcin to acute treatment effects, such as the effects of large doses of intravenous methylprednisolone.[230] During teriparatide treatment, ALP is not increased as early or as much as procollagen propeptides or osteocalcin (see Figure 52-28).[108]

ALP and BALP are stable in serum in vitro and do not require special specimen handling. Because of its long half-life, ALP has a long half-life in serum and is relatively unaffected by diurnal variation. BALP is more useful than osteocalcin (see later) in individuals with impaired renal function because it is not cleared by glomerular filtration.

Because 1,25-dihydroxyvitamin D regulates the synthesis of BALP and osteocalcin, both of these markers may be misleading in patients treated with calcitriol and in those with abnormal concentrations of this hormone.

Measurement of Bone Alkaline Phosphatase

Measurement of the enzymatic activities of total and bone ALP was described in Chapter 22. Although internal standards for ALP isoenzymes have been used to increase assay precision in assays of BALP activity,[83] the assays tend to be technically complicated and labor intensive, imprecise, insensitive, and inaccurate. Heat denaturation has been criticized because of its irreproducibility or variability. A method using wheat germ agglutinin (WGA) to precipitate BALP has been criticized because WGA does not precipitate all BAP from serum from Paget disease patients and fails to completely separate bone and liver activity.[158] Lot-to-lot variability of the lectin is also evident.[29]

Several immunoassays have been reported for BALP. However, none of the monoclonal antibodies used is completely specific for bone or liver ALP.[191] Two commercially available immunoassays use monoclonal antibodies against BALP from SaOS-2 cells. One immunoassay is an IRMA using two monoclonal antibodies—a capture antibody and a radioiodinated signal antibody—preferentially reacting with BAP. This two-site immunoassay measures the mass of BALP in μg/L. Subsequently, an immunoenzymatic method was developed by replacing the signal antibody with direct measurement of the activity of immobilized BALP.[38] A modification of this method is available on an automated immunoassay analyzer using chemiluminescence detection. The other assay uses a single monoclonal antibody against BALP. Microtiter plates are coated with this antibody and are used to separate BALP from other isoforms and isoenzymes. After immunoseparation, the activity (U/L) of BALP is determined with a *p*-nitrophenyl phosphate substrate.

The analytical and clinical performances of these BALP immunoassays have been characterized in a series of articles. Unfortunately, current immunoassays are not completely specific for BALP and exhibit 7 to 17% cross-reactivity with ALP from liver.[38,234] It has been difficult to exactly determine cross-reactivity with the liver isoform because of limitations of existing preparations and incomplete understanding of the exact nature of circulating isoforms. BALP immunoassays provide greater sensitivity and specificity for bone formation than does the measurement of total ALP. Current methods for BALP are not reliable in patients with liver disease with increased concentrations of the liver isoform,[191] and BALP may be misleading in liver disease because of this cross-reactivity of current methods with liver ALP.

Reference Intervals

Serum concentrations of BALP are influenced by age and gender. Concentrations are higher in men and increase with age in both men and women, consistent with the age-related increase in bone turnover. The reference interval of BALP with the IRMA is 5 to 20 μg/L. With the immunoabsorption assay, it is 15.0 to 41.3 U/L for men and 11.6 to 29.6 U/L for premenopausal women. For the automated chemiluminescent immunoenzymatic method, the 95th percentile limit is reported to be 14.3 μg/L for men and 20.1 μg/L for premenopausal women. Children have much higher concentrations, especially during growth spurts.[192,241]

Osteocalcin

Osteocalcin (OC), also known as bone gla protein (BGP), is the most abundant noncollagenous protein of human bone. It is a small protein of 49 amino acids with a molecular mass of 5669 Da; its gene, symbol *BGLAP*, is located in chromosome 1. 1,25$(OH)_2$D upregulates OC synthesis. OC contains three glutamyl residues at amino acid positions 17, 21, and 24 (Figure 52-30), which may be converted to γ-carboxyglutamyl residues by a post-translational, vitamin K–dependent enzymatic carboxylation. These unique carboxylated amino acids bind calcium ions and are found in various proteins involved in blood coagulation and in calcium transport, deposition, and homeostasis. OC binds calcium and hydroxyapatite, suggesting a physiologic role in bone mineralization.[118]

Osteocalcin knockout mice have increased bone formation compared with wild-type mice.[74] They develop a phenotype marked by higher bone mass and bones of improved functional quality by 6 to 9 months. This could indicate an inhibitory function of OC on osteoblast activity, but further study has demonstrated that osteocalcin has a small role in bone and dentine mineralization, in contrast to another γ-carboxylated protein of bone, matrix gla protein.[211]

Instead of bone formation defects, these knockout mice show decreased insulin and adiponectin secretion, insulin

Osteocalcin [Bone Gla Protein (BGP)]

1				5					10
Tyr	Leu	Tyr	Gln	Trp	Leu	Gly	Ala	Pro	Val
11				15					20
Pro	Tyr	Pro	Asp	Pro	Leu	**Gla**	Pro	Arg	Arg
21				25					30
Gla	Val	Cys	**Gla**	Leu	Asn	Pro	Asp	Cys	Asp
31				35					40
Glu	Leu	Ala	Asp	His	Ile	Gly	Phe	Gln	Glu
41				45				49	
Ala	Tyr	Arg	Arg	Phe	Tyr	Gly	Pro	Val	

Figure 52-30 Structure of human osteocalcin. Three glutamyl residues at positions 17, 21, and 24 can be carboxylated in a post-translational, vitamin K–dependent, enzymatic step producing γ-carboxyglutamyl (Gla) residues. A disulfide bond formed between cysteines in positions 23 and 29 stabilizes two antiparallel α-helical structures representing 40% of the overall structure.

resistance, higher serum glucose concentrations, and increased adiposity.[176] Osteocalcin in fact may be an osteoblast-secreted hormone regulating insulin secretion and sensitivity.[58,94] Leptin formed in adipose tissues, on the other hand, regulates synthesis of osteocalcin in osteoblasts. Adipose cells can also produce osteocalcin.[89]

Both in mice and in men, osteocalcin can be present in the serum in carboxylated and undercarboxylated forms; it is the undercarboxylated form of osteocalcin that acts as a hormone. The undercarboxylated fraction represents 16 to 21% of the total OC.[324]

Serum OC is cleared by the kidneys and has a half-life of approximately 5 minutes. OC concentrations are increased in individuals with renal failure. OC exhibits a diurnal variation with a nocturnal peak, dropping by as much as 50% to a morning nadir. Circulating OC is heterogenous; in addition to the intact molecule, several fragments are the result of proteolysis at arginine residues in positions 19, 20, 43, and 44 (see Figure 52-30). Intact OC has been estimated to account for about 35% of total OC, N-terminal/midregion for about 30%, and other fragments for much less in the circulation.[103] These proportions are different in some conditions (e.g., osteoporosis).

Clinical Significance

The concentration of OC changes rapidly in situations that affect bone turnover. During teriparatide treatment, OC increases rapidly but less pronouncedly than PINP and continues to increase until the end of the first month of treatment (see Figure 52-28).[108] OC will rapidly decrease in patients who get large doses of methylprednisolone intravenously.[230] Thus OC is increased in metabolic bone disease with increased bone formation, including osteoporosis, hyperparathyroidism, renal osteodystrophy, and thyrotoxicosis, and in individuals with fractures, acromegaly, and bone metastases. OC is decreased in hypoparathyroidism, hypothyroidism, and growth hormone deficiency, and during estrogen therapy and treatment with glucocorticoids, bisphosphonates, and calcitonin.

OC concentrations may be misleading in several situations. They increase in patients with impaired renal function without a similar increase in bone formation, because OC is cleared by the kidneys. OC may be increased during bed rest without an increase in bone formation. Serum OC may not reflect bone formation in patients treated with $1,25(OH)_2D$ or those with abnormalities in this hormone, because OC is regulated by $1,25(OH)_2D$.

About 10 to 30% of OC synthesized by the osteoblast is released into the circulation. OC is not a pure marker of bone formation: freshly synthesized OC is secreted in part into the bloodstream and is incorporated in part into the bone matrix.[235] Osteocalcin is also released from the bone matrix during bone resorption; these fragments of OC may contribute to circulating concentrations of osteocalcin. Thus, serum osteocalcin may be considered a marker of bone turnover rather than bone formation.[149] Measurements of OC are used more in research than in clinical practice.

Measurement of Osteocalcin

Many immunoassay methods have been developed for OC since the first assay was reported in 1980.[235] Early OC assays were competitive immunoassays, but noncompetitive methods have been developed.[175] Noncompetitive methods measuring intact OC, especially those measuring both intact OC plus the N-terminal/midregion (1-43) fragment, are of particular interest. These assays do not measure smaller fragments of OC that can be produced during bone resorption. OC concentrations are more stable when measured with assays that recognize both intact hormone (1-49) and the N-terminal/midregion (1-43), because this fragment is produced in vitro by hydrolysis of intact OC.[255]

For most assays, specificities with respect to carboxylated and undercarboxylated forms of OC are not known. An ELISA assay for N-terminal midfragment is independent of the degree of γ-carboxylation of human OC.[255] If the serum sample is precipitated with hydroxyapatite[203] or barium sulfate,[289] the supernatant contains undercarboxylated OC.

The circulating concentration of OC measured in healthy subjects varies widely between methods and laboratories. One study reported that mean values for healthy individuals ranged from 3 to 27 ng/mL.[69] Such variability may be a consequence of differences in specificities and sensitivities of antisera/antibodies used in the assays, and in the purity, potency, and immunoreactivity of OC calibrators. Another important source of variation between methods may be their dependence on, or independence of, calcium concentration in the assay. Calcium binding to γ-carboxyglutamyl residues induces a conformational change in OC. Although EDTA is added to some assays to eliminate this effect, other assays require the addition of calcium.

An immunoassay for the undercarboxylated form of osteocalcin has also been developed. This assay uses recombinant human undercarboxylated OC for calibration and two monoclonal antibodies[324]; one of these specifically recognizes the 14-30 sequence, in which the three glutamic acid residues are not carboxylated.

Specimen Requirements

Osteocalcin is rapidly degraded in blood samples at room temperature or at 4 °C.[13,24,103] Measured serum OC concentrations are more stable when assessed with methods measuring both intact OC and the N-terminal/midregion fragment (1-43): measured concentrations were unchanged after 3 hours at room temperature and after 24 hours at 4 °C.[24,103]

Reference Intervals

OC concentrations are influenced by age, gender, and diurnal variation. Men have somewhat higher concentrations of OC than women. OC concentrations have been reported to increase, decrease, or remain unchanged with advancing age as a probable consequence of the heterogeneity of circulating OC and differences in immunoassay specificity. OC concentrations generally are increased during menopause. In a commercially available OC ELISA, the reference interval is 9.6 to 40.8 μg/L in men, 8.4 to 33.9 μg/L in premenopausal women, and 12.8 to 55.0 μg/L in postmenopausal women. Concentrations are higher in children; the highest concentrations are observed during periods of rapid growth.[192,241]

Biochemical Markers of Bone Resorption

Most markers of bone resorption reflect aspects of the degradation of type I collagen. These markers were initially measured in urine, but serum-based methods have been developed. An osteoclast-derived enzyme, serum tartrate-resistant acid phosphatase (TRAP5b), has also been used to assess bone resorption. Bone resorption markers are listed in Box 52-13.

Collagen Cross-Links

Procollagen undergoes extensive intracellular post-translational processing, including hydroxylation of proline and lysine residues, glycosylation of hydroxylysine residues, and formation of the collagenous triple helix.[247] After it is secreted, procollagen is converted to collagen during extracellular processing, with enzymatic removal of PINP and PICP (see Figure 52-26).

Extracellularly, type I collagen molecules are assembled into immature fibrils with limited tensile strength, which then are modified by formation of intramolecular and intermolecular covalent bonds or cross-links.[162] Intermolecular cross-linking sites have been located in short non–triple-helical domains at each end of the type I collagen molecule, called *telopeptides* (see Figure 52-26). Two hydroxylysine and/or lysine residues in the telopeptide at the amino-terminal end (N-telopeptide) can be linked to a helical site at amino acid 930, and two C-telopeptides can be linked to a helical site at amino acid 87. The activities of two enzymes—intracellular lysyl hydroxylase 2b and extracellular lysyl oxidase—regulate which variant structures of cross-links are formed (Figure 52-31).[265] Lysyl hydroxylase 2b forms hydroxylysine in telopeptide sequences, and lysyl oxidase deaminates the ε-amino group of lysine or hydroxylysine to produce allysine or hydroxyallysine. After this enzymatic processing of telopeptides, the other reactions are spontaneous, leading to a series of divalent and later trivalent cross-links. Of the latter, pyridinoline and deoxypyridinoline (Figure 52-32) are stable even in acid hydrolysis, whereas the pyrrole variants are quite unstable (see Figure 52-31). Trivalent cross-links are found in soft tissues and in collagen types other than type I (type II, III, etc.).

In soft tissues, only mature, trivalent cross-links are found, but bone contains immature, divalent cross-links because mineralization occurs at the same locations as telopeptide cross-links. C-terminal telopeptide isolated from human bone contains un–cross-linked as well as divalently and trivalently cross-linked telopeptides.[81] Pyridinolines were the first mature cross-links to be identified, but their quantity in bone is relatively low—≈1 per 3 to 5 collagen molecules—compared with the quantity of their divalent precursors—1 per collagen molecule.[10,125] The pyrrole cross-links are concentrated at the N-terminal end of human bone collagen.[125] More pyrrole is produced if the activity of lysyl hydroxylase 2b is low in the osteoblast.[10]

Both telopeptides have a sequence with an aspartic acid residue, which as the result of a nonenzymatic reaction, can undergo racemization and β-isomerization.[31,86] Immunoassays detect only one form of these structures, thus decreasing the amount or concentration of antigen detected and creating the possibility that changes in concentration (e.g., with treatment) are due in part to changes in the fine structure of the antigen, rather than to changes in total concentration.

Degradation of Bone Collagen

Cathepsin K is the main enzyme that degrades bone collagen within the lacuna of the osteoclast. Its activity alone is sufficient to completely dissolve insoluble collagen of adult human cortical bone.[98] Osteoclasts also produce other proteases, notably several matrix metalloproteinase (MMP) enzymes (e.g., MMP-9, MMP-10, MMP-12, MMP-14).[67] Cross-linked telopeptides are released from type I collagen during bone resorption because cross-links resist proteolysis of adjacent

BOX 52-13 Biochemical Markers of Bone Resorption

Type I Collagen Telopeptides
- N-telopeptide (NTX)
- C-telopeptide (CTX)
- ICTP

Pyridinium Cross-links
- Free deoxypyridinoline
- Free deoxypyridinoline and pyridinoline
- Total deoxypyridinoline and pyridinoline

Tartrate-Resistant Acid Phosphatase

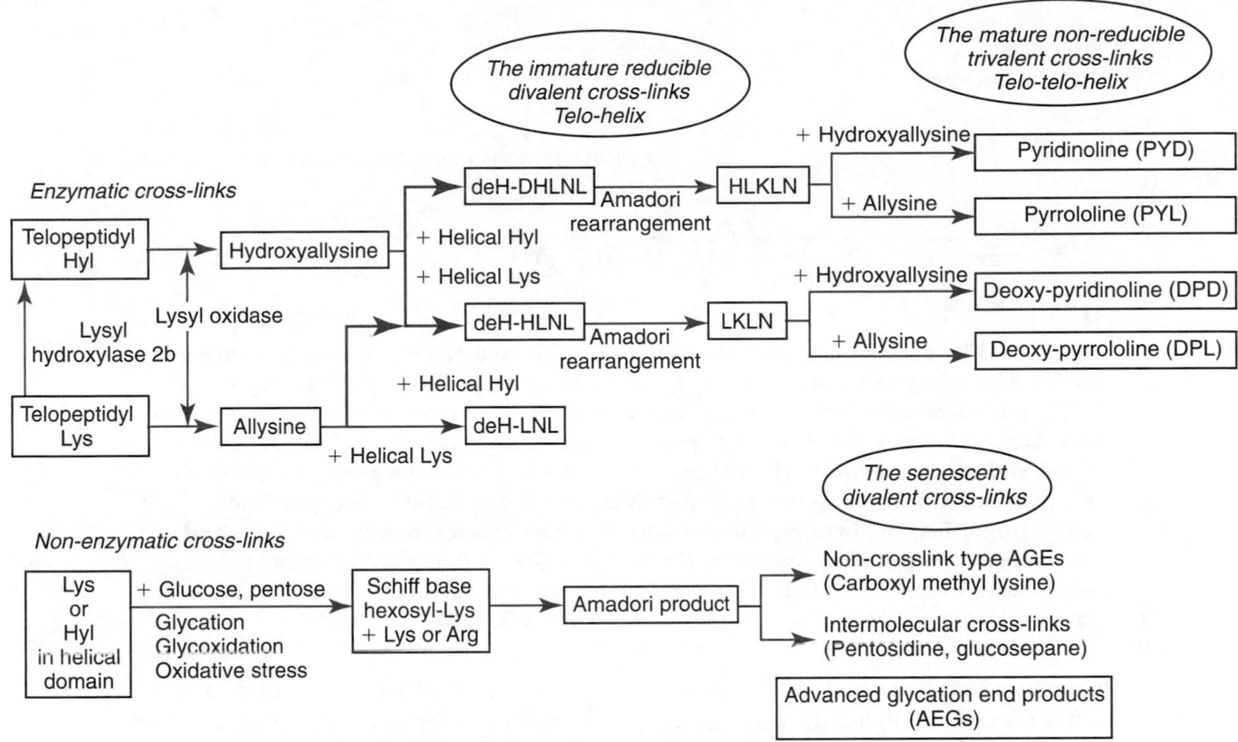

Figure 52-31 Pathways of enzymatic and nonenzymatic cross-link formation in bone collagen. Lysyl hydroxylase 2b– and lysyl oxidase–controlled reactions are the first steps for enzymatic cross-linking within collagen fibers. *deH-DHLNL*, Dehydrodihydroxylysinonorleucine; *deH-HLNL*, dehydrohydroxylysinonorleucine; *deH-LNL*, dehydrolysinonorleucine; *HLKNL*, hydroxylysino-5-ketonorleucine; *LKNL*, lysino-5-ketonorleucine. *(Modified from Saito M, Marumo K. Collagen cross-links as a determinant of bone quality: a possible explanation for bone fragility in aging, osteoporosis, and diabetes mellitus. Osteoporosis Int 2010;21:195-214.)*

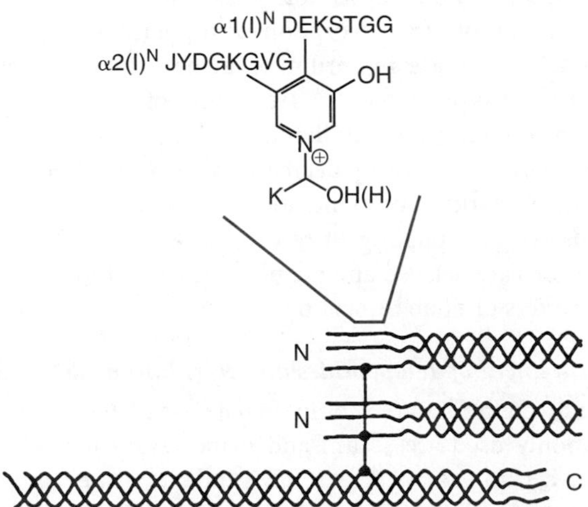

Figure 52-32 Structure and molecular origin of the N-telopeptide (NTX) epitope in type I collagen fibrils. The peptides excreted in urine consist of two telopeptide fragments still linked to the cross-linking residue, which can have a deoxypyridinoline *(as shown here)*, a pyridinoline, or a pyrrole structure. *(Modified from Atley LM, Mort JS, Lalumiere M, Eyre DR. Proteolysis of human bone collagen by cathepsin K: characterization of the cleavage sites generating the cross-linked N-telopeptide neoepitope. Bone 2000;26:241-7.)*

polypeptide chains. This may lead to generation of a neoepitope such as NTX that can be detected by an immunoassay (see Figure 52-32).[9]

For C-terminal telopeptides, two distinct immunoassays—ICTP and CTX—reflect different enzymatic pathways of bone breakdown.[100] Cathepsin K releases CTX antigen but destroys reactivity in the ICTP assay (Figure 52-33). ICTP antigen is stable after MMP-1, MMP-9, and MMP-13 digestion.[269] It has been suggested that the ICTP assay could be called the *CTX-MMP assay.*[68] The importance of MMPs is demonstrated by pycnodysostosis, a lysosomal disease caused by cathepsin K deficiency.[107] In this disease, ICTP is the major fragment released during bone resorption.[218]

NTX and CTX reflect normal osteoclastic function,[133] whereas ICTP detects pathologic degradation of bone and soft connective tissue as seen in multiple myeloma, bone metastasis, and rheumatoid arthritis.[248] Thus, in rheumatoid arthritis, CTX is generally within the reference interval, whereas ICTP is increased, correlating with markers of inflammation (CRP and ESR).[268] It seems that MMPs are important in this condition because lack of cathepsin K activity does not abolish erosion.[4]

Excretion of hydroxyproline has been used to assess bone turnover or bone resorption, but it is rarely used today. It is

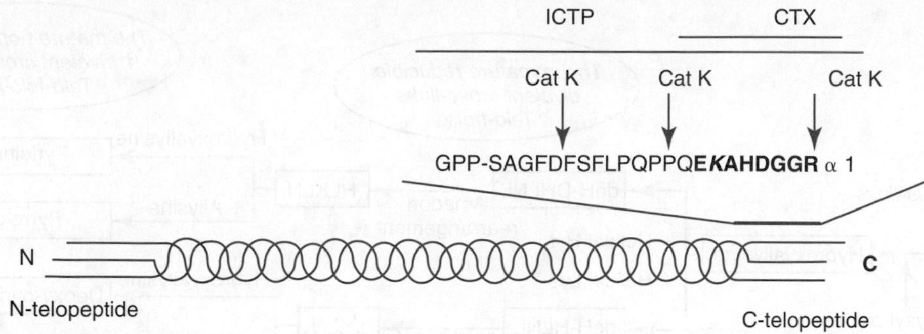

Figure 52-33 Schematic representation of the CTX and ICTP epitopes and cathepsin K (Cat K) cleavage sites in the carboxy-terminal telopeptide of type I collagen. The CTX epitope corresponds to an 8 amino acid sequence in the telopeptide part of an α1(I) chain, whereas the ICTP epitope is a larger conformational epitope, requiring telopeptide parts of two α1(I) chains, both of which contain the phenylalanine-rich region. As shown in the figure, cathepsin K degrades the ICTP phenotype, while generating CTX. The hydroxylysine residue (K) participates in intramolecular and intermolecular covalent cross-links. *(Modified from Garnero P, Ferreras M, Karsdal MA, Nicamhlaoibh R, Risteli J, Borel O, et al. The type I collagen fragments ICTP and CTX reveal distinct enzymatic pathways of bone collagen degradation. J Bone Miner Res 2003;18:859-67.)*

found mainly in collagens, where it accounts for about 13% of total amino acids. It is needed to stabilize the triple-helical structure at body temperature. When the helical collagenous sequence is degraded, this amino acid is released and about 90% of it is catabolized in the liver to urea and carbon dioxide. About 10% is excreted in urine, where it can be analyzed by any one of several methods. However, hydroxyproline is not specific for collagen in that other proteins also contain it (e.g., complement C1q). In addition, the amino-terminal propeptides of type I and III procollagens, markers of collagen synthesis, include in their structure a triple-helical part, which contains hydroxyproline (see Figure 52-26). In addition, ingestion of meat or gelatin increases hydroxyproline excretion.

Comparison of Urine and Serum Analyses

Urine used to be the sample of choice for measuring bone collagen degradation. Urine hydroxyproline analysis was replaced by the more sensitive and specific cross-link and telopeptide assays. Urine measurement needs to be corrected for creatinine excretion to adjust for effects of urine concentration or dilution. This includes a second analyte, which has its own analytical variation that adds to the uncertainty of the result.

Serum and urine telopeptide assays have been compared in several studies; correlation coefficients have varied from 0.6 to 0.9.[134] Kidneys are involved in further degradation of cross-linked peptides; as a result, ≈40% of total cross-links in the urine are free (i.e., not peptide bound).[256] The mean fractional excretion of NTX (0.22) is lower than that of CTX (0.44), indicating that renal degradation is greater for the former analyte.[82]

During antiresorptive treatment, urinary telopeptide assessment may overestimate the decrease in bone resorption because the renal metabolism of these peptides can change. The response to antiresorptive therapy is generally greatest when measured with telopeptide assays, intermediate with total DPD assay, and lowest with free DPD assay.[102,155] Fractional excretion of conjugated cross-links is less than 1, whereas that of the free fraction is greater than 1.[57] It is likely that serum assays will replace urine assays.

Clinical Significance of Telopeptides and Cross-links

Increased urinary telopeptides and deoxypyridinoline have been reported in osteoporosis, Paget disease of bone, primary and secondary hyperparathyroidism, hyperthyroidism, and other diseases (e.g., carcinoma metastases, multiple myeloma), with increased bone resorption or osteolysis.

Inhibition of bone resorption with pharmacologic agents leads to a decrease in serum or urinary telopeptides and urinary deoxypyridinoline. Treatment of postmenopausal women or osteoporotic individuals with bisphosphonates or other antiresorptive drugs decreases bone resorption markers. Although markers of bone formation are also decreased because of the coupling of resorption and formation, their reductions are delayed and are not as great as those observed for markers of bone resorption.

Measurement of Telopeptides and Pyridinium Cross-Links

Several methods are commercially available; the most commonly used are serum and urine assays for NTX and CTX, serum assay for ICTP, and a urine assay for deoxypyridinoline.

N-Telopeptide. NTX in urine is measured with a commercially available ELISA, which uses a monoclonal antibody against the NTX fraction isolated from the urine of healthy adolescents.[126] The antibody recognizes a conformational epitope of the cross-linked α_2(I)N-telopeptide containing the sequence QYDGKGVG, which is a product of osteoclastic proteolysis (see Figure 52-32). It does not recognize a precursor that is not cross-linked, but it does measure both pyridolines and pyrroles.[125] Because the assay does not measure precursors of cross-links, only degradation of mature collagen is measured, just as with the pyridinolines. Measurement of NTX provides considerable specificity for bone because DPD cross-links primarily involve the α_2(I) chain. By contrast, α_1(I) predominates in other tissues. Moreover, two thirds of deoxypyridinoline cross-links in bone collagen are at the NTX site, whereas one third are at the CTX site. On the other hand, about 85% of the pyrroles are located in the N-telopeptide. The lability and reactivity of pyrroles and their potential for oxidation and hydrolytic ring opening explain the difficulties encountered in isolating and characterizing these structures from NTX antigen.[125] When urine is treated with UV light for 3 days, the apparent concentration of urinary NTX unexpectedly increases by ≈30%, which probably indicates dissolution of aggregated N-telopeptides.[23]

The commercially available urinary NTX ELISA assay measures only nonisomerized α_2(I) N-telopeptide.[31] However, in adult urine, the amount of β-isomerized NTX-peptide is about 10-fold that of nonisomerized forms.

The NTX method has been adapted for the measurement of N-telopeptides in serum.[54] The use of serum eliminates the need to measure urine creatinine to correct for urine concentration and can significantly reduce within-subject day-to-day variation in NTX measurements. Experimental and clinical data have demonstrated this serum assay to provide a useful index of bone resorption; however, mostly for technical reasons, the serum assay has not become as widely used as the assay for NTX in urine.[134]

C-Telopeptide CTX Assay. The first CTX immunoassays were based on a polyclonal antibody produced in rabbits against a synthetic peptide corresponding to residues 15C to 22C (EKAHDGGR) of the α_1(I) chain of type I collagen.[26] This region includes the cross-linking hydroxylysine at residue 16C. Subsequently, several other methods were developed for measuring CTX in urine and serum. The most widely used methods recognize the β-isomer, formed during aging of bone by transfer of the peptide backbone from the α-carboxyl group of aspartic acid to the β-carboxyl group of the same amino acid. In healthy human bone, ≈70 to 80% of C-telopeptides have this β-isomerization, but in Paget disease, it accounts for only about 50 to 60%.[101] This fact introduces additional uncertainly in that β-isomerization and racemization may vary between individuals.[247] All CTX methods require the C-terminal amino acid to be a free arginine.

Serum CTX is measured using two monoclonal antibodies.[254] With two α_1(I) chain telopeptides in each collagen molecule, the use of two antibodies directed against the β-isomer ensures that only the ββ-forms are measured. A modification of this method is now available on an automated immunoassay analyzer using electrochemiluminescence detection.[99]

C-Telopeptide ICTP Assay. A radioimmunoassay for the C-terminal telopeptide of type I collagen (ICTP) detects collagen degradation fragments in serum.[246] Rabbit antibodies were raised against a cross-linked C-telopeptide of type I collagen produced by collagenase digestion of human bone. The epitope measured is vulnerable to digestion by cathepsin K (see Figure 52-33); this method is relatively insensitive to changes in bone resorption caused by normal bone turnover.[100] However, the method is suitable for detecting the osteolytic processes taking place in multiple myeloma[77] or metastatic bone disease, as well as the erosion process in rheumatoid arthritis.

Deoxypyridinoline and Pyridinoline. DPD and PYD were originally measured by HPLC. Today, DPD is measured primarily by immunoassay using automated analyzers or manual ELISA. Unlike most HPLC methods, which measure total DPD and total PYD, the immunoassays for DPD or DPD/PYD measure primarily free, but not peptide-bound, forms. In urine, approximately 40% of PYD and DPD is free and 60% is protein bound.

Comparisons of free and total DPD and PYD suggest that the ratio of free to total pyridinolines varies with physiology, pathophysiology, and treatment.[102,155] Total DPD has been reported to be increased more than free DPD in individuals with disorders involving increased bone resorption (e.g., postmenopausal women; women with osteoporosis, Paget disease, hyperthyroidism). Furthermore, short-term bisphosphonate treatment of patients with Paget disease or osteoporosis reduces the total but not the free DPD.

One commercially available ELISA measures both PYD and DPD with equimolar cross-reactivity.[111] Of greater interest for monitoring bone resorption is the commercially available ELISA that measures DPD but not PYD.[251] This method, a competitive ELISA, uses a streptavidin-coated microtiter plate and biotinylated deoxypyridinoline as the solid phase. Sample or calibrator and the monoclonal antibody against DPD are added and incubated. After washing, a second antibody, goat antimouse immunoglobulin (Ig)G conjugated to ALP, is added. Bound antibody-antibody-enzyme conjugate is measured after addition of *p*-nitrophenyl phosphate.

More recently, automated immunoanalyzer methods for DPD have become commercially available. The most widely used is a solid-phase, competitive EIA with chemiluminescence detection. The solid-phase antibody is incubated with serum or calibrator and ALP conjugated to DPD. After washing, antibody-antigen-enzyme complexes are determined after the addition of substrate.

DPD and PYD can be measured by HPLC with fluorescence detection.[151] Because ≈60% of the pyridinolines in urine are contained in peptides, most methods use acid hydrolysis to generate free amino acids. The hydrolysate is fractionated by column chromatography before resolution of the pyridinolines by reverse-phase chromatography. Because the pyridinolines are highly polar at acid pH, ion-pairing agents have been used to increase their retention by reverse-phase columns. Although most methods have used gradient elution, simpler isocratic methods have been described.[151] Fluorometric detection is used to quantify these naturally occurring fluorescent pyridinium compounds. Lack of synthetic calibrators, controversy over the molar fluorescence yield of pyridinolines, and variability of acid hydrolysis have been suggested as factors contributing to differences observed between laboratories.[250]

Specimen Requirements

Serum is collected after overnight fasting. Both timed and random urine tests have been used for pyridinolines and telopeptides. Although early studies used 24 hour urine samples, timed or early-morning voided urine has also been used. A second morning void, collected by 1000, is most commonly recommended.[37] For treatment monitoring, the specimens should be collected at the same time as the baseline specimen. Peak urinary excretion of pyridinolines occurs at about 0500 to 0800, reflecting the nocturnal peak in bone turnover. Urinary pyridinolines reach a nadir between 1400 and 2300.

DPD and telopeptides are relatively stable in urine. Exposure to UV light, but not laboratory lighting, decreases DPD and PYD.[23] Free pyridinolines are especially vulnerable to UV lighting. It is recommended that prolonged exposure to light and exposure to direct sunlight should be avoided.

Reference Intervals

Concentrations of collagen cross-links are influenced by age and gender. Reference intervals for NTX, CTX, ICTP, and DPD are listed in Table 52-7. Concentrations are markedly higher in children, with highest concentrations observed during early infancy and adolescence—periods of rapid bone growth. In adults, concentrations of collagen cross-links are relatively constant between the ages of 30 and 45, but they increase significantly after menopause in women. Age-related increases have also been reported in men.

Tartrate-Resistant Acid Phosphatase (TRACP5b)

Osteoclasts produce and secrete a tartrate-resistant acid phosphatase (see Figure 52-2) during bone resorption (EC 3.1.3.2).[233] In cell culture, its activity is used to detect and enumerate osteoclasts.[133] Osteoclast number can be elevated in bone disorders and is decreased by antiresorptive treatment (such as bisphosphonates and selective estrogen receptor modulators).[340] The activity of this acid phosphatase in serum has been measured by a number of methods, but most previous methods failed to distinguish between two isoforms: TRACP5b produced by the osteoclasts, and TRACP5a produced by inflammatory macrophages and dendritic cells. These isoforms differ in their carbohydrate content: 5a contains a sialic acid and mannose, but 5b only mannose. In addition, isoform 5b is a dimer, whereas 5a is a monomer. Only about 10% of TRACP circulates in enzymatically active form, and the remaining 90% circulates as inactive fragments.[122]

Several approaches may be used to measure only TRACP5b activity. In a kinetic method, TRACP5b activity is estimated by subtracting tartrate-resistant fluoride-resistant acid phosphatase activity from total activity.[212] Two commercial immunoassays are also available for TRACP5b. In one of them, monoclonal antibody (O1A) binds both isoforms but no inactive fragments; the activity of bound enzymes is then detected with *p*-nitrophenyl phosphate as a substrate at pH 6.1, which is selective for TRACP5b activity.[120,121] In another assay, two monoclonal antibodies are used. One antibody binds the active 5b isoforms of 5b; the other binds inactive fragments, and the activity of bound enzyme is then detected with the TRACP 5b-selective substrate, 2-chloro-4-nitrophenyl phosphate.[224] The two assays have similar TRACP5b specificity and clinical performance in monitoring antiresorptive treatment.[340]

Specimen Requirements

The preferred sample for measuring TRACP5b is serum. Diurnal variation is minor, probably indicating that the half-life of TRACP5b is longer than those of the other markers of bone resorption.[124] TRACP5b may be relatively unstable on storage, although it has been shown that TRACP5b can be stored for up to 8 hours at room temperature and up to 3 days at 4 °C. For long-term storage, it is essential that samples be

TABLE 52-7 Reference Intervals of Type I Collagen Telopeptides and Deoxypyridinoline Cross-links

Test	Premenopausal Women	Men
N-Telopeptide		
Serum, nmol BCE/L	8.7-19.8	10.7-22.9
Urine, µmol BCE/mol creatinine	10-110	11-103
C-Telopeptide		
Serum,* ng/L	≤573	≤584
Urine, mg/mol creatinine	220 (128)†	249 (128)†
ICTP		
Serum, µg/L	1.5-5.0	1.5-5.0
Deoxypyridinoline, Free (µmol/mol creatinine)	3.0-7.4	2.3-5.4

BCE Bone Collagen Equivalent.[126]
*CTX by automated immunoassay with electrochemiluminescence detection.
†Mean (SD).

stored at −80 °C.[121] Six months' storage at −20 °C reduces activity by at least 40%.[121]

Clinical Significance

In response to alendronate, TRACP5b decreased by a mean (SE) of 39% (4%), compared with 49% (4%) to 69% (5%) for urinary telopeptides (CTX and NTX), and 75% (8%) for serum CTX.[124] TRACP5b activity changes in children; boys aged 13 to 17 years have higher concentrations than girls in the same age groups.[241]

Reference Interval

An immunoassay for TRACP5b has upper limits of reference intervals of 4.15 U/L for women and 4.82 U/L for men.

Preanalytical and Analytical Variables of Bone Turnover Marker

Controllable sources of preanalytical variability include sampling time, sample preservation procedures, and food intake. Bone marker concentrations in urine and serum vary with the time of day because of the diurnal variation of bone resorption and formation. Because of the nocturnal peak in bone turnover, most bone markers peak in the early morning hours (0400 to 0800) and reach their nadir in the afternoon (1300 to 2300). The amplitude of this variation is greatest for resorption markers, with nadir values averaging 70% of peak values. Consequently, specimens should be collected at a standardized time of day to minimize the impact of diurnal variability. For urinary markers, collection of the second morning void is often recommended.

Concentrations of urinary resorption markers are usually normalized by dividing by the urinary creatinine concentration. Variability (within- and between-method) in creatinine measurements, within-subject variability in urinary creatinine, and its dependence on muscle mass contribute to the overall variability of urinary resorption markers.

Long-term, within-individual variability of urine markers is generally higher (15 to 60%) than that of serum markers (5 to 10%). Compared with other bone markers, BALP and TRACP5b do not demonstrate much diurnal variation because of their long half-lives in serum.

Food intake has a marked effect only on serum CTX concentration.[56] The diurnal variation of serum CTX has a magnitude of about ±40% around the 24 hour mean; the only variable that has been recognized as influencing circadian variation is fasting, which reduces variation to about one fourth.[237] With other bone markers, the clinical impact of feeding versus fasting is small. However, in clinical practice, collection of samples in the fasting state is standard practice.

METABOLIC BONE DISEASES

Metabolic bone disease results from a partial uncoupling or imbalance between bone resorption and formation. Decreased bone mass, or *osteopenia,* is more common than abnormal increases in bone mass. The most prevalent metabolic bone diseases are osteoporosis, osteomalacia and rickets, and renal osteodystrophy. Osteoporosis, the most prevalent metabolic bone disease in developed countries, is characterized by loss of bone mass, microarchitectural deterioration of bone tissue, and increased risk of fracture. Rickets and osteomalacia, which are more common in the less-developed countries, are characterized by defective mineralization of bone matrix. Renal osteodystrophy is a complex condition that develops in response to abnormalities of the endocrine and excretory functions of the kidneys. In addition to these three diseases that affect the skeleton in general, two diseases characterized by localized bone involvement are discussed here: Paget disease of bone and bone metastases.

Osteoporosis

Osteoporosis, the most prevalent metabolic bone disease in the United States, results in 1.5 million fractures each year.[128] Osteoporosis is associated with increased risk for vertebral, hip, and distal forearm fractures. At age 50, women have a lifetime fracture risk (at any of these three sites) of about 40%. Men have a lifetime fracture risk of approximately one third that of women. Because trabecular bone turns over at five to seven times the rate of cortical bone, fractures of bones that are predominantly trabecular (vertebra and distal forearm) occur earlier in life. One third of women who are older than 65 years suffer vertebral crush fractures. Vertebral crush fractures can occur acutely and result in disabling pain and discomfort. Long-term complications include immobility and loss of height. Secondary problems include protuberant abdomen, chronic constipation, and loss of self-esteem. Many mild vertebral fractures may be clinically silent when they occur, only to manifest much later as an incidental finding on an x-ray.

Fractures of bone with more cortical bone (proximal femur or hip) occur later in life. For women, the lifetime risk of hip fracture is 15% and for men 3%. The mortality rate accompanying hip fracture may be as high as 20%. Hip fracture mortality is higher in men than in women, increases with age, and is higher for those with coexisting illness and poor prefracture functional status.[128] Twenty-five percent of survivors are confined to long-term care in nursing homes. The cost of medical care for osteoporosis in the United States is estimated to be close to $20 billion.

Peak bone mass normally is attained by 30 years of age and begins to decrease slowly after age 40 in both men and women. The amount of bone attained during growth is an important determinant of whether clinical osteoporosis develops later in life. Exercise and adequate nutrition play important roles in attaining and maintaining skeletal mass. During early adult life, bone formation is coupled with bone resorption so that bone mass remains stable. Aging is a major risk factor for bone loss because after 40 years of age, bone resorption slightly exceeds bone formation, so that approximately 0.5% of the skeletal mass is lost per year. In women, the decrease in sex steroids at menopause accelerates bone loss (postmenopausal osteoporosis) to about 2% per year. Osteoporosis is usually due to inadequate bone formation

BOX 52-14 Causes of Osteoporosis

Failure to develop normal skeletal mass during growth and development because of poor nutrition or inadequate exercise
Endocrine deficiency or excess
- Estrogen or testosterone deficiency
- Cushing syndrome
- Hyperthyroidism
- Hyperparathyroidism

Immobilization or weightlessness
Hematologic malignancies (multiple myeloma)
Inherited defects of collagen synthesis (osteogenesis imperfecta)
Systemic mastocytosis
Heparin therapy
Rheumatoid arthritis
Idiopathic juvenile osteoporosis

during growth or a pathophysiologic process that impairs osteoblastic bone formation or increases bone resorption. Clinically, osteoporosis is most commonly encountered in postmenopausal women. Advanced age, female gender, and sex steroid deficiency are prominent risk factors. Other risk factors include a family history of osteoporosis, alcohol abuse, smoking, and chronic disease.

After decreased bone mass is documented by bone mass measurements, the diagnostic work-up is directed at determining the cause (Box 52-14). Most often, the cause is attributed to age ("senile" osteoporosis), postmenopausal osteoporosis, or both, but it may be secondary to chronic disease, drug therapy, or other causes. If osteoporosis is inconsistent with age or gender (such as in a middle-aged man or a premenopausal woman), laboratory testing should be performed to exclude other secondary causes of osteoporosis, including hyperthyroidism, Cushing syndrome, hypogonadism, primary hyperparathyroidism, and multiple myeloma. Chronic excess of thyroid hormone, cortisol, or PTH may cause osteoporosis. Long-standing hyperthyroidism or excessive thyroid hormone replacement increases bone resorption to a greater extent than is seen with formation leading to osteoporosis. Cortisol markedly decreases bone formation and causes an increase in bone resorption. Patients with Cushing syndrome may have severe osteoporosis. More commonly, patients receiving glucocorticoid therapy for diseases like asthma and rheumatoid arthritis may have disabling osteoporosis. Hyperparathyroidism occurs most commonly in postmenopausal women and may lead to osteoporosis. Multiple myeloma not uncommonly presents with vertebral crush fracture, and osteoporosis must be considered in these patients.

Bone markers can be used to assess bone turnover in patients with osteoporosis, because the rate of bone turnover (spontaneous or modified by the therapy) is considered an important determinant of bone fragility in postmenopausal and older women.[301] Elevated markers of bone turnover indicate increased bone turnover but are not diagnostic for osteoporosis. Markers for both bone resorption and bone formation can, because of coupling of bone formation and resorption, be useful in monitoring the effects of antiresorptive therapy.[21,301] Teriparatide treatment is best monitored by PINP or osteocalcin, but resorption markers may change later during therapy (see Figure 52-28). International Osteoporosis Foundation and IFCC recommend one bone formation marker (serum PINP) and one bone resorption marker (serum CTX) to be used as reference markers.[323A]

Prevention of osteoporosis is an important goal. Adequate nutrition and exercise during growth allow achievement of optimal bone mass. High calcium intake (1000 to 1500 mg/d), adequate vitamin D (at least 400 to 800 U/d), sufficient protein intake, and a regular exercise program are helpful in maintaining bone mass and preventing osteoporosis.

Treatment of osteoporosis depends on the cause. In secondary osteoporosis, treatment is directed at the underlying condition. Most therapies for the treatment of postmenopausal osteoporosis are directed at decreasing osteoclastic bone resorption. Antiresorptive therapies approved by the U.S. Food and Drug Administration (FDA) in the United States include bisphosphonates (alendronate and risedronate, ibandronate, and zoledronic acid), selective estrogen receptor modulators (raloxifene), and calcitonin (nasal spray or injection). Estrogen is approved for management of menopausal symptoms and has an effect on slowing down early postmenopausal bone loss that appears as robust as that of the bisphosphonates. Recombinant hPTH(1-34), also known as teriparatide, is the only FDA-approved therapy for stimulating bone formation, but strontium ranelate has been approved for this purpose in Europe and in several other countries.

Osteomalacia and Rickets

Osteomalacia and rickets are caused by a mineralization defect that occurs during bone formation, resulting in an increase in osteoid, the unmineralized organic matrix of bone.[185] Defective mineralization produces rickets in children and osteomalacia in adults. Osteomalacia or rickets is usually due to vitamin D deficiency or phosphate depletion.

The causes of decreased 25(OH)D and $1,25(OH)_2D$ are listed in Boxes 52-9 and 52-10, respectively. Vitamin D deficiency may be secondary to dietary deprivation and/or inadequate exposure to sunlight, vitamin D malabsorption, disorders of vitamin D metabolism, or end-organ resistance to the action of vitamin D. In spite of supplementation of milk, bread, and some cereals with vitamin D, vitamin D insufficiency may be more common than was previously thought, in both North America and Europe.[46,186] Breast-fed infants, the elderly, strict vegetarians, and individuals with darker skin pigmentation are at increased risk. Although clinical osteomalacia caused by vitamin D deficiency appears to be uncommon, the prevalence of subclinical or mild osteomalacia in the overall population is unknown. Subclinical osteomalacia may coexist with osteoporosis in elderly patients with poor diets and little exposure to sunlight. It has also been shown that mild to moderate vitamin D deficiency may be associated with reduced muscle strength, impaired physical performance, and falls—all factors contributing to osteoporotic fracture.[185] Vitamin D deficiency may develop in patients with malabsorption caused by postgastrectomy syndrome, small bowel disease (e.g., celiac sprue), hepatobiliary disease, or pancreatic insufficiency.

Vitamin D resistance is rare. Vitamin D–dependent rickets type I is an inherited defect in 25(OH)D-1α-hydroxylase that causes impaired formation of $1,25(OH)_2D$.[185] The disease is manifested in infancy and can be treated with physiologic doses of $1,25(OH)_2D$. Vitamin D–dependent rickets type II is an inherited disorder that is characterized by very high serum concentrations of $1,25(OH)_2D$.[185] This syndrome is caused by resistance to $1,25(OH)_2D$, secondary to defects in the $1,25(OH)_2D$ receptor.

Osteomalacia and rickets may also occur as the result of phosphate depletion. The most common cause of rickets in the United States is hypophosphatemic osteomalacia (also known as *hypophosphatemic vitamin D–resistant rickets* and *vitamin D–resistant rickets*).[260] This disorder is an X-linked dominant inherited trait characterized by renal phosphate wasting. Tubular phosphate wasting can also occur sporadically in adults and as part of Fanconi syndrome. Certain rare mesenchymal tumors may produce a phosphaturic factor (phosphatonin or FGF-23), resulting in renal phosphate wasting and osteomalacia.

In developing countries, dietary calcium deprivation may lead to the clinical picture of rickets, without clear vitamin D or phosphate deficiency.[223]

Drugs have also been associated with osteomalacia. Anticonvulsants increase the hepatic catabolism of vitamin D metabolites and also produce end-organ resistance. Phosphate-binding antacids used for treatment of peptic ulcer disease cause osteomalacia by preventing the intestinal absorption of phosphate. Etidronate treatment (e.g., of Paget disease, osteoporosis, hypercalcemia of malignancy) can cause a mineralization defect, resulting in osteomalacia.

Clinical manifestations of rickets and osteomalacia are a consequence of the defect in mineralization. Rachitic manifestations include bowing of the extremities, short stature, costochondral junction swelling, indentation of the lower ribs, and flattening of the skull. In adults, bone pain is the most common symptom, and stress fractures and frank skeletal fractures may occur. X-rays show classic findings in rickets, such as cupping and fraying of the epiphyseal and diaphyseal ends of the long bone. Pseudofractures are common among adults.

Vitamin D deficiency is diagnosed by measuring serum 25(OH)D (see Table 52-5). Other laboratory findings in rickets and osteomalacia include increased serum ALP, with other alterations in bone and mineral metabolism dependent on the cause and severity of the disorder. ALP is usually increased because of increased osteoblastic activity associated with producing unmineralized osteoid. Calcium may be low-normal or low in vitamin D deficiency, depending on the severity of the disease. Phosphate may be normal or low but falls with the development of secondary hyperparathyroidism. Serum calcium and PTH concentrations are usually normal in renal tubular defects of phosphate transport. Renal phosphate defects can be best assessed through determination of the renal phosphate threshold.

Treatment of rickets and osteomalacia is dictated by the cause of the disorder. Nutritional rickets and osteomalacia are healed by treatment with physiologic doses of vitamin D, whereas higher doses may be required in malabsorption. Adequate dietary intakes of calcium and phosphorus are critical during therapy. Renal phosphate-wasting syndromes require frequent pharmacologic administration of oral phosphorus.

Disorders of Bone and Mineral in Chronic Kidney Disease (Renal Osteodystrophy)

Chronic renal failure is associated with a multitude of disorders of bone and mineral metabolism.[113,145] Renal bone diseases include both high-turnover bone disease (osteitis fibrosa or secondary hyperparathyroidism) and low-turnover bone disease (osteomalacia and adynamic bone disease). Quantitative histomorphometric analysis of bone biopsies, measurement of bone formation by double tetracycline labeling, and special stains are often necessary for correct diagnosis of patients with osteitis fibrosa, osteomalacia, adynamic bone disease, and mixed bone disease of renal osteodystrophy.

Osteitis fibrosa (hyperparathyroid bone disease) is the most common high-turnover bone disease. This disorder is caused by high concentrations of serum PTH in secondary hyperparathyroidism. Secondary hyperparathyroidism is a consequence of the hypocalcemia associated with hyperphosphatemia and $1,25(OH)_2D$ deficiency. Hyperphosphatemia is a result of the inability of the kidneys to excrete phosphate. $1,25(OH)_2D$ deficiency results from the inability of the kidneys to synthesize $1,25(OH)_2D$ because of decreased renal mass and suppression of 25(OH)D-1α-hydroxylase activity by high concentrations of phosphate. Deficiency of $1,25(OH)_2D$ leads to reduced intestinal absorption of calcium and reduced inhibition of PTH secretion by $1,25(OH)_2D$. Skeletal resistance to PTH also contributes to hypocalcemia and secondary hyperparathyroidism.

Low-turnover bone diseases include osteomalacia and adynamic (also known as *aplastic*) bone disease. Osteomalacia and adynamic bone disease are distinguished by the extent of unmineralized bone matrix or osteoid: osteoid is increased in osteomalacia and normal or low in adynamic bone disease. Osteomalacia in chronic renal failure may reflect vitamin D deficiency caused by decreased renal synthesis of $1,25(OH)_2D$ (see "Osteomalacia and Rickets") or aluminum-related disease. In the 1970s and 1980s, aluminum intoxication was a significant contributing factor to the development of osteomalacia and adynamic bone disease. Aluminum intoxication was commonly caused by aluminum contamination of dialysis water and by therapeutic use of oral aluminum-containing antacids to reduce serum phosphate by binding phosphate and preventing its intestinal absorption. The inability of patients with renal failure to excrete aluminum leads to high concentrations in serum (see section on aluminum toxicity in Chapter 48) and deposition in bone, inhibiting bone cell function and bone mineralization. Aluminum-related disease is less common today because of reduced use of aluminum-containing antacids and the use of effective means to decrease the concentrations of aluminum in dialysis water. Other causes of adynamic renal bone disease include calcium supplementation, excessive vitamin D administration, treatment of hyperparathyroidism, advanced age and osteoporosis, diabetes, corticosteroid therapy, and immobilization. Today, oversuppression of parathyroid function (brought about by the use of oral calcium carbonate to control hyperphosphatemia and treatment with vitamin D and dialysate solutions containing high calcium to control hyperparathyroidism) is believed to be the main cause of adynamic renal bone disease.

Amyloid deposition may be noted in bone and in other tissues. It is thought to result from reduced degradation of α_2-microglobulin by the kidneys. The amyloid in renal failure is primarily composed of α_2-microglobulin. The fraction of patients with amyloidosis increases with the duration of dialysis therapy; 70 to 80% of patients have clinical features of amyloidosis after 10 or more years of hemodialysis. Amyloidosis may coexist with high-turnover or low-turnover bone disease.

Bone pain is the most common complaint of patients with renal osteodystrophy. The weight-bearing bones are the site of greatest discomfort, with leg and hip pain and back pain being common. If the patient is a growing child, skeletal deformities may result, with bowing of the extremities, kyphoscoliosis, and slipped femoral epiphyses. Extracellular calcification is also commonly found in periarticular areas, in the medial layer of arteries, and in internal organs (lungs, heart muscle, and other tissue).

The central role of serum PTH in guiding therapy requires that the PTH assay used can be relied on to measure only the active hormone. This is not true for any of the assay generations (see "Parathyroid Hormone, Measurement of PTH"), and kidney disease leads to accumulation of inactive PTH fragments well above the concentrations seen in healthy individuals. Treatment guidelines take this problem into account, but inconsistencies among assays can still lead to situations in which opposite therapeutic decisions could be made for a single patient, depending on the assay used.[292] Studies are clearly needed to test whether modern biomarkers of bone turnover, when used with measurements of circulating PTH concentrations, could more adequately define the type of osteodystrophy.[145]

Biochemical findings in chronic renal failure include hyperphosphatemia and hypocalcemia. The measured concentration of immunoreactive PTH is generally increased, often dramatically, and $1,25(OH)_2D$ is decreased. Serum ALP is increased in patients with hyperparathyroidism or osteomalacia. Because magnesium is cleared by the kidney, modest elevations (2 to 4 mg/dL or 0.08 to 0.16 mmol/L) are common, especially in those taking magnesium-containing antacids.

Early management of renal failure calls for dietary restriction of phosphate and administration of phosphate-binding agents. Calcium supplements added to the diet to prevent secondary hyperparathyroidism may also serve as phosphate binders. Administration of $1,25(OH)_2D$ or other active forms of vitamin D enhances intestinal calcium absorption and may act directly on the parathyroid gland to reduce PTH secretion. Ultimately, dialysis or renal transplantation may be necessary.

Paget Disease of Bone

Paget disease is a localized disease of bone characterized by osteoclastic bone resorption, followed by replacement of bone in a chaotic fashion.[284,285] This disease has a restricted geographic distribution; it is most common in Europe, North America, Australia, and New Zealand in persons of Anglo-Saxon descent—the prevalence may be up to 4% among people older than 40 years—whereas it is extremely uncommon in Asia, Africa, and Scandinavia. Its origin has been linked to genetics, as a family history of Paget disease is reported by 20 to 30% of patients, but also to environmental factors, in particular to a possible viral infection. The disease typically has late onset, spotty involvement, and inclusions that resemble viral nucleocapsids in the nuclei of osteoclasts. An apparent decline in the frequency and severity of the disease has been reported; this change is too rapid to be explained by genetics alone.[59,285]

Paget disease may affect one bone or several bones. Signs and symptoms depend on which skeletal site is affected; the skull, femur, pelvis, and vertebrae are most commonly affected. In most affected individuals in the United States, the disease is diagnosed from radiographs or laboratory tests (ALP) performed for another reason. With more extensive disease, localized bone pain and increased warmth may be noted in or over the affected bone. Advanced disease can produce deformities such as skull enlargement and bowing of the weight-bearing bones (femur and tibia). Complications of deformed bone include arthritic symptoms, nerve compression, deafness, spinal nerve compression, and, in rare cases, osteogenic sarcoma.

Laboratory and other findings include increased markers of bone turnover[278] and abnormal radiographs and bone scans. Radiologic examination demonstrates the characteristic findings of Paget disease: lytic areas in sites of active osteoclastic bone resorption and thickened, expanded, and sclerotic areas in the sites where osteoblasts have formed woven bone. The radioisotopic bone scan is the most sensitive test for detecting small, early lesions. The most common finding leading to the diagnosis of Paget disease is increased serum ALP (up to 10-fold and higher).

Other biochemical markers of bone formation and degradation give information about the pathologic process taking place. Discrepancies have been noted between the formation markers that reflect different phases of the normal osteoblast phenotype: PINP and total and bone ALP all perform similarly,[278] whereas osteocalcin is less consistently elevated. Paget disease leads to a disproportionate increase in serum PINP compared with that of PICP.[279] This finding is yet to be explained.

Increases in biochemical markers of bone resorption reflect the osteoclastic nature of the disease. In untreated Paget disease, the αCTX derived from relatively newly formed collagen, is raised more (16-fold) than the βCTX (threefold), which dominates in diseases with generally increased resorption of normal bone such as hyperparathyroidism or hyperthyroidism.[278]

Bone markers are used in diagnosis and therapeutic monitoring. Total ALP (TALP) is usually sufficient, but in patients with hepatocellular injury, a measurement of bone ALP (BALP) or PINP may be helpful.[285]

Therapy is directed at decreasing osteoclastic bone resorption. Bisphosphonates and calcitonin are effective in decreasing bone pain, serum ALP, and other biochemical markers of bone turnover. Patients occasionally may need surgery for skeletal deformity that limits mobility or for arthritic changes, fractures, or nerve compression.

Involvement of Bone in Malignancies

Bone metastases are the most common skeletal complication of malignancy, occurring in up 70% of patients with advanced breast or prostate cancer, and in 15 to 30% of patients with carcinoma of lung, colon, stomach, bladder, uterus, rectum, thyroid, or kidney.[252] Metastases can have a markedly osteolytic or osteoblastic character, but often they are mixed. Most patients with breast cancer have predominantly osteolytic lesions,[116] but about 15 to 20% of metastases have a predominantly osteoblastic nature. Metastases of prostate cancer are generally regarded as osteoblastic.[117] In most carcinoma metastases, however, both bone degradation and formation take place to some extent. The lesions of multiple myeloma are purely osteolytic; the tumor cells secrete factors that suppress bone formation; generalized osteoporosis is also a feature of the disease (see Box 52-14).[197,253]

Many biochemical bone markers, reflecting bone formation or bone resorption, have been investigated for their potential for early detection or treatment monitoring of bone metastases and myeloma.[276] In addition to localized malignant lesions, generalized osteoporosis can complicate the interpretation of most resorption markers, with the possible exception of ICTP. In multiple myeloma, serum ICTP and urinary NTX are the most sensitive tools for estimating increased bone breakdown and may be clinically useful for identifying patients with increased risk of progression of bone disease.[77,132] Resorption markers [e.g., deoxypyridinoline (DPD)] respond promptly to antiresorptive therapy (e.g., with bisphosphonates) for multiple myeloma,[276] whereas serum ICTP has been reported to predict the overall clinical outcome.[77] TRACP5b activity is increased in various carcinomas with bone involvement,[53,120] but evidence for its clinical value is still quite limited.

In carcinomas with predominantly or partially osteoblastic metastases, bone formation markers such as PINP can help in early detection of skeletal involvement.[160,161,164]

REFERENCES

1. Abernethy MH, Fowler RT. Micellar improvement of the calmagite compleximetric measurement of magnesium in plasma. Clin Chem 1982;28:520-2.
2. Adami S. Calcitonin. In: Rosen CJ, Compston JE, Lian JB, eds. Primer on the metabolic bone diseases and disorders of mineral metabolism, 7th edition. Washington, DC: American Society for Bone and Mineral Research, 2008:250-1.
3. Adams JS, Hewison M. Update in vitamin D. J Clin Endocrinol Metab 2010;95:471-8.
4. Ainola M, Valleala H, Nykänen P, Risteli J, Hanemaaijer R, Konttinen YT. Erosive arthritis in a patient with pycnodysostosis: an experiment of nature. Arthritis Rheum 2008;58:3394-401.
5. Almaden Y, Hernandez A, Torregrosa V, Canalejo A, Sabate L, Fernandez Cruz L, et al. High phosphate level directly stimulates parathyroid hormone secretion and synthesis by human parathyroid tissue in vitro. J Am Soc Nephrol 1998;9:1845-52.
6. Alvarez JC, De Mazancourt P. Rapid and sensitive high-performance liquid chromatographic method for simultaneous determination of retinol, alpha-tocopherol, 25-hydroxyvitamin D3 and 25-hydroxyvitamin D2 in human plasma with photodiode-array ultraviolet detection. J Chromatogr B Biomed Sci Appl 2001;755: 129-35.
7. Anderson HC, Sipe JB, Hessle L, Dhanyamraju R, Atti E, Camacho NP, et al. Impaired calcification around matrix vesicles of growth plate and bone in alkaline phosphatase-deficient mice. Am J Pathol 2004;164:841-7.
8. Anh DJ, Dimai HP, Hall SL, Farley JR. Skeletal alkaline phosphatase activity is primarily released from human osteoblasts in an insoluble form, and the net release is inhibited by calcium and skeletal growth factors. Calcif Tissue Int 1998;62:332-40.
9. Atley LM, Mort JS, Lalumiere M, Eyre DR. Proteolysis of human bone collagen by cathepsin K: characterization of the cleavage sites generating by cross-linked N-telopeptide neoepitope. Bone 2000;26: 241-7.
10. Bailey AJ, Knott L. Molecular changes in bone collagen in osteoporosis and osteoarthritis in the elderly. Exp Gerontol 1999;34: 337-51.
11. Baird GS, Rainey PM, Wener M, Chandler W. Reducing routine ionized calcium measurement. Clin Chem 2009;55:533-40.
12. Baldwin T, Chernow B. Hypocalcemia in the ICU: coping with the causes and consequences. J Crit Illness 1987;2:9-16.
13. Banfi G, Daverio R. In vitro stability of osteocalcin. Clin Chem 1994;40:833-4.
14. Barbour HM, Davidson W. Studies on measurement of plasma magnesium: application of the Magon dye method to the "Monarch" centrifugal analyzer. Clin Chem 1988;34:2103-5.
15. Basuyau JP, Mallet E, Leroy M, Brunelle P. Reference intervals for serum calcitonin in men, women, and children. Clin Chem 2004;50: 1828-30.
16. Beilby J, Randall A, Davis J. Variable citrate interference in arsenazo III dye assays of total calcium in serum. Clin Chem 1990;36:824-5.
17. Ben Rayana MC, Burnett RW, Covington AK, D'Orazio P, Fogh-Andersen N, Jacobs E, et al. IFCC guideline for sampling, measuring and reporting ionized magnesium in plasma. Clin Chem Lab Med 2008;46:21-6.
18. Berth M, Delanghe J. Protein precipitation as a possible important pitfall in the clinical chemistry analysis of blood samples containing monoclonal immunoglobulins: 2 case reports and a review of the literature. Acta Clin Belg 2004;59:263-73.
19. Bieglmayer C, Vierhapper H, Dudczak R, Niederle B. Measurement of calcitonin by immunoassay analyzers. Clin Chem Lab Med 2007; 45:662-6.
20. Bikle D, Adams J, Christakos S. Vitamin D: production metabolism, mechanism of action, and clinical requirements. In: Rosen CJ, Compston JE, Lian JB, eds. Primer on the metabolic bone diseases and disorders of mineral metabolism, 7th edition. Washington, DC: American Society for Bone and Mineral Research, 2008:141-9.

20A. Bilezikian JP, Khan AA, Potts JT. Guidelines for the management of asymptomatic primary hyperparathyroidism: summary statement from the third international workshop. J Endocrinol Metab 2009;94: 335-9.
21. Bilezikian JP, Rubin MR. Monitoring anabolic treatment. In: Seibel MJ, Robins SP, Bilezikian JP, eds. Dynamics of bone and cartilage metabolism, 2nd edition. San Diego, Calif: Academic Press, 2006: 629-47.
22. Birnbaum J, Van Herle AJ. Immunoheterogeneity of parathyroid hormone in parathyroid cysts: diagnostic implications. J Endocrinol Invest 1989;12:831-6.
23. Blumsohn A, Colwell A, Naylor K, Eastell R. Effect of light and gamma-irradiation on pyridinolines and telopeptides of type I collagen in urine. Clin Chem 1995;41:1195-7.
24. Blumsohn A, Hannon RA, Eastell R. Apparent instability of osteocalcin in serum as measured with different commercially available immunoassays. Clin Chem 1995;41:318-9.
25. Boink AB, Buckley BM, Christiansen TF, Covington AK, Maas AH, Muller-Plathe O, et al. IFCC recommendation on sampling, transport and storage for the determination of the concentration of ionized calcium in whole blood, plasma and serum. J Automat Chem 1991; 13:235-9.
26. Bonde M, Qvist P, Fledelius C, Riis BJ, Christiansen C. Immunoassay for quantifying type I collagen degradation products in urine evaluated. Clin Chem 1994;40:2022-5.
27. Boudou P, Ibrahim F, Cormier C, Chabas A, Sarfati E, Souberbielle JC. Third- or second-generation parathyroid hormone assays: a remaining debate in the diagnosis of primary hyperparathyroidism. J Clin Endocrinol Metab 2005;90:6370-2.
28. Bouillon R, Carmeliet G, Verlinden L, van Etten E, Verstuyf A, Luderer HF, et al. Vitamin D and human health: lessons from vitamin D receptor null mice. Endocr Rev 2008;29:726-76.
29. Bouman AA, Scheffer PG, Ooms ME, Lips P, Netelenbos C. Two bone alkaline phosphatase assays compared with osteocalcin as a marker of bone formation in healthy elderly women. Clin Chem 1995;41:196-9.
30. Bowers GN Jr, Brassard C, Sena SF. Measurement of ionized calcium in serum with ion-selective electrodes: a mature technology that can meet the daily service needs. Clin Chem 1986;32:1437-47.
31. Brady JD, Ju J, Robins SP. Isoaspartyl bond formation within N-terminal sequences of collagen type I: implications for their use as markers of collagen degradation. Clin Sci (Lond) 1999;96:209-15.
32. Brandt J, Krogh TN, Jensen CH, Frederiksen JK, Teisner B. Thermal instability of the trimeric structure of the N-terminal propeptide of human procollagen type I in relation to assay technology. Clin Chem 1999;45:47-53.
33. Bringhurst FR. Circulating forms of parathyroid hormone: peeling back the onion. Clin Chem 2003;49:1973-5.
34. Brossard JH, Cloutier M, Roy L, Lepage R, Gascon-Barre M, D'Amour P. Accumulation of a non-(1-84) molecular form of parathyroid hormone (PTH) detected by intact PTH assay in renal failure: importance in the interpretation of PTH values. J Clin Endocrinol Metab 1996;81:3923-9.
35. Brown EM. Ca^{2+}-sensing receptor. In: Rosen CJ, Compston JE, Lian JB, eds. Primer on the metabolic bone diseases and disorders of mineral metabolism, 7th edition. Washington, DC: American Society for Bone and Mineral Research, 2008:134-41.
36. Brown EM. Calcium receptor and regulation of parathyroid hormone secretion. Rev Endocr Metab Disord 2000;1:307-15.
37. Brown JP, Albert C, Nassar BA, Adachi JD, Cole D, Davison KS, et al. Bone turnover markers in the management of postmenopausal osteoporosis. Clin Biochem 2009;42:929-42.
38. Broyles DL, Nielsen RG, Bussett EM, Lu WD, Mizrahi IA, Nunnelly PA, et al. Analytical and clinical performance characteristics of Tandem-MP Ostase, a new immunoassay for serum bone alkaline phosphatase. Clin Chem 1998;44:2139-47.
39. Bucht E, Rong H, Sjöberg HE, Sjöstedt U, Granberg B, Tørring O. Serum calcitonin forms and concentrations in young and elderly healthy females. Calcif Tissue Int 1995;56:32-7.
40. Buckley BM, Russell LJ. The measurement of ionised calcium in blood plasma. Ann Clin Biochem 1988;25(Pt 5):447-65.
41. Burnett RW, Christiansen TF, Covington AK, Fogh-Andersen N, Kulpmann WR, Lewenstam A, et al. IFCC recommended reference method for the determination of the substance concentration of ionized calcium in undiluted serum, plasma or whole blood. Clin Chem Lab Med 2000;38:1301-14.
42. Burnett RW, Covington AK, Fogh-Andersen N, Külpman WR, Maas AH, Müller-Plathe O, et al. Recommendations on whole blood sampling, transport, and storage for simultaneous determination of pH, blood gases, and electrolytes. International Federation of Clinical Chemistry Scientific Division. J Int Fed Clin Chem 1994;6:115-20.
43. Burtis WJ. Parathyroid hormone-related protein: structure, function, and measurement. Clin Chem 1992;38:2171-83.
44. Cali JP, Bowers GN Jr, Young DS. A referee method for the determination of total calcium in serum. Clin Chem 1973;19: 1208-13.
45. Calvo MS, Eastell R, Offord KP, Bergstralh EJ, Burritt MF. Circadian variation in ionized calcium and intact parathyroid hormone: evidence for sex differences in calcium homeostasis. J Clin Endocrinol Metab 1991;72:69-76.
46. Calvo MS, Whiting SJ. Prevalence of vitamin D insufficiency in Canada and the United States: importance to health status and efficacy of current food fortification and dietary supplement use. Nutr Rev 2003;61:107-13.
47. Cao Z, Tongate C, Elin RJ. Evaluation of AVL988/4 analyzer for measurement of ionized magnesium and ionized calcium. Scand J Clin Lab Invest 2001;61:389-94.
48. Cardenas-Rivero N, Chernow B, Stoiko MA, Nussbaum SR, Todres ID. Hypocalcemia in critically ill children. J Pediatr 1989;114:946-51.
49. Carmeliet G, Verstuyf A, Maes C, Eelen G, Bouillon R. The vitamin D hormone and its nuclear receptor: mechanisms involved in bone biology. In: Seibel MJ, Robins SP, Bilezikian JP, eds. Dynamics of bone and cartilage metabolism, 2nd edition. San Diego, Calif: Academic Press, 2006:307-25.
50. Carter AB, Howanitz PJ. Intraoperative testing for parathyroid hormone: a comprehensive review of the use of the assay and the relevant literature. Arch Pathol Lab Med 2003;127:1424-42.
51. Carter GD, Carter CR, Gunter E, Jones J, Jones G, Makin HL, et al. Measurement of vitamin D metabolites: an international perspective on methodology and clinical interpretation. J Steroid Biochem Mol Biol 2004;89-90:467-71.
52. Cecco SA, Hristova EN, Rehak NN, Elin RJ. Clinically important intermethod differences for physiologically abnormal ionized magnesium results. Am J Clin Pathol 1997;108:564-9.
53. Chao TY, Wu YY, Janckila AJ. Tartrate-resistant acid phosphatase isoform 5b (TRACP 5b) as a serum maker for cancer with bone metastasis. Clin Chim Acta 2010;411:1553-64.
54. Clemens JD, Herrick MV, Singer FR, Eyre DR. Evidence that serum NTx (collagen-type I N-telopeptides) can act as an immunochemical marker of bone resorption. Clin Chem 1997;43:2058-63.
55. Clemens TL, Cormier S, Eichinger A, Endlich K, Fiaschi-Taesch N, Fischer E, et al. Parathyroid hormone-related protein and its receptors: nuclear functions and roles in the renal and cardiovascular systems, the placental trophoblasts and the pancreatic islets. Br J Pharmacol 2001;134:1113-36.
56. Clowes JA, Hannon RA, Yap TS, Hoyle NR, Blumsohn A, Eastell R. Effect of feeding on bone turnover markers and its impact on biological variability of measurements. Bone 2002;30:886-90.
57. Colwell A, Eastell R. The renal clearance of free and conjugated pyridinium cross-links of collagen. J Bone Miner Res 1996;11: 1976-80.
58. Confavreux CB, Levine RL, Karsenty G. A paradigm of integrative physiology, the crosstalk between bone and energy metabolisms. Mol Cell Endocrinol 2009;310:21-9.
59. Cooper C, Harvey NC, Dennison EM, van Staa TP. Update on the epidemiology of Paget's disease of bone. J Bone Miner Res 2006; 21(suppl 2):P3-8.

60. Corns CM, Ludman CJ. Some observations on the nature of the calcium-cresolphthalein complex: one reaction and its relevance to the clinical laboratory. Ann Clin Biochem 1987;24:345-51.
61. Cowley DM, Mottram BM, Haling NB, Sinton TJ. Improved linearity of the calcium-cresolphthalein complex one reaction with sodium acetate. Clin Chem 1986;32:894-5.
62. Crofton PM, Evans N, Taylor MR, Holland CV. Procollagen type I amino-terminal propeptide: pediatric reference data and relationship with procollagen type I carboxyl-terminal propeptide. Clin Chem 2004;50:2173-6.
63. Cummings SR, San Martin J, McClung MR, Siris ES, Eastell R, Reid IR, et al. Denosumab for prevention of fractures in postmenopausal women with osteoporosis. N Engl J Med 2009;361:756-65.
64. D'Amour P, Brossard JH, Rousseau L, Roy L, Gao P, Cantor T. Amino-terminal form of parathyroid hormone (PTH) with immunologic similarities to hPTH(1-84) is overproduced in primary and secondary hyperparathyroidism. Clin Chem 2003;49:2037-44.
65. Davidson W, Barbour HM. Determination of urine magnesium using the magon dye method on the "Monarch" centrifugal analyser. Ann Clin Biochem 1990;27:595-6.
66. Davis CD. Vitamin D and cancer: current dilemmas and future research needs. Am J Clin Nutr 2008;88:565S-9S.
67. Delaissé JM, Andersen TL, Engsig MT, Henriksen K, Troen T, Blavier L. Matrix metalloproteinases (MMP) and cathepsin K contribute differently to osteoclastic activities. Microsc Res Tech 2003;61:504-13.
68. Delmas PD. Standardization of bone marker nomenclature. Clin Chem 2001;47:1497.
69. Delmas PD, Christiansen C, Mann KG, Price PA. Bone Gla protein (osteocalcin) assay standardization report. J Bone Miner Res 1990;5:5-11.
70. DeLuca HF. Overview of general physiologic features and functions of vitamin D. Am J Clin Nutr 2004;80:1689S-96S.
71. Dimeski G, Badrick T, John AS. Ion selective electrodes (ISEs) and interferences—a review. Clin Chim Acta 2010;411:309-17.
72. Divieti P, John MR, Juppner H, Bringhurst FR. Human PTH-(7-84) inhibits bone resorption in vitro via actions independent of the type 1 PTH/PTHrP receptor. Endocrinology 2002;143:171-6.
73. Donhowe JM, Freier EF, Wong ET, Steffes MW. Factitious hypophosphatemia related to mannitol therapy. Clin Chem 1981;27:1765-9.
74. Ducy P, Desbois C, Boyce B, Pinero G, Story B, Dunstan C, et al. Increased bone formation in osteocalcin-deficient mice. Nature 1996;382:448-52.
75. Eastell R, Chen P, Saag KG, Burshell AL, Wong M, Warner MR, et al. Bone formation markers in patients with glucocorticoid-induced osteoporosis treated with teriparatide or alendronate. Bone 2010;46:929-34.
76. Eknoyan G, Levin A, Levin NW. Bone metabolism and disease in chronic kidney disease. Am J Kidney Dis 2003;42(suppl):1-201.
77. Elomaa I, Virkkunen P, Risteli L, Risteli J. Serum concentration of the cross-linked carboxyterminal telopeptide of type I collagen (ICTP) is a useful prognostic indicator in multiple myeloma. Br J Cancer 1992;66:337-41.
78. Endres DB, Morgan CH, Garry PJ, Omdahl JL. Age-related changes in serum immunoreactive parathyroid hormone and its biological action in healthy men and women. J Clin Endocrinol Metab 1987;65:724-31.
79. Endres DB, Villanueva R, Sharp CF Jr, Singer FR. Immunochemiluminometric and immunoradiometric determinations of intact and total immunoreactive parathyrin: performance in the differential diagnosis of hypercalcemia and hypoparathyroidism. Clin Chem 1991;37:162-8.
80. Engelbach M, Görges R, Forst T, Pfützner A, Dawood R, Heerdt S, et al. Improved diagnostic methods in the follow-up of medullary thyroid carcinoma by highly specific calcitonin measurements. J Clin Endocrinol Metab 2000;85:1890-4.
81. Eriksen HA, Sharp CA, Robins SP, Sassi ML, Risteli L, Risteli J. Differently cross-linked and uncross-linked carboxy-terminal telopeptides of type I collagen in human mineralised bone. Bone 2004;34:720-7.
82. Fall PM, Kennedy D, Smith JA, Seibel MJ, Raisz LG. Comparison of serum and urine assays for biochemical markers of bone resorption in postmenopausal women with and without hormone replacement therapy and in men. Osteoporos Int 2000;11:481-5.
83. Farley JR, Hall SL, Herring S, Libanati C, Wergedal JE. Reference standards for quantification of skeletal alkaline phosphatase activity in serum by heat inactivation and lectin precipitation. Clin Chem 1993;39:1878-84.
84. Favus MJ, Goltzman D. Regulation of calcium and magnesium. In: Rosen CJ, Compston JE, Lian JB, eds. Primer on the metabolic bone diseases and disorders of mineral metabolism, 7th edition. Washington, DC: American Society for Bone and Mineral Research, 2008:104-8.
85. Fitzpatrick L, Bilezikian JP. Parathyroid hormone: structure, function, and dynamic actions. In: Seibel MJ, Robins SP, Bilezikian JP, eds. Dynamics of bone and cartilage metabolism, 2nd edition. San Diego, Calif: Academic Press, 2006:273-91.
86. Fledelius C, Johnsen AH, Cloos PA, Bonde M, Qvist P. Characterization of urinary degradation products derived from type I collagen: identification of a beta-isomerized Asp-Gly sequence within the C-terminal telopeptide (alpha 1) region. J Biol Chem 1997;272:9755-63.
87. Fleisher M, Gladstone M, Crystal D, Schwartz MK. Two whole-blood multi-analyte analyzers evaluated. Clin Chem 1989;35:1532-5.
88. Fogh-Andersen N, Bjerrum PJ, Siggaard-Andersen O. Ionic binding, net charge, and Donnan effect of human serum albumin as a function of pH. Clin Chem 1993;39:48-52.
89. Foresta C, Strapazzon G, De Toni L, Gianesello L, Calcagno A, Pilon C, et al. Evidence for osteocalcin production by adipose tissue and its role in human metabolism. J Clin Endocrinol Metab 2010;95:3502-6.
90. Fraser CG. The application of theoretical goals based on biological variation data in proficiency testing. Arch Pathol Lab Med 1988;112:404-15.
91. Fraser WD, Robinson J, Lawton R, Durham B, Gallacher SJ, Boyle IT, et al. Clinical and laboratory studies of a new immunoradiometric assay of parathyroid hormone-related protein. Clin Chem 1993;39:414-9.
92. Fritchie K, Zedek D, Grenache DG. The clinical utility of parathyroid hormone-related peptide in the assessment of hypercalcemia. Clin Chim Acta 2009;402:146-9.
93. Fujita T, Kawakami Y, Kohda S, Takata S, Sunahara Y, Arisue K. Assay of magnesium in serum and urine with use of only one enzyme, isocitrate dehydrogenase (NADP+). Clin Chem 1995;41:1302-5.
94. Fukumoto S, Martin TJ. Bone as an endocrine organ. Trends Endocrinol Metab 2009;20:230-6.
95. Gao P, D'Amour P. Evolution of the parathyroid hormone (PTH) assay—importance of circulating PTH immunoheterogeneity and of its regulation. Clin Lab 2005;51:21-9.
96. Gao P, Scheibel S, D'Amour P, John MR, Rao SD, Schmidt-Gayk H, et al. Development of a novel immunoradiometric assay exclusively for biologically active whole parathyroid hormone 1-84: implications for improvement of accurate assessment of parathyroid function. J Bone Miner Res 2001;16:605-14.
97. Garber CC, Miller RC. Revisions of the 1963 semidine HC1 standard method for inorganic phosphorus. Clin Chem 1983;29:184-8.
98. Garnero P, Borel O, Byrjalsen I, Ferreras M, Drake FH, McQueney MS, et al. The collagenolytic activity of cathepsin K is unique among mammalian proteinases. J Biol Chem 1998;273:32347-52.
99. Garnero P, Borel O, Delmas PD. Evaluation of a fully automated serum assay for C-terminal cross-linking telopeptide of type I collagen in osteoporosis. Clin Chem 2001;47:694-702.
100. Garnero P, Ferreras M, Karsdal MA, Nicamhlaoibh R, Risteli J, Borel O, et al. The type I collagen fragments ICTP and CTX reveal distinct enzymatic pathways of bone collagen degradation. J Bone Miner Res 2003;18:859-67.

101. Garnero P, Fledelius C, Gineyts E, Serre CM, Vignot E, Delmas PD. Decreased beta-isomerization of the C-terminal telopeptide of type I collagen alpha 1 chain in Paget's disease of bone. J Bone Miner Res 1997;12:1407-15.
102. Garnero P, Gineyts E, Arbault P, Christiansen C, Delmas PD. Different effects of bisphosphonate and estrogen therapy on free and peptide-bound bone cross-link excretion. J Bone Miner Res 1995;10:641-9.
103. Garnero P, Grimaux M, Seguin P, Delmas PD. Characterization of immunoreactive forms of human osteocalcin generated in vivo and in vitro. J Bone Miner Res 1994;9:255-64.
104. Garnero P, Vergnaud P, Hoyle N. Evaluation of a fully automated serum assay for total N-terminal propeptide of type I collagen in postmenopausal osteoporosis. Clin Chem 2008;54:188-96.
105. Gauci C, Moranne O, Fouqueray B, de la Faille R, Maruani G, Haymann JP, et al. Pitfalls of measuring total blood calcium in patients with CKD. J Am Soc Nephrol 2008;19:1592-8.
106. Gawoski JM, Walsh D. Citrate interference in assays of total calcium in serum. Clin Chem 1989;35:2140-1.
107. Gelb BD, Shi GP, Chapman HA, Desnick RJ. Pycnodysostosis, a lysosomal disease caused by cathepsin K deficiency. Science 1996;273:1236-8.
108. Glover SJ, Eastell R, McCloskey EV, Rogers A, Garnero P, Lowery J, et al. Rapid and robust response of biochemical markers of bone formation to teriparatide therapy. Bone 2009;45:1053-8.
109. Glover SJ, Gall M, Schoenborn-Kellenberger O, Wagener M, Garnero P, Boonen S, et al. Establishing a reference interval for bone turnover markers in 637 healthy, young, premenopausal women from the United Kingdom, France, Belgium, and the United States. J Bone Miner Res 2009;24:389-97.
110. Goltzman D. Interaction of parathyroid hormone-related peptide with the skeleton. In: Seibel MJ, Robins SP, Bilezikian JP, eds. Dynamics of bone and cartilage metabolism, 2nd edition. San Diego, Calif: Academic Press, 2006:293-305.
111. Gomez B Jr, Ardakani S, Evans BJ, Merrell LD, Jenkins DK, Kung VT. Monoclonal antibody assay for free urinary pyridinium cross-links. Clin Chem 1996;42:1168-75.
112. Gomez P, Coca C, Vargas C, Acebillo J, Martinez A. Normal reference-intervals for 20 biochemical variables in healthy infants, children, and adolescents. Clin Chem 1984;30:407-12.
113. Gonzalez EA, Al Aly Z, Martin KJ. Assessment of bone and joint diseases: renal osteodystrophy. In: Seibel MJ, Robins SP, Bilezikian JP, eds. Dynamics of bone and cartilage metabolism, 2nd edition. San Diego, Calif: Academic Press, 2006:755-65.
114. Goodman WG, Jüppner H, Salusky IB, Sherrard DJ. Parathyroid hormone (PTH), PTH-derived peptides, and new PTH assays in renal osteodystrophy. Kidney Int 2003;63:1-11.
115. Gosling P. Analytical reviews in clinical biochemistry: calcium measurement. Ann Clin Biochem 1986;23:146-56.
116. Guise TA. Breaking down bone: new insight into site-specific mechanisms of breast cancer osteolysis mediated by metalloproteinases. Genes Dev 2009;23:2117-23.
117. Guise TA, Mohammad KS, Clines G, Stebbins EG, Wong DH, Higgins LS, et al. Basic mechanisms responsible for osteolytic and osteoblastic bone metastases. Clin Cancer Res 2006;12:6213s-6s.
118. Gundberg CM. Matrix proteins. Osteoporos Int 2003;14(suppl 5):S37-40.
119. Haddad JG. Plasma vitamin D-binding protein (Gc-globulin): multiple tasks. J Steroid Biochem Mol Biol 1995;53:579-82.
120. Halleen JM, Alatalo SL, Janckila AJ, Woitge HW, Seibel MJ, Väänänen HK. Serum tartrate-resistant acid phosphatase 5b is a specific and sensitive marker of bone resorption. Clin Chem 2001;47:597-600.
121. Halleen JM, Alatalo SL, Suominen H, Cheng S, Janckila AJ, Väänänen HK. Tartrate-resistant acid phosphatase 5b: a novel serum marker of bone resorption. J Bone Miner Res 2000;15:1337-45.
122. Halleen JM, Hentunen TA, Karp M, Käkönen SM, Pettersson K, Väänänen HK. Characterization of serum tartrate-resistant acid phosphatase and development of a direct two-site immunoassay. J Bone Miner Res 1998;13:683-7.
123. Halling Linder C, Narisawa S, Millan JL, Magnusson P. Glycosylation differences contribute to distinct catalytic properties among bone alkaline phosphatase isoforms. Bone 2009;45:987-93.
124. Hannon RA, Clowes JA, Eagleton AC, Al Hadari A, Eastell R, Blumsohn A. Clinical performance of immunoreactive tartrate-resistant acid phosphatase isoform 5b as a marker of bone resorption. Bone 2004;34:187-94.
125. Hanson DA, Eyre DR. Molecular site specificity of pyridinoline and pyrrole cross-links in type I collagen of human bone. J Biol Chem 1996;271:26508-16.
126. Hanson DA, Weis MA, Bollen AM, Maslan SL, Singer FR, Eyre DR. A specific immunoassay for monitoring human bone resorption: quantitation of type I collagen cross-linked N-telopeptides in urine. J Bone Miner Res 1992;7:1251-8.
127. Harmey D, Hessle L, Narisawa S, Johnson KA, Terkeltaub R, Millan JL. Concerted regulation of inorganic pyrophosphate and osteopontin by akp2, enpp1, and ank: an integrated model of the pathogenesis of mineralization disorders. Am J Pathol 2004;164:1199-209.
128. Harvey NC, Dennison EM, Cooper C. Epidemiology of osteoporotic fractures. In: Rosen CJ, Compston JE, Lian JB, eds. Primer on the metabolic bone diseases and disorders of mineral metabolism, 7th edition. Washington, DC: American Society for Bone and Mineral Research, 2008:198-203.
129. Haverstick DM, Brill LB 2nd, Scott MG, Bruns DE. Preanalytical variables in measurement of free (ionized) calcium in lithium heparin-containing blood collection tubes. Clin Chim Acta 2009;403:102-4.
130. Heaney RP, Horst RL, Cullen DM, Armas LA. Vitamin D3 distribution and status in the body. J Am Coll Nutr 2009;28:252-6.
131. Heath H 3rd, Earll JM, Schaaf M, Piechocki JT, Li TK. Serum ionized calcium during bed rest in fracture patients and normal men. Metabolism 1972;21:633-40.
132. Heider U, Fleissner C, Zavrski I, Kaiser M, Hecht M, Jakob C, et al. Bone markers in multiple myeloma. Eur J Cancer 2006;42:1544-53.
133. Henriksen K, Tanko LB, Qvist P, Delmas PD, Christiansen C, Karsdal MA. Assessment of osteoclast number and function: application in the development of new and improved treatment modalities for bone diseases. Osteoporos Int 2007;18:681-5.
134. Herrmann M, Seibel MJ. The amino- and carboxyterminal cross-linked telopeptides of collagen type I, NTX-I and CTX-I: a comparative review. Clin Chim Acta 2008;393:57-75.
135. Hessle L, Johnson KA, Anderson HC, Narisawa S, Sali A, Goding JW, et al. Tissue-nonspecific alkaline phosphatase and plasma cell membrane glycoprotein-1 are central antagonistic regulators of bone mineralization. Proc Natl Acad Sci U S A 2002;99:9445-9.
136. Hodsman AB, Bauer DC, Dempster DW, Dian L, Hanley DA, Harris ST, et al. Parathyroid hormone and teriparatide for the treatment of osteoporosis: a review of the evidence and suggested guidelines for its use. Endocr Rev 2005;26:688-703.
136A. Holick MF, Binkley NC, Bischoff-Ferrari HA, Gordon CM, Hanley DA, Heaney RP, et al. Evaluation, treatment, and prevention of vitamin D deficiency: an Endocrine Society clinical practice guideline. J Clin Endocrinol Metab 2011;96:1911-30.
137. Hollis BW. 1,25-Dihydroxyvitamin D3-26,23-lactone interferes in determination of 1,25-dihydroxyvitamin D by RIA after immunoextraction. Clin Chem 1995;41:1313-4.
138. Hollis BW. Assessment of circulating 25(OH)D and 1,25(OH)2D: emergence as clinically important diagnostic tools. Nutr Rev 2007;65:S87-90.
139. Hollis BW. Comparison of commercially available (125)I-based RIA methods for the determination of circulating 25-hydroxyvitamin D. Clin Chem 2000;46:1657-61.
140. Hollis BW. Measuring 25-hydroxyvitamin D in a clinical environment: challenges and needs. Am J Clin Nutr 2008;88:507S-10S.
141. Hollis BW, Kamerud JQ, Kurkowski A, Beaulieu J, Napoli JL. Quantification of circulating 1,25-dihydroxyvitamin D by radioimmunoassay with 125I-labeled tracer. Clin Chem 1996;42:586-92.

142. Hollis BW, Kamerud JQ, Selvaag SR, Lorenz JD, Napoli JL. Determination of vitamin D status by radioimmunoassay with an 125I-labeled tracer. Clin Chem 1993;39:529-33.
143. Horwitz MJ, Hodak SP, Stewart AF. Non-parathyroid hypercalcemia. In: Rosen CJ, Compston JE, Lian JB, eds. Primer on the metabolic bone diseases and disorders of mineral metabolism, 7th edition. Washington, DC: American Society for Bone and Mineral Research, 2008:307-12.
144. Hristova EN, Cecco S, Niemela JE, Rehak NN, Elin RJ. Analyzer-dependent differences in results for ionized calcium, ionized magnesium, sodium, and pH. Clin Chem 1995;41:1649-53.
145. Hruska KA, Mathew S. Chronic kidney disease mineral bone disorder (CKD-MBD). In: Rosen CJ, Compston JE, Lian JB, eds. Primer on the metabolic bone diseases and disorders of mineral metabolism, 7th edition. Washington, DC: American Society for Bone and Mineral Research, 2008:343-9.
146. Huijgen HJ, Sanders R, Cecco SA, Rehak NN, Sanders GT, Elin RJ. Serum ionized magnesium: comparison of results obtained with three ion-selective analyzers. Clin Chem Lab Med 1999;37:465-70.
147. Hyppönen E, Power C. Hypovitaminosis D in British adults at age 45 y: nationwide cohort study of dietary and lifestyle predictors. Am J Clin Nutr 2007;85:860-8.
148. Iqbal SJ, Whittaker P, Bourke J, Mumford R, Huthinson P, Le Van LW. Possible interference with calcipotriol on new IDS RIA for 1,25 dihydroxyvitamin D. Clin Chem 1996;42:112-3.
149. Ivaska KK, Hentunen TA, Vääräniemi J, Ylipahkala H, Pettersson K, Väänänen HK. Release of intact and fragmented osteocalcin molecules from bone matrix during bone resorption in vitro. J Biol Chem 2004;279:18361-9.
150. Jain A, Bhayana S, Vlasschaert M, House A. A formula to predict corrected calcium in haemodialysis patients. Nephrol Dial Transplant 2008;23:2884-8.
151. James IT, Walne AJ, Perrett D. The measurement of pyridinium crosslinks: a methodological overview. Ann Clin Biochem 1996; 33(Pt 5):397-420.
152. James MT, Zhang J, Lyon AW, Hemmelgarn BR. Derivation and internal validation of an equation for albumin-adjusted calcium. BMC Clin Pathol 2008;8:12.
153. Johnson KA, Hessle L, Vaingankar S, Wennberg C, Mauro S, Narisawa S, et al. Osteoblast tissue-nonspecific alkaline phosphatase antagonizes and regulates PC-1. Am J Physiol Regul Integr Comp Physiol 2000; 279:R1365-77.
154. Jukkola A, Tähtelä R, Tholix E, Vuorinen K, Blanco G, Risteli L, et al. Aggressive breast cancer leads to discrepant serum levels of the type I procollagen propeptides PINP and PICP. Cancer Res 1997;57:5517-20.
154A. Jüppner H. Phosphate and FGF-23. Kidney Int 2011;79(Suppl 121): S24–S27.
155. Kamel S, Brazier M, Neri V, Picard C, Samson L, Desmet G, et al. Multiple molecular forms of pyridinoline cross-links excreted in human urine evaluated by chromatographic and immunoassay methods. J Bone Miner Res 1995;10:1385-92.
156. Kang HP, Scott MG, Joe BN, Narra V, Heiken J, Parvin CA. Model for predicting the impact of gadolinium on plasma calcium measured by the o-cresolphthalein method. Clin Chem 2004;50:741-6.
157. Kearns AE, Khosla S, Kostenuik PJ. Receptor activator of nuclear factor kappaB ligand and osteoprotegerin regulation of bone remodeling in health and disease. Endocr Rev 2008;29:155-92.
158. Klein G, Bodenmuller H. Standards required for quantification of skeletal alkaline phosphatase. Clin Chem 1996;42:480-2.
159. Klein GL, Wadlington EL, Collins ED, Catherwood BD, Deftos LJ. Calcitonin levels in sera of infants and children: relations to age and periods of bone growth. Calcif Tissue Int 1984;36:635-8.
160. Klepzig M, Jonas D, Oremek GM. Procollagen type 1 amino-terminal propeptide: a marker for bone metastases in prostate carcinoma. Anticancer Res 2009;29:671-3.
161. Klepzig M, Sauer-Eppel H, Jonas D, Oremek GM. Value of procollagen type 1 amino-terminal propeptide in patients with renal cell carcinoma. Anticancer Res 2008;28:2443-6.
162. Knott L, Bailey AJ. Collagen cross-links in mineralizing tissues: a review of their chemistry, function, and clinical relevance. Bone 1998;22:181-7.
163. Koivula MK, Ruotsalainen V, Björkman M, Nurmenniemi S, Ikäheimo R, Savolainen K, et al. Difference between total and intact assays for N-terminal propeptide of type I procollagen reflects degradation of pN-collagen rather than denaturation of intact propeptide. Ann Clin Biochem 2010;47:67-71.
164. Koopmans N, de Jong IJ, Breeuwsma AJ, van der Veer E. Serum bone turnover markers (PINP and ICTP) for the early detection of bone metastases in patients with prostate cancer: a longitudinal approach. J Urol 2007;178:849-53.
165. Kovacs CS. Fetal calcium metabolism. In: Rosen CJ, Compston JE, Lian JB, eds. Primer on the metabolic bone diseases and disorders of mineral metabolism, 7th edition. Washington, DC: American Society for Bone and Mineral Research, 2008:108-12.
166. Kovacs CS, Kronenberg HM. Maternal-fetal calcium and bone metabolism during pregnancy, puerperium, and lactation. Endocr Rev 1997;18:832-72.
167. Kovacs CS, Kronenberg HM. Pregnancy and lactation. In: Rosen CJ, Compston JE, Lian JB, eds. Primer on the metabolic bone diseases and disorders of mineral metabolism, 7th ed. Washington, DC: American Society for Bone and Mineral Research, 2008:90-5.
168. Kragh-Hansen U, Vorum H. Quantitative analyses of the interaction between calcium ions and human serum albumin. Clin Chem 1993; 39:202-8.
169. Kumar V, Barnidge DR, Chen LS, Twentyman JM, Cradic KW, Grebe SK, et al. Quantification of serum 1-84 parathyroid hormone in patients with hyperparathyroidism by immunocapture in situ digestion liquid chromatography-tandem mass spectrometry. Clin Chem 2010;56:306-13.
170. Kutuzova GD, Akhter S, Christakos S, Vanhooke J, Kimmel-Jehan C, Deluca HF. Calbindin D(9k) knockout mice are indistinguishable from wild-type mice in phenotype and serum calcium level. Proc Natl Acad Sci U S A 2006;103:12377-81.
171. Landt M, Hortin GL, Smith CH, McClellan A, Scott MG. Interference in ionized calcium measurements by heparin salts. Clin Chem 1994; 40:565-70.
172. Larner AJ. Pseudohyperphosphatemia. Clin Biochem 1995;28:391-3.
173. Larsson L, Ohman S. Effect of silicone-separator tubes and storage time on ionized calcium in serum. Clin Chem 1985;31:169-70.
174. Leary NO, Pembroke A, Duggan PF. Single stable reagent (Arsenazo III) for optically robust measurement of calcium in serum and plasma. Clin Chem 1992;38:904-8.
175. Lee AJ, Hodges S, Eastell R. Measurement of osteocalcin. Ann Clin Biochem 2000;37(Pt 4):432-46.
176. Lee NK, Sowa H, Hinoi E, Ferron M, Ahn JD, Confavreux C, et al. Endocrine regulation of energy metabolism by the skeleton. Cell 2007;130:456-69.
177. Leicht E, Biro G. Mechanisms of hypocalcaemia in the clinical form of severe magnesium deficit in the human. Magnes Res 1992;5:37-44.
178. Lensmeyer GL, Binkley N, Drezner MK. New horizons for assessment of vitamin D status in man. In: Seibel MJ, Robins SP, Bilezikian JP, eds. Dynamics of bone and cartilage metabolism, 2nd edition. San Diego, Calif: Academic Press, 2006:513-27.
179. Lepage R, Roy L, Brossard JH, Rousseau L, Dorais C, Lazure C, et al. A non-(1-84) circulating parathyroid hormone (PTH) fragment interferes significantly with intact PTH commercial assay measurements in uremic samples. Clin Chem 1998;44:805-9.
180. Lewenstam A. Design and pitfalls of ion selective electrodes. Scand J Clin Lab Invest Suppl 1994;217:11-9.
181. Lian JB, Stein GS. Development of the osteoblast phenotype: molecular mechanisms mediating osteoblast growth and differentiation. Iowa Orthop J 1995;15:118-40.
182. Liedtke RJ, Kroon G. Automated calmagite compleximetric measurement of magnesium in serum, with sequential addition of EDTA to eliminate endogenous interference. Clin Chem 1984;30: 1801-4.

183. Lips P. Relative value of 25(OH)D and 1,25(OH)2D measurements. J Bone Miner Res 2007;22:1668-71.
184. Lips P. Which circulating level of 25-hydroxyvitamin D is appropriate? J Steroid Biochem Mol Biol 2004;89-90:611-4.
185. Lips P, van Schoor NM, Bravenboer N. Vitamin D-related disorders. In: Rosen CJ, Compston JE, Lian JB, eds. Primer on the metabolic bone diseases and disorders of mineral metabolism, 7th edition. Washington, DC: American Society for Bone and Mineral Research, 2008:329-35.
186. Looker AC, Dawson-Hughes B, Calvo MS, Gunter EW, Sahyoun NR. Serum 25-hydroxyvitamin D status of adolescents and adults in two seasonal subpopulations from NHANES III. Bone 2002;30:771-7.
187. Lopez MF, Rezai T, Sarracino DA, Prakash A, Krastins B, Athanas M, et al. Selected reaction monitoring—mass spectrometric immunoassay responsive to parathyroid hormone and related variants. Clin Chem 2010;56:281-90.
188. Lumachi F, Brunello A, Roma A, Basso U. Cancer-induced hypercalcemia. Anticancer Res 2009;29:1551-5.
189. Lyon ME, Guajardo M, Laha T, Malik S, Henderson PJ, Kenny MA. Electrolyte balanced heparin may produce a bias in the measurement of ionized calcium concentration in specimens with abnormally low protein concentration. Clin Chim Acta 1995;233:105-13.
190. Maeda SS, Fortes EM, Oliveira UM, Borba VC, Lazaretti-Castro M. Hypoparathyroidism and pseudohypoparathyroidism. Arq Bras Endocrinol Metabol 2006;50:664-73.
191. Magnusson P, Arlestig L, Paus E, Di Mauro S, Testa MP, Stigbrand T, et al. Monoclonal antibodies against tissue-nonspecific alkaline phosphatase. Report of the ISOBM TD9 Workshop. Tumour Biol 2002;23:228-48.
192. Magnusson P, Hager A, Larsson L. Serum osteocalcin and bone and liver alkaline phosphatase isoforms in healthy children and adolescents. Pediatr Res 1995;38:955-61.
193. Malluche HH, Mawad H, Trueba D, Monier-Faugere MC. Parathyroid hormone assays–evolution and revolutions in the care of dialysis patients. Clin Nephrol 2003;59:313-8.
193A. Marin L, Koivula MK, Jukkola-Vuorinen A, Leino A, Risteli J. Comparison of total and intact aminoterminal propeptide of type I procollagen assays in patients with breast cancer with or without bone metastases. Ann Clin Biochem 2011 doi: 10.1258.
194. Martin KJ, Gonzalez EA. The evolution of assays for parathyroid hormone. Curr Opin Nephrol Hypertens 2001;10:569-74.
195. Martin MT, Shapiro R. Atomic absorption spectrometry of magnesium. Methods Enzymol 1988;158:365-70.
196. Masters PW, Payne RB. Comparison of hypertonic and isotonic reference electrode junctions for measuring ionized calcium in whole blood: a clinical study. Clin Chem 1993;39:1082-5.
197. Matsumoto T, Abe M. Bone destruction in multiple myeloma. Ann N Y Acad Sci 2006;1068:319-26.
198. Maunsell Z, Wright DJ, Rainbow SJ. Routine isotope-dilution liquid chromatography-tandem mass spectrometry assay for simultaneous measurement of the 25-hydroxy metabolites of vitamins D2 and D3. Clin Chem 2005;51:1683-90.
199. Meier C, Seibel MJ, Kraenzlin ME. Use of bone turnover markers in the real world: are we there yet? J Bone Miner Res 2009;24: 386-8.
200. Melkko J, Hellevik T, Risteli L, Risteli J, Smedsrød B. Clearance of NH2-terminal propeptides of types I and III procollagen is a physiological function of the scavenger receptor in liver endothelial cells. J Exp Med 1994;179:405-12.
201. Melkko J, Kauppila S, Niemi S, Risteli L, Haukipuro K, Jukkola A, et al. Immunoassay for intact amino-terminal propeptide of human type I procollagen. Clin Chem 1996;42:947-54.
202. Melkko J, Niemi S, Risteli L, Risteli J. Radioimmunoassay of the carboxyterminal propeptide of human type I procollagen. Clin Chem 1990;36:1328-32.
203. Merle B, Delmas PD. Normal carboxylation of circulating osteocalcin (bone Gla-protein) in Paget's disease of bone. Bone Miner 1990;11: 237-45.
204. Miller WG, Myers GL, Ashwood ER, Killeen AA, Wang E, Ehlers GW, et al. State of the art in trueness and interlaboratory harmonization for 10 analytes in general clinical chemistry. Arch Pathol Lab Med 2008;132:838-46.
205. Misra M, Pacaud D, Petryk A, Collett-Solberg PF, Kappy M. Vitamin D deficiency in children and its management: review of current knowledge and recommendations. Pediatrics 2008;122:398-417.
206. Mitchell DM, Jüppner H. Regulation of calcium homeostasis and bone metabolism in the fetus and neonate. Curr Opin Endocrinol Diabetes Obes 2010;17:25-30.
207. Mittendorf EA, McHenry CR. Parathyroid carcinoma. J Surg Oncol 2005;89:136-42.
208. Miyauchi A, Matsumoto T, Sugimoto T, Tsujimoto M, Warner MR, Nakamura T. Effects of teriparatide on bone mineral density and bone turnover markers in Japanese subjects with osteoporosis at high risk of fracture in a 24-month clinical study: 12-month, randomized, placebo-controlled, double-blind and 12-month open-label phases. Bone 2010;47:493-502.
209. Monier-Faugere MC, Geng Z, Mawad H, Friedler RM, Gao P, Cantor TL, et al. Improved assessment of bone turnover by the PTH-(1-84)/ large C-PTH fragments ratio in ESRD patients. Kidney Int 2001;60: 1460-8.
210. Murray TM, Rao LG, Divieti P, Bringhurst FR. Parathyroid hormone secretion and action: evidence for discrete receptors for the carboxyl-terminal region and related biological actions of carboxyl-terminal ligands. Endocr Rev 2005;26:78-113.
211. Murshed M, Schinke T, McKee MD, Karsenty G. Extracellular matrix mineralization is regulated locally: different roles of two gla-containing proteins. J Cell Biol 2004;165:625-30.
212. Nakanishi M, Yoh K, Miura T, Ohasi T, Rai SK, Uchida K. Development of a kinetic assay for band 5b tartrate-resistant acid phosphatase activity in serum. Clin Chem 2000;46:469-73.
213. Naveh-Many T. Minireview: the play of proteins on the parathyroid hormone messenger ribonucleic acid regulates its expression. Endocrinology 2010;151:1398-402.
214. NCCLS. Ionized calcium determinations: precollection variables, specimen choice, collection, and handling: approved guideline C31-A2E, 2nd edition. Wayne, Pa: NCCLS, 2001.
215. Neer RM, Arnaud CD, Zanchetta JR, Prince R, Gaich GA, Reginster JY, et al. Effect of parathyroid hormone (1-34) on fractures and bone mineral density in postmenopausal women with osteoporosis. N Engl J Med 2001;344:1434-41.
216. Nguyen-Yamamoto L, Rousseau L, Brossard JH, Lepage R, Gao P, Cantor T, et al. Origin of parathyroid hormone (PTH) fragments detected by intact-PTH assays. Eur J Endocrinol 2002;147:123-31.
217. Nikolakakis NI, De Francisco AM, Rodger RS, Gaiger E, Goodship TH, Ward MK. Effect of storage on measurement of ionized calcium in serum of uremic patients. Clin Chem 1985;31:287-9.
218. Nishi Y, Atley L, Eyre DE, Edelson JG, Superti-Furga A, Yasuda T, et al. Determination of bone markers in pycnodysostosis: effects of cathepsin K deficiency on bone matrix degradation. J Bone Miner Res 1999;14:1902-8.
219. Nissenson RA, Jüppner H. Parathyroid hormone. In: Rosen CJ, Compston JE, Lian JB, eds. Primer on the metabolic bone diseases and disorders of mineral metabolism, 7th edition. Washington, DC: American Society for Bone and Mineral Research, 2008:123-7.
220. Normann PT, Froysa A, Svaland M. Interference of gadodiamide injection (OMNISCAN) on the colorimetric determination of serum calcium. Scand J Clin Lab Invest 1995;55:421-6.
221. Nosjean O, Koyama I, Goseki M, Roux B, Komoda T. Human tissue non-specific alkaline phosphatases: sugar-moiety-induced enzymic and antigenic modulations and genetic aspects. Biochem J 1997; 321(Pt 2):297-303.
222. Oesch U, Ammann D, Simon W. Ion-selective membrane electrodes for clinical use. Clin Chem 1986;32:1448-59.
223. Oginni LM, Sharp CA, Badru OS, Risteli J, Davie MW, Worsfold M. Radiological and biochemical resolution of nutritional rickets with calcium. Arch Dis Child 2003;88:812-7.

224. Ohashi T, Igarashi Y, Mochizuki Y, Miura T, Inaba N, Katayama K, et al. Development of a novel fragment absorbed immunocapture enzyme assay system for tartrate-resistant acid phosphatase 5b. Clin Chim Acta 2007;376:205-12.
225. Orum O, Hansen M, Jensen CH, Sørensen HA, Jensen LB, Hørslev-Petersen K, et al. Procollagen type I N-terminal propeptide (PINP) as an indicator of type I collagen metabolism: ELISA development, reference interval, and hypovitaminosis D induced hyperparathyroidism. Bone 1996;19:157-63.
226. Pandian MR, Morgan CH, Carlton E, Segre GV. Modified immunoradiometric assay of parathyroid hormone-related protein: clinical application in the differential diagnosis of hypercalcemia. Clin Chem 1992;38:282-8.
227. Papazachariou IM, Martinez-Isla A, Efthimiou E, Williamson RC, Girgis SI. Magnesium deficiency in patients with chronic pancreatitis identified by an intravenous loading test. Clin Chim Acta 2000;302:145-54.
228. Partridge NC, Li X, Qin L. Understanding parathyroid hormone action. Ann N Y Acad Sci 2006;1068:187-93.
229. Payne RB, Jones DP. Protein interferes with ionised calcium measurement at the reference electrode liquid junction. Ann Clin Biochem 1987;24(Pt 4):400-7.
230. Peretz A, Moris M, Willems D, Bergmann P. Is bone alkaline phosphatase an adequate marker of bone metabolism during acute corticosteroid treatment? Clin Chem 1996;42:102-3.
231. Poupon-Fleuret C, Chapuis-Cellier C. Monoclonal immunoglobulin interferences in measurement of serum inorganic phosphate with a new modified reagent. Clin Chem 1996;42:1298-300.
232. Prentice A, Goldberg GR, Schoenmakers I. Vitamin D across the lifecycle: physiology and biomarkers. Am J Clin Nutr 2008;88:500S-6S.
233. Price CP, Kirwan A, Vader C. Tartrate-resistant acid phosphatase as a marker of bone resorption. Clin Chem 1995;41:641-3.
234. Price CP, Milligan TP, Darte C. Direct comparison of performance characteristics of two immunoassays for bone isoform of alkaline phosphatase in serum. Clin Chem 1997;43:2052-7.
235. Price PA, Nishimoto SK. Radioimmunoassay for the vitamin K-dependent protein of bone and its discovery in plasma. Proc Natl Acad Sci U S A 1980;77:2234-8.
236. Pybus J, Feldman FJ, Bowers GN Jr. Measurement of total calcium in serum by atomic absorption spectrophotometry, with use of a strontium internal reference. Clin Chem 1970;16:998-1007.
237. Qvist P, Christgau S, Pedersen BJ, Schlemmer A, Christiansen C. Circadian variation in the serum concentration of C-terminal telopeptide of type I collagen (serum CTx): effects of gender, age, menopausal status, posture, daylight, serum cortisol, and fasting. Bone 2002;31:57-61.
238. Raisz LG. Pathogenesis of osteoporosis: concepts, conflicts, and prospects. J Clin Invest 2005;115:3318-25.
239. Ramasamy I. Recent advances in physiological calcium homeostasis. Clin Chem Lab Med 2006;44:237-73.
240. Ratcliffe WA, Norbury S, Stott RA, Heath DA, Ratcliffe JG. Immunoreactivity of plasma parathyrin-related peptide: three region-specific radioimmunoassays and a two-site immunoradiometric assay compared. Clin Chem 1991;37:1781-7.
241. Rauchenzauner M, Schmid A, Heinz-Erian P, Kapelari K, Falkensammer G, Griesmacher A, et al. Sex- and age-specific reference curves for serum markers of bone turnover in healthy children from 2 months to 18 years. J Clin Endocrinol Metab 2007;92:443-9.
242. Rayana MC, Burnett RW, Covington AK, D'Orazio P, Fogh-Andersen N, Jacobs E, et al. Guidelines for sampling, measuring and reporting ionized magnesium in undiluted serum, plasma or blood. International Federation of Clinical Chemistry and Laboratory Medicine (IFCC): IFCC Scientific Division, Committee on Point of Care Testing. Clin Chem Lab Med 2005;43:564-9.
243. Rehak NN, Cecco SA, Niemela JE, Hristova EN, Elin RJ. Linearity and stability of the AVL and Nova magnesium and calcium ion-selective electrodes. Clin Chem 1996;42:880-7.
244. Reichel H, Esser A, Roth HJ, Schmidt-Gayk H. Influence of PTH assay methodology on differential diagnosis of renal bone disease. Nephrol Dial Transplant 2003;18:759-68.
245. Renoe BW, McDonald JM, Ladenson JH. The effects of stasis with and without exercise on free calcium, various cations, and related parameters. Clin Chim Acta 1980;103:91-100.
246. Risteli J, Elomaa I, Niemi S, Novamo A, Risteli L. Radioimmunoassay for the pyridinoline cross-linked carboxy-terminal telopeptide of type I collagen: a new serum marker of bone collagen degradation. Clin Chem 1993;39:635-40.
247. Risteli J, Risteli L. Products of bone collagen metabolism. In: Seibel MJ, Robins SP, Bilezikian JP, eds. Dynamics of bone and cartilage metabolism, 2nd edition. San Diego, Calif: Academic Press, 2006: 391-405.
248. Risteli J, Risteli L. Serum-based test of the pathologic breakdown of type I collagen fibers. Clin Chem 2009;55:1032-3.
249. Rizzoli R, Bonjour J-P. Physiology of calcium and phosphate homeostasis. In: Seibel MJ, Robins SP, Bilezikian JP, eds. Dynamics of bone and cartilage metabolism, 2nd edition. San Diego, Calif: Academic Press, 2006:345-60.
250. Robins SP, Duncan A, Wilson N, Evans BJ. Standardization of pyridinium crosslinks, pyridinoline and deoxypyridinoline, for use as biochemical markers of collagen degradation. Clin Chem 1996;42: 1621-6.
251. Robins SP, Woitge H, Hesley R, Ju J, Seyedin S, Seibel MJ. Direct, enzyme-linked immunoassay for urinary deoxypyridinoline as a specific marker for measuring bone resorption. J Bone Miner Res 1994;9:1643-9.
252. Roodman GD. Mechanisms of bone metastasis. N Engl J Med 2004; 350:1655-64.
253. Roodman GD. Osteoblast function in myeloma. Bone 2011;48: 135-40.
254. Rosenquist C, Fledelius C, Christgau S, Pedersen BJ, Bonde M, Qvist P, et al. Serum CrossLaps One Step ELISA: first application of monoclonal antibodies for measurement in serum of bone-related degradation products from C-terminal telopeptides of type I collagen. Clin Chem 1998;44:2281-9.
255. Rosenquist C, Qvist P, Bjarnason N, Christiansen C. Measurement of a more stable region of osteocalcin in serum by ELISA with two monoclonal antibodies. Clin Chem 1995;41:1439-45.
256. Rubinacci A, Melzi R, Zampino M, Soldarini A, Villa I. Total and free deoxypyridinoline after acute osteoclast activity inhibition. Clin Chem 1999;45:1510-6.
257. Rude RK. Magnesium deficiency: a cause of heterogeneous disease in humans. J Bone Miner Res 1998;13:749-58.
258. Rude RK. Magnesium depletion and hypermagnesemia. In: Rosen CJ, Compston JE, Lian JB, eds. Primer on the metabolic bone diseases and disorders of mineral metabolism, 7th edition. Washington, DC: American Society for Bone and Mineral Research, 2008:325-8.
259. Rude RK, Singer FR, Gruber HE. Skeletal and hormonal effects of magnesium deficiency. J Am Coll Nutr 2009;28:131-41.
260. Ruppe M, Jan de Beur S. Disorders of phosphate homeostasis. In: Rosen CJ, Compston JE, Lian JB, eds. Primer on the metabolic bone diseases and disorders of mineral metabolism, 7th edition. Washington, DC: American Society for Bone and Mineral Research, 2008:317-25.
261. Russwurm S, Reinhart K. Procalcitonin mode of action: new pieces in a complex puzzle. Crit Care Med 2004;32:1801-2.
262. Saag KG, Shane E, Boonen S, Marin F, Donley DW, Taylor KA, et al. Teriparatide or alendronate in glucocorticoid-induced osteoporosis. N Engl J Med 2007;357:2028-39.
263. Sachs C, Chaneac M, Rabouine P, Kindermans C, Dechaux M. Inadequate algorithm: a cause for 'incorrect pH 7.40 correction' in ionized calcium analysers. Scand J Clin Lab Invest 1989;49:561-5.
264. Saggese G, Baroncelli GI, Bertelloni S. Determination of intact parathyrin by immunoradiometric assay evaluated in normal children and in patients with various disorders of calcium metabolism. Clin Chem 1991;37:1999-2001.

265. Saito M, Marumo K. Collagen cross-links as a determinant of bone quality: a possible explanation for bone fragility in aging, osteoporosis, and diabetes mellitus. Osteoporos Int 2010;21:195-214.
266. Sanders GT, Huijgen HJ, Sanders R. Magnesium in disease: a review with special emphasis on the serum ionized magnesium. Clin Chem Lab Med 1999;37:1011-33.
267. Saris NE, Mervaala E, Karppanen H, Khawaja JA, Lewenstam A. Magnesium: an update on physiological, clinical and analytical aspects. Clin Chim Acta 2000;294:1-26.
268. Sassi ML, Åman S, Hakala M, Luukkainen R, Risteli J. Assay for cross-linked carboxyterminal telopeptide of type I collagen (ICTP) unlike CrossLaps assay reflects increased pathological degradation of type I collagen in rheumatoid arthritis. Clin Chem Lab Med 2003;41: 1038-44.
269. Sassi ML, Eriksen H, Risteli L, Niemi S, Mansell J, Gowen M, et al. Immunochemical characterization of assay for carboxyterminal telopeptide of human type I collagen: loss of antigenicity by treatment with cathepsin K. Bone 2000;26:367-73.
270. Savory J, Margrey KS, Shipe JR Jr, Savory MG, Margrey MH, Mifflin TE, et al. Stabilization of the calmagite reagent for automated measurement of magnesium in serum and urine. Clin Chem 1985;31: 487-8.
270A. Schlingmann KP, Kaufmann M, Weber S, Irwin A, Goos C, John U, et al. Mutations in *CYP24A1* and idiopathic infantile hypercalcemia. N Engl J Med 2011;365:410-21.
271. Schluter KD. PTH and PTHrP: similar structures but different functions. News Physiol Sci 1999;14:243-9.
272. Schmidt-Gayk H. Measurement of calcium, phosphate and magnesium. In: Seibel MJ, Robins SP, Bilezikian JP, eds. Dynamics of bone and cartilage metabolism, 2nd edition. San Diego, Calif: Academic Press, 2006:487-505.
273. Schwalfenberg GK, Genuis SJ, Hiltz MN. Addressing vitamin D deficiency in Canada: a public health innovation whose time has come. Public Health 2010;124:350-9.
274. Schytte S, Hansen M, Møller S, Junker P, Henriksen JH, Hillingso J, et al. Hepatic and renal extraction of circulating type I procollagen aminopropeptide in patients with normal liver function and in patients with alcoholic cirrhosis. Scand J Clin Lab Invest 1999;59:627-33.
275. Seibel MJ. Biochemical markers of bone turnover part II: clinical applications in the management of osteoporosis. Clin Biochem Rev 2006;27:123-38.
276. Seibel MJ. Clinical use of markers of bone turnover in metastatic bone disease. Nat Clin Pract Oncol 2005;2:504-17.
277. Sena SF, Bowers GN Jr. Measurement of ionized calcium in biological fluids: ion-selective electrode method. Methods Enzymol 1988;158: 320-34.
278. Shankar S, Hosking DJ. Biochemical assessment of Paget's disease of bone. J Bone Miner Res 2006;21(suppl 2):P22-7.
279. Sharp CA, Davie MW, Worsfold M, Risteli L, Risteli J. Discrepant blood concentrations of type I procollagen propeptides in active Paget disease of bone. Clin Chem 1996;42:1121-2.
280. Sharp CA, Linder C, Magnusson P. Analysis of human bone alkaline phosphatase isoforms: comparison of isoelectric focusing and ion-exchange high-performance liquid chromatography. Clin Chim Acta 2007;379:105-12.
281. Sherman SS, Hollis BW, Tobin JD. Vitamin D status and related parameters in a healthy population: the effects of age, sex, and season. J Clin Endocrinol Metab 1990;71:405-13.
282. Silverberg SJ, Bilezikian JP. Primary hyperparathyroidism. In: Seibel MJ, Robins SP, Bilezikian JP, eds. Dynamics of bone and cartilage metabolism, 2nd edition. San Diego, Calif: Academic Press, 2006: 767-77.
283. Silverberg SJ, Gao P, Brown I, LoGerfo P, Cantor TL, Bilezikian JP. Clinical utility of an immunoradiometric assay for parathyroid hormone (1-84) in primary hyperparathyroidism. J Clin Endocrinol Metab 2003;88:4725-30.
283A. Singh RJ, Taylor RL, Reddy GS, Grebe SK. C3-epimers can account for a significant proportion of total circulating 25-hydroxyvitamin D in infants, complicating accurate measurement and interpretation of vitamin D status. J Clin Endocrinol Metab 2006;91:3055-61.
284. Siris ES. Paget's disease of bone. J Bone Miner Res 1998;13:1061-5.
285. Siris ES, Roodman GD. Paget's disease of bone. In: Rosen CJ, Compston JE, Lian JB, eds. Primer on the metabolic bone diseases and disorders of mineral metabolism, 7th edition. Washington, DC: American Society for Bone and Mineral Research, 2008:335-43.
286. Slatopolsky E, Finch J, Clay P, Martin D, Sicard G, Singer G, et al. A novel mechanism for skeletal resistance in uremia. Kidney Int 2000;58:753-61.
287. Smedsrød B, Melkko J, Risteli L, Risteli J. Circulating C-terminal propeptide of type I procollagen is cleared mainly via the mannose receptor in liver endothelial cells. Biochem J 1990;271:345-50.
288. Snellman G, Melhus H, Gedeborg R, Byberg L, Berglund L, Wernroth L, et al. Determining vitamin D status: a comparison between commercially available assays. PLoS One 2010;5:e11555.
289. Sokoll LJ, O'Brien ME, Camilo ME, Sadowski JA. Undercarboxylated osteocalcin and development of a method to determine vitamin K status. Clin Chem 1995;41:1121-8.
290. Sokoll LJ, Wians FH Jr, Remaley AT. Rapid intraoperative immunoassay of parathyroid hormone and other hormones: a new paradigm for point-of-care testing. Clin Chem 2004;50:1126-35.
291. Sorva A, Tähtelä R, Risteli J, Risteli L, Laitinen K, Juntunen-Backman K, et al. Familial high serum concentrations of the carboxyl-terminal propeptide of type I procollagen. Clin Chem 1994;40:1591-3.
292. Souberbielle JC, Boutten A, Carlier MC, Chevenne D, Coumaros G, Lawson-Body E, et al. Inter-method variability in PTH measurement: implication for the care of CKD patients. Kidney Int 2006;70:345-50.
293. Standing Committee on the Scientific Evaluation of Dietary Reference Intakes, FaNB, Institute of Medicine. Dietary reference intakes for calcium, phosphorus, magnesium, vitamin D, and fluoride. Washington, DC: National Academies Press, 1997.
294. Stewart AF. Clinical practice: hypercalcemia associated with cancer. N Engl J Med 2005;352:373-9.
295. Stewart AF, Adler M, Byers CM, Segre GV, Broadus AE. Calcium homeostasis in immobilization: an example of resorptive hypercalciuria. N Engl J Med 1982;306:1136-40.
296. Stone MJ, Chowdrey PE, Miall P, Price CP. Validation of an enzymatic total magnesium determination based on activation of modified isocitrate dehydrogenase. Clin Chem 1996;42:1474-7.
297. Strewler GJ. The parathyroid hormone-related protein. Endocrinol Metab Clin North Am 2000;29:629-45.
298. Strewler GJ. The physiology of parathyroid hormone-related protein. N Engl J Med 2000;342:177-85.
299. Suvanto-Luukkonen E, Risteli L, Sundström H, Penttinen J, Kauppila A, Risteli J. Comparison of three serum assays for bone collagen formation during postmenopausal estrogen-progestin therapy. Clin Chim Acta 1997;266:105-16.
300. Swanson JR, Heeter C, Limbocker M, Sullivan M. Bias of ionized calcium results from blood gas syringes. Clin Chem 1994;40:669-70.
301. Szulc P, Delmas P. Biochemical markers of bone turnover in osteoporosis. In: Rosen CJ, Compston JE, Lian JB, eds. Primer on the metabolic bone diseases and disorders of mineral metabolism, 7th edition. Washington, DC: American Society for Bone and Mineral Research, 2008:174-9.
302. Tabata M, Kido T, Totani M, Murachi T. Direct spectrophotometry of magnesium in serum after reaction with hexokinase and glucose-6-phosphate dehydrogenase. Clin Chem 1985;31:703-5.
303. Tähtelä R, Turpeinen M, Sorva R, Karonen SL. The aminoterminal propeptide of type I procollagen: evaluation of a commercial radioimmunoassay kit and values in healthy subjects. Clin Biochem 1997;30:35-40.
304. Takeda S, Karsenty G. Molecular bases of the sympathetic regulation of bone mass. Bone 2008;42:837-40.
305. Takeda S, Karsenty G. Molecular bases of the sympathetic regulation of bone mass. Bone 2008;42:837-40.
306. Thode J. Actual ionized calcium and pH in blood collected in capillary or evacuated tubes. Scand J Clin Lab Invest 1986;46:89-93.

307. Thode J, Fogh-Andersen N, Aas F, Siggaard-Andersen O. Sampling and storage of blood for determination of ionized calcium. Scand J Clin Lab Invest 1985;45:131-8.
308. Thode J, Holmegaard SN, Transbol I, Fogh-Andersen N, Siggaard-Andersen O. Adjusted ionized calcium (at pH 7.4) and actual ionized calcium (at actual pH) in capillary blood compared for clinical evaluation of patients with disorders of calcium metabolism. Clin Chem 1990;36:541-4.
309. Thode J, Juul-Jorgensen B, Bhatia HM, Kjaerulf-Nielsen M, Bartels PD, Fogh-Andersen N, et al. Comparison of serum total calcium, albumin-corrected total calcium, and ionized calcium in 1213 patients with suspected calcium disorders. Scand J Clin Lab Invest 1989;49: 217-23.
310. Thuvasethakul P, Wajjwalku W. Serum magnesium determined by use of methylthymol blue. Clin Chem 1987;33:614-5.
311. Toffaletti J. Use of novel preparations of heparin to eliminate interference in ionized calcium measurements: have all the problems been solved? Clin Chem 1994;40:508-9.
312. Toffaletti J, Abrams B, Bird C, Schwing M. Clinical validation of an automated thin-film reflectance method for measurement of magnesium in serum and urine. Magnesium 1988;7:84-90.
313. Toffaletti J, Blosser N, Kirvan K. Effects of storage temperature and time before centrifugation on ionized calcium in blood collected in plain vacutainer tubes and silicone-separator (SST) tubes. Clin Chem 1984;30:553-6.
314. Toffaletti J, Ernst P, Hunt P, Abrams B. Dry electrolyte-balanced heparinized syringes evaluated for determining ionized calcium and other electrolytes in whole blood. Clin Chem 1991;37:1730-3.
315. Toffaletti J, Lee KM. Preparation and use of serum-based material as control and calibrator in evaluating ion-selective electrodes for calcium. Clin Chem 1985;31:1349-52.
316. Toffaletti J, Thompson T. Effects of blended lithium-zinc heparin on ionized calcium and general clinical chemistry tests. Clin Chem 1995;41:328-9.
317. Toivonen J, Tähtelä R, Laitinen K, Risteli J, Välimäki MJ. Markers of bone turnover in patients with differentiated thyroid cancer with and following withdrawal of thyroxine suppressive therapy. Eur J Endocrinol 1998;138:667-73.
318. Tommasi M, Raspanti S. Comparison of calcitonin determinations by polyclonal and monoclonal IRMAs. Clin Chem 2007;53:798-9.
319. Tommasi M, Raspanti S. Hook effect in calcitonin immunoradiometric assay. Clin Chem Lab Med 2007;45:1073-4.
320. Tong GM, Rude RK. Magnesium deficiency in critical illness. J Intensive Care Med 2005;20:3-17.
321. Torres PU. The need for reliable serum parathyroid hormone measurements. Kidney Int 2006;70:240-3.
322. Truong NU, deB Edwardes MD, Papavasiliou V, Goltzman D, Kremer R. Parathyroid hormone-related peptide and survival of patients with cancer and hypercalcemia. Am J Med 2003;115: 115-21.
323. Turpeinen U, Hohenthal U, Stenman UH. Determination of 25-hydroxyvitamin D in serum by HPLC and immunoassay. Clin Chem 2003;49:1521-4.
323A. Vasikaran S, Cooper C, Eastell R, Griesmacher A, Morris HA, Trenti T, et al. International Osteoporosis Foundation and International Federation of Clinical Chemisrty and Laboratory Medicine position on bone marker standards in osteoporosis. Clin Chem Lab Med 2011; May 24 [Epub ahead of print].
324. Vergnaud P, Garnero P, Meunier PJ, Breart G, Kamihagi K, Delmas PD. Undercarboxylated osteocalcin measured with a specific immunoassay predicts hip fracture in elderly women: the EPIDOS Study. J Clin Endocrinol Metab 1997;82:719-24.
325. Vieira JG, Kunii I, Nishida S. Evolution of PTH assays. Arq Bras Endocrinol Metabol 2006;50:621-7.
326. Vogeser M, Kyriatsoulis A, Huber E, Kobold U. Candidate reference method for the quantification of circulating 25-hydroxyvitamin D3 by liquid chromatography-tandem mass spectrometry. Clin Chem 2004; 50:1415-7.
327. Wacker WE. Measurement of magnesium in human tissues and fluids: a historical perspective. Magnesium 1987;6:61-4.
328. Walton RJ, Bijvoet OL. Nomogram for derivation of renal threshold phosphate concentration. Lancet 1975;2:309-10.
329. Wandrup J. Critical analytical and clinical aspects of ionized calcium in neonates. Clin Chem 1989;35:2027-33.
330. Wandrup J, Kancir C, Hyltoft Petersen P. Ionized calcium and acid-base status in arterial and venous whole blood during general anaesthesia. Scand J Clin Lab Invest 1988;48:115-22.
331. Wang S, McDonnell EH, Sedor FA, Toffaletti JG. pH effects on measurements of ionized calcium and ionized magnesium in blood. Arch Pathol Lab Med 2002;126:947-50.
332. Weisinger JR, Bellorin-Font E. Magnesium and phosphorus. Lancet 1998;352:391-6.
333. Welch MW, Hamar DW, Fettman MJ. Method comparison for calcium determination by flame atomic absorption spectrophotometry in the presence of phosphate. Clin Chem 1990;36:351-4.
334. Wennberg C, Hessle L, Lundberg P, Mauro S, Narisawa S, Lerner UH, et al. Functional characterization of osteoblasts and osteoclasts from alkaline phosphatase knockout mice. J Bone Miner Res 2000;15: 1879-88.
335. Wilhite TR, Smith CH, Landt M. Interference of zinc heparin anticoagulant in determination of plasma magnesium. Clin Chem 1994;40:848-9.
336. Wills MR, Sunderman FW, Savory J. Methods for the estimation of serum magnesium in clinical laboratories. Magnesium 1986;5:317-27.
337. Woodrow JP, Sharpe CJ, Fudge NJ, Hoff AO, Gagel RF, Kovacs CS. Calcitonin plays a critical role in regulating skeletal mineral metabolism during lactation. Endocrinology 2006;147:4010-21.
338. Wysolmerski JJ. Parathyroid hormone-related protein. In: Rosen CJ, Compston JE, Lian JB, eds. Primer on the metabolic bone diseases and disorders of mineral metabolism, 7th edition. Washington, DC: American Society for Bone and Mineral Research, 2008:127-33.
339. Yamashita H, Gao P, Noguchi S, Cantor T, Uchino S, Watanabe S, et al. Role of cyclase activating parathyroid hormone (1-84 PTH) measurements during parathyroid surgery: potential improvement of intraoperative PTH assay. Ann Surg 2002;236:105-11.
340. Ylipahkala H, Fagerlund KM, Janckila AJ, Houston B, Laurie D, Halleen JM. Specificity and clinical performance of two commercial TRACP 5b immunoassays. Clin Lab 2009;55:223-8.
341. Zaloga GP, Chernow B. Hypocalcemia in critical illness. JAMA 1986;256:1924-9.
342. Zidehsarai MP, Moe SM. Review article: chronic kidney disease-mineral bone disorder: have we got the assays right? Nephrology (Carlton) 2009;14:374-82.

ADDITIONAL READING

Bilezikian JP, Marcus R, Levine MA. The parathyroids: basic and clinical concepts, 2nd edition. San Diego, Calif: Academic Press, 2001.
Rosen C, Compston J, Lian JB, eds. Primer on the metabolic bone diseases and disorders of mineral metabolism, 7th edition. Washington, DC: American Society for Bone and Mineral Research, 2008.
Seibel MJ, Robins SP, Bilezikian JP, eds. Dynamics of bone and cartilage metabolism: principles and clinical applications, 2nd edition. San Diego, Calif: Academic Press, 2006.

CHAPTER 53

Pituitary Function and Pathophysiology

*William E. Winter, M.D., Ishwarlal Jialal, M.D., Ph.D., F.R.C.Path(London), D.A.B.C.C., Mary Lee Vance, M.D., and Roger L. Bertholf, Ph.D.**

The pituitary gland (also called the *hypophysis*) regulates the endocrine system by integrating chemical signals from the brain with feedback from the concentration of circulating hormones to stimulate intermittent hormone release from target endocrine glands.[115,156] The pituitary clearly serves as the master gland in maintaining homeostasis by orchestrating the many processes necessary for survival of the individual, as well as for survival of the species.

The hypophysis is composed of the adenohypophysis (the anterior lobe of the pituitary; ≈75% of the mass of the pituitary) and the neurohypophysis (the posterior lobe of the pituitary, ≈25% of the mass of the pituitary; also called the pars nervosa) (Figure 53-1).[10] In turn, the adenohypophysis has three parts: (1) the pars distalis, where most hormone-producing cells are located; (2) the pars tuberalis, which is part of the hypophyseal stalk; and (3) the pars intermedia. The pars intermedia may be referred to as the intermediate lobe of the pituitary, although it is really part of the adenohypophysis.

The biology of the adenohypophysis is distinctly different from that of the neurohypophysis: the adenohypophysis is controlled by the hypothalamus via releasing or inhibiting hormones, whereas the cell bodies of the neurohypophysis are anatomically located in hypothalamic nuclei, with oxytocin or antidiuretic hormone (ADH) reaching the neurohypophysis through neurohypophyseal nerve axons.[96] Thus the neurohypophysis is not a discrete endocrine organ, but rather functions as a reservoir for these two hormones.

The roles of the various hormones secreted by the pituitary are exceedingly diverse and include regulation of (1) the body's response to stress [adrenocorticotropic hormone (ACTH, or corticotropin) and growth hormone (GH)], (2) the metabolic rate [thyroid-stimulating hormone (TSH, or thyrotropin)], (3) growth (TSH and GH), (4) reproduction [luteinizing hormone (LH) and follicle-stimulating hormone (FSH)], (5) nourishment for the newborn and infant (prolactin), (6) parturition and milk let-down during breast feeding (oxytocin), and (7) fluid balance (ADH, or vasopressin). Some of the pituitary hormones have specific targets (e.g., ACTH, TSH, LH, or FSH), whereas other hormones have multiple targets (e.g., GH, prolactin, oxytocin, and ADH).

A newly recognized product of the pituitary gland detected in some perimenopausal and postmenopausal women is human chorionic gonadotropin (hCG).[185] Usually, hCG is associated with pregnancy or gestational trophoblastic disease. In early pregnancy, hCG doubles approximately every 48 hours, whereas the concentration of hCG from pituitary or gestational trophoblastic disease origin is relatively stable and does not increase in the pattern seen in pregnancy. If an elevated hCG of 5 to 14 IU/L is detected in a postmenopausal woman, it is likely to be of pituitary origin if (1) the FSH is elevated (>45 IU/L), (2) the hCG is suppressed after 2 weeks of estrogen replacement, and (3) gestational trophoblastic disease has been excluded.

The placenta produces several hormones that are similar to pituitary hormones: hCG has functional and structural similarity to LH; human placental lactogen (hPL, or somatomammotropin) has actions similar to prolactin and GH; placental GH becomes the predominant maternal GH during gestation; and placental corticotropin-releasing hormone (CRH) concentration rises in the fetus throughout gestation.[131] Placental GH (GH-V) differs from pituitary GH in 13 of 191 amino acids. Furthermore, GH-V exists in glycosylated and nonglycosylated forms, whereas pituitary GH is not glycosylated. The site of glycosylation in GH-V is asparagine at residue 140.

ANATOMY

The pituitary is located at the base of the brain and is protected anteriorly, inferiorly, and posteriorly by the bony sella turcica. Inferior and anterior to the sella is the air-containing

The authors gratefully acknowledge the contributions of Ronald J. Whitley, A. Wayne Meikle, Nelson B. Watts, and Laurence M. Demers, on which portions of this chapter are based.

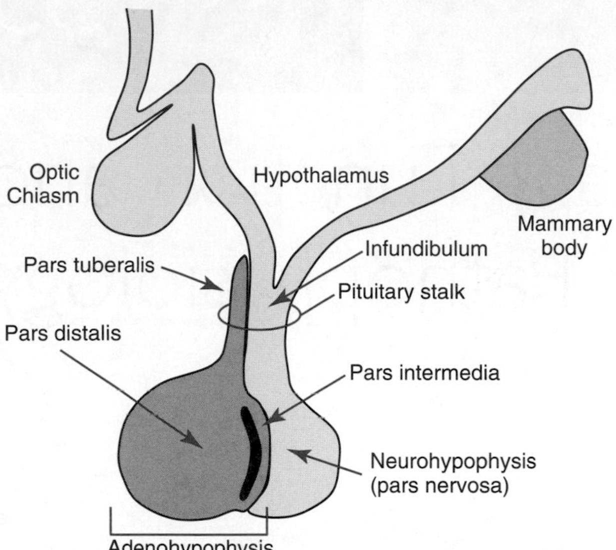

Figure 53-1 The hypophysis (pituitary gland) is composed of the adenohypophysis (the anterior lobe of the pituitary) and the neurohypophysis (the posterior lobe of the pituitary; pars nervosa). The adenohypophysis has three parts: the pars distalis, where most of the hormone-producing cells are located; the pars tuberalis, which is part of the pituitary stalk; and the pars intermedia.

sphenoid sinus, which communicates with the nasopharynx. Neurosurgeons take advantage of the proximity of the sphenoid sinus to the pituitary; the preferred surgical route to the pituitary is transsphenoidal (an incision is made in the mucosa of the oral cavity above the gum line, and the skin covering the upper lip and lower nose is dissected free of the underlying tissue; next the nasal septum is removed with entry into the sphenoid sinus; by removal of the floor of the sella, the pituitary is exposed).

The pituitary weighs only 0.5 to 0.6 g. The gland is larger in women than in men; its size increases during pregnancy, and it is largest in multiparous women. At the completion of pregnancy, when the pituitary is largest, it is susceptible to infarction if hypovolemic shock develops from hemorrhage following delivery, producing a postpartum hypopituitarism called *Sheehan syndrome.*

If the pituitary is greatly reduced in size or is apparently absent on magnetic resonance imaging (MRI) studies, the sella is said to be "empty."[125] In the empty sella syndrome, the sella may be normal in size or enlarged. An incompetent diaphragma sella with compression of the pituitary gland by herniating arachnoid can cause an empty sella, or the pituitary may be reduced in size as the result of some form of injury, radiotherapy, or surgery.

Arterial blood is supplied to the pituitary via the superior and inferior hypophyseal arteries, both of which are branches of the carotid arteries. The superior hypophyseal arteries supply the anterior pituitary and hypophyseal stalk, whereas the inferior hypophyseal arteries supply the posterior pituitary.

Direct delivery of hypothalamic regulatory hormones to the adenohypophysis occurs through the hypothalamic-pituitary portal system, which invests the adenohypophysis (pars distalis). A portal system is a vascular apparatus in which blood that initially passes through one capillary network (e.g., the hypothalamus) is collected into vessels that subsequently supply a second capillary network (e.g., the anterior pituitary). In this way, the hypothalamus controls the secretion of adenohypophyseal hormones via delivery of hypothalamic venous blood to the anterior pituitary gland. There is also retrograde flow from the pituitary to the hypothalamus via the portal system.

Via the lateral hypophyseal veins, pituitary venous drainage is moved to the cavernous and intercavernous sinuses. The cavernous sinus drains to the superior and inferior petrosal sinuses, which join the transverse sinus to form the jugular vein. This anatomic relationship is clinically important because access to pituitary secretions can be afforded by cannulation of the inferior petrosal venous sinuses.[193] Usually, the neuroradiologist places a catheter into a femoral vein that traverses an iliac vein, inferior vena cava, or superior vena cava to the jugular vein to enter the inferior petrosal venous sinus. Inferior petrosal venous sinus sampling can be helpful in the evaluation of patients with Cushing syndrome, to differentiate between Cushing disease (an anterior pituitary corticotropinoma) and ectopic ACTH syndrome.

The internal carotid arteries are located laterally to the pituitary. Above the pituitary is the diaphragma sella, which comprises circular (intercavernous) sinuses containing venous blood. Anterior and superior to the pituitary is the optic chiasm. These relations are clinically important because pituitary neoplasms can invade or compress these structures, as well as the bony sella turcica. For example, expanding anterior pituitary adenomas can compress the optic chiasm, producing bilateral hemianopsia.[202] In this condition, both lateral visual fields are lost. While walking, affected patients will bump into lateral structures in the environment because of loss of their lateral vision.

PITUITARY EMBRYOLOGY

The adenohypophysis develops in utero from a dorsal evagination of the roof of the stomodeum, which becomes the Rathke pouch.[204] The superior portion of the Rathke pouch constitutes the pars tuberalis (see earlier), whereas the posterior portion of the Rathke pouch develops into the pars intermedia (or intermediate lobe). Transcription factors that regulate the development of the anterior pituitary gland include HESX, LHX3, LHX4, SOX3, Pit-1, PROP1, RIEG, and GLI2.[54,55,117] The pars intermedia, which is active only late in pregnancy and in utero, secretes alpha-, beta-, and gamma-melanocyte stimulating hormone (MSH), corticotropin-like intermediate lobe peptide (CLIP), gamma-lipotropin, and beta-endorphin. MSH is believed to promote melanin synthesis. Lipotropins mobilize fat from adipose tissue, and endorphins are endogenous opioids.[128] The clinical significance of these products as causes of disease is not well understood.

TABLE 53-1 Hypothalamic Releasing or Inhibiting Hormones, Their Target Cells, and the Hormone That Is Regulated

Hypothalamic Hormone/ Abbreviation	Amino Acids	Anterior Pituitary Target Cell	Hormone Regulated	Amino Acids	MW
Corticotropin-releasing hormone (CRH)	41	Corticotroph	ACTH	39	4.5 kDa
Thyrotropin-releasing hormone (TRH)	3	Thyrotroph	TSH*	alpha: 92 beta: 118	28 kDa
Growth hormone–releasing hormone (GHRH)	44	Somatotroph	GH	191 176	22 kDa 20 kDa
Somatotropin release–inhibiting hormone† (SRIH)	14	Somatotroph	GH		(see above)
Gonadotropin-releasing hormone (GnRH)	10	Gonadotroph	LH*	alpha: 92 beta: 121	32 kDa
			FSH*	alpha: 92 beta: 111	30 kDa
Prolactin release-inhibiting hormone (PRIH)	1	Lactotroph	Prolactin	199	22 kDa

*All alpha glycoprotein chains are identical, including the alpha chain of human chorionic gonadotropin (hCG).
†a.k.a. somatostatin.
MW, Molecular weight.

Regulation of Function of the Adenohypophysis

The synthesis and release of the following anterior pituitary hormones are stimulated by hypothalamic releasing hormones: ACTH, TSH, GH, LH, and FSH.[96] Prolactin is the sole anterior pituitary hormone whose release is predominantly regulated through suppression. Corticotrophs secrete ACTH, thyrotrophs secrete TSH, somatotrophs secrete GH, gonadotrophs secrete both LH and FSH, and lactotrophs (or mammotrophs) secrete prolactin. Except for LH and FSH, each hormone is normally produced by a unique cell type. However in pathologic circumstances, both GH and prolactin may be secreted by an anterior pituitary adenoma. The molecular composition of the anterior pituitary hormones is summarized in Table 53-1.

Multiple levels of control of the hypothalamic-pituitary-end organ-hormone axis are known (Figure 53-2).[42] Except for prolactin and LH at the midpoint of the menstrual cycle, negative feedback controls secretion of the adenohypophyseal hormones. The long feedback loop involves suppression of the hypothalamic releasing hormone and the anterior pituitary trophic hormone by the hormonal product of the target tissue. The major site of negative feedback for cortisol (regulated by ACTH), insulin-like growth factor-I (IGF-I; regulated by GH), and sex steroids and inhibins (regulated by LH and FSH) is the hypothalamus. In contrast, for thyroid hormone (regulated by TSH), the major site of negative feedback is the anterior pituitary. Retrograde flow from the pituitary to the hypothalamus via the portal system permits the existence of short negative feedback loops where pituitary hormones suppress the secretion of hypothalamic releasing hormones. Ultra-short feedback loops also exist in which pituitary hormones inhibit their own secretion.

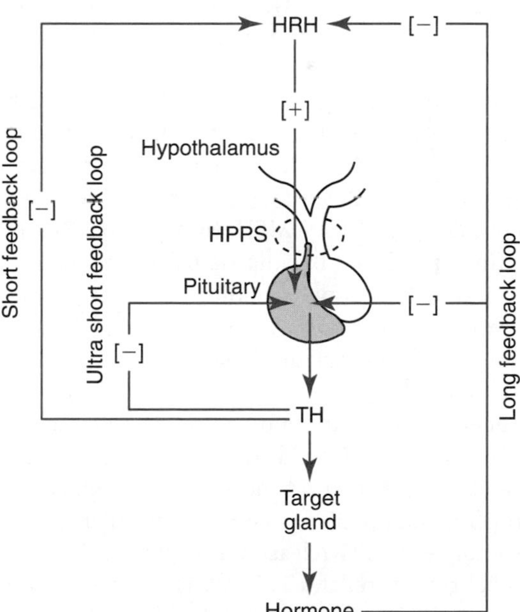

Figure 53-2 Many anterior pituitary trophic hormones (THs) (e.g., ACTH, TSH, GH, LH, FSH) are regulated by hypothalamic releasing hormones (HRHs). Releasing hormones secreted by the hypothalamus reach the pituitary via the hypothalamic-pituitary portal system (HPPS). Long feedback loops involve negative feedback of the target cell hormone at the pituitary gland and hypothalamus. The short feedback loop involves the anterior pituitary trophic hormone feeding back at the hypothalamus, whereas the ultra-short feedback loop involves the anterior pituitary hormone feeding back at the anterior pituitary. [+], Stimulation; [−], suppression.

HYPOTHALAMIC REGULATION

The hypothalamus is an area of the brain that produces hormones that control a number of bodily functions including the release of hormones from the pituitary gland. It is located in the middle of the base of the brain, and encapsulates the ventral portion of the third ventricle.

Hormones released by the hypothalmus that regulate the anterior pituitary hormones are listed in Table 53-1. With the exception of ACTH, hypothalamic hormones are structurally smaller than all of the anterior pituitary hormones.

CRH has wide distribution throughout the brain and brainstem.[86] In the hypothalamus, it is released by the paraventricular nucleus (PVN). CRH secretion is stimulated by systemic physiologic stress via (1) neurons of subfornical origin, (2) neurons of the nucleus tractus solitarius (NTS), (3) hypothalamic glutamatergic neurons, and (4) 5-hydroxytryptamine–secreting neurons of the raphe nucleus. Neurogenic stress to release CRH also acts via hypothalamic glutamatergic neurons. Stress inhibits hypothalamic GABAergic neurons of the PVN that otherwise would suppress CRH release. GABA (gamma-aminobutyric acid) serves as an inhibitory neurotransmitter. GABAergic neurons that innervate CRH-secreting neurons also originate from the lateral septum and the bed nucleus of the stria terminalis (BST). ACTH release is stimulated by serotonin, endorphins, and acetylcholine, and suppressed by GABA. Physiologically, stress, inflammation, and hypoglycemia stimulate ACTH release.

Thyrotropin-releasing hormone (TRH) is a tripeptide the product of the PVN of the hypothalamus.[155] TRH-secreting neurons in the PVN are innervated by axons that release (1) norepinephrine, (2) leptin, (3) neuropeptide Y, (4) agouti-related protein (AgRP), (5) MSH, (6) CRH, or (7) somatostatin. Leptin is produced by adipose tissue and acts to reduce appetite and raise energy expenditure as body fat stores rise. Leptin receptors are expressed in the ventromedial nucleus (VMN) of the hypothalamus. Neuropeptide Y and AgRP promote food intake.

The energy state and temperature of the organism influence TRH secretion. In addition to TRH, TSH secretion is suppressed by (1) thyroid hormone, (2) glucocorticoids, (3) estrogens, and possibly (4) GH. Acute inflammatory cytokines stimulate ACTH release but suppress TRH and TSH. Norepinephrine stimulates TSH release, whereas endorphins, serotonin, and dopamine suppress TSH.

Growth hormone–releasing hormone (GHRH) is produced by neurons in the arcuate nucleus of the medial basal hypothalamus. Simulators of GHRH include dopamine- and galanin-secreting neurons, and brainstem neurons with catecholaminergic inputs.[143] Galanin is a neuropeptide that is widely expressed in the endocrine, central nervous, and peripheral nervous systems. Hypothalamic somatostatin release–inhibiting hormone (SRIH) suppresses both GHRH release and anterior pituitary GH release. Leptin from adipose tissue and ghrelin from the stomach overall have the effect of increasing GHRH secretion and directly increasing GH concentrations. However, the clinical relevance of these influences and of other growth hormone–releasing peptides (e.g., GHRP-6) is not well understood. Ghrelin binds to GH secretogogue receptors (GHS-R) that increases food intake. Hormones that affect GH secretion include estrogen, testosterone, and glucocorticoids. Physiologically, amino acids and hypoglycemia stimulate GH release. In turn, the secretion of IGF-I in response to GH is influenced by nutrition, sex steroids, thyroid hormone, and the presence of chronic disease. Dopamine, endorphins, serotonin, and norepinephrine stimulate GH secretion.

Gonadotropin-releasing hormone (GnRH) regulation is complicated by the fact that GnRH must differentially control LH and FSH secretion, which vary greatly during the menstrual cycle in women.[129] GnRH-secreting neurons are not located in a discrete nucleus, but instead are diffusely distributed in the hypothalamus. Embryologically, these neurons are unusual in that they originate outside the central nervous system. GnRH secretion is stimulated by neurons that secrete (1) galanin-like peptide (GALP), (2) kisspeptin, (3) glutamate, (4) neuropeptide Y, and (5) norepinephrine. Kisspeptin is a neuropeptide that regulates puberty and reproduction. Neurons secreting GABA, beta-endorphins, and CRH inhibit GnRH. Gonadotropin release is stimulated by norepinephrine, GABA, and acetylcholine, and is suppressed by endorphins, dopamine, and serotonin.

GnRH pulsatility is essential to gonadotroph responsiveness. Tonic release of GnRH will downregulate GnRH receptors on gonadotrophs, leading to hypogonadism. Therapeutically, downregulation is accomplished with a long-acting GnRH agonist such as leuprolide acetate (Lupron Depot, Abbott Laboratories, Abbott Park, Ill) in the treatment of central precocious puberty in children, or the induction of hypogonadism in males with prostate cancer. Conversely, pulsatile GnRH administration is used to initiate puberty and to induce ovulation or spermatogenesis in GnRH deficiency. The rate of pulsatility may influence the relative secretion of LH and FSH. In primate studies, GnRH at one pulse per hour preferentially released LH, whereas one pulse every 3 hours caused a decline in LH and a mild rise in FSH.

Anterior Pituitary

In the anterior pituitary, (1) CRH receptors are expressed on corticotrophs, (2) TRH receptors are expressed on thyrotrophs, (3) GHRH receptors are expressed on somatotrophs, (4) GnRH receptors are expressed on gonadotrophs, and (5) prolactin-inhibiting hormone (PRIH) receptors are expressed on lactotrophs. In pathologically high concentrations, TRH stimulates the release of LH and prolactin. Otherwise, TRH does not appear to play a major role in regulating LH or prolactin secretion.

Corticotrophs are stimulated by high concentrations of proinflammatory cytokines such as interleukin (IL)-1, IL-6, and tumor necrosis factor (TNF)-alpha.[209] This emphasizes the interrelationship of the endocrine and immune systems in a hypothalamic-pituitary-adrenal-immune system axis. Through vasopressin type 3 receptors (V1b receptors), high

TABLE 53-2 Hypothalamic Hormones, Anterior Pituitary Hormones That They Regulate, Target Organ or Tissues Regulated by the Anterior Pituitary Hormone, and Hormonal Product of the Target Organ or Tissues

Hypothalamic Hormone(S)	Anterior Pituitary Hormone	Target Organ/Tissue	Target Hormone
CRH	ACTH	Adrenal cortex: zona fasiculata and zona reticularis	Cortisol
TRH	TSH	Thyroid follicular cell	Thyroxine (T_4) and 3,5,3′-triiodothyronine (T_3)
GHRH and SRIH	GH	Liver and many tissues of the body	Insulin-like growth factor-I (IGF-I), IGF binding protein-3 (IGFBP-3), and acid-labile subunit (ALS)
GnRH	LH, FSH	Gonad	Sex steroids and inhibins
PRIH	Prolactin	Breast	Not applicable

concentrations of ADH stimulate corticotrophs to release ACTH.

The hormonal products of each anterior pituitary target cell (if applicable) are listed in Table 53-2 along with a summary of each system. Many of these hormones display circadian (daily), ultradian (>daily) or infradian (<daily) variation that reflects changes in hypothalamic control. Deficiency of an individual pituitary hormone is typically called *hypopituitarism*,[13,179,194] whereas deficiency of all anterior pituitary hormones is termed *panhypopituitarism*.

Growth Hormone and Insulin-like Growth Factors

Linear growth is the consequence of (1) genetic potential, (2) nutrition, (3) the presence or absence of disease, and (4) hormonal effects.[212] Many hormones influence growth, but the most important are GH, thyroid hormone, and sex steroids. Excess glucocorticoids can impair growth in children. GH deficiency produces disease in adults, thus GH is essential for health throughout life.

Growth Hormone–Releasing Hormone (GHRH)

PreproGHRH is a polypeptide chain of 108 amino acids (12.4 kDa). Removal of the 20 amino acid signal (leader) sequence yields the 88 amino acid proGHRH. Cleavage of the 11 amino acid N-terminal pro-sequence and the 31 amino acid C-terminal pro-sequence, with release of 2 free amino acids (positions 76-77 with reference to preproGHRH), produces the 44 amino acid mature GHRH. The terminal leucine of GHRH is amidated. Alternative splicing of the mRNA (isoform 2) produces a preproGHRH protein of 107 amino acids, which is missing amino acid 103.

Somatotropin Release–Inhibiting Hormone

Somatotropin release–inhibiting hormone (SRIH) also is known as *somatostatin*.[195] It is widely distributed throughout the body (CNS, gut, and delta cells of the islets of Langerhan) and produces multiple physiologic effects. Somatostatin receptors are widely distributed (see later). Somatostatin that functions as SRIH is produced by the paraventricular nucleus of the hypothalamus. In the islets, somatostatin suppresses glucagon and insulin secretion, whereas somatostatin release is stimulated by both of these hormones. In this way, delta cell somatostatin modulates islet function by smoothing out extremes in the secretion of glucagon and insulin to maintain a stable blood glucose concentration. Somatostatin in the gut is found in highest concentration in the duodenum and jejunum.

Expression of the somatostatin gene produces the 116 amino acid polypeptide preprosomatostatin. Cleavage of the signal sequence (24 amino acids) produces prosomatostatin (92 amino acids), and subsequent cleavage of the N-terminal pro-sequence (64 amino acids) yields a 28 amino acid form of somatostatin (SST-28). SST-28 has an intrachain disulfide bond between amino acids 17 and 28. In many tissues, SST-28 undergoes cleavage to a 14 amino acid form (SST-14) through removal of the N-terminal 14 amino acid sequence by the enzymes prohormone convertase 1/prohormone convertase 2 (PC1/PC2) and carboxypeptidase E (CPE). SST-14 is the major form of somtatostatin in the CNS and delta cells, whereas SST-28 is the major form in the gastrointestinal tract. SST-28 is also the major circulating form of somatostatin. Therefore, somatostatin measurements in peripheral blood do not reflect SRIH secretion. Somatostatin is highly conserved in nature: all vertebrates have the identical sequence for SST-14.[195]

In addition to GH suppression, somatostatin also suppresses TRH, TSH, CRH, and ACTH. However, the effect of somatostatin on regulation of the adrenal cortical and thyroid axes ordinarily is minor. In the gastrointestinal tract, somatostatin reduces the secretion of multiple hormones including (1) gastrin, (2) secretin, (3) cholecystokinin, (4) vasoactive intestinal polypeptide, (5) motilin, (6) neurotensin, and (7) pepsin and reduces gastric pH, intestinal motility, ion and nutrient absorption, and proliferation of the mucosa (see Chapter 51). Calcitonin, catecholamines, renin, and pancreatic exocrine function are suppressed by somatostatin. Somatostatin analogs (e.g., octreotide) are used pharmacologically to suppress a variety of hormone overproduction conditions.[28]

TABLE 53-3 Biology of the Somatostatin Receptors

SSTR	Gene Location	Amino Acids/ Molecular Wt	SST Binding	Distribution
SSTR1	14q1	391 aa 42.7 kDa	SST-14 > SST-28	Fetal kidney, fetal liver, adult pancreas, brain, lung, jejunum, stomach
SSTR2	17q2	369 aa 41.3 kDa	SST14 and SST-28	Cerebrum, kidney
SSTR3	22q13.1	418 aa 45.8 kDa	SST-14 and SST-28	Brain, pituitary, pancreas
SSTR4	20p11.2	388 aa 42 kDa	SST-14	Fetal and adult brain, lung, stomach, less in kidney, pituitary, adrenals
SSTR5	16p13.3	364 aa 39.2 kDa	SST-28 > SST-14	Adult pituitary, heart, small intestine, adrenal, cerebellum, fetal hypothalamus

Growth Hormone–Releasing Hormone Receptor (GHRHR)

The anterior pituitary somatotroph GHRH receptor (GHRHR) is a member of family B-III of the G-coupled receptor superfamily (the "secretin" family).[7] Receptors for (1) secretin, (2) vasoactive intestinal polypeptide (VIP), (3) parathyroid hormone (PTH), and (4) calcitonin share partial sequence identity with GHRHR.

PreGHRHR is a 423 amino acid polypeptide that is converted to the mature 401 amino acid form of GHRHR by removal of the 22 amino acid signal peptide. The N-terminal extracellular domain is 110 amino acids. GHRHR has seven transmembrane domains and a 42 amino acid cytoplasmic domain. Amino acid 50 may be glycosylated.

Somatostatin (SRIH) Receptor

Throughout the body, there are five receptors for somatostatin (SSTR1 through SSTR5; Table 53-3). Each receptor is encoded by a gene located on a separate chromosome. SSTR2 has two alternatively spliced isoforms. All of the SSTR receptors have seven transmembrane domains, and are coupled with a pertussis toxin–sensitive G protein. SSTR3, SSTR4, and SSTR5 are expressed in the pituitary.

Growth Hormone (GH)

GH has two disulfide bridges (amino acids 54 and 165, and amino acids 182 and 189).[59] Structurally, GH has four main alpha-helices, and within the connecting loops three mini-helices. Two circulating forms of GH are present: a 22 kDa form that is a 191 amino acid chain (full-length GH) representing 85 to 90% of circulating GH, and a 20 kDa GH that lacks amino acids 32 through 46.[184] The 20 kDa form of GH results from alternative splicing of the GH mRNA transcript. In addition to the 22 kDa and 20 kDa forms, circulating GH exists as aggregates and oligomers. "Big GH" is a dimer of GH monomers, and "big-big GH" is GH associated with its binding protein (GHBP). GHBP is the external domain of the GH receptor (GHR), which binds GH with high affinity and is produced by cleavage of the GHR. Approximately 55% of all circulating GH forms are monomeric; big GH and big-big GH represent ≈27% and ≈18% of circulating GH, respectively. Approximately 50% of GH is not bound to GHBP, ≈45% is bound to GHBP, and the remaining 5% of GH is bound to low-affinity binding proteins. Considering the multiple forms of GH, it is not surprising that significant analytical biases are observed between different immunoassays for GH.

The gene for GH (chromosome 17q24.2) is a member of the GH subfamily that includes (–5′ to 3′ direction) (1) GH (the *GH1* gene), (2) a chorionic somatomammotropin (human placental lactogen) pseudogene designated *CSHP*, (3) a chorionic somatomammotropin-A designated *CSH1*, (4) the placentally produced 22 kDa GH variant (GH-V; gene designation *GH2*), and (5) chorionic somatomammotropin-B (gene designation *CSH2*).[40] Somatomammotropin (hPL) is a placental hormone with growth-promoting properties. Prolactin (199 amino acids) shares a homologous amino acid sequence with GH, but prolactin, encoded on chromosome 6p22, is not part of the GH complex on 17q24.2.

GH has both direct and indirect activity. Its direct actions will be described in the following sections.[118] The indirect activity of GH is mediated by IGF-I. To initiate its direct and indirect activity, GH binds to tissue receptors (GHR) that appear to be expressed by all tissues.

Growth Hormone Receptor (GHR)

The GHR is a member of the class 1 hematopoietic cytokine family.[142] Other members of this family include receptors for erythropoietin, granulocyte-macrophage colony-stimulating factor, and various interferons. Structurally, the GHR is a single-chain, 620 amino acid protein (130 kDa). PreGHR includes an 18 amino acid leader sequence. The GHR structure includes an extracellular domain (246 amino acids), a transmembrane domain (24 amino acids), and a cytoplasmic domain (350 amino acids).[31] When the extracellular portion of the GHR is shed, the 55 kDa GHBP moiety is released into the circulation.

Four isoforms of the GHR are expressed by alternative splicing of the nascent mRNA. Isoform 1 is the full-length receptor. Isoform 2 differs in the sequence of amino acids 292-297 (with reference to preGHR) and lacks amino acids

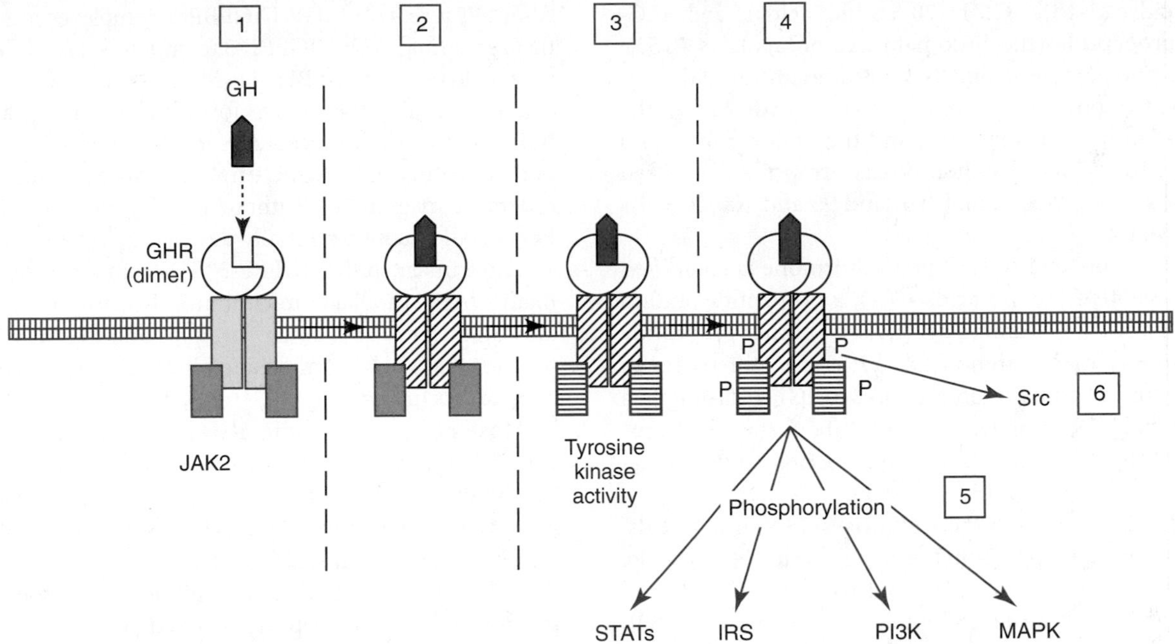

Figure 53-3 The growth hormone receptor (GHR) exists as a cell surface dimer in its inactive state. With GH binding to the GHR *[1]*, the GHR recruits or activates Janus-associated kinase molecules (JAK2) *[2]*. JAK2 then achieves tyrosine kinase activity *[3]*, and JAK2 and the GHR are phosphorylated *[4]*. Activated JAK2 now triggers several intracellular pathways involving STATs (signal transducers and activators of transcription), the insulin receptor substrate (IRS), phosphatidylinositol 3′-kinase (PI3K), and a mitogen-activated protein kinase (MAPK) *[5]*. Independent of JAK2, GHR signaling can proceed via Src *[6]*.

298-638. Isoform 3 differs in the sequence of amino acids 292-294 and lacks amino acids 295-638. An alanine at position four is replaced by aspartic acid, and amino acids 25 to 46 are missing in isoform 4.

The GHR exists as a cell surface dimer in its inactive state (Figure 53-3). When GH binds to the GHR, the receptor recruits or activates 120 kDa Janus-associated kinase enzymes (JAK2, a type of adapter tyrosine kinase). JAK2 then exerts tyrosine kinase activity by phosphorylating itself and the GHR.[132] Phosphorylation activates JAK2, which triggers several intracellular pathways involving (1) STATs (signal transducers and activators of transcription), (2) the insulin receptor substrate (IRS), (3) phosphatidylinositol 3′-kinase (PI3K), and (4) a mitogen-activated protein kinase (MAPK). STAT5b is involved, but it is unclear whether STAT5a is also involved. In its role as a transcription factor, phosphorylated, dimerized STAT5b enters the nucleus to promote gene transcription. Independent of JAK2, GHR signaling can be effected via Src, which is a tyrosine kinase. (*Note:* Src is the Rous sarcoma virus proto-oncogene.)

Insulin-like Growth Factors

IGF-I is a member of the insulin-related peptide family whose other members include IGF-II, insulin, and relaxin. Stimulated by hCG during pregnancy, relaxin is produced by the corpus luteum verum (the corpus luteum of pregnancy), the decidua (the uterine lining during pregnancy), and the placenta. Relaxin increases collagenase activity to soften and lengthen the cervix and pubic symphysis and facilitate parturition. Relaxin also reduces uterine contractility by inhibiting myosin kinase activity. In humans, there are three nonallelic relaxin genes: *RLN1, RLN2,* and *RLN3.*

Proinsulin, IGF-I, IGF-II, and relaxin are all composed of two domains (A and B) joined by a connecting domain. The connecting domains vary in sequence and length much more than the A and B domains. The connecting domain of proinsulin is cleaved to release C-peptide (connecting peptide), producing insulin A and B chains. Insulin, IGF-I, IGF-II, and relaxin have two disulfide bridges. IGF-I and IGF-II share 62% homology, and they each share 50% homology with insulin.

The 110 amino acid sequence of preproinsulin includes a signal peptide (amino acids 1-24), the insulin B chain (amino acids 25-54), C-peptide (amino acids 57-87), and the insulin A chain (amino acids 90-110). The two interchain disulfide bonds are between amino acids 31 and 96, and 43 and 109. The single intrachain disulfide bond is between amino acids 95 and 100.

Two forms of prepro-IGF-I are expressed as a consequence of alternative mRNA splicing: IGF-IA and IGF-IB. The IGF-IA preprohormone is 153 amino acids, including a signal peptide (amino acids 1-21), an N-terminal propeptide (amino acids 22-48), IGF-I (70 amino acids), and a C-terminal propeptide (the E domain, amino acids 119-153). The IGF-I polypeptide includes the B domain (amino acids 49-77), the C (connecting) domain (amino acids 78-89), the A domain (amino acids 90-110), and the D domain (amino acids 111-118). Three disulfide bonds are present between amino acids 54 and 96, 66 and 109, and 95 and 100. IGF-I is not glycosylated.

The 195 amino acid IGF-IB preprohormone is composed of a signal peptide (amino acids 1-21), a propeptide (amino acids 22-48), IGF-I (70 amino acids), and another propeptide region (the E domain, amino acids 119-195). Differences in the D versus E domain of the prepro-IGF-I distinguish IGF-IA from IGF-IB; the tertiary structure of the IGF-I proteins and the placement of disulfide bonds are identical between IGF-IA and IGF-IB.

The IGF-II preprohormone comprises 180 amino acids. The first 24 residues constitute the signal (or leader) peptide. After their removal, IGF-II is derived from pro-IGF-II after cleavage of the C-terminal E peptide (amino acids 92-180). Therefore, amino acids 25 to 91 include the B region (amino acids 25-52), the C region (amino acids 53-64), the A region (amino acids 65-85), and the D region (amino acids 86-91) of IGF-II. Isoform I is the full-length prepro-IGF-II (180 amino acids). Formed by alternative splicing, isoform II lacks amino acid 25 (alanine) and is therefore 179 amino acids in length. IGF-II is glycosylated at amino acid 99 and has three intrachain disulfide bonds between amino acids 33 and 71, 45 and 84, and 70 and 75. A potential glycosylation site is amino acid 163.

Prorelaxin is a 185 amino acid protein that contains a signal sequence (amino acids 1-22), a B chain (amino acids 23-53), a connecting propeptide (amino acids 56-158), and an A chain (amino acids 163-185). A-B interchain disulfide bonds can occur between amino acids 35 and 172, and 47 and 185. An additional disulfide bridge may occur between amino acids 171 and 176.

IGF-I and IGF-II circulate together with an IGF binding protein, IGFBP (specifically IGFBP-3), and the acid-labile subunit (ALS) to form a 150 kDa trimeric protein complex. About 75 to 80% of IGF-I/IGFBP-3 complexes are trimeric; the remaining IGF-I/IGFBP-3 complexes are dimeric and may include other IGFBPs. Less than 1% of the total IGF-I is free (the biologically active form). The binding affinity of IGF-I for the insulin receptor is low (≈7% of insulin affinity), but circulating IGF-I concentrations exceed insulin by three orders of magnitude. Without binding proteins, therefore, IGF-I could cause potentially devastating hypoglycemia.

The trimeric IGF-I-IGFBP-3-ALS complexes do not normally cross capillary membranes because of their size. However, the 50 kDa binary complex and free IGF-I are able to enter the interstitium, where binding to type I IGF receptors can occur.

Most of the circulating IGF-I is produced by hepatocytes.[139] However, IGF-I is also produced locally throughout the body and thus acts as a paracrine and an autocrine hormone. The possible endocrine (systemic) influence of IGF-I on growth is discussed later.

Similar to IGF-I, IGF-II does not normally produce hypoglycemia. However, reports have described tumors that secrete a larger than normal form of IGF-II. This big IGF-II did not bind normally to IGFBP-3, and therefore the free IGF-II concentration was greatly elevated. As a result of IGF-II binding to the insulin receptor, the clinical syndrome was similar to hypoglycemia caused by hyperinsulinism (i.e., free fatty acids were not elevated, ketones were absent, and lactate and alanine were not elevated), yet insulin itself was suppressed because the beta cells were normal. Removal of the tumor resolved the patient's hypoglycemia.[44]

Insulin-like Growth Factor Binding Proteins

Because of their very high affinity (K_d 10^{-10} to 10^{-11} M) for IGFs, IGFBPs are regarded as inhibitors of IGF action.[136] IGFBPs have higher affinity for IGFs than the IGF receptors. Currently under study is the possibility that IGFBPs may directly influence growth. Receptors for IGFBPs have been described. Proteolysis of IGFBPs releases IGF-I; therefore IGFBP proteases can influence free IGF-I concentrations. Table 53-4 summarizes the features of the seven known IGFBPs.

TABLE 53-4 Characteristics of Insulin-like Growth Factor Binding Proteins (IGFBPs)

IGFBP	Chromosome Gene Location	Amino Acids	Affinity for IGF-I vs. IGF-II	Specific Features
1	7p13	234	1 = 2	RGD sequence*
2	2q3	289	1 < 2	RGD sequence*
3	7p13	264	1 = 2	N-glycosylation
4	17q	237	1 = 2	Extra cysteines
5	2q3	252	1 < 2	Ternary complex with ALS
6	12q13	216	1 < 2	O-glycosylation
7	4q12	282	†	Stimulates prostacyclin production

*RGD sequence = Arg-Gly-Asp.
†Binds IGF-I and IGF-II with low affinity.
ALS, Acid-labile subunit.

Receptors for Insulin-like Growth Factors

Two types of receptors for IGFs have been identified: the type I IGF receptor and the type II IGF receptor (Figure 53-4).[134] Structurally, the type I IGF receptor is similar to the insulin receptor. Because this receptor does not exclusively bind IGF-I, the terminology "IGF-I receptor" is not recommended. The type I receptor is derived from a single precursor protein of 1367 amino acids that includes the 30 amino acid signal peptide. The 706 amino acid (130 kDa) alpha chain is extracellular and is bound by a disulfide bond to the transmembrane 90 kDa (627 amino acids) beta chain. Cleavage of the alpha and beta chains releases a tetrapeptide (707 to 710: arginine-lysine-arginine-arginine). Beta chain amino acids 906 to 929 form a transmembrane domain. The receptor exists as a homodimer (beta-alpha-alpha-beta) with the two alpha chains bound to each other by two disulfide bonds. Similar to the type I IGF receptor, the insulin receptor is a homodimer of two 135 kDa alpha chains and two 95 kDa beta chains.

Tyrosine kinase activity in the cytoplasmic portion of the type I IGF receptor beta chain results from binding of an IGF molecule to the cysteine-rich portion of the alpha chains (amino acids 148-302), which causes conformational changes in both alpha and beta chains. Intracellular signaling involves autophosphorylation and phosphorylation of the 185 kDa insulin receptor substrate 1 (IRS1), which is the predominant target of the active type I IGF receptor. The type I IGF receptor binds IGF-I with higher affinity than IGF-II, and affinity for insulin is lower than the affinity of the receptor for IGF-I or IGF-II. The affinities of the insulin receptor are the opposite: insulin >> IGF-II > IGF-I.

The type II IGF receptor is structurally dissimilar from the type I IGF receptor and the insulin receptor. The 270 kDa, 2451 amino acid, type II IGF receptor is a monomeric protein that is similar to the epidermal growth factor (EGF) receptor.

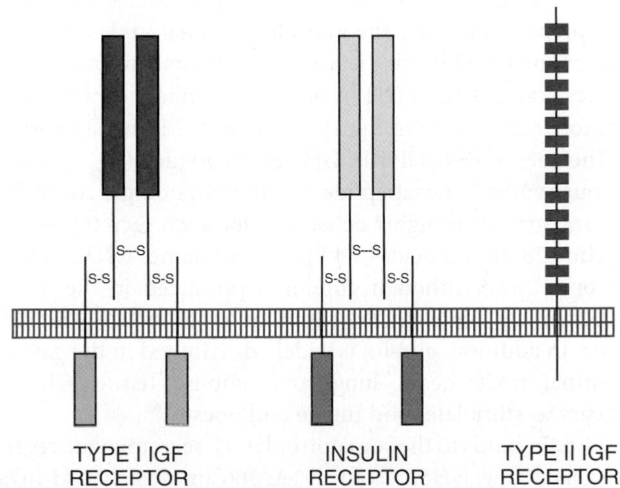

Figure 53-4 The type I IGF receptor is structurally similar to the insulin receptor. The structure of the type II IGF receptor is similar to that of the epidermal growth factor receptor.

(*Note:* The leader sequence is 40 amino acids.) The EGF receptor itself is also known as ErbB1 or HER1. The external portion of the receptor is 2264 amino acids, the transmembrane domain is 23 amino acids, and the cytoplasmic domain is 164 amino acids. Beginning at the N-terminus, thirteen ≈150 amino acid repeats and a 47 amino acid fibronectin type II domain are followed by two more repeats. Evidence indicates at least five glycosylation sites: amino acids 112 (with preference for the pre-type II IGF receptor), 581, 626, 747, and 1246. Two disulfide bonds are found between amino acids 1903 and 1927, and between amino acids 1917 and 1942.

Ligand binding to EGF receptors results in dimerization and tyrosine kinase activation. The external ligand-binding domain of EGFs is composed of numerous short amino acid repeats. The type II IGF receptor removes IGF-II from the circulation, and its engagement leads to activation of transforming growth factor (TGF)-beta. The type II IGF receptor binds mannose-6-phosphate, in addition to IGFs, permitting the uptake and intracellular movement of mannose-6-phosphate–containing lysosomal enzymes. The binding sites for IGFs and mannose-6-phosphate are found on different parts of the receptor. The affinities of the type II IGF receptor are as follows: IGF-II >> IGF-I > insulin. Because this receptor does not exclusively bind IGF-II, the terminology "IGF-II receptor" is not recommended.

A hybrid receptor consisting of the alpha-beta chain of the insulin receptor and the alpha-beta chain of the type I IGF receptor has been described. It has been suggested that these hybrid receptors may allow cancers to respond to insulin.[23] Increasing evidence suggests that IGF-I may enhance the growth of many tumors. Thus, the casual use of IGF-I injections in children to enhance growth in short but otherwise normal children is problematic and potentially carcinogenic.

Regulation of Growth Hormone (GH) Secretion

GH ultimately stimulates release of IGF-I, which negatively feeds back to regulate GH release via two hypothalamic hormones: somatotropin-release inhibiting hormone (SRIH, or somatostatin; from the hypothalamic paraventricular nucleus) and growth hormone–releasing hormone (GHRH; from the hypothalamic infundibular nucleus) (Figure 53-5). These hypothalamic GH-regulating hormones are carried to the anterior pituitary via the specialized hypothalamic-pituitary portal vascular system. Somatotrophs of the anterior pituitary gland have receptors for both hormones. Somatostatin inhibits GH release, whereas GHRH promotes the release of GH. However, GH release is the predominant hypothalamic effect, because surgical interruption of the pituitary stalk with destruction of the hypothalamic-pituitary portal system leads to GH deficiency, not excess. In addition to its hypothalamic negative feedback effects, IGF-I directly suppresses pituitary release of GH.

Physiologically, GH secretion is episodic.[138] Consequently, random measurements cannot exclude GH deficiency; between pulses, GH concentrations can be quite low and do

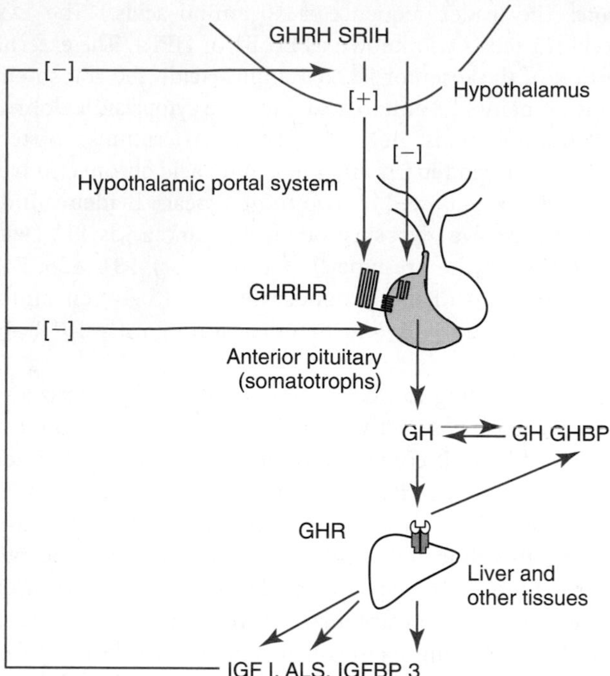

Figure 53-5 The hypothalamus secretes growth hormone–releasing hormone (GHRH) and somatotropin release–inhibiting hormone (SRIH; somatostatin), which regulate growth hormone (GH) release. The receptor for GHRH (GHRHR) is illustrated because mutations in this receptor can cause some forms of inherited GH deficiency. GH circulates unbound and bound to its binding protein (GHBP). GHBP is the extracellular domain of the GHR, which is cleaved from the GHR to circulate in the plasma. GH releases insulin-like growth factor-I (IGF-I), insulin-like growth factor binding protein 3 (IGFBP-3) and the acid-labile subunit (ALS). IGF-I negatively feeds back at the anterior pituitary somatotrophs and at the hypothalamus. Because transection of the pituitary stalk leads to GH deficiency, the predominant hypothalamic control of GH is stimulatory via GHRH.

not distinguish GH insufficiency from normal production of the hormone. During daytime hours, the plasma concentration of GH in healthy adults remains stable and relatively low (<2 μg/L), with several secretory spikes occurring approximately 3 hours after meals (particularly meals high in protein and arginine) and after exercise. In contrast, during the evening hours, adults and children show a marked rise in GH secretory activity ≈90 minutes after the onset of sleep; GH concentrations reach a peak value during the period of deepest sleep. This pattern of GH secretion may be important for anabolic and repair processes, and for proper skeletal growth. GH is also increased by psychologic or physical stress and hypoglycemia. Normal GH secretion requires thyroxine and age-appropriate concentrations of testosterone or estrogen.

GH is suppressed by elevations in blood glucose. One of the tests for GH excess measures GH following an oral glucose load; the normal response is a GH concentration of less than

BOX 53-1 Protocol for Glucose Suppression of Growth Hormone Test

Rationale

Normal subjects show suppression of serum growth hormone (GH) concentrations after oral administration of glucose. Subjects with acromegaly fail to exhibit appropriate GH suppression.

Procedure

The test should be performed after an overnight fast with the patient maintained at bed rest. After a baseline blood specimen is collected for GH and glucose measurement, a solution of 75 g of glucose is given orally. Glucose and serum GH are measured again on specimens collected 30, 60, 90, and 120 minutes later.

Interpretation

Serum GH concentrations in normal individuals fall to less than 1 to 2 μg/L (i.e., below the lower limit of detection of the GH assay used). Subjects with acromegaly fail to show this suppression and sometimes show a paradoxical increase in GH concentration. Patients with liver disease, uremia, or heroin addiction may have false-positive results with this test (failure to suppress serum GH concentrations after oral glucose load).

1 to 2 μg/L, depending on the lower limit of detection of the GH immunoassay (Box 53-1). GH also declines with increases in free fatty acid concentrations, rapid eye movement sleep, and aging. In the presence of abnormally high concentrations of glucocorticoids, GH secretion is suppressed. In addition, circulating GH is thought to influence the release of hypothalamic hormones through the short feedback loop. Other hypothalamic hormones, such as TRH and GnRH, do not affect GH release in normal subjects but may provoke GH release in patients with acromegaly.

Age-associated decline in GH production has spawned an industry of dietary supplements purported to "support" growth hormone secretion.[97] These supplements are amino acid preparations that theoretically stimulate release of the subject's own GH. Such dietary supplements have no proven medical value. Use of GH by athletes to enhance strength or promote recovery from injury is prohibited in most sports.

The role of non-GHRH GH secretogogues (e.g., ghrelin, various synthetic hexapeptides) in the physiologic control of GH and growth is highly debated.[6] One such secretogogue is ghrelin (28 amino acids, 3.4 kDa; gene name: *GHRL;* chromosome 3p2). Although ghrelin is produced in the hypothalamus, its highest concentration is found in stomach tissue. In addition, ghrelin is widely distributed in the gastrointestinal tract, heart, lung, and adipose tissue. Ghrelin appears to stimulate food intake and obesity.[65]

Ghrelin binds to the somatotroph GH-secretogogue receptor (gene name: *GHSR;* isoform 1A: 366 amino acids, 41 kDa; isoform 1B: 289 amino acids, 32 kDa; chromosome 3q26.31), which is distinct from the GHRHR. *GHRL,* the gene that encodes ghrelin, also encodes the 23 amino acid peptide obestatin. Obestatin may decrease food intake and increase satiety, but this has been debated. Obestatin is a ligand for the orphan GPR39 receptor (453 amino acids, 51 kDa; chromosome 2q21). However, despite obestatin binding to the GPR39 receptor, receptor activation may not follow.[133]

Physiologic Actions

GH effects can be classified as indirect or direct.[173] GH directly raises blood glucose by stimulating gluconeogenesis and reducing insulin sensitivity. Also, it causes adipose tissue lipolysis and the resulting GH-induced elevations in free fatty acids provide an alternative energy source that serves to spare glucose for CNS utilization. Therefore when glucose and free fatty acid concentrations are raised at times of stress, in partnership with epinephrine, glucagon, and cortisol, fuels for the fight-or-flight response are provided. GH has other effects on intermediary metabolism: GH stimulates the uptake of nonesterified fatty acids by muscle and accelerates the mobilization and metabolism of fat from adipose tissue to the liver.

At the epiphysis of growing bone, GH promotes epiphyseal prechondrocyte differentiation. GH directly stimulates the production of IGF-I, IGFBP-3, and the acid labile subunit (ALS). In turn, after entering the interstitium, unbound IGF-I binds to type I IGF receptors.

Indirect effects of GH are mediated through IGF-I production, which (together with GH) is necessary for linear growth in childhood. IGF-I is mitogenic and antiapoptotic. Epiphyseal prechondrocyte differentiation stimulated by GH, along with the local effects of IGF-I (also under the control of GH), stimulates the clonal expansion of differentiating chondrocytes.

Thus, the overall effect of GH is to promote growth in soft tissue, cartilage, and bone. This action results from stimulation of protein synthesis that is induced in part by an increase in amino acid transport through cell membranes. The effects of GH on bone and muscle are exerted both directly and through the effects of IGF-I under the influence of GH. Increased growth of soft tissue and the skeleton is accompanied by changes in electrolyte metabolism, including positive nitrogen and phosphorous balance, a rise in plasma phosphorous concentration, and a fall in blood urea and amino acid concentrations. Additional responses to GH include increased intestinal absorption of calcium and decreased urinary excretion of sodium and potassium. The metabolic changes most likely are caused by increased uptake of these ions by growing tissue.

IGF-I increases glucose oxidation in adipose tissue and stimulates glucose and amino acid transport into diaphragmatic muscle and heart muscle. Synthesis of collagen and proteoglycans is enhanced by IGF-I, which also has positive effects on calcium, magnesium, and potassium homeostasis. The insulin-like effects of this growth factor have been ascribed in part to its structural similarity to insulin.

Evidence indicates that the local effects of IGF-I (autocrine or paracrine) are predominant in stimulating growth, when compared with the systemic effects of IGF-I produced by the liver. When the hepatic *IGF-I* gene was knocked out in mice (although nonhepatic tissues expressed IGF-I), growth was normal, and IGFBP-3 and ALS concentrations were low. IGF-I may function as a growth factor in utero; however, its secretion in utero is not under the control of GH.

In the absence of GH, IGF-I is not as effective a growth stimulant as it is when both are present. IGF-I treatment alone is not recommended as therapy for GH deficiency; IGF-I therapy is reserved for cases of GH resistance due to GHR deficiency.[95]

GH (through IGF-I) and insulin induce growth in a similar manner because both have protein anabolic effects and stimulate the transport of amino acids into peripheral cells. Their respective effects on glucose homeostasis, however, oppose each other. Most growth-promoting GH effects are delayed rather than immediate and are exerted primarily through IGF-I.

IGF-I concentrations vary widely with age and gender.[83] IGF-I rises during childhood, and during puberty, IGF-I concentrations can be two to three times the adult concentration. Following adolescence, IGF-I concentrations show a gradual decline, reaching a steady state in the third decade of life.

GH is not the only determinant of IGF-I concentration in the circulation. Transformation of the GH stimulus to IGF-I production and secretion is modulated by (1) nutrition, (2) the presence or absence of chronic inflammation, (3) thyroid function, (4) glucocorticoids, and (5) sex steroids. IGF-I secretion is reduced by (1) malnutrition, (2) malabsorption (e.g., inflammatory bowel disease), (3) celiac disease, (4) cystic fibrosis, (5) chronic disease, (6) hypothyroidism (e.g., Hashimoto thyroiditis), and (7) sex hormone deficiency during adolescence. Therefore a decreased IGF-I concentration is not necessarily synonymous with GH deficiency.

In cases of acquired GH resistance and genetic GH resistance (*GHR* mutation or signaling disorder), GH concentrations will rise, and high concentrations of GH produce hyperlipidemia and hyperglycemia.[75] Cases of acquired GH resistance are not treated with GH or IGF-I, but instead are treated through resolution of the underlying disorder.

The actions and regulation of IGF-II have been debated.[160] IGF-II is believed to be important for intrauterine growth. Mice display intrauterine growth retardation when the IGF-II gene is knocked out. Although IGF-II–producing tumors are very rare, such tumors can produce hypoglycemia. The tumors produce an aberrant form of IGF- II ("big" IGF-II) that does not associate normally with IGFBPs. The production of big IGF-II, in combination with a reduction in an IGFBP concentration, results in higher concentrations of free IGF-II, which causes hypoglycemia by associating with the insulin receptor. Both IGF-I and IGF-II are of great interest to cancer researchers, but a detailed discussion of this topic is beyond the scope of this chapter.

Clinical Significance

Clinically important states of GH excess or deficiency are uncommon and are often difficult to diagnose.[90] GH concentrations vary widely under normal circumstances; therefore random measurements of GH, in general, are not diagnostically useful. A single GH measurement cannot distinguish between normal fluctuations and the low or high concentrations that are typical of various diseases. GH measurements are best determined as part of dynamic testing: physiologic or pharmacologic provocative stimuli are used to help diagnose GH deficiency, whereas GH suppression (or lack thereof) following glucose administration is useful in evaluating GH excess.[71] IGF-I concentrations often correlate better with the clinical severity of acromegaly than with glucose-suppressed or basal GH concentrations.[49]

In contrast to GH, a single measurement of IGF-I is considered to be an accurate reflection of GH-IGF-I production, irrespective of the time of the day or meals. IGF-I has a much longer half-life than GH, so its concentration is more stable. The half-life of GH is slightly longer than 15 minutes, whereas the half-life of the trimeric IGF-I-IGFBP-3-ALS complex is 17 to 22 hours. The half-life of unbound IGF-I is only 10 to 20 minutes, but the unbound form of the hormone accounts for less than 1% of the total concentration. Serum concentrations of IGF-I are influenced by (1) age, (2) gender, (3) degree of sexual maturity, (4) thyroid status, and (5) nutritional status. As mentioned previously, IGF-I concentrations are low in GH deficiency and in patients with acute or chronic protein or caloric deprivation. In pediatric endocrinology, measurements of IGFBP-3 have been used in addition to IGF-I measurements to assess GH; however, the value of this approach has not been established. The diagnostic use of GH to stimulate IGF-I production is controversial and is not currently included in standard medical practice.[161]

Growth Hormone Excess

Acromegaly is the rare clinical syndrome in adults that results from GH excess.[57,214] Even less common is gigantism, which results from GH excess in childhood. The clinical features of acromegaly involve overgrowth of the skeleton and soft tissue, producing (1) acral enlargement (enlargement of the extremities), (2) organomegaly (enlarged heart and/or liver), (3) facial coarsening, (4) intestinal polyposis, (5) premature cardiovascular disease, (6) hyperhidrosis (increased sweating), (7) skin tags, (8) joint disease, (9) myopathy with weakness, (10) insulin resistance, and often (11) diabetes mellitus. Premature cardiovascular disease is the most common cause of death in individuals with acromegaly. Gigantism is characterized by extreme tall stature, in addition to the clinical features of acromegaly, as pathologic GH excess occurs before epiphyseal fusion is complete.

Most cases of acromegaly (≈95%) result from anterior pituitary GH-secreting tumors (somatotropinomas).[58] Somatotropinomas are usually large macroadenomas (>10 mm in diameter); approximately 75% of these tumors are visualized by computed tomography (CT) or magnetic resonance imaging (MRI) (the preferred method for pituitary imaging is MRI). Some anterior pituitary tumors secrete both GH and prolactin (somatomammotropinomas). Approximately 5% of acromegaly cases result from GHRH-secreting hypothalamic tumors, and less than 1% of cases result from extrapituitary somatotropinomas, GHRH-secreting islet cells, or lung or breast tumors.

In severe or advanced cases of GH excess, the diagnosis may be nearly certain on the basis of physical appearance alone. However, in less severe or early cases, the physical changes may be subtle and gradual, so a high degree of clinical suspicion is needed to make an early diagnosis. The reversibility of tissue changes depends largely on the duration of the disease. In addition to soft tissue changes, acromegaly may cause severe disability or death from cardiac, pulmonary, and/or neurologic sequelae. The most important requirement for the diagnosis of acromegaly is the demonstration of inappropriate and excessive GH secretion.[150]

As many as 10% of patients with active acromegaly have random serum GH concentrations that fall within the normal reference interval. Essentially all patients with acromegaly have an abnormal GH response to oral glucose (53-1). Patients with acromegaly typically show no change in their basal concentration of GH or demonstrate a paradoxical increase in GH[70]; normal individuals, on the other hand, show suppression of GH concentrations to less than 1.0 μg/L after the oral glucose load. Serum IGF-I concentrations are also elevated in active acromegaly, and often correlate better with the clinical severity of acromegaly than do glucose-suppressed or basal GH concentrations.

Growth Hormone Deficiency and Growth Retardation

In children, short stature with a normal growth velocity (≥4 to 5 cm/y) results from (1) familial short stature, (2) primordial growth failure (prenatal-onset growth failure), or (3) constitutional delay in growth and adolescence (delayed maturation). Short stature with a low growth velocity (<4 to 5 cm/y) results from genetic short stature, chronic illness, malnutrition, deprivation (nutritional or psychologic), Turner syndrome in girls, or endocrine disorders (e.g., hypothyroidism, disorders of the GHRH-GH-IGF-I axis, poorly controlled diabetes, rickets, pseudohypoparathyroidism, pseudopseudohypoparathyroidism, and Cushing syndrome).[167]

GH deficiency is not a common cause of growth retardation. About one half of children evaluated for growth retardation have no specific organic cause; about 15% have an endocrine disorder, of which approximately half (about 8% of all children with short stature) have GH deficiency. However, short children with low growth velocities with no clear explanation should be screened for GH deficiency once hypothyroidism has been excluded.

GH deficiency in children is characterized by (1) short stature, (2) low growth (3) velocity, (4) immature facial appearance, (5) retarded bone age on radiologic examination, and (6) increased adiposity. In cases of congenital GH deficiency, size at birth is usually normal because in utero, IGF-I does not appear to be under GH control. Micropenis (an abnormally short penis) is evident in some boys with congenital GH deficiency and will resolve with GH replacement in childhood. Adults with GH deficiency experience (1) reduced muscle mass, (2) increased adiposity, (3) osteoporosis with decreased bone density, (4) an increase in fracture risk, (5) decreased quality of life, (6) dyslipidemia,

TABLE 53-5 GH Deficiency of Genetic Etiology

Gene/Classification/Inheritance	Mutation	Phenotype
GH1; IA; AR	Deletion, FS, NS	Absent GH expression; immune resistance to GH treatment is common
GH1; IB; AR	Splicing?	Reduced GH; responds to GH treatment*
GHRHR; IB; AR	Possible MS	Reduced GH; responds to GH treatment*
GH1; II; AD	DN	Reduced GH; responds to GH treatment; MPHD is possible
Unknown; III; XLR	—	Reduced GH; responds to GH treatment; agammaglobulinemia is possible

*One third of heterozygotes may be short.
AD, Autosomal dominant inheritance; *AR,* autosomal recessive inheritance; *DN,* dominant negative; *FS,* frameshift; *MS,* missense mutation; *NS,* nonsense mutation (stop codon); *XLR,* X-linked recessive; *?,* otherwise not defined.

and (7) an increased risk for cardiovascular disease.[113] GH deficiency is probably the most common identifiable abnormality in adults with large pituitary adenomas[33] and in patients who have undergone pituitary irradiation. Thus GH replacement therapy is an important clinical intervention in GH-deficient adults and children and is considered the standard of care.

GH insufficiency can be a consequence of (1) hypothalamic disease, (2) disruption of the portal system between hypothalamic nuclei and the anterior pituitary, (3) GHRHR loss-of-function mutations, or (4) somatotroph disease. GH deficiency can occur in isolation [isolated GH deficiency] or together with other pituitary deficiencies [multiple pituitary hormone deficiencies (MPHD) or combined pituitary hormone deficiencies (CPHD)]. Patients with isolated GH deficiency should be followed clinically for the development of other pituitary hormone deficiencies because MPHD can evolve over time. Biochemical testing is necessary to establish the diagnosis of GH deficiency, growth hormone resistance, or MPHD. In most affected children, the cause of GH deficiency is unknown [idiopathic GH deficiency].[159] Approximately one in four children with proven GH deficiency has an organic origin for their GH deficiency; half of these children will be diagnosed with a CNS tumor.

Any type of hypothalamic disease or dysfunction can lead to GHRH deficiency, including (1) tumor, (2) inflammation, (3) previous infection, (4) trauma (including previous surgery),[124] (5) bleeding, (6) irradiation, and (7) malformation [septo-optic dysplasia (SOD)].[116] Low-dose irradiation of the hypothalamus/pituitary can cause idiopathic GH deficiency, whereas higher doses of irradiation can cause MPHD. SOD is defined by the triad of (1) midline brain defects such as agenesis of the septum pellucidum and/or corpus callosum, (2) hypoplasia of the optic nerve, and (3) anterior and/or posterior pituitary hormone abnormalities. A small number of cases of SOD are explained by mutations in *HESX1, SOX2,* and *SOX3,* all of which are transcription factors. *HEXS1* (chromosome 3p14.3) is a paired-like homeobox gene, *SOX2* (chromosome 3q26.3) is the SRY (sex-determining region on the Y chromosome) box 2 gene, and *SOX3* (chromosome Xq27.1) is the SRY box 3 gene. Midline brain tumors, such as meningiomas, gliomas, germinomas, third ventricle colloid cysts, ependymomas, and optic nerve gliomas, also affect the hypothalamus. Disruptions in the hypothalamic-pituitary portal system can result from tumor, inflammation, previous infection, trauma (including previous surgery), and irradiation.

Congenital GH deficiency from pituitary disease has many causes, including *GHRHR* gene mutations (idiopathic GH deficiency type IB), *GH1* mutations (idiopathic GH deficiency types IA, IB, II, and III, and bioinactive GH), and transcription factor mutations (usually causing MPHD: *LHX3, LHX4, PROP1, Pit-1, RIEG*) and malformations (anencephaly and holoprosencephaly) (Table 53-5).[168] Homozygous *LHX3* mutations have caused panhypopituitarism, with the exception that ACTH was not affected. Heterozygous *LHX4* mutations have caused deficiencies of GH, TSH, and ACTH. *PROP1* (name derived from "PROphet of Pit-1"; POU1F1; Pit-1 stands for "paired-like homeodomain transcription factor")[157] mutations causes deficiencies of GH, prolactin, TSH, and gonadotropins. ACTH deficiency has also occurred in some families. *PROP1* gene mutations are inherited as autosomal recessive traits. *Pit-1* gene mutations cause GH, prolactin, and variable degrees of TSH deficiency. These transcription factor mutations may be inherited as autosomal recessive or dominant traits. Heterozygous *RIEG* gene mutations (*PITX2,* a paired-like homeobox gene) are the cause of Rieger syndrome, which may include GH deficiency. Features of Rieger syndrome encompass developmental abnormalities of teeth, the anterior chamber of the eye, and the umbilicus. Mutations in *GLI1, GLI2, Shh, ZIC2, SIX3, tgif, PATCHED1, DGF1,* and *FAST1* have variously been cited as causes of holoprosencephaly.[88] Children with midline facial clefts (cleft lip, cleft palate, or combined) or a single central incisor can exhibit GH deficiency. Two *GH1* gene mutations have been identified to cause bioinactive GH.[189] In these mutations, GH does not have full biological activity but retains normal immunoreactivity. Therefore, in contrast to other forms of pituitary or hypothalamic disease, the GH concentration is not deficient. At least one reference laboratory provides *GHRHR, GH1,* and *GHR* gene sequencing services (Athena Diagnostics, Worcester, Mass).[7,62,207]

Acquired causes of pituitary disease include (1) tumor (craniopharyngioma, Rathke cleft cyst, arachnoid cyst, or anterior pituitary adenoma), (2) infiltrative disease—amyloidosis, (3) inflammation (autoimmune hypophysitis and granulomatous inflammation), (4) infection, (5) trauma (including surgery), (6) bleeding, (7) irradiation, (8) infarction (pituitary apoplexy from Sheehan syndrome), and (9) metabolic derangement (hemochromatosis, iron overload from long-term transfusion therapy, or certain anemias, such as sideroblastic anemia).[5] Hemochromatosis does not cause hypopituitarism until many decades have passed.[35] Some investigators believe that all patients with "idiopathic" hypopituitarism should be screened for hemochromatosis.[141]

A staged approach to the evaluation of GH secretion is advised.[166] Initial screening can involve one of the following tests: (1) measurement of IGF-I (with or without IGFBP-3), (2) GH measurement following exercise, or (3) pharmacologic GH screening. All forms of GH testing should be performed after the subject has fasted overnight. If a GH screening test is abnormal, definitive testing should be pursued.[201] If GH adequacy is demonstrated by GH screening tests, definitive GH testing need not be performed unless there is a very high index of suspicion for GH deficiency. In children, the likelihood of a falsely abnormal GH screening test can be reduced by pretreatment of both boys and girls with a short course of sex steroids [ethinylestradiol: for body weights <50 lb, 20 μg/dose 18 hours, 12 hours, and 1 hour before testing; for body weights ≥50 lb: 50 μg/dose 18, 12, and 1 hour before testing, or 100 μg/d for 3 days; Premarin: for body weights <30 lb: 2.5 mg twice daily for 3 days; for body weights ≥30 lb, 5 mg twice daily for 3 days; diethylstilbestrol (DES): 5 mg/d for 3 days; or, exclusively in boys, testosterone enanthate 50 mg injected intramuscularly 2 or 3 weeks before testing]. The mechanism is unclear; however, sex steroids appear to play a major role in increasing the response of IGF-I to GH at the time of puberty. From clinical experience, GH deficiency is overdiagnosed in some peripubertal children who are tested without the benefit of sex hormone priming.

Exercise physiologically enhances GH release.[72] Typically, in the fasting state, the subject exercises vigorously for ≈20 minutes (e.g., running up and down stairs, running on a treadmill). At the completion of the exercise, when the subject is tachycardic and sweating, a sample is collected for GH measurement (Box 53-2). A baseline GH measurement is not required. A GH concentration may also be obtained 40 minutes after exercise, in case of delayed GH release. Finally, screening for GH deficiency can be performed by measuring GH 60 to 90 minutes following clonidine, glucagon, or L-dopa administration. (*Note:* L-dopa is not currently available in the United States.) Doses of clonidine, glucagon, and L-dopa are identical to doses used in formal GH testing scenarios (see later).

It has been argued that measuring GH during sleep is a physiologic assessment of the hypothalamic-somatotroph-GH axis. Some authorities suggest electroencephalographic (EEG) monitoring with GH measured during deep sleep (e.g., stage III, stage IV). More simply, GH could be measured 1 hour after the onset of sleep. However, in reality these types of sleep studies are cumbersome because they require hospitalization or overnight boarding in a sleep laboratory. In practice, this is rarely done. Furthermore, the high cost of hospitalization or the sleep laboratory suggests that an exercise tolerance test or a simple pharmacologic stimulus would be a more cost-effective approach to initial GH testing.

BOX 53-2 Protocol for the Exercise Stimulation Test for Growth Hormone

Rationale

Brisk exercise normally causes an increase in serum growth hormone (GH) concentrations.

Procedure

The test is best performed in the morning after an overnight fast, but may be done at any time. Vigorous physical exercise (running or calisthenics) is performed for 20 minutes. A venous blood specimen for determination of GH is drawn immediately after termination of exercise.

Interpretation

If the serum GH concentration is 7 to 10 μg/L or greater (depending on the specific GH immunoassay used), GH deficiency is unlikely in children. A normal response in adults is a GH concentration of 5 μg/L or greater. In children, a single subnormal response is not diagnostic for GH deficiency and should be confirmed with a second provocative test.

Reference intervals for IGF-I and IGFBP-3 are age and gender dependent.[73] If IGF-I is within its reference interval for age and gender in children, GH deficiency is excluded. If IGF-I is low, definitive GH testing is required. Because IGF-I concentrations can be depressed in states of (1) malnutrition, (2) malabsorption, (3) chronic disease, (4) hypothyroidism, and (5) sex hormone deficiency, a low IGF-I concentration does not confirm GH deficiency. IGFBP-3 is less dependent on good nutrition to achieve normal concentrations, so it may be a superior marker of GH deficiency compared with IGF-I. However, one study failed to demonstrate that measuring IGFBP-3 alone or together with free IGF-I was superior to measuring IGF-I alone as a screening test for GH deficiency.[48] In another study, only ≈50% of GH-deficient children had a low IGFBP-3 concentration; this finding calls into question its value as a sensitive screening test.[198]

Analytical advantages of IGFBP-3 over IGF-I include the following: (1) IGF-I must be separated from its binding proteins to be measured, but IGFBP-3 does not require a dissociation step; (2) IGFBP-3 is present in higher concentration than IGF-I; and (3) less age dependency is seen for IGFBP-3 compared with IGF-I.[47] Because of their stability over the course of a day, IGF-I and IGFBP-3 measurements may be obtained randomly. However, some researchers have concluded that IGFBP-3 measurements are too nonspecific to be used for the evaluation of GH deficiency.[45] Furthermore, reports indicate that IGF-I and

BOX 53-3 Protocol for the Insulin-Induced Hypoglycemia Stimulation Test [Insulin Tolerance Test (ITT)]

Rationale

The stress of insulin-induced hypoglycemia triggers the release of growth hormone (GH) and adrenocorticotropin hormone (ACTH) from the pituitary gland in normal subjects. The GH response is measured directly. Cortisol is measured as the indication of the ACTH response.

Procedure

The test is done after an overnight fast with the patient at bed rest. An indwelling intravenous line is inserted. Sampling is begun after a 30 minute rest period. Baseline samples are drawn for determination of glucose, GH, and cortisol. Regular insulin, 0.1 to 0.15 units/kg body weight, is injected intravenously. Samples are then obtained at +10, +20, +40, and +60 minutes for glucose, GH, and cortisol determinations. Optional time points are +30, +75, +90, and +120 minutes. To be confident that adequate stress has been applied, the patient must become symptomatic (exhibit sweating or tremor), or the glucose concentration must fall to below 40 to 45 mg/dL. Additional IV insulin may be given if this has not occurred by 30 minutes, in which case sampling should be prolonged by 30 minutes. The physician should be in attendance throughout the test, and 50% dextrose for IV administration should be kept on hand to be used in the event of severe hypoglycemic reaction and after adequate hypoglycemia has been documented. Glucagon (1 mg) should be available for parenteral administration in case IV access is lost. The test is contraindicated in patients with seizure disorder, ischemic heart disease, or cardiovascular insufficiency.

Interpretation

The serum cortisol concentration should increase to a peak value of 18 to 20 µg/dL or greater. The serum GH concentration should rise to a peak value of 7 to 10 ng/mL or greater. No response or inadequate response may be due to pituitary hormone deficiency or a hypothalamic lesion.

IGFBP-3 exhibit imperfect sensitivity and specificity for the diagnosis of GH deficiency.[169]

IGF-I measurements in adults often are not diagnostically helpful.[130] For reasons that are unclear, IGF-I concentrations can be normal in GH-deficient adults. Therefore, a normal IGF-I does not rule out adult GH deficiency. If the IGF-I concentration is very low and suspicion for GH deficiency is high (MPHD or childhood-onset severe GH deficiency), some experts would diagnose GH deficiency in the absence of GH testing.[87]

GH responses to insulin-induced hypoglycemia [insulin tolerance test (ITT); Box 53-3] and GH responses to centrally acting pharmacologic or biological agents (Box 53-4) are considered definitive tests. The stimuli can be sequential or administered on different days. The classical diagnosis of pediatric GH deficiency requires that GH responses to two different stimuli (Table 53-6) be deficient. In research settings, GHRH and GHRP-6 have been used to stimulate GH

BOX 53-4 Protocol for the Arginine Stimulation Test for Growth Hormone

Rationale

In normal subjects, IV administration of arginine hydrochloride stimulates growth hormone (GH) release.

Procedure

The test should be done after an overnight fast with the patient maintained at bed rest. A 10% solution of arginine hydrochloride, 0.5 g/kg body weight (maximum dose = 30 g), is infused intravenously over 30 minutes. Blood samples are drawn for determination of GH before the infusion is started, and 30, 60, and 90 minutes after the infusion is begun. Optional time points are +15 and +120 minutes.

Interpretation

The serum GH concentration should rise to a peak value of 7 to 10 ng/mL or greater. A subnormal response is seen in GH-deficient subjects, but a single subnormal GH response is not diagnostic for GH deficiency and should be confirmed with a second provocative test.

TABLE 53-6 Growth Hormone (GH) Stimuli

GH Stimulus	Dose	GH Sampling, Minutes*
Glucagon	0.03-0.1 mg/kg, IM, max 1 mg	0, 30, 60, 90, 120, 150, 180, ±240 (maximum response ≈2-3 hours)
L-dopa	500 mg/M² (15 mg/kg) max 500 mg (or) <15 kg: 125 mg 15-30 kg: 250 mg >30 kg: 500 mg	0, 40, 60, 90, 120
Clonidine	0.15 mg/M² <30 lb: 0.05 mg >30 lb: 0.1 mg (0.1 mg/tab)	0, 30, 60, 90
Arginine HCl	0.5 g/kg, max 30 g (10% solution IV over 30 min)	0, ±15, 30, 60, 90, ±120
Insulin tolerance test (ITT)	0.1 U/kg (0.05-0.15) IV push insulin	0, 10, 20, ±30, 40, 60, ±75, ±90, ±120
Arginine-insulin tolerance test (AITT)	Arginine: begin at time zero, give insulin at +60 minutes	0, 30, 60, 70, 80, 100, 120

*Experts may differ on the best interval of GH measurements; ± indicates an optional time point.

release. However, because these agents are not available for clinical use, they are not included in Table 53-6. Note that many variations of these protocols are available because endocrinologists often customize these tests. Diazepam and pentagastrin have been studied as GH secretogogues; however, experience with these agents is limited, and they are not included in Table 53-6.

Of children with appropriate stature for age, approximately 80% will have normal GH responses to one stimulus, and at least 95% will have normal GH responses to at least one of two stimuli. This is why two stimuli are generally recommended—to avoid overdiagnosis of GH deficiency. However, the GH Research Society advises that a single definitive abnormal test is adequate to diagnose GH deficiency if the child has (1) confirmed CNS pathology, (2) a history of CNS irradiation, (3) multiple pituitary hormone deficiencies, or (4) a genetic defect.[1]

A history of childhood GH deficiency, CNS disease, trauma, or irradiation is an indication to test adults for GH deficiency.[39,190] Retesting of adults with the diagnosis of childhood GH deficiency is necessary because not all adults with childhood GH deficiency remain deficient as adults. In adults, a single abnormal GH response to a stimulus is diagnostic of GH deficiency if the deficiency is congenital or genetic, or if multiple pituitary hormone deficiencies are due to organic disease. Guidelines published in 2009 recommended that a low IGF-I concentration in a patient with three or more pituitary hormone deficiencies is sufficient to diagnose GH deficiency.[8] Unfortunately GH testing is not very reproducible.[103]

Insulin-induced hypoglycemia (ITT) is often considered to be the "gold standard" stimulus when hypoglycemia is indeed achieved (glucose <40 to 45 mg/dL).[112] The risk associated with this type of test is that untreated severe hypoglycemia can be life threatening. Venous access for infusion of glucose is very important during the ITT. Should vascular access be lost during the ITT, glucagon should be readily available for IM injection (the dose of glucagon is 1 mg). If intravenous access cannot be ensured, stimuli other than insulin should be considered. In general, GH stimulation tests are not conducted by laboratory personnel because of the risks and complexities of testing. Arginine infusion presents the danger of acidosis and even death.[183]

Stimulated GH concentration less than 7 to 10 µg/L defines GH deficiency in children.[26] In adults, GH deficiency is present when stimulated GH is less than 5 µg/L. GH deficiency in adults can be parsed according to the stimulus. For ITTs, a deficient peak GH response is less than 3 µg/L. For GHRH plus arginine, a deficient peak GH response is less than 11 µg/L when the body mass index (BMI) is less than 25 kg/m^2. However if the BMI is 25 to 30 kg/m^2, deficient is defined as less than 8 µg/L, and for BMI greater than 30 kg/m^2, deficient is identified at less than 4 µg/L. Because GHRH is not commercially available, and clonidine and arginine alone are not helpful in defining GH deficiency in adults, the ITT remains the best test of GH secretion in adults.

Controversy continues as to what constitutes a "normal" GH response to stimuli, because insulin-induced hypoglycemia is considered by some to be a nonphysiologic stimulus. Discordance between normal stimulated GH concentration and a deficient spontaneous rise in GH concentration has been described as neurosecretory GH deficiency.[53] Neurosecretory GH deficiency can result from CNS or hypothalamic disease. The diagnosis of neurosecretory GH deficiency requires overnight, every 20 minute blood sampling with GH measurements—a protocol that ordinarily requires hospitalization. The combined costs of GH assays, physician fees, and inpatient services would exceed several thousand dollars.

The definition of *partial GH deficiency* is especially problematic because the definition of *simple GH deficiency* is itself controversial.[91,110] Eliminating GH stimulation testing has been proposed, with the diagnosis of GH deficiency based on growth parameter, IGF-I and IGFBP-3 measurements, neuroradiologic investigation, and genetic considerations.[14,137,211]

Growth Hormone Resistance

In children with short stature and low growth velocity, if IGF-I is (1) below the reference interval for the child's bone age and gender, (2) if the GH concentration is normal or elevated, and (3) if non–GH-dependent causes of IGF-I deficiency (malnutrition, malabsorption, chronic disease, hypothyroidism, and sex hormone deficiency compared with the patient's bone age) have been excluded, GH resistance should be considered.[171] As uncommon as GH deficiency is in the general pediatric population (1 in 10,000 children), GH resistance as a primary problem is far less frequent.

GH resistance can be congenital, resulting from loss-of-function *GHR* mutations or GHR signaling defects (*STAT5b* mutations),[123,215] or from defects in the production of IGF-I itself. Most *GHR* mutations involve the extracellular domain that involves GH binding to the GHR. Some *GHR* mutations affect homodimerization. Loss of the intracellular GHR domain can result from splice-site mutations. GHR is not expressed on the cell surface if the transmembrane domain is defective. Recall that circulating GHBP is derived from the extracellular domain of the GHR. Most cases of GHR deficiency display low or absent concentrations of GHBP. STAT5b is necessary for normal GH-GHR signaling to the cell nucleus. These are autosomal recessive disorders. Size at birth is normal because in utero IGF-I production is independent of GH.

IGF-I gene inactivating mutations or deletions are rare, and only two such mutations have been described. In contrast to GH receptor and signaling defects, when IGF-I itself cannot be produced because of intrinsic *IGF-I* gene mutations, intrauterine growth retardation will result, in addition to extrauterine growth failure. Other consequences of *IGF-I* gene mutations include severe mental retardation, deafness, and micrognathia (mandibular hypoplasia).[206,216]

IGF-I and IGFBP-3 concentrations are very low in rare cases of ALS deficiency, while baseline and poststimulation

GH concentrations are normal.[67] Although adolescence was delayed, adult stature was nearly normal in persons with ALS deficiency.

Acquired GH resistance is far more common than congenital GH resistance. In cases of acquired GH resistance, the IGF-I is low (despite sufficient GH secretion) because of malnutrition, malabsorption, chronic disease, hypothyroidism, or sex hormone deficiency. An acquired form of GH resistance is also observed in patients with idiopathic GH deficiency type I, who develop GH-inhibitory antibodies when treated with exogenous GH. Because GH is absent in this form of congenital GH deficiency, exogenous GH is seen by the immune system as foreign. Apparently, the resulting antibodies directed against exogenous GH bind to, and inactivate, the GH. This is reminiscent of the development of factor VIII antibodies in some boys with severe hemophilia A, who are treated with exogenous factor VIII.

A number of criteria for GH resistance have been proposed, including (1) height more than 3 standard deviations below the mean for age; (2) basal GH greater than 2.5 ng/mL; (3) basal IGF-I less than 50 ng/mL; (4) basal IGFBP-3 more than 2 standard deviations below the mean for age; (5) an increase in IGF-I of less than 15 ng/mL after 4 days of GH treatment (0.05 mg/kg/d); and (6) increase in IGFBP-3 of less than 0.4 μg/mL after GH treatment. The largest concentrations of subjects with GH resistance are found in Israel and southern Ecuador.[170]

IGF-I Resistance

Even less common than GH resistance as a cause of growth failure is IGF-I resistance.[3,76] IGF-I resistance is characterized by growth failure despite elevations in GH and IGF-I. In contrast to GH deficiency and GH resistance states, and in common with *IGF-I* gene mutations, IGF-I resistance causes intrauterine growth retardation and growth failure in childhood. IGF-I resistance can result from mutations in the type I IGF receptor (IGFR), or from downstream signaling mutations.

Rare cases of familial short stature have been ascribed to hemizygosity for the type I IGF receptor gene.[205] Approximately 1 in 50 children with intrauterine growth retardation, short stature, and normal IGF-I concentrations have heterozygous type I IGF receptor mutations.

Measurement of Growth Hormone in Blood

Development of immunochemical methods for measuring GH has followed the same path as those for most other peptide hormones, progressing from radioimmunoassay to immunoradiometric assay, and then to nonisotopic methods involving two antibodies and enzyme, fluorescent, or chemiluminescent labels. Today, a variety of isotopic and nonisotopic assays are commercially available; most of the modern GH assays use mouse monoclonal antibodies and recombinant-derived GH as the competing (labeled) antigens, or as calibrators. Gravimetrically prepared international reference preparations (IRPs), such as the World Health Organization (WHO) international standard of IRP 80/505 human growth hormone recombinant (hGHr), which has a potency of 3.3 IU/mg of r-hGH, or other reference preparations, such as WHO IRP 66/217 or 88/624, have been developed. An international collaborative group currently recommends use of the WHO IRP 98/574 to harmonize GH assays,[196] and at least one commercially available two-site noncompetitive immunoassay has been harmonized to this IRP.[17]

Noncompetitive two-site immunoassays for GH are widely available; most include monoclonal antibodies coupled to an enzyme, chemiluminescent, or fluorescent label. The most sensitive of these GH assays have a detection limit of 1 to 2 μg/L. Of note, although GH is filtered in the glomerulus and excreted in the urine, measurement of urinary GH concentration is not clinically useful.

Analytical Challenges

GH is not a single molecular species, but instead exists in the circulation as a heterogeneous mixture of structural isoforms, including monomeric, dimeric, and oligomeric forms, as well as post-translationally modified monomers with molecular weights ranging from 20 to 22 kDa.[163] Two genes on chromosome 17q code human GH: the product of one is designated GH-N (or GH1) and is expressed primarily in the pituitary; the other is designated GH-V (or GH2) and is derived from the placenta. Both products are 22 kDa proteins, but they differ at 13 residues, and the GH-N isoform is susceptible to deletion of an internal 15 amino acid sequence, producing a 20 kDa GH isoform that accounts for 5 to 10% of the total GH and has a propensity to dimerize. Normally, the human gene for GH that directs the synthesis of a monomeric 22 kDa protein accounts for most of the GH found in the circulation. The 20 kDa variant has less biological activity and does not react with some GH assays, but antibodies that specifically recognize the 20 kDa variant are available.[140] No clinical indications are known for measuring the 20 kDa form of GH, but it has been suggested that it can be used to detect GH doping in sports (see later). Because recombinant GH is the 22 kDa isoform, and exogenous GH suppresses endogenous secretion of the hormone, administration of the recombinant hormone should suppress production of the 20 kDa variant; this effect has been demonstrated.[208] The immunoreactivity of the oligomeric (up to pentameric) isoforms of GH has not been well characterized, although it is known that they have reduced bioactivity and clearance. Approximately half of circulating GH is bound to GHBP derived from the extracellular domain of the GH receptor,[18,19] and a small amount (5 to 8%) is bound to a low-affinity protein.[127] Generally, anti-GH antibodies have sufficiently higher affinity for GH to compete with GH-binding proteins when enough time is allowed for the GH-protein complexes to dissociate. Therefore, immunoassays provide a good approximation of total hormone concentration. Assays for measuring unbound (free) GH also have been developed.[84] Free GH concentrations are proportional to total GH and are inversely proportional to

GH-binding protein, but the clinical usefulness of free GH measurements has not been established.

Variability between GH immunoassays has been reviewed,[26] and it is apparent that significant challenges remain.

Detecting GH Doping in Athletes

Because GH promotes anabolic and lipolytic activities, it has been used by athletes to enhance their physical size, strength, and endurance. In response, the World Anti-Doping Agency has banned the use of GH by athletes competing in sanctioned events. Detecting GH use is challenging, however, because recombinant forms of the hormone are available that are identical to endogenous GH, and normal GH concentrations vary significantly because of the pulsatile nature of hormone release from the pituitary.[74] Although suppression of the 20 kDa GH isoform has showed some promise as a marker of GH doping, most current strategies focus on secondary markers, including IGF and IGFBP.[2]

Specimen Collection and Storage

The preferred specimen is serum; plasma with ethylenediaminetetraacetic acid (EDTA) or heparin added to prevent coagulation may also be used, but values are method dependent. Serum specimens should be stored at 2 to 8 °C if they are not to be tested within 8 hours. If specimens must be stored for longer periods, they should be frozen at −20 °C or colder.

Comments

A single basal or random concentration of GH provides limited diagnostic information. As has been discussed earlier in this chapter, secretion of GH by the pituitary gland is both episodic and pulsatile, and transient concentrations of up to 40 µg/L have been observed in normal, healthy subjects. Serum concentrations are low between pulses in healthy individuals, and some immunoassays are not sensitive enough to distinguish patients with abnormally low concentrations from healthy individuals who have concentrations that happen to fall in the low-normal reference interval. In some individuals, spontaneous GH secretion is better monitored by using a continuous withdrawal pump or by drawing specimens for GH assay every 20 to 30 minutes over a 12 to 24 hour period (e.g., during evaluation of neurogenic GH deficiency). Several stimulation tests have been developed to assess the adequacy of GH secretion (as discussed previously), including the ITT, arginine and GHRH, GHRH and GH-releasing peptide (GHRP), and glucagon stimulation tests. Consensus guidelines have been published for diagnosis of GH deficiency; the commonly accepted ITT cutoff for GH deficiency in adults is less than 3 µg/L following insulin suppression of glucose concentrations to less than 40 mg/dL.[104]

Measurement of Insulin-like Growth Factors

Insulin-like growth factor I (IGF-I; somatomedin C) produced in the liver in response to GH represents the major source of circulating IGF-I. However, it is the autocrine and paracrine production of IGF-I (as controlled by GH) that is responsible for growth. Thus IGF-I is the principal mediator of somatotropic activity of GH.

IGF-I has a longer biological half-life than GH, so its measurement provides an integrated estimate of GH secretion; it is also a more sensitive measure of GH excess in acromegaly. IGF-II is a fetal growth hormone, and the clinical usefulness of measuring IGF-II is very limited.

Historically, radioisotope-based immunoassays for IGF-I were double-antibody methods (competitive or noncompetitive) that used ^{125}I as the tracer. Older IGF-I methods were calibrated with hormone isolated from human serum, but recombinant IGF-I is now available and is used in most procedures. Current IGF-I methods should use a reference material that is traceable to the International Reference Preparation IGF-I 87/518, or the newer WHO First International Standard 02/254.[36] To avoid interference from IGF-binding proteins, many assays isolate IGF using a variety of extraction methods, including (1) gel filtration, (2) acid-ethanol precipitation, (3) cryoprecipitation, (4) C-18 column extraction, or (5) reversed-phase chromatography.[32] Direct (no extraction) procedures are also available, but extraction methods prevent the formation of complexes with carrier proteins and serum proteases. Moreover, extraction procedures are better able to discriminate between GH-deficient patients and age-matched controls. Commercial assays that include chemiluminescent labels are available for measuring IGF-I, usually with minimal cross-reactivity to IGF-II (0 to 3%). It is important to establish age-related reference intervals for IGF-I because of marked differences in hormone concentrations between adults and children.

IGF-binding protein 3 (IGFBP-3) is the major protein carrier of circulating IGF-I and is an indirect measure of GH activity. IGFBP-3 measurements therefore provides additional evidence in cases of suspected GH deficiency. This protein has been measured in unextracted plasma by radioimmunoassay (RIA) using rabbit antihuman IGFBP-3; cross-reactivity with other binding proteins is less than 0.2%.[27]

Measurement of IGF-I has become a staple in the evaluation of growth hormone abnormalities, but problems with interassay agreement remain, mostly related to binding proteins. The availability of reliable reference materials against which immunoassays for IGF-I may be calibrated has been problematic. These difficulties have been reviewed.[85]

Specimen Collection and Storage

Serum or plasma (with heparin or EDTA added to prevent coagulation) is used, depending on the assay method. Samples should be centrifuged within 1 hour of collection and stored frozen at −20 °C or colder for up to 30 days. Some procedures use dried whole blood or serum collected on filter paper.[151]

Prolactin

Prolactin is secreted by lactotrophs of the adenohypophysis.[92] Prolactin stimulates and sustains lactation in postpartum mammals after the mammary glands have been prepared by other hormones, including estrogens, progesterone, growth hormone, corticosteroids, and insulin.

Biochemistry

Hypothalamic prolactin release inhibitory hormone (PRIH) is dopamine, which is a product of the tuberoinfundibular cells and the hypothalamic tuberohypophyseal dopaminergic system. In lactotrophs, dopamine binds to the type 2 dopamine (D2) receptor, one of five dopamine receptors. Dopamine receptors are located in the caudate putamen, nucleus accumbens, and olfactory tubercle, affecting (1) locomotion, (2) learning, (3) memory, (4) reward, and (5) reinforcement.

The gene for the D2 receptor is located on chromosome 11q2, contains 443 amino acids, and has a mass of 50.6 kDa. The extracellular domain is 37 amino acids, and seven transmembrane domains are present, along with a 14 amino acid cytoplasmic domain. A large extracellular loop is evident between amino acids 211 and 373. Three potential sites of N-glycosylation are noted: amino acids 5, 17, and 23. A disulfide bridge may occur between amino acids 107 and 182. Three isoforms of the D2 receptor have been identified: the full-length isoform is referred to as D2 (long); isoform 2 is D2 (short) and lacks amino acids 242-270; isoform 3, D2 (longer), contains a val → trp-glu substitution at position 270. Mutations in the D2 receptor cause dystonia type 11 (myoclonus dystonia, or alcohol-responsive dystonia).

The gene that encodes prolactin was described in the section concerning the *GH1* gene. Initially, preprolactin is synthesized (227 amino acids), and following cleavage of the leader sequence, the 199 amino acid prolactin hormone is liberated. Amino acid 59 is the site of putative N-glycosylation. Intra-chain disulfide bonds are located between amino acids 32 and 39, 86 and 202, and 219 and 227.

Circulating prolactin exists in several forms: monomeric prolactin (23 kDa, "little" prolactin), dimeric prolactin (48-56 kDa, "big" prolactin), and polymeric prolactin (>100 kDa, "big, big" prolactin). Occasionally, and independent of the presence or absence of disease, immunoglobulin G (IgG) autoantibodies against prolactin can bind to prolactin, forming macroprolactin. The presence of macroprolactin elevates the total prolactin concentration, as the result of lower clearance, in the absence of excess prolactin secretion by the anterior pituitary lactotrophs. Failure to recognize macroprolactin can lead to the inappropriate diagnosis of hyperprolactinemia. In nature, many examples of macroproteins resulting from the complex of an antibody and a protein can be found, including macro-creatine kinase, macroamylase, macro-lactate dehydrogenase, and macro-aspartate aminotransferase.

The gene for the prolactin receptor *(PRLR)* is located at chromosome 5p13.2. Pre-PRLR is 622 amino acids (69.5 kDa). Upon removal of the signal peptide, the full-length PRLR is released (598 amino acids). The first 210 amino acids of the receptor are extracellular, 24 amino acids are present in the transmembrane domain, and the cytoplasmic domain consists of 364 amino acids. Amino acids 27-121 (with reference to preprolactin) represent a fibronectin type III-1 domain, whereas amino acids 127-227 represent a fibronectin type III-2 domain. Amino acids 215-219 display a WSXWS motif, and amino acids 267-275 display a box 1 motif. The WSXWS motif is the tryptophan-serine-wild card-tryptophan-serine sequence located near the lipid bilayer. Box 1 motifs are expressed in the cytoplasmic domain of receptors that engage in Janus kinase 2 (Jak2) receptor signaling. Glycosylation may occur at amino acids 59, 104, and 233, and intrachain disulfide bonds occur between amino acids 36 and 46, and 75 and 86. The PRLR forms a homodimer upon binding prolactin.

Eight isoforms of the PRLR have been described. Isoform 1 is the full-length PRLR. In isoform 2, amino acids 24 to 124 are missing. In isoform 3, amino acids 229 (aspartate) and 230 (phenylalanine) are replaced, respectively, by alanine and tryptophan (amino acids 231 to 622 are missing; therefore this protein lacks a transmembrane domain and the protein is soluble). This isoform has been reported as the product of a breast cancer cell line. Isoform 4 has changes in the amino acid sequence of amino acids 338-376, with the remaining amino acids deleted, and is nonfunctional. Because of a deletion of part of exon 10, and a frameshift mutation, the sequence of isoform 5 is altered among amino acids 337-349; thereafter the remaining amino acids are absent. In isoform 6, amino acids 286-288 (lysine-glycine-lysine) are replaced, respectively, by valine, tyrosine, and proline, and the amino acids distal to 288 are absent; this receptor is nonfunctional. Isoform 7 is secreted with changes in amino acids 229 to 268, and amino acids 269-622 are absent. Last, isoform 8 begins at amino acid 72, and amino acids 286-288 are replaced, respectively, by valine, tyrosine, and proline; the amino acids distal to 288 are absent, as in isoform 6.

Physiology

The biological importance of prolactin in men is unclear.[180] In women, prolactin is necessary for lactation following delivery of the newborn. Prolactin is stimulated by breast-feeding, chest wall disease, and stress. Although prolactin is higher during the day than at night, and a night-to-day prolactin ratio greater than 1 : 2 is considered normal, the ratio has no diagnostic value. Prolactin is measured in its basal state without stimulatory or suppressive manipulation. As with other adenohypophyseal hormones, the release of prolactin is episodic and varies predictably during the day, with lowest concentrations found at midday and highest values shortly after the onset of deep sleep.

Receptors for prolactin are located in the hypothalamus, breast, and ovary. Breast development during puberty can occur in the absence of prolactin, but estrogen is required, along with GH and GH-stimulated IGF-I. Fetal breast development is stimulated by parathyroid hormone–related peptide (PTHrP), which shares the N-terminal active domain of parathyroid hormone but has extraparathyroidal origins.

Prolactin secretion by lactotrophs is controlled predominantly through suppression by PRIH.[80] In addition, prolactin may provide feedback centrally to stimulate PRIH in a short negative feedback loop, but this has been difficult to confirm. An ultra-short feedback loop is present where prolactin suppresses its own release. Besides very high concentrations of TRH, other factors that may stimulate prolactin secretion include oxytocin, VIP, basic fibroblast growth factor, EGF, hypothalamic prolactin-releasing peptide (PrRP), galanin, and neurotensin. Identified in the hypothalamus, amygdala, basal ganglia, and dorsal gray matter of the spinal cord, neurotensin is a 13 amino acid peptide neurotransmitter. Neurotensin affects gastrointestinal function and has a role in pain perception.

Estrogen increases prolactin gene transcription and secretion; this explains why prolactin concentrations are higher in women than in men. The upper limit of the prolactin reference interval for women is 20 ng/mL, whereas in men it is 10 ng/mL. Prolactin is lowest while awake and highest during sleep. Prolactin rises during pregnancy because of elevated concentrations of sex steroids (predominantly estradiol). The average serum prolactin during pregnancy is approximately 200 ng/mL. Because of increased lactotrophs, the pituitary approximately doubles in size during pregnancy.

The breast is prepared for lactation during pregnancy through the actions of (1) estrogen, (2) progesterone, (3) prolactin, (4) GH-V, (5) hPL, and possibly (6) IGF-I.[102] Just as the visible size of the breast increases during pregnancy, many microscopic changes occur in breast tissue. Typically, lactation is not active until after delivery, when estrogen and progesterone concentrations have declined. Prolactin increases amino acid and glucose uptake by breast tissue, and synthesis of alpha-lactalbumin and beta-casein, lactose, and milk fats is increased.

Postpartum, a positive feedback loop is seen between suckling and milk production. Transmitted via nerve fibers from the nipple to the CNS, suckling reduces PRIH, which increases prolactin release. With suckling, prolactin can rise by more than eightfold over baseline. The positive feedback loop of suckling, prolactin secretion, and milk production is a "stimulus-secretion" reflex. However, with continued breast-feeding, prolactin concentration declines. One report observed mean prolactin concentrations of 162 ng/mL 2 to 4 weeks postpartum, 130 ng/mL 5 to 14 weeks postpartum, and 77 ng/mL 15 to 24 weeks postpartum. Suckling also stimulates oxytocin release, which is discussed in the section of this chapter concerning the posterior pituitary.

Because elevated prolactin concentrations reduce LH and FSH by inhibiting GnRH release (a short feedback loop between prolactin and the hypothalamus), breast-feeding delays the onset of menses following delivery.[148] Lactation amenorrhea is beneficial because it temporarily ensures that the mother can adequately breast-feed her newborn before she becomes pregnant again. It is understood that oligomenorrhea, amenorrhea, and infertility in hyperprolactinemic women, and impotence and oligospermia in hyperprolactinemic men, result from prolactin suppression of GnRH secretion. Prolactin has direct effects on prolactin receptors in the ovary.

The role of prolactin in the immune system is controversial. At this time, it is difficult to ascribe any major, specific immune function to prolactin.

Hyperprolactinemia

Hyperprolactinemia is the most common hypothalamic-pituitary disorder encountered in clinical endocrinology.[114] Prolactin concentrations may be elevated in women who have only subtle alterations in fertility, such as (1) anovulation with or without menstrual irregularity, (2) amenorrhea and galactorrhea, or (3) galactorrhea alone. Prolactin excess in men is frequently manifested as oligospermia, or impotence, or both. Hyperprolactinemia can also cause galactorrhea in men. In addition, men with prolactin-secreting pituitary adenomas more often than women present with macroadenomas and visual field disturbances resulting from a large tumor pressing on the optic chiasm. Men, of course, do not have the subtle symptom of an irregular menstrual period that frequently reveals a microadenoma (≤10 mm in diameter) in women. Elevated prolactin concentrations are observed in as many as 30% of women with polycystic ovarian syndrome and patients with clinically silent pituitary adenoma. If a borderline elevation of prolactin is found, it is advisable to repeat the measurement on at least two other occasions, taking care to obtain a morning specimen under conditions of minimal excitement or stress to the patient, that is, no trauma and no breast stimulation. The patient should not be on any medication that could stimulate prolactin release. The differential diagnosis of hyperprolactinemia is extensive (Table 53-7).

An extremely important cause of hyperprolactinemia is a prolactinoma.[50,78] The higher the prolactin concentration, the greater is the likelihood that hyperprolactinemia is the result of a prolactinoma. Hyperprolactinemia due to a macroprolactinoma (>10 mm in diameter) can produce prolactin concentrations into the tens of thousands (ng/mL). Prolactin

TABLE 53-7 Differential Diagnosis of Hyperprolactinemia

PRIH (dopamine) deficiency	Hypothalamic disease Interruption in the hypothalamic-pituitary portal system
Drugs	Dopamine antagonists Cholinergic antagonists Serotonergic antagonists
Hormones	Estrogen, pregnancy
Neurogenic	Nursing (nipple stimulation) Chest wall disease Spinal cord injury
Other diseases	Hypothyroidism (pathologically elevated TRH can release prolactin) Chronic renal disease Cirrhosis

concentrations greater than 200 ng/mL usually indicate a macroprolactinoma. Prolactinomas are diagnostically challenging. Because any degree of hyperprolactinemia can be seen in cases of prolactinoma, if hyperprolactinemia is otherwise not explained, a thorough search for a prolactinoma, including MRI imaging, should be undertaken. Mass displacement effects from an anterior pituitary tumor include destruction of the sella turcica, invasion of other structures, compression of the stalk, or optic nerve compression with bitemporal hemianopsia.

Early diagnosis of a prolactinoma is critical because therapy with dopamine agonists, such as bromocriptine, can reduce tumor size and control tumor progression.[108] Surgical excision of a prolactinoma usually is considered only when a destructive invasion of adjacent structures and/or serious optic nerve compression occurs.

Macroprolactinemia is a common cause of an elevated plasma prolactin concentration; this benign condition should be ruled out before additional diagnostic studies are performed.[101] Macroprolactinemia can result from elevated circulating concentrations of the polymeric forms of prolactin and/or from prolactin-immunoglobulin complexes with molecular masses in excess of 100 kDa.

Polymeric forms of prolactin lack biological activity; thus, none of the sequelae associated with an elevated prolactin concentration (sexual dysfunction and galactorrhea) are present. In addition, macroprolactinemia is not associated with negative or positive feedback effects at the hypothalamus. Because macroprolactin is formed outside of lactotrophs, it is not found in pituitary tissue, and its size prevents entry into the cerebrospinal fluid. Therefore, macroprolactin appears to be confined to the vascular compartment.

Macroprolactinemia, although asymptomatic, is troublesome for clinicians and the laboratory because it is detected by most prolactin immunoassays. In one report, almost 20% of patients who presented for a clinical work-up for prolactinoma had hyperprolactinemia attributable to the presence of macroprolactin. Although the prevalence of macroprolactinemia was approximately 1.5% in the population studied, the report suggested that macroprolactinemia is more common than was previously realized. Thus, clinical laboratories must be able to rule out the presence of a macroprolactin.[188] Macroprolactin can be precipitated by the addition of polyethylene glycol (PEG) to serum; this is the most common laboratory approach to detecting macroprolactin.[192]

Another diagnostic challenge in the investigation of hyperprolactinemia is the presence of a pituitary incidentaloma in a patient with elevated prolactin that could potentially lead to inappropriate surgery.[152-154] A lesion identified by MRI cannot unequivocally be associated with hyperprolactinemia because of the possibility of an incidentaloma. Compression of the optic chiasm, or destruction of bone, argues against an incidentaloma, but mild to modest elevations in prolactin concentration (50 to 200 ng/mL) are possible when other anterior pituitary tumors compress the hypothalamic-pituitary portal system, impairing the delivery of PRIH to the lactotrophs; these conditions are called *pseudoprolactinomas.* Treatment with a dopamine agonist should lower prolactin concentration in cases of a true prolactinoma, but will not reduce prolactin concentration with pseudoprolactinoma. Prolactin measurements are also susceptible to a high-dose hook effect that may lead to a missed diagnosis of hyperprolactinemia. If a macroadenoma is present by MRI yet the prolactin is only modestly elevated, clinicians may request that the prolactin be remeasured at 1 to 10 and 1 to 100 dilution. If a hook effect is present, the concentration of the diluted sample will be significantly greater than that of the undiluted sample.

MRI of the pituitary gland is performed as part of the clinical assessment when a prolactinoma is suspected. Unless a pituitary tumor can be demonstrated by MRI, prolactin-secreting microadenoma (≤10 mm in diameter) is diagnosed by exclusion. Because half of all prolactin-secreting microadenomas are too small to be detected by imaging methods, differentiating between a small pituitary tumor, prolactin-cell hyperplasia, and idiopathic hyperprolactinemia may not be possible without surgical exploration.

Medications that stimulate prolactin release (through PRIH suppression) are the most common cause of hyperprolactinemia in otherwise healthy individuals.[41] When significant elevation of prolactin is confirmed, a careful history should rule out the possibility that medications are the cause. In addition to estrogens, dopamine receptor blockers (such as the phenothiazines) and dopamine antagonists (such as metoclopramide and domperidone used to treat gastrointestinal diseases) cause significant increases in prolactin. Certain psychiatric drugs, including haloperidol and risperidone, cause elevated prolactin. Antihypertensive agents (such as beta blockers and calcium channel blockers) and antihistamines (such as cimetidine and ranitidine) are associated with modest elevations in prolactin. Thyrotropin (TSH) measurements should be considered in patients suspected of a prolactinoma, to rule out primary hypothyroidism; in rare cases of severe primary hypothyroidism, TRH will promote release of prolactin. A pregnancy test should be performed in women of reproductive age because pregnancy is a cause of hyperprolactinemia.

Prolactin Deficiency

Prolactin is of great clinical importance in the postpartum period, because prolactin is required for lactation.[175] Without the availability of infant formulas or wet nurses, failure of maternal lactation can be fatal to the newborn. Other than the necessity of breast-feeding, however, prolactin deficiency in humans does not appear to have adverse consequences.

Measurement of Prolactin

Similar to most hormone assays, RIA was the first practical method for measuring prolactin, but performance of the early assays was variable, and they have been mostly replaced by nonisotopic methods. Modern prolactin assays typically involve noncompetitive, heterogeneous "sandwich" techniques that make use of two antibodies that recognize different epitopes on the prolactin polypeptide.

Structural variations in circulating prolactin result in biases between immunoassays for this hormone. Monomeric prolactin accounts for more than 85% of the total circulating hormone, but glycosylated and inactive complexed forms (sometimes referred to as "big" and "big-big" prolactin, respectively) constitute a significant fraction, and immunoreactivity of these prolactin complexes is variable. IgG-bound prolactin, now referred to as *macroprolactin,* is a relatively common finding in healthy patients and, according to one study, may account for up to 10% of misdiagnoses in hyperprolactinemic patients,[188] because renal clearance of the immunoglobulin-bound hormone is reduced. IgG-bound prolactin can be separated by gel chromatography, or more conveniently by precipitation of immunoglobulin complexes with the addition of PEG. PEG precipitation removes a small fraction of monomeric prolactin as well, but remains a useful method for distinguishing between clinical hyperprolactinemia and prolactin elevations due to prolactin-IgG complexes.[24]

Prolactin methods should be calibrated against reference materials with known international unit potency, such as the WHO first IRP 75/504, the second international standard (IS) 83/562, or the third IS 84/500, to allow assay-to-assay comparison. Despite the heterogeneity of prolactin, immunoassays correlate well with bioassay-validated prolactin standards.

Specimen Collection and Storage

Prolactin is measured in serum or plasma, although individual assays may recommend serum only. Special handling procedures are not necessary; specimens can be stored at 4 °C for at least 24 hours, but should be frozen if analysis is delayed for longer than 24 hours. Prolactin concentrations rise rapidly during sleep and peak in the early morning hours, so attention should be given to the appropriate reference interval. Emotional stress, exercise, ambulation, and a protein-rich diet all stimulate prolactin secretion; thus specimens collected after an overnight fast when the patient is resting provide the most reliable prolactin concentrations.

Adrenocorticotropic Hormone and Related Peptides

Adrenocorticotropic hormone (ACTH; corticotropin) is secreted by the adenohypophysis as a derivative of pro-opiomelanocortin (POMC).[186,213] ACTH acts primarily on the adrenal cortex, stimulating its growth and the secretion of corticosteroids (specifically cortisol). ACTH production is increased during physiologic or psychologic stress.

Biochemistry

The biochemistry of ACTH, with its origin from POMC and POMC-derived peptides, is described in detail in Chapter 54.

Regulation of ACTH Secretion

Many variables affect the secretion of ACTH, which is both pulsatile and circadian in nature. Thus, regulation of pituitary secretion of ACTH by the hypothalamus is complex. The control of ACTH release by the pituitary is an integral part of the neuroendocrine regulation of stress homeostasis.

Cortisol is the major negative feedback hormone for the tonic inhibition of hypothalamic CRH and pituitary ACTH secretion. However, endogenous opioids such as met-enkephalin and beta-endorphin, produced by the adrenal glands, have a downregulatory effect on the hypothalamic-pituitary-ACTH axis as well. Regulation of ACTH is discussed at length in Chapter 54.

Clinical Significance

Because ACTH synthesis originates from the POMC precursor peptide, its production by the pituitary is closely linked with the secretion of endogenous opioid peptides, such as beta-endorphin.[178] The physiologic effects of endogenous opiates include (1) sedation; (2) an increased threshold of pain; and (3) autonomic regulation of respiration, blood pressure, and heart rate. These peptides are also involved in modifying endocrine responses to stress and water balance, and may play a role in the regulation of reproduction and the immune system.

Gonadotropin secretion by the pituitary is under inhibitory control by opioid peptides, as is evident by the effects of beta-endorphin analogs on the pulse frequency and amplitude of pituitary LH release. In contrast, beta-endorphin antagonists (such as naloxone) can elicit an increase in the amount and pattern of gonadotropin secretion. ACTH secretion is similarly downregulated by endogenous opioid peptides; therefore naloxone causes an increase in plasma ACTH concentrations.

No diseases have been clearly associated with disordered metabolism of opioid peptides, but changes in their plasma concentrations may accompany other disorders, such as Cushing disease and depression (increased beta-endorphin concentrations)[60] or pheochromocytoma (increased enkephalin concentrations). Altered concentrations of opioids in cerebrospinal fluid may reflect disorders such as chronic pain syndrome, schizophrenia, and depression.

In summary, the only POMC derivative that is measured in the diagnosis of certain human disease states is ACTH. Further discussion of adrenal disorders, including disorders of ACTH secretion, is found in Chapter 54.

Measurement of ACTH

ACTH has been measured by bioassay, receptor assay, and immunoassay. Previous editions of this textbook contain details of bioassays and receptor assays for ACTH, which now are mostly of historical interest.

Immunoassays that measure the concentration of ACTH are more common than bioassays or receptor assays. Competitive binding RIAs have been developed for ACTH; they differ in (1) the choice of radioactive label (^{125}I is most common), (2) separation system (charcoal adsorption, PEG, or second-antibody precipitation), (3) antibody (N-terminal or C-terminal specificity), and (4) whether pre-extraction of ACTH is required. Most polyclonal antibodies recognize a segment of the biologically active N-terminal portion of the molecule and react with intact ACTH (amino acids 1-39), N-terminal ACTH fragments (amino acids 1-24), and ACTH precursors such as POMC and pro-ACTH.

Immunoradiometric ACTH assays that use labeled monoclonal antibodies in noncompetitive formats have also been developed.[79] In these assays, two monoclonal antibodies (or a polyclonal/monoclonal combination) are directed toward different sites on the ACTH molecule (e.g., the N-terminal and C-terminal domains). These double antibody (sandwich) immunoassays can detect ACTH concentrations of 1 to 4 pg/mL. Monoclonal immunoassays have improved analytical specificity for intact ACTH but may not recognize biologically active precursors and fragments.[165] Less specific ACTH immunoassays are sometimes used to detect the presence of these peptide fragments in patients with cancer-related syndromes (e.g., ectopic ACTH Cushing syndrome); a two-site IRMA has been developed for measuring ACTH precursors in plasma.[52] A direct (unextracted) immunoradiometric test kit for ACTH is commercially available that uses a polyclonal antibody–monoclonal antibody sandwich to detect ACTH; the monoclonal antibody is radiolabeled with ^{125}I. A nonisotopic time-resolved immunofluorometric method has also been reported.[66] ACTH assays have been developed for automated immunoassay platforms using chemiluminescent labels. These methods are more precise than manual methods [coefficients of variation (CVs) <8%], and, analytically, they are sensitive enough to distinguish between low-normal and suppressed hormone secretion.

Quantitative results from different ACTH immunoassays may demonstrate bias as the result of calibration. Currently, manufacturers of commercial ACTH immunoassays usually calibrate their assays with ACTH preparations obtained from research centers, such as human purified ACTH 1-39 (MRC 74/555, 6.2 IU/25 μg), supplied by the National Institute for Biological Standards and Control (United Kingdom), or synthetic ACTH 1-39 (4.71 IU/50 μg), supplied by the U.S. National Hormone and Pituitary Program, which was formerly known as the National Pituitary Agency. For comparison between assays, the calibrators used in a particular assay system must be clearly specified.

Specimen Collection and Storage

Some precautions are necessary in the collection, transportation, and storage of specimens. ACTH is easily oxidized, adsorbs to glass surfaces, and is rapidly degraded by plasma proteases into nonreactive fragments during freezing and thawing of the specimen. Factors that influence plasma ACTH, such as prior administration of corticosteroids, the time of day at which the specimen is collected (diurnal variation), and stress from the venipuncture procedure, should be taken into account. To minimize these problems, it is recommended that blood specimens should be collected into prechilled polystyrene (plastic) tubes containing EDTA, immediately placed on ice, and centrifuged at 4 °C. Some laboratories recommend the use of protease inhibitors, such as aprotinin (Trasylol). The plasma should be transferred to another plastic tube and frozen at −20 °C or colder if analysis is delayed. Antioxidants, such as mercaptoethanol, may be used to stabilize ACTH. Immediately before the ACTH assay is set up, frozen specimens should be thawed and centrifuged to remove any fibrin clots that can interfere with the assay.

Measurement of Endogenous Opioid Peptides

Beta-endorphin is a cleavage product of POMC, which is also the precursor to ACTH and beta-lipotropin. Both RIAs and immunoradiometric assays (IRMAs) have been developed for measurement of beta-endorphin. Commercial assays are widely available, and most reference laboratories offer beta-endorphin assays. The concentration of beta-endorphin is usually very low or undetectable in healthy subjects, and some analytical methods require extraction procedures to detect meaningful concentrations in plasma. The specificity of commercial antibodies for beta-endorphin (relative to beta-lipotropin) can be variable, and some assays cross-react as much as 50% with beta-lipotropin. Assays based on polyclonal antibodies may produce spuriously high results as the consequence of cross-reactivity with serum IgG (e.g., in patients with an IgG myeloma).[99]

Met-enkephalin shares a 5 amino acid N-terminal sequence with beta-endorphin but is thought to be derived from pro-enkephalin, rather than POMC. Measurement of met-enkephalin in plasma is difficult because of its very short half-life (2.5 minutes at 37 °C). Even if blood is immediately chilled on ice and centrifuged under refrigeration, about 50% of met-enkephalin is lost unless the specimen is collected in 23 mmol/L of citric acid. Commercial assays for met-enkephalin have been developed, and anti-enkephalin antibodies are available.

Gonadotropins (Follicle-Stimulating Hormone, Luteinizing Hormone)

Luteinizing hormone and follicle-stimulating hormone are synthesized by gonadotrophs in the adenohypophysis. The actions of FSH are to (1) stimulate the growth and maturation of ovarian follicles, (2) stimulate estrogen secretion (estradiol), (3) promote via estrogen the endometrial changes characteristic of the first portion (proliferative or follicular phase) of the menstrual cycle, and (4) stimulate spermatogenesis in males. FSH is also called *follitropin*.

LH and FSH act synergistically to promote ovulation and secretion of androgens (androstenedione) and progesterone. The actions of LH are to (1) promote and maintain the second (secretory or luteal) portion of the menstrual cycle; (2) in females, to assist in the formation of the corpus luteum; and (3) in males, to stimulate the development and functional activity of testicular Leydig cells that produce testosterone. LH is also called *interstitial cell–stimulating hormone (ICSH)*, or *lutropin*.

Biochemistry

Under the generic term *gonadotropins*, LH and FSH control the functional activity of gonads. In males and females, gonadotropin secretion is regulated via GnRH.[51] Pituitary gonadotropin secretion is controlled by feedback from the gonadotropic hormones. In females, estrogen and inhibin regulate LH and FSH secretion, respectively, and in males, testosterone and inhibin regulate LH and FSH release.

Two *GnRH* genes are present: *GnRH1,* located at chromosome 8p21, and *GnRH2,* located at chromosome 20p13. PreproGnRH1 is a 92 amino acid, 10.4 kDa polypeptide with a 23 amino acid leader sequence. Removal of the leader sequence produces ProGnRH1, which comprises 69 amino acids. Release of the C-terminal GnRH-associated peptide-1 yields *GnRH1* (amino acids 24-33). Amino acid 24 is modified as a pyrrolidone carboxylic acid, and amino acid 33 is modified as a glycine amide.

GnRH2 is expressed in higher concentrations outside than within the CNS. GnRH2 is principally produced in the prostate, bone marrow, and kidney. PreproGnRH2 is a 120 amino acid (12.9 kDa) polypeptide. Cleavage of the 23 amino acid leader sequence generates proGnRH2, which is 97 amino acids in length. Release of the C-terminal GnRH-associated peptide 2 yields GnRH2 (amino acids 24-33). Similar to GnRH1, amino acid 24 is modified as a pyrrolidone carboxylic acid, and amino acid 33 is modified as a glycine amide. GnRH2 has three isoforms: isoform 1 is the full-length protein; isoform 2 lacks amino acids 52-59; and isoform 3 is missing amino acids 52-58.

The receptor for GnRH (GnRHR) is expressed on anterior pituitary gonadotropic cells. The gene for GnRHR is located at chromosome 4q. GnRHR is a 328 amino acid protein; the first 38 amino acids are extracellular, and seven transmembrane domains are present. Only two amino acids are cytoplasmic. The GnRHR is possibly glycosylated at amino acids 18 and 102, and a disulfide bond is probably present between amino acids 114 and 196. Two isoforms of GnRHR are expressed: the full-length protein (isoform 1) and isoform 2, which differs in the amino acid sequence between residues 176 and 328. A putative second GnRHR (GnRH2R) exists, comprising 178 amino acids. However, the gene for GnRH2R (located on chromosome 1) may be a pseudogene.

Both LH and FSH are secreted by gonadotrophs. Similar to TSH and hCG, LH and FSH are glycoprotein alpha/beta heterodimers.[77] The alpha chain is shared among all four hormones. The glycoprotein alpha chain gene is located on chromosome 6q1. The alpha chain includes 116 amino acids and weighs 13.1 kDa, including a leader sequence of 24 amino acids; the secreted chain is 92 amino acids. Amino acids 76 and 102 in the alpha chain are glycosylated. Five disulfide bonds are present at amino acids 31-55, 34-84, 52-106, 56-108, and 83-111.

The gene for the LH beta chain is located at chromosome 19q13.3. The leader sequence (amino acids 1-20) is followed by the 121 amino acid beta chain, which is the secreted form. The beta chain is glycosylated at amino acid 50, and six disulfide bonds are present at amino acids 29-77, 43-92, 46-130, 54-108, 58-110, and 113-120.

The gene for the FSH beta chain is located at chromosome 11p1. The 129 amino acid pre-FSH beta chain is 14.7 kDa, including an 18 amino acid leader sequence; the secreted FSH beta chain is 111 amino acids. FSH-β is glycosylated at amino acids 25 and 42 and contains six disulfide bonds at amino acids 21-69, 35-84, 38-122, 46-100, 50-102, and 105-112. Isolated alpha-subunits are devoid of biological activity; the beta-subunit of FSH may have slight intrinsic biological activity, but full activity is attained when alpha- and beta-subunits are recombined. This suggests that the presence of both alpha- and beta-subunits is important for specific receptor recognition, and that the beta-subunit is responsible for eliciting the specific biological response.

In men, the LH receptor (LHR) is expressed by Leydig cells, whereas in women, the LHR is expressed on theca cells and is induced by FSH on granulosa cells during the follicular phase of the menstrual cycle. The gene for the LHR is located at chromosome 2p21. The pre-LHR protein is 699 amino acids (78.6 kDa). After removal of the leader sequence, LHR comprises 673 amino acids. The extracellular domain is 337 amino acids, followed by seven transmembrane domains and a cytoplasmic domain of 72 amino acids. Seven leucine-rich repeats are present at amino acids 48-71, 97-121, 122-147, 149-171, 172-196, 197-220, and 221-244. Cysteines at positions 643 and 644 are lipidated to S-palmitoyl cysteine. Potential glycosylation sites exist at amino acids 99, 174, 195, 291, 299, and 313. A disulfide bond is likely between amino acids 439 and 514. Two isoforms of LHR are expressed: the long isoform is the full-length LHR, and the short isoform lacks amino acids 227-289.

The FSH receptor (FSHR) is expressed on Sertoli cells in men and on granulosa cells in women. Following the 17 amino acid leader sequence is the 678 amino acid FSHR. The extracellular domain is 349 amino acids, with seven transmembrane domains. The cytoplasmic domain is 65 amino acids. Ten leucine-rich repeats are present at amino acids 18-48, 49-72, 73-97, 98-118, 119-143, 144-169, 170-192, 193-216, 217-240, and 241-259. The FSHR has four proven or suspected sites of glycosylation at amino acids 191, 199, 293, and 318; two definitive disulfide bonds (amino acids 18-25 and 23-32); and one possible disulfide bond (amino acids 442-517). Two isoforms of the FSHR are expressed: isoform 1 is the full-length FSHR, and isoform 2 lacks amino acids 224-285.

Physiologic Activity

In men, LH stimulates testosterone synthesis and secretion by Leydig cells. In response to FSH, Sertoli cells nourish developing sperm during spermatogenesis.

Based on the two-cell model of estradiol and progesterone production by the adult ovary, androstenedione is produced by theca cells in response to LH stimulation (Figure 53-6). Granulosa cells do not have direct access to the circulation; therefore low-density lipoprotein cholesterol is not readily available to granulosa cells in the follicular phase of the menstrual cycle. Consequently, granulosa cell synthesis of sex steroids is dependent on theca cell androstenedione. Granulosa cells initially respond to FSH, and later to FSH plus LH.

FSH has several effects on the ovary during the follicular phase of the menstrual cycle (see Chapter 56). When bound to granulosa cell FSHRs, FSH stimulates granulosa cell

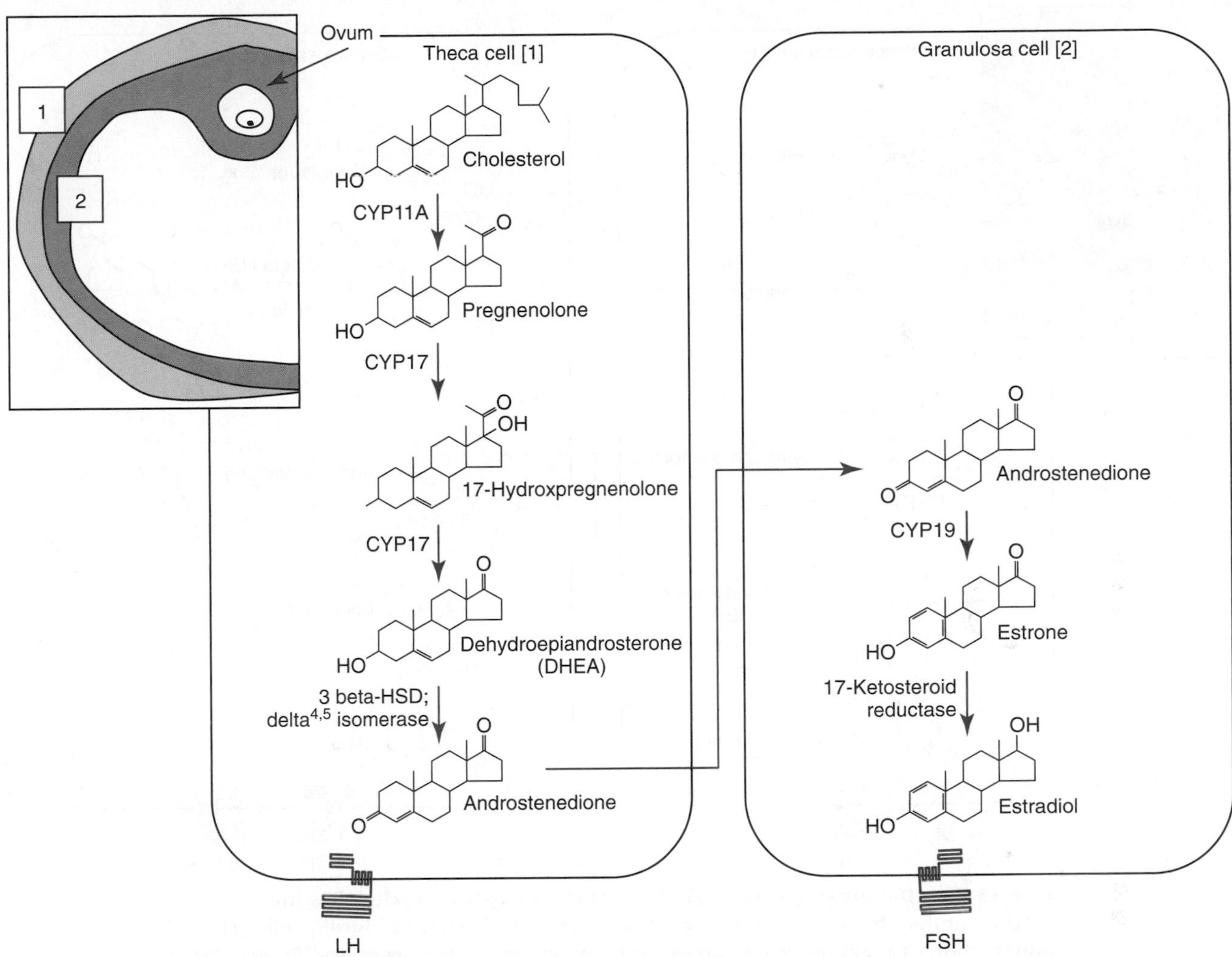

Figure 53-6 In the follicular (proliferative) phase of the menstrual cycle, under the influence of luteinizing hormone (LH), theca cells *[1]* produce androstenedione from cholesterol (the intermediary steps are illustrated). Under the influence of follicle-stimulating hormone (FSH), granulosa cells utilize the androstenedione produced by the theca cells to synthesize estradiol (the intermediary steps are illustrated) *[2]*. *3 Beta-HSD,* 3 Beta-hydroxysteroid dehydrogenase; *CYP11A,* 20,22 desmolase; *CYP17,* 17-hydroxylase activity; and *CYP19,* aromatase.

proliferation. As a result, a dominant follicle develops containing the ovum that will be expelled midcycle (ovulation). When stimulated by FSH, granulosa cells use theca cell androstenedione as the precursor for estradiol synthesis. FSH also stimulates the expression of LHRs on the granulosa cells. Estradiol and inhibins from the ovary provide negative feedback for hypothalamic release of GnRH.

At midcycle, as a consequence of the LH surge, the follicle ruptures with release of the ovum (ovulation). The corpus luteum of the ovary (Figure 53-7) is formed from the remaining theca and granulosa cells. The theca cells (responsive to LH) become the theca lutein cells, and the granulosa cells (now responsive to LH and FSH) are converted to the granulosa lutein cells, which now are vascularized and gain access to low-density lipoprotein (LDL) cholesterol from the circulation. With an adequate supply of cholesterol from LDL, the granulosa lutein cells generate progesterone and estradiol. Estradiol and progesterone convert the proliferative endometrium of the first half of the menstrual cycle to the secretory endometrium of the second (luteal) half of the menstrual cycle.

In the absence of pregnancy (i.e., in the absence of hCG), progesterone concentrations decline and menstruation occurs because the corpus luteum atrophies to become the corpus albicans. However, if a fertilized ovum implants in the uterine wall, the syncytiotrophoblast, via hCG, will maintain the corpus luteum, and menstruation is avoided because of continued secretion of estradiol and progesterone. The corpus luteum (supported by hCG) then becomes the corpus luteum of pregnancy.

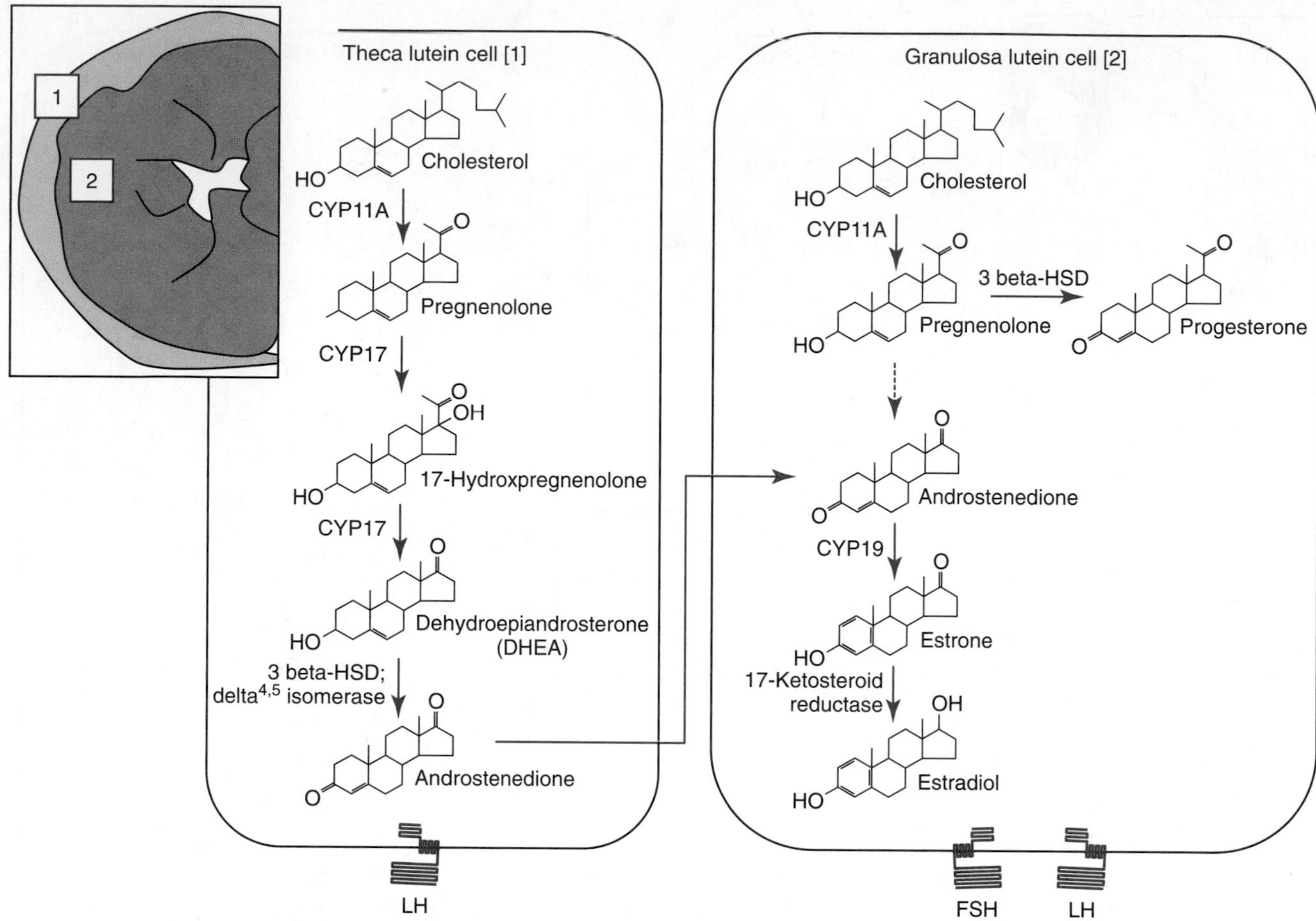

Figure 53-7 In the luteal (secretory) phase of the menstrual cycle following ovulation, under the influence of luteinizing hormone (LH), theca lutein cells *[1]* produce androstenedione from cholesterol (the intermediary steps are illustrated). Under the influence of follicle-stimulating hormone (FSH) and LH, granulosa lutein cells utilize androstenedione produced by the theca cells to synthesize estradiol, and utilize cholesterol available from LDL to synthesize progesterone (the intermediary steps are illustrated) *[2]*. *3 Beta-HSD,* 3 Beta-hydroxysteroid dehydrogenase; *CYP11A,* 20,22 desmolase; *CYP17,* 17-hydroxylase activity; *CYP19,* aromatase; and *LDL,* low-density lipoprotein.

Regulation and Clinical Significance

In hypogonadal patients, if gonadotropin concentrations are greatly elevated, hypergonadotropic hypogonadism is diagnosed, indicating that gonadal (end-organ) failure has occurred.[46] Alternatively, if gonadotropin concentrations are consistently low in hypogonadal patients, the diagnosis of hypogonadotropic hypogonadism is likely. To ensure that the pituitary is unable to respond to GnRH, a GnRH stimulation test can be performed.[107,174] In children (especially boys), in whom hypogonadotropic hypogonadism versus constitutional delay in growth and adolescence (delayed puberty) is a diagnostic dilemma, and basal LH and FSH may be low, GnRH testing should be performed. If basal LH and FSH concentrations are low, but LH and FSH rise substantially following GnRH stimulation, constitutional delay in growth and adolescence is likely, and hypogonadotropic hypogonadism can be excluded. The therapeutic approach to these two conditions is very different. Children with constitutional delay in growth and adolescence eventually will enter puberty (although later than their peers), whereas hypogonadotropic hypogonadism will require sex hormone replacement therapy for initiation of puberty. If hypogonadotropic hypogonadism is diagnosed, a thorough search for its cause (e.g., a CNS tumor) is essential. Induction of fertility in patients with hypogonadotropic hypogonadism requires gonadotropin replacement. A protocol for performance of the GnRH test is discussed in the following section.

Hypogonadotropic hypogonadism has also been found to result from loss-of-function mutations in the *GnRHR* gene.[22] Isolated FSH deficiency can result from mutations in the FSH beta chain. However, isolated FSH deficiency is a rare cause of infertility in men or women. Men with FSH deficiency (but LH sufficiency) will have normal testosterone concentrations because LH and responding Leydig cells are normal.

Gain-of-function mutations in the LHR cause a hypogonadotropic, familial, male precocious puberty, in which the testes autonomously and prematurely produce testosterone (testotoxicosis).[181] Leydig cell adenomas with *LHR* mutations can cause precocious puberty.

LHR loss-of-function mutations cause Leydig cell hypoplasia and inadequate virilization of males in utero, leading to ambiguous genitalia.[217] In females, *LHR* loss-of-function mutations cause oligomenorrhea, amenorrhea, or infertility. *FSHR* loss-of-function mutations in females result in ovarian dysgenesis.

Central precocious puberty occurs with early activation of the hypothalamic-pituitary-gonadal axis, leading to gonadotropin-driven early puberty (onset of breast development or pubic hair before age 8 years or menses before age 9.5 years in girls, and puberty onset in boys before age 9).[38] In most girls (≈95%), no specific cause is identified (idiopathic precocious puberty). Central precocious puberty is uncommon in boys. However, when central precocious puberty occurs in boys, the likelihood of CNS pathology is greater than in girls.

Other details concerning the regulation and clinical significance of LH and FSH are discussed in Chapter 56.

Measurement of LH and FSH

The alpha subunit of LH and FSH is a member of the "cystine knot" superfamily of polypeptides that includes growth hormone, chorionic gonadotropin, and thyrotropin. Therefore, analytical methods for measuring LH and FSH must recognize the unique beta subunits of these hormones, because the alpha subunit is shared among several homologous pituitary products.

Two-site (double antibody) heterogeneous immunoassays are currently the most common methods for measuring gonadotropins, and a wide variety of assays have been adapted to automated platforms. Some commercially available methods attach a capture antibody to the surface of test tubes or plastic beads, whereas others use a paramagnetic label or a microparticle to capture the antibody-antigen complexes. Numerous labels have been used for the second antibody, including radioisotopes, enzymes,[82] fluorophores,[120] and chemiluminescent molecules. In modern immunometric assays, hCG interference has been mostly eliminated (<0.008% cross-reactivity), better assay precision has been achieved (between-assay CVs <10%), and sensitivity has been improved (detection limits <0.2 IU/L).[21] The analytical sensitivity of LH assays is especially important in the evaluation of prepubertal children and patients with hypothalamic disorders, because LH concentrations are very low.

Calibration of gonadotropin assays is difficult because LH and FSH undergo post-translational modifications that produce a mixture of closely related compounds. The earliest reference material used for calibration of LH and FSH assays was the second IRP for human menopausal gonadotropins, isolated from the urine of postmenopausal women. Alterations during metabolism and excretion, however, limited the comparability of this preparation with circulating forms of the hormones, and subsequent calibrators were prepared from extracts derived from the human pituitary gland. Purified pituitary extracts, such as the first and second IRPs for FSH and LH, were available for many years but have been replaced by highly purified extracts that have minimal contamination with cross-reacting glycoproteins. Manufacturers of older immunoassays for LH and FSH used one or more pituitary-derived reference materials for their working calibrators, but recombinant gonadotropin calibrators are now available.

Biases in analytical results still exist between different immunoassay systems (most notably in LH assays), and results can differ by more than 50%, even when calibrated with the same reference preparation.[203,210] The most likely explanation for the bias is the specificity of the antibodies used in each method. Gonadotropic hormones are glycosylated, and this affects their antigenicity.[105] For example, LH immunoassays using monoclonal antibodies generate considerably lower LH concentrations than RIAs using polyclonal antibodies, presumably because of the greater specificity of monoclonal antibodies, which may recognize only a subset of LH isoforms and epitopes. Other factors that contribute to method-dependent biases include differences in calibration procedures and the assay matrix itself.

Specimen Collection and Storage

Serum is the preferred specimen for gonadotropin measurements. Hemolyzed, lipemic, and/or icteric specimens should not be used. Both hormones are stable for 8 days at room temperature, and for 2 weeks at 4 °C; for longer periods, the serum specimen should be frozen at or below −20 °C. Because of episodic, circadian, and cyclic variations in the secretion of gonadotropins, meaningful clinical evaluation of these hormones may require determinations in pooled blood specimens, multiple serial blood specimens, or timed urine specimens. Urine specimens should not contain preservatives; storage at or below −20 °C is recommended.

Measurement of Urinary FSH and LH

Clinically, the pulsatile and episodic release of gonadotropins makes a single blood concentration of FSH or LH difficult to interpret. In adults, concentrations of gonadotropins in blood, particularly LH, may differ as much as threefold between blood specimens collected from the same individual 20 minutes apart. In addition, the lower detection limit of many FSH and LH immunoassays may be within the reference interval for these hormones in normal adults. In prepubertal children, most blood assays are not capable of measuring normal concentrations because they are so low. To optimize detection limits for gonadotropin assays in children, urinary FSH or LH assays have been used.[177] Some pediatric endocrinologists favor urine assays when investigating pubertal disorders of gonadotropin secretion.

Thyroid-Stimulating Hormone (TSH)

TSH (thyrotropin), which is synthesized in thyrotrophs of the adenohypophysis, promotes the growth of thyroid follicular cells and sustains and stimulates the hormonal secretion of thyroid gland hormones 3,5,3′,5′ tetraiodothyronine (thyroxine; T_4) and 3,5,3′-triiodothyronine (T_3).[121]

Biochemistry and Physiology

TSH binds to TSH receptors (TSHRs) located on the surfaces of thyroid follicular cells.[126] TSH (1) stimulates growth and vascularity of the thyroid gland, (2) stimulates growth of thyroid follicular cells, (3) promotes thyroid hormone synthesis by increasing the uptake of iodine (via the sodium-iodide transporter), (4) promotes the organification (reduction) of iodine, (5) promotes the coupling of tyrosines, and (6) promotes the proteolytic release of stored thyroid hormone from thyroglobulin. TSH release is stimulated by TRH and is suppressed by thyroid hormone (principally, circulating T_4).

TRH is a modified tripeptide produced by the hypothalamus. The thyroid-releasing hormone receptor (TRHR) is expressed on anterior pituitary thyrotrophs. TRHR is a 398 amino acid protein, and 28 of its amino acids constitute an extracellular domain. Seven transmembrane domains are present, along with a 79 amino acid cytoplasmic domain. Two possible glycosylation sites exist at amino acids 3 and 10, and a disulfide bridge is present between amino acids 98 and 179. Details of TRH and TRHR production are discussed in Chapter 55.

The glycoprotein alpha chain, shared with FSH, LH, and hCG, was described earlier in this chapter. The beta chain of TSH is encoded on chromosome 1p13. Following removal of the 20 amino acid leader sequence, the proTSH beta chain consists of 118 amino acids. Cleavage of the six C-terminal residues released from the propeptide yields the TSH beta chain (112 amino acids). TSH is glycosylated at residue 43, and disulfide bonds are likely at amino acids 22-72, 36-87, 39-125, 47-103, 51-105, and 108-115.

Regulation, Clinical Significance, and Analytical Methods

Details concerning the regulation, clinical significance, and measurement of TSH are discussed in Chapter 55.

Assessment of Anterior Pituitary Lobe Reserve

Evaluation of endocrine function is an important part of the management of patients with pituitary disease.[25,34] Detection of hormone deficiencies before and after treatment and recognition of hormone-producing tumors are the two objectives of testing of pituitary function in patients with pituitary disease.[56]

Assessment of anterior and posterior pituitary function in patients with a pituitary tumor is important in the identification of clinically significant hormone deficiency states caused by the tumor, and in the re-evaluation of patients after pituitary surgery or irradiation to detect hormone deficiencies that occur as a result of invasive treatment. Testing of pituitary function usually is performed under basal conditions, but it can be performed under provocative conditions to expose subtle or mild deficiencies observed in disorders of the adrenal gland or gonads. The primary relevance of prolactin deficiency relates to Sheehan syndrome, in which postpartum hemorrhage results in pituitary infarction and panhypopituitarism; this is still an important problem in developing countries.

The lower detection limits of the newer two-site immunoassays for the measurement of pituitary hormones make it possible to distinguish an abnormally low value from the lower end of the normal reference interval. Although assessment of a particular aspect of pituitary function should include clinical signs and symptoms of hormone deficiency and measurement of hormones secreted by the pertinent endocrine gland (e.g., T_4, cortisol, testosterone), newer, ultrasensitive assays for TSH, FSH, LH, and ACTH allow accurate distinction between a pathologically low result and a low-normal result. A scheme for testing of pituitary reserve is proposed in Box 53-5.

BOX 53-5 Assessment of Pituitary Reserve in Surgical Patients

Before Pituitary Surgery

Adrenal function: measurement of morning serum cortisol concentration or cosyntropin stimulation test

Thyroid function: free T_4

Gonadal function: sex hormone determinations (estradiol in women and testosterone in men) and gonadotropins (LH and FSH) if sex steroids are low

Shortly After Pituitary Surgery (2 to 4 Days After Surgery)

Adrenal function: morning serum cortisol concentration

Thyroid function: deferred

Gonadal function: deferred

One Month After Pituitary Surgery

Adrenal function: cosyntropin stimulation test or insulin tolerance test (ITT)

Thyroid function: free T_4

Gonadal function: sex hormone determinations (estradiol in women and testosterone in men)

Hypothalamic-Pituitary-Adrenal Axis

A morning serum cortisol concentration in excess of 18 to 20 µg/dL usually provides adequate evidence that the hypothalamic-pituitary-adrenal (HPA) axis is intact and is functioning properly. A typical reference interval for morning cortisol is 7 to 25 µg/dL. Therefore, a morning cortisol results can fall within the reference interval, yet may not prove that the patient has a normal HPA axis.

If AM cortisol is frankly low (<5 µg/dL) or equivocal (5 to <17 µg/dL), or if a strong clinical suspicion of adrenal insufficiency is present, the cosyntropin stimulation test is helpful (see Box 54-1). Cosyntropin provocation of cortisol release is performed by obtaining a baseline blood specimen for cortisol followed by intravenous (IV) administration of 250 µg of cosyntropin (an active ACTH analog). Blood specimens are collected 30 and 60 minutes after IV administration of cosyntropin. A normal response to cosyntropin is a peak cortisol of 18 to 20 µg/dL or greater, with an increase in cortisol over the baseline of 7 µg/dL or greater. When the two criteria are compared, the absolute cortisol concentration is believed to be more important. A lower-dose cosyntropin test (1.0 µg IV) has been proposed as a more sensitive test of impaired pituitary reserve, but its utility is still unclear and controversial.[81]

Tests of the entire HPA axis, such as the insulin tolerance test (also called the insulin-induced hypoglycemia stimulation test; see Box 53-3), occasionally are abnormal in patients who have (1) a normal morning cortisol result, (2) a normal response to cosyntropin, and (3) no signs of adrenal insufficiency. Although an abnormality in these sensitive tests suggests some diminution of ACTH reserve, the clinical significance is most relevant when the patient encounters a major stress, such as gastroenteritis. These tests should be reserved for patients who are strongly suspected of having adrenal insufficiency, or whose morning cortisol concentration or response to ACTH has been found to be abnormal. Standard protocols for the performance and interpretation of these tests have been published. These tests involve some patient risk and discomfort and should be performed only under the direct supervision of an experienced physician.

Measurement of ACTH in blood collected at baseline or after stimulation with insulin adds little to the utility of the tests discussed previously and generally is not recommended. In fact, in patients who have undergone pituitary surgery, the cortisol negative feedback loop to ACTH secretion may take time to normalize. ACTH and cortisol measurements after administration of CRH potentially are a direct test of pituitary ACTH reserve. The insulin-induced hypoglycemia test is currently the definitive test of ACTH and/or cortisol reserve; however, this test is contraindicated in patients with a history of coronary heart disease, seizure disorder, or general debility. Metyrapone testing is discussed in Chapter 55 as another test of pituitary ACTH reserve.

Hypothalamic-Pituitary-Thyroid Axis

Because the current generation of TSH assays provide limits of detection extending to 0.01 IU/mL or less, which is sufficient to distinguish between low-normal and pathologically suppressed TSH secretion, TRH testing usually is not required for assessment of thyroid function.[158] Pharmaceutical TRH currently is not available in the United States.

The sole value of the TRH test is in the diagnosis of a TSH-secreting tumor in a patient presenting with increased free T_4 and an inappropriately elevated TSH.[9] In these patients, the TSH response to TRH is impaired. Such patients may also have elevated concentrations of free alpha subunits.

TRH testing involves the bolus IV administration of TRH (1 µg/kg, 100 µg/m^2, or 500 µg total in adults), along with the measurement of TSH at baseline and at 30 minutes. (*Note:* Some protocols extend TSH measurements to 45 and 60 minutes.) The expected (normal) response is an increase in TSH concentration over baseline of 5 to 30 IU/mL. Some sources report that a normal response to TRH is a fivefold to tenfold increase in serum TSH concentration within 60 minutes after TRH administration. A TSH change less than 5 uIU/mL indicates TSH suppression (primary hyperthyroidism) or inability of the pituitary to respond (secondary hypothyroidism). TSH responses greater than 30 IU/mL are consistent with primary hypothyroidism. In tertiary hypothyroidism, TSH will rise slowly in a delayed response pattern.

Hypothalamic-Pituitary-Gonadal Axis

History and physical examination are extremely helpful in evaluating the status of the hypothalamic-pituitary-gonadal axis, particularly in women during their reproductive years.[12,146] Normal menstrual cycles usually indicate an intact hypothalamic-pituitary-gonadal axis in women of reproductive age. A serum progesterone concentration greater than 10 ng/mL during the luteal phase of the menstrual cycle supports ovulation.

Baseline laboratory assessment for hypothalamic-pituitary-gonadal dysregulation should include measurement of serum gonadotropins (LH and FSH) and sex steroids (estradiol in females and testosterone in males). Provocative testing of this axis with GnRH administration and measurements of FSH and LH (Box 53-6) are useful in selected patients. However, the definition of an appropriate response to GnRH is controversial and depends on the stage of sexual maturation of the subject. Following GnRH injection, LH normally rises more than FSH. Two shortened variations of

BOX 53-6 Protocol for the Gonadotropin-Releasing Hormone Stimulation Test for Luteinizing Hormone and Follicle-Stimulating Hormone Reserve

Rationale

The hypothalamic releasing hormone GnRH stimulates the pituitary release of both LH and FSH in normal individuals. Subnormal responses are seen in some patients with pituitary or hypothalamic disorders. However, the magnitude of LH and FSH responses to GnRH is usually predictable from basal LH and FSH concentrations. This test may be useful in patients in whom the clinical picture and basal gonadotropin measurements are inconclusive.

Procedure

The test may be performed without regard to previous feeding or time of day. After baseline specimens are obtained for LH and FSH measurement, 100 µg or 2.5 µg/kg (to a maximum of 100 µg) GnRH is given intravenously. Samples for LH and FSH determination should be drawn every 15 to 20 minutes for 1 to 2 hours.

Interpretation

LH response should increase by threefold to tenfold. The FSH response is of lesser magnitude (usually a 1.5- to 3-fold increase). Peak responses for both LH and FSH occur between 15 and 30 minutes.

the GnRH test are available: in one variation, leuprolide (a GnRH agonist; 500 μg or 20 μg/kg) is injected subcutaneously, and LH and FSH are measured 3 hours later; in the other variant, 100 μg of GnRH is injected subcutaneously, and LH and FSH are measured 40 minutes later. These tests, however, can be unreliable in differentiating pituitary disorders from hypothalamic dysfunction; the physician usually is dependent on an accurate determination of gonadotropins and sex steroids, along with clinical judgment, in differentiating hypothalamic from pituitary disease.

Pituitary Assessment in Surgical Patients

Initial Assessment

Preoperative testing is indicated in patients with large pituitary tumors or specific clinical indications such as suspected ACTH deficiency, when glucocorticoids may be required preoperatively (see Box 53-5), but the gonadal axis may be compromised in patients with microadenomas as well. In addition to the history and physical examination, patients at risk for pituitary insufficiency should be evaluated for endocrine function before surgery is performed, including laboratory measurements of serum prolactin, free T_4, LH, FSH, sex steroids (testosterone in males and estradiol in females), serum sodium, and urine specific gravity (or serum and urine osmolality), and a morning serum cortisol or cosyntropin stimulation test.

Perioperative Assessment

The optimum time for retesting endocrine function after pituitary surgery is not known. Many protocols (often based on sparse data) explain how potential cortisol deficiency is managed in the perioperative period. Some neurosurgeons provide "stress" doses (high doses) of glucocorticoids immediately before, during, and after surgery. If the patient had ACTH deficiency preoperatively, IV glucocorticoids can be substituted with oral replacement doses (e.g., the equivalent of 12 mg/m^2 per day of hydrocortisone in children, or 20 to 30 mg in adults in divided doses) after 2 to 3 days. If the patient had normal adrenal function preoperatively, exogenous glucocorticoids can be discontinued on the second or third postoperative day. Morning cortisol should be measured 24 hours later; if the result is less than 5 μg/dL, ACTH deficiency is likely and glucocorticoid replacement is indicated. If the 24 hour postoperative cortisol is 10 μg/dL or greater, the HPA axis is normal and glucocorticoid replacement is not required. If cortisol is between 5 and 10 μg/dL, the patient should be treated with glucocorticoids, or provocative testing (ITT) should be performed; the ITT can be used concurrently to assess GH deficiency.

Some neurosurgeons do not treat with glucocorticoids if preoperative adrenal function is normal,[106] instead assessing the patient's postoperative morning cortisol concentration. If cortisol concentration is less than 3.6 μg/dL, ACTH deficiency is present and glucocorticoid treatment is necessary. If cortisol is greater than 16 μg/dL, ACTH deficiency is not present and glucocorticoid treatment is not required. Definitive testing is indicated only for patients with a morning cortisol of 3.6 to 16 μg/dL; pituitary function in these patients can be evaluated with an ITT or glucagon stimulation test. Patients with a morning cortisol between 3.6 and 9 μg/dL usually receive daily glucocorticoid treatment, whereas those with an AM cortisol between 9 and 16 μg/dL are treated only at times of stress.

In the first 4 weeks after pituitary surgery, the cosyntropin test may not be a reliable indicator of HPA axis integrity. During this period, the adrenal response to cosyntropin may be normal, yet endogenous ACTH may be insufficient in the basal state or at times of stress to avoid glucocorticoid insufficiency. Once the adrenal gland atrophies from a deficiency of endogenous ACTH (which may take ≈4 weeks), the cosyntropin challenge becomes abnormal, reflecting endogenous ACTH deficiency.

Postoperative Assessment

It is advisable to wait until 1 month after surgery to evaluate thyroid function (TSH and free T_4) and gonadal function (testosterone in males and estradiol in females; see Box 53-5). Early treatment of thyroid and gonadal deficiencies is not critical, and misleading test results might be observed in the early postoperative period. Adrenal function should be reassessed with a 250 μg cosyntropin stimulation test 1 month after surgery even if immediate results are subnormal, because ACTH deficiency after pituitary surgery is often transient. Periodic clinical follow-up and laboratory assessment should be tailored to individual circumstances.

Stimulation tests for the secretion of ACTH, GH, and GnRH can be combined. For example, the ITT can be combined with the GnRH stimulation test. The ITT assesses GH and ACTH secretion, whereas the GnRH stimulation test assesses the ability of the anterior pituitary to secrete gonadotropins in response to GnRH.

After pituitary irradiation, patients should be evaluated every 6 months with measurement of free T_4, sex steroids, cortisol, and cosyntropin stimulation.

The Neurohypophysis

The neurohypophysis (posterior pituitary) is derived from the brain neuroectodermis. Embryologically, ventral evagination of the floor of the third ventricle forms the neurohypophysis.[63] Antidiuretic hormone (ADH; vasopressin) and oxytocin are secreted from the neurohypophysis, the cell bodies of which are located in hypothalamic supraoptic and paraventricular nuclei. These neurons are located in, and travel through, the median eminence and pituitary stalk, with nerve endings projecting to the posterior lobe of the pituitary gland.

Antidiuretic Hormone

Disorders of ADH involve excess hormone [syndrome of inappropriate ADH (SIADH)] or deficient ADH action [diabetes insipidus (DI)]. DI can result from ADH deficiency, ADH resistance, or renal tubular disease; the latter two conditions are termed *nephrogenic DI*. Disorders of oxytocin secretion have not been described.

Biochemistry

Both ADH and oxytocin are nonapeptides consisting of a cyclic hexapeptide and a 3 amino acid side chain (Figure 53-8). At the physiologic pH of plasma, ADH and oxytocin circulate mainly as unbound (free) hormones.

The gene for ADH is located at chromosome 20p13. PreproADH consists of 164 amino acids (17.3 kDa). The gene also encodes neurophysin 2 and copeptin. The first 19 amino acids of preproADH are the leader sequence. Amino acids 20-28 constitute the ADH nonapeptide hormone; amino acids 32-124 represent neurophysin 2; and amino acids 126-164 represent copeptin (C-terminal provasopressin). The glycine residue at position 28 is amidated, and amino acid 131 is glycosylated. Disulfide bonds are definitive or possible at amino acids 20-25, 41-85, 44-58, 52-75, 59-65, 92-104, 98-116, and 105-110. The disulfide bridge at residues 20-25 is within ADH.

The ADH receptor in the renal tubules (specifically the collecting ducts) is termed the *arginine vasopressin receptor 2 (V2 receptor)*. The V2 receptor is a member of the seven-transmembrane domain G-protein–coupled receptor (GPCR) superfamily, whose other members include the V1a and V1b vasopressin receptors and the oxytocin receptor.

The gene for the V2 receptor is located on chromosome Xq28. The receptor is 371 amino acids (40.3 kDa), including a 38 amino acid extracellular domain, seven transmembrane domains, and a 43 amino acid cytoplasmic domain. Amino acid 22 may be glycosylated, and amino acids 341 and 342 are lipidated as S-palmitoyl cysteines. Two isoforms of the V2 receptor are known: isoform 1 is the full-length receptor, whereas isoform 2 varies in the sequence of amino acids 305 to 309, and amino acids 310 to 371 are absent.

The V1a receptor (V1 receptor) gene is located at chromosome 12q14. The protein is 418 amino acids and weighs 46.8 kDa. A 52 amino acid extracellular domain is present, along with seven transmembrane domains and a 67 amino acid cytoplasmic domain. Glycosylation is possible at amino acids 27 and 196. Amino acids 365 and 366 may be lipidated as S-palmitoyl cysteines. A serine residue at position 404 may be phosphorylated to phosphoserine, and a disulfide bond is likely between amino acids 124 and 203.

The V1b receptor (V3 receptor) is encoded by a gene located on chromosome 1q32. The V3 receptor is composed of 424 amino acids (47.0 kDa). A 35 amino acid extracellular domain is present, along with seven transmembrane domains and an 83 amino acid cytoplasmic domain. The receptor is possibly glycosylated at amino acid 21, and a disulfide bond is likely between amino acids 107 and 186.

Aquaporin-2 is a 271 amino acid protein (28.8 kDa).[100] The gene encoding aquaporin-2 is located on chromosome 12q1. The external domain contains 16 amino acids, along with seven transmembrane domains and a 47 amino acid cytoplasmic domain. Phosphoserines are possible or definitive at amino acids 256, 261, and 264, and amino acid 123 is a possible site of glycosylation. Amino acids 68-70 and 184-186 are NPA (asparagine-proline-alanine) motifs.

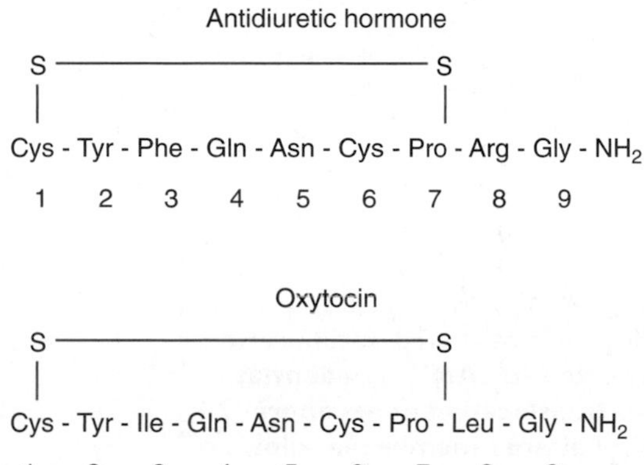

Figure 53-8 The amino acid sequences of antidiuretic hormone (ADH) and oxytocin are compared.

Regulation of ADH Secretion

ADH secretion is controlled predominantly by plasma osmolality (tonicity).[16] Plasma osmolality is sensed by osmoreceptors located in cell bodies in or near the magnocellular nuclei of the hypothalamus. Increased osmolality results in ADH release; even relatively small changes in osmolality affect ADH secretion. A 2% increase in extracellular fluid osmolality can stimulate the osmoreceptor to release ADH. Plasma osmolality above 280 mOsm/kg is thought to be the osmotic threshold for triggering ADH release.

In addition to the osmoreceptor mechanism of vasopressin release, physiologic regulation of ADH secretion involves a pressure-volume mechanism that is distinct from the osmotic sensor. High-pressure arterial baroreceptors of the aortic arch and carotid sinus, and low pressure volume receptors in the pulmonary venous system and atria, also regulate ADH release. Therefore, ADH is secreted in response to decreased circulating blood volume, or decreased blood pressure. Other nonosmotic stimuli for ADH release include pain, stress, nausea and vomiting, sleep, exercise, and chemical agents such as catecholamines, angiotensin II, opiates, prostaglandins, anesthetics, nicotine, and barbiturates.

The thirst center is regulated by many of the same factors that determine ADH release. This center has a higher set point than the osmoreceptors and responds to osmolalities above 290 mOsm/kg. Responses involving ADH, thirst, and renal reabsorption of sodium and water are coordinated in a complex scheme that maintains plasma osmolality in healthy individuals within a narrow interval (284 to 295 mOsm/kg).

Physiologic Activity

Both ADH and neurophysin 2 are present in secretory vesicles that reach the terminal portion of the axon 12 to 14 hours after they are synthesized (this is also true for oxytocin and neurophysin 1). Upon nerve stimulation, release of neurohypophyseal hormones into the portal circulation occurs via calcium-dependent exocytosis. When a stimulus for secretion of ADH or oxytocin occurs, the stimulus acts on the appropriate magnocellular cell body in the hypothalamus, sending an action potential down the long axon to the posterior pituitary, causing an influx of calcium and the release of hormone from neurosecretory granules.

The exact role of the neurophysins is unclear, but their proper synthesis is necessary for ADH secretion. The biological role of copeptin is unknown. Because of analytical difficulties in measuring ADH, some investigators have suggested measuring copeptin as a surrogate for ADH, because copeptin is secreted in amounts stoichiometrically equivalent to ADH, and copeptin is stable in plasma.

The actions of ADH are to conserve free water (via V2 receptors) and stimulate vasoconstriction (via V1a receptors).[30] These effects combine to maintain proper osmolality of the extracellular space (the major action of ADH) and blood pressure through maintenance of circulating blood volume and prevention of dehydration and excessive loss of water.

ADH increases the permeability of renal collecting ducts to water, thereby increasing water reabsorption and concentrating the urine (Figure 53-9).

An alternative name for ADH is *vasopressin* (or *arginine vasopressin*), which emphasizes the vasoconstrictive effects of high concentrations of ADH.[197] These vasoconstrictive effects are manifested when ADH binds to V1a receptors on arterial smooth muscle cells. Note that the major endocrine system regulating blood pressure is the renin-angiotensin-aldosterone system. ADH, however, is believed to play an important role in the maintenance of arterial blood pressure during blood loss. Release of ADH into the pituitary portal system also augments the release of ACTH from the adenohypophysis, but does not appear to affect the release of other anterior pituitary hormones.

ADH binding to the V1a receptor stimulates the secretion of vascular endothelial growth factor (VEGF). The V1a receptor may also affect platelet aggregation, coagulation factor release, and glycogenolysis by its expression on platelets and hepatocytes.

The V1b receptor (V3 receptor) is expressed in the CNS. In this way, ADH can release ACTH to aid in the response to stress. The V1b receptor also has been reported to be expressed in islet cells, influencing insulin secretion.

Clinical Significance

Disorders of ADH activity have been divided into hypofunction (DI) and hyperfunction (SIADH) (Figure 53-10).[176,182]

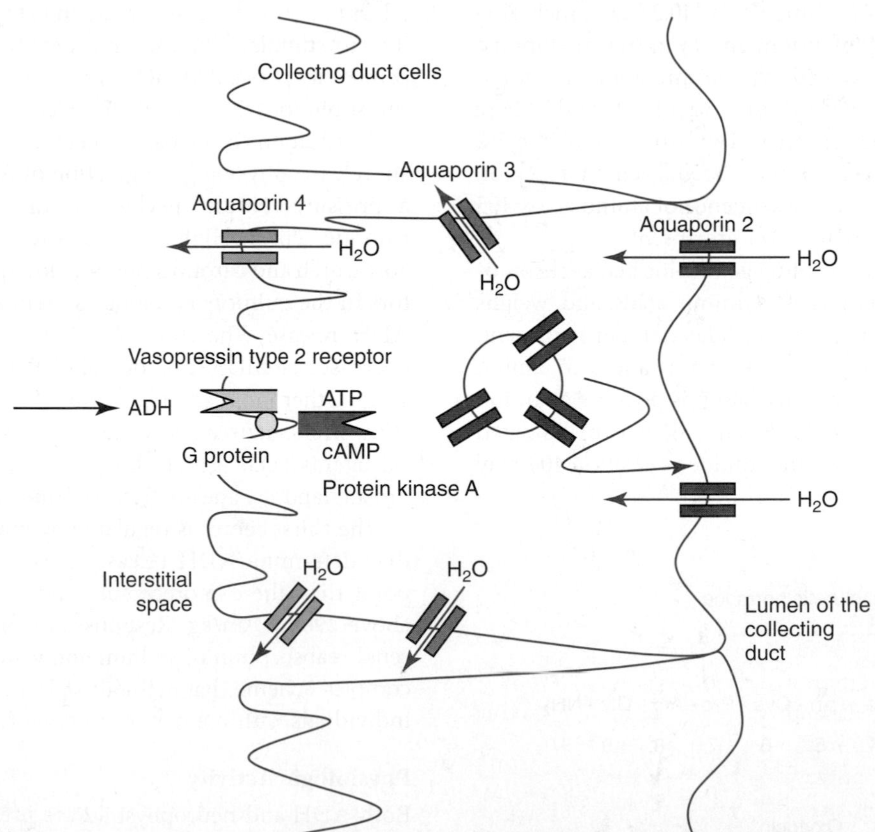

Figure 53-9 Vasopressin type 2 receptors on collecting duct cells bind antidiuretic hormone (ADH). Via a G-protein system, ATP is converted to cAMP via adenylate cyclase with protein kinase A activation. This leads to translocation of aquaporin-2 water channels from an intracellular pool to the apical plasma membrane, allowing free water uptake by cells of the collecting duct. Via the basolateral plasma membrane aquaporin-3 and aquaporin-4 water channels, free water then leaves these cells.

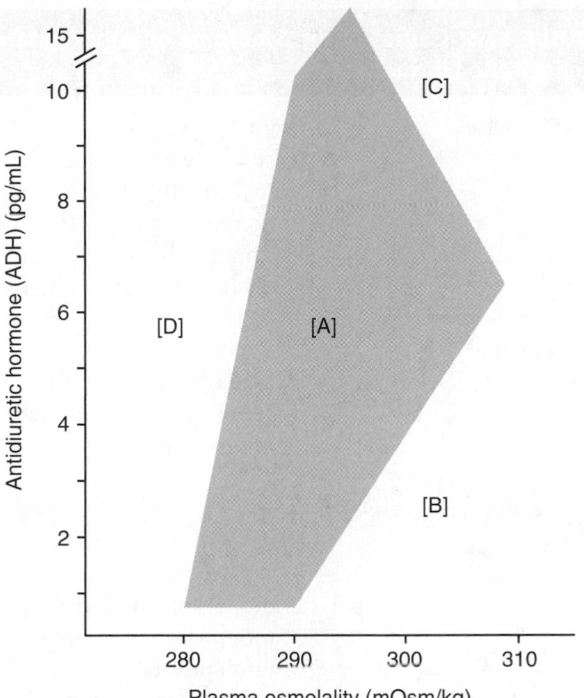

Figure 53-10 The relationship of plasma antidiuretic hormone (ADH) to plasma osmolality. Region *[A]* is the reference interval and the results observed in subjects with psychogenic polydipsia and excessive water intake. Region *[B]* represents findings in central diabetes insipidus, whereas region *[C]* represents findings in nephrogenic diabetes insipidus. Region *[D]* represents findings in the syndrome of inappropriate ADH (SIADH) secretion. *(Modified and abstracted from Zerbe RL, Robertson GL. A comparison of plasma vasopressin measurements with a standard indirect test in the differential diagnosis of polyuria. N Engl J Med 1981;305:1539-46.)*

TABLE 53-8 Causes of Central Diabetes Insipidus

Congenital	Midline malformations: septo-optic dysplasia, holoprosencephaly, single central incisor, cleft lip and/or palate
	Malformation of the pituitary (ectopia or hypogenesis)
	Diabetes insipidus-diabetes mellitus-optic atrophy syndrome (DIDMOA; Wolfram syndrome)
	Familial diabetes insipidus (autosomal dominant and recessive forms)
Acquired	Tumors (craniopharyngioma, germinoma, pinealoma, optic glioma, pituitary adenoma, metastatic tumor, leukemia)
	Trauma (e.g., stalk section)
	Infarction (e.g., septic shock, Sheehan syndrome, hypoxic injury)
	Infiltrative disease (sarcoidosis, hypophysitis, histiocytosis)
	Cysts and aneurysms
	Drugs (opiates, alcohol, phenytoin, alpha-adrenergic agents, etc.)
	Infection
	Increased metabolism of ADH (vasopressinase in pregnancy)

Polyuric states are divided into two main categories: (1) deficient ADH action, producing DI (sometimes called "water diabetes"), and (2) excessive oral water intake (psychogenic polydipsia).[191] Inadequate ADH activity can result from ADH deficiency or ADH resistance. An osmotic diuresis may also produce polyuria and polydipsia. Uncontrolled diabetes mellitus with a high glucose load to the kidney is a common cause of osmotic diuresis.

In DI, polyuria results from excessive loss of water into the urine.[147] Under normal circumstances, urine output is mostly dependent on fluid intake; thus an arbitrary upper limit for normal urine output cannot be defined. When urine output is greater than 2.5 L/d, an investigation is usually indicated. In the absence of ADH, urine output may approach 1 L/h. Increased osmolality normally stimulates thirst. Therefore if a patient with DI has an intact thirst mechanism and free access to water, excessive urinary loss of water will be matched by excessive intake of fluids. This is why DI patients report polydipsia in addition to polyuria. The major laboratory finding is urine of low osmolality and serum sodium within the upper half of the reference interval, with a corresponding high-normal serum osmolality. If water is not available, or the individual with DI is physically impaired or lacks a normal thirst mechanism, serum osmolality rises, serum sodium rises (producing hypernatremia), urine osmolality remains low, and polyuria continues. With dehydration, weight loss is acute (because of fluid loss) and blood pressure falls, inducing tachycardia.

Central DI can result from any destructive hypothalamic lesion or infundibular lesion (Table 53-8). DI resulting from such lesions can equally be termed *hypothalamic, neurogenic, central,* or *cranial DI.* Central DI is caused by failure of the posterior pituitary gland to secrete appropriate amounts of ADH in response to rising plasma osmolality. Increased fluid intake promoted by thirst mechanisms usually prevents dehydration. When the thirst center is also abnormal, severe dehydration can occur. Destruction of 80% of ADH-secreting neurons is required to produce central DI. Surgical or traumatic injury to the neurohypophysis may cause transient DI.

The incidence of central DI is about 1 in 25,000 people. In 30% of patients, central DI occurs without apparent cause. Remaining cases are associated with (1) neoplastic disease, (2) neurologic surgery, (3) head trauma, (4) ischemic or hypoxic disorder, (5) granulomatous disease, (6) infection, or (7) autoimmune disorder. A hereditary form of the disorder is transmitted as an autosomal dominant trait. Inborn errors in the ADH gene cause deficiency of the hormone.

Individuals with familial neurohypophyseal diabetes insipidus (FNHDI) are typically recognized before the age of 6 years and display worsening polyuria and compensatory polydipsia.[43] More than 50 mutations have been identified as causes of FNHDI. Although rare, diabetes insipidus can develop during pregnancy as a result of high circulating concentrations of the enzyme cysteine aminopeptidase (vasopressinase), which inactivates ADH.[111] The vasopressinase may be of placental origin.

DI can result from tubular diseases that affect the responsiveness of renal tubules to ADH (nephrogenic DI). In X-linked congenital diabetes insipidus, an inactivating mutation of the V2 receptor is noted.[187] Loss-of-function mutations in aquaporin-2 cause autosomal recessive and autosomal dominant forms of congenital nephrogenic DI.[144] Chronic hypokalemia and hypercalcemia produce a form of nephrogenic DI that results from downregulation of aquaporin-2 expression.[119]

In the broadest sense, any form of tubular injury with impaired water reabsorption including (1) polycystic kidney disease, (2) medullary cystic kidney, (3) chronic pyelonephritis, (4) acute tubular necrosis, (5) obstructive uropathy, (6) sickle cell nephropathy, and (7) renal amyloidosis causes nephrogenic DI. A large number of drugs can cause nephrogenic DI, including (1) lithium, (2) various antimicrobials (amphotericin B, rifampin, methicillin, demeclocycline, and foscarnet), and (3) several antineoplastic drugs (cisplatin and ifosfamide). In psychogenic polydipsia (primary polydipsia), excessive water intake eventually begins to impair the concentrating ability of the kidney.

Pathologic ADH excess produces SIADH (Table 53-9).[20] SIADH causes excessive water retention, resulting in reduced plasma osmolality, hyponatremia, elevated urine osmolality, and reduced urine output. Water retention can cause edema. Presumably because of suppression of the renin-angiotensin-aldosterone system from relative fluid overload, urinary sodium loss is not restricted, and the usual urinary sodium concentration in SIADH is 20 to 40 mEq/L. By contrast, dehydration fully activates the renin-angiotensin-aldosterone system, and urinary sodium is usually less than 10 mEq/L. Causes of SIADH are legion (see Table 53-9). A rare form of nephrogenic SIADH results from a gain-of-function mutation in the V2 receptor.

TABLE 53-9 Causes of the Syndrome of Inappropriate Antidiuretic Hormone

CNS disease	Brain tumor Infection (e.g., meningitis, encephalitis, abscess) Prolonged seizure Psychiatric disease Stress (e.g., prolonged nausea)
Non-CNS tumor (e.g., leukemia)	
Pulmonary disease	Hypoxia (e.g., neonatal) Infection (e.g., pneumonia, emphysema)
Nonpulmonary infection (e.g., AIDS)	
Drugs	Drugs with CNS effects (anticonvulsants, antiparkinsonian drugs, antipsychotics, antipyretics, antidepressants) Angiotensin-converting enzyme (ACE) inhibitors Antineoplastic drugs First-generation sulfonylureas

Diagnostic Studies

ADH usually is not measured for diagnostic purposes because ADH excess and deficiency are evident in changes in serum and urine osmolality, serum sodium, and urine volume.[64] Less precise measures of fluid balance include clinical evaluation for dehydration, blood pressure (supine and upright), heart rate, and body weight. Hormone concentration is not measured in some endocrine disorders because the consequent metabolic abnormality is more important. The best example is diabetes mellitus. Diagnosis and management of diabetes mellitus center on measurement of glucose (and now hemoglobin A_{1c})—not on measurement of insulin or C-peptide.

Serum osmolality can be estimated from serum sodium, glucose, and urea (BUN), but is more reliably measured directly by freezing point depression. Various formulas are available for estimating serum osmolality; all are based on the fact that sodium represents approximately half of all the ions in serum (each sodium is balanced by an anion, and sodium accounts for almost 95% of all cations); among all nonionic solutes, only glucose and urea have high enough concentrations to substantially affect (alone) osmolality. Hence, osmolality can be estimated by adding together twice the sodium, the glucose, and the urea concentrations (in the United States, glucose and BUN, measured in mg/dL, must be converted to mmol/L by dividing their concentrations by 18 and 2.8, respectively).

Several variations may be seen in the calculation of serum osmolality (see Chapters 28 and 49). The simple equation,

$$\text{mOsmol/kg} = 2\times[Na^+] + \frac{[Glu]}{18} + \frac{[BUN]}{2.8}$$

underestimates the true osmolality by 5 to 10 mOsm/kg because of the remaining constituents in serum that do not, individually, have significant concentrations, but when combined contribute approximately that amount. Some laboratories provide a reference interval that accounts for the difference, whereas others add an average factor (often 8 or 9 mOsm/kg) (and use a different reference interval) to make the calculated osmolality a closer estimate of measured osmolality. The equation assumes that the activity coefficient for Na^+ is 1.0, and this is not the case. Regression analysis of sodium versus measured osmolality produces a slope that corresponds to a factor of approximately 1.86, so some calculations of osmolality (particularly automated calculations) use that factor instead of 2, which results in a bias of approximately 5% between the two equations. As discussed in Chapter 28, the following equations are often recommended:

$$\text{mOsmol/kg} = 1.86[\text{Na}^+(\text{mmol/L})] + \text{Glucose}(\text{mmol/L}) + \text{Urea}(\text{mmol/L}) + 9$$

or

$$\text{mOsmol/kg} = 1.86[\text{Na}^+(\text{mmol/L})] + \text{Glucose}(\text{mg/dL}) + \text{Urea}(\text{mg/dL})/2.8 + 9$$

In the absence of proteinuria, hematuria, glycosuria, and other osmotically active substances (such as radiocontrast dyes), urine specific gravity is a rough estimate of urine osmolality.

Investigation of Polyuria

Assuming that diabetes mellitus is excluded, a differential diagnosis of polyuric states can be made using measurements of plasma and urine osmolality and plasma ADH concentrations (if the findings are equivocal).[89] A recommended strategy is shown in Box 53-7. A screening test for ADH sufficiency is measurement of the urine specific gravity in the first morning-voided urine sample. The specific gravity should be 1.010 or greater in patients with adequate ADH secretion. Failure to demonstrate an appropriate urine specific gravity in a subject with a history of polyuria and polydipsia should trigger assessment of a basic metabolic panel, urinalysis, serum osmolality, and urine osmolality. Hyperglycemia or glycosuria would suggest diabetes mellitus (see Chapter 46).

Urine osmolality below 300 mOsm/kg combined with serum osmolality above 300 mOsm/kg (or with hypernatremia) is diagnostic for diabetes insipidus. If urine osmolality is above 600 mOsm/kg and serum osmolality is below 270 mOsm/kg, DI is unlikely.

If the diagnosis of DI is unclear, a water deprivation test should be performed, although this is rarely needed.[4] Prior to a water deprivation test, uncontrolled diabetes mellitus should be corrected, and thyroid and adrenal function should be normal (or treated if deficient). Water deprivation testing should not be carried out if the subject is dehydrated at baseline or has renal insufficiency. The overnight water deprivation test is usually conducted in a hospital setting because of immediate concerns of profound hypotension and possible mortality.[149,164] Hypertonic saline infusion testing is dangerous and is not used clinically.

The water deprivation test is usually begun on the morning after an overnight fast, unless the history describes large volumes of water ingested and urine produced, in which case the test should begin after breakfast. The subject remains fasting throughout the entire test. A heparin lock is inserted intravenously, so that serial blood samples are obtained easily. Baseline laboratory tests include (1) sodium, (2) potassium, (3) chloride, (4) serum CO_2, (5) BUN, (6) creatinine, (7) glucose, (8) calcium, and (9) serum osmolality. Potassium and calcium are measured to exclude hypokalemia and hypercalcemia as causes of nephrogenic DI (see later).

Measurements of serum sodium, chloride, CO_2, and urine pH provide an assessment of the patient's renal tubular acid-base function.[93] Renal function and hydration status are evaluated with creatinine and BUN measurements. A urine specimen is obtained for measurement of urine sodium, urine osmolality, and urine specific gravity. Body weight and vital signs at baseline are recorded. Thereafter, each hour, serum and urine tests are repeated with measurement of hourly urine output, body weight, and urine volume. If ADH measurements are requested, they can be performed at the beginning, middle, and completion of the test; however, ADH measurements are not required for making the diagnosis of DI. The test is continued for 8 to 10 hours unless the diagnosis of DI is confirmed before the full time has elapsed.

One approach that reduces laboratory charges is to perform serum and urine measurements every 4 hours until plasma osmolality reaches 280 mOsm/kg, when the frequency is increased to every 2 hours. When plasma osmolality reaches 290 mOsm/kg (or serum sodium exceeds 140 mEq/L, or weight loss nears 3%), the tests are performed hourly. During the water deprivation test, if urine osmolality exceeds 600 mOsm/kg on two samples 1 hour apart, or a single urine sample exceeds 1000 mOsm, DI is effectively ruled out, and the test can be concluded. If urine osmolality is below 600 mOsm and serum osmolality is above 300 mOsm/kg, DI is diagnosed and the test can be concluded. If serum osmolality does not exceed 300 mOsm/kg, the test should be

BOX 53-7 Diagnosis of Diabetes Insipidus (DI)

Document polyuria (urine volume >2.5 L/d in adults) and exclude glycosuria. If desired, creatinine excretion can be measured as an estimate of the completeness of the urine collection. Substances that influence antidiuretic hormone (ADH) secretion should be avoided (e.g., nicotine, alcohol, caffeine). If plasma osmolality is greater than 295 mOsm/kg, or if the serum sodium concentration is greater than 145 mEq/L, primary polydipsia is unlikely. If the diagnosis of DI is unclear, proceed with the overnight water deprivation test (see text for a description of this test).

Overnight water deprivation test: If the ratio of urine to plasma osmolality is less than 1.5 at the end of the test, primary polydipsia is unlikely. Measure plasma and urine osmolalities and plasma ADH concentrations at the end of the test; use these relationships to differentiate normal, nephrogenic, and hypothalamic diabetes insipidus, as well as psychogenic polydipsia. If urine osmolality is greater than 400 mOsm/kg at the end of the test, give 5 U of aqueous vasopressin subcutaneously (minimum, 1 U/m^2). If urine osmolality increases by more than 10%, central diabetes insipidus is probable; if urine osmolality does not increase, nephrogenic diabetes insipidus is highly probable.

continued. If mental status changes or hypotension occurs, or weight loss exceeds 3%, the test should be terminated.

If DI is diagnosed during a water deprivation test, aqueous vasopressin is injected subcutaneously (1 U/m^2), or desamino-D-arginine vasopressin (dDAVP, desmopressin) is given IV or IM (2 μg). A decline in urine volume with doubling of urine osmolality over the next 1 to 2 hours identifies the DI as central in origin with the patient ADH deficient. Following exogenous ADH administration, some references define an increase in urine osmolality of 10% or greater over 60 minutes as evidence of ADH deficiency. Failure to respond to exogenous ADH defines nephrogenic DI. Most patients with psychogenic polydipsia have normal urine osmolality after water deprivation, but some fail to produce concentrated urine unless the water deprivation is prolonged. When psychogenic polydipsia is suspected, the patient should be given a minimum of 1 L of normal saline IV to re-establish the renal medullary concentrating gradient, so that the patient can respond appropriately to ADH.

The diagnosis of "partial" DI, in which test results fall between normal and frank DI, is difficult, because no clear-cut boundaries are evident between normal and partial DI, or between partial DI and complete DI.[200] In some cases, measurement of ADH in plasma or urine may be required to reach the correct diagnosis. After water deprivation, patients with central DI have low or inappropriately normal plasma ADH concentrations relative to high plasma osmolality or low urine osmolality, whereas patients with nephrogenic DI have high plasma concentrations of ADH when plasma osmolality exceeds 300 mOsm/kg and urine osmolality is low. Patients with primary polydipsia have normal concentrations of ADH relative to their plasma osmolality. Because ADH concentrations are most discriminatory when plasma osmolality is high, in the past ADH was measured after hypertonic saline was administered to the patient. However, this saline infusion test is potentially dangerous and currently is not used by clinical endocrinologists.

Syndrome of Inappropriate Antidiuretic Hormone Secretion (SIADH)

The autonomous, sustained production of ADH in the absence of recognized and appropriate stimuli (such as hyperosmolality) is termed *SIADH.*[15] In this syndrome, plasma ADH concentrations are "inappropriately" elevated relative to decreased plasma osmolality, and relative to normal or increased plasma volume.

SIADH may be the result of one of several factors including (1) production of ADH by a malignancy (such as small cell carcinoma of the lung), (2) the presence of acute or chronic disease of the central nervous system, (3) pulmonary disorders, or it may occur as (4) a side effect of certain drug therapies. In addition, as many as 10% of patients undergoing pituitary surgery have transient SIADH (for 2 to 3 days) approximately 8 to 9 days after surgery (typically when the patient is at home) that responds to water restriction and resolves spontaneously. This may represent the release of ADH from the posterior pituitary or hypothalamus following surgical trauma.

In SIADH, primary excess of ADH, coupled with unrestricted fluid intake, promotes increased reabsorption of water by the kidney. The consequences are decreased urine volume and increased urine osmolality. As a result of water retention, patients become modestly volume expanded. The increase in intravascular volume causes hemodilution accompanied by dilutional hyponatremia and low plasma osmolality. Volume expansion also decreases renal sodium reabsorption, thus the urine sodium concentration is increased.

SIADH is a common cause of hyponatremia in hospitalized patients.[11] However, other disorders can cause dilutional hyponatremia and must be differentiated from SIADH. These conditions include (1) congestive heart failure, (2) renal insufficiency, (3) nephrotic syndrome, (4) liver cirrhosis, and (5) hypothyroidism. Excessive administration of hypotonic fluids and treatment with drugs that stimulate ADH (chlorpropamide, vincristine, carbamazepine, nicotine, phenothiazines, and cyclophosphamide) can also cause dilutional hyponatremia. Additionally, hyponatremia may occur from renal or extrarenal sodium loss (depletional hyponatremia) as a result of vomiting, diarrhea, excessive sweating, diuretic abuse, salt-losing nephropathy, or mineralocorticoid deficiency. In these latter conditions, plasma BUN is generally increased. Hyponatremia is increasingly recognized as a marker of disease severity.[172] However, selectively increasing the patient's plasma sodium through fluid manipulation will not improve the outcome; it is the underlying disorder that most likely is responsible for the hyponatremia.

Clinical manifestations of hyponatremia are nonspecific and include weakness and apathy in mild cases, and CNS changes such as lethargy, coma, and seizures in more severe cases.[68] No signs or symptoms are specific for SIADH. History, physical examination, and routine laboratory test results often suggest that hyponatremia is dilutional (decreased BUN, hemoglobin, or albumin) or depletional (increased BUN, hemoglobin, or albumin).

Measurements of sodium and osmolality in blood and urine, combined with clinical assessment of volume status, usually permit the appropriate differential diagnosis of hyponatremic conditions (Box 53-8). The diagnosis of SIADH usually is explored solely on the basis of the clinical scenario and the routine laboratory studies discussed previously.[61] SIADH is diagnosed when hyponatremia (<135 mEq/L) and reduced serum osmolality (<270 to 280 mOsm/kg) are present, together with an inappropriately concentrated urine (urine osmolality >100 mOsm/kg). Maximally dilute urine normally is 50 to 80 mOsm/kg, and this is expected in the setting of hyponatremia and hypo-osmolality. However in SIADH, despite serum hypo-osmolality, urine osmolality is typically 250 to 1400 mOsm/kg. It is important to point out that the urine osmolality does not need to exceed the serum osmolality for the diagnosis of SIADH to be made: the urine need only be inappropriately concentrated with respect to the

BOX 53-8 Diagnosis of the Syndrome of Inappropriate Antidiuretic Hormone

Document plasma hypo-osmolality (≤275 mOsm/kg) and hyponatremia (sodium concentration ≤130 mEq/L). Use the history, physical examination, and appropriate laboratory tests to exclude cardiac, hepatic, renal, thyroid, or adrenal failure, along with the effects of pituitary surgery, diuretic therapy, or medications known to stimulate ADH release. (SIADH cannot be diagnosed unless these factors are corrected.) Measure the urine sodium concentration and osmolality. Urine osmolality greater than plasma osmolality and without correspondingly low urine sodium concentration (usually greater than 40 to 60 mEq/L) indicates that SIADH is probable (see the text for details). If the cause of DI is unclear, consider measuring plasma ADH and plasma renin concentrations. SIADH is characterized by high ADH concentration and low renin concentration. If both plasma ADH and renin concentrations are low, a primary defect in renal water excretion is present.

serum. Urine sodium in SIADH is usually 40 to 60 mEq/L or greater.

Patients with dilutional hyponatremia resulting from excess water intake (psychogenic polydipsia) have a hypotonic plasma, an unremarkable urine sodium concentration (<20 mEq/L), and a dilute urine (urine osmolality less than that of plasma).[69] Patients with depletional hyponatremia caused by extrarenal sodium loss have hypotonic plasma, a low urine sodium concentration (usually <10 to 20 mEq/L), and urine osmolality greater than that of plasma. Patients with depletional hyponatremia caused by impaired renal sodium conservation have similar results, except that their urine sodium concentrations are inappropriately elevated in the setting of volume depletion.

Water load testing is not recommended in cases of suspected SIADH, as it may cause acute hyponatremia with significant adverse consequences. Water load testing involves the administration of water orally (20 mL/kg to 1.5 L maximum) with subsequent observation of the volume of urine passed over the next 4 hours (normal response: >90% of ingested volume excreted). With SIADH, less than 70% of the volume is excreted.

Measurement of ADH

Measurement of ADH typically requires extracting and concentrating the hormone from biological fluids because of its low (pmol/L) concentration and the presence of potentially interfering compounds. ADH can be extracted into acetone, petroleum ether, or ethanol,[37] or it can be chromatographically isolated using octadecyl silica (C-18) columns.[29,122,218] Although nonisotopic (enzyme) immunoassays have been described,[98,199] most laboratories measure ADH by RIA. Most ADH RIA methods are noncompetitive, and separation of bound and free ligand is commonly achieved using second-antibody precipitation techniques.

An ADH method described by Kluge and colleagues[122] extracts the hormone from 0.5 mL of acidified plasma onto a C-18 column preconditioned with methanol/water. After washing with 0.67 mol/L acetic acid, ADH is eluted from the column with 1.0 g/L trifluoracetic acid in methanol. The extract is dried and reconstituted in 0.25 mL of phosphate buffer containing 2.5 g/L bovine serum albumin, 0.01 mol/L EDTA, and 1 g/L neomycin sulfate. A 100 μL aliquot of reconstituted extract is mixed with 25 μL of polyclonal ADH antisera, and after incubation for 24 hours at 4 °C, ^{125}I-labeled ADH is added, followed by incubation for 16 hours. Antigen-antibody complexes are adsorbed on activated charcoal, and following centrifugation, radioactivity is measured in the pellet. This method had an average CV of 3.4% over an analytical range of 0.25 to 5.1 ng/L and a minimum detectable concentration of 0.06 ng/L, determined by 3 SD above the mean result for an ADH-free calibrator.

Specimen Collection and Storage

Blood specimens for ADH should be collected into prechilled tubes containing EDTA as an anticoagulant. Most procedures recommend that specimens be delivered to the laboratory on ice and centrifuged at 4 °C within 30 minutes of collection. The plasma is then removed and stored or shipped frozen at −20 °C until analysis is performed. Random urine specimens may be collected without preservatives; alternatively, complete 24 hour urine specimens may be collected in 10 mL of 6 mol/L hydrochloric acid.[162] Significant deterioration of ADH occurs after prolonged storage.

Oxytocin

Oxytocin is a nonapeptide secreted by the magnocellular neurons of the hypothalamus and stored in the neurohypophysis along with ADH. It promotes uterine contractions and milk ejection and contributes to the second stage of labor.[135]

Biochemistry

The structure of oxytocin is similar to that of ADH (see Figure 53-8), but with a phenylalanine → isoleucine substitution at residue 3, and an arginine → leucine substitution at residue 8.

The gene for oxytocin is located on chromosome 20p13. Prepro-oxytocin is 125 amino acids (12.7 kDa). Similar to the ADH gene, the oxytocin gene encodes two proteins: oxytocin and neurophysin 1. In contrast to preproADH, prepro-oxytocin lacks a sequence analogous to copeptin in ADH. Following the leader sequence of 19 amino acids, the nonapeptide oxytocin is encoded, followed by the 94 amino acid C-terminal propeptide neurophysin 1. The glycine residue at position 28 is amidated. Suspected or definitive disulfide bonds are at amino acids 20-25 (within oxytocin), 41-85, 44-58, 52-75, 59-65, 92-104, and 105-110. ADH and oxytocin are highly conserved throughout a variety of species, suggesting that mutations in the genes that encode them are likely to produce serious consequences.

Oxytocin receptors are expressed in the uterine myometrium and myoepithelial cells of the breast. More myometrial receptors are expressed toward the end of pregnancy. The gene for the oxytocin receptor is encoded on chromosome 3p25. Of its 389 amino acids (42.8 kDa), the first 38 amino acids are extracellular, followed by seven transmembrane domains and a 57 amino acid cytoplasmic domain. Three potential sites of glycosylation are known: amino acids 8, 15, and 26. A disulfide bond may be found between amino acids 112 and 187. Oxytocin receptors occur throughout the CNS, and it is thought that these receptors affect behaviors related to stress, socialization, and maternity.

Regulation of Oxytocin Secretion and Physiologic Activity

Oxytocin is present in both males and females, but its physiologic effects are known only for females.[145] Afferent nerve fibers from the uterus and cervix (and possibly the vagina) communicate with the paraventricular (PVN) and supraoptic nuclei (SON) in the hypothalamus; these are the sites of cell bodies that synthesize oxytocin. Near the conclusion of pregnancy, mechanical stimulation of the cervix by the growing fetus stimulates stretch mechanoreceptors that, in turn, promote oxytocin release from the hypothalamus. Next, uterine contractions during labor trigger additional release of oxytocin. The effect of oxytocin is to increase the strength of uterine contractions, providing positive feedback to oxytocin release until the time of delivery of the fetus. For the myometrium to respond to oxytocin, it must be estrogen primed. Thus, increasing responsiveness of the myometrium to oxytocin is noted near term. Increased sensitivity to oxytocin in the myometrium may reflect changes in oxytocin receptor number and/or responsiveness. Centrally, estrogens enhance the response of oxytocin to these stimuli. The influence of oxytocin on other parts of the brain has been reported. For example, emotional stress inhibits lactation.

With delivery of the newborn and placenta, declining concentrations of sex steroids allow prolactin to trigger active lactation. The role of oxytocin is to stimulate the smooth muscle cells of the breast to propel the milk toward the nipple. These smooth muscle cells (myoepithelial cells) surround the milk-producing cells. With suckling, afferent fibers that travel to the PVN and SON trigger oxytocin release. Contraction of the myoepithelial cells causes "milk let-down" (milk ejection), and milk can leak from the nipple if suckling is not continued.

In summary, oxytocin stimulates uterine smooth muscle contraction during labor and milk duct constriction during suckling that propels milk toward the nipple. Therefore oxytocin is critical for delivery of the newborn. Likewise, oxytocin is exceedingly important for nourishment and hydration of the newborn and infant.

Clinical disorders involving oxytocin have not been reported. However, oxytocin and its derivatives (pitocin) are used as pharmaceuticals to increase the intensity of uterine contractions during labor (e.g., as treatment for prolonged or failed labor) and to prevent or treat postdelivery uterine hemorrhage.

TABLE 53-10 Disorders of Overproduction and Underproduction of Pituitary Hormones

Pituitary Hormone	Consequences of Hormone Excess	Consequences of Hormone Deficiency
ACTH	Cushing disease	Cortisol deficiency
TSH	Central hyperthyroidism	Central hypothyroidism
GH	Children: gigantism	Children: short stature
	Adults: acromegaly	Adults: adult GHD
LH, FSH	Alpha chain overproduction	Hypogonadism
Prolactin	Galactorrhea, hypogonadism	Inadequate lactation or lactation failure in mothers after delivery
ADH	SIADH	DI

Measurement of Oxytocin

Immunoassays for measuring oxytocin in plasma or urine have been developed but are mostly of research interest, because no clinical indications for measuring oxytocin are known. With most plasma oxytocin assays, a preliminary extraction procedure is required to concentrate the hormone and remove interfering substances.

SUMMARY OF PITUITARY RELATED DISORDERS

Disorders that result from overproduction or underproduction of pituitary hormones are tremendously diverse (Table 53-10). Pituitary adenomas may be secretory or nonsecretory.[109] Corticotropinomas secrete ACTH; somatotropinomas secrete GH; and prolactinomas secrete prolactin. Gonadotropinomas usually do not secrete intact LH and/or FSH but may secrete free alpha subunits.[94] These topics are reviewed in depth in many chapters in this textbook. Understanding pituitary function and the various diseases that result from pituitary dysfunction is a fundamental and essential aspect of clinical and laboratory medicine practice.

REFERENCES

1. A consensus guideline for the diagnosis and treatment of growth hormone (GH) deficiency in childhood and adolescence: summary statement of the GH Research Society. J Clin Endocrinol Metab 2000;11:3990-3.
2. Abellan R, Ventura R, Palmi I, di Carlo S, Bacosi A, Bellver M, et al. Immunoassays for the measurement of IGF-II, IGFBP-2 and -3, and ICTP as indirect biomarkers of recombinant human growth hormone

misuse in sport: values in selected population of athletes. J Pharm Biomed Anal 2008;3:844-52.
3. Abuzzahab MJ, Schneider A, Goddard A, Grigorescu F, Lautier C, Keller E, et al. IGF-I receptor mutations resulting in intrauterine and postnatal growth retardation. N Engl J Med 2003;23:2211-22.
4. Agha A, Thornton E, O'Kelly P, Tormey W, Phillips J, Thompson CJ. Posterior pituitary dysfunction after traumatic brain injury. J Clin Endocrinol Metab 2004;12:5987-92.
5. Aimaretti G, Ambrosio MR, Benvenga S, Borretta G, De Marinis L, De Menis E, et al. Hypopituitarism and growth hormone deficiency (GHD) after traumatic brain injury (TBI). Growth Horm IGF Res 2004;14(suppl A):S114-7.
6. Aimaretti G, Bellone S, Baldelli R, Grottoli S, Bona G, Ghigo E. Growth hormone stimulation tests in pediatrics. Review. The Endocrinologist 2004;4:216-21.
7. Alba M, Salvatori R. Familial growth hormone deficiency and mutations in the GHRH receptor gene. Vitam Horm 2004;69: 209-20.
8. Alexopoulou O, Abs R, Maiter D. Treatment of adult growth hormone deficiency: who, why and how? A review. Acta Clin Belg 2010;1:13-22.
9. Allahabadia A, Weetman AP. Dynamic thyroid stimulating hormone tests: do they still have a role? J Endocrinol Invest 2003;7(suppl):31-8.
10. Amar AP, Weiss MH. Pituitary anatomy and physiology. Neurosurg Clin N Am 2003;1:11-23.
11. Anderson RJ, Chung HM, Kluge R, Schrier RW. Hyponatremia: a prospective analysis of its epidemiology and the pathogenetic role of vasopressin. Ann Intern Med 1985;2:164-8.
12. Apter D. Development of the hypothalamic-pituitary-ovarian axis. Ann N Y Acad Sci 1997;816:9-21.
13. Ascoli P, Cavagnini F. Hypopituitarism. Pituitary 2006;4:335-42.
14. Badaru A, Wilson DM. Alternatives to growth hormone stimulation testing in children. Trends Endocrinol Metab 2004;6:252-8.
15. Bagshaw SM, Townsend DR, McDermid RC. Disorders of sodium and water balance in hospitalized patients. Can J Anaesth 2009;2:151-67.
16. Ball SG. Vasopressin and disorders of water balance: the physiology and pathophysiology of vasopressin. Ann Clin Biochem 2007;(Pt 5):417-31.
17. Barth JH, Sibley PE. Standardization of the IMMULITE systems growth hormone assay with the recombinant IS 98/574. Ann Clin Biochem 2008;(Pt 6):598-600.
18. Baumann G. Growth hormone binding to a circulating receptor fragment—the concept of receptor shedding and receptor splicing. Exp Clin Endocrinol Diabetes 1995;1:2-6.
19. Baumann G, Amburn K, Shaw MA. The circulating growth hormone (GH)-binding protein complex: a major constituent of plasma GH in man. Endocrinology 1988;3:976-84.
20. Baylis PH. The syndrome of inappropriate antidiuretic hormone secretion. Int J Biochem Cell Biol 2003;11:1495-9.
21. Beastall GH, Ferguson KM, O'Reilly DS, Seth J, Sheridan B. Assays for follicle stimulating hormone and luteinising hormone: guidelines for the provision of a clinical biochemistry service. Ann Clin Biochem 1987;24(Pt 3):246-62.
22. Bedecarrats GY, Kaiser UB. Mutations in the human gonadotropin-releasing hormone receptor: insights into receptor biology and function. Semin Reprod Med 2007;5:368-78.
23. Belfiore A. The role of insulin receptor isoforms and hybrid insulin/IGF-I receptors in human cancer. Curr Pharm Des 2007;7:671-86.
24. Beltran L, Fahie-Wilson MN, McKenna TJ, Kavanagh L, Smith TP. Serum total prolactin and monomeric prolactin reference intervals determined by precipitation with polyethylene glycol: evaluation and validation on common immunoassay platforms. Clin Chem 2008;10: 1673-81.
25. Benbow SJ, Foy P, Jones B, Shaw D, MacFarlane IA. Pituitary tumours presenting in the elderly: management and outcome. Clin Endocrinol (Oxf) 1997;6:657-60.
26. Bidlingmaier M, Freda PU. Measurement of human growth hormone by immunoassays: current status, unsolved problems and clinical consequences. Growth Horm IGF Res 2010;1:19-25.
27. Blum WF, Ranke MB, Kietzmann K, Gauggel E, Zeisel HJ, Bierich JR. A specific radioimmunoassay for the growth hormone (GH)-dependent somatomedin-binding protein: its use for diagnosis of GH deficiency. J Clin Endocrinol Metab 1990;5:1292-8.
28. Bodei L, Ferone D, Grana CM, Cremonesi M, Signore A, Dierckx RA, et al. Peptide receptor therapies in neuroendocrine tumors. J Endocrinol Invest 2009;4:360-9.
29. Bodola F, Benedict CR. Rapid, simplified radioimmunoassay of arginine-vasopressin and atrial natriuretic peptide in plasma. Clin Chem 1988;5:970-3.
30. Boone M, Deen PM. Physiology and pathophysiology of the vasopressin-regulated renal water reabsorption. Pflugers Arch 2008;6:1005-24.
31. Bougneres P, Goffin V. The growth hormone receptor in growth. Endocrinol Metab Clin North Am 2007;1:1-16.
32. Breier BH, Gallaher BW, Gluckman PD. Radioimmunoassay for insulin-like growth factor-I: solutions to some potential problems and pitfalls. J Endocrinol 1991;3:347-57.
33. Buatti JM, Marcus RB Jr. Pituitary adenomas: current methods of diagnosis and treatment. Oncology (Williston Park) 1997;6:791-6.
34. Bulatov AA, Martynov AV, Grigor'ian AL, Komolov IS. [Molecular forms of human growth hormone and prolactin, secreted by cultured pituitary tumor cells]. Biokhimiia 1995;10:1637-46.
35. Burke W, Press N, McDonnell SM. Hemochromatosis: genetics helps to define a multifactorial disease. Clin Genet 1998;1:1-9.
36. Burns C, Rigsby P, Moore M, Rafferty B. The first international standard for insulin-like growth factor-1 (IGF-1) for immunoassay: preparation and calibration in an international collaborative study. Growth Horm IGF Res 2009;5:457-62.
37. Camps J, Martinez-Vea A, Perez-Ayuso RM, Arroyo V, Gaya JM, Rivera-Fillat F. Radioimmunoassay for arginine-vasopressin in cold ethanol extracts of plasma. Clin Chem 1983;5:882-4.
38. Carel JC, Leger J. Clinical practice: precocious puberty. N Engl J Med 2008;22:2366-77.
39. Casanueva FF, Castro AI, Micic D, Kelestimur F, Dieguez C. New guidelines for the diagnosis of growth hormone deficiency in adults. Horm Res 2009;71(suppl 1):112-5.
40. Cattini PA, Yang X, Jin Y, Detillieux KA. Regulation of the human growth hormone gene family: possible role for Pit-1 in early stages of pituitary-specific expression and repression. Neuroendocrinology 2006;3-4:145-53.
41. Chahal J, Schlechte J. Hyperprolactinemia. Pituitary 2008;2:141-6.
42. Chiamolera MI, Wondisford FE. Minireview: thyrotropin-releasing hormone and the thyroid hormone feedback mechanism. Endocrinology 2009;3:1091-6.
43. Christensen JH, Rittig S. Familial neurohypophyseal diabetes insipidus—an update. Semin Nephrol 2006;3:209-23.
44. Christofilis MA, Remacle-Bonnet M, Atlan-Gepner C, Garrouste F, Vialettes B, Fuentes P, et al. Study of serum big-insulin-like growth factor (IGF)-II and IGF binding proteins in two patients with extrapancreatic tumor hypoglycemia, using a combination of Western blotting methods. Eur J Endocrinol 1998;3:317-22.
45. Cianfarani S, Liguori A, Germani D. IGF-I and IGFBP-3 assessment in the management of childhood onset growth hormone deficiency. Endocr Dev 2005;9:66-75.
46. Ciccone NA, Kaiser UB. The biology of gonadotroph regulation. Curr Opin Endocrinol Diabetes Obes 2009;4:321-7.
47. Clemmons DR. Quantitative measurement of IGF-I and its use in diagnosing and monitoring treatment of disorders of growth hormone secretion. Endocr Dev 2005;9:55-65.
48. Clemmons DR. Value of insulin-like growth factor system markers in the assessment of growth hormone status. Endocrinol Metab Clin North Am 2007;1:109-29.
49. Clemmons DR, Van Wyk JJ, Ridgway EC, Kliman B, Kjellberg RN, Underwood LE. Evaluation of acromegaly by radioimmunoassay of somatomedin-C. N Engl J Med 1979;21:1138-42.
50. Colao A. Pituitary tumours: the prolactinoma. Best Pract Res Clin Endocrinol Metab 2009;5:575-96.

51. Conn PM, Janovick JA, Stanislaus D, Kuphal D, Jennes L. Molecular and cellular bases of gonadotropin-releasing hormone action in the pituitary and central nervous system. Vitam Horm 1995;50:151-214.
52. Crosby SR, Stewart MF, Ratcliffe JG, White A. Direct measurement of the precursors of adrenocorticotropin in human plasma by two-site immunoradiometric assay. J Clin Endocrinol Metab 1988;6:1272-7.
53. Darzy KH, Shalet SM. Pathophysiology of radiation-induced growth hormone deficiency: efficacy and safety of GH replacement. Growth Horm IGF Res 2006;16(suppl A):S30-40.
54. Dattani M, Preece M. Growth hormone deficiency and related disorders: insights into causation, diagnosis, and treatment. Lancet 2004;9425:1977-87.
55. Dattani MT. Growth hormone deficiency and combined pituitary hormone deficiency: does the genotype matter? Clin Endocrinol (Oxf) 2005;2:121-30.
56. Davies MJ, Howlett TA. A survey of the current methods used in the UK to assess pituitary function. J R Soc Med 1996;3:159P-64P.
57. de Herder WW. Acromegaly and gigantism in the medical literature: case descriptions in the era before and the early years after the initial publication of Pierre Marie (1886). Pituitary 2009;3:236-44.
58. de Jager CM, de Heide LJ, van den Berg G, Wolthuis A, van Schelven WD. Acromegaly caused by a growth hormone-releasing hormone secreting carcinoid tumour of the lung: the effect of octreotide treatment. Neth J Med 2007;7:263-6.
59. De Palo EF, De Filippis V, Gatti R, Spinella P. Growth hormone isoforms and segments/fragments: molecular structure and laboratory measurement. Clin Chim Acta 2006;1-2:67-76.
60. Dean B, Kolavcic M, Tizian L, Harrison L. Should plasma beta-endorphin be measured in patients with disorders of the hypothalamic-pituitary-adrenal axis? Clin Chem 1986;5:895.
61. Decaux G, Musch W. Clinical laboratory evaluation of the syndrome of inappropriate secretion of antidiuretic hormone. Clin J Am Soc Nephrol 2008;4:1175-84.
62. Desai MP, Upadhye PS, Kamijo T, Yamamoto M, Ogawa M, Hayashi Y, et al. Growth hormone releasing hormone receptor (GHRH-r) gene mutation in Indian children with familial isolated growth hormone deficiency: a study from western India. J Pediatr Endocrinol Metab 2005;10:955-73.
63. di Iorgi N, Secco A, Napoli F, Calandra E, Rossi A, Maghnie M. Developmental abnormalities of the posterior pituitary gland. Endocr Dev 2009;14:83-94.
64. Diederich S, Eckmanns T, Exner P, Al-Saadi N, Bahr V, Oelkers W. Differential diagnosis of polyuric/polydipsic syndromes with the aid of urinary vasopressin measurement in adults. Clin Endocrinol (Oxf) 2001;5:665-71.
65. Dimaraki EV, Jaffe CA. Role of endogenous ghrelin in growth hormone secretion, appetite regulation and metabolism. Rev Endocr Metab Disord 2006;4:237-49.
66. Dobson S, White A, Hoadley M, Lovgren T, Ratcliffe J. Measurement of corticotropin in unextracted plasma: comparison of a time-resolved immunofluorometric assay and an immunoradiometric assay, with use of the same monoclonal antibodies. Clin Chem 1987;10:1747-51.
67. Domene HM, Hwa V, Argente J, Wit JM, Camacho-Hubner C, Jasper HG, et al. Human acid-labile subunit deficiency: clinical, endocrine and metabolic consequences. Horm Res 2009;3:129-41.
68. Douglas I. Hyponatremia: why it matters, how it presents, how we can manage it. Cleve Clin J Med 2006;73(suppl 3):S4-12.
69. Dundas B, Harris M, Narasimhan M. Psychogenic polydipsia review: etiology, differential, and treatment. Curr Psychiatry Rep 2007;3:236-41.
70. Earll JM, Sparks LL, Forsham PH. Glucose suppression of serum growth hormone in the diagnosis of acromegaly. JAMA 1967;8:628-30.
71. Eddy RL, Gilliland PF, Ibarra JD Jr, McMurry JF Jr, Thompson JQ. Human growth hormone release: comparison of provocative test procedures. Am J Med 1974;2:179-85.
72. Eliakim A, Nemet D. Exercise provocation test for growth hormone secretion: methodologic considerations. Pediatr Exerc Sci 2008;4:370-8.
73. Elmlinger MW, Kuhnel W, Weber MM, Ranke MB. Reference ranges for two automated chemiluminescent assays for serum insulin-like growth factor I (IGF-I) and IGF-binding protein 3 (IGFBP-3). Clin Chem Lab Med 2004;6:654-64.
74. Erotokritou-Mulligan I, Eryl BE, Cowan D, Bartlett C, Milward P, Sartorio A, et al. The use of growth hormone (GH)-dependent markers in the detection of GH abuse in sport: physiological intra-individual variation of IGF-I, type 3 pro-collagen (P-III-P) and the GH-2000 detection score. Clin Endocrinol (Oxf) 2010;72:520-6.
75. Fan Y, Menon RK, Cohen P, Hwang D, Clemens T, DiGirolamo DJ, et al. Liver-specific deletion of the growth hormone receptor reveals essential role of growth hormone signaling in hepatic lipid metabolism. J Biol Chem 2009;30:19937-44.
76. Fang P, Schwartz ID, Johnson BD, Derr MA, Roberts CT Jr, Hwa V, et al. Familial short stature caused by haploinsufficiency of the insulin-like growth factor I receptor due to nonsense-mediated messenger ribonucleic acid decay. J Clin Endocrinol Metab 2009;5:1740-7.
77. Fares F. The role of O-linked and N-linked oligosaccharides in the structure-function of glycoprotein hormones: development of agonists and antagonists. Biochim Biophys Acta 2006;4:560-7.
78. Fideleff HL, Boquete HR, Suarez MG, Azaretzky M. Prolactinoma in children and adolescents. Horm Res 2009;4:197-205.
79. Findling JW, Engeland WC, Raff H. The use of immunoradiometric assay for the measurement of ACTH in human plasma. Trends Endocrinol Metab 1990;6:283-7.
80. Fitzgerald P, Dinan TG. Prolactin and dopamine: what is the connection? A review article. J Psychopharmacol 2008;(2 suppl):12-9.
81. Fleseriu M, Gassner M, Yedinak C, Chicea L, Delashaw JB Jr, Loriaux DL. Normal hypothalamic-pituitary-adrenal axis by high-dose cosyntropin testing in patients with abnormal response to low-dose cosyntropin stimulation: a retrospective review. Endocr Pract 2010;1:64-70.
82. Ford KA, Baker HN, Baar JG, Balay D, Marlewski D, Venetucci M, et al. Automated enzyme immunoassay for lutropin with the Abbott IMx analyzer. Clin Chem 1989;12:2333-5.
83. Friedrich N, Krebs A, Nauck M, Wallaschofski H. Age- and gender-specific reference ranges for serum insulin-like growth factor I (IGF-I) and IGF-binding protein-3 concentrations on the Immulite 2500: results of the Study of Health in Pomerania (SHIP). Clin Chem Lab Med 2010;1:115-20.
84. Frystyk J, Andreasen CM, Fisker S. Determination of free growth hormone. J Clin Endocrinol Metab 2008;8:3008-14.
85. Frystyk J, Freda P, Clemmons DR. The current status of IGF-I assays—a 2009 update. Growth Horm IGF Res 2010;1:8-18.
86. Gallagher JP, Orozco-Cabal LF, Liu J, Shinnick-Gallagher P. Synaptic physiology of central CRH system. Eur J Pharmacol 2008;2-3:215-25.
87. Gasco V, Corneli G, Rovere S, Croce C, Beccuti G, Mainolfi A, et al. Diagnosis of adult GH deficiency. Pituitary 2008;2:121-8.
88. Geng X, Oliver G. Pathogenesis of holoprosencephaly. J Clin Invest 2009;6:1403-13.
89. Ghirardello S, Garre ML, Rossi A, Maghnie M. The diagnosis of children with central diabetes insipidus. J Pediatr Endocrinol Metab 2007;3:359-75.
90. Giustina A, Barkan A, Chanson P, Grossman A, Hoffman A, Ghigo E, et al. Guidelines for the treatment of growth hormone excess and growth hormone deficiency in adults. J Endocrinol Invest 2008;9:820-38.
91. Gleeson HK, Gattamaneni HR, Smethurst L, Brennan BM, Shalet SM. Reassessment of growth hormone status is required at final height in children treated with growth hormone replacement after radiation therapy. J Clin Endocrinol Metab 2004;2:662-6.
92. Goffin V, Binart N, Touraine P, Kelly PA. Prolactin: the new biology of an old hormone. Annu Rev Physiol 2002;64:47-67.
93. Green R, Hatton TM. Renal tubular function in gestation. Am J Kidney Dis 1987;4:265-9.
94. Greenman Y, Stern N. Non-functioning pituitary adenomas. Best Pract Res Clin Endocrinol Metab 2009;5:625-38.

95. Guevara-Aguirre J, Rosenbloom AL, Vasconez O, Martinez V, Gargosky SE, Allen L, et al. Two-year treatment of growth hormone (GH) receptor deficiency with recombinant insulin-like growth factor I in 22 children: comparison of two dosage levels and to GH-treated GH deficiency. J Clin Endocrinol Metab 1997;2:629-33.
96. Guillemin R. Hypothalamic hormones a.k.a. hypothalamic releasing factors. J Endocrinol 2005;1:11-28.
97. Harridge SD, Velloso CP. IGF-I and GH: potential use in gene doping. Growth Horm IGF Res 2009;4:378-82.
98. Hashida S, Tanaka K, Yamamoto N, Uno T, Yamaguchi K, Ishikawa E. Detection of one attomole of [Arg8]-vasopressin by novel noncompetitive enzyme immunoassay (hetero-two-site complex transfer enzyme immunoassay). J Biochem 1991;4:486-92.
99. Hashimoto T, Miyabo S, Nishibu M, Matsubara F, Migita S. Interference of immunoglobulins in the radioimmunoassay of human beta-endorphin. J Clin Chem Clin Biochem 1990;12:937-41.
100. Hasler U, Leroy V, Martin PY, Feraille E. Aquaporin-2 abundance in the renal collecting duct: new insights from cultured cell models. Am J Physiol Renal Physiol 2009;1:F10-8.
101. Hattori N. Macroprolactinemia: a new cause of hyperprolactinemia. J Pharmacol Sci 2003;3:171-7.
102. Heinrichs M, Meinlschmidt G, Neumann I, Wagner S, Kirschbaum C, Ehlert U, et al. Effects of suckling on hypothalamic-pituitary-adrenal axis responses to psychosocial stress in postpartum lactating women. J Clin Endocrinol Metab 2001;10:4798-804.
103. Hilczer M, Smyczynska J, Lewinski A. Limitations of clinical utility of growth hormone stimulating tests in diagnosing children with short stature. Endocr Regul 2006;3:69-75.
104. Ho KK. Consensus guidelines for the diagnosis and treatment of adults with GH deficiency II: a statement of the GH Research Society in association with the European Society for Pediatric Endocrinology, Lawson Wilkins Society, European Society of Endocrinology, Japan Endocrine Society, and Endocrine Society of Australia. Eur J Endocrinol 2007;6:695-700.
105. Howanitz JH. Review of the influence of polypeptide hormone forms on immunoassay results. Arch Pathol Lab Med 1993;4:369-72.
106. Inder WJ, Hunt PJ. Glucocorticoid replacement in pituitary surgery: guidelines for perioperative assessment and management. J Clin Endocrinol Metab 2002;6:2745-50.
107. Isidori AM, Giannetta E, Lenzi A. Male hypogonadism. Pituitary 2008;2:171-80.
108. Ivan G, Szigeti-Csucs N, Olah M, Nagy GM, Goth MI. Treatment of pituitary tumors: dopamine agonists. Endocrine 2005;1:101-10.
109. Jaffe CA. Clinically non-functioning pituitary adenoma. Pituitary 2006;4:317-21.
110. Juul A, Bernasconi S, Clayton PE, Kiess W, DeMuinck-Keizer SS. European audit of current practice in diagnosis and treatment of childhood growth hormone deficiency. Horm Res 2002;5:233-41.
111. Kalelioglu I, Kubat UA, Yildirim A, Ozkan T, Gungor F, Has R. Transient gestational diabetes insipidus diagnosed in successive pregnancies: review of pathophysiology, diagnosis, treatment, and management of delivery. Pituitary 2007;1:87-93.
112. Kano T, Sugihara H, Sudo M, Nagao M, Harada T, Ishizaki A, et al. Comparison of pituitary-adrenal responsiveness between insulin tolerance test and growth hormone-releasing peptide-2 test: a pilot study. Peptides 2010;4:657-61.
113. Kato Y, Murakami Y, Sohmiya M, Nishiki M. Regulation of human growth hormone secretion and its disorders. Intern Med 2002;1:7-13.
114. Kaye TB. Hyperprolactinemia: causes, consequences, and treatment options. Postgrad Med 1996;5:265-8.
115. Keenan DM, Roelfsema F, Biermasz N, Veldhuis JD. Physiological control of pituitary hormone secretory-burst mass, frequency, and waveform: a statistical formulation and analysis. Am J Physiol Regul Integr Comp Physiol 2003;3:R664-73.
116. Kelberman D, Dattani MT. Septo-optic dysplasia: novel insights into the aetiology. Horm Res 2008;5:257-65.
117. Kelberman D, Rizzoti K, Lovell-Badge R, Robinson IC, Dattani MT. Genetic regulation of pituitary gland development in human and mouse. Endocr Rev 2009;7:790-829.
118. Kelly PA, Finidori J, Moulin S, Kedzia C, Binart N. Growth hormone receptor signalling and actions in bone growth. Horm Res 2001; 55(suppl 2):14-7.
119. Khanna A. Acquired nephrogenic diabetes insipidus. Semin Nephrol 2006;3:244-8.
120. Khosravi MJ, Morton RC, Diamandis EP. Sensitive, rapid procedure for time-resolved immunofluorometry of lutropin. Clin Chem 1988;8:1640-4.
121. Kirsten D. The thyroid gland: physiology and pathophysiology. Neonatal Netw 2000;8:11-26.
122. Kluge M, Riedl S, Erhart-Hofmann B, Hartmann J, Waldhauser F. Improved extraction procedure and RIA for determination of arginine8-vasopressin in plasma: role of premeasurement sample treatment and reference values in children. Clin Chem 1999;1:98-103.
123. Kofoed EM, Hwa V, Little B, Woods KA, Buckway CK, Tsubaki J, et al. Growth hormone insensitivity associated with a STAT5b mutation. N Engl J Med 2003;12:1139-47.
124. Kokshoorn NE, Wassenaar MJ, Biermasz NR, Roelfsema F, Smit JW, Romijn JA, et al. Hypopituitarism following traumatic brain injury: prevalence is affected by the use of different dynamic tests and different normal values. Eur J Endocrinol 2010;1:11-8.
125. Komada H, Yamamoto M, Okubo S, Nagai K, Iida K, Nakamura T, et al. A case of hypothalamic panhypopituitarism with empty sella syndrome: case report and review of the literature. Endocr J 2009;4:585-9.
126. Kopp P. The TSH receptor and its role in thyroid disease. Cell Mol Life Sci 2001;9:1301-22.
127. Kratzsch J, Selisko T, Birkenmeier G. Identification of transformed alpha 2-macroglobulin as a growth hormone-binding protein in human blood. J Clin Endocrinol Metab 1995;2:585-90.
128. Krieger DT, Yamaguchi H, Liotta AS. Human plasma ACTH, lipotropin, and endorphin. Adv Biochem Psychopharmacol 1981;28:541-56.
129. Krsmanovic LZ, Hu L, Leung PK, Feng H, Catt KJ. The hypothalamic GnRH pulse generator: multiple regulatory mechanisms. Trends Endocrinol Metab 2009;8:402-8.
130. Kwan AY, Hartman ML. IGF-I measurements in the diagnosis of adult growth hormone deficiency. Pituitary 2007;2:151-7.
131. Lacroix MC, Guibourdenche J, Frendo JL, Pidoux G, Evain-Brion D. Placental growth hormones. Endocrine 2002;1:73-9.
132. Lanning NJ, Carter-Su C. Recent advances in growth hormone signaling. Rev Endocr Metab Disord 2006;4:225-35.
133. Lauwers E, Landuyt B, Arckens L, Schoofs L, Luyten W. Obestatin does not activate orphan G protein-coupled receptor GPR39. Biochem Biophys Res Commun 2006;1:21-5.
134. Lawrence MC, McKern NM, Ward CW. Insulin receptor structure and its implications for the IGF-1 receptor. Curr Opin Struct Biol 2007;6:699-705.
135. Lee HJ, Macbeth AH, Pagani JH, Young WS III. Oxytocin: the great facilitator of life. Prog Neurobiol 2009;2:127-51.
136. Lelbach A, Muzes G, Feher J. The insulin-like growth factor system: IGFs, IGF-binding proteins and IGFBP-proteases. Acta Physiol Hung 2005;2:97-107.
137. Lemaire P, Brauner N, Hammer P, Trivin C, Souberbielle JC, Brauner R. Improved screening for growth hormone deficiency using logical analysis data. Med Sci Monit 2009;1:MT5-10.
138. Lengyel AM. From growth hormone-releasing peptides to ghrelin: discovery of new modulators of GH secretion. Arq Bras Endocrinol Metabol 2006;1:17-24.
139. LeRoith D. Clinical relevance of systemic and local IGF-I: lessons from animal models. Pediatr Endocrinol Rev 2008;5(suppl 2):739-43.
140. Leung KC, Howe C, Gui LY, Trout G, Veldhuis JD, Ho KK. Physiological and pharmacological regulation of 20-kDa growth hormone. Am J Physiol Endocrinol Metab 2002;4:E836-43.

141. Lewis AS, Courtney CH, Atkinson AB. All patients with "idiopathic" hypopituitarism should be screened for hemochromatosis. Pituitary 2009;3:273-5.
142. Lichanska AM, Waters MJ. New insights into growth hormone receptor function and clinical implications. Horm Res 2008;3:138-45.
143. Lin-Su K, Wajnrajch MP. Growth hormone releasing hormone (GHRH) and the GHRH receptor. Rev Endocr Metab Disord 2002;4: 313-23.
144. Loonen AJ, Knoers NV, van Os CH, Deen PM. Aquaporin 2 mutations in nephrogenic diabetes insipidus. Semin Nephrol 2008;3: 252-65.
145. Macdonald K, Macdonald TM. The peptide that binds: a systematic review of oxytocin and its prosocial effects in humans. Harv Rev Psychiatry 2010;1:1-21.
146. Magiakou MA, Mastorakos G, Webster E, Chrousos GP. The hypothalamic-pituitary-adrenal axis and the female reproductive system. Ann N Y Acad Sci 1997;816:42-56.
147. Majzoub JA, Srivatsa A. Diabetes insipidus: clinical and basic aspects. Pediatr Endocrinol Rev 2006;4(suppl 1):60-5.
148. McNeilly AS. Lactational control of reproduction. Reprod Fertil Dev 2001;7-8:583-90.
149. Miller M, Dalakos T, Moses AM, Fellerman H, Streeten DH. Recognition of partial defects in antidiuretic hormone secretion. Ann Intern Med 1970;5:721-9.
150. Mims RB, Bethune JE. Acromegaly with normal fasting growth hormone concentrations but abnormal growth hormone regulation. Ann Intern Med 1974;6:781-4.
151. Mitchell ML, Hermos RJ, Schoepfer A, Orson JM. Reference ranges for insulin-like growth factor-1 in healthy children and adolescents, determined with filter-paper blood specimens. Clin Chem 1990;12: 2138-9.
152. Molitch ME. Pituitary incidentalomas. Endocrinol Metab Clin North Am 1997;4:725-40.
153. Molitch ME. Nonfunctioning pituitary tumors and pituitary incidentalomas. Endocrinol Metab Clin North Am 2008;1:151-71, xi.
154. Molitch ME. Pituitary tumours: pituitary incidentalomas. Best Pract Res Clin Endocrinol Metab 2009;5:667-75.
155. Monga V, Meena CL, Kaur N, Jain R. Chemistry and biology of thyrotropin-releasing hormone (TRH) and its analogs. Curr Med Chem 2008;26:2718-33.
156. Moore HP, Andresen JM, Eaton BA, Grabe M, Haugwitz M, Wu MM, et al. Biosynthesis and secretion of pituitary hormones: dynamics and regulation. Arch Physiol Biochem 2002;1-2:16-25.
157. Mullis PE. Genetics of growth hormone deficiency. Endocrinol Metab Clin North Am 2007;1:17-36.
158. Nakamoto J. Laboratory diagnosis of multiple pituitary hormone deficiencies: issues with testing of the growth and thyroid axes. Pediatr Endocrinol Rev 2009;6(suppl 1):291-7.
159. Nathan BM, Allen DB. Growth hormone treatment. In: Lifshitz F, ed. Pediatric endocrinology. New York, NY: Informa Healthcare, 2007: 117.
160. O'Dell SD, Day IN. Insulin-like growth factor II (IGF-II). Int J Biochem Cell Biol 1998;7:767-71.
161. Obara-Moszynska M, Kedzia A, Korman E, Niedziela M. Usefulness of growth hormone (GH) stimulation tests and IGF-I concentration measurement in GH deficiency diagnosis. J Pediatr Endocrinol Metab 2008;6:569-79.
162. Panzali A, Signorini C, Ferrari R, Albertini A. Direct determination of arginine-vasopressin in urine. Clin Chem 1990;2:384-5.
163. Popii V, Baumann G. Laboratory measurement of growth hormone. Clin Chim Acta 2004;1-2:1-16.
164. Price JD, Lauener RW. Serum and urine osmolalities in the differential diagnosis of polyuric states. J Clin Endocrinol Metab 1966;2:143-8.
165. Raff H, Findling JW. A new immunoradiometric assay for corticotropin evaluated in normal subjects and patients with Cushing's syndrome. Clin Chem 1989;4:596-600.
166. Richmond EJ, Rogol AD. Growth hormone deficiency in children. Pituitary 2008;2:115-20.
167. Romero CJ, Nesi-Franca S, Radovick S. The molecular basis of hypopituitarism. Trends Endocrinol Metab 2009;10:506-16.
168. Romero CJ, Nesi-Franca S, Radovick S. The molecular basis of hypopituitarism. Trends Endocrinol Metab 2009;10:506-16.
169. Rosenbloom AL, Connor EL. Hypopituitarism and other disorders of the growth hormone-insulin-like growth factor-I axis. In: Lifshitz F, ed. Pediatric endocrinology. New York, NY: Informa Healthcare, 2007:65-99.
170. Rosenbloom AL, Guevara AJ, Rosenfeld RG, Fielder PJ. The little women of Loja—growth hormone-receptor deficiency in an inbred population of southern Ecuador. N Engl J Med 1990;20:1367-74.
171. Rosenfeld RG, Hwa V. New molecular mechanisms of GH resistance. Eur J Endocrinol 2004;151(suppl 1):S11-5.
172. Rosner MH, Ronco C. Dysnatremias in the intensive care unit. Contrib Nephrol 2010;165:292-8.
173. Ross J, Czernichow P, Biller BM, Colao A, Reiter E, Kiess W. Growth hormone: health considerations beyond height gain. Pediatrics 2010;4: e906-18.
174. Rothman MS, Wierman ME. Female hypogonadism: evaluation of the hypothalamic-pituitary-ovarian axis. Pituitary 2008;2:163-9.
175. Saito T, Tojo K, Oki Y, Sakamoto N, Matsudaira T, Sasaki T, et al. A case of prolactin deficiency with familial puerperal alactogenesis accompanying impaired ACTH secretion. Endocr J 2007;1:59-62.
176. Samarasinghe S, Vokes T. Diabetes insipidus. Expert Rev Anticancer Ther 2006;6(suppl 9):S63-74.
177. Santner SJ, Santen RJ, Kulin HE, Demers LM. A model for validation of radioimmunoassay kit reagents: measurement of follitropin and lutropin in blood and urine. Clin Chem 1981;11:1892-5.
178. Schick R, Schusdziarra V. Physiological, pathophysiological and pharmacological aspects of exogenous and endogenous opiates. Clin Physiol Biochem 1985;1:43-60.
179. Schneider HJ, Aimaretti G, Kreitschmann-Andermahr I, Stalla GK, Ghigo E. Hypopituitarism. Lancet 2007;9571:1461-70.
180. Seo Y, Jeong B, Kim JW, Choi J. Plasma concentration of prolactin, testosterone might be associated with brain response to visual erotic stimuli in healthy heterosexual males. Psychiatry Investig 2009;3: 194-203.
181. Shenker A. Activating mutations of the lutropin choriogonadotropin receptor in precocious puberty. Receptors Channels 2002;1:3-18.
182. Shirland L. SIADH: a case review. Neonatal Netw 2001;1:25-9.
183. Silverstein JH, Malasanos TH, Valladares A. Arginine overdose: death in a child: case report. Reactions Weekly 2008;8.
184. Smith CR, Norman MR. Prolactin and growth hormone: molecular heterogeneity and measurement in serum. Ann Clin Biochem 1990; 27(Pt 6):542-50.
185. Snyder JA, Haymond S, Parvin CA, Gronowski AM, Grenache DG. Diagnostic considerations in the measurement of human chorionic gonadotropin in aging women. Clin Chem 2005;10:1830-5.
186. Solomon S. POMC-derived peptides and their biological action. Ann N Y Acad Sci 1999;85:22-40.
187. Spanakis E, Milord E, Gragnoli C. AVPR2 variants and mutations in nephrogenic diabetes insipidus: review and missense mutation significance. J Cell Physiol 2008;3:605-17.
188. Suliman AM, Smith TP, Gibney J, McKenna TJ. Frequent misdiagnosis and mismanagement of hyperprolactinemic patients before the introduction of macroprolactin screening: application of a new strict laboratory definition of macroprolactinemia. Clin Chem 2003;9:1504-9.
189. Takahashi Y, Chihara K. Clinical significance and molecular mechanisms of bioinactive growth hormone (review). Int J Mol Med 1998;3:287-91.
190. Thomas JD, Monson JP. Adult GH deficiency throughout lifetime. Eur J Endocrinol 2009;161(suppl 1):S97-106.
191. Thompson CJ. Polyuric states in man. Baillieres Clin Endocrinol Metab 1989;2:473-97.
192. Toldy E, Locsei Z, Szabolcs I, Goth MI, Kneffel P, Szoke D, et al. Macroprolactinemia: the consequences of a laboratory pitfall. Endocrine 2003;3:267-73.

193. Tomycz ND, Horowitz MB. Inferior petrosal sinus sampling in the diagnosis of sellar neuropathology. Neurosurg Clin N Am 2009;3: 361-7.
194. Toogood AA, Stewart PM. Hypopituitarism: clinical features, diagnosis, and management. Endocrinol Metab Clin North Am 2008;1:235-61, x.
195. Tostivint H, Lihrmann I, Vaudry H. New insight into the molecular evolution of the somatostatin family. Mol Cell Endocrinol 2008;1-2: 5-17.
196. Trainer PJ, Barth J, Sturgeon C, Wieringaon G. Consensus statement on the standardisation of GH assays. Eur J Endocrinol 2006;1:1-2.
197. Treschan TA, Peters J. The vasopressin system: physiology and clinical strategies. Anesthesiology 2006;3:599-612.
198. Trivin C, Souberbielle JC, Aubertin G, Lawson-Body E, Adan L, Brauner R. Diagnosis of idiopathic growth hormone deficiency: contributions of data on the acid-labile subunit, insulin-like growth factor (IGF)-I and-II, and IGF binding protein-3. J Pediatr Endocrinol Metab 2006;4:481-9.
199. Uno T, Uehara K, Motomatsu K, Ishikawa E, Kato K. Enzyme immunoassay for arginine vasopressin. Experientia 1982;7:786-7.
200. Valtin H. Differential diagnosis and pathophysiology of diabetes insipidus. Nippon Jinzo Gakkai Shi 1995;11:601-9.
201. van Vught AJ, Nieuwenhuizen AG, Gerver WJ, Veldhorst MA, Brummer RJ, Westerterp-Plantenga MS. Pharmacological and physiological growth hormone stimulation tests to predict successful GH therapy in children. J Pediatr Endocrinol Metab 2009;8:679-94.
202. Vance ML. Pituitary adenoma: a clinician's perspective. Endocr Pract 2008;6:757-63.
203. Vermes I, Bonte HA, Sluijs VG, Schoemaker J. Interpretations of five monoclonal immunoassays of lutropin and follitropin: effects of normalization with WHO standard. Clin Chem 1991;3:415-21.
204. Wagner J, Thomas P. Genetic determinants of mammalian pituitary morphogenesis. Front Biosci 2007;12:125-34.
205. Walenkamp MJ, de Muinck Keizer-Schrama SM, de Mos M, Kalf ME, van Duyvenvoorde HA, Boot AM, et al. Successful long-term growth hormone therapy in a girl with haploinsufficiency of the insulin-like growth factor-I receptor due to a terminal 15q26.2 >qter deletion detected by multiplex ligation probe amplification. J Clin Endocrinol Metab 2008;6:2421-5.
206. Walenkamp MJ, Karperien M, Pereira AM, Hilhorst-Hofstee Y, van Doorn J, Chen JW, et al. Homozygous and heterozygous expression of a novel insulin-like growth factor-I mutation. J Clin Endocrinol Metab 2005;5:2855-64.
207. Walenkamp MJ, Wit JM. Genetic disorders in the growth hormone-insulin-like growth factor-I axis. Horm Res 2006;5:221-30.
208. Wallace JD, Cuneo RC, Bidlingmaier M, Lundberg PA, Carlsson L, Boguszewski CL, et al. Changes in non-22-kilodalton (kDa) isoforms of growth hormone (GH) after administration of 22-kDa recombinant human GH in trained adult males. J Clin Endocrinol Metab 2001;4: 1731-7.
209. Webster EL, Torpy DJ, Elenkov IJ, Chrousos GP. Corticotropin-releasing hormone and inflammation. Ann N Y Acad Sci 1998;840: 21-32.
210. Wheeler MJ, D'Souza A, Horn AN. Evaluation of test kits for gonadotropins. Lancet 1989;8663:616-7.
211. Wilson DM, Frane J. A brief review of the use and utility of growth hormone stimulation testing in the NCGS: do we need to do provocative GH testing? Growth Horm IGF Res 2005;15 (suppl A):S21-5.
212. Winter WE, Hardt NS. Laboratory evaluation of short stature in children. In: Winter WE, Sokoll L, Jialal I, eds. Handbook of diagnostic endocrinology. Washington, DC: AACC Press, 2008: 139-74.
213. Winter WE, Harris NS. Laboratory approaches to diseases of the adrenal cortex and adrenal medulla. In: Winter WE, Sokoll L, Jialal I, eds. Handbook of diagnostic endocrinology. Washington, DC: AACC Press, 2008:75-138.
214. Wong NA, Ahlquist JA, Camacho-Hubner C, Goodwin CJ, Dattani M, Marshall NJ, et al. Acromegaly or chronic renal failure: a diagnostic dilemma. Clin Endocrinol (Oxf) 1997;2:221-6.
215. Woods K. Genetic defects of the growth-hormone-IGF axis associated with growth hormone insensitivity. Endocr Dev 2007;11:6-15.
216. Woods KA, Camacho-Hubner C, Barter D, Clark AJ, Savage MO. Insulin-like growth factor I gene deletion causing intrauterine growth retardation and severe short stature. Acta Paediatr Suppl 1997;423: 39-45.
217. Wu SM, Chan WY. Male pseudohermaphroditism due to inactivating luteinizing hormone receptor mutations. Arch Med Res 1999;6: 495-500.
218. Ysewijn-Van Brussel KA, De Leenheer AP. Development and evaluation of a radioimmunoassay for Arg8-vasopressin, after extraction with Sep-Pak C18. Clin Chem 1985;6:861-3.

CHAPTER 54

The Adrenal Cortex

*Roger L. Bertholf, Ph.D., Ishwarlal Jialal, M.D., Ph.D., F.R.C.Path(London), D.A.B.C.C., and William E. Winter, M.D.**

The adrenal cortex and gonads produce steroid hormones. Steroids are a class of organic compounds that contain the cyclopentanoperhydrophenanthrene nucleus that is characterized by four aliphatic rings produced by the biosynthetic cyclization of a linear triterpene, squalene, which is produced by the mevalonate pathway (Figure 54-1). Three rings (A, B, and C) are made up of six carbons, and one ring (ring D) is made up of five carbons. Sterols are steroids that have been hydroxylated at position 3 on the A ring; cholesterol is a sterol. Cholesterol has a double bond between carbons 5 and 6 and contains an eight carbon aliphatic side group at position 17. Cholesterol is the precursor for all human steroid hormones. In humans, cholesterol is derived from both dietary sources and de novo synthesis, and is transported principally in low-density lipoproteins (LDLs). As cellular cholesterol concentrations rise, LDL receptor (LDLR) expression declines in an autoregulatory fashion. The synthesis of cholesterol is reviewed in Chapter 27.

ANATOMY

The adrenal glands are pyramidal in shape, 2 to 3 cm wide, 4 to 6 cm long, and about 1 cm thick. Because each gland sits atop the kidney, the adrenal glands are also referred to as the *suprarenal glands.* Arterial blood is supplied to the adrenal gland by (1) the superior adrenal (or suprarenal) artery from the inferior phrenic artery (a branch of the aorta); (2) the middle adrenal artery, which is directly from the aorta; and (3) the inferior adrenal artery, a branch of the renal artery. Possibly of more clinical importance than the arterial supply, especially when adrenal function is assessed via catheterization, is the venous drainage of the adrenal gland. Adrenal veins are present for each gland: the right adrenal vein enters directly into the vena cava at an acute angle, whereas the left adrenal vein enters into the left renal vein.

The adrenal cortex and the gonads share many metabolic pathways in the synthesis of steroid hormones because both are embryologically derived from nearby mesodermal anlagen.[148] Two important transcription factors in development of the adrenal cortex are steroidogenic factor-1 (SF-1) and the dosage-sensitive sex reversal adrenal hypoplasia congenita (AHC) on the X-chromosome gene 1 *(DAX-1).*[78] SF-1 regulates *DAX-1.*

The postnatal adrenal cortex is composed of three layers: the glomerulosa (10 to 15% of the cortex), the fasciculata (up to 75% of the cortex), and the reticularis (5 to 10% of the cortex). The fetal adrenal gland is proportionately much larger than adrenal glands observed later in life because of the presence of the fetal cortex (which wanes by 18 months of age). The fetal adrenal layer is situated between the definitive cortex and the medulla, and is characterized by large steroid-secreting cells arranged in a reticular pattern. At birth, the adrenal gland is nearly equal in weight to that of an adult (8 to 12 grams). The large size of the fetal adrenal (≈250 mg/100 g body weight) may explain the propensity of the gland to be occasionally traumatized during delivery. Between 3 and 18 months of age, the adrenal glands involute to approximately half their size at birth. Later in life, the adrenal glands are less susceptible to trauma and represent less than 50 mg/100 g of body weight. Adult adrenal glands weigh 4 to 6 g each.

Table 54-1 shows the location and action of major products of the adrenal gland.

STEROID BIOCHEMISTRY

Major hormones produced by the adrenal cortex include (1) mineralcorticoids, (2) glucocorticoids, and (3) adrenal androgens.

Mineralocorticoids (Aldosterone)

Mineralocorticoids bind to the mineralocorticoid receptor (MR) in the distal convoluted tubule and collecting duct of the nephron, the colon, and the salivary glands to promote sodium reabsorption and potassium and hydrogen ion excretion.[352] Similar to receptors for other steroid hormones and thyroid hormone, the MR functions as a transcription factor. When mineralocorticoid binds to the cytoplasmic MRs, the mineralocorticoid-MR complex relocates to the nucleus, where it influences cellular DNA regulating gene transcription. The principal mineralocorticoid is aldosterone, but

**The authors gratefully acknowledge the contribution of Professor Laurence M. Demers to the previous edition of this textbook, on which portions of this chapter are based.*

other compounds with mineralocorticoid activity include 11-desoxycorticosterone (DOC), 18-hydroxycorticosterone, corticosterone, and cortisol.

The *MR* gene encodes a 107 kDa protein and is officially labeled nuclear receptor subfamily 3, group C, member 2 (NR3C2), located on chromosome 4q31.1-31.2. Alternative splicing yields an alpha and beta MR mRNA. Aldosterone stimulates epithelial sodium channel (ENaC) activity via serum and glucocorticoid-induced kinase (SGK) and K-ras, increases expression of mitochondrial ATP-producing genes, and stimulates the basolateral Na^+/K^+-ATPase pump. ENaC, a highly selective epithelial sodium channel that is amiloride sensitive (amiloride is a K^+-sparing diuretic), has three subunits: the alpha subunit (most important of the three subunits: the sodium channel, non–voltage-gated protein 1, alpha coded by *SCNN1A,* chromosome 12p13), the beta subunit (sodium channel, non–voltage-gated 1, beta *SCNN1B,* chromosome 16p13-p12), and the gamma subunit (sodium channel, non–voltage-gated 1, gamma *SCNN1G,* chromosome 16p13-p12).[178] All ENaC subunits are similar and contain a large N-terminal extracellular domain, two transmembrane spanning domains (M1 and M2), and a C-terminal, short intracellular domain.[140] Although the binding of aldosterone to the MR occurs in the cytoplasm with transit of the complex to the nucleus, some free MR is present in the nucleus. The MR binds cortisol and 11-desoxycorticosterone with affinity equal to that of aldosterone. However, the MR is protected from cortisol and 11-desoxycorticosterone by 11 beta-hydroxysteroid dehydrogenase-2 (HSD11B2), where, for example, HSD11B2 catalyzes the conversion of cortisol to cortisone (Figure 54-2). Cortisone does not bind to the MR. Variations in HSD11B2 may be involved in some cases of otherwise "essential" hypertension.[86] Chronic elevations in angiotensin, which controls aldosterone synthesis and release, produces pathologic changes in the heart and kidney by eliciting myocardial fibrosis and inflammatory changes in the renal vasculature.[139] The actions of mineralocorticoids are summarized in Table 54-2.

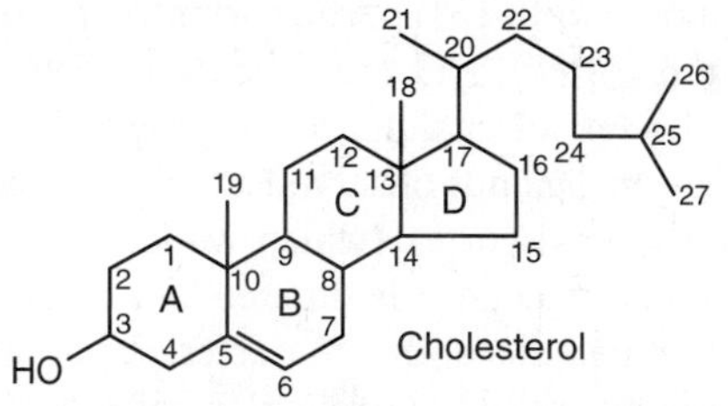

Figure 54-1 Steroids are a class of compounds that are characterized by four interconnected rings labeled *A* to *D*. The carbons are numbered in a standard fashion as illustrated. A sterol is a type of steroid wherein a hydroxyl group is attached to the ring (e.g., cholesterol where the hydroxyl group is attached to carbon 3). Cholesterol has a double bond between carbons 5 and 6 and contains an eight-carbon R group.

Glucocorticoids (Cortisol)

Glucocorticoids bind to the glucocorticoid receptor (GR) located in a large number of tissues, including lymphocytes, hepatocytes, and bone.[34] The *GR* gene contains 10 exons (exons 1 through 8 plus 9 alpha and 9 beta). Alternative splicing yields GR alpha and GR beta transcripts. Because of the wide distribution of the GR, glucocorticoid effects are diverse, including changes in intermediary metabolism and immunoregulation. Glucocorticoids raise blood glucose concentrations by enhancing the synthesis of gluconeogenic enzymes

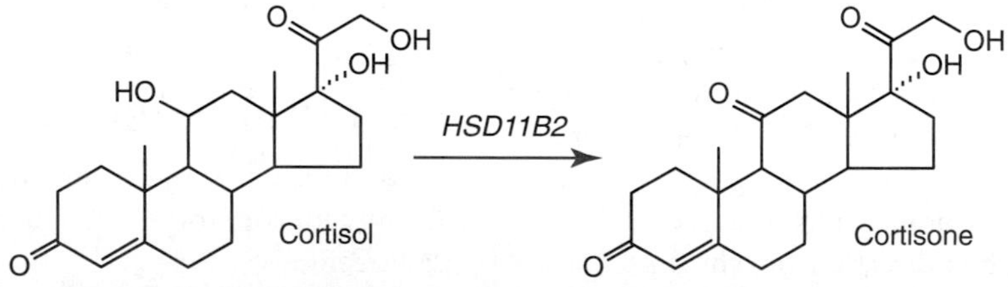

Figure 54-2 Normally, the mineralocorticoid receptor is protected from cortisol by 11 beta-hydroxysteroid dehydrogenase-2 (HSD11B2), which inactivates cortisol to cortisone. Cortisone does not bind to the mineralocorticoid receptor.

TABLE 54-1 Anatomy and Products of the Adrenal Gland

Adrenal Layer	Major Product(s)	Action
Cortex		
Zona glerulosa	Aldosterone	Mineralocorticoid
Zona fasciculata	Cortisol	Glucocorticoid
Zona reticularis	Dehydroepiandrosterone Androstenedione	Adrenal androgen
Medulla	Epinephrine	Catecholamine

(e.g., glucose-6-phosphatase and phosphoenol pyruvate carboxykinase), increase liver glycogen content through activation of glycogen synthase, and inhibit glycogen phosphorylase, producing insulin resistance in both muscle and adipose tissue that further raises blood glucose concentrations. Excessive catabolism of skeletal muscle causes myopathy and consequent weakness. Protein catabolism causes thinning of the skin and loss of strength in connective tissues. With excess glucocorticoids, bone loss may result from collagen catabolism and loss of osteoid, which can lead to fractures and compressed vertebrae.

Glucocorticoids cause adipose tissue redistribution centrally to the trunk, neck, and face, increased adipocyte differentiation, and promotion of lipogenesis in these tissues. Insulin resistance raises very low-density lipoprotein (VLDL) and triglyceride concentrations and lowers high-density lipoprotein (HDL) concentrations. The activity of adipose tissue hormone-sensitive lipase (HSL) is decreased because of insulin resistance, allowing triglyceride breakdown to free fatty acids and increased free fatty acid delivery to the liver, which provides substrate for hepatic triglyceride resynthesis and VLDL production and export. Glucocorticoids increase appetite, and a subsequent increase in caloric intake causes weight gain.

TABLE 54-2 Major Actions of Mineralocorticoids

Action	Adverse Outcome Excessive Action	Deficient Action
Sodium retention*	Hypertension	Hypotension
Urinary potassium wasting	Hypokalemia	Hyperkalemia
Urinary hydrogen ion wasting	Alkalosis	

*With consequent H_2O retention.

When glucocorticoids bind to the cytoplasmic GR, heat shock proteins (HSPs) are released (HSP70 and HSP90).[63] Glucocorticoids are powerful anti-inflammatory hormones that inhibit nuclear factor kappaB (NFkappaB) through the induction of IkappaB synthesis.[91] IkappaB binds to NFkappaB in the cytoplasm, impairing the entrance of NFkappaB into the nucleus. Within the nucleus, the GR-cortisol complex binds NFkappaB, preventing its binding to DNA. Finally, within the nucleus, GR-cortisol and NFkappaB compete for cofactors that are available in limited quantities. Although IkappaB synthesis is enhanced, many proinflammatory genes are repressed, such as cyclo-oxygenase 2 (COX-2), inducible nitric oxide synthase (iNOS), various interleukins (IL-1, IL-2, and IL-6), tumor necrosis factor-alpha, interferon-gamma, and E-selectin. Adrenocorticotropic hormone (ACTH) also stimulates the release of IL-1, IL-6, and tumor necrosis factor-alpha.[275]

Glucocorticoids help maintain vascular tone and cardiac output, and stabilize lysosomal membranes.[44] Glucocorticoids suppress hypersensitivity responses by inhibiting the production of histamine by basophils and mast cells. Modest doses of glucocorticoids may improve one's mood, yet in pharmacologic concentrations, they may produce psychosis. Pathologically elevated concentrations of glucocorticoids are discussed further under the heading of "Cushing syndrome." The relative potencies of corticosteroids in terms of glucocorticoid and mineralocorticoid activity are given in Table 54-3. The actions of glucocorticoids are summarized in Table 54-4.

Adrenal Androgens (DHEA and Androstenedione)

The adrenal androgens dehydroepiandrosterone (DHEA), dehydroepiandrosterone sulfate (DHEA-S), and androstenedione provide androgenic effects through their peripheral conversion to testosterone, which in turn binds to the androgen receptor (AR) that is described in Chapter 56.[149] Between ages 7 and 8, the urinary excretion of 17-ketosteroids (the breakdown products of adrenal androgens) increases as an early sign that puberty will begin in the coming 3 to 5 years.[239]

TABLE 54-3 Relative Potencies of Corticosteroids

Corticosteroid	Glucocorticoid Activity	Mineralocorticoid Activity
Aldosterone	0.1	400
Corticosterone	0.2	2
Cortisol	1	1
Cortisone	0.7	0.7
Dexamethasone*	50-150	2
11-Deoxycorticosterone	0	20
Fludrocortisone*	10	400
6α-Methylprednisolone*	5	0.5
Prednisolone*	4	0.7
Prednisone*	4	0.7
Triamcinolone*	3	0

*Synthetic.

TABLE 54-4 Major Targets of Glucocorticoid Action and Adverse Consequences of Excesses and Deficiencies

	Adverse Outcome	
Target Tissue	**Excessive Action**	**Deficient Action**
Central Nervous System	Polyphagia	Anorexia
	Depression or psychosis	Depression
Endocrine System		
Carbohydrate metabolism	Hyperglycemia	Hypoglycemia
Glycogen synthesis, gluconeogenesis, insulin resistance	Increased	Decreased
Free fatty acids, triglycerides	Increased	NSE
Body weight	Increased	Decreased
Fat distribution	Centripital	NSE
Pituitary	Decreased TSH	NSE
Musculoskeletal and Connective Tissue		
Muscle	Atrophy (catabolism)	NSE
Skin	Thinning (catabolism)	NSE
Bone	Osteoporosis	NSE
Immune System	Immunosuppression	NSE

NSE, No specific effect.

In males, adrenal androgens, such as DHEA and androstenedione, are normally of negligible importance because testosterone is a much more potent androgen. However, adrenal androgens are important in pubertal and adult women because they produce axillary and pubic hair. Women with Turner syndrome are an excellent example of the effects of adrenal androgens in women. Because of streak gonads (hypoplastic and dysfunctioning gonads mainly composed of fibrous tissue), adolescents with Turner syndrome do not experience gonadarchy (the period during which the gonads begin to secrete sex hormones) because all of their ovarian follicles are atretic before birth. Estrogen deficiency during adolescence is manifest in lack of breast development, primary amenorrhea, and failure of fat redistribution to the hips and buttocks. However, because adrenarchy (the increase in activity of the adrenal glands preceding puberty) is normal in adolescents with Turner syndrome, they will develop axillary and pubic hair despite their lack of estrogenization.

Throughout life, DHEA is sulfated, and circulating concentrations of DHEA-S exceed those of DHEA by 100-fold or more. For example, a typical DHEA reference interval in males is 180 to 1250 ng/dL, whereas the DHEA-S reference interval is 125 to 619 μg/dL.

PHYSIOLOGY AND REGULATION OF ADRENOCORTICAL HORMONES

Steroid hormones are not stored in hormone-producing cells and therefore must be produced as needed. As lipophilic molecules, steroids pass through cell membranes to exit the hormone-producing cells, enter the circulation to be distributed throughout the body, and enter target cells passing through the target cell membrane into the cytoplasm, where they bind to receptors. Translocation of the hormone-receptor complex to the nucleus initiates the action of the hormone. Growing evidence suggests that steroid hormones may concurrently act independently of their effect on DNA transcription. In the circulation, steroids exist as free and bound species. This is discussed in greater detail in Chapter 56.

Aldosterone

Aldosterone production and secretion are controlled through the renin-angiotensin system (Figure 54-3).[216,342] The rate-limiting component in this system is renin release, which is regulated by the juxtaglomerular apparatus. Anatomically, the juxtaglomerular apparatus is composed of (1) the juxtaglomerular cells of the afferent arteriole that immediately leads to the glomerulus, (2) lacis cells (extraglomerular mesangial cells located at the vascular pole of the renal corpuscle), and (3) the macula densa.

The juxtaglomerular cells are modified smooth muscle cells that synthesize and secrete renin. Preprorenin is a 406 amino acid protein. Removal of the 20 amino acid presequence yields prorenin (386 amino acids). Cleavage of the 46 amino acid pro-segment produces the active hormone (340 amino acids, 37 kDa). Both prorenin and renin are released by the juxtaglomerular cells, which function as baroreceptors that detect arterial wall stretch produced by renal perfusion pressure. Therefore, decreased renal perfusion leads to renin release. This is the most important mechanism regulating renin concentrations in the circulation.

The macula densa consists of specialized cells that line the distal convoluted tubule (DCT). Compared with other tubular cells, these cells are unique in that their nuclei are near the apical (luminal) pole of the cell, whereas the Golgi apparatus is near the basolateral pole of the cell. Acting as

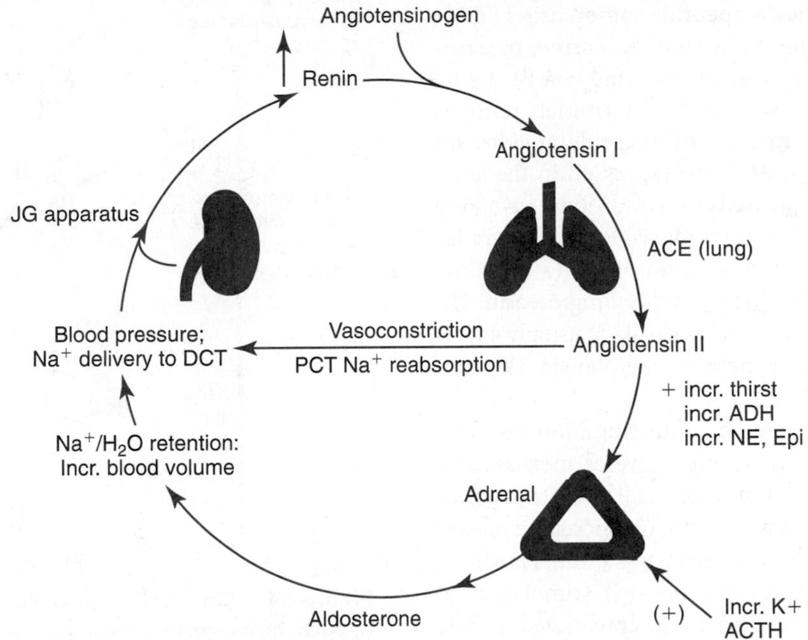

Figure 54-3 The juxtaglomerular (JG) apparatus monitors the perfusion pressure of the glomerulus and the sodium concentration in the distal convoluted tubule (DCT). Renin is released in cases of decreased renal perfusion or decreased sodium concentration in the DCT. Renin cleaves angiotensinogen to angiotensin I. Angiotensin-converting enzyme (ACE) converts angiotensin I to angiotensin II predominantly in the lung. Angiotensin II has direct vasoconstrictive effects, stimulates sodium reabsorption by the proximal convoluted tubule (PCT), and stimulates thirst, antidiuretic hormone (ADH) release, catecholamine release (*Epi,* epinephrine; *NE,* norepinephrine), and aldosterone synthesis and secretion. Aldosterone increases sodium reabsorption, and as water follows salt, blood volume increases along with blood pressure. Overall these effects act to restore renal perfusion. Adrenocorticotropic hormone (ACTH) and increased potassium have minor effects in stimulating aldosterone synthesis and secretion.

a chemoreceptor, the macula densa monitors the sodium concentration in the DCT. If a decline in sodium concentration occurs in the DCT, the macula densa signals the juxtaglomerular cells via prostacyclin to release renin. Anatomically, the DCT passes between the afferent and efferent arterioles of the nephron, which, respectively, supply blood to and drain blood from the glomerular capillaries.

Decreased sodium delivery to the DCT occurs in states of decreased renal perfusion. Decreased sodium delivery to the DCT can result from hyponatremia or a decreased glomerular filtration rate, both of which would elicit renin release. Sympathetic innervation of the juxtaglomerular cells also influences renin secretion via beta$_1$-adrenoreceptors. For this reason, norepinephrine and dopamine stimulate renin release. Thus, with upright posture and catecholamine release, renin release is enhanced. Potassium also directly stimulates renin release. Overall, renin is physiologically released in response to hypovolemia, reduced cardiac output, systemic vasodilatation, selectively reduced renal perfusion, hyponatremia, and stress (mediated by catecholamines).

Angiotensinogen (≈60 kDa) is an alpha$_2$-globulin synthesized in hepatocytes.[211] Renin acts as an aspartyl proteolytic enzyme cleaving the 10 N-terminal amino acids of

TABLE 54-5 Angiotensinogen and Derived Peptides

Molecule	Size (Amino Acids; Abbreviation)
Angiotensinogen	485
↓	
↓ Renin	
↓	
Angiotensin I	10 (A1-10)
↓	
↓ Angiotensin-converting enzyme (ACE)	
↓	
Angiotensin II	8 (A1-8)
↓	
↓ Amino peptidase A	
↓	
Angiotensin III	7 (A2-8)
↓	
↓ Arginyl aminopeptidase	
↓	
Angiotensin IV	6 (A3-8)

angiotensinogen to form the decapeptide angiotensin I (Table 54-5). Angiotensin I has no endocrine, paracrine, or autocrine effects. Angiotensin-converting enzyme (ACE), a zinc metallopeptidase, removes the two C-terminal residues from angiotensin I to generate the octapeptide angiotensin II.[315] High concentrations of ACE are expressed in the lung. ACE is pathologically expressed in conditions involving macrophage activation such as sarcoidosis. Further degradation of angiotensin II by aminopeptidase A (a glutamyl aminopeptidase) yields the heptapeptide angiotensin III. The ratio of angiotensin II to angiotensin III is usually 4 to 1. An arginyl aminopeptidase generates angiotensin IV from angiotensin III.

Angiotensin II acts to preserve circulating blood volume and maintain blood pressure through several mechanisms: (1) stimulation of aldosterone synthase (CYP11B2) to produce aldosterone; (2) direct vasoconstriction; (3) increased release of epinephrine and norepinephrine from the adrenal medulla, which will also act as vasoconstrictors; (4) stimulation of sodium reabsorption in the proximal convoluted tubule (PCT); (5) stimulation of thirst; and (6) stimulated release of antidiuretic hormone (ADH). Angiotensin III has equivalent potency in stimulating aldosterone secretion.

The best characterized of the angiotensin receptors are AT1 and AT2 that involve multiple second messenger systems.[134] Most functions of angiotensin II are mediated via the AT1 receptor. Some actions of the stimulated AT2 receptor oppose those of the AT1 receptor (e.g., AT2 receptor engagement causes vasodilatation).

CORTISOL

Cortisol is controlled through a traditional hypothalamic-pituitary-end organ negative feedback system (Figure 54-4). Corticotropin-releasing hormone (CRH) is released by stress, exercise, and hypoglycemia. Examples of physiologic stress include pain, trauma, surgery, and hemorrhage. Examples of psychologic stress include severe anxiety and major depression. Prolonged administration of supraphysiologic doses of glucocorticoids orally or parenterally will suppress the hypothalamic-pituitary-adrenal axis, leading to adrenal atrophy. As a result, abrupt termination of exogenous steroids may induce an acute and possibly life-threatening glucocorticoid insufficiency.

CRH is produced by the paraventricular nucleus of the hypothalamus. Prohormone convertase-1 (PC1) and PC2 liberate a C-terminal, 43 amino acid CRH precursor from the 196 amino acid preprohormone. Peptidylglycine alpha-amidating mono-oxygenase (PAM) removes the two C-terminal residues and adds an amine group, producing the 41 amino acid polypeptide, CRH.

Following hypothalamic secretion, CRH reaches the anterior pituitary gland through the hypothalamic pituitary portal system.[244] Corticotrophs represent about 20% of functional anterior pituitary cells and express receptors for CRH that promote synthesis, storage, and release of corticotropin (ACTH; 4.5 kDa).[110] ACTH is also released by ADH stimulation but to a lesser degree than CRH. The proinflammatory

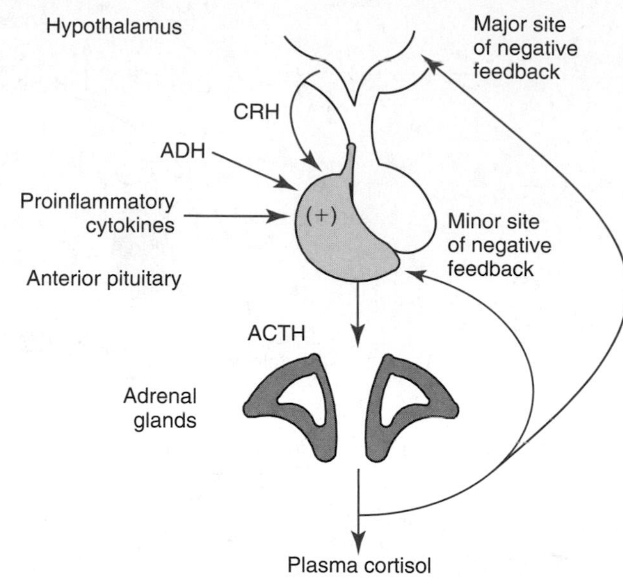

Figure 54-4 Cortisol is controlled through a traditional hypothalamic-pituitary-end organ negative feedback system. Corticotropin-releasing hormone (CRH) is released from the hypothalamus and is delivered to the anterior pituitary via the hypothalamic-pituitary portal system. CRH releases adrenocorticotropic hormone (ACTH) from anterior pituitary corticotrophs. Increased concentrations of antidiuretic hormone (ADH) and proinflammatory cytokines (e.g., IL-1, IL-6, and tumor necrosis factor-alpha) can also stimulate ACTH release. ACTH stimulates the synthesis and release of cortisol from the adrenal cortex. Cortisol feeds back negatively at the pituitary, but the major site of negative feedback is the hypothalamus.

cytokines IL-1, IL-6, and tumor necrosis factor-alpha also release ACTH. There are two CRH receptors (CRH-R1 and CRH-R2) and three splice variants of CRH-2 (CRH-2alpha, CRH-2beta, and CRH-2gamma). CRH mediates its effects on corticotrophs exclusively through CRH-R1. CRH and its receptors are widely distributed throughout the central nervous system (CNS).

ACTH is released from its 32 kDa precursor protein, 266 amino acid pro-opiomelanocortin (POMC; gene: 8 kb; chromosome 2p23), by proteolysis (Figure 54-5).[133,159] In the corticotrophs, subtilisin-like proprotein convertase (PC1/3) cleaves POMC into two fragments: the 22 kDa pro-ACTH fragment and beta-lipotropin (amino acids 42-134), whose function remains poorly understood. Next, PC1/3 releases ACTH (amino acids 1-39) from pro-ACTH. The resulting N-terminal fragment is further cleaved to pro-gamma-melanocyte-stimulating hormone (MSH) and a joining peptide (JP). ACTH is not further cleaved in corticotrophs.

The action of PC2 in the hypothalamus, skin, and melanotrophs of the intermediate lobe is to release gamma-MSH from pro-opiocortin (N-POC); alpha-melanocyte-stimulating hormone (alpha-MSH; amino acids 1-13) and corticotropin-like intermediate lobe peptide (CLIP; amino acids 18-39) from ACTH; and gamma-lipotropin (amino

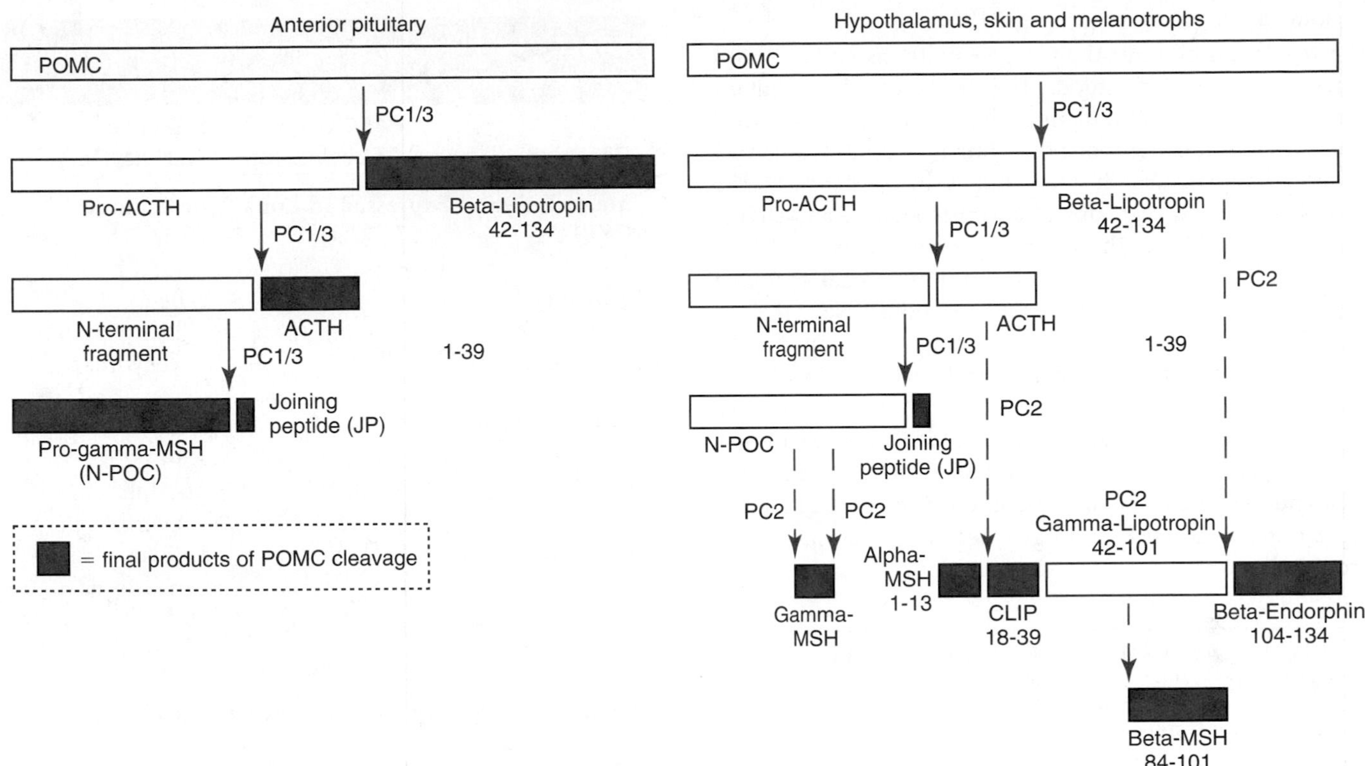

Figure 54-5 Adrenocorticotropic hormone (ACTH) is derived from pro-opiomelanocortin (POMC) by proteolysis. In the corticotrophs through the action of subtilisin-like proprotein convertase PC1/3, POMC is first cleaved into two fragments: the 22 kDa pro-ACTH fragment and beta-lipotropin (amino acids 42-134), whose function remains poorly understood. Next, PC1/3 releases ACTH (amino acids 1-39) from pro-ACTH. The resulting N-terminal fragment is further cleaved to pro-gamma-MSH (a.k.a. N-POC) and a joining peptide (JP). ACTH is not further cleaved in corticotrophs. In the hypothalamus, skin, and melanotrophs, further processing of N-POC, ACTH, and beta-lipotropin occurs. The action of PC2 in the hypothalamus, skin, and melanotrophs of the intermediate lobe of the pituitary is to release gamma-MSH from N-POC; alpha-melanocyte stimulating hormone (alpha-MSH; amino acids 1-13) and corticotropin-like intermediate lobe peptide (CLIP, amino acids 18-39) from ACTH; and gamma-lipotropin (amino acids 42-101) and beta-endorphin (amino acids 104-134) from beta-lipotropin. Last, beta-MSH (amino acids 84-101) is derived from gamma-lipotropin via PC2.

acids 42-101) and beta-endorphin (amino acids 104-134) from beta-lipotropin (see Figure 54-5). Last, beta-MSH (amino acids 84-101) is derived from gamma-lipotropin via PC2.

Hyperpigmentation that occurs with ACTH excess appears to be a direct consequence of the MSH-like activity of ACTH and not ACTH cleavage into alpha-MSH.[349] Whereas (1) a gamma-MSH sequence is contained within the N-terminal fragment, (2) alpha-MSH is contained within ACTH, and (3) beta-MSH is contained within gamma-lipotropin (a fragment of beta-lipotropin), MSH is not released by the human anterior pituitary gland.

ACTH circulates systemically to bind to ACTH receptors located on cells within the adrenal cortex. The ACTH receptor is the G-protein–coupled melanocortin-2 receptor (MC2R; gene location: chromosome 18p11.2).[77] The second messenger system involves adenyl cyclase and the generation of cyclic AMP. The actions of ACTH are then triggered via protein kinase A and protein kinase C, leading to steroidogenesis, increased size and number of adrenocortical cells, and increased size and functional complexity of cellular organelles. Cortisol is then synthesized and released. Cortisol feeds back centrally at the hypothalamus and to a lesser degree feeds back negatively at the pituitary to suppress CRH and ACTH secretion.[158] Other negative feedback loops include ACTH suppression of hypothalamic CRH and an ultra-short feedback loop whereby ACTH suppresses its own release.

Pulses of CRH cause the release of ACTH, which stimulates cortisol secretion. A wide diurnal variation in the secretion of cortisol is noted, with highest concentrations in the early morning (≈2 hours before awakening) and lowest concentrations near midnight (assuming that the individual is asleep overnight).

Adrenal Androgens

The regulation of adrenal androgen synthesis and secretion remains poorly understood. The existence of a pituitary adrenal androgen–stimulating hormone or a cortical androgen–stimulating hormone remains doubtful despite many years of research that sought its existence.[116] The best characterized regulator of androstenedione and DHEA secretion is ACTH. This is not surprising, as CYP17 is regulated by ACTH. A diurnal rhythm in adrenal androgen concentrations parallels cortisol variations. Nevertheless, ACTH regulation of adrenal androgens does not explain the normal prepubertal and pubertal increases in adrenal androgen synthesis that occurs in both boys and girls: ACTH does not increase prior to puberty. Evidence indicates that sympathetic innervation of the zona reticularis may exist and may regulate adrenal androgen secretion. Immune regulation of adrenal androgen secretion has also been proposed.

BIOSYNTHESIS OF ADRENOCORTICAL HORMONES[100]

An overview of steroid biosynthesis is provided in Figure 54-6, and the steroidogenic enzymes are listed in Table 54-6.

Aldosterone

Within the cytoplasm of steroid-producing cells, cholesterol ester is hydrolyzed to free cholesterol and a free fatty acid via the ACTH-responsive steroidogenesis activator protein, which is functionally a cholesterol esterase. Free cholesterol is then transported across the outer mitochondrial membrane by a sterol transfer protein into the mitochondrial intermembranous space. The 30 kDa steroidogenic acute regulatory protein (StAR) next transports cholesterol across the inner membrane into the mitochondria.[205,301] StAR-mediated transport of cholesterol into the mitochondria is a rate-limiting step in steroid hormone synthesis. StAR synthesis is enhanced by rising concentrations of cyclic AMP resulting from ACTH binding to its receptor. In the mitochondria, cholesterol is converted to pregnenolone by the action of CYP11A, which is the cytochrome P450 sidechain cleavage enzyme (P450ssc; gene location: chromosome 15q23-24) that is functionally a 20,22-desmolase that releases isocaproaldehyde. CYP11A therefore initiates the conversion of the C_{27} steroid cholesterol to the other C_{21} steroids (the subscript indicates the number of carbons in the compound).

Pregnenolone moves from the mitochondrion to the lumen of the endoplasmic reticulum. In the zona glomerulosa, CYP17 (P450c17) activity is not expressed; therefore pregnenolone is converted to progesterone via the non-P450 enzyme, 3-beta-hydroxysteroid dehydrogenase type 2 (3 beta-HSD; gene location: chromosome 1p13.1). The conversion of pregnenolone to progesterone also requires delta(5)-ketosteroid isomerase, which "moves" the double bond from the 5 position to the 4 position. Indeed, pregnenolone, 17-hydroxypregnenolone, and DHEA are characterized as delta(5) steroids, whereas progesterone, 17-hydroxyprogesterone, and androstenedione are characterized as delta(4) steroids based on the location of their double bond.

TABLE 54-6 Major Steroidogenic Enzymes Expressed in Adrenal Cortex

Protein*	P450 Abbreviation	Enzyme Activity(ies)
Major Enzymes Expressed in Zona Glomerulosa		
CYP11A	P450ssc	20,22-Desmolase (20,22-Lyase)
3-Beta HSD (type 2) (gene name: *HSD3B2*)	—	3-Beta hydroxysteroid dehydrogenase
Delta^5-ketosteroid isomerase	—	Delta^5-ketosteroid isomerase
CYP21	P450c21	21-Alpha hydroxylase
CYP11B2	P450 aldo	11-Beta hydroxylase 18-Hydroxylase 18-Oxidase
Major Enzymes Expressed in Zona Fasciculata and Reticularis		
CYP11A	P450ssc	20,22-Desmolase (20,22-Lyase)
3-Beta HSD (type 2) (gene name: *HSD3B2*)	—	3-Beta hydroxysteroid dehydrogenase
Delta^5-ketosteroid isomerase	—	Delta^5-ketosteroid isomerase
CYP17	P450c17	17-Hydroxylase 17,20-Lyase (ZR > ZF)
CYP21	P450c21	21-Alpha hydroxylase
CYP11B1	P450c11	11-Beta hydroxylase

*Usually these terms when italicized refer to the gene name. However, because different sources refer to these enzymes in a variety of ways (gene name vs. enzyme activity), the gene name un-italicized will be used to name the protein. *ZF*, Zona fasciculata; *ZR*, zona reticularis.

CYP21, a P450 21 alpha-hydroxylase (P450c21; gene location: chromosome 6p21.3) also expressed in the zona fasciculata, converts progesterone to 11-desoxycorticosterone (DOC). DOC migrates back into the mitochondrion, where CYP11B2 (P450 aldo; gene location: 8q24.3) catalyzes the conversion of DOC ultimately to aldosterone. Normally, little CYP11B1 (P450c11; gene location: 8q24.3) activity occurs in the zona glomerulosa.

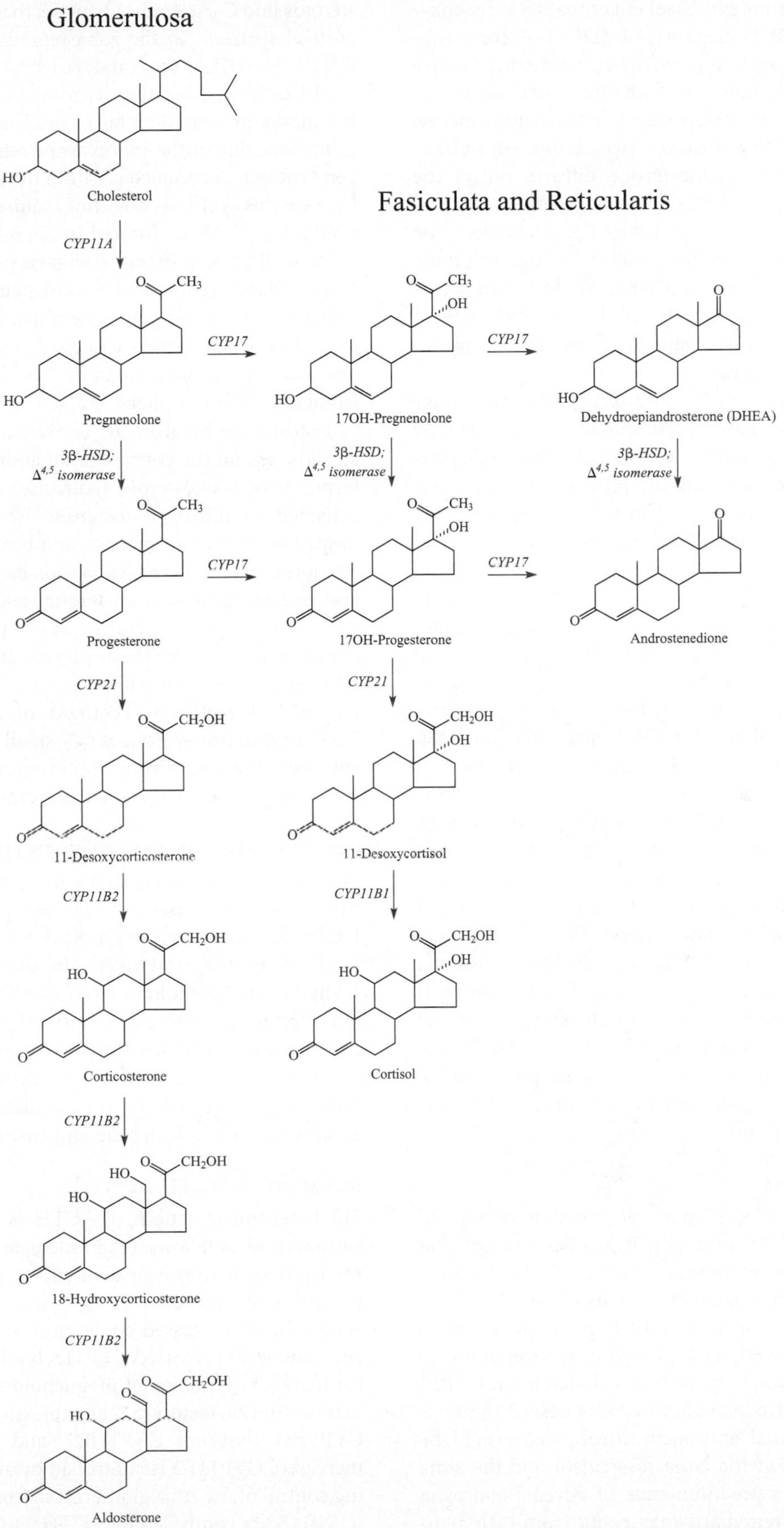

Glomerulosa

Fasiculata and Reticularis

Cholesterol

CYP11A

Pregnenolone → CYP17 → 17OH-Pregnenolone → CYP17 → Dehydroepiandrosterone (DHEA)

3β-HSD; $\Delta^{4,5}$ isomerase

Progesterone → CYP17 → 17OH-Progesterone → CYP17 → Androstenedione

CYP21

11-Desoxycorticosterone

11-Desoxycortisol

CYP11B2

CYP11B1

Corticosterone

Cortisol

CYP11B2

18-Hydroxycorticosterone

CYP11B2

Aldosterone

Figure 54-6 The zona glomerulosa is the site of aldosterone synthesis. CYP11B2 is under the predominant control of angiotensin II, which controls aldosterone synthesis and secretion. In the fasciculata and reticularis layers, cortisol and the adrenal androgens DHEA and androstenedione are produced. CYP11A, 3 beta-HSD, CYP17, CYP21, and CYP11B1 are controlled by ACTH.

CYP11B2 (aldosterone synthase) encompasses three enzymatic activities: (1) an 11-hydroxylase (DOC → corticosterone), (2) an 18-hydroxylase [corticosterone methyl oxidase I (CMOI); corticosterone → 18-hydroxycorticosterone], and (3) an 18-hydroxydehydrogenase [corticosterone methyl oxidase II (CMOII); 18-hydroxycorticosterone → aldosterone; see Figure 54-6].[234] Aldosterone diffuses out of the mitochondrion into the cytoplasm and across the cell membrane to enter the interstitium and then the circulation. The aldosterone secretion rate per day is 100 to 150 μg, with some estimates varying up to 200 μg. Thus the aldosterone secretion rate is approximately one tenth the secretion rate of cortisol on a weight basis. The half-life of circulating aldosterone is less than 15 minutes.

Whereas CYP11A, CYP17, and CYP11B1 are under ACTH control, CYP11B2 is predominantly controlled by angiotensin II. In this way, control of aldosterone synthesis is mostly independent of the anterior pituitary. Cortisol and adrenal androgens are not formed in the zona glomerulosa because the zona glomerulosa lacks expression of CYP17.

Cortisol

Cortisol production increases within minutes of an increase in circulating ACTH concentrations. In the zona fasciculata, where CYP17 (P450c17; gene location: chromosome 10q24.3) is expressed, CYP17 hydroxylates pregnenolone to 17-hydroxypregnenolone.[206] CYP17 also includes P450 17,20-lyase activity, which is important for the formation of adrenal androgens. 3-Beta-HSD and delta(5)-4-isomerase next catalyze the conversion of 17-hydroxypregnenolone to 17-hydroxyprogesterone. The last step outside of the mitochondrion involves CYP21 that 21-hydroxylates 17-hydroxyprogesterone to 11-desoxycortisol. 11-Desoxycortisol travels back to the mitochondrion, where CYP11B1 (P450c11) catalyzes the conversion of 11-desoxycortisol to cortisol via its 11-beta hydroxylase activity. Little CYP11B2 activity is seen in the zona fasciculata. Similar to aldosterone, cortisol diffuses out of the cell to ultimately enter the circulation. The normal cortisol secretion rate is 6 to 14 mg/m^2 per 24 hours. In adults, this is approximately 10 to 20 mg/d, with some estimates as high as 25 mg/d.

Adrenal Androgens

Debate continues as to the anatomic location of adrenal androgen synthesis.[258] Traditionally, it has been taught that adrenal androgens are synthesized exclusively in the zona reticularis. However, the enzymatic activity of the 17,20-lyase (17,20-desmolase) that converts 17-hydroxypregnenolone to DHEA [a delta(5) steroid] and 17-hydroxyprogesterone to androstenedione [a delta(4) steroid] is included in the CYP17 protein, whose 17-hydroxylase activity was described previously. Therefore, adrenal androgens theoretically could be synthesized within both the zona fasciculata and the zona reticularis. However, a predominance of adrenal androgen synthesis in the zona reticularis may result from high cytochrome 5b expression, which increases the 17,20-lyase activity of CYP17. The 17,20-lyase activity of CYP17 converts C_{21} steroids into C_{19} steroids. Likewise, there is nothing to prevent cortisol synthesis in the zona reticularis. The conversion of DHEA to DHEA-S is catalyzed by DHEA sulfotransferase (SULT2A1; gene location: chromosome 19q13.3). Based on the model presented so far of enzymes partitioned into the mitochondrion or the endoplasmic reticulum, adrenal androgen synthesis is completed within the endoplasmic reticulum because this synthesis does not require CYP21, CYP11B1, or CYP11B2, which are located in the mitochondrion.

A small amount of testosterone is produced by the adrenal cortex. DHEA is converted to androstenediol by 17-ketosteroid reductase (17 beta-hydroxysteroid dehydrogenase, 17 beta-OHSD); this is followed by conversion of androstenediol to testosterone via the actions of 3-beta HSD and delta(4)-5-isomerase. The peripheral conversion of adrenal androgens to testosterone involves the conversion of DHEA to androstenedione and the conversion of androstenedione to testosterone via 17-ketosteroid reductase. Finally, testosterone is activated to dihydrotestosterone by 5-alpha reductase in target tissues (penis, scrotum, and beard). Peripheral aromatization of androstenedione yields estrone, whereas peripheral aromatization of testosterone yields estradiol.

Adrenal androgens are the major product of the adrenal cortex, whose total synthesis exceeds 20 to 25 mg/d. The adult adrenal secretes approximately 6 to 8 mg/d of DHEA, 8 to 16 mg/d of DHEA-S, 1.5 mg/d of androstenedione, and 0.05 mg/d of testosterone. Only small amounts of the estrogens estradiol and estrone and insignificant amounts of progesterone and other precursor steroids are produced.

Adrenal Steroid Synthesis in the Fetus

The fetal adrenal lacks adult concentrations of 3-beta-HSD expression with resulting elevated production of DHEA, DHEA-S, and 16-hydroxy DHEA-S (from hydroxylation of DHEA-S in the fetal liver). In utero, pregnenolone and 17-hydroxypregnenolone from the fetal adrenal enter the fetal circulation to be converted in the placenta, respectively, into progesterone and 17-hydroxyprogesterone via placental 3-beta-HSD. Progesterone and 17-hydroxyprogesterone then return to the adrenal (via the circulation), where they serve as substrates for aldosterone and cortisol, respectively.[225]

Summary of ACTH Activity

The biochemical actions of ACTH on the adrenal cortex is summarized as follows: (1) immediate ACTH effects via steroidogenesis activator protein and StAR; (2) increased cholesterol esterase activity; (3) decreased cholesterol ester synthesis; (4) increased cholesterol transport into the mitochondrion; (5) increased CYP11A binding of cholesterol; and (6) increased synthesis of pregnenolone. Through the action of transcription factors (SF-1), expression of CYP11A, CYP17, CYP11B1 (but not CYP11B2), and the LDL receptor is increased. CYP11B2 is controlled by angiotensin II, separating control of the zona glomerulosa from the zona fasciculata (CYP11B2 is controlled by ACTH). In addition, ACTH and other factors yet not discovered control adrenal androgen synthesis.

ADRENOCORTICAL HORMONES IN THE CIRCULATION

Steroid hormones are 90 to 98% bound to specific carrier proteins or albumin. Steroids that are sulfated or glucuronidated circulate unbound in the plasma. Aldosterone is carried primarily by albumin as cortisol, corticosterone, and 17-hydroxyprogesterone occupy most of the binding sites on corticosteroid-binding globulin (CBG; transcortin), a 58 kDa, 383 amino acid alpha-1 globulin.[111,266] Normal concentrations of total cortisol exceed the normal concentrations of aldosterone by many-fold, explaining why little aldosterone is carried on CBG. CBG is a member of the serine protease inhibitor superfamily, specifically, SERPINA6 (clade A—alpha-1 antiprotease, antitrypsin—member 6; gene location: chromosome 14q3).[168]

Between 80 and 90% of cortisol is carried by CBG, 7% of cortisol is loosely bound to albumin, and 2 to 3% is unbound (free). When total cortisol rises in Cushing syndrome (see later), the increased proportion of plasma free cortisol readily spills into the urine, increasing the urinary free cortisol (UFC) excretion.[176] Typically, only 0.25 to 0.5% of total cortisol is excreted in the urine.

Because more cortisol than aldosterone is bound to CBG, the half-life of cortisol is longer (60 to 80 minutes) than the half-life of aldosterone (20 to 30 minutes).[61] In addition to cortisol, progestins are carried by CBG. *Progestin* is a generic term for any substance that produces some or all of the biological effects of progesterone.

CBG concentrations rise in response to estrogens. In pregnancy, CBG may rise two- to threefold. Some patients with chronic active hepatitis may display increased CBG concentrations. Alternatively, CBG concentrations are reduced in (1) nephrosis (as a result of CBG loss in the urine), (2) cirrhosis (because of decreased production), and (3) hyperthyroidism (as caused by increased metabolism), and with glucocorticoid treatment (probably as a result of catabolism). Even with changes in total cortisol due to changes in CBG, the concentration of free cortisol remains stable if the hypothalamic-pituitary-adrenal axis is functioning normally.

DHEA and its sulfated form, DHEA-S, and estradiol are predominantly carried by albumin. In contrast, testosterone and dihydrotestosterone (DHT) are carried by sex hormone–binding globulin (SHBG), an ≈100 kDa homodimer (each monomer is ≈50 kDa; 373 amino acids; gene location: chromosome 17p1).[254] Estrogens and thyroid hormone increase SHBG concentrations, whereas insulin, growth hormone, glucocorticoids, androgens, and progestins lower SHBG concentrations. SHBG concentrations are higher in children than in adults.

METABOLISM OF ADRENAL STEROIDS[7]

The liver is the major site of steroid metabolism via P450 enzyme systems, with the kidney playing less of a metabolic role but an important excretory role. Clearance of steroid hormones involves (1) hydroxylation, (2) dehydrogenation, (3) reduction of double bonds, and (4) conjugation to sulfates or glucuronides. The reduction in steroid concentrations increases their solubility and provides functional sites (such as hydroxyl groups) for their conjugation to sulfate or glucuronic acid; this increases their solubility in urine, promoting their excretion. Approximately 90% of conjugated steroids are excreted by the kidney.

ALDOSTERONE[20]

Aldosterone is reduced to tetrahydroaldosterone. Glucuronidation produces tetrahydroaldosterone 3-glucuronide, which can be excreted by the kidney. Aldosterone is 3 alpha- and 5 alpha-reduced, or 3 alpha- and 5 beta-reduced (Figure 54-7). Only ≈0.5% of aldosterone is excreted unchanged in the urine. Aldosterone is glucuronidated at the carbon 18 position. Cirrhosis, severe congestive heart failure, and ascites impair hepatic aldosterone clearance.

CORTISOL[311]

Cortisone is formed from cortisol via 11 beta-hydroxysteroid dehydrogenase type 2 (see Figure 54-7). In this reaction, the 11-hydroxyl group is converted to an 11-oxo group by removal of two hydrogens. Cortisone lacks glucocorticoid activity. [*Note:* When cortisone is used as a drug, it can be activated back to cortisol in the liver via 11-beta hydroxysteroid dehydrogenase type 1, an nicotinamide adenine dinucleotide phosphate (NADPH)-dependent oxo-reductase.] Reduction of the double bonds at carbons 4-5 via delta(4)-5-beta reductase or delta(4)-5-alpha reductase yields dihydrocortisol and dihydrocortisone (DHE). Metabolism with reduction of the ketone groups at carbon 3 results in tetrahydrocortisol (THF) and tetrahydrocortisone (THE), which account for the major portion of cortisol clearance (≈50%). The only difference in the outcome of delta(4)-5-beta reductase versus delta(4)-5-alpha reductase activity is the alpha or beta orientation of the hydrogen (5 beta-THF or 5-alpha-THF). Normally, the beta metabolite predominates (5-beta THF:5-alpha-THF ratio = 2 : 1).

Further metabolism of THF and THE via 20-alpha-hydroxysteroid dehydrogenase or 20-beta-hydroxysteroid dehydrogenase produces alpha and beta cortol and cortolone (the cortoic acids), which account for ≈30% of cortisol excretion. Opening the carbon 17-20 bond creates a ketone and gives rise to 11 beta-hydroxyetiocholanolone and 11-ketoetiocholanolone, representing ≈10% of cortisol excretion. Only about 1% of cortisol is normally excreted as free cortisol or cortisone. Minor cortisol metabolites include (1) 20 alpha-hydroxycortisol and 20 beta-hydroxycortisol, which result from reduction of the carbon 20 ketone, and (2) 6 beta-hydroxycortisol, which results from hydroxylation of carbon 6. Oxidation of carbon 17 in THF and THE yields oxo or hydroxy metabolites (Figure 54-8). Minor cortisone metabolites are shown in Figure 54-8.

Of the many cortisol metabolites, more than 95% are conjugated at carbon 3 to glucuronic acid, or sulfated at the C-21 position. Proportionately, the glucuronide metabolites predominate over sulfated metabolites.

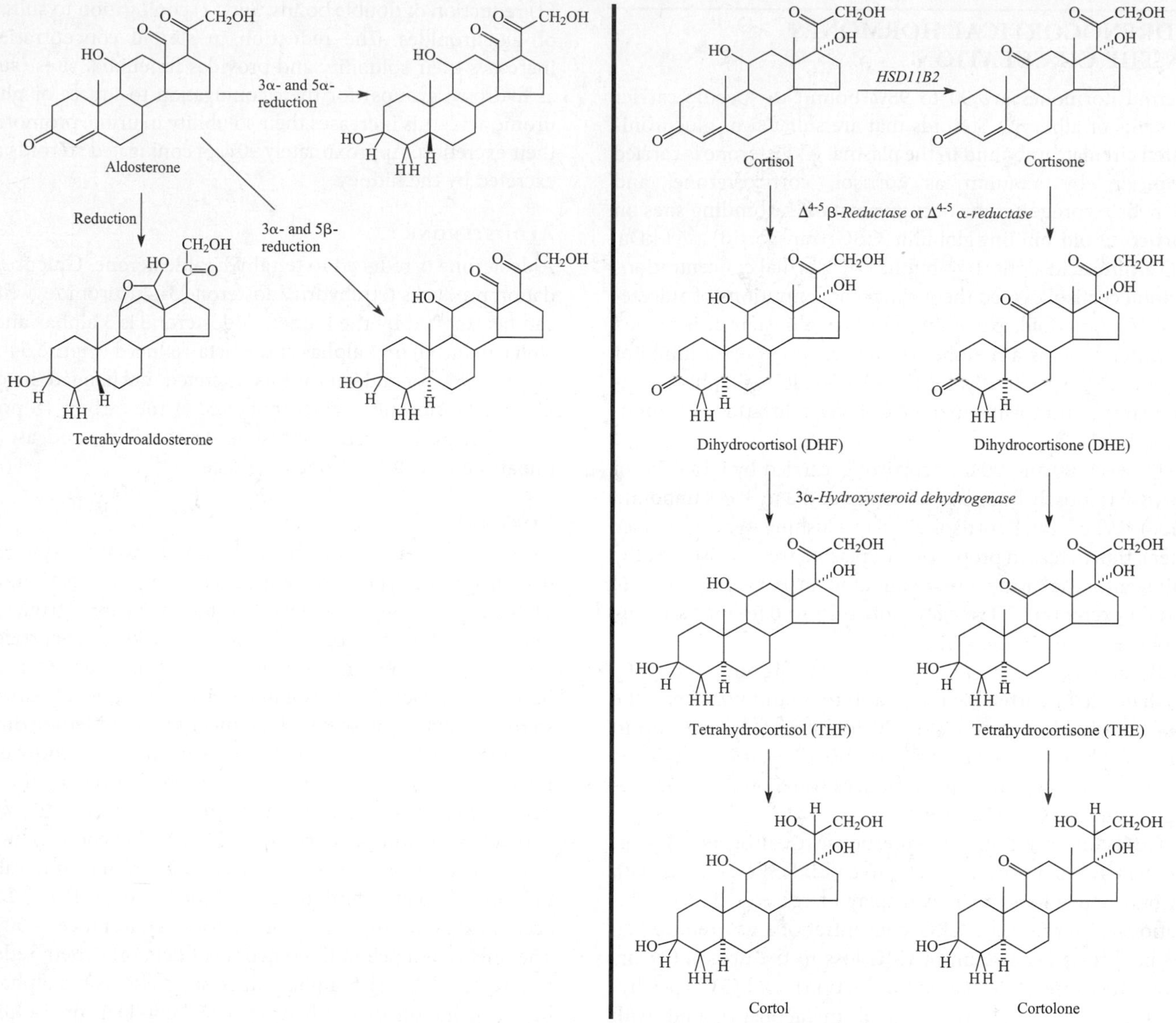

Figure 54-7 *Left panel:* Aldosterone metabolism: Aldosterone is reduced to tetrahydroaldosterone. Aldosterone can be 3 alpha- and 5 alpha-reduced or 3 alpha- and 5 beta-reduced. *Right panel:* Cortisol metabolism: Cortisone is formed from cortisol via 11-beta hydroxysteroid dehydrogenase-2 (HSD11B2). Reduction of the double bonds at carbons 4-5 via delta(4)-5 beta reductase or delta(4)-5 alpha reductase yields dihydrocortisol (DHF) and dihydrocortisone (DHE). Metabolism with reduction of the ketone groups at carbon 3 results in tetrahydrocortisol (THF) and tetrahydrocortisone (THE), which account for the major portion of cortisol clearance (≈50%). Further metabolism of THF and THE via 20-alpha hydroxysteroid dehydrogenase or 20-beta hydroxysteroid dehydrogenase produces alpha and beta cortol and cortolone (the cortoic acids), which account for ≈30% of cortisol excretion.

Adrenal Androgens[100]

Regarding the metabolism of the adrenal androgens, DHEA is sulfated to DHEA-S (Figure 54-9). These compounds are 7 alpha-hydroxylated or 16-alpha-hydroxylated. Alternatively, 17-ketosteroid reductase reduces the ketone at carbon 17 to a hydroxyl group, yielding androstenediol from DHEA and androstenediol sulfate from DHEA-S. Androstenedione is converted to androsterone via 3-alpha- and 5-alpha-reduction, whereas 3-alpha- and 5-beta-reduction yields etiocholanolone (see Figure 54-9). Similar to metabolites of cortisol, metabolites of the adrenal androgens are glucuronidated or sulfated for urinary excretion.

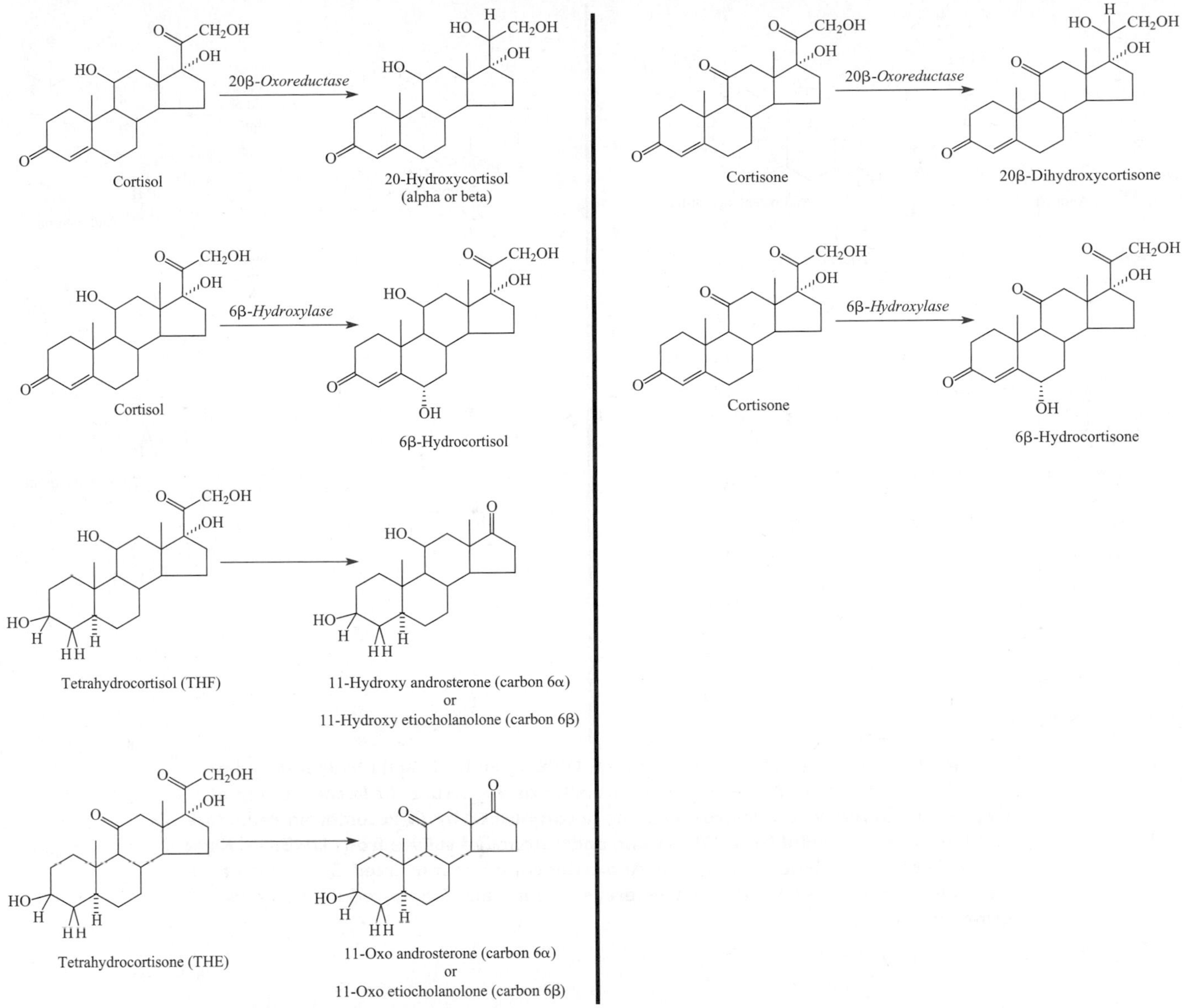

Cortisol → 20β-*Oxoreductase* → 20-Hydroxycortisol (alpha or beta)

Cortisone → 20β-*Oxoreductase* → 20β-Dihydroxycortisone

Cortisol → 6β-*Hydroxylase* → 6β-Hydrocortisol

Cortisone → 6β-*Hydroxylase* → 6β-Hydrocortisone

Tetrahydrocortisol (THF) → 11-Hydroxy androsterone (carbon 6α) or 11-Hydroxy etiocholanolone (carbon 6β)

Tetrahydrocortisone (THE) → 11-Oxo androsterone (carbon 6α) or 11-Oxo etiocholanolone (carbon 6β)

Figure 54-8 ***Left panel:*** **Minor cortisol metabolites include (1) 20-alpha-hydroxycortisol and 20-beta-hydroxycortisol, which result from reduction of the carbon 20 ketone, and (2) 6-beta-hydroxycortisol, which results from hydroxylation of carbon 6. Oxidation of carbon 17 in THF and THE yields oxo or hydroxy metabolites, as listed in the Figure.** ***Right panel:*** **Minor cortisone metabolites include 20 beta-dihydrocortisone and 6 beta-hydrocortisone.**

Urinary Metabolites

Whereas measurement of biliary excretion of adrenal steroids is not clinically useful, measurement of the urinary excretion of these compounds is common in the laboratory assessment of adrenal disease. Immunoassays for the major circulating steroid hormones are widely available.

Biochemically17-hydroxyprogesterone is reduced to pregnanetriol, which is measured in urine. The reduction converts keto groups at the 3-position and the 20-position to hydroxyl groups, giving the molecule three hydroxyl groups (hence the term *triol*). Hydroxylation helps solubilize the compound for renal excretion. Before the development of immunoassays for 17-hydroxyprogesterone, a 24 hour urine was collected for measurement of pregnanetriol excretion in cases of congenital adrenal hyperplasia (CAH) due to CYP21 or CYP11B1 deficiency. If these forms of CAH were managed appropriately, ideally the pregnanetriol excretion would return to within it's reference interval.

The urinary metabolites of 11-desoxycortisol and cortisol are classified as 17-hydroxycorticosteroids (17-OHCS). Analytically, 17-OHCS are photometrically determined by the reaction of 17,21-dihydroxy-20-oxosteroids with a phenylhydrazine-ethanol-sulfuric acid reagent, producing yellow phenylhydrazones that are termed *Porter-Silber*

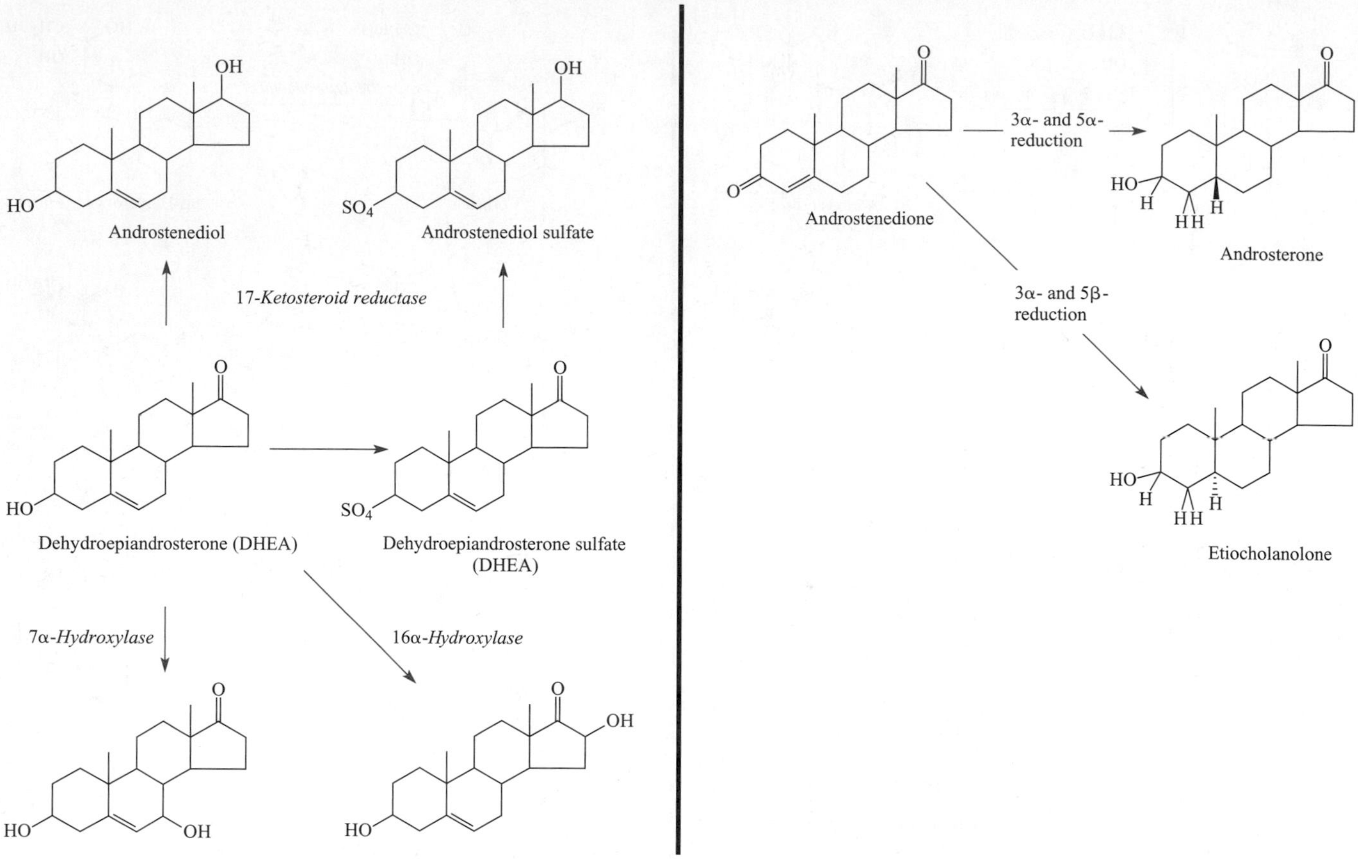

Figure 54-9 ***Left panel:*** **DHEA metabolism: DHEA can be 7 alpha-hydroxylated or 16 alpha-hydroxylated. Alternatively, conversion of the carbon 17 ketone group of DHEA and DHEA-S to a hydroxyl can be accomplished by 17-ketosteroid reductase, yielding androstenediol from DHEA and androstenediol sulfate from DHEA-S.** ***Right panel:*** **Androstenedione metabolism: Androstenedione is converted to androsterone via 3-alpha- and 5-alpha-reduction, whereas 3-alpha- and 5-beta-reduction yields etiocholanolone.**

chromogens. Measurements of 17-OHCS have been used to differentiate CYP21 deficiency from CYP11B1 deficiency. In CYP21 deficiency, 17-OHCS would not be elevated because both 11-desoxycortisol and cortisol are low. However, because CYP11B1 deficiency increases 11-desoxycortisol (the metabolic block is between 11-desoxycortisol and cortisol), 17-OHCS would be elevated in untreated or undertreated CYP11B1 deficiency. Also, CYP11B1 deficiency and CYP21 deficiency are differentiated by the greatly elevated plasma 11-desoxycortisol concentrations in the former.

The urinary metabolites of 17-hydroxyprogesterone, 11-desoxycortisol, and cortisol are 17-ketogenic steroids (17-KGS) because oxidation of these compounds yields a keto group at the 17 position. Ketogenic steroids have been measured using the Zimmermann reaction, in which an alkaline solution of meta-dinitrobenzene reacts with methylene groups at carbon-16 of the 17-ketosteroids. In CYP17 deficiency, 17-KGS would not be elevated. However, in both CYP21 and CYP11B1 deficiencies, when untreated or undertreated, 17-KGS are elevated.

DHEA and androstenedione metabolites are measured in the same way as 17-ketosteroids because both have keto groups in the C-17 position. Because testosterone has a hydroxyl group at the C-17 position, it is not a 17-ketosteroid. DHEA and androstenedione are elevated in untreated and undertreated CYP21 and CYP11B1 deficiencies. Figure 54-10 summarizes these urine steroid measurements.

Factors Affecting Adrenal Steroid Metabolism

Cortisol clearance (or metabolism) affects cortisol concentrations. If the clearance of cortisol is reduced, plasma cortisol concentrations can increase, whereas enhanced clearance of cortisol decreases its concentration. Rifampin-induced Addisonian crisis from increased cortisol metabolism has been reported. However, in most cases, cortisol, free cortisol, and ACTH are normal in these conditions, presumably because alterations in the free cortisol concentration will be sensed by the hypothalamus, which will respond by secreting CRH to ultimately return the free cortisol concentration to within it's

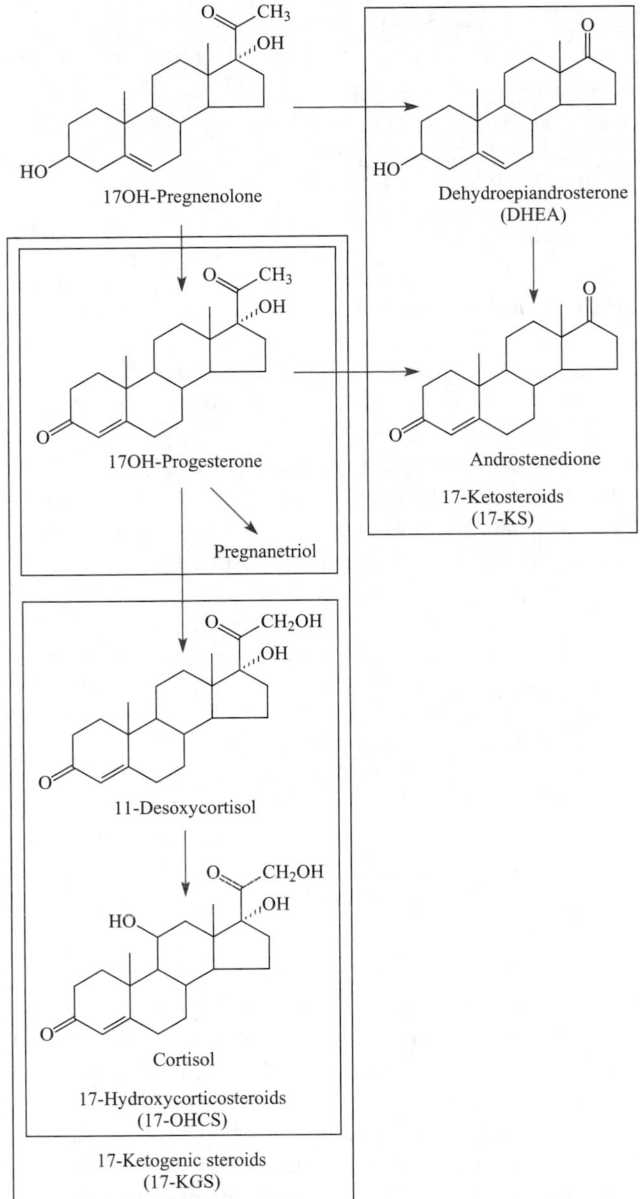

Figure 54-10 This figure summarizes the urinary metabolites generated from steroids involved in cortisol and adrenal androgen synthesis.

reference interval. Table 54-7 lists a number of conditions that affect cortisol concentrations.

DYNAMIC TESTS OF ADRENAL FUNCTION

Several strategies are used to assess adrenal function. These tests are typically designed to differentiate between primary and secondary causes of disease, or to detect abnormalities that may not be apparent in the results of static, baseline laboratory measurements. For example, provocative stimulation tests are useful in documenting hyposecretion of adrenocortical hormones.[226] A specific stimulus is applied, and the release of a given hormone over a specific time frame is measured. Also, suppression tests are used to document hypersecretion of the adrenocortical hormones.[76]

BOX 54-1 Protocol for the 1 Hour (Rapid) Cosyntropin Stimulation Test

Rationale

Administration of ACTH to normal subjects results in a rapid rise in the serum cortisol concentration. Patients with adrenal destruction (e.g., Addison disease) show no change or an inadequate change in serum cortisol concentration after ACTH injection. Patients with atrophy of the adrenal cortex caused by exogenous glucocorticoid treatment or dysfunction of the pituitary gland or hypothalamus may show a slight rise in serum cortisol concentration, but not one of normal magnitude.

Procedure

A baseline blood sample is drawn for determination of serum cortisol concentration; then 250 μg of cosyntropin is given intramuscularly or intravenously. Additional samples for serum cortisol determination are drawn 30 and 60 minutes after injection.

Interpretation

A peak serum cortisol concentration of 18 to 20 μg/dL or greater is a normal response. The expected change in cortisol concentration is 7 to 10 μg/dL (the delta cortisol). The peak cortisol value is more important than the incremental change. The incremental change may not be seen in patients who are tested at times of stress, when their adrenal output of cortisol is already maximally stimulated by endogenous ACTH.

ACTH Stimulation (Cosyntropin) Test

ACTH stimulation tests, sometimes referred to as the *cosyntropin tests,* are designed to document the functional capacity of the adrenal glands to synthesize cortisol (Boxes 54-1 and 54-2). Cosyntropin (Cortrosyn) is a synthetic polypeptide that is the N-terminal 24 amino acid sequence of ACTH, which contains the biologically active domain. Another name for cosyntropin is *tetracosactrin* (Synacthen). Cosyntropin, a potent stimulator of cortisol secretion, has a very brief half-life and minimal antigenicity. The protocols for 1 hour and multiple-day ACTH stimulation tests are shown in Box 54-1.

Investigators have sought to determine whether a lower dose of cosyntropin (1 μg vs. 250 μg) in the 1 hour stimulation test might be more sensitive for the detection of adrenal insufficiency from ACTH deficiency or primary adrenal failure.[143] Some patients have normal responses to 250 μg of ACTH yet inadequate responses to 1 μg of ACTH. This remains a point of controversy, and the 1 μg ACTH dose has not been universally accepted as superior to the 250 μg dose in detecting glucocorticoid deficiency.[89,218,317]

TABLE 54-7 Conditions That Affect Cortisol Clearance

Endocrinopathy	Cortisol Clearance	Mechanism
Hyperthyroidism	Incr	Inhibition of hepatic 11-beta HSDI and stimulation of 5-alpha reductase and 5-beta reductase
Hypothyroidism	Decr	Stimulation of hepatic 11-beta HSDI and inhibition of 5-alpha reductase and 5-beta reductase
Acromegaly	Incr	Inhibition of hepatic 11-beta HSDI
Cushing syndrome	Incr	Induction of 6 beta-hydroxylase
Solid Organ Dysfunction		
Chronic liver disease (disease including alcoholic cirrhosis)	Decr	Decreased cortisol metabolism
Renal disease	Decr	Reduced renal conversion: cortisol → cortisone
Drugs/Toxins		
Acute alcohol ingestion	Decr	—
Rifampin	Incr	Induction of 6 beta-hydroxylase
Phenytoin	Incr	Induction of 6 beta-hydroxylase
Phenobarbital	Incr	Induction of hepatic mixed-function oxidases
Other		
Aging	Decr	*Note:* Decreased clearance is balanced by decreased synthesis; therefore cortisol concentrations and responses to ACTH are normal.
Starvation	Decr	Balanced by decreased production
Anorexia nervosa	Decr	—

—, Not defined; *decr,* decreased; *incr,* increased.

CRH Stimulation Test

A direct and selective test of pituitary gland function is the CRH stimulation test (Box 54-3).[119,179] Injection of ovine CRH stimulates ACTH secretion in normal subjects within 60 to 180 minutes; glucocorticoids inhibit this effect (as in cases of Cushing syndrome resulting from an adrenal adenoma or ectopic ACTH secretion by a tumor). However, in Cushing disease, the corticotropinoma can respond to exogenous CRH with a normal or exaggerated response. This test may be used in the differential diagnosis of adrenocortical hyperfunction and hypofunction. CRH stimulation is also used in the differential diagnosis of endogenous Cushing syndrome and in distinguishing secondary from tertiary ACTH deficiency.

A variation of the CRH stimulation test measures ACTH in blood samples drawn from the two inferior petrosal venous sinuses (IPSs) to differentiate pituitary-dependent Cushing disease from ectopic ACTH syndrome.[237,305] Blood samples are collected from both right and left IPS veins and from a peripheral vein (e.g., the inferior vena cava) at −30, 0, +2, +5, +10, and +30 minutes after intravenous administration of ovine CRH (1 μg/kg body weight) over 20 to 60 seconds. The ratio of the IPS concentration to the peripheral venous concentration of plasma ACTH is used to predict the location of excess ACTH secretion. An IPS-to-peripheral vein ratio greater than 2.0 is consistent with a pituitary lesion (Cushing disease) as the cause of Cushing syndrome, whereas a ratio less than 1.4 to 1.7 supports the diagnosis of an ectopic ACTH syndrome. Some endocrinologists claim that IPS sampling is the best test for distinguishing ACTH-dependent forms of Cushing syndrome (ectopic ACTH syndrome vs. Cushing disease) when performed in the setting of long-standing hypercortisolism. ACTH concentrations are suppressed in patients with primary adrenal tumors compared with patients with Cushing syndrome or the ectopic ACTH syndrome.[138,312] Imaging studies cannot yet replace laboratory testing for Cushing disease.[9] Even when ectopic ACTH syndrome is diagnosed, localization of the source tumor can be very difficult.[107,297]

Insulin-Induced Hypoglycemia Stimulation Test

To test the integrity of the hypothalamic-pituitary-adrenal axis, other indirect tests of ACTH secretion rely on the adrenal response to maneuvers that stimulate endogenous ACTH release. In the insulin-induced hypoglycemia stimulation test, insulin is given to stimulate the release of CRH through hypoglycemia, and plasma ACTH or cortisol concentrations are measured.[79] This test involves the risk of hypoglycemia (obtundation, seizure, coma, and death) and should be performed only with an experienced physician in

BOX 54-2 Protocol for the Multiple-Day Adrenocorticotropic Hormone (ACTH) Stimulation Test

Rationale
Multiple-day ACTH stimulation testing for assessment of adrenal cortex function is required occasionally to evaluate adrenal cortisol responsiveness. A common situation is the diagnosis of adrenal insufficiency, which is treated with glucocorticosteroids before a cause has been established. Prolonged ACTH stimulation is used to distinguish primary from secondary and/or tertiary (central) causes of adrenal insufficiency.

Procedure
A total of 250 μg of cosyntropin is injected daily for 3 days. This is followed by an 8 hour infusion of 250 μg of cosyntropin. Urinary free cortisol and serum cortisol are measured daily.

Interpretation
Serum cortisol values of 18 to 20 μg/dL or greater exclude primary adrenal insufficiency. Glucocorticoid withdrawal would be required before assessment of secondary or tertiary adrenal insufficiency in such cases. Little or no increase in cortisol secretion is seen in primary adrenal failure even over successive days. A progressive staircase rise is seen over 2 to 3 days in adrenal insufficiency caused by pituitary or hypothalamic disease or steroid concentration suppression. Little or no response is seen in congenital adrenal hyperplasia (CAH) caused by 21- and 17-hydroxylase deficiencies. The 2 day and 5 day variations of this test have been employed in clinical practice.

BOX 54-3 Protocol for the Corticotropin-Releasing Hormone (CRH) Stimulation Test

Rationale
Exogenous CRH stimulates the secretion of ACTH from the anterior pituitary gland in normal subjects. The subsequent cortisol concentration is an indicator of the ACTH response.

Procedure
Synthetic ovine CRH (corticorelin ovine triflutate), 1 μg/kg body weight, is administered intravenously in bolus form at 0900 or 2000 hours. Blood samples for cortisol and ACTH assays are collected 15 minutes and immediately before and 5, 15, 30, 60, 120, and 180 minutes after CRH injection.

Interpretation
In normal subjects, plasma ACTH concentrations peak 30 minutes after CRH injection (80 ± 7 pg/mL at 0930 h; 29 ± 2.6 pg/mL at 2030 h), and serum cortisol peaks at 60 minutes (13 ± 1 μg/dL at 1000 h; 17 ± 0.7 μg/dL at 2100 h). Patients with pituitary ACTH deficiency (secondary adrenal insufficiency) have decreased ACTH and cortisol responses. Patients with hypothalamic disease have prolonged ACTH responses and subnormal cortisol responses. Most patients with Cushing syndrome caused by adrenal tumors or nonendocrine ACTH-producing tumors do not respond to CRH injection. Most patients with Cushing disease respond with a normal or excessive increase in ACTH. Responses usually are normal in patients with depression.

attendance. It is contraindicated in patients with a seizure disorder or coronary artery disease. Venous access must be maintained during the procedure to ensure a ready avenue for the rapid administration of glucose should hypoglycemia not spontaneously resolve or a hypoglycemia-induced seizure occur requiring immediate administration of intravenous glucose.

Metyrapone Stimulation Test

A less risky indirect test of hypothalamic-pituitary-adrenal axis function involves the administration of metyrapone, an inhibitor of the 11 beta-hydroxylase enzyme that converts 11-desoxycortisol to cortisol.[24] Several protocols have been designed for metyrapone stimulation testing; one that is simple and relatively safe for outpatient testing is described in Box 54-4.

Dexamethasone Suppression Test

In normal individuals, an elevation in the blood concentration of cortisol inhibits ACTH release from the pituitary gland. This results in decreased production of cortisol and other ACTH-dependent adrenal steroids from the adrenal cortex. The integrity of this feedback mechanism has been tested by administering a potent glucocorticoid, such as

BOX 54-4 Protocol for the Overnight Single-Dose Metyrapone Stimulation Test

Rationale
Metyrapone inhibits 11-beta-hydroxylase (CYP11B1), the enzyme that catalyzes the step immediately preceding cortisol synthesis. As the blood concentration of cortisol falls, the negative feedback effect is diminished, causing the release of ACTH from the pituitary gland. The stimulatory effect of ACTH on the adrenal cortex leads to a rise in 11-deoxycortisol, the compound immediately preceding cortisol in the biosynthetic pathway.

Procedure
Metyrapone (30 mg/kg body weight) is given orally at midnight with milk or a snack (to delay absorption). At 0800 hours the following morning, blood is drawn for determination of 11-deoxycortisol, cortisol, and ACTH concentrations.

Interpretation
In normal subjects, 11-desoxycortisol increases from less than 1 μg/dL to greater than 7 μg/dL after metyrapone stimulation, and ACTH values exceed 150 pg/mL. No response or an impaired response may be seen in pituitary or hypothalamic disease combined with inadequate enzyme blockade (plasma cortisol >3 μg/dL) or with Cushing syndrome caused by adrenal tumors or nonendocrine ACTH-secreting tumors. Exaggerated responses may be seen in pituitary Cushing syndrome.

Note: This test is not recommended in cases of suspected Addison disease for fear that suppression of cortisol production might precipitate an Addisonian crisis. That being said, patients with Addison disease have an inadequate rise in 11-desoxycortisol in response to metyrapone.

BOX 54-5 Protocol for the Overnight Low-Dose Dexamethasone Suppression Test

Rationale

In low doses, dexamethasone, a synthetic glucocorticoid and cortisol analog, suppresses ACTH and cortisol production in normal subjects, but not in patients with Cushing syndrome.

Procedure

One milligram of dexamethasone is given orally between 2200 and 2400. Blood is drawn for determination of serum cortisol at 0800 hours the next morning.

Interpretation

In normal subjects, the serum cortisol concentration is suppressed to 2 µg/dL or less after administration of 1 mg of dexamethasone. A postdexamethasone 0800 hours cortisol cutoff of less than 5 µg/dL is more sensitive for the detection of Cushing syndrome but is less specific. Most patients with Cushing syndrome do not show adequate suppression, and 0800 hours cortisol concentrations are usually 10 µg/dL or greater. Serum cortisol greater than 2 µg/dL may be seen in cases of stress, obesity, infection, acute or chronic illness, alcohol abuse, severe depression, oral contraceptive use, pregnancy, estrogen therapy, failure to take dexamethasone, or treatment with phenytoin or phenobarbital (which can enhance dexamethasone metabolism).

dexamethasone, and judging suppression of ACTH secretion by measuring serum or urine cortisol concentrations. Several dexamethasone suppression tests are available for clinical use (Boxes 54-5 through 54-7). Dexamethasone is chosen for suppression testing because it does not significantly cross-react in cortisol immunoassays. Therefore the secreted endogenous glucocorticoid, cortisol, can be distinguished from the exogenous glucocorticoid, dexamethasone.

A low dose of dexamethasone (1 mg in adults, 0.3 mg/m^2 in children) is used initially to document true hypersecretion of cortisol (see Box 54-5).[345] Patients with Cushing syndrome of any cause will fail to suppress their morning cortisol concentration to less than 5 µg/dL with a low dose of dexamethasone.[98] It should be emphasized that this is a screening test, and confirmation of Cushing syndrome requires repeat testing or measurement of urinary cortisol on at least two separate days or some other combination of tests (e.g., midnight cortisol <5 µg/dL, salivary cortisol <0.112 µg/dL).[151,166] A 0.5 mg dose variant of the overnight dexamethasone suppression test has been described and validated.[235] On the other hand, a 2 mg dexamethasone dose has been used to exclude Cushing syndrome in obese individuals.[274]

Higher doses of dexamethasone given over 48 hours are used to resolve the differential diagnosis of an ACTH-secreting pituitary adenoma (a corticotropinoma causing Cushing disease) versus an ectopic ACTH source. Suppression of basal urinary cortisol excretion by less than 50% is a response consistent with Cushing disease, but not ectopic

BOX 54-6 Protocol for the Classic Low-Dose/ High-Dose Dexamethasone Suppression Test

Rationale

Normal subjects show a decline in urinary free cortisol concentrations under conditions of low-dose dexamethasone suppression. However, patients with excess cortisol production, regardless of the cause, do not suppress on low-dose dexamethasone. Patients with Cushing syndrome caused by an ACTH-producing pituitary adenoma (e.g., Cushing disease from a corticotropinoma) may show suppression of cortisol excretion with high-dose dexamethasone. Patients with Cushing syndrome from other causes (adrenocortical adenoma or carcinoma, or ectopic production of ACTH or CRH) usually do not demonstrate cortisol suppression with high-dose dexamethasone treatment.

Procedure

Twenty-four hour urine samples are collected daily for 6 consecutive days. Free cortisol and creatinine are measured in each 24 hour urine sample. Urinary free cortisol (UFC) is regarded as a more specific measure of cortisol secretion than 17-hydroxycorticosteroids. The first 2 days provide baseline measurements of the excretion of cortisol. Dexamethasone 0.5 mg ("low-dose dexamethasone") is given orally every 6 hours starting at 0800 hours on day 3 (for a total of eight doses: days 3 and 4). Dexamethasone 2.0 mg ("high-dose dexamethasone") is then given orally every 6 hours starting at 0800 hours on day 5 (for a total of eight doses: days 5 and 6).

Interpretation

On the first 2 days, urinary excretion of cortisol (i.e., the baseline measurements) should be elevated in cases of Cushing syndrome. In cases of true endogenous Cushing syndrome, baseline UFC is usually at least two to three times higher than the upper limit of the reference interval. In normal individuals, baseline UFC excretion should be within the reference interval. Should a normal individual be stressed, psychologically or physiologically, and the baseline UFC is elevated, UFC on days 3 and 4 should be suppressed to less than 50% of the baseline level (e.g., "UFC suppression was achieved"). All subjects with true endogenous hypercortisolism should not suppress on day 3 or 4. If suppression of UFC excretion occurs on days 5 and 6 or on day 6, Cushing disease is diagnosed. However, not all cases of Cushing disease suppress on high-dose dexamethasone. Therefore failure to suppress on high-dose dexamethasone leaves three diagnostic possibilities: Cushing disease, adrenal adenoma (or, less commonly, adrenal carcinoma), and ectopic ACTH or CRH syndrome. Those patients taking phenytoin or phenobarbital, or both, may metabolize dexamethasone more rapidly than normal subjects and may not show appropriate suppression.

ACTH syndrome or primary adrenal pathology for hypercortisolism, in which ACTH is not suppressed by high doses of dexamethasone.

The classic (or "formal") low dose-high dose dexamethasone suppression test is detailed in Box 54-6. On high-dose dexamethasone, suppression will occur in about 60% of patients with Cushing disease. Thus, the high-dose stage may

BOX 54-7 Protocol for the High-Dose Overnight Dexamethasone Suppression Test

Rationale

The rationale for this test is similar to the rationale for the multiple high-dose dexamethasone suppression test.

Procedure

Dexamethasone 4 mg is given orally at 2300 and 2400 hours. Blood is drawn for determination of plasma cortisol at 0700 hours or 0800 hours the next morning, or 8 to 9 hours after dexamethasone is given.

Interpretation

Most patients with Cushing syndrome show suppression of baseline cortisol concentration of at least 50%. If suppression is not greater than 50%, the test should be repeated with 8 to 24 mg of dexamethasone.

allow identification of Cushing disease. However, failure of suppression on high-dose dexamethasone does not distinguish Cushing disease from the other causes of Cushing syndrome, and other diagnostic approaches must be pursued, such as IPS sampling.

Failure of cortisol suppression by dexamethasone has been observed in patients with (1) depression, (2) severe stress, (3) uncontrolled diabetes mellitus, (4) anorexia nervosa with estrogen administration; and (5) in subjects receiving medications (such as phenytoin) that induce the hepatic cytochrome P450 enzymes that metabolize dexamethasone.[325] If noncompliance or hypermetabolism of dexamethasone is a clinical consideration in patients who do not suppress their cortisol during the dexamethasone suppression test, dexamethasone can be measured in reference laboratories.

Mineralocorticoid Stimulation Tests

The renin-angiotensin-aldosterone system responds to electrolyte balance (and imbalance).[104] Sodium excretion and extracellular fluid volume are inversely correlated with plasma renin and aldosterone concentrations. The sodium (Na)-to-creatinine (Cr) ratio in a urine specimen is used as a marker for sodium volume status. As well, the fractional excretion of sodium (FENa) provides insights into the patient's sodium status. The equation for the fractional excretion of sodium is given below:

$$FENa = \frac{[U_{Na^+}][S_{Cr}]}{[S_{Na^+}][U_{Cr}]} \times 100$$

Percent sodium excreted is the unit reported. FENa is typically less than 1%. The FENa has been observed to exceed 1% with tubular disease or injury with sodium wasting. The calculation of the FENa is not valid when patients are treated with diuretics. Procedures for stimulating the renin-angiotensin system are based on volume depletion maneuvers, such as sodium restriction, upright posture, or diuretic administration.

BOX 54-8 Protocol for the Furosemide Stimulation Test

Rationale

Plasma renin activity (PRA) varies with the patient's state of hydration and sodium intake. Administration of furosemide, a potent diuretic, provides a stimulus to increase plasma renin secretion.

Procedure

Furosemide (Lasix; Hoechst-Roussel Pharmaceuticals, Somerville, NJ) 40 to 80 mg is given orally after an overnight fast. The subject is maintained in an upright posture (sitting, standing, or walking) throughout the test. Blood is drawn for determination of PRA before and 4 hours after furosemide administration.

Interpretation

Responses must be defined for the assay technique used. Patients with renin-dependent forms of hypertension (e.g., renovascular hypertension) show values that are approximately five times normal. Increased PRA following furosemide is seen in patients with high-renin essential hypertension, pheochromocytoma, and Bartter syndrome. Patients with hypertension from mineralocorticoid excess (e.g., primary hyperaldosteronism) usually display PRA below the lower limit of detection for the PRA assay. Patients with hyporeninemic hypoaldosteronism usually have low concentrations of plasma renin and low aldosterone concentrations.

In the furosemide stimulation test, oral or intravenous furosemide (40 to 80 mg) is administered, followed by 4 hours of upright posture (Box 54-8). This test does not require hospitalization or special diets, although it is recommended that the patient maintain a diet with a normal salt intake.[23] The typical response to this diuretic is a twofold to threefold rise in plasma renin. Another simple and convenient stimulation test consists of sodium restriction and upright posture. Dietary sodium is restricted to less than 20 mmol/d for 3 to 5 days; urine is collected for creatinine and sodium measurements until equilibrium with the new diet is established. Then, plasma renin activity is obtained after 2 hours of standing. A typical response is a twofold to threefold increase in plasma renin.

Mineralocorticoid Suppression Tests

Mineralocorticoid suppression tests have been designed that are based on salt loading. For example, (1) saline infusion, (2) oral salt loading, or (3) mineralocorticoid administration has been used to suppress the secretion of aldosterone by the adrenal gland. In healthy individuals, acute expansion of plasma volume with salt increases renal perfusion, suppresses renin release, and decreases aldosterone secretion.

The protocol for the saline suppression test is shown in Box 54-9. This test should not be performed in the setting of severe hypertension or heart failure. Administration of fludrocortisone, a synthetic mineralocorticoid, normally produces comparable suppression of aldosterone secretion (see

BOX 54-9 Protocol for the Saline Suppression Test

Rationale
Rapid volume expansion with intravenous saline should suppress plasma aldosterone in normal subjects, but not in patients with primary hyperaldosteronism.

Procedure
Care must be taken to ensure that the subject is not hypokalemic before beginning the test. The subject is awakened at 0600 hours and is kept in an upright posture for 2 hours. Blood is drawn for determination of plasma aldosterone at 0800 hours. The subject then assumes a supine position, and 2 L of isotonic saline 0.9 g/dL is infused over a 4 hour period. Blood is drawn for plasma aldosterone determination at noon.

Interpretation
Normal subjects show a plasma aldosterone concentration of 5 ng/dL (140 pmol/L) or less after saline infusion. Concentrations greater than 10 ng/dL are usually seen in patients with autonomously functioning aldosterone-secreting tumors.

BOX 54-10 Protocol for the Fludrocortisone Suppression Test

Rationale
Fludrocortisone, a potent mineralocorticoid, suppresses aldosterone production in normal subjects, but not in subjects with primary hyperaldosteronism.

Procedure
Hypokalemia must be corrected before starting this test, and serum potassium must be monitored during the test. Fludrocortisone 0.1 mg every 6 hours is given for 3 days. Plasma is collected for aldosterone determination after a standing position has been maintained for 2 hours (for baseline measurement) and at the end of fludrocortisone administration. Twenty-four hour urine collections for measurement of aldosterone are obtained 1 day before fludrocortisone administration is started and on day 3 of the test course.

Interpretation
Normal subjects show suppression of plasma aldosterone to less than 4 ng/dL (111 pmol/L); urine aldosterone is 20 µg/d or greater on day 3.

fludocortisone suppression test; Box 54-10). Fludrocortisone should be administered with caution in patients with hypokalemia and heart or renal failure. An alternate suppression test uses the ACE inhibitor captopril.[182] This test is recommended when risks from volume overload (e.g., the development of pulmonary edema or hypertension) preclude the use of other procedures. Captopril inhibits the conversion of angiotensin I to angiotensin II, removing the angiotensin II stimulus for aldosterone secretion.

Adrenal Androgen Stimulation Tests

The response of adrenal androgen secretion to ACTH stimulation is variable. Plasma DHEA and androstenedione are increased threefold to fourfold after 90 minutes of stimulation with ACTH (10 µg/m^2). DHEA-S, on the other hand, is increased by 30 to 50% with ACTH administration. ACTH stimulation studies are not considered useful in evaluating hypoandrogenic disorders.[246]

Adrenal Androgen Suppression Tests

Overnight suppression using dexamethasone produces small changes in adrenal androgen concentration compared with those of cortisol. Dexamethasone, 0.75 mg, administered at midnight for several days reliably suppresses adrenal androgen concentrations measured in blood. Tissue stores of these androgens may account in part for the delay in response.[201]

DISORDERS OF THE ADRENAL CORTEX

Thomas Addison first reported hypofunction of the adrenal cortex in 1855.[248] However, only over the past 65 years have many of the diseases associated with abnormal adrenal function been discovered and studied.[217] In general, diseases of this organ are classified as resulting from hypofunction or hyperfunction of the adrenal cortex.[321] Nonfunctional adrenal tumors are diagnosed histologically.

Although circulating concentrations of adrenal androgens decline with advancing age, it is unclear whether this simply reflects physiologic changes associated with aging, or if it is a pathologic condition that should be treated.[33] Most experts believe the former and do not prescribe adrenal androgens as "treatment" for aging.[209] Adrenal androgen deficiency does occur as part of primary adrenal failure, but it has no clear pathologic consequences.[4] Excess prenatal adrenal androgens have been known to produce ambiguous genitalia in females. Excess postnatal adrenal androgens can lead to precocious pseudopuberty in boys and hirsutism or virilization in girls. *Pseudopuberty* involves pubertal changes that result from autonomous gonadal or adrenal hypersecretion of sex steroids, independent of the CNS. In central precocious puberty, gonadotropins drive early sexual development.

Adrenal Insufficiency (Addison Disease)[156]

Adrenal insufficiency causing combined mineralocorticoid and glucocorticoid deficiency is a rare disorder with a prevalence of only 4 to 11 cases per 100,000.[80] If untreated, adrenal insufficiency can be fatal.[74] Cortisol deficiency is classified as (1) primary, (2) secondary, or (3) tertiary.[333]

Primary adrenal insufficiency, also known as Addison disease, results from progressive destruction or dysfunction of the adrenal glands by (1) an autoimmune process, (2) some systemic disorder, (3) an inborn error of metabolism (endogenous causes), or (4) by an exogenous cause such as infection (Table 54-8).[130] Worldwide, infectious disease is the most common cause of primary adrenal insufficiency and may include tuberculosis, fungal infection (histoplasmosis, cryptococcosis, North and South American blastomycosis,

TABLE 54-8 Causes of Primary Adrenal Insufficiency or Failure of Aldosterone Production

Endogenous Causes	
Autoimmune disease	Sporadic Autoimmune polyglandular syndrome type 1 (Addison's disease, candidiasis, hypoparathyroidism, and primary gonadal failure) Autoimmune polyglandular syndrome type 2 (Addison's disease, primary hypothyroidism, primary hypogonadism, diabetes, and pernicious anemia)
Inborn errors	Congenital adrenal hyperplasia Congenital adrenal hypoplasia (*DAX-1* mutation) Demyelinating disorders: adrenoleukodystrophies Childhood X-linked recessive adrenoleukodystrophy (Brown-Schilder disease) Neonatal autosomal recessive adrenoleukodystrophy X-linked recessive adrenomyeloneuropathy (sudanophilic leukodystrophy) Familial (isolated) glucocorticoid deficiency (degeneration of fasciculata-reticularis layers) Wolman disease (lysosomal acid lipase deficiency) Steroidogenic factor-1 (SF-1) mutations Mitochondrial forms of Addison disease (Kearns-Sayre syndrome) Smith-Lemli-Opitz syndrome (sterol delta-7-reductase mutations) ACTH resistance syndromes
Vascular disorders	Intra-adrenal hemorrhage (Waterhouse-Friderichsen syndrome): infection (caused by *Neisseria meningitidis, Pseudomonas aeruginosa, Haemophilus influenzae, Streptococcus pyogenes, Streptococcus pneumoniae*) or anticoagulants
Glandular infiltration	Neoplastic Leukemia, lymphoma, carcinoma of the lung, carcinoma of the breast Non-neoplastic Amyloid Hemochromatosis
Exogenous Causes	
Infection	Granulomatous disease Tuberculosis, sarcoidosis, histoplasmosis, cryptococcosis, blastomycosis (North and South American), sporotrichosis, and coccidiomycosis Other infections Cytomegalovirus, HIV
Drugs	Blockers of steroid synthesis: mitotane, aminoglutethimide, trilostane, ketoconazole, metyrapone Glucocorticoid receptor blockers: RU-486
Abdominal Irradiation	
Bilateral adrenalectomy	Intra-adrenal thrombosis: renal vein thrombosis in neonates, heparin-induced thrombocytopenia, the antiphospholipid syndrome
Causes of Deficient Mineralocorticoid Activity	
Failure of Aldosterone Production (Decreased Aldosterone)	
Hyperreninemia hypoaldosteronism (synthetic deficiency)	Primary adrenal insufficiency (see Table 54-10) Selective aldosterone deficiency Inborn errors (e.g., *CYP11B2* mutations) Drug-induced aldosterone suppression Heparin (direct inhibition of aldosterone secretion) Angiotensin-converting enzyme (ACE) inhibitors Angiotensin receptor blockers (ARBs) Hypoaldosteronism in critical illness/hypotension (e.g., selective zona glomerulosa injury)
Hyporeninemia hypoaldosteronism (deficient aldosterone stimulation)	Renin deficiency (e.g., diabetes, renal failure)

Continued

TABLE 54-8 Causes of Primary Adrenal Insufficiency or Failure of Aldosterone Production—cont'd

Causes of Deficient Mineralocorticoid Activity—cont'd	
Deficient Aldosterone Action (Resistance to Aldosterone; Elevated Aldosterone)	
Pseudohypoaldosteronism, type 1	Renal Multiple target organ defects Early childhood hyperkalemia

sporotrichosis, and coccidiomycosis), and cytomegalovirus infection. Syphilis can produce a syphilitic gumma (a fibrotic and granulomatous lesion) that destroys the adrenal gland. Human immunodeficiency virus (HIV) infection increases the risk of adrenalitis.[93] Autoimmune adrenalitis accounts for more than 70% of cases reported in the Western world, with adrenal autoantibodies measurable in more than 75% of cases.[193] The adrenal glands are atrophic, with loss of cortical cells but an intact medulla. Patients with autoimmune adrenalitis can also have pluriglandular autoimmune deficiency syndromes, as described in detail later.

The most common inborn steroidogenic defects involve the synthesis of cortisol with or without concurrent aldosterone deficiency, producing congenital adrenal hyperplasia.[230] Because such disorders commonly lead to excessive adrenal androgen overproduction, they are discussed in a later section concerning hyperfunction of the adrenal cortex, although such patients present a mixed picture of cortisol deficiency and possible aldosterone deficiency plus adrenal androgen overproduction.

Because the entire adrenal cortex is affected in primary adrenal insufficiency, all classes of adrenal steroids are deficient. The onset of clinical manifestations is usually gradual, and the degree and severity of symptoms depend on the extent of adrenal failure.[64] In early or mild expressions of primary adrenal insufficiency, hypofunction may not be evident unless the patient is under stress (e.g., following trauma or surgery). Complete glucocorticoid deficiency can manifest in a variety of ways, including fatigue, weakness, weight loss, gastrointestinal disturbance, and fasting hypoglycemia. Mineralocorticoid deficiency leads to dehydration with hypotension, acidosis, hyponatremia, and hyperkalemia. Excessive pituitary release of ACTH, unchecked by the negative feedback system, may cause hyperpigmentation of the skin and mucous membranes.[228]

Measurement of basal ACTH and cortisol concentrations along with ACTH stimulation testing (see Box 54-1) is recommended if primary adrenal insufficiency is suspected from the patient's clinical history and symptoms.[39] Basal plasma ACTH concentrations greater than 150 pg/mL, along with serum cortisol concentrations less than 5 μg/dL, are diagnostic of adrenal insufficiency (Figure 54-11). A subnormal cortisol response in the cosyntropin stimulation test supports the diagnosis of primary adrenal insufficiency (Figure 54-12). A normal cortisol response to cosyntropin stimulation establishes that the adrenal cortex is capable of releasing cortisol in a normal fashion and excludes primary adrenal failure. A

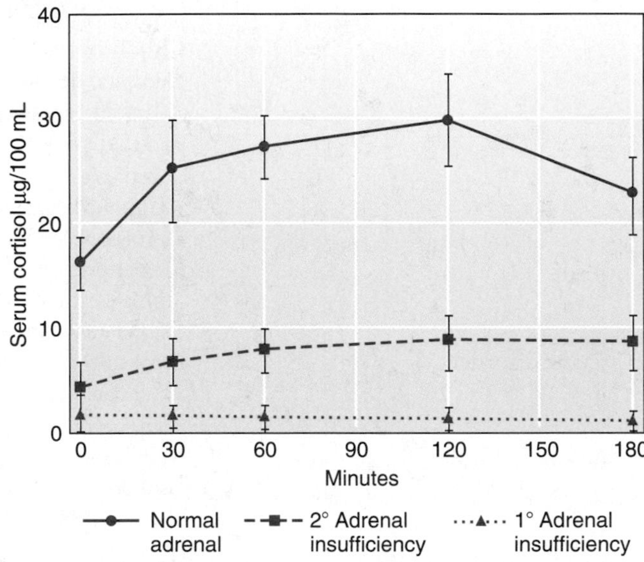

Figure 54-11 Serum cortisol response to 0.25 mg of cosyntropin (ACTH) in nine normal individuals (normal adrenal), eight patients with hypopituitarism (secondary adrenal insufficiency), and seven patients with Addison's disease (primary adrenal insufficiency).

subnormal response to cosyntropin stimulation suggests the diagnosis of primary, secondary, or tertiary adrenal failure. The clinical presentation usually assists in the differentiation of primary (hyperpigmentation and hypotension) from secondary or tertiary hypoadrenalism (other trophic hormone deficiencies may be present, such as growth hormone or thyroid-stimulating hormone, but hyperpigmentation and hyperkalemia are absent). If needed, a plasma ACTH concentration can help differentiate primary from secondary and tertiary hypoadrenalism.

It is important to note that both mineralocortioid and glucocorticoid deficiency may occur in cases of primary adrenal insufficiency. In contrast, when ACTH deficiency (secondary or tertiary) is the cause of adrenal hypofunction, mineralocorticoid secretion is essentially normal.[8] A rare cause of isolated glucocorticoid deficiency of adrenal origin is familial glucocorticoid deficiency. In this autosomal recessive disorder, resistance to the effects of ACTH is caused by mutations in *MCR2* or melanocortin 2 receptor accessory protein (MRAP), although some cases are currently unexplained.[54]

In secondary and tertiary adrenal insufficiency, inadequate cortisol production may be due to destructive processes in

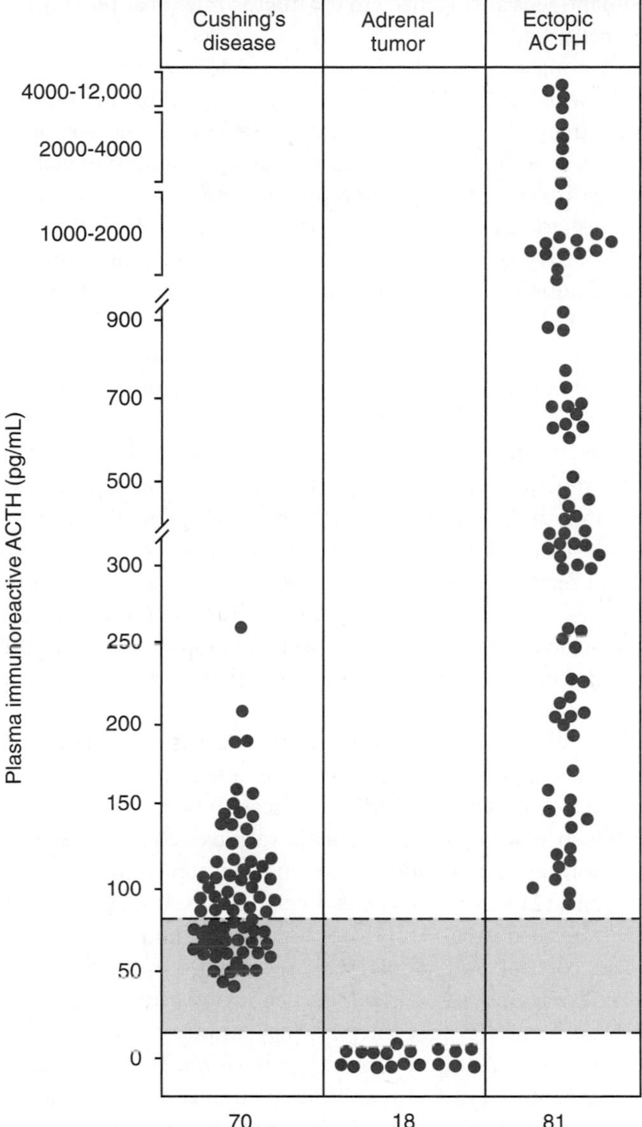

Figure 54-12 Basal plasma ACTH concentrations in patients with spontaneous Cushing's syndrome. *(From Scott AP. Pituitary adrenocorticotrophin and the melanocyte stimulating hormones. In: Parsons JA, ed. Peptide hormones. Baltimore: University Park Press, 1979.)*

TABLE 54-9 Causes of Central Glucocorticoid Deficiency

Hypothalamic causes of CRH deficiency	Destructive tumor Inflammation Status post infection Trauma (including surgery) Bleeding Irradiation Malformations (e.g., septo-optic dysplasia)
Disorders of the hypothalamic-pituitary portal system	Trauma Destruction via compression (e.g., tumor)
Pituitary causes of ACTH deficiency	Tumors (e.g., destructive adenoma, craniopharyngioma) Infiltrative disease (e.g., amyloidosis) Inflammation (e.g., autoimmunity: hypophysitis; granuloma) Status post infection Trauma (including surgery) Bleeding Irradiation Infarction (pituitary apoplexy, e.g., Sheehan syndrome) Metabolic (e.g., hemochromatosis) Malformations: transcription factor mutations (e.g., *Pit-1, PROP-1*)

the hypothalamus and/or pituitary that result in a decreased ability to secrete CRH (tertiary) or ACTH (secondary) (Table 54-9).[350] However, the most common cause of tertiary insufficiency is long-term pharmacologic administration of glucocorticoids that suppress CRH. This leads to a decrease in both ACTH release and cortisol secretion. Clinical features of secondary and tertiary adrenal insufficiency are similar to those of primary insufficiency, except that hyperpigmentation is not present and hypotension is less severe. Mineralocorticoid deficiency, hyperkalemia, and ACTH excess are not seen in secondary or tertiary adrenal insufficiency.

The cosyntropin stimulation test (see Box 54-1) may be used to demonstrate adrenal insufficiency in patients with secondary and tertiary adrenal insufficiency. When results of this test are abnormal, however, the cosyntropin stimulation test does not identify the cause of adrenal failure. Mild to moderate dysfunction of ACTH secretion may go undetected. Some patients with partial ACTH deficiency maintain sufficient ACTH to prevent adrenal atrophy, but are unable to augment ACTH secretion in response to stress or hypoglycemia. In these cases, pituitary ACTH reserve can be investigated with a metyrapone test (see Box 54-4) or an insulin-induced hypoglycemia test. Neither test, however, should be performed if primary adrenal insufficiency is suspected, because of the danger of precipitating Addisonian crisis. Subnormal responses to these tests suggest that pituitary ACTH release is inadequate, thus supporting a diagnosis of secondary or tertiary adrenal insufficiency.

ACTH and cortisol concentrations often are not useful for establishing the diagnosis of secondary adrenal insufficiency. Episodic secretion and circadian variation result in ACTH and cortisol concentrations that overlap between normal subjects and individuals with secondary or tertiary adrenal insufficiency. Elevated basal plasma ACTH in a patient with an abnormal response to acute ACTH stimulation suggests primary adrenal failure, whereas low ACTH and subnormal response to the cosyntropin stimulation test suggest a hypothalamic or pituitary disorder.

The multiple-day cosyntropin stimulation test is used to distinguish primary and central (i.e., secondary or tertiary) causes of adrenal insufficiency (see Box 54-2). It is particularly useful when patients have been receiving glucocorticoid therapy. In primary adrenal insufficiency, the damaged adrenal glands do not respond to exogenous cosyntropin administration even with several days of repeated cosyntropin stimulation. Patients with secondary or tertiary adrenal insufficiency usually have an inadequate or absent cortisol response at first because the adrenal glands have been unstimulated for some time and steroidogenesis requires the trophic priming of ACTH. Eventually, a delayed or staircase response is seen, indicating reactivation of the normal steroidogenic pathways, as the adrenal gland benefits from the trophic actions of ACTH. This test, however, is not used as frequently in this situation because of the availability of better and sensitive ACTH immunoassays that more accurately determine ACTH concentrations at baseline. In primary adrenal insufficiency, the ACTH concentration is disproportionately elevated compared with the decreased plasma cortisol concentration.

The CRH stimulation test (see Box 54-3) is used to differentiate tertiary from secondary adrenal insufficiency.[237] Those individuals with tertiary disease show an elevation in ACTH following CRH administration, whereas individuals with secondary disease show only minimal changes in ACTH concentration.

Although subnormal basal plasma concentrations of DHEA-S occur in primary, secondary, and tertiary forms of adrenal insufficiency, DHEA-S measurements are of little value in the diagnosis of adrenal insufficiency; low concentrations of adrenal androgens are normally observed in young children (before ages 7 to 9) and in the elderly. Patients with HIV infection have been shown to have reduced concentrations of DHEA-S.[200] DHEA-S concentrations are usually determined in the management of women with hirsutism or patients suspected of having adrenal tumors, or sometimes in the adrenogenital syndrome (e.g., congenital adrenal hyperplasia).[341]

Measurement of adrenal autoantibodies has been shown to be useful in evaluating patients suspected of adrenal insufficiency.[131] Antibodies against the adrenal cytoplasm or the 21 alpha-hydroxylase enzyme have been used in this regard and are diagnostic for autoimmune adrenal destruction in the setting of primary adrenal insufficiency.[279]

The first assay for adrenal autoantibodies utilized indirect immunofluorescence with human adrenal gland as substrate. Fluorescence of the cortex indicates the presence of adrenal cytoplasmic autoantibodies (ACAs) in the serum.[264] Usually all layers of the adrenal cortex fluoresce, whereas the medulla rarely fluoresces, because the adrenal cortical cytoplasmic autoantigens are localized to the microsomes of adrenal cortical cells.[41,72]

Among new-onset patients with Addison disease, 60 to 70% will express ACA. Studies in the 1990s established that target adrenal autoantigens were enzymes whose expression was limited to steroid-producing endocrine glands: 17-hydroxylase and 21-alpha-hydroxylase.[21,22,160,214] Autoantibodies to 21-alpha-hydroxylase (P450c21, CYP21) and 17-hydroxylase (P450c17, CYP17) has been detected by immunoprecipitation or enzyme-linked immunosorbent assay (ELISA) techniques. At least one vendor has developed commercial assays for the detection of autoantibodies to 21-alpha-hydroxylase. In many comparison studies, the ACA and 21-alpha-hydroxylase autoantibody immunoassays performed similarly in identifying humoral adrenal autoimmunity in patients with Addison disease. Once the diagnosis of Addison disease has been established, testing for adrenal antibodies can be undertaken to resolve the underlying cause. In the absence of adrenal autoantibodies, testing for the presence of very long-chain free fatty acids (VLCFAs) is now performed in search of adrenoleukodystrophy (ALD). In the absence of abnormalities of VLCFA, other diagnoses must be considered.[343]

In otherwise asymptomatic individuals, the detection of ACAs or of 21-alpha-hydroxylase autoantibodies predicts the development of Addison disease.[27] The evolution of Addison disease passes through various sequential stages: (1) normal to low aldosterone and elevated renin concentrations, (2) a deficient cortisol response to ACTH injection, (3) increased basal ACTH concentrations, and (4) deficient basal cortisol and aldosterone secretion.[29] Autoantibodies directed against the adrenal cortical cytoplasm or steroidogenic enzymes precede the initial appearance of clinical manifestations of Addison disease[28,55]; however, their predictive power is more evident in children than in adults.[30,31] Autoantibodies of higher titer are also more predictive of progression to clinical disease.[32,167] Approaches to the diagnosis of Addison disease are provided in Figures 54-13 and 54-14.

Hypoaldosteronism

Deficient aldosterone production occurs in conditions other than Addison disease (see Table 54-8).[323] Isolated aldosterone deficiency accompanied by normal cortisol production is seen in patients with (1) inadequate production of renin by the kidney, which leads to secondary aldosterone deficiency (hyporeninemic hypoaldosteronism); (2) inherited enzyme defects in aldosterone biosynthesis (e.g., CYP11B2 deficiency; CYP11B2 = P450 aldo); and (3) acquired forms of primary aldosterone deficiency (heparin therapy and post surgery).[324] The resulting metabolic changes are hyperkalemia and hyponatremia, often with hypochloremic acidosis. Mild or moderate volume depletion, often with postural or unprovoked hypotension, may also occur. Hyporeninemic hypoaldosteronism can be established by demonstrating failure of both plasma renin and aldosterone to increase in response to furosemide stimulation or upright posture (see Box 54-8). This

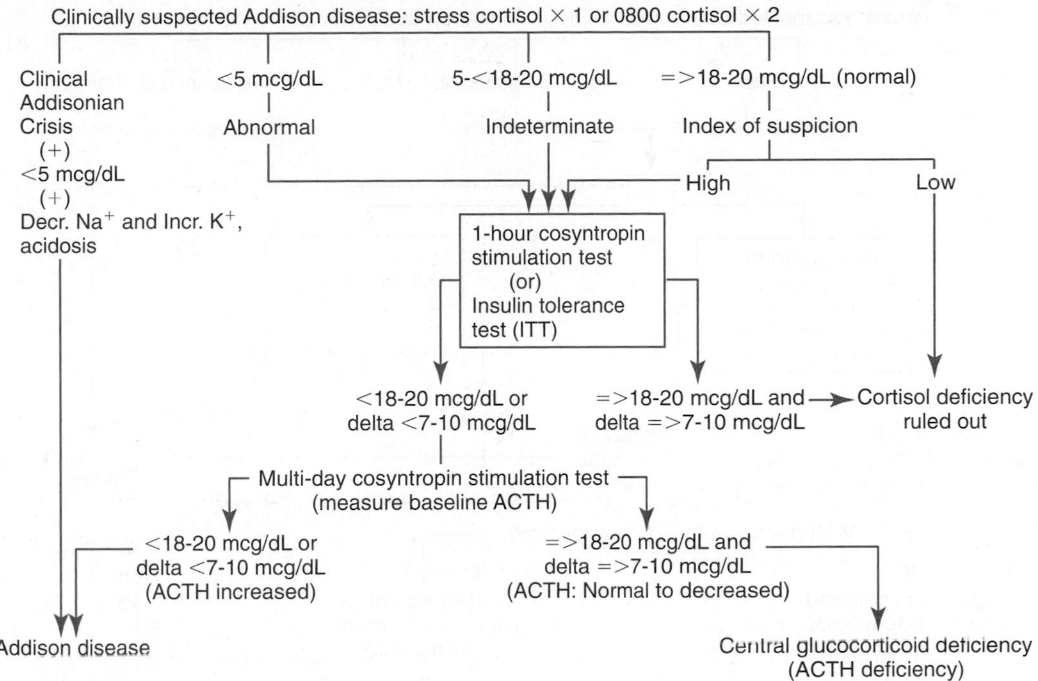

Figure 54-13 In cases of clinically suspected Addison disease, at the time of an Addisonian crisis with compatible hyponatremia, hyperkalemia, and acidosis, cortisol concentrations less than 5 µg/dL are diagnostic for Addison disease. Otherwise, further testing guided by the cortisol concentration is required (either the "stress" cortisol concentration or the average of two 0800 cortisol levels). Further testing can include the 1 hour cosyntropin stimulation test or an insulin tolerance test (ITT). If the "stress" or average AM cortisol is 18 to 20 µg/dL or greater, and the index of suspicion for Addison disease is low, no further testing is required. However, if the index of suspicion for Addison disease is high despite a "stress" or average AM cortisol of 18 to 20 µg/dL or greater, further testing should be considered. As depicted, results of the 1 hour cosyntropin stimulation test or the ITT determine whether cortisol deficiency is excluded or, alternatively, a multiple-day cosyntropin stimulation test is indicated. Failure to demonstrate increased cortisol production in response to multiple-day cosyntropin stimulation supports the diagnosis of Addison disease (primary adrenal insufficiency). Not shown, but of importance: an elevated ACTH in the setting of proven cortisol deficiency also supports the diagnosis of Addison disease. If cortisol rises in response to prolonged cosyntropin stimulation, ACTH deficiency is evident (e.g., central ACTH deficiency).

disorder is more common in older patients and in individuals with diabetes mellitus and nephropathy. These patients have a hyperkalemic acidosis with low renin and aldosterone concentrations and may have hypertension.

Patients with primary adrenal insufficiency almost always suffer from aldosterone deficiency, in addition to cortisol deficiency.[3] Most endocrinologists, however, do not ordinarily conduct tests to confirm aldosterone deficiency in such patients, because coexistent electrolyte abnormalities (e.g., hyperkalemia) and hypotension support the diagnosis of primary adrenal insufficiency in the setting of cortisol deficiency, an elevated ACTH, and hyperpigmentation.

Hyperfunction of the adrenal cortex produces clinical syndromes of mineralocorticoid excess, glucocorticoid excess, and androgen excess.

Glucocorticoid Excess (Cushing Syndrome)[56]

Endogenous Cushing syndrome is the result of autonomous excessive production of cortisol, leading to the classic symptoms that are characteristic of this disorder (Table 54-10). The clinical picture includes (1) truncal obesity, (2) moon face, (3) a "buffalo" hump on the upper back below the neck, (4) supraclavicular fat pads, (5) purple striae, (6) myopathy, (7) hypertension, (8) hirsutism, (9) hypokalemic alkalosis, (10) carbohydrate intolerance, (11) disturbed reproductive function, and (12) neuropsychiatric symptoms.[37] Exogenous Cushing syndrome is caused by excessive oral or parenteral glucocorticoid therapy.

Endogenous disorders that cause hypersecretion of cortisol and Cushing syndrome may be classified as ACTH dependent or ACTH independent (Table 54-11 and Figure

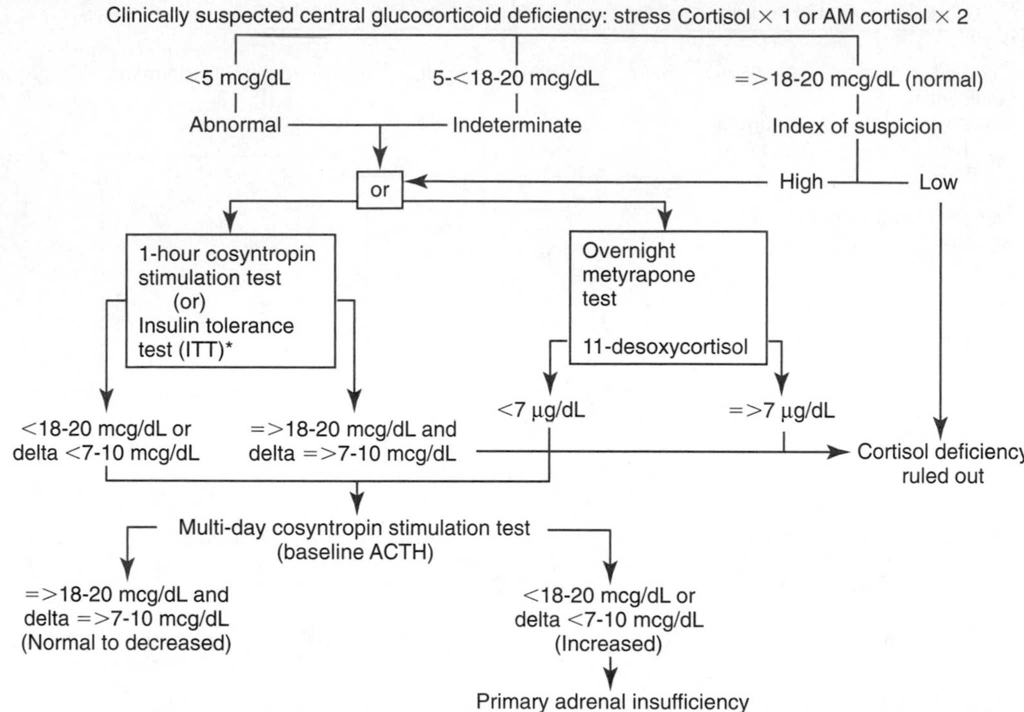

Figure 54-14 In cases of clinically suspected ACTH deficiency (e.g., central glucocorticoid deficiency), unless the 0800 cortisol is 18 to 20 µg/dL or greater, and the index of suspicion for ACTH deficiency is low, the 1 hour cosyntropin stimulation test, an insulin tolerance test (ITT), or an overnight metyrapone test is performed. (*Note:* Metyrapone is not currently available in the United States.) Normal responses to such tests rule out cortisol deficiency. An abnormal response to such testing triggers testing via the multiple-day cosyntropin stimulation test. If cortisol rises in response to prolonged cosyntropin stimulation, ACTH deficiency is evident. Failure to respond to prolonged cosyntropin stimulation indicates primary adrenal failure, and concurrent mineralocorticoid deficiency should be investigated.

TABLE 54-10 Incidence of Clinical Manifestations in Cushing Syndrome

Clinical Manifestation	Incidence, %
Obesity	90
Hypertension	85
Hyperglycemia and decreased glucose tolerance	80
Menstrual and sexual dysfunction	76
Hirsutism, acne, plethora	72
Striae, atrophic skin	67
Weakness, proximal myopathy	65
Osteoporosis	55
Easy bruisability	55
Psychiatric disturbances	50
Edema	46
Polyuria, polyphagia	16
Ocular changes and exophthalmos	8

TABLE 54-11 Causes of Spontaneous Cushing Syndrome

Etiology	Incidence, %
ACTH Dependent	
Cushing disease	68
Ectopic ACTH-secreting tumor	15
ACTH Independent	
Adenoma	5
Carcinoma	3
Nodular adrenal hyperplasia	9
Adrenocortical rest tumor	<1

54-15).[282] Cushing disease is the pituitary-dependent form of Cushing syndrome.[313A] In Cushing disease, hypersecretion of ACTH by a pituitary microadenoma is the primary defect that leads to bilateral adrenal hyperplasia and cortisol overproduction.[26] In the ectopic ACTH syndrome, nonendocrine tumors develop the ability to secrete ACTH, resulting in bilateral adrenal hyperplasia, unregulated cortisol secretion, and suppression of pituitary ACTH release.[229] Rarely, ectopic secretion of CRH occurs. In ectopic ACTH syndrome, the patient's clinical presentation is usually dominated by the presence of cancer, and the patient may not display classic clinical findings of Cushing syndrome such as centripetal obesity.

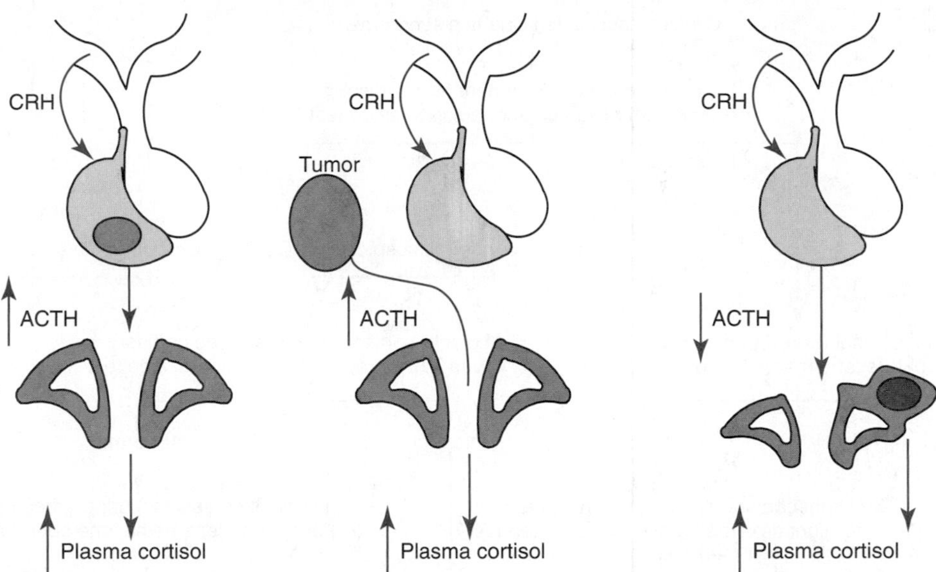

Figure 54-15 Endogenous Cushing syndrome can be classified as Cushing disease *(left panel)*, ectopic ACTH syndrome *(middle panel)*, or adrenal Cushing syndrome *(right panel)*. ACTH is elevated in cases of Cushing disease and ectopic ACTH syndrome. ACTH is suppressed in cases of adrenal Cushing syndrome.

Multiple endocrine neoplasia type 1 (MEN1) can cause Cushing syndrome through (1) hypersecretion of ACTH from a pituitary microadenoma, (2) an ectopic ACTH-secreting tumor of the pancreas, or (3) medullary thyroid carcinoma.[5] Cushing syndrome caused by primary adrenal disease suppresses both CRH and ACTH, resulting in atrophy of the nontumorous adrenal zona fasciculata and zona reticularis.[109]

Glucocorticoid-producing adenomas are usually unilateral, circumscribed, brown-yellow in color, and homogeneous in consistency, and weigh less than 30 g.[126] Histologically, the cells appear normal. Glucocorticoid-producing carcinomas are usually irregular in shape and histologically display (1) hemorrhage, (2) necrosis, (3) nuclear pleomorphism, (4) mitotic figures, and (5) capsular and blood vessel invasion. The clinical history is more acute (4 to 6 months) than in cases of functional adenoma. Adrenal carcinomas have been known to exceed 100 g and may be palpable, and metastases can produce hepatomegaly. Adrenal carcinoma also occur in the Li-Fraumeni syndrome (*p53* loss-of-function mutations),[318] along with sarcoma, brain tumor, leukemia, lymphoma, and early-onset breast cancer.

Less common than adenomas, adrenal hyperplasia can cause cortisol excess.[303] In bilateral micronodular hyperplasia (also called *primary nodular hyperplasia* or *adrenocortical dysplasia*), nodules of 0.1 to 0.3 cm diameter are observed that may be pigmented. The clinical outcome is similar to that of adrenal adenoma. Bilateral micronodular hyperplasia can be observed in the Carney complex, which includes (1) growth hormone–producing anterior pituitary adenoma, (2) Sertoli cell tumor, (3) atrial or ventricular myxoma, (4) mammary fibroadenoma, and (5) cutaneous myxoma.[36,304] Affected patients can display a spotty skin pigmentation pattern. In bilateral macronodular hyperplasia (also called *massive macronodular hyperplasia* or *macronodular adrenal dysplasia*), large nodules of 0.2 to larger than 4 cm diameter are evident. Adrenal weight can exceed 100 g. Because of aberrant expression of a receptor for gastric-inhibitory polypeptide on the surface of tumor cells, hypercortisolism may follow meals. Activating mutations of the G_s protein postreceptor signaling molecule have also been reported.

Screening Tests for Cushing Syndrome

Cushing syndrome is an uncommon disorder, but many of the usual signs and symptoms of this syndrome are seen in patients with normal adrenal function.[276] The initial diagnosis of Cushing syndrome, particularly in mild or early disease, rests on laboratory evidence of excessive and autonomous cortisol production.[251,294] Three simple screening tests are available for detecting Cushing syndrome. One test is the measurement of 24 hour urinary free cortisol. Under normal circumstances, less than 2% of secreted cortisol appears in urine as free cortisol. In general, a 24 hour urinary free cortisol concentration less than 50 µg/d excludes the diagnosis of Cushing syndrome (Figure 54-16). Diagnostic accuracy is greater than 90% when the test is properly performed.[60] An elevated rate of excretion documents overproduction of cortisol. However, (1) improper timing of the urine specimen (e.g., collection over more than 24 hours), (2) concomitant use of a diuretic, (3) high salt intake, (4) depression, and (5) stress have been observed to cause false-positive (abnormal) test results. Any single test that exhibits cortisol excess should not, in itself, be used to definitively diagnose Cushing syndrome, so that the patient will not

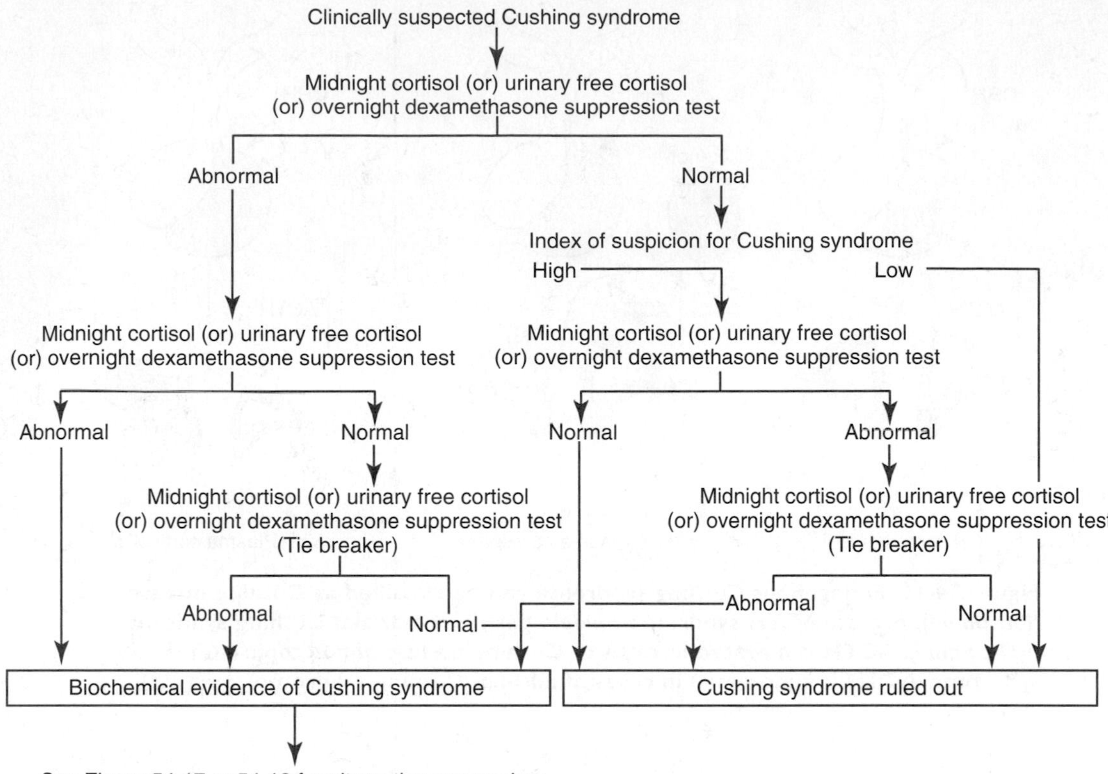

Figure 54-16 The first challenge in diagnosing Cushing syndrome is establishing whether hypercortisolism truly exists. Three screening tests are commonly applied: the overnight dexamethasone suppression test, measurement of the 24 hour urinary free cortisol excretion, and a midnight cortisol measurement (plasma or salivary cortisol). Hypercortisolism is present when two out of two, or two out of three, of any combination of these tests are abnormal.

have to undergo highly invasive therapy (e.g., transsphenoidal neurosurgery for a suspected pituitary adenoma) without proper evaluation.[249]

Another reliable and convenient screening test for Cushing syndrome is the overnight low-dose dexamethasone suppression test, wherein 1 mg of dexamethasone is taken orally between 2200 and 2400 (see Box 54-5). Cortisol concentrations at 0800 suppressed to below 5 μg/dL (<140 nmol/L) are normal and make the diagnosis of Cushing syndrome less likely. A cortisol concentration less than 2 μg/dL essentially rules out Cushing syndrome. Cortisol values greater than 10 μg/dL significantly favor the diagnosis of hypercortisolism and require further evaluation.

A multiple low-dose test may also be used (see Box 54-6 regarding low-dose dexamethasone suppression). Following low-dose dexamethasone (0.5 mg every 6 hours for 48 hours), plasma cortisol is usually suppressed to less than 2.2 μg/dL and urine free cortisol is suppressed to less than 25 μg/d. Diagnostic accuracy of 90% has been achieved with the simultaneous measurement of cortisol and dexamethasone (with assurance that dexamethasone was taken and taken in proper dose), although this approach is rarely used. Incorrect dosing and alterations in the clearance of dexamethasone are detected by measuring dexamethasone; thus both false-negative and false-positive suppression test results can be identified.

Examination of the circadian rhythm of cortisol secretion has been used in the past to screen for Cushing syndrome, although this is considerably less helpful than measurement of urinary cortisol, measurement of the morning cortisol concentration following dexamethasone, or cortisol measurements taken at 2400 (serum or salivary). Elevations in the night cortisol (e.g., concentrations >9 μg/dL) suggest loss of diurnal variation. The later in the night that cortisol can be measured, the more helpful the test will be. Some patients with Cushing syndrome do not exhibit loss of diurnal variation even with elevations in both morning and night and cortisol concentrations. Therefore loss of diurnal variation is not a consistent finding in Cushing syndrome. In general, measuring cortisol at 0800 as a screening test for Cushing syndrome is not recommended. If a single cortisol measurement is to be taken, this should be done near 2400.[227] Salivary cortisol can also be measured at 2400. Because of the ease of obtaining saliva, some endocrinologists favor this screening approach. However, analysis in a reference laboratory is usually required because salivary cortisol concentration is much lower than plasma cortisol concentration.

Differential Diagnosis of Cushing Syndrome

When findings are abnormal, the screening tests discussed support the diagnosis of endogenous Cushing syndrome by revealing hypercortisolism. More definitive testing should then be performed to determine the source of the overproduction of cortisol (Table 54-12 and Figures 54-17 and 54-18). Plasma ACTH concentrations are low in patients with adrenal tumor (<10 pg/mL) and are normal or moderately elevated in patients with Cushing disease (generally >50 pg/mL). Plasma concentrations of ACTH are very often markedly elevated in patients with nonendocrine ACTH-secreting tumors (ectopic ACTH syndrome), because the tumor source of the ACTH does not respond to negative feedback from cortisol. On the other hand, we can consider the ACTH-secreting pituitary adenoma of Cushing disease as having an elevated set point for negative feedback; if the cortisol (or other glucocorticoid) concentration is elevated high enough, some measure of negative feedback will occur (e.g., 60% of patients with Cushing disease achieve ACTH and urinary free cortisol suppression when treated with high-dose dexamethasone). Plasma ACTH concentrations greater than 300 pg/mL are usually suggestive of a nonendocrine ACTH-secreting tumor (ectopic ACTH syndrome).

High-dose dexamethasone suppression testing (overnight high dose or multiple-day high dose; see Boxes 54-6 and 54-7) is useful in differentiating Cushing syndrome caused by adrenal tumor and nonendocrine ACTH-secreting tumor from pituitary Cushing disease.

Some patients with Cushing disease may fail to suppress cortisol (plasma or urinary) on high-dose dexamethasone, as would be expected in cases of Cushing disease. Such test results can be assessed by administering 1.0 mg (low dose) or 8 mg (high dose) of dexamethasone at midnight (overnight dexamethasone suppression test). Serum is collected at 0800 hours for the measurement of cortisol. In the overnight dexamethasone suppression test, 1 mg of dexamethasone should not suppress cortisol in any form of Cushing syndrome. In patients with adrenal tumor and, with a few exceptions, in those patients with nonendocrine ACTH-secreting tumor, suppression does not occur after the high-dose 8 mg dexamethasone administration. Furthermore, with high-dose dexamethasone testing, less than 10% of patients with Cushing disease fail to show some degree of suppression, although most patients show only 50 to 60% suppression. Failure to suppress in response to high-dose dexamethasone has occurred in patients with accelerated clearance of dexamethasone in response to hepatic cytochrome P450–inducing drugs, such as phenytoin and rifampicin. In these patients, measurements of plasma dexamethasone can be useful in gauging the effective blood concentration.

The CRH stimulation test (see Box 54-3) produces exaggerated ACTH or cortisol response, or both, in about 90% of patients with Cushing disease. Usually plasma cortisol increases by 20% and plasma ACTH increases by 50% following CRH (1.0 µg/kg). Poor responses occur in patients with adrenal tumor and in most patients with nonendocrine ACTH-secreting tumor (usually those having elevated basal concentrations of plasma ACTH). Patients with depression and anorexia nervosa usually do not exhibit an exaggerated ACTH response to CRH injection.

If the cause of Cushing syndrome is uncertain, measurement of ACTH from inferior petrosal venous sinus specimens before and after CRH stimulation can be helpful.[237] When ACTH concentrations in inferior petrosal venous sinus specimens are similar to those of simultaneously obtained peripheral vein plasma specimens (e.g., from the inferior vena cava), the diagnosis of a nonpituitary source of ACTH is evident. In virtually all patients with ectopic production of ACTH, the ratio of ACTH concentrations between the inferior petrosal venous sinus and a peripheral venous specimen is less than 1.4 : 1. In contrast, patients with Cushing disease have a ratio greater than 2.0, and an average ratio near 15.[180] Inferior petrosal venous sinus sampling is not useful in delineating the side of the lesion because venous drainage can cross over.[305,353] Table 54-13 provides examples of ACTH

TABLE 54-12 Differentiating the Causes of Cushing Syndrome

	Cushing Disease	Ectopic ACTH Syndrome	Adrenal Tumor
Biochemical Evaluation			
ACTH	Nl, Incr	Nl, Incr	Decr
UFC response to high-dose dexamethasone	Usually declines by >50%	Does not decline by >50%	Does not decline by 50%
Basal and post-CRH ACTH levels	IPS > peripheral	IPS = peripheral	Not performed
Radiologic Evaluation			
CT or MRI			
Pituitary	Abn	Nl	Nl
Adrenal	Nl	Nl	Abn
Other location	Nl	Abn	Nl

Abn, Abnormal; *CT,* computed tomography; *decr,* decreased; *incr,* increased; *IPS,* inferior petrosal sinus; *MRI,* magnetic resonance imaging; *Nl,* normal.

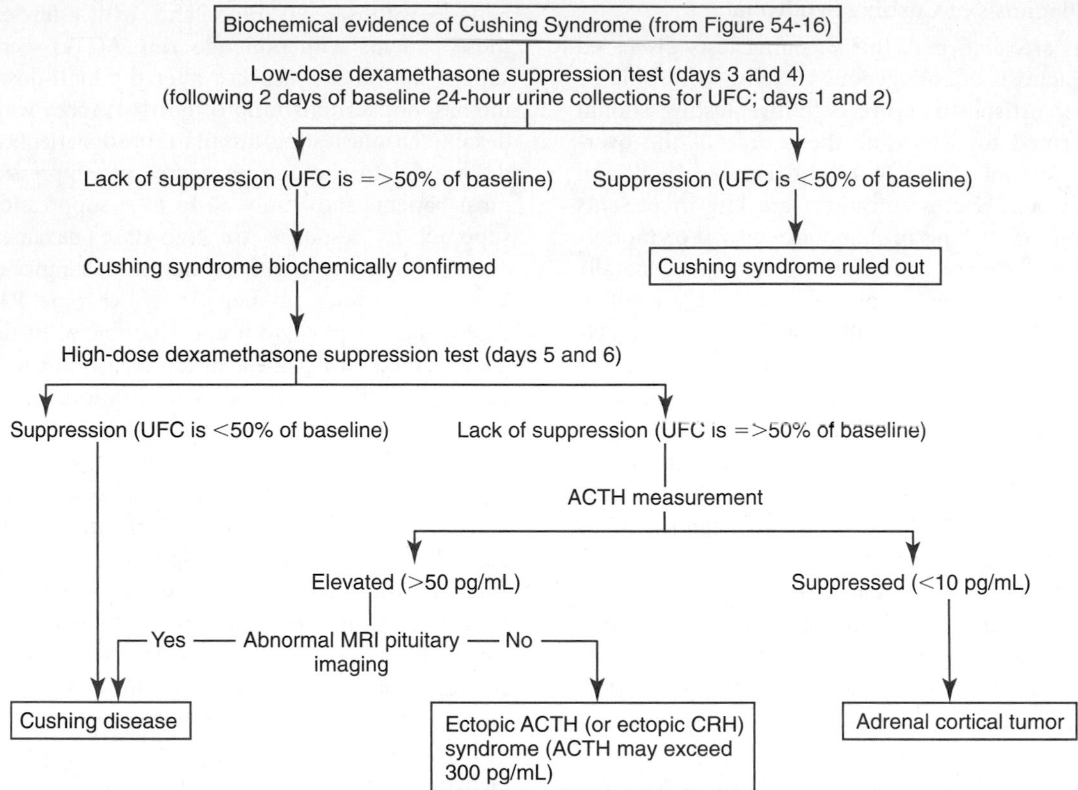

Figure 54-17 Once the diagnosis of hypercortisolism is established, low-dose/high-dose dexamethasone suppression testing can be carried out. Suppression of urinary free cortisol (UFC) on low-dose dexamethasone excludes cortisol excess. Suppression on high-dose dexamethasone establishes the diagnosis of Cushing disease, but not all patients with Cushing disease are suppressed on high-dose dexamethasone. Lack of suppression on high-dose dexamethasone triggers the measurement of ACTH. Suppressed ACTH establishes the diagnosis of adrenal Cushing syndrome (e.g., a cortisol-secreting adrenal cortical tumor). If ACTH is elevated, the pituitary is studied radiologically (and via inferior petrosal venous sinus sampling) to distinguish Cushing disease from ectopic ACTH (or ectopic CRH) syndrome. ACTH levels are usually higher in ectopic ACTH syndrome than in Cushing disease.

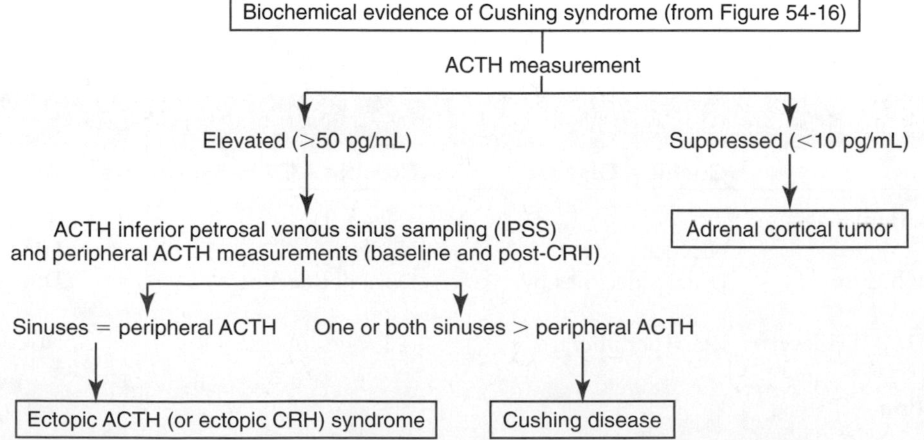

Figure 54-18 In an alternative diagnostic approach, once hypercortisolism is confirmed, ACTH is measured. A suppressed ACTH establishes the diagnosis of adrenal Cushing syndrome (i.e., a cortisol-secreting adrenal cortical tumor). If ACTH is elevated, the pituitary is examined via inferior petrosal venous sinus sampling (and MRI scanning) to resolve Cushing disease versus ectopic ACTH syndrome.

TABLE 54-13 An Example of Inferior Petrosal Venous Sinus Sampling Testing in an Individual With Cushing Disease

Time	ACTH, pg/mL, Peripheral	ACTH, pg/mL, IPSS-R*	ACTH, pg/mL, IPSS-L†	ACTH Ratio: IPSS-R/ Peripheral	ACTH Ratio: IPSS-L/ Peripheral	ACTH Ratio: IPSS-R/ IPSS-L	Cortisol, μg/dL
−15	15	170	13	11.3	0.87	13.1	10
0	20	285	18	14.2	0.90	15.8	8.8
+3	21	836	48	39.8	2.3	17.4	8.3
+5	40	729	78	18.2	1.95	9.3	7.5
+10	45	585	56	13.0	1.24	10.4	12.6
+15	70	747	81	10.7	1.16	9.2	18.8
+30	94	797	105	8.5	1.12	7.6	26.3
+60	132	784	221	5.9	1.67	3.5	30.8

**IPSS-R,* Right inferior petrosal sinus sample.
†*IPSS-L,* Left inferior petrosal sinus sample.

concentrations from IPS testing in a patient proven to have Cushing disease.

Adrenal androgens and plasma DHEA-S are measured in the differential diagnosis of hirsutism without Cushing syndrome.[92] In patients with Cushing syndrome, plasma DHEA-S concentrations are usually normal or moderately elevated (plasma DHEA-S ≈5 μg/mL). Patients with an adrenal adenoma usually have low age-adjusted concentrations of DHEA-S. The concentrations for plasma DHEA-S in patients with nonendocrine ACTH-secreting tumors range from normal to elevated. In patients with congenital adrenal hyperplasia (CAH), adrenal androgens are suppressed normally with administration of 0.75 mg of dexamethasone for 2 to 3 weeks, but suppression does not occur in patients with adrenal tumors and nonendocrine ACTH-secreting tumors.

CRH stimulation of ACTH after dexamethasone suppression has been used for the detection of hypercortisolism. The concept is that a normal individual were exposed to dexamethasone, would secrete reduced amounts of ACTH in response to CRH compared with a patient with Cushing syndrome. In a 2007 paper it was reported that a post-CRH ACTH concentration of 28 pg/mL or greater yielded clinical sensitivity of 95% and specificity of 97% for the recognition of Cushing syndrome, and a 15 minute cortisol of 2.6 μg/dL or greater was 90% sensitive and 90% specific.[81] Such combined testing (i.e., dexamethasone suppressed, post-CRH ACTH measurements) is being used in a variety of psychiatric evaluations.[289]

In addition to suppression and stimulation testing, methods of tumor localization should be used to document the cause of Cushing syndrome. Computed tomography (CT) of the adrenal glands has been helpful in localizing adrenal tumors, macronodular hyperplasia, and bilateral hyperplasia of the adrenal glands.[106] CT in combination with magnetic resonance imaging (MRI) of the pituitary gland can help to detect pituitary microadenomas.[273] However as mentioned elsewhere, anatomic abnormalities are not always related to functional abnormalities. For this reason, when an adrenal source of excess cortisol is suggested by CT scanning or MRI, it is prudent that the patient undergo venography with measurement of cortisol in each adrenal vein. In the case of a cortisol-secreting adrenal adenoma, the cortisol should be significantly higher (e.g., 50% higher) in one adrenal vein compared with the other adrenal vein. In the case of bilateral hyperplasia causing hypercortisolism, no significant difference (<50%) between sides should be noted. The search for ectopic sources of ACTH can require conventional radiography, ultrasonography, and CT scanning or MRI for the detection of suspected neoplasms.

Especially challenging are cases of episodic Cushing syndrome, wherein hypercortisolism is not always present. Some rare cortisol-secreting adrenal tumors have been reported that express incretin receptors.[25] In these cases, hypercortisolism occurs only with meals.

Conditions That Mimic Cushing Syndrome

Alcohol abuse has been known to induce a "pseudo-Cushing syndrome" that mimics the clinical and biochemical features of the actual disease. The abnormalities are all reversible when alcohol abuse by the patient is stopped. The clinician therefore must use considerable judgment in detecting the cause of Cushing syndrome before therapy is initiated.[85,332] HIV, anorexia nervosa, and depression are associated with elevated serum cortisol concentrations, and patients with these disorders may have abnormal low-dose, overnight dexamethasone suppression tests (morning cortisol ≥5 μg/dL). Cortisol measurements at 2400 may help exclude Cushing syndrome in these circumstances.[245] However, the clinical features of patients with HIV and anorexia nervosa are not typical of patients with Cushing syndrome. Measurement of urinary free cortisol and plasma cortisol with the dexamethasone suppression test improves the predictive value in the diagnosis of both Cushing syndrome and depression.[199] In patients with depression, it is best to repeat testing after the depression has been treated.

Obese patients have also presented with clinical features that mimic true Cushing syndrome.[19] Truncal obesity,

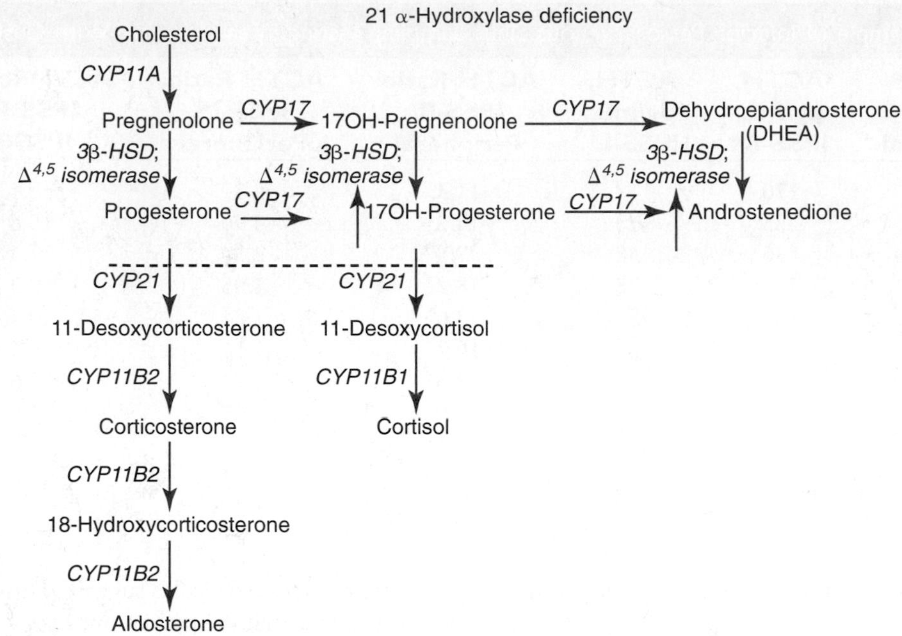

Figure 54-19 In 21 alpha-hydroxylase deficiency (CYP21; *dashed line*), cortisol deficiency and possibly aldosterone deficiency are present. Elevations in 17-hydroxyprogesterone and androstenedione are observed. The normal major pathway of cortisol synthesis is noted by the *bold arrows*.

striae, and excretion of elevated concentrations of 17-hydroxycorticosteroids are features of Cushing syndrome that occur in normal, obese subjects. Urinary free cortisol, however, is normal in the obese individual and can effectively differentiate normal subjects from those with true Cushing syndrome.[255] Likewise, 48 hours of low-dose dexamethasone (0.5 mg orally every 6 hours) should suppress urinary free cortisol excretion by more than 50% in obese subjects.

Congenital Adrenal Hyperplasia

Congenital adrenal hyperplasia (CAH) is the most common cause of adrenocortical insufficiency in newborns.[337] However, CAH is discussed under adrenal hormone overproduction syndromes because CAH commonly leads to overproduction of adrenal androgens. Thus, as noted previously, CAH presents a mixed picture of cortisol deficiency (hypofunction) and adrenal androgen overproduction (hyperfunction).

CAH results from loss-of-function mutations in specific adrenocortical enzymes that are responsible for the synthesis of cortisol.[10] These disorders are inherited as autosomal recessive traits. Rarely, traumatic adrenal hemorrhage or adrenal hemorrhage from sepsis causes adrenal failure in newborns. Six enzymes are necessary for the conversion of cholesterol into cortisol: CYP11A (a 20,22-desmolase; sometimes called a 20 alpha-hydroxylase), CYP17 (a 17-hydroxylase), 3 beta-hydroxysteroid dehydrogenase, delta(4)-5-isomerase, CYP21 (a 21-alpha-hydroxylase), and CYP11B1 (an 11-beta-hydroxylase).

With insufficient cortisol production, ACTH concentrations increase and anatomically stimulate the adrenal hyperplasia in utero for which CAH is named.[102,223,224]

21-Alpha-hydroxylase deficiency (CYP21 deficiency; Figure 54-19) and 11-beta-hydroxylase deficiency (CYP11B1 deficiency); are the two most common causes of CAH (Figure 54-20). A total of 95% of CAH cases result from 21-alpha-hydroxylase deficiency, and 11-beta-hydroxylase deficiency accounts for most of the remaining CAH cases. Other causes of CAH are rare. The incidence of 21-alpha-hydroxylase CAH in Western societies varies from 1 in 5000 to 15,000 live births.[1]

Screening for 21-alpha-hydroxylase–deficient and 11-beta-hydroxylase–deficient CAH in newborns by measuring 17-alpha-hydroxyprogesterone (17-OHP) is standard practice in the United States and many other countries.[123,299,300,320] The application of methods based on tandem mass spectrometry for steroid analysis may decrease false-positive 17-alpha-hydroxyprogesterone CAH screens.[163,192]

The metabolic block in cortisol biosynthesis leads to an accumulation of precursors including adrenal androgens.[203] Therefore, measurements of the precursor steroids in blood are useful for identifying the specific enzyme defect and for monitoring response to cortisol replacement therapy. A partial block may cause marked or subtle clinical manifestations, whereas a complete enzyme block can be incompatible with life. The closer the enzyme block is to the final cortisol product, the less life threatening are the symptoms.

Because CAH produces elevations of adrenal androgens (DHEA and androstenedione) in utero, virilization of the external genitalia of the female fetus occurs, producing sexual ambiguity (ambiguous genitalia). Only rarely does CAH lead to inadequate male sexual development (see 3-beta-hydroxysteroid reductase deficiency, later).

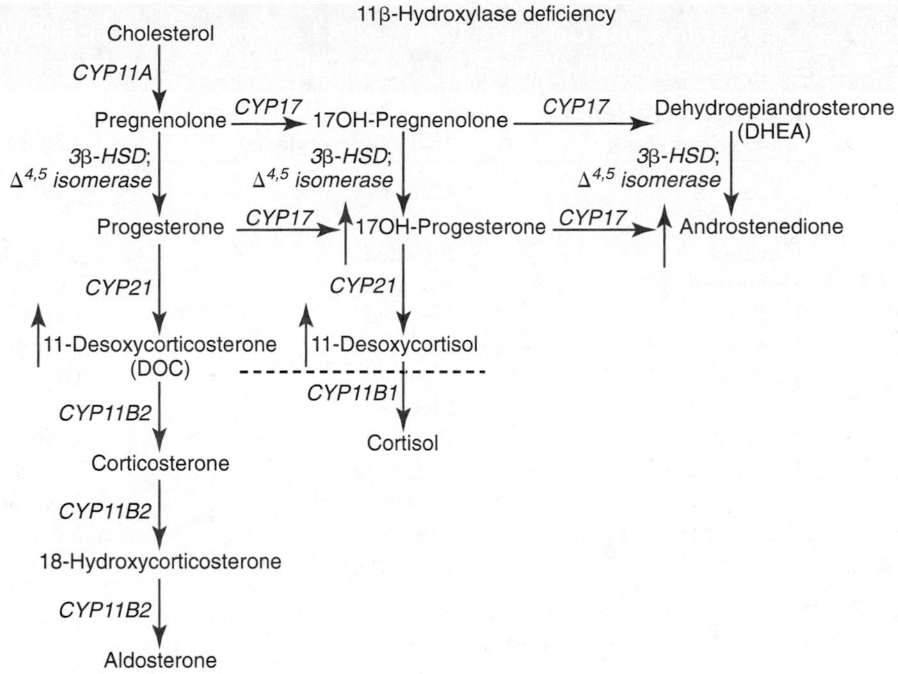

Figure 54-20 In 11 beta-hydroxylase deficiency (CYP11B1) *(dashed line)*, cortisol production is deficient. Elevations in 11-desoxycortisol, 17-hydroxyprogesterone, androstenedione, and 11-desoxycorticosterone concentrations are observed. The normal major pathway of cortisol synthesis is noted by the *bold arrows*.

Cortisol deficiency in affected individuals leads to (1) malaise, (2) failure to thrive, (3) hypoglycemia, and (4) vascular instability. In approximately one half of infants afflicted with 21-alpha-hydroxylase–deficient CAH, in addition to inadequate cortisol production, insufficient aldosterone production can cause (1) hyponatremia, (2) hyperkalemia, (3) acidosis, (4) dehydration, and (5) hypotension. In its most severe form, this type of "salt-losing" 21-alpha-hydroxylase–deficient CAH clinically presents at 10 to 14 days of age with Addisonian crisis. Untreated, mortality is very high in salt-losing 21-alpha-hydroxylase deficiency. The non–salt-losing form of this disease is customarily referred to as *simple virilizing* 21 alpha-hydroxylase–deficient CAH.

Before newborn screening for CAH with 17-alpha-hydroxyprogesterone measurements was available, the diagnosis of CAH was more common in girls than in boys.[247] The lower number of males diagnosed with CAH appeared to be the result of deaths of undiagnosed males afflicted with salt-losing CAH. The cause of death could have been erroneously ascribed to sepsis or idiopathic dehydration and not to Addisonian crisis. Presently, with newborn CAH screening, the male and female incidences of CAH are approximately equal, which is characteristic of an autosomal recessive condition.

In 21-alpha-hydroxylase deficiency and 11-beta-hydroxylase deficiency, the excess of ACTH and the metabolic block in cortisol biosynthesis result in overproduction of the adrenal androgens DHEA, DHEA-S, and androstenedione.[202] In females, overproduction of the adrenal androgens induces virilization of the external genitalia in utero, producing ambiguous genitalia [intersex or a disorder of sexual development (DSD)]. Virilization in females varies from mild fusion of the labia, to marked labial fusion with clitoromegaly, to complete masculinization with apparent male external genitalia. (*Note:* Such newborns can be incorrectly categorized as males with bilaterally undescended testes.) Untreated, postnatal females who survive will continue to virilize. Because salt-losing 21-alpha-hydroxylase deficiency is a more severe expression of the inborn error than is non–salt-losing 21-alpha-hydroxylase deficiency, the salt-losing form of CAH is associated with more severe degrees of virilization in females.

In males, adrenal androgen overproduction produces precocious pseudopuberty and some degree of hyperpigmentation of the male external genitalia. Untreated, postnatal males will experience early-onset puberty with advanced secondary sex characteristics, and, despite an early acceleration in their growth rate and tall stature, they may ultimately suffer from short stature because of premature closure of their epiphyses.[129] The more profound the defect in cortisol biosynthesis, the greater is the degree of precocious pseudopuberty in males. True precocious puberty is driven by the pituitary gonadotropins luteinizing hormone (LH) and follicle-stimulating hormone (FSH), as evidenced in testicular enlargement. In contrast, CAH-induced pseudopuberty does not produce testicular enlargement until true puberty occurs (which likely will be early because of the boys' advanced biological age). If adrenal rests are adherent to the testes, they can enlarge with untreated or undertreated CAH (a *rest* is a

TABLE 54-14 Comparisons of 21-Hydroxylase Deficiency Congenital Adrenal Hyperplasia, 11 Beta-Hydroxylase Deficiency Congenital Adrenal Hyperplasia, and 17 Alpha-Hydroxylase Deficiency Congenital Adrenal Hyperplasia

	Enzyme Deficiency 21-Hydroxylase	11β-Hydroxylase	17α-Hydroxylase
Gene	*CYP21*	*CYP11B1*	*CYP17*
Concentrations			
17-OHP	Elevated	Elevated	Depressed
DOC	Depressed	Elevated	Elevated
11-Desoxy-cortisol	Depressed	Elevated	Depressed
Cortisol*	Depressed	Depressed	Depressed
17-KGS	Elevated	Elevated	Depressed
17-OHCS	Depressed	Elevated	Depressed
17-KS	Elevated	Elevated	Depressed
Ambiguous genitalia	In females	In females	In males
Precocious puberty	In boys	In boys	None
Salt loss	Present in ≈¾ of patients	None	None
Hypertension	None	Late childhood/adolescence	Late childhood/adolescence

*In mild forms of CAH, cortisol may be low-normal from a compensatory elevation in ACTH.
17-KGS, 17-Ketogenic steroids; *17-KS,* 17-ketosteroids; *17-OHCS,* 17-hydroxycorticosteroids.

group of cells that has become displaced and lies embedded in another tissue).

In summary, females with 21-alpha-hydroxylase deficiency CAH can present with ambiguous genitalia and postnatal virilization, and may display neonatal salt-losing Addisonian crisis. Males present with precocious pseudopuberty during infancy or childhood, or present in the neonatal period with salt-losing crisis.

In the case of 11-beta-hydroxylase deficiency CAH from *CYP11B1* mutations, mineralocorticoid deficiency does not occur.[145] This is expected because the conversion of DOC to corticosterone in the zona glomerulosa is predominantly catalyzed by CYP11B2 (aldosterone synthase, P450 aldo) which is not affected in 11-beta-hydroxylase (CYP11B1) deficiency CAH. Also, elevated ACTH may have some effect in stimulating DOC production, and DOC is reported to be elevated in CYP11B1 11-beta-hydroxylase deficiency CAH.[231] Because 11-beta-hydroxylase activity of CYP11B2 is normal in CYP11B1 11-beta-hydroxylase deficiency CAH, DOC may be elevated by the small amount of 11-beta-hydroxylase activity of CYP11B1 that is normally present in the zona glomerulosa.

Whereas girls with CYP11B1 11-beta-hydroxylase deficiency present with ambiguous genitalia and boys display precocious pseudopuberty, salt loss does not occur in CYP11B1 11-beta-hydroxylase deficiency. Thus, electrolyte disturbances and acidosis do not occur, nor does Addisonian crisis develop, in the newborn period or later. However, later in childhood, hypertension, with or without hypokalemia, can develop. The incidence of CYP11B1 11-beta hydroxylase CAH is approximately 1 in 100,000.

The diagnosis of 21-alpha-hydroxylase deficiency and CYP-11B1 11-beta-hydroxylase deficiency is dependent on finding elevated concentrations of 17-OHP in plasma or serum (see Figures 54-19 and 54-20). These two conditions are differentiated by several findings: patients with CYP-11B1 11-beta-hydroxylase deficiency do not exhibit hypotension and may develop hypokalemic hypertension during childhood (Table 54-14). Biochemically, 17-OHCS are elevated in CYP11B1 11-beta-hydroxylase deficiency (i.e., 11-desoxycortisol is elevated and contributes to 17-OHCS), whereas 17-OHCS are low in 21-hydroxylase deficiency (both 11-desoxycortisol and cortisol are low). 11-Desoxycortisol and its urinary metabolite tetrahydrodesoxycortisol (THS) will be elevated in CYP-11B1 11-beta-hydroxylase deficiency, as will the ratio of plasma 11-desoxycortisol to plasma cortisol and the ratio of their urinary metabolites, THS to tetrahydrocortisol (THF). In 21-alpha-hydroxylase deficiency the synthesis of both 11-desoxyocortisol and cortisol is impaired and the ratio of urinary THS to THF is not elevated.

Once a proband child in a family is diagnosed with CAH, fetal DNA testing in subsequent pregnancies allows prenatal diagnosis of CAH.[247] The importance of prenatal diagnosis is that maternal treatment with high-dose dexamethasone can suppress excess fetal adrenal androgen production. This prevents ambiguous genitalia in females, as well as the androgenizing effects of excess fetal adrenal androgens on the fetal brain.[189,232]

A "late-onset" or "attenuated" (nonclassical) form of 21-alpha-hydroxylase deficiency can present in female adolescents as hirsutism or virilization associated with (1) menstrual irregularities, (2) oligomenorrhea, (3) amenorrhea, and (4) a polycystic ovary–like syndrome.[52,162] Thus, late-onset 21-alpha-hydroxylase deficiency CAH is much milder than the classical ("virilizing") form of 21-alpha-hydroxylase deficiency of prenatal onset. Whereas baseline and post-ACTH 17-OHP concentrations in attenuated 21-alpha-hydroxylase–deficient CAH are higher than in controls, the values are not

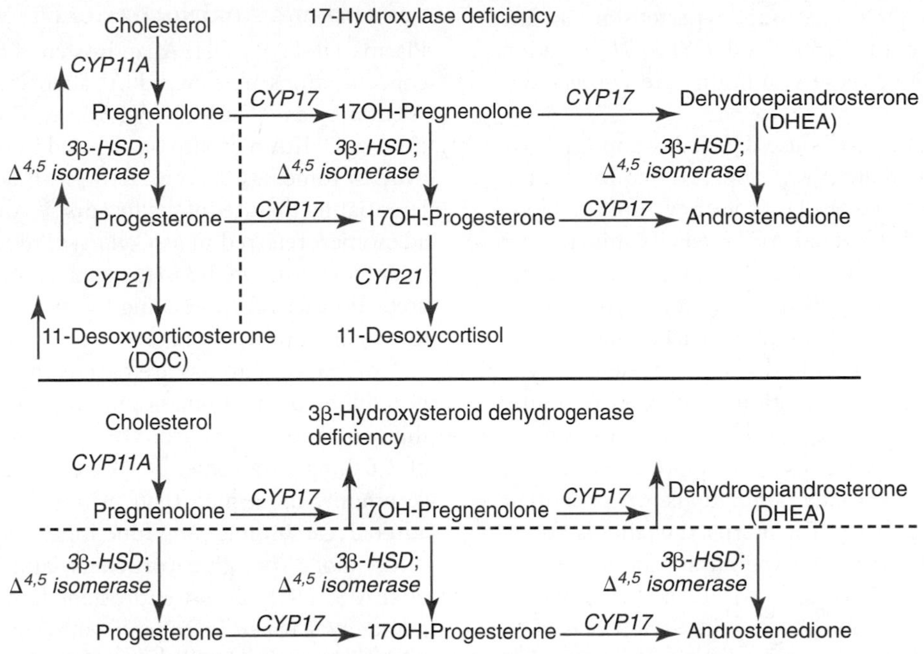

Figure 54-21 ***Top panel:*** **In 17-hydroxylase (CYP17) deficiency** ***(dashed line),*** **cortisol and adrenal androgens are deficient. Increased concentrations of pregnenolone, progesterone, and 11-desoxycorticosterone are recognized.** ***Bottom panel:*** **In 3 beta-hydroxysteroid dehydrogenase deficiency** ***(dashed line),*** **delta(5) steroids are not appropriately converted to delta(4) steroids. DHEA is overproduced, and aldosterone and cortisol are deficient. Increased concentrations of pregnenolone, 17-hydroxypregnenolone, and DHEA are recognized.**

as high as those seen in classical 21-alpha-hydroxylase deficiency CAH. Nomograms are available in the literature that allow basal 17-OHP to be plotted against post-ACTH 17-OHP in diagnosing CAH gene carriers versus attenuated 21-alpha-hydroxylase deficiency versus classical 21-alpha-hydroxylase deficiency. Gene carriers (individuals heterozygous for a wild-type allele and a mutant allele) usually have normal basal concentrations of 17-OHP but excessive 17-OHP responses to a cosyntropin challenge.

Measurements of early morning 17-OHP or random androstenedione are used to assess the CAH patient's response to glucocorticoid replacement.[10] With adequate glucocorticoid replacement, 17-OHP or androstenedione should not be elevated above the upper limit of the reference interval for age and sex. Insufficient glucocorticoid replacement permits excess adrenal production of androgens. Alternatively, overtreatment with glucocorticoids can suppress growth through the induction of a mild state of iatrogenic Cushing syndrome. Some investigators have questioned whether patients with CAH should undergo adrenalectomy to "ablate" adrenal hyperandrogenism. However, this would be fraught with danger, as it would produce frank Addison disease.

In patients with 21-alpha-hydroxylase deficiency CAH, aldosterone is replaced with oral fludrocortisone (Fluorinef). Adequacy of mineralocorticoid replacement is assessed by measuring the patient's blood pressure and renin. Inadequate replacement may result in hypertension from elevated renin that increases angiotensin II, causing vasoconstriction despite possible volume depletion. However, mineralocorticoid overdosage can also induce hypertension through excess sodium retention. Hypokalemia and alkalosis are possible consequences of over-replacement with fludrocortisone. The effectiveness of treatment is judged on the basis of the presence or absence of normal linear growth, normal sexual development, and suppression of 17-OHP and/or adrenal androgen concentrations into the reference intervals.

Medically, 17-Alpha-hydroxylase deficiency (CYP17, P450c17) is a rare cause of CAH (Figure 54-21).[15] Normally, 17-alpha-hydroxylase converts pregnenolone to 17-hydroxypregnenelone and progesterone to 17-alpha-hydroxyprogesterone in the zona glomerulosa and the zona reticularis. In the absence of 17-alpha-hydroxylase activity, there exists an obstruction to cortisol biosynthesis. *CYP17* mutations will also influence sex steroid production in males in utero and in females at the time of puberty, as this gene provides zona reticularis and gonadal 17,20-desmolase (lyase) activity. 17,20-Desmolase converts 17-hydroxypregnenelone to DHEA and 17-hydroxyprogesterone to androstenedione. In turn, in the gonad, the adrenal androgen DHEA is the precursor of androstenediol, which is the immediate precursor of testosterone. Thus, in addition to interference in cortisol biosynthesis, *CYP17* mutations preclude sex steroid production of both androgens and estrogens. In contrast, the aldosterone pathway remains intact and salt-wasting does not occur with elevated DOC, causing hypertension in later childhood. Because both *CYP17* and *CYP11B1* mutations can cause hypertension, these conditions are compared in Table 54-14.

Similar to 21-alpha-hydroxylase deficiency and CYP11B1 11-beta-hydroxylase deficiency, ACTH concentrations increase because of cortisol deficiency in 17-alpha-hydroxylase deficiency. Elevated ACTH elicits mineralocorticoid overproduction in the zona glomerulosa. Salt and water retention can then suppress aldosterone synthesis and secretion. Because of excess mineralocorticoid activity, salt-wasting is not present in 17-alpha-hydroxylase deficiency; in fact, excessive salt and water retention from excessive mineralocorticoid activity frequently produces hypertension in childhood. Because sex steroids are not produced, genetic males will appear as sexually ambiguous or phenotypic females with delayed puberty. The uterus, the fallopian tubes, and the upper one third of the vagina are absent because of Müllerian inhibiting hormone (MIH, or anti-Müllerian hormone, AMH) that is elaborated by the Sertoli cells of the testes. Virilization of the external genitalia is reduced or absent in males in utero because of the block in testosterone biosynthesis. In genetic females, the genitalia are not ambiguous; however, puberty and menses will not occur spontaneously because estrogens will not be produced.

Another rare form of CAH causing cortisol deficiency is 3-beta-hydroxysteroid dehydrogenase deficiency (see Figure 54-21).[293] This non-P450 enzyme converts ^{5}delta to ^{4}delta steroids such as pregnenolone to progesterone, 17-hydroxypregnenolone to 17-OHP, and DHEA to androstenedione. Because the gonads share these pathways with the adrenal glands, male fetuses are undervirilized as the result of deficient testosterone production, and female fetuses are overvirilized because of excessive adrenal androgen production (overproduction of DHEA). In 3-beta-hydroxysteroid dehydrogenase deficiency, the ratios of (1) pregnenolone to progesterone, (2) 17-hydroxypregnenolone to 17-OHP, and (3) DHEA to androstenedione are elevated. A late-onset form has been described in patients with premature pubarche with hirsutism, acne, and menstrual irregularities. Biochemically, 17-ketosteroid reductase deficiency affects sex steroid synthesis in the gonads, but it does not affect aldosterone or cortisol biosynthesis.[243] Therefore, 17-ketosteroid reductase deficiency causes in utero testosterone deficiency with sexual ambiguity in males, and primary amenorrhea and failure to enter puberty in girls.

The least common (but most severe) form of CAH is not an enzyme deficiency but a disorder involving steroidogenic acute regulatory protein (StAR).[187] StAR mediates the transport of cholesterol across the inner mitochondrial membrane. A deficiency of StAR is potentially lethal and causes congenital lipoid adrenal hyperplasia when the adrenal glands are packed with cholesterol and cholesterol esters that are not further metabolized because of the inborn error. In this disorder, deficiencies of all steroid hormones are present. Failure of androgen production in males is expressed as ambiguous genitalia.

Functioning Adrenocortical Tumors[298]

Plasma DHEA-S, DHEA, androstenedione, and testosterone concentrations are elevated in patients with virilizing adrenal adenomas and Cushing syndrome. The plasma concentrations of DHEA may also be elevated in women with virilizing ovarian tumors. CT scans along with MRI are useful in differentiating the sites of the tumors.[287] Aldosterone-producing adenomas, referred to as *Conn syndrome,* are typically small microadenomas found in the zona glomerulosa that hypersecrete aldosterone, producing the syndrome characterized by low renin hypertension.[174]

Adrenal carcinomas are rare, with an incidence of only 1 per million population; they usually are larger than 4 cm, and they may cause only virilization, and not the typical features of Cushing syndrome.[329] Adrenal carcinomas occur more commonly in women than in men, by a 2.5:1 ratio. Most adrenal carcinomas are functional, producing glucocorticoids alone or glucocorticoids and androgens. Plasma DHEA-S, DHEA, and androstenedione concentrations are markedly elevated in patients with functional adrenal carcinomas. The peripheral conversion of adrenal androgens to testosterone results in hirsutism and virilization. Concentrations of DHEA-S can often exceed 10 μg/mL in patients with adrenal carcinoma and usually are diagnostic for this malignancy. High-dose glucocorticoids do not suppress the elevated androgen concentrations.

Feminizing adrenocortical carcinomas are also rare.[210,288] These tumors result in elevations of plasma DHEA-S, DHEA, androstenedione, estrone, and estradiol concentrations. Gynecomastia and sexual dysfunction occur in males, and precocious pseudopuberty occurs in females. Steroid hormone production fails to decrease normally after treatment with dexamethasone.

Nonfunctioning Adrenocortical Tumors

Approximately 2% of the population has an adrenal tumor; most of these tumors are nonfunctioning and benign and are called *incidentalomas* (or *incidentomas*) when found by accident.[6,57] The tumors usually are found when CT or MRI scans of the abdomen are performed that easily detect tumors 1 cm in diameter or 5 g in weight. No virilizing tumors smaller than 1 cm in diameter have been reported. Carcinomas usually weigh more than 30 g.

The challenge occurs when CT or MRI of the abdomen reveals an adrenal mass in a patient lacking clinical evidence of adrenal hyperfunction.[307] The CT or MRI might have been ordered for evaluation of undiagnosed "chronic abdominal pain," for example. Upon finding an unexpected adrenal mass, the clinician generally is obliged to exclude subclinical adrenal disease by screening for (1) Cushing syndrome, (2) hypermineralocorticoidism, and (3) pheochromocytoma. Screening for Cushing syndrome is as described earlier with a 24 hour urinary free cortisol measurement, an overnight 1 mg dexamethasone suppression test, or a midnight plasma or salivary cortisol measurement. Diagnostically challenging cases with possibly mild hypercortisolism may be revealed.[308] Screening for hypermineralocorticoidism could be accomplished by measuring the patient's blood pressure and serum potassium (assuming that the patient has not previously been diagnosed with hypertension, and the patient is not on potassium-wasting diuretics). Because adrenal androgen- or estrogen-secreting tumors are very rare, it is argued that these may be detected solely by taking a history and performing a physical examination with attention to evidence of androgen or estrogen excess. Screening for pheochromocytoma involves measuring plasma free metanephrine or 24 hour urinary metanephrines and/or catecholamines.

Mineralocorticoid Excess (Hyperaldosteronism)

Primary hyperaldosteronism, commonly referred to as *Conn syndrome,* is a syndrome of hypersecretion of the aldosterone.[198] In primary hyperaldosteronism, excessive aldosterone production originates within the adrenal gland; in secondary hyperaldosteronism, a stimulus outside the adrenal gland activates the renin-angiotensin system. (*Note:* The term *aldosteronism* is often used synonymously with *hyperaldosteronism.*) The interaction of renin, angiotensin, and aldosterone is important in the regulation of extracellular fluid volume and blood pressure, and in the balance of sodium and potassium ions as well as acid-base balance.

Control of renin release from the kidney is influenced by (1) the specialized distal convoluted tubule, where chemoreceptor macula densa cells monitor the sodium concentration of fluid in the distal tubules; (2) the pressure-transducer juxtaglomerular cells, which monitor renal perfusion pressure; (3) the sympathetic nervous system, which supplies the kidney and controls catecholamine release; and (4) humoral factors such as potassium, atrial natriuretic peptides, and angiotensin II. Secondary events that disturb the normal equilibrium of renin release are much more common than primary abnormalities of renin secretion (Table 54-15). For example, a decrease in effective plasma volume or mean arterial pressure from sudden blood loss leads to release of renin from the juxtaglomerular cells of the kidneys; more angiotensin I and angiotensin II are formed, and production of aldosterone by the adrenal glands is increased. Angiotensin II also causes increased sodium reabsorption in the proximal convoluted tubule, increased thirst, increased release of ADH, and release of catecholamines. These events result in retention of sodium and water, an increase in extracellular volume, hydrogen ion wasting, and a decrease in the serum potassium ion concentration as renal potassium excretion increases. This state of secondary hyperaldosteronism is commonly present in patients with (1) congestive heart failure, (2) nephrotic syndrome, (3) cirrhosis of the liver, (4) other hypoproteinemic states, or (5) conditions of chronic depletion of plasma volume.

Secondary hyperaldosteronism is suspected in patients with volume depletion, edema, and hypokalemic alkalosis. Whereas hypertension is present in primary hyperaldosteronism, it is usually absent in secondary hyperaldosteronism, unless the patient has a reninoma or renal artery stenosis. Measurements of renin and aldosterone concentrations are seldom needed in cases of secondary hyperaldosteronism, because precipitating circumstances that explain the patient's hypokalemia and alkalosis (e.g., secondary hyperaldosteronism is expected in congestive heart failure) are apparent. Renin and aldosterone measurements are invaluable, however, in the investigation of primary disturbances in the renin-angiotensin-aldosterone system, in the assessment of renal artery stenosis, and in the genesis and maintenance of arterial hypertension.

TABLE 54-15 Causes of Functional Hypermineralocorticoidism

Hyperaldosteronism	Primary (hyporeninemic) • Aldosterone-producing adenoma • Aldosterone-producing carcinoma • Idiopathic adrenal hyperplasia • Unilaternal adrenocortical hyperplasia • Glucocorticoid remediable hypertension Secondary (hyperreninemic) • Renin-secreting tumors • Renovascular hypertension • Compensatory (nephrosis, cirrhosis, CHF) • Bartter syndrome • Gitelman syndrome
Desoxycorticosterone (DOC) excess	DOC-secreting adrenal adenoma 11 Beta-hydroxylase (CYP11B1) deficiency 17-Hydroxylase (CYP17) deficiency
Glucocorticoid excess	Cushing syndrome Cortisol resistance
Increased mineralocorticoid action without circulating mineralocorticoid excess	Apparent mineralocorticoid excess (HSD11B2 deficiency) Acquired HSD11B2 inhibition (glycyrrhizic acid induced) • Liddle syndrome (type 1 pseudohyperaldosteronism) • MR gain-of-function mutation (type 2 pseudohyperaldosteronism)

CHF, Congestive heart failure; *MR,* mineralocorticoid receptor.

Primary Hyperaldosteronism

Primary hyperaldosteronism, which was first described by Conn in 1955, is characterized by an elevated plasma concentration of aldosterone and a suppressed renin concentration, along with hypertension and hypokalemic alkalosis. Historically, it has been taught that no more than 1% of hypertensive patients have primary hyperaldosteronism. However, results from a 2007 study identified primary hyperaldosteronism in 10% or more of cases of otherwise defined "essential" hypertension.[269]

Clinical indications for a formal evaluation of hyperaldosteronism (measurement of the aldosterone-to-renin ratio)[268] include hypokalemia that is unprovoked by diuretics and the patient's lack of response to conventional antihypertensive drug treatment.[262] However, not all patients with primary hyperaldosteronism are hypokalemic.

Overproduction of aldosterone may be due to autonomous and inappropriate secretion of aldosterone by (1) an adenoma of one adrenal gland [aldosterone-producing adrenal adenoma (APA), or Conn syndrome], (2) hyperplasia of aldosterone-producing cells in both glands [bilateral idiopathic adrenal hyperplasia (IAH)], (3) an aldosterone-producing adrenal carcinoma, or (4) a rare familial condition known as *glucocorticoid-suppressible hyperaldosteronism* (familial hyperaldosteronism type 1).[215,238] Familial hyperaldosteronism type 2 is the rare occurrence of familial APA, familial hyperaldosteronism from IAH, or combined familial APA and hyperplasia. A rare cause of hyperaldosteronism is unilateral adrenocortical zona glomerulosa hyperplasia, which can be micronodular or macronodular. Very rarely, does primary hyperaldosteronism result from ectopic aldosterone secretion from the ovary or kidney.

Clinical features of primary hyperaldosteronism generally are related to the consequences of aldosterone overproduction. Increased retention of sodium through the effects of aldosterone on the renal tubular handling of sodium (increased ENaC activity), expansion of extracellular fluid volume, and increased tubular secretion of potassium and hydrogen ions constitute the cardinal manifestations of primary hyperaldosteronism. Hypokalemic alkalosis is a consequence of progressive renal depletion of body potassium and hydrogen ions. As a consequence of sodium retention, a modest expansion of extracellular fluid volume occurs, along with an increase in arterial blood pressure.

Diagnosis and Treatment of Primary Hyperaldosteronism

Hypokalemia is the principal clue that primary hyperaldosteronism may be present in a patient with diastolic hypertension. To confirm the diagnosis, it is necessary to demonstrate (1) hyposecretion of renin, which is not appropriately elevated during volume depletion, and (2) hypersecretion of aldosterone, which fails to suppress appropriately during volume expansion.[38] Figure 54-22 shows a suggested scheme for evaluating patients with suspected excessive mineralocorticoid action causing hypertension.

Most patients with autonomous aldosterone overproduction are hypokalemic, but most patients with hypokalemia do not have primary hyperaldosteronism. Because not all patients with primary hyperaldosteronism are hypokalemic, primary hyperaldosteronism as a cause of hypertension may be under-recognized. In hyperaldosteronism, urinary potassium excretion is inappropriately high, and a random urine potassium greater than 30 mmol/L is usually indicative of primary hyperaldosteronism, or some form of mineralocorticoid excess. If hypokalemia can be shown to be due to nonrenal potassium loss, the diagnosis of hyperaldosteronism does not need to be considered further.

In primary hyperaldosteronism, low renin activity and elevated aldosterone concentration are expected.[101,283] Many other factors, however, influence the secretion of renin and aldosterone, and these factors must be considered before testing.[164] Because drugs such as ACE inhibitors, beta blockers, and spironolactone alter renin release, patients should be withdrawn from these medications for several weeks before the plasma aldosterone-to-renin ratio is determined. When patients with suspected primary hyperaldosteronism are evaluated, it is helpful, for example, (1) to compare ambulatory PRA activity versus the patient's urinary sodium excretion, or (2) to stimulate renin production with a potent diuretic such as furosemide. An elevated plasma renin activity could be due to secondary hyperaldosteronism (e.g., renovascular hypertension, pheochromocytoma). Low renin activity, on the other hand, suggests primary hyperaldosteronism or low-renin hypertension. The latter may be caused by exogenous or endogenous mineralocorticoids that mimic the action of aldosterone, producing expanded plasma volume, hypertension, and hypokalemia.

The ACE inhibitor captopril has been used for the diagnosis of primary hyperaldosteronism.[348] In individuals who are normotensive or have essential hypertension, acute inhibition of ACE decreases angiotensin-mediated aldosterone production to less than 15 ng/dL, whereas autonomous aldosterone production from an aldosterone-producing adenoma is unaffected by the ACE inhibitor. The determination of plasma renin responsiveness, however, is not sufficient in diagnosing primary aldosteronism because suppressed renin activity also occurs in about 25% of patients with essential hypertension. Recently, losartan (an angiotensin II receptor antagonist drug marketed under the name Cozaar) suppression of aldosterone was found to be superior to captopril suppression in the diagnosis of primary hyperaldosteronism.[347]

Primary hyperaldosteronism is differentiated from other hypermineralocorticoid states on the basis of inappropriate secretion of aldosterone.[97] Demonstration of an elevated concentration of aldosterone in blood or urine in a patient with an unequivocally suppressed renin concentration (a plasma aldosterone-to-renin ratio >25 to 30) is presumptive evidence of primary hyperaldosteronism.[233,283] Because hypokalemia has a suppressive effect on aldosterone secretion, the potassium deficit should be replaced before aldosterone measurements are performed. To establish aldosterone autonomy, aldosterone production may be suppressed with rapid volume expansion using the saline suppression test (see Box 54-9)[146] with a potent mineralocorticoid such as fludrocortisone (see Box 54-10)[35] or pharmacologically with captopril. Failure of aldosterone to be suppressed by these maneuvers confirms the diagnosis of primary hyperaldosteronism.

Once the diagnosis of primary hyperaldosteronism is established, it is necessary to distinguish between APA and bilateral IAH. This differentiation is vital because most

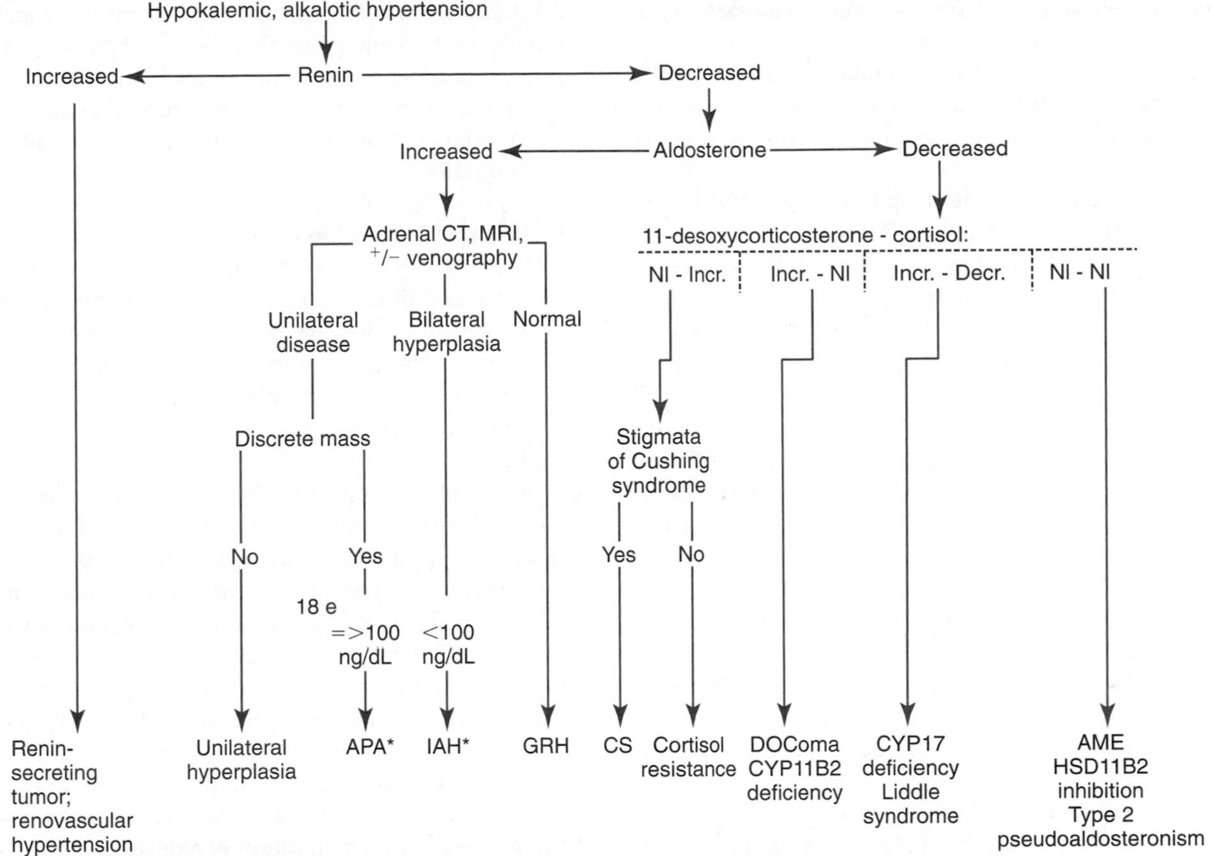

Figure 54-22 This figure provides a reasonable approach to the differential diagnosis of hypokalemic, alkalotic hypertension. If the concentration of renin is elevated, diagnostic considerations include a juxtaglomerular renin-secreting tumor (a reninoma) and renovascular hypertension (assuming that intrinsic renal disease has been ruled out, which can cause elevated renin and aldosterone, leading to hypertension). If renin is suppressed and aldosterone is elevated (an aldosterone-to-renin ratio >20 to 25), Imaging and venography can help separate unilateral disease without a discrete mass (rare unilateral adrenal hyperplasia), unilateral disease with a discrete mass (aldosteronoma), bilateral idiopathic adrenal hyperplasia (IAH), or the rare condition of glucocorticoid-remediable hyperaldosteronism, with no masses or hyperplasia (see text for details). If aldosterone is not elevated, 11-desoxycorticosterone (DOC) and cortisol should be assayed, allowing the discrimination of several entities: Cushing syndrome or cortisol resistance (normal DOC and elevated cortisol), DOComa (DOC-secreting adrenal adenoma) or CYP11B2 (aldosterone synthase) deficiency (increased DOC and normal cortisol), deficiency of CYP17 (17-hydroxylase deficiency) (increased DOC and decreased cortisol), and end-organ disorders (normal DOC and cortisol).* In familial hyperaldosteronism type 2, aldosterone-producing adrenal adenoma (APA), IAH, or combined disease can be observed. *AME,* Apparent mineralocorticoid excess; *decr,* decrease; *incr,* increase; *Nl,* normal.

patients with adrenal adenoma respond favorably to surgical removal of the tumor, whereas those with adrenal hyperplasia do not respond favorably and are managed medically.[177] Localization using imaging techniques[144] [spiral CT scans,[124,287] ultrasonography, and adrenal scanning with NP-59 (^{125}I-6-iodomethyl-19-norcholesterol)] can be helpful, and adrenal venography with or without selective adrenal venous sampling for aldosterone measurements is used to determine whether the right or left adrenal is hypersecreting aldosterone. This is valuable when tumors are too small to be detected by imaging techniques. However, when CT or MRI findings are equated with a functional APA, mistakes can be made (e.g., the visualized mass was an incidentaloma and was not the APA).[147] This was discovered when surgery did not cure the patient's hypertension and hyperaldosteronism. Therefore, it has been argued that venography with aldosterone measurements should always be completed before adrenal surgery for a suspected APA, to confirm the laterality suggested by CT or MRI. Also if venography is performed, it is prudent to consider measuring cortisol in the adrenal veins and inferior vena cava (in addition to aldosterone) to confirm the anatomic identification of the vein, in case one of the adrenal veins is not truly cannulated. The usual ratio of cortisol in the adrenal veins to the inferior vena cava is 10 to 1. Adrenal carcinomas are rare causes of primary hyperaldosteronism.[334]

Numerous biochemical clues help in the differential diagnosis of APA versus bilateral IAH. Aldosterone hypersecretion and plasma renin suppression are usually greater with adrenal adenoma. After sodium depletion, or after 2 to 4 hours of upright posture, patients with APA usually show no change or a paradoxical fall in plasma aldosterone, whereas patients with IAH typically show a rise in plasma aldosterone (presumably because the hyperplastic glands are sensitive to increases in the PRA, and adenomas are insensitive to increases in the PRA).[117] Elevated plasma concentrations of 18-hydroxycorticosterone (>100 ng/dL) are observed in most patients with APA, but not in patients with IAH (see Figure 54-22).

Adrenal vein catheterization is considered the gold standard for differentiation of an aldosteronoma versus IAH. To correct for variations in cortisol and aldosterone concentrations induced by the stress of venography, a cosyntropin intravenous infusion of 50 µg/h can be provided during the procedure. When the aldosterone-to-cortisol ratio of one side versus the aldosterone-to-cortisol ratio of the other side is studied, aldosteronomas display a mean side-to-side ratio of 18, whereas the ratio in patients with IAH averages 1.8. The consensus is that side-to-side aldosterone-to-cortisol ratios of 4 or greater are consistent with aldosteronoma, whereas side-to-side ratios of 3 or less are consistent with IAH. Ratios greater than 3 and less than 4 fall into a gray zone, and other techniques must be relied upon to differentiate aldosteronoma and IAH.

A small percentage of patients with hypermineralocorticoidism respond to dexamethasone treatment (e.g., rare glucocorticoid-remediable hyperaldosteronism, also called *dexamethasone-suppressible hypertension*) with normalization of their blood pressure and correction of their biochemical abnormalities.[96,175,263] Dexamethasone treatment should be attempted before surgery, particularly in young patients, or when the normal fall in plasma aldosterone concentration after salt depletion and standing does not occur and no unilateral lesion is seen on CT/MRI. Also, a trial treatment of spironolactone, an aldosterone antagonist, usually normalizes blood pressure in patients who are likely to have a good response to surgery. In glucocorticoid-remediable hyperaldosteronism, concentrations of 18-oxocortisol and 18-hydroxycortisol are increased as a result of the gene fusion between CYP11B1, the 11-beta-hydroxylase (P450c11) of the zona fasciculata/reticularis, and CYP11B2 (aldosterone synthase, P450 aldo).

Adrenocortical carcinomas have been found to produce excess mineralocorticoid and cause hypertension with hypokalemia.[286] Aldosterone or DOC, or both, may be produced in excess.[219,313,327] Mineralocorticoid concentrations do not respond to glucocorticoid therapy or alterations in salt status. CT scans are helpful; adrenal carcinomas are usually large tumors that weigh more than 30 g, whereas aldosterone-producing adenomas are usually much smaller. Carcinomas are similar to adenomas in that furosemide stimulation or upright posture should not elevate renin or aldosterone concentrations.

Other Causes of Excessive Mineralocorticoid Action

Unusual conditions that suggest aldosterone excess but do not involve disorders of renin, angiotensin II, or aldosterone[285] include (1) apparent mineralocorticoid excess, (2) type 1 pseudohyperaldosteronism (Liddle syndrome), (3) type 2 pseudohyperaldosteronism, and (4) cortisol resistance.[190]

Apparent mineralocorticoid excess (AME) results from 11-beta-hydroxysteroid dehydrogenase-2 (HSD11B2) deficiency or inhibition.[292] Normally, HSD11B2 protects the MR from cortisol by converting cortisol to cortisone in tissues expressing the MR. Cortisone does not bind to the MR. Impaired conversion of cortisol to cortisone allows cortisol to bind to the MR, producing a mineralocorticoid effect in the absence of elevations in aldosterone or DOC. Therefore, 11-beta-hydroxysteroid dehydrogenase-2 (HSD11B2) deficiency is described as an "apparent" excess of mineralocorticoid because patients can manifest hypertension, hypokalemia, and alkalosis without elevation of aldosterone nor DOC.

Apparent mineralocorticoid excess is inherited as an autosomal recessive trait and presents in childhood. Spironolactone is used to treat hypertension because spironolactone blocks the MR. Through feedback inhibition of ACTH to suppress cortisol production, dexamethasone sometimes corrects hypokalemia; however, this treatment does not consistently lower the patient's blood pressure.[204] Glycyrrhetinic acid, which is found in black licorice, inhibits 11-beta-hydroxysteroid dehydrogenase-2, causing an acquired form of apparent mineralocorticoid excess.[339] Apparent mineralocorticoid excess is diagnosed by an increased ratio of cortisol to cortisone and an increased ratio of urinary tetrahydrocortisol to urinary tetrahydrocorticosterone.[240]

Liddle syndrome (type 1 pseudohyperaldosteronism) results from gain-of-function mutations in the beta or gamma subunit of the amiloride-sensitive ENaC.[112,241,291] Consequences include (1) excessive sodium reabsorption, (2) expanded blood volume, (3) hypertension, (4) hypokalemia, and (5) alkalosis. Because the activity of ENaC is autonomous, both renin and aldosterone are suppressed. This disorder responds to triamterene but not to spironolactone (which blocks the MR). Triamterene is believed to inhibit ENaC through a mechanism similar to the action of amiloride. Type 2 pseudohyperaldosteronism is a gain-of-function mutation in the MR.

Loss-of-function mutations in the GR cause cortisol resistance.[272] In response to decreased cortisol action, CRH and ACTH concentrations rise, increasing the circulating cortisol to a sufficient concentration that functional cortisol deficiency is not present. However, the protective action of

TABLE 54-16 Renal Tubule Disorders Characterized by Loss of Sodium Chloride That Lead to Secondary Hyperaldosteronism*

Subtype	Channel/Transporter	Site of Expression	Gene	Gene Location
Bartter syndrome, classic, 3	Renal chloride channel	ALH	*CLCNKB*	1p36
Bartter syndrome, neonatal, 1	Na^+-K^+-$2Cl^-$ cotransporter	ALH	*NKCC2*	15q15-q21.1
Bartter syndrome, neonatal, 2	Potassium channel (ROMK)	ALH	*KCNJ1*	11q24-q25
Gitelman	Thiazide-sensitive sodium-chloride cotransporter (TSC; a.k.a. NCCT)	DCT	*SLC12A3*	16q13

*Pseudohypoaldosteronism type 1 is not included in this table.
ALH, Ascending loop of Henle; *DCT,* distal convoluted tubule.

HSD11B2 in converting cortisol to cortisone is overwhelmed, resulting in increased binding of cortisol to the MR and excessive mineralocorticoid effects. This is treated with a mineralocorticoid receptor blocker such as spironolactone or dexamethasone, which suppresses ACTH.

Non–Mineralocorticoid-Deficient Causes of Urinary Sodium Loss

Bartter syndrome is a consequence of sodium loss from dysfunction of the ascending, thick loop of Henle or the distal convoluted tubule.[336] Loss of sodium evokes a compensatory secondary hyperaldosteronism (with increased renin and aldosterone), producing hypokalemia and alkalosis. Although affected adults may be asymptomatic, infants can display (1) failure to thrive, (2) salt craving, (3) polyuria, and (4) polydipsia. Potassium depletion elicits prostaglandin-induced vasodilatation that can further worsen the attempted compensatory hyperaldosteronism. A variety of gene mutations cause urinary sodium loss that leads to secondary hyperaldosteronism with hypokalemia and alkalosis (Table 54-16).

In pseudohypoaldosteronism (resistance to aldosterone), the clinical view of hypoaldosteronism is seen (acidosis, hyperkalemia, possible hypotension) concurrent with elevated concentrations of aldosterone. Pseudohypoaldosteronism (PHA) may be classified as (1) renal type 1 PHA, (2) multiple target organ defects type 1 PHA, (3) early childhood hyperkalemia type 1 PHA, (4) Spitzer-Weinstein syndrome (adolescent hyperkalemic syndrome, (5) subtype 3 RTA [renal tubular acidosis] IV type 2 PHA), and (6) Gordon syndrome (mineralocorticoid-resistant hyperkalemia, chloride shunt syndrome type 2 PHA).

Renal type 1 PHA results from reduced numbers or function of the renal MR. This occurs as an autosomal dominant or sporadic disorder, and usually the child is asymptomatic by age 2. In multiple target organ defects type 1 PHA (an autosomal recessive disorder), a loss-of-function mutation in ENaC affects the sweat glands, salivary glands, and colon, in addition to the kidney, throughout the patient's life. Early childhood hyperkalemia type 1 PHA is milder than renal type 1 PHA, and its cause is unknown. The child usually has "outgrown" this disorder by age 5.

Whereas renin and aldosterone are elevated in PHA type 1, in PHA type 2 renin and aldosterone are normal to low. Type 2 PHA results from a defect in the distal nephron consequent to absent WNK1 or WNK4 kinase function. Some researchers have speculated that Gordon syndrome is caused by increased generalized activity of the bumetanide-sensitive Na^+-K^+-$2Cl^-$ cotransporter, but this requires formal study.

Plasma Renin in Renovascular Hypertension

When used as a screening test, elevated plasma renin after furosemide stimulation, or when correlated with urinary sodium excretion, suggests renal artery stenosis as the cause of hypertension.[165,340] If arteriographic evidence indicates the presence of renal artery stenosis, measurement of plasma renin in specimens obtained from selective renal vein catheterization is helpful in predicting the response to surgical correction of the renal vascular lesion or nephrectomy.[103] Lateralization of renin in the renal vein to the radiographically involved side, especially after sodium depletion, is predictive of a good response to surgery in 90% of cases (Box 54-11).[197] Comparison of renin activity in the renal artery with that in the renal vein can allow a further distinction.[322]

LABORATORY EVALUATION OF ADRENOCORTICAL FUNCTION

Laboratory evaluation of adrenal cortex function centers on measurement of (1) cortisol, the primary corticosteroid; (2) aldosterone, the primary mineralocorticoid; and (3) sex hormones, of which the adrenal cortex is a secondary source. Chromaffin cells in the adrenal medulla are a source of catecholamines, which are discussed in Chapter 30. Underproduction or overproduction of cortisol and aldosterone gives rise to characteristic clinical syndromes, and genetic defects in steroid hormone biosynthesis produce abnormalities in

BOX 54-11 Protocol for the Differential Renal Vein Renin Test

Rationale

In renovascular hypertension, plasma renin activity (PRA) is significantly higher in the renal vein on the involved side.

Procedure

The patient should be on a low-sodium, high-potassium diet and receiving a diuretic for 3 days before the procedure. Under fluoroscopic guidance, percutaneous catheterization is performed, and blood samples are obtained from both renal veins and the inferior vena cava for determination of PRA.

Interpretation

Various criteria have been suggested for interpretation. A ratio of PRA (affected side to unaffected side) that is greater than 1.5 suggests functionally significant renovascular disease.

sex hormone concentrations that are associated with clinical symptoms as well. Therefore, measurement of steroid hormones produced in the adrenal cortex is essential to the clinical diagnosis of a variety of endocrine disorders.

Steroid hormones such as those produced in the adrenal cortex share considerable structural similarity based on their terpenoid sterane core, which is modified by functional groups at various locations on the tetracyclic backbone. In general, steroids are lipophilic compounds, but they require additional modification—esterification to fatty acids—to facilitate their transport across cellular membranes. Transport in the bloodstream typically involves carrier proteins (e.g., transcortin, SHBG). These properties influence the choice of analytical methods for measuring steroid hormone concentrations; most procedures begin with enzymatic or chemical hydrolysis of steroid esters and displacement of the steroid from carrier proteins through addition of a protein-binding agent such as 8-anilino-1-naphthalene-sulfonic acid (ANS) or salicylate. Photometric and fluorometric measurements of steroids lack specificity unless extraction and purification procedures are used. Immunoassays are practical for the measurement of steroid hormones and are widely available on a variety of automated instrumental platforms, but cross-reactivity with structurally similar hormones often results in bias between various immunochemical methods. Endogenous interferences also occur, for example, near the time of birth, when placental steroid concentrations are very high. Steroids can be extracted into organic solvents and analyzed, however, chromatographic methods coupled with mass spectrometric detection provide sensitive and specific quantitative results for these compounds. In contrast to peptide hormones, most of which exhibit considerable heterogeneity as the result of post-translational modifications, steroid hormones constitute a relatively homogenous group of compounds that are calibrated against gravimetrically validated synthetic calibrators.

Episodic secretion and circadian variation limit the clinical diagnostic accuracy of basal serum cortisol concentrations.[67] Serum cortisol concentrations are highest in the early morning hours and vary between 7 and 25 μg/dL at between 0400 and 1200 hours. Late afternoon concentrations are about half the morning concentrations and frequently are less than 5 μg/dL at between 2200 and 0200 hours. A midnight cortisol less than 5 μg/dL is considered normal. Serum cortisol combined with plasma ACTH improves the diagnostic accuracy of basal values, although ACTH concentrations display even greater variation throughout the day than cortisol concentrations.

Choice of Specimen

Steroid hormones have been measured in urine, blood, saliva, and recently, hair.[309] The choice of specimen depends on the application. For clinical assessment of adrenal function, blood (plasma) measurements are convenient, but conditions that cause the binding protein concentration to increase have been known to produce clinically irrelevant elevations in the total cortisol concentration. Urinary concentrations are helpful in determining time-integrated hormone production and provide useful estimates of free hormone concentrations in blood, if an appropriately timed urine specimen collection is available. Measurement of steroid hormones in saliva has been proposed as an alternative to urinary hormone assays to estimate free hormone concentrations in blood, the principal advantage being ease of collection. Hair analysis may be useful for assessing adrenal hormone production over an extended time, but currently hair testing is not in widespread use.

Urine

Urinary excretion of a hormone, or its metabolites, provides an approximation of the amount secreted over the time the urine is collected, typically 24 hours. Thus, urinary hormone or metabolite measurements are useful when the hormone has a very short biological half-life and/or its secretion is pulsatile or varies in predictable cycles. Timed urine collections suffer variability associated with factors such as completeness of collection and impaired renal function. Urinary metabolites may reflect only a fraction of the active steroid hormones; these metabolites, in turn, may be affected by metabolic disease, as well as diet and medications. Even with these limitations, urinary free cortisol and measurement of urinary free estradiol, estrone, and testosterone are useful for estimating the rates at which these steroids are produced, and are not affected by variations in the concentrations of proteins that bind hormones, such as corticosteroid-binding globulin (CBG) and albumin. Use of the term *urinary free cortisol*, or *UFC*, is common, although it is somewhat redundant; only the uncomplexed fraction of blood cortisol is filtered in the glomerulus, so urinary cortisol is, by definition, the free hormone.

UFC obtained from a 24 hour urine collection, an integrated measure of plasma free cortisol, eliminates the circadian influence on cortisol secretion.[46] With increases in total cortisol and stable concentrations of CBG, the serum free cortisol fraction rises substantially and is cleared into the urine. UFC measurements therefore are considered a superior screening test for cortisol excess. In Cushing syndrome, UFC is two to three times the upper limit of the reference interval. The UFC excretion rate in normal subjects is less than 50 μg/d when assayed by high-performance liquid chromatography (HPLC).

Blood

Circulating concentrations of steroids in the blood provide the most direct measure of endocrine activity mediated by these hormones. Immunoassays and chromatographic methods have been developed for measuring most of the clinically relevant steroids in blood. Provocative testing (stimulation and suppression tests, discussed earlier) may require blood samples because of the rapid changes that occur in hormone activity when stimulus or suppression is applied. Many of the steroid hormones are released in a pulsatile or rhythmic fashion, so their concentrations in an isolated blood specimen should take into account these variables.

Mineralocorticoid and adrenal androgen secretion is circadian and episodic in nature, but the dynamic swings in concentration are not as pronounced as with cortisol. It is usually recommended, however, that blood samples for adrenal steroids should be collected in the 0700 to 1000 hour time frame for consistency in interpreting the results.

Steroid hormone concentrations in serum and plasma are nearly the same. It has been suggested that steroid hormone concentrations may change in unseparated blood specimens as the result of 17β-hydroxysteroid dehydrogenase activity in red blood cells and macrophages, but stability studies of estradiol, cortisol, testosterone, progesterone, 17α-hydroxyprogesterone, androstenedione, and DHEA-S have failed to reveal any clinically significant changes in these hormones in whole blood specimens stored at room temperature for up to 1 week.[69]

Saliva

Most steroids of clinical interest have been measured in saliva, and for some steroids, such as cortisol, estriol, and progesterone, salivary concentrations appear to correlate with the free hormone concentration in plasma.[326] For other steroids (e.g., testosterone, 17α-hydroxyprogesterone, estradiol, aldosterone), the clinical usefulness of salivary measurements has not been established.

Measurement of steroids in saliva is attractive because specimens are simple to collect; this consideration is particularly important in pediatric patients. Several saliva collection devices using absorbent materials have been designed to collect a sufficient volume of saliva for steroid analysis. However, recovery of cortisol from these devices has been questioned. Using cotton swabs, cotton ropes, and hydrocellulose microsponges, Harmon and colleagues demonstrated that recovery of both the volume of saliva specimen and the cortisol concentration was variable, relative to a directly collected ("passive drool") saliva specimen.[114]

Hair

Hair grows at an average rate of 1 cm per month; therefore it can reveal historical blood concentrations of substances that are deposited in the forming hair matrix. Also it has been used as an alternative to urine specimens for the detection of illicit drug use, because a number drugs are detectable in urine for only a few days following exposure.[95] Several reports describe methods for measuring steroid hormones in hair.[53,152,309,351] These methods have shown potential as diagnostic tools but will require additional validation studies before they can be applied generally.

Basal Peptide and Steroid Hormone Concentrations

Concentrations of adrenal mineralocorticoids and elements of the renin-angiotensin system are routinely measured in body fluids by various immunoassay and mass spectrometric methods.[270,271] As with cortisol, aldosterone is secreted episodically, with the highest circulating concentrations near the time of awakening, and the lowest concentrations shortly after sleep onset. Aldosterone concentrations, however, are only modestly stimulated by ACTH secretion. In healthy subjects, consuming a low-sodium diet, maintaining an upright posture, and using diuretics all increase plasma aldosterone concentrations, whereas consuming a high-sodium diet and lying in the supine position decrease aldosterone secretion. Standardized procedures for obtaining blood and urine specimens are required for proper interpretation of test results. It is useful to interpret aldosterone concentrations together with urinary sodium excretion, because salt intake can profoundly influence the aldosterone concentration. Normally, the aldosterone concentration is inversely proportional to the urinary sodium concentration.

Because it has enzymatic activity, renin is measured by its activity or its mass, and both methods are available. Plasma renin activity (PRA) is determined by the generation of angiotensin I, which is measured using immunoassay techniques.[13] The relative merits of activity and mass assays of renin are discussed in the following paragraphs.

Renin release is controlled by many physiologic factors. Consuming low-sodium diets, maintaining an upright posture, and using diuretic medications increase renin release (causing a rise in aldosterone) and should be controlled or eliminated before testing of the renin-angiotensin-aldosterone axis is begun. Because plasma renin varies with sodium balance, it is helpful to interpret ambulatory renin measurements together with urinary sodium excretion. An inverse relationship exists (similar to aldosterone), allowing the identification of low-, normal-, and high-plasma renin groups from a standard nomogram.

Age, estrogen therapy, and diabetes mellitus without renal failure affect plasma renin results.[1] Patients older than 55 years and those with diabetes have PRA results that are about 50% of normal. Estrogen causes an increase in the hepatic synthesis of angiotensinogen, thereby increasing the endogenous substrate concentration for the renin enzyme. This causes inappropriately elevated renin activity for the urinary sodium concentration. Several medications may affect plasma renin activities. Angiotensin-converting enzyme (ACE) inhibitors and spironolactone raise renin concentrations, whereas beta blockers and nonsteroidal anti-inflammatory agents block renin release.

Even when time of sampling, posture, drug intake, and diet are controlled, it is often difficult to identify disorders of mineralocorticoid secretion on the basis of basal hormone concentrations alone.[43] A variety of dynamic tests have been developed to assess hypersecretion or hyposecretion of aldosterone and renin.

The diagnosis of adrenal insufficiency in the setting of critical illness has become highly controversial.[11,40,153,191,257] On one hand, if the diagnosis of cortisol deficiency or combined cortisol and aldosterone deficiencies is missed and replacement medication is not administered, the patient can die from Addisonian crisis, as might occur in Waterhouse-Friderichsen syndrome. However, inappropriate administration of cortisol in the setting of sepsis could produce immunosuppression that may be fatal. Some investigators believe that free cortisol measurements would be of diagnostic help because CBG concentrations frequently decline from liver disease or acute malnutrition that could lead to overdiagnosis of cortisol deficiency. In equivocal cases of adrenal insufficiency, some authors caution that a single low cortisol concentration should not be used to make the diagnosis of cortisol deficiency.[257] Just as free testosterone can be estimated from total testosterone and SHBG concentrations, a free cortisol index has been described as the simple ratio of total cortisol to CBG.[169]

Free Versus Bound Steroids

Many hormones circulate in the blood bound to carrier proteins. Hormone-binding proteins serve two functions: (1) they solubilize lipophilic compounds such as steroid hormones to facilitate their transport in the primarily aqueous circulatory environment, and (2) they buffer the concentration of free, active hormone in tissue. Protein-bound hormones are not ordinarily active, but the protein-bound reservoir provides a relatively constant, buffered concentration of the free hormone for activity at tissue receptors. However, for hormones that are highly protein bound, the concentration of the binding protein is the principal determinant of the total concentration of hormone. Therefore, total hormone concentration vary significantly, while the free, active hormone concentration remains within physiologically appropriate limits. Measurement of free (unbound) hormone concentrations provides the best indicator of hormone activity, but analytical methods that isolate free hormone concentrations without disrupting the free/bound equilibrium are sometimes difficult to design. Antibodies that recognize steroid hormones may have binding affinities that compete with binding proteins and detect portions, if not all, of the bound fraction. Preanalytical methods to separate bound and free fractions often disrupt the physiologic equilibrium between bound and free hormone. Urinary and salivary steroid hormone measurements have been widely used to estimate free hormone concentrations; specific applications are discussed later.

Analytical Methods

In contrast to peptide hormones, which may exhibit considerable structural heterogeneity, steroids present less of a challenge in the design of specific analytical methods because these compounds, for the most part, are homogeneous. Sensitive immunometric methods for measuring steroid hormones have been available for decades, and methodological approaches include most, if not all, of the common labels (radioisotope, enzyme, fluorescent, chemiluminescent) and immunoassay designs (heterogeneous, homogeneous, competitive, noncompetitive). Currently, a participant survey from a 2009 College of American Pathologists proficiency challenge revealed that, among participating clinical laboratories reporting cortisol results, a vast majority use heterogeneous chemiluminescent or electrochemiluminescent immunoassays.

Measurement of Cortisol

Approximately 90% of circulating cortisol is bound to plasma proteins, primarily to CBG (corticosteroid binding globulin, or transcortin). Cortisol also binds weakly to albumin. The concentration of CBG in the plasma rises in hyperestrogenic states, including pregnancy and oral contraceptive use; therefore total cortisol in serum is increased in these conditions, although free cortisol remains normal. Analytical methods involving organic solvent extraction or protein precipitation estimate both free and protein-bound cortisol in the circulation, but immunoassays for direct measurement of cortisol have mostly replaced extraction/chromatographic methods for routine cortisol determinations.

Historical methods for the quantitative estimation of total cortisol in blood include the Porter-Silber color reaction,[222,253] in which dihydroxyacetone groups at carbons 19, 20, and 21 of 17-hydroxycorticosteroids react with phenylhydrazine to produce a yellow adduct and sulfuric acid–induced fluorescence.[150,196] However, immunoassays and chromatographic assays are now used in most clinical laboratories for the quantitative determination of cortisol in serum or urine. Methods for measuring cortisol in clinical laboratories have been reviewed.[99]

Chromatographic Methods

Gas chromatography (GC),[142,346] thin-layer chromatography (TLC),[83] and HPLC[135,176,194,213,236] have been used to measure cortisol. GC and HPLC coupled to mass spectrophotometric detectors (GC/MS, LC/MS, and LC/MS-MS) provide the most specific methods for measuring corticosteroids.[70,290] Cortisol methods based on capillary electrophoresis are also available.[157,281] All of these methods demonstrate high specificity for cortisol but have relatively low throughput and require sample preparation steps before analysis. For example, most HPLC methods require preanalytical extraction of cortisol with solid-phase extraction columns[319] or liquid-liquid extraction[181] prior to separation and detection by reversed- or normal-phase HPLC and a fluorescence or ultraviolet absorption detector.[113] A reference method for serum cortisol using isotope dilution GC/MS has been proposed.[142] GC/MS methods for cortisol typically require extraction of the hormone from plasma and conversion to the methoxime-trimethylsilyl derivative prior to analysis. Deuterated cortisol is available for use as the internal standard.

Although GC/MS has long been considered the standard for reference methods measuring organic compounds, liquid chromatography-tandem mass spectrometry (LC/MS-MS) methods are becoming increasingly common. Liquid chromatography has the advantage of not requiring volatile derivatives, so specimen preparation can be vastly simplified. LC/MS-MS methods have been developed that measure cortisol,[195,331] cortisol and corticosterone,[90] and multiple corticosteroids.[49,108,259,260] LC/MS-MS appears poised to become the method of choice for corticosteroid profiling.

Immunoassay

In routine laboratory practice, immunoassays are the most common methods used for measuring cortisol in serum and urine, and are widely available on various automated immunoassay platforms. Most cortisol immunoassays in routine use are heterogeneous, competitive-binding assays that require no initial extraction of steroids from the specimen. Cortisol is displaced from CBG and other endogenous binding proteins by (1) protein-binding agents such as ANS or salicylate, (2) low pH, or (3) heat treatment. The efficiency of cortisol displacement from proteins by agents such as ANS may be influenced by the concentration of binding proteins in the specimen. For example, the amount of ANS that is adequate for plasma obtained from healthy men and nonpregnant women may be insufficient to displace cortisol from CBG in pregnancy, when CBG concentrations are elevated.

Isotopic Methods

Radioimmunoassays (RIAs) for cortisol are predominantly of historical interest, having been widely replaced by nonisotopic assays. The tracer most commonly used in RIAs for total cortisol was iodine-125 (^{125}I). A variety of formats have been used in cortisol RIAs, including both solid- and liquid-phase capture antibodies, and a variety of methods for immobilizing antibodies (e.g., coated tube, glass beads, paramagnetic particles). Some commercial RIA kits for serum cortisol use liquid-phase double-antibody separations or solid-phase antibody suspensions. In double-antibody systems, a second antibody is used to precipitate the primary antibody after incubation with specimen and labeled antigen. Solid-phase suspension systems use antibodies bound to small particles that remain suspended in the reaction medium. After incubation, the suspended particles are separated by centrifugation and the radioactivity in the precipitate is measured.

Almost all commercial RIA methods for serum cortisol demonstrate some cross-reactivity with prednisolone, which is a metabolic product of prednisone. Therefore, these methods should be used with caution to measure cortisol in patients on prednisone therapy. The degree of cross-reactivity with 11-desoxycorticosterone, corticosterone, and prednisone varies from 1 to 5%, depending on the particular assay.[127] In patients with high plasma concentrations of 11-desoxycorticosterone (such as in 11α-hydroxylase deficiency or after administration of metyrapone), extraction with carbon tetrachloride to remove this steroid may be necessary to avoid significant interference.

Nonisotopic Methods

Most contemporary automated cortisol immunoassays use nonisotopic labels. Enzyme labels used in these immunoassays include horseradish peroxidase, alkaline phosphatase, or β-galactosidase, and enzyme activity has been measured using photometric,[136,161,172] fluorescent,[171] or chemiluminescent substrates.[354] Nonenzymatic approaches involve fluorescent and chemiluminescent[335] labels; these are the most common methods currently in use.[265] Both heterogeneous and homogeneous designs have been developed. Most current heterogeneous immunoassays for cortisol involve chemiluminescent labels and magnetic separation. Homogeneous immunoassays for cortisol include fluorescence polarization immunoassay (FPIA), enzyme-multiplied immunoassay technique (EMIT),[335] and the cloned enzyme donor immunoassay (CEDIA).[59] These assays do not require separation of bound and free fractions. Most immunoassay methods for cortisol are available on fully automated immunoassay systems.[265]

Other Methods

A highly sensitive method for measuring salivary cortisol using a biosensor based on nanolinking and surface plasmon resonance detection has been described.[207] This method had a detection limit of 49 pg/mL in human saliva, and the technology eventually may give rise to point-of-care instruments that measure salivary cortisol.

Specimen Collection and Storage[338]

Cortisol can be measured in serum, heparinized plasma, or ethylenediaminetetraacetic acid (EDTA) plasma, although some methods recommend against using EDTA plasma because of assay interference. In serum or plasma specimens, cortisol is stable for 7 days at room temperature or refrigerated, and is stable for 3 months frozen at −20 °C.

Comments

Blood cortisol concentrations parallel ACTH concentrations, with episodic and diurnal minima and maxima observed throughout the day. The cortisol concentration in the evening is normally less than 50% of the morning cortisol concentration. Increased cortisol is associated with (1) stress, (2) glucocorticoid therapy, (3) pregnancy, (4) depression, (5) hypoglycemia, and (6) hyperthyroidism. No significant difference in cortisol concentrations has been noted between men and women, and reference intervals for cortisol are not age dependent. The half-life of cortisol in the circulation is approximately 60 minutes,[338] so concentrations of this hormone in blood can change rapidly. In newborns, a transient rise in cortisol occurs immediately after delivery, but after 12 to 48 hours, cortisol declines to concentrations below umbilical cord blood concentrations; it then increases to a stable reference interval by about 1 week of age. Renal failure does not directly affect serum cortisol, but metabolites that are not cleared in the urine have the potential to cross-react with immunoassays, causing overestimation of blood cortisol concentrations. Extraction of cortisol into an organic solvent may eliminate interference from hydrophilic metabolites. Celite chromatography has been used to "clear" the sample of possible interference before immunoassay measurements are carried out in patients with renal failure.

Measurement of Free Cortisol

Free or unbound cortisol is the biologically active form of the circulating hormone; its concentration is buffered by the large reservoir bound to its transport proteins, CBG and albumin. Various methods have been developed to measure the free fraction of cortisol in serum, including ultrafiltration, equilibrium dialysis, and gel filtration, but these assays are technically demanding and expensive, and are not in general use.[99] Algorithms have been suggested for estimating the free cortisol concentration on the basis of CBG and albumin concentrations.[18,58,71]

Measurement of urinary cortisol provides an estimate of the free hormone concentration and for many years has been considered the gold standard screening test for Cushing disease,[37] although salivary cortisol has been recommended as the first-line diagnostic test.[227] Approximately 2% of total cortisol is excreted into the urine, and urinary cortisol may be used as a screening test for cortisol hypersecretion. However, β-hydroxycortisol also appears in the urine and may interfere with some immunoassays used to measure cortisol in urine.[170]

Measurement of cortisol in saliva (or oral fluid) is a practical and convenient way to assess the free hormone.[14,256] Salivary cortisol reflects the concentration of free cortisol in blood because CBG and albumin, the primary cortisol-binding proteins, do not appear in saliva. Most immunoassay kits for total serum cortisol can be used for the measurement of cortisol in saliva[221]; extraction is not required because saliva contains virtually no cortisol-binding proteins or other cortisol metabolites. The glycoproteins in saliva is precipitated by freezing and thawing followed by centrifugation, producing a clear fluid that is free of protein interference. At this point, the challenge in measuring salivary cortisol involves achieving an adequate lower limit of detection, because the concentration of cortisol in saliva is less than in serum or plasmal.

Immunoassays designed to measure total serum cortisol can be used to measure urinary (free) cortisol if cortisol metabolites and conjugates that cross-react with the anticortisol antibodies are removed. Because most interfering substances are more soluble in the aqueous urine matrix than cortisol, it can be partitioned into an organic solvent such as dichloromethane or ethyl acetate. Typically, the urine specimen is thoroughly mixed with the organic solvent; the two phases separate, and the organic layer containing the cortisol is removed. The organic solvent is evaporated to dryness, and the residue is resuspended in a buffer before analysis is begun. Extraction efficiency can be assessed by adding known amounts of cortisol (the method of standard additions) prior to extraction. Radiolabeled cortisol can be used to assess recovery of cortisol during the extraction procedure.

Unextracted urine may be assayed for cortisol if the antibody has sufficient selectivity, although reference values may differ from those seen in methods that include an extraction step.[208] Even with solvent extraction, most commercial assays for cortisol in urine are subject to interference and imprecision. Chromatographic procedures (such as HPLC) are more specific than immunoassays for measuring urinary cortisol; LC/MS-MS is emerging as the preferred method.[49,90,331]

Specimen Collection and Storage

A 24 hour urine specimen should be collected with 10 g of boric acid to maintain the urine pH below 7.5, and the urine should be refrigerated. After the total volume is measured, a thoroughly mixed aliquot may be stored at −20 °C prior to analysis. Care should be taken to ensure an appropriately timed, complete 24 hour collection because an incorrectly timed sample is the largest source of error with this method. Cortisol measurements on randomly collected urines are not useful. A 2009 report described falsely elevated urinary cortisol results attributed to interference from carbamazepine.[310] The drug interfered with the liquid chromatography method used for measuring urinary cortisol. It was also speculated that CYP3A4 induction by carbamazepine affected the results of the low-dose dexamethasone suppression test through enhanced metabolism of dexamethasone.

Cortisol is stable in saliva for 1 week at 4 °C and for 4 months when stored frozen. Freezing of specimens is recommended because it leads to precipitation of salivary glycoproteins and produces a nonviscous liquid supernatant that makes volumetric transfer by pipette more reliable.[208]

Measurement of urinary creatinine sometimes is used to assess the completeness of the collection, or to adjust concentrations of urinary constituents in spot urine collections for changes in urine specific gravity related to water intake. Diurnal variations in cortisol production, however, place greater importance on the integrity of the 24 hour urine specimen, in that daily cortisol excretion is what correlates with the functional adrenal status of the patient. Salivary cortisol measurements serve as a practical and convenient method to assess cortisol secretion in many patients. Morning salivary cortisol concentration is decreased in adrenal insufficiency; evening values are increased in Cushing syndrome.

Measurement of Aldosterone

Measurement of aldosterone is technically challenging, because the concentration of this hormone in blood is very low, nearly one thousandth that of the cortisol concentration. Immunoassays for measuring aldosterone in blood and urine are available. Radioimmunoassay methods for measuring aldosterone ordinarily use antibodies generated against an aldosterone-3-mono-oxime-bovine serum albumin (BSA) conjugate, an ^{125}I-labeled ligand, and ANS at pH 3.6 to displace aldosterone from binding proteins (primarily albumin). Although RIA methods for measuring aldosterone remain relatively common, nonisotopic immunoassays are becoming increasingly available.[302]

The cross-reactivity of antialdosterone antibodies with other adrenal steroids (e.g., DOC, corticosterone) is relatively low (<0.01%). Nevertheless, the concentration of potentially cross-reacting steroids sometimes is very high, requiring some purification of aldosterone before measurement. Unconjugated plasma aldosterone will extract into an organic solvent and can be purified by chromatography. The addition of tritiated aldosterone as an internal standard corrects for incomplete extraction. In urine, unconjugated steroids first are extracted into an organic solvent such as ethyl acetate or methylene chloride after acid hydrolysis of the conjugates. The solvent is evaporated, and the dried extract is reconstituted in a buffer before analysis. Whether the specimen requires purification depends on the diagnostic kit being used and the type of patient being evaluated. For example, specificity is not a significant concern in hypertensive adults without adrenal disease, whereas greater specificity may be needed for newborns and young infants, patients with adrenal disease, and pregnant women, in whom high concentrations of potentially interfering steroids are likely.

An automated heterogeneous immunoassay for aldosterone involving a monoclonal antialdosterone antibody and a chemiluminescent tracer has been validated against three RIA methods.[280] This method displays minimal (<0.05) cross-reactivity with corticosterone, cortisol, 11-desoxycorticosterone, 18-hydroxycorticosterone, and dexamethasone, and a linear range of 15 to 1200 ng/L. A time-resolved fluorescence immunoassay for measuring aldosterone in saliva was described in 2010.[188] LC/MS-MS has also been applied to aldosterone measurements[306]; these results were in close agreement with RIA measurements. The LC/MS-MS method has a detection limit of 69 pmol/L and a linearity up to 5.5 nmol/L.

Specimen Collection and Storage[338,355]

If possible, the patient should be in an upright position (standing or seated) for at least 2 hours before collection. Plasma (heparin or EDTA) or serum is suitable for aldosterone measurement, although EDTA plasma is preferred. The aldosterone concentration in specimens stored at room temperature begins to decline after 24 hours, although little change in aldosterone was observed in unseparated blood specimens stored at 32 °C for 24 hours. The aldosterone concentration in refrigerated or frozen specimens is stable for at least 4 days. For urine assays, a 24 hour urine specimen should be collected with boric acid as a preservative.

Measurement of 17-Hydroxyprogesterone

The most common cause of congenital adrenal hyperplasia (CAH) is a deficiency in the 21α-hydroxylase enzyme (CYP21), which converts 17-hydroxyprogesterone (17-OHP) to 11-desoxycortisol. 17-OHP is also elevated in CYP11B1-11-beta-hydroxylase deficiency CAH. Therefore, measurement of serum or plasma 17-OHP can be used to diagnose almost all cases of CAH. In 21α-hydroxylase deficiency, 17-OHP concentrations may reach several hundred times the upper limit of normal.

Radioimmunoassays for 17-OHP that use antibodies against 17-hydroxyprogesterone-3-carboxymethyloxime-BSA are available; these methods can be used with serum, plasma, saliva, and even amniotic fluid. Monoclonal antibody–based methods have also been described.[50] In addition to radioiodinated tracers,[73,123,328] nonisotopic labels used in 17-OHP immunoassays include enzymes with photometric, fluorescent, or chemiluminescent substrates,[50,51,184,314] and fluorescence-based immunoassays using fluorescein or streptavidin-europium labels,[75] and chemiluminescent labels.[12] Despite the use of highly specific antisera, most immunoassays are susceptible to interference by other corticosteroids that may be present in neonatal and infant plasma specimens.[186,344]

Methods for measuring 17-OHP in serum by gas chromatography/mass spectrometry[185] and LC/MS-MS[82,261,316] have been described. For chromatographic analysis, 17-OHP is typically extracted using a liquid-liquid (diethylether/diethylacetate,[316] methyl-tert-butyl-ether[267]), solid-phase,[82] or on-line[108,261] extraction procedure; these methods have detection limits below 1 nmol/L. LC/MS-MS methods for measuring 17-OHP in dried blood spots obtained from neonates[121,137] and in urine[49] are also available.

Specimen Collection and Storage

Most reports of analytical methods for measuring 17-OHP use serum, although plasma has also been used. Specimens have been stored at 4 °C for up to 4 days or at −20 °C for up to 1 month. 17-OHP was stable in unseparated blood at room temperature for 1 week.[69]

Screening newborns for 21α-hydroxylase deficiency has been possible since the introduction of 17-OHP immunoassays in 1977.[242] Neonatal specimens can be obtained by heel puncture and collected in capillary tubes or on filter paper. Dried blood specimens are stable and easily transported and are widely used to screen newborns for metabolic defects. It has been reported that the presence of EDTA in dried blood specimens may interfere with 17-OHP results measured by immunometric methods based on lanthanide fluorescence.[125] The utility of salivary 17-OHP measurements has been reviewed,[220] and the principal advantage is ease of collection.[105]

Measurement of 11-Desoxycortisol

Serum or plasma 11-desoxycortisol (compound S) measurements are used to detect 11β-hydroxylase (or C-11 hydroxylase) deficiency or as part of the metyrapone stimulation test. Metyrapone inhibits the 11β-hydroxylase enzyme, and a 40- to 80-fold increase in plasma 11-desoxycortisol is observed after metyrapone stimulation in patients with normal pituitary-adrenal reserve. As a consequence, analytical methods for 11-desoxycortisol in metyrapone stimulation tests do not require particularly high sensitivity.

Radioimmunoassay methods for the direct determination of plasma 11-desoxycortisol are available.[250] Antiserum raised against 11-desoxycortisol-3-carboxymethyloxime-BSA has provided appropriate specificity with minimal cross-reactivity against other adrenal steroids. Some radioimmunoassay methods include an extraction step or column chromatography, or both.[66,84] Nonisotopic methods for measuring 11-desoxycortisol in serum have been described, including enzyme immunoassays,[155,173] fluorometric methods,[88,330] and fluorescence polarization.[2] One method[132] for measurement of 11-desoxycortisol involves the "open-sandwich enzyme immunoassay" technique, which is based on the reassociation of two cloned antibody variable regions) by a bridging antigen.

Liquid chromatography/tandem mass spectrometry methods for measuring 11-desoxycortisol have been described, mostly as part of corticosteroid profiles.[49,108,259,260,267] These methods typically involve liquid-liquid extraction into an organic solvent, although solid-phase extraction has been used as well.[49]

Specimen Collection and Storage

Most of the methods used for measuring 11-desoxycortisol have used serum, although use of plasma and urine are also used. Data in the literature on the stability of 11-desoxycortisol in stored specimens are lacking.

Measurement of Renin

Methods for measuring renin have been the subject of two reviews,[45,277] upon which most of the following discussion is based.

Circulating concentrations of prorenin may be as many as 100-fold greater than the concentration of renin (although a 10:1 ratio of prorenin to renin is more common); therefore even minimal cross-reactivity of prorenin with antirenin antibodies used in immunoassays to measure renin can be problematic. Assays exist to measure plasma renin activity (by monitoring the production of angiotensin I) or the mass of renin by immunoassay. Each approach has advantages and disadvantages.

Measuring Renin Activity

Measuring renin activity (traditionally called "plasma renin activity," or PRA) provides an indication of the biologically active fraction of renin in the specimen, because it measures the primary function of the enzyme, which is the conversion of angiotensinogen to angiotensin I. Renin activity measurements, however, are difficult to standardize, and two general approaches are used to measure renin activity. In the classic PRA method, first described in 1975,[94] inhibitors of angiotensinase and angiotensin-converting enzyme (ACE) are added to prevent the conversion of angiotensin I to angiotensin II (some methods "trap" angiotensin I with an antibody to prevent its conversion to angiotensin II), the specimen is incubated at 37 °C, and production of angiotensin I is measured. The rate of the reaction is influenced by pH, incubation time, and, most important, the endogenous angiotensinogen concentration in the specimen (which can be increased in pregnancy, glucocorticoid excess, and estrogen administration). Because the angiotensinogen concentration in blood does not ordinarily exceed the K_m for the renin-angiotensinogen complex, its concentration is rate limiting. Therefore, the classic PRA method produces results that vary significantly, depending on the endogenous concentration of angiotensinogen. An ELISA method has been described to measure angiotensinogen.[141] PRA procedures are also susceptible to variability associated with storage conditions.[42]

Although several variations of the classic PRA method exist, a typical approach involves the preparation of two aliquots of plasma. One of the aliquots is incubated at 37 °C for 3 hours, and the other is kept at 4 °C (renin is not active at cold temperature). Following the incubation period, angiotensin I is measured by RIA in both aliquots, and the difference between the two reflects the renin activity, expressed as pg of angiotensin I per mL of plasma. The specificity of the PRA assay can be validated using plasma from anephric patients or deangiotensinized plasma.[68]

A second approach to measuring renin activity uses exogenous angiotensinogen as substrate and thereby avoids the variability associated with endogenous angiotensinogen concentrations. This approach is sometimes called *plasma renin concentration assay,*[45,277] which is a confusing term in that the assay still involves the measurement of activity, rather than concentration. Furthermore, the term is not consistently applied; *plasma renin concentration* has been used in reference to immunoassays that measure the renin concentration, rather than activity.[16,42]

These renin activity methods use angiotensinogen derived from plasma collected from nephrectomized sheep; it is added at a concentration that is several times the K_m for the renin-angiotensinogen complex, ensuring that the reaction rate is limited by renin activity alone. The advantage of using a consistent source of angiotensinogen is that the activity assays can be calibrated against renin reference materials; an International Reference Preparation of human renin (68/356), validated by bioassay, has been available since 1975.[17]

Prorenin exists in two forms, depending on whether the 46 amino acid "pro" segment is in an "open" or "closed" conformation. The open conformation of prorenin has the active site of the enzyme exposed, so this form is enzymatically active. In the blood, approximately 2% of prorenin is in the open conformation, but assay conditions such as cooling and low pH can cause the closed conformation of prorenin to open, which results in an overestimate of physiologic renin activity. Incubation of plasma at 22 °C for 24 hours reversibly activates (unfolds) approximately 5% of prorenin,[65] although incubation at 37 °C promotes refolding of the "pro" segment to its closed form.[252] In some assays, the closed prorenin is deliberately opened by acidification (pH 3.3) or incubation with trypsin, which removes the "pro" segment from prorenin altogether. These assays measure total renin and prorenin by activating all of the prorenin and following with a standard renin activity assay.[284]

Care must be taken when measuring and interpreting renin activity in patients who are taking renin inhibitors, a relatively new class of drugs used to treat essential hypertension. Aliskiren was the first member of this class of drugs to be approved by the U.S. Food and Drug Administration (FDA). Renin activity will be suppressed in these patients, although renin and prorenin concentrations will be high.[45,277]

Measuring Angiotensin I and II

All renin activity assays rely on angiotensin I as a direct measure of renin activity and a surrogate marker for angiotensin II, which is the active form of the hormone. Angiotensin II has a very short half-life (1 to 2 minutes), and is difficult to measure.[48] Monoclonal antibodies with high affinity and specificity have been produced against angiotensin II. These have been used to develop a direct radioimmunoassay; as little as 0.8 fmol of angiotensin II in 2 mL of plasma has been detected without interference from angiotensin I.[296] When angiotensinogen and ACE are in sufficient supply, however, the concentration of the prohormone angiotensin I is a reliable estimate of renin activity and angiotensin II concentration in blood.[45] Most angiotensin I methods involve radioimmunoassay, but enzyme immunoassays,[128,278] HPLC,[154] and fluorescence polarization methods[183] have also been described. A 2009 report described a homogeneous immunoassay for angiotensin I that is based on luminescent oxygen channeling, a technology involving chemiluminescence stimulated by photoexcited singlet oxygen.[47]

Angiotensin I and angiotensin II have poor immunogenicity because of their small molecular size. They must be conjugated to proteins such as albumin, hemocyanin, or succinylated polylysine to be sufficiently immunogenic to elicit antibodies. Polyclonal antisera usually lack sufficient specificity to distinguish between the decapeptide, heptapeptide, and hexapeptide angiotensins. Problems associated with immunoassay of angiotensins have been reviewed.[284] Angiotensins are labile oligopeptides in plasma and can be generated in vitro even in frozen plasma. Therefore great care must be taken in the collection and storage of specimens for angiotensin assays.[118]

With continued improvement and availability of nonisotopic immunometric assays for direct measurement of the concentration of renin, activity assays may soon be replaced by direct mass assays for routine assessment of plasma renin. However, because physicians are so familiar with PRA testing results, renin mass assays will require realignment of physician practices.

Measuring Renin Concentration

As an alternative to the PRA assay, the concentration of renin can be measured by immunoassay (these methods are sometimes called *direct renin assays* or *mass assays*). As discussed previously, immunoassays for renin cross-react with prorenin in both closed and open conformations, and assays based on monoclonal antibodies are likely to have the highest specificity for renin. A variety of monoclonal immunoradiometric assays (IRMAs) for renin have been developed, some of which measure renin and prorenin in the open configuration, and others that measure all forms of renin and prorenin.[45] An example of a two-site IRMA was described by Simon and coworkers.[295] This assay uses two monoclonal antibodies, and the specificity of the assay was verified by immunoprecipitation of prorenin with a monoclonal antibody directed to the "pro" sequence. The method had a limit of detection of 3.5 ng/L and is linear from 7 to 270 ng/L. Immunochemiluminometric (ICL) methods for renin are also available, and the results of these assays have been correlated with IRMA results. One such assay[62] involves a biotinylated capture antibody (which recognizes both renin and prorenin) immobilized to streptavidin-coated magnetic particles, and an acridinium ester–labeled signal antibody that recognizes only renin.[120] The chemiluminescent assay had a limit of detection of less than 0.1 mU/L and a functional sensitivity (CV <20%) of 2.6 mU/L.

Direct renin immunoassays (both IRMA and ICL) have been compared with renin activity assays.[115] With direct renin results expressed in mIU/L, and PRA results expressed in $ng \bullet mL^{-1} \bullet h^{-1}$, the overall correlation coefficient was 0.98, and the standard error of the residuals was 11.8 mU/L. Better interlaboratory agreement with direct renin assay results compared with PRA has been reported.[212]

The aldosterone-to-renin ratio (ARR), based on aldosterone concentration and PRA, was proposed[122] in 1981 as a sensitive screening test for primary hyperaldosteronism in normokalemic patients. The screening thresholds for ARR have been re-established using measurements of renin concentration, rather than activity.[87]

Specimen Collection and Storage

EDTA plasma is typically used for PRA assays. After centrifugation, plasma should be removed and frozen at −20 °C or lower, although the renin concentration is stable in unseparated blood at room temperature for up to 6 hours. Plasma for PRA can be stored frozen up to 1 month before assay, but freeze-thaw cycles should be avoided because of the possible activation of prorenin. At the time of collection, blood should not be chilled or placed on ice because irreversible cryoactivation of prorenin can occur, leading to falsely high estimates of PRA. Serum or plasma collected in another anticoagulant can also be used as long as EDTA is added (3 mmol/L) before incubation, because it inhibits ACE. Cryoactivation of prorenin, however, is more likely in serum than in plasma. Hemolyzed specimens should not be used because red blood cells contain angiotensinases.

The patient should be ambulatory for 2 hours before blood collection. A 24 hour urine specimen for sodium is often collected on the day before the renin test to reference the result to salt intake. Specimens with high renin activity can generate considerable amounts of angiotensin I before and during storage even at −20 °C. This will not affect results, however, because angiotensin I is determined with and without the incubation step.

REFERENCES

1. Ahmed SB, Fisher ND, Stevanovic R, Hollenberg NK. Body mass index and angiotensin-dependent control of the renal circulation in healthy humans. Hypertension 2005;6:1316-20.
2. Al-Ansari AA, Massoud M, Perry LA, Smith DS. Polarization fluoroimmunoassay of 11-deoxycortisol in serum and saliva. Clin Chem 1983;10:1803-5.
3. al-Jubouri MA. Isolated aldosterone deficiency progressing to Addison's disease in a 4-year-old girl. Ann Clin Biochem 1994;31 (Pt 4):391-2.
4. Alkatib AA, Cosma M, Elamin MB, Erickson D, Swiglo BA, Erwin PJ, et al. A systematic review and meta-analysis of randomized placebo-controlled trials of DHEA treatment effects on quality of life in women with adrenal insufficiency. J Clin Endocrinol Metab 2009;10:3676-81.
5. Alzahrani AS, Al-Khaldi N, Shi Y, Al-Rijjal RA, Zou M, Baitei EY, et al. Diagnosis by serendipity: Cushing syndrome attributable to cortisol-producing adrenal adenoma as the initial manifestation of multiple endocrine neoplasia type 1 due to a rare splicing site MEN1 gene mutation. Endocr Pract 2008;5:595-602.
6. Anagnostis P, Karagiannis A, Tziomalos K, Kakafika AI, Athyros VG, Mikhailidis DP. Adrenal incidentaloma: a diagnostic challenge. Hormones (Athens) 2009;3:163-84.
7. Andrew R. Clinical measurement of steroid metabolism. Best Pract Res Clin Endocrinol Metab 2001;1:1-16.
8. Andrioli M, Pecori GF, Cavagnini F. Isolated corticotrophin deficiency. Pituitary 2006;4:289-95.
9. Andrioli M, Pecori GF, De Martin M, Cattaneo A, Carzaniga C, Cavagnini F. Differential diagnosis of ACTH-dependent hypercortisolism: imaging versus laboratory. Pituitary 2009;4:294-6.
10. Antal Z, Zhou P. Congenital adrenal hyperplasia: diagnosis, evaluation, and management. Pediatr Rev 2009;7:e49-57.
11. Arafah BM. Hypothalamic pituitary adrenal function during critical illness: limitations of current assessment methods. J Clin Endocrinol Metab 2006;10:3725-45.
12. Arakawa H, Maeda M, Tsuji A. Chemiluminescence enzyme immunoassay of 17 alpha-hydroxyprogesterone using glucose oxidase and bis(2,4,6-trichlorophenyl) oxalate-fluorescent dye system. Chem Pharm Bull (Tokyo) 1982;8:3036-9.
13. Asbert M, Jimenez W, Gaya J, Gines P, Arroyo V, Rivera F, et al. Assessment of the renin-angiotensin system in cirrhotic patients: comparison between plasma renin activity and direct measurement of immunoreactive renin. J Hepatol 1992;1-2:179-83.
14. Atkinson KR, Lo KR, Payne SR, Mitchell JS, Ingram JR. Rapid saliva processing techniques for near real-time analysis of salivary steroids and protein. J Clin Lab Anal 2008;6:395-402.
15. Auchus RJ. The genetics, pathophysiology, and management of human deficiencies of P450c17. Endocrinol Metab Clin North Am 2001;1: 101-19, vii.
16. Azizi M, Menard J. Measurement of plasma renin: a critical review of methodology. J Renin Angiotensin Aldosterone Syst 2010;11: 89-90.
17. Bangham DR, Robertson I, Robertson JI, Robinson CJ, Tree M. An international collaborative study of renin assay: establishment of the international reference preparation of human renin. Clin Sci Mol Med Suppl 1975;2:135a-59s.
18. Barsano CP, Baumann G. Simple algebraic and graphic methods for the apportionment of hormone (and receptor) into bound and free fractions in binding equilibria; or how to calculate bound and free hormone? Endocrinology 1989;3:1101-6.
19. Batista DL, Courcoutsakis N, Riar J, Keil MF, Stratakis CA. Severe obesity confounds the interpretation of low-dose dexamethasone test combined with the administration of ovine corticotrophin-releasing hormone in childhood Cushing syndrome. J Clin Endocrinol Metab 2008;11:4323-30.
20. Batlle DC, Kurtzman NA. Clinical disorders of aldosterone metabolism. Dis Mon 1984;8:1-55.
21. Baumann-Antczak A, Wedlock N, Bednarek J, Kiso Y, Krishnan H, Fowler S, et al. Autoimmune Addison's disease and 21-hydroxylase. Lancet 1992;8816:429-30.
22. Bednarek J, Furmaniak J, Wedlock N, Kiso Y, Baumann-Antczak A, Fowler S, et al. Steroid 21-hydroxylase is a major autoantigen involved in adult onset autoimmune Addison's disease. FEBS Lett 1992;1:51-5.
23. Benchetrit S, Bernheim J, Podjarny E. Normokalemic hyperaldosteronism in patients with resistant hypertension. Isr Med Assoc J 2002;1:17-20.
24. Berneis K, Staub JJ, Gessler A, Meier C, Girard J, Muller B. Combined stimulation of adrenocorticotropin and compound-S by single dose metyrapone test as an outpatient procedure to assess hypothalamic-pituitary-adrenal function. J Clin Endocrinol Metab 2002;12:5470-5.
25. Bertagna X, Groussin L, Luton JP, Bertherat J. Aberrant receptor-mediated Cushing's syndrome. Horm Res 2003;59(suppl 1):99-103.
26. Bertagna X, Guignat L, Groussin L, Bertherat J. Cushing's disease. Best Pract Res Clin Endocrinol Metab 2009;5:607-23.
27. Betterle C, Coco G, Zanchetta R. Adrenal cortex autoantibodies in subjects with normal adrenal function. Best Pract Res Clin Endocrinol Metab 2005;1:85-99.
28. Betterle C, Scalici C, Pedini B, Mantero F. [Addison's disease: principal clinical associations and description of natural history of the disease.] Ann Ital Med Int 1989;3:195-206.
29. Betterle C, Scalici C, Presotto F, Pedini B, Moro L, Rigon F, et al. The natural history of adrenal function in autoimmune patients with adrenal autoantibodies. J Endocrinol 1988;3:467-75.
30. Betterle C, Volpato M, Rees SB, Furmaniak J, Chen S, Greggio NA, et al. I. Adrenal cortex and steroid 21-hydroxylase autoantibodies in adult patients with organ-specific autoimmune diseases: markers of low progression to clinical Addison's disease. J Clin Endocrinol Metab 1997;3:932-8.
31. Betterle C, Volpato M, Rees SB, Furmaniak J, Chen S, Zanchetta R, et al. II. Adrenal cortex and steroid 21-hydroxylase autoantibodies in children with organ-specific autoimmune diseases: markers of high progression to clinical Addison's disease. J Clin Endocrinol Metab 1997;3:939-42.
32. Betterle C, Zanette F, Zanchetta R, Pedini B, Trevisan A, Mantero F, et al. Complement-fixing adrenal autoantibodies as a marker for predicting onset of idiopathic Addison's disease. Lancet 1983;8336: 1238-41.
33. Bhagra S, Nippoldt TB, Nair KS. Dehydroepiandrosterone in adrenal insufficiency and ageing. Curr Opin Endocrinol Diabetes Obes 2008; 3:239-43.
34. Biddie SC, Hager GL. Glucocorticoid receptor dynamics and gene regulation. Stress 2009;3:193-205.
35. Biglieri EG, Stockigt JR, Schambelan M. A preliminary evaluation for primary aldosteronism. Arch Intern Med 1970;6:1004-7.
36. Boikos SA, Stratakis CA. Carney complex: the first 20 years. Curr Opin Oncol 2007;1:24-9.
37. Boscaro M, Arnaldi G. Approach to the patient with possible Cushing's syndrome. J Clin Endocrinol Metab 2009;9:3121-31.
38. Boscaro M, Ronconi V, Turchi F, Giacchetti G. Diagnosis and management of primary aldosteronism. Curr Opin Endocrinol Diabetes Obes 2008;4:332-8.
39. Bouillon R. Acute adrenal insufficiency. Endocrinol Metab Clin North Am 2006;4:767-75, ix.
40. Bourne RS, Webber SJ, Hutchinson SP. Adrenal axis testing and corticosteroid replacement therapy in septic shock patients—local and national perspectives. Anaesthesia 2003;6:591-6.
41. Bright GM, Singh I. Adrenal autoantibodies bind to adrenal subcellular fractions enriched in cytochrome-c reductase and 5′-nucleotidase. J Clin Endocrinol Metab 1990;1:95-9.
42. Brossaud J, Corcuff JB. Pre-analytical and analytical considerations for the determination of plasma renin activity. Clin Chim Acta 2009;1-2: 90-2.
43. Brunner HR, Nussberger J, Waeber B. Responsiveness of renin secretion: a key mechanism in the maintenance of blood pressure. J Hypertens Suppl 1986;4:S89-94.

44. Burry LD, Wax RS. Role of corticosteroids in septic shock. Ann Pharmacother 2004;3:464-72.
45. Campbell DJ, Nussberger J, Stowasser M, Danser AH, Morganti A, Frandsen E, et al. Activity assays and immunoassays for plasma renin and prorenin: information provided and precautions necessary for accurate measurement. Clin Chem 2009;5:867-77.
46. Canalis E, Reardon GE, Caldarella AM. A more specific, liquid-chromatographic method for free cortisol in urine. Clin Chem 1982;12:2418-20.
47. Cauchon E, Liu S, Percival MD, Rowland SE, Xu D, Binkert C, et al. Development of a homogeneous immunoassay for the detection of angiotensin I in plasma using AlphaLISA acceptor beads technology. Anal Biochem 2009;1:134-9.
48. Cawood ML. Measurement of plasma renin activity. Methods Mol Biol 2006;324:187-96.
49. Cho HJ, Kim JD, Lee WY, Chung BC, Choi MH. Quantitative metabolic profiling of 21 endogenous corticosteroids in urine by liquid chromatography-triple quadrupole-mass spectrometry. Anal Chim Acta 2009;1:101-8.
50. Chong H, Cheah SH, Ragavan M, Johgalingam VT. Production and characterization of monoclonal antibodies against 17alpha-hydroxyprogesterone. Hybridoma (Larchmt) 2006;1:34-40.
51. Chong H, Cheah SH, Ragavan M, Johgalingam VT. Development of an indirect enzyme immunoassay using monoclonal antibodies for the measurement of 17alpha-hydroxyprogesterone in human serum. J Immunoassay Immunochem 2009;2:166-79.
52. Chrousos GP, Loriaux DL, Mann D, Cutler GB Jr. Late-onset 21-hydroxylase deficiency is an allelic variant of congenital adrenal hyperplasia characterized by attenuated clinical expression and different HLA haplotype associations. Horm Res 1982;4:193-200.
53. Cirimele V, Kintz P, Dumestre V, Goulle JP, Ludes B. Identification of ten corticosteroids in human hair by liquid chromatography-ion spray mass spectrometry. Forensic Sci Int 2000;1-3:381-8.
54. Clark AJ, Chan LF, Chung TT, Metherell LA. The genetics of familial glucocorticoid deficiency. Best Pract Res Clin Endocrinol Metab 2009;2:159-65.
55. Coco G, Dal PC, Presotto F, Albergoni MP, Canova C, Pedini B, et al. Estimated risk for developing autoimmune Addison's disease in patients with adrenal cortex autoantibodies. J Clin Endocrinol Metab 2006;5:1637-45.
56. Contreras P, Araya V. [Cushing's syndrome: review of a national caseload.] Rev Med Chil 1995;3:350-62.
57. Conzo G, Tricarico A, Belli G, Candela S, Corcione F, Del GG, et al. Adrenal incidentalomas in the laparoscopic era and the role of correct surgical indications: observations from 255 consecutive adrenalectomies in an Italian series. Can J Surg 2009;6:E281-5.
58. Coolens JL, Van BH, Heyns W. Clinical use of unbound plasma cortisol as calculated from total cortisol and corticosteroid-binding globulin. J Steroid Biochem 1987;2:197-202.
59. Coty WA, Loor R, Bellet N, Khanna PL, Kaspar P, Baier M. CEDIA—homogeneous immunoassays for the 1990s and beyond. Wien Klin Wochenschr Suppl 1992;191:5-11.
60. Crapo L. Cushing's syndrome: a review of diagnostic tests. Metabolism 1979;9:955-77.
61. Czock D, Keller F, Rasche FM, Haussler U. Pharmacokinetics and pharmacodynamics of systemically administered glucocorticoids. Clin Pharmacokinet 2005;1:61-98.
62. de Bruin RA, Bouhuizen A, Diederich S, Perschel FH, Boomsma F, Deinum J. Validation of a new automated renin assay. Clin Chem 2004;11:2111-6.
63. De Bosscher K, Haegeman G. Minireview: latest perspectives on antiinflammatory actions of glucocorticoids. Mol Endocrinol 2009;3:281-91.
64. De Rosa G, Corsello SM, Cecchini L, Della CS, Testa A. A clinical study of Addison's disease. Exp Clin Endocrinol 1987;2:232-42.
65. Deinum J, Derkx FH, Schalekamp MA. Improved immunoradiometric assay for plasma renin. Clin Chem 1999;6(Pt 1):847-54.
66. Demers LM, Ebright L, Derck DD. Improved radioimmunoassay for 11-deoxycortisol (compound S) in plasma. Clin Chem 1979;10:1704-7.
67. Deuschle M, Schweiger U, Weber B, Gotthardt U, Korner A, Schmider J, et al. Diurnal activity and pulsatility of the hypothalamus-pituitary-adrenal system in male depressed patients and healthy controls. J Clin Endocrinol Metab 1997;1:234-8.
68. Dillon MJ. Measurement of plasma renin activity by semi-micro radioimmunoassay of generated angiotensin I. J Clin Pathol 1975;8:625-30.
69. Diver MJ, Hughes JG, Hutton JL, West CR, Hipkin LJ. The long-term stability in whole blood of 14 commonly-requested hormone analytes. Ann Clin Biochem 1994;31(Pt 6):561-5.
70. Dodds HM, Taylor PJ, Cannell GR, Pond SM. A high-performance liquid chromatography-electrospray-tandem mass spectrometry analysis of cortisol and metabolites in placental perfusate. Anal Biochem 1997;2:342-7.
71. Dorin RI, Pai HK, Ho JT, Lewis JG, Torpy DJ, Urban FK III, et al. Validation of a simple method of estimating plasma free cortisol: role of cortisol binding to albumin. Clin Biochem 2009;1-2:64-71.
72. Drexhage HA. Autoimmune adrenocortical failure. In: Volpe R, ed. Contemporary endocrinology: autoimmune endocrinopathies. Totowa, NJ: Humana Press, 1999:309-36.
73. Dyas J, Read GF, Guha-Maulik T, Hughes IA, Riad-Fahmy D. A rapid assay for 17 alpha OH-progesterone in plasma, saliva and amniotic fluid using a magnetisable solid-phase antiserum. Ann Clin Biochem 1984;21(Pt 5):417-24.
74. Ebeling PR. Death after failure to diagnose Addison disease. Aust Fam Physician 2008;1-2:6.
75. el-Gamal BA, Eremin SA, Smith DS, Landon J. Development of a direct fluoroimmunoassay for serum levels of 17-hydroxyprogesterone. Ann Clin Biochem 1988;48:35-41.
76. Elamin MB, Murad MH, Mullan R, Erickson D, Harris K, Nadeem S, et al. Accuracy of diagnostic tests for Cushing's syndrome: a systematic review and metaanalyses. J Clin Endocrinol Metab 2008;5:1553-62.
77. Elias LL, Clark AJ. The expression of the ACTH receptor. Braz J Med Biol Res 2000;10:1245-8.
78. Else T, Hammer GD. Genetic analysis of adrenal absence: agenesis and aplasia. Trends Endocrinol Metab 2005;10:458-68.
79. Endert E, Ouwehand A, Fliers E, Prummel MF, Wiersinga WM. Establishment of reference values for endocrine tests. Part IV. Adrenal insufficiency. Neth J Med 2005;11:435-43.
80. Erichsen MM, Lovas K, Skinningsrud B, Wolff AB, Undlien DE, Svartberg J, et al. Clinical, immunological, and genetic features of autoimmune primary adrenal insufficiency: observations from a Norwegian registry. J Clin Endocrinol Metab 2009;12:4882-90.
81. Erickson D, Natt N, Nippoldt T, Young WF Jr, Carpenter PC, Petterson T, et al. Dexamethasone-suppressed corticotropin-releasing hormone stimulation test for diagnosis of mild hypercortisolism. J Clin Endocrinol Metab 2007;8:2972-6.
82. Etter ML, Eichhorst J, Lehotay DC. Clinical determination of 17-hydroxyprogesterone in serum by LC-MS/MS: comparison to Coat-A-Count RIA method. J Chromatogr B Analyt Technol Biomed Life Sci 2006;1:69-74.
83. Fenske M. Determination of cortisol in human plasma by thin-layer chromatography and fluorescence derivatization with isonicotinic acid hydrazide. J Chromatogr Sci 2008;1:1-3.
84. Fernandes VT, Ribeiro-Neto LM, Lima SB, Vieira JG, Verreschi IT, Kater CE. Reversed-phase high performance liquid chromatography separation of adrenal steroids prior to radioimmunoassay: application in congenital adrenal hyperplasia. J Chromatogr Sci 2003;5:251-4.
85. Fernandez-Real JM, Ricart-Engel W, Simo R. Pre-clinical Cushing's syndrome: report of three cases and literature review. Horm Res 1994;5-6:230-5.
86. Ferrari P, Krozowski Z. Role of the 11beta-hydroxysteroid dehydrogenase type 2 in blood pressure regulation. Kidney Int 2000;4:1374-81.

87. Ferrari P, Shaw SG, Nicod J, Saner E, Nussberger J. Active renin versus plasma renin activity to define aldosterone-to-renin ratio for primary aldosteronism. J Hypertens 2004;2:377-81.
88. Fiet J, Giton F, Boudou P, Villette JM, Soliman H, Morineau G, et al. A new specific and sensitive time resolved-fluoroimmunoassay of 11-deoxycortisol in serum. J Steroid Biochem Mol Biol 2001;2-3:143-50.
89. Fleseriu M, Gassner M, Yedinak C, Chicea L, Delashaw JB Jr, Loriaux DL. Normal hypothalamic-pituitary-adrenal axis by high-dose cosyntropin testing in patients with abnormal response to low-dose cosyntropin stimulation: a retrospective review. Endocr Pract 2010;1:64-70.
90. Fong BM, Tam S, Leung KS. Improved liquid chromatography-tandem mass spectrometry method in clinical utility for the diagnosis of Cushing's syndrome. Anal Bioanal Chem 2010;2:783-90.
91. Franchimont D. Overview of the actions of glucocorticoids on the immune response: a good model to characterize new pathways of immunosuppression for new treatment strategies. Ann N Y Acad Sci 2004;1024:124-37.
92. Freeman DA. Steroid hormone-producing tumors in man. Endocr Rev 1986;2:204-20.
93. Fujii K, Morimoto I, Wake A, Okada Y, Inokuchi N, Ishida O, et al. Adrenal insufficiency in a patient with acquired immunodeficiency syndrome. Endocr J 1994;1:13-8.
94. Fyhrquist F, Soveri P, Puutula L, Stenman UH. Radioimmunoassay of plasma renin activity. Clin Chem 1976;2:250-6.
95. Gallardo E, Queiroz JA. The role of alternative specimens in toxicological analysis. Biomed Chromatogr 2008;8:795-821.
96. Ganguly A. New insights and questions about glucocorticoid-suppressible hyperaldosteronism. Am J Med 1982;6:851-4.
97. Ganguly A. Distinguishing unilateral aldosteronoma from bilateral disease. J Clin Endocrinol Metab 2001;8:4004-5.
98. Garcia C, Biller BM, Klibanski A. The role of the clinical laboratory in the diagnosis of Cushing syndrome. Am J Clin Pathol 2003; 120(suppl):S38-45.
99. Gatti R, Antonelli G, Prearo M, Spinella P, Cappellin E, De Palo EF. Cortisol assays and diagnostic laboratory procedures in human biological fluids. Clin Biochem 2009;12:1205-17.
100. Ghayee HK, Auchus RJ. Basic concepts and recent developments in human steroid hormone biosynthesis. Rev Endocr Metab Disord 2007;4:289-300.
101. Giacchetti G, Mulatero P, Mantero F, Veglio F, Boscaro M, Fallo F. Primary aldosteronism, a major form of low renin hypertension: from screening to diagnosis. Trends Endocrinol Metab 2008;3:104-8.
102. Goncalves J, Friaes A, Moura L. Congenital adrenal hyperplasia: focus on the molecular basis of 21-hydroxylase deficiency. Expert Rev Mol Med 2007;11:1-23.
103. Goonasekera CD, Shah V, Wade AM, Dillon MJ. The usefulness of renal vein renin studies in hypertensive children: a 25-year experience. Pediatr Nephrol 2002;11:943-9.
104. Gradman AH. Evolving understanding of the renin-angiotensin-aldosterone system: pathophysiology and targets for therapeutic intervention. Am Heart J 2009;6(suppl):S1-6.
105. Groschl M, Rauh M, Dorr HG. Cortisol and 17-hydroxyprogesterone kinetics in saliva after oral administration of hydrocortisone in children and young adolescents with congenital adrenal hyperplasia due to 21-hydroxylase deficiency. J Clin Endocrinol Metab 2002;3:1200-4.
106. Gross MD, Djekidel M, Hay RV, Rubello D. Scintigraphic localization of adrenal tumors. Minerva Endocrinol 2009;2:171-84.
107. Grossman AB, Kelly P, Rockall A, Bhattacharya S, McNicol A, Barwick T. Cushing's syndrome caused by an occult source: difficulties in diagnosis and management. Nat Clin Pract Endocrinol Metab 2006; 11:642-7.
108. Guo T, Taylor RL, Singh RJ, Soldin SJ. Simultaneous determination of 12 steroids by isotope dilution liquid chromatography-photospray ionization tandem mass spectrometry. Clin Chim Acta 2006;1-2:76-82.
109. Hackman KL, Davis AL, Curnow PA, Serpell JW, McLean CA, Topliss DJ. Cushing syndrome in a young woman due to primary pigmented nodular adrenal disease. Endocr Pract 2010;1:84-8.
110. Hadley ME, Haskell-Luevano C. The proopiomelanocortin system. Ann N Y Acad Sci 1999;885:1-21.
111. Hammond GL, Smith CL, Underhill DA. Molecular studies of corticosteroid binding globulin structure, biosynthesis and function. J Steroid Biochem Mol Biol 1991;4-6:755-62.
112. Hansson JH, Nelson-Williams C, Suzuki H, Schild L, Shimkets R, Lu Y, et al. Hypertension caused by a truncated epithelial sodium channel gamma subunit: genetic heterogeneity of Liddle syndrome. Nat Genet 1995;1:76-82.
113. Hariharan M, Naga S, VanNoord T, Kindt EK. Simultaneous assay of corticosterone and cortisol in plasma by reversed-phase liquid chromatography. Clin Chem 1992;3:346-52.
114. Harmon AG, Hibel LC, Rumyantseva O, Granger DA. Measuring salivary cortisol in studies of child development: watch out—what goes in may not come out of saliva collection devices. Dev Psychobiol 2007;5:495-500.
115. Hartman D, Sagnella GA, Chesters CA, Macgregor GA. Direct renin assay and plasma renin activity assay compared. Clin Chem 2004;11: 2159-61.
116. Havelock JC, Auchus RJ, Rainey WE. The rise in adrenal androgen biosynthesis: adrenarche. Semin Reprod Med 2004;4:337-47.
117. Herf SM, Teates DC, Tegtmeyer CJ, Vaughan ED Jr, Ayers CR, Carey RM. Identification and differentiation of surgically correctable hypertension due to primary aldosteronism. Am J Med 1979;3: 397-402.
118. Hermann K, Ganten D, Unger T, Bayer C, Lang RE. Measurement and characterization of angiotensin peptides in plasma. Clin Chem 1988;6: 1046-51.
119. Hermus AR, Pieters GF, Pesman GJ, Smals AG, Benraad TJ, Kloppenborg PW. ACTH and cortisol responses to ovine corticotrophin-releasing factor in patients with primary and secondary adrenal failure. Clin Endocrinol (Oxf) 1985;6:761-9.
120. Heusser CH, Bews JP, Alkan SS, Dietrich FM, Wood JM, de Gasparo M, et al. Monoclonal antibodies to human renin: properties and applications. Clin Exp Hypertens A 1987;8-9:1259-75.
121. Higashi T, Nishio T, Uchida S, Shimada K, Fukushi M, Maeda M. Simultaneous determination of 17alpha-hydroxypregnenolone and 17alpha-hydroxyprogesterone in dried blood spots from low birth weight infants using LC-MS/MS. J Pharm Biomed Anal 2008;1: 177-82.
122. Hiramatsu K, Yamada T, Yukimura Y, Komiya I, Ichikawa K, Ishihara M, et al. A screening test to identify aldosterone-producing adenoma by measuring plasma renin activity: results in hypertensive patients. Arch Intern Med 1981;12:1589-93.
123. Hofman LF, Klaniecki JE, Smith EK. Direct solid-phase radioimmunoassay for screening 17 alpha-hydroxyprogesterone in whole-blood samples from newborns. Clin Chem 1985;7:1127-30.
124. Hogan MJ, McRae J, Schambelan M, Biglieri EG. Location of aldosterone-producing adenomas with 131I-19-iodocholesterol. N Engl J Med 1976;8:410-4.
125. Holtkamp U, Klein J, Sander J, Peter M, Janzen N, Steuerwald U, et al. EDTA in dried blood spots leads to false results in neonatal endocrinologic screening. Clin Chem 2008;3:602-5.
126. Hsiao HP, Kirschner LS, Bourdeau I, Keil MF, Boikos SA, Verma S, et al. Clinical and genetic heterogeneity, overlap with other tumor syndromes, and atypical glucocorticoid hormone secretion in adrenocorticotropin-independent macronodular adrenal hyperplasia compared with other adrenocortical tumors. J Clin Endocrinol Metab 2009;8:2930-7.
127. Huang CM, Zweig M. Evaluation of a radioimmunoassay of urinary cortisol without extraction. Clin Chem 1989;1:125-6.
128. Hubl W, Haussig K, Hofmann F, Buchner M, Rohde W, Dorner G. Enzyme immunoassay and radioimmunoassay for plasma renin activity. I. Comparison of the methods. Endokrinologie 1981;3: 333-40.

129. Hughes IA. Congenital adrenal hyperplasia: a lifelong disorder. Horm Res 2007;68(suppl 5):84-9.
130. Husebye E, Lovas K. Pathogenesis of primary adrenal insufficiency. Best Pract Res Clin Endocrinol Metab 2009;2:147-57.
131. Husebye ES, Lovas K. Immunology of Addison's disease and premature ovarian failure. Endocrinol Metab Clin North Am 2009;2: 389-405, ix.
132. Ihara M, Suzuki T, Kobayashi N, Goto J, Ueda H. Open-sandwich enzyme immunoassay for one-step noncompetitive detection of corticosteroid 11-deoxycortisol. Anal Chem 2009;20:8298-304.
133. Imura H, Nakai Y, Nakao K, Oki S, Fukata J, Tanaka I. Biosynthesis and distribution of ACTH and related peptides. Acta Physiol Pol 1981;32:15-35.
134. Inagami T, Kambayashi Y, Ichiki T, Tsuzuki S, Eguchi S, Yamakawa T. Angiotensin receptors: molecular biology and signalling. Clin Exp Pharmacol Physiol 1999;7:544-9.
135. Inoue S, Inokuma M, Harada T, Shibutani Y, Yoshitake T, Charles B, et al. Simultaneous high-performance liquid chromatographic determination of 6 beta-hydroxycortisol and cortisol in urine with fluorescence detection and its application for estimating hepatic drug-metabolizing enzyme induction. J Chromatogr B Biomed Appl 1994;1:15-23.
136. Izquierdo JM, Quiros A, Alvarez-Uria J, Sotorrio P. Homogeneous enzyme immunoassay for cortisol with a centrifugal analyzer. Clin Chem 1984;11:1824-6.
137. Janzen N, Peter M, Sander S, Steuerwald U, Terhardt M, Holtkamp U, et al. Newborn screening for congenital adrenal hyperplasia: additional steroid profile using liquid chromatography-tandem mass spectrometry. J Clin Endocrinol Metab 2007;7:2581-2.
138. Jehle S, Walsh JE, Freda PU, Post KD. Selective use of bilateral inferior petrosal sinus sampling in patients with adrenocorticotropin-dependent Cushing's syndrome prior to transsphenoidal surgery. J Clin Endocrinol Metab 2008;12:4624-32.
139. Kai H, Kudo H, Takayama N, Yasuoka S, Kajimoto H, Imaizumi T. Large blood pressure variability and hypertensive cardiac remodeling—role of cardiac inflammation. Circ J 2009;12:2198-203.
140. Kashlan OB, Maarouf AB, Kussius C, Denshaw RM, Blumenthal KM, Kleyman TR. Distinct structural elements in the first membrane-spanning segment of the epithelial sodium channel. J Biol Chem 2006;41:30455-62.
141. Katsurada A, Hagiwara Y, Miyashita K, Satou R, Miyata K, Ohashi N, et al. Novel sandwich ELISA for human angiotensinogen. Am J Physiol Renal Physiol 2007;3:F956-60.
142. Kawaguchi M, Takatsu A. Development of a candidate reference measurement procedure for the analysis of cortisol in human serum samples by isotope dilution-gas chromatography-mass spectrometry. Anal Sci 2009;8:989-92.
143. Kazlauskaite R, Evans AT, Villabona CV, Abdu TA, Ambrosi B, Atkinson AB, et al. Corticotropin tests for hypothalamic-pituitary-adrenal insufficiency: a metaanalysis. J Clin Endocrinol Metab 2008; 11:4245-53.
144. Kehlet H, Blichert-Toft M, Hancke S, Pedersen JF, Kristensen JK, Efsen F, et al. Comparative study of ultrasound, 131I-19-iodocholesterol scintigraphy, and aortography in localising adrenal lesions. Br Med J 1976;6037:665-7.
145. Kelestimur F. Non-classic congenital adrenal hyperplasia. Pediatr Endocrinol Rev 2006;3(suppl 3):451-4.
146. Kem DC, Weinberger MH, Mayes DM, Nugent CA. Saline suppression of plasma aldosterone in hypertension. Arch Intern Med 1971;3:380-6.
147. Kempers MJ, Lenders JW, van Outheusden L, van der Wilt GJ, Schultze Kool LJ, Hermus AR, et al. Systematic review: diagnostic procedures to differentiate unilateral from bilateral adrenal abnormality in primary aldosteronism. Ann Intern Med 2009;5:329-37.
148. Kempna P, Fluck CE. Adrenal gland development and defects. Best Pract Res Clin Endocrinol Metab 2008;1:77-93.
149. Kerkhofs S, Denayer S, Haelens A, Claessens F. Androgen receptor knockout and knock-in mouse models. J Mol Endocrinol 2009;1:11-7.
150. Khveshchuk PF, Rudakova AV. [Analysis of glucocorticoids in biological objects using spectrofluorometry.] Klin Lab Diagn 1995;4:33-5.
151. Kiess W, Meidert A, Dressendorfer RA, Schriever K, Kessler U, Konig A, et al. Salivary cortisol levels throughout childhood and adolescence: relation with age, pubertal stage, and weight. Pediatr Res 1995;4(Pt 1):502-6.
152. Kirschbaum C, Tietze A, Skoluda N, Dettenborn L. Hair as a retrospective calendar of cortisol production: increased cortisol incorporation into hair in the third trimester of pregnancy. Psychoneuroendocrinology 2009;1:32-7.
153. Klaff LS, Wisse BE. Current controversy related to glucocorticoid and insulin therapy in the intensive care unit. Endocr Pract 2007;5:542-9.
154. Klickstein LB, Wintroub BU. Separation of angiotensins and assay of angiotensin-generating enzymes by high-performance liquid chromatography. Anal Biochem 1982;1:146-50.
155. Kobayashi Y, Mukai H, Tsubota N, Watanabe F. Enzyme immunoassay of 11-deoxycortisol. J Steroid Biochem 1984;4A:913-5.
156. Kong MF, Jeffcoate W. Eighty-six cases of Addison's disease. Clin Endocrinol (Oxf) 1994;6:757-61.
157. Koutny LB, Schmalzing D, Taylor TA, Fuchs M. Microchip electrophoretic immunoassay for serum cortisol. Anal Chem 1996;1: 18-22.
158. Kretz O, Reichardt HM, Schutz G, Bock R. Corticotropin-releasing hormone expression is the major target for glucocorticoid feedback-control at the hypothalamic level. Brain Res 1999;2:488-91.
159. Krieger DT, Liotta AS, Brownstein MJ, Zimmerman EA. ACTH, beta-lipotropin, and related peptides in brain, pituitary, and blood. Recent Prog Horm Res 1980;36:277-344.
160. Krohn K, Uibo R, Aavik E, Peterson P, Savilahti K. Identification by molecular cloning of an autoantigen associated with Addison's disease as steroid 17 alpha-hydroxylase. Lancet 1992;8796:770-3.
161. Kronkvist K, Lovgren U, Svenson J, Edholm LE, Johansson G. Competitive flow injection enzyme immunoassay for steroids using a post-column reaction technique. J Immunol Methods 1997;1-2:145-53.
162. Labarta JI, Bello E, Ruiz-Echarri M, Rueda C, Martul P, Mayayo E, et al. Childhood-onset congenital adrenal hyperplasia: long-term outcome and optimization of therapy. J Pediatr Endocrinol Metab 2004;17(suppl 3):411-22.
163. Lacey JM, Minutti CZ, Magera MJ, Tauscher AL, Casetta B, McCann M, et al. Improved specificity of newborn screening for congenital adrenal hyperplasia by second-tier steroid profiling using tandem mass spectrometry. Clin Chem 2004;3:621-5.
164. Lamarre-Cliche M, de Champlain J, Lacourciere Y, Poirier L, Karas M, Larochelle P. Effects of circadian rhythms, posture, and medication on renin-aldosterone interrelations in essential hypertensives. Am J Hypertens 2005;1:56-64.
165. Laragh JH, Sealey J, Brunner HR. The control of aldosterone secretion in normal and hypertensive man: abnormal renin-aldosterone patterns in low renin hypertension. Am J Med 1972;5:649-63.
166. Laudat MH, Cerdas S, Fournier C, Guiban D, Guilhaume B, Luton JP. Salivary cortisol measurement: a practical approach to assess pituitary-adrenal function. J Clin Endocrinol Metab 1988;2:343-8.
167. Laureti S, De Bellis A, Muccitelli VI, Calcinaro F, Bizzarro A, Rossi R, et al. Levels of adrenocortical autoantibodies correlate with the degree of adrenal dysfunction in subjects with preclinical Addison's disease. J Clin Endocrinol Metab 1998;10:3507-11.
168. Law RH, Zhang Q, McGowan S, Buckle AM, Silverman GA, Wong W, et al. An overview of the serpin superfamily. Genome Biol 2006;5:216.
169. le Roux CW, Sivakumaran S, Alaghband-Zadeh J, Dhillo W, Kong WM, Wheeler MJ. Free cortisol index as a surrogate marker for serum free cortisol. Ann Clin Biochem 2002;(Pt 4):406-8.
170. Lee C. 6-Beta-hydroxycortisol interferes with immunoassay of urinary free cortisol. Clin Chem 1996;8(Pt 1):1290-1.
171. Lentjes EG, Romijn F, Maassen RJ, de Graaf L, Gautier P, Moolenaar AJ. Free cortisol in serum assayed by temperature-controlled ultrafiltration before fluorescence polarization immunoassay. Clin Chem 1993;12:2518-1.

172. Letellier M, Levesque A, Daigle F, Grant A. Performance evaluation of automated immunoassays on the Technicon Immuno 1 system. Clin Chem 1996;10:1695-701.
173. Lewis JG, Yeo KH, Elder PA. A competitive enzyme-linked immunosorbent assay for plasma 11-deoxycortisol (17,21-dihydroxy-4-pregnene-3,20-dione). Steroids 1986;6:365-72.
174. Li JT, Shu SG, Chi CS. Aldosterone-secreting adrenal cortical adenoma in an 11-year-old child and collective review of the literature. Eur J Pediatr 1994;10:715-7.
175. Lifton RP, Dluhy RG, Powers M, Rich GM, Gutkin M, Fallo F, et al. Hereditary hypertension caused by chimaeric gene duplications and ectopic expression of aldosterone synthase. Nat Genet 1992;1:66-74.
176. Lin CL, Wu TJ, Machacek DA, Jiang NS, Kao PC. Urinary free cortisol and cortisone determined by high performance liquid chromatography in the diagnosis of Cushing's syndrome. J Clin Endocrinol Metab 1997;1:151-5.
177. Lo CY, Tam PC, Kung AW, Lam KS, Wong J. Primary aldosteronism: results of surgical treatment. Ann Surg 1996;2:125-30.
178. Loffing J, Korbmacher C. Regulated sodium transport in the renal connecting tubule (CNT) via the epithelial sodium channel (ENaC). Pflugers Arch 2009;1:111-35.
179. Loriaux DL, Nieman L. Corticotropin-releasing hormone testing in pituitary disease. Endocrinol Metab Clin North Am 1991;2:363-9.
180. Loriaux L. Tests of adrenocortical function. In: Becker KL, ed. Principles and practice of endocrinology and metabolism. Philadelphia, Pa: JB Lippincott, 1995:665-6.
181. Lovgren U, Johansson M, Kronkvist K, Edholm LE. Biocompatible sample pretreatment for immunochemical techniques using micellar liquid chromatography for separation of corticosteroids. J Chromatogr B Biomed Appl 1995;1:33-44.
182. Luderer JR, Demers LM, Harrison TS, Hayes AH Jr. Converting enzyme inhibition with captopril in patients with primary hyperaldosteronism. Clin Pharmacol Ther 1982;3:305-11.
183. Maeda H, Nakayama M, Iwaoka D, Sato T. Assay of angiotensin I by fluorescence polarization method. Adv Exp Med Biol 1979;120A: 203-11.
184. Maeda M, Arakawa H, Tsuji A, Yamagami Y, Isozaki A, Takahashi T, et al. Enzyme-linked immunosorbent assay for 17 alpha-hydroxyprogesterone in dried blood spotted on filter paper. Clin Chem 1987;6:761-4.
185. Magnisali P, Dracopoulou M, Mataragas M, Dacou-Voutetakis A, Moutsatsou P. Routine method for the simultaneous quantification of 17alpha-hydroxyprogesterone, testosterone, dehydroepiandrosterone, androstenedione, cortisol, and pregnenolone in human serum of neonates using gas chromatography-mass spectrometry. J Chromatogr A 2008;2:166-77.
186. Makela SK, Ellis G. Nonspecificity of a direct 17 alpha-hydroxyprogesterone radioimmunoassay kit when used with samples from neonates. Clin Chem 1988;10:2070-5.
187. Manna PR, Stocco DM. Regulation of the steroidogenic acute regulatory protein expression: functional and physiological consequences. Curr Drug Targets Immune Endocr Metabol Disord 2005;1:93-108.
188. Manolopoulou J, Gerum S, Mulatero P, Rossignol P, Plouin PF, Reincke M, et al. Salivary aldosterone as a diagnostic aid in primary aldosteronism. Horm Metab Res 2010;42:400-5.
189. Manson JE. Prenatal exposure to sex steroid hormones and behavioral/cognitive outcomes. Metabolism 2008;57(suppl 2): S16-21.
190. Mantero F, Palermo M, Petrelli MD, Tedde R, Stewart PM, Shackleton CH. Apparent mineralocorticoid excess: type I and type II. Steroids 1996;4:193-6.
191. Marik PE. Mechanisms and clinical consequences of critical illness associated adrenal insufficiency. Curr Opin Crit Care 2007;4:363-9.
192. Marsden D, Larson CA. Emerging role for tandem mass spectrometry in detecting congenital adrenal hyperplasia. Clin Chem 2004;3:467-8.
193. Marzotti S, Falorni A. Addison's disease. Autoimmunity 2004;4:333-6.
194. Mason SR, Ward LC, Reilly PE. Fluorometric detection of serum corticosterone using high-performance liquid chromatography. J Chromatogr 1992;2:267-71.
195. Matsui F, Koh E, Yamamoto K, Sugimoto K, Sin HS, Maeda Y, et al. Liquid chromatography-tandem mass spectrometry (LC-MS/MS) assay for simultaneous measurement of salivary testosterone and cortisol in healthy men for utilization in the diagnosis of late-onset hypogonadism in males. Endocr J 2009;9:1083-93.
196. Mattlingly D. A simple fluorometric method for the estimation of free 11-hydroxycorticoids in human plasma. J Clin Pathol 1962;15: 374-9.
197. Maxwell MH, Marks LS, Lupu AN, Cahill PJ, Franklin SS, Kaufman JJ. Predictive value of renin determinations in renal artery stenosis. JAMA 1977;24:2617-20.
198. McKenzie TJ, Lillegard JB, Young WF Jr, Thompson GB. Aldosteronomas—state of the art. Surg Clin North Am 2009;5:1241-53.
199. Meikle AW. Dexamethasone suppression tests: usefulness of simultaneous measurement of plasma cortisol and dexamethasone. Clin Endocrinol (Oxf) 1982;4:401-8.
200. Meikle AW, Daynes RA, Araneo BA. Adrenal androgen secretion and biologic effects. Endocrinol Metab Clin North Am 1991;2:381-400.
201. Meikle AW, Odell WD. Effect of short- and long-term dexamethasone on 3 alpha-androstanediol glucuronide in hirsute women. Fertil Steril 1986;2:227-31.
202. Merke DP, Bornstein SR. Congenital adrenal hyperplasia. Lancet 2005; 9477:2125-36.
203. Migeon CJ, Donohoue PA. Congenital adrenal hyperplasia caused by 21-hydroxylase deficiency: its molecular basis and its remaining therapeutic problems. Endocrinol Metab Clin North Am 1991;2: 277-96.
204. Milford DV. Investigation of hypertension and the recognition of monogenic hypertension. Arch Dis Child 1999;5:452-5.
205. Miller WL. Steroidogenic enzymes. Endocr Dev 2008;13:1-18.
206. Miller WL, Auchus RJ, Geller DH. The regulation of 17,20 lyase activity. Steroids 1997;1:133-42.
207. Mitchell JS, Lowe TE, Ingram JR. Rapid ultrasensitive measurement of salivary cortisol using nano-linker chemistry coupled with surface plasmon resonance detection. Analyst 2009;2:380-6.
208. Moore A, Aitken R, Burke C, Gaskell S, Groom G, Holder G, et al. Cortisol assays: guidelines for the provision of a clinical biochemistry service. Ann Clin Biochem 1985;22(Pt 5):435-54.
209. Morales A, Black A, Emerson L, Barkin J, Kuzmarov I, Day A. Androgens and sexual function: a placebo-controlled, randomized, double-blind study of testosterone vs. dehydroepiandrosterone in men with sexual dysfunction and androgen deficiency. Aging Male 2009;4: 104-12.
210. Moreno S, Guillermo M, Decoulx M, Dewailly D, Bresson R, Proye C. Feminizing adreno-cortical carcinomas in male adults: a dire prognosis. Three cases in a series of 801 adrenalectomies and review of the literature. Ann Endocrinol (Paris) 2006;1:32-8.
211. Morgan L, Broughton PF, Kalsheker N. Angiotensinogen: molecular biology, biochemistry and physiology. Int J Biochem Cell Biol 1996;11: 1211-22.
212. Morganti A, Pelizzola D, Mantero F, Gazzano G, Opocher G, Piffanelli A. Immunoradiometric versus enzymatic renin assay: results of the Italian Multicenter Comparative Study. Italian Multicenter Study for Standardization of Renin Measurement. J Hypertens 1995;1:19-26.
213. Mueller HW, Eitel J. Quality control in the determination of cortisol in plasma/serum by using, on every sample, two different three-step separation methods including ultrafiltration, restricted-access high-performance liquid chromatography and reversed-phase high-performance liquid chromatography, and contrasting results to immunoassays. J Chromatogr B Biomed Appl 1996;2:137-50.
214. Muir A, Maclaren NK. Autoimmune diseases of the adrenal glands, parathyroid glands, gonads, and hypothalamic-pituitary axis. Endocrinol Metab Clin North Am 1991;3:619-44.

215. Mulatero P, Bertello C, Verhovez A, Rossato D, Giraudo G, Mengozzi G, et al. Differential diagnosis of primary aldosteronism subtypes. Curr Hypertens Rep 2009;3:217-23.
216. Mulrow PJ. Adrenal renin: regulation and function. Front Neuroendocrinol 1992;1:47-60.
217. Munver R, Volfson IA. Adrenal insufficiency: diagnosis and management. Curr Urol Rep 2006;1:80-5.
218. Mushtaq T, Shakur F, Wales JK, Wright NP. Reliability of the low dose synacthen test in children undergoing pituitary function testing. J Pediatr Endocrinol Metab 2008;12:1129-32.
219. Mussig K, Wehrmann M, Horger M, Maser-Gluth C, Haring HU, Overkamp D. Adrenocortical carcinoma producing 11-deoxycorticosterone: a rare cause of mineralocorticoid hypertension. J Endocrinol Invest 2005;1:61-65.
220. Mylonas PG, Makri M, Georgopoulos NA, Theodoropoulou A, Leglise M, Vagenakis AG, et al. Adequacy of saliva 17-hydroxyprogesterone determination using various collection methods. Steroids 2006;3: 273-6.
221. Nahoul K, Patricot MC, Bressot N, Penes MC, Revol A. [Measurement of salivary cortisol with four commercial kits.] Ann Biol Clin (Paris) 1996;2:75-82.
222. Nelson DH, Samuels LT. A method for the determination of 17-hydroxycorticosteroids in blood: 17-hydroxycorticosterone in the peripheral circulation. J Clin Endocrinol Metab 1952;5:519-26.
223. New MI. Inborn errors of adrenal steroidogenesis. Mol Cell Endocrinol 2003;1-2:75-83.
224. New MI. An update of congenital adrenal hyperplasia. Ann N Y Acad Sci 2004;1038:14-43.
225. Nguyen AD, Conley AJ. Adrenal androgens in humans and nonhuman primates: production, zonation and regulation. Endocr Dev 2008;13:33-54.
226. Nieman LK. Dynamic evaluation of adrenal hypofunction. J Endocrinol Invest 2003;7(suppl):74-82.
227. Nieman LK, Biller BM, Findling JW, Newell-Price J, Savage MO, Stewart PM, et al. The diagnosis of Cushing's syndrome: an Endocrine Society Clinical Practice Guideline. J Clin Endocrinol Metab 2008;5: 1526-40.
228. Nieman LK, Chanco Turner ML. Addison's disease. Clin Dermatol 2006;4:276-80.
229. Nijhoff MF, Dekkers OM, Vleming LJ, Smit JW, Romijn JA, Pereira AM. ACTH-producing pheochromocytoma: clinical considerations and concise review of the literature. Eur J Intern Med 2009;7:682-5.
230. Nimkarn S, Lin-Su K, New MI. Steroid 21 hydroxylase deficiency congenital adrenal hyperplasia. Endocrinol Metab Clin North Am 2009;4:699-718.
231. Nimkarn S, New MI. Steroid 11beta- hydroxylase deficiency congenital adrenal hyperplasia. Trends Endocrinol Metab 2008;3: 96-9.
232. Nimkarn S, New MI. Prenatal diagnosis and treatment of congenital adrenal hyperplasia due to 21-hydroxylase deficiency. Mol Cell Endocrinol 2009;1-2:192-6.
233. Nishizaka MK, Pratt-Ubunama M, Zaman MA, Cofield S, Calhoun DA. Validity of plasma aldosterone-to-renin activity ratio in African American and white subjects with resistant hypertension. Am J Hypertens 2005;6:805-12.
234. Okamoto M, Nonaka Y, Takemori H, Doi J. Molecular identity and gene expression of aldosterone synthase cytochrome P450. Biochem Biophys Res Commun 2005;1:325-30.
235. Oki Y, Hashimoto K, Hirata Y, Iwasaki Y, Nigawara T, Doi M, et al. Development and validation of a 0.5 mg dexamethasone suppression test as an initial screening test for the diagnosis of ACTH-dependent Cushing's syndrome. Endocr J 2009;7:897-904.
236. Okumura T, Nakajima Y, Takamatsu T, Matsuoka M. Column-switching high-performance liquid chromatographic system with a laser-induced fluorometric detector for direct, automated assay of salivary cortisol. J Chromatogr B Biomed Appl 1995;1:11-20.
237. Oldfield EH, Doppman JL, Nieman LK, Chrousos GP, Miller DL, Katz DA, et al. Petrosal sinus sampling with and without corticotropin-releasing hormone for the differential diagnosis of Cushing's syndrome. N Engl J Med 1991;13:897-905.
238. Opocher G, Rocco S, Carpene G, Armanini D, Mantero F. [Primary hyperaldosteronism.] Minerva Endocrinol 1995;1:49-54.
239. Orentreich N, Brind JL, Rizer RL, Vogelman JH. Age changes and sex differences in serum dehydroepiandrosterone sulfate concentrations throughout adulthood. J Clin Endocrinol Metab 1984;3:551-5.
240. Palermo M, Shackleton CH, Mantero F, Stewart PM. Urinary free cortisone and the assessment of 11 beta-hydroxysteroid dehydrogenase activity in man. Clin Endocrinol (Oxf) 1996;5:605-11.
241. Palmer BF, Alpern RJ. Liddle's syndrome. Am J Med 1998;3:301-9.
242. Pang S, Hotchkiss J, Drash AL, Levine LS, New MI. Microfilter paper method for 17 alpha-hydroxyprogesterone radioimmunoassay: its application for rapid screening for congenital adrenal hyperplasia. J Clin Endocrinol Metab 1977;5:1003-8.
243. Pang SY, Softness B, Sweeney WJ III, New MI. Hirsutism, polycystic ovarian disease, and ovarian 17-ketosteroid reductase deficiency. N Engl J Med 1987;21:1295-301.
244. Papadimitriou A, Priftis KN. Regulation of the hypothalamic-pituitary-adrenal axis. Neuroimmunomodulation 2009;5:265-71.
245. Papanicolaou DA, Yanovski JA, Cutler GB Jr, Chrousos GP, Nieman LK. A single midnight serum cortisol measurement distinguishes Cushing's syndrome from pseudo-Cushing states. J Clin Endocrinol Metab 1998;4:1163-7.
246. Parker LN. Control of adrenal androgen secretion. Endocrinol Metab Clin North Am 1991;2:401-21.
247. Pass KA, Neto EC. Update: newborn screening for endocrinopathies. Endocrinol Metab Clin North Am 2009;4:827-37.
248. Pearce JM. Thomas Addison (1793-1860). J R Soc Med 2004;6: 297-300.
249. Pecori GF. Recent challenges in the diagnosis of Cushing's syndrome. Horm Res 2009;123-7.
250. Perry LA, Al-Dujaili EA, Edwards CR. A direct radioimmunoassay for 11-deoxycortisol. Steroids 1982;2:115-28.
251. Perry LA, Grossman AB. The role of the laboratory in the diagnosis of Cushing's syndrome. Ann Clin Biochem 1997;34(Pt 4):345-59.
252. Pitarresi TM, Rubattu S, Heinrikson R, Sealey JE. Reversible cryoactivation of recombinant human prorenin. J Biol Chem 1992;17:11753-9.
253. Porter CC, Silber RH. A quantitative color reaction for cortisone and related 17,21-dihydroxy-20-ketosteroids. J Biol Chem 1950;1:201-7.
254. Pugeat M, Crave JC, Tourniaire J, Forest MG. Clinical utility of sex hormone-binding globulin measurement. Horm Res 1996;3-5:148-55.
255. Putignano P, Toja P, Dubini A, Pecori GF, Corsello SM, Cavagnini F. Midnight salivary cortisol versus urinary free and midnight serum cortisol as screening tests for Cushing's syndrome. J Clin Endocrinol Metab 2003;9:4153-7.
256. Raff H. Utility of salivary cortisol measurements in Cushing's syndrome and adrenal insufficiency. J Clin Endocrinol Metab 2009;10:3647-55.
257. Rai R, Cohen J, Venkatesh B. Assessment of adrenocortical function in the critically ill. Crit Care Resusc 2004;2:123-9.
258. Rainey WE, Nakamura Y. Regulation of the adrenal androgen biosynthesis. J Steroid Biochem Mol Biol 2008;3-5:281-6.
259. Rauh M. Steroid measurement with LC-MS/MS in pediatric endocrinology. Mol Cell Endocrinol 2009;1-2:272-81.
260. Rauh M. Steroid measurement with LC-MS/MS: application examples in pediatrics. J Steroid Biochem Mol Biol 2009;121:520-7.
261. Rauh M, Groschl M, Rascher W, Dorr HG. Automated, fast and sensitive quantification of 17 alpha-hydroxy-progesterone, androstenedione and testosterone by tandem mass spectrometry with on-line extraction. Steroids 2006;6:450-8.
262. Ribeiro MJ, Figueiredo Neto JA, Memoria EV, Lopes MC, Faria MS, Salgado FN, et al. Prevalence of primary hyperaldosteronism in a systemic arterial hypertension league. Arq Bras Cardiol 2009;1:39-45.

263. Rich GM, Ulick S, Cook S, Wang JZ, Lifton RP, Dluhy RG. Glucocorticoid-remediable aldosteronism in a large kindred: clinical spectrum and diagnosis using a characteristic biochemical phenotype. Ann Intern Med 1992;10:813-20.
264. Riley WJ, Maclaren NK, Neufeld M. Adrenal autoantibodies and Addison disease in insulin-dependent diabetes mellitus. J Pediatr 1980;2:191-5.
265. Roberts RF, Roberts WL. Performance characteristics of five automated serum cortisol immunoassays. Clin Biochem 2004;6: 489-93.
266. Rosner W. Plasma steroid-binding proteins. Endocrinol Metab Clin North Am 1991;4:697-720.
267. Rossi C, Calton L, Hammond G, Brown HA, Wallace AM, Sacchetta P, et al. Serum steroid profiling for congenital adrenal hyperplasia using liquid chromatography-tandem mass spectrometry. Clin Chim Acta 2010;3-4:222-8.
268. Rossi GP, Seccia TM, Palumbo G, Belfiore A, Bernini G, Caridi G, et al. Within-patient reproducibility of the aldosterone: renin ratio in primary aldosteronism. Hypertension 2010;1:83-9.
269. Rossi GP, Seccia TM, Pessina AC. Clinical use of laboratory tests for the identification of secondary forms of arterial hypertension. Crit Rev Clin Lab Sci 2007;1:1-85.
270. Rossi GP, Seccia TM, Pessina AC. Primary aldosteronism. Part I. Prevalence, screening, and selection of cases for adrenal vein sampling. J Nephrol 2008;4:447-54.
271. Rossi GP, Seccia TM, Pessina AC. Primary aldosteronism. Part II. Subtype differentiation and treatment. J Nephrol 2008;4:455-62.
272. Ruiz M, Lind U, Gafvels M, Eggertsen G, Carlstedt-Duke J, Nilsson L, et al. Characterization of two novel mutations in the glucocorticoid receptor gene in patients with primary cortisol resistance. Clin Endocrinol (Oxf) 2001;3:363-71.
273. Sahdev A, Reznek RH, Evanson J, Grossman AB. Imaging in Cushing's syndrome. Arq Bras Endocrinol Metabol 2007;8: 1319-28.
274. Sahin M, Kebapcilar L, Taslipinar A, Azal O, Ozgurtas T, Corakci A, et al. Comparison of 1 mg and 2 mg overnight dexamethasone suppression tests for the screening of Cushing's syndrome in obese patients. Intern Med 2009;1:33-9.
275. Sapolsky R, Rivier C, Yamamoto G, Plotsky P, Vale W. Interleukin-1 stimulates the secretion of hypothalamic corticotropin-releasing factor. Science 1987;4826:522-4.
276. Savage MO, Chan LF, Grossman AB, Storr HL. Work-up and management of paediatric Cushing's syndrome. Curr Opin Endocrinol Diabetes Obes 2008;4:346-51.
277. Schalekamp MA, Derkx FH, Deinum J, Danser AJ. Newly developed renin and prorenin assays and the clinical evaluation of renin inhibitors. J Hypertens 2008;5:928-37.
278. Scharpe S, Verkerk R, Sasmito E, Theeuws M. Enzyme immunoassay of angiotensin I and renin. Clin Chem 1987;10:1774-7.
279. Schatz DA, Winter WE. Autoimmune polyglandular syndrome. II. Clinical syndrome and treatment. Endocrinol Metab Clin North Am 2002;2:339-52.
280. Schirpenbach C, Seiler L, Maser-Gluth C, Beuschlein F, Reincke M, Bidlingmaier M. Automated chemiluminescence-immunoassay for aldosterone during dynamic testing: comparison to radioimmunoassays with and without extraction steps. Clin Chem 2006;9:1749-55.
281. Schmalzing D, Nashabeh W, Yao XW, Mhatre R, Regnier FE, Afeyan NB, et al. Capillary electrophoresis-based immunoassay for cortisol in serum. Anal Chem 1995;3:606-612.
282. Schuff KG. Issues in the diagnosis of Cushing's syndrome for the primary care physician. Prim Care 2003;4:791-9.
283. Schwartz GL, Turner ST. Screening for primary aldosteronism in essential hypertension: diagnostic accuracy of the ratio of plasma aldosterone concentration to plasma renin activity. Clin Chem 2005;2: 386-94.
284. Sealey JE. Plasma renin activity and plasma prorenin assays. Clin Chem 1991;10(Pt 2):1811-9.
285. Sebastian A, Hulter HN, Kurtz I, Maher T, Schambelan M. Disorders of distal nephron function. Am J Med 1982;2:289-307.
286. Seccia TM, Fassina A, Nussdorfer GG, Pessina AC, Rossi GP. Aldosterone-producing adrenocortical carcinoma: an unusual cause of Conn's syndrome with an ominous clinical course. Endocr Relat Cancer 2005;1:149-59.
287. Sheaves R, Goldin J, Reznek RH, Chew SL, Dacie JE, Lowe DG, et al. Relative value of computed tomography scanning and venous sampling in establishing the cause of primary hyperaldosteronism. Eur J Endocrinol 1996;3:308-13.
288. Shen WT, Sturgeon C, Duh QY. From incidentaloma to adrenocortical carcinoma: the surgical management of adrenal tumors. J Surg Oncol 2005;3:186-92.
289. Sher L. Combined dexamethasone suppression-corticotropin-releasing hormone stimulation test in studies of depression, alcoholism, and suicidal behavior. Scientific World Journal 2006;6:1398-404.
290. Shibasaki H, Furuta T, Kasuya Y. Quantification of corticosteroids in human plasma by liquid chromatography-thermospray mass spectrometry using stable isotope dilution. J Chromatogr B Biomed Sci Appl 1997;1:7-14.
291. Shimkets RA, Warnock DG, Bositis CM, Nelson-Williams C, Hansson JH, Schambelan M, et al. Liddle's syndrome: heritable human hypertension caused by mutations in the beta subunit of the epithelial sodium channel. Cell 1994;3:407-14.
292. Shimojo M, Stewart PM. Apparent mineralocorticoid excess syndromes. J Endocrinol Invest 1995;7:518-32.
293. Simard J, Ricketts ML, Gingras S, Soucy P, Feltus FA, Melner MH. Molecular biology of the 3beta-hydroxysteroid dehydrogenase/ delta5-delta4 isomerase gene family. Endocr Rev 2005;4:525-82.
294. Simard M. The biochemical investigation of Cushing syndrome. Neurosurg Focus 2004;4:E4.
295. Simon D, Hartmann DJ, Badouaille G, Caillot G, Guyenne TT, Corvol P, et al. Two-site direct immunoassay specific for active renin. Clin Chem 1992;10:1959-62.
296. Simon D, Romestand B, Huang H, Badouaille G, Fehrentz JA, Pau B, et al. Direct, simplified, and sensitive assay of angiotensin II in plasma extracts performed with a high-affinity monoclonal antibody. Clin Chem 1992;10:1963-7.
297. Singer J, Werner F, Koch CA, Bartels M, Aigner T, Lincke T, et al. Ectopic Cushing's syndrome caused by a well differentiated ACTH-secreting neuroendocrine carcinoma of the ileum. Exp Clin Endocrinol Diabetes 2010;118:524-9.
298. Sloan DA, Schwartz RW, McGrath PC, Kenady DE. Diagnosis and management of adrenal tumors. Curr Opin Oncol 1996;1:30-6.
299. Speiser PW. Improving neonatal screening for congenital adrenal hyperplasia. J Clin Endocrinol Metab 2004;8:3685-6.
300. Speiser PW. Prenatal and neonatal diagnosis and treatment of congenital adrenal hyperplasia. Horm Res 2007;68(suppl 5):90-2.
301. Stocco DM. Intramitochondrial cholesterol transfer. Biochim Biophys Acta 2000;1:184-97.
302. Stowasser M, Gordon RD. Aldosterone assays: an urgent need for improvement. Clin Chem 2006;9:1640-2.
303. Stratakis CA. Cushing syndrome caused by adrenocortical tumors and hyperplasias (corticotropin-independent Cushing syndrome). Endocr Dev 2008;13:117-32.
304. Stratakis CA. New genes and/or molecular pathways associated with adrenal hyperplasias and related adrenocortical tumors. Mol Cell Endocrinol 2009;1-2:152-7.
305. Tabarin A, Greselle JF, San-Galli F, Leprat F, Caille JM, Latapie JL, et al. Usefulness of the corticotropin-releasing hormone test during bilateral inferior petrosal sinus sampling for the diagnosis of Cushing's disease. J Clin Endocrinol Metab 1991;1:53-9.
306. Taylor PJ, Cooper DP, Gordon RD, Stowasser M. Measurement of aldosterone in human plasma by semiautomated HPLC-tandem mass spectrometry. Clin Chem 2009;6:1155-62.
307. Terzolo M, Bovio S, Pia A, Reimondo G, Angeli A. Management of adrenal incidentaloma. Best Pract Res Clin Endocrinol Metab 2009;2:233-43.

308. Terzolo M, Bovio S, Reimondo G, Pia A, Osella G, Borretta G, et al. Subclinical Cushing's syndrome in adrenal incidentalomas. Endocrinol Metab Clin North Am 2005;2:423-39.
309. Thomson S, Koren G, Fraser LA, Rieder M, Friedman TC, Van Uum SH. Hair analysis provides a historical record of cortisol levels in Cushing's syndrome. Exp Clin Endocrinol Diabetes 2010;2:133-8.
310. Tiong K, Falhammar H. Carbamazepine and falsely positive screening tests for Cushing's syndrome. N Z Med J 2009;1288:100-2.
311. Tomlinson JW, Stewart PM. Cortisol metabolism and the role of 11beta-hydroxysteroid dehydrogenase. Best Pract Res Clin Endocrinol Metab 2001;1:61-78.
312. Tomycz ND, Horowitz MB. Inferior petrosal sinus sampling in the diagnosis of sellar neuropathology. Neurosurg Clin N Am 2009;3: 361-7.
313. Toyoda Y, Mizukoshi M, Umemoto M, Kuchii M, Ueyama K, Tomimoto S, et al. Adrenal tumor producing 11-deoxycorticosterone, 18-hydroxy-11-deoxycorticosterone and aldosterone. Intern Med 1996;2:123-8.
313A. Tritos NA, Biller BM, Swearingen B. Medscape. Management of Cushing disease. Nat Rev Endocrinol 2011;7:279-89.
314. Tsuji A, Maeda M, Arakawa H, Shimizu S, Ikegami T, Sudo Y, et al. Fluorescence and chemiluminescence enzyme immunoassays of 17 alpha-hydroxyprogesterone in dried blood spotted on filter paper. J Steroid Biochem 1987;1-3:33-40.
315. Turner AJ, Hooper NM. The angiotensin-converting enzyme gene family: genomics and pharmacology. Trends Pharmacol Sci 2002;4: 177-83.
316. Turpeinen U, Itkonen O, Ahola L, Stenman UH. Determination of 17alpha-hydroxyprogesterone in serum by liquid chromatography-tandem mass spectrometry and immunoassay. Scand J Clin Lab Invest 2005;1:3-12.
317. Unluhizarci K, Kelestimur F, Guven M, Bayram F, Colak R. The value of low dose (1 microg) ACTH stimulation test in the investigation of non-classic adrenal hyperplasia due to 11beta-hydroxylase deficiency. Exp Clin Endocrinol Diabetes 2002;8:381-5.
318. Upton B, Chu Q, Li BD. Li-Fraumeni syndrome: the genetics and treatment considerations for the sarcoma and associated neoplasms. Surg Oncol Clin N Am 2009;1:145-56, ix.
319. van der Hoeven RA, Hofte AJ, Frenay M, Irth H, Tjaden UR, van der Greef J, et al. Liquid chromatography mass spectrometry with on-line solid-phase extraction by a restricted-access C18 precolumn for direct plasma and urine injection. J Chromatogr A 1997;1-2:193-200.
320. van der Kamp HJ, Wit JM. Neonatal screening for congenital adrenal hyperplasia. Eur J Endocrinol 2004;151(suppl 3):U71-5.
321. Vaughan ED Jr. Diseases of the adrenal gland. Med Clin North Am 2004;2:443-66.
322. Vaughan ED Jr, Buhler FR, Laragh JH, Sealey JE, Baer L, Bard RH. Renovascular hypertension: renin measurements to indicate hypersecretion and contralateral suppression, estimate renal plasma flow, and score for surgical curability. Am J Med 1973;3:402-14.
323. Veldhuis JD, Kulin HE, Santen RJ, Wilson TE, Melby JC. Inborn error in the terminal step of aldosterone biosynthesis: corticosterone methyl oxidase tpe II deficiency in a North American pedigree. N Engl J Med 1980;3:117-21.
324. Veldhuis JD, Melby JC. Isolated aldosterone deficiency in man: acquired and inborn errors in the biosynthesis or action of aldosterone. Endocr Rev 1981;4:495-517.
325. Vilar L, Freitas MC, Faria M, Montenegro R, Casulari LA, Naves L, et al. Pitfalls in the diagnosis of Cushing's syndrome. Arq Bras Endocrinol Metabol 2007;8:1207-16.
326. Vining RF, McGinley RA. The measurement of hormones in saliva: possibilities and pitfalls. J Steroid Biochem 1987;1-3:81-94.
327. Wada N, Kubo M, Kijima H, Yamane Y, Nishikawa T, Sasano H, et al. A case of deoxycorticosterone-producing adrenal adenoma. Endocr J 1995;5:637-42.
328. Wallace AM, Beastall GH, Cook B, Currie AJ, Ross AM, Kennedy R, et al. Neonatal screening for congenital adrenal hyperplasia: a programme based on a novel direct radioimmunoassay for 17-hydroxyprogesterone in blood spots. J Endocrinol 1986;2: 299-308.
329. Wandoloski M, Bussey KJ, Demeure MJ. Adrenocortical cancer. Surg Clin North Am 2009;5:1255-67.
330. Watanabe F, Tsubota N, Kobayashi Y, Miyata O, Ninomiya I, Miyai K. Solid phase fluoroimmunoassay for 11-deoxycortisol in serum using 21-amino-17-hydroxyprogesterone. Steroids 1982;4:393-401.
331. Wear JE, Owen LJ, Duxbury K, Keevil BG. A simplified method for the measurement of urinary free cortisol using LC-MS/MS. J Chromatogr B Analyt Technol Biomed Life Sci 2007;1-2:27-31.
332. Weber A, Trainer PJ, Grossman AB, Afshar F, Medbak S, Perry LA, et al. Investigation, management and therapeutic outcome in 12 cases of childhood and adolescent Cushing's syndrome. Clin Endocrinol (Oxf) 1995;1:19-28.
333. Webster JB, Bell KR. Primary adrenal insufficiency following traumatic brain injury: a case report and review of the literature. Arch Phys Med Rehabil 1997;3:314-8.
334. Weingartner K, Gerharz EW, Bittinger A, Rosai J, Leppek R, Riedmiller H. Isolated clinical syndrome of primary aldosteronism in a patient with adrenocortical carcinoma: case report and review of the literature. Urol Int 1995;4:232-5.
335. Westerhuis LW. Measurement of cortisol with EMIT and Amerlite immunoassays. Clin Chem 1988;11:2374.
336. White MG. Bartter's syndrome: a manifestation of renal tubular defects. Arch Intern Med 1972;1:41-7.
337. White PC, New MI, Dupont B. Congenital adrenal hyperplasia (2). N Engl J Med 1987;25:1580-6.
338. World Health Organization. Use of anticoagulants in diagnostic laboratory investigations and stability of blood, plasma and serum samples. Geneva, Switzerland: WHO, 2002.
339. Whorwood CB, Sheppard MC, Stewart PM. Licorice inhibits 11 beta-hydroxysteroid dehydrogenase messenger ribonucleic acid levels and potentiates glucocorticoid hormone action. Endocrinology 1993; 6:2287-92.
340. Wilcox CS. Functional testing: renin studies. Semin Nephrol 2000;5: 432-6.
341. Wild RA, Applebaum-Bowden D, Demers LM, Bartholomew M, Landis JR, Hazzard WR, et al. Lipoprotein lipids in women with androgen excess: independent associations with increased insulin and androgen. Clin Chem 1990;2:283-9.
342. Willenberg HS, Schinner S, Ansurudeen I. New mechanisms to control aldosterone synthesis. Horm Metab Res 2008;7:435-41.
343. Winter WE, Harris NS. Laboratory approaches to diseases of the adrenal cortex and adrenal medulla. In: Winter WE, Sokoll L, Jialal I, eds. Handbook of diagnostic endocrinology. Washington, DC: AACC Press, 2008:75-138.
344. Wong T, Shackleton CH, Covey TR, Ellis G. Identification of the steroids in neonatal plasma that interfere with 17 alpha-hydroxyprogesterone radioimmunoassays. Clin Chem 1992;9: 1830-7.
345. Wood PJ, Barth JH, Freedman DB, Perry L, Sheridan B. Evidence for the low dose dexamethasone suppression test to screen for Cushing's syndrome—recommendations for a protocol for biochemistry laboratories. Ann Clin Biochem 1997;34(Pt 3):222-9.
346. Wotiz HH, Chattoraj SC. The role of gas-liquid chromatography in steroid hormone analysis. J Chromatogr Sci 1973;4:167-74.
347. Wu VC, Chang HW, Liu KL, Lin YH, Chueh SC, Lin WC, et al. Primary aldosteronism: diagnostic accuracy of the losartan and captopril tests. Am J Hypertens 2009;8:821-7.
348. Wu VC, Kuo CC, Chang HW, Tsai CT, Lin CY, Lin LY, et al. Diagnosis of primary aldosteronism: comparison of post-captopril active renin concentration and plasma renin activity. Clin Chim Acta 2010;411: 657-63.
349. Yamaguchi Y, Hearing VJ. Physiological factors that regulate skin pigmentation. Biofactors 2009;2:193-9.
350. Yamamoto T, Fukuyama J, Hasegawa K, Sugiura M. Isolated corticotropin deficiency in adults: report of 10 cases and review of literature. Arch Intern Med 1992;8:1705-12.

351. Yang HZ, Lan J, Meng YJ, Wan XJ, Han DW. A preliminary study of steroid reproductive hormones in human hair. J Steroid Biochem Mol Biol 1998;5-6:447-50.
352. Yang J, Young MJ. The mineralocorticoid receptor and its coregulators. J Mol Endocrinol 2009;2:53-64.
353. Yanovski JA, Cutler GB Jr, Doppman JL, Miller DL, Chrousos GP, Oldfield EH, et al. The limited ability of inferior petrosal sinus sampling with corticotropin-releasing hormone to distinguish Cushing's disease from pseudo-Cushing states or normal physiology. J Clin Endocrinol Metab 1993;2:503-9.
354. Yatscoff RW, Chapelsky L, Morrish D. Analytical and clinical evaluation of an automated cortisol assay on the ACS:180. Clin Biochem 1996;4:315-9.
355. Zhang DJ, Elswick RK, Miller WG, Bailey JL. Effect of serum-clot contact time on clinical chemistry laboratory results. Clin Chem 1998;6(Pt 1):1325-33.

CHAPTER 55

The Thyroid: Pathophysiology and Thyroid Function Testing

*William E. Winter, M.D., Desmond Schatz, M.D., and Roger L. Bertholf, Ph.D.**

The thyroid is a butterfly-shaped gland located in the front of the neck, just above the trachea. The fully developed thyroid gland in a human is composed of two lobes connected by a thin band of tissue, the isthmus, which gives the gland the appearance of a butterfly. The gland is closely attached to the trachea in the anterior aspect of the neck. Anatomically and embryologically, the thyroid gland is two glands in one: the thyroid follicular cells produce thyroid hormones and the parafollicular (or C) cells secrete calcitonin.[21]

THYROID GLAND: STRUCTURAL AND FUNCTIONAL ONTOGENY

Embryologically at day 24, the thyroid gland develops from an anterior outpouching of the foregut. From this thyroid diverticulum, the thyroid gland descends, and the process is usually complete at 7 weeks. Failure of descent can produce (1) a lingual thyroid gland (located at the base of the tongue), (2) an ectopic gland, or (3) a hypoplastic or aplastic gland. Coincident with thyroid development, the parafollicular (C cells) cells (producing calcitonin) develop.

The fetus is dependent on the transplacental passage of maternal thyroid hormone for the first half of gestation.[26,29,65,225] Although only minute amounts of maternal thyroid hormone cross the placenta, maternal hypothyroidism in the first 20 weeks of gestation may adversely impact fetal central nervous system (CNS) development, leading to neuropsychologic impairment in infants and children.[178] Worldwide, the most common cause of hypothyroidism during pregnancy is iodine deficiency. Conversely, in developed countries, where iodine fortification is widespread, the most common cause of primary hypothyroidism is Hashimoto thyroiditis (chronic autoimmune thyroiditis/inflammation of the thyroid gland).

Hypothalamic thyrotropin-releasing hormone (TRH) stimulates thyrotropin [thyroid-stimulating hormone (TSH)], which in turn stimulates thyroid hormone synthesis. By 10 weeks, fetal thyroid follicles and thyroxine synthesis are demonstrable. By the mid second trimester, maturation of the hypothalamic-pituitary-thyroid axis occurs, so that by 20 weeks, the fetus is becoming responsible for its own production of thyroid hormone. Thyroxine-binding globulin (TBG) and thyroxine are first detectable in fetal serum at 8 to 10 weeks' gestation and increase thereafter until they plateau at 35 to 37 weeks (Figure 55-1). Thyroxine [tetraiodothyronine (T_4); see Table 55-1 for nomenclature and abbreviations) and TSH rise until birth, with T_4 near ≈10 μg/dL and TSH reaching a concentration of 7 to 10 mIU/L. Beginning at ≈30 weeks, T_4 is converted to triiodothyronine (T_3) by increased activity of the type 1 deiodinase (D1), so that T_3 concentrations rise, while reverse T_3 (rT_3) concentrations decline. At 30 weeks, T_3 is less than 15 ng/dL; at term, T_3 is ≈50 ng/dL.

Within hours of birth, TSH, T_4, and T_3 rise rapidly (Figure 55-2).[52] Cold stress is believed to be responsible for the massive TSH surge to concentrations of 70 to 100 mIU/L. By 2 to 3 days, the TSH concentration falls in most cases to less than 20 mIU/L. Total T_4 peaks near ≈17 μg/dL. T_4 then falls to adult concentrations by 1 to 2 months of age. The postbirth rise in T_3 results from increased thyroid gland release in response to the rising TSH concentration and increased conversion of T_4 to T_3 due to maturation of the type 1 deiodinase enzyme (D1).

*The authors gratefully acknowledge the previous contributions of L. M. Demers and C. Spencer, on which portions of this chapter are based.

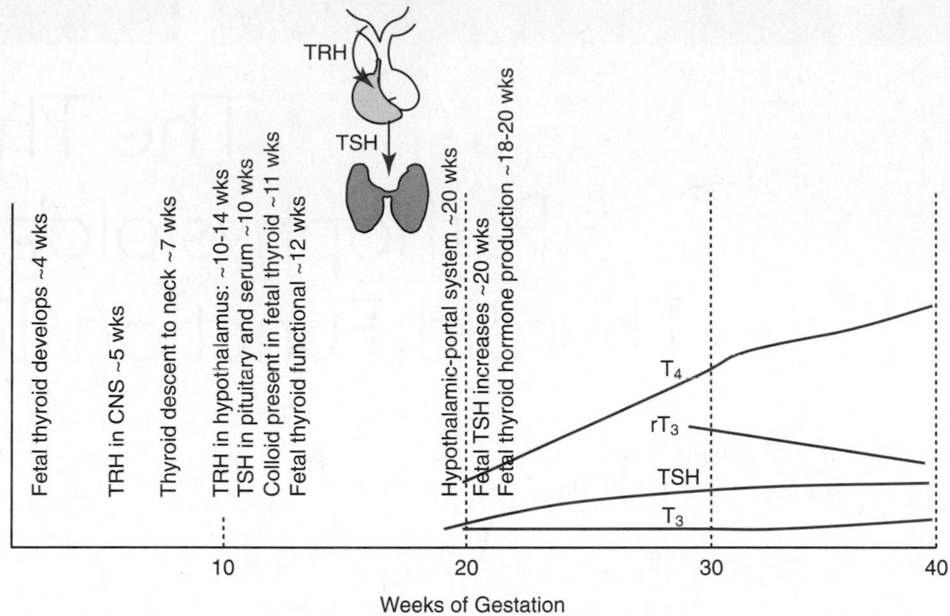

Figure 55-1 Changes in fetal thyroid function during gestation. During the first half of gestation, the fetus is dependent on transplacental passage of thyroid hormone. After mid gestation, the fetus produces its own thyroid hormone.

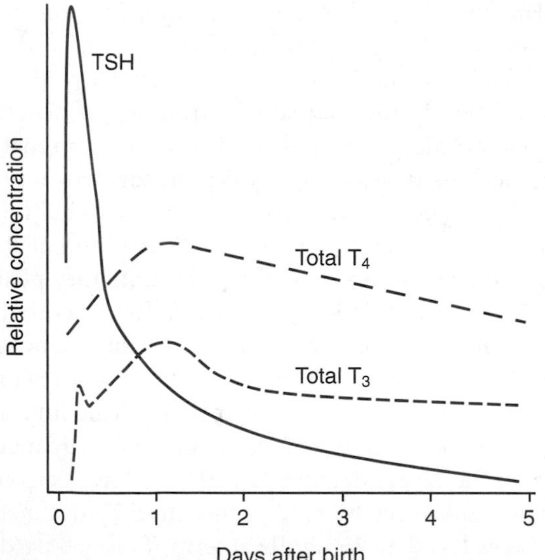

Figure 55-2 Concentrations of thyroid hormones for 5 days after birth. After birth, an immediate TSH surge peaks at ~30 minutes. T_3 and T_4 rapidly rise, peaking at ≈24 hours after delivery. The greater initial rise in T_3 as compared with T_4 in the first 24 hours of life likely represents acutely increased conversion of T_4 to T_3. Following their peak concentrations, T_4 and T_3 decline to stable concentrations.

THYROID GLAND ANATOMY

The adult thyroid gland weighs between 15 and 20 g. However, in disease states, the gland can attain a weight of several hundred grams. The thyroid gland is normally bilobed, with the right lobe somewhat larger than the left lobe. In adults, the lobes are ≈2.0 to 2.5 cm thick by ≈2.0 to 2.5 cm wide by ≈4 cm high. The lobes are connected by the isthmus, which is ≈0.5 cm thick by ≈2.0 cm wide by ≈1 to 2 cm high.

Microscopically, the thyroid gland is composed of follicles or acini (Figure 55-3, *A*). The outside of the follicular unit/acinus is enveloped by a basement membrane. Along the inside of the basement membrane are squamous or cuboidal epithelial follicular cells. The height of the follicular cells reflects their biochemical activity: the greater their height, the more thyroid hormone synthetic activity is occurring. The basal pole of the follicular cell is oriented toward the basement membrane, and the apical pole is oriented toward the center of the follicle (Figure 55-3, *B*). In the center of the follicle, lined by the apical aspects of the follicular cells, is the lacuna, which contains colloid composed predominantly of thyroglobulin.

On average, follicles are ≈200 microns wide (compared with a normal red blood cell diameter of 7 microns). The parafollicular cells usually are located below the basement membrane but are not adjacent to the lumen (lacuna) of the follicle. Without immunohistochemical staining for calcitonin, the parafollicular cells are very difficult to identify.

Branches of the common carotid artery (the superior thyroid arteries) and the subclavian arteries (the inferior thyroid arteries) supply the thyroid. It is surprising to note that on a per gram basis, the thyroid gland receives more blood than the kidney: 4 to 6 mL/min/g of thyroid tissue versus 3 mL/min/g of kidney. In cases of hyperthyroidism, blood flow to the entire thyroid gland can exceed 1000 mL/min, which is ≈20% of the normal cardiac output of an adult.

TABLE 55-1 Nomenclature and Abbreviations for Thyroid Tests

Name	Abbreviation
Hormones	
Total thyroxine	T_4
Total triiodothyronine (3,5,3′-triiodothyronine)	T_3
Free thyroxine	FT_4
Free triiodothyronine	FT_3
Thyrotropin (thyroid-stimulating hormone)	TSH
Reverse T_3 (3,3′,5′-triiodothyronine)	rT_3
Serum-Binding Proteins	
Thyroxine-binding globulin	TBG
Thyroxine-binding prealbumin (transthyretin)	TBPA
Thyroxine-binding proteins	TBP
Tests for Autoimmune Thyroid Disease	
Thyroglobulin autoantibodies	TGA
Thyroid microsomal autoantibodies	TMA
Thyroperoxidase autoantibodies	TPOA
TSH receptor autoantibodies	TRA
Thyroid-stimulating immunoglobulins	TSI
Thyrotropin-binding inhibitory immunoglobulin	TBII
Other Hormones, Thyroid-Related Proteins, and Conditions	
Thyrotropin-releasing hormone	TRH
Thyroglobulin	Tg
Thyroid hormone receptor	TR
Thyroperoxidase	TPO
TSH receptor autoantibodies	TRA
Thyroid hormone receptor-alpha	THRA
Thyroid hormone receptor-beta	THRB
Autoimmune thyroid disease	AITD
Calcitonin	CT

BIOLOGICAL FUNCTION

Thyroid hormones (T_4 and T_3) bind to intranuclear receptors that function as transcription factors and thereby regulate gene expression. Thyroid hormones have ubiquitous effects on growth and development in the fetus, child, and adolescent, and they regulate calorigenesis and metabolic rate throughout life. At a molecular level, thyroid hormones (1) increase oxygen consumption within tissues via increased membrane transport (cycling of sodium/potassium ATPase with increased synthesis and consumption of adenosine triphosphate), (2) enhance mitochondrial metabolism (stimulation of mitochondrial respiration and oxidative phosphorylation), (3) increase sensitivity to catecholamines with increased heart rate and myocardial contractility, (4) stimulate protein synthesis and carbohydrate metabolism, (5) increase synthesis and degradation of cholesterol and triglycerides (e.g., regulation of low density lipoprotein receptor expression by the liver), (6) increase vitamin requirements, and (7) regulate calcium and phosphorous metabolism.

Thyroid hormones maintains the basal metabolic rate and thus regulates the metabolism of endogenous and exogenous substances. Hypothyroidism impairs the excretion of many drugs, with hyperthyroidism accelerating their clearance.

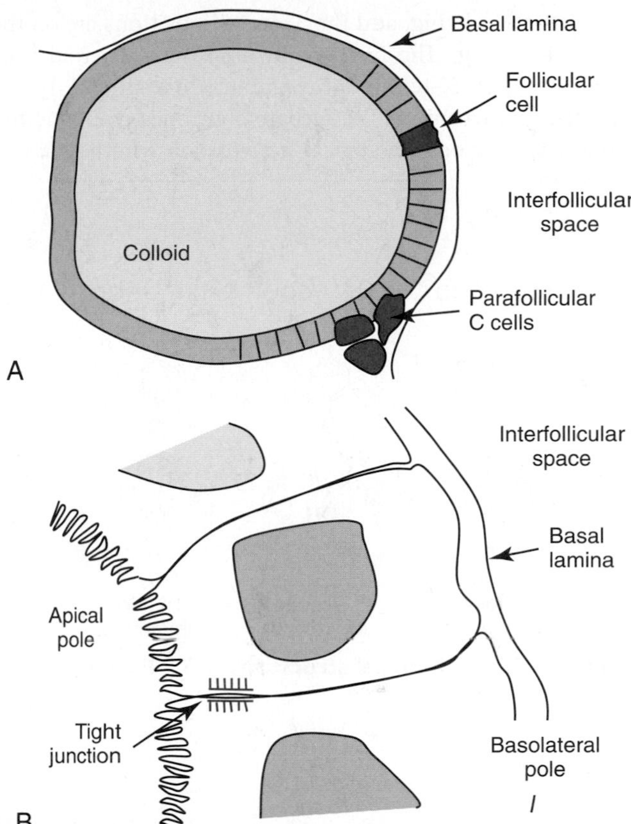

Figure 55-3 A, Basic unit of the thyroid gland. The follicle is the basic unit of the thyroid gland. It is composed of thyroid follicular cells surrounding the colloid. Outside the follicular cells is a basal lamina. B, Apical and basolateral poles of the follicular cells and tight junctions between the follicular cells. Parafollicular (C cells) that secrete calcitonin can be found beneath or outside the basal lamina. Not pictured between the follicles are capillaries and fibroblasts.

BIOCHEMISTRY

Thyroid hormone is derived from the amino acid tyrosine. Thyronine is produced by substitution of a second phenol moiety for the phenolic hydrogen on tyrosine, producing a diphenyl ether having two phenol rings attached to one another through an ether linkage (Figure 55-4).

There are four possible sites for iodine attachment to thyronine at the meta positions on both phenyl rings, designated the 3, 5, 3′, and 5′ positions. The 3 and 5 positions are on the alpha (inner) ring, and the 3′ and 5′ positions are on the beta (outer) ring. The biologically important thyroid hormones are 3,5,3′,5′-tetraiodothyronine [thyroxine (T_4)] and 3,5,3′-triiodothyronine (T_3). Debate continues over whether T_4 has any intrinsic biological activity, or whether it is a prohormone.

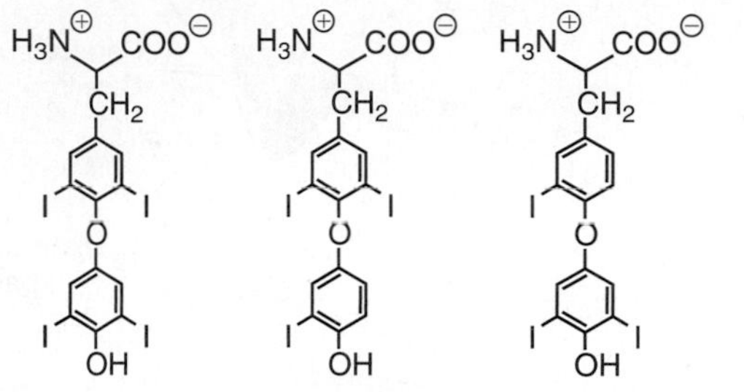

T_4 Tetraiodo-thyronine (Thyroxine) | T_3 3,5,3′ Triiodo-thyronine | rT_3 3,3′,5′ Triiodo-thyronine

Figure 55-4 Chemical structures of T_4, T_3, and rT_3.

Iodination of tyrosine to ultimately produce T_4 and T_3 involves the tyrosine residues on thyroglobulin.[86] An isomer of T_3 is reverse T_3 (rT_3), in which the alpha ring is monoiodinated and the beta ring is di-iodinated, producing 3,3′,5′-L-tri-iodothyronine. Reverse T_3 is not biologically active. Almost all rT_3 is formed by the extrathyroidal conversion of T_4 to rT_3, and approximately 80% of T_3 is formed by extrathyroidal monodeiodination of T_4 to T_3.

Thyroid hormone biosynthesis begins with the active transport of iodide (I^-) into the thyroid gland via the Na^+/I^- (sodium-iodide) symporter (NIS, SLC5A; SLC = solute carrier; chromosome 19p12-13.2; Figure 55-5).[20] Iodide transport is inhibited by lithium, which competes with sodium, but the NIS transports other anions besides iodide. In the follicular cells, the iodine concentration is 30- to 40-fold greater than the circulating concentration. When the thyroid gland is stimulated by TSH, even larger iodide concentration gradients can result. Antithyroid drugs such as propylthiouracil and methimazole inhibit iodination and coupling; this can lead to an 800-fold difference in the concentration of iodide in the thyroid gland versus the plasma.

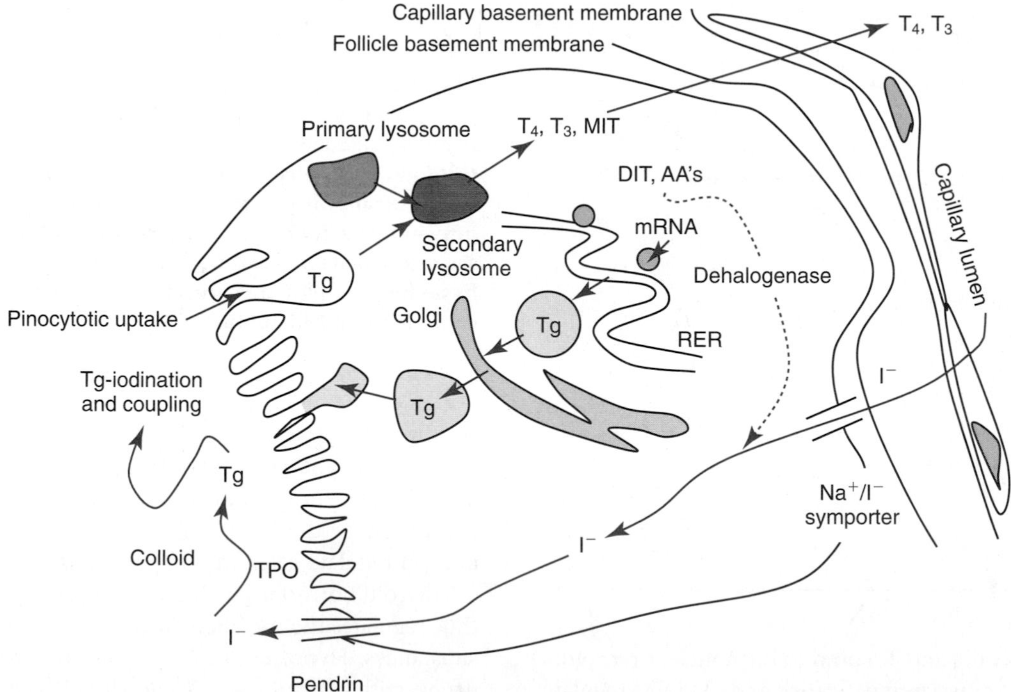

Figure 55-5 Synthesis of thyroid hormones begins with absorption of iodide by the thyroid follicular cell and the Na^+/I^- symporter (NIS). From the cytoplasm, iodide moves into the lacunae via pendrin. Within the lacunae, thyroperoxidase (TPO) and the dual oxidases [DUOX (not depicted)] convert iodide to iodine, leading to iodination of tyrosine residues on thyroglobulin (Tg). Tg is synthesized in the cell and exported to the lacunae. TPO is responsible for the coupling of monoiodotyrosine (MIT) and di-iodotyrosine (DIT) to form T_3, and di-iodotyrosine and di-iodotyrosine to form T_4. Upon uptake of iodinated Tg (containing T_4 and T_3) and fusion of this phagosome-like vesicle with a primary lysosome, Tg is degraded in a secondary lysosome, releasing T_4 and T_3 into the circulation and MIT and DIT undergo deiodination via a dehalogenase to recycle the iodine for new thyroid hormone synthesis.

Once in the thyroid follicular cells, cytoplasmic iodide moves into the lacuna (colloid) via pendrin (*SLC26A4* gene on chromosome 7q21-34) (see Figure 55-5).[88] Pendrin is a passive iodide-transporting glycoprotein identified during studies of patients with Pendred syndrome. Pendred syndrome is an autosomal recessive disorder of dyshormonogenesis that is characterized by goiter and sensorineural deafness.

Thyroglobulin (Tg) is necessary for thyroid hormone synthesis. Similar to other proteins, Tg is synthesized in follicular epithelial cells by ribosomes located on the endoplasmic reticulum (see Figure 55-5). Tg may represent up to 50% of protein synthesis in the thyroid gland and may account for 75% of glandular total protein.

The 42-exon gene encoding Tg is located on chromosome 8q24 and spans 250 kilobases. Tg is a glycoprotein homodimer of 660 kDa. A total of 134 tyrosine residues are found in the homodimer, and 25 to 30 of these residues are iodinated. However, T_4 is formed only at residues 5, 1290, and 2553, and T_3 is formed only at residue 2746. The Tg sedimentation coefficient of 19S is similar to that of circulating pentameric IgM, reflecting the large size of Tg. TSH is the principal stimulator of Tg synthesis. Thyroid transcription factor 1 (TTF1) interacts with the Tg promoter to stimulate Tg mRNA synthesis.

Although most Tg is secreted into the follicular lumen, a small amount of Tg is released from the follicular cells without transport into the colloid, and this Tg is not iodinated. Of consequence in autoimmune thyroid disease, iodination increases the immunogenicity of Tg. Increased dietary iodine exposure is associated with the development or expression of Hashimoto thyroiditis.[112]

Once in the lacuna, iodide is oxidized ("organified") to an iodine radical by the thyroperoxidase (TPO) enzyme. Hydrogen peroxide (H_2O_2) serves as the terminal electron acceptor, forming $H_2O_2^-$.[185] Hydrogen peroxide is generated at the apical membrane by the action of DUOX1 and DUOX2 (DUOX was previously known as THOX, or thyroid oxidase). DUOX is a dual oxidase that has domains analogous to the domains found in nicotinamide adenine dinucleotide phosphate (NADPH) oxidoreductases. Hypothyroidism due to *DUOX* mutations has been reported.[130]

TPO catalyzes the monoiodination of Tg tyrosines to monoiodotyrosine (MIT) (Figure 55-6). Di-iodination of tyrosine forms di-iodotyrosine (DIT) (Figure 55-6). After Tg is iodinated to form MIT and DIT, TPO catalyzes the coupling reaction to produce T_4 (Figure 55-7) and T_3 (Figure 55-8). In the coupling reaction, T_3 (bound to Tg) is formed from one DIT and one MIT residue with the transfer of one monoiodinated phenolic group to a DIT residue. T_4 (bound to Tg) is formed from two DIT residues with the transfer of one di-iodinated phenolic group to another DIT residue.

Tg, along with its T_3 and T_4 residues, remains in the colloid, providing a reservoir of thyroid hormone. With TSH stimulation, the apical pole of the follicular cell releases colloid into a vesicle by pinocytosis (see Figure 55-5). The follicular cell digests the intravesicular colloid containing Tg after fusion of the phagosome body with a primary lysosome. Fusion of the endocytosed Tg with the primary lysosome forms a secondary lysosome, in which digestion of Tg occurs, releasing T_4, T_3, MIT, DIT, and amino acids. By diffusion, the lipophilic T_4 and T_3 molecules exit the lysosome and cross the follicular cell plasma membrane to be captured in thyroid capillaries, where the vast majority of thyroid hormone is protein bound. Only 0.03% of total T_4 is free (unbound and bioactive), and only 0.3% of total T_3 is unbound and bioactive.

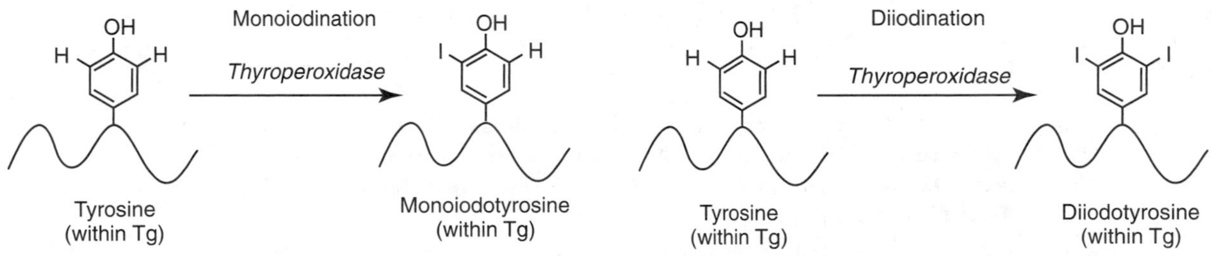

Figure 55-6 Monoiodination and di-iodination of tyrosine.

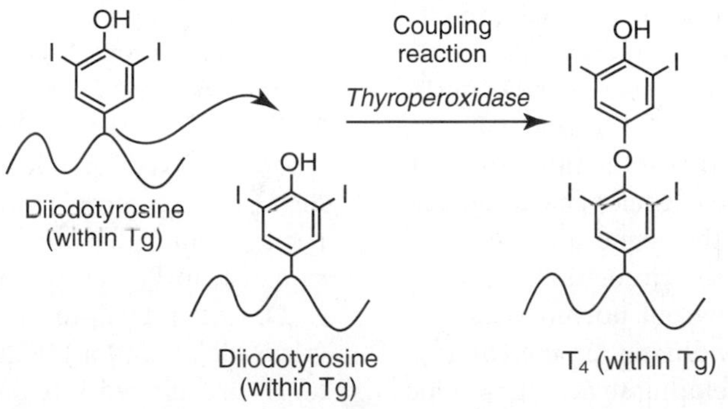

Figure 55-7 Chemical coupling of two molecules of di-iodotyrosine to produce a molecule of T_4 (thyroxine). The reaction is catalyzed by thyroperoxidase.

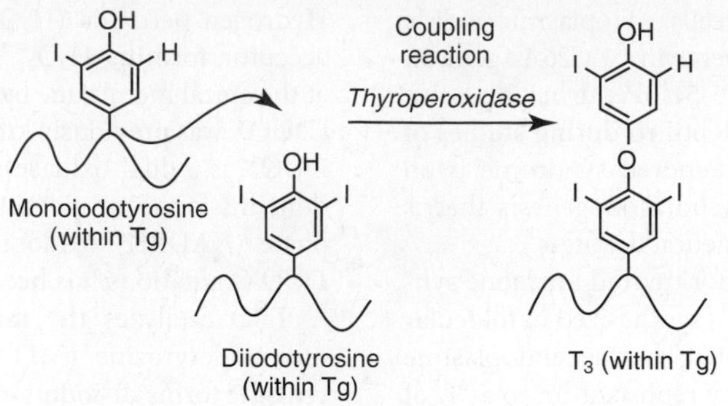

Figure 55-8 Chemical coupling of one molecule of monoiodotyrosine and one molecule of di-iodotyrosine to produce one molecule of T_3. The reaction is catalyzed by thyroperoxidase.

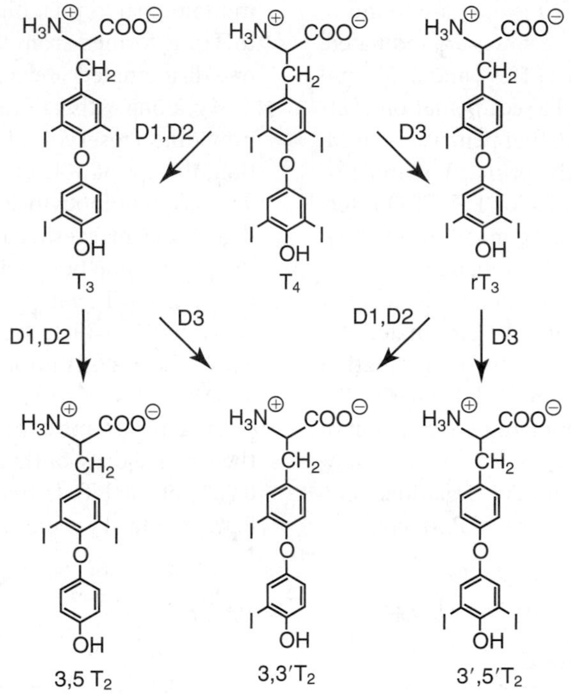

Figure 55-9 Metabolic pathways of T_4. Type 1 deiodinase (D1) converts T_4 to T_3 or rT_3. D1 then converts T_3 to 3,3′-T_2, while D1 converts rT_3 to 3,3′-T_2. Type 2 deiodinase (D2) converts T_4 to T_3 and rT_3 to 3,3′-T_2. Type 3 deiodinase (D3) converts T_4 to rT_3 and T_3 to 3,3′-T_2.

Within the cytoplasm of the follicular cell, the released MIT and DIT are stripped of iodine by dehalogenase (Dhal) to produce free iodide ions, which can be recycled immediately for the synthesis of new thyroid hormone.[64] Two dehalogenase genes have been described: *Dhal1* and *Dhal1b*. Normally, only negligible amounts of MIT and DIT are released from the thyroid gland into the circulation. However, loss-of-function mutations in the dehalogenase enzyme potentially lead to iodine loss in the urine and increased concentrations of DIT and MIT in the circulation.

The peripheral metabolism of thyroid hormones is very complex.[191] Three homodimeric deiodinases are present: type 1 (D1), with inner and outer ring deiodinase activities found in liver, kidney, thyroid, and possibly the anterior pituitary gland (Figure 55-9); type 2 (D2), with outer ring deiodinase activity expressed in the CNS, anterior pituitary, brown fat, placenta, heart, skeletal muscle, and thyroid; and type 3 (D3), with inner ring deiodinase activity identified in CNS, liver, endometrium, and placenta. Approximately 40% of T_4 is deiodinated to T_3 by D1 or D2, and ≈45% is deiodinated to rT_3 by D1 or D3. About 80% of circulating T_3 comes from 5′-deiodination of T_4; only ≈20% of T_3 is released directly from the thyroid gland (Figure 55-9). Almost all circulating rT_3 results from 5-deiodination of T_4. By regulating the conversion of T_4 to T_3, the body, in part, regulates the metabolic rate.

D1 converts T_4 to rT_3 (via 5-deiodination) and T_4 to T_3 (via 5′-deiodination) (Figure 55-10). The preferred substrates for D1 are sulfated T_3 (converted to 3,3′-T_2 via 5-deiodination) and rT_3 (converted to 3,3′-T_2 via 5′-deiodination). D1 activity is stimulated by thyroid hormone through increased gene transcription. Thus, increased D1 activity promotes peripheral conversion of T_4 to T_3 in hyperthyroidism. Therapeutically, D1 is inhibited by propylthiouracil, which is used to treat hyperthyroidism. In contrast to the effect of thyroid hormone on D1, D2 expression is suppressed by thyroid hormone. The K_m for the D1-T4 complex is approximately 1000-fold greater than the corresponding K_m for D2 or D3. Regulation of the $T_4 \rightarrow T_3$ and $T_4 \rightarrow rT_3$ conversions is dependent on the tissue distribution of D1, D2, and D3. The free T_3 (FT_3)-to-T_4 (FT_4) ratio is affected by a genetic polymorphism in the D1 gene (*DIO1;* the single-nucleotide polymorphism rs2235544).[143]

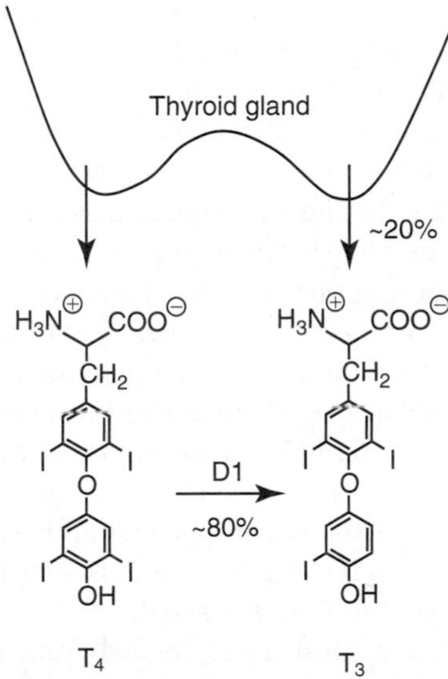

Figure 55-10 Metabolic sources of T_4 and T_3. The only source of T_4 is the thyroid gland. However, most T_3 (≈80%) comes from peripheral monodeiodination of T_4 to T_3 [catalyzed by type I deiodinase (D1) and type 2 deiodinase (D2)] with only a minority of T_3 (≈20%) coming directly from the thyroid gland.

Each of the deiodinase enzymes has a single transmembrane domain. The deiodinases are attached to the inner plasma membrane (D1 and D3) or endoplasmic reticulum (D2), and the active site of the enzyme is on the cytoplasmic domain. Therefore, thyroid hormone must enter the cytoplasm of cells to be metabolized. In addition to thyroid hormone metabolism via deiodination, small amounts of T_4 are glucuronidated or sulfated and excreted in the bile. Intestinal cleavage of glucuronidated T_4 releases T_4 that can then be reabsorbed from the intestine back into the circulation.

Until recently it was believed that both T_4 and T_3 entered cells by passive diffusion across the plasma membrane. However, evidence has shown that thyroid hormones cross plasma membranes using specific transporters.[74] One important thyroid hormone transporter is monocarboxylate transporter 8 (MCT8).[118] The solute carrier family of monocarboxylate transporters has 14 members (MCT1 through MCT14); examples of other monocarboxylates transported by these carriers are lactate and pyruvate.

It has been shown that MCT10 (*SLC16A10;* chromosome 6q) transports iodothyronines and aromatic amino acids across membranes, and MCT10 is likely more preferential than MCT8 in transporting T_3 over T_4 across plasma membranes. Organic anion transporting polypeptide 1C1 (OATP1C1) also has high affinity for thyroid hormone and may be an important component of the transport of T_3 and T_4.

Transport of thyroid hormone into neurons is especially critical for normal CNS development and function (Figure 55-11). OATP1C1 may be responsible for thyroid hormone uptake and release by astrocytes, although this has not yet

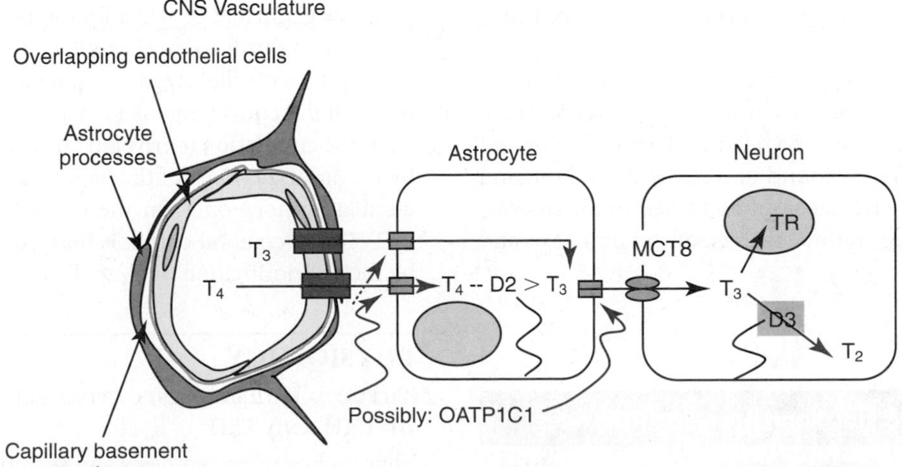

Figure 55-11 Transport of thyroid hormones to neurons. Before thyroid hormones are transported to neurons, T_4 and T_3 pass through endothelial cells and astrocytes. Organic anion–transporting polypeptide 1C1 (OATP1C1) may allow astrocyte uptake of T_4 and T_3. Within the astrocyte, T_4 may be converted to T_3 via type 2 deiodinase (D2). T_3 then may leave the astrocyte via OATP1C1 to enter neurons via monocarboxylate transporter 8 (MCT8). Within the neuron, T_3 can interact with a thyroid hormone receptor (TR) or can be converted to 3,3′-T_2 via type 3 deiodinase (D3).

been definitively demonstrated. Within the astrocyte, T_4 is converted to T_3 via D2 attached to the astrocyte membrane. T_3 may exit the astrocyte via OATP1C1 to be taken up by neurons via MCT8. Within the neuron, T_3 can interact with the intranuclear thyroid hormone receptor (TR), or can be converted to 3,3′-T_2 via membrane-attached D3.

Although T_4 is converted to T_3 outside of target organs (the liver converts T_4 to T_3 and then releases T_3 back into the circulation), target organs can also deiodinate T_4 to T_3 so that T_3 can bind to TRs. The liver, kidney, brain, brown fat, anterior pituitary, pineal, heart, skeletal muscle, and placenta all express a 5′-deiodinase capable of deriving T_3 from T_4.

T_3 binds to specific intranuclear TRs to exert its hormonal effects. In humans (and various animals), thyroid hormone upregulates the expression of growth hormone,[110] myelin basic protein, the alpha-myosin heavy chain, and a sarcoplasmic reticulum calcium ATPase, while downregulating the expression of the TSH beta chain and the beta-myosin heavy chain. In part, suppression of TSH beta chain synthesis contributes to negative feedback.

TRs are members of the steroid hormone supergene family and serve as transcription factors that include domains for DNA binding, T_3 binding, and transactivation. T_3 binds to the TRs with 15-fold greater affinity than T_4. The TRs form heterodimers with the retinoid X receptor (RXR) to interact with the thyroid response elements (TREs) in DNA. Monomers and homodimers of TRs can also bind to the TREs. TRs have zinc-finger structures that form alpha helices for interaction with the response elements.

Two types of TRs are known: TRα and TRβ (Table 55-2).[218] TRα is encoded by the thyroid hormone receptor-alpha *(THRA)* gene on chromosome 17q11.2. Of its two expressed isoforms (TRα1 and TRα2), only TRα1 binds thyroid hormone. A TRα3 isoform produced by alternative splicing has also been reported. TRα1 is expressed throughout the body, but its mRNA is in highest concentrations in the heart, brain, liver, and kidneys.

TRβ is encoded by 11 exons on the thyroid hormone receptor-beta *(THRB)* gene on chromosome 3p24.3. Three isoforms of TRβ exist: TRβ1, TRβ2, and TRβ3. The highest concentrations of TRβ1 are found in heart, kidney, liver, and brain. Expression of TRβ2 has been identified in the anterior pituitary, hypothalamus, retina, cochlea of the inner ear, and developing brain. Defects in TRβ1 can produce resistance to thyroid hormone; defects in TRα have not been reported.

Within most cells, ≈90% of T_3 is cytosolic and ≈10% is intranuclear. An exception is seen in the pituitary gland, where T_3 is distributed approximately equally between the cytoplasm and the nucleus. A T_3-binding protein (CTBP, or C-T_3BP) has been identified that may influence the intracellular distribution of thyroid hormone; however, this protein does not exhibit receptor activity.

It is important to consider the comparative biological activity of circulating T_4 and T_3. On a molar basis, there is ≈100 times as much circulating T_4 as T_3. Typical reference intervals for T_4 and T_3 are 60 to 135 nmol/Land 1 to 3.5, nmol/L, respectively. The difference in T_4 and T_3 concentrations narrows, however, to a 10-fold excess of free (active) T_4, compared with unbound T_3, in the circulation. Because T_3 is 4 to 15 times as biologically active as T_4, the difference in effectiveness narrows further. It is debated whether the effects of T_4 exceed those of T_3, or whether they equally influence the tissues. Within the cells of the anterior pituitary, large intracellular amounts of T_3 are derived from monodeiodination of T_4, so circulating FT_4 appears to be the major regulator of pituitary TSH secretion. This is an important concept that explains why TSH remains normal in the early stages of the sick euthyroid syndrome, when FT_4 is normal, preventing a rise in TSH, yet the T_3 is decreased.

In the pituitary, most T_3 is derived from intrapituitary conversion of T_4 to T_3. Within target tissues, if more T_3 comes from T_4 (via target cell 5′-deiodination) than from the circulation itself, T_4 has a major effect on tissues. Nevertheless because most T_3 is derived from T_4, within the circulation or within a target cell, T_4 is often considered to be a prohormone in the generation of T_3.

Compared with the kidney, liver, and cerebral cortex, much higher concentrations of TRs are found in the anterior pituitary gland and brown adipose tissue. In both of the latter tissues, two thirds to three quarters of the receptors are occupied by T_3, with slightly more than half of the T_3 derived from intracellular conversion of T_4 to T_3 via D2, versus T_3 taken up from the circulation (derived from T_4 outside the target tissue by D1 and D2). Most of the hepatic and renal T_3 comes from circulating hormone. On the other hand, the vast majority of T_3 in the cerebral cortex is derived intracellularly from T_4 by monodeiodination of T_4 to T_3.

TABLE 55-2 Thyroid Hormone Receptor (TR) Sizes

	Amino Acids	kDa
TRα1	410	47
TRα2	490*	55
TRβ1	461	53
TRβ2	514†	58

*Extended C-terminal region (does not bind T_3).
†Extended N-terminal region.

PHYSIOLOGY

Thyroid Hormone Negative Feedback Control of TRH and TSH

Thyroid hormone synthesis and secretion are controlled by a negative feedback system involving the hypothalamus, the pituitary, and the thyroid follicular cells (Figure 55-12).[30] In contrast to other hypothalamic-anterior pituitary target organ systems that utilize a negative feedback system, however, the major site of thyroid hormone feedback is at the level of the anterior pituitary thyrotrophs—not at the level of the hypothalamus.

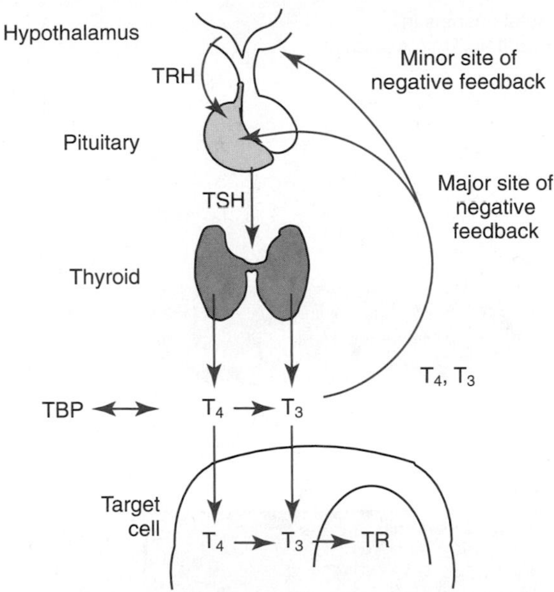

Figure 55-12 Metabolic control of thyroid hormones. Thyrotropin-releasing hormone (TRH) from the hypothalamus enters the hypothalamic-pituitary portal system to release thyroid-stimulating hormone (TSH; thyrotropin) from anterior pituitary thyrotrophs. TSH stimulates the release of T_4 and T_3 from the thyroid gland, although most T_3 comes from peripheral monodeiodination of T_4 to T_3. More than 99% of T_4 and T_3 is bound to various thyroid hormone–binding proteins. T_4 and T_3 negatively feed back on the hypothalamus and, more powerfully, the pituitary. T_4 and T_3 enter into target tissues, where T_4 is converted to T_3 with T_3 binding to the thyroid hormone receptor (TR).

(pyro)Glu-His-Pro(NH_2)

Figure 55-13 Chemical structure of thyrotropin-releasing hormone (TRH). Note that TRH is a tripeptide (L-pyroglutamyl-L-histidyl-L-prolinamide).

Hypothalamic Physiology

Thyrotropin-releasing hormone (TRH; thyrotropin-releasing factor, thyroliberin, or protirelin) is encoded on chromosome 3, and the modified tripeptide L-pyroglutamyl-L-histidyl-L-prolinamide is secreted by the paraventricular nuclei (PVN) in the hypothalamus (Figure 55-13). Cyclization of the glutamate terminus is required for TRH bioactivity. The PVN are located in the anterior hypothalamus, rostral to the optic chiasm. TRH concentrations rise in thyroid hormone deficiency with TRH declining when thyroid hormone is in excess. TRH is delivered to the anterior pituitary gland via the hypothalamic-pituitary portal system.

Anterior Pituitary Thyrotroph Physiology

Thyrotrophs, the anterior pituitary cells that secrete thyroid-stimulating hormone (TSH; thyrotropin), express TRH receptors, which are G-protein–coupled receptors with seven transmembrane domains. When TRH binds to its receptor, the thyrotroph depolarizes, triggering calcium influx. Consequently, increased free cytosolic calcium activates the Ca^{2+}-phosphatidylinositol cascade, effecting TSH release, synthesis, and glycosylation of alpha and beta TSH subunits. In relative terms, TRH has a greater effect on TSH glycosylation than hormone release.[165] However, glycosylation of TSH is necessary for normal TSH bioactivity. When TRH is deficient, TSH may lack potency as the result of insufficient glycosylation, yet nonglycosylated TSH may retain much of its immunoreactivity. Therefore, immunoassays for TSH may not reflect the activity of the hormone when injury or disease results in a TRH deficiency.

TRH modifies the sensitivity of the thyrotroph to thyroid hormone negative feedback; increased TRH makes the thyrotroph less sensitive to inhibition with decreasing TRH makes the thyrotroph more sensitive to negative feedback. The mechanism for TRH control involves reduced expression of TRs in the thyrotroph following TRH stimulation. When the thyrotroph is less sensitive to negative feedback from thyroid hormone, TSH release is potentiated. Therefore, TSH secretion rises in thyroid hormone deficiency and declines in thyroid hormone excess. An inverse logarithmic relationship exists between TSH and FT_4 concentrations (Figure 55-14); a 50% decline in FT_4 concentration results in a 100-fold increase in TSH.

TSH is a 30 kDa heterodimeric glycoprotein that shares a subunit with luteinizing hormone (LH), follicular stimulating hormone (FSH), and human chorionic gonadotropin (hCG).[174] All four hormones contain a 14.7 kDa alpha subunit (gene location: chromosome 6q21.1-q23). Each of these hormones has a unique beta subunit that is responsible for the specific activity of the hormone. The 15.6 kDa TSH beta chain is encoded by a three-exon gene located on chromosome 1p. The alpha chain contains two oligosaccharides, and the TSH beta subunit contains one oligosaccharide modification.

Thyroid Follicular Cell Physiology

The effects of TSH on the thyroid follicular cell are mediated through TSH receptor (TSHR)–G-protein–adenyl cyclase–coupled synthesis of intracellular cyclic adenosine monophosphate (cAMP).[197] At supraphysiologic concentrations (100× normal), TSH will signal through the inositol-phosphate diacylglycerol cascade, activating phospholipase C (PLC) and raising intracellular calcium concentrations, with

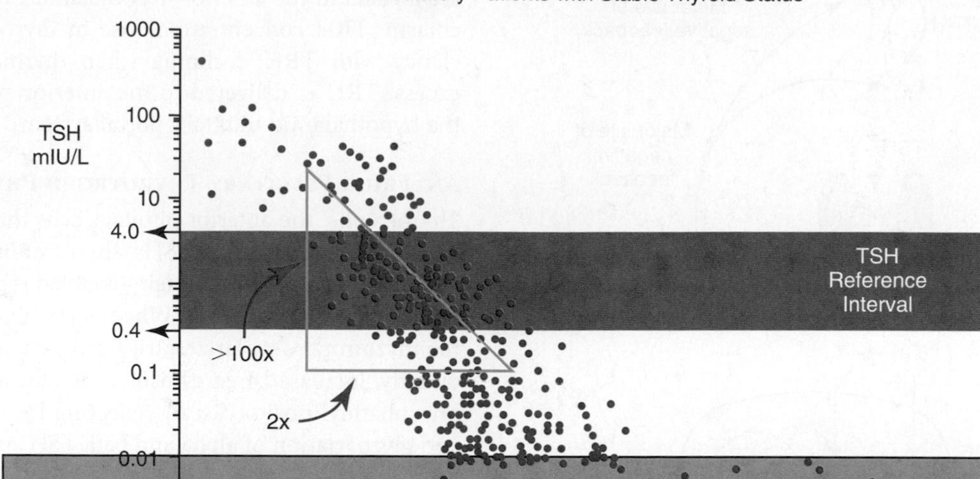

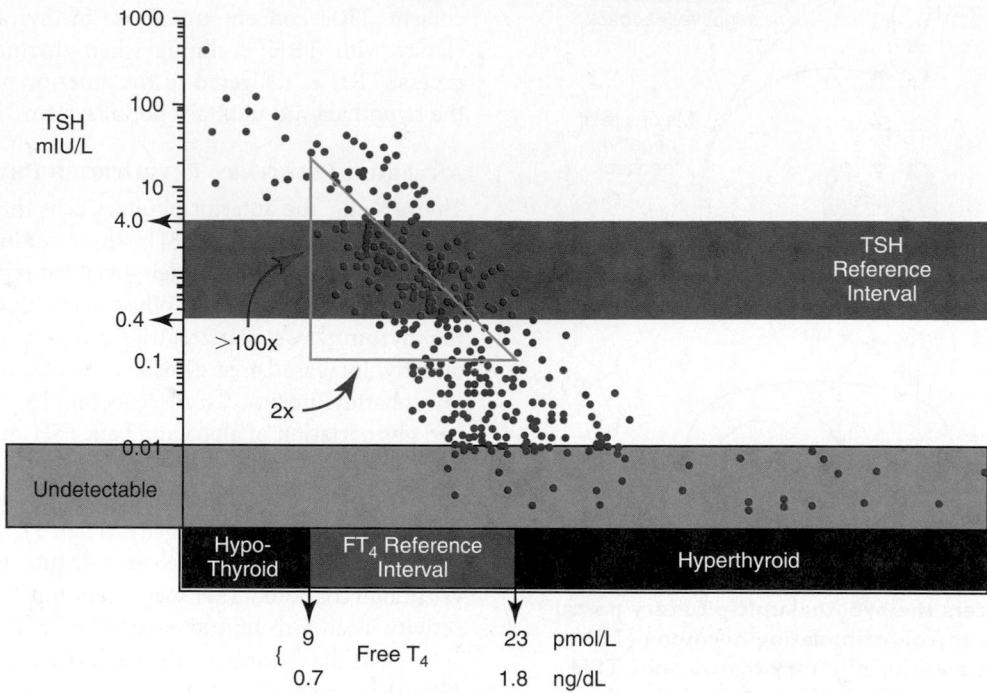

Figure 55-14 The log-linear relationship between thyroid-stimulating hormone (TSH) and FT_4. A twofold change in TSH is associated with an approximate 100-fold change in circulating FT_4 concentrations. *(Modified from Spencer CA, LoPresti JS, Patel A, Guttler RB, Eigen A, Shen D, et al. Applications of a new chemiluminometric thyrotropin assay to subnormal measurement. J Clin Endocrinol Metab 1990;70:453-60. Copyright © 1990, The Endocrine Society.)*

subsequent stimulation of H_2O_2 generation and iodide efflux into the follicular lumen.

The TSHR is a 743 amino acid, 84.5 kDa protein generated after cleavage of a 21 amino acid pre- (or leader) sequence. After post-translational glycosylation, the TSHR is ≈100 kDa. The first nine exons encode the 398 amino acid N-terminal extracellular domain. The extracellular domain contains six N-glycosylation sites that make up the TSH-binding domain. The TSHR may be in either of two conformations: the "on" conformation, with active signaling, or the "off" conformation, where signaling does not occur. TSH binding to the TSHR puts it in the "on" conformation, leading to stimulation of the thyroid gland.

Within the TSH-stimulated thyroid follicular cell, the activity of the sodium-iodine symporter increases; increased synthesis of thyroglobulin (Tg) and TPO, increased generation of hydrogen peroxide and NADPH, and pinocytosis of colloid with consequent degradation and release of T_4 and T_3 from Tg are also noted. Replication of thyroid follicular cells is stimulated by cAMP, phospholipase C, insulin-like growth factor-I (IGF-I), and a fibroblastic growth factor (FGF)-mediated kinase. TSH stimulation increases the size and number of thyroid follicular cells. Likewise, follicular cellular hyperplasia is seen in Graves' disease, when an agonistic autoantibody stimulates the TSH receptor.

THYROID HORMONES IN THE CIRCULATION

Both T_4 and T_3 are highly bound to plasma proteins in circulation. Protein-bound T_4 and T_3 serve as thyroid hormone reservoirs within plasma. In the thyroid gland, Tg serves as a reservoir. The unbound fraction of circulating thyroid hormone is the biologically active form, so FT_4 concentrations correlate more closely with the clinical status of the patient than do total T_4 concentrations.[15,142] However, elevations in FT_3 usually correlate with the clinical status of the patient, low FT_3 concentrations do not always equate with clinical hypothyroidism, as evidenced in the sick euthyroid syndrome (see later). Similarly, elevated free concentrations of T_4 or T_3 do not always correlate with hyperthyroidism because of the possibility of peripheral thyroid hormone resistance syndromes and rare MCT8 loss-of-function mutations. Alterations in the concentrations of thyroid hormone–binding proteins can profoundly affect the total concentrations of T_4 and T_3 without significant changes in the free hormone concentrations.

T_4 binds to thyroxine-binding globulin (TBG; a 54 kDa α_1-globulin), thyroxine-binding prealbumin (TBPA, or transthyretin; 54 kDa), and albumin. T_3 binds almost exclusively to TBG and albumin; TBPA binds only negligible amounts of T_3 (Table 55-3).[176] On serum protein electrophoresis, TBPA migrates in the prealbumin region (hence, its name). TBG (chromosome Xq11-23) is a 395 amino acid acidic glycoprotein with one iodothyronine-binding site. TBG has 4 heterosaccharide sidechains with 5 to 9 sialic acid moieties. As the degree of sialylation increases (an effect of estrogen), the half-life of TBG increases, thus raising TBG concentrations.

Increased concentrations of TBG raise total T_4, yet FT_4 remains within the euthyroid interval as the result of negative feedback (see Figure 55-12). Similarly, decreased TBG concentrations lower total T_4 while maintaining normal FT_4.

Causes of elevations and depressions in thyroid hormone–binding protein (TBP) are shown in Box 55-1. In congenital TBG excess (an X-linked dominant condition), male hemizygotes display threefold to fivefold elevations in TBG concentration, while female heterozygotes typically have twofold to threefold elevations in TBG. Abnormal forms of albumin (familial dysalbuminemic hyperthyroxinemia) and TBPA (familial euthyroid thyroid excess) alter the concentrations of total T_4, yet do not affect FT_4, total T_3, or FT_3. These conditions are discussed later, along with antithyroid hormone autoantibodies that raise total thyroid hormone concentrations. Isolated euthyroid hypertriiodothyroninemia (with all other thyroid parameters normal) caused by a rare form of dysalbuminemia has been reported.

TABLE 55-3 Thyroid Hormone Transport in Plasma

TBP	TBG	TTR	Albumin
Concentration	4-5.4 mg/dL	10-20 mg/dL	3.5-5 g/dL
Affinity for T_4	High	Modest	Low
T_4 capacity, mcg/dL	22	120	1000
Distribution			
T_4	67%	20%	13%
T_3	53%	1%	46%

BOX 55-1 Alterations in the Concentration or Affinity of Thyroid Hormone–Binding Proteins

Increases in

A. Thyroxine-binding globulin (TBG) concentration (or affinity)
   1. Genetic (inherited) causes
   2. Nonthyroidal illness (HIV infection, infectious and chronic active hepatitis, estrogen-producing tumors, acute intermittent porphyria)
   3. Normal physiology (pregnancy, newborn)
   4. Drug use (oral contraceptives, estrogens, tamoxifen, methadone)

B. Prealbumin binding (familial euthyroid thyroxine excess)

C. Albumin binding (familial dysalbuminemic hyperthyroxinemia)

D. T_4 binding by antibodies (autoimmune thyroid disease, hepatocellular carcinoma)

Decreases in

A. TBG concentration
   1. Genetic (inherited) determination
   2. Nonthyroidal illness (major illness or surgical stress, chronic liver disease, protein-losing enteropathy, nephrotic syndrome)
   3. Drug use (androgens, anabolic steroids, large doses of glucocorticoids)

B. TBG-binding capacity (drugs bound to TBG such as salicylates and phenytoin)

C. Prealbumin concentration

RADIOGRAPHIC THYROID TESTING

Thyroid gland location, anatomy, and function is also assessed radiographically. For example, thyroidal uptake of radioactive iodine (I-123 or I-131) or technetium pertechnetate (^{99m}Tc-pertechnetate; TcO_4^-) is assessed over time as an index of thyroid function.[116]

The degree of uptake of an exogenously administered radioactive tracer versus time reflects the activity of the thyroid gland (Figure 55-15). Radioactive iodine or technetium pertechnetate can be used. The radioactive iodine uptake (RAIU) is typically expressed as the counts measured (via scanning of the thyroid gland) divided by the total counts administered. The reference interval for the RAIU is usually 5 to 25%, which means that 5 to 25% of administered radioactive tracers are present in the thyroid gland at the time of the scan (usually at 24 hours).

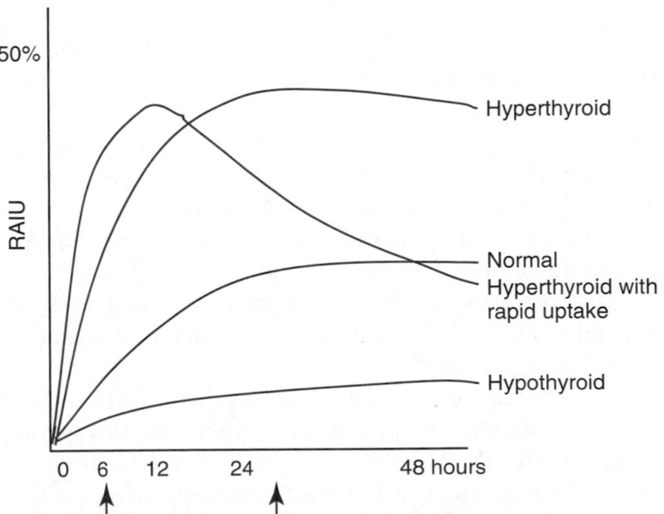

Figure 55-15 Radioactive iodine uptake (RAIU) as a function of time. RAIU is dependent on the activity of the thyroid gland. In hyperthyroidism, excessive uptake of radioactive iodine occurs. In hypothyroidism, uptake of radioactive iodine is deficient. In cases of severe hyperthyroidism, RAIU may peak before 24 hours and a 6 hour measurement is necessary to detect an elevated uptake.

In most endogenous hyperthyroid states, the RAIU is increased; in hypothyroid states, the RAIU is decreased. In thyrotoxicosis, measurement of the RAIU at 6 hours may be helpful because a hyperactive thyroid gland takes up the radioiodine at a very rapid rate and may have released some of the tracer by 24 hours. Otherwise, scanning at 24 hours alone might reveal a falsely lower measurement of the RAIU. As iodine has become more plentiful in the diet, the reference interval for the RAIU has declined.

Thyroid Scans

Administration of radioactive iodine or technetium pertechnetate allows visualization of thyroid tissue in the neck and throughout the body. In such studies, the scanner provides an image of the thyroid gland that can reveal low uptake, high uptake, and anatomic disorders such as (1) hemithyroid, a toxic (hyperactive) nodule; (2) a cold nodule (a nodule that fails to take up the radioactive tracer); or (3) ectopic thyroid tissue. Thyroid scans have been used after thyroidectomy to detect residual thyroid tissue at the surgical site, as well as differentiated thyroid cancer metastases.

Perchlorate Discharge

Normally, iodide is rapidly transported into the thyroid gland via the NIS. Within minutes of entry into the thyroid gland, intracellular iodide is transported into the lacunae via pendrin and undergoes oxidation, leading to iodination of tyrosine residues on thyroglobulin. DUOX and thyroperoxidase are responsible for the formation of organified iodine, and thyroperoxidase is responsible for the iodination of tyrosine. TPO couples MIT and DIT to produce T_3, and DIT and DIT to produce T_4. The NIS also concentrates other anions within the thyroid gland, such as thiocyanate (SCN^-), pertechnetate (TcO_4^-), and perchlorate (ClO_4^-).

The *perchlorate discharge test* is used to detect defects in thyroid gland iodide oxidation or iodination of Tg. Radioactive iodine is administered prior to perchlorate, and any radioiodine still in the follicular cells that has not yet been incorporated into colloidal Tg is released.[227] Perchlorate does not block iodination of Tg. If the NIS has transported radioiodide into the thyroid gland, but the iodide is not yet incorporated into Tg after perchlorate administration, a supranormal amount of radioiodine is released from the thyroid gland (an increase in the perchlorate discharge of radioiodine occurs).

Causes of increased radioiodide discharge after perchlorate administration include defects in pendrin, thyroperoxidase, and DUOX. Alternatively, if an inborn error is present in the NIS (e.g., a loss-of-function mutation), release of radioiodide is not increased after perchlorate because radioiodide was not initially taken up by the thyroid gland.

CLINICAL CONDITIONS

Because the signs and symptoms of thyroid dysfunction are extremely variable, thyroid function studies are often measured in clinical practice.[36,41] An enlarged thyroid gland (goiter) is typically evaluated by measurement of TSH and thyroid hormones, and on the basis of (1) history, (2) physical examination, and (3) laboratory results; patients may be classified as (1) euthyroid, (2) hypothyroid, or (3) hyperthyroid.[95,125,153]

Patients presenting with a thyroid mass are typically euthyroid. Suspicious masses are typically followed by ultrasound-guided fine-needle aspiration of the mass with cytologic examination. A thorough discussion of all forms of thyroid cancer is beyond the scope of this chapter, although the role of Tg measurements will be examined as a tumor marker for differentiated thyroid cancers.[67]

If clinical findings do not suggest an abnormality in the hypothalamic-pituitary thyroid axis, laboratory evaluation is begun with measurement of TSH (Figure 55-16).[4,95A] If TSH is within the reference interval, thyroid dysfunction generally can be excluded. If TSH is below the reference interval, measurement of FT_4 is indicated. If TSH is depressed and FT_4 is elevated, the biochemical diagnosis of primary hyperthyroidism is established. Although total T_3 can be measured at this point (and is expected to be greatly elevated), this value should not change the diagnosis or the initial therapy. If TSH is depressed and FT_4 is within the reference interval, T_3 should be measured in search of T_3 toxicosis. The authors favor total T_3 measurements over FT_3 measurements because total T_3 measurements are both more accurate and less expensive than FT_3 measurements. If TSH is depressed and both FT_4 and T_3 are normal on more than one occasion, subclinical hyperthyroidism is diagnosed. This assumes that causes of TSH suppression such as high-dose glucocorticoids and dopamine have been excluded. If TSH is depressed, FT_4 is normal, and T_3 is elevated, the diagnosis of T_3 toxicosis is established.[50]

If TSH is above the reference interval, FT_4 should be measured. If FT_4 is depressed, the biochemical diagnosis of primary hypothyroidism is established. Measurement of T_3 (or FT_3) provides no essential or additional information when hypothyroidism is a clinical consideration. Furthermore, in primary hypothyroidism, T_3 declines later than T_4 because elevated TSH concentrations in primary hypothyroidism stimulate T_3 production more than T_4 production. Whether this is due to limited availability of iodine during an attempt at increased thyroid hormone production or the increased "speed" of synthesis (T_3 synthesis requires only one iodination versus two for T_4 synthesis) is unknown.

If TSH is elevated and FT_4 is within the reference interval on more than one occasion in an asymptomatic patient, subclinical hypothyroidism is diagnosed (assuming that heterophilic antibodies have been excluded as a cause of TSH elevation).[8,145] Elevated TSH and FT_4 raise the possibility of central hyperthyroidism or thyroid hormone resistance. These disorders are differentiated clinically: patients with thyroid hormone resistance usually are euthyroid or, at worst, mildly hypothyroid, however, those with true hyperthyroidism clinically manifest thyrotoxicosis (see later). Because of the log-linear relationship of TSH to FT_4, FT_4 usually is normal as long as TSH is between 0.5 and 10 mcIU/mL.

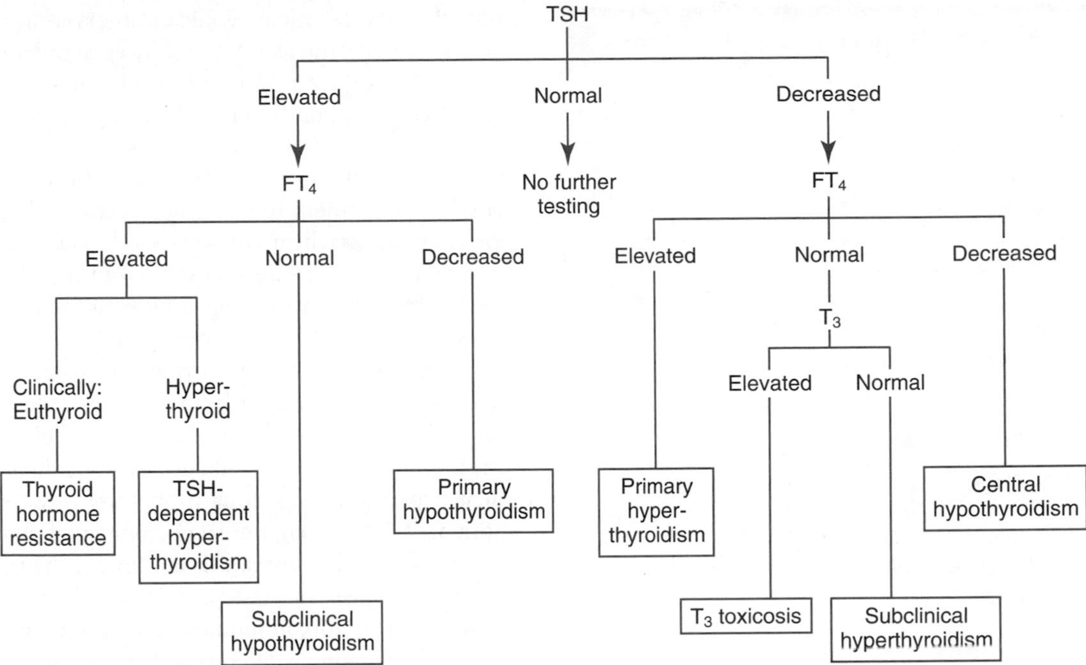

Figure 55-16 Suggested algorithm for the laboratory evaluation of thyroid function.

If hypothalamic or pituitary disease is suspected, initial testing requires measurement of both TSH and FT_4 (with FT_4 being more important). FT_4 is used to establish the presence of the biochemical euthyroid state, hypothyroidism, or hyperthyroidism. When FT_4 is low and TSH is low or normal, central hypothyroidism may be present. If FT_4 is low with only a mild elevation in TSH, central hypothyroidism is still possible because of discordance in the ratio of immunoreactivity to bioactivity, with a decrement in bioactivity from abnormal TSH glycosylation from pituitary disease or TRH deficiency. In the setting of clinical hyperthyroidism, central hyperthyroidism is diagnosed with an elevated FT_4 and normal or elevated TSH.

HYPOTHYROIDISM

Hypothyroidism is defined as a deficiency in thyroid hormone secretion and action that produces a variety of clinical signs and symptoms of hypometabolism.[73,84,198] This common disorder occurs in 2 to 15% of the population, more commonly in women than in men. The risk of developing hypothyroidism increases with age.[39]

Clinical symptoms suggesting hypothyroidism include (1) mental dullness (including mental retardation in children with untreated or undertreated congenital hypothyroidism), (2) somnolence, (3) increased sleeping, (4) lethargy, (5) easy fatigability, (6) hoarseness or deepening of the voice, (7) hair loss, (8) weight gain, (9) cold intolerance, (10) menstrual irregularities, (11) infertility, (12) growth failure, (13) delayed puberty in adolescents, (14) constipation, (15) muscle weakness or cramps, and (16) depressed affect or frank clinical depression.[171] Physical signs compatible with hypothyroidism include (1) bradycardia, (2) decreased pulse pressure, (3) cool and/or dry skin, (4) puffy eyes, (5) loss of the outer lateral eyebrows, (6) delayed relaxation phase of reflexes ("hung-up" reflexes), (7) myopathy, (8) carotenemia, (9) occasional galactorrhea, and (10) radiologic evidence of delayed bone age in children. In cases of severe hypothyroidism, congestive heart failure or coma may develop.[90] In children with untreated congenital hypothyroidism, severe growth failure and mental retardation ensue. The development of biological and biochemical processes is delayed in cases of congenital hypothyroidism. For example, affected infants often have prolonged jaundice as the result of immaturity of UDP-glucuronyl transferase.

A rare (and controversial) manifestation of Hashimoto thyroiditis is encephalopathy.[216] However, no definitive clinical test is available to diagnose encephalopathy resulting from Hashimoto thyroiditis. The diagnosis is considered when encephalopathy of unknown origin is associated with autoantibodies against the thyroid gland.

Laboratory evidence compatible with hypothyroidism encompasses hyponatremia, a normocytic or macrocytic anemia, elevated creatine kinase (from myopathy), and hypercholesterolemia and/or hypertriglyceridemia [from decreased lipoprotein-lipase activity and decreased low-density lipoprotein (LDL) receptor expression]. Anatomically, stimulation of the TSH receptor can cause follicular cell hyperplasia and goiter. Goiter can also be caused by glandular infiltration (e.g., Hashimoto thyroiditis, in which the gland is heavily infiltrated by lymphocytes).

Based on TSH and FT_4, the causes of hypothyroidism are classified as primary thyroid gland failure (low FT_4 and increased TSH; primary hypothyroidism) or central hypothyroidism (low FT_4 and usually a normal or low TSH concentration). Central hypothyroidism results from pituitary

BOX 55-2 Causes of Primary Hypothyroidism

Endogenous Disorders
Autoimmune thyroid disease
  Hashimoto thyroiditis
  Atrophic thyroiditis
  Late-stage Graves' disease
  Postpartum thyroiditis
Inborn errors in thyroid hormone biosynthesis (dyshormonogenesis)
  Na^+/iodide pump dysfunction
  Inadequate organification/iodination—thyroperoxidase dysfunction
  Defective thyroglobulin
  Deiodinase deficiency
  Pendred syndrome—hypothyroidism and deafness
Developmental disorders involving the thyroid gland
  Congenital hypothyroidism: aplasia, hypoplasia
  Ectopic thyroid: lingual thyroid, thyroglossal duct cyst
Consumptive hypothyroidism

Exogenous Disorders
Iodine excess/deficiency
Drugs
Thionamides
Lithium
Nitroprusside
Amiodarone
Biologicals (e.g., interferon, interleukin-2)
Dietary goitrogens
Radiation-induced hypothyroidism
Surgical removal of the thyroid gland
Viral or bacterial thyroiditis

disease (secondary hypothyroidism from TSH deficiency) or hypothalamic disease (tertiary hypothyroidism from TRH deficiency).

Primary Hypothyroidism

The causes of primary hypothyroidism are classified as endogenous or exogenous (Box 55-2).[38] Endogenous disorders are conditions that develop within the patient such as autoimmune thyroid gland dysfunction, inborn errors, and developmental abnormalities. Exogenous disorders are conditions that originate outside the patient such as iodine deficiency or excess, goitrogen or drug effects, and postsurgical hypothyroidism or hypothyroidism following radioactive iodine treatment.

Autoimmune Hypothyroidism

Excluding the newborn period, autoimmune thyroid disease (AITD) is the most common cause of thyroid disease and primary hypothyroidism.[111,148,203] Hashimoto thyroiditis (chronic lymphocytic thyroiditis) leads to destruction of the thyroid follicular cells through a cell-mediated autoimmune process.[102] Histologically, the gland is infiltrated with lymphocytes and plasma cells to the extent that secondary lymphoid follicles develop within the thyroid gland that are similar to the secondary follicles observed in normal lymph nodes. Initially, the gland is usually enlarged. Over time, with destruction of the gland, the gland can atrophy or become firm. In the rare condition of Riedel thyroiditis (Riedel disease or struma, ligneous struma, ligneous thyroiditis, chronic fibrous thyroiditis), the thyroid gland becomes fibrotic with possible attachment to adjacent structures that can produce, for example, tracheal compression.[144] Subacute (viral) thyroiditis may also cause Riedel thyroiditis.[31] Not all cases of Riedel thyroiditis are presaged by Hashimoto thyroiditis.

Although atrophy may occur in Hashimoto thyroiditis, atrophic thyroiditis may also occur when autoantibodies against the TSH receptor bind to the receptor and block the action of endogenous TSH. TSH receptor blocking autoantibodies can cross the placenta during pregnancy, causing transient hyperthyrotropinemia in infants (elevated TSH with a normal T_4) or even transient congenital hypothyroidism. Therefore atrophic thyroiditis falls under the rubric of AITD.

The diagnosis of Hashimoto thyroiditis is supported by recognition of autoantibodies against TPO or Tg.[113] Ninety percent of patients with chronic lymphocytic thyroiditis (the histologic description of Hashimoto thyroiditis) have antithyroperoxidase autoantibodies (TPOA), antithyroid microsomal autoantibodies (TMA), and/or antithyroglobulin autoantibodies (TgA), making these autoantibodies excellent markers for Hashimoto thyroiditis.[182] TPOA testing was initially pursued by testing for TMA (see section on thyroid autoantibody testing). TMA testing is being replaced by specific testing for TPOA using TPO as the antigen in the immunoassay. TPOA/TMA positivity is more common at the time of diagnosis than TgA positivity with TgA usually appearing later in the disease process. TgA overall are less common than TMA or TPOA. Ultrasound has limited value and is not routinely used to detect Hashimoto thyroiditis.

In many families, AITD appears to be inherited in an autosomal dominant pattern although some family members develop Hashimoto thyroiditis and other family members develop Graves' disease. Several genetic loci have been associated with susceptibility to Hashimoto thyroiditis (or AITD): HLA-DR, CTLA-4, CD40, FCRL3, Tg, the TSH receptor, PTPN22, and the IL-2 receptor. However, no single Mendelian locus explains the apparent autosomal dominant pattern of inheritance of AITD.[66] It is most appropriate to describe AITD as polygenic and multifactorial, indicating that both environment and multiple genes provide susceptibility to these very common disorders.

Nonendocrine and endocrine autoimmune disorders can occur with increased frequency in people with AITD. Chronic lymphocytic gastritis causing pernicious anemia may accompany AITD, particularly in older patients. AITD also occurs commonly in association with type 1 diabetes and pernicious anemia.[61,91,104] Another, less common, association is AITD and Addison disease.[82]

AITD can occur as part of autoimmune polyglandular syndrome type 2 (APS 2) and, more rarely, APS 1.[161,175] APS 2 affects women more often than men with onset in childhood or early adulthood and is diagnosed when Addison disease (or adrenal autoantibodies) occurs together with AITD and/or type 1 diabetes. In contrast to the polygenic nature of APS 2, mutations in AIRE (the autoimmune regulator gene that is a transcription factor; gene location: chromosome 21q22.3) produce autoimmune polyglandular syndrome type 1 (APS 1), which is inherited in an autosomal recessive pattern, thus affecting males and females equally.[18,93]

Another variant of AITD is postpartum thyroiditis (PPT).[192] PPT develops presumably as a consequence of a decline in the natural immunosuppression of pregnancy following delivery. PPT follows ≈5% of all pregnancies and ≈10% of pregnancies in women with type 1 diabetes. The clinical phenotype of PPT is transient hypothyroidism, hyperthyroidism, or both (one following the other) with a return to the euthyroid state by approximately 1 year postpartum. Women with thyroid autoantibodies are at highest risk for PPT. Later in life, permanent clinical evidence of AITD can develop in women afflicted with PPT. Thyroid autoimmunity, even in the absence of hypothyroidism, may impair fertility in women and increase the risk of spontaneous abortion in those women who do become pregnant.[154] Therefore an indication for thyroid autoantibody testing in the absence of hypothyroidism would be female infertility or recurrent miscarriage. Convincing data suggest that T_4 treatment of pregnant women who are positive for thyroid autoantibodies (especially TPOA) leads to a higher frequency of miscarriage (13.8%) than is seen in pregnant women who lack TPOA (2.4% rate of miscarriage), and that T_4 treatment of the TPOA-positive group reduces the rate of miscarriage to approximately 3.5%.[136]

Inborn Errors in Thyroid Hormone Biosynthesis

Inborn errors in thyroid hormone biosynthesis (dyshormonogenesis) are rare causes of primary hypothyroidism. These defects usually present early in life and can appear in newborns as a goiter. In very rare cases, asphyxia from tracheal compression has been reported.[213] Biochemical defects include iodine transport defects from loss-of-function mutations in the NIS (no increase in the perchlorate discharge); defects in thyroperoxidase, DUOX2,[130] and pendrin (with increased perchlorate discharge); thyroglobulin deficiency; and iodotyrosine dehalogenase mutations (potentially causing iodine deficiency through loss of MIT, DIT, and iodine in the urine).[129]

Developmental Hypothyroidism Disorders

Developmental causes of primary hypothyroidism involve aplasia or hypoplasia of the thyroid gland and ectopic and lingual thyroid glands.[202] These disorders account for ≈75% of cases of congenital hypothyroidism. Other causes of congenital hypothyroidism include thyroid dyshormonogenesis (10% of cases; see earlier), hypothalamic or pituitary abnormalities (5% of cases). Ten percent of cases of congenital hypothyroidism are transient.

Rare causes of congenital hypothyroidism involve loss-of-function mutations in the pituitary TRH receptor,[23] the TSH beta chain,[128] and the TSH receptor.[19,58] Mutations in anterior pituitary transcription factors (HESX1, LHX3, LHX4, PROP1, PIT1) can lead to TSH deficiency. Causes of transient congenital hypothyroidism include (1) severe maternal iodine deficiency, (2) acute iodine exposure, (3) transplacental passage of thionamides taken for treatment of maternal hyperthyroidism, (4) transplacental transfer of TSH receptor blocking antibodies, (5) hypothyroxinemia of prematurity, and (6) heterozygosity for a DUOX2 mutation.

Dried blood spot (DBS) screening for congenital hypothyroidism in North America reveals a general population frequency of congenital hypothyroidism of ≈1 in 4000. Congenital hypothyroidism is more common in Hispanic infants, less common in Caucasian infants, and least common in African American infants. The male-to-female ratio is 1 : 2. A higher frequency of congenital hypothyroidism is seen in infants with Down syndrome (≈1 in 140).

Clinically, fewer than 1 in 20 hypothyroid babies are recognized in the newborn nursery by physicians. This emphasizes the critical need for newborn biochemical screening. Early intervention improves clinical outcomes in these cases. However, some studies report that even with rapid treatment after birth, the IQ of affected children may be ≈10 points below that of their unaffected siblings. An increased frequency of neuropsychologic deficits has been reported in children with appropriately treated congenital hypothyroidism.

In North America, screening for congenital hypothyroidism is carried out predominantly by measuring total T_4 on DBSs. A common practice is to measure TSH in babies who have the lowest 10% of T_4's measured on the day of testing. Usually if the TSH is 60 mcIU/mL or greater (after the first 24 to 48 hours of life), a presumptive diagnosis of primary hypothyroidism is made, and the infant is transferred to a referral center emergently to be evaluated and started on thyroxine replacement therapy (e.g., 10 to 15 μg/kg/d). If the TSH is between 20 and 59 mIU/L, the infant is clinically evaluated and repeat thyroid function testing is performed before thyroid hormone replacement is started. If the TSH is less than 20 mIU/L, primary hypothyroidism is excluded. Screening with "T_4 only testing" will lead to missed rare cases of central hypothyroidism (1/100,000) and cases of hypothyroidism wherein TSH is elevated but T_4 is not yet depressed. In Europe, many screening programs use a TSH-first strategy. Although TSH screening will detect subclinical hypothyroidism (see later), cases of central hypothyroidism will be missed. Transcription factor mutations involving *TTF-1* and *Pax8* have been recognized in some children with congenital hypothyroidism. It is not clear whether molecular testing will prove useful in future screening programs for congenital hypothyroidism.

Hypothyroidism Caused by Iodine Deficiency or Excess

Worldwide, the most common cause of goiter is iodine deficiency. In iodine-deficient areas, especially mountainous areas, iodine deficiency produces "endemic" goiter. Frank hypothyroidism, however, is far less common because with iodine deficiency, more T_3 is synthesized than T_4, and within the thyroid gland, more T_4 is converted to T_3 to maintain the euthyroid state overall. Endemic goiters can develop nodularity (with or without hemorrhage into the nodule); in such cases, neoplasia must be excluded. Large goiters can produce dysphagia, obstruction of the trachea, or compression of the recurrent laryngeal nerves. A rare cause of iodine deficiency is nephrotic syndrome, with increased urinary loss of iodine often in the form of thyroid hormone.[53,114]

A significant danger of iodine deficiency is maternal hypothyroidism leading to an insufficient supply of thyroid hormone to the fetus in the first half of gestation, when the fetus is entirely dependent on maternal thyroid hormone. Thus maternal hypothyroidism can produce a reduction in the IQ of the affected child. Maternal iodine deficiency will produce fetal iodine deficiency.

Although it is logical that iodine deficiency would produce hypothyroidism because iodine is a necessary component in the synthesis of thyroid hormone, it is ironic that excess iodine can interfere with normal thyroid gland function.[106] However, excessive iodine does suppress thyroid gland function. High doses of iodine [super-saturated potassium iodide (SSKI) or Lugol's solution] are routinely used before planned surgical thyroidectomy for Graves' disease, to inhibit further thyroid hormone release and decrease the vascularity of the gland to reduce surgical blood loss.

Excess iodine reduces thyroid hormone release and inhibits organification of iodine and iodination of Tg (the *Wolff-Chaikoff effect*). The Wolff-Chaikoff effect can speculatively be interpreted as an autoregulatory response of the thyroid gland to avoid excessive production of thyroid hormone when exposed to high doses of exogenous iodine. Nondietary sources of excess iodine include amiodarone (an antiarrhythmic drug), povidone-iodine (used to disinfect the skin before surgery), and radiologic contrast agents that contain iodine. Excess iodine does not usually cause permanent thyroid dysfunction because the gland normally recovers ("escapes") from suppression after approximately 10 days of high-dose iodine administration. However, if the patient has underlying disease that may involve the thyroid (e.g., Hashimoto thyroiditis, Graves' disease), escape from the Wolff-Chaikoff effect is less likely and permanent hypothyroidism can develop.

Drug-Induced Hypothyroidism

Various drugs affect thyroid gland function (Table 55-4).[63] Collectively known as thionamides or thioureas, propylthiouracil (PTU), methimazole, and carbimazole inhibit the oxidation of iodide and the subsequent binding of iodine to tyrosine residues in Tg. Other drugs with thionamide-like activity include ethionamide, aminoglutethimide, phenylbutazone, and para-aminosalicylic acid. Evidence suggests an immunosuppressive effect of thionamides on thyroid autoimmunity.

PTU, methimazole, and carbimazole are commonly used to treat hyperthyroidism. (*Note:* Carbimazole is not available in the United States.) When large doses of PTU are used, the

TABLE 55-4 Effects of Some Drugs on Tests of Thyroid Function

Cause	Drug	Effect
Inhibit TSH secretion	Dopamine L-dopa Glucocorticoids Somatostatin	↓ T_4; ↓ T_3; ↓ TSH
Inhibit thyroid hormone synthesis or release	Iodine Lithium	↓ T_4; ↓ T_3; ↑ TSH
Inhibit conversion of T_4 to T_3	Amiodarone Glucocorticoids Propranolol Propylthiouracil Radiographic contrast agents	↓ T_3; ↑ rT_3; ↓, ⇌, ↑ T_4 and FT_4; ⇌, ↑ TSH
Inhibit binding of T_4/T_3 to serum proteins	Salicylates Phenytoin Carbamazepine Furosemide Nonsteroidal anti-inflammatory agents Heparin (in vitro effect)	↓ T_4; ↓ T_3; ↓ FT_4E, ⇌, ↑ FT_4; ⇌ TSH
Stimulate metabolism of iodothyronines	Phenobarbital Phenytoin Carbamazepine Rifampicin	↓ T_4; ↓ FT_4; ⇌ TSH
Inhibit absorption of ingested T_4	Aluminum hydroxide Ferrous sulfate Cholestyramine Colestipol Iron sucralfate Soybean preparations Kayexalate	↓ T_4; ↓ FT_4; ↑ TSH
Increase in concentration of T_4-binding proteins	Estrogen Clofibrate Opiates (heroin, methadone) 5-Fluorouracil Perphenazine	↑ T_4; ↑ T_3; ⇌ FT_4; ⇌ TSH
Decrease in concentration of T_4-binding proteins	Androgens Glucocorticoids	↓ T_4; ↓ T_3; ⇌ FT_4; ⇌ TSH

Data from Smallridge RD. Chapter 33. Thyroid function tests. In: Becker KL, ed. Principles and practice of endocrinology and metabolism, 7th edition. Philadelphia, Pa: JB Lippincott, 1995:299-306; Stockigt JR. Thyroid hormone changes in critical illness: the sick euthyroid "syndrome." Diagn Endo Metab 1997;15:39-46.

↓, Reduced serum concentration; ↑, increased serum concentration; ⇌, no change.

drug decreases peripheral conversion of T_4 to T_3 through inhibition of the D1 deiodinase. Because of this effect (in addition to the direct suppressive effect of PTU on the thyroid gland), some endocrinologists argue that PTU should be chosen over methimazole for the treatment of hyperthyroidism. However, recognition of serious or even fatal liver disease in a small (but significant) number of children treated with PTU is increasing.[100] Therefore, many pediatric endocrinologists discourage the routine use of PTU for the treatment of hyperthyroidism in children. Reduced granulocyte counts and subsequent infections are serious but uncommon side effects of thionamides. Therefore the white blood cell count and the differential count should be monitored during such therapy.

A potential advantage of methimazole over PTU is its longer half-life (PTU $t_{1/2}$ = 1.5 hours and methimazole $t_{1/2}$ = 6 hours). Both PTU and methimazole cross the placenta, can interfere with fetal thyroid function, and can cause goiter. Additionally, methimazole has been associated with aplasia cutis and choanal atresia. Therefore during pregnancy, PTU is the preferred drug in the treatment of maternal hyperthyroidism.

A variety of other drugs have been known to cause hypothyroidism. For example, lithium, which is used in the treatment of bipolar disorder (manic-depressive illness), can induce hypothyroidism.[85] The action of lithium appears similar to that of high-dose iodine, inhibiting thyroid hormone release and organification of iodine. Prolonged use of nitroprusside, a drug used to treat acute-onset, severe hypertension or severe heart failure by inducing preload and afterload reduction, may lead to hypothyroidism. Cyanide (CN^-) released from nitroprusside is metabolically converted to thiocyanate (SCN^-), which inhibits iodide uptake by the thyroid gland. Fortunately, nitroprusside only rarely causes hypothyroidism. Amiodarone is an antiarrhythmic drug that contains two iodine atoms per molecule and can induce hypothyroidism or hyperthyroidism.[22,204] Various recombinant DNA-derived biologicals (e.g., interferon-alpha, interleukin-2) used to treat chronic viral hepatitis or cancer have been found to cause thyroid dysfunction (hypothyroidism or hyperthyroidism).[124]

Surgical and Radiation-Induced Hypothyroidism

Surgical removal of the thyroid gland will produce hypothyroidism. External irradiation of the thyroid gland (e.g., treatment of lymphoma or Hodgkin disease) or ingestion of radioactive iodine can ablate the gland, causing hypothyroidism.[123] Administration of radioactive iodine to pregnant women can lead to ablation of the fetal thyroid gland, causing congenital hypothyroidism.

Viral or Bacterial Thyroiditis

Only rarely do viral or bacterial infections of the thyroid gland occur. Even more rarely do these entities damage the thyroid gland sufficiently to produce hypothyroidism. Viral infection of the thyroid gland is termed *subacute thyroiditis* (de Quervain, granulomatous, or giant cell thyroiditis) and can produce generalized thyroid gland tenderness. Bacterial infection of the thyroid gland is termed *acute thyroiditis* and can produce a thyroid abscess.[3]

Central Hypothyroidism

In a patient with clinical evidence of hypothyroidism, supported by laboratory findings of a low FT_4, if TSH is not elevated to the extent predicted (by FT_4), or if TSH is within or below the reference interval, central hypothyroidism should be considered.[92,229] Isolated pituitary TSH deficiency is rare, as most patients with secondary hypothyroidism also have other anterior pituitary hormone deficiencies (panhypopituitarism). Causes of central hypothyroidism (hypothalamic or pituitary disease) include (1) tumor, (2) hemorrhage, (3) trauma, (4) malformation, (5) postinfectious damage, and (6) postsurgical damage. Also, several rare autosomal recessive or dominant hereditary disorders involving transcription factor mutations can cause hypopituitarism and TSH deficiency: examples include paired-like homeodomain transcription factor-1 (Pit-1) and PROphet of Pit-1 *(PROP1)* mutations.[131]

Subclinical Hypothyroidism

Subclinical hypothyroidism is defined by a persistent elevation in TSH (6 to 12 weeks or longer) in the setting of FT_4 concentrations that are repeatedly found within the reference interval.[49] Other conditions wherein TSH is elevated but FT_4 is normal encompass recent reinstitution of thyroid hormone replacement therapy (FT_4 returns to normal before TSH declines), poor compliance with treatment in primary hypothyroidism, recovery from nonthyroidal illness, positively interfering heterophilic antibodies [e.g., human antimouse antibodies (HAMA)] in double-antibody immunoassays, and thyroid hormone resistance.

Subclinical hypothyroidism is very common, affecting 3 to 8% of the general population. By the sixth decade of life, 10% of the population exhibits laboratory findings consistent with subclinical hypothyroidism. Consequences of subclinical hypothyroidism include a high risk of progression to clinical hypothyroidism, dyslipidemia, vascular endothelial dysfunction, increased risk of cardiovascular disease and death, and possible neurocognitive deficits. The general consensus is that if TSH is repeatedly 10 mIU/L or greater, thyroid hormone replacement therapy is warranted. It is controversial whether thyroid hormone therapy is beneficial when TSH is less than 10 mIU/L, except during pregnancy, wherein any persistent TSH elevation requires treatment.

Controversy is ongoing over the appropriate upper limit of the reference interval for TSH. Basing the TSH reference interval on the central 95% of the general, healthy population results in an upper limit of normal between 4.0 and 5.0 mIU/L for many TSH assays. If patients with thyroid autoantibodies such as TPOA, a family history of thyroid disease, or an abnormal thyroid gland ultrasound are excluded from the reference population, the upper limit of the reference interval declines to approximately 2.5 to 3.0 mIU/L. Therefore, an upper limit of 2.5 to 3.0 mIU/L for TSH may be a truer definition of normal, because the reference population mostly excludes individuals with endogenous thyroid disease or propensity to develop thyroid disease. However, it is unclear how patients with TSH concentrations between 2.5/3.0 mIU/L and 4.0/5.0 mIU/L should be managed. It has been argued that lowering the upper limit of the reference interval will provide no clear patient benefit and inevitably will lead to confusion and possible overtreatment of subclinical hypothyroidism. Overtreatment carries the risk of predisposing the patient to osteoporosis and atrial fibrillation. As noted previously, the value of treatment when TSH is between 4.0/5.0 and 9.9 mIU/L is currently debated. Another component of the TSH reference interval debate is that according to National Health and Nutrition Examination Survey (NHANES) data,[9,134A,209] TSH rises as populations age. For example, in healthy adults age 80 and older, the upper limit of the reference interval for TSH is 7.5 mIU/L.

Thyroid Hormone Monitoring During Replacement Therapy

The thyroid hormone replacement of choice is Na^+-L-thyroxine (levothyroxine; T_4). Several brands of T_4 are available, including Synthroid (Abbott, North Chicago, Ill), Levothroid (Forest, St Louis, Mo) and Levoxyl (King, Bristol, Tenn). USP (United States Pharmacopeia) Thyroid or mixtures of T_4 and T_3 should not be used for thyroid hormone replacement. USP Thyroid is a desiccated extract of whole animal thyroid containing variable proportions of T_3 and T_4. Because its exact formulation is highly variable and is not standardized, USP Thyroid will not produce stable concentrations of thyroid hormone over the long term, leading to periods of excess or deficient thyroid hormone replacement. Despite many trials, fixed mixtures of T_3 plus T_4—examples include Naturethroid (RLC, Tempe, Ariz) and Thyrolar (Forest)—have not been shown to be clinically superior to T_4 replacement alone. Administering T_4 alone allows the body to regulate the production of T_3. Recall that normally 80% of T_3 comes from peripheral monodeiodination of T_4 to T_3. The sodium salt of T_3 (liothyronine) is available in tablet (Cytomel, King) and injectable (Triostat, King) forms. Considerable controversy surrounds whether generic preparations of T_4 are as effective as brand name preparations because of variable consistency and/or absorption from the gastrointestinal tract. Anecdotal reports have suggested that brand name preparations are clinically superior to generics.

Thyroxine should be taken at the same time of day for clinical consistency. The timing of FT_4 measurements should also be standardized because FT_4 may rise abruptly within hours of oral thyroxine ingestion. Thyroxine is best absorbed without food. A 2009 study demonstrated that TSH was lowest when thyroxine was taken in the fasting state (mean TSH, 1.06 mIU/L) versus when taken with breakfast (2.93 mIU/L) or at bedtime (2.19 mIU/L).[12] Many reasons have been put forth for variations in TSH measurements over time,[52] including intraindividual variation of 15 to 35%.[6] The 2003 National Academy of Clinical Biochemistry Laboratory Practice Management Guideline on thyroid function testing reported intraindividual coefficients of variation for TSH of 19.3% for 1 week, 20.6% for 6 weeks, and 22.4% for 1 year.[13] A significant source of biological variation in TSH is the pulsatile pattern of secretion and the fairly short half-life of TSH (approximately 1 to 2 hours).[80] In one study, TSH was released in approximately 18 pulses over the course of a day, and TSH half-life was 60 to 90 minutes. The half-life of TSH may vary between individuals, depending on interindividual differences in the degree of sialylation and sulfation of TSH.[47,149]

FT_4 and TSH are usually measured approximately 6 weeks after the beginning of thyroxine treatment for hypothyroidism. The dose of thyroxine should be titrated upward until FT_4 is in the upper half of the reference interval. TSH returns to the reference interval more slowly than the rise of FT_4 into the reference interval occurs in response to therapy. Ideally during treatment, TSH should be maintained within the reference interval. As the dose of thyroxine is increased during the initial months of therapy, some endocrinologists will allow TSH to be slightly suppressed (but >0.02 to 0.04 mIU/L) if the patient feels substantially better. It can be argued that, particularly in women, it is prudent to measure bone mineral density by dual-energy x-ray absorptiometry (DEXA) scan at least once a year to screen for bone loss that could result from overtreatment with thyroxine. Overtreatment of hypothyroidism is not uncommon.[7]

HYPERTHYROIDISM

Hyperthyroidism, also known as thyrotoxicosis, is the clinical syndrome that results from elevated concentrations of free thyroid hormone in the plasma, associated with clinical evidence of hypermetabolism.[135,139,178A] Symptoms of thyrotoxicosis include (1) nervousness, (2) erratic behavior, (3) emotional lability, (4) restlessness, 5) sleeplessness, (6) difficulty concentrating, (7) smooth and/or shiny hair and/or skin, (8) weight loss, (9) excessive sweating, (10) heat intolerance, (11) menstrual irregularities, and (12) diarrhea or frequent bowel movements. Physical signs compatible with hyperthyroidism include tachycardia, atrial arrhythmias, systolic murmurs, increased pulse pressure, a bounding pulse, warm and/or damp skin, softened texture of the skin, tremor, increased reflexes, eyelid retraction (and other signs of ophthalmopathy in Graves' disease), and hypocholesterolemia.

Based on TSH and FT_4, the causes of hyperthyroidism may be classified as primary (elevated FT_4 and decreased TSH) or central (elevated FT_4 and normal to elevated TSH). Central hyperthyroidism can be further parsed into pituitary (secondary hyperthyroidism from TSH excess) and hypothalamic (tertiary hyperthyroidism from TRH excess) causes. In primary hyperthyroidism, TSH is typically less than 0.05 mIU/L. With current assays, a TSH concentration within the reference interval nearly always excludes the diagnosis of primary hyperthyroidism.

Causes of Hyperthyroidism

The causes of hyperthyroidism are listed in Box 55-3. Endogenous disorders causing hyperthyroidism include intrinsic thyroid disease (primary hyperthyroidism), ectopic thyroid tissue (struma ovarii),[166] and disorders of the hypothalamus or pituitary causing excess TSH secretion (secondary hyperthyroidism). Exogenous causes of hyperthyroidism (disease related to external factors) encompass infectious origins (thyroid gland inflammation and destruction), iodine-induced hyperthyroidism, and thyroid hormone ingestion (thyrotoxicosis factitia).

The first line of treatment for primary hyperthyroidism is controversial. Administration of radioactive iodine is the first choice in many adults and older children with Graves' disease. When medical therapy is chosen, thionamides are used to suppress thyroid gland hyperactivity.[195] In the immediate period following the start of thionamide therapy, TSH measurements may poorly reflect the patient's thyroid status because TSH can remain suppressed for months even after the patient becomes clinically euthyroid. This is similar to the treatment of hypothyroidism, where 6 weeks or more can elapse before TSH returns to normal even with adequate thyroxine replacement.

After 1 to 2 years of thionamide therapy, if disease remission has not occurred, radioactive iodine is usually advised.[71] An alternative therapy is thyroidectomy, particularly in specialized centers with extensive surgical experience. However, with radioactive iodine ablation of the gland, there is no surgical risk of inadvertent parathyroidectomy or recurrent laryngeal nerve injury. As a consequence of radioactive iodine treatment or thyroidectomy, primary hypothyroidism can subsequently develop, necessitating surveillance for hypothyroidism with yearly TSH measurements.

BOX 55-3 Causes of Hyperthyroidism

Endogenous Thyroid Disorders
- Autoimmune thyroid disease
- Graves' disease
- Hashitoxicosis
- Postpartum thyroiditis
- Gain-of-function mutation in the TSH receptor
- Toxic nodule

Toxic multinodular goiter
- Toxic adenoma
- Familial
- Struma ovarii
- hCG-induced hyperthyroidism

Gestational transient thyrotoxicosis
TSH receptor sensitivity to hCG
hCG-secreting tumors
- Secondary hyperthyroidism (e.g., central hyperthyroidism)

Exogenous Disorders
Thyroid destruction from viral or bacterial thyroiditis
Iodine-induced hyperthyroidism
Thyroid hormone ingestion (thyrotoxicosis factitia)

T_3 Toxicosis

T_3 toxicosis is defined by the presence of clinical hyperthyroidism in a patient with suppressed TSH, normal FT_4, and elevated T_3 (or FT_3).[50] FT_4 may be normal in early hyperthyroidism when a very mild excess of thyroid hormone is causing increased thyroidal and peripheral deiodination of T_4 to T_3, raising the latter but not the former. Recall that D1 conversion of T_4 to T_3 is enhanced in hyperthyroidism. T_3 toxicosis is also possible when hyperthyroidism occurs in the presence of mild iodine deficiency, when iodine is sufficient to synthesize excessive amounts of T_3 but not T_4. Last, it is known that stimulation of the TSHR enhances the production of T_3 more than T_4. T_3 toxicosis is not a unique or individual disease, but rather can be considered a phase in the natural progression of primary hyperthyroidism that may or may not be recognized by the clinician.

Graves' Disease

Graves' disease affects approximately 0.4% of the U.S. population and results from agonistic autoantibodies that bind to, and activate, the TSH receptor, producing excess release of thyroid hormone and subsequent clinical hyperthyroidism.[24] Women are more frequently affected by Graves' disease than men, by a 5:1 ratio.

The classical clinical triad observed in patients with Graves' disease consists of (1) goiter and biochemical hyperthyroidism, (2) exophthalmos, and (3) nonpitting pretibial myxedema.[220] The presence of exophthalmos strongly suggests Graves' disease in a hyperthyroid patient. Exophthalmos appears to have an autoimmune cause. Retro-orbital tissues may express TSH receptors, and consequent to stimulatory TSH receptor autoantibodies, retro-orbital tissue hyperplasia occurs, producing exophthalmos.[17] Myxedema is the accumulation of mucopolysaccharides in subcutaneous tissue that cause visible and palpable swelling. The potential finding of myxedema in both Graves' disease and Hashimoto thyroiditis (with hypothyroidism) is not readily explained.

Similar to Hashimoto thyroiditis, genetic susceptibility to Graves' disease is polygenic.[66] In practice, Hashimoto thyroiditis is often associated with HLA-DR5 while Graves' disease is associated with HLA-DR3.

TPOA (including TMA) and TgA are seen in both Hashimoto thyroiditis and Graves' disease but usually are found in higher concentrations in Hashimoto thyroiditis. However, these autoantibodies do not distinguish between the two conditions. Testing for TSH receptor autoantibodies should be reserved for cases where the diagnosis of Graves' disease is in doubt. TSH receptor autoantibody (TRA) testing is available for stimulatory autoantibodies [TSH receptor stimulatory autoantibodies (TSI)] and receptor-binding autoantibodies [thyrotropin-binding inhibitory immunoglobulins (TBII)]. Usually, both TSI and TBII tests are positive in patients with Graves' disease.

Hashitoxicosis and Postpartum Thyroiditis

During the clinical course of Hashimoto thyroiditis, if a period of accelerated destruction of thyroid follicular cells occurs, subsequent release of thyroid hormone can produce a transient interval of hyperthyroidism, termed *Hashitoxicosis.*[133] Hashitoxicosis should be differentiated from Graves' disease because the treatments for these two conditions are different. Hashitoxicosis is self-limited, and if any treatment is required, β-blockers (such as propranolol) are used to suppress the effects of excess catecholamines, such as tachycardia. TRA are usually positive in patients with Graves' disease and negative in Hashitoxicosis. In addition, the RAIU is elevated in Graves' disease but is not elevated in Hashitoxicosis. Patients with postpartum thyroiditis can experience a period of transient, usually self-limited, hyperthyroidism from accelerated breakdown of thyroid tissue. Subacute or acute thyroiditis can produce a period of transient hyperthyroidism.

Toxic Nodular or Multinodular Goiter

A subset of patients with nodular or multinodular goiter can develop hyperthyroidism.[35,155,181] When hyperthyroidism is caused by these lesions, the term *toxic* has been used *(toxic multinodular goiter).* In the older literature, toxic multinodular goiter is referred to as Plummer disease.

The cause of nodular or multinodular goiter is not well characterized. One theory is that these disorders arise from colloid goiters.[37] A colloid goiter itself is a disorder of unknown origin, in which the thyroid gland enlarges because of increased size of the follicular lacunae.[5] Microscopically, the enlarged lacunae display wide variation in size. However, colloid goiters do not display the follicular cell hyperplasia typical of Graves' disease. Patients with colloid goiter lack thyroid autoantibodies, and no evidence suggests a defect in thyroid hormone biosynthesis. Over many years, some regions of colloid goiters undergo further hypertrophy, while other areas atrophy, producing nodules that may become palpable. TRA are negative in toxic multinodular goiter.[214]

In some cases of nodular or multinodular goiter, the hyperactive tissue can display a somatic gain-of-function mutation in the TSH receptor or G_s protein, so that the receptor is perpetually in the "on" confirmation or functions as though it is in the "on" position, in the absence of TSH binding to the receptor.[201] This mutation occurs in at least 60% of cases of nodular or multinodular goiter with hyperthyroidism. However, in the other 40% of cases, the cause of the hyperthyroidism is unknown. Somatically acquired gain-of-function mutations in the G_s alpha subunit produce many of the symptoms of McClune-Albright syndrome, including thyrotoxicosis.

Sometimes follicular adenomas are autonomously hyperactive, producing hyperthyroidism (toxic adenomas).[87] Other than elevated FT_4 and depressed TSH from hyperthyroidism, no specific laboratory tests can diagnose nodular or multinodular goiter, or a toxic adenoma. Toxic (hyperactive, or "hot") nodules are very rarely carcinomas. Cold nodules (nodules that do not synthesize thyroid hormone and do not take up radioactive iodine or technetium) may result from TSH receptor loss-of-function mutations. Any nodule that is not "hot" may be cancerous, and fine-needle aspiration biopsy should be strongly considered.

Gain-of-Function Mutations in the TSH Receptor

A familial, autosomal dominant form of non–Graves' disease hyperthyroidism that is due to gain-of-function mutations in the TSH receptor has been described.[89] The gain-of-function mutation places the TSH receptor in the "on" position in the absence of ligand (TSH) binding. In infants homozygous for such mutations, neonatal thyrotoxicosis, even requiring emergency thyroidectomy, has been observed. Certain heterozygous mutations have caused infantile hyperthyroidism.[217]

Central Hyperthyroidism

TSH-secreting anterior pituitary adenomas are very rare.[103] This diagnosis is suggested by (1) clinical hyperthyroidism, (2) elevated FT_4, (3) normal to elevated TSH concentration, and (4) evidence of a pituitary mass on computed tomography (CT) scan or magnetic resonance imaging (MRI). Incidentalomas of the pituitary are found in approximately 5% of the general population; therefore a CT or MRI anomaly is not pathognomonic for a pituitary adenoma. A thyrotropinoma can produce a mass displacement effect, resulting in deficiencies of other anterior pituitary hormones caused by compression of pituitary tissue.[96]

Rarely, selective pituitary resistance to the effects of thyroid hormone is present, yet peripheral sensitivity is normal.[226] This condition produces clinical hyperthyroidism because only elevated concentrations of thyroid hormones suppress TSH. The subsequent rise in TSH promotes thyroid hormone synthesis and release from the thyroid gland, producing clinical hyperthyroidism because the peripheral tissues have normal responsiveness to thyroid hormone. Selective pituitary resistance to thyroid hormone feedback is suggested when the pituitary CT scan or MRI is normal. Unique mutations in TRβ causing selective pituitary resistance have been described.[169]

Hyperthyroidism Due to Human Chorionic Gonadotropin

Human chorionic gonadotropin (hCG)–induced hyperthyroidism is observed in gestational transient thyrotoxicosis, TSH receptor sensitivity to appropriate hCG concentrations during pregnancy, and hCG-secreting tumors.[94,97,163] Gestational transient thyrotoxicosis occurs in 2 to 3% of all pregnancies, and results from activation of TSH receptors by hCG, which is greatly elevated during pregnancy. The degree of hyperthyroidism is typically mild, and treatment is not usually required. In contrast to Graves' disease, thyroid autoantibodies are negative. If PTU or methimazole is used, fetal monitoring for thyroid dysfunction is important, because these drugs cross the placenta, potentially causing fetal hypothyroidism and goiter.

Fetal thyroid gland suppression by thionamides is a concern when any pregnant woman with hyperthyroidism is treated. The size of the fetal thyroid gland can be monitored by ultrasound. TSH and T_4 can be measured in fetal blood obtained by cordocentesis (a high-risk procedure) or in the amniotic fluid.[34] Besides the analytical challenge of measuring the very low concentrations of these hormones in nonplasma body fluids, finding an appropriate reference interval can be difficult. Also, it is unlikely that many laboratories have validated measurements of thyroid hormone or TSH in amniotic fluid. Hyperemesis gravidarum (severe vomiting during pregnancy) has been associated with gestational transient thyrotoxicosis and may be related to very high hCG concentrations.[147]

Tumors that secrete hCG, such as choriocarcinoma, hydatidiform mole, or metastatic embryonal carcinoma, have caused hyperthyroidism through hCG stimulation of the TSH receptor.[212]

Iodine-Induced Hyperthyroidism

In a patient with iodine deficiency and underlying Graves' disease or nodular/multinodular goiter, iodine administration may lead to hyperthyroidism.[132] Before iodine replenishment is provided, hyperthyroidism is likely to be kept in check by iodine deficiency.[193] The phenomenon of iodine-induced hyperthyroidism is termed the *Jod-Basedow syndrome* (or phenomenon). Distinct from these two disorders (iodine-induced hyperthyroidism in iodine-deficient Graves' disease and nodular/multinodular goiter) are rare patients without underlying thyroid disease who paradoxically develop hyperthyroidism with iodine treatment.[10,101]

Sources of iodine besides the diet include administered iodinated radiocontrast dyes, Lugol's solution, topical antiseptics, iodine-containing expectorants, and amiodarone.[152] The typical intake of iodine in the United States is 150 to 200 µg/d, one 200 mg tablet of amiodarone contains 75 mg of iodine, of which 6 mg is liberated (corresponding to at least 30 times the usual daily intake!).

Other Exogenous Causes of Hyperthyroidism

Thyroid gland destruction from any cause, including nonautoimmune thyroiditis from viral (subacute) or bacterial (acute) causes, can release excessive amounts of thyroid hormone, producing hyperthyroidism.[179,180] Intentional or unintentional ingestion of excess thyroid hormone can also produce hyperthyroidism.[76] In one interesting report, hyperthyroidism developed in people who ate hamburger meat that included bovine thyroid glands added during the grinding process.[146]

When thyroid hormone is ingested or released from an inflamed or damaged thyroid gland, subsequent suppression of TSH reduces thyroidal iodine uptake, which is reflected in a reduction in the RAIU test. Likewise, glandular suppression will lower circulating Tg concentrations. If T_3 is ingested (e.g., Cytomel), hyperthyroidism can ensue, producing an unusual set of biochemical abnormalities: suppressed TSH, suppressed FT_4 (and total T_4, because of TSH suppression), and elevated total T_3 (and FT_3).

Maternal Graves' disease can cause fetal (and transient neonatal) hyperthyroidism from the transplacental passage of TSI.[89] In these cases, neonatal hyperthyroidism, although potentially serious and possibly fatal if not recognized and appropriately treated, is usually self-limited.

Thyroid Storm and Apathic Hyperthyroidism

Thyroid storm (also, *thyrotoxic crisis*) is an uncommon syndrome of severe and accelerating hyperthyroidism potentially manifested in (1) tachycardia, (2) restlessness, (3) high-output congestive heart failure, (4) fever greater than 41 °C, (5) extreme irritability, (6) delirium or coma, (7) hypotension, and (8) vomiting or diarrhea.[134] Although laboratory tests reveal suppressed TSH and elevated FT_4 and T_3 concentrations, thyroid storm remains a clinical diagnosis. Thyroid storm cannot be diagnosed on the basis of the magnitude of FT_4 or T_3 concentrations, or of changes observed in these hormones compared with previous measurements.

In older individuals, an unusual variant of hyperthyroidism is termed *apathetic hyperthyroidism.*[127] In this disorder, biochemical evidence of thyroid hormone excess is observed in the absence of any clinical evidence of hyperthyroidism. Alternatively, only a single organ system may be affected.

Subclinical Hyperthyroidism

A persistent depression in TSH when FT_4 and T_3 concentrations are normal identifies subclinical hyperthyroidism.[55] Patients with subclinical hyperthyroidism have increased frequencies of atrial fibrillation and osteoporosis. In the absence of a clinically compatible cardiac arrhythmia or significantly reduced bone mineral density, there is little justification for placing a patient with subclinical hyperthyroidism on thionamide therapy. The treatment of patients with asymptomatic hyperthyroidism is much more controversial than the treatment of those with asymptomatic hypothyroidism.

Nonthyroidal Illness (Sick Euthyroid Syndrome)

Any type of significant nutritional deprivation, acute severe illness, or chronic illness can result in thyroid function changes characterized as *nonthyroidal illness* (NTI; "sick euthyroid syndrome"; low T_3 syndrome; Table 55-5).[1] Suppressed peripheral conversion of T_4 to T_3 by D1 and D2 leads to decreased circulating T_3 (and FT_3), while diminished degradation of rT_3 by D1 raises circulating rT_3 concentrations (Figure 55-17). In experimental systems, interleukin (IL)-1 and IL-6 have been shown to impair D1 activity. T_3 can decline by as much as 50% with a twofold to threefold increase in rT_3. Poorly controlled diabetes mellitus and drugs such as glucocorticoids and β-blockers can also inhibit the conversion of T_4 to T_3. As mentioned previously, one effect of propylthiouracil is to block D1, inhibiting the conversion of T_4 to T_3.

Decreased T_3 reduces oxygen and nutritional demands and is considered to be an adaptive and beneficial response to illness. The recognition that NTI does not represent hypothyroidism is important because thyroid hormone replacement therapy of patients affected with NTI does not improve clinical outcome and may be detrimental.[48,79,207]

Because FT_4 concentrations are usually normal in NTI (at least in the early stages), and D2 activity is sustained in the

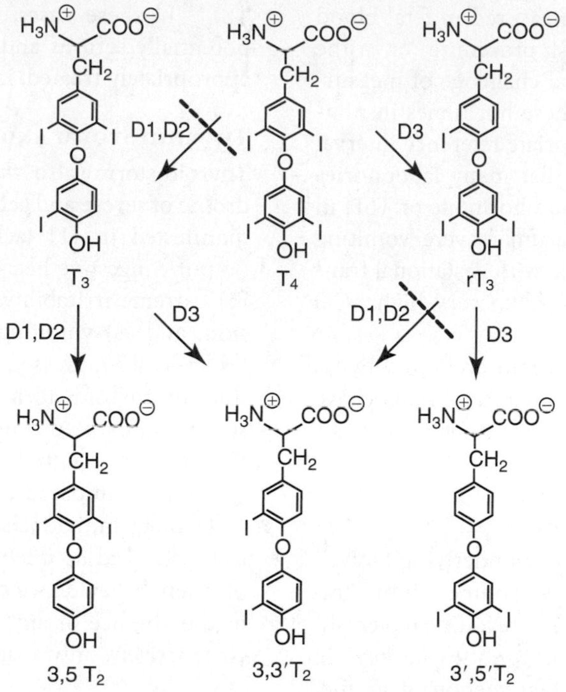

Figure 55-17 Effects of altered deiodination. In states of nonthyroidal illness (e.g., the sick euthyroid syndrome), thyroid hormone deiodination patterns are altered, with reduced T_3 concentrations and elevated concentrations of rT_3.

TABLE 55-5 Nonthyroidal Illness

	Initial	Mid Course	Prolonged	Resolution
TSH	Nl	Nl, Decr	Decr	Incr
T_4	Nl	Variable	Decr	Decr
T_3	Decr (−)	Decr (− −)	Decr (− − −)	Decr (−)
rT_3	Incr (+)	Incr (+ +)	Incr (+)	Incr (+)

Note: The severity of decreased T_3 is proportional to the number of (−) signs. The degree of increase in rT_3 is proportional to the number of (+) signs.

pituitary, the pituitary is exposed to adequate concentrations of T_3 from intrapituitary conversion of T_4 to T_3. Therefore, although plasma T_3 may decline in NTI, TSH concentrations do not rise (at least not before the recovery stage of NTI). The pulsatility of TSH is attenuated, yet TSH typically remains within the reference interval. Occasionally, paradoxical increases in FT_4 result from T_4 displacement from thyroxine-binding proteins caused by elevated free fatty acid concentrations, as well as other uncharacterized substances that rise in concentration in NTI.

With prolonged NTI, disordered hypothalamic-pituitary function causes a decline in TSH concentration, which results in a concurrent decline in FT_4. During recovery, TSH can rise above the reference interval and remain elevated until FT_4 and T_3 return to normal, usually after 1 to 2 months. The sequential stages in NTI are illustrated in Table 55-5.

Because of NTI, it can be very difficult to interpret thyroid function abnormalities in hospitalized patients. Thus, thyroid function testing in inpatients should be carried out only when there is the legitimate suspicion that thyroid dysfunction is contributing to the patient's acute need for hospitalization (such as cardiovascular disease, heart failure, or coma).

In a hospitalized patient, thyroid replacement therapy should be considered only if the TSH is significantly elevated (≥20 mIU/L). When modest elevations in TSH are observed (5 to 19 mIU/L), measurement of rT_3 may be helpful; rT_3 is low in hypothyroidism, but elevated in NTI. However, rT_3 measurements usually are not essential to the diagnosis of NTI. If a long-term hospitalized patient without hypothalamic or pituitary disease has TSH less than 0.05 mIU/L, hyperthyroidism is a possibility. With hospitalized patents, a cooperative dialogue between the clinician and the laboratorian can be helpful in deciding the proper diagnosis and management of the patient.

Thyroid Hormone Resistance

Loss-of-function mutations in the TRβ chain (the intranuclear thyroid hormone receptor, beta chain) lead to the rare syndrome of thyroid hormone resistance.[2] In this autosomal dominant condition, supraphysiologic concentrations of T_3

and T_4 (and FT_3 and FT_4) are required to maintain the euthyroid state. Therefore, in the absence of clinical hyperthyroidism, if the biochemical picture of elevated T_4, FT_4, T_3, and FT_3 is present with TSH in the upper reference interval or mildly elevated, thyroid hormone resistance is likely. Because of TSH stimulation of the thyroid, glandular enlargement may be seen because there is no resistance to TSH. Some affected patients may, in fact, have mild clinical findings of hypothyroidism. If patients with thyroid hormone resistance are incorrectly treated with thyroid-suppressing drugs, clinical hypothyroidism may be induced.

Another form of thyroid hormone resistance results from defective conversion of T_4 to T_3. This condition results from a mutation in the sequence-binding protein 2 (gene name: *SECISBP2*), which influences the synthesis of cellular deiodinases.

Euthyroid Hyperthyroxinemia

Euthyroid hyperthyroxinemia exists when total T_4 is elevated yet the patient is clinically euthyroid.[158,205] Because FT_4 measurements have supplanted total T_4 measurements, euthyroid hyperthyroxinemia is not commonly encountered in modern clinical practice.

Besides TBG elevations and the thyroid hormone resistance syndromes, euthyroid hyperthyroxinemia can also result from acute illness (through a mechanism that is not well understood) or abnormalities in albumin and transthyretin. Familial dysalbuminemic hyperthyroxinemia is an autosomal dominant disorder characterized by an albumin variant that has a greater binding affinity for T_4 (but not T_3).[16,28] Although TSH, FT_4, and total T_3 (and FT_3) are all normal, total T_4 is elevated. Mutations in transthyretin can lead to familial euthyroid thyroxine excess, an autosomal dominant disorder producing abnormal thyroid function tests similar to what is observed in familial dysalbuminemic hyperthyroxinemia.[14] These two disorders can be distinguished from conditions involving overproduction of TBG by measuring TBG concentration.

MCT8 Mutations

Loss-of-function mutations in MCT8, causing a rare form of X-linked mental retardation, have been reported.[74,211] Because MCT8 is important for the transport of thyroid hormone into neurons, there are profound adverse effects on the development of the nervous system in affected males. In addition to mental retardation and hypotonia, an unusual pattern of thyroid function abnormalities occurs, with increased T_3, normal to decreased T_4 (and FT_4), normal to elevated TSH, and low rT_3 concentrations.

Defective cellular uptake of T_3 can, in part, explain elevated T_3 concentrations in the blood. However, evidence indicates that not all tissues display equivalent defects in thyroid hormone uptake, and this may explain the decline in T_4 and rT_3. Increased T_3 concentrations in the liver may also promote T_4 and rT_3 clearance. If the pituitary or hypothalamus is less sensitive to negative feedback from thyroid hormones (because T_3 does not normally enter thyrotrophs or the hypothalamic PVN), theoretically, TSH concentrations would rise. The elevation in TSH may further contribute to elevated T_3 concentrations caused by increased T_3 production by the thyroid gland. The observation that MCT8 mutations exist requires recognition of a new pattern of thyroid function studies. Various patterns of thyroid function tests are shown in Table 55-6.

SCREENING FOR THYROID DYSFUNCTION

Other than newborn screening for congenital hypothyroidism, the value of thyroid function testing in asymptomatic individuals is highly controversial.[72,196,210] Excluding newborn screening for congenital hypothyroidism, so far no compelling data show that screening asymptomatic individuals,

TABLE 55-6 Patterns of Thyroid Dysfunction

	TSH	FT_4	Comments
Primary hypothyroidism	Increased	Decreased	-----
Subclinical primary hypothyroidism	Increased	Normal	-----
Primary hyperthyroidism	Decreased	Increased	T_3: increased
T_3 toxicosis	Decreased	Normal	T_3: increased
Subclinical primary hyperthyroidism	Decreased	Normal	T_3: normal
Thyroid hormone resistance due to defects in the thyroid hormone receptor	Normal to increased	Increased	T_3: increased; rT_3: increased
Thyroid hormone resistance due to defects in thyroid hormone metabolism	Mildly increased	Increased	T_3: decreased; rT_3: increased
Thyroid hormone resistance due to defects in thyroid hormone transport into cells	Normal to increased	Normal to decreased	T_3: increased; rT_3: decreased

including pregnant women or the elderly, improves the clinical outcome of the patient.

DRUG EFFECTS ON THYROID FUNCTION

Various drugs alter thyroid function in a large number of ways.[60,170] For example, dopamine, L-dopa, glucocorticoids, and somatostatin all depress TSH, potentially leading to a fall in thyroid hormone concentrations. As noted previously, iodine (including amiodarone) and lithium impair thyroid hormone synthesis or release, causing primary hypothyroidism.[85]

Many drugs inhibit conversion of T_4 to T_3, including amiodarone, glucocorticoids, β-blockers, propylthiouracil, and radiographic contrast agents. While T_3 declines and rT_3 rises, FT_4 may increase, decrease, or remain unchanged. Other drugs can displace T_4 and T_3 from thyroid hormone–binding proteins; salicylates, phenytoin, carbamazepine, furosemide, nonsteroidal anti-inflammatory agents, and heparin (in vitro effect) lower total T_4 and T_3 by occupying binding sites on proteins, yet FT_4 remains within the reference interval or rises.

Increased metabolism of thyroid hormone lowers T_4 and T_3. Phenobarbital, phenytoin, carbamazepine, and rifampicin can lower T_4 and T_3. Because (1) aluminum hydroxide, (2) ferrous sulfate, (3) cholestyramine, (4) colestipol, (5) iron sucralfate, (6) soybean preparations, and (7) Kayexalate all inhibit thyroid hormone absorption, their effects should be considered in any patient being treated with thyroxine replacement.

THYROGLOBULIN

The biology of Tg was extensively reviewed in the biochemistry section of this chapter. Some Tg normally enters the circulation by direct exocytosis from thyroid follicular cells without being iodinated. Tg is normally detected in the circulation in concentrations between 3 and 40 ng/mL. The highest Tg concentrations are in cord blood and are noted during the first weeks of life. Between 2 and 6 weeks of age, Tg concentrations are between 10 and 250 ng/mL,[51] and they decline until adulthood.[141] Three factors influence the concentration of Tg in the plasma: (1) the degree of thyroid gland stimulation via the TSH receptor, (2) the mass of thyroid tissue present in the individual, and (3) the presence of thyroid disease or damage, which leads to increased release of Tg into the circulation.

When TSH is within the reference interval, each gram of thyroid tissue provides approximately 1 ng/mL of Tg to the circulation. At TSH concentrations less than 0.1 mIU/L, each gram of thyroid tissue releases only about 0.5 ng/dL of Tg into the plasma. Trauma to the thyroid gland, inflammation (such as subacute thyroiditis or amiodarone-induced thyroiditis), surgical removal, or irradiation produces elevated Tg concentrations. Following fine-needle aspiration, Tg can be elevated for up to 3 weeks. Tg is typically decreased in acquired hypothyroidism, congenital hypothyroidism (from thyroid hypoplasia), factitious hyperthyroidism (because of TSH suppression), and following thyroidectomy.

Clinical Utility of Thyroglobulin Measurements

Thyroid cancer is classified according to the cell of origin (follicular vs. parafollicular) and the degree of differentiation (cancers of follicular origin, including differentiated papillary, follicular, or Hürthle cell carcinoma, vs. anaplastic thyroid cancer). Following surgery for differentiated thyroid carcinoma, the completeness of tumor excision can be assessed by measuring serum Tg concentrations.[54,67] If thyroglobulin autoantibodies are present (see later), Tg measurements are unreliable.

Following thyroidectomy and/or radioactive iodine therapy, plasma Tg should be undetectable unless residual thyroid tissue or metastatic lesions are present. To ensure that any remnant thyroid, or metastatic tumor, tissue is stimulated to produce Tg, the patient's TSH must not be suppressed (postoperative thyroid hormone replacement must be discontinued), or, alternatively, exogenous recombinant DNA-produced TSH (thyrogen-alpha; Thyrogen, Genzyme, Cambridge, Mass) may be given.[140] Exogenous TSH administration normally stimulates at least a fivefold increase in Tg if responsive tissue is present. With a local thyroid tumor remnant (following incomplete thyroidectomy) or a well-differentiated thyroid tumor, TSH can stimulate a tenfold increase in Tg concentration.[188] With poorly differentiated tumors, Tg rises less than threefold after TSH. One caveat is that the differentiated thyroid cancer should be shown to produce Tg before surgery is performed, lest the patient be judged to be in remission following surgery but his or her cancer is a rare non–Tg-secreting differentiated thyroid carcinoma.

Tg measurements have other clinical uses. For example, the absence of detectable Tg in the serum of an infant with congenital hypothyroidism supports the diagnosis of thyroid dysgenesis. In cases of congenital hypothyroidism where Tg is undetectable, but thyroid gland tissue is identified by thyroid scan, a Tg gene mutation should be considered. In cases of suspected factitious hyperthyroidism (hyperthyroidism caused by exogenous thyroid hormone ingestion), Tg will be suppressed; in Graves' disease, Tg is measurable.

ANALYTICAL METHODS

The approach to the laboratory assessment of thyroid function has changed considerably over the past 2 decades. This change was driven by two technologic advances: (1) a roughly 100-fold improvement in the lower detection limits of analytical methods to measure TSH, and (2) widespread availability of free (unbound) T_4 assays on automated platforms. An unfortunate consequence of this change, however, was the emergence of a confusing array of terms used to describe the analytical methods that measure thyroid hormones. Terms such as "direct," "indirect," "index," "one-step," and "two-step" are used in nonstandard and often inconsistent ways in reference to FT_4 assays.[120] In addition, the term "analog" (or "analogue," in the UK) is often used to describe FT_4 immunoassays, as though these methods involve a technology that is unique from other competitive and noncompetitive binding immunoassays that make use of a chemically modified antigen, when the approach basically is the same. Finally, "generational" numbers have been applied to TSH immunoassays to designate the analytical sensitivity. In other analytes (such as troponin T), generational numbers mostly refer to improvements in specificity, and more sensitive assays for analytes such as C-reactive protein are simply designated as "high sensitivity." Except where helpful to establish historical relationships, use of these terms will be avoided in favor of more standard immunoassay terminology.

Measurement of Thyrotropin (TSH)

Human thyrotropin [thyroid-stimulating hormone (TSH)] is a 28 to 30 kDa dimeric glycoprotein consisting of a 92 amino acid alpha subunit (identical to the alpha subunit of human chorionic gonadotropin, follicle-stimulating hormone, and luteinizing hormone) and a 112 to 118 amino acid beta subunit. Functionally important domains are present on both alpha and beta subunits; neither is active alone. Residues 113 to 118 of the beta subunit undergo post-translational proteolytic cleavage without affecting hormonal activity, so the C-terminal end of the beta subunit apparently is not necessary for receptor binding.

Although bioassays are available for measurement of TSH activity, and radioimmunoassay (RIA) has been used as well, nearly all modern TSH methods are two-site "sandwich" heterogeneous immunoassays involving an enzyme or chemiluminescent label. Migration to more sensitive TSH methods about 2 decades ago prompted a change in the strategy for laboratory investigation of thyroid dysfunction, establishing TSH as its foundation. Sensitivity was the essential catalyst of this change because TSH concentrations may be decreased in nonthyroidal illness, and the lower limit of detection was necessary to distinguish between nonthyroidal causes of suppressed TSH and thyrotoxicosis, which is associated with TSH concentrations less than 0.01 mIU/L.

The "generational" classification divides TSH methods by analytical sensitivities separated by roughly one log unit. Thus, first-, second-, and third-generation methods have functional sensitivities of 1.0, 0.1, and 0.01 mIU/L, respectively. Some methods claim a detection limit of 0.001 mIU/L and, following this convention, are called fourth-generation methods. These definitions are not formal but were loosely adopted by manufacturers of TSH assays and are used more for marketing purposes than to express analytical performance by standard criteria.

In 1991, the Nomenclature Committee of the American Thyroid Association recommended that the *functional detection limit* of serum TSH assays should be determined on the basis of low-end interassay precision characteristics.[69] The Committee recommended that precision [coefficient of variation (CV)] at the lower reporting limit should be 10 to 15%, but no worse than 20%. Currently, functional sensitivity is defined as the lowest concentration of TSH at which an interassay CV of 20% or less can be achieved.[168,190] The American Thyroid Association determined that only TSH assays with third-generation (≤0.01 mIU/L) functional sensitivity are sufficient for use as screening tests for hyperthyroidism; their recommendation is consistent with the National Academy of Clinical Biochemistry Laboratory Medicine Practice Guideline[13] for assessment of thyroid function.

An additional complication in defining the analytical performance of TSH assays is that the hormone is subject to structural heterogeneity because of genetic polymorphisms and post-translational modifications affecting the carbohydrate content, as well as proteolytic removal of the six C-terminal beta subunit residues. There was poor agreement between various TSH immunoassays until an International Reference Preparation (IRP) isolated from pituitary tissue was made available in the 1980s. In 1999, a recombinant human TSH IRP was created,[157] but significant differences have been noted between recombinant TSH and isolates from pituitary tissue, primarily as the result of modifications of polysaccharide moieties on TSH, which are highly cell specific. Pituitary-derived TSH contains polysaccharides that are mostly sulfated, however the recombinant hormone is primarily sialylated.[157] These modifications produce epitopic diversity and change the antigenic profile of the protein. Efforts have been made to chemically modify recombinant TSH to more closely resemble the circulating form of the hormone. This approach eventually may result in better agreement between various TSH immunoassays.[40]

Principles of TSH Immunoassays

Modern automated TSH immunoassays typically involve a double-antibody approach [for which the enzyme-linked immunosorbent assay (ELISA) is the prototype], with the capture antibody directed toward the alpha subunit and a signal antibody that recognizes an epitope on the unique beta subunit.

Heterogeneous immunoassays differ in the method used to separate bound and free fractions before application of the signal antibody. The various designs of automated heterogeneous immunoassays are discussed in Chapter 16.

As noted previously, TSH immunoassays are calibrated with a reference preparation of TSH (World Health Organization Second International Reference Preparation, 2nd IRP 80/558) and are expressed as milli-international units of biological activity per liter of serum (mIU/L), a value established by bioassay. In contrast to the inverse dose-response curve produced in radioimmunoassay, immunometric assays generate a proportional dose-response curve, with larger signals corresponding to higher concentrations of analyte. Because the physiologic interval of TSH concentrations is typically three orders of magnitude, high-dose hook effects are rarely encountered with TSH immunoassays. Automated heterogeneous immunoassays for TSH offer improved sensitivity and rapid turnaround time, along with a wider linear measurement range, when compared with traditional competitive immunoassays such as RIA.

A wide variety of TSH methods are now available. Most TSH methods use a detection antibody labeled with a chemiluminescent (or electrochemiluminescent) tracer.[119,156] Some assays use peroxidase, alkaline phosphatase, photometric, and fluorescent[167] labels. Other TSH methods are based on fluorescent labels using europium chelates,[78] chemiluminescent compounds such as acridinium esters or ruthenium, or bioluminescent molecules such as recombinant aequorin.

Chemiluminescence-based immunoassays are available in several configurations.[109] For example, one assay involves a polystyrene tube coated with a monoclonal capture antibody and a polyclonal detection antibody conjugated to an acridinium ester; the acridinium ester emits a photon when reacted with hydrogen peroxide in alkaline solution.[189] Another approach uses an antibody-coated tube, a polyclonal antibody conjugated to alkaline phosphatase, and an adamantyl dioxetane phosphate ester as substrate; on dephosphorylation, the substrate decomposes and emits a sustained glow of light.[25] Cross-reactivity of this TSH assay with luteinizing hormone, follicle-stimulating hormone, human chorionic gonadotropin, or the free beta subunit of glycoprotein hormones is less than 0.001%.

Specimen Collection and Storage

Serum or plasma may be used for TSH measurements. TSH is stable for 5 days at 2 to 8 °C, and for at least 1 month when stored frozen. For newborn screening, whole blood may be collected by heel puncture 48 to 72 hours after birth.

Comments on TSH Measurements

Secretion of TSH is circadian; peak concentrations of TSH occur between 0200 and 0400, and the nadir occurs between 1700 and 1800. Low-amplitude oscillations occur throughout the day. The nocturnal increase in TSH is lost in critical illness and after surgery. TSH surges immediately after birth, reaching a peak of 25 to 160 mIU/L within 30 minutes, and declining back to cord blood concentrations by postpartum day 3. TSH concentrations stabilize to near adult concentrations within the first few weeks of life. In the first trimester of pregnancy, TSH concentrations decline as hCG stimulates the maternal thyroid gland to produce thyroid hormone, sometimes leading to a TSH concentration that is just below the lower limit of the reference interval. Reference intervals for adult TSH concentrations are the same for men and women, and no significant racial influence on concentrations of this hormone has been noted. The distribution of TSH concentrations in healthy populations is log-Gaussian (or log-normal); reference intervals should be determined nonparametrically.

Measurement of Total Thyroxine (T_4)

Thyroxine [3,5,3′,5′-tetraiodothyronine (T_4)] is the principal hormone secreted by the thyroid gland (see Figure 55-4), and its circulating concentration is under the influence of TSH. The hormone is synthesized from tyrosine residues on thyroglobulin in the colloid of the thyroid gland. Circulating T_4 is highly (>99.9%) protein bound, and the fraction that is bound to protein is biologically inactive.

Instrument-Based Methods

Electron capture gas chromatography,[150] high-performance liquid chromatography,[68] and isotope dilution tandem mass spectrometry[126,183,184A] have been used in measuring T_4 in human serum. The latter method has been suggested as a reference method for assay of T_4. With this technique, tritium-labeled T_4 is added as an internal standard before extraction, derivatization, and quantitation of T_4 by combined gas chromatography–mass spectrometry.

Immunoassays

Most clinical laboratories measure total T_4 by using an automated competitive immunoassay. Many T_4 immunoassays use high-affinity polyclonal antibodies produced against an albumin-T_4 conjugate. These polyclonal antibodies are highly specific and display minimal cross-reactivity with T_3. Thyroglobulin sometimes has been used as the immunogen because it contains iodinated tyrosine residues that are the precursors of T_4 and T_3. Monoclonal antibodies against T_4 have also been developed.

Immunoassays of total T_4 measure both free and protein-bound hormone. Accurate measurement of total T_4 therefore requires dissociation of the hormone from serum proteins (thyroxine-binding globulin, albumin, and transthyretin) that bind more than 99.9% of circulating T_4. Dissociation of T_4 from albumin is not a concern because the association constant of T_4 for anti-T_4 antibodies (usually $\geq 10^9$ L/mol) is several orders of magnitude higher than the association constant for albumin-bound T_4 (approximately 1.6×10^6 L/mol). However, association constants for T_4 binding to thyroxine-binding globulin (TBG) and transthyretin are higher: 2×10^{10} L/mol and 2×10^8 L/mol, respectively. T_4 can be dissociated from transthyretin by the addition of barbital, which competitively inhibits T_4 binding to this protein. Various blocking agents have been used to dissociate T_4 from TBG. The most common of these blocking agents is 8-anilino-1-naphthalene-sulfonic acid (ANS), although salicylate, thimerosal, and phenytoin have been used to displace T_4 from TBG. In some assays, proportional bias has been attributed to incomplete release of T_4 from serum-binding proteins.[138]

Considerable effort has been directed toward the development of immunoassays that do not require the use and measurement of radioactivity, and nonisotopic assays for T_4 are widely available for use on various automated immunoassay systems, or adaptable to automated chemistry platforms. In recent College of American Pathologists Ligand Assay Surveys, the number of participants using RIA to measure total T_4 was insufficient to report as a peer group. A variety of different labels have been used in the design of nonisotopic immunoassays. Enzymes such as horseradish peroxidase, alkaline phosphatase, and alpha-D-galactosidase are popular, in addition to fluorescent and chemiluminescent labels.

Heterogeneous enzyme immunoassays for T_4 often involve solid-phase separation systems. Some methods immobilize the anti-T_4 antibodies on a plastic surface (e.g., polystyrene beads, test tubes, microwells) so that bound and free analyte may be separated by decanting and washing. For example, one automated assay uses test tubes that contain polystyrene beads coated with a monoclonal anti-T_4 capture antibody.[11] T_4 in the specimen is liberated from binding proteins by ANS and competes with a T_4–alkaline phosphatase conjugate for binding sites on antibodies attached to the polystyrene beads. After the unbound label is rinsed away, the bound enzyme is measured using a chemiluminescent substrate. This combination of an enzyme label with a chemiluminescent substrate has been applied to other automated T_4 procedures as well. An antibody-coated tube enzyme immunoassay has been devised for measurement of T_4 and includes a peroxidase-T_4 conjugate with a photometric substrate.

Several enzyme immunoassays attach paramagnetic particles to the anti-T_4 antibodies so that free and bound T_4 can be separated magnetically. In one automated scheme, plastic cups contain magnetic beads coated with a T_4 antibody. Endogenous T_4, displaced from its binding proteins by ANS, competes with alkaline phosphatase–labeled T_4 for a limited number of binding sites on the immobilized antibody. The magnetized beads are washed to remove unbound enzyme-labeled T_4 and then are incubated with a fluorogenic substrate. As with all competitive immunoassays, the amount of enzyme-labeled T_4 captured on the magnetic beads is inversely proportional to the T_4 concentration in the specimen.

Homogeneous enzyme immunoassays have been developed for measuring serum T_4 concentration. Chapter 16 discusses several approaches to homogeneous immunoassays. In the enzyme-multiplied immunoassay technique (EMIT) for T_4, glucose-6-phosphate dehydrogenase (G-6-PDH) is covalently linked to T_4 as the enzyme label. When T_4-specific antibodies bind to the enzyme-labeled T_4, enzyme activity is inhibited as the result of steric obstruction of the substrate-binding site. The cloned enzyme donor immunoassay (CEDIA) technique for measuring T_4 is based on the use of cloned fragments of alpha-galactosidase, a tetrameric hydrolase enzyme that converts alpha-galactosides into galactose. The CEDIA approach involves two fragments of the monomeric subunit of alpha-galactosidase, the larger of which is called the *acceptor*, and the smaller of which is called the *donor*. In solution, the two fragments spontaneously associate to form a monomeric subunit, which subsequently associates with three other monomers to form the active enzyme. In the CEDIA method, T_4 is labeled with the donor fragment of alpha-galactosidase monomer, and antibody binding to the labeled T_4 prevents association with the acceptor fragment; hence, enzyme activity is lost.

Fluorescent probes have been used to measure T_4, and both heterogeneous and homogeneous immunoassays based on fluorescent labels are available. An example of the latter is the fluorescence polarization immunoassay (FPIA). In the FPIA, fluorescein-labeled T_4 competes with unlabeled hormone in the patient specimen for binding sites on anti-T_4 antibodies. Polarized excitation light (485 nm) induces fluorescence of the fluorescein tracer. Polarization of the emitted light (525 to 550 nm) requires that the orientation of the tracer remain fixed for the time interval between excitation and fluorescence; this interval is typically nanoseconds. The unbound T_4-fluorescein conjugate has a rotational frequency of femtoseconds^{-1}, so the orientation of the uncomplexed tracer is randomized between excitation and fluorescence, and polarization is lost. However, when fluorescein-labeled T_4 is bound to antibody, the rotational frequency is several orders of magnitude slower, so excitation and fluorescence occur in the same plane, and polarization is maintained.

Heterogeneous fluorescent immunoassays for T_4 based on lanthanide rare earth elements and time-resolved fluorescence are also available. The use of europium chelates as fluorescent probes is particularly attractive because of their wide Stokes shifts and long fluorescence decay times, which improve the specificity of the measurement by limiting interference from scattered excitation light and endogenous fluorophores. In a typical competitive immunoassay design, T_4 in the specimen competes with europium-labeled T_4 for a limited number of binding sites on monoclonal T_4 antibodies. Antibody-bound and free antigen fractions are separated by adsorption of T_4 antibodies to the surface of a microwell coated with antimouse immunoglobulin (Ig)G. After incubation and washing, the europium ions are dissociated from the bound phase, converted into a highly fluorescent chelate, and measured in a fluorometer with time resolution capability. A variation on this technique involves attachment of biotin to a monoclonal T_4 antibody and streptavidin coupled to the europium chelate.

Most contemporary automated immunoassays for measuring total T_4 use chemiluminescent labels. In one design, endogenous T_4 competes with T_4 coupled to paramagnetic particles for binding sites on a mouse monoclonal antibody labeled with acridinium ester. After incubation, the labeled T_4 is captured on a magnetized surface that is subsequently washed to remove the unbound label. The antibody-bound labeled T_4 is quantified in a luminometer after hydrogen peroxide is added to initiate the chemiluminescence reaction.

Electrochemiluminescence has also been applied to total T_4 measurement. In this technology, a ruthenium tris(bipyridyl) [$Ru(bpy)_3^{2+}$] complex is used as the antibody label. In the presence of tripropylamine and an applied electrical potential, the ruthenium complex undergoes a chemiluminescent reaction.

Particle-enhanced immunoassays involving turbidimetric measurements have been developed for measuring T_4 in serum. These homogeneous immunoassays are based on competition between T_4 in the specimen and a T_4-ficoll conjugate for binding sites on a monoclonal antibody coupled to microparticles. The rate of formation of cross-linked complexes is inhibited by competing T_4 and is measured turbidimetrically by the change in absorbance at 600 nm.

Dry-chemistry immunoassay systems, which do not require liquid reagents or sample pretreatment, have also been developed for T_4. One such system uses a thin-film multilayer test module consisting of three distinct layers mounted on a plastic support. The serum specimen is applied to the top layer of film, which contains phenoxynaphthalene sulfonic acid, to displace T_4 from binding proteins. The released T_4 passes through an iron oxide screen into the detection layer, where the hormone competes with rhodamine-labeled T_4 for binding sites on immobilized T_4 antibodies. Unbound fluorescent-labeled T_4 diffuses into the opaque layers above the screen, where it cannot be detected. The fluorescent signal of the remaining antibody-bound labeled T_4 fraction is measured fluorometrically. This signal is inversely proportional to the concentration of T_4 in the specimen.

Specimen Collection and Storage

Serum is the preferred specimen for the measurement of T_4, but plasma with EDTA or heparin as anticoagulant has also been used. Plasma may form fibrin clots after freezing and thawing, however, and may produce spurious results in methods that are susceptible to changes in specimen viscosity. Gel barrier collection devices do not have any apparent adverse effect on T_4 methods. T_4 is a stable analyte with no appreciable change in concentration for up to 7 days at room temperature, or 30 days when frozen. As with most analytes, repeated freezing and thawing of specimens should be avoided because it can produce concentration gradients that require vigorous mixing to alleviate. Mild to moderate hemolysis and lipemia do not significantly affect most T_4 immunoassays; however, grossly hemolyzed specimens should be avoided because of dilutional effects. Intracellular T_4 concentrations are very low because thyroxine-binding proteins are mostly extracellular. T_4 autoantibodies interfere with some immunoassays and may produce erroneously low or high results, depending on the method.[215]

Heelstick capillary specimens have been used for T_4 measurement, as have dried blood specimens collected on filter paper. Dried blood specimens are stable and easily transported and are widely used in the United States to screen neonates for congenital hypothyroidism.[115] When this collection technique is used, a one eighth inch dot is punched out from the blood-saturated filter paper and T_4 is extracted into a buffer before the assay is performed. The filter paper should not be exposed to extreme heat or light.

Comments on Total T_4 Measurements

Total T_4 concentration alone provides limited clinical information, because it reflects mostly inactive (protein-bound) hormone. In fact, it is reasonable to question whether isolated measurements of total T_4 currently have any value in the assessment of thyroid disease. In conjunction with free hormone measurements, total T_4 may reveal protein-binding abnormalities that influence the ratio of bound to free hormone, and total T_4 should inversely correlate with TSH activity in the absence of protein-binding abnormalities. In patients with normal serum thyroxine-binding capacity (normal albumin, TBG, and transthyretin), total T_4 is proportional to the active free hormone concentration. Methods for measuring free T_4 are widely available and largely supplant the need for total T_4 measurements. As discussed later, free (unbound) T_4 measurements are more useful clinically, except in unusual circumstances.

Cord blood T_4 concentrations are lower in preterm than in full-term neonates, and they correlate positively with birth weight in full-term infants. At birth, serum total T_4 concentrations are higher in neonates because of the maternal estrogen-induced increase in serum TBG; free T_4 concentrations are near adult concentrations. Total T_4 rises abruptly in the first few hours after birth and declines gradually until adolescence. In males, T_4 production declines as they mature sexually, but this phenomenon is not observed in females.

Analytical performance goals have been recommended for thyroid hormone assays.[13] When total T_4 is used to diagnose thyroid disease, the suggested goals for maximum bias and imprecision (coefficient of variation) are 2.9% and 5.7%, respectively. When the T_4 assay is used to monitor changes in an individual over time, bias and imprecision goals are 1.3% and 2.6%, respectively.

Measurement of Triiodothyronine (T_3)

Triiodothyronine [3,5,3′-triiodothyronine (T_3)] is the principal active thyroid hormone, and although a small amount of T_3 is secreted directly by the thyroid gland, most of this hormone is produced by deiodination of T_4 in the peripheral tissues, primarily in the liver. Similar to T_4, T_3 is highly bound to protein, with less than 1% of the total concentration as free active hormone. Total T_3 measurements have limited clinical use in that the T_3 concentration usually reflects its progenitor, T_4. However, clinical conditions are known that affect peripheral conversion of T_4 to T_3 (discussed earlier), resulting in a clinical hypothyroid state in the presence of normal or elevated T_4, with normal (or even elevated) TSH. Compared with T_4, T_3 is less tightly bound to serum proteins by about an order of magnitude, so displacement of bound T_3 from proteins is essentially complete in the presence of conventional blocking agents such as ANS. T_3 does not ordinarily displace T_4 from thyroid hormone–binding proteins.

Radioimmunoassays

Numerous commercial RIA kits have been introduced for measuring total T_3 concentrations in serum. These methods are similar to the RIAs previously described for T_4, except that a ^{125}I-T_3 tracer and T_3-specific antibody are used. Most analytical designs incorporate antibodies bound to a solid phase, such as the wall of a cuvette or paramagnetic particles. As with T_4 methods, ANS can be used to release the hormone from proteins without disturbing T_3 binding to antibody.

Nonisotopic Immunoassays

Nonisotopic immunoassays for T_3 are similar to total T_4 methods. Many of the T_3 methods have been developed for use on automated immunoassay systems, and some are compatible with chemistry platforms. Many commercial methods use enzyme labels, such as peroxidase or alkaline phosphatase, conjugated to T_3 or anti-T_3 antibodies. Enzyme activity is determined by using a variety of sensitive photometric,[99] fluorescent, or chemiluminescent substrates. Immunoassays for T_3 that use fluorescent and chemiluminescent labels are also available, and as with T_4 assays, chemiluminescence-based methods on automated platforms dominate the present clinical laboratory market. Both heterogeneous and homogeneous immunoassays for T_3 have been described.[81]

Specimen Collection and Storage

Serum is the preferred specimen, but plasma with ethylenediaminetetraacetic acid (EDTA) or heparin as anticoagulant may be used. Serum specimens should be tested within 24 hours of collection, or stored at 2 to 8 °C if tested beyond 24 hours. Frozen specimens are stable for at least 30 days. Repeated freezing and thawing of the specimens should be avoided for reasons described earlier. Turbid samples may require centrifugation before testing.

Comments on Total T_3 Measurements

Significant discrepancies have been observed when the results of different T_3 immunoassays were compared using reference sera. Interlaboratory quality assurance (proficiency testing) results also demonstrate higher analytical variance for T_3 compared with T_4 methods. Among the factors that have been suggested to account for the poorer analytical performance of T_3 immunoassays are the lower concentration of T_3 in serum, the greater antibody cross-reactivity, protein interferences, and the different assay limits of detection. Performance goals for bias and precision have been suggested for T_3.[13] When a total T_3 assay is used for diagnosis, the suggested goals for maximum bias and imprecision are 5.7% and 11.5% (CV), respectively. For therapeutic guidance, bias and imprecision goals are 2.6% and 5.2%, respectively. Total T_3 measurements are useful in the diagnosis and monitoring of hyperthyroid patients with suppressed TSH and normal free T_4 concentrations ("T_3-thyrotoxicosis"); T_3 measurements have only limited value in euthyroid and hypothyroid patients.[83] Thyroid hormone replacement for hypothyroid patients is based on TSH and FT_4 measurements.

Measurement of Reverse Triiodothyronine (rT_3)

Reverse T_3 is produced by monodeiodination of the alpha ring of T_4 to 3,3′,5′-triiodothyronine and is biologically inert. Several radioimmunoassay methods for measuring rT_3 have been developed. Antibodies to rT_3 generally are obtained by immunizing rabbits with rT_3-human serum albumin (HSA) [or bovine serum albumin (BSA)] conjugates.[32] Cross-reactivity of anti-rT_3 antibodies with T_4 varies between 0.01% and 0.15%, and insignificant cross-reactivity of these antibodies with monoiodinated and di-iodinated thyronines is noted.[117] Similar to T_3 and T_4, rT_3 is highly bound to TBG, transthyretin, and albumin in serum but is displaced by ethanol extraction or ANS.

Commercial assays for measurement of rT_3 are available, but none has been adapted to an automated platform because rT_3 measurement has limited diagnostic value.

Specimen Collection and Storage

Specimen requirements for rT_3 are essentially the same as those previously described for T_3.

Comments on rT_3 Measurements

Reverse T_3 in serum is produced almost exclusively from peripheral deiodination of T_4 by 5-deiodinase (D1 or D3) enzymes. Although deiodination of T_4 in the peripheral tissues produces roughly equal amounts of T_3 and rT_3, the serum concentration of rT_3 is typically lower than that of T_3 because it is metabolized and cleared more rapidly. Serum rT_3 concentrations are elevated at birth, but decrease to stable concentrations by about the fifth day of life. Reverse T_3 in amniotic fluid decreases with increasing gestational age. The use of rT_3 to diagnose sick euthyroid syndrome has been questioned because of its poor sensitivity. Renal failure is associated with low rT_3 concentrations.

Measurement of Free Thyroid Hormones

No practical methods are available for measuring the exact concentration of unbound, active thyroid hormones. Bioassays can measure the activity of T_3 and T_4 but are imprecise and are not easily adapted to automated chemistry analyzers. Direct potentiometry measures the activity of various electrolytes, independent of the inactive bound fraction, but electrodes that respond to thyroid hormones have not been developed. Methods that remove unbound T_4 inevitably disrupt the equilibrium between bound and free hormone; therefore at best, FT_4 methods only approximate the true active concentration of the hormone.

In physiologic systems, proteins often act in much the same way as the conjugate acid or base in a pH buffered solution, providing a large reservoir of bound, inactive ligand that protects against precipitous changes in the total concentration of a hormone resulting from variations in glandular output. In principle, the free, active concentration of T_4 or T_3 could be mathematically derived by measuring the total T_4 concentration in a manner analogous to the way blood gas analyzers use the Henderson-Hasselbalch equation to calculate the bicarbonate concentration from measured pH and PCO_2 (from which the undissociated acid is estimated). The cumulative dissociation constant for T_4 from its binding proteins is approximately 10^{-5}, which is similar to the K_a of a weak acid, producing a free T_4 concentration that is approximately 0.03% of the total T_4 concentration. However, this approach is not satisfactory for two reasons: (1) T_4 binds to at least three different proteins, the concentrations of which change in a variety of clinical conditions, and only one (albumin) is routinely measured in clinical laboratories; and (2) the affinities of T_4-binding proteins for the hormone can be altered by competing ligands, as well as by genetic polymorphisms that alter the protein structure and thyroid hormone–binding affinities.

Clinical assessment of thyroid function in symptomatic patients with normal TSH, or asymptomatic patients with low or high TSH, has focused on measuring FT_4, because this can reveal whether TSH activity is consistent with the concentration of active hormone, regardless of abnormalities in binding protein concentrations or affinities.

Analytical strategies for measuring FT_4 have followed one of two basic paths: (1) separate the bound and free fractions and measure the concentration of T_4 (immunometrically or gravimetrically) in the free fraction; or (2) assay the free fraction using a competitive T_4 analog that does not bind to albumin, TBG, or transthyretin. The former category includes equilibrium dialysis and ultrafiltration (coupled with a variety of immunochemical or mass spectrometric methods for measuring T_4 and T_3 in the free fraction), and the latter comprises an assortment of competitive and noncompetitive immunoassays available on automated systems. The term *direct method* has been used to describe FT_4 methods that measure the concentration of free hormone (i.e., equilibrium dialysis and ultrafiltration). Alternatively, the *indirect method* often refers to an immunoassay that measures quantities of both bound and free fractions, relying on calibration against specimens with FT_4 concentrations verified by "direct" methods. Neither of these terms is consistently used, however, and both approaches, to a greater or lesser degree, only approximate the FT_4 concentration.

The analytical validity and clinical utility of FT_4 methods have been debated for longer than 2 decades.[43-45,121,122,222-224] Special reports from the Nomenclature Committee of the American Thyroid Association of the National Academy of Clinical Biochemistry[69] the Clinical and Laboratory Standards Institute (CLSI) [formerly National Committee for Clinical Laboratory Standards (NCCLS)] review some of the issues and concerns regarding free thyroid hormone measurements.

Direct (Reference) Methods

Direct measurement of FT_4 (and FT_3) in serum is technically challenging because the amount of free hormone in normal serum is exceedingly small—typically less than 100 pmol/L (or ng/L). The most reliable methods for measuring FT_4 and FT_3 in serum involve separation of free and bound hormone fractions by equilibrium dialysis or ultrafiltration, and subsequent measurement of the free concentration by a sensitive analytical method such as immunoassay or mass spectrometry. In equilibrium dialysis, the dialysis buffer dilutes the specimen, so there is some effect on the equilibrium between bound and free hormones, but the effect is minimal. Similarly, ultrafiltration changes the concentration of T_4-binding proteins in the retentate, changing the bound/free equilibrium.

Equilibrium Dialysis

In a equilibrium dialysis method for FT_4 and FT_3 described in 2008,[230] 200 μL aliquots of serum were dialyzed against 200 μL of a HEPES buffer containing physiologic concentrations of sodium, chloride, potassium, magnesium, sulfate, phosphate, calcium, and urea, with sodium azide added as a preservative using a cellulose membrane (5 kDa molecular weight cutoff). Specimens were dialyzed at 37 °C for approximately 20 hours. After the addition of ^{13}C-labeled internal standards, T_3 and T_4 were extracted from the dialysate onto a C5 guard column, and then were eluted into a polar LC column [solid-phase extraction-liquid chromatography (SPE-LC)] before analysis by tandem mass spectrometry. The upper and lower limits of quantitation, using the criterion of ±15% total bias, were 400 and 1.0 ng/L, respectively. FT_4 results using this method correlated well with equilibrium dialysis/RIA. FT_3 results by the SPE-LC-MS/MS method were compared with equilibrium tracer dialysis (see later), and a bias of 38 to 53% was observed. Others have reported similar equilibrium dialysis methods using LC-MS/MS to quantify FT_4.[208]

Ultrafiltration

A second method for separating protein bound and free fractions of T_4 is ultrafiltration, which is significantly less time-consuming than dialysis.[200] In an ultrafiltration method described by Soldin and coworkers,[184] the serum specimen was filtered through a 30 K MW cutoff filter by centrifugation for 1 hour at 25 °C and 2900 rpm in a fixed-angle rotor. T_4 was measured in the ultrafiltrate by isotope dilution LC/MS-MS. Results using this ultrafiltration method correlated closely with equilibrium dialysis and immunoassay. In a 2009 report,[77] performance of this method was assessed in four different patient populations: (1) pediatric, (2) euthyroid adults with thyroid disease (both before and after thyroidectomy), (3) healthy nonpregnant women, and (4) pregnant women. In all of these groups, FT_4 values measured by ultrafiltration and LC-MS/MS correlated inversely with log-transformed TSH concentrations.

Equilibrium Tracer Dialysis

Equilibrium tracer dialysis is a variation of equilibrium dialysis, except that isotopically labeled T_4 or T_3 "tracer" is added to the specimen before dialysis is performed. When equilibrium is established, concentrations of the tracer on both sides of the dialysis membrane are used to calculate the ratio of bound to free hormone, so the FT_4 (or FT_3) concentration can be calculated based on the total T_4 (or T_3) concentration. If the amount of tracer added to the specimen is small in comparison with the endogenous hormone concentration, minimal disruption of free/bound hormone is noted. This method is thought to provide the best estimate of FT_4 concentration, because radioassay methods for measuring T_4 have very low limits of detection, and displacement of hormone from binding proteins in the retentate is not required. However, equilibrium tracer dialysis involves the use of radioactive isotopes, a lengthy dialysis step, and instrumentation for measuring radioactivity. These considerations limit its use for routine measurement of FT_4 and FT_3.

Comments on Free Hormone Measurements Using Separation Techniques

Ultrafiltration provides a faster (an hour or less) means for separating protein-bound and free hormone fractions compared with equilibrium dialysis, which ordinarily requires 24 hours. Mass action, however, suggests that ultrafiltration disrupts free/bound equilibrium concentrations, as the protein concentration increases in the retentate during filtration. Some ultrafiltration methods are performed at physiologic temperature because of concerns about temperature-related changes in the equilibrium concentration of free hormone, but it is interesting to note that Soldin and associates found that ultrafiltration at 25 °C produced FT_4 results that correlated better with equilibrium dialysis (at 37 °C) than with ultrafiltration at 37 °C.[184]

The reliability of ultrafiltration as a method for quantitatively separating free T_3 and T_4 fractions in serum has been questioned. In a 2007 study, Fritz and colleagues[56] demonstrated poor recovery of isotopically labeled T_4 and T_3 when reference materials prepared in protein-free serum filtrates were passed through four commercially available ultrafiltration devices. Tritiated water was used as the internal standard and was evenly distributed between ultrafiltrate and retentate in all cases. However, large discrepancies between labeled hormone concentrations in the filtrate and retentate were observed. The authors of the study conclude that ultrafiltration "is complex, poorly characterized, and incompletely understood." Whether such anomalies also affect the results of equilibrium dialysis, which is similarly based on the presumption that free hormone equilibrates across a semipermeable membrane, has not been studied.

Free Thyroid Hormone Immunoassays

Many free thyroid hormone assays are commercially available for use on automated chemistry and immunoassay platforms. Before the advent of automated methods for measuring free T_4, strategies emerged to approximate free hormone by measuring the total T_4 concentration and using an indirect method to assess protein-binding capacity. These methods are no longer useful because immunoassays to measure the FT_4 concentration are widely available. Even though FT_4 immunoassays (both one- and two-step) are susceptible to bias when serum proteins that bind the hormone deviate significantly from normal concentrations, or when binding affinity is altered by genetic polymorphisms or competing ligands, in the vast number of patients, these assays provide reliable estimates of FT_4 concentration. Therefore, "index" methods that estimate free hormone concentrations based on protein-binding capacity are mostly obsolete. For more information on index methods, see the previous edition of this textbook.

General Considerations

Immunochemical methods for measuring FT_4 follow two basic strategies: (1) noncompetitive assays involve adsorption of free hormone on immobilized anti-T_4 antibodies, removal of the supernatant, and quantitation of the unoccupied solid-phase binding sites through addition of labeled T_4; the captured amount of labeled T_4 is inversely proportional to the FT_4 concentration; (2) alternatively, competitive immunoassays involve a labeled T_4 derivative (often called "analog," the distinguishing feature of which is significantly reduced affinity for T_4-binding proteins) that is added to serum along with anti-T_4 antibodies, and after isolation of the antibody fraction, the amount of labeled T_4 analog captured by the antibody will be inversely proportional to the endogenous FT_4 concentration. This approach is sometimes called "one-step," because only one separation of bound and free ligand is involved, in contrast to "two-step" methods, which remove the soluble protein fraction before the addition of the labeled ligand. Another approach is to immobilize T_4 analogs on a solid support and measure the amount of labeled antibody adsorbed on the solid support; in this design, captured label will be inversely proportional to the concentration of FT_4, which competes for binding sites on the labeled antibody.

Analog methods measure the distribution of labeled T_4 between endogenous binding proteins (TBP, transthyretin, and albumin) and an anti-T_4 antibody. Therefore, these methods produce only an estimate of the FT_4 concentration, because the introduction of an exogenous binding protein—the T_4 antibody—disrupts the equilibrium between free and bound hormones in the specimen. If the assay is calibrated with calibrators that have similar T_4 protein–binding capacity to the specimen being assayed, and if the calibrators have been validated using a reference method (such as equilibrium dialysis), then the results provide a good estimate of FT_4 concentration. However, biases will be introduced when the concentrations, or affinities, of T_4-binding proteins deviate significantly from expected values, because calibration of these methods assumes a normal serum T_4-binding capacity. The serum protein-binding capacity for thyroid hormones can be affected by physiological variations in protein synthesis (as in pregnancy and infancy), proteinopathies resulting from liver dysfunction (such as hypoalbuminemia), nonthyroidal disease, genetic factors that produce proteins with diminished or enhanced T_4 binding, competing ligands, and the presence of T_4 autoantibodies. With the exceptions of pregnancy and infancy—most notably, prematurity—most of these conditions are relatively rare.

Another source of bias in FT_4 immunoassays that involve a T_4 analog is the binding of analog to serum proteins, which has been demonstrated to occur.[137] Because analog methods are based on the theoretical principle of competition between free analog and free endogenous T_4 for binding sites on the capture antibody, significant binding of the hormone analog to serum proteins invalidates the theoretical model. The extent to which these limitations affect the FT_4 estimates obtained by one-step analog methods has been debated (see earlier).

Two-Step FT_4 Immunoassays

The key feature of the two-step method is that the labeled hormone is added only after serum-binding proteins have been removed, ensuring that no competition exists between antibody and serum proteins for binding of tracer. This does not ensure that the assay is not susceptible to changes in serum protein-binding capacity, because the initial step involves equilibration of labeled FT_4 between the capture antibody and serum hormone-binding proteins. However, results using this approach correlate well with reference (equilibrium or ultrafiltration) methods across a wide variety of clinical disorders.

The first commercially available two-step immunoassay for FT_4 was introduced in 1979. Subsequently, a number of manual and automated procedures were developed for FT_4 (and FT_3). The earliest methods used radioactive labels and antibody-coated tubes or microbeads, but these have been largely replaced by automated methods involving nonisotopic labels and a variety of solid-phase formats. Automated "one-step" homogeneous FT_4 immunoassays have largely supplanted the use of these methods.

One-Step FT_4 Immunoassays

"One-step" FT_4 immunoassay is a slightly confusing misnomer, because homogeneous immunoassays are typically "one-step," in that no separation is required. However, all "one-step" approaches to immunochemical measurement of FT_4 and FT_3 are competitive, heterogeneous immunoassays, requiring separation of bound and free ligand prior to measurement of signal. These FT_4 methods are, for the most part, variations on the prototypical ELISA described in Chapter 16. Two common approaches consist of one involving labeled ligand, and the other using a labeled antibody.

In the labeled ligand scheme, anti-T_4 antibody may be immobilized to a solid support or bound to a paramagnetic particle, which can be used to capture the antibody-ligand complex. Free T_4 in the specimen and the labeled T_4 analog compete for binding sites on the anti-T_4 antibodies, and the amount of label adsorbed by the antibody is inversely proportional to the endogenous T_4 concentration. Of course, capture of endogenous T_4 will disrupt the equilibrium between protein-bound and free T_4, so the assay really measures the competition between thyroid hormone–binding proteins and the anti-T_4 antibody. Typical assays of this type remove 1 to 2% of the protein-bound T_4 fraction—a quantity that exceeds the true FT_4 concentration by at least two orders of magnitude. Theoretical arguments have been made that removal of such a small amount of the total T_4 causes minimal disruption of the bound/free ratio; therefore a properly calibrated method should produce a close estimate of the actual FT_4 concentration.[33,121,122]

Another analytical strategy for measuring FT_4 is to immobilize a modified T_4 analog to a solid support (or paramagnetic particle), and allow a labeled anti-T_4 antibody to equilibrate between endogenous FT_4 and the immobilized analog. Evidence suggests that immobilized T_4 analog has less affinity for T_4-binding proteins than the labeled free analog described earlier,[231] which makes the labeled antibody methods less susceptible to bias resulting from binding of the T_4 analog to endogenous proteins. In the labeled antibody method, after the unbound fraction is removed, the signal is measured in the solid (or immobilized) phase and will be inversely proportional to the FT_4 concentration. As with labeled ligand methods, substantially more endogenous T_4 is bound to antibody than is contained in the original free fraction as the result of re-equilibration after free T_4 binds to antibody, but the fraction removed from binding proteins is small (1 to 2%) compared with the total T_4 concentration, so the equilibrium bound/free ratio is not significantly affected. These methods are calibrated with reference materials containing normal quantities of T_4-binding proteins, and in which FT_4 (or FT_3) has been measured by a reference method such as equilibrium dialysis or ultrafiltration.

Many commercially available FT_4 and FT_3 assays follow one or the other of the labeled ligand or labeled antibody schemes, differing only in (1) the label, (2) the analog, and (3) the chemical method for immobilizing antibody or analog. Radioactive isotopes, enzymes, fluorophores, and chemiluminescent and electrochemiluminescent labels have been used in FT_4 immunoassays, but most modern methods use one of the latter two. The structure of the analog, which is a modified form of T_4 designed to have limited affinity for thyroxine-binding protein, albumin, and transthyretin, is often proprietary, although T_4 analogs involving protein conjugates have been described in the literature.[231] In these experiments, T_4 was conjugated to rabbit gamma globulin, thyroglobulin, transferrin-1 (and -2), and ferritin. The antibody or analog are immobilized by biotin-avidin (or streptavidin) or paramagnetic particles.

Selection of Tests for Measuring Free Thyroid Hormones

Immunoassays that estimate FT_4 and FT_3 using the approaches just described generally produce reliable results in healthy subjects, hyperthyroid and hypothyroid patients, and patients with mild protein-binding abnormalities. Hence, for most clinical situations, selection of a specific FT_4 or FT_3 method can be based on factors such as (1) technical convenience, (2) turnaround time, (3) commercial availability, and (4) cost. In certain clinical conditions, however, free hormone estimates may produce results with significant bias compared with reference methods. Table 54-4 summarizes the types of bias that have been observed between reference and estimate methods for FT_4 in patients with thyroid hormone–binding protein abnormalities. One study[172] examined the bias between nine commercially available FT_4 immunoassays and equilibrium dialysis in patient specimens with low, normal, and high concentrations of T_4-binding proteins. Relative to specimens with normal concentrations of binding proteins, the low group had a mean TBG concentration 21% lower, and the high group had a mean TBG concentration 167% higher. Although little bias was observed for high-concentration TBG specimens, significant negative bias was observed in low-TBG concentration specimens. A 2009 study[98] compared FT_4 measured by two immunoassays in nonpregnant women and pregnant women subdivided by trimester. Although results were not compared with FT_4 measured by a reference method, a large number (5 to 67%) of pregnant subjects had FT_4 concentrations below the assay manufacturer's lower reference limit, although all specimens had normal total T_4 concentrations.

In addition to pregnancy, other clinical conditions may produce unreliable FT_4 results. In patients with familial dysalbuminemic hyperthyroxinemia (estimated incidence among Caucasians: 1:10,000), a normally minor albumin variant with a high affinity for T_4 is overexpressed, resulting in a larger fraction of albumin-bound T_4 and elevated total T_4. The affinity of the albumin variant for T_3 is not significantly different from normal albumin. Patients with familial dysalbuminemic hyperthyroxinemia are clinically euthyroid, and free hormone concentrations are normal as measured by reference methods and by most two-step immunoassays. However, one-step immunoassays are likely to produce erroneously high FT_4 estimates as the result of binding of the T_4 analog to the variant albumin. Patients with circulating T_4 autoantibodies, or with increased transthyretin, will produce similarly elevated FT_4 results by these immunoassays, because both conditions result in enhanced T_4-binding capacity in the serum.

FT_4 and FT_3 methods may not be reliable in patients with congenital TBG excess or deficiency, because the immunoassay methods are calibrated with reference materials containing normal amounts of TBG, and most of the circulating hormone is bound to this protein. Patients with these conditions are clinically euthyroid, and their FT_4 and FT_3 are usually within their reference interval when measured by reference methods (and sometimes by two-step immunoassays).

Estimates of FT_4 and FT_3 may be affected by medications that displace hormones from binding sites on serum proteins. The free hormone concentration will rise in the presence of such drugs, and in patients with normal thyroid function, TSH will be suppressed and production of T_4 will decrease, resulting in lower total T_4 with (after delay) normalized FT_4. With methods that use undiluted serum (ultrafiltration and equilibrium dialysis), measurement of FT_4 and FT_3 in the presence of competing drugs should be reliable. However, methods that dilute the specimen diminish the effects of inhibitors, and free hormone concentration may be underestimated.

BOX 55-4 Alterations in the Concentration or Affinity of Thyroid Hormone–Binding Proteins

Increases in
- A. Thyroxine-binding globulin (TBG) concentration (or affinity)
  1. Genetic (inherited) causes
  2. Nonthyroidal illness (HIV infection, infectious and chronic active hepatitis, estrogen-producing tumors, acute intermittent porphyria)
  3. Normal physiology (pregnancy, newborn)
  4. Drug use (oral contraceptives, estrogens, tamoxifen, methadone)
- B. Prealbumin concentration
- C. Albumin binding (familial dysalbuminemic hyperthyroxinemia)
- D. T_4 binding by antibodies (autoimmune thyroid disease, hepatocellular carcinoma)

Decreases in
- A. TBG concentration
  1. Genetic (inherited) determination
  2. Nonthyroidal illness (major illness or surgical stress, nephrotic syndrome)
  3. Drug use (androgens, anabolic steroids, large doses of glucocorticoids)
- B. TBG-binding capacity (drugs bound to TBG such as salicylates and phenytoin)
- C. Prealbumin concentration

Measurement of Thyroxine-Binding Globulin (TBG) and Other Thyroid Hormone–Binding Proteins

Thyroxine-binding globulin (TBG) is a 54 kDa protein that binds T_4 and T_3 with high affinity ($K_a \cong 10^{10}$). Although TBG has the lowest concentration of any of the three proteins that bind T_4, and its hormone binding sites are normally only 25% saturated, about 70% of the total T_4 and 80% of the total T_3 is bound to TBG. Therefore, TBG concentration is the primary regulator of total and free T_4 and T_3 concentrations. Estrogen-induced TBG excess and congenital TBG deficiency are the most significant TBG abnormalities that affect the interpretation of thyroid function test results (Box 55-4).

Methods for Measuring TBG

Historical methods measured TBG indirectly by competition between unlabeled and radiolabeled T_4 for binding sites on TBG, while blocking T_4-binding sites on transthyretin and albumin with a barbital buffer. After removal of the unbound hormone, radioactivity retained in the protein fraction was proportional to the TBG concentration. The presence of various drugs that inhibit T_4 binding to TBG, or abnormal transthyretin and albumin concentration or affinity, can interfere with these assays and produce artificially low TBG measurements.

Modern TBG methods measure the protein concentration directly using a variety of immunochemical approaches. One competitive, heterogeneous method measures the competition between endogenous TBG and labeled TBG for binding to an immobilized anti-TBG antibody. After incubation, bound and free fractions are separated by a variety of standard methods, and the concentration of label in the bound fraction is inversely proportional to endogenous TBG concentration. A competitive chemiluminescence enzyme immunoassay for TBG uses peroxidase-labeled TBG and anti-TBG antibody that is captured by a solid-phase second antibody; bound conjugate is measured by chemiluminescence after the addition of luminol and hydrogen peroxide. Another immunoassay for TBG is based on enhanced microparticle turbidimetry, in which the presence of endogenous antigen inhibits the cross-linking of antigen-microparticle complexes by anti-TBG antibody, reducing the turbidity of the reaction mixture.

Specimen Collection and Storage

Serum is the preferred specimen; plasma with EDTA or heparin as anticoagulant may also be used. Serum specimens are best stored at 2 to 8 °C if they will not be tested within 24 hours. If longer periods of storage are necessary, freezing the specimens is recommended. Frozen specimens are stable for at least 30 days. Repeated freezing and thawing of the specimens should be avoided. Turbid samples should be centrifuged before testing.

Thyroglobulin Measurement

Both competitive and noncompetitive immunoassays have been applied to Tg measurement.[190,228] Present-day competitive immunoassays typically incubate the serum with anti-Tg antibody; this is followed by the addition of ^{125}I-labeled Tg. The Tg–anti-Tg complex is precipitated by a second antibody, separating antibody-bound from free ^{125}I-labeled Tg. Longer incubation generally enhances the sensitivity of the assay.

Noncompetitive (sandwich) immunoassays for Tg have been developed using a variety of labels (radioactive isotope, enzyme, chemiluminescent, and electrochemiluminescent). The capture antibody and the labeled (or signal) antibody recognize different epitopes on Tg that do not sterically interfere with one another. The capture antibody can be attached to a polystyrene bead or a paramagnetic bead to separate bound and free fractions of antigen. Another variation is to attach an antibody to biotin and separate the biotin-antibody-Tg complex using avidin bound to a solid phase.

For most Tg double-antibody assays, the lower limit of detection is near 0.5 to 1 ng/mL, with a coefficient of variation of ≈20%. Day-to-day coefficients of variation are usually less than 6% near the center of the reportable interval but can rise to 15% at very low or very high Tg concentrations.

A Tg reference preparation developed by the European Community Bureau of Reference is used in many present-day immunometric assays. With this reference preparation, interassay variability is ≈30%, which exceeds intraindividual biological variability by a factor of three. Because of such variability between different Tg assays, Tg monitoring requires that the same assay be used longitudinally. Alternatively, if a new Tg assay is introduced, the baseline Tg concentration for the patient should be re-established with the new assay.

Technical challenges in Tg measurement include poor interassay agreement, hook effects, interassay calibration variability, and the need to reduce the lower limits of detection of Tg immunoassays for improved detection of residual thyroid cancer, metastasis, or recurrence.[75] A new generation of Tg assays with enhanced lower limits of detection may eliminate the need to withdraw thyroid hormone replacement or administer rDNA TSH before Tg testing is performed.[62]

Thyroglobulin Assay Interferences

Interference from human antimouse antibodies (HAMA), other heterophile antibodies, or rheumatoid factor can affect almost any immunoassay. Thyroglobulin autoantibodies (TGA) in the patient's blood also interfere with accurate measurement of Tg.[187] Unfortunately, anti-Tg autoantibodies are much more common in thyroid cancer patients than in the general population. TGA are reported in 15 to 35% of thyroid cancer patients.

It is standard practice to search for TGA whenever Tg is measured. The TGA assay should be sensitive to low concentrations of TGA. TGA tend to decrease Tg measurements in noncompetitive assays. Although some laboratories might use polyethylene glycol to precipitate TGA-bound Tg to measure the nonbound Tg fraction, practically speaking, if TGA are detected, the Tg determination is not reliable. Therefore, Tg measurements should not be used as tumor markers in the clinical management of patients with demonstrated TGA.

The interference of TGA with various two-site sandwich immunoassays is unpredictable. TGA increase Tg concentrations in some assays. In other assays, TGA may result in negative bias. Recovery studies generally are not useful for determining whether TGA influences the Tg concentration.[107,186]

When TGA are detected, their concentration may be useful as a secondary marker of the mass of thyroid tissue present in the patient. If TGA concentrations reflect the degree of antigenic stimulation of B cells, higher TGA concentrations should correlate with greater amounts of thyroid tissue in the patient. Therefore, in differentiated thyroid cancers where TGA are positive, higher TGA concentrations suggest more residual thyroid tissue and/or local or distal spread of the tumor. Because of the uncertainty that TGA positivity introduces into the interpretation of any Tg assay, however, clinicians should rely principally on thyroid scans to detect residual thyroid tissue in cases of differentiated thyroid cancer when TGA are present.

Specimen Collection and Storage

The preferred specimen for Tg measurement is serum, but EDTA or heparinized plasma may also be used. If not tested within 24 hours, serum specimens are best stored at 2 to 8 °C. If testing is delayed beyond a few days, the specimen should be frozen until it is analyzed. Frozen specimens are stable for at least 30 days. Repeated freeze-thaw cycles should be avoided. Turbid samples should be centrifuged before testing.

Reference Interval

The reference interval for Tg in euthyroid individuals varies from a lower limit of 0.5 to 2 ng/mL to an upper limit of 20 to 42 ng/mL, depending on the method. One major reference laboratory provides the following reference intervals: 0 to 11 months: 0.6 to 5.5 ng/mL; 1 to 11 years: 0.6 to 40.0 ng/mL; and 12 years and older: 1.3 to 31.8 ng/mL. For patients lacking a thyroid gland who are not receiving T_4 replacement therapy, Tg should not be detectable regardless of the patient's TSH concentration.

Novel Markers of Thyroid Tissue in the Management of Differentiated Thyroid Carcinoma

Another approach to the detection of residual thyroid cancer is the measurement of Tg mRNA in the circulation.[164] This may be helpful when Tg cannot be measured because of TGA.

This procedure involves reverse-transcriptase polymerase chain reaction amplification of mRNA in serum.[159] This nucleic acid approach may be valuable as an early marker of relapse.[160] However, the value of Tg mRNA detection is controversial because of problems with both sensitivity and specificity.[46,57] Thyroperoxidase and TSH receptor mRNAs are alternative markers that are under investigation.[162] In research studies, the detection of minimal residual disease in thyroid cancer has also included polymerase chain reaction detection of cytokeratin 20.[219]

Thyroid Autoantibodies

Multiple autoantigens are targeted in AITD, including thyroperoxidase, thyroglobulin, the TSH receptor, a thyroid colloidal antigen, the NIS, and megalin.[105,177] Autoantibodies that appear to promote thyroid growth have also been described.[206] These antibodies stimulate tritiated thymidine uptake, a measure of cellular proliferation, without increasing cAMP generation—a measure of TSH-like stimulation. Autoantibodies against T_4 and T_3 have also been described; and these may interfere with measurement of these hormones but do not appear to cause clinical disease.[151,173]

Thyroid microsomal autoantibodies (TMAs), thyroperoxidase autoantibodies (TPOAs), and thyroglobulin autoantibodies (TGAs) can be detected by a variety of methods, including (1) indirect immunofluorescence, (2) the agar gel diffusion precipitin technique, (3) agglutination (hemagglutination or latex particle agglutination), (4) radioimmunoassay, (5) complement fixation, (6) ELISA techniques, and (7) chemiluminescence-based immunometric assays.[27,221] Modern assays have reduced the lower limits of detection of these autoantibodies. With the older agglutination techniques, red blood cells denatured with tannic acid treatment were coated with microsomal antigen isolated from human hyperplastic thyroid glands. TMA-positive sera would agglutinate the "tanned" RBCs. Serial dilutions were performed until agglutination was not detected. The last dilution before the disappearance of agglutination represented the "titer." Newer immunoassays are more sensitive and can detect lower concentrations of these autoantibodies. For example, some assays attach TPOs to a solid support, and, with the addition of patient serum, TPOA bind to the immobilized TPOs. A labeled antihuman immunoglobulin antibody is added to detect the TPOAs. Similar assays for TGAs are available. Because of the interference of TGAs with Tg measurements, TGAs assays with excellent low-end sensitivity are very important.

It was initially believed that TGAs developed because thyroglobulin was released into the circulation following thyroid follicular cell damage, thus exposing the immune system to a previously sequestered antigen. However, as discussed previously, sensitive radioimmunoassays demonstrated that Tg was present in normal serum; thus Tg does not appear to be a sequestered antigen.

Two assay formats are commonly used for measuring thyroid receptor autoantibodies (TRAs): measurement of (1) thyroid-stimulating immunoglobulins (TSIs), and (2) thyrotropin-binding inhibitory immunoglobulins (TBIIs). TRAs are detected using bioassays for TSIs and radioreceptor assays for TBII. A report published in 2009 describes an automated assay for TBIIs.[59] In most patients with Graves' disease, TSIs can be detected.[194]

TSIs are measured by adding patient serum to thyroid follicular cells and assessing the release of T_4 or cAMP (the secondary messenger generated by stimulation of the TSH receptor), or by observing colloid mobilization.[199] A variety of sources of thyroid follicular cells have been used, such as thyroid slices or cultured human thyroid cell monolayers (FRTL-5).

TBIIs are measured in a radioreceptor assay format.[70] Patient serum is added to a solution containing TSH receptors. Competition then occurs between ^{125}I-labeled TSH and TRAs in the patient serum for binding to TSH receptors. As the concentration of TRAs rise in a patient's serum, less ^{125}I-labeled TSH will bind to TSH receptors present in the assay. The TBIIs assay does not distinguish agonistic from antagonistic TRAs. Therefore, TBIIs typically are positive in both Graves' disease and atrophic thyroiditis, and negative in Hashimoto thyroiditis. However, TSIs are negative in atrophic thyroiditis. TSIs and TBIIs should be measured in pregnant women with Graves' disease (past or present) to assess the risk of fetal or neonatal thyrotoxicosis from maternal IgG that has crossed the placenta: if TSIs are present in high concentration, the risk for the development of fetal or neonatal thyrotoxicosis is increased. TSIs are detected in 95% of patients with untreated Graves' disease. Several studies have shown that higher TSIs concentrations predict relapse and lower rates of remission. In atrophic thyroiditis in pregnant women, TBIIs can cross the placenta, and this may result in transient congenital hypothyroidism or transient hyperthyrotropinemia.[108] On the other hand, TPOAs/TMAs and TGAs are not associated with congenital hypothyroidism, indicating that these autoantibodies are not pathogenic.[42]

REFERENCES

1. Adler SM, Wartofsky L. The nonthyroidal illness syndrome. Endocrinol Metab Clin North Am 2007;3:657-72, vi.
2. Agrawal NK, Goyal R, Rastogi A, Naik D, Singh SK. Thyroid hormone resistance. Postgrad Med J 2008;995:473-7.
3. Al-Dajani N, Wootton SH. Cervical lymphadenitis, suppurative parotitis, thyroiditis, and infected cysts. Infect Dis Clin North Am 2007;2:523-41, viii.
4. Allahabadia A, Weetman AP. Dynamic thyroid stimulating hormone tests: do they still have a role? J Endocrinol Invest 2003;7(suppl):31-8.
5. Alter CA, Moshang T Jr. Diagnostic dilemma: the goiter. Pediatr Clin North Am 1991;3:567-78.
6. Andersen S, Bruun NH, Pedersen KM, Laurberg P. Biologic variation is important for interpretation of thyroid function tests. Thyroid 2003; 11:1069-78.
7. Aoki Y, Belin RM, Clickner R, Jeffries R, Phillips L, Mahaffey KR. Serum TSH and total T4 in the United States population and their association with participant characteristics: National Health and Nutrition Examination Survey (NHANES 1999-2002). Thyroid 2007; 12:1211-23.
8. Arrigo T, Wasniewska M, Crisafulli G, Lombardo F, Messina MF, Rulli I, et al. Subclinical hypothyroidism: the state of the art. J Endocrinol Invest 2008;1:79-84.

9. Atzmon G, Barzilai N, Hollowell JG, Surks MI, Gabriely I. Extreme longevity is associated with increased serum thyrotropin. J Clin Endocrinol Metab 2009;4:1251-4.
10. Azizi F, Hedayati M, Rahmani M, Sheikholeslam R, Allahverdian S, Salarkia N. Reappraisal of the risk of iodine-induced hyperthyroidism: an epidemiological population survey. J Endocrinol Invest 2005;1: 23-9.
11. Babson AL, Olson DR, Palmieri T, Ross AF, Becker DM, Mulqueen PJ. The IMMULITE assay tube: a new approach to heterogeneous ligand assay. Clin Chem 1991;9:1521-2.
12. Bach-Huynh TG, Nayak B, Loh J, Soldin S, Jonklaas J. Timing of levothyroxine administration affects serum thyrotropin concentration. J Clin Endocrinol Metab 2009;10:3905-12.
13. Baloch Z, Carayon P, Conte-Devolx B, Demers LM, Feldt-Rasmussen U, Henry JF, et al. Laboratory medicine practice guidelines: laboratory support for the diagnosis and monitoring of thyroid disease. Thyroid 2003;1:3-126.
14. Barlow JW, Csicsmann JM, White EL, Funder JW, Stockigt JR. Familial euthyroid thyroxine excess: characterization of abnormal intermediate affinity thyroxine binding to albumin. J Clin Endocrinol Metab 1982;2:244-50.
15. Bartalena L, Bogazzi F, Brogioni S, Burelli A, Scarcello G, Martino E. Measurement of serum free thyroid hormone concentrations: an essential tool for the diagnosis of thyroid dysfunction. Horm Res 1996;3-5:142-7.
16. Bartalena L, Robbins J. Variations in thyroid hormone transport proteins and their clinical implications. Thyroid 1992;3:237-45.
17. Bartalena L, Tanda ML. Clinical practice: Graves' ophthalmopathy. N Engl J Med 2009;10:994-1001.
18. Betterle C, Zanchetta R. Update on autoimmune polyendocrine syndromes (APS). Acta Biomed 2003;1:9-33.
19. Biebermann H, Schoneberg T, Krude H, Schultz G, Gudermann T, Gruters A. Mutations of the human thyrotropin receptor gene causing thyroid hypoplasia and persistent congenital hypothyroidism. J Clin Endocrinol Metab 1997;10:3471-80.
20. Bizhanova A, Kopp P. Minireview: the sodium-iodide symporter NIS and pendrin in iodide homeostasis of the thyroid. Endocrinology 2009;3:1084-90.
21. Bliss RD, Gauger PG, Delbridge LW. Surgeon's approach to the thyroid gland: surgical anatomy and the importance of technique. World J Surg 2000;8:891-7.
22. Bogazzi F, Bartalena L, Gasperi M, Braverman LE, Martino E. The various effects of amiodarone on thyroid function. Thyroid 2001;5: 511-9.
23. Bonomi M, Busnelli M, Beck-Peccoz P, Costanzo D, Antonica F, Dolci C, et al. A family with complete resistance to thyrotropin-releasing hormone. N Engl J Med 2009;7:731-4.
24. Brent GA. Clinical practice: Graves' disease. N Engl J Med 2008;24: 2594-605.
25. Bronstein I, Voyta JC, Thorpe GH, Kricka LJ, Armstrong G. Chemiluminescent assay of alkaline phosphatase applied in an ultrasensitive enzyme immunoassay of thyrotropin. Clin Chem 1989;7:1441-6.
26. Burrow GN, Fisher DA, Larsen PR. Maternal and fetal thyroid function. N Engl J Med 1994;16:1072-8.
27. Carle A, Laurberg P, Knudsen N, Perrild H, Ovesen L, Rasmussen LB, et al. Thyroid peroxidase and thyroglobulin auto-antibodies in patients with newly diagnosed overt hypothyroidism. Autoimmunity 2006;6:497-503.
28. Cartwright D, O'Shea P, Rajanayagam O, Agostini M, Barker P, Moran C, et al. Familial dysalbuminemic hyperthyroxinemia: a persistent diagnostic challenge. Clin Chem 2009;5:1044-6.
29. Chan SY, Vasilopoulou E, Kilby MD. The role of the placenta in thyroid hormone delivery to the fetus. Nat Clin Pract Endocrinol Metab 2009;1:45-54.
30. Chiamolera MI, Wondisford FE. Minireview: thyrotropin-releasing hormone and the thyroid hormone feedback mechanism. Endocrinology 2009;3:1091-6.
31. Cho MH, Kim CS, Park JS, Kang ES, Ahn CW, Cha BS, et al. Riedel's thyroiditis in a patient with recurrent subacute thyroiditis: a case report and review of the literature. Endocr J 2007;4:559-62.
32. Chopra IJ. A radioimmunoassay for measurement of 3,3′,5′-triiodothyronine (reverse T3). J Clin Invest 1974;3:583-92.
33. Christofides ND, Sheehan CP, Midgley JE. One-step, labeled-antibody assay for measuring free thyroxin. I. Assay development and validation. Clin Chem 1992;1:11-18.
34. Davidson KM, Richards DS, Schatz DA, Fisher DA. Successful in utero treatment of fetal goiter and hypothyroidism. N Engl J Med 1991;8:543-6.
35. Day TA, Chu A, Hoang KG. Multinodular goiter. Otolaryngol Clin North Am 2003;1:35-54.
36. DeBoer MD, Lafranchi SH. Pediatric thyroid testing issues. Pediatr Endocrinol Rev 2007;5(suppl 1):570-7.
37. Derwahl M, Studer H. Multinodular goitre: 'much more to it than simply iodine deficiency.' Baillieres Best Pract Res Clin Endocrinol Metab 2000;4:577-600.
38. Devdhar M, Ousman YH, Burman KD. Hypothyroidism. Endocrinol Metab Clin North Am 2007;3:595-615, v.
39. Dominguez LJ, Bevilacqua M, Dibella G, Barbagallo M. Diagnosing and managing thyroid disease in the nursing home. J Am Med Dir Assoc 2008;1:9-17.
40. Donadio S, Pascual A, Thijssen JH, Ronin C. Feasibility study of new calibrators for thyroid-stimulating hormone (TSH) immunoprocedures based on remodeling of recombinant TSH to mimic glycoforms circulating in patients with thyroid disorders. Clin Chem 2006;2:286-97.
41. Dufour DR. Laboratory tests of thyroid function: uses and limitations. Endocrinol Metab Clin North Am 2007;3:579-94, v.
42. Dussault JH, Fisher DA. Thyroid function in mothers of hypothyroid newborns. Obstet Gynecol 1999;1:15-20.
43. Ekins R. Validity of analog free thyroxin immunoassays. Clin Chem 1987;12:2137-44.
44. Ekins R. Measurement of free hormones in blood. Endocr Rev 1990;1: 5-46.
45. Ekins R. The free hormone hypothesis and measurement of free hormones. Clin Chem 1992;7:1289-93.
46. Eszlinger M, Neumann S, Otto L, Paschke R. Thyroglobulin mRNA quantification in the peripheral blood is not a reliable marker for the follow-up of patients with differentiated thyroid cancer. Eur J Endocrinol 2002;5:575-82.
47. Fares F. The role of O-linked and N-linked oligosaccharides on the structure-function of glycoprotein hormones: development of agonists and antagonists. Biochim Biophys Acta 2006;4:560-7.
48. Farwell AP. Thyroid hormone therapy is not indicated in the majority of patients with the sick euthyroid syndrome. Endocr Pract 2008;9: 1180-7.
49. Fatourechi V. Subclinical hypothyroidism: an update for primary care physicians. Mayo Clin Proc 2009;1:65-71.
50. Ferrari C, Romussi M, Rampini P, Benco R, Boghen M, Paracchi A, et al. Serum free thyroid hormones in T3-toxicosis: a study of 35 patients. J Endocrinol Invest 1983;1:55-8.
51. Fisher DA. Disorders of the thyroid in the newborn and infant. In: Sperling MA, ed. Pediatric endocrinology. Philadelphia, Pa: Saunders, 1996:51-70.
52. Fisher DA, Klein AH. Thyroid development and disorders of thyroid function in the newborn. N Engl J Med 1981;12:702-12.
53. Fonseca V, Thomas M, Katrak A, Sweny P, Moorhead JF. Can urinary thyroid hormone loss cause hypothyroidism? Lancet 1991;8765:475-6.
54. Francis Z, Schlumberger M. Serum thyroglobulin determination in thyroid cancer patients. Best Pract Res Clin Endocrinol Metab 2008;6: 1039-46.
55. Franklyn JA. Subclinical thyroid disorders—consequences and implications for treatment. Ann Endocrinol (Paris) 2007;4:229-30.
56. Fritz KS, Weiss RM, Nelson JC, Wilcox RB. Unequal concentrations of free T3 and free T4 after ultrafiltration. Clin Chem 2007;7: 1384-5.

57. Fugazzola L, Mihalich A, Persani L, Cerutti N, Reina M, Bonomi M, et al. Highly sensitive serum thyroglobulin and circulating thyroglobulin mRNA evaluations in the management of patients with differentiated thyroid cancer in apparent remission. J Clin Endocrinol Metab 2002;7:3201-8.
58. Gagne N, Parma J, Deal C, Vassart G, Van VG. Apparent congenital athyreosis contrasting with normal plasma thyroglobulin levels and associated with inactivating mutations in the thyrotropin receptor gene: are athyreosis and ectopic thyroid distinct entities? J Clin Endocrinol Metab 1998;5:1771-5.
59. Gassner D, Stock W, Golla R, Roth HJ. First automated assay for thyrotropin receptor autoantibodies. Clin Chem Lab Med 2009;9: 1091-5.
60. George J, Joshi SR. Drugs and thyroid. J Assoc Physicians India 2007; 55:215-23.
61. Gilani BB, MacGillivray MH, Voorhess ML, Mills BJ, Riley WJ, MacLaren NK. Thyroid hormone abnormalities at diagnosis of insulin-dependent diabetes mellitus in children. J Pediatr 1984;2: 218-22.
62. Giovanella L. Highly sensitive thyroglobulin measurements in differentiated thyroid carcinoma management. Clin Chem Lab Med 2008;8:1067-73.
63. Gittoes NJ, Franklyn JA. Drug-induced thyroid disorders. Drug Saf 1995;1:46-55.
64. Gnidehou S, Caillou B, Talbot M, Ohayon R, Kaniewski J, Noel-Hudson MS, et al. Iodotyrosine dehalogenase 1 (DEHAL1) is a transmembrane protein involved in the recycling of iodide close to the thyroglobulin iodination site. FASEB J 2004;13:1574-6.
65. Gyamfi C, Wapner RJ, D'Alton ME. Thyroid dysfunction in pregnancy: the basic science and clinical evidence surrounding the controversy in management. Obstet Gynecol 2009;3:702-7.
66. Hadj-Kacem H, Rebuffat S, Mnif-Feki M, Belguith-Maalej S, Ayadi H, Peraldi-Roux S. Autoimmune thyroid diseases: genetic susceptibility of thyroid-specific genes and thyroid autoantigen contributions. Int J Immunogenet 2009;2:85-96.
67. Harish K. Thyroglobulin: current status in differentiated thyroid carcinoma (review). Endocr Regul 2006;2:53-67.
68. Hay ID, Annesley TM, Jiang NS, Gorman CA. Simultaneous determination of D- and L-thyroxine in human serum by liquid chromatography with electrochemical detection. J Chromatogr 1981;2:383-90.
69. Hay ID, Bayer MF, Kaplan MM, Klee GG, Larsen PR, Spencer CA. American Thyroid Association assessment of current free thyroid hormone and thyrotropin measurements and guidelines for future clinical assays. The Committee on Nomenclature of the American Thyroid Association. Clin Chem 1991;11:2002-8.
70. Heberling HJ, Bierwolf B, Kuhlmann E, Lohmann D. Measurement of TSH-binding-inhibiting immunoglobulins (TBII) using a radioreceptor-assay (TRAK) in patients with and without thyroid disease. Radiobiol Radiother (Berl) 1987;5:582-5.
71. Hegedus L. Treatment of Graves' hyperthyroidism: evidence-based and emerging modalities. Endocrinol Metab Clin North Am 2009;2: 355-71, ix.
72. Helfand M. Screening for subclinical thyroid dysfunction in nonpregnant adults: a summary of the evidence for the U.S. Preventive Services Task Force. Ann Intern Med 2004;2:128-41.
73. Hennessey JV, Scherger JE. Evaluating and treating the patient with hypothyroid disease. J Fam Pract 2007;8(suppl Hot Topics):S31-9.
74. Heuer H, Visser TJ. Minireview: pathophysiological importance of thyroid hormone transporters. Endocrinology 2009;3:1078-83.
75. Iervasi A, Iervasi G, Carpi A, Zucchelli GC. Serum thyroglobulin measurement: clinical background and main methodological aspects with clinical impact. Biomed Pharmacother 2006;8:414-24.
76. Ioos V, Das V, Maury E, Baudel JL, Guechot J, Guidet B, et al. A thyrotoxicosis outbreak due to dietary pills in Paris. Ther Clin Risk Manag 2008;6:1375-9.
77. Jonklaas J, Kahric-Janicic N, Soldin OP, Soldin SJ. Correlations of free thyroid hormones measured by tandem mass spectrometry and immunoassay with thyroid-stimulating hormone across 4 patient populations. Clin Chem 2009;7:1380-8.
78. Kaihola HL, Irjala K, Viikari J, Nanto V. Determination of thyrotropin in serum by time-resolved fluoroimmunoassay evaluated. Clin Chem 1985;10:1706-9.
79. Kaptein EM, Beale E, Chan LS. Thyroid hormone therapy for obesity and nonthyroidal illnesses: a systematic review. J Clin Endocrinol Metab 2009;10:3663-75.
80. Keenan DM, Roelfsema F, Biermasz N, Veldhuis JD. Physiological control of pituitary hormone secretory-burst mass, frequency, and waveform: a statistical formulation and analysis. Am J Physiol Regul Integr Comp Physiol 2003;3:R664-73.
81. Keffer JH. Preanalytical considerations in testing thyroid function. Clin Chem 1996;1:125-34.
82. Ketchum CH, Riley WJ, MacLaren NK. Adrenal dysfunction in asymptomatic patients with adrenocortical autoantibodies. J Clin Endocrinol Metab 1984;6:1166-70.
83. Klee GG. Clinical usage recommendations and analytic performance goals for total and free triiodothyronine measurements. Clin Chem 1996;1:155-9.
84. Klein I, Levey GS. Unusual manifestations of hypothyroidism. Arch Intern Med 1984;1:123-8.
85. Kleiner J, Altshuler L, Hendrick V, Hershman JM. Lithium-induced subclinical hypothyroidism: review of the literature and guidelines for treatment. J Clin Psychiatry 1999;4:249-5.
86. Knobel M, Medeiros-Neto G. An outline of inherited disorders of the thyroid hormone generating system. Thyroid 2003;8:771-801.
87. Kohn B, Grasberger H, Lam LL, Ferrara AM, Refetoff S. A somatic gain-of-function mutation in the thyrotropin receptor gene producing a toxic adenoma in an infant. Thyroid 2009;2:187-91.
88. Kopp P, Pesce L, Solis-S JC. Pendred syndrome and iodide transport in the thyroid. Trends Endocrinol Metab 2008;7:260-8.
89. Kratzsch J, Pulzer F. Thyroid gland development and defects. Best Pract Res Clin Endocrinol Metab 2008;1:57-75.
90. Kwaku MP, Burman KD. Myxedema coma. J Intensive Care Med 2007;4:224-31.
91. Lam-Tse WK, Batstra MR, Koeleman BP, Roep BO, Bruining MG, Aanstoot HJ, et al. The association between autoimmune thyroiditis, autoimmune gastritis and type 1 diabetes. Pediatr Endocrinol Rev 2003;1:22-37.
92. Lania A, Persani L, Beck-Peccoz P. Central hypothyroidism. Pituitary 2008;2:181-6.
93. Lankisch TO, Jaeckel E, Strassburg CP. The autoimmune polyendocrinopathy-candidiasis-ectodermal dystrophy or autoimmune polyglandular syndrome type 1. Semin Liver Dis 2009;3: 307-14.
94. Lao TT. Thyroid disorders in pregnancy. Curr Opin Obstet Gynecol 2005;2:123-7.
95. Laurberg P, Andersen S, Bulow P, Carle A. Hypothyroidism in the elderly: pathophysiology, diagnosis and treatment. Drugs Aging 2005;1:23-38.
95A. Laurberg P, Andersen S, Carlé A, Karmisholt J, Knudsen N, Pedersen IB. The TSH upper reference limit: where are we at? Nat Rev Endocrinol 2011;7:232-9.
96. Laws ER, Vance ML, Jane JA Jr. TSH adenomas. Pituitary 2006;4: 313-5.
97. Lazarus JH. Hyperthyroidism during pregnancy: etiology, diagnosis and management. Womens Health (Lond Engl) 2005;1:97-104.
98. Lee RH, Spencer CA, Mestman JH, Miller EA, Petrovic I, Braverman LE, et al. Free T4 immunoassays are flawed during pregnancy. Am J Obstet Gynecol 2009;3:260-6.
99. Letellier M, Levesque A, Daigle F, Grant A. Performance evaluation of automated immunoassays on the Technicon Immuno 1 system. Clin Chem 1996;10:1695-701.
100. Levy M. Propylthiouracil hepatotoxicity: a review and case presentation. Clin Pediatr (Phila) 1993;1:25-9.
101. Lewinski A, Szybinski Z, Bandurska-Stankiewicz E, Grzywa M, Karwowska A, Kinalska I, et al. Iodine-induced hyperthyroidism—an

epidemiological survey several years after institution of iodine prophylaxis in Poland. J Endocrinol Invest 2003;2(suppl):57-62.
102. Lorini R, Gastaldi R, Traggiai C, Perucchin PP. Hashimoto's thyroiditis. Pediatr Endocrinol Rev 2003;1(suppl 3):205-11.
103. Losa M, Fortunato M, Molteni L, Peretti E, Mortini P. Thyrotropin-secreting pituitary adenomas: biological and molecular features, diagnosis and therapy. Minerva Endocrinol 2008;4:329-40.
104. MacLaren NK, Riley WJ. Thyroid, gastric, and adrenal autoimmunities associated with insulin-dependent diabetes mellitus. Diabetes Care 1985;8:34-8.
105. Marino M, Chiovato L, Friedlander JA, Latrofa F, Pinchera A, McCluskey RT. Serum antibodies against megalin (GP330) in patients with autoimmune thyroiditis. J Clin Endocrinol Metab 1999;7:2468-74.
106. Markou K, Georgopoulos N, Kyriazopoulou V, Vagenakis AG. Iodine-induced hypothyroidism. Thyroid 2001;5:501-10.
107. Massart C, Maugendre D. Importance of the detection method for thyroglobulin antibodies for the validity of thyroglobulin measurements in sera from patients with Graves' disease. Clin Chem 2002;1:102-7.
108. Matsuura N, Yamada Y, Nohara Y, Konishi J, Kasagi K, Endo K, et al. Familial neonatal transient hypothyroidism due to maternal TSH-binding inhibitor immunoglobulins. N Engl J Med 1980;13: 738-41.
109. McCapra F, Watmore D, Sumun F, Patel A, Beheshti I, Ramakrishnan K, et al. Luminescent labels for immunoassay—from concept to practice. J Biolumin Chemilumin 1989;1:51-8.
110. McDonald NQ, Hendrickson WA. A structural superfamily of growth factors containing a cystine knot motif. Cell 1993;3:421-4.
111. McGrogan A, Seaman HE, Wright JW, de Vries CS. The incidence of autoimmune thyroid disease: a systematic review of the literature. Clin Endocrinol (Oxf) 2008;5:687-96.
112. McLachlan SM, Rapoport B. Why measure thyroglobulin autoantibodies rather than thyroid peroxidase autoantibodies? Thyroid 2004;7:510-20.
113. McLachlan SM, Rapoport B. Thyroid peroxidase as an autoantigen. Thyroid 2007;10:939-48.
114. McLean RH, Kennedy TL, Rosoulpour M, Ratzan SK, Siegel NJ, Kauschansky A, et al. Hypothyroidism in the congenital nephrotic syndrome. J Pediatr 1982;1:72-5.
115. Mei JV, Alexander JR, Adam BW, Hannon WH. Use of filter paper for the collection and analysis of human whole blood specimens. J Nutr 2001;5:1631S-6S.
116. Meier DA, Kaplan MM. Radioiodine uptake and thyroid scintiscanning. Endocrinol Metab Clin North Am 2001;2:291-313, viii.
117. Meinhold H, Visser TJ. International survey of the radioimmunological measurement of serum reverse triiodothyronine. Clin Chim Acta 1980;3:343-50.
118. Merezhinskaya N, Fishbein WN. Monocarboxylate transporters: past, present, and future. Histol Histopathol 2009;2:243-64.
119. Mestman JH, Goodwin TM, Montoro MM. Thyroid disorders of pregnancy. Endocrinol Metab Clin North Am 1995;1:41-71.
120. Midgley JE. Direct and indirect free thyroxine assay methods: theory and practice. Clin Chem 2001;8:1353-63.
121. Midgley JE, Christofides ND. Point: legitimate and illegitimate tests of free-analyte assay function. Clin Chem 2009;3:439-41.
122. Midgley JE, Moon CR, Wilkins TA. Validity of analog free thyroxin immunoassays. Part II. Clin Chem 1987;12:2145-52.
123. Miller MC, Agrawal A. Hypothyroidism in postradiation head and neck cancer patients: incidence, complications, and management. Curr Opin Otolaryngol Head Neck Surg 2009;2:111-5.
124. Miossec P. Cytokine-induced autoimmune disorders. Drug Saf 1997;2:93-104.
125. Mistry N, Wass J, Turner MR. When to consider thyroid dysfunction in the neurology clinic. Pract Neurol 2009;3:145-56.
126. Moller B, Falk O, Bjorkhem I. Isotope dilution—mass spectrometry of thyroxin proposed as a reference method. Clin Chem 1983;12: 2106-10.
127. Mooradian AD. Asymptomatic hyperthyroidism in older adults: is it a distinct clinical and laboratory entity? Drugs Aging 2008;5:371-80.
128. Morales AE, Shi JD, Wang CY, She JX, Muir A, Novel TSH. Beta subunit gene mutation causing congenital central hypothyroidism in a newborn male. J Pediatr Endocrinol Metab 2004;3:355-9.
129. Moreno JC, Klootwijk W, van Toor H, Pinto G, D'Alessandro M, Leger A, et al. Mutations in the iodotyrosine deiodinase gene and hypothyroidism. N Engl J Med 2008;17:1811-8.
130. Moreno JC, Visser TJ. New phenotypes in thyroid dyshormonogenesis: hypothyroidism due to DUOX2 mutations. Endocr Dev 2007;10:99-117.
131. Mullis PE. Genetics of growth hormone deficiency. Endocrinol Metab Clin North Am 2007;1:17-36.
132. Mussig K, Thamer C, Bares R, Lipp HP, Haring HU, Gallwitz B. Iodine-induced thyrotoxicosis after ingestion of kelp-containing tea. J Gen Intern Med 2006;6:C11-4.
133. Nabhan ZM, Kreher NC, Eugster EA. Hashitoxicosis in children: clinical features and natural history. J Pediatr 2005;4:533-6.
134. Nayak B, Burman K. Thyrotoxicosis and thyroid storm. Endocrinol Metab Clin North Am 2006;4:663-86, vii.
134A. National Health and Nutrition Examination Survey: NHANES 2009-2010. National Center for Health Statistics, Hyattsville, MD 20782.
135. Nayak B, Hodak SP. Hyperthyroidism. Endocrinol Metab Clin North Am 2007;3:617-56, v.
136. Negro R, Formoso G, Mangieri T, Pezzarossa A, Dazzi D, Hassan H. Levothyroxine treatment in euthyroid pregnant women with autoimmune thyroid disease: effects on obstetrical complications. J Clin Endocrinol Metab 2006;7:2587-91.
137. Nelson JC, Wang R, Asher DT, Wilcox RB. Underestimates and overestimates of total thyroxine concentrations caused by unwanted thyroxine-binding protein effects. Thyroid 2005;1:12-15.
138. Nelson JC, Wilcox RB. Analytical performance of free and total thyroxine assays. Clin Chem 1996;1:146-54.
139. Nygaard B. Hyperthyroidism. Am Fam Physician 2007;7:1014-6.
140. Pacini F, Castagna MG. Diagnostic and therapeutic use of recombinant human TSH (rhTSH) in differentiated thyroid cancer. Best Pract Res Clin Endocrinol Metab 2008;6:1009-21.
141. Pacini F, Pinchera A. Serum and tissue thyroglobulin measurement: clinical applications in thyroid disease. Biochimie 1999;5:463-7.
142. Palha JA. Transthyretin as a thyroid hormone carrier: function revisited. Clin Chem Lab Med 2002;12:1292-300.
143. Panicker V, Cluett C, Shields B, Murray A, Parnell KS, Perry JR, et al. A common variation in deiodinase 1 gene DIO1 is associated with the relative levels of free thyroxine and triiodothyronine. J Clin Endocrinol Metab 2008;8:3075-81.
144. Papi G, LiVolsi VA. Current concepts on Riedel thyroiditis. Am J Clin Pathol 2004;121(suppl):S50-63.
145. Papi G, Uberti ED, Betterle C, Carani C, Pearce EN, Braverman LE, et al. Subclinical hypothyroidism. Curr Opin Endocrinol Diabetes Obes 2007;3:197-208.
146. Parmar MS, Sturge C. Recurrent hamburger thyrotoxicosis. CMAJ 2003;5:415-7.
147. Patil-Sisodia K, Mestman JH. Graves' hyperthyroidism and pregnancy: a clinical update. Endocr Pract 2009;16:1-36.
148. Pearce EN, Farwell AP, Braverman LE. Thyroiditis. N Engl J Med 2003;26:2646-55.
149. Persani L, Borgato S, Romoli R, Asteria C, Pizzocaro A, Beck-Peccoz P. Changes in the degree of sialylation of carbohydrate chains modify the biological properties of circulating thyrotropin isoforms in various physiological and pathological states. J Clin Endocrinol Metab 1998;7: 2486-92.
150. Petersen BA, Hanson RN, Giese RW, Karger BL. Picogram analysis of free triiodothyronine and free thyroxine hormones in serum by equilibrium dialysis and electron capture gas chromatography. J Chromatogr 1976;126:503-16.
151. Pietras SM, Safer JD. Diagnostic confusion attributable to spurious elevation of both total thyroid hormone and thyroid hormone uptake

measurements in the setting of autoantibodies: case report and review of related literature. Endocr Pract 2008;6:738-42.
152. Piga M, Serra A, Boi F, Tanda ML, Martino E, Mariotti S. Amiodarone-induced thyrotoxicosis: a review. Minerva Endocrinol 2008;3:213-28.
153. Pimentel L, Hansen KN. Thyroid disease in the emergency department: a clinical and laboratory review. J Emerg Med 2005;2:201-9.
154. Poppe K, Velkeniers B, Glinoer D. The role of thyroid autoimmunity in fertility and pregnancy. Nat Clin Pract Endocrinol Metab 2008;7:394-405.
155. Porterfield JR Jr, Thompson GB, Farley DR, Grant CS, Richards ML. Evidence-based management of toxic multinodular goiter (Plummer's disease). World J Surg 2008;7:1278-84.
156. Preissner CM, Klee GG, Krco CJ. Nonisotopic "sandwich" immunoassay of thyroglobulin in serum by the biotin-streptavidin technique: evaluation and comparison with an immunoradiometric assay. Clin Chem 1988;9:1794-8.
157. Rafferty B, Gaines DR. Comparison of pituitary and recombinant human thyroid-stimulating hormone (rhTSH) in a multicenter collaborative study: establishment of the first World Health Organization reference reagent for rhTSH. Clin Chem 1999;12: 2207-15.
158. Rajatanavin R, Braverman LE. Euthyroid hyperthyroxinemia. J Endocrinol Invest 1983;6:493-505.
159. Ringel MD, Balducci-Silano PL, Anderson JS, Spencer CA, Silverman J, Sparling YH, et al. Quantitative reverse transcription-polymerase chain reaction of circulating thyroglobulin messenger ribonucleic acid for monitoring patients with thyroid carcinoma. J Clin Endocrinol Metab 1999;11:4037-42.
160. Ringel MD, Ladenson PW, Levine MA. Molecular diagnosis of residual and recurrent thyroid cancer by amplification of thyroglobulin messenger ribonucleic acid in peripheral blood. J Clin Endocrinol Metab 1998;12:4435-42.
161. Robles DT, Fain PR, Gottlieb PA, Eisenbarth GS. The genetics of autoimmune polyendocrine syndrome type II. Endocrinol Metab Clin North Am 2002;2:353-vii.
162. Roddiger SJ, Bojunga J, Klee V, Stanisch M, Renneberg H, Lindhorst E, et al. Detection of thyroid peroxidase mRNA in peripheral blood of patients with malignant and benign thyroid diseases. J Mol Endocrinol 2002;3:287-95.
163. Rodien P, Jordan N, Lefevre A, Royer J, Vasseur C, Savagner F, et al. Abnormal stimulation of the thyrotrophin receptor during gestation. Hum Reprod Update 2004;2:95-105.
164. Rodrigo JP, Rinaldo A, Devaney KO, Shaha AR, Ferlito A. Molecular diagnostic methods in the diagnosis and follow-up of well-differentiated thyroid carcinoma. Head Neck 2006;11:1032-9.
165. Rose SR. Disorders of thyrotropin synthesis, secretion, and function. Curr Opin Pediatr 2000;4:375-81.
166. Roth LM, Talerman A. The enigma of struma ovarii. Pathology 2007;1:139-46.
167. Rugg JA, Flaa CW, Dawson SR, Rigl CT, Leung KS, Evans SA. Automated quantification of thyrotropin by radial partition immunoassay. Clin Chem 1988;1:118-22.
168. Sadler WA, Murray LM, Turner JG. What does "functional sensitivity" mean? Clin Chem 1996;12:2051-2.
169. Safer JD, O'Connor MG, Colan SD, Srinivasan S, Tollin SR, Wondisford FE. The thyroid hormone receptor-beta gene mutation R383H is associated with isolated central resistance to thyroid hormone. J Clin Endocrinol Metab 1999;9:3099-109.
170. Saikia UK, Saikia M. Drug-induced thyroid disorders. J Indian Med Assoc 2006;10:583, 585-7, 600.
171. Samuels MH. Cognitive function in untreated hypothyroidism and hyperthyroidism. Curr Opin Endocrinol Diabetes Obes 2008;5: 429-33.
172. Sapin R, d'Herbomez M. Free thyroxine measured by equilibrium dialysis and nine immunoassays in sera with various serum thyroxine-binding capacities. Clin Chem 2003;9:1531-5.
173. Sapin R, Gasser F, Schlienger JL. Familial dysalbuminemic hyperthyroxinemia and thyroid hormone autoantibodies: interference in current free thyroid hormone assays. Horm Res 1996;3-5:139-41.
174. Sato A, Perlas E, Ben-Menahem D, Kudo M, Pixley MR, Furuhashi M, et al. Cystine knot of the gonadotropin alpha subunit is critical for intracellular behavior but not for in vitro biological activity. J Biol Chem 1997;29:18098-103.
175. Schatz DA, Winter WE. Autoimmune polyglandular syndrome. II. Clinical syndrome and treatment. Endocrinol Metab Clin North Am 2002;2:339-52.
176. Schussler GC. The thyroxine-binding proteins. Thyroid 2000;2:141-9.
177. Seissler J, Wagner S, Schott M, Lettmann M, Feldkamp J, Scherbaum WA, et al. Low frequency of autoantibodies to the human Na(+)/I(−) symporter in patients with autoimmune thyroid disease. J Clin Endocrinol Metab 2000;12:4630-4.
178. Setian NS. Hypothyroidism in children: diagnosis and treatment. J Pediatr (Rio J) 2007;5(suppl):S209-16.
178A. Sharma M, Aronow WS, Patel L, Gandhi K, Desai H. Hyperthyroidism. Med Sci Monit 2011;17:RA85-91.
179. Sherman SI, Ladenson PW. Subacute thyroiditis causing thyroid storm. Thyroid 2007;3:283.
180. Sicilia V, Mezitis S. A case of acute suppurative thyroiditis complicated by thyrotoxicosis. J Endocrinol Invest 2006;11:997-1000.
181. Siegel RD, Lee SL. Toxic nodular goiter: toxic adenoma and toxic multinodular goiter. Endocrinol Metab Clin North Am 1998;1: 151-68.
182. Sinclair D. Clinical and laboratory aspects of thyroid autoantibodies. Ann Clin Biochem 2006;(Pt 3):173-83.
183. Soldin OP, Hilakivi-Clarke L, Weiderpass E, Soldin SJ. Trimester-specific reference intervals for thyroxine and triiodothyronine in pregnancy in iodine-sufficient women using isotope dilution tandem mass spectrometry and immunoassays. Clin Chim Acta 2004;1-2:181-9.
184. Soldin SJ, Soukhova N, Janicic N, Jonklaas J, Soldin OP. The measurement of free thyroxine by isotope dilution tandem mass spectrometry. Clin Chim Acta 2005;1-2:113-8.
184A. Soldin OP, Soldin SJ. Thyroid hormone testing by tandem mass spectrometry. Clin Biochem 2011;44:89-94.
185. Song Y, Driessens N, Costa M, De Deken X, Detours V, Corvilain B, et al. Roles of hydrogen peroxide in thyroid physiology and disease. J Clin Endocrinol Metab 2007;10:3764-73.
186. Spencer CA. Recoveries cannot be used to authenticate thyroglobulin (Tg) measurements when sera contain Tg autoantibodies. Clin Chem 1996;5:661-3.
187. Spencer CA, LoPresti JS. Measuring thyroglobulin and thyroglobulin autoantibody in patients with differentiated thyroid cancer. Nat Clin Pract Endocrinol Metab 2008;4:223-33.
188. Spencer CA, LoPresti JS, Fatemi S, Nicoloff JT. Detection of residual and recurrent differentiated thyroid carcinoma by serum thyroglobulin measurement. Thyroid 1999;5:435-41.
189. Spencer CA, LoPresti JS, Patel A, Guttler RB, Eigen A, Shen D, et al. Applications of a new chemiluminometric thyrotropin assay to subnormal measurement. J Clin Endocrinol Metab 1990;2:453-60.
190. Spencer CA, Takeuchi M, Kazarosyan M. Current status and performance goals for serum thyroglobulin assays. Clin Chem 1996;1:164-73.
191. St Germain DL, Galton VA, Hernandez A. Minireview: defining the roles of the iodothyronine deiodinases: current concepts and challenges. Endocrinology 2009;3:1097-107.
192. Stagnaro-Green A. Postpartum thyroiditis. Best Pract Res Clin Endocrinol Metab 2004;2:303-16.
193. Stanbury JB, Ermans AE, Bourdoux P, Todd C, Oken E, Tonglet R, et al. Iodine-induced hyperthyroidism: occurrence and epidemiology. Thyroid 1998;1:83-100.
194. Strakosch CR, Wenzel BE, Row VV, Volpe R. Immunology of autoimmune thyroid diseases. N Engl J Med 1982;24:1499-507.
195. Streetman DD, Khanderia U. Diagnosis and treatment of Graves' disease. Ann Pharmacother 2003;7-8:1100-9.

196. Surks MI, Ortiz E, Daniels GH, Sawin CT, Col NF, Cobin RH, et al. Subclinical thyroid disease: scientific review and guidelines for diagnosis and management. JAMA 2004;2:228-38.
197. Szkudlinski MW, Fremont V, Ronin C, Weintraub BD. Thyroid-stimulating hormone and thyroid-stimulating hormone receptor structure-function relationships. Physiol Rev 2002;2:473-502.
198. Tachman ML, Guthrie GP Jr. Hypothyroidism: diversity of presentation. Endocr Rev 1984;3:456-65.
199. Takasu N, Oshiro C, Akamine H, Komiya I, Nagata A, Sato Y, et al. Thyroid-stimulating antibody and TSH-binding inhibitor immunoglobulin in 277 Graves' patients and in 686 normal subjects. J Endocrinol Invest 1997;8:452-61.
200. Tikanoja SH, Liewendahl BK. New ultrafiltration method for free thyroxin compared with equilibrium dialysis in patients with thyroid dysfunction and nonthyroidal illness. Clin Chem 1990;5:800-4.
201. Tonacchera M, Chiovato L, Pinchera A, Agretti P, Fiore E, Cetani F, et al. Hyperfunctioning thyroid nodules in toxic multinodular goiter share activating thyrotropin receptor mutations with solitary toxic adenoma. J Clin Endocrinol Metab 1998;2:492-8.
202. Topaloglu AK. Athyreosis, dysgenesis, and dyshormonogenesis in congenital hypothyroidism. Pediatr Endocrinol Rev 2006;3(suppl 3): 498-502.
203. Topliss DJ, Eastman CJ. 5. Diagnosis and management of hyperthyroidism and hypothyroidism. Med J Aust 2004;4:186-93.
204. Ursella S, Testa A, Mazzone M, Gentiloni SN. Amiodarone-induced thyroid dysfunction in clinical practice. Eur Rev Med Pharmacol Sci 2006;5:269-78.
205. Uy HL, Reasner CA. Elevated thyroxine levels in a euthyroid patient: a search for the cause of euthyroid hyperthyroxinemia. Postgrad Med 1994;5:195-202.
206. Valente WA, Vitti P, Rotella CM, Vaughan MM, Aloj SM, Grollman EF, et al. Antibodies that promote thyroid growth: a distinct population of thyroid-stimulating autoantibodies. N Engl J Med 1983;17:1028-34.
207. van Wassenaer AG, Kok JH, de Vijlder JJ, Briet JM, Smit BJ, Tamminga P, et al. Effects of thyroxine supplementation on neurologic development in infants born at less than 30 weeks' gestation. N Engl J Med 1997;1:21-6.
208. Van UK, Stockl D, Ross HA, Thienpont LM. Use of frozen sera for FT4 standardization: investigation by equilibrium dialysis combined with isotope dilution-mass spectrometry and immunoassay. Clin Chem 2006;9:1817-21.
209. Vanderpas J. Nutritional epidemiology and thyroid hormone metabolism. Annu Rev Nutr 2006;26:293-322.
210. Villar HC, Saconato H, Valente O, Atallah AN. Thyroid hormone replacement for subclinical hypothyroidism. Cochrane Database Syst Rev 2007;3:CD003419.
211. Visser WE, Friesema EC, Jansen J, Visser TJ. Thyroid hormone transport in and out of cells. Trends Endocrinol Metab 2008;2:50-6.
212. Voigt W, Maher G, Wolf HH, Schmoll HJ. Human chorionic gonadotropin-induced hyperthyroidism in germ cell cancer—a case presentation and review of the literature. Onkologie 2007;6:330-4.
213. Vono-Toniolo J, Kopp P. Thyroglobulin gene mutations and other genetic defects associated with congenital hypothyroidism. Arq Bras Endocrinol Metabol 2004;1:70-82.
214. Wallaschofski H, Kuwert T, Lohmann T. TSH-receptor autoantibodies—differentiation of hyperthyroidism between Graves' disease and toxic multinodular goitre. Exp Clin Endocrinol Diabetes 2004;4:171-4.
215. Ward G, McKinnon L, Badrick T, Hickman PE. Heterophilic antibodies remain a problem for the immunoassay laboratory. Am J Clin Pathol 1997;4:417-21.
216. Watemberg N, Greenstein D, Levine A. Encephalopathy associated with Hashimoto thyroiditis: pediatric perspective. J Child Neurol 2006;1:1-5.
217. Watkins MG, Dejkhamron P, Huo J, Vazquez DM, Menon RK. Persistent neonatal thyrotoxicosis in a neonate secondary to a rare thyroid-stimulating hormone receptor activating mutation: case report and literature review. Endocr Pract 2008;4:479-83.
218. Webb P. Another story of mice and men: the types of RTH. Proc Natl Acad Sci U S A 2009;23:9129-30.
219. Weber T, Klar E. Minimal residual disease in thyroid carcinoma. Semin Surg Oncol 2001;4:272-7.
220. Weetman AP. Graves' disease. N Engl J Med 2000;17:1236-48.
221. Weetman AP. Autoimmune thyroid disease. Autoimmunity 2004;4: 337-40.
222. Wilcox RB, Nelson JC. Counterpoint: legitimate and illegitimate tests of free-analyte assay function: we need to identify the factors that influence free-analyte assay results. Clin Chem 2009;3:442-4.
223. Wilkins TA. Albumin in analog FT4 assay reagents: the facts. Clin Chem 1987;7:1293.
224. Wilkins TA, Midgley JE. Albumin-dependence of free thyroxin in nonthyroidal illness. Clin Chem 1987;8:1494-6.
225. Williams GR. Neurodevelopmental and neurophysiological actions of thyroid hormone. J Neuroendocrinol 2008;6:784-94.
226. Winter WE, Signorino MR. Review: molecular thyroidology. Ann Clin Lab Sci 2001;3:221-44.
227. Wolff J. Perchlorate and the thyroid gland. Pharmacol Rev 1998;1: 89-105.
228. Wong J, Lu Z, Doery J, Fuller P. Lessons from a review of thyroglobulin assays in the management of thyroid cancer. Intern Med J 2008;6:441-4.
229. Yamada M, Mori M. Mechanisms related to the pathophysiology and management of central hypothyroidism. Nat Clin Pract Endocrinol Metab 2008;12:683-94.
230. Yue B, Rockwood AL, Sandrock T, La'ulu SL, Kushnir MM, Meikle AW. Free thyroid hormones in serum by direct equilibrium dialysis and online solid-phase extraction—liquid chromatography/tandem mass spectrometry. Clin Chem 2008;4:642-51.
231. Zacharopoulou AD, Christofidis I, Kakabakos SE, Koupparis MA. Free thyroxine solid-analog immunoassays: investigation of the albumin effect on the antibody binding to immobilized thyroxine-protein conjugates. J Immunoassay Immunochem 2002;1:95-105.

CHAPTER 56

Reproductive Endocrinology and Related Disorders

*T. Scott Isbell, Ph.D., Emily Jungheim, M.D., and Ann M. Gronowski, Ph.D.**

Reproductive endocrinology encompasses the hormones of the hypothalamic-pituitary-gonadal axis, as well as the adrenal glands (see Chapter 54). These hormones are crucial for reproductive function and include gonadotropin-releasing hormone (GnRH), luteinizing hormone (LH), follicle-stimulating hormone (FSH), and a multitude of sex steroids. The sex steroids are synthesized by the ovaries, testes, and adrenal glands and are responsible for the manifestation of primary and secondary sex characteristics. This chapter is divided into four sections: Male Reproductive Biology, Female Reproductive Biology, Infertility, and Methods.

MALE REPRODUCTIVE BIOLOGY

The mature testes synthesize both sperm and androgens. The testes contain a structured network of tightly packed seminiferous tubules. The lumina of the seminiferous tubules are lined by maturing germ cells and Sertoli cells. Sertoli cells play a crucial role in sperm maturation and secrete *inhibin*, a glycoprotein that inhibits the pituitary secretion of FSH. Surrounding the seminiferous tubules are the interstitial Leydig cells, the primary site of androgen production. The principal androgen in man is testosterone, which serves a central role in reproductive physiology. Testosterone is required for sexual differentiation, spermatogenesis, and promotion and maintenance of sexual maturity at puberty. At the cellular level, these effects are mediated by binding of testosterone or its more potent metabolite dihydrotestosterone (DHT) to the androgen receptor or via aromatization to estradiol and subsequent binding to the estrogen receptor. Testicular function is under the control of the hypothalamic-pituitary-gonadal axis.

Hypothalamic-Pituitary-Gonadal Axis

Gonadotropin-releasing hormone (GnRH) is a decapeptide synthesized in the hypothalamus and transported to the anterior pituitary gland, where it stimulates the release of both FSH and LH (see also Chapter 53).

In adult men, GnRH and thus LH and FSH are secreted in pulsatile patterns. A circadian rhythm is present, with higher concentrations found in the early morning hours and lower concentrations in the late evening.[302] LH acts on Leydig cells to stimulate the conversion of cholesterol to pregnenolone. FSH acts on Sertoli cells and spermatocytes and is central to the initiation (in puberty) and maintenance (in adulthood) of spermatogenesis.[297] Sex steroids and inhibin (a 32 kDa protein secreted by the Sertoli cells) provide negative feedback control of LH and FSH secretion, respectively. LH secretion is inhibited by testosterone and by its metabolites, estradiol and DHT. FSH may be elevated in disorders in which Sertoli cell numbers (and hence inhibin concentrations) are reduced. Likewise, a reduction in the number of Leydig cells (and hence testosterone secretion) leads to increased LH concentrations.

Androgens

Androgens are a group of C-19 steroids (Figure 56-1) responsible for masculinization of the genital tract and development and maintenance of male secondary sex characteristics. Testosterone is the principle androgen secreted in men.

Biosynthesis of Testosterone

Testosterone is synthesized primarily by the Leydig cells of the testes (95%) and, to a lesser extent (≈5%) via peripheral conversion from the precursors dehydroepiandrosterone (DHEA) and androstenedione (which are synthesized in the

**The authors gratefully acknowledge the original contribution of R. J. Whitley, A. W. Meikle, and N. B. Watts, on which portions of this chapter are based.*

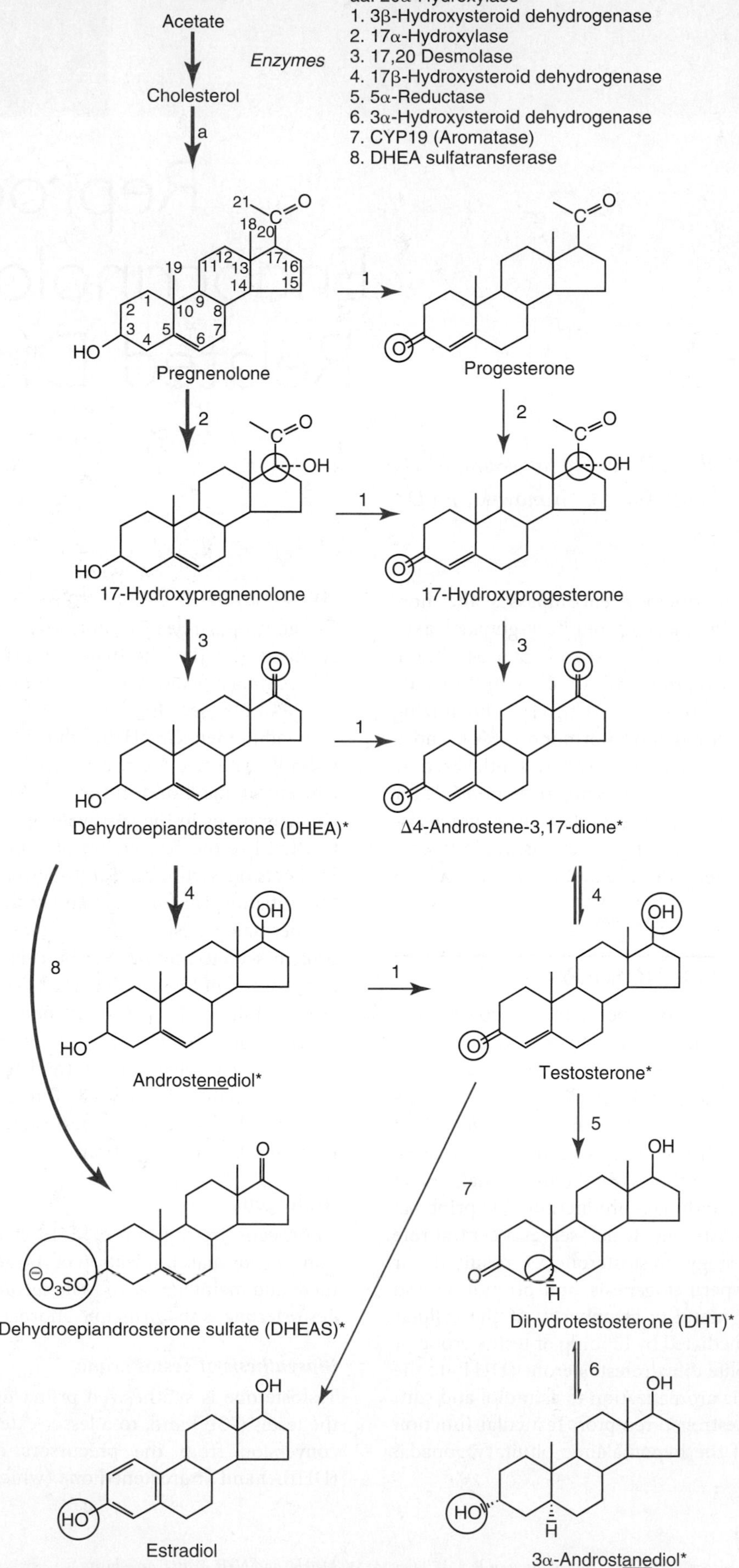

Figure 56-1 Biosynthesis of androgens (adrenal glands and testis). The *heavy arrows* indicate the preferred pathway. The *enclosed area* represents the site of chemical change. *Denotes androgens.

zona reticularis of the adrenal glands). Synthesis of androgens begins with mobilization of cholesterol derived from lipoprotein cholesterol or by de novo synthesis.[84,124] Cholesterol released from the lipid droplets migrates to the inner mitochondrial membrane, where pregnenolone formation is catalyzed by the cholesterol sidechain cleavage enzyme, CYP11A1. Conversion of cholesterol to pregnenolone is the rate-limiting step in testosterone synthesis[113,281]; however, it is thought that the rate of steroidogenesis is determined not by the activity of CYP11A1, but rather by delivery of cholesterol to the enzyme in the inner mitochondrial membrane by the steroidogenic regulatory protein (StAR)—a process thought to be regulated by LH.[282] Following the formation of pregnenolone, four additional enzymatic steps are required to convert cholesterol to testosterone. The pathway for testosterone formation is shown in Figure 56-1, with the preferred pathway defined by heavy red arrows.

Androgen Transport in Blood

Testosterone and DHT circulate in plasma freely (≈2 to 3%) or bound to plasma proteins. Binding proteins include the specific sex hormone–binding globulin (SHBG) and nonspecific proteins such as albumin. SHBG is an α-globulin that has low capacity for steroids but binds with very high affinity ($K_a = 1 \times 10^8$ to 1×10^9), whereas albumin has high capacity but low affinity ($K_a = 1 \times 10^4$ to 1×10^6).[281] SHBG has the highest affinity for DHT and the lowest for estradiol. In men, testosterone circulates bound 44 to 65% to SHBG and 33 to 50% to albumin, whereas in women, testosterone is bound 66 to 78% to SHBG and 20 to 30% to albumin.[222,230]

The biologically active fraction includes free testosterone; some have suggested that albumin-bound testosterone may also be available for tissue uptake.[63,229] Therefore, the bioavailable testosterone is equal to ≈35% of the total quantity (free + albumin-bound). Whether albumin-bound testosterone dissociates sufficiently fast to enter tissues is controversial.[192,200] However, concentrations of bioavailable testosterone correlate with those of free testosterone.[209,306]

Testosterone and SHBG exhibit rhythmic variation in their circulating concentrations. Testosterone concentrations peak at approximately 0400 to 0800 hours, and nadir concentrations occur at between 1600 and 2000 hours.[262,298] Daily variations in SHBG concentrations are similar to those of other proteins and albumin in serum, with major changes related to posture.[298] Concentrations of SHBG are elevated with hyperthyroidism and in hypogonadal men.

Metabolism of Testosterone

Circulating testosterone serves as a precursor for the formation of two additional active metabolites: DHT and estradiol (Figure 56-2). In one pathway, 5α-reductase converts 6 to 8% of testosterone to DHT. Both testosterone and DHT bind the androgen receptor, but DHT binds with higher affinity. In an alternative pathway, testosterone and androstenedione are converted to estrogens (≈0.3%) through aromatase (CYP19). DHT is formed in androgen target tissues such as the skin and prostate, whereas aromatization occurs in many tissues, especially the liver and adipose tissue. Peripheral aromatization occurs primarily in adipose tissue (of both men and women) because of the high concentration of aromatase in this tissue. The rate of extraglandular aromatization therefore increases with body fat.

Dihydrotestosterone is metabolized to 3α-androstanediol (see Figure 56-1) and then is conjugated to form 3α-androstanediol glucuronide. These metabolites have been used as markers of DHT production in peripheral tissues. Serum concentrations of 3α-androstanediol glucuronide or 3α-androstanediol reflect the production of DHT in peripheral tissues such as skin.[138,183] However, DHT may also arise from precursors other than testosterone. The reduction in serum 3α-androstanediol glucuronide concentrations noted in patients treated with glucocorticoids that suppress adrenal glucocorticoid and androgen production supports this conclusion.[199]

The main excretory metabolites of androstenedione, testosterone, and DHEA are shown in Figure 56-3. Except for epitestosterone, these catabolites constitute a group of

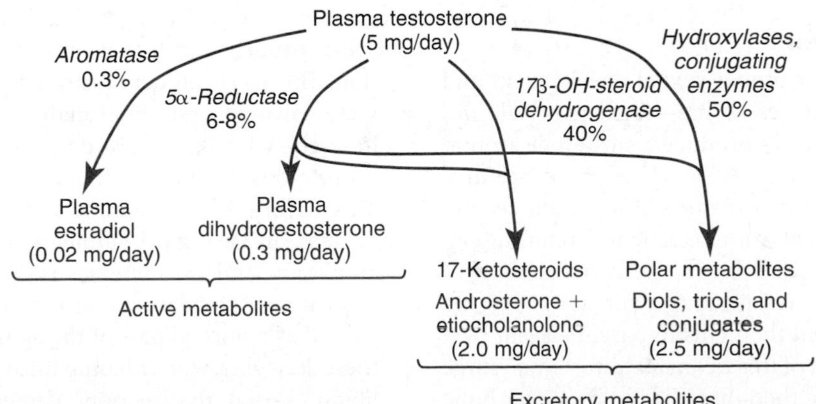

Figure 56-2 Pathways of peripheral metabolism of plasma testosterone. Testosterone can be metabolized to active metabolites or to excretory metabolites. *(From Griffin JE, Wilson JD. The testis. In: Bondy PK, Rosenberg LE, eds. Metabolic control and disease, 8th edition. Philadelphia, Pa: WB Saunders, 1980:1535-78; used with permission.)*

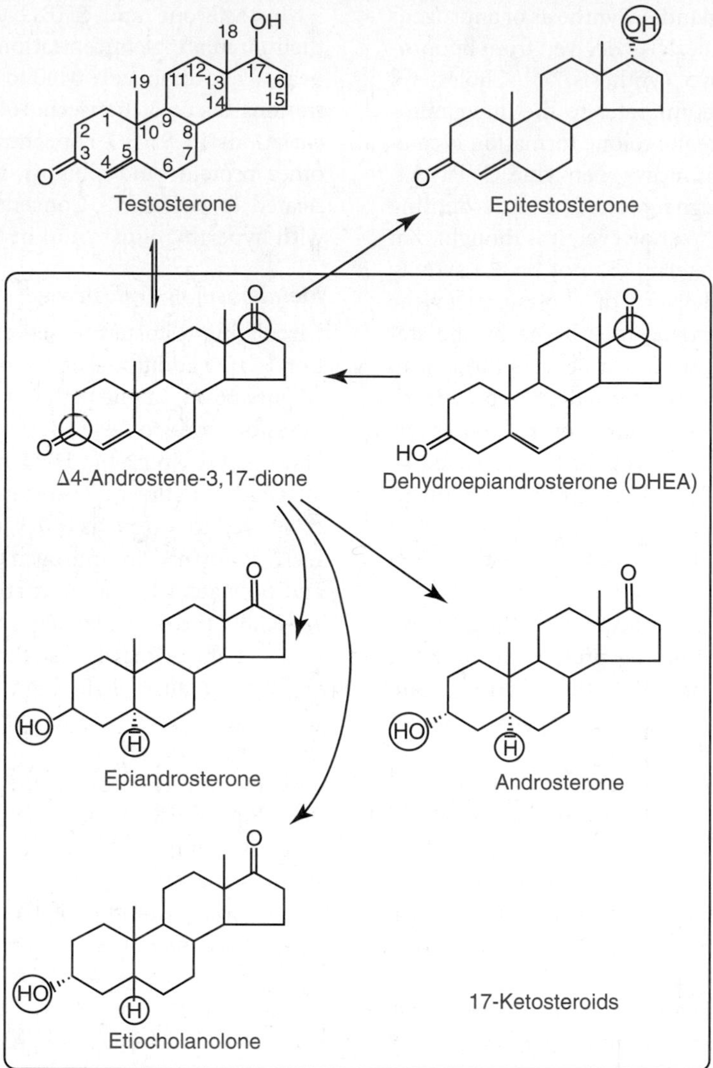

Figure 56-3 Catabolism of $C_{19}O_2$ androgens. The *circled area* represents the site of chemical change.

steroids known as *17-ketosteroids* (17-KS); they are excreted primarily in the urine.

Testosterone Concentrations

Testosterone is required for proper sexual development and function throughout all stages of life—fetal, pubertal, and adult (Figure 56-4). Fetal testes produce testosterone around the seventh week of gestation with peak serum concentrations of ≈250 ng/dL observed at the beginning of the second trimester, and with concentrations gradually returning to baseline by birth. Shortly after birth, the concentration of testosterone begins to increase, peaking again at ≈250 ng/dL at 2 to 3 months of age, and then falls to baseline again by 6 to 12 months. The function of this neonatal testosterone surge is not entirely clear, but it is thought to be important for bone growth and remodeling[272] and development of external male genitalia.[32] The concentration of testosterone remains low (<50 ng/dL) until puberty, when the concentration of testosterone rises to 500 to 700 ng/dL. Testosterone remains elevated through adulthood until around the third to fourth decade.

Men beyond the age of 30 to 40 years experience an age-dependent decrease in circulating testosterone concentration. This has been demonstrated consistently in both cross-sectional and longitudinal analyses. Collectively these studies have shown a 0.5 to 2% decrease per year in total serum testosterone from about the fourth decade onward.[93,126,208,304] This decline in testosterone is thought to be due to (1) a decrease in Leydig cell numbers, (2) decreased GnRH pulse amplitude, and (3) increases in SHBG.[208] In the past, these decreases in circulating concentrations of testosterone were viewed as a normal part of the aging process. Now, however, these decreases, when accompanied by symptoms of decreased libido, sexual dysfunction, decreased energy levels, and decreased muscle mass, are regarded as a syndrome with a variety of names, such as (1) androgen deficiency in the aging male (ADAM), (2) partial androgen deficiency of the aging male (PADAM), (3) late-onset hypogonadism (LOH),

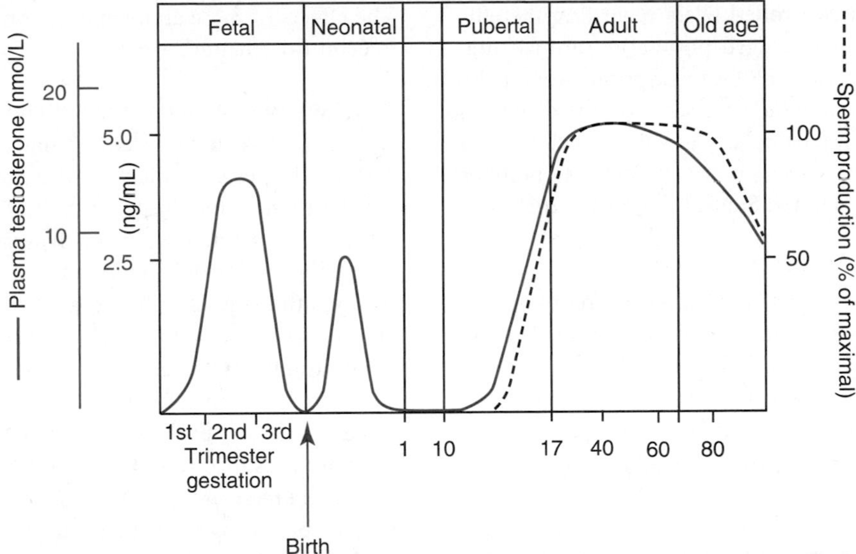

Figure 56-4 Schematic diagram of different phases of male sexual function during life as indicated by mean plasma testosterone concentration and sperm production at different ages. *[From Griffin JE, Wilson JD. The testis. In: Bondy PK, Rosenberg LE (eds). Metabolic control and disease, 8th edition. Philadelphia, Pa: WB Saunders, 1980:1535-78.]*

and, erroneously, (4) andropause. The name *andropause* is inaccurate and misleading, given that in contrast to menopause in women, concentrations of sex steroids in men do not decrease sharply with secondary cessation of reproductive function. A name put forward more recently is *testosterone deficiency syndrome (TDS)*, highlighting a specific deficit in testosterone as part of the clinical picture.[207,294]

Diagnosis of LOH (TDS) should be based on both clinical and laboratory assessment.[40] Clinically, patients should exhibit symptoms suggestive of testosterone deficiency, such as (1) decreased libido, (2) erectile dysfunction, (3) decreased muscle mass and strength, (4) decreased bone mineral density, and (5) changes in mood. Patients should exhibit one to three of these symptoms with a concomitant low concentration of serum testosterone to fit various diagnostic criteria. Total serum testosterone is the most widely used biochemical parameter for assessment of hypogonadism; although there is no agreed upon lower limit of normal, recently published consensus recommendations drafted by five professional andrology/urology societies concur that total testosterone above 12 nmol/L (350 ng/dL) does not require testosterone supplementation, whereas patients whose concentrations fall below 8 nmol/L (230 ng/dL) may benefit from testosterone replacement. This value is similar to the 200 ng/dL intent-to-treat cutoff published in the 2002 practice guidelines of the American Association of Clinical Endocrinology.[234] The joint societies further recommend, for those patients falling in the gray zone between 8 and 12 nmol/L, repeat measurement of serum total testosterone with measurement of SHBG to calculate free testosterone, or direct measurement of free testosterone by equilibrium dialysis (if available). Measurement of free or bioavailable testosterone should be considered when total testosterone is not diagnostic despite the clinical presentation of hypogonadism.[101]

This is particularly true in the setting of obesity and advanced age, where concentrations of SHBG have been shown to be elevated. High concentrations of SHBG may mask a true deficit in testosterone. Transient decreases in testosterone secondary to acute illness should be excluded during this assessment. Moreover, underlying chronic disease that lowers concentrations of testosterone should be taken into consideration and treated appropriately. To assess whether hypogonadism is primary or secondary, serum LH should be measured; a serum prolactin measurement is indicated when serum testosterone concentrations are lower than 5.2 nmol/L (150 ng/dL), or when secondary hypogonadism is suspected.[312-314] In sum, no absolute cutoffs or specific tests (total vs. bioavailable vs. free testosterone) are available for the laboratory diagnosis of hypogonadism in the aging male. Each patient's laboratory results should be interpreted on an individual basis, with particular attention given to those parameters of the biochemistry of testosterone (e.g., obesity, age, comorbidities, medications) that may affect the findings.

Patients who meet these criteria may be candidates for treatment with testosterone replacement therapy (TRT). The goal of therapy is to improve the symptoms and signs associated with testosterone deficiency. For more information on TRT, readers may consult recently published guidelines and position statements.[312-314] Considerable controversy surrounds TRT, primarily regarding potential adverse effects, specifically, the effects of TRT on prostate and cardiovascular health. TRT in younger patients diagnosed with hypogonadism has proved both safe and effective. However, data from prospective randomized controlled trials regarding the efficacy and safety of TRT in the aged population are lacking. Despite this lack of evidence, TRT prescriptions are on the rise; thus a sustained role for the laboratory in the diagnosis of LOH becomes evident, particularly given a growing aging population of males older than 65 years, projected to number some 31.3 million in the United States by the year 2030.[137]

Male Reproductive Abnormalities

A wide variety of abnormalities affect the male reproductive system before birth, in childhood, or in adulthood. For the purposes of this chapter, they have been divided into categories of (1) hypogonadotropic hypogonadism, (2) hypergonadotropic hypogonadism, (3) defects in androgen action (Box 56-1), (4) erectile dysfunction, and (5) gynecomastia.

BOX 56-1 Male Reproductive Abnormalities

Hypogonadotropic Hypogonadism

- Panhypopituitarism (congenital or acquired)
- Hypothalamic syndrome (acquired or congenital)
  - Structural defects (neoplastic, inflammatory, and infiltrative)
  - Prader-Willi syndrome
  - Laurence-Moon-Biedl syndrome
- GnRH deficiency (Kallmann syndrome)
- Hyperprolactinemia (prolactinoma or drugs)
- Malnutrition and anorexia nervosa
- Drug-induced suppression of luteinizing hormone (androgens, estrogens, tranquilizers, antidepressants, antihypertensives, barbiturates, cimetidine, GnRH analogs, and opiates)

Hypergonadotropic Hypogonadism

- Acquired (irradiation, mumps orchitis, castration, and cytotoxic drugs)
- Chromosome defects
  - Klinefelter syndrome (47,XXY) and mosaics
  - Autosomal and sex chromosomes, polyploidies
  - True hermaphroditism
- Defective androgen biosynthesis
  - 20α-Hydroxylase (cholesterol 20,22-desmolase) deficiency
  - 17,20-Lyase deficiency
  - 3β-Hydroxysteroid dehydrogenase deficiency
  - 17α-Hydroxylase deficiency
  - 17β-Hydroxysteroid dehydrogenase deficiency
- Testicular agenesis
- Selective seminiferous tubular disease
- Miscellaneous
  - Noonan syndrome (short stature, pulmonary valve stenosis, hypertelorism, and ptosis)
  - Streak gonads
  - Myotonia dystrophica
- Acute and chronic disease

Defects in Androgen Action

- Complete androgen insensitivity *(testicular feminization)*
- Partial androgen sensitivity
  - 5α-Reductase deficiency

GnRH, Gonadotropin-releasing hormone.

The effects of these abnormalities on infertility are discussed later in this chapter.

Hypogonadotropic Hypogonadism

Male hypogonadism is a condition caused by decreased function of the testes, which can lead to retardation of sexual development if manifested early in life. The disorder is classified as *hypo*gonadotropic or *hyper*gonadotropic.

Hypogonadotropic hypogonadism occurs when defects in the hypothalamus or pituitary prevent normal gonadal stimulation. Causative factors include congenital or acquired panhypopituitarism, hypothalamic syndromes, GnRH deficiency, hyperprolactinemia, malnutrition or anorexia, and iatrogenic causes. All of these abnormalities are associated with decreased testosterone and gonadotropin concentrations.

Kallmann syndrome, the most common form of hypogonadotropic hypogonadism, results from a deficiency of GnRH in the hypothalamus during embryonic development.[119] It is characterized by hypogonadism and anosmia (loss of the sense of smell) in male or female patients, and is inherited as an autosomal dominant trait with variable penetrance.[50,262] This syndrome arises from a defect in the migration of GnRH neurons to the hypothalamus. The pituitary disorders are characterized by isolated gonadotropin deficiency with or without growth hormone deficiency. Patients with isolated gonadotropin deficiency display sexual infantilism and long arms and legs; those with combined deficiency do not have long arms and legs. These patients must be distinguished from those with growth delay. In all of these patients, LH, FSH, and testosterone concentrations are lower than normal. However, heterogeneity exists in the degree of gonadotropin deficiency; hence concentrations of LH, FSH, and testosterone have been shown to differ among affected patients.

Hypergonadotropic Hypogonadism

Hypergonadotropic hypogonadism results from a primary gonadal disorder. Patients with primary testicular failure have increased concentrations of LH and FSH and decreased concentrations of testosterone. Causes for primary hypogonadism are categorized as (1) acquired causes (irradiation, castration, mumps orchitis, or cytotoxic drugs), (2) chromosome defects (Klinefelter syndrome), (3) defective androgen synthesis (20α-hydroxylase deficiency), (4) testicular agenesis, (5) seminiferous tubular disease, and (6) other miscellaneous causes. Aging is associated with gonadal failure, specifically, decreased Leydig cell mass and reserve capacity with reduction in pulsatile secretion of GnRH by the hypothalamus, leading to decreased testosterone secretion.[191]

Defects in Androgen Action

The most common and severe defect in androgen action is *androgen insensitivity syndrome* (AIS), a disorder arising from mutations in the androgen receptor gene (AR). AIS may be classified as complete (CAIS) or partial (PAIS), depending on the amount of residual receptor function. Individuals with complete AIS (formerly known as testicular feminization) have a male karyotype (46,XY) with female external genitalia (labia, clitoris, and vaginal opening). The testes are present intra-abdominally, and because they produce anti-Müllerian hormone (AMH) (also known as Müllerian inhibitory substance), no uterus, fallopian tubules, or proximal vagina is present. The circulating concentration of testosterone in these patients is greater than or equal to that of a healthy male.[145] Concentrations of LH are increased, presumably because of resistance of the hypothalamic-pituitary system to androgen inhibition.

Males with *5α-reductase deficiency* (5-ARD) do not convert testosterone to the more potent DHT. Because DHT leads to masculinization of external genitalia in utero, males are born with ambiguous genitalia.[325] High ratios of the circulating concentrations of testosterone to DHT are indicative of 5-ARD. Moreover, evidence indicates that DHT formation is deficient in the tissues of the urogenital tract in these patients.[145]

In patients with cryptorchidism or ambiguous genitalia, identification of abdominal gonads is essential for proper diagnosis and treatment. The presence of testicular tissue has traditionally been detected by measurement of Leydig cell testosterone production after stimulation with hCG. A growing appreciation of assessment of Sertoli cell function has been noted. Inhibin and AMH reflect Sertoli cell function and may offer a noninvasive evaluation of seminiferous tubular integrity.[99,174,206,244] In one study, the mean plasma AMH concentration in anorchid patients was 0.8 ng/mL, compared with 48.2 ng/mL in patients with normal testes.[174] AMH concentrations are also elevated in boys with delayed puberty and partial androgen insensitivity. Inhibin B may be used as a basal serum marker for the presence and function of testicular tissue in boys with nonpalpable testicles.[12,118,164]

Studies have shown that boys with anorchia have undetectable serum inhibin B concentrations.[164] Boys with severe testicular damage or gonadal dysgenesis also have undetectable or very low concentrations of inhibin B, whereas normal serum inhibin B concentrations are observed among boys with abdominal "normal" testes.[164]

Erectile Dysfunction

Erectile dysfunction (formerly referred to as impotence) is the persistent inability to develop or maintain a penile erection that is sufficient for intercourse and ejaculation in 50% or more of attempts.[163,262] A wide variety of organic and psychological abnormalities may cause changes in sexual drive and in the ability to have an erection or to ejaculate. Psychogenic erectile dysfunction is the most common diagnosis. Other causes include vascular disease, diabetes mellitus, hypertension, uremia, neurologic disease, hypogonadism, hyperthyroidism and hypothyroidism, neoplasms, and drugs. The physician must pursue a careful evaluation of possible psychological factors, neuropathy, or vascular abnormalities that may be interfering with proper sexual function. If no obvious explanation for erectile dysfunction can be found, measurement of morning serum testosterone, LH, and thyroid-stimulating hormone (TSH) concentrations has been suggested.[111,262] Elevated gonadotropin concentrations indicate primary hypogonadism. Total and even free testosterone concentrations may be within normal reference intervals, yet still may be subnormal for a given patient if found in the presence of elevated LH or FSH. Hyperprolactinemia is an infrequent cause of erectile dysfunction but should be considered in unusual situations.

Sildenafil (sold under the trade names Viagra, Revatio, and others) was approved by the U.S. Food and Drug Administration (FDA) in April 1998 for use as an oral therapeutic agent for male erectile dysfunction.[33,34,130,212,264] This agent and the drugs tadalafil (Cialis) and vardenafil (Levitra) are selective inhibitors of phosphodiesterase 5 (PDE5).[34] By inhibiting PDE5 in the corpus cavernosum of the penis, these drugs block degradation of cyclic guanosine monophosphate (GMP), which is increased during sexual arousal. Increased cyclic GMP results in relaxation of vascular smooth muscle and increased inflow of blood. A high-performance liquid chromatography (HPLC) method for sildenafil has been developed.[62]

Gynecomastia

Gynecomastia, the benign growth of glandular breast tissue in men, is a common finding among males of varied ages.[39,103,194] Gynecomastia, which is associated with an increase in the estrogen/androgen ratio, is commonly associated with three distinct periods of life. First, transient gynecomastia can be found in 60 to 90% of all newborns because of high estrogen concentrations that cross the placenta. The second peak occurs during puberty in 50 to 70% of normal boys. It is usually self limited and may be due to low serum testosterone, low DHT, or a high estrogen/androgen ratio. The last peak is found in the adult population, most frequently among men aged 50 to 80 years. Gynecomastia may be due to testicular failure, resulting in an increased estrogen/androgen ratio, or to increased body fat, resulting in increased peripheral aromatization of testosterone to estradiol.[39,103,194]

Gynecomastia may also develop as the result of iatrogenic causes, hyperthyroidism, or liver disease. Liver disease impairs estrogen clearance and SHBG production, leading to increased bioavailable estrogen and subsequent gynecomastia. Finally, germinal cell or nonendocrine tumors that produce human chorionic gonadotropin (hCG), as well as estrogen-producing tumors of the adrenal glands, the testes, or the liver, will cause gynecomastia. hCG stimulates testicular aromatase activity and estrogen production, resulting in gynecomastia.[103] In cases of striking gynecomastia in which history and physical examination point to no specific disorder, measurements of hCG, plasma estradiol, testosterone, and LH concentrations are appropriate.[39] It is important to note that prolactin plays an important role in *galactorrhea* (milk production), but only an indirect role in gynecomastia.

FEMALE REPRODUCTIVE BIOLOGY

The ovaries produce ova and secrete the sex hormones progesterone and estrogen. Every healthy female neonate possesses approximately 400,000 primordial follicles, each containing an immature ovum. During the reproductive life span of an adult woman, 300 to 400 follicles will reach maturity.[97,110] A single mature follicle is produced during each normal menstrual cycle at approximately day 14. Surrounding the oocyte of the mature follicle are three distinct cell layers: (1) *theca externa,* (2) *theca interna,* and (3) *granulosa cells.* The theca interna cells are the primary source of androgens, which are transported to adjacent granulosa cells, where they are aromatized to estrogens.[50]

The mature follicle undergoes ovulation by the process of rupture, thereby releasing the oocyte into the proximity of the fallopian tubes. The follicle then fills with blood to form the corpus hemorrhagicum. The granulosa and theca cells of the follicle lining quickly proliferate to form lipid-rich luteal cells, replacing the clotted blood and forming the *corpus luteum* (yellow body). The luteal cells produce estrogen and progesterone. If fertilization and pregnancy occur, the corpus luteum persists and continues to produce estrogen and progesterone. If no pregnancy occurs, the corpus luteum regresses, and the next menstrual cycle begins.

The uterine cavity is lined by the endometrium. The endometrium undergoes cyclic changes in preparation for implantation and pregnancy in response to cyclic changes in estrogen and progesterone. During the follicular phase, the endometrial lining increases in thickness and vascularity in response to increasing circulating concentrations of estrogen; after regression of the corpus luteum, menstruation begins, and the endometrium is shed in response to the withdrawal of progesterone.

Hypothalamic-Pituitary-Gonadal Axis

In adult women, a tightly coordinated feedback system exists between hypothalamus, anterior pituitary, and ovaries to orchestrate menstruation. FSH serves to stimulate follicular growth, and LH stimulates ovulation and progesterone secretion from the developing corpus luteum. These actions are discussed in greater depth later in this chapter.

Estrogens

Estrogens are responsible for the development and maintenance of female sex organs and female secondary sex characteristics. In conjunction with progesterone, they participate in regulation of the menstrual cycle and of breast and uterine growth, and in the maintenance of pregnancy.

Estrogens affect calcium homeostasis and have a beneficial effect on bone mass. They decrease bone resorption, and in prepubertal girls, estrogen accelerates linear bone growth, resulting in epiphyseal closure. Long-term estrogen depletion is associated with loss of bone mineral content, an increase in stress fractures, and postmenopausal osteoporosis.

Estrogens also have well-established effects on plasma proteins that influence endocrine testing. They increase concentrations of SHBG, corticosteroid-binding globulin, and thyroxine-binding globulin. Hence, boys and girls have comparable concentrations of SHBG, but adult men have SHBG concentrations that are about one half those of adult women. Concentrations of plasma proteins that bind copper and iron

Estrane Estrone (E_1) 17β-Estradiol (E_2) Estriol (E_3)

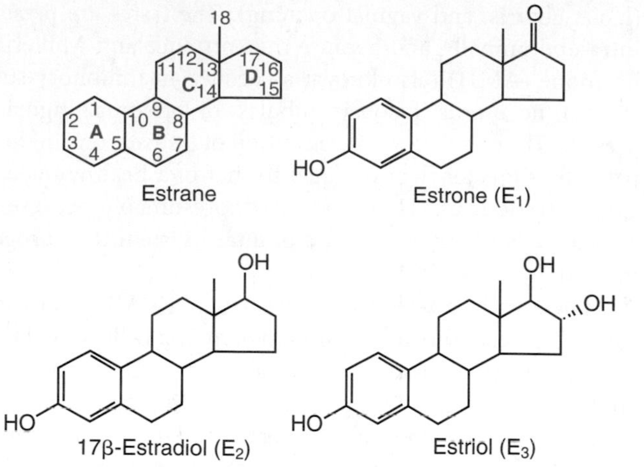

Figure 56-5 Biologically active estrogens.

are also elevated in response to estrogen, as are those of high-density and very high-density lipoproteins. In addition, estrogens are believed to play a preventive role in coronary heart disease.[114]

Chemistry

The three most biologically active estrogens in order of potency are estrone (E_1), estradiol (E_2), and estriol (E_3) (Figure 56-5). Structurally, estrogens are derivatives of the parent hydrocarbon *estrane,* which is an 18-carbon molecule with an aromatic ring A and a methyl group at C-13.[50,333] All estrogens possess a phenolic hydroxyl group at C-3, which gives the compounds acidic properties, and lack a methyl group at C-10. In addition, estrogens may possess a ketone (estrone) or hydroxyl group (estradiol) at position C-17. The phenolic ring A and the hydroxyl group at C-17 are essential for biological activity.

Biosynthesis

The biochemical pathway illustrating aromatization of testosterone to estradiol and androstenedione to estrone is shown in Figure 56-6. The role of estrogens in normal and abnormal menstrual cycles is described later in this chapter.

Estrogens are secreted primarily in healthy women by the ovarian follicles and the corpus luteum, and during pregnancy by the placenta. The adrenal glands and testes (in men) are also believed to secrete minute quantities of estrogens. The ovary synthesizes estrogens via aromatization of androgens. Synthesis of estrogens begins in the theca interna cells with the enzymatic synthesis of androstenedione from cholesterol. Androstenedione is then transported to the granulosa cells, where it is further metabolized directly to estrone (androstenedione → estrone), or first to testosterone and then to estradiol (androstenedione → testosterone → estradiol). These conversions are catalyzed by the enzyme aromatase. The healthy human ovary produces all three classes of sex steroids: estrogens, progestagens, and androgens; however, estradiol and progesterone are its primary secretory products. Because the ovary lacks

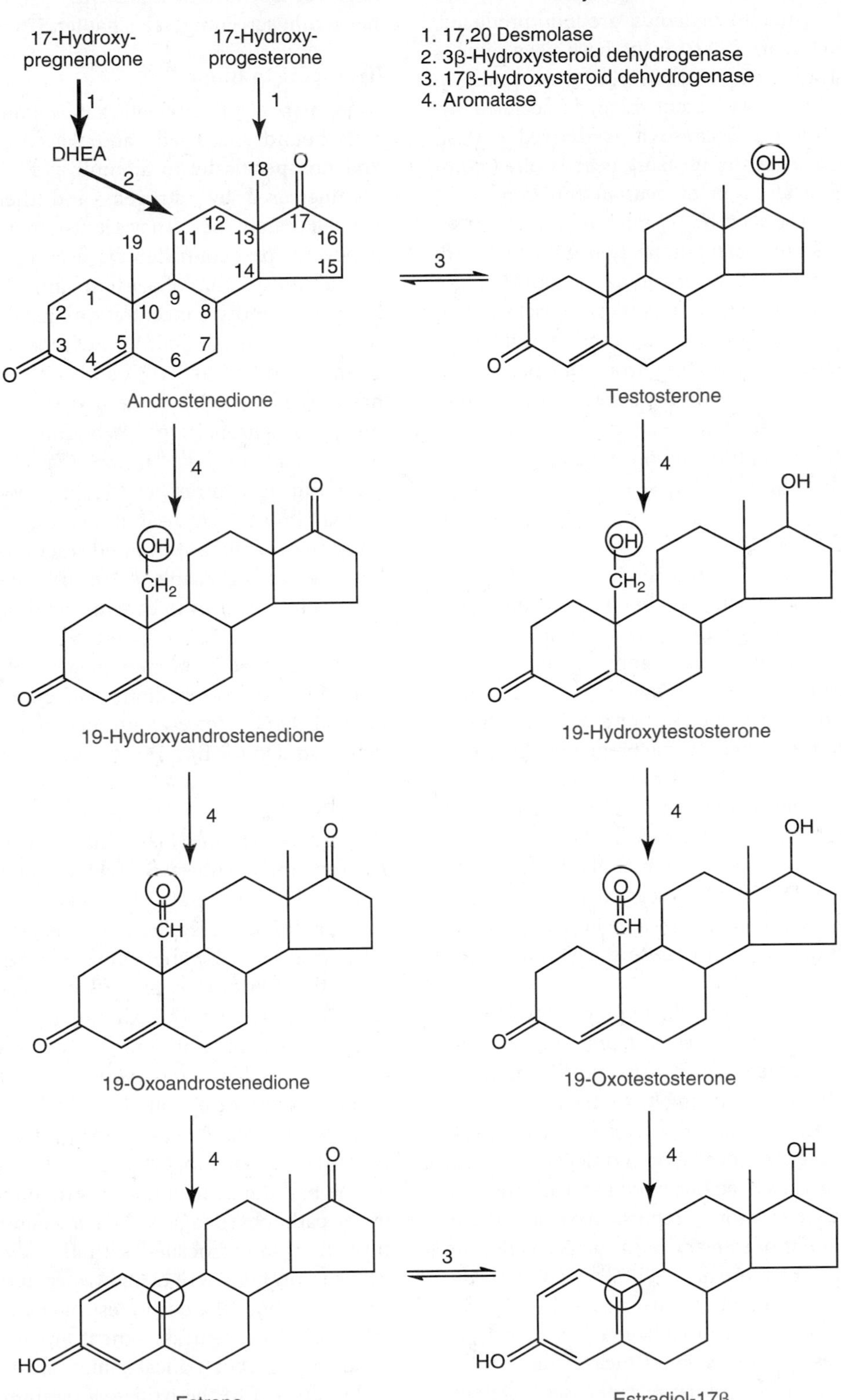

Figure 56-6 Biosynthesis of estrogens. ***Heavy arrows*** **indicate the Δ5-3β-hydroxy pathway. The** ***circled area*** **represents the site of chemical change. See Figure 56-1 for early synthetic steps.**

both the 21-hydroxylase and 11β-hydroxylase enzymes, glucocorticoids and mineralocorticoids are not produced in the ovary.[50,333] More than 20 estrogens have been identified, but only 17β-estradiol (E_2) and estriol (E_3) are routinely measured clinically. The most potent estrogen secreted by the ovary is 17β-estradiol. Because it is derived almost exclusively from the ovaries, its measurement is often considered sufficient for evaluation of ovarian function.

Estrogens are also produced by peripheral aromatization of androgens, primarily androstenedione. In healthy men and women, ≈1% of secreted androstenedione is converted to estrone.[50,333] Although the ovaries of postmenopausal women do not secrete estrogens, these women have significant blood concentrations of estrone originating from the peripheral conversion of adrenal androstenedione. Because a major site of this conversion is adipose tissue, estrone is increased in obese postmenopausal women, sometimes yielding enough estrogen to produce bleeding.[50,333,336]

Biosynthesis During Pregnancy

Research has shown that biosynthesis of estrogens differs qualitatively and quantitatively in pregnant women compared with nonpregnant ones. In pregnant women, the major source of estrogens is the placenta, whereas in nonpregnant women, the ovaries are the main site of synthesis.[50,333,336] In contrast to the microgram quantities secreted by nonpregnant women, the quantity of estrogens secreted during pregnancy increases to milligram amounts. The major estrogen secreted by the ovary is estradiol (E_2), whereas the major product secreted by the placenta is estriol (E_3). E_3 is formed in the placenta by sequential desulfation and aromatization of plasma dehydroepiandrosterone sulfate (DHEA-S). Except during pregnancy, measurements of E_3 have little clinical value because in nonpregnant women, E_3 is derived almost exclusively from E_2 (see also Chapter 57).

E_3 is the predominant hormone of late pregnancy. Maternal E_3 is almost entirely (≈90%) derived from fetal and placental sources. It is first detected during the ninth gestational week and gradually increases during the first and second trimesters. Plasma and salivary E_3 concentrations peak approximately 3 to 5 weeks before labor and delivery.[108] This characteristic surge in E_3 has been observed in term, preterm, and post-term pregnancies. Some reports have suggested utility in the measurement of salivary E_3 in the prediction of risk for spontaneous preterm birth.[107,132-134,167,195] This test has a high negative predictive value but a low positive predictive value. Consequently, the American College of Obstetricians and Gynecologists does not now suggest measuring salivary E_3 concentrations, except for research purposes.[2] Details regarding techniques used to determine serum and salivary E_3 concentrations are discussed later in the section on analytical methods.

Serum unconjugated E_3 measurements, along with alpha fetoprotein, hCG, and inhibin A, are commonly used as part of the "quad" maternal screens for Down syndrome–affected fetuses. On average, unconjugated E_3 is 0.72 times less than normal (median value at 16 weeks: 0.30 to 1.50 μg/L) when fetal Down syndrome is present.[47,198,287,309] For more on maternal serum screening, see Chapter 57.

Transport in Blood

More than 97% of circulating E_2 is bound to plasma proteins. It is bound specifically and with high affinity to SHBG, and nonspecifically to albumin.[222,281] SHBG concentrations are increased by estrogens and therefore are higher in women than in men. They are also increased during (1) pregnancy, (2) oral contraceptive use, (3) hyperthyroidism, and (4) administration of certain antiepileptic drugs such as dilantoin. SHBG concentrations may decrease in hypothyroidism, obesity, or androgen excess. In women, E_2 circulates bound 40 to 60% to SHBG, and 40 to 60% to albumin. SHBG has a higher affinity for testosterone than E_2; therefore, in men, E_2 circulates 20 to 30% bound to SHBG, and 70 to 80% bound to albumin.[222,230] Only 2 to 3% of total E_2 circulates in free form. In contrast, estrone and estrone sulfate circulate bound almost exclusively to albumin. As with testosterone, both free and albumin-bound fractions of E_2 are thought to be biologically available,[230] but measurement of this fraction has not been shown to be clinically important.

Diurnal variation in blood estrone concentrations occurs in postmenopausal women, presumably reflecting the variation in the androstenedione precursor that originates in the adrenal glands. However, no such diurnal rhythms have been demonstrated for E_2.

Metabolism

The metabolism of E_2 is chiefly an oxidative process dominated by three pathways, of which the fastest is oxidation of the β-hydroxy group at C-17 to a ketone (estradiol → estrone). This process is reversible; however, equilibrium favors the estrone species. Estrone is further oxidized along two pathways: the *2-hydroxylation pathway,* leading to formation of catechol estrogens (2-hydroxyestrone, 2-hydroxyestradiol, and 2-hydroxyestriol and their corresponding methoxy derivatives), and the *16α-hydroxylation pathway,* leading predominantly to formation of E_3[50,333] (Figure 56-7).

Normally, blood estrone concentrations parallel E_2 concentrations throughout the menstrual cycle, but at one third to one half their magnitude. Estrone metabolism is affected by the pathophysiologic state. For example, obesity and hypothyroidism are associated with an increase in E_3 formation, whereas low body weight and hyperthyroidism are associated with formation of catechol estrogens.[50] Although assays for catechol estrogen measurement are available,[55,196] they have no known current clinical value.

In addition to the oxidative pathways already described, formation of estrogen conjugates has been reported as a major route of estrogen metabolism. The most abundant circulating estrogen conjugates are the sulfates, followed by the glucuronides, with estrone sulfate circulating at concentrations tenfold higher than unconjugated estrone.[236] Initially, it was thought that sulfate conjugation would lead to an increase in polarity, making the compound more readily excretable; however, estrogen sulfates actually exhibit a longer half-life

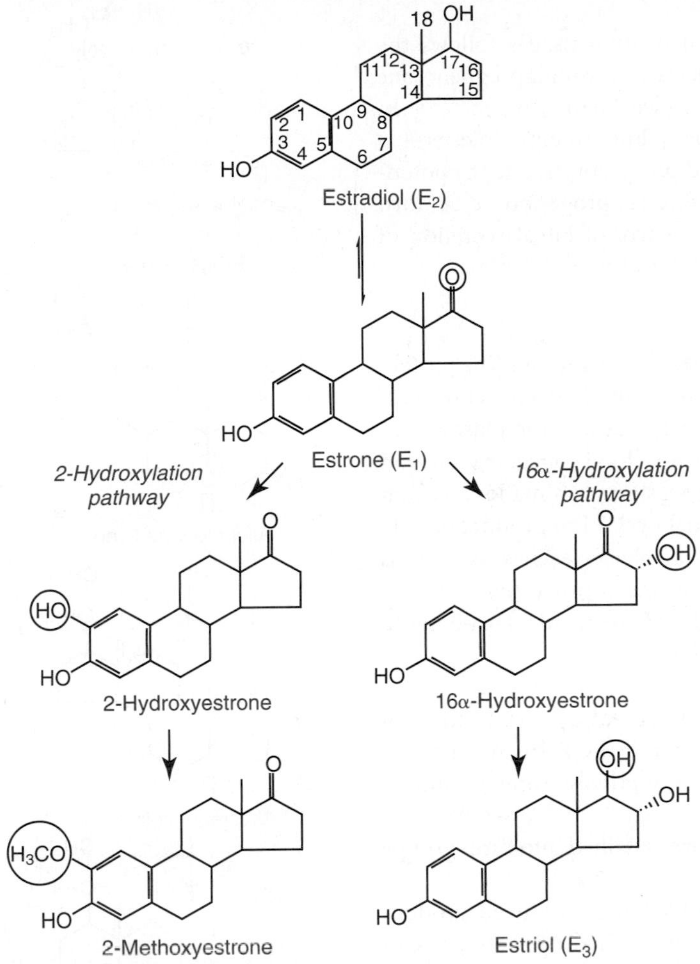

Figure 56-7 Main pathways of estradiol metabolism in humans. The *circled area* represents the site of chemical change.

than do parent estrogens.[236] These observations have led to the idea that estrone sulfate may serve as a precursor for the bioactive estrogens via desulfation and conversion to E_2 by 17β-hydroxysteroid dehydrogenase. In contrast to estrogen sulfates, glucuronidation of estrogens generally is accepted to serve a classic excretory role. Estrogen glucuronides are detectable in both urine and bile.

Progesterone

Progesterone, similar to the estrogens, is a female sex hormone. In conjunction with estrogens, it helps to regulate the accessory organs during the menstrual cycle.[333,336] This hormone is especially important in preparing the uterus for implantation of the blastocyst and in maintaining pregnancy. In nonpregnant women, progesterone is secreted mainly by the corpus luteum. During pregnancy, the placenta becomes the major source of this hormone. Minor sources are the adrenal cortex in both sexes and the testes in men.

Chemistry

The structural formula of progesterone, a C_{21} compound, is shown in Figure 56-8. Similar to the corticosteroids and testosterone, progesterone (pregn-4-ene-3,20-dione) contains a

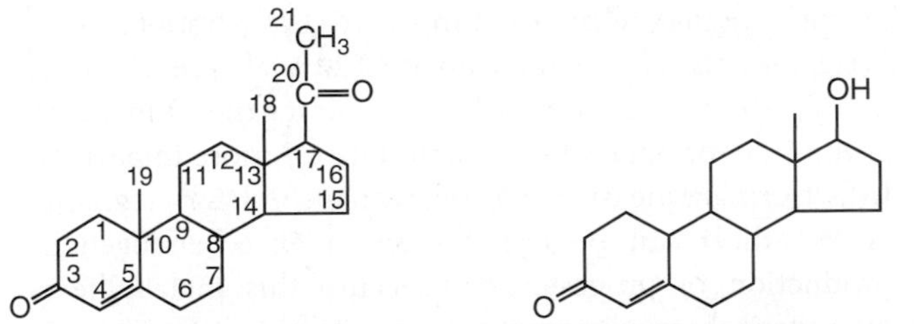

Figure 56-8 Structural formulas of progesterone and 19-nortestosterone.

keto group (at C-3) and a double bond between C-4 and C-5 (Δ^4); both structural characteristics are essential for progestational activity. The two-carbon sidechain (CH_3CO) on C-17 does not seem to be very important for its physiologic action. Indeed, the synthetic compound 19-nortestosterone (see Figure 56-8) and its derivatives, which are widely used as oral contraceptives, are more potent progestational agents than progesterone itself.

Biosynthesis

Biosynthesis of progesterone in ovarian tissues follows the same path from acetate to cholesterol through pregnenolone as it does in the adrenal cortex (see Figure 56-1).[50,333,335] In luteal tissue, however, low-density lipoprotein cholesterol is thought to serve as the preferred precursor despite the potential of the corpus luteum to synthesize progesterone de novo from acetate.[271] Initiation and control of luteal secretion of progesterone are regulated by LH and FSH.[50,283,333]

Transport

Progesterone does not have a specific plasma-binding protein but, similar to cortisol, is found bound to corticosteroid-binding globulin. Reported concentrations for plasma free progesterone vary from 2% to 10% of total concentration, and the percentage of unbound progesterone remains constant throughout the normal menstrual cycle. The production rate of progesterone during the luteal phase reaches as high as 30 mg/d, whereas the production rate of progesterone by the placenta during the third trimester of pregnancy is ≈300 mg/d.

Metabolism

The important metabolic events leading to inactivation of progesterone are reduction and conjugation. The main metabolic pathway for the metabolism of progesterone is outlined in Figure 56-9.

Metabolites of progesterone are classified into three groups based on the degree of reduction:

1. *Pregnanediones.* The C4-5 double bond is reduced, producing two compounds: pregnanedione (hydrogen atom at C-5 is in β-orientation) and allopregnanedione (hydrogen atom at C-5 is in α-orientation).
2. *Pregnanolones.* The keto group at C-3 is reduced, producing hydroxyl groups in α- or β-orientation. However, most urinary pregnanolones exist in the α-configuration.
3. *Pregnanediols.* The keto group at C-20 is also reduced. As in the previous case, metabolites containing the 20-hydroxyl group in α-orientation are quantitatively more important. In fact, urinary measurement of pregnanediol (5β-pregnane-3α,20α-diol) can be used as an index of endogenous production of progesterone, because this metabolite is quantitatively very significant, and its concentration correlates with most clinical conditions.

Reduced metabolites are eventually conjugated with glucuronic acid and excreted as water-soluble glucuronides.

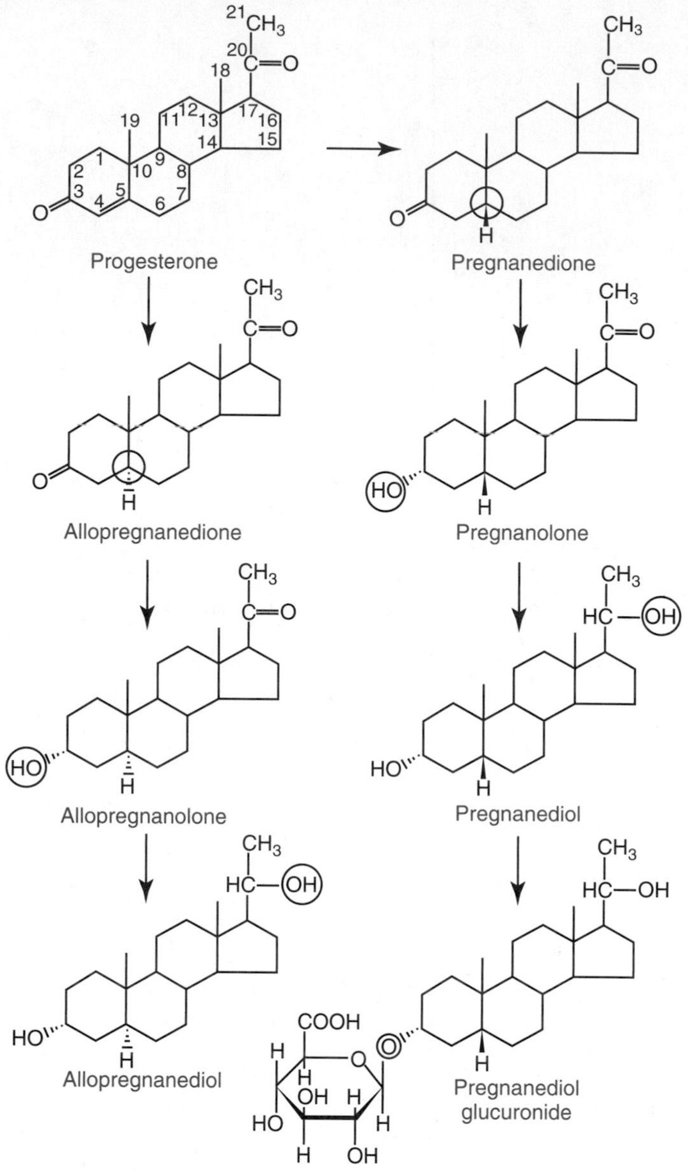

Female Reproductive Development

Reproductive development begins with anatomy during the fetal period, a postnatal period of adaptation to reduced maternal sex steroids, and finishes with sexual maturation during puberty. Normal females remain fertile and menstruating until menopause.

Fetal

In the genotypic female, lack of testosterone and AMH causes regression of the wolffian ducts and maintenance of the Müllerian ducts, thus forming the female reproductive tract.

Figure 56-9 Metabolism of progesterone. The *circled area* represents the site of chemical change.

Gonadotropin activity in utero is suppressed because of high concentrations of circulating estrogens derived from the mother.[50,333]

Postnatal

When the placenta separates, concentrations of fetal sex steroids drop abruptly. Serum E_2 in neonates is decreased to basal concentrations within 5 to 7 days after birth and persists at this concentration until puberty. The negative feedback action of steroids is now removed, and gonadotropins are released. Postnatal peaks of LH and FSH are measurable for a few months after birth, peaking at 2 to 5 months and then dropping to basal concentrations. During childhood, circulating concentrations of sex steroids and gonadotropins are low and are similar for both sexes. However, in patients with hypogonadism (Turner syndrome), LH and FSH concentrations are higher than in healthy children.[50,333]

Puberty

The transition from sexual immaturity appears to begin with diminished sensitivity of the pituitary gland or hypothalamus, or both, to the negative feedback effect of sex steroids. The mechanism for this change is unclear. As puberty approaches, nocturnal secretion of gonadotropins occurs. Concentrations for LH, FSH, and gonadal steroids rise gradually over several years before stabilizing at adult concentrations when full sexual maturity is reached. In girls, puberty is considered precocious if onset of pubertal development (secondary sex characteristics) occurs before the age of 8 years (see later section on precocious puberty), and delayed if no development has occurred by the age of 13 years, or if menarche has not occurred by age 16.5 years.[67,205] It was reported in 2003 that the median age of menarche in the United States is 12.43 years, which is 0.34 year earlier than that reported in 1973.[57,189] This study also found that the median age at menarche of non-Hispanic black (12.06 years) girls is significantly earlier than that of non-Hispanic white (12.55 years) and Mexican-American (12.25 years) girls.[57]

Adrenarche precedes puberty by a few years. In girls, the rise in adrenal androgen concentrations (DHEA, DHEA-S, and androstenedione) begins at age 6 to 7 years.[231] This rise in adrenal androgen concentrations lasts until late puberty. A cortical androgen-stimulating hormone may contribute to the rise in adrenal androgens at puberty in both sexes.[231] In girls, puberty is associated with elevations in estrogen secretion by the ovary in response to gonadotropin concentrations that increase in response to GnRH. Estrogen secretion by the ovary increases, causing enlargement of the uterus and breasts. In the breast, estrogen enhances growth of ducts; progesterone augments this effect. As the breast develops, estrogen increases adipose tissue around the lactiferous duct system, contributing to the further enlargement of breast tissue.[50,333] These physiologic and physical processes associated with puberty in girls culminate in *menarche*—the beginning of menstrual function and the first menstrual period.

Normal Menstrual Cycle

During a normal menstrual cycle, a closely coordinated interplay of feedback effects occurs between the hypothalamus, the anterior lobe of the pituitary gland, and the ovaries. In addition, cyclic hormone changes lead to functional and structural changes in the ovaries (follicle maturation, ovulation, and corpus luteum development), uterus (preparation of the endometrium for possible implantation of the fertilized ovum), cervix (to permit transport of sperm), and vagina (Figure 56-10).

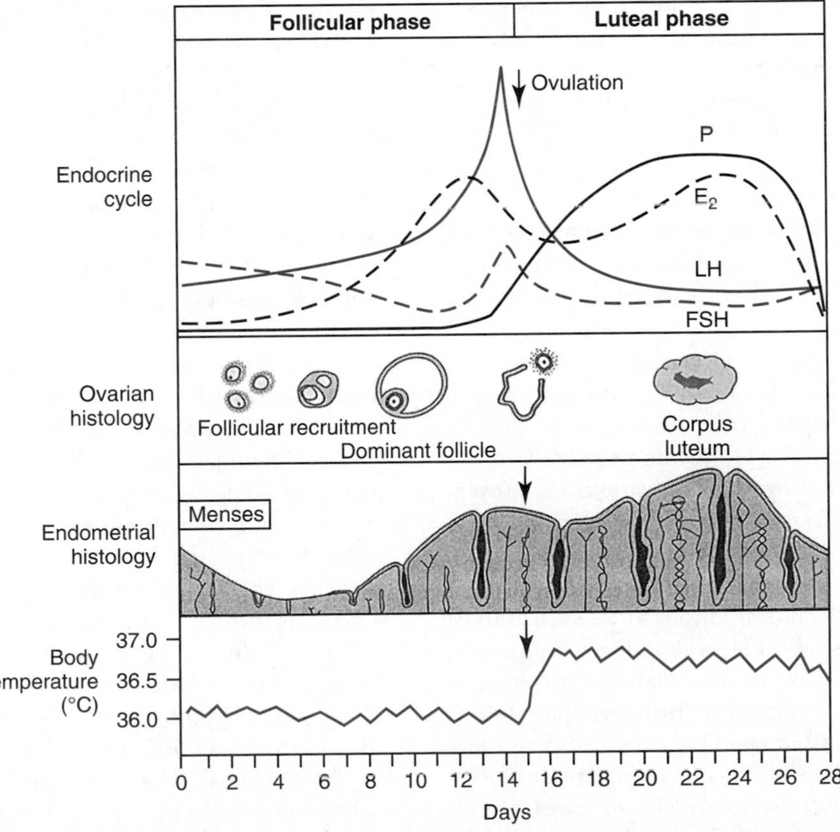

Figure 56-10 Hormonal, ovarian, endometrial, and basal body temperature changes throughout the normal menstrual cycle. *(From Carr BR, Bradshaw KD. Disorders of the ovary and female reproductive tract. In: Braunwald E, Fauci A, Kasper D, Hauser SL, Longo DL, Jameson JL, eds. Harrison's principles of internal medicine, 15th ed. New York, NY: McGraw-Hill, 2001:2158; used with permission.)*

Phases

The menstrual cycle is measured beginning on day 1 as the first day of menstrual bleeding. Each cycle consists of a follicular phase followed by ovulation and then a luteal phase.

Follicular Phase. The *follicular phase,* that is, the initiation of follicular growth, actually begins during the last few days of the previous luteal phase and terminates at ovulation (see Figure 56-10). During the early part of the follicular phase, concentrations of FSH are elevated, but they decline up until ovulation (see Figure 56-10). LH secretion begins to increase around the middle of the follicular phase. Just before ovulation, estrogen secretion by the follicle increases dramatically; this positively stimulates the hypothalamus and triggers the LH surge. The LH surge is a reliable predictor of ovulation, with onset of the surge for 90% of women occurring 16 to 58 hours before, and the peak occurring 3 to 36 hours before, ovulation.[50] Ovulation occurs around day 14 of the menstrual cycle.

Luteal Phase. The *luteal phase,* the last half of the cycle, is characterized by increasing production of progesterone and estrogen from the corpus luteum with consequent gradual lowering of LH and FSH concentrations. The concentration of progesterone reaches a peak at about 8 days post ovulation. If ovulation does not occur, the corpus luteum fails to form, and a cyclic rise in progesterone is subnormal. If ovulation and pregnancy occurs, hCG maintains the corpus luteum and progesterone continues to rise. In the absence of conception, the corpus luteum resolves, resulting in a decrease in estrogen and progesterone concentrations and a breakdown of the endometrium. The average duration of menstrual flow is 4 to 6 days, and average menstrual blood loss is 30 mL.[50]

Role of Individual Hormones

To explain further the intricacies of the normal menstrual cycle, fluctuations in each major hormone are discussed separately in the following sections with regard to control and effects (see Figure 56-10).

Gonadotropin-Releasing Hormone. Gonadotropin-releasing hormone triggers the surge of LH that precedes ovulation.[50,333,336] There appear to be two separate feedback centers in the hypothalamus: (1) a tonic negative feedback center in the basal medial hypothalamus, and (2) a cyclic positive feedback center in the anterior regions of the hypothalamus. Low concentrations of E_2, such as those that are present during the follicular phase, affect the negative feedback center, whereas high concentrations of E_2, such as those seen just before the midcycle LH peak, trigger the positive feedback center. Progesterone, in combination with estrogen, affects the negative feedback center in the luteal phase. GnRH is released in a pulsatile fashion and has a self-priming effect; the first dose potentiates the effects of subsequent doses. The magnitude of the LH response to GnRH increases steadily through the follicular phase and is greatest at the time of the preovulatory surge of LH, after which it declines again.

Follicle-Stimulating Hormone. A few days before day 1 of the cycle, FSH shows a slight but important peak (see Figure 56-10), probably triggered by a fall in E_2 concentration that briefly eliminates the negative feedback effect.[50,333,336] This peak in FSH initiates the growth and maturation of a cohort of ovarian follicles. LH and FSH release is pulsatile throughout the cycle; therefore, the values shown in Figure 56-10 represent integrated concentrations. As estrogen is released from the growing follicles, FSH concentrations fall again and remain low through the follicular phase. By days 5 to 7, a single follicle is selected for further growth. The effect of FSH on the maturing follicle is increased through estradiol-induced changes in FSH receptors. FSH, aided by E_2, acts on the cells of the follicle to increase the responsiveness of LH receptors by the time of the midcycle surge. FSH and LH receptors respond with an increase in their number or in their affinity for corresponding gonadotropin. A rise in FSH at midcycle is triggered by progesterone. The function of this peak is not entirely known, but it is thought to stimulate plasminogen activator and increase granulosa cell LH receptors.[50] During the luteal phase, FSH is suppressed by negative feedback from E_2 until a lesser FSH peak, occurring near the end of the cycle, starts off the follicular maturation of the next cycle.

Luteinizing Hormone. Luteinizing hormone secretion is suppressed in the follicular phase by negative feedback from E_2.[50,333,336] As E_2 production by the developing follicle increases, the effect of E_2 on the positive feedback center becomes important. Increasing release of GnRH from the hypothalamus and increasing the sensitivity of the anterior lobe of the pituitary gland to GnRH lead to the midcycle surge of LH. Ovarian follicle receptors for LH, sensitized by FSH and E_2, transmit the stimulus to enhance differentiation of the theca cell and production of progesterone by the developing corpus luteum. LH production is suppressed during the luteal phase by negative feedback from progesterone combined with E_2, but a low concentration of LH is probably necessary to prolong corpus luteum function.

Estradiol. E_2 production by the ovary decreases near the end of a cycle but begins to increase again under the influence of FSH (see Figure 56-10).[50,333,336] E_2 enhances the FSH effect on a maturing follicle through changes in FSH receptors of the follicular cells, but it suppresses pituitary FSH and LH release during the follicular phase through negative feedback. Before the mid–follicular phase, estrogen concentrations are less than 50 pg/mL, but they increase rapidly as the follicle matures. E_2 production increases, reaching a midcycle peak at between 250 and 500 pg/mL.[281] E_2 concentrations decrease abruptly after ovulation but increase again as the corpus luteum is formed, reaching concentrations of approximately 125 pg/mL during the luteal phase.[281] Progesterone produced by the corpus luteum, combined with E_2, exerts a negative effect on the hypothalamus and anterior lobe of the pituitary gland. As a result, LH and FSH secretion is suppressed again during the luteal phase. E_2 is essential for the development of proliferative endometrium and is synergistic with progesterone for the development of changes in the endometrium that initiate shedding; the decrease in negative feedback from E_2 on the anterior lobe of the pituitary gland triggers the FSH surge that begins the development of an ovarian follicle for the next cycle.

Changes in androgen production also occur during the menstrual cycle, with a peak at midcycle. E_2 is not the only estrogen produced; estrone secretion, mainly from peripheral sources, also is increased throughout the cycle. Estrogen and progesterone have visible effects on vaginal cytology and cervical mucus, and progesterone elevates body temperature (as discussed later).

Progesterone. Progesterone is not produced in significant amounts until the midcycle LH surge and ovulation. LH enhances theca cell differentiation and progesterone production, which increase by a factor of 10 to 20 to a maximum about 8 days after the midcycle peak of LH. Progesterone is thought to stimulate the ovulatory peak of FSH and to promote the growth of secretory endometrium, which is necessary for implantation of the fertilized ovum.[50]

Ovulation

An intricate interplay of endocrine events contributes to follicular maturation. Growth of ovarian follicles appears to be continuous. How an individual follicle is singled out for each menstrual cycle is not known; however, the late-cycle peak in FSH concentration is likely important in this process. Once a follicle has been stimulated, E_2 production causes that specific follicle to be more receptive to effects of FSH. The high concentration of E_2 just before midcycle is responsible for triggering positive feedback in the hypothalamus that leads to the midcycle LH surge. After ovulation, LH is suppressed by progesterone and E_2, but the effect of LH on the corpus luteum is increased.[50,283,333,336] In the event of successful fertilization and implantation, corpus luteum function is sustained by hCG produced by trophoblastic cells of the developing embryo with high molecular homology to LH, and is capable of binding and stimulating LH receptors. Otherwise, the declining concentration of E_2 leads to regression of the corpus luteum and to the late-cycle FSH peak that starts the process again.

Menopause

Menopause is defined as the permanent cessation of menstruation resulting from loss of ovarian follicular activity.[10] It begins with the ovaries failing to produce adequate amounts of estrogen and inhibin; as a result, gonadotropin production is increased in a continued attempt to stimulate the ovary (Figure 56-11). The mean age of menopause in the United States is 51 years but varies considerably.[41,50,112,146] Ovarian failure may occur at any age, but menopause before age 40 years is considered premature.[68]

Hormonal changes begin about 5 years before the actual menopause, as the response of the ovary to gonadotropins begins to decrease and menstrual cycles become increasingly irregular.[112,146,278] The term *perimenopausal* refers to the time interval from onset of these menstrual irregularities to menopause itself. This transition phase will last from 2 to 8 years.[112,278] At this time, FSH concentrations increase and E_2 concentrations decrease, whereas LH and progesterone concentrations remain unchanged, indicating that menstrual cycles are ovulatory. As estrogen continues to decline, an associated decrease in prolactin concentrations is noted. The

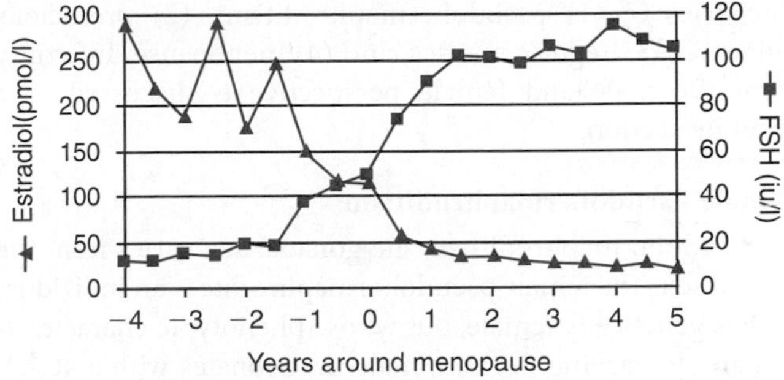

Figure 56-11 Geometric means for follicle-stimulating hormone (FSH) and estradiol in relation to the final menstrual period (FMP). The horizontal axis represents time (y) with respect to the FMP (0); negative (positive) numbers represent time before (after) the FMP. *(From Burger HG, Dudley EC, Hopper JL, Groome N, Guthrie JR, Green A, et al. Prospectively measured levels of serum follicle-stimulating hormone, estradiol, and the dimeric inhibins during the menopausal transition in a population-based cohort of women. J Clin Endocrinol Metab 1999;84:4025-30; Figure 1A, used with permission.)*

decrease in estrogen concentrations gives rise to vasomotor instability and "hot flashes."

After menopause, the ovary continues to produce androgens, particularly testosterone and androstenedione, as a result of increased LH concentrations. In addition, the adrenal gland continues to secrete androgens. The resulting decrease in the estrogen/androgen ratio is the cause of the hirsutism often seen in postmenopausal women.[146] Prolonged estrogen deficiency results in increased resorption and bone remodeling, leading to accelerated bone loss and osteoporosis in postmenopausal women. Estrogen replacement therapy reduces bone loss and has been reported to reduce fracture risk by half.[112,146] The issue of hormone replacement treatment for (1) menopausal symptoms, (2) osteoporosis, (3) various cardiac problems, and (4) other disorders has received a great deal of attention, and data concerning the benefits and risks have changed ideas about indications and contraindications.[70,106,263] No single, reliable hormonal marker of menopause status is available for a given woman. Physicians should diagnose menopausal status on the basis of menstrual history and age without relying on laboratory test results.[27,45]

It is important to note that perimenopausal and postmenopausal women secrete pituitary hCG.[13,22,35,173] Serum concentrations generally are low (<13 IU/L), but positive hCG results often causes confusion and can delay important diagnostic tests or treatments. Pituitary versus placental hCG has been confirmed by measuring serum LH (concentrations of LH >45 IU/L are consistent with menopause and make pregnancy unlikely) or by 2 weeks of hormone replacement therapy (hormone replacement therapy should decrease LH, FSH, and hCG concentrations).[60,116]

Female Reproductive Abnormalities

A wide variety of abnormalities affect the female reproductive system and have been classified in a variety of ways. For the purposes of this chapter, they have been divided into categories of (1) pseudohermaphroditism, (2) precocious puberty, (3) irregular menses, and (4) menopause. Infertility from the male and female perspective is discussed in a separate section.

Female Pseudohermaphroditism

In pseudohermaphroditism, the gonadal sex varies from the genital sex. The female pseudohermaphrodite is an individual who is genetically female, but whose phenotypic characteristics are, to varying degrees, male. In neonates with a 46,XX karyotype and ambiguous genitalia, *congenital adrenal hyperplasia* (CAH) should be considered. CAH is a family of autosomal recessive disorders of adrenal steroidogenesis (see Chapter 54). Each disorder has a specific pattern of hormonal abnormalities resulting in deficiency or excess of androgens. The molecular genetics of CAH is discussed in detail in several reviews.[64,140,141,169,322] In female fetuses, exposure to androgens before the 12th week of gestation causes ambiguous genitalia; after 13 weeks, it results in clitoral enlargement.[50,262] Because androgen excess occurs before the 12th week of gestation in those with CAH, ambiguous genitalia are almost always present. Only deficiencies of 21-hydroxylase and 11β-hydroxylase are predominantly virilizing disorders. Deficiency of 3β-hydroxysteroid dehydrogenase is rare, but when it occurs, affected girls may exhibit virilization.

Diagnosis of *21-hydroxylase deficiency* is made in infants and children with excess excretion of urinary 17-KS and pregnanetriol (a metabolite of 17-hydroxyprogesterone; see Chapter 54) and elevated concentrations of plasma 17-hydroxyprogesterone and androstenedione.[119,141,218] However, sick and premature infants may have elevated concentrations of 17-hydroxyprogesterone and androstenedione.[119,141] Elevation of 17-hydroxyprogesterone concentrations in early infancy (>3000 ng/dL) confirms the diagnosis of this disorder.[119,310] Additionally, molecular diagnostic testing is now available for detection of the mutations that account for most cases (80 to 90%) of 21-hydroxylase deficiency.[279]

An *11β-hydroxylase deficiency* is confirmed by finding elevated plasma concentrations of 11–deoxycortisol and deoxycorticosterone, increased concentrations of their metabolites in urine, and their suppression by glucocorticoid therapy (see Chapter 54). Plasma renin activity and aldosterone concentrations are low in this deficiency.[119,169,235]

Elevated plasma concentrations of 17-hydroxypregnenolone, DHEA, and DHEA-S are found in patients with 3β-*hydroxysteroid dehydrogenase deficiency* (see Chapter 54). Plasma concentrations of 17-hydroxyprogesterone may be elevated as a result of peripheral conversion of 17-hydroxypregnenolone. The ratio of 17-hydroxypregnenolone to 17-hydroxyprogesterone is strikingly elevated in these patients.[119,169,226]

Precocious Puberty

Precocious puberty is the development of secondary sexual characteristics in girls younger than 8 years old and boys younger than 9 years old.[247] In 1999, the Lawson Wilkins Pediatric Society issued new recommendations to lower the age standards at which puberty should be considered precocious from 8 to 7 in white girls and to 6 in black girls.[151] These recommendations have been met with criticism because they are based solely on a single epidemiologic study performed by Herman-Giddens and collaborators in 1997.[135] Many argue that the decreased age standards will result in underdiagnosis of this condition.[177,203,249]

Despite the debate over the age of onset, pediatric endocrinologists agree that it is important to distinguish between benign advanced pubertal conditions and true precocious puberty.[51,144,159,172,176,201] Early puberty is manifested by the appearance of secondary sexual characteristics such as premature thelarche (premature breast development), premature adrenarche (premature sexual hair development), or phallic enlargement. When presented as isolated cases, these secondary sexual characteristics are not considered to be pathologic, as none progresses to full-blown puberty, nor are they associated with increased rates of bone growth and maturation. However, if a child has at least two signs of puberty and also demonstrates increased rates of bone growth and maturation, the many causes of true precocious puberty must be considered.[201]

Precocious puberty has been classified as GnRH dependent or independent.[51,144,159,201] GnRH-dependent precocious puberty (also called *central precocious puberty*) is due to precocious activation of the hypothalamic-pituitary-gonadal axis. In girls, the cause is most commonly idiopathic (90%); however, idiopathic cases account for less than 10% of central precocious puberty in boys. Central nervous system tumors also have been known to cause central precocious puberty, the most common being hypothalamic hamartoma. Neurofibromatosis has been documented to lead to GnRH-dependent precocious puberty.

GnRH-independent precocious puberty (also called *pseudoprecocious puberty*) refers to precocious sex steroid secretion that is independent of pituitary gonadotropin release. Congenital adrenal hyperplasias (CAH) are a common cause of pseudoprecocious puberty. Classic forms of CAH present with virilization, growth acceleration, and accelerated bone maturation. Nonclassic or late-onset forms usually present in childhood or adolescence with premature adrenarche and acne. In fact, 5 to 10% of children who present with premature adrenarche have late-onset adrenal hyperplasia. Tumors of the adrenal gland, ovaries, and testes that secrete androgens or estrogens may result in GnRH-independent precocious puberty. Signs of puberty exhibited in males around 2 years of age are characteristic of testotoxicosis, a familial male-limited form of precocious puberty. This autosomal dominant disorder is due to activating mutations affecting LH receptors. The McCune-Albright syndrome is due to mutation of the *GNAS1* gene, which is involved in the signaling of G-proteins associated with gonadotropin receptors. The mutation causes the gonads to function as if both FSH and LH receptors are constitutively activated. Although this mutation results in GnRH-independent precocious puberty in both sexes, it is most common in girls. Precocious puberty, polyostotic fibrous dysplasia, and café au lait pigmentation are hallmarks for McCune-Albright syndrome. Severe hypothyroidism is also associated with GnRH-independent precocious puberty, likely caused by intrinsic FSH activity of high circulating concentrations of TSH. Unlike the other causes, hypothyroid-induced precocious puberty is associated with skeletal and growth delays.

Diagnosis of precocious puberty is based on (1) clinical presentation, (2) a thorough pubertal history, (3) bone age determinations, and (4) laboratory tests performed to assess gonadotropin concentrations and response to exogenous GnRH.* The GnRH stimulation test is the gold standard for diagnosis of GnRH-dependent precocious puberty. Pubertal responses of LH and FSH to GnRH stimulation are considered diagnostic of precocious puberty when chronological age is inappropriate for the hormone response. The GnRH stimulation test is also used to monitor the effectiveness of GnRH agonist therapy.[170,258,259] Typically, an IV bolus of exogenous GnRH is administered (100 µg or 2.5 µg/kg, maximal dose 100 µg), followed by a single measurement (at 40 to 45 minutes) or serial measurements of LH and FSH concentrations.† A predominant LH response correlates with a pubertal pattern, and cutoffs vary depending on the assay, with sex differences noted. A typical pubertal response is characterized by a rise in LH to 8 IU/L or greater after IV administration of 100 µg GnRH.[205] In girls, peak LH/FSH ratios (>0.66 to 1.0) have been proposed to be diagnostic of central precocious puberty.[223,308] Highly sensitive fluorometric[43] and chemiluminetric[216] immunoassays are now available for use in measuring basal LH concentrations. Basal LH concentrations have been used instead of the GnRH stimulation test for diagnosis of central precocious puberty. A fluorometric assay resulting in a basal concentration of LH greater than 0.6 IU/L in either sex indicates a pubertal pattern and is consistent with precocious puberty. Values less than 0.6 IU/L have been seen with all forms of precocious puberty and require follow-up with a GnRH stimulation test.[43] A similar pattern is observed for immunochemiluminometric assays using a cutoff of 0.3 IU/L.[215,216]

Response to exogenous GnRH is suppressed and LH and FSH concentrations are low in individuals with GnRH-independent precocious puberty. The diagnosis of GnRH-independent precocious puberty must exclude nonclassic adrenal hyperplasia (NCAH). Basal 17-hydroxyprogesterone concentrations of early morning samples have been used to screen for 21-OH–deficient NCAH. A basal 17-hydroxyprogesterone concentration less than 6.0 nmol/L (200 ng/dL) almost always rules out 21-OH–deficient NCAH. Patients with intermediate (200 to 500 ng/dL) basal 17-hydroxyprogesterone concentrations should undergo an ACTH stimulation test to confirm the presence of 21-OH–deficient NCAH. This is achieved by measuring the 17-hydroxyprogesterone response to ACTH stimulation. An exaggerated response is expected in cases of NCAH. Guidelines (1983) use a 17-hydroxyprogesterone diagnostic cutoff of greater than 30 nmol/L (1000 ng/dL).[219] However, some argue that the cutoff should be raised to greater than 45 (1500 ng/dL) or 60 nmol/L (2000 ng/dL), as the value of 30 nmol/L was set before molecular genotyping became available, and studies have indicated that several nonaffected carriers exhibit 17-hydroxyprogesterone concentrations above 30 nmol/L.[15,16,18]

Therapy for precocious puberty is dependent on the presenting symptoms and underlying causes.[159,172,176,201,232] Isolated premature thelarche or adrenarche does not require therapy. Patients with premature thelarche should be followed for 3 to 6 months and require further evaluation for precocious puberty. Cases of premature adrenarche should be evaluated for NCAH and/or polycystic ovary syndrome in girls with determined insulin resistance. GnRH-dependent precocious puberty is treated with GnRH agonists to inhibit normal gonadotropin release, thereby slowing pubertal progression. Therapy for GnRH-independent precocious puberty is determined by the underlying cause.

*References 51, 144, 159, 172, 176, and 201.

†References 53, 85, 144, 160, 175, 215, and 216.

Estrogens and Breast Cancer

Suspicions of estrogen-based causes in the development of human breast cancer stem from epidemiologic and experimental observations.[142,186] Early menarche and later natural menopause are associated with increased risk of breast cancer. A two-stage mechanism has been postulated: (1) initiation of a precancerous state by ovarian activity during the early reproductive years; and (2) continuation of ovarian activity in later years as a promoting influence on already initiated tumor cells. Ovarian estrogen has been assumed to be the causative factor because administration of estrogen negates the protective effects of early oophorectomy. Moreover, treatment of men with estrogen for prostatic cancer or after transsexual operations is associated with increased risk of breast cancer.

Low risk for breast cancer has consistently been connected with high parity. Increased risk is associated with early menarche, late (>30 years of age) first full-term pregnancy, and late menopause. Pregnancy occurring before age 25 to 30 years has a protective effect.

According to the theory, relative concentrations of individual estrogen fractions (E_1, E_2, and E_3) produced in the first decade or so after puberty are important determinants of a woman's lifetime risk of breast cancer.[61] In particular, pregnancy at a young age is associated with both favorable estrogen fraction ratios and decreased risk. Further discussion of the role of estrogen in the genesis of breast cancer is found in monographs and review articles.[59,127-129,153,154,182]

The rationale for using endocrine therapy in women with breast carcinoma is based on the fact that estrogen stimulates biochemical processes in cells of the uterus, pituitary gland, hypothalamus, and breast that normally contain the estrogen receptor. A reduction in circulating estrogen concentrations would be expected to decrease the biochemical activity of these cells. Approximately one third of women with metastatic breast carcinoma experience an objective remission after various types of endocrine therapy directed at lowering their estrogen concentrations. Such therapy includes oophorectomy, hypophysectomy, and adrenalectomy (ablative therapy), as well as administration of antiestrogens, androgens, and aromatase inhibitors (additive therapy).[29,46,168,245]

Cytoplasmic estrogen receptors are important prognostic indicators that are now routinely measured in samples of breast tissue after surgical removal of the tumor. Sixty percent of patients with carcinoma of the breast have tumors that are estrogen receptor positive. Approximately two thirds of patients with estrogen receptor–positive tumors respond to endocrine therapy; 95% of those with estrogen receptor–negative tumors fail to respond. Therefore, the greater the estrogen receptor content of the tumor, the higher is the response rate to endocrine therapy and the lower is the incidence of recurrence.

Irregular Menses

Healthy women display considerable variation in cycle length ranging from 25 to 30 days (28 days on average).[50] Amenorrhea, the absence of menstrual bleeding, is traditionally categorized as primary (women who have never menstruated) or secondary (women in whom menstruation is present for a variable time and then ceases). Amenorrhea is a relatively common disorder, with an estimated prevalence of 5% in the general population and as high as 8.5% in an unselected adolescent postpubescent population.[193]

Primary Amenorrhea

Primary amenorrhea is defined as failure to establish spontaneous periodic menstruation by the age of 16 years regardless of whether secondary sex characteristics have developed.[67,156,197] About 40% of phenotypic females who have primary amenorrhea (nearly always associated with absence of development of secondary sex characteristics) have *Turner syndrome* (45,X karyotype) or *pure gonadal dysgenesis* (46,XX or XY karyotype).[50,335] *Müllerian duct agenesis* or *dysgenesis* with absence of the vagina or uterus is the second most common manifestation, and the third most common is *androgen insensitivity syndrome* (androgen receptor deficiency and normal or elevated plasma testosterone concentrations if the patient is past puberty and is karyotype XY).

A *17α-hydroxylase deficiency* is a rare form of CAH that is associated with delayed puberty, primary amenorrhea, and hypertension. Patients have a 46,XX karyotype with elevated gonadotropins, low sex steroids, hypertension, and hypokalemia.[67,169]

Another rare cause of amenorrhea is the so called *resistant ovary syndrome.* This primary hypogonadal condition is associated with increased concentrations of plasma FSH and LH, and ovaries that contain predominantly primordial follicles. It is thought to arise from a defect in FSH receptors.[50] This disorder can be diagnosed only by examination of an ovarian biopsy specimen, which will exhibit functioning ovarian follicles despite the presence of amenorrhea. Ovulation sometimes is induced in these patients with administration of high doses of gonadotropins.

As discussed earlier, *Kallmann syndrome* involves hypogonadotropic hypogonadism associated with anosmia or hyposmia and is caused by a defect in the formation and migration of GnRH neurons. Sexual infantilism is the prominent manifestation, and primary amenorrhea is common.[50,335] Finally, delayed pubertal development should be considered.

Evaluation. When puberty is delayed in a girl, serum gonadotropins should be measured. Low concentrations may indicate pituitary failure, whereas concentrations elevated into the postmenopausal interval indicate definite gonadal failure.[50,238,335] In the latter case, chromosome studies are indicated. In the former case, pituitary function testing and radiography may be helpful. Patients with short stature without Turner syndrome but with primary amenorrhea may have multiple deficiencies of pituitary hormone secretion. In these patients, a craniopharyngioma or pituitary tumor should be suspected.

The diagnosis of *17α-hydroxylase deficiency* is made when the concentration of (1) serum progesterone is greater than 3 ng/mL; (2) 17α-hydroxyprogesterone is less than 0.2 ng/mL; (3) aldosterone is low; and (4) 11-deoxycorticosterone is elevated. Plasma concentrations of 11-deoxycortisol, testosterone, E_2, and DHEA-S are also low. The diagnosis is confirmed with an *ACTH stimulation test* in which baseline concentrations of progesterone and 17α-hydroxyprogesterone are measured first, followed by administration of 0.25 mg ACTH. Diagnosis is made if serum concentrations of progesterone are significantly elevated and 17α-hydroxyprogesterone concentrations are unchanged at 60 minutes after ACTH administration.[67,224]

Secondary Amenorrhea

Secondary amenorrhea is defined as absence of periodic menstruation for at least 6 months in women who have previously experienced menses.[68,156,197,241,316] *Oligomenorrhea* is infrequent menstruation that occurs fewer than nine times per year.[250] With few exceptions, the causes of primary and secondary amenorrhea overlap (Box 56-2). Pregnancy, the most common cause of secondary amenorrhea, must be considered first and ruled out.[156,197,316] Elevated concentrations of prolactin—iatrogenic or induced by a prolactin-secreting tumor—have been found to result in oligomenorrhea or amenorrhea.[156,197,316] About one third of women with no obvious cause of amenorrhea have elevated prolactin concentrations.[156] It is thought that hyperprolactinemia inhibits the release of LH and FSH.[161] Both hyperthyroidism and hypothyroidism are associated with a variety of menstrual disorders because of their effects on metabolism and interconversion of androgens and estrogens.[156,197,334] In practice, it is helpful to separate patients with secondary amenorrhea into those with and without signs of hirsutism and androgen excess.

Evaluation. Evaluation of women with amenorrhea should begin with a careful history that includes a complete description of menstrual patterns. In addition, the patient should be evaluated for (1) galactorrhea, (2) hot flashes, (3) symptoms of hypothyroidism, (4) hirsutism, (5) prior

BOX 56-2 Causes of Amenorrhea

Primary Amenorrhea
- Lower tract defects
  - Vaginal aplasia
  - Imperforate hymen
  - Congenital vaginal atresia
- Uterine disorders
  - Congenital absence of the uterus
  - Endometritis
  - Müllerian agenesis (Mayer-Rokitansky-Kuster-Hauser syndrome)
- Ovarian disorders
  - XO gonadal and X dysgenesis and variants
  - XX gonadal dysgenesis
  - Turner syndrome
  - Androgen insensitivity syndrome (AIS)
  - 17-Hydroxylase deficiency of the ovaries and adrenal glands
  - Autoimmune oophoritis
  - Resistant ovary syndrome
  - Polycystic ovary syndrome
- Adrenal disorders (congenital adrenal hyperplasia)
- Thyroid disorders (hypothyroidism)
- Pituitary-hypothalamic disorders
  - Hypopituitarism
  - Constitutional delay in the onset of menses (physiologic)
  - Nutritional disorders
  - Kallmann syndrome

Secondary Amenorrhea
- Pregnancy/lactation
- Uterine disorders
  - Post-traumatic uterine synechiae (Asherman syndrome)
  - Progestational agents
- Ovarian disorders
  - Polycystic ovary syndrome (hypothalamic)
  - Ovarian tumor
  - Primary ovarian insufficiency (idiopathic, autoimmune, chemotherapy, radiation, injury)
  - Antimetabolite therapy
- Adrenal disorders
  - Late-onset adrenal hyperplasia
  - Cushing syndrome
  - Virilizing adrenal tumors
  - Adrenocorticoid insufficiency
- Thyroid disorders
  - Hypothyroidism
  - Hyperthyroidism
- Pituitary disorders
  - Acquired hypopituitarism (trauma, tumor, Sheehan syndrome, lymphocytic hypophysitis)
  - Physiologic or pathologic hyperprolactinemia
- Hypothalamic disorders
  - Tumor and infiltrative disease
  - Nutritional disorders
  - Hypophysitis
  - Excessive exercise
  - Stress
- Iatrogenic
  - Antipsychotics (phenothiazines, haloperidol, clozapine, pimozide)
  - Antidepressants (tricyclics, monoamine oxidase inhibitors)
  - Antihypertensives (calcium channel blockers, methyldopa, reserpine)
  - Drugs with estrogenic activity (digitalis, flavonoids, marijuana, oral contraceptives)
  - Drugs with ovarian toxicity (busulfan, chlorambucil, cisplatin, cyclophosphamide, fluorouracil)

abdominal surgery, (6) pelvis or uterus trauma, (7) medications prescribed, (8) nutritional history, (9) patterns of exercise, (10) previous contraceptive use, (11) weight changes, (12) stress, and (13) chronic disease. The physical examination should determine the visual fields, thyroid size and function, cushingoid appearance, galactorrhea, hirsutism, abdominal masses, pelvic masses, clitoral enlargement, and evidence of malnutrition. Serum or urine β-hCG should be measured to rule out pregnancy. Because both hypothyroidism and hyperprolactinemia have been known to cause amenorrhea, they are easily excluded by measuring concentrations of serum thyroid-stimulating hormone and prolactin.

A 24 hour urine sample for cortisol measurement or an overnight dexamethasone suppression test is performed in those patients suspected of having Cushing syndrome (see Chapter 54). On the basis of the preliminary assessment, computed tomography of the sella turcica should be performed in patients with evidence of pituitary or hypothalamic disease. A GnRH stimulation test with measurement of LH and FSH concentrations in those patients with gonadotropin deficiency assists in differentiating hypothalamic disease from pituitary disease. For diagnosis of polycystic ovary disease (PCOS), see the later section, "Laboratory Evaluation of Hirsutism/Virilization."

Progesterone Challenge for Evaluating Amenorrhea

When the cause of amenorrhea is unclear after the initial assessment, relative estrogen status should be determined. Serum E_2 can be measured, or a *progesterone challenge* may be performed.[50,335] Women with an estrogen-primed uterus have withdrawal vaginal bleeding after treatment with oral progestin (medroxyprogesterone acetate; Provera), 30 mg daily for 3 days, or 10 mg daily for 5 to 10 days, or 100 to 200 mg of progesterone in oil given intramuscularly. If estrogen concentrations are adequate and the outflow tract is intact, menstrual bleeding should occur within a week of treatment. In patients with withdrawal bleeding, the plasma

E_2 concentration is usually greater than 40 pg/mL.[50,68] Measurement of serum E_2 can be made instead of the progesterone challenge but is not preferred because estrogen concentrations fluctuate throughout the day, and withdrawal bleeding is an indication of a normal outflow tract.

If bleeding fails to occur after progestin challenge, then additional laboratory tests are indicated, including measurement of LH and FSH to localize the problem to the follicle, pituitary, or hypothalamus. High gonadotropin and low estrogen concentrations indicate that the ovarian follicle is not responding to gonadotropin stimulation. A single measurement of LH or FSH greater than 50 mIU/mL is a reliable indicator of ovarian failure. Because of the association of *primary ovarian insufficiency* (POI) with thyroid, parathyroid, or adrenal insufficiency secondary to autoimmune disease, it has been suggested that patients younger than 35 years should be screened for thyroid antibodies.[68] The differential diagnosis for evaluation of amenorrhea is listed in Table 56-1. As indicated by the clinical presentation, special additional testing may be required.

If the patient demonstrates withdrawal bleeding after the progestin challenge test, this indicates that the ovaries are producing sufficient estrogen to cause endometrial proliferation, and no anatomic obstruction is present. Most of these women have a history of oral contraceptive use, stress, weight loss, or excessive exercise.

Androgen Excess

Amenorrhea due to androgen excess can be due to (1) adult-onset CAH, (2) corticotropin-dependent Cushing syndrome, or (3) polycystic ovary syndrome (PCOS). Patients with androgen excess often will present with acne, obesity, and variable degrees of excess hair on the face, chest, abdomen, and thighs. Some individuals with 21-hydroxylase deficiency

TABLE 56-1 Differential Diagnosis of Amenorrhea

Causes	FSH	LH	Estrogen (E_2)	Uterine Bleeding After Progesterone
Hypothalamic				
CNS—hypothalamic dysfunction				
Idiopathic	N	N	N	+
Secondary to medications	N	N	N	+
Secondary to stress	N	N	N	+
CNS—hypothalamic dysfunction or failure due to exercise	↓ or N	↓ or N	↓ or N	±
CNS—hypothalamic dysfunction or failure due to weight loss				
Simple weight loss	↓ or N	↓ or N	↓ or N	±
Anorexia nervosa	↓	↓	↓	–
CNS—hypothalamic failure				
Lesions	↓	↓	↓	–
Idiopathic	↓	↓	↓	–
CNS—hypothalamic–adreno-ovarian dysfunction (polycystic ovary syndrome) or hyperandrogen chronic anovulation	N	↑*	N	+
Pituitary				
Destructive lesions (Sheehan syndrome)	↓	↓	↓	–
Tumor	↓	↓	↓	–
Ovarian				
Premature ovarian failure	↑	↑	↓	–
Loss of ovarian function (oophorectomy, infection, cystic degeneration, chemotherapy, radiation)	↑	↑	↓	–
Uterine				
Uterine synechiae (Asherman syndrome)	N	N	N	–

CNS, Central nervous system; *FSH,* follicle-stimulating hormone; *LH,* luteinizing hormone; *N,* value within normal reference interval; ↓, value below normal reference interval; ↑, value above normal reference interval; ↑*, >25 mIU/mL, less than menopausal concentration; ±, positive or negative bleeding response to progesterone.

From Davajan V, Kletzky OA. Amenorrhea. In: Mishell DR, Davajan V, Lobo RA, eds. Infertility, contraception and reproductive endocrinology, 3rd edition. Boston, Mass: Blackwell Scientific Publications, 1991:373.

do not manifest any developmental abnormalities or salt wasting, but they present with signs of androgen excess. This clinical syndrome, referred to as *nonclassic, adult-onset,* or *late-onset CAH,* may be clinically indistinguishable from PCOS.[15,79,100]

PCOS occurs in ≈4% of premenopausal women, and its basic pathophysiologic defect is not known.[50,109,280,337] PCOS is clinically defined by hyperandrogenism with chronic anovulation in women with no other cause.[123] This syndrome is characterized by (1) infertility, (2) hirsutism, (3) obesity (in approximately half of those affected), and (4) various menstrual disturbances ranging from amenorrhea to irregular vaginal bleeding (Table 56-2). These women have an increased prevalence of diabetes, along with increased risk for coronary heart disease and endometrial cancer. Although this syndrome is associated with polycystic ovaries, they often are not present in women with this syndrome. The name is actually a misnomer in that the ovaries are covered with follicles, not cysts. Relatively low FSH and disproportionately high LH concentrations are common in PCOS. Serum androstenedione and testosterone concentrations (total and free concentrations) are elevated, with mean concentrations 50 to 150% higher than normal.[26,50,100]

PCOS patients have substantial estrogen production because of the peripheral conversion of androgens to estrogens. Abnormal bleeding patterns seen in PCOS are due to chronic anovulation and lack of progesterone stimulation and withdrawal. Chronic estrogen exposure without progesterone may predispose patients to endometrial cancer. Some attempt has been made to link PCOS to *leptin,* a hormone that is secreted by adipocytes and is thought to play a role in regulating food intake and metabolism.[44] Animals that lack leptin are infertile; leptin injection increases gonadotropin secretion and restores fertility.[23,56] However, the literature suggests that leptin concentrations are normal in patients with PCOS.[49] Veldhuis and collaborators note that although serum leptin concentrations were the same in PCOS patients and controls, the pattern of leptin secretion was abnormal in girls with PCOS.[303] For PCOS patients who are not interested in conceiving, the mainstay of therapy is oral contraceptive pills. For those who are overweight or obese, weight loss and exercise are essential. For women with PCOS who wish to conceive, treatment is aimed at ovulation induction. Weight reduction should be attempted first in those women who are overweight, as it often helps to promote ovulation. If ovulation does not occur, then medications such as clomiphene citrate, metformin, and aromatase inhibitors may be useful.[123] *Ovarian hyperthecosis,* a non-neoplastic lesion of the ovary characterized by the presence of islands of luteinized thecal cells in the ovarian stroma, is sometimes confused with PCOS. Features that distinguish it from PCOS include higher concentrations of testosterone, androstenedione, and DHT derived from ovarian secretion. Thus, androgenization is greater than is usually observed in patients with PCOS. Both LH and FSH concentrations are low or low-normal. Insulin resistance and hyperinsulinism are present to a greater degree than in PCOS. Finally, patients with ovarian hyperthecosis fail to ovulate when treated with an antiestrogen such as clomiphene citrate.[337]

TABLE 56-2 Clinical Features of the Polycystic Ovary Syndrome*

Clinical Feature	Frequency, %
Hirsutism	65
Acne	26
Obesity	37
Infertility	48
Amenorrhea	35
Oligomenorrhea	42
Regular menstrual cycle	20

*Data were compiled from three studies. Two used ultrasonography as the primary method of diagnosis, one used ovarian histology. Total $N = 1935$. Modified from Franks S. Polycystic ovary syndrome. N Engl J Med 1995;333:853.

Hirsutism and Virilization

Hirsutism is defined as excessive growth of terminal hair in women and children in a distribution similar to that occurring in postpubertal men.[14,246,257] True hirsutism, which is androgen responsive, has to be distinguished from hypertrichosis, which consists of excessive growth of vellus or non–androgen-responsive hair. Vellus is fine, downy hair that is usually unpigmented, whereas terminal hairs are thick and are found in androgen-responsive areas of the skin.[251,257] Growth of vellus hair diffusely over the trunk and face may be familial or drug induced, and is treatable only by mechanical hair removal or withdrawal of the inducing drug. Women with androgen-dependent hirsutism may have exposure to excess androgens or may have heightened sensitivity to normal circulating concentrations of androgen. As a consequence, vellus follicles develop into terminal hair follicles in areas of androgen-sensitive skin.

The causes of hirsutism are listed in Box 56-3. The estimated prevalence for idiopathic hirsutism ranges from 6 to 50% of women evaluated for hirsutism, depending on the definition.[17,48,257,261] Typically, idiopathic hirsutism is defined by normal physical and laboratory findings in hirsute women. However, it has been reported that the prevalence of idiopathic hirsutism changes drastically, whether or not factors such as ovulatory function and androgen concentrations are considered.[17] It is thought that increased sensitivity of the hair follicle to normal circulating androgens causes the excess hair growth.[257] Non-neoplastic forms of hirsutism are slow to progress and usually manifest at the time of puberty, when circulating concentrations of androgens increase, or after a period of weight gain, or when oral contraceptives have been stopped.[246] Rapid onset of hirsutism suggests an iatrogenic cause or, if associated with virilization, a neoplastic source of androgens. The most common cause of androgen hypersecretion in women is PCOS; 70 to 80% of hirsute women are

BOX 56-3 Causes of Hirsutism

Ovarian
- Severe insulin resistance
- Hyperthecosis, hilus cell or stromal cell hyperplasia
- Androgen-producing ovarian tumor
- Menopause

Adrenal
- Classic congenital hyperplasia
  - 21-Hydroxylase deficiency
  - 11-Hydroxylase deficiency
  - 3β-Hydroxysteroid dehydrogenase deficiency
- Adult or attenuated adrenal hyperplasia
- Androgen-producing adrenal tumor

Familial Hirsutism

Endocrine Disorders
- Polycystic ovary syndrome
- Hyperprolactinemia
- Acromegaly
- Cushing syndrome

Idiopathic Hirsutism (includes increased skin sensitivity to androgens)

Iatrogenic
- Androgens
- Dilantin
- Diazoxide
- Minoxidil
- Streptomycin
- Cyclosporine
- Danazol
- Metyrapone
- Phenothiazides
- Progestagens (19-nonsteroid derivatives)

reportedly afflicted with this disorder.[261] Hyperandrogenism usually arises from both ovaries and the adrenal glands (for more on PCOS, see previous section). Late-onset CAH (see Chapter 54), acromegaly, hyperprolactinemia, menopause (see earlier section, "Menopause"), and ACTH-dependent Cushing syndrome have been observed to cause hirsutism.

Virilization is characterized by clitoral hypertrophy, deepening of the voice, temporal hair recession, baldness, increased libido, decreased body fat, and menstrual irregularities or amenorrhea. Hirsutism is usually associated with normal or slightly elevated serum androgens, whereas virilization is associated with marked increases in ovarian or adrenal androgen production.[50]

Laboratory Evaluation of Hirsutism/Virilization

The two most important screening tests used in the evaluation of women for hirsutism and virilization are serum total or free testosterone and DHEA-S.[50,251] Elevation of DHEA-S concentration suggests an adrenal origin of androgens, whereas elevations in testosterone indicate an adrenal or ovarian source. Neoplastic disease is unlikely if the serum testosterone concentration is less than 2 ng/mL, the DHEA-S concentration is less than 700 μg/dL, or 17-KS concentrations are less than 30 mg/d.[50,100,257] Regardless of the source of excess androgen production, the androstanediol glucuronide concentration is elevated in more than 90% of women with hirsutism, because it is a marker of excessive DHT production in skin. Because concentrations of SHBG can be decreased in hirsute women, there has been some debate over whether total testosterone or bioavailable testosterone (free and weakly bound testosterone) is more clinically informative in diagnosing hirsutism. The reader is directed to a review by Wheeler that discusses many of these issues.[319]

Polycystic ovary syndrome is primarily a clinical diagnosis, and few laboratory tests are needed. Given a history of androgen excess and chronic anovulation (usually since menarche), the only condition that needs to be excluded is 21-hydroxylase–deficient nonclassic CAH; this can be done by measuring 17-hydroxyprogesterone (early morning; follicular phase). If the result is less than 2 ng/mL, nonclassic CAH can be excluded. Serum testosterone measurement is not necessary if clear hirsutism is present. Testosterone concentrations greater than 60 ng/dL are consistent with PCOS.[123] FSH concentrations are often disproportionately normal or low. It has been suggested that a ratio of LH to FSH greater than 2 or 2.5 indicates the presence of PCOS.[50,257] However, because of the pulsatile nature of gonadotropins, this ratio is insensitive. Patients with PCOS usually have E_2 concentrations greater than 40 pg/mL and therefore experience withdrawal bleeding in response to a progestin challenge.

Morning plasma 17α-hydroxyprogesterone concentrations are measured to evaluate *nonclassic* or *late-onset 21-hydroxylase deficiency* (NCAH). A concentration less than 200 ng/dL (6.1 nmol/L) excludes this diagnosis, and a concentration greater than 1500 ng/dL (30 nmol/L) in nonpregnant women is confirmatory. When basal concentrations between 200 and 1500 ng/dL are found, an ACTH stimulation test should be performed. NCAH typically has a 17α-hydroxyprogesterone concentration greater than 1500 ng/dL, and classic CAH has a response over 2000 ng/dL.[205,246,251] Patients with attenuated forms of CAH usually have normal concentrations of FSH and LH. About one half have elevated testosterone and androstenedione concentrations.[336] Most of these patients also have increased concentrations of DHEA-S, and more than 90% have supranormal concentrations of androstanediol glucuronide.[199,227]

Other Factors

Many other factors or conditions have been observed to cause secondary amenorrhea, including disorders of the ovary, uterus, pituitary, and hypothalamus, and the use of drugs.

Disorders of the ovary, such as *primary ovarian insufficiency (POI)* [formerly referred to as premature ovarian failure (POF)] and loss of ovarian function, have been known to cause amenorrhea. POI has been defined as failure of ovarian estrogen production that occurs in a hypergonadotropic state at any age between menarche and 40 years.[50,68,156,316] If the patient is younger than 25 years, karyotyping should be performed to rule out the presence of a variety of chromosomal abnormalities involving duplications or absence of the X chromosome or the presence of a Y chromosome. Screening for the fragile X premutation *(FMR1)* should also be performed.[217] Patients with POI may present with symptoms of hypoestrogenism, including hot flashes and high gonadotropin concentrations. Autoimmune disorders have been associated with 20 to 40% of cases of POI that result in destruction of the ovary and in amenorrhea.[50,68,156,316] Patients also may have antibodies to other endocrine and nonendocrine tissues. Other causes for ovarian failure include (1) oophorectomy, (2) cystic degeneration, (3) trauma, (4) infection, (5) interference with blood supply, (6) radiotherapy treatment, and (7) treatment with cytotoxic chemotherapeutic agents. In rare patients, ovarian resistance to gonadotropins may be evident.[50,316]

Secondary amenorrhea is also caused by uterine failure. The patient with a uterine problem is normal hormonally but does not menstruate. *Asherman syndrome*, or intrauterine adhesions, is the most common outflow tract abnormality that causes amenorrhea. Endometrial damage may occur in response to a dilatation and curettage, and to infection of the endometrium.[68,156] Pituitary dysfunction will also cause secondary amenorrhea. This is most often due to intrinsic pituitary tumors. However, Sheehan syndrome and pituitary apoplexy will also result in hormone deficiency. Empty sella syndrome has been reported in 4 to 16% of patients with amenorrhea and galactorrhea.[156]

Hypothalamic dysfunction consists of those disorders that disrupt the frequency or amplitude of GnRH. Rarely is this due to a lesion or tumor. However, most commonly, disruption occurs in response to psychological stress, depression, severe weight loss, anorexia nervosa, or strenuous exercise.[68,156] A syndrome known as the *female athletic triad* has been described. This syndrome is prevalent in women who exercise vigorously, and is associated with amenorrhea, disordered eating, and osteoporosis. Competitive long-distance runners, gymnasts, and professional ballet dancers appear to be at highest risk. Although the mechanism for the disturbance is unclear, symptoms and laboratory profiles are similar to those of other forms of hypothalamic amenorrhea. LH and FSH concentrations are normal or low, and E_2 concentrations are low. As a result of chronic low estrogen, bone mineral content is low and the incidence of stress fractures is increased.[68,193]

Several hormone-producing tumors of the ovary, pituitary gland, and adrenal glands occur in combination with amenorrhea.[50,185,296,335] This amenorrhea may be confused with pregnancy if the tumors produce hCG. Choriocarcinoma of the uterus or ovary may produce large amounts of hCG that cause hyperthyroidism, because of the slight thyrotropic action of hCG. Granulosa–theca cell tumors are usually associated with estrogen secretion that results in amenorrhea and irregular menses and, rarely, excessive androgen with associated virilization.[50,335]

Many drugs produce amenorrhea (see Box 56-2), particularly phenothiazines and other psychotropic drugs such as haloperidol, pimozide, or clozapine.[156] Phenothiazine-induced amenorrhea is usually associated with hyperprolactinemia and galactorrhea. Drugs that affect the normal pathway of dopamine secretion will produce amenorrhea by decreasing the secretion of norepinephrine. Because norepinephrine is important in controlling the synthesis and secretion of GnRH, any alteration in its synthesis or secretion will result in menstrual abnormalities.[68,161] Amenorrhea may follow discontinuation of contraceptive steroids—so-called *post-pill amenorrhea*. Contraceptive steroids have a suppressive effect on the pituitary that sometimes persists after medication has been discontinued. In most women, menses resumes within 6 months after discontinuation of oral contraceptives.[68] If menses has not resumed within this time frame, evaluation is warranted. If other causes of amenorrhea are suspected, evaluation should not be delayed.

INFERTILITY

Infertility is defined as the inability to conceive after 1 year of unprotected intercourse.[24,50,307] It has been estimated that 93% of healthy couples practicing unprotected intercourse should expect to conceive within 1 year, and 100% will be successful within 2 years.[91] A specific cause of infertility is identified in ≈80% of couples: one third are due to female factors alone, one third to male factors alone, and one third to a combination of problems.

Primary infertility refers to couples or patients who have had no previous successful pregnancies. Secondary infertility encompasses patients who have previously conceived, but are currently unable to conceive. These types of infertility generally share common causes.

Infertility problems often arise as a result of hormonal dysfunction of the hypothalamic-pituitary-gonadal axis. Measurements of peptide and steroid hormones in the serum are therefore essential aspects of the evaluation of infertility. This section focuses on hormonal and biochemical aspects of evaluating infertility.

Male Infertility

A list of the most common male infertility factors is given in Box 56-4. One algorithm for the evaluation of male infertility is shown in Figure 56-12. Initial evaluation of male infertility should include a detailed history and physical examination. The physical examination should pay particular attention to (1) the external genitalia—for evidence of proper androgenization, (2) hair pattern—degree of virilization, (3) breast abnormalities—gynecomastia and or discharge, and (4) neurologic findings—sense of smell and visual impairments. The history must include (1) reproductive history, including living children and any pregnancies that resulted in miscarriage, (2) prescribed medications, (3) recreational and performance-enhancing drug and alcohol use, (4) systemic illness, and (5) potential toxin exposure. Sexual history should include sexual technique,

BOX 56-4 Male Infertility Factors

Endocrine Disorders
Hypothalamic dysfunction (Kallmann syndrome)
Pituitary failure (tumor, radiation, surgery)
Hyperprolactinemia (drug, tumor)
Exogenous androgens
Thyroid disorders
Adrenal hyperplasia
Testicular failure

Anatomic
Congenital absence of vas deferens
Obstructed vas deferens
Congenital abnormalities of ejaculatory system
Varicocele
Retrograde ejaculation

Abnormal Spermatogenesis
Unexplained azoospermia
Chromosomal abnormalities
Mumps orchitis
Cryptorchidism
Chemical or radiation exposure

Abnormal Motility
Absent cilia (Kartagener syndrome)
Antibody formation

Psychosocial
Unexplained impotence
Decreased libido

Modified from Morell V. Basic infertility assessment. Primary Care 1997;24:195-204.

TABLE 56-3 Normal Seminal Fluid Values

Parameter	Value
Ejaculate volume	>2 mL*
Sperm density	>20 million/mL*
Total sperm count	>40 million/ejaculate*
Motility	>50% with forward progression or >25% with rapid progression within 60 minutes of ejaculation*
Morphology	>30% normal*
pH	7.2-8.0*
Color	Gray-white-yellow
Liquefaction	Within 40 minutes
Fructose	>1200 μg/mL
Acid phosphatase	100-300 μg/mL
Citric acid	>3 mg/mL
Inositol	>1 mg/mL
Zinc	>75 μg/mL
Magnesium	>70 μg/mL
Prostaglandins (PGE_1 + PGE_2)	30-200 μg/mL
Glycerylphosphorylcholine	>650 μg/mL
Carnitine	>250 μg/mL
Glucosidase	>20 mU per ejaculate

*Values from World Health Organization. Laboratory manual for the examination of human semen and semen–cervical mucus penetration, 3rd edition. Cambridge, UK: Cambridge University Press, 1992.
From Glezerman M, Bartoov B. Semen analysis. In: Insler V, Lunenfeld B, eds. Infertility: male and female, 2nd edition. New York, NY: Churchill Livingstone, 1993:285-315.

frequency of intercourse, and use of any lubricants. Issues of potency must be distinguished from those of infertility or subfertility. All abnormalities in the history and physical examination should be pursued. Testosterone should be measured, especially when the patient history or physical examination suggests deficient development of secondary sex characteristics.

Laboratory evaluation of male infertility should begin with evaluation of semen, which should be followed by evaluation of endocrine parameters.

Evaluation of Semen

Semen analysis measures ejaculate volume, pH, sperm count, motility, forward progression, and morphology. Semen should be analyzed within 1 hour after collection. Although semen analysis is not a test for infertility, it is considered the most important laboratory test in the evaluation of male fertility. Controversy exists as to what constitutes a "normal" semen profile. With the exception of the *azoospermic* male (defined as no sperm in the ejaculate), the lines between fertility and infertility are blurred and are intimately associated with the status of the female partner's reproductive function. However, clinical studies of infertile men and World Health Organization (WHO) guidelines have helped establish limits of adequacy (Table 56-3).[11,95] If semen analysis is normal, it is unlikely that other laboratory testing will be useful. If semen analysis is abnormal, it should be repeated in ≈6 weeks. A new approach to semen analysis for investigation of infertility uses a monoclonal antibody to sperm protein SP-10. A version of the test is available to check the success of vasectomy. A home-use version (http://www.contravac.com/) was cleared by the FDA in 2010 as substantially equivalent to a sperm count and is expected to be marketed widely.

Evaluation of Obstruction

Obstruction of the male reproductive tract will result in male infertility, and analysis of specific semen parameters has proved a useful adjunct to physical examination in the evaluation of male reproductive tract obstruction. Testosterone produced after administration of hCG causes the seminal vesicles, epididymis, and prostate to increase the volume of ejaculate. An appropriate increase in serum testosterone without change in the ejaculate volume may indicate mechanical blockage. Absence of, or a decrease in, specific biochemical markers such as acid phosphatase and citric acid (from

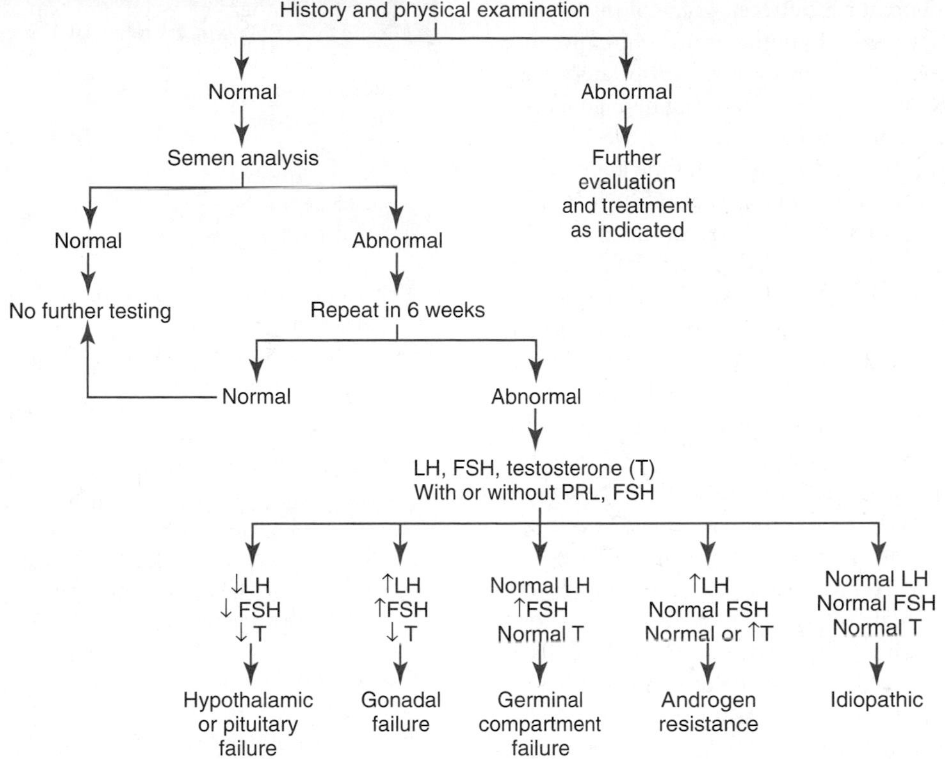

Figure 56-12 Algorithm for the evaluation of male infertility. *FSH,* Follicle-stimulating hormone; *LH,* luteinizing hormone; *T,* testosterone.

prostate), fructose, and prostaglandins (from seminal vesicles) can assist determination of the location of blockage.[104] Low seminal glucosidase concentrations, in the presence of testes of normal size and consistency, normal semen volume, and normal serum FSH, have been used as an indication of obstruction (usually in the epididymis) or congenital bilateral absence of the vas deferens (a condition associated with mutations of the cystic fibrosis gene).[6]

Evaluation of Endocrine Parameters

If severe oligospermia or azoospermia is found, then measurement of serum testosterone, LH, and FSH concentrations is warranted, with or without measurement of prolactin and TSH. Hyperprolactinemia is a cause of secondary testicular dysfunction.[113] Prolactin excess likely causes hypogonadism by impairing GnRH release. It also leads to underandrogenization and erectile dysfunction (see earlier section, "Erectile Dysfunction"). If hyperprolactinemia is found, it is imperative to check for hypothyroidism, because elevated TRH concentrations can result in hyperprolactinemia. Pituitary adenomas and drugs such as anxiolytics, antihypertensives, serotonergics, and histamine H_2 receptor antagonists also increase serum prolactin.[332] Hyperthyroidism and hypothyroidism will alter spermatogenesis. Hyperthyroidism affects both pituitary and testicular function, with alterations in the secretion of releasing hormones and increased conversion of androgens to estrogens.

Patients with borderline or suppressed testosterone concentrations can be evaluated with an *hCG stimulation test.* With this test, an injection of 5000 IU hCG is administered intramuscularly following collection of a basal, early morning testosterone sample. Serum testosterone is measured 72 hours later. Hypogonadal men show a depressed rise in testosterone concentration in response to this challenge. Doubling of testosterone concentration over baseline is consistent with normal Leydig cell function. Failure to increase testosterone to greater than 150 ng/dL indicates primary hypogonadism.[147]

Testosterone is essential for normal sperm development (see Figure 56-4). Therefore, any disorder that results in hypogonadism (and hence low testosterone concentrations) results in infertility. Among the causes are hypogonadotropic and hypergonadotropic hypogonadism.

Hypergonadotropic Hypogonadism

Measurement of the concentration of FSH is indicated in men with sperm count lower than 5 to 10 million/mL. Elevated concentrations of FSH indicate Sertoli cell dysfunction and, in azoospermic men, primary germinal cell failure, Sertoli cell–only syndrome, or genetic conditions such as Klinefelter syndrome.[105] Elevated FSH (>120 mIU/mL) in the setting of decreased testosterone (<200 ng/dL) and oligospermia indicate primary testicular failure.

Hypogonadotropic Hypogonadism

Decreased concentrations of testosterone (<200 ng/dL) and decreased concentrations of FSH (<10 mIU/mL) are suggestive of hypogonadotropic hypogonadism. Administering

GnRH may help to distinguish between gonadal insufficiencies caused by pituitary versus hypothalamic failure. Because the pituitary is sensitive to sex steroids for appropriate gonadotropin secretion, patients with long-standing hypogonadism should be given exogenous testosterone for 1 week before the GnRH stimulation test is administered. One approach to this test involves the intravenous injection of 100 µg of GnRH with measurement of FSH and LH concentrations at 0, 30, 60, 120, and 180 minutes after injection. Results of the GnRH test are classified as follows. An increase in serum gonadotropins of 10 mIU/mL or more over baseline is normal. If little to no increase in gonadotropins is seen, pituitary disease is likely. Patients with hypothalamic disease will demonstrate a delayed but significant increase of 7 mIU/mL or more within 180 minutes.[147] The most common cause of hypothalamic hypogonadism is *congenital idiopathic hypogonadotropic hypogonadism* (IHH) or its variant, Kallmann syndrome (see earlier section, "Male Reproductive Abnormalities").[220] An adult-onset form of IHH has been recognized as a potentially treatable form of male infertility.[213] Molecular diagnosis using fluorescence in situ hybridization (FISH) analysis is now offered to families with X-linked Kallmann syndrome. This is the most common type of testing performed, but it will detect only major deletions in the *KAL* gene. Genome microarray analysis and prenatal diagnosis also are now available.

Mutations in the X chromosome gene, *Dax1*, also have been known to cause hypogonadotropic hypogonadism in association with congenital adrenal hypoplasia. This gene encodes an orphan nuclear hormone receptor that has a critical role in development of the hypothalamus, pituitary, adrenal, and gonads.[105] FISH analysis is also available for the diagnosis of *Dax1* mutations.

Y-Chromosome Microdeletions

Deletions in either of the azoospermia factor regions (AZF1 and AZF2) on the long arm of the Y chromosome are associated with an inability to make sperm. In addition, genes such as *SRY* (sex-determining region Y) are on the short arm of chromosome Y. Deletion of these regions is associated with azoospermia or, less frequently, oligospermia. The incidence of Y microdeletions in idiopathic nonobstructive azoospermic men is 8% to 18%.[105] Testing for Y-chromosome microdeletions includes polymerase chain reaction (PCR) of specific regions of the Y chromosome to identify microdeletions. Tests should span AZFa and AZF2 and other regions thought to encode putative spermatogenesis genes.[105]

Immunologic Parameters

Antibodies to sperm surface antigens have been explored as a cause of infertility. They are thought to impair fertility by decreasing motility, increasing agglutination, and impairing the ability of sperm to penetrate human ova.[295] However, this is controversial, and laboratory testing for antisperm antibodies is rarely performed. The reader is directed to the previous edition of this chapter for further details about methods.[131]

BOX 56-5 Female Infertility Factors

Ovarian or Hormonal Factors
- Metabolic disease
  - Thyroid
  - Liver
  - Obesity
  - Androgen excess
  - Polycystic ovarian syndrome
- Hypergonadotropic hypogonadism
  - Menopause
  - Luteal phase deficiency
  - Gonadal dysgenesis
  - Primary ovarian insufficiency (autoimmune, cytotoxic, chemotherapy, radiation, tumor)
  - Resistant ovary syndrome
- Hypogonadotropic hypogonadism
  - Hyperprolactinemia (tumor, drugs)
  - Hypothalamic insufficiency (Kallmann syndrome)
  - Pituitary insufficiency (tumor, necrosis, thrombosis, stress, exercise, anorexia)

Tubal Factors
- Occlusion or scarring
- Salpingitis isthmica nodosa
- Infectious salpingitis

Cervical Factors
- Stenosis
- Inflammation or infection
- Abnormal mucous viscosity

Uterine Factors
- Leiomyomata
- Congenital malformation
- Adhesions
- Endometritis or abnormal endometrium

Psychosocial Factors
- Decreased libido
- Anorgasmia

Iatrogenic

Immunologic (Antisperm Antibodies)

Modified from Morell V. Basic infertility assessment. Primary Care 1997;24:195-204.

Female Infertility

Evaluating female infertility is more complex than evaluating infertility of the male. A list of the most common female infertility factors is given in Box 56-5. One algorithm for the evaluation of female infertility is shown in Figure 56-13. This evaluation should be considered after 1 year of unprotected intercourse in women with regular menses younger than 35. If a woman is over the age of 35, or if the woman or her partner has a history of issues that would contribute to infertility, this work-up should ensue sooner. Examples of issues that would prompt earlier work-up include (1) irregular menses, (2) history of pelvic inflammatory disease or

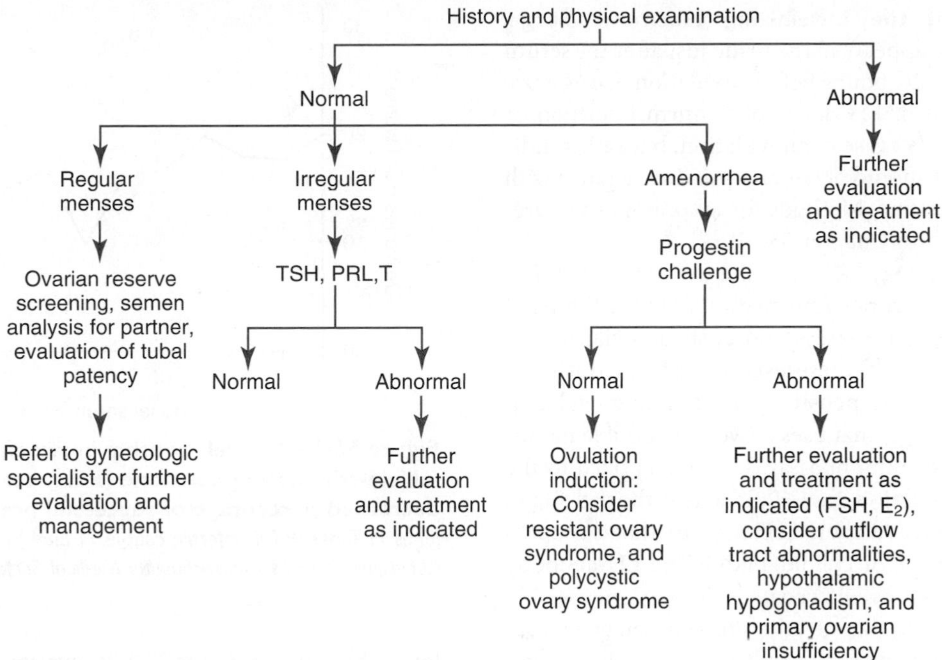

Figure 56-13 Algorithm for the evaluation of female infertility. ***FSH,*** **Follicle-stimulating hormone;** ***LH,*** **luteinizing hormone;** ***PRL,*** **prolactin;** ***T,*** **testosterone;** ***TSH,*** **thyroid-stimulating hormone.**

(3) sexually transmitted infection, and (4) history of exposure to gonadotoxic agents.

Initial Evaluation of Female Infertility

The initial evaluation of female infertility should include a detailed history and physical examination. The physical examination should include evaluation of (1) the external genitalia and hair pattern (for signs of androgen excess, including clitoromegaly, hirsutism, and virilization), (2) the pelvis (for masses, nodularity, or tenderness), (3) the breasts (for signs of galactorrhea), (4) neurologic findings (sense of smell and visual impairments), (5) the thyroid (for enlargement or nodules), and (6) body mass index. All abnormalities in the history and physical examination should be pursued. A thorough medical and surgical history is also necessary, including an assessment of the patient's (1) gravidity and parity, (2) coital frequency, (3) duration of infertility, and (4) prior work-up and treatment for infertility. History of sexually transmitted infections, assessment of previous cervical cytologic and human papillomavirus (HPV) testing and treatment, and a menstrual history also should be obtained. Concentrations of TSH, testosterone, and prolactin should be measured if menstrual cycles are absent or irregular, or if signs of galactorrhea or thyroid abnormalities are present. Ovulation reserve testing as discussed here should be considered in cases where diminished ovarian reserve is suspected.

Evaluation of Ovulation

In the menstruating woman, the next step would be to determine whether ovulation occurs. No current laboratory tests will confirm ovum release. However, measurement of the concentration of mid-luteal plasma progesterone does indicate that a corpus luteum was formed. Other methods such as measurement of the LH surge (to predict ovulation) and basal body temperature (to detect a rise in progesterone) have been used to assess ovulation.

Progesterone Measurement. Measurement of the concentration of serum progesterone is the primary assay used for the evaluation of ovulation.[149,265] It is important to note that an increase in progesterone concentration indicates that a corpus luteum has been formed, but does not confirm that the egg was actually released. Beginning immediately after ovulation, serum progesterone concentrations rise (see Figure 56-10); they peak within 5 to 9 days during the mid-luteal phase (days 21 to 23).[265] If ovulation does not occur, the corpus luteum fails to form, and the expected cyclic rise in progesterone concentration is subnormal. If pregnancy occurs, hCG maintains the corpus luteum, and progesterone production continues to rise. Mid-luteal progesterone concentrations greater than 3 ng/mL indicate that ovulation has taken place, although concentrations of 10 ng/mL or more are more common in conception cycles. Concentrations less than 10 ng/mL indicate the possibility of inadequate luteal phase progesterone production, or inappropriate timing of sample collection.[323]

Basal Body Temperature. Basal body temperature charts have long been accepted as simple, cost-effective indicators of ovulation. Ovulation is associated with a rapid rise in body temperature (by 0.5 °F), which persists through the luteal phase. The rise in temperature is due to increased progesterone concentration. However, similar to progesterone, the rise in body temperature is evident only retrospectively and therefore does not predict imminent ovulation in a way helpful for timing intercourse.

Measurement of the Luteinizing Hormone Surge. Luteinizing hormone appears in the urine just after the serum LH surge and 24 to 36 hours before ovulation (see Figure 56-10). Measurement of LH does not confirm ovulation or provide insight into the cause of anovulation, but rather indicates when ovulation should occur and provides a guide with which to time intercourse. Methods for laboratory measurement of LH are given in Chapter 53.

Monoclonal technology has led to the use of *home LH kits* that not only provide accurate information as to the timing of ovulation, but may reduce stress and costs associated with infertility programs, because these tests are performed at home and are comparatively inexpensive.[171] Most home ovulation kits consist of a "dipstick" that uses a two-site, double monoclonal enzyme-linked immunoassay. Urine is applied to the test pad, and capillary action draws fluid across the pad. LH in the urine first is bound to an anti-LH antibody that is coupled to an enzyme conjugate, or colloidal gold. The LH-antibody complex then migrates to a region coated with a second anti-LH antibody. Once bound to this site, the substrate-enzyme reaction or colloidal gold complexes result in a color change that is proportional to the amount of LH present. A reference region is provided. A test result that matches or is darker in color than the reference region is considered a positive result, indicating that the LH surge is occurring. These tests effectively predict ovulation in 70% of women.[86] In one study of 26 normal women, home LH kits had a 92% positive predictive value for ovulation to occur within 48 hours of a positive urine LH screen.[204] The clinical utility of these devices is controversial, however,[225] and no studies have been performed to determine whether the use of home LH devices alters outcomes in women not being treated for infertility. A few studies have been published to look at outcomes in infertility patients, but the results are mixed when compared with serum LH testing or basal body temperature.[225]

Evaluation of Endocrine Parameters

Disorders of hypothalamus, pituitary, and ovary are endocrine causes of infertility.

Hypergonadotropic Hypogonadism

Premature ovarian failure is indicated by repeatedly elevated basal FSH concentrations (>30 IU/L) or a single elevation of greater than 40 IU/L in a woman younger than 40 years. These patients are hypoestrogenic (E_2 < 20 IU/L)[265] and do not respond to a progestin challenge because their endometrium is atrophic (see earlier section on evaluation of secondary amenorrhea). Basal serum FSH has been used as an indicator of relative ovarian reserve. Figure 56-14 shows the relationship between rising serum FSH and the reduced rate of successful pregnancy. A precipitous drop occurs at concentrations greater than 20 IU/L.

Assessing Ovarian Reserve

Women in their mid to late 30s and early 40s with infertility constitute the largest portion of the total infertility population. These women are also at increased risk for pregnancy

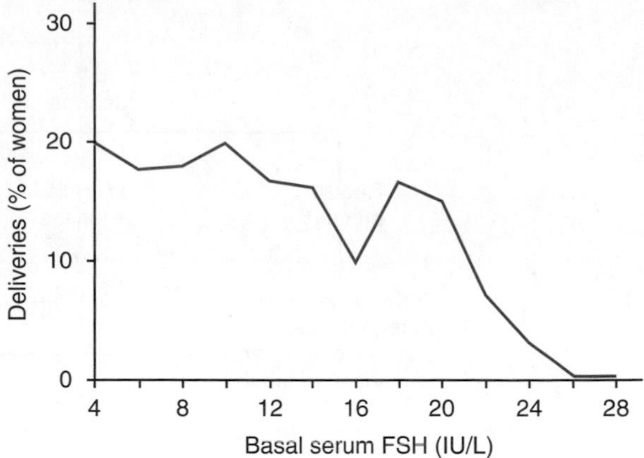

Figure 56-14 The relationship between increasing follicle-stimulating hormone (FSH) concentrations and decreased percentage of successful pregnancies. *(From Jones H, Toner JP. The infertile couple. N Engl J Med 1993;329:1710-5. Copyright © 1993 Massachusetts Medical Society. All rights reserved.)*

loss. This reflects a diminished ovarian reserve as a result of follicular depletion and a decline in oocyte quality. As women age, serum FSH concentrations in the early follicular phase begin to increase. It has been suggested that this is due to a decline in the number of small follicles secreting inhibin B.

Basal serum FSH and E_2 measurements are a popular screening test for assessing ovarian reserve before fertility treatment is initiated. The rise in basal FSH is an excellent indicator of ovarian aging. In general, day 3 FSH concentrations greater than 20 to 25 IU/L are considered to be elevated and associated with poor reproductive outcome.[158] Concomitant measurement of serum E_2 concentration adds to the predictive power of an isolated FSH determination. Basal E_2 concentrations greater than 75 to 80 pg/mL are associated with poor response to ovarian stimulation and pregnancy outcome.[181]

Inhibin B is produced by developing follicles, and concentrations peak during the follicular phase. Concentrations of inhibin B can be used in conjunction with serum FSH and E_2 to assess ovarian function. Because inhibin is produced by gonadal tissue, it is thought to be a more direct marker of gonadal activity and ovarian reserve than pituitary hormones alone. In addition, cycle day 3 inhibin B concentrations may demonstrate a decrease before day 3 FSH concentrations.[268]

It has been reported that women undergoing in vitro fertilization (IVF) with day 3 inhibin B concentration less than 45 pg/mL had a pregnancy rate of 7% and a spontaneous abortion rate of 33% as compared with a pregnancy rate of 26% and an abortion rate of 3% in women with day 3 inhibin B concentrations greater than 45 pg/mL.[267] However, measurement of inhibin adds little to the more established use of serum FSH and E_2 and transvaginal ultrasound. Measurement of inhibins, therefore, remains of research interest only.

Anti-Müllerian hormone (AMH) [also known as Müllerian-inhibiting substance (MIS)] has been promoted as a marker of ovarian reserve and decline in reproductive capacity,[30,92,300,301] as well as response to assisted reproductive technologies.[166,178] Although assays are commercially available, cutoffs have yet to be established.

Increasing evidence indicates that young women with spontaneous premature ovarian failure are at increased risk of developing autoimmune adrenal insufficiency.[20,31,65,217] It has been suggested that adrenal antibodies (21-hydroxylase antibodies or adrenal cortex autoantibodies) should be measured as a screening test for all women with spontaneous premature ovarian failure. Patients with antibodies present and patients with signs and symptoms of adrenal insufficiency should be tested using a standard ACTH stimulation test.

Luteal phase deficiency is diagnosed when the time between ovulation and menses is 10 days or less. The most specific diagnostic information may be gained from an endometrial biopsy obtained on day 26 of a 28 day cycle.[318] If peak progesterone concentrations are repetitively below 10 ng/mL, it is possible to diagnose luteal phase deficiency without an endometrial biopsy. Decreased progesterone production is presumed to be responsible, but this may follow (1) insufficient follicular phase FSH secretion, (2) abnormal LH surge, or (3) other endocrine abnormalities.[277] Some studies show that luteal phase deficiency is no more prevalent in infertile women than in normal women.[273,317] Other studies have shown an association with increased risk of infertility, ectopic pregnancy, and spontaneous abortion.[28,122] Luteal phase dysfunction may be secondary to excess androgen production, which suppresses follicle development. Prolactin excess may also contribute to the development of this disorder.[283]

Hypogonadotropic Hypogonadism

In hypogonadotropic hypogonadism, serum E_2 concentrations are less than 40 pg/mL (110 pmol/L); therefore, there is no withdrawal bleeding with a progestin challenge.[255] Decreased LH (<10 IU/L) and decreased FSH (<10 IU/L) are also present.[265] Hyperprolactinemia can cause hypergonadotropic hypogonadic infertility. The upper limit of normal plasma prolactin in an amenorrheic, hypoestrogenic, nonpregnant woman is 400 to 500 mIU/mL (20 to 25 ng/mL). If estrogen status is normal, maximum prolactin concentrations vary from 600 to 800 mIU/mL (30 to 40 ng/mL).[179] Thyroid-stimulating hormone should be measured to exclude hypothyroidism. Prolactin concentrations can be elevated in patients with PCOS and those taking medications such as antidepressants, cimetidine, and methyldopa, and in stressful conditions. Radiographic imaging of the pituitary is indicated to rule out pituitary adenoma or empty sella syndrome.

Ovulatory Factors

Ovulatory dysfunction is difficult to diagnose because it will manifest in the presence or absence of normal menses. Metabolic diseases of many types affect ovulatory function, including those that result in androgen excess. PCOS, which results in androgen excess, is the most common cause of anovulation and was discussed in detail earlier in the chapter. In women with hirsutism, CAH should be considered. 21-Hydroxylase deficiency or 3-β-hydroxysteroid deficiency may be present in up to 26% of cases.[228] Elevated serum follicular 17-hydroxyprogesterone concentrations require further evaluation for these conditions. In addition, it is possible for ovulatory dysfunction to be secondary to liver or thyroid disorders.

As with male infertility, hypogonadism (hypergonadotropic or hypogonadotropic) results in female infertility. Causes of hypergonadotropic hypogonadism include (1) primary ovarian insufficiency (POI), (2) gonadal dysgenesis, (3) resistant ovary syndrome, (4) menopause, and (5) luteal phase deficiency. Causes of hypogonadotropic hypogonadism include pituitary or hypothalamic insufficiency and hyperprolactinemia. Many of these pathologic states have been discussed in the earlier section, "Irregular Menses."

Ovulation with inadequate luteinization and reduced progesterone secretion during the luteal phase has been termed *luteal phase deficiency*. The contribution of luteal insufficiency to infertility is controversial. It is manifested by a short luteal phase, in which the interval between LH peak and onset of menses is 10 days or longer, or is a luteal phase of normal length with reduced progesterone secretion.[50] Decreased progesterone production is presumed to be responsible, but this may follow insufficient follicular phase FSH secretion, abnormal LH surge, or other endocrine abnormalities.[277] The most specific diagnostic information may be gained from an endometrial biopsy obtained on day 26 of a 28 day cycle.[318] Some studies show luteal phase deficiency to be no more prevalent in infertile women than in normal women.[273,317] Other studies have shown an association with increased risk of infertility, ectopic pregnancy, and spontaneous abortion.[28,122] Luteal phase dysfunction may also be secondary to excess androgen production, which suppresses follicle development. Prolactin excess may contribute to the development of this disorder.[283] An inadequate luteal phase and a deficit of progesterone lead to poor proliferation of the endometrium and, therefore, an unsuitable environment for the early embryo.[50,336] Luteal dysfunction is believed to cause infertility in 5% of infertile women. It is found periodically in 30% of women and is not considered to contribute to infertility unless diagnosed twice in separate cycles.[307]

Postcoital Test

The postcoital test has been used historically to evaluate infertility; however, it has been shown to have limited utility. The reader is directed to the previous edition of this chapter for further reading on this test.[131]

Immunologic Factors

Antisperm antibodies have been proposed to contribute to female infertility. However, this topic is controversial, and laboratory testing for antisperm antibodies is rarely performed. The reader is directed to the previous edition of this chapter for further details about methods.[131]

Assisted Reproduction

Couples with a multitude of infertility problems, including unidentified causes and persistent infertility despite standard treatments, may benefit from assisted reproductive techniques. If no definable cause is identified, standard initial therapy consists of ovulation induction and artificial insemination for at least 6 months before progression to more expensive and exotic techniques. If very low sperm counts or tubal pathology is present, it may be reasonable to proceed directly to in vitro fertilization.

The laboratory plays an important role in the process of ovulation induction. The principle involves administration of gonadotropins to stimulate follicular growth, followed by hCG to stimulate ovulation follicular maturation. Clinical, laboratory, and ultrasound monitoring of the treatment cycle is necessary to (1) identify the dose and length of therapy, (2) determine when or whether to administer hCG, and (3) obtain an adequate ovulatory response while avoiding hyperstimulation.[266]

Infertility treatments involve procedures that deliver a concentrated sperm sample directly to the uterus (artificial insemination) or assisted reproductive techniques. The latter are techniques that involve acquiring fertile ova using transvaginal ultrasound and assisting fertilization in the laboratory with conventional IVF or intracytoplasmic sperm injection (ICSI) in the fallopian tubes using gamete intrafallopian transfer (GIFT) or zygote intrafallopian transfer (ZIFT).[210] In vitro fertilization then requires embryo transfer back into the uterus. Very few GIFT or ZIFT procedures are performed today owing to the availability of improved embryo culture techniques. The latest successful techniques include direct ovum fertilization using direct micropipette ICSI of the sperm.[269] This procedures provides hope to even the azoospermic man for whom testicular aspiration may yield a few nonmotile sperm. ICSI is widely used today for non–male factor infertility cases as well, and is employed in about 50% to 60% of IVF cycles.

ANALYTICAL METHODS FOR REPRODUCTIVE HORMONES

A variety of methods are available for measuring sex steroids in body fluids. Currently, the most common method is nonisotopic immunoassay. However, use of mass spectrometry to measure sex steroids is increasing. Advantages and disadvantages will be discussed in this chapter. Methods used for reproductive protein hormones are discussed in Chapters 53 and 57. Methods used for reproductive steroid hormones are discussed here.

Methods for Determination of Total Testosterone in Blood

Circulating testosterone comprises three different forms or pools: (1) a non–protein-bound or "free" form, (2) a weakly bound form, and (3) a tightly bound form. The weakly bound form is associated with albumin, and the tightly bound form with sex hormone-binding globulin (SHBG), which is also known as testosterone/estradiol-binding globulin. The term *total testosterone* refers to serum measurements of free testosterone, albumin-bound testosterone, and SHBG-bound testosterone. Bioavailable testosterone includes circulating free testosterone and albumin-bound testosterone. Testosterone bound to SHBG is not biologically active, whereas the free form is available for target cells. Albumin-bound testosterone is also available to target tissues because testosterone can dissociate from the albumin carrier and rapidly diffuse into target cells.[192]

Methods

A 2008 College of American Pathologists (CAP) survey reports that nonisotopic enzyme immunoassays have replaced radioimmunoassay (RIA) as the most widely used technique for measuring the concentration of circulating testosterone (both protein-bound and non–protein-bound forms).[3]

For more about RIAs for testosterone, the reader is directed to the previous edition of this chapter.[131]

Direct (no extraction required) immunoassay methods have been developed for the determination of testosterone in serum or plasma.[143,157] The steroid must be displaced from its binding proteins (albumin and SHBG). In this method, results of the assay depend on the effectiveness of the displacement. Methods used to release testosterone from endogenous binding proteins include use of (1) salicylates, (2) surfactants, (3) pH alterations, (4) temperature changes, and (5) competing steroids such as estrone or estradiol. Most of the direct immunologic methods use antisera generated against a C_{19} testosterone-protein conjugate. These assays have demonstrated variable precision agreement with mass spectrophotometry and established RIA methods.[96,260,321] However, most routine immunoassays are not sensitive enough to measure very low testosterone concentrations such as those found in women, children, or hypogonadal men. The Endocrine Society recommends use of a highly sensitive method such as a liquid chromatography/mass spectrometry/mass spectrometry (LC/MS/MS) method whenever low testosterone concentrations are suspected.[254]

Gas chromatography combined with mass spectrometry (GC-MS) remains the reference method for testosterone measurement and is often used to assess the bias of routine immunoassay methods.[83,94,96] Several mass spectrometry–based methods have been described.[270,291] The use of mass spectrometry is discussed in greater detail in Chapter 14 and later in this section.

Regardless of immunoassay type, almost all testosterone antisera show some degree of cross-reactivity with DHT (typically 3 to 5%) but show negligible cross-reactivity with other androgens. Assays that use antisera generated against the C-19 position provide maximum analytical specificity with respect to endogenous steroids. However, cross-reactions with 19-nonsteroids used in contraceptive preparations sometimes cause a problem. In most clinical situations, estimation of testosterone without prior separation of DHT is permitted because plasma concentrations of DHT are only 10 to 20% of those for testosterone. Moreover, testosterone and DHT are the two most important androgens in the systemic circulation; even when a method measures the concentrations of both, clinically useful information about the total androgen load is obtained. DHEA-S has been reported to cross-react in some testosterone assays.[202] If specific estimation of testosterone concentration is required, mass spectrometry is recommended.

Specimen Collection and Storage

Serum or heparinized plasma is used to measure total testosterone. Testosterone is subject to diurnal variation, reaching a peak concentration at between 0400 and 0800 hours. Therefore, morning specimens are preferred. Serum/plasma samples are stable for up to 24 hours at room temperature, up to 1 week refrigerated, and up to 1 year frozen at −20 °C.[80,121] DHEA supplementation should be avoided before testing.[320]

Reference Intervals

Reference intervals for total testosterone in serum are listed in Table 56-4.[9,293]

Comments

Estimation of SHBG in serum is useful for interpreting blood concentrations of total testosterone and for calculating androgen index and bioavailable testosterone. Immunoassays for measurement of SHBG in the routine laboratory have been developed.[148] SHBG concentrations change with age.[88]

Methods for the Determination of Free and Bioavailable Testosterone in Blood

In cases where SHBG concentrations are altered, as in women, aging men, and illness, measurements of free or bioavailable testosterone are thought to more accurately reflect androgen status. Excellent reviews of various methods used to measure this fraction of testosterone are available.[319]

Various methods are available for determining the concentrations of free or bioavailable forms of testosterone in serum or plasma. They include the following:

1. Estimation of the free testosterone fraction by equilibrium dialysis or ultrafiltration.
2. Estimation of free hormone using a direct (analog tracer) radioimmunoassay.
3. Estimation of combined free and weakly bound (bioavailable) testosterone fractions by selective precipitation of the tightly bound form.
4. Calculation of the androgen index using indices that reflect the ratios of testosterone pools.
5. Calculation of free and weakly bound testosterone concentrations by mathematical modeling.

Each approach will be discussed in turn in the following sections. Reference intervals for free testosterone and percent free testosterone in serum are listed in Table 56-5. Reference intervals for bioavailable testosterone in serum are listed in Table 56-6.

Equilibrium Dialysis/Ultrafiltration

Only a small fraction (1 to 2%) of unconjugated testosterone exists in the free state (non–protein-bound) in serum or plasma. None of the conventional assay methods, including

TABLE 56-4 Reference Intervals for Total Testosterone in Serum

Testosterone (method: LC/MS/MS)	ng/dL	nmol/L
Adults		
18-69 y, males	250-1100	8.7-38.2
females		
70-89 y, males	2-45	0.07-1.6
70-94 y, females	90-890	3.1-30.9
1st-trimester pregnancy	2-40	0.07-1.4
2nd-trimester pregnancy	20-135	0.7-4.7
3rd-trimester pregnancy	11-153	0.4-5.3
Children	11-146	0.4-5.1
Cord blood, males	17-61	0.6-2.1
females	16-44	0.6-1.5
1-10 d, males	≤187	≤6.5
females	≤24	≤0.8
1-3 mo, males	72-344	2.5-11.9
females	≤17	≤0.59
3-5 mo, males	≤201	≤7.0
females	≤12	≤0.4
5-7 mo, males	≤59	≤2.1
females	≤13	≤0.5
7-12 mo, males	≤16	≤0.6
females	≤11	≤0.4
1-5.9 y, males	≤5	≤0.2
females	≤8	≤0.3
6-7.9 y, males	≤25	≤0.9
females	≤20	≤0.7
8-10.9 y, males	≤42	≤1.5
females	≤35	≤1.2
11-11.9 y, males	≤260	≤9.0
females	≤40	≤1.4
12-13.9 y, males	≤420	≤14.6
females	≤40	≤1.4
14-17.9 y, males	≤1000	≤34.7
females	≤40	≤1.4
Tanner stages		
I, males	≤5	≤0.2
females	≤8	≤0.3
II, males	≤167	≤5.8
females	≤24	≤0.8
III, males	21-719	0.7-25.0
females	≤28	≤1.0
IV, males	25-912	0.9-31.7
females	≤31	≤1.1
V, males	110-975	3.8-33.8
females	≤33	≤1.2

From Fisher DA, ed. The Quest Diagnostics manual: endocrinology, test selection and interpretation, 4th edition. Capistrano, Calif: Quest Diagnostics/Nichols Institute, 2007.

TABLE 56-5 Reference Intervals for Free Testosterone in Serum

Free Testosterone (method: tracer equilibrium dialysis)	pg/mL	pmol/L	Free Fraction, % of Total
Men			
18-69 y	35.0-155.0	121-538	1.5-2.2
70-89 y	30.0-135.0	104-468	1.5-2.2
Women			
18-69 y	0.1-6.4	0.4-22.2	0.5-2.0
70-89 y	0.2-3.7	0.7-12.8	0.5-2.0
Pregnancy			
1st trimester	0.5-6.0	1.7-20.8	0.15-0.66
2nd trimester	0.2-3.1	0.7-10.8	0.10-0.34
3rd trimester	0.2-4.1	0.7-14.2	0.15-0.51
Children, males			
5-9 y	≤5.3	≤18.4	0.44-1.78
10-13 y	0.7-52.0	2.4-180	0.53-3.33
14-17 y	18.0-111.0	62-385	1.05-2.91

From Fisher DA, ed. The Quest Diagnostics manual: endocrinology, test selection and interpretation, 4th edition. Capistrano, Calif: Quest Diagnostics/Nichols Institute, 2007.

TABLE 56-6 Reference Intervals for Bioavailable Testosterone in Serum

Bioavailable Testosterone (method: calculation)	ng/dL	nmol/L
Adults		
18-69 y, males	110-575	3.8-20.0
females	0.5-8.5	0.02-0.3
70-89 y, males	15-150	0.5-5.2
females	0.5-8.8	0.02-0.3
Children		
1-11.9 y, males	≤5.4	≤0.2
females	≤3.4	≤0.1
12-13.9 y, males	≤140	≤4.9
females	≤3.4	≤0.1
14-17.9 y, males	8.0-210	0.3-7.3
females	≤7.8	≤0.3

From Fisher DA, ed. The Quest Diagnostics manual: endocrinology, test selection and interpretation, 4th edition. Capistrano, Calif: Quest Diagnostics/Nichols Institute, 2007.

RIA, is sufficiently sensitive to quantify free steroid directly in a protein-free ultrafiltrate of plasma. Instead, free steroid is estimated in plasma by adding a known amount of radiolabeled compound to the sample and allowing labeled and unlabeled compounds to reach equilibrium in their competition for the same binding sites on proteins. Bound and free radiolabeled fractions are then separated, and the ratio of free labeled to total labeled compound is determined. At equilibrium, this ratio is taken as a measure of the free testosterone fraction. An estimate of serum free testosterone can be calculated by multiplying the free testosterone fraction by the total testosterone concentration. A detailed procedure for the equilibrium dialysis method is included in the third edition of this textbook.[117]

Most of the problems with this procedure have involved tracer impurities and separation of bound and free labeled fractions. Several separation techniques have been used, including (1) equilibrium dialysis, (2) membrane ultrafiltration, and (3) steady-state gel filtration. Deficiencies associated with these techniques include (1) a requirement for a large sample volume, (2) the need for complicated correction of sample volume changes that occur during the separation, and (3) difficulties involved in collecting and measuring radioactivity in numerous fractions of each sample. Equilibrium dialysis has been used most often in the past, but serious errors often arise from the sample dilution required by this method.[305] Symmetric dialysis of undiluted samples is reported to be less susceptible to tracer contamination and dilution effects.[284] Ultrafiltration appears to overcome these problems and to obviate errors due to dilution.[125]

Direct (Analog Tracer) Radioimmunoassay

Several RIA procedures are commercially available for the direct estimation of free testosterone.[157,209,256,319,326] These assays use a labeled derivative (analog) of testosterone that, in theory, retains the ability to react with exogenous antitestosterone antibodies but is restricted from interacting with testosterone-binding proteins in the serum sample.

Advantages of RIA analog methods include a small sample requirement, relatively rapid results, a simple procedure, and the option to measure free testosterone without the need to measure total testosterone.[157,209,306,326] Thus, RIA analog assays are the most commonly used method for determining free testosterone. Although there is reportedly good correlation between values obtained by RIA and equilibrium dialysis, some have reported that RIAs are grossly inaccurate, underestimating free testosterone concentrations by manyfold.[209,252,253,306] For example, one study in females revealed that free testosterone concentrations obtained by two different analog assays were 15 to 35% and 25 to 30% of those obtained by ultrafiltration.[120] Calculated free testosterone is considered more reliable than values obtained by the RIA method.

Selective Precipitation

Selective precipitation of SHBG with ammonium sulfate is also used to measure bioavailable testosterone. With this technique, aliquots of serum or plasma are first incubated with radiolabeled testosterone. Testosterone bound to SHBG is then precipitated with 50% ammonium sulfate. The samples are centrifuged, and aliquots of the supernatant containing free and albumin-bound testosterone (also known as *non-SHBG-bound testosterone*) are radioactively counted. The percentage of radio label not bound to SHBG is subsequently multiplied by the total testosterone concentration to obtain the bioavailable testosterone.[319] The amount of bioavailable testosterone also is measured directly, by RIA, in the supernatants of plasma after ammonium sulfate precipitation and solvent extraction.[74] An indirect method using a commercially available enzyme immunoassay to measure bioavailable testosterone has been described.[69] Alternatively, it is possible to estimate the fraction of testosterone not bound to SHBG by a technique that involves saturating SHBG-binding sites with 5α-DHT, the natural steroid bound with highest affinity by SHBG. Then the non–protein-bound fraction is measured in treated and untreated samples by centrifugal ultrafiltration dialysis[233] or by semiautomated equilibrium dialysis.[25]

Androgen Index

This index is a ratio of testosterone and SHBG multiplied by 100.[319] Although this is only an indicator of free testosterone, some have found it to be useful in the evaluation of hirsutism.[214] Other reports have indicated that the free androgen index is not a reliable parameter of free testosterone because of its variability as a function of SHBG concentration.[152,209,306]

Mathematical Modeling

Methods based on mathematical modeling use algorithms to derive non–SHBG-bound testosterone. These algorithms assume that when concentrations of total testosterone, SHBG, and albumin and the constants for binding of testosterone to SHBG and albumin are known, free testosterone and bioavailable testosterone are calculated. These calculations are based on a proper estimation of the association constant for binding of testosterone to SHBG and albumin. However, various association constants for SHBG have been reported. The reader is directed to the previous edition of this book and other references for further details on this method.[131,274,319] Conditions resulting in abnormal plasma protein concentrations such as nephritic syndrome, cirrhosis, and pregnancy require adjustments in the assumption for albumin concentration.

Other algorithms based on concentrations measured with a gold standard technique have been proposed.[89,187,211]

Algorithms for calculating bioavailable testosterone are available free on the Internet (http://www.issam.ch/freetesto.htm); however, these sources do not always provide a reference for which an algorithm is being used.

In practice, it should be noted that no consensus has been reached about the use of these bioavailable testosterone algorithms. de Ronde and associates compared five algorithms and concluded that they are not transferable to samples from other laboratories unless revalidation using laboratory-specific assays has been performed.[71] Likewise, Giton and colleagues reported that instead of using theoretical association constants, optimal paired association constants should be determined for each studied population.[102] Because this is impossible for the average clinician to do, these authors suggest using ammonium sulfate precipitation. Finally, Dechaud and coworkers reported an age-associated discrepancy between calculated and measured bioavailable testosterone, suggesting that a simplified law of mass action cannot predict variations in steroid distribution in serum.[73] These authors state that consensus is needed regarding the proper measurement of bioavailable testosterone for therapeutic decisions.

Methods for the Determination of Testosterone Precursors and Metabolites in Blood

Several biosynthetic precursors and metabolites of testosterone are measured using (1) specific immunoassays (directly or after sample extraction), (2) chromatography, or (3) LC-MS/MS.[239,270,275,288] Examples include DHT, 3α-androstanediol glucuronide, and androstenedione.

Reference intervals for these analytes in serum are listed in Table 56-7.

Methods for the Determination of Dehydroepiandrosterone and Its Sulfate

Measurements of DHEA or its sulfated conjugate, DHEA-S, in serum and plasma are important for investigations of adrenal androgen production, such as assessment of (1) adrenal hyperplasia, (2) adrenal tumors, (3) adrenarche, (4) delayed puberty, or (5) hirsutism. DHEA-S in circulation originates primarily from the adrenal glands, although in men some may be derived from the testes; none is produced by the ovaries. DHEA is secreted almost entirely by the adrenal glands.

DHEA concentrations exhibit a circadian rhythm that reflects the secretion of ACTH; these concentrations vary during the menstrual cycle. DHEA-S concentrations, however, do not exhibit a circadian rhythm because of their longer circulating half-life.[224] Concentrations in serum are increased in cord blood and drop precipitously at birth. Concentrations in premature infants in general are much higher than those in full-term infants. Pregnancy and oral contraceptives induce a modest reduction, and glucocorticoids a marked decrease. Patients with polycystic ovary disease often have elevated concentrations of DHEA-S, suggesting an adrenal androgen contribution to the defect in this disorder.[221] Concentrations of DHEA-S are also elevated in CAH and with adrenal cortical tumors (concentrations higher with adrenal carcinoma than with adrenal adenoma).[224] However, concentrations are not elevated in women with virilizing ovarian tumors. Glucocorticoid administration for several days suppresses concentrations in patients with adrenal hyperplasia. DHEA is commercially available in health food stores; therefore, increased serum concentrations may be due to exogenous use.

Methods

Although both isotopic and nonisotopic methods are available, according to a 2008 CAP survey, the latter are most frequently utilized for measurement of DHEA-S.[11] Other methods include competitive protein-binding assays[40,42,248] and GC-MS.[330,339] Immunoassays for DHEA-S demonstrate significant cross-reactivity with DHEA, androstenedione, and androsterone, yet the relative concentrations of these steroids have a minimal effect on assay performance.

TABLE 56-7 Reference Intervals for Dihydrotestosterone (DHT), 3α-Androstanediol Glucuronide, and Androstenedione in Serum

	ng/dL	nmol/L
Dihydrotestosterone (DHT) (method: RIA)		
Adult men	25-75	0.09-2.6
Adult women	5-30	0.17-1.0
Children (prepubertal)		
Cord blood, males	<2-8	<0.07-0.28
females	<2-5	<0.07-0.17
1-6 mo, males	12-85	0.41-2.9
females	<5	<0.2
Prepubertal, males	<5	<0.2
females	<5	<0.2
Tanner II-III, males	3-33	0.10-1.1
females	5-19	0.2-0.7
Tanner IV-V, males	22-75	0.76-2.6
females	3-30	0.1-1.0
3α-Androstanediol Glucuronide (method: RIA)		
Men	260-1500	5.5-32
Women	60-300	1.3-6.4
Children		
Prepubertal	10-60	0.2-1.3
Tanner II-III		
Males	19-164	0.4-4.5
Females	33-244	0.7-5.2
Androstenedione (method: LC/MS/MS)		
Men		
18-30 y	50-220	1.7-7.7
31-50 y	40-190	1.4-6.6
51-60 y	50-220	1.7-7.7
Women		
Follicular	35-250	1.2-8.7
Midcycle	60-285	2.1-9.9
Luteal	30-235	1.0-8.2
Postmenopausal	20-75	0.7-2.6
Children		
1-12 mo	6-78	0.2-2.7
1-4 y	5-51	0.2-1.8
5-9 y	6-115	0.2-4.0
10-13 y	12-221	0.4-7.7
14-17 y	22-225	0.8-7.9
Tanner II-III		
Males	17-82	0.6-2.9
Females	43-180	1.5-6.3
Tanner IV-V		
Males	57-150	2.0-5.2
Females	73-220	2.6-7.7

From Fisher DA, ed. The Quest Diagnostics manual: endocrinology, test selection and interpretation, 4th edition. Capistrano, Calif: Quest Diagnostics/Nichols Institute, 2007.

Specimen Collection and Storage

Serum or plasma [preserved with ethylenediaminetetraacetic acid (EDTA)] is suitable for DHEA or DHEA-S immunoassays.[4,7] Early morning collection, before 1030 hours, is preferred for DHEA.[4,8] DHEA-S specimens are stable for at least 1 day at room temperature. Refrigerated serum/plasma samples (4 to 8 °C) are stable for up to 14 days, and those frozen at −20 °C are stable for longer than 1 year.[80,121,338]

Reference Intervals

Reference intervals for serum concentrations of DHEA-S and DHEA are listed in Table 56-8.[7,293]

Comments

Analysis of DHEA by immunoassay usually requires pretreatment of serum samples because the serum concentration of DHEA is 1000-fold lower than that of DHEA-S. Several extraction and chromatographic procedures have been suggested for this purpose. Celite is the preferred adsorbent, and dichloromethane and ethyl acetate are common choices for extraction solvents. Commercial RIA kits using solid-phase separation techniques and ^{125}I-labeled DHEA are widely available for convenient measurement of serum concentrations. A typical kit method will detect as little as 3 ng/dL (0.1 nmol/L) of DHEA.[4] Cross-reactivity of antisera with related steroids is relatively low, with some exceptions (androstanediol, about 6%; androstenedione, about 2%; and testosterone, about 1%). Interextraction precision, expressed as a coefficient of variation, is less than ±12% at a DHEA concentration of 120 ng/dL (4.1 nmol/L).

Determination of 17-Ketosteroids in Urine

The 17-ketosteroids (KS) are metabolites of steroids that contain a keto group at C-17 and include (1) androsterone, (2) epiandrosterone, (3) etiocholanolone, (4) DHEA, (5) 11-keto- and 11β-hydroxyandrosterone, and (6) 11-keto- and 11β-hydroxyetiocholanolone. In men, approximately one third of total urinary 17-KS represents metabolites of testosterone secreted by the testes, whereas most of the remaining two thirds is derived from steroids produced by the adrenal glands. In women, who normally excrete smaller quantities than men, total 17-KS concentrations are derived almost exclusively from the adrenal glands. Thus, the main purpose of measuring these steroid metabolites is to assess adrenal androgen production.

Measurement of DHEA-S in serum serves as a more convenient marker for adrenal androgen production than does urinary 17-KS excretion because 24 hour urine collection is not required, and because many drugs interfere with the 17-KS assay.[184] For these reasons, many clinicians now prefer concentrations for plasma DHEA-S to those for urinary 17-KS. For a description of the method used to measure 17-KS in urine, please refer to the fourth edition of this textbook.[131]

TABLE 56-8 Reference Intervals for Dehydroepiandrosterone Sulfate (DHEA-S) and Unconjugated Dehydroepiandrosterone (DHEA) in Serum

Dehydroepiandrosterone Sulfate (DHEA-S) (method: immunochemiluminometric assay)	μg/dL	μmol/L
Men		
18-29 y	110-510	3.0-14.0
30-39 y	110-370	3.0-10.0
40-49 y	45-345	1.2-9.4
50-59 y	25-240	0.7-6.5
60-69 y	25-95	0.7-2.6
70-90 y	≤75	≤2.0
Women		
18-29 y	45-320	1.2-8.7
30-39 y	40-325	1.1-8.8
40-49 y	25-220	0.7-6.0
50-59 y	15-170	0.4-4.6
60-69 y	≤185	≤5.0
70-90 y	≤90	≤2.4
Children	Male	
0-1 mo, male	≤316	≤8.6
female	15-261	0.4-7.1
1-6 mo, male	≤58	≤1.6
female	≤74	≤2.0
7-12 mo, male	≤26	≤0.7
female	≤26	≤0.7
1-3 y, male	≤15	≤0.4
female	≤22	≤0.6
4-6 y, male	≤27	≤0.7
female	≤34	≤0.9
7-9 y, male	≤91	≤2.5
female	≤92	≤2.5
10-13 y, male	≤138	≤3.7
female	≤148	≤4.0
14-16 y, male	38-340	1.0-9.2
female	37-307	1.0-8.3
Tanner stages		
I, male	≤89	≤2.4
female	≤46	≤1.2
II, male	≤81	≤2.2
female	15-113	0.4-3.1
III, male	22-126	0.6-3.4
female	42-162	1.1-4.4
IV, male	33-177	0.9-4.8
female	42-241	1.1-6.5
V, male	110-510	3.0-13.8
female	45-320	1.2-8.7

Dehydroepiandrosterone (DHEA) (method: LC/MS/MS)	ng/dL	nmol/L
Men	61-1636	2.1-56.4
Women	102-1185	3.5-40.9
Children		
1-5 y	≤377	≤13.0
6-9 y	19-592	0.7-20.4
10-13 y	42-1067	1.4-36.8
14-17 y	137-1489	4.7-51.3

From Fisher DA, ed. The Quest Diagnostics manual: endocrinology, test selection and interpretation, 4th edition. Capistrano, Calif: Quest Diagnostics/Nichols Institute, 2007.

Methods for the Detection of Anabolic Steroids

Detection of exogenous steroids used to improve athletic performance poses a challenge for the laboratory given the variety of exogenous anabolic steroids, which include both natural and synthetic testosterone analogs. Since the 1980s, GC-MS has been the method of choice to detect anabolic steroids.[38] The ratio of testosterone to epitestosterone (17 α-epimer) in urine has been used as a screening test for the detection of anabolic steroid abuse. A ratio of testosterone to epitestosterone greater than 6:1 suggests exogenous steroid use, and further testing should be performed for confirmation.[52] Others have suggested the ratio of testosterone to LH in the urine as an indication of testosterone doping. Detailed studies of these ratios are available.[155] For a more in-depth discussion of analytical considerations around drug monitoring in athletes, the reader is referred to the review by Bowers.[38]

Methods for the Determination of Estradiol in Blood

Both chromatography-mass spectrometry and immunoassay-based methods are used to measure estrogens in blood. GC-MS methods utilizing isotope dilution provide the most accurate and reliable measurement of E_2.[75,269,292,329] The main steps in these reference methods include solvent extraction, chromatographic fractionation, and chemical derivatization before analysis. Validation of immunoassay methods by this technique has become important in many external quality assurance programs.

Immunoassays consist of both indirect (extraction required) and direct (no extraction required) methods. The most common antigen used to prepare antibodies for E_2 assays is estradiol-6-(*O*-carboxymethyl)oxime conjugated to bovine serum albumin.[237] Cross-reactivity with other C-18 steroids is usually very minor because the 3- and 17-hydroxyl groups are left free. A 2008 CAP survey reported that direct enzyme immunoassays have largely replaced RIAs for routine measurement of E_2 concentrations.[11] For more information about RIA assays, the reader is directed to the previous edition of this chapter.[131] Evaluation of estrogen concentrations in men, postmenopausal women, and children requires the use of more sensitive RIA- or mass spectrometry–based methods.

To measure E_2 directly without extraction and chromatography, the steroid must be displaced from its binding proteins. The displacing agents used in commercial methods often are not disclosed, but in some systems, effective displacement is achieved by adding 8-anilino-1-naphthalene sulfonic acid (ANS) or a large excess of a competing steroid such as dihydrotestosterone to the sample.[237]

Caution should be exercised when assaying samples from subjects who are receiving oral contraceptives or estrogen replacement therapy because cross-reacting steroids may cause elevated results. Most notably, cross-reactivity with estrone is as high as 10% for some assays, but much lower (<1%) for others. This is likely due to a difference in the specificity of the antibody used for E_2. Similar effects have been observed for metabolites conjugated at the 3 position, such as estrone-3-sulfate and estrone-3-glucuronide.[136,180]

Several immunoassays for E_2 have been developed and adapted for use on fully automated immunoassay systems.[331] All are heterogeneous assays (separation step needed), but most are direct assays and do not require preliminary extraction. Most procedures offer the convenience of solid-phase separation methods. For routine clinical applications, the greatest experience is with enzyme immunoassays. Most commercial enzyme immunoassays use horseradish peroxidase or alkaline phosphatase to label E_2 antigens; enzyme activity is determined using a variety of photometric,[37,115,180] fluorescent,[19,21,240,242] or chemiluminescent substrates.[66] A semiautomated "ultrasensitive" chemiluminescent immunoassay for E_2 has been described.[90] This method is advantageous because it is reportedly capable of accurately measuring low concentrations (<50 pmol/L) of E_2 observed in perimenopausal and postmenopausal women, healthy men, and children.

Taieb and coworkers compared detection limits and functional sensitivities of nine automated E_2 immunoassays.[285] They concluded that functional sensitivities, defined as the lowest concentration of analyte that can be measured with a run-to-run imprecision of 20%, were twofold to fourfold higher than detection limits of the tests. It is also important to note that none of the assays analyzed in this study had the functional sensitivity required for evaluation of serum E_2 measurements in men, menopausal women, and children.[81] Functional sensitivities ranged from 20 to 169 pmol/L (5.5 to 46 pg/mL). These assays have been optimized for clinical applications such as monitoring of ovarian stimulation for IVF, in which high E_2 concentrations are expected, but the values obtained depend on the method used.[286] The authors suggest that until E_2 assays are better standardized, reference intervals and cutoff points used as clinical decision criteria must be evaluated and modified, if necessary, for each assay.

Specimen Collection and Storage

Serum have plasma (with EDTA or heparin as anticoagulant) have been used. Specimens should be centrifuged and separated within 24 hours. Serum/plasma specimens may be stored at room temperature for 1 day, refrigerated for 3 days, or frozen for up to 1 year.[80,121,338] Oral contraceptives have been known to alter E_2 concentrations.

Reference Intervals

Reference intervals for serum concentrations of E_2 are listed in Table 56-9.

Methods for the Determination of Estriol in Blood

Except for purposes of fetal aneuploidy screening, measurement of E_3 has little clinical value because in nonpregnant women, E_3 is derived almost exclusively from E_2. Both RIA and nonisotopic immunoassay methods for E_3 measurement in serum and plasma are commercially available. A 2008 CAP survey reports that automated enzymatic immunoassay methods account for all unconjugated E_3 measurements.[11] Several of these assays have been validated for use in maternal serum screening.[162,190]

Specimen Collection and Storage

E_3 serum or plasma specimens are stable at room temperature for 24 hours; they can be refrigerated for 2 days and frozen at −20 °C for up to 1 year.[121]

Methods for the Determination of Estrone in Blood

Estrone determinations have limited clinical utility. Normally, blood estrone concentrations parallel E_2 concentrations throughout the menstrual cycle, but at slightly lower concentrations. For a specific analysis of estrone, the interested reader is directed to other references.[58,82]

Methods for the Determination of Progesterone in Blood

A 2008 CAP survey reports that enzyme immunoassays account for most of the progesterone assays used today.[11] Initial immunoassays for serum progesterone measurement used organic solvents to remove the steroid from endogenous binding proteins such as corticosteroid-binding globulin and albumin. Direct (nonextraction) measurement of progesterone in serum or plasma is considered the method of choice for routine applications. Various antigens have been used to prepare antisera for progesterone assays. Cross-reactivity is most prominent with 5α-pregnanediol ranging from 6% to 11%. Both RIAs and nonisotopic immunoassays are available for measuring progesterone. For details on RIAs, the reader is directed to the previous edition of this chapter.[131]

Several immunoassays are available on fully automated immunoassay systems.[87,243,289,324] All are heterogeneous assays that require separation of free and antibody-bound fractions. Enzymes appear to be the most widely used nonradioactive label. Alkaline phosphatase and horseradish peroxidase

TABLE 56-9 Reference Intervals for Estradiol (E_2) in Serum

Estradiol (method: LC/MS/MS)	pg/mL	pmol/L
Men	≤29	≤106
Women		
Follicular	39-375	143-1377
Midcycle peak	94-762	345-2797
Luteal phase	48-440	176-1615
Postmenopausal	≤10	≤37
Children		
Prepubertal (1-9 y), males	≤4	≤15
females	≤16	≤59
10-11 y, males	≤12	≤44
females	≤65	≤239
12-14 y, males	≤24	≤88
females	≤142	≤521
15-17 y, males	≤31	≤114
females	≤283	≤1040

From Fisher DA, ed. The Quest Diagnostics manual: endocrinology, test selection and interpretation, 4th edition. Capistrano, Calif: Quest Diagnostics/Nichols Institute, 2007.

coupled to progesterone or antiprogesterone antibodies are particularly popular. An assortment of photometric,[139,180,299] fluorescent,[98,243,324] and luminescent[36,188] substrates are available for monitoring the enzyme activity of the antibody-bound fraction. Direct time-resolved fluoroimmunoassays for progesterone have been described.[72,150]

Although automated immunoassays are less labor intensive than RIAs and yield results in less time without the need for radioactivity, these assays do not have adequate functional sensitivity for the measurement of low progesterone concentrations in men, postmenopausal women, and children. Taieb and coworkers analyzed the detection limits and functional sensitivities of eight automated progesterone methods.[285] They reported that functional sensitivities (0.32 to 1.43 nmol/L), defined as the lowest concentration of analyte that could be measured with a run-to-run imprecision of 20%, ranged from twofold to fourfold higher than the manufacturer-stated detection limit (0.19 to 0.48 nmol/L). Automated progesterone assays have been optimized for use in in vitro fertilization protocols as a rapid, cost-effective way to evaluate ovarian stimulation and monitor ovulation.

Double-isotope derivative methods[328] and competitive protein-binding assays[78] have been applied to the measurement of serum progesterone, but these methods require extensive purification of the steroid and are labor intensive. GC procedures using flame ionization, electron capture, or nitrogen detection have been used to improve the accuracy of progesterone analysis.[42,78] However, these methods are time-consuming and often require solvent extraction, chromatography, and derivatization before the steroid is quantitated. GC-MS has been recommended as a reference method for progesterone determination. The GC-MS method of Thienpont and associates[290] makes use of heptafluorobutyric ester derivatives and 19-$^2H_3$-progesterone as internal standards. Mass spectrophotometry is discussed further later in this chapter.

Plasma concentrations of 17α-hydroxyprogesterone are measured to evaluate 21-hydroxylase deficiency. For specific methods regarding this analyte, the reader is referred to a review by Wallace.[310]

Specimen Collection and Storage

Serum or plasma (with heparin or EDTA as anticoagulant) is used and should be separated within 24 hours.[7] The patient need not be fasting, and no special handling procedures are necessary.[1,5] Serum/plasma specimens may be stored at room temperature for 24 hours and refrigerated at 4 to 8 °C for up to 3 days or at 20 °C for up to 1 year.[80,121,338]

Reference Intervals

Reference intervals for serum concentrations of progesterone are listed in Table 56-10.[293]

Measurement of Sex Steroids by Mass Spectrometry

Although immunoassays are the predominant method for the detection and measurement of sex steroids (E_2, testosterone, progesterone, etc.), they are associated with considerable analytical problems. For example, automated immunoassays (nonisotopic) have accuracy and imprecision problems, particularly at the low end of detectability. Studies by Wang and associates comparing testosterone measurement by the four most commonly used automated direct immunoassay platforms against an LC-MS/MS reference method indicate acceptable correlation only in the adult male range.[311] Immunoassay methods failed to accurately and precisely detect concentrations of testosterone below 100 ng/dL (3.47 nmol/L).[311] Because concentrations of testosterone in women, children, and hypogonadal men typically fall below 100 ng/dL (3.47 nmol/L), measurement by immunoassay is not recommended. In addition, there is a clinical demand for the measurement of low concentrations of E_2 (<25 pg/mL or <90 pmol/L), for example, in the setting of breast cancer risk assessment among postmenopausal women or following response to aromatase inhibitor treatment.[77] Again, these demands are met by current automated immunoassays and call for a more sensitive approach.

Mass spectrometry–based methods have been described for several of the sex steroids, including testosterone, DHT, E_2, and progesterone.[165,270,290,291,315] In addition, methods are available to measure precursors and metabolites, including DHEA, DHEA-S, androstenedione, and androstenedione glucoronide.[239,275,288] Tandem mass spectrometry coupled with liquid chromatography (HPLC) offers several advantages over traditional immunoassays, including lower limits of detection, enhanced specificity, small sample size, and the possibility of analyzing multiple steroids within the same sample. This ability to simultaneously measure a variety of

TABLE 56-10 Reference Intervals for Progesterone in Serum

Progesterone (method: LC/MS/MS)	ng/mL	nmol/L
Men		
18-29 y	≤0.3	≤1.0
30-39 y	≤0.2	≤0.6
40-49 y	≤0.2	≤0.6
50-59 y	≤0.2	≤0.6
Women		
Follicular phase	≤2.7	≤8.6
Luteal phase	≤31.4	≤100
Postmenopausal	≤0.2	≤0.6
Children		
5-9 y, male	≤0.7	≤2.2
female	≤0.6	≤1.9
10-13 y, male	≤1.2	≤3.8
female	≤10.2	≤32.4
14-17 y, male	≤0.8	≤2.5
female	≤11.9	≤38

From Fisher DA, ed. The Quest Diagnostics manual: endocrinology, test selection and interpretation, 4th edition. Capistrano, Calif: Quest Diagnostics/Nichols Institute, 2007.

analytes provides the opportunity for steroid profiling, which may enhance diagnostic capabilities. For a more thorough discussion of tandem mass spectrometry and steroid analysis, the reader is directed to a review by Soldin and Soldin.[276] However, this technology has some disadvantages, including lack of standardization, high costs of equipment and maintenance, and the requirement for highly trained personnel. Despite these disadvantages, professional societies are beginning to recognize the utility of mass spectrometry. For example, the Endocrine Society suggested using extraction and chromatography followed by MS or MS/MS as a potential gold standard for measurement of testosterone.[254]

Measurement of Salivary Sex Steroids

Measurement of salivary concentrations of steroids has the potential to serve as a noninvasive and convenient procedure for the assessment of "serum free" steroid concentrations. However, primarily because of rapid fluctuations in salivary concentration necessitating the collection of multiple samples, salivary testing for sex steroids is not commonplace. For example, Chatterton and colleagues showed that salivary E_2 concentrations in individual women reflected a pulsatile pattern over a 60 to 90 minute window, thereby requiring serial sampling for accurate measurement of E_2.[54] Fluctuations have also been observed for progesterone, with studies indicating that salivary progesterone shows much greater 24 hour variation than is seen with serum concentrations.[76] Similarly, salivary testosterone has been noted to fluctuate. Consequently, single salivary samples are not considered informative. For a more complete discussion of salivary steroid measurements, the reader is referred to a review by Wood.[327]

REFERENCES

1. Anonymous. Abbott Laboratories: package insert for progesterone on AxSym. Abbott Park, Ill: Abbott Laboratories, 1996.
2. Anonymous. ACOG practice bulletin. Assessment of risk factors for preterm birth: clinical management guidelines for obstetrician-gynecologists, number 31, October 2001 (replaces technical bulletin number 206, June 1995; Committee Opinion number 172, May 1996; Committee Opinion number 187, September 1997; Committee Opinion number 198, February 1998; and Committee Opinion number 251, January 2001). Obstet Gynecol 2001;98:709-16.
3. Anonymous. College of American Pathologists. Y-B ligands (special) survey. Northfield, Ill: College of American Pathologists, 2008.
4. Anonymous. Diagnostic Products Corporation: package insert for Coat-A-Count DHEA kit. Los Angeles, Calif: Diagnostic Products Corporation, 1992.
5. Anonymous. Diagnostic Products Corporation: package insert for Coat-A-Count progesterone kit. Los Angeles, Calif: Diagnostic Products Corporation, 1997.
6. Anonymous. ESHRE Capri Workshop. Infertility revisited: the state of the art today and tomorrow. Hum Reprod 1996;11:1179-807.
7. Anonymous. InterScience Institute. Current unique and rare endocrine assays. Inglewood, Calif: InterScience Institute, 1997.
8. Anonymous. Mayo Medical Laboratories. Interpretive handbook. Rochester, Minn: Mayo Medical Laboratories, 1997.
9. Anonymous. Quest Diagnostics/Nichols Institute. The Corning endocrine manual. Capistrano, Calif: Quest Diagnostics/Nichols Institute, 1996.
10. Anonymous. Research on the menopause in the 1990s. Technical report, Scr 866. Geneva, Switzerland: World Health Organization, 1996.
11. Anonymous. WHO. Laboratory manual for the examination of human semen and semen-cervical mucus penetration, 4th edition. Cambridge, UK: Cambridge University Press, 1999.
12. Andersson AM, Skakkebaek NE. Serum inhibin B levels during male childhood and puberty. Mol Cell Endocrinol 2001;180:103-7.
13. Armstrong EG, Ehrlich PH, Birken S, Schlatterer JP, Siris E, Hembree WC, et al. Use of a highly sensitive and specific immunoradiometric assay for detection of human chorionic gonadotropin in urine of normal, nonpregnant, and pregnant individuals. J Clin Endocrinol Metab 1984;59:867-74.
14. Azziz R. The evaluation and management of hirsutism. Obstet Gynecol 2003;101:995-1007.
15. Azziz R, Dewailly D, Owerbach D. Clinical review 56: nonclassic adrenal hyperplasia: current concepts. J Clin Endocrinol Metab 1994;78:810-5.
16. Azziz R, Hincapie LA, Knochenhauer ES, Dewailly D, Fox L, Boots LR. Screening for 21-hydroxylase-deficient nonclassic adrenal hyperplasia among hyperandrogenic women: a prospective study. Fertil Steril 1999;72:915-25.
17. Azziz R, Waggoner WT, Ochoa T, Knochenhauer ES, Boots LR. Idiopathic hirsutism: an uncommon cause of hirsutism in Alabama. Fertil Steril 1998;70:274-8
18. Bachega TA, Brenlha EM, Billerbeck AE, Marcondes JA, Madureira G, Arnhold IJ, et al. Variable ACTH-stimulated 17-hydroxyprogesterone values in 21-hydroxylase deficiency carriers are not related to the different CYP21 gene mutations. J Clin Endocrinol Metab 2002; 87:786-90.
19. Bahar I, Case A, Jackson M. Rapid self-contained immunoassay for estradiol. Clin Chem 1992;38:954-5.
20. Bakalov VK, Vanderhoof VH, Bondy CA, Nelson LM. Adrenal antibodies detect asymptomatic auto-immune adrenal insufficiency in young women with spontaneous premature ovarian failure. Hum Reprod 2002;17:2096-100.
21. Baker HN, Massei MK, Ramp SK, Trach P, Starup-Brynes I, Massei MK et al. Development of a fully automated immunoassay for estradiol on the Abbott IMxTM automated immunoassay system. Clin Chem 1991;37:1036 Abstract #0601.

22. Bandi ZL, Schoen I, Waters M. An algorithm for testing and reporting serum choriogonadotropin at clinically significant decision levels with use of "pregnancy test" reagents. Clin Chem 1989;35:545-51.
23. Barash IA, Cheung CC, Weigle DS, Ren H, Kabigting EB, Kuijper JL, et al. Leptin is a metabolic signal to the reproductive system. Endocrinol 1996;137:3144-7.
24. Barbieri RL. Infertility. In: Yen SSC, Jaffe RB, Barbieri RL, eds. Reproductive endocrinology: physiology, pathophysiology, and clinical management, 4th edition. Philadelphia, Pa: WB Saunders, 1999:562-93.
25. Barini A, Liberale I, Menini E. Simultaneous determination of free testosterone and testosterone bound to non-sex-hormone-binding globulin by equilibrium dialysis. Clin Chem 1993;39:938-41.
26. Barontini M, Garcia-Rudaz MC, Veldhuis JD. Mechanisms of hypothalamic-pituitary-gonadal disruption in polycystic ovarian syndrome. Arch Med Res 2001;32:544-52.
27. Bastian LA, Smith CM, Nanda K. Is this woman perimenopausal? JAMA 2003;289:895-902.
28. Batista MC, Cartledge TP, Zellmer AW, Merino MJ, Nieman LK, Loriaux DL, et al. A prospective controlled study of luteal and endometrial abnormalities in an infertile population. Fertil Steril 1996;65:495-502.
29. Benson JR, Pitsinis V. Update on clinical role of tamoxifen. Curr Opin Obstet Gynecol 2003;15:13-23.
30. Berin I, Teixeira J. Utility of serum antimüllerian hormone/ Mullerian-inhibiting substance for predicting ovarian reserve in older women. Menopause 2008;15:824-6.
31. Betterle C, Coco G, Zanchetta R. Adrenal cortex autoantibodies in subjects with normal adrenal function. Best Pract Res Clin Endocrinol Metab 2005;19:85-99.
32. Boas M, Boisen KA, Virtanen HE, Kaleva M, Suomi AM, Schmidt IM, et al. Postnatal penile length and growth rate correlate to serum testosterone levels: a longitudinal study of 1962 normal boys. Eur J Endocrinol 2006;154:125-9.
33. Boolell M, Allen MJ, Ballard SA, Gepi-Attee S, Muirhead GJ, Naylor AM. Sildenafil: an orally active type 5 cyclic GMP-specific phosphodiesterase inhibitor for the treatment of penile erectile dysfunction. Int J Impot Res 1996;8:47-52.
34. Boolell M, Gepi-Attee S, Gingell JC, Allen MJ. Sildenafil, a novel effective oral therapy for male erectile dysfunction. Brit J Urol 1996;78:257-61.
35. Borkowski A, Puttaert V, Gyling M, Muquardt C, Body JJ. Human chorionic gonadotropin-like substance in plasma of normal nonpregnant subjects and women with breast cancer. J Clin Endocrinol Metab 1984;58:1171-8.
36. Bouma S, Worobec S, Baker A, Dubler R, Frias E, Ginsburg S, et al. Performance of automated chemiluminescent paramagnetic microparticle immunoassays for estradiol, progesterone, and testosterone on the Abbott i2000 system. Clin Chem 1997;43: S171.
37. Bouve J, De Boever J, Leyseele D, Bosmans E, Dubois P, Kohen F, et al. Direct enzyme immunoassay of estradiol in serum of women enrolled in an in vitro fertilization and embryo transfer program. Clin Chem 1992;38:1409-13.
38. Bowers L. The analytical chemistry of drug monitoring in athletes. Ann Rev Anal Chem 2009;2:485-507.
39. Braunstein GD. Gynecomastia. N Engl J Med 1993;328:490-5.
40. Bremner WJ, Vitiello MV, Prinz PN. Loss of circadian rhythmicity in blood testosterone levels with aging in normal men. J Clin Endocrinol Metab 1983;56:1278-81.
41. Brenner PF, Mishell DR. Menopause. In: Mishell DR, Davajan V, Lobo RA, eds. Infertility, contraception and reproductive endocrinology. Boston, Mass: Blackwell Scientific Publications, 1993:241-53.
42. Breuer H, Hamel D, Kruskemper H, eds. Methods of hormone analysis. New York, NY: John Wiley & Sons Inc., 1976.
43. Brito VN, Batista MC, Borges MF, Latronico AC, Kohek MB, Thirone AC, et al. Diagnostic value of fluorometric assays in the evaluation of precocious puberty. J Clin Endocrinol Metab 1999;84:3539-44.
44. Brzechffa PR, Jakimiuk AJ, Agarwal SK, Weitsman SR, Buyalos RP, Magoffin DA. Serum immunoreactive leptin concentrations in women with polycystic ovary syndrome. J Clin Endocrinol Metab 1996; 81:4166-9.
45. Burger HG, Dudley EC, Hopper JL, Groome N, Guthrie JR, Green A, et al. Prospectively measured levels of serum follicle-stimulating hormone, estradiol, and the dimeric inhibins during the menopausal transition in a population-based cohort of women. J Clin Endocrinol Metab 1999;84:4025-30.
46. Buzdar A. Anastrozole as adjuvant therapy for early-stage breast cancer: implications of the ATAC trial. Clin Breast Cancer 2003;4(suppl 1):S42-8.
47. Canick JA, Knight GJ, Palomaki GE, Haddow JE, Cuckle HS, Wald NJ. Low second trimester maternal serum unconjugated oestriol in pregnancies with Down's syndrome. Br J Obstet Gynaecol 1988;95:330-3.
48. Carmina E. Prevalence of idiopathic hirsutism. Eur J Endocrinol 1998;139:421-3.
49. Caro JF. Leptin is normal in PCOS, an editorial about three "negative" papers. J Clin Endocrinol Metab 1997;82:1685-6.
50. Carr BR. Disorders of the ovary and female reproductive tract. In: Williams RH, Foster DW, Kronenberg HM, Larsen PR, Wilson JD, eds. Williams textbook of endocrinology, 9th edition. Philadelphia, Pa: WB Saunders, 1998:751-817.
51. Cassio A, Cacciari E, Zucchini S, Balsamo A, Diegoli M, Orsini F. Central precocious puberty: clinical and imaging aspects. J Pediatr Endocrinol Metab 2000;13(suppl 1):703-8.
52. Catlin DH, Hatton CK, Starcevic SH. Issues in detecting abuse of xenobiotic anabolic steroids and testosterone by analysis of athletes' urine. Clin Chem 1997;43:1280-8.
53. Cavallo A, Richards GE, Busey S, Michaels SE. A simplified gonadotrophin-releasing hormone test for precocious puberty. Clin Endocrinol (Oxf) 1995;42:641-6.
54. Chatterton RT Jr, Mateo ET, Hou N, Rademaker AW, Acharya S, Jordan VC et al. Characteristics of salivary profiles of oestradiol and progesterone in premenopausal women. J Endocrinol 2005; 186:77-84.
55. Chattoraj SC, Turner AK, Pinkus JL, Charles D. The significance of urinary free cortisol and progesterone in normal and anencephalic pregnancy. Am J Obstet Gynecol 1976;124:848-54.
56. Chehab FF, Lim ME, Lu R. Correction of the sterility defect in homozygous obese female mice by treatment with the human recombinant leptin. Nat Genet 1996;12:318-20.
57. Chumlea WC, Schubert CM, Roche AF, Kulin HE, Lee PA, Himes JH, et al. Age at menarche and racial comparisons in US girls. Pediatrics 2003;111:110-3.
58. Ciotti PM, Franceschetti F, Bulletti C, Jasonni VM, Bolelli GF. Rapid and specific RIA of serum estrone sulfate with selective solid phase extraction. J Steroid Biochem 1989;32:473-4.
59. Clemons M, Goss P. Estrogen and the risk of breast cancer. N Engl J Med 2001;344:276-85.
60. Cole LA, Sasaki Y, Muller CY. Normal production of human chorionic gonadotropin in menopause. N Engl J Med 2007;356: 1184-6.
61. Cole P, MacMahon B. Oestrogen fractions during early reproductive life in the aetiology of breast cancer. Lancet 1969;1:604-6.
62. Cooper JD, Muirhead DC, Taylor JE, Baker PR. Development of an assay for the simultaneous determination of sildenafil (Viagra) and its metabolite (UK-103,320) using automated sequential trace enrichment of dialysates and high-performance liquid chromatography. J Chromatogr B Biomed Sci Appl 1997;701: 87-95.
63. Cumming DC, Wall SR. Non-sex hormone-binding globulin-bound testosterone as a marker for hyperandrogenism. J Clin Endocrinol Metab 1985;61:873-6.
64. Dacou-Voutetakis C, Maniati-Christidi M, Dracopoulou-Vabouli M. Genetic aspects of congenital adrenal hyperplasia. J Pediatr Endocrinol Metab 2001;14(suppl 5):1303-8; discussion 1317.

65. Dal Pra C, Chen S, Furmaniak J, Smith BR, Pedini B, Moscon A, et al. Autoantibodies to steroidogenic enzymes in patients with premature ovarian failure with and without Addison's disease. Eur J Endocrinol 2003;148:565-70.
66. Dancoine F, Couplet G, Buvat J, Guittard C, Marcolin G, Fourlinnie JC, et al. Analytical and clinical evaluation of the Immulite estradiol assay in serum from patients undergoing in vitro fertilization: estradiol increase in mature follicles. Clin Chem 1997;43:1165-71.
67. Davajan V, Kletzky OA. Primary amenorrhea: phenotypic female external genitalia. In: Mishell DR, Davajan V, Lobo RA, eds. Infertility, contraception and reproductive endocrinology, 3rd edition. Boston, Mass: Blackwell Scientific Publications, 1993:356-71.
68. Davajan V, Kletzky OA. Secondary amenorrhea without galactorrhea or androgen excess. In: Mishell DR, Davajan V, Lobo RA, eds. Infertility, contraception and reproductive endocrinology, 3rd edition. Boston, Mass: Blackwell Scientific Publications, 1993:372-95.
69. Davies R, Collier C, Raymond M, Heaton J, Clark A. Indirect measurement of bioavailable testosterone with the Bayer Immuno 1 system. Clin Chem 2002;48:388-90.
70. Davison S, Davis SR. Hormone replacement therapy: current controversies. Clin Endocrinol (Oxf) 2003;58:249-61.
71. de Ronde W, van der Schouw YT, Pols HA, Gooren LJ, Muller M, Grobbee DE, et al. Calculation of bioavailable and free testosterone in men: a comparison of 5 published algorithms. Clin Chem 2006;52:1777-84.
72. Dechaud H, Bador R, Claustrat F, Desuzinges C, Mallein R. New approach to competitive lanthanide immunoassay: time-resolved fluoroimmunoassay of progesterone with labeled analyte. Clin Chem 1988;34:501-4.
73. Dechaud H, Denuziere A, Rinaldi S, Bocquet J, Lejeune H, Pugeat M. Age-associated discrepancy between measured and calculated bioavailable testosterone in men. Clin Chem 2007;53:723-8.
74. Dechaud H, Lejeune H, Garoscio-Cholet M, Mallein R, Pugeat M. Radioimmunoassay of testosterone not bound to sex-steroid-binding protein in plasma. Clin Chem 1989;35:1609-14.
75. Dehennin L. Estradiol-17 beta determined in plasma by gas chromatography-mass spectrometry with selected ion monitoring of mixed silyl ether-perfluoroacyl ester derivatives and use of various stable-isotope-labeled internal standards. Clin Chem 1989;35:532-6.
76. Delfs TM, Klein S, Fottrell P, Naether OG, Leidenberger FA, Zimmermann RC. 24-Hour profiles of salivary progesterone. Fertil Steril 1994;62:960-6.
77. Demers LM. Testosterone and estradiol assays: current and future trends. Steroids 2008;73:1333-8.
78. Demetriou J. Progesterone. In: Pesce A, Kaplan L, eds. Methods in clinical chemistry. St Louis, Mo: CV Mosby, 1987:253-7.
79. Dewailly D. Nonclassic 21-hydroxylase deficiency. Semin Reprod Med 2002;20:243-8.
80. Diver MJ, Hughes JG, Hutton JL, West CR, Hipkin LJ. The long-term stability in whole blood of 14 commonly-requested hormone analytes. Ann Clin Biochem 1994;31(Pt 6):561-5.
81. Diver MJ, Nisbet JA. Warning on plasma oestradiol measurement. Lancet 1987;2:1097.
82. Dobson H, Dean PD. Radioimmunoassay of oestrone, oestradiol-17alpha and -17beta in bovine plasma during the oestrous cycle and last stages of pregnancy. J Endocrinol 1974;61:479-86.
83. Dorgan JF, Fears TR, McMahon RP, Aronson Friedman L, Patterson BH, Greenhut SF. Measurement of steroid sex hormones in serum: a comparison of radioimmunoassay and mass spectrometry. Steroids 2002;67:151-8.
84. Dufau ML, Winters CA, Hattori M, Aquilano D, Baranao JL, Nozu K, et al. Hormonal regulation of androgen production by the Leydig cell. J Steroid Biochem 1984;20:161-73.
85. Eckert KL, Wilson DM, Bachrach LK, Anhalt H, Habiby RL, Olney RC, et al. A single-sample, subcutaneous gonadotropin-releasing hormone test for central precocious puberty. Pediatrics 1996;97:517-9.
86. Elkind-Hirsch K, Goldzieher JW, Gibbons WE, Besch PK. Evaluation of the OvuSTICK urinary luteinizing hormone kit in normal and stimulated menstrual cycles. Obstet Gynecol 1986;67:450-3.
87. Elmlinger MW, Kuhnel W, Ranke MB. Reference ranges for serum concentrations of lutropin (LH), follitropin (FSH), estradiol (E_2), prolactin, progesterone, sex hormone-binding globulin (SHBG), dehydroepiandrosterone sulfate (DHEAS), cortisol and ferritin in neonates, children and young adults. Clin Chem Lab Med 2002;40:1151-60.
88. Elmlinger MW, Kuhnel W, Ranke MB. Reference intervals for testosterone, androstenedione and SHBG levels in healthy females and males from birth until old age. Clin Lab 2005;51:625-32.
89. Emadi-Konjin P, Bain J, Bromberg IL. Evaluation of an algorithm for calculation of serum "bioavailable" testosterone (BAT). Clin Biochem 2003;36:591-6.
90. England BG, Parsons GH, Possley RM, McConnell DS, Midgley AR. Ultrasensitive semiautomated chemiluminescent immunoassay for estradiol. Clin Chem 2002;48:1584-6.
91. Evers JL. Female subfertility. Lancet 2002;360:151-9.
92. Fanchin R, Schonauer LM, Righini C, Guibourdenche J, Frydman R, Taieb J. Serum anti-Müllerian hormone is more strongly related to ovarian follicular status than serum inhibin B, estradiol, FSH and LH on day 3. Hum Reprod 2003;18:323-7.
93. Feldman HA, Longcope C, Derby CA, Johannes CB, Araujo AB, Coviello AD, et al. Age trends in the level of serum testosterone and other hormones in middle-aged men: longitudinal results from the Massachusetts male aging study. J Clin Endocrinol Metab 2002;87:589-98.
94. Finlay EM, Gaskell SJ. Determination of testosterone in plasma from men by gas chromatography/mass spectrometry, with high-resolution selected-ion monitoring and metastable peak monitoring. Clin Chem 1981;27:1165-70.
95. Fisch H, Lipshultz LI. Diagnosing male factors of infertility. Arch Path Lab Med 1992;116:398-405.
96. Fitzgerald RL, Herold DA. Serum total testosterone: immunoassay compared with negative chemical ionization gas chromatography-mass spectrometry. Clin Chem 1996;42:749-55.
97. Forabosco A, Sforza C, De Pol A,Vizzotto L, Marzona L, Ferrario VF. Morphometric study of the human neonatal ovary. Anat Rec 1991;231:201-8.
98. Ford K, Caplan DE, Tobias DD, Turn JE, Osikowicz E. Automated direct enzyme immunoassay of progesterone on the Abbott IMx analyzer. Clin Chem 1990;36:1099.
99. Forest MG. Serum müllerian inhibiting substance assay—a new diagnostic test for disorders of gonadal development. N Engl J Med Commentary 1997;336:1519-21.
100. Franks S. Polycystic ovary syndrome. N Engl J Med 1995;333:853-61.
101. Gheorghiu I, Moshyk A, Lepage R, Ahnadi CE, Grant AM. When is bioavailable testosterone a redundant test in the diagnosis of hypogonadism in men? Clin Biochem 2005;38:813-8.
102. Giton F, Fiet J, Guechot J, Ibrahim F, Bronsard F, Chopin D, et al. Serum bioavailable testosterone: assayed or calculated? Clin Chem 2006;52:474-81.
103. Glass AR. Gynecomastia. Endocrinol Metab Clin North Am 1994;23:825-37.
104. Glezerman M, Bartoov B. Semen analysis. In: Insler V, Lunenfeld B, eds. Infertility: male and female. New York, NY: Churchill Livingstone, 1993:285-315.
105. Glezerman M, Lunenfeld B. Diagnosis of male infertility. In: Insler V, Lunenfeld B, eds. Infertility: male and female, 2nd edition. New York, NY: Churchill Livingstone, 1993:317-22.
106. Gnatuk CL. The controversy over estrogen replacement therapy: an update on clinical trials. Curr Womens Health Rep 2002;2:89-94.
107. Goffinet F, Maillard F, Fulla Y, Cabrol D. Biochemical markers (without markers of infection) of the risk of preterm delivery: implications for clinical practice. Eur J Obstet Gynecol Reprod Biol 2001;94:59-68.

108. Goodwin TM. A role for estriol in human labor, term and preterm. Am J Obstet Gynecol 1999;180:S208-13.
109. Gordon CM. Menstrual disorders in adolescents: excess androgens and the polycystic ovary syndrome. Pediatr Clin North Am 1999;46:519-43.
110. Gougeon A, Ecochard R, Thalabard JC. Age-related changes of the population of human ovarian follicles: increase in the disappearance rate of non-growing and early-growing follicles in aging women. Biol Reprod 1994;50:653-63.
111. Govier FE, McClure RD, Kramer-Levien D. Endocrine screening for sexual dysfunction using free testosterone determinations. J Urol 1996;156:405-8.
112. Greendale GA, Lee NP, Arriola ER. The menopause. Lancet 1999;353:571-80.
113. Griffin JE, Wilson JD. Disorders of the testes and male reproductive tract. In: Williams RH, Foster DW, Kronenberg HM, Larsen PR, Wilson JD, eds. Williams textbook of endocrinology, 9th edition. Philadelphia, Pa: WB Saunders, 1998:819-75.
114. Grodstein F, Stampfer M. The epidemiology of coronary heart disease and estrogen replacement in postmenopausal women. Prog Cardiovasc Dis 1995;38:199-210.
115. Grol M, Stock W, Ebert C. Fully automated steroid determination on the immuno-analyzer ES 300: development and performance of a new direct highly sensitive enzyme immunoassay for serum estradiol. Clin Chem 1991;37:1027.
116. Gronowski AM, Fantz CR, Parvin CA, Sokoll LJ, Wiley CL, Wener MH, et al. Use of serum FSH to identify perimenopausal women with pituitary hCG. Clin Chem 2008;54:652-6.
117. Gronowski AM, Landau-Levine M. Reproductive endocrine function. In: Burtis CA, Ashwood ER, eds. Tietz textbook of clinical chemistry, 3rd edition. Philadelphia, Pa: WB Saunders, 1999:1601-41.
118. Groome NP, Evans LW. Does measurement of inhibin have a clinical role? Ann Clin Biochem 2000;37(Pt 4):419-31.
119. Grumbach MM, Conte FA. Disorders of sex differentiation. In: Williams RH, Foster DW, Kronenberg HM, Larsen PR, Wilson JD, eds. Williams textbook of endocrinology, 8th edition. Philadelphia, Pa: WB Saunders, 1998:1303-425.
120. Gruschke A, Kuhl H. Validity of radioimmunological methods for determining free testosterone in serum. Fertil Steril 2001;76:576-82.
121. Guder WG, Narayanan H, Wisser H, Zawata B. List of analytes and preanalytical variables. In: Guder W, Narayanan H, Wisser H, Zawata B, eds. Samples: from the patient to the laboratory: the impact of preanalytical variables on the quality of laboratory results. Darmstadt, Germany: Git Verlag GmBH, 1996:1-48.
122. Guillaume AJ, Benjamin F, Sicuranza B, Deutsch S, Spitzer M. Luteal phase defects and ectopic pregnancy. Fertil Steril 1995;63:30-3.
123. Guzick DS. Polycystic ovary syndrome. Obstet Gynecol 2004;103: 181-93.
124. Hall PF. Testicular steroid synthesis: organization and regulation. In: Knobil E, Neill JD, eds. The physiology of reproduction. New York, NY: Raven Press, 1988:975-98.
125. Hammond GL, Nisker JA, Jones LA, Siiteri PK. Estimation of the percentage of free steroid in undiluted serum by centrifugal ultrafiltration-dialysis. J Biol Chem 1980;255:5023-6.
126. Harman SM, Metter EJ, Tobin JD, Pearson J, Blackman MR. Longitudinal effects of aging on serum total and free testosterone levels in healthy men. Baltimore Longitudinal Study of Aging. J Clin Endocrinol Metab 2001;86:724-31.
127. Harris JR, Lippman ME, Veronesi U, Willett W. Breast cancer (I). N Engl J Med 1992;327:319-28.
128. Harris JR, Lippman ME, Veronesi U, Willett W. Breast cancer (II). N Engl J Med 1992;327:390-8.
129. Harris JR, Lippman ME, Veronesi U, Willett W. Breast cancer (III). N Engl J Med 1992;327:473-80.
130. Hawton K. Integration of treatments for male erectile dysfunction. Lancet 1998;351:7-8.
131. Haymond S, Gronowski AM. Reproductive related disorders. In: Burtis CA, Ashwood ER, Bruns DD, eds. Tietz textbook of clinical chemistry and molecular diagnostics, 4th edition. St Louis, Mo: Elsevier Saunders, 2006:2097-152.
132. Hedriana HL, Munro CJ, Eby-Wilkens EM, Lasley BL. Changes in rates of salivary estriol increases before parturition at term. Am J Obstet Gynecol 2001;184:123-30.
133. Heine RP, McGregor JA, Dullien VK. Accuracy of salivary estriol testing compared to traditional risk factor assessment in predicting preterm birth. Am J Obstet Gynecol 1999;180:S214-8.
134. Heine RP, McGregor JA, Goodwin TM, Artal R, Hayashi RH, Robertson PA, et al. Serial salivary estriol to detect an increased risk of preterm birth. Obstet Gynecol 2000;96:490-7.
135. Herman-Giddens ME, Slora EJ, Wasserman RC, Bourdony CJ, Bhapkar MV, Koch GG, et al. Secondary sexual characteristics and menses in young girls seen in office practice: a study from the Pediatric Research in Office Settings network. Pediatrics 1997; 99:505-12.
136. Hershlag A, Zinger M, Lesser M, Scholl G, Bjornson L. Is chemiluminescent immunoassay an appropriate substitution for radioimmunoassay in monitoring estradiol levels? Fertil Steril 2000;73:1174-8.
137. Hijazi RA, Cunningham GR. Andropause: is androgen replacement therapy indicated for the aging male? Annu Rev Med 2005;56: 117-37.
138. Horton R, Lobo R, Hawks D. Androstanediol glucuronide in plasma, a marker of androgen action in men and women. Clin Res 1982;30: 491A.
139. Hoyle N, Ebert C. Fully automated determination on the immunoanalyzer ES 300: performance of serum progesterone and testosterone assays. Clin Chem 1991;37:1020.
140. Hughes I. Congenital adrenal hyperplasia: phenotype and genotype. J Pediatr Endocrinol Metab 2002;15(suppl 5):1329-40.
141. Hughes IA. Congenital adrenal hyperplasia: 21-hydroxylase deficiency in the newborn and during infancy. Semin Reprod Med 2002; 20:229-42.
142. Hulka BS. Epidemiologic analysis of breast and gynecologic cancers. Prog Clin Biol Res 1997;396:17-29.
143. Hunter WM, Corrie JET, eds. Immunoassays for clinical chemistry, 2nd edition. Edinburgh, Scotland: Churchill Livingstone, 1983.
144. Iughetti L, Predieri B, Ferrari M, Gallo C, Livio L, Milioli S, et al. Diagnosis of central precocious puberty: endocrine assessment. J Pediatr Endocrinol Metab 2000;13(suppl 1):709-15.
145. Jaffe RB. Disorders of sexual development. In: Yen SSC, Jaffe RB, Barbieri RL, eds. Reproductive endocrinology: physiology, pathophysiology, and clinical management, 4th edition. Philadelphia, Pa: WB Saunders, 1999:363-87.
146. Jaffe RB. Menopause and aging. In: Yen SSC, Jaffe RB, Barbieri RL, eds. Reproductive endocrinology: physiology, pathophysiology, and clinical management, 4th edition. Philadelphia, Pa: WB Saunders, 1999:301-62.
147. Jialal I, Winter WE, Chan DW, eds. Handbook of diagnostic endocrinology. Washington, DC: AACC Press, 1999.
148. Jin M, Wener MH, Bankson DD. Evaluation of automated sex hormone binding globulin immunoassays. Clin Biochem 2006;39:91-4.
149. Jones HW Jr, Toner JP. The infertile couple. N Engl J Med 1993;329:1710-5.
150. Kakabakos SE, Khosravi MJ. Direct time-resolved fluorescence immunoassay of progesterone in serum involving the biotin-streptavidin system and the immobilized-antibody approach. Clin Chem 1992;38:725-30.
151. Kaplowitz PB, Oberfield SE. Reexamination of the age limit for defining when puberty is precocious in girls in the United States: implications for evaluation and treatment. Drug and Therapeutics and Executive Committees of the Lawson Wilkins Pediatric Endocrine Society. Pediatrics 1999;104:936-41.
152. Kapoor P, Luttrell BM, Williams D. The free androgen index is not valid for adult males. J Steroid Biochem Mol Biol 1993;45: 325-6.

153. Kelsey JL, Gammon MD. Epidemiology of breast cancer. Epidemiol Rev 1990;12:228-40.
154. Key TJ, Verkasalo PK, Banks E. Epidemiology of breast cancer. Lancet Oncol 2001;2:133-40.
155. Kicman AT, Brooks RV, Collyer SC, Cowan DA, Nanjee MN, Southan GJ, et al. Criteria to indicate testosterone administration. Brit J Sports Med 1990;24:253-64.
156. Kiningham RB, Apgar BS, Schwenk TL. Evaluation of amenorrhea. Am Fam Physician 1996;53:1185-94.
157. Klee GG, Heser DW. Techniques to measure testosterone in the elderly. Mayo Clin Proc 2000;75(suppl):S19-25.
158. Klein J, Sauer MV. Assessing fertility in women of advanced reproductive age. Am J Obstet Gynecol 2001;185:758-70.
159. Klein KO. Precocious puberty: who has it? Who should be treated? J Clin Endocrinol Metab 1999;84:411-4.
160. Klein KO, Baron J, Colli MJ, McDonnell DP, Cutler GB Jr. Estrogen levels in childhood determined by an ultrasensitive recombinant cell bioassay. J Clin Invest 1994;94:2475-80.
161. Kletzky OA, Davajan V. Hyperprolactinemia. In: Mishell DR, Davajan V, eds. Infertility, contraception and reproductive endocrinology, 3rd edition. Boston, Mass: Blackwell Scientific Publications, 1993:372-95.
162. Koenn ME, Ndah BV. Method comparison studies for prostate specific antigen and unconjugated estriol immunoassays. Clin Lab Sci 2003;16:94-8.
163. Korenman SG. Sexual function and dysfunction. In: Williams RH, Foster DW, Kronenberg HM, Larsen PR, Wilson JD, eds. Williams textbook of endocrinology, 9th edition. Philadelphia, Pa: WB Saunders, 1998:927-38.
164. Kubini K, Zachmann M, Albers N, Hiort O, Bettendorf M, Wolfle J, et al. Basal inhibin B and the testosterone response to human chorionic gonadotropin correlate in prepubertal boys. J Clin Endocrinol Metab 2000;85:134-8.
165 Kushnir MM, Rockwood AL, Bergquist J, Varshavsky M, Roberts WL, Yue B, et al. High-sensitivity tandem mass spectrometry assay for serum estrone and estradiol. Am J Clin Pathol 2008;129: 530-9.
166. La Marca A, Giulini S, Tirelli A, Bertucci E, Marsella T, Xella S, et al. Anti-Müllerian hormone measurement on any day of the menstrual cycle strongly predicts ovarian response in assisted reproductive technology. Hum Reprod 2007;22:766-71.
167. Lachelin GC, McGarrigle HH. A comparison of saliva, plasma unconjugated and plasma total oestriol levels throughout normal pregnancy. Br J Obstet Gynaecol 1984;91:1203-9.
168. Lake DE, Hudis C. Aromatase inhibitors in breast cancer: an update. Cancer Control 2002;9:490-8.
169. Laue L, Rennert OM. Congenital adrenal hyperplasia: molecular genetics and alternative approaches to treatment. Adv Pediatr 1995;42:113-43.
170. Lawson ML, Cohen N. A single sample subcutaneous luteinizing hormone (LH)-releasing hormone (LHRH) stimulation test for monitoring LH suppression in children with central precocious puberty receiving LHRH agonists. J Clin Endocrinol Metab 1999;84:4536-40.
171. Leader LR, Russell T, Clifford K, Stenning B. The clinical value of Clearplan home ovulation detection kits in infertility practice. Aust N Z J Obstet Gynaecol 1991;31:142-4.
172. Lebrethon MC, Bourguignon JP. Management of central isosexual precocity: diagnosis, treatment, outcome. Curr Opin Pediatr 2000;12:394-9.
173. Lee C L, Iles RK, Shepherd JH, Hudson CN, Chard T. The purification and development of a radioimmunoassay for beta-core fragment of human chorionic gonadotrophin in urine: application as a marker of gynaecological cancer in premenopausal and postmenopausal women. J Endocrinol 1991;130:481-9.
174. Lee MM, Donahoe PK, Silverman BL, Hasegawa T, Hasegawa Y, Gustafson ML, et al. Measurements of serum müllerian inhibiting substance in the evaluation of children with nonpalpable gonads. N Engl J Med 1997;336:1480-6.
175. Lee PA. Laboratory monitoring of children with precocious puberty. Arch Pediatr Adolesc Med 1994;148:369-76.
176. Lee PA. Central precocious puberty: an overview of diagnosis, treatment, and outcome. Endocrinol Metab Clin North Am 1999;28:901-18, xi.
177. Lee PA, Kulin HE, Guo SS. Age of puberty among girls and the diagnosis of precocious puberty. Pediatrics 2001;107:1493.
178. Lee TH, Liu CH, Huang CC, Wu YL, Shih YT, Ho HN, et al. Serum anti-Müllerian hormone and estradiol levels as predictors of ovarian hyperstimulation syndrome in assisted reproduction technology cycles. Hum Reprod 2008;23:160-7.
179. Lenton EA, Sulaiman R, Sobowale O, Cooke ID. The human menstrual cycle: plasma concentrations of prolactin, LH, FSH, oestradiol and progesterone in conceiving and non-conceiving women. J Reprod Fertil 1982;65:131-9.
180. Levesque A, Letellier M, Dillon PW, Grant A. Analytical performance of Bayer Immuno 1 estradiol and progesterone assays. Clin Chem 1997;43:1601-9.
181. Licciardi FL, Liu HC, Rosenwaks Z. Day 3 estradiol serum concentrations as prognosticators of ovarian stimulation response and pregnancy outcome in patients undergoing in vitro fertilization. Fertil Steril 1995;64:991-4.
182. Lippman ME. Endocrine-responsive cancers. In: Williams RH, Foster DW, Kronenberg HM, Larsen PR, Wilson JD, eds. Williams textbook of endocrinology, 9th edition. Philadelphia, Pa: WB Saunders, 1998:1675-92.
183. Lobo RA, Goebelsmann U, Horton R. Evidence for the importance of peripheral tissue events in the development of hirsutism in polycystic ovary syndrome. J Clin Endocrinol Metab 1983;57:393-7.
184. Lobo RA, Paul WL, Goebelsmann U. Dehydroepiandrosterone sulfate as an indicator of adrenal androgen function. Obstet Gynecol 1981;57:69-73.
185. Loriaux DL, Malinak LR, Noall MW. The contribution of plasma dehydroepiandrosterone sulfate to testosterone in a virilized patient with an arrhenoblastoma. J Clin Endocrinol Metab 1970;31:702-4.
186. Lupulescu A. Estrogen use and cancer incidence: a review. Cancer Invest 1995;13:287-95.
187. Ly LP, Handelsman DJ. Empirical estimation of free testosterone from testosterone and sex hormone-binding globulin immunoassays. Eur J Endocrinol 2005;152:471-8.
188. Mabbett S, McIntyre A, Thompson W, Montague D. Development of an enhanced luminescence immunoassay for progesterone. Clin Chem 1989;35:1149. Abstract #393
189. MacMahon B. Age at menarche, United States. series 11, 133NCHS. Washington, DC: National Center for Health Statistics, 1973.
190. MacRae AR, Gardner HA, Allen LC, Tokmakejian S, Lepage N. Outcome validation of the Beckman Coulter access analyzer in a second-trimester Down syndrome serum screening application. Clin Chem 2003;49:69-76.
191. Mahmoud A, Comhaire FH. Mechanisms of disease: late-onset hypogonadism. Nat Clin Pract Urol 2006;3:430-8.
192. Manni A, Pardridge WM, Cefalu W, Nisula BC, Bardin CW, Santner SJ, et al. Bioavailability of albumin-bound testosterone. J Clin Endocrinol Metab 1985;61:705-10.
193. Marshall LA. Clinical evaluation of amenorrhea in active and athletic women. Clin Sports Med 1994;13:371-87.
194. Mathur R, Braunstein GD. Gynecomastia: pathomechanisms and treatment strategies. Horm Res 1997;48:95-102.
195. McGregor JA, Jackson GM, Lachelin GC, Goodwin TM, Artal R, Hastings C, et al. Salivary estriol as risk assessment for preterm labor: a prospective trial. Am J Obstet Gynecol 1995;173:1337-42.
196. McGuinness BJ, Power MJ, Fottrell PF. Radioimmunoassay of 2-hydroxyestrone in urine. Clin Chem 1994;40:80-5.
197. McIver B, Romanski SA, Nippoldt TB. Evaluation and management of amenorrhea. Mayo Clin Proc 1997;72:1161-9.
198. Meier C, Huang T, Wyatt PR, Summers AM. Accuracy of expected risk of Down syndrome using the second-trimester triple test. Clin Chem 2002;48:653-5.

199. Meikle AW, Odell WD. Effect of short- and long-term dexamethasone on 3 alpha-androstanediol glucuronide in hirsute women. Fertil Steril 1986;46:227-31.
200. Mendel CM. The free hormone hypothesis: a physiologically based mathematical model. Endocr Rev 1989;10:232-74.
201. Merke DP, Cutler GB Jr. Evaluation and management of precocious puberty. Arch Dis Child 1996;75:269-71.
202. Middle JG. Dehydroepiandrostenedione sulphate interferes in many direct immunoassays for testosterone. Ann Clin Biochem 2007;44:173-7.
203. Midyett LK, Moore WV, Jacobson JD. Are pubertal changes in girls before age 8 benign? Pediatrics 2003;111:47-51.
204. Miller PB, Soules MR. The usefulness of a urinary LH kit for ovulation prediction during menstrual cycles of normal women. Obstet Gynecol 1996;87:13-7.
205. Miller WL, Styne DM. Female puberty and its disorders. In: Yen SSC, Jaffe RB, Barbieri RL, eds. Reproductive endocrinology: physiology, pathophysiology, and clinical management, 4th edition. Philadelphia, Pa: WB Saunders, 1999:388-412.
206. Misra M, MacLaughlin DT, Donahoe PK, Lee MM. Measurement of Müllerian inhibiting substance facilitates management of boys with microphallus and cryptorchidism. J Clin Endocrinol Metab 2002;87:3598-602.
207. Morales A, Schulman CC, Tostain J, and Wu FCW. Testosterone deficiency syndrome (TDS) needs to be named appropriately—the importance of accurate terminology. Eur Urol 2006;50: 407-9.
208. Morley JE, Kaiser FE, Perry HM 3rd, Patrick P, Morley PM, Stauber PM, et al. Longitudinal changes in testosterone, luteinizing hormone, and follicle-stimulating hormone in healthy older men. Metabolism 1997;46:410-3.
209. Morley JE, Patrick P, Perry HM 3rd. Evaluation of assays available to measure free testosterone. Metabolism 2002;51:554-9.
210. Morrell V. Basic infertility assessment. Primary Care Women's Health 1997;24:195-204.
211. Morris PD, Malkin CJ, Channer KS, Jones TH. A mathematical comparison of techniques to predict biologically available testosterone in a cohort of 1072 men. Eur J Endocrinol 2004;151:241-9.
212. Mulhall J. Sildenafil: a novel effective oral therapy for male erectile dysfunction. Brit J Urol 1997;79:663-4.
213. Nachtigall LB, Boepple PA, Pralong FP, Crowley WF Jr. Adult-onset idiopathic hypogonadotropic hypogonadism—a treatable form of male infertility. N Engl J Med 1997;336:410-5.
214. Nanjee MN, Wheeler MJ. Plasma free testosterone—is an index sufficient? Ann Clin Biochem 1985;22(Pt 4):387-90.
215. Neely EK, Hintz RL, Wilson DM, Lee PA, Gautier T, Argente J, et al. Normal ranges for immunochemiluminometric gonadotropin assays. J Pediatr 1995;127:40-6.
216. Neely EK, Wilson DM, Lee PA, Stene M, Hintz RL. Spontaneous serum gonadotropin concentrations in the evaluation of precocious puberty. J Pediatr 1995;127:47-52.
217. Nelson LM. Clinical practice: primary ovarian insufficiency. N Engl J Med 2009;360:606-14.
218. New MI. Antenatal diagnosis and treatment of congenital adrenal hyperplasia. Curr Urol Rep 2001;2:11-8.
219. New MI, Lorenzen F, Lerner AJ, Kohn B, Oberfield SE, Pollack MS, et al. Genotyping steroid 21-hydroxylase deficiency: hormonal reference data. J Clin Endocrinol Metab 1983;57:320-6.
220. Nieschlag E. Care for the infertile male. Clin Endocrinol 1993;38:123-33.
221. Norman RJ, Dewailly D, Legro RS, Hickey TE. Polycystic ovary syndrome. Lancet 2007;370:685-97.
222. O'Malley B, Strott CA. Steroid hormones: metabolism and mechanism of action. In: Yen SSC, Jaffe RB, Barbieri RL, eds. Reproductive endocrinology: physiology, pathophysiology, and clinical management, 4th edition. Philadelphia, Pa: WB Saunders, 1999:110-33.
223. Oerter KE, Uriarte MM, Rose SR, Barnes KM, Cutler GB Jr. Gonadotropin secretory dynamics during puberty in normal girls and boys. J Clin Endocrinol Metab 1990;71:1251-8.
224. Orth DN, Kovacs WJ. The adrenal cortex. In: Williams RH, Foster DW, Kronenberg HM, Larsen PR, Wilson JD, eds. Williams textbook of endocrinology, 9th edition. Philadelphia, Pa: WB Saunders, 1998:517-664.
225. Palmer OM, Grenache DG, Gronowski AM. The NACB Laboratory Medicine practice guidelines for point of care reproductive testing. Point of Care 2007;6:265-72.
226. Pang S. Congenital adrenal hyperplasia owing to 3 beta-hydroxysteroid dehydrogenase deficiency. Endocrinol Metab Clin North Am 2001;30:81-99, vi-vii.
227. Pang S, Wang M, Jeffries S, Riddick L, Clark A, Estrada E. Normal and elevated 3 alpha-androstanediol glucuronide concentrations in women with various causes of hirsutism and its correlation with degree of hirsutism and androgen levels. J Clin Endocrinol Metab 1992;75:243-8.
228. Pang SY, Lerner AJ, Stoner E, Levine LS, Oberfield SE, Engel I, et al. Late-onset adrenal steroid 3 beta-hydroxysteroid dehydrogenase deficiency. I. A cause of hirsutism in pubertal and postpubertal women. J Clin Endocrinol Metab 1985;60:428-39.
229. Pardridge WM. Receptor-mediated peptide transport through the blood-brain barrier. Endocr Rev 1986;7:314-30.
230. Pardridge WM. Serum bioavailability of sex steroid hormones. Clin Endocrinol Metab 1986;15:259-78.
231. Parker LN. Control of adrenal androgen secretion. Endocrinol Metab Clin North Am 1991;20:401-21.
232. Partsch CJ, Sippell WG. Treatment of central precocious puberty. Best Pract Res Clin Endocrinol Metab 2002;16:165-89.
233. Pearce S, Dowsett M, Jeffcoate SL. Three methods compared for estimating the fraction of testosterone and estradiol not bound to sex-hormone-binding globulin. Clin Chem 1989;35:632-5.
234. Petak SM, Nankin HR, Spark RF, Swerdloff RS, Rodriguez-Rigau LJ. American Association of Clinical Endocrinologists Medical Guidelines for clinical practice for the evaluation and treatment of hypogonadism in adult male patients—2002 update. Endocr Pract 2002;8:440-56.
235. Peter M. Congenital adrenal hyperplasia: 11beta-hydroxylase deficiency. Semin Reprod Med 2002;20:249-54.
236. Raftogianis R, Creveling C, Weinshilboum R, Weisz J. Estrogen metabolism by conjugation. J Natl Cancer Inst Monogr 2000;27:113-24.
237. Ratcliffe WA, Carter GD, Dowsett M, Hillier SG, Middle JG, Reed MJ. Oestradiol assays: applications and guidelines for the provision of a clinical biochemistry service. Ann Clin Biochem 1988;25(Pt 5): 466-83.
238. Rebar RW. Practical evaluation of hormonal status. In: Yen SSC, Jaffe RB, Barbieri RL, eds. Reproductive endocrinology: physiology, pathophysiology, and clinical management, 4th edition. Philadelphia, Pa: WB Saunders, 1999:709-48.
239. Reddy DS, Venkatarangan L, Chien B, Ramu K. A high-performance liquid chromatography-tandem mass spectrometry assay of the androgenic neurosteroid 3alpha-androstanediol (5alpha-androstane-3alpha,17beta-diol) in plasma. Steroids 2005;70:879-85.
240. Regan J, Mahmood N, Alvarez W, Gamble J, Sissors D, Knez R, et al. Automated quantification of estradiol by radial partition immunoassay. Clin Chem 1991;37:936. Abstract #0128
241. Reindollar RH, Novak M, Tho SP, McDonough PG. Adult-onset amenorrhea: a study of 262 patients. Am J Obstet Gynecol 1986;155:531-43.
242. Reinsberg J, Jost E. Analytical performance of the fully automated AxSYM estradiol assay. Clin Chem Lab Med 2000;38: 51-5.
243. Reinsberg J, Jost E, van der Ven H. Performance of the fully automated progesterone assays on the Abbott AxSYM and the Technicon Immuno 1 analyser compared with the radioimmunoassay Progesterone MAIA. Clin Biochem 1997;30:469-71.

244. Rey R. How to evaluate gonadal function in the cryptorchid boy: lessons from new testicular markers. J Pediatr Endocrinol Metab 2003;16:357-64.
245. Riggs BL, Hartmann LC. Selective estrogen-receptor modulators—mechanisms of action and application to clinical practice. N Engl J Med 2003;348:618-29.
246. Rittmaster RS. Hirsutism. Lancet 1997;349:191-5.
247. Rogol A, Blizzard RM. Variations and disorders of pubertal development. In: Kappy MS, Blizzard RM, Migeon CJ, eds. Wilkins' the diagnosis and treatment of endocrine disorders in childhood and adolescence, 4th edition. Springfield, Ill: Charles C Thomas, 1994:857-917.
248. Rosenfield RL. A competitive protein binding method for the measurement of unconjugated and sulfate-conjugated dehydroepiandrosterone in peripheral plasma. Steroids 1971;17:689-96.
249. Rosenfield RL, Bachrach LK, Chernausek SD, Gertner JM, Gottschalk M, Hardin DS, et al. Current age of onset of puberty. Pediatrics 2000;106:622-3.
250. Rosenfield RL, Barnes RB. Menstrual disorders in adolescence. Endocrinol Metab Clin North Am 1993;22:491-505.
251. Rosenfield RL, Lucky AW. Acne, hirsutism, and alopecia in adolescent girls: clinical expressions of androgen excess. Endocrinol Metab Clin North Am 1993;22:507-32.
252. Rosner W. Errors in the measurement of plasma free testosterone. J Clin Endocrinol Metab 1997;82:2014-5.
253. Rosner W. An extraordinarily inaccurate assay for free testosterone is still with us. J Clin Endocrinol Metab 2001;86:2903.
254. Rosner W, Auchus RJ, Azziz R, Sluss PM, Raff H. Position statement: utility, limitations, and pitfalls in measuring testosterone: an Endocrine Society position statement. J Clin Endocrinol Metab 2007;92:405-13.
255. Rowe PJ, Comhaire FH, Hargreave TB, Mellows HJ. WHO manual for the standardizing investigation of the infertile couple. Cambridge, UK: Cambridge University Press, 1993.
256. Said El Shami A, Ito T, Durham A. First solid-phase radioimmunoassay for free testosterone by the analog method. Clin Chem 1985;31:910.
257. Sakiyama R. Approach to patients with hirsutism. Western J Med 1996;165:386-91.
258. Salerno M, Di Maio S, Gasparini N, Mariano A, Macchia V, Tenore A. Central precocious puberty: a single blood sample after gonadotropin-releasing hormone agonist administration in monitoring treatment. Horm Res 1998;50:205-11.
259. Salerno M, Di Maio S, Tenore A. Monitoring therapy for central precocious puberty. Pediatrics 2002;110:1255; author reply 1255.
260. Sanchez-Carbayo M, Mauri M, Alfayate R, Miralles C, and Soria F. Elecsys testosterone assay evaluated. Clin Chem 1998;44:1744-6.
261. Sanchez LA, Knochenhauer ES, Gatlin R, Moran C, Azziz R. Differential diagnosis of clinically evident hyperandrogenism: experience with over 1000 consecutive patients. Fertil Steril 2001;76:S111.
262. Santen RJ. The testis: function and dysfunction. In: Yen SSC, Jaffe RB, Barbieri RL, eds. Reproductive endocrinology: physiology, pathophysiology, and clinical management, 4th edition. Philadelphia, Pa: WB Saunders, 1999:632-68.
263. Santoro NF, Col NF, Eckman MH, Wong JB, Pauker SG, Cauley JA, et al. Therapeutic controversy: hormone replacement therapy—where are we going? J Clin Endocrinol Metab 1999;84:1798-812.
264. Schultheiss D, Stief CG, Truss MC, Jonas U. Pharmacological therapy in erectile dysfunction—current standards and new viewpoints. Wien Med Wochenschr 1997;147:102-4.
265. Scott MG, Ladenson JH, Green ED, Gast MJ. Hormonal evaluation of female infertility and reproductive disorders. Clin Chem 1989;35:620-9.
266. Seibel MM. Ovulation induction with follicle-stimulating hormone. In: Seibel MM, ed. Infertility: a comprehensive text, 2nd edition. Stamford, Conn: Appleton & Lange, 1997:525-36.
267. Seifer DB, Lambert-Messerlian G, Hogan JW, Gardiner AC, Blazar AS, Berk CA. Day 3 serum inhibin-B is predictive of assisted reproductive technologies outcome. Fertil Steril 1997;67:110-4.
268. Seifer DB, Scott RT Jr, Bergh PA, Abrogast LK, Friedman CI, Mack CK, et al. Women with declining ovarian reserve may demonstrate a decrease in day 3 serum inhibin B before a rise in day 3 follicle-stimulating hormone. Fertil Steril 1999;72:63-5.
269. Shane JM. Evaluation and treatment of infertility. Clin Adv Pediatr Symp 1993;45:2-32.
270. Shiraishi S, Lee PW, Leung A, Goh VH, Swerdloff RS, Wang C. Simultaneous measurement of serum testosterone and dihydrotestosterone by liquid chromatography-tandem mass spectrometry. Clin Chem 2008;54:1855-63.
271. Simpson ER. Initiation of parturition, prevention of prematurity. In: MacDonald PC, Hasselmeyer EC, eds. Report of the Fourth Ross Conference on Obstetric Research. Columbus, OH: Ross Laboratories, 1983:94.
272. Sims NA, Brennan K, Spaliviero J, Handelsman DJ, Seibel MJ. Perinatal testosterone surge is required for normal adult bone size but not for normal bone remodeling. Am J Physiol Endocrinol Metab 2006;290:E456-62.
273. Smith SK, Lenton EA, Landgren BM, Cooke ID. The short luteal phase and infertility. Brit J Obstet Gynaecol 1984;91:1120-2.
274. Sodergard R, Backstrom T, Shanbhag V, Carstensen H. Calculation of free and bound fractions of testosterone and estradiol-17 beta to human plasma proteins at body temperature. J Steroid Biochem 1982;16:801-10.
275. Soldin OP, Guo T, Weiderpass E, Tractenberg RE, Hilakivi-Clarke L, Soldin SJ. Steroid hormone levels in pregnancy and 1 year postpartum using isotope dilution tandem mass spectrometry. Fertil Steril 2005;84:701-10.
276. Soldin SJ, Soldin OP. Steroid hormone analysis by tandem mass spectrometry. Clin Chem 2009;55:1061-6.
277. Soules MR, McLachlan RI, Ek M, Dahl KD, Cohen NL, Bremner WJ. Luteal phase deficiency: characterization of reproductive hormones over the menstrual cycle. J Clin Endocrinol Metab 1989;69:804-12.
278. Soules MR, Sherman S, Parrott E, Rebar R, Santoro N, Utian W, et al. Executive summary: Stages of Reproductive Aging Workshop (STRAW). Fertil Steril 2001;76:874-8.
279. Speiser PW. Molecular diagnosis of CYP21 mutations in congenital adrenal hyperplasia: implications for genetic counseling. Am J Pharmacogenomics 2001;1:101-10.
280. Stafford DE, Gordon CM. Adolescent androgen abnormalities. Curr Opin Obstet Gynecol 2002;14:445-51.
281. Stanczyk FZ. Steroid hormones. In: Mishell DR, Davajan V, Lobo RA, eds. Infertility, contraception and reproductive endocrinology, 3rd edition. Boston, Mass: Blackwell Scientific Publications, 1993:53-76.
282. Stocco DM. The steroidogenic acute regulatory (StAR) protein two years later: an update. Endocrine 1997;6:99-109.
283. Strauss JF, Coutifaris C. The endometrium and myometrium: regulation and dysfunction. In: Yen SSC, Jaffe RB, Barbieri RL, eds. Reproductive endocrinology: physiology, pathophysiology, and clinical management, 4th edition. Philadelphia, Pa: WB Saunders, 1999:218-56.
284. Swinkels LM, Ross H, Benraad TJ. A symmetric dialysis method for the determination of free testosterone in human plasma. Clin Chim Acta 1978;165:341-9.
285. Taieb J, Benattar C, Birr AS, and Lindenbaum A. Limitations of steroid determination by direct immunoassay. Clin Chem 2002;48:583-5.
286. Taieb J, Benattar C, Diop R, Birr AS, and Lindenbaum A. Use of the Architect-i2000 estradiol immunoassay during in vitro fertilization. Clin Chem 2003;49:183-6.
287. Tanski S, Rosengren SS, Benn PA. Predictive value of the triple screening test for the phenotype of Down syndrome. Am J Med Genet 1999;85:123-6.

288. Taylor RL, Machacek D, Singh RJ. Validation of a high-throughput liquid chromatography-tandem mass spectrometry method for urinary cortisol and cortisone. Clin Chem 2002;48:1511-9.
289. Tello FL, Hernandez DM. Performance evaluation of nine hormone assays on the Immulite 2000 immunoassay system. Clin Chem Lab Med 2000;38:1039-42.
290. Thienpont L, Siekmann L, Lawson A, Colinet E, De Leenheer A. Development, validation, and certification by isotope dilution gas chromatography-mass spectrometry of lyophilized human serum reference materials for cortisol (CRM 192 and 193) and progesterone (CRM 347 and 348). Clin Chem 1991;37:540-6.
291. Thienpont LM, Van Uytfanghe K, Blincko S, Ramsay CS, Xie H, Doss RC, et al. State-of-the-art of serum testosterone measurement by isotope dilution-liquid chromatography-tandem mass spectrometry. Clin Chem 2008;54:1290-7.
292. Thienpont LM, Verhaeghe PG, Van Brussel KA, De Leenheer AP. Estradiol-17 beta quantified in serum by isotope dilution-gas chromatography-mass spectrometry: reversed-phase C18 high-performance liquid chromatography compared with immuno-affinity chromatography for sample pretreatment. Clin Chem 1988;34:2066-9.
293. Tietz NW, ed. Clinical guide to laboratory tests, 3rd edition. Philadelphia, Pa: WB Saunders, 1995.
294. Tostain JL, Blanc F. Testosterone deficiency: a common, unrecognized syndrome. Nat Clin Pract Urol 2008;5:388-96.
295. Tsukui S, Noda Y, Fukuda A, Matsumoto H, Tatsumi K, Mori T. Blocking effect of sperm immobilizing antibodies on sperm penetration of human zonae pellucidae. J In Vitro Fertil Embryo Transfer 1988;5:123-8.
296. Tulchinsky D, Chopra IJ. Estrogen-androgen imbalance in patients with hirsutism and amenorrhea. J Clin Endocrinol Metab 1974;39:164-9.
297. Turek PJ. Male infertility. In: Tanagho E, McAninch J, eds. Smith's general urology, 17th edition. New York, NY: McGraw-Hill, 2008.
298. Valero-Politi J, Fuentes-Arderiu X. Daily rhythmic and non-rhythmic variations of follitropin, lutropin, testosterone, and sex-hormone-binding globulin in men. Eur J Clin Chem Clin Biochem 1996;34:455-62.
299. Vallejo R, Cavanaugh A, Price JA, Lawruk T, Parente M, Simon F, et al. Development of an enzyme immunoassay for the direct measurement of serum progesterone using monoclonal antibodies. Clin Chem 1988;34:1162.
300. van Rooij IA, Broekmans FJ, Scheffer GJ, Looman CW, Habbema JD, de Jong FH, et al. Serum antimüllerian hormone levels best reflect the reproductive decline with age in normal women with proven fertility: a longitudinal study. Fertil Steril 2005;83:979-87.
301. van Rooij IA, Broekmans FJ, te Velde ER, Fauser BC, Bancsi LF, de Jong FH, et al. Serum anti-Müllerian hormone levels: a novel measure of ovarian reserve. Hum Reprod 2002;17:3065-71.
302. Veldhuis JD. The male hypothalamic-pituitary-gonadal axis. In: Yen SSC, Jaffe RB, Barbieri RL, eds. Reproductive endocrinology: physiology, pathophysiology, and clinical management, 4th edition. Philadelphia, Pa: WB Saunders, 1999:622-31.
303. Veldhuis JD, Pincus SM, Garcia-Rudaz MC, Ropelato MG, Escobar ME, Barontini M. Disruption of the synchronous secretion of leptin, LH, and ovarian androgens in nonobese adolescents with the polycystic ovarian syndrome. J Clin Endocrinol Metab 2001;86:3772-8.
304. Vermeulen A. Androgen replacement therapy in the aging male—a critical evaluation. J Clin Endocrinol Metab 2001;86:2380-90.
305. Vermeulen A, Stoica T, Verdonck L. The apparent free testosterone concentration, an index of androgenicity. J Clin Endocrinol Metab 1971;33:759-67.
306. Vermeulen A, Verdonck L, Kaufman JM. A critical evaluation of simple methods for the estimation of free testosterone in serum. J Clin Endocrinol Metab 1999;84:3666-72.
307. Viniker DA. Investigations for infertility management. In: Viniker DA, ed. Practical guide to reproductive medicine. New York, NY: Parthenon Publishing Group Ltd., 1997:93-110.
308. Wacharasindhu S, Srivuthana S, Aroonparkmongkol S, Shotelersuk V. A cost-benefit of GnRH stimulation test in diagnosis of central precocious puberty (CPP). J Med Assoc Thai 2000;83:1105-11.
309. Wald NJ, Densem JW, Smith D, Klee GG. Four-marker serum screening for Down's syndrome. Prenat Diagn 1994;14:707-16.
310. Wallace AM. Analytical support for the detection and treatment of congenital adrenal hyperplasia. Ann Clin Biochem 1995;32(Pt 1): 9-27.
311. Wang C, Catlin DH, Demers LM, Starcevic B, Swerdloff RS. Measurement of total serum testosterone in adult men: comparison of current laboratory methods versus liquid chromatography-tandem mass spectrometry. J Clin Endocrinol Metab 2004;89:534-43.
312. Wang C, Nieschlag E, Swerdloff R, Behre HM, Hellstrom WJ, Gooren LJ, et al. Investigation, treatment, and monitoring of late-onset hypogonadism in males: ISA, ISSAM, EAU, EAA, and ASA recommendations. J Androl 2009;30:1-9.
313. Wang C, Nieschlag E, Swerdloff R, Behre HM, Hellstrom WJ, Gooren LJ, et al. ISA, ISSAM, EAU, EAA and ASA recommendations: investigation, treatment and monitoring of late-onset hypogonadism in males. Int J Impot Res 2009;21:1-8.
314. Wang C, Nieschlag E, Swerdloff R, Behre HM, Hellstrom WJ, Gooren LJ, et al. ISA, ISSAM, EAU, EAA and ASA recommendations: investigation, treatment and monitoring of late-onset hypogonadism in males. Aging Male 2009;12:5-12.
315. Wang C, Shiraishi S, Leung A, Baravarian S, Hull L, Goh V, et al. Validation of a testosterone and dihydrotestosterone liquid chromatography tandem mass spectrometry assay: interference and comparison with established methods. Steroids 2008;73:1345-52.
316. Warren MP. Clinical review 77: evaluation of secondary amenorrhea. J Clin Endocrinol Metab 1996;81:437-42.
317. Wentz AC. Diagnosing luteal phase inadequacy. Fertil Steril 1982;37:334-5.
318. Wentz AC, Kossoy LR, Parker RA. The impact of luteal phase inadequacy in an infertile population. Am J Obstet Gynecol 1990;162:937-43.
319. Wheeler MJ. The determination of bio-available testosterone. Ann Clin Biochem 1995;32:345-57.
320. Wheeler MJ, Barnes SC. Measurement of testosterone in the diagnosis of hypogonadism in the ageing male. Clin Endocrinol (Oxf) 2008;69:515-25.
321. Wheeler MJ, D'Souza A, Matadeen J, Croos P. Ciba Corning ACS:180 testosterone assay evaluated. Clin Chem 1996;42:1445-9.
322. White PC. Genetic diseases of steroid metabolism. Vitam Horm 1994;49:131-95.
323. Williams C, Giannopoulos T, Sherriff EA. ACP best practice no. 170: investigation of infertility with the emphasis on laboratory testing and with reference to radiological imaging. J Clin Pathol 2003;56: 261-7.
324. Wilson DH, Groskopf W, Hsu S, Caplan D, Langner T, Baumann M, et al. Rapid, automated assay for progesterone on the Abbott AxSYM analyzer. Clin Chem 1998;44:86-91.
325. Wilson JD, George FW, Griffin JE. The hormonal control of sexual development. Science 1981;211:1278-84.
326. Winters SJ, Kelley DE, Goodpaster B. The analog free testosterone assay: are the results in men clinically useful? Clin Chem 1998; 44:2178-82.
327. Wood P. Salivary steroid assays: research or routine? Ann Clin Biochem 2009;46:183-96.
328. Woolever C, Goldfien A. A double isotope derivative method for plasma progesterone assay. Int J Appl Radiat 1963;14:163-71.
329. Wu H, Ramsay C, Ozaeta P, Liu L, Aboleneen H. Serum estradiol quantified by isotope dilution-gas chromatography/mass spectrometry. Clin Chem 2002;48:364-6.
330. Wudy SA, Wachter UA, Homoki J, Teller WM. Determination of dehydroepiandrosterone sulfate in human plasma by gas chromatography/mass spectrometry using a deuterated internal standard: a method suitable for routine clinical use. Horm Res 1993;39:235-40.

331. Yang DT, Owen WE, Ramsay CS, Xie H, Roberts WL. Performance characteristics of eight estradiol immunoassays. Am J Clin Pathol 2004;122:332-7.
332. Yazigi RA, Quintero CH, Salameh WA. Prolactin disorders. Fertil Steril 1997;67:215-25.
333. Yeh J, Adashi EY. The ovarian life cycle. In: Yen SSC, Jaffe RB, Barbieri RL, eds. Reproductive endocrinology: physiology, pathophysiology, and clinical management, 4th edition. Philadelphia, Pa: WB Saunders, 1999:153-90.
334. Yen SSC. Chronic anovulation caused by peripheral endocrine disorders. In: Yen SSC, Jaffe RB, Barbieri RL, eds. Reproductive endocrinology: physiology, pathophysiology, and clinical management, 4th edition. Philadelphia, Pa: WB Saunders, 1999:479-515.
335. Yen SSC. Chronic anovulation due to CNS-hypothalamic-pituitary dysfunction. In: Yen SSC, Jaffe RB, Barbieri RL, eds. Reproductive endocrinology: physiology, pathophysiology, and clinical management, 4th edition. Philadelphia, Pa: WB Saunders, 1999:516-61.
336. Yen SSC. The human menstrual cycle: neuroendocrine regulation. In: Yen SSC, Jaffe RB, Barbieri RL, eds. Reproductive endocrinology: physiology, pathophysiology, and clinical management, 4th edition. Philadelphia, Pa: WB Saunders, 1999:191-217.
337. Yen SSC. Polycystic ovary syndrome: hyperandrogenic chronic anovulation. In: Yen SSC, Jaffe RB, Barbieri RL, eds. Reproductive endocrinology: physiology, pathophysiology, and clinical management, 4th edition. Philadelphia, Pa: WB Saunders, 1999:436-78.
338. Young D. Effects of preanalytical variables on clinical laboratory tests. Washington, DC: AACC Press, 1993.
339. Zemaitis MA, Kroboth PD. Simplified procedure for measurement of serum dehydroepiandrosterone and its sulfate with gas chromatography-ion trap mass spectrometry and selected reaction monitoring. J Chromatogr B Biomed Sci Appl 1998;716:19-26.

CHAPTER 57

Pregnancy and Its Disorders

*Edward R. Ashwood, M.D., David G. Grenache, Ph.D., M.T.(A.S.C.P.), D.A.B.C.C., F.A.C.B., and Geralyn Lambert-Messerlian, Ph.D.**

The clinical laboratory has an important role in managing pregnancy.[25] In contrast to most clinical situations, when treating an expectant mother, a physician must simultaneously care for more than one patient. The health of the mother and that of her fetus are intertwined, each affecting the other; thus pregnancy management must consider both. This chapter reviews the biology of pregnancy and discusses laboratory tests used to detect, evaluate, and monitor both normal and abnormal pregnancies. Included are common tests, such as (1) chorionic gonadotropin (CG); (2) hematocrit; (3) blood type; (4) glucose tolerance testing; (5) prenatal testing and screening and diagnosis of fetal aneuplodies; and (6) esoteric tests, such as fetal lung maturity tests and amniotic fluid bilirubin examination.

HUMAN PREGNANCY

To appreciate the role of laboratory tests in pregnancy health care, it is necessary to understand fundamental topics such as (1) conception, embryo development, and fetal growth; (2) the role of the placenta; (3) the importance and composition of amniotic fluid; (4) maternal adaptation to pregnancy; and (5) functional maturation of the fetus.

Conception, Embryo, and Fetus

Normal human pregnancy (i.e., gestation) lasts approximately 40 weeks, as measured from the first day of the last normal menstrual period, a date commonly represented by the abbreviations LMP or LNMP. The anticipated date of birth of an infant is commonly referred to as the *expected date of confinement*, or EDC. During pregnancy, a woman undergoes dramatic physiologic and hormonal changes. When talking with patients, physicians customarily divide pregnancy into four time intervals. The first three time intervals are called *trimesters,* each of which is ≈13 weeks. The last time interval, 37 to 42 weeks, is coined *term.* By convention, the first trimester, 0 to 13 weeks, begins on the first day of the last menses.

Ovulation occurs on approximately the 14th day of the regular menstrual cycle (see Chapter 56). If conception occurs, the ovum is fertilized, usually in the fallopian tube, and becomes a *zygote,* which is then carried down the tube into the uterus. The zygote divides, becoming a *morula.* After 50 to 60 cells are present, the morula develops a cavity, the primitive *yolk sac,* and thus becomes a *blastocyst,* which implants into the uterine wall about 5 days after fertilization. The cells on the exterior wall of the blastocyst, *trophoblasts,* synergistically invade the uterine endometrium and develop into chorionic villi, creating the placenta. Trophoblasts are subdivided into syncytiotrophoblasts and cytotrophoblasts, depending on location and cellular morphology.

At this stage, the product of conception is referred to as an *embryo.* A cavity called the *amnion* forms and enlarges with the accumulation of *liquor amnii,* commonly referred to as *amniotic fluid.* Nourished by the placenta and protected by the amniotic fluid, an embryo undergoes rapid cell division, differentiation, and growth. From combinations of three primary cell types, *ectoderm, mesoderm,* and *endoderm,* organs begin to form through a process called *organogenesis.* At 10 weeks, an embryo has developed most major structures and is now referred to as a *fetus.* At 13 weeks, the fetus weighs approximately 13 g and is ≈8 cm long.

Rapid fetal growth occurs during the 13 to 26 weeks of the second trimester. By the end of the second trimester, the fetus weighs approximately 700 g and is 30 cm long. Many fetal organs begin to mature. The 26 to 38 weeks of the third trimester is the period in which fetal organs complete their prenatal maturation. During this trimester, the growth rate decelerates. At the end of the third trimester, the fetus weighs approximately 3200 g and is about 50 cm long. *Term* is the interval from 37 to 42 weeks. Normal labor, rhythmic uterine contractions, and birth occur during this period.

**The authors gratefully acknowledge the original contributions of George J. Knight, upon which portions of this chapter are based.*

Placenta

The placenta and the umbilical cord form the primary link between fetus and mother. The placenta grows throughout pregnancy and is normally delivered through the birth canal immediately after the birth of the infant.

Function

The placenta (1) keeps the maternal and fetal circulation systems separate, (2) nourishes the fetus, (3) eliminates fetal wastes, and (4) produces hormones vital to pregnancy. It is composed of large collections of fetal vessels called *villi,* which are surrounded by intervillous spaces in which maternal blood flows. For substances to move from the maternal circulation to the fetal circulation, they must cross through the trophoblasts and several membranes. The transfer of any substance depends largely on the (1) concentration gradient between the maternal and fetal circulatory systems, (2) presence or absence of circulating binding proteins, (3) lipid solubility of the substance, and (4) presence of facilitated transport, such as ion pumps or receptor-mediated endocytosis (Box 57-1). The placenta is an effective barrier to the movement of large proteins and hydrophobic compounds bound to plasma proteins. Maternal immunoglobulin (Ig)G crosses the placenta via receptor-mediated endocytosis. Because of its long half-life, maternally produced IgG protects a newborn for the first 6 months of life. Antibody assays with low limits of detection may be positive in infants up to age 18 months because of maternal antibodies.

Placental Hormones

The placenta produces several protein and steroid hormones (Figure 57-1). The major protein hormones are CG and placental lactogen (PL). The steroids include progesterone, estradiol, estriol, and estrone. The placenta secretes most of its products into the maternal circulation; only small amounts reach the fetal circulation. Close proximity of the maternal blood vessels to the site of placental hormone production may explain some of this preferential accumulation of hormones in the maternal blood circulation. Generally, hormone production by the placenta increases in proportion to the increase in placental mass. Therefore concentrations of hormones derived from the placenta, such as PL, increase in maternal peripheral blood as the placenta increases in size. CG, which peaks at the end of the first trimester, is an exception.

Chorionic Gonadotropin

One of the most important placental hormones is CG. It stimulates the ovary to produce progesterone, which, in turn, prevents menstruation, thereby protecting the pregnancy. The chemistry, biochemistry, and methods for CG are discussed later in this chapter.

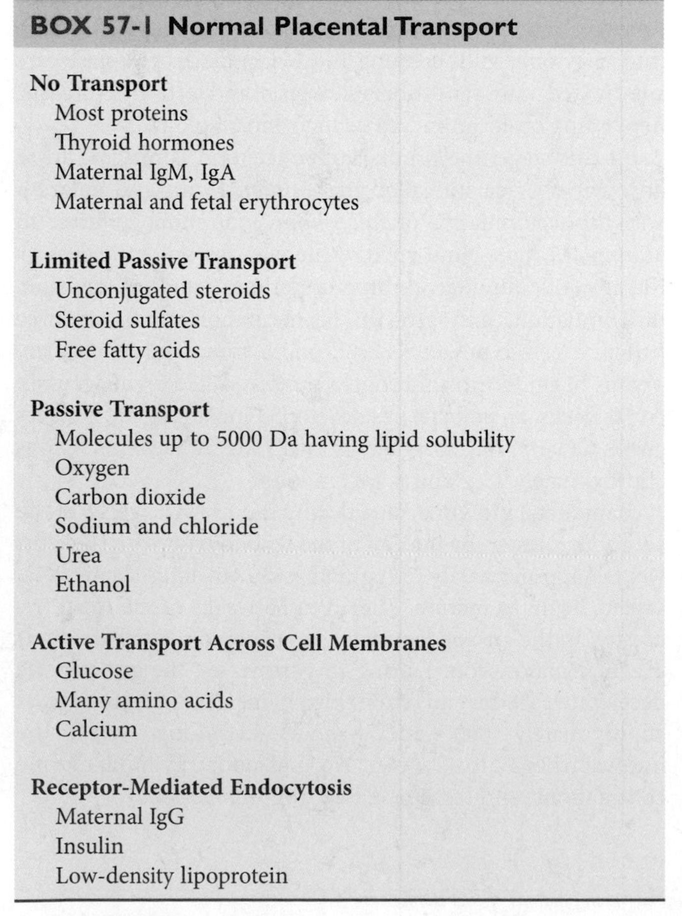

BOX 57-1 Normal Placental Transport

No Transport
- Most proteins
- Thyroid hormones
- Maternal IgM, IgA
- Maternal and fetal erythrocytes

Limited Passive Transport
- Unconjugated steroids
- Steroid sulfates
- Free fatty acids

Passive Transport
- Molecules up to 5000 Da having lipid solubility
- Oxygen
- Carbon dioxide
- Sodium and chloride
- Urea
- Ethanol

Active Transport Across Cell Membranes
- Glucose
- Many amino acids
- Calcium

Receptor-Mediated Endocytosis
- Maternal IgG
- Insulin
- Low-density lipoprotein

Ig, Immunoglobulin.

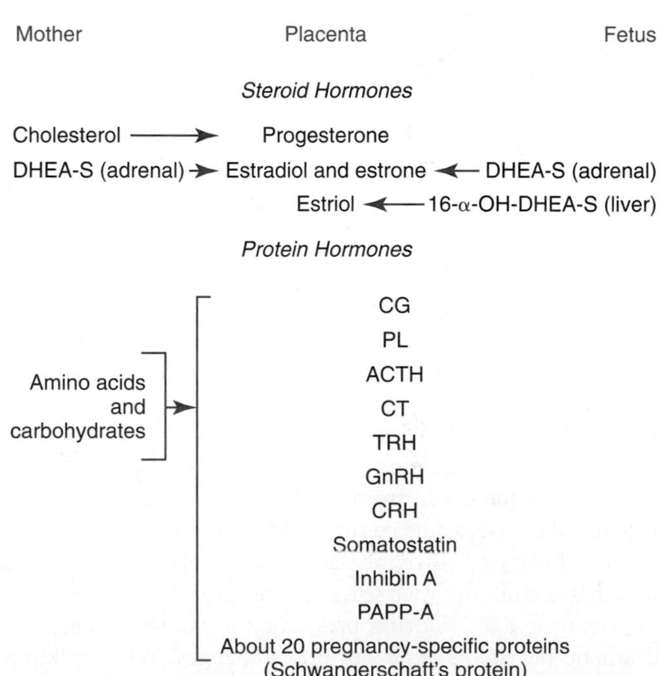

Figure 57-1 Schematic representation of steroid and protein hormone production by the placenta. ***ACTH,*** **Adrenocorticotropic hormone;** ***CG,*** **chorionic gonadotropin;** ***CRH,*** **corticotropin-releasing hormone;** ***CT,*** **chorionic thyrotropin;** ***DHEA-S,*** **dehydroepiandrosterone sulfate;** ***GnRH,*** **gonadotropin-releasing hormone;** ***PAPP-A,*** **pregnancy-associated plasma protein-A;** ***PL,*** **placental lactogen;** ***TRH,*** **thyroid-stimulating hormone.**

Placental Lactogen

PL, also known as human placental lactogen (hPL) and human chorionic somatomammotropin (hCS), is a single polypeptide chain of 191 amino acids having two intramolecular disulfide bridges and a molecular mass of 22,279 Da. The structure of PL is exceptionally homologous (96%) with growth hormone (GH) and less so with prolactin (67%). Also, PL has potent growth and lactogenic properties. Five genes on chromosome 17 compose a gene family that codes for both GH and PL.[279] PL production has been localized by immunofluorescence studies to the syncytiotrophoblast cells of the placenta. The increase in maternal serum PL concentration with advancing gestational age is directly correlated with the increasing mass of placental tissue and of functional syncytiotrophoblast tissue.[333] Placental secretion near term is 1 to 2 g/d, the largest of any known human hormone.

PL has many biological activities, including (1) lactogenic, (2) metabolic, (3) somatotropic, (4) luteotropic, (5) erythropoietic, and (6) aldosterone-stimulating effects. In addition, either directly or in synergism with prolactin, PL has a significant role in preparing the mammary glands for lactation. The many metabolic activities of PL closely resemble those of GH, including (1) inhibition of glucose uptake, (2) enhanced lipolysis leading to increased mobilization of free fatty acids, and (3) enhancement of nitrogen retention. Because glucose is the primary energy substrate for a fetus, it has been suggested that the glucose-sparing action of PL may provide a strategy to direct maternal metabolism toward greater use of fat for the mother's requirements, thereby sparing maternal glucose for fetal use. Rare normal pregnancies have been reported in which complete absence of PL was noted. Although PL was used in the past to evaluate fetal well-being, currently no apparent clinical reason exists to measure PL.[101]

Placental Steroids

The placenta produces a wide variety of steroid hormones, including estrogen and progesterone with large amounts of estrogens produced at term. The chemistry of these steroids is described in Chapter 56. Maternal cholesterol is the main precursor for placental progesterone production. Biosynthesis of estrogens by the placenta differs from that of the ovaries because the placenta has no 17α-hydroxylase. Thus, each of the estrogens—estrone (E_1), estradiol (E_2), and estriol (E_3)—must be synthesized from C-19 intermediates that already have a hydroxyl group at position 17. In nonpregnant women, the ovaries secrete 100 to 600 μg/d of estradiol, of which about 10% is metabolized to estriol. During late pregnancy, the placenta produces 50 to 150 mg/d of estriol and 15 to 20 mg/d of estradiol and estrone. Secretion of estrogens and progesterone throughout pregnancy ensures (1) appropriate development of the endometrium, (2) uterine growth, (3) adequate uterine blood supply, and (4) preparation of the uterus for labor. Although measurement of estriol in the third trimester was used in the past to assess fetal well-being, most obstetricians now consider this practice obsolete.[100] Estriol measurements in the second trimester of pregnancy are useful in predicting fetal trisomy 21 and 18 (see later discussion on maternal serum screening for fetal defects).

Amniotic Fluid

Throughout intrauterine life, the fetus lives within a fluid-filled compartment. The amniotic fluid provides a medium in which a fetus readily moves; it cushions a fetus against possible injury and helps maintain a constant temperature. This fluid is a dynamic medium whose volume and chemical composition are controlled within relatively narrow limits.

Volume and Dynamics

The volume of amniotic fluid increases progressively until 34 weeks' gestation, when it decreases slightly through the 40th week and then more sharply declines until the 42nd week.[312] The volume is 200 to 300 mL at 16 weeks, 400 to 1400 mL at 26 weeks, 300 to 2000 mL at 34 weeks, and 300 to 1400 mL at 40 weeks. The volume at any given moment is a function of several interrelated fluid fluxes. Direct measurements in primates and indirect measurements in humans have been used to derive a mathematical model of amniotic fluid volume.[239] At term, total fluid fluxes into and out of the amniotic cavity are large (≈60 mL/h) and result in complete exchange of the amniotic fluid volume twice per day. Gross unidirectional fluid volume shifts occur episodically: into the amniotic cavity by fetal urination and out of the cavity by fetal swallowing. These unidirectional shifts begin at the end of the first trimester and increase linearly until approximately 30 weeks. Fetal swallowing and urination then exponentially increase, peaking at term at about 1000 mL/d. Bidirectional water exchanges—so-called intramembranous fluxes—occur across the following surfaces: (1) placenta (mother-fetus); (2) umbilical vessels, through the substance of the umbilical cord (fetus–amniotic fluid); (3) fetal skin (fetus–amniotic fluid); and (4) fetal membranes (amniotic fluid–mother). These exchanges increase in a linear fashion throughout pregnancy. At term, they are approximately 400 mL/d. The fetal tracheobronchial tree is filled with amniotic fluid. Although lung fluid transport contributes a small volume, fetal breathing of this fluid is the mechanism of surfactant transport from the fetal lungs into the amniotic fluid.

Pathologic decreases and increases in amniotic fluid volume are encountered frequently in clinical practice. Intrauterine growth retardation and anomalies of the fetal urinary tract, such as bilateral renal agenesis or obstruction of the urethra, are associated with *oligohydramnios,* an abnormally low amniotic fluid volume. Increased fluid volume is known as *hydramnios* (also termed *polyhydramnios*). Conditions associated with hydramnios include (1) maternal diabetes mellitus, (2) severe Rh isoimmune disease, (3) fetal esophageal atresia, (4) multifetal pregnancy, (5) anencephaly, and (6) spina bifida.

Composition

Early in gestation, the composition of the amniotic fluid resembles a complex dialysate of the maternal serum. As a fetus grows, the amniotic fluid changes in several ways

TABLE 57-1 Composition of Amniotic Fluid (Mean Values)

Component	Gestational Age, Wk		
	15	25	40
Sodium, mmol/L	136	138	126
Potassium, mmol/L	3.9	4.0	4.3
Chloride, mmol/L	111	109	103
Bicarbonate, mmol/L	16	18	16
Urea nitrogen, mg/dL (mmol urea/L)	11 (3.9)	11 (3.9)	18 (6.4)
Creatinine, mg/dL (µmol/L)	0.8 (71)	0.9 (80)	2.2 (194)
Glucose, mg/dL (mmol/L)	47 (2.6)	39 (2.2)	32 (1.8)
Uric acid, mg/dL (mmol/L)	4.0 (0.24)	5.7 (0.34)	10.4 (0.61)
Total protein, g/dL (g/L)	0.5 (5)	0.8 (8)	0.3 (3)
Bilirubin, mg/dL (µmol/L)	0.13 (2.2)	0.14 (2.4)	0.04 (0.7)
Osmolality, mOsm/kg H_2O	272	272	255

From Benzie RJ, Doran TA, Harkins JL, Owen VM, Porter CJ. Composition of the amniotic fluid and maternal serum in pregnancy. Am J Obstet Gynecol 1974;119:798-810.

(Table 57-1). Most notably, sodium concentration and osmolality decrease and concentrations of urea, creatinine, and uric acid increase.[39] The activities of many enzymes in amniotic fluid have been studied with respect to both gestational age and fetal status but have not been found to be clinically useful. The major lipids of interest are the phospholipids, whose type and concentrations reflect fetal lung maturity (discussed further later). Numerous steroid and protein hormones are also present in amniotic fluid.[418] Concentrations of androgens and estrogens have been measured in futile attempts to predict fetal sex. The rare syndrome of congenital adrenal hyperplasia (CAH) has been diagnosed antenatally by measuring 17-hydroxyprogesterone and pregnanetriol in the amniotic fluid near term.[190] Measurements of thyroid-stimulating hormone (TSH) and thyroxine in amniotic fluid may be useful in cases of fetal thyroid disease.[348] No other diagnostic uses for amniotic fluid hormone measurements are in common use. Prostaglandins E_1, E_2, $F_{1\alpha}$, and $F_{2\alpha}$ all are found in low concentrations in amniotic fluid and increase gradually during pregnancy. PGE_2 and $PGF_{2\alpha}$ concentrations are very high during active labor.[109] Attempts to demonstrate an acute rise in PGE_2 or $PGF_{2\alpha}$ immediately before the onset of labor, at the initiation of parturition, have been unsuccessful.

Early in pregnancy, little or no particulate matter is found in the amniotic fluid. By 16 weeks of gestation, large numbers of cells are present, having been shed from the surfaces of the amnion, skin, and tracheobronchial tree. These cells have proved to be of great utility in antenatal diagnosis. As pregnancy continues to progress, scalp hair and *lanugo* (fine hair on the body of the fetus) are shed into the fluid and contribute to its turbidity. Production of surfactant particles in the lung, termed *lamellar bodies,* greatly increases the haziness of the fluid. At term, amniotic fluid contains gross particles of *vernix caseosa,* the oily substance composed of sebum and desquamated epithelial cells covering the fetal skin.

Normal fetuses do not defecate during pregnancy. If severely stressed, a fetus may pass stool that is called *meconium.* This heterogeneous material contains many bile pigments and therefore stains the amniotic fluid green. Meconium-stained amniotic fluid is a sign of fetal stress.

Maternal Adaptation

During pregnancy, a woman undergoes dramatic physiologic and hormonal changes. The large quantities of estrogen, progesterone, PL, and corticosteroids produced during pregnancy affect various metabolic, physiologic, and endocrinologic systems. In addition, the woman experiences (1) an increase in resistance to angiotensin; (2) a predominance of lipid metabolism over glucose use; and (3) increased synthesis by the liver of thyroid- and steroid-binding proteins, fibrinogen, and other proteins characteristic of pregnancy. As a result of such changes, many of the laboratory reference intervals for nonpregnant patients are not appropriate for pregnant patients. Lockitch[229] has developed reference intervals for more than 70 analytes in normal pregnancy. Her study group included 29 pregnant subjects tested from 16 weeks to term and also postpartum. Mean values for selected tests expressed as a percentage of control means are presented in Table 57-2.

Hematologic Changes

Maternal blood volume increases during pregnancy by an average of 45%. Plasma volume increases more rapidly than red blood cell mass; therefore, despite augmented erythropoiesis, hemoglobin concentration, erythrocyte count, and hematocrit decrease during normal pregnancy. Hemoglobin concentrations at term average 12.6 g/dL, compared with 13.3 g/dL for the nonpregnant state. The leukocyte count varies considerably during pregnancy, from 4000 to 13,000/µL. During labor and puerperium (the interval immediately after delivery), leukocyte counts may be markedly elevated.

The concentrations of several blood coagulation factors are increased during pregnancy. For example, plasma fibrinogen increases by approximately 65%, from 275 to 450 mg/dL; this increase contributes to the increase in sedimentation rate. Other clotting factors also increase, including factors VII, VIII, IX, and X. Prothrombin and factors V and XII do not change, whereas factors XI and XIII decrease slightly. Even though the platelet count remains unchanged in most

TABLE 57-2 Mean Serum and Plasma Laboratory Values During Normal Pregnancies Expressed as a Percentage of the Nonpregnant Mean ($n = 29$)

Analyte	Time of Gestation 12 Wk	32 Wk	Term
Sodium	97	98	97
Potassium	95	95	100
Bicarbonate	85	85	81
Chloride	98	100	99
Urea nitrogen	77	63	77
Creatinine	71	74	81
Fasting glucose	98	94	94
Bilirubin, unconjugated	56	67	78
Albumin	93	78	78
Protein	92	83	83
Uric acid	68	92	120
Calcium	98	94	97
Free ionized calcium	99	101	102
Parathyroid hormone, intact	—	—	140
1,25-Dihydroxyvitamin D	—	—	400
Phosphate	108	97	96
Magnesium	92	87	87
Alkaline phosphatase	90	203	347
Creatine kinase	87	86	135
α_1-Antitrypsin	129	174	191
Transferrin	105	160	170
Cholesterol	100	144	156
HDL-cholesterol	121	119	130
LDL-cholesterol	80	118	146
Fasting triglycerides	141	300	349
Iron	112	94	94
Iron-binding capacity	95	139	144
Transferrin saturation	136	68	64
Zinc protoporphyrin	107	109	144
Ferritin	81	33	59
Thyroxine	103	107	100
Triiodothyronine	100	121	121
Free thyroxine	98	72	74
Thyroxine-binding globulin	114	155	182
Thyroid-stimulating hormone	111	122	139
Cortisol	111	301	309
Aldosterone	—	—	1500
Prolactin	—	—	800
Hemoglobin	95	90	96
Hematocrit	94	91	97
Leukocyte count	144	167	240
Prothrombin time	99	97	97
Activated partial thromboplastin time	95	91	93
Platelet count	98	96	100
Fibrinogen	119	154	165

Data from Lockitch G, ed. Handbook of diagnostic biochemistry and hematology in normal pregnancy. Boca Raton, Fla: CRC Press, 1993.
HDL, High-density lipoprotein; *LDL*, low-density lipoprotein.

women and prothrombin time and activated partial thromboplastin time shorten slightly (see Table 57-2), pregnancy increases the risk of thromboembolism to up to five times that of nonpregnant women.

Biochemical Changes

During pregnancy, electrolytes show little change, but an approximately 40% increase in serum triglycerides, cholesterol, phospholipids, and free fatty acids is seen. Plasma albumin is decreased to an average of 3.4 g/dL in late pregnancy; plasma globulin concentrations increase slightly. Several of the plasma transport proteins, including thyroxine-binding globulin (TBG), cortisol-binding globulin (CBG), and sex hormone-binding globulin (SHBG), increase markedly. Serum cholinesterase activity is reduced, whereas alkaline phosphatase activity in serum is tripled, mainly as the result of an increase in very heat-stable alkaline phosphatase of placental origin. In addition, creatine kinase can markedly increase upon delivery.

Renal Function

Pregnancy increases the glomerular filtration rate (GFR) to about 170 mL/min/1.73 m^2 by 20 weeks, and therefore increases the clearance of urea, creatinine, and uric acid. Concentrations of these three analytes are slightly decreased in serum for much of the pregnancy. As term approaches, GFR begins to return to nonpregnant values. Urea and creatinine concentrations rise slightly during the last 4 weeks. During this time, tubular reabsorption of uric acid increases dramatically, which increases serum uric acid compared with the nonpregnant state. Glucosuria, up to 1000 mg/d, may be present owing to increased GFR, which presents more fluid to the tubules and therefore lowers the renal glucose threshold. Protein loss in the urine can increase to up to 300 mg/d.

Endocrine Changes

The action of progesterone prevents menses and thus allows pregnancy to continue. In early pregnancy, progesterone is produced by the corpus luteum of the maternal ovary in response to CG. In later stages, the placenta directly produces enough progesterone to maintain the pregnancy.

Throughout pregnancy, the plasma parathyroid hormone (PTH) is increased by approximately 40%, with almost no change in the plasma free ionized calcium fraction, thus suggesting a new set point for the secretion of PTH. Calcitonin does not increase predictably during pregnancy, whereas 1,25-dihydroxyvitamin D is increased during pregnancy and promotes increased intestinal calcium absorption. These changes permit the transfer of large amounts of calcium to the developing fetus.

Elevated estrogen concentration stimulates increased hepatic production of CBG. The hepatic clearance of cortisol decreases. Thus, the absolute plasma concentrations of both total and free cortisol are several times higher during pregnancy. The diurnal rhythm of cortisol, higher in the morning and lower in the evening, is maintained. Increased plasma aldosterone and deoxycorticosterone concentrations are observed.

Increasing estrogen concentrations throughout pregnancy increase the secretion of prolactin up to tenfold. Conversely, high estrogen concentrations during pregnancy suppress the secretion of luteinizing hormone (LH) and follicle-stimulating hormone (FSH) below the detection limit. Baseline concentrations of other pituitary hormones such as TSH remain nearly unchanged (see Table 57-2), but the GH response to provocative stimuli is blunted.

Although normal pregnancy is a euthyroid state, many changes occur in thyroid function. High concentrations of TBG raise the concentration of total thyroxine (T_4) and triiodothyronine (T_3), but a slight decrease in free T_4 concentration occurs during the second and third trimesters. A slight reciprocal increase in TSH was reported by Lockitch.[229] Thyroglobulin is significantly increased, especially in the third trimester.[151] Very few (<0.2%) pregnant individuals develop hyperthyroidism, and hypothyroidism is very rare.[67] Postpartum thyroid dysfunction is common and is frequently unrecognized. The fetal thyroid-pituitary axis functions independently from the mother's axis in most cases. However, if the mother has preexisting Graves disease (hyperthyroidism caused by autoantibodies that stimulate the thyroid), those antibodies can cross the placenta, causing hyperthyroidism in the fetus. If the mother has anti-TSH autoantibodies, the infant can develop transient hypothyroidism.[229]

Functional Development of the Fetus

Fetal organs mature during the third trimester but not at the same rate. This section reviews the lung, liver, and kidneys, and blood maturation, in the fetus.

Lungs and Pulmonary Surfactant

In normal air-breathing lungs, a substance called *pulmonary surfactant* coats the alveolar epithelium and responds to alveolar volume changes by reducing surface tension in the alveolar wall during expiration. Surfactant is needed because surface tension is an inverse function of the radius of the airway. Thus small alveoli have a higher collapsing force than larger alveoli. Surfactant opposes the force and keeps the small alveoli from collapsing. Specialized alveolar cells called *type II granular pneumocytes* synthesize pulmonary surfactant and package it into laminated storage granules called *lamellar bodies*.[186,351] These storage granules are 1 to 5 μm in diameter and contain phospholipids, cholesterol, and protein.[276] Production starts as early as 20 weeks' gestation,[351] but adequate amounts do not accumulate until about 36 weeks. Exudation of pulmonary fluid (via the trachea) and fetal breathing movements transport lamellar bodies into the amniotic fluid. The internal structure of the particles is rearranged into a formation described as *tubular myelin* by those using electron microscopy.[186] The newborn lung contains 100 times more surfactant per cm^3 than the adult lung. Excessive surfactant is needed at birth as the newborn is transformed from breathing water to breathing air. Surfactant overcomes the surface tension produced in water-filled alveoli that are admitting air for the first time.

Pulmonary surfactant is a complex mixture of lipids and proteins; less than 5% is composed of carbohydrates. Most of the lipid is phospholipid, and most of that is lecithin (phosphatidylcholine).[65] Unlike lecithin from other tissues, pulmonary lecithin has two saturated fatty acids, usually palmitoyl groups. Other lipids present are phosphatidylglycerol (PG), phosphatidylinositol (PI), and phosphatidylethanolamine (see Chapter 27). Sphingomyelin is present in very small amounts (<2%). The protein fraction of lamellar bodies is approximately 4% and is composed of four surfactant-specific proteins: SP-A, SP-B, SP-C, and SP-D.[177,297]

Type II pneumocytes synthesize phosphatidylcholine in a manner quite different from that seen in other cells. Most other cells synthesize phosphatidylserine from cytidine diphosphate diacylglycerol and serine. The phosphatidylserine then is decarboxylated to yield phosphatidyl ethanolamine. The final step is the successive donation of three methyl groups via *S*-adenosylmethionine to form phosphatidylcholine. The pulmonary biosynthetic pathway is shown in Figure 57-2. The enzyme choline phosphotransferase forms PC directly from cytidine diphosphocholine and diacylglycerol. Phosphatidylinositol formation peaks at about 35 weeks. As PI decreases in concentration, PG begins to increase.

Liver

Hematopoiesis occurs in the liver during the first two trimesters and is transferred to the fetal bone marrow during the third trimester. The liver is also responsible for production of specific proteins (such as albumin and clotting factors), metabolism and detoxification of many compounds, and secretion of substances such as bilirubin. A clinically useful protein produced by the liver is alpha fetoprotein (AFP). Detoxification and bilirubin secretion mechanisms are immature until late in pregnancy and even in the first few months after birth. Thus premature infants often have high serum bilirubin concentrations and metabolize drugs poorly.

Kidneys

Toward the end of the first trimester, the fetal kidneys begin to produce urine, which is the main component of amniotic fluid. Early nephrons cannot produce concentrated urine, and pH regulation is also limited. Complete maturation occurs after birth. Although kidneys are not required for fetal survival, amniotic fluid is required. Without fluid to breathe, the fetal lungs fail to properly develop. Thus newborns without kidneys die of pulmonary failure.

Fetal Blood Development

Fetal blood is produced first by the embryonic yolk sac, then by the liver, and finally by the fetal bone marrow. The yolk sac produces three embryonic hemoglobins: Portland ($\zeta_2\gamma_2$), Gower-1 ($\zeta_2\varepsilon_2$), and Gower-2 ($\alpha_2\varepsilon_2$). These normal embryonic hemoglobins are of little importance in clinical chemistry because they are present in fetal blood only in the first trimester.

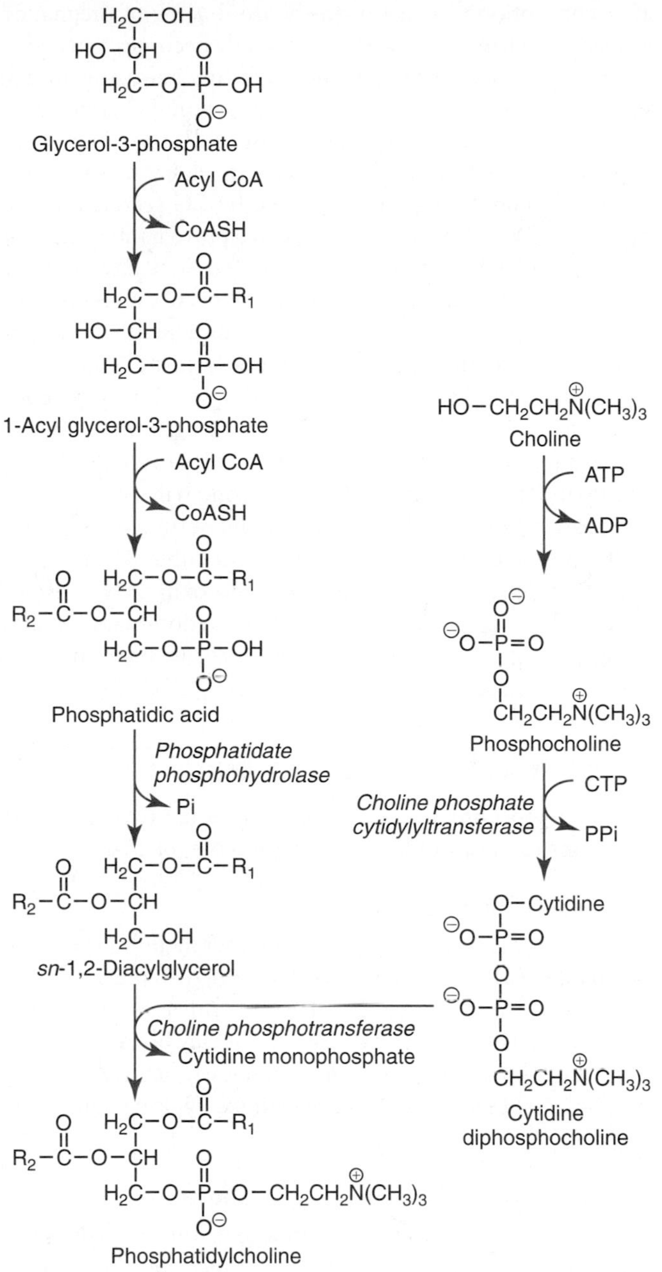

Glycerol-3-phosphate

Acyl CoA → CoASH

1-Acyl glycerol-3-phosphate

Acyl CoA → CoASH

Phosphatidic acid

Phosphatidate phosphohydrolase → Pi

sn-1,2-Diacylglycerol

Choline phosphotransferase → Cytidine monophosphate

Phosphatidylcholine

Choline

ATP → ADP

Phosphocholine

Choline phosphate cytidylyltransferase CTP → PPi

Cytidine diphosphocholine

Figure 57-2 The biosynthetic pathway for phosphatidylcholine in type 2 pneumocytes.

With the switch of erythropoiesis to the fetal liver and spleen, fetal hemoglobin (Hb F) production begins. Hb F consists of two α- and two γ-chains ($\alpha_2\gamma_2$). Small amounts of adult hemoglobin, Hb A ($\alpha_2\beta_2$), are also produced, but Hb F predominates during the remainder of fetal life.

As the fetal bone marrow begins red cell production, Hb A production increases. At birth, fetal blood contains 75% Hb F and 25% Hb A. Hb F production rapidly diminishes during the first year of postnatal life. In normal adults, less than 1% of hemoglobin is Hb F. The difference between fetal and adult hemoglobin is very significant as Hb F has a higher affinity for oxygen than does Hb A. Thus in the placenta, oxygen is released from the maternal Hb A, diffuses into the chorionic villi, and binds to the fetal Hb F. In addition, 2,3-diphosphoglycerate (2,3-DPG) does not bind Hb F and therefore cannot decrease its affinity for oxygen.

MATERNAL AND FETAL HEALTH ASSESSMENT

For optimum healthcare during pregnancy, a woman should consult her physician before conception.[8,253] Unfortunately, 49% of pregnancies in the United States are unintended—higher for unmarried women.[179] Preconception evaluation should include a medical, reproductive, and family history; physical examination; and laboratory tests.

Laboratory Testing

The following laboratory tests are recommended as part of a preconception evaluation: (1) hematocrit, (2) blood type and Rh compatibility, (3) erythrocyte antibody screen, (4) Papanicolaou smear [or human papillomavirus (HPV) test], (5) urinalysis, (6) rubella titer, (7) Rapid Plasma Reagin (RPR) test, (8) gonococcal and chlamydia DNA test, (9) cystic fibrosis carrier status,[162] (10) human immunodeficiency virus (HIV) antibody,[7] and (11) hepatitis B surface antigen.[14] Depending on demographic risks, genetic testing for disorders such as Tay-Sachs disease, thalassemia, and sickle cell disease may be offered.[13] A careful diet history is warranted. Folic acid supplementation should be recommended to reduce the risk of neural tube defects.[248] Women at high risk for diabetes mellitus should be screened for this disorder (see Chapter 46).

Most individuals consult a physician a few days after a missed menses if they suspect they might be pregnant. Many laboratory tests are useful for managing normal and abnormal pregnancies. A urine pregnancy test result is positive (meaning that the test can detect a CG concentration of about 25 IU/L) in about half of pregnant females at the beginning of the missed menses—at about 2 weeks after conception.[90] Screening for fetal neural tube defects and Down syndrome should be offered to all pregnant patients. Until 2002, screening was recommended at 16 to 18 weeks' gestation,[10] but Down syndrome screening can now be performed as early as 10 weeks.[400] Depending on diabetes risk, glucose tolerance testing should be performed immediately or at 24 to 28 weeks (see Chapter 46 for details). Some physicians screen selected patients for preterm labor risk at 24 to 30 weeks using fetal fibronectin.[18] Although PL and estriol measurements were used previously to predict fetal well-being, both tests are now obsolete for this purpose.[100,101] Maternal observation and recording of fetal movements,[9] ultrasound examination, and tests that monitor the fetal heart rate[17] during random uterine contractions or fetal movement are the currently accepted methods for monitoring fetal well-being.

Clinical Specimens

Many different samples are used in clinical laboratory analysis before and during pregnancy. These include (1) paternal saliva, serum, and blood; (2) maternal saliva, serum, blood, and urine; (3) amniotic fluid obtained by amniocentesis[101,347] or from pools of fluid in the vagina after rupture of the fetal membranes; (4) chorionic villi; (5) fetal blood obtained by percutaneous umbilical blood sampling; and (6) fetal tissue obtained by biopsy.[105]

The technique of amniocentesis is described in Chapter 7. Additional information is found in the section on tests for evaluating fetal lung maturity, later in this chapter.

Diagnosis and Dating of Pregnancy

The most important aspects of pregnancy management are detection of pregnancy and establishing accurate estimates of fetal age. Obstetricians measure the length of pregnancy in terms of *weeks,* not trimesters. The most useful test for detecting pregnancy is the CG test.

Qualitative tests for CG in blood or urine are used primarily to screen for pregnancy. Urine CG tests usually suffice to diagnose normal pregnancy when it has progressed beyond the first week after the first missed period. However, qualitative serum pregnancy tests may detect pregnancy earlier, and quantitative serum tests can help reveal problems in early pregnancy. False-positive or increased serum CG test results have been obtained from qualitative and quantitative assays when human antimouse antibodies (HAMA) or heterophile antibodies are present.[91,157] If suspected, investigative experiments include testing a urine specimen for the presence of CG, serially diluting the serum to confirm an appropriate dose response, testing the serum using a different CG method, and retesting the serum after treatment with interfering antibody blocking agents.

To establish accurate dates, obstetricians rely on (1) menstrual history, (2) physical examination, (3) fetal heart tones, (4) ultrasonography, and (5) detection and quantification of CG. In the first 8 weeks of pregnancy, the CG concentration in maternal serum rises geometrically (Figure 57-3). Detectable amounts (≈5 IU/L) are present in the serum 8 to 11 days after conception,[234] which is in the third week of pregnancy as measured from the LMP.[221] CG usually becomes detectable in the urine 1 to 3 days later, although this interval is highly variable.[234] For women aged 13 to 40, serum CG concentrations of 5 IU/L or greater are consistent with pregnancy. Higher values are infrequently seen in older, nonpregnant women and are thought to be caused by CG secreted by the pituitary gland.[350] Concentrations in approximately half of pregnant women reach 25 IU/L on the first day of their missed period. The peak concentration occurs at about 8 to 10 weeks and is about 100,000 IU/L. Subsequently, CG concentrations start to decline in serum and urine, and by the end of the second trimester, a 90% reduction from peak concentration has usually occurred. In the first trimester, maternal serum CG is about 96% to 98% intact, 1% to 3% β subunit, and up to 1% α subunit. During the second trimester, subunit synthesis becomes unbalanced and the serum distribution shifts to 92% to 98% intact, 1% to 7% α subunit, and up to 1% β subunit.[280] Concentrations are approximately constant during the third trimester, with the predominant species being intact CG. The presence of twins approximately doubles CG concentrations.[389]

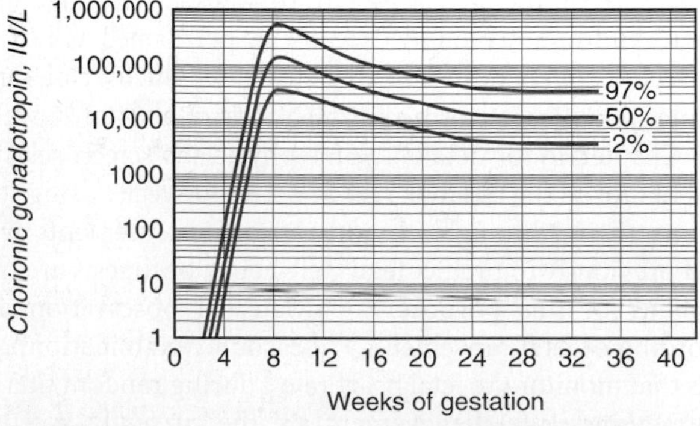

Figure 57-3 Concentration of chorionic gonadotropin (CG) in maternal serum as a function of gestational age. Lines represent the 2nd, 50th, and 97th percentiles. Maternal serum values from 14 to 25 weeks are medians calculated from 24,229 pregnancies from testing performed at ARUP Laboratories Inc. from January to October 1997. *(Redrawn from Ashwood ER. Evaluating health and maturation of the unborn: the role of the clinical laboratory. Clin Chem 1992;38:1523-9. Permission granted from Clinical Chemistry.)*

COMPLICATIONS OF PREGNANCY

Although most pregnancies progress without problems, complications can arise in the mother, placenta, or fetus.

Abnormal Pregnancies

Conditions arising primarily in the mother include (1) ectopic pregnancy, (2) hyperemesis gravidarum, (3) preeclampsia, (4) HELLP syndrome (see later), (5) liver disease, (6) Graves disease, and (7) hemolytic disease of the newborn. The clinician must distinguish abnormal changes in laboratory tests from normal physiologic changes induced by pregnancy (see Table 57-2).

Ectopic Pregnancy and Threatened Abortion

When a fertilized egg implants in a location other than the body of the uterus, the condition is called an *ectopic pregnancy.* Most abnormal implantations occur in the fallopian tube; they can also occur in the abdomen, although this is rare. Tubal rupture and hemorrhage are common serious complications of ectopic pregnancy. About 25% of individuals with an ectopic pregnancy have three classic symptoms: lower abdominal pain, vaginal bleeding, and an adnexal mass.[332] Of all individuals with these symptoms, about 15% have an ectopic pregnancy, and a smaller percentage have incomplete or complete spontaneous abortion. In 2006, the United States had 13.3 pregnancy-related deaths per 100,000 live births[257]—3% caused by ectopic pregnancy.[181] A pregnant patient has about a 1 in 200 chance of dying from an ectopic pregnancy.[155] Management of ectopic pregnancy is surgical (by laparoscopy) or medical (with intramuscular administration of methotrexate).[15,21] Early detection and proper management of ectopic pregnancy are the most effective means of preventing maternal morbidity and mortality. Some have suggested that asymptomatic women at high risk for ectopic pregnancy should be screened with the use of ultrasound and laboratory tests.[69]

Ultrasound examination is used to evaluate women with symptoms. When ultrasound is nondiagnostic, quantitative measurements of serum CG are used to identify women with ectopic pregnancy or abnormal intrauterine pregnancy. These conditions frequently produce abnormal CG concentrations and slow rates of increase.[58]

An accurate gestational age is the best predictor of when an intrauterine pregnancy should be detected with transvaginal ultrasound. Failure to detect a gestational sac by sonography 24 days or longer after conception provides presumptive evidence of an ectopic pregnancy or fetal demise.[193] In the absence of an accurate gestational age, a serum CG concentration is required to assist in interpreting a nondiagnostic ultrasound. An intrauterine pregnancy should be visible by ultrasonography at a CG concentration of 1500 to 2000 IU/L, but this concentration has a clinical sensitivity of only 42% and a clinical specificity of 81% for the detection of ectopic pregnancy when no intrauterine gestational sac is visualized.[205]

When CG concentrations are less than 1500 IU/L and ultrasonography is nondiagnostic, serial testing of CG may be very helpful. In normal intrauterine pregnancy, during the second through fifth weeks, the CG doubles every 1.5 days. After 5 weeks' gestation, the doubling time gradually lengthens to 2 to 3 days.[305] Before 7 weeks, calculation of the slope of log(CG) versus time in days is useful for identifying normal pregnancies.[192] At least two CG determinations should be obtained from specimens collected 1 to 7 days apart. The log-linear slope, Δlog(CG)/Δtime [in log(IU/L)/d], is greater than 0.11 in the vast majority of normal pregnancies. In cases of ectopic pregnancy or spontaneous abortion, the slope is usually less than 0.11, and the CG concentrations often decrease. An increase in CG of at least 53% over 48 hours is 99% specific for excluding an ectopic pregnancy,[33] but as many as 35% of ectopic gestations produce an increase greater than this.[345]

Serum progesterone concentration is often low in mothers with abnormal pregnancy.[314] For example, a serum progesterone less than 6 ng/mL predicts an abnormal pregnancy outcome with 81% confidence for asymptomatic women within 8 weeks of their last menses,[106] but average serum progesterone in nonviable pregnancies is 10 ng/mL. For women with clinical symptoms of abnormal pregnancy, measurement of both CG and progesterone is more predictive of abnormal pregnancy than a single CG measurement. In a large outcome study, 97% of patients with CG less than 3000 IU/L and progesterone less than 12.6 ng/mL had an abnormal pregnancy outcome, whereas those with CG greater than 3000 IU/L or progesterone greater than 12.6 ng/mL had a normal pregnancy.[272] McCord and associates[242] reported that in women at risk for ectopic pregnancy, a progesterone cutoff of 17.5 ng/mL detected 92% of ectopic cases (clinical sensitivity) but had a very poor clinical specificity of about 14%. Investigators concluded that patients with progesterone greater than 17.5 ng/mL needed no additional laboratory tests. Finally, in symptomatic patients, Stewart and colleagues[362] reported a clinical sensitivity of 99% and a clinical specificity of 65% when a Δlog(CG)/Δtime greater than 0.14 is used to distinguish normal intrauterine pregnancy from ectopic pregnancy combined with inevitable abortion. A progesterone cutoff above 8 ng/mL had a clinical sensitivity of 81% and a clinical specificity of 88%.

Preeclampsia and Eclampsia

Preeclampsia is a pregnancy condition characterized by hypertension, proteinuria, and often edema, usually occurring late in the second trimester or early in the third trimester, and affecting 5 to 10% of pregnancies. It is a major cause of maternal and perinatal mortality. If the mother develops convulsions, the condition is called *eclampsia*. The cause has not been elucidated,[359] but research suggests that increased circulating soluble fms-like tyrosine kinase 1 (sFlt-1) may have a role.[222]

The disorder manifests with placental ischemia and endothelial dysfunction that leads to intravascular deposition of fibrin with subsequent end-organ damage.[320] Most maternal deaths are due to central nervous system complications, but ischemic liver damage may also occur. The only cure for preeclampsia is delivery of the placenta.[359]

HELLP Syndrome

The HELLP syndrome (**h**emolysis, **e**levated **l**iver enzymes, and **l**ow **p**latelet counts in association with preeclampsia) is a life-threatening obstetric complication that occurs in 0.1% of pregnancies. Its most prominent features are thrombocytopenia and disseminated intravascular coagulation (DIC; see Chapter 59). Most cases occur between the 27th and 36th weeks of pregnancy, but the syndrome also may occur postpartum. Women typically present with epigastric or right upper quadrant pain, malaise, nausea, vomiting, and headache.[240,343] Jaundice occurs in 5% of patients. Lactate dehydrogenase (LD) concentrations may be very high, and alanine aminotransferase (ALT) and aspartate aminotransferase (AST) are usually 2 to 10 times their upper reference limits. Treatment is delivery. Postpartum management of the patient may require plasmapheresis or organ transplantation. Recurrence rates are 3 to 27%.

Liver Disease

Several liver disorders are unique to pregnancy.[191,204] These include (1) hyperemesis gravidarum, (2) cholestasis of pregnancy, and (3) fatty liver of pregnancy. These disorders must be distinguished from the normal physiologic changes of pregnancy (see Table 57-2). Significant changes normally seen in pregnancy include a dilutional decrease in serum albumin and elevation of alkaline phosphatase (from the placenta). Notably, total bilirubin; 5′-nucleotidase, gamma-glutamyltranspeptidase (GGT), ALT, and AST are unchanged in mothers with a normal pregnancy. Changes in these analytes reflect hepatobiliary disease. Also discussed in this section are (1) non–pregnancy-related liver disease in pregnancy, (2) differential diagnosis, and (3) effect of pregnancy on preexisting liver disease.

Hyperemesis Gravidarum

Hyperemesis gravidarum is characterized by nausea and vomiting and, in severe cases, dehydration and malnutrition. It typically occurs in the first trimester. When hyperemesis is severe enough to cause dehydration, abnormal liver enzyme values—usually less than four times the upper reference limit—are seen in approximately 50% of patients.[191] Mild hyperbilirubinemia may occur. However, significant liver disease does not occur, and liver biopsy results are normal. Low birth weight babies are common, especially for women who develop malnutrition.

Cholestasis of Pregnancy

Cholestasis of pregnancy usually occurs in the third trimester and is manifested clinically by diffuse pruritus and, in 10% of patients, jaundice. Typical features of cholestasis, including pale stools and dark urine, are present and last until delivery. Women who experience cholestasis while taking oral contraceptives usually develop cholestasis of pregnancy. Serum bilirubin rarely exceeds 5 mg/dL. Alkaline phosphatase is typically two to four times the upper reference limit. Aminotransferase enzyme concentrations are mildly elevated. Prothrombin time may be elevated because of vitamin K malabsorption. Although many clinicians order serum bile acids in this setting,[130] this test is offered by only a few clinical laboratories and is rarely necessary for diagnosis. The condition itself is benign, but is associated with increased risk of premature birth and fetal death. It recurs with subsequent pregnancies.[317]

Fatty Liver of Pregnancy

Fatty liver of pregnancy occurs in approximately 1 in 10,000 pregnancies and is characterized by accumulation of microvesicular fat in the hepatocytes.[77] Many cases of this maternal disorder are caused by an inherited mitochondrial fatty acid oxidation disorder in the fetus, long-chain 3-hydroxyacyl-CoA dehydrogenase deficiency (LCHAD).[379] Mothers carrying fetuses with this disorder are 50 times more likely to develop fatty liver of pregnancy.[66] The disease typically occurs at week 37 and is manifested clinically by rapid onset of malaise, nausea, vomiting, and abdominal pain. Mild elevations in aminotransferase enzyme concentrations occur, with the AST elevation typically greater than the ALT elevation but with both less than six times the upper reference limit. Serum bilirubin is usually greater than 6 mg/dL. Life-threatening hypoglycemia may occur.[320] Hyperuricemia, presumably from tissue destruction and renal failure, is characteristic. Liver histology shows acute fatty infiltration with little necrosis or inflammation. The fat is microvesicular and pericentral in the cell, similar to what is seen in Reye syndrome. If untreated, fulminant hepatic failure with hepatic encephalopathy ensues. Treatment is immediate termination of the pregnancy, at which time rapid recovery usually occurs. Infant and maternal mortality is approximately 50% and 20%.

Non–Pregnancy-Related Liver Disease in Pregnancy

Pregnancy does not preclude the acquisition or aggravation of non–pregnancy-related liver disease. Thus, cholestasis during pregnancy may reflect the presence of (1) hepatotoxicity from drugs, (2) primary biliary cirrhosis, (3) Dubin-Johnson syndrome, or (4) cholelithiasis (see Chapter 50). Abdominal ultrasound, endoscopic retrograde cholangiography, or liver biopsy may be necessary to exclude these conditions.

Viral hepatitis occurs with the same frequency in pregnancy as would be expected in a comparable age group.[323] It is manifested by malaise, nausea, vomiting, dark urine, and mild fever. AST and ALT are virtually always more than 10 times the upper reference limit and are usually greater than 20 times the upper reference limit. The prognosis, with the exception of hepatitis E and herpes simplex, is the same as in nonpregnant women. Hepatitis E, an enteric infection occurring in India, Africa, the Middle East, and Central America, has a mortality rate of 15 to 20% in the pregnant patient.[208] Herpes simplex hepatitis, usually accompanied by oral or vulvar vesicles, has a mortality rate of 43%.[201] Distinguishing features include mild bilirubin elevation and marked aminotransferase elevations. Liver biopsy is usually required for diagnosis and demonstrates typical intranuclear inclusions and the other usual features of viral hepatitis. Antiviral therapy greatly improves the prognosis.

Women who acquire hepatitis B late in pregnancy or who are chronic carriers are likely to transmit the disease to their babies. This is especially so if the mother is hepatitis B e antigen (HBeAg) positive (see Chapter 50). The outcome in the infant varies from fulminant hepatitis (rare and usually in anti–HBe-positive mothers) to mild hepatitis to chronic hepatitis (the usual outcome in 90% of chronically infected woman). All pregnant women should be screened for hepatitis B with hepatitis B surface antigen (HBsAg).[14] If positive, their babies should be immunized with hepatitis B immune globulin and hepatitis B vaccine. Babies born to hepatitis C–positive mothers usually have the passively transmitted antibody for several months, but transmission of active hepatitis is unusual.[372] Because there is no known treatment for the newborn, screening is not recommended for hepatitis C virus infection.

Differential Diagnosis

It is often difficult to distinguish the various liver diseases of pregnancy from each other and from naturally occurring liver diseases. Acute fatty liver is suggested when nausea, vomiting, and abdominal pain are followed by jaundice, and encephalopathy occurs in the presence of a small or normal-sized liver. The white blood cell count is usually elevated above 15,000 cells/μL, and ALT concentrations are typically four to six times the upper reference limit. Hypoalbuminemia, hyperuricemia, hypoglycemia, and DIC are typical. Hepatic ultrasound and computed tomography (CT) usually demonstrate fatty liver when present. In preeclampsia and the HELLP syndrome, the liver is usually enlarged, ALT concentrations are usually lower, and bilirubin concentrations are mildly elevated or normal. Hyperuricemia is uncommon. Marked elevations in aminotransferase enzyme concentrations suggest hepatic infarction or viral hepatitis. Liver biopsy may be needed to differentiate non–pregnancy-related causes of liver disease, but should not be used to differentiate acute fatty liver from preeclampsia or HELLP syndrome because treatment is the same for all of these conditions—delivery of the infant.[249]

Effect of Pregnancy on Preexisting Liver Disease

Conception and full-term parturition do not usually occur in women who have cirrhosis. However, liver disease is not a reason for termination. The hypervolemia associated with pregnancy may aggravate cirrhosis and predispose to bleeding from esophageal varices.[61]

Autoimmune chronic hepatitis is usually associated with amenorrhea, but pregnancy may occur after treatment to remission with corticosteroids. Steroids should be continued during pregnancy. Pregnancy should be avoided in patients being treated with azathioprine.

Neonatal Thyroid Function

During the first trimester of pregnancy, the fetus is dependent on the mother for its supply of thyroid hormone. Low maternal thyroid hormone concentrations (overt or subclinical hypothyroidism) have been associated with adverse outcomes, such as preterm delivery,[76] fetal death, and a reduced intelligence quotient (IQ) in children.[4,168] Women with untreated thyroid deficiency in pregnancy are more likely to have permanent hypothyroidism after pregnancy (64%) than are euthyroid mothers.[168]

Later in pregnancy, the fetal thyroid-pituitary axis functions independently from the mother's axis in most cases. However, if the mother has preexisting Graves disease (see Chapter 55), her autoantibodies can cross the placenta and stimulate the fetal thyroid gland. Thus the fetus can develop hyperthyroidism. Measurement of thyrotropin-binding inhibitory immunoglobulins (TBII) is useful for assessing risk of fetal or neonatal Graves disease.

Thyroid screening in pregnancy is recommended for high-risk women but is controversial for others.[19,146] Regardless, when tested, thyroid hormone results should be interpreted using pregnancy-specific reference values.[213]

Hemolytic Disease of the Newborn

Hemolytic disease of the newborn (HDN) is a fetal hemolytic disorder caused by maternal antibodies directed against antigen on fetal erythrocytes. Commonly used synonyms for this disorder are *isoimmunization disease, Rh isoimmune disease, Rh disease,* and *D isoimmunization.* Any of a large number of erythrocyte surface antigens—Rh(CcDEc), A, B, Kell, Duffy, Kidd, and others—may be responsible for isoimmune hemolysis. When severe, the disorder is known as *erythroblastosis fetalis* and is life threatening to fetus and newborn. In the past, disease severity was assessed by measuring the amount of bilirubin in the amniotic fluid (AF). Presently ultrasonographic determination of middle fetal cerebral artery velocity is replacing AF bilirubin. Pioneering work by Bevis[44-47] uncovered the association between amniotic fluid bilirubin and D isoimmunization. Liley[224] extended this work by noting an association between gestational age, severity of the disease, and amniotic fluid bilirubin concentration.

Rh Blood Groups

Two genes, *RhD* and *RhCE,* encode for erythrocyte membrane proteins that are antigenic. Both are located on chromosome 1p about 30 kb apart. Approximately 15% of Caucasians, 5% of Africans, and less than 1% of Asians are RhD negative. The most prevalent RhD-negative allele is a deletion.[31] Exon 5 of *RhCE* has two common polymorphisms producing *E* or *e* antigen. Exon 2 of *RhCE* has two common polymorphisms producing *C* or *c* antigen.

Etiology

Maternal sensitization may occur in response to blood transfusion or a pregnancy in which the fetus has a blood cell antigen that the mother lacks. Antibodies against RhD are the most common cause of HDN, although antibodies against other erythrocyte antigens can also cause disease.

The resulting antibodies are actively transported across the placenta and into the fetus, where they cause destruction of fetal erythrocytes. The severity of the resulting hemolysis is influenced by antibody specificity, titer, and transfer rate, as well as by the functional maturity of the fetal spleen in which sensitized erythrocytes are destroyed.

Destruction of fetal erythrocytes, which is the central problem, produces several other problems. For example, fetal anemia imposes an extra burden on the fetal heart to provide an adequate oxygen supply to fetal tissues. Anemia stimulates the fetal marrow and extramedullary erythropoiesis in the liver and spleen to replace destroyed erythrocytes. Extramedullary erythropoiesis destroys hepatocytes and leads to decreased production of serum albumin and decreased oncotic pressure in the intravascular space.

When severe, these changes lead to congestive heart failure and generalized fetal edema, a condition referred to as *hydrops fetalis,* which carries a very grave prognosis. Without therapeutic intervention, intrauterine demise soon follows.

If a fetus survives, the newborn will encounter a number of problems. In utero, the placenta and the mother perform the functions of respiration and removal of bilirubinoid pigments resulting from hemolysis. Newborns must assume these functions for themselves in the presence of hydrops. The lungs are edematous, and pleural effusions and ascites physically restrict their ability to expand. The damaged liver is unable to conjugate and excrete bilirubin adequately. When bilirubin accumulates in the blood to excessive concentrations, it passes through the blood-brain barrier to deposit in the brain and destroy brain cells. This form of brain damage is termed *kernicterus.* Although kernicterus was not a concern in the hydropic fetus, it is a significant concern in these sick newborns. A severely erythroblastotic baby can be one of the most challenging cases in a neonatal intensive care unit.

Prophylaxis

An anti-RhD immune globulin, RhoGAM (Ortho Clinical Diagnostics, Raritan, NJ), has been used in the United States since 1968[56]; other similar products were introduced in 1971 and later. A 300 µg dose is administered intramuscularly to a mother potentially exposed to 15 mL or less of RhD-positive fetal erythrocytes following abortion, fetomaternal hemorrhage, amniocentesis, chorionic villi sampling (CVS), or delivery.[11] Use of anti-RhD immune globulin has been responsible for the dramatic reduction in the incidence of HDN. In addition to recognized fetomaternal hemorrhage, undetected transplacental fetomaternal bleeding during an apparently normal pregnancy can lead to antepartum sensitization. This would not be prevented by immediate postpartum administration of RhD immunoglobulin; therefore antepartum administration at 28 weeks' gestation is recommended for RhD-negative women. Despite this immune prophylaxis, a small number of sensitized pregnancies continue to occur.

Clinical Management of Sensitized Mothers

To identify sensitized women, an alloantibody screen is performed at the first prenatal visit.[250] If an antibody to an erythrocyte antigen is identified, the titer is determined.[11] The critical anti-RhD titer, defined as the titer associated with risk for fetal hydrops, is usually 1:8 to 1:32, although studies of critical titer are quite disparate.[159] For all sensitized women, the paternal erythrocyte phenotype is determined. If the father is RhD negative, then no follow-up studies are required. If he is D positive, then zygosity is determined. Although this has historically been estimated from Rh antigen phenotypes (D, C/c, E/e) in conjunction with gene frequency tables based on race, DNA testing for RhD zygosity is more reliable. If the father is homozygous, all of his offspring can be assumed to be RhD positive, negating the need for fetal RhD testing. Fetal RhD genotyping from cultured amniocytes is required if the father is heterozygous or is not available for testing. To guard against a false negative caused by a paternal RhD gene rearrangement (occurring in about 1.5% of Caucasians), the father can also be genotyped. A frequent occurrence in those of African ancestry is an RhD pseudogene; the patient is RhD negative by serology, but RhD positive on genotype. If the fetus is RhD genotype positive, the mother (who is RhD negative serologically) should be tested for RhD genotype. Laboratories have begun to offer fetal Rh genotyping using cell-free fetal DNA that circulates in maternal blood (see Chapter 45).[133]

For sensitized mothers with an at-risk fetus, serial titers are performed on maternal serum every month until 24 weeks' gestation, then every 2 weeks thereafter. If a critical titer anti-D is detected, ultrasound Doppler measurements are used to determine the peak velocity of blood flow in the fetal middle cerebral artery. Higher velocity is a strong indicator of fetal anemia. If Doppler velocimetry is not available, amniocentesis is performed every 10 to 14 days to assess the bilirubin concentration in amniotic fluid. The procedure was originally called ΔOD_{450},[224] but the preferred clinical chemistry term is ΔA_{450}. This method is described later in the chapter in the section entitled "Laboratory Tests." Serial testing is indicated every 10 to 14 days. Decreasing values are reassuring and indicate an unaffected or RhD-negative fetus. Values that plateau or increase suggest active hemolysis, which may require therapeutic intervention including ultrasound-guided umbilical blood sampling to determine fetal blood type, hemoglobin, antibody screen, reticulocyte count, and total bilirubin. Intrauterine intravascular blood transfusion can be performed if indicated. If fetal pulmonary maturation has occurred (usually 35 weeks or greater), delivery is indicated.

Trophoblastic Disease

Serum CG determinations are very useful for monitoring patients with germ cell–derived neoplasms or other CG-producing tumors, such as lung carcinoma. Use of CG in these diseases is discussed in Chapter 24.

Fetal Anomalies

Open neural tube defects, Down syndrome, trisomy 18 and the Smith-Lemli-Opitz syndrome (discussed separately later) are fetal anomalies that are partially detectable by prenatal screening. However, because of the large number of pregnancies screened and the interest in other fetal conditions and their possible association with abnormal maternal serum analyte concentrations, a wealth of associations between rarer conditions and screening results has been published. These findings are never diagnostic and are reported rarely by the screening laboratory. In certain circumstances, however, the healthcare provider may recommend pursuing a more extensive medical evaluation.

Neural Tube Defects

Neural tube defects are serious abnormalities that occur early in embryonic development. By 19 days after fertilization, the area that is to form the central nervous system (brain and spinal cord) has differentiated into a plate of cells. The flat plate then rolls up, and its edges fuse into a hollow neural tube that drops into the embryo to develop just underneath what will become the skin of the back. Neural tube formation is normally complete 4 weeks after fertilization. Failure of neural tube fusion leads to permanent developmental defects of the brain, spinal cord, or both. These defects are called *anencephaly, meningomyelocele* (which is commonly called *spina bifida*), and *encephalocele*. Although many heterogeneous causes are known, about 90% fall into the classification of multifactorial inheritance.[183] Folic acid deficiency is clearly associated with increased frequency of neural tube closure defects.[387] The cause in these cases may be derangement of homocysteine metabolism caused by folate deficiency.[358] Estimates attribute 70% or more of all neural tube defects to folate deficiency.[394] Since 1997, grain products in the United States and Canada have been fortified with 140 µg folic acid/100 g,[383] but the amount added is unlikely to be sufficient to reduce birth prevalence by more than about 30%—the reduction that is commonly reported in observational trials.[290] Organizations such as the March of Dimes are conducting vigorous campaigns to educate women about the need for folic acid supplementation before becoming pregnant, as recommended by the Centers for Disease Control and Prevention.[79] Most vitamin supplements contain 400 µg of folic acid, which is what is recommended daily by authorities.[256] Data published in 2009 suggest that vitamin B_{12} is also necessary.[251]

The birth prevalence of open neural tube defects varies with factors such as (1) geographic location (higher in the Eastern United States, lower in the West), (2) race (lower in African Americans), (3) ethnicity (higher in Scotch-Irish), (4) family history (higher with prior births of affected individuals),[96] and (5) maternal weight (higher in obese women).[335,403] An average figure for the United States is 1 open neural tube defect per 1000 pregnancies (about 1 in 2000 for each individual defect). Almost all cases of anencephaly and about 95% of meningomyeloceles are open, with no overlying skin, and therefore are in direct communication with the amniotic fluid. Thus fetal serum proteins normally present in amniotic fluid at low concentrations gain access in large quantities to the amniotic fluid. The elevated amniotic fluid AFP concentration leads to increased amounts in the maternal circulation. Only open neural tube defects are detected by maternal serum AFP screening.[390]

Down Syndrome

Down syndrome is the most common serious disorder of the autosomal chromosomes, occurring in 1 in 700 live births. An extra copy of the long arm region q22.1 to q22.3 of chromosome 21 results in a phenotype consisting of moderate to severe mental retardation, hypotonia, congenital heart defects, and a flat facial profile. Chromosome 21 is the smallest chromosome, making up about 1.7% of the human genome. Most often an affected child has three copies of chromosome 21 (i.e., trisomy 21), but 5% of cases are caused by translocations and 1% of cases are mosaics. The risk increases slowly up to age 30 and then steadily increases between ages 30 and 45 (Figure 57-4) to a plateau.[255]

Trisomy 18

Trisomy 18 (Edwards syndrome) is caused by a nondisjunction event during meiosis that results in a fetus having an extra copy of chromosome 18. Although it occurs in only 1 in 8000 births, it is probably the most common chromosome defect at the time of conception. The dramatic change in prevalence is due to the very high fetal loss rate both before 8 weeks (>80%) and during the second and third trimesters (≈70%). Approximately 25% of affected fetuses have meningomyelocele (spina bifida) or omphalocele (abdominal wall defect). A high cesarean section rate has been reported for undiagnosed cases.[284] Following birth, half of infants die within the first 5 days and 90% die within 100 days.[75]

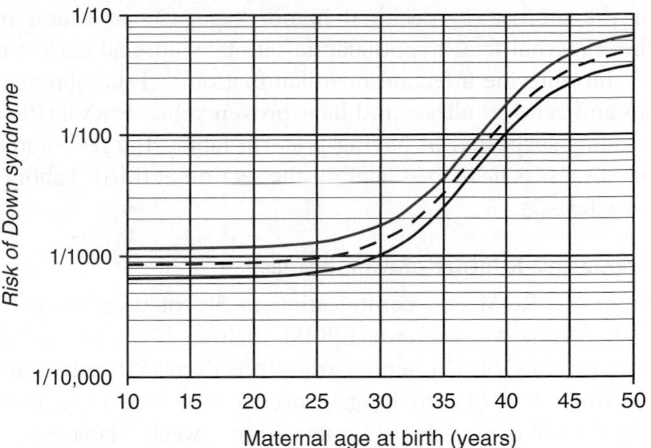

Figure 57-4 The relationship of maternal age to the risk of having a pregnancy affected with Down syndrome. ***Dashed line,*** **Second trimester risk;** ***red line,*** **first-trimester risk;** ***solid black line,*** **term risk. The term risk is calculated from $1/[1 + \exp(7.33 - 4.211/\{1 + \exp[-0.2815 \times (\text{age} - 37.23 - 0.5)]\})]$.[255]**

Smith-Lemli-Opitz Syndrome

Smith-Lemli-Opitz syndrome (SLOS) is caused by a defect in cholesterol synthesis. SLOS is inherited as an autosomal recessive mutation and occurs rarely, in about 1 of every 100,000 Caucasian pregnancies.[95] Children affected with SLOS have mental and growth deficiencies and other structural malformations of the skeleton, kidneys, genitals, lungs, and heart.[199]

Preterm Delivery

The leading cause of neonatal morbidity and mortality in the United States is preterm delivery, defined as delivery before 37 weeks' gestation. Approximately 300,000 to 500,000 preterm births occur each year.[16] Rupture of the fetal membranes before the onset of uterine contractions is known as premature rupture of membranes (PROM). When this occurs at less than 37 completed weeks' gestation, it is referred to as preterm PROM and is responsible for nearly one third of preterm deliveries.[245]

Infants born before 37 weeks' gestation are usually of low birth weight (<2500 g) and are vulnerable to numerous complications, including (1) infection, (2) necrotizing enterocolitis, and (3) intraventricular hemorrhage, and often develop (4) *respiratory distress syndrome* (RDS). Some are of very low birth weight (<1500 g). According to the National Center for Health Statistics,[181] in 2006, 8.2% of all U.S. live-born infants were of low birth weight and 1.5% were of very low birth weight. Most of these infants will spend time in intensive care units at a cost of up to $3500 per day.

The cause of preterm labor is unknown, but it is likely that many factors are involved and several mechanisms have been supported by a considerable amount of clinical and experimental evidence. These include (1) pathologic distention of the uterus, (2) decidual hemorrhage, (3) activation of the maternal-fetal hypothalamic-pituitary-adrenal axis, and (4) intrauterine infection or inflammation.[346] Fetal fibronectin and cervical ultrasound have proven value for evaluating patients suspected of having preterm labor. The fetal fibronectin test is described later, in the section entitled "Laboratory Tests."

Premature Rupture of Membranes

Preterm PROM is a complication in 3% of pregnancies.[245] Risk factors for preterm PROM include (1) a history of preterm PROM, (2) genital tract infection, (3) antepartum bleeding, and (4) smoking. Most women who experience PROM will deliver their infants within 1 week. Management of preterm PROM varies according to the gestational age of the fetus and the presence or absence of maternal/fetal infection. When PROM occurs at 34 to 36 weeks' gestation, the infant should be delivered, as this has been shown to reduce maternal and fetal infection rates compared with expectant management.[246] When it occurs at 32 to 33 weeks, fetal lung maturity should be determined and the infant delivered if maturity is indicated. If the fetal lungs are immature, conservative management with close fetal monitoring is necessary in conjunction with antibiotic therapy and administration of corticosteroids to accelerate lung development.[245] Because of the high risk of severe neonatal morbidity and mortality, women with PROM at less than 32 weeks' gestation must be managed conservatively in an attempt to prolong pregnancy to 32 weeks. Interventions include antibiotic therapy, administration of tocolytics, and fetal monitoring.[245]

The diagnosis of PROM is often difficult, and commonly used observations or tests to detect it lack clinical sensitivity and specificity.[265,282] These include (1) direct observation of fluid leaking from the cervix or pooling in the posterior fornix of the vagina, (2) ultrasound for the detection of oligohydramnios, and (3) nitrazine (pH), and (4) fern tests. An immunochromatographic test for the rapid detection of placental alpha microglobulin-1 protein in amniotic fluid is described later, in the section entitled "Laboratory Tests."

Fetal Lung Maturity

RDS, also called *hyaline membrane disease,* is the most common critical problem encountered in clinical management of preterm newborns. The worldwide incidence of RDS is 1% of live births and 10 to 15% of live preterm births (<37 weeks or <2500 g).[261] The risk of RDS is affected strongly by gestational age at the time of birth: 1% at 37 weeks, 20% at 34 weeks, and 60% at 29 weeks.[129] In 2006, RDS killed over 800 infants in the United States.[181] Affected infants require supplemental oxygen and mechanical ventilation to remain properly oxygenated. The disorder is caused by a deficiency of *pulmonary surfactant.* In normal lungs, surfactant coats the alveolar epithelium and responds to alveolar volume changes by reducing surface tension in the alveolar wall during expiration. When the quantity of surfactant is deficient, many of the alveoli collapse on expiration and thereby overinflate the remaining airways. This process is known as *focal atelectasis.* The lungs become progressively noncompliant (stiff), and blood flowing through the capillary beds of collapsed alveoli fails to oxygenate. During the first few hours of life, affected infants develop tachypnea with or without cyanosis, nasal flaring, expiratory grunting, and intercostal retractions. The disease worsens during the next few days and usually is worse on the third or fourth day of life. Infants at risk for developing RDS have been treated with intratracheal administration of exogenous surfactant immediately at birth.[174]

Very rarely is the respiratory distress in a term newborn caused by a mutation in the gene encoding for SP-B.[268] This condition, termed *congenital alveolar proteinosis,* is often fatal. A significant derangement in lamellar body production occurs in these cases. Study of the genetic variation suggests that there may be mild, nonfatal cases of this disorder.[113]

PRENATAL SCREENING FOR FETAL DEFECTS

Prenatal screening is the process of identifying pregnancies at sufficiently high risk of a serious birth defect such as an open neural tube defect or Down syndrome. Before 2003, most obstetricians offered amniocentesis for fetal karyotype determination to all mothers who would be 35 years of age or older at the time of birth. However, in 2002, almost 14% of pregnant women in the United States were 35 or older, and these women accounted for 51% of Down syndrome pregnancies.[316] Therefore, if maternal age alone were used for screening, half of Down syndrome pregnancies would not be detected, and no cases in younger women would be identified. The risk for Down syndrome calculated using screening tests is more accurate than the use of maternal age alone, and it is now recommended by the American College of Obstetricians and Gynecologists (ACOG) to offer screening to women of all ages.[12]

Terminology and Method of Risk Calculation in Prenatal Screening

Calculation of risk in prenatal screening depends on the pregnancy's prior risk and the pattern of test results.

Multiple of the Median

Understanding the published literature and clinical screening requires an understanding of the multiple of the median (MoM), the statistic used to normalize analyte values. The initial step in calculating an MoM is to develop a set of median values for each week (or day) of gestation, using the laboratory's own assay values measured on the population to be screened. Individual test results are then expressed as MoM by dividing each individual test result by the median for the relevant gestational age. This convention was originally developed to take into account large differences among centers in AFP assay values seen in the 1977 U.K. collaborative study.[390] The MoM is now universally used as a common factor for converting analyte values into an

TABLE 57-3 Estimated Down Syndrome Detection Rates (DRs), False-Positive Rates (FPRs), and Odds of Being Affected Given a Positive Result (OAPR) at Three Risk Cutoff Values for Selected Combinations of Maternal Serum Marker and Two Methods of Dating

Second Trimester							
Risk Cutoff (Term), 1 in	Maternal Age and Serum Markers	DR, %		FPR, %		OAPR, 1:N	
		LMP	US	LMP	US	LMP	US
150 (200)	AFP, uE_3, CG	61	67	3.6	3.7	43	40
	AFP, uE_3, CG, inhA	68	71	2.8	2.9	30	29
190 (250)	AFP, uE_3, CG	65	70	4.6	4.7	51	49
	AFP, uE_3, CG, inhA	71	74	3.5	3.7	36	36
270 (350)	AFP, uE_3, CG	70	74	6.6	6.5	69	64
	AFP, uE_3, CG, inhA	75	78	5.0	5.1	48	48

AFP, Alpha fetoprotein; *CG,* chorionic gonadotropin; *inhA,* inhibin A; *LMP,* gestational age estimated from last menstrual period; *uE_3,* unconjugated estriol; *US,* gestational age estimated from ultrasound measurements.

interpretative unit and serves as the starting point for calculating screening results for neural tube defects, Down syndrome, and trisomy 18.[284,391,393]

Calculating Individualized Patient-Specific Risks Using Multiple Biochemical Measurements

Measurements of each analyte are made on a serum sample, and the results in mass units are converted to MoM for the appropriate week (or day) of gestation. This MoM value is then adjusted for other variables, such as maternal weight and race (as described later in this chapter). Patient-specific Down syndrome risks are calculated using adjusted MoM values along with the woman's maternal age at expected delivery by employing an algorithm for multivariate analysis that uses overlapping log Gaussian distributions.

The individualized risk (patient-specific risk) for any given condition is determined by multiplying the a priori risk for that condition by a likelihood ratio that is calculated using the woman's analyte measurements (i.e., Patient risk = A priori risk × Likelihood ratio). This basic equation is used to calculate patient-specific risk for neural tube defects, Down syndrome, trisomy 18, or any other condition in which the distributions of analytes for the unaffected and the affected population have been determined. The a priori risk is obtained from large epidemiologic studies that ascertain the prevalence for the condition under consideration. For example, a woman's age is used to define her a priori risk for having a fetus with Down syndrome. Furthermore, because of spontaneous fetal loss during pregnancy, age-related risks are higher in the first trimester than at term. The likelihood ratio is determined by calculating the ratio of the heights of the affected and unaffected overlapping population distributions for any specified MoM value. When multiple tests are used, a single likelihood ratio is calculated using the overlapping distributions for each test but with the correlation between tests taken into account. This final risk, rather than the analyte concentrations themselves, is the screening variable upon which clinical decisions are made. The final risk should indicate the trimester for which it was calculated (i.e., 1 in 100 first-trimester risk).

The test performance (detection and false-positive rates) achievable depends on many factors, including (1) the analyte combination chosen, (2) the risk cutoff chosen, (3) the method of dating used to establish gestational age, and (4) the maternal ages of the women being tested. Table 57-3 summarizes the impact of these factors in a hypothetical cohort of women having the maternal age distribution found in the United States in 2000.[171] The table demonstrates how choices of a second-trimester test combination and risk cutoff affect detection and screen-positive rates.

Reporting Individual Results

The maternal serum screening report should contain the following information: (1) the concentrations and MoM values for measured analytes, (2) an interpretation as screen positive or screen negative, (3) the Down syndrome risk estimate (along with risks for other abnormalities such as trisomy 18), and (4) recommendations for possible further action. Physician-provided information should include (1) the specimen collection date, (2) identification as a first or second specimen, (3) the date of LMP or gestational age confirmed by ultrasound, and maternal birth date (or age), (4) relevant pregnancy history, (5) number of fetuses (if known), (6) maternal race, and (7) the presence or absence of preconceptional maternal diabetes requiring insulin therapy.

Second-Trimester Screening Tests

Maternal serum screening began in the 1970s with the use of second-trimester serum specimens for neural tube defects and progressed to include screening for Down syndrome.

Neural Tube Defects

In the early 1970s, Brock and colleagues demonstrated increased AFP concentrations in the amniotic fluid of mothers carrying fetuses affected with an open neural tube defect (NTD, e.g., anencephaly, open spina bifida).[64] Subsequently,

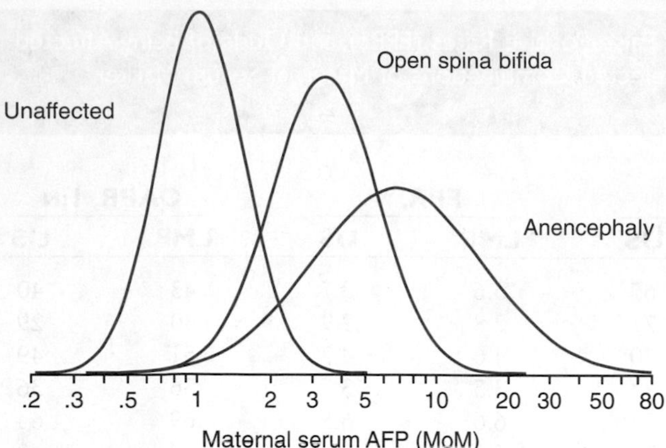

Figure 57-5 Distribution of maternal serum alpha fetoprotein (AFP) measurements in unaffected pregnancies and pregnancies affected with open spina bifida or anencephaly.

it was shown that AFP concentrations also were increased in maternal serum (in the second trimester).[62] Concentrations in serum in affected and unaffected pregnancies overlapped considerably, however, indicating that maternal serum AFP would be useful only as an initial screening test to identify women at high risk for having an affected fetus (Figure 57-5). These women would then need to be referred for diagnostic procedures (e.g., high-resolution ultrasound and, if indicated, amniocentesis for measurement of AFP and acetylcholinesterase in amniotic fluid) to determine whether the fetus had an open neural tube defect. A large collaborative study conducted in the United Kingdom in 1977 showed that maternal serum AFP screening for open neural tube defects in the second trimester of pregnancy was feasible. The final report provided estimates of screening performance in terms of detection and false-positive rates.[390] A family history of neural tube defects in either parent increases the risk that the fetus is affected 5-fold to 15-fold, but more than 90% of all infants with neural tube defects are born to unsuspecting parents who have no recognized risk factor for the disorder.[138,378] Maternal serum AFP testing thus provided a screening method that was available to all women to identify pregnancies at high risk, or to estimate the numeric risk of having a fetus with an open neural tube defect.[391] In the 1980s, the use of maternal serum AFP to screen for open neural tube defects became a standard of care in the United States. The ACOG,[12] the American Society of Human Genetics,[20] and the American Academy of Pediatrics[5] have issued official statements supporting its use.

Optimal screening occurs at between 16 and 18 completed weeks' gestation—a time when the distributions of results for affected and unaffected pregnancies are maximally different, and when time for follow-up studies is adequate. Screening at 15 weeks is acceptable, but screening for open neural tube defects before 14 weeks is difficult to justify.[390,394] Although a patient-specific risk can be used when screening for open neural tube defects,[391] nearly all laboratories define a screen-positive result as AFP at or above a fixed MoM cutoff. The two most commonly used AFP MoM cutoffs in the United States are 2.0 and 2.5 MoM, yielding initial screen-positive rates of 3% to 5% and 1% to 3%, respectively. Observed rates are more likely to be at the lower end of the cited ranges if many pregnancies are dated by ultrasound. This improvement is a result of the finding that increased AFP values attributable to underestimated gestational age, fetal demise, and twin gestation usually will have been identified. The lower initial positive rate at 2.5 MoM is associated with a reduced detection rate for open spina bifida: 70% to 75% as compared with 80% to 85% at 2.0 MoM.[102,390] Nearly all cases of anencephaly are detecting with maternal serum AFP screening.

Down Syndrome

In 1984, a major expansion of biochemical prenatal screening became possible when an association between second-trimester maternal serum AFP and fetal Down syndrome was reported.[247] Maternal serum AFP concentrations are about 25% lower in Down syndrome than in unaffected pregnancies. The association of AFP and Down syndrome was found to be independent of maternal age.[99] Before this discovery, the only available screening test for Down syndrome involved asking a woman her age. Women 35 years or older at the time of delivery would be offered amniocentesis and fetal karyotyping. Down syndrome screening using maternal age is based on the well-documented increase in risk for having a baby with Down syndrome as maternal age increases (see Figure 57-4). The independence of maternal serum AFP measurements and maternal age established that it was possible to offer a screening method to younger women, in whom most cases of Down syndrome occur. Maternal serum AFP screening for Down syndrome also introduced the concept of using risk, rather than analyte concentration, as the screening variable for identifying high-risk women.[99] The effectiveness of maternal serum AFP screening in younger women was subsequently established.[264]

The discovery that a protein produced in pregnancy could be altered in the presence of a fetal chromosomal defect stimulated a search for other substances in pregnancy serum that would have predictive value. Of the many that were examined, two additional analytes emerged quickly as sufficiently discriminatory and independent to be useful additions in screening for Down syndrome in the second trimester. Unconjugated estriol (uE_3),[71] a product of the fetoplacental unit, is about 25% lower in pregnancies with Down syndrome. In contrast, concentrations of CG were found to be about twice as high.[52] In 1988, a method was proposed for combining maternal age with measurements of these three analytes (the triple test) into a single Down syndrome risk estimate.[393] A fourth analyte, inhibin A (inhA), was introduced as a clinical marker for Down syndrome screening in the late 1990s. Concentrations are two times higher in Down syndrome versus unaffected pregnancies.[398] The "quadruple test" is commonly offered and provides approximately 80% detection at a 5% false-positive rate. Two large trials have confirmed its performance.[36,397] Table 57-4 shows general

TABLE 57-4 Conditions Associated With Various Maternal Serum Screening Result Patterns

	Second Trimester				**First Trimester**		
Condition	**AFP**	**CG**	**uE$_3$**	**InhA**	**PAPP-A**	**CG**	**NT**
Amniocentesis	Normal to high	—	—	—	—	—	—
Anencephaly	Very high	—	Very low	—	—	—	—
Congenital nephrosis, duodenal atresia, encephalocele, esophageal atresia, gastroschisis, hydrocephalus, Meckel syndrome, omphalocele, sacrococcygeal teratoma	High	—	—	—	—	—	—
Cystic hygroma	High	—	—	—	—	—	Increased
Down syndrome	Low	High	Low	High	Low	High	Increased
Fetal blood contamination	High to very high	Unchanged	Unchanged	Unchanged	—	—	—
Molar pregnancy	Very low	Very high	Very low	Normal	—	—	—
Molar pregnancy (partial)	Low to normal	Very high	Low to normal	Normal	—	—	—
Myelomeningocele (open spina bifida)	High	—	—	—	—	—	—
Normal pregnancy	Low, normal, or high	Low, normal, or high	Low, normal, or high	Low, normal, or high	—	—	—
Overestimated gestational age	Low	High	Low	Normal	—	—	—
Preeclampsia	Normal to high	High	—	—	—	—	—
Pseudocyesis (imaginary pregnancy)	Undetectable	Undetectable	Undetectable	Undetectable	—	—	—
Smith-Lemli-Opitz syndrome	Low	Low	Very low	—	—	—	—
Spontaneous or impending pregnancy loss	Variable	Low or high	Low	Low or high	—	—	—
Steroid sulfatase deficiency (fetal)	Unchanged	Unchanged	Very low	Unchanged	—	—	—
Triploidy (paternal)	Variable	High	Low	High	Variable	Very high	—
Triploidy (maternal)	Variable	Low	Low	Low	Variable	Very low	—
Trisomy 13	Variable	Variable	Variable	Variable	Very low	Low	High
Trisomy 18	Low	Low	Very low	Normal	Very low	Very low	High
Turner syndrome without hydrops	Low	Low	Very low	Low	Variable	Variable	High
Turner syndrome with hydrops	Low	High	Very low	High	Variable	Variable	High
Twins and other multiple gestations	High	High	High	High	High	High	—
Underestimated gestational age	High	Low	High	Normal	—	—	—

AFP, Alpha fetoprotein; *CG,* chorionic gonadotropin; *inhA,* inhibin A; *NT,* nuchal translucency; *PAPP-A,* pregnancy-associated plasma protein-A; *uE$_3$,* unconjugated estriol.

patterns of first- and second-trimester analytes associated with various disorders.[72,142]

Trisomy 18

Prenatal screening studies have found that fetal trisomy 18 has a distinctive triple marker pattern that is different from the Down syndrome pattern (see Table 57-4).[74] It is, however, the least common of the three disorders considered for second-trimester maternal serum screening. It also is the one that is least compatible with life. For these reasons, a screening program exclusively devoted to the prenatal identification of trisomy 18 is unjustified. However, given that serum analytes are already being measured to screen for Down syndrome and open neural tube defects, an additional interpretation of these analytes to quantify the risk of fetal trisomy 18 is warranted. Because the birth prevalence of trisomy 18 is one tenth that of Down syndrome,[284] the percentage of women identified as screen positive must be correspondingly lower than that for Down syndrome.

In trisomy 18 pregnancies, AFP (median = 0.65 MoM) and uE_3 (0.43 MoM) concentrations are low, but CG concentrations (0.36 MoM) are also very low.[284] A method for trisomy 18 risk calculation was published and is often included in prenatal screening programs.[37,284] The risk-based algorithm showed that at a second-trimester risk cutoff of 1:100, 60% of trisomy 18 pregnancies could be identified, with about 0.5% of women having an initial positive screen.[284]

SLOS

Second-trimester risk assessment for the Smith-Lemli-Opitz syndrome is possible using a multivariate Gaussian algorithm specific for this disorder. The marker pattern in affected pregnancies includes low AFP and hCG (median = 0.72 and 0.76 MoM, respectively), with very low unconjugated estriol (0.21 MoM) concentrations (see Table 57-4).[283] Only pregnancies with a very high risk (1 in 50 or greater) are classified as screen positive for SLOS and are recommended for diagnostic testing by amniocentesis. In this manner, 83% of SLOS cases can be identified at a 0.3% positive rate.[95] It is noteworthy that there is a high rate of fetal loss and other chromosomal (3.3%) or structural abnormalities (5.8%) among false-positive patients.

Other Aneuplodies

Although chromosome disorders other than trisomies 21 and 18 are not part of routine screening, the marker patterns exhibited in maternal serum for some aneuploidies are similar. In particular, hydropic Turner syndrome and triploidy of paternal origin have serum marker patterns resembling that of Down syndrome pregnancy and sometimes are identified as high risk using this algorithm. Similarly, Turner syndrome without hydrops and triploidy of maternal origin are sometimes identified by the trisomy 18 risk algorithm. The pattern for trisomy 13 is variable (see Table 57-4).

Newer Screening Algorithms

Following extensive use of screening tests in the second trimester, new tests have been introduced that use serum collected in the first trimester.

First-Trimester Combined Test

For patients seeking early diagnosis, screening for Down syndrome in the first trimester (10 to 13 weeks' gestation) is available. First-trimester screening involves measurement of maternal serum pregnancy-associated plasma protein-A (PAPP-A) concentration, which is relatively low in Down syndrome pregnancy (median = 0.4 to 0.5 MoM between 10 and 13 weeks), and CG (free beta subunit or total) concentration, which is relatively high in Down syndrome (median = 1.7 to 2.2 MoM).[287] In combination with maternal age, these two serum tests yield a detection rate of 60% at a 5% false-positive rate.[172] A third marker used to improve first-trimester screening performance is the ultrasound measurements of nuchal translucency (NT), the subcutaneous space between the skin and the cervical spine; this marker has been shown to be increased (about 2.0 MoM) in fetuses with Down syndrome.[266,368] Increased NT measurements are also a nonspecific finding for many fetal structural abnormalities,[404] and therefore are useful only as a screening test.[281] NT measurement alone detects 60% or more of Down syndrome cases at a 5% screen-positive rate, making NT the best single screening test described to date.[395]

However, neither ultrasound findings nor serum tests in the first trimester have sufficient predictive power to be used alone. In 2003 and 2005, two independent large multicenter trials demonstrated that a combination of NT and serum tests (the combined test) was comparable or slightly better than the second-trimester quadruple test for Down syndrome screening, detecting about 85% of cases at a 5% false-positive rate. These trials were critical in proving the efficacy of first-trimester screening because they accounted for fetal losses between the first and second trimesters. The National Screening Committee of the U.K. National Health Service advocates use of the combined test for Down syndrome prenatal screening.[258]

Reports have described trisomy 18 detection using first-trimester combined screening.[382] The pattern of markers in affected pregnancies consists of an increased NT measurement (median about 3.2 MoM), with reduced PAPP-A (0.18 MoM) and CG (0.28 MoM) in the first trimester.[382] Estimates for the performance of first-trimester combined testing in the detection of trisomy 18 are varied, likely as the result of a high fetal loss rate and difficulties in complete ascertainment. The most optimistic estimates suggest that 90 to 100% of trisomy 18 cases can be detected, with only 0.2 to 2.0% being called screen positive,[194,296] but a large multicenter study with more comprehensive outcome tracking suggests that detection rates are closer to 80% for a 0.3% positive rate.[59]

Although first-trimester screening has obvious advantages, it also has limitations. First, unlike the second-trimester screening test, detection and false-positive rates are dependent on the gestational week of testing, as shown in Table

TABLE 57-5 Expected Down Syndrome False-Positive Rates (FPRs) for a Detection Rate of 85% During the First Trimester

Test Combinations*	Weeks' Gestation 11	12	13	11 to 13 Combined
NT	27	37	54	39
PAPP-A	43	51	60	51
Free CGβ	56	50	42	50
Total CG	72	61	45	60
NT, PAPP-A, and free CGβ	5.3	6.1	7.6	6.3
NT, PAPP-A, and total CG	6.8	7.2	7.3	7.1

*Maternal age is used with each test combination.
CG, Chorionic gonadotropin; *NT*, nuchal translucency; *PAPP-A*, pregnancy-associated plasma protein-A.
(Adapted from Palomaki GE, Lambert-Messerlian GM, Canick JA. A summary analysis of Down syndrome markers in the late first trimester. Adv Clin Chem 2007;43:177-210.)

57-5. Screening performance of PAPP-A and CG measurements improves with advancing gestational age within the first trimester, while the performance of NT sonography decreases. If these markers are used simultaneously, first-trimester screening performance is optimal at 12 to 13 weeks' gestation. Second, immunoassays for PAPP-A and the free beta subunit of CG are currently available on a limited basis in the United States because they have not been cleared by the U.S. Food and Drug Administration (FDA). This has been a particular difficulty for the free beta CG assay—a problem that has been addressed in some laboratories by the use of total CG immunoassay during gestational weeks 11 to 13 as an alternative.[73] Furthermore, to be reliable, NT measurements must be performed at specialized referral centers that employ sonographers who have undergone rigorous training and participate in ongoing quality control programs. Routine office ultrasound is unsuitable for obtaining NT measurements. Therefore, access for women in some rural areas is limited. NT measurements are relatively expensive, as first-trimester ultrasound examinations are not routine, and third party payers may be reluctant to reimburse these costs. The ACOG[12] recommends that first-trimester screening should be offered only with appropriately trained sonographers, a quality assurance program for NT, and access to diagnosis by chorionic villus samplings (CVS). Last, routine screening for open neural tube defects using maternal serum AFP would still need to be performed, as such screening is not effective in the first trimester.[390,394]

Adding First- and Second-Trimester Markers Into a Single Integrated Screening Test

The integrated test takes advantage of first- and second-trimester markers and avoids most of the limitations of stand-alone first-trimester screening.[402] With this approach, measurements of NT and PAPP-A are made in the first trimester but are not interpreted or acted upon until testing in the second trimester is complete. In the second trimester, a serum is drawn and a quadruple test performed. Results from all six tests (NT, PAPP-A, AFP, uE_3, CG, and inhA) are then combined into a single risk estimate. This approach detects 85% of Down syndrome cases with only a 1% false-positive rate.[402] Studies involving more than 47,000 and 38,000 pregnancies at multiple centers, obtained results consistent with this estimate.[237,400]

Given the low false-positive rate of the integrated test, it may be considered the safest maternal serum screening test. Because fewer amniocenteses are needed, fewer fetal losses occur per Down syndrome case diagnosed. The integrated test has been shown to be a cost-effective approach to Down syndrome screening, again on the basis of fewer costly diagnostic tests and affected liveborns.[399] Most of the cost in integrated screening comes from the NT ultrasound. Although NT alone is the best univariate screening marker, integrated screening can be offered effectively and at a lower cost by using a modified test based only on serum markers (serum integrated). Maternal serum PAPP-A concentrations are measured at 10 to 13 weeks and combined with a second-trimester quad test for a five-marker screening panel. The serum integrated test gives 85% detection of Down syndrome cases with about a 4% false-positive rate. The relative performance of first-trimester, second-trimester, and integrated screening tests is shown in Figure 57-6.

An alternative approach to integrated screening is the sequential integrated test, in which women at the very highest risk for Down syndrome pregnancy (e.g. 1 in 25 or higher) after the first-trimester phase are alerted and recommended for diagnostic testing.[289,401] All remaining women (≈98%) proceed to second-trimester blood collection for a full integrated risk analysis. The advantages of this approach are that very high risk women are afforded the opportunity for early diagnosis, and most patients have the safest and most effective screening strategy. The sequential integrated test offers an 85% detection rate with a 2 to 3% false-positive rate. This assumes that all patients have a first-trimester NT scan because a serum PAPP-A alone in the first trimester is not sufficient for calculation of interim risk. Contingent screening has been proposed, whereby patients at very high and at very low risk receive results in the first trimester, while those with an interim risk go on to have the second part of the full integrated screening test.[289,401] It should be noted, however, that this protocol has yet to be evaluated using an intervention trial.

Follow-up Testing for Women With Screen-Positive Results

Recommended follow-up testing depends on the types of positive results obtained.

Neural Tube Defects

Women who have a positive screening test result for an open neural tube defect should be offered genetic counseling and further testing. A low-resolution ultrasound examination

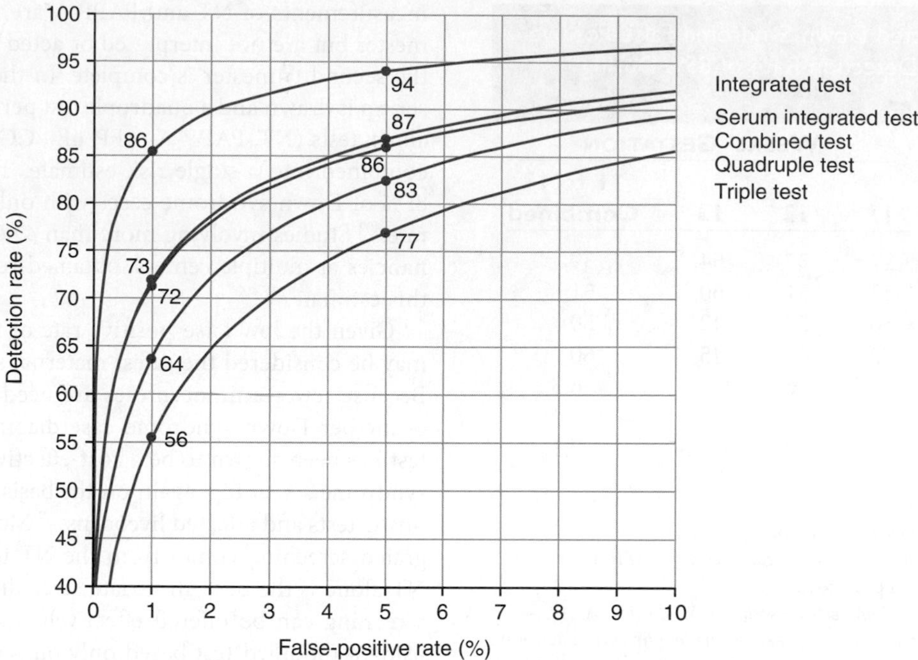

Figure 57-6 Receiver operating characteristic curves for tests used to screen for Down syndrome. *(Reprinted with permission from Wald NJ, Rodeck C, Hackshaw AK, Rudnicka A. SURUSS in perspective. Semin Perinatol 2005;29:225-35.)*

may verify gestational age and identify other possible reasons for the increased AFP test results (e.g., inaccurate gestational dating, recent fetal demise, twins). Patients who have an unexplained high maternal serum AFP result are offered high-resolution ultrasound, amniocentesis for measurement of amniotic fluid AFP and acetylcholinesterase (AChE), or both.

Compared with maternal serum, the distribution of amniotic fluid AFP concentrations in pregnancies affected by open neural tube defects is far more separated from unaffected pregnancies.[388] However, amniotic fluid AFP measurements are not by themselves diagnostic because of rare false-positive results. If the amniotic fluid is contaminated with even a small amount of fetal blood, as many as 2 to 3% of results can be falsely positive.[388] All abnormal amniotic fluid AFP results must be confirmed by measurement of amniotic fluid AChE. The combination of amniotic fluid AFP and AChE is virtually diagnostic for an open neural tube defect.[315,388]

High-resolution ultrasound will almost always confirm a chemical diagnosis of a neural tube defect. Anencephaly is readily identifiable, and ultrasound diagnosis of open spina bifida is considerably enhanced by the presence of two cranial signs (known as fruit signs) resulting from the Arnold-Chiari malformation associated with this defect.[110,267] The first sign is a "pinched" skull in the frontal region, resulting in a "lemon" shape compared with the normal egg shape. The second sign is a reduction in the transverse diameter of the cerebellum, causing the two cerebellar hemispheres to assume a bow shape—the "banana sign." Ultrasound diagnosis of open neural tube defects is now so reliable that it is sometimes used for diagnosis in women with elevated maternal serum AFP without waiting for amniotic fluid measurements.

Down Syndrome

Women who have a positive screening test result for increased risk of Down syndrome are usually referred for genetic counseling and further testing. A low-resolution ultrasound examination may be offered as a way to verify gestational age and to identify other possible reasons for the positive test result. One of the most common reasons for increased Down syndrome risk is overestimated gestational age. Up to one third of women with positive second-trimester Down syndrome screening results who are dated by the last menstrual period will be found to be too early in their pregnancies for reliable screening (<15 weeks) or will be reclassified as low risk after ultrasound revision of gestational age.[173] Women who are still at increased risk after the ultrasound examination should be offered amniocentesis to obtain fetal cells for karyotyping. Although some second-trimester ultrasound findings are associated with Down syndrome (e.g., nuchal fold and shortened femur and humeral length), these findings are not diagnostic.[342] The only way to diagnose Down syndrome is via fetal karyotype. However, the benefits of accurately diagnosing a chromosome abnormality in gestation must be weighed against the potential for harming a normal fetus during amniocentesis. This invasive procedure carries a small but real risk of harming the fetus or causing spontaneous abortion. Even amniocentesis performed by an experienced obstetrician using ultrasonography for guidance may have a procedure-related rate of fetal loss as high as 1 in 200.[347] Given that about 1 in 30 women with an initial screen-positive test result (high risk) will have a fetus with a chromosome abnormality, the offer of the invasive procedure is justifiable.

Women who have a screen-positive result in the first trimester may be offered CVS to diagnose Down syndrome. This procedure is performed between the 10th and 12th weeks, carries a slightly higher risk of fetal loss than amniocentesis,[366] and is not available to patients in some geographic regions.

Trisomy 18

In contrast to screening protocols for open neural tube defects and Down syndrome, a dating ultrasound is not recommended as the first step after a finding of increased risk of trisomy 18. The second-trimester serum marker pattern is not consistent with incorrect gestational dating, and amniocentesis should be offered.[131,286] A high proportion of fetuses with trisomy 18 will have abnormal but nondiagnostic second-trimester ultrasound findings (e.g., heart defects and clenched fists).[32] CVS may be offered to patients at high risk of trisomy 18 based on first-trimester screening results.

SLOS

Patients at risk for SLOS should be offered genetic counseling to discuss the risks and benefits of diagnosis by amniocentesis. High amniotic fluid concentrations of the precursor 7-dehydrocholesterol are diagnostic of the disorder.[1]

Adjustments for Factors That Influence Analyte Measurements

Prenatal screening for both open neural tube defects and Down syndrome is optimized when each woman's analyte concentration is compared with those of other women (the reference group) who are "similar" to her in many respects.[169] In addition to gestational age, this "similarity" extends to other factors that have been shown to affect analyte concentrations, including (1) maternal weight, (2) race, (3) insulin-dependent diabetes (IDD), and (4) multiple pregnancy. Taking into account these factors enhances the accuracy of the interpretation.

Maternal Weight

As maternal weight increases, the average concentration of analyte values decreases, because a fixed amount of analyte is diluted in an increased maternal blood volume. For example, heavier women have, on average, lower AFP values and are less likely than lighter-weight women to be screen positive for neural tube defects. Without taking maternal weight into account, screening is less effective in heavier women because their MoM values are inappropriately low. The importance of adjusting AFP MoM values for weight is reinforced by studies showing that heavier women have about a twofold to fourfold increased risk for open spina bifida.[335,403] No association between maternal weight and Down syndrome has been reported. The weight effect is also significant for CG, inhA, and PAPP-A, but less so for uE_3. Maternal weight is taken into account for all serum markers by adjusting each woman's MoM values by a factor corresponding to the expected MoM value (Figure 57-7) for women with her weight. These factors are empirically derived from the screened population in a manner that is similar to deriving median analyte concentrations for each gestational age. Optimally, each laboratory should derive its own maternal weight adjustment factors for each analyte, because the average maternal weight may differ from that seen in other laboratories. These adjustment factors should be applied only over the maternal weight range in which they have been shown to be appropriate. For example, if few or no data are available to derive adjustment factors for women weighing more than 300 pounds, then the laboratory should be careful in extrapolating factors to these women from data on women of lower weight. Laboratories should limit the range of adjustment using upper (and lower) truncation limits. If a woman's weight is outside these limits, adjustment should be applied as if the woman were at the respective limit. An effective model for all analytes is a linear reciprocal model. Maternal weights are stratified into weight groups and are regressed against the reciprocal of maternal weight. This model and its application have been described in detail elsewhere.[169,263] Distributions of maternal weight vary within each racial group, with Asian women tending to have lower maternal weights than Caucasians, and with African Americans weighing more. It is optimal to apply adjustment equations for each racial group to correct marker concentrations for weight.

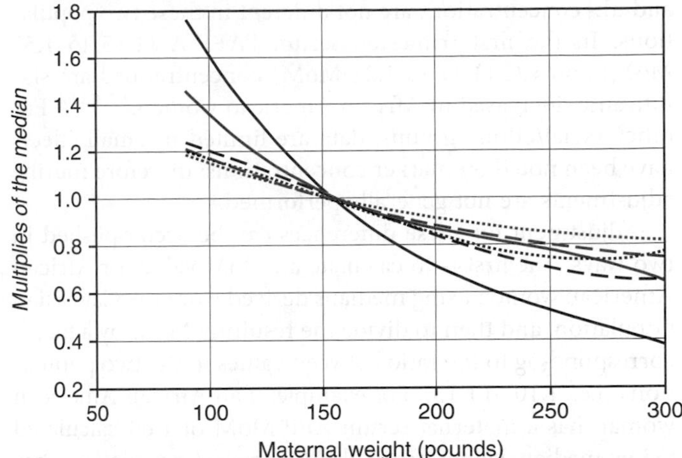

Figure 57-7 The relationship of AFP, uE_3, CG, inhA, and PAPP-A [expressed as multiples of the median (MoM)] and maternal weight. The horizontal line at 1.0 MoM is the value found for a woman of average weight. *Red solid line*, AFP; *red dashed line*, inhA; *red dotted line*, uE_3; *black solid line*, PAPP-A; *black dashed line*, first-trimester CG; *black dotted line*, second-trimester CG.

Maternal Race

For second-trimester markers, African American women have maternal serum AFP and CG concentrations that are 10 to 15% higher than those found in Caucasian women.[169] InhA concentrations are about 8% lower in African Americans,[406] and uE_3 concentrations are not different in these two populations. In the first trimester, serum PAPP-A (1.35 to 1.57 MoM) and CG (1.11 to 1.21 MoM) concentrations are significantly increased in African American women.[207,353,356] For other racial/ethnic groups, data are limited or small effects have been noted on marker concentrations; therefore routine adjustments are not generally performed.

Adjustment for these differences can be accomplished in two ways. The first is to calculate an MoM value for African American women using medians derived from the Caucasian population, and then to divide the resulting MoM by a factor corresponding to the ratio between values in the two populations (i.e., 1.10 to 1.15). For example, if an African American woman has a maternal serum AFP MoM of 1.60 calculated using median values from the Caucasian population, her adjusted MoM is 1.45 (1.60/1.10). The second approach is to calculate a separate set of medians using values measured on the African American population.

Strong evidence suggests that the birth prevalence of open neural tube defects in African American women is half or less than that in Caucasian women from the same geographic region.[156] Thus, at any given maternal serum AFP MoM, an African American woman has half the risk of a Caucasian woman of having a pregnancy affected by an open neural tube defect. Limited information is available on AFP concentrations in African American women with an open neural tube defect, but what is published indicates that screening in this population should be equally effective. The prevalence of neural tube defects has declined since the practice of folic acid fortification was introduced, particularly in African American women.[80] Data from California suggest that Hispanic women have the highest rates of NTD (0.112%) as compared with Caucasians (0.096%) and Black or Asian women (0.075%).[132]

Insulin-Dependent Diabetes

Maternal serum AFP values in women who require insulin before pregnancy (type 1) have been reported to be systematically lower by about 20% (0.88 MoM).[187] Women with type 2 diabetes, taking insulin or other oral agents, or on dietary restriction before pregnancy, also show reduced second-trimester maternal serum AFP concentrations.[374] However, controversy is ongoing regarding the need for adjustment of AFP concentrations in diabetic women when weight correction has been applied.[124] Some studies show that reduced AFP concentrations persist in diabetic women even after weight adjustment[374]; others suggest that reduced AFP concentrations can be completely explained by weight effects.[124] Debate also continues regarding whether the degree of glycemic control has an impact on maternal serum AFP concentrations in diabetic mothers.[327]

Second-trimester concentrations of uE_3 were also significantly reduced (0.95 MoM) in women with preexisting diabetes and may warrant adjustment. In contrast, alterations of second-trimester CG and inhA concentrations are small, and whether or not they are taken into account will have little impact on the resulting Down syndrome risk. Similarly, first-trimester PAPP-A and CG concentrations were not significantly altered in women with IDD.[214]

No compelling evidence indicates that the rate of Down syndrome births in women with IDD is substantially different from that in the general population.[189] However, evidence suggests that birth prevalence of open neural tube defects is higher by up to a factor of 5.[2] Thus at a given AFP MoM concentration, women with IDD are at substantially higher risk of open neural tube defects than the general population. This can be taken into account by lowering the AFP MoM cutoff from, for example, 2.0 to 1.5. It is not possible to define the associated detection rate for diabetic mothers because no large series of maternal serum AFP measurements in IDD women with a fetus affected with an open neural tube defect have been published.

Twin Pregnancy

Maternal serum AFP concentrations in twin pregnancies are about twice the concentration found in singleton pregnancies (i.e., ≈2.0 MoM).[169] Among singleton pregnancies with open spina bifida, the median serum AFP MoM is about 3.5.[390] Thus the expected maternal serum AFP in the average twin pregnancy affected with open spina bifida is thought to be around 4.5 MoM (1.0 MoM contributed by the unaffected fetus, and 3.5 MoM from the fetus with open spina bifida). Screening performance in twin pregnancies therefore will not be as effective as in singleton pregnancies because the AFP distributions are less separated. Although most affected twin pregnancies are discordant for open neural tube defects, if both twins are affected (seen in about 5% of affected twin pregnancies), screening performance can be expected to approach that in singleton pregnancies.

Calculation of Down syndrome risk requires that the distribution of analyte values for all tests in both unaffected and affected pregnancies is known. These distributions are well defined for AFP, uE_3, CG, inhA, and PAPP-A in singleton pregnancies; thus reliable risks can be calculated. The distributions of these analytes also are available for twin pregnancy unaffected by Down syndrome; the median MoMs in unaffected twin pregnancy for AFP, uE_3, CG, inhA, and PAPP-A are about 2.0, 1.7, 1.9, 2.0, and 1.8, respectively.[169,214,356] Fewer data are available for concentrations of these analytes in twin pregnancies affected with Down syndrome. A further complication is that in approximately one third of pregnancies, both twins will be affected (monozygotic), and in two thirds of pregnancies, only one twin will be affected (dizygotic). Screening will be less effective when only one twin is affected. Reports suggest that first-trimester serum marker concentrations differ in monozygotic and dizygotic twin pregnancies, with lower values in the former group.[226,355] Another difficulty is that the prevalence of Down syndrome is not well defined in twin pregnancies. Based on the rate of monozygotic and dizygotic twins, the prevalence of Down syndrome would be predicted to be 1.67 times higher in twin pregnancies. However, published data indicate that the prevalence of Down syndrome in twin pregnancies is actually similar to that found in singleton pregnancies.[117,143]

Given these limitations, calculation of only an approximate risk (sometimes called a *pseudorisk*) for twin pregnancy is possible.[262] This is accomplished by dividing the MoM value for each analyte by the corresponding median found in unaffected twin pregnancies. The twin pregnancy risk is then computed in the same way as for singleton pregnancies. If fetus-specific nuchal translucency measurements are available, adjusted serum marker results are used with *each* NT value to get a fetus-specific risk. The overall risk for the pregnancy is then calculated by adding the risk for each fetus in a dichorionic (presumed dizygotic) pregnancy, and averaging them for a monochorionic (presumed monozgotic) pregnancy. The resulting pseudorisk is compared with the same risk cutoff used for women with singleton pregnancies to identify twin pregnancies as screen positive. This twin screening protocol will (1) correctly rank pregnancies from highest to lowest risk, and (2) yield a screen-positive rate similar to the rate found for singleton pregnancies at any given screening cutoff. The Down syndrome pseudorisk, however, may not be correct. Screen-positive women with twin pregnancies can be informed that their test results place them in a high-risk group, but that their actual risk is uncertain. Interpretation of risk for triplets and higher gestations is not recommended because of limited available data. Additional factors that need to be considered when such screening is offered are the increased difficulty and fetal loss associated with multiple needle insertions required during amniocentesis, and loss of the unaffected twin should an affected twin be identified and selectively terminated.[123]

Pregnancies Achieved by Assisted Reproductive Technologies

As women are choosing pregnancy at more advanced chronological ages, the use of assisted reproductive technologies (ART), such as in vitro fertilization (IVF), for conception is increasing. Previous studies have shown that women who achieve pregnancy by IVF are about twice as likely to have a positive result after second-trimester Down syndrome screening than are women who achieve pregnancy spontaneously.[140] The increased rate is avoided with adjustment of certain MoM values. In particular, concentrations of uE_3 tend to be reduced (0.9 MoM), and CG and inhA increased (1.1 to 1.2 MoM), in pregnancies achieved by IVF.[140,212] Correction of these MoMs restores an appropriate screen-positive rate. Pregnancies achieved by intrauterine insemination, with or without ovulation induction, show a similar trend in marker concentrations; however, this reproductive technology is less often reported to screening programs and therefore is difficult to take into account for risk analysis. In contrast, IVF pregnancies involving donation of oocytes have a unique marker pattern with relatively elevated maternal serum AFP and inhA concentrations. Because these results provide opposing effects on risk, screen-positive rates are not increased and adjustment is not needed.[212]

The effects of ART on first-trimester screening markers are less pronounced. Although serum PAPP-A and CG concentrations are slightly altered in IVF pregnancies[212] (PAPP-A = 0.9 MoM; CG = 1.1 MoM) relative to spontaneously achieved pregnancies, most studies show that these changes are not sufficient to lead to increased screen-positive rates.[212,415] Adjustment of first-trimester screening markers for ART pregnancies is less critical than adjustment of second-trimester markers and, if done, would provide only a minimal improvement in screening performance. Expected and observed screen-positive rates in various ART pregnancies are shown in Table 57-6.[212]

Use of Epidemiologic Monitoring in Quality Control

In prenatal screening, the interpretative unit for each analyte is the MoM, which takes into account variables such as gestational age, maternal weight, race, and other factors. Expressing these results in MoMs allows the calculation of a patient-specific risk for Down syndrome. One of the most common causes of poor laboratory performance is the use of incorrect median values, either because those values are inappropriate for the kit being used, or because systematic

TABLE 57-6 Screen-Positive Rates (%) Observed (95% Confidence Intervals) and Expected for Assisted Reproductive Technologies

Type of Assisted Reproductive Technology	N	First Trimester		Second Trimester	
		Observed	Expected	Observed	Expected
In vitro fertilization with ovulation induction	277	8.6 (5.3 to 11.9)	5.5	20.2 (15.4 to 25.0)	14.7
Intrauterine insemination with ovulation induction	323	3.4 (1.4 to 5.4)	4.2	21.2 (16.6 to 25.7)	11.9
Intrauterine insemination without ovulation induction	247	6.1 (3.1 to 9.1)	4.3	19.1 (14.1 to 24.0)	12.3
In vitro fertilization with ovulation induction and egg donation	59	3.4 (0.0 to 8.0)	2.5	12.3 (3.8 to 20.8)	7.4
In vitro fertilization with egg donation	56	1.8 (0.0 to 5.3)	1.0	7.4 (0.4 to 14.4)	3.9

Adapted from Lambert-Messerlian G, Dugoff L, Vidaver J, Canick JA, Malone FD, Ball RH, et al. First- and second-trimester Down syndrome screening markers in pregnancies achieved through assisted reproductive technologies (ART): a FASTER trial study. Prenat Diagn 2006;26:672-8.

shifts in assay values have occurred. Poor analytical performance also occurs when an assay is nonspecific or relatively inaccurate. Ensuring that median values (and by extension, MoM values) are accurate is one of the most important responsibilities of the screening laboratory. The following discussions are adapted from Knight and Palomaki,[202] a publication that discusses in detail the process of epidemiologic monitoring.

Definition of Epidemiologic Monitoring

A powerful method for evaluating and monitoring the appropriateness of medians is epidemiologic monitoring. This process involves gathering data from the screened population to calculate detection (proportion of affected pregnancies with positive test results) and screen-positive (proportion of screened pregnancies with a positive test result) rates. These rates are then to be compared with expectations based on the maternal age distribution of the population studied. Obtaining a detection rate is difficult because complete ascertainment of all pregnancy outcomes is required, and it can take years before a sufficient number of affected pregnancies occur to allow reliable estimates. In practice, the screen-positive rate is used for epidemiologic monitoring because a reliable estimate can be calculated in a short time, and it is not necessary to have outcome information. For prenatal screening, the positive rate is defined as the proportion of women with test results falling at or above a specified AFP MoM (for open neural tube defect screening), or a specified risk cutoff (Down syndrome screening). These rates are in fact similar to false-positive rates because few screen-positive individuals have true-positive results (i.e., they do have an affected fetus). For this reason, the term *initial positive rate (IPR)* has been suggested, because it more accurately describes what is being calculated. The IPR can be used to assess whether medians are appropriate, because it will be shifted upward or downward if medians are incorrect for the population being screened. Further, once the IPR is shown to be within acceptable limits, continuous monitoring can help detect shifts in assay values.

Establishing Assay-Specific and Population-Specific Median Values

Another important responsibility of the prenatal screening laboratory is to establish kit-specific and population-specific median values for each analyte used in screening, or to show that median values obtained from another source are appropriate. Relatively small errors in median values have a disproportionate impact on both the accuracy of the calculated risk and the number of women identified as screen positive. Values measured on the same patients and the same proficiency testing samples have been known to differ among methods by 5 to 200%, depending on the analyte measured.[92] Median values therefore are not directly transferable between reagent sets from different methods. Median values sometimes differ among laboratories even when the same method is employed. This difference is caused by such factors as the reliability of gestational dating, race, maternal weight, and even apparently subtle differences in assay instrumentation, or changes in manufacturer lot numbers of reagents or calibrators.[122]

Median values must be routinely monitored and updated as necessary. Median values provided in package inserts are not acceptable for many of the reasons already given. It has been recommended that median values should be established using at least 100 values for each week of gestation in the screening period. In practice, however, obtaining 100 serum samples for each gestational week is very difficult even for large laboratories. Given these constraints, the following strategies are recommended for obtaining reliable median values, categorized according to whether a laboratory is implementing a screening test for the first time, or is updating an existing set of median values.

Two alternatives are available when a laboratory is establishing median values for the first time. The first and optimal method is to obtain measurements on 300 to 500 patient specimens using the assay selected for screening. Establishing that all of these samples come from unaffected singleton pregnancies is not necessary, because the prevalence of conditions that produce abnormal values (e.g., twins, fetal demise, open fetal defects) is small and will have minimal impact.[169] Data are used to derive median values for each completed week of gestation. Appropriate weighted regression analysis is then used to fit the observed data. The regression equation is used to predict "smoothed" medians for each week of gestation. Usually the median value is found at each completed week and is regressed against the average gestational age for that week. This technique helps reduce the effects of outliers. Weighting takes into account the reliability of these summary estimates and usually is based on the square root of the number of samples observed at each week.

Measurements of the concentrations AFP, uE_3, and PAPP-A increase by a constant proportion—about 15% per week for AFP, 25% per week for uE_3 measurements, and 50% for PAPP-A. A log-linear model best fits this relationship [log of the measurements (y-axis) is regressed against gestational age (x-axis)]. The regression model for CG versus gestational age fits an exponential model similar to that used for radioactive decay. Measurements of inhA are relatively flat, but experience has shown that a cubic model fits the data, with a minimum found between 16 and 18 weeks' gestation.[396] Figures 57-8 to 57-11 are graphical representations of weighted regression equations and resulting smoothed medians for the second-trimester markers (the legends contain the respective median regression equations). The data are provided in Table 57-7. Figure 57-12 shows medians and weighted regression lines for first trimester PAPP-A and total CG.

Some laboratories use "day-specific" medians rather than weekly medians where a different median value is used for each day of pregnancy. Although individual pregnancies cannot be reliably dated to within 1 day, a consistent day-by-day change in analyte concentrations is noted when data from a group of pregnant women is observed. Table 57-8 shows observed and regressed medians for uE_3 for a group of

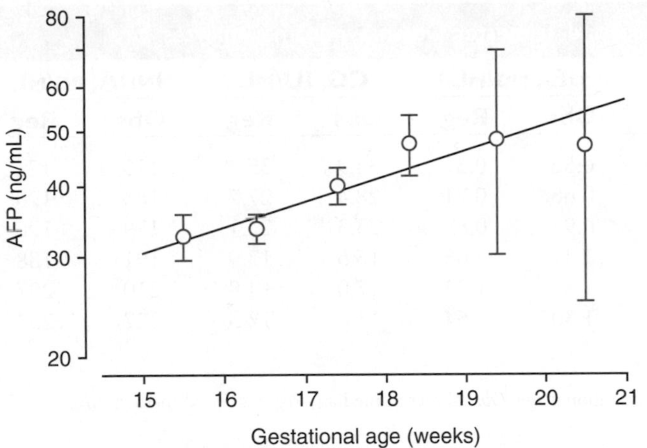

Figure 57-8 Computation of median values for maternal serum alpha fetoprotein (AFP) in the second trimester. The observed average gestational age from Table 57-7 is plotted on the horizontal axis and the median of that week's AFP measurements on the vertical logarithmic axis. The thin vertical lines represent 95% confidence intervals of the medians. The line represents the results of a linear regression analysis of log AFP versus age weighted by the square root of the number of samples. The equation of that line in completed weeks is median AFP = $10^{0.04465 \times (\text{weeks}) + 0.8334}$. The corresponding equation for day-specific medians is median AFP = $10^{0.006378 \times (\text{days}) + 0.8142}$.

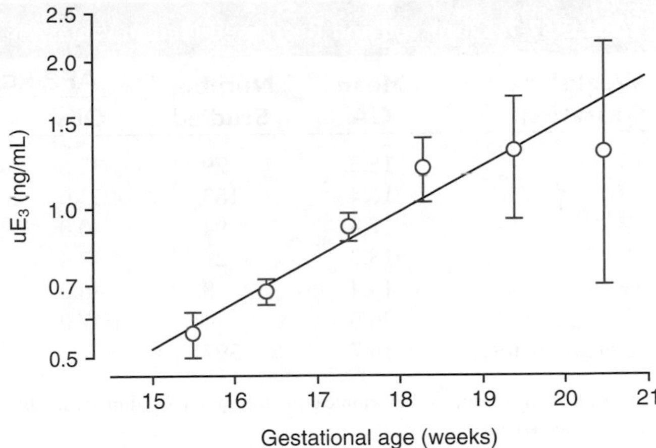

Figure 57-9 Computation of median values for maternal serum unconjugated estriol (uE_3) in the second trimester. The observed average gestational age from Table 57-7 is plotted on the horizontal axis and the median of that week's uE_3 measurements on the vertical logarithmic axis. The thin vertical lines represent 95% confidence intervals of the medians. The line represents the results of a linear regression analysis of log uE_3 versus age weighted by the square root of the number of samples. The equation of that line in completed weeks is median $uE_3 = 10^{0.09165 \times (\text{weeks}) - 1.618}$. The corresponding equation for day-specific medians is median $uE_3 = 10^{0.01309 \times (\text{days}) - 1.657}$.

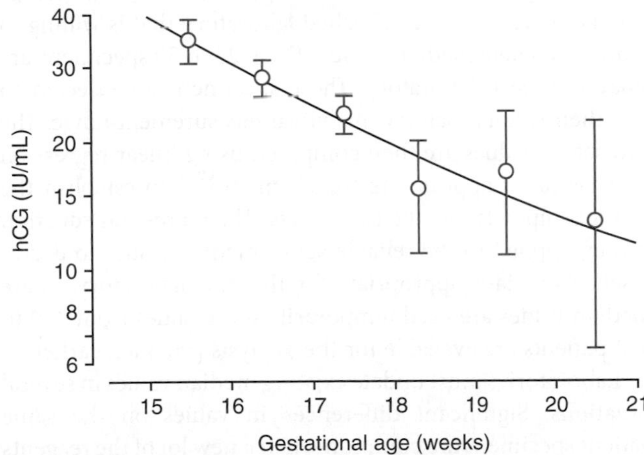

Figure 57-10 Computation of median values for maternal serum chorionic gonadotropin (CG) in the second trimester. The observed average gestational age from Table 57-7 is plotted on the horizontal axis and the median of that week's CG measurements on the vertical logarithmic axis. The thin vertical lines represent the 95% confidence intervals of the medians. The line represents the results of a nonlinear regression analysis weighted by the square root of the number of samples. The equation of that curve in completed weeks is CG median = 39.69 $\times e^{-0.3001 \times (\text{weeks} - 14)} + 5.93$. The corresponding equation for day-specific medians is CG median = $45.14 \times e^{-0.04287 \times (\text{days})} + 5.93$.

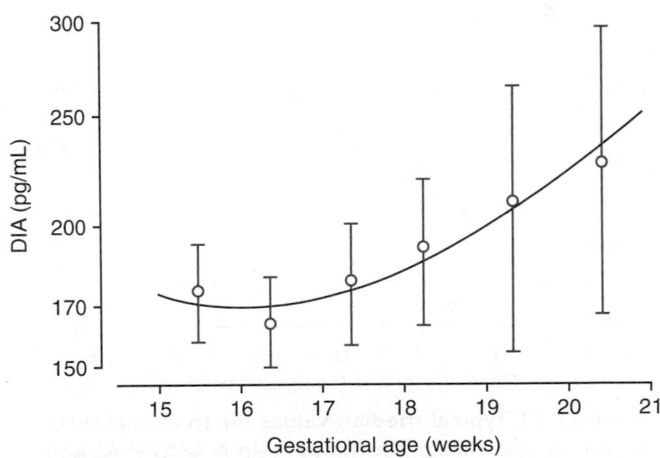

Figure 57-11 Computation of median values for maternal serum dimeric inhibin A (inhA) in the second trimester. The observed average gestational age from Table 57-7 is plotted on the horizontal axis and the median of that week's inhA measurements on the vertical logarithmic axis. The thin vertical lines represent 95% confidence intervals of the medians. The line represents the results of a quadratic regression analysis weighted by the square root of the number of samples. The equation of that curve in completed weeks is inhA median = $3.404 \times \text{weeks}^2 - 106.7 \times \text{weeks} + 1005.7$. The corresponding equation for day-specific medians is inhA median = $0.06947 \times \text{days}^2 - 15.66 \times \text{days} + 1052$.

TABLE 57-7 Observed and Regressed Median Values for Four Second-Trimester Down Syndrome Analytes

Weeks' Gestation	Mean GA	Number Studied	AFP, NG/ML		uE_3, NG/ML		CG, IU/ML		INHA, PG/ML	
			Obs	Reg	Obs	Reg	Obs	Reg	Obs	Reg
15	15.5	79	32.6	31.8	0.56	0.57	34.9	35.3	175	171
16	16.4	183	33.6	35.3	0.68	0.71	28.4	27.7	164	170
17	17.4	94	40.0	39.1	0.92	0.87	23.3	22.1	179	176
18	18.3	29	47.4	43.4	1.21	1.08	15.5	17.9	191	188
19	19.4	8	48.2	48.0	1.31	1.33	17.0	14.8	210	207
20	20.5	4	47.0	53.2	1.30	1.64	13.0	12.5	227	233
Average or total	16.7	397								

AFP, Alpha fetoprotein; *CG,* chorionic gonadotropin; *DIA,* dimeric inhibin A; *GA,* gestational age; *Obs,* observed median; *Reg,* regressed median; *uE_3,* unconjugated estriol.

TABLE 57-8 Observed and Regressed Day-Specific Medians for Unconjugated Estriol During the 17th Week of Gestation

Gestational Age, week, day	Number of Observations	uE_3, ng/mL, Observed	Regressed
16, 0	195	0.67	0.68
16, 1	225	0.69	0.70
16, 2	228	0.71	0.72
16, 3	219	0.76	0.74
16, 4	186	0.78	0.76
16, 5	191	0.80	0.79
16, 6	175	0.78	0.81

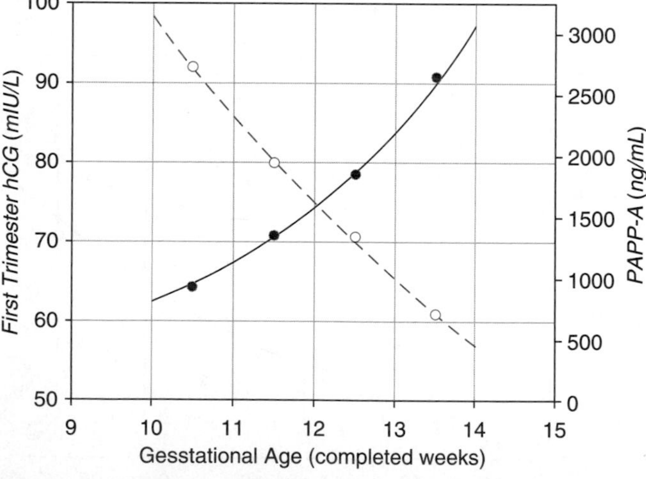

Figure 57-12 Typical median values for maternal serum pregnancy associated plasma protein-A (PAPP-A) and total CG in the first trimester. The observed average gestational age is plotted on the horizontal axis and the median of that week's PAPP-A or total CG measurements on the vertical logarithmic axis. The PAPP-A median = $10^{(1.4633 + 0.144501 \times \text{weeks})}$. The total CG median = 385.1 × 0.98069^{days}.

ultrasound-dated women in their 17th week of gestation. The observed median concentrations clearly increase during that week. The regressed median for 16 weeks, 0 days, is quite different from the median for 16 weeks, 6 days. If weekly medians were to have been used instead, all of these samples would have been interpreted against a single median—≈0.74 ng/mL (0.74 µg/L).

An acceptable alternative for the generation of new median data is to identify an established laboratory that is willing to share its reliable median values. Then, 25 to 50 specimens are assayed at each laboratory. These specimens are selected so that their results span the analytical measurement range. The two sets of values are then compared using linear regression analysis (after appropriate transformations) to establish the relationship between the two assays. The regression equation is then applied to the reliable set of median values to derive a set of medians appropriate for the new laboratory. These median values are used temporarily until values from 300 to 500 patients are available for the analysis provided earlier.

Laboratories must update existing median values in several situations. Significant differences in values on the same patient specimens are common when a new lot of the reagents or reagents from a different manufacturer are used. In this situation, the relationship between new and old methods is established by regression analysis of values measured on the same patient specimens. If a periodic adjustment is required, the laboratory should carefully choose the characteristics of the population to be used (e.g., race, method of dating, time period) and should verify that the assay has been providing consistent results over the time period of interest. This is done by routinely monitoring the median MoM over time (epidemiologic monitoring), as is discussed in greater detail later in this chapter. Resulting data are then analyzed, as described previously.

Epidemiologic Monitoring of Open Neural Tube Defect Screening

In maternal serum AFP screening for open neural tube defects, the IPR is the proportion of women with values above the specified MoM cutoff. For example, at a screening cutoff of 2.5 MoM, IPRs should be 1 to 3%. When new medians are implemented, the IPR can be used to determine whether the medians are appropriate by comparing the expected with the observed IPRs. If the IPR falls outside the expected range, it is possible that the medians are incorrect for the assay being used or for the population being screened. For example, if the IPR at a cutoff of 2.5 MoM is 5%, median values may be too low, resulting in too many high MoMs and too many women having screen-positive results.

Once the IPR is shown to be within an acceptable range, ongoing monitoring of this rate serves as a check on shifts in assay calibration caused by changes in (1) kit lots, (2) reagent deterioration, (3) poor technical performance, and (4) other factors. Simultaneous monitoring of the IPR and the results of quality control samples can facilitate identification of shifts in assay values. If, for instance, the IPR at a 2.5 AFP MoM cutoff increases from 2 to 4%, and at the same time some or all of the values of quality control (QC) samples shift significantly upward by 10% or more, the change is consistent with an upward shift in assay calibration. The IPR increases when assay values increase, because individual AFP values are interpreted by using medians generated from data gathered in the past. In the example given previously, it may be necessary to calculate new medians or to adjust existing median values to take into account the assay shift.

It is difficult to establish an absolute rule as to how large a change in the IPR is sufficient to warrant recomputing medians. Factors other than the assay can affect the IPR. For example, a significant increase in the number of pregnancies dated by ultrasound will reduce the IPR, because incorrectly dated pregnancies will be identified before the AFP test is done. However, consider that an upward shift in AFP values of just 10% can increase the IPR by more than 50% (e.g., from 2 to 3%) with little gain in detection. In effect, more interventions (ultrasound examinations or amniocenteses or both) will be required to detect each case of neural tube defect. Therefore, if a change in the IPR of 50% or more occurs simultaneously with an identifiable shift in assay values of 10% or more, medians need to be recalculated. Laboratories may wish to have stricter warning limits (e.g., shifts of 25% or more in the IPR occurring simultaneously with a change of 7% or more in quality control samples). When these rules are applied, enough values should be used to ensure that a reliable IPR can be calculated (generally 300 to 500 values will ensure reliability) and that observed changes are statistically significant. Further, the change should occur over several kit lots. Otherwise the laboratory may be tracking random error. The IPR can also be calculated using a moving window to improve reliability. For example, consider a laboratory that screens 300 women per month. In addition to calculating a monthly IPR, the laboratory could calculate a cumulative 3-month moving window by adding the current month's data and dropping data from the oldest month. The actual time period for both the individual and a cumulative moving window will be determined by how many samples are screened per unit time by any given laboratory.

Epidemiologic Monitoring of Down Syndrome Screening

In screening for Down syndrome, the IPR is the proportion of women with a risk at or above the cutoff. In contrast to neural tube defect screening, the IPR for Down syndrome screening is influenced by each of the analytes used in the risk calculation. Therefore, monitoring the IPR does not provide information on which assay(s) might be responsible when an inappropriate IPR is obtained. Consequently, it is necessary to monitor each assay separately. Individual monitoring of each assay can be accomplished according to the following rationale. When individual MoM values are calculated for each patient using gestational age–specific medians, MoM values can be analyzed collectively without regard for the gestational week. If the medians are appropriate, the resulting distribution of MoM values will have a grand median MoM of 1.00. The center of the distribution is typically expressed as the median, rather than the mean, because MoM distributions are not Gaussian on the linear scale.

Initial application of the grand MoM is done to ensure that when medians are first implemented, they are appropriate for the assay and the population being screened. This is accomplished by calculating the grand MoM using values from 300 to 500 individuals screened after the new set of medians is implemented. The grand MoM should be 1.00, within statistical limits. A convenient approach is to plot the grand MoM values on a graph, thus facilitating the detection of trends. IPR observations can be plotted on the same graph. If the IPR begins to trend in a positive or negative direction, the grand MoM for each assay can be examined to determine whether one of the analytes is paralleling the IPR change. If a significant change in one of the assays has occurred, corrective action should be taken (e.g., recalculating medians). For example, suppose the IPR shows a significant upward trend (e.g., from 6 to 9%), and over the same time period, the median MoM of the uE_3 assay significantly decreases (e.g., from 1.03 to 0.91). Because low uE_3 values are associated with increased risk for fetal Down syndrome, it is probable that the change in the uE_3 assay is responsible for the increase in IPR. The next step would be to examine quality control specimen values to determine whether a corresponding downward shift in values has occurred. If a shift has occurred, it is appropriate to recalculate and implement a new set of uE_3 medians using data collected after the time when the change in the uE_3 assay occurred (or to apply an adjustment factor to the old medians). A simultaneous change in two assays can complicate monitoring because the IPR might not change if the shift in one analyte value increases risk and the shift in the other analyte decreases risk. Simultaneous monitoring of the IPR and the median MoM for each analyte is recommended. IPRs should be calculated only when sufficient patient values are available (typically, 300 to 500 samples) to ensure a statistically reliable rate. Further, a single IPR or median MoM that deviates from expected should serve only as a warning to examine quality control data more closely.

Laboratories need to have an action limit in place to determine how much variability is to be allowed in the grand MoM. To accomplish this, one should consider the impact on the Down syndrome detection rate and the IPR of a 10% downward shift in uE_3 values (grand MoM of 0.90). This is simulated by recalculating MoM values after assay values are artificially shifted down by 10%, followed by mathematical modeling of the detection rate and the associated IPR. Such an assay shift effectively changes the MoM for any given sample, because current assay values are interpreted using reference data collected in the past. When uE_3 values shift downward by 10%, the detection rate increases only slightly from 59 to 62%. However, the IPR increases from 4.8 to 6.7%—a 40% increase. Thus, what might be viewed as a small shift in assay values has a large impact on the IPR, with little corresponding gain in detection. Relatively large changes in the IPR accompanying small shifts in assay values are one of the primary reasons for closely monitoring assays to ensure that the amniocentesis referral rate is maintained within reasonable limits. Given these facts, screening laboratories should consider important, as a minimum, a consistent deviation of 10% from 1.00 MoM (range, 0.90 to 1.10). Laboratories may wish to consider setting up stricter warning limits, such as 7% (assuming that this percentage is based on sufficient numbers of samples to yield statistically significant results). With this limit, median MoM values outside the range of 0.93 to 1.07 would be considered sufficiently deviant to warrant further investigation to determine whether a problem exists.

Although the IPR for laboratories screening for Down syndrome using multiple tests is generally about 5% in an unselected pregnancy population, it may be affected by various factors (other than incorrect medians), including the type of tests used, the screening cutoff chosen, and the maternal age distribution of the screened population. For example, if screening is applied primarily to older women, the IPR will be substantially higher, because older women are collectively more likely to be screen positive as a result of their higher age-specific risks. For example, if the triple test is being used to screen women age 35 and older at a term risk cutoff of 1:250, approximately 25% of women will be screen positive.[170] The method of gestational dating will also affect the IPR. Laboratories with a high percentage of pregnancies dated by the first day of the LMP will have a higher IPR than do laboratories where most gestational ages have been provided from ultrasound measurements because there is more variability in the accuracy of dating a population by LMP than by ultrasound.[173]

Epidemiologic Monitoring of NT Measurements

The introduction of ultrasound measurement of NT as part of the Down syndrome screening test has led to a new era in epidemiologic monitoring. Although serum screening analytes are under the day-to-day control of the laboratory, NT ultrasound is performed outside of the laboratory, at multiple locations and by many individuals. This situation is comparable to trying to report uniform screening results with each patient's AFP measurement being run in a different laboratory using a different assay and kit lot.

To bring uniformity to NT measurements, credentialing agencies have been established to train and certify sonographers. Examples of these agencies include the Fetal Medicine Foundation and the Nuchal Translucency Quality Review program, a subsidiary organization of the Society for Maternal-Fetal Medicine (SMFM). Certification involves didactic and hands-on training, along with image review. NT should be used in screening by sonographers only after training has been provided and when quality assurance measures are in place.[12] Previous studies have clearly shown that without such training, the performance of NT as a marker for Down syndrome is erratic, with anywhere from 0 to 100% of cases detected prenatally.[172]

The laboratory has the responsibility to establish NT median data for each sonographer and to monitor performance over time. To determine a median equation, preliminary data should be submitted to the laboratory that includes a series of paired NT and crown-rump length (CRL) measurements. Regression analysis as described earlier provides an appropriate median equation. NT data should fit a log-linear regression and should increase by about 25% per gestational week (Figure 57-13).[330] A single median equation may be used for all sonographers but is not likely to provide optimal interpretations for each individual sonographer. Even when all sonographers are trained using a single method, median NT results often show marked variation.[328] A better approach is to generate an NT median equation for each sonographer or each group of sonographers for whom measurements are similar. Improved screening performance is observed when median data are made more specific.[166,238]

The task of monitoring NT performance over time is daunting given the variable relationship between sonography

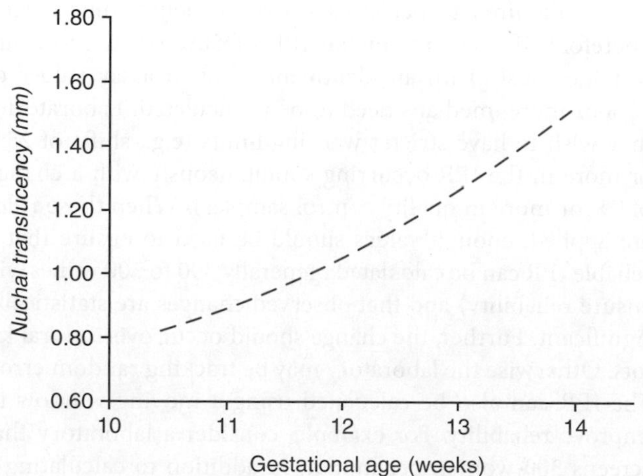

Figure 57-13 Typical medians for nuchal translucency during the first trimester.

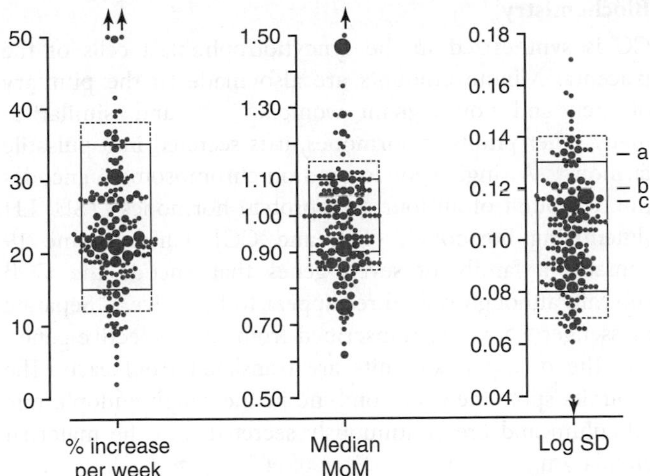

Figure 57-14 Summary of quality assessment parameters for 140 sonographers, showing the increase per week *(left column)*, the median NT MoM *(center column)*, and logarithmic standard deviation *(right column)*. *[Reprinted from Palomaki GE, Neveux LM, Donnenfeld A, Lee JF, McDowell G, Canick JA, et al. Quality assessment of routine nuchal translucency measurements: a North American laboratory perspective. Genet Med 2008;10:131-8.]*

and laboratory staff at different institutions and the sheer numbers of sonographers who may be submitting data to one laboratory. A further complication is that a single sonographer may submit very few data points to a laboratory, and long time intervals may be required before it is possible to conduct a meaningful review of results. Nevertheless, objective criteria upon which sonography data should be judged have been identified. As with serum markers, NT data, once normalized for gestational age, should center at a median of 1.0 MoM. The distribution of NT values in unaffected pregnancies generally has a standard deviation of the log MoM in the range of 0.1. The rate of increase with advancing gestational age between 10 and 13 weeks' gestation should be about 25% per week, as shown in Figure 57-14.[288] Examination of NT data over time can be performed in-house or obtained externally through services provided to laboratories by the Nuchal Translucency Quality Review (NTQR) (www.ntqr.org/ accessed August 26, 2011) or the NT Monitor (www.ipmms.org/ accessed August 26, 2011) program. Regardless of method, ongoing quality assessment of NT data is essential for screening accuracy.[104]

External Proficiency Testing

All laboratories performing prenatal screening should participate in an external proficiency testing program that distributes unknown specimens reflecting the concentrations of analytes found in pregnancy. These programs will evaluate the laboratory's ability to convert analyte values into a MoM using the laboratory's own median equations, to make screening recommendations, to adjust for variables that influence analyte values, and to calculate patient-specific risks. In the United States, the College of American Pathologists (CAP) provides a second-trimester program (CAP Maternal Screening Survey FP) with approximately 200 enrolled laboratories. Five second-trimester serum and two amniotic fluid proficiency samples are distributed three times each year. The CAP program has information on its Website (www.cap.org/ accessed September 23, 2011) that assists participants with risk calculation verification depending on the parameter set used. New York State also has an external proficiency testing program that is required for laboratories serving New York State residents. Five serum and five amniotic fluid samples are distributed three times each year. A similar interlaboratory proficiency program for first-trimester screening markers is available through the Women and Infants Hospital of Rhode Island at www.ipmms.org/ accessed August 26, 2011.

New Techniques

In 1997, fetal DNA was found to circulate in small amounts, along with maternal DNA, as fee fragments in maternal plasma. This led to the measurement of Y-chromosome sequences as an aid in the diagnosis of gender-linked fetal disorders.[182] Noninvasive determination of fetal Rhesus factor status in RhD-negative mothers has also been implemented clinically.[137] Active research is under way to find a method for the detection of fetal Down syndrome and other aneuploidies, using only maternal blood. Early studies described separation of fetal cells and cell-free fetal nucleic acids in maternal blood (see reviews[334,417]). Application of newer, sophisticated molecular techniques such as (1) massive sequencing of DNA fragments in maternal blood with chromosome quantification,[86,126] (2) selective amplification of placental methylated DNA with quantification by mass spectrometry,[270] and (3) calculation of haplotype ratios using tandem single-nucleotide polymorphisms[145] hold promise for high-quality noninvasive screening or diagnosis of Down syndrome in the near future. A more detailed discussion is provided by Lo and Chiu in Chapter 45.

LABORATORY TESTS

In this section of the chapter, we review methods for measurement of (1) CG, (2) AFP, (3) uE_3, (4) inhA, (5) PAPP-A, (6) fetal fibronectin, (7) amniotic fluid bilirubin, and (8) six tests for fetal lung maturity.

Chorionic Gonadotropin

Measurement of CG is used to (1) detect pregnancy and its abnormalities (e.g., ectopic and molar pregnancies), (2) screen for Down syndrome and trisomy 18, and (3) monitor the course of a patient with a CG-producing cancer. Because CG has these diverse uses, many assays are used, including qualitative urine and serum kits and quantitative serum assays.

This hormone is commonly called *human chorionic gonadotropin* and often is abbreviated as hCG or HCG. This term and its abbreviations should be abandoned because the adjective "human" is superfluous. Nonetheless, when communicating with clinicians (at least in the United States), hCG is the preferable term to avoid misunderstanding.

Chemistry

CG is a glycoprotein containing a protein core with branched carbohydrate sidechains that usually terminate with sialic acid. The hormone is a heterodimer composed of two non-identical, non–covalently bound glycoprotein subunits—alpha (α) and beta (β). When the CG dimer is dissociated, hormone activity is lost. However, a major part of the original activity is restored by equimolar recombination of the two subunits. The CGα subunit contains 92 amino acids, 2 carbohydrate sidechains, and 5 disulfide bridges. The molecular mass of the α subunit is estimated to be 14,900 Da, of which 10,200 is the protein component. CGβ consists of 145 amino acids and has 6 carbohydrate sidechains and 6 disulfide bridges. The molecular mass of the β subunit is estimated to be 23,000. Thus the heterodimer has a molecular weight of approximately 37,900 Da and a higher carbohydrate proportion than any other human hormone.

The CG carbohydrate composition changes as pregnancy progresses. In the first few weeks of pregnancy, more than 80% of immunoreactive CG is a large molecular mass form (Mr 41,000 to 42,000 Da), with additional monosaccharides in its carbohydrate chains, called *hyperglycosylated CG* (CG-H).[271] Serum concentrations of CG-H decline rapidly after the fourth week, and the 37,900 Da molecular mass form predominates for the remainder of the pregnancy.[88] In addition to CG and CG-H, maternal serum includes numerous other CG variants. To avoid confusion, the International Federation of Clinical Chemistry (IFCC) has recommended specific nomenclature for the identification of intact CG (hCG) and its variants.[60] These include (1) nicked CG (hCGn), (2) the free α subunit (hCGα), (3) the free β subunit (hCGβ), (4) the nicked free β subunit (hCGβn), and (5) the beta core fragment (hCGβcf). CGn is produced from enzymatic cleavage of peptide bonds in CGβ at position 44-45 (and, after prolonged incubation, at position 51-52).[197] Nicking inactivates the hormone and may reduce the ability to bind some CG antibodies. Other nicking sites are at β44-45, β47-48, and α70-71.[49] CGβcf is the terminal degradation product of CGβ and represents the 73 amino acid core of CGβ. It is composed of two pieces of the β subunit, residues 6-40, and residues 55-92, held together by disulfide bridges.[48] CGβcf is detected only in urine and has a molecular mass of 13,000 Da.

Urine contains predominantly CGβcf and to a lesser degree unmodified CG and CGn. Clearance occurs both in the liver and through the kidneys and varies for the different CG forms. Hepatic clearance[407] is approximately 2 mL/min/m^2, and renal clearance is approximately 0.4 mL/min/m^2; thus early morning urine specimens have CG concentrations comparable with those in serum. A study using highly specific immunoassays for CG, CGβ, and CGα found that disappearance after term pregnancy was triphasic.[206] Rapid, medium, and slow half-lives were, respectively, CG, 3.6, 18, and 53 hours; CGβ, 1.0, 23, and 194 hours; and CGα, 0.63, 6, and 22 hours.

Biochemistry

CG is synthesized in the syncytiotrophoblast cells of the placenta. Minute amounts are also made in the pituitary of men and nonpregnant women,[50,350,361] and, similar to many other pituitary hormones, it is secreted in a pulsatile fashion.[273] A single gene located on chromosome 6 encodes the α subunit of all four glycoprotein hormones [TSH, LH (luteinizing hormone), FSH, and CG]. Chromosome 19 contains a family of seven genes that encode the CGβ subunit, although only three appear to be active.[306] Separate messenger RNAs are transcribed from the respective genes, and the α and β subunits are translated from each. The subunits spontaneously combine in the rough endoplasmic reticulum and are continuously secreted into the maternal circulation.

Synthesis of CGβ peaks at about 8 to 10 weeks, but production of the α subunit continues to increase and appears to be a function of the mass of the placenta. The production of CGβ in the syncytiotrophoblasts may be under paracrine control of gonadotropin-releasing hormone (GnRH) produced in cytotrophoblasts. Studies suggest that the cytotrophoblasts produce inhibin, which stimulates CG production.[299] The number of cytotrophoblasts peaks at about the same time the CGβ production peaks. In the second trimester, more than 99% of CG is the dimer form; only a small amount circulates as free CGβ.[280]

Extensive homology exists between the peptide portions of CGβ and LHβ subunits. Investigators have proposed that a single base pair deletion in the ancestral LHβ gene lengthened the subunit from 115 amino acids to 145 amino acids; 80% of the first 115 amino acids in both β subunits are identical, but 20 additional amino acid residues are unique in CGβ.[371]

Physiology

CG stimulates the corpus luteum in the ovary to make progesterone during the first weeks of pregnancy. The placenta makes inadequate amounts of progesterone during this time. No specific receptor for CG is known; it binds to and activates the LH receptor in cells of the corpus luteum in the maternal ovary. Species other than primates and horses use LH for this function. Glycation of the α subunit has a dominant role[325] in signal transduction—an increase in intracellular cyclic adenosine monophosphate (cAMP). The cAMP increase in turn stimulates the production of progesterone, a steroid that prevents menses and thus facilitates pregnancy. CG binds weakly to TSH receptors in the maternal thyroid, and extremely elevated CG concentrations have the potential to be thyrotropic. A study of 63 women with a CG concentration greater than 400,000 IU/L revealed that TSH was suppressed and free thyroxine was increased in 100 and 80% of specimens, respectively. However, only four women had clinical signs and symptoms of hyperthyroidism.[232]

CG-H is synthesized by invasive cytotrophoblast cells and appears to have an autocrine function that modulates cytotrophoblast invasion of the myometrium in early pregnancy.[89]

CG Assays

Many assay techniques have been used to determine CG, and all modern techniques are based on immunoassay.

Of historical note, Vaitukaitis and colleagues took advantage of the uniqueness of CGβ to produce the first specific assay for CG, which used polyclonal antibodies raised against the β subunit.[384] Subsequently, highly specific monoclonal antibodies have been produced that recognize epitopes on the CG dimer and CGβ. The molecular epitope structure and the specificities of some of these antibodies have been described.[40]

Currently, bioassays, receptor assays, and agglutination inhibition assays are obsolete for detecting pregnancy. The historical bioassays are interesting, however, because they exploit the physiologic effect of CG.[78,83,120,329,375]

Qualitative CG Tests

Numerous tests for the qualitative detection of CG in urine or serum are available as over-the-counter (home) or point-of-care (POC) devices, and their use for the rapid identification of pregnancy is well established. Qualitative detection of CG in urine is a test granted waived status under the Clinical Laboratory Improvement Amendments of 1988 (CLIA '88); therefore this is performed at home and at the POC. In contrast, the use of serum as a sample matrix is considered a moderately complex test, even when the test device itself is approved for use with urine or serum. The difference in test complexity status is due to the requirement that serum, rather than whole blood, should be analyzed, and that centrifugation of the specimen is necessary. As such, most qualitative serum CG tests are performed in laboratories—not at home nor in POC situations.

POC devices are single-use tests that utilize immunochromatography for the rapid qualitative detection of CG when its concentration exceeds a detection threshold, frequently 25 IU/L. Cervinski and associates[81] evaluated the analytical lower limit of detection of 12 different brands of qualitative CG tests (6 over-the-counter and 6 point-of-care devices) using urine specimens collected from 10 women in early pregnancy (within 10 days of expected menses). Detection limits varied from 6 to 100 IU/L for POC devices and from 0.5 to 25 IU/L for over-the-counter devices.[81] Considerable variation was noted across devices tested with a single specimen and within a device tested with different specimens; this was attributed to the heterogeneous mixture of CG variants in pregnancy urine. The lower analytical limits of detection of over-the-counter devices was thought to be a function of the specimen volume used to perform those tests, which is approximately five times greater than volumes required for POC CG tests.

Because qualitative CG tests are used for the detection of pregnancy, they are designed to detect dimeric CG using a combination of anti-CGα and anti-CGβ antibodies. However, some devices detect nondimeric CG variants[81,344]—a fact that may be due to incompletely characterized reagent antibodies. Because of its relative abundance in early pregnancy, it has been suggested that qualitative CG tests should be designed to preferentially detect CG-H, a suggestion that was based on data derived from the addition of CG-H to CG-free urine.[68] Given the analytical performance that is currently observed using urine obtained during early pregnancy,[81] such a modification appears to be unnecessary.

First-morning specimens are preferred for qualitative POC urine pregnancy tests because they are concentrated and contain abundant CG. Urine applied to the device is absorbed into a nitrocellulose bed. CG is concentrated into a narrow band as the urine migrates. A dye- or latex bead–labeled anti-CG antibody in the device binds to the migrating CG and passes through a zone having solid-phase capture antibody to CG. The appearance of a colored line indicates a positive test. An area of solid-phase antibody with specificity for the labeled anti-CG antibody is located separate from the test band and controls for the addition of adequate specimen volume. False-positive results may occur because of the presence in serum of interfering substances such as interfering antibodies.[157] The test area of some devices may darken over time even in the absence of CG; therefore delayed interpretation of the test band has been known to produce a false-positive result. False-negative results are more commonly encountered and occur if the CG concentration is below the detection threshold (e.g., a dilute urine), or if it is extremely elevated as a result of the high-dose hook effect. False-negative results have also been caused by elevated concentrations of CGβcf because of its ability to bind one of the two anti-CG reagent antibodies, thus preventing the binding of dimeric CG.[163] Because CGβcf is a predominant CG variant in urine after the fifth week of pregnancy, this CG "variant effect" is an important consideration in healthcare settings where qualitative pregnancy tests are often performed beyond the first few weeks of pregnancy.

Exactly how soon after fertilization and implantation CG becomes detectable in the urine varies considerably between women. Wilcox and colleagues[413] demonstrated that 90% of pregnancies could be detected on the day of the missed menses, and 100% were detected 11 or more days later using a highly sensitive quantitative CG test.

The simplicity and speed with which results are obtained make these tests valuable for pregnancy confirmation, but they may miss the diagnosis of a very early or abnormal pregnancy. Qualitative *serum* assays are available and have better analytical performance.

Quantitative CG Tests

All commonly used quantitative CG tests are high-performance immunometric assays designed to measure CG over a wide range of concentrations. Upper limits of detection vary from 400 to 15,000 IU/L, and so specimen dilution is frequently required to obtain an absolute measurement. The lowest detectable concentration of these assays is from 1 to 2 IU/L.

Measurement of CG is complicated by its molecular heterogeneity, and considerable variation in measured CG concentrations is observed between the different assays. One reason for this variation is the use of different antibody pairs in different CG assays. Antibodies to CG will recognize epitopes on the α subunit, the β subunit, or the αβ heterodimer,[40] and so analytical specificity is dependent on the specific pair of antibodies utilized. Another source of variation is the reference material used to calibrate CG assays. Most CG assays are calibrated against the World Health Organization (WHO) Third (75/537) or Fourth (75/589) International Standard, which contains purified urinary hCG with an activity value of 9300 IU/mg determined by bioassay.[70,363] However, these reference materials also contain substantial amounts of CGn and CGβ; this is problematic in that some CG assays over- or under-recognize these variants or may not detect them at all. As such, CG assays lack harmonization. Exacerbating this problem is the use of secondary CG reference materials that vary greatly in terms of the purity that assay manufacturers provide to the end-user for assay calibration. As a consequence, results from different CG assays are not the same and cannot be directly compared.[164,364,410]

In an effort to address some of these problems, the IFCC established the Working Group for the Standardization of hCG in 1994. This group prepared highly purified standards for 6 CG variants and calibrated them in molar concentration.[49,60] These preparations are designated *reference reagents* (RR) and contain CG (99/688), CGn (99/642), CGα (99/650), CGβn (99/692), CGβcf, and CGα (99/720). The impact of using RR for assay calibration and harmonization is under study.

Because of variation between CG assays, median CG values calculated for maternal serum screening are not transferable and should be considered method specific. CG measurements in early pregnancy generally are expressed as international units per liter (IU/L). A typical CG concentration at 16 weeks is approximately 30,000 IU/L, and many screening laboratories express CG concentrations in international units per milliliter (e.g., 30,000 IU/L is expressed as 30 IU/mL) (see Figure 57-3). A simple alternative is to use kilo-international units per liter, consistent with the international system for SI units, in which concentrations are expressed per liter.

Immunoassays specific for free CGβ are commercially available outside the United States (see las.perkinelmer.com/Catalog/accessed Sept. 23, 2011) and may be preferred for first-trimester screening.[73]

Specimen Collection and Handling

Serum is used for quantitative CG assays and are obtained from fasting or nonfasting women by standard phlebotomy techniques. Blood specimens are collected into suitable tubes without anticoagulants, are allowed to clot at room temperature, and are centrifuged to obtain clear serum. CG is stable in maternal serum and can be shipped at ambient temperature and stored at 4 to 8 °C for 1 week.[216] If testing is to be delayed beyond 1 week, serum should be stored at −20 °C. As with most biological materials, repeated freezing and thawing of the specimen should be avoided. Serum specimens showing gross hemolysis, gross lipemia, or turbidity should be avoided.

Specificity of CG Assays

Modern CG immunoassays should have little or no cross-reactivity with LH. Testing of serum samples with high physiologic LH concentrations has been used to ascertain that this hormone does not significantly influence the CG results. Serum from postmenopausal women is a convenient source of specimens with high LH.

As discussed earlier, considerable variation has been noted between different CG assays regarding their detection of specific CG variants. CG assays are classified on the basis of their analytical specificity into those that (1) detect only dimeric CG, (2) detect CG and CGβ, and (3) detect CG, CGβ, and CGβcf.[364,410]

Clinical Significance

Measurement of CG assists in diagnosing and dating pregnancy, identifying ectopic pregnancies and other abnormalities, managing certain neoplasms, and predicting the risk of Down syndrome and trisomy 18. Each of these clinical uses was discussed earlier in this chapter or in Chapter 24. Typical values during pregnancy are shown in Figure 57-3.

Alpha Fetoprotein

Measurement of AFP in maternal serum and amniotic fluid is used extensively throughout the United States and the United Kingdom for prenatal detection of some serious fetal anomalies. Use of AFP in nonpregnant patients for monitoring certain cancers is described in Chapter 24.

Chemistry

A fetal protein having α-electrophoretic motility was discovered in 1956 by Bergstrand and Czar.[41] Gitlin subsequently named this substance *α-fetoprotein*.[150,218] This glycoprotein has a molecular mass of ≈70,000 Da. The gene, located within q11-22 on chromosome 4, is part of a family of genes that also codes for albumin and vitamin D–binding protein (also called *group-specific component* and *Gc globulin*).[176] The protein is composed of carbohydrate and a single polypeptide chain containing 591 amino acids. The complete amino acid sequence was reported in 1987.[148] The carbohydrate composition varies depending on the organ of synthesis, the length of gestation, and the source of the specimen (fetal serum vs. amniotic fluid).[108] Although determination of the carbohydrate content does not appear to be useful diagnostically in the setting of pregnancy, it may be useful in the diagnosis of hepatocellular carcinoma.[307] Heterogeneity has been demonstrated by electrophoresis and dissimilar binding to various lectins, such as concanavalin A.

Biochemistry

AFP is produced initially by the fetal yolk sac in small quantities, and then by the fetal liver in larger quantities as the yolk sac degenerates. Trace amounts are also produced in the fetal gut and kidneys. Early in embryonic life, this protein has a high concentration in fetal serum, reaching about one tenth the concentration of albumin. Maximal concentration in fetal serum—≈3 million μg/L—is reached at about 9 weeks'

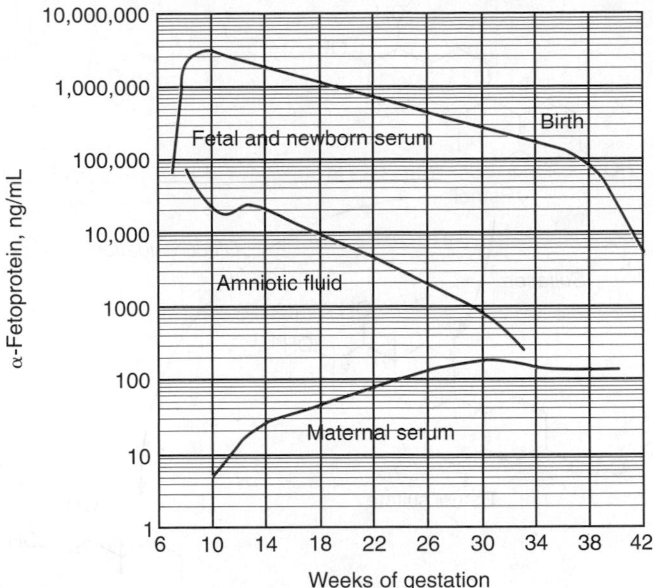

Figure 57-15 Concentrations of alpha fetoprotein (AFP) in fetal and newborn serum, maternal serum, and amniotic fluid. Maternal serum values are medians calculated from 24,232 pregnancies, and amniotic fluid values are medians calculated from 1544 pregnancies from testing performed at ARUP Laboratories Inc. from January to October 1997. Fetal serum values are from Gitlin.[150] Newborn serum values are from Wu et al.[419]

gestation. The concentration then declines steadily to about 20,000 µg/L at term (Figure 57-15).[150] The increase and decrease in concentration of AFP in the amniotic fluid roughly parallel those in the fetal serum, but the concentration is two to three orders of magnitude lower (≈15,000 µg/L at 16 weeks' gestation). The relationship with respect to maternal serum concentration is slightly more complicated because of several factors, including (1) fetal-maternal transfer, (2) rapid growth of the fetus, (3) relatively constant size of the mother, (4) maternal clearance of the protein, and (5) variation of the volume of distribution in the mother with maternal weight. AFP is first detectable (≈5 µg/L) in maternal serum at about the 10th week of gestation. The concentration increases about 15% per week to a peak of approximately 180 µg/L at about 25 weeks. A typical 16 week concentration is approximately 35 µg/L (see Figure 57-8).[169] The concentration in maternal serum then subsequently declines slowly until term. After birth, the maternal serum AFP rapidly decreases to less than 2 µg/L. In an infant, serum AFP declines exponentially to reach adult concentrations by the 10th month of life.[419]

The distribution of serum AFP concentrations in a population of pregnant mothers is Gaussian after logarithmic transformation.[390] Factors that affect the concentration of AFP in maternal serum include (1) gestational age, (2) maternal weight, (3) the presence of insulin-dependent maternal diabetes mellitus, (4) maternal race, (5) the number of fetuses present, (6) fetal renal disorders that cause proteinuria, and (7) fetal structural anomalies.

Amniotic fluid AFP has been measured as early as 8 weeks.[405] It rapidly decreases to its lowest point at 11 weeks, then increases to reach a second maximum at 13 weeks. The concentration then falls in a log-linear fashion until 25 weeks, when the decline steepens. Several studies have shown that AChE used in combination with amniotic fluid AFP can aid in the detection of open neural tube defects from 13 to 25 weeks of pregnancy.[97]

Methods for Determining Alpha Fetoprotein

Although AFP was traditionally measured by radioimmunoassay (RIA), newer methods use immunoenzymometric assay (IEMA) or chemiluminescent immunoassay (CIA) because of their (1) lower detection limits, (2) increased precision, (3) speed, (4) avoidance of radioactivity, and (5) ease of automation.[51] As indicated in a CAP survey, in 2010, most laboratories in the United States measure AFP by using automated systems available from a number of vendors. Judging from the results of proficiency testing offered by the College of American Pathologists (Survey FP), all of these systems perform satisfactorily.[92]

Calibration

Although two essentially equivalent international reference materials [WHO Reference Preparation for AFP (72-225) and British Standard (72-227)]—both calibrated in international units—are available, most laboratories in the United States report AFP in nanograms per milliliter (i.e., micrograms per liter). The relationship between nanograms and international units usually is given as 1.21 ng = 1 IU, but conversion factors may vary by manufacturer, perhaps reflecting differences in the carbohydrate content of respective calibrators.[22]

Specimen Collection and Handling

Serum specimens are obtained from nonfasting women through standard phlebotomy techniques. AFP is very stable in maternal serum and can be shipped at ambient temperature and stored at 4 to 8 °C for 1 week or at −20 °C for years.[216]

Clinical Significance

Maternal serum and amniotic fluid AFP are useful tests for detecting some serious fetal anomalies. Maternal serum AFP is elevated in 85 to 95% of cases of fetal open neural tube defect[390] and is low in about 30% of cases of fetal Down syndrome.[99,247] Because maternal serum screening for fetal defects involves multiple tests, this subject was discussed earlier under "Second-Trimester Maternal Serum Screening Tests." It is noteworthy that AFP is not even required for healthy pregnancy. For example, a mutation of the AFP gene, which resulted in the complete absence of this protein in maternal serum or amniotic fluid, was not associated with fetal malformations or pregnancy complications.[298]

Measuring Amniotic Fluid Alpha Fetoprotein

Amniotic fluid AFP is measured using the same immunoassays as for maternal serum AFP after a suitable dilution (usually 1:50 to 1:200). Results are expressed in nanograms per milliliter, micrograms per liter, or kilo IU per liter, and most laboratories use mass units. AFP in amniotic fluid is less stable than in serum, and leaving samples at room temperature for prolonged periods, such as might occur during processing for chromosome analysis, results in degradation of amniotic fluid AFP. Refrigeration of amniotic fluid will compromise the chromosome analysis. Therefore a portion of the collected fluid should be placed in the refrigerator as soon as possible after collection. Samples sent to reference laboratories should be shipped for next day delivery at ambient temperature or on ice packs if the outside temperature is high. The presence of fetal blood in amniotic fluid samples has been known to increase AFP results, and laboratories should note the presence of blood on the report. In the event of an increased amniotic fluid AFP result (usually >2.0 or 2.5 MoM), the laboratory should test for the presence of fetal blood, or should refer this reflex test to another laboratory. Laboratories that measure amniotic fluid AFP need to establish medians for each week between 13 and 25 weeks' gestation. A method has been published that allows extrapolation to 13 weeks using data from 14 to 25 weeks.[285] Medians from ARUP Laboratories (Salt Lake City, Utah) are shown graphically in Figure 57-15.

Measuring Amniotic Fluid Acetylcholinesterase. AChE is an essential confirmatory test for samples with elevated amniotic fluid AFP. Normal amniotic fluid contains a group of nonspecific cholinesterases referred to as *pseudocholinesterase (PChE).* Cerebrospinal fluid contains high concentrations of the neural enzyme AChE, and in cases of fetal open neural tube defects (and in about 80% of cases with defects of the abdominal wall), fluid leaks from the open lesion, allowing AChE to enter the amniotic fluid.

The usual technique for identification of AChE is fractionation by polyacrylamide gel electrophoresis followed by incubation of the gel with the substrate acetylcholine and copper ions. AChE migrates more rapidly than PChE and appears as a distinct white precipitate band below the PChE band. That the second band is AChE is documented by inhibition of enzyme activity in the band by the specific AChE inhibitor 1,5-bis(4-allyldimethylammoniumphenyl)pentan-3-one dibromide—BW284C51. Because no method is available commercially, laboratories have to develop their own assay systems using published methods.[63,167] Enzyme immunoassay using a monoclonal antibody specific for neurally derived AChE has also been used.[269]

Unconjugated Estriol

Measurement of urinary and serum estriol (E_3), once used to assess fetal well-being, is no longer recommended for that purpose.[101] Measurement of unconjugated estriol (uE_3) is now used routinely by most U.S. laboratories that provide screening for Down syndrome. This steroid, rather than total estriol (unconjugated plus conjugated estriol), is the most specific of the estrogens for identifying a fetus with Down syndrome.

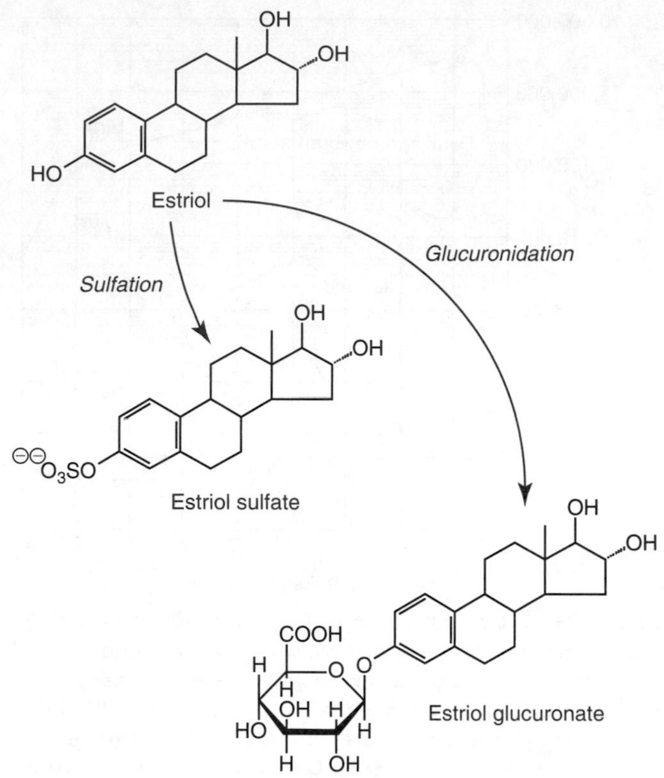

Estriol
Sulfation
Glucuronidation
Estriol sulfate
Estriol glucuronate

Figure 57-16 Forms of estriol present in maternal serum. Glucuronidation and sulfation can also occur at the other hydroxyl positions.

Chemistry

Estriol is an estrogen with hydroxyl groups at positions 3, 16, and 17 (see Chapter 56). Its systematic name is 1,3,5(10)-estriene-3,16-α,17-β-triol. Although present in nonpregnant patients in very low concentrations, during late pregnancy this estrogen predominates. Only a minor amount (≈10%) of the hormone circulates in plasma unconjugated[295] and, because of its low solubility, this form is strongly bound to SHBG. The majority exists as conjugates of glucuronate and sulfate (Figure 57-16). Conjugation occurs in the maternal liver, makes the hormone more soluble, and thus permits renal clearance.

Biochemistry

Estriol is produced in very large amounts during the last trimester of pregnancy. The biosynthetic pathway requires three organs to be fully functioning: fetal adrenal, fetal liver, and placenta (Figure 57-17). The fetal adrenal cortex possesses a unique zone for the production of steroids. The demand for estriol is so great that the fetal adrenal is massive compared with that of an adult. The fetal cortex accounts for approximately 80% of adrenal weight. The fetal adrenal avidly binds low-density lipoprotein to take in cholesterol, which is converted to two major steroid intermediates: pregnenolone sulfate and dehydroepiandrosterone sulfate (DHEA-S). These intermediates are secreted into the fetal circulation. The fetal liver, possessing 16α-hydroxylase, converts DHEA-S

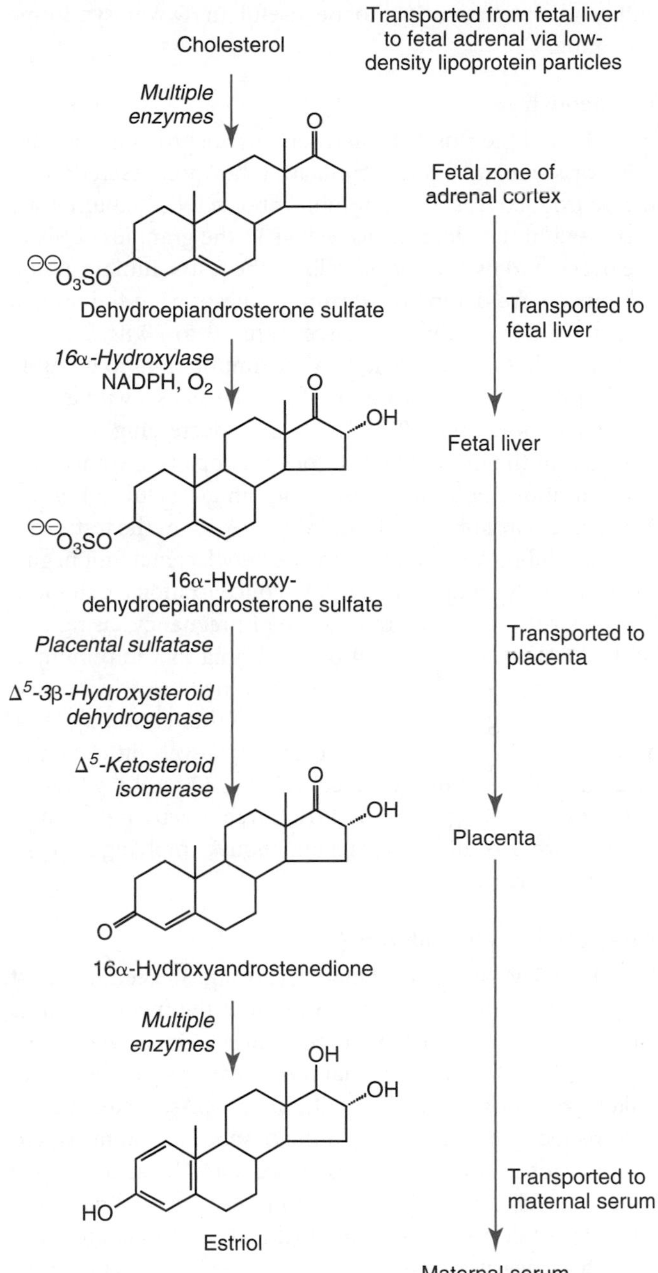

Figure 57-17 Biosynthetic pathway for estriol during pregnancy.

to 16α-hydroxy-DHEA-S, which is secreted back into the fetal circulation. Finally the placenta synthesizes estriol from 16α-hydroxy-DHEA-S. Approximately 90% of maternal serum estriol is derived from this pathway. A minor amount is made using precursors from the maternal ovary. The relationship of maternal serum uE_3 to gestational age in the second trimester is log-linear, increasing at a rate of 20 to 25% per gestational week[169] (Figure 57-18). Concentrations typical for the second trimester of pregnancy are 0.70 to 2.50 μg/L, depending on the assay used. Serum concentrations of estriol conjugates are fivefold to tenfold higher than serum concentrations of uE_3 during pregnancy.

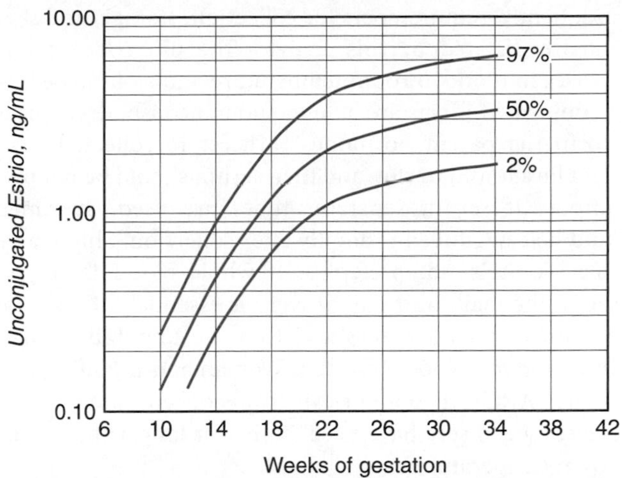

Figure 57-18 Concentration of unconjugated estriol (uE_3) in maternal serum as a function of gestational age. Lines represent the 2nd, 50th, and 97th percentiles. Maternal serum values from 14 to 25 weeks are medians calculated from 11,309 pregnancies from testing performed at ARUP Laboratories Inc. from January to October 1997.

Methods for Determining Unconjugated Estriol

Determination of uE_3 is made difficult by its low concentration. Until 2002, uE_3 was measured by ultrasensitive RIA methods [primarily the assay available from Diagnostic Systems Laboratories (DSL, Webster, Texas, no longer available)] that have been clinically validated extensively by case-control and intervention studies. Subsequently, nonisotopic assays became available, usually as part of automated systems. The correlation between these methods and RIA methods is generally only fair ($r^2 = 0.8$), and most have not been clinically validated. A clinical outcome study using a nonisotopic method yielded screening performance equivalent to a previously validated RIA.[236] In addition, concentrations of estrone, estriol-3-sulfate, and estriol-3-glucuronide up to 1000 ng/mL cross-react less than 0.03% in current assays. Values obtained with various uE_3 assays vary widely as judged using the CAP proficiency testing survey FP.[92] Conversion to MoM reduces between-method differences, but uE_3 is still the most variable of the screening analytes.

Calibration

Assays for uE_3 are calibrated by the use of chemically pure estriol. Estriol values are reported in mass units (nanograms per milliliter or micrograms per liter) or SI units (nanomoles per liter). The equation for converting mass to SI units is 1 nmol/L = 3.47 ng/mL = 3.47 μg/L. Although pure uE_3 is available for calibrating uE_3 assays, commercial kits yield values on clinical specimens that differ by factors of 2 to 3.[92]

Specimen Collection and Handling

Maternal serum specimens are obtained from nonfasting women by standard phlebotomy techniques. Of the four analytes currently used for screening, uE_3 is the least stable, and consequently, requirements for collection, storage, and shipment are dictated by this analyte. The uE_3 concentration increases in blood at room temperature and at 4 °C, because the conjugated forms are able to spontaneously deconjugate to form the parent hormone.[169] Therefore collected blood should be allowed to clot, and then serum should be removed promptly. If serum separator tubes are used, specimens should be centrifuged promptly after collection. Shipment of whole blood is not preferred. If whole blood is shipped through the mail, next day delivery is essential. uE_3 is stable in serum for up to 7 days at 2 to 4 °C (unpublished data, Foundation for Blood Research, Woman and Infant's Hospital, and ARUP Laboratories). The concentration of uE_3 increases when sera have been stored for longer than 4 days at room temperature.

Clinical Significance

Any disruption in the biosynthetic pathway will lead to very low maternal serum uE_3. Conditions that cause disruption include (1) fetal anencephaly, (2) placental sulfatase deficiency, (3) fetal death, (4) chromosome abnormalities, (5) molar pregnancy, and (6) Smith-Lemli-Opitz syndrome.[57,376] Placental sulfatase deficiency presents in the infant as X-linked ichthyosis. It is present in approximately 1 in every 2000 males. Because of the lack of uE_3, the mother often has delayed onset of labor, and the cesarean section rate is significantly higher in these mothers. SLOS is a serious, rare birth defect that is the result of an inborn error in cholesterol metabolism, 7-dehydrosterol-7-reductase deficiency. Down syndrome leads to a modest decrease in uE_3. Screening for Down syndrome is now the most common application of uE_3 measurements.[392]

Inhibin A

Inhibins are members of the transforming growth factor-β (TGFβ) superfamily of proteins. As described in Chapter 56, inhibin is a negative feedback regulator of FSH secretion in both males and females. Inhibin A and B are proven bioactive forms. The placenta produces large quantities of inhibin A that completely suppress FSH.

Chemistry

Inhibins are proteins consisting of dimers of dissimilar subunits (α and β) linked by disulfide bridges. The β subunit occurs in two closely related forms (β_A and β_B), leading to two types of dimeric inhibin (dimeric inhibin A, $\alpha\beta_A$, and dimeric inhibin B, $\alpha\beta_B$). The mature form of inhibin, which has a molecular mass of approximately 30,000 Da, is produced by cleavage of larger precursor forms. In follicular fluid and serum, mature inhibins, precursors of inhibins (particularly the processed form of the free α subunit, pro-αC), and intermediate molecules of varying molecular weight are present.[373] Another group of related molecules, the activins, are dimers consisting of just the β subunits.[291] Inhibin/activin β_C, β_D, and β_E subunits have also been identified, but are less well understood. Inhibin A is the only form within the inbibin/activin family of proteins that provides sufficient discrimination to be useful in Down syndrome screening.[215]

Biochemistry

Inhibins and the closely related activins are proteins that suppress or stimulate follicle-stimulating hormone secretion. In the reproductive system, inhibin and activin subunits are expressed in the placenta, as well as in the granulosa cells of the ovary, and by the Sertoli cells of the testis. Inhibin A and inhibin B have distinctive serum profiles during the human menstrual cycle. Inhibin A rises from 10 to 20 ng/L in the follicular phase of the cycle to a maximum of 40 to 60 ng/L. Inhibin B is maximal in the midfollicular phase, with a peak at ovulation (about 60 ng/L), before decreasing to basal amounts in the luteal phase. In postmenopausal women, the concentrations of both forms of inhibin are below 5 ng/L.[233] Men secrete inhibin B, but not inhibin A, from the testis into serum. Inhibin A is produced by the fetoplacental unit beginning in early pregnancy. InhA concentrations exhibit a complex pattern during the course of pregnancy, rising to a peak at 8 to 10 weeks' gestation, declining to a minimum at 17 weeks of pregnancy, and then resuming to slowly increase at term (see Figure 57-11). Unlike the other screening tests, average inhibin concentrations change relatively little from 15 to 20 weeks' gestation. A typical value at 17 weeks' gestation is 175 ng/L (175 pg /mL). In 2010, inhibin/activin β_C and β_E subunits were localized in placental tissues, implying a potential role in pregnancy.[149,409]

Assay Methods for Inhibin A

Inhibin assays used for Down syndrome screening must measure only dimeric inhibin A and not the free α subunits and the precursors of higher molecular weight, which also circulate in blood. The original inhibin assays were enzyme-linked immunosorbent assay (ELISA) or RIAs, used antibodies directed against epitopes on the α-subunit, and measured all forms of inhibin, including precursors. These assays are referred to as total inhibin or immunoreactive inhibin assays. Highly specific assays using monoclonal antibodies are available that measure only dimeric inhibin A. Specific inhA assays provide better screening performance than the nonspecific total inhibin assays.[215] The widely used inhA method, originally from Diagnostic Systems Laboratories (Webster, Tex, now available from Beckman Coulter, Brea, Calif), has been clinically validated[203] and performs well in the College of American Pathologists Maternal Survey FP.[92] An automated method for inhibin A measurement was released by Beckman Coulter in 2007 and has been shown to have acceptable analytical and clinical performance.[217] Typical values in the second trimester of pregnancy range from 50 to 400 pg/mL (50 to 400 ng/L), as shown in Figure 57-11.

Specimen and Sampling Handling

Serum specimens are obtained from nonfasting women by standard phlebotomy techniques. InhA is stable in maternal serum and has been shipped at ambient temperature and stored at 4 to 8 °C for 1 week.[216]

Clinical Significance

In addition to the usefulness of inhA as a predictor of Down syndrome risk as discussed previously, inhibin A and B measurements have found applications in (1) ovarian cancer monitoring, (2) disorders of ovulation, (3) early detection of viable pregnancy following in vitro fertilization, and (4) evaluation of male infertility.[215,318]

Pregnancy-Associated Plasma Protein-A

Pregnancy-associated plasma protein A is a unique serum marker for Down syndrome pregnancy in that concentrations are low in the first trimester (median = 0.34 MoM) but are unchanged in the second trimester (1.11 MoM).[400] PAPP-A concentrations in the maternal serum of women during the first trimester of pregnancy are associated with fetal and placental health and development.

Chemistry

The human PAPP-A gene is found on chromosome 9 and consists of 22 exons. It is translated into a 1626 amino acid product, of which 1546 amino acids compose the mature protein. Circulating PAPP-A is part of a larger molecular complex that includes two subunits of PAPP-A covalently bound to two subunits of pro major basic protein (pro MBP), forming a heterotetramer (Figure 57-19).[53] The PAPP-A complex has a molecular mass of about 500 kDa.

Biochemistry

PAPP-A is a zinc-containing metalloproteinase glycoprotein. It is expressed at low concentrations in all tissues, but high amounts of PAPP-A protein and mRNA are localized in placental tissues throughout gestation. PAPP-A immunoreactivity is found in syncytiotrophoblast cells,[54] and the eosinophil major basic protein (pro-MBP) subunit is found in cytotrophoblast cells. Maternal serum PAPP-A concentrations increase as gestation proceeds to term. Concentrations of PAPP-A are critical to normal fetal growth because of its role as an insulin-like growth factor binding protein (IGFBP) protease. PAPP-A regulates the action of insulin-like growth factor II (IGF-II) by cleaving its binding protein and thereby increasing bioavailable forms. PAPP-A predominantly cleaves IGFBP-4, a reaction that is dependent on the presence of IGF-II.[53]

Of note, the pro MBP subunits are inactive precursor forms of MBP that are found in eosinophil crystalloid bodies and function in inflammatory responses.

Assay Methods for PAPP-A

PAPP-A was initially measured in pregnancy serum using antibody pairs in an ELISA format,[235] and was later optimized for limit of detection[310] and detection of the PAPP-A–pro MBP complex.[308]

PAPP-A immunoassays are now commercially available in the United States, for research use only, in both manual and automated formats. Outside the United States, other PAPP-A assay methods are available.[225,278,353,414]

Specimen and Sampling Handling

Serum specimens are obtained from nonfasting women by standard phlebotomy techniques. A small increase in PAPP-A concentrations has been reported for collection in plastic versus glass tubes,[349] along with a significant decrease in heparin or EDTA plasma tubes versus serum.[354] PAPP-A was

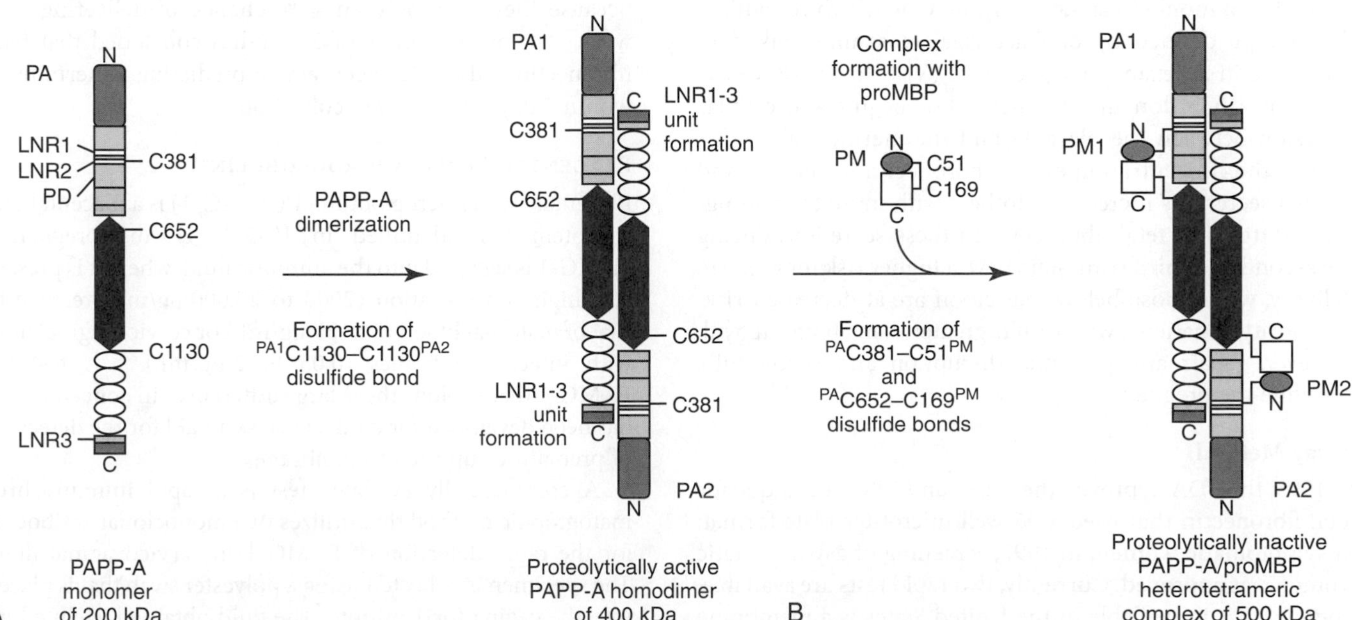

Figure 57-19 PAPP-A monomer, homodimer, and heterotetrameric complex. *[Reprinted from Boldt HB, Conover CA. Pregnancy-associated plasma protein-A (PAPP-A): a local regulator of IGF bioavailability through cleavage of IGFBPs. Growth Horm IGF Res 2007;17:10-8.]*

stable with up to nine freeze-thaw cycles.[43] First-trimester serum PAPP-A concentrations are stable in serum at 4 °C for 1 week or longer, depending on the assay used for testing.[94,216]

Clinical Significance

Low PAPP-A concentrations early in pregnancy have been associated with (1) Down syndrome, (2) a high rate of fetal loss, and (3) other adverse pregnancy outcomes, including (4) poor fetal growth [intrauterine growth retardation (IUGR)], (5) premature delivery, (6) hypertension, and (7) preeclampsia.[121,352] Low PAPP-A concentrations have been reported in the second trimester of pregnancies with Cornelia de Lange syndrome, a serious developmental malformation syndrome of unknown origin.[3]

In addition to placental tissues, PAPP-A has been localized in (1) colon, (2) kidney, (3) endometrium,[277] (4) ovary, (5) fibroblasts, (6) vascular smooth muscle cells, and (7) osteoblasts.[53] Functional roles for PAPP-A in bone formation[311] and wound healing[84] have been described. Furthermore, ultrasensitive cardiac-specific measurements of PAPP-A have utility in the detection of acute coronary syndromes,[309] with higher concentrations indicative of a relatively poor prognosis.[34,198]

Fetal Fibronectin

Determining the risk of preterm labor would help clinicians manage those at high risk more aggressively, thereby lowering the incidence of preterm delivery. In 1991, fetal fibronectin concentration in cervical and vaginal secretions was proposed as a test to aid in predicting preterm delivery.[230]

Fibronectin is a term for a family of ubiquitous adhesive glycoproteins that cross-link to collagen to bind cells together. These proteins are found on cell surfaces and in plasma and amniotic fluid. The fetus has a unique fibronectin that is defined by a monoclonal antibody, FDC-6, which recognizes the epitope defined by α-*N*-acetylgalactosamine linked to threonine in a hexapeptide sequence (Val-Thr-His-Pro-Gly-Tyr), the IIICS domain.[241] When labor begins and cellular adhesion between the placenta and the uterine wall is disrupted, the concentration of fetal fibronectin in cervical and vaginal secretions increases. Mothers with more than 50 ng/mL (50 μg/L) of fetal fibronectin in these secretions during the second and third trimesters have a higher risk for preterm delivery, while those below that cutoff are at decreased risk. A majority of patients with results greater than 50 ng/mL will, however, repair any placental disruption and successfully continue the pregnancy.[153]

Assay Method

In 1995, the FDA approved the use of an ELISA technique for fetal fibronectin that used a 96-well microtiter plate format; in symptomatic women; in 1997, screening of asymptomatic women was approved. Currently, two rapid tests are available. The one that is available in the United States is a membrane immunoassay. The test utilizes a solid-phase polyclonal goat anti-fFN antibody and an enzyme-labeled monoclonal anti-fFN, FDC-6 detection antibody. The specimen is obtained by collecting cervical or vaginal mucus with a Dacron polyester swab. The fully saturated swab contains approximately 150 μL of fluid. The swab is placed into 750 μL of buffer, creating a 1:5 dilution. An aliquot of the specimen is added to the cassette containing the antibodies. Absorbance of the developed color is measured photometrically.

Asymptomatic Patients

In screening asymptomatic women, testing should take place sometime between 22 and 31 weeks' gestation. Women with a positive result (>50 ng/mL) have been shown to have a ninefold higher risk for delivery at or before 34 weeks.[154] A negative test following a positive test lowers the risk, and a second subsequent negative test returns the risk to baseline.[153] A systematic review revealed that among asymptomatic women, positive fFN results have a likelihood ratio of 4.01 (95% confidence interval, 2.93 to 5.49) for predicting birth before 34 weeks' gestation. For negative fFN results, the corresponding likelihood ratio is 0.78 (0.72 to 0.84).[185] The ACOG does not recommend routine screening of low-risk, asymptomatic women.[18]

Symptomatic Patients

In screening symptomatic women, testing should take place sometime between 24 and 35 weeks' gestation. Symptoms of preterm labor include (1) regular uterine contractions, (2) low back pain, (3) lower abdominal cramping, (4) vaginal bleeding, and (5) increased vaginal discharge. A systematic review revealed that among symptomatic women, positive fFN results have a likelihood ratio of 5.42 (95% confidence interval, 4.36 to 6.74) for predicting delivery before 34 weeks' gestation or within the next 7 days. For negative fFN results, the corresponding likelihood ratio is 0.25 (0.20 to 0.31).[185] Those patients with a negative test can safely return home because they have only an ≈1% chance of delivering in 1 week.[293] A meta-analysis of 32 studies concluded that fetal fibronectin had limited accuracy in predicting preterm birth within 7 days of specimen collection.[326]

Placental Alpha Microglobulin-1

Placental alpha microglobulin-1 (PAMG-1) is a placental glycoprotein first identified in 1977.[300] During pregnancy, PAMG-1 is secreted into the amniotic fluid, where it is present at a high concentration (2000 to 25,000 ng/mL) relative to that of maternal blood (5 to 25 ng/mL) or cervicovaginal fluid with intact membranes (0.05 to 2 ng/mL).[220] A test for PAMG-1 that exploits these large differences in concentration has been developed for clinical use as an aid for the detection of premature rupture of membranes.

A commercially available test is a rapid immunochromatographic method that utilizes two monoclonal antibodies for the rapid detection of PAMG-1 in cervicovaginal fluid. The specimen is collected using a polyester swab that is placed into the vagina for 1 minute. The fluid obtained is eluted off the swab by rinsing it in a vial containing a buffer solution for 1 minute. A test strip is then placed into the buffer for 10 minutes. The test result is determined by visual inspection of a test and a control line on the lateral flow device. The analytical limit of detection of the test is 5 ng/mL.

Two studies have reported that this test is more sensitive and specific for the detection of PROM than clinical assessment or the nitrazine or ferning test.[93,220] A study by Cousins et al[93] included 203 women presenting with suspected PROM. The diagnosis of PROM was based on two positive results from a retrospective review of patient medical records and had to include two positive results from visual pooling of amniotic fluid, nitrazine testing, or fern testing. The clinical sensitivity of the test was 99% with a specificity of 100%.

In a prospective study of 184 women with suspected PROM, Lee et al[220] evaluated this test against conventional clinical criteria. Women were diagnosed with PROM if amniotic fluid was observed leaking from the cervix, or if any two of the following were true: (1) pooling of amniotic fluid in the posterior fornix, (2) positive nitrazine test, or (3) detection of microscopic ferning. The definitive diagnosis of PROM was made after delivery and was based on a review of the clinical record. The test was noted to be 99% sensitive and 88% specific compared with 87% and 100%, respectively, for the conventional assessment. Three false-positive results were unexplained, but it was speculated that they may have been caused by small leakages of amniotic fluid that were clinically unapparent. Compared with the nitrazine test alone, this test was significantly more sensitive (99% vs. 88%) with the same specificity (88%).

Contamination with large amounts of blood will cause a false-positive result. False-negative results may occur if the specimen is collected 12 or more hours after a rupture that is subsequently obstructed by the fetus or is resealed.

Amniotic Fluid Bilirubin (ΔA_{450})

The concentration of bilirubin in amniotic fluid is generally too low (≈0.01 to 0.03 mg/dL; 0.17 to 0.51 μmol/L) to be measured by standard photometric techniques. It is possible, however, to rapidly, accurately, and directly measure amniotic bilirubin by absorption spectrophotometry.[224] Maximal absorbance of bilirubin is at 450 nm. In the absence of significant amounts of bilirubin, however, the absorbance spectrum for amniotic fluid between 365 and 550 nm defines a nearly exponential curve (Figure 57-20). On log-linear axes, the height of the curve at 450 nm above the straight line is linearly proportional to the concentration of bilirubin in the amniotic fluid. This is the difference in absorbance at 450 nm (ΔA_{450}), which is still occasionally referred to in the clinical literature as the ΔOD_{450} (change in optical density). Normally a small amount of bilirubin is present in amniotic fluid, and this amount changes with gestational age (Figure 57-21). Therefore, to interpret properly the ΔA_{450}, it is necessary to know the gestational age.

Interpretation

The Liley or the Queenan chart is used for interpretation of ΔA_{450} data and their relationship to the gestational age of the pregnancy for unaffected and affected fetuses. The Liley chart (see Figure 57-21) was created in 1961 from data collected between 27 and 40 weeks' gestation.[224] Because of advances in neonatal care, it became necessary to utilize the Liley chart at gestational ages earlier than 27 weeks, and use of an extrapolated curve became widespread despite the fact that this modified curve was never validated. Consequently, Queenan

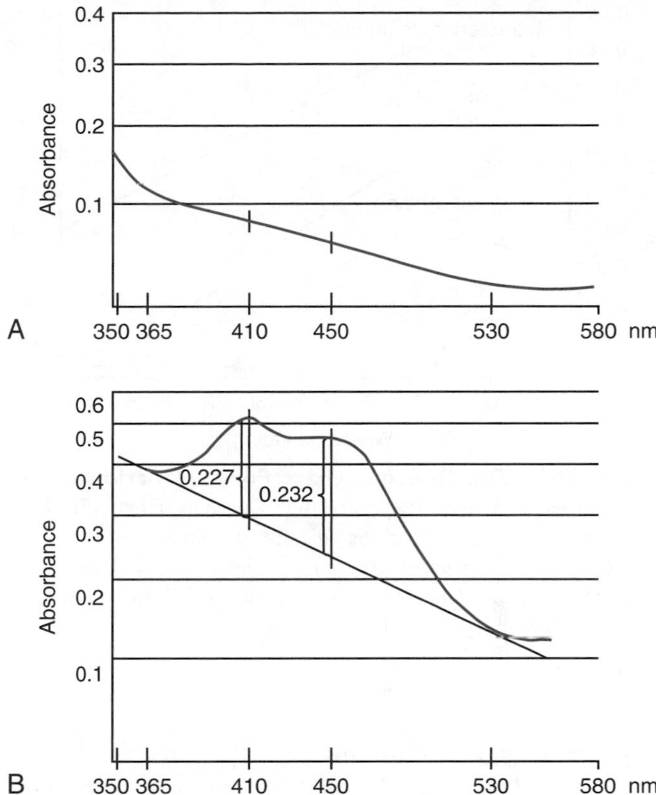

Figure 57-20 A, Normal amniotic fluid. Note near linearity of the curve when plotted on log-linear graph. B, Amniotic fluid showing the bilirubin peak at 450 nm and the oxyhemoglobin peak at approximately 410 nm. Note the baseline drawn between linear parts of the curve, from 530 and 365 nm.

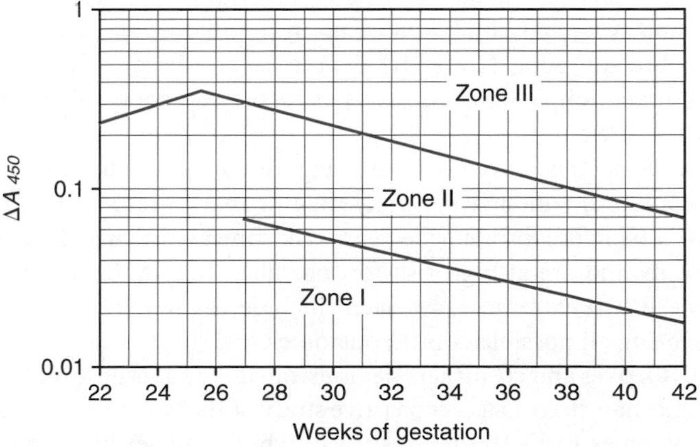

Figure 57-21 Liley's three-zone chart (with modification) for interpretation of amniotic fluid ΔA_{450}. For explanation of the three zones, see text. *(Modified from Liley AW. Liquor amnii analysis in the management of the pregnancy complicated by rhesus sensitization. Am J Obstet Gynecol 1961;82:1359-70.)*

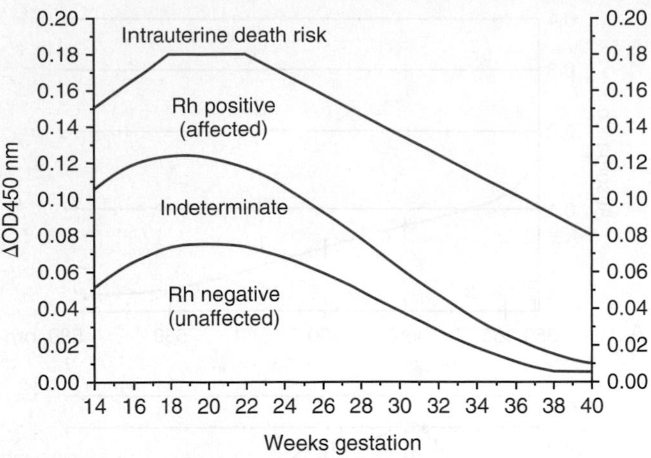

Figure 57-22 The Queenan chart. For explanation of the four zones, see text. *(Reprinted from Queenan JT, Tomai TP, Ural SH, King JC. Deviation in amniotic fluid optical density at a wavelength of 450 nm in Rh-immunized pregnancies from 14 to 40 weeks' gestation: a proposal for clinical management. Am J Obstet Gynecol 1993;168:1370-6.)*

published an alternative to the Liley chart in 1993 that was developed from data obtained between 14 and 40 weeks' gestation.[313]

Values that fall into Liley's bottom zone are considered to represent an unaffected or very mildly affected fetus. Values in the middle zone are still compatible with a minimally affected fetus, but as values rise within this zone, it is increasingly likely that the fetus is suffering moderate to marked hemolysis. Depending on the trend with time and the clinical circumstances, some clinicians recommend intervention when ΔA_{450} has climbed 80% up in the middle zone. Values in the top zone (zone III) denote severe disease. Without intervention, a fetus with values in the top zone will most likely die.[224]

Using the Queenan chart (Figure 57-22), values in the unaffected zone may be unaffected or may have mild HDN. Results in the intrauterine death risk zone tend to have severe HDN and are at high risk for mortality. Results in between these two extreme zones often include many fetuses representing all possible clinical outcomes.

Oepkes and coworkers demonstrated the superiority of the Queenan chart in a comparative study of the two charts using outcomes from 165 fetuses, 74 of which had severe anemia defined as a hemoglobin more than 5 standard deviations below the mean.[274] The Queenan and Liley charts were 81% and 76% clinically sensitive, respectively, for detecting severe anemia, with specificities of 81% and 77%, respectively. The Queenan chart is now considered the preferred chart for interpreting the ΔA_{450} result.

Contamination of an amniotic fluid specimen with fetal blood from an affected fetus with a high serum bilirubin concentration could introduce a substantial error, the magnitude of which cannot accurately be predicted. Blood contamination of amniotic fluid should be obvious from the red color and the presence of erythrocytes in the pellet after centrifugation. It is important to minimize hemolysis of the erythrocytes in such samples (by rapid processing) because the hemoglobin will interfere with the test. If the amniotic fluid remaining within the amniotic cavity has been contaminated with blood by traumatic amniocentesis, these erythrocytes lyse and contaminate the fluid with hemoglobin and bilirubinoid pigments. It takes 2 to 3 weeks for these pigments to be cleared, and for the fluid to return to the original state. Both mathematical corrections and chloroform extraction have been used for bloody specimens.[135]

Meconium staining of amniotic fluid increases the ΔA_{450} with a broad and variable peak at 400 to 415 nm[223] and it is not possible to compensate quantitatively for meconium contamination. Clearance of meconium from a single episode of passage into the amniotic fluid requires about 3 weeks.

In a pregnancy with twins within separate sacs, the individual sacs must be sampled. Inadvertent sampling of maternal urine is always a possibility,[223] although the risk of this error is reduced when ultrasonography is used.

Tests for Evaluating Fetal Lung Maturity

Fetal lung maturity (FLM) tests help a clinician decide whether the best perinatal survival will be achieved in utero or in the nursery. The most common situation in which a fetal lung maturity test is ordered is before repeat cesarean delivery when the age of gestation is uncertain. Another major indication is anticipated early delivery because of some medical or obstetrical indication, such as (1) preterm labor, (2) premature rupture of the membranes, (3) worsening maternal hypertension, (4) severe renal disease, (5) intrauterine growth retardation, or (6) fetal distress. Results indicating immaturity of the fetal lungs might cause postponement of elective delivery or prompt active interventions to suppress preterm labor. Pharmacologic administration of corticosteroids is recommended for women between 24 and 34 weeks' gestation who are likely to deliver in the next week.[6] This therapy is thought to accelerate pulmonary maturation and prevent respiratory distress syndrome. If delivery of an infant is inevitable, transfer to a tertiary healthcare center is appropriate.

Numerous tests of amniotic fluid for FLM have been developed. Tests that measure lamellar bodies directly, the surfactant they contain, or the biophysical property of surfactant are the most useful for evaluating FLM. Methods still in clinical use today include (1) fluorescence polarization, (2) lamellar body count (LBC), (3) detection of the phosphatidylglycerol lecithin/sphingomyelin (L/S) ratio, and (4) foam stability.

In a survey of laboratories that offered FLM testing, a commercial fluorescence polarization test was the most widely offered FLM test.[161] This was followed by rapid detection of phophatidylglycerol (21% of laboratories), L/S ratio (18% of laboratories), and LBC (13% of laboratories), and the detection of phosphatidylglycerol by thin-layer chromatography (TLC) (7% of laboratories) and the foam stability test (1% of laboratories).

The number of FLM tests performed each year in the United States is declining. Surveys of obstetricians suggest that the primary reason for the decline in utilization is that physicians feel the tests are not medically necessary for patient care.[161,244] The impact that removal of the TDx FLM II test will have on the utilization of FLM tests is uncertain. Faced with its loss, physicians have indicated that they would order the L/S ratio or the lamellar body count (LBC); however, few laboratories are currently offering either test.[161] The LBC is a logical replacement for the TDx FLM II test.

Standards of laboratory practice for FLM testing were published in 1997[25] and 2006[340] that made several recommendations regarding specimen collection, handling, centrifugation, and mixing that remain valid today. Hospital laboratories should offer a rapid test in their laboratory or from a reference laboratory, such as fluorescence polarization, phosphatidylglycerol, or LBC. These should be available daily on both a routine and emergency basis. Requests for L/S ratios may be sent to a reference laboratory. Analysts should communicate the results of any FLM test immediately to the ordering location, because the patient's status may be changing and the information might assist with management of labor.

In 2008, the ACOG issued a revised practice bulletin on fetal lung maturity.[16] This bulletin encourages the assessment of FLM prior to a scheduled delivery at less than 39 weeks' gestation, unless it could be inferred from clinical history. It also acknowledges the high negative (mature) predictive value of all FLM tests and encourages test selection based on sample quality. Readers may want to carefully read that bulletin, because many obstetricians rely on it.

Collection and Handling of Amniotic Fluid for Fetal Lung Maturity Assessment

Before the details of individual methods are given, details of the specimen and specimen handling are described. These topics are common to many methods.

Specimen Collection and Processing

Amniotic fluid is obtained by transabdominal amniocentesis, usually during real-time sonographic visualization (see Chapter 7). In a multifetal pregnancy, there are usually separate sacs, each of which should be sampled. Vaginal pool specimens are rarely adequate for testing. Clinicians should seriously consider amniocentesis in patients with ruptured membranes.[25]

Whenever possible, the fluid should be tested immediately. If there is to be a delay of a few hours, the fluid should be refrigerated at 4 °C.[331] The total phospholipid content of amniotic fluid does not change significantly during at least a week of storage,[385] and lamellar bodies are stable for at least 30 days.[231] If testing will be delayed longer than 1 week (e.g., fluids kept for research studies), fluids should be stored frozen at −20 or −70 °C. It should be noted that a single freeze-thaw cycle will decrease the LBC.[231] Immediately before the fluid is tested, it should be gently inverted 20 times to obtain a uniform suspension. At least 2 minutes on a test tube rocker is recommended.[25]

Procedures for measuring fetal lung maturity include a centrifugation step to remove debris. Careful attention to technique is needed to obtain reproducible results. Any centrifugation removes some pulmonary surfactant from the specimen. Accidentally prolonged centrifugation has been found to reduce recovery of the phospholipids to less than 50%.[275] For best results, the specimen should be well mixed, lightly centrifuged, decanted, and mixed again.

Fluorescence Polarization Fetal Lung Maturity Tests[30,134,370]

Fluorescence polarization is a dimensionless ratio with values from 0.000 to 0.500 for dilute solutions containing fluorescing compounds (see Chapter 10).[211] Polarization (P) measures the rotational diffusion of the fluorophore relative to its fluorescent half-life. If the half-life is short compared with the rate of rotational diffusion, P will be high. In contrast, if molecular rotation is faster than the excited state decay, then P will be low.

The test was originally described in 1976 by Shinitzky and colleagues, who used diphenylhexatriene (DPH) as the fluorescent dye and proposed that for amniotic fluid, lower polarization values reflected a decrease in the microviscosity of surfactant phospholipids.[341] The fluidity of these phospholipids paralleled the change in lipid composition with maturation of the fetal lungs.[341] Several disadvantages prevented widespread use of DPH fluorescence polarization in clinical laboratories. Tait and associates[370] improved the technique by using a more stable fluorescent dye, NBD-PC, and a commercial polarimeter. NBD-PC binds to albumin and to surfactant; thus the resulting polarization is a function of the surfactant/albumin ratio.[26] Russell[321] developed a commercial version of the assay using a slightly different dye, PC-16.[302]

TDx FLM II Method

The commercial fluorescence polarization test, TDx FLM II (Abbott Laboratories), is to be retired by the manufacturer at the end of 2011. It has an analytical measurement range of 0 to 160 mg surfactant/g albumin. Uncentrifuged amniotic fluid is used for this method. If specimens have been accidentally centrifuged, the surfactant should be resuspended before testing.[160] The TDx FLM II assay uses 25 μL of filtered amniotic fluid. Imprecision (CV) is 4 to 5% at 20 and 115 mg/g.

A first-generation instrument that was commercially available[184,322,360,416] recommended a maturity cutoff of 70 mg phospholipid/g of albumin or greater, a second-generation instrument with values less than or equal to 39 mg/g are considered immature, those greater than or equal to 55 mg/g mature, and others (40 to 54 mg/g) intermediate. Several clinical outcome studies of the first-generation test suggested that the upper cutoff could be lowered without impacting the sensitivity for RDS.[23,180,360] Similar studies of second generation machine showed that ≈45 mg/g could be used as a cut point, which will improve assay specificity to 85%, while maintaining sensitivity for clinically significant respiratory distress syndrome at 95 to 100%.[127,200]

Several investigators have recommended that FLM should be interpreted as a function of gestational age.[195,292,303] Instead of changing the decision limits for each gestational age, the authors recommend reporting the RDS risk for a given FLM result at a specific gestational age. Calculated absolute risks, however, will vary with the prevalence of RDS in the tested population.[165] This restricts their usefulness to populations that have an RDS prevalence similar to that from which the risks were derived. One study reported odds ratios that were independent of RDS prevalence at each gestational age and therefore are more broadly applicable.[292]

Most twins are delivered preterm, and many suffer from preterm complications. If those complications are excluded, twins have the same RDS incidence as singletons matched for gestational age.[139] After 31 weeks' gestation, however, average FLM results from twin pregnancies are 22 mg/g higher than those from singleton pregnancies.[243] Sampling both sacs is recommended when testing before 32 weeks' gestation.[411]

Several studies have concluded that diabetes does not affect the reference values of FLM.[112,227]

NBD-PC Fluorescence Polarization Method

The NBD-PC method is also called FPol. The specimen is amniotic fluid that has been centrifuged at 400 ×g for 2 minutes. Results are expressed using artificial units of millipolarization (P × 1000, mP). The analytical measurement range is 150 to 350 mP. No calibrators are used, but use of a Triton ×100 control ensures that the temperature is correct, and that the dye is not degraded. Comparison of the NBD-PC assay with a similar assay reveals, a strong nonlinear, inverse correlation.[24,28]

An NBD-PC fluorescence polarization value of less than 260 mP is considered mature, values between 260 and 290 mP are considered transitional, and values greater than 290 mP are considered immature.[85,369] Using 260 mP as the cutoff, this test has a clinical sensitivity of 94% and a clinical specificity of 84%. Supplemental use of the L/S ratio for those patients with transitional results is of little benefit. The 260 mP cutoff is appropriate for high-risk pregnancies. In the setting of a patient who needs a cesarean section at term, when there is no penalty for delaying delivery, a cutoff of 230 mP is more appropriate.

If there is less than 0.5% blood in the amniotic fluid, the results are not affected. Contamination with more than this amount tends to increase low results and decrease high results.[370] Results that are clearly mature (<230 mP) or immature (>290 mP) are reliable for predicting fetal lung status. Results between these values cannot be interpreted.

Because of improved pregnancy management, very few infants with RDS are born to women with diabetes. Thus exact estimates of clinical sensitivity and specificity are not available in this clinical setting. The predictive value of mature status in a patient with diabetes mellitus appears to be equivalent to that in a patient without diabetes.[85,112,227]

Lamellar Body Counts

Lamellar bodies have been counted directly using the platelet channel of most whole blood cell counters.[119] This technique is termed the lamellar body count (LBC).[29] None of the manufacturers of whole blood cell counters have claims to support the use of their instruments for the LBC, and so the test is considered a laboratory-developed test (LDT).

Lamellar bodies have a broad size distribution, ranging from 0.2 to 10 fL.[29] Whole blood cell counters used during development of the LBC method used a size gate from 2 to 20 fL. Therefore only a portion of lamellar bodies are counted in these instruments. Because the LBC is a direct reflection of surfactant concentration in amniotic fluid, fetal urination lowers the LBC.

Centrifugation of amniotic fluid should be omitted.[25,118,259] Mixing of the fluid is critical—2 minutes is recommended on a tube rocker or at least 20 inversions immediately before analysis.[259] Typical LBC results vary from 0 to 150,000/μL.

Because of different platelet identification algorithms, counts will be lower or higher on different instruments. Instruments that use similar algorithms (e.g., impedance) will show greater concordance than those that use different algorithms.[158,231,365]

Specimens containing mucus produce erratic results.[259] Contamination of the fluid with whole blood will decrease the LBC by presumably trapping them in a fibrin matrix, which occurs when the number of red blood cells exceeds 31,000/μL.[231] Even small amounts of meconium have been observed to produce dramatic increases in the LBC.[231]

Interpretation

Most outcome studies that have evaluated the LBC as a test of fetal lung maturity have utilized Beckman Coulter brand cell counters. Results of these studies support the consensus maturity cutoff of 50,000/μL.[259] However, given the variation in LBC results between cell counters, this cutoff should not be adopted by a laboratory without validation, because studies using different brands of cell counters have suggested different cutoffs for maturity.[82,188]

All clinical outcomes studies* have reported that LBC has high clinical sensitivity (95 to 100%) but low clinical specificity (about 70%) for prediction of RDS. A meta-analysis[412] reported that at a fixed clinical sensitivity of 95%, the LBC specificity was 80%, whereas the L/S ratio specificity was 70%.

Studies of the diagnostic accuracy of LBC assays for diabetic mothers have not been conducted. An assay comparison study of LBC, L/S ratio, and PG, however, reported good agreement among the tests for 90 diabetic subjects with no cases of RDS.[114] Similarly, in a study of 187 women, 22% of whom had inadequate glycemic control (defined as arithmetic glucose mean greater than 120 mg/dL from all

*References 27, 35, 55, 107, 115, 119, 125, 158, 178, 188, 196, 219, 260, and 294.

glucose tests performed during the third trimester), no significant differences in the LBC were observed between those with adequate and inadequate glucose control.[111]

Determination of Lecithin/Sphingomyelin Ratio and Saturated Phosphatidylcholine[357,377]

The major surface active component of the lung surfactant is palmitate disaturated-phosphatidylcholine (DSPC), which represents 85% of total lecithins. Its concentration in amniotic fluid tends to rise with increasing gestational age. Most of the DSPC in amniotic fluid comes from the fetal lungs via tracheal effluent. The concentration of DSPC in amniotic fluid is measured directly and is correlated with FLM, or its concentration is related to another lipid, sphingomyelin, and that ratio used to predict lung maturity. Although sphingomyelin is a minor component of pulmonary surfactant, it is ubiquitously distributed in cell membranes, especially those of erythrocytes, and is also found in plasma. Nearly all of the sphingomyelin in amniotic fluid is derived from nonlung sources; thus it has no role in the surfactant system in the lungs. The concentration of lecithin relative to sphingomyelin, the L/S ratio, tends to rise with increasing gestational age. This is not a uniform gradual increase; a rather sudden increase occurs at 34 to 36 weeks' gestation and correlates with the development of fetal lung maturity.[152]

Most laboratories use a commercially available method for L/S determination. However, because many techniques are available, laboratories should be very careful when establishing medical decision limits.[65,357,377] Some methods measure all phosphatidylcholine species, both saturated and unsaturated. Different staining methods will differentially stain phosphatidylcholine compared with the biological internal standard, sphingomyelin. The L/S ratio is a labor intensive test that has poor within- and between-laboratory precision, which may be why only 13% of laboratories perform it.[161]

Interpretation

The original maturity decision limit for the L/S ratio was 2.0 or greater.[380,381] Most laboratories use a method that omits the acetone precipitation step, which will produce slightly higher values. A conservative reference interval for lung maturity is an L/S ratio of 2.5 or greater. About 1% of babies delivered within 24 hours of obtaining an L/S ratio greater than 2.5 are expected to develop RDS; thus 99% of babies predicted to be mature are and will not develop RDS. Almost half of infants with L/S ratios between 1.5 and 2.5, however, will not develop RDS. Thus in contrast to the high degree of reliability of a prediction of maturity, only one third of babies predicted to be immature will in fact develop RDS.

Before the use of tight glycemic control during pregnancy, babies of diabetic mothers more frequently developed RDS.[319] A number of investigators have reported that infants of diabetic mothers more frequently develop RDS despite mature L/S ratios,[98] but other studies have reported no delay in lung maturity for infants of diabetic mothers.[141,367] In poorly controlled diabetic cases, both maturation delay[304] and lack of delay[252] have been reported. Although no RDS outcome studies exist, other studies of well-controlled diabetic mothers report no effect on the relationship between L/S ratio and gestational age.[42,252] For this reason, separate reference intervals are not recommended for well-controlled diabetic pregnancies.[25,340]

For multifetus pregnancies, separate specimens should be analyzed for each fetus. Infrequently, more than one fetus shares an amniotic fluid cavity. In this situation, a mature result is less predictive of maturity, because it represents a mixture of pulmonary surfactant from multiple fetuses. In the case of twins, the smaller one is more likely to develop RDS than the larger one.[254]

Serum has a large concentration of lecithin and sphingomyelin. The serum ratio varies between 1.5 and 2.0, depending on the individual. Values of blood-contaminated specimens therefore tend to be drawn into that range from higher or lower values. A high L/S ratio in the presence of even substantial blood contamination can safely be interpreted as reflecting mature lungs.[147] Similarly, contaminated samples with very low ratios clearly reflect immature lungs. Borderline values of bloody specimens should not be interpreted, because they may represent very immature values falsely elevated or mature values falsely depressed. Various effects of meconium contamination have been reported, including some evidence that the L/S ratio may be changed in the absence of contamination that is visible to the eye.[386] The chromatograms of fluids heavily contaminated with meconium are not interpretable.

Vaginal contamination of specimens obtained from a pool of fluid that has been present in the vagina for a relatively brief period does not affect either test.[116,301]

Phosphatidylglycerol

The detection of phosphatidylglycerol is a commonly used qualitative method used to assess FLM. Measurement of PG was classically performed in conjunction with the L/S ratio, and the combination of the two tests is known as the *lung profile*.[210] The rapid detection of phosphatidylglycerol is accomplished using a commercially available immunochemical test.

The concentration of PG in amniotic fluid increases with gestational age. Most TLC techniques are positive when PG exceeds about 2 μmol/L. At this cutoff, results indicating maturity are almost always correct, but results indicating immaturity are frequently incorrect.

AmnioStat-FLM

Most laboratories that offer PG testing use a qualitative rapid agglutination test (AmnioStat-FLM-PG, Irvine Scientific, Santa Ana, Calif). This test utilizes polyclonal anti-PG antibodies to agglutinate microscopic PG-containing lamellar bodies into macroscopic clusters. The test is simple to perform and is accomplished by mixing equal volumes of amniotic fluid and a lecithin/cholesterol reagent with a buffer solution. An aliquot of this mixture is combined with anti-PG antibody reagent on a laminated card, and is mixed and rotated on a serologic rotator at 60 revolutions per minute (rpm) for 10 minutes. Agglutination is determined by visible inspection and indicates the presence of PG. Results for this test are reported as negative (immature) or positive (mature). Note that this nomenclature is opposite that used for other FLM tests, with positive meaning immature. RDS rarely develops in an infant when a positive PG result is obtained.

Interpretation

Several clinical outcome studies using AmnioStat have been reported.[128,136,144,175,228,408] Although positive PG results are about 99% predictive of maturity, negative results are highly unpredictive (RDS develops in about 25% of cases with a negative PG, depending on the population) and therefore are not useful clinically. A positive PG result is very useful in low-risk pregnancies that require cesarean section. Determination of PG is also useful for specimens contaminated with blood or meconium. PG is not found in blood nor meconium; therefore results are not affected by the presence of either of these contaminants.[38,128]

Many clinicians rely on PG whenever they need to assess FLM in a diabetic patient.[118] However, no modern studies support this practice. In normal pregnancy, PG is detected by TLC or AmnioStat-FLM-PG at approximately 35 weeks' gestation. In diabetic patients, regardless of glycemic control, PG is detected about 1.5 weeks later.[103,252,381] Many diabetic patients will deliver term infants unaffected by RDS before any PG is detected.[304] The diabetic status of the patient does not affect the method of detection.[324]

Determination of the Lung Profile[209,210]

This method for assessing FLM was invented by Marie Kulovich and Louis Gluck in the early 1970s. Although it is still offered by some reference laboratories, most hospital laboratories have converted to newer techniques. The pattern of L/S ratio, PI, and PG are used to determine the status of fetal pulmonary maturation.

Foam Stability Index[337]

When pulmonary surfactant is present in amniotic fluid in sufficient concentrations, the fluid is able to form a highly stable surface film that supports bubbles. Other substances in the fluid, including proteins, bile salts, and salts of free fatty acids, are also capable of forming stable bubbles, but they can be removed from the film by ethanol, which competes with the other substrates for a position in the surface film.[87] The test makes use of the principle that more surfactant activity is necessary to support a stable foam as the fraction of ethanol in the mixture is increased.[336-339] Therefore a fixed volume of undiluted amniotic fluid is mixed with increasing volumes of ethanol, and the largest fraction of ethanol in which the amniotic fluid is still capable of supporting a foam is determined. The highest fraction of ethanol at which a positive reading is obtained is the foam stability index (FSI). In practice, however, the FSI is not recommended because of several disadvantages. Evaluation of the meniscus for a stable ring of bubbles is a subjective test, and amniotic fluid samples contaminated with blood or meconium have been observed to produce false-mature results. Additionally, the use of hygroscopic ethanol presents a challenge, as it readily absorbs water from the atmosphere and decreases the relative percentage of ethanol in the reagent. This presents a considerable challenge to laboratories that wish to continue to offer this LDT.

Interpretation

An FSI value of 0.47 or greater is interpreted as mature. Several studies have demonstrated that the risk of RDS increases with decreasing FSI.[336-338] Similar to other tests of lung maturity, the FSI has excellent clinical sensitivity but frequently produces false-immature results from infants who do not develop RDS.

Tubes and stoppers must be clean and free of detergents to prevent false-positive readings. The final concentration of ethanol is critical. Ethanol is hygroscopic; therefore careful attention must be paid to its preparation and storage. Specimens contaminated with blood or meconium tend to give a falsely mature result.

REFERENCES

1. Abuelo DN, Tint GS, Kelley R, Batta AK, Shefer S, Salen G. Prenatal detection of the cholesterol biosynthetic defect in the Smith-Lemli-Opitz syndrome by the analysis of amniotic fluid sterols. Am J Med Genet 1995;56:281-5.
2. Adams MJ Jr, Windham GC, James LM, Greenberg F, Clayton-Hopkins JA, Reimer CB, et al. Clinical interpretation of maternal serum alpha-fetoprotein concentrations. Am J Obstet Gynecol 1984;148:241-54.
3. Aitken DA, Ireland M, Berry E, Crossley JA, Macri JN, Burn J, et al. Second-trimester pregnancy associated plasma protein-A levels are reduced in Cornelia de Lange syndrome pregnancies. Prenat Diagn 1999;19:706-10.
4. Allan WC, Haddow JE, Palomaki GE, Williams JR, Mitchell ML, Hermos RJ, et al. Maternal thyroid deficiency and pregnancy complications: implications for population screening. J Med Screen 2000;7:127-30.
5. American Academy of Pediatrics Committee on Genetics. Maternal serum alpha-fetoprotein screening. Pediatrics 1991;88:1282-3.
6. American College of Obstetricians and Gynecologists. ACOG Committee Opinion No. 402. Antenatal corticosteroid therapy for fetal maturation. Obstet Gynecol 2008;111:805-7.
7. American College of Obstetricians and Gynecologists. ACOG Committee Opinion No. 418. Prenatal and perinatal human immunodeficiency virus testing: expanded recommendations. Obstet Gynecol 2008;112:739-42.
8. American College of Obstetricians and Gynecologists. ACOG Committee Opinion No. 313, September 2005. The importance of preconception care in the continuum of women's health care. Obstet Gynecol 2005;106:665-6.
9. American College of Obstetricians and Gynecologists. ACOG Committee Opinion No. 172, May 1996 (replaces No. 115, September 1992). Committee on Obstetric Practice. Home uterine activity monitoring. Int J Gynaecol Obstet 1996;54:71-7.

10. American College of Obstetricians and Gynecologists. ACOG Educational Bulletin No. 228, September 1996 (replaces No. 154, April 1991). Committee on Educational Bulletins of the American College of Obstetricians and Gynecologists. Maternal serum screening. Int J Gynaecol Obstet 1996;55:299-308.
11. American College of Obstetricians and Gynecologists. ACOG Practice Bulletin No. 75. Management of alloimmunization. Obstet Gynecol 2006;108:457-64.
12. American College of Obstetricians and Gynecologists. ACOG Practice Bulletin No. 77. Screening for fetal chromosomal abnormalities. Obstet Gynecol 2007;109:217-27.
13. American College of Obstetricians and Gynecologists. ACOG Practice Bulletin No. 78. Hemoglobinopathies in pregnancy. Obstet Gynecol 2007;109:229-37.
14. American College of Obstetricians and Gynecologists. ACOG Practice Bulletin No. 86. Viral hepatitis in pregnancy. Obstet Gynecol 2007; 110:941-56.
15. American College of Obstetricians and Gynecologists. ACOG Practice Bulletin No. 94. Medical management of ectopic pregnancy. Obstet Gynecol 2008;111:1479-85.
16. American College of Obstetricians and Gynecologists. ACOG Practice Bulletin No. 97. Fetal lung maturity. Obstet Gynecol 2008;112:717-26.
17. American College of Obstetricians and Gynecologists. ACOG Practice Bulletin No. 9, October 1999 (replaces Technical Bulletin No. 188, January 1994). Antepartum fetal surveillance: clinical management guidelines for obstetrician-gynecologists. Int J Gynaecol Obstet 2000;68:175-85.
18. American College of Obstetricians and Gynecologists. ACOG Practice Bulletin. Assessment of risk factors for preterm birth. Obstet Gynecol 2001;98:709-16.
19. American College of Obstetricians and Gynecologists. ACOG Practice Bulletin No. 37, August 2002 (replaces Practice Bulletin No. 32, November 2001). Thyroid disease in pregnancy: clinical management guidelines for obstetrician-gynecologists. Obstet Gynecol 2002;100: 387-96.
20. American Society of Human Genetics. American Society of Human Genetics policy statement for maternal serum alpha-fetoprotein screening programs and quality control for laboratories performing maternal serum and amniotic fluid alpha-fetoprotein assays. Am J Hum Genet 1987;40:75-82.
21. Ander DS, Ward KR. Medical management of ectopic pregnancy—the role of methotrexate. J Emerg Med 1997;15:177-82.
22. Anonymous. Equivalence between international units and mass units of alpha-foetoprotein: report of a collaborative study. Clin Chim Acta 1979;96:59-65.
23. Apple FS, Bilodeau L, Preese LM, Benson P. Clinical implementation of a rapid, automated assay for assessing fetal lung maturity. J Reprod Med 1994;39:883-7.
24. Ashwood ER. Markers of fetal lung maturity. In: Gronowski AM, ed. Handbook of clinical laboratory testing during pregnancy. Totowa, NJ: Humana Press, 2004:55-70.
25. Ashwood ER. Standards of laboratory practice: evaluation of fetal lung maturity. National Academy of Clinical Biochemistry. Clin Chem 1997;43:211-4.
26. Ashwood ER, Chamberlain BV. Binding of fluorescent phosphatidylcholine in amniotic fluid. Obstet Gynecol 1988;71:370-4.
27. Ashwood ER, Oldroyd RG, Palmer SE. Measuring the number of lamellar body particles in amniotic fluid. Obstet Gynecol 1990;75: 289-92.
28. Ashwood ER, Palmer SE, Lenke RR. Rapid fetal lung maturity testing: commercial versus NBD-phosphatidylcholine assay. Obstet Gynecol 1992;80:1048-53.
29. Ashwood ER, Palmer SE, Taylor JS, Pingree SS. Lamellar body counts for rapid fetal lung maturity testing. Obstet Gynecol 1993;81:619-24.
30. Ashwood ER, Tait JF, Foerder CA, Franklin RW, Benedetti TJ. Improved fluorescence polarization assay for use in evaluating fetal lung maturity. III. Retrospective clinical evaluation and comparison with the lecithin/sphingomyelin ratio. Clin Chem 1986;32:260-4.
31. Avent ND. Molecular biology of the Rh blood group system. J Pediatr Hematol Oncol 2001;23:394-402.
32. Bahado-Singh RO, Choi SJ, Oz U, Mendilcioglu I, Rowther M, Persutte W. Early second-trimester individualized estimation of trisomy 18 risk by ultrasound. Obstet Gynecol 2003;101:463-8.
33. Barnhart K, Sammel MD, Chung K, Zhou L, Hummel AC, Guo W. Decline of serum human chorionic gonadotropin and spontaneous complete abortion: defining the normal curve. Obstet Gynecol 2004; 104:975-81.
34. Bayes-Genis A, Conover CA, Overgaard MT, Bailey KR, Christiansen M, Holmes DR Jr, et al. Pregnancy-associated plasma protein A as a marker of acute coronary syndromes. N Engl J Med 2001;345:1022-9.
35. Beinlich A, Fischass C, Kaufmann M, Schlosser R, Dericks-Tan JS. Lamellar body counts in amniotic fluid for prediction of fetal lung maturity. Arch Gynecol Obstet 1999;262:173-80.
36. Benn PA, Fang M, Egan JF, Horne D, Collins R. Incorporation of inhibin-A in second-trimester screening for Down syndrome. Obstet Gynecol 2003;101:451-4.
37. Benn PA, Leo MV, Rodis JF, Beazoglou T, Collins R, Horne D. Maternal serum screening for fetal trisomy 18: a comparison of fixed cutoff and patient-specific risk protocols. Obstet Gynecol 1999;93: 707-11.
38. Benoit J, Merrill S, Rundell C, Meeker CI. Amniostat-FLM: an initial clinical trial with both vaginal pool and amniocentesis samples. Am J Obstet Gynecol 1986;154:65-8.
39. Benzie RJ, Doran TA, Harkins JL, Owen VM, Porter CJ. Composition of the amniotic fluid and maternal serum in pregnancy. Am J Obstet Gynecol 1974;119:798-810.
40. Berger P, Sturgeon C, Bidart J-M, Paus E, Gerth R, Niang M, et al. The ISOBM TD-7 Workshop on hCG and related molecules. Towards user-oriented standardization of pregnancy and tumor diagnosis: assignment of epitopes to the three-dimensional structure of diagnostically and commercially relevant monoclonal antibodies directed against human chorionic gonadotropin and derivatives. Tumour Biol 2002;23:1-38.
41. Bergstrand CG, Czar B. Paper electrophoretic study of human fetal serum proteins with demonstration of a new protein fraction. Scand J Clin Lab Invest 1957;9:277-86.
42. Berkowitz K, Reyes C, Saadat P, Kjos SL. Fetal lung maturation: comparison of biochemical indices in gestational diabetic and nondiabetic pregnancies. J Reprod Med 1997;42:793-800.
43. Bersinger NA, Marguerat P, Pescia G, Schneider H. Pregnancy-associated plasma protein A (PAPP-A): measurement by highly sensitive and specific enzyme immunoassay, importance of first-trimester serum determinations, and stability studies. Reprod Fertil Dev 1995;7:1419-23.
44. Bevis DC. The antenatal prediction of haemolytic disease of the newborn. Lancet 1952;1:395-8.
45. Bevis DC. Blood pigments in haemolytic disease of the newborn. J Obstet Gynaecol Br Emp 1956;63:68-75.
46. Bevis DC. Composition of liquor amnii in haemolytic disease of newborn. Lancet 1950;2:443.
47. Bevis DC. The composition of liquor amnii in haemolytic disease of the newborn. J Obstet Gynaecol Br Emp 1953;60:244-51.
48. Birken S, Armstrong EG, Kolks MA, Cole LA, Agosto GM, Krichevsky A, et al. Structure of the human chorionic gonadotropin beta-subunit fragment from pregnancy urine. Endocrinology 1988;123:572-83.
49. Birken S, Berger P, Bidart JM, Weber M, Bristow A, Norman R, et al. Preparation and characterization of new WHO reference reagents for human chorionic gonadotropin and metabolites. Clin Chem 2003;49: 144-54.
50. Birken S, Maydelman Y, Gawinowicz MA, Pound A, Liu Y, Hartree AS. Isolation and characterization of human pituitary chorionic gonadotropin. Endocrinology 1996;137:1402-11.
51. Bock JL. Current issues in maternal serum alpha-fetoprotein screening. Am J Clin Pathol 1992;97:541-54.

52. Bogart MH, Pandian MR, Jones OW. Abnormal maternal serum chorionic gonadotropin levels in pregnancies with fetal chromosome abnormalities. Prenat Diagn 1987;7:623-30.
53. Boldt HB, Conover CA. Pregnancy-associated plasma protein-A (PAPP-A): a local regulator of IGF bioavailability through cleavage of IGFBPs. Growth Horm IGF Res 2007;17:10-8.
54. Bonno M, Oxvig C, Kephart GM, Wagner JM, Kristensen T, Sottrup-Jensen L, et al. Localization of pregnancy-associated plasma protein-A and colocalization of pregnancy-associated plasma protein-A messenger ribonucleic acid and eosinophil granule major basic protein messenger ribonucleic acid in placenta. Lab Invest 1994; 71:560-6.
55. Bowie LJ, Shammo J, Dohnal JC, Farrell E, Vye MV. Lamellar body number density and the prediction of respiratory distress. Am J Clin Pathol 1991;95:781-6.
56. Bowman J. Thirty-five years of Rh prophylaxis. Transfusion 2003;43: 1661-6.
57. Bradley LA, Canick JA, Palomaki GE, Haddow JE. Undetectable maternal serum unconjugated estriol levels in the second trimester: risk of perinatal complications associated with placental sulfatase deficiency. Am J Obstet Gynecol 1997;176:531-5.
58. Braunstein GD, Karow WG, Gentry WC, Rasor J, Wade ME. First-trimester chorionic gonadotropin measurements as an aid in the diagnosis of early pregnancy disorders. Am J Obstet Gynecol 1978; 131:25-32.
59. Breathnach FM, Malone FD, Lambert-Messerlian G, Cuckle HS, Porter TF, Nyberg DA, et al. First- and second-trimester screening: detection of aneuploidies other than Down syndrome. Obstet Gynecol 2007;110:651-7.
60. Bristow A, Berger P, Bidart J-M, Birken S, Norman R, Stenman U-H, et al. Establishment, value assignment, and characterization of new WHO reference reagents for six molecular forms of human chorionic gonadotropin. Clinical Chemistry 2005;51:177-82.
61. Britton RC. Pregnancy and esophageal varices. Am J Surg 1982;143: 421-5.
62. Brock DJ, Bolton AE, Monaghan JM. Prenatal diagnosis of anencephaly through maternal serum-alphafetoprotein measurement. Lancet 1973;2:923-4.
63. Brock DJ, Hayward C. Gel electrophoresis of amniotic fluid acetylcholinesterase as an aid to the prenatal diagnosis of fetal defects. Clin Chim Acta 1980;108:135-41.
64. Brock DJ, Sutcliffe RG. Alpha-fetoprotein in the antenatal diagnosis of anencephaly and spina bifida. Lancet 1972;2:197-9.
65. Brown LM, Duck-Chong CG. Methods of evaluating fetal lung maturity. Crit Rev Clin Lab Sci 1982;16:85-159.
66. Browning MF, Levy HL, Wilkins-Haug LE, Larson C, Shih VE. Fetal fatty acid oxidation defects and maternal liver disease in pregnancy. Obstet Gynecol 2006;107:115-20.
67. Burrow GN. The management of thyrotoxicosis in pregnancy. N Engl J Med 1985;313:562-5.
68. Butler SA, Khanlian SA, Cole LA. Detection of early pregnancy forms of human chorionic gonadotropin by home pregnancy test devices. Clin Chem 2001;47:2131-6.
69. Cacciatore B, Stenman UH, Ylostalo P. Early screening for ectopic pregnancy in high-risk symptom-free women. Lancet 1994;343: 517-8.
70. Canfield RE, Ross GT. A new reference preparation of human chorionic gonadotrophin and its subunits. Bull World Health Organ 1976;54:463-72.
71. Canick JA, Knight GJ, Palomaki GE, Haddow JE, Cuckle HS, Wald NJ. Low second trimester maternal serum unconjugated oestriol in pregnancies with Down's syndrome. Br J Obstet Gynaecol 1988;95: 330-3.
72. Canick JA, Lambert-Messerlian GM, Farina A. Laboratory issues related to maternal serum screening for Down syndrome. Available at: www.uptodate.com (accessed on May 29, 2009).
73. Canick JA, Lambert-Messerlian GM, Palomaki GE, Neveux LM, Malone FD, Ball RH, et al. Comparison of serum markers in first-trimester Down syndrome screening. Obstet Gynecol 2006;108: 1192-9.
74. Canick JA, Palomaki GE, Osathanondh R. Prenatal screening for trisomy 18 in the second trimester. Prenat Diagn 1990;10:546-8.
75. Carter PE, Pearn JH, Bell J, Martin N, Anderson NG. Survival in trisomy 18: life tables for use in genetic counselling and clinical paediatrics. Clin Genet 1985;27:59-61.
76. Casey B. Environmental contaminants and maternal thyroid function. Am J Obstet Gynecol 2005;193:1889-90.
77. Castro MA, Fassett MJ, Reynolds TB, Shaw KJ, Goodwin TM. Reversible peripartum liver failure: a new perspective on the diagnosis, treatment, and cause of acute fatty liver of pregnancy, based on 28 consecutive cases. Am J Obstet Gynecol 1999;181: 389-95.
78. Catt KJ, Dufau ML, Tsuruhara T. Radioligand-receptor assay of luteinizing hormone and chorionic gonadotropin. J Clin Endocrinol Metab 1972;34:123-32.
79. Centers for Disease Control and Prevention. Recommendations for the use of folic acid to reduce the number of cases of spina bifida and other neural tube defects. MMWR Recomm Rep 1992;41:1-7.
80. Centers for Disease Control and Prevention (CDC). Racial/ethnic differences in the birth prevalence of spina bifida—United States, 1995-2005. MMWR Morb Mortal Wkly Rep 2009;57:1409-13.
81. Cervinski MA, Lockwood CM, Ferguson AM, Odem RR, Stenman UH, Alfthan H, et al. Qualitative point-of-care and over-the-counter urine hCG devices differentially detect the hCG variants of early pregnancy. Clin Chim Acta 2009;406:81-5.
82. Chapman JF, Ashwood ER, Feld R, Wu AH. Evaluation of two-dimensional cytometric lamellar body counts on the ADVIA 120 hematology system for estimation of fetal lung maturation. Clin Chim Acta 2004;340:85-92.
83. Chayen J, Daly JR, Loveridge N, Bitensky L. The cytochemical bioassay of hormones. Recent Prog Horm Res 1976;32:33-79.
84. Chen BK, Leiferman KM, Pittelkow MR, Overgaard MT, Oxvig C, Conover CA. Localization and regulation of pregnancy-associated plasma protein a expression in healing human skin. J Clin Endocrinol Metab 2003;88:4465-71.
85. Chen C, Roby PV, Weiss NS, Wilson JA, Benedetti TJ, Tait JF. Clinical evaluation of the NBD-PC fluorescence polarization assay for prediction of fetal lung maturity. Obstet Gynecol 1992;80:688-92.
86. Chiu RW, Chan KC, Gao Y, Lau VY, Zheng W, Leung TY, et al. Noninvasive prenatal diagnosis of fetal chromosomal aneuploidy by massively parallel genomic sequencing of DNA in maternal plasma. Proc Natl Acad Sci U S A 2008;105:20458-63.
87. Clements JA, Platzker AC, Tierney DF, Hobel CJ, Creasy RK, Margolis AJ, et al. Assessment of the risk of the respiratory-distress syndrome by a rapid test for surfactant in amniotic fluid. N Engl J Med 1972; 286:1077-81.
88. Cole LA. Hyperglycosylated hCG. Placenta 2007;28:977-86.
89. Cole LA, Khanlian SA. Hyperglycosylated hCG: a variant with separate biological functions to regular hCG. Mol Cell Endocrinol 2007;260:228-36.
90. Cole LA, Khanlian SA, Sutton JM, Davies S, Rayburn WF. Accuracy of home pregnancy tests at the time of missed menses. Am J Obstet Gynecol 2004;190:100-5.
91. Cole LA, Shahabi S, Butler SA, Mitchell H, Newlands ES, Behrman HR, et al. Utility of commonly used commercial human chorionic gonadotropin immunoassays in the diagnosis and management of trophoblastic diseases. Clin Chem 2001;47:308-15.
92. College of American Pathologists. CAP surveys, maternal screening survey, set FP-A. Northfield, Ill: College of American Pathologists, 2010.
93. Cousins LM, Smok DP, Lovett SM, Poeltler DM. AmniSure placental alpha microglobulin-1 rapid immunoassay versus standard diagnostic methods for detection of rupture of membranes. Am J Perinatol 2005; 22:317-20.
94. Cowans NJ, Stamatopoulou A, Hellstrom J, Makela MM, Spencer K. PAPP-A and free ss-hCG stability in first trimester serum using

PerkinElmer AutoDELFIA and DELFIA Xpress systems. Prenat Diagn 2010;30:127-32.
95. Craig WY, Haddow JE, Palomaki GE, Kelley RI, Kratz LE, Shackleton CH, et al. Identifying Smith-Lemli-Opitz syndrome in conjunction with prenatal screening for Down syndrome. Prenat Diagn 2006;26:842-9.
96. Crandall BF. Prenatal screening for the detection of neural tube defects. In: Simpson JL, Elias S, eds. Essentials of prenatal diagnosis. New York: Churchill Livingstone, 1993:253-74.
97. Crandall BF, Chua C. Risks for fetal abnormalities after very and moderately elevated AF-AFPs. Prenat Diagn 1997;17:837-41.
98. Cruz AC, Buhi WC, Birk SA, Spellacy WN. Respiratory distress syndrome with mature lecithin/sphingomyelin ratios: diabetes mellitus and low Apgar scores. Am J Obstet Gynecol 1976;126:78-82.
99. Cuckle HS, Wald NJ, Lindenbaum RH. Maternal serum alpha-fetoprotein measurement: a screening test for Down syndrome. Lancet 1984;1:926-9.
100. Cunningham FG, MacDonald PC, Gant NF. The placental hormones. In: Williams obstetrics, 18th edition. Norwark, Conn: Appleton & Lange, 1989:67-85.
101. Cunningham FG, MacDonald PC, Gant NF. Techniques to evaluate fetal health. In: Williams obstetrics, 18th edition. Norwark, Conn: Appleton & Lange, 1989:277-305.
102. Cunningham GC, Tompkinison DG. Cost and effectiveness of the California triple marker prenatal screening program. Genet Med 1999;1:199-206.
103. Cunningham MD, McKean HE, Gillispie DH, Greene JW Jr. Improved prediction of fetal lung maturity in diabetic pregnancies: a comparison of chromatographic methods. Am J Obstet Gynecol 1982;142:197-204.
104. D'Alton ME, Cleary-Goldman J, Lambert-Messerlian G, Ball RH, Nyberg DA, Comstock CH, et al. Maintaining quality assurance for sonographic nuchal translucency measurement: lessons from the FASTER Trial. Ultrasound Obstet Gynecol 2009;33:142-6.
105. D'Alton ME, DeCherney AH. Prenatal diagnosis. N Engl J Med 1993;328:114-20.
106. Daily CA, Laurent SL, Nunley WC Jr. The prognostic value of serum progesterone and quantitative beta-human chorionic gonadotropin in early human pregnancy. Am J Obstet Gynecol 1994;171:380-3; discussion 383-4.
107. Dalence CR, Bowie LJ, Dohnal JC, Farrell EE, Neerhof MG. Amniotic fluid lamellar body count: a rapid and reliable fetal lung maturity test. Obstet Gynecol 1995;86:235-9.
108. Dallaire L, Belanger L, Smith CJ, Kelleher PC. Origin of amniocentesis-induced rises of alpha-fetoprotein concentrations in maternal serum. Br J Obstet Gynaecol 1980;87:856-9.
109. Dawood MY. Hormones in amniotic fluid. Am J Obstet Gynecol 1977;128:576-83.
110. de Courcy-Wheeler RH, Pomeranz MM, Wald NJ, Nicolaides KH. Small fetal transverse cerebellar diameter: a screening test for spina bifida. Br J Obstet Gynaecol 1994;101:904-5.
111. De Luca AKC, Nakazawa CY, Azevedo BC, Rudge MVC, De Araújo Costa RA, Calderon IMP. Influence of glycemic control on fetal lung maturity in gestations affected by diabetes or mild hyperglycemia. Acta Obstet Gynecol Scand 2009;88:1036-40.
112. Del Valle GO, Adair CD, Ramos EE, Gaudier FL, Sanchez-Ramos L, Morales R. Interpretation of the TDx-FLM fluorescence polarization assay in pregnancies complicated by diabetes mellitus. Am J Perinatol 1997;14:241-4.
113. deMello DE, Nogee LM, Heyman S, Krous HF, Hussain M, Merritt TA, et al. Molecular and phenotypic variability in the congenital alveolar proteinosis syndrome associated with inherited surfactant protein B deficiency. J Pediatr 1994;125:43-50.
114. DeRoche ME, Ingardia CJ, Guerette PJ, Wu AH, LaSala CA, Mandavilli SR. The use of lamellar body counts to predict fetal lung maturity in pregnancies complicated by diabetes mellitus. Am J Obstet Gynecol 2002;187:908-12.
115. Dilena BA, Ku F, Doyle I, Whiting MJ. Six alternative methods to the lecithin/sphingomyelin ratio in amniotic fluid for assessing fetal lung maturity. Ann Clin Biochem 1997;34(Pt 1):106-8.
116. Dombroski RA, MacKenna J, Brame RG. Comparison of amniotic fluid lung maturity profiles in paired vaginal and amniocentesis specimens. Am J Obstet Gynecol 1981;140:461-4.
117. Doyle PE, Beral V, Botting B, Wale CJ. Congenital malformations in twins in England and Wales. J Epidemiol Community Health 1991;45:43-8.
118. Dubin SB. Assessment of fetal lung maturity: practice parameter. Am J Clin Pathol 1998;110:723-32.
119. Dubin SB. Characterization of amniotic fluid lamellar bodies by resistive-pulse counting: relationship to measures of fetal lung maturity. Clin Chem 1989;35:612-6.
120. Dufau ML, Mendelson CR, Catt KJ. A highly sensitive in vitro bioassay for luteinizing hormone and chorionic gonadotropin: testosterone production by dispersed Leydig cells. J Clin Endocrinol Metab 1974;39:610-3.
121. Dugoff L, Hobbins JC, Malone FD, Porter TF, Luthy D, Comstock CH, et al. First-trimester maternal serum PAPP-A and free-beta subunit human chorionic gonadotropin concentrations and nuchal translucency are associated with obstetric complications: a population-based screening study (the FASTER Trial). Am J Obstet Gynecol 2004;191:1446-51.
122. Erickson JA, Ashwood ER, Gin CA. Evaluation of a dimeric inhibin-A assay for assessing fetal Down syndrome: establishment, comparison, and monitoring of median concentrations for normal pregnancies. Arch Pathol Lab Med 2004;128:415-20.
123. Evans MI, Berkowitz RL, Wapner RJ, Carpenter RJ, Goldberg JD, Ayoub MA, et al. Improvement in outcomes of multifetal pregnancy reduction with increased experience. Am J Obstet Gynecol 2001;184:97-103.
124. Evans MI, Harrison HH, O'Brien JE, Dvorin E, Huang X, Krivchenia EL, et al. Correction for insulin-dependent diabetes in maternal serum alpha-fetoprotein testing has outlived its usefulness. Am J Obstet Gynecol 2002;187:1084-6.
125. Fakhoury G, Daikoku NH, Benser J, Dubin NH. Lamellar body concentrations and the prediction of fetal pulmonary maturity. Am J Obstet Gynecol 1994;170:72-6.
126. Fan HC, Blumenfeld YJ, Chitkara U, Hudgins L, Quake SR. Noninvasive diagnosis of fetal aneuploidy by shotgun sequencing DNA from maternal blood. Proc Natl Acad Sci U S A 2008;105:16266-71.
127. Fantz CR, Powell C, Karon B, Parvin CA, Hankins K, Dayal M, et al. Assessment of the diagnostic accuracy of the TDx-FLM II to predict fetal lung maturity. Clin Chem 2002;48:761-5.
128. Farquharson J, Jamieson EC, Berry E, Buchanan R, Logan RW. Assessment of the AmnioStat-FLM immunoagglutination test for phosphatidylglycerol in amniotic fluid. Clin Chim Acta 1986;156:271-7.
129. Farrell PM, Avery ME. Hyaline membrane disease. Am Rev Respir Dis 1975;111:657-88.
130. Favre N, Bourdel N, Sapin V, Abergel A, Gallot D. [Importance of bile acids for intra-hepatic cholestasis of pregnancy]. Gynecol Obstet Fertil 2010;38:293-5.
131. Feuchtbaum LB, Currier RJ, Lorey FW, Cunningham GC. Prenatal ultrasound findings in affected and unaffected pregnancies that are screen-positive for trisomy 18: the California experience. Prenat Diagn 2000;20:293-9.
132. Feuchtbaum LB, Currier RJ, Riggle S, Roberson M, Lorey FW, Cunningham GC. Neural tube defect prevalence in California (1990-1994): eliciting patterns by type of defect and maternal race/ethnicity. Genet Test 1999;3:265-72.
133. Finning K, Martin P, Daniels G. A clinical service in the UK to predict fetal Rh (Rhesus) D blood group using free fetal DNA in maternal plasma. Ann N Y Acad Sci 2004;1022:119-23.
134. Foerder CA, Tait JF, Franklin RW, Ashwood ER. Improved fluorescence polarization assay for use in evaluating fetal lung

maturity. II. Analytical evaluation and comparison with the lecithin/sphingomyelin ratio. Clin Chem 1986;32:255-9.

135. Foster K, Moore J, Hankins K, Parvin CA, Gronowski AM. Effect of blood contamination on delta 450 bilirubin measurement: an in vitro comparison of two corrective methods. Clin Chem 2004;50:1420-2.

136. Francoual J, Cohen H, Benattar C, Papiernik E, Leluc R. [Phosphatidylglycerol in amniotic fluid: value of rapid determination using an immunologic technic]. J Gynecol Obstet Biol Reprod (Paris) 1985;14:879-82.

137. Freeman K, Szczepura A, Osipenko L. Non-invasive fetal RHD genotyping tests: a systematic review of the quality of reporting of diagnostic accuracy in published studies. Eur J Obstet Gynecol Reprod Biol 2009;142:91-8.

138. Frey L, Hauser WA. Epidemiology of neural tube defects. Epilepsia 2003;44(suppl 3):4-13.

139. Friedman SA, Schiff E, Kao L, Kuint J, Sibai BM. Do twins mature earlier than singletons? Results from a matched cohort study. Am J Obstet Gynecol 1997;176:1193-6; discussion 1196-9.

140. Frishman GN, Canick JA, Hogan JW, Hackett RJ, Kellner LH, Saller DN Jr. Serum triple-marker screening in in vitro fertilization and naturally conceived pregnancies. Obstet Gynecol 1997;90:98-101.

141. Gabbe SG, Lowensohn RI, Mestman JH, Freeman RK, Goebelsmann U. Lecithin/sphingomyelin ratio in pregnancies complicated by diabetes mellitus. Am J Obstet Gynecol 1977;128:757-60.

142. Gagnon A, Wilson RD, Audibert F, Allen VM, Blight C, Brock JA, et al. Obstetrical complications associated with abnormal maternal serum markers analytes. J Obstet Gynaecol Can 2008;30:918-49.

143. Garchet-Beaudron A, Dreux S, Leporrier N, Oury JF, Muller F. Second-trimester Down syndrome maternal serum marker screening: a prospective study of 11,040 twin pregnancies. Prenat Diagn 2008;28: 1105-9.

144. Garite TJ, Yabusaki KK, Moberg LJ, Symons JL, White T, Itano M, et al. A new rapid slide agglutination test for amniotic fluid phosphatidylglycerol: laboratory and clinical correlation. Am J Obstet Gynecol 1983;147:681-6.

145. Ghanta S, Mitchell ME, Ames M, Hidestrand M, Simpson P, Goetsch M, et al. Non-invasive prenatal detection of trisomy 21 using tandem single nucleotide polymorphisms. PLoS One 2010;5:e131-84.

146. Gharib H, Tuttle RM, Baskin HJ, Fish LH, Singer PA, McDermott MT. Consensus statement #1. Subclinical thyroid dysfunction: a joint statement on management from the American Association of Clinical Endocrinologists, the American Thyroid Association, and The Endocrine Society. Thyroid 2005;15:24-8; response 32-3.

147. Gibbons JM Jr, Huntley TE, Corral AG. Effect of maternal blood contamination on amniotic fluid analysis. Obstet Gynecol 1974;44: 657-60.

148. Gibbs PE, Zielinski R, Boyd C, Dugaiczyk A. Structure, polymorphism, and novel repeated DNA elements revealed by a complete sequence of the human alpha-fetoprotein gene. Biochemistry 1987;26:1332-43.

149. Gingelmaier A, Bruning A, Kimmich T, Makovitzky J, Bergauer F, Schiessl B, et al. Inhibin/activin-betaE subunit is expressed in normal and pathological human placental tissue including chorionic carcinoma cell lines. Arch Gynecol Obstet 2010 Jan 6. [Epub ahead of print].

150. Gitlin D. Normal biology of alpha-fetoprotein. Ann N Y Acad Sci 1975;259:7-16.

151. Glinoer D, de Nayer P, Bourdoux P, Lemone M, Robyn C, van Steirteghem A, et al. Regulation of maternal thyroid during pregnancy. J Clin Endocrinol Metab 1990;71:276-87.

152. Gluck L, Kulovich MV. Lecithin-sphingomyelin ratios in amniotic fluid in normal and abnormal pregnancy. Am J Obstet Gynecol 1973;115:539-46.

153. Goldenberg RL, Mercer BM, Iams JD, Moawad AH, Meis PJ, Das A, et al. The preterm prediction study: patterns of cervicovaginal fetal fibronectin as predictors of spontaneous preterm delivery. National Institute of Child Health and Human Development Maternal-Fetal Medicine Units Network. Am J Obstet Gynecol 1997;177:8-12.

154. Goldenberg RL, Mercer BM, Meis PJ, Copper RL, Das A, McNellis D. The preterm prediction study: fetal fibronectin testing and spontaneous preterm birth. NICHD Maternal Fetal Medicine Units Network. Obstet Gynecol 1996;87:643-8.

155. Goldner TE, Lawson HW, Xia Z, Atrash HK. Surveillance for ectopic pregnancy—United States, 1970-1989. MMWR CDC Surveill Summ 1993;42:73-85.

156. Greenberg F, James LM, Oakley GP Jr. Estimates of birth prevalence rates of spina bifida in the United States from computer-generated maps. Am J Obstet Gynecol 1983;145:570-3.

157. Greene DN, Hall BJ, Grenache DG. An unlikely pregnancy. Clin Chem 2010;56:1645-6.

158. Greenspoon JS, Rosen DJ, Roll K, Dubin SB. Evaluation of lamellar body number density as the initial assessment in a fetal lung maturity test cascade. J Reprod Med 1995;40:260-6.

159. Grenache DG. Hemolytic disease of the newborn. In: Gronowski AM, ed. Handbook of clinical laboratory testing during pregnancy. Totowa, NJ: Humana Press, 2004:219-43.

160. Grenache DG, Parvin CA, Gronowski AM. Preanalytical factors that influence the Abbott TDx Fetal Lung Maturity II assay. Clin Chem 2003;49:935-9.

161. Grenache DG, Wilson AR, Gross GA, Gronowski AM. Clinical and laboratory trends in fetal lung maturity testing. Clin Chim Acta 2010;411:1746-9.

162. Grody WW, Cutting GR, Klinger KW, Richards CS, Watson MS, Desnick RJ. Laboratory standards and guidelines for population-based cystic fibrosis carrier screening. Genet Med 2001;3:149-54.

163. Gronowski AM, Cervinski M, Stenman U-H, Woodworth A, Ashby L, Scott MG. False-negative results in point-of-care qualitative human chorionic gonadotropin (hCG) devices due to excess hCGbeta core fragment. Clin Chem 2009;55:1389-94.

164. Gronowski AM, Grenache DG. Characterization of the hCG variants recognized by different hCG immunoassays: an important step toward standardization of hCG measurements. Clin Chem 2009;55: 1447-9.

165. Gronowski AM, Parvin CA. Prediction of risk for respiratory distress syndrome using gestational age and the TDx-FLM II assay. Am J Obstet Gynecol 2003;189:1511-2; author reply 1513-4.

166. Gyselaers WJ, Vereecken AJ, Van Herck EJ, Straetmans DP, Ombelet WU, Nijhuis JG. Nuchal translucency thickness measurements for fetal aneuploidy screening: log NT-MoM or delta-NT, performer-specific medians and ultrasound training. J Med Screen 2006;13:4-7.

167. Haddow JE, Morin ME, Holman MS, Miller WA. Acetylcholinesterase and fetal malformations: modified qualitative technique for diagnosis of neural tube defects. Clin Chem 1981;27:61-3.

168. Haddow JE, Palomaki GE, Allan WC, Williams JR, Knight GJ, Gagnon J, et al. Maternal thyroid deficiency during pregnancy and subsequent neuropsychological development of the child. N Engl J Med 1999;341:549-55.

169. Haddow JE, Palomaki GE, Knight GJ, Canick JA. Variables which influence levels of AFP, uE3, and hCG and/or risk for Down syndrome. In: Foundation for Blood Research handbook, vol II: screening for Down syndrome. Scarborough, Maine: Foundation for Blood Research, 1998:1-48.

170. Haddow JE, Palomaki GE, Knight GJ, Cunningham GC, Lustig LS, Boyd PA. Reducing the need for amniocentesis in women 35 years of age or older with serum markers for screening. N Engl J Med 1994; 330:1114-8.

171. Haddow JE, Palomaki GE, Knight GJ, Foster DL, Neveux LM. Second trimester screening for Down's syndrome using maternal serum dimeric inhibin A. J Med Screen 1998;5:115-9.

172. Haddow JE, Palomaki GE, Knight GJ, Williams J, Miller WA, Johnson A. Screening of maternal serum for fetal Down's syndrome in the first trimester. N Engl J Med 1998;338:955-61.

173. Haddow JE, Palomaki GE, Knight GJ, Williams J, Pulkkinen A, Canick JA, et al. Prenatal screening for Down's syndrome with use of maternal serum markers. N Engl J Med 1992;327:588-93.

174. Hallman M, Merritt TA, Jarvenpaa AL, Boynton B, Mannino F, Gluck L, et al. Exogenous human surfactant for treatment of severe respiratory distress syndrome: a randomized prospective clinical trial. J Pediatr 1985;106:963-9.
175. Halvorsen PR, Gross TL. Laboratory and clinical evaluation of a rapid slide agglutination test for phosphatidylglycerol. Am J Obstet Gynecol 1985;151:1061-6.
176. Harper ME, Dugaiczyk A. Linkage of the evolutionarily-related serum albumin and alpha-fetoprotein genes within q11-22 of human chromosome 4. Am J Hum Genet 1983;35:565-72.
177. Hawgood S, Clements JA. Pulmonary surfactant and its apoproteins. J Clin Invest 1990;86:1-6.
178. Haymond S, Luzzi VI, Parvin CA, Gronowski AM. A direct comparison between lamellar body counts and fluorescent polarization methods for predicting respiratory distress syndrome. Am J Clin Pathol 2006;126:894-9.
179. Henshaw SK. Unintended pregnancy in the United States. Fam Plann Perspect 1998;30:24-9, 46.
180. Herbert WN, Chapman JF, Schnoor MM. Role of the TDx FLM assay in fetal lung maturity. Am J Obstet Gynecol 1993;168:808-12.
181. Heron MP, Hoyert DL, Murphy SL, Xu JQ, Kochanek KD, Tejada-Vera B. Deaths: final data for 2006. National vital statistics reports, vol 57-14. Hyattsville, Md: National Center for Health Statistics, 2009.
182. Hill M, Finning K, Martin P, Hogg J, Meaney C, Norbury G, et al. Non-invasive prenatal determination of fetal sex: translating research into clinical practice. Clin Genet 2011;80:68-75.
183. Holmes LB, Driscoll SG, Atkins L. Etiologic heterogeneity of neural-tube defects. N Engl J Med 1976;294:365-9.
184. Holt JA, Ryan DF, Russell JC. Automated rapid assessment of surfactant and fetal lung maturity. Lab Med 1990;21:359-66.
185. Honest H, Bachmann LM, Gupta JK, Kleijnen J, Khan KS. Accuracy of cervicovaginal fetal fibronectin test in predicting risk of spontaneous preterm birth: systematic review. BMJ 2002;325:301.
186. Hook GE, Gilmore LB, Tombropoulos EG, Fabro SE. Fetal lung lamellar bodies in human amniotic fluid. Am Rev Respir Dis 1978;117:541-50.
187. Huttly W, Rudnicka A, Wald NJ. Second-trimester prenatal screening markers for Down syndrome in women with insulin-dependent diabetes mellitus. Prenat Diagn 2004;24:804-7.
188. Janicki MB, Dries LM, Egan JFX, Zelop CM. Determining a cutoff for fetal lung maturity with lamellar body count testing. J Matern Fetal Neonatal Med 2009;22:419-22.
189. Janssen PA, Rothman I, Schwartz SM. Congenital malformations in newborns of women with established and gestational diabetes in Washington State, 1984-91. Paediatr Perinat Epidemiol 1996;10: 52-63.
190. Jeffcoate TN, Fliegner JR, Russell SH, Davis JC, Wade AP. Diagnosis of the adrenogenital syndrome before birth. Lancet 1965;2:553-5.
191. Joshi D, James A, Quaglia A, Westbrook RH, Heneghan MA. Liver disease in pregnancy. Lancet 2010;375:594-605.
192. Kadar N, Bohrer M, Kemman E, Shelden R. A prospective, randomized study of the chorionic gonadotropin-time relationship in early gestation: clinical implications. Fertil Steril 1993;60:409-12.
193. Kadar N, Bohrer M, Kemmann E, Shelden R. The discriminatory human chorionic gonadotropin zone for endovaginal sonography: a prospective, randomized study. Fertil Steril 1994;61:1016-20.
194. Kagan KO, Wright D, Maiz N, Pandeva I, Nicolaides KH. Screening for trisomy 18 by maternal age, fetal nuchal translucency, free beta-human chorionic gonadotropin and pregnancy-associated plasma protein-A. Ultrasound Obstet Gynecol 2008;32:488-92.
195. Kaplan LA, Chapman JF, Bock JL, Santa Maria E, Clejan S, Huddleston DJ, et al. Prediction of respiratory distress syndrome using the Abbott FLM-II amniotic fluid assay. Clin Chim Acta 2002;326:61-8.
196. Karcher R, Sykes E, Batton D, Uddin Z, Ross G, Hockman E, et al. Gestational age-specific predicted risk of neonatal respiratory distress syndrome using lamellar body count and surfactant-to-albumin ratio in amniotic fluid. Am J Obstet Gynecol 2005;193:1680-4.
197. Kardana A, Cole LA. Polypeptide nicks cause erroneous results in assays of human chorionic gonadotropin free beta-subunit. Clin Chem 1992;38:26-33.
198. Kavsak PA, Wang X, Henderson M, Ko DT, MacRae AR, Jaffe AS. PAPP-A as a marker of increased long-term risk in patients with chest pain. Clin Biochem 2009;42:1012-8.
199. Kelley RI, Hennekam RC. The Smith-Lemli-Opitz syndrome. J Med Genet 2000;37:321-35.
200. Kesselman EJ, Figueroa R, Garry D, Maulik D. The usefulness of the TDx/TDxFLx fetal lung maturity II assay in the initial evaluation of fetal lung maturity. Am J Obstet Gynecol 2003;188:1220-2.
201. Klein NA, Mabie WC, Shaver DC, Latham PS, Adamec TA, Pinstein ML, et al. Herpes simplex virus hepatitis in pregnancy: two patients successfully treated with acyclovir. Gastroenterology 1991;100:239-44.
202. Knight GJ, Palomaki GE. Epidemiologic monitoring of prenatal screening for neural tube defects and Down syndrome. Clin Lab Med 2003;23:531-51, xi.
203. Knight GJ, Palomaki GE, Neveux LM, Haddow JE, Lambert-Messerlian GM. Clinical validation of a new dimeric inhibin-A assay suitable for second trimester Down's syndrome screening. J Med Screen 2001;8:2-7.
204. Knox TA, Olans LB. Liver disease in pregnancy. N Engl J Med 1996; 335:569-76.
205. Kohn MA, Kerr K, Malkevich D, O'Neil N, Kerr MJ, Kaplan BC. Beta-human chorionic gonadotropin levels and the likelihood of ectopic pregnancy in emergency department patients with abdominal pain or vaginal bleeding. Acad Emerg Med 2003;10:119-26.
206. Korhonen J, Alfthan H, Ylostalo P, Veldhuis J, Stenman UH. Disappearance of human chorionic gonadotropin and its alpha- and beta-subunits after term pregnancy. Clin Chem 1997;43:2155-63.
207. Krantz DA, Hallahan TW, Macri VJ, Macri JN. Maternal weight and ethnic adjustment within a first-trimester Down syndrome and trisomy 18 screening program. Prenat Diagn 2005;25:635-40.
208. Krawczynski K. Hepatitis E. Hepatology 1993;17:932-41.
209. Kulovich MV, Gluck L. The lung profile. II. Complicated pregnancy. Am J Obstet Gynecol 1979;135:64-70.
210. Kulovich MV, Hallman MB, Gluck L. The lung profile. I. Normal pregnancy. Am J Obstet Gynecol 1979;135:57-63.
211. Lakowicz JR. Fluorescence polarization: principles of fluorescence spectroscopy. New York, NY: Plenum Press, 1983:111-53.
212. Lambert-Messerlian G, Dugoff L, Vidaver J, Canick JA, Malone FD, Ball RH, et al. First- and second-trimester Down syndrome screening markers in pregnancies achieved through assisted reproductive technologies (ART): a FASTER trial study. Prenat Diagn 2006;26: 672-8.
213. Lambert-Messerlian G, McClain M, Haddow JE, Palomaki GE, Canick JA, Cleary-Goldman J, et al. First- and second-trimester thyroid hormone reference data in pregnant women: a FaSTER (First- and Second-Trimester Evaluation of Risk for aneuploidy) Research Consortium study. Am J Obstet Gynecol 2008;199:62 e1-6.
214. Lambert-Messerlian G, Palomaki GE, Canick JA. Adjustment of serum markers in first trimester screening. J Med Screen 2009;16: 102-3.
215. Lambert-Messerlian GM, Canick JA, Palomaki GE, Schneyer AL. Second trimester levels of maternal serum inhibin A, total inhibin, alpha inhibin precursor, and activin in Down's syndrome pregnancy. J Med Screen 1996;3:58-62.
216. Lambert-Messerlian GM, Eklund EE, Malone FD, Palomaki GE, Canick JA, D'Alton ME. Stability of first- and second-trimester serum markers after storage and shipment. Prenat Diagn 2006;26:17-21.
217. Lambert-Messerlian GM, Palomaki GE, Canick JA. Inhibin A measurement using an automated assay platform. Prenat Diagn 2008;28:399-403.
218. Lau HL, Linkins SE. Alpha-fetoprotein. Am J Obstet Gynecol 1976; 124:533-54.
219. Lee IS, Cho YK, Kim A, Min WK, Kim KS, Mok JE. Lamellar body count in amniotic fluid as a rapid screening test for fetal lung maturity. J Perinatol 1996;16:176-80.

220. Lee SE, Park JS, Norwitz ER, Kim KW, Park HS, Jun JK. Measurement of placental alpha-microglobulin-1 in cervicovaginal discharge to diagnose rupture of membranes. Obstet Gynecol 2007;109:634-40.
221. Lenton EA, Neal LM, Sulaiman R. Plasma concentrations of human chorionic gonadotropin from the time of implantation until the second week of pregnancy. Fertil Steril 1982;37:773-8.
222. Levine RJ, Maynard SE, Qian C, Lim KH, England LJ, Yu KF, et al. Circulating angiogenic factors and the risk of preeclampsia. N Engl J Med 2004;350:672-83.
223. Liley AW. Errors in the assessment of hemolytic disease from amniotic fluid. Am J Obstet Gynecol 1963;86:485-94.
224. Liley AW. Liquor amnil analysis in the management of the pregnancy complicated by resus sensitization. Am J Obstet Gynecol 1961;82: 1359-70.
225. Linskens IH, Levitus M, Frans A, Schielen PC, van Vugt JM, Blankenstein MA, et al. Performance of free beta-human chorionic gonadotrophin (free beta-hCG) and pregnancy associated plasma protein-A (PAPP-A) analysis between Delfia Xpress and AutoDelfia systems in The Netherlands. Clin Chem Lab Med 2009;47:222-6.
226. Linskens IH, Spreeuwenberg MD, Blankenstein MA, van Vugt JM. Early first-trimester free beta-hCG and PAPP-A serum distributions in monochorionic and dichorionic twins. Prenat Diagn 2009;29:74-8.
227. Livingston EG, Herbert WN, Hage ML, Chapman JF, Stubbs TM. Use of the TDx-FLM assay in evaluating fetal lung maturity in an insulin-dependent diabetic population. The Diabetes and Fetal Maturity Study Group. Obstet Gynecol 1995;86:826-9.
228. Lockitch G, Wittmann BK, Mura SM, Hawkley LC. Evaluation of the Amniostat-FLM assay for assessment of fetal lung maturity. Clin Chem 1984;30:1233-7.
229. Lockitch GM, ed. Handbook of diagnostic biochemistry and hematology in normal pregnancy. Boca Raton, Fla: CRC Press, 1993.
230. Lockwood CJ, Senyei AE, Dische MR, Casal D, Shah KD, Thung SN, et al. Fetal fibronectin in cervical and vaginal secretions as a predictor of preterm delivery. N Engl J Med 1991;325:669-74.
231. Lockwood CM, Crompton JC, Riley JK, Landeros K, Dietzen DJ, Grenache DG, et al. Validation of lamellar body counts using three hematology analyzers. Am J Clin Pathol 2010;134:420-8.
232. Lockwood CM, Grenache DG, Gronowski AM. Serum human chorionic gonadotropin concentrations greater than 400,000 IU/L are invariably associated with suppressed serum thyrotropin concentrations. Thyroid 2009;19:863-8.
233. Lockwood GM, Muttukrishna S, Ledger WL. Inhibins and activins in human ovulation, conception and pregnancy. Hum Reprod Update 1998;4:284-95.
234. Lohstroh PN, Overstreet JW, Stewart DR, Nakajima ST, Cragun JR, Boyers SP, et al. Secretion and excretion of human chorionic gonadotropin during early pregnancy. Fertil Steril 2005;83:1000-11.
235. MacDonald DJ, Mehta HC, Mack DS, Duffy T, Glen AC. Enzyme immunoassay for pregnancy-associated plasma protein-A. Clin Chem 1984;30:1848-50.
236. MacRae AR, Gardner HA, Allen LC, Tokmakejian S, Lepage N. Outcome validation of the Beckman Coulter access analyzer in a second-trimester Down syndrome serum screening application. Clin Chem 2003;49:69-76.
237. Malone FD, Canick JA, Ball RH, Nyberg DA, Comstock CH, Bukowski R, et al. First-trimester or second-trimester screening, or both, for Down's syndrome. N Engl J Med 2005;353:2001-11.
238. Malone FD, Wald NJ, Canick JA. Use of overall population, center-specific, and sonographer-specific nuchal translucency medians in Down syndrome screening: which is best? (results from the FaSTER trial). Am J Obstet Gynecol 2003;189:S232.
239. Mann SE, Nijland MJ, Ross MG. Mathematic modeling of human amniotic fluid dynamics. Am J Obstet Gynecol 1996;175:937-44.
240. Martin JN Jr, Blake PG, Perry KG Jr, McCaul JF, Hess LW, Martin RW. The natural history of HELLP syndrome: patterns of disease progression and regression. Am J Obstet Gynecol 1991;164:1500-9; discussion 1509-13.
241. Matsuura H, Greene T, Hakomori S. An alpha-N-acetylgalactosaminylation at the threonine residue of a defined peptide sequence creates the oncofetal peptide epitope in human fibronectin. J Biol Chem 1989;264:10472-6.
242. McCord ML, Muram D, Buster JE, Arheart KL, Stovall TG, Carson SA. Single serum progesterone as a screen for ectopic pregnancy: exchanging specificity and sensitivity to obtain optimal test performance. Fertil Steril 1996;66:513-6.
243. McElrath TF, Norwitz ER, Robinson JN, Tanasijevic MJ, Lieberman ES. Differences in TDx fetal lung maturity assay values between twin and singleton gestations. Am J Obstet Gynecol 2000;182:1110-2.
244. McGinnis KT, Brown JA, Morrison JC. Changing patterns of fetal lung maturity testing. J Perinatol 2008;28:20-3.
245. Mercer BM. Preterm premature rupture of the membranes: current approaches to evaluation and management. Obstet Gynecol Clin North Am 2005;32:411-28.
246. Mercer BM, Crocker LG, Boe NM, Sibai BM. Induction versus expectant management in premature rupture of the membranes with mature amniotic fluid at 32 to 36 weeks: a randomized trial. Am J Obstet Gynecol 1993;169:775-82.
247. Merkatz IR, Nitowsky HM, Macri JN, Johnson WE. An association between low maternal serum alpha-fetoprotein and fetal chromosomal abnormalities. Am J Obstet Gynecol 1984;148:886-94.
248. Milunsky A, Jick H, Jick SS, Bruell CL, MacLaughlin DS, Rothman KJ, et al. Multivitamin/folic acid supplementation in early pregnancy reduces the prevalence of neural tube defects. JAMA 1989;262: 2847-52.
249. Minakami H, Takahashi T, Tamada T. Should routine liver biopsy be done for the definite diagnosis of acute fatty liver of pregnancy? Am J Obstet Gynecol 1991;164:1690-1.
250. Moise KJ Jr. Management of rhesus alloimmunization in pregnancy. Obstet Gynecol 2002;100:600-11.
251. Molloy AM, Kirke PN, Troendle JF, Burke H, Sutton M, Brody LC, et al. Maternal vitamin B12 status and risk of neural tube defects in a population with high neural tube defect prevalence and no folic acid fortification. Pediatrics 2009;123:917-23.
252. Moore TR. A comparison of amniotic fluid fetal pulmonary phospholipids in normal and diabetic pregnancy. Am J Obstet Gynecol 2002;186:641-50.
253. Moos MK, Cefalo RC. Preconceptional health promotion: a focus for obstetric care. Am J Perinatol 1987;4:63-7.
254. Morales WJ, O'Brien WF, Knuppel RA, Gaylord S, Hayes P. The effect of mode of delivery on the risk of intraventricular hemorrhage in nondiscordant twin gestations under 1500 g. Obstet Gynecol 1989; 73:107-10.
255. Morris JK, Mutton DE, Alberman E. Revised estimates of the maternal age specific live birth prevalence of Down's syndrome. J Med Screen 2002;9:2-6.
256. Moss AJ, Levy AS, Kim I, Park YK. Use of vitamin and mineral supplements in the United States: current users, types of products, and nutrients. Advance data no. 174. Hyattsville, Md: National Center for Health Statistics, 1989.
257. National Center for Health Statistics. Health, United States, 2009 (with special feature on medical technology). Hyattsville, Md: National Center for Health Statistics, 2010.
258. National Institute for Health and Clinical Excellence. NICE clinical guideline 62. Antenatal care, routine care for the healthy pregnant woman. London, UK: RCOG Press, 2008.
259. Neerhof MG, Dohnal JC, Ashwood ER, Lee IS, Anceschi MM. Lamellar body counts: a consensus on protocol. Obstet Gynecol 2001;97:318-20.
260. Neerhof MG, Haney EI, Silver RK, Ashwood ER, Lee IS, Piazze JJ. Lamellar body counts compared with traditional phospholipid analysis as an assay for evaluating fetal lung maturity. Obstet Gynecol 2001;97:305-9.
261. Nelson GH, McPherson JCJ. Respiratory distress syndrome in various cultures and a possible role of diet. In: Nelson GH, ed. Pulmonary

development: transition from intrauterine to extrauterine life. New York, NY: Marcel Dekker Inc., 1985:159-78.

262. Neveux LM, Palomaki GE, Knight GJ, Haddow JE. Multiple marker screening for Down syndrome in twin pregnancies. Prenat Diagn 1996;16:29-34.
263. Neveux LM, Palomaki GE, Larrivee DA, Knight GJ, Haddow JE. Refinements in managing maternal weight adjustment for interpreting prenatal screening results. Prenat Diagn 1996;16:1115-9.
264. New England Regional Genetics Group Prenatal Collaborative Study of Down Syndrome Screening. Combining maternal serum alpha-fetoprotein measurements and age to screen for Down syndrome in pregnant women under age 35. Am J Obstet Gynecol 1989;160: 575-81.
265. Nichols JH. Evidenced-based practice for point-of-care testing: National Academy of Clinical Biochemistry Laboratory Medicine practice guidelines. Washington, DC: National Academy of Clinical Biochemistry, 2006:1-187.
266. Nicolaides KH, Azar G, Byrne D, Mansur C, Marks K. Fetal nuchal translucency: ultrasound screening for chromosomal defects in first trimester of pregnancy. BMJ 1992;304:867-9.
267. Nicolaides KH, Campbell S, Gabbe SG, Guidetti R. Ultrasound screening for spina bifida: cranial and cerebellar signs. Lancet 1986;2: 72-4.
268. Nogee LM, Garnier G, Dietz HC, Singer L, Murphy AM, deMello DE, et al. A mutation in the surfactant protein B gene responsible for fatal neonatal respiratory disease in multiple kindreds. J Clin Invest 1994; 93:1860-3.
269. Norgaard-Pedersen B, Hangaard J, Bjerrum OJ. Quantitative enzyme antigen immunoassay of acetylcholinesterase in amniotic fluid. Clin Chem 1983;29:1061-4.
270. Nygren AO, Dean J, Jensen TJ, Kruse S, Kwong W, van den Boom D, et al. Quantification of fetal DNA by use of methylation-based DNA discrimination. Clin Chem 2010;56:1627-35.
271. O'Connor JF, Ellish N, Kakuma T, Schlatterer J, Kovalevskaya G. Differential urinary gonadotrophin profiles in early pregnancy and early pregnancy loss. Prenat Diagn 1998;18:1232-40.
272. O'Leary P, Nichols C, Feddema P, Lam T, Aitken M. Serum progesterone and human chorionic gonadotrophin measurements in the evaluation of ectopic pregnancy. Aust N Z J Obstet Gynaecol 1996;36:319-23.
273. Odell WD, Griffin J. Pulsatile secretion of human chorionic gonadotropin in normal adults. N Engl J Med 1987;317:1688-91.
274. Oepkes D, Seaward PG, Vandenbussche FP, Windrim R, Kingdom J, Beyene J, et al. Doppler ultrasonography versus amniocentesis to predict fetal anemia. N Engl J Med 2006;355:156-64.
275. Oulton M. The role of centrifugation in the measurement of surfactant in amniotic fluid. Am J Obstet Gynecol 1979;135: 337-43.
276. Oulton M, Martin TR, Faulkner GT, Stinson D, Johnson JP. Developmental study of a lamellar body fraction isolated from human amniotic fluid. Pediatr Res 1980;14:722-8.
277. Overgaard MT, Oxvig C, Christiansen M, Lawrence JB, Conover CA, Gleich GJ, et al. Messenger ribonucleic acid levels of pregnancy-associated plasma protein-A and the proform of eosinophil major basic protein: expression in human reproductive and nonreproductive tissues. Biol Reprod 1999;61:1083-9.
278. Owen WE, Rawlins ML, La'ulu SL, Roberts WL. Performance characteristics of the Access pregnancy-associated plasma protein-A assay. Clin Chim Acta 2008;398:165-7.
279. Owerbach D, Rutter WJ, Martial JA, Baxter JD, Shows TB. Genes for growth hormone, chorionic somatommammotropin, and growth hormone-like gene on chromosome 17 in humans. Science 1980;209: 289-92.
280. Ozturk M, Bellet D, Manil L, Hennen G, Frydman R, Wands J. Physiological studies of human chorionic gonadotropin (hCG), alpha hCG, and beta hCG as measured by specific monoclonal immunoradiometric assays. Endocrinology 1987;120:549-58.
281. Pajkrt E, Mol BW, Bleker OP, Bilardo CM. Pregnancy outcome and nuchal translucency measurements in fetuses with a normal karyotype. Prenat Diagn 1999;19:1104-8.
282. Palmer OM, Grenache DG, Gronowski AM. The NACB laboratory medicine practice guidelines for point-of-care reproductive testing. Point of Care 2007;6:265-72.
283. Palomaki GE, Bradley LA, Knight GJ, Craig WY, Haddow JE. Assigning risk for Smith-Lemli-Opitz syndrome as part of 2nd trimester screening for Down's syndrome. J Med Screen 2002;9:43-4.
284. Palomaki GE, Haddow JE, Knight GJ, Wald NJ, Kennard A, Canick JA, et al. Risk-based prenatal screening for trisomy 18 using alpha-fetoprotein, unconjugated oestriol and human chorionic gonadotropin. Prenat Diagn 1995;15:713-23.
285. Palomaki GE, Knight GJ, Haddow JE. Calculating amniotic fluid alpha-fetoprotein median values in the first trimester. Prenat Diagn 1993;13:887-9.
286. Palomaki GE, Knight GJ, Haddow JE, Canick JA, Saller DN Jr, Panizza DS. Prospective intervention trial of a screening protocol to identify fetal trisomy 18 using maternal serum alpha-fetoprotein, unconjugated oestriol, and human chorionic gonadotropin. Prenat Diagn 1992;12:925-30.
287. Palomaki GE, Lambert-Messerlian GM, Canick JA. A summary analysis of Down syndrome markers in the late first trimester. Adv Clin Chem 2007;43:177-210.
288. Palomaki GE, Neveux LM, Donnenfeld A, Lee JE, McDowell G, Canick JA, et al. Quality assessment of routine nuchal translucency measurements: a North American laboratory perspective. Genet Med 2008;10:131-8.
289. Palomaki GE, Steinort K, Knight GJ, Haddow JE. Comparing three screening strategies for combining first- and second-trimester Down syndrome markers. Obstet Gynecol 2006;107:367-75.
290. Palomaki GE, Williams J, Haddow JE. Comparing the observed and predicted effectiveness of folic acid fortification in preventing neural tube defects. J Med Screen 2003;10:52-3.
291. Pangas SA, Woodruff TK. Activin signal transduction pathways. Trends Endocrinol Metab 2000;11:309-14.
292. Parvin CA, Kaplan LA, Chapman JF, McManamon TG, Gronowski AM. Predicting respiratory distress syndrome using gestational age and fetal lung maturity by fluorescent polarization. Am J Obstet Gynecol 2005;192:199-207.
293. Peaceman AM, Andrews WW, Thorp JM, Cliver SP, Lukes A, Iams JD, et al. Fetal fibronectin as a predictor of preterm birth in patients with symptoms: a multicenter trial. Am J Obstet Gynecol 1997;177:13-8.
294. Pearlman ES, Baiocchi JM, Lease JA, Gilbert J, Cooper JH. Utility of a rapid lamellar body count in the assessment of fetal maturity. Am J Clin Pathol 1991;95:778-80.
295. Penney LL, Klenke WJ. Variability in unconjugated and total estriol in serum during normal third trimester pregnancy. Clin Chem 1980;26: 1800-3.
296. Perni SC, Predanic M, Kalish RB, Chervenak FA, Chasen ST. Clinical use of first-trimester aneuploidy screening in a United States population can replicate data from clinical trials. Am J Obstet Gynecol 2006;194:127-30.
297. Persson A, Chang D, Crouch E. Surfactant protein D is a divalent cation-dependent carbohydrate-binding protein. J Biol Chem 1990; 265:5755-60.
298. Petit FM, Hebert M, Picone O, Brisset S, Maurin ML, Parisot F, et al. A new mutation in the AFP gene responsible for a total absence of alpha feto-protein on second trimester maternal serum screening for Down syndrome. Eur J Hum Genet 2009;17:387-90.
299. Petraglia F, Sawchenko P, Lim AT, Rivier J, Vale W. Localization, secretion, and action of inhibin in human placenta. Science 1987;237: 187-9.
300. Petrunin DD, Griaznova IM, Petrunina Iu A, Tatarinov Iu S. Immunochemical identification of organ specific human placental alphal-globulin and its concentration in amniotic fluid. Akush Ginekol (Mosk) 1977:62-4.

301. Phillippe M, Acker D, Torday J, Schiff I, Frigoletto FD. The effects of vaginal contamination on two pulmonary phospholipid assays. J Reprod Med 1982;27:283-6.
302. Pinette MG. Prediction of risk for respiratory distress syndrome using gestational age and the TDx-FLM II assay (reply). Am J Obstet Gynecol 2003;189:1513-4.
303. Pinette MG, Blackstone J, Wax JR, Cartin A. Fetal lung maturity indices—a plea for gestational age-specific interpretation: a case report and discussion. Am J Obstet Gynecol 2002;187:1721-2.
304. Piper JM, Langer O. Does maternal diabetes delay fetal pulmonary maturity? Am J Obstet Gynecol 1993;168:783-6.
305. Pittaway DE, Reish RL, Wentz AC. Doubling times of human chorionic gonadotropin increase in early viable intrauterine pregnancies. Am J Obstet Gynecol 1985;152:299-302.
306. Policastro P, Ovitt CE, Hoshina M, Fukuoka H, Boothby MR, Boime I. The beta subunit of human chorionic gonadotropin is encoded by multiple genes. J Biol Chem 1983;258:11492-9.
307. Poon TC, Mok TS, Chan AT, Chan CM, Leong V, Tsui SH, et al. Quantification and utility of monosialylated alpha-fetoprotein in the diagnosis of hepatocellular carcinoma with nondiagnostic serum total alpha-fetoprotein. Clin Chem 2002;48:1021-7.
308. Qin QP, Christiansen M, Oxvig C, Pettersson K, Sottrup-Jensen L, Koch C, et al. Double-monoclonal immunofluorometric assays for pregnancy-associated plasma protein A/proeosinophil major basic protein (PAPP-A/proMBP) complex in first-trimester maternal serum screening for Down syndrome. Clin Chem 1997;43:2323-32.
309. Qin QP, Kokkala S, Lund J, Tamm N, Qin X, Lepantalo M, et al. Immunoassays developed for pregnancy-associated plasma protein-A (PAPP-A) in pregnancy may not recognize PAPP-A in acute coronary syndromes. Clin Chem 2006;52:398-404.
310. Qin QP, Nguyen TH, Christiansen M, Larsen SO, Norgaard-Pedersen B. Time-resolved immunofluorometric assay of pregnancy-associated plasma protein A in maternal serum screening for Down's syndrome in first trimester of pregnancy. Clin Chim Acta 1996;254:113-29.
311. Qin X, Wergedal JE, Rehage M, Tran K, Newton J, Lam P, et al. Pregnancy-associated plasma protein-A increases osteoblast proliferation in vitro and bone formation in vivo. Endocrinology 2006;147:5653-61.
312. Queenan JT, Thompson W, Whitfield CR, Shah SI. Amniotic fluid volumes in normal pregnancies. Am J Obstet Gynecol 1972;114:34-8.
313. Queenan JT, Tomai TP, Ural SH, King JC. Deviation in amniotic fluid optical density at a wavelength of 450 nm in Rh-immunized pregnancies from 14 to 40 weeks' gestation: a proposal for clinical management. Am J Obstet Gynecol 1993;168:1370-6.
314. Radwanska E, Frankenberg J, Allen EI. Plasma progesterone levels in normal and abnormal early human pregnancy. Fertil Steril 1978;30:398-402.
315. Rasmussen Loft AG, Nanchahal K, Cuckle HS, Wald NJ, Hulten M, Leedham P, et al. Amniotic fluid acetylcholinesterase in the prenatal diagnosis of open neural tube defects and abdominal wall defects: a comparison of gel electrophoresis and a monoclonal antibody immunoassay. Prenat Diagn 1990;10:449-59.
316. Resta RG. Changing demographics of advanced maternal age (AMA) and the impact on the predicted incidence of Down syndrome in the United States: implications for prenatal screening and genetic counseling. Am J Med Genet A 2005;133A:31-6.
317. Reyes H. The spectrum of liver and gastrointestinal disease seen in cholestasis of pregnancy. Gastroenterol Clin North Am 1992;21:905-21.
318. Risbridger GP, Schmitt JF, Robertson DM. Activins and inhibins in endocrine and other tumors. Endocr Rev 2001;22:836-58.
319. Robert MF, Neff RK, Hubbell JP, Taeusch HW, Avery ME. Association between maternal diabetes and the respiratory-distress syndrome in the newborn. N Engl J Med 1976;294:357-60.
320. Rolfes DB, Ishak KG. Liver disease in toxemia of pregnancy. Am J Gastroenterol 1986;81:1138-44.
321. Russell JC. A calibrated fluorescence polarization assay for assessment of fetal lung maturity. Clin Chem 1987;33:1177-84.
322. Russell JC, Cooper CM, Ketchum CH, Torday JS, Richardson DK, Holt JA, et al. Multicenter evaluation of TDx test for assessing fetal lung maturity. Clin Chem 1989;35:1005-10.
323. Rustgi VK, Hoofnagle JH. Viral hepatitis during pregnancy. Semin Liver Dis 1987;7:40-6.
324. Saad SA, Fadel HE, Fahmy K, Nelson GH, Moustafa M, Davis HC. The reliability and clinical use of a rapid phosphatidylglycerol assay in normal and diabetic pregnancies. Am J Obstet Gynecol 1987;157:1516-20.
325. Sairam MR, Bhargavi GN. A role for glycosylation of the alpha subunit in transduction of biological signal in glycoprotein hormones. Science 1985;229:65-7.
326. Sanchez-Ramos L, Delke I, Zamora J, Kaunitz AM. Fetal fibronectin as a short-term predictor of preterm birth in symptomatic patients: a meta-analysis. Obstet Gynecol 2009;114:631-40.
327. Sancken U, Bartels I. Biochemical screening for chromosomal disorders and neural tube defects (NTD): is adjustment of maternal alpha-fetoprotein (AFP) still appropriate in insulin-dependent diabetes mellitus (IDDM)? Prenat Diagn 2001;21:383-6.
328. Schielen PC, van Leeuwen-Spruijt M, Belmouden I, Elvers LH, Jonker M, Loeber JG. Multi-centre first-trimester screening for Down syndrome in the Netherlands in routine clinical practice. Prenat Diagn 2006;26:711-8.
329. Schneck P. [Selmar Aschheim (1878-1965) and Bernhard Zondek (1891-1966). On the fate of 2 Jewish physicians and researchers at the Berlin Charite Hospital]. Z Arztl Fortbild Qualitatssich 1997;91:187-94.
330. Schuchter K, Hafner E, Stangl G, Metzenbauer M, Hofinger D, Philipp K. The first trimester 'combined test' for the detection of Down syndrome pregnancies in 4939 unselected pregnancies. Prenat Diagn 2002;22:211-5.
331. Schwartz DB, Engle MJ, Brown DJ, Farrell PM. The stability of phospholipids in amniotic fluid. Am J Obstet Gynecol 1981;141:294-8.
332. Schwartz RO, Di Pietro DL. Beta-hCG as a diagnostic aid for suspected ectopic pregnancy. Obstet Gynecol 1980;56:197-203.
333. Sciarra JJ, Sherwood LM, Varma AA, Lundberg WB. Human placental lactogen (HPL) and placental weight. Am J Obstet Gynecol 1968;101:413-6.
334. Sekizawa A, Purwosunu Y, Matsuoka R, Koide K, Okazaki S, Farina A, et al. Recent advances in non-invasive prenatal DNA diagnosis through analysis of maternal blood. J Obstet Gynaecol Res 2007;33:747-64.
335. Shaw GM, Velie EM, Schaffer D. Risk of neural tube defect-affected pregnancies among obese women. JAMA 1996;275:1093-6.
336. Sher G, Statland BE. Assessment of fetal pulmonary maturity by the Lumadex Foam Stability Index Test. Obstet Gynecol 1983;61:444-9.
337. Sher G, Statland BE, Freer DE. Clinical evaluation of the quantitative foam stability index test. Obstet Gynecol 1980;55:617-20.
338. Sher G, Statland BE, Freer DE, Kraybill EN. Assessing fetal lung maturation by the foam stability index test. Obstet Gynecol 1978;52:673-7.
339. Sher G, Statland BE, Knutzen VK. Diagnostic reliability of the lecithin/sphingomyelin ratio assay and the quantitative foam stability index test: results of a comparative study. J Reprod Med 1982;27:51-5.
340. Sherwin JE, Lockitch G, Rosenthal P, Ashwood ER, Geaghan S, Magee LA. Maternal-fetal risk assessment and reference values in pregnancy. National Academy of Clinical Biochemistry Laboratory Medicine practice guidelines. Washington, DC: National Academy of Clinical Biochemistry, 2006:1-75.
341. Shinitzky M, Goldfisher A, Bruck A, Goldman B, Stern E, Barkai G, et al. A new method for assessment of fetal lung maturity. Br J Obstet Gynaecol 1976;83:838-44.
342. Shipp TD, Benacerraf BR. Second trimester ultrasound screening for chromosomal abnormalities. Prenat Diagn 2002;22:296-307.
343. Sibai BM. The HELLP syndrome (hemolysis, elevated liver enzymes, and low platelets): much ado about nothing? Am J Obstet Gynecol 1990;162:311-6.

344. Sigel CS, Grenache DG. Detection of unexpected isoforms of human chorionic gonadotropin by qualitative tests. Clin Chem 2007;53: 989-90.

345. Silva C, Sammel MD, Zhou L, Gracia C, Hummel AC, Barnhart K. Human chorionic gonadotropin profile for women with ectopic pregnancy. Obstet Gynecol 2006;107:605-10.

346. Simhan HN, Caritis SN. Prevention of preterm delivery. N Engl J Med 2007;357:477-87.

347. Simpson JL. Genetic counseling and prenatal diagnosis. In: Gabbe SG, Niebyl JR, Simpson JL, eds. Obstetrics: normal and problem pregnancies, 2nd edition. New York, NY: Churchill Livingstone, 1991:269-98.

348. Singh PK, Parvin CA, Gronowski AM. Establishment of reference intervals for markers of fetal thyroid status in amniotic fluid. J Clin Endocrinol Metab 2003;88:4175-9.

349. Smets EM, Dijkstra-Lagemaat JE, Blankenstein MA. Influence of blood collection in plastic vs. glass evacuated serum-separator tubes on hormone and tumour marker levels. Clin Chem Lab Med 2004;42: 435-9.

350. Snyder JA, Haymond S, Parvin CA, Gronowski AM, Grenache DG. Diagnostic considerations in the measurement of human chorionic gonadotropin in aging women. Clin Chem 2005;51:1830-5.

351. Snyder JM, Mendelson CR, Johnston JM. The morphology of lung development in the human fetus. In: Nelson GH, ed. Pulmonary development: transition from intrauterine to extrauterine life, New York: Marcel Dekker, 1985:19-46.

352. Spencer CA, Allen VM, Flowerdew G, Dooley K, Dodds L. Low levels of maternal serum PAPP-A in early pregnancy and the risk of adverse outcomes. Prenat Diagn 2008;28:1029-36.

353. Spencer K. First trimester maternal serum screening for Down's syndrome: an evaluation of the DPC Immulite 2000 free beta-hCG and pregnancy-associated plasma protein-A assays. Ann Clin Biochem 2005;42:30-40.

354. Spencer K. The influence of different sample collection types on the levels of markers used for Down's syndrome screening as measured by the Kryptor Immunosassay system. Ann Clin Biochem 2003;40: 166-8.

355. Spencer K, Kagan KO, Nicolaides KH. Screening for trisomy 21 in twin pregnancies in the first trimester: an update of the impact of chorionicity on maternal serum markers. Prenat Diagn 2008;28:49-52.

356. Spencer K, Ong CY, Liao AW, Nicolaides KH. The influence of ethnic origin on first trimester biochemical markers of chromosomal abnormalities. Prenat Diagn 2000;20:491-4.

357. Spillman T, Cotton DB, Lynn SC Jr, Bretaudiere JP. Influence of phospholipid saturation on classical thin-layer chromatographic detection methods and its effect on amniotic fluid lecithin/ sphingomyelin ratio determinations. Clin Chem 1983;29:250-5.

358. Steegers-Theunissen RP, Boers GH, Blom HJ, Nijhuis JG, Thomas CM, Borm GF, et al. Neural tube defects and elevated homocysteine levels in amniotic fluid. Am J Obstet Gynecol 1995;172:1436-41.

359. Steegers EA, von Dadelszen P, Duvekot JJ, Pijnenborg R. Pre-eclampsia. Lancet 2010;376;631-44.

360. Steinfeld JD, Samuels P, Bulley MA, Cohen AW, Goodman DB, Senior MB. The utility of the TDx test in the assessment of fetal lung maturity. Obstet Gynecol 1992;79:460-4.

361. Stenman UH, Alfthan H, Ranta T, Vartiainen E, Jalkanen J, Seppala M. Serum levels of human chorionic gonadotropin in nonpregnant women and men are modulated by gonadotropin-releasing hormone and sex steroids. J Clin Endocrinol Metab 1987;64:730-6.

362. Stewart BK, Nazar-Stewart V, Toivola B. Biochemical discrimination of pathologic pregnancy from early, normal intrauterine gestation in symptomatic patients. Am J Clin Pathol 1995;103:386-90.

363. Storring PL, Gaines-Das RE, Bangham DR. International reference preparation of human chorionic gonadotrophin for immunoassay: potency estimates in various bioassay and protein binding assay systems; and international reference preparations of the alpha and beta subunits of human chorionic gonadotrophin for immunoassay. J Endocrinol 1980;84:295-310.

364. Sturgeon CM, Berger P, Bidart JM, Birken S, Burns C, Norman RJ, et al. Differences in recognition of the 1st WHO international reference reagents for hCG-related isoforms by diagnostic immunoassays for human chorionic gonadotropin. Clin Chem 2009;55:1484-91.

365. Szallasi A, Gronowski AM, Eby CS. Lamellar body count in amniotic fluid: a comparative study of four different hematology analyzers. Clin Chem 2003;49:994-7.

366. Tabor A, Vestergaard CH, Lidegaard O. Fetal loss rate after chorionic villus sampling and amniocentesis: an 11-year national registry study. Ultrasound Obstet Gynecol 2009;34:19-24.

367. Tabsh KM, Brinkman CR 3rd, Bashore RA. Lecithin:sphingomyelin ratio in pregnancies complicated by insulin-dependent diabetes mellitus. Obstet Gynecol 1982;59:353-8.

368. Taipale P, Hiilesmaa V, Salonen R, Ylostalo P. Increased nuchal translucency as a marker for fetal chromosomal defects. N Engl J Med 1997;337:1654-8.

369. Tait JF, Foerder CA, Ashwood ER, Benedetti TJ. Prospective clinical evaluation of an improved fluorescence polarization assay for predicting fetal lung maturity. Clin Chem 1987;33:554-8.

370. Tait JF, Franklin RW, Simpson JB, Ashwood ER. Improved fluorescence polarization assay for use in evaluating fetal lung maturity. I. Development of the assay procedure. Clin Chem 1986;32:248-54.

371. Talmadge K, Vamvakopoulos NC, Fiddes JC. Evolution of the genes for the beta subunits of human chorionic gonadotropin and luteinizing hormone. Nature 1984;307:37-40.

372. Thaler MM, Park CK, Landers DV, Wara DW, Houghton M, Veereman-Wauters G, et al. Vertical transmission of hepatitis C virus. Lancet 1991;338:17-8.

373. Thirunavukarasu P, Stephenson T, Forray J, Stanton PG, Groome N, Wallace E, et al. Changes in molecular weight forms of inhibin A and pro-alpha C in maternal serum during human pregnancy. J Clin Endocrinol Metab 2001;86:5794-804.

374. Thornburg LL, Knight KM, Peterson CJ, McCall KB, Mooney RA, Pressman EK. Maternal serum alpha-fetoprotein values in type 1 and type 2 diabetic patients. Am J Obstet Gynecol 2008;199:135 e1-5.

375. Tietz NW. Comparative study of immunologic and biologic pregnancy tests in early pregnancy. Obstet Gynecol 1965;25:197-200.

376. Tint GS, Irons M, Elias ER, Batta AK, Frieden R, Chen TS, et al. Defective cholesterol biosynthesis associated with the Smith-Lemli-Opitz syndrome. N Engl J Med 1994;330:107-13.

377. Torday J, Carson L, Lawson EE. Saturated phosphatidylcholine in amniotic fluid and prediction of the respiratory-distress syndrome. N Engl J Med 1979;301:1013-8.

378. Toriello HV, Higgins JV. Occurrence of neural tube defects among first-, second-, and third-degree relatives of probands: results of a United States study. Am J Med Genet 1983;15:601-6.

379. Treem WR. Mitochondrial fatty acid oxidation and acute fatty liver of pregnancy. Semin Gastrointest Dis 2002;13:55-66.

380. Tsai MY, Cain M, Josephson MW. Improved thin-layer chromatography of disaturated phosphatidylcholine in amniotic fluid. Clin Chem 1981;27:239-42.

381. Tsai MY, Shultz EK, Williams PP, Bendel R, Butler J, Farb H, et al. Assay of disaturated phosphatidylcholine in amniotic fluid as a test of fetal lung maturity: experience with 2000 analyses. Clin Chem 1987; 33:1648-51.

382. Tul N, Spencer K, Noble P, Chan C, Nicolaides K. Screening for trisomy 18 by fetal nuchal translucency and maternal serum free beta-hCG and PAPP-A at 10-14 weeks of gestation. Prenat Diagn 1999;19:1035-42.

383. U.S. Food and Drug Administration. Food standards: amendment of standards of identity for enrichment of grain products to require addition of folic acid. Vol 61: Federal Register 1996:8781-97.

384. Vaitukaitis JL, Braunstein GD, Ross GT. A radioimmunoassay which specifically measures human chorionic gonadotropin in the presence of human luteinizing hormone. Am J Obstet Gynecol 1972;113:751-8.

385. van Voorst tot Voorst EJ. Effects of centrifugation, storage, and contamination of amniotic fluid on its total phospholipid content. Clin Chem 1980;26:232-4.
386. Wagstaff TI, Whyley GA, Freedman G. Factors influencing the measurement of the lecithin sphingomyelin ration in amniotic fluid. J Obstet Gynaecol Br Commonw 1974;81:264-77.
387. Wald N. Folic acid and the prevention of neural tube defects. Ann N Y Acad Sci 1993;678:112-29.
388. Wald N, Cuckle H, Nanchahal K. Amniotic fluid acetylcholinesterase measurement in the prenatal diagnosis of open neural tube defects: second report of the Collaborative Acetylcholinesterase Study. Prenat Diagn 1989;9:813-29.
389. Wald N, Cuckle H, Wu TS, George L. Maternal serum unconjugated oestriol and human chorionic gonadotrophin levels in twin pregnancies: implications for screening for Down's syndrome. Br J Obstet Gynaecol 1991;98:905-8.
390. Wald NJ, Cuckle H, Brock JH, Peto R, Polani PE, Woodford FP. Maternal serum-alpha-fetoprotein measurement in antenatal screening for anencephaly and spina bifida in early pregnancy: report of U.K. collaborative study on alpha-fetoprotein in relation to neural-tube defects. Lancet 1977;1:1323-32.
391. Wald NJ, Cuckle HS. Estimating an individual's risk of having a fetus with open spina bifida and the value of repeat alpha-fetoprotein testing. J Epidemiol Community Health 1982;36:87-95.
392. Wald NJ, Cuckle HS, Densem JW, Nanchahal K, Canick JA, Haddow JE, et al. Maternal serum unconjugated oestriol as an antenatal screening test for Down's syndrome. Br J Obstet Gynaecol 1988;95: 334-41.
393. Wald NJ, Cuckle HS, Densem JW, Nanchahal K, Royston P, Chard T, et al. Maternal serum screening for Down's syndrome in early pregnancy. BMJ 1988;297:883-7.
394. Wald NJ, Hackshaw A, Stone R, Densem J. Serum alpha-fetoprotein and neural tube defects in the first trimester of pregnancy. MRC Vitamin Study Research Group. Prenat Diagn 1993;13:1047-50.
395. Wald NJ, Hackshaw AK. Combining ultrasound and biochemistry in first-trimester screening for Down's syndrome. Prenat Diagn 1997;17: 821-9.
396. Wald NJ, Huttly WJ, Bestwick JP. Inhibin-A concentrations between 14 and 22 weeks of gestation. Prenat Diagn 2008;28:360-1.
397. Wald NJ, Huttly WJ, Hackshaw AK. Antenatal screening for Down's syndrome with the quadruple test. Lancet 2003;361:835-6.
398. Wald NJ, Kennard A, Hackshaw A, McGuire A. Antenatal screening for Down's syndrome. J Med Screen 1997;4:181-246.
399. Wald NJ, Rodeck C, Hackshaw AK, Rudnicka A. SURUSS in perspective. Semin Perinatol 2005;29:225-35.
400. Wald NJ, Rodeck C, Hackshaw AK, Walters J, Chitty L, Mackinson AM. First and second trimester antenatal screening for Down's syndrome: the results of the Serum, Urine and Ultrasound Screening Study (SURUSS). J Med Screen 2003;10:56-104.
401. Wald NJ, Rudnicka AR, Bestwick JP. Sequential and contingent prenatal screening for Down syndrome. Prenat Diagn 2006;26:769-77.
402. Wald NJ, Watt HC, Hackshaw AK. Integrated screening for Down's syndrome on the basis of tests performed during the first and second trimesters. N Engl J Med 1999;341:461-7.
403. Waller DK, Mills JL, Simpson JL, Cunningham GC, Conley MR, Lassman MR, et al. Are obese women at higher risk for producing malformed offspring? Am J Obstet Gynecol 1994;170:541-8.
404. Wapner R, Thom E, Simpson JL, Pergament E, Silver R, Filkins K, et al. First-trimester screening for trisomies 21 and 18. N Engl J Med 2003;349:1405-13.
405. Wathen NC, Campbell DJ, Kitau MJ, Chard T. Alphafetoprotein levels in amniotic fluid from 8 to 18 weeks of pregnancy. Br J Obstet Gynaecol 1993;100:380-2.
406. Watt HC, Wald NJ, Smith D, Kennard A, Densem J. Effect of allowing for ethnic group in prenatal screening for Down's syndrome. Prenat Diagn 1996;16:691-8.
407. Wehmann RE, Nisula BC. Metabolic and renal clearance rates of purified human chorionic gonadotropin. J Clin Invest 1981;68:184-94.
408. Weinbaum PJ, Richardson D, Schwartz JS, Gabbe SG. Amniostat FLM: a new technique for detection of phosphatidylglycerol in amniotic fluid. Am J Perinatol 1985;2:88-92.
409. Weissenbacher T, Bruning A, Kimmich T, Makovitzky J, Gingelmaier A, Mylonas I. Immunohistochemical labeling of the inhibin/activin betaC subunit in normal human placental tissue and chorionic carcinoma cell lines. J Histochem Cytochem 2010;58:751-7.
410. Whittington J, Fantz CR, Gronowski AM, McCudden C, Mullins R, Sokoll L, et al. The analytical specificity of human chorionic gonadotropin assays determined using WHO International Reference Reagents. Clin Chim Acta 2010;411:81-5.
411. Whitworth NS, Magann EF, Morrison JC. Evaluation of fetal lung maturity in diamniotic twins. Am J Obstet Gynecol 1999;180:1438-41.
412. Wijnberger LD, Huisjes AJ, Voorbij HA, Franx A, Bruinse HW, Mol BW. The accuracy of lamellar body count and lecithin/sphingomyelin ratio in the prediction of neonatal respiratory distress syndrome: a meta-analysis. BJOG 2001;108:583-8.
413. Wilcox AJ, Baird DD, Dunson D, McChesney R, Weinberg CR. Natural limits of pregnancy testing in relation to the expected menstrual period. JAMA 2001;286:1759-61.
414. Wojdemann KR, Larsen SO, Rode L, Shalmi A, Sundberg K, Christiansen M, et al. First trimester Down syndrome screening: distribution of markers and comparison of assays for quantification of pregnancy-associated plasma protein-A. Scand J Clin Lab Invest 2006;66:101-11.
415. Wojdemann KR, Larsen SO, Shalmi A, Sundberg K, Christiansen M, Tabor A. First trimester screening for Down syndrome and assisted reproduction: no basis for concern. Prenat Diagn 2001;21:563-5.
416. Wong SS, Schenkel O, Qutishat A. Strategic utilization of fetal lung maturity tests. Scand J Clin Lab Invest 1996;56:525-32.
417. Wright CF, Burton H. The use of cell-free fetal nucleic acids in maternal blood for non-invasive prenatal diagnosis. Hum Reprod Update 2009;15:139-51.
418. Wu CH, Mennuti MT, Mikhail G. Free and protein-bound steroids in amniotic fluid of midpregnancy. Am J Obstet Gynecol 1979;133: 666-72.
419. Wu JT, Roan Y, Knight JA. Serum AFP levels in normal infants: their clinical and physiological significance. In: Mizejewski G, Porter IH, eds. Alpha-fetoprotein and congenital disorders, Orlando, Fla: Academic Press, 1985:111-21.

CHAPTER 58

Newborn Screening and Inborn Errors of Metabolism

*Marzia Pasquali, Ph.D., F.A.C.M.G., and Nicola Longo, M.D., Ph.D.**

An inborn error of metabolism (IEM) is a genetically determined biochemical disorder that affects an individual's ability to convert nutrients or to use them for energy production. Typically, IEMs present in the newborn period or in infancy. Some diseases, however, such as fatty acid oxidation defects or milder variants of classic metabolic disorders, may not be detected until adulthood. Despite the long asymptomatic period, their consequences can still be devastating and may lead to death. Therefore identification and treatment of these diseases before irreversible damage occurs is critical. Clinical biochemical genetics is the discipline that deals with the diagnosis and treatment of patients with inborn errors of metabolism. In contrast to other, more common diseases, treatment of IEMs is lifelong and requires frequent monitoring. The biochemical diagnosis of IEMs and treatment monitoring involve analysis of (1) metabolites, (2) enzymatic activity, and/or (3) molecular structure. Because of technological advances [such as the introduction of tandem mass spectrometry (MS/MS), allowing the simultaneous detection of multiple analytes] and improved outcomes of patients with IEMs identified and treated early, many IEMs are now included in newborn screening programs.

CLINICAL PRESENTATION

Inborn errors of metabolism, which are due to impaired activity of enzymes, transporters, or cofactors, result in accumulation of abnormal metabolites (substrates) proximal to the metabolic block, or lack of necessary products. Figure 58-1 shows a hypothetical metabolic pathway in which the substrate A needs to be converted into the product D, with arrows representing individual enzymes. If an enzyme is defective (vertical rectangle), the concentration of substrate A will increase and the concentration of product D will decrease. It is then possible that high concentrations of substrate A will accumulate and become a source of substrate for enzymes not usually involved in its metabolism, thereby producing abnormal byproducts (E and F) through alternative pathways. Accumulation of specific metabolites and their byproducts within organs and tissues and/or the lack of reaction products are the chemical bases of the pathology observed in different inborn errors of metabolism. At the same time, measurement of some of these metabolites or their byproducts serves as the basis of biochemical diagnostic testing for inborn errors of metabolism and early detection by newborn screening programs.

Symptoms of inborn errors of metabolism usually appear early in infancy, although several types become symptomatic in late childhood or adulthood. Signs and symptoms include (1) failure to thrive, (2) seizures, (3) mental retardation, (4) organ failure, and even (5) death. Inborn errors of metabolism have been divided into three broad categories, based on the effects of their metabolic derangement[55]:

1. Intoxication effect: IEMs in this category are the result of metabolites accumulating in the body that produce a toxic effect on different organs. The patient may become acutely ill after a symptom-free period, usually 24 to 72 hours, and concomitantly with ingestion of metabolites that are not metabolized, such as proteins or sugars. Types of IEMs that belong in this group include (1) aminoacidopathies (e.g., phenylketonuria, maple syrup urine disease, homocystinuria), (2) urea cycle defects (e.g., citrullinemia, argininosuccinic aciduria, ornithine transcarbamylase deficiency), (3) organic acidemias (e.g., propionic acidemia, methylmalonic acidemia, glutaric acidemia type I), and (4) disorders of sugar metabolism (galactosemia, hereditary fructose intolerance). Some of these disorders, such as phenylketonuria, affect primarily the brain, causing severe mental retardation but without acute decompensation. In other

**The authors gratefully acknowledge the contributions of Drs. Piero Rinaldo, Si Houn Hahn, and Dietrich Matern to the previous edition of this text, on which portions of this chapter are based.*

disorders (e.g., organic acidemias), symptoms appear shortly after protein intake (usually after the first few feedings) and include vomiting, lethargy, seizures, and coma leading rapidly to death if not recognized and treated appropriately.

2. Energy deficiency: Symptoms of disorders in this category are due to impaired energy production. In some cases, patients may be asymptomatic for a long time, until energy requirements are increased as the result of involuntary fasting, illness, infection, or strenuous exercise. A classic example of these disorders involves fatty acid oxidation (e.g., medium chain acyl–coenzyme A [CoA] dehydrogenase deficiency, very long chain acyl-CoA dehydrogenase deficiency, carnitine uptake defect, carnitine palmitoyl transferase deficiency I and II), although in this case, the block in the metabolic pathway, in addition to impairment in energy production, leads to the accumulation of intermediates that cause an intoxication effect.[52] Other diseases in this group include glycogen storage disorders, in which hypoglycemia can occur in the presence or absence of any stress, mitochondrial disorders, and congenital lactic acidosis, in which the clinical course is progressive even in the absence of triggering conditions.[43]

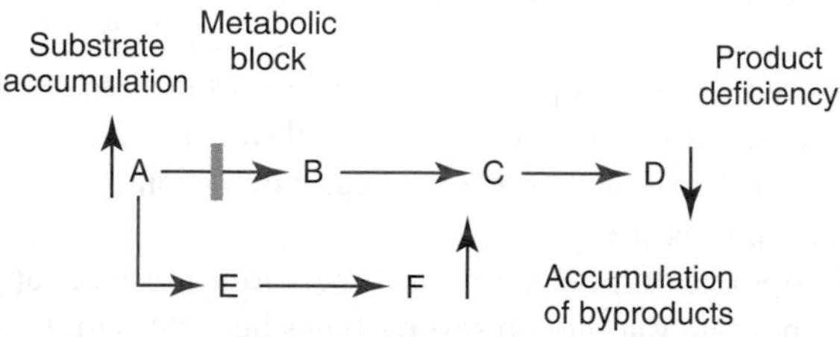

Figure 58-1 Schematic of metabolic pathway. The substrate *A* is converted by a series of reactions into product *D*. If one of the enzymes *(red arrows)* is defective (metabolic block), the substrate of the reaction will accumulate (*A* in this case) and can enter alternative pathways of metabolism, leading to the formation of byproducts (*E* and *F* in this case). At the same time, the concentration of the product of the reaction *(D)* will decrease.

3. Disorders of complex molecules: These disorders result from defects in the synthesis or catabolism of complex molecules. They are progressive, are independent of intercurrent events, and are not related to food intake. The metabolism of complex molecules is altered in all (1) lysosomal disorders, (2) peroxisomal disorders, and (3) disorders of intracellular trafficking and processing. For some of these disorders, a therapy is now available that is usually more effective if initiated before irreversible organ damage has occurred. For this reason, some of these conditions are also being considered for newborn screening.

DIAGNOSIS

With few exceptions, the diagnosis of IEM is primarily a laboratory process. For example, routine laboratory tests in the symptomatic IEM patient and a high index of suspicion often point the clinician toward a specific IEM. For example, (1) hyperammonemia without metabolic acidosis suggests a defect of the urea cycle; (2) hypoketotic hypoglycemia usually with hyperammonemia to various degrees suggests fatty acid oxidation impairment; and (3) hyperammonemia with metabolic acidosis and ketosis is suggestive of an organic acidemia (Table 58-1). The diagnosis of IEMs requires specific tests that usually are performed in Biochemical Genetics Laboratories. The core group of tests necessary for the diagnosis of IEMs includes (1) amino acid analysis in plasma, urine (in few cases), and cerebrospinal fluid (in even fewer cases), (2) organic acid analysis in urine, and (3) carnitine and acylcarnitine profile in plasma.

In contrast to common chemistry tests, biochemical genetics tests are complex and require specialized personnel to perform the tests and interpret the results. For example, it is recommended that each profile be interpreted in the context of clinical history, physical signs, and other laboratory studies by a board-certified doctoral scientist or physician with specialized training in metabolic disease and analytical testing. When the results are suggestive of a metabolic disorder, interpretation should include information about the disease and should suggest additional tests to confirm the diagnosis, when appropriate.

TABLE 58-1 Biochemical Findings in Disorders of Amino Acid, Fatty Acid, and Organic Acid Metabolism

	Organic Acidurias	Fatty Acid Oxidation Disorders	Urea Cycle Disorders	MSUD	NKHG
Neurologic distress	I	I/ED	I	I	I
Metabolic acidosis	+++	–	+	+	–
Ketonuria (ketone bodies)	+++	–	–	+	–
Hyperammonemia	+	+	+++	–	–
Hypoglycemia (fasting)	+	+++	–	–	–
Lactic acidemia	++	+	–	–	–

ED, Energy deficiency; *I,* intoxication type of neurologic distress (see text); *MSUD,* maple syrup urine disease; *NKHG,* nonketotic hyperglycinemia.
+, possibly present; ++, frequently present; +++, typically present with high diagnostic significance; –, not typically present.

Some metabolic disorders are treated by dietary modifications usually consisting of a life-long dietary regimen in which the nutrient in question is restricted, with supplementation of vitamins, cofactors, and, in some cases, medications. Because of the excellent outcomes of metabolic patients when treatment is initiated before symptoms or any damage has occurred, a major focus of Biochemical Genetics is on early identification of IEMs, prenatally and especially in the newborn period, through universal newborn screening.

Prenatal Diagnosis

Despite constant progress in medical treatment, several IEMs result in severe morbidity and inevitable mortality early in life. Most of these disorders are inherited as autosomal recessive traits (Table 58-2); therefore the recurrence risk in subsequent pregnancies of the same couple is 25%. Genetic counseling of parents consists of a balanced assessment of (1) familial risk factors (parental consanguinity and ethnic origin), (2) risk of pregnancy loss as a consequence of the sampling procedure [0.5 to 1% by chorionic villus sampling (CVS), 0.5% by amniocentesis], (3) risk of maternal complications,[53] (4) clinical validity of the prenatal test, (5) the burden of the disease, and (6) variable phenotypic expression of the disease even within the same family.

Methods used for prenatal diagnosis of IEMs have different requirements in terms of timing, sample collection, and options for independent confirmation. CVS is performed at 10 to 13 weeks' gestational age, has a higher risk of fetal loss as compared with classic amniocentesis, and might not provide accurate results because of possible contamination with maternal tissue. Alternatively, certain enzymes, such as those of the glycine cleavage pathway defective in glycine encephalopathy, are expressed only in cells of chorionic villi, rendering this procedure the only possibility when DNA testing is not possible.[4] Amniocentesis is performed later in pregnancy (14 to 20 weeks) and provides both amniocytes and amniotic fluid to be used for independent and complementary diagnostic methods. Reliance on separate tests based on independent methods performed by laboratories with adequate prior experience is strongly encouraged to avoid incorrect or inconclusive results. In some IEMs (e.g., organic acidemias), amniotic fluid is tested for the presence or absence of specific metabolites, in addition to providing amniocytes for enzyme assay, DNA analysis, or both. The combination of at least two independent tests (e.g., enzyme assay + DNA; metabolite analysis + enzyme or DNA) enhances confidence in establishing a prenatal diagnosis. Before entertaining a prenatal diagnosis, one should ensure that the proband (individual first brought to medical attention in whom the diagnosis was established) related to the index case has a diagnosis confirmed by traditional methods, including enzymology when appropriate. If DNA analysis is considered, mutations of the index case should be known and confirmed as causative of the disease. Major advantages of direct metabolite analysis in amniotic fluid include independence from tissue expression and rapid turnaround time. However, analysis of direct metabolites in amniotic fluid has been reported for only a very limited number of diseases.

Newborn Screening

Newborn screening is a public health activity aimed at early identification of conditions for which timely intervention is expected to result in elimination or reduction of morbidity, mortality, and disabilities. It is an important and effective component of preventive medicine. Originally instituted in the 1960s for the early detection of phenylketonuria (PKU), the number of diseases screened for in the newborn period has dramatically increased with the introduction of MS/MS multiplex analyses of acylcarnitine and amino acid profiles.[13] Inclusion of IEMs as a whole in newborn screening panels has been controversial, because with few exceptions, their incidence, natural history, and prospective screening experience, as well as the effectiveness of treatment, have not yet been defined.[10] However, implementation of this expanded screening allows collection of these data leading to a better understanding of these diseases. The complexity of the interpretation of MS/MS newborn screening results has prompted the development of algorithms for proper confirmatory testing and differential diagnosis of all detectable IEMs (http://www.acmg.net/resources/policies/ACT/condition-analyte-links.htm/accessed September 29, 2011).

Although metabolic disorders identified by MS/MS represent the largest group of diseases identifiable by newborn screening, other IEMs and endocrine and hematologic disorders (such as galactosemia, biotinidase deficiency, cystic fibrosis, congenital hypothyroidism, congenital adrenal hyperplasia, and hemoglobinopathies) are identifiable through more traditional screening methods (e.g., enzyme assays, immunoassays, electrophoresis). Advances in therapeutic interventions for IEMs are continuously expanding the role of newborn screening. Newborn screening does not identify all metabolic disorders, and some patients can be missed by newborn screening. Therefore a symptomatic patient, at any age, should be investigated despite normal newborn screening results.

Evaluation of Symptomatic Patients

The most informative samples are collected from patients during acute metabolic decompensation. When possible, urine and blood should be collected at the same time. In several diseases, especially in fatty acid oxidation disorders, diagnostic abnormalities may not be detected when the patient has recovered from the acute episode. Urine and plasma/serum samples are stored at −20 °C until the need for specialized tests has been determined. Quantitative profiling of amino acids, carnitine, acylcarnitines, and fatty acids in plasma, and organic acids and acylglycines in urine, is the biochemical investigation necessary to diagnose these disorders. Alternatively, a blood spot on filter paper may provide enough material for one or more of the investigations described in this chapter. In case of death, collection of body fluid and tissue should be secured according to available protocols.[12,54]

Text continued on page 2052

TABLE 58-2 Clinical and Laboratory Characteristics of Disorders of Amino Acid Metabolism

Common Name	OMIM* No.	Inheritance	Enzyme/Transport Defect	Incidence (USA)	Major Clinical Features	Major Biochemical Marker(s)
Disorders of Aromatic Amino Acid Metabolism						
Classic phenylketonuria (PKU)	261600	AR	Phenylalanine hydroxylase	>1:25,000	Mental retardation, fair complexion and pigmentation	Phenylalanine (B), phenylpyruvic (U), phenyllactic (U), 2-OH phenylacetic (U)
Defect of biopterin cofactor biosynthesis	233910	AR	GTP cyclohydrolase I	<1:100,000	Progressive mental retardation, seizures, muscle tone abnormalities, microcephaly, movement disorder	Phenylalanine (B), low neopterin and biopterin (U), low 5-HIAA and HVA (CSF)
Defect of biopterin cofactor biosynthesis	261640	AR	6-Pyruvoyltetrahydropterin synthase	<1:100,000	Progressive mental retardation, seizures, muscle tone abnormalities, microcephaly, movement disorder	Phenylalanine (B), high neopterin, low biopterin (U), low 5-HIAA, HVA (CSF)
Defect of biopterin cofactor regeneration	261630	AR	Dihydropterin reductase (DHPR)	<1:100,000	Progressive mental retardation, spasticity, dystonia, myoclonus, microcephaly, movement disorder	Phenylalanine (B), high biopterin (U), low 5-HIAA, HVA (CSF), low DHPR activity in DBS
Defect of biopterin cofactor regeneration	264070	AR	Pterin-4a-carbinolamine dehydratase	<1:100,000	Transient muscle tone abnormalities, long-term outcome usually benign	Phenylalanine (B), high neopterin and primapterin (U)
Tyrosinemia type I	276700	AR	Fumarylacetoacetase	<1:100,000	Cirrhosis, hepatocellular carcinoma, rickets, renal Fanconi syndrome, neuropathic pain	Tyrosine (B), succinylacetone (U), 4-OH phenylpyruvic, 4-OH phenyllactic (U)
Tyrosinemia type II	276600	AR	Tyrosine aminotransferase	<1:100,000	Corneal ulcers, keratosis on palms and soles, photophobia, pain to extremities	Tyrosine (B), 4-OH phenylpyruvic, 4-OH phenyllactic (U)
Tyrosinemia type III	276710	AR	4-Hydroxyphenylpyruvate dioxygenase	<1:100,000	Developmental delay	Tyrosine (B), 4-OH phenylpyruvic, 4-OH phenyllactic (U)

Hawkinsinuria	140350	AD	4-Hydroxyphenylpyruvate dioxygenase	<1:100,000	Failure to thrive, hepatocellular dysfunction	2-Cystenyl-1,4-dihydrocyclohexenylacetate (U), 4-hydroxycyclohexylacetic acid (U)
Disorders of Branched-Chain Amino Acid Metabolism						
Maple syrup urine disease (MSUD IA, IB, II)	248600	AR	Branched-chain ketoacid dehydrogenase complex	<1:100,000 (1:378 Mennonite)	Hypotonia, lethargy, seizures, coma, vomiting, ketosis, pancreatitis, brain edema	Branched-chain amino acids (B), allo isoleucine (B), branched-chain 2-ketoacids, and branched-chain 2-hydroxy acids (U)
E3 deficiency	246900	AR	Dihydrolipoyl dehydrogenase (E3)	<1:100,000	Failure to thrive, hypotonia, developmental delay, seizures, coma, lactic acidosis, hypoglycemia	Branched-chain amino acids (B), allo isoleucine (B), lactic and pyruvic acids (B,U), 2-ketoglutaric acid, branched-chain 2-ketoacids, and branched-chain 2-hydroxy acids (U)
Disorders of Sulfur Amino Acid Metabolism						
Hypermethioninemia	250850	AR	Methionine adenosyltransferase	<1:100,000	Fetid breath, demyelination	Methionine (B)
S-Adenosylhomocysteine hydrolase deficiency	180960	AR	*S*-Adenosylhomocysteine hydrolase	Unknown	Developmental delay, hypotonia, hepatocellular dysfunction, white matter atrophy, abnormal myelination	Methionine (B), total plasma homocysteine, mildly elevated (B), elevated *S*-adenosylhomocysteine, and *S*-adenosylmethionine (B)
Glycine-*N*-methyltransferase deficiency	606664	AR	Glycine *N*-methyltransferase	Unknown	Hepatomegaly	Methionine (B), *S*-adenosylmethionine (B)
Homocystinuria	236200	AR	Cystathionine beta-synthase	<1:100,000	Mental retardation, ectopia lentis, skeletal anomalies	Free homocystine, total homocysteine, and methionine (B,U)
Sulfite oxidase deficiency	272300	AR	Sulfite oxidase	<1:100,000	Mental retardation, seizures, ectopia lentis, dysmorphic features, muscle tone abnormalities	*S*-sulfocysteine and taurine (B,U); low cystine (B,U)

Continued

TABLE 58-2 Clinical and Laboratory Characteristics of Disorders of Amino Acid Metabolism—cont'd

Common Name	OMIM* No.	Inheritance	Enzyme/Transport Defect	Incidence (USA)	Major Clinical Features	Major Biochemical Marker(s)
Molybdenum cofactor deficiency	252150	AR	Sulfite oxidase, xanthine dehydrogenase, aldehyde oxidase	<1 : 100,000	Mental retardation, seizures, ectopia lentis, dysmorphic features, muscle tone abnormalities	*S*-sulfocysteine and taurine (B,U); low cystine (B,U); elevated hypoxanthine and xanthine (U); low uric acid (B)
Urea Cycle Disorders						
N-Acetylglutamate synthase deficiency	237310	AR	*N*-Acetylglutamate synthase	<1 : 100,000	Hyperammonemia, lethargy, hypothermia, apnea, brain edema, coma	Glutamine, alanine (B), low citrulline and arginine (B)
CPS-I deficiency	237300	AR	Carbamoylphosphate I synthetase	<1 : 100,000	Hyperammonemia, lethargy, hypothermia, apnea, brain edema, coma	Glutamine, alanine (B), low citrulline and arginine (B)
OTC deficiency	311250	X-linked	Ornithine transcarbamylase	>1 : 50,000	Hyperammonemia, lethargy, hypothermia, apnea, brain edema, coma	Orotic (U), glutamine, alanine (B), low citrulline, arginine (B)
Citrullinemia	603470	AR	Argininosuccinate synthase	>1 : 75,000	Hyperammonemia, lethargy, hypothermia, apnea, brain edema, coma	Citrulline (B), orotic (U)
Citrullinemia type II (citrin deficiency)	603471 (adult onset); 605814 (neonatal onset)	AR	Aspartate/glutamate mitochondrial exchanger	<1 : 100,000	Cholestatic jaundice, hepatocellular dysfunction, episodic hyperammonemia, neurologic/psychiatric symptoms	Citrulline, methionine, lysine (B), orotic (U), elevated galactose (B) in neonatal onset
Argininosuccinic acidemia	207900	AR	Argininosuccinate lyase	<1 : 100,000	Hyperammonemia, lethargy, hypothermia, apnea, brain edema, coma, trichorrhexis nodosa	Argininosuccinic (B,U), citrulline (B), low arginine (B)
Argininemia	207800	AR	Arginase	<1 : 100,000	Progressive spasticity, mental retardation	Arginine (B, CSF), orotic acid (U)

HHH syndrome	238970	AR	Mitochondrial ornithine transporter	<1:100,000	Mental retardation, seizures, pyramidal signs, compromised sense of vibration, episodic hyperammonemia	Ornithine (B,U), homocitrulline (U)
Miscellaneous Disorders of Amino Acid Metabolism						
Nonketotic hyperglycinemia	605899	AR	Glycine cleavage system (P, H, T, L proteins)	<1:100,000	Lethargy, seizures, myoclonic jerks, hypotonia, hiccups	Glycine (B,CSF,U), CSF Gly/Plasma Gly ratio >0.09
Gyrate atrophy of the choroid and retina	258870	AR	Ornithine aminotransferase	<1:100,000	Myopia, night blindness, progressive loss of peripheral vision	Ornithine (B)
Hyperprolinemia type I	239500	AR	Proline oxidase	<1:100,000	Clinically benign (most likely); renal disease, neurologic manifestations (disputed)	Proline (B,U), Hydroxyproline, glycine (U)
Hyperprolinemia type II	239510	AR	Delta 1-pryrroline-5-carboxylate dehydrogenase	<1:100,000	Mental retardation, pyridoxine-responsive seizures	Proline (B,U), pyrroline 5-carboxylic (U)
Disorders of Amino Acid Membrane Transport						
Cystinuria	220100	AR	Absorption of cystine and dibasic amino acids in renal tubule and GI tract	>1:25,000	Nephrolithiasis	Cystine, lysine, ornithine, arginine (U)
Lysinuric protein intolerance (LPI)	222700	AR	Cationic amino acid transporter (SLC7A7)	<1:100,000	Failure to thrive, alveolar proteinosis, hepatosplenomegaly, pancreatitis, diarrhea, osteoporosis, hypotonia, postprandial hyperammonemia	Lysine, arginine, ornithine (U), orotic acid (U)
Hartnup disease	234500	AR	Neutral amino acid transporter 1 (SLC6A19)	>1:50,000	Ataxia, seizures, photodermatitis (pellagra-like)	Hyperexcretion of ALA, SER, THR, VAL, LEU, ILE, PHE, TYR, TRP, HIS, GLN, ASN (U)

*OMIM, Online Mendelian Inheritance in Man (www.ncbi.nlm.nih.gov/entrez/query.fcgi?db=OMIM/accessed September 29, 2011).

AD, Autosomal dominant; *AR*, autosomal recessive; *DBS*, dried blood spot; *NBS*, newborn screening; *5-HIAA*, 5-hydroxyindoleacetic acid; *HVA*, homovanillic acid.

Postmortem Screening

Among IEMs, fatty acid oxidation (FAO) disorders are those recognized more often after the diagnosis of an affected sibling or as a cause of sudden death.[5] Early reports attributed up to 5% of cases of sudden death in children younger than 5 years to FAO,[7] and mounting evidence indicates that some of these disorders can cause mortality in adults as well.[38] The postmortem evaluation of unexpected death, independent of age, especially when evidence of acute illness or infection is found, should consider FAO as a cause. This is accomplished by analysis of acylcarnitines in blood and bile spots (Figure 58-2).[52] Reference intervals for acylcarnitines in postmortem blood and bile spots are listed in Table 58-3.

Blood and bile are collected on filter paper identical to the cards used for newborn screening; once properly dried they are shipped to the laboratory at room temperature. In cases with a higher index of suspicion, an effort should be made to collect and freeze a specimen of liver[7] and to collect a skin biopsy for establishing the fibroblast culture to be used, if needed, to confirm a diagnosis. Although fatty infiltration of the liver and/or other organs (e.g., heart, muscle, kidneys) is a common observation in FAO disorders, the finding of macroscopic steatosis should not be used as the only criterion in deciding whether to investigate a possible underlying FAO disorder during postmortem evaluation of a case of sudden death. Sudden death from cardiac arrhythmia can be the only finding in fatty acid oxidation defects, and the absence of obvious physical findings on autopsy does not exclude this, especially in adults. In cases of sudden infant death, if parental permission to perform an autopsy is not granted, any leftover specimens or unused portions of blood spots collected for newborn screening, if still available, could be useful samples in obtaining a diagnosis.

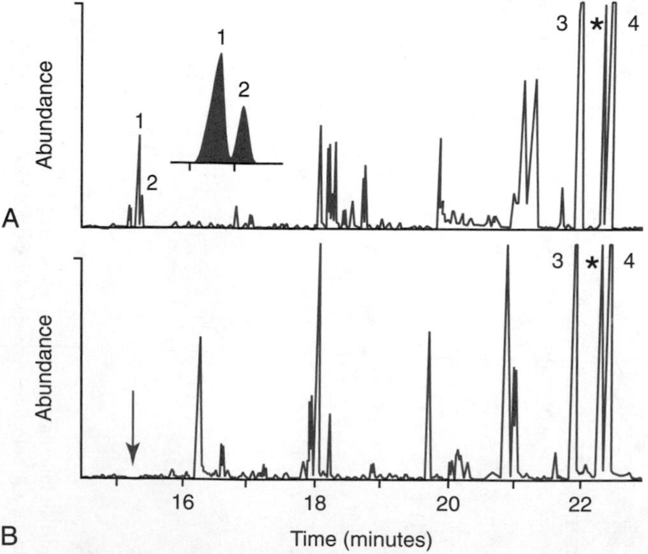

Figure 58-2 Partial urine organic acid profiles. A, Profile of acutely ill patient. Peaks 1 and 2 are derivatives of succinylacetone. B, Reference profile of 15 month old patient. Note * marks the peak of internal standard. *(From Rinaldo P, Matern D, Bennett MJ. Fatty acid oxidation disorders. Ann Rev Physiol 2002;64:477-502.)*

Biochemical Genetics Tests: Analytical Considerations

In addition to clinical presentation and routine laboratory tests, the diagnosis of patients with inborn errors of metabolism relies on specific tests such as ion-exchange chromatography and liquid chromatography with tandem mass spectrometry (LC-MS/MS) for amino acid analysis, gas chromatography/mass spectrometry (GC/MS) for organic acid analysis, tandem mass spectrometry (MS/MS) with (LC-MS/MS) or without liquid chromatographic separation for acylcarnitine profiles, and LC-MS/MS or GC/MS for acylglycine profiles. The combination of these tests, with the use of different specimen types, is the key to biochemical confirmation of metabolic disorders, whose diagnosis is then definitively confirmed using DNA testing or enzyme/transporter assays.

Analysis of (1) plasma amino acids, (2) urine organic acids, and (3) plasma acylcarnitines is the mainstay for the diagnosis of most amino acidopathies, organic acidemias, and disorders of fatty acid oxidation. Because of the early identification of asymptomatic patients by newborn screening, the sensitivity and specificity of these methods need to be very high to detect even low concentrations of diagnostic metabolites. Furthermore, the availability of age-appropriate reference intervals is necessary, because the concentrations of several metabolites (e.g., acylcarnitines) change rapidly with age.

Amino Acid Analysis by Ion-Exchange Chromatography

Several methods have been used in the analysis of amino acids in biological fluids such as plasma, urine, and cerebrospinal fluid. All involve chromatographic separation of amino acids with precolumn [high-performance liquid chromatography (HPLC), GC methods] or postcolumn (ion-exchange chromatography) derivatization, followed by detection by ultraviolet (UV), fluorescence, or mass spectrometry.[1,35,61,65,77,78] The gold standard for analysis of amino acids remains ion-exchange chromatography (IEC), even though recent work using tandem mass spectrometry is showing promising results. The challenge with amino acid analysis includes the need (1) to cover a wide dynamic range, (2) to have a very low detection limit, and (3) to have a high upper limit of linearity. In addition to these analytical requirements, isomers need to be separated and quantified. With ion-exchange chromatography, the sample (plasma/urine/CSF) is deproteinized and injected onto an ion-exchange column (typically a lithium cation-exchange column). Amino acids are separated on the basis of their pK_a by changing the pH and ionic strength of eluting buffers and the temperature of the column. Acidic amino acids are eluted first, followed by neutral then basic amino acids. After their elution from the column, amino acids are mixed with ninhydrin at 135 °C to form a colored adduct. The intensity of their absorbance is proportional to the concentration of the amino acid. Absorbance is read at

TABLE 58-3 Acylcarnitine Reference Intervals in Postmortem Blood and Bile Dried Spots

		Blood ($n = 448$)		**Bile ($n = 525$)**	
		Median	**5-95%ile**	**Median**	**5-95%ile**
		μmol/L			
Acetylcarnitine	C2	73.87	23.55-181.22	87.34	20.44-245.72
Acrylylcarnitine	C3:1	0.03	0.01-0.12	0.07	0.02-0.30
Propionylcarnitine	C3	2.95	0.55-8.01	2.07	0.36-8.10
Iso-/Butyrylcarnitine	C4	4.24	0.79-14.49	1.81	0.50-5.75
Tiglylcarnitine	C5:1	0.07	0.02-0.21	0.13	0.03-0.53
Isovaleryl/2-CH_3 butyrylcarnitine	C5	0.65	0.18-1.73	0.85	0.19-2.90
3-OH-butyrylcarnitine	C4-OH	1.97	0.35-6.25	0.65	0.12-2.26
Hexanoylcarnitine	C6	0.61	0.12-1.58	0.56	0.12-3.31
3-OH-isovalerylcarnitine	C5-OH	0.28	0.10-0.74	0.22	0.06-0.67
Heptanoylcarnitine	C7	0.05	0.01-0.14	0.12	0.03-0.75
3-OH-hexanoylcarnitine	C6-OH	0.14	0.03-0.45	0.16	0.03-0.59
Octenoylcarnitine	C8:1	0.16	0.03-0.48	2.56	0.18-36.01
Octanoylcarnitine	C8	0.35	0.19-1.02	0.63	0.19-6.46
Malonylcarnitine	C3-DC	0.12	0.03-0.32	0.22	0.04-0.96
Decadienoylcarnitine	C10:2	0.03	0.01-0.08	0.26	0.03-3.93
Decenoylcarnitine	C10:1	0.05	0.01-0.15	0.58	0.06-11.80
Decanoylcarnitine	C10	0.09	0.02-0.37	0.35	0.05-6.47
Methylmalonylcarnitine	C4-DC	0.29	0.09-0.81	0.30	0.06-0.92
3-OH-decenoylcarnitine	C10:1-OH	0.05	0.02-0.14	0.18	0.04-1.97
Glutarylcarnitine (3-OH-C10)	C5-DC	0.07	0.02-0.21	0.18	0.04-1.53
Dodecenoylcarnitine	C12:1	0.03	0.01-0.13	0.30	0.03-13.50
Dodecanoylcarnitine	C12	0.17	0.07-0.61	0.49	0.08-7.40
3-OH-dodecenoylcarnitine	C12:1-OH	0.04	0.01-0.11	0.24	0.04-4.86
3-OH-dodecanoylcarnitine	C12-OH	0.04	0.01-0.18	0.28	0.03-2.28
Tetradecadienoylcarnitine	C14:2	0.06	0.01-0.26	0.36	0.04-9.49
Tetradecenoylcarnitine	C14:1	0.07	0.02-0.30	0.30	0.03-12.49
Tetradecanoylcarnitine	C14	0.14	0.04-0.47	0.25	0.04-3.81
3-OH-tetradecenoylcarnitine	C14:1-OH	0.04	0.01-0.10	0.15	0.03-2.60
3-OH-tetradecanoylcarnitine	C14-OH	0.03	0.01-0.08	0.11	0.02-1.15
Hexadecenoylcarnitine	C16:1	0.07	0.02-0.28	0.15	0.03-2.73
Hexadecanoylcarnitine	C16	0.53	0.10-1.74	0.42	0.09-3.39
3-OH-hexadecenoylcarnitine	C16:1-OH	0.06	0.02-0.24	0.24	0.04-1.45
3-OH-hexadecanoylcarnitine	C16-OH	0.04	0.01-0.12	0.27	0.03-1.48
Octadecadienoylcarnitine	C18:2	0.18	0.03-0.55	0.22	0.03-2.93
Octadecenoylcarnitine	C18:1	0.53	0.11-1.69	0.38	0.07-3.75
Octadecanoylcarnitine	C18	0.43	0.12-1.34	0.36	0.06-2.13
3-OH-octadecadienoylcarnitine	C18:2-OH	0.03	0.01-0.08	0.09	0.01-0.55
3-OH-octadecenoylcarnitine	C18:1-OH	0.04	0.01-0.11	0.10	0.02-1.01
3-OH-octadecanoylcarnitine	C18-OH	0.03	0.01-0.10	0.07	0.00-0.66

From Rinaldo P, Hahn S, Matern D. Inborn errors of amino acid, organic acid, and fatty acid metabolism. In: Burtis CA, Ashwood ER, Bruns DE, eds. Tietz textbook of clinical chemistry and molecular diagnostics, 4th edition. St. Louis, Elsevier Saunders, 2006:2241.

two different wavelengths: 570 nm (maximum absorbance for amino acids) and 440 nm (maximum absorbance for imino acids, such as proline and hydroxyproline). The concentration of amino acids is calculated using an internal standard and external calibration. Identification of individual amino acids relies on retention time, ratio of absorbance at the two wavelengths (440/570 nm), and, in case of doubt, spiking of the sample with a standard.

Plasma collected under fasting conditions is the specimen of choice. In infants and small children, the sample should be collected at least 2 hours after the last feeding. Collection of serum should be avoided because of artifacts deriving from the clotting process. Blood should be collected with an anticoagulant (lithium/sodium heparin) and immediately separated and frozen until the time of analysis. Storage of samples at inappropriate temperature, at room temperature, or refrigerated has been known to result in deamination of glutamine and binding of sulfur amino acids to protein. The concentration of most amino acids in red blood cells is very similar to their concentration in plasma; however, some amino acids (e.g., aspartic acid, taurine, glutamic acid) are present at higher concentrations in red blood cells; therefore, hemolysis will result in an artificially increased concentration of those amino acids. In addition, red blood cells contain the enzyme arginase, which converts arginine to ornithine and urea. Hemolysis may release this enzyme, resulting in decreased concentrations of arginine and increased concentrations of ornithine. Results of plasma amino acid analysis are usually expressed in micromoles/liter.

Urine amino acids are useful only in the investigation of disorders of amino acid transport (e.g., cystinuria, lysinuric protein intolerance, Hartnup disorder) or of prolidase deficiency. A random urine sample, without preservative, is usually sufficient. Specific reabsorption studies may require a timed (24 hour) urine collection. The sample should be collected without preservative and kept refrigerated until the end of the collection. Urine samples, like plasma, should be frozen as soon as possible and kept frozen until analysis. Results are usually normalized to the concentration of creatinine in the specimen.

Analysis of cerebrospinal fluid (CSF) amino acids is performed for very specific cases, such as in the diagnostic investigation of glycine encephalopathy (nonketotic hyperglycinemia) and in disorders of serine metabolism. CSF should be collected while avoiding blood contamination; it should be frozen immediately and kept frozen until the time of analysis. Measurements of CSF amino acids are expressed in micromoles/liter. Amino acid results, independent of specimen type, should be correlated with clinical status, diet, and medications.

Urine Organic Acid Analysis by Gas Chromatography/Mass Spectrometry

The label *organic acids* includes metabolites of almost all pathways of intermediary metabolism and exogenous compounds. Organic acids analyzed by gas chromatography/mass spectrometry (GC/MS) are separated on the basis of their volatility and solubility in the stationary nonpolar liquid phase of the capillary gas chromatography column. Before GC/MS analysis is performed, organic acids must be (1) extracted, usually with an organic solvent; (2) converted to volatile trimethylsilyl (TMS) derivatives; and (3) dissolved in organic solvents.[40,78] With this technique, the mass spectrometer is employed as a detector, thus allowing positive identification of organic acids both by retention time and by their characteristic fragmentation spectrum. A random urine specimen is routinely used for this analysis; however, the most informative samples for the diagnosis of IEM are collected during acute metabolic decompensation. Organic acid analysis in blood or CSF usually is not informative to establish a diagnosis. Their interpretation is challenging because hundreds of compounds will be present in a specimen. Key factors in correct interpretation of results include (1) recognition of abnormal patterns and possible interferences due to dietary or medication artifacts, (2) knowledge about metabolic disorders and their presentation, and (3) information about the clinical status of patients.

Plasma Acylcarnitine Profile

Acylcarnitines derive from conjugation of carnitine with acyl-CoA. Carnitine [3-hydroxy-4-(trimethylazaniumyl) butanoate] is a water-soluble molecule that is essential in the transfer of long-chain fatty acids inside mitochondria for beta-oxidation. In addition, carnitine binds acyl residues accumulating in several organic acidemias and in fatty acid oxidation disorders, to facilitate their excretion. In the presence of a metabolic block (organic acidemia or fatty acid oxidation disorder), specific acylcarnitines, derived from conjugation of carnitine with acyl-CoA upstream of the metabolic block, accumulate, producing a pattern that is characteristic for each disease or group of diseases, so acylcarnitine analysis plays an essential role in the diagnosis of metabolic disorders (see Figure 58-2). Such an analysis is usually performed by tandem mass spectrometry (MS/MS) with or without liquid chromatographic separation prior to MS/MS detection.[39,41] Plasma/serum is the biological fluid of choice, and whole blood spotted on filter paper is used for screening of newborns. Concentrations of acylcarnitines in plasma differ from concentrations in whole blood, especially for long-chain acylcarnitines. This is thought to be due to binding of long-chain acylcarnitines to the membranes of blood cells, resulting in reduced long-chain species in plasma. Plasma for analysis of acylcarnitines should be separated immediately after collection and kept frozen until analysis. Hemolysis has been known to result in elevated long-chain acylcarnitines, misleading the diagnosis. Storage of the sample at room temperature or even refrigerated may result in hydrolysis and, consequently, reduced concentrations of acylcarnitines. Urine acylcarnitine analysis is performed only in the diagnostic work-up of specific disorders, such as glutaric acidemia type I, and only if equivocal results are obtained with other tests. Quantification of acylcarnitines is typically performed using stable isotope dilution. However, some deuterated internal standards are not available for all identified acylcarnitine species. Caution should be taken when acylcarnitine results from different laboratories are compared, because the values may change depending on the internal standards used.[14]

Reference Intervals

Age-appropriate reference intervals should be used in the interpretation of biochemical genetics tests. Reference intervals for urine organic acids, urine acylglycines, plasma, and urine acylcarnitines are listed in Tables 58-4, 58-5, and 58-6.

Enzyme Assay and DNA Testing

Several inborn errors of metabolism produce a characteristic pattern of metabolites that is not observed in other conditions. For most, however, the diagnosis needs to be confirmed by a more specific method involving measurement of the activity of the putatively defective enzyme/transporter and/or DNA testing. This confirmation is very critical, in that for many conditions, specific therapy, if available, needs to be continued for life or is very aggressive (organ or bone marrow transplant). In addition, for some metabolic disorders, genotype-phenotype correlation with specific mutations

TABLE 58-4 Reference Intervals of Selected Organic Acids and Acylglycines in Urine, mmol/mol Creatinine*

Age Groups	0-1 Month	1-6 Months	6 Months-5 Years	>5 Years
Acetylaspartic acid†	nd-13	nd-13	nd-13	nd-13
cis-Aconitic acid	5-31	10-97	10-97	3-44
Adipic acid	9-37	9-37	nd-15	nd-5
Azelaic acid	nd-1	nd-1	nd-1	nd-1
Butyrylglycine†	0.1-2	0.1-2	0.1-2	0.1-2
trans-Cinnamoylglycine†	0.1-8	0.1-8	0.1-8	0.1-8
Citric acid	nd-1045	104-268	0-656	87-639
Dodecanedioic acid†	nd-0.05	nd-0.05	nd-0.05	nd-0.05
Ethylmalonic acid†	0.4-17	0.4-17	0.4-17	0.4-17
Fumaric acid	10-45	4-45	1-27	2-4
Glutaric acid†	0.5-13	0.5-13	0.5-13	0.5-13
Glyceric acid†	nd-39	nd-184	nd-70	0-60
Glycolic acid†	nd-62	nd-104	3-121	nd-166
Glyoxylic acid†	nd-13	0-16	nd-7	nd-9
Hexadecanedioic acid†	nd-0.4	nd-0.4	nd-0.4	nd-0.4
Hexanoylglycine†	0.1-1.2	0.1-1.2	0.1-1.2	0.1-1.2
Homogentisic acid	nd-10	nd-10	nd-10	nd-10
Homovanillic acid†	nd-22	nd-22	nd-8	nd-7
3-Hydroxybutyric acid	nd-5	nd-5	nd-5	nd-10
2-Hydroxyglutaric acid	nd-15	nd-15	nd-15	nd-15
5-Hydroxyindoleacetic acid†	nd-12	nd-12	nd-12	nd-9
4-Hydroxyphenyllactic acid	nd-50	nd-10	nd-10	nd-10
4-Hydroxyphenylpyruvic acid	nd-20	nd-5	nd-5	nd-5
Isobutyrylglycine†	nd-9	0-9	0-9	0-9
Isocitric acid	0-368	0-67	0-77	16-99
Isovalerylglycine†	0.2-10	0.2-10	0.2-10	0.2-10
2-Ketoglutaric acid	22-567	63-552	36-103	41-82
Lactic acid	46-348	57-346	21-38	20-101
Malic acid	0-52	8-73	4-57	17-47
2-Methylbutyrylglycine†	0.2-5	0.2-5	0.2-5	0.2-5
Methylmalonic acid†	nd-3.6	nd-3.6	nd-3.6	nd-3.6
Methylsuccinic acid†	0-12	0-12	0-12	0-12
Octanoylglycine†	0.1-1.2	0.1-1.2	0.1-1.2	0.1-1.2
Orotic acid	1.4-5.3	1.0-3.2	0.5-3.3	0.4-1.2
Oxalic acid†	51-931	7-567	7-352	nd-187
3-Phenylpropionylglycine†	nd-0.6	nd-0.6	nd-0.6	nd-0.6
Pimelic acid	nd-1	nd-1	nd-1	nd-1
Pyroglutamic acid	nd-61	nd-61	nd-61	nd-61
Pyruvic acid	24-123	8-90	3-19	6-9
Sebacic acid	3-16	3-16	nd-8	nd-8
Suberic acid	4-20	4-20	nd-8	nd-8
Suberylglycine†	nd-5.4	nd-5.4	nd-5.4	nd-5.4
Succinic acid	35-547	34-156	16-118	29-87
Tetradecanedioic acid†	nd-0.40	nd-0.40	nd-0.40	nd-0.40
Uracil†	nd-32	nd-32	nd-21	nd-17
Uric acid†	359-2644	359-2644	185-1134	199-1034
Vanillylmandelic acid†	nd-15	nd-10	nd-7	nd-5

From Rinaldo P, Hahn S, Matern D. Inborn errors of amino acid, organic acid, and fatty acid metabolism. In: Burtis CA, Ashwood ER, Bruns DE, eds. Tietz textbook of clinical chemistry and molecular diagnostics, 4th edition. St. Louis, Elsevier Saunders, 2006:2238.

*TIC detection limit: 0.1 mmol/mol creatinine; SIM detection limit (with stable isotope labeled internal standard): 0.01 mmol/mol creatinine.

†Measured using a stable isotope-labeled internal standard.

nd, Not detected.

TABLE 58-5 Acylcarnitine Reference Intervals in Plasma

		0 to 7 Days (n = 143)		8 Days to 7 Years (n = 2677)		>7 Years (n = 834)	
		Median	**5-95%ile**	**Median**	**5-95%ile**	**Median**	**5-95%ile**
		μmol/L					
Acetylcarnitine	C2	8.37	2.82-19.67	10.45	4.70-33.66	8.45	3.29-25.72
Acrylylcarnitine	C3:1	0.01	0.00-0.03	0.01	0.00-0.03	0.01	0.00-0.03
Propionylcarnitine	C3	0.34	0.07-1.85	0.49	0.17-1.27	0.45	0.17-1.49
Iso-/Butyrylcarnitine	C4	0.27	0.13-0.70	0.31	0.16-0.74	0.30	0.15-1.05
Tiglylcarnitine	C5:1	0.01	0.00-0.06	0.01	0.00-0.05	0.02	0.00-0.10
Isovaleryl/2-CH_3 butyrylcarnitine	C5	0.15	0.04-0.42	0.15	0.05-0.44	0.14	0.06-0.51
3-OH-butyrylcarnitine	C4-OH	0.04	0.01-0.15	0.04	0.01-0.29	0.03	0.01-0.19
Hexanoylcarnitine	C6	0.05	0.01-0.49	0.06	0.02-0.20	0.05	0.02-0.21
3-OH-isovalerylcarnitine	C5-OH	0.03	0.01-0.15	0.02	0.01-0.07	0.02	0.01-0.19
Heptanoylcarnitine	C7	0.01	0.00-0.05	0.01	0.00-0.04	0.01	0.00-0.06
3-OH-hexanoylcarnitine	C6-OH	0.02	0.00-0.07	0.02	0.01-0.06	0.02	0.00-0.07
Octenoylcarnitine	C8:1	0.18	0.03-0.45	0.19	0.06-0.53	0.19	0.06-0.72
Octanoylcarnitine	C8	0.16	0.08-1.40	0.15	0.08-0.41	0.16	0.08-0.45
Malonylcarnitine	C3-DC	0.03	0.01-0.08	0.03	0.01-0.09	0.04	0.01-0.17
Decadienoylcarnitine	C10:2	0.03	0.01-0.07	0.02	0.01-0.07	0.02	0.01-0.11
Decenoylcarnitine	C10:1	0.09	0.03-0.41	0.12	0.04-0.37	0.14	0.03-0.46
Decanoylcarnitine	C10	0.10	0.02-0.51	0.13	0.04-0.44	0.14	0.03-0.58
Methylmalonylcarnitine	C4-DC	0.01	0.00-0.03	0.01	0.00-0.03	0.01	0.00-0.06
3-OH-decenoylcarnitine	C10:1-OH	0.03	0.01-0.11	0.02	0.01-0.05	0.03	0.01-0.11
Glutarylcarnitine (3-OH-C10)	C5-DC	0.02	0.00-0.11	0.02	0.00-0.06	0.02	0.00-0.12
Dodecenoylcarnitine	C12:1	0.04	0.01-0.29	0.05	0.01-0.19	0.06	0.01-0.21
Dodecanoylcarnitine	C12	0.07	0.02-0.33	0.07	0.03-0.18	0.06	0.02-0.18
3-OH-dodecenoylcarnitine	C12:1-OH	0.02	0.00-0.07	0.01	0.00-0.05	0.02	0.00-0.08
3-OH-dodecanoylcarnitine	C12-OH	0.02	0.00-0.08	0.01	0.00-0.03	0.01	0.00-0.04
Tetradecadienoylcarnitine	C14:2	0.03	0.01-0.12	0.03	0.01-0.12	0.03	0.01-0.12
Tetradecenoylcarnitine	C14:1	0.05	0.01-0.39	0.05	0.01-0.23	0.05	0.01-0.24
Tetradecanoylcarnitine	C14	0.04	0.01-0.23	0.03	0.01-0.10	0.02	0.01-0.12
3-OH-tetradecenoylcarnitine	C14:1-OH	0.02	0.01-0.08	0.02	0.01-0.05	0.02	0.01-0.07
3-OH-tetradecanoylcarnitine	C14-OH	0.01	0.00-0.06	0.01	0.00-0.03	0.01	0.00-0.04
Hexadecenoylcarnitine	C16:1	0.04	0.01-0.24	0.03	0.01-0.10	0.03	0.01-0.09
Hexadecanoylcarnitine	C16	0.17	0.05-0.67	0.10	0.04-0.23	0.09	0.04-0.21
3-OH-hexadecenoylcarnitine	C16:1-OH	0.01	0.00-0.30	0.01	0.00-0.05	0.01	0.00-0.04
3-OH-hexadecanoylcarnitine	C16-OH	0.01	0.00-0.08	0.01	0.00-0.03	0.01	0.00-0.03
Octadecadienoylcarnitine	C18:2	0.04	0.01-0.12	0.05	0.02-0.16	0.06	0.02-0.15
Octadecenoylcarnitine	C18:1	0.12	0.03-0.38	0.13	0.05-0.35	0.14	0.04-0.33
Octadecanoylcarnitine	C18	0.04	0.01-0.20	0.05	0.02-0.11	0.05	0.02-0.10
3-OH-octadecadienoylcarnitine	C18:2-OH	0.01	0.00-0.04	0.01	0.00-0.02	0.01	0.00-0.02
3-OH-octadecenoylcarnitine	C18:1-OH	0.01	0.00-0.04	0.01	0.00-0.03	0.01	0.00-0.03
3-OH-octadecanoylcarnitine	C18-OH	0.01	0.00-0.03	0.01	0.00-0.02	0.01	0.00-0.02

From Rinaldo P, Hahn S, Matern D. Inborn errors of amino acid, organic acid, and fatty acid metabolism. In: Burtis CA, Ashwood ER, Bruns DE, eds. Tietz textbook of clinical chemistry and molecular diagnostics, 4th edition. St. Louis, Elsevier Saunders, 2006:2239.

affects the overall prognosis. For some diseases, such as phenylketonuria, the mutant enzyme is expressed only in the liver, and it is not practical and is very invasive to obtain diagnostic confirmation by enzyme assay. DNA testing (by sequencing of the whole gene) in this case is often more useful. For several other conditions, the missing enzyme is expressed in blood cells or in fibroblasts obtained by skin biopsy. It must be noted that with decreased costs of DNA testing, this technology is widely used to provide final diagnostic confirmation. The major limitation of DNA sequencing is that for certain conditions, the same biochemical abnormality is caused by deficiency of any of a number of genes (e.g., in methylmalonic acidemia), or multiple genes might be required to encode all subunits of a single enzyme (such as in maple syrup urine disease). Further, DNA sequencing (1) might not identify all mutations causing a disease,

TABLE 58-6 Acylcarnitine Reference Intervals in Urine

		0 to 7 Days (n = 20)		8 Days to 7 Years (n = 20)		>7 Years (n = 20)	
		Mean	Range	Mean	Range	Mean	Range
		mmol/mol Creatinine					
Acetylcarnitine	C2	1.13	0.19-2.92	4.30	0.07-16.46	0.35	0.04-1.26
Acrylylcarnitine	C3:1	0.02	0.00-0.06	0.01	0.00-0.04	0.00	0.00-0.00
Propionylcarnitine	C3	0.06	0.01-0.20	0.23	0.01-1.20	0.02	0.00-0.06
Iso-/Butyrylcarnitine	C4	0.14	0.02-0.36	0.79	0.02-2.74	0.10	0.01-0.29
Tiglylcarnitine	C5:1	0.05	0.01-0.14	0.10	0.00-0.34	0.01	0.00-0.03
Isovaleryl/2-CH_3 butyrylcarnitine	C5	0.09	0.00-0.25	0.39	0.00-1.53	0.03	0.00-0.07
3-OH-butyrylcarnitine	C4-OH	0.03	0.01-0.06	0.09	0.00-0.26	0.01	0.00-0.03
Hexanoylcarnitine	C6	0.03	0.01-0.06	0.05	0.00-0.16	0.01	0.00-0.04
3-OH-isovalerylcarnitine	C5-OH	0.09	0.00-0.19	0.17	0.01-0.52	0.02	0.01-0.05
Benzoylcarnitine	BZC	0.02	0.00-0.05	0.11	0.01-0.37	0.01	0.00-0.04
Heptanoylcarnitine	C7	0.02	0.00-0.06	0.04	0.00-0.15	0.00	0.00-0.01
3-OH-hexanoylcarnitine	C6-OH	0.02	0.01-0.06	0.08	0.00-0.32	0.00	0.00-0.01
Octenoylcarnitine	C8:1	0.12	0.01-0.36	0.84	0.02-4.30	0.09	0.01-0.23
Octanoylcarnitine	C8	0.26	0.02-0.82	0.14	0.01-0.61	0.02	0.00-0.05
Malonylcarnitine	C3-DC	0.10	0.02-0.22	0.13	0.01-0.50	0.02	0.00-0.04
Decadienoylcarnitine	C10:2	0.04	0.00-0.09	0.17	0.01-0.48	0.03	0.01-0.08
Decenoylcarnitine	C10:1	0.05	0.01-0.13	0.24	0.01-0.65	0.03	0.01-0.07
Decanoylcarnitine	C10	0.03	0.01-0.08	0.04	0.00-0.21	0.01	0.00-0.02
Methylmalonylcarnitine	C4-DC	0.14	0.03-0.25	0.15	0.02-0.57	0.02	0.01-0.05
3-OH-decenoylcarnitine	C10:1-OH	0.12	0.01-0.25	0.08	0.01-0.26	0.01	0.00-0.03
Glutarylcarnitine (3-OH-C10)	C5-DC	0.14	0.03-0.31	0.13	0.01-0.37	0.03	0.01-0.06
Dodecenoylcarnitine	C12:1	0.01	0.00-0.03	0.03	0.00-0.07	0.00	0.00-0.01
Dodecanoylcarnitine	C12	0.05	0.01-0.10	0.05	0.00-0.19	0.01	0.00-0.02
Adipoylcarnitine	C6-DC	0.17	0.04-0.40	0.19	0.01-0.81	0.03	0.00-0.13
3-OH-dodecenoylcarnitine	C12:1-OH	0.07	0.01-0.25	0.07	0.00-0.27	0.01	0.00-0.03
3-OH-dodecanoylcarnitine	C12-OH	0.05	0.01-0.12	0.05	0.00-0.16	0.01	0.00-0.01
Tetradecadienoylcarnitine	C14:2	0.12	0.01-0.55	0.01	0.00-0.02	0.00	0.00-0.00
Tetradecenoylcarnitine	C14:1	0.05	0.00-0.24	0.05	0.00-0.21	0.01	0.00-0.01
Tetradecanoylcarnitine	C14	0.05	0.01-0.11	0.09	0.00-0.39	0.01	0.00-0.02
3-OH-tetradecenoylcarnitine	C14:1-OH	0.04	0.01-0.10	0.04	0.00-0.14	0.01	0.00-0.01
3-OH-tetradecanoylcarnitine	C14-OH	0.03	0.01-0.07	0.03	0.00-0.09	0.00	0.00-0.02
Hexadecenoylcarnitine	C16:1	0.01	0.00-0.03	0.01	0.00-0.04	0.00	0.00-0.00
Hexadecanoylcarnitine	C16	0.05	0.01-0.13	0.05	0.00-0.18	0.01	0.00-0.02
3-OH-hexadecenoylcarnitine	C16:1-OH	0.32	0.00-2.06	0.01	0.00-0.02	0.00	0.00-0.00
3-OH-hexadecanoylcarnitine	C16-OH	0.05	0.00-0.24	0.01	0.00-0.05	0.00	0.00-0.00
Octadecadienoylcarnitine	C18:2	0.08	0.00-0.37	0.01	0.00-0.02	0.00	0.00-0.00
Octadecenoylcarnitine	C18:1	0.01	0.00-0.03	0.01	0.00-0.02	0.00	0.00-0.00
Octadecanoylcarnitine	C18	0.01	0.00-0.02	0.01	0.00-0.05	0.00	0.00-0.00
3-OH-octadecadienoylcarnitine	C18:2-OH	0.01	0.00-0.02	0.00	0.00-0.01	0.00	0.00-0.00
3-OH-octadecenoylcarnitine	C18:1-OH	0.01	0.00-0.03	0.01	0.00-0.03	0.00	0.00-0.00
3-OH-octadecanoylcarnitine	C18-OH	0.01	0.00-0.03	0.01	0.00-0.02	0.00	0.00-0.00

From Rinaldo P, Hahn S, Matern D. Inborn errors of amino acid, organic acid, and fatty acid metabolism. In: Burtis CA, Ashwood ER, Bruns DE, eds. Tietz textbook of clinical chemistry and molecular diagnostics, 4th edition. St. Louis, Elsevier Saunders, 2006:2240.

(2) can miss single exon deletions/duplications, and (3) can identify new variations whose clinical significance is unclear because they have not been reported in other affected patients. For these reasons, biochemical and molecular investigations need to be performed together to confirm or exclude the diagnosis of a metabolic disorder.

DISORDERS OF AMINO ACID METABOLISM

Concentrations of individual amino acids in physiologic fluids reflect a balance between their intake, their release from the catabolism of endogenous proteins, their filtration and reabsorption by the kidney, and their utilization by the body to synthesize proteins or to produce energy. Changes in any of these processes can affect protein and amino acid metabolism through accumulation or excessive loss of one or more amino acids.

Inborn errors of amino acid metabolism can present at any time in a person's life; most become evident in infancy and early childhood. Affected patients may have failure to thrive, neurologic symptoms, digestive problems, psychomotor retardation, and a wide spectrum of laboratory findings. If not diagnosed promptly and treated properly, these disorders can result in poor growth, mental retardation, and death.

Table 58-2 provides a summary of the most common disorders of amino acid metabolism and transport and their characteristics. Several of these disorders are discussed in the following sections.

Classic Phenylketonuria and Other Hyperphenylalaninemias

Hyperphenylalaninemias result from the impaired conversion of phenylalanine to tyrosine, leading to an increased concentration of phenylalanine in body fluids. They are caused by a primary deficiency of phenylalanine hydroxylase, the enzyme that converts phenylalanine to tyrosine (Figure 58-3), or, in rare cases (<2% of total cases in the United States), by a defect in synthesis (Figure 58-4) or recycling (Figure 58-5) of the essential cofactor tetrahydrobiopterin. The combined incidence of these conditions is about 1 : 10,000

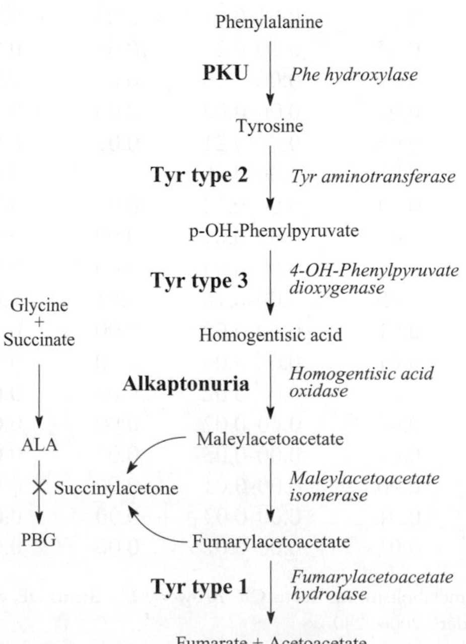

Figure 58-3 Metabolism of phenylalanine and tyrosine. Many different enzymes are required for the conversion of phenylalanine to fumarate and acetoacetate that can be subsequently oxidized to CO_2 and water. The disease caused by deficiency of any of these enzymes is indicated at the left of the arrows representing the function of the enzyme. In humans, no deficiency of maleylacetoacetate isomerase has been reported.

to 1 : 20,000 live births. In PKU, accumulation of phenylalanine and other metabolites such as phenyllactate and phenylpyruvate (phenylketones) occurs. Elevated phenylalanine interferes with neurotransmitter synthesis and uptake, leading to clinical symptoms of phenylketonuria.[63]

Patients with phenylketonuria appear healthy at birth, apart from an increased incidence of gastroesophageal reflux in patients with very high phenylalanine concentrations. Delays in development, chronic eczema, and acquired microcephaly become evident after a few months of life. Abnormal brain development results in mental retardation. This and all other problems are prevented by a special diet low in phenylalanine that needs to be initiated before 3 weeks of age. Therefore, all infants are screened at birth for this condition. In utero, phenylalanine is removed from the child by the placenta. After birth, phenylalanine accumulates as the child initiates feedings and is exposed to proteins. Therefore, for optimal results, infants should be screened after 24 hours of life, when at least one feeding has occurred, to ensure an adequate rise in phenylalanine concentrations. The diagnosis of phenylketonuria is confirmed by plasma amino acid analysis. In each infant with even minimally elevated serum phenylalanine, cofactor defects need to be excluded by measuring the urine pterin profile and activity of dihydropteridine reductase (DHPR) in blood cells. Hyperphenylalaninemia due to phenylalanine hydroxylase deficiency is biochemically diagnosed when plasma phenylalanine concentrations are above the normal reference interval with a normal urine pterin profile and normal DHPR activity. Phenylalanine hydroxylase is expressed only in the liver, and confirmation of the diagnosis by enzyme assay is not routinely performed. DNA sequencing of the causative gene, however, will definitively confirm the diagnosis, if needed.

In patients with PKU due to phenylalanine hydroxylase deficiency, dietary treatment with a special formula without phenylalanine should be started as soon as possible—ideally before 3 weeks of age.[63] Diet needs to be continued for life. Phenylalanine concentrations are monitored periodically and should remain between 60 and 360 μmol/L (reference interval, 30 to 80 μmol/L) to ensure adequate brain development. If the concentration of phenylalanine is too low, growth of the child is compromised; if it is too high, executive functioning is impaired. High concentrations of phenylalanine in the first years of life lead to mental retardation. Phenylalanine at high concentrations is teratogenic and, depending on the concentration and the period of exposure during pregnancy, will cause (1) increased risk of spontaneous abortion, (2) congenital heart defects, (3) facial dysmorphism, (4) microcephaly, and (5) developmental delay (even in the absence of microcephaly) in the fetuses of women with PKU. Adverse pregnancy outcomes in pregnant women with PKU are minimized by maintaining phenylalanine concentrations less than 360 μmol/L.[37]

In approximately 2% of cases, hyperphenylalaninemia is due to a deficiency of biosynthesis (see Figure 58-4) or recycling (see Figure 58-5) of the cofactor tetrahydrobiopterin (BH_4). BH_4 is also a cofactor for tyrosine and tryptophan

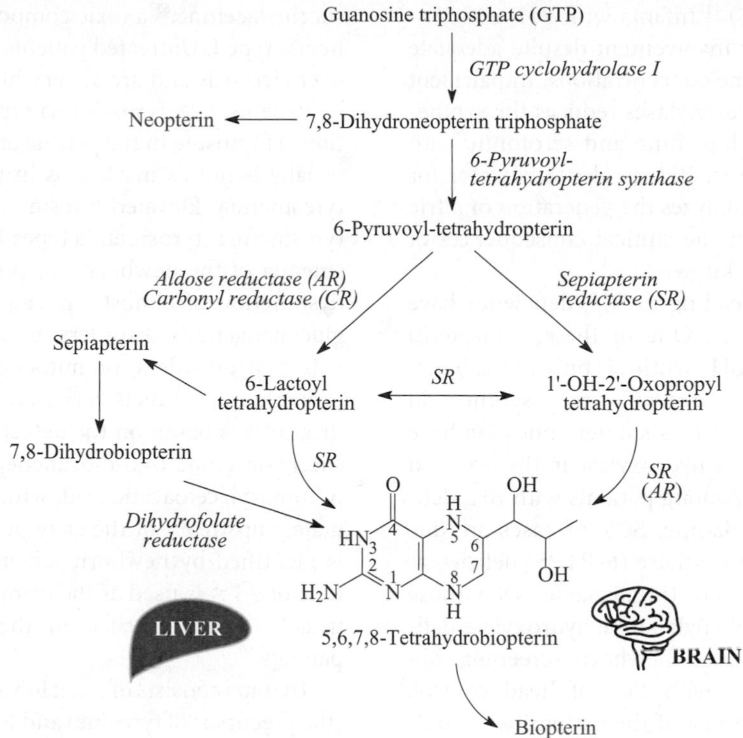

Figure 58-4 Biosynthesis of tetrahydrobiopterin (BH_4). BH_4 synthesis requires three different enzymes: GTP-cyclohydrolase I, 6-pyruvoyltetrahydropterin synthase, and sepiapterin reductase. Some steps can be performed differently in the brain, which is strongly dependent on sepiapterin reductase, as compared with the liver, which can perform the same reaction through the combined action of different enzymes. This leads to tetrahydrohydrobiopterin deficiency only in the brain in sepiapterin reductase deficiency without an increase in plasma phenylalanine, because sufficient synthesis of the cofactor is retained in the liver. The origin of the commonly measured neopterin, biopterin, and sepiapterin is indicated. *(From Longo N. Disorders of biopterin metabolism. J Inherit Metab Dis 2009;32:333-42.)*

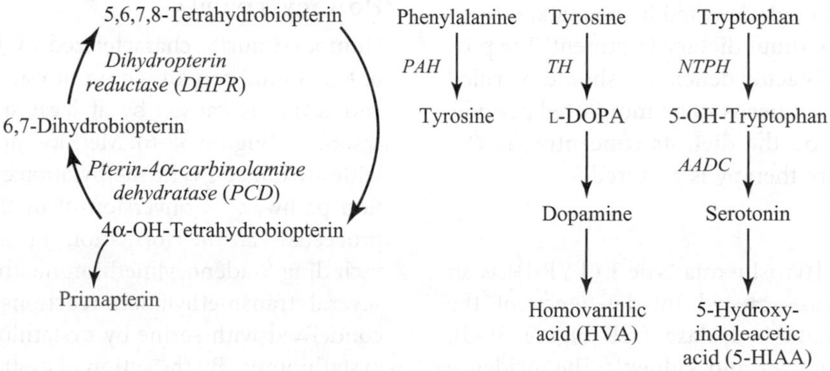

Figure 58-5 Regeneration of tetrahydrobiopterin. Tetrahydrobiopterin provides electrons for the hydroxylation of phenylalanine, tyrosine, and tryptophan by the action of phenylalanine hydroxylase (PAH), tyrosine hydroxylase (TH), and neuronal tryptophan hydroxylase (NTPH), respectively. Reduction of 4α-OH-tetrahydrobiopterin back to the active form requires the sequential action of pterin-4α-carbinolamine dehydratase and dihydropteridine reductase. In the absence of pterin-4α-carbinolamine dehydratase, the substrate is spontaneously converted to primapterin, which can be detected in urine. *(From Longo N. Disorders of biopterin metabolism. J Inherit Metab Dis 2009;32:333-42.)*

hydroxylases (see Figure 58-5).[42] Infants with BH_4 deficiencies show signs of neurologic involvement despite adequate dietary control of phenylalanine concentrations. Impairment of tyrosine and tryptophan hydroxylases reduces the synthesis of the neurotransmitters dopamine and serotonin, with severe neurologic consequences. BH_4 is also a cofactor for nitric oxide synthase, which catalyzes the generation of nitric oxide from arginine, although the clinical consequences of this latter impairment are not known.

Five enzyme deficiencies leading to BH_4 deficiency have been reported (see Table 58-2). One of these, sepiapterin reductase deficiency, impairs BH_4 synthesis only in the brain, because alternative pathways are available for its synthesis in the liver. As a result, patients with this latter condition have normal activity of phenylalanine hydroxylase in the liver and no hyperphenylalaninemia.[21] Among patients with BH_4 deficiencies and elevated phenylalanine, 50% of cases are due to 6-pyruvoyltetrahydropterin synthase (6-PTPS) deficiency. These patients are clinically indistinguishable from those with classic PKU (caused by phenylalanine hydroxylase deficiency), when diagnosed through newborn screening, but they progressively deteriorate with loss of head control, truncal hypotonia with hypertonia of the extremities, drooling, swallowing difficulties, and myoclonic seizures at between 2 and 6 months of age.[42] Treatment of these patients requires BH_4, which usually normalizes the concentration of phenylalanine (except in some cases of DHPR deficiency), and neurotransmitter precursors (L-dopa/carbidopa and 5-OH-tryptophan), which obviate the need for tyrosine and tryptophan hydroxylase.

Infants with benign hyperphenylalaninemia (phenylalanine <300 μmol/L) occasionally are identified by newborn screening because of a moderately elevated blood concentration of phenylalanine. These patients have a partial deficiency of phenylalanine hydroxylase with residual enzyme activity up to 35% of normal. Although detected by neonatal screening, they remain healthy without dietary treatment. The possibility of an underlying cofactor deficiency should be ruled out. Phenylalanine, however, needs to be monitored periodically because, depending on the diet, its concentration can increase to the point where therapy is required.

Tyrosinemia Type I

Hepatorenal tyrosinemia [tyrosinemia type I (TYR-I)] is an autosomal recessive disease caused by deficiency of the enzyme fumarylacetoacetate hydrolase (see Figure 58-3), expressed primarily in the liver and kidney.[62] The incidence of TYR-I is approximately 1 in 100,000, with a clustering of cases in the Lac-St. Jean region of Quebec (Canada). Patients with tyrosinemia type I present before 6 months of age with severe liver involvement, or after 6 months of age with (1) chronic failure to thrive, (2) mild hepatocellular dysfunction, (3) renal involvement, and (4) rickets due to renal Fanconi syndrome.[62] They have extreme irritability caused by peripheral neuropathy mimicking acute intermittent porphyria. This is caused by accumulation of 5-aminolevulinic acid (ALA) as the result of inhibition of ALA dehydratase by succinylacetone,[62] a toxic compound accumulating in tyrosinemia type I. Untreated patients have been known to develop liver cirrhosis and are at very high risk for liver cancer.

Patients with tyrosinemia type I have elevated concentrations of tyrosine in the plasma amino acids, but this elevation usually is not as marked as in patients with other forms of tyrosinemia. Elevated tyrosine is seen in (1) other forms of tyrosinemia (tyrosinemia types II and III), (2) transient tyrosinemia of the newborn, (3) prematurity, (4) hepatocellular dysfunction of almost any cause (including that caused by gluconeogenesis disorders, galactosemia, fructosemia, peroxisomal disorders, or mitochondrial DNA depletion syndrome), and (5) diets very rich in proteins. The biochemical diagnosis is based on the detection in urine organic acids of succinylacetone (4,6-dioxaneheptanoic acid), the byproduct of fumarylacetoacetic acid, which is the intermediate immediately upstream of the enzyme defect.[62] Tyrosinemia type I is identified by newborn screening only when succinylacetone or ALA is used as the primary marker, because tyrosine usually is not elevated in the newborn period in these patients.[60]

Therapy consists of a diet low in tyrosine and phenylalanine (the precursor of tyrosine) and NTBC [2-(2-nitro-4-trifluoromethylbenzoyl)-1,3-cyclohexanedione], an inhibitor of 4-hydroxyphenylpyruvate dioxygenase, the enzyme located upstream of fumarylacetoacetate hydrolase (see Figure 58-3). NTBC prevents the synthesis of succinylacetone, which disappears almost immediately from urine organic acids after initiation of treatment. The adequacy of the diet is monitored by plasma amino acids. Measurement of alpha fetoprotein is also used to monitor these patients, because liver cancer is a complication of this condition. Liver transplantation is indicated in patients who progress to liver failure and in those acquiring liver cancer.[62]

Homocystinuria

Homocystinuria, characterized by increased concentrations of the sulfur-containing amino acid homocystine in blood and urine, is caused by at least seven genetically different disorders (Figure 58-6). Methionine, homocysteine, and cysteine are linked by the methylation cycle and the transsulfuration pathway.[49] Conversion of methionine to homocysteine proceeds via the formation of *S*-adenosyl intermediates including *S*-adenosylmethionine, the methyl group donor in several transmethylation reactions. Homocysteine is then condensed with serine by cystathionine β-synthase to form cystathionine. By the action of cystathionase, cysteine is generated and participates in protein, glutathione, or taurine synthesis. Homocysteine is also remethylated back to methionine by the action of methionine synthase, an enzyme that requires methylfolate and methylcobalamin as cofactors. Defects in any of these steps can result in homocystinuria. The most common form, classic homocystinuria, is caused by reduced activity of cystathionine β -synthase. The worldwide incidence is approximately 1 : 300,000 live births[64] with a very high incidence in Qatar (1 : 1800).[26] Clinical manifestations are nonspecific at first and may include failure to thrive and

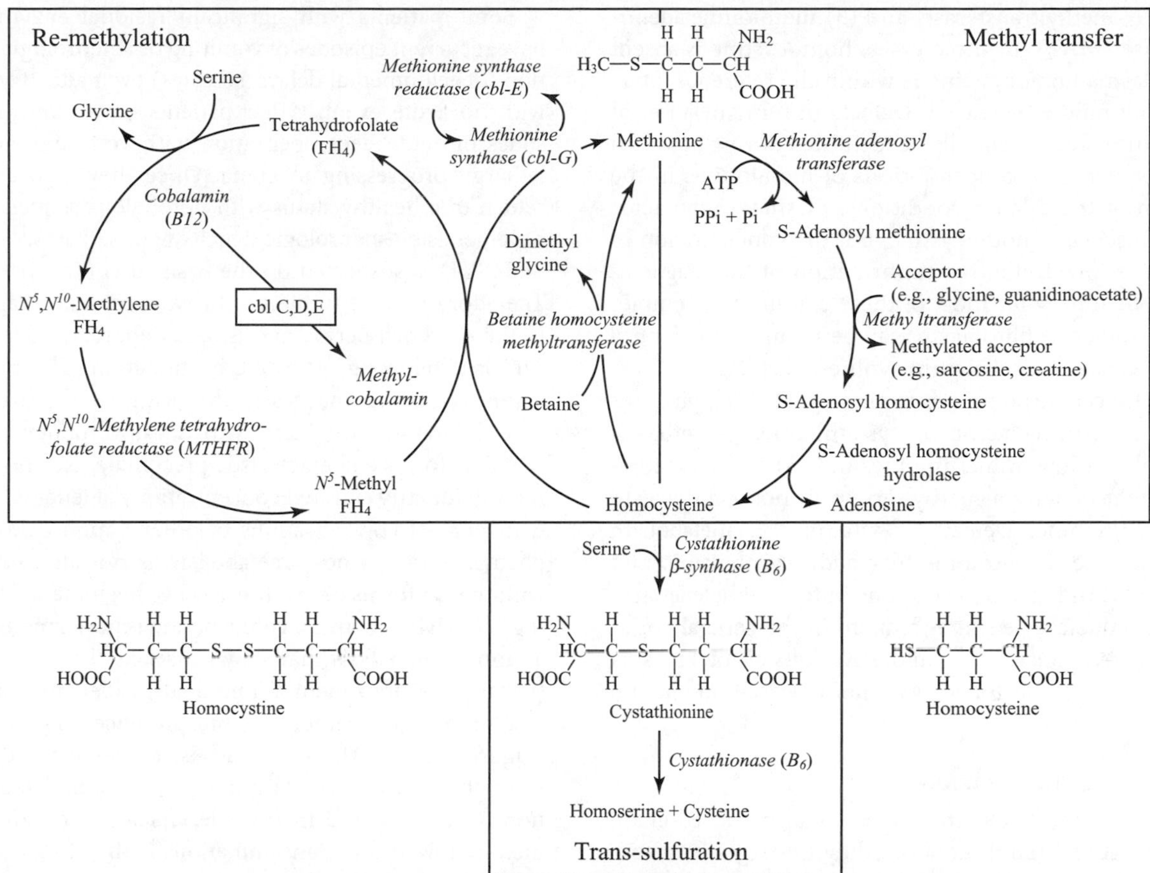

Figure 58-6 Sulfur amino acid metabolism. Methionine transfers a methyl group during its conversion to homocysteine. Defects in methyl transfer or in the subsequent metabolism of homocysteine by the pyridoxal phosphate (vitamin B_6)–dependent cystathionine beta-synthase increase plasma methionine concentrations. Homocysteine is transformed into methionine via remethylation. This occurs through methionine synthase, a reaction requiring methylcobalamin and folic acid. Deficiencies in these enzymes or lack of cofactors is associated with decreased or normal methionine concentrations. In an alternative pathway, homocysteine can be remethylated by betaine:homocysteine methyl transferase. The chemical structures of homocystine (detected by plasma amino acids) and homocysteine (detected by a separate test) are also shown.

developmental delay. Patients present during childhood or adolescence with (1) ophthalmologic problems such as downward dislocation of the lens and myopia, (2) bone abnormalities with marfanoid habitus and pectus excavatum, (3) osteoporosis, (4) mental retardation, and (5) psychiatric disturbances. Thromboembolic episodes have been seen even in children and are a major cause of morbidity and mortality.

The biochemical diagnosis is obtained by plasma amino acid analysis showing increased plasma concentrations of methionine (especially in children) and the presence of the disulfide homocystine. Total plasma homocysteine (measured after reduction of all disulfide bonds and release of homocysteine from proteins) is also markedly increased in this condition; this is measured by immunoassays, by high-performance liquid chromatography, or by tandem mass spectrometry. Increased homocystine and elevated total plasma homocysteine are observed in defects of homocysteine remethylation such as deficiency of (1) 5,10-methylene-tetrahydrofolate reductase, (2) methionine synthase *(cblG)* and methionine synthase reductase *(cblE)*, (3) 5-methyl-tetrahydrofolate-homocysteine-methyltransferase, and (4) vitamin B_{12}, and in disorders of cobalamin metabolism (*cblC, cblD,* and *cblF*). Patients with *cblC* and *cblF* and some with *cblD* defects have methylmalonic aciduria, in addition to homocystinuria, because the synthesis of adenosylcobalamin (the cofactor of methylmalonyl CoA mutase) is impaired, as is the synthesis of methylcobalamin (the cofactor of methionine synthase).[25]

Classic homocystinuria is detected in newborn screening by elevated methionine concentration. Methionine is also increased in liver disease, in diets rich in proteins, and in other more rare disorders of sulfur amino acid metabolism such as deficiency of (1) *S*-adenosylhomocysteine hydrolase,

(2) glycine *N*-methyltransferase, and (3) methionine adenosyltransferase (MAT). In these cases, homocystine is absent and total plasma homocysteine is within the reference interval or is only mildly increased. Defects in remethylation of homocysteine could potentially be identified during newborn screening by very low concentrations of methionine. In the severe form of these latter conditions, plasma amino acids show the presence of homocystine, but the concentration of methionine is low. Definitive confirmation of the diagnosis requires DNA testing for most of these conditions. Complementation studies in fibroblasts may be required to identify the specific cause of a cobalamin synthetic defect.

Therapy for classic homocystinuria requires (1) high doses of pyridoxine (the cofactor of cystathionine β-synthase), (2) a special diet low in methionine, and (3) administration of betaine that donates a methyl group to homocysteine to generate methionine. Defects of vitamin B_{12} metabolism require high doses of intramuscular hydroxycobalamin and oral betaine.[49] Mild genetic variations in the methylenetetrahydrofolate reductase gene are frequent in the general population and are responsible for mild elevations of total plasma homocysteine, a risk factor for vascular disease[16] and neural tube defects.[69]

Maple Syrup Urine Disease

Leucine, isoleucine, and valine are essential branched-chain amino acids. After transamination, they undergo decarboxylation by branched-chain α-keto acid dehydrogenase (BCKD), a complex enzyme that requires thiamine pyrophosphate as a cofactor.[17] This complex is composed of four subunits: $E_1\alpha$, $E_1\beta$, E_2, and E_3. The E_3 subunit is shared by two other dehydrogenases: pyruvate dehydrogenase and 2-oxoglutarate dehydrogenase.[17] A defect of any component of the complex causes maple syrup urine disease (MSUD), an autosomal recessive disorder with an incidence of approximately 1:250,000 live births. Several forms of this disease may occur, depending on the severity of the mutations: (1) the classic form, which is the most severe, is characterized by very high plasma concentrations of branched-chain amino acids; (2) some forms that are responsive to pharmacologic amounts of thiamine (thiamine-responsive MSUD)[23]; (3) intermediate or intermittent forms that are triggered by high consumption of proteins or a catabolic state (in which endogenous proteins released mostly by the muscle are degraded to produce energy); and (4) E_3 deficiency which is seen with combined deficiency of pyruvate and 2-oxoglutarate dehydrogenase.[15]

Classic MSUD presents with poor feeding and vomiting during the first week of life followed by lethargy and coma within a few days. This usually follows a normal birth and an uneventful first few days of life, during which branched-chain amino acids, especially leucine, increase to toxic concentrations. Leucine accumulates within the brain, causing cerebral edema, which is responsible for the progressive worsening of neurologic symptoms. Routine laboratory work is mostly unremarkable except for the presence of ketones in urine.

Some patients with significant residual enzyme activity have recurrent episodes of vomiting or a neurologic presentation (developmental delays, seizures) even after 1 year of age with no acute event. Other patients have intermittent episodes of acute decompensation with vomiting, ataxia, and lethargy progressing to coma. Once they recover, patients return to a healthy status with no obvious sequelae, or they have persistent neurologic deficits with seizures.[15]

MSUD is suspected on the basis of clinical presentation. The odor of maple syrup is not always present or appreciated in the newborn period and is better appreciated by smelling ear wax following otoscopic examination. The presence of ketones in urine analysis further suggests the diagnosis, in that the rapid urine test with 2,4-dinitrophenylhydrazine (DNPH) forms a characteristic precipitate. Newborn screening will identify elevated concentrations of leucine/isoleucine with normal concentrations of other amino acids (such as phenylalanine), whose metabolism is not affected. Patients with milder forms of the disease have been missed by screening.[6] Initial biochemical confirmation is performed by plasma amino acid analysis that shows marked elevation of leucine (usually the prominent amino acid), isoleucine, and valine, in addition to the pathognomonic presence of L-alloisoleucine (Figure 58-7). Alloisoleucine is a stereoisomer derived through stepwise racemization and keto-enol tautomerization of (2*S*) 2-oxo-3-methylvaleric acid to its (2*R*) enantiomer, followed by transamination.[58] The 2-oxo acids, the substrates immediately upstream of the enzyme block, are responsible for the positive DNPH test; their respective hydroxy analogs are detectable by urine organic acid analysis after stabilization of the 2-oxo groups via oximation. Urine organic acids show the presence of characteristic branched-chain oxoacids and increased excretion of 2-hydroxyisovaleric acid during episodes of decompensation (see Figure 58-7).

Cornerstones of treatment include dietary restriction of branched-chain amino acids, high-dose thiamine (in responsive cases), valine, and isoleucine supplements. Acute episodes are life threatening and require aggressive treatment of brain edema with intravenous mannitol, careful maintenance of sodium concentrations at above 135 mmol/L with administration of 3% sodium chloride, administration of sufficient calories with intravenous glucose, and use of lipids to block catabolism. Dialysis is sometimes necessary to rapidly remove excess leucine.[47]

Urea Cycle Defects

The urea cycle disposes of the nitrogen groups of amino acids before their carbon skeleton is metabolized to gluconeogenic (most amino acids) or ketogenic precursors (leucine and lysine), or both (isoleucine, phenylalanine, tyrosine, and tryptophan). This cycle requires the combined action of different enzymes and mitochondrial transporters (Figure 58-8). Ornithine enters mitochondria through a specific transporter, ORC1; there it combines with carbamyl phosphate by the action of ornithine transcarbamylase (OTC). Synthesis of carbamyl phosphate requires the ammonia generated from the nitrogen group of amino acids, CO_2, two molecules of ATP,

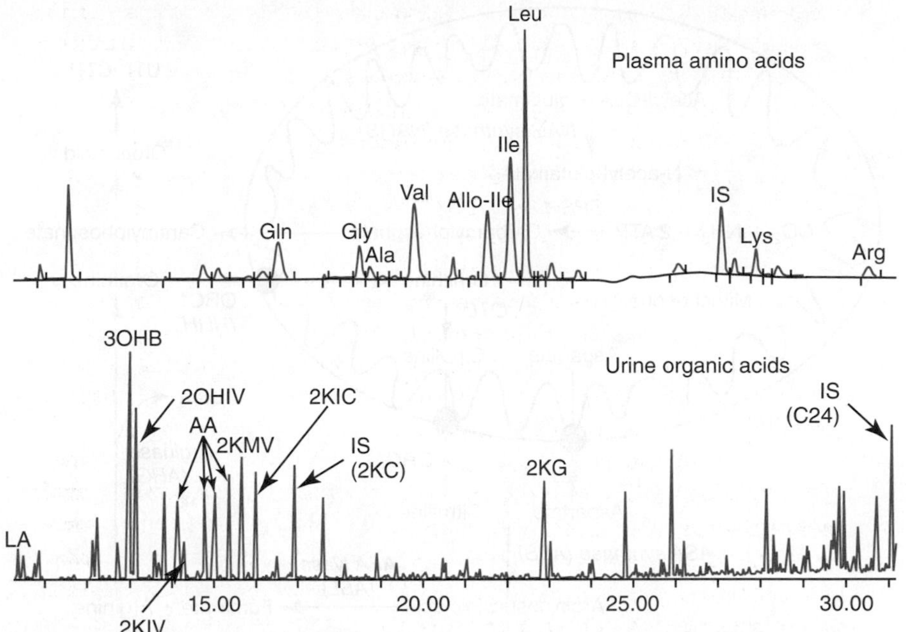

Figure 58-7 Plasma amino acids (by Ion-exchange chromatography) and urine organic acids (by gas chromatography/mass spectrometry) in maple syrup urine disease (branched-chain ketoacid dehydrogenase deficiency). ***Top,*** **All three branched-chain amino acids (leucine, valine, and isoleucine) become elevated in maple syrup urine disease. Alloisoleucine, an amino acid not normally present, is also seen in this condition.** ***Bottom,*** **Urine organic acids show the presence of the characteristic metabolites 2-OH-isovaleric acid (2OHIV), 2-ketoisovaleric acid (2KIV), 2-ketomethylvaleric acid (2KMV), and 2-ketoisocaproic (2KIC). Lactic acid (LA) and ketones [3-OH-butyric acid (3OHB) and acetoacetate (AA)] are also increased in the catabolic state. 2-Ketocaproic acid (2KC) and tetracosane (C24) are used as internal standards (IS).**

and the action of carbamyl phosphate synthase 1 (CPS-1). The activity of this enzyme is dependent on an allosteric activator, *N*-acetylglutamate, which is synthesized by *N*-acetylglutamate synthase (NAGS). The reaction between ornithine and carbamyl phosphate generates citrulline, which exits mitochondria through the ornithine/citrulline exchanger (ORC1).[50] In the cytoplasm, citrulline combines with aspartate that is exported from mitochondria by the citrin transporter (aspartate/glutamate exchanger) through the action of argininosuccinate synthase (ASS). Argininosuccinate is cleaved by a lyase (ASL) into arginine and fumarate. Finally, arginase (ARG) generates urea and ornithine to restart the cycle. Deficiency of any of these enzymes or transporters will impair the function of the urea cycle, causing hyperammonemia. Newborn screening identifies elevated citrulline in citrullinemia type 1 (ASS deficiency) or 2 (citrin deficiency) and, in addition to argininosuccinate, in argininosuccinate lyase deficiency (ASL deficiency). Elevated ornithine and homocitrulline theoretically are the markers for hyperammonemia, hyperornithinemia, and homocitrullinuria syndrome (ORC1 deficiency/HHH syndrome), but it is unclear whether newborns with this condition show elevations of these amino acids. Low concentrations of citrulline with elevated glutamine have been found in NAGS, CPS-1, and OTC deficiency, although appropriate cutoffs have not yet been established for consistent identification of these conditions.

Patients with urea cycle defects may present at any age.[66] In the neonatal period, there is usually a brief interval between birth and clinical manifestations, with the most severe cases presenting before the results of newborn screening are available.[48] Hyperammonemia and the accumulation of glutamine in the brain lead to (1) poor feeding, (2) vomiting, (3) lethargy, or (4) irritability progressing to coma and death. This is caused by the toxic effects of ammonia and by the brain edema caused by glutamine/glutamate accumulation. Milder cases, in which the enzymatic block is not complete, present later in life, many times triggered by excess protein intake or a catabolic state secondary to fasting/infection. In infancy, the symptoms are similar to the neonatal period, but less severe and more variable. Neurologic abnormalities also include ataxia and irritability. Patients are often misdiagnosed as having gastrointestinal disorders, food allergies, behavioral problems, or nonspecific hepatitis. In children and adults, chronic neurologic problems are characterized by (1) learning difficulties, (2) mental retardation, (3) behavioral problems, and (4) recurrent vomiting, which occasionally deteriorates to acute decompensation with severe encephalopathy.[66] Arginase deficiency differs by the usually milder

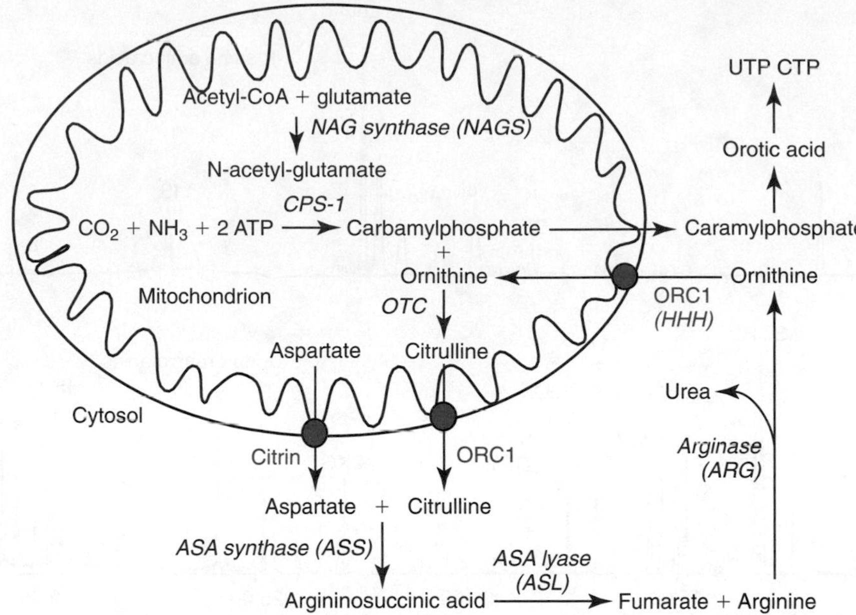

Figure 58-8 The urea cycle leads to the formation of urea starting from ammonia (NH_3). It requires many enzymes and mitochondrial transporters, any of which can be defective and may impair the function of the urea cycle. *ASL,* Arginino succinate lyase; *ASS,* argininosuccinate synthase; *ARG,* arginase; *citrin,* aspartate/glutamate exchanger; *CP,* carbamylphosphate; *CPS-1,* carbamyl phosphate synthase 1; *CTP,* cytidine triphosphate; *NAGS,* N-acetylglutamate synthase; *ORC1,* ornithine/citrulline mitochondrial transporter; *OTC,* ornithine transcarbamylase; *UTP,* uridine triphosphate.

hyperammonemia and by a clinical picture of spastic diplegia, frequently diagnosed as cerebral palsy.[56]

Dominant laboratory findings in urea cycle defects include hyperammonemia and abnormalities of liver function, with variably elevated transaminases and an abnormal prothrombin time (PT)/partial thromboplastin time (PTT) ratio. Plasma amino acids, urine orotic acid, and, in some cases, urine amino acids are necessary for the diagnosis of these disorders. Other conditions that cause hyperammonemia, such as organic acidemias and fatty acid oxidation defects, are excluded by measuring urine organic acid concentrations and observing a plasma acylcarnitine profile. Elevated concentrations of glutamine and alanine, seen when plasma amino acid analysis is performed, are a common finding in all urea cycle defects. Citrulline is the amino acid key to the diagnosis of specific defects. Citrulline is low or undetectable in proximal defects of the urea cycle (NAGS, CPS-1, or OTC deficiency). The concentration of urine orotic acid is elevated in OTC deficiency, but it is within the reference interval or low in NAGS and CPS-1 deficiency. A marked increase in the concentration of plasma citrulline is found in argininosuccinic acid synthase deficiency, a condition commonly known as citrullinemia type 1. A twofold to fivefold elevation of the concentration of plasma citrulline in the presence of argininosuccinic acid is indicative of argininosuccinic acid lyase deficiency. Mild elevation of the concentration of plasma citrulline without elevation of argininosuccinic acid concentration is also seen in citrin deficiency (citrullinemia type 2) or, with other biochemical abnormalities and a severe clinical picture, in the neonatal variant of pyruvate carboxylase deficiency.

Acute hyperammonemia should be treated promptly as a medical emergency. Calories should be provided as intravenous glucose and lipids, with insulin used if possible to reverse the catabolic state. A variety of conjugating agents (benzoate, phenylacetate, phenylbutyrate) are used to deplete the nitrogen pool via excretion of their glycine and glutamine conjugates. Citrulline and/or arginine supplementation provides substrates of the urea cycle downstream to the specific block to allow protein synthesis to resume. If these therapies along with reversal of catabolism fail to effectively reduce blood ammonia within hours, hemodialysis must be instituted. Long-term therapy consists of a diet low in proteins supplemented with citrulline (in OTC, or CPS-1, deficiency) or arginine (ASS; ASL deficiency) and the oral administration of ammonia scavengers (phenylbutyrate, benzoate).[48,66] NAGS deficiency responds to therapy with oral *N*-carbamylglutamate, a precursor of *N*-acetylglutamate.[27]

Glycine Encephalopathy (Nonketotic Hyperglycinemia)

Glycine, the simplest amino acid, is metabolized by several different pathways. The major catabolic pathway for glycine is through the glycine cleavage system, a four peptide complex (protein P, H, T, and L) attached to the inner mitochondrial membrane in liver, brain, kidney, and placenta.[4,36] One carbon is converted to carbon dioxide, and the other is transferred to tetrahydrofolate to form hydroxymethyltetrahydrofolate, which may react with another mole of glycine to produce serine or to form methyltetrahydrofolate, which serves as a methyl donor.[4,20,36]

Glycine encephalopathy or nonketotic hyperglycinemia (NKHG) is a severe condition caused, in most cases, by a defect in P, T, and H proteins of the glycine cleavage system.[20] Patients with the classic form of the disease present within the first days of life with (1) lethargy, (2) poor sucking, (3) severe hypotonia, (4) hiccups, (5) seizures, and (6) apnea. Most of these patients die in the first few months of life or survive with profound developmental delays. Few patients have been described with transient NKHG that disappears within the first 6 months of life. Atypical variants of NKHG have been diagnosed in patients with rather disparate manifestations who have in common in most cases seizures and delays of different degrees of severity.[20]

Patients with these conditions have no defined abnormalities on routine laboratory testing. Newborn screening is not reliable in identifying patients affected by this condition. The disease is characterized by elevated concentrations of plasma (Figure 58-9) and CSF glycine with no other notable abnormalities, and by unremarkable concentrations of urine organic acids and plasma acylcarnitine profile (to exclude ketotic hyperglycinemia, caused by organic acidemias such as propionic or methylmalonic acidemia). The concentration of glycine will vary in plasma from mildly to markedly elevated, but it is always elevated in the CSF (>30 μmol/L). The calculated CSF : plasma glycine concentration ratio (>0.08, reference interval <0.04) is critical in the diagnosis of this condition,[4] but caution should be used in interpreting the ratio when plasma and CSF specimens are not collected simultaneously or no more than 1 hour apart. Individuals with organic acidemias, such as propionic and methylmalonic acidemia, have been known to present with elevated plasma and CSF glycine in the concentrations observed in NKHG. In this case, analysis of urine organic acids should reveal the metabolites characteristic of the organic acidemia. Contamination of CSF with blood results in increased concentrations of glycine; however, when this occurs, other unrelated amino acids are also elevated. Seizure medications, such as valproate, inhibit the glycine cleavage system, resulting in elevated plasma and CSF glycine. The diagnosis of NKHG is confirmed by enzyme assay or molecular analysis,[4] although some atypical, late-onset cases might have no identifiable mutations in the P, H, or T gene.[20]

No effective treatment is known. Sodium benzoate binds glycine and decreases its concentration. It might help in milder forms of the disease. Treatment of seizures is indicated, although there is no treatment to prevent progression of the disease in severe cases.

ORGANIC ACIDEMIAS

Organic acidemias are inborn errors of metabolism characterized by the accumulation of intermediates in the catabolic pathways of amino acids. These intermediates are water-soluble compounds containing one or more carboxyl groups (organic acids) and other functional groups (-keto, -hydroxy). They may be physiologic metabolites present in excessive amounts, or metabolites not normally present but derived

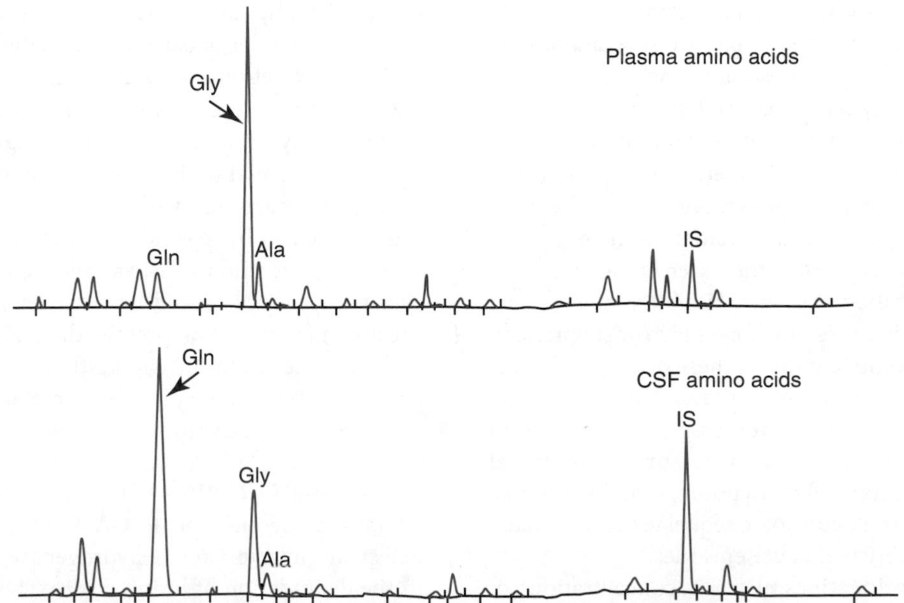

Figure 58-9 **Plasma *(top)* and cerebrospinal fluid (CSF) *(bottom)* amino acids (by ion-exchange chromatography) in glycine encephalopathy. Glycine becomes the predominant amino acid in the plasma amino acids *(top)* and is much higher than normal in the cerebrospinal fluid *(bottom)* as compared with glutamine, which physiologically is the predominant amino acid.**

from activation of alternative pathways in response to a specific metabolic block. They have heterogeneous clinical presentations, with many of them causing the accumulation of organic compounds resulting in metabolic acidosis (pH = 6.85 to 7.3) with low bicarbonate (<5 to 15 mmol/L) and sometimes hyperammonemia. They differ from renal tubular acidosis by the presence of a significant anion gap, represented by organic anions not measured in routine chemistry panels. The biochemical diagnosis of organic acidemia is accomplished via urine organic acid analysis by gas chromatography-mass spectrometry (GC/MS), in addition to plasma amino acid and plasma acylcarnitine analysis.

Table 58-7 summarizes the most common organic acidemias. Several of these are discussed later.

Disorders of Propionate Metabolism

Propionyl-CoA is an intermediate in the catabolism of isoleucine, valine, threonine, methionine, pyrimidines (uracil and thymine), and cholesterol, and is the final product of the β-oxidation of odd-chain fatty acids. Propionyl-CoA is converted by a biotin-dependent carboxylase (propionyl-CoA carboxylase) to methylmalonyl-CoA, which is converted to succinyl-CoA by an adenosylcobalamin-dependent mutase (methylmalonyl-CoA mutase) for oxidation in the tricarboxylic acid cycle.[18] Primary or secondary defects of these two enzymes were among the first organic acidurias to be discovered; their natural history has been characterized in greater detail than any other inborn error of organic acid metabolism.[18]

The combined incidence of propionic acidemia (PA) and methylmalonic acidemia (MMA) varies considerably, with estimates ranging from 1:2000 to 1:5000 (Saudi Arabia and Greenland)[51] to 1:100,000. Patients with PA and MMA typically are born at term with no pregnancy complications and present with an intoxication type of picture several hours to days after birth. Prominent manifestations include (1) vomiting, (2) hypotonia or hypertonia, (3) lethargy, (4) apnea, (5) hypothermia, and (6) rapid onset of coma. Routine laboratory investigations show severe metabolic acidosis and ketonuria (a finding of critical significance never to be overlooked in the newborn period); lactic acidemia and hyperammonemia are often present[18] with the latter being extremely severe, as in defects of the urea cycle. Similarly, neutropenia and thromobocytopenia caused by bone marrow suppression have been observed. Complications of these disorders include (1) cardiomyopathy (mostly in propionic acidemia), (2) acute and chronic pancreatitis, and (3) progressive renal failure (in methylmalonic acidemia).[18] Patients who survive the initial event have developmental delay, hypotonia or hypertonia, and variable cognitive and neurologic sequelae that are linked to the number and severity of acute episodes.

Newborn screening identifies elevated concentrations of C3 carnitine in both propionic and methylmalonic acidemias, with higher concentrations usually seen in PA. Second-tier methods,[46] performed on the same blood spot used for the initial newborn screening, are available for measurement of methylmalonic and methylcitric acids. Mildly elevated C3 carnitine concentrations have been observed in patients with vitamin B_{12} deficiency and sometimes with hyperbilirubinemia. Diagnosis is confirmed by measurement of urine organic acids showing elevated concentrations of 2-methylcitric acid and other propionate metabolites in propionic acidemia and markedly elevated concentrations of methylmalonic acid in methylmalonic acidemia (Figure 58-10). Variant forms of propionic acidemia, in which the presentation is neurologic, without ketosis or acidosis, are known. In these cases, the only abnormal metabolite is 2-methylcitric acid. With plasma amino acid analysis, hyperglycinemia is observed, although patients with PA in the neonatal period may have normal concentrations of glycine. Acylcarnitine analysis reveals elevated concentrations of propionylcarnitine in both PA and MMA, sometimes associated with carnitine deficiency. Treatment is based on restriction of precursor amino acids and supplementation with carnitine and cofactors—biotin or hydroxycobalamin—as indicated.

Isovaleric Acidemia

Isovaleric acidemia (IVA) is a disorder of leucine catabolism caused by deficiency of isovaleryl-CoA dehydrogenase.[75] Clinical presentation includes both severe metabolic acidosis and hyperammonemia leading to death shortly after birth. Milder variants present with vomiting and failure to thrive, evolving into acute presentation triggered by fever or other illnesses. One revealing feature of this IEM is the characteristic odor of "sweaty feet." Newborn screening by MS/MS reveals elevated concentrations of C5-carnitine (Figure 58-11). The diagnosis is confirmed by urine organic acid analysis showing elevated concentrations of isovalerylglycine as the major byproduct and 3-hydroxyisovaleric acid (see Figure 58-11). Elevated concentrations of C5-carnitine also reflect 2-methyl-butyryl-CoA dehydrogenase deficiency, an inherited disorder of isoleucine metabolism characterized by variable excretion of 2-methylbutyrylglycine. In these patients, analysis of urine organic acids may not detect 2-methylbutyrylglycine; therefore acylglycine analysis should also be performed in the investigation of elevated concentrations of C5-carnitine with normal concentrations of urine organic acids. In several patients identified by newborn screening, excretion of isovalerylglycine is only moderately elevated, possibly caused by a milder form of the disease.[75] Treatment with a low-protein diet, glycine (250 mg/kg/d), and carnitine (50 to 100 mg/kg/d) supplements allows a good prognosis, but acute episodes of metabolic decompensation could be life threatening at any age.

Glutaric Acidemia Type 1

Glutaric acidemia type 1 (GA-1) results from an inherited defect in glutaryl-CoA dehydrogenase, an enzyme involved in the degradation of lysine, hydroxylysine, and tryptophan. Affected individuals may have macrocephaly at birth or may develop it in the first year of life.[30] They can have mild hypotonia, and some develop acute dystonia and spasticity, with metabolic decompensation usually triggered by fever

Text continued on page 2071

TABLE 58-7 Clinical and Laboratory Characteristics of Disorders of Organic Acid Metabolism

Common Name	OMIM* No.	Inheritance	Enzyme/Transport Defect	Incidence (USA)	Major Clinical Features	Major Biochemical Marker(s)
Disorders of Propionate Metabolism and Related Cofactors						
Propionic acidemia	232000, 232050	AR	Propionyl-CoA carboxylase (subunit alpha, beta)	>1:75,000	Failure to thrive, developmental delay, hypotonia, neutropenia, lethargy progressing to coma, vomiting, hyperammonemia, metabolic acidosis	GLY (not in the neonatal period), propionylcarnitine (B), methylcitric acid, 3-OH-propionic acid, propionylglycine, tiglylglycine (U)
Multiple carboxylase deficiency	253270	AR	Holocarboxylase synthase	<1:100,000	Alopecia, perioral skin erosions, hearing loss, developmental delay, hypotonia, seizures, breathing problems, dehydration, ketoacidosis, lactic acidemia	Lactic acid, C5-OH-carnitine, C3-carnitine (B), 3-OH-isovaleric acid, 3-methylcrotonylglycine, 3-OH-propionic acid, methylcitric acid, lactate, tiglylglycine (U)
Methylmalonic acidemia (mut 0 and mut–)	251000	AR	Methylmalonyl-CoA mutase	>1:75,000	Failure to thrive, anorexia, developmental delay, hypotonia, dehydration, ketoacidosis, vomiting, hyperammonemia	GLY, MMA, propionylcarnitine (B), MMA, methylcitric acid, 3-OH-propionic acid (U)
Methylmalonic acidemia (cblA and cblB)	251100	AR	Mitochondrial cobalamin reductase	<1:100,000	Failure to thrive, anorexia, developmental delay, hypotonia, dehydration, ketoacidosis	MMA, propionylcarnitine (B), MMA, methylcitric acid (U)
Methylmalonic acidemia (cblC): combined methylmalonic acidemia/ homocystinuria	277400	AR	Methionine synthase; methylmalonyl-CoA mutase	<1:100,000	Failure to thrive, developmental delay, hypotonia, megaloblastic anemia, hemolytic-uremic syndrome, apnea, seizures, dehydration, ketoacidosis	MMA, tHcy, propionylcarnitine (B), MMA, methylcitric acid (U)
Methylmalonic acidemia (cblD): combined methylmalonic acidemia/ homocystinuria; variant 1: homocystinuria only; variant 2: methylmalonic acidemia only	277410	AR	Methionine synthase; methylmalonyl-CoA mutase	<1:100,000	Failure to thrive, developmental delay, hypotonia, megaloblastic anemia, hemolytic-uremic syndrome, apnea, seizures, dehydration, ketoacidosis	MMA, tHcy, propionylcarnitine (B), MMA, methylcitric acid (U)

Continued

TABLE 58-7 Clinical and Laboratory Characteristics of Disorders of Organic Acid Metabolism—cont'd

Common Name	OMIM* No.	Inheritance	Enzyme/Transport Defect	Incidence (USA)	Major Clinical Features	Major Biochemical Marker(s)
Disorders of Propionate Metabolism and Related Cofactors—cont'd						
Methylmalonic acidemia (cblF)	277380	AR	Vitamin B_{12} lysosomal release	<1:100,000	Failure to thrive, developmental delay, hypotonia	MMA (B,U); tHCy (B,U)
Other Disorders of Branched-Chain Amino Acid Metabolism						
Isovaleric acidemia	243500	AR	Isovaleryl-CoA dehydrogenase	<1:100,000	Episodic vomiting, lethargy, coma, sweaty feet odor, dehydration, ketoacidosis	Isovalerylcarnitine (B), 3-OH-isovaleric acid, isovalerylglycine (U)
3-Methylcrotonylglycinuria	210200	AR	3-Methylcrotonyl-CoA carboxylase	>1:60,000	Episodic vomiting, lethargy, coma, dehydration, ketoacidosis	C5-OH-carnitine (B), 3-OH-isovaleric acid, 3-methylcrotonylglycine (U)
3-Methylglutaconic aciduria	250950	AR	3-Methylglutaconyl-CoA hydratase	<1:100,000	Speech defect, mental retardation, hypertonia, spasticity, hypoglycemia, acidosis	C5-OH-carnitine (B), 3-OH-isovaleric acid, 3-methylglutaconic acid (U)
3-Hydroxy-3-methylglutaric aciduria	246450	AR	3-Hydroxy-3-methylglutaryl-CoA lyase	<1:100,000	Episodic vomiting, hypotonia, hypoglycemia, metabolic acidosis, hepatomegaly	C5-OH-carnitine (B), 3-OH-isovaleric acid, 3-methylglutaconic acid, 3-OH-3-methylglutaric acid (U)
2-Methylbutyrylglycinuria	600301	AR	2-Methylbutyryl-CoA dehydrogenase	<1:100,000 (1:500 Hmong)	Developmental delay, seizures, progressive muscle weakness, hypoglycemia, acidosis. Lack of symptoms also possible.	C5-carnitine (B), 2-methylbutyrylglycine (U)
2-Methyl-3-hydroxybutyric aciduria	300438	X-linked	2-Methyl-3-hydroxybutyryl-CoA dehydrogenase	<1:100,000	Progressive loss of mental and motor skills, acidosis	C5-OH-carnitine, C5:1-carnitine (B), 2-methyl-3-OH-butyric acid, tiglylglycine (U)
Beta-ketothiolase deficiency	203750	AR	Beta-ketothiolase	<1:100,000	Episodic vomiting, lethargy, hypotonia, mental retardation, speech problems, ketoacidosis, seizures	C5-OH-carnitine, C5:1-carnitine (B), 2-methyl-3-OH-butyric acid, 2-methylacetoacetic, tiglylglycine (U)

Isobutyrylglycinuria	611283	AR	Isobutyryl-CoA dehydrogenase	<1:100,000	Anemia, dilated cardiomyopathy	C4-carnitine (B), isobutyrylglycine (U)
3-Hydroxyisobutyric aciduria	Pending	AR	3-Hydroxyisobutyryl-CoA dehydrogenase or methylmalonic semialdehyde dehydrogenase	<1;100,000	Congenital anomalies, short stature, hypotonia, episodic ketoacidosis	3-OH-isobutyric acid, 2-ethylhydracrylic acid (U)
Miscellaneous Disorders of Organic Acid Metabolism						
Alkaptonuria	203500	AR	Homogentisic dioxygenase	<1:100,000	Arthritis, ochronosis, heart valvulitis	Homogentisic acid (U)
Biotinidase deficiency	253260	AR	Biotinidase	>1:75,000	Alopecia, periorificial skin rash, conjunctivitis, developmental delay, hypotonia	Low biotinidase activity (B); 3-OH-isovaleric acid and 3-methylcrotonylglycine (U) and C5-OH-carnitine (B) may be elevated
4-OH-butyric aciduria	271980	AR	Succinic semialdehyde dehydrogenase	<1:100,000	Developmental delay, ataxia, hypotonia, seizures, hyperkinetic behavior	4-OH-butyric acid (U)
Canavan disease	271900	AR	*N*-aspartoacylase	<1:100,000 (1:5000 Ashkenazi)	Hypotonia, developmental delay, macrocephaly, optic atrophy, seizures, progressive neurologic degeneration	*N*-acetyl aspartic acid(U)
Ethylmalonic encephalopathy	602473	AR	Mitochondrial matrix protein (ETHE1)	<1:100,000	Hypotonia, spastic tetraparesis, petechiae, orthostatic acrocyanosis, diarrhea, lactic acidosis, developmental delay	C4-, C5-carnitines (B), EMA, lactic acid, isobutyrylglycine, 2-methylbutyrylglycine (U)
Glutaric acidemia type I	231670	AR	Glutaryl-CoA dehydrogenase	>1:75,000 (1:500 Amish)	Macrocephaly, hypotonia, abnormal movement, frontotemporal atrophy, basal ganglia lesions	C5-DC-carnitine (B,U), glutaric acid, 3-OH-glutaric acid (U)
Glyceroluria	307030	X-linked	Glycerol kinase	<1:100,000	Failure to thrive, episodic vomiting, developmental delay, bone fracture, acidosis, adrenal insufficiency	Pseudo-hypertriglyceridemia (B), glycerol (B, U)

Continued

TABLE 58-7 Clinical and Laboratory Characteristics of Disorders of Organic Acid Metabolism—cont'd

Common Name	OMIM* No.	Inheritance	Enzyme/Transport Defect	Incidence (USA)	Major Clinical Features	Major Biochemical Marker(s)
Miscellaneous Disorders of Organic Acid Metabolism—cont'd						
Hyperoxaluria type I	259900	AR	Alanine: glyoxylate aminotransferase	<1:100,000	Urolithiasis, nephrocalcinosis, renal failure	Oxalic acid, glycolic acid (U)
Hyperoxaluria type II	260000	AR	D-Glyceric dehydrogenase	<1:100,000	Urolithiasis, hematuria, urinary tract infection, rarely nephrocalcinosis and renal failure	Oxalic acid, glyceric acid (U)
Malonic acidemia	248360	AR	Malonyl-CoA decarboxylase	<1:100,000	Short stature, cardiomyopathy, GI symptoms, hypotonia, developmental delay, hypoglycemia, acidosis	C3-DC-carnitine (B), malonic acid, methylmalonic acid (U)
Pyroglutamic aciduria	266130	AR	Glutathione synthase	<1:100,000	Mental retardation, ataxia, spastic tetraparesis, seizures, acidosis, hemolytic anemia, neutropenia	Pyroglutamic (U)
Mevalonic aciduria	251170	AR	Mevalonate kinase	<1:100,000	Failure to thrive, developmental delay, ataxia, hypotonia, hepatosplenomegaly, skin rash, diarrhea	Mevalonic acid, mevalonolactone (U)

*OMIM: Online Mendelian Inheritance in Man (www.ncbi.nlm.nih.gov/entrez/query.fcgi?db=OMIM/accessed September 29, 2011).

EMA, Ethylmalonic acid; *MMA*, methylmalonic acid; *NAA*, *N*-acetylaspartic acid; *NBS*, newborn screening; *RFLP*, restriction fragment length polymorphism.

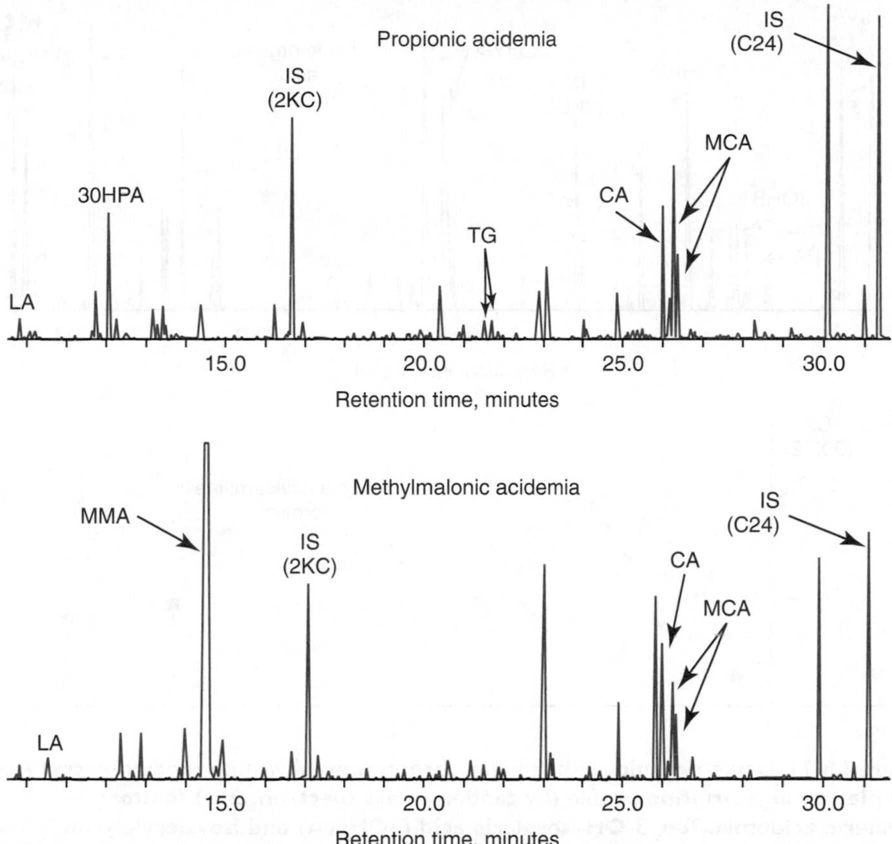

Figure 58-10 Urine organic acids (by gas chromatography/mass spectrometry) in propionic *(top)* and methylmalonic *(bottom)* acidemia. *Top,* Methylcitric acid (MCA) is the characteristic metabolite of propionic acidemia and is present in excess even in milder forms of this condition. Other metabolites are 3-OH-propionic acid (3OHPA), tiglylglycine (TG), and propionylglycine (not seen in this chromatogram). *Bottom,* Methylmalonic acid (MMA) is markedly increased in patients with methylmalonic acidemia. Methylcitric acid can also be present in excess. *IS,* Internal standard; *LA,* lactic acid.

or other illnesses. Brain imaging of affected individuals demonstrates frontotemporal atrophy and, after a crisis, the characteristic sequelae of acute striatal degeneration and shrinkage of the caudate and putamen.[30] Hypotonia followed by spasticity, abnormal movement, seizures, mild hypoglycemia, and metabolic acidosis has been associated with acute events.

Diagnosis of this condition is confirmed by analysis for urine organic acids indicating excretion of massive quantities of glutaric and 3-hydroxyglutaric acids. This is associated with increased concentrations of glutarylcarnitine in plasma. Some patients, referred to as low excretors, show a more subtle biochemical phenotype with normal or mildly elevated glutaric acid and mildly increased excretion of 3-hydroxyglutaric acid.[30] In these patients, the concentration of plasma glutarylcarnitine is sometimes normal, although they tend to have elevated urinary excretion of glutarylcarnitine.[73] Infants with GA-1 usually have elevated concentrations of glutarylcarnitine identifiable by newborn screening, although low excretors are sometimes missed. Concentrations of glutarylcarnitine are also elevated in patients with kidney failure, but usually in association with other acylcarnitine species.

Treatment consists of a diet restricted in lysine and tryptophan and carnitine supplementation. Prompt treatment of infection or other illness and prevention of metabolic decompensation are critical components in the treatment of this disease.

DISORDERS OF THE CARNITINE CYCLE AND FATTY ACID OXIDATION

Carnitine [3-hydroxy-4-(trimethylazaniumyl)butanoate] plays an essential role in the transport of long-chain fatty acids inside mitochondria for β-oxidation. During periods of fasting or high energy demand, the main substrates for energy production in the liver, cardiac muscle, and skeletal muscle are fatty acids, which are released by adipose tissue. The brain is unable to utilize fatty acids because they cannot cross the blood-brain barrier; however, it is capable of oxidizing ketone bodies derived from β-oxidation of fatty acids in the liver.[44] If fatty acid oxidation is impaired, fatty acids

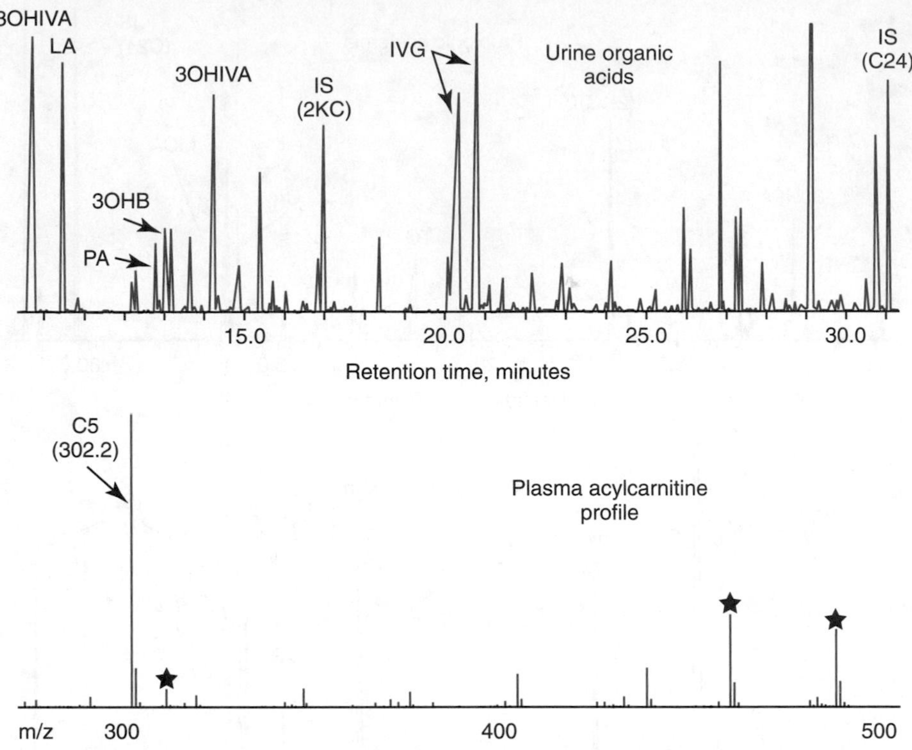

Figure 58-11 Urine organic acids (by gas chromatography/mass spectrometry) *(top)* and plasma acylcarnitine profile (by tandem mass spectrometry) *(bottom)* in isovaleric acidemia. *Top,* 3-OH-isovaleric acid (3OHIVA) and isovalerylglycine (IVG) are the characteristic metabolites of isovaleric acidemia. In this sample, lactic acid (LA), propionic acid (PA), and 3-OH-butyric acid (3OHB) were also increased. *IS,* Internal standard. *Bottom,* C5 (Isovaleryl)-carnitine is markedly increased in patients with classic isovaleric acidemia. Internal standards are indicated with a star.

will still be released by adipose tissue during fasting or high energy demands, but they accumulate in the liver, heart, and skeletal muscle. In the liver, impaired oxidation of fatty acids will result in steatosis and decreased production of ketones. Ketones are used by the heart, skeletal muscle, and brain as energy sources sparing glucose; in the liver, increased acetyl-CoA, derived from β-oxidation of fatty acids, stimulates gluconeogenesis (production of glucose), mostly from the carbon skeleton of amino acids released from the muscle. Excessive utilization of glucose and lack of gluconeogenesis cause hypoglycemia, which, in addition to decreased availability of ketones, decreases the energy supply to the brain, causing loss of consciousness, seizures, and coma. Fats also accumulate in the heart and skeletal muscle, causing cardiomyopathy and myopathy, in addition to fatal arrhythmias.

Long-chain fatty acids, released from adipose tissue, enter mitochondria for subsequent β-oxidation through the carnitine cycle (Figure 58-12). This cycle requires enzymes and transporters that (1) accumulate carnitine within the cell (OCTN2 carnitine transporter), (2) conjugate it with long-chain fatty acids to form long-chain acylcarnitines [carnitine palmitoyl transferase 1 (CPT-1)], (3) transfer acylcarnitines across the inner plasma membrane [carnitine-acylcarnitine translocase (CACT)], and (4) conjugate fatty acids back to coenzyme A for subsequent β-oxidation [carnitine palmitoyl transferase 2 (CPT-2)]. Medium- and short-chain fatty acids also cross the mitochondrial membrane independent of the carnitine cycle. In the mitochondrial matrix, long-chain fatty acids undergo a series of enzymatic reactions to progressively shorten their chain by two carbon units (acetyl-CoA). Several dehydrogenases are present, each with different carbon chain length specificity from C18 to C4. These enzymes introduce a double bond between carbons C2 and C3 of a given fatty acid (Figure 58-13) and include (1) very long-chain acyl CoA dehydrogenase (VLCAD), (2) long-chain acyl CoA dehydrogenase (LCAD), (3) medium-chain acyl CoA dehydrogenase (MCAD), and (4) short-chain acyl CoA dehydrogenase (SCAD). A trifunctional protein (TFP) adds water and cleaves two carbon atoms from the long-chain fatty acid. This is done through the sequential action of a hydratase (enoyl-CoA hydratase), a β-hydroxyacyl-CoA dehydrogenase [long-chain 3-OH-acyl-CoA dehydrogenase (LCHAD)], and a thiolase (acyl-CoA acetyltransferase). The two-carbon units generated are completely oxidized in the muscle to CO_2 or generate ketone bodies in the liver that are transported to other organs, where they serve as an energy source.

Deficiency in any of these steps leads to impaired energy production, in most cases aggravated by fasting or a catabolic state. Characteristics of disorders of the carnitine cycle and

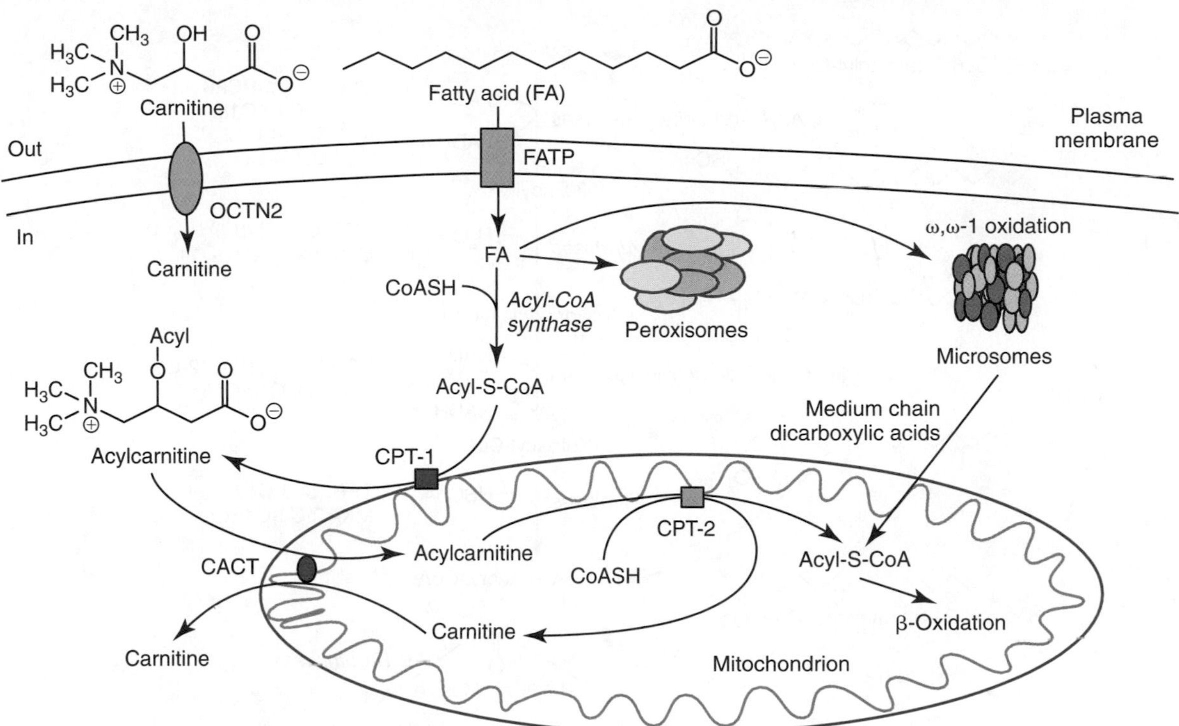

Figure 58-12 The carnitine cycle in fatty acid oxidation. The carnitine cycle is responsible for delivering long-chain fatty acid to the mitochondrial matrix for subsequent beta oxidation. *CACT*, Carnitine acyl carnitine translocase; *CPT-1*, carnitine palmitoyl transferase 1; *CPT-2*, carnitine palmitoyl transferase 2; *FA*, fatty acid; *FATP*, fatty acid transporter protein. *(Modified from Longo N, Amat di San Filippo C, Pasquali M. Disorders of carnitine transport and the carnitine cycle. Am J Med Genet C Semin Med Genet 2006;142:77-85.)*

of fatty acid oxidation are summarized in Table 58-8 and are discussed in greater detail in the following sections.

Carnitine Uptake Defect

Carnitine uptake defect (CUD), or primary carnitine deficiency (OMIM 212140), is an autosomal recessive disorder of the carnitine cycle affecting fatty acid oxidation. It is caused by lack of functional OCTN2 carnitine transporter. Primary carnitine deficiency has a frequency of about 1:40,000 newborns in the general population, but a much higher incidence in the Faroe Islands (1:720).[45] Lack of the plasma membrane carnitine transporter results in urinary carnitine wasting, low serum carnitine concentrations (0 to 9 μmol/L, reference interval 25 to 50 μmol/L), and decreased intracellular carnitine accumulation. Patients with primary carnitine deficiency lose significant amounts (50 to 95%) of filtered carnitine in urine, and their heterozygous parents lose two to three times the normal amount, which explains their mildly reduced plasma carnitine concentrations.[57] Patients typically present with hepatic encephalopathy or cardiomyopathy triggered by fasting or infection. Routine laboratory studies show hypoglycemia with minimal or no ketones in urine, hyperammonemia with variably elevated liver transaminase activities, and, occasionally, elevated creatine kinase activity. Some patients have been completely asymptomatic all of their life and are diagnosed only following the birth of an affected child.[59] Other children, diagnosed because of an affected sibling, had only mild developmental delays. Newborn screening is used to identify reduced concentrations of free carnitine in blood spots. Low carnitine concentrations are also seen in the newborn blood spots of infants of mothers with low carnitine due to a carnitine uptake defect or secondary to an undiagnosed organic acidemia or fatty acid oxidation defect. Diagnosis is further suspected with the finding of extremely reduced concentrations of free, total, and acylated carnitine (free carnitine <9 μmol/L, reference interval 25 to 50 μmol/L) with unremarkable concentrations of urine organic acids. In symptomatic patients, urine organic acid concentrations may reveal a nonspecific dicarboxylic aciduria. Diagnosis is confirmed by demonstrating reduced carnitine transport (<15% of normal) in skin fibroblasts and/or by performing DNA testing, which, however, can fail to identify some of the causative mutations. Therapy consists of lifelong carnitine (100 to 300 mg/kg/d) supplementation.

Carnitine Palmitoyl Transferase 1 Deficiency

Carnitine palmitoyl transferase 1 (CPT-1) conjugates fatty acids to carnitine, allowing their subsequent mitochondrial import (see Figure 58-12). Three different isoforms of CPT-1 have tissue-specific expression encoded by different genes:

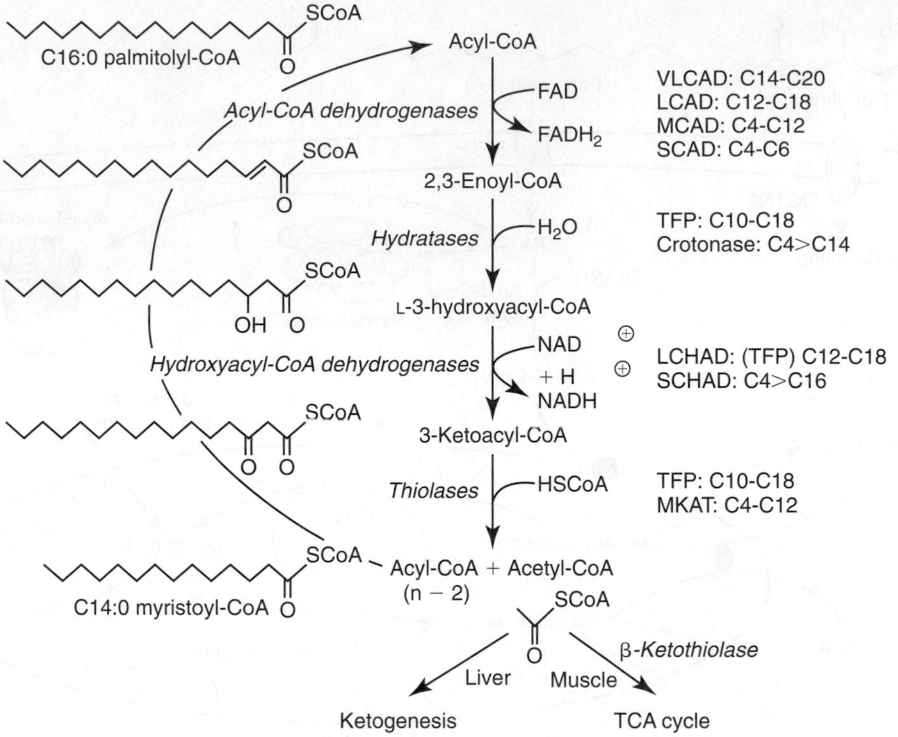

Figure 58-13 Beta oxidation of fatty acids. In the mitochondrial matrix, long-chain fatty acids undergo a series of steps to progressively shorten the fatty acids of two carbon units (acetyl-CoA) through a series of enzymatic reactions. Dehydrogenases with different carbon chain length specificity (*LCAD,* long-chain acyl-CoA dehydrogenase; *MCAD,* medium-chain acyl-CoA dehydrogenase; *SCAD,* short-chain acyl-CoA dehydrogenase; *VLCAD,* very long-chain acyl-CoA dehydrogenase) introduce a double bond between C2 and C3. A trifunctional protein (TFP) adds water and cleaves two carbon atoms from the long-chain fatty acid. This is done through sequential action of a hydratase (enoyl-CoA hydratase), a L-3-hydroxyacyl-CoA dehydrogenase (*LCHAD,* long-chain 3-OH-acyl-CoA dehydrogenase), and a thiolase (acyl-CoA acetyltransferase). The two carbon units generated can be completely oxidized in the muscle to CO_2 or can generate ketone bodies in the liver that may be exported to provide energy to other organs.

liver type (CPT-1A), encoded by a gene on 11q13; muscle type (CPT-1B), encoded by a gene on 22q13; and brain type (CPT-1C), whose gene maps to 19q13.[9] Only deficiency of the liver type, CPT-1A, has been demonstrated in humans. CPT-1 deficiency (OMIM* 255120) is usually triggered by fasting or viral illness. Affected children present, usually between birth and 18 months of age, with altered mental status and hepatomegaly. Routine laboratory evaluation indicates nonketotic hypoglycemia, mild hyperammonemia, elevated liver function tests, and elevated concentrations of free fatty acids. Newborn screening is used to identify elevated concentrations of free carnitine with low concentrations of long-chain acylcarnitines (C16 and C18) and an elevated free carnitine/(C16+C18) ratio. This latter ratio allows discrimination of elevated free carnitine caused by carnitine supplements from CPT-1 deficiency.[24] Plasma carnitine concentrations are usually increased in classic cases, but they generally fall within the reference intervals in milder cases. In these cases, DNA testing or assay of CPT-1 activity in fibroblasts is required to confirm or exclude the diagnosis. Therapy consists of avoidance of fasting, benefitting from night-time feeds with uncooked cornstarch and a low-fat diet rich in medium-chain triglycerides, which do not need the carnitine cycle for β-oxidation in liver mitochondria.

Carnitine-Acylcarnitine Translocase Deficiency

Carnitine-acylcarnitine translocase (CACT) is responsible for transporting both carnitine and carnitine-fatty acid complexes across the inner mitochondrial membrane (see Figure 58-12). CACT deficiency (OMIM 212138) presents most often in the neonatal period with (1) seizures, (2) irregular heartbeat, and (3) apnea. Frequently, these episodes are triggered by fasting or by the physiologic stress of birth. Patients

*Online Mendelian Inheritance in Man. OMIM is a comprehensive, authoritative, and timely compendium of human genes and genetic phenotypes (http://www.ncbi.nlm.nih.gov/omim/accessed September 29, 2011).

TABLE 58-8 Clinical and Laboratory Characteristics of Fatty Acid Oxidation Disorders

Common Name	OMIM* No.	Inheritance	Enzyme/ Transport Defect	Incidence (USA)	Major Clinical Features	Major Biochemical Marker(s)
Carnitine uptake defect	212140	AR	Carnitine transporter	1:40,000	Hypoglycemia, cardiomyopathy, fasting intolerance, hypoketotic hypoglycemia, sudden death	Low free carnitine (B), low long-chain acylcarnitines (B), decreased urinary carnitine reabsorption
CPT-1A deficiency (liver)	255120	AR	Carnitine palmitoyl transferase I	<1:100,000	Liver disease, hypotonia, renal tubular acidosis, fasting intolerance, hypoketotic hypoglycemia	High free carnitine (B), low long-chain acylcarnitines (B)
Translocase deficiency	212138	AR	Carnitine acylcarnitine translocase	<1:100,000	Cardiomyopathy, liver disease, fasting intolerance, hypoketotic hypoglycemia	C16/C18 acylcarnitines (B)
CPT-2 deficiency	600649 608836 255110	AR	Carnitine palmitoyl transferase II	<1:100,000	Cardiomyopathy, liver disease, congenital anomalies, adult-onset myopathy, fasting/exercise/ cold intolerance, myoglobinuria	C16/C18 acylcarnitines (B)
VLCAD deficiency	201475	AR	Very long-chain acyl-CoA dehydrogenase	>1:75,000	Spectrum from early-onset cardiomyopathy, coma, liver disease, fasting intolerance, hypoketotic hypoglycemia to adult-onset myopathy	C14:1-carnitine (B)
LCHAD deficiency	600890	AR	Long-chain 3-hydroxyacyl-CoA dehydrogenase	>1:75,000	Cardiomyopathy, liver disease, retinopathy, peripheral neuropathy, fasting intolerance, hypoketotic hypoglycemia, myoglobinuria, maternal AFLP/ HELLP syndrome	C16-OH/C18-OH acylcarnitines (B); C6-C14 3-OH-dicarboxylic acids (U)

Continued

TABLE 58-8 Clinical and Laboratory Characteristics of Fatty Acid Oxidation Disorders—cont'd

Common Name	OMIM* No.	Inheritance	Enzyme/ Transport Defect	Incidence (USA)	Major Clinical Features	Major Biochemical Marker(s)
TFP deficiency	600890 143450	AR	Trifunctional protein	<1:100,000	Cardiomyopathy, liver disease, retinopathy, peripheral neuropathy, fasting intolerance, hypoketotic hypoglycemia, myoglobinuria, maternal AFLP/ HELLP syndrome	C16-OH/C18-OH acylcarnitines (B); C6-C14 3-OH-dicarboxylic acids (U)
Glutaric acidemia type II	231680	AR	Electron transfer flavoprotein (ETF), ETF ubiquinone oxidoreductase	<1:100,000	Cardiomyopathy, liver disease, congenital anomalies, adult-onset myopathy, hypoketotic hypoglycemia, myoglobinuria	C4 to C18 acylcarnitines (B); C5-C10 dicarboxylic acid, ethylmalonic acid, C4-C8 acylglycines (U)
MCAD deficiency	201450	AR	Medium-chain acyl-CoA dehydrogenase	>1:15,000	Liver disease, fasting intolerance, hypoketotic hypoglycemia	C6, C8, and C10 acylcarnitines (B); suberic acid, hexanoylglycine, suberylglycine (U)
M/SCHAD deficiency	609975 231530		Medium/ short-chain 3-hydroxyacyl-CoA dehydrogenase	<1:100,000	Liver disease, hyperinsulinemia, hypoglycemia	C4-OH-carnitine (B), insulin (B)
SCAD deficiency	201470		Short-chain acyl-CoA dehydrogenase	>1:50,000	Mostly benign; developmental delay, hypotonia, seizures (may be observed)	C4-carnitine (B); ethylmalonic acid, methylsuccinic acid, butyrylglycine (U)

*OMIM: Online Mendelian Inheritance in Man (www.ncbi.nlm.nih.gov/entrez/query.fcgi?db=OMIM).
AFLP, Acute fatty liver of pregnancy; *HELLP syndrome*, hemolysis, elevated liver enzymes, and low platelet count; *NBS*, newborn screening.

with milder cases present in childhood with attacks triggered by fever, infection, and fasting as other fatty acid oxidation defects. Fasting hypoglycemia and seizures have been reported in these patients.

In neonatal cases and during acute attacks, routine laboratory testing reveals nonketotic hypoglycemia and hyperammonemia with elevated activities of creatine kinase (CK) and abnormal liver function tests. This disease is identified upon newborn screening by elevated concentrations of C16- and C18:1-carnitine, often in addition to low concentrations of free carnitine. Diagnosis is confirmed by a plasma acylcarnitine profile demonstrating a marked increase in concentrations of long-chain acylcarnitines and decreased concentrations of free carnitine. This abnormal profile, however, is not distinguishable from that of neonatal CPT-2 deficiency and direct assay of carnitine-acylcarnitine translocase in fibroblasts or DNA analysis is needed for diagnostic confirmation. Therapy consists of frequent feedings of a diet (1) rich in carbohydrates, (2) low in fat, most of which should be medium-chain triglycerides, and (3) supplemented with carnitine. This therapy improves the acylcarnitine profile and prevents additional attacks of hypoglycemia and arrhythmia.[32]

Carnitine Palmitoyl Transferase 2 Deficiency

Carnitine palmitoyl transferase 2 (CPT-2) deficiency presents most frequently in adolescents and young adults (OMIM 255110) with muscle pain with or (in most cases) without myoglobinuria, accompanied by elevated activities of serum creatine kinase precipitated by strenuous exercise, cold, fever, or prolonged fasting. Myoglobinuria can cause kidney failure and death. CPT-2 deficiency also presents in infancy (OMIM 600649) and in the neonatal period (OMIM 608836).[9] The neonatal form, which is rapidly fatal, presents shortly after birth (a few hours to 4 days) with (1) respiratory distress, (2) seizures, (3) hepatomegaly, (4) cardiomegaly, (5) cardiac arrhythmia, and, in many cases, (6) dysmorphic features, (7) renal dysgenesis, and (8) neuronal migration defects. The infantile variety usually presents between 6 and 24 months of age with recurrent attacks of hypoketotic hypoglycemia causing loss of consciousness and seizures, liver failure, and transient hepatomegaly. Some children have heart involvement with cardiomyopathy and arrhythmia. Episodes are triggered by infection, fever, and fasting.

Routine laboratory testing usually indicates hyperammonemia, metabolic acidosis, and hypoketotic hypoglycemia with elevated activities of creatine kinase. Newborn screening reveals the same elevation of long-chain acylcarnitines (C16, C18:1) seen in CACT deficiency, with carnitine deficiency being absent in patients with milder forms. Diagnosis is confirmed by an abnormal plasma acylcarnitine profile and by enzyme assay in fibroblasts and/or DNA analysis to differentiate from CACT deficiency. Late-onset CPT-2 deficiency responds to exercise limitation, restriction of fat and long-chain fatty acids with increased dietary carbohydrates, and avoidance of fasting.

Very Long-Chain Acyl-CoA Dehydrogenase Deficiency

Very long-chain acyl-CoA dehydrogenase (VLCAD) catalyzes the first step of the fatty acid β-oxidation spiral (see Figure 58-13). In the mid 1980s, patients with VLCAD deficiency were initially described as having long-chain acyl-CoA dehydrogenase (LCAD) deficiency.[29] However, affected patients were subsequently shown to have VLCAD deficiency.[67] The severity of the phenotype correlates with the genotype[3] with earlier and more severe presentation observed in patients with the most severe deficiency. Patients with VLCAD deficiency present in infancy with (1) cardiomyopathy, (2) cardiac arrest, (3) hypoglycemia, and (4) other hepatic symptoms. This form is rapidly fatal. Older children present with hypoketotic hypoglycemia, and hepatomegaly with or without cardiomyopathy. The milder form presents in adolescents or adults with muscle weakness and pain without cardiac and hepatic involvement.[28]

Routine laboratory testing during acute episodes reveals hypoketotic hypoglycemia and elevated activities of creatine kinase and transaminases. Elevated concentration of C14:1-carnitine in the first newborn screen blood spot is often the only abnormality detected, and it may no longer be present in subsequent screens or diagnostic tests (plasma acylcarnitine profile). For this reason, in all infants with elevated concentrations of C14:1-carnitine on newborn screening, the diagnosis of VLCAD deficiency needs to be confirmed or excluded by specific enzyme assay or fatty acid oxidation studies in vitro, and/or by molecular genetic analysis of the VLCAD gene.[8] Therapy for this condition consists of avoidance of fasting, prompt treatment of infection, and a low-fat diet with medium-chain triglycerides providing most of the calories from lipids. Low-dose carnitine supplements (25 mg/kg/d) are sometimes given. Figure 58-14 shows a characteristic plasma acylcarnitine profile of VLCAD deficiency.

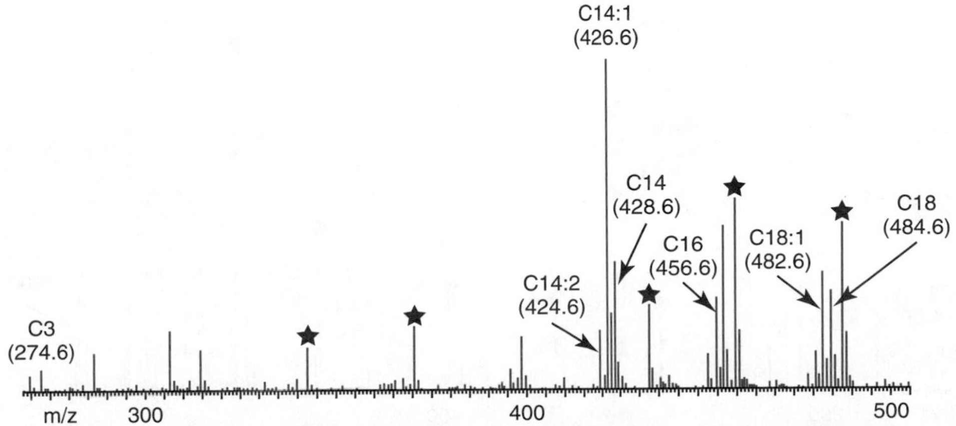

Figure 58-14 Plasma acylcarnitine profile (by tandem mass spectrometry) in very long-chain acyl-CoA dehydrogenase (VLCAD) deficiency. C14:1-carnitine is the diagnostic metabolite in VLCAD deficiency with elevation of other long-chain acylcarnitines (C14-, C16-, C18-, C14:2-, and C18:1-carnitine). Internal standards are indicated with a star.

Trifunctional Protein and Long-Chain 3-Hydroxy-Acyl-CoA Dehydrogenase Deficiencies

The trifunctional protein (TFP) is a hetero-octamer containing four α- and four β-subunits encoded by two different genes.[11] The α-subunit harbors the activities of the second and third steps of fatty acid β-oxidation, long-chain enoyl-CoA hydratase (LCEH), and long-chain 3-hydroxy-acyl-CoA dehydrogenase (LCHAD). The β-subunit harbors the activity of long-chain 3-oxoacyl-CoA dehydrogenase (LCKAT), which catalyzes the last step in β-oxidation of long-chain fatty acids. Mutations in either gene may cause complete TFP deficiency, and a prevalent mutation in the *HADHA* gene encoding the α-subunit (c.G1528C, p.E474Q) causes isolated LCHAD deficiency.[68] A genotype-phenotype correlation has emerged for TFP deficiency, with residual enzyme activity being associated with a milder, later-onset phenotype. Three clinical phenotypes are known: (1) a severe neonatal presentation with cardiomyopathy, Reye-like symptoms, and early death; (2) a hepatic form with recurrent hypoketotic hypoglycemia; and (3) a milder, later-onset neuromyopathic phenotype with episodic myoglobinuria. Patients with LCHAD/TFP deficiencies may also develop pigmentary retinopathy and peripheral neuropathy, whose pathophysiology remains obscure. In addition, mothers of these patients can have significant complications with acute fatty liver of pregnancy or hemolysis, elevated liver enzymes, and low platelet (HELLP) syndrome,[70] possibly due to the transplacental passage of 3-OH-fatty acids and related acylcarnitines.[22] This complication occurs in mothers independently of the fetal phenotype.[68]

Newborn screening identifies elevated concentrations of C16:OH- and C18:1-OH-carnitines in blood spots of infants with LCHAD/TFP deficiency. An abnormal plasma acylcarnitine profile identifies the same abnormalities with elevation of additional long-chain acylcarnitines (Figure 58-15). Urine organic acids collected at the time of an acute episode show hypoketotic C6-C10-dicarboxylic aciduria and C6-C14-3-hydroxydicarboxylic aciduria with prominent unsaturated species. Concentrations of urine organic acids rapidly normalize with therapy and fall within the reference interval in asymptomatic patients. Therapy for these conditions consists of avoidance of fasting, prompt treatment of infection, and a low-fat diet with medium-chain triglycerides providing most of the calories from lipids. Low-dose carnitine supplements (25 mg/kg/d) may be given.

Medium-chain Acyl-CoA Dehydrogenase Deficiency

Medium-chain acyl-CoA dehydrogenase (MCAD) deficiency is the most common disorder of fatty acid oxidation, with an estimated frequency of 1:6000 to 1:10,000 Caucasian births.[19,31] Symptoms of the disease are variable, from completely asymptomatic patients to those with hypoglycemia, lethargy, coma, or sudden death. Symptoms usually are triggered by prolonged fasting or illness. Although most patients present in the first year of life, clinical symptoms have been known to occur at any time, and as many as 20% of patients die before diagnosis.[33]

Patients with MCAD deficiency are identified by MS/MS newborn screening because of their characteristic acylcarnitine profile, with increased concentrations of C6- (hexanoyl), C8- (octanoyl), and C10:1-(decenoyl) carnitine, and elevated C8/C2 and C8/C10 ratios (Figure 58-16). Urine organic acid and urine acylglycine analyses during metabolic crisis show (1) increased excretion of dicarboxylic acids (adipic, suberic, sebacic)—saturated and unsaturated, (2) few or absent ketones, and (3) increased excretion of hexanoylglycine and suberylglycine. Phenylpropionylglycine may be present, although usually in older patients. When patients are metabolically stable, the urinary concentration of these analytes is greatly reduced, although concentrations of hexanoylglycine and suberylglycine remain detectable. The abnormal plasma

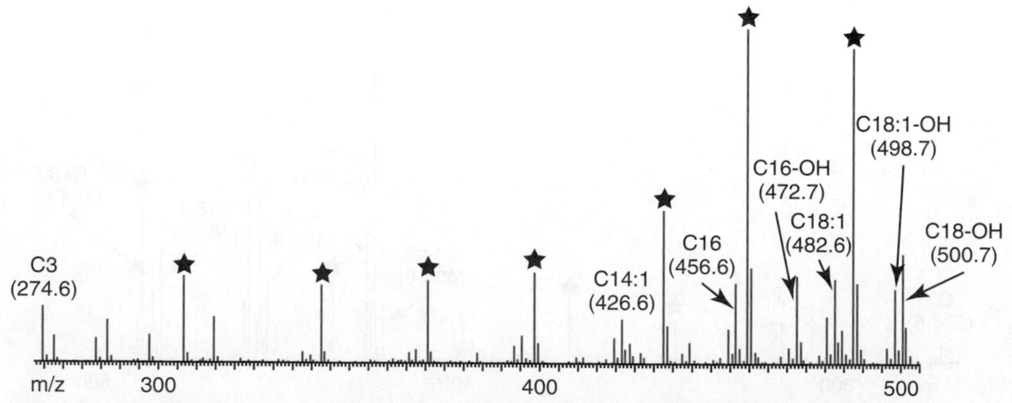

Figure 58-15 Plasma acylcarnitine profile (by tandem mass spectrometry) in trifunctional protein (TFP)/long-chain 3-OH-acyl-CoA dehydrogenase (LCHAD) deficiency. 3-OH-long-chain acylcarnitines (C16-OH-, C18-OH-, and C18:1-OH-carnitine), in addition to long-chain acylcarnitines, become elevated in both TFP and LCHAD deficiency. Internal standards are indicated by a star.

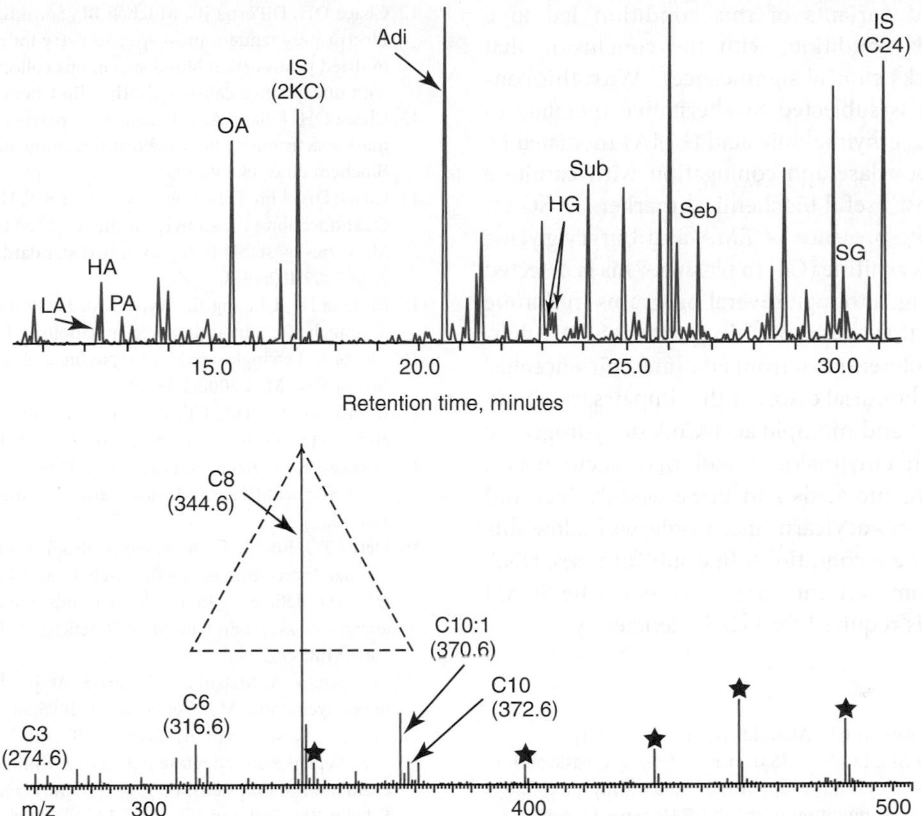

Figure 58-16 Urine organic acids (by gas chromatography/mass spectrometry) *(top)* and plasma acylcarnitine profile (by tandem mass spectrometry) *(bottom)* in medium-chain acyl-CoA dehydrogenase (MCAD) deficiency. Patients with MCAD deficiency can have dicarboxylic aciduria [increased excretion of adipic (Adi), suberic (Sub), and sebacic (Seb) acids, usually in a descending pattern, with adipic being the most increased] during episodes of decompensation or fasting. Hexanoic acid (HA) and octanoic acid (OA) can also be present during decompensation. Hexanoylglycine (HG) and suberylglycine (SG) are the diagnostic metabolites that usually remain present even when the patient is well compensated. Phenylpropionylglycine can appear in older patients as well. Urine acylglycine analysis is more effective than urine organic acid analysis for their quantification. *IS,* Internal standard; *LA,* lactic acid; *PA,* pyruvic acid. *Bottom,* The plasma acylcarnitine profile is characterized by elevated C8-, C6-, and C10:1-carnitine, with the C8-carnitine peak at the vertex of a triangle over the other two elevated species *(indicated by the dashed lines).* In carriers for this condition, C8-carnitine can be elevated, but it is not usually the highest peak on visual inspection. Internal standards are indicated with a star.

acylcarnitine profile is almost always present. Follow-up of an abnormal newborn screening for MCAD deficiency should include analysis of urine organic acids, urine acylglycines, and the plasma acylcarnitine profile. Diagnosis is confirmed by DNA analysis. Among patients presenting with clinical symptoms, 98% carry at least one copy of the common *p.K304E* mutation, with 80% being homozygous for this mutation.[2] In newborns detected prospectively by newborn screening, the *p.Y42H* mutation has been found frequently in association with the common *p.K304E* mutation.[2] The *p.Y42H* mutation has not yet been reported in patients with clinical symptoms[2] and is associated with lower concentrations of diagnostic metabolites in blood and urine.[76]

Treatment consists of avoidance of fasting, low-fat diet, carnitine supplementation, and institution of an emergency plan in case of illness or other metabolic stress. Early diagnosis through newborn screening and early initiation of treatment lead to improved outcomes.

Short-Chain Acyl-CoA Dehydrogenase Deficiency

Short-chain acyl-CoA dehydrogenase (SCAD) deficiency has been associated with a variety of clinical phenotypes, ranging from catastrophic illness in the neonatal period, to hypotonia, developmental delay, seizures, myopathy, and others.[34,74] Lack of a consistent phenotype and the large number of infants identified with mild variants of this condition led to a re-evaluation of this condition, with the conclusion that SCAD deficiency lacks clinical significance.[74] With this condition, butyryl-CoA is subjected to alternative metabolism with carboxylation to ethylmalonic acid (EMA) mediated by propionyl-CoA carboxylase and conjugation with carnitine and glycine. The most useful biochemical markers of SCAD deficiency include the presence of EMA and butyrylglycine in urine, and butyrylcarnitine (C4) in plasma. This is detected by newborn screening, although several programs in Europe no longer screen for this condition.[74] In practice, SCAD deficiency needs to be differentiated from ethylmalonic encephalopathy, a fatal mitochondrial disorder that impairs the ability to remove sulfide,[71,72] and multiple acyl-CoA dehydrogenase deficiency (in which ethylmalonic acid may accumulate). Analysis of urine organic acids and urine acylglycines and completion of a plasma acylcarnitine profile will allow differentiation among these conditions. In doubtful cases, DNA analysis identifies common and rare variants of the SCAD gene. No treatment is required for SCAD deficiency.

REFERENCES

1. Al-Dirbashi OY, Abu-Amero KK, Alswaid AF, Hoffmann GF, Al-Qahtani K, Rashed MS. LC-MS/MS determination of dibasic amino acids for the diagnosis of cystinuria: application in a family affected by a novel splice-acceptor site mutation in the SLC7A9 gene. J Inherit Metab Dis 2007;30:611.
2. Andresen BS, Dobrowolski SF, O'Reilly L, Muenzer J, McCandless SE, Frazier DM, et al. Medium-chain acyl-CoA dehydrogenase (MCAD) mutations identified by MS/MS-based prospective screening of newborns differ from those observed in patients with clinical symptoms: identification and characterization of a new, prevalent mutation that results in mild MCAD deficiency. Am J Hum Genet 2001;68:1408-18.
3. Andresen BS, Olpin S, Poorthuis BJ, Scholte HR, Vianey-Saban C, Wanders R, et al. Clear correlation of genotype with disease phenotype in very-long-chain acyl-CoA dehydrogenase deficiency. Am J Hum Genet 1999;64:479-94.
4. Applegarth DA, Toone JR. Nonketotic hyperglycinemia (glycine encephalopathy): laboratory diagnosis. Mol Genet Metab 2001;74: 139-46.
5. Bennett MJ, Rinaldo P. The metabolic autopsy comes of age. Clin Chem 2001;47:1145-6.
6. Bhattacharya K, Khalili V, Wiley V, Carpenter K, Wilcken B. Newborn screening may fail to identify intermediate forms of maple syrup urine disease. J Inherit Metab Dis 2006;29:586.
7. Boles RG, Buck EA, Blitzer MG, Platt MS, Cowan TM, Martin SK, et al. Retrospective biochemical screening of fatty acid oxidation disorders in postmortem livers of 418 cases of sudden death in the first year of life. J Pediatr 1998;132:924-33.
8. Boneh A, Andresen BS, Gregersen N, Ibrahim M, Tzanakos N, Peters H, et al. VLCAD deficiency: pitfalls in newborn screening and confirmation of diagnosis by mutation analysis. Mol Genet Metab 2006;88:166-70.
9. Bonnefont JP, Djouadi F, Prip-Buus C, Gobin S, Munnich A, Bastin J. Carnitine palmitoyltransferases 1 and 2: biochemical, molecular and medical aspects. Mol Aspects Med 2004;25:495-520.
10. Botkin JR. Research for newborn screening: developing a national framework. Pediatrics 2005;116:862-71.
11. Carpenter K, Pollitt RJ, Middleton B. Human liver long-chain 3-hydroxyacyl-coenzyme A dehydrogenase is a multifunctional membrane-bound beta-oxidation enzyme of mitochondria. Biochem Biophys Res Commun 1992;183:443-8.
12. Chace DH, DiPerna JC, Mitchell BL, Sgroi B, Hofman LF, Naylor EW. Electrospray tandem mass spectrometry for analysis of acylcarnitines in dried postmortem blood specimens collected at autopsy from infants with unexplained cause of death. Clin Chem 2001;47:1166-82.
13. Chace DH, Kalas TA. A biochemical perspective on the use of tandem mass spectrometry for newborn screening and clinical testing. Clin Biochem 2005;38:296-309.
14. Chace DH, Lim T, Hansen CR, Adam BW, Hannon WH. Quantification of malonylcarnitine in dried blood spots by use of MS/MS varies by stable isotope internal standard composition. Clin Chim Acta 2009;402:14-8.
15. Chuang DT, Chuang JL, Wynn RM. Lessons from genetic disorders of branched-chain amino acid metabolism. J Nutr 2006;136:243S-9S.
16. Clarke R, Lewington S. Homocysteine and coronary heart disease. Semin Vasc Med 2002;2:391-9.
17. Danner DJ, Doering CB. Human mutations affecting branched chain alpha-ketoacid dehydrogenase. Front Biosci 1998;3:d517-24.
18. Deodato F, Boenzi S, Santorelli FM, Dionisi-Vici C. Methylmalonic and propionic aciduria. Am J Med Genet C Semin Med Genet 2006;142C: 104-12.
19. Derks TG, Boer TS, van Assen A, Bos T, Ruiter J, Waterham HR, et al. Neonatal screening for medium-chain acyl-CoA dehydrogenase (MCAD) deficiency in The Netherlands: the importance of enzyme analysis to ascertain true MCAD deficiency. J Inherit Metab Dis 2008;31:88-96.
20. Dinopoulos A, Matsubara Y, Kure S. Atypical variants of nonketotic hyperglycinemia. Mol Genet Metab 2005;86:61-9.
21. Echenne B, Roubertie A, Assmann B, Lutz T, Penzien JM, Thony B, et al. Sepiapterin reductase deficiency: clinical presentation and evaluation of long-term therapy. Pediatr Neurol 2006;35:308-13.
22. Eskelin PM, Laitinen KA, Tyni TA. Elevated hydroxyacylcarnitines in a carrier of LCHAD deficiency during acute liver disease of pregnancy: a common feature of the pregnancy complication? Mol Genet Metab 2010;100:204-6.
23. Fernhoff PM, Lubitz D, Danner DJ, Dembure PP, Schwartz HP, Hillman R, et al. Thiamine response in maple syrup urine disease. Pediatr Res 1985;19:1011-6.
24. Fingerhut R, Roschinger W, Muntau AC, Dame T, Kreischer J, Arnecke R, et al. Hepatic carnitine palmitoyltransferase I deficiency: acylcarnitine profiles in blood spots are highly specific. Clin Chem 2001;47:1763-8.
25. Finkelstein JD, Martin JJ. Homocysteine. Int J Biochem Cell Biol 2000;32:385-9.
26. Gan-Schreier H, Kebbewar M, Fang-Hoffmann J, Wilrich J, Abdoh G, Ben-Omran T, et al. Newborn population screening for classic homocystinuria by determination of total homocysteine from Guthrie cards. J Pediatr 2010;156:427-32.
27. Gessler P, Buchal P, Schwenk HU, Wermuth B. Favourable long-term outcome after immediate treatment of neonatal hyperammonemia due to N-acetylglutamate synthase deficiency. Eur J Pediatr 2010;169: 197-9.
28. Gregersen N, Andresen BS, Corydon MJ, Corydon TJ, Olsen RK, Bolund L, et al. Mutation analysis in mitochondrial fatty acid oxidation defects: exemplified by acyl-CoA dehydrogenase deficiencies, with special focus on genotype-phenotype relationship. Hum Mutat 2001;18: 169-89.
29. Hale DE, Stanley CA, Coates PM. The long-chain acyl-CoA dehydrogenase deficiency. Prog Clin Biol Res 1990;321:303-11.
30. Hedlund GL, Longo N, Pasquali M. Glutaric acidemia type 1. Am J Med Genet C Semin Med Genet 2006;142C:86-94.
31. Horvath GA, Davidson AG, Stockler-Ipsiroglu SG, Lillquist YP, Waters PJ, Olpin S, et al. Newborn screening for MCAD deficiency: experience of the first three years in British Columbia, Canada. Can J Public Health 2008;99:276-80.
32. Iacobazzi V, Pasquali M, Singh R, Matern D, Rinaldo P, Amat di San Filippo C, et al. Response to therapy in carnitine/acylcarnitine translocase (CACT) deficiency due to a novel missense mutation. Am J Med Genet A 2004;126A:150-5.

33. Iafolla AK, Thompson RJ Jr, Roe CR. Medium-chain acyl-coenzyme A dehydrogenase deficiency: clinical course in 120 affected children. J Pediatr 1994;124:409-15.
34. Jethva R, Bennett MJ, Vockley J. Short-chain acyl-coenzyme A dehydrogenase deficiency. Mol Genet Metab 2008;95:195-200.
35. Kaspar H, Dettmer K, Chan Q, Daniels S, Nimkar S, Daviglus ML, et al. Urinary amino acid analysis: a comparison of iTRAQ-LC-MS/MS, GC-MS, and amino acid analyzer. J Chromatogr B Analyt Technol Biomed Life Sci 2009;877:1838-46.
36. Kikuchi G, Motokawa Y, Yoshida T, Hiraga K. Glycine cleavage system: reaction mechanism, physiological significance, and hyperglycinemia. Proc Jpn Acad Ser B Phys Biol Sci 2008;84:246-63.
37. Koch R, Hanley W, Levy H, Matalon K, Matalon R, Rouse B, et al. The Maternal Phenylketonuria International Study: 1984-2002. Pediatrics 2003;112:1523-9.
38. Lang TF. Adult presentations of medium-chain acyl-CoA dehydrogenase deficiency (MCADD). J Inherit Metab Dis 2009;32: 675-83.
39. Liu A, Johnson DW, Pasquali M. Addition of formic acid improves acetonitrile extraction of dicarboxylic acylcarnitines. Clin Chim Acta 2009;404:169-70.
40. Liu A, Kushnir MM, Roberts WL, Pasquali M. Solid phase extraction procedure for urinary organic acid analysis by gas chromatography mass spectrometry. J Chromatogr B Analyt Technol Biomed Life Sci 2004;806:283-7.
41. Liu A, Pasquali M. Acidified acetonitrile and methanol extractions for quantitative analysis of acylcarnitines in plasma by stable isotope dilution tandem mass spectrometry. J Chromatogr B Analyt Technol Biomed Life Sci 2005;827:193-8.
42. Longo N. Disorders of biopterin metabolism. J Inherit Metab Dis 2009;32:333-42.
43. Longo N. Mitochondrial encephalopathy. Neurol Clin 2003;21:817-31.
44. Longo N, Amat di San Filippo C, Pasquali M. Disorders of carnitine transport and the carnitine cycle. Am J Med Genet C Semin Med Genet 2006;142C:77-85.
45. Lund AM, Joensen F, Hougaard DM, Jensen LK, Christensen E, Christensen M, et al. Carnitine transporter and holocarboxylase synthetase deficiencies in The Faroe Islands. J Inherit Metab Dis 2007;30:341-9.
46. Matern D, Tortorelli S, Oglesbee D, Gavrilov D, Rinaldo P. Reduction of the false-positive rate in newborn screening by implementation of MS/MS-based second-tier tests: the Mayo Clinic experience (2004-2007). J Inherit Metab Dis 2007;30:585-92.
47. Morton DH, Strauss KA, Robinson DL, Puffenberger EG, Kelley RI. Diagnosis and treatment of maple syrup disease: a study of 36 patients. Pediatrics 2002;109:999-1008.
48. Nassogne MC, Heron B, Touati G, Rabier D, Saudubray JM. Urea cycle defects: management and outcome. J Inherit Metab Dis 2005;28: 407-14.
49. Orendac M, Zeman J, Stabler SP, Allen RH, Kraus JP, Bodamer O, et al. Homocystinuria due to cystathionine beta-synthase deficiency: novel biochemical findings and treatment efficacy. J Inherit Metab Dis 2003; 26:761-73.
50. Palmieri F. Diseases caused by defects of mitochondrial carriers: a review. Biochim Biophys Acta 2008;1777:564-78.
51. Ravn K, Chloupkova M, Christensen E, Brandt NJ, Simonsen H, Kraus JP, et al. High incidence of propionic acidemia in greenland is due to a prevalent mutation, 1540insCCC, in the gene for the beta-subunit of propionyl CoA carboxylase. Am J Hum Genet 2000;67:203-6.
52. Rinaldo P, Matern D, Bennett MJ. Fatty acid oxidation disorders. Annu Rev Physiol 2002;64:477-502.
53. Rinaldo P, Studinski AL, Matern D. Prenatal diagnosis of disorders of fatty acid transport and mitochondrial oxidation. Prenat Diagn 2001;21:52-4.
54. Rinaldo P, Yoon HR, Yu C, Raymond K, Tiozzo C, Giordano G. Sudden and unexpected neonatal death: a protocol for the postmortem diagnosis of fatty acid oxidation disorders. Semin Perinatol 1999;23: 204-10.
55. Saudubray JM, Nassogne MC, de Lonlay P, Touati G. Clinical approach to inherited metabolic disorders in neonates: an overview. Semin Neonatol 2002;7:3-15.
56. Scaglia F, Lee B. Clinical, biochemical, and molecular spectrum of hyperargininemia due to arginase I deficiency. Am J Med Genet C Semin Med Genet 2006;142C:113-20.
57. Scaglia F, Wang Y, Singh RH, Dembure PP, Pasquali M, Fernhoff PM, et al. Defective urinary carnitine transport in heterozygotes for primary carnitine deficiency. Genet Med 1998;1:34-9.
58. Schadewaldt P, Bodner-Leidecker A, Hammen HW, Wendel U. Formation of L-alloisoleucine in vivo: an L-[13C]isoleucine study in man. Pediatr Res 2000;47:271-7.
59. Schimmenti LA, Crombez EA, Schwahn BC, Heese BA, Wood TC, Schroer RJ, et al. Expanded newborn screening identifies maternal primary carnitine deficiency. Mol Genet Metab 2007;90:441-5.
60. Schlump JU, Mayatepek E, Spiekerkoetter U. Significant increase of succinylacetone within the first 12 h of life in hereditary tyrosinemia type 1. Eur J Pediatr 2009;169:569-72.
61. Schwarz EL, Roberts WL, Pasquali M. Analysis of plasma amino acids by HPLC with photodiode array and fluorescence detection. Clin Chim Acta 2005;354:83-90.
62. Scott CR. The genetic tyrosinemias. Am J Med Genet C Semin Med Genet 2006;142C:121-6.
63. Scriver CR, Kaufman S. Hyperphenylalaninemia: phenylalanine hydroxylase deficiency. In: Scriver CR, Sly WS, Valle D, eds. The metabolic and molecular bases of inherited disease, 8th edition. New York, NY: McGraw-Hill, 2001:1667-724.
64. Shinawi M. Hyperhomocysteinemia and cobalamin disorders. Mol Genet Metab 2007;90:113-21.
65. Slocum RH. Amino acid analysis of physiological samples. In: Hommes FA, ed. Techniques in diagnostic human biochemical genetics. New York, NY: Wiley-Liss, 1991:87-126.
66. Smith W, Kishnani PS, Lee B, Singh RH, Rhead WJ, Sniderman King L, et al. Urea cycle disorders: clinical presentation outside the newborn period. Crit Care Clin 2005;21:S9-17.
67. Souri M, Aoyama T, Orii K, Yamaguchi S, Hashimoto T. Mutation analysis of very-long-chain acyl-coenzyme A dehydrogenase (VLCAD) deficiency: identification and characterization of mutant VLCAD cDNAs from four patients. Am J Hum Genet 1996;58:97-106.
68. Spiekerkoetter U, Sun B, Khuchua Z, Bennett MJ, Strauss AW. Molecular and phenotypic heterogeneity in mitochondrial trifunctional protein deficiency due to beta-subunit mutations. Hum Mutat 2003;21: 598-607.
69. Steegers-Theunissen RP, Boers GH, Trijbels FJ, Eskes TK. Neural-tube defects and derangement of homocysteine metabolism. N Engl J Med 1991;324:199-200.
70. Strauss AW, Bennett MJ, Rinaldo P, Sims HF, O'Brien LK, Zhao Y, et al. Inherited long-chain 3-hydroxyacyl-CoA dehydrogenase deficiency and a fetal-maternal interaction cause maternal liver disease and other pregnancy complications. Semin Perinatol 1999;23:100-12.
71. Tiranti V, D'Adamo P, Briem E, Ferrari G, Mineri R, Lamantea E, et al. Ethylmalonic encephalopathy is caused by mutations in ETHE1, a gene encoding a mitochondrial matrix protein. Am J Hum Genet 2004;74: 239-52.
72. Tiranti V, Viscomi C, Hildebrandt T, Di Meo I, Mineri R, Tiveron C, et al. Loss of ETHE1, a mitochondrial dioxygenase, causes fatal sulfide toxicity in ethylmalonic encephalopathy. Nat Med 2009;15:200-5.
73. Tortorelli S, Hahn SH, Cowan TM, Brewster TG, Rinaldo P, Matern D. The urinary excretion of glutarylcarnitine is an informative tool in the biochemical diagnosis of glutaric acidemia type I. Mol Genet Metab 2005;84:137-43.
74. van Maldegem BT, Duran M, Wanders RJ, Niezen-Koning KE, Hogeveen M, Ijlst L, et al. Clinical, biochemical, and genetic heterogeneity in short-chain acyl-coenzyme A dehydrogenase deficiency. JAMA 2006;296:943-52.
75. Vockley J, Ensenauer R. Isovaleric acidemia: new aspects of genetic and phenotypic heterogeneity. Am J Med Genet C Semin Med Genet 2006;142C:95-103.

76. Waddell L, Wiley V, Carpenter K, Bennetts B, Angel L, Andresen BS, et al. Medium-chain acyl-CoA dehydrogenase deficiency: genotype-biochemical phenotype correlations. Mol Genet Metab 2006;87: 32-9.
77. Waterval WA, Scheijen JL, Ortmans-Ploemen MM, Habets-van der Poel CD, Bierau J. Quantitative UPLC-MS/MS analysis of underivatised amino acids in body fluids is a reliable tool for the diagnosis and follow-up of patients with inborn errors of metabolism. Clin Chim Acta 2009;407:36-42.
78. Woontner M, Goodman SI. Chromatographic analysis of amino and organic acids in physiological fluids to detect inborn errors of metabolism. Curr Protoc Hum Genet 2006;Chapter 17:Unit 172:1-19.

CHAPTER 59

Hemostasis

Russell A. Higgins, M.D., Steve Kitchen, Ph.D.,
and John D. Olson, M.D., Ph.D.

Hemostasis is the mechanism by which animals with a vascular system protect themselves from exsanguination following an injury. The mechanism is designed to form the hemostatic plug at the site of an injury. It is well recognized that the process may hypofunction, leading to a bleeding diathesis (i.e., predisposition or tendency to bleed), or it may hyperfunction, leading to intravascular coagulation or formation of a potentially life-threatening blood clot in a blood vessel (thrombosis). For purposes of discussion, normal hemostasis is often divided into three parts: (1) vascular, (2) platelet (cellular), and (3) plasma coagulation components. It is important to remember that these three contributors **do not act** separately, but are simultaneously activated and are mutually dependent upon one another.

VASCULAR

At the time of an injury, small and medium vessels contract in response to mechanical, neural, and chemical (platelet secretory products) stimuli, in a remarkably successful effort to prevent blood loss. In addition, the endothelial cell plays a key role in the procoagulant and anticoagulant regulation of platelet function and plasma coagulation. Endothelial cells support platelet function through the synthesis and secretion of von Willebrand factor (VWF) and down regulates function by secretion of the potent inhibitor, prostacyclin (PgI_2). Anticoagulant functions occurring at the endothelial surface include (1) binding of thrombin to thrombomodulin (TM); (2) conversion of protein C to activated protein C; and (3) clearance of activated coagulation factors by antithrombin (AT). The endothelium also contributes to activation and regulation of fibrinolysis by secretion of tissue plasminogen activator (tPA) and plasminogen activator inhibitors.[93] Tissue factor (TF) is found in many tissues in the body, but of particular interest is its presence in the vascular smooth muscle and pericytes that surround the vessel. This vascular distribution of TF has been referred to as the hemostatic envelope.[34,39] Figure 59-1 depicts the procoagulant and regulatory roles of the endothelium in hemostasis.

PLATELETS

Platelets are key cellular elements in the hemostatic process.[77] They are anuclear fragments of the megakaryocyte, produced in the bone marrow and released into the bone marrow sinusoids. They normally circulate for approximately ten days. The functions of the platelet include (Table 59-1): *(1). adhesion* of the platelet to surfaces at the site of injury—the platelet recognizes non-endothelial surfaces and adheres to those surfaces in an initial step in the hemostatic process; *(2). aggregation* of platelets at the site of an injury—platelets recognize one another and aggregate, building a structure of platelets at the site of injury; *(3) secretion* of the two types of granules, alpha granules (contain such proteins as fibrinogen and von Willebrand factor) and dense bodies (contain non-protein components like epinephrine, adenine nucleotides, serotonin and others)—upon platelet activation, granule contents are secreted into the microenvironment, contributing to vascular smooth muscle contraction, further platelet activation and support of plasma coagulation; *(4) support of plasma coagulation* at the site of the injury—macromolecular enzyme complexes are assembled on the surface of the platelet, greatly accelerating the production of thrombin and, consequently, fibrin; *(5) clot retraction* may be thought of as the in vivo suture—the platelet contains contractile proteins that shrink the clot by drawing the edges of small injuries closer together, a function that may be an early step in the healing process; *(6) support of the injured endothelial cell* occurs with the fusion of platelets to damaged endothelium—the platelet becomes a part of the endothelium, helping to support its function.[5] Platelet function testing parallels these activities of the platelet.

COAGULATION

Blood coagulation is a complex biological process that occurs as conversion of the soluble molecule, fibrinogen, to the insoluble molecule, fibrin. The cascade of enzymatic reactions leading to the formation of fibrin allows for amplification of the initial signal from injury and regulation of the process.

The process of coagulation has three pathways: extrinsic, intrinsic, and common. The extrinsic pathway (also known

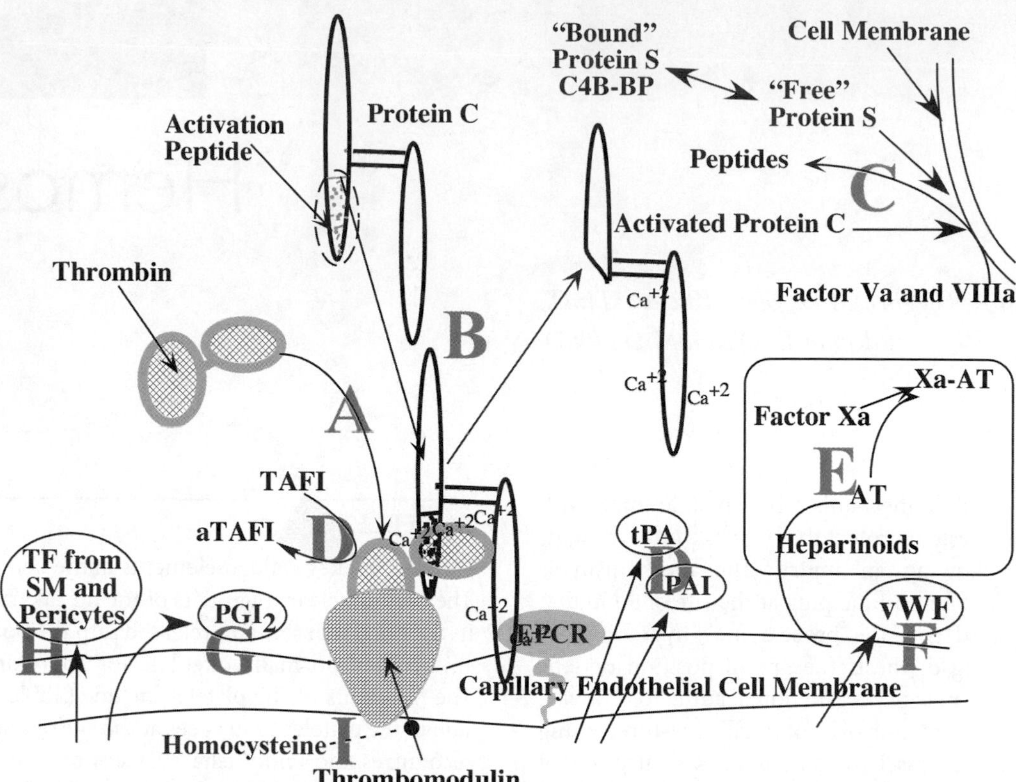

Figure 59-1 Role of the Endothelium in Hemostasis. [A] Thrombin released into the circulation at the site of an injury binds to thrombomodulin (TM), an endothelial cell membrane protein. Bound to TM, thrombin does not cleave fibrinogen. [B] Protein C, bound to the endothelium by endothelial cell protein C receptor (EPCR), is cleaved by thrombin bound to thrombomodulin; the activation peptide is removed and activated protein C (APC) released. [C] At a distant site of coagulation, APC with its cofactor, the free form of protein S, cleaves factors Va and VIIIa, inactivating them and downregulating coagulation at the site. [D] Fibrinolysis is also regulated by actions at the surface of the endothelium by the release of tissue plasminogen activator (tPA) and plasminogen activator inhibitors (PAI), as well as the activation of thrombin-activatable fibrinolysis inhibitor by thrombin bound to TM. [E] Antithrombin (AT) associated with heparin-like compounds in the endothelial cell membrane binds to activated serine proteases such as factor Xa, inhibiting their function through covalent linkage, allowing clearance from the circulation by the liver. [F] VWF, a key molecule in platelet adhesion, is synthesized by the endothelial cell and secreted both into the blood and abluminally into the subendothelial basement membrane. [G] Prostaglandin synthesis in the endothelial cells produces PGI_2, a potent platelet inhibitor, and secretes it into the blood. [H] Tissue factor (TF) is synthesized in the smooth muscle and pericytes of small vessels forming the hemostatic envelope. [I] Homocysteine in the endothelial cell inhibits the expression of TM in the endothelial cell membrane.

as the tissue factor pathway) is initiated by release of TF and F is measured by the prothrombin time (PT). The intrinsic pathway (also known as the contact activation pathway) is initiated by activation of the "contact factors" of plasma and is measured by the activated partial thromboplastin time (aPTT) test. The common pathway results from merging of the extrinsic and intrinsic pathways and includes the final steps before a clot is formed. The individual pathways and their interactions are shown in Figure 59-2 and will be discussed later in the chapter.

The process of coagulation in vivo proceeds through stages of initiation, amplification, and propagation (Figure 59-3). The initial action of TF and factor VIIa generates small amounts of thrombin, which serve to amplify the reaction through (1) activation of platelets, (2) activation of platelet membrane-bound factors V and VIII, and (3) assembly of macromolecular enzyme complexes on the platelet surface. This leads to amplified generation of thrombin that will feed back to activate factors XI, VIII, and V, propagating the reaction.[84] Thrombin plays two key roles in these final

TABLE 59-1 Platelet Functions

Function	Description
Adhesion	Upon activation, the platelet recognizes surfaces other than normal endothelium and adheres to those surfaces.
Aggregation	Upon activation, the platelet recognizes and attaches (aggregates) to other platelets.
Secretion	Upon activation, the platelet secretes the contents of the alpha granules and dense bodies (delta granules).
Support of plasma coagulation	At the site of injury, the platelet serves as a surface upon which macromolecular enzyme complexes form and plasma coagulation is accelerated.
Clot retraction	Following clot formation, the filapodia of platelets attach to the fibrin strands and, through contraction, reduce clot size and express serum in vitro and juxtapose edges of the injury in vivo.
Support of damaged endothelium	Platelets adhere to damaged endothelium, fuse with the membrane, and become incorporated with the endothelial cytoplasm.

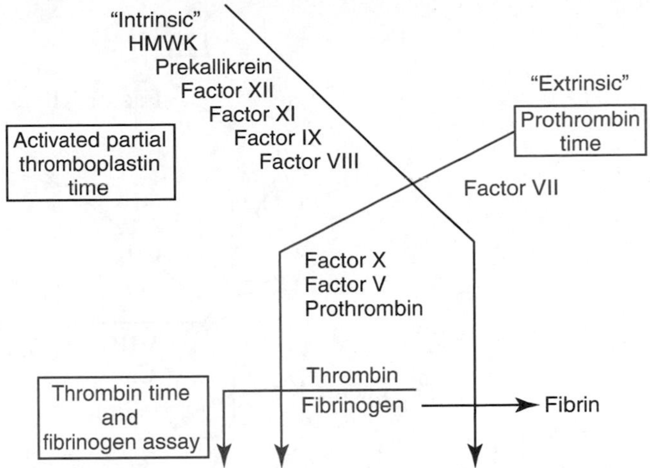

Figure 59-2 Extrinsic, intrinsic, and common pathways of coagulation. (See text for details.)

steps in the formation of fibrin. First, it is the procoagulant enzyme that cleaves fibrinogen, forming fibrin monomer; second, following fibrin monomer polymerization, thrombin activates factor XIII. Activated factor XIII is a transglutaminase that cross-links the polymer via formation of bonds between lysine and glutamine near the carboxyl end of the $\gamma\gamma$ chains (within the strands) and bonding between the $\alpha\gamma$ chains. It is important to keep the process localized to the site of injury, a process that involves regulation of reactions at the site, as well as inactivation of any circulating activated factors on the endothelial surface in the downstream capillary bed. Localization of the process is facilitated by the platelet serving as the template for reactions and by the presence of natural inhibitors like tissue factor pathway inhibitor that neutralize excess enzyme.[40,106] Thrombin that is released also binds to TM in the endothelial cell membrane in the capillary bed and activates protein C, which, with cofactor protein S, inhibits excess enzyme generation through inactivation of factors Va and VIIIa. As fibrin is formed at the site of injury, platelets contract, drawing fibrin strands closer together and helping to stabilize the clot and juxtaposing edges of the wound in anticipation of healing. Note: The in vitro (Figure 59-2) and the in vivo (Figure 59-3) coagulation mechanisms are not identical. In vitro, high molecular weight kininogen, prekallikreln and factor XII play a key role in coagulation activation, while these same factors play no role in coagulation in vivo.

Fibrinolysis is the process of converting insoluble fibrin to soluble products that are then cleared from the circulation by the liver. The zymogen plasminogen, which is closely associated with fibrin in the clot via molecular sites of recognition, is converted to the enzyme plasmin by urokinase or tPA (Figure 59-4). Plasmin cleaves fibrin to form fibrin degradation products, most commonly measured in the plasma as D-dimer.[11,25A]

When some procoagulant factors are increased, or regulatory proteins are decreased, patients are at increased risk for the development of thrombosis. Thus, acquired or inherited disorders affecting one or more of the many elements involved in hemostasis can lead to an increased risk of thrombosis.

This chapter describes the tests that are most commonly used in evaluating the hemostatic process, along with a brief description of disorders as they relate to those tests.

PRIMARY HEMOSTASIS

Primary hemostasis is characterized by vascular contraction, platelet adhesion, and formation of a platelet thrombus. It begins immediately after endothelial disruption with platelets being a key cellular component in the hemostatic process.[77] Platelets are anuclear fragments of the megakaryocyte cytoplasm, produced in the bone marrow and released into the bone marrow sinusoids. They normally circulate for approximately 10 days. Functions of the platelet are listed in Table 59-1.[63] Platelet function testing parallels these activities of the platelet.

Clinical testing is used to evaluate key aspects of platelets, including (1) number of platelets in a volume of blood, (2) microscopic structure of platelets, (3) global function of platelets, (4) platelet adhesion, (5) platelet aggregation

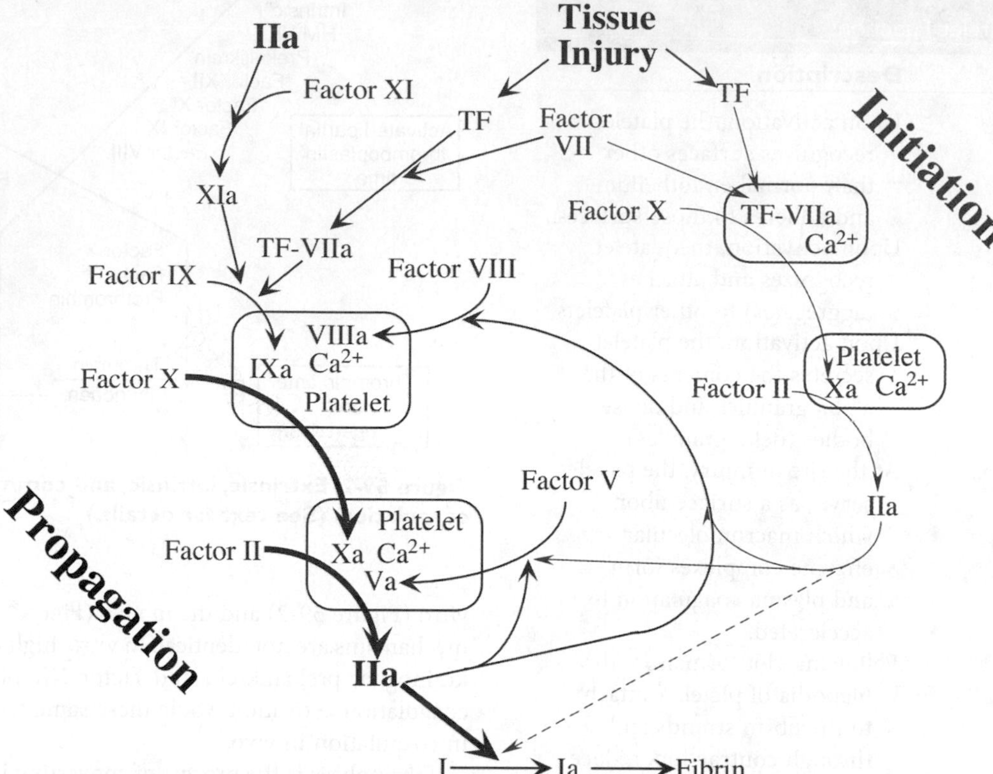

Figure 59-3 Model of the In Vivo Activation of Coagulation. At the site of injury, tissue factor (TF) is released and binds to and activates factor VII. In the presence of calcium (Ca^{2+}), the complex activates factor X. A macromolecular complex is formed on phospholipid (surface of the platelet) with the cofactor, factor V, and initial limited quantities of thrombin (IIa) are produced from prothrombin. This process has been called *extrinsic coagulation* and is the initiation of the coagulation process. This small amount of thrombin serves to activate platelets at the site, activate factor V, activate factor VIII, and activate factor XI. This feedback activation leads to acceleration of the cascading activation of enzymes on the surface of the activated platelet with a resulting burst of IIa generation and the formation of fibrin. The activities enclosed in the boxes depict the formation of macromolecular enzyme complexes that involve vitamin K–dependent coagulation factors (II, VII, IX, and X) and their cofactors (VIIIa and Va), joining with Ca^{2+} on the surface of the platelet.

and secretion, (6) platelet support of plasma coagulation, (7) platelet retraction, and (8) molecules on the platelet surface that are observable by flow cytometry.

Evaluating Platelet Number

The number of platelets in a whole blood sample is counted using automated or manual techniques. The number is usually expressed as thousands of platelet per microliter of blood.

Automated Platelet Counting

Automated methods are effective in counting normal numbers of platelets in a background of normal blood cells. Initial platelet counts are nearly always performed using automated methods.[10] The specimen that is used is whole blood that has been collected into a tube containing ethylenediaminetetraacetic acid (EDTA). In addition to preventing coagulation, the high affinity of EDTA for calcium inhibits platelet activation. Automated cell counters rely on two basic methods to count platelets in whole blood, both of which exploit the small size of the cell in comparison with other normal cells. In the first of these methods, diluted cells are aspirated through a small aperture across which there is an electrical potential. The lipid envelope of the cell causes a change in the potential when it passes the aperture. Thus, the cell is counted by measuring this change in potential, with the magnitude of the change being proportional to the volume of the cell. Platelets are distinguished from other cells on the basis of their small size. For samples with high platelet counts, statistical adjustments are made to the raw count to adjust for the coincidence of more than one cell passing the aperture simultaneously.

In a second automated method, diluted cell suspensions are passed through a cuvette that is slightly larger than a capillary. Laminar flow within the cuvette causes cells to pass through single file. A laser beam passes through the cuvette to a detector. As each cell passes through the path of the laser,

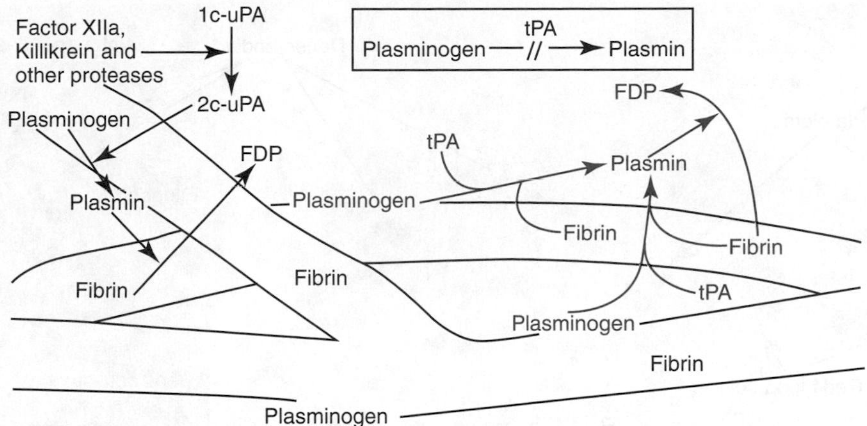

Figure 59-4 Activation of Plasminogen and Fibrinolysis. In vivo, plasminogen is activated to the plasmin (a serine protease) by two pathways. First, *(shown in black)* single-change urokinase (1c-uPA) is converted to active two-chain urokinase (2c-uPA) by contact activation factors and other proteases. Then 2c-uPA cleaves plasminogen to form plasmin. Second, tissue plasminogen activator (tPA) *(shown in red)* converts plasminogen to plasmin only in the presence of its cofactor, fibrin. Fibrin as a cofactor for this reaction is of interest because it is also the substrate for the enzyme being generated. Without fibrin, conversion of plasminogen to plasmin is too inefficient to be physiologically relevant.

the event is counted, and the size and complexity of the cell cytoplasm is determined by the degree of forward and side light scatter, respectively. As varying types of cells pass the laser, they are distinguished from one another on the basis of size and cytoplasmic complexity.

Manual Platelet Counting

At extremes of platelet count and in conditions with red blood cell or white blood cell cytoplasmic fragmentation, the platelets in a specimen are counted manually. This requires manual dilution of the blood and visual counting of the cells in a hemocytometer chamber that holds a defined volume of blood. Alternatively, the proportion of platelets to red blood cells is determined on a blood film using a method similar to that used to count reticulocytes. The platelet count is then determined by using the ratio of platelets to red blood cells and calculating from the red blood cell count which can be determined by manual or automated counting.

Evaluating Platelet Structure

Platelet structures that are morphologically evaluated for their role in hemostasis include alpha particles and dense bodies.

Evaluating Alpha Granules

The alpha secretory granule, the most common organelle of the platelet, contains a number of proteins (von Willebrand factor, fibrinogen, and many others) that are secreted when the platelet is activated. These granules (proteins) are a deep purple color when stained with Wright-Giemsa stain and give the platelets their delicate granular structure when a routine blood film is examined. Figure 59-5 demonstrates the light microscopic appearance of alpha granules.

Evaluating Dense Bodies (Delta Granules)

The dense secretory granule of the platelet contains nonprotein molecules (adenine and guanine nucleotides, vasoactive amines, and many others) that are secreted upon activation. These granules have a high content of calcium ion, making them electron dense (see Figure 59-5). Platelets in platelet-rich plasma adhere when placed on a transmission electron microscopy (TEM) grid, where they are then visualized using TEM.[144] The method, called *whole mount TEM,* is rapid and reliably demonstrates the 5 to 10 delta granules seen normally in platelets. Figure 59-5 demonstrates whole mount and thin-section electron microscopy of a normal platelet.

Thin-section TEM, although used less frequently than whole mount TEM, provides greater detail of platelet structure and may be helpful in determining the cause of hemorrhage related to abnormal platelet activity.[143]

Evaluating Global Platelet and Vascular Function

Various techniques are used to evaluate platelet and vascular function, including bleeding time and the PFA-100 analyzer (Siemens Healthcare Diagnostics, Deerfield, Ill).

Bleeding Time

Over the past century, many iterations of bleeding time have been employed. Currently, the test is performed on the volar aspect (the surface of the arm on the same side as the palm) of the forearm. A blood pressure cuff is applied at 40 mm Hg to provide uniform intravascular pressure at the site of the incision. A small incision (≈1 cm long and 1 mm deep) is made using a disposable template that provides a uniform incision from test to test. The result is influenced by the

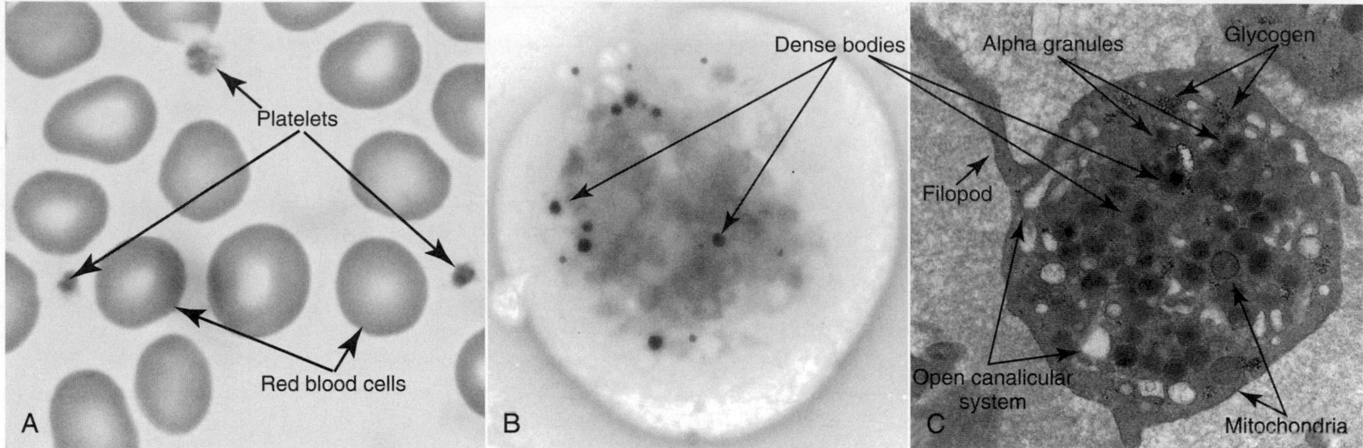

Figure 59-5 Platelet Morphology. A is a photo of a Wright-Giemsa–stained blood film with several red blood cells and three platelets. Normally, the platelets demonstrate some variation in size and shape, as seen here. Variable staining of the cytoplasm of the platelet is due to the alpha granules, the proteins of which stain deep purple. B is an electron micrograph of a whole mount of a platelet. The purpose of the preparation is to demonstrate the dense bodies (electron dense because of the high concentration of calcium). Visualization of other organelles requires thin-section preparation. C is a thin-section electron micrograph demonstrating many of the platelet organelles.

direction of incision, with a shorter time obtained if the incision is parallel to the sides of the forearm compared with a perpendicular incision. Blood at the site of injury is gently blotted with a filter paper every 30 seconds until no blood is detectable on the paper (time required ≈4 to 8 minutes). The test is not very sensitive, exhibits high intertechnologist imprecision, and has fallen out of favor, being replaced with other global tests of platelet function like the PFA-100. This may be appropriate for testing of platelet function; but, in most laboratories, bleeding time remains the only method by which to assess the vascular contribution to hemostasis and may continue to be useful for this purpose.[19,82] In the United States, many institutions no longer perform the test.

Platelet Function Analyzer (PFA-100 and PFA-200)

Platelets exposed to shear stress, such as occurs at the site of injury, are activated. This characteristic is exploited in the PFA-100 analyzer, a global test of platelet function. The analyzer utilizes a whole blood specimen containing 109 mmol/L trisodium citrate as an anticoagulant. After blood is drawn through a capillary tube, platelets pass through a small perforation in a membrane with embedded activators [collagen/epinephrine and collagen/adenosine diphosphate (ADP)]. The time required for adhering and aggregating platelets to close the perforation is measured (the closure time) (Figure 59-6). The collagen/epinephrine test is sensitive, and if it is found to be normal, the collagen/ADP test usually is not performed. If the collagen/epinephrine test is abnormal, it is followed by the collagen/ADP test. If the collagen/ADP test is normal, the problem is likely related to aspirin or another medication that affects platelet function. If the collagen/ADP test is abnormal, the problem is likely related to an inherited or acquired disorder of platelet function (Table 59-2). The test is affected by anemia and thrombocytopenia (any disorder in which there is an abnormally low number of platelets) and is not performed if the patient has either or both of those conditions. Similar to the test for bleeding time, the test is not sensitive.[54] The PFA-200 also provides a method to evaluate the effect of the platelet function-inhibiting thienopyridine drugs on platelets.

TABLE 59-2 Expected Results of the PFA-100 Analyzer

Condition	Collagen/ Epinephrine Cartridge Closure Time	Collagen/ADP Cartridge Closure Time
Normal	Normal	Normal
Medication (aspirin effect)	Prolonged	Normal
Platelet function defect	Prolonged	Prolonged

PFA-100 Platelet Function Analyzer, Siemens Healthcare Diagnostics, Deerfield, Ill.
ADP, Adenosine diphosphate.

Evaluating Platelet Adhesion

Various assays are used to evaluate platelet adhesion. They include assays for (1) ristocetin-induced platelet aggregation (RIPA), (2) von Willebrand factor–ristocetin cofactor, (3) von Willebrand factor–collagen binding, (4) von Willebrand factor immunoactivity, (5) von Willebrand antigen, (6) VWF multimer, and (7) ADAMTS13.

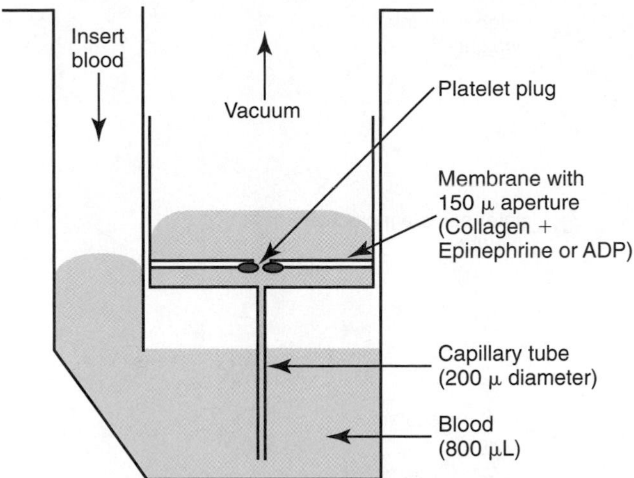

Figure 59-6 Schematic of the PFA-100 Analyzer. The PFA-100 analyzer provides a global measure of platelet function in a whole blood specimen. Blood anticoagulated with citrate is pipetted into the cuvette with a reaction membrane with collagen/epinephrine or collagen/ADP. Using a vacuum (syringe suction), blood is aspirated through the capillary tube at a rate sufficient to produce a wall shear rate of 1000 seconds^{-1}. Blood containing shear stress–activated platelets enters a small chamber and passes through the aperture of the membrane. At the aperture, the platelets adhere and aggregate until the aperture is closed and flow is obstructed. The time to achieve closure is referred to as *closure time*.

Ristocetin-Induced Platelet Aggregation Assay

Ristocetin is an antibiotic that was originally derived from cultures of *Norcardia lurida*. It was found to cause in vivo and in vitro aggregation of platelets. Aggregation induced by ristocetin is mediated by VWF. When aggregation is induced by ristocetin, the test will reflect both the activity of VWF in the plasma and function of the receptor for VWF in the platelet membrane (GP Ib-V-IX complex). The methods used to detect aggregation of the platelets are the same as those described in the section on platelet aggregation (see later). Testing is done at a high concentration of ristocetin to detect VWF ristocetin cofactor (VWF:RCo) activity, and at low concentration to detect possible increased affinity of VWF:RCo for its receptor on the platelet. The value of this is discussed later.[45,79]

von Willebrand Factor–Ristocetin Cofactor Assay (VWF:RCo)

The most common of the assays for VWF, it exploits the binding of VWF to platelets in the presence of ristocetin.[99] Platelets are prepared free of VWF using gel filtration or washing. Platelets are used fresh for the assay or, as is done for commercial assays, are lyophilized for longer storage and then are reconstituted with a buffer for the assay. Platelets are used in an agglutination reaction with ristocetin as the agonist. The specimen used is platelet-poor plasma (PPP) harvested from whole blood anticoagulated with 109 mmol/L trisodium citrate. Using dilutions of normal pooled plasma, a calibration curve is developed based on the rate or extent of agglutination. The rate or extent of agglutination of the patient's specimen is then compared with the calibration curve, and the value extrapolated. This original method for determining the activity of VWF is very labor intense, but despite difficulty with imprecision, it remains the gold standard for the development and validation of other methods.

von Willebrand Factor–Collagen-Binding Assay (VWF:CB)

The binding of VWF to collagen matrix initiates the process of platelet adhesion and the hemostatic process. VWF activity is quantified using the collagen-binding function.[43] The specimen used is PPP harvested from whole blood containing 109 mmol/L trisodium citrate as an anticoagulant. The methods available are primarily enzyme-linked immunosorbent assay (ELISA)-type assays in which VWF binds to stationary phase collagen (collagen types I and III—alone or in combination—derived from human, equine, or bovine tendon), followed by quantification of the bound VWF. The concentration of VWF:CB tends to parallel that of VWF:RCo in most settings. Some assays of VWF:CB are more sensitive to high molecular weight VWF multimers and may detect type 2 VWD (see later) more readily.

von Willebrand Factor Immunoactivity Assay (VWF:IA)

Monoclonal antibodies to functional epitopes in the VWF (e.g., GP Ib-binding site) have been developed. A homogeneous immunoturbidometric assay with antibody-coated latex beads shows a direct correlation of the degree of agglutination with VWF activity in the plasma.[122] These assays have been correlated with other functional assays of VWF. For additional details regarding this type of immunoassay, see Chapter 16.

von Willebrand Antigen Assays (VWF:Ag)

The specimen used is PPP harvested from whole blood anticoagulated with 109 mmol/L trisodium citrate. The original assay for VWF:Ag was the immunoelectrophoretic method of Laurell (referred to as Laurell rocket assay).[81] With this method, polyclonal monospecific antibody to VWF is uniformly distributed in a porous agarose gel. Controls and patient specimens are electrophoresed into the gel, the distance of a precipitin "rocket" from the sample well being proportional to the quantity of VWF protein. This method is labor-intensive and time-consuming and has been replaced by classic ELISA assays (see Chapter 16 for description of enzyme-linked immunosorbent and related assays). To simplify the assay and allow for easier automation, currently popular microparticle agglutination assays were developed and are most commonly used. Monoclonal antibody to VWF is coated on microparticles [latex immunoassay (LIA)]. VWF directly agglutinates the microparticles with the end point measured by turbidometric or nephelometric methods. Acceptable correlation of the classic ELISA with the LIA has been noted, and although LIA assays may give higher results

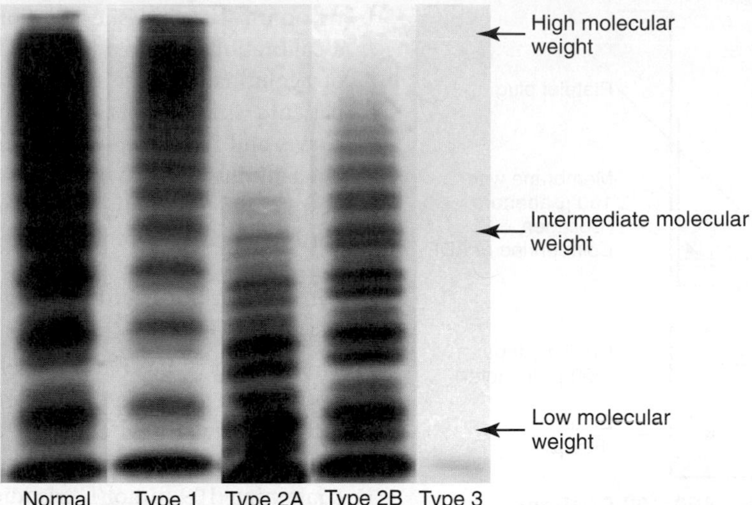

Figure 59-7 Multimeric Analysis of VWF-Ag. Plasma is electrophoresed into a porous gel of agarose or agarose and acrylamide, the multimers are separated, and the VWF:Ag multimers are radiolabeled with antibody to VWF:Ag. Typical patterns of normal and VWD types 1, 2A, 2B, and 3 are shown in the autoradiograph. The pattern seen in type 2M is like that of type 1. *(Image courtesy M. R. Ledford-Kraemer.)*

than the ELISA, good agreement among results is currently obtained with different methods in proficiency testing exercises.[44]

VWF:Multimer Assay

In megakaryocytes and endothelial cells, the *VWF* gene codes for a subunit protein of approximately 220 kDa. Post-ribosomally, carbohydrate is added to the subunit, dimers of the subunits are formed, and the dimers undergo polymerization. The VWF secreted is a population of molecules varying in size from 500 kDa to as large as 20,000 kDa or more. The size of these VWF multimers is controlled in the plasma by a metalloprotease, ADAMTS13 (see later), the size of the multimers being related to the function of the molecule. These multimers are qualitatively detected in the plasma using electrophoresis in a porous gel, followed by visualization with a radiolabeled or enzymatically labeled antibody to VWF.[42,117] Analysis of the multimer patterns is subjective (Figure 59-7). The specimen used is PPP harvested from whole blood containing 109 mmol/L trisodium citrate as an anticoagulant. Loss of the high molecular weight multimers is associated with reduced function (type 2A or 2B VWD), as described later.

ADAMTS13 Assay

ADAMTS13 is **a** **d**isintegrin **a**nd **m**etalloproteinase with a **t**hrombo**s**pondin type 1 motif, member **13**. It also is known as the VWF-cleaving protease and is the enzyme that depolymerizes VWF after secretion from the endothelial cell. When ADAMTS13 is absent or inhibited by autoantibody, thrombotic thrombocytopenic purpura (TTP) can result. The available functional assay for this molecule is based on the ability of the patient's plasma to cleave the high molecular weight multimers of VWF. It requires lengthy incubation followed by VWF multimer analysis, taking up to 2 days. TTP is a condition of clinical urgency; the current assay is not timely enough for diagnostic purposes, being used only for confirmation after treatment has begun. New assays have become available, including the fluorescence resonance energy transfer (FRET) assay[74] and the ELISA,[146] which are proving to be of greater diagnostic usefulness.

Evaluating Platelet Aggregation and Secretion

Platelet aggregation and secretion is evaluated by using aggregation and secretion studies.

Platelet Aggregation Studies

The original platelet aggregation studies were described more than 40 years ago. In the presence of agonist, platelets will stick to each other in a reaction that is mediated primarily by fibrinogen. After more than 45 years, light transmission aggregometry (LTA), with minimal modification, remains the "gold standard" method for evaluating platelet aggregation.[12] For LTA, the specimen used is platelet-rich plasma (PRP) harvested from whole blood containing 109 mmol/L trisodium citrate as an anticoagulant. It is also necessary to harvest PPP because the limit of detection of the aggregometer is adjusted with the patient's own PPP for maximum light transmission, and PRP for minimum light transmission. LTA is a simple turbidometric measurement, the PRP is placed in the light path (37 °C, continuous stirring), and, after the agonist is added, increased transmission of light is recorded over time as the platelets aggregate (Figure 59-8). An alternative method has been developed that allows the use of anticoagulated whole blood. In this case, an electric probe is placed in the specimen and an alternating current passed through the blood. Upon activation, platelets are attracted to the electrodes to which they attach. As more platelets

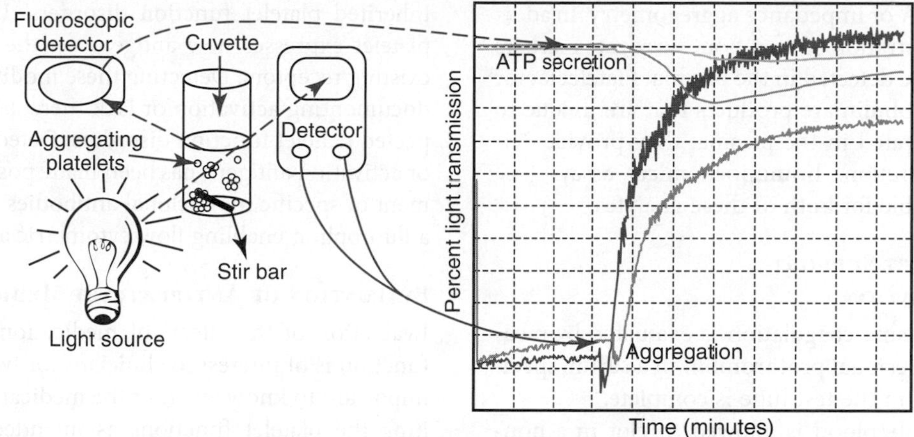

Figure 59-8 Platelet Aggregation. Platelet-rich plasma harvested from whole blood collected in citrate anticoagulant is stirred continuously at a constant rate at 37 °C. Increasing absorbance (loss of turbidity) following addition of an agonist is measured. The gain of the detector is set using the patient's platelet-rich plasma and platelet-poor plasma. The reaction may be quantified by measuring its rate or extent. Measuring secreted adenosine triphosphate (ATP) reflects secretion of platelet-dense bodies from the platelet. Luciferin and luciferase are added to the aggregation reaction. Luciferase converts luciferin to its product in a reaction that is absolutely dependent on ATP and emits photons. Fluorescence is measured, and secretion is quantified as a function of the quantity of ATP released.

TABLE 59-3 Commonly Used Platelet Aggregation Agonists

Collagen	Activates receptor GP VI
ADP	Activates receptors P_2Y_1 and P_2Y_{12}
TRAP	Activates the thrombin receptors PAR_1 and PAR_4
Epinephrine	Activates the alpha 2 receptor
Arachidonic acid	Activates the cyclooxygenase pathway
Ristocetin	Activates VWF binding to GP Ib/V/IX

ADP, Adenosine diphosphate; *TRAP*, thrombin receptor activation peptide.

attach, the flow of current is impeded—a change that is plotted over time. Although LTA remains the "gold standard" for platelet aggregation, advantages of the impedance method include (1) testing in the presence of other blood cells, (2) reduced artifact from preparation, and (3) a smaller sample size requirement.[89] Regardless of the method used to measure the end point, the agonists used to assess aggregation function are the same. The commonly used agonists are summarized in Table 59-3.

Platelet Secretion

Platelets secrete a wide variety of products into the microenvironment following activation. These products are stored in the platelet delta granules (dense bodies) and alpha granules (Table 59-4). Initial evaluation of platelet secretory function requires a morphologic evaluation (see earlier) to determine whether these granules are present and morphologically adequate. The function of secretion was originally evaluated by exploiting the ability of platelets to take up radioactively labeled serotonin in the laboratory and then measuring release of the label following stimulation of the platelets. The method is very labor-intensive and requires the use of radioisotopes. However it remains the method of choice for evaluation of heparin-induced thrombocytopenia (see later). This method has been replaced in all other clinical settings with the use of the lumi-aggregometer, in which luciferin and luciferase are added to the patient specimen before the agonist is added.[145] Conversion of luciferin to its product by luciferase is dependent on adenosine triphosphate (ATP), the only source of which is release from the platelets. In the conversion of luciferin to its product, photons are emitted and are detected by a fluorometer in a quantity that correlates with the ATP released. This method allows for the simultaneous assessment of aggregation and secretion in the same reaction. The method

TABLE 59-4 Representative Contents of Alpha Granules and Dense Bodies in Platelets

Representative alpha granule contents	Adhesion proteins Chemokines Coagulation factors Growth factors Immunoglobulins
Representative dense body contents	Amines Nucleotides Ions Transmitters

is conducted using LTA or impedance aggregometry. In addition to in vitro demonstration of secretion, surrogate markers of in vivo release can be detected in the plasma. Platelet factor 4 and beta-thromboglobulin are products that are unique to the platelet; when elevated in the plasma, they provide evidence of in vivo secretion. Immunochemical assays (see Chapter 16) are available for both of these analytes.

Evaluating Platelet Support of Plasma Coagulation

Platelet support of plasma coagulation is evaluated by measuring the amount of residual prothrombin in a serum specimen after coagulation in the test tube is complete.

When normal whole blood is allowed to clot in a nonsiliconized glass tube, the combined function of platelets and plasma coagulation will efficiently convert nearly all of the available prothrombin to thrombin (prothrombin consumption). Abnormality of any of the coagulation factors or platelets will reduce the efficiency of this process, and some prothrombin will be left in the serum. This prothrombin is then quantified and compared with the starting plasma prothrombin, allowing an assessment of the percentage of prothrombin that is consumed. If the patient's prothrombin time and activated partial thromboplastin time are normal, prothrombin consumption reflects the contribution of the platelet to fibrin generation. The test suffers from lack of reproducibility and is not in widespread use, but it can provide information on platelet support of plasma coagulation. It is most frequently abnormal in acquired platelet function disorders such as paraproteinemias and uremia.[13]

Evaluating Platelet Contractile Function

Platelet contractile function is evaluated by determining clot retraction.

Upon activation, platelets form filapodia, slender projections from the surface of the cell that attach to fibrin strands. Platelet actin tethers to membrane receptors and organizes with cytoplasmic myosin within these filapodia, forming a rudimentary muscle that contracts at the conclusion of the hemostatic process. This has been described as the in vivo suture, drawing the edges of the injury closer together as healing is initiated. This phenomenon is seen (and is measured qualitatively) by observing the formation of serum in a tube without anticoagulant; the clot shrinks (an active process that depends on the platelet), expressing the serum. This clot retraction is dependent on the contractile function of the platelet, and methods have been described to quantify it. Although not widely used, the technique remains useful, particularly if the more specific information provided by platelet aggregometry is not available.[13,125]

Evaluation of Platelets Using Flow Cytometry

Flow cytometry is a useful adjunct in evaluating platelet function in selected situations. Agonist receptors and other membrane proteins are detected on the resting platelet. Study of a specific receptor to determine whether it is present and to assess its surface density is used to identify some of the inherited platelet function disorders. Upon activation, the platelet expresses new antigens on the surface or modifies existing receptors. Detecting these modifications is helpful in documenting activation or lack thereof in patients with suspected platelet function disorders. Detection of these surface or activation antigens has been made possible by the development of specific monoclonal antibodies that are labeled with a fluorophor, enabling flow cytometric analysis.[92]

Evaluation of Antiplatelet Medication

Evaluation of the effects of medications that affect platelet function is of interest to clinicians for two reasons. First, it is important to know whether the medication is actually inhibiting the platelet functions as intended for the patient to receive the desired reduced risk of thrombosis. Second, many patients who are taking antiplatelet medications need emergency or elective procedures and may be at increased risk for hemorrhage during those procedures. Increased risk of hemorrhage in patients taking antiplatelet medications has been demonstrated but is widely variable among patients. Unfortunately, tests of the medication effect on platelet function do not accurately predict whether there will be a hemorrhagic outcome.

Several techniques are used to measure the effects that medications have on platelet function. They include the PFA-100 and PFA-200 analyzers and the Verify Now and platelet aggregation assays.

PFA-100

The PFA-100 was described earlier in the chapter. It has been shown to be effective in detecting aspirin resistance in many cases and may detect the reduced platelet function caused by aspirin. It is not useful in the evaluation of other antiplatelet medications, but the PFA-200 offers a method to evaluate the thienopyridines.

Verify Now

Verify Now (Accumetrics, San Diego, Calif) is a rapid turbidometric assay that exploits the affinity of activated platelets for fibrinogen. With it, a whole blood specimen is pipetted into a disposable cartridge containing fibrinogen-coated microparticles. By using cartridges with different agonists, the effect of antiplatelet medication is assessed: (1) for glycoprotein IIb/IIIa (GP IIb/IIIa) antagonist drugs, (2) for activation with thrombin receptor activation peptide (TRAP); (3) for aspirin, activation with arachidonic acid; and (4) for thienopyridine drugs, activation with ADP.[88] The specimen used is whole blood containing 109 mmol/L trisodium citrate as an anticoagulant, collected into a special plastic 2 mL vacutainer tube. Currently, this method is used only for evaluation of medication effect.[76]

Platelet Aggregation

The "gold standard" for medication effect on platelet function is platelet aggregation using LTA or impedance with the appropriate agonist for the medication (ADP for the thienopyridines; arachidonic acid or collagen for aspirin). Other

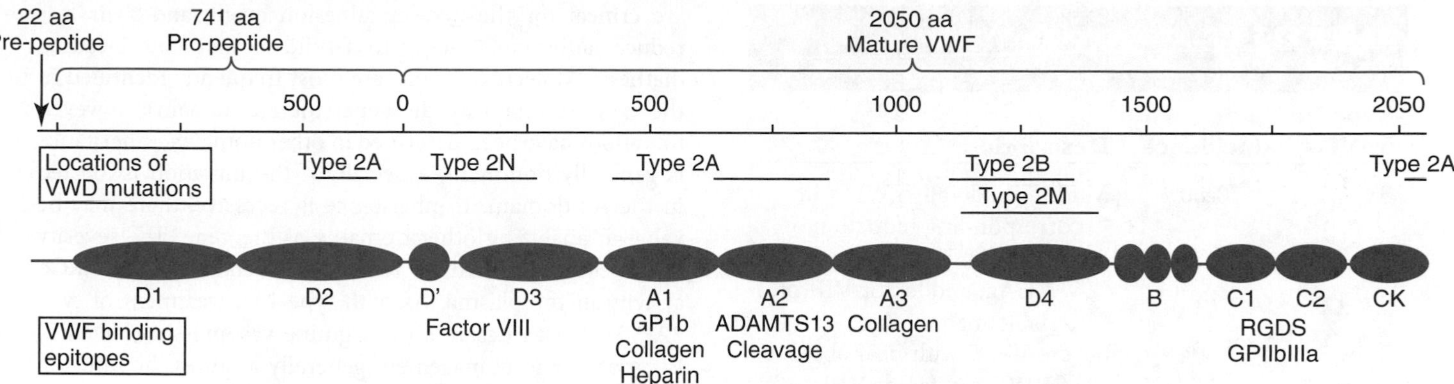

Figure 59-9 VWF Protein. The VWF gene, residing in chromosome 12p13.2, is approximately 178 kilobases with 52 exons. The product of the gene is a protein of 2813 amino acids. There is a 22 amino acid pre-peptide and a larger 741 amino acid pro-peptide, both of which are cleaved from the molecule leaving the mature VWF (2050 amino acids). VWF contains four types of repeated molecular domains. The figure depicts the domains, the locations of functional epitopes, and the locations of the most common mutations in the types of VWD. The protein forms dimers by linkage of the amino terminal end with subsequent formation of multimers via polymerization of the dimers.

methods can be compared against this reference method. LTA and impedance are cumbersome, labor-intense methods that do not lend themselves well to urgent or routine testing, leading to the development of Verify Now and PFA-100. Of interest, agreement is still lacking regarding the appropriate concentrations of agonists to be used when evaluating medication effects.[76]

Clinical Use of Laboratory Tests for Platelet Disorders

The assays and devices discussed earlier are used to detect both inherited and acquired platelet disorders.

Inherited Disorders

Inherited disorders of platelet function include (1) von Willebrand disease, (2) the Bernard-Soulier syndrome, (3) Glanzmann thrombasthenia, and (4) other disorders.

von Willebrand Disease

VWD is the most common of the inherited bleeding disorders. Its exact frequency is not accurately defined. Some have estimated the prevalence to be as high as 1 : 100; however, in clinical practice it does not appear that high. This is a disorder of platelet function that is caused by the absence or abnormality of a plasma protein, VWF. The function of the platelet itself is normal. A second important role for VWF is the binding and stabilizing of coagulation factor VIII in the circulation. The *VWF* gene, residing in chromosome 12p13.2, is approximately 178 kilobases with 52 exons. The product of the gene is a protein of 2813 amino acids. There is a 22 amino acid pre-peptide and a larger 741 amino acid pro-peptide, both of which are cleaved from the molecule, leaving the mature VWF (2050 amino acids). VWF contains four types of repeated molecular domains.[50] Figure 59-9 shows a schematic of the VWF domains and their related functional epitopes. Currently, 526 mutations have been catalogued (http://www.vwf.group.shef.ac.uk/). Analysis of the mutations associated with VWD was initially undertaken to understand the structure and function of the *VWF* gene, the mRNA, and VWF protein; however, some mutation analysis has now become a part of clinical diagnosis. Details of the mutations are beyond the scope of this chapter. For more information, the reader is referred to Sadler and Blinder.[119] The classification of VWD is defined by (1) the quantity of VWF, (2) the relationship of the VWF activity : antigen ratio, (3) the concentration of factor VIII, and (4) the multimeric structure of the VWF:Ag.[120] Types 1 and 3 represent quantitative reductions in the factor, and type 2 (2A, 2B, 2M, 2N) represents dysfunctional factor. Table 59-5 summarizes the classification.

Type 3 VWD is the most severe form of the disorder and the least common, occurring in approximately 0.5 to 5 : 1,000,000 in the population. VWF activity and antigen are usually undetectable, and factor VIII is commonly 0.05 U/mL or less. Patients manifest a severe bleeding disorder and often require treatment with VWF-containing products. Multimeric analysis is not performed because VWAg is essentially absent. The condition is inherited as a recessive trait in which patients are homozygous or doubly heterozygous. Mutations, mostly deletions, do not occur in a localized portion of the gene, but are distributed between exons 3 and 52. Because VWF is essentially absent, the amount of factor VIII will also be severely reduced, because factor VIII needs VWF to stabilize it in the circulation. As in all types of VWD, management is focused on replacement of VWF; however, platelet transfusion may also play a role. Alpha granules of platelets of patients with type 3 VWD contain no VWF, the secretion of which is important in adhesion. Thus, in contrast to all other types of VWD, these patients may benefit from platelet transfusion.[120]

TABLE 59-5 Classification of Von Willebrand Disease (VWD)

Type of VWD	Incidence	Description
Type 1	70-80%	Mild to moderate VWD with corresponding reduction of VWF:RCo, VWF:CB, and VWF:Ag, and factor VIII of variable magnitude
Type 3	<1%	Severe VWD with near absence of VWF and factor VIII
Type 2A	10-15%	Dysfunctional VWF with reduced high molecular weight VWF:Ag multimers
Type 2B	5%	Dysfunctional VWF with reduced high molecular weight VWF:Ag multimers and increased affinity of VWF for the GP Ib-IX-V receptor on the platelet
Type 2M	<1%	Dysfunctional VWF with normal distribution of VWF:Ag multimers
Type 2N	<1%	Dysfunctional VWF with reduced binding of factor VIII manifesting as reduced circulating factor VIII and normal platelet function

Type 2 VWD occurs as the result of an abnormal or dysfunctional VWF and, as a group, accounts for 20 to 30% of cases of VWD. As might be expected, with a multifunctional, large protein, mutations have led to a number of variations in the dysfunction of the molecule. The classification requires analysis of the VWF multimers because the loss of high molecular weight multimers is associated with dysfunction in two of the subtypes of VWD—2A and 2B. Current subtypes of the dysfunction of the molecule are listed in Table 59-5, and each are discussed below.

Type 2 VWD is suspected when there is a discrepancy between VWF activity and the VWF antigen. Ratios of $\frac{\text{VWF:RCo}}{\text{VWF:Ag}}$ of 0.5 to 0.6 or less indicate a dysfunctional molecule and serve as an indication to test further, as described later, to subtype the disorder. In general, the ratio $\frac{\text{VWF:CB}}{\text{VWF:Ag}}$ will be lower than the ratio $\frac{\text{VWF:RCo}}{\text{VWF:Ag}}$ in type 2A and 2B, but the reverse is true in type 2M.[120]

Type 2A VWD is associated with abnormal multimer analysis and loss of high molecular weight multimers. It is the most common of the type 2 subtypes, accounting for 10 to 15% of cases of VWD. High molecular weight multimers are critical for the platelet adhesion event, and their loss reduces adhesion, leading to a mild to moderate bleeding diathesis. Molecular lesions are most frequently identified in the exon 28 region of the gene (the A2 domain); however, mutations have been described in other domains. Inheritance is generally dominant, especially if the mutation is located in the A2 domain. If inheritance is recessive, there may be value in analyzing other domains of the gene. The severity of the bleeding diathesis tends to be related to VWF:RCo activity in the plasma. As with type 2M, treatment of type 2A VWD with desamino-D-arginine vasopressin (DDAVP) is variable, and management generally requires the infusion of VWF-containing products. Platelet transfusion is not recommended.[120]

Type 2B VWD is associated with loss of the high molecular weight multimers of VWF:Ag; however, the proportion of those multimers that are missing is often less than that seen in type 2A. Type 2B VWD is uncommon, accounting for less than 5% of cases of VWD. The mutations that have been described are also in exon 28 (the A2 domain), at or near the GP Ib binding epitope of the mature protein. The abnormality gives the VWF protein a higher affinity for the GP Ib receptor on the platelet surface. This increased affinity is detected in the laboratory by demonstrating RIPA at a low concentration of ristocetin (usually ≤0.5 mg/mL)—a concentration that will not induce aggregation in the presence of normal VWF. This testing is indicated whenever multimeric analysis shows loss of the high molecular weight VWF:Ag multimers and is the method used to distinguish type 2A from type 2B VWD. In type 2B VWD, binding of VWF to platelets in vivo may occur spontaneously or with minimal stimulus, causing in vivo aggregation and clearance of the platelets. Thus, thrombocytopenia is a common finding in patients with this disorder, and consumption of VWF in this manner contributes to decreased amounts of VWF. Patients with type 2B VWD present with a mild to moderate bleeding diathesis. Management is generally limited to infusion of VWF-containing products. Use of DDAVP is not recommended because of the possibility that the release of VWF may induce in vivo platelet agglutination and precipitate a thrombotic complication. Platelet transfusion is not recommended.[120] Platelet-type VWD (pseudo-VWD) is a syndrome with reduced high molecular weight multimers due to increased affinity in the receptor for VWF on the platelet. VWD type 2B and platelet-type VWD are difficult to distinguish clinically. See the discussion of the Bernard Soulier syndrome, later.

Type 2M VWD comprises those patients in whom the VWF activity-to-antigen ratio is low and multimeric analysis of the VWF:Ag shows a normal distribution of the multimers (with M indicating normal multimers). This type of VWD is rare and the prevalence has not been well characterized. Mutations of the gene are most frequently found in exon 28 (the A2 domain of the gene). The tendency to bleed is generally mild to moderate. Management generally consists of infusion with VWF-containing products. The response to DDAVP is variable, and a trial with DDAVP may be useful. Platelet transfusion is not recommended.

Type 2N VWD results in a decrease in plasma factor VIII but normal VWF-mediated platelet function. Thus, the phenotype of the disorder is similar to that of hemophilia but shows autosomal inheritance. All testing of VWF functions and antigen is normal. Mutations in the *VWF* gene occur in exons 20 to 28 (the D′ domain), which code for the epitope in the VWF protein that binds to factor VIII. A few specialty laboratories are able to measure the binding of factor VIII to patient VWF, confirming the diagnosis. Distinguishing type 2N VWD from hemophilia is important because treatment of the disorders requires the infusion of different products.[120]

Type 1 VWD is the most prevalent form of VWD, accounting for approximately 70 to 80% of cases.[101] Inheritance of type 1 VWD is autosomal; however, the phenotype of the associated bleeding tendency is quite variable, with many patients manifesting a mild to moderate bleeding disorder, while others with similar laboratory values do not manifest a bleeding tendency. With laboratory analysis, one generally finds a concomitant reduction in VWF activity, VWF antigen, and factor VIII. Values vary from below 0.2 IU/mL to as high as 0.5 IU/mL. Genetic analysis of patients is complex. European and Canadian reports of the molecular analysis of patients with type 1 VWD show that of those patients with clearly normal multimer analysis, only 55 to 63% had an identifiable mutation, and that those mutations were not localized in the gene.[21,52] There is a relationship between the concentration of VWF in the plasma and the probability of detecting a mutation in the gene. Of those with 0.15 IU/mL or less VWF protein, 95% had a mutation, while only 50% of those with 0.45 IU/mL or greater VWF protein had mutations. Among those who have mutations, 10 to 15% have more than one mutation identified.[50] What of those patients with reduced VWF and no identifiable mutation? Carboxylation of the VWF protein is closely associated with the ABO blood group of normal individuals. Those with blood group O have lower circulating VWF than those who have the A and/or B antigen. It is thought that carboxylation may influence the half-life of the molecule.[49] Analysis of the blood groups of patients with type 1 VWD shows a significantly higher number of patients with blood group O. Thus, changes in the postribosomal carboxylation of VWF may account for VWD without mutations in the *VWF* gene. Management of bleeding in type 1 VWD depends on the severity and expected duration of the hemorrhagic challenge. Those with a mild challenge of short duration can receive DDAVP, while those with more extensive challenge require infusion with VWF-containing products.[119]

Bernard-Soulier Syndrome

The Bernard-Soulier syndrome (BSS) is a disorder of platelet function that is related to the function of VWF; however, in this condition, the amount of VWF protein is normal, with the lesion being in the VWF receptor on the surface of the platelet, GP Ib/V/IX. The disorder is inherited as an autosomal recessive trait with bleeding seen only in homozygotes, and it is seen most frequently in consanguineous relations. It is a rare disorder, with a prevalence of less than 1 : 1,000,000 in the general population. Mutations have been reported in the genes coding for GP Iba (gene symbol *GP1BA*) and GP IX *(GP9)*, but not GP V *(GP5)*. For further details, see http://www.bernard-soulier.org/mutations. It is one of the giant platelet syndromes with concurrent thrombocytopenia and is associated with moderate to severe bleeding. Bleeding episodes are managed with platelet transfusions. While discussing mutations of the GP Ib/V/IX receptor, it is useful to mention platelet-type or pseudo-VWD. This is also an inherited bleeding syndrome in which there is a normal *VWF* gene and protein, but a lesion in the platelet receptor causes an increased affinity with VWF. This disorder is difficult to distinguish from type 2B VWD. The diagnosis relies on demonstration that the VWF is normal in the plasma and that the platelets are abnormal (complex mixing studies are done in some laboratories), or the differential diagnosis is made with mutation analysis. The distinction is important because the condition is managed with platelet transfusion.[78]

Glanzmann Thrombasthenia

Absence or abnormality of the platelet integrin, GP IIb/IIIa, the receptor for fibrinogen in aggregation, is the cause of Glanzmann thrombasthenia (GT). Mutations (deletions or other mutations) in the genes for GP IIb or GP IIIa membrane proteins have been identified. The disorder is inherited as an autosomal recessive trait that leads to a mild to moderate bleeding diathesis. It is a rare disorder, affecting approximately 1 : 1,000,000 in the general population; however, it may be more prevalent in populations with consanguineous relations. Platelet count is normal; however, platelet aggregation with all agonists except ristocetin is abnormal. In addition, the bleeding time is prolonged, the PFA-100 value is prolonged, and clot retraction is abnormal. Bleeding episodes are treated with platelet transfusion.[98]

Other Disorders

Many other functions of the platelet such as those related to (1) binding of collagen, (2) formation of secretory granules, (3) mechanisms of secretion, and (4) others have rare inherited disorders that affect these specific functions. Only a small number of laboratories are capable of evaluating these rare disorders, and the ability to make diagnoses of this type is often complicated by the need to evaluate fresh platelets to evaluate function. Molecular approaches have not yet been documented sufficiently to be of clinical diagnostic usefulness.

Acquired Disorders

Factors that affect acquired disorders include medications, degree of renal failure, paraproteinemia, and primary bone marrow disorder.

Medication

Many medications affect platelet function. For example, drugs such as aspirin, thienopyridines, and monoclonal inhibitors of GP IIb/IIIa are used specifically to reduce function when inhibition of thrombosis, particularly arterial thrombosis, is

TABLE 59-6 Examples of Medications Affecting Platelet Function

Class of Medication	Examples
Nonsteroidal anti-inflamatory	Aspirin, naproxen, ibuprofen, indomethacin
GP IIb/IIIa antagonists (antibodies)	Abciximab, eptifibatide, tirofiban
Thienopyridines	Clopidogrel, ticlopidine
Increase cAMP and/or cGMP	Iloprost, dipyridamole, prostacyclin
Cardiovascular medications	Many
Volume expanders	Dextran, hydroxyethyl starch
Chemotherapeutic agents	Mitomycin, daunorubicin, BCNU
Psychotropic medications	Many
Others	Antihistamines, clofibrate, rad contrast agents

desired. In other cases, the effects on platelet function are adverse complications of the medication. These effects generally are not enough to lead to a bleeding complication; however, if the medication is used in patients with inherited or acquired platelet disorders or other disorders of hemostasis, the effect may increase bleeding. Examples of medications that affect platelet function are listed in Table 59-6.[8]

Renal Failure

In patients with renal failure, organic acids such as guanidinosuccinic and phenolic acids are abnormally retained in the blood. These acids have a deleterious effect on all platelet functions and are often associated with a bleeding diathesis. Neither creatinine nor urea has a significant effect on platelet function, but they provide a useful surrogate marker for other retained products. Platelet functions tend to be affected at urea nitrogen of ≈60 mg/dL or greater and creatinine of 3 to 4 mg/dL. In vitro studies have confirmed the deleterious effects of organic acids and the rapid rate at which normal platelets demonstrate loss of function. For this reason, the use of platelet transfusion in managing hemorrhage in uremic patients is ineffective. Management is difficult; however, treatment with dialysis to reduce retained acids is often effective. In addition, the use of DDAVP has proven of some value.[139] Treatment of anemia by keeping the hemoglobin above 10 g/dL using erythropoietin and transfusion has a beneficial effect in managing bleeding.[95]

Paraproteinemia

Patients with multiple myeloma or Waldenström macroglobulinemia often have remarkably elevated concentrations of immunoglobulins. These immunoglobulins are associated with hemorrhage via two basic mechanisms. First, the paraproteins interfere with fibrin-monomer polymerization, which is reflected in prolonged thrombin time. Second, the proteins adsorb nonspecifically to the surface of the platelet, masking the receptors on the surface of the platelet and reducing platelet activity. These problems are managed by reducing the concentration of the protein through management of the underlying malignancy. In acute situations, plasmapheresis is effective in reducing paraprotein concentrations, but only for short-term management.[38]

Primary Bone Marrow Disorder

In myeloproliferative and myelodysplasplastic syndromes, the megakaryocyte, similar to other cell lines, is affected by malignant transformation. The effects of malignant megakaryocyte production of platelets on platelet function are widely variable. These effects may include but are not limited to (1) increased or decreased platelet counts, (2) reduced granules, (3) reduced or abnormal membrane receptors, (4) adsorption of high molecular weight VWF multimers, causing an acquired type 2 von Willebrand disease (VWD), or (5) abnormal signal transduction mechanisms. As a result of these variable effects, patients may manifest abnormal bleeding or, paradoxically, thrombosis. Bleeding episodes may be managed with platelet transfusion; however, in patients with thrombocytosis, it is difficult to determine whether the risk to the patient is bleeding or thrombosis. Patients at thrombotic risk may benefit from treatment with antiplatelet medication.[109]

GENERAL CONSIDERATIONS IN COAGULATION TESTING

Special considerations in coagulation testing include (1) preanalytical variables, (2) optical versus mechanical end point detection, and (3) chromogenic assays.

Preanalytical Variables for Coagulation-Based Assays

Control of preanalytical issues in coagulation testing is paramount to good laboratory performance. In addition to the common issues of hemolyzed, icteric, or lipemic samples, some preanalytical factors of particular importance in coagulation testing include (1) clotted specimens, (2) improper blood-to-anticoagulant ratio, and (3) contamination with heparin or other anticoagulants. Traumatic venipuncture, activation of blood within the collection device, or improper mixing of the anticoagulant with blood may result in clotting, which consumes coagulation factors, making testing unreliable. Blood for coagulation testing should be collected by standard venipuncture techniques into 109 mmol/L (3.2%) trisodium citrate, such that the final ratio of blood to anticoagulant is 9:1. Blood is commonly collected into commercially available tubes with prealiquoted trisodium citrate and a line indicating the appropriate volume of blood to be drawn. Collection of a volume of specimen less than the recommended volume ("a short draw") will result in excess anticoagulant and prolonged clotting times. Likewise, samples with high hematocrit (>55%) will require a decreased volume of anticoagulant because of a lower plasma volume. Some coagulation testing, such as activated clotting time, may be performed on whole blood; however, most routine clot-based assays are performed on platelet-poor plasma. To avoid interference from phospholipid and other platelet-derived substances such as platelet factor 4, platelet-poor plasma is prepared by centrifugation, typically at 1500 g for at least 15 minutes. Phospholipids are important for the spatial orientation of coagulation molecules and have a significant impact on the activated partial thromboplastin time. Platelet factor 4 binds heparin and may alter clot-based tests. Centrifugation and testing should occur as soon as possible, usually within 24 hours for prothrombin time (PT), or within 4 hours for aPTT. Centrifuged samples may be stored at 18 to 24 °C, whereas colder temperatures should be avoided because of possible activation of factor VII. When testing is delayed, the plasma should be separated from the cells and kept below −20 °C or at −70 °C for longer storage.[25] Household grade freezers with autodefrost cycles are not suitable.

Optical versus Mechanical End Point Detection

Clot-based tests, among which PT/international normalized ratio (INR) and aPTT are common, are based on detecting the time interval from initiation of coagulation to clot formation. Detection of clot formation as an end point has been accomplished in a number of ways. Early methods used a tilt-tube technique that depended on visually identifying clot formation in plasma samples. A water bath was necessary to keep the temperature at 37 °C. Currently, this time-intensive manual method is used only to develop international standards for thromboplastin.

As a result of high-volume testing, most coagulation testing is now performed on automated instruments that control the temperature of the reaction and detect end points by use of any one of several methods. Most methods detect a change in physical/mechanical properties or a change in the light transmission produced by polymerized fibrin. Numerous approaches for mechanical end point detection have been developed. One mechanical method consists of a metal ball at the bottom of a sample cuvette that is sent into a back-and-forth motion by a magnet; the end point is detected when fibrin monomers polymerize into fibrin strands and impede the motion of the ball. Another mechanical detection system uses a magnet to hold a ball to the side of a rotating cuvette until fibrin strands physically displace the ball. Optical detection (usually nephelometric but occasionally turbidometric, Chapter 10, Optical Techniques) is the most commonly employed method, detecting a decrease in light transmission or increased light scatter as fibrin monomers are polymerized into fibrin strands.[124] Optical end points may occur at preset thresholds; however, other instruments use the kinetics, such as maximum acceleration of fibrin polymerization, to define end points. Light sources have traditionally been halogen lamps or lasers, but newer instruments may use light-emitting diodes (LEDs) that increase longevity and allow measurement at wavelengths that have less overlap with interfering substances. Differences are expected between end point detection systems. An advantage of mechanical over optical end point detection is the ability to measure clots in the presence of substances such as hemoglobin, bilirubin or lipid that interfere with optical methods.

Chromogenic Assays

Chromogenic assays have been used to bypass the complexity of the clotting cascade, including the effects of elevated coagulation factors, anticoagulant medications, and lupus anticoagulants (discussed later). In these assays, serine proteases (such as thrombin, factor Xa, factor IXa, factor XIa, and factor XIIa) of the clotting cascade cleave oligopeptide substrates, releasing chromogens that are then detected optically at 405 nm:

$$\text{Serine Protease} + \text{Chromogenic Substrate} \rightarrow p\text{-nitroaniline (detected at 405 nm)}$$

The chromogenic method is commonly applied to assays that measure (1) factor VIII, (2) factor X, (2) protein C, (3) antithrombin, and (4) heparin concentration (anti-Xa method). However, numerous other applications are possible. The 405-nm wavelength is advantageous because of less spectral overlap with common interfering substances.

SECONDARY HEMOSTASIS

As opposed to primary hemostasis, which involves the processes of vascular contraction and platelet function, secondary hemostasis is defined as "the formation of fibrin through the coagulation cascade" (http://ahdc.vet.cornell.edu/clinpath/modules/coags/second.htm).

Vitamin K–Dependent Factors

Activity of coagulation factors II, VII, IX, and X and natural anticoagulants, protein C, and protein S, is dependent on the action of vitamin K (see Chapter 31). Vitamin K–dependent carboxylases convert glutamic acid residues to gamma-carboxyglutamic acid residues on vitamin K–dependent coagulation factors, imparting calcium binding function to these factors. Reduced vitamin K is regenerated through the action of a vitamin K epoxide reductase. Deficiencies of vitamin K result in inactive coagulation factors as the result of inadequate gamma carboxylation with resultant loss of calcium binding capability. Vitamin K deficiency, therefore, may lead to an acquired bleeding disorder.

Oral vitamin K antagonists (VKAs), such as warfarin, are used for individuals who require sustained anticoagulation. VKA inhibits vitamin K epoxide reductase that is responsible for regenerating the active vitamin K cofactor necessary for gamma carboxylation. Because protein C is a vitamin K–dependent natural anticoagulant with a short half-life, patients treated with VKA alone have an initial risk of thrombosis until the other vitamin K–dependent procoagulants are also reduced. For this reason, anticoagulant effect is first achieved with heparin, and then oral VKA is overlapped with heparin therapy for 3 to 5 days. A study comparing combined VKA and heparin therapy against VKA therapy alone for proximal vein thrombosis was terminated early because of an increased rate of symptomatic extension or recurrence of venous thromboembolism in the group treated with VKA alone.[15]

Evaluation of Secondary Hemostasis

Tests used to evaluate secondary hemostasis include (1) prothrombin time and international normalized ratio, (2) activated partial thromboplastin time, (3) fibrinogen assays (Clauss and derived), (4) mixing studies, (5) factor assays, (6) inhibitor assays, (7) factor XIII assays, and (8) thrombin time.

Prothrombin Time/International Normalized Ratio (PT/INR)

The PT is a clot-based assay that reflects the activity of *extrinsic and common pathway* factors of the coagulation cascade. The PT is initiated by the addition of a thromboplastin reagent containing tissue factor, calcium, and phospholipid. The PT cannot be compared among different laboratories because the specific thromboplastin/instrument combination determines the responsiveness of the test. The INR, which is derived mathematically from the PT, allows harmonization of PT across laboratories for the purpose of monitoring VKA. All results are standardized using the international sensitivity index (ISI) for the particular thromboplastin/instrument combination used to perform the test.[127] ISI is based on the slope of the relationship between log PT values obtained with a test thromboplastin reagent and a reference thromboplastin, using samples from normal individuals and patients on VKA. The INR is then calculated as follows:

$$INR = \left[\frac{\text{PT (patient)}}{\text{PT (geometric mean of normal)}}\right]^{ISI}$$

The PT/INR is performed on platelet-poor plasma at 37 °C. The tissue factor in the reagent initiates the extrinsic pathway of the coagulation cascade (see Figure 59-2), the phospholipids provide a surface for assembly of coagulation factors, and the calcium chloride counteracts the binding of plasma calcium by citrate, making calcium available for the coagulation process. The timer is started when reagent is added, and the end point occurs when fibrin monomer polymerization is detected.

Patient plasma + Thromboplastin (Tissue factor and Phospholipid) + $CaCl_2$ → Fibrin clot

The addition of tissue factor activates the extrinsic pathway much like the natural process; however, clotting occurs before the intrinsic pathway is significantly propagated, as occurs with in vivo coagulation. Consequently, the PT/INR is not sensitive to factor VIII or other intrinsic coagulation factors, and PT/INR could be considered a test of the initiation phase of coagulation.

The PT/INR is used to identify deficiencies or inhibitors of factors VII, X, V, and II and fibrinogen. Expected results of clotting assays, including PT/INR, are shown in Table 59-7 for key inherited and acquired disorders.

The sensitivity of PT/INR reagents to the deficiency of coagulation factors varies with the specific reagent and instrument combination. Therefore, it is useful for laboratories to determine the sensitivity of a given PT/INR system to factors VII, X, V, and II. This is accomplished by measuring the PT/INR in a dilutional series of factor-deficient plasma with normal pooled plasma. The activity at which the PT/INR is prolonged beyond the upper limit of the reference interval signifies the sensitivity of the assay to the factor being tested (Figure 59-10; for illustration, this example uses the aPTT test rather than PT/INR). If a reagent is overly sensitive to decreases in a factor (e.g., 0.5 IU/mL factor VII), the laboratory may detect clinically insignificant prolongations of the PT/INR. Needless laboratory evaluations and delays in surgical interventions may be avoided if reagents are selected carefully.

The PT/INR has been used to monitor vitamin K antagonist therapy because it is sensitive to vitamin K–dependent factors, II, VII, IX, and X. Monitoring during bridging or conversion of patients from heparin therapy to therapy with VKAs is made possible by the addition of heparin-neutralizing substances. Vitamin K antagonist therapy and its monitoring are addressed in greater detail later.

Activated Partial Thromboplastin Time (aPTT)

The aPTT is a clot-based assay that is initiated by activation of contact factors and reflects the activity of the intrinsic and common coagulation pathways (see Figure 59-2). Activation of contact factors [high molecular weight kininogen (HMWK), prekallikrein, and factors XII, and XI] is achieved by the addition of one of a wide variety of activators, most having in common a negatively charged surface. Activators including kaolin, celite, and micronized silica have been used extensively when mechanical end points are determined by coagulometers (see earlier); however, if an optical detection is used, micronized silica or the soluble chemical activator, ellagic acid, is used because they do not interfere with light transmission.

The aPTT is carried out in two stages. First, reagent containing an activator and phospholipids is added and incubated with the citrated plasma at 37 °C for several minutes (varies with the method). Second, the plasma is recalcified with calcium chloride, which is required for subsequent activation of downstream coagulation factors, and the timer is started. The timer is stopped when the end point is detected.

Patient plasma + Activator + Phospholipid → Factor XIIa + Factor XIa (stage 1)

$CaCl_2$ + Factor XIIa + Factor XIa + Other Coagulation Factors → Fibrin Clot (stage 2)

The aPTT is sensitive to activities of the intrinsic and common pathway factors (1) HMWK, (2) prekallikrein, (3) XII, (4) XI, (5) IX, (6) VIII, (7) X, (8) V, (9) II, and (10) fibrinogen.[14] Common uses of the aPTT include monitoring of heparin therapy and screening for deficiencies or

TABLE 59-7 Clinical Settings and Coagulation Tests

	Presentation	aPTT	PT	TT	Fibrinogen
Inherited Disorders					
Contact factor deficiencies (HMWK, prekallikrein, and factor XII)	None	↑	Nl	Nl	Nl
Intrinsic pathway procoagulant deficiencies (factor XI, IX, and VIII)	Bleeding	↑	Nl	Nl	Nl
Extrinsic pathway procoagulant deficiencies (factor VII)	Bleeding	Nl	↑	Nl	Nl
Common pathway deficiencies (factor X, V, and II)	Bleeding	↑	↑	Nl	Nl
Congenital hypofibrinogenemia	Bleeding	↑	↑	↑	↓
Congenital dysfibrinogenemia	Bleeding/Thrombosis	Nl	Nl	↑	Nl
Natural anticoagulant deficiencies (protein C, protein S, and antithrombin)	Thrombosis	Nl	Nl	Nl	Nl
von Willebrand disease	Bleeding	Nl or ↑	Nl	Nl	Nl
Glanzmann thrombasthenia	Bleeding	Nl	Nl	Nl	Nl
Bernard-Soulier syndrome	Bleeding	Nl	Nl	Nl	Nl
Acquired Disorders					
Liver disease	Bleeding/Thrombosis	Nl or ↑†	↑	↑	Nl or ↓
Disseminated intravascular coagulation	Bleeding/Thrombosis	Nl or ↑†	↑	↑	↓¶
Vitamin K deficiency	Bleeding	Nl or ↑†	↑	Nl	Nl
Lupus anticoagulant	Thrombosis*	↑	Nl§	Nl	Nl
Specific intrinsic pathway factor inhibitors (factor XI, IX, and VIII)	Bleeding	Nl	↑	Nl	Nl
Specific common pathway factor inhibitors (factor X, V, and II)	Bleeding	↑	↑	Nl	Nl
Medications					
Unfractionated heparin		↑	Nl or ↑‖	↑	Nl
Low molecular weight heparin		↑‡	Nl or ↑‖	↑	Nl
Direct thrombin inhibitor		↑	↑	↑	**
Anti–vitamin K (warfarin)		Nl or ↑†	↑	Nl	Nl

*Thrombosis associated with antiphospholipid syndrome.
†Prolongation of aPTT depends on the sensitivity of the reagents and the degree of factor deficiency.
‡aPTT is not predictably prolonged by low molecular weight heparin.
§Rare lupus anticoagulants prolong PT in addition to aPTT.
‖PT reagents may contain heparin-neutralizing reagents (usually up to 1 U/mL).
¶Fibrinogen decreased with overt DIC.
**Direct thrombin inhibitors may cause underestimation of fibrinogen by the Clauss method.
Nl, Normal.

inhibitors of intrinsic and common pathway factors. The use of aPTT for monitoring heparin therapy is discussed later. The response of aPTT reagents to (1) heparin,[71] (2) factor deficiency, (3) specific factor inhibitors, and (4) lupus anticoagulants[16] varies widely. If a clinical laboratory intends to use aPTT to detect factor deficiencies, it is important to know the threshold of factor deficiency that prolongs the aPTT. The response of aPTT to factor VIII and factor IX is particularly important because of the prevalence of hemophilias A and B. Determining this responsiveness is accomplished by measuring the aPTT in a dilutional series of factor-deficient plasma with normal pooled plasma. The activity at which the aPTT is prolonged beyond the upper limit of the reference interval signifies the sensitivity of the assay to the factor being tested (see Figure 59-10). In general, the desired response to factors VIII, IX, and XI should be approximately 0.3 IU/mL. Very sensitive or insensitive reagents may create problems.

The aPTT is prolonged in a variety of clinically significant and insignificant scenarios. Table 59-7 summarizes some causes of prolonged aPTT and/or PT/INR. Seven general potential causes of isolated prolongation of aPTT include (1) a procoagulant deficiency that may be associated with a bleeding history—may include multiple factor deficiencies; (2) a contact factor deficiency without bleeding risk (XII, prekallikrein, HMWK); (3) a specific inhibitor acquired as an alloimmune or autoimmune phenomenon (e.g., factor VIII inhibitor); (4) a nonspecific inhibitor such as a lupus anticoagulant; (5) a medication effect or contamination (e.g.,

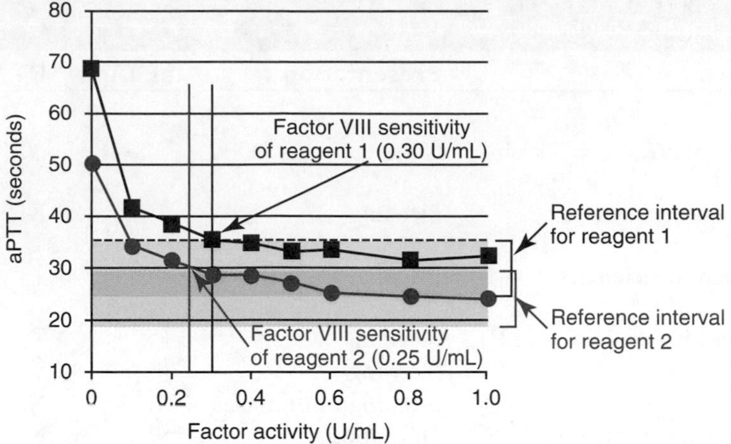

Figure 59-10 Relationship of aPTT to Factor VIII Activity. The graph demonstrates typical relationships of factor activity to clotting time. Response curves are shown for two aPTT reagents. Reference intervals for the reagents are represented as gray and red shaded areas for reagent 1 and reagent 2, respectively. The factor activity at which aPTT prolongs above the reference interval is the limit of detection of the reagent *(shown as black or red arrows)*. The graph demonstrates that aPTT reagents vary in their response to coagulation factors. Reagent 2 has a lower sensitivity than reagent 1 for factor VIII and may be less useful in detecting mild hemophilia A. PT reagents (and instrument combinations) also vary in their responses to extrinsic and common pathway factors and are assessed in a similar manner.

heparin, direct thrombin inhibitor); (6) a spurious result; and (7) an extreme of the population in which the aPTT may be minimally increased outside the upper limit of the reference interval, usually defined by two standard deviations, which includes only 95% of the population.

Although activated partial *thromboplastin* time implies the addition of thromboplastin, this is not the case. This ambiguity is a result of use of the term "partial" thromboplastin by Langdell and associates[80] to describe a group of reagents that produced clotting that was less rapid in hemophiliac plasma than in normal plasma. This was contrasted with "complete" thromboplastin reagents used in the prothrombin time assay, which did not discriminate normal and hemophiliac plasmas. Partial thromboplastin activity was achieved by replacing thromboplastin with cephalin or diluting thromboplastin; however, the overall effect of the dilutions was to remove the thromboplastin activity, making the contribution of the intrinsic pathway measurable. Subsequently, the addition of activators led to the aPTT that we recognize.

aPTT may be prolonged in patients who are not at risk for bleeding, such as those with deficiency of factor XII, prekallikrein, or HMWK. In fact, the intrinsic pathway is best considered a laboratory phenomenon, and in vivo coagulation is better considered in terms of initiation, amplification, and propagation (see Figures 59-2 and 59-3). In vivo, the initiation phase of coagulation is rapidly inhibited by tissue factor pathway inhibitor, with accompanying feedback by thrombin that initiates the propagation phase of coagulation. The aPTT reflects clinically significant deficiencies of factors in the propagation phase (factors XI, IX, and VIII) of in vivo coagulation and is an important test for identifying these deficiencies.

Fibrinogen (Clauss and Derived)

Coagulation ultimately depends on the conversion of fibrinogen to fibrin monomer by thrombin (see Figure 59-2). The Clauss method[24] is the most common method used to measure fibrinogen concentration. Initial dilution of plasma (usually 1:10) to dilute fibrinogen with addition of excess thrombin results in a clotting assay that is dependent on the functional fibrinogen concentration. Thrombin (final concentration 30 to 100 U/mL) is added to the diluted plasma. With the enzyme (thrombin) at saturation, and the substrate (fibrinogen) at limiting concentration, the rate of fibrin formation depends on the concentration of fibrinogen:

$$\text{Citrated patient plasma (diluted)} + \text{Thrombin (30 to 100 U/mL)} \rightarrow \text{Fibrin clot}$$

The fibrin end point is used to determine fibrinogen concentration from a calibration curve. The calibration curve is generated using plasma with a known fibrinogen concentration. Five dilutions of the calibrator are made, and a calibration curve is generated by plotting fibrinogen concentration against the rate of fibrin clot formation.

Another method of fibrinogen determination is PT-derived fibrinogen, or PT-fibrinogen. The fibrinogen concentration is proportional to the change in absorbance in an optical PT/INR measurement. A calibrator is used to create a calibration curve relating the change of absorbance of PT/INR to the fibrinogen concentration. The PT-fibrinogen assay may overestimate fibrinogen concentration in (1) patients with disseminated intravascular coagulation, (2) patients on fibrinolytic therapy, and (3) many patients with dysfibrinogenemia. In addition, some fibrinogen calibrators contribute more turbidity and may not be optimal for PT-fibrinogen measurements. The Clauss method is considered by many to provide a more meaningful fibrinogen measurement because fibrinogen degradation products are not detected, whereas PT-fibrinogen methods are more sensitive to fibrinogen degradation products. Fibrinogen degradation products prolong some clot-based tests by interfering with fibrin monomer polymerization but may also clinically act as anticoagulants and may contribute to hemorrhage in disseminated intravascular coagulation (see later).[86]

Mixing Studies

Mixing studies are performed on abnormally prolonged clot-based assays such as aPTT and PT. The purpose of mixing studies is to determine whether prolonged clotting times are due to factor deficiency or inhibitor activity. Mixing studies are useful for guiding the coagulation work-up, but they lack clinical sensitivity and specificity. Hence, the results of mixing studies are followed up with (1) lupus anticoagulant tests, (2) factor assays, and (3) possibly functional inhibitor studies for confirmation. Inhibitors are categorized as nonspecific or specific types. Nonspecific inhibitors (e.g., heparin, lupus anticoagulant) have activity against multiple procoagulants, while specific inhibitors are directed at a single factor. Lupus anticoagulants are a heterogeneous group of immunoglobulins with phospholipid-dependent activity against coagulation factors; they are discussed in greater detail later. Acquired factor VIII inhibitors are specific inhibitors that prolong the aPTT and clinically manifest as bleeding. These are usually seen as alloantibodies in the setting of hemophilia A treated with factor VIII concentrates, but they may be seen in nonhemophiliac patients as an autoantibody. Although rare, specific inhibitors may occur against any factor, and a high degree of clinical suspicion is needed when bleeding is otherwise unexplained.

Mixing studies are useful when clotting time (e.g., aPTT, PT) is unexpectedly prolonged outside of the reference interval. They are also recommended for lupus anticoagulant testing (see section on DRVVT and lupus anticoagulant studies later) to confirm the inhibitor effect. Citrate-anticoagulated patient plasma is mixed in a 1:1 ratio with normal pooled plasma, and then the clotting assay is repeated *immediately*. Normal pooled plasma should be derived from a sufficient number of apparently healthy individuals to ensure a quantity of 1 IU/mL of all factors. If a factor deficiency in the patient plasma exists, the resulting 1:1 mix supplies the factors needed to correct the clotting time back into the reference interval. If an inhibitor is present, the mixed specimen will not correct the clotting time into the reference interval.

The utility of mixing studies largely depends on the patient population and the clinical setting. For example, aPTT mixing studies are performed more frequently than PT/INR mixing studies because lupus anticoagulants, which are common, affect aPTT much more frequently than PT. When aPTT is prolonged and mixing studies fail to adequately correct into the reference interval, an inhibitor is suspected. If the patient is asymptomatic or has a history of thrombosis, the next step should be to look for lupus anticoagulant rather than to measure factor VIII, IX, and XI concentrations. Conversely, if the patient has a bleeding presentation, a specific inhibitor may be suspected and factor concentrations should be measured. PT/INR mixing studies may be helpful at times. Inhibitors and deficiencies of factor VII and the common pathway factors are rare and can be investigated with PT/INR or aPTT mixing studies.

Immediate aPTT mixing studies that correct to the reference interval require incubated mixing to assess for *time-dependent inhibitors*. In such studies, the patient's plasma is mixed with normal pooled plasma and they are incubated *together* for 1 or 2 hours at 37 °C. The aPTT is then repeated and compared with a control. The control consists of patient plasma and normal pooled plasma incubated at 37 °C *separately,* followed by mixing and aPTT. This step is important because it controls for loss of labile factors during the incubation process (Figure 59-11). One approach to interpretation is to consider a 10% difference between the test and the control to indicate a time-dependent inhibitor. Acquired alloantibodies to factor VIII are frequently time dependent; however, up to 15% of lupus anticoagulant measurements are also time dependent.[26] Considering the high prevalence of lupus anticoagulant relative to the low prevalence of acquired factor VIII inhibitors in hemophilia patients (1 to 2 per million of population per year), laboratories are more likely to encounter time-dependent lupus anticoagulants than time-dependent acquired factor VIII inhibitors (Table 59-8).

The performance characteristics of mixing studies as tests to detect lupus anticoagulants depend on the (1) phospholipid content of reagents; (2) factor and phospholipid content of normal pooled plasma (NPP); (3) titer and strength of the lupus anticoagulant; (4) presence of multiple factor deficiencies; (5) heparin contamination; and (6) criteria for interpretation. Weak inhibitors or very sensitive aPTT reagents

TABLE 59-8 Prevalence of Time-Dependent Inhibitors in a Population of 300 Million*

Inhibitor Type	Population	Prevalence of Inhibitor	% Time Dependence	Number of Time-Dependent Inhibitors
Lupus anticoagulants	300×10^6	3%	10%	900,000
Factor VIII inhibitor in hemophilia A	30,000	15%	90%	4050

*Time-dependent inhibitors are 222 times more likely to be due to LA than to specific factor VIII inhibitor.

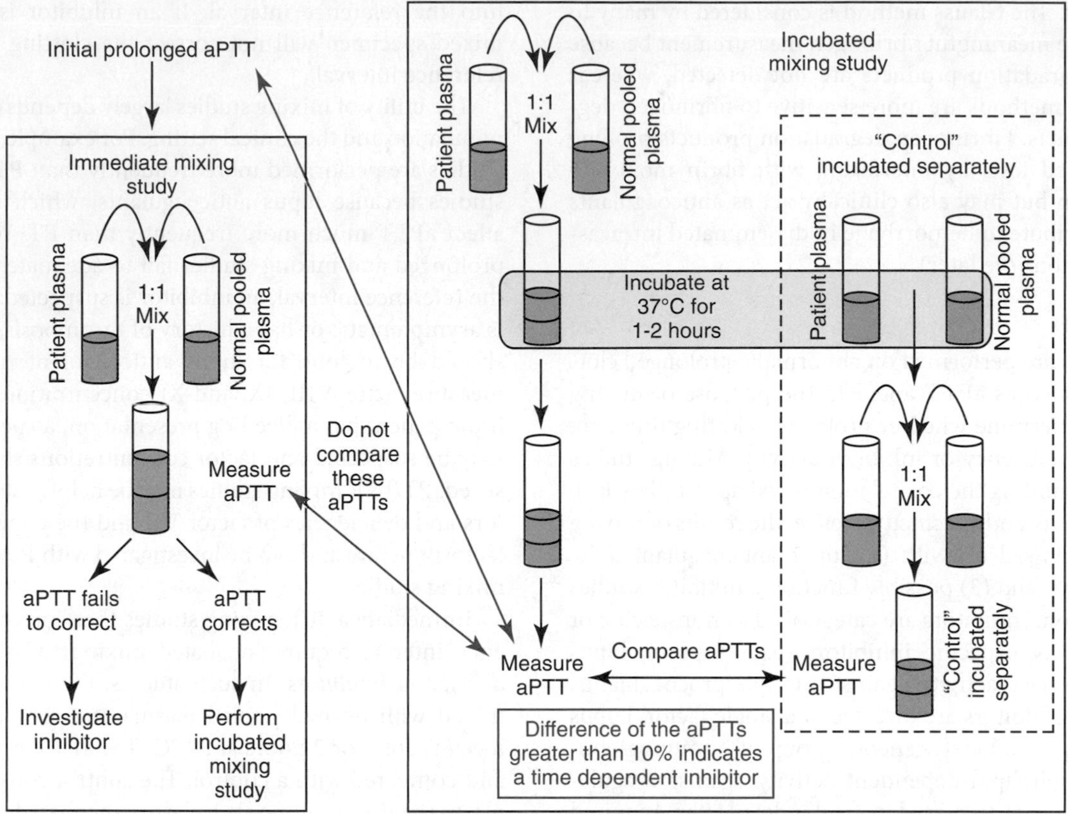

Figure 59-11 Sequence for the Performance of Mixing Studies. In this example, a 1:1 mixing study is used. An immediate mixing study is shown on the left. Equal volumes of patient plasma and normal pooled plasma are mixed, and then the aPTT is measured. If aPTT fails to correct (e.g., into the reference interval), then there is evidence of an inhibitor and the mixing study is complete. If the immediate mixing study corrects, then an incubated mixing study is needed to exclude a time-dependent inhibitor. The incubated mixing study starts with mixing equal volumes of patient plasma and normal pooled plasma. The 1:1 mix is incubated for 37 °C for 1 to 2 hours, and then an aPTT is performed. Interpretation of the incubated mixing study relies on the control shown in the *dashed black box,* in which patient plasma and normal pooled plasma are incubated separately (i.e., mixed after incubation) to control for loss of labile factors. The control aPTT is used for comparison with the incubated mixing study; neither the initial aPTT nor the aPTT of the immediate mix should be used for comparison.

may cause substantial difficulties. Phospholipid-poor assay reagents are more sensitive to lupus anticoagulants, so perhaps weaker lupus anticoagulants are detected before mixing, but they are rapidly diluted out by 1:1 mixing. *If the aPTT is only minimally elevated (e.g., <5 seconds above the reference interval), then 1:1 mixing studies are not useful, because the clotting times may correct despite the presence of an inhibitor.* Some laboratories use an alternative mixing study with four parts patient and one part NPP to improve sensitivity for these weak inhibitors.[23] Mixing studies certainly are not quantitative, and the clinical significance of these "weak" inhibitors is not known. NPP should be prepared from at least 20 apparently healthy individuals to ensure 1.0 IU/mL of all factors. It is also important that NPP be platelet poor because contamination, especially in frozen aliquots, may contribute to phospholipid content that will neutralize lupus anticoagulants. In some instances, 1:1 mixing may not correct when multiple factors are deficient. Heparin or direct thrombin inhibitors may confound interpretation and should be suspected with prolonged or unmeasurable thrombin time.

Interpretation of mixing studies is not always straightforward, and criteria for interpretation may vary somewhat from laboratory to laboratory. Although we have considered correction of the immediate 1:1 mix to be into the reference interval (+2 standard deviations), many variations are used (e.g., +3 standard deviations of the mean aPTT). Rosner and colleagues[116] suggested an index, and Chang and coworkers demonstrated improved performance when using a percent correction and a 4:1 mix.[23] In summary, there is no uniformity in the performance of mixing studies, nor are there uniform criteria for interpretation; ultimately, the laboratory director must decide the appropriate approach and each result should be accompanied with an interpretation.

Factor Assays

The most commonly performed factor assay is the one-stage factor assay. One-stage assays are based on the aPTT or the PT, depending on which factor is being measured. The assay is performed on dilutions of patient plasma into factor-deficient plasma. Factor-deficient plasma is deficient in a single factor but contains essentially 1.0 IU/mL of all other factors. Plasma from severe hemophiliacs has been used historically; factor-deficient plasmas manufactured by immunodepletion methods are now commercially available. Dilution of patient plasma into deficient plasma ensures that clotting times are dependent on the factor being measured. aPTT-based one-stage assays are used to measure factor activity of intrinsic factors, and PT/INR-based assays are used to measure factor activity of factor VII. aPTT- or PT/INR-based assays have been used to measure the activity of common pathway factors (factor II, V, or X). Factor activity is then determined from a calibration curve created by plotting the clotting time (PT or aPTT) in seconds versus the concentration of factor (Figure 59-12).

The aPTT-based one-stage factor VIII assay consists of a dilutional series of patient plasma into factor VIII–deficient plasma, starting with a 1:10 dilution. The initial dilution serves to prolong the aPTT into a steeper part of the relationship between clotting time and factor activity (see Figure 59-12). The aPTTs of the dilutional series are used to extrapolate factor VIII activity from the calibration line. The 1:10 dilution is considered the starting point for comparison with the calibration line, which also starts with a 1:10 dilution. Each subsequent dilution in the series needs to be multiplied by a dilution factor to achieve the equivalent of the 1:10 dilution. This procedure also is used to measure the intrinsic and common pathway factors by substituting the appropriate factor-deficient plasma.

Various mathematical transformations, most commonly log transformation, are employed to create a straight calibration line. Factor activity should be determined with at least three dilutions to enhance accuracy and allow for the detection of inhibitors by assessing parallelism. Because one-stage assays are aPTT or PT in INR dependent, they may be affected

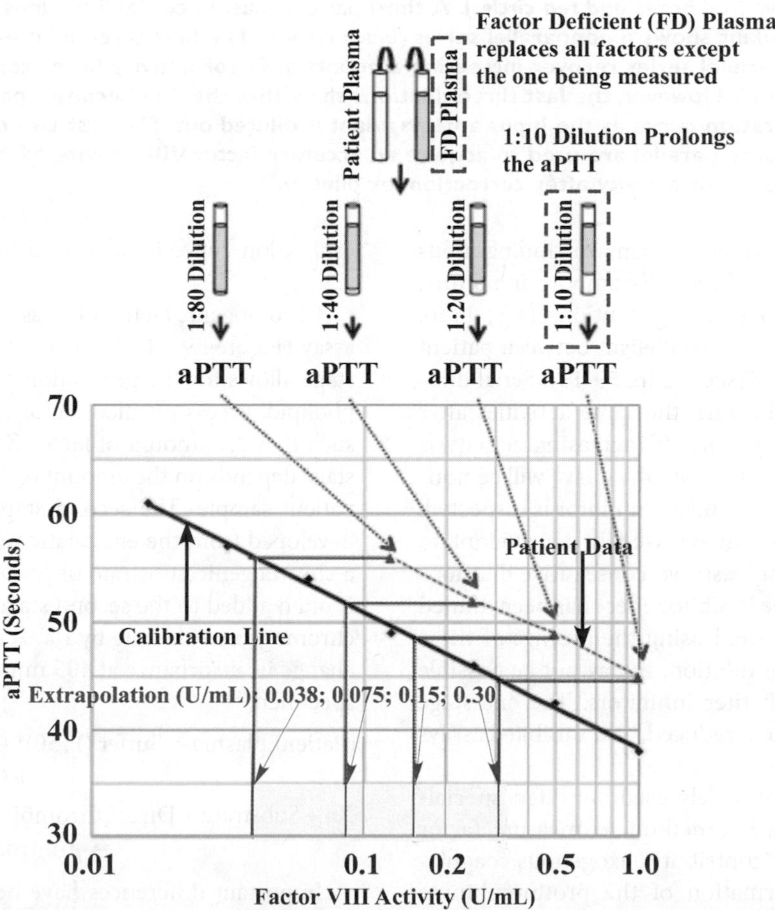

Figure 59-12 aPTT-Based One-Stage Factor VIII Assay. Dilutions of patient plasma into factor VIII–deficient plasma are made by starting with a 1:10 dilution. The aPTT of diluted plasmas is used to extrapolate factor VIII activity from the calibration curve. The 1:10 dilution is considered the starting point for comparison with the calibration line, which also starts with a 1:10 dilution. Each subsequent dilution in the series needs to be multiplied by a dilution factor to achieve the equivalent of the 1:10 dilution.

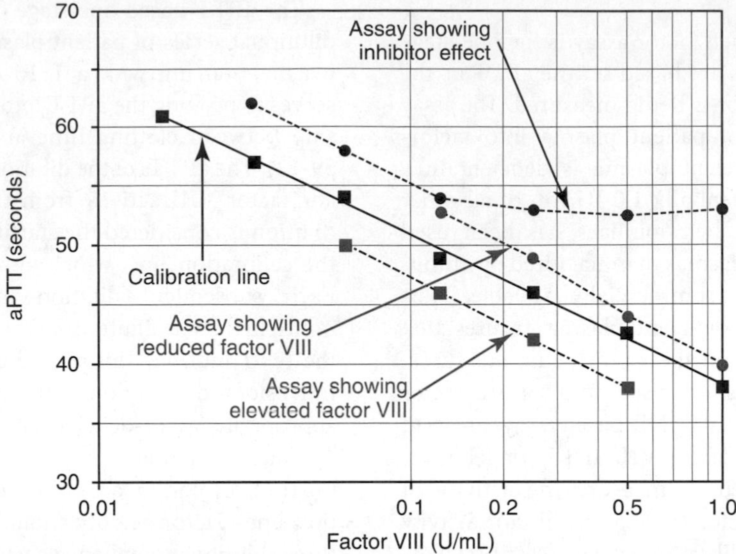

Figure 59-13 Factor VIII Assay Demonstrating the Effect of an Inhibitor. Parallelism should be demonstrated to ensure accurate measurement of factor activity. The dilutional series of three separate patient plasmas are shown. Parallelism between the calibration curve and the patient plasma dilutions is seen in two of the factor VIII assays *(red boxes and red circles)*. A third patient plasma containing lupus anticoagulant shows a nonparallel series *(black circles)*. The first three dilutions of the nonparallel series recover increasing amounts of factor activity (after correction for dilution). However, the last three dilutions show that the line becomes parallel to the calibration curve as the lupus anticoagulant is diluted out. The first two dilutions that become parallel are used to acquire an accurate factor VIII activity, by averaging factor activity after correction for dilution.

by inhibitors present n the patient's plasma including lupus anticoagulant, heparin, or direct thrombin inhibitors. Multiple determinations at increasing dilutions (e.g., 1:10, 1:20, 1:40) allow assessment of parallelism between patient data and the calibration curve (see Figure 59-13). Serial dilutions, when parallel, should return the same activities after multiplying by the dilution factors. If increasing activity is obtained as dilutions increase, the patient's curve will be nonparallel to the calibration curve, and an inhibitor is suspected. Additional higher dilutions can be used in an attempt to dilute the inhibitor. When at least two consecutive dilutions produce similar activities, the inhibitor effect has been diluted out; the activity is then reported using the average of these activities, after correction for dilution. It may not be possible to dilute out strong or high titer inhibitors. The one-stage factor assay depicting elevated, reduced, and inhibited assays is shown in Figure 59-13.

The two-stage assay is not widely used but offers specialized laboratories an alternative method to measure factor VIII activity. The first stage contributes exogenous coagulation factors needed for formation of the prothrombinase complex, except for factor VIII. In this first stage, the formation of Xa depends on the amount of factor VIII in the patient's plasma. In the second stage, normal pooled plasma is added to the reaction (now containing factor Xa) as a source of prothrombin and fibrinogen so that fibrin clotting will occur. The clotting time in the second step is proportional to the amount of factor VIII in the patient sample. A calibration curve is then used to determine the factor VIII activity.[5]

Chromogenic factor VIII assays are based on the two-stage assay (Figure 59-14). Similar to the two-stage assay, the first stage allows for the generation of factor Xa. Calcium, phospholipid, excess purified factor IXa, and factor X are added such that the amount of factor Xa generated during this first stage depends on the amount of factor VIII received from the patient sample. The second stage measures the absorbance developed from the enzymatic release of *p*-nitroaniline from a chromogenic substrate of Xa. A direct thrombin inhibitor is often added to the second stage to decrease cleavage of the chromogenic substrate by IIa. A calibration curve relates the change in absorbance at 405 nm to factor VIII activity in the specimen.[70]

$$[\text{Patient plasma} + \text{Buffer } (1:50)] + [\text{IXa and X (in excess)}] + CaCl_2 + \text{Phospholipid} \rightarrow \text{Xa}$$

$$\text{Xa} + \text{Substrate} + \text{Direct thrombin inhibitor} \rightarrow p\text{-nitroaniline (detected at 405 nm)}$$

Important differences have been observed in factor VIII activity depending on the method used. Two-stage assays and chromogenic assays are less sensitive to lupus anticoagulants[32] because of the higher initial plasma dilutions employed. Some chromogenic assays include thrombin to fully activate factor VIII to VIIIa; others rely on feedback activation of factor VIII by thrombin generation analogous to the in vivo propagation phase of coagulation. One-stage assays sometimes will

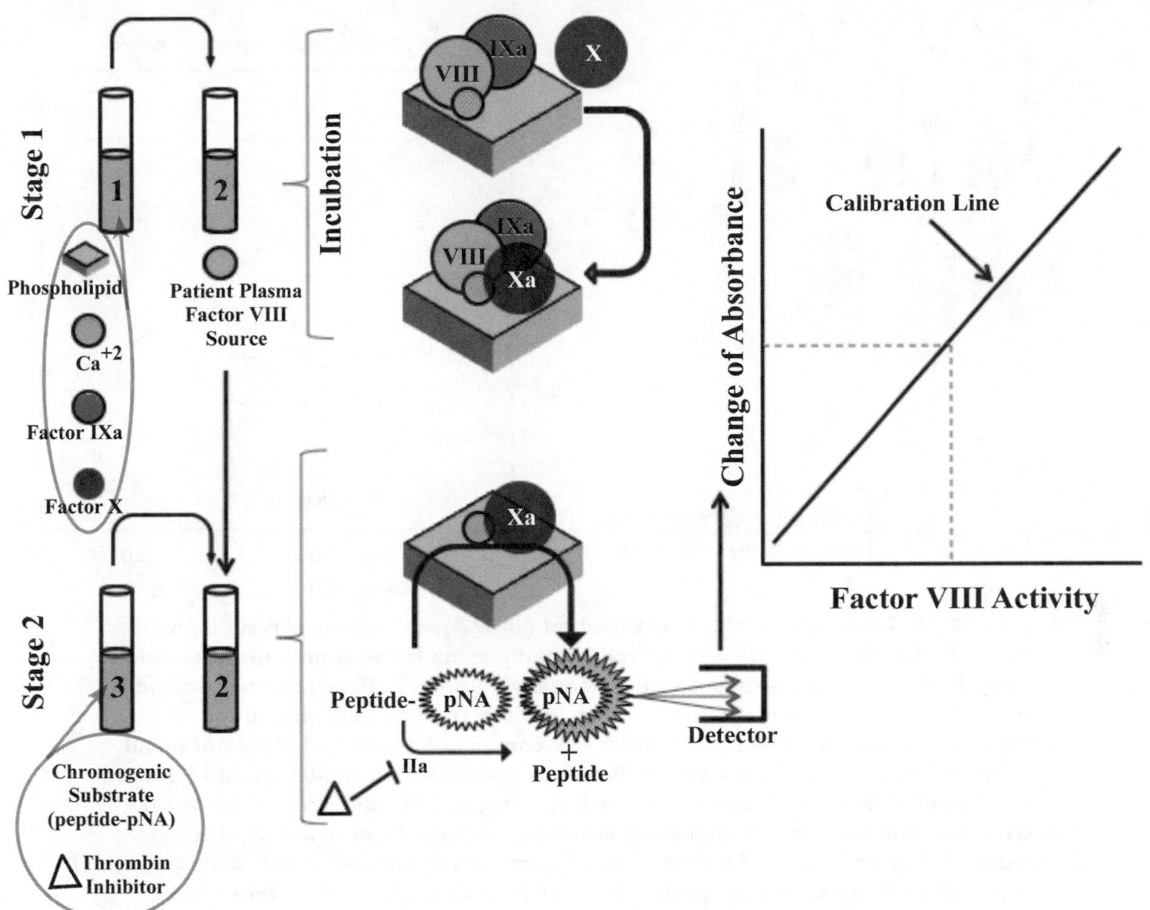

Figure 59-14 Schematic of the Chromogenic Assay for Factor VIII. The chromogenic factor VIII assay is modeled after the classic two-stage factor VIII assay. The patient sample *(tube 2)* is highly diluted with buffer, allowing measurement in the presence of lupus anticoagulant. During the first stage, substrates *(tube 1)* are added to the diluted patient plasma to allow formation of the tenase complex and subsequent conversion of factor X to factor Xa. Conversion of factor X to factor Xa is dependent on factor VIII activity supplied by patient plasma. The second stage starts when chromogenic substrate is added to tube 2. Factor Xa generated during the first stage hydrolyzes the chromogenic peptide substrate and releases para-nitroaniline. A thrombin inhibitor prevents nonspecific hydrolysis of the chromogenic substrate by thrombin. Absorbance resulting from the release of para-nitroaniline is detected at 405 nm and is used to extrapolate factor VIII activity from the calibration curve. *pNA*, Para-nitroaniline.

overestimate factor VIII activity when compared with two-stage or chromogenic assays.[36,100] It is important to keep this in mind because a one-stage assay may not exclude a mild hemophilia A, and clinical correlation with bleeding symptoms and family history may be needed. Less frequently, two-stage assays will recover more factor VIII activity.

Factor Inhibitor Assays

Inhibitors are quantified by using a functional inhibitor assay. The Bethesda assay established the framework for functional inhibitor assays and defined the Bethesda unit.[65] The primary focus of this assay and unit was to create uniformity in the measurement of factor VIII inhibitors in patients with hemophilia A. This is accomplished by creating an incubated mix of patient plasma (containing the inhibitor) with NPP (containing approximately 1.0 IU/mL factor VIII activity) and then measuring the remaining factor VIII activity. Strong inhibitors reduce the resultant factor VIII activity more than weak inhibitors do. Titration of this effect is possible by using serial dilutions of patient plasma before mixing.

The Bethesda assay begins with undiluted patient plasma or dilutions of patient plasma with imidazole buffer. The patient sample is then mixed with NPP. The mixed sample is incubated for 2 hours at 37 °C, and then factor VIII is assayed. A reference mix, consisting of a 1 : 1 incubated mix of imidazole buffer and NPP, is crucial to control for loss of labile factors. The residual factor activity is calculated as follows:

$$\text{Residual Factor Activity (IU/mL)} = \frac{\text{Patient Mix Factor Activity (IU/mL)}}{\text{Reference Mix Factor Activity (IU/mL)}}$$

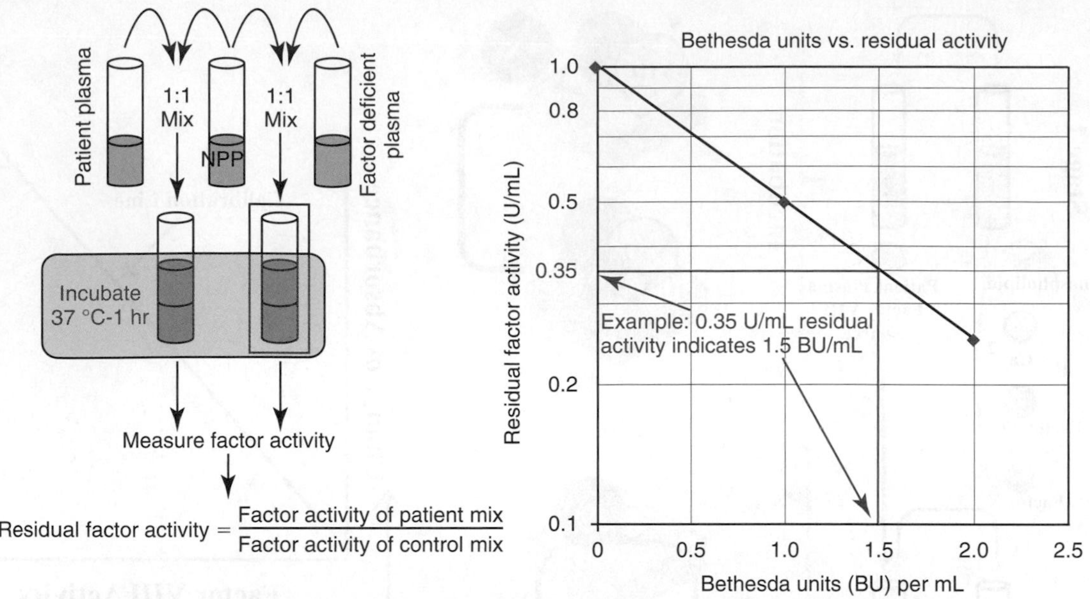

Figure 59-15 Schematic of the Functional Inhibitor Assay. Patient plasma is the source of inhibitor, and buffered normal pooled plasma is the source of coagulation factors. Patient plasma is mixed with an equal volume of buffered normal pooled plasma. The mix is then incubated for 1 to 2 hours at 37 °C, allowing time-dependent inhibitors to work. A control mix consists of an incubated mix of equal volumes of factor (e.g., factor VIII)-deficient plasma (without inhibitor) and buffered normal pooled plasma. One-stage factor assays are used to determine the factor activities of the patient mix and the control mix. Residual factor activity is then calculated. The definition of a Bethesda unit provides a calibration line, and residual factor activity is used to extrapolate the titer in Bethesda units/mL. When high titers of inhibitor are present, initial dilutions of the patient plasma into factor-deficient plasma are required *(not shown).*

Finally the residual factor activity is translated into Bethesda units. One Bethesda unit (BU) per milliliter is defined as the inhibitor activity producing a residual factor activity of 0.5 IU/mL. A value of 2 BU/mL is then the inhibitor activity producing a residual factor activity of 0.25 IU/mL. A log-linear graph of factor activity and BU/mL is drawn according to this definition (Figure 59-15). For ease of use, a chart relating residual factor to BU/mL is constructed. Parallelism of dilutions should be expected to confirm the precision of the result. To assay other factor inhibitors, the factor VIII–deficient plasma used in the assay is replaced with the corresponding factor-deficient plasma.

Nijmejen modifications of the Bethesda assay improve specificity near the low analytical limit of detection.[137] The Nijmejen modifications are that (1) factor-deficient plasma is used for dilutions instead of imidazole buffer and (2) NPP is buffered at pH 7.4. Both of these changes reduce loss of factor VIII during incubation. Buffering the NPP prevents increasing pH, and diluting with factor-deficient plasma normalizes protein concentrations in the reference plasma. Many laboratories in the North American Specialized Coagulation Laboratory (NASCOLA) survey were found to be using a hybrid of the classic Bethesda and Nijmejen procedures in which a commercially available buffered NPP was used but imidazole buffer was used for dilutions of patient plasma. The high coefficient of variation (CV) and the variation in laboratory procedures make standard treatment guidelines based on BU/mL difficult.[102]

The behaviors of inhibitors in laboratory tests are not uniform. Although most inhibitors demonstrate an expected increase in residual factor VIII activity with increasing dilutions (type I inhibitor), some inhibitors (type II inhibitors) lack this relationship. Type II inhibitors lack parallelism to the calibration curve and may be difficult to titer. In these cases, dilutions of patient plasma corresponding to approximately 0.5 IU/mL residual activity are used to estimate BU/mL.[136] In addition, some factor VIII inhibitors increase factor VIII clearance but do not affect factor VIII activity. These non-neutralizing factor VIII inhibitors cannot be detected with a mixing study, nor can they be titered with a functional inhibitor assay. ELISA assays for detecting factor VIII antibodies would be a more appropriate alternative for non-neutralizing types of inhibitors.

Factor XIII Assays

Plasma factor XIII is a zymogen that is activated by thrombin in a calcium-dependent reaction. The active enzyme catalyzes the covalent cross-linking of fibrin molecules and polymers, producing a stable clot (Figure 59-16). Factor XIIIa is a transglutaminase that links glutamine residues to lysine residues via the transfer of an acyl group and the release of ammonia. Factor XIIIa activity is not reflected in clot-based assays such

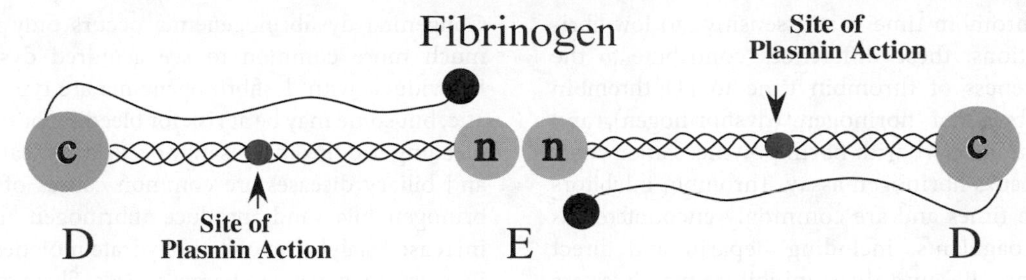

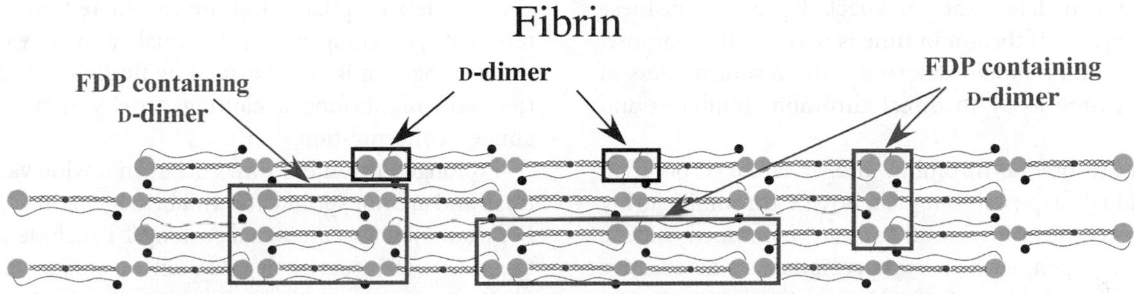

Figure 59-16 Fibrinogen, Fibrin and the Formation of D-dimer. The primary substrate for the enzyme thrombin is fibrinogen (340kDa). When activated by thrombin, an N terminus peptide is cleaved from the Aα and Bβ, fibrinopeptides A and B, forming fibrin monomer. Fibrin monomer polymerizes end to end and side to side forming a fiber, fibrin, in a process that is not enzymatically driven. As depicted, the polymerization of fibrin monomer occurs with the association of the *D* domains of two fibrin monomers (referred to as D-dimer) with the *E* domain of a third. Crosslinking occurs with the action of a transamidase, factor XIIIa, forming the stable fibrin clot. Fibrinolysis occurs upon the activation of plasminogen to plasmin, a serine protease the initially cleaves the fibrin molecule between the *D* and *E* domains. Soluble fragments of fibrin (fibrin degradation products) that contain variable numbers of the *D-D* domains (D-dimer) are produced.

as aPTT and PT/INR, which depend on fibrin polymerization as an end point, because non–covalently linked, polymerized fibrin monomer is sufficiently stable to support the mechanical end point in the tests.

The urea solubility screen, or a variation thereof, is the most common screening method for factor XIII deficiency. Before the actions of factor XIIIa take place, fibrin polymer structure is held together by hydrogen bonds and is soluble when subjected to weak alkalis and acids[114] or to high concentrations of solute such as urea. This is the basis of factor XIII screening methods. In the urea solubility screen, fibrin clot is formed from citrated patient plasma and then is suspended in 6 mol/L urea. The clot is visually observed at intervals for dissolution. Covalently linked fibrin clots do not dissolve. Non–covalently linked fibrin clots are dissolved after 1 to 3 hours in severe factor XIII–deficient plasmas. A fibrin clot prepared from NPP serves as the control. This method detects only very severe factor deficiency; very little factor XIIIa activity is required to stabilize a fibrin clot.

Data from U.K. National External Quality Assessment Scheme (NEQUAS) Surveys demonstrated variability in screening methods.[62] Fibrin clots were achieved with calcium alone, calcium and thrombin, or thrombin alone; moreover, when thrombin was used, the concentration was not uniform. Acetic acid, urea, and monochloroacetic acid were used as solvents. Altogether 15 different combinations of solvents and clot preparations were used, contributing to variable responses. Further evaluation of plasmas spiked with factor XIII confirmed that a combination of thrombin and acetic acid provided the best sensitivity, which was in the interval of 0.01 to 0.05 IU/mL factor XIII. Positive solubility screens for factor XIII need confirmation by quantitative methods that may be factor XIII antigen assays or factor XIII activity assays. For a full description of quantitative assays, see Reference 64.

Thrombin Time

Thrombin time (TT) is a clot-based assay reflecting two steps: (1) conversion of fibrinogen to fibrin monomer by thrombin, and (2) polymerization of fibrin monomers. A low concentration of thrombin (final concentration of 0.1 to 0.3 U/mL; concentration depends on the source of thrombin) is added to citrated plasma, fibrin is generated, and the time it takes to form the clot is measured.

Citrated patient plasma (undiluted)
+ Thrombin (low concentration) → Fibrin clot

Note that TT is different from the Clauss fibrinogen measurement because, in the Clauss fibrinogen method, the patient plasma is diluted and a higher concentration of thrombin is used. Although thrombin time is still sensitive to low fibrinogen concentrations, these differences contribute to the greater responsiveness of thrombin time to (1) thrombin inhibitors, (2) abnormal fibrinogen (dysfibrinogen), and (3) substances that interfere with fibrin polymerization compared with the Clauss fibrinogen assay. Thrombin inhibitors prolong thrombin times and are commonly encountered as therapeutic anticoagulants, including heparin and direct thrombin inhibitors. Because these inhibitors may interfere with other clot-based tests, some laboratories use thrombin time as a tool to detect the unexpected presence of these therapeutic agents. If thrombin time is used for this purpose, then the laboratory should determine the responsiveness of its thrombin time assay to direct thrombin inhibitors and heparin.

Inhibitors to bovine thrombin and/or factor V occur in some individuals exposed to topical bovine thrombin during surgical procedures. Bovine thrombin combined with a source of fibrinogen, such as cryoprecipitate, is an effective hemostatic agent. However, topical bovine thrombin preparations also contain bovine factor V, so inhibitors to both bovine II and V can be produced. Bovine factor V inhibitors may cross-react with human factor V to produce bleeding, but cross-reactivity of bovine thrombin inhibitors with human thrombin is rare. There is, however, prolongation of the thrombin time if bovine thrombin is used for thrombin time assays instead of human thrombin; this will be confirmed by a normal thrombin time using human thrombin.

Thrombin time may be prolonged in the presence of structurally abnormal fibrinogens, called *dysfibrinogens.* Congenital dysfibrinogenemia occurs only rarely, and it is much more common to see acquired dysfibrinogenemia. Individuals with dysfibrinogenemia are typically asymptomatic, but some may be at risk for bleeding or thrombosis. Both bleeding and thrombosis may occur in the same patient. Liver and biliary diseases are common causes of acquired dysfibrinogenemia and produce fibrinogen molecules with increased sialylation of carbohydrate moieties. As a result, an increase in negative charge retards fibrin polymerization[31] and prolongs the thrombin time. Thrombin time and the closely related reptilase time are considered initial screening tests for dysfibrinogenemia. The final laboratory diagnosis of dysfibrinogenemia is confirmed by finding a discrepancy in the ratio of fibrinogen clotting activity to the fibrinogen antigen concentration.[28]

Prolonged thrombin times occur in a wide variety of settings and are not specific for dysfibrinogenemia (Table 59-9). For example, substances that prolong TT include (1) paraproteins, (2) fibrin(ogen) degradation products, and (3) high fibrinogen concentrations. Paraproteins affecting thrombin times may be of any heavy chain and are seen in the clinical setting of Waldenström macroglobulinemia or multiple myeloma. Paraproteins may affect other tests of hemostasis, including aPTT and bleeding time.[104] These patients may even have clinical symptoms of bleeding, but it is not possible to predict bleeding based on any laboratory test. Increased fibrin degradation products and increased fibrinogen, by virtue of their structural similarities to fibrin, may prolong the thrombin time by competing with normal fibrin monomers in the polymerization process. High concentrations of

TABLE 59-9 Thrombin Time in Various Clinical Settings

Clinical Settings	Thrombin Time	Mechanism
Inherited dysfibrinogenemia	Prolonged	Inhibition of fibrinopeptide A and B Inhibition of fibrin monomer polymerization
Acquired dysfibrinogenemia	Prolonged*	Inhibition of fibrin monomer polymerization
AL amyloidosis	Prolonged	Unknown
Monoclonal immunoglobulins	Prolonged	Inhibition of thrombin Inhibition of fibrin monomer polymerization
Fibrin degradation products	Prolonged	Inhibition of fibrin monomer polymerization
Low fibrinogen	Prolonged	Decreased fibrinogen substrate
Elevated fibrinogen	Prolonged	Interference with fibrin-monomer polymerization
Medications/Iatrogenic Settings		
Argatroban	Prolonged	Inhibition of thrombin
Hirudin and related medications	Prolonged	Inhibition of thrombin
Unfractionated heparin	Prolonged	Inhibition of thrombin
Fractionated heparin	Prolonged	Inhibition of thrombin
Bovine thrombin, topical	Prolonged	Development of alloantibodies to thrombin*
Dextran	Shortened	Increased rate of fibrin monomer polymerization
Hydroxyethyl starch	Shortened	Unknown
Thrombolytics (urokinase, tissue plasminogen activator)	Prolonged	Inhibition of fibrin monomer polymerization due to fibrin degradation products
Radiocontrast agents	Prolonged	Inhibition of fibrin monomer generation and polymerization

*Thrombin time is most commonly affected when bovine thrombin is used as a reagent.

Modified after Cunningham MT, Brandt JT, Laposata M, Olson JD. Laboratory diagnosis of dysfibrinogenemia. Arch Pathol Lab Med 2002;126:499-505.

fibrin degradation products are seen in disseminated intravascular coagulation and after fibrinolytic therapy. High concentrations of fibrinogen are commonly encountered as part of an acute-phase reaction in hospitalized patients. Thus fibrinogen assays are useful in the evaluation of prolonged thrombin time.

Clinical Use of Laboratory Tests for Disorders of Secondary Hemostasis

Laboratory tests described earlier are used in the diagnosis and evaluation of inherited and acquired disorders of secondary hemostasis.

Inherited Disorders

The most common inheritable bleeding disorders due to coagulation factor deficiencies include (1) hemophilia A (factor VIII deficiency), (2) hemophilia B (factor IX deficiency), and (3) factor XI deficiency (historically referred to as hemophilia C). The pathophysiologic consequence of these deficiencies is a defect in the propagation phase of coagulation. As discussed earlier, the clot-based tests, aPTT and PT artificially separate coagulation into intrinsic, extrinsic, and common pathways (see Figure 59-2) that only loosely resemble physiologic coagulation, wherein the pathways do not operate independently. In the laboratory, deficiencies of the intrinsic pathway produce isolated prolongation of aPTT. Mixing studies are indicated to help guide further laboratory evaluation toward factor deficiency or the presence of inhibition. Together, correction of the immediate aPTT mixing study and lack of prolongation after incubation suggest factor deficiency. Measurement of intrinsic factor activities is then indicated, usually starting with factor VIII, factor IX, and factor XI, because of their clinical association with bleeding. Measurement of factor XII, prekallikrein, and HMWK is helpful in explaining prolonged aPTT in the absence of deficiency of factor VIII, factor IX, or factor XI, particularly if there is no clinical bleeding history.

Inherited deficiencies of factors VII, X, V, and II and fibrinogen are rare but present with bleeding phenotypes. Factor VII deficiency causes isolated prolongation in PT/INR without prolongation of the aPTT. A mixing study of the PT/INR indicates a deficiency, and factor VII activity is low, usually in the 0 to 20% range in significant deficiency. Inherited deficiencies of X, V, and II and fibrinogen prolong PT and aPTT. aPTT mixing studies show a factor deficiency, and factor activity is markedly decreased. Inherited afibrinogenemia or hypofibrinogenemia causes prolongation of PT/INR and aPTT, which correct with mixing studies. A functional fibrinogen assay shows markedly decreased fibrinogen. In all cases of inherited deficiency, clinical correlation with a bleeding and family history is needed to make a diagnosis.

Factor XIII deficiency is a rare disorder of secondary hemostasis with a bleeding phenotype and normal PT/INR, aPTT, TT, and fibrinogen. A urea solubility test demonstrates dissolution of fibrin clot in 1 to 2 hours. Low factor XIII can be confirmed with antigen or activity assays. Platelet function and studies of fibrinolysis are normal.

Factor VIII Deficiency (Hemophilia A)

Factor VIII deficiency is an X-linked recessive genetic disorder with an incidence of 1 in 5000 live male births. Because one third of mutations occur spontaneously, a family history is not always present. Severity of bleeding correlates with the amount of factor VIII with activities of (1) less than 0.01 IU/mL, (2) 0.01 to 0.05 IU/mL, and (3) 0.05 to 0.40 IU/mL associated with severe, moderate, and mild hemophilia A, respectively.[142]

Laboratory studies of individuals with factor VIII deficiency show isolated prolongation of aPTT and normal PT. A normal thrombin time is helpful to exclude heparin contamination as a cause for prolonged aPTT. Mixing studies should help identify a factor deficiency. Factor activities of the intrinsic pathway should be measured to confirm suspicion of an intrinsic pathway deficiency. In a male patient, factor VIII, IX, and XI activity should be measured. Female carriers may have mildly reduced factor VIII activity and mild bleeding symptoms, but investigation of factor XI deficiency and VWD is probably best considered first in females. Decreased factor VIII activity with normal activity of factors IX and XI is expected in hemophilia A. Patients with *von Willebrand disease also present with an isolated prolonged aPTT and low factor VIII activity, so evaluation of von Willebrand disease is warranted in some cases before a diagnosis is rendered.* Correlation with the family and clinical history completes the diagnosis of factor VIII deficiency. The distinction of hemophilia A from type 2N VWD is difficult. Type 2N VWD is caused by decreased affinity of VWF for Factor VIII. The patients thus have decreased factor VIII because it is not protected by binding to VWF. The distinction of type 2N VWD and hemophilia A can be accomplished with a careful family history and a VWF:VIII binding assay, which is performed only at very specialized laboratories. A family history of hemophilia may be absent in up to 30% of infant males with hemophilia A due to spontaneous mutations. Genetic testing to identify a specific factor VIII mutation may be useful in prenatal testing of carrier females.

Factor VIII activity is used to follow factor VIII replacement therapy—the mainstay of prophylaxis and of management of an acute bleed. When postinfusion recovery of factor VIII activity is lower than anticipated or the patient fails to respond clinically, a factor VIII inhibitor is suspected. The aPTT is prolonged, but in this case, mixing studies suggest an inhibitor. Most factor VIII inhibitors are time dependent; thus, an immediate aPTT mixing study may correct the prolonged aPTT. However, an incubated aPTT mixing study reveals prolongation compared with the appropriate control. Factor VIII inhibitor is quantified in BU/mL with a Bethesda assay or a variation thereof. The titer is used to guide therapeutic decisions. An inhibitor titer of less than 5 BU/mL may respond to high doses of factor replacement, although higher titers are not likely to respond and require alternative treatment. Anamnestic responses may occur, in which low or undetectable inhibitor titers rise 4 to 7 days after re-exposure to factor VIII. Inhibitors have been reported in 10 to 25% of patients and are associated with certain molecular defects in the *F8* (for factor VIII) gene. Inhibitors may occur in mild disease. Alternative treatments for patients with inhibitors have included replacement with porcine factor VIII (previously available as a plasma-derived concentrate and currently in trials as a recombinant product) or products with factor VIII-bypassing activity such as recombinant activated factor VIIa concentrate or activated prothrombin complex concentrates.[67] These latter two products activate factor X without factor VIII or IX.

Factor IX Deficiency (Hemophilia B)

Factor IX deficiency, also known as hemophilia B or Christmas disease, is a heritable X-linked recessive bleeding disorder. The incidence is approximately 1 in 30,000 males. Clinically, the bleeding manifestations relate closely to the amount of factor IX. This is similar to hemophilia A, but a lower proportion of these patients inherit severe deficiency.

The laboratory approach to diagnosis is similar to that for hemophilia A. When an isolated prolonged aPTT is present, investigation with mixing studies helps identify a factor deficiency. Measured factor IX activity is low with normal factor VIII and XI activity.

The mainstay of treatment for bleeding episodes with these patients is infusion of factor IX concentrates. The amount infused depends on (1) the severity of bleeding, (2) the site of the bleeding, and (3) the size of the patient. In susceptible individuals, infusion may induce the development of alloantibodies to factor IX. The incidence of inhibitor formation in hemophilia B is approximately 1 to 3%—much lower than that in hemophilia A. The development of inhibitors can be preceded or accompanied by an allergic or anaphylactic reaction. Bleeding episodes with a factor IX inhibitor titer less than 5 BU/mL in low responders and those that do not produce a significant anamnestic reaction are treated with factor IX concentrates. Higher inhibitor titers (≥5 BU/mL) and high responders require infusion of products that bypass factor IX (e.g., recombinant factor VIIa).

Factor XI Deficiency (Hemophilia C)

Factor XI deficiency is a rare autosomal recessive disorder with a high incidence in the Ashkenazi Jewish population. Terms for this disorder include (1) plasma thromboplastin antecedent (PTA) deficiency, (2) Rosenthal syndrome, and (3) hemophilia C. More recently, autosomal dominant forms have been described. The bleeding symptoms are heterogeneous, and, in contrast to factor VIII or IX deficiency, bleeding severity does not correlate well with plasma factor concentration. Bleeding at mucosal sites or after surgical challenges is common, so deficiency is not discovered until adulthood in some cases.

aPTT is prolonged and factor XI activity is low. Two mutations are responsible for most (88%) of the classic autosomal recessive disease in the Ashkenazi Jewish population; combinations of these mutations produce factor XI activities in the 0.01 to 0.1 IU/mL interval.[53] Mixing studies of aPTT suggest a deficiency. Inhibitors may occur after treatment with plasma and may be titered with functional inhibitor assays. Inhibitors occur frequently in patients with low factor XI concentrations when exposed to plasma as replacement therapy.[123] Plasma concentrates and recombinant products are not available.

Factor XIII Deficiency

Inherited deficiency of factor XIII is rare with an estimated prevalence of 1 to 2 per million.[3] The classic presentation of (1) umbilical stump bleeding, (2) excessive bleeding after trauma, and (3) abnormal scar formation was described in 1960.[35] Severe factor XIII deficiency is associated with recurrent spontaneous abortion.[58] Bleeding risk is expected when factor XIII activity falls below 0.03 IU/mL. Severe factor XIII deficiency is treated with fresh frozen plasma (FFP) or cryoprecipitate.

A limited number of clinical settings may warrant detection of factor XIII above 0.05 to 0.1 IU/mL. Monitoring with quantitative assays may be helpful in demonstrating recovery and in timing doses. Monitoring may also be helpful during pregnancy in women with factor XIII deficiency because a factor XIII concentration of 0.1 IU/mL has been suggested to support pregnancy.[3,58] Rarely, acquired deficiencies or inhibitors of factor XIII have been encountered that may be associated with amounts of factor XIII greater than that of classic factor XIII deficiency. Some less sensitive solubility-based screening methods may not detect these mild to moderate factor XIII deficiencies, so quantitative methods may be desirable when these clinical scenarios are evaluated. Overall experience with quantitative assays is still somewhat limited.

Acquired Disorders

Many conditions cause acquired disorders of secondary hemostasis that manifest as hemorrhage (see Table 59-7). Lupus anticoagulants are associated with thrombosis and will be discussed later. Specific factor inhibitors, except for factor XII inhibitor, cause a bleeding phenotype. Specific factor inhibitors prolong PT, aPTT, or both, depending on the targeted factor. The work-up includes demonstration of an inhibitor with mixing studies, demonstration of decreased factor, measurement of the inhibitor titer, and clinical correlation with a bleeding phenotype.

Unfractionated heparin, low molecular weight heparin, and direct thrombin inhibitors are examples of pharmacologic inhibitors that prolong PT and aPTT. Unfractionated heparin below 1.0 IU/mL does not affect many commercially available PT reagents because a heparin neutralizing substance is added. Mixing studies typically demonstrate an inhibitor. A complication of anticoagulant therapy is hemorrhage. Monitoring is required for some anticoagulants to ensure that coagulation is within a therapeutic interval. See the later section on monitoring anticoagulation therapy for a detailed discussion.

Acquired factor deficiencies usually involve deficiency of multiple coagulation factors. A notable exception is the rare association of AL amyloidosis with factor X deficiency. Vitamin K deficiency and VKA therapy (discussed earlier) decrease activities of factors II, VII, IX, and X. Disseminated intravascular coagulation (DIC; discussed in greater detail later under "Fibrinolysis") is a pathologic disorder that consumes fibrinogen and multiple coagulation factors. Because many coagulation factors are synthesized in the hepatocytes, liver disease is associated with multiple factor deficiencies.[132] Dilutional coagulopathy in patients receiving aggressive fluid replacement or massive transfusions of cellular components without sufficient plasma replacement is another example of acquired deficiency of multiple coagulation factors. These acquired deficiencies of multiple coagulation factors can cause isolated prolongation of PT/INR or prolongation of both PT/INR and aPTT. aPTT mixing studies can be difficult to interpret in multiple factor deficiency because a 1 : 1 mix may not correct the aPTT to the reference interval. In these cases, clinical correlation and additional laboratory tests, including TT and measurements of D-dimer, fibrinogen, and specific factors, are often helpful.

Liver Disease

Traditionally, severe chronic liver disease was thought to be associated with impairment of secondary hemostasis resulting in a bleeding phenotype. Because procoagulants are synthesized in the liver, cirrhosis is associated with prolongation of clotting tests. A notable exception is factor VIII, an acute-phase reactant that is increased in liver disease. PT/INR and aPTT are indeed prolonged in cirrhosis, and PT/INR in particular has been used to assess bleeding risk and to guide therapy with FFP before procedures are undertaken. Unfortunately, PT/INR does not reliably predict bleeding risk in severe liver disease.

It has been suggested that bleeding risk in cirrhosis may be partially attributed to hyperfibrinolysis due to deficiencies of naturally occurring fibrinolysis inhibitors that are produced in the liver such as (1) thrombin-activatable fibrinolysis inhibitor (TAFI), (2) α_2-antiplasmin, and (3) plasminogen activator inhibitor-1 (PAI-1). Similarly, thrombotic complications in cirrhosis have been attributed to deficiencies of natural anticoagulants (e.g., protein C, protein S) or plasminogen, all of which are produced by the liver. Clotting assays do not reflect the contributions of these liver-derived molecules to in vivo hemostasis. Likewise, measurement of individual components of fibrinolysis or secondary hemostasis may not be informative in isolation. More recent models of hemostasis in severe liver disease suggest that it is the summative balance of secondary hemostasis and fibrinolysis that determines risk.[135]

Moderate to severe thrombocytopenia associated with cirrhosis also may contribute to bleeding risk. Following platelet count is an important part of assessing bleeding risk in cirrhotic patients.

INR is used in the model for end-stage liver disease (MELD) score, an index of severity of liver disease used to prioritize liver transplantation. The current INR system was designed to monitor patients on VKA therapy. As a consequence, the ISI does not harmonize INRs among laboratories for the purpose of monitoring liver disease. Interlaboratory variation in PT/INR systems contributes to variation in MELD scores. Harmonizing results with liver-specific ISIs is effective,[7,133] but currently, laboratories are poorly equipped to handle two INR systems, and commercial thromboplastins do not have an assigned ISI for liver disease.

Vitamin K Deficiency

Vitamin K deficiency may manifest with bleeding or may be identified incidentally with an isolated prolonged PT/INR or prolonged PT/INR and aPTT in a nonbleeding patient. TT and fibrinogen are normal. Measuring vitamin K–dependent factors can help confirm the diagnosis. It is helpful to measure several vitamin K–dependent factors along with at least one non–vitamin K–dependent factor for comparison. Mixing studies can potentially be useful, but multiple-factor deficiency may not correct after mixing. The utility of PT/INR mixing studies or factor assays is also limited because vitamin K deficiency is very common and may be investigated clinically by treating with vitamin K. If vitamin K therapy fails to restore the PT/INR, then mixing studies and factor assays are performed to evaluate for possible inherited deficiency or acquired inhibitor.

Without vitamin K prophylaxis, neonates are at risk for vitamin K deficiency. Neonatal risk of vitamin K deficiency is due to a combination of inadequate vitamin K intake and lack of intestinal flora—an important source of vitamin K. Bleeding from neonatal vitamin K deficiency is easily avoided by treating neonates with vitamin K, but this problem is still encountered in developing countries. Adult vitamin K deficiency may be due to drugs that affect vitamin K metabolism, inadequate intake, liver or biliary disease, or inadequate intestinal adsorption. Postsurgical patients receiving parenteral nutrition are at risk of acquired deficiency because the vitamin K stored in the liver can be depleted in a short time. Antibiotic therapy that alters the intestinal flora may lead to deficiency of vitamin K.

FIBRINOLYSIS

Fibrinolysis is a regulated mechanism for the enzymatic degradation of existing cross-linked fibrin clots (see Figure 59-4). Plasmin, a key enzyme of fibrinolysis, cleaves the insoluble, cross-linked fibrin clot into soluble fibrin degradation products (See Figure 59-16 and further description below under the heading *D-Dimer Assays*) of varying molecular weights and compositions. Fibrinolysis serves to balance the activity of coagulation. Perturbations in coagulation or fibrinolysis disrupt the balance and create risk for thrombosis or hemorrhage.

Fibrinolysis is limited to the site of injury/thrombosis by the local production of tPA by endothelial cells and by circulating inhibitors in the plasma. Fibrinolysis is downregulated by (1) PAI-1, (2) α_2-antiplasmin, and (3) thrombin activatable fibrinolysis inhibition (TAFI). PAI-1 irreversibly binds and inhibits tPA. α_2-Antiplasmin is found free in the circulating plasma or covalently bound to fibrin, through the action of factor XIIIa. α_2-Antiplasmin binds to and then cleaves plasmin, resulting in an inactivated plasmin/α_2-antiplasmin complex. Circulating plasmin is more rapidly neutralized than fibrin-bound plasmin, further contributing to the localization of fibrinolysis.

TAFI provides a regulatory link between coagulation and fibrinolysis. In the presence of thrombomodulin, thrombin converts TAFI to TAFIa. TAFIa cleaves C-terminal lysines on fibrin at potential binding sites of plasminogen. Consequently, plasminogen is less available for plasmin generation, thus delaying fibrinolysis.[113]

Evaluation of Fibrinolytic Activity

Various tests are used to evaluate fibrinolytic activity, including (1) thrombin time, (2) fibrin(ogen) degradation product (FDP) assays, (3) D-dimer assays, (4) PAI-1 assays, (5) α_2-antiplasmin assays, and (6) plasminogen assays.

Thrombin Time

Thrombin time was discussed in detail earlier in relation to secondary hemostasis testing. However, thrombin time also is used in evaluation of fibrinolytic activity. Thrombin time may be prolonged by increased fibrin degradation products in settings of increased fibrinolysis such as disseminated intravascular coagulation and thrombolytic therapy.

FDP Assays

Under normal physiologic conditions, plasmin cleaves cross-linked fibrin into soluble fibrin degradation products of various molecular weights and compositions. If plasmin activity exceeds the capacity of antiplasmin activity in the circulation, fibrinogen may be cleaved into fibrinogen degradation products. Fibrinogen is cleaved into high molecular weight fragments, known as X and Y fragments. Further enzymatic degradation yields lower molecular weight D and E fragments.[85] Collectively, fibrin and fibrinogen products are referred to as FDP. FDP titers are determined by immunoassays, usually manual semiquantitative latex-agglutination immunoassays using monoclonal antibodies raised against FDP. Serum is tested in assays that employ antibodies that are reactive against fibrinogen; plasma or serum may be used in assays employing antibodies without fibrinogen reactivity.

When increased plasmin activity (e.g., from increased urokinase after prostate surgery) is the prevailing pathology, the process is referred to as *primary fibrin(ogen)olysis* and may be associated with bleeding. The clinical utility of FDP assays is limited because of their poor low end sensitivity compared to many current quantitative D-dimer assays.

D-Dimer Assays

D-Dimer moieties are formed specifically by the cross-linkage of D-domain subunits of fibrin strands by factor XIIIa (see Figure 59-16). D-Dimers are detected in plasma after plasmin has enzymatically cleaved cross-linked fibrin clot. Therefore, detection of D-dimer in plasma signifies cleavage of cross-linked fibrin, but not cleavage of fibrinogen, fibrin monomers, or non–cross-linked fibrin strands. D-Dimer assays are useful for the evaluation of disseminated intravascular coagulation and, if the assay has sufficient negative predictive value and diagnostic sensitivity, for the evaluation of patients in whom deep vein thrombosis or thromboembolism is suspected.

Immunoassays used to measure concentrations of D-dimer include (1) ELISA, (2) immunoturbidometric assay, (3) latex immunoassay techniques, and (4) luminescence immunoassay. Fragments of fibrin degradation containing D-dimer moieties are not uniform, and various dimer, trimer, and tetramer species of fragments occur. Also, monoclonal antibodies vary in their ability to recognize the wide variety of D-dimer species, and calibrators vary in their content of these D-dimer species. This variability has led to considerable difficulty in standardizing D-dimer assays. Therefore, rather than standardization, international efforts have focused on harmonization of D-dimer testing. Further difficulty has arisen from inconsistency in reported D-dimer units. It is imperative that both the unit type and the unit of concentration are reported correctly. D-Dimer units may be D-dimer units (D-DU) or fibrinogen equivalent units (FEU). D-DU (185 kDa) is approximately one half the weight of FEU (340 kDa). The appropriate unit type (D-DU vs. FEU) and unit of concentration (e.g., ng/mL; µg/L; etc.) are determined by the calibrator used in the assay and should be available in the package insert. Using the wrong units may result in poor interlaboratory accuracy (failed proficiency testing) and, more important, improper laboratory thresholds for excluding deep vein thrombosis (DVT) and pulmonary embolism (PE).

Quantitative D-dimer is widely used to exclude DVT and PE. Clinicians use the D-dimer concentration combined with the degree of clinical suspicion of DVT or PE (low, moderate, or high pretest probability) to decide whether diagnostic imaging is indicated. The value of the D-dimer assay for this purpose derives from its high sensitivity and negative predictive value. A D-dimer concentration below the established threshold, in a patient with low or moderate pretest probability, strongly suggests that DVT or PE is not present, and imaging studies are not pursued. Patients with high pretest probability require diagnostic imaging, and D-dimer should not be measured. Only quantitative D-dimer assays meeting criteria for negative predictive value and sensitivity, established in large clinical studies for evaluation of DVT and PE, should be used to exclude thromboembolism. The minimum performance criteria at the threshold D-dimer value for excluding thromboembolism are as follows: (1) 0.98 negative predictive value with the one-sided lower confidence interval at 0.95, and (2) 0.98 sensitivity with the one-sided lower confidence interval at 0.90. In most instances, laboratories cannot establish their own threshold values and must rely on clinical studies performed by manufacturers of commercial D-dimer kits. Semiquantitative tests by latex agglutination generally lack sensitivity and are inappropriate for evaluation of thromboembolism.

Plasminogen Activator Inhibitor Type 1 Assays

PAI-1 deficiency has been reported as a congenital defect but may be acquired as well. Congenital PAI-1 deficiency is associated with bleeding risk, but experience is limited and the prevalence is unknown. High concentrations of PAI-1 have been associated with risk of arterial thrombosis. PAI-1 assays are not widely performed in clinical laboratories but may be useful after common causes of bleeding have been conclusively ruled out. As with other enzymes of coagulation and fibrinolysis, qualitative and quantitative defects of PAI-1 have been reported, and a functional assay for screening purposes is desirable.

A specific chromogenic substrate for plasmin simplifies functional assays for PAI-1, plasminogen, and α_2-antiplasmin. A general scheme for PAI-1 functional assays is to add a known amount of plasminogen activator (tPA or urokinase) to citrated patient plasma, followed by excess plasminogen. Plasmin activity is measured by its cleavage of a chromogenic substrate. Residual plasmin activity is inversely proportional to the PAI-1 of the subject plasma. Inhibitors of α_2-antiplasmin and other plasmin inhibitors are added to prevent interference.[27]

PAI-1 activity assays were developed to detect increased PAI-1, and the available assays do not perform acceptably at low concentrations. Zero activity has been included in the reference interval with this strategy. Agren and associates[1] modified a PAI-1 activity assay by adding calibration points to the low end of the calibration curve. The same group has suggested that the reference cutoff for PAI-1 activity for this method is around 1U/mL.

PAI-1 deficiency is an important consideration in patients with convincing bleeding histories because antifibrinolytic therapies may be beneficial. PAI-1 deficiency is a difficult diagnosis to make and requires exclusion of more common hemorrhagic diatheses before it is entertained. Data on PAI-1 are difficult to interpret because of their diurnal variation and their elevation as an acute-phase reactant. PAI-1 activity may be combined with PAI-1 antigen assays to assist interpretation of results. Strict clinical correlation and sometimes studies of family members are needed to make a diagnosis.

α_2-Antiplasmin

Congenital α_2-antiplasmin deficiency is a rare disorder associated with bleeding. Bleeding symptoms may be delayed, reminiscent of other deficiencies affecting clot stability, such as factor XIII deficiency or PAI-1 deficiency. Acquired deficiencies also occur with liver disease. Similar to other rare disorders of fibrinolysis, careful clinical and laboratory exclusion of more common bleeding disorders is required before a diagnosis of α_2-antiplasmin deficiency is pursued. Quantitative and qualitative types of α_2-antiplasmin deficiency have been reported.[20]

For functional α_2-antiplasmin assays, excess plasmin is added to citrated patient plasma. α_2-Antiplasmin from the patient sample will form inactive plasmin-antiplasmin complexes. Residual plasmin activity is measured by the addition of a chromogenic substrate. Residual plasmin is inversely proportional to antiplasmin in the patient plasma. A calibration curve relates the absorbance change due to plasmin activity to α_2-antiplasmin activity of the test plasma. Antigen assays may be considered in individuals with decreased functional activity to substantiate findings or to define qualitative deficiency.

Plasminogen Assay

Plasminogen deficiency is a rare congenital disorder. Originally, plasminogen deficiency was reported to be associated with thrombosis, but other reports challenge its importance as an independent risk factor. More important, severe congenital plasminogen deficiency can result in the unusual clinical finding of fibrin pseudomembranes at various mucosal surfaces. The most common site of pseudomembrane deposition is the eye, referred to as *ligneous conjunctivitis.* Quantitative and qualitative deficiencies have been identified, but pseudomembrane deposition is thought to be associated with quantitative deficiencies. Acquired plasminogen deficiency (e.g., in liver disease) may occur, but the clinical importance is not clear.[91]

Excess tissue plasminogen activator is added to citrated patient plasma. Plasmin activity is then measured chromogenically, and the plasminogen is extrapolated from a calibration curve. Antigenic assays are also available.

Clinical Use of Laboratory Tests for Disorders of Fibrinolysis—Disseminated Intravascular Coagulation

Overt disseminated intravascular coagulation (DIC) is an excessive uncontrolled thrombin generation and fibrinolysis, exceeding the regulatory capacity of the endothelium and plasma inhibitors. Fibrin thrombi are formed in the microvasculature, trapping platelets and shearing red blood cells (RBCs) into schistocytes as they pass through the fibrin strands. Ultimately DIC consumes (1) coagulation factors, (2) inhibitors, (3) platelets, and (4) RBCs. Clinically, patients with DIC present with bleeding and thrombosis, although thrombosis may not be as readily apparent because these clots primarily occur in the microvasculature. Ecchymosis, petechiae, and oozing from intravenous access sites or surgical incisions are frequent hemorrhagic presentations. In addition, occlusion of small vessels leads to end-organ damage. DIC is not a disease, but rather a manifestation of a wide variety of possible underlying disorders (Table 59-10). The clinical diagnosis begins with recognizing the thrombohemorrhagic picture, which should then trigger a search for the underlying disease process. Compensated DIC, or nonovert DIC, may precede overt DIC or may occur in isolation. In nonovert DIC, the regulatory mechanisms are not completely overwhelmed, and consumption of RBCs, platelets, and hemostatic factors is not complete. Nonovert DIC can also occur in chronic clinical conditions such as cancer, often with predominantly prothrombotic manifestations. Treatment is supportive and relies on clinical management of the underlying cause.

Stereotypical laboratory data for overt DIC include (1) prolonged clotting times (aPTT, PT, and TT), (2) low fibrinogen, (3) elevated FDP, (4) elevated D-dimer, (5) thrombocytopenia, and (6) anemia, often with schistocytes on a peripheral smear. Clotting times may be prolonged because

TABLE 59-10 International Society of Thrombosis and Hemostasis Criteria for Diagnosis of Overt Disseminated Intravascular Coagulation (DIC)

Clinical Conditions Associated With DIC	Diagnostic Algorithm for the Diagnosis of Overt DIC
Sepsis/severe infection Trauma/burns/surgery Organ destruction Malignancy Obstetric calamities Vascular abnormalities Severe hepatic failure Severe toxic or immunologic reactions	1. Risk assessment: Does the patient have an underlying disorder known to be associated with overt DIC (from column to left)? If yes: Proceed to 2. If no: Do not use this algorithm. 2. Order global coagulation tests (PLT count, PT, fibrinogen, soluble fibrin monomers or fibrin degradation products). 3. Score global coagulation test results. PLT count (>100 = 0; <100 = 1; <50 = 2) Elevated fibrin-related marker (e.g., FDP, D-dimer) (no increase = 0; moderate increase = 2; strong increase = 3) Prolonged PT (<3 s = 0; >3 s but <6 s = 1; >6 s = 2) Fibrinogen level (>1 g/L = 0; <1 g/L = 1) 4. Calculate score. 5. If ≥5: Compatible with overt DIC; repeat score daily. If <5: Suggestive (not affirmative) for nonovert DIC; repeat score next 1 to 2 days.

Modified after Taylor FB Jr, Toh CH, Hoots WK, Wada H, Levi M. Towards definition, clinical and laboratory criteria, and a scoring system for disseminated intravascular coagulation. Thromb Haemost 2001;86:1327-30.

of hypofibrinogenemia, interference from FDPs, or consumption of coagulation factors. Prolongation of clotting assays, however, is not always present in DIC because circulating activated factors partially degrade fibrinogen and shorten clotting times. Fibrinogen concentrations may be low from consumption but are not low in every case. Likewise, platelet count varies significantly in DIC patients, and schistocytes are not always present. Nonetheless, clotting assays, fibrinogen assays, platelet counts, and reviews of peripheral smears are important tests for evaluating DIC.

The International Society on Thrombosis and Haemostasis (ISTH) has published a scoring system for the diagnosis of overt DIC (see Table 59-10).[130] This scoring system subsequently was prospectively validated. The ISTH has also provided an approach to nonovert DIC. The diagnosis of nonovert DIC is more difficult, relying on the daily trend of laboratory test results, not on a single set of laboratory data.

THROMBOSIS

Thrombosis is defined as "the formation or presence of a blood clot in a blood vessel." The vessel may be any vein or artery as, for example, in deep vein thrombosis or coronary (artery) thrombosis. The clot itself is termed a *thrombus.* If the clot breaks loose and travels through the bloodstream, it is a thromboembolism (http://www.medterms.com).

REGULATION

Fibrin generation is controlled by several mechanisms involving a number of different inhibitors and pathways, including (1) control over the initiation phase, whereby tissue factor/factor VII (TF/FVII) drives the generation of factor Xa; (2) inhibition of several activated clotting factors principally by antithrombin; and (3) control of cofactor functions of factors V and VIII through the protein C pathway.

Initiation of coagulation is controlled by tissue factor pathway inhibitor (TFPI), which inhibits factor Xa and also the TF-FVIIa-phospholipid complex in a two-step process. First, TFPI binds to factor Xa, whose action is then inhibited. The TFPI-Xa complex then binds to TF/VIIa through a different part of the TFPI molecule. Both factor Xa and factor VIIa are inactive in this quaternary complex. TFPI therefore shuts down the initiation stage, and only if sufficient activation of factor X overcomes this inhibition does the process of coagulation proceed. About 80% of TFPI is associated with the endothethial cell membranes and is not normally available in plasma for measurement in laboratory assays. The remainder circulates in plasma, but about ¾ of plasma TFPI is bound to low-density lipoproteins, and perhaps half of the free TFPI is inactive. Protein S facilitates the effect of TFPI by enhancing the formation of the TFPI-FXa complex.[51] This anticoagulant effect of protein S is a more recent discovery than the identification of protein S as an anticoagulant component of the protein C pathway (see later). Determination of TFPI in plasma does not currently have a role beyond continuing research, and available assays are probably too crude in view of the complex relationships involved, although genetic knockout of the gene *TFPI* (which codes for TFPI) in mice is lethal, so this is undoubtedly a physiologically important protein.

As was discussed earlier, when coagulation is initiated, various enzyme reactions (nearly all serine proteases) lead to

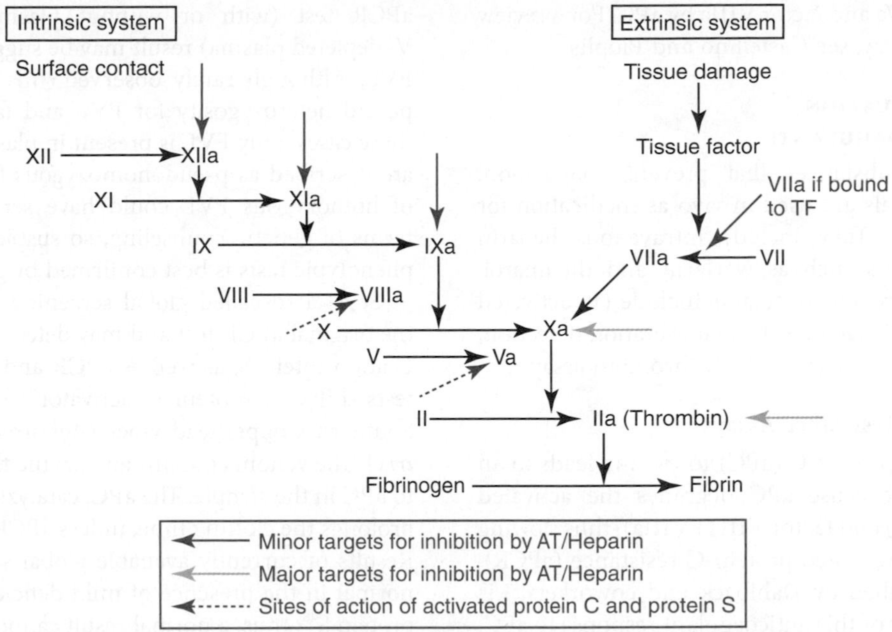

Figure 59-17 Points at Which Natural Inhibitors Affect the Coagulation Cascade. AT inhibits the activity of serine proteases. The primary effect is inhibition of factor Xa and thrombin (IIa); however, other factors are also inhibited, including plasmin *(not shown)*. Factor XIII is not a serine protease; it is a transglutaminase and is not inhibited by AT. Protein C and protein S inhibit coagulation through cleavage of the activated forms of factors V and VIII.

a cascading activation of coagulation factors to generate thrombin. These are subject to control by the serine protease inhibitors collectively termed *serpins,* the most important of which is AT. Activated clotting factors inhibited by AT are shown in Figure 59-17. Serpins, including AT, first bind to their target and form a final covalent complex, whereby the protease is irreversibly trapped in an inactive state. AT predominantly inhibits thrombin, factor Xa, and factor IXa, but it also inhibits other coagulation proteases. The anticoagulant action of AT is dependent on its cofactor, heparin. In vivo, several types of heparin-like glycosaminoglycans function as cofactors for AT; these include heparan sulfate on the endothelial cell surface. It is the interaction with AT and this heparan sulfate that localizes the activity of AT to the vessel wall. When the vessel wall is lost or damaged, this reaction does not occur, allowing thrombin to accelerate coagulation unchecked. Thrombin that is bound to fibrin in the clot is protected from inhibition by AT, which is synthesized in the liver and circulates with a half-life of approximately 3 days. A second serpin, whose action is enhanced by the presence of heparan or dermatan sulfate, is named heparin cofactor II (HC II). In contrast to AT, HC II inhibits thrombin whether clot bound or not. It has no action against other coagulation serine proteases. About a quarter of thrombin inhibition occurs via HC II. AT deficiency is highly associated with thrombophilia, but HC II deficiency is not. The primary function of HC II may relate to the role of thrombin outside of hemostasis. For a review of AT and HC II, see Rau and colleagues.[110]

The critical complexes that lead to generation of factor Xa and of thrombin have several features in common. Both are formed by calcium-mediated assembly of clotting factor complexes on the surface of phospholipid. Both complexes require a cofactor for reaction rates to be sufficiently enhanced for enzyme generation to overcome the control mechanisms ranged against them. Factor VIII after its conversion to factor VIIIa is the cofactor that facilitates activation of factor X; factor V after conversion to factor Va performs a similar function, leading to the formation of thrombin. Both factor Va and factor VIIIa are regulated by the protein C pathway (see Figure 59-1).

Protein C is a vitamin K–dependent protein produced in the liver. Activation of PC to activated protein C (aPC) is driven by thrombin in complex with thrombomodulin, a protein located in the endothelial cell surface. This process is mediated through PC binding to an endothelial cell PC receptor (EPCR) that presents PC to the thrombin-thrombomodulin complex. When thrombin is complexed with thrombomodulin, it loses its normal procoagulant functions and takes on an anticoagulant role via activation of PC, because aPC then inactivates factor Va and factor VIIIa through proteolytic degradation in the presence of calcium, phospholipid, and its cofactor protein S. Similar to protein C, protein S is a vitamin K–dependent factor. It is produced in the liver, endothelial cells, and megakaryocytes. Approximately 60 to 70% of plasma protein S is bound to C4b binding protein (C4bBP) and has no significant role in hemostasis. The remainder is termed free protein S and functions as a cofactor for the degradation of factor Va and factor VIIIa by aPC. For a review of the protein C pathway, see Castellino and Ploplis.[22]

Tests for the Evaluation of Natural Anticoagulants

Anticoagulants are substances that prevent coagulation. Various pharmaceuticals are used in vivo as medication for thrombotic disorders. They include intravenous heparin and oral anticoagulants such as warfarin and dicumarol. Assays used to measure anticoagulants include (1) activated protein C resistance, (2) factor V Leiden mutation detection, (3) protein C, (4) protein S, and (5) antithrombin assays.

Activated Protein C Resistance Assays

Addition of activated protein C (aPC) to plasma leads to an anticoagulant effect, because aPC degrades the activated forms of factor V (FVa) and factor VIII (FVIIIa), thus slowing the clotting process. Activated protein C resistance (aPCR), which was first described by Dahlback and coworkers,[29] is defined as impairment of this anticoagulant response to aPC. These authors reported that aPCR was associated with a predisposition to thrombosis. Activated protein C cleaves factor Va, and a vast majority of patients with familial aPCR have a point mutation at the cleavage site.[9] This abnormal factor V protein, in which the arginine at position 506 is replaced with a glutamine (Arg506Gln or R506Q), has been named factor V Leiden (FVL).[9]

The first assay established for determination of aPCR measured aPTT with and without purified human aPC in the calcium chloride reagent. The aPTT with aPC is divided by the baseline aPTT and the quotient is called the aPCR ratio. A low ratio indicates the presence of aPCR. A number of tests are now available to detect the abnormal phenotype or the presence of the genetic defect.

Because phenotypic aPCR tests may be influenced by in vitro platelet activation and platelet contamination, plasma should be double-centrifuged at 2000 ×g for 15 minutes to reduce the residual platelet count to a minimum. Other factors that affect the test include reduced concentrations of clotting factor II or factor X (decreased ratio) and increased quantities of factor VIII (increased ratio). The presence of lupus anticoagulant (LAC) has been known to increase aPCR. The original aPCR test[115] should not be used during VKA anticoagulant therapy and is unreliable if the patient has a prolonged PT/INR or aPTT for other reasons. Increased aPCR has been observed to occur in the absence of FVL and has been reported to increase the risk of thrombosis.[33] The original test detects both FVL- and non–FVL-related causes of aPCR, but many centers use a modified version that is more sensitive and more specific for the presence of FVL. This involves the dilution of patient plasma in factor V–depleted plasma. A normal result in this modified aPCR test result excludes the presence of FVL and is not affected by clotting factor concentrations.

Good separations of aPCR results are often noted in (1) normal subjects, (2) patients with heterozygous deficiency of FVL, and (3) homozygous individuals. Thus, a very low aPCR test (with or without plasma dilution in factor V–depleted plasma) result may be suggestive of homozygous FVL. Although rarely observed, this may be due to compound heterozygosity for FVL and factor V deficiency. In these cases, only FVL is present in plasma, and such patients are described as pseudohomozygous for FVL. Misdiagnosis of homozygous FVL could have serious consequences in terms of genetic counseling, so suspicion of FVL based on phenotypic tests is best confirmed by genetic analysis.

Several so-called global screening tests are variations of the original aPCR test and may detect deficiencies of protein C and protein S, as well as aPCR and FVL. Several of these tests utilize a protein C activator from the venom of the Southern Copperhead viper *(Agkistrodon contortrix contortrix)*. The venom contains an enzyme that converts protein C to aPC in the sample. The aPC, catalyzed by protein S, greatly prolongs the clotting time, unless aPCR and FVL are present. Results of currently available global screening tests may be normal in the presence of mild deficiency of protein C and protein S[48]; thus, a normal result cannot be used to exclude a deficiency of these factors.

Factor V Leiden Mutation Detection

FVL is the most common cause of inherited thrombophilia in many countries in Western Europe and in North America, and some variability among different populations has been noted. Heterozygous FVL has a prevalence of around 3% in Caucasians but is more prevalent still in the area of Sweden where the defect was first identified. It is practically absent from some Eastern populations and the black populations of Africa.

FVL was originally detected using amplification of *F5* gene DNA by use of the polymerase chain reaction, where DNA fragments were amplified before digestion with a restriction enzyme.[9] Such assays using restriction enzyme digestion of DNA are labor-intensive compared with other methods and may include hazardous components. Alternative methods include the allele-refractory mutation system (ARMS) and real-time polymerase chain reaction with melting analysis of the products. Details of molecular methods are found in Section IV of this book, "Molecular Diagnostics and Genetics."

External quality assurance is available for FVL and prothrombin G20210A analysis with an error rate of 3 to 6% among approximately 50 centers performing such tests.[108] Errors identified include sample mismatching, equipment malfunction, and transcription errors. Similar results have been reported in other programs. Genetic tests are generally considered to be definitive, and mistakes are serious errors. It is prudent to confirm FVL homozygous genotypes on a separate sample.

Protein C Assays

Heritable protein C deficiency has a prevalence of about 1 in 700 in the general population and of 2 to 4% in selected subjects with a personal history of venous thrombosis. Protein C deficiency is associated with a fivefold to 10-fold increased risk of venous thromboembolism, although some kindreds appear to have no such increased risk. Combined defects with coinheritance of protein C deficiency and FVL markedly increase thrombotic risk, beyond that caused by inheritance of either defect alone.[72]

Protein C concentration is very low in the newborn. Protein C concentrations may only reach adult values at 16 years of age, with further increases occurring up until about 30 years of age.[129] Protein C concentrations may be reduced in patients with (1) liver disease and (2) vitamin K deficiency, and (3) by vitamin K antagonists such as warfarin. In vitamin K deficiency, the protein C assay result depends on the measurement system. When a low concentration of protein C is detected, physiologic, clinical, and pharmacologic causes should be excluded. PT/INR should be performed as an indication of normal liver function. Not all cases with genetic defects of protein C have reduced activity by protein C assay. Some carriers have protein C concentrations within the normal reference interval.

On initiation of warfarin therapy, protein C concentrations fall with a half-life of around 4 to 6 hours, similar to factor VII, but much shorter than other vitamin K–dependent clotting factors such as IX, X, and II. It should be noted that it is not possible to diagnose protein C deficiency in subjects who are in the induction phase of warfarin therapy and testing is not recommended in patients on stable VKA therapy.

Clotting, chromogenic, and antigenic assays are available for measuring protein C concentrations. Clotting-based protein C assays require the addition of test sample to protein C–depleted plasma, then Southern Copperhead viper activator converts protein C to aPC, which prolongs clotting time through destruction of factors Va and VIIIa. The clotting end point is based on aPTT, PT/INR, or the addition of snake vemons. Assays based on aPTT may be influenced by the phospholipid composition of the reagent and by the concentration of factor VIII.

Protein C assays based on aPTT may underestimate protein C in samples with high concentrations of factor VIII. The presence of FVL, particularly homozygous FVL, may falsely reduce concentrations of protein C reported by clotting-based assays because FVL is resistant to destruction by aPC, and clotting time does not fully reflect aPC activity. Predilution of patient plasma in protein C–depleted plasma may reduce or remove the influence of FVL.[61] Protein C can be overestimated through the anticoagulant influence of LAC. The advantage of clotting-based assays is that they may detect rare heritable functional defects that remain undetected by other techniques.

Chromogenic assays of protein C generally utilize Southern Copperhead viper activator conversion of protein C to aPC. However, currently available chromogenic substrates for protein C measurement lack complete specificity and are cleaved by a variety of proteases. Partially clotted samples and serum may give falsely high chromogenic protein C activity results because of background protease activity. Some Southern Copperhead viper activator-based chromogenic assays are unable to detect all patients with type II protein C deficiency, where there is disparity between antigen and functional activity.

Protein C antigen is now typically determined by ELISA-based assays, which are relatively precise and very sensitive to low concentrations of protein C. These have been used to differentiate type I and II deficiency. About ¾ of patients recorded as having protein C deficiency have type I deficiency (low antigen and function), with most of the rest having type II deficiency which is characterized by normal concentrations of protein but low protein C as measured by both clotting and chromogenic assays.

Protein S

Protein S is a glycoprotein whose amino acid sequence is coded by the *PROS1* gene. Deficiency of protein S is associated with a fivefold increased risk of venous thrombosis, and the combination of the FV Leiden mutation and the protein S deficiency is associated with a high risk for thrombosis.[73] The incidence of familial protein S deficiency is around 1 in 700 to 1 in 3000 of the general population in the United Kingdom.[37]

Heritable protein S deficiency is classified as type I, II, or III. Type I is defined by reduced concentrations of total protein S antigen (total PS) and free protein S antigen (free PS) and reduced protein S activity. Type II deficiency is characterized by isolated deficiency of protein S activity. Type III deficiency displays normal concentrations of total PS, but a reduced concentration of free PS and reduced activity of PS. Type III protein S deficiency, however, may not be a separate disorder because it has occurred with some of the same gene mutations that cause type I deficiency in other family members. Protein S concentrations are lower in women than in men and may be further decreased by certain oral contraceptives; its quantities are particularly low in the newborn. Gender-specific reference intervals are therefore useful. Low total protein S with normal concentrations of free protein S occur in patients with low concentrations of C4bBP. Pregnancy, acute phase reactions, oral contraceptives, and hormone replacement therapy may reduce concentrations of total protein S, but not free protein S. Again similar to protein C, protein S concentrations are reduced in (1) liver disease, (2) vitamin K deficiency, and (3) VKA therapy. Testing of patients while they are anticoagulated is problematic. Measurement of total protein S antigen probably is not helpful in most cases, and an assay that measures the concentration of free protein S is preferred. In normal subjects, the free protein S antigen concentration reflects the functional protein S activity in plasma. Free protein S has been measured by ELISA but is increasingly measured using latex-based assays in automated analyzers. Many of these methods have removed the need to first separate free PS from that bound to C4bBP, usually by precipitation of bound PS using polyethylene glycol. Measurement of free PS has been shown to be better at detecting protein S deficiency in subjects with *PROS1* gene defects than measurement of total protein S.[83]

Functional assays of protein S are based on the ability of protein S to act as cofactor in aPC-mediated destruction of activated V and/or VIII. This anticoagulant activity may be detected through PT, aPTT, or venom-based clotting time. Functional assays of protein S may be sensitive to type II defects, which are missed by antigenic assay. However, problems arise when many functional assays are used. Some patients were incorrectly diagnosed as having type II protein S deficiency when aPC resistance resulted in underestimation of protein S by functional assay.[41] Results obtained in proficiency testing surveys indicate that even in normal subjects, activity results determined using different assays are not interchangeable. As with protein C, protein S can be overestimated through the additive anticoagulant influence of LAC. Consequently, many laboratories currently avoid use of functional assays because of these problems.

Antithrombin Assays

Antithrombin deficiency may be inherited as the result of a molecular defect, but it may also be acquired (1) through decreased production (e.g., liver disease), (2) through increased turnover (e.g., consumption, heparin therapy), or (3) by renal loss in nephrotic syndrome. The in vivo half-life of plasma antithrombin is around 65 hours, although it may be shorter for antithrombin infused as replacement therapy.

Two main categories of antithrombin deficiency are known: type I, which is characterized by parallel reduction in activity and antigen concentration, and type II, in which activity and antigen concentration are discordant. Three types of qualitative functional defects have been identified, including (1) those in the heparin-binding site (HBS), (2) those in the reactive site, and (3) pleiotropic/multiple effects. Heritable antithrombin deficiency has a prevalence of around 1 in 3000 of the population and is associated with a 10- to 50-fold increased risk of venous thrombosis. Not all defects are equally thrombotic, and individuals with heterozygous HBS defects may have no increased risk.

Because antigen concentrations are normal in many type 2 defects, a functional antithrombin assay is essential. Most experts prefer an assay sensitive to all type II defects. The reference interval for antithrombin concentration is narrow, and accurate assays are required to distinguish normal from abnormal. Suitable chromogenic assays are available based on the ability of the sample to inhibit generation of color by the action of either thrombin or factor Xa (in the reagent) on a chromogenic substrate specific for the protease (thrombin or Xa).

Antithrombin variants may react poorly with one enzyme (thrombin or Xa) and normally with another; this pattern may vary in the presence and absence of heparin. Heparin cofactor II, whose activity is enhanced by heparin, is an additional protein that neutralizes human thrombin. The presence of heparin cofactor II in plasma may reduce the specificity of antithrombin assays, particularly those utilizing human thrombin, where there is an assay incubation time with thrombin of longer than 30 seconds.[131] This problem is partially solved by using bovine thrombin or factor Xa. Thrombin-based antithrombin assays should not be used in patients receiving direct thrombin inhibitors when concentrations can be substantially overestimated.

Results obtained with different assays vary, so that in some defects normal results occur in one assay type, whereas activity is low in another. Many variant AT defects have been described when these problems occur, so results should be interpreted only with knowledge about the assay characteristics.

Chromogenic substrate assays are preferred for measurement of antithrombin concentration. These generally involve the incubation of enzyme (thrombin or factor Xa) with diluted plasma in the presence of heparin before a chromogenic substrate is added; para-nitroaniline (pNA) release from the substrate is monitored at 405 nm. Antithrombin inhibits the enzyme, and the decrease in absorbance at 405 nm with sample compared with no sample is proportional to the antithrombin concentration. Precision varies among different assays. For example, bovine-thrombin–based assays typically show a CV of approximately 1.5%, whereas factor Xa–based assays tend to have a CV of about 2.5%. The determination of the reference interval (to include the 2.5 to 97.5 percentile) for antithrombin should use non-parametric methods because the distribution of results is not Gaussian. Factors such as (1) age, (2) sex, (3) oral contraceptive use, and (4) circadian rhythm influence antithrombin concentrations to varying degrees. However, for practical purposes, it is acceptable to use a single (adult) reference interval that includes similar numbers of men and women. Antithrombin concentrations are low in neonates. Antithrombin is consumed during clotting, and artificially low concentrations are found in clotted samples, whereas genuinely low concentrations may occur as a consequence of recent massive thrombosis. Because liver disease and heparin therapy will reduce AT concentrations, a PT/INR should be performed on specimens with low antithrombin concentration to assess whether the sample is clotted or the patient has liver disease.

When a congenital deficiency is suspected, antithrombin antigen is measured to differentiate type I from type II antithrombin deficiency. Antithrombin antigen is measured by immunoassays such as ELISA, immunoelectrophoresis (IEP), radial immunodiffusion (RID), and immunoturbidometry (ITB). Genetic analysis is useful to identify the defect at a molecular level because different defects are associated with different thrombotic risk.

Evaluating Excess Procoagulants

Many substances are precursors of the various blood factors that promote coagulation of blood. They are known as procoagulants and include substances such as (1) prothrombin 20210, (2) factor VIII and von Willebrand factor, (3) fibrinogen, and (4) factor XIII.

Prothrombin *G20210A* Detection

The prothrombin *G20210A* mutation is a genetic defect that leads to an increase in the concentration of factor II in plasma and confers an increased risk of venous thrombosis.

This defect *(PT G20210A)* occurs in around 2 to 3% of Caucasians and leads to a twofold to threefold increased risk of venous thromboembolism (VTE).[107] Increased prothrombin concentration alone will not reliably identify carriers of the genetic defect. Details of molecular methods are found in Section IV of this book, "Molecular Diagnostics and Genetics."

Factor VIII and von Willebrand Factor

It has been reported that elevated activity of factor VIII is an independent risk factor for venous thrombosis.[75] For example, elevated activities of factor VIII are found in approximately 20% of subjects with VTE. The elevation is independent of the acute-phase response (which causes transient but marked increases in factor VIII). The risk increases as factor VIII rises above 150 IU/dL, with an eightfold increase in risk above 270 IU/dL. Elevated activities of factor VIII, however, do occur in a number of other situations, and activities above 150 IU/dL are found in 10 to 30% of apparently healthy subjects. For this reason, many laboratories do not routinely include factor VIII determination in the standard panel of tests used to investigate patients for heritable thrombophilia; it is not recommended in some countries, such as the United Kingdom.[4]

It has been reported that risk of VTE is increased as the activity of von Willebrand factor is increased.[96] One function of VWF is to transport factor VIII in plasma, forming a relationship between the two molecules. Higher quantities of VWF lead to greater quantities of factor VIII, and when multivariate analysis is performed, factor VIII is shown to be an independent risk factor, whereas VWF is not; increased risk of thrombosis is a consequence of the increased quantities of factor VIII.[75]

Fibrinogen

Numerous studies have shown that the concentration of fibrinogen is associated with risk of coronary heart disease and stroke, and a meta-analysis of 31 such studies has confirmed this.[30] It remains unclear, however, whether higher fibrinogen causes coronary heart disease, and no consensus has been reached on whether measurement of the concentration of fibrinogen is clinically useful for assessing risk in individual patients. Currently it seems likely that the independent effect of fibrinogen is small. At present most experts would suggest that it is not cost-effective to consider population-wide screening of fibrinogen concentrations.

Factor XIII

As discussed earlier, factor XIII is a tetrameric transglutaminase consisting of two A subunits, which form the active site, and two B subunits, which protect the A subunits from degradation. Once activated by thrombin to factor XIIIa, the A subunits dissociate from the B subunits in the presence of calcium, revealing the active site. Factor XIIIa then covalently cross-links fibrin to produce a clot with high mechanical strength and increased resistance to fibrinolysis. There is a molecular defect of factor XIII in which a G-to-T transition leads to a leucine in place of a valine at amino acid 34.[128,140] This factor XIII *Val34Leu* variant behaves differently than wild-type factor XIII and is activated two to three times more quickly. The resulting clot has a different structure from that which occurs in the presence of wild-type factor XIIIa. A meta-analysis of 12 studies (which included more than 3000 objectively diagnosed VTE cases) has confirmed that the presence of this factor XIII Leu allele confers a small but significant protective effect against VTE (about a 15% reduction in risk among heterozygotes).[140] More studies related to arterial thrombosis are available, and a meta-analysis of more than 200 publications has confirmed that the risk of acute myocardial infarction is reduced by about 20% in patients heterozygous for this defect.[128]

Monitoring Anticoagulant Therapy

Several guidelines are available from the American College of Chest Physicians on the monitoring of anticoagulant therapy. They address anticoagulants such as (1) argatroban, (2) bivalirudin, (3) fondaparinux, (4) hirudin, (5) low molecular weight heparin, (6) unfractionated heparin,[55,56] and (7) vitamin K antagonists.[2] Details of several of these substances are discussed in the following sections.

Unfractionated Heparin

Heparin is a highly sulfated polysaccharide used as an anticoagulant for the treatment and prevention of thromboembolic disease. For many years, clinical preparations were unfractionated, containing mixtures of polysaccharide chains of different lengths. Such unfractionated materials typically have average molecular weights of 12,000 to 15,000 Da.

The anticoagulant effect of unfractionated heparin (UFH) is exerted after binding to a cofactor, AT, referred to in the older literature as antithrombin III. After binding to heparin, the AT undergoes a conformational change, facilitating very rapid inactivation of thrombin and several other activated clotting factors, which, like thrombin, have serine in their active site (so-called serine proteases). These include factor Xa, factor IXa, factor XIa, and factor XIIa. The number of saccharide units in the polysaccharide chain of heparin influences these reactions. At least 5 saccharide units are required for some anticoagulant activity. Polymers measuring less than 5 saccharide units in length have no anticoagulant activity. For inhibition of thrombin, heparin chains must bind to both AT and thrombin and thus need to be 18 or more units in length. Simultaneous binding is not required for neutralization of factor Xa, and chains between 5 and 17 units long catalyze neutralization of Xa without affecting thrombin directly. So-called low molecular weight heparins (LMWHs), containing a more uniform population of these shorter polysaccharides, are manufactured from UFH by controlled depolymerization. LMWH is discussed later. Laboratory monitoring of treatment doses of UFH therapy is compulsory because the dose needed for protection from thrombosis varies between subjects, and overdose is associated with hemorrhagic risk.

aPTT for Monitoring UFH

The most widely used test for monitoring UFH is the aPTT (discussed above). In an early study, it was demonstrated that the risk of VTE was reduced when the aPTT ratio (patient/control value) was greater than 1.5, and a therapeutic reference interval of 1.5 to 2.5 was suggested.[6] However, several subsequent studies have shown marked differences among aPTT reagents and methods in terms of heparin responsiveness.[18] Thus, a specific reference interval of 1.5 to 2.5 is not appropriate for all reagents. For each aPTT method, it is necessary to establish a therapeutic reference interval by measurement of aPTT and heparin concentration by protamine titration or anti-Xa assay. For example, for the early studies,[6] an aPTT reference interval of 1.5 to 2.5 was found to be equivalent to 0.2 to 0.4 International Units (IU) of heparin/mL by protamine titration assay or 0.3 to 0.7 IU/mL by anti-Xa assay.[55] (Note that IU of heparin are completely distinct from the saccharide units that make up the molecules of heparin. The IU are based on anticlotting activity, whereas the saccharide units are structures.) Titration or heparin assay, regression analysis is used to calculate the reference intervals of aPTT ratios equivalent to the above heparin concentrations.[18] This should not be done using plasmas spiked with heparin in vitro because the reference interval established may be different from that determined using ex vivo samples. (*Note:* Such a reference interval should be established using between 30 and 60 such samples, although some have suggested that several hundred specimens may be needed.)

If the aPTT ratio is used, it should be calculated using the midpoint of the normal reference interval as the denominator. It should be noted that there is a poor correlation between aPTT and heparin concentration, possibly reflecting the poor specificity of aPTT for heparin effect. The aPTT is influenced by the concentrations of other clotting factors, including those affected (1) by warfarin (see later) or (2) by factor XII, or (3) especially by the quantity of factor VIII, which will change dramatically as a patient with acute thrombosis recovers, that is, as the acute-phase response changes. Because of variability in the process, the therapeutic reference interval should be checked for all new lot numbers of aPTT reagent. In practice, laboratories often sequester large amounts of a single reagent lot to avoid the labor-intensive process of calibrating the aPTT assay for new lots. Preanalytical variables dramatically affect the results of aPTT in samples containing UFH. For example, when citrate is used as anticoagulant, platelets in the blood sample are activated, leading to release of a granule constituent, platelet factor 4, which neutralizes heparin. The aPTT therefore decreases over time by perhaps 30% within 4 to 5 hours, depending on the reagent. Therefore, citrate samples should be analyzed within 2 to 3 hours to minimize this problem. The problem with citrated samples is particularly marked if a blood sample has a large air space within the tube, with much more rapid and marked loss of heparin.[112] The problem is avoided if blood samples are collected into an anticoagulant cocktail comprising citrate, theophylline, adenosine, and dipyridamole (CTAD) that is commercially available and that inhibits platelets, thereby avoiding this problem. Such samples are stable with respect to aPTT for much longer than 4 hours.

If UFH is given by intravenous infusion or by subcutaneous injection, the sample should be collected 4 to 6 hours after initiation of therapy or after any dose adjustment, to allow steady state to be reached.

On various occasions, the aPTT is inappropriate for monitoring UFH because of lack of specificity. Thus, the aPTT may be within the therapeutic reference interval despite suboptimal heparin concentrations because of (1) the presence of lupus anticoagulant (LA); (2) combined UFH and VKA; (3) combined UFH and thrombolytic therapy; and (4) congenital or acquired factor deficiency. The effect of UFH is rapidly reversed by infusion of protamine sulfate.

Heparin Assays for Monitoring UFH

Historically, a heparin assay based on protamine titration was used in North America to establish the therapeutic reference interval for UFH therapy (see aPTT section earlier). However, this assay was (1) poorly standardized, (2) not commercially available, (3) not well suited to automation, and (4) practically obsolete in terms of current usage. Currently, the most popular assays used to measure heparin activity are based on the ability of heparin to neutralize factor Xa that has been added to the test sample. They are known as anti-Xa assays and measure the ability of heparin-accelerated AT to inhibit Xa with residual Xa activity measured through its ability to clot plasma or more often by the amidolytic cleavage of a small chromogenic substrate. In the latter assay, a peptide substrate is cleaved to release para-nitroaniline with the change in absorbance being inversely proportional to heparin concentration. Some anti-Xa assays include the addition of exogenous AT to the test sample, ensuring an excess of AT. Other heparin assays do not add exogenous AT, the rationale being that the assay should reflect the ability of heparin to exert an anticoagulant effect, regardless of the quantity of AT present in the patient's plasma. Therefore, these assays may be more likely to correlate with clinical efficacy. This is especially important in that infusion of UFH could lead to a reduction in the quantity of the patient's AT through increased clearance and a shorter half-life. Similar available assays employ thrombin (FIIa) in place of factor Xa; they are therefore anti-IIa assays. Both anti-Xa and anti-IIa assays for UFH need to be calibrated with a heparin that has itself been calibrated against a World Health Organization (WHO) international standard.

Thrombin Time for Monitoring UFH

Thrombin-clotting time (TCT) is prolonged by UFH, the magnitude of which depends on the reagents, the method, and the concentration of heparin. Although it has been proposed as suitable for monitoring therapy, the test is rarely selected for this purpose. One problem is that for many methods, the TCT becomes difficult to measure at doses of heparin within or just above the upper limit of the therapeutic reference interval. This problem is removed by the use of higher concentrations of thrombin, or by the inclusion of calcium in the thrombin time reagent, which may improve the correlation between TCT and concentration of UFH. However, some versions of TCT methods are useful even at low concentrations of heparin. Such methods are useful in the detection/exclusion of heparin as a cause of prolonged aPTT, where clinical information is lacking, or where contamination of heparin in a sample is suspected.

Activated Clotting Time for Monitoring UFH

UFH is used in high doses during cardiopulmonary bypass at concentrations of 3 to 10 U/mL or more; this causes aPTT and TCT to be unmeasurable by all available conventional methods. The test of choice for monitoring in this setting is activated clotting time (ACT). A variety of instruments and methods are available for this purpose, and currently no consensus has been reached on whether one particular method should be recommended. It is important to keep in mind that results obtained using different methods are not interchangeable,[141] despite the fact that there are similarities in the terminology used for reporting results. With most techniques, the ACT employs an activator such as celite or kaolin to accelerate clotting during the operative and perioperative periods. The activator affects the ACT; however, celite-activated ACT is prolonged relative to an ACT determined using kaolin. In addition, ACT may be prolonged by the hypothermia and hemodilution that may accompany cardiopulmonary bypass procedures. Thus, a poor correlation has been noted between heparin concentration as measured in specific assays and results obtained by ACT. Aprotinin prolongs celite-activated ACT in a dose-dependent way independently of heparin, and if aprotinin is used, ACT should be maintained at a higher result to ensure adequate heparinization, perhaps with twofold higher ACT results. When all factors are taken into account, management protocols often need to be device and anticoagulant specific.

ACT results are affected by the quantities of several clotting factors. For example, if the patient has severe deficiency of factor XII, HMWK, or prekallikrein, then the contact phase is compromised and the baseline value is grossly prolonged to similar values as those achieved by the high-dose heparin used for anticoagulation during cardiopulmonary bypass and other procedures. In these cases, the test cannot be used safely, so tests specific for the action of heparin such as anti-Xa assay must be considered. Therefore, a preheparinization baseline ACT is needed to exclude the presence of such an abnormality.

Low Molecular Weight Heparin

Evidence-based practice guidelines for anticoagulant therapy were published in 2008.[55] As mentioned previously, LMWHs are derived from UFH by depolymerization of the polysaccharide chains. The ratio of activity against factor Xa to activity against thrombin is high but varies among different preparations. LMWHs are favored over UFH as the treatment of choice in a number of clinical situations for several reasons, including (1) a better benefit-to-risk ratio, (2) more predictable dose response with reduced requirement for monitoring, and (3) a lower incidence of heparin-induced thrombocytopenia. Most LMWHs have an average molecular weight below 5000 Da, and their bioavailability is approximately 90% after subcutaneous injection, with a half-life of between 3 and 6 hours. Prophylactic doses are given as fixed doses or weight-adjusted doses; therapeutic doses are weight-based. For most patients, monitoring is not necessary, but some experts recommend monitoring in special populations including (1) obese patients (less reliable dose-response relationship), (2) pediatric patients, (3) patients with renal insufficiency (LMWHs are cleared by the kidney), and (4) pregnant women. When creatinine clearance is less than 30 mL/min, 50% of the normal recommended dose of LMWH has been recommended.[55] The test of choice if monitoring is performed is the anti-Xa assay. If twice-daily doses of enoxaparin are used, the target for therapy is a peak concentration of 0.6 to 1.0 IU/mL for samples taken 4 hours after injection.[55] For once-daily treatment doses, anti-Xa activity 4 hours after injection is often more than 1 U/mL and may be closer to 2 U/mL. Evidence-based guidance on expected concentrations in such patients is lacking. Anti-Xa assays should be calibrated with an LMWH preparation that has itself been calibrated against a WHO international standard for LMWH; even then differences between results of different assays are noted. Clotting-based anti-Xa assays are unsuitable for monitoring LMWH. The anti-Xa activity of LMWH is poorly reversed by protamine sulfate.

Fondaparinux

Fondaparinux (trade name Arixtra) is a synthetic pentasaccharide with a molecular weight of ≈1700 Da that binds AT with higher affinity than does heparin. It has a half-life of ≈17 hours after subcutaneous injection. A predictable anticoagulant response allows once-daily subcutaneous injection in fixed doses without the need for laboratory monitoring. It is contraindicated in renal insufficiency. In circumstances where it may be useful to determine the activity of fondaparinux, the assay of choice is anti-Xa, but in this case, the assay must be calibrated using fondaparinux in the standard plasma—not LMWH. Expected concentrations following 2.5 mg and 7.5 mg daily doses are 0.2 to 0.4 μg/mL and 0.5 to 1.5 μg/mL, respectively, although the therapeutic reference interval has not been established.[55] Fondaparinux is not reversed by protamine sulfate.

Direct Thrombin Inhibitors

The most widely used oral and parenteral anticoagulants including VKA, UFH, and LMWH have a number of limitations that have led to the development of newer alternatives. Several direct thrombin inhibitors have now been licensed for use in particular clinical settings. For example, recombinant hirudin is licensed for treatment of arterial or venous thrombosis where heparin-induced thrombocytopenia (HIT) is present (see later discussion of HIT), and for use in cardiopulmonary bypass. In most studies, increased bleeding compared with alternatives has restricted its use somewhat. A synthetic hirudin analog named bivalirudin is also available and may be useful in certain settings.

New Anticoagulants

Rivaroxaban and dabigatran are two new anticoagulant drugs that have been released for clinical use.

Rivaroxaban (**Xarelto**) is an oral direct factor Xa inhibitor already licensed in Europe and Canada for VTE prophylaxis in adults undergoing elective hip or knee replacement surgery.[118] Laboratory monitoring is not required. The half-life is 7 to 11 hours. Bioavailability is 80 to 100% for oral doses with predictable pharmacokinetics and pharmacodynamics. Excretion is about ⅔ via the renal route, primarily as an unchanged drug. Rivaroxaban has been shown to be more effective than enoxaparin in preventing VTE after knee replacement.[57]

Dabigatran extexilate (Pradaxa in Australia, Europe and USA; Pradax in Canada; Prazaxa in Japan) is a new anticoagulant at an advanced stage of clinical development.[126] This oral prodrug is converted to dabigatran. The plasma half-life of dabigatran is 14 to 17 hours, with excretion largely through the kidneys. It was found to be equivalent to enoxaparin therapy after hip or knee replacement, with similar efficacy and safety.[57] In 2009, it was shown to be equivalent to warfarin over a 6 month treatment course in the prevention of recurrent VTE, when dabigatran etexilate was given in fixed doses with no monitoring; however, warfarin was dose-adjusted to achieve and maintain an INR of 2 to 3.[126]

Satifactory assays for rivaroxaban and dabigatran are not yet available. Despite the fact the monitoring is not required for these anticoagulants, there are many clinical circumstances in which the clinician will want to know if the drug is at an appropriate level, as in the patient with bleeding complication or recurrent thrombosis. Efforts to develop assays are underway at the time of this writing.

Hepatic toxicity was a concern in relation to a recently withdrawn, newly developed anticoagulant, ximelagatran, which is a prodrug of a direct thrombin inhibitor, melagatran. Such problems are more likely to occur with longer-term use.[90] Currently available data suggest that the type of hepatotoxicity seen with ximelagatran may not occur with rivaroxaban or dabigatran etexilate, but this remains to be fully established.

Most experts predict that use of VKA and widely used parenteral anticoagulants will decline, to be replaced by some of the newer anticoagulants that are given orally, safely, effectively, and without laboratory monitoring. For a review, see Garcia and coworkers.[47]

Therapy With Vitamin K Antagonists

Vitamin K antagonists such as warfarin are used (1) as oral drugs for the treatment of VTE; and (2) as prophylaxis in patients with atrial fibrillation, artificial heart valves, or various thrombophilic states. The number of patients requiring long-term VKA therapy continues to grow and is estimated at 750,000 to 1 million at present in the United Kingdom, with a similar prevalence in many developed Western populations. This number is expected to continue to rise, even though possible new anticoagulant drugs are being investigated in clinical trials.

VKAs function as an anticoagulant by interfering with the vitamin K cycle, which is needed for the postribosomal modification of clotting factors II, VII, IX, and X, as well as the anticoagulant proteins PC, PS, and protein Z. A consequence of VKA therapy is that these factors are no longer fully functional. Typically in the clotting process, several amino acids in these factors are carboxylated in a way that facilitates binding of the factors to calcium and phospholipid surfaces. Without these modifications, binding is reduced and clotting proceeds much more slowly. The problem is that the dose response is variable, so dosage must be very closely monitored to avoid over- or under-anticoagulation.

Many different types of VKA are used; warfarin (also known as Coumadin, Jantoven, Marevan, Lawarin, and Waran) is most common in North America and the United Kingdom. Numerous drugs affect the action of VKA in an unpredictable fashion, making monitoring necessary. Indeed, optimal oral anticoagulant therapy requires regular monitoring to ensure an appropriate balance between antithrombotic effects and unwanted hemorrhagic side effects. As discussed earlier, the test of choice for this monitoring in most countries is measurement of PT. Because of variability in different lots of thromboplastins, a normalization model has been developed that is based on expression of results using the INR.

As discussed in greater detail earlier in this chapter, the INR is based on the source of thromboplastins, and series of international standard thromboplastins are available from the WHO. Commercial thromboplastins are calibrated against the WHO reference thromboplastin by determination of paired prothombin times performed with the reference and commercial thromboplastin on a series of plasma specimens from healthy normal subjects and plasmas from patients stabilized on VKA therapy. The $\log_{10}$ of paired PTs is plotted and a regression line fitted through the data. The slope of the line indicates the responsiveness of the commercial thromboplastin relative to the WHO international standard. This is used to derive the ISI. The ISI is then used to convert PT into INR using the equation presented earlier.

The ISI is influenced by the analyzer used to perform testing; thus a single thromboplastin may have different ISIs when used with different analyzers. The reagent manufacturer, therefore, provides specific ISI values for different models. It has been reported that some analyzers of the same model type vary to the extent that local calibration of the ISI may be needed. For a full review, see Tripodi.[134] When the INR system is used, the same result should be obtained, irrespective of the methods that have been used to derive the value, but on some occasions, this does not occur. For example, this is a particular problem when INRs are elevated substantially above the therapeutic reference interval. It may also occur when patients have LAC where prolongation of PT/INR is a combination of VKA therapy and interference with the test by LAC. Some reagents and certain patients are particularly prone to this problem. To monitor VKA

TABLE 59-11 Some PT/INR-POC Devices

	End Point Detection	Memory Storage	Sample Volume	Quality Control Available	Sample Type	Tests Other Than INR
CoaguChek S (Roche)	Iron oxide particles	60	10 µL	Liquid QC	Capillary/venous native whole blood	No
CoaguChek XS (Roche)	Electrochemical cleavage	100	10 µL	Built-in QC	Capillary/venous native whole blood	No
CoaguChek XS Plus (Roche)	Electrochemical cleavage	500	10 µL	Liquid and built-in QC	Capillary/venous native whole blood	No
Hemochron Signature Series (ITC/Thoratec Corporation)	Blood flow through a restriction channel	200+ basic model 600+ top model	50 µL	Liquid QC	Native or citrated capillary/ venous whole blood	Yes
i-STAT (Abbott Diagnostics)	Electrochemical cleavage	5000	20 µL	Liquid QC	Native whole blood	Yes
INRatio (HemoSense/ Inverness Medical)	Electric impedance	60	15 µL	Built-in QC	Native capillary whole blood	No
ProTime (ITC/Thoratec Corporation)	Photoptic detection of decreased blood flow	50	27 µL	Liquid and built-in QC	Capillary/venous native whole blood	No

therapy when the PT/INR is affected by LAC, it is necessary to select a PT/INR system (perhaps by sending samples to other laboratories) that is not responsive to the LAC effect in that patient (as evidenced by a normal PT/INR before commencement of VKA therapy). For clinical recommendations on targets for INR in VKA therapy, see Ansell and associates.[2]

Point of Care for Monitoring VKA Therapy

Much of the testing for monitoring anticoagulant therapy continues to be performed in core or reference clinical laboratories, but there is a trend toward performing such measurements near the patient.[105] This type of testing is known as point-of-care (POC) testing[68] (see Chapter 20), and POC devices are now available that allow the patient to measure INR at home.[87] Consequently, the patient is able to adjust his or her VKA dose, and guidelines and recommendations have been established for self-testing and self-management of oral anticoagulation.[17,46] However, it should be noted that results from a 2010 study did not support the superiority of self-testing over clinic testing in reducing the risk of stroke, major bleeding episodes, and death among patients taking warfarin therapy.[87]

Determination of INR with POC instruments involves insertion of an individual test strip or cartridge into the monitor, followed by addition of the patient's blood sample. The blood reconstitutes dried thromboplastin reagent and initiates clotting reactions in the presence of calcium, leading to clot formation, which is detected as an end point. Within POC-INR devices are many types of end-point detection systems. For some systems, electronic quality control (QC) is available, whereby an electronic device is inserted into the monitor in place of the test strip, and an electronic signal is produced that tests the electronic system within the POC monitor. Table 59-11 provides a list of currently used POC-INR systems.

Some manufacturers of POC-INR systems produce test strips for INR determination with built-in quality control. For example, the CoaguChek XS and CoaguChek XS Plus devices (Roche Diagnostics Corp., Indianapolis, Ind) have a test strip integrity check. With these devices, a test strip containing a compound (Resazurin) that is sensitive to factors such as light, humidity, and temperature is analyzed. Chemical changes that occur are measured electrochemically, and the patient INR is displayed only if the test strip integrity check is acceptable. In addition to internal QC checks, external quality assurance (QA) is available for POC-INR testing in the United States and Europe.[69]

It should be noted that POC-INR results may not agree with those generated in local clinical laboratories, particularly when values are beyond the therapeutic interval. As part of the quality control process, a venous sample is collected at the same time as the POC test and is analyzed in an appropriate laboratory. Some patients show discrepancies between INRs determined by two different techniques, despite being stabilized on oral anticoagulant therapy. One cause of this is the presence of LAC, although discrepancies also occur without an LAC.

In a 2008 study, Murray and colleagues[97] concluded that patients could successfully participate in a formal external quality assurance (EQA) program utilizing the same freeze-dried test samples as are used in conventional laboratory EQA programs. The same study demonstrated that comparing the patient POC device with a reference device was an effective form of EQA.

Heparin-Induced Thrombocytopenia

Heparin-induced thrombocytopenia (HIT) is a serious complication of heparin therapy because patients with HIT have a substantially increased thrombotic risk. HIT is thought to be caused by the development of antibodies that recognize neoantigens formed from complexes of platelet factor 4 and heparin. Thrombocytopenia or thrombosis without the presence of heparin-dependent antibodies is not HIT, nor is the isolated presence of such antibodies without thrombocytopenia or thrombosis. The diagnosis of HIT is therefore based on both clinical and laboratory features. The frequency of HIT is greater in surgical than medical patients and is greater with UFH than LMWH. In orthopedic patients given prophylactic subcutaneous heparin, the incidence is around 5%, which is approximately 10-fold higher than the incidence with LMWH in this group. For medical patients on therapeutic UFH, the incidence is around 0.5 to 1%. When HIT develops, the platelet count decreases 5 to 14 days following initiation of therapy in patients who were not previously exposed to heparin therapy. If patients have had heparin in the previous 3 months, preexisting antibodies may appear as soon as heparin is used. Because the platelet count decreases by more than 50%, it must be checked regularly to identify those at risk of HIT with associated thombosis. Severe thrombocytopenia ($<15 \times 10^9$ cells/L) is rare. Approximately half of patients who develop HIT will have associated thrombosis. The initial assessment is clinical and is based on a system that has been termed the 4 T's system (**t**hrombocytopenia; **t**iming of fall in platelets; **t**hrombosis; o**t**her causes of thrombocytopenia not evident). This system generates a pretest probability score. If the score is high, then heparin therapy must be terminated and alternative anticoagulants used.

It is important to remember that diagnosis and management of HIT are clinical, with the laboratory used only for confirmatory purposes. Several laboratory tests available for these purposes are based on platelet activation (functional) or immunologic assays using PF4-heparin complexes as an antigen. Platelet activation assays require a healthy subject as a source of donor platelets, and not all subjects are suitable because responsiveness to HIT antibodies varies. Such assays are improved by washing of platelets, but overall these assays are technically difficult and are not widely used. Alternatively, commercial ELISA assays are available from several manufacturers, as are rapid gel agglutination techniques. Antigen assays available at the time of this writing have clinical sensitivity in the range of 80 to 100% but low specificity. False positives are common. The degree of positivity is important in that strong positivity is associated with thrombosis. Some experts believe that only immunoglobulin (Ig)G antibodies cause the clinical disorder. Many commercial antigen assays detect IgM and IgA antibodies, as well as IgG. For full reviews and guidance, see Warkentin and coworkers[138] and Keeling and associates.[66]

Antiphospholipid Antibodies and Lupus Anticoagulant

Antiphospholipid antibodies (APAs), including lupus anticoagulant antibodies, anticardiolipin antibodies, and β_2 glycoprotein-1 antibodies, occur in the antiphospholipid syndrome (APS). This is a disorder of the immune system that is characterized by excessive clotting of blood and/or certain complications of pregnancy [i.e., premature miscarriage, unexplained fetal death, or premature birth (http://www.medicinenet.com)]. It is an acquired problem with immune pathogenesis that has been known to cause thrombosis and pregnancy loss. APS is diagnosed when particular clinical symptoms coincide with the presence of APA in laboratory tests. Some antibodies are transient; thus a diagnosis of APS requires repeat testing for confirmation after 12 weeks. The most common thrombotic symptoms are venous thromboembolism and ischemic stroke, with some patients having thrombocytopenia. Types of pregnancy failure that are consistent with APS include (1) three or more unexplained consecutive abortions before 10 weeks, (2) unexplained death of a morphologically normal fetus at or after 10 weeks, and (3) premature birth before 34 weeks due to severe preeclampsia or placental insufficiency. Internationally, classification criteria have been published.[94]

At present the degree of standardization of tests for APA is poor, and the limitations of such tests must be kept in mind when patients are assessed for possible APS. Several types of APA are undoubtedly linked to thrombosis and pregnancy loss. These include (1) anti-β_2-glycoprotein-1(anti-β_2-GP-1), (2) lupus anticoagulant (LA), and (3) anticardiolipin antibodies (ACAs). Other types of APA have been reported to be linked to APS, but currently no consensus has been reached on their clinical relevance.

It has long been recognized that some individuals with systemic lupus erythematosus (SLE) have prolonged aPTTs. This was shown to be due to the presence of an in vitro inhibitor called lupus anticoagulant (LAC). These inhibitors previously were thought to work against phospholipid but were found to be active against proteins that bind to lipids; these proteins include β_2-glycoprotein-1, prothrombin, annexin V, and others.[59,111,121] Antibodies that prolong phospholipid-dependent clotting tests are collectively termed LAC. This group is very heterogeneous in relation to clinical picture and laboratory features. It should be noted that although some SLE individuals are positive for LAC, most cases of LAC are not associated with SLE, even though the term *lupus anticoagulant* has continued to be used. In addition, it should be noted that not all antiphospholipid antibodies prolong these clotting tests. Some cases with detectable LA do not have clinical features and therefore are not classified as APS. The aPTT, however, is not prolonged in all cases where LA is present, and most cases with LA and prolonged aPTT have no bleeding symptoms but may have thrombosis as described previously. Only rarely is LA associated with bleeding, usually when acquired prothrombin deficiency is a consequence of high concentrations of antiprothrombin antibody.

The guidelines for LAC detection were updated by the Scientific and Standardization Committee (SSC) of the ISTH in 2009.[103] This update addresses a number of important aspects of standardization. For example, the quality of the sample affects results of LA tests, and if there are residual platelets, they can rupture during the testing, leading to loss of antibody and false-negative results. This is a particular problem if plasmas are frozen before testing; therefore, double centrifugation is required before deep freezing. Filtering to remove residual platelets, however, is not recommended. The guidelines also recommend that the dilute Russell's viper venom time (DRVVT) should be the first test performed, and the second test should be a sensitive aPTT-based test. The DRVVT is a clot-based test that is initiated by the addition of a Russell viper venom that directly activates factor X, thereby bypassing effects of extrinsic and intrinsic pathways. For an aPTT test to be sensitive to the presence of LAC, the aPTT reagent should have a low phospholipid concentration. Only the DRVVT or the aPTT test needs to be positive to be considered evidence of LAC, although in most cases, both will be positive. In addition, a confirmatory step is required for each individual LAC test to confirm the phospholipid-dependent nature of the inhibitor. This confirmation is achieved by repeating the test with a higher phospholipid concentration to neutralize the phospholipid-dependent inhibitors. There is also a role for performing a mixing study of LAC tests to help differentiate between a clotting factor deficiency (which may be associated with bleeding) and a lupus inhibitor (more likely associated with thrombosis than bleeding).

As a consequence of thrombosis, many patients with LAC require VKA therapy. Interpretation of LAC tests is difficult during VKA therapy because reductions in the quantities of various coagulation factors during VKA therapy will affect the DRVVT and aPTT tests. The SSC LAC guideline recommends that such testing should be done 1 to 2 weeks after discontinuation of VKA therapy.[103] If testing is necessary at the time of VKA therapy, it is recommended that (1) the DRVVT should be performed when the INR is less than 1.5, (2) testing should not be done when the INR is greater than 3.5, and (3) a mix of test and normal plasma should be considered when the INR is between these limits. In addition, the SSC guideline does not recommend use of (1) dilute prothrombin time, (2) assays based on snake venoms, or (3) kaolin-clotting time for LAC detection.

Various solid-phase ELISA tests are available for the detection of APA. These include tests for ACA for which commercial kits have been available for many years. Standardization of such kits, however, is rather poor, and comparisons consistently demonstrate that even concordance as to whether a sample is positive or negative is frequently absent when testing is done with two or more different kits.[60] Both IgG and IgM forms of ACA occur. Evidence that the IgM isotype is of clinical relevance is weak, and many laboratories test only for IgG. Some but not all ACA assays incorporate β_2-glycoprotein-1 in the reagents so that cardiolipin bound to the surface of a microtiter plate will be associated with β_2-glycoprotein-1. Some ACA kits detect only β_2-glycoprotein-1–dependent antibodies, whereas others detect non–β_2-glycoprotein-1–dependent antibodies. Evidence suggests that it is the β_2-glycoprotein-1–dependent antibodies that have the greatest clinical significance in APS, and a number of specific anti-β_2-glycoprotein-1 antibody kits are in use. As for ACA kits, standardization of APS kits is poor, and there will be patients with APS who are negative by one kit and positive by another.[60]

REFERENCES

1. Agren A, Wiman B, Stiller V, Lindmarker P, Sten-Linder M, Carlsson A, et al. Evaluation of low PAI-1 activity as a risk factor for hemorrhagic diathesis. J Thromb Haemost 2006;4:201-8.
2. Ansell J, Hirsh J, Hylek E, Jacobson A, Crowther M, Palareti G. Pharmacology and management of the vitamin K antagonists: American College of Chest Physicians evidence-based clinical practice guidelines, 8th edition. Chest 2008;133:160S-98S.
3. Asahina T, Kobayashi T, Takeuchi K, Kanayama N. Congenital blood coagulation factor XIII deficiency and successful deliveries: a review of the literature. Obstet Gynecol Surv 2007;62:255-60.
4. Baglin T, Gray E, Greaves M, Hunt B, Keeling D, Machin S, et al. Clinical guidelines for testing for heritable thrombophilia. Available at: http://www.bcshguidelines.com/pdf/ThrombophiliaGuideline_101209.pdf (accessed on September 29, 2011).
5. Barrowcliffe TW. Methodology of the two-stage assay of factor VIII (VIII:C). Scand J Haematol Suppl 1984;41:25-38.
6. Basu D, Gallus A, Hirsh J, Cade J. A prospective study of the value of monitoring heparin treatment with the activated partial thromboplastin time. N Engl J Med 1972;287:324-7.
7. Bellest L, Eschwege V, Poupon R, Chazouilleres O, Robert A. A modified international normalized ratio as an effective way of prothrombin time standardization in hepatology. Hepatology 2007; 46:528-34.
8. Bennett J. Acquired platelet function defects. Cambridge: Cambridge University Press, 2002.
9. Bertina RM, Koeleman BP, Koster T, Rosendaal FR, Dirven RJ, de Ronde H, et al. Mutation in blood coagulation factor V associated with resistance to activated protein C. Nature 1994;369:64-7.
10. Bessman JD. Automated cell counts and differentials. Baltimore, Md: Johns Hopkins University Press, 1986.
11. Booth NA, Bachmann F. Plasminogen-plasmin system. In: Colman RW, Marder VJ, Clowes AW, George JN, Goldhaber SZ, eds. Hemostasis and thrombosis: basic principles and clinical practice, 5th edition. Philadelphia, Pa: JB Lippincott Williams and Wilkins, 2006: 335-64.
12. Born GVR. Aggregation of blood platelets with adenosine diphosphate and its reversal. Nature 1962;194:927-9.
13. Bowie EJW, Thompson JH, Didisheim P, Owen CA. Mayo Clinic laboratory manual of hemostasis. Philadelphia, Pa: WB Saunders, 1971.
14. Bowyer A, Kitchen S, Makris M. The responsiveness of different APTT reagents to mild factor VIII, IX and XI deficiencies. Int J Lab Hematol 2010;33:154-8.
15. Brandjes DP, Heijboer H, Buller HR, de Rijk M, Jagt H, ten Cate JW. Acenocoumarol and heparin compared with acenocoumarol alone in the initial treatment of proximal-vein thrombosis. N Engl J Med 1992;327:1485-9.
16. Brandt JT, Triplett DA, Musgrave K, Orr C. The sensitivity of different coagulation reagents to the presence of lupus anticoagulants. Arch Pathol Lab Med 1987;111:120-4.

17. Briggs C, Guthrie D, Hyde K, Mackie I, Parker N, Popek M, et al. Guidelines for POC testing: haematology, 2008. Available at: http://www.bcshguidelines.com/pdf/POCT_guidelines_310707.pdf (accessed on September 29, 2011).
18. Brill-Edwards P, Ginsberg JS, Johnston M, Hirsh J. Establishing a therapeutic range for heparin therapy. Ann Intern Med 1993;119:104-9.
19. Burns ER, Lawrence C. Bleeding time: a guide to its diagnostic and clinical utility. Arch Pathol Lab Med 1989;113:1219-24.
20. Carpenter SL, Mathew P. Alpha2-antiplasmin and its deficiency: fibrinolysis out of balance. Haemophilia 2008;14:1250-4.
21. Castaman G, Tosetto A, Goodeve A, Federici AB, Lethagen S, Budde U, et al. The impact of bleeding history, von Willebrand factor and PFA-100 on the diagnosis of type 1 von Willebrand disease: results from the European study MCMDM-1VWD. Br J Haematol 2010;151:245-51.
22. Castellino FJ, Ploplis VA. The protein C pathway and pathologic processes. J Thromb Haemost 2009;7(suppl 1):140-5.
23. Chang SH, Tillema V, Scherr D. A "percent correction" formula for evaluation of mixing studies. Am J Clin Pathol 2002;117:62-73.
24. Clauss A. [Rapid physiological coagulation method in determination of fibrinogen]. Acta Haematol 1957;17:237-46.
25. Clinical and Laboratory Standards Institute. Transport and processing of blood specimens for testing plasma-based coagulation assays: approved guideline H21-A4, 5th edition. Wayne, Pa: Clinical and Laboratory Standards Institute, 2008.
25A. Clinical and Laboratory Standards Institute. Quantitative D-dimer for the exclusion of venous thromboembolic disease; approved guideline. H59-A. Wayne, Pa: Clinical and Laboratory Standards Institute, 2012.
26. Clyne LP, White PF. Time dependency of lupuslike anticoagulants. Arch Intern Med 1988;148:1060-3.
27. Contant G, Nicham F, Marinoli JL. Determination of plasminogen activator inhibitor (PAI) by a new venom-based assay. Fibrinolysis 1992;S6:85-6.
28. Cunningham MT, Brandt JT, Laposata M, Olson JD. Laboratory diagnosis of dysfibrinogenemia. Arch Pathol Lab Med 2002;126: 499-505.
29. Dahlback B, Carlsson M, Svensson PJ. Familial thrombophilia due to a previously unrecognized mechanism characterized by poor anticoagulant response to activated protein C: prediction of a cofactor to activated protein C. Proc Natl Acad Sci U S A 1993;90:1004-8.
30. Danesh J, Lewington S, Thompson SG, Lowe GD, Collins R, Kostis JB, et al. Plasma fibrinogen level and the risk of major cardiovascular diseases and nonvascular mortality: an individual participant meta-analysis. JAMA 2005;294:1799-809.
31. Dang CV, Shin CK, Bell WR, Nagaswami C, Weisel JW. Fibrinogen sialic acid residues are low affinity calcium-binding sites that influence fibrin assembly. J Biol Chem 1989;264:15104-8.
32. de Maistre E, Wahl D, Perret-Guillaume C, Regnault V, Clarac S, Briquel ME, et al. A chromogenic assay allows reliable measurement of factor VIII levels in the presence of strong lupus anticoagulants. Thromb Haemost 1998;79:237-8.
33. de Visser MC, Rosendaal FR, Bertina RM. A reduced sensitivity for activated protein C in the absence of factor V Leiden increases the risk of venous thrombosis. Blood 1999;93:1271-6.
34. Drake TA, Morrissey JH, Edgington TS. Selective cellular expression of tissue factor in human tissues: implications for disorders of hemostasis and thrombosis. Am J Pathol 1989;134:1087-97.
35. Duckert F, Jung E, Shmerling DH. A hitherto undescribed congenital haemorrhagic diathesis probably due to fibrin stabilizing factor deficiency. Thromb Diath Haemorrh 1960;5:179-86.
36. Duncan EM, Duncan BM, Tunbridge LJ, Lloyd JV. Familial discrepancy between the one-stage and two-stage factor VIII methods in a subgroup of patients with haemophilia A. Br J Haematol 1994;87:846-8.
37. Dykes AC, Walker ID, McMahon AD, Islam SI, Tait RC. A study of protein S antigen levels in 3788 healthy volunteers: influence of age, sex and hormone use, and estimate for prevalence of deficiency state. Br J Haematol 2001;113:636-41.
38. Eby C, Blinder M. Hemostatic complications associated with paraproteinemias. Curr Hematol Rep 2003;2:388-94.
39. Eilertsen KE, Osterud B. Tissue factor: (patho)physiology and cellular biology. Blood Coagul Fibrinolysis 2004;15:521-38.
40. Esmon CT. The protein C pathway. Chest 2003;124:26S-32S.
41. Faioni EM, Franchi F, Asti D, Sacchi E, Bernardi F, Mannucci PM. Resistance to activated protein C in nine thrombophilic families: interference in a protein S functional assay. Thromb Haemost 1993;70: 1067-71.
42. Fass DN, Knutson GJ, Bowie EJ. Porcine Willebrand factor: a population of multimers. J Lab Clin Med 1978;91:307-20.
43. Favaloro EJ. An update on the von Willebrand factor collagen binding assay: 21 years of age and beyond adolescence but not yet a mature adult. Semin Thromb Hemost 2007;33:727-44.
44. Favaloro EJ. Detection of von Willebrand disorder and identification of qualitative von Willebrand factor defects: direct comparison of commercial ELISA-based von Willebrand factor activity options. Am J Clin Pathol 2000;114:608-18.
45. Favaloro EJ. Laboratory identification of von Willebrand disease: technical and scientific perspectives. Semin Thromb Hemost 2006;32: 456-71.
46. Fitzmaurice DA, Gardiner C, Kitchen S, Mackie I, Murray ET, Machin SJ. An evidence-based review and guidelines for patient self-testing and management of oral anticoagulation. Br J Haematol 2005;131:156-65.
47. Garcia D, Libby E, Crowther MA. The new oral anticoagulants. Blood 2010;115:15-20.
48. Gardiner C, Cooper PC, Makris M, Mackie IJ, Malia RG, Machin SJ. An evaluation of screening tests for defects in the protein C pathway: commercial kits lack sensitivity and specificity. Blood Coagul Fibrinolysis 2002;13:155-63.
49. Gill JC, Endres-Brooks J, Bauer PJ, Marks WJ Jr, Montgomery RR. The effect of ABO blood group on the diagnosis of von Willebrand disease. Blood 1987;69:1691-5.
50. Goodeve A, Peake I. Laboratory analysis of von Willebrand disease: molecular analysis. In: Kitchen S, Olson JD, Preston FE, eds. Quality in laboratory hemostasis and thrombosis. Hoboken, NJ: Wiley-Blackwell, 2009:137-46.
51. Hackeng TM, Maurissen LF, Castoldi E, Rosing J. Regulation of TFPI function by protein S. J Thromb Haemost 2009;7(suppl 1):165-8.
52. Hampshire DJ, Burghel GJ, Goudemand J, Bouvet L, Eikenboom JC, Schneppenheim R, et al. Polymorphic variation within the VWF gene contributes to the failure to detect mutations in patients historically diagnosed with type 1 VWD from the MCMDM-1VWD cohort. Haematologica 2010;95:2163-5.
53. Hancock JF, Wieland K, Pugh RE, Martinowitz U, Schulman S, Kakkar VV, et al. A molecular genetic study of factor XI deficiency. Blood 1991;77:1942-8.
54. Hayward CP, Harrison P, Cattaneo M, Ortel TL, Rao AK. Platelet function analyzer (PFA)-100 closure time in the evaluation of platelet disorders and platelet function. J Thromb Haemost 2006;4:312-9.
55. Hirsh J, Bauer KA, Donati MB, Gould M, Samama MM, Weitz JI. Parenteral anticoagulants: American College of Chest Physicians evidence-based clinical practice guidelines, 8th edition. Chest 2008;133:141S-59S.
56. Hirsh J, Guyatt G, Albers GW, Harrington R, Schunemann HJ, American College of Chest Physicians. Antithrombotic and thrombolytic therapy: American College of Chest Physicians evidence-based clinical practice guidelines, 8th edition. Chest 2008;133:110S-2S.
57. Huisman MV, Quinlan DJ, Dahl OE, Schulman S. Enoxaparin versus dabigatran or rivaroxaban for thromboprophylaxis after hip or knee arthroplasty: results of separate pooled analyses of phase III multicenter randomized trials. Circ Cardiovasc Qual Outcomes 2010;3:652-60.
58. Inbal A, Muszbek L. Coagulation factor deficiencies and pregnancy loss. Semin Thromb Hemost 2003;29:171-4.
59. Iverson GM, Victoria EJ, Cockerill KA, Linnik MD. Advances in understanding what we measure when detecting anticardiolipin autoantibodies. Clin Chim Acta 2004;343:37-44.

60. Jennings I, Greaves M, Mackie IJ, Kitchen S, Woods TA, Preston FE. Lupus anticoagulant testing: improvements in performance in a UK NEQAS proficiency testing exercise after dissemination of national guidelines on laboratory methods. Br J Haematol 2002;119:364-9.
61. Jennings I, Kitchen S, Cooper PC, Rimmer JE, Woods TA, Preston FE. Further evidence that activated protein C resistance affects protein C coagulant activity assays. Thromb Haemost 2000;83:171-2.
62. Jennings I, Kitchen S, Woods TA, Preston FE. Problems relating to the laboratory diagnosis of factor XIII deficiency: a UK NEQAS study. J Thromb Haemost 2003;1:2603-8.
63. Johnson SA, Balboa RS, Dessel BH, Monto RW, Siegesmund KA, Greenwalt TJ. The mechanism of the endothelial supporting function of intact platelets. Exp Mol Pathol 1964;34:115-27.
64. Karimi M, Bereczky Z, Cohan N, Muszbek L. Factor XIII deficiency. Semin Thromb Hemost 2009;35:426-38.
65. Kasper CK, Aledort L, Aronson D, Counts R, Edson JR, van Eys J, et al. Proceedings: a more uniform measurement of factor VIII inhibitors. Thromb Diath Haemorrh 1975;34:612.
66. Keeling D, Davidson S, Watson H. The management of heparin-induced thrombocytopenia. Br J Haematol 2006;133:259-69.
67. Kempton CL, White GC 2nd. How we treat a hemophilia A patient with a factor VIII inhibitor. Blood 2009;113:11-7.
68. Kitchen S, Hayward C, Negrier C, Dargaud Y. New developments in laboratory diagnosis and monitoring. Haemophilia 2010;16(suppl 5): 61-6.
69. Kitchen S, Kitchen DP, Jennings I, Woods TA, Walker ID, Preston FE. Point-of-care international normalised ratios: UK NEQAS experience demonstrates necessity for proficiency testing of three different monitors. Thromb Haemost 2006;96:590-6.
70. Kitchen S, Preston FE. Assay of factor VIII and other clotting factors. In: Kitchen S, Olson JD, Preston FE, eds. Quality in laboratory hemostasis and thrombosis. Hoboken, NJ: Wiley-Blackwell, 2009: 81-9.
71. Kitchen S, Preston FE. The therapeutic range for heparin therapy: relationship between six activated partial thromboplastin time reagents and two heparin assays. Thromb Haemost 1996;75:734-9.
72. Koeleman BP, Reitsma PH, Allaart CF, Bertina RM. Activated protein C resistance as an additional risk factor for thrombosis in protein C-deficient families. Blood 1994;84:1031-5.
73. Koeleman BP, van Rumpt D, Hamulyak K, Reitsma PH, Bertina RM. Factor V Leiden: an additional risk factor for thrombosis in protein S deficient families? Thromb Haemost 1995;74:580-3.
74. Kokame K, Nobe Y, Kokubo Y, Okayama A, Miyata T. FRETS-VWF73, a first fluorogenic substrate for ADAMTS13 assay. Br J Haematol 2005; 129:93-100.
75. Koster T, Blann AD, Briet E, Vandenbroucke JP, Rosendaal FR. Role of clotting factor VIII in effect of von Willebrand factor on occurrence of deep-vein thrombosis. Lancet 1995;345:152-5.
76. Kottke-Marchant K. Antiplatelet agents. In: Kottke-Marchant K, ed. An algorithmic approach to hemostasis testing. Northfield, Ill: College of American Pathologists, 2008:333-46.
77. Kottke-Marchant K. Platelet structure and function. In: Kottke-Marchant K, ed. An algorithmic approach to hemostasis testing. Northfield, Ill: College of American Pathologists, 2008:13-27.
78. Kunishima S, Kamiya T, Saito H. Genetic abnormalities of Bernard-Soulier syndrome. Int J Hematol 2002;76:319-27.
79. Laffan M, Brown SA, Collins PW, Cumming AM, Hill FG, Keeling D, et al. The diagnosis of von Willebrand disease: a guideline from the UK Haemophilia Centre Doctors' Organization. Haemophilia 2004; 10:199-217.
80. Langdell RD, Wagner RH, Brinkhous KM. Effect of antihemophilic factor on one-stage clotting tests; a presumptive test for hemophilia and a simple one-stage antihemophilic factor assay procedure. J Lab Clin Med 1953;41:637-47.
81. Laurell CB. Quantitative estimation of proteins by electrophoresis in agarose gel containing antibodies. Anal Biochem 1966;15:45-52.
82. Lind SE. The bleeding time does not predict surgical bleeding. Blood 1991;77:2547-52.
83. Makris M, Leach M, Beauchamp NJ, Daly ME, Cooper PC, Hampton KK, et al. Genetic analysis, phenotypic diagnosis, and risk of venous thrombosis in families with inherited deficiencies of protein S. Blood 2000;95:1935-41.
84. Mann KG. Biochemistry and physiology of blood coagulation. Thromb Haemost 1999;82:165-74.
85. Marder VJ, Shulman NR, Carroll WR. High molecular weight derivatives of human fibrinogen produced by plasmin. I. Physicochemical and immunological characterization. J Biol Chem 1969;244:2111-9.
86. Marder VJ, Shulman NR. High molecular weight derivatives of human fibrinogen produced by plasmin. II. Mechanism of their anticoagulant activity. J Biol Chem 1969;244:2120-4.
87. Matchar DB, Jacobson A, Dolor R, Edson R, Uyeda L, Phibbs CS, et al. Effect of home testing of international normalized ratio on clinical events. N Engl J Med 2010;363:1608-20.
88. McGlasson DL, Fritsma GA. Comparison of four laboratory methods to assess aspirin sensitivity. Blood Coagul Fibrinolysis 2008;19:120-3.
89. McGlasson DL, Fritsma GA. Whole blood platelet aggregometry and platelet function testing. Semin Thromb Hemost 2009;35:168-80.
90. Medi C, Hankey GJ, Freedman SB. Stroke risk and antithrombotic strategies in atrial fibrillation. Stroke. 2010;41:2705-13.
91. Mehta R, Shapiro AD. Plasminogen deficiency. Haemophilia 2008;14: 1261-8.
92. Michelson AD, Linden MD, Barnard MR, Furman MI, Frelinger AL. Flow cytometry. In: Michelson AD, ed. Platelets, 2nd edition. San Diego, Calif: Academic Press, 2007:545-63.
93. Michiels C. Endothelial cell functions. J Cell Physiol 2003;196:430-43.
94. Miyakis S, Lockshin MD, Atsumi T, Branch DW, Brey RL, Cervera R, et al. International consensus statement on an update of the classification criteria for definite antiphospholipid syndrome (APS). J Thromb Haemost 2006;4:295-306.
95. Moia M, Mannucci PM, Vizzotto L, Casati S, Cattaneo M, Ponticelli C. Improvement in the haemostatic defect of uraemia after treatment with recombinant human erythropoietin. Lancet 1987;2:1227-9.
96. Motykie GD, Zebala LP, Caprini JA, Lee CE, Arcelus JI, Reyna JJ, et al. A guide to venous thromboembolism risk factor assessment. J Thromb Thrombolysis 2000;9:253-62.
97. Murray ET, Jennings I, Kitchen D, Kitchen S, Fitzmaurice DA. Quality assurance for oral anticoagulation self management: a cluster randomized trial. J Thromb Haemost 2008;6:464-9.
98. Nair S, Ghosh K, Kulkarni B, Shetty S, Mohanty D. Glanzmann's thrombasthenia: updated. Platelets 2002;13:387-93.
99. Olson JD, Brockway WJ, Fass DN, Magnuson MA, Bowie EJ. Evaluation of ristocetin-Willebrand factor assay and ristocetin-induced platelet aggregation. Am J Clin Pathol 1975;63:210-8.
100. Parquet-Gernez A, Mazurier C, Goudemand M. Functional and immunological assays of FVIII in 133 haemophiliacs—characterization of a subgroup of patients with mild haemophilia A and discrepancy in 1- and 2-stage assays. Thromb Haemost 1988;59:202-6.
101. Peake I, Goodeve A. Type 1 von Willebrand disease. J Thromb Haemost 2007(5 suppl 1):7-11.
102. Peerschke EI, Castellone DD, Ledford-Kraemer M, Van Cott EM, Meijer P. Laboratory assessment of factor VIII inhibitor titer: the North American Specialized Coagulation Laboratory Association experience. Am J Clin Pathol 2009;131:552-8.
103. Pengo V, Tripodi A, Reber G, Rand JH, Ortel TL, Galli M, et al. Update of the guidelines for lupus anticoagulant detection. J Thromb Haemost 2009;7:1737-40.
104. Perkins HA, MacKenzie MR, Fudenberg HH. Hemostatic defects in dysproteinemias. Blood 1970;35:695-707.
105. Perry DJ, Fitzmaurice DA, Kitchen S, Mackie IJ, Mallett S. Point-of-care testing in haemostasis. Br J Haematol 2010;150: 501-14.
106. Piro O, Broze GJ Jr. Comparison of cell-surface TFPIalpha and beta. J Thromb Haemost 2005;3:2677-83.
107. Poort SR, Rosendaal FR, Reitsma PH, Bertina RM. A common genetic variation in the 3′-untranslated region of the prothrombin

gene is associated with elevated plasma prothrombin levels and an increase in venous thrombosis. Blood 1996;88:3698-703.

108. Preston FE, Kitchen S, Jennings I, Woods TA. A UK National External Quality Assessment scheme (UK Neqas) for molecular genetic testing for the diagnosis of familial thrombophilia. Thromb Haemost 1999;82: 1556-7.
109. Raman BK, Van Slyck EJ, Riddle J, Sawdyk MA, Abraham JP, Saeed SM. Platelet function and structure in myeloproliferative disease, myelodysplastic syndrome, and secondary thrombocytosis. Am J Clin Pathol 1989;91:647-55.
110. Rau JC, Beaulieu LM, Huntington JA, Church FC. Serpins in thrombosis, hemostasis and fibrinolysis. J Thromb Haemost 2007;5(suppl 1):102-15.
111. Rand JH, Wu XX, Quinn AS, Taatjes DJ. The annexin A5-mediated pathogenic mechanism in the antiphospholipid syndrome: role in pregnancy losses and thrombosis. Lupus 2010;19:460-9.
112. Ray MJ. An artefact related to the ratio of sample volume to the blood collection vial size which effects the APTTs of specimens taken to monitor heparin therapy. Thromb Haemost 1991;66:387-8.
113. Rijken DC, Lijnen HR. New insights into the molecular mechanisms of the fibrinolytic system. J Thromb Haemost 2009;7:4-13.
114. Robbins KC. A study on the conversion of fibrinogen to fibrin. Am J Physiol 1944;142:581-8.
115. Rosen S, Johansson K, Lindberg K, Dahlback B. Multicenter evaluation of a kit for activated protein C resistance on various coagulation instruments using plasmas from healthy individuals. The APC Resistance Study Group. Thromb Haemost 1994;72:255-60.
116. Rosner E, Pauzner R, Lusky A, Modan M, Many A. Detection and quantitative evaluation of lupus circulating anticoagulant activity. Thromb Haemost 1987;57:144-7.
117. Ruggeri ZM, Zimmerman TS. Variant von Willebrand's disease: characterization of two subtypes by analysis of multimeric composition of factor VIII/von Willebrand factor in plasma and platelets. J Clin Invest 1980;65:1318-25.
118. Rupprecht HJ, Blank R. Clinical pharmacology of direct and indirect factor Xa inhibitors. Drugs 2010;70:2153-70.
119. Sadler JE, Blinder M. Von Willebrand disease: diagnosis, classification and treatment. In: Colman RW, Marder VJ, Clowes AW, George JN, Goldhaber SZ, eds. Hemostasis and thrombosis: basic principles and clinical practice, 5th edition. Philadelphia, Pa: JB Lippincott Williams and Wilkins, 2006:905-21.
120. Sadler JE, Budde U, Eikenboom JC, Favaloro EJ, Hill FG, Holmberg L, et al. Update on the pathophysiology and classification of von Willebrand disease: a report of the Subcommittee on von Willebrand Factor. J Thromb Haemost 2006;4:2103-14.
121. Saigal R, Kansal A, Mittal M, Singh Y, Ram H. Antiphospholipid antibody syndrome. J Assoc Physicians India 2010;58:176-84.
122. Salem RO, Van Cott EM. A new automated screening assay for the diagnosis of von Willebrand disease. Am J Clin Pathol 2007;127:730-5.
123. Salomon O, Zivelin A, Livnat T, Dardik R, Loewenthal R, Avishai O, et al. Prevalence, causes, and characterization of factor XI inhibitors in patients with inherited factor XI deficiency. Blood 2003;101:4783-8.
124. Schlueter A, Olson JD. Coagulation instrumentation: hospital laboratory to the home. In: Rowan RM, van Assendelft OW, Preston FE, eds. Advanced laboratory methods in haematology. London, UK: Arnold, 2002:316-36.
125. Schoenwaelder SM, Yuan Y, Cooray P, Salem HH, Jackson SP. Calpain cleavage of focal adhesion proteins regulates the cytoskeletal attachment of integrin alphaIIbbeta3 (platelet glycoprotein IIb/IIIa) and the cellular retraction of fibrin clots. J Biol Chem 1997;272: 1694-702.
126. Schulman S, Kearon C, Kakkar AK, Mismetti P, Schellong S, Eriksson H, et al. Dabigatran versus warfarin in the treatment of acute venous thromboembolism. N Engl J Med 2009;361:2342-52.
127. Sermon AM, Smith JM, Maclean R, Kitchen S. An international sensitivity index (ISI) derived from patients with abnormal liver function improves agreement between INRs determined with different reagents. Thromb Haemost 2010;103:757-65.
128. Shafey M, Anderson JL, Scarvelis D, Doucette SP, Gagnon F, Wells PS. Factor XIII Val34Leu variant and the risk of myocardial infarction: a meta-analysis. Thromb Haemost 2007;97:635-41.
129. Tait RC, Walker ID, Islam SI, Mitchell R, Conkie JA, McCall F, et al. Age related changes in protein C activity in healthy adult males. Thromb Haemost 1991;65:326-7.
130. Taylor FB Jr, Toh CH, Hoots WK, Wada H, Levi M. Towards definition, clinical and laboratory criteria, and a scoring system for disseminated intravascular coagulation. Thromb Haemost 2001;86: 1327-30.
131. Tran TH, Duckert F. Influence of heparin cofactor II (HCII) on the determination of antithrombin III (AT). Thromb Res 1985;40: 571-6.
132. Tripodi A, Baglin T, Robert A, Kitchen S, Lisman T, Trotter JF. Reporting prothrombin time results as international normalized ratios for patients with chronic liver disease. Subcommittee on Control of Anticoagulation of the Scientific and Standardisation Committee of the International Society on Thrombosis and Haemostasis. J Thromb Haemost 2010;8:1410-2.
133. Tripodi A, Chantarangkul V, Primignani M, Fabris F, Dell'Era A, Sei C, et al. The international normalized ratio calibrated for cirrhosis [INR(liver)] normalizes prothrombin time results for model for end-stage liver disease calculation. Hepatology 2007; 46:520-7.
134. Tripodi A. Monitoring oral anticoagulant therapy. In: Kitchen S, Olson JD, Preston FE, eds. Quality in laboratory hemostasis and thrombosis, vol 1. Hoboken, NJ: Wiley-Blackwell, 2009.
135. Tripodi A. Tests of coagulation in liver disease. Clin Liver Dis 2009; 13:55-61.
136. Verbruggen B, Novakova I, van Heerde W. Detection and quantifying functional inhibitors in hemostasis. In: Kitchen S, Olson JD, Preston FE, eds. Quality in laboratory hemostasis and thrombosis. Hoboken, NJ: Wiley-Blackwell, 2009:203.
137. Verbruggen B, Novakova I, Wessels H, Boezeman J, van den Berg M, Mauser-Bunschoten E. The Nijmegen modification of the Bethesda assay for factor VIII:C inhibitors: improved specificity and reliability. Thromb Haemost 1995;73:247-51.
138. Warkentin TE, Greinacher A, Koster A, Lincoff AM. Treatment and prevention of heparin-induced thrombocytopenia: American College of Chest Physicians evidence-based clinical practice guidelines, 8th edition. Chest 2008;133:340S-80S.
139. Weigert AL, Schafer AI. Uremic bleeding: pathogenesis and therapy. Am J Med Sci 1998;316:94-104.
140. Wells PS, Anderson JL, Scarvelis DK, Doucette SP, Gagnon F. Factor XIII Val34Leu variant is protective against venous thromboembolism: a HuGE review and meta-analysis. Am J Epidemiol 2006;164:101-9.
141. Welsby IJ, McDonnell E, El-Moalem H, Stafford-Smith M, Toffaletti JG. Activated clotting time systems vary in precision and bias and are not interchangeable when following heparin management protocols during cardiopulmonary bypass. J Clin Monit Comput 2002;17:287-92.
142. White GC 2nd, Rosendaal F, Aledort LM, Lusher JM, Rothschild C, Ingerslev J. Definitions in hemophilia: recommendation of the Scientific Subcommittee on Factor VIII and Factor IX of the Scientific and Standardization Committee of the International Society on Thrombosis and Haemostasis. Thromb Haemost 2001;85:560.
143. White JG. Platelet structure. In: Michelson AD, ed. Platelets. Boston, Mass: Elsevier, 2007:45-73.
144. White JG. The dense bodies of human platelets. In: Meyers KM, Barnes CD, eds. The platelet amine storage granule. Boca Raton, Fla: CRC Press, 1992:31-50.
145. White MM, Foust JT, Mauer AM, Robertson JT, Jennings LK. Assessment of lumiaggregometry for research and clinical laboratories. Thromb Haemost 1992;67:572-7.
146. Yagi H, Ito S, Kato S, Hiura H, Matsumoto M, Fujimura Y. Plasma levels of ADAMTS13 antigen determined with an enzyme immunoassay using a neutralizing monoclonal antibody parallel ADAMTS13 activity levels. Int J Hematol 2007;85:403-7.

SECTION VI

Appendix

CHAPTER 60

Reference Information for the Clinical Laboratory

William L. Roberts, M.D., Ph.D., Gwendolyn A. McMillin, Ph.D., D.A.B.C.C.(C.C., T.C.), Carl A. Burtis, Ph.D., and David E. Bruns, M.D.*

CONTENTS

TABLE 60-1 Reference Intervals and Values

Results of laboratory tests have little practical utility until clinical studies have ascribed various states of health and disease to intervals of values. Reference intervals are useful because they attempt to describe the typical results found in a defined population of apparently healthy people. Different methods may yield different values, depending on calibration and other technical considerations. Hence, different reference intervals and results may be obtained in different laboratories. Variability among methods is particularly characteristic of methods that use antibodies to detect the material of interest, and when results are reported as relative units of activity. Values from apparently "healthy" and diseased people may overlap significantly. Therefore reference intervals, although useful as a guide for clinicians, should not be used as absolute indicators of health and disease (see Chapter 5). The reference intervals presented in this chapter are for **general informational purposes only.** Guidelines for defining and determining reference intervals have been discussed in Chapter 5 and published in the 2010 CLSI C28-A3 guideline ("How to Define and Determine Reference Intervals in the Clinical Laboratory; Approved Guideline—Third Edition"). As stated in several chapters in this textbook, each individual laboratory should generate its own set of reference intervals.

Where both exist, reference intervals are listed in both conventional and international units and are for use in adults in the fasting state unless otherwise stated. Values for other age groups, when included, are clearly identified. Most of the values listed were obtained from chapters in this book. Some were extracted, however, from WU Alan H. B. *Tietz clinical guide to laboratory tests,* 4th edition. Philadelphia, WB Saunders, 2006; and Burtis CA, Ashwood ER, Bruns DE. *Tietz textbook of clinical chemistry and molecular diagnostics,* 4th edition. Philadelphia, WB Saunders, 2006. For several of the specific proteins, reference intervals—obtained after calibration of the analytical system with the international protein reference RPPHS/CRM-470—are listed in Chapter 21.

A valuable source for reference intervals for older methods is http://cclnprod.cc.nih.gov/dlm/testguide.nsf/ (accessed August 18, 2011).

For convenience and to preserve space, we have used standard abbreviations commonly used in laboratory medicine. Less common abbreviations and some nonstandard abbreviations are given below:

Continued

The authors gratefully acknowledge the contributions of Pennell C. Painter, June Y. Cope, and Jane L. Smith upon which portions of this chapter are based.

TABLE 60-1 Reference Intervals and Values—cont'd

Amf	Amniotic fluid
CSF	Cerebrospinal fluid
EDTA	Ethylenediaminetetraacetic acid
F^-	Fluoride ion
F^-/Ox	Fluoride ion and oxalate
Hep	Heparin
Occup. exp.	Occupational exposure
Ox	Oxalate
P	Plasma
Plt	Platelets
RBC	Red blood cells
S	Serum
Sal	Saliva
U	Urine
WB	Whole blood

			Reference Intervals		
Analyte	**Specimen**	**Condition**	**Conventional Units**	**Conversion Factor**	**Si Units**
Acetaldehyde			mg/dL		µmol/L
	WB (F^-/Ox)		<0.2	22.7	<4.5
		Occup. exp.	<0.5		<11.4
		Toxic	1-2		22.7-45.4
Acetylaspartic acid					mmol/mol creatinine
		U			<14
α_1-Acid glycoprotein			mg/dL		g/L
	S	Adult (20-60 y)	50-120	0.01	0.5-1.2
cis-Aconitic acid					mmol/mol creatinine
	U	0-1 mo			5-31
		1-6 mo			10-97
		6 mo-5 y			10-97
		>5 y			3-44
Adipic acid					mmol/mol creatinine
	U	0-6 mo			9-37
		6 mo-5 y			<16
		>5 y			<6
Adipoylcarnitine					mmol/mol creatinine
	U	0-7 d			0.04-0.40
		8 d-7 y			0.01-0.81
		>7 y			0.00-0.13
Adrenocorticotropic hormone			pg/mL		pmol/L
	P, EDTA	Cord	50-570	0.22	11-125
		Newborn	10-185		2.2-41
		Adult (0800-0900)	<120		<26
		Adult (24 h, supine)	<85		<19
Alanine			mg/dL		µmol/L
	P	Premature, 1 d	2.44-4.24	112.2	274-476
		Newborn, 1 d	2.10-3.65		236-410
		1-3 mo	1.19-3.71		134-416
		2-6 mo	1.58-3.68		177-413
		9 mo-2 y	0.88-2.79		99-313
		3-10 y	1.22-2.71		137-305
		6-18 y	1.72-4.85		193-545
		Adult	1.87-5.88		210-661

TABLE 60-1 Reference Intervals and Values—cont'd

Analyte	Specimen	Condition	Reference Intervals: Conventional Units	Conversion Factor	SI Units
Alanine—*cont'd*	U, 24 h		mg/d		µmol/d
		10 d-7 wk	4.1-9.3	11.2	46-104
		3-12 y	9.1-39.2		102-439
		Adult	7.9-48.3		88-541
			µmol/g creatinine		µmol/mol creatinine
		0-1 mo	554-2957	0.113	62.6-334.1
		1-6 mo	613-2874		59.3-324.8
		6 mo-1 y	428-2064		48.4-233.2
		1-2 y	389-1497		44.0-169.2
		2-3 y	255-1726		28.8-195.0
β-Alanine			mg/dL		µmol/L
	P		<0.44	112.2	<49
			<0.26		<29
			mg/d		µmol/d
	U, 24 h	3-16 y	<3.8	11.2	<42
		Adult	<8.3		<93
			mg/g creatinine		mmol/mol creatinine
			11	1.27	14
Alanine aminotransferase	S		U/L		µkat/L
(ALT, SGPT)		Adult male	<45	0.017	<0.77
IFCC, 37 °C		Adult female	<34		<0.58
Albumin			g/dL		g/L
	S	0-4 d	2.8-4.4	10	28-44
		4 d-14 y	3.8-5.4		38-54
		14-18 y	3.2-4.5		32-45
		Adult (20-60 y)	3.5-5.2		35-52
		60-90 y	3.2-4.6		32-46
		>90 y	2.9-4.5		29-45
			mg/d		mg/d
	U, 24 h		3.9-24.4	1	3.9-24.4
			mg/dL		mg/L
	CSF, lumbar		17.7-25.1	10	177-251
Aldolase			U/L		µkat/L
	S	Child			
		10-24 mo	10-40	0.017	0.17-0.68
		25 mo-16 y	5-20		0.09-0.34
		Adult	2.5-10.0		0.04-0.13
Aldosterone			ng/dL		nmol/L
	S	Cord blood	40-200	0.0277	1.11-5.54
		Premature infants	19-141		0.53-3.91
		Full-term infants			
		3 d	7-184		0.19-5.10
		1 wk	5-175		0.03-4.85
		1-12 mo	5-90		0.14-2.49
		1-2 y	7-54		0.19-1.50
		2-10 y (supine)	3-35		0.08-0.97
		2-10 y (upright)	5-80		0.14-2.22
		10-15 y (supine)	2-22		0.06-0.61
		10-15 y (upright)	4-48		0.11-1.33
		Adults			
		(supine)	3-16		0.08-0.44
		(upright)	7-30		0.19-0.83

Continued

TABLE 60-1 Reference Intervals and Values—cont'd

Analyte	Specimen	Condition	Conventional Units	Conversion Factor	Si Units
			REFERENCE INTERVALS		
Aldosterone—*cont'd*	U, 24 h		μg/d	nmol/d	μg/g creatinine
		Newborns (1-3 d)	0.5-5	2.771-14	20-140
		Prepubertal children 4-10 y	1-8	3-22	4-22
		Adults	3-19	8-51	1.5-20
Aluminum			μg/L		μmol/L
	S, P		<5.51	0.0371	<0.2
		Patients on hemodialysis	20-550		0.74-20.4
		Al medication	<30		<1.11
	U		5-30		0.19-1.11
Ammonia nitrogen	P (Hep)		μg N/dL		μmol N/L
		Newborn	90-150	0.714	64-107
		0-2 wk	79-129		56-92
		>1 mo	29-70		21-50
		Adult	15-45		11-32
	U, 24 h		mg N/d		mmol N/d
		Infant	560-2900	0.0714	40-207
		Adult	140-1500		10-107
Amylase	S		U/L		μkat/L
IFCC, 37 °C		Adult	28-100	0.017	0.48-1.70
3α-Androstanediol glucuronide			ng/dL		nmol/L
	S	Child, prepubertal	10-60	0.0213	0.2-1.3
		Adult, M	260-1500		5.5-32
		Adult, F	60-300		1.3-6.4
Androstenedione			ng/dL		nmol/L
	S	Child, prepubertal	<5	0.0349	<0.2
		Adults	75-205		2.6-7.2
		Adult, F postmenopausal	82-275		3.0-9.6
Antidiuretic hormone (ADH)	P, EDTA	mOsm/kg	ng/L		pmol/L
		270-280	<1.5	0.926	<1.4
		280-285	<2.5		<2.3
		285-290	1-5		0.9-4.6
		290-294	2-7		1.9-6.5
		295-300	4-12		3.7-11.1
Antimony		μg/dL			nmol/L
	P (Hep)		0.014-0.090	82.1	1.15-7.39
			μg/L		nmol/L
	U		<10	8.21	<82.1
			mg/L		μmol/L
		Toxic	>1		>8.21
α_1-Antitrypsin	S		mg/dL		g/L
		Adult (20-60 y)	90-200	0.01	0.9-2.0

TABLE 60-1 Reference Intervals and Values—cont'd

Analyte	Specimen	Condition		Conventional Units	Conversion Factor	Si Units
				REFERENCE INTERVALS		
Apolipoprotein A-1				mg/dL		g/L
	S	4-5 y	M	109-172	0.01	1.09-1.72
			F	104-163		1.04-1.63
		6-11 y	M	111-177		1.11-1.77
			F	110-166		1.10-1.66
		12-19 y	M	99-165		0.99-1.65
			F	105-180		1.05-1.80
		20-29 y	M	105-173		1.05-1.73
			F	111-209		1.11-2.09
		30-39 y	M	105-173		1.05-1.73
			F	110-189		1.10-1.89
		40-49 y	M	103-178		1.03-1.78
			F	115-195		1.15-1.95
		50-59 y	M	107-173		1.07-1.73
			F	117-211		1.17-2.11
		60-69 y	M	111-184		1.11-1.84
			F	120-205		1.20-2.05
		>69 y	M	109-180		1.09-1.80
			F	118-199		1.18-1.99
Apolipoprotein B				mg/dL		g/L
	S	4-5 y	M	58-103	0.01	0.58-1.03
			F	58-104		0.58-1.04
		6-11 y	M	56-105		0.56-1.05
			F	57-113		0.57-1.13
		12-19 y	M	55-110		0.55-1.10
			F	53-119		0.53-1.19
		20-29 y	M	59-130		0.59-1.30
			F	59-132		0.59-1.32
		30-39 y	M	63-143		0.63-1.43
			F	70-132		0.70-1.32
		40-49 y	M	71-152		0.71-1.52
			F	75-136		0.75-1.36
		50-59 y	M	75-160		0.75-1.60
			F	75-168		0.75-1.68
		60-69 y	M	81-156		0.81-1.56
			F	75-173		0.75-1.73
		>69 y	M	73-152		0.73-1.52
			F	79-168		0.79-1.68
Arginine				mg/dL		μmol/L
	P	Premature, 1 d		0.17-1.57	57.4	10-90
		Newborn, 1 d		0.38-1.53		22-88
		1-3 mo		0.38-1.30		22-74
		2-6 mo		0.98-2.47		56-142
		9 mo-2 y		0.19-1.13		11-65
		3-10 y		0.40-1.50		23-86
		6-18 y		0.77-2.26		44-130
		Adult		0.37-2.40		21-138
	U, 24 h			mg/d		μmol/d
		10 d-7 wk		<1.2	5.74	<7
		3-12 y		<5.1		<29
		Adult		<50.2		<288
				mg/g creatinine		mmol/mol creatinine
		Adult		0-4	0.65	0-2.7

Continued

TABLE 60-1 Reference Intervals and Values—cont'd

Analyte	Specimen	Condition	Conventional Units	Conversion Factor	Si Units
			Reference Intervals		
Arsenic			μg/L		μmol/L
	WB (Hep)		2-23	0.0133	0.03-0.31
		Chronic poisoning	100-500		1.33-6.65
		Acute poisoning	600-9300		7.98-124
			μg/d		μmol/d
	U, 24 h		5-50		0.07-0.67
Ascorbic acid (see Vitamin C)					
Asparagine			mg/dL		μmol/L
	P	1-3 mo	0.08-0.44	75.7	6-33
		3 mo-6 y	0.95-1.90		72-144
		6-18 y	0.42-0.82		32-62
		Adult	0.40-0.91		30-69
			mg/d		μmol/d
	U, 24 h	Adult	4.5-13.2	7.57	34-100
			mg/g creatinine		mmol/mol creatinine
		Adult	2-10	0.86	1.8-8.6
Aspartate aminotransferase (AST, SGOT) IFCC, 37 °C	S		U/L		μkat/L
		Adult male	<35	0.017	<0.60
		Adult female	<31		<0.53
Aspartic acid			mg/dL		μmol/L
	P	Premature, 1 d	0-0.39	75.1	0-30
		Newborn, 1 d	<0.21		<16
		1-3 mo	0-0.15		0-8
		9 mo-2 y	<0.12		<9
		19 mo-10 y	<0.27		<20
		6-18 y	<0.19		<14
		Adult	<0.32		<24
	U, 24 h		mg/d		μmol/d
		3-12 y	<5.1	7.51	<38
		Adult	<26.2		<197
			mg/g creatinine		mmol/mol creatinine
		Adult	0-4	0.85	0.1-3.7
Azelaic acid					mmol/mol creatinine
	U				<1.1
Beryllium	U, 24 h		μg/L		μmol/L
		Negative	None detected	0.111	None detected
		Toxic	>20		>2.22
Bilirubin			mg/dL		μmol/L
Total	S	Cord (premature)	<2.0	17.1	<34.2
		Cord (full term)	<2.0		<34.2
		0-1 d (premature)	1.0-8.0		17-187
		0-1 d (full term)	2.0-6.0		34-103
		1-2 d (premature)	6.0-12.0		103-205
		1-2 d (full term)	6.0-10.0		103-171
		3-5 d (premature)	10.0-14.0		171-240
		3-5 d (full term)	4.0-8.0		68-137
		Adult	0-2.0		0-34
	U		Negative		Negative

TABLE 60-1 Reference Intervals and Values—cont'd

Analyte	Specimen	Condition	Reference Intervals: Conventional Units	Conversion Factor	SI Units
Bilirubin—*cont'd*	Amf	28 wk	<0.075		<1.28
			ΔA_{450} <0.048		
		40 wk	<0.025		<0.43
			ΔA_{450} <0.02		
Conjugated	S		0.0-0.2		0.0-3.4
Biotin	WB	Healthy			0.5-2.20 nmol/L
		Deficiency			<0.5 nmol/L
BNP (see Chapter 47)					
	U				0.1-2.0
Cadmium	WB (Hep)		μg/L		nmol/L
		Nonsmokers	0.3-1.2	8.897	2.7-10.7
		Smokers	0.6-3.9		5.3-34.7
			μg/L		μmol/L
	U, 24 h	Toxic range	100-3000		0.9-26.7
Calcitonin	S, P		pg/mL		ng/L
		Men	<8.8	1.0	<8.8
		Women	<5.8		<5.8
		Athyroidal	<0.5		<0.5
Calcium, ionized (free)	S, P (Hep)		mg/dL		mmol/L
		Adults	4.6-5.3	0.25	1.15-1.33
Calcium, total	S, P (Hep)		mg/dL		mmol/L
		Adults	8.6-10.2	0.25	2.15-2.55
β-Carotene	S		μg/dL		μmol/L
HPLC			10-85	0.0186	0.19-1.58
Cancer antigen 15-3			U/mL		kU/L
	S		<30	1.0	<30
Cancer antigen 19-9			U/mL		kU/L
	S		<37	1.0	<37
Cancer antigen 27.29			U/mL		kU/L
	S		<37.7	1.0	<37.7
Cancer antigen 50			U/mL		kU/L
	S		<14-20	1.0	<14-20
Cancer antigen 72-4			U/mL		kU/L
	S		<6	1.0	<6
Cancer antigen 125			U/mL		kU/L
	S		<35	1.0	<35
Cancer antigen 242			U/mL		kU/L
	S		<20	1.0	<20
Cancer antigen 549			U/mL		kU/L
	S		<11	1.0	<11
Carbon dioxide, partial pressure			mm Hg		kPa
PCO_2	WB, arterial (Hep)	Newborn	27-40	0.133	3.59-5.32
		Infant	27-41		3.59-5.45
		Adult M	35-48		4.66-6.38
		Adult F	32-45		4.26-5.99
Carbon dioxide, total (tCO_2)			mEq/L		mmol/L
	Cord blood		14-22	1.0	14-22
	P, S	Adult	23-29		23-29
		>60 y	23-31		23-31
		>90 y	20-29		20-29

Continued

TABLE 60-1 Reference Intervals and Values—cont'd

Analyte	Specimen	Condition	Reference Intervals: Conventional Units	Conversion Factor	SI Units
Carbon dioxide, total (tCO_2)—*cont'd*	P, Capillary	Premature, 1 wk	14-27		14-27
		Newborn	13-22		13-22
		Infant	20-28		20-28
		Child	20-28		20-28
		Adult	22-28		22-28
	Whole blood				
	Arterial		19-24		19-24
	Venous		22-26		22-26
Carbon monoxide	WB (EDTA)		% HbCO		HbCO fraction
		Nonsmokers	0.5-1.5	0.01	0.005-0.015
		Smokers			
		1-2 packs/d	4-5		0.04-0.05
		>2 packs/d	8-9		0.08-0.09
		Toxic	>20		>0.20
		Lethal	>50		>0.5
Carcinoembryonic antigen (CEA)			ng/mL		μg/L
	S	Nonsmokers	<3	1.0	<3
		Smokers	<5		<5
Catecholamines					
Epinephrine	P	Adults	pg/mL		pmol/L
		Supine (30 min)	<50	5.46	<273
		Sitting (15 min)	<60		<328
		Standing (30 min)	<90		<491
Norepinephrine	P	Adults	pg/mL		pmol/L
		Supine (30 min)	110-410	5.91	650-2423
		Sitting (15 min)	120-680		709-4019
		Standing (30 min)	125-700		739-4137
Dopamine	P	Adults	pg/mL		pmol/L
		Supine (30 min)	<87	6.53	<475
		Sitting (15 min)	<87		<475
		Standing (30 min)	<87		<475
Epinephrine	U, 24 h		μg/d		nmol/d
		0-1 y	0-2.5	5.46	0-14
		1-2 y	0-3.5		0-19
		2-4 y	0-6.0		0-33
		4-7 y	0.2-10		1-55
		7-10 y	0.2-10		1-55
		10-15 y	0.5-20		3-109
		>15 y	0.5-20		3-109
Norepinephrine	U, 24 h		μg/d		nmol/d
		0-1 y	0-10	5.91	0-59
		1-2 y	1-17		6-100
		2-4 y	4-29		24-171
		4-7 y	8-45		47-266
		7-10 y	13-65		77-384
		10-15 y	15-80		89-473
		>15 y	15-80		89-473
Dopamine	U, 24 h		μg/d		nmol/d
		0-1 y	0-85	6.53	0-555
		1-2 y	10-140		65-914
		2-4 y	40-260		261-1697
		4-7 y	65-400		424-2612
		7-10 y	65-400		424-2612
		10-15 y	65-400		424-2612
		>15 y	65-400		424-2612

TABLE 60-1 Reference Intervals and Values—cont'd

Analyte	Specimen	Condition		Conventional Units	Conversion Factor	Si Units
				REFERENCE INTERVALS		
Ceruloplasmin				mg/L		g/L
	P	Cord (term)		50-330	0.001	0.050-0.33
		Birth-4 mo		150-560		0.15-0.56
		5-6 mo		260-830		0.26-0.83
		7-36 mo		310-900		0.31-0.90
		4-12 y		250-450		0.25-0.45
		13-19 y (male)		150-370		0.15-0.37
		13-19 y (female)		220-500		0.22-0.50
		Adult (male		220-400		0.22-0.40
		Adult (female) no contraceptive		250-600		0.25-0.60
		Adult (female) contraceptives (estrogen)		270-660		0.27-0.66
		Adult, pregnant female		300-1200		0.30-1.20
				mg/dL		g/L
	S	Adult (20-60 y)		20-60	0.01	0.2-0.6
Chloride (Cl)	S, P			mEq/L		mmol/L
		Cord		96-104	1.0	96-104
		Premature		95-110		95-110
		0-30 d		98-113		98-113
		Adult		98-107		98-107
		>90 y		98-111		98-111
				mEq/d		mmol/d
	U, 24 h	Infant		2-10		2-10
		Child <6 y		15-40		15-40
		6-10 y				
		M		36-110		36-110
		F		18-74		18-74
		10-14 y				
		M		64-176		64-176
		F		36-173		36-173
		Adult		110-250		110-250
		>60 y		95-195		95-195
	Sweat (iontophoresis)			mEq/L		mmol/L
		Normal		5-35		5-35
		Marginal		30-70		30-70
		Cystic fibrosis		60-200		60-200
Cholesterol				mg/dL 5th-95th percentile		mmol/L 5th-95th percentile
	S	0-4 y	M	114-203	0.0259	2.96-5.26
			F	112-200		2.90-5.18
		5-9 y	M	125-189		3.23-4.89
			F	131-197		3.39-5.10
		10-14 y	M	124-204		3.21-5.29
			F	125-205		3.24-5.31
		15-19 y	M	118-191		3.06-4.95
			F	119-208		3.08-5.39
		20-24 y	M	118-212		3.06-5.49
			F	121-237		3.14-6.14

Continued

TABLE 60-1 Reference Intervals and Values—cont'd

Analyte	Specimen	Condition		Conventional Units	Conversion Factor	Si Units
				Reference Intervals		
Cholesterol—*cont'd*		25-29 y	M	130-234		3.37-6.06
			F	130-231		3.37-5.99
		30-34 y	M	142-258		3.68-6.68
			F	133-227		3.45-5.87
		35-39 y	M	147-267		3.81-6.92
			F	139-249		3.60-6.45
		40-44 y	M	150-260		3.89-6.74
			F	146-259		3.78-6.71
		45-49 y	M	163-275		4.22-7.12
			F	148-268		3.83-6.94
		50-54 y	M	156-274		4.04-7.10
			F	163-281		4.22-7.28
		55-59 y	M	161-280		4.17-7.25
			F	167-294		4.33-7.61
		60-64 y	M	163-287		4.22-7.43
			F	172-300		4.46-7.77
		65-69 y	M	166-288		4.30-7.46
			F	167-291		4.33-7.54
		>69 y	M	144-265		3.73-6.87
			F	173-280		4.48-7.25
	Coronary heart disease risk					
	Child	Desirable		<170		<4.4
		Borderline high		170-199		4.40-5.15
		High		>199		>5.15
	Adult	Desirable		<200		<5.18
		Borderline high		200-239		5.18-6.19
		High		>239		>6.19
Cholinesterase (37 °C)				U/L		µkat/L
	S	Male		40-78	0.017	0.68-1.33
		Female		33-76		0.56-1.29
Chorionic gonadotropin intact molecule				mIU/mL		IU/L
	S	Male and nonpregnant female		<5.0	1.0	<5.0
		Female				
		Pregnancy (weeks of gestation)				
		4 wk		5-100		5-100
		5 wk		200-3000		200-3000
		6 wk		10,000-80,000		10,000-80,000
		7-14 wk		90,000-500,000		90,000-500,000
		15-26 wk		5000-80,000		5000-80,000
		27-40 wk		3000-15,000		3000-15,000
				Values based on the Second International Standard for CG		
		Trophoblastic disease		>100,000		>100,000

TABLE 60-1 Reference Intervals and Values—cont'd

Analyte	Specimen	Condition	Reference Intervals: Conventional Units	Conversion Factor	SI Units
Chorionic gonadotropin intact molecule—*cont'd*	U		Negative One half of pregnancies are detected on the first day of the missed menstrual period		Negative One half of pregnancies are detected on the first day of the missed menstrual period
Chromium			μg/L		nmol/L
	WB (Hep)		0.7-28.0	19.23	14-538
	S		0.1-0.2		2-3
			μg/d		nmol/d
	U, 24 h		0.1-2.0		1.9-38.4
			μg/L		nmol/L
	RBC		20-36		384-692
Chymotrypsin (37 °C)	F		12 U/g stool	1	12 U/g stool
trans-Cinnamoylglycine					mmol/mol creatinine
	U				0.1-8.0
Citric acid					mmol/mol creatinine
	U	0-1 mo			<1046
		1-6 mo			104-268
		6 mo-5 y			0-656
		>5 y			87-639
Cobalt			μg/L		nmol/L
	S		0.11-0.45	16.97	1.9-7.6
	U		1-2		17.0-34.0
			μg/kg		nmol/kg
	RBC		16-46		272-781
Complement C3	S		mg/dL		g/L
		Adult (20-60 y)	90-180	0.01	0.9-1.8
Complement C4	S		mg/dL		g/L
		Adult (20-60 y)	10-40		0.1-0.4
Copper	S		μg/dL		μmol/L
		Birth-6 mo	20-70	0.157	3.14-10.99
		Deficiency	<30		<5
		6 y	90-190		14.13-29.83
		12 y	80-160		12.56-25.12
		Adult			
		Male	70-140		10.99-21.98
		Female	80-155		12.56-24.34
		Deficiency	50		8
		Pregnancy, at term	118-302		18.53-47.41
		Blacks	Blacks 8-12% higher		Blacks 8-12% higher
	U, 24 h	Adults	<60 μg/24 h	0.0157	1.0 μmol/24 h
		Wilson disease	>200 μg/24 h		>3 μmol/24 h

Continued

TABLE 60-1 Reference Intervals and Values—cont'd

			Reference Intervals		
Analyte	**Specimen**	**Condition**	**Conventional Units**	**Conversion Factor**	**SI Units**
Cortisol, free			μg/dL		nmol/L
	S	0800 h	0.6-1.6	27.6	17-44
		1600 h	0.2-0.9		6-25
			ng/mL		nmol/L
	Sal	0700 h	1.4-10.1	2.76	4-30
		2200 h	0.7-2.2		2-6
			μg/d		nmol/d
	U, 24 h	Child			
		1-10 y	2-27		6-74
		2-11 y	1-21		3-58
		11-20 y	5-55		14-152
		12-16 y	2-38		6-105
		Adult			
		Extracted	20-90		55-248
		Unextracted	75-270		207-745
Cortisol, total			μg/dL		nmol/L
	S	Cord blood	5-17	27.6	138-469
		Infant (1-7 d)	2-11		55-304
		Child (1-16 y)			
		0800 h	3-21		83-580
		Adult			
		0800 h	5-23		138-635
		1600 h	3-16		83-441
		2000 h	<50% of 0800 values		<50% of 0800 values
CKMB, mass (see Chapter 47)					
C-reactive protein (CRP)	S		mg/dL		mg/L
		Adult (20-60 y)	<0.5	10	<5
CRP (high-sensitivity)	S		mg/L		mg/L
		American males	0.3-8.6	1.0	0.3-8.6
		White American males	0.2-12.3		0.2-12.3
		African American males	0.1-8.2		0.1-8.2
		Mexican American males	0.2-6.3		0.2-6.3
		European males	0.3-8.6		0.3-8.6
		Japanese males	<7.8		<7.8
		American females	0.2-9.1		0.2-9.1
		European females	0.3-8.8		0.3-8.8
Creatine kinase (CK)	S		U/L		μkat/L
IFCC, 37 °C		Male	46-171	0.017	0.78-2.90
		Female	34-145		0.58-2.47
Creatine kinase isoenzymes	S	Fraction 2 (MB)	<5.0 μg/L	1.0	<5.0 μg/L
		Relative index	<3.9%	0.01	<0.039
		MB/total CK			Fractional activity
Creatine kinase isoforms	S		% Total activity		Fractional activity
		CK-3_1	42-75	0.01	0.42-0.75
		CK-3_2	18-51		0.18-0.51
		CK-3_3	2-14		0.02-0.14

TABLE 60-1 Reference Intervals and Values—cont'd

Analyte	Specimen	Condition	Reference Intervals: Conventional Units	Reference Intervals: Conversion Factor	Reference Intervals: Si Units
Creatinine					
Enzymatic	S		mg/dL		μmol/L
		0-1 y	0.04-0.33		4-29
		2-5 y	0.04-0.45		4-40
		6-9 y	0.20-0.52		18-46
		10 y	0.22-0.59		19-52
		Adult male	0.62-1.10		55-96
		Adult female	0.45-0.75		40-66
Jaffe	S		mg/dL		μmol/L
		Cord	0.6-1.2	88.4	53-106
		Newborn (1-4 d)	0.3-1.0		27-88
		Infant	0.2-0.4		18-35
		Child	0.3-0.7		27-62
		Adolescent	0.5-1.0		44-88
		18-60 y			
		Male	0.9-1.3		80-115
		Female	0.6-1.1		53-97
		60-90 y			
		Male	0.8-1.3		71-115
		Female	0.6-1.2		53-106
		>90 y			
		Male	1.0-1.7		88-150
		Female	0.6-1.3		53-115
Jaffe, manual	U, 24 h		mg/kg/d		μmol/kg/d
		Infant	8-20	8.84	71-177
		Child	8-22		71-194
		Adolescent	8-30		71-265
		Adult			
		Male	14 26		124-230
		Female	11-20		97-177
Creatinine clearance (see Glomerular filtration rate)					
C-Telopeptide	S		ng/L		ng/L
		Men	<1009	1.0	<1009
		Premenopausal women	<574		<574
			mg/mol creatinine		mg/mol creatinine
	U	Men	0-505		0-505
		Premenopausal women	0-476		0-476
Cyanide	WB (Ox)		mg/L		μmol/L
		Nonsmokers	<0.2	38.5	<7.7
		Smokers	<0.4		<15.4
		Nitroprusside therapy	Up to 100 without toxicity		Up to 3850
		Toxic	>1		>38.5

Continued

TABLE 60-1 Reference Intervals and Values—cont'd

Analyte	Specimen	Condition	Reference Intervals: Conventional Units	Conversion Factor	Si Units
Cystine			mg/dL		μmol/L
	S	Premature, 1 d	0.54-1.02	83.3	45-85
		Newborn, 1 d	0.43-1.01		36-84
		1-3 mo	0.15-1.15		13-96
		2-6 mo	0.64-0.97		53-81
		3-10 y	0.54-0.92		45-77
		6-18 y	0.43-0.70		36-58
		Adult	0.40-1.40		33-117
	U, 24 h		mg/d		μmol/d
		10 d-7 wk	2.16-3.37	8.33	18-28
		3-12 y	4.9-30.9		41-257
		Adult	<38.1		<317
			mg/g creatinine		mmol/mol creatinine
		Adult	2-14	0.94	1.9-13.1
Dehydroepiandrosterone, unconjugated			ng/dL		nmol/L
	S	Children			
		6-9 y, M	13-187	0.0347	0.45-6.49
		6-9 y, F	18-189		0.62-6.55
		10-11 y, M	31-205		1.07-7.11
		10-11 y, F	112-224		3.88-7.77
		12-14 y, M	83-258		2.88-8.95
		12-14 y, F	98-360		3.40-12.5
		Adult			
		M	180-1250		6.25-43.4
		F	130-980		4.51-34.0
Dehydroepiandrosterone sulfate			μg/dL		μmol/L
	S	Children			
		1-5 d, M	12-254	0.027	0.3-6.9
		1-5 d, F	10-248		0.3-6.7
		1 mo-5 y, M	1-41		0.03-1.1
		1 mo-5 y, F	5-55		0.1-1.5
		6-9 y, M	2.5-145		0.07-3.9
		6-9 y, F	2.5-140		0.07-3.8
		10-11 y, M	15-115		0.4-3.1
		10-11 y, F	15-260		0.4-7.0
		12-17 y, M	20-555		0.5-15.0
		12-17 y, F	20-535		0.5-14.4
		Pubertal levels, Tanner stage			
		1 M	5-265		0.1-7.2
		1 F	5-125		0.1-3.4
		2 M	15-380		0.4-10.3
		2 F	15-150		0.4-4.0
		3 M	60-505		1.6-13.6
		3 F	20-535		0.5-14.4
		4 M	65-560		1.8-15.1
		4 F	35-485		0.9-13.1
		5 M	165-500		4.4-13.5
		5 F	75-530		2.0-14.3

TABLE 60-1 Reference Intervals and Values—cont'd

Analyte	Specimen	Condition	REFERENCE INTERVALS Conventional Units	Conversion Factor	Si Units
Dehydroepiandrosterone sulfate—*cont'd*		Adults			
		18-30 y, M	125-619		3.4-16.7
		18-30 y, F	45-380		1.2-10.3
		31-50 y, M	5-532		1.6-12.2
		31-50 y, F	12-379		0.8-10.2
		51-60 y, M	20-413		0.5-11.1
		61-83 y, M	10-285		0.3-7.7
		Postmenopausal F	30-260		0.8-7.0
11-Deoxycortisol			ng/dL		nmol/L
	S	Cord blood	295-554	0.0289	9-16
		Children and adults	20-158		0.6-4.6
Deoxypyridinoline			μmol/mol creatinine		μmol/mol creatinine
	U	Men	2.3-5.4	1.0	2.3-5.4
		Premenopausal women	3.0-7.4		3.0-7.4
Dihydrotestosterone			ng/dL		nmol/L
	S	Child, prepubertal	<3	0.0344	<0.10
		Adult, M	30-85		1.03-2.92
		Adult, F	4-22		0.14-0.76
Dodecanedioic acid					mmol/mol creatinine
	U				<0.06
Dopamines	P, S	Normotensive adults	pg/mL		nmol/L
L-Dopa (L-dodecenoylcarnitine)			1042-2366	0.0051	5.3-12.0
DOPAC (3, 4-dihydroxyphenylacetic acid)			674-2636	0.0059	4.0-15.7
DHPG (3, 4-dihydroxyphenylglycol)			797-1208	0.0059	4.7-7.1
DU-PAN-2			U/mL		kU/L
			<401	1.0	<401
Estradiol			pg/mL		pmol/L
	S	Children			
		1-5 y, M	3-10	3.69	11-37
		1-5 y, F	5-10		18-37
		6-9 y, M	3-10		11-37
		6-9 y, F	5-60		18-220
		10-11 y, M	5-10		18-37
		10-11 y, F	5-300		18-1100
		12-14 y, M	5-30		18-110
		12-14 y, F	24-410		92-1505
		15-17 y, M	5-45		18-165
		12-17 y, F	40-410		147-1505
		Adults			
		M	10-50		37-184
		F			
		Early follicular phase	20-150		73-550
		Late follicular phase	40-350		147-1285
		Midcycle	150-750		550-2753
		Luteal phase	30-450		110-1652
		Postmenopausal	<21		<74

Continued

TABLE 60-1 Reference Intervals and Values—cont'd

			REFERENCE INTERVALS		
Analyte	**Specimen**	**Condition**	**Conventional Units**	**Conversion Factor**	**Si Units**
Estradiol—*cont'd*		Pubertal levels, Tanner stage			
		1, M	3-15		11-35
		1, F	5-10		18-37
		2, M	3-10		11-37
		2, F	5-115		18-422
		3, M	5-15		18-55
		3, F	5-180		18-660
		4, M	3-40		11-147
		4, F	25-345		92-1267
		5, M	15-45		55-165
		5, F	25-410		92-1505
Estriol, free (unconjugated, uE_3)			ng/mL		nmol/L
	S	Males and nonpregnant females	<2.0	3.47	<6.9
		Pregnancy (weeks of gestation)			
		16	0.30-1.05		1.04-3.64
		18	0.63-2.30		2.19-7.98
		34	5.3-18.3		18.4-63.5
		35	5.2-26.4		18.0-91.6
		36	8.2-28.1		28.4-97.5
		37	8.0-30.1		27.8-104.0
		38	8.6-38.0		29.8-131.9
		39	7.2-34.3		25.0-119.0
		40	9.6-28.9		33.3-100.3
	Amf	Pregnancy (weeks of gestation)			
		16-20	1.0-3.2		3.5-11
		20-24	2.1-7.8		7.3-27
		24-28	2.1-7.8		7.3-27
		28-32	4.0-13.6		14-47
		32-36	3.6-15.5		12-54
		36-38	4.6-18.0		16-62
		38-40	5.4-19.8		19-69
Estriol, total (E_3)			ng/mL		nmol/L
	S	Pregnancy (weeks of gestation)			
		34	38-140	3.47	132-486
		35	31-140		108-486
		36	35-330		121-1145
		37	45-260		156-902
		38	48-350		167-1215
		39	59-570		205-1978
		40	95-460		330-1596

TABLE 60-1 Reference Intervals and Values—cont'd

Analyte	Specimen	Condition	Conventional Units	Conversion Factor	SI Units
			Reference Intervals		
Estriol, total (E_3)—*cont'd*			μg/d		nmol/d
	U, 24 h	Male	1.0-11.0	3.47	3.5-38.2
		Female			
		Follicular phase	0-15.0		0-52.0
		Ovulatory phase	13.0-54.0		45.1-187.4
		Luteal phase	8.0-60.0		27.8-208.2
		Postmenopausal	0-11.0		0-38.2
		Pregnancy			
		1st trimester	0-800		0-2776
		2nd trimester	800-12,000		2776-41,640
		3rd trimester	5000-50,000		17,350-173,500
			ng/mL		nmol/L
	Amf	Weeks of gestation			
		21-32	5-50		17-174
		33-35	90-240		312-833
		36-41	150-213		521-739
Estrone			pg/mL		pmol/L
	S	Male	15-65	3.69	55-240
		Female	15-150		55-555
		Early follicular phase	100-250		370-925
		Late follicular phase			
		Luteal phase	15-200		55-740
		Postmenopausal	15-55		55-204
Ethanol	WB (Ox)		mg/dL		mmol/L
		Impairment	50-100	0.217	11-22
		Depression of CNS	>100		>21.7
		Fatalities reported	>400		>86.8
Ethylmalonic acid					mmol/mol creatinine
	U				0.4-17
Ferritin	S		ng/mL		μg/L
		Newborn	25-200	1.0	25-200
		1 mo	200-600		200-600
		2-5 mo	50-200		50-200
		6 mo-15 y	7-140		7-140
		Adult			
		Male	20-250		20-250
		Female	10-120		10-120
α-Fetoprotein (AFP)	S		mg/L		g/L
		Fetal, 1st trimester	200-400	0.01	2.0-4.0
		Cord blood	<5		<0.05
			ng/mL		μg/L
		Child, 1 y	<30	1.0	<30
		Adult (85% of population)	<8.5		<8.5
		Adult (100% of population)	<15		<15

Continued

TABLE 60-1 Reference Intervals and Values—cont'd

			Reference Intervals		
Analyte	**Specimen**	**Condition**	**Conventional Units**	**Conversion Factor**	**Si Units**
α-Fetoprotein (AFP)—*cont'd*			ng/mL		μg/L
	Maternal serum	Weeks of gestation	(median)		(median)
		14	25.6		25.6
		15	29.9		29.9
		16	34.8		34.8
		17	40.6		40.6
		18	47.3		47.3
		19	55.1		55.1
		20	64.3		64.3
		21	74.9		74.9
	S	Tumor marker	ng/mL		μg/L
		Early marker	10-20		10-20
		Cancer	>1000		>1000
			μg/mL		mg/L
	Amf	Weeks of gestation	(median)		(median)
		15	16.3		16.3
		16	14.5		14.5
		17	13.4		13.4
		18	12.0		12.0
		19	10.7		10.7
		20	8.1		8.1
Fluoride	S		mg/L		μmol/L
			0.2-3.2	52.6	10.5-168
Folate			μg/L		nmol/L
	S		2.6-12.2	2.265	6.0-28.0
	Erythrocyte		103-411		237-948
	S Deficiency		<1.4		<3.2
	Erythrocyte deficiency		<110		<252
Follicle-stimulating hormone (FSH)			mIU/mL		IU/L
	S	Males (23-70 y)	1.4-15.4	1.0	1.4-15.4
		Female			
		Follicular phase	1.4-9.9		1.4-9.9
		Midcycle peak	0.2-17.2		0.2-17.2
		Luteal phase	1.1-9.2		1.1-9.2
		Postmenopausal	19.3-100.6		19.3-100.6
Fructosamine	S	Child	5% below adult levels		
		Adult	205-285 μmol/L	1.0	205-285 μmol/L
Fumaric acid					mmol/mol creatinine
	U	0-1 mo			10-45
		1-6 mo			4-45
		6 mo-5 y			1-27
		>5 y			2-4

TABLE 60-1 Reference Intervals and Values—cont'd

Analyte	Specimen	Condition	Reference Intervals: Conventional Units	Conversion Factor	SI Units
Glomerular filtration rate (endogenous)			mL/ min/1.73 m^2		mL/s/m^2
	S or P and U	Males			
		17-24 y	93-131	0.00963	0.90-1.26
		25-34 y	78-146		0.75-1.41
		35-44 y	74-138		0.71-1.33
		45-54 y	74-129		0.72-1.24
		55-64 y	69-122		0.67-1.18
		65-74 y	61-114		0.59-1.10
		75-84 y	52-102		0.50-0.98
		Females			
		40-49 y	65-123		0.63-1.19
		50-59 y	58-110		0.56-1.06
		60-69 y	50-111		0.48-1.07
		70-79 y	46-105		0.44-1.01
		80+ y	48-85		0.46-0.82
Glucagon			ng/L		ng/L
	P (Hep or EDTA)	Adult	70-180	1.0	70-180
	Amf	Midgestation	23-63		23-63
		Term	41-193		41-193
Glucose	S, fasting		mg/dL		mmol/L
		Cord	45-96	0.0555	2.5-5.3
		Premature	20-60		1.1-3.3
		Neonate	30-60		1.7-3.3
		Newborn			
		1 d	40-60		2.2-3.3
		>1 d	50-80		2.8-4.5
		Child	60-100		3.3-5.6
		Adult	74-100		4.1-5.6
		>60 y	82-115		4.6-6.4
		>90 y	75-121		4.2-6.7
	WB (Hep)	Adult	65-95		3.5-5.3
	CSF	Infant, child	60-80		3.3-4.5
		Adult	40-70		2.2-3.9
	U		1-15		0.1-0.8
	U, 24 h		<0.5 g/d	5.55	<2.8 mmol/d
Glucose-6-phosphate dehydrogenase (G-6-PD) in erythrocytes, WHO, and ICSH	WB (ACD, EDTA, or Hep)		7.9-16.3 U/g Hb	64.5	510-1050 U/ mmol Hb
			230-470 U/10^{12} RBC	10^{-3}	0.23-0.47 nU/ RBC
			2.69-5.53 U/ mL RBC	1.0	2.69-5.53 kU/L RBC
Glutamic acid			mg/dL		µmol/L
	P	Premature, 1 d	0-1.98	68.0	0-135
		Newborn, 1 d	0.29-1.57		20-107
		6 mo-3 y	0.28-1.47		19-100
		3-10 y	0.34-3.68		23-250
		6-18 y	0.10-0.96		7-65
		Adult	0.21-2.82		14-192

Continued

TABLE 60-1 Reference Intervals and Values—cont'd

			REFERENCE INTERVALS		
Analyte	**Specimen**	**Condition**	**Conventional Units**	**Conversion Factor**	**Si Units**
Glutamic acid—*cont'd*	U, 24 h		mg/d		μmol/d
		10 d-7 wk	0.3-1.5	6.80	2-10
		Adult	<33.8		<230
			mg/g creatinine		mmol/mol creatinine
		Adult	2-6	0.77	1.5-4.7
Glutamine	P		mg/dL		μmol/L
		3 mo-6 y	6.93-10.89	68.5	475-746
		6-18 y	5.26-10.80		360-740
		Adult	5.78-10.38		396-711
	U, 24 h		mg/d		μmol/d
		10 d-7 wk	12.4-25.8	6.85	85-177
		3-12 y	20.4-113.7		140-779
		Adult	43.8-151.8		300-1040
			mg/g creatinine		mmol/mol creatinine
		Adult	2-78	0.77	2-60
γ-Glutamyltransferase IFCC, 37 °C	S		U/L		μkat/L
		Male	<55	0.017	<0.94
		Female	<38		<0.65
Glutaric acid					mmol/mol creatinine
	U				0.5-13
Glycated hemoglobin (HbA_{1c})			% Total Hb		Hb fraction
	WB (EDTA, Hep, or Ox)	Cut off for diagnosis	<6.5 (NGSP)		<6.5
			4-5.6		4-5.6
Glyceric acid					mmol/mol creatinine
	U	0-1 mo			<40
		1-6 mo			<185
		6 mo-5 y			<71
		>5 y			<61
Glycine			mg/dL		μmol/L
	P	Premature 1 d	0-7.57	133.3	0-1010
		Newborn 1 d	1.68-3.86		224-514
		1-3 mo	0.79-1.67		106-222
		2-6 mo	1.31-2.22		175-296
		9 mo-2 y	0.42-2.31		56-308
		3-10 y	0.88-1.67		117-223
		6-18	1.18-2.27		158-302
		Adult	0.90-4.16		120-554
			mg/d		μmol/d
	U, 24 h	10 d-7 wk	14.6-59.2	13.3	194-787
		3-12 y	12.4-106.8		165-1420
		Adult	59.0-294.6		785-3918
			mg/g creatinine		mmol/mol creatinine
		Adult	12-108	1.51	18.2-163
Glycolic acid					mmol/mol creatinine
	U	0-1 mo			<63
		1-6 mo			<105
		6 mo-5 y			3-121
		>5 y			<167

TABLE 60-1 Reference Intervals and Values—cont'd

Analyte	Specimen	Condition		Conventional Units (Reference Intervals)	Conversion Factor (Reference Intervals)	Si Units (Reference Intervals)
Glyoxylic acid						mmol/mol creatinine
	U	0-1 mo				<14
		1-6 mo				<17
		6 mo-5 y				<8
		>5 y				<10
Growth hormone	S			ng/mL		µg/L
		Basal		2-5	1.0	2-5
		Insulin tolerance test		>10		>10
		Arginine		>7.5		>7.5
		L-Dopa		>7.5		>7.5
Haptoglobin	S			mg/dL		g/L
		Children		20-160	0.01	0.2-1.6
		Adult (20-60 y)		30-200		0.3-2.0
High-density lipoprotein cholesterol (HDL-C)				mg/dL		mmol/L
				5th-95th percentile		5th-95th percentile
	S	5-9 y	M	38-75	0.0259	0.99-1.94
			F	36-73		0.93-1.89
		10-14 y	M	37-74		0.96-1.92
			F	37-70		0.96-1.82
		15-19 y	M	30-63		0.78-1.63
			F	35-74		0.91-1.92
		20-24 y	M	30-63		0.78-1.63
			F	33-79		0.86-2.05
		25-29 y	M	31-63		0.81-1.63
			F	37-83		0.96-2.15
		30-34 y	M	28-63		0.73-1.63
			F	36-77		0.94-2.00
		35-39 y	M	29-62		0.75-1.61
			F	34-82		0.88-2.13
		40-44 y	M	27-67		0.70-1.74
			F	34-88		0.88-2.28
		45-49 y	M	30-64		0.78-1.66
			F	34-87		0.88-2.26
		50-54 y	M	28-63		0.73-1.63
			F	37-92		0.96-2.39
		55-59 y	M	28-71		0.73-1.84
			F	37-91		0.96-2.36
		60-64 y	M	30-74		0.78-1.92
			F	38-92		0.99-2.39
		65-69 y	M	30-75		0.78-1.95
			F	35-96		0.91-2.49
		>69 y	M	31-75		0.80-1.95
			F	33-92		0.86-2.39
	ATP III classification			mg/dL		g/L
	S	Low		<40	0.01	<0.40
		High		>59		>0.59

Continued

TABLE 60-1 Reference Intervals and Values—cont'd

			Reference Intervals		
Analyte	**Specimen**	**Condition**	**Conventional Units**	**Conversion Factor**	**Si Units**
Histidine			mg/dL		μmol/L
	P	Premature, 1 d	0.16-1.40	64.5	10-90
		Newborn, 1 d	0.76-1.77		49-114
		1-3 mo	0.66-1.30		43-83
		2-6 mo	1.49-2.12		96-137
		9 mo-2 y	0.37-1.74		24-112
		3-10 y	0.37-1.32		24-85
		6-18 y	0.99-1.64		64-106
		Adult	0.50-1.66		32-107
	U, 24 h		mg/d		μmol/d
		10 d-7 wk	16.0-38.6	6.45	103-249
		3-12 y	47.4-199.2		306-1285
		Adult	72.9-440.8		470-2843
			mg/g creatinine		mmol/mol creatinine
		Adult	1-141	0.73	1-103
Homocysteine, total			μmol/L		μmol/L
	S, P	Folate supplemented diet			
		<15 y	<8	1.0	<8
		15-65 y	<12		<12
		>65 y	<16		<16
		No folate supplementation			
		<15 y	<10		<10
		15-65 y	<15		<15
		>65 y	<20		<20
Homogentisic acid					mmol/mol creatinine
	U				<11
Homovanillic acid (HVA)	U, 24 h		mg/d		μmol/d
		3-6 y	1.4-4.3	5.49	8-24
		6-10 y	2.1-4.7		12-26
		10-16 y	2.4-8.7		13-48
		16-83 y	1.4-8.8		8-48
	U		mg/g creatinine		mmol/mol creatinine
		0-6 mo	<40	0.571	<23
		6 mo-5 y	<10		<6
		3-6 y	5.4-15.5		3.4-9.6
		6-10 y	4.4-11.5		2.7-7.1
		10-16 y	3.3-10.3		2.0-6.4
3-Hydroxybutyric acid					mmol/mol creatinine
	U	0-5 y			<6
		>5 y			<11
2-Hydroxyglutaric acid					mmol/mol creatinine
	U				<16
5-Hydroxyindoleacetic acid			ng/L		nmol/L
	P		5.2-13.4	5.23	27-70

TABLE 60-1 Reference Intervals and Values—cont'd

			Reference Intervals		
Analyte	**Specimen**	**Condition**	**Conventional Units**	**Conversion Factor**	**Si Units**
5-Hydroxyindoleacetic acid—*cont'd*			mg/g creatinine		mmol/mol creatinine
	U	0-5 y	<21	0.592	<13
		>5 y	<16		<10
4-Hydroxyphenyllactic acid					mmol/mol creatinine
	U	0-1 mo			<51
		>1 mo			<11
4-Hydroxyphenylpyruvic acid					mmol/mol creatinine
	U	0-1 mo			<21
		>1 mo			<6
17-Hydroxyprogesterone			ng/dL		nmol/L
		Cord blood	900-5000	0.03	27.3-151.5
		Premature	26-568		0.8-17.0
		Newborn, 3 d	7-77		0.2-2.7
		Prepubertal child	3-90		0.1-2.7
		Puberty			
		Tanner stage			
		1. Male	3-90		0.1-2.7
		Female	3-82		0.1-2.5
		2. Male	5-115		0.2-3.5
		Female	11-98		0.3-3.0
		3. Male	10-139		0.3-4.2
		Female	11-155		0.3-4.7
		4. Male	29-180		0.9-5.4
		Female	18-230		0.5-7.0
		5. Male	24-175		0.7-5.3
		Female	20-267		0.6-8.0
		Adults			
		Male	27-199		0.8-6.0
		Female			
		Follicular phase	15-70		0.4-2.1
		Luteal phase	35-290		1.0-8.7
		Pregnancy[186]	200-1200		6.0-36.0
		Post ACTH	<320		<9.6
		Postmenopausal	<70		<2.1
Hydroxyproline			mg/dL		μmol/L
	P	Premature, 1 d	0-1.56	76.3	0-120
		6-18 y (M)	<0.66		<50
		6-18 y (F)	<0.58		<44
		Adult (M)	<0.55		<42
		Adult (F)	<0.45		<34
			mg/d		μmol/d
	U, 24 h	Adult	<1.4	7.63	<11
			μg/g creatinine		mmol/mol creatinine
		Adult	19-36	0.863	16-31
Immunoglobulin A			mg/dL		g/L
	S	Neonate (4 d)	0-2.2	0.01	0.0-0.02
		Adult (20-60 y)	70-400		0.7-4.0
		Adult (>60 y)	90-410		0.9-4.1

Continued

TABLE 60-1 Reference Intervals and Values—cont'd

Analyte	Specimen	Condition	Reference Intervals: Conventional Units	Conversion Factor	Si Units
Immunoglobulin A—*cont'd*	CSF		0.0-0.6		0.0-0.006
	Saliva		<11		<0.11
Immunoglobulin D			IU/mL		kIU/L
	S	Adult (20-60 y)	0-160	1.0	0-160
			ng/mL		μg/L
			0-384	1.0	0-384
Immunoglobulin E			kIU/L		μg/L
	S	Adult (20-60 y)	0-160	2.4	0-380
Immunoglobulin G			mg/dL		g/L
	S	Newborn (4 d)	700-1480	0.01	7.0-14.8
		Adult (20-60 y)	700-1600		7.0-16.0
		Adult (>60 y)	600-1560		6.0-15.6
	CSF		0-5.5		0-0.055
Immunoglobulin M			mg/dL		g/L
	S	Newborn (4 d)	5-30	0.01	0.05-0.30
		Adult (20-60 y)	40-230		0.4-2.3
		Adult (>60 y)	30-360		0.3-3.6
	CSF		0.0-1.3		0.0-0.013
Inhibin A			pg/mL		ng/L
	S	Males	1.0-3.6	1.0	1.0-3.6
		Females (Cycling; days of cycle)			
		Early follicular phase (–14 to –10 d)	5.5-28.2		5.5-28.2
		Midfollicular phase (–9 to –4 d)	7.9-34.5		7.9-34.5
		Late follicular phase (–3 to –1 d)	19.5-102.3		19.5-102.3
		Midcycle (day 0)	49.9-155.5		49.9-155.5
		Early luteal (1 to 3 d)	35.9-132.7		35.9-132.7
		Midluteal (4 to 11 d)	13.2-159.6		13.2-159.6
		Late luteal (12 to 14 d)	7.3-89.9		7.3-89.9
		IVF, peak levels	354-1690		354-1690
		PCOS, ovulatory	5.7-16.0		5.7-16.0
		Postmenopausal	1.0-3.9		1.0-3.9
	S, maternal	Pregnancy, wk	pg/mL (median)		ng/L (median)
		15	174		174
		16	170		170
		17	173		173
		18	182		182
		19	198		198
		20	222		222
Insulin	S		μIU/mL		pmol/L
		Adult	2-25	6.00	12-150

TABLE 60-1 Reference Intervals and Values—cont'd

Analyte	Specimen	Condition	Reference Intervals: Conventional Units	Conversion Factor	SI Units
Insulin-like growth factor-I	S		ng/mL		μg/L
		1-2 y			
		Male	31-160	1.0	31-160
		Female	11-206		11-206
		3-6 y			
		Male	16-288		16-288
		Female	70-316		70-316
		7-10 y			
		Male	136-385		136-385
		Female	123-396		123-396
		11-12 y			
		Male	136-440		136-440
		Female	191-462		191-462
		13-14 y			
		Male	165-616		165-616
		Female	286-660		286-660
		15-18 y			
		Male	134-836		134-836
		Female	152-660		152-660
		19-25 y			
		Male	202-433		202-433
		Female	231-550		231-550
		Adult (25-85 y)			
		Male	135-449		135-449
		Female	135-449		135-449
Insulin-like growth factor-II	S		ng/mL		μg/L
		Child			
		Prepubertal	334-642	1.0	334-642
		Pubertal	245-737		245-737
		Adult	288-736		288-736
		GH deficiency	51-299		51-299
Iron	It is advised that a laboratory independently define its own reference intervals (see Chapter 31).				
Isocitric acid					mmol/mol creatinine
	U	0-1 mo			0-368
		1-6 mo			0-67
		6 mo-5 y			0-77
		>5 y			16-99
Isoleucine			mg/dL		μmol/L
	P	Premature, 1 d	0.26-0.78	76.3	20-60
		Newborn, 1 d	0.35-0.69		27-53
		1-3 mo	0.59-0.95		45-73
		2-6 mo	0.50-1.61		38-123
		9 mo-2 y	0.34-1.23		26-94
		3-10 y	0.37-1.10		28-84
		6-18 y	0.50-1.24		38-95
		Adult	0.48-1.28		37-98

Continued

TABLE 60-1 Reference Intervals and Values—cont'd

Analyte	Specimen	Condition	Reference Intervals: Conventional Units	Conversion Factor	Si Units
Isoleucine—*cont'd*			mg/d		µmol/d
	U	10 d-7 wk	Trace-0.4	7.62	Trace-3
		3-12 y	2-7		15-53
		Adult	5-24		38-183
			mg/g creatinine		mmol/mol creatinine
		Adult	1-5	0.86	0.8-4.4
L-Lactate			mg/dL		mmol/L
	WB (Hep)	At bed rest	5-12	0.111	0.56-1.39
		Venous	3-7		0.36-0.75
		Arterial	16-17		1.78-1.88
	CSF	Child	496-1982 mg/d	0.0111	5.5-22 mmol/d
	U, 24 h	Adult			
					mmol/mol creatinine
		0-1 mo			46-348
		1-6 mo			57-346
		6 mo-5 y			21-38
		>5 y			20-101
	Gastric fluid		Negative		Negative
Lactate dehydrogenase (LD)			U/L		µkat/L
Total L →P	S	24 mo-12 y	180-360	0.017	3.1-6.1
IFCC, 37 °C		12-60 y	125-220		2.1-3.7
Lead			µg/dL		µmol/L
	WB (Hep)	Child	<25	0.0483	<1.21
		Adult	<25		<1.21
		Toxic	>99		>4.78
			µg/L		µmol/L
	U, 24 h		<80		<0.39
Leucine			mg/dL		µmol/L
	P	Premature, 1 d	0.26-1.58	76.3	20-120
		Newborn, 1 d	0.62-1.43		47-109
		1-3 mo	10.58-2.14		44-164
		9 mo-2 y	0.59-2.03		45-155
		3-10 y	0.73-2.33		56-178
		6-18 y	1.03-2.28		79-174
		Adult	0.98-2.29		75-175
	U, 24 h		mg/d		µmol/d
		10 d-7 wk	0.9-2.0	7.624	7-15
		3-12 y	3-11		23-84
		Adult	2.6-8.1		20-62
			mg/g creatinine		mmol/mol creatinine
		Adult	0-8	0.86	0-6.8
Lipase, 37 °C			U/L		µkat/L
	S	Adult	<38	0.017	<0.65

TABLE 60-1 Reference Intervals and Values—cont'd

Analyte	Specimen	Condition		Conventional Units	Conversion Factor	Si Units
				REFERENCE INTERVALS		
Low-density lipoprotein cholesterol (LDL-C)				mg/dL		mmol/L
				5th-95th percentile		5th-95th percentile
	S	5-9 y	M	63-129	0.0259	1.63-3.34
			F	68-140		1.76-3.63
		10-14 y	M	64-133		1.66-3.44
			F	68-136		1.76-3.52
		15-19 y	M	62-130		1.61-3.37
			F	59-137		1.53-3.55
		20-24 y	M	66-147		1.53-3.81
			F	57-159		1.48-4.12
		25-29 y	M	70-165		1.81-4.27
			F	71-164		1.84-4.25
		30-34 y	M	78-185		2.02 4.79
			F	70-156		1.81-4.04
		35-39 y	M	81-189		2.10-4.90
			F	75-172		1.94-4.45
		40-44 y	M	87-186		2.25-4.82
			F	74-174		1.92-4.51
		45-49 y	M	97-202		2.51-5.23
			F	79-186		2.05-4.82
		50-54 y	M	89-197		2.31-5.10
			F	88-201		2.28-5.21
		55-59 y	M	88-203		2.28-5.26
			F	89-210		2.31-5.44
		60-64 y	M	83-210		2.15-5.44
			F	100-224		2.59-5.81
		65-69 y	M	98-210		2.54-5.44
			F	92-221		2.39-5.73
		>69 y	M	88-186		2.28-4.82
			F	96-206		2.49-5.34
	Risk coronary heart disease			mg/dL		mmol/L
		Optimal		<100	0.0259	<2.59
		Near/above optimal		100-129		2.59-3.34
		Borderline high		130-159		3.37-4.12
		High		160-189		4.15-4.90
		Very high		>189		>4.90
L/S ratio	Amf			Ratio		Ratio
		State of fetal maturity				
		Immature		<1.5	1.0	<1.5
		Transitional		1.6-2.4		1.6-2.4
		Mature		>2.5		>2.5
		Diabetic		>2.5		>2.5
Luteinizing hormone (LH)				mIU/mL		IU/L
		Males (23-70 y)		1.2-7.8	1.0	1.2-7.8
		Female				
		Follicular phase		1.7-15.0		1.7-15.0
		Midcycle peak		21.9-56.6		21.9-56.6
		Luteal phase		0.6-16.3		0.6-16.3
		Postmenopausal		14.2-52.3		14.2-52.3

Continued

TABLE 60-1 Reference Intervals and Values—cont'd

Analyte	Specimen	Condition	Reference Intervals: Conventional Units	Conversion Factor	SI Units
Lysine			mg/dL		μmol/L
	P	Premature, 1 d	1.01-4.53	68.5	70-310
		Newborn, 1 d	1.66-3.93		114-269
		1-3 mo	0.54-2.46		37-169
		9 mo-2 y	0.66-2.10		45-144
		3-10 y	1.04-2.20		71-151
		6-18 y	1.58-3.40		108-233
		Adult	1.21-3.47		83-238
	U, 24 h		mg/d		μmol/d
		10 d-7 wk	5.7-10.9	6.85	39-75
		3-12 y	9.3-93.7		64-642
		Adult	3.1-153.0		21-1048
			mg/g creatinine		mmol/mol creatinine
		Adult	4-12	0.77	3.2-9.2
α_2-Macroglobulin	S		mg/dL		g/L
		Adult (20-60 y)	130-300	0.01	1.3-3.0
Magnesium AAS			mg/dL		mmol/L
	S	Newborn, 2-4 d	1.5-2.2	0.4114	0.62-0.91
		5 mo-6 y	1.7-2.3		0.70-0.95
		6-12 y	1.7-2.1		0.70-0.86
		>12 y	1.6-2.6		0.66-1.07
	U, 24 h		12-291 mg/24h	0.083	1.0-24.0 mEq/24h
Magnesium, free	S		mmol/L		mmol/L
			0.45-0.60	1.0	0.45-0.60
Malic acid					mmol/mol creatinine
	U	0-1 mo			0-52
		1-6 mo			8-73
		6 mo-5 y			4-57
		>5 y			17-47
Manganese			μg/L		nmol/L
	WSB (Hep)		5-15	18.0	90-270
	S		0.5-1.3		9-24
	U, collect in metal free container		0.5-9.8		9.1-178
		Toxic conc.	>19		>342
Mercury			μg/L		nmol/L
	WB (EDTA)		0.6-59	4.99	3.0-294.4
	U, 24 h		<20		<99.8
		Toxic conc.	>150		>748.5
		Lethal conc.	>800		>3992
Metanephrines					
Free normetanephrine	S, P		pg/mL		nmol/L
		Hypertensive adults	24-145	0.0054	0.13-0.79
		Normotensive adults	18-101		0.10-0.55
		Normotensive children	22-83		0.12-0.45

TABLE 60-1 Reference Intervals and Values—cont'd

Analyte	Specimen	Condition	Conventional Units	Conversion Factor	Si Units
			REFERENCE INTERVALS		
Metanephrines—*cont'd*					
Metanephrine	S, P		pg/mL		nmol/L
		Hypertensive adults	12-72	0.0050	0.06-0.37
		Normotensive adults	12-67		0.06-0.34
		Normotensive children	10-95		0.05-0.48
Total normetanephrine	S, P		pg/mL		nmol/L
		Hypertensive adults	755-5623	0.0054	4.1-30.7
		Normotensive adults	624-3041		3.4-16.6
		Normotensive children	851-2398		4.7-13.1
Metanephrine	S, P		pg/mL		nmol/L
		Hypertensive adults	327-2042	0.0050	1.7-10.4
		Normotensive adults	328-1837		1.7-9.3
		Normotensive children	380-1995		1.9-10.1
Metanephrines (total)					
Metanephrine	U, 24 h		μg/d		nmol/d
		0-3 mo	5.9-37	5.07	30-188
		4-6 mo	6.1-42		31-213
		7-9 mo	12-41		61-210
		10-12 mo	8.5-101		43-510
		1-2 y	6.7-52		34-264
		2-6 y	11-99		56-501
		6-10 y	54-138		275-701
		10-16 y	39-242		200-1231
		Adult	74-297		375-1506
Metanephrine	U		μg/g creatinine		mmol/mol creatinine
		0-3 mo	202-708	0.574	116-407
		4-6 mo	156-572		89-328
		7-9 mo	150-526		86-302
		10-12 mo	148-651		85-374
		1-2 y	40-526		23-302
		2-6 y	74-504		42-289
		6-10 y	121-319		69-183
		10-16 y	46-307		26-176
Normetanephrine	U, 24 h		μg/d		nmol/d
		0-3 mo	47-156	5.46	257-852
		4-6 mo	31-111		171-607
		7-9 mo	42-109		230-595
		10-12 mo	23-103		127-562
		1-2 y	32-118		175-647
		2-6 y	50-111		274-604
		6-10 y	47-176		255-964
		10-16 y	53-290		289-1586
		Adult	105-354		573-1933

Continued

TABLE 60-1 Reference Intervals and Values—cont'd

Analyte	Specimen	Condition	Conventional Units	Conversion Factor	SI Units
Metanephrines (total)—*cont'd*					
Normetanephrine	U		μg/g creatinine		mmol/mol creatinine
		0-3 mo	1535-3355	0.617	947-2070
		4-6 mo	737-2194		454-1354
		7-9 mo	592-1046		365-645
		10-12 mo	271-1117		167-689
		1-2 y	350-1275		216-787
		2-6 y	104-609		64-376
		6-10 y	103-452		63-279
		10-16 y	96-411		59-254
Methanol			mg/L		mmol/L
	WB (F^-/Ox)		<1.5	0.0312	<0.05
		Toxic	>200		>6.24
	U	Occup. exp.	<50		<1.56
			ppm		mmol/L
	Breath		0.8		0.03
		Occup. exp.	2.5		0.08
Methemoglobin (MetHb)			g/dL		μmol/L
	WB (EDTA, Hep, or ACD)		0.06-0.24	155	9.3-37.2
			% of total HB		Mass fraction of total HB
			0.04-1.52	0.01	0.0004-0.0152
Methionine			mg/dL		μmol/L
	P	Premature, 1 d	0.38-0.66	67.7	25-45
		Newborn, 1 d	0.13-0.61		9-41
		1-3 mo	0.05-0.57		3-39
		2-6 mo	0.24-0.73		16-49
		9 mo-2 y	0.04-0.43		3-29
		3-10 y	0.16-0.24		11-16
		6-18 y	0.24-0.55		16-37
		Adult	0.09-0.60		6-40
			mg/d		μmol/d
	U, 24 h	10 d-7 wk	0.1-1.9	6.70	0.7-13
		3-12 y	3-14		20-95
		Adult	<9.1		<63
			mg/g creatinine		mmol/mol creatinine
		Adult	0-9.5	0.76	0-7.2
2-Methylbutyrylglycine					mmol/mol creatinine
	U				0.2-5
Methylsuccinic acid					mmol/mol creatinine
	U				0-12
β_2-Microglobulin			mg/dL (mean)		mg/L (mean)
	S	Neonates	0.30	10	3.0
		0-59 y	0.19		1.9
		60-69 y	0.21		2.1
		>70 y	0.24		2.4
Molybdenum			μg/L		nmol/L
	S		0.1-3.0	10.42	1.0-31.3
	U, 24 h		40-60 μg/d		416-625 nmol/d

TABLE 60-1 Reference Intervals and Values—cont'd

Analyte	Specimen	Condition	Reference Intervals: Conventional Units	Conversion Factor	SI Units
Mucin-like carcinoma-associated antigen (MCA)			U/mL		kU/L
	S		<14	1.0	<14
Niacin			mg/d		μmol/d
	U, 24 h		2.4-6.4	7.30	17.5-46.7
Nickel			μg/L		nmol/L
	S or P (Hep)		0.14-1.0	17	2.4-17.0
	WB		1.0-28.0		17-476
			μg/d		nmol/d
	U, 24 h		0.1-10		2-170
N-telopeptide (BCE = bone collagen equivalents)			nmol BCE/L		nmol BCE/L
	S	Men	5.4-24.2	1.0	5.4-24.2
		Premenopausal women	6.2-19.0		6.2-19.0
			nmol BCE/mmol creatinine		nmol BCE/mmol creatinine
	U	Men	3-63		3-63
		Premenopausal women	5-65		5-65
Nuclear matrix protein 22 (NMP-22)			U/mL		kU/L
		S	<10	1.0	<10
Orotic acid					mmol/mol creatinine
	U	0-1 mo			1.4-5.3
		1-6 mo			1.0-3.2
		6 mo-5 y			0.5-3.3
		>5 y			0.4-1.2
Osteocalcin			ng/mL		μg/L
	S	Adult male	3.0-13.0	1.0	3.0-13.0
		Adult female			
		Premenopausal	0.4-8.2		0.4-8.2
		Postmenopausal	1.5-11.0		1.5-11.0
Oxalic acid					mmol/mol creatinine
	U	0-1 mo			51-931
		1-6 mo			7-567
		6 mo-5 y			7-352
		>5 y			<188
2-Oxoglutaric acid	S	0-1 mo			mmol/mol creatinine
					22-567
		1-6 mo			63-552
		6 mo-5 y			36-103
		>5 y			41-82
Oxygen, partial pressure (PO_2)			mm Hg		kPa
	Cord blood				
	Arterial		5.7-30.5	0.133	0.8-4.0
	Venous		17.4-41.0		2.3-5.5

Continued

TABLE 60-1 Reference Intervals and Values—cont'd

Analyte	Specimen	Condition	Conventional Units	Conversion Factor	Si Units
			Reference Intervals		
Oxygen, partial pressure (PO_2)—*cont'd*	WB, arterial				
		Birth	8-24		1.06-3.19
		5-10 min	33-75		4.39-9.96
		30 min	31-85		4.12-11.31
		1 h	55-80		7.32-10.64
		1 d	54-95		7.18-12.64
		2 d-60 y	83-108		11.04-14.36
		>60 y	>80		>10.64
		>70 y	>70		>9.31
		>80 y	>60		>7.98
		>90 y	>50		>6.65
Oxygen, saturation (sO_2)	WB, arterial		Percent saturation		Fraction saturation
		Newborn	40-90	0.01	0.40-0.90
		Thereafter	94-98		0.94-0.98
Oxytocin	P, EDTA		μU/mL		mU/L
		Males	1.1-1.9	1.0	1.0-1.9
		Females			
		Nonpregnant	1.0-1.8		1.0-1.8
		Second stage of labor	3.2-5.3		3.2-5.3
Pantothenic acid	WB		344-583 μg/L	0.0046	1.57-2.66 μmol/L
	U, 24 h		1-15 mg/d	4.53	5-68 μmol/d
Parathyroid hormone, intact	S		pg/mL		ng/L
			10-65	1.0	10-65
Parathyroid hormone, (1-84)	S		pg/mL		ng/L
			6-40	1.0	6-40
Parathyroid hormone-related peptide (PTHrP)	S		pmol/L		pmol/L
			<1.4		<1.4
pH (37 °C)	WB, arterial		pH		pH
		Cord blood			
		Arterial	7.18-7.38	1.0	7.18-7.38
		Venous	7.25-7.45		7.25-7.45
		Newborn			
		Premature, 48 h	7.35-7.50		7.35-7.50
		Full term			
		Birth	7.11-7.36		7.11-7.36
		5-10 min	7.09-7.30		7.09-7.30
		30 min	7.21-7.38		7.21-7.38
		1 h	7.26-7.49		7.26-7.49
		1 d	7.29-7.45		7.29-7.45
		Children, adults			
		Arterial	7.35-7.45		7.35-7.45
		Venous	7.32-7.43		7.32-7.43
		Adults			
		60-90 y	7.31-7.42		7.31-7.42
		>90 y	7.26-7.43		7.26-7.43
Phenylalanine			mg/dL		μmol/L
	WB on filter paper		<2.1	60.5	<122

TABLE 60-1 Reference Intervals and Values—cont'd

			REFERENCE INTERVALS		
Analyte	**Specimen**	**Condition**	**Conventional Units**	**Conversion Factor**	**Si Units**
Phenylalanine—*cont'd*	P	Premature	2.0-7.5		121-454
		Newborn	1.2-3.4		73-205
		Phenylketonuric 2-3 d	>4.5		>272
		Phenylketonuric untreated	15-30		907-1815
		Adult	0.8-1.8		48-109
			mg/d		µmol/d
	U, 24 h	10 d-7 wk	1.2-1.7	6.05	7-10
		3-13 y	4.0-17.5		24-106
		Adult	<16.5		<100
			mg/g creatinine		mmol/mol creatinine
		Adult	2-10	0.68	1.3-6.9
3-Phenylpropionylglycine					mmol/mol creatinine
	U				<0.7
Phosphate	S, P (Hep)		mg/dL		mmol/L
		Children	4.0-7.0	0.323	1.29-2.26
		Adults	2.5-4.5		0.81-1.45
	U, 24 h		g/d		mmol/d
		Adults	0.4-1.3	32.3	12.9-42.0
Phosphatase, acid tartrate resistant 37 °C	S		U/L		µkat/L
		Children	3.4-9.0	0.017	0.05-0.15
		Adult	1.5-4.5		0.03-0.08
Phosphatase, alkaline			U/L		µkat/L
IFCC, 37 °C	S	4-15 y (male)	54-369	0.017	0.91-6.23
		4-15 y (female)	54-369		0.91-6.23
		20-50 y (male)	53-128		0.90-2.18
		20-50 y (female)	42-98		0.71-1.67
		>60 y (male)	56-119		0.95-2.02
		>60 y (female)	53-141		0.90-2.40
Phosphatase, alkaline (bone specific, by immunoabsorption)			U/L		U/L
	S	Men	15.0-41.3	1.0	15.0-41.3
		Premenopausal women	11.6-29.6		11.6-29.6
Phosphatase, alkaline isoenzymes					
Percentage of total activity	<1 y	1-15 y	Adult	Pregnant women	Postmenopausal women
Biliary	3-6	2-5	1-3	1-3	0-12
Liver	20-34	22-34	17-35	5-17	17-48
Bone	20-30	21-30	13-19	8-14	8-21
Placental	8-19	5-17	13-21	53-69	7-15
Renal	1-3	0-1	0-2	3-6	0-2
Intestinal	0-2	0-1	0-1	0-1	0-1
Fraction activity	<1 y	1-15 y	Adult	Pregnant women	Postmenopausal women
Biliary	0.03-0.06	0.02-0.05	0.01-0.03	0.01-0.03	0.0-0.12
Liver	0.20-0.34	0.22-0.34	0.17-0.35	0.05-0.17	0.17-0.48
Bone	0.20-0.30	0.21-0.30	0.13-0.19	0.08-0.14	0.08-0.21

Continued

TABLE 60-1 Reference Intervals and Values—cont'd

Analyte	Specimen	Condition	Reference Intervals: Conventional Units	Conversion Factor	Si Units
Phosphatase, alkaline isoenzymes—*cont'd*					
Placental	0.08-0.19	0.05-0.17	0.13-0.21	0.53-0.69	0.07-0.15
Renal	0.01-0.03	0.0-0.01	0.0-0.02	0.03-0.06	0.0-0.02
Intestinal	0.0-0.02	0.0-0.01	0.0-0.01	0.0-0.01	0.0-0.01
Pimelic acid					mmol/mol creatinine
	U				<1.1
Porphobilinogen			mg/L		µmol/L
	U, 24 h		<2.26	4.42	<10
Porphyrins, total					nmol/L
	U, 24 h				20-320
					nmol/L g dry wt
	Feces				10-200
					µmol/L erythrocytes
	Erythrocytes				0.4-1.7
Potassium (K)			mEq/L		mmol/L
	S	Premature cord	5.0-10.2	1.0	5.0-10.2
		Premature, 48 h	3.0-6.0		3.0-6.0
		Newborn cord	5.6-12.0		5.6-12.0
		Newborn	3.7-5.9		3.7-5.9
		Infant	4.1-5.3		4.1-5.3
		Child	3.4-4.7		3.4-4.7
		Adults	3.5-5.1		3.5-5.1
	P (Hep)	Male	3.5-4.5		3.5-4.5
		Female	3.4-4.4		3.4-4.4
			mEq/d		mmol/d
	U, 24 h	6-10 y			
		M	17-54		17-54
		F	8-37		8-37
		10-14 y			
		M	22-57		22-57
		F	18-58		18-58
		Adult	25-125		25-125
Proinsulin	S		pmol/L		pmol/L
			1.1-6.9	1.0	1.1-6.9
Prolactin			ng/mL		µg/L
	S	Cord blood	45-539	1.0	45-539
		Children, Tanner stage 1			
		Male	<10		<10
		Female	3.6-12		3.6-12
		Children, Tanner stage 2-3			
		Male	<6.1		<6.1
		Female	2.6-18		2.6-18
		Children, Tanner stage 4-5			
		Male	2.8-11		2.8-11
		Female	3.2-20		3.2-20
		Adult			
		Male	3.0-14.7		3.0-14.7
		Female	3.8-23.0		3.8-23.0
		Pregnancy, third trimester	95-473		95-473

TABLE 60-1 Reference Intervals and Values—cont'd

Analyte	Specimen	Condition	Conventional Units (Reference Intervals)	Conversion Factor (Reference Intervals)	SI Units (Reference Intervals)
Proline			mg/dL		µmol/L
	P	Premature, 1 d	0.92-4.36	86.9	80-380
		Newborn, 1 d	1.23-3.18		107-277
		1-3 mo	0.89-3.73		77-325
		9 mo-2 y	0.59-2.13		51-185
		3-10 y	0.78-1.70		68-148
		6-18 y	0.67-3.72		58-324
		Adult	1.17-3.86		102-336
	U, 24 h		mg/d		µmol/d
		10 d-7 wk	3.2-11.0	8.69	28-96
		3-12 y	Trace		Trace
		Adult	Trace		Trace
			µmol/g creatinine		µmol/mol creatinine
		0-1 mo	70-2300	0.113	7.91-259.9
		1-6 mo	<600		<67.8
		6 mo-1 y	<300		<33.9
		1-2 y	<270		<30.5
		2-3 y	<220		<24.9
Propionylcarnitine					µmol/L
	P	0-7 d			0.07-1.85
		8 d-7 y			0.17-1.27
		>7 y			0.17-1.49
	WB spots				0.55-8.01
	Bile spots				0.36-8.10
					mmol/mol creatinine
	U	0-7 d			0.01-0.20
		8 d-7 y			0.01-1.20
		>7 y			0.00-0.06
Prostate-specific antigen (PSA)			ng/mL		µg/L
	S	Males			
		40-49 y	0-2.5	1.0	0-2.5
		50-59 y	0-3.5		0-3.5
		60-69 y	0-4.5		0-4.5
		70-79 y	0-6.5		0-6.5
Protein, total			g/dL		g/L
	S	Cord	4.8-8.0	10	48-80
		Premature	3.6-6.0		36-60
		Newborn	4.6-7.0		46-70
		1 wk	4.4-7.6		44-76
		7 mo-1 y	5.1-7.3		51-73
		1-2 y	5.6-7.5		56-75
		>2 y	6.0-8.0		60-80
		Adult, ambulatory	6.4-8.3		64-83
		Adult, recumbent	6.0-7.8		60-78
		>60 y	Lower by <0.2		Lower by <2.0
			mg/dL		mg/L
	U, 24 h	Adult	1-14		10-140
		Excretion	mg/d		g/d
		Adult	<100	0.001	<0.1
		Pregnancy	<150		<0.15

Continued

TABLE 60-1 Reference Intervals and Values—cont'd

Analyte	Specimen	Condition	Reference Intervals: Conventional Units	Conversion Factor	SI Units
Protein, total—*cont'd*			mg/dL		g/L
	CSF	Premature	15-130	10	150-1300
		Full-term newborn	40-120		400-1200
		<1 mo	20-80		200-800
		>1 mo	15-40		150-400
		Ventricular fluid	5-15		50-150
		Cisternal fluid	15-25		150-250
			g/dL		g/L
	Amf	Early pregnancy	0.2-1.7		2.0-17.0
		Late pregnancy	0.175-0.705		1.8-7.1
Pyroglutamic acid					mmol/mol creatinine
	U				<62
Pyruvic acid			mg/dL		μmol/L
	WB, arterial	Adult	0.2-0.7	0.114	0.02-0.08
	WB, venous	Adult	0.3-0.9		0.03-0.10
	CSF	Adult	0.5-1.7		0.06-0.19
	U, 24 h	Adult			<1.1 mmol/d
					mmol/mol creatinine
	U	0-1 mo			24-123
		1-6 mo			8-90
		6 mo-5 y			3-19
		>5 y			6-9
Retinol-binding protein (RBP)			mg/dL		g/L
	S	Birth	1.1-3.4	0.01	0.011-0.034
		6 mo	1.8-5.0		0.018-0.05
		Adult	3.0-6.0		0.03-0.06
Reverse triiodothyronine (rT_3)			ng/dL		nmol/L
	S	Cord (>37 wk)	130-300	0.0154	2.00-4.62
		Children			
		1 d	83-194		1.28-2.99
		2 d	107-209		1.65-3.22
		3 d	102-166		1.57-2.56
		1 mo-20 y	10-35		0.15-0.54
		Adult	10-28		0.15-0.43
		Maternal serum (15-40 wk)	11-33		0.17-0.51
		Amniotic serum (17-22 wk)	163-599		2.51-9.22
Riboflavin (vitamin B_2)			μg/dL		nmol/L
	S		4-24	26.6	106-638
	Erythrocytes		10-50		266-1330
	U		>80 μg/g creatinine	0.3	>24 μmol/mol creatinine
	U, 24 h		>100 μg/d	2.66	>266 nmol/L
Sebacic acid					mmol/mol creatinine
	U	0-1 mo			3-16
		1-6 mo			3-26
		>6 mo			<9

TABLE 60-1 Reference Intervals and Values—cont'd

Analyte	Specimen	Condition	Reference Intervals: Conventional Units	Conversion Factor	Si Units
Selenium			μg/L		μmol/L
	S	Neonates	<8.0 (deficiency)	0.0127	<0.10 (deficiency)
		<2 y	16-71		0.2-0.9
		2-4 y	40-103		0.5-1.3
		4-16 y	55-134		0.7-1.7
		Adults	63-160		0.8-2.0
	WB (Hep)		58-234		0.74-2.97
	U, 24 h		7-160		0.09-2.03
		Toxic conc.	>400		>5.08
Serine			mg/dL		μmol/L
	P	Newborn, 1 d	0.99-2.55	95.2	94-243
		1-3 mo	0.8-1.60		76-152
		9 mo-2 y	0.35-1.34		33-128
		3-10 y	0.83-1.18		79-112
		6-18 y	0.75-1.90		71-181
		Adult	0.68-2.03		65-193
	U, 24 h		mg/d		μmol/d
		10 d-7 wk	6.2-24.7	9.52	59-235
		3-12 y	16.3-56.7		155-540
		Adult	13.6-145.7		129-1387
			mg/g creatinine		mmol/mol creatinine
		Adult	0-47	1.08	0-50.8
Serotonin			ng/mL		nmol/L
	WB		50-200	5.68	280-1140
			ng/10^9 platelets		nmol/10^9 platelets
	WB		88-1230	0.00568	0.5-7.0
			ng/mL		nmol/L
	S		30-200	5.68	170-1140
			μg/d		nmol/d
	U, 24 h		60-167		340-950
			μg/g creatinine		μmol/mol creatinine
	U		38-101	0.653	25-66
			ng/mL		nmol/L
	CSF		1.0-2.1	5.68	5.7-12.0
			ng/10^9 platelets		nmol/10^9 platelets
	Platelet-rich serum		370-970	0.00568	2.07-5.55
			ng/10^9 platelets		nmol/10^9 platelets
	Isolated platelets		154-1086		0.88-6.16
			ng/mL		nmol/L
	Platelet-poor plasma		0-3.60	5.68	0-22.5

Continued

TABLE 60-1 Reference Intervals and Values—cont'd

Analyte	Specimen	Condition	Conventional Units (Reference Intervals)	Conversion Factor	Si Units
Sodium (Na)			mEq/L		mmol/L
		Premature cord	116-140	1.0	116-140
		Premature, 48 h	128-148		128-148
		Newborn cord	126-166		126-166
		Newborn	133-146		133-146
		Infant	139-146		139-146
		Child	138-145		138-145
		Adult	136-145		136-145
		>90 y	132-146		132-146
	U, 24 h	6-10 y	mEq/d		mmol/L
		M	41-115		41-115
		F	20-69		20-69
		10-14 y			
		M	63-177		63-177
		F	48-168		48-168
		Adult			
		M	40-220		40-220
		F	27-287		27-287
Suberic acid					mmol/mol creatinine
	U	0-6 mo			4-20
		>6 mo			<9
Succinic acid					mmol/mol creatinine
	U	0-1 mo			35-547
		1-6 mo			34-156
		6 mo-5 y			16-118
		>5 y			29-87
Testosterone, bioavailable	S		ng/dL		nmol/L
		Adult, M	66-417	0.0347	2.29-14.5
		Adult, F	0.6-5.0		0.02-0.17
Testosterone, free	S		pg/mL		pmol/L
		Cord, M	5-22	3.47	17.4-76.3
		Cord, F	4-19		13.9-55.5
		Newborn, 1-15 d, M	1.5-31.0		5.2-107.5
		Newborn, 1-15 d, F	0.5-2.5		1.7-8.7
		1-3 mo, M	3.3-8.0		11.5-62.5
		1-3 mo, F	0.1-1.3		0.3-4.5
		3-5 mo, M	0.7-14.0		2.4-48.6
		3-5 mo, F	0.3-1.1		1.0-3.8
		5-7 mo, M	0.4-4.8		1.4-16.6
		5-7 mo, F	0.2-0.6		0.7-2.1
		6-9 y, M	0.1-3.2		0.3-11.1
		6-9 y, F	0.1-0.9		0.3-3.1
		10-11 y, M	0.6-5.7		2.1-19.8
		10-11 y, F	1.0-5.2		3.5-18.0
		12-14 y, M	1.4-156		4.9-541
		12-14 y, F	1.0-5.2		3.5-18.0
		15-17 y, M	80-159		278-552
		15-17 y, F	1.0-5.2		3.5-18.0
		Adult, M	50-210		174-729
		Adult, F	1.0-8.5		3.5-29.5

TABLE 60-1 Reference Intervals and Values—cont'd

Analyte	Specimen	Condition	Conventional Units	Conversion Factor	Si Units
			REFERENCE INTERVALS		
Testosterone, total			ng/dL		nmol/L
	S	Cord, M	13-55	0.0347	0.45-1.91
		Cord, F	5-45		0.17-1.56
		Premature, M	37-198		1.28-6.87
		Premature, F	5-22		0.17-0.76
		Newborn, M	75-400		2.6-13.9
		Newborn, F	20-64		0.69-2.22
		Prepubertal child			
		1-5 mo M	1-177		0.03-6.14
		1-5 mo F	1-5		0.03-0.17
		6-11 mo M	2-7		0.07-0.24
		6-11 mo F	2-5		0.07-0.17
		1-5 y M	2-25		0.07-0.87
		1-5 y F	2-10		0.07-0.35
		6-9 y M	3-30		0.10-1.04
		6-9 y F	2-20		0.07-0.69
		Puberty, Tanner stage			
		1, M	2-23		0.07-0.80
		1, F	2-10		0.07-0.35
		2, M	5-70		0.17-2.43
		2, F	5-30		0.17-1.04
		3, M	15-280		0.52-9.72
		3, F	10-30		0.35-1.04
		4, M	105-545		3.64-18.91
		4, F	15-40		0.52-1.39
		5, M	65-800		9.19-27.76
		5, F	10-40		0.35-1.39
		Adult M	260-1000		9-34.72
		Adult F	15-70		0.52-2.43
Tetradecanedioic acid					mmol/mol creatinine
	U				<0.5
Thallium			μg/L		nmol/L
	WB (Hep)		<5	4.89	<24.5
			mg/L		μmol/L
		Toxic	0.1-8.0		0.5-390
			μg/L		nmol/L
	U, 24 h		<2.0		<9.8
			mg/L		μmol/L
		Toxic	1.0-20.0		4.9-97.8
Thiocyanate			mg/dL		μmol/L
	S	Nonsmokers	<0.4	172.4	<69
		Smokers	<1.2		<207
		Nitroprusside therapy	0.6-2.9		103-500
		Toxic	>5		>862
Threonine			mg/dL		μmol/L
	P	Premature, 1 d	1.14-3.98	84.0	95-335
		Newborn, 1 d	1.36-3.99		114-335
		1-3 mo	0.75-2.67		64-224
		2-6 mo	2.27-4.33		191-364
		3-10 y	0.50-1.13		42-95
		6-18 y	0.88-2.40		74-202
		Adult	0.94-2.30		79-193

Continued

TABLE 60-1 Reference Intervals and Values—cont'd

			Reference Intervals		
Analyte	**Specimen**	**Condition**	**Conventional Units**	**Conversion Factor**	**Si Units**
Threonine—*cont'd*	U, 24 h		mg/d		µmol/d
		10 d-7 wk	1.5-11.9	8.40	13-100
		3-12 y	10.1-29.6		85-249
		Adult	14.3-46.7		120-392
			mg/g creatinine		mmol/mol creatinine
		Adult	0-28	0.95	0-27
Thyroglobulin (Tg)			ng/mL		µg/L
	S	Adult euthyroid	3-42	1.0	3-42
		Athyroidic patient	<5		<5
Thyrotropin (thyroid-stimulating hormone) (TSH)			µIU/mL		mIU/L
	S	Premature, 28-36 wk	0.7-27.0	1.0	0.7-27.0
		Cord blood (>37 wk)	2.3-13.2		2.3-13.2
		Children			
		Birth-4 d	1.0-39.0		1.0-39.0
		2-20 wk	1.7-9.1		1.7-9.1
		21 wk-20 y	0.7-6.4		0.7-6.4
		Adults			
		21-54 y	0.4-4.2		0.4-4.2
		55-87 y	0.5-8.9		0.5-8.9
		Pregnancy			
		First trimester	0.3-4.5		0.3-4.5
		Second trimester	0.5-4.6		0.5-4.6
		Third trimester	0.8-5.2		0.8-5.2
	Whole blood (heel puncture)	Newborn screen	<20		<20
Thyroxine-binding globulin (TBG)			mg/dL		mg/L
	S	Cord	3.6-9.6	10	36-96
		Children			
		4-12 mo	3.1-5.6		31-56
		1-5 y	2.9-5.4		29-54
		5-10 y	2.5-5.0		25-50
		10-15 y	2.1-4.6		21-46
		Adult			
		Male	1.2-2.5		12-25
		Female	1.4-3.0		14-30
		Female (oral contraceptive)	1.5-5.5		15-55
Thyroxine (T_4)			µg/dL		nmol/L
	S	Cord	7.4-13.1	12.9	95-168
		Children			
		1-3 d	11.8-22.6		152-292
		1-2 wk	9.9-16.6		126-214
		1-4 mo	7.2-14.4		93-186
		4-12 mo	7.8-16.5		101-213
		1-5 y	7.3-15.0		94-194
		5-10 y	6.4-13.3		83-172
		1-15 y	5.6-11.7		72-151
		Adults (15-60 y)			
		Males	4.6-10.5		59-135
		Females	5.5-11.0		65-138
		>60 y	5.0-10.7		65-138
		Newborn screen			
		1-5 d	>7.5		>97
		6 d	>6.5		>84

TABLE 60-1 Reference Intervals and Values—cont'd

Analyte	Specimen	Condition		Conventional Units	Conversion Factor	SI Units
				REFERENCE INTERVALS		
Thyroxine, free (FT_4)				ng/dL		pmol/L
	S	Newborns (1-4 d)		2.2-5.3	12.9	28.4-68.4
		Children (2 wk-20 y)		0.8-2.0		10.3-25.8
		Adults (21-87 y)		0.8-2.7		10.3-34.7
		Pregnancy				
		First trimester		0.7-2.0		9.0-25.7
		Second and third trimesters		0.5-1.6		6.4-20.6
Thyroxine, free index (FT_4 I)				µg/dL		nmol/L
	S	Cord		6.0-13.2	12.9	77-170
		Infants				
		1-3 d		9.9-17.5		128-226
		1 wk		7.5-15.1		97-195
		1-12 mo		5.0-13.0		65-168
		Children				
		1-10 y		5.4-12.8		70-165
		Pubertal child and adult		4.2-13.0		54-168
Transferrin	S			mg/dL		g/L
		Newborn		117-250	0.01	1.17-2.5
		20-60 y		200-360		2.0-3.6
		>60 y		160-340		1.6-3.4
Transketolase, erythrocyte	Erythrocytes			0.75-1.30 U/g Hb	64.53	48.4-83.9 kU/mol Hb
Transthyretin (prealbumin)	S			mg/dL		g/L
		Adult (20-60 y)		20-40	0.01	0.2-0.4
Triglycerides				mg/dL 5th-95th percentile		mmol/L 5th-95th percentile
	S	0-4 y	M	29-99	0.0113	0.33-1.12
			F	34-112		0.39-1.27
		5-9 y	M	28-85		0.32-0.96
			F	32-126		0.36-1.43
		10-14 y	M	33-111		0.38-1.26
			F	39-120		0.44-1.36
		15-19 y	M	38-143		0.43-1.62
			F	36-126		0.41-1.43
		20-24 y	M	44-165		0.50-1.87
			F	37-168		0.42-1.90
		25-29 y	M	45-204		0.57-2.31
			F	42-159		0.48-1.80
		30-34 y	M	46-253		0.52-2.86
			F	40-163		0.45-1.84
		35-39 y	M	52-316		0.59-3.57
			F	40-205		0.45-2.32
		40-44 y	M	56-318		0.63-3.60
			F	45-191		0.51-2.16
		45-49 y	M	56-279		0.64-3.16
			F	44-223		0.50-2.52
		50-54 y	M	63-313		0.71-3.54
			F	53-223		0.60-2.52
		55-59 y	M	60-261		0.68-2.95
			F	59-279		0.67-3.16

Continued

TABLE 60-1 Reference Intervals and Values—cont'd

Analyte	Specimen	Condition		Conventional Units	Conversion Factor	Si Units
				REFERENCE INTERVALS		
Triglycerides—*cont'd*		60-64 y	M	56-240		0.64-2.71
			F	57-256		0.65-2.90
		65-69 y	M	54-256		0.61-2.90
			F	56-260		0.64-2.94
		>69 y	M	63-239		0.71-2.70
			F	60-289		0.68-3.27
	Recommended cutoff points			mg/dL		mmol/L
		Normal		<150	0.0113	<1.70
		High		150-199		1.70-2.25
		Hypertriglyceridemic		200-499		2.26-5.64
		Very high		>499		>5.64
Triiodothyronine (T_3), free				pg/dL		pmol/L
	S	Cord		15-391	0.0154	0.2-6.0
		Child and adult		210-440		3.2-6.8
		Pregnancy		200-380		3.1-5.9
Triiodothyronine (T_3), total				ng/dL		nmol/L
	S	Cord (>37 wk)		5-141	0.0154	0.08-2.17
		Children				
		1-3 d		100-740		1.54-11.40
		1-11 mo		105-245		1.62-3.77
		1-5 y		105-269		1.62-4.14
		6-10 y		94-241		1.44-3.28
		11-15 y		82-213		1.26-3.28
		Adolescents				
		16-20 y		80-210		1.23-3.23
		Adults				
		20-50 y		70-204		1.08-3.14
		50-90 y		40-181		0.62-2.79
		Pregnancy				
		First trimester		81-190		1.25-2.93
		Second and third trimesters		100-260		1.54-4.00
Troponins (see Chapter 47)						
Tryptophan				mg/dL		μmol/L
	P	Premature, 1 d		0-1.23	49.0	0-60
		Newborn, 1 d		<1.37		<67
		1-16 y		0.49-1.61		24-79
		>16 y		0.41-1.94		20-95
				mg/d		μmol/d
	U, 24 h	Adult		5-39	4.90	25-191
				mg/g creatinine		mmol/mol creatinine
		Adult		<30	0.55	<16.5
Tumor-associated trypsin inhibitor (TATI)				ng/mL		μg/L
	S			3-21	1.0	3-21
	U			7-51		7-51

TABLE 60-1 Reference Intervals and Values—cont'd

Analyte	Specimen	Condition	Reference Intervals: Conventional Units	Conversion Factor	Si Units
Tyrosine			mg/dL		mmol/L
	P	Premature, 1 d	0-5.79	55.2	0-320
		Newborn, 1 d	0.76-1.79		42-99
		1-3 mo	0.54-2.42		30-134
		2-6 mo	1.30-3.91		72-216
		9 mo-2 y	0.20-2.21		11-122
		3-10 y	0.56-1.29		31-71
		6-18 y	0.78-1.59		43-88
		Adult	0.40-1.58		22-87
			mg/d		μmol/d
	U, 24 h	10 d-7 wk	4.0-7.2	5.52	22-40
		3-12 y	7.2-30.4		40-168
		Adult	12.0-55.1		66-304
			mg/g creatinine		mmol/mol creatininc
		Adult	0-23	0.62	0-14.2
Uracil					mmol/mol creatinine
	U	0-6 mo			<33
		6 mo-5 y			<22
		>5 y			<18
Urea nitrogen	S		mg/dL		mmol/L
		Cord	21-40	0.357	7.5-14.3
		Premature (1 wk)	3-25		1.1-8.9
		Newborn	4-12		1.4-4.3
		Infant/child	5-18		1.8-6.4
		Adult	6-20		2.1-7.1
		Adult >60 y	8-23		2.9-8.2
			g/d		mol/d
	U, 24 h		10-20	0.0357	0.43-0.71
Uric acid					
Phosphotungstate	S		mg/dL		mmol/L
		Adult			
		Male	4.4-7.6	0.059	0.26-0.45
		Female	2.3-6.6		0.13-0.39
		>60 y			
		Male	4.2-8.0		0.25-0.47
		Female	3.5-7.3		0.20-0.43
Uricase		Child	2.0-5.0	0.060	0.12-0.32
		Adult			
		Male	3.5-7.2		0.21-0.42
		Female	2.6-6.0		0.15-0.35
	U, 24 h		mg/d		mmol/L
		Purine-free diet			
		Male	<420	0.0059	<2.48
		Female	Slightly lower		Slightly lower
		Low-purine diet			
		Male	<480		<2.83
		Female	<400		<2.36
		High-purine diet	<1000		<5.90
		Average diet	250-750		1.48-4.43

Continued

TABLE 60-1 Reference Intervals and Values—cont'd

			Reference Intervals		
Analyte	**Specimen**	**Condition**	**Conventional Units**	**Conversion Factor**	**Si Units**
Uricase—*cont'd*	U				mmol/mol creatinine
		0-1 mo			359-2644
		1-6 mo			359-2644
		6 mo-5 y			185-1134
		>5 y			199-1034
Valine			mg/dL		µmol/L
	P	Premature, 1 d	0.34-2.70	85.5	30-230
		Newborn, 1 d	0.94-2.88		80-246
		1-3 mo	1.13-3.41		96-292
		9 mo-2 y	0.67-3.07		57-262
		3-10 y	1.50-3.31		128-283
		6-18 y	1.83-3.37		156-288
		Adult	1.65-3.71		141-317
			mg/d		µmol/d
	U	10 d-7 wk	1.4-3.2	8.55	12-27
		3-12 y	1.8-6.0		15-51
		Adult	2.5-11.9		21-102
			mg/g creatinine		mmol/mol creatinine
		Adult	2-6	0.97	1.9-5.9
Vanillylmandelic acid (VMA)	U, 24 h		mg/d		µmol/d
		3-6 y	1-2.6	5.05	5-13
		6-10 y	2.0-3.2		10-16
		10-16 y	2.3-5.2		12-26
		16-83 y	1.4-6.5		7-33
	U		mg/g creatinine		mmol/mol creatinine
		0-1 mo	<27	0.571	<16
		1-6 mo	<19		<11
		6 mo-5 y	<13		<8
		3-6 y	4.0-10.8		2.3-6.2
		6-10 y	4.0-7.5		2.3-4.3
		10-16 y	3.0-8.8		1.7-5.0
Vitamin A	S		µg/dL		µmol/L
		1-6 y	20-40	0.0349	0.70-1.40
		7-12 y	26-49		0.91-1.71
		13-19 y	26-72		0.91-2.51
		Adult	30-80		1.05-2.8
Vitamin B_1 (thiamine diphosphate)	WB		90-140 nmol/L	1.0	90-140 nmol/L
	Erythrocytes		280-590 ng/g Hb	0.146	40.3-85.0 µmol/mol Hb
Vitamin B_2 (see Riboflavin)					
Vitamin B_6	P (EDTA)		ng/mL		nmol/L
			5-30	4.046	20-121
		Deficiency	<5		<20.2
Vitamin B_{12}			ng/L		pmol/L
	S		206-678	0.733	151-497
		Acceptable (WHO)	>201		>147
		Deficiency (WHO)	<150		<110

TABLE 60-1 Reference Intervals and Values—cont'd

			Reference Intervals		
Analyte	**Specimen**	**Condition**	**Conventional Units**	**Conversion Factor**	**Si Units**
Vitamin C (ascorbic acid)			mg/dL		μmol/L
	S		0.4-1.5	56.78	23-85
		Deficiency	<0.2		<11
	Leukocyte		20-53 μg/10^8 leukocytes	0.057	1.14-3.01 fmol/10^8 leukocytes
		Deficiency	<10 μg/10^8 leukocytes		<0.57 fmol/10^8 leukocytes
Vitamin D 25(OH)D	S		ng/mL		nmol/L
			10-65	2.50	25-162
			pg/mL		pmol/L
1,25$(OH)_2$D			15-60	2.4	36-144
Vitamin E	S		mg/dL		μmol/L
		Premature neonates	0.1-0.5	23.2	2.3-11.6
		Children	0.3-0.9		7-21
		Teenagers	0.6-1.0		14-23
		Adults	0.5-1.8		12-42
Vitamin K	S		ng/mL		nmol/L
			0.13-1.19	2.22	0.29-2.64
Zinc			μg/dL		μmol/L
	S		80-120	0.153	12-18
		Deficiency	<30		<5
	U, 24 h		0.2-1.3 mg/24 h	15.3	3-21 μmol/24 h

TABLE 60-2 Therapeutic and Toxic Levels of Drugs

Therapeutic drug monitoring and detection of drug overdose have become increasingly important aspects of the r laboratory in patient care. The information given for drugs in this table has been gathered from published sources. Thes are intended to complement Chapter 34 of this book, and do not represent all drugs for which drug testing may be useful. knowledge and drug measurement methodologies are continuously improving; therefore it may be necessary to su information given here with information obtained from other sources as it becomes available for these and other drug analysis information depends on a well-coordinated sample collection, assay methodology characteristi associated considerations such as age, disease state, concomitant drug administration, and clinical procedures tha have undergone. In practice, each organization should have its own set of therapeutic and toxic levels for the dr

Many tests for therapeutic drugs require careful timing between administration and sample collection if the is to be of optimal use clinically. Drugs are listed by their chemical or generic name, followed by an example of name for the drug (where appropriate). Unless otherwise indicated, target concentrations reflect steady-st sampling. These targets, as well as toxic thresholds provided, are intended to serve as guidelines and should drug dosing independently of clinical factors. See Chapter 34 for detailed information about therapeutic dr these and additional drugs.

Conversion factors provided represent the free-base form of the parent drug only—not metabolites, Active metabolites are indicated for many drugs as "+," but therapeutic or toxic concentrations are not r calculated conversions to SI units are rounded, unless the value is less than 1.0. For convenience an abbreviations commonly used in laboratory medicine are used. Less common abbreviations and so are given in the following paragraph. Whenever plasma or whole blood is indicated, the recommen be EDTA, although heparin may be acceptable. Separator gel blood collection tubes for serum or p drug testing because of possible adsorption of drugs and/or drug metabolites to the gel itself, co drug concentrations. Some drugs (e.g., busulfan, olanzapine) are labile and require special hand data and current literature sources for specific handling recommendations and anticipated sta

TABLE 60-2 Therapeutic and Toxic Levels of Drugs—cont'd

Abbreviation	Term
AUC	Area under the plasma drug concentration versus time curve
EDTA	Ethylenediaminetetraacetic acid
MIC	Minimum inhibitory concentration
P	Plasma
S	Serum
Therap	Therapeutic
U	Urine
WB	Whole blood

REFERENCES

Drug information handbook, 19th edition. Hudson, OH: Lexi-Comp, 2010.
http://www.drugbank.ca/accessed August 23, 2011.
O'Neil MJ ed. The Merck index: An encyclopedia of chemicals, drugs, and biologicals. Whitehouse Station: NJ; Merck & Co, 2006.
Physicians desk reference, 65th edition. Montvale: NJ: Thomson, 2011.
Porter RS, ed. The Merck manual of diagnosis and therapy, Whitehouse Station: NJ; Merck & Co, 2011.
Schulz M, Schmoldt A. Therapeutic and toxic blood concentrations of more than 800 drugs and other xenobiotics. Pharmazie 2003;58:447-74.
Snozek CLH, McMillin GA, Moyer TP. Chapter 34. Therapeutic drugs and their management. In: Burtis CA, Ashwood ER, Bruns DE, eds. Tietz textbook of clinical chemistry and molecular diagnostics 5th edition, St Louis: MO, 2011, 1057-108.

			REFERENCE VALUES		
Drug	**Specimen**	**Status**	**Conventional Units**	**Conversion Factor**	**SI Units**
Acetaminophen (Tylenol)	S or P		μg/mL	6.62	μmol/L
		Therap	10-30		66-199
		Toxic			
		4 h after dose	>200		>1324
		12 h after dose	>50		>331
Amikacin (Amikin)	S or P		μg/mL	1.71	μmol/L
		Therap			
		Peak	25-35		43-60
		Trough			
		Less severe infection	1-4		2-7
		Severe infection	4-8		7-14
		Toxic			
		Peak	>40		>68
		Trough	>10		>17
		Peak/MIC	>10		>17
minocaproic acid (Amicar)	S or P		μg/mL	7.62	μmol/L
		Therap			
		Trough	100-400		762-3048
iodarone (Cordarone)	S or P		μg/mL	1.47	μmol/L
		Therap	0.5-2.0		1-3
		Toxic	>2.5		>4
triptyline (Elavil) + rtriptyline	S or P		ng/mL	3.61	nmol/L
		Therap	80-200		289-722
		Toxic	>500 (sum)		>1805
rbital (Amytal)	S or P		μg/mL	4.42	μmol/L
		Therap	1-5		4-22
		Toxic	>10		>44
ine (Asendin) +8- y amoxapine	S or P		ng/mL	3.19	nmol/L
		Therap	200-600		638-1914
		Toxic	>600		>1914

TABLE 60-2 Therapeutic and Toxic Levels of Drugs—cont'd

Drug	Specimen	Status	Reference Values: Conventional Units	Reference Values: Conversion Factor	Reference Values: SI Units
Amphetamine (Adderall)	S or P		ng/mL	7.40	nmol/L
		Therap	20-30		148-222
		Toxic	>200		>1480
Bromide as bromine	S or P		μg/mL	0.0125	mmol/L
		Therap	750-1500		9-19
		Toxic	>1250		>16
Bupropion (Wellbutrin, Zyban)	S or P		ng/mL	3.62	nmol/L
		Therap	25-100		91-362
		Toxic	>100		>362
Caffeine	S or P		μg/mL	5.15	μmol/L
		Therap	8-20		41-103
		Toxic	>20		>103
Carbamazepine (Tegretol)	S or P		μg/mL	4.23	μmol/L
		Therap	4-12		17-51
		Toxic	>15		>63
Carbamazepine-10,11-epoxide (carbamazepine metabolite)	S or P		μg/mL	3.97	μmol/L
		Therap	0.4-4		2-16
		Toxic	>8		>32
Carbenicillin (Geopen)	S or P		μg/mL	2.64	μmol/L
		Therap	Dependent on MIC of specific organism		
		Toxic	>250 (neurotoxicity)		>660
Chloral hydrate (Noctec) as trichloroethanol	S or P		μg/mL	6.69	μmol/L
		Therap	2-12		13-80
		Toxic	>20		>134
Chloramphenicol (Chloromycetin)	S or P		μg/mL	3.09	μmol/L
		Therap	10-25		31-77
		Toxic	>25		>77
		Gray baby syndrome	>40		>124
Chlordiazepoxide (Librium) + nordiazepine	S or P		ng/mL	0.003	μmol/L
		Therap	700-1000		2-3
		Toxic	>5000		>17
Chlorpromazine (Thorazine)	S or P		ng/mL	3.14	nmol/L
		Therap			
		Adult	30-300		94-942
		Child	40-80		126-251
		Toxic	>750		>2355
Cimetidine (Tagamet)	S or P		μg/mL	3.96	μmol/L
		Therap			
		Trough	0.5-1.2		2-5
		Toxic	>1.3		>5

Continued

TABLE 60-2 Therapeutic and Toxic Levels of Drugs—cont'd

Drug	Specimen	Status	Reference Values: Conventional Units	Conversion Factor	SI Units
Ciprofloxacin (Cipro)	S or P		μg/mL	3.02	μmol/L
		Therap			
		Peak (oral dose)	0.5-1.5		2-5
		Peak (IV dose)	<5.0		<15
		Toxic	>5.0		>15
		Gram-positive AUC/MIC	>30		
		Gram-negative AUC/MIC	>125		
Clomipramine (Anafranil) + norclomipramine	S or P		ng/mL	3.18	nmol/L
		Therap	175-450		556-1431
		Toxic	>400 (sum)		>1272
Clonazepam (Klonopin)	S or P		ng/mL	3.17	nmol/L
		Therap	20-70		63-222
		Toxic	>80		>254
Clonidine (Catapres)	S or P		ng/mL	4.35	nmol/L
		Therap	1.0-2.0		4-9
Clorazepate (Tranxene) (see Nordiazepam)					
Clozapine (Clozaril)	S or P		ng/mL	3.06	nmol/L
		Therap	350-600		1071-1836
		Toxic	>900		>2754
Codeine	S or P		ng/mL	3.34	nmol/L
		Therap	10-100		33-334
		Toxic	>1100		>3340
Cyclosporin A (Sandimmune)	WB	Therap	ng/mL	0.83	nmol/L
		12 h after dose	50-350		42-291
		Toxic	>350		>291
Delavirdine (Rescriptor)			μg/mL	1.80	μmol/L
	S or P	Therap			
		Trough	3-8		5-14
		Peak	14-16		25-29
		Toxic	>16		>29
Desipramine (Norpramin)	S or P				
			ng/mL	3.75	nmol/L
		Therap	100-300		375-1126
		Toxic	>400		>1502
Diazepam (Valium) + nordiazepine	S or P		ng/mL	3.51	nmol/L
		Therap	100-1000		351-3512
		Toxic	>5000		>17,559
Digitoxin	S or P		ng/mL	1.31	nmol/L
	≥8 h after dose	Therap	10-30		13-39
		Toxic	>45		>59
Digoxin (Lanoxin)	S or P		ng/mL	1.28	nmol/L
	≥12 h after dose	Therap	0.5-2.0		0.6-3
		In heart failure	0.5-0.8		0.6-1
		Toxic	>1.5		>2

TABLE 60-2 Therapeutic and Toxic Levels of Drugs—cont'd

			REFERENCE VALUES		
Drug	**Specimen**	**Status**	**Conventional Units**	**Conversion Factor**	**SI Units**
Disopyramide (Norpace)	S or P		μg/mL	2.95	μmol/L
		Therap	2.8-7.5		8-22
		Toxic	>5		>15
Doxepin (Sinequan, Adapin) + nordoxepin	S or P		ng/mL	3.58	nmol/L
		Therap	50-150		179-537
		Toxic	>500		>1790
Efavirenz (Sustiva)	S or P		μg/mL	3.16	μmol/L
		Therap	1-4		3-13
		Toxic	>4		>13
Ephedrine (Ectasule)	S or P		μg/mL	6.05	μmol/L
		Therap	0.05-0.10		0.3-0.6
		Toxic	>2		>12
Ethchlorvynol (Placidyl)	S or P		μg/mL	6.92	μmol/L
		Therap	2-8		14-55
		Toxic	>20		>138
Ethosuximide (Zarontin)	S or P		μg/mL	7.08	μmol/L
		Therap	40-100		283-708
		Toxic	>150		>1062
Everolimus (Zortress)	WB		ng/mL	1.04	nmol/L
		Therap	3-15		3-16
		Toxic	>15		>16
Felbamate (Felbatol)	S or P		μg/mL	4.20	μmol/L
		Therap	30-60		126-252
		Toxic	>120		>504
Fenoprofen (Nalfon)	S or P		μg/mL	4.12	μmol/L
		Therap	20-65		82-268
Flecainide (Tambocor)	S or P		μg/mL	2.41	μmol/L
		Therap	0.2-1.0		0.5-2
		Toxic	>1.0		>2
5-Flucytosine (Ancobon)	S or P		μg/mL	7.75	μmol/L
		Peak	>25		>194
		Toxic	>100		>775
Fluoxetine (Prozac) + norfluoxetine	S or P		ng/mL	3.23	nmol/L
		Therap	120-300		388-969
		Toxic	>1000		>3230
Fluphenazine (Modecate)	S or P		ng/mL	2.29	nmol/L
		Therap	0.5-2		1-5
		Toxic	>100		>229
Flurazepam (Dalmane)	S or P		μg/mL	2.58	μmol/L
		Toxic	>0.2		>0.5
Gabapentin (Neurontin)	S or P		μg/mL	5.84	μmol/L
		Therap	2-20		12-117
		Toxic	>12		>70

Continued

TABLE 60-2 Therapeutic and Toxic Levels of Drugs—cont'd

			Reference Values		
Drug	**Specimen**	**Status**	**Conventional Units**	**Conversion Factor**	**SI Units**
Gentamicin (Garamycin)	S or P		µg/mL	2.09	µmol/L
		Therap			
		Peak			
		Less severe infection	5-8		11-17
		Severe infection	8-10		17-21
		Trough			
		Less severe infection	<1		<2
		Moderate infection	<2		<4
		Severe infection	<4		<8
		Toxic			
		Peak	>10		>21
		Trough	>2		>4
		Peak/MIC	>10		>21
Glutethimide (Doriden)	S or P		µg/mL	4.60	µmol/L
		Therap	2-6		9-28
		Toxic	>5		>23
Haloperidol (Haldol)	S or P		ng/mL	2.66	nmol/L
		Therap	5-17		13-45
		Toxic	>42		>112
Hydromorphone (Dilaudid)	S or P		ng/mL	3.50	nmol/L
		Therap	1-3		4-11
		Toxic	>100		>350
Ibuprofen (Motrin)	S or P		µg/mL	4.85	µmol/L
		Therap	10-50		49-243
		Toxic	>200		>970
Imipramine (Tofranil) + desipramine	S or P		ng/mL	3.57	nmol/L
		Therap	150-300		536-1071
		Toxic	>400 (sum)		>1428
Indinavir (Crixivan)	S or P		µg/mL	1.41	µmol/L
		Therap			
		Trough	>0.1		>0.14
		Peak	8-10		11-14
		Toxic	>10		>14
Isoniazid (Hyzyd, Nydrazid)	S or P		µg/mL	7.29	µmol/L
		Therap	1-7		7-51
		Toxic	>20		>146
Itraconazole (Sporanox) + hydroxyitraconazole	S or P		µg/mL	1.42	µmol/L
		Therap	>1.5		>2
Kanamycin (Kantrex)	S or P		µg/mL	2.06	µmol/L
		Therap			
		Peak	25-35		52-72
		Trough			
		Less severe infection	1-4		2-8
		Severe infection	4-8		8-17
		Toxic			
		Peak	>35		>72
		Trough	>10		>21
		Peak/MIC	>10		>21

TABLE 60-2 Therapeutic and Toxic Levels of Drugs—cont'd

Drug	Specimen	Status	Reference Values: Conventional Units	Reference Values: Conversion Factor	Reference Values: SI Units
Lamivudine (Epivir, 3TC)	S or P		μg/mL	4.36	μmol/L
		Therap	>0.4		>2
Lamotrigine (Lamictal)	S or P		μg/mL	3.91	μmol/L
		Therap	2.5-15		10-59
Levetiracetam (Keppra)	S or P		μg/mL	5.88	μmol/L
		Therap	12-46		71-270
Lidocaine (Xylocaine)	S or P		μg/mL	4.27	μmol/L
	≥45 min following bolus dose	Therap	1.5-5		6-21
		Toxic	>6		>26
Lithium (Eskalith)	S or P		mEq/L	1.0	mmol/L
		Therap	0.5-1.2		0.5-1
		Toxic	>2		>2
Lorazepam (Ativan)	S or P		ng/mL	3.11	nmol/L
		Therap dose	50-240		156-746
Maprotiline (Ludiomil)	S or P		ng/mL	3.60	nmol/L
		Therap	125-200		450-720
		Toxic	>300		>1080
Meperidine (Demerol)	S or P		ng/mL	4.04	nmol/L
		Therap	70-500		283-2020
		Toxic	>1000		>4004
Mephobarbital (Mebaral)	S or P		μg/mL	4.06	μmol/L
		Therap	1-7		4-28
		Toxic	>15		>61
Meprobamate (Equanil)	S or P		μg/mL	4.58	μmol/L
		Therap	6-12		28-55
		Toxic	>60		>275
Methadone (Dolophine)	S or P		ng/mL	3.23	nmol/L
		Therap	100-400		320-1280
		Toxic	>2000		>6460
Methamphetamine (Desoxyn)	S or P		μg/mL	6.70	μmol/L
		Therap	0.01-0.05		0.07-0.34
		Toxic	>0.5		>3
Methaqualone (Quaalude)	S or P		μg/mL	4.00	μmol/L
		Therap	2-3		8-12
		Toxic	>10		>40
Methotrexate (Trexall, Rheumatrex)	S or P		μmol/L	2.20	μmol/L
		Toxic			
		24 h after high-dose therapy	≥10		≥22
		48 h after high-dose therapy	≥1		≥2
		72 h after high-dose therapy	≥0.1		≥0.2
Methsuximide (Celontin) as normethsuximide	S or P		μg/mL	5.29	μmol/L
		Therap	10-40		53-212
		Toxic	>40		>212

Continued

TABLE 60-2 Therapeutic and Toxic Levels of Drugs—cont'd

			REFERENCE VALUES		
Drug	**Specimen**	**Status**	**Conventional Units**	**Conversion Factor**	**SI Units**
Methyldopa (Aldomet)	S or P		μg/mL	4.73	μmol/L
		Therap	1-5		5-24
		Toxic	>7		>33
Methyprylon (Noludar)	S or P		μg/mL	5.46	μmol/L
		Therap	8-10		43-55
		Toxic	>50		273
Mexiletine (Mexitil)	S or P		μg/mL	5.58	μmol/L
		Therap	0.5-2		3-11
		Toxic	>2.0		>11
Morphine	S or P		ng/mL	3.50	nmol/L
		Therap	10-80		35-280
		Toxic	>200		>700
Mycophenolate mofetil (CellCept) as mycophenolic acid	S or P		μg/mL	3.12	μmol/L
		Therap	1.3-3.5		4-11
		Toxic	>12		>38
Nefazodone (Serzone)	S or P		ng/mL	2.13	nmol/L
		Therap	25-2500		53-5325
		Toxic	>2500		>5325
Nelfinavir (Viracept)	S or P		μg/mL	1.76	μmol/L
		Therap	>1		>2
		Toxic	>6		>11
Netilmicin (Netromycin)	S or P		μg/mL	2.10	μmol/L
		Therap			
		Peak			
		Less severe infection	5-8		10-17
		Severe infection	8-10		17-21
		Trough			
		Less severe infection	<1		<2
		Moderate infection	<2		<4
		Severe infection	<4		<8
		Toxic			
		Peak	>10		>21
		Trough	>2		>4
Nevirapine (Viramune)	S or P		μg/mL	3.76	μmol/L
		Therap	>3.5		<13.2
		Toxic	>12		>45.1
Nordiazepine, active metabolite of several benzodiazepines	S or P		ng/mL	3.76	nmol/L
	S or P	Therap	100-500		376-1880
		Toxic	>500		>1880
Nortriptyline (Aventyl)	S or P		ng/mL	3.80	nmol/L
		Therap	70-170		266-646
		Toxic	>500		>1900
Olanzapine (Zyprexa)	S or P		ng/mL	3.20	nmol/L
		Therap	20-80		64-256
		Toxic	>1000		>3200
Oxazepam (Serax)	S or P		μg/mL	3.49	μmol/L
		Therap	0.2-1.4		0.7-5

TABLE 60-2 Therapeutic and Toxic Levels of Drugs—cont'd

			REFERENCE VALUES		
Drug	**Specimen**	**Status**	**Conventional Units**	**Conversion Factor**	**SI Units**
Oxcarbazepine (Trileptal) as monohydroxyoxcarbazepine (MHD)	S or P		μg/mL	3.97	μmol/L
	S or P	Therap	3-35		12-139
		Toxic	>40		>159
Oxycodone (Percodan)	S or P		ng/mL	3.17	nmol/L
		Therap	10-100		32-317
		Toxic	>200		>634
Paraldehyde (Paral)	S or P		μg/mL	7.57	μmol/L
		Therap			
		Sedation	10-100		76-757
		Anesthesia	>200		>1514
		Toxic	>200		>1514
		Lethal	>500		>3785
Paroxetine (Paxil)	S or P		ng/mL	3.04	nmol/L
		Therap	70-120		213-365
Pentazocine (Talwin)	S or P		μg/mL	3.5	μmol/L
		Therap	0.05-0.2		0.2-0.7
		Toxic	>1.0		>4
Pentobarbital (Nembutal)	S or P		μg/mL	4.42	μmol/L
		Therap			
		Hypnotic	1-5		4-22
		Therap coma	20-50		88-221
		Toxic	>10		>44
Perphenazine (Apo-Perphenazine)	S or P		μg/mL	2.48	μmol/L
		Therap	0.6-2.4		2-6
		Toxic	>12		>30
Phenacetin	S or P		μg/mL	5.58	μmol/L
		Therap	1-30		6-167
		Toxic	50-250		279-1395
Phenobarbital (Luminal)	S or P		μg/mL	4.31	μmol/L
		Therap	10-40		43-173
		Toxic			
		Slowness, ataxia, nystagmus	35-80		151-345
		Coma, with reflexes	65-117		280-504
		Coma, without reflexes	>100		>431
Phensuximide (Milontin) + norphensuximide	S or P		μg/mL	5.29	μmol/L
		Therap	40-60		212-317
Phenylbutazone (Butazolidin)	S or P		μg/mL	3.24	μmol/L
		Therap	50-100		162-324
		Toxic	>100		>324
Phenytoin (Dilantin)	S or P		μg/mL	3.96	μmol/L
		Therap	10-20		40-79
		Free	1.0-2.0		4-8
		Toxic	>20		>79
Posaconazole (Noxafil)	S or P		μg/mL	1.43	μmol/L
		Therap	>1.25		>2

Continued

TABLE 60-2 Therapeutic and Toxic Levels of Drugs—cont'd

Drug	Specimen	Status	Reference Values: Conventional Units	Conversion Factor	SI Units
Primidone (Mysoline) + phenobarbital	S or P		μg/mL	4.58	μmol/L
		Therap	5-10		23-46
		Toxic	>15		>69
Procainamide (Pronestyl) + *N*-acetylprocainamide (NAPA)	S or P		μg/mL	4.25	μmol/L
		Therap	4-10		17-42
			12-18 (NAPA)	3.61	43-65
		Toxic	>12		>51
			>40 (NAPA)		>144
Propafenone (Rythmol)	S or P		μg/mL	2.93	μmol/L
		Therap	0.5-2.0		1.5-6
		Toxic	>2		>6
Propoxyphene (Darvon)	S or P		μg/mL	2.95	μmol/L
		Therap	0.1-0.4		0.3-1
		Toxic	>0.5		>2
Propranolol (Inderal)	S or P		ng/mL	3.86	nmol/L
		Therap	20-100		77-386
Protriptyline (Vivactil)	S or P		ng/mL	3.80	nmol/L
		Therap	70-260		266-988
		Toxic	>500		>1900
Quetiapine (Seroquel)	S or P		mg/L	2.58	μmol/L
		Therap	0.7-1.7		2-4
		Toxic	>200		>516
Quinidine (BioQuin)	S or P		μg/mL	3.08	μmol/L
		Therap	2-5		6-15
		Toxic	>6		>19
Risperidone (Risperdal) + 9-hydroxyrisperidone	S or P		ng/mL	2.44	nmol/L
		Therap	20-60		49-146
Ritonavir (Norvir)	S or P		μg/mL	1.39	μmol/L
		Therap	>2		>3
		Toxic	>22		>31
Salicylates as salicylic acid	S or P		μg/mL	0.00727	mmol/L
		Therap			
		Analgesia, antipyresis	<100		<0.7
		Anti-inflammatory	150-300		1-2
		Toxic	>100		>0.7
		Lethal, 24+ h after a dose or with chronic ingestion	>500		>4
Saquinavir (Fortovase, Invirase)	S or P		μg/mL	1.49	μmol/L
		Therap	>0.25		>0.4
		Toxic	>6.0		>9
Secobarbital (Seconal)	S or P		μg/mL	4.20	μmol/L
		Therap	1-2		4.2-8.4
		Toxic	>5		>21.0

TABLE 60-2 Therapeutic and Toxic Levels of Drugs—cont'd

Drug	Specimen	Status	Reference Values: Conventional Units	Reference Values: Conversion Factor	Reference Values: SI Units
Sertraline (Zoloft)	S or P		ng/mL	3.27	nmol/L
		Therap	10-50		33-164
		Toxic	>300		>981
Sirolimus (Rapamune, Rapamycin)	WB		ng/mL	1.10	nmol/L
		Therap	4-20		4-22
		Toxic	>20		>22
Sotalol (Betapace, Sorine)	S or P		µg/mL	3.67	µmol/L
		Therap	1-3		4-11
Streptomycin	S or P		µg/mL	1.72	
		Therap			
		Trough	<5		<9
		Peak	20-30		34-52
		Peak/MIC	>10		>17.2
		Toxic	>50		>86
Sulfonamides as sulfanilamide	S or P		mg/mL	5.81	mmol/L
		Therap	5-15		29-87
		Toxic	>20		>116
Tacrolimus (FK 506, Prograf)	WB		ng/mL	1.24	nmol/L
		Therap	3-20		4-25
		Toxic	>20		>25
Teicoplanin (Targocid)	S or P		µg/mL	0.53	µmol/L
		Peak	>10		>5
Theophylline (Uniphyl)	S or P		µg/mL	5.55	µmol/L
		Therap			
		Bronchodilator	8-20		44-111
		Prem apnea	6-13		33-72
		Toxic	>20		>111
Thiopental (Pentothal)	S or P		µg/mL	4.13	µmol/L
		Hypnotic	1-5		4-21
		Coma	30-100		124-413
		Anesthesia	7-130		29-536
		Toxic	>10		>41
Thioridazine (Mellaril)	S or P		µg/mL	2.70	µmol/L
		Therap	0.2-2.0		0.5-5
		Toxic	>10		>27
Tiagabine (Gabitril)	S or P		ng/mL	2.66	nmol/L
		Therap	20-200		53-532
		Toxic	>520		>1383
Tobramycin (Nebcin)	S or P		µg/mL	2.14	µmol/L
		Therap			
		Peak			
		Less severe infection	5-8		11-17
		Severe infection	8-10		17-21
		Trough			
		Less severe infection	<1		<2
		Moderate infection	<2		<4
		Severe infection	<4		<9

Continued

TABLE 60-2 Therapeutic and Toxic Levels of Drugs—cont'd

			Reference Values		
Drug	**Specimen**	**Status**	**Conventional Units**	**Conversion Factor**	**SI Units**
Tobramycin (Nebcin)—*cont'd*		Toxic			
		Peak	>10		>21
		Trough	>2		>4
		Peak/MIC	>10		>21
Tocainide (Tonocard)	S or P		μg/mL	5.20	μmol/L
		Therap	6-15		31-78
		Toxic	>15		>78
Tolbutamide (Orinase)	S or P		μg/mL	3.70	μmol/L
		Therap	90-240		333-888
		Toxic	>640		>2368
Topiramate (Topamax)	S or P		μg/mL	2.95	μmol/L
		Therap	5-20		15-59
		Toxic	>12		>36
Trazodone (Desyrel)	S or P		ng/mL	2.68	nmol/L
		Therap	650-1500		1748-4020
		Toxic	>4000		>10,720
Trimipramine (Surmontil)	S or P		ng/mL	3.40	nmol/L
		Therap	150-350		510-1190
		Toxic	>500		>1700
Valproic acid (Depakene)	S or P		μg/mL	6.93	μmol/L
		Therap	50-100		346-693
		Toxic	>100		>693
Vancomycin (Vancocin)	S or P		μg/mL	0.69	μmol/L
		Therap			
		Peak	20-40		14-28
		Trough	>10		>7
		Toxic	>80		>55
Venlafaxine (Effexor) + desmethylvenlafaxine	S or P		ng/mL	3.61	nmol/L
		Therap	195-400		704-1444
		Toxic	>1000 (sum)		>3610
Vigabatrin (Sabril)	S or P		μg/mL	7.74	μmol/L
		Therap	0.8-36		6-279
Voriconazole (Vfend)	S or P		μg/mL	2.86	μmol/L
		Therap	1-6		3-17
		Toxic	>6		>17
Warfarin (Coumadin)	S or P		μg/mL	3.24	μmol/L
		Therap	1-10		3-32
		Toxic	>10		>32
Zidovudine (AZT, Retrovir)	S or P		μg/mL	3.74	μmol/L
		Therap	>0.2		>0.8
Zonisamide (Zonegran)	S or P		μg/mL	4.71	μmol/L
		Therap	10-40		47-188

TABLE 60-3 Critical Values

Critical values, also known as panic or alert values, are laboratory results that indicate a life-threatening situation for the patient. Because of their critical nature, urgent notification of a critical value to the appropriate healthcare professional is necessary. Table 60-3 has been adapted from extensive national surveys. The median or average critical limit determined by these surveys is shown. In practice, each organization should have its own set of critical limits and physician notification policy.

Test	Units	Lower Limit	Upper Limit	Comments
Blood Gases				
pH		7.2	7.6	Arterial, capillary
PCO_2	mm Hg	20	70	Arterial, capillary
PO_2	mm Hg	40	—	Arterial
PO_2 (children)	mm Hg	45	125	Arterial
PO_2 (newborn)	mm Hg	35	90	Arterial
Chemistry				
Albumin (children)	g/dL	1.7	6.8	Serum or plasma
Ammonia (children)	μmol/L	—	109	Plasma
Bilirubin (newborn)	mg/dL	—	15	Serum or plasma
Calcium	mg/dL	6.0	13	Serum or plasma
Calcium (children)	mg/dL	6.5	12.7	Serum or plasma
Calcium, ionized	mmol/L	0.75	1.6	Plasma
Carbon dioxide, total	mmol/L	10	40	Serum or plasma
Chloride	mmol/L	80	120	Serum or plasma
Creatinine	mg/dL	—	5.0	Serum or plasma
Creatinine (children)	mg/dL	—	3.8	Serum or plasma
Glucose	mg/dL	40	450	Serum or plasma
Glucose (children)	mg/dL	46	445	Serum or plasma
Glucose (newborn)	mg/dL	30	325	Serum or plasma
Glucose, CSF	mg/dL	40	200	CSF
Glucose, CSF (children)	mg/dL	31	—	CSF
Lactate	mmol/L	—	3.4	Plasma
Lactate (children)	mmol/L	—	4.1	Plasma
Magnesium	mg/dL	1.0	4.7	Serum or plasma
Osmolality	mOsm/kg	250	325	Serum or plasma
Phosphorus	mg/dL	1.0	8.9	Serum or plasma
Potassium	mmol/L	2.8	6.2	Serum or plasma
Potassium (newborn)	mmol/L	2.8	7.8	Serum or plasma
Protein (children)	g/dL	3.4	9.5	Serum or plasma
Protein, CSF (children)	mg/dL	—	188	CSF
Sodium	mmol/L	120	160	Serum or plasma
Urea nitrogen	mg/dL	—	80	Serum or plasma
Urea nitrogen (children)	mg/dL	—	55	Serum or plasma
Uric acid	mg/dL	—	13	Serum or plasma
Uric acid (children)	mg/dL	—	12	Serum or plasma
Hematology				
Hematocrit				
Adult	%	20	60	First report only
Newborn	%	33	71	
Hemoglobin				
Adult	g/dL	7	20	First report only
Newborn	g/dL	10	22	
WBC				
Adult	∞10^3/μL	2.0	30	First report only
Children	∞10^3/μL	2.0	43	
Platelets	∞10^3/μL	40	1000	
Blasts	Any seen (first report only)			
Drepanocytes	Presence of sickle cells or aplastic crisis			

Continued

TABLE 60-3 Critical Values—cont'd

Test	Units	Lower Limit	Upper Limit	Comments
Coagulation				
Fibrinogen	mg/dL	100	800	
Prothrombin time	s	—	30	
Partial thromboplastin time	s	—	78	
Urinalysis	Presence of pathological crystals (urate, cysteine, leucine, or tyrosine)			
Microscopic	Strongly positive glucose and ketones			
Chemical				
Cerebrospinal Fluid				
WBC (0-1 y)	Cells per μL	—	>30	
WBC (1-4 y)	Cells per μL	—	>20	
WBC (5-17 y)	Cells per μL	—	>10	
WBC (>17 y)	Cells per μL	—	>5	
Malignant cells, blasts, or microorganisms		Any	Applies to other sterile body fluids	

REFERENCES

Dighe AS, Rao A, Coakley AB, Lewandrowski KB. Analysis of laboratory critical value reporting at a large academic medical center. Am J Clin Pathol 2006;12:758-64.

Emancipator K. Critical values: ASCP practice parameter. Am J Clin Path 1997;108:247-53.

Genzen JR, Tormey CA. Pathology consultation on reporting of critical values. Am J Clin Pathol 2011;135:505-13.

Hortin GL, Csako G. Critical values, panic values, or alert values? Am J Clin Pathol 1998;109:496-8.

Howanitz PJ, Steindel SJ, Heard NV. Laboratory critical values policies and procedures: a College of American Pathologists Q-probes study in 623 institutions. Arch Pathol Lab Med 2002;126:663-9.

Kost GJ. Critical limits for urgent clinician notification at US medical centers. JAMA 1990;263:701-7.

Kost GJ. Critical limits for emergency clinician notification at United States children's hospitals. Pediatrics 1991;88:597-603.

Kost GJ. Using critical limits to improve patient outcome. Med Lab Observ 1993;23:22-7.

Kost GJ. The significance of ionized calcium in cardiac and critical care: availability and critical limits at U.S. medical centers and children's hospitals. Arch Pathol Lab Med 1993;117:890-6.

Parl FF, O'Leary MF, Kaiser AB, Paulett JM, Statnikova K, Shultz EK. Implementation of a closed-loop reporting system for critical values and clinical communication in compliance with goals of The Joint Commission. Clin Chem 2010;56:417-23.

Piva E, Sciacovelli L, Zaninotto M, Laposata, M, Plebani, M. Evaluation of effectiveness of a computerized notification system for reporting critical values. Am J Clin Pathol 2011;131:432-41.

Tillman J, Barth JH; ACB National Audit Group. A survey of laboratory 'critical (alert) limits' in the UK. Ann Clin Biochem 2003;40:181-4.

Index

Note: Page numbers followed by "f" refer to illustrations; page numbers followed by "t" refer to tables; page numbers followed by "b" refer to boxes.

B

D

H

J

K

T

U

V

W